ICD-10-CM 2020

The Complete Official Codebook

AMA publications fund initiatives that drive improvements in patient health, practice innovation and medical education.

AMAstore.com

Publisher's Notice

The *ICD-10-CM: The Complete Official Codebook* is designed to be an accurate and authoritative source regarding coding and every reasonable effort has been made to ensure accuracy and completeness of the content. However, the American Medical Association (AMA) makes no guarantee, warranty, or representation that this publication is accurate, complete or without errors. It is understood that the AMA is not rendering any legal or other professional services or advice in this publication and that the AMA bears no liability for any results or consequences that may arise from the use of this book.

Our Commitment to Accuracy

The AMA is committed to producing accurate and reliable materials.

AMA product updates, errata, and addenda can be found at amaproductupdates.org.

To report corrections, please call the AMA Unified Service Center at (800) 621-8335.

To purchase additional copies, contact the AMA at 800 621-8335 or visit the AMA store at amastore.com. Refer to product number OP201420.

Acknowledgments

Marianne Randall, CPC, *Product Manager*
Karen Schmidt, BSN, *Technical Director*
Anita Schmidt, BS, RHIA, AHIMA-approved ICD-10-CM/PCS Trainer, *Clinical Technical Editor*
Leanne Patterson, CPC, *Clinical Technical Editor*
Karen Krawzik, RHIT, CCS, AHIMA-approved ICD-10-CM/PCS Trainer, *Clinical Technical Editor*
LaJuana Green, RHIA, CCS, *Clinical Technical Editor*
Peggy Willard, CCS, AHIMA-approved ICD-10-CM/PCS Trainer, *Clinical Technical Editor*
Dr. Vikas Kumar, BHMS, CPC, CPC-H, *Clinical Technical Editor*
Stacy Perry, *Manager, Desktop Publishing*
Lisa Singley, *Project Manager*
Tracy Betzler, *Senior Desktop Publishing Specialist*
Hope M. Dunn, *Senior Desktop Publishing Specialist*
Katie Russell, *Desktop Publishing Specialist*
Kate Holden, *Editor*

Anita Schmidt, BS, RHIA, AHIMA-approved ICD-10-CM/PCS Trainer

Ms. Schmidt has expertise in ICD-10-CM/PCS, DRG, and CPT with more than 15 years' experience in coding in multiple settings, including inpatient, observation, and same-day surgery. Her experience includes analysis of medical record documentation, assignment of ICD-10-CM and PCS codes, and DRG validation. She has conducted training for ICD-10-CM/PCS and electronic health record. She has also collaborated with clinical documentation specialists to identify documentation needs and potential areas for physician education. Most recently she has been developing content for resource and educational products related to ICD-10-CM, ICD-10-PCS, DRG, and CPT. Ms. Schmidt is an AHIMA-approved ICD-10-CM/PCS trainer and is an active member of the American Health Information Management Association (AHIMA) and the Minnesota Health Information Management Association.

Leanne Patterson, CPC

Ms. Patterson has more than 15 years of experience in the healthcare profession. She has an extensive background in professional component coding, with expertise in E/M coding and auditing, and HIPAA compliance. Her experience includes general surgery coding, serving as Director of Compliance, conducting chart-to-claim audits, and physician education. She has been responsible for coding and denial management in large multi-specialty physician practices, and most recently has been part of a team developing content for educational products related to ICD-10-CM. Ms. Patterson is credentialed by the American Academy of Professional Coders (AAPC) as a Certified Professional Coder (CPC).

Contents

Contents

Preface

ICD-10-CM Official Preface

This FY 2020 update of the International Statistical Classification of Diseases and Related Health Problems, 10th revision, Clinical Modification (ICD-10-CM) is being published by the United States government in recognition of its responsibility to promulgate this classification throughout the United States for morbidity coding. The International Statistical Classification of Diseases and Related Health Problems, 10th Revision (ICD-10), published by the World Health Organization (WHO), is the foundation of ICD-10-CM. ICD-10 continues to be the classification used in cause-of-death coding in the United States. The ICD-10-CM is comparable with the ICD-10. The WHO Collaborating Center for the Family of International Classifications in North America, housed at the Centers for Disease Control and Prevention's National Center for Health Statistics (NCHS), has responsibility for the implementation of ICD and other WHO-FIC classifications and serves as a liaison with the WHO, fulfilling international obligations for comparable classifications and the national health data needs of the United States. The historical background of ICD and ICD-10 can be found in the Introduction to the International Classification of Diseases and Related Health Problems (ICD-10), 2010, World Health Organization, Geneva, Switzerland.

ICD-10-CM is the United States' clinical modification of the World Health Organization's ICD-10. The term "clinical" is used to emphasize the modification's intent: to serve as a useful tool in the area of classification of morbidity data for indexing of health records, medical care review, and ambulatory and other health care programs, as well as for basic health statistics. To describe the clinical picture of the patient the codes must be more precise than those needed only for statistical groupings and trend analysis.

Characteristics of ICD-10-CM

ICD-10-CM far exceeds its predecessors in the number of concepts and codes provided. The disease classification has been expanded to include health-related conditions and to provide greater specificity at the sixth and seventh character level. The sixth and seventh characters are not optional and are intended for use in recording the information documented in the clinical record.

ICD-10-CM extensions, interpretations, modifications, addenda, or errata other than those approved by the Centers for Disease Control and Prevention are not to be considered official and should not be utilized. Continuous maintenance of the ICD-10-CM is the responsibility of the aforementioned agencies. However, because the ICD-10-CM represents the best in contemporary thinking of clinicians, nosologists, epidemiologists, and statisticians from both public and private sectors, when future modifications are considered, advice will be sought from all stakeholders.

All official authorized addenda since the last complete update (October 1, 2019) have been included in this revision. For more detailed information please see the complete official authorized addenda to ICD-10-CM, including the "ICD-10-CM Official Guidelines for Coding and Reporting," and a description of the ICD-10-CM updating and maintenance process.

How to Use ICD-10-CM: The Complete Official Codebook 2020

Introduction

ICD-10-CM: The Complete Official Codebook 2020 is your definitive coding resource, combining the work of the National Center for Health Statistics (NCHS), Centers for Medicare and Medicaid Services (CMS), American Hospital Association (AHA), and Publisher experts to provide the information you need for coding accuracy.

The International Classification of Diseases, 10th Revision, Clinical Modification (ICD-10-CM), is an adaptation of ICD-10, copyrighted by the World Health Organization (WHO). The development and maintenance of this clinical modification (CM) is the responsibility of the NCHS as authorized by WHO. Any new concepts added to ICD-10-CM are based on an established update process through the collaboration of WHO's Update and Revision Committee and the ICD-10-CM Coordination and Maintenance Committee.

In addition to the ICD-10-CM classification, other official government source information has been included in this manual. Depending on the source, updates to information may be annual or quarterly. This manual provides the most current information that was available at the time of publication. For updates to the source documents that may have occurred after this manual was published, please refer to the following:

- **National Center for Health Statistics (NCHS), International Classification of Diseases, Tenth Revision, Clinical Modification (ICD-10-CM)**

    https://www.cdc.gov/nchs/icd/icd10cm.htm

    https://www.cms.gov/Medicare/Coding/ICD10/2019-ICD-10-CM.html

- **Centers for Medicare and Medicaid Services (CMS) Integrated Outpatient Code Editor (IOCE), version 20.2**

    https://www.cms.gov/Medicare/Coding/OutpatientCodeEdit/OCEQtrReleaseSpecs.html

- **Centers for Medicare & Medicaid Services (CMS) Risk Adjustment Model, version 24**

    https://www.cms.gov/Medicare/Health-Plans/MedicareAdvtgSpecRateStats/Risk-Adjustors.html

- **Centers for Medicare & Medicaid Services (CMS) Quality Payment Program (QPP)**

    https://qpp.cms.gov/mips/explore-measures/quality-measures?py=2019#measures

- **American Hospital Association (AHA) Coding Clinics**

    https://www.codingclinicadvisor.com/

The official NCHS ICD-10-CM classification includes three main sections: the guidelines, the indexes, and the tabular list, all of which make up the bulk of this coding manual. To complement the classification, Optum360's coding experts have incorporated Medicare-related coding edits and proprietary features, such as supplementary notations, coding tools, and appendixes, into a comprehensive and easy-to-use reference. This publication is organized as follows:

What's New for 2020

This section provides a high-level overview of the changes made to the ICD-10-CM official code set for fiscal 2020, identifying codes that have been added and deleted from the classification, codes that had validity changes as a result of these additions and deletions, as well as codes that had revisions to their descriptions. All changes are based on the 2020 official addendum, posted June 20, 2019, by the National Center for Health Statistics (NCHS), the agency charged with maintaining and updating ICD-10-CM. NCHS is part of the Centers for Disease Control and Prevention (CDC).

Conversion Table

The conversion table was developed by National Center for Healthcare Statistics (NCHS) to help facilitate data retrieval as new codes are added to the ICD-10-CM classification. This table provides a crosswalk from each FY 2020 new code to the equivalent code(s) assigned prior to October 1, 2019, for that particular diagnosis or condition. For the full conversion table, including code crosswalks before October 1, 2019, refer to the 2020 Conversion Table zip file at https://www.cms.gov/Medicare/Coding/ICD10/2020-ICD-10-CM.html.

10 Steps to Correct Coding

This step-by-step tutorial walks the coder through the process of finding the correct code — from locating the code in the official indexes to verifying the code in the tabular section — while following applicable conventions, guidelines, and instructional notes. Specific examples are provided with detailed explanations of each coding step along with advice for proper sequencing.

Official ICD-10-CM Guidelines for Coding and Reporting

This section provides the full official conventions and guidelines regulating the appropriate assignment and reporting of ICD-10-CM codes. These conventions and guidelines are published by the U.S. Department of Health and Human Services (DHHS) and approved by the cooperating parties (American Health Information Management Association [AHIMA], National Center for Health Statistics [NCHS], Centers for Disease Control and Prevention [CDC], and the American Hospital Association [AHA]).

Indexes

Index to Diseases and Injuries

The Index to Diseases and Injuries is arranged in alphabetic order by terms specific to a disease, condition, illness, injury, eponym, or abbreviation as well as terms that describe circumstances other than a disease or injury that may require attention from a health care professional.

Neoplasm Table

The Neoplasm Table is arranged in alphabetic order by anatomical site. Codes are then listed in individual columns based upon the histological behavior (malignant, in situ, benign, uncertain, or unspecified) of the neoplasm.

Table of Drugs and Chemicals

The Table of Drugs and Chemicals is arranged in alphabetic order by the specific drug or chemical name. Codes are listed in individual columns based upon the associated intent (poisoning, adverse effect, or underdosing).

External Causes Index

The External Causes Index is arranged in alphabetic order by main terms that describe the cause, the intent, the place of occurrence, the activity, and the status of the patient at the time the injury occurred or health condition arose.

Index Notations

With

The word "with" or "in" should be interpreted to mean "associated with" or "due to." The classification presumes a causal relationship between the two conditions linked by these terms in the index. These conditions should be coded as related even in the absence of provider documentation explicitly linking them unless the documentation clearly states the conditions are unrelated or when another guideline specifically requires a documented linkage between two conditions (e.g., the sepsis guideline for "acute organ dysfunction that is not clearly associated with the sepsis"). For conditions not specifically linked by these relational terms in the classification or when a guideline requires explicit documentation of a linkage between two conditions, provider documentation must link the conditions to code them as related.

The word "with" in the index is sequenced immediately following the main term, not in alphabetical order.

> **Dermatopolymyositis** M33.90
> with
> myopathy M33.92
> respiratory involvement M33.91
> specified organ involvement NEC M33.99
> in neoplastic disease — *see also* Neoplasm D49.9 *[M36.0]*

See

When the instruction "see" follows a term in the index, it indicates that another term must be referenced to locate the correct code.

> **Hematoperitoneum** — *see* Hemoperitoneum

See Also

The instructional note "see also" simply provides alternative terms the coder may reference that may be useful in determining the correct code but are not necessary to follow if the main term supplies the appropriate code.

> **Hematinuria** — *see also* Hemaglobinuria
> malarial B50.8

Default Codes

In the index, the default code is the code listed next to the main term and represents the condition most commonly associated with that main term. This code may be assigned when documentation does not support reporting a more specific code. Alternatively, it may provide an unspecified code for the condition.

> **Headache** R51
> allergic NEC G44.89
> associated with sexual activity G44.82
> chronic daily R51

Parentheses

Parentheses in the indexes enclose nonessential modifiers, supplementary words that may be present or absent in the statement of a disease without affecting the code.

> **Pseudomeningocele** (cerebral) (infective) (post-traumatic) G96.19
> postprocedural (spinal) G97.82

Brackets

ICD-10-CM has a coding convention addressing code assignment for manifestations that occur as a result of an underlying condition. This convention requires the underlying condition to be sequenced first, followed by the code or codes for the associated manifestation. In the index, italicized codes in brackets identify manifestation codes.

> **Polyneuropathy** (peripheral) G62.9
> alcoholic G62.1
> amyloid (Portuguese) E85.1 *[G63]*
> transthyretin-related (ATTR) familial E85.1 *[G63]*

Shaded Guides

Exclusive vertical shaded guides in the Index to Diseases and Injuries and External Causes Index help the user easily follow the indent levels for the subentries under a main term. Sequencing rules may apply depending on the level of indent for separate subentries.

> **Hemicrania**
> congenital malformation Q00.0
> continua G44.51
> meaning migraine — *see also* Migraine G43.909
> paroxysmal G44.039
> chronic G44.049
> intractable G44.041
> not intractable G44.049
> episodic G44.039
> intractable G44.031
> not intractable G44.039
> intractable G44.031
> not intractable G44.039

Following References

The Index to Diseases and Injuries includes following references to assist in locating out-of-sequence codes in the tabular list. Out-of-sequence codes contain an alphabetic character (letter) in the third- or 4th-character position. These codes are placed according to the classification rules — according to condition — not according to alphabetic or numeric sequencing rules.

> **Carcinoma** (malignant) — *see also* Neoplasm, by site, malignant
> neuroendocrine — *see also* Tumor, neuroendocrine
> high grade, any site C7A.1 (*following* C75)
> poorly differentiated, any site C7A.1 (*following* C75)

Additional Character Required

The Index to Diseases and Injuries, Neoplasm Table, and External Causes Index provide an icon after certain codes to signify to the user that additional characters are required to make the code valid. The tabular list should be consulted for appropriate character selection.

> **Fall, falling** (accidental) W19 ☑
> building W20.1 ☑

Tabular List of Diseases

ICD-10-CM codes and descriptions are arranged numerically within the tabular list of diseases with 19 separate chapters providing codes associated with a particular body system or nature of injury or disease. There is also a chapter providing codes for external causes of an injury or health conditions and finally a chapter for codes that address encounters with healthcare facilities for circumstances other than a disease or injury.

Code and Code Descriptions

ICD-10-CM is an alphanumeric classification system that contains categories, subcategories, and valid codes. The first character is always a letter with any additional characters represented by either a letter or number. A three-character category without further subclassification is equivalent to a valid three-character code. Valid codes may be three, four, five, six, or seven characters in length, with each level of subdivision after a three-character category representing a subcategory. The final level of subdivision is a valid code.

Boldface

Boldface type is used for all codes and descriptions in the tabular list.

Italics

Italicized type is used to identify manifestation codes, those codes that should not be reported as first-listed diagnoses.

Deleted Text

~~Strikethrough~~ on a code and code description indicates a deletion from the classification for the current year.

Key Word

Green font is used throughout the Tabular List of Diseases to differentiate the key words that appear in similar code descriptions in a given category or subcategory. The key word convention is used only in those categories in which there are multiple codes with very similar descriptions with only a few words that differentiate them.

For example, refer to the list of codes below from category H55:

✓4ᵗʰ	**H55**	**Nystagmus and other irregular eye movements**
✓5ᵗʰ	**H55.0**	**Nystagmus**
	H55.00	**Unspecified nystagmus**
	H55.01	**Congenital nystagmus**
	H55.02	**Latent nystagmus**
	H55.03	**Visual deprivation nystagmus**
	H55.04	**Dissociated nystagmus**
	H55.09	**Other forms of nystagmus**

The portion of the code description that appears in **green font** in the tabular list helps the coder quickly identify the key terms and the correct code. This convention is especially useful when the codes describe laterality, such as the following codes from subcategory H40.22:

✓6ᵗʰ	**H40.22**	**Chronic angle-closure glaucoma**
		Chronic primary angle-closure glaucoma
✓7ᵗʰ	**H40.221**	**Chronic angle-closure glaucoma, right eye**
✓7ᵗʰ	**H40.222**	**Chronic angle-closure glaucoma, left eye**
✓7ᵗʰ	**H40.223**	**Chronic angle-closure glaucoma, bilateral**
✓7ᵗʰ	**H40.229**	**Chronic angle-closure glaucoma, unspecified eye**

Tabular Notations

Official parenthetical notes as well as Optum360's supplementary notations are provided at the chapter, code block, category, subcategory, and individual code level to help the user assign proper codes. The information in the notation can apply to one or more codes depending on where the citation is placed.

Official Notations

Includes Notes

The word INCLUDES appears immediately under certain categories to further define, clarify, or give examples of the content of a code category.

Inclusion Terms

Lists of inclusion terms are included under certain codes. These terms indicate some of the conditions for which that code number may be used. Inclusion terms may be synonyms with the code title, or, in the case of "other specified" codes, the terms may also provide a list of various conditions included within a classification code. The inclusion terms are not exhaustive. The index may provide additional terms that may also be assigned to a given code.

Excludes Notes

ICD-10-CM has two types of excludes notes. Each note has a different definition for use. However, they are similar in that they both indicate that codes excluded from each other are independent of each other.

Excludes 1

An EXCLUDES 1 note is a "pure" excludes. It means "NOT CODED HERE!" An Excludes 1 note indicates mutually exclusive codes: two conditions that cannot be reported together. An Excludes1 note indicates that the code excluded should never be used at the same time as the code above the Excludes1 note. An Excludes1 is used when two conditions cannot occur together, such as a congenital form versus an acquired form of the same condition.

An exception to the Excludes 1 definition is when the two conditions are unrelated to each other. If it is not clear whether the two conditions involving an Excludes 1 note are related or not, query the provider. For example, code F45.8 Other somatoform disorders, has an Excludes 1 note for "sleep related teeth grinding (G47.63)" because "teeth grinding" is an inclusion term under F45.8. Only one of these two codes should be assigned for teeth grinding. However psychogenic dysmenorrhea is also an inclusion term under F45.8, and a patient could have both this condition and sleep-related teeth grinding. In this case, the two conditions are clearly unrelated to each other, so it would be appropriate to report F45.8 and G47.63 together.

Excludes 2

An EXCLUDES 2 note means "NOT INCLUDED HERE." An Excludes 2 note indicates that although the excluded condition is not part of the condition it is excluded from, a patient may have both conditions at the same time. Therefore, when an Excludes 2 note appears under a code, it may be acceptable to use both the code and the excluded code together if supported by the medical documentation.

Note

The term "NOTE" appears as an icon and precedes the instructional information. These notes function as alerts to highlight coding instructions within the text.

Code First/Use additional code

These instructional notes provide sequencing instruction. They may appear independently of each other or to designate certain etiology/manifestation paired codes. These instructions signal the coder that an additional code should be reported to provide a more complete picture of that diagnosis.

In etiology/manifestation coding, ICD-10-CM requires the underlying condition to be sequenced first, followed by the manifestation. In these situations, codes with "In diseases classified elsewhere" in the code description are never permitted as a first-listed or principal diagnosis code and must be sequenced following the underlying condition code.

Code Also

A "code also" note alerts the coder that more than one code may be required to fully describe the condition. The sequencing depends on the circumstances of the encounter. Factors that may determine sequencing include severity and reason for the encounter.

Revised Text

The revised text ▶◀ "bow ties" alert the user to changes in official notations for the current year. Revised text may include the following:

- A change in a current parenthetical description
- A change in the code(s) associated with a current parenthetical note
- A change in how a current parenthetical note is classified (e.g., an Excludes 1 note that changed to an Excludes 2 note)
- Addition of a new parenthetical note(s) to a code

Deleted Text

~~Strikethrough~~ on official notations indicate a deletion from the classification for the current year.

Publisher Notations

AHA Coding Clinic Citations

Coding Clinics are official American Hospital Associated (AHA) publications that provide coding advice specific to ICD-10-CM and ICD-10-PCS.

These citations identify the year, quarter, and page number of one or more Coding Clinic publications that may have coding advice relevant to a particular code or group of codes. With the most current citation listed first, these notations are preceded by the symbol **AHA:** and appear in purple type.

> **I15.1 Hypertension secondary to** other renal disorders
> **AHA:** 2016, 3Q, 22

Definitions

Definitions explain a specific term, condition, or disease process in layman's terms. These notations are preceded by the symbol **DEF:** and appear in purple type.

> ☑5ᵗʰ **M51.4 Schmorl's nodes**
> **DEF:** Irregular bone defect in the margin of the vertebral body that causes herniation into the end plate of the vertebral body.

Coding Tips

The tips in the tabular list offer coding advice that is not readily available within the ICD-10-CM classification. It may relate official coding guidelines, indexing nuances, or advice from *AHA's Coding Clinic for ICD-10-CM/PCS*. These notations are preceded by the symbol **TIP:** and appear in brown type.

> **P15.8 Other specified birth injuries**
> **TIP:** Use for any injury of newborn from scalpel.

Icons

Note: The following icons are placed to the left of the code.

●   **New Code**
Codes that have been added to the classification system for the current year.

▲   **Revised Code Title**
Codes that have had a change to their description or validity change for the current year. For additional information on codes with validity changes, see the "What's New" section.

☑ Additional Characters Required

☑4ᵗʰ This symbol indicates that the code requires a 4th character.

☑5ᵗʰ This symbol indicates that the code requires a 5th character.

☑6ᵗʰ This symbol indicates that the code requires a 6th character.

☑7ᵗʰ This symbol indicates that the code requires a 7th character.

> ☑5ᵗʰ **H60.3 Other infective otitis externa**
> ☑6ᵗʰ **H60.31** Diffuse otitis externa
>   **H60.311** Diffuse otitis externa, right ear
>   **H60.312** Diffuse otitis externa, left ear
>   **H60.313** Diffuse otitis externa, bilateral
>   **H60.319** Diffuse otitis externa, unspecified ear

☑x7ᵗʰ Placeholder Alert

This symbol indicates that the code requires a 7th character following the placeholder "X". Codes with fewer than six characters that require a 7th character must contain placeholder "X" to fill in the empty character(s).

> ☑x7ᵗʰ **T16.1 Foreign body in** right ear

Note: The following icons are placed to the right of the code description.

Age Edits

Codes intended for a specific age group based on CMS IOCE designations, v20.2.

N   **Newborn Age: 0**
These diagnoses are intended for newborns and neonates and the patient's age must be 0 years.

> **N47.0 Adherent prepuce, newborn**   N♂

P   **Pediatric Age: 0-17**
These diagnoses are intended for children and the patient's age must be between 0 and 17 years.

> **L21.1 Seborrheic** infantile dermatitis   P

M   **Maternity Age: 12-55**
These diagnoses are intended for childbearing patients between the age of 12 and 55 years.

> **O02.9 Abnormal product of conception, unspecified**   M♀

A   **Adult Age: 15-124**
These diagnoses are intended for patients between the age of 15 and 124 years.

> **R54 Age-related physical debility**   A
>   Frailty
>   Old age
>   Senescence
>   Senile asthenia
>   Senile debility
>   **EXCLUDES 1** *age-related cognitive decline (R41.81)*
>   *sarcopenia (M62.84)*
>   *senile psychosis (F03)*
>   *senility NOS (R41.81)*

Sex Edits

Codes intended for a specific sex based on CMS IOCE designations, v20.2.

♂   **Male diagnosis only**

> **Q98.0 Klinefelter syndrome karyotype 47, XXY**   ♂

♀   **Female diagnosis only**

> **N35.12 Postinfective urethral stricture, not elsewhere classified,** female   ♀

HCC   **CMS-HCC Condition**

This icon identifies conditions that are considered a CMS-HCC (hierarchical condition category) diagnosis.

The HCC codes represented in this manual have been updated to reflect the 2020 Initial ICD-10-CM Mappings for CMS-HCC Model v24. Midyear final mappings were not available at the time this publication went to print; refer to the following CMS website for final mappings: https://www.cms.gov/Medicare/Health-Plans/MedicareAdvtgSpecRateStats/Risk-Adjustors.html.

> **Y62.2**   **Failure of sterile precautions during kidney dialysis and other perfusion**   **HCC**

Q   **QPP Condition**

This icon identifies conditions recognized as a quality measure for claims-based reporting under CMS's Merit-based Incentive Payment System (MIPS).

> **G44.52**   **New daily persistent headache (NDPH)**   **Q**

PDx   **Z-code as First-Listed Diagnosis**

Identify Z codes that generally are for use as a first-listed diagnosis only but may be used as an additional diagnosis if the patient has more than one encounter on the same day or there is more than one reason for the encounter.

The instructions for Z code use contained in the ICD-10-CM official coding guidelines identify those Z codes that can be used only as a PDx. All other Z codes may either be SDx or PDx, depending upon circumstances of the encounter, by meeting the definition of first-listed or principal diagnosis, and by following any specific Z code guidelines in section I.C.21 a-c. The responsibility of those assigning the Z codes as PDx is to make sure the circumstances of the encounter meet the definition of first-listed or principal diagnosis, follow all coding instructions, and follow the Z code specific guidelines. Optum360 does not include any SDx edit since there is no official source for it and the Z code use is determined by circumstances of the encounter.

Note: Please note that the symbols indicating the Z code "principal or first-listed only" designation and the Z codes that may be principal or first-listed diagnoses included in the official coding guidelines [section I.C.21.c.16] are consistent with reporting guidelines for health care encounters *excluding acute care inpatient admissions*. These Z code edits are often in conflict with the inpatient prospective payment system (IPPS) edits. For example, code Z34.90 Encounter for supervision of normal pregnancy, unspecified, unspecified trimester, may be an appropriate primary reason for an outpatient encounter. However, supervision for a normal pregnancy is not an acceptable principal diagnosis or reason for an inpatient admission and will have an unacceptable principal diagnosis edit under the inpatient prospective payment system (IPPS).

> **Z51.12**   **Encounter for antineoplastic immunotherapy**   **PDx**

Color Bars

Manifestation Code

Codes defined as manifestation codes based on CMS IOCE designations v20.2, appear in italic type, with a blue color bar over the code description. A manifestation cannot be reported as a first-listed code; it is sequenced as a secondary diagnosis with the underlying disease code listed first.

> *G32.89*   *Other specified degenerative disorders of nervous system in diseases classified elsewhere*
> Degenerative encephalopathy in diseases classified elsewhere

Unspecified Diagnosis

Codes that appear with a gray color bar over the alphanumeric code identify unspecified diagnoses. These codes should be used in limited circumstances, when neither the diagnostic statement nor the documentation provides enough information to assign a more specific diagnosis code. The abbreviation NOS, "not otherwise specified," in the tabular list may be interpreted as "unspecified."

> **G03.9**   **Meningitis, unspecified**
> Arachnoiditis (spinal) NOS

Footnotes

Certain codes in the tabular section have a numerical superscript located to the upper left of the code. This numerical superscript corresponds to a specific footnote description.

For example:

> [1] **✓7th** **M48.51**   **Collapsed vertebra, not elsewhere classified, occipito-atlanto-axial region**   **HCC**

For convenience, the footnote descriptions are provided on the front cover.

The following list also provides the footnote descriptions of all numerical superscripts found in the Tabular List of Diseases:

1   These codes are considered an HCC when reported as an initial encounter (7th character A, B, or C).

2   These codes are considered an HCC when reported as an initial encounter (7th character A or B) OR sequela (7th character S).

3   These codes are considered an HCC when reported as a sequela (7th character S).

Chapter-Level Notations

Chapter-specific Guidelines with Coding Examples

Each chapter begins with the Official Guidelines for Coding and Reporting specific to that chapter, where provided. Coding examples specific to outpatient care settings have been provided to illustrate the coding and/or sequencing guidance in these guidelines.

Muscle and Tendon Table

ICD-10-CM categorizes certain muscles and tendons in the upper and lower extremities by their action (e.g., extension or flexion) as well as their anatomical location. The Muscle/Tendon table is provided at the beginning of chapter 13 and chapter 19 to help users when code selection depends on the action of the muscle and/or tendon.

Note: This table is not all-inclusive, and proper code assignment should be based on the provider's documentation.

Appendixes

The additional resources described below have been included as appendixes for this book. These resources further instruct the professional coder on the appropriate application of the ICD-10-CM code set.

Appendix A: Valid 3-character ICD-10-CM Codes

The user may consult this table to confirm that no further specificity, such as the use of 4th, 5th, 6th, or 7th characters or placeholders (X), is necessary. All ICD-10-CM codes that are valid at the three-character level are listed.

Appendix B: Pharmacology List 2020

This reference is a comprehensive but not all-inclusive list of pharmacological agents used to treat acute and/or chronic conditions. Drugs are listed in alphabetical order by their brand and/or generic names along with their drug action and indications for which they may commonly be prescribed. Some drugs have also been mapped to their appropriate Z code for long-term drug use.

Appendix C: Z Codes for Long-Term Drug Use with Associated Drugs
This resource correlates Z codes that are used to identify current long-term drug use with a list of drugs that are typically categorized to that class of drug.

Note: These tables are not all-inclusive but list some of the more commonly used drugs.

Appendix D: Z Codes Only as Principal/First-Listed Diagnosis
Chapter 21, "Factors Influencing Health Status and Contact with Health Services," provides codes to deal with encounters for circumstances other than a disease or injury. Many of these codes may be reported *only* as the principal/first-listed diagnosis. This resource lists all of these codes in one table for quick and easy reference to ensure accurate reporting.

Appendix E: Centers for Medicare & Medicaid Services Hierarchical Condition Categories (CMS-HCC)
This resource provides the framework behind the Centers for Medicare and Medicaid Services' (CMS) Medicare Advantage (MA) program, a risk-adjustment model developed as a means of compensating health care plans with large numbers of Medicare Part C beneficiaries. It includes

a brief synopsis of the evolution of the program from its inception; insight into the various elements needed to predict risk, including the principles used to develop the hierarchical condition categories (HCCs), which make up one of the fundamental components of the risk-adjustment model. This appendix also outlines the audit process used to ensure the accuracy of payments made to MA plans.

Appendix F: Centers for Medicare & Medicaid Services Quality Payment Program
This resource provides an overview of the Medicare Access and CHIP Reauthorization Act (MACRA), which replaced Medicare's sustainable growth rate (SGR) methodology with the Quality Payment Program (QPP). It summarizes the Merit-based Incentive Payment System (MIPS) track used by those who opt to participate in traditional Medicare and not an advanced alternative payment model (APM). This includes eligibility requirements and an overview of the four performance categories that combine to make up the MIPS.

Illustrations

This section includes illustrations of normal anatomy with ICD-10-CM-specific terminology.

What's New for 2020

Official Updates

The official ICD-10-CM addendum was posted to the Centers for Medicare and Medicaid Services (CMS) website on June 20, 2019, identifying the changes to the ICD-10-CM code set for fiscal 2020, effective October 1, 2019, to September 30, 2020. These changes were made by the agency charged with maintaining and updating the ICD-10-CM code set, the National Center for Health Statistics (NCHS), a section of the Centers for Disease Control and Prevention (CDC). A summary of the changes is provided below:

15 Codes with a Change in Validity

Note: Validity changes are the result of codes being added to or deleted from the classification. Codes that change from valid to invalid allow the creation of a new subcategory to which new codes can be assigned that provide greater detail about the condition. Codes that change from invalid to valid are the result of subcategory codes being deleted from the classification, when the detail provided in those codes is no longer required.

Valid to Invalid

D81.3	I48.1	I48.2	Q66.0	Q66.1
Q66.21	Q66.22	Q66.3	Q66.4	Q66.7
Q66.9	Q79.6	Q87.1	R82.8	

Invalid to Valid
H81.4

7 Codes Deleted from the Classification

H81.41	Vertigo of central origin, right ear
H81.42	Vertigo of central origin, left ear
H81.43	Vertigo of central origin, bilateral
H81.49	Vertigo of central origin, unspecified ear
T67.0XXA	Heatstroke and sunstroke, initial encounter
T67.0XXD	Heatstroke and sunstroke, subsequent encounter
T67.0XXS	Heatstroke and sunstroke, sequela

273 New Codes Added to the Classification

D75.A	Glucose-6-phosphate dehydrogenase (G6PD) deficiency without anemia
D81.30	Adenosine deaminase deficiency, unspecified
D81.31	Severe combined immunodeficiency due to adenosine deaminase deficiency
D81.32	Adenosine deaminase 2 deficiency
D81.39	Other adenosine deaminase deficiency
I26.93	Single subsegmental pulmonary embolism without acute cor pulmonale
I26.94	Multiple subsegmental pulmonary emboli without acute cor pulmonale
I48.11	Longstanding persistent atrial fibrillation
I48.19	Other persistent atrial fibrillation
I48.20	Chronic atrial fibrillation, unspecified
I48.21	Permanent atrial fibrillation
I80.241	Phlebitis and thrombophlebitis of right peroneal vein
I80.242	Phlebitis and thrombophlebitis of left peroneal vein
I80.243	Phlebitis and thrombophlebitis of peroneal vein, bilateral
I80.249	Phlebitis and thrombophlebitis of unspecified peroneal vein
I80.251	Phlebitis and thrombophlebitis of right calf muscular vein
I80.252	Phlebitis and thrombophlebitis of left calf muscular vein
I80.253	Phlebitis and thrombophlebitis of calf muscular vein, bilateral
I80.259	Phlebitis and thrombophlebitis of unspecified calf muscular vein
I82.451	Acute embolism and thrombosis of right peroneal vein
I82.452	Acute embolism and thrombosis of left peroneal vein
I82.453	Acute embolism and thrombosis of peroneal vein, bilateral
I82.459	Acute embolism and thrombosis of unspecified peroneal vein
I82.461	Acute embolism and thrombosis of right calf muscular vein
I82.462	Acute embolism and thrombosis of left calf muscular vein
I82.463	Acute embolism and thrombosis of calf muscular vein, bilateral
I82.469	Acute embolism and thrombosis of unspecified calf muscular vein
I82.551	Chronic embolism and thrombosis of right peroneal vein
I82.552	Chronic embolism and thrombosis of left peroneal vein
I82.553	Chronic embolism and thrombosis of peroneal vein, bilateral
I82.559	Chronic embolism and thrombosis of unspecified peroneal vein
I82.561	Chronic embolism and thrombosis of right calf muscular vein
I82.562	Chronic embolism and thrombosis of left calf muscular vein
I82.563	Chronic embolism and thrombosis of calf muscular vein, bilateral
I82.569	Chronic embolism and thrombosis of unspecified calf muscular vein
L89.006	Pressure-induced deep tissue damage of unspecified elbow
L89.016	Pressure-induced deep tissue damage of right elbow
L89.026	Pressure-induced deep tissue damage of left elbow
L89.106	Pressure-induced deep tissue damage of unspecified part of back
L89.116	Pressure-induced deep tissue damage of right upper back
L89.126	Pressure-induced deep tissue damage of left upper back
L89.136	Pressure-induced deep tissue damage of right lower back
L89.146	Pressure-induced deep tissue damage of left lower back
L89.156	Pressure-induced deep tissue damage of sacral region
L89.206	Pressure-induced deep tissue damage of unspecified hip
L89.216	Pressure-induced deep tissue damage of right hip
L89.226	Pressure-induced deep tissue damage of left hip
L89.306	Pressure-induced deep tissue damage of unspecified buttock
L89.316	Pressure-induced deep tissue damage of right buttock
L89.326	Pressure-induced deep tissue damage of left buttock
L89.46	Pressure-induced deep tissue damage of contiguous site of back, buttock and hip
L89.506	Pressure-induced deep tissue damage of unspecified ankle
L89.516	Pressure-induced deep tissue damage of right ankle
L89.526	Pressure-induced deep tissue damage of left ankle

L89.606	Pressure-induced deep tissue damage of unspecified heel
L89.616	Pressure-induced deep tissue damage of right heel
L89.626	Pressure-induced deep tissue damage of left heel
L89.816	Pressure-induced deep tissue damage of head
L89.896	Pressure-induced deep tissue damage of other site
L89.96	Pressure-induced deep tissue damage of unspecified site
N63.15	Unspecified lump in the right breast, overlapping quadrants
N63.25	Unspecified lump in the left breast, overlapping quadrants
N99.85	Post endometrial ablation syndrome
Q66.00	Congenital talipes equinovarus, unspecified foot
Q66.01	Congenital talipes equinovarus, right foot
Q66.02	Congenital talipes equinovarus, left foot
Q66.10	Congenital talipes calcaneovarus, unspecified foot
Q66.11	Congenital talipes calcaneovarus, right foot
Q66.12	Congenital talipes calcaneovarus, left foot
Q66.211	Congenital metatarsus primus varus, right foot
Q66.212	Congenital metatarsus primus varus, left foot
Q66.219	Congenital metatarsus primus varus, unspecified foot
Q66.221	Congenital metatarsus adductus, right foot
Q66.222	Congenital metatarsus adductus, left foot
Q66.229	Congenital metatarsus adductus, unspecified foot
Q66.30	Other congenital varus deformities of feet, unspecified foot
Q66.31	Other congenital varus deformities of feet, right foot
Q66.32	Other congenital varus deformities of feet, left foot
Q66.40	Congenital talipes calcaneovalgus, unspecified foot
Q66.41	Congenital talipes calcaneovalgus, right foot
Q66.42	Congenital talipes calcaneovalgus, left foot
Q66.70	Congenital pes cavus, unspecified foot
Q66.71	Congenital pes cavus, right foot
Q66.72	Congenital pes cavus, left foot
Q66.90	Congenital deformity of feet, unspecified, unspecified foot
Q66.91	Congenital deformity of feet, unspecified, right foot
Q66.92	Congenital deformity of feet, unspecified, left foot
Q79.60	Ehlers-Danlos syndrome, unspecified
Q79.61	Classical Ehlers-Danlos syndrome
Q79.62	Hypermobile Ehlers-Danlos syndrome
Q79.63	Vascular Ehlers-Danlos syndrome
Q79.69	Other Ehlers-Danlos syndromes
Q87.11	Prader-Willi syndrome
Q87.19	Other congenital malformation syndromes predominantly associated with short stature
R11.15	Cyclical vomiting syndrome unrelated to migraine
R82.81	Pyuria
R82.89	Other abnormal findings on cytological and histological examination of urine
S02.121A	Fracture of orbital roof, right side, initial encounter for closed fracture
S02.121B	Fracture of orbital roof, right side, initial encounter for open fracture
S02.121D	Fracture of orbital roof, right side, subsequent encounter for fracture with routine healing
S02.121G	Fracture of orbital roof, right side, subsequent encounter for fracture with delayed healing

S02.121K	Fracture of orbital roof, right side, subsequent encounter for fracture with nonunion
S02.121S	Fracture of orbital roof, right side, sequela
S02.122A	Fracture of orbital roof, left side, initial encounter for closed fracture
S02.122B	Fracture of orbital roof, left side, initial encounter for open fracture
S02.122D	Fracture of orbital roof, left side, subsequent encounter for fracture with routine healing
S02.122G	Fracture of orbital roof, left side, subsequent encounter for fracture with delayed healing
S02.122K	Fracture of orbital roof, left side, subsequent encounter for fracture with nonunion
S02.122S	Fracture of orbital roof, left side, sequela
S02.129A	Fracture of orbital roof, unspecified side, initial encounter for closed fracture
S02.129B	Fracture of orbital roof, unspecified side, initial encounter for open fracture
S02.129D	Fracture of orbital roof, unspecified side, subsequent encounter for fracture with routine healing
S02.129G	Fracture of orbital roof, unspecified side, subsequent encounter for fracture with delayed healing
S02.129K	Fracture of orbital roof, unspecified side, subsequent encounter for fracture with nonunion
S02.129S	Fracture of orbital roof, unspecified side, sequela
S02.831A	Fracture of medial orbital wall, right side, initial encounter for closed fracture
S02.831B	Fracture of medial orbital wall, right side, initial encounter for open fracture
S02.831D	Fracture of medial orbital wall, right side, subsequent encounter for fracture with routine healing
S02.831G	Fracture of medial orbital wall, right side, subsequent encounter for fracture with delayed healing
S02.831K	Fracture of medial orbital wall, right side, subsequent encounter for fracture with nonunion
S02.831S	Fracture of medial orbital wall, right side, sequela
S02.832A	Fracture of medial orbital wall, left side, initial encounter for closed fracture
S02.832B	Fracture of medial orbital wall, left side, initial encounter for open fracture
S02.832D	Fracture of medial orbital wall, left side, subsequent encounter for fracture with routine healing
S02.832G	Fracture of medial orbital wall, left side, subsequent encounter for fracture with delayed healing
S02.832K	Fracture of medial orbital wall, left side, subsequent encounter for fracture with nonunion
S02.832S	Fracture of medial orbital wall, left side, sequela
S02.839A	Fracture of medial orbital wall, unspecified side, initial encounter for closed fracture
S02.839B	Fracture of medial orbital wall, unspecified side, initial encounter for open fracture
S02.839D	Fracture of medial orbital wall, unspecified side, subsequent encounter for fracture with routine healing
S02.839G	Fracture of medial orbital wall, unspecified side, subsequent encounter for fracture with delayed healing
S02.839K	Fracture of medial orbital wall, unspecified side, subsequent encounter for fracture with nonunion
S02.839S	Fracture of medial orbital wall, unspecified side, sequela

S02.841A	Fracture of lateral orbital wall, right side, initial encounter for closed fracture
S02.841B	Fracture of lateral orbital wall, right side, initial encounter for open fracture
S02.841D	Fracture of lateral orbital wall, right side, subsequent encounter for fracture with routine healing
S02.841G	Fracture of lateral orbital wall, right side, subsequent encounter for fracture with delayed healing
S02.841K	Fracture of lateral orbital wall, right side, subsequent encounter for fracture with nonunion
S02.841S	Fracture of lateral orbital wall, right side, sequela
S02.842A	Fracture of lateral orbital wall, left side, initial encounter for closed fracture
S02.842B	Fracture of lateral orbital wall, left side, initial encounter for open fracture
S02.842D	Fracture of lateral orbital wall, left side, subsequent encounter for fracture with routine healing
S02.842G	Fracture of lateral orbital wall, left side, subsequent encounter for fracture with delayed healing
S02.842K	Fracture of lateral orbital wall, left side, subsequent encounter for fracture with nonunion
S02.842S	Fracture of lateral orbital wall, left side, sequela
S02.849A	Fracture of lateral orbital wall, unspecified side, initial encounter for closed fracture
S02.849B	Fracture of lateral orbital wall, unspecified side, initial encounter for open fracture
S02.849D	Fracture of lateral orbital wall, unspecified side, subsequent encounter for fracture with routine healing
S02.849G	Fracture of lateral orbital wall, unspecified side, subsequent encounter for fracture with delayed healing
S02.849K	Fracture of lateral orbital wall, unspecified side, subsequent encounter for fracture with nonunion
S02.849S	Fracture of lateral orbital wall, unspecified side, sequela
S02.85XA	Fracture of orbit, unspecified, initial encounter for closed fracture
S02.85XB	Fracture of orbit, unspecified, initial encounter for open fracture
S02.85XD	Fracture of orbit, unspecified, subsequent encounter for fracture with routine healing
S02.85XG	Fracture of orbit, unspecified, subsequent encounter for fracture with delayed healing
S02.85XK	Fracture of orbit, unspecified, subsequent encounter for fracture with nonunion
S02.85XS	Fracture of orbit, unspecified, sequela
T50.911A	Poisoning by multiple unspecified drugs, medicaments and biological substances, accidental (unintentional), initial encounter
T50.911D	Poisoning by multiple unspecified drugs, medicaments and biological substances, accidental (unintentional), subsequent encounter
T50.911S	Poisoning by multiple unspecified drugs, medicaments and biological substances, accidental (unintentional), sequela
T50.912A	Poisoning by multiple unspecified drugs, medicaments and biological substances, intentional self-harm, initial encounter
T50.912D	Poisoning by multiple unspecified drugs, medicaments and biological substances, intentional self-harm, subsequent encounter
T50.912S	Poisoning by multiple unspecified drugs, medicaments and biological substances, intentional self-harm, sequela
T50.913A	Poisoning by multiple unspecified drugs, medicaments and biological substances, assault, initial encounter
T50.913D	Poisoning by multiple unspecified drugs, medicaments and biological substances, assault, subsequent encounter
T50.913S	Poisoning by multiple unspecified drugs, medicaments and biological substances, assault, sequela
T50.914A	Poisoning by multiple unspecified drugs, medicaments and biological substances, undetermined, initial encounter
T50.914D	Poisoning by multiple unspecified drugs, medicaments and biological substances, undetermined, subsequent encounter
T50.914S	Poisoning by multiple unspecified drugs, medicaments and biological substances, undetermined, sequela
T50.915A	Adverse effect of multiple unspecified drugs, medicaments and biological substances, initial encounter
T50.915D	Adverse effect of multiple unspecified drugs, medicaments and biological substances, subsequent encounter
T50.915S	Adverse effect of multiple unspecified drugs, medicaments and biological substances, sequela
T50.916A	Underdosing of multiple unspecified drugs, medicaments and biological substances, initial encounter
T50.916D	Underdosing of multiple unspecified drugs, medicaments and biological substances, subsequent encounter
T50.916S	Underdosing of multiple unspecified drugs, medicaments and biological substances, sequela
T67.01XA	Heatstroke and sunstroke, initial encounter
T67.01XD	Heatstroke and sunstroke, subsequent encounter
T67.01XS	Heatstroke and sunstroke, sequela
T67.02XA	Exertional heatstroke, initial encounter
T67.02XD	Exertional heatstroke, subsequent encounter
T67.02XS	Exertional heatstroke, sequela
T67.09XA	Other heatstroke and sunstroke, initial encounter
T67.09XD	Other heatstroke and sunstroke, subsequent encounter
T67.09XS	Other heatstroke and sunstroke, sequela
Y35.009A	Legal intervention involving unspecified firearm discharge, unspecified person injured, initial encounter
Y35.009D	Legal intervention involving unspecified firearm discharge, unspecified person injured, subsequent encounter
Y35.009S	Legal intervention involving unspecified firearm discharge, unspecified person injured, sequela
Y35.019A	Legal intervention involving injury by machine gun, unspecified person injured, initial encounter
Y35.019D	Legal intervention involving injury by machine gun, unspecified person injured, subsequent encounter
Y35.019S	Legal intervention involving injury by machine gun, unspecified person injured, sequela
Y35.029A	Legal intervention involving injury by handgun, unspecified person injured, initial encounter
Y35.029D	Legal intervention involving injury by handgun, unspecified person injured, subsequent encounter
Y35.029S	Legal intervention involving injury by handgun, unspecified person injured, sequela
Y35.039A	Legal intervention involving injury by rifle pellet, unspecified person injured, initial encounter
Y35.039D	Legal intervention involving injury by rifle pellet, unspecified person injured, subsequent encounter

Y35.039S Legal intervention involving injury by rifle pellet, unspecified person injured, sequela

Y35.049A Legal intervention involving injury by rubber bullet, unspecified person injured, initial encounter

Y35.049D Legal intervention involving injury by rubber bullet, unspecified person injured, subsequent encounter

Y35.049S Legal intervention involving injury by rubber bullet, unspecified person injured, sequela

Y35.099A Legal intervention involving other firearm discharge, unspecified person injured, initial encounter

Y35.099D Legal intervention involving other firearm discharge, unspecified person injured, subsequent encounter

Y35.099S Legal intervention involving other firearm discharge, unspecified person injured, sequela

Y35.109A Legal intervention involving unspecified explosives, unspecified person injured, initial encounter

Y35.109D Legal intervention involving unspecified explosives, unspecified person injured, subsequent encounter

Y35.109S Legal intervention involving unspecified explosives, unspecified person injured, sequela

Y35.119A Legal intervention involving injury by dynamite, unspecified person injured, initial encounter

Y35.119D Legal intervention involving injury by dynamite, unspecified person injured, subsequent encounter

Y35.119S Legal intervention involving injury by dynamite, unspecified person injured, sequela

Y35.129A Legal intervention involving injury by explosive shell, unspecified person injured, initial encounter

Y35.129D Legal intervention involving injury by explosive shell, unspecified person injured, subsequent encounter

Y35.129S Legal intervention involving injury by explosive shell, unspecified person injured, sequela

Y35.199A Legal intervention involving other explosives, unspecified person injured, initial encounter

Y35.199D Legal intervention involving other explosives, unspecified person injured, subsequent encounter

Y35.199S Legal intervention involving other explosives, unspecified person injured, sequela

Y35.209A Legal intervention involving unspecified gas, unspecified person injured, initial encounter

Y35.209D Legal intervention involving unspecified gas, unspecified person injured, subsequent encounter

Y35.209S Legal intervention involving unspecified gas, unspecified person injured, sequela

Y35.219A Legal intervention involving injury by tear gas, unspecified person injured, initial encounter

Y35.219D Legal intervention involving injury by tear gas, unspecified person injured, subsequent encounter

Y35.219S Legal intervention involving injury by tear gas, unspecified person injured, sequela

Y35.299A Legal intervention involving other gas, unspecified person injured, initial encounter

Y35.299D Legal intervention involving other gas, unspecified person injured, subsequent encounter

Y35.299S Legal intervention involving other gas, unspecified person injured, sequela

Y35.309A Legal intervention involving unspecified blunt objects, unspecified person injured, initial encounter

Y35.309D Legal intervention involving unspecified blunt objects, unspecified person injured, subsequent encounter

Y35.309S Legal intervention involving unspecified blunt objects, unspecified person injured, sequela

Y35.319A Legal intervention involving baton, unspecified person injured, initial encounter

Y35.319D Legal intervention involving baton, unspecified person injured, subsequent encounter

Y35.319S Legal intervention involving baton, unspecified person injured, sequela

Y35.399A Legal intervention involving other blunt objects, unspecified person injured, initial encounter

Y35.399D Legal intervention involving other blunt objects, unspecified person injured, subsequent encounter

Y35.399S Legal intervention involving other blunt objects, unspecified person injured, sequela

Y35.409A Legal intervention involving unspecified sharp objects, unspecified person injured, initial encounter

Y35.409D Legal intervention involving unspecified sharp objects, unspecified person injured, subsequent encounter

Y35.409S Legal intervention involving unspecified sharp objects, unspecified person injured, sequela

Y35.419A Legal intervention involving bayonet, unspecified person injured, initial encounter

Y35.419D Legal intervention involving bayonet, unspecified person injured, subsequent encounter

Y35.419S Legal intervention involving bayonet, unspecified person injured, sequela

Y35.499A Legal intervention involving other sharp objects, unspecified person injured, initial encounter

Y35.499D Legal intervention involving other sharp objects, unspecified person injured, subsequent encounter

Y35.499S Legal intervention involving other sharp objects, unspecified person injured, sequela

Y35.819A Legal intervention involving manhandling, unspecified person injured, initial encounter

Y35.819D Legal intervention involving manhandling, unspecified person injured, subsequent encounter

Y35.819S Legal intervention involving manhandling, unspecified person injured, sequela

Y35.831A Legal intervention involving a conducted energy device, law enforcement official injured, initial encounter

Y35.831D Legal intervention involving a conducted energy device, law enforcement official injured, subsequent encounter

Y35.831S Legal intervention involving a conducted energy device, law enforcement official injured, sequela

Y35.832A Legal intervention involving a conducted energy device, bystander injured, initial encounter

Y35.832D Legal intervention involving a conducted energy device, bystander injured, subsequent encounter

Y35.832S Legal intervention involving a conducted energy device, bystander injured, sequela

Y35.833A Legal intervention involving a conducted energy device, suspect injured, initial encounter

Y35.833D Legal intervention involving a conducted energy device, suspect injured, subsequent encounter

Y35.833S Legal intervention involving a conducted energy device, suspect injured, sequela

Y35.839A	Legal intervention involving a conducted energy device, unspecified person injured, initial encounter
Y35.839D	Legal intervention involving a conducted energy device, unspecified person injured, subsequent encounter
Y35.839S	Legal intervention involving a conducted energy device, unspecified person injured, sequela
Y35.99XA	Legal intervention, means unspecified, unspecified person injured, initial encounter
Y35.99XD	Legal intervention, means unspecified, unspecified person injured, subsequent encounter
Y35.99XS	Legal intervention, means unspecified, unspecified person injured, sequela
Z01.020	Encounter for examination of eyes and vision following failed vision screening without abnormal findings
Z01.021	Encounter for examination of eyes and vision following failed vision screening with abnormal findings
Z11.7	Encounter for testing for latent tuberculosis infection
Z22.7	Latent tuberculosis
Z71.84	Encounter for health counseling related to travel
Z86.002	Personal history of in-situ neoplasm of other and unspecified genital organs
Z86.003	Personal history of in-situ neoplasm of oral cavity, esophagus and stomach
Z86.004	Personal history of in-situ neoplasm of other and unspecified digestive organs
Z86.005	Personal history of in-situ neoplasm of middle ear and respiratory system
Z86.006	Personal history of melanoma in-situ
Z86.007	Personal history of in-situ neoplasm of skin
Z86.15	Personal history of latent tuberculosis infection
Z96.82	Presence of neurostimulator

30 Code Descriptions Revised

Note: Each code is listed with its revised description only. Please refer to the full FY 2020 official addenda code files at https://www.cms.gov/Medicare/Coding/ICD10/2020-ICD-10-CM.html for the specific changes made to the codes listed.

B96.21	Shiga toxin-producing Escherichia coli [E. coli] [STEC] O157 as the cause of diseases classified elsewhere
B96.22	Other specified Shiga toxin-producing Escherichia coli [E. coli] [STEC] as the cause of diseases classified elsewhere
B96.23	Unspecified Shiga toxin-producing Escherichia coli [E. coli] [STEC] as the cause of diseases classified elsewhere
G43.A0	Cyclical vomiting, in migraine, not intractable
G43.A1	Cyclical vomiting, in migraine, intractable
I70.238	Atherosclerosis of native arteries of right leg with ulceration of other part of lower leg
I70.248	Atherosclerosis of native arteries of left leg with ulceration of other part of lower leg

J44.0	Chronic obstructive pulmonary disease with (acute) lower respiratory infection
M50.120	Mid-cervical disc disorder, unspecified level
M66.88	Spontaneous rupture of other tendons, other sites
M67.839	Other specified disorders of synovium and tendon, unspecified wrist
M77.50	Other enthesopathy of unspecified foot and ankle
M77.51	Other enthesopathy of right foot and ankle
M77.52	Other enthesopathy of left foot and ankle
N35.814	Other anterior urethral stricture, male
R82.993	Hyperuricosuria
T40.906A	Underdosing of unspecified psychodysleptics [hallucinogens], initial encounter
T40.906D	Underdosing of unspecified psychodysleptics [hallucinogens], subsequent encounter
T40.906S	Underdosing of unspecified psychodysleptics [hallucinogens], sequela
T40.996A	Underdosing of other psychodysleptics [hallucinogens], initial encounter
T40.996D	Underdosing of other psychodysleptics [hallucinogens], subsequent encounter
T40.996S	Underdosing of other psychodysleptics [hallucinogens], sequela
T44.1X6A	Underdosing of other parasympathomimetics [cholinergics], initial encounter
T44.1X6D	Underdosing of other parasympathomimetics [cholinergics], subsequent encounter
T44.1X6S	Underdosing of other parasympathomimetics [cholinergics], sequela
V43.13XA	Car passenger injured in collision with pick-up truck in nontraffic accident, initial encounter
V43.13XD	Car passenger injured in collision with pick-up truck in nontraffic accident, subsequent encounter
V43.13XS	Car passenger injured in collision with pick-up truck in nontraffic accident, sequela
Z45.42	Encounter for adjustment and management of neurostimulator
Z68.43	Body mass index (BMI) 50.0-59.9, adult

Proprietary Updates

The following proprietary features have also been added:

- 40+ new definitions that describe, in lay terms, a specific condition or disease process

- 40+ new coding tips that provide coding advice beyond the code classification

- Updated *AHA Coding Clinic* references through second quarter 2019

- Conversion table of ICD-10-CM codes

Conversion Table of ICD-10-CM Codes

Code Assignment Beginning 10/1/2019	Previous Code(s) Assignment	Code Assignment Beginning 10/1/2019	Previous Code(s) Assignment	Code Assignment Beginning 10/1/2019	Previous Code(s) Assignment
D75.A	D55.0	L89.316	L89.310	S02.121A	S02.19A*
D81.30	D81.3	L89.326	L89.320	S02.121B	S02.19B*
D81.31	D81.3	L89.46	L89.45	S02.121D	S02.19D*
D81.32	D81.3	L89.506	L89.500	S02.121G	S02.19G*
D81.39	D81.3	L89.516	L89.510	S02.121K	S02.19K*
H81.4	H81.41–H81.43; H81.49	L89.526	L89.520	S02.121S	S02.19S*
I26.93	I26.99	L89.606	L89.600	S02.122A	S02.19A*
I26.94	I26.99	L89.616	L89.610	S02.122B	S02.19B*
I48.11	I48.1	L89.626	L89.620	S02.122D	S02.19D*
I48.19	I48.1	L89.816	L89.810	S02.122G	S02.19G*
I48.20	I48.2	L89.896	L89.890	S02.122K	S02.19K*
I48.21	I48.2	L89.96	L89.95	S02.122S	S02.19S*
I80.241	I80.291	N63.15	N63.11–N63.14	S02.129A	S02.19A*
I80.242	I80.292	N63.25	N63.21–N63.24	S02.129B	S02.19B*
I80.243	I80.293	N99.85	N99.89	S02.129D	S02.19D*
I80.249	I80.299	Q66.00	Q66.0	S02.129G	S02.19G*
I80.251	I80.291	Q66.01	Q66.0	S02.129K	S02.19K*
I80.252	I80.292	Q66.02	Q66.0	S02.129S	S02.19S*
I80.253	I80.293	Q66.10	Q66.1	S02.831A	S02.81XA
I80.259	I80.299	Q66.11	Q66.1	S02.831B	S02.81XB
I82.451	I80.491	Q66.12	Q66.1	S02.831D	S02.81XD
I82.452	I80.492	Q66.211	Q66.21	S02.831G	S02.81XG
I82.453	I80.493	Q66.212	Q66.21	S02.831K	S02.81XK
I82.459	I80.499	Q66.219	Q66.21	S02.831S	S02.81XS
I82.461	I80.491	Q66.221	Q66.22	S02.832A	S02.82XA
I82.462	I80.492	Q66.222	Q66.22	S02.832B	S02.82XB
I82.463	I80.493	Q66.229	Q66.22	S02.832D	S02.82XD
I82.469	I80.499	Q66.30	Q66.3	S02.832G	S02.82XG
I82.551	I80.591	Q66.31	Q66.3	S02.832K	S02.82XK
I82.552	I80.592	Q66.32	Q66.3	S02.832S	S02.82XS
I82.553	I80.593	Q66.40	Q66.4	S02.839A	S02.80XA
I82.559	I80.599	Q66.41	Q66.4	S02.839B	S02.80XB
I82.561	I80.591	Q66.42	Q66.4	S02.839D	S02.80XD
I82.562	I80.592	Q66.70	Q66.7	S02.839G	S02.80XG
I82.563	I80.593	Q66.71	Q66.7	S02.839K	S02.80XK
I82.569	I80.599	Q66.72	Q66.7	S02.839S	S02.80XS
L89.006	L89.000	Q66.90	Q66.9	S02.841A	S02.81XA
L89.016	L89.010	Q66.91	Q66.9	S02.841B	S02.81XB
L89.026	L89.020	Q66.92	Q66.9	S02.841D	S02.81XD
L89.106	L89.100	Q79.60	Q79.6	S02.841G	S02.81XG
L89.116	L89.110	Q79.61	Q79.6	S02.841K	S02.81XK
L89.126	L89.120	Q79.62	Q79.6	S02.841S	S02.81XS
L89.136	L89.130	Q79.63	Q79.6	S02.842A	S02.82XA
L89.146	L89.140	Q79.69	Q79.6	S02.842B	S02.82XB
L89.156	L89.150	Q87.11	Q87.1	S02.842D	S02.82XD
L89.206	L89.200	Q87.19	Q87.1	S02.842G	S02.82XG
L89.216	L89.210	R11.15	K31.89 and a code from R11-	S02.842K	S02.82XK
L89.226	L89.220	R82.81	R82.8	S02.842S	S02.82XS
L89.306	L89.300	R82.89	R82.8	S02.849A	S02.80XA
				S02.849B	S02.80XB

Conversion Table of ICD-10-CM Codes

Code Assignment Beginning 10/1/2019	Previous Code(s) Assignment	Code Assignment Beginning 10/1/2019	Previous Code(s) Assignment	Code Assignment Beginning 10/1/2019	Previous Code(s) Assignment
S02.849D	S02.80XD	Y35.029A	None	Y35.409D	None
S02.849G	S02.80XG	Y35.029D	None	Y35.409S	None
S02.849K	S02.80XK	Y35.029S	None	Y35.419A	None
S02.849S	S02.80XS	Y35.039A	None	Y35.419D	None
S02.85XA	S02.80XA	Y35.039D	None	Y35.419S	None
S02.85XB	S02.80XB	Y35.039S	None	Y35.499A	None
S02.85XD	S02.80XD	Y35.049A	None	Y35.499D	None
S02.85XG	S02.80XG	Y35.049D	None	Y35.499S	None
S02.85XK	S02.80XK	Y35.049S	None	Y35.819A	None
S02.85XS	S02.80XS	Y35.099A	None	Y35.819D	None
T50.911A	T50.991A	Y35.099D	None	Y35.819S	None
T50.911D	T50.991D	Y35.099S	None	Y35.831A	Y35.891A
T50.911S	T50.991S	Y35.109A	None	Y35.831D	Y35.891D
T50.912A	T50.992A	Y35.109D	None	Y35.831S	Y35.891S
T50.912D	T50.992D	Y35.109S	None	Y35.832A	Y35.892A
T50.912S	T50.992S	Y35.119A	None	Y35.832D	Y35.892D
T50.913A	T50.993A	Y35.119D	None	Y35.832S	Y35.892S
T50.913D	T50.993D	Y35.119S	None	Y35.833A	Y35.893A
T50.913S	T50.993S	Y35.129A	None	Y35.833D	Y35.893D
T50.914A	T50.994A	Y35.129D	None	Y35.833S	Y35.893S
T50.914D	T50.994D	Y35.129S	None	Y35.839A	None
T50.914S	T50.994S	Y35.199A	None	Y35.839D	None
T50.915A	T50.995A	Y35.199D	None	Y35.839S	None
T50.915D	T50.995D	Y35.199S	None	Y35.99XA	None
T50.915S	T50.995S	Y35.209A	None	Y35.99XD	None
T50.916A	T50.996A	Y35.209D	None	Y35.99XS	None
T50.916D	T50.996D	Y35.209S	None	Z01.020	Z01.00
T50.916S	T50.996S	Y35.219A	None	Z01.021	Z01.01
T67.01XA	T67.0XXA	Y35.219D	None	Z11.7	Z11.1
T67.01XD	T67.0XXD	Y35.219S	None	Z22.7	R76.11
T67.01XS	T67.0XXS	Y35.299A	None	Z71.84	Z71.89
T67.02XA	T67.0XXA	Y35.299D	None	Z86.002	Z86.008
T67.02XD	T67.0XXD	Y35.299S	None	Z86.003	Z86.008
T67.02XS	T67.0XXS	Y35.309A	None	Z86.004	Z86.008
T67.09XA	T67.0XXA	Y35.309D	None	Z86.005	Z86.008
T67.09XD	T67.0XXD	Y35.309S	None	Z86.006	Z86.008
T67.09XS	T67.0XXS	Y35.319A	None	Z86.007	Z86.008
Y35.009A	None	Y35.319D	None	Z86.15	R76.11
Y35.009D	None	Y35.319S	None	Z96.82	Z96.89
Y35.009S	None	Y35.399A	None		
Y35.019A	None	Y35.399D	None		
Y35.019D	None	Y35.399S	None		
Y35.019S	None	Y35.409A	None		

* These codes are listed exactly as found in the official conversion table from the CDC.

10 Steps to Correct Coding

Follow the 10 steps below to correctly code encounters for health care services.

Step 1: Identify the reason for the visit or encounter (i.e., a sign, symptom, diagnosis and/or condition).
The medical record documentation should accurately reflect the patient's condition, using terminology that includes specific diagnoses and symptoms or clearly states the reasons for the encounter.

Choosing the main term that best describes the reason chiefly responsible for the service provided is the most important step in coding. If symptoms are present and documented but a definitive diagnosis has not yet been determined, code the symptoms. *For outpatient cases, do not code conditions that are referred to as "rule out," "suspected," "probable," or "questionable."* Diagnoses often are not established at the time of the initial encounter/visit and may require two or more visits to be established. Code only what is documented in the available outpatient records and only to the highest degree of certainty known at the time of the patient's visit. For inpatient medical records, uncertain diagnoses may be reported if documented at the time of discharge.

Step 2: After selecting the reason for the encounter, consult the alphabetic index.
The most critical rule is to begin code selection in the alphabetic index. Never turn first to the tabular list. The index provides cross-references, essential and nonessential modifiers, and other instructional notations that may not be found in the tabular list.

Step 3: Locate the main term entry.
The alphabetic index lists conditions, which may be expressed as nouns or eponyms, with critical use of adjectives. Some conditions known by several names have multiple main entries. Reasons for encounters may be located under general terms such as admission, encounter, and examination. Other general terms such as history, status (post), or presence (of) can be used to locate other factors influencing health.

Step 4: Scan subterm entries.
Scan the subterm entries, as appropriate, being sure to review continued lines and additional subterms that may appear in the next column or on the next page. Shaded vertical guidelines in the index indicate the indentation level for each subterm in relation to the main terms.

Step 5: Pay close attention to index instructions.
- Parentheses ( ) enclose nonessential modifiers, terms that are supplementary words or explanatory information that may or may not appear in the diagnostic statement and do not affect code selection.

- Brackets [ ] enclose manifestation codes that can be used only as secondary codes to the underlying condition code immediately preceding it. If used, manifestation codes must be reported with the appropriate etiology codes.

- Default codes are listed next to the main term and represent the condition most commonly associated with the main term or the unspecified code for the main term.

- "*See*" cross-references, identified by italicized type and "code by" cross-references indicate that another term *must be referenced* to locate the correct code.

- "*See also*" cross-references, identified by italicized type, provide alternative terms that may be useful to look up but *are not mandatory*.

- "Omit code" cross-references identify instances when a code is not applicable depending on the condition being coded.

- "With" subterms are listed out of alphabetic order and identify a presumed causal relationship between the two conditions they link.

- "Due to" subterms identify a relationship between the two conditions they link.

- "NEC," abbreviation for "not elsewhere classified," follows some main terms or subterms and indicates that there is no specific code for the condition even though the medical documentation may be very specific.

- "NOS," abbreviation for "not otherwise specified," follows some main terms or subterms and is the equivalent of unspecified; NOS signifies that the information in the medical record is insufficient for assigning a more specific code.

- *Following* references help coders locate alphanumeric codes that are out of sequence in the tabular section.

- Check-additional-character symbols flag codes that require additional characters to make the code valid; the characters available to complete the code should be verified in the tabular section.

Step 6: Choose a potential code and locate it in the tabular list.
To prevent coding errors, always use both the alphabetic index (to identify a code) and the tabular list (to verify a code), as the index does not include the important instructional notes found in the tabular list. An added benefit of using the tabular list, which groups like things together, is that while looking at one code in the list, a coder might see a more specific one that would have been missed had the coder relied solely on the alphabetic index. Additionally, many of the codes require a fourth, fifth, sixth, or seventh character to be valid, and many of these characters can be found only in the tabular list.

Step 7: Read all instructional material in the tabular section.
The coder must follow any Includes, Excludes 1 and Excludes 2 notes, and other instructional notes, such as "Code first" and "Use additional code," listed in the tabular list for the chapter, category, subcategory, and subclassification levels of code selection that direct the coder to use a different or additional code. Any codes in the tabular range A00.0- through T88.9- may be used to identify the diagnostic reason for the encounter. The tabular list encompasses many codes describing disease and injury classifications (e.g., infectious and parasitic diseases, neoplasms, symptoms, nervous and circulatory system etc.).

Codes that describe symptoms and signs, as opposed to definitive diagnoses, should be reported when an established diagnosis has not been made (confirmed) by the physician. Chapter 18 of the ICD-10-CM code book, "Symptoms, Signs, and Abnormal Clinical and Laboratory Findings, Not Elsewhere Classified" (codes R00.--R99), contains many, but not all, codes for symptoms.

ICD-10-CM classifies encounters with health care providers for circumstances other than a disease or injury in chapter 21, "Factors Influencing Health Status and Contact with Health Services" (codes Z00–Z99). Circumstances other than a disease or injury often are recorded as chiefly responsible for the encounter.

A code is invalid if it does not include the full number of characters (greatest level of specificity) required. Codes in ICD-10-CM can contain from three to seven alphanumeric characters. A three-character code is to be used only if the category is not further subdivided into four-, five-, six-, or seven-character codes. Placeholder character X is used as part of an alphanumeric code to allow for future expansion and as a placeholder for empty characters in a code that requires a seventh character but has no fourth, fifth, or sixth character. Note that certain categories require seventh characters that apply to all codes in that category. Always check the category level for applicable seventh characters for that category.

Step 8: Consult the official ICD-10-CM conventions and guidelines.

The *ICD-10-CM Official Guidelines for Coding and Reporting* govern the use of certain codes. These guidelines provide both general and chapter-specific coding guidance.

Step 9: Confirm and assign the code.

Having reviewed all relevant information concerning the possible code choices, assign the code that most completely describes the condition.

Repeat steps 1 through 9 for all additional documented conditions that meet the following criteria:

- They exist at the time of the visit *AND*
- They require or affect patient care, treatment, or management

Step 10: Sequence codes correctly.

Sequencing is the order in which the codes are listed on the claim. List first the ICD-10-CM code for the diagnosis, condition, problem, or other reason for the encounter/visit that is shown in the medical record to be chiefly responsible for the services provided. List additional codes that describe any coexisting conditions. Follow the official coding guidelines (see the guidelines, section II, "Selection of Principal Diagnosis"; section III, "Reporting Additional Diagnoses"; and section IV, "Diagnostic Coding and Reporting Guidelines for Outpatient Services") on proper sequencing of codes.

Coding Examples

Diagnosis: Anorexia

Step 1: The reason for the encounter was the condition, anorexia.

Step 2: Consult the alphabetic index.

Step 3: Locate the main term "Anorexia."

Step 4: Two possible subterms are available, "hysterical" and "nervosa." Neither is documented in this instance, however, so they cannot be used in code selection.

Step 5: The code listed next to the main term is called the default code selection. Because the two subentries (essential modifiers) do not apply in this instance, the default code (R63.0) should be used.

Step 6: Turn to code R63.0 in the tabular list and read all instructional notes.

Step 7: The Excludes 1 note at code R63.0 indicates that anorexia nervosa and loss of appetite determined to be of nonorganic origin should be reported with a code from chapter 5. The diagnostic statement does not describe the condition as anorexia nervosa, however, and does not indicate that the anorexia is of a nonorganic origin. There is no further division of the category past the fourth-character subcategory. Therefore, code R63.0 is at the highest level of specificity.

Step 8: Review of official guideline I.C.18 indicates that a symptom code is appropriate when a more definitive diagnosis is not documented.

Step 9: The default code, R63.0 Anorexia, is the correct code selection.

Repeat steps 1 through 9 for any concomitant diagnoses.

Step 10: Since anorexia is listed as the chief reason for the health care encounter, the first-listed, or principal, diagnosis is R63.0. Note that this is a chapter 18 symptom code but can be assigned for both inpatient and outpatient records since the provider did not establish a more definitive diagnosis, according to sections II.A and IV.D.

Diagnosis: Acute bronchitis

Step 1: The reason for the encounter was the condition, acute bronchitis.

Step 2: Consult the alphabetic index.

Step 3: Locate the main term "Bronchitis."

Step 4: There is a subterm for "acute or subacute." Additional subterms are not included in the diagnostic statement.

Step 5: Review the instructional notes. Nonessential modifiers (with bronchospasm or obstruction) are terms that do not affect code assignment. Since no other subterms indented under "acute" apply here, the code listed next to this subentry—in this case J20.9—should be chosen.

Step 6: Turn to code J20.9 in the tabular list and read all instructional notes.

Step 7: The Includes note under category J20 lists alternative terms for acute bronchitis. Note that the list is not exhaustive but is only a representative selection of diagnoses that are included in the subcategory. The Excludes 1 note refers to category J40 for bronchitis and tracheobronchitis NOS. There are several conditions in the Excludes 2 notes that, if applicable, can be coded in addition to this code.

Note that the codes included in J20 represent acute bronchitis due to various infectious organisms that could be selected if identified in the documentation. In this case, the organism was not identified and there is no further division of the category past the fourth character subcategory. Therefore, code J20.9 is at the highest level of specificity.

Step 8: Review of official guideline I.C.10 provides no additional information affecting the code selected.

Step 9: Assign code J20.9 Acute bronchitis, unspecified.

Repeat steps 1 through 9 for any concomitant diagnoses.

Step 10: In the absence of additional diagnoses that may affect sequencing, code J20.9 should be sequenced as the first-listed, or principal, diagnosis.

Diagnosis: Cerebellar ataxia in myxedema

Step 1: The reason for the encounter was the condition, cerebellar ataxia.

Step 2: Consult the alphabetic index.

Step 3: Locate the main term "Ataxia."

Step 4: Available subterms include "cerebellar (hereditary)," with additional indented subterms for "in" and "myxedema," all essential modifiers that are included in the diagnostic statement. Two codes are provided, E03.9 and G13.2, the latter of which is in brackets.

Step 5: Note the nonessential modifier (in parentheses) after the subterm cerebellar includes the term "hereditary." Because it is in parentheses, this term is not required in the diagnostic statement for this subentry to apply. The brackets around G13.2 identify this code as a manifestation of the condition described by code E03.9 and indicate that the two must be reported together and sequencing rules apply.

Step 6: Locate codes E03.9 and G13.2 in the tabular list, and read all instructional notes.

Step 7: For code E03.9, there are no instructional notes in the tabular list at the category E03 or code level that indicate that this condition should be coded elsewhere in the classification or that additional codes are required. Without further information from the diagnostic statement, myxedema, not otherwise specified (NOS), is appropriately reported with code E03.9 Hypothyroidism, unspecified, according to the inclusion term at this code.

Code G13.2 in the tabular list has an instructional note to "Code first underlying disease," which includes conditions found in category E03.-. Based on this note, codes E03.9 and G13.2 are to be coded together, with G13.2 listed only as a secondary diagnosis. This correlates with what the alphabetic index indicated. As there is no further division of codes in category G13 beyond the fourth character, G13.2 is at the highest level of specificity.

Step 8: Although there are some general conventions, such as how to interpret brackets in the alphabetic index, no chapter-specific guidelines apply to this coding scenario.

Step 9: Assign codes E03.9 Hypothyroidism, unspecified, and G13.2 Systemic atrophy primarily affecting the central nervous system in myxedema.

Repeat steps 1 through 9 for any concomitant diagnoses.

Step 10: Based on the alphabetic index and tabular instructional notations, code E03.9 should be sequenced as the first-listed, or principal, diagnosis followed by G13.2 as a secondary diagnosis.

Diagnosis: Decubitus ulcer of right elbow with skin loss and necrosis of subcutaneous tissue

Step 1: The reason for the encounter was the condition, decubitus ulcer.

Step 2: Consult the alphabetic index.

Step 3: Locate the main term "Ulcer."

Step 4: For the subterm "decubitus," there is no code provided or additional subterms indented, but a cross-reference is listed.

Step 5: The italicized cross-reference instructs the coder to "*see* Ulcer, pressure, by site."

Repeat steps 3 through 5 for the cross-reference.

Step 3: Locate the main term "Ulcer."

Step 4: Review the subentries for the subterm "pressure." The next level of indent lists either the site of the ulcer or the specific stage of the ulcer (stage 1–4, unstageable, and unspecified stages). The diagnostic statement provides the site, right elbow, and the extent of tissue damage (skin loss and necrosis of subcutaneous tissue) but does not specifically state that the ulcer is stage 1, stage 2, etc. Nonessential modifiers (in parentheses) at each stage include a description of the typical extent of damage at each stage. For example, stage 1 describes "pre-ulcer skin changes limited to persistent focal edema." Based on the documentation in the record, the coder can correlate the documentation to the nonessential modifiers and choose the specific stage from the index. The coder can also go directly to the body site, choosing the stage of the ulcer after reviewing the code options and instructional notations in the tabular list.

The diagnostic statement indicates that the extent of the damage to the elbow includes skin loss and necrosis of subcutaneous tissue, coinciding with the nonessential modifier next to the subentry "stage 3." The body site of elbow (L89.0-) is listed as another level of indent with other body sites.

Step 5: Note that code L89.0 is followed by a dash and an additional-character-required icon, which indicate that more characters are needed to complete the code. From here, the tabular listing for L89.0- can be consulted.

Step 6: Locate code L89.0- in the tabular list and read all instructional notes.

Step 7: The tabular listing at category L89 has an Includes note for "decubitus ulcer," which confirms that category L89 is the appropriate category to represent what is documented in the diagnostic statement.

Several Excludes 2 notes are also listed at the category level. Excludes 2 notes represent conditions that can occur concomitantly with the decubitus ulcer and can be coded in addition to code L89, if supported by the documentation.

The subcategory codes under L89.0 indicate that the fifth character describes laterality. Locate the right elbow at subcategory L89.01. See that an additional sixth character to specify the stage of the ulcer is now needed to complete the code. The stage can be determined either by the specific documentation of the stage (e.g., stage 1, stage 2) or, in this case, a description that matches one of the inclusion terms that follow

each stage code. For example, the diagnostic description in this case of "skin loss and necrosis of the subcutaneous tissue" matches the inclusion term under L89.013 Pressure ulcer of right elbow, stage 3. No additional characters are required because code L89.013 is at its highest level of specificity.

Step 8: The official guidelines contain quite a bit of information relating to pressure ulcers in chapter-specific guideline I.C.12 as well as information in general guideline I.B.14. These and any other pertinent guidelines should be reviewed to ensure appropriate code assignment.

Step 9: Assign code L89.013 Pressure ulcer of right elbow, stage 3.

Repeat steps 1 through 9 for any concomitant diagnoses.

Step 10: Since the decubitus ulcer is listed as the chief reason for the health care encounter, the first-listed, or principal, diagnosis is L89.013. However, according to the code first instructional note at the L89 category level, gangrene (I96) would be sequenced before the pressure ulcer if it were documented.

Diagnosis: Emergency department visit for bimalleolar fracture of the right ankle due to trauma

Step 1: The reason for the encounter was the condition, bimalleolar fracture.

Step 2: Consult the alphabetic index.

Step 3: Locate the main term "Fracture." Note that many main terms represent fractures: "Fracture, burst," "Fracture, chronic," "Fracture, insufficiency," "Fracture, nontraumatic NEC," "Fracture, pathological," and "Fracture, traumatic." Since the diagnostic statement specifically states that this fracture was the result of trauma, the main term "Fracture, traumatic" should be used.

Step 4: Subterms that should be referenced are "ankle" and "bimalleolar (displaced)," which lists code S82.84-.

Step 5: A nonessential modifier (in parentheses) next to the term bimalleolar for "displaced" indicates that S82.84- is the default category unless the fracture is specifically identified as "nondisplaced."

Note that code S82.84- is followed by a dash and an additional-character icon, both of which indicate that more characters are required. From here, the tabular list can be consulted.

Step 6: Locate code S82.84- in the tabular list and read all instructional notes.

Step: 7 The instructional notes at category S82 indicate that fractures not specified as displaced or nondisplaced default to displaced and that fractures not designated as open or closed default to closed. Additional instructional notes can be found at the category level but none pertain to the current scenario.

Read through the subcategory codes under S82.84, and note that the sixth character specifies displaced or nondisplaced and laterality. Based on the index nonessential modifier (displaced) and the code note at category S82, code selection should identify a displaced fracture of the right side. A displaced bimalleolar fracture of the right lower leg is coded to S82.841.

To complete the code, a seventh character must be assigned to identify the type of encounter (initial, subsequent, or sequela) and whether the fracture is open or closed. Most of the codes in category S82 require a seventh character represented in the list at the category level. However, it is important to note that some subcategories have their own specific set of seventh characters. In this instance, subcategory S82.84- does not have a unique set of seventh characters and the list provided at the category level should be used. Without documentation of the fracture being open, the tabular notation indicates that the default is closed. Character A, representing "initial encounter for closed fracture," listed in the box at the category level is the most appropriate option.

Step 8: Assign code S82.841A Displaced bimalleolar fracture of right lower leg, initial encounter for closed fracture.

Repeat steps 1 through 9 for any concomitant diagnoses.

Step 9: Review chapter-specific guideline I.C.19. and any other official conventions or guidelines to ensure appropriate code assignment.

Step 10: Additional codes can be applied to relate the specific cause of the injury, the place of occurrence, the activity of the patient at the time of the injury, and the patient's status, when this information is available in the record. However, coding this information is voluntary and

reporting requirements depend on state mandates and/or facility-specific reporting requirements. If assigned, the external cause codes should be reported as secondary diagnoses only with the injury (fracture) sequenced first. Most codes in chapter 20, "External Causes of Morbidity," require a seventh character to identify the type of encounter. The seventh character assigned to an external cause code should match the seventh character of the code assigned for the associated injury or condition for the encounter.

2020 ICD-10-CM Official Guidelines for Coding and Reporting

Narrative changes appear in **bold** text

Items underlined have been moved within the guidelines since the FY 2019 version

Italics are used to indicate revisions to heading changes

The Centers for Medicare and Medicaid Services (CMS) and the National Center for Health Statistics (NCHS), two departments within the U.S. Federal Government's Department of Health and Human Services (DHHS) provide the following guidelines for coding and reporting using the International Classification of Diseases, 10th Revision, Clinical Modification (ICD-10-CM). These guidelines should be used as a companion document to the official version of the ICD-10-CM as published on the NCHS website. The ICD-10-CM is a morbidity classification published by the United States for classifying diagnoses and reason for visits in all health care settings. The ICD-10-CM is based on the ICD-10, the statistical classification of disease published by the World Health Organization (WHO).

These guidelines have been approved by the four organizations that make up the Cooperating Parties for the ICD-10-CM: the American Hospital Association (AHA), the American Health Information Management Association (AHIMA), CMS, and NCHS.

These guidelines are a set of rules that have been developed to accompany and complement the official conventions and instructions provided within the ICD-10-CM itself. The instructions and conventions of the classification take precedence over guidelines. These guidelines are based on the coding and sequencing instructions in the Tabular List and Alphabetic Index of ICD-10-CM, but provide additional instruction. Adherence to these guidelines when assigning ICD-10-CM diagnosis codes is required under the Health Insurance Portability and Accountability Act (HIPAA). The diagnosis codes (Tabular List and Alphabetic Index) have been adopted under HIPAA for all healthcare settings. A joint effort between the healthcare provider and the coder is essential to achieve complete and accurate documentation, code assignment, and reporting of diagnoses and procedures. These guidelines have been developed to assist both the healthcare provider and the coder in identifying those diagnoses that are to be reported. The importance of consistent, complete documentation in the medical record cannot be overemphasized. Without such documentation accurate coding cannot be achieved. The entire record should be reviewed to determine the specific reason for the encounter and the conditions treated.

The term encounter is used for all settings, including hospital admissions. In the context of these guidelines, the term provider is used throughout the guidelines to mean physician or any qualified health care practitioner who is legally accountable for establishing the patient's diagnosis. Only this set of guidelines, approved by the Cooperating Parties, is official.

The guidelines are organized into sections. Section I includes the structure and conventions of the classification and general guidelines that apply to the entire classification, and chapter-specific guidelines that correspond to the chapters as they are arranged in the classification. Section II includes guidelines for selection of principal diagnosis for non-outpatient settings. Section III includes guidelines for reporting additional diagnoses in non-outpatient settings. Section IV is for outpatient coding and reporting. It is necessary to review all sections of the guidelines to fully understand all of the rules and instructions needed to code properly.

2020 ICD-10-CM Official Guidelines for Coding and Reporting *(vertical left margin)*

Section I. Conventions, general coding guidelines and chapter specific guidelines

The conventions, general guidelines and chapter-specific guidelines are applicable to all health care settings unless otherwise indicated. The conventions and instructions of the classification take precedence over guidelines.

A. Conventions for the ICD-10-CM

The conventions for the ICD-10-CM are the general rules for use of the classification independent of the guidelines. These conventions are incorporated within the Alphabetic Index and Tabular List of the ICD-10-CM as instructional notes.

1. The Alphabetic Index and Tabular List
The ICD-10-CM is divided into the Alphabetic Index, an alphabetical list of terms and their corresponding code, and the Tabular List, a structured list of codes divided into chapters based on body system or condition. The Alphabetic Index consists of the following parts: the Index of Diseases and Injury, the Index of External Causes of Injury, the Table of Neoplasms and the Table of Drugs and Chemicals.

See Section I.C2. General guidelines

See Section I.C.19. Adverse effects, poisoning, underdosing and toxic effects

2. Format and Structure:
The ICD-10-CM Tabular List contains categories, subcategories and codes. Characters for categories, subcategories and codes may be either a letter or a number. All categories are 3 characters. A three-character category that has no further subdivision is equivalent to a code. Subcategories are either 4 or 5 characters. Codes may be 3, 4, 5, 6 or 7 characters. That is, each level of subdivision after a category is a subcategory. The final level of subdivision is a code. Codes that have applicable 7th characters are still referred to as codes, not subcategories. A code that has an applicable 7th character is considered invalid without the 7th character.

The ICD-10-CM uses an indented format for ease in reference.

3. Use of codes for reporting purposes
For reporting purposes only codes are permissible, not categories or subcategories, and any applicable 7th character is required.

4. Placeholder character
The ICD-10-CM utilizes a placeholder character "X". The "X" is used as a placeholder at certain codes to allow for future expansion. An example of this is at the poisoning, adverse effect and underdosing codes, categories T36-T50.

Where a placeholder exists, the X must be used in order for the code to be considered a valid code.

5. 7th Characters
Certain ICD-10-CM categories have applicable 7th characters. The applicable 7th character is required for all codes within the category, or as the notes in the Tabular List instruct. The 7th character must always be the 7th character in the data field. If a code that requires a 7th character is not 6 characters, a placeholder X must be used to fill in the empty characters.

6. Abbreviations
a. Alphabetic Index abbreviations
NEC "Not elsewhere classifiable"

This abbreviation in the Alphabetic Index represents "other specified." When a specific code is not available for a condition, the Alphabetic Index directs the coder to the "other specified" code in the Tabular List.

NOS "Not otherwise specified"

This abbreviation is the equivalent of unspecified.

b. Tabular List abbreviations
NEC "Not elsewhere classifiable"

This abbreviation in the Tabular List represents "other specified". When a specific code is not available for a condition, the Tabular List includes an NEC entry under a code to identify the code as the "other specified" code.

NOS "Not otherwise specified"

This abbreviation is the equivalent of unspecified.

7. Punctuation
[ ] Brackets are used in the Tabular List to enclose synonyms, alternative wording or explanatory phrases. Brackets are used in the Alphabetic Index to identify manifestation codes.

( ) Parentheses are used in both the Alphabetic Index and Tabular List to enclose supplementary words that may be present or absent in the statement of a disease or procedure without affecting the code number to which it is assigned. The terms within the parentheses are referred to as nonessential modifiers. The nonessential modifiers in the Alphabetic Index to Diseases apply to subterms following a main term except when a nonessential modifier and a subentry are mutually exclusive, the subentry takes precedence. For example, in the ICD-10-CM Alphabetic Index under the main term Enteritis, "acute" is a nonessential modifier and "chronic" is a subentry. In this case, the nonessential modifier "acute" does not apply to the subentry "chronic".

: Colons are used in the Tabular List after an incomplete term which needs one or more of the modifiers following the colon to make it assignable to a given category.

8. Use of "and"
See Section I.A.14. Use of the term "And"

9. Other and Unspecified codes
a. "Other" codes
Codes titled "other" or "other specified" are for use when the information in the medical record provides detail for which a specific code does not exist. Alphabetic Index entries with NEC in the line designate "other" codes in the Tabular List. These Alphabetic Index entries represent specific disease entities for which no specific code exists so the term is included within an "other" code.

b. "Unspecified" codes
Codes titled "unspecified" are for use when the information in the medical record is insufficient to assign a more specific code. For those categories for which an unspecified code is not provided, the "other specified" code may represent both other and unspecified.

See Section I.B.18 Use of Signs/Symptom/Unspecified Codes

10. Includes Notes
This note appears immediately under a three character code title to further define, or give examples of, the content of the category.

11. Inclusion terms
List of terms is included under some codes. These terms are the conditions for which that code is to be used. The terms may be synonyms of the code title, or, in the case of "other specified" codes, the terms are a list of the various conditions assigned to that code. The inclusion terms are not necessarily exhaustive. Additional terms found only in the Alphabetic Index may also be assigned to a code.

12. Excludes Notes
The ICD-10-CM has two types of excludes notes. Each type of note has a different definition for use but they are all similar in that they indicate that codes excluded from each other are independent of each other.

a. Excludes1
A type 1 Excludes note is a pure excludes note. It means "NOT CODED HERE!" An Excludes1 note indicates that the code excluded should never be used at the same time as the code above the Excludes1 note. An Excludes1 is used when two conditions cannot occur together, such as a congenital form versus an acquired form of the same condition.

An exception to the Excludes1 definition is the circumstance when the two conditions are unrelated to each other. If it is not clear whether the two conditions involving an Excludes1 note are related or not, query the provider. For example, code F45.8, Other somatoform disorders, has an Excludes1 note for "sleep related teeth grinding (G47.63)," because "teeth grinding" is an inclusion term under F45.8. Only one of these two codes should be assigned for teeth grinding. However psychogenic dysmenorrhea is also an inclusion term under F45.8, and a patient could have both this condition and sleep related teeth grinding. In this case, the two conditions are clearly unrelated to each other, and so it would be appropriate to report F45.8 and G47.63 together.

b. Excludes2

A type 2 Excludes note represents "Not included here." An excludes2 note indicates that the condition excluded is not part of the condition represented by the code, but a patient may have both conditions at the same time. When an Excludes2 note appears under a code, it is acceptable to use both the code and the excluded code together, when appropriate.

13. Etiology/manifestation convention ("code first", "use additional code" and "in diseases classified elsewhere" notes)

Certain conditions have both an underlying etiology and multiple body system manifestations due to the underlying etiology. For such conditions, the ICD-10-CM has a coding convention that requires the underlying condition be sequenced first, if applicable, followed by the manifestation. Wherever such a combination exists, there is a "use additional code" note at the etiology code, and a "code first" note at the manifestation code. These instructional notes indicate the proper sequencing order of the codes, etiology followed by manifestation.

In most cases the manifestation codes will have in the code title, "in diseases classified elsewhere." Codes with this title are a component of the etiology/ manifestation convention. The code title indicates that it is a manifestation code. "In diseases classified elsewhere" codes are never permitted to be used as first-listed or principal diagnosis codes. They must be used in conjunction with an underlying condition code and they must be listed following the underlying condition. See category F02, Dementia in other diseases classified elsewhere, for an example of this convention.

There are manifestation codes that do not have "in diseases classified elsewhere" in the title. For such codes, there is a "use additional code" note at the etiology code and a "code first" note at the manifestation code, and the rules for sequencing apply.

In addition to the notes in the Tabular List, these conditions also have a specific Alphabetic Index entry structure. In the Alphabetic Index both conditions are listed together with the etiology code first followed by the manifestation codes in brackets. The code in brackets is always to be sequenced second.

An example of the etiology/manifestation convention is dementia in Parkinson's disease. In the Alphabetic Index, code G20 is listed first, followed by code F02.80 or F02.81 in brackets. Code G20 represents the underlying etiology, Parkinson's disease, and must be sequenced first, whereas code F02.80 and F02.81 represent the manifestation of dementia in diseases classified elsewhere, with or without behavioral disturbance.

"Code first" and "Use additional code" notes are also used as sequencing rules in the classification for certain codes that are not part of an etiology/ manifestation combination.

See Section I.B.7. Multiple coding for a single condition.

14. "And"

The word "and" should be interpreted to mean either "and" or "or" when it appears in a title.

For example, cases of "tuberculosis of bones", "tuberculosis of joints" and "tuberculosis of bones and joints" are classified to subcategory A18.0, Tuberculosis of bones and joints.

15. "With"

The word "with" or "in" should be interpreted to mean "associated with" or "due to" when it appears in a code title, the Alphabetic Index (either under a main term or subterm), or an instructional note in the Tabular List. The classification presumes a causal relationship between the two conditions linked by these terms in the Alphabetic Index or Tabular List. These conditions should be coded as related even in the absence of provider documentation explicitly linking them, unless the documentation clearly states the conditions are unrelated or when another guideline exists that specifically requires a documented linkage between two conditions (e.g., sepsis guideline for "acute organ dysfunction that is not clearly associated with the sepsis").

For conditions not specifically linked by these relational terms in the classification or when a guideline requires that a linkage between two conditions be explicitly documented, provider documentation must link the conditions in order to code them as related.

The word "with" in the Alphabetic Index is sequenced immediately following the main term **or subterm**, not in alphabetical order.

16. "See" and "See Also"

The "see" instruction following a main term in the Alphabetic Index indicates that another term should be referenced. It is necessary to go to the main term referenced with the "see" note to locate the correct code.

A "see also" instruction following a main term in the Alphabetic Index instructs that there is another main term that may also be referenced that may provide additional Alphabetic Index entries that may be useful. It is not necessary to follow the "see also" note when the original main term provides the necessary code.

17. "Code also" note

A "code also" note instructs that two codes may be required to fully describe a condition, but this note does not provide sequencing direction. The sequencing depends on the circumstances of the encounter.

18. Default codes

A code listed next to a main term in the ICD-10-CM Alphabetic Index is referred to as a default code. The default code represents that condition that is most commonly associated with the main term, or is the unspecified code for the condition. If a condition is documented in a medical record (for example, appendicitis) without any additional information, such as acute or chronic, the default code should be assigned.

19. Code assignment and Clinical Criteria

The assignment of a diagnosis code is based on the provider's diagnostic statement that the condition exists. The provider's statement that the patient has a particular condition is sufficient. Code assignment is not based on clinical criteria used by the provider to establish the diagnosis.

B. General Coding Guidelines

1. Locating a code in the ICD-10-CM

To select a code in the classification that corresponds to a diagnosis or reason for visit documented in a medical record, first locate the term in the Alphabetic Index, and then verify the code in the Tabular List. Read and be guided by instructional notations that appear in both the Alphabetic Index and the Tabular List.

It is essential to use both the Alphabetic Index and Tabular List when locating and assigning a code. The Alphabetic Index does not always provide the full code. Selection of the full code, including laterality and any applicable 7th character can only be done in the Tabular List. A dash (-) at the end of an Alphabetic Index entry indicates that additional characters are required. Even if a dash is not included at the Alphabetic Index entry, it is necessary to refer to the Tabular List to verify that no 7th character is required.

2. Level of Detail in Coding

Diagnosis codes are to be used and reported at their highest number of characters available.

ICD-10-CM diagnosis codes are composed of codes with 3, 4, 5, 6 or 7 characters. Codes with three characters are included in ICD-10-CM as the heading of a category of codes that may be further subdivided by the use of fourth and/or fifth characters and/or sixth characters, which provide greater detail.

A three-character code is to be used only if it is not further subdivided. A code is invalid if it has not been coded to the full number of characters required for that code, including the 7th character, if applicable.

3. Code or codes from A00.0 through T88.9, Z00-Z99.8

The appropriate code or codes from A00.0 through T88.9, Z00-Z99.8 must be used to identify diagnoses, symptoms, conditions, problems, complaints or other reason(s) for the encounter/visit.

4. Signs and symptoms

Codes that describe symptoms and signs, as opposed to diagnoses, are acceptable for reporting purposes when a related definitive diagnosis has not been established (confirmed) by the provider. Chapter 18 of ICD-10-CM, Symptoms, Signs, and Abnormal Clinical and Laboratory Findings, Not Elsewhere Classified (codes R00.0 - R99) contains many, but not all, codes for symptoms.

See Section I.B.18 Use of Signs/Symptom/Unspecified Codes

5. Conditions that are an integral part of a disease process

Signs and symptoms that are associated routinely with a disease process should not be assigned as additional codes, unless otherwise instructed by the classification.

6. Conditions that are not an integral part of a disease process

Additional signs and symptoms that may not be associated routinely with a disease process should be coded when present.

7. **Multiple coding for a single condition**

In addition to the etiology/manifestation convention that requires two codes to fully describe a single condition that affects multiple body systems, there are other single conditions that also require more than one code. "Use additional code" notes are found in the Tabular List at codes that are not part of an etiology/manifestation pair where a secondary code is useful to fully describe a condition. The sequencing rule is the same as the etiology/manifestation pair, "use additional code" indicates that a secondary code should be added, if known.

For example, for bacterial infections that are not included in chapter 1, a secondary code from category B95, Streptococcus, Staphylococcus, and Enterococcus, as the cause of diseases classified elsewhere, or B96, Other bacterial agents as the cause of diseases classified elsewhere, may be required to identify the bacterial organism causing the infection. A "use additional code" note will normally be found at the infectious disease code, indicating a need for the organism code to be added as a secondary code.

"Code first" notes are also under certain codes that are not specifically manifestation codes but may be due to an underlying cause. When there is a "code first" note and an underlying condition is present, the underlying condition should be sequenced first, if known.

"Code, if applicable, any causal condition first" notes indicate that this code may be assigned as a principal diagnosis when the causal condition is unknown or not applicable. If a causal condition is known, then the code for that condition should be sequenced as the principal or first-listed diagnosis.

Multiple codes may be needed for sequela, complication codes and obstetric codes to more fully describe a condition. See the specific guidelines for these conditions for further instruction.

8. **Acute and Chronic Conditions**

If the same condition is described as both acute (subacute) and chronic, and separate subentries exist in the Alphabetic Index at the same indentation level, code both and sequence the acute (subacute) code first.

9. **Combination Code**

A combination code is a single code used to classify:

    Two diagnoses, or

    A diagnosis with an associated secondary process (manifestation)

    A diagnosis with an associated complication

Combination codes are identified by referring to subterm entries in the Alphabetic Index and by reading the inclusion and exclusion notes in the Tabular List.

Assign only the combination code when that code fully identifies the diagnostic conditions involved or when the Alphabetic Index so directs. Multiple coding should not be used when the classification provides a combination code that clearly identifies all of the elements documented in the diagnosis. When the combination code lacks necessary specificity in describing the manifestation or complication, an additional code should be used as a secondary code.

10. **Sequela (Late Effects)**

A sequela is the residual effect (condition produced) after the acute phase of an illness or injury has terminated. There is no time limit on when a sequela code can be used. The residual may be apparent early, such as in cerebral infarction, or it may occur months or years later, such as that due to a previous injury. Examples of sequela include: scar formation resulting from a burn, deviated septum due to a nasal fracture, and infertility due to tubal occlusion from old tuberculosis. Coding of sequela generally requires two codes sequenced in the following order: the condition or nature of the sequela is sequenced first. The sequela code is sequenced second.

An exception to the above guidelines are those instances where the code for the sequela is followed by a manifestation code identified in the Tabular List and title, or the sequela code has been expanded (at the fourth, fifth or sixth character levels) to include the manifestation(s). The code for the acute phase of an illness or injury that led to the sequela is never used with a code for the late effect.

See Section I.C.9. Sequelae of cerebrovascular disease

See Section I.C.15. Sequelae of complication of pregnancy, childbirth and the puerperium

See Section I.C.19. Application of 7th characters for Chapter 19

11. **Impending or Threatened Condition**

Code any condition described at the time of discharge as "impending" or "threatened" as follows:

    If it did occur, code as confirmed diagnosis.

If it did not occur, reference the Alphabetic Index to determine if the condition has a subentry term for "impending" or "threatened" and also reference main term entries for "Impending" and for "Threatened."

If the subterms are listed, assign the given code.

If the subterms are not listed, code the existing underlying condition(s) and not the condition described as impending or threatened.

12. **Reporting Same Diagnosis Code More than Once**

Each unique ICD-10-CM diagnosis code may be reported only once for an encounter. This applies to bilateral conditions when there are no distinct codes identifying laterality or two different conditions classified to the same ICD-10-CM diagnosis code.

13. **Laterality**

Some ICD-10-CM codes indicate laterality, specifying whether the condition occurs on the left, right or is bilateral. If no bilateral code is provided and the condition is bilateral, assign separate codes for both the left and right side. If the side is not identified in the medical record, assign the code for the unspecified side.

When a patient has a bilateral condition and each side is treated during separate encounters, assign the "bilateral" code (as the condition still exists on both sides), including for the encounter to treat the first side. For the second encounter for treatment after one side has previously been treated and the condition no longer exists on that side, assign the appropriate unilateral code for the side where the condition still exists (e.g., cataract surgery performed on each eye in separate encounters). The bilateral code would not be assigned for the subsequent encounter, as the patient no longer has the condition in the previously-treated site. If the treatment on the first side did not completely resolve the condition, then the bilateral code would still be appropriate.

14. **Documentation *by Clinicians Other than the Patient's Provider***

Code assignment is based on the documentation by patient's provider (i.e., physician or other qualified healthcare practitioner legally accountable for establishing the patient's diagnosis). There are a few exceptions, such as codes for the Body Mass Index (BMI), depth of non-pressure chronic ulcers, pressure ulcer stage, coma scale, and NIH stroke scale (NIHSS) codes, code assignment may be based on medical record documentation from clinicians who are not the patient's provider (i.e., physician or other qualified healthcare practitioner legally accountable for establishing the patient's diagnosis), since this information is typically documented by other clinicians involved in the care of the patient (e.g., a dietitian often documents the BMI, a nurse often documents the pressure ulcer stages, and an emergency medical technician often documents the coma scale). However, the associated diagnosis (such as overweight, obesity, acute stroke, or pressure ulcer) must be documented by the patient's provider. If there is conflicting medical record documentation, either from the same clinician or different clinicians, the patient's attending provider should be queried for clarification.

For social determinants of health, such as information found in categories Z55-Z65, Persons with potential health hazards related to socioeconomic and psychosocial circumstances, code assignment may be based on medical record documentation from clinicians involved in the care of the patient who are not the patient's provider since this information represents social information, rather than medical diagnoses.

The BMI, coma scale, NIHSS codes and categories Z55-Z65 should only be reported as secondary diagnoses.

15. **Syndromes**

Follow the Alphabetic Index guidance when coding syndromes. In the absence of Alphabetic Index guidance, assign codes for the documented manifestations of the syndrome. Additional codes for manifestations that are not an integral part of the disease process may also be assigned when the condition does not have a unique code.

16. **Documentation of Complications of Care**

Code assignment is based on the provider's documentation of the relationship between the condition and the care or procedure, unless otherwise instructed by the classification. The guideline extends to any complications of care, regardless of the chapter the code is located in. It is important to note that not all conditions that occur during or following medical care or surgery are classified as complications. There must be a cause-and-effect relationship between the care provided and the condition, and an indication in the documentation that it is a complication. Query the provider for clarification, if the complication is not clearly documented.

17. Borderline Diagnosis

If the provider documents a "borderline" diagnosis at the time of discharge, the diagnosis is coded as confirmed, unless the classification provides a specific entry (e.g., borderline diabetes). If a borderline condition has a specific index entry in ICD-10-CM, it should be coded as such. Since borderline conditions are not uncertain diagnoses, no distinction is made between the care setting (inpatient versus outpatient). Whenever the documentation is unclear regarding a borderline condition, coders are encouraged to query for clarification.

18. Use of Sign/Symptom/Unspecified Codes

Sign/symptom and "unspecified" codes have acceptable, even necessary, uses. While specific diagnosis codes should be reported when they are supported by the available medical record documentation and clinical knowledge of the patient's health condition, there are instances when signs/symptoms or unspecified codes are the best choices for accurately reflecting the healthcare encounter. Each healthcare encounter should be coded to the level of certainty known for that encounter.

If a definitive diagnosis has not been established by the end of the encounter, it is appropriate to report codes for sign(s) and/or symptom(s) in lieu of a definitive diagnosis. When sufficient clinical information isn't known or available about a particular health condition to assign a more specific code, it is acceptable to report the appropriate "unspecified" code (e.g., a diagnosis of pneumonia has been determined, but not the specific type). Unspecified codes should be reported when they are the codes that most accurately reflect what is known about the patient's condition at the time of that particular encounter. It would be inappropriate to select a specific code that is not supported by the medical record documentation or conduct medically unnecessary diagnostic testing in order to determine a more specific code.

19. Coding for Healthcare Encounters in Hurricane Aftermath

a. Use of External Cause of Morbidity Codes

An external cause of morbidity code should be assigned to identify the cause of the injury(ies) incurred as a result of the hurricane. The use of external cause of morbidity codes is supplemental to the application of ICD-10-CM codes. External cause of morbidity codes are never to be recorded as a principal diagnosis (first-listed in non-inpatient settings). The appropriate injury code should be sequenced before any external cause codes. The external cause of morbidity codes capture how the injury or health condition happened (cause), the intent (unintentional or accidental; or intentional, such as suicide or assault), the place where the event occurred, the activity of the patient at the time of the event, and the person's status (e.g., civilian, military). They should not be assigned for encounters to treat hurricane victims' medical conditions when no injury, adverse effect or poisoning is involved. External cause of morbidity codes should be assigned for each encounter for care and treatment of the injury. External cause of morbidity codes may be assigned in all health care settings. For the purpose of capturing complete and accurate ICD-10-CM data in the aftermath of the hurricane, a healthcare setting should be considered as any location where medical care is provided by licensed healthcare professionals.

b. Sequencing of External Causes of Morbidity Codes

Codes for cataclysmic events, such as a hurricane, take priority over all other external cause codes except child and adult abuse and terrorism and should be sequenced before other external cause of injury codes. Assign as many external cause of morbidity codes as necessary to fully explain each cause. For example, if an injury occurs as a result of a building collapse during the hurricane, external cause codes for both the hurricane and the building collapse should be assigned, with the external causes code for hurricane being sequenced as the first external cause code. For injuries incurred as a direct result of the hurricane, assign the appropriate code(s) for the injuries, followed by the code X37.0-, Hurricane (with the appropriate 7th character), and any other applicable external cause of injury codes. Code X37.0- also should be assigned when an injury is incurred as a result of flooding caused by a levee breaking related to the hurricane. Code X38.-, Flood (with the appropriate 7th character), should be assigned when an injury is from flooding resulting directly from the storm. Code X36.0.-, Collapse of dam or man-made structure, should not be assigned when the cause of the collapse is due to the hurricane. Use of code X36.0- is limited to collapses of man-made structures due to earth surface movements, not due to storm surges directly from a hurricane.

c. Other External Causes of Morbidity Code Issues

For injuries that are not a direct result of the hurricane, such as an evacuee that has incurred an injury as a result of a motor vehicle accident, assign the appropriate external cause of morbidity code(s) to

describe the cause of the injury, but do not assign code X37.0-, Hurricane. If it is not clear whether the injury was a direct result of the hurricane, assume the injury is due to the hurricane and assign code X37.0-, Hurricane, as well as any other applicable external cause of morbidity codes. In addition to code X37.0-, Hurricane, other possible applicable external cause of morbidity codes include:

W54.0-, Bitten by dog

X30-, Exposure to excessive natural heat

X31-, Exposure to excessive natural cold

X38-, Flood

d. Use of Z codes

Z codes (other reasons for healthcare encounters) may be assigned as appropriate to further explain the reasons for presenting for healthcare services, including transfers between healthcare facilities. The ICD-10-CM Official Guidelines for Coding and Reporting identify which codes maybe assigned as principal or first-listed diagnosis only, secondary diagnosis only, or principal/first-listed or secondary (depending on the circumstances). Possible applicable Z codes include:

Z59.0,   Homelessness

Z59.1,   Inadequate housing

Z59.5,   Extreme poverty

Z75.1,   Person awaiting admission to adequate facility elsewhere

Z75.3,   Unavailability and inaccessibility of health-care facilities

Z75.4,   Unavailability and inaccessibility of other helping agencies

Z76.2,   Encounter for health supervision and care of other healthy infant and child

Z99.12, Encounter for respirator [ventilator] dependence during power failure

The external cause of morbidity codes and the Z codes listed above are not an all-inclusive list. Other codes may be applicable to the encounter based upon the documentation. Assign as many codes as necessary to fully explain each healthcare encounter. Since patient history information may be very limited, use any available documentation to assign the appropriate external cause of morbidity and Z codes.

C. Chapter-Specific Coding Guidelines

In addition to general coding guidelines, there are guidelines for specific diagnoses and/or conditions in the classification. Unless otherwise indicated, these guidelines apply to all health care settings. Please refer to Section II for guidelines on the selection of principal diagnosis.

1. Chapter 1: Certain Infectious and Parasitic Diseases (A00-B99)

a. Human Immunodeficiency Virus (HIV) Infections

1) Code only confirmed cases

Code only confirmed cases of HIV infection/illness. This is an exception to the hospital inpatient guideline Section II, H.

In this context, "confirmation" does not require documentation of positive serology or culture for HIV; the provider's diagnostic statement that the patient is HIV positive, or has an HIV-related illness is sufficient.

2) Selection and sequencing of HIV codes

(a) Patient admitted for HIV-related condition

If a patient is admitted for an HIV-related condition, the principal diagnosis should be B20, Human immunodeficiency virus [HIV] disease followed by additional diagnosis codes for all reported HIV-related conditions.

(b) Patient with HIV disease admitted for unrelated condition

If a patient with HIV disease is admitted for an unrelated condition (such as a traumatic injury), the code for the unrelated condition (e.g., the nature of injury code) should be the principal diagnosis. Other diagnoses would be B20 followed by additional diagnosis codes for all reported HIV-related conditions.

(c) Whether the patient is newly diagnosed

Whether the patient is newly diagnosed or has had previous admissions/encounters for HIV conditions is irrelevant to the sequencing decision.

(d) Asymptomatic human immunodeficiency virus

Z21, Asymptomatic human immunodeficiency virus [HIV] infection status, is to be applied when the patient without any documentation of symptoms is listed as being "HIV positive," "known HIV," "HIV test positive," or similar terminology. Do not use this code if the term "AIDS" is used or if the patient is treated for any HIV-related illness or is described as having any condition(s) resulting from his/her HIV positive status; use B20 in these cases.

(e) Patients with inconclusive HIV serology

Patients with inconclusive HIV serology, but no definitive diagnosis or manifestations of the illness, may be assigned code R75, Inconclusive laboratory evidence of human immunodeficiency virus [HIV].

(f) Previously diagnosed HIV-related illness

Patients with any known prior diagnosis of an HIV-related illness should be coded to B20. Once a patient has developed an HIV-related illness, the patient should always be assigned code B20 on every subsequent admission/encounter. Patients previously diagnosed with any HIV illness (B20) should never be assigned to R75 or Z21, Asymptomatic human immunodeficiency virus [HIV] infection status.

(g) HIV Infection in Pregnancy, Childbirth and the Puerperium

During pregnancy, childbirth or the puerperium, a patient admitted (or presenting for a health care encounter) because of an HIV-related illness should receive a principal diagnosis code of O98.7-, Human immunodeficiency [HIV] disease complicating pregnancy, childbirth and the puerperium, followed by B20 and the code(s) for the HIV-related illness(es). Codes from Chapter 15 always take sequencing priority.

Patients with asymptomatic HIV infection status admitted (or presenting for a health care encounter) during pregnancy, childbirth, or the puerperium should receive codes of O98.7- and Z21.

(h) Encounters for testing for HIV

If a patient is being seen to determine his/her HIV status, use code Z11.4, Encounter for screening for human immunodeficiency virus [HIV]. Use additional codes for any associated high risk behavior.

If a patient with signs or symptoms is being seen for HIV testing, code the signs and symptoms. An additional counseling code Z71.7, Human immunodeficiency virus [HIV] counseling, may be used if counseling is provided during the encounter for the test.

When a patient returns to be informed of his/her HIV test results and the test result is negative, use code Z71.7, Human immunodeficiency virus [HIV] counseling.

If the results are positive, see previous guidelines and assign codes as appropriate.

b. Infectious agents as the cause of diseases classified to other chapters

Certain infections are classified in chapters other than Chapter 1 and no organism is identified as part of the infection code. In these instances, it is necessary to use an additional code from Chapter 1 to identify the organism. A code from category B95, Streptococcus, Staphylococcus, and Enterococcus as the cause of diseases classified to other chapters, B96, Other bacterial agents as the cause of diseases classified to other chapters, or B97, Viral agents as the cause of diseases classified to other chapters, is to be used as an additional code to identify the organism. An instructional note will be found at the infection code advising that an additional organism code is required.

c. Infections resistant to antibiotics

Many bacterial infections are resistant to current antibiotics. It is necessary to identify all infections documented as antibiotic resistant. Assign a code from category Z16, Resistance to antimicrobial drugs, following the infection code only if the infection code does not identify drug resistance.

d. Sepsis, Severe Sepsis, and Septic Shock

1) Coding of Sepsis and Severe Sepsis

(a) Sepsis

For a diagnosis of sepsis, assign the appropriate code for the underlying systemic infection. If the type of infection or causal organism is not further specified, assign code A41.9, Sepsis, unspecified organism.

A code from subcategory R65.2, Severe sepsis, should not be assigned unless severe sepsis or an associated acute organ dysfunction is documented.

(i) Negative or inconclusive blood cultures and sepsis

Negative or inconclusive blood cultures do not preclude a diagnosis of sepsis in patients with clinical evidence of the condition; however, the provider should be queried.

(ii) Urosepsis

The term urosepsis is a nonspecific term. It is not to be considered synonymous with sepsis. It has no default code in the Alphabetic Index. Should a provider use this term, he/she must be queried for clarification.

(iii) Sepsis with organ dysfunction

If a patient has sepsis and associated acute organ dysfunction or multiple organ dysfunction (MOD), follow the instructions for coding severe sepsis.

(iv) Acute organ dysfunction that is not clearly associated with the sepsis

If a patient has sepsis and an acute organ dysfunction, but the medical record documentation indicates that the acute organ dysfunction is related to a medical condition other than the sepsis, do not assign a code from subcategory R65.2, Severe sepsis. An acute organ dysfunction must be associated with the sepsis in order to assign the severe sepsis code. If the documentation is not clear as to whether an acute organ dysfunction is related to the sepsis or another medical condition, query the provider.

(b) Severe sepsis

The coding of severe sepsis requires a minimum of 2 codes: first a code for the underlying systemic infection, followed by a code from subcategory R65.2, Severe sepsis. If the causal organism is not documented, assign code A41.9, Sepsis, unspecified organism, for the infection. Additional code(s) for the associated acute organ dysfunction are also required.

Due to the complex nature of severe sepsis, some cases may require querying the provider prior to assignment of the codes.

2) Septic shock

(a) Septic shock generally refers to circulatory failure associated with severe sepsis, and, therefore, it represents a type of acute organ dysfunction.

For cases of septic shock, the code for the systemic infection should be sequenced first, followed by code R65.21, Severe sepsis with septic shock or code T81.12, Postprocedural septic shock. Any additional codes for the other acute organ dysfunctions should also be assigned. As noted in the sequencing instructions in the Tabular List, the code for septic shock cannot be assigned as a principal diagnosis.

3) Sequencing of severe sepsis

If severe sepsis is present on admission, and meets the definition of principal diagnosis, the underlying systemic infection should be assigned as principal diagnosis followed by the appropriate code from subcategory R65.2 as required by the sequencing rules in the Tabular List. A code from subcategory R65.2 can never be assigned as a principal diagnosis.

When severe sepsis develops during an encounter (it was not present on admission), the underlying systemic infection and the appropriate code from subcategory R65.2 should be assigned as secondary diagnoses.

Severe sepsis may be present on admission, but the diagnosis may not be confirmed until sometime after admission. If the documentation is not clear whether severe sepsis was present on admission, the provider should be queried.

4) Sepsis *or* severe sepsis with a localized infection

If the reason for admission is sepsis or severe sepsis and a localized infection, such as pneumonia or cellulitis, a code(s) for the underlying systemic infection should be assigned first and the code for the localized infection should be assigned as a secondary diagnosis. If the patient has severe sepsis, a code from subcategory R65.2 should also be assigned as a secondary diagnosis. If the patient is admitted with a localized infection, such as pneumonia, and sepsis/severe sepsis doesn't develop until after admission, the localized infection should be assigned first, followed by the appropriate sepsis/severe sepsis codes.

5) **Sepsis due to a postprocedural infection**

(a) **Documentation of causal relationship**
As with all postprocedural complications, code assignment is based on the provider's documentation of the relationship between the infection and the procedure.

(b) **Sepsis due to a postprocedural infection**
For infections following a procedure, a code from T81.40, to T81.43 Infection following a procedure, or a code from O86.00 to O86.03, Infection of obstetric surgical wound, that identifies the site of the infection should be coded first, if known. Assign an additional code for sepsis following a procedure (T81.44) or sepsis following an obstetrical procedure (O86.04). Use an additional code to identify the infectious agent. If the patient has severe sepsis, the appropriate code from subcategory R65.2 should also be assigned with the additional code(s) for any acute organ dysfunction.

For infections following infusion, transfusion, therapeutic injection, or immunization, a code from subcategory T80.2, Infections following infusion, transfusion, and therapeutic injection, or code T88.0-, Infection following immunization, should be coded first, followed by the code for the specific infection. If the patient has severe sepsis, the appropriate code from subcategory R65.2 should also be assigned, with the additional codes(s) for any acute organ dysfunction.

(c) **Postprocedural infection and postprocedural septic shock**
If a postprocedural infection has resulted in postprocedural septic shock, assign the codes indicated above for sepsis due to a postprocedural infection, followed by code T81.12-, Postprocedural septic shock. Do not assign code R65.21, Severe sepsis with septic shock. Additional code(s) should be assigned for any acute organ dysfunction.

6) **Sepsis and severe sepsis associated with a noninfectious process (condition)**
In some cases a noninfectious process (condition), such as trauma, may lead to an infection which can result in sepsis or severe sepsis. If sepsis or severe sepsis is documented as associated with a noninfectious condition, such as a burn or serious injury, and this condition meets the definition for principal diagnosis, the code for the noninfectious condition should be sequenced first, followed by the code for the resulting infection. If severe sepsis is present, a code from subcategory R65.2 should also be assigned with any associated organ dysfunction(s) codes. It is not necessary to assign a code from subcategory R65.1, Systemic inflammatory response syndrome (SIRS) of non-infectious origin, for these cases.

If the infection meets the definition of principal diagnosis, it should be sequenced before the non-infectious condition. When both the associated non-infectious condition and the infection meet the definition of principal diagnosis, either may be assigned as principal diagnosis.

Only one code from category R65, Symptoms and signs specifically associated with systemic inflammation and infection, should be assigned. Therefore, when a non-infectious condition leads to an infection resulting in severe sepsis, assign the appropriate code from subcategory R65.2, Severe sepsis. Do not additionally assign a code from subcategory R65.1, Systemic inflammatory response syndrome (SIRS) of non-infectious origin.

See Section I.C.18. SIRS due to non-infectious process

7) **Sepsis and septic shock complicating abortion, pregnancy, childbirth, and the puerperium**
See Section I.C.15. Sepsis and septic shock complicating abortion, pregnancy, childbirth and the puerperium

8) **Newborn sepsis**
See Section I.C.16. f. Bacterial sepsis of Newborn

e. **Methicillin Resistant Staphylococcus aureus (MRSA) Conditions**

1) **Selection and sequencing of MRSA codes**

(a) **Combination codes for MRSA infection**
When a patient is diagnosed with an infection that is due to methicillin resistant *Staphylococcus aureus* (MRSA), and that infection has a combination code that includes the causal organism (e.g., sepsis, pneumonia) assign the appropriate combination code for the condition (e.g., code A41.02, Sepsis due to Methicillin resistant Staphylococcus aureus or code J15.212, Pneumonia due to Methicillin resistant Staphylococcus aureus). Do not assign code B95.62, Methicillin resistant Staphylococcus aureus infection as the cause of diseases classified elsewhere, as an additional code, because the combination code includes the type of infection and the MRSA organism. Do not assign a code from subcategory Z16.11, Resistance to penicillins, as an additional diagnosis.

See Section C.1. for instructions on coding and sequencing of sepsis and severe sepsis.

(b) **Other codes for MRSA infection**
When there is documentation of a current infection (e.g., wound infection, stitch abscess, urinary tract infection) due to MRSA, and that infection does not have a combination code that includes the causal organism, assign the appropriate code to identify the condition along with code B95.62, Methicillin resistant Staphylococcus aureus infection as the cause of diseases classified elsewhere for the MRSA infection. Do not assign a code from subcategory Z16.11, Resistance to penicillins.

(c) **Methicillin susceptible Staphylococcus aureus (MSSA) and MRSA colonization**
The condition or state of being colonized or carrying MSSA or MRSA is called colonization or carriage, while an individual person is described as being colonized or being a carrier. Colonization means that MSSA or MSRA is present on or in the body without necessarily causing illness. A positive MRSA colonization test might be documented by the provider as "MRSA screen positive" or "MRSA nasal swab positive".

Assign code Z22.322, Carrier or suspected carrier of Methicillin resistant Staphylococcus aureus, for patients documented as having MRSA colonization. Assign code Z22.321, Carrier or suspected carrier of Methicillin susceptible Staphylococcus aureus, for patients documented as having MSSA colonization. Colonization is not necessarily indicative of a disease process or as the cause of a specific condition the patient may have unless documented as such by the provider.

(d) **MRSA colonization and infection**
If a patient is documented as having both MRSA colonization and infection during a hospital admission, code Z22.322, Carrier or suspected carrier of Methicillin resistant Staphylococcus aureus, and a code for the MRSA infection may both be assigned.

f. **Zika virus infections**

1) **Code only confirmed cases**
Code only a confirmed diagnosis of Zika virus (A92.5, Zika virus disease) as documented by the provider. This is an exception to the hospital inpatient guideline Section II, H. In this context, "confirmation" does not require documentation of the type of test performed; the **provider's** diagnostic statement that the condition is confirmed is sufficient. This code should be assigned regardless of the stated mode of transmission.

If the provider documents "suspected", "possible" or "probable" Zika, do not assign code A92.5. Assign a code(s) explaining the reason for encounter (such as fever, rash, or joint pain) or Z20.821, Contact with and (suspected) exposure to Zika virus.

2. **Chapter 2: Neoplasms (C00-D49)**
General guidelines
Chapter 2 of the ICD-10-CM contains the codes for most benign and all malignant neoplasms. Certain benign neoplasms, such as prostatic adenomas, may be found in the specific body system chapters. To properly code a neoplasm it is necessary to determine from the record if the neoplasm is benign, in-situ, malignant, or of uncertain histologic behavior. If malignant, any secondary (metastatic) sites should also be determined.

Primary malignant neoplasms overlapping site boundaries

A primary malignant neoplasm that overlaps two or more contiguous (next to each other) sites should be classified to the subcategory/code .8 ('overlapping lesion'), unless the combination is specifically indexed elsewhere. For multiple neoplasms of the same site that are not contiguous such as tumors in different quadrants of the same breast, codes for each site should be assigned.

Malignant neoplasm of ectopic tissue

Malignant neoplasms of ectopic tissue are to be coded to the site of origin mentioned, e.g., ectopic pancreatic malignant neoplasms involving the stomach are coded to malignant neoplasm of pancreas, unspecified (C25.9).

The neoplasm table in the Alphabetic Index should be referenced first. However, if the histological term is documented, that term should be referenced first, rather than going immediately to the Neoplasm Table, in order to determine which column in the Neoplasm Table is appropriate. For example, if the documentation indicates "adenoma," refer to the term in the Alphabetic Index to review the entries under this term and the instructional note to "see also neoplasm, by site, benign." The table provides the proper code based on the type of neoplasm and the site. It is important to select the proper column in the table that corresponds to the type of neoplasm. The Tabular List should then be referenced to verify that the correct code has been selected from the table and that a more specific site code does not exist.

See Section I.C.21. Factors influencing health status and contact with health services, Status, for information regarding Z15.0, codes for genetic susceptibility to cancer.

a. Treatment directed at the malignancy

If the treatment is directed at the malignancy, designate the malignancy as the principal diagnosis.

The only exception to this guideline is if a patient admission/encounter is solely for the administration of chemotherapy, immunotherapy or external beam radiation therapy, assign the appropriate Z51.-- code as the first-listed or principal diagnosis, and the diagnosis or problem for which the service is being performed as a secondary diagnosis.

b. Treatment of secondary site

When a patient is admitted because of a primary neoplasm with metastasis and treatment is directed toward the secondary site only, the secondary neoplasm is designated as the principal diagnosis even though the primary malignancy is still present.

c. Coding and sequencing of complications

Coding and sequencing of complications associated with the malignancies or with the therapy thereof are subject to the following guidelines:

1) Anemia associated with malignancy

When admission/encounter is for management of an anemia associated with the malignancy, and the treatment is only for anemia, the appropriate code for the malignancy is sequenced as the principal or first-listed diagnosis followed by the appropriate code for the anemia (such as code D63.0, Anemia in neoplastic disease).

2) Anemia associated with chemotherapy, immunotherapy and radiation therapy

When the admission/encounter is for management of an anemia associated with an adverse effect of the administration of chemotherapy or immunotherapy and the only treatment is for the anemia, the anemia code is sequenced first followed by the appropriate codes for the neoplasm and the adverse effect (T45.1X5-, Adverse effect of antineoplastic and immunosuppressive drugs).

When the admission/encounter is for management of an anemia associated with an adverse effect of radiotherapy, the anemia code should be sequenced first, followed by the appropriate neoplasm code and code Y84.2, Radiological procedure and radiotherapy as the cause of abnormal reaction of the patient, or of later complication, without mention of misadventure at the time of the procedure.

3) Management of dehydration due to the malignancy

When the admission/encounter is for management of dehydration due to the malignancy and only the dehydration is being treated (intravenous rehydration), the dehydration is sequenced first, followed by the code(s) for the malignancy.

4) Treatment of a complication resulting from a surgical procedure

When the admission/encounter is for treatment of a complication resulting from a surgical procedure, designate the complication as the principal or first-listed diagnosis if treatment is directed at resolving the complication.

d. Primary malignancy previously excised

When a primary malignancy has been previously excised or eradicated from its site and there is no further treatment directed to that site and there is no evidence of any existing primary malignancy at that site, a code from category Z85, Personal history of malignant neoplasm, should be used to indicate the former site of the malignancy. Any mention of extension, invasion, or metastasis to another site is coded as a secondary malignant neoplasm to that site. The secondary site may be the principal or first-listed **diagnosis** with the Z85 code used as a secondary code.

e. Admissions/Encounters involving chemotherapy, immunotherapy and radiation therapy

1) Episode of care involves surgical removal of neoplasm

When an episode of care involves the surgical removal of a neoplasm, primary or secondary site, followed by adjunct chemotherapy or radiation treatment during the same episode of care, the code for the neoplasm should be assigned as principal or first-listed diagnosis.

2) Patient admission/encounter solely for administration of chemotherapy, immunotherapy and radiation therapy

If a patient admission/encounter is solely for the administration of chemotherapy, immunotherapy or external beam radiation therapy assign code Z51.0, Encounter for antineoplastic radiation therapy, or Z51.11, Encounter for antineoplastic chemotherapy, or Z51.12, Encounter for antineoplastic immunotherapy as the first-listed or principal diagnosis. If a patient receives more than one of these therapies during the same admission more than one of these codes may be assigned, in any sequence.

The malignancy for which the therapy is being administered should be assigned as a secondary diagnosis.

If a patient admission/encounter is for the insertion or implantation of radioactive elements (e.g., brachytherapy) the appropriate code for the malignancy is sequenced as the principal or first-listed diagnosis. Code Z51.0 should not be assigned.

3) Patient admitted for radiation therapy, chemotherapy or immunotherapy and develops complications

When a patient is admitted for the purpose of external beam radiotherapy, immunotherapy or chemotherapy and develops complications such as uncontrolled nausea and vomiting or dehydration, the principal or first-listed diagnosis is Z51.0, Encounter for antineoplastic radiation therapy, or Z51.11, Encounter for antineoplastic chemotherapy, or Z51.12, Encounter for antineoplastic immunotherapy followed by any codes for the complications.

When a patient is admitted for the purpose of insertion or implantation of radioactive elements (e.g., brachytherapy) and develops complications such as uncontrolled nausea and vomiting or dehydration, the principal or first-listed diagnosis is the appropriate code for the malignancy followed by any codes for the complications.

f. Admission/encounter to determine extent of malignancy

When the reason for admission/encounter is to determine the extent of the malignancy, or for a procedure such as paracentesis or thoracentesis, the primary malignancy or appropriate metastatic site is designated as the principal or first-listed diagnosis, even though chemotherapy or radiotherapy is administered.

g. Symptoms, signs, and abnormal findings listed in Chapter 18 associated with neoplasms

Symptoms, signs, and ill-defined conditions listed in Chapter 18 characteristic of, or associated with, an existing primary or secondary site malignancy cannot be used to replace the malignancy as principal or first-listed diagnosis, regardless of the number of admissions or encounters for treatment and care of the neoplasm.

See section I.C.21. Factors influencing health status and contact with health services, Encounter for prophylactic organ removal.

h. Admission/encounter for pain control/management

See Section I.C.6. for information on coding admission/encounter for pain control/management.

i. **Malignancy in two or more noncontiguous sites**

A patient may have more than one malignant tumor in the same organ. These tumors may represent different primaries or metastatic disease, depending on the site. Should the documentation be unclear, the provider should be queried as to the status of each tumor so that the correct codes can be assigned.

j. **Disseminated malignant neoplasm, unspecified**

Code C80.0, Disseminated malignant neoplasm, unspecified, is for use only in those cases where the patient has advanced metastatic disease and no known primary or secondary sites are specified. It should not be used in place of assigning codes for the primary site and all known secondary sites.

k. **Malignant neoplasm without specification of site**

Code C80.1, Malignant (primary) neoplasm, unspecified, equates to Cancer, unspecified. This code should only be used when no determination can be made as to the primary site of a malignancy. This code should rarely be used in the inpatient setting.

l. **Sequencing of neoplasm codes**

1) **Encounter for treatment of primary malignancy**

If the reason for the encounter is for treatment of a primary malignancy, assign the malignancy as the principal/first-listed diagnosis. The primary site is to be sequenced first, followed by any metastatic sites.

2) **Encounter for treatment of secondary malignancy**

When an encounter is for a primary malignancy with metastasis and treatment is directed toward the metastatic (secondary) site(s) only, the metastatic site(s) is designated as the principal/first-listed diagnosis. The primary malignancy is coded as an additional code.

3) **Malignant neoplasm in a pregnant patient**

When a pregnant woman has a malignant neoplasm, a code from subcategory O9A.1-, Malignant neoplasm complicating pregnancy, childbirth, and the puerperium, should be sequenced first, followed by the appropriate code from Chapter 2 to indicate the type of neoplasm.

4) **Encounter for complication associated with a neoplasm**

When an encounter is for management of a complication associated with a neoplasm, such as dehydration, and the treatment is only for the complication, the complication is coded first, followed by the appropriate code(s) for the neoplasm.

The exception to this guideline is anemia. When the admission/encounter is for management of an anemia associated with the malignancy, and the treatment is only for anemia, the appropriate code for the malignancy is sequenced as the principal or first-listed diagnosis followed by code D63.0, Anemia in neoplastic disease.

5) **Complication from surgical procedure for treatment of a neoplasm**

When an encounter is for treatment of a complication resulting from a surgical procedure performed for the treatment of the neoplasm, designate the complication as the principal/first-listed diagnosis. See **the** guideline regarding the coding of a current malignancy versus personal history to determine if the code for the neoplasm should also be assigned.

6) **Pathologic fracture due to a neoplasm**

When an encounter is for a pathological fracture due to a neoplasm, and the focus of treatment is the fracture, a code from subcategory M84.5, Pathological fracture in neoplastic disease, should be sequenced first, followed by the code for the neoplasm.

If the focus of treatment is the neoplasm with an associated pathological fracture, the neoplasm code should be sequenced first, followed by a code from M84.5 for the pathological fracture.

m. **Current malignancy versus personal history of malignancy**

When a primary malignancy has been excised but further treatment, such as an additional surgery for the malignancy, radiation therapy or chemotherapy is directed to that site, the primary malignancy code should be used until treatment is completed.

When a primary malignancy has been previously excised or eradicated from its site, there is no further treatment (of the malignancy) directed to that site, and there is no evidence of any existing primary malignancy at that site, a code from category Z85, Personal history of malignant neoplasm, should be used to indicate the former site of the malignancy.

Subcategories Z85.0 – Z85.7 should only be assigned for the former site of a primary malignancy, not the site of a secondary malignancy. Codes from subcategory Z85.8-, may be assigned for the former site(s) of either a primary or secondary malignancy included in this subcategory.

See Section I.C.21. Factors influencing health status and contact with health services, History (of)

n. **Leukemia, Multiple Myeloma, and Malignant Plasma Cell Neoplasms in remission versus personal history**

The categories for leukemia, and category C90, Multiple myeloma and malignant plasma cell neoplasms, have codes indicating whether or not the leukemia has achieved remission. There are also codes Z85.6, Personal history of leukemia, and Z85.79, Personal history of other malignant neoplasms of lymphoid, hematopoietic and related tissues. If the documentation is unclear as to whether the leukemia has achieved remission, the provider should be queried.

See Section I.C.21. Factors influencing health status and contact with health services, History (of)

o. **Aftercare following surgery for neoplasm**

See Section I.C.21. Factors influencing health status and contact with health services, Aftercare

p. **Follow-up care for completed treatment of a malignancy**

See Section I.C.21. Factors influencing health status and contact with health services, Follow-up

q. **Prophylactic organ removal for prevention of malignancy**

See Section I.C. 21, Factors influencing health status and contact with health services, Prophylactic organ removal

r. **Malignant neoplasm associated with transplanted organ**

A malignant neoplasm of a transplanted organ should be coded as a transplant complication. Assign first the appropriate code from category T86.-, Complications of transplanted organs and tissue, followed by code C80.2, Malignant neoplasm associated with transplanted organ. Use an additional code for the specific malignancy.

3. **Chapter 3: Disease of the blood and blood-forming organs and certain disorders involving the immune mechanism (D50-D89)**

Reserved for future guideline expansion

4. **Chapter 4: Endocrine, Nutritional, and Metabolic Diseases (E00-E89)**

a. **Diabetes mellitus**

The diabetes mellitus codes are combination codes that include the type of diabetes mellitus, the body system affected, and the complications affecting that body system. As many codes within a particular category as are necessary to describe all of the complications of the disease may be used. They should be sequenced based on the reason for a particular encounter. Assign as many codes from categories E08 – E13 as needed to identify all of the associated conditions that the patient has.

1) **Type of diabetes**

The age of a patient is not the sole determining factor, though most type 1 diabetics develop the condition before reaching puberty. For this reason type 1 diabetes mellitus is also referred to as juvenile diabetes.

2) **Type of diabetes mellitus not documented**

If the type of diabetes mellitus is not documented in the medical record the default is E11.-, Type 2 diabetes mellitus.

3) **Diabetes mellitus and the use of insulin and oral hypoglycemics**

If the documentation in a medical record does not indicate the type of diabetes but does indicate that the patient uses insulin, code E11-, Type 2 diabetes mellitus, should be assigned. An additional code should be assigned from category Z79 to identify the long-term (current) use of insulin or oral hypoglycemic drugs. If the patient is treated with both oral medications and insulin, only the code for long-term (current) use of insulin should be assigned. Code Z79.4 should not be assigned if insulin is given temporarily to bring a type 2 patient's blood sugar under control during an encounter.

4) **Diabetes mellitus in pregnancy and gestational diabetes**

See Section I.C.15. Diabetes mellitus in pregnancy.

See Section I.C.15. Gestational (pregnancy induced) diabetes

5) **Complications due to insulin pump malfunction**

(a) **Underdose of insulin due to insulin pump failure**
An underdose of insulin due to an insulin pump failure should be assigned to a code from subcategory T85.6, Mechanical complication of other specified internal and external prosthetic devices, implants and grafts, that specifies the type of pump malfunction, as the principal or first-listed code, followed by code T38.3X6-, Underdosing of insulin and oral hypoglycemic [antidiabetic] drugs. Additional codes for the type of diabetes mellitus and any associated complications due to the underdosing should also be assigned.

(b) **Overdose of insulin due to insulin pump failure**
The principal or first-listed code for an encounter due to an insulin pump malfunction resulting in an overdose of insulin, should also be T85.6-, Mechanical complication of other specified internal and external prosthetic devices, implants and grafts, followed by code T38.3X1-, Poisoning by insulin and oral hypoglycemic [antidiabetic] drugs, accidental (unintentional).

6) **Secondary diabetes mellitus**
Codes under categories E08, Diabetes mellitus due to underlying condition, E09, Drug or chemical induced diabetes mellitus, and E13, Other specified diabetes mellitus, identify complications/manifestations associated with secondary diabetes mellitus. Secondary diabetes is always caused by another condition or event (e.g., cystic fibrosis, malignant neoplasm of pancreas, pancreatectomy, adverse effect of drug, or poisoning).

(a) **Secondary diabetes mellitus and the use of insulin or oral hypoglycemic drugs**
For patients with secondary diabetes mellitus who routinely use insulin or oral hypoglycemic drugs, an additional code from category Z79 should be assigned to identify the long-term (current) use of insulin or oral hypoglycemic drugs. If the patient is treated with both oral medications and insulin, only the code for long-term (current) use of insulin should be assigned. Code Z79.4 should not be assigned if insulin is given temporarily to bring a secondary diabetic patient's blood sugar under control during an encounter.

(b) **Assigning and sequencing secondary diabetes codes and its causes**
The sequencing of the secondary diabetes codes in relationship to codes for the cause of the diabetes is based on the Tabular List instructions for categories E08, E09 and E13.

(i) **Secondary diabetes mellitus due to pancreatectomy**
For postpancreatectomy diabetes mellitus (lack of insulin due to the surgical removal of all or part of the pancreas), assign code E89.1, Postprocedural hypoinsulinemia. Assign a code from category E13 and a code from subcategory Z90.41, Acquired absence of pancreas, as additional codes.

(ii) **Secondary diabetes due to drugs**
Secondary diabetes may be caused by an adverse effect of correctly administered medications, poisoning or sequela of poisoning.
See section I.C.19.e for coding of adverse effects and poisoning, and section I.C.20 for external cause code reporting.

5. **Chapter 5: Mental, Behavioral and Neurodevelopmental disorders (F01–F99)**

a. **Pain disorders related to psychological factors**
Assign code F45.41, for pain that is exclusively related to psychological disorders. As indicated by the Excludes 1 note under category G89, a code from category G89 should not be assigned with code F45.41.

Code F45.42, Pain disorders with related psychological factors, should be used with a code from category G89, Pain, not elsewhere classified, if there is documentation of a psychological component for a patient with acute or chronic pain.
See Section I.C.6. Pain

b. **Mental and behavioral disorders due to psychoactive substance use**

1) **In Remission**
Selection of codes for "in remission" for categories F10-F19, Mental and behavioral disorders due to psychoactive substance use (categories F10-F19 with -.11, -.21) requires the provider's clinical judgment. The appropriate codes for "in remission" are assigned only on the basis of provider documentation (as defined in the Official Guidelines for Coding and Reporting), unless otherwise instructed by the classification.

Mild substance use disorders in early or sustained remission are classified to the appropriate codes for substance abuse in remission, and moderate or severe substance use disorders in early or sustained remission are classified to the appropriate codes for substance dependence in remission.

2) **Psychoactive Substance Use, Abuse and Dependence**
When the provider documentation refers to use, abuse and dependence of the same substance (e.g. alcohol, opioid, cannabis, etc.), only one code should be assigned to identify the pattern of use based on the following hierarchy:
- If both use and abuse are documented, assign only the code for abuse
- If both abuse and dependence are documented, assign only the code for dependence
- If use, abuse and dependence are all documented, assign only the code for dependence
- If both use and dependence are documented, assign only the code for dependence.

3) **Psychoactive Substance Use, Unspecified**
As with all other unspecified diagnoses, the codes for unspecified psychoactive substance use (F10.9-, F11.9-, F12.9-, F13.9-, F14.9-, F15.9-, F16.9-, F18.9-, F19.9-) should only be assigned based on provider documentation and when they meet the definition of a reportable diagnosis (see Section III, Reporting Additional Diagnoses). These codes are to be used only when the psychoactive substance use is associated with a physical, mental or behavioral disorder, and such a relationship is documented by the provider.

c. **Factitious Disorder**
Factitious disorder imposed on self or Munchausen's syndrome is a disorder in which a person falsely reports or causes his or her own physical or psychological signs or symptoms. For patients with documented factitious disorder on self or Munchausen's syndrome, assign the appropriate code from subcategory F68.1-, Factitious disorder imposed on self.

Munchausen's syndrome by proxy (MSBP) is a disorder in which a caregiver (perpetrator) falsely reports or causes an illness or injury in another person (victim) under his or her care, such as a child, an elderly adult, or a person who has a disability. The condition is also referred to as "factitious disorder imposed on another" or "factitious disorder by proxy." The perpetrator, not the victim, receives this diagnosis. Assign code F68.A, Factitious disorder imposed on another, to the perpetrator's record. For the victim of a patient suffering from MSBP, assign the appropriate code from categories T74, Adult and child abuse, neglect and other maltreatment, confirmed, or T76, Adult and child abuse, neglect and other maltreatment, suspected.
See Section I.C.19.f. Adult and child abuse, neglect and other maltreatment

6. **Chapter 6: Diseases of the Nervous System (G00-G99)**

a. **Dominant/nondominant side**
Codes from category G81, Hemiplegia and hemiparesis, and subcategories G83.1, Monoplegia of lower limb, G83.2, Monoplegia of upper limb, and G83.3, Monoplegia, unspecified, identify whether the dominant or nondominant side is affected. Should the affected side be documented, but not specified as dominant or nondominant, and the classification system does not indicate a default, code selection is as follows:
- For ambidextrous patients, the default should be dominant.
- If the left side is affected, the default is non-dominant.
- If the right side is affected, the default is dominant.

b. **Pain - Category G89**

1) **General coding information**
Codes in category G89, Pain, not elsewhere classified, may be used in conjunction with codes from other categories and

chapters to provide more detail about acute or chronic pain and neoplasm-related pain, unless otherwise indicated below.

If the pain is not specified as acute or chronic, post-thoracotomy, postprocedural, or neoplasm-related, do not assign codes from category G89.

A code from category G89 should not be assigned if the underlying (definitive) diagnosis is known, unless the reason for the encounter is pain control/ management and not management of the underlying condition.

When an admission or encounter is for a procedure aimed at treating the underlying condition (e.g., spinal fusion, kyphoplasty), a code for the underlying condition (e.g., vertebral fracture, spinal stenosis) should be assigned as the principal diagnosis. No code from category G89 should be assigned.

(a) Category G89 Codes as Principal or First-Listed Diagnosis
Category G89 codes are acceptable as principal diagnosis or the first-listed code:

- When pain control or pain management is the reason for the admission/encounter (e.g., a patient with displaced intervertebral disc, nerve impingement and severe back pain presents for injection of steroid into the spinal canal). The underlying cause of the pain should be reported as an additional diagnosis, if known.

- When a patient is admitted for the insertion of a neurostimulator for pain control, assign the appropriate pain code as the principal or first-listed diagnosis. When an admission or encounter is for a procedure aimed at treating the underlying condition and a neurostimulator is inserted for pain control during the same admission/encounter, a code for the underlying condition should be assigned as the principal diagnosis and the appropriate pain code should be assigned as a secondary diagnosis.

(b) Use of Category G89 Codes in Conjunction with Site Specific Pain Codes

(i) Assigning Category G89 and Site-Specific Pain Codes
Codes from category G89 may be used in conjunction with codes that identify the site of pain (including codes from chapter 18) if the category G89 code provides additional information. For example, if the code describes the site of the pain, but does not fully describe whether the pain is acute or chronic, then both codes should be assigned.

(ii) Sequencing of Category G89 Codes with Site-Specific Pain Codes
The sequencing of category G89 codes with site-specific pain codes (including chapter 18 codes), is dependent on the circumstances of the encounter/admission as follows:

- If the encounter is for pain control or pain management, assign the code from category G89 followed by the code identifying the specific site of pain (e.g., encounter for pain management for acute neck pain from trauma is assigned code G89.11, Acute pain due to trauma, followed by code M54.2, Cervicalgia, to identify the site of pain).

- If the encounter is for any other reason except pain control or pain management, and a related definitive diagnosis has not been established (confirmed) by the provider, assign the code for the specific site of pain first, followed by the appropriate code from category G89.

2) Pain due to devices, implants and grafts
See Section I.C.19. Pain due to medical devices

3) Postoperative Pain
The provider's documentation should be used to guide the coding of postoperative pain, as well as *Section III. Reporting Additional Diagnoses and Section IV. Diagnostic Coding and Reporting in the Outpatient Setting.*

The default for post-thoracotomy and other postoperative pain not specified as acute or chronic is the code for the acute form.

Routine or expected postoperative pain immediately after surgery should not be coded.

(a) Postoperative pain not associated with specific postoperative complication
Postoperative pain not associated with a specific postoperative complication is assigned to the appropriate postoperative pain code in category G89.

(b) Postoperative pain associated with specific postoperative complication
Postoperative pain associated with a specific postoperative complication (such as painful wire sutures) is assigned to the appropriate code(s) found in Chapter 19, Injury, poisoning, and certain other consequences of external causes. If appropriate, use additional code(s) from category G89 to identify acute or chronic pain (G89.18 or G89.28).

4) Chronic pain
Chronic pain is classified to subcategory G89.2. There is no time frame defining when pain becomes chronic pain. The provider's documentation should be used to guide use of these codes.

5) Neoplasm Related Pain
Code G89.3 is assigned to pain documented as being related, associated or due to cancer, primary or secondary malignancy, or tumor. This code is assigned regardless of whether the pain is acute or chronic.

This code may be assigned as the principal or first-listed code when the stated reason for the admission/encounter is documented as pain control/pain management. The underlying neoplasm should be reported as an additional diagnosis.

When the reason for the admission/encounter is management of the neoplasm and the pain associated with the neoplasm is also documented, code G89.3 may be assigned as an additional diagnosis. It is not necessary to assign an additional code for the site of the pain.

See Section I.C.2 for instructions on the sequencing of neoplasms for all other stated reasons for the admission/encounter (except for pain control/pain management).

6) Chronic pain syndrome
Central pain syndrome (G89.0) and chronic pain syndrome (G89.4) are different than the term "chronic pain," and therefore codes should only be used when the provider has specifically documented this condition.

See Section I.C.5. Pain disorders related to psychological factors

7. Chapter 7: Diseases of the Eye and Adnexa (H00-H59)
a. Glaucoma
1) Assigning Glaucoma Codes
Assign as many codes from category H40, Glaucoma, as needed to identify the type of glaucoma, the affected eye, and the glaucoma stage.

2) Bilateral glaucoma with same type and stage
When a patient has bilateral glaucoma and both eyes are documented as being the same type and stage, and there is a code for bilateral glaucoma, report only the code for the type of glaucoma, bilateral, with the seventh character for the stage.

When a patient has bilateral glaucoma and both eyes are documented as being the same type and stage, and the classification does not provide a code for bilateral glaucoma (i.e. subcategories H40.10 and H40.20) report only one code for the type of glaucoma with the appropriate seventh character for the stage.

3) Bilateral glaucoma stage with different types or stages
When a patient has bilateral glaucoma and each eye is documented as having a different type or stage, and the classification distinguishes laterality, assign the appropriate code for each eye rather than the code for bilateral glaucoma.

When a patient has bilateral glaucoma and each eye is documented as having a different type, and the classification does not distinguish laterality (i.e. subcategories H40.10 and H40.20), assign one code for each type of glaucoma with the appropriate seventh character for the stage.

When a patient has bilateral glaucoma and each eye is documented as having the same type, but different stage, and the classification does not distinguish laterality (i.e. subcategories H40.10 and H40.20), assign a code for the type of glaucoma for each eye with the seventh character for the specific glaucoma stage documented for each eye.

4) Patient admitted with glaucoma and stage evolves during the admission

If a patient is admitted with glaucoma and the stage progresses during the admission, assign the code for highest stage documented.

5) Indeterminate stage glaucoma

Assignment of the seventh character "4" for "indeterminate stage" should be based on the clinical documentation. The seventh character "4" is used for glaucomas whose stage cannot be clinically determined. This seventh character should not be confused with the seventh character "0", unspecified, which should be assigned when there is no documentation regarding the stage of the glaucoma.

b. Blindness

If "blindness" or "low vision" of both eyes is documented but the visual impairment category is not documented, assign code H54.3, Unqualified visual loss, both eyes. If "blindness" or "low vision" in one eye is documented but the visual impairment category is not documented, assign a code from H54.6-, Unqualified visual loss, one eye. If "blindness" or "visual loss" is documented without any information about whether one or both eyes are affected, assign code H54.7, Unspecified visual loss.

8. Chapter 8: Diseases of the Ear and Mastoid Process (H60-H95)

Reserved for future guideline expansion

9. Chapter 9: Diseases of the Circulatory System (I00-I99)

a. Hypertension

The classification presumes a causal relationship between hypertension and heart involvement and between hypertension and kidney involvement, as the two conditions are linked by the term "with" in the Alphabetic Index. These conditions should be coded as related even in the absence of provider documentation explicitly linking them, unless the documentation clearly states the conditions are unrelated.

For hypertension and conditions not specifically linked by relational terms such as "with," "associated with" or "due to" in the classification, provider documentation must link the conditions in order to code them as related.

1) Hypertension with Heart Disease

Hypertension with heart conditions classified to I50.- or I51.4-I51.7, I51.89, I51.9, are assigned to a code from category I11, Hypertensive heart disease. Use additional code(s) from category I50, Heart failure, to identify the type(s) of heart failure in those patients with heart failure.

The same heart conditions (I50.-, I51.4-I51.7, I51.89, I51.9) with hypertension are coded separately if the provider has documented they are unrelated to the hypertension. Sequence according to the circumstances of the admission/encounter.

2) Hypertensive Chronic Kidney Disease

Assign codes from category I12, Hypertensive chronic kidney disease, when both hypertension and a condition classifiable to category N18, Chronic kidney disease (CKD), are present. CKD should not be coded as hypertensive if the provider indicates the CKD is not related to the hypertension.

The appropriate code from category N18 should be used as a secondary code with a code from category I12 to identify the stage of chronic kidney disease.

See Section I.C.14. Chronic kidney disease.

If a patient has hypertensive chronic kidney disease and acute renal failure, an additional code for the acute renal failure is required.

3) Hypertensive Heart and Chronic Kidney Disease

Assign codes from combination category I13, Hypertensive heart and chronic kidney disease, when there is hypertension with both heart and kidney involvement. If heart failure is present, assign an additional code from category I50 to identify the type of heart failure.

The appropriate code from category N18, Chronic kidney disease, should be used as a secondary code with a code from category I13 to identify the stage of chronic kidney disease.

See Section I.C.14. Chronic kidney disease.

The codes in category I13, Hypertensive heart and chronic kidney disease, are combination codes that include hypertension, heart disease and chronic kidney disease. The Includes note at I13 specifies that the conditions included at I11 and I12 are included together in I13. If a patient has hypertension, heart disease and chronic kidney disease, then a code from I13 should be used, not individual codes for hypertension, heart disease and chronic kidney disease, or codes from I11 or I12.

For patients with both acute renal failure and chronic kidney disease, an additional code for acute renal failure is required.

4) Hypertensive Cerebrovascular Disease

For hypertensive cerebrovascular disease, first assign the appropriate code from categories I60-I69, followed by the appropriate hypertension code.

5) Hypertensive Retinopathy

Subcategory H35.0, Background retinopathy and retinal vascular changes, should be used with a code from category I10- I15, Hypertensive disease to include the systemic hypertension. The sequencing is based on the reason for the encounter.

6) Hypertension, Secondary

Secondary hypertension is due to an underlying condition. Two codes are required: one to identify the underlying etiology and one from category I15 to identify the hypertension. Sequencing of codes is determined by the reason for admission/encounter.

7) Hypertension, Transient

Assign code R03.0, Elevated blood pressure reading without diagnosis of hypertension, unless patient has an established diagnosis of hypertension. Assign code O13.-, Gestational [pregnancy-induced] hypertension without significant proteinuria, or O14.-, Pre-eclampsia, for transient hypertension of pregnancy.

8) Hypertension, Controlled

This diagnostic statement usually refers to an existing state of hypertension under control by therapy. Assign the appropriate code from categories I10-I15, Hypertensive diseases.

9) Hypertension, Uncontrolled

Uncontrolled hypertension may refer to untreated hypertension or hypertension not responding to current therapeutic regimen. In either case, assign the appropriate code from categories I10-I15, Hypertensive diseases.

10) Hypertensive Crisis

Assign a code from category I16, Hypertensive crisis, for documented hypertensive urgency, hypertensive emergency or unspecified hypertensive crisis. Code also any identified hypertensive disease (I10-I15). The sequencing is based on the reason for the encounter.

11) Pulmonary Hypertension

Pulmonary hypertension is classified to category I27, Other pulmonary heart diseases. For secondary pulmonary hypertension (I27.1, I27.2-), code also any associated conditions or adverse effects of drugs or toxins. The sequencing is based on the reason for the encounter, except for adverse effects of drugs (See Section I.C.19.e.)

b. Atherosclerotic Coronary Artery Disease and Angina

ICD-10-CM has combination codes for atherosclerotic heart disease with angina pectoris. The subcategories for these codes are I25.11, Atherosclerotic heart disease of native coronary artery with angina pectoris and I25.7, Atherosclerosis of coronary artery bypass graft(s) and coronary artery of transplanted heart with angina pectoris.

When using one of these combination codes it is not necessary to use an additional code for angina pectoris. A causal relationship can be assumed in a patient with both atherosclerosis and angina pectoris, unless the documentation indicates the angina is due to something other than the atherosclerosis.

If a patient with coronary artery disease is admitted due to an acute myocardial infarction (AMI), the AMI should be sequenced before the coronary artery disease.

See Section I.C.9. Acute myocardial infarction (AMI)

c. Intraoperative and Postprocedural Cerebrovascular Accident

Medical record documentation should clearly specify the cause-and-effect relationship between the medical intervention and the cerebrovascular accident in order to assign a code for intraoperative or postprocedural cerebrovascular accident.

Proper code assignment depends on whether it was an infarction or hemorrhage and whether it occurred intraoperatively or postoperatively. If it was a cerebral hemorrhage, code assignment depends on the type of procedure performed.

d. Sequelae of Cerebrovascular Disease

1) Category I69, Sequelae of Cerebrovascular disease

Category I69 is used to indicate conditions classifiable to categories I60-I67 as the causes of sequela (neurologic deficits), themselves classified elsewhere. These "late effects" include neurologic deficits that persist after initial onset of conditions classifiable to categories I60-I67. The neurologic deficits caused by cerebrovascular disease may be present from the onset or may arise at any time after the onset of the condition classifiable to categories I60-I67.

Codes from category I69, Sequelae of cerebrovascular disease, that specify hemiplegia, hemiparesis and monoplegia identify whether the dominant or nondominant side is affected. Should the affected side be documented, but not specified as dominant or nondominant, and the classification system does not indicate a default, code selection is as follows:

- For ambidextrous patients, the default should be dominant.
- If the left side is affected, the default is non-dominant.
- If the right side is affected, the default is dominant.

2) Codes from category I69 with codes from I60-I67

Codes from category I69 may be assigned on a health care record with codes from I60-I67, if the patient has a current cerebrovascular disease and deficits from an old cerebrovascular disease.

3) Codes from category I69 and Personal history of transient ischemic attack (TIA) and cerebral infarction (Z86.73)

Codes from category I69 should not be assigned if the patient does not have neurologic deficits.

See Section I.C.21. 4. History (of) for use of personal history codes

e. Acute myocardial infarction (AMI)

1) Type 1 ST elevation myocardial infarction (STEMI) and non-ST elevation myocardial infarction (NSTEMI)

The ICD-10-CMcodes for type 1 acute myocardial infarction (AMI) identify the site, such as anterolateral wall or true posterior wall. Subcategories I21.0-I21.2 and code I21.3 are used for type 1 ST elevation myocardial infarction (STEMI). Code I21.4, Non-ST elevation (NSTEMI) myocardial infarction, is used for type 1 non ST elevation myocardial infarction (NSTEMI) and nontransmural MIs.

If a type 1 NSTEMI evolves to STEMI, assign the STEMI code. If a type 1 STEMI converts to NSTEMI due to thrombolytic therapy, it is still coded as STEMI.

For encounters occurring while the myocardial infarction is equal to, or less than, four weeks old, including transfers to another acute setting or a postacute setting, and the myocardial infarction meets the definition for "other diagnoses" (see Section III, Reporting Additional Diagnoses), codes from category I21 may continue to be reported. For encounters after the 4 week time frame and the patient is still receiving care related to the myocardial infarction, the appropriate aftercare code should be assigned, rather than a code from category I21. For old or healed myocardial infarctions not requiring further care, code I25.2, Old myocardial infarction, may be assigned.

2) Acute myocardial infarction, unspecified

Code I21.9, Acute myocardial infarction, unspecified, is the default for unspecified acute myocardial infarction or unspecified type. If only type 1 STEMI or transmural MI without the site is documented, assign code I21.3, ST elevation (STEMI) myocardial infarction of unspecified site.

3) AMI documented as nontransmural or subendocardial but site provided

If an AMI is documented as nontransmural or subendocardial, but the site is provided, it is still coded as a subendocardial AMI.

See Section I.C.21.3 for information on coding status post administration of tPA in a different facility within the last 24 hours.

4) Subsequent acute myocardial infarction

A code from category I22, Subsequent ST elevation (STEMI) and non-ST elevation (NSTEMI) myocardial infarction, is to be used when a patient who has suffered a type 1 or unspecified AMI has a new AMI within the 4 week time frame of the initial AMI. A code from category I22 must be used in conjunction with a code from category I21. The sequencing of the I22 and I21 codes depends on the circumstances of the encounter.

Do not assign code I22 for subsequent myocardial infarctions other than type 1 or unspecified. For subsequent type 2 AMI assign only code I21.A1. For subsequent type 4 or type 5 AMI, assign only code I21.A9.

If a subsequent myocardial infarction of one type occurs within 4 weeks of a myocardial infarction of a different type, assign the appropriate codes from category I21 to identify each type. Do not assign a code from category I22. Codes from category I22 should only be assigned if both the initial and subsequent myocardial infarctions are type 1 or unspecified.

5) Other Types of Myocardial Infarction

The ICD-10-CM provides codes for different types of myocardial infarction. Type 1 myocardial infarctions are assigned to codes I21.0-I21.4.

Type 2 myocardial infarction (myocardial infarction due to demand ischemia or secondary to ischemic **im**balance), is assigned to code I21.A1, Myocardial infarction type 2 with the underlying cause **coded first**. Do not assign code I24.8, Other forms of acute ischemic heart disease, for the demand ischemia. **If** a type 2 AMI is described as NSTEMI or STEMI, only assign code I21.A1. Codes I21.01-I21.4 should only be assigned for type 1 AMIs.

Acute myocardial infarctions type 3, 4a, 4b, 4c and 5 are assigned to code I21.A9, Other myocardial infarction type.

The "Code also" and "Code first" notes should be followed related to complications, and for coding of postprocedural myocardial infarctions during or following cardiac surgery.

10. Chapter 10: Diseases of the Respiratory System (J00-J99)

a. Chronic Obstructive Pulmonary Disease [COPD] and Asthma

1) Acute exacerbation of chronic obstructive bronchitis and asthma

The codes in categories J44 and J45 distinguish between uncomplicated cases and those in acute exacerbation. An acute exacerbation is a worsening or a decompensation of a chronic condition. An acute exacerbation is not equivalent to an infection superimposed on a chronic condition, though an exacerbation may be triggered by an infection.

b. Acute Respiratory Failure

1) Acute respiratory failure as principal diagnosis

A code from subcategory J96.0, Acute respiratory failure, or subcategory J96.2, Acute and chronic respiratory failure, may be assigned as a principal diagnosis when it is the condition established after study to be chiefly responsible for occasioning the admission to the hospital, and the selection is supported by the Alphabetic Index and Tabular List. However, chapter-specific coding guidelines (such as obstetrics, poisoning, HIV, newborn) that provide sequencing direction take precedence.

2) Acute respiratory failure as secondary diagnosis

Respiratory failure may be listed as a secondary diagnosis if it occurs after admission, or if it is present on admission, but does not meet the definition of principal diagnosis.

3) Sequencing of acute respiratory failure and another acute condition

When a patient is admitted with respiratory failure and another acute condition, (e.g., myocardial infarction, cerebrovascular accident, aspiration pneumonia), the principal diagnosis will not be the same in every situation. This applies whether the other acute condition is a respiratory or nonrespiratory condition. Selection of the principal diagnosis will be dependent on the circumstances of admission. If both the respiratory failure and the other acute condition are equally responsible for occasioning the admission to the hospital, and there are no chapter-specific sequencing rules, the guideline regarding two or more diagnoses that equally meet the definition for principal diagnosis *(Section II, C.)* may be applied in these situations.

If the documentation is not clear as to whether acute respiratory failure and another condition are equally responsible for occasioning the admission, query the provider for clarification.

c. Influenza due to certain identified influenza viruses

Code only confirmed cases of influenza due to certain identified influenza viruses (category J09), and due to other identified influenza virus (category J10). This is an exception to the hospital inpatient guideline Section II, H. (Uncertain Diagnosis).

In this context, "confirmation" does not require documentation of positive laboratory testing specific for avian or other novel influenza A or other identified influenza virus. However, coding should be based on the provider's diagnostic statement that the patient has avian influenza, or other novel influenza A, for category J09, or has another particular identified strain of influenza, such as H1N1 or H3N2, but not identified as novel or variant, for category J10.

If the provider records "suspected" or "possible" or "probable" avian influenza, or novel influenza, or other identified influenza, then the appropriate influenza code from category J11, Influenza due to unidentified influenza virus, should be assigned. A code from category J09, Influenza due to certain identified influenza viruses, should not be assigned nor should a code from category J10, Influenza due to other identified influenza virus.

d. Ventilator associated Pneumonia
   1) Documentation of Ventilator associated Pneumonia
   As with all procedural or postprocedural complications, code assignment is based on the provider's documentation of the relationship between the condition and the procedure.

   Code J95.851, Ventilator associated pneumonia, should be assigned only when the provider has documented ventilator associated pneumonia (VAP). An additional code to identify the organism (e.g., Pseudomonas aeruginosa, code B96.5) should also be assigned. Do not assign an additional code from categories J12-J18 to identify the type of pneumonia.

   Code J95.851 should not be assigned for cases where the patient has pneumonia and is on a mechanical ventilator and the provider has not specifically stated that the pneumonia is ventilator-associated pneumonia. If the documentation is unclear as to whether the patient has a pneumonia that is a complication attributable to the mechanical ventilator, query the provider.

   2) Ventilator associated Pneumonia Develops after Admission
   A patient may be admitted with one type of pneumonia (e.g., code J13, Pneumonia due to Streptococcus pneumonia) and subsequently develop VAP. In this instance, the principal diagnosis would be the appropriate code from categories J12-J18 for the pneumonia diagnosed at the time of admission. Code J95.851, Ventilator associated pneumonia, would be assigned as an additional diagnosis when the provider has also documented the presence of ventilator associated pneumonia.

11. Chapter 11: Diseases of the Digestive System (K00-K95)
   Reserved for future guideline expansion

12. Chapter 12: Diseases of the Skin and Subcutaneous Tissue (L00-L99)
   a. Pressure ulcer stage codes
      1) Pressure ulcer stages
      Codes **in** category L89, Pressure ulcer, identify the site **and stage** of the pressure ulcer.

      The ICD-10-CM classifies pressure ulcer stages based on severity, which is designated by stages 1-4, **deep tissue pressure injury,** unspecified stage and unstageable.

      Assign as many codes from category L89 as needed to identify all the pressure ulcers the patient has, if applicable.

      See Section I.B.14 for pressure ulcer stage documentation by clinicians other than patient's provider

      2) Unstageable pressure ulcers
      Assignment of the code for unstageable pressure ulcer (L89.--0) should be based on the clinical documentation. These codes are used for pressure ulcers whose stage cannot be clinically determined (e.g., the ulcer is covered by eschar or has been treated with a skin or muscle graft). This code should not be confused with the codes for unspecified stage (L89.--9). When there is no documentation regarding the stage of the pressure ulcer, assign the appropriate code for unspecified stage (L89.--9).

      3) Documented pressure ulcer stage
      Assignment of the pressure ulcer stage code should be guided by clinical documentation of the stage or documentation of the terms found in the Alphabetic Index. For clinical terms describing the stage that are not found in the Alphabetic Index, and there is no documentation of the stage, the provider should be queried.

      4) Patients admitted with pressure ulcers documented as healed
      No code is assigned if the documentation states that the pressure ulcer is completely healed **at the time of admission**.

   5) Pressure ulcers documented as healing
   Pressure ulcers described as healing should be assigned the appropriate pressure ulcer stage code based on the documentation in the medical record. If the documentation does not provide information about the stage of the healing pressure ulcer, assign the appropriate code for unspecified stage.

   If the documentation is unclear as to whether the patient has a current (new) pressure ulcer or if the patient is being treated for a healing pressure ulcer, query the provider.

   For ulcers that were present on admission but healed at the time of discharge, assign the code for the site and stage of the pressure ulcer at the time of admission.

   6) Patient admitted with pressure ulcer evolving into another stage during the admission
   If a patient is admitted to an inpatient hospital with a pressure ulcer at one stage and it progresses to a higher stage, two separate codes should be assigned: one code for the site and stage of the ulcer on admission and a second code for the same ulcer site and the highest stage reported during the stay.

   7) Pressure-induced deep tissue damage
   For pressure-induced deep tissue damage or deep tissue pressure injury, assign only the appropriate code for pressure-induced deep tissue damage (L89.--6).

b. Non-Pressure Chronic Ulcers
   1) Patients admitted with non-pressure ulcers documented as healed
   No code is assigned if the documentation states that the non-pressure ulcer is completely healed **at the time of admission**.

   2) Non-pressure ulcers documented as healing
   Non-pressure ulcers described as healing should be assigned the appropriate non-pressure ulcer code based on the documentation in the medical record. If the documentation does not provide information about the severity of the healing non-pressure ulcer, assign the appropriate code for unspecified severity.

   If the documentation is unclear as to whether the patient has a current (new) non-pressure ulcer or if the patient is being treated for a healing non-pressure ulcer, query the provider.

   For ulcers that were present on admission but healed at the time of discharge, assign the code for the site and severity of the non-pressure ulcer at the time of admission.

   3) Patient admitted with non-pressure ulcer that progresses to another severity level during the admission
   If a patient is admitted to an inpatient hospital with a non-pressure ulcer at one severity level and it progresses to a higher severity level, two separate codes should be assigned: one code for the site and severity level of the ulcer on admission and a second code for the same ulcer site and the highest severity level reported during the stay.

   See Section I.B.14 for pressure ulcer stage documentation by clinicians other than patient's provider

13. Chapter 13: Diseases of the Musculoskeletal System and Connective Tissue (M00-M99)
   a. Site and laterality
   Most of the codes within Chapter 13 have site and laterality designations. The site represents the bone, joint or the muscle involved. For some conditions where more than one bone, joint or muscle is usually involved, such as osteoarthritis, there is a "multiple sites" code available. For categories where no multiple site code is provided and more than one bone, joint or muscle is involved, multiple codes should be used to indicate the different sites involved.

      1) Bone versus joint
      For certain conditions, the bone may be affected at the upper or lower end, (e.g., avascular necrosis of bone, M87, Osteoporosis, M80, M81). Though the portion of the bone affected may be at the joint, the site designation will be the bone, not the joint.

   b. Acute traumatic versus chronic or recurrent musculoskeletal conditions
   Many musculoskeletal conditions are a result of previous injury or trauma to a site, or are recurrent conditions. Bone, joint or muscle conditions that are the result of a healed injury are usually found in chapter 13. Recurrent bone, joint or muscle conditions are also usually found in chapter 13. Any current, acute injury should be coded to the

appropriate injury code from chapter 19. Chronic or recurrent conditions should generally be coded with a code from chapter 13. If it is difficult to determine from the documentation in the record which code is best to describe a condition, query the provider.

c. Coding of Pathologic Fractures

7th character A is for use as long as the patient is receiving active treatment for the fracture. While the patient may be seen by a new or different provider over the course of treatment for a pathological fracture, assignment of the 7th character is based on whether the patient is undergoing active treatment and not whether the provider is seeing the patient for the first time.

7th character D is to be used for encounters after the patient has completed active treatment for the fracture and is receiving routine care for the fracture during the healing or recovery phase. The other 7th characters, listed under each subcategory in the Tabular List, are to be used for subsequent encounters for treatment of problems associated with the healing, such as malunions, nonunions, and sequelae.

Care for complications of surgical treatment for fracture repairs during the healing or recovery phase should be coded with the appropriate complication codes.

See Section I.C.19. Coding of traumatic fractures.

d. Osteoporosis

Osteoporosis is a systemic condition, meaning that all bones of the musculoskeletal system are affected. Therefore, site is not a component of the codes under category M81, Osteoporosis without current pathological fracture. The site codes under category M80, Osteoporosis with current pathological fracture, identify the site of the fracture, not the osteoporosis.

1) Osteoporosis without pathological fracture

Category M81, Osteoporosis without current pathological fracture, is for use for patients with osteoporosis who do not currently have a pathologic fracture due to the osteoporosis, even if they have had a fracture in the past. For patients with a history of osteoporosis fractures, status code Z87.310, Personal history of (healed) osteoporosis fracture, should follow the code from M81.

2) Osteoporosis with current pathological fracture

Category M80, Osteoporosis with current pathological fracture, is for patients who have a current pathologic fracture at the time of an encounter. The codes under M80 identify the site of the fracture. A code from category M80, not a traumatic fracture code, should be used for any patient with known osteoporosis who suffers a fracture, even if the patient had a minor fall or trauma, if that fall or trauma would not usually break a normal, healthy bone.

14. Chapter 14: Diseases of Genitourinary System (N00-N99)

a. Chronic kidney disease

1) Stages of chronic kidney disease (CKD)

The ICD-10-CM classifies CKD based on severity. The severity of CKD is designated by stages 1-5. Stage 2, code N18.2, equates to mild CKD; stage 3, code N18.3, equates to moderate CKD; and stage 4, code N18.4, equates to severe CKD. Code N18.6, End stage renal disease (ESRD), is assigned when the provider has documented end-stage-renal disease (ESRD).

If both a stage of CKD and ESRD are documented, assign code N18.6 only.

2) Chronic kidney disease and kidney transplant status

Patients who have undergone kidney transplant may still have some form of chronic kidney disease (CKD) because the kidney transplant may not fully restore kidney function. Therefore, the presence of CKD alone does not constitute a transplant complication. Assign the appropriate N18 code for the patient's stage of CKD and code Z94.0, Kidney transplant status. If a transplant complication such as failure or rejection or other transplant complication is documented, see section I.C.19.g for information on coding complications of a kidney transplant. If the documentation is unclear as to whether the patient has a complication of the transplant, query the provider.

3) Chronic kidney disease with other conditions

Patients with CKD may also suffer from other serious conditions, most commonly diabetes mellitus and hypertension. The sequencing of the CKD code in relationship to codes for other contributing conditions is based on the conventions in the Tabular List.

See I.C.9. Hypertensive chronic kidney disease.

See I.C.19. Chronic kidney disease and kidney transplant complications.

15. Chapter 15: Pregnancy, Childbirth, and the Puerperium (O00-O9A)

a. General Rules for Obstetric Cases

1) Codes from chapter 15 and sequencing priority

Obstetric cases require codes from chapter 15, codes in the range O00-O9A, Pregnancy, Childbirth, and the Puerperium. Chapter 15 codes have sequencing priority over codes from other chapters. Additional codes from other chapters may be used in conjunction with chapter 15 codes to further specify conditions. Should the provider document that the pregnancy is incidental to the encounter, then code Z33.1, Pregnant state, incidental, should be used in place of any chapter 15 codes. It is the provider's responsibility to state that the condition being treated is not affecting the pregnancy.

2) Chapter 15 codes used only on the maternal record

Chapter 15 codes are to be used only on the maternal record, never on the record of the newborn.

3) Final character for trimester

The majority of codes in Chapter 15 have a final character indicating the trimester of pregnancy. The timeframes for the trimesters are indicated at the beginning of the chapter. If trimester is not a component of a code, it is because the condition always occurs in a specific trimester, or the concept of trimester of pregnancy is not applicable. Certain codes have characters for only certain trimesters because the condition does not occur in all trimesters, but it may occur in more than just one.

Assignment of the final character for trimester should be based on the provider's documentation of the trimester (or number of weeks) for the current admission/encounter. This applies to the assignment of trimester for pre-existing conditions as well as those that develop during or are due to the pregnancy. The provider's documentation of the number of weeks may be used to assign the appropriate code identifying the trimester.

Whenever delivery occurs during the current admission, and there is an "in childbirth" option for the obstetric complication being coded, the "in childbirth" code should be assigned.

4) Selection of trimester for inpatient admissions that encompass more than one trimester

In instances when a patient is admitted to a hospital for complications of pregnancy during one trimester and remains in the hospital into a subsequent trimester, the trimester character for the antepartum complication code should be assigned on the basis of the trimester when the complication developed, not the trimester of the discharge. If the condition developed prior to the current admission/encounter or represents a pre-existing condition, the trimester character for the trimester at the time of the admission/encounter should be assigned.

5) Unspecified trimester

Each category that includes codes for trimester has a code for "unspecified trimester." The "unspecified trimester" code should rarely be used, such as when the documentation in the record is insufficient to determine the trimester and it is not possible to obtain clarification.

6) 7th character for Fetus Identification

Where applicable, a 7th character is to be assigned for certain categories (O31, O32, O33.3 - O33.6, O35, O36, O40, O41, O60.1, O60.2, O64, and O69) to identify the fetus for which the complication code applies.

Assign 7th character "0":

- For single gestations
- When the documentation in the record is insufficient to determine the fetus affected and it is not possible to obtain clarification.
- When it is not possible to clinically determine which fetus is affected.

b. Selection of OB Principal or First-listed Diagnosis

1) Routine outpatient prenatal visits

For routine outpatient prenatal visits when no complications are present, a code from category Z34, Encounter for supervision of normal pregnancy, should be used as the first-listed diagnosis. These codes should not be used in conjunction with chapter 15 codes.

2) Supervision of High-Risk Pregnancy
Codes from category O09, Supervision of high-risk pregnancy, are intended for use only during the prenatal period. For complications during the labor or delivery episode as a result of a high-risk pregnancy, assign the applicable complication codes from Chapter 15. If there are no complications during the labor or delivery episode, assign code O80, Encounter for full-term uncomplicated delivery.

For routine prenatal outpatient visits for patients with high-risk pregnancies, a code from category O09, Supervision of high-risk pregnancy, should be used as the first-listed diagnosis. Secondary chapter 15 codes may be used in conjunction with these codes if appropriate.

3) Episodes when no delivery occurs
In episodes when no delivery occurs, the principal diagnosis should correspond to the principal complication of the pregnancy which necessitated the encounter. Should more than one complication exist, all of which are treated or monitored, any of the complication codes may be sequenced first.

4) When a delivery occurs
When an obstetric patient is admitted and delivers during that admission, the condition that prompted the admission should be sequenced as the principal diagnosis. If multiple conditions prompted the admission, sequence the one most related to the delivery as the principal diagnosis. A code for any complication of the delivery should be assigned as an additional diagnosis. In cases of cesarean delivery, if the patient was admitted with a condition that resulted in the performance of a cesarean procedure, that condition should be selected as the principal diagnosis. If the reason for the admission was unrelated to the condition resulting in the cesarean delivery, the condition related to the reason for the admission should be selected as the principal diagnosis.

5) Outcome of delivery
A code from category Z37, Outcome of delivery, should be included on every maternal record when a delivery has occurred. These codes are not to be used on subsequent records or on the newborn record.

c. Pre-existing conditions versus conditions due to the pregnancy
Certain categories in Chapter 15 distinguish between conditions of the mother that existed prior to pregnancy (pre-existing) and those that are a direct result of pregnancy. When assigning codes from Chapter 15, it is important to assess if a condition was pre-existing prior to pregnancy or developed during or due to the pregnancy in order to assign the correct code.

Categories that do not distinguish between pre-existing and pregnancy-related conditions may be used for either. It is acceptable to use codes specifically for the puerperium with codes complicating pregnancy and childbirth if a condition arises postpartum during the delivery encounter.

d. Pre-existing hypertension in pregnancy
Category O10, Pre-existing hypertension complicating pregnancy, childbirth and the puerperium, includes codes for hypertensive heart and hypertensive chronic kidney disease. When assigning one of the O10 codes that includes hypertensive heart disease or hypertensive chronic kidney disease, it is necessary to add a secondary code from the appropriate hypertension category to specify the type of heart failure or chronic kidney disease.

See Section I.C.9. Hypertension.

e. Fetal Conditions Affecting the Management of the Mother
1) Codes from categories O35 and O36
Codes from categories O35, Maternal care for known or suspected fetal abnormality and damage, and O36, Maternal care for other fetal problems, are assigned only when the fetal condition is actually responsible for modifying the management of the mother, i.e., by requiring diagnostic studies, additional observation, special care, or termination of pregnancy. The fact that the fetal condition exists does not justify assigning a code from this series to the mother's record.

2) In utero surgery
In cases when surgery is performed on the fetus, a diagnosis code from category O35, Maternal care for known or suspected fetal abnormality and damage, should be assigned identifying the fetal condition. Assign the appropriate procedure code for the procedure performed.

No code from Chapter 16, the perinatal codes, should be used on the mother's record to identify fetal conditions. Surgery performed in utero on a fetus is still to be coded as an obstetric encounter.

f. HIV Infection in Pregnancy, Childbirth and the Puerperium
During pregnancy, childbirth or the puerperium, a patient admitted because of an HIV-related illness should receive a principal diagnosis from subcategory O98.7-, Human immunodeficiency [HIV] disease complicating pregnancy, childbirth and the puerperium, followed by the code(s) for the HIV-related illness(es).

Patients with asymptomatic HIV infection status admitted during pregnancy, childbirth, or the puerperium should receive codes of O98.7- and Z21, Asymptomatic human immunodeficiency virus [HIV] infection status.

g. Diabetes mellitus in pregnancy
Diabetes mellitus is a significant complicating factor in pregnancy. Pregnant women who are diabetic should be assigned a code from category O24, Diabetes mellitus in pregnancy, childbirth, and the puerperium, first, followed by the appropriate diabetes code(s) (E08-E13) from Chapter 4.

h. Long term use of insulin and oral hypoglycemics
See section I.C.4.a.3 for information on the long term use of insulin and oral hypoglycemic.

i. Gestational (pregnancy induced) diabetes
Gestational (pregnancy induced) diabetes can occur during the second and third trimester of pregnancy in women who were not diabetic prior to pregnancy. Gestational diabetes can cause complications in the pregnancy similar to those of pre-existing diabetes mellitus. It also puts the woman at greater risk of developing diabetes after the pregnancy. Codes for gestational diabetes are in subcategory O24.4, Gestational diabetes mellitus. No other code from category O24, Diabetes mellitus in pregnancy, childbirth, and the puerperium, should be used with a code from O24.4.

The codes under subcategory O24.4 include diet controlled, insulin controlled, and controlled by oral hypoglycemic drugs. If a patient with gestational diabetes is treated with both diet and insulin, only the code for insulin-controlled is required. If a patient with gestational diabetes is treated with both diet and oral hypoglycemic medications, only the code for "controlled by oral hypoglycemic drugs" is required. Code Z79.4, Long-term (current) use of insulin or code Z79.84, Long term (current) use of oral hypoglycemic drugs, should not be assigned with codes from subcategory O24.4.

An abnormal glucose tolerance in pregnancy is assigned a code from subcategory O99.81, Abnormal glucose complicating pregnancy, childbirth, and the puerperium.

j. Sepsis and septic shock complicating abortion, pregnancy, childbirth and the puerperium
When assigning a chapter 15 code for sepsis complicating abortion, pregnancy, childbirth, and the puerperium, a code for the specific type of infection should be assigned as an additional diagnosis. If severe sepsis is present, a code from subcategory R65.2, Severe sepsis, and code(s) for associated organ dysfunction(s) should also be assigned as additional diagnoses.

k. Puerperal sepsis
Code O85, Puerperal sepsis, should be assigned with a secondary code to identify the causal organism (e.g., for a bacterial infection, assign a code from category B95-B96, Bacterial infections in conditions classified elsewhere). A code from category A40, Streptococcal sepsis, or A41, Other sepsis, should not be used for puerperal sepsis. If applicable, use additional codes to identify severe sepsis (R65.2-) and any associated acute organ dysfunction.

l. Alcohol, tobacco and drug use during pregnancy, childbirth and the puerperium
1) Alcohol use during pregnancy, childbirth and the puerperium
Codes under subcategory O99.31, Alcohol use complicating pregnancy, childbirth, and the puerperium, should be assigned for any pregnancy case when a mother uses alcohol during the pregnancy or postpartum. A secondary code from category F10, Alcohol related disorders, should also be assigned to identify manifestations of the alcohol use.

2) Tobacco use during pregnancy, childbirth and the puerperium
Codes under subcategory O99.33, Smoking (tobacco) complicating pregnancy, childbirth, and the puerperium, should

be assigned for any pregnancy case when a mother uses any type of tobacco product during the pregnancy or postpartum. A secondary code from category F17, Nicotine dependence, should also be assigned to identify the type of nicotine dependence.

3) **Drug use during pregnancy, childbirth and the puerperium**
Codes under subcategory O99.32, Drug use complicating pregnancy, childbirth, and the puerperium, should be assigned for any pregnancy case when a mother uses drugs during the pregnancy or postpartum. This can involve illegal drugs, or inappropriate use or abuse of prescription drugs. Secondary code(s) from categories F11-F16 and F18-F19 should also be assigned to identify manifestations of the drug use.

m. **Poisoning, toxic effects, adverse effects and underdosing in a pregnant patient**
A code from subcategory O9A.2, Injury, poisoning and certain other consequences of external causes complicating pregnancy, childbirth, and the puerperium, should be sequenced first, followed by the appropriate injury, poisoning, toxic effect, adverse effect or underdosing code, and then the additional code(s) that specifies the condition caused by the poisoning, toxic effect, adverse effect or underdosing.
See Section I.C.19. Adverse effects, poisoning, underdosing and toxic effects.

n. **Normal Delivery, Code O80**
1) **Encounter for full term uncomplicated delivery**
Code O80 should be assigned when a woman is admitted for a full-term normal delivery and delivers a single, healthy infant without any complications antepartum, during the delivery, or postpartum during the delivery episode. Code O80 is always a principal diagnosis. It is not to be used if any other code from chapter 15 is needed to describe a current complication of the antenatal, delivery, or **postnatal** period. Additional codes from other chapters may be used with code O80 if they are not related to or are in any way complicating the pregnancy.

2) **Uncomplicated delivery with resolved antepartum complication**
Code O80 may be used if the patient had a complication at some point during the pregnancy, but the complication is not present at the time of the admission for delivery.

3) **Outcome of delivery for O80**
Z37.0, Single live birth, is the only outcome of delivery code appropriate for use with O80.

o. **The Peripartum and Postpartum Periods**
1) **Peripartum and Postpartum periods**
The postpartum period begins immediately after delivery and continues for six weeks following delivery. The peripartum period is defined as the last month of pregnancy to five months postpartum.

2) **Peripartum and postpartum complication**
A postpartum complication is any complication occurring within the six-week period.

3) **Pregnancy-related complications after 6 week period**
Chapter 15 codes may also be used to describe pregnancy-related complications after the peripartum or postpartum period if the provider documents that a condition is pregnancy related.

4) **Admission for routine postpartum care following delivery outside hospital**
When the mother delivers outside the hospital prior to admission and is admitted for routine postpartum care and no complications are noted, code Z39.0, Encounter for care and examination of mother immediately after delivery, should be assigned as the principal diagnosis.

5) **Pregnancy associated cardiomyopathy**
Pregnancy associated cardiomyopathy, code O90.3, is unique in that it may be diagnosed in the third trimester of pregnancy but may continue to progress months after delivery. For this reason, it is referred to as peripartum cardiomyopathy. Code O90.3 is only for use when the cardiomyopathy develops as a result of pregnancy in a woman who did not have pre-existing heart disease.

p. **Code O94, Sequelae of complication of pregnancy, childbirth, and the puerperium**
1) **Code O94**
Code O94, Sequelae of complication of pregnancy, childbirth, and the puerperium, is for use in those cases when an initial

complication of a pregnancy develops a sequelae requiring care or treatment at a future date.

2) **After the initial postpartum period**
This code may be used at any time after the initial postpartum period.

3) **Sequencing of Code O94**
This code, like all sequela codes, is to be sequenced following the code describing the sequelae of the complication.

q. **Termination of Pregnancy and Spontaneous abortions**
1) **Abortion with Liveborn Fetus**
When an attempted termination of pregnancy results in a liveborn fetus, assign code Z33.2, Encounter for elective termination of pregnancy and a code from category Z37, Outcome of Delivery.

2) **Retained Products of Conception following an abortion**
Subsequent encounters for retained products of conception following a spontaneous abortion or elective termination of pregnancy, without complications are assigned O03.4, Incomplete spontaneous abortion without complication, or code O07.4, Failed attempted termination of pregnancy without complication. This advice is appropriate even when the patient was discharged previously with a discharge diagnosis of complete abortion. If the patient has a specific complication associated with the spontaneous abortion or elective termination of pregnancy in addition to retained products of conception, assign the appropriate complication **code (e.g., O03.-, O04.-, O07.-)** instead of code O03.4 or O07.4

3) **Complications leading to abortion**
Codes from Chapter 15 may be used as additional codes to identify any documented complications of the pregnancy in conjunction with codes in categories in O04, O07 and O08.

r. **Abuse in a pregnant patient**
For suspected or confirmed cases of abuse of a pregnant patient, a code(s) from subcategories O9A.3, Physical abuse complicating pregnancy, childbirth, and the puerperium, O9A.4, Sexual abuse complicating pregnancy, childbirth, and the puerperium, and O9A.5, Psychological abuse complicating pregnancy, childbirth, and the puerperium, should be sequenced first, followed by the appropriate codes (if applicable) to identify any associated current injury due to physical abuse, sexual abuse, and the perpetrator of abuse.
See Section I.C.19. Adult and child abuse, neglect and other maltreatment.

16. **Chapter 16: Certain Conditions Originating in the Perinatal Period (P00-P96)**
For coding and reporting purposes the perinatal period is defined as before birth through the 28th day following birth. The following guidelines are provided for reporting purposes.

a. **General Perinatal Rules**
1) **Use of Chapter 16 Codes**
Codes in this chapter are <u>never</u> for use on the maternal record. Codes from Chapter 15, the obstetric chapter, are never permitted on the newborn record. Chapter 16 codes may be used throughout the life of the patient if the condition is still present.

2) **Principal Diagnosis for Birth Record**
When coding the birth episode in a newborn record, assign a code from category Z38, Liveborn infants according to place of birth and type of delivery, as the principal diagnosis. A code from category Z38 is assigned only once, to a newborn at the time of birth. If a newborn is transferred to another institution, a code from category Z38 should not be used at the receiving hospital.

A code from category Z38 is used only on the newborn record, not on the mother's record.

3) **Use of Codes from other Chapters with Codes from Chapter 16**
Codes from other chapters may be used with codes from chapter 16 if the codes from the other chapters provide more specific detail. Codes for signs and symptoms may be assigned when a definitive diagnosis has not been established. If the reason for the encounter is a perinatal condition, the code from chapter 16 should be sequenced first.

4) **Use of Chapter 16 Codes after the Perinatal Period**
Should a condition originate in the perinatal period, and continue throughout the life of the patient, the perinatal code should continue to be used regardless of the patient's age.

5) Birth process or community acquired conditions

If a newborn has a condition that may be either due to the birth process or community acquired and the documentation does not indicate which it is, the default is due to the birth process and the code from Chapter 16 should be used. If the condition is community-acquired, a code from Chapter 16 should not be assigned.

6) Code all clinically significant conditions

All clinically significant conditions noted on routine newborn examination should be coded. A condition is clinically significant if it requires:

- clinical evaluation; or
- therapeutic treatment; or
- diagnostic procedures; or
- extended length of hospital stay; or
- increased nursing care and/or monitoring; or
- has implications for future health care needs

Note: The perinatal guidelines listed above are the same as the general coding guidelines for "additional diagnoses," except for the final point regarding implications for future health care needs. Codes should be assigned for conditions that have been specified by the provider as having implications for future health care needs.

b. Observation and Evaluation of Newborns for Suspected Conditions not Found

1) Use of Z05 codes

Assign a code from category Z05, Observation and evaluation of newborns and infants for suspected conditions ruled out, to identify those instances when a healthy newborn is evaluated for a suspected condition that is determined after study not to be present. Do not use a code from category Z05 when the patient has identified signs or symptoms of a suspected problem; in such cases code the sign or symptom.

2) Z05 on other than the birth record

A code from category Z05 may also be assigned as a principal or first-listed code for readmissions or encounters when the code from category Z38 code no longer applies. Codes from category Z05 are for use only for healthy newborns and infants for which no condition after study is found to be present.

3) Z05 on a birth record

A code from category Z05 is to be used as a secondary code after the code from category Z38, Liveborn infants according to place of birth and type of delivery.

c. Coding Additional Perinatal Diagnoses

1) Assigning codes for conditions that require treatment

Assign codes for conditions that require treatment or further investigation, prolong the length of stay, or require resource utilization.

2) Codes for conditions specified as having implications for future health care needs

Assign codes for conditions that have been specified by the provider as having implications for future health care needs.

Note: This guideline should not be used for adult patients.

d. Prematurity and Fetal Growth Retardation

Providers utilize different criteria in determining prematurity. A code for prematurity should not be assigned unless it is documented. Assignment of codes in categories P05, Disorders of newborn related to slow fetal growth and fetal malnutrition, and P07, Disorders of newborn related to short gestation and low birth weight, not elsewhere classified, should be based on the recorded birth weight and estimated gestational age.

When both birth weight and gestational age are available, two codes from category P07 should be assigned, with the code for birth weight sequenced before the code for gestational age.

e. Low birth weight and immaturity status

Codes from category P07, Disorders of newborn related to short gestation and low birth weight, not elsewhere classified, are for use for a child or adult who was premature or had a low birth weight as a newborn and this is affecting the patient's current health status.

See Section I.C.21. Factors influencing health status and contact with health services, Status.

f. Bacterial Sepsis of Newborn

Category P36, Bacterial sepsis of newborn, includes congenital sepsis. If a perinate is documented as having sepsis without documentation

of congenital or community acquired, the default is congenital and a code from category P36 should be assigned. If the P36 code includes the causal organism, an additional code from category B95, Streptococcus, Staphylococcus, and Enterococcus as the cause of diseases classified elsewhere, or B96, Other bacterial agents as the cause of diseases classified elsewhere, should not be assigned. If the P36 code does not include the causal organism, assign an additional code from category B96. If applicable, use additional codes to identify severe sepsis (R65.2-) and any associated acute organ dysfunction.

g. Stillbirth

Code P95, Stillbirth, is only for use in institutions that maintain separate records for stillbirths. No other code should be used with P95. Code P95 should not be used on the mother's record.

17. Chapter 17: Congenital malformations, deformations, and chromosomal abnormalities (Q00-Q99)

Assign an appropriate code(s) from categories Q00-Q99, Congenital malformations, deformations, and chromosomal abnormalities when a malformation/deformation or chromosomal abnormality is documented. A malformation/deformation/or chromosomal abnormality may be the principal/first-listed diagnosis on a record or a secondary diagnosis.

When a malformation/deformation or chromosomal abnormality does not have a unique code assignment, assign additional code(s) for any manifestations that may be present.

When the code assignment specifically identifies the malformation/deformation or chromosomal abnormality, manifestations that are an inherent component of the anomaly should not be coded separately. Additional codes should be assigned for manifestations that are not an inherent component.

Codes from Chapter 17 may be used throughout the life of the patient. If a congenital malformation or deformity has been corrected, a personal history code should be used to identify the history of the malformation or deformity. Although present at birth, **a** malformation/deformation/or chromosomal abnormality may not be identified until later in life. Whenever the condition is diagnosed by the **provider**, it is appropriate to assign a code from codes Q00-Q99. For the birth admission, the appropriate code from category Z38, Liveborn infants, according to place of birth and type of delivery, should be sequenced as the principal diagnosis, followed by any congenital anomaly codes, Q00- Q99.

18. Chapter 18: Symptoms, signs, and abnormal clinical and laboratory findings, not elsewhere classified (R00-R99)

Chapter 18 includes symptoms, signs, abnormal results of clinical or other investigative procedures, and ill-defined conditions regarding which no diagnosis classifiable elsewhere is recorded. Signs and symptoms that point to a specific diagnosis have been assigned to a category in other chapters of the classification.

a. Use of symptom codes

Codes that describe symptoms and signs are acceptable for reporting purposes when a related definitive diagnosis has not been established (confirmed) by the provider.

b. Use of a symptom code with a definitive diagnosis code

Codes for signs and symptoms may be reported in addition to a related definitive diagnosis when the sign or symptom is not routinely associated with that diagnosis, such as the various signs and symptoms associated with complex syndromes. The definitive diagnosis code should be sequenced before the symptom code.

Signs or symptoms that are associated routinely with a disease process should not be assigned as additional codes, unless otherwise instructed by the classification.

c. Combination codes that include symptoms

ICD-10-CM contains a number of combination codes that identify both the definitive diagnosis and common symptoms of that diagnosis.

When using one of these combination codes, an additional code should not be assigned for the symptom.

d. Repeated falls

Code R29.6, Repeated falls, is for use for encounters when a patient has recently fallen and the reason for the fall is being investigated.

Code Z91.81, History of falling, is for use when a patient has fallen in the past and is at risk for future falls. When appropriate, both codes R29.6 and Z91.81 may be assigned together.

e. Coma scale

The coma scale codes (R40.2-) can be used in conjunction with traumatic brain injury codes, acute cerebrovascular disease or sequelae of cerebrovascular disease codes. These codes are primarily for use by trauma registries, but they may be used in any setting where this information is collected. The coma scale may also be used to assess the status of the central nervous system for other non-trauma conditions, such as monitoring patients in the intensive care unit regardless of medical condition. The coma scale codes should be sequenced after the diagnosis code(s).

These codes, one from each subcategory, are needed to complete the scale. The 7th character indicates when the scale was recorded. The 7th character should match for all three codes.

At a minimum, report the initial score documented on presentation at your facility. This may be a score from the emergency medicine technician (EMT) or in the emergency department. If desired, a facility may choose to capture multiple coma scale scores.

Assign code R40.24, Glasgow coma scale, total score, when only the total score is documented in the medical record and not the individual score(s).

Do not report codes for individual or total Glasgow coma scale scores for a patient with a medically induced coma or a sedated patient.

See Section I.B.14 for coma scale documentation by clinicians other than patient's provider

f.   Functional quadriplegia

GUIDELINE HAS BEEN DELETED EFFECTIVE OCTOBER 1, 2017

g.   SIRS due to Non-Infectious Process

The systemic inflammatory response syndrome (SIRS) can develop as a result of certain non-infectious disease processes, such as trauma, malignant neoplasm, or pancreatitis. When SIRS is documented with a noninfectious condition, and no subsequent infection is documented, the code for the underlying condition, such as an injury, should be assigned, followed by code R65.10, Systemic inflammatory response syndrome (SIRS) of non-infectious origin without acute organ dysfunction, or code R65.11, Systemic inflammatory response syndrome (SIRS) of non-infectious origin with acute organ dysfunction. If an associated acute organ dysfunction is documented, the appropriate code(s) for the specific type of organ dysfunction(s) should be assigned in addition to code R65.11. If acute organ dysfunction is documented, but it cannot be determined if the acute organ dysfunction is associated with SIRS or due to another condition (e.g., directly due to the trauma), the provider should be queried.

h.   Death NOS

Code R99, Ill-defined and unknown cause of mortality, is only for use in the very limited circumstance when a patient who has already died is brought into an emergency department or other healthcare facility and is pronounced dead upon arrival. It does not represent the discharge disposition of death.

i.   NIHSS Stroke Scale

The NIH stroke scale (NIHSS) codes (R29.7- -) can be used in conjunction with acute stroke codes (I63) to identify the patient's neurological status and the severity of the stroke. The stroke scale codes should be sequenced after the acute stroke diagnosis code(s).

At a minimum, report the initial score documented. If desired, a facility may choose to capture multiple stroke scale scores.

See Section I.B.14 for NIHSS stroke scale documentation by clinicians other than patient's provider

19. Chapter 19: Injury, poisoning, and certain other consequences of external causes (S00-T88)

a.   Application of 7th Characters in Chapter 19

Most categories in chapter 19 have a 7th character requirement for each applicable code. Most categories in this chapter have three 7th character values (with the exception of fractures): A, initial encounter, D, subsequent encounter and S, sequela. Categories for traumatic fractures have additional 7th character values. While the patient may be seen by a new or different provider over the course of treatment for an injury, assignment of the 7th character is based on whether the patient is undergoing active treatment and not whether the provider is seeing the patient for the first time.

For complication codes, active treatment refers to treatment for the condition described by the code, even though it may be related to an earlier precipitating problem. For example, code T84.50XA, Infection and inflammatory reaction due to unspecified internal joint prosthesis, initial encounter, is used when active treatment is provided for the infection, even though the condition relates to the prosthetic device, implant or graft that was placed at a previous encounter.

7th character "A", initial encounter is used for each encounter where the patient is receiving active treatment for the condition.

7th character "D" subsequent encounter is used for encounters after the patient has completed active treatment of the condition and is receiving routine care for the condition during the healing or recovery phase.

The aftercare Z codes should not be used for aftercare for conditions such as injuries or poisonings, where 7th characters are provided to identify subsequent care. For example, for aftercare of an injury, assign the acute injury code with the 7th character "D" (subsequent encounter).

7th character "S", sequela, is for use for complications or conditions that arise as a direct result of a condition, such as scar formation after a burn. The scars are sequelae of the burn. When using 7th character "S", it is necessary to use both the injury code that precipitated the sequela and the code for the sequela itself. The "S" is added only to the injury code, not the sequela code. The 7th character "S" identifies the injury responsible for the sequela. The specific type of sequela (e.g. scar) is sequenced first, followed by the injury code.

See Section I.B.10 Sequelae, (Late Effects)

b.   Coding of Injuries

When coding injuries, assign separate codes for each injury unless a combination code is provided, in which case the combination code is assigned. Codes from category T07, Unspecified multiple injuries should not be assigned in the inpatient setting unless information for a more specific code is not available. Traumatic injury codes (S00-T14.9) are not to be used for normal, healing surgical wounds or to identify complications of surgical wounds.

The code for the most serious injury, as determined by the provider and the focus of treatment, is sequenced first.

1)   Superficial injuries

Superficial injuries such as abrasions or contusions are not coded when associated with more severe injuries of the same site.

2)   Primary injury with damage to nerves/blood vessels

When a primary injury results in minor damage to peripheral nerves or blood vessels, the primary injury is sequenced first with additional code(s) for injuries to nerves and spinal cord (such as category S04), and/or injury to blood vessels (such as category S15). When the primary injury is to the blood vessels or nerves, that injury should be sequenced first.

3)   Iatrogenic injuries

Injury codes from Chapter 19 should not be assigned for injuries that occur during, or as a result of, a medical intervention. Assign the appropriate complication code(s).

c.   Coding of Traumatic Fractures

The principles of multiple coding of injuries should be followed in coding fractures. Fractures of specified sites are coded individually by site in accordance with both the provisions within categories S02, S12, S22, S32, S42, S49, S52, S59, S62, S72, S79, S82, S89, S92 and the level of detail furnished by medical record content.

A fracture not indicated as open or closed should be coded to closed. A fracture not indicated whether displaced or not displaced should be coded to displaced.

More specific guidelines are as follows:

1)   Initial vs. subsequent encounter for fractures

Traumatic fractures are coded using the appropriate 7th character for initial encounter (A, B, C) for each encounter where the patient is receiving active treatment for the fracture. The appropriate 7th character for initial encounter should also be assigned for a patient who delayed seeking treatment for the fracture or nonunion.

Fractures are coded using the appropriate 7th character for subsequent care for encounters after the patient has completed active treatment of the fracture and is receiving routine care for the fracture during the healing or recovery phase.

Care for complications of surgical treatment for fracture repairs during the healing or recovery phase should be coded with the appropriate complication codes.

Care of complications of fractures, such as malunion and nonunion, should be reported with the appropriate 7th character for subsequent care with nonunion (K, M, N,) or subsequent care with malunion (P, Q, R).

Malunion/nonunion: The appropriate 7th character for initial encounter should also be assigned for a patient who delayed seeking treatment for the fracture or nonunion.

The open fracture designations in the assignment of the 7th character for fractures of the forearm, femur and lower leg, including ankle are based on the Gustilo open fracture classification. When the Gustilo classification type is not specified for an open fracture, the 7th character for open fracture type I or II should be assigned (B, E, H, M, Q).

A code from category M80, not a traumatic fracture code, should be used for any patient with known osteoporosis who suffers a fracture, even if the patient had a minor fall or trauma, if that fall or trauma would not usually break a normal, healthy bone.

See Section I.C.13. Osteoporosis.

The aftercare Z codes should not be used for aftercare for traumatic fractures. For aftercare of a traumatic fracture, assign the acute fracture code with the appropriate 7th character.

2) Multiple fractures sequencing
Multiple fractures are sequenced in accordance with the severity of the fracture.

3) Physeal fractures
For physeal fractures, assign only the code identifying the type of physeal fracture. Do not assign a separate code to identify the specific bone that is fractured.

d. Coding of Burns and Corrosions
The ICD-10-CM makes a distinction between burns and corrosions. The burn codes are for thermal burns, except sunburns, that come from a heat source, such as a fire or hot appliance. The burn codes are also for burns resulting from electricity and radiation. Corrosions are burns due to chemicals. The guidelines are the same for burns and corrosions.

Current burns (T20-T25) are classified by depth, extent and by agent (X code). Burns are classified by depth as first degree (erythema), second degree (blistering), and third degree (full-thickness involvement). Burns of the eye and internal organs (T26-T28) are classified by site, but not by degree.

1) Sequencing of burn and related condition codes
Sequence first the code that reflects the highest degree of burn when more than one burn is present.

a.   When the reason for the admission or encounter is for treatment of external multiple burns, sequence first the code that reflects the burn of the highest degree.

b.   When a patient has both internal and external burns, the circumstances of admission govern the selection of the principal diagnosis or first-listed diagnosis.

c.   When a patient is admitted for burn injuries and other related conditions such as smoke inhalation and/or respiratory failure, the circumstances of admission govern the selection of the principal or first-listed diagnosis.

2) Burns of the same anatomic site
Classify burns of the same anatomic site and on the same side but of different degrees to the subcategory identifying the highest degree recorded in the diagnosis (e.g., for second and third degree burns of right thigh, assign only code T24.311-).

3) Non-healing burns
Non-healing burns are coded as acute burns.
Necrosis of burned skin should be coded as a non-healed burn.

4) Infected *burn*
For any documented infected burn site, use an additional code for the infection.

5) Assign separate codes for each burn site
When coding burns, assign separate codes for each burn site. Category T30, Burn and corrosion, body region unspecified is extremely vague and should rarely be used.

Codes for burns of "multiple sites" should only be assigned when the medical record documentation does not specify the individual sites.

6) Burns and corrosions classified according to extent of body surface involved
Assign codes from category T31, Burns classified according to extent of body surface involved, or T32, Corrosions classified according to extent of body surface involved, when the site of the burn is not specified or when there is a need for additional data. It is advisable to use category T31 as additional coding when needed to provide data for evaluating burn mortality, such as that needed by burn units. It is also advisable to use category T31 as an additional code for reporting purposes when there is mention

of a third-degree burn involving 20 percent or more of the body surface.

Categories T31 and T32 are based on the classic "rule of nines" in estimating body surface involved: head and neck are assigned nine percent, each arm nine percent, each leg 18 percent, the anterior trunk 18 percent, posterior trunk 18 percent, and genitalia one percent. Providers may change these percentage assignments where necessary to accommodate infants and children who have proportionately larger heads than adults, and patients who have large buttocks, thighs, or abdomen that involve burns.

7) Encounters for treatment of sequela of burns
Encounters for the treatment of the late effects of burns or corrosions (i.e., scars or joint contractures) should be coded with a burn or corrosion code with the 7th character "S" for sequela.

8) Sequelae with a late effect code and current burn
When appropriate, both a code for a current burn or corrosion with 7th character "A" or "D" and a burn or corrosion code with 7th character "S" may be assigned on the same record (when both a current burn and sequelae of an old burn exist). Burns and corrosions do not heal at the same rate and a current healing wound may still exist with sequela of a healed burn or corrosion.

See Section I.B.10 Sequela (Late Effects)

9) Use of an external cause code with burns and corrosions
An external cause code should be used with burns and corrosions to identify the source and intent of the burn, as well as the place where it occurred.

e. Adverse Effects, Poisoning, Underdosing and Toxic Effects
Codes in categories T36-T65 are combination codes that include the substance that was taken as well as the intent. No additional external cause code is required for poisonings, toxic effects, adverse effects and underdosing codes.

1) Do not code directly from the Table of Drugs
Do not code directly funderosinrom the Table of Drugs and Chemicals. Always refer back to the Tabular List.

2) Use as many codes as necessary to describe
Use as many codes as necessary to describe completely all drugs, medicinal or biological substances.

3) If the same code would describe the causative agent
If the same code would describe the causative agent for more than one adverse reaction, poisoning, toxic effect or underdosing, assign the code only once.

4) If two or more drugs, medicinal or biological substances
If two or more drugs, medicinal or biological substances are **taken**, code each individually unless a combination code is listed in the Table of Drugs and Chemicals.

If multiple unspecified drugs, medicinal or biological substances were taken, assign the appropriate code from subcategory T50.91, Poisoning by, adverse effect of and underdosing of multiple unspecified drugs, medicaments and biological substances.

5) The occurrence of drug toxicity is classified in ICD-10-CM as follows:

(a) Adverse Effect
When coding an adverse effect of a drug that has been correctly prescribed and properly administered, assign the appropriate code for the nature of the adverse effect followed by the appropriate code for the adverse effect of the drug (T36-T50). The code for the drug should have a 5th or 6th character "5" (for example T36.0X5-) Examples of the nature of an adverse effect are tachycardia, delirium, gastrointestinal hemorrhaging, vomiting, hypokalemia, hepatitis, renal failure, or respiratory failure.

(b) Poisoning
When coding a poisoning or reaction to the improper use of a medication (e.g., overdose, wrong substance given or taken in error, wrong route of administration), first assign the appropriate code from categories T36-T50. The poisoning codes have an associated intent as their 5th or 6th character (accidental, intentional self-harm, assault and undetermined. If the intent of the poisoning is unknown or unspecified, code the intent as accidental intent. The undetermined

intent is only for use if the documentation in the record specifies that the intent cannot be determined. Use additional code(s) for all manifestations of poisonings.

If there is also a diagnosis of abuse or dependence of the substance, the abuse or dependence is assigned as an additional code.

Examples of poisoning include:

(i) Error was made in drug prescription
Errors made in drug prescription or in the administration of the drug by provider, nurse, patient, or other person.

(ii) Overdose of a drug intentionally taken
If an overdose of a drug was intentionally taken or administered and resulted in drug toxicity, it would be coded as a poisoning.

(iii) Nonprescribed drug taken with correctly prescribed and properly administered drug
If a nonprescribed drug or medicinal agent was taken in combination with a correctly prescribed and properly administered drug, any drug toxicity or other reaction resulting from the interaction of the two drugs would be classified as a poisoning.

(iv) Interaction of drug(s) and alcohol
When a reaction results from the interaction of a drug(s) and alcohol, this would be classified as poisoning.

See Section I.C.4. if poisoning is the result of insulin pump malfunctions.

(c) Underdosing

Underdosing refers to taking less of a medication than is prescribed by a provider or a manufacturer's instruction. Discontinuing the use of a prescribed medication on the patient's own initiative (not directed by the patient's provider) is also classified as an underdosing. For underdosing, assign the code from categories T36-T50 (fifth or sixth character "6").

Codes for underdosing should never be assigned as principal or first-listed codes. If a patient has a relapse or exacerbation of the medical condition for which the drug is prescribed because of the reduction in dose, then the medical condition itself should be coded.

Noncompliance (Z91.12-, Z91.13- and Z91.14-) or complication of care (Y63.6-Y63.9) codes are to be used with an underdosing code to indicate intent, if known.

(d) Toxic Effects

When a harmful substance is ingested or comes in contact with a person, this is classified as a toxic effect. The toxic effect codes are in categories T51-T65.

Toxic effect codes have an associated intent: accidental, intentional self-harm, assault and undetermined.

f. Adult and child abuse, neglect and other maltreatment

Sequence first the appropriate code from categories T74, Adult and child abuse, neglect and other maltreatment, confirmed) or T76, Adult and child abuse, neglect and other maltreatment, suspected) for abuse, neglect and other maltreatment, followed by any accompanying mental health or injury code(s).

If the documentation in the medical record states abuse or neglect it is coded as confirmed (T74.-). It is coded as suspected if it is documented as suspected (T76.-).

For cases of confirmed abuse or neglect an external cause code from the assault section (X92-Y09) should be added to identify the cause of any physical injuries. A perpetrator code (Y07) should be added when the perpetrator of the abuse is known. For suspected cases of abuse or neglect, do not report external cause or perpetrator code.

If a suspected case of abuse, neglect or mistreatment is ruled out during an encounter code Z04.71, Encounter for examination and observation following alleged physical adult abuse, ruled out, or code Z04.72, Encounter for examination and observation following alleged child physical abuse, ruled out, should be used, not a code from T76.

If a suspected case of alleged rape or sexual abuse is ruled out during an encounter code Z04.41, Encounter for examination and observation following alleged adult rape or code Z04.42, Encounter for examination and observation following alleged child rape, should be used, not a code from T76.

If a suspected case of forced sexual exploitation or forced labor exploitation is ruled out during an encounter, code Z04.81, Encounter

for examination and observation of victim following forced sexual exploitation, or code Z04.82, Encounter for examination and observation of victim following forced labor exploitation, should be used, not a code from T76.

See Section I.C.15. Abuse in a pregnant patient.

g. Complications of care

1) General guidelines for complications of care

(a) Documentation of complications of care

See Section I.B.16. for information on documentation of complications of care.

2) Pain due to medical devices

Pain associated with devices, implants or grafts left in a surgical site (for example painful hip prosthesis) is assigned to the appropriate code(s) found in Chapter 19, Injury, poisoning, and certain other consequences of external causes. Specific codes for pain due to medical devices are found in the T code section of the ICD-10-CM. Use additional code(s) from category G89 to identify acute or chronic pain due to presence of the device, implant or graft (G89.18 or G89.28).

3) Transplant complications

(a) Transplant complications other than kidney

Codes under category T86, Complications of transplanted organs and tissues, are for use for both complications and rejection of transplanted organs. A transplant complication code is only assigned if the complication affects the function of the transplanted organ. Two codes are required to fully describe a transplant complication: the appropriate code from category T86 and a secondary code that identifies the complication.

Pre-existing conditions or conditions that develop after the transplant are not coded as complications unless they affect the function of the transplanted organs.

See I.C.21. for transplant organ removal status

See I.C.2. for malignant neoplasm associated with transplanted organ.

(b) Kidney transplant complications

Patients who have undergone kidney transplant may still have some form of chronic kidney disease (CKD) because the kidney transplant may not fully restore kidney function. Code T86.1- should be assigned for documented complications of a kidney transplant, such as transplant failure or rejection or other transplant complication. Code T86.1- should not be assigned for post kidney transplant patients who have chronic kidney (CKD) unless a transplant complication such as transplant failure or rejection is documented. If the documentation is unclear as to whether the patient has a complication of the transplant, query the provider.

Conditions that affect the function of the transplanted kidney, other than CKD, should be assigned a code from subcategory T86.1, Complications of transplanted organ, Kidney, and a secondary code that identifies the complication.

For patients with CKD following a kidney transplant, but who do not have a complication such as failure or rejection, *see section I.C.14. Chronic kidney disease and kidney transplant status.*

4) Complication codes that include the external cause

As with certain other T codes, some of the complications of care codes have the external cause included in the code. The code includes the nature of the complication as well as the type of procedure that caused the complication. No external cause code indicating the type of procedure is necessary for these codes.

5) Complications of care codes within the body system chapters

Intraoperative and postprocedural complication codes are found within the body system chapters with codes specific to the organs and structures of that body system. These codes should be sequenced first, followed by a code(s) for the specific complication, if applicable.

Complication codes from the body system chapters should be assigned for intraoperative and postprocedural complications (e.g., the appropriate complication code from chapter 9 would be assigned for a vascular intraoperative or postprocedural complication) unless the complication is specifically indexed to a T code in chapter 19.

20. Chapter 20: External Causes of Morbidity (V00-Y99)

The external causes of morbidity codes should never be sequenced as the first-listed or principal diagnosis.

External cause codes are intended to provide data for injury research and evaluation of injury prevention strategies. These codes capture how the injury or health condition happened (cause), the intent (unintentional or accidental; or intentional, such as suicide or assault), the place where the event occurred the activity of the patient at the time of the event, and the person's status (e.g., civilian, military).

There is no national requirement for mandatory ICD-10-CM external cause code reporting. Unless a provider is subject to a state-based external cause code reporting mandate or these codes are required by a particular payer, reporting of ICD-10-CM codes in Chapter 20, External Causes of Morbidity, is not required. In the absence of a mandatory reporting requirement, providers are encouraged to voluntarily report external cause codes, as they provide valuable data for injury research and evaluation of injury prevention strategies.

a. General External Cause Coding Guidelines

1) Used with any code in the range of A00.0-T88.9 Z00-Z99

An external cause code may be used with any code in the range of A00.0-T88.9, Z00-Z99, classification that represents a health condition due to an external cause. Though they are most applicable to injuries, they are also valid for use with such things as infections or diseases due to an external source, and other health conditions, such as a heart attack that occurs during strenuous physical activity.

2) External cause code used for length of treatment

Assign the external cause code, with the appropriate 7th character (initial encounter, subsequent encounter or sequela) for each encounter for which the injury or condition is being treated.

Most categories in chapter 20 have a 7th character requirement for each applicable code. Most categories in this chapter have three 7th character values: A, initial encounter, D, subsequent encounter and S, sequela. While the patient may be seen by a new or different provider over the course of treatment for an injury or condition, assignment of the 7th character for external cause should match the 7th character of the code assigned for the associated injury or condition for the encounter.

3) Use the full range of external cause codes

Use the full range of external cause codes to completely describe the cause, the intent, the place of occurrence, and if applicable, the activity of the patient at the time of the event, and the patient's status, for all injuries, and other health conditions due to an external cause.

4) Assign as many external cause codes as necessary

Assign as many external cause codes as necessary to fully explain each cause. If only one external code can be recorded, assign the code most related to the principal diagnosis.

5) The selection of the appropriate external cause code

The selection of the appropriate external cause code is guided by the Alphabetic Index of External Causes and by Inclusion and Exclusion notes in the Tabular List.

6) External cause code can never be a principal diagnosis

An external cause code can never be a principal (first-listed) diagnosis.

7) Combination external cause codes

Certain of the external cause codes are combination codes that identify sequential events that result in an injury, such as a fall which results in striking against an object. The injury may be due to either event or both. The combination external cause code used should correspond to the sequence of events regardless of which caused the most serious injury.

8) No external cause code needed in certain circumstances

No external cause code from Chapter 20 is needed if the external cause and intent are included in a code from another chapter (e.g. T36.0X1- Poisoning by penicillins, accidental (unintentional)).

b. Place of Occurrence Guideline

Codes from category Y92, Place of occurrence of the external cause, are secondary codes for use after other external cause codes to identify the location of the patient at the time of injury or other condition.

Generally, a place of occurrence code is assigned only once, at the initial encounter for treatment. However, in the rare instance that a new injury occurs during hospitalization, an additional place of occurrence code may be assigned. No 7th characters are used for Y92.

Do not use place of occurrence code Y92.9 if the place is not stated or is not applicable.

c. Activity Code

Assign a code from category Y93, Activity code, to describe the activity of the patient at the time the injury or other health condition occurred.

An activity code is used only once, at the initial encounter for treatment. Only one code from Y93 should be recorded on a medical record.

The activity codes are not applicable to poisonings, adverse effects, misadventures or sequela.

Do not assign Y93.9, Unspecified activity, if the activity is not stated.

A code from category Y93 is appropriate for use with external cause and intent codes if identifying the activity provides additional information about the event.

d. Place of Occurrence, Activity, and Status Codes Used with other External Cause Code

When applicable, place of occurrence, activity, and external cause status codes are sequenced after the main external cause code(s). Regardless of the number of external cause codes assigned, generally there should be only one place of occurrence code, one activity code, and one external cause status code assigned to an encounter. However, in the rare instance that a new injury occurs during hospitalization, an additional place of occurrence code may be assigned.

e. If the Reporting Format Limits the Number of External Cause Codes

If the reporting format limits the number of external cause codes that can be used in reporting clinical data, report the code for the cause/intent most related to the principal diagnosis. If the format permits capture of additional external cause codes, the cause/intent, including medical misadventures, of the additional events should be reported rather than the codes for place, activity, or external status.

f. Multiple External Cause Coding Guidelines

More than one external cause code is required to fully describe the external cause of an illness or injury. The assignment of external cause codes should be sequenced in the following priority:

If two or more events cause separate injuries, an external cause code should be assigned for each cause. The first-listed external cause code will be selected in the following order:

External codes for child and adult abuse take priority over all other external cause codes.

See Section I.C.19., Child and Adult abuse guidelines.

External cause codes for terrorism events take priority over all other external cause codes except child and adult abuse.

External cause codes for cataclysmic events take priority over all other external cause codes except child and adult abuse and terrorism.

External cause codes for transport accidents take priority over all other external cause codes except cataclysmic events, child and adult abuse and terrorism.

Activity and external cause status codes are assigned following all causal (intent) external cause codes.

The first-listed external cause code should correspond to the cause of the most serious diagnosis due to an assault, accident, or self-harm, following the order of hierarchy listed above.

g. Child and Adult Abuse Guideline

Adult and child abuse, neglect and maltreatment are classified as assault. Any of the assault codes may be used to indicate the external cause of any injury resulting from the confirmed abuse.

For confirmed cases of abuse, neglect and maltreatment, when the perpetrator is known, a code from Y07, Perpetrator of maltreatment and neglect, should accompany any other assault codes.

See Section I.C.19. Adult and child abuse, neglect and other maltreatment

h. Unknown or Undetermined Intent Guideline

If the intent (accident, self-harm, assault) of the cause of an injury or other condition is unknown or unspecified, code the intent as accidental intent. All transport accident categories assume accidental intent.

1) Use of undetermined intent
External cause codes for events of undetermined intent are only for use if the documentation in the record specifies that the intent cannot be determined.

i. Sequelae (Late Effects) of External Cause Guidelines

1) Sequelae external cause codes
Sequela are reported using the external cause code with the 7th character "S" for sequela. These codes should be used with any report of a late effect or sequela resulting from a previous injury.
See Section I.B.10 Sequela (Late Effects)

2) Sequela external cause code with a related current injury
A sequela external cause code should never be used with a related current nature of injury code.

3) Use of sequela external cause codes for subsequent visits
Use a late effect external cause code for subsequent visits when a late effect of the initial injury is being treated. Do not use a late effect external cause code for subsequent visits for follow-up care (e.g., to assess healing, to receive rehabilitative therapy) of the injury when no late effect of the injury has been documented.

j. Terrorism Guidelines

1) Cause of injury identified by the Federal Government (FBI) as terrorism
When the cause of an injury is identified by the Federal Government (FBI) as terrorism, the first-listed external cause code should be a code from category Y38, Terrorism. The definition of terrorism employed by the FBI is found at the inclusion note at the beginning of category Y38. Use additional code for place of occurrence (Y92.-). More than one Y38 code may be assigned if the injury is the result of more than one mechanism of terrorism.

2) Cause of an injury is suspected to be the result of terrorism
When the cause of an injury is suspected to be the result of terrorism a code from category Y38 should not be assigned. Suspected cases should be classified as assault.

3) Code Y38.9, Terrorism, secondary effects
Assign code Y38.9, Terrorism, secondary effects, for conditions occurring subsequent to the terrorist event. This code should not be assigned for conditions that are due to the initial terrorist act.

It is acceptable to assign code Y38.9 with another code from Y38 if there is an injury due to the initial terrorist event and an injury that is a subsequent result of the terrorist event.

k. External Cause Status
A code from category Y99, External cause status, should be assigned whenever any other external cause code is assigned for an encounter, including an Activity code, except for the events noted below. Assign a code from category Y99, External cause status, to indicate the work status of the person at the time the event occurred. The status code indicates whether the event occurred during military activity, whether a non-military person was at work, whether an individual including a student or volunteer was involved in a non-work activity at the time of the causal event.

A code from Y99, External cause status, should be assigned, when applicable, with other external cause codes, such as transport accidents and falls. The external cause status codes are not applicable to poisonings, adverse effects, misadventures or late effects.

Do not assign a code from category Y99 if no other external cause codes (cause, activity) are applicable for the encounter.

An external cause status code is used only once, at the initial encounter for treatment. Only one code from Y99 should be recorded on a medical record.

Do not assign code Y99.9, Unspecified external cause status, if the status is not stated.

21. Chapter 21: Factors influencing health status and contact with health services (Z00-Z99)
Note: The chapter specific guidelines provide additional information about the use of Z codes for specified encounters.

a. Use of Z Codes in Any Healthcare Setting
Z codes are for use in any healthcare setting. Z codes may be used as either a first-listed (principal diagnosis code in the inpatient setting) or secondary code, depending on the circumstances of the encounter. Certain Z codes may only be used as first-listed or principal diagnosis.

b. Z Codes Indicate a Reason for an Encounter
Z codes are not procedure codes. A corresponding procedure code must accompany a Z code to describe any procedure performed.

c. Categories of Z Codes

1) Contact/Exposure
Category Z20 indicates contact with, and suspected exposure to, communicable diseases. These codes are for patients who do not show any sign or symptom of a disease but are suspected to have been exposed to it by close personal contact with an infected individual or are in an area where a disease is epidemic.

Category Z77, Other contact with and (suspected) exposures hazardous to health, indicates contact with and suspected exposures hazardous to health.

Contact/exposure codes may be used as a first-listed code to explain an encounter for testing, or, more commonly, as a secondary code to identify a potential risk.

2) Inoculations and vaccinations
Code Z23 is for encounters for inoculations and vaccinations. It indicates that a patient is being seen to receive a prophylactic inoculation against a disease. Procedure codes are required to identify the actual administration of the injection and the type(s) of immunizations given. Code Z23 may be used as a secondary code if the inoculation is given as a routine part of preventive health care, such as a well-baby visit.

3) Status
Status codes indicate that a patient is either a carrier of a disease or has the sequelae or residual of a past disease or condition. This includes such things as the presence of prosthetic or mechanical devices resulting from past treatment. A status code is informative, because the status may affect the course of treatment and its outcome. A status code is distinct from a history code. The history code indicates that the patient no longer has the condition.

A status code should not be used with a diagnosis code from one of the body system chapters, if the diagnosis code includes the information provided by the status code. For example, code Z94.1, Heart transplant status, should not be used with a code from subcategory T86.2, Complications of heart transplant. The status code does not provide additional information. The complication code indicates that the patient is a heart transplant patient.

For encounters for weaning from a mechanical ventilator, assign a code from subcategory J96.1, Chronic respiratory failure, followed by code Z99.11, Dependence on respirator [ventilator] status.

The status Z codes/categories are:

Z14	Genetic carrier

Genetic carrier status indicates that a person carries a gene, associated with a particular disease, which may be passed to offspring who may develop that disease. The person does not have the disease and is not at risk of developing the disease.

Z15	Genetic susceptibility to disease

Genetic susceptibility indicates that a person has a gene that increases the risk of that person developing the disease.

Codes from category Z15 should not be used as principal or first-listed codes. If the patient has the condition to which he/she is susceptible, and that condition is the reason for the encounter, the code for the current condition should be sequenced first. If the patient is being seen for follow-up after completed treatment for this condition, and the condition no longer exists, a follow-up code should be sequenced first, followed by the appropriate personal history and genetic susceptibility codes. If the purpose of the encounter is genetic counseling associated with procreative management, code Z31.5, Encounter for genetic counseling, should be assigned as the first-listed code, followed by a code from category Z15. Additional codes should be assigned for any applicable family or personal history.

Z16	Resistance to antimicrobial drugs

This code indicates that a patient has a condition that is resistant to antimicrobial drug treatment. Sequence the infection code first.

Z17	Estrogen receptor status
Z18	Retained foreign body fragments

Z19	Hormone sensitivity malignancy status
Z21	Asymptomatic HIV infection status

This code indicates that a patient has tested positive for HIV but has manifested no signs or symptoms of the disease.

Z22	Carrier of infectious disease

Carrier status indicates that a person harbors the specific organisms of a disease without manifest symptoms and is capable of transmitting the infection.

Z28.3	Underimmunization status
Z33.1	Pregnant state, incidental

This code is a secondary code only for use when the pregnancy is in no way complicating the reason for visit. Otherwise, a code from the obstetric chapter is required.

Z66	Do not resuscitate

This code may be used when it is documented by the provider that a patient is on do not resuscitate status at any time during the stay.

Z67	Blood type
Z68	Body mass index (BMI)

BMI codes should only be assigned when **there is an associated, reportable diagnosis (such as obesity).** Do not assign BMI codes during pregnancy.

See Section I.B.14 for BMI documentation by clinicians other than the patient's provider.

Z74.01	Bed confinement status
Z76.82	Awaiting organ transplant status
Z78	Other specified health status

Code Z78.1, Physical restraint status, may be used when it is documented by the provider that a patient has been put in restraints during the current encounter. Please note that this code should not be reported when it is documented by the provider that a patient is temporarily restrained during a procedure.

Z79	Long-term (current) drug therapy

Codes from this category indicate a patient's continuous use of a prescribed drug (including such things as aspirin therapy) for the long-term treatment of a condition or for prophylactic use. It is not for use for patients who have addictions to drugs. This subcategory is not for use of medications for detoxification or maintenance programs to prevent withdrawal symptoms in patients with drug dependence (e.g., methadone maintenance for opiate dependence). Assign the appropriate code for the drug dependence instead.

Assign a code from Z79 if the patient is receiving a medication for an extended period as a prophylactic measure (such as for the prevention of deep vein thrombosis) or as treatment of a chronic condition (such as arthritis) or a disease requiring a lengthy course of treatment (such as cancer). Do not assign a code from category Z79 for medication being administered for a brief period of time to treat an acute illness or injury (such as a course of antibiotics to treat acute bronchitis).

Z88	Allergy status to drugs, medicaments and biological substances

Except: Z88.9, Allergy status to unspecified drugs, medicaments and biological substances status

Z89	Acquired absence of limb
Z90	Acquired absence of organs, not elsewhere classified
Z91.0-	Allergy status, other than to drugs and biological substances
Z92.82	Status post administration of tPA (rtPA) in a different facility within the last 24 hours prior to admission to a current facility

Assign code Z92.82, Status post administration of tPA (rtPA) in a different facility within the last 24 hours prior to admission to current facility, as a secondary diagnosis when a patient is received by transfer into a facility and documentation indicates they were administered tissue plasminogen activator (tPA) within the last 24 hours prior to admission to the current facility.

This guideline applies even if the patient is still receiving the tPA at the time they are received into the current facility.

The appropriate code for the condition for which the tPA was administered (such as cerebrovascular disease or myocardial infarction) should be assigned first.

Code Z92.82 is only applicable to the receiving facility record and not to the transferring facility record.

Z93	Artificial opening status
Z94	Transplanted organ and tissue status
Z95	Presence of cardiac and vascular implants and grafts
Z96	Presence of other functional implants
Z97	Presence of other devices
Z98	Other postprocedural states

Assign code Z98.85, Transplanted organ removal status, to indicate that a transplanted organ has been previously removed. This code should not be assigned for the encounter in which the transplanted organ is removed. The complication necessitating removal of the transplant organ should be assigned for that encounter.

See section I.C19. for information on the coding of organ transplant complications.

Z99	Dependence on enabling machines and devices, not elsewhere classified

Note: Categories Z89-Z90 and Z93-Z99 are for use only if there are no complications or malfunctions of the organ or tissue replaced, the amputation site or the equipment on which the patient is dependent.

4) **History (of)**

There are two types of history Z codes, personal and family. Personal history codes explain a patient's past medical condition that no longer exists and is not receiving any treatment, but that has the potential for recurrence, and therefore may require continued monitoring.

Family history codes are for use when a patient has a family member(s) who has had a particular disease that causes the patient to be at higher risk of also contracting the disease.

Personal history codes may be used in conjunction with follow-up codes and family history codes may be used in conjunction with screening codes to explain the need for a test or procedure. History codes are also acceptable on any medical record regardless of the reason for visit. A history of an illness, even if no longer present, is important information that may alter the type of treatment ordered.

The history Z code categories are:

Z80	Family history of primary malignant neoplasm
Z81	Family history of mental and behavioral disorders
Z82	Family history of certain disabilities and chronic diseases (leading to disablement)
Z83	Family history of other specific disorders
Z84	Family history of other conditions
Z85	Personal history of malignant neoplasm
Z86	Personal history of certain other diseases
Z87	Personal history of other diseases and conditions
Z91.4-	Personal history of psychological trauma, not elsewhere classified
Z91.5	Personal history of self-harm
Z91.81	History of falling
Z91.82	Personal history of military deployment
Z92	Personal history of medical treatment

Except: Z92.0, Personal history of contraception

Except: Z92.82, Status post administration of tPA (rtPA) in a different facility within the last 24 hours prior to admission to a current facility

5) **Screening**

Screening is the testing for disease or disease precursors in seemingly well individuals so that early detection and treatment can be provided for those who test positive for the disease (e.g., screening mammogram).

The testing of a person to rule out or confirm a suspected diagnosis because the patient has some sign or symptom is a diagnostic examination, not a screening. In these cases, the sign or symptom is used to explain the reason for the test.

A screening code may be a first-listed code if the reason for the visit is specifically the screening exam. It may also be used as an additional code if the screening is done during an office visit for other health problems. A screening code is not necessary if the screening is inherent to a routine examination, such as a pap smear done during a routine pelvic examination.

Should a condition be discovered during the screening then the code for the condition may be assigned as an additional diagnosis.

The Z code indicates that a screening exam is planned. A procedure code is required to confirm that the screening was performed.

The screening Z codes/categories:

Z11 Encounter for screening for infectious and parasitic diseases

Z12 Encounter for screening for malignant neoplasms

Z13 Encounter for screening for other diseases and disorders
Except: Z13.9, Encounter for screening, unspecified

Z36 Encounter for antenatal screening for mother

6) Observation

There are three observation Z code categories. They are for use in very limited circumstances when a person is being observed for a suspected condition that is ruled out. The observation codes are not for use if an injury or illness or any signs or symptoms related to the suspected condition are present. In such cases the diagnosis/symptom code is used with the corresponding external cause code.

The observation codes are to be used as principal diagnosis only. The only exception to this is when the principal diagnosis is required to be a code from category Z38, Liveborn infants according to place of birth and type of delivery. Then a code from category Z05, Encounter for observation and evaluation of newborn for suspected diseases and conditions ruled out, is sequenced after the Z38 code. Additional codes may be used in addition to the observation code, but only if they are unrelated to the suspected condition being observed.

Codes from subcategory Z03.7, Encounter for suspected maternal and fetal conditions ruled out, may either be used as a first-listed or as an additional code assignment depending on the case. They are for use in very limited circumstances on a maternal record when an encounter is for a suspected maternal or fetal condition that is ruled out during that encounter (for example, a maternal or fetal condition may be suspected due to an abnormal test result). These codes should not be used when the condition is confirmed. In those cases, the confirmed condition should be coded. In addition, these codes are not for use if an illness or any signs or symptoms related to the suspected condition or problem are present. In such cases the diagnosis/symptom code is used.

Additional codes may be used in addition to the code from subcategory Z03.7, but only if they are unrelated to the suspected condition being evaluated.

Codes from subcategory Z03.7 may not be used for encounters for antenatal screening of mother. *See Section I.C.21. Screening.*

For encounters for suspected fetal condition that are inconclusive following testing and evaluation, assign the appropriate code from category O35, O36, O40 or O41.

The observation Z code categories:

Z03 Encounter for medical observation for suspected diseases and conditions ruled out

Z04 Encounter for examination and observation for other reasons
Except: Z04.9, Encounter for examination and observation for unspecified reason

Z05 Encounter for observation and evaluation of newborn for suspected diseases and conditions ruled out

7) Aftercare

Aftercare visit codes cover situations when the initial treatment of a disease has been performed and the patient requires continued care during the healing or recovery phase, or for the long-term consequences of the disease. The aftercare Z code should not be used if treatment is directed at a current, acute disease. The diagnosis code is to be used in these cases. Exceptions to this rule are codes Z51.0, Encounter for antineoplastic radiation therapy, and codes from subcategory Z51.1, Encounter for antineoplastic chemotherapy and immunotherapy. These codes are to be first-listed, followed by the diagnosis code when a patient's encounter is solely to receive radiation therapy, chemotherapy, or immunotherapy for the treatment of a neoplasm. If the reason for the encounter is more than one type of antineoplastic therapy, code Z51.0 and a code from subcategory Z51.1 may be assigned together, in which case one of these codes would be reported as a secondary diagnosis.

The aftercare Z codes should also not be used for aftercare for injuries. For aftercare of an injury, assign the acute injury code with the appropriate 7th character (for subsequent encounter).

The aftercare codes are generally first-listed to explain the specific reason for the encounter. An aftercare code may be used as an additional code when some type of aftercare is provided in addition to the reason for admission and no diagnosis code is applicable. An example of this would be the closure of a colostomy during an encounter for treatment of another condition.

Aftercare codes should be used in conjunction with other aftercare codes or diagnosis codes to provide better detail on the specifics of an aftercare encounter visit, unless otherwise directed by the classification. The sequencing of multiple aftercare codes depends on the circumstances of the encounter.

Certain aftercare Z code categories need a secondary diagnosis code to describe the resolving condition or sequelae. For others, the condition is included in the code title.

Additional Z code aftercare category terms include fitting and adjustment, and attention to artificial openings.

Status Z codes may be used with aftercare Z codes to indicate the nature of the aftercare. For example, code Z95.1, Presence of aortocoronary bypass graft, may be used with code Z48.812, Encounter for surgical aftercare following surgery on the circulatory system, to indicate the surgery for which the aftercare is being performed. A status code should not be used when the aftercare code indicates the type of status, such as using Z43.0, Encounter for attention to tracheostomy, with Z93.0, Tracheostomy status.

The aftercare Z category/codes:

Z42 Encounter for plastic and reconstructive surgery following medical procedure or healed injury

Z43 Encounter for attention to artificial openings

Z44 Encounter for fitting and adjustment of external prosthetic device

Z45 Encounter for adjustment and management of implanted device

Z46 Encounter for fitting and adjustment of other devices

Z47 Orthopedic aftercare

Z48 Encounter for other postprocedural aftercare

Z49 Encounter for care involving renal dialysis

Z51 Encounter for other aftercare and medical care

8) Follow-up

The follow-up codes are used to explain continuing surveillance following completed treatment of a disease, condition, or injury. They imply that the condition has been fully treated and no longer exists. They should not be confused with aftercare codes, or injury codes with a 7th character for subsequent encounter, that explain ongoing care of a healing condition or its sequelae. Follow-up codes may be used in conjunction with history codes to provide the full picture of the healed condition and its treatment. The follow-up code is sequenced first, followed by the history code.

A follow-up code may be used to explain multiple visits. Should a condition be found to have recurred on the follow-up visit, then the diagnosis code for the condition should be assigned in place of the follow-up code.

The follow-up Z code categories:

Z08   Encounter for follow-up examination after completed treatment for malignant neoplasm

Z09   Encounter for follow-up examination after completed treatment for conditions other than malignant neoplasm

Z39   Encounter for maternal postpartum care and examination

9) Donor

Codes in category Z52, Donors of organs and tissues, are used for living individuals who are donating blood or other body tissue. These codes are only for individuals donating for others, not for self-donations. They are not used to identify cadaveric donations.

10) Counseling

Counseling Z codes are used when a patient or family member receives assistance in the aftermath of an illness or injury, or when support is required in coping with family or social problems.

The counseling Z codes/categories:

Z30.0-   Encounter for general counseling and advice on contraception

Z31.5   Encounter for procreative genetic counseling

Z31.6-   Encounter for general counseling and advice on procreation

Z32.2   Encounter for childbirth instruction

Z32.3   Encounter for childcare instruction

Z69   Encounter for mental health services for victim and perpetrator of abuse

Z70   Counseling related to sexual attitude, behavior and orientation

Z71   Persons encountering health services for other counseling and medical advice, not elsewhere classified

Note: Code Z71.84, Encounter for health counseling related to travel, is to be used for health risk and safety counseling for future travel purposes.

Z76.81   Expectant mother prebirth pediatrician visit

11) Encounters for Obstetrical and Reproductive Services

See Section I.C.15. Pregnancy, Childbirth, and the Puerperium, for further instruction on the use of these codes.

Z codes for pregnancy are for use in those circumstances when none of the problems or complications included in the codes from the Obstetrics chapter exist (a routine prenatal visit or postpartum care). Codes in category Z34, Encounter for supervision of normal pregnancy, are always first-listed and are not to be used with any other code from the OB chapter.

Codes in category Z3A, Weeks of gestation, may be assigned to provide additional information about the pregnancy. Category Z3A codes should not be assigned for pregnancies with abortive outcomes (categories O00-O08), elective termination of pregnancy (code Z33.2), nor for postpartum conditions, as category Z3A is not applicable to these conditions. The date of the admission should be used to determine weeks of gestation for inpatient admissions that encompass more than one gestational week.

The outcome of delivery, category Z37, should be included on all maternal delivery records. It is always a secondary code. Codes in category Z37 should not be used on the newborn record.

Z codes for family planning (contraceptive) or procreative management and counseling should be included on an obstetric record either during the pregnancy or the postpartum stage, if applicable.

Z codes/categories for obstetrical and reproductive services:

Z30   Encounter for contraceptive management

Z31   Encounter for procreative management

Z32.2   Encounter for childbirth instruction

Z32.3   Encounter for childcare instruction

Z33   Pregnant state

Z34   Encounter for supervision of normal pregnancy

Z36   Encounter for antenatal screening of mother

Z3A   Weeks of gestation

Z37   Outcome of delivery

Z39   Encounter for maternal postpartum care and examination

Z76.81   Expectant mother prebirth pediatrician visit

12) Newborns and Infants

See Section I.C.16. Newborn (Perinatal) Guidelines, for further instruction on the use of these codes.

Newborn Z codes/categories:

Z76.1   Encounter for health supervision and care of foundling

Z00.1-   Encounter for routine child health examination

Z38   Liveborn infants according to place of birth and type of delivery

13) Routine and Administrative Examinations

The Z codes allow for the description of encounters for routine examinations, such as, a general check-up, or, examinations for administrative purposes, such as, a pre-employment physical. The codes are not to be used if the examination is for diagnosis of a suspected condition or for treatment purposes. In such cases the diagnosis code is used. During a routine exam, should a diagnosis or condition be discovered, it should be coded as an additional code. Pre-existing and chronic conditions and history codes may also be included as additional codes as long as the examination is for administrative purposes and not focused on any particular condition.

Some of the codes for routine health examinations distinguish between "with" and "without" abnormal findings. Code assignment depends on the information that is known at the time the encounter is being coded. For example, if no abnormal findings were found during the examination, but the encounter is being coded before test results are back, it is acceptable to assign the code for "without abnormal findings." When assigning a code for "with abnormal findings," additional code(s) should be assigned to identify the specific abnormal finding(s).

Pre-operative examination and pre-procedural laboratory examination Z codes are for use only in those situations when a patient is being cleared for a procedure or surgery and no treatment is given.

The Z codes/categories for routine and administrative examinations:

Z00   Encounter for general examination without complaint, suspected or reported diagnosis

Z01   Encounter for other special examination without complaint, suspected or reported diagnosis

Z02   Encounter for administrative examination

Except: Z02.9, Encounter for administrative examinations, unspecified

Z32.0-   Encounter for pregnancy test

14) Miscellaneous Z *Codes*

The miscellaneous Z codes capture a number of other health care encounters that do not fall into one of the other categories. Certain of these codes identify the reason for the encounter; others are for use as additional codes that provide useful information on circumstances that may affect a patient's care and treatment.

Prophylactic Organ Removal

For encounters specifically for prophylactic removal of an organ (such as prophylactic removal of breasts due to a genetic susceptibility to cancer or a family history of cancer), the principal or first-listed code should be a code from category Z40, Encounter for prophylactic surgery, followed by the appropriate codes to identify the associated risk factor (such as genetic susceptibility or family history).

If the patient has a malignancy of one site and is having prophylactic removal at another site to prevent either a new primary malignancy or metastatic disease, a code for the malignancy should also be assigned in addition to a code from subcategory Z40.0, Encounter for prophylactic surgery for risk factors related to malignant neoplasms. A Z40.0 code should not be assigned if the patient is having organ removal for treatment of a malignancy, such as the removal of the testes for the treatment of prostate cancer.

Miscellaneous Z codes/categories:

Z28 Immunization not carried out

Except: Z28.3, Underimmunization status

Z29 Encounter for other prophylactic measures

Z40 Encounter for prophylactic surgery

Z41 Encounter for procedures for purposes other than remedying health state

Except: Z41.9, Encounter for procedure for purposes other than remedying health state, unspecified

Z53 Persons encountering health services for specific procedures and treatment, not carried out

Z55 Problems related to education and literacy

Z56 Problems related to employment and unemployment

Z57 Occupational exposure to risk factors

Z58 Problems related to physical environment

Z59 Problems related to housing and economic circumstances

Z60 Problems related to social environment

Z62 Problems related to upbringing

Z63 Other problems related to primary support group, including family circumstances

Z64 Problems related to certain psychosocial circumstances

Z65 Problems related to other psychosocial circumstances

Z72 Problems related to lifestyle

Note: These codes should be assigned only when the documentation specifies that the patient has an associated problem

Z73 Problems related to life management difficulty

Z74 Problems related to care provider dependency

Except: Z74.01, Bed confinement status

Z75 Problems related to medical facilities and other health care

Z76.0 Encounter for issue of repeat prescription

Z76.3 Healthy person accompanying sick person

Z76.4 Other boarder to healthcare facility

Z76.5 Malingerer [conscious simulation]

Z91.1- Patient's noncompliance with medical treatment and regimen

Z91.83 Wandering in diseases classified elsewhere

Z91.84- Oral health risk factors

Z91.89 Other specified personal risk factors, not elsewhere classified

See Section I.B.14 for Z55-Z65 Persons with potential health hazards related to socioeconomic and psychosocial circumstances, documentation by clinicians other than the patient's provider.

15) **Nonspecific Z** *Codes*

Certain Z codes are so non-specific, or potentially redundant with other codes in the classification, that there can be little justification for their use in the inpatient setting. Their use in the outpatient setting should be limited to those instances when there is no further documentation to permit more precise coding. Otherwise, any sign or symptom or any other reason for visit that is captured in another code should be used.

Nonspecific Z codes/categories:

Z02.9 Encounter for administrative examinations, unspecified

Z04.9 Encounter for examination and observation for unspecified reason

Z13.9 Encounter for screening, unspecified

Z41.9 Encounter for procedure for purposes other than remedying health state, unspecified

Z52.9 Donor of unspecified organ or tissue

Z86.59 Personal history of other mental and behavioral disorders

Z88.9 Allergy status to unspecified drugs, medicaments and biological substances status

Z92.0 Personal history of contraception

16) **Z Codes That May Only be Principal/First-Listed Diagnosis**

The following Z codes/categories may only be reported as the principal/first-listed diagnosis, except when there are multiple encounters on the same day and the medical records for the encounters are combined:

Z00 Encounter for general examination without complaint, suspected or reported diagnosis

Except: Z00.6

Z01 Encounter for other special examination without complaint, suspected or reported diagnosis

Z02 Encounter for administrative examination

Z03 Encounter for medical observation for suspected diseases and conditions ruled out

Z04 Encounter for examination and observation for other reasons

Z33.2 Encounter for elective termination of pregnancy

Z31.81 Encounter for male factor infertility in female patient

Z31.83 Encounter for assisted reproductive fertility procedure cycle

Z31.84 Encounter for fertility preservation procedure

Z34 Encounter for supervision of normal pregnancy

Z39 Encounter for maternal postpartum care and examination

Z38 Liveborn infants according to place of birth and type of delivery

Z40 Encounter for prophylactic surgery

Z42 Encounter for plastic and reconstructive surgery following medical procedure or healed injury

Z51.0 Encounter for antineoplastic radiation therapy

Z51.1- Encounter for antineoplastic chemotherapy and immunotherapy

Z52 Donors of organs and tissues

Except: Z52.9, Donor of unspecified organ or tissue

Z76.1 Encounter for health supervision and care of foundling

Z76.2 Encounter for health supervision and care of other healthy infant and child

Z99.12 Encounter for respirator [ventilator] dependence during power failure

Section II. Selection of Principal Diagnosis

The circumstances of inpatient admission always govern the selection of principal diagnosis. The principal diagnosis is defined in the Uniform Hospital Discharge Data Set (UHDDS) as "that condition established after study to be chiefly responsible for occasioning the admission of the patient to the hospital for care."

The UHDDS definitions are used by hospitals to report inpatient data elements in a standardized manner. These data elements and their definitions can be found in the July 31, 1985, Federal Register (Vol. 50, No, 147), pp. 31038-40.

Since that time the application of the UHDDS definitions has been expanded to include all non-outpatient settings (acute care, short term, long term care and psychiatric hospitals; home health agencies; rehab facilities; nursing homes, etc). The UHDDS definitions also apply to hospice services (all levels of care).

In determining principal diagnosis, coding conventions in the ICD-10-CM, the Tabular List and Alphabetic Index take precedence over these official coding guidelines.

(See Section I.A., Conventions for the ICD-10-CM)

The importance of consistent, complete documentation in the medical record cannot be overemphasized. Without such documentation the application of all coding guidelines is a difficult, if not impossible, task.

A. **Codes for symptoms, signs, and ill-defined conditions**

Codes for symptoms, signs, and ill-defined conditions from Chapter 18 are not to be used as principal diagnosis when a related definitive diagnosis has been established.

B. **Two or more interrelated conditions, each potentially meeting the definition for principal diagnosis.**

When there are two or more interrelated conditions (such as diseases in the same ICD-10-CM chapter or manifestations characteristically associated with a certain disease) potentially meeting the definition of principal diagnosis, either condition may be sequenced first, unless the circumstances of the admission, the therapy provided, the Tabular List, or the Alphabetic Index indicate otherwise.

C. Two or more diagnoses that equally meet the definition for principal diagnosis

In the unusual instance when two or more diagnoses equally meet the criteria for principal diagnosis as determined by the circumstances of admission, diagnostic workup and/or therapy provided, and the Alphabetic Index, Tabular List, or another coding guidelines does not provide sequencing direction, any one of the diagnoses may be sequenced first.

D. Two or more comparative or contrasting conditions

In those rare instances when two or more contrasting or comparative diagnoses are documented as "either/or" (or similar terminology), they are coded as if the diagnoses were confirmed and the diagnoses are sequenced according to the circumstances of the admission. If no further determination can be made as to which diagnosis should be principal, either diagnosis may be sequenced first.

E. A symptom(s) followed by contrasting/comparative diagnoses

GUIDELINE HAS BEEN DELETED EFFECTIVE OCTOBER 1, 2014

F. Original treatment plan not carried out

Sequence as the principal diagnosis the condition, which after study occasioned the admission to the hospital, even though treatment may not have been carried out due to unforeseen circumstances.

G. Complications of surgery and other medical care

When the admission is for treatment of a complication resulting from surgery or other medical care, the complication code is sequenced as the principal diagnosis. If the complication is classified to the T80-T88 series and the code lacks the necessary specificity in describing the complication, an additional code for the specific complication should be assigned.

H. Uncertain Diagnosis

If the diagnosis documented at the time of discharge is qualified as "probable," "suspected," "likely," "questionable," "possible," or "still to be ruled out," **"compatible with," "consistent with,"** or other similar terms indicating uncertainty, code the condition as if it existed or was established. The bases for these guidelines are the diagnostic workup, arrangements for further workup or observation, and initial therapeutic approach that correspond most closely with the established diagnosis.

Note: This guideline is applicable only to inpatient admissions to short-term, acute, long-term care and psychiatric hospitals.

I. Admission from Observation Unit

1. Admission Following Medical Observation

When a patient is admitted to an observation unit for a medical condition, which either worsens or does not improve, and is subsequently admitted as an inpatient of the same hospital for this same medical condition, the principal diagnosis would be the medical condition which led to the hospital admission.

2. Admission Following Post-Operative Observation

When a patient is admitted to an observation unit to monitor a condition (or complication) that develops following outpatient surgery, and then is subsequently admitted as an inpatient of the same hospital, hospitals should apply the Uniform Hospital Discharge Data Set (UHDDS) definition of principal diagnosis as "that condition established after study to be chiefly responsible for occasioning the admission of the patient to the hospital for care."

J. Admission from Outpatient Surgery

When a patient receives surgery in the hospital's outpatient surgery department and is subsequently admitted for continuing inpatient care at the same hospital, the following guidelines should be followed in selecting the principal diagnosis for the inpatient admission:

- If the reason for the inpatient admission is a complication, assign the complication as the principal diagnosis.
- If no complication, or other condition, is documented as the reason for the inpatient admission, assign the reason for the outpatient surgery as the principal diagnosis.
- If the reason for the inpatient admission is another condition unrelated to the surgery, assign the unrelated condition as the principal diagnosis.

K. Admissions/Encounters for Rehabilitation

When the purpose for the admission/encounter is rehabilitation, sequence first the code for the condition for which the service is being performed. For example, for an admission/encounter for rehabilitation for right-sided dominant hemiplegia following a cerebrovascular infarction, report code I69.351, Hemiplegia and hemiparesis following cerebral infarction affecting right dominant side, as the first-listed or principal diagnosis.

If the condition for which the rehabilitation service is being provided is no longer present, report the appropriate aftercare code as the first-listed or principal diagnosis, unless the rehabilitation service is being provided following an injury. For rehabilitation services following active treatment of an injury, assign the injury code with the appropriate seventh character for subsequent encounter as the first-listed or principal diagnosis. For example, if a patient with severe degenerative osteoarthritis of the hip, underwent hip replacement and the current encounter/admission is for rehabilitation, report code Z47.1, Aftercare following joint replacement surgery, as the first-listed or principal diagnosis. If the patient requires rehabilitation post hip replacement for right intertrochanteric femur fracture, report code S72.141D, Displaced intertrochanteric fracture of right femur, subsequent encounter for closed fracture with routine healing, as the first-listed or principal diagnosis.

See Section I.C.21.c.7, Factors influencing health states and contact with health services, Aftercare.

See Section I.C.19.a for additional information about the use of 7th characters for injury codes.

Section III. Reporting Additional Diagnoses

GENERAL RULES FOR OTHER (ADDITIONAL) DIAGNOSES

For reporting purposes the definition for "other diagnoses" is interpreted as additional conditions that affect patient care in terms of requiring:

> clinical evaluation; or
> therapeutic treatment; or
> diagnostic procedures; or
> extended length of hospital stay; or
> increased nursing care and/or monitoring.

The UHDDS item #11-b defines Other Diagnoses as "all conditions that coexist at the time of admission, that develop subsequently, or that affect the treatment received and/or the length of stay. Diagnoses that relate to an earlier episode which have no bearing on the current hospital stay are to be excluded." UHDDS definitions apply to inpatients in acute care, short-term, long term care and psychiatric hospital setting. The UHDDS definitions are used by acute care short-term hospitals to report inpatient data elements in a standardized manner. These data elements and their definitions can be found in the July 31, 1985, Federal Register (Vol. 50, No, 147), pp. 31038-40.

Since that time the application of the UHDDS definitions has been expanded to include all non-outpatient settings (acute care, short term, long term care and psychiatric hospitals; home health agencies; rehab facilities; nursing homes, etc). The UHDDS definitions also apply to hospice services (all levels of care).

The following guidelines are to be applied in designating "other diagnoses" when neither the Alphabetic Index nor the Tabular List in ICD-10-CM provide direction. The listing of the diagnoses in the patient record is the responsibility of the attending provider.

A. Previous conditions

If the provider has included a diagnosis in the final diagnostic statement, such as the discharge summary or the face sheet, it should ordinarily be coded. Some providers include in the diagnostic statement resolved conditions or diagnoses and status-post procedures from previous admission that have no bearing on the current stay. Such conditions are not to be reported and are coded only if required by hospital policy.

However, history codes (categories Z80-Z87) may be used as secondary codes if the historical condition or family history has an impact on current care or influences treatment.

B. Abnormal findings

Abnormal findings (laboratory, x-ray, pathologic, and other diagnostic results) are not coded and reported unless the provider indicates their clinical significance. If the findings are outside the normal range and the attending provider has ordered other tests to evaluate the condition or prescribed treatment, it is appropriate to ask the provider whether the abnormal finding should be added.

Please note: This differs from the coding practices in the outpatient setting for coding encounters for diagnostic tests that have been interpreted by a provider.

C. Uncertain Diagnosis

If the diagnosis documented at the time of discharge is qualified as "probable," "suspected," "likely," "questionable," "possible," or "still to be ruled out," **"compatible with," "consistent with,"** or other similar terms indicating uncertainty, code the condition as if it existed or was established. The bases for these guidelines are the diagnostic workup, arrangements for further workup or observation, and initial therapeutic approach that correspond most closely with the established diagnosis.

Note: This guideline is applicable only to inpatient admissions to short-term, acute, long-term care and psychiatric hospitals.

Section IV. Diagnostic Coding and Reporting Guidelines for Outpatient Services

These coding guidelines for outpatient diagnoses have been approved for use by hospitals/ providers in coding and reporting hospital-based outpatient services and provider-based office visits. Guidelines in Section I, Conventions, general coding guidelines and chapter-specific guidelines, should also be applied for outpatient services and office visits.

Information about the use of certain abbreviations, punctuation, symbols, and other conventions used in the ICD-10-CM Tabular List (code numbers and titles), can be found in Section IA of these guidelines, under "Conventions Used in the Tabular List." Section I.B. contains general guidelines that apply to the entire classification. Section I.C. contains chapter-specific guidelines that correspond to the chapters as they are arranged in the classification. Information about the correct sequence to use in finding a code is also described in Section I.

The terms encounter and visit are often used interchangeably in describing outpatient service contacts and, therefore, appear together in these guidelines without distinguishing one from the other.

Though the conventions and general guidelines apply to all settings, coding guidelines for outpatient and provider reporting of diagnoses will vary in a number of instances from those for inpatient diagnoses, recognizing that:

The Uniform Hospital Discharge Data Set (UHDDS) definition of principal diagnosis does not apply to hospital-based outpatient services and provider-based office visits.

Coding guidelines for inconclusive diagnoses (probable, suspected, rule out, etc.) were developed for inpatient reporting and do not apply to outpatients.

A. Selection of first-listed condition
In the outpatient setting, the term first-listed diagnosis is used in lieu of principal diagnosis.

In determining the first-listed diagnosis the coding conventions of ICD-10-CM, as well as the general and disease specific guidelines take precedence over the outpatient guidelines.

Diagnoses often are not established at the time of the initial encounter/visit. It may take two or more visits before the diagnosis is confirmed.

The most critical rule involves beginning the search for the correct code assignment through the Alphabetic Index. Never begin searching initially in the Tabular List as this will lead to coding errors.

1. Outpatient Surgery
When a patient presents for outpatient surgery (same day surgery), code the reason for the surgery as the first-listed diagnosis (reason for the encounter), even if the surgery is not performed due to a contraindication.

2. Observation Stay
When a patient is admitted for observation for a medical condition, assign a code for the medical condition as the first-listed diagnosis.

When a patient presents for outpatient surgery and develops complications requiring admission to observation, code the reason for the surgery as the first reported diagnosis (reason for the encounter), followed by codes for the complications as secondary diagnoses.

B. Codes from A00.0 through T88.9, Z00-Z99
The appropriate code(s) from A00.0 through T88.9, Z00-Z99 must be used to identify diagnoses, symptoms, conditions, problems, complaints, or other reason(s) for the encounter/visit.

C. Accurate reporting of ICD-10-CM diagnosis codes
For accurate reporting of ICD-10-CM diagnosis codes, the documentation should describe the patient's condition, using terminology which includes specific diagnoses as well as symptoms, problems, or reasons for the encounter. There are ICD-10-CM codes to describe all of these.

D. Codes that describe symptoms and signs
Codes that describe symptoms and signs, as opposed to diagnoses, are acceptable for reporting purposes when a diagnosis has not been established (confirmed) by the provider. Chapter 18 of ICD-10-CM, Symptoms, Signs, and Abnormal Clinical and Laboratory Findings Not Elsewhere Classified (codes R00-R99) contain many, but not all codes for symptoms.

E. Encounters for circumstances other than a disease or injury
ICD-10-CM provides codes to deal with encounters for circumstances other than a disease or injury. The Factors Influencing Health Status and Contact with Health Services codes (Z00-Z99) are provided to deal with occasions when circumstances other than a disease or injury are recorded as diagnosis or problems.

See Section I.C.21. Factors influencing health status and contact with health services.

F. Level of Detail in Coding

1. ICD-10-CM codes with 3, 4, 5, 6 or 7 characters
ICD-10-CM is composed of codes with 3, 4, 5, 6 or 7 characters. Codes with three characters are included in ICD-10-CM as the heading of a category of codes that may be further subdivided by the use of fourth, fifth, sixth or seventh characters to provide greater specificity.

2. Use of full number of characters required for a code
A three-character code is to be used only if it is not further subdivided. A code is invalid if it has not been coded to the full number of characters required for that code, including the 7th character, if applicable.

G. ICD-10-CM code for the diagnosis, condition, problem, or other reason for encounter/visit
List first the ICD-10-CM code for the diagnosis, condition, problem, or other reason for encounter/visit shown in the medical record to be chiefly responsible for the services provided. List additional codes that describe any coexisting conditions. In some cases the first-listed diagnosis may be a symptom when a diagnosis has not been established (confirmed) by the **provider**.

H. Uncertain diagnosis
Do not code diagnoses documented as "probable", "suspected," "questionable," "rule out," **"compatible with," "consistent with,"** or "working diagnosis" or other similar terms indicating uncertainty. Rather, code the condition(s) to the highest degree of certainty for that encounter/visit, such as symptoms, signs, abnormal test results, or other reason for the visit.

Please note: This differs from the coding practices used by short-term, acute care, long-term care and psychiatric hospitals.

I. Chronic diseases
Chronic diseases treated on an ongoing basis may be coded and reported as many times as the patient receives treatment and care for the condition(s)

J. Code all documented conditions that coexist
Code all documented conditions that coexist at the time of the encounter/visit, and require or affect patient care treatment or management. Do not code conditions that were previously treated and no longer exist. However, history codes (categories Z80-Z87) may be used as secondary codes if the historical condition or family history has an impact on current care or influences treatment.

K. Patients receiving diagnostic services only
For patients receiving diagnostic services only during an encounter/visit, sequence first the diagnosis, condition, problem, or other reason for encounter/visit shown in the medical record to be chiefly responsible for the outpatient services provided during the encounter/visit. Codes for other diagnoses (e.g., chronic conditions) may be sequenced as additional diagnoses.

For encounters for routine laboratory/radiology testing in the absence of any signs, symptoms, or associated diagnosis, assign Z01.89, Encounter for other specified special examinations. If routine testing is performed during the same encounter as a test to evaluate a sign, symptom, or diagnosis, it is appropriate to assign both the Z code and the code describing the reason for the non-routine test.

For outpatient encounters for diagnostic tests that have been interpreted by a physician, and the final report is available at the time of coding, code any confirmed or definitive diagnosis(es) documented in the interpretation. Do not code related signs and symptoms as additional diagnoses.

Please note: This differs from the coding practice in the hospital inpatient setting regarding abnormal findings on test results.

L. Patients receiving therapeutic services only
For patients receiving therapeutic services only during an encounter/visit, sequence first the diagnosis, condition, problem, or other reason for encounter/visit shown in the medical record to be chiefly responsible for the outpatient services provided during the encounter/visit. Codes for other diagnoses (e.g., chronic conditions) may be sequenced as additional diagnoses.

The only exception to this rule is that when the primary reason for the admission/encounter is chemotherapy or radiation therapy, the appropriate Z code for the service is listed first, and the diagnosis or problem for which the service is being performed listed second.

M. Patients receiving preoperative evaluations only

For patients receiving preoperative evaluations only, sequence first a code from subcategory Z01.81, Encounter for pre-procedural examinations, to describe the pre-op consultations. Assign a code for the condition to describe the reason for the surgery as an additional diagnosis. Code also any findings related to the pre-op evaluation.

N. Ambulatory surgery

For ambulatory surgery, code the diagnosis for which the surgery was performed. If the postoperative diagnosis is known to be different from the preoperative diagnosis at the time the diagnosis is confirmed, select the postoperative diagnosis for coding, since it is the most definitive.

O. Routine outpatient prenatal visits

See Section I.C.15. Routine outpatient prenatal visits.

P. Encounters for general medical examinations with abnormal findings

The subcategories for encounters for general medical examinations, Z00.0- and encounter for routine child health examination, Z00.12-, provide codes for with and without abnormal findings. Should a general medical examination result in an abnormal finding, the code for general medical examination with abnormal finding should be assigned as the first-listed diagnosis. An examination with abnormal findings refers to a condition/diagnosis that is newly identified or a change in severity of a chronic condition (such as uncontrolled hypertension, or an acute exacerbation of chronic obstructive pulmonary disease) during a routine physical examination. A secondary code for the abnormal finding should also be coded.

Q. Encounters for routine health screenings

See Section I.C.21. Factors influencing health status and contact with health services, Screening

Appendix I. Present on Admission Reporting Guidelines

Introduction

These guidelines are to be used as a supplement to the *ICD-10-CM Official Guidelines for Coding and Reporting* to facilitate the assignment of the Present on Admission (POA) indicator for each diagnosis and external cause of injury code reported on claim forms (UB-04 and 837 Institutional).

These guidelines are not intended to replace any guidelines in the main body of the *ICD-10-CM Official Guidelines for Coding and Reporting.* The POA guidelines are not intended to provide guidance on when a condition should be coded, but rather, how to apply the POA indicator to the final set of diagnosis codes that have been assigned in accordance with Sections I, II, and III of the official coding guidelines. Subsequent to the assignment of the ICD-10-CM codes, the POA indicator should then be assigned to those conditions that have been coded.

As stated in the Introduction to the *ICD-10-CM Official Guidelines for Coding and Reporting,* a joint effort between the healthcare provider and the coder is essential to achieve complete and accurate documentation, code assignment, and reporting of diagnoses and procedures. The importance of consistent, complete documentation in the medical record cannot be overemphasized. Medical record documentation from any provider involved in the care and treatment of the patient may be used to support the determination of whether a condition was present on admission or not. In the context of the official coding guidelines, the term "provider" means a physician or any qualified healthcare practitioner who is legally accountable for establishing the patient's diagnosis.

These guidelines are not a substitute for the provider's clinical judgment as to the determination of whether a condition was/was not present on admission. The provider should be queried regarding issues related to the linking of signs/symptoms, timing of test results, and the timing of findings.

Please see the CDC website for the detailed list of ICD-10-CM codes that do not require the use of a POA indicator (https://www.cdc.gov/nchs/icd/icd10cm.htm). The codes and categories on this exempt list are for circumstances regarding the healthcare encounter or factors influencing health status that do not represent a current disease or injury or that describe conditions that are always present on admission.

General Reporting Requirements

All claims involving inpatient admissions to general acute care hospitals or other facilities that are subject to a law or regulation mandating collection of present on admission information.

Present on admission is defined as present at the time the order for inpatient admission occurs -- conditions that develop during an outpatient encounter, including emergency department, observation, or outpatient surgery, are considered as present on admission.

POA indicator is assigned to principal and secondary diagnoses (as defined in Section II of the Official Guidelines for Coding and Reporting) and the external cause of injury codes.

Issues related to inconsistent, missing, conflicting or unclear documentation must still be resolved by the provider.

If a condition would not be coded and reported based on UHDDS definitions and current official coding guidelines, then the POA indicator would not be reported.

Reporting Options

    Y - Yes

    N - No

    U - Unknown

    W – Clinically undetermined

    Unreported/Not used – (Exempt from POA reporting)

Reporting Definitions

    Y = present at the time of inpatient admission

    N = not present at the time of inpatient admission

    U = documentation is insufficient to determine if condition is present on admission

    W = provider is unable to clinically determine whether condition was present on admission or not

Timeframe for POA Identification and Documentation

There is no required timeframe as to when a provider (per the definition of "provider" used in these guidelines) must identify or document a condition to be present on admission. In some clinical situations, it may not be possible for a provider to make a definitive diagnosis (or a condition may not be recognized or reported by the patient) for a period of time after admission. In some cases it may be several days before the provider arrives at a definitive diagnosis. This does not mean that the condition was not present on admission. Determination of whether the condition was present on admission or not will be based on the applicable POA guideline as identified in this document, or on the provider's best clinical judgment.

If at the time of code assignment the documentation is unclear as to whether a condition was present on admission or not, it is appropriate to query the provider for clarification.

Assigning the POA Indicator

Condition is on the "Exempt from Reporting" list

    Leave the "present on admission" field blank if the condition is on the list of ICD-10-CM codes for which this field is not applicable. This is the only circumstance in which the field may be left blank.

POA Explicitly Documented

    Assign Y for any condition the provider explicitly documents as being present on admission.

    Assign N for any condition the provider explicitly documents as not present at the time of admission.

Conditions diagnosed prior to inpatient admission

    Assign "Y" for conditions that were diagnosed prior to admission (example: hypertension, diabetes mellitus, asthma)

Conditions diagnosed during the admission but clearly present before admission

    Assign "Y" for conditions diagnosed during the admission that were clearly present but not diagnosed until after admission occurred.

    Diagnoses subsequently confirmed after admission are considered present on admission if at the time of admission they are documented as suspected, possible, rule out, differential diagnosis, or constitute an underlying cause of a symptom that is present at the time of admission.

Condition develops during outpatient encounter prior to inpatient admission

    Assign Y for any condition that develops during an outpatient encounter prior to a written order for inpatient admission.

Documentation does not indicate whether condition was present on admission

    Assign "U" when the medical record documentation is unclear as to whether the condition was present on admission. "U" should not be routinely assigned and used only in very limited circumstances. Coders are encouraged to query the providers when the documentation is unclear.

Documentation states that it cannot be determined whether the condition was or was not present on admission

> Assign "W" when the medical record documentation indicates that it cannot be clinically determined whether or not the condition was present on admission.

Chronic condition with acute exacerbation during the admission

> If a single code identifies both the chronic condition and the acute exacerbation, see POA guidelines pertaining to codes that contain multiple clinical concepts.

> If a single code only identifies the chronic condition and not the acute exacerbation (e.g., acute exacerbation of chronic leukemia), assign "Y."

Conditions documented as possible, probable, suspected, or rule out at the time of discharge

> If the final diagnosis contains a possible, probable, suspected, or rule out diagnosis, and this diagnosis was based on signs, symptoms or clinical findings suspected at the time of inpatient admission, assign "Y."

> If the final diagnosis contains a possible, probable, suspected, or rule out diagnosis, and this diagnosis was based on signs, symptoms or clinical findings that were not present on admission, assign "N."

Conditions documented as impending or threatened at the time of discharge

> If the final diagnosis contains an impending or threatened diagnosis, and this diagnosis is based on symptoms or clinical findings that were present on admission, assign "Y".

> If the final diagnosis contains an impending or threatened diagnosis, and this diagnosis is based on symptoms or clinical findings that were not present on admission, assign "N".

Acute and Chronic Conditions

> Assign "Y" for acute conditions that are present at time of admission and N for acute conditions that are not present at time of admission.

> Assign "Y" for chronic conditions, even though the condition may not be diagnosed until after admission.

> If a single code identifies both an acute and chronic condition, see the POA guidelines for codes that contain multiple clinical concepts.

Codes That Contain Multiple Clinical Concepts

> Assign "N" if at least one of the clinical concepts included in the code was not present on admission (e.g., COPD with acute exacerbation and the exacerbation was not present on admission; gastric ulcer that does not start bleeding until after admission; asthma patient develops status asthmaticus after admission).

> Assign "Y" if all of the clinical concepts included in the code were present on admission (e.g., duodenal ulcer that perforates prior to admission).

> For infection codes that include the causal organism, assign "Y" if the infection (or signs of the infection) were present on admission, even though the culture results may not be known until after admission (e.g., patient is admitted with pneumonia and the provider documents Pseudomonas as the causal organism a few days later).

Same Diagnosis Code for Two or More Conditions

> When the same ICD-10-CM diagnosis code applies to two or more conditions during the same encounter (e.g. two separate conditions classified to the same ICD-10-CM diagnosis code):

> Assign "Y" if all conditions represented by the single ICD-10-CM code were present on admission (e.g. bilateral unspecified age-related cataracts).

> Assign "N" if any of the conditions represented by the single ICD-10-CM code was not present on admission (e.g. traumatic secondary and recurrent hemorrhage and seroma is assigned to a single code T79.2, but only one of the conditions was present on admission).

Obstetrical conditions

> Whether or not the patient delivers during the current hospitalization does not affect assignment of the POA indicator. The determining factor for POA assignment is whether the pregnancy complication or obstetrical condition described by the code was present at the time of admission or not.

> If the pregnancy complication or obstetrical condition was present on admission (e.g., patient admitted in preterm labor), assign "Y".

> If the pregnancy complication or obstetrical condition was not present on admission (e.g., 2nd degree laceration during delivery, postpartum hemorrhage that occurred during current hospitalization, fetal distress develops after admission), assign "N".

> If the obstetrical code includes more than one diagnosis and any of the diagnoses identified by the code were not present on admission assign "N". (e.g., Category O11, Pre-existing hypertension with pre-eclampsia)

Perinatal conditions

> Newborns are not considered to be admitted until after birth. Therefore, any condition present at birth or that developed in utero is considered present at admission and should be assigned "Y". This includes conditions that occur during delivery (e.g., injury during delivery, meconium aspiration, exposure to streptococcus B in the vaginal canal).

Congenital conditions and anomalies

> Assign "Y" for congenital conditions and anomalies except for categories Q00-Q99, Congenital anomalies, which are on the exempt list. Congenital conditions are always considered present on admission.

External cause of injury codes

> Assign "Y" for any external cause code representing an external cause of morbidity that occurred prior to inpatient admission (e.g., patient fell out of bed at home, patient fell out of bed in emergency room prior to admission)

> Assign "N" for any external cause code representing an external cause of morbidity that occurred during inpatient hospitalization (e.g., patient fell out of hospital bed during hospital stay, patient experienced an adverse reaction to a medication administered after inpatient admission).

A

arskog's syndrome Q87.19
bandonment — *see* Maltreatment
basia (-astasia) (hysterical) F44.4
bderhalden-Kaufmann-Lignac syndrome (cystinosis) E72.04
bdomen, abdominal — *see also* condition
  muscle deficiency syndrome Q79.4
  angina K55.1
    acute R10.0
bdominalgia — *see* Pain, abdominal
bduction contracture, hip or other joint — *see* Contraction, joint
berrant (congenital) — *see also* Malposition, congenital
  hepatic duct Q44.5
  endocrine gland NEC Q89.2
  breast Q83.8
  artery (peripheral) Q27.8
    basilar NEC Q28.1
    cerebral Q28.3
    coronary Q24.5
    digestive system Q27.8
    eye Q15.8
    lower limb Q27.8
    precerebral Q28.1
    pulmonary Q25.79
    renal Q27.2
    retina Q14.1
    specified site NEC Q27.8
    subclavian Q27.8
    upper limb Q27.8
    vertebral Q28.1
  adrenal gland Q89.1
  pancreas Q45.3
  parathyroid gland Q89.2
  pituitary gland Q89.2
  sebaceous glands, mucous membrane, mouth, congenital Q38.6
  spleen Q89.09
  subclavian artery Q27.8
  thymus (gland) Q89.2
  thyroid gland Q89.2
  vein (peripheral) NEC Q27.8
    cerebral Q28.3
    digestive system Q27.8
    lower limb Q27.8
    precerebral Q28.1
    specified site NEC Q27.8
    upper limb Q27.8
berration
  distantial — *see* Disturbance, visual
  mental F99
betalipoproteinemia E78.6
biotrophy R68.89
blatio, ablation
  retinae — *see* Detachment, retina
blepharia, ablepharon Q10.3
Abnormal, abnormality, abnormalities — *see also* Anomaly
  acid-base balance (mixed) E87.4
  albumin R77.0
  alphafetoprotein R77.2
  alveolar ridge K08.9
  anatomical relationship Q89.9
  apertures, congenital, diaphragm Q79.1
  auditory perception H93.29- ☑
    diplacusis — *see* Diplacusis
    hyperacusis — *see* Hyperacusis
    recruitment — *see* Recruitment, auditory
    threshold shift — *see* Shift, auditory threshold
  autosomes Q99.9
    fragile site Q95.5
  basal metabolic rate R94.8
  biosynthesis, testicular androgen E29.1
  bleeding time R79.1
  blood level (of)
    cobalt R79.0
    copper R79.0
    iron R79.0
    lithium R78.89
    magnesium R79.0

Abnormal, abnormality, abnormalities — *continued*
  blood level — *continued*
    mineral NEC R79.0
    zinc R79.0
  blood pressure
    elevated R03.0
    low reading (nonspecific) R03.1
  blood sugar R73.09
  blood-gas level R79.81
  bowel sounds R19.15
    absent R19.11
    hyperactive R19.12
  brain scan R94.02
  breathing R06.9
  caloric test R94.138
  cerebrospinal fluid R83.9
    cytology R83.6
    drug level R83.2
    enzyme level R83.0
    hormones R83.1
    immunology R83.4
    microbiology R83.5
    nonmedicinal level R83.3
    specified type NEC R83.8
  chemistry, blood R79.9
    C-reactive protein R79.82
    drugs — *see* Findings, abnormal, in blood
    gas level R79.81
    minerals R79.0
    pancytopenia D61.818
    PTT R79.1
    specified NEC R79.89
    toxins — *see* Findings, abnormal, in blood
  chest sounds (friction) (rales) R09.89
  chromosome, chromosomal Q99.9
    with more than three X chromosomes, female Q97.1
    analysis result R89.8
      bronchial washings R84.8
      cerebrospinal fluid R83.8
      cervix uteri NEC R87.89
      nasal secretions R84.8
      nipple discharge R89.8
      peritoneal fluid R85.89
      pleural fluid R84.8
      prostatic secretions R86.8
      saliva R85.89
      seminal fluid R86.8
      sputum R84.8
      synovial fluid R89.8
      throat scrapings R84.8
      vagina R87.89
      vulva R87.89
      wound secretions R89.8
    dicentric replacement Q93.2
    ring replacement Q93.2
    sex Q99.8
      female phenotype Q97.9
        specified NEC Q97.8
      male phenotype Q98.9
        specified NEC Q98.8
      structural male Q98.6
    specified NEC Q99.8
  clinical findings NEC R68.89
  coagulation D68.9
    newborn, transient P61.6
    profile R79.1
    time R79.1
  communication — *see* Fistula
  conjunctiva, vascular H11.41- ☑
  coronary artery Q24.5
  cortisol-binding globulin E27.8
  course, eustachian tube Q17.8
  creatinine clearance R94.4
  cytology
    anus R85.619
      atypical squamous cells cannot exclude high grade squamous intraepithelial lesion (ASC-H) R85.611
      atypical squamous cells of undetermined significance (ASC-US) R85.610
      cytologic evidence of malignancy R85.614

Abnormal, abnormality, abnormalities — *continued*
  cytology — *continued*
    anus — *continued*
      high grade squamous intraepithelial lesion (HGSIL) R85.613
      human papillomavirus (HPV) DNA test
        high risk positive R85.81
        low risk postive R85.82
      inadequate smear R85.615
      low grade squamous intraepithelial lesion (LGSIL) R85.612
      satisfactory anal smear but lacking transformation zone R85.616
      specified NEC R85.618
      unsatisfactory smear R85.615
    female genital organs — *see* Abnormal, Papanicolaou (smear)
  dark adaptation curve H53.61
  dentofacial NEC — *see* Anomaly, dentofacial
  development, developmental Q89.9
    central nervous system Q07.9
  diagnostic imaging
    abdomen, abdominal region NEC R93.5
    biliary tract R93.2
    bladder R93.41
    breast R92.8
    central nervous system NEC R90.89
    cerebrovascular NEC R90.89
    coronary circulation R93.1
    digestive tract NEC R93.3
    gastrointestinal (tract) R93.3
    genitourinary organs R93.89
    head R93.0
    heart R93.1
    intrathoracic organ NEC R93.89
    kidney R93.42- ☑
    limbs R93.6
    liver R93.2
    lung (field) R91.8
    musculoskeletal system NEC R93.7
    renal pelvis R93.41
    retroperitoneum R93.5
    site specified NEC R93.89
    skin and subcutaneous tissue R93.89
    skull R93.0
    testis R93.81- ☑
    ureter R93.41
    urinary organs specified NEC R93.49
  direction, teeth, fully erupted M26.30
  ear ossicles, acquired NEC H74.39- ☑
    ankylosis — *see* Ankylosis, ear ossicles
    discontinuity — *see* Discontinuity, ossicles, ear
    partial loss — *see* Loss, ossicles, ear (partial)
  Ebstein Q22.5
  echocardiogram R93.1
  echoencephalogram R90.81
  echogram — *see* Abnormal, diagnostic imaging
  electrocardiogram [ECG] [EKG] R94.31
  electroencephalogram [EEG] R94.01
  electrolyte — *see* Imbalance, electrolyte
  electromyogram [EMG] R94.131
  electro-oculogram [EOG] R94.110
  electrophysiological intracardiac studies R94.39
  electroretinogram [ERG] R94.111
  erythrocytes
    congenital, with perinatal jaundice D58.9
  feces (color) (contents) (mucus) R19.5
  finding — *see* Findings, abnormal, without diagnosis
  fluid
    amniotic — *see* Abnormal, specimen, specified
    cerebrospinal — *see* Abnormal, cerebrospinal fluid
    peritoneal — *see* Abnormal, specimen, digestive organs
    pleural — *see* Abnormal, specimen, respiratory organs
    synovial — *see* Abnormal, specimen, specified
    thorax (bronchial washings) (pleural fluid) — *see* Abnormal, specimen, respiratory organs
    vaginal — *see* Abnormal, specimen, female genital organs
  form
    teeth K00.2

Abnormal, abnormality, abnormalities —
continued
  form — *continued*
    uterus — *see* Anomaly, uterus
  function studies
    auditory R94.120
    bladder R94.8
    brain R94.09
    cardiovascular R94.30
    ear R94.128
    endocrine NEC R94.7
    eye NEC R94.118
    kidney R94.4
    liver R94.5
    nervous system
      central NEC R94.09
      peripheral NEC R94.138
    pancreas R94.8
    placenta R94.8
    pulmonary R94.2
    special senses NEC R94.128
    spleen R94.8
    thyroid R94.6
    vestibular R94.121
  gait — *see* Gait
    hysterical F44.4
  gastrin secretion E16.4
  globulin R77.1
    cortisol-binding E27.8
    thyroid-binding E07.89
  glomerular, minor — *see also* N00-N07 with fourth
      character .0 N05.0
  glucagon secretion E16.3
  glucose tolerance (test) (non-fasting) R73.09
  gravitational (G) forces or states (effect of) T75.81 ☑
  hair (color) (shaft) L67.9
    specified NEC L67.8
  hard tissue formation in pulp (dental) K04.3
  head movement R25.0
  heart
    rate R00.9
      specified NEC R00.8
    shadow R93.1
    sounds NEC R01.2
  hemoglobin (disease) — *see also* Disease, hemoglobin
      D58.2
    trait — *see* Trait, hemoglobin, abnormal
  histology NEC R89.7
  immunological findings R89.4
    in serum R76.9
      specified NEC R76.8
  increase in appetite R63.2
  involuntary movement — *see* Abnormal, movement,
      involuntary
  jaw closure M26.51
  karyotype R89.8
  kidney function test R94.4
  knee jerk R29.2
  leukocyte (cell) (differential) NEC D72.9
  liver function test R94.5
  loss of
    height R29.890
    weight R63.4
  mammogram NEC R92.8
    calcification (calculus) R92.1
    microcalcification R92.0
  Mantoux test R76.11
  movement (disorder) — *see also* Disorder, movement
    head R25.0
    involuntary R25.9
      fasciculation R25.3
      of head R25.0
      spasm R25.2
      specified type NEC R25.8
      tremor R25.1
  myoglobin (Aberdeen) (Annapolis) R89.7
  neonatal screening P09
  oculomotor study R94.113
  palmar creases Q82.8
  Papanicolaou (smear)
    anus R85.619
      atypical squamous cells cannot exclude high
          grade squamous intraepithelial lesion
          (ASC-H) R85.611
      atypical squamous cells of undetermined signif-
          icance (ASC-US) R85.610
      cytologic evidence of malignancy R85.614

Abnormal, abnormality, abnormalities —
continued
  Papanicolaou — *continued*
    anus — *continued*
      high grade squamous intraepithelial lesion
          (HGSIL) R85.613
      human papillomavirus (HPV) DNA test
        high risk positive R85.81
        low risk postive R85.82
      inadequate smear R85.615
      low grade squamous intraepithelial lesion (LGSIL)
          R85.612
      satisfactory anal smear but lacking transforma-
          tion zone R85.616
      specified NEC R85.618
      unsatisfactory smear R85.615
    bronchial washings R84.6
    cerebrospinal fluid R83.6
    cervix R87.619
      atypical squamous cells cannot exclude high
          grade squamous intraepithelial lesion
          (ASC-H) R87.611
      atypical squamous cells of undetermined signif-
          icance (ASC-US) R87.610
      cytologic evidence of malignancy R87.614
      high grade squamous intraepithelial lesion
          (HGSIL) R87.613
      inadequate smear R87.615
      low grade squamous intraepithelial lesion (LGSIL)
          R87.612
      non-atypical endometrial cells R87.618
      satisfactory cervical smear but lacking transfor-
          mation zone R87.616
      specified NEC R87.618
      thin preparaton R87.619
      unsatisfactory smear R87.615
    nasal secretions R84.6
    nipple discharge R89.6
    peritoneal fluid R85.69
    pleural fluid R84.6
    prostatic secretions R86.6
    saliva R85.69
    seminal fluid R86.6
    sites NEC R89.6
    sputum R84.6
    synovial fluid R89.6
    throat scrapings R84.6
    vagina R87.629
      atypical squamous cells cannot exclude high
          grade squamous intraepithelial lesion
          (ASC-H) R87.621
      atypical squamous cells of undetermined signif-
          icance (ASC-US) R87.620
      cytologic evidence of malignancy R87.624
      high grade squamous intraepithelial lesion
          (HGSIL) R87.623
      inadequate smear R87.625
      low grade squamous intraepithelial lesion (LGSIL)
          R87.622
      specified NEC R87.628
      thin preparation R87.629
      unsatisfactory smear R87.625
    vulva R87.69
    wound secretions R89.6
  partial thromboplastin time (PTT) R79.1
  pelvis (bony) — *see* Deformity, pelvis
  percussion, chest (tympany) R09.89
  periods (grossly) — *see* Menstruation
  phonocardiogram R94.39
  plantar reflex R29.2
  plasma
    protein R77.9
      specified NEC R77.8
    viscosity R70.1
  pleural (folds) Q34.0
  posture R29.3
  product of conception O02.9
    specified type NEC O02.89
  prothrombin time (PT) R79.1
  pulmonary
    artery, congenital Q25.79
    function, newborn P28.89
    test results R94.2
  pulsations in neck R00.2
  pupillary H21.56- ☑
    function (reaction) (reflex) — *see* Anomaly, pupil,
        function
  radiological examination — *see* Abnormal, diagnostic
      imaging

Abnormal, abnormality, abnormalities —
continued
  red blood cell(s) (morphology) (volume) R71.8
  reflex — *see* Reflex
  renal function test R94.4
  response to nerve stimulation R94.130
  retinal correspondence H53.31
  retinal function study R94.111
  rhythm, heart — *see also* Arrhythmia
  saliva — *see* Abnormal, specimen, digestive organs
  scan
    kidney R94.4
    liver R93.2
    thyroid R94.6
  secretion
    gastrin E16.4
    glucagon E16.3
  semen, seminal fluid — *see* Abnormal, specimen, male
      genital organs
  serum level (of)
    acid phosphatase R74.8
    alkaline phosphatase R74.8
    amylase R74.8
    enzymes R74.9
      specified NEC R74.8
    lipase R74.8
    triacylglycerol lipase R74.8
  shape
    gravid uterus — *see* Anomaly, uterus
  sinus venosus Q21.1
  size, tooth, teeth K00.2
  spacing, tooth, teeth, fully erupted M26.30
  specimen
    digestive organs (peritoneal fluid) (saliva) R85.9
      cytology R85.69
      drug level R85.2
      enzyme level R85.0
      histology R85.7
      hormones R85.1
      immunology R85.4
      microbiology R85.5
      nonmedicinal level R85.3
      specified type NEC R85.89
    female genital organs (secretions) (smears) R87.9
      cytology R87.69
        cervix R87.619
          human papillomavirus (HPV) DNA test
            high risk positive R87.810
            low risk positive R87.820
          inadequate (unsatisfactory) smear
              R87.615
          non-atypical endometrial cells R87.618
          specified NEC R87.618
        vagina R87.629
          human papillomavirus (HPV) DNA test
            high risk positive R87.811
            low risk positive R87.821
          inadequate (unsatisfactory) smear
              R87.625
        vulva R87.69
      drug level R87.2
      enzyme level R87.0
      histological R87.7
      hormones R87.1
      immunology R87.4
      microbiology R87.5
      nonmedicinal level R87.3
      specified type NEC R87.89
    male genital organs (prostatic secretions) (semen)
        R86.9
      cytology R86.6
      drug level R86.2
      enzyme level R86.0
      histological R86.7
      hormones R86.1
      immunology R86.4
      microbiology R86.5
      nonmedicinal level R86.3
      specified type NEC R86.8
    nipple discharge — *see* Abnormal, specimen, spec-
        ified
    respiratory organs (bronchial washings) (nasal secre-
        tions) (pleural fluid) (sputum) R84.9
      cytology R84.6
      drug level R84.2
      enzyme level R84.0
      histology R84.7
      hormones R84.1
      immunology R84.4

2

☑ **Additional Character Required** — **Refer to the Tabular List for Character Selection**   ▽ **Subterms under main terms may continue to next column or page**

bnormal, abnormality, abnormalities — *continued*
  specimen — *continued*
    respiratory organs — *continued*
      microbiology R84.5
      nonmedicinal level R84.3
      specified type NEC R84.8
    specified organ, system and tissue NOS R89.9
      cytology R89.6
      drug level R89.2
      enzyme level R89.0
      histology R89.7
      hormones R89.1
      immunology R89.4
      microbiology R89.5
      nonmedicinal level R89.3
      specified type NEC R89.8
    synovial fluid — *see* Abnormal, specimen, specified
    thorax (bronchial washings) (pleural fluids) — *see* Abnormal, specimen, respiratory organs
    vagina (secretion) (smear) R87.629
    vulva (secretion) (smear) R87.69
    wound secretion — *see* Abnormal, specimen, specified
  spermatozoa — *see* Abnormal, specimen, male genital organs
  sputum (amount) (color) (odor) R09.3
  stool (color) (contents) (mucus) R19.5
    bloody K92.1
    guaiac positive R19.5
  synchondrosis Q78.8
  thermography — *see also* Abnormal, diagnostic imaging R93.89
  thyroid-binding globulin E07.89
  tooth, teeth (form) (size) K00.2
  toxicology (findings) R78.9
  transport protein E88.09
  tumor marker NEC R97.8
  ultrasound results — *see* Abnormal, diagnostic imaging
  umbilical cord complicating delivery O69.9 ☑
  urination NEC R39.198
  urine (constituents) R82.90
    bile R82.2
    cytological examination R82.89
    drugs R82.5
    fat R82.0
    glucose R81
    heavy metals R82.6
    hemoglobin R82.3
    histological examination R82.89
    ketones R82.4
    microbiological examination (culture) R82.79
    myoglobin R82.1
    positive culture R82.79
    protein — *see* Proteinuria
    specified substance NEC R82.998
      chromoabnormality NEC R82.91
    substances nonmedical R82.6
  uterine hemorrhage — *see* Hemorrhage, uterus
  vectorcardiogram R94.39
  visually evoked potential (VEP) R94.112
  white blood cells D72.9
    specified NEC D72.89
  X-ray examination — *see* Abnormal, diagnostic imaging

Abnormity (any organ or part) — *see* Anomaly

Abocclusion M26.29

Abo
  hemolytic disease (newborn) P55.1
  incompatibility reaction ABO — *see* Complication(s), transfusion, incompatibility reaction, ABO

Abolition, language R48.8

Aborter, habitual or recurrent — *see* Loss (of), pregnancy, recurrent

Abortion (complete) (spontaneous) O03.9
  with
    retained products of conception — *see* Abortion, incomplete
  attempted (elective) (failed) O07.4
    complicated by O07.30
      afibrinogenemia O07.1
      cardiac arrest O07.36
      chemical damage of pelvic organ(s) O07.34
      circulatory collapse O07.31
      cystitis O07.38
      defibrination syndrome O07.1
      electrolyte imbalance O07.33
      embolism (air) (amniotic fluid) (blood clot) (fat) (pulmonary) (septic) (soap) O07.2
      endometritis O07.0

Abortion — *continued*
  attempted — *continued*
    complicated by — *continued*
      genital tract and pelvic infection O07.0
      hemolysis O07.1
      hemorrhage (delayed) (excessive) O07.1
      infection
        genital tract or pelvic O07.0
        urinary tract tract O07.38
      intravascular coagulation O07.1
      laceration of pelvic organ(s) O07.34
      metabolic disorder O07.33
      oliguria O07.32
      oophoritis O07.0
      parametritis O07.0
      pelvic peritonitis O07.0
      perforation of pelvic organ(s) O07.34
      renal failure or shutdown O07.32
      salpingitis or salpingo-oophoritis O07.0
      sepsis O07.37
      shock O07.31
      specified condition NEC O07.39
      tubular necrosis (renal) O07.32
      uremia O07.32
      urinary tract infection O07.38
      venous complication NEC O07.35
        embolism (air) (amniotic fluid) (blood clot) (fat) (pulmonary) (septic) (soap) O07.2
  complicated (by) (following) O03.80
    afibrinogenemia O03.6
    cardiac arrest O03.86
    chemical damage of pelvic organ(s) O03.84
    circulatory collapse O03.81
    cystitis O03.88
    defibrination syndrome O03.6
    electrolyte imbalance O03.83
    embolism (air) (amniotic fluid) (blood clot) (fat) (pulmonary) (septic) (soap) O03.7
    endometritis O03.5
    genital tract and pelvic infection O03.5
    hemolysis O03.6
    hemorrhage (delayed) (excessive) O03.6
    infection
      genital tract or pelvic O03.5
      urinary tract O03.88
    intravascular coagulation O03.6
    laceration of pelvic organ(s) O03.84
    metabolic disorder O03.83
    oliguria O03.82
    oophoritis O03.5
    parametritis O03.5
    pelvic peritonitis O03.5
    perforation of pelvic organ(s) O03.84
    renal failure or shutdown O03.82
    salpingitis or salpingo-oophoritis O03.5
    sepsis O03.87
    shock O03.81
    specified condition NEC O03.89
    tubular necrosis (renal) O03.82
    uremia O03.82
    urinary tract infection O03.88
    venous complication NEC O03.85
      embolism (air) (amniotic fluid) (blood clot) (fat) (pulmonary) (septic) (soap) O03.7
  failed — *see* Abortion, attempted
  habitual or recurrent N96
    with current abortion — *see* categories O03-O04
    without current pregnancy N96
    care in current pregnancy O26.2- ☑
  incomplete (spontaneous) O03.4
    complicated (by) (following) O03.30
      afibrinogenemia O03.1
      cardiac arrest O03.36
      chemical damage of pelvic organ(s) O03.34
      circulatory collapse O03.31
      cystitis O03.38
      defibrination syndrome O03.1
      electrolyte imbalance O03.33
      embolism (air) (amniotic fluid) (blood clot) (fat) (pulmonary) (septic) (soap) O03.2
      endometritis O03.0
      genital tract and pelvic infection O03.0
      hemolysis O03.1
      hemorrhage (delayed) (excessive) O03.1
      infection
        genital tract or pelvic O03.0
        urinary tract O03.38
      intravascular coagulation O03.1
      laceration of pelvic organ(s) O03.34

Abortion — *continued*
  incomplete — *continued*
    complicated — *continued*
      metabolic disorder O03.33
      oliguria O03.32
      oophoritis O03.0
      parametritis O03.0
      pelvic peritonitis O03.0
      perforation of pelvic organ(s) O03.34
      renal failure or shutdown O03.32
      salpingitis or salpingo-oophoritis O03.0
      sepsis O03.37
      shock O03.31
      specified condition NEC O03.39
      tubular necrosis (renal) O03.32
      uremia O03.32
      urinary infection O03.38
      venous complication NEC O03.35
        embolism (air) (amniotic fluid) (blood clot) (fat) (pulmonary) (septic) (soap) O03.2
  induced (encounter for) Z33.2
    complicated by O04.80
      afibrinogenemia O04.6
      cardiac arrest O04.86
      chemical damage of pelvic organ(s) O04.84
      circulatory collapse O04.81
      cystitis O04.88
      defibrination syndrome O04.6
      electrolyte imbalance O04.83
      embolism (air) (amniotic fluid) (blood clot) (fat) (pulmonary) (septic) (soap) O04.7
      endometritis O04.5
      genital tract and pelvic infection O04.5
      hemolysis O04.6
      hemorrhage (delayed) (excessive) O04.6
      infection
        genital tract or pelvic O04.5
        urinary tract O04.88
      intravascular coagulation O04.6
      laceration of pelvic organ(s) O04.84
      metabolic disorder O04.83
      oliguria O04.82
      oophoritis O04.5
      parametritis O04.5
      pelvic peritonitis O04.5
      perforation of pelvic organ(s) O04.84
      renal failure or shutdown O04.82
      salpingitis or salpingo-oophoritis O04.5
      sepsis O04.87
      shock O04.81
      specified condition NEC O04.89
      tubular necrosis (renal) O04.82
      uremia O04.82
      urinary tract infection O04.88
      venous complication NEC O04.85
        embolism (air) (amniotic fluid) (blood clot) (fat) (pulmonary) (septic) (soap) O04.7
  missed O02.1
  spontaneous — *see* Abortion (complete) (spontaneous)
    threatened O20.0
  threatened (spontaneous) O20.0
  tubal O00.10- ☑
    with intrauterine pregnancy O00.11- ☑

Abortus fever A23.1

Aboulomania F60.7

Abrami's disease D59.8

Abramov-Fiedler myocarditis (acute isolated myocarditis) I40.1

Abrasion T14.8 ☑
  abdomen, abdominal (wall) S30.811 ☑
  alveolar process S00.512 ☑
  ankle S90.51- ☑
  antecubital space — *see* Abrasion, elbow
  anus S30.817 ☑
  arm (upper) S40.81- ☑
  auditory canal — *see* Abrasion, ear
  auricle — *see* Abrasion, ear
  axilla — *see* Abrasion, arm
  back, lower S30.810 ☑
  breast S20.11- ☑
  brow S00.81 ☑
  buttock S30.810 ☑
  calf — *see* Abrasion, leg
  canthus — *see* Abrasion, eyelid
  cheek S00.81 ☑
    internal S00.512 ☑
  chest wall — *see* Abrasion, thorax
  chin S00.81 ☑

Abrasion — *continued*
- clitoris S30.814 ☑
- cornea S05.0- ☑
- costal region — *see* Abrasion, thorax
- dental K03.1
- digit(s)
  - foot — *see* Abrasion, toe
  - hand — *see* Abrasion, finger
- ear S00.41- ☑
- elbow S50.31- ☑
- epididymis S30.813 ☑
- epigastric region S30.811 ☑
- epiglottis S10.11 ☑
- esophagus (thoracic) S27.818 ☑
  - cervical S10.11 ☑
- eyebrow — *see* Abrasion, eyelid
- eyelid S00.21- ☑
- face S00.81 ☑
- finger(s) S60.41- ☑
  - index S60.41- ☑
  - little S60.41- ☑
  - middle S60.41- ☑
  - ring S60.41- ☑
- flank S30.811 ☑
- foot (except toe(s) alone) S90.81- ☑
  - toe — *see* Abrasion, toe
- forearm S50.81- ☑
  - elbow only — *see* Abrasion, elbow
- forehead S00.81 ☑
- genital organs, external
  - female S30.816 ☑
  - male S30.815 ☑
- groin S30.811 ☑
- gum S00.512 ☑
- hand S60.51- ☑
- head S00.91 ☑
  - ear — *see* Abrasion, ear
  - eyelid — *see* Abrasion, eyelid
  - lip S00.511 ☑
  - nose S00.31 ☑
  - oral cavity S00.512 ☑
  - scalp S00.01 ☑
  - specified site NEC S00.81 ☑
- heel — *see* Abrasion, foot
- hip S70.21- ☑
- inguinal region S30.811 ☑
- interscapular region S20.419 ☑
- jaw S00.81 ☑
- knee S80.21- ☑
- labium (majus) (minus) S30.814 ☑
- larynx S10.11 ☑
- leg (lower) S80.81- ☑
  - knee — *see* Abrasion, knee
  - upper — *see* Abrasion, thigh
- lip S00.511 ☑
- lower back S30.810 ☑
- lumbar region S30.810 ☑
- malar region S00.81 ☑
- mammary — *see* Abrasion, breast
- mastoid region S00.81 ☑
- mouth S00.512 ☑
- nail
  - finger — *see* Abrasion, finger
  - toe — *see* Abrasion, toe
- nape S10.81 ☑
- nasal S00.31 ☑
- neck S10.91 ☑
  - specified site NEC S10.81 ☑
  - throat S10.11 ☑
- nose S00.31 ☑
- occipital region S00.01 ☑
- oral cavity S00.512 ☑
- orbital region — *see* Abrasion, eyelid
- palate S00.512 ☑
- palm — *see* Abrasion, hand
- parietal region S00.01 ☑
- pelvis S30.810 ☑
- penis S30.812 ☑
- perineum
  - female S30.814 ☑
  - male S30.810 ☑
- periocular area — *see* Abrasion, eyelid
- phalanges
  - finger — *see* Abrasion, finger
  - toe — *see* Abrasion, toe
- pharynx S10.11 ☑

Abrasion — *continued*
- pinna — *see* Abrasion, ear
- popliteal space — *see* Abrasion, knee
- prepuce S30.812 ☑
- pubic region S30.810 ☑
- pudendum
  - female S30.816 ☑
  - male S30.815 ☑
- sacral region S30.810 ☑
- scalp S00.01 ☑
- scapular region — *see* Abrasion, shoulder
- scrotum S30.813 ☑
- shin — *see* Abrasion, leg
- shoulder S40.21- ☑
- skin NEC T14.8 ☑
- sternal region S20.319 ☑
- submaxillary region S00.81 ☑
- submental region S00.81 ☑
- subungual
  - finger(s) — *see* Abrasion, finger
  - toe(s) — *see* Abrasion, toe
- supraclavicular fossa S10.81 ☑
- supraorbital S00.81 ☑
- temple S00.81 ☑
- temporal region S00.81 ☑
- testis S30.813 ☑
- thigh S70.31- ☑
- thorax, thoracic (wall) S20.91 ☑
  - back S20.41- ☑
  - front S20.31- ☑
- throat S10.11 ☑
- thumb S60.31- ☑
- toe(s) (lesser) S90.416 ☑
  - great S90.41- ☑
- tongue S00.512 ☑
- tooth, teeth (dentifrice) (habitual) (hard tissues) (occupational) (ritual) (traditional) K03.1
- trachea S10.11 ☑
- tunica vaginalis S30.813 ☑
- tympanum, tympanic membrane — *see* Abrasion, ear
- uvula S00.512 ☑
- vagina S30.814 ☑
- vocal cords S10.11 ☑
- vulva S30.814 ☑
- wrist S60.81- ☑

Abrism — *see* Poisoning, food, noxious, plant

Abruptio placentae O45.9- ☑
- with
  - afibrinogenemia O45.01- ☑
  - coagulation defect O45.00- ☑
    - specified NEC O45.09- ☑
  - disseminated intravascular coagulation O45.02- ☑
  - hypofibrinogenemia O45.01- ☑
- specified NEC O45.8- ☑

Abruption, placenta — *see* Abruptio placentae

Abscess (connective tissue) (embolic) (fistulous) (infective) (metastatic) (multiple) (pernicious) (pyogenic) (septic) L02.91
- with
  - diverticular disease (intestine) K57.80
    - with bleeding K57.81
    - large intestine K57.20
      - with
        - bleeding K57.21
        - small intestine K57.40
          - with bleeding K57.41
    - small intestine K57.00
      - with
        - bleeding K57.01
        - large intestine K57.40
          - with bleeding K57.41
  - lymphangitis — *code by* site under Abscess
- abdomen, abdominal
  - cavity K65.1
  - wall L02.211
- abdominopelvic K65.1
- accessory sinus — *see* Sinusitis
- adrenal (capsule) (gland) E27.8
- alveolar K04.7
  - with sinus K04.6
- amebic A06.4
  - brain (and liver or lung abscess) A06.6
  - genitourinary tract A06.82
  - liver (without mention of brain or lung abscess) A06.4
  - lung (and liver) (without mention of brain abscess) A06.5

Abscess — *continued*
- amebic — *continued*
  - specified site NEC A06.89
  - spleen A06.89
- anerobic A48.0
- ankle — *see* Abscess, lower limb
- anorectal K61.2
- antecubital space — *see* Abscess, upper limb
- antrum (chronic) (Highmore) — *see* Sinusitis, maxillar
- anus K61.0
- apical (tooth) K04.7
  - with sinus (alveolar) K04.6
- appendix K35.33
- areola (acute) (chronic) (nonpuerperal) N61.1
  - puerperal, postpartum or gestational — *see* Infection, nipple
- arm (any part) — *see* Abscess, upper limb
- artery (wall) I77.89
- atheromatous I77.2
- auricle, ear — *see* Abscess, ear, external
- axilla (region) L02.41- ☑
  - lymph gland or node L04.2
- back (any part, except buttock) L02.212
- Bartholin's gland N75.1
  - with
    - abortion — *see* Abortion, by type complicated by, sepsis
    - ectopic or molar pregnancy O08.0
  - following ectopic or molar pregnancy O08.0
- Bezold's — *see* Mastoiditis, acute
- bilharziasis B65.1
- bladder (wall) — *see* Cystitis, specified type NEC
- bone (subperiosteal) — *see also* Osteomyelitis, specified type NEC
  - accessory sinus (chronic) — *see* Sinusitis
  - chronic or old — *see* Osteomyelitis, chronic
  - jaw (lower) (upper) M27.2
  - mastoid — *see* Mastoiditis, acute, subperiosteal
  - petrous — *see* Petrositis
  - spinal (tuberculous) A18.01
    - nontuberculous — *see* Osteomyelitis, vertebra
- bowel K63.0
- brain (any part) (cystic) (otogenic) G06.0
  - amebic (with abscess of any other site) A06.6
  - gonococcal A54.82
  - pheomycotic (chromomycotic) B43.1
  - tuberculous A17.81
- breast (acute) (chronic) (nonpuerperal) N61.1
  - newborn P39.0
  - puerperal, postpartum, gestational — *see* Mastitis, obstetric, purulent
- broad ligament N73.2
  - acute N73.0
  - chronic N73.1
- Brodie's (localized) (chronic) M86.8X- ☑
- bronchi J98.09
- buccal cavity K12.2
- bulbourethral gland N34.0
- bursa M71.00
  - ankle M71.07- ☑
  - elbow M71.02- ☑
  - foot M71.07- ☑
  - hand M71.04- ☑
  - hip M71.05- ☑
  - knee M71.06- ☑
  - multiple sites M71.09
  - pharyngeal J39.1
  - shoulder M71.01- ☑
  - specified site NEC M71.08
  - wrist M71.03- ☑
- buttock L02.31
- canthus — *see* Blepharoconjunctivitis
- cartilage — *see* Disorder, cartilage, specified type NEC
- cecum K35.33
- cerebellum, cerebellar G06.0
  - sequelae G09
- cerebral (embolic) G06.0
  - sequelae G09
- cervical (meaning neck) L02.11
  - lymph gland or node L04.0
- cervix (stump) (uteri) — *see* Cervicitis
- cheek (external) L02.01
  - inner K12.2
- chest J86.9
  - with fistula J86.0
  - wall L02.213
- chin L02.01
- choroid — *see* Inflammation, chorioretinal

☑ **Additional Character Required** — **Refer to the Tabular List for Character Selection**   ▽ **Subterms under main terms may continue to next column or page**

Abscess — *continued*
circumtonsillar J36
cold (lung) (tuberculous) — *see also* Tuberculosis, abscess, lung
  articular — *see* Tuberculosis, joint
colon (wall) K63.Ø
colostomy K94.Ø2
conjunctiva — *see* Conjunctivitis, acute
cornea H16.31- ☑
corpus
  cavernosum N48.21
  luteum — *see* Oophoritis
Cowper's gland N34.Ø
cranium GØ6.Ø
cul-de-sac (Douglas') (posterior) — *see* Peritonitis, pelvic, female
cutaneous — *see* Abscess, by site
dental KØ4.7
  with sinus (alveolar) KØ4.6
dentoalveolar KØ4.7
  with sinus KØ4.6
diaphragm, diaphragmatic K65.1
Douglas' cul-de-sac or pouch — *see* Peritonitis, pelvic, female
Dubois A5Ø.59
ear (middle) — *see also* Otitis, media, suppurative
  acute — *see* Otitis, media, suppurative, acute
  external H6Ø.Ø- ☑
entamebic — *see* Abscess, amebic
enterostomy K94.12
epididymis N45.4
epidural GØ6.2
  brain GØ6.Ø
  spinal cord GØ6.1
epiglottis J38.7
epiploon, epiploic K65.1
erysipelatous — *see* Erysipelas
esophagus K2Ø.8
ethmoid (bone) (chronic) (sinus) J32.2
external auditory canal — *see* Abscess, ear, external
extradural GØ6.2
  brain GØ6.Ø
    sequelae GØ9
  spinal cord GØ6.1
extraperitoneal K68.19
eye — *see* Endophthalmitis, purulent
eyelid HØØ.Ø3- ☑
face (any part, except ear, eye and nose) LØ2.Ø1
fallopian tube — *see* Salpingitis
fascia M72.8
fauces J39.1
fecal K63.Ø
femoral (region) — *see* Abscess, lower limb
filaria, filarial — *see* Infestation, filarial
finger (any) — *see also* Abscess, hand
  nail — *see* Cellulitis, finger
foot LØ2.61- ☑
forehead LØ2.Ø1
frontal sinus (chronic) J32.1
gallbladder K81.Ø
genital organ or tract
  female (external) N76.4
  male N49.9
    multiple sites N49.8
    specified NEC N49.8
gestational mammary O91.11- ☑
gestational subareolar O91.11- ☑
gingival — *see* Periodontitis, localized
gland, glandular (lymph) (acute) — *see* Lymphadenitis, acute
gluteal (region) LØ2.31
gonorrheal — *see* Gonococcus
groin LØ2.214
gum — *see* Periodontitis, localized
hand LØ2.51- ☑
head NEC LØ2.811
  face (any part, except ear, eye and nose) LØ2.Ø1
heart — *see* Carditis
heel — *see* Abscess, foot
helminthic — *see* Infestation, helminth
hepatic (cholangitic) (hematogenic) (lymphogenic) (pylephlebitic) K75.Ø
  amebic AØ6.4
hip (region) — *see* Abscess, lower limb
horseshoe K61.31
ileocecal K35.33
ileostomy (bud) K94.12
iliac (region) LØ2.214

Abscess — *continued*
iliac — *continued*
  fossa K35.33
infraclavicular (fossa) — *see* Abscess, upper limb
inguinal (region) LØ2.214
  lymph gland or node LØ4.1
intersphincteric K61.4
intestine, intestinal NEC K63.Ø
  rectal K61.1
intra-abdominal — *see also* Abscess, peritoneum K65.1
  following procedure T81.43 ☑
    obstetrical O86.Ø3
  postprocedural T81.49 ☑
    retroperitoneal K68.11
intracranial GØ6.Ø
intramammary — *see* Abscess, breast
intramuscular, following procedure T81.42 ☑
  obstetrical O86.Ø2
intraorbital — *see* Abscess, orbit
intraperitoneal K65.1
intrasphincteric (anus) K61.4
intraspinal GØ6.1
intratonsillar J36
ischiorectal (fossa) (specified NEC) K61.39
jaw (bone) (lower) (upper) M27.2
joint — *see* Arthritis, pyogenic or pyemic
  spine (tuberculous) A18.Ø1
    nontuberculous — *see* Spondylopathy, infective
kidney N15.1
  with calculus N2Ø.Ø
    with hydronephrosis N13.6
  puerperal (postpartum) O86.21
knee — *see also* Abscess, lower limb
  joint MØØ.9
labium (majus) (minus) N76.4
lacrimal
  caruncle — *see* Inflammation, lacrimal, passages, acute
  gland — *see* Dacryoadenitis
  passages (duct) (sac) — *see* Inflammation, lacrimal, passages, acute
lacunar N34.Ø
larynx J38.7
lateral (alveolar) KØ4.7
  with sinus KØ4.6
leg (any part) — *see* Abscess, lower limb
lens H27.8
lingual K14.Ø
  tonsil J36
lip K13.Ø
Littre's gland N34.Ø
liver (cholangitic) (hematogenic) (lymphogenic) (pylephlebitic) (pyogenic) K75.Ø
  amebic (due to Entamoeba histolytica) (dysenteric) (tropical) AØ6.4
    with
      brain abscess (and liver or lung abscess) AØ6.6
      lung abscess AØ6.5
loin (region) LØ2.211
lower limb LØ2.41- ☑
lumbar (tuberculous) A18.Ø1
  nontuberculous LØ2.212
lung (miliary) (putrid) J85.2
  with pneumonia J85.1
    due to specified organism (see Pneumonia, in (due to))
  amebic (with liver abscess) AØ6.5
    with
      brain abscess AØ6.6
      pneumonia AØ6.5
lymph, lymphatic, gland or node (acute) — *see also* Lymphadenitis, acute
  mesentery I88.Ø
malar M27.2
mammary gland — *see* Abscess, breast
marginal, anus K61.Ø
mastoid — *see* Mastoiditis, acute
maxilla, maxillary M27.2
  molar (tooth) KØ4.7
    with sinus KØ4.6
  premolar KØ4.7
  sinus (chronic) J32.Ø
mediastinum J85.3
meibomian gland — *see* Hordeolum
meninges GØ6.2
mesentery, mesenteric K65.1
mesosalpinx — *see* Salpingitis
mons pubis LØ2.215

Abscess — *continued*
mouth (floor) K12.2
muscle — *see* Myositis, infective
myocardium I4Ø.Ø
nabothian (follicle) — *see* Cervicitis
nasal J32.9
nasopharyngeal J39.1
navel LØ2.216
  newborn P38.9
    with mild hemorrhage P38.1
    without hemorrhage P38.9
neck (region) LØ2.11
  lymph gland or node LØ4.Ø
nephritic — *see* Abscess, kidney
nipple N61.1
  associated with
    lactation — *see* Pregnancy, complicated by
    pregnancy — *see* Pregnancy, complicated by
nose (external) (fossa) (septum) J34.Ø
  sinus (chronic) — *see* Sinusitis
omentum K65.1
operative wound T81.49 ☑
orbit, orbital — *see* Cellulitis, orbit
otogenic GØ6.Ø
ovary, ovarian (corpus luteum) — *see* Oophoritis
oviduct — *see* Oophoritis
palate (soft) K12.2
  hard M27.2
palmar (space) — *see* Abscess, hand
pancreas (duct) — *see* Pancreatitis, acute
parafrenal N48.21
parametric, parametrium N73.2
  acute N73.Ø
  chronic N73.1
paranephric N15.1
parapancreatic — *see* Pancreatitis, acute
parapharyngeal J39.Ø
pararectal K61.1
parasinus — *see* Sinusitis
parauterine — *see also* Disease, pelvis, inflammatory N73.2
paravaginal — *see* Vaginitis
parietal region (scalp) LØ2.811
parodontal — *see* Periodontitis, aggressive, localized
parotid (duct) (gland) K11.3
  region K12.2
pectoral (region) LØ2.213
pelvis, pelvic
  female — *see* Disease, pelvis, inflammatory
  male, peritoneal K65.1
penis N48.21
  gonococcal (accessory gland) (periurethral) A54.1
perianal K61.Ø
periapical KØ4.7
  with sinus (alveolar) KØ4.6
periappendicular K35.33
pericardial I3Ø.1
pericecal K35.33
pericemental — *see* Periodontitis, aggressive, localized
pericholecystic — *see* Cholecystitis, acute
pericoronal — *see* Periodontitis, aggressive, localized
peridental — *see* Periodontitis, aggressive, localized
perimetric — *see also* Disease, pelvis, inflammatory N73.2
perinephric, perinephritic — *see* Abscess, kidney
perineum, perineal (superficial) LØ2.215
  urethra N34.Ø
periodontal (parietal) — *see* Periodontitis, aggressive, localized
  apical KØ4.7
periosteum, periosteal — *see also* Osteomyelitis, specified type NEC
  with osteomyelitis — *see also* Osteomyelitis, specified type NEC
  acute — *see* Osteomyelitis, acute
  chronic — *see* Osteomyelitis, chronic
peripharyngeal J39.Ø
peripleuritic J86.9
  with fistula J86.Ø
periprostatic N41.2
perirectal K61.1
perirenal (tissue) — *see* Abscess, kidney
perisinuous (nose) — *see* Sinusitis
peritoneum, peritoneal (perforated) (ruptured) K65.1
  with appendicitis — *see also* Appendicitis K35.33
  pelvic
    female — *see* Peritonitis, pelvic, female
    male K65.1

▽ **Subterms under main terms may continue to next column or page**   ☑ **Additional Character Required — Refer to the Tabular List for Character Selection**   5

Abscess — Abscess

Index

Abscess — *continued*
peritoneum, peritoneal — *continued*
  postoperative T81.49 ☑
  puerperal, postpartum, childbirth O85
  tuberculous A18.31
peritonsillar J36
perityphlic K35.33
periureteral N28.89
periurethral N34.0
  gonococcal (accessory gland) (periurethral) A54.1
periuterine — *see also* Disease, pelvis, inflammatory N73.2
perivesical — *see* Cystitis, specified type NEC
petrous bone — *see* Petrositis
phagedenic NOS L02.91
  chancroid A57
pharynx, pharyngeal (lateral) J39.1
pilonidal L05.01
pituitary (gland) E23.6
pleura J86.9
  with fistula J86.0
popliteal — *see* Abscess, lower limb
postcecal K35.33
postlaryngeal J38.7
postnasal J34.0
postoperative (any site) — *see also* Infection, postoperative wound T81.49 ☑
  retroperitoneal K68.11
postpharyngeal J39.0
posttonsillar J36
post-typhoid A01.09
pouch of Douglas — *see* Peritonitis, pelvic, female
premammary — *see* Abscess, breast
prepatellar — *see* Abscess, lower limb
prostate N41.2
  gonococcal (acute) (chronic) A54.22
psoas muscle K68.12
puerperal — *code by* site under Puerperal, abscess
pulmonary — *see* Abscess, lung
pulp, pulpal (dental) K04.01
  irreversible K04.02
  reversible K04.01
rectovaginal septum K63.0
rectovesical — *see* Cystitis, specified type NEC
rectum K61.1
renal — *see* Abscess, kidney
retina — *see* Inflammation, chorioretinal
retrobulbar — *see* Abscess, orbit
retrocecal K65.1
retrolaryngeal J38.7
retromammary — *see* Abscess, breast
retroperitoneal NEC K68.19
  postprocedural K68.11
retropharyngeal J39.0
retrouterine — *see* Peritonitis, pelvic, female
retrovesical — *see* Cystitis, specified type NEC
root, tooth K04.7
  with sinus (alveolar) K04.6
round ligament — *see also* Disease, pelvis, inflammatory N73.2
rupture (spontaneous) NOS L02.91
sacrum (tuberculous) A18.01
  nontuberculous M46.28
salivary (duct) (gland) K11.3
scalp (any part) L02.811
scapular — *see* Osteomyelitis, specified type NEC
sclera — *see* Scleritis
scrofulous (tuberculous) A18.2
scrotum N49.2
seminal vesicle N49.0
septal, dental K04.7
  with sinus (alveolar) K04.6
serous — *see* Periostitis
shoulder (region) — *see* Abscess, upper limb
sigmoid K63.0
sinus (accessory) (chronic) (nasal) — *see also* Sinusitis
  intracranial venous (any) G06.0
Skene's duct or gland N34.0
skin — *see* Abscess, by site
specified site NEC L02.818
spermatic cord N49.1
sphenoidal (sinus) (chronic) J32.3
spinal cord (any part) (staphylococcal) G06.1
  tuberculous A17.81
spine (column) (tuberculous) A18.01
  epidural G06.1
  nontuberculous — *see* Osteomyelitis, vertebra
spleen D73.3

Abscess — *continued*
spleen — *continued*
  amebic A06.89
stitch T81.41 ☑
  following an obstetrical procedure O86.01
subarachnoid G06.2
  brain G06.0
  spinal cord G06.1
subareolar — *see* Abscess, breast
subcecal K35.33
subcutaneous — *see also* Abscess, by site
  following procedure T81.41 ☑
    obstetrical O86.01
  pheomycotic (chromomycotic) B43.2
subdiaphragmatic K65.1
subdural G06.2
  brain G06.0
    sequelae G09
  spinal cord G06.1
sub-fascial, following an obstetrical procedure O86.02
subgaleal L02.811
subhepatic K65.1
sublingual K12.2
  gland K11.3
submammary — *see* Abscess, breast
submandibular (region) (space) (triangle) K12.2
  gland K11.3
submaxillary (region) L02.01
  gland K11.3
submental L02.01
  gland K11.3
subperiosteal — *see* Osteomyelitis, specified type NEC
subphrenic K65.1
  following an obstetrical procedure O86.03
  postoperative T81.43 ☑
suburethral N34.0
sudoriparous L75.8
supraclavicular (fossa) — *see* Abscess, upper limb
supralevator K61.5
suprapelvic, acute N73.0
suprarenal (capsule) (gland) E27.8
sweat gland L74.8
tear duct — *see* Inflammation, lacrimal, passages, acute
temple L02.01
temporal region L02.01
temporosphenoidal G06.0
tendon (sheath) M65.00
  ankle M65.07- ☑
  foot M65.07- ☑
  forearm M65.03- ☑
  hand M65.04- ☑
  lower leg M65.06- ☑
  pelvic region M65.05- ☑
  shoulder region M65.01- ☑
  specified site NEC M65.08
  thigh M65.05- ☑
  upper arm M65.02- ☑
testis N45.4
thigh — *see* Abscess, lower limb
thorax J86.9
  with fistula J86.0
throat J39.1
thumb — *see also* Abscess, hand
  nail — *see* Cellulitis, finger
thymus (gland) E32.1
thyroid (gland) E06.0
toe (any) — *see also* Abscess, foot
  nail — *see* Cellulitis, toe
tongue (staphylococcal) K14.0
tonsil(s) (lingual) J36
tonsillopharyngeal J36
tooth, teeth (root) K04.7
  with sinus (alveolar) K04.6
  supporting structures NEC — *see* Periodontitis, aggressive, localized
trachea J39.8
trunk L02.219
  abdominal wall L02.211
  back L02.212
  chest wall L02.213
  groin L02.214
  perineum L02.215
  umbilicus L02.216
tubal — *see* Salpingitis
tuberculous — *see* Tuberculosis, abscess
tubo-ovarian — *see* Salpingo-oophoritis
tunica vaginalis N49.1
umbilicus L02.216

Abscess — *continued*
upper
  limb L02.41- ☑
  respiratory J39.8
urethral (gland) N34.0
urinary N34.0
uterus, uterine (wall) — *see also* Endometritis
  ligament — *see also* Disease, pelvis, inflammatory N73.2
  neck — *see* Cervicitis
uvula K12.2
vagina (wall) — *see* Vaginitis
vaginorectal — *see* Vaginitis
vas deferens N49.1
vermiform appendix K35.33
vertebra (column) (tuberculous) A18.01
  nontuberculous — *see* Osteomyelitis, vertebra
vesical — *see* Cystitis, specified type NEC
vesico-uterine pouch — *see* Peritonitis, pelvic, female
vitreous (humor) — *see* Endophthalmitis, purulent
vocal cord J38.3
von Bezold's — *see* Mastoiditis, acute
vulva N76.4
vulvovaginal gland N75.1
web space — *see* Abscess, hand
wound T81.49 ☑
wrist — *see* Abscess, upper limb
Absence (of) (organ or part) (complete or partial)
adrenal (gland) (congenital) Q89.1
  acquired E89.6
albumin in blood E88.09
alimentary tract (congenital) Q45.8
  upper Q40.8
alveolar process (acquired) — *see* Anomaly, alveolar
ankle (acquired) Z89.44- ☑
anus (congenital) Q42.3
  with fistula Q42.2
aorta (congenital) Q25.41
appendix, congenital Q42.8
arm (acquired) Z89.20- ☑
  above elbow Z89.22- ☑
    congenital (with hand present) — *see* Agenesis, arm, with hand present
      and hand — *see* Agenesis, forearm, and hand
  below elbow Z89.21- ☑
    congenital (with hand present) — *see* Agenesis, arm, with hand present
      and hand — *see* Agenesis, forearm, and hand
  congenital — *see* Defect, reduction, upper limb
  shoulder (following explantation of shoulder joint prosthesis) (joint) (with or without presence of antibiotic-impregnated cement spacer) Z89.23- ☑
    congenital (with hand present) — *see* Agenesis, arm, with hand present
artery (congenital) (peripheral) Q27.8
  brain Q28.3
  coronary Q24.5
  pulmonary Q25.79
  specified NEC Q27.8
  umbilical Q27.0
atrial septum (congenital) Q21.1
auditory canal (congenital) (external) Q16.1
auricle (ear), congenital Q16.0
bile, biliary duct, congenital Q44.5
bladder (acquired) Z90.6
  congenital Q64.5
bowel sounds R19.11
brain Q00.0
  part of Q04.3
breast(s) (and nipple(s)) (acquired) Z90.1- ☑
  congenital Q83.8
broad ligament Q50.6
bronchus (congenital) Q32.4
canaliculus lacrimalis, congenital Q10.4
cerebellum (vermis) Q04.3
cervix (acquired) (with uterus) Z90.710
  with remaining uterus Z90.712
  congenital Q51.5
chin, congenital Q18.8
cilia (congenital) Q10.3
  acquired — *see* Madarosis
clitoris (congenital) Q52.6
coccyx, congenital Q76.49
cold sense R20.8
congenital
  lumen — *see* Atresia
  organ or site NEC — *see* Agenesis

Absence — continued
  congenital — continued
    septum — see Imperfect, closure
    corpus callosum Q04.0
    cricoid cartilage, congenital Q31.8
    diaphragm (with hernia), congenital Q79.1
    digestive organ(s) or tract, congenital Q45.8
      acquired NEC Z90.49
      upper Q40.8
    ductus arteriosus Q28.8
    duodenum (acquired) Z90.49
      congenital Q41.0
    ear, congenital Q16.9
      acquired H93.8- ☑
      auricle Q16.0
      external Q16.0
      inner Q16.5
      lobe, lobule Q17.8
      middle, except ossicles Q16.4
        ossicles Q16.3
      ossicles Q16.3
    ejaculatory duct (congenital) Q55.4
    endocrine gland (congenital) NEC Q89.2
      acquired E89.89
    epididymis (congenital) Q55.4
      acquired Z90.79
    epiglottis, congenital Q31.8
    esophagus (congenital) Q39.8
      acquired (partial) Z90.49
    eustachian tube (congenital) Q16.2
    extremity (acquired) Z89.9
      congenital Q73.0
      knee (following explantation of knee joint prosthesis) (joint) (with or without presence of antibiotic-impregnated cement spacer) Z89.52- ☑
      lower (above knee) Z89.619
        below knee Z89.51- ☑
      upper — see Absence, arm
    eye (acquired) Z90.01
      congenital Q11.1
      muscle (congenital) Q10.3
    eyeball (acquired) Z90.01
    eyelid (fold) (congenital) Q10.3
      acquired Z90.01
    face, specified part NEC Q18.8
    fallopian tube(s) (acquired) Z90.79
      congenital Q50.6
    family member (causing problem in home) NEC — see also Disruption, family Z63.32
    femur, congenital — see Defect, reduction, lower limb, longitudinal, femur
    fibrinogen (congenital) D68.2
      acquired D65
    finger(s) (acquired) Z89.02- ☑
      congenital — see Agenesis, hand
    foot (acquired) Z89.43- ☑
      congenital — see Agenesis, foot
    forearm (acquired) — see Absence, arm, below elbow
    gallbladder (acquired) Z90.49
      congenital Q44.0
    gamma globulin in blood D80.1
      hereditary D80.0
    genital organs
      acquired (female) (male) Z90.79
      female, congenital Q52.8
        external Q52.71
        internal NEC Q52.8
      male, congenital Q55.8
    genitourinary organs, congenital NEC
      female Q52.8
      male Q55.8
    globe (acquired) Z90.01
      congenital Q11.1
    glottis, congenital Q31.8
    hand and wrist (acquired) Z89.11- ☑
      congenital — see Agenesis, hand
    head, part (acquired) NEC Z90.09
    heat sense R20.8
    hip (following explantation of hip joint prosthesis) (joint) (with or without presence of antibiotic-impregnated cement spacer) Z89.62- ☑
    hymen (congenital) Q52.4
    ileum (acquired) Z90.49
      congenital Q41.2
    immunoglobulin, isolated NEC D80.3
      IgA D80.2
      IgG D80.3
      IgM D80.4

Absence — continued
  incus (acquired) — see Loss, ossicles, ear
    congenital Q16.3
  inner ear, congenital Q16.5
  intestine (acquired) (small) Z90.49
    congenital Q41.9
      specified NEC Q41.8
    large Z90.49
      congenital Q42.9
        specified NEC Q42.8
  iris, congenital Q13.1
  jejunum (acquired) Z90.49
    congenital Q41.1
  joint
    acquired
      hip (following explantation of hip joint prosthesis) (with or without presence of antibiotic-impregnated cement spacer) Z89.62- ☑
      knee (following explantation of knee joint prosthesis) (with or without presence of antibiotic-impregnated cement spacer) Z89.52- ☑
      shoulder (following explantation of shoulder joint prosthesis) (with or without presence of antibiotic-impregnated cement spacer) Z89.23- ☑
    congenital NEC Q74.8
  kidney(s) (acquired) Z90.5
    congenital Q60.2
      bilateral Q60.1
      unilateral Q60.0
  knee (following explantation of knee joint prosthesis) (joint) (with or without presence of antibiotic-impregnated cement spacer) Z89.52- ☑
  labyrinth, membranous Q16.5
  larynx (congenital) Q31.8
    acquired Z90.02
  leg (acquired) (above knee) Z89.61- ☑
    below knee (acquired) Z89.51- ☑
    congenital — see Defect, reduction, lower limb
  lens (acquired) — see also Aphakia
    congenital Q12.3
    post cataract extraction Z98.4- ☑
  limb (acquired) — see Absence, extremity
  lip Q38.6
  liver (congenital) Q44.7
  lung (fissure) (lobe) (bilateral) (unilateral) (congenital) Q33.3
    acquired (any part) Z90.2
  menstruation — see Amenorrhea
  muscle (congenital) (pectoral) Q79.8
    ocular Q10.3
  neck, part Q18.8
  neutrophil — see Agranulocytosis
  nipple(s) (with breast(s)) (acquired) Z90.1- ☑
    congenital Q83.2
  nose (congenital) Q30.1
    acquired Z90.09
  organ
    of Corti, congenital Q16.5
    or site, congenital NEC Q89.8
      acquired NEC Z90.89
  osseous meatus (ear) Q16.4
  ovary (acquired)
    bilateral Z90.722
    congenital
      bilateral Q50.02
      unilateral Q50.01
    unilateral Z90.721
  oviduct (acquired)
    bilateral Z90.722
    congenital Q50.6
    unilateral Z90.721
  pancreas (congenital) Q45.0
    acquired Z90.410
      complete Z90.410
      partial Z90.411
      total Z90.410
  parathyroid gland (acquired) E89.2
    congenital Q89.2
  patella, congenital Q74.1
  penis (congenital) Q55.5
    acquired Z90.79
  pericardium (congenital) Q24.8
  pituitary gland (congenital) Q89.2
    acquired E89.3
  prostate (acquired) Z90.79
    congenital Q55.4

Absence — continued
  pulmonary valve Q22.0
  punctum lacrimale (congenital) Q10.4
  radius, congenital — see Defect, reduction, upper limb, longitudinal, radius
  rectum (congenital) Q42.1
    with fistula Q42.0
    acquired Z90.49
  respiratory organ NOS Q34.9
  rib (acquired) Z90.89
    congenital Q76.6
  sacrum, congenital Q76.49
  salivary gland(s), congenital Q38.4
  scrotum, congenital Q55.29
  seminal vesicles (congenital) Q55.4
    acquired Z90.79
  septum
    atrial (congenital) Q21.1
    between aorta and pulmonary artery Q21.4
    ventricular (congenital) Q20.4
  sex chromosome
    female phenotype Q97.8
    male phenotype Q98.8
  skull bone (congenital) Q75.8
    with
      anencephaly Q00.0
      encephalocele — see Encephalocele
      hydrocephalus Q03.9
        with spina bifida — see Spina bifida, by site, with hydrocephalus
      microcephaly Q02
  spermatic cord, congenital Q55.4
  spine, congenital Q76.49
  spleen (congenital) Q89.01
    acquired Z90.81
  sternum, congenital Q76.7
  stomach (acquired) (partial) Z90.3
    congenital Q40.2
  superior vena cava, congenital Q26.8
  teeth, tooth (congenital) K00.0
    acquired (complete) K08.109
      class I K08.101
      class II K08.102
      class III K08.103
      class IV K08.104
      due to
        caries K08.139
          class I K08.131
          class II K08.132
          class III K08.133
          class IV K08.134
        periodontal disease K08.129
          class I K08.121
          class II K08.122
          class III K08.123
          class IV K08.124
        specified NEC K08.199
          class I K08.191
          class II K08.192
          class III K08.193
          class IV K08.194
        trauma K08.119
          class I K08.111
          class II K08.112
          class III K08.113
          class IV K08.114
      partial K08.409
        class I K08.401
        class II K08.402
        class III K08.403
        class IV K08.404
        due to
          caries K08.439
            class I K08.431
            class II K08.432
            class III K08.433
            class IV K08.434
          periodontal disease K08.429
            class I K08.421
            class II K08.422
            class III K08.423
            class IV K08.424
          specified NEC K08.499
            class I K08.491
            class II K08.492
            class III K08.493
            class IV K08.494
          trauma K08.419
            class I K08.411

Absence — *continued*
  teeth, tooth — *continued*
    acquired — *continued*
      partial — *continued*
        due to — *continued*
          trauma — *continued*
            class II K08.412
            class III K08.413
            class IV K08.414
  tendon (congenital) Q79.8
  testis (congenital) Q55.0
    acquired Z90.79
  thumb (acquired) Z89.01- ☑
    congenital — *see* Agenesis, hand
  thymus gland Q89.2
  thyroid (gland) (acquired) E89.0
    cartilage, congenital Q31.8
    congenital E03.1
  toe(s) (acquired) Z89.42- ☑
    with foot — *see* Absence, foot and ankle
    congenital — *see* Agenesis, foot
    great Z89.41- ☑
  tongue, congenital Q38.3
  trachea (cartilage), congenital Q32.1
  transverse aortic arch, congenital Q25.49
  tricuspid valve Q22.4
  umbilical artery, congenital Q27.0
  upper arm and forearm with hand present, congenital
    — *see* Agenesis, arm, with hand present
  ureter (congenital) Q62.4
    acquired Z90.6
  urethra, congenital Q64.5
  uterus (acquired) Z90.710
    with cervix Z90.710
    with remaining cervical stump Z90.711
    congenital Q51.0
  uvula, congenital Q38.5
  vagina, congenital Q52.0
  vas deferens (congenital) Q55.4
    acquired Z90.79
  vein (peripheral) congenital NEC Q27.8
    cerebral Q28.3
    digestive system Q27.8
    great Q26.8
    lower limb Q27.8
    portal Q26.5
    precerebral Q28.1
    specified site NEC Q27.8
    upper limb Q27.8
  vena cava (inferior) (superior), congenital Q26.8
  ventricular septum Q20.4
  vertebra, congenital Q76.49
  vulva, congenital Q52.71
  wrist (acquired) Z89.12- ☑
Absorbent system disease I87.8
Absorption
  carbohydrate, disturbance K90.49
  chemical — *see* Table of Drugs and Chemicals
    through placenta (newborn) P04.9
      environmental substance P04.6
      nutritional substance P04.5
      obstetric anesthetic or analgesic drug P04.0
  drug NEC — *see* Table of Drugs and Chemicals
    addictive
      through placenta (newborn) — *see also* New-
        born, affected by, maternal, use of P04.40
        cocaine P04.41
        hallucinogens P04.42
        specified drug NEC P04.49
    medicinal
      through placenta (newborn) P04.19
    through placenta (newborn) P04.19
      obstetric anesthetic or analgesic drug P04.0
  fat, disturbance K90.49
    pancreatic K90.3
  noxious substance — *see* Table of Drugs and Chemicals
  protein, disturbance K90.49
  starch, disturbance K90.49
  toxic substance — *see* Table of Drugs and Chemicals
  uremic — *see* Uremia
Abstinence symptoms, syndrome
  alcohol F10.239
    with delirium F10.231
  cocaine F14.23
  neonatal P96.1
  nicotine — *see* Dependence, drug, nicotine, with,
    withdrawal
  opioid F11.93

Abstinence symptoms, syndrome — *continued*
  opioid — *continued*
    with dependence F11.23
  psychoactive NEC F19.939
    with
      delirium F19.931
      dependence F19.239
        with
          delirium F19.231
          perceptual disturbance F19.232
        uncomplicated F19.230
      perceptual disturbance F19.932
    uncomplicated F19.930
  sedative F13.939
    with
      delirium F13.931
      dependence F13.239
        with
          delirium F13.231
          perceptual disturbance F13.232
        uncomplicated F13.230
      perceptual disturbance F13.932
    uncomplicated F13.930
  stimulant NEC F15.93
    with dependence F15.23
Abulia R68.89
Abulomania F60.7
Abuse
  adult — *see* Maltreatment, adult
    as reason for
      couple seeking advice (including offender) Z63.0
  alcohol (non-dependent) F10.10
    with
      anxiety disorder F10.180
      intoxication F10.129
        with delirium F10.121
        uncomplicated F10.120
      mood disorder F10.14
      other specified disorder F10.188
      psychosis F10.159
        delusions F10.150
        hallucinations F10.151
      sexual dysfunction F10.181
      sleep disorder F10.182
      unspecified disorder F10.19
    counseling and surveillance Z71.41
    in remission (early) (sustained) F10.11
  amphetamine (or related substance) — *see also* Abuse,
    drug, stimulant NEC
    stimulant NEC F15.10
      with
        anxiety disorder F15.180
        intoxication F15.129
          with
            delirium F15.121
            perceptual disturbance F15.122
  analgesics (non-prescribed) (over the counter) F55.8
  antacids F55.0
  antidepressants — *see* Abuse, drug, psychoactive NEC
  anxiolytic — *see* Abuse, drug, sedative
  barbiturates — *see* Abuse, drug, sedative
  caffeine — *see* Abuse, drug, stimulant NEC
  cannabis, cannabinoids — *see* Abuse, drug, cannabis
  child — *see* Maltreatment, child
  cocaine — *see* Abuse, drug, cocaine
  drug NEC (non-dependent) F19.10
    with sleep disorder F19.182
    amphetamine type — *see* Abuse, drug, stimulant
      NEC
    analgesics (non-prescribed) (over the counter) F55.8
    antacids F55.0
    antidepressants — *see* Abuse, drug, psychoactive
      NEC
    anxiolytics — *see* Abuse, drug, sedative
    barbiturates — *see* Abuse, drug, sedative
    caffeine — *see* Abuse, drug, stimulant NEC
    cannabis F12.10
      with
        anxiety disorder F12.180
        intoxication F12.129
          with
            delirium F12.121
            perceptual disturbance F12.122
          uncomplicated F12.120
        other specified disorder F12.188
        psychosis F12.159
          delusions F12.150
          hallucinations F12.151

Abuse — *continued*
  drug — *continued*
    cannabis — *continued*
      with — *continued*
        unspecified disorder F12.19
      in remission (early) (sustained) F12.11
    cocaine F14.10
      with
        anxiety disorder F14.180
        intoxication F14.129
          with
            delirium F14.121
            perceptual disturbance F14.122
          uncomplicated F14.120
        mood disorder F14.14
        other specified disorder F14.188
        psychosis F14.159
          delusions F14.150
          hallucinations F14.151
        sexual dysfunction F14.181
        sleep disorder F14.182
        unspecified disorder F14.19
      in remission (early) (sustained) F14.11
    counseling and surveillance Z71.51
    hallucinogen F16.10
      with
        anxiety disorder F16.180
        flashbacks F16.183
        intoxication F16.129
          with
            delirium F16.121
            perceptual disturbance F16.122
          uncomplicated F16.120
        mood disorder F16.14
        other specified disorder F16.188
        perception disorder, persisting F16.183
        psychosis F16.159
          delusions F16.150
          hallucinations F16.151
        unspecified disorder F16.19
      in remission (early) (sustained) F16.11
    hashish — *see* Abuse, drug, cannabis
    herbal or folk remedies F55.1
    hormones F55.3
    hypnotics — *see* Abuse, drug, sedative
    in remission (early) (sustained) F19.11
    inhalant F18.10
      with
        anxiety disorder F18.180
        dementia, persisting F18.17
        intoxication F18.129
          with delirium F18.121
          uncomplicated F18.120
        mood disorder F18.14
        other specified disorder F18.188
        psychosis F18.159
          delusions F18.150
          hallucinations F18.151
        unspecified disorder F18.19
      in remission (early) (sustained) F18.11
    laxatives F55.2
    LSD — *see* Abuse, drug, hallucinogen
    marihuana — *see* Abuse, drug, cannabis
    morphine type (opioids) — *see* Abuse, drug, opioid
    opioid F11.10
      with
        intoxication F11.129
          with
            delirium F11.121
            perceptual disturbance F11.122
          uncomplicated F11.120
        mood disorder F11.14
        other specified disorder F11.188
        psychosis F11.159
          delusions F11.150
          hallucinations F11.151
        sexual dysfunction F11.181
        sleep disorder F11.182
        unspecified disorder F11.19
      in remission (early) (sustained) F11.11
    PCP (phencyclidine) (or related substance) — *see*
      Abuse, drug, hallucinogen
    psychoactive NEC F19.10
      with
        amnestic disorder F19.16
        anxiety disorder F19.180
        dementia F19.17
        intoxication F19.129

Abuse — continued
  drug — continued
    psychoactive — continued
      with — continued
        intoxication — continued
          with
            delirium F19.121
            perceptual disturbance F19.122
          uncomplicated F19.120
        mood disorder F19.14
        other specified disorder F19.188
        psychosis F19.159
          delusions F19.150
          hallucinations F19.151
        sexual dysfunction F19.181
        sleep disorder F19.182
        unspecified disorder F19.19
    sedative, hypnotic or anxiolytic F13.10
      with
        anxiety disorder F13.180
        intoxication F13.129
          with delirium F13.121
          uncomplicated F13.120
        mood disorder F13.14
        other specified disorder F13.188
        psychosis F13.159
          delusions F13.150
          hallucinations F13.151
        sexual dysfunction F13.181
        sleep disorder F13.182
        unspecified disorder F13.19
      in remission (early) (sustained) F13.11
    solvent — see Abuse, drug, inhalant
    steroids F55.3
    stimulant NEC F15.10
      with
        anxiety disorder F15.180
        intoxication F15.129
          with
            delirium F15.121
            perceptual disturbance F15.122
          uncomplicated F15.120
        mood disorder F15.14
        other specified disorder F15.188
        psychosis F15.159
          delusions F15.150
          hallucinations F15.151
        sexual dysfunction F15.181
        sleep disorder F15.182
        unspecified disorder F15.19
      in remission (early) (sustained) F15.11
    tranquilizers — see Abuse, drug, sedative
    vitamins F55.4
  hallucinogens — see Abuse, drug, hallucinogen
  hashish — see Abuse, drug, cannabis
  herbal or folk remedies F55.1
  hormones F55.3
  hypnotic — see Abuse, drug, sedative
  inhalant — see Abuse, drug, inhalant
  laxatives F55.2
  LSD — see Abuse, drug, hallucinogen
  marihuana — see Abuse, drug, cannabis
  morphine type (opioids) — see Abuse, drug, opioid
  non-psychoactive substance NEC F55.8
    antacids F55.0
    folk remedies F55.1
    herbal remedies F55.1
    hormones F55.3
    laxatives F55.2
    steroids F55.3
    vitamins F55.4
  opioids — see Abuse, drug, opioid
  PCP (phencyclidine) (or related substance) — see
    Abuse, drug, hallucinogen
  physical (adult) (child) — see Maltreatment
  psychoactive substance — see Abuse, drug, psychoactive NEC
  psychological (adult) (child) — see Maltreatment
  sedative — see Abuse, drug, sedative
  sexual — see Maltreatment
  solvent — see Abuse, drug, inhalant
  steroids F55.3
  vitamins F55.4
Acalculia R48.8
  developmental F81.2
Acanthamebiasis (with) B60.10
  conjunctiva B60.12
  keratoconjunctivitis B60.13

Acanthamebiasis — continued
  meningoencephalitis B60.11
  other specified B60.19
Acanthocephaliasis B83.8
Acanthocheilonemiasis B74.4
Acanthocytosis E78.6
Acantholysis L11.9
Acanthosis (acquired) (nigricans) L83
  benign Q82.8
  congenital Q82.8
  seborrheic L82.1
    inflamed L82.0
  tongue K14.3
Acapnia E87.3
Acarbia E87.2
Acardia, acardius Q89.8
Acardiacus amorphus Q89.8
Acardiotrophia I51.4
Acariasis B88.0
  scabies B86
Acarodermatitis (urticarioides) B88.0
Acarophobia F40.218
Acatalasemia, acatalasia E80.3
Acathisia (drug induced) G25.71
Accelerated atrioventricular conduction I45.6
Accentuation of personality traits (type A) Z73.1
Accessory (congenital)
  adrenal gland Q89.1
  anus Q43.4
  appendix Q43.4
  atrioventricular conduction I45.6
  auditory ossicles Q16.3
  auricle (ear) Q17.0
  biliary duct or passage Q44.5
  bladder Q64.79
  blood vessels NEC Q27.9
    coronary Q24.5
  bone NEC Q79.8
  breast tissue, axilla Q83.1
  carpal bones Q74.0
  cecum Q43.4
  chromosome(s) NEC (nonsex) Q92.9
    with complex rearrangements NEC Q92.5
      seen only at prometaphase Q92.8
    13 — see Trisomy, 13
    18 — see Trisomy, 18
    21 — see Trisomy, 21
    partial Q92.9
    sex
      female phenotype Q97.8
  coronary artery Q24.5
  cusp(s), heart valve NEC Q24.8
    pulmonary Q22.3
  cystic duct Q44.5
  digit(s) Q69.9
  ear (auricle) (lobe) Q17.0
  endocrine gland NEC Q89.2
  eye muscle Q10.3
  eyelid Q10.3
  face bone(s) Q75.8
  fallopian tube (fimbria) (ostium) Q50.6
  finger(s) Q69.0
  foreskin N47.8
  frontonasal process Q75.8
  gallbladder Q44.1
  genital organ(s)
    female Q52.8
      external Q52.79
      internal NEC Q52.8
    male Q55.8
  genitourinary organs NEC Q89.8
    female Q52.8
    male Q55.8
  hallux Q69.2
  heart Q24.8
    valve NEC Q24.8
      pulmonary Q22.3
  hepatic ducts Q44.5
  hymen Q52.4
  intestine (large) (small) Q43.4
  kidney Q63.0
  lacrimal canal Q10.6
  leaflet, heart valve NEC Q24.8
  ligament, broad Q50.6
  liver Q44.7
    duct Q44.5
  lobule (ear) Q17.0
  lung (lobe) Q33.1

Accessory — continued
  muscle Q79.8
  navicular of carpus Q74.0
  nervous system, part NEC Q07.8
  nipple Q83.3
  nose Q30.8
  organ or site not listed — see Anomaly, by site
  ovary Q50.31
  oviduct Q50.6
  pancreas Q45.3
  parathyroid gland Q89.2
  parotid gland (and duct) Q38.4
  pituitary gland Q89.2
  preauricular appendage Q17.0
  prepuce N47.8
  renal arteries (multiple) Q27.2
  rib Q76.6
    cervical Q76.5
  roots (teeth) K00.2
  salivary gland Q38.4
  sesamoid bones Q74.8
    foot Q74.2
    hand Q74.0
  skin tags Q82.8
  spleen Q89.09
  sternum Q76.7
  submaxillary gland Q38.4
  tarsal bones Q74.2
  teeth, tooth K00.1
  tendon Q79.8
  thumb Q69.1
  thymus gland Q89.2
  thyroid gland Q89.2
  toes Q69.2
  tongue Q38.3
  tooth, teeth K00.1
  tragus Q17.0
  ureter Q62.5
  urethra Q64.79
  urinary organ or tract NEC Q64.8
  uterus Q51.28
  vagina Q52.10
  valve, heart NEC Q24.8
    pulmonary Q22.3
  vertebra Q76.49
  vocal cords Q31.8
  vulva Q52.79
Accident
  birth — see Birth, injury
  cardiac — see Infarct, myocardium
  cerebral I63.9
  cerebrovascular (embolic) (ischemic) (thrombotic) I63.9
    aborted I63.9
    hemorrhagic — see Hemorrhage, intracranial, intracerebral
    old (without sequelae) Z86.73
      with sequelae (of) — see Sequelae, infarction, cerebral
  coronary — see Infarct, myocardium
  craniovascular I63.9
  vascular, brain I63.9
Accidental — see condition
Accommodation (disorder) — see also condition
  hysterical paralysis of F44.89
  insufficiency of H52.4
  paresis — see Paresis, of accommodation
  spasm — see Spasm, of accommodation
Accouchement — see Delivery
Accreta placenta O43.21- ☑
Accretio cordis (nonrheumatic) I31.0
Accretions, tooth, teeth K03.6
Acculturation difficulty Z60.3
Accumulation secretion, prostate N42.89
Acephalia, acephalism, acephalus, acephaly Q00.0
Acephalobrachia monster Q89.8
Acephalochirus monster Q89.8
Acephalogaster Q89.8
Acephalostomus monster Q89.8
Acephalothorax Q89.8
Acerophobia F40.298
Acetonemia R79.89
  in Type 1 diabetes E10.10
    with coma E10.11
Acetonuria R82.4
Achalasia (cardia) (esophagus) K22.0
  congenital Q39.5
  pylorus Q40.0
  sphincteral NEC K59.8

▼ Subterms under main terms may continue to next column or page   ☑ Additional Character Required — Refer to the Tabular List for Character Selection   9

Abuse — Achalasia

Ache(s) — *see* Pain
Acheilia Q38.6
Achillobursitis — *see* Tendinitis, Achilles
Achillodynia — *see* Tendinitis, Achilles
Achlorhydria, achlorhydric (neurogenic) K31.83
   anemia D50.8
   diarrhea K31.83
   psychogenic F45.8
   secondary to vagotomy K91.1
Achluophobia F40.228
Acholia K82.8
Acholuric jaundice (familial) (splenomegalic) — *see also*
   Spherocytosis
   acquired D59.8
Achondrogenesis Q77.0
Achondroplasia (osteosclerosis congenita) Q77.4
Achroma, cutis L80
Achromat (ism), achromatopsia (acquired) (congenital)
   H53.51
Achromia, congenital — *see* Albinism
Achromia parasitica B36.0
Achylia gastrica K31.89
   psychogenic F45.8
Acid
   burn — *see* Corrosion
   deficiency
      amide nicotinic E52
      ascorbic E54
      folic E53.8
      nicotinic E52
      pantothenic E53.8
   intoxication E87.2
   peptic disease K30
   phosphatase deficiency E83.39
   stomach K30
      psychogenic F45.8
Acidemia E87.2
   argininosuccinic E72.22
   isovaleric E71.110
   metabolic (newborn) P19.9
      first noted before onset of labor P19.0
      first noted during labor P19.1
      noted at birth P19.2
   methylmalonic E71.120
   pipecolic E72.3
   propionic E71.121
Acidity, gastric (high) K30
   psychogenic F45.8
Acidocytopenia — *see* Agranulocytosis
Acidocytosis D72.1
Acidopenia — *see* Agranulocytosis
Acidosis (lactic) (respiratory) E87.2
   in Type 1 diabetes E10.10
      with coma E10.11
   kidney, tubular N25.89
   lactic E87.2
   metabolic NEC E87.2
      with respiratory acidosis E87.4
      hyperchloremic, of newborn P74.421
      late, of newborn P74.0
   mixed metabolic and respiratory, newborn P84
   newborn P84
   renal (hyperchloremic) (tubular) N25.89
   respiratory E87.2
      complicated by
         metabolic
            acidosis E87.4
            alkalosis E87.4
Aciduria
   4-hydroxybutyric E72.81
   argininosuccinic E72.22
   gamma-hydroxybutyric E72.81
   glutaric (type I) E72.3
      type II E71.313
      type III E71.5- ☑
   orotic (congenital) (hereditary) (pyrimidine deficiency)
      E79.8
      anemia D53.0
Acladiosis (skin) B36.0
Aclasis, diaphyseal Q78.6
Acleistocardia Q21.1
Aclusion — *see* Anomaly, dentofacial, malocclusion
Acne L70.9
   artificialis L70.8
   atrophica L70.2
   cachecticorum (Hebra) L70.8
   conglobata L70.1
   cystic L70.0

Acne — *continued*
   decalvans L66.2
   excoriée (des jeunes filles) L70.5
   frontalis L70.2
   indurata L70.0
   infantile L70.4
   keloid L73.0
   lupoid L70.2
   necrotic, necrotica (miliaris) L70.2
   neonatal L70.4
   nodular L70.0
   occupational L70.8
   picker's L70.5
   pustular L70.0
   rodens L70.2
   rosacea L71.9
   specified NEC L70.8
   tropica L70.3
   varioliformis L70.2
   vulgaris L70.0
Acnitis (primary) A18.4
Acosta's disease T70.29 ☑
Acoustic — *see* condition
Acousticophobia F40.298
Acquired — *see also* condition
   immunodeficiency syndrome (AIDS) B20
Acrania Q00.0
Acroangiodermatitis I78.9
Acroasphyxia, chronic I73.89
Acrobystitis N47.7
Acrocephalopolysyndactyly Q87.0
Acrocephalosyndactyly Q87.0
Acrocephaly Q75.0
Acrochondrohyperplasia — *see* Syndrome, Marfan's
Acrocyanosis I73.89
   newborn P28.2
      meaning transient blue hands and feet — *omit code*
Acrodermatitis L30.8
   atrophicans (chronica) L90.4
   continua (Hallopeau) L40.2
   enteropathica (hereditary) E83.2
   Hallopeau's L40.2
   infantile papular L44.4
   perstans L40.2
   pustulosa continua L40.2
   recalcitrant pustular L40.2
Acrodynia — *see* Poisoning, mercury
Acromegaly, acromegalia E22.0
Acromelalgia I73.81
Acromicria, acromikria Q79.8
Acronyx L60.0
Acropachy, thyroid — *see* Thyrotoxicosis
Acroparesthesia (simple) (vasomotor) I73.89
Acropathy, thyroid — *see* Thyrotoxicosis
Acrophobia F40.241
Acroposthitis N47.7
Acroscleriasis, acroscleroderma, acrosclerosis — *see*
   Sclerosis, systemic
Acrosphacelus I96
Acrospiroma, eccrine — *see* Neoplasm, skin, benign
Acrostealgia — *see* Osteochondropathy
Acrotrophodynia — *see* Immersion
ACTH ectopic syndrome E24.3
Actinic — *see* condition
Actinobacillosis, actinobacillus A28.8
   mallei A24.0
   muris A25.1
Actinomyces israelii (infection) — *see* Actinomycosis
Actinomycetoma (foot) B47.1
Actinomycosis, actinomycotic A42.9
   with pneumonia A42.0
   abdominal A42.1
   cervicofacial A42.2
   cutaneous A42.89
   gastrointestinal A42.1
   pulmonary A42.0
   sepsis A42.7
   specified site NEC A42.89
Actinoneuritis G62.82
Action, heart
   disorder I49.9
   irregular I49.9
      psychogenic F45.8
Activated protein C resistance D68.51
Activation
   mast cell (disorder) (syndrome) D89.40
      idiopathic D89.42

Activation — *continued*
   mast cell — *continued*
      monoclonal D89.41
      secondary D89.43
      specified type NEC D89.49
Active — *see* condition
Acute — *see also* condition
   abdomen R10.0
   gallbladder — *see* Cholecystitis, acute
Acyanotic heart disease (congenital) Q24.9
Acystia Q64.5
Adair-Dighton syndrome (brittle bones and blue sclera,
   deafness) Q78.0
Adamantinoblastoma — *see* Ameloblastoma
Adamantinoma — *see also* Cyst, calcifying odontogeni
   long bones C40.90
      lower limb C40.2- ☑
      upper limb C40.0- ☑
   malignant C41.1
      jaw (bone) (lower) C41.1
      upper C41.0
   tibial C40.2- ☑
Adamantoblastoma — *see* Ameloblastoma
Adams-Stokes (-Morgagni) disease or syndrome I45.9
Adaption reaction — *see* Disorder, adjustment
Addiction — *see also* Dependence F19.20
   alcohol, alcoholic (ethyl) (methyl) (wood) (without re
      mission) F10.20
      with remission F10.21
   drug — *see* Dependence, drug
   ethyl alcohol (without remission) F10.20
      with remission F10.21
   heroin — *see* Dependence, drug, opioid
   methyl alcohol (without remission) F10.20
      with remission F10.21
   methylated spirit (without remission) F10.20
      with remission F10.21
   morphine (-like substances) — *see* Dependence, drug,
      opioid
   nicotine — *see* Dependence, drug, nicotine
   opium and opioids — *see* Dependence, drug, opioid
   tobacco — *see* Dependence, drug, nicotine
Addison-Biermer anemia (pernicious) D51.0
Addisonian crisis E27.2
Addison's
   anemia (pernicious) D51.0
   disease (bronze) or syndrome E27.1
      tuberculous A18.7
   keloid L94.0
Addison-Schilder complex E71.528
Additional — *see also* Accessory
   chromosome(s) Q99.8
      21 — *see* Trisomy, 21
      sex — *see* Abnormal, chromosome, sex
Adduction contracture, hip or other joint — *see*
   Contraction, joint
Adenitis — *see also* Lymphadenitis
   acute, unspecified site L04.9
   axillary I88.9
      acute L04.2
      chronic or subacute I88.1
   Bartholin's gland N75.8
   bulbourethral gland — *see* Urethritis
   cervical I88.9
      acute L04.0
      chronic or subacute I88.1
   chancroid (Hemophilus ducreyi) A57
   chronic, unspecified site I88.1
   Cowper's gland — *see* Urethritis
   due to Pasteurella multocida (P. septica) A28.0
   epidemic, acute B27.09
   gangrenous L04.9
   gonorrheal NEC A54.89
   groin I88.9
      acute L04.1
      chronic or subacute I88.1
   infectious (acute) (epidemic) B27.09
   inguinal I88.9
      acute L04.1
      chronic or subacute I88.1
   lymph gland or node, except mesenteric I88.9
      acute — *see* Lymphadenitis, acute
      chronic or subacute I88.1
   mesenteric (acute) (chronic) (nonspecific) (subacute)
      I88.0
   parotid gland (suppurative) — *see* Sialoadenitis
   salivary gland (any) (suppurative) — *see* Sialoadenitis
   scrofulous (tuberculous) A18.2

☑ **Additional Character Required** — **Refer to the Tabular List for Character Selection**
▽ **Subterms under main terms may continue to next column or page**

denitis — *continued*
  Skene's duct or gland — *see* Urethritis
  strumous, tuberculous A18.2
  subacute, unspecified site I88.1
  sublingual gland (suppurative) — *see* Sialoadenitis
  submandibular gland (suppurative) — *see* Sialoadenitis
  submaxillary gland (suppurative) — *see* Sialoadenitis
  tuberculous — *see* Tuberculosis, lymph gland
  urethral gland — *see* Urethritis
  Wharton's duct (suppurative) — *see* Sialoadenitis
denoacanthoma — *see* Neoplasm, malignant, by site
denoameloblastoma — *see* Cyst, calcifying odontogenic
denocarcinoid (tumor) — *see* Neoplasm, malignant, by site
denocarcinoma — *see also* Neoplasm, malignant, by site
  acidophil
    specified site — *see* Neoplasm, malignant, by site
    unspecified site C75.1
  adrenal cortical C74.0- ☑
  alveolar — *see* Neoplasm, lung, malignant
  apocrine
    breast — *see* Neoplasm, breast, malignant
    in situ
      breast D05.8- ☑
      specified site NEC — *see* Neoplasm, skin, in situ
      unspecified site D04.9
    specified site NEC — *see* Neoplasm, skin, malignant
    unspecified site C44.99
  basal cell
    specified site — *see* Neoplasm, skin, malignant
    unspecified site C08.9
  basophil
    specified site — *see* Neoplasm, malignant, by site
    unspecified site C75.1
  bile duct type C22.1
    liver C22.1
    specified site NEC — *see* Neoplasm, malignant, by site
    unspecified site C22.1
  bronchiolar — *see* Neoplasm, lung, malignant
  bronchioloalveolar — *see* Neoplasm, lung, malignant
  ceruminous C44.29- ☑
  cervix, in situ — *see also* Carcinoma, cervix uteri, in situ D06.9
  chromophobe
    specified site — *see* Neoplasm, malignant, by site
    unspecified site C75.1
  diffuse type
    specified site — *see* Neoplasm, malignant, by site
    unspecified site C16.9
  duct
    infiltrating
      with Paget's disease — *see* Neoplasm, breast, malignant
      specified site — *see* Neoplasm, malignant, by site
      unspecified site (female) C50.91- ☑
        male C50.92- ☑
    specified site — *see* Neoplasm, malignant, by site
    unspecified site
      female C56.9
      male C61
  eosinophil
    specified site — *see* Neoplasm, malignant, by site
    unspecified site C75.1
  follicular
    with papillary C73
    moderately differentiated C73
    specified site — *see* Neoplasm, malignant, by site
    trabecular C73
    unspecified site C73
    well differentiated C73
  Hurthle cell C73
  in
    adenomatous
      polyposis coli C18.9
  infiltrating duct
    with Paget's disease — *see* Neoplasm, breast, malignant
    specified site — *see* Neoplasm, by site, malignant
    unspecified site (female) C50.91- ☑
      male C50.92- ☑
  inflammatory
    specified site — *see* Neoplasm, by site, malignant
    unspecified site (female) C50.91- ☑

Adenocarcinoma — *continued*
  inflammatory — *continued*
    unspecified site — *continued*
      male C50.92- ☑
  intestinal type
    specified site — *see* Neoplasm, by site, malignant
    unspecified site C16.9
  intracystic papillary
  intraductal
    breast D05.1- ☑
    noninfiltrating
      breast D05.1- ☑
      papillary
        with invasion
          specified site — *see* Neoplasm, by site, malignant
          unspecified site (female) C50.91- ☑
            male C50.92- ☑
        breast D05.1- ☑
        specified site NEC — *see* Neoplasm, in situ, by site
        unspecified site D05.1- ☑
      specified site NEC — *see* Neoplasm, in situ, by site
      unspecified site D05.1- ☑
    papillary
      with invasion
        specified site — *see* Neoplasm, malignant, by site
        unspecified site (female) C50.91- ☑
          male C50.92- ☑
      breast D05.1- ☑
      specified site — *see* Neoplasm, in situ, by site
      unspecified site D05.1- ☑
    specified site NEC — *see* Neoplasm, in situ, by site
    unspecified site D05.1- ☑
  islet cell
    with exocrine, mixed
      specified site — *see* Neoplasm, malignant, by site
      unspecified site C25.9
    pancreas C25.4
    specified site NEC — *see* Neoplasm, malignant, by site
    unspecified site C25.4
  lobular
    in situ
      breast D05.0 ☑
      specified site NEC — *see* Neoplasm, in situ, by site
      unspecified site D05.0- ☑
    specified site — *see* Neoplasm, malignant, by site
    unspecified site (female) C50.91- ☑
      male C50.92- ☑
  mucoid — *see also* Neoplasm, malignant, by site
    cell
      specified site — *see* Neoplasm, malignant, by site
      unspecified site C75.1
  nonencapsulated sclerosing C73
  papillary
    with follicular C73
    follicular variant C73
    intraductal (noninfiltrating)
      with invasion
        specified site — *see* Neoplasm, malignant, by site
        unspecified site (female) C50.91- ☑
          male C50.92- ☑
      breast D05.1- ☑
      specified site NEC — *see* Neoplasm, in situ, by site
      unspecified site D05.1- ☑
    serous
      specified site — *see* Neoplasm, malignant, by site
      unspecified site C56.9
  papillocystic
    specified site — *see* Neoplasm, malignant, by site
    unspecified site C56.9
  pseudomucinous
    specified site — *see* Neoplasm, malignant, by site
    unspecified site C56.9
  renal cell C64- ☑
  sebaceous — *see* Neoplasm, skin, malignant
  serous — *see also* Neoplasm, malignant, by site

Adenocarcinoma — *continued*
  serous — *see also* Neoplasm, malignant, by site — *continued*
    papillary
      specified site — *see* Neoplasm, malignant, by site
      unspecified site C56.9
  sweat gland — *see* Neoplasm, skin, malignant
  water-clear cell C75.0
Adenocarcinoma-in-situ — *see also* Neoplasm, in situ, by site
  breast D05.9- ☑
Adenofibroma
  clear cell — *see* Neoplasm, benign, by site
  endometrioid D27.9
    borderline malignancy D39.10
    malignant C56- ☑
  mucinous
    specified site — *see* Neoplasm, benign, by site
    unspecified site D27.9
  papillary
    specified site — *see* Neoplasm, benign, by site
    unspecified site D27.9
  prostate — *see* Enlargement, enlarged, prostate
  serous
    specified site — *see* Neoplasm, benign, by site
    unspecified site D27.9
  specified site — *see* Neoplasm, benign, by site
  unspecified site D27.9
Adenofibrosis
  breast — *see* Fibroadenosis, breast
  endometrioid N80.0
Adenoiditis (chronic) J35.02
  with tonsillitis J35.03
  acute J03.90
    recurrent J03.91
    specified organism NEC J03.80
      recurrent J03.81
    staphylococcal J03.80
      recurrent J03.81
    streptococcal J03.00
      recurrent J03.01
Adenoids — *see* condition
Adenolipoma — *see* Neoplasm, benign, by site
Adenolipomatosis, Launois-Bensaude E88.89
Adenolymphoma
  specified site — *see* Neoplasm, benign, by site
  unspecified site D11.9
Adenoma — *see also* Neoplasm, benign, by site
  acidophil
    specified site — *see* Neoplasm, benign, by site
    unspecified site D35.2
  acidophil-basophil, mixed
    specified site — *see* Neoplasm, benign, by site
    unspecified site D35.2
  adrenal (cortical) D35.00
    clear cell D35.00
    compact cell D35.00
    glomerulosa cell D35.00
    heavily pigmented variant D35.00
    mixed cell D35.00
  alpha-cell
    pancreas D13.7
    specified site NEC — *see* Neoplasm, benign, by site
    unspecified site D13.7
  alveolar D14.30
  apocrine
    breast D24- ☑
    specified site NEC — *see* Neoplasm, skin, benign, by site
    unspecified site D23.9
  basal cell D11.9
  basophil
    specified site — *see* Neoplasm, benign, by site
    unspecified site D35.2
  basophil-acidophil, mixed
    specified site — *see* Neoplasm, benign, by site
    unspecified site D35.2
  beta-cell
    pancreas D13.7
    specified site NEC — *see* Neoplasm, benign, by site
    unspecified site D13.7
  bile duct D13.4
    common D13.5
    extrahepatic D13.5
    intrahepatic D13.4
    specified site NEC — *see* Neoplasm, benign, by site
    unspecified site D13.4

Adenoma — *continued*
  black D35.00
  bronchial D38.1
    cylindroid type — *see* Neoplasm, lung, malignant
  ceruminous D23.2- ☑
  chief cell D35.1
  chromophobe
    specified site — *see* Neoplasm, benign, by site
    unspecified site D35.2
  colloid
    specified site — *see* Neoplasm, benign, by site
    unspecified site D34
  duct
  eccrine, papillary — *see* Neoplasm, skin, benign
  endocrine, multiple
    single specified site — *see* Neoplasm, uncertain
      behavior, by site
    two or more specified sites D44- ☑
    unspecified site D44.9
  endometrioid — *see also* Neoplasm, benign
    borderline malignancy — *see* Neoplasm, uncertain
      behavior, by site
  eosinophil
    specified site — *see* Neoplasm, benign, by site
    unspecified site D35.2
  fetal
    specified site — *see* Neoplasm, benign, by site
    unspecified site D34
  follicular
    specified site — *see* Neoplasm, benign, by site
    unspecified site D34
  hepatocellular D13.4
  Hurthle cell D34
  islet cell
    pancreas D13.7
    specified site NEC — *see* Neoplasm, benign, by site
    unspecified site D13.7
  liver cell D13.4
  macrofollicular
    specified site — *see* Neoplasm, benign, by site
    unspecified site D34
  malignant, malignum — *see* Neoplasm, malignant, by
    site
  microcystic
    pancreas D13.6
    specified site NEC — *see* Neoplasm, benign, by site
    unspecified site D13.6
  microfollicular
    specified site — *see* Neoplasm, benign, by site
    unspecified site D34
  mucoid cell
    specified site — *see* Neoplasm, benign, by site
    unspecified site D35.2
  multiple endocrine
    single specified site — *see* Neoplasm, uncertain
      behavior, by site
    two or more specified sites D44- ☑
    unspecified site D44.9
  nipple D24- ☑
  papillary — *see also* Neoplasm, benign, by site
    eccrine — *see* Neoplasm, skin, benign, by site
  Pick's tubular
    specified site — *see* Neoplasm, benign, by site
    unspecified site
      female D27.9
      male D29.20
  pleomorphic
    carcinoma in — *see* Neoplasm, salivary gland, ma-
      lignant
    specified site — *see* Neoplasm, malignant, by
      site
    unspecified site C08.9
  polypoid — *see also* Neoplasm, benign
    adenocarcinoma in — *see* Neoplasm, malignant, by
      site
    adenocarcinoma in situ — *see* Neoplasm, in situ, by
      site
  prostate — *see* Neoplasm, benign, prostate
  rete cell D29.20
  sebaceous — *see* Neoplasm, skin, benign
  Sertoli cell
    specified site — *see* Neoplasm, benign, by site
    unspecified site
      female D27.9
      male D29.20
  skin appendage — *see* Neoplasm, skin, benign
  sudoriferous gland — *see* Neoplasm, skin, benign
  sweat gland — *see* Neoplasm, skin, benign

Adenoma — *continued*
  testicular
    specified site — *see* Neoplasm, benign, by site
    unspecified site
      female D27.9
      male D29.20
  tubular — *see also* Neoplasm, benign, by site
    adenocarcinoma in — *see* Neoplasm, malignant, by
      site
    adenocarcinoma in situ — *see* Neoplasm, in situ, by
      site
    Pick's
      specified site — *see* Neoplasm, benign, by site
      unspecified site
        female D27.9
        male D29.20
  tubulovillous — *see also* Neoplasm, benign, by site
    adenocarcinoma in — *see* Neoplasm, malignant, by
      site
    adenocarcinoma in situ — *see* Neoplasm, in situ, by
      site
  villous — *see* Neoplasm, uncertain behavior, by site
    adenocarcinoma in — *see* Neoplasm, malignant, by
      site
    adenocarcinoma in situ — *see* Neoplasm, in situ, by
      site
  water-clear cell D35.1
Adenomatosis
  endocrine (multiple) E31.20
    single specified site — *see* Neoplasm, uncertain
      behavior, by site
  erosive of nipple D24- ☑
  pluriendocrine — *see* Adenomatosis, endocrine
  pulmonary D38.1
    malignant — *see* Neoplasm, lung, malignant
  specified site — *see* Neoplasm, benign, by site
  unspecified site D12.6
Adenomatous
  goiter (nontoxic) E04.9
    with hyperthyroidism — *see* Hyperthyroidism, with,
      goiter, nodular
    toxic — *see* Hyperthyroidism, with, goiter, nodular
Adenomyoma — *see also* Neoplasm, benign, by site
  prostate — *see* Enlarged, prostate
Adenomyometritis N80.0
Adenomyosis N80.0
Adenopathy (lymph gland) R59.9
  generalized R59.1
  inguinal R59.0
  localized R59.0
  mediastinal R59.0
  mesentery R59.0
  syphilitic (secondary) A51.49
  tracheobronchial R59.0
    tuberculous A15.4
      primary (progressive) A15.7
  tuberculous — *see also* Tuberculosis, lymph gland
    tracheobronchial A15.4
      primary (progressive) A15.7
Adenosalpingitis — *see* Salpingitis
Adenosarcoma — *see* Neoplasm, malignant, by site
Adenosclerosis I88.8
Adenosis (sclerosing) breast — *see* Fibroadenosis, breast
Adenovirus, as cause of disease classified elsewhere
  B97.0
Adentia (complete) (partial) — *see* Absence, teeth
Adherent — *see also* Adhesions
  labia (minora) N90.89
  pericardium (nonrheumatic) I31.0
    rheumatic I09.2
  placenta (with hemorrhage) O72.0
    without hemorrhage O73.0
  prepuce, newborn N47.0
  scar (skin) L90.5
  tendon in scar L90.5
Adhesions, adhesive (postinfective) K66.0
  with intestinal obstruction K56.50
    complete K56.52
    incomplete K56.51
    partial K56.51
  abdominal (wall) — *see* Adhesions, peritoneum
  appendix K38.8
  bile duct (common) (hepatic) K83.8
  bladder (sphincter) N32.89
  bowel — *see* Adhesions, peritoneum
  cardiac I31.0
    rheumatic I09.2
  cecum — *see* Adhesions, peritoneum

Adhesions, adhesive — *continued*
  cervicovaginal N88.1
    congenital Q52.8
    postpartal O90.89
      old N88.1
  cervix N88.1
  ciliary body NEC — *see* Adhesions, iris
  clitoris N90.89
  colon — *see* Adhesions, peritoneum
  common duct K83.8
  congenital — *see also* Anomaly, by site
    fingers — *see* Syndactylism, complex, fingers
    omental, anomalous Q43.3
    peritoneal Q43.3
    tongue (to gum or roof of mouth) Q38.3
  conjunctiva (acquired) H11.21- ☑
    congenital Q15.8
  cystic duct K82.8
  diaphragm — *see* Adhesions, peritoneum
  due to foreign body — *see* Foreign body
  duodenum — *see* Adhesions, peritoneum
  ear
    middle H74.1- ☑
  epididymis N50.89
  epidural — *see* Adhesions, meninges
  epiglottis J38.7
  eyelid H02.59
  female pelvis N73.6
  gallbladder K82.8
  globe H44.89
  heart I31.0
    rheumatic I09.2
  ileocecal (coil) — *see* Adhesions, peritoneum
  ileum — *see* Adhesions, peritoneum
  intestine — *see also* Adhesions, peritoneum
    with obstruction K56.50
      complete K56.52
      incomplete K56.51
      partial K56.51
  intra-abdominal — *see* Adhesions, peritoneum
  iris H21.50- ☑
    anterior H21.51- ☑
    goniosynechiae H21.52- ☑
    posterior H21.54- ☑
    to corneal graft T85.898 ☑
  joint — *see* Ankylosis
    knee M23.8X ☑
    temporomandibular M26.61- ☑
  labium (majus) (minus), congenital Q52.5
  liver — *see* Adhesions, peritoneum
  lung J98.4
  mediastinum J98.59
  meninges (cerebral) (spinal) G96.12
    congenital Q07.8
    tuberculous (cerebral) (spinal) A17.0
  mesenteric — *see* Adhesions, peritoneum
  nasal (septum) (to turbinates) J34.89
  ocular muscle — *see* Strabismus, mechanical
  omentum — *see* Adhesions, peritoneum
  ovary N73.6
    congenital (to cecum, kidney or omentum) Q50.3
  paraovarian N73.6
  pelvic (peritoneal)
    female N73.6
      postprocedural N99.4
    male — *see* Adhesions, peritoneum
    postpartal (old) N73.6
    tuberculous A18.17
  penis to scrotum (congenital) Q55.8
  periappendiceal — *see also* Adhesions, peritoneum
  pericardium (nonrheumatic) I31.0
    focal I31.8
    rheumatic I09.2
    tuberculous A18.84
  pericholecystic K82.8
  perigastric — *see* Adhesions, peritoneum
  periovarian N73.6
  periprostatic N42.89
  perirectal — *see* Adhesions, peritoneum
  perirenal N28.89
  peritoneum, peritoneal (postinfective) K66.0
    with obstruction (intestinal) K56.50
      complete K56.52
      incomplete K56.51
      partial K56.51
    congenital Q43.3
    pelvic, female N73.6
      postprocedural N99.4

Adhesions, adhesive — *continued*
  peritoneum, peritoneal — *continued*
    postpartal, pelvic N73.6
    postprocedural K66.0
    to uterus N73.6
  peritubal N73.6
  periureteral N28.89
  periuterine N73.6
  perivesical N32.89
  perivesicular (seminal vesicle) N50.89
  pleura, pleuritic J94.8
    tuberculous NEC A15.6
  pleuropericardial J94.8
  postoperative (gastrointestinal tract) K66.0
    with obstruction — *see also* Obstruction, intestine, postoperative K91.30
    due to foreign body accidentally left in wound — *see* Foreign body, accidentally left during a procedure
    pelvic peritoneal N99.4
    urethra — *see* Stricture, urethra, postprocedural
    vagina N99.2
  postpartal, old (vulva or perineum) N90.89
  preputial, prepuce N47.5
  pulmonary J98.4
  pylorus — *see* Adhesions, peritoneum
  sciatic nerve — *see* Lesion, nerve, sciatic
  seminal vesicle N50.89
  shoulder (joint) — *see* Capsulitis, adhesive
  sigmoid flexure — *see* Adhesions, peritoneum
  spermatic cord (acquired) N50.89
    congenital Q55.4
  spinal canal G96.12
  stomach — *see* Adhesions, peritoneum
  subscapular — *see* Capsulitis, adhesive
  temporomandibular M26.61- ☑
  tendinitis (*see also* Tenosynovitis, specified type NEC)
    shoulder — *see* Capsulitis, adhesive
  testis N44.8
  tongue, congenital (to gum or roof of mouth) Q38.3
    acquired K14.8
  trachea J39.8
  tubo-ovarian N73.6
  tunica vaginalis N44.8
  uterus N73.6
    internal N85.6
    to abdominal wall N73.6
  vagina (chronic) N89.5
    postoperative N99.2
  vitreomacular H43.82- ☑
  vitreous H43.89
  vulva N90.89

Adiaspiromycosis B48.8
Adie (-Holmes) **pupil or syndrome** — *see* Anomaly, pupil, function, tonic pupil
Adiponecrosis neonatorum P83.88
Adiposis — *see also* Obesity
  cerebralis E23.6
  dolorosa E88.2
Adiposity — *see also* Obesity
  heart — *see* Degeneration, myocardial
  localized E65
Adiposogenital dystrophy E23.6
Adjustment
  disorder — *see* Disorder, adjustment
  implanted device — *see* Encounter (for), adjustment (of)
  prosthesis, external — *see* Fitting
  reaction — *see* Disorder, adjustment
Administration of tPA (rtPA) in a different facility within the last 24 hours prior to admission to current facility Z92.82
Admission (for) — *see also* Encounter (for)
  adjustment (of)
    artificial
      arm Z44.00- ☑
        complete Z44.01- ☑
        partial Z44.02- ☑
      eye Z44.2 ☑
      leg Z44.10- ☑
        complete Z44.11- ☑
        partial Z44.12- ☑
    brain neuropacemaker Z46.2
      implanted Z45.42
    breast
      implant Z45.81 ☑
      prosthesis (external) Z44.3 ☑

Admission — *continued*
  adjustment — *continued*
    colostomy belt Z46.89
    contact lenses Z46.0
    cystostomy device Z46.6
    dental prosthesis Z46.3
    device NEC
      abdominal Z46.89
      implanted Z45.89
        cardiac Z45.09
          defibrillator (with synchronous cardiac pacemaker) Z45.02
          pacemaker (cardiac resynchronization therapy (CRT-P)) Z45.018
            pulse generator Z45.010
          resynchronization therapy defibrillator (CRT-D) Z45.02
        hearing device Z45.328
          bone conduction Z45.320
          cochlear Z45.321
        infusion pump Z45.1
        nervous system Z45.49
          CSF drainage Z45.41
          hearing device — *see* Admission, adjustment, device, implanted, hearing device
          neuropacemaker Z45.42
          visual substitution Z45.31
        specified NEC Z45.89
        vascular access Z45.2
        visual substitution Z45.31
    nervous system Z46.2
      implanted — *see* Admission, adjustment, device, implanted, nervous system
    orthodontic Z46.4
    prosthetic Z44.9
      arm — *see* Admission, adjustment, artificial, arm
      breast Z44.3 ☑
      dental Z46.3
      eye Z44.2 ☑
      leg — *see* Admission, adjustment, artificial, leg
      specified type NEC Z44.8
    substitution
      auditory Z46.2
        implanted — *see* Admission, adjustment, device, implanted, hearing device
      nervous system Z46.2
        implanted — *see* Admission, adjustment, device, implanted, nervous system
      visual Z46.2
        implanted Z45.31
    urinary Z46.6
  hearing aid Z46.1
    implanted — *see* Admission, adjustment, device, implanted, hearing device
  ileostomy device Z46.89
  intestinal appliance or device NEC Z46.89
  neuropacemaker (brain) (peripheral nerve) (spinal cord) Z46.2
    implanted Z45.42
  orthodontic device Z46.4
  orthopedic (brace) (cast) (device) (shoes) Z46.89
  pacemaker (cardiac resynchronization therapy (CRT-P))
    cardiac Z45.018
      pulse generator Z45.010
    nervous system Z46.2
      implanted Z45.42
  portacath (port-a-cath) Z45.2
  prosthesis Z44.9
    arm — *see* Admission, adjustment, artificial, arm
    breast Z44.3 ☑
    dental Z46.3
    eye Z44.2 ☑
    leg — *see* Admission, adjustment, artificial, leg
    specified NEC Z44.8
  spectacles Z46.0
  aftercare — *see also* Aftercare Z51.89
    postpartum
      immediately after delivery Z39.0
      routine follow-up Z39.2
    radiation therapy (antineoplastic) Z51.0
  attention to artificial opening (of) Z43.9
    artificial vagina Z43.7
    colostomy Z43.3
    cystostomy Z43.5

Admission — *continued*
  attention to artificial opening — *continued*
    enterostomy Z43.4
    gastrostomy Z43.1
    ileostomy Z43.2
    jejunostomy Z43.4
    nephrostomy Z43.6
    specified site NEC Z43.8
      intestinal tract Z43.4
      urinary tract Z43.6
    tracheostomy Z43.0
    ureterostomy Z43.6
    urethrostomy Z43.6
  breast augmentation or reduction Z41.1
  breast reconstruction following mastectomy Z42.1
  change of
    dressing (nonsurgical) Z48.00
    neuropacemaker device (brain) (peripheral nerve) (spinal cord) Z46.2
      implanted Z45.42
    surgical dressing Z48.01
  circumcision, ritual or routine (in absence of diagnosis) Z41.2
  clinical research investigation (control) (normal comparison) (participant) Z00.6
  contraceptive management Z30.9
  cosmetic surgery NEC Z41.1
  counseling — *see also* Counseling
    dietary Z71.3
    gestational carrier Z31.7
    HIV Z71.7
    human immunodeficiency virus Z71.7
    nonattending third party Z71.0
    procreative management NEC Z31.69
  delivery, full-term, uncomplicated O80
    cesarean, without indication O82
  desensitization to allergens Z51.6
  dietary surveillance and counseling Z71.3
  ear piercing Z41.3
  examination at health care facility (adult) — *see also* Examination Z00.00
    with abnormal findings Z00.01
    clinical research investigation (control) (normal comparison) (participant) Z00.6
    dental Z01.20
      with abnormal findings Z01.21
    donor (potential) Z00.5
    ear Z01.10
      with abnormal findings NEC Z01.118
    eye Z01.00
      with abnormal findings Z01.01
      following failed vision screening Z01.020
        with abnormal findings Z01.021
    general, specified reason NEC Z00.8
    hearing Z01.10
      with abnormal findings NEC Z01.118
      infant or child (over 28 days old) Z00.129
        with abnormal findings Z00.121
    postpartum checkup Z39.2
    psychiatric (general) Z00.8
      requested by authority Z04.6
    vision Z01.00
      with abnormal findings Z01.01
      following failed vision screening Z01.020
        with abnormal findings Z01.021
      infant or child (over 28 days old) Z00.129
        with abnormal findings Z00.121
  fitting (of)
    artificial
      arm — *see* Admission, adjustment, artificial, arm
      eye Z44.2 ☑
      leg — *see* Admission, adjustment, artificial, leg
    brain neuropacemaker Z46.2
      implanted Z45.42
    breast prosthesis (external) Z44.3 ☑
    colostomy belt Z46.89
    contact lenses Z46.0
    cystostomy device Z46.6
    dental prosthesis Z46.3
    dentures Z46.3
    device NEC
      abdominal Z46.89
      nervous system Z46.2
        implanted — *see* Admission, adjustment, device, implanted, nervous system
      orthodontic Z46.4
      prosthetic Z44.9
        breast Z44.3 ☑

Admission — *continued*
  fitting — *continued*
    device — *continued*
      prosthetic — *continued*
        dental Z46.3
        eye Z44.2 ☑
      substitution
        auditory Z46.2
          implanted — *see* Admission, adjustment,
            device, implanted, hearing device
        nervous system Z46.2
          implanted — *see* Admission, adjustment,
            device, implanted, nervous system
        visual Z46.2
          implanted Z45.31
    hearing aid Z46.1
    ileostomy device Z46.89
    intestinal appliance or device NEC Z46.89
    neuropacemaker (brain) (peripheral nerve) (spinal
      cord) Z46.2
      implanted Z45.42
    orthodontic device Z46.4
    orthopedic device (brace) (cast) (shoes) Z46.89
    prosthesis Z44.9
      arm — *see* Admission, adjustment, artificial, arm
      breast Z44.3 ☑
      dental Z46.3
      eye Z44.2 ☑
      leg — *see* Admission, adjustment, artificial, leg
      specified type NEC Z44.8
    spectacles Z46.0
  follow-up examination Z09
  intrauterine device management Z30.431
    initial prescription Z30.014
  mental health evaluation Z00.8
    requested by authority Z04.6
  observation — *see* Observation
  Papanicolaou smear, cervix Z12.4
    for suspected malignant neoplasm Z12.4
  plastic and reconstructive surgery following medical
    procedure or healed injury NEC Z42.8
  plastic surgery, cosmetic NEC Z41.1
  postpartum observation
    immediately after delivery Z39.0
    routine follow-up Z39.2
  poststerilization (for restoration) Z31.0
    aftercare Z31.42
  procreative management Z31.9
  prophylactic (measure) — *see also* Encounter, prophy-
    lactic measures
    organ removal Z40.00
      breast Z40.01
      fallopian tube(s) Z40.03
        with ovary(s) Z40.02
      ovary(s) Z40.02
      specified organ NEC Z40.09
      testes Z40.09
  vaccination Z23
  psychiatric examination (general) Z00.8
    requested by authority Z04.6
  radiation therapy (antineoplastic) Z51.0
  reconstructive surgery following medical procedure or
    healed injury NEC Z42.8
  removal of
    cystostomy catheter Z43.5
    drains Z48.03
    dressing (nonsurgical) Z48.00
    implantable subdermal contraceptive Z30.46
    intrauterine contraceptive device Z30.432
    neuropacemaker (brain) (peripheral nerve) (spinal
      cord) Z46.2
      implanted Z45.42
    staples Z48.02
    surgical dressing Z48.01
    sutures Z48.02
    ureteral stent Z46.6
  respirator [ventilator] use during power failure Z99.12
  restoration of organ continuity (poststerilization) Z31.0
    aftercare Z31.42
  sensitivity test — *see also* Test, skin
    allergy NEC Z01.82
    Mantoux Z11.1
  tuboplasty following previous sterilization Z31.0
    aftercare Z31.42
  vasoplasty following previous sterilization Z31.0
    aftercare Z31.42
  vision examination Z01.00
    with abnormal findings Z01.01

Admission — *continued*
  vision examination — *continued*
    following failed vision screening Z01.020
      with abnormal findings Z01.021
    infant or child (over 28 days old) Z00.129
      with abnormal findings Z00.121
  waiting period for admission to other facility Z75.1
Adnexitis (suppurative) — *see* Salpingo-oophoritis
Adolescent X-linked adrenoleukodystrophy E71.521
Adrenal (gland) — *see* condition
Adrenalism, tuberculous A18.7
Adrenalitis, adrenitis E27.8
  autoimmune E27.1
  meningococcal, hemorrhagic A39.1
Adrenarche, premature E27.0
Adrenocortical syndrome — *see* Cushing's, syndrome
Adrenogenital syndrome E25.9
  acquired E25.8
  congenital E25.0
  salt loss E25.0
Adrenogenitalism, congenital E25.0
Adrenoleukodystrophy E71.529
  neonatal E71.511
  X-linked E71.529
    Addison only phenotype E71.528
    Addison-Schilder E71.528
    adolescent E71.521
    adrenomyeloneuropathy E71.522
    childhood cerebral E71.520
    other specified E71.528
Adrenomyeloneuropathy E71.522
Adventitious bursa — *see* Bursopathy, specified type
    NEC
Adverse effect — *see* Table of Drugs and Chemicals,
    categories T36-T50, with 6th character 5
Advice — *see* Counseling
Adynamia (episodica) (hereditary) (periodic) G72.3
Aeration lung imperfect, newborn — *see* Atelectasis
Aerobullosis T70.3 ☑
Aerocele — *see* Embolism, air
Aerodermectasia
  subcutaneous (traumatic) T79.7 ☑
Aerodontalgia T70.29 ☑
Aeroembolism T70.3 ☑
Aerogenes capsulatus infection A48.0
Aero-otitis media T70.0 ☑
Aerophagy, aerophagia (psychogenic) F45.8
Aerophobia F40.228
Aerosinusitis T70.1 ☑
Aerotitis T70.0 ☑
Affection — *see* Disease
Afibrinogenemia — *see also* Defect, coagulation D68.8
  acquired D65
  congenital D68.2
  following ectopic or molar pregnancy O08.1
  in abortion — *see* Abortion, by type, complicated by,
    afibrinogenemia
  puerperal O72.3
African
  sleeping sickness B56.9
  tick fever A68.1
  trypanosomiasis B56.9
    gambian B56.0
    rhodesian B56.1
Aftercare — *see also* Care Z51.89
  following surgery (for) (on)
    amputation Z47.81
    attention to
      drains Z48.03
      dressings (nonsurgical) Z48.00
        surgical Z48.01
      sutures Z48.02
    circulatory system Z48.812
    delayed (planned) wound closure Z48.1
    digestive system Z48.815
    explantation of joint prosthesis (staged procedure)
      hip Z47.32
      knee Z47.33
      shoulder Z47.31
    genitourinary system Z48.816
    joint replacement Z47.1
    neoplasm Z48.3
    nervous system Z48.811
    oral cavity Z48.814
    organ transplant
      bone marrow Z48.290
      heart Z48.21
      heart-lung Z48.280

Aftercare — *continued*
  following surgery — *continued*
    organ transplant — *continued*
      kidney Z48.22
      liver Z48.23
      lung Z48.24
      multiple organs NEC Z48.288
      specified NEC Z48.298
    orthopedic NEC Z47.89
    planned wound closure Z48.1
    removal of internal fixation device Z47.2
    respiratory system Z48.813
    scoliosis Z47.82
    sense organs Z48.810
    skin and subcutaneous tissue Z48.817
    specified body system
      circulatory Z48.812
      digestive Z48.815
      genitourinary Z48.816
      nervous Z48.811
      oral cavity Z48.814
      respiratory Z48.813
      sense organs Z48.810
      skin and subcutaneous tissue Z48.817
      teeth Z48.814
    specified NEC Z48.89
    spinal Z47.89
    teeth Z48.814
  fracture — *code to* fracture with seventh character D
  involving
    removal of
      drains Z48.03
      dressings (nonsurgical) Z48.00
      staples Z48.02
      surgical dressings Z48.01
      sutures Z48.02
    neuropacemaker (brain) (peripheral nerve) (spinal cord)
      Z46.2
      implanted Z45.42
    orthopedic NEC Z47.89
  postprocedural — *see* Aftercare, following surgery
After-cataract — *see* Cataract, secondary
Agalactia (primary) O92.3
  elective, secondary or therapeutic O92.5
Agammaglobulinemia (acquired (secondary) (nonfamil
    ial) D80.1
  with
    immunoglobulin-bearing B-lymphocytes D80.1
    lymphopenia D81.9
  autosomal recessive (Swiss type) D80.0
  Bruton's X-linked D80.0
  common variable (CVAgamma) D80.1
  congenital sex-linked D80.0
  hereditary D80.0
  lymphopenic D81.9
  Swiss type (autosomal recessive) D80.0
  X-linked (with growth hormone deficiency) (Bruton)
    D80.0
Aganglionosis (bowel) (colon) Q43.1
Age (old) — *see* Senility
Agenesis
  adrenal (gland) Q89.1
  alimentary tract (complete) (partial) NEC Q45.8
    upper Q40.8
  anus, anal (canal) Q42.3
    with fistula Q42.2
  aorta Q25.41
  appendix Q42.8
  arm (complete) Q71.0- ☑
    with hand present Q71.1- ☑
  artery (peripheral) Q27.9
    brain Q28.3
    coronary Q24.5
    pulmonary Q25.79
    specified NEC Q27.8
    umbilical Q27.0
  auditory (canal) (external) Q16.1
  auricle (ear) Q16.0
  bile duct or passage Q44.5
  bladder Q64.5
  bone Q79.9
  brain Q00.0
    part of Q04.3
  breast (with nipple present) Q83.8
    with absent nipple Q83.0
  bronchus Q32.4
  canaliculus lacrimalis Q10.4
  carpus — *see* Agenesis, hand

☑ **Additional Character Required** — Refer to the Tabular List for Character Selection   ▽ **Subterms under main terms may continue to next column or page**

Agenesis — *continued*
cartilage Q79.9
cecum Q42.8
cerebellum Q04.3
cervix Q51.5
chin Q18.8
cilia Q10.3
circulatory system, part NOS Q28.9
clavicle Q74.0
clitoris Q52.6
coccyx Q76.49
colon Q42.9
  specified NEC Q42.8
corpus callosum Q04.0
cricoid cartilage Q31.8
diaphragm (with hernia) Q79.1
digestive organ(s) or tract (complete) (partial) NEC Q45.8
  upper Q40.8
ductus arteriosus Q28.8
duodenum Q41.0
ear Q16.9
  auricle Q16.0
  lobe Q17.8
ejaculatory duct Q55.4
endocrine (gland) NEC Q89.2
epiglottis Q31.8
esophagus Q39.8
eustachian tube Q16.2
eye Q11.1
  adnexa Q15.8
eyelid (fold) Q10.3
face
  bones NEC Q75.8
  specified part NEC Q18.8
fallopian tube Q50.6
femur — *see* Defect, reduction, lower limb, longitudinal, femur
fibula — *see* Defect, reduction, lower limb, longitudinal, fibula
finger (complete) (partial) — *see* Agenesis, hand
foot (and toes) (complete) (partial) Q72.3- ☑
forearm (with hand present) — *see* Agenesis, arm, with hand present
  and hand Q71.2- ☑
gallbladder Q44.0
gastric Q40.2
genitalia, genital (organ(s))
  female Q52.8
    external Q52.71
    internal NEC Q52.8
  male Q55.8
glottis Q31.8
hair Q84.0
hand (and fingers) (complete) (partial) Q71.3- ☑
heart Q24.8
  valve NEC Q24.8
    pulmonary Q22.0
hepatic Q44.7
humerus — *see* Defect, reduction, upper limb
hymen Q52.4
ileum Q41.2
incus Q16.3
intestine (small) Q41.9
  large Q42.9
    specified NEC Q42.8
iris (dilator fibers) Q13.1
jaw M26.09
jejunum Q41.1
kidney(s) (partial) Q60.2
  bilateral Q60.1
  unilateral Q60.0
labium (majus) (minus) Q52.71
labyrinth, membranous Q16.5
lacrimal apparatus Q10.4
larynx Q31.8
leg (complete) Q72.0- ☑
  with foot present Q72.1- ☑
  lower leg (with foot present) — *see* Agenesis, leg, with foot present
    and foot Q72.2- ☑
lens Q12.3
limb (complete) Q73.0
  lower — *see* Agenesis, leg
  upper — *see* Agenesis, arm
lip Q38.0
liver Q44.7
lung (fissure) (lobe) (bilateral) (unilateral) Q33.3

Agenesis — *continued*
mandible, maxilla M26.09
metacarpus — *see* Agenesis, hand
metatarsus — *see* Agenesis, foot
muscle Q79.8
  eyelid Q10.3
  ocular Q15.8
musculoskeletal system NEC Q79.8
nail(s) Q84.3
neck, part Q18.8
nerve Q07.8
nervous system, part NEC Q07.8
nipple Q83.2
nose Q30.1
nuclear Q07.8
organ
  of Corti Q16.5
  or site not listed — *see* Anomaly, by site
osseous meatus (ear) Q16.1
ovary
  bilateral Q50.02
  unilateral Q50.01
oviduct Q50.6
pancreas Q45.0
parathyroid (gland) Q89.2
parotid gland(s) Q38.4
patella Q74.1
pelvic girdle (complete) (partial) Q74.2
penis Q55.5
pericardium Q24.8
pituitary (gland) Q89.2
prostate Q55.4
punctum lacrimale Q10.4
radioulnar — *see* Defect, reduction, upper limb
radius — *see* Defect, reduction, upper limb, longitudinal, radius
rectum Q42.1
  with fistula Q42.0
renal Q60.2
  bilateral Q60.1
  unilateral Q60.0
respiratory organ NEC Q34.8
rib Q76.6
roof of orbit Q75.8
round ligament Q52.8
sacrum Q76.49
salivary gland Q38.4
scapula Q74.0
scrotum Q55.29
seminal vesicles Q55.4
septum
  atrial Q21.1
  between aorta and pulmonary artery Q21.4
  ventricular Q20.4
shoulder girdle (complete) (partial) Q74.0
skull (bone) Q75.8
  with
    anencephaly Q00.0
    encephalocele — *see* Encephalocele
    hydrocephalus Q03.9
      with spina bifida — *see* Spina bifida, by site, with hydrocephalus
    microcephaly Q02
spermatic cord Q55.4
spinal cord Q06.0
spine Q76.49
spleen Q89.01
sternum Q76.7
stomach Q40.2
submaxillary gland(s) (congenital) Q38.4
tarsus — *see* Agenesis, foot
tendon Q79.8
testicle Q55.0
thymus (gland) Q89.2
thyroid (gland) E03.1
  cartilage Q31.8
tibia — *see* Defect, reduction, lower limb, longitudinal, tibia
tibiofibular — *see* Defect, reduction, lower limb, specified type NEC
toe (and foot) (complete) (partial) — *see* Agenesis, foot
tongue Q38.3
trachea (cartilage) Q32.1
ulna — *see* Defect, reduction, upper limb, longitudinal, ulna
upper limb — *see* Agenesis, arm
ureter Q62.4
urethra Q64.5

Agenesis — *continued*
urinary tract NEC Q64.8
uterus Q51.0
uvula Q38.5
vagina Q52.0
vas deferens Q55.4
vein(s) (peripheral) Q27.9
  brain Q28.3
  great NEC Q26.8
  portal Q26.5
vena cava (inferior) (superior) Q26.8
vermis of cerebellum Q04.3
vertebra Q76.49
vulva Q52.71
Ageusia R43.2
Agitated — *see* condition
Agitation R45.1
Aglossia (congenital) Q38.3
Aglossia-adactylia syndrome Q87.0
Aglycogenosis E74.00
Agnosia (body image) (other senses) (tactile) R48.1
  developmental F88
  verbal R48.1
    auditory R48.1
      developmental F80.2
    developmental F80.2
  visual (object) R48.3
Agoraphobia F40.00
  with panic disorder F40.01
  without panic disorder F40.02
Agrammatism R48.8
Agranulocytopenia — *see* Agranulocytosis
Agranulocytosis (chronic) (cyclical) (genetic) (infantile) (periodic) (pernicious) — *see also* Neutropenia D70.9
  congenital D70.0
  cytoreductive cancer chemotherapy sequela D70.1
  drug-induced D70.2
    due to cytoreductive cancer chemotherapy D70.1
  due to infection D70.3
  secondary D70.4
    drug-induced D70.2
      due to cytoreductive cancer chemotherapy D70.1
Agraphia (absolute) R48.8
  with alexia R48.0
  developmental F81.81
Ague (dumb) — *see* Malaria
Agyria Q04.3
Ahumada-del Castillo syndrome E23.0
Aichomophobia F40.298
AIDS (related complex) B20
Ailment heart — *see* Disease, heart
Ailurophobia F40.218
AIN — *see* Neoplasia, intraepithelial, anal
Ainhum (disease) L94.6
AIPHI (acute idiopathic pulmonary hemorrhage in infants (over 28 days old)) R04.81
Air
  anterior mediastinum J98.2
  compressed, disease T70.3 ☑
  conditioner lung or pneumonitis J67.7
  embolism (artery) (cerebral) (any site) T79.0 ☑
    with ectopic or molar pregnancy O08.2
    due to implanted device NEC — *see* Complications, by site and type, specified NEC
    following
      abortion — *see* Abortion by type, complicated by, embolism
      ectopic or molar pregnancy O08.2
      infusion, therapeutic injection or transfusion T80.0 ☑
    in pregnancy, childbirth or puerperium — *see* Embolism, obstetric
    traumatic T79.0 ☑
  hunger, psychogenic F45.8
  rarefied, effects of — *see* Effect, adverse, high altitude
  sickness T75.3 ☑
Airplane sickness T75.3 ☑
Akathisia (drug-induced) (treatment-induced) G25.71
  neuroleptic induced (acute) G25.71
  tardive G25.71
Akinesia R29.898
Akinetic mutism R41.89
Akureyri's disease G93.3
Alactasia, congenital E73.0
Alagille's syndrome Q44.7
Alastrim B03

Albers-Schönberg syndrome Q78.2
Albert's syndrome — see Tendinitis, Achilles
Albinism, albino E70.30
  with hematologic abnormality E70.339
    Chédiak-Higashi syndrome E70.330
    Hermansky-Pudlak syndrome E70.331
    other specified E70.338
  I E70.320
  II E70.321
  ocular E70.319
    autosomal recessive E70.311
    other specified E70.318
    X-linked E70.310
  oculocutaneous E70.329
    other specified E70.328
    tyrosinase (ty) negative E70.320
    tyrosinase (ty) positive E70.321
  other specified E70.39
Albinismus E70.30
Albright (-McCune)(-Sternberg) syndrome Q78.1
Albuminous — see condition
Albuminuria, albuminuric (acute) (chronic) (subacute)
  — see also Proteinuria R80.9
  complicating pregnancy — see Proteinuria, gestational
  with
    gestational hypertension — see Pre-eclampsia
    pre-existing hypertension — see Hypertension,
      complicating pregnancy, pre-existing,
      with, pre-eclampsia
  gestational — see Proteinuria, gestational
  with
    gestational hypertension — see Pre-eclampsia
    pre-existing hypertension — see Hypertension,
      complicating pregnancy, pre-existing,
      with, pre-eclampsia
  orthostatic R80.2
  postural R80.2
  pre-eclamptic — see Pre-eclampsia
  scarlatinal A38.8
Albuminurophobia F40.298
Alcaptonuria E70.29
Alcohol, alcoholic, alcohol-induced
  addiction (without remission) F10.20
    with remission F10.21
  amnestic disorder, persisting F10.96
    with dependence F10.26
  anxiety disorder F10.980
  bipolar and related disorder F10.94
  brain syndrome, chronic F10.97
    with dependence F10.27
  cardiopathy I42.6
  counseling and surveillance Z71.41
    family member Z71.42
  delirium (acute) (tremens) (withdrawal) F10.231
    with intoxication F10.921
      in
        abuse F10.121
        dependence F10.221
  dementia F10.97
    with dependence F10.27
  depressive disorder F10.94
  deterioration F10.97
    with dependence F10.27
  hallucinosis (acute) F10.951
    in
      abuse F10.151
      dependence F10.251
  insanity F10.959
  intoxication (acute) (without dependence) F10.129
    with
      delirium F10.121
      dependence F10.229
        with delirium F10.221
        uncomplicated F10.220
      uncomplicated F10.120
  jealousy F10.988
  Korsakoff's, Korsakov's, Korsakow's F10.26
  liver K70.9
    acute — see Disease, liver, alcoholic, hepatitis
  major neurocognitive disorder, amnestic-confabulatory
    type F10.96
  major neurocognitive disorder, nonamnestic-confabu-
    latory type F10.97
  mania (acute) (chronic) F10.959
  mild neurocognitive disorder F10.988
  paranoia, paranoid (type) psychosis F10.950
  pellagra E52

Alcohol, alcoholic, alcohol-induced — continued
  poisoning, accidental (acute) NEC — see Table of Drugs
    and Chemicals, alcohol, poisoning
  psychosis — see Psychosis, alcoholic
  psychotic disorder F10.959
  sexual dysfunction F10.981
  sleep disorder F10.982
  withdrawal (without convulsions) F10.239
    with delirium F10.231
Alcoholism (chronic) (without remission) F10.20
  with
    psychosis — see Psychosis, alcoholic
    remission F10.21
  Korsakov's F10.96
    with dependence F10.26
Alder (-Reilly) **anomaly or syndrome** (leukocyte granulation) D72.0
Aldosteronism E26.9
  familial (type I) E26.02
  glucocorticoid-remediable E26.02
  primary (due to (bilateral) adrenal hyperplasia) E26.09
  primary NEC E26.09
  secondary E26.1
  specified NEC E26.89
Aldosteronoma D44.10
Aldrich (-Wiskott) **syndrome** (eczema-thrombocytopenia) D82.0
Alektorophobia F40.218
Aleppo boil B55.1
Aleukemic — see condition
Aleukia
  congenital D70.0
  hemorrhagica D61.9
    congenital D61.09
  splenica D73.1
Alexia R48.0
  developmental F81.0
  secondary to organic lesion R48.0
Algoneurodystrophy M89.00
  ankle M89.07- ☑
  foot M89.07- ☑
  forearm M89.03- ☑
  hand M89.04- ☑
  lower leg M89.06- ☑
  multiple sites M89.0- ☑
  shoulder M89.01- ☑
  specified site NEC M89.08
  thigh M89.05- ☑
  upper arm M89.02- ☑
Algophobia F40.298
Alienation, mental — see Psychosis
Alkalemia E87.3
Alkalosis E87.3
  metabolic E87.3
    with respiratory acidosis E87.4
    of newborn P74.41
  respiratory E87.3
Alkaptonuria E70.29
Allen-Masters syndrome N83.8
Allergy, allergic (reaction) (to) T78.40 ☑
  air-borne substance NEC (rhinitis) J30.89
  alveolitis (extrinsic) J67.9
    due to
      Aspergillus clavatus J67.4
      Cryptostroma corticale J67.6
      organisms (fungal, thermophilic actinomycete)
        growing in ventilation (air conditioning)
        systems J67.7
    specified type NEC J67.8
  anaphylactic reaction or shock T78.2 ☑
  angioneurotic edema T78.3 ☑
  animal (dander) (epidermal) (hair) (rhinitis) J30.81
  bee sting (anaphylactic shock) — see Toxicity, venom,
    arthropod, bee
  biological — see Allergy, drug
  colitis — see also Colitis, allergic K52.29
  dander (animal) (rhinitis) J30.81
  dandruff (rhinitis) J30.81
  dental restorative material (existing) K08.55
  dermatitis — see Dermatitis, contact, allergic
  diathesis — see History, allergy
  drug, medicament & biological (any) (external) (inter-
    nal) T78.40 ☑
    correct substance properly administered — see Ta-
      ble of Drugs and Chemicals, by drug, adverse
      effect

Allergy, allergic — continued
  drug, medicament & biological — continued
    wrong substance given or taken NEC (by accident)
      — see Table of Drugs and Chemicals, by drug
      poisoning
  due to pollen J30.1
  dust (house) (stock) (rhinitis) J30.89
    with asthma — see Asthma, allergic extrinsic
  eczema — see Dermatitis, contact, allergic
  epidermal (animal) (rhinitis) J30.81
  feathers (rhinitis) J30.89
  food (any) (ingested) NEC T78.1 ☑
    anaphylactic shock — see Shock, anaphylactic, du
      to food
    dermatitis — see Dermatitis, due to, food
    dietary counseling and surveillance Z71.3
    in contact with skin L23.6
    rhinitis J30.5
    status (without reaction) Z91.018
      eggs Z91.012
      milk products Z91.011
      peanuts Z91.010
      seafood Z91.013
      specified NEC Z91.018
  gastrointestinal — see also specific type of allergic re
    action
    meaning colitis — see also Colitis, allergic K52.29
    meaning gastroenteritis — see also Gastroenteritis
      allergic K52.29
    meaning other adverse food reaction not elsewhere
      classified T78.1 ☑
  grain J30.1
  grass (hay fever) (pollen) J30.1
    asthma — see Asthma, allergic extrinsic
  hair (animal) (rhinitis) J30.81
  history (of) — see History, allergy
  horse serum — see Allergy, serum
  inhalant (rhinitis) J30.89
    pollen J30.1
  kapok (rhinitis) J30.89
  medicine — see Allergy, drug
  milk protein — see also Allergy, food Z91.011
    anaphylactic reaction T78.07 ☑
    dermatitis L27.2
    enterocolitis syndrome K52.21
    enteropathy K52.22
    gastroenteritis K52.29
    gastroesophageal reflux — see also Reaction, ad-
      verse, food K21.9
      with esophagitis K21.0
    proctocolitis K52.82
  nasal, seasonal due to pollen J30.1
  pneumonia J82
  pollen (any) (hay fever) J30.1
    asthma — see Asthma, allergic extrinsic
  primrose J30.1
  primula J30.1
  proctocolitis K52.82
  purpura D69.0
  ragweed (hay fever) (pollen) J30.1
    asthma — see Asthma, allergic extrinsic
  rose (pollen) J30.1
  seasonal NEC J30.2
  Senecio jacobae (pollen) J30.1
  serum — see also Reaction, serum T80.69 ☑
    anaphylactic shock T80.59 ☑
  shock (anaphylactic) T78.2 ☑
    due to
      administration of blood and blood products
        T80.51 ☑
      adverse effect of correct medicinal substance
        properly administered T88.6 ☑
      immunization T80.52 ☑
      serum NEC T80.59 ☑
      vaccination T80.52 ☑
  specific NEC T78.49 ☑
  tree (any) (hay fever) (pollen) J30.1
    asthma — see Asthma, allergic extrinsic
  upper respiratory J30.9
  urticaria L50.0
  vaccine — see Allergy, serum
  wheat — see Allergy, food
Allescheriasis B48.2
Alligator skin disease Q80.9
Allocheiria, allochiria R20.8
Almeida's disease — see Paracoccidioidomycosis
Alopecia (hereditaria) (seborrheica) L65.9

☑ **Additional Character Required** — Refer to the Tabular List for Character Selection   ▽ **Subterms under main terms may continue to next column or page**

Alopecia — *continued*
androgenic L64.9
  drug-induced L64.0
  specified NEC L64.8
areata L63.9
  ophiasis L63.2
  specified NEC L63.8
  totalis L63.0
  universalis L63.1
cicatricial L66.9
  specified NEC L66.8
circumscripta L63.9
congenital, congenitalis Q84.0
due to cytotoxic drugs NEC L65.8
mucinosa L65.2
postinfective NEC L65.8
postpartum L65.0
premature L64.8
specific (syphilitic) A51.32
specified NEC L65.8
syphilitic (secondary) A51.32
totalis (capitis) L63.0
universalis (entire body) L63.1
X-ray L58.1
Alpers' disease G31.81
Alpine sickness T70.29 ☑
Alport syndrome Q87.81
ALTE (apparent life threatening event) **in newborn and infant** R68.13
Alteration (of), Altered
awareness
  transient R40.4
  unintended under general anesthesia, during procedure T88.53 ☑
mental status R41.82
pattern of family relationships affecting child Z62.898
sensation
  following
    cerebrovascular disease I69.998
      cerebral infarction I69.398
      intracerebral hemorrhage I69.198
      nontraumatic intracranial hemorrhage NEC I69.298
      specified disease NEC I69.898
      subarachnoid hemorrhage I69.098
Alternating — *see* condition
Altitude, high (effects) — *see* Effect, adverse, high altitude
Aluminosis (of lung) J63.0
Alveolitis
allergic (extrinsic) — *see* Pneumonitis, hypersensitivity
due to
  Aspergillus clavatus J67.4
  Cryptostroma corticale J67.6
fibrosing (cryptogenic) (idiopathic) J84.112
jaw M27.3
sicca dolorosa M27.3
Alveolus, alveolar — *see* condition
Alymphocytosis D72.810
thymic (with immunodeficiency) D82.1
Alymphoplasia, thymic D82.1
Alzheimer's disease or sclerosis — *see* Disease, Alzheimer's
Amastia (with nipple present) Q83.8
with absent nipple Q83.0
Amathophobia F40.228
Amaurosis (acquired) (congenital) — *see also* Blindness
fugax G45.3
hysterical F44.6
Leber's congenital H35.50
uremic — *see* Uremia
Amaurotic idiocy (infantile) (juvenile) (late) E75.4
Amaxophobia F40.248
Ambiguous genitalia Q56.4
Amblyopia (congenital) (ex anopsia) (partial) (suppression) H53.00- ☑
anisometropic — *see* Amblyopia, refractive
deprivation H53.01- ☑
hysterical F44.6
nocturnal — *see also* Blindness, night
  vitamin A deficiency E50.5
refractive H53.02- ☑
strabismic H53.03- ☑
suspect H53.04- ☑
tobacco H53.8
toxic NEC H53.8
uremic — *see* Uremia
Ameba, amebic (histolytica) — *see also* Amebiasis

Ameba, amebic — *continued*
abscess (liver) A06.4
Amebiasis A06.9
with abscess — *see* Abscess, amebic
acute A06.0
chronic (intestine) A06.1
  with abscess — *see* Abscess, amebic
cutaneous A06.7
cutis A06.7
cystitis A06.81
genitourinary tract NEC A06.82
hepatic — *see* Abscess, liver, amebic
intestine A06.0
nondysenteric colitis A06.2
skin A06.7
specified site NEC A06.89
Ameboma (of intestine) A06.3
Amelia Q73.0
lower limb — *see* Agenesis, leg
upper limb — *see* Agenesis, arm
Ameloblastoma — *see also* Cyst, calcifying odontogenic
long bones C40.9- ☑
  lower limb C40.2- ☑
  upper limb C40.0- ☑
malignant C41.9
  jaw (bone) (lower) C41.1
    upper C41.0
tibial C40.2- ☑
Amelogenesis imperfecta K00.5
nonhereditaria (segmentalis) K00.4
Amenorrhea N91.2
hyperhormonal E28.8
primary N91.0
secondary N91.1
Amentia — *see* Disability, intellectual
Meynert's (nonalcoholic) F04
American
leishmaniasis B55.2
mountain tick fever A93.2
Ametropia — *see* Disorder, refraction
AMH (asymptomatic microscopic hematuria) R31.21
Amianthosis J61
Amimia R48.8
Amino-acid disorder E72.9
anemia D53.0
Aminoacidopathy E72.9
Aminoaciduria E72.9
Amnesia R41.3
anterograde R41.1
auditory R48.8
dissociative F44.0
  with dissociative fugue F44.1
hysterical F44.0
postictal in epilepsy — *see* Epilepsy
psychogenic F44.0
retrograde R41.2
transient global G45.4
Amnes(t)ic syndrome (post-traumatic) F04
induced by
  alcohol F10.96
    with dependence F10.26
  psychoactive NEC F19.96
    with
      abuse F19.16
      dependence F19.26
  sedative F13.96
    with dependence F13.26
Amnion, amniotic — *see* condition
Amnionitis — *see* Pregnancy, complicated by
Amok F68.8
Amoral traits F60.89
Amphetamine (or other stimulant) **-induced**
anxiety disorder F15.980
bipolar and related disorder F15.94
delirium F15.921
depressive disorder F15.94
obsessive-compulsive and related disorder F15.988
psychotic disorder F15.959
sexual dysfunction F15.981
sleep disorder F15.982
stimulant withdrawal F15.23
Ampulla
lower esophagus K22.8
phrenic K22.8
Amputation — *see also* Absence, by site, acquired
neuroma (postoperative) (traumatic) — *see* Complications, amputation stump, neuroma

Amputation — *continued*
stump (surgical)
  abnormal, painful, or with complication (late) — *see* Complications, amputation stump
  healed or old NOS Z89.9
traumatic (complete) (partial)
  arm (upper) (complete) S48.91- ☑
    at
      elbow S58.01- ☑
        partial S58.02- ☑
      shoulder joint (complete) S48.01- ☑
        partial S48.02- ☑
    between
      elbow and wrist (complete) S58.11- ☑
        partial S58.12- ☑
      shoulder and elbow (complete) S48.11- ☑
        partial S48.12- ☑
    partial S48.92- ☑
  breast (complete) S28.21- ☑
    partial S28.22- ☑
  clitoris (complete) S38.211
    partial S38.212
  ear (complete) S08.11- ☑
    partial S08.12- ☑
  finger (complete) (metacarpophalangeal) S68.11- ☑
    index S68.11- ☑
    little S68.11- ☑
    middle S68.11- ☑
    partial S68.12- ☑
      index S68.12- ☑
      little S68.12- ☑
      middle S68.12- ☑
      ring S68.12- ☑
    ring S68.11- ☑
    thumb — *see* Amputation, traumatic, thumb
    transphalangeal (complete) S68.61- ☑
      index S68.61- ☑
      little S68.61- ☑
      middle S68.61- ☑
      partial S68.62- ☑
        index S68.62- ☑
        little S68.62- ☑
        middle S68.62- ☑
        ring S68.62- ☑
      ring S68.61- ☑
  foot (complete) S98.91- ☑
    at ankle level S98.01- ☑
      partial S98.02- ☑
    midfoot S98.31- ☑
      partial S98.32- ☑
    partial S98.92- ☑
  forearm (complete) S58.91- ☑
    at elbow level (complete) S58.01- ☑
      partial S58.02- ☑
    between elbow and wrist (complete) S58.11- ☑
      partial S58.12- ☑
    partial S58.92- ☑
  genital organ(s) (external)
    female (complete) S38.211 ☑
      partial S38.212 ☑
    male
      penis (complete) S38.221 ☑
        partial S38.222 ☑
      scrotum (complete) S38.231 ☑
        partial S38.232 ☑
      testes (complete) S38.231 ☑
        partial S38.232 ☑
  hand (complete) (wrist level) S68.41- ☑
    finger(s) alone — *see* Amputation, traumatic, finger
    partial S68.42- ☑
    thumb alone — *see* Amputation, traumatic, thumb
    transmetacarpal (complete) S68.71- ☑
      partial S68.72- ☑
  head
    ear — *see* Amputation, traumatic, ear
    nose (partial) S08.812 ☑
      complete S08.811 ☑
    part S08.89 ☑
      scalp S08.0 ☑
  hip (and thigh) (complete) S78.91- ☑
    at hip joint (complete) S78.01- ☑
      partial S78.02- ☑
    between hip and knee (complete) S78.11- ☑
      partial S78.12- ☑

▽ **Subterms under main terms may continue to next column or page**   ☑ **Additional Character Required — Refer to the Tabular List for Character Selection**   **17**

Alopecia — Amputation

Amputation — continued
  traumatic — continued
    hip — continued
      partial S78.92- ☑
    labium (majus) (minus) (complete) S38.21- ☑
      partial S38.21- ☑
    leg (lower) S88.91- ☑
      at knee level S88.01- ☑
        partial S88.02- ☑
      between knee and ankle S88.11- ☑
        partial S88.12- ☑
      partial S88.92- ☑
    nose (partial) S08.812 ☑
      complete S08.811 ☑
    penis (complete) S38.221 ☑
      partial S38.222 ☑
    scrotum (complete) S38.231 ☑
      partial S38.232 ☑
    shoulder — see Amputation, traumatic, arm
      at shoulder joint — see Amputation, traumatic, arm, at shoulder joint
    testes (complete) S38.231 ☑
      partial S38.232 ☑
    thigh — see Amputation, traumatic, hip
    thorax, part of S28.1
      breast — see Amputation, traumatic, breast
    thumb (complete) (metacarpophalangeal) S68.01- ☑
      partial S68.02- ☑
      transphalangeal (complete) S68.51- ☑
        partial S68.52- ☑
    toe (lesser) S98.13- ☑
      great S98.11- ☑
        partial S98.12- ☑
      more than one S98.21- ☑
        partial S98.22- ☑
      partial S98.14- ☑
    vulva (complete) S38.211 ☑
      partial S38.212 ☑
Amputee (bilateral) (old) Z89.9
Amsterdam dwarfism Q87.19
Amusia R48.8
  developmental F80.89
Amyelencephalus, amyelencephaly Q00.0
Amyelia Q06.0
Amygdalitis — see Tonsillitis
Amygdalolith J35.8
Amyloid heart (disease) E85.4 [I43]
Amyloidosis (generalized) (primary) E85.9
  with lung involvement E85.4 [J99]
  familial E85.2
  genetic E85.2
  heart E85.4 [I43]
  hemodialysis-associated E85.3
  light chain (AL) E85.81
  liver E85.4 [K77]
  localized E85.4
  neuropathic heredofamilial E85.1
  non-neuropathic heredofamilial E85.0
  organ limited E85.4
  Portuguese E85.1
  pulmonary E85.4 [J99]
  secondary systemic E85.3
  senile systemic (SSA) E85.82
  skin (lichen) (macular) E85.4 [L99]
  specified NEC E85.89
  subglottic E85.4 [J99]
  wild-type transthyretin-related (ATTR) E85.82
Amylopectinosis (brancher enzyme deficiency) E74.03
Amylophagia — see Pica
Amyoplasia congenita Q79.8
Amyotonia M62.89
  congenita G70.2
Amyotrophia, amyotrophy, amyotrophic G71.8
  congenita Q79.8
  diabetic — see Diabetes, amyotrophy
  lateral sclerosis G12.21
  neuralgic G54.5
  spinal progressive G12.25
Anacidity, gastric K31.83
  psychogenic F45.8
Anaerosis of newborn P28.89
Analbuminemia E88.09
Analgesia — see Anesthesia
Analphalipoproteinemia E78.6
Anaphylactic
  purpura D69.0

Anaphylactic — continued
  shock or reaction — see Shock, anaphylactic
Anaphylactoid shock or reaction — see Shock, anaphylactic
Anaphylactoid syndrome of pregnancy O88.01- ☑
Anaphylaxis — see Shock, anaphylactic
Anaplasia cervix — see also Dysplasia, cervix N87.9
Anaplasmosis, human A77.49
Anarthria R47.1
Anasarca R60.1
  cardiac — see Failure, heart, congestive
  lung J18.2
  newborn P83.2
  nutritional E43
  pulmonary J18.2
  renal N04.9
Anastomosis
  aneurysmal — see Aneurysm
  arteriovenous ruptured brain I60.8
    intracerebral I61.8
    intraparenchymal I61.8
    intraventricular I61.5
    subarachnoid I60.8
  intestinal K63.89
    complicated NEC K91.89
      involving urinary tract N99.89
  retinal and choroidal vessels (congenital) Q14.8
Anatomical narrow angle H40.03- ☑
Ancylostoma, ancylostomiasis (braziliense) (caninum) (ceylanicum) (duodenale) B76.0
  Necator americanus B76.1
Andersen's disease (glycogen storage) E74.09
Anderson-Fabry disease E75.21
Andes disease T70.29 ☑
Andrews' disease (bacterid) L08.89
Androblastoma
  benign
    specified site — see Neoplasm, benign, by site
    unspecified site
      female D27.9
      male D29.20
  malignant
    specified site — see Neoplasm, malignant, by site
    unspecified site
      female C56.9
      male C62.90
  specified site — see Neoplasm, uncertain behavior, by site
  tubular
    with lipid storage
      specified site — see Neoplasm, benign, by site
      unspecified site
        female D27.9
        male D29.20
    specified site — see Neoplasm, benign, by site
    unspecified site
      female D27.9
      male D29.20
  unspecified site
    female D39.10
    male D40.10
Androgen insensitivity syndrome — see also Syndrome, androgen insensitivity E34.50
Androgen resistance syndrome — see also Syndrome, androgen insensitivity E34.50
Android pelvis Q74.2
  with disproportion (fetopelvic) O33.3 ☑
    causing obstructed labor O65.3
Androphobia F40.290
Anectasis, pulmonary (newborn) — see Atelectasis
Anemia (essential) (general) (hemoglobin deficiency) (infantile) (primary) (profound) D64.9
  with (due to) (in)
    disorder of
      anaerobic glycolysis D55.2
      pentose phosphate pathway D55.1
    koilonychia D50.9
  achlorhydric D50.8
  achrestic D53.1
  Addison (-Biermer) (pernicious) D51.0
  agranulocytic — see Agranulocytosis
  amino-acid-deficiency D53.0
  aplastic D61.9
    congenital D61.09
    drug-induced D61.1
    due to
      drugs D61.1
      external agents NEC D61.2

Anemia — continued
  aplastic — continued
    due to — continued
      infection D61.2
      radiation D61.2
    idiopathic D61.3
    red cell (pure) D60.9
      chronic D60.0
      congenital D61.01
      specified type NEC D60.8
      transient D60.1
    specified type NEC D61.89
    toxic D61.2
  aregenerative
    congenital D61.09
  asiderotic D50.9
  atypical (primary) D64.9
  Baghdad spring D55.0
  Balantidium coli A07.0
  Biermer's (pernicious) D51.0
  blood loss (chronic) D50.0
    acute D62
  bothriocephalus B70.0 [D63.8]
  brickmaker's B76.9 [D63.8]
  cerebral I67.89
  childhood D58.9
  chlorotic D50.8
  chronic
    blood loss D50.0
    hemolytic D58.9
      idiopathic D59.9
    simple D53.9
  chronica congenita aregenerativa D61.09
  combined system disease NEC D51.0 [G32.0]
    due to dietary vitamin B12 deficiency D51.3 [G32.]
  complicating pregnancy, childbirth or puerperium – see Pregnancy, complicated by (management affected by), anemia
  congenital P61.4
    aplastic D61.09
    due to isoimmunization NOS P55.9
    dyserythropoietic, dyshematopoietic D64.4
    following fetal blood loss P61.3
    Heinz body D58.2
    hereditary hemolytic NOS D58.9
    pernicious D51.0
    spherocytic D58.0
  Cooley's (erythroblastic) D56.1
  cytogenic D51.0
  deficiency D53.9
    2, 3 diphosphoglycurate mutase D55.2
    2, 3 PG D55.2
    6 phosphogluconate dehydrogenase D55.1
    6-PGD D55.1
    amino-acid D53.0
    combined B12 and folate D53.1
    enzyme D55.9
      drug-induced (hemolytic) D59.2
      glucose-6-phosphate dehydrogenase (G6PD) D55.0
      glycolytic D55.2
      nucleotide metabolism D55.3
      related to hexose monophosphate (HMP) shur pathway NEC D55.1
      specified type NEC D55.8
    erythrocytic glutathione D55.1
    folate D52.9
      dietary D52.0
      drug-induced D52.1
    folic acid D52.9
      dietary D52.0
      drug-induced D52.1
    G SH D55.1
    G6PD D55.0
    GGS-R D55.1
    glucose-6-phosphate dehydrogenase D55.0
    glutathione reductase D55.1
    glyceraldehyde phosphate dehydrogenase D55.2
    hexokinase D55.2
    iron D50.9
      secondary to blood loss (chronic) D50.0
    nutritional D53.9
      with
        poor iron absorption D50.8
        specified deficiency NEC D53.8
    phosphofructo-aldolase D55.2
    phosphoglycerate kinase D55.2
    PK D55.2
    protein D53.0

Anemia — continued
  deficiency — continued
    pyruvate kinase D55.2
    transcobalamin II D51.2
    triose-phosphate isomerase D55.2
    vitamin B12 NOS D51.9
      dietary D51.3
      due to
        intrinsic factor deficiency D51.0
        selective vitamin B12 malabsorption with
          proteinuria D51.1
      pernicious D51.0
      specified type NEC D51.8
  Diamond-Blackfan (congenital hypoplastic) D61.01
  dibothriocephalus B70.0 [D63.8]
  dimorphic D53.1
  diphasic D53.1
  Diphyllobothrium (Dibothriocephalus) B70.0 [D63.8]
  due to (in) (with)
    antineoplastic chemotherapy D64.81
    blood loss (chronic) D50.0
      acute D62
    chemotherapy, antineoplastic D64.81
    chronic disease classified elsewhere NEC D63.8
    chronic kidney disease D63.1
    deficiency
      amino-acid D53.0
      copper D53.8
      folate (folic acid) D52.9
        dietary D52.0
        drug-induced D52.1
      molybdenum D53.8
      protein D53.0
      zinc D53.8
    dietary vitamin B12 deficiency D51.3
    disorder of
      glutathione metabolism D55.1
      nucleotide metabolism D55.3
    drug — see Anemia, by type — see also Table of
      Drugs and Chemicals
    end stage renal disease D63.1
    enzyme disorder D55.9
    fetal blood loss P61.3
    fish tapeworm (D.latum) infestation B70.0 [D63.8]
    hemorrhage (chronic) D50.0
      acute D62
    impaired absorption D50.9
    loss of blood (chronic) D50.0
      acute D62
    myxedema E03.9 [D63.8]
    Necator americanus B76.1 [D63.8]
    prematurity P61.2
    selective vitamin B12 malabsorption with protein-
      uria D51.1
    transcobalamin II deficiency D51.2
  Dyke-Young type (secondary) (symptomatic) D59.1
  dyserythropoietic (congenital) D64.4
  dyshematopoietic (congenital) D64.4
  Egyptian B76.9 [D63.8]
  elliptocytosis — see Elliptocytosis
  enzyme-deficiency, drug-induced D59.2
  epidemic — see also Ancylostomiasis B76.9 [D63.8]
  erythroblastic
    familial D56.1
    newborn — see also Disease, hemolytic P55.9
    of childhood D56.1
  erythrocytic glutathione deficiency D55.1
  erythropoietin-resistant anemia (EPO resistant anemia)
    D63.1
  Faber's (achlorhydric anemia) D50.9
  factitious (self-induced blood letting) D50.0
  familial erythroblastic D56.1
  Fanconi's (congenital pancytopenia) D61.09
  favism D55.0
  fish tapeworm (D. latum) infestation B70.0 [D63.8]
  folate (folic acid) deficiency D52.9
  glucose-6-phosphate dehydrogenase (G6PD) deficiency
    D55.0
  glutathione-reductase deficiency D55.1
  goat's milk D52.0
  granulocytic — see Agranulocytosis
  Heinz body, congenital D58.2
  hemolytic D58.9
    acquired D59.9
      with hemoglobinuria NEC D59.6
      autoimmune NEC D59.1
      infectious D59.4
      specified type NEC D59.8

Anemia — continued
  hemolytic — continued
    acquired — continued
      toxic D59.4
    acute D59.9
      due to enzyme deficiency specified type NEC
        D55.8
      Lederer's D59.1
    autoimmune D59.1
      drug-induced D59.0
    chronic D58.9
      idiopathic D59.9
    cold type (secondary) (symptomatic) D59.1
    congenital (spherocytic) — see Spherocytosis
    due to
      cardiac conditions D59.4
      drugs (nonautoimmune) D59.2
        autoimmune D59.0
      enzyme disorder D55.9
        drug-induced D59.2
      presence of shunt or other internal prosthetic
        device D59.4
    familial D58.9
    hereditary D58.9
      due to enzyme disorder D55.9
        specified type NEC D55.8
      specified type NEC D58.8
    idiopathic (chronic) D59.9
    mechanical D59.4
    microangiopathic D59.4
    nonautoimmune D59.4
      drug-induced D59.2
    nonspherocytic
      congenital or hereditary NEC D55.8
        glucose-6-phosphate dehydrogenase deficien-
          cy D55.0
        pyruvate kinase deficiency D55.2
        type
          I D55.1
          II D55.2
      type
        I D55.1
        II D55.2
    secondary D59.4
      autoimmune D59.1
    specified (hereditary) type NEC D58.8
    Stransky-Regala type — see also Hemoglobinopathy
      D58.8
    symptomatic D59.4
      autoimmune D59.1
    toxic D59.4
    warm type (secondary) (symptomatic) D59.1
  hemorrhagic (chronic) D50.0
    acute D62
  Herrick's D57.1
  hexokinase deficiency D55.2
  hookworm B76.9 [D63.8]
  hypochromic (idiopathic) (microcytic) (normoblastic)
    D50.9
    due to blood loss (chronic) D50.0
      acute D62
    familial sex-linked D64.0
    pyridoxine-responsive D64.3
    sideroblastic, sex-linked D64.0
  hypoplasia, red blood cells D61.9
    congenital or familial D61.01
  hypoplastic (idiopathic) D61.9
    congenital or familial (of childhood) D61.01
  hypoproliferative (refractive) D61.9
  idiopathic D64.9
    aplastic D61.3
    hemolytic, chronic D59.9
  in (due to) (with)
    chronic kidney disease D63.1
    end stage renal disease D63.1
    failure, kidney (renal) D63.1
    neoplastic disease — see also Neoplasm D63.0
  intertropical — see also Ancylostomiasis D63.8
  iron deficiency D50.9
    secondary to blood loss (chronic) D50.0
      acute D62
    specified type NEC D50.8
  Joseph-Diamond-Blackfan (congenital hypoplastic)
    D61.01
  Lederer's (hemolytic) D59.1
  leukoerythroblastic D61.82
  macrocytic D53.9
    nutritional D52.0
    tropical D52.8

Anemia — continued
  malarial — see also Malaria B54 [D63.8]
  malignant (progressive) D51.0
  malnutrition D53.9
  marsh — see also Malaria B54 [D63.8]
  Mediterranean (with other hemoglobinopathy) D56.9
  megaloblastic D53.1
    combined B12 and folate deficiency D53.1
    hereditary D51.1
    nutritional D52.0
    orotic aciduria D53.0
    refractory D53.1
    specified type NEC D53.1
  megalocytic D53.1
  microcytic (hypochromic) D50.9
    due to blood loss (chronic) D50.0
      acute D62
    familial D56.8
  microdrepanocytosis D57.40
  microelliptopoikilocytic (Rietti-Greppi- Micheli) D56.9
  miner's B76.9 [D63.8]
  myelodysplastic D46.9
  myelofibrosis D75.81
  myelogenous D64.89
  myelopathic D64.89
  myelophthisic D61.82
  myeloproliferative D47.Z9 (following D47.4)
  newborn P61.4
    due to
      ABO (antibodies, isoimmunization, maternal/fetal
        incompatibility) P55.1
      Rh (antibodies, isoimmunization, maternal/fetal
        incompatibility) P55.0
    following fetal blood loss P61.3
    posthemorrhagic (fetal) P61.3
  nonspherocytic hemolytic — see Anemia, hemolytic,
    nonspherocytic
  normocytic (infectional) D64.9
    due to blood loss (chronic) D50.0
      acute D62
    myelophthisic D61.82
  nutritional (deficiency) D53.9
    with
      poor iron absorption D50.8
      specified deficiency NEC D53.8
    megaloblastic D52.0
  of prematurity P61.2
  orotaciduric (congenital) (hereditary) D53.0
  osteosclerotic D64.89
  ovalocytosis (hereditary) — see Elliptocytosis
  paludal — see also Malaria B54 [D63.8]
  pernicious (congenital) (malignant) (progressive) D51.0
  pleochromic D64.89
    of sprue D52.8
  posthemorrhagic (chronic) D50.0
    acute D62
    newborn P61.3
  postoperative (postprocedural)
    due to (acute) blood loss D62
      chronic blood loss D50.0
    specified NEC D64.9
  postpartum O90.81
  pressure D64.89
  progressive D64.9
    malignant D51.0
    pernicious D51.0
  protein-deficiency D53.0
  pseudoleukemica infantum D64.89
  pure red cell D60.9
    congenital D61.01
  pyridoxine-responsive D64.3
  pyruvate kinase deficiency D55.2
  refractory D46.4
    with
      excess of blasts D46.20
        1 (RAEB 1) D46.21
        2 (RAEB 2) D46.22
        in transformation (RAEB T) — see Leukemia,
          acute myeloblastic
      hemochromatosis D46.1
      sideroblasts (ring) (RARS) D46.1
    megaloblastic D53.1
    sideroblastic D46.1
    sideropenic D50.9
    without ring sideroblasts, so stated D46.0
    without sideroblasts without excess of blasts D46.0
  Rietti-Greppi-Micheli D56.9
  scorbutic D53.2

Anemia — *continued*
  secondary to
    blood loss (chronic) D50.0
      acute D62
    hemorrhage (chronic) D50.0
      acute D62
  semiplastic D61.89
  sickle-cell — *see* Disease, sickle-cell
  sideroblastic D64.3
    hereditary D64.0
    hypochromic, sex-linked D64.0
    pyridoxine-responsive NEC D64.3
    refractory D46.1
    secondary (due to)
      disease D64.1
      drugs and toxins D64.2
    specified type NEC D64.3
  sideropenic (refractory) D50.9
    due to blood loss (chronic) D50.0
      acute D62
  simple chronic D53.9
  specified type NEC D64.89
  spherocytic (hereditary) — *see* Spherocytosis
  splenic D64.89
  splenomegalic D64.89
  stomatocytosis D58.8
  syphilitic (acquired) (late) A52.79 *[D63.8]*
  target cell D64.89
  thalassemia D56.9
  thrombocytopenic — *see* Thrombocytopenia
  toxic D61.2
  tropical B76.9 *[D63.8]*
    macrocytic D52.8
  tuberculous A18.89 *[D63.8]*
  vegan D51.3
  vitamin
    B12 deficiency (dietary) pernicious D51.0
    B6-responsive D64.3
  von Jaksch's D64.89
  Witts' (achlorhydric anemia) D50.8
Anemophobia F40.228
Anencephalus, anencephaly Q00.0
Anergasia — *see* Psychosis, organic
Anesthesia, anesthetic R20.0
  complication or reaction NEC — *see also* Complications, anesthesia T88.59 ☑
    due to
      correct substance properly administered — *see* Table of Drugs and Chemicals, by drug, adverse effect
      overdose or wrong substance given — *see* Table of Drugs and Chemicals, by drug, poisoning
      unintended awareness under general anesthesia during procedure T88.53 ☑
        personal history of Z92.84
  cornea H18.81- ☑
  dissociative F44.6
  functional (hysterical) F44.6
  hyperesthetic, thalamic G89.0
  hysterical F44.6
  local skin lesion R20.0
  sexual (psychogenic) F52.1
  shock (due to) T88.2 ☑
  skin R20.0
  testicular N50.9
Anetoderma (maculosum) (of) L90.8
  Jadassohn-Pellizzari L90.2
  Schweniger-Buzzi L90.1
Aneurin deficiency E51.9
Aneurysm (anastomotic) (artery) (cirsoid) (diffuse) (false) (fusiform) (multiple) (saccular) I72.9
  abdominal (aorta) I71.4
    ruptured I71.3
    syphilitic A52.01
  aorta, aortic (nonsyphilitic) I71.9
    abdominal I71.4
      ruptured I71.3
    arch I71.2
      ruptured I71.1
    arteriosclerotic I71.9
      ruptured I71.8
    ascending I71.2
      ruptured I71.1
    congenital Q25.43
    descending I71.9
      abdominal I71.4
        ruptured I71.3

Aneurysm — *continued*
  aorta, aortic — *continued*
    descending — *continued*
      ruptured I71.8
      thoracic I71.2
        ruptured I71.1
    root Q25.43
    ruptured I71.8
    sinus, congenital Q25.43
    syphilitic A52.01
    thoracic I71.2
      ruptured I71.1
    thoracoabdominal I71.6
      ruptured I71.5
    thorax, thoracic (arch) I71.2
      ruptured I71.1
    transverse I71.2
      ruptured I71.1
    valve (heart) — *see also* Endocarditis, aortic I35.8
  arteriosclerotic I72.9
    cerebral I67.1
      ruptured — *see* Hemorrhage, intracranial, subarachnoid
  arteriovenous (congenital) — *see also* Malformation, arteriovenous
    acquired I77.0
      brain I67.1
        ruptured — *see* Aneurysm, arteriovenous, brain, ruptured
      coronary I25.41
      pulmonary I28.0
    brain Q28.2
      ruptured I60.8
        intracerebral I61.8
        intraparenchymal I61.8
        intraventricular I61.5
        subarachnoid I60.8
    peripheral — *see* Malformation, arteriovenous, peripheral
    precerebral vessels Q28.0
    specified site NEC — *see also* Malformation, arteriovenous
      acquired I77.0
  basal — *see* Aneurysm, brain
  basilar (trunk) I72.5
  berry (congenital) (nonruptured) I67.1
    ruptured I60.7
  brain I67.1
    arteriosclerotic I67.1
      ruptured — *see* Hemorrhage, intracranial, subarachnoid
    arteriovenous (congenital) (nonruptured) Q28.2
      acquired I67.1
        ruptured — *see* Aneurysm, arteriovenous, brain, ruptured I60.8
      ruptured — *see* Aneurysm, arteriovenous, brain, ruptured I60.8
    berry (congenital) (nonruptured) I67.1
      ruptured — *see also* Hemorrhage, intracranial, subarachnoid I60.7
    congenital Q28.3
      ruptured I60.7
    meninges I67.1
      ruptured I60.8
    miliary (congenital) (nonruptured) I67.1
      ruptured — *see also* Hemorrhage, intracranial, subarachnoid I60.7
    mycotic I33.0
    ruptured — *see* Aneurysm, arteriovenous, brain, ruptured I60.8
    syphilitic (hemorrhage) A52.05
  cardiac (false) — *see also* Aneurysm, heart I25.3
  carotid artery (common) (external) I72.0
    internal (intracranial) I67.1
      extracranial portion I72.0
      ruptured into brain I60.0- ☑
      syphilitic A52.09
        intracranial A52.05
  cavernous sinus I67.1
    arteriovenous (congenital) (nonruptured) Q28.3
      ruptured I60.8
  celiac I72.8
  central nervous system, syphilitic A52.05
  cerebral — *see* Aneurysm, brain
  chest — *see* Aneurysm, thorax
  circle of Willis I67.1
    congenital Q28.3
      ruptured I60.6

Aneurysm — *continued*
  circle of Willis — *continued*
    ruptured I60.6
  common iliac artery I72.3
  congenital (peripheral) Q27.8
    aorta (root) (sinus) Q25.43
    brain Q28.3
      ruptured I60.7
    coronary Q24.5
    digestive system Q27.8
    lower limb Q27.8
    pulmonary Q25.79
    retina Q14.1
    specified site NEC Q27.8
    upper limb Q27.8
  conjunctiva — *see* Abnormality, conjunctiva, vascula
  conus arteriosus — *see* Aneurysm, heart
  coronary (arteriosclerotic) (artery) I25.41
    arteriovenous, congenital Q24.5
    congenital Q24.5
    ruptured — *see* Infarct, myocardium
    syphilitic A52.06
    vein I25.89
  cylindroid (aorta) I71.9
    ruptured I71.8
    syphilitic A52.01
  ductus arteriosus Q25.0
  endocardial, infective (any valve) I33.0
  femoral (artery) (ruptured) I72.4
  gastroduodenal I72.8
  gastroepiploic I72.8
  heart (wall) (chronic or with a stated duration of over 4 weeks) I25.3
    valve — *see* Endocarditis
  hepatic I72.8
  iliac (common) (artery) (ruptured) I72.3
  infective I72.9
    endocardial (any valve) I33.0
  innominate (nonsyphilitic) I72.8
    syphilitic A52.09
  interauricular septum — *see* Aneurysm, heart
  interventricular septum — *see* Aneurysm, heart
  intrathoracic (nonsyphilitic) I71.2
    ruptured I71.1
    syphilitic A52.01
  lower limb I72.4
  lung (pulmonary artery) I28.1
  mediastinal (nonsyphilitic) I72.8
    syphilitic A52.09
  miliary (congenital) I67.1
    ruptured — *see* Hemorrhage, intracerebral, subarachnoid, intracranial
  mitral (heart) (valve) I34.8
  mural — *see* Aneurysm, heart
  mycotic I72.9
    endocardial (any valve) I33.0
    ruptured, brain — *see* Hemorrhage, intracerebral, subarachnoid
  myocardium — *see* Aneurysm, heart
  neck I72.0
  pancreaticoduodenal I72.8
  patent ductus arteriosus Q25.0
  peripheral NEC I72.8
    congenital Q27.8
      digestive system Q27.8
      lower limb Q27.8
      specified site NEC Q27.8
      upper limb Q27.8
  popliteal (artery) (ruptured) I72.4
  precerebral
    congenital (nonruptured) Q28.1
    specified site, NEC I72.5
  pulmonary I28.1
    arteriovenous Q25.72
      acquired I28.0
    syphilitic A52.09
    valve (heart) — *see* Endocarditis, pulmonary
  racemose (peripheral) I72.9
    congenital — *see* Aneurysm, congenital
  radial I72.1
  Rasmussen NEC A15.0
  renal (artery) I72.2
  retina — *see also* Disorder, retina, microaneurysms
    congenital Q14.1
    diabetic — *see* E08-E13 with .3-
  sinus of Valsalva Q25.49
  specified NEC I72.8
  spinal (cord) I72.8

20

☑ Additional Character Required — Refer to the Tabular List for Character Selection   ▽ Subterms under main terms may continue to next column or page

Anemia — Aneurysm

neurysm — *continued*
  spinal — *continued*
    syphilitic (hemorrhage) A52.09
  splenic I72.8
  subclavian (artery) (ruptured) I72.8
    syphilitic A52.09
  superior mesenteric I72.8
  syphilitic (aorta) A52.09
    central nervous system A52.05
    congenital (late) A50.54 [I79.0]
    spine, spinal A52.09
  thoracoabdominal (aorta) I71.6
    ruptured I71.5
    syphilitic A52.01
  thorax, thoracic (aorta) (arch) (nonsyphilitic) I71.2
    ruptured I71.1
    syphilitic A52.01
  traumatic (complication) (early), specified site — *see* Injury, blood vessel
  tricuspid (heart) (valve) I07.8
  ulnar I72.1
  upper limb (ruptured) I72.1
  valve, valvular — *see* Endocarditis
  venous — *see also* Varix I86.8
    congenital Q27.8
      digestive system Q27.8
      lower limb Q27.8
      specified site NEC Q27.8
      upper limb Q27.8
  ventricle — *see* Aneurysm, heart
  vertebral artery I72.6
  visceral NEC I72.8
Angelman syndrome Q93.51
Anger R45.4
Angiectasis, angiectopia I99.8
Angiitis I77.6
  allergic granulomatous M30.1
  hypersensitivity M31.0
  necrotizing M31.9
    specified NEC M31.8
  nervous system, granulomatous I67.7
Angina (attack) (cardiac) (chest) (heart) (pectoris) (syndrome) (vasomotor) I20.9
  with
    atherosclerotic heart disease — *see* Arteriosclerosis, coronary (artery),
    documented spasm I20.1
  abdominal K55.1
  accelerated — *see* Angina, unstable
  agranulocytic — *see* Agranulocytosis
  angiospastic — *see* Angina, with documented spasm
  aphthous B08.5
  crescendo — *see* Angina, unstable
  croupous J05.0
  cruris I73.9
  de novo effort — *see* Angina, unstable
  diphtheritic, membranous A36.0
  equivalent I20.8
  exudative, chronic J37.0
  following acute myocardial infarction I23.7
  gangrenous diphtheritic A36.0
  intestinal K55.1
  Ludovici K12.2
  Ludwig's K12.2
  malignant diphtheritic A36.0
  membranous J05.0
    diphtheritic A36.0
    Vincent's A69.1
  mesenteric K55.1
  monocytic — *see* Mononucleosis, infectious
  of effort — *see* Angina, specified NEC
  phlegmonous J36
    diphtheritic A36.0
  post-infarctional I23.7
  pre-infarctional — *see* Angina, unstable
  Prinzmetal — *see* Angina, with documented spasm
  progressive — *see* Angina, unstable
  pseudomembranous A69.1
  pultaceous, diphtheritic A36.0
  spasm-induced — *see* Angina, with documented spasm
  specified NEC I20.8
  stable I20.8
  stenocardia — *see* Angina, specified NEC
  stridulous, diphtheritic A36.2
  tonsil J36
  trachealis J05.0
  unstable I20.0
  variant — *see* Angina, with documented spasm

Angina — *continued*
  Vincent's A69.1
  worsening effort — *see* Angina, unstable
Angioblastoma — *see* Neoplasm, connective tissue, uncertain behavior
Angiocholecystitis — *see* Cholecystitis, acute
Angiocholitis — *see also* Cholecystitis, acute K83.09
Angiodysgenesis spinalis G95.19
Angiodysplasia (cecum) (colon) K55.20
  with bleeding K55.21
  duodenum (and stomach) K31.819
    with bleeding K31.811
  stomach (and duodenum) K31.819
    with bleeding K31.811
Angioedema (allergic) (any site) (with urticaria) T78.3 ☑
  hereditary D84.1
Angioendothelioma — *see* Neoplasm, uncertain behavior, by site
  benign D18.00
    intra-abdominal D18.03
    intracranial D18.02
    skin D18.01
    specified site NEC D18.09
  bone — *see* Neoplasm, bone, malignant
  Ewing's — *see* Neoplasm, bone, malignant
Angioendotheliomatosis C85.8- ☑
Angiofibroma — *see also* Neoplasm, benign, by site
  juvenile
    specified site — *see* Neoplasm, benign, by site
    unspecified site D10.6
Angiohemophilia (A) (B) D68.0
Angioid streaks (choroid) (macula) (retina) H35.33
Angiokeratoma — *see* Neoplasm, skin, benign
  corporis diffusum E75.21
Angioleiomyoma — *see* Neoplasm, connective tissue, benign
Angiolipoma — *see also* Lipoma
  infiltrating — *see* Lipoma
Angioma — *see also* Hemangioma, by site
  capillary I78.1
  hemorrhagicum hereditaria I78.0
  intra-abdominal D18.03
  intracranial D18.02
  malignant — *see* Neoplasm, connective tissue, malignant
  plexiform D18.00
    intra-abdominal D18.03
    intracranial D18.02
    skin D18.01
    specified site NEC D18.09
  senile I78.1
  serpiginosum L81.7
  skin D18.01
  specified site NEC D18.09
  spider I78.1
  stellate I78.1
  venous Q28.3
Angiomatosis Q82.8
  bacillary A79.89
  encephalotrigeminal Q85.8
  hemorrhagic familial I78.0
  hereditary familial I78.0
  liver K76.4
Angiomyolipoma — *see* Lipoma
Angiomyoliposarcoma — *see* Neoplasm, connective tissue, malignant
Angiomyoma — *see* Neoplasm, connective tissue, benign
Angiomyosarcoma — *see* Neoplasm, connective tissue, malignant
Angiomyxoma — *see* Neoplasm, connective tissue, uncertain behavior
Angioneurosis F45.8
Angioneurotic edema (allergic) (any site) (with urticaria) T78.3 ☑
  hereditary D84.1
Angiopathia, angiopathy I99.9
  cerebral I67.9
    amyloid E85.4 [I68.0]
  diabetic (peripheral) — *see* Diabetes, angiopathy
  peripheral I73.9
    diabetic — *see* Diabetes, angiopathy
    specified type NEC I73.89
  retinae syphilitica A52.05
  retinalis (juvenilis)
    diabetic — *see* Diabetes, retinopathy
    proliferative — *see* Retinopathy, proliferative
Angiosarcoma — *see also* Neoplasm, connective tissue, malignant

Angiosarcoma — *continued*
  liver C22.3
Angiosclerosis — *see* Arteriosclerosis
Angiospasm (peripheral) (traumatic) (vessel) I73.9
  brachial plexus G54.0
  cerebral G45.9
  cervical plexus G54.2
  nerve
    arm — *see* Mononeuropathy, upper limb
      axillary G54.0
      median — *see* Lesion, nerve, median
      ulnar — *see* Lesion, nerve, ulnar
    axillary G54.0
    leg — *see* Mononeuropathy, lower limb
    median — *see* Lesion, nerve, median
    plantar — *see* Lesion, nerve, plantar
    ulnar — *see* Lesion, nerve, ulnar
Angiospastic disease or edema I73.9
Angiostrongyliasis
  due to
    Parastrongylus
      cantonensis B83.2
      costaricensis B81.3
  intestinal B81.3
Anguillulosis — *see* Strongyloidiasis
Angulation
  cecum — *see* Obstruction, intestine
  coccyx (acquired) — *see also* subcategory M43.8 ☑
    congenital NEC Q76.49
  femur (acquired) — *see also* Deformity, limb, specified type NEC, thigh
    congenital Q74.2
  intestine (large) (small) — *see* Obstruction, intestine
  sacrum (acquired) — *see also* subcategory M43.8 ☑
    congenital NEC Q76.49
  sigmoid (flexure) — *see* Obstruction, intestine
  spine — *see* Dorsopathy, deforming, specified NEC
  tibia (acquired) — *see also* Deformity, limb, specified type NEC, lower leg
    congenital Q74.2
  ureter N13.5
    with infection N13.6
  wrist (acquired) — *see also* Deformity, limb, specified type NEC, forearm
    congenital Q74.0
Angulus infectiosus (lips) K13.0
Anhedonia R45.84
  sexual F52.0
Anhidrosis L74.4
Anhydration E86.0
Anhydremia E86.0
Anidrosis L74.4
Aniridia (congenital) Q13.1
Anisakiasis (infection) (infestation) B81.0
Anisakis larvae infestation B81.0
Aniseikonia H52.32
Anisocoria (pupil) H57.02
  congenital Q13.2
Anisocytosis R71.8
Anisometropia (congenital) H52.31
Ankle — *see* condition
Ankyloblepharon (eyelid) (acquired) — *see also* Blepharophimosis
  filiforme (adnatum) (congenital) Q10.3
  total Q10.3
Ankyloglossia Q38.1
Ankylosis (fibrous) (osseous) (joint) M24.60
  ankle M24.67- ☑
  arthrodesis status Z98.1
  cricoarytenoid (cartilage) (joint) (larynx) J38.7
  dental K03.5
  ear ossicles H74.31- ☑
  elbow M24.62- ☑
  foot M24.67- ☑
  hand M24.64- ☑
  hip M24.65- ☑
  incostapedial joint (infectional) — *see* Ankylosis, ear ossicles
  jaw (temporomandibular) M26.61- ☑
  knee M24.66- ☑
  lumbosacral (joint) M43.27
  postoperative (status) Z98.1
  produced by surgical fusion, status Z98.1
  sacro-iliac (joint) M43.28
  shoulder M24.61- ☑
  spine (joint) — *see also* Fusion, spine
    spondylitic — *see* Spondylitis, ankylosing

Ankylosis — *continued*
  surgical Z98.1
  temporomandibular M26.61- ☑
  tooth, teeth (hard tissues) K03.5
  wrist M24.63- ☑
Ankylostoma — *see* Ancylostoma
Ankylostomiasis — *see* Ancylostomiasis
Ankylurethria — *see* Stricture, urethra
Annular — *see also* condition
  detachment, cervix N88.8
  organ or site, congenital NEC — *see* Distortion
  pancreas (congenital) Q45.1
Anodontia (complete) (partial) (vera) K00.0
  acquired K08.10 ☑
Anomaly, anomalous (congenital) (unspecified type)
    Q89.9
  abdominal wall NEC Q79.59
  acoustic nerve Q07.8
  adrenal (gland) Q89.1
  Alder (-Reilly) (leukocyte granulation) D72.0
  alimentary tract Q45.9
    upper Q40.9
  alveolar M26.70
    hyperplasia M26.79
      mandibular M26.72
      maxillary M26.71
    hypoplasia M26.79
      mandibular M26.74
      maxillary M26.73
    ridge (process) M26.79
    specified NEC M26.79
  ankle (joint) Q74.2
  anus Q43.9
  aorta (arch) NEC Q25.40
    coarctation (preductal) (postductal) Q25.1
  aortic cusp or valve Q23.9
  appendix Q43.8
  apple peel syndrome Q41.1
  aqueduct of Sylvius Q03.0
    with spina bifida — *see* Spina bifida, with hydro-
        cephalus
  arm Q74.0
  arteriovenous NEC
    coronary Q24.5
    gastrointestinal Q27.33
      acquired — *see* Angiodysplasia
  artery (peripheral) Q27.9
    basilar NEC Q28.1
    cerebral Q28.3
    coronary Q24.5
    digestive system Q27.8
    eye Q15.8
    great Q25.9
      specified NEC Q25.8
    lower limb Q27.8
    peripheral Q27.9
      specified NEC Q27.8
    pulmonary NEC Q25.79
    renal Q27.2
    retina Q14.1
    specified site NEC Q27.8
    subclavian Q27.8
      origin Q25.48
    umbilical Q27.0
    upper limb Q27.8
    vertebral NEC Q28.1
  aryteno-epiglottic folds Q31.8
  atrial
    bands or folds Q20.8
    septa Q21.1
  atrioventricular
    excitation I45.6
    septum Q21.0
  auditory canal Q17.8
  auricle
    ear Q17.8
      causing impairment of hearing Q16.9
    heart Q20.8
  Axenfeld's Q15.0
  back Q89.9
  band
    atrial Q20.8
    heart Q24.8
    ventricular Q24.8
  Bartholin's duct Q38.4
  biliary duct or passage Q44.5
  bladder Q64.70
    absence Q64.5

Anomaly, anomalous — *continued*
  bladder — *continued*
    diverticulum Q64.6
    exstrophy Q64.10
      cloacal Q64.12
      extroversion Q64.19
      specified type NEC Q64.19
      supravesical fissure Q64.11
    neck obstruction Q64.31
    specified type NEC Q64.79
  bone Q79.9
    arm Q74.0
    face Q75.9
    leg Q74.2
    pelvic girdle Q74.2
    shoulder girdle Q74.0
    skull Q75.9
      with
        anencephaly Q00.0
        encephalocele — *see* Encephalocele
        hydrocephalus Q03.9
          with spina bifida — *see* Spina bifida, by
              site, with hydrocephalus
        microcephaly Q02
  brain (multiple) Q04.9
    vessel Q28.3
  breast Q83.9
  broad ligament Q50.6
  bronchus Q32.4
  bulbus cordis Q21.9
  bursa Q79.9
  canal of Nuck Q52.4
  canthus Q10.3
  capillary Q27.9
  cardiac Q24.9
    chambers Q20.9
      specified NEC Q20.8
    septal closure Q21.9
      specified NEC Q21.8
    valve NEC Q24.8
      pulmonary Q22.3
  cardiovascular system Q28.8
  carpus Q74.0
  caruncle, lacrimal Q10.6
  cascade stomach Q40.2
  cauda equina Q06.3
  cecum Q43.9
  cerebral Q04.9
    vessels Q28.3
  cervix Q51.9
  Chédiak-Higashi (-Steinbrinck) (congenital gigantism
      of peroxidase granules) E70.330
  cheek Q18.9
  chest wall Q67.8
    bones Q76.9
  chin Q18.9
  chordae tendineae Q24.8
  choroid Q14.3
    plexus Q07.8
  chromosomes, chromosomal Q99.9
    D (1) — *see* condition, chromosome 13
    E (3) — *see* condition, chromosome 18
    G — *see* condition, chromosome 21
    sex
      female phenotype Q97.8
      gonadal dysgenesis (pure) Q99.1
      Klinefelter's Q98.4
      male phenotype Q98.9
      Turner's Q96.9
    specified NEC Q99.8
  cilia Q10.3
  circulatory system Q28.9
  clavicle Q74.0
  clitoris Q52.6
  coccyx Q76.49
  colon Q43.9
  common duct Q44.5
  communication
    coronary artery Q24.5
    left ventricle with right atrium Q21.0
  concha (ear) Q17.3
  connection
    portal vein Q26.5
    pulmonary venous Q26.4
      partial Q26.3
      total Q26.2
    renal artery with kidney Q27.2
  cornea (shape) Q13.4
  coronary artery or vein Q24.5

Anomaly, anomalous — *continued*
  cranium — *see* Anomaly, skull
  cricoid cartilage Q31.8
  cystic duct Q44.5
  dental
    alveolar — *see* Anomaly, alveolar
    arch relationship M26.20
      specified NEC M26.29
  dentofacial M26.9
    alveolar — *see* Anomaly, alveolar
    dental arch relationship M26.20
      specified NEC M26.29
    functional M26.50
      specified NEC M26.59
    jaw size M26.00
      macrogenia M26.05
      mandibular
        hyperplasia M26.03
        hypoplasia M26.04
      maxillary
        hyperplasia M26.01
        hypoplasia M26.02
      microgenia M26.06
      specified type NEC M26.09
    jaw-cranial base relationship M26.10
      asymmetry M26.12
        maxillary M26.11
      specified type NEC M26.19
    malocclusion M26.4
      dental arch relationship NEC M26.29
      jaw size — *see* Anomaly, dentofacial, jaw size
      jaw-cranial base relationship — *see* Anomaly,
          dentofacial, jaw-cranial base relationship
    specified type NEC M26.89
  temporomandibular joint M26.60- ☑
    adhesions M26.61- ☑
    ankylosis M26.61- ☑
    arthralgia M26.62- ☑
    articular disc M26.63- ☑
    specified type NEC M26.69
  tooth position, fully erupted M26.30
    specified NEC M26.39
  dermatoglyphic Q82.8
  diaphragm (apertures) NEC Q79.1
  digestive organ(s) or tract Q45.9
    lower Q43.9
    upper Q40.9
  distance, interarch (excessive) (inadequate) M26.25
  distribution, coronary artery Q24.5
  ductus
    arteriosus Q25.0
    botalli Q25.0
  duodenum Q43.9
  dura (brain) Q04.9
    spinal cord Q06.9
  ear (external) Q17.9
    causing impairment of hearing Q16.9
    inner Q16.5
    middle (causing impairment of hearing) Q16.4
    ossicles Q16.3
  Ebstein's (heart) (tricuspid valve) Q22.5
  ectodermal Q82.9
  Eisenmenger's (ventricular septal defect) Q21.8
  ejaculatory duct Q55.4
  elbow Q74.0
  endocrine gland NEC Q89.2
  epididymis Q55.4
  epiglottis Q31.8
  esophagus Q39.9
  eustachian tube Q17.8
  eye Q15.9
    anterior segment Q13.9
      specified NEC Q13.89
    posterior segment Q14.9
      specified NEC Q14.8
    ptosis (eyelid) Q10.0
    specified NEC Q15.8
  eyebrow Q18.8
  eyelid Q10.3
    ptosis Q10.0
  face Q18.9
    bone(s) Q75.9
  fallopian tube Q50.6
  fascia Q79.9
  femur NEC Q74.2
  fibula NEC Q74.2
  finger Q74.0
  fixation, intestine Q43.3

☑ **Additional Character Required** — Refer to the Tabular List for Character Selection   ▽ **Subterms under main terms may continue to next column or page**

Anomaly, anomalous — *continued*
flexion (joint) NOS Q74.9
  hip or thigh Q65.89
foot NEC Q74.2
  varus (congenital) Q66.3- ☑
foramen
  Botalli Q21.1
  ovale Q21.1
forearm Q74.0
forehead Q75.8
form, teeth K00.2
fovea centralis Q14.1
frontal bone — *see* Anomaly, skull
gallbladder (position) (shape) (size) Q44.1
Gartner's duct Q52.4
gastrointestinal tract Q45.9
genitalia, genital organ(s) or system
  female Q52.9
    external Q52.70
    internal NOS Q52.9
  male Q55.9
    hydrocele P83.5
    specified NEC Q55.8
genitourinary NEC
  female Q52.9
  male Q55.9
Gerbode Q21.0
glottis Q31.8
granulation or granulocyte, genetic (constitutional)
  (leukocyte) D72.0
gum Q38.6
gyri Q07.9
hair Q84.2
hand Q74.0
hard tissue formation in pulp K04.3
head — *see* Anomaly, skull
heart Q24.9
  auricle Q20.8
  bands or folds Q24.8
  fibroelastosis cordis I42.4
  obstructive NEC Q22.6
  patent ductus arteriosus (Botalli) Q25.0
  septum Q21.9
    auricular Q21.1
    interatrial Q21.1
    interventricular Q21.0
      with pulmonary stenosis or atresia, dextraposition of aorta and hypertrophy of right ventricle Q21.3
    specified NEC Q21.8
    ventricular Q21.0
      with pulmonary stenosis or atresia, dextraposition of aorta and hypertrophy of right ventricle Q21.3
  tetralogy of Fallot Q21.3
  valve NEC Q24.8
    aortic
      bicuspid valve Q23.1
      insufficiency Q23.1
      stenosis Q23.0
        subaortic Q24.4
    mitral
      insufficiency Q23.3
      stenosis Q23.2
    pulmonary Q22.3
      atresia Q22.0
      insufficiency Q22.2
      stenosis Q22.1
        infundibular Q24.3
        subvalvular Q24.3
    tricuspid
      atresia Q22.4
      stenosis Q22.4
  ventricle Q20.8
heel NEC Q74.2
Hegglin's D72.0
hemianencephaly Q00.0
hemicephaly Q00.0
hemicrania Q00.0
hepatic duct Q44.5
hip NEC Q74.2
hourglass stomach Q40.2
humerus Q74.0
hydatid of Morgagni
  female Q50.5
  male (epididymal) Q55.4
    testicular Q55.29
hymen Q52.4
hypersegmentation of neutrophils, hereditary D72.0

Anomaly, anomalous — *continued*
hypophyseal Q89.2
ileocecal (coil) (valve) Q43.9
ileum Q43.9
ilium NEC Q74.2
integument Q84.9
  specified NEC Q84.8
interarch distance (excessive) (inadequate) M26.25
intervertebral cartilage or disc Q76.49
intestine (large) (small) Q43.9
  with anomalous adhesions, fixation or malrotation Q43.3
iris Q13.2
ischium NEC Q74.2
jaw — *see* Anomaly, dentofacial
  alveolar — *see* Anomaly, alveolar
jaw-cranial base relationship — *see* Anomaly, dentofacial, jaw-cranial base relationship
jejunum Q43.8
joint Q74.9
  specified NEC Q74.8
Jordan's D72.0
kidney(s) (calyx) (pelvis) Q63.9
  artery Q27.2
  specified NEC Q63.8
Klippel-Feil (brevicollis) Q76.1
knee Q74.1
labium (majus) (minus) Q52.70
labyrinth, membranous Q16.5
lacrimal apparatus or duct Q10.6
larynx, laryngeal (muscle) Q31.9
  web (bed) Q31.0
lens Q12.9
leukocytes, genetic D72.0
  granulation (constitutional) D72.0
lid (fold) Q10.3
ligament Q79.9
  broad Q50.6
  round Q52.8
limb Q74.9
  lower NEC Q74.2
    reduction deformity — *see* Defect, reduction, lower limb
  upper Q74.0
lip Q38.0
liver Q44.7
  duct Q44.5
lower limb NEC Q74.2
lumbosacral (joint) (region) Q76.49
  kyphosis — *see* Kyphosis, congenital
  lordosis — *see* Lordosis, congenital
lung (fissure) (lobe) Q33.9
mandible — *see* Anomaly, dentofacial
maxilla — *see* Anomaly, dentofacial
May (-Hegglin) D72.0
meatus urinarius NEC Q64.79
meningeal bands or folds Q07.9
  constriction of Q07.8
  spinal Q06.9
meninges Q07.9
  cerebral Q04.8
  spinal Q06.9
meningocele Q05.9
mesentery Q45.9
metacarpus Q74.0
metatarsus NEC Q74.2
middle ear Q16.4
  ossicles Q16.3
mitral (leaflets) (valve) Q23.9
  insufficiency Q23.3
  specified NEC Q23.8
  stenosis Q23.2
mouth Q38.6
Müllerian — *see also* Anomaly, by site
  uterus NEC Q51.818
multiple NEC Q89.7
muscle Q79.9
  eyelid Q10.3
musculoskeletal system, except limbs Q79.9
myocardium Q24.8
nail Q84.6
narrowness, eyelid Q10.3
nasal sinus (wall) Q30.8
neck (any part) Q18.9
nerve Q07.9
  acoustic Q07.8
  optic Q07.8
nervous system (central) Q07.9

Anomaly, anomalous — *continued*
nipple Q83.9
nose, nasal (bones) (cartilage) (septum) (sinus) Q30.9
  specified NEC Q30.8
ocular muscle Q15.8
omphalomesenteric duct Q43.0
opening, pulmonary veins Q26.4
optic
  disc Q14.2
  nerve Q07.8
opticociliary vessels Q13.2
orbit (eye) Q10.7
organ Q89.9
  of Corti Q16.5
origin
  artery
    innominate Q25.8
    pulmonary Q25.79
    renal Q27.2
    subclavian Q25.48
osseous meatus (ear) Q16.1
ovary Q50.39
oviduct Q50.6
palate (hard) (soft) NEC Q38.5
pancreas or pancreatic duct Q45.3
papillary muscles Q24.8
parathyroid gland Q89.2
paraurethral ducts Q64.79
parotid (gland) Q38.4
patella Q74.1
Pelger-Huët (hereditary hyposegmentation) D72.0
pelvic girdle NEC Q74.2
pelvis (bony) NEC Q74.2
  rachitic E64.3
penis (glans) Q55.69
pericardium Q24.8
peripheral vascular system Q27.9
Peter's Q13.4
pharynx Q38.8
pigmentation L81.9
  congenital Q82.8
pituitary (gland) Q89.2
pleural (folds) Q34.0
portal vein Q26.5
  connection Q26.5
position, tooth, teeth, fully erupted M26.30
  specified NEC M26.39
precerebral vessel Q28.1
prepuce Q55.69
prostate Q55.4
pulmonary Q33.9
  artery NEC Q25.79
  valve Q22.3
    atresia Q22.0
    insufficiency Q22.2
    specified type NEC Q22.3
    stenosis Q22.1
      infundibular Q24.3
      subvalvular Q24.3
  venous connection Q26.4
    partial Q26.3
    total Q26.2
pupil Q13.2
  function H57.00
    anisocoria H57.02
    Argyll Robertson pupil H57.01
    miosis H57.03
    mydriasis H57.04
    specified type NEC H57.09
    tonic pupil H57.05- ☑
pylorus Q40.3
radius Q74.0
rectum Q43.9
reduction (extremity) (limb)
  femur (longitudinal) — *see* Defect, reduction, lower limb, longitudinal, femur
  fibula (longitudinal) — *see* Defect, reduction, lower limb, longitudinal, fibula
  lower limb — *see* Defect, reduction, lower limb
  radius (longitudinal) — *see* Defect, reduction, upper limb, longitudinal, radius
  tibia (longitudinal) — *see* Defect, reduction, lower limb, longitudinal, tibia
  ulna (longitudinal) — *see* Defect, reduction, upper limb, longitudinal, ulna
  upper limb — *see* Defect, reduction, upper limb
refraction — *see* Disorder, refraction
renal Q63.9

Anomaly, anomalous — *continued*
renal — *continued*
artery Q27.2
pelvis Q63.9
specified NEC Q63.8
respiratory system Q34.9
specified NEC Q34.8
retina Q14.1
rib Q76.6
cervical Q76.5
Rieger's Q13.81
rotation — *see* Malrotation
hip or thigh Q65.89
round ligament Q52.8
sacroiliac (joint) NEC Q74.2
sacrum NEC Q76.49
kyphosis — *see* Kyphosis, congenital
lordosis — *see* Lordosis, congenital
saddle nose, syphilitic A50.57
salivary duct or gland Q38.4
scapula Q74.0
scrotum — *see* Malformation, testis and scrotum
sebaceous gland Q82.9
seminal vesicles Q55.4
sense organs NEC Q07.8
sex chromosomes NEC — *see also* Anomaly, chromosomes
female phenotype Q97.8
male phenotype Q98.9
shoulder (girdle) (joint) Q74.0
sigmoid (flexure) Q43.9
simian crease Q82.8
sinus of Valsalva Q25.49
skeleton generalized Q78.9
skin (appendage) Q82.9
skull Q75.9
with
anencephaly Q00.0
encephalocele — *see* Encephalocele
hydrocephalus Q03.9
with spina bifida — *see* Spina bifida, by site,
with hydrocephalus
microcephaly Q02
specified organ or site NEC Q89.8
spermatic cord Q55.4
spine, spinal NEC Q76.49
column NEC Q76.49
kyphosis — *see* Kyphosis, congenital
lordosis — *see* Lordosis, congenital
cord Q06.9
nerve root Q07.8
spleen Q89.09
agenesis Q89.01
stenonian duct Q38.4
sternum NEC Q76.7
stomach Q40.3
submaxillary gland Q38.4
tarsus NEC Q74.2
tendon Q79.9
testis — *see* Malformation, testis and scrotum
thigh NEC Q74.2
thorax (wall) Q67.8
bony Q76.9
throat Q38.8
thumb Q74.0
thymus gland Q89.2
thyroid (gland) Q89.2
cartilage Q31.8
tibia NEC Q74.2
saber A50.56
toe Q74.2
tongue Q38.3
tooth, teeth K00.9
eruption K00.6
position, fully erupted M26.30
spacing, fully erupted M26.30
trachea (cartilage) Q32.1
tragus Q17.9
tricuspid (leaflet) (valve) Q22.9
atresia or stenosis Q22.4
Ebstein's Q22.5
Uhl's (hypoplasia of myocardium, right ventricle) Q24.8
ulna Q74.0
umbilical artery Q27.0
union
cricoid cartilage and thyroid cartilage Q31.8
thyroid cartilage and hyoid bone Q31.8
trachea with larynx Q31.8

Anomaly, anomalous — *continued*
upper limb Q74.0
urachus Q64.4
ureter Q62.8
obstructive NEC Q62.39
cecoureterocele Q62.32
orthotopic ureterocele Q62.31
urethra Q64.70
absence Q64.5
double Q64.74
fistula to rectum Q64.73
obstructive Q64.39
stricture Q64.32
prolapse Q64.71
specified type NEC Q64.79
urinary tract Q64.9
uterus Q51.9
with only one functioning horn Q51.4
uvula Q38.5
vagina Q52.4
valleculae Q31.8
valve (heart) NEC Q24.8
coronary sinus Q24.5
inferior vena cava Q24.8
pulmonary Q22.3
sinus coronario Q24.5
venae cavae inferioris Q24.8
vas deferens Q55.4
vascular Q27.9
brain Q28.3
ring Q25.45
vein(s) (peripheral) Q27.9
brain Q28.3
cerebral Q28.3
coronary Q24.5
developmental Q28.3
great Q26.9
specified NEC Q26.8
vena cava (inferior) (superior) Q26.9
venous — *see* Anomaly, vein(s)
venous return Q26.8
ventricular
bands or folds Q24.8
septa Q21.0
vertebra Q76.49
kyphosis — *see* Kyphosis, congenital
lordosis — *see* Lordosis, congenital
vesicourethral orifice Q64.79
vessel(s) Q27.9
optic papilla Q14.2
precerebral Q28.1
vitelline duct Q43.0
vitreous body or humor Q14.0
vulva Q52.70
wrist (joint) Q74.0
Anomia R48.8
Anonychia (congenital) Q84.3
acquired L60.8
Anophthalmos, anophthalmus (congenital) (globe)
Q11.1
acquired Z90.01
Anopia, anopsia H53.46- ☑
quadrant H53.46- ☑
Anorchia, anorchism, anorchidism Q55.0
Anorexia R63.0
hysterical F44.89
nervosa F50.00
atypical F50.9
binge-eating type F50.2
with purging F50.02
restricting type F50.01
Anorgasmy, psychogenic (female) F52.31
male F52.32
Anosmia R43.0
hysterical F44.6
postinfectional J39.8
Anosognosia R41.89
Anosteoplasia Q78.9
Anovulatory cycle N97.0
Anoxemia R09.02
newborn P84
Anoxia (pathological) R09.02
altitude T70.29 ☑
cerebral G93.1
complicating
anesthesia (general) (local) or other sedation
T88.59 ☑
in labor and delivery O74.3

Anoxia — *continued*
cerebral — *continued*
complicating — *continued*
anesthesia or other sedation — *continued*
in pregnancy O29.21- ☑
postpartum, puerperal O89.2
delivery (cesarean) (instrumental) O75.4
during a procedure G97.81
newborn P84
resulting from a procedure G97.82
due to
drowning T75.1 ☑
high altitude T70.29 ☑
heart — *see* Insufficiency, coronary
intrauterine P84
myocardial — *see* Insufficiency, coronary
newborn P84
spinal cord G95.11
systemic (by suffocation) (low content in atmospher
— *see* Asphyxia, traumatic
Anteflexion — *see* Anteversion
Antenatal
care (normal pregnancy) Z34.90
screening (encounter for) of mother — *see also* Encounter, antenatal screening Z36.9
Antepartum — *see* condition
Anterior — *see* condition
Antero-occlusion M26.220
Anteversion
cervix — *see* Anteversion, uterus
femur (neck), congenital Q65.89
uterus, uterine (cervix) (postinfectional) (postpartal,
old) N85.4
congenital Q51.818
in pregnancy or childbirth — *see* Pregnancy, con
plicated by
Anthophobia F40.228
Anthracosilicosis J60
Anthracosis (lung) (occupational) J60
lingua K14.3
Anthrax A22.9
with pneumonia A22.1
cerebral A22.8
colitis A22.2
cutaneous A22.0
gastrointestinal A22.2
inhalation A22.1
intestinal A22.2
meningitis A22.8
pulmonary A22.1
respiratory A22.1
sepsis A22.7
specified manifestation NEC A22.8
Anthropoid pelvis Q74.2
with disproportion (fetopelvic) O33.0
Anthropophobia F40.10
generalized F40.11
Antibodies, maternal (blood group) — *see* Isoimmuniza
tion, affecting management of pregnancy
anti-D — *see* Isoimmunization, affecting managemer
of pregnancy, Rh
newborn P55.0
Antibody
anticardiolipin R76.0
with
hemorrhagic disorder D68.312
hypercoagulable state D68.61
antiphosphatidylglycerol R76.0
with
hemorrhagic disorder D68.312
hypercoagulable state D68.61
antiphosphatidylinositol R76.0
with
hemorrhagic disorder D68.312
hypercoagulable state D68.61
antiphosphatidylserine R76.0
with
hemorrhagic disorder D68.312
hypercoagulable state D68.61
antiphospholipid R76.0
with
hemorrhagic disorder D68.312
hypercoagulable state D68.61
Anticardiolipin syndrome D68.61
Anticoagulant, circulating (intrinsic) — *see also* Disor
der, hemorrhagic D68.318
drug-induced (extrinsic) — *see also* Disorder, hemor
rhagic D68.32

Anticoagulant, circulating — *continued*
  iatrogenic D68.32
Antidiuretic hormone syndrome E22.2
Antimonial cholera — *see* Poisoning, antimony
Antiphospholipid
  antibody
    with hemorrhagic disorder D68.312
    syndrome D68.61
Antisocial personality F60.2
Antithrombinemia — *see* Circulating anticoagulants
Antithromboplastinemia D68.318
Antithromboplastinogenemia D68.318
Antitoxin complication or reaction — *see* Complications, vaccination
Antlophobia F40.228
Antritis J32.0
  maxilla J32.0
    acute J01.00
      recurrent J01.01
  stomach K29.60
    with bleeding K29.61
Antrum, antral — *see* condition
Anuria R34
  calculous (impacted) (recurrent) — *see also* Calculus, urinary N20.9
  following
    abortion — *see* Abortion by type complicated by, renal failure
    ectopic or molar pregnancy O08.4
  newborn P96.0
  postprocedural N99.0
  postrenal N13.8
  traumatic (following crushing) T79.5 ☑
Anus, anal — *see* condition
Anusitis K62.89
Anxiety F41.9
  depression F41.8
  episodic paroxysmal F41.0
  generalized F41.1
  hysteria F41.8
  neurosis F41.1
  panic type F41.0
  reaction F41.1
  separation, abnormal (of childhood) F93.0
  specified NEC F41.8
  state F41.1
Aorta, aortic — *see* condition
Aortectasla — *see* Ectasla, aorta
  with aneurysm — *see* Aneurysm, aorta
Aortitis (nonsyphilitic) (calcific) I77.6
  arteriosclerotic I70.0
  Doehle-Heller A52.02
  luetic A52.02
  rheumatic — *see* Endocarditis, acute, rheumatic
  specific (syphilitic) A52.02
  syphilitic A52.02
    congenital A50.54 [I79.1]
Apathetic thyroid storm — *see* Thyrotoxicosis
Apathy R45.3
Apeirophobia F40.228
Apepsia K30
  psychogenic F45.8
Aperistalsis, esophagus K22.0
Apertognathia M26.29
Apert's syndrome Q87.0
Aphagia R13.0
  psychogenic F50.9
Aphakia (acquired) (postoperative) H27.0- ☑
  congenital Q12.3
Aphasia (amnestic) (global) (nominal) (semantic) (syntactic) R47.01
  acquired, with epilepsy (Landau-Kleffner syndrome) — *see* Epilepsy, specified NEC
  auditory (developmental) F80.2
  developmental (receptive type) F80.2
    expressive type F80.1
    Wernicke's F80.2
  following
    cerebrovascular disease I69.920
      cerebral infarction I69.320
      intracerebral hemorrhage I69.120
      nontraumatic intracranial hemorrhage NEC I69.220
      specified disease NEC I69.820
      subarachnoid hemorrhage I69.020
  primary progressive G31.01 [F02.80]
    with behavioral disturbance G31.01 [F02.81]
  progressive isolated G31.01 [F02.80]

Aphasia — *continued*
  progressive isolated — *continued*
    with behavioral disturbance G31.01 [F02.81]
  sensory F80.2
  syphilis, tertiary A52.19
  Wernicke's (developmental) F80.2
Aphonia (organic) R49.1
  hysterical F44.4
  psychogenic F44.4
Aphthae, aphthous — *see also* condition
  Bednar's K12.0
  cachectic K14.0
  epizootic B08.8
  fever B08.8
  oral (recurrent) K12.0
  stomatitis (major) (minor) K12.0
  thrush B37.0
  ulcer (oral) (recurrent) K12.0
    genital organ(s) NEC
      female N76.6
      male N50.89
    larynx J38.7
Apical — *see* condition
Apiphobia F40.218
Aplasia — *see also* Agenesis
  abdominal muscle syndrome Q79.4
  alveolar process (acquired) — *see* Anomaly, alveolar
    congenital Q38.6
  aorta (congenital) Q25.41
  axialis extracorticalis (congenita) E75.29
  bone marrow (myeloid) D61.9
    congenital D61.01
  brain Q00.0
    part of Q04.3
  bronchus Q32.4
  cementum K00.4
  cerebellum Q04.3
  cervix (congenital) Q51.5
  congenital pure red cell D61.01
  corpus callosum Q04.0
  cutis congenita Q84.8
  erythrocyte congenital D61.01
  extracortical axial E75.29
  eye Q11.1
  fovea centralis (congenital) Q14.1
  gallbladder, congenital Q44.0
  iris Q13.1
  labyrinth, membranous Q16.5
  limb (congenital) Q73.8
    lower — *see* Defect, reduction, lower limb
    upper — *see* Agenesis, arm
  lung, congenital (bilateral) (unilateral) Q33.3
  pancreas Q45.0
  parathyroid-thymic D82.1
  Pelizaeus-Merzbacher E75.29
  penis Q55.5
  prostate Q55.4
  red cell (with thymoma) D60.9
    acquired D60.9
      due to drugs D60.9
    adult D60.9
    chronic D60.0
    congenital D61.01
    constitutional D61.01
    due to drugs D60.9
    hereditary D61.01
    of infants D61.01
    primary D61.01
    pure D61.01
      due to drugs D60.9
    specified type NEC D60.8
    transient D60.1
  round ligament Q52.8
  skin Q84.8
  spermatic cord Q55.4
  spleen Q89.01
  testicle Q55.0
  thymic, with immunodeficiency D82.1
  thyroid (congenital) (with myxedema) E03.1
  uterus Q51.0
  ventral horn cell Q06.1
Apnea, apneic (of) (spells) R06.81
  newborn NEC P28.4
    obstructive P28.4
    sleep (central) (obstructive) (primary) P28.3
  prematurity P28.4
  sleep G47.30
    central (primary) G47.31

Apnea, apneic — *continued*
  sleep — *continued*
    central — *continued*
      idiopathic G47.31
      in conditions classified elsewhere G47.37
    obstructive (adult) (pediatric) G47.33
      hypopnea G47.33
    primary central G47.31
    specified NEC G47.39
Apneumatosis, newborn P28.0
Apocrine metaplasia (breast) — *see* Dysplasia, mammary, specified type NEC
Apophysitis (bone) — *see also* Osteochondropathy
  calcaneus M92.8
  juvenile M92.9
Apoplectiform convulsions (cerebral ischemia) I67.82
Apoplexia, apoplexy, apoplectic
  adrenal A39.1
  heart (auricle) (ventricle) — *see* Infarct, myocardium
  heat T67.01 ☑
  hemorrhagic (stroke) — *see* Hemorrhage, intracranial
  meninges, hemorrhagic — *see* Hemorrhage, intracranial, subarachnoid
  uremic N18.9 [I68.8]
Appearance
  bizarre R46.1
  specified NEC R46.89
  very low level of personal hygiene R46.0
Appendage
  epididymal (organ of Morgagni) Q55.4
  intestine (epiploic) Q43.8
  preauricular Q17.0
  testicular (organ of Morgagni) Q55.29
Appendicitis (pneumococcal) (retrocecal) K37
  with
    gangrene K35.891
    perforation NOS K35.32
    peritoneal abscess K35.33
    peritonitis NEC K35.33
      generalized (with perforation or rupture) K35.20
        with abscess K35.21
      localized K35.30
        with
          gangrene K35.31
          perforation K35.32
            and abscess K35.33
    rupture (with localized peritonitis) K35.32
  acute (catarrhal) (fulminating) (gangrenous) (obstructive) (retrocecal) (suppurative) K35.80
    with
      gangrene K35.891
      peritoneal abscess K35.33
      peritonitis NEC K35.33
        generalized (with perforation or rupture) K35.20
          with abscess K35.21
        localized K35.30
          with
            gangrene K35.31
            perforation K35.32
              and abscess K35.33
    specified NEC K35.890
      with gangrene K35.891
  amebic A06.89
  chronic (recurrent) K36
  exacerbation — *see* Appendicitis, acute
  gangrenous — *see* Appendicitis, acute
  healed (obliterative) K36
  interval K36
  neurogenic K36
  obstructive K36
  recurrent K36
  relapsing K36
  ruptured NOS (with localized peritonitis) K35.32
  subacute (adhesive) K36
  subsiding K36
  suppurative — *see* Appendicitis, acute
  tuberculous A18.32
Appendicopathia oxyurica B80
Appendix, appendicular — *see also* condition
  epididymis Q55.4
  Morgagni
    female Q50.5
    male (epididymal) Q55.4
    testicular Q55.29
  testis Q55.29
Appetite
  depraved — *see* Pica

Appetite — *continued*
excessive R63.2
lack or loss — *see also* Anorexia R63.0
nonorganic origin F50.89
psychogenic F50.89
perverted (hysterical) — *see* Pica
Apple peel syndrome Q41.1
Apprehension state F41.1
Apprehensiveness, abnormal F41.9
Approximal wear K03.0
Apraxia (classic) (ideational) (ideokinetic) (ideomotor)
(motor) (verbal) R48.2
following
cerebrovascular disease I69.990
cerebral infarction I69.390
intracerebral hemorrhage I69.190
nontraumatic intracranial hemorrhage NEC
I69.290
specified disease NEC I69.890
subarachnoid hemorrhage I69.090
oculomotor, congenital H51.8
Aptyalism K11.7
Apudoma — *see* Neoplasm, uncertain behavior, by site
Aqueous misdirection H40.83- ☑
Arabicum elephantiasis — *see* Infestation, filarial
Arachnitis — *see* Meningitis
Arachnodactyly — *see* Syndrome, Marfan's
Arachnoiditis (acute) (adhesive) (basal) (brain) (cere-
brospinal) — *see* Meningitis
Arachnophobia F40.210
Arboencephalitis, Australian A83.4
Arborization block (heart) I45.5
ARC (AIDS-related complex) B20
Arch
aortic Q25.49
bovine Q25.49
Arches — *see* condition
Arcuate uterus Q51.810
Arcuatus uterus Q51.810
Arcus (cornea) senilis — *see* Degeneration, cornea, senile
Arc-welder's lung J63.4
Areflexia R29.2
Areola — *see* condition
Argentaffinoma — *see also* Neoplasm, uncertain behav-
ior, by site
malignant — *see* Neoplasm, malignant, by site
syndrome E34.0
Argininemia E72.21
Arginosuccinic aciduria E72.22
Argyll Robertson phenomenon, pupil or syndrome
(syphilitic) A52.19
atypical H57.09
nonsyphilitic H57.09
Argyria, argyriasis
conjunctival H11.13- ☑
from drug or medicament — *see* Table of Drugs and
Chemicals, by substance
Argyrosis, conjunctival H11.13- ☑
Arhinencephaly Q04.1
Ariboflavinosis E53.0
Arm — *see* condition
Arnold-Chiari disease, obstruction or syndrome (type
II) Q07.00
with
hydrocephalus Q07.02
with spina bifida Q07.03
spina bifida Q07.01
with hydrocephalus Q07.03
type III — *see* Encephalocele
type IV Q04.8
Aromatic amino-acid metabolism disorder E70.9
specified NEC E70.8
Arousals, confusional G47.51
Arrest, arrested
cardiac I46.9
complicating
abortion — *see* Abortion, by type, complicated
by, cardiac arrest
anesthesia (general) (local) or other sedation —
see Table of Drugs and Chemicals, by drug
in labor and delivery O74.2
in pregnancy O29.11- ☑
postpartum, puerperal O89.1
delivery (cesarean) (instrumental) O75.4
due to
cardiac condition I46.2
specified condition NEC I46.8

Arrest, arrested — *continued*
cardiac — *continued*
intraoperative I97.71- ☑
newborn P29.81
personal history, successfully resuscitated Z86.74
postprocedural I97.12- ☑
obstetric procedure O75.4
cardiorespiratory — *see* Arrest, cardiac
circulatory — *see* Arrest, cardiac
deep transverse O64.0 ☑
development or growth
bone — *see* Disorder, bone, development or growth
child R62.50
tracheal rings Q32.1
epiphyseal
complete
femur M89.15- ☑
humerus M89.12- ☑
tibia M89.16- ☑
ulna M89.13- ☑
forearm M89.13- ☑
specified NEC M89.13- ☑
ulna — *see* Arrest, epiphyseal, by type, ulna
lower leg M89.16- ☑
specified NEC M89.168
tibia — *see* Arrest, epiphyseal, by type, tibia
partial
femur M89.15- ☑
humerus M89.12- ☑
tibia M89.16- ☑
ulna M89.13- ☑
specified NEC M89.18
granulopoiesis — *see* Agranulocytosis
growth plate — *see* Arrest, epiphyseal
heart — *see* Arrest, cardiac
legal, anxiety concerning Z65.3
physeal — *see* Arrest, epiphyseal
respiratory R09.2
newborn P28.81
sinus I45.5
spermatogenesis (complete) — *see* Azoospermia
incomplete — *see* Oligospermia
transverse (deep) O64.0 ☑
Arrhenoblastoma
benign
specified site — *see* Neoplasm, benign, by site
unspecified site
female D27.9
male D29.20
malignant
specified site — *see* Neoplasm, malignant, by site
unspecified site
female C56.9
male C62.90
specified site — *see* Neoplasm, uncertain behavior, by
site
unspecified site
female D39.10
male D40.10
Arrhythmia (auricle) (cardiac) (juvenile) (nodal) (reflex)
(sinus) (supraventricular) (transitory) (ventricle) I49.9
block I45.9
extrasystolic I49.49
newborn
bradycardia P29.12
occurring before birth P03.819
before onset of labor P03.810
during labor P03.811
tachycardia P29.11
psychogenic F45.8
specified NEC I49.8
vagal R55
ventricular re-entry I47.0
Arrillaga-Ayerza syndrome (pulmonary sclerosis with
pulmonary hypertension) I27.0
Arsenical pigmentation L81.8
from drug or medicament — *see* Table of Drugs and
Chemicals
Arsenism — *see* Poisoning, arsenic
Arterial — *see* condition
Arteriofibrosis — *see* Arteriosclerosis
Arteriolar sclerosis — *see* Arteriosclerosis
Arteriolith — *see* Arteriosclerosis
Arteriolitis I77.6
necrotizing, kidney I77.5
renal — *see* Hypertension, kidney
Arteriolosclerosis — *see* Arteriosclerosis

Arterionephrosclerosis — *see* Hypertension, kidney
Arteriopathy I77.9
cerebral autosomal dominant, with subcortical infarcts
and leukoencephalopathy (CADASIL) I67.850
Arteriosclerosis, arteriosclerotic (diffuse) (obliterans)
(of) (senile) (with calcification) I70.90
aorta I70.0
arteries of extremities — *see* Arteriosclerosis, extremities
brain I67.2
bypass graft
coronary — *see* Arteriosclerosis, coronary, bypass
graft
extremities — *see* Arteriosclerosis, extremities, bypass graft
cardiac — *see* Disease, heart, ischemic, atherosclerotic
cardiopathy — *see* Disease, heart, ischemic,
atherosclerotic
cardiorenal — *see* Hypertension, cardiorenal
cardiovascular — *see* Disease, heart, ischemic,
atherosclerotic
carotid — *see also* Occlusion, artery, carotid I65.2- ☑
central nervous system I67.2
cerebral I67.2
cerebrovascular I67.2
coronary (artery)
due to
calcified coronary lesion (severely) I25.84
lipid rich plaque I25.83
bypass graft I25.810
with
angina pectoris I25.709
with documented spasm I25.701
specified type NEC I25.708
unstable I25.700
ischemic chest pain I25.709
autologous artery I25.810
with
angina pectoris I25.729
with documented spasm I25.721
specified type I25.728
unstable I25.720
ischemic chest pain I25.729
autologous vein I25.810
with
angina pectoris I25.719
with documented spasm I25.711
specified type I25.718
unstable I25.710
ischemic chest pain I25.719
nonautologous biological I25.810
with
angina pectoris I25.739
with documented spasm I25.731
specified type I25.738
unstable I25.730
ischemic chest pain I25.739
specified type NEC I25.810
with
angina pectoris I25.799
with documented spasm I25.791
specified type I25.798
unstable I25.790
ischemic chest pain I25.799
native vessel
with
angina pectoris I25.119
with documented spasm I25.111
specified type NEC I25.118
unstable I25.110
ischemic chest pain I25.119
transplanted heart I25.811
bypass graft I25.812
with
angina pectoris I25.769
with documented spasm I25.761
specified type I25.768
unstable I25.760
ischemic chest pain I25.769
native coronary artery I25.811
with
angina pectoris I25.759
with documented spasm I25.751
specified type I25.758
unstable I25.750
ischemic chest pain I25.759
extremities (native arteries) I70.209
bypass graft I70.309

☑ **Additional Character Required** — Refer to the Tabular List for Character Selection ▽ **Subterms under main terms may continue to next column or page**

Arteriosclerosis, arteriosclerotic — *continued*
  extremities — *continued*
    bypass graft — *continued*
      autologous vein graft I70.409
        leg I70.409
          with
            gangrene (and intermittent claudication, rest pain and rest pain) I70.469
            intermittent claudication I70.419
            rest pain (and intermittent claudication) I70.429
        bilateral I70.403
          with
            gangrene (and intermittent claudication, rest pain and ulcer) I70.463
            intermittent claudication I70.463
            rest pain (and intermittent claudication) I70.423
          specified type NEC I70.493
        left I70.402
          with
            gangrene (and intermittent claudication, rest pain and ulcer) I70.462
            intermittent claudication I70.412
            rest pain (and intermittent claudication) I70.422
            ulceration (and intermittent claudication and rest pain) I70.449
              ankle I70.443
              calf I70.442
              foot site NEC I70.445
              heel I70.444
              lower leg NEC I70.448
              midfoot I70.444
              thigh I70.441
          specified type NEC I70.492
        right I70.401
          with
            gangrene (and intermittent claudication, rest pain and ulcer) I70.461
            intermittent claudication I70.411
            rest pain (and intermittent claudication) I70.421
            ulceration (and intermittent claudication and rest pain) I70.439
              ankle I70.433
              calf I70.432
              foot site NEC I70.435
              heel I70.434
              lower leg NEC I70.438
              midfoot I70.434
              thigh I70.431
          specified type NEC I70.491
        specified type NEC I70.499
      specified NEC I70.408
        with
          gangrene (and intermittent claudication, rest pain and ulcer) I70.468
          intermittent claudication I70.418
          rest pain (and intermittent claudication) I70.428
          ulceration (and intermittent claudication and rest pain) I70.45
        specified type NEC I70.498
      leg I70.309
        with
          gangrene (and intermittent claudication, rest pain and ulcer) I70.369
          intermittent claudication I70.319
          rest pain (and intermittent claudication) I70.329
        bilateral I70.303
          with
           gangrene (and intermittent claudication, rest pain and ulcer) I70.363
           intermittent claudication I70.313
           rest pain (and intermittent claudication) I70.323
         specified type NEC I70.393
        left I70.302
          with
           gangrene (and intermittent claudication, rest pain and ulcer) I70.362
           intermittent claudication I70.312
           rest pain (and intermittent claudication) I70.322

Arteriosclerosis, arteriosclerotic — *continued*
  extremities — *continued*
    bypass graft — *continued*
      leg — *continued*
        left — *continued*
          with — *continued*
            ulceration (and intermittent claudication and rest pain) I70.349
              ankle I70.343
              calf I70.342
              foot site NEC I70.345
              heel I70.344
              lower leg NEC I70.348
              midfoot I70.344
              thigh I70.341
          specified type NEC I70.392
        right I70.301
          with
            gangrene (and intermittent claudication, rest pain and ulcer) I70.361
            intermittent claudication I70.311
            rest pain (and intermittent claudication) I70.321
            ulceration (and intermittent claudication and rest pain I70.339
              ankle I70.333
              calf I70.332
              foot site NEC I70.335
              heel I70.334
              lower leg NEC I70.338
              midfoot I70.334
              thigh I70.331
          specified type NEC I70.391
        specified type NEC I70.399
      nonautologous biological graft I70.509
        leg I70.509
          with
           gangrene (and intermittent claudication, rest pain and ulcer) I70.569
           intermittent claudication I70.519
           rest pain (and intermittent claudication) I70.529
        bilateral I70.503
          with
           gangrene (and intermittent claudication, rest pain and ulcer) I70.563
           intermittent claudication I70.513
           rest pain (and intermittent claudication) I70.523
         specified type NEC I70.593
        left I70.502
          with
           gangrene (and intermittent claudication, rest pain and ulcer) I70.562
           intermittent claudication I70.512
           rest pain (and intermittent claudication) I70.522
           ulceration (and intermittent claudication and rest pain) I70.549
            ankle I70.543
            calf I70.542
            foot site NEC I70.545
            heel I70.544
            lower leg NEC I70.548
            midfoot I70.544
            thigh I70.541
         specified type NEC I70.592
        right I70.501
          with
           gangrene (and intermittent claudication, rest pain and ulcer) I70.561
           intermittent claudication I70.511
           rest pain (and intermittent claudication) I70.521
           ulceration (and intermittent claudication and rest pain) I70.539
            ankle I70.533
            calf I70.532
            foot site NEC I70.535
            heel I70.534
            lower leg NEC I70.538
            midfoot I70.534
            thigh I70.531
         specified type NEC I70.591
        specified type NEC I70.599
      specified NEC I70.508

Arteriosclerosis, arteriosclerotic — *continued*
  extremities — *continued*
    bypass graft — *continued*
      nonautologous biological graft — *continued*
        specified — *continued*
          with
           gangrene (and intermittent claudication, rest pain and ulcer) I70.568
           intermittent claudication I70.518
           rest pain (and intermittent claudication) I70.528
           ulceration (and intermittent claudication and rest pain) I70.55
        specified type NEC I70.598
      nonbiological graft I70.609
        leg I70.609
          with
           gangrene (and intermittent claudication, rest pain and ulcer) I70.669
           intermittent claudication I70.619
           rest pain (and intermittent claudication) I70.629
        bilateral I70.603
          with
           gangrene (and intermittent claudication, rest pain and ulcer) I70.663
           intermittent claudication I70.613
           rest pain (and intermittent claudication) I70.623
         specified type NEC I70.693
        left I70.602
          with
           gangrene (and intermittent claudication, rest pain and ulcer) I70.662
           intermittent claudication I70.612
           rest pain (and intermittent claudication) I70.622
           ulceration (and intermittent claudication and rest pain) I70.649
            ankle I70.643
            calf I70.642
            foot site NEC I70.645
            heel I70.644
            lower leg NEC I70.648
            midfoot I70.644
            thigh I70.641
         specified type NEC I70.692
        right I70.601
          with
           gangrene (and intermittent claudication, rest pain and ulcer) I70.661
           intermittent claudication I70.611
           rest pain (and intermittent claudication) I70.621
           ulceration (and intermittent claudication and rest pain) I70.639
            ankle I70.633
            calf I70.632
            foot site NEC I70.635
            heel I70.634
            lower leg NEC I70.638
            midfoot I70.634
            thigh I70.631
         specified type NEC I70.691
        specified type NEC I70.699
      specified NEC I70.608
        with
          gangrene (and intermittent claudication, rest pain and ulcer) I70.668
          intermittent claudication I70.618
          rest pain (and intermittent claudication) I70.628
          ulceration (and intermittent claudication and rest pain) I70.65
        specified type NEC I70.698
      specified graft NEC I70.709
        leg I70.709
          with
           gangrene (and intermittent claudication, rest pain and ulcer) I70.769
           intermittent claudication I70.719
           rest pain (and intermittent claudication) I70.729
        bilateral I70.703

Arteriosclerosis, arteriosclerotic — *continued*
  extremities — *continued*
    bypass graft — *continued*
      specified graft — *continued*
        leg — *continued*
          bilateral — *continued*
            with
              gangrene (and intermittent claudication, rest pain and ulcer) I70.763
              intermittent claudication I70.713
              rest pain (and intermittent claudication) I70.723
              specified type NEC I70.793
          left I70.702
            with
              gangrene (and intermittent claudication, rest pain and ulcer) I70.762
              intermittent claudication I70.712
              rest pain (and intermittent claudication) I70.722
              ulceration (and intermittent claudication and rest pain) I70.749
                ankle I70.743
                calf I70.742
                foot site NEC I70.745
                heel I70.744
                lower leg NEC I70.748
                midfoot I70.744
                thigh I70.741
            specified type NEC I70.792
          right I70.701
            with
              gangrene (and intermittent claudication, rest pain and ulcer) I70.761
              intermittent claudication I70.711
              rest pain (and intermittent claudication) I70.721
              ulceration (and intermittent claudication and rest pain) I70.739
                ankle I70.733
                calf I70.732
                foot site NEC I70.735
                heel I70.734
                lower leg NEC I70.738
                midfoot I70.734
                thigh I70.731
            specified type NEC I70.791
        specified type NEC I70.799
      specified NEC I70.708
        with
          gangrene (and intermittent claudication, rest pain and ulcer) I70.768
          intermittent claudication I70.718
          rest pain (and intermittent claudication) I70.728
          ulceration (and intermittent claudication and rest pain) I70.75
          specified type NEC I70.798
      specified NEC I70.308
        with
          gangrene (and intermittent claudication, rest pain and ulcer) I70.368
          intermittent claudication I70.318
          rest pain (and intermittent claudication) I70.328
          ulceration (and intermittent claudication and rest pain) I70.35
          specifiec type NEC I70.398
    leg I70.209
      with
        gangrene (and intermittent claudication, rest pain and ulcer) I70.269
        intermittent claudication I70.219
        rest pain (and intermittent claudication) I70.229
      bilateral I70.203
        with
          gangrene (and intermittent claudication, rest pain and ulcer) I70.263
          intermittent claudication I70.213
          rest pain (and intermittent claudication) I70.223
          specified type NEC I70.293
      left I70.202

Arteriosclerosis, arteriosclerotic — *continued*
  extremities — *continued*
    leg — *continued*
      left — *continued*
        with
          gangrene (and intermittent claudication, rest pain and ulcer) I70.262
          intermittent claudication I70.212
          rest pain (and intermittent claudication) I70.222
          ulceration (and intermittent claudication and rest pain) I70.249
            ankle I70.243
            calf I70.242
            foot site NEC I70.245
            heel I70.244
            lower leg NEC I70.248
            midfoot I70.244
            thigh I70.241
        specified type NEC I70.292
      right I70.201
        with
          gangrene (and intermittent claudication, rest pain and ulcer) I70.261
          intermittent claudication I70.211
          rest pain (and intermittent claudication) I70.221
          ulceration (and intermittent claudication and rest pain) I70.239
            ankle I70.233
            calf I70.232
            foot site NEC I70.235
            heel I70.234
            lower leg NEC I70.238
            midfoot I70.234
            thigh I70.231
        specified type NEC I70.291
      specified type NEC I70.299
    specified site NEC I70.208
      with
        gangrene (and intermittent claudication, rest pain and ulcer) I70.268
        intermittent claudication I70.218
        rest pain (and intermittent claudication) I70.228
        ulceration (and intermittent claudication and rest pain) I70.25
        specified type NEC I70.298
  generalized I70.91
  heart (disease) — *see* Arteriosclerosis, coronary (artery),
  kidney — *see* Hypertension, kidney
  medial — *see* Arteriosclerosis, extremities
  mesenteric (artery) K55.1
  Mönckeberg's — *see* Arteriosclerosis, extremities
  myocarditis I51.4
  peripheral (of extremities) — *see* Arteriosclerosis, extremities
  pulmonary (idiopathic) I27.0
  renal (arterioles) — *see also* Hypertension, kidney
    artery I70.1
  retina (vascular) I70.8 [H35.0-] ☑
  specified artery NEC I70.8
  spinal (cord) G95.19
  vertebral (artery) I67.2
Arteriospasm I73.9
Arteriovenous — *see* condition
Arteritis I77.6
  allergic M31.0
  aorta (nonsyphilitic) I77.6
    syphilitic A52.02
  aortic arch M31.4
  brachiocephalic M31.4
  brain I67.7
    syphilitic A52.04
  cerebral I67.7
    in systemic lupus erythematosus M32.19
    listerial A32.89
    syphilitic A52.04
    tuberculous A18.89
  coronary (artery) I25.89
    rheumatic I01.8
      chronic I09.89
    syphilitic A52.06
  cranial (left) (right), giant cell M31.6
  deformans — *see* Arteriosclerosis
  giant cell NEC M31.6
    with polymyalgia rheumatica M31.5
  necrosing or necrotizing M31.9

Arteritis — *continued*
  necrosing or necrotizing — *continued*
    specified NEC M31.8
  nodosa M30.0
  obliterans — *see* Arteriosclerosis
  pulmonary I28.8
  rheumatic — *see* Fever, rheumatic
  senile — *see* Arteriosclerosis
  suppurative I77.2
  syphilitic (general) A52.09
    brain A52.04
    coronary A52.06
    spinal A52.09
  temporal, giant cell M31.6
  young female aortic arch syndrome M31.4
Artery, arterial — *see also* condition
  abscess I77.89
  single umbilical Q27.0
Arthralgia (allergic) — *see also* Pain, joint
  in caisson disease T70.3 ☑
  temporomandibular M26.62- ☑
Arthritis, arthritic (acute) (chronic) (nonpyogenic) (subacute) M19.90
  allergic — *see* Arthritis, specified form NEC
  ankylosing (crippling) (spine) — *see also* Spondylitis, ankylosing
    sites other than spine — *see* Arthritis, specified form NEC
  atrophic — *see* Osteoarthritis
    spine — *see* Spondylitis, ankylosing
  back — *see* Spondylopathy, inflammatory
  blennorrhagic (gonococcal) A54.42
  Charcot's — *see* Arthropathy, neuropathic
    diabetic — *see* Diabetes, arthropathy, neuropathic
    syringomyelic G95.0
  chylous (filarial) — *see also* category M01 B74.9
  climacteric (any site) NEC — *see* Arthritis, specified form NEC
  crystal (-induced) — *see* Arthritis, in, crystals
  deformans — *see* Osteoarthritis
  degenerative — *see* Osteoarthritis
  due to or associated with
    acromegaly E22.0
    brucellosis — *see* Brucellosis
    caisson disease T70.3 ☑
    diabetes — *see* Diabetes, arthropathy
    dracontiasis — *see also* category M01 B72
    enteritis NEC
      regional — *see* Enteritis, regional
    erysipelas — *see also* category M01 A46
    erythema
      epidemic A25.1
      nodosum L52
    filariasis NOS B74.9
    glanders A24.0
    helminthiasis — *see also* category M01 B83.9
    hemophilia D66 *[M36.2]*
    Henoch- (Schönlein) purpura D69.0 *[M36.4]*
    human parvovirus — *see also* category M01 B97.6
    infectious disease NEC M01 ☑
    leprosy (see also category M01) — *see also* Leprosy A30.9
    Lyme disease A69.23
    mycobacteria — *see also* category M01 A31.8
    parasitic disease NEC — *see also* category M01 B89
    paratyphoid fever (see also category M01) — *see also* Fever, paratyphoid A01.4
    rat bite fever — *see also* category M01 A25.1
    regional enteritis — *see* Enteritis, regional
    respiratory disorder NOS J98.9
    serum sickness — *see also* Reaction, serum T80.69 ☑
    syringomyelia G95.0
    typhoid fever A01.04
  epidemic erythema A25.1
  febrile — *see* Fever, rheumatic
  gonococcal A54.42
  gouty (acute) — *see* Gout
  in (due to)
    acromegaly — *see also* subcategory M14.8- E22.0
    amyloidosis — *see also* subcategory M14.8- E85.4
    bacterial disease — *see also* subcategory M01 A49.9
    Behçet's syndrome M35.2
    caisson disease — *see also* subcategory M14.8- T70.3 ☑
    coliform bacilli (Escherichia coli) — *see* Arthritis, in, pyogenic organism NEC

28 ☑ **Additional Character Required** — Refer to the Tabular List for Character Selection   ▽ **Subterms under main terms may continue to next column or page**

Arteriosclerosis, arteriosclerotic — Arthritis, arthritic

Arthritis, arthritic — *continued*
  in — *continued*
    crystals M11.9
      dicalcium phosphate — *see* Arthritis, in, crystals, specified type NEC
      hydroxyapatite M11.0- ☑
      pyrophosphate — *see* Arthritis, in, crystals, specified type NEC
      specified type NEC M11.80
        ankle M11.87- ☑
        elbow M11.82- ☑
        foot joint M11.87- ☑
        hand joint M11.84- ☑
        hip M11.85- ☑
        knee M11.86- ☑
        multiple sites M11.8- ☑
        shoulder M11.81- ☑
        vertebrae M11.88
        wrist M11.83- ☑
    dermatoarthritis, lipoid E78.81
    dracontiasis (dracunculiasis) — *see also* category M01 B72
    endocrine disorder NEC — *see also* subcategory M14.8- E34.9
    enteritis, infectious NEC — *see also* category M01 A09
      specified organism NEC — *see also* category M01 A08.8
    erythema
      multiforme — *see also* subcategory M14.8- L51.9
      nodosum — *see also* subcategory M14.8- L52
    gout — *see* Gout
    helminthiasis NEC — *see also* category M01 B83.9
    hemochromatosis — *see also* subcategory M14.8- E83.118
    hemoglobinopathy NEC D58.2 *[M36.3]*
    hemophilia NEC D66 *[M36.2]*
    Hemophilus influenzae M00.8- ☑ *[B96.3]*
    Henoch (-Schönlein) purpura D69.0 *[M36.4]*
    hyperparathyroidism NEC — *see also* subcategory M14.8- E21.3
    hypersensitivity reaction NEC T78.49 ☑ *[M36.4]*
    hypogammaglobulinemia — *see also* subcategory M14.8- D80.1
    hypothyroidism NEC — *see also* subcategory M14.8- E03.9
    infection — *see* Arthritis, pyogenic or pyemic
      spine — *see* Spondylopathy, infective
    infectious disease NEC M01 ☑
    leprosy — *see also* category M01 A30.9
    leukemia NEC C95.9- ☑ *[M36.1]*
    lipoid dermatoarthritis E78.81
    Lyme disease A69.23
    Mediterranean fever, familial — *see also* subcategory M14.8- M04.1
    Meningococcus A39.83
    metabolic disorder NEC — *see also* subcategory M14.8- E88.9
    multiple myelomatosis C90.0- ☑ *[M36.1]*
    mumps B26.85
    mycosis NEC — *see also* category M01 B49
    myelomatosis (multiple) C90.0- ☑ *[M36.1]*
    neurological disorder NEC G98.0
    ochronosis — *see also* subcategory M14.8- E70.29
    O'nyong-nyong — *see also* category M01 A92.1
    parasitic disease NEC — *see also* category M01 B89
    paratyphoid fever — *see also* category M01 A01.4
    Pseudomonas — *see* Arthritis, pyogenic, bacterial NEC
    psoriasis L40.50
    pyogenic organism NEC — *see* Arthritis, pyogenic, bacterial NEC
    Reiter's disease — *see* Reiter's disease
    respiratory disorder NEC — *see also* subcategory M14.8- J98.9
    reticulosis, malignant — *see also* subcategory M14.8- C86.0
    rubella B06.82
    Salmonella (arizonae) (cholerae-suis) (enteritidis) (typhimurium) A02.23
    sarcoidosis D86.86
    specified bacteria NEC — *see* Arthritis, pyogenic, bacterial NEC
    sporotrichosis B42.82
    syringomyelia G95.0
    thalassemia NEC D56.9 *[M36.3]*
    tuberculosis — *see* Tuberculosis, arthritis

Arthritis, arthritic — *continued*
  in — *continued*
    typhoid fever A01.04
    urethritis, Reiter's — *see* Reiter's disease
    viral disease NEC — *see also* category M01 B34.9
  infectious or infective — *see also* Arthritis, pyogenic or pyemic
    spine — *see* Spondylopathy, infective
  juvenile M08.90
    with systemic onset — *see* Still's disease
    ankle M08.97- ☑
    elbow M08.92- ☑
    foot joint M08.97- ☑
    hand joint M08.94- ☑
    hip M08.95- ☑
    knee M08.96- ☑
    multiple site M08.99
    pauciarticular M08.40
      ankle M08.47- ☑
      elbow M08.42- ☑
      foot joint M08.47- ☑
      hand joint M08.44- ☑
      hip M08.45- ☑
      knee M08.46- ☑
      shoulder M08.41- ☑
      vertebrae M08.48
      wrist M08.43- ☑
    psoriatic L40.54
    rheumatoid — *see* Arthritis, rheumatoid, juvenile
    shoulder M08.91- ☑
    specified type NEC M08.80
      ankle M08.87- ☑
      elbow M08.82- ☑
      foot joint M08.87- ☑
      hand joint M08.84- ☑
      hip M08.85- ☑
      knee M08.86- ☑
      multiple site M08.89
      shoulder M08.81- ☑
      specified joint NEC M08.88
      vertebrae M08.88
      wrist M08.83- ☑
    wrist M08.93- ☑
  meaning osteoarthritis — *see* Osteoarthritis
  meningococcal A39.83
  menopausal (any site) NEC — *see* Arthritis, specified form NEC
  mutilans (psoriatic) L40.52
  mycotic NEC — *see also* category M01 B49
  neuropathic (Charcot) — *see* Arthropathy, neuropathic
    diabetic — *see* Diabetes, arthropathy, neuropathic
    nonsyphilitic NEC G98.0
    syringomyelic G95.0
  ochronotic — *see also* subcategory M14.8- E70.29
  palindromic (any site) — *see* Rheumatism, palindromic
  pneumococcal M00.10
    ankle M00.17- ☑
    elbow M00.12- ☑
    foot joint — *see* Arthritis, pneumococcal, ankle
    hand joint M00.14- ☑
    hip M00.15- ☑
    knee M00.16- ☑
    multiple site M00.19
    shoulder M00.11- ☑
    vertebra M00.18
    wrist M00.13- ☑
  postdysenteric — *see* Arthropathy, postdysenteric
  postmeningococcal A39.84
  postrheumatic, chronic — *see* Arthropathy, postrheumatic, chronic
  primary progressive — *see also* Arthritis, specified form NEC
    spine — *see* Spondylitis, ankylosing
  psoriatic L40.50
  purulent (any site except spine) — *see* Arthritis, pyogenic or pyemic
    spine — *see* Spondylopathy, infective
  pyogenic or pyemic (any site except spine) M00.9
    bacterial NEC M00.80
      ankle M00.87- ☑
      elbow M00.82- ☑
      foot joint — *see* Arthritis, pyogenic, bacterial NEC, ankle
      hand joint M00.84- ☑
      hip M00.85- ☑
      knee M00.86- ☑
      multiple site M00.89

Arthritis, arthritic — *continued*
  pyogenic or pyemic — *continued*
    bacterial — *continued*
      shoulder M00.81- ☑
      vertebra M00.88
      wrist M00.83- ☑
    pneumococcal — *see* Arthritis, pneumococcal
    spine — *see* Spondylopathy, infective
    staphylococcal — *see* Arthritis, staphylococcal
    streptococcal — *see* Arthritis, streptococcal NEC
      pneumococcal — *see* Arthritis, pneumococcal
  reactive — *see* Reiter's disease
  rheumatic — *see also* Arthritis, rheumatoid
    acute or subacute — *see* Fever, rheumatic
  rheumatoid M06.9
    with
      carditis — *see* Rheumatoid, carditis
      endocarditis — *see* Rheumatoid, carditis
      heart involvement NEC — *see* Rheumatoid, carditis
      lung involvement — *see* Rheumatoid, lung
      myocarditis — *see* Rheumatoid, carditis
      myopathy — *see* Rheumatoid, myopathy
      pericarditis — *see* Rheumatoid, carditis
      polyneuropathy — *see* Rheumatoid, polyneuropathy
      rheumatoid factor — *see* Arthritis, rheumatoid, seropositive
      splenoadenomegaly and leukopenia — *see* Felty's syndrome
      vasculitis — *see* Rheumatoid, vasculitis
      visceral involvement NEC — *see* Rheumatoid, arthritis, with involvement of organs NEC
    juvenile (with or without rheumatoid factor) M08.00
      ankle M08.07- ☑
      elbow M08.02- ☑
      foot joint M08.07- ☑
      hand joint M08.04- ☑
      hip M08.05- ☑
      knee M08.06- ☑
      multiple site M08.09
      shoulder M08.01- ☑
      vertebra M08.08
      wrist M08.03- ☑
    seronegative M06.00
      ankle M06.07- ☑
      elbow M06.02- ☑
      foot joint M06.07- ☑
      hand joint M06.04- ☑
      hip M06.05- ☑
      knee M06.06- ☑
      multiple site M06.09
      shoulder M06.01- ☑
      vertebra M06.08
      wrist M06.03- ☑
    seropositive M05.9
      specified NEC M05.80
        ankle M05.87- ☑
        elbow M05.82- ☑
        foot joint M05.87- ☑
        hand joint M05.84- ☑
        hip M05.85- ☑
        knee M05.86- ☑
        multiple sites M05.89
        shoulder M05.81- ☑
        vertebra — *see* Spondylitis, ankylosing
        wrist M05.83- ☑
      without organ involvement M05.70
        ankle M05.77- ☑
        elbow M05.72- ☑
        foot joint M05.77- ☑
        hand joint M05.74- ☑
        hip M05.75- ☑
        knee M05.76- ☑
        multiple sites M05.79
        shoulder M05.71- ☑
        vertebra — *see* Spondylitis, ankylosing
        wrist M05.73- ☑
    specified type NEC M06.80
      ankle M06.87- ☑
      elbow M06.82- ☑
      foot joint M06.87- ☑
      hand joint M06.84- ☑
      hip M06.85- ☑
      knee M06.86- ☑
      multiple site M06.89

Arthritis, arthritic — *continued*
  rheumatoid — *continued*
    specified type — *continued*
      shoulder M06.81- ☑
      vertebra M06.88
      wrist M06.83- ☑
    spine — *see* Spondylitis, ankylosing
  rubella B06.82
  scorbutic — *see also* subcategory M14.8- E54
  senile or senescent — *see* Osteoarthritis
  septic (any site except spine) — *see* Arthritis, pyogenic or pyemic
    spine — *see* Spondylopathy, infective
  serum (nontherapeutic) (therapeutic) — *see* Arthropathy, postimmunization
  specified form NEC M13.80
    ankle M13.87- ☑
    elbow M13.82- ☑
    foot joint M13.87- ☑
    hand joint M13.84- ☑
    hip M13.85- ☑
    knee M13.86- ☑
    multiple site M13.89
    shoulder M13.81- ☑
    specified joint NEC M13.88
    wrist M13.83- ☑
  spine — *see also* Spondylopathy, inflammatory
    infectious or infective NEC — *see* Spondylopathy, infective
    Marie-Strümpell — *see* Spondylitis, ankylosing
    pyogenic — *see* Spondylopathy, infective
    rheumatoid — *see* Spondylitis, ankylosing
    traumatic (old) — *see* Spondylopathy, traumatic
    tuberculous A18.01
  staphylococcal M00.00
    ankle M00.07- ☑
    elbow M00.02- ☑
    foot joint — *see* Arthritis, staphylococcal, ankle
    hand joint M00.04- ☑
    hip M00.05- ☑
    knee M00.06- ☑
    multiple site M00.09
    shoulder M00.01- ☑
    vertebra M00.08
    wrist M00.03- ☑
  streptococcal NEC M00.20
    ankle M00.27- ☑
    elbow M00.22- ☑
    foot joint — *see* Arthritis, streptococcal, ankle
    hand joint M00.24- ☑
    hip M00.25- ☑
    knee M00.26- ☑
    multiple site M00.29
    shoulder M00.21- ☑
    vertebra M00.28
    wrist M00.23- ☑
  suppurative — *see* Arthritis, pyogenic or pyemic
  syphilitic (late) A52.16
    congenital A50.55 *[M12.80]*
  syphilitica deformans (Charcot) A52.16
  temporomandibular M26.69
  toxic of menopause (any site) — *see* Arthritis, specified form NEC
  transient — *see* Arthropathy, specified form NEC
  traumatic (chronic) — *see* Arthropathy, traumatic
  tuberculous A18.02
    spine A18.01
  uratic — *see* Gout
  urethritica (Reiter's) — *see* Reiter's disease
  vertebral — *see* Spondylopathy, inflammatory
  villous (any site) — *see* Arthropathy, specified form NEC

Arthrocele — *see* Effusion, joint
Arthrodesis status Z98.1
Arthrodynia — *see also* Pain, joint
Arthrodysplasia Q74.9
Arthrofibrosis, joint — *see* Ankylosis
Arthrogryposis (congenital) Q68.8
  multiplex congenita Q74.3
Arthrokatadysis M24.7
Arthropathy — *see also* Arthritis M12.9
  Charcot's — *see* Arthropathy, neuropathic
    diabetic — *see* Diabetes, arthropathy, neuropathic
    syringomyelic G95.0
  cricoarytenoid J38.7
  crystal (-induced) — *see* Arthritis, in, crystals
  diabetic NEC — *see* Diabetes, arthropathy

Arthropathy — *continued*
  distal interphalangeal, psoriatic L40.51
  enteropathic M07.60
    ankle M07.67- ☑
    elbow M07.62- ☑
    foot joint M07.67- ☑
    hand joint M07.64- ☑
    hip M07.65- ☑
    knee M07.66- ☑
    multiple site M07.69
    shoulder M07.61- ☑
    vertebra M07.68
    wrist M07.63- ☑
  following intestinal bypass M02.00
    ankle M02.07- ☑
    elbow M02.02- ☑
    foot joint M02.07- ☑
    hand joint M02.04- ☑
    hip M02.05- ☑
    knee M02.06- ☑
    multiple site M02.09
    shoulder M02.01- ☑
    vertebra M02.08
    wrist M02.03- ☑
  gouty — *see also* Gout
    in (due to)
      Lesch-Nyhan syndrome E79.1 *[M14.8-]* ☑
      sickle-cell disorders D57- *[M14.8-]* ☑
  hemophilic NEC D66 *[M36.2]*
    in (due to)
      hyperparathyroidism NEC E21.3 *[M14.8-]* ☑
      metabolic disease NOS E88.9 *[M14.8-]* ☑
  in (due to)
    acromegaly E22.0 *[M14.8-]* ☑
    amyloidosis E85.4 *[M14.8-]* ☑
    blood disorder NOS D75.9 *[M36.3]*
    diabetes — *see* Diabetes, arthropathy
    endocrine disease NOS E34.9 *[M14.8-]* ☑
    erythema
      multiforme L51.9 *[M14.8-]* ☑
      nodosum L52 *[M14.8-]* ☑
    hemochromatosis E83.118 *[M14.8-]* ☑
    hemoglobinopathy NEC D58.2 *[M36.3]*
    hemophilia NEC D66 *[M36.2]*
    Henoch-Schönlein purpura D69.0 *[M36.4]*
    hyperthyroidism E05.90 *[M14.8-]* ☑
    hypothyroidism E03.9 *[M14.8-]* ☑
    infective endocarditis I33.0 *[M12.80]*
    leukemia NEC C95.9- ☑ *[M36.1]*
    malignant histiocytosis C96.A *[M36.1]*
    metabolic disease NOS E88.9 *[M14.8-]* ☑
    multiple myeloma C90.0- ☑ *[M36.1]*
    neoplastic disease NOS (*see also* Neoplasm) D49.9 *[M36.1]*
    nutritional deficiency — *see also* subcategory M14.8- E63.9
    psoriasis NOS L40.50
    sarcoidosis D86.86
    syphilis (late) A52.77
      congenital A50.55 *[M12.80]*
    thyrotoxicosis — *see also* subcategory M14.8- E05.90
    ulcerative colitis K51.90 *[M07.60]*
    viral hepatitis (postinfectious) NEC B19.9 *[M12.80]*
    Whipple's disease — *see also* subcategory M14.8- K90.81
  Jaccoud — *see* Arthropathy, postrheumatic, chronic
  juvenile — *see* Arthritis, juvenile
    psoriatic L40.54
  mutilans (psoriatic) L40.52
  neuropathic (Charcot) M14.60
    ankle M14.67- ☑
    diabetic — *see* Diabetes, arthropathy, neuropathic
    elbow M14.62- ☑
    foot joint M14.67- ☑
    hand joint M14.64- ☑
    hip M14.65- ☑
    knee M14.66- ☑
    multiple site M14.69
    nonsyphilitic NEC G98.0
    shoulder M14.61- ☑
    syringomyelic G95.0
    vertebra M14.68
    wrist M14.63- ☑
  osteopulmonary — *see* Osteoarthropathy, hypertrophic, specified NEC

Arthropathy — *continued*
  postdysenteric M02.10
    ankle M02.17- ☑
    elbow M02.12- ☑
    foot joint M02.17- ☑
    hand joint M02.14- ☑
    hip M02.15- ☑
    knee M02.16- ☑
    multiple site M02.19
    shoulder M02.11- ☑
    vertebra M02.18
    wrist M02.13- ☑
  postimmunization M02.20
    ankle M02.27- ☑
    elbow M02.22- ☑
    foot joint M02.27- ☑
    hand joint M02.24- ☑
    hip M02.25- ☑
    knee M02.26- ☑
    multiple site M02.29
    shoulder M02.21- ☑
    vertebra M02.28
    wrist M02.23- ☑
  postinfectious NEC B99 ☑ *[M12.80]*
    in (due to)
      enteritis due to Yersinia enterocolitica A04.6 *[M12.80]*
      syphilis A52.77
      viral hepatitis NEC B19.9 *[M12.80]*
  postrheumatic, chronic (Jaccoud) M12.00
    ankle M12.07- ☑
    elbow M12.02- ☑
    foot joint M12.07- ☑
    hand joint M12.04- ☑
    hip M12.05- ☑
    knee M12.06- ☑·
    multiple site M12.09
    shoulder M12.01- ☑
    specified joint NEC M12.08
    vertebrae M12.08
    wrist M12.03- ☑
  psoriatic NEC L40.59
    interphalangeal, distal L40.51
  reactive M02.9
    in (due to)
      infective endocarditis I33.0 *[M02.9]*
    specified type NEC M02.80
      ankle M02.87- ☑
      elbow M02.82- ☑
      foot joint M02.87- ☑
      hand joint M02.84- ☑
      hip M02.85- ☑
      knee M02.86- ☑
      multiple site M02.89
      shoulder M02.81- ☑
      vertebra M02.88
      wrist M02.83- ☑
  specified form NEC M12.80
    ankle M12.87- ☑
    elbow M12.82- ☑
    foot joint M12.87- ☑
    hand joint M12.84- ☑
    hip M12.85- ☑
    knee M12.86- ☑
    multiple site M12.89
    shoulder M12.81- ☑
    specified joint NEC M12.88
    vertebrae M12.88
    wrist M12.83- ☑
  syringomyelic G95.0
  tabes dorsalis A52.16
  tabetic A52.16
  transient — *see* Arthropathy, specified form NEC
  traumatic M12.50
    ankle M12.57- ☑
    elbow M12.52- ☑
    foot joint M12.57- ☑
    hand joint M12.54- ☑
    hip M12.55- ☑
    knee M12.56- ☑
    multiple site M12.59
    shoulder M12.51- ☑
    specified joint NEC M12.58
    vertebrae M12.58
    wrist M12.53- ☑
Arthropyosis — *see* Arthritis, pyogenic or pyemic

☑ **Additional Character Required** — Refer to the Tabular List for Character Selection   ▽ **Subterms under main terms may continue to next column or page**

Arthrosis (deformans) (degenerative) (localized) — *see also* Osteoarthritis M19.90
  spine — *see* Spondylosis
Arthus' phenomenon or reaction T78.41 ☑
  due to
    drug — *see* Table of Drugs and Chemicals, by drug
Articular — *see* condition
Articulation, reverse (teeth) M26.24
Artificial
  insemination complication — *see* Complications, artificial, fertilization
  opening status (functioning) (without complication) Z93.9
    anus (colostomy) Z93.3
    colostomy Z93.3
    cystostomy Z93.50
      appendico-vesicostomy Z93.52
      cutaneous Z93.51
      specified NEC Z93.59
    enterostomy Z93.4
    gastrostomy Z93.1
    ileostomy Z93.2
    intestinal tract NEC Z93.4
    jejunostomy Z93.4
    nephrostomy Z93.6
    specified site NEC Z93.8
    tracheostomy Z93.0
    ureterostomy Z93.6
    urethrostomy Z93.6
    urinary tract NEC Z93.6
    vagina Z93.8
  vagina status Z93.8
Arytenoid — *see* condition
Asbestosis (occupational) J61
Ascariasis B77.9
  with
    complications NEC B77.89
    intestinal complications B77.0
    pneumonia, pneumonitis B77.81
Ascaridosis, ascaridiasis — *see* Ascariasis
Ascaris (infection) (infestation) (lumbricoides) — *see* Ascariasis
Ascending — *see* condition
ASC-H (atypical squamous cells cannot exclude high grade squamous intraepithelial lesion on cytologic smear)
  anus R85.611
  cervix R87.611
  vagina R87.621
Aschoff's bodies — *see* Myocarditis, rheumatic
Ascites (abdominal) R18.8
  cardiac — *see also* Failure, heart, right I50.810
  chylous (nonfilarial) I89.8
    filarial — *see* Infestation, filarial
  due to
    cirrhosis, alcoholic K70.31
    hepatitis
      alcoholic K70.11
      chronic active K71.51
    S. japonicum B65.2
  heart — *see also* Failure, heart, right I50.810
  malignant R18.0
  pseudochylous R18.8
  syphilitic A52.74
  tuberculous A18.31
ASC-US (atypical squamous cells of undetermined significance on cytologic smear)
  anus R85.610
  cervix R87.610
  vagina R87.620
Aseptic — *see* condition
Asherman's syndrome N85.6
Asialia K11.7
Asiatic cholera — *see* Cholera
Asimultagnosia (simultanagnosia) R48.3
Askin's tumor — *see* Neoplasm, connective tissue, malignant
Asocial personality F60.2
Asomatognosia R41.4
Aspartylglucosaminuria E77.1
Asperger's disease or syndrome F84.5
Aspergilloma — *see* Aspergillosis
Aspergillosis (with pneumonia) B44.9
  bronchopulmonary, allergic B44.81
  disseminated B44.7
  generalized B44.7
  pulmonary NEC B44.1
    allergic B44.81
    invasive B44.0

Aspergillosis — *continued*
  specified NEC B44.89
  tonsillar B44.2
Aspergillus (flavus) (fumigatus) (infection) (terreus) — *see* Aspergillosis
Aspermatogenesis — *see* Azoospermia
Aspermia (testis) — *see* Azoospermia
Asphyxia, asphyxiation (by) R09.01
  antenatal P84
  birth P84
  bunny bag — *see* Asphyxia, due to, mechanical threat to breathing, trapped in bed clothes
  crushing S28.0
  drowning T75.1 ☑
  gas, fumes, or vapor — *see* Table of Drugs and Chemicals
  inhalation — *see* Inhalation
  intrauterine P84
  local I73.00
    with gangrene I73.01
  mucus — *see also* Foreign body, respiratory tract, causing asphyxia
  newborn P84
  pathological R09.01
  postnatal P84
    mechanical — *see* Asphyxia, due to, mechanical threat to breathing
  prenatal P84
  reticularis R23.1
  strangulation — *see* Asphyxia, due to, mechanical threat to breathing
  submersion T75.1 ☑
  traumatic T71.9 ☑
    due to
      crushed chest S28.0
      foreign body (in) — *see* Foreign body, respiratory tract, causing asphyxia
      low oxygen content of ambient air T71.20 ☑
        due to
          being trapped in
            low oxygen environment T71.29 ☑
            in car trunk T71.221 ☑
              circumstances undetermined T71.224 ☑
              done with intent to harm by
                another person T71.223 ☑
                self T71.222 ☑
            in refrigerator T71.231 ☑
              circumstances undetermined T71.234 ☑
              done with intent to harm by
                another person T71.233 ☑
                self T71.232 ☑
      cave-in T71.21 ☑
    mechanical threat to breathing (accidental) T71.191 ☑
      circumstances undetermined T71.194 ☑
      done with intent to harm by
        another person T71.193 ☑
        self T71.192 ☑
      hanging T71.161 ☑
        circumstances undetermined T71.164 ☑
        done with intent to harm by
          another person T71.163 ☑
          self T71.162 ☑
      plastic bag T71.121 ☑
        circumstances undetermined T71.124 ☑
        done with intent to harm by
          another person T71.123 ☑
          self T71.122 ☑
      smothering
        in furniture T71.151 ☑
          circumstances undetermined T71.154 ☑
          done with intent to harm by
            another person T71.153 ☑
            self T71.152 ☑
        under
          another person's body T71.141 ☑
            circumstances undetermined T71.144 ☑
            done with intent to harm T71.143 ☑
          pillow T71.111 ☑
            circumstances undetermined T71.114 ☑
            done with intent to harm by another person T71.113 ☑

Asphyxia, asphyxiation — *continued*
  traumatic — *continued*
    due to — *continued*
      mechanical threat to breathing — *continued*
        smothering — *continued*
          under — *continued*
            pillow — *continued*
              done with intent to harm by — *continued*
                self T71.112 ☑
          trapped in bed clothes T71.131 ☑
            circumstances undetermined T71.134 ☑
            done with intent to harm by
              another person T71.133 ☑
              self T71.132 ☑
  vomiting, vomitus — *see* Foreign body, respiratory tract, causing asphyxia
Aspiration
  amniotic (clear) fluid (newborn) P24.10
    with
      pneumonia (pneumonitis) P24.11
      respiratory symptoms P24.11
  blood
    newborn (without respiratory symptoms) P24.20
      with
        pneumonia (pneumonitis) P24.21
        respiratory symptoms P24.21
      specified age NEC — *see* Foreign body, respiratory tract
  bronchitis J69.0
  food or foreign body (with asphyxiation) — *see* Asphyxia, food
  liquor (amnii) (newborn) P24.10
    with
      pneumonia (pneumonitis) P24.11
      respiratory symptoms P24.11
  meconium (newborn) (without respiratory symptoms) P24.00
    with
      pneumonitis (pneumonitis) P24.01
      respiratory symptoms P24.01
  milk (newborn) (without respiratory symptoms) P24.30
    with
      pneumonia (pneumonitis) P24.31
      respiratory symptoms P24.31
    specified age NEC — *see* Foreign body, respiratory tract
  mucus — *see also* Foreign body, by site, causing asphyxia
    newborn P24.10
      with
        pneumonia (pneumonitis) P24.11
        respiratory symptoms P24.11
      neonatal P24.9
      specific NEC (without respiratory symptoms) P24.80
        with
          pneumonia (pneumonitis) P24.81
          respiratory symptoms P24.81
    newborn P24.9
      specific NEC (without respiratory symptoms) P24.80
        with
          pneumonia (pneumonitis) P24.81
          respiratory symptoms P24.81
  pneumonia J69.0
  pneumonitis J69.0
  syndrome of newborn — *see* Aspiration, by substance, with pneumonia
  vernix caseosa (newborn) P24.80
    with
      pneumonia (pneumonitis) P24.81
      respiratory symptoms P24.81
  vomitus — *see also* Foreign body, respiratory tract
    newborn (without respiratory symptoms) P24.30
      with
        pneumonia (pneumonitis) P24.31
        respiratory symptoms P24.31
Asplenia (congenital) Q89.01
  postsurgical Z90.81
Assam fever B55.0
Assault, sexual — *see* Maltreatment
Assmann's focus NEC A15.0
Astasia (-abasia) (hysterical) F44.4
Asteatosis cutis L85.3
Astereognosia, astereognosis R48.1
Asterixis R27.8
  in liver disease K71.3
Asteroid hyalitis — *see* Deposit, crystalline
Asthenia, asthenic R53.1

Asthenia, asthenic — continued
cardiac — see also Failure, heart I50.9
  psychogenic F45.8
cardiovascular — see also Failure, heart I50.9
  psychogenic F45.8
heart — see also Failure, heart I50.9
  psychogenic F45.8
hysterical F44.4
myocardial — see also Failure, heart I50.9
  psychogenic F45.8
nervous F48.8
neurocirculatory F45.8
neurotic F48.8
psychogenic F48.8
psychoneurotic F48.8
psychophysiologic F48.8
reaction (psychophysiologic) F48.8
senile R54
Asthenopia — see also Discomfort, visual
hysterical F44.6
psychogenic F44.6
Asthenospermia — see Abnormal, specimen, male
  genital organs
Asthma, asthmatic (bronchial) (catarrh) (spasmodic)
  J45.909
with
  chronic obstructive bronchitis J44.9
    with
      acute lower respiratory infection J44.0
      exacerbation (acute) J44.1
  chronic obstructive pulmonary disease J44.9
    with
      acute lower respiratory infection J44.0
      exacerbation (acute) J44.1
  exacerbation (acute) J45.901
  hay fever — see Asthma, allergic extrinsic
  rhinitis, allergic — see Asthma, allergic extrinsic
  status asthmaticus J45.902
allergic extrinsic J45.909
  with
    exacerbation (acute) J45.901
    status asthmaticus J45.902
atopic — see Asthma, allergic extrinsic
cardiac — see Failure, ventricular, left
cardiobronchial I50.1
childhood J45.909
  with
    exacerbation (acute) J45.901
    status asthmaticus J45.902
chronic obstructive J44.9
  with
    acute lower respiratory infection J44.0
    exacerbation (acute) J44.1
collier's J60
cough variant J45.991
detergent J69.8
due to
  detergent J69.8
  inhalation of fumes J68.3
eosinophilic J82
extrinsic, allergic — see Asthma, allergic extrinsic
grinder's J62.8
hay — see Asthma, allergic extrinsic
heart I50.1
idiosyncratic — see Asthma, nonallergic
intermittent (mild) J45.20
  with
    exacerbation (acute) J45.21
    status asthmaticus J45.22
intrinsic, nonallergic — see Asthma, nonallergic
Kopp's E32.8
late-onset J45.909
  with
    exacerbation (acute) J45.901
    status asthmaticus J45.902
mild intermittent J45.20
  with
    exacerbation (acute) J45.21
    status asthmaticus J45.22
mild persistent J45.30
  with
    exacerbation (acute) J45.31
    status asthmaticus J45.32
Millar's (laryngismus stridulus) J38.5
miner's J60
mixed J45.909
  with
    exacerbation (acute) J45.901

Asthma, asthmatic — continued
mixed — continued
  with — continued
    status asthmaticus J45.902
moderate persistent J45.40
  with
    exacerbation (acute) J45.41
    status asthmaticus J45.42
nervous — see Asthma, nonallergic
nonallergic (intrinsic) J45.909
  with
    exacerbation (acute) J45.901
    status asthmaticus J45.902
persistent
  mild J45.30
    with
      exacerbation (acute) J45.31
      status asthmaticus J45.32
  moderate J45.40
    with
      exacerbation (acute) J45.41
      status asthmaticus J45.42
  severe J45.50
    with
      exacerbation (acute) J45.51
      status asthmaticus J45.52
platinum J45.998
pneumoconiotic NEC J64
potter's J62.8
predominantly allergic J45.909
psychogenic F54
pulmonary eosinophilic J82
red cedar J67.8
Rostan's I50.1
sandblaster's J62.8
sequoiosis J67.8
severe persistent J45.50
  with
    exacerbation (acute) J45.51
    status asthmaticus J45.52
specified NEC J45.998
stonemason's J62.8
thymic E32.8
tuberculous — see Tuberculosis, pulmonary
Wichmann's (laryngismus stridulus) J38.5
wood J67.8
Astigmatism (compound) (congenital) H52.20- ☑
irregular H52.21- ☑
regular H52.22- ☑
Astraphobia F40.220
Astroblastoma
specified site — see Neoplasm, malignant, by site
unspecified site C71.9
Astrocytoma (cystic)
anaplastic
  specified site — see Neoplasm, malignant, by site
  unspecified site C71.9
fibrillary
  specified site — see Neoplasm, malignant, by site
  unspecified site C71.9
fibrous
  specified site — see Neoplasm, malignant, by site
  unspecified site C71.9
gemistocytic
  specified site — see Neoplasm, malignant, by site
  unspecified site C71.9
juvenile
  specified site — see Neoplasm, malignant, by site
  unspecified site C71.9
pilocytic
  specified site — see Neoplasm, malignant, by site
  unspecified site C71.9
piloid
  specified site — see Neoplasm, malignant, by site
  unspecified site C71.9
protoplasmic
  specified site — see Neoplasm, malignant, by site
  unspecified site C71.9
specified site NEC — see Neoplasm, malignant, by site
subependymal D43.2
  giant cell
    specified site — see Neoplasm, uncertain behavior, by site
    unspecified site D43.2
  specified site — see Neoplasm, uncertain behavior, by site
  unspecified site D43.2
unspecified site C71.9

Astroglioma
specified site — see Neoplasm, malignant, by site
unspecified site C71.9
Asymbolia R48.8
Asymmetry — see also Distortion
between native and reconstructed breast N65.1
face Q67.0
jaw (lower) — see Anomaly, dentofacial, jaw-cranial base relationship, asymmetry
Asynergia, asynergy R27.8
ventricular I51.89
Asystole (heart) — see Arrest, cardiac
At risk
for
  dental caries Z91.849
    high Z91.843
    low Z91.841
    moderate Z91.842
  falling Z91.81
Ataxia, ataxy, ataxic R27.0
acute R27.8
brain (hereditary) G11.9
cerebellar (hereditary) G11.9
  with defective DNA repair G11.3
  alcoholic G31.2
  early-onset G11.1
  in
    alcoholism G31.2
    myxedema E03.9 [G13.2]
    neoplastic disease — see also Neoplasm D49.9 [G32.81]
    specified disease NEC G32.81
  late-onset (Marie's) G11.2
cerebral (hereditary) G11.9
congenital nonprogressive G11.0
family, familial — see Ataxia, hereditary
following
  cerebrovascular disease I69.993
    cerebral infarction I69.393
    intracerebral hemorrhage I69.193
    nontraumatic intracranial hemorrhage NEC I69.293
    specified disease NEC I69.893
    subarachnoid hemorrhage I69.093
Friedreich's (heredofamilial) (cerebellar) (spinal) G11.1
gait R26.0
  hysterical F44.4
general R27.8
gluten M35.9 [G32.81]
  with celiac disease K90.0 [G32.81]
hereditary G11.9
  with neuropathy G60.2
  cerebellar — see Ataxia, cerebellar
  spastic G11.4
  specified NEC G11.8
  spinal (Friedreich's) G11.1
heredofamilial — see Ataxia, hereditary
Hunt's G11.1
hysterical F44.4
locomotor (progressive) (syphilitic) (partial) (spastic) A52.11
  diabetic — see Diabetes, ataxia
Marie's (cerebellar) (heredofamilial) (late-onset) G11.2
nonorganic origin F44.4
nonprogressive, congenital G11.0
psychogenic F44.4
Roussy-Lévy G60.0
Sanger-Brown's (hereditary) G11.2
spastic hereditary G11.4
spinal
  hereditary (Friedreich's) G11.1
  progressive (syphilitic) A52.11
spinocerebellar, X-linked recessive G11.1
telangiectasia (Louis-Bar) G11.3
Ataxia-telangiectasia (Louis-Bar) G11.3
Atelectasis (massive) (partial) (pressure) (pulmonary) J98.11
newborn P28.10
  due to resorption P28.11
  partial P28.19
  primary P28.0
  secondary P28.19
primary (newborn) P28.0
tuberculous — see Tuberculosis, pulmonary
Atelocardia Q24.9
Atelomyelia Q06.1

☑ **Additional Character Required — Refer to the Tabular List for Character Selection**   ▽ **Subterms under main terms may continue to next column or page**

Atheroembolism
- of
  - extremities
    - lower I75.02- ☑
    - upper I75.01- ☑
  - kidney I75.81
  - specified NEC I75.89

Atheroma, atheromatous — *see also* Arteriosclerosis I70.90
- aorta, aortic I70.0
  - valve — *see also* Endocarditis, aortic I35.8
- aorto-iliac I70.0
- artery — *see* Arteriosclerosis
- basilar (artery) I67.2
- carotid (artery) (common) (internal) I67.2
- cerebral (arteries) I67.2
- coronary (artery) I25.10
  - with angina pectoris — *see* Arteriosclerosis, coronary (artery),
  - degeneration — *see* Arteriosclerosis
- heart, cardiac — *see* Disease, heart, ischemic, atherosclerotic
- mitral (valve) I34.8
- myocardium, myocardial — *see* Disease, heart, ischemic, atherosclerotic
- pulmonary valve (heart) — *see also* Endocarditis, pulmonary I37.8
- tricuspid (heart) (valve) I36.8
- valve, valvular — *see* Endocarditis
- vertebral (artery) I67.2

Atheromatosis — *see* Arteriosclerosis

Atherosclerosis — *see also* Arteriosclerosis
- coronary
  - artery I25.10
    - with angina pectoris — *see* Arteriosclerosis, coronary (artery),
    - due to
      - calcified coronary lesion (severely) I25.84
      - lipid rich plaque I25.83
    - transplanted heart I25.811
      - bypass graft I25.812
        - with angina pectoris — *see* Arteriosclerosis, coronary (artery),
      - native coronary artery I25.811
        - with angina pectoris — *see* Arteriosclerosis, coronary (artery),

Athetosis (acquired) R25.8
- bilateral (congenital) G80.3
- congenital (bilateral) (double) G80.3
- double (congenital) G80.3
- unilateral R25.8

Athlete's
- foot B35.3
- heart I51.7

Athrepsia E41

Athyrea (acquired) — *see also* Hypothyroidism
- congenital E03.1

Atonia, atony, atonic
- bladder (sphincter) (neurogenic) N31.2
- capillary I78.8
- cecum K59.8
  - psychogenic F45.8
- colon — *see* Atony, intestine
- congenital P94.2
- esophagus K22.8
- intestine K59.8
  - psychogenic F45.8
- stomach K31.89
  - neurotic or psychogenic F45.8
- uterus (during labor) O62.2
  - with hemorrhage (postpartum) O72.1
  - postpartum (with hemorrhage) O72.1
    - without hemorrhage O75.89

Atopy — *see* History, allergy

Atransferrinemia, congenital E88.09

Atresia, atretic
- alimentary organ or tract NEC Q45.8
  - upper Q40.8
- ani, anus, anal (canal) Q42.3
  - with fistula Q42.2
- aorta (ring) Q25.29
- aortic (orifice) (valve) Q23.0
  - arch Q25.21
    - congenital with hypoplasia of ascending aorta and defective development of left ventricle (with mitral stenosis) Q23.4
  - in hypoplastic left heart syndrome Q23.4
- aqueduct of Sylvius Q03.0

Atresia, atretic — *continued*
- aqueduct of Sylvius — *continued*
  - with spina bifida — *see* Spina bifida, with hydrocephalus
- artery NEC Q27.8
  - cerebral Q28.3
  - coronary Q24.5
  - digestive system Q27.8
  - eye Q15.8
  - lower limb Q27.8
  - pulmonary Q25.5
  - specified site NEC Q27.8
  - umbilical Q27.0
  - upper limb Q27.8
- auditory canal (external) Q16.1
- bile duct (common) (congenital) (hepatic) Q44.2
  - acquired — *see* Obstruction, bile duct
- bladder (neck) Q64.39
  - obstruction Q64.31
- bronchus Q32.4
- cecum Q42.8
- cervix (acquired) N88.2
  - congenital Q51.828
  - in pregnancy or childbirth — *see* Anomaly, cervix, in pregnancy or childbirth
    - causing obstructed labor O65.5
- choana Q30.0
- colon Q42.9
  - specified NEC Q42.8
- common duct Q44.2
- cricoid cartilage Q31.8
- cystic duct Q44.2
  - acquired K82.8
    - with obstruction K82.0
- digestive organs NEC Q45.8
- duodenum Q41.0
- ear canal Q16.1
- ejaculatory duct Q55.4
- epiglottis Q31.8
- esophagus Q39.0
  - with tracheoesophageal fistula Q39.1
- eustachian tube Q17.8
- fallopian tube (congenital) Q50.6
  - acquired N97.1
- follicular cyst N83.0- ☑
- foramen of
  - Luschka Q03.1
    - with spina bifida — *see* Spina bifida, with hydrocephalus
  - Magendie Q03.1
    - with spina bifida — *see* Spina bifida, with hydrocephalus
- gallbladder Q44.1
- genital organ
  - external
    - female Q52.79
    - male Q55.8
  - internal
    - female Q52.8
    - male Q55.8
- glottis Q31.8
- gullet Q39.0
  - with tracheoesophageal fistula Q39.1
- heart valve NEC Q24.8
  - pulmonary Q22.0
  - tricuspid Q22.4
- hymen Q52.3
  - acquired (postinfective) N89.6
- ileum Q41.2
- intestine (small) Q41.9
  - large Q42.9
    - specified NEC Q42.8
- iris, filtration angle Q15.0
- jejunum Q41.1
- lacrimal apparatus Q10.4
- larynx Q31.8
- meatus urinarius Q64.33
- mitral valve Q23.2
  - in hypoplastic left heart syndrome Q23.4
- nares (anterior) (posterior) Q30.0
- nasopharynx Q34.8
- nose, nostril Q30.0
  - acquired J34.89
- organ or site NEC Q89.8
- osseous meatus (ear) Q16.1
- oviduct (congenital) Q50.6
  - acquired N97.1
- parotid duct Q38.4
  - acquired K11.8

Atresia, atretic — *continued*
- pulmonary (artery) Q25.5
  - valve Q22.0
- pulmonic Q22.0
- pupil Q13.2
- rectum Q42.1
  - with fistula Q42.0
- salivary duct Q38.4
  - acquired K11.8
- sublingual duct Q38.4
  - acquired K11.8
- submandibular duct Q38.4
  - acquired K11.8
- submaxillary duct Q38.4
  - acquired K11.8
- thyroid cartilage Q31.8
- trachea Q32.1
- tricuspid valve Q22.4
- ureter Q62.10
  - pelvic junction Q62.11
  - vesical orifice Q62.12
- ureteropelvic junction Q62.11
- ureterovesical orifice Q62.12
- urethra (valvular) Q64.39
  - stricture Q64.32
- urinary tract NEC Q64.8
- uterus Q51.818
  - acquired N85.8
- vagina (congenital) Q52.4
  - acquired (postinfectional) (senile) N89.5
- vas deferens Q55.3
- vascular NEC Q27.8
  - cerebral Q28.3
  - digestive system Q27.8
  - lower limb Q27.8
  - specified site NEC Q27.8
  - upper limb Q27.8
- vein NEC Q27.8
  - digestive system Q27.8
  - great Q26.8
  - lower limb Q27.8
  - portal Q26.5
  - pulmonary Q26.4
    - partial Q26.3
    - total Q26.2
  - specified site NEC Q27.8
  - upper limb Q27.8
- vena cava (inferior) (superior) Q26.8
- vesicourethral orifice Q64.31
- vulva Q52.79
  - acquired N90.5

Atrichia, atrichosis — *see* Alopecia

Atrophia — *see also* Atrophy
- cutis senilis L90.8
  - due to radiation L57.8
- gyrata of choroid and retina H31.23
- senilis R54
  - dermatological L90.8
    - due to radiation (nonionizing) (solar) L57.8
- unguium L60.3
  - congenita Q84.6

Atrophie blanche (en plaque) (de Milian) L95.0

Atrophoderma, atrophodermia (of) L90.9
- diffusum (idiopathic) L90.4
- maculatum L90.8
  - et striatum L90.8
    - due to syphilis A52.79
  - syphilitic A51.39
- neuriticum L90.8
- Pasini and Pierini L90.3
- pigmentosum Q82.1
- reticulatum symmetricum faciei L66.4
- senile L90.8
  - due to radiation (nonionizing) (solar) L57.8
- vermiculata (cheeks) L66.4

Atrophy, atrophic (of)
- adrenal (capsule) (gland) E27.49
  - primary (autoimmune) E27.1
- alveolar process or ridge (edentulous) K08.20
- anal sphincter (disuse) N81.84
- appendix K38.8
- arteriosclerotic — *see* Arteriosclerosis
- bile duct (common) (hepatic) K83.8
- bladder N32.89
  - neurogenic N31.8
- blanche (en plaque) (of Milian) L95.0
- bone (senile) NEC — *see also* Disorder, bone, specified type NEC

Atrophy, atrophic — *continued*
  bone — *see also* Disorder, bone, specified type —
      continued
    due to
      tabes dorsalis (neurogenic) A52.11
  brain (cortex) (progressive) G31.9
    frontotemporal circumscribed G31.01 *[F02.80]*
      with behavioral disturbance G31.01 *[F02.81]*
    senile NEC G31.1
  breast N64.2
    obstetric — *see* Disorder, breast, specified type NEC
  buccal cavity K13.79
  cardiac — *see* Degeneration, myocardial
  cartilage (infectional) (joint) — *see* Disorder, cartilage,
      specified NEC
  cerebellar — *see* Atrophy, brain
  cerebral — *see* Atrophy, brain
  cervix (mucosa) (senile) (uteri) N88.8
    menopausal N95.8
  Charcot-Marie-Tooth G60.0
  choroid (central) (macular) (myopic) (retina) H31.10- ☑
    diffuse secondary H31.12- ☑
    gyrate H31.23
    senile H31.11- ☑
  ciliary body — *see* Atrophy, iris
  conjunctiva (senile) H11.89
  corpus cavernosum N48.89
  cortical — *see* Atrophy, brain
  cystic duct K82.8
  Déjérine-Thomas G23.8
  disuse NEC — *see* Atrophy, muscle
  Duchenne-Aran G12.21
  ear H93.8- ☑
  edentulous alveolar ridge K08.20
  endometrium (senile) N85.8
    cervix N88.8
  enteric K63.89
  epididymis N50.89
  eyeball — *see* Disorder, globe, degenerated condition,
      atrophy
  eyelid (senile) — *see* Disorder, eyelid, degenerative
  facial (skin) L90.9
  fallopian tube (senile) N83.32- ☑
    with ovary N83.33- ☑
  fascioscapulohumeral (Landouzy- Déjérine) G71.02
  fatty, thymus (gland) E32.8
  gallbladder K82.8
  gastric K29.40
    with bleeding K29.41
  gastrointestinal K63.89
  glandular I89.8
  globe H44.52- ☑
  gum — *see* Recession, gingival
  hair L67.8
  heart (brown) — *see* Degeneration, myocardial
  hemifacial Q67.4
    Romberg G51.8
  infantile E41
    paralysis, acute — *see* Poliomyelitis, paralytic
  intestine K63.89
  iris (essential) (progressive) H21.26- ☑
    specified NEC H21.29
  kidney (senile) (terminal) — *see also* Sclerosis, renal
      N26.1
    congenital or infantile Q60.5
      bilateral Q60.4
      unilateral Q60.3
    hydronephrotic — *see* Hydronephrosis
  lacrimal gland (primary) H04.14- ☑
    secondary H04.15- ☑
  Landouzy-Déjérine G71.02
  laryngitis, infective J37.0
  larynx J38.7
  Leber's optic (hereditary) H47.22
  lip K13.0
  liver (yellow) K72.90
    with coma K72.91
    acute, subacute K72.00
      with coma K72.01
    chronic K72.10
      with coma K72.11
  lung (senile) J98.4
  macular (dermatological) L90.8
    syphilitic, skin A51.39
      striated A52.79
  mandible (edentulous) K08.20
    minimal K08.21
    moderate K08.22

Atrophy, atrophic — *continued*
  mandible — *continued*
    severe K08.23
  maxilla K08.20
    minimal K08.24
    moderate K08.25
    severe K08.26
  muscle, muscular (diffuse) (general) (idiopathic) (primary) M62.50
    ankle M62.57- ☑
    Duchenne-Aran G12.21
    foot M62.57- ☑
    forearm M62.53- ☑
    hand M62.54- ☑
    infantile spinal G12.0
    lower leg M62.56- ☑
    multiple sites M62.59
    myelopathic — *see* Atrophy, muscle, spinal
    myotonic G71.11
    neuritic G58.9
    neuropathic (peroneal) (progressive) G60.0
    pelvic (disuse) N81.84
    peroneal G60.0
    progressive (bulbar) G12.21
      adult G12.1
      infantile (spinal) G12.0
      spinal G12.25
        adult G12.1
        infantile G12.0
    pseudohypertrophic G71.02
    shoulder region M62.51- ☑
    specified site NEC M62.58
    spinal G12.9
      adult form G12.1
      Aran-Duchenne G12.21
      childhood form, type II G12.1
      distal G12.1
      hereditary NEC G12.1
      infantile, type I (Werdnig-Hoffmann) G12.0
      juvenile form, type III (Kugelberg- Welander)
          G12.1
      progressive G12.25
      scapuloperoneal form G12.1
      specified NEC G12.8
    syphilitic A52.78
    thigh M62.55- ☑
    upper arm M62.52- ☑
  myocardium — *see* Degeneration, myocardial
  myometrium (senile) N85.8
    cervix N88.8
  myopathic NEC — *see* Atrophy, muscle
  myotonia G71.11
  nail L60.3
  nasopharynx J31.1
  nerve — *see also* Disorder, nerve
    abducens — *see* Strabismus, paralytic, sixth nerve
    accessory G52.8
    acoustic or auditory H93.3 ☑
    cranial G52.9
      eighth (auditory) H93.3 ☑
      eleventh (accessory) G52.8
      fifth (trigeminal) G50.8
      first (olfactory) G52.0
      fourth (trochlear) — *see* Strabismus, paralytic,
          fourth nerve
      second (optic) H47.20
      sixth (abducens) — *see* Strabismus, paralytic,
          sixth nerve
      tenth (pneumogastric) (vagus) G52.2
      third (oculomotor) — *see* Strabismus, paralytic,
          third nerve
      twelfth (hypoglossal) G52.3
    hypoglossal G52.3
    oculomotor — *see* Strabismus, paralytic, third nerve
    olfactory G52.0
    optic (papillomacular bundle)
      syphilitic (late) A52.15
        congenital A50.44
    pneumogastric G52.2
    trigeminal G50.8
    trochlear — *see* Strabismus, paralytic, fourth nerve
    vagus (pneumogastric) G52.2
  neurogenic, bone, tabetic A52.11
  nutritional E41
  old age R54
  olivopontocerebellar G23.8
  optic (nerve) H47.20
    glaucomatous H47.23- ☑

Atrophy, atrophic — *continued*
  optic — *continued*
    hereditary H47.22
    primary H47.21- ☑
    specified type NEC H47.29- ☑
    syphilitic (late) A52.15
      congenital A50.44
  orbit H05.31- ☑
  ovary (senile) N83.31- ☑
    with fallopian tube N83.33- ☑
  oviduct (senile) — *see* Atrophy, fallopian tube
  palsy, diffuse (progressive) G12.22
  pancreas (duct) (senile) K86.89
  parotid gland K11.0
  pelvic muscle N81.84
  penis N48.89
  pharynx J39.2
  pluriglandular E31.8
    autoimmune E31.0
  polyarthritis M15.9
  prostate N42.89
  pseudohypertrophic (muscle) G71.02
  renal — *see also* Sclerosis, renal N26.1
  retina, retinal (postinfectional) H35.89
  rhinitis J31.0
  salivary gland K11.0
  scar L90.5
  sclerosis, lobar (of brain) G31.09 *[F02.80]*
    with behavioral disturbance G31.09 *[F02.81]*
  scrotum N50.89
  seminal vesicle N50.89
  senile R54
    due to radiation (nonionizing) (solar) L57.8
  skin (patches) (spots) L90.9
    degenerative (senile) L90.8
    due to radiation (nonionizing) (solar) L57.8
    senile L90.8
  spermatic cord N50.89
  spinal (acute) (cord) G95.89
    muscular — *see* Atrophy, muscle, spinal
    paralysis G12.20
      acute — *see* Poliomyelitis, paralytic
      meaning progressive muscular atrophy G12.25
  spine (column) — *see* Spondylopathy, specified NEC
  spleen (senile) D73.0
  stomach K29.40
    with bleeding K29.41
  striate (skin) L90.6
    syphilitic A52.79
  subcutaneous L90.9
  sublingual gland K11.0
  submandibular gland K11.0
  submaxillary gland K11.0
  Sudeck's — *see* Algoneurodystrophy
  suprarenal (capsule) (gland) E27.49
    primary E27.1
  systemic affecting central nervous system
    in
      myxedema E03.9 *[G13.2]*
      neoplastic disease — *see also* Neoplasm
          D49.9 *[G13.1]*
      specified disease NEC G13.8
  tarso-orbital fascia, congenital Q10.3
  testis N50.0
  thenar, partial — *see* Syndrome, carpal tunnel
  thymus (fatty) E32.8
  thyroid (gland) (acquired) E03.4
    with cretinism E03.1
    congenital (with myxedema) E03.1
  tongue (senile) K14.8
    papillae K14.4
  trachea J39.8
  tunica vaginalis N50.89
  turbinate J34.89
  tympanic membrane (nonflaccid) H73.82- ☑
    flaccid H73.81- ☑
  upper respiratory tract J39.8
  uterus, uterine (senile) N85.8
    cervix N88.8
    due to radiation (intended effect) N85.8
      adverse effect or misadventure N99.89
  vagina (senile) N95.2
  vas deferens N50.89
  vascular I99.8
  vertebra (senile) — *see* Spondylopathy, specified NEC
  vulva (senile) N90.5
  Werdnig-Hoffmann G12.0
  yellow — *see* Failure, hepatic

☑ **Additional Character Required — Refer to the Tabular List for Character Selection**   ▽ **Subterms under main terms may continue to next column or page**

Attack, attacks
   with alteration of consciousness (with automatisms)
      — see Epilepsy, localization-related, symptomat-
      ic, with complex partial seizures
   Adams-Stokes I45.9
   akinetic — see Epilepsy, generalized, specified NEC
   angina — see Angina
   atonic — see Epilepsy, generalized, specified NEC
   benign shuddering G25.83
   cataleptic — see Catalepsy
   coronary — see Infarct, myocardium
   cyanotic, newborn P28.2
   drop NEC R55
   epileptic — see Epilepsy
   heart — see infarct, myocardium
   hysterical F44.9
   jacksonian — see Epilepsy, localization-related, symp-
      tomatic, with simple partial seizures
   myocardium, myocardial — see Infarct, myocardium
   myoclonic — see Epilepsy, generalized, specified NEC
   panic F41.0
   psychomotor — see Epilepsy, localization-related,
      symptomatic, with complex partial seizures
   salaam — see Epilepsy, spasms
   schizophreniform, brief F23
   shuddering, benign G25.83
   Stokes-Adams I45.9
   syncope R55
   transient ischemic (TIA) G45.9
      specified NEC G45.8
   unconsciousness R55
      hysterical F44.89
   vasomotor R55
   vasovagal (paroxysmal) (idiopathic) R55
   without alteration of consciousness — see Epilepsy,
      localization-related, symptomatic, with simple
      partial seizures
Attention (to)
   artificial
      opening (of) Z43.9
         digestive tract NEC Z43.4
            colon Z43.3
            ilium Z43.2
            stomach Z43.1
         specified NEC Z43.8
         trachea Z43.0
         urinary tract NEC Z43.6
            cystostomy Z43.5
            nephrostomy Z43.6
            ureterostomy Z43.6
            urethrostomy Z43.6
      vagina Z43.7
   colostomy Z43.3
   cystostomy Z43.5
   deficit disorder or syndrome F98.8
      with hyperactivity — see Disorder, attention-deficit
         hyperactivity
   gastrostomy Z43.1
   ileostomy Z43.2
   jejunostomy Z43.4
   nephrostomy Z43.6
   surgical dressings Z48.01
   sutures Z48.02
   tracheostomy Z43.0
   ureterostomy Z43.6
   urethrostomy Z43.6
Attrition
   gum — see Recession, gingival
   tooth, teeth (excessive) (hard tissues) K03.0
Atypical, atypism — see also condition
   cells (on cytolgocial smear) (endocervical) (endometrial)
      (glandular)
      cervix R87.619
      vagina R87.629
   cervical N87.9
   endometrium N85.9
      hyperplasia N85.00
   parenting situation Z62.9
Auditory — see condition
Aujeszky's disease B33.8
Aurantiasis, cutis E67.1
Auricle, auricular — see also condition
   cervical Q18.2
Auriculotemporal syndrome G50.8
Austin Flint murmur (aortic insufficiency) I35.1
Australian
   Q fever A78
   X disease A83.4

Autism, autistic (childhood) (infantile) F84.0
   atypical F84.9
   spectrum disorder F84.0
Autodigestion R68.89
Autoerythrocyte sensitization (syndrome) D69.2
Autographism L50.3
Autoimmune
   disease (systemic) M35.9
   inhibitors to clotting factors D68.311
   lymphoproliferative syndrome [ALPS] D89.82
   thyroiditis E06.3
Autointoxication R68.89
Automatism G93.89
   with temporal sclerosis G93.81
   epileptic — see Epilepsy, localization-related, symp-
      tomatic, with complex partial seizures
   paroxysmal, idiopathic — see Epilepsy, localization-
      related, symptomatic, with complex partial
      seizures
Autonomic, autonomous
   bladder (neurogenic) N31.2
   hysteria seizure F44.5
Autosensitivity, erythrocyte D69.2
Autosensitization, cutaneous L30.2
Autosome — see condition by chromosome involved
Autotopagnosia R48.1
Autotoxemia R68.89
Autumn — see condition
Avellis' syndrome G46.8
Aversion
   oral R63.3
      newborn P92.- ☑
      nonorganic origin F98.2 ☑
   sexual F52.1
Aviator's
   disease or sickness — see Effect, adverse, high altitude
   ear T70.0 ☑
Avitaminosis (multiple) — see also Deficiency, vitamin
      E56.9
   B E53.9
      with
         beriberi E51.11
         pellagra E52
   B2 E53.0
   B6 E53.1
   B12 E53.8
   D E55.9
      with rickets E55.0
   G E53.0
   K E56.1
   nicotinic acid E52
AVNRT (atrioventricular nodal re-entrant tachycardia)
      I47.1
AVRT (atrioventricular nodal re-entrant tachycardia) I47.1
Avulsion (traumatic)
   blood vessel — see Injury, blood vessel
   bone — see Fracture, by site
   cartilage — see also Dislocation, by site
      symphyseal (inner), complicating delivery O71.6
   external site other than limb — see Wound, open, by
      site
   eye S05.7- ☑
   head (intracranial)
      external site NEC S08.89 ☑
      scalp S08.0 ☑
   internal organ or site — see Injury, by site
   joint — see also Dislocation, by site
      capsule — see Sprain, by site
   kidney S37.06- ☑
   ligament — see Sprain, by site
   limb — see also Amputation, traumatic, by site
      skin and subcutaneous tissue — see Wound, open,
         by site
   muscle — see Injury, muscle
   nerve (root) — see Injury, nerve
   scalp S08.0 ☑
   skin and subcutaneous tissue — see Wound, open, by
      site
   spleen S36.032 ☑
   symphyseal cartilage (inner), complicating delivery
      O71.6
   tendon — see Injury, muscle
   tooth S03.2 ☑
Awareness of heart beat R00.2
Axenfeld's
   anomaly or syndrome Q15.0
   degeneration (calcareous) Q13.4

Axilla, axillary — see also condition
   breast Q83.1
Axonotmesis — see Injury, nerve
Ayerza's disease or syndrome (pulmonary artery scle-
      rosis with pulmonary hypertension) I27.0
Azoospermia (organic) N46.01
   due to
      drug therapy N46.021
      efferent duct obstruction N46.023
      infection N46.022
      radiation N46.024
      specified cause NEC N46.029
      systemic disease N46.025
Azotemia R79.89
   meaning uremia N19
Aztec ear Q17.3
Azygos
   continuation inferior vena cava Q26.8
   lobe (lung) Q33.1

B

Baastrup's disease — see Kissing spine
Babesiosis B60.0
Babington's disease (familial hemorrhagic telangiecta-
      sia) I78.0
Babinski's syndrome A52.79
Baby
   crying constantly R68.11
   floppy (syndrome) P94.2
Bacillary — see condition
Bacilluria R82.71
Bacillus — see also Infection, bacillus
   abortus infection A23.1
   anthracis infection A22.9
   coli infection — see also Escherichia coli B96.20
   Flexner's A03.1
   mallei infection A24.0
   Shiga's A03.0
   suipestifer infection — see Infection, salmonella
Back — see condition
Backache (postural) M54.9
   sacroiliac M53.3
   specified NEC M54.89
Backflow — see Reflux
Backward reading (dyslexia) F81.0
Bacteremia R78.81
   with sepsis — see Sepsis
Bactericholia — see Cholecystitis, acute
Bacterid, bacteride (pustular) L40.3
Bacterium, bacteria, bacterial
   agent NEC, as cause of disease classified elsewhere
      B96.89
   in blood — see Bacteremia
   in urine — see Bacteriuria
Bacteriuria, bacteruria R82.71
   asymptomatic R82.71
Bacteroides
   fragilis, as cause of disease classified elsewhere B96.6
Bad
   heart — see Disease, heart
   trip
      due to drug abuse — see Abuse, drug, hallucinogen
      due to drug dependence — see Dependence, drug,
         hallucinogen
Baelz's disease (cheilitis glandularis apostematosa) K13.0
Baerensprung's disease (eczema marginatum) B35.6
Bagasse disease or pneumonitis J67.1
Bagassosis J67.1
Baker's cyst — see Cyst, Baker's
Bakwin-Krida syndrome (metaphyseal dysplasia) Q78.5
Balancing side interference M26.56
Balanitis (circinata) (erosiva) (gangrenosa) (phagedenic)
      (vulgaris) N48.1
   amebic A06.82
   candidal B37.42
   due to Haemophilus ducreyi A57
   gonococcal (acute) (chronic) A54.23
   xerotica obliterans N48.0
Balanoposthitis N47.6
   gonococcal (acute) (chronic) A54.23
   ulcerative (specific) A63.8
Balanorrhagia — see Balanitis
Balantidiasis, balantidiosis A07.0
Bald tongue K14.4
Baldness — see also Alopecia
   male-pattern — see Alopecia, androgenic

☑ **Additional Character Required** — Refer to the Tabular List for Character Selection   ▽ **Subterms under main terms may continue to next column or page**

▽ Subterms under main terms may continue to next column or page   ☑ Additional Character Required — Refer to the Tabular List for Character Selection   37

Bifurcation — Bite

Bite(s) — *continued*
foot(s alone) — *continued*
superficial — *continued*
insect S90.86- ☑
toe — *see* Bite, toe
forearm S51.85- ☑
elbow only — *see* Bite, elbow
superficial NEC S50.87- ☑
insect S50.86- ☑
forehead — *see* Bite, head, specified site NEC
genital organs, external
female S31.552 ☑
superficial NEC S30.876 ☑
insect S30.866 ☑
vagina and vulva — *see* Bite, vulva
male S31.551 ☑
penis — *see* Bite, penis
scrotum — *see* Bite, scrotum
superficial NEC S30.875 ☑
insect S30.865 ☑
testes — *see* Bite, testis
groin — *see* Bite, abdomen, wall
gum — *see* Bite, oral cavity
hand S61.45- ☑
finger — *see* Bite, finger
superficial NEC S60.57- ☑
insect S60.56- ☑
thumb — *see* Bite, thumb
head S01.95 ☑
cheek — *see* Bite, cheek
ear — *see* Bite, ear
eyelid — *see* Bite, eyelid
lip — *see* Bite, lip
nose — *see* Bite, nose
oral cavity — *see* Bite, oral cavity
scalp — *see* Bite, scalp
specified site NEC S01.85 ☑
superficial NEC S00.87 ☑
insect S00.86 ☑
superficial NEC S00.97 ☑
insect S00.96 ☑
temporomandibular area — *see* Bite, cheek
heel — *see* Bite, foot
hip S71.05- ☑
superficial NEC S70.27- ☑
insect S70.26- ☑
hymen S31.45 ☑
hypochondrium — *see* Bite, abdomen, wall
hypogastric region — *see* Bite, abdomen, wall
inguinal region — *see* Bite, abdomen, wall
insect — *see* Bite, by site, superficial, insect
instep — *see* Bite, foot
interscapular region — *see* Bite, thorax, back
jaw — *see* Bite, head, specified site NEC
knee S81.05- ☑
superficial NEC S80.27- ☑
insect S80.26- ☑
labium (majus) (minus) — *see* Bite, vulva
lacrimal duct — *see* Bite, eyelid
larynx S11.015 ☑
superficial NEC S10.17 ☑
insect S10.16 ☑
leg (lower) S81.85- ☑
ankle — *see* Bite, ankle
foot — *see* Bite, foot
knee — *see* Bite, knee
superficial NEC S80.87- ☑
insect S80.86- ☑
toe — *see* Bite, toe
upper — *see* Bite, thigh
lip S01.551 ☑
superficial NEC S00.571 ☑
insect S00.561 ☑
lizard (venomous) — *see* Venom, bite, reptile
loin — *see* Bite, abdomen, wall
lower back — *see* Bite, back, lower
lumbar region — *see* Bite, back, lower
malar region — *see* Bite, head, specified site NEC
mammary — *see* Bite, breast
marine animals (venomous) — *see* Toxicity, venom, marine animal
mastoid region — *see* Bite, head, specified site NEC
mouth — *see* Bite, oral cavity
nail
finger — *see* Bite, finger
toe — *see* Bite, toe

Bite(s) — *continued*
nape — *see* Bite, neck, specified site NEC
nasal (septum) (sinus) — *see* Bite, nose
nasopharynx — *see* Bite, head, specified site NEC
neck S11.95 ☑
involving
cervical esophagus — *see* Bite, esophagus, cervical
larynx — *see* Bite, larynx
pharynx — *see* Bite, pharynx
thyroid gland S11.15 ☑
trachea — *see* Bite, trachea
specified site NEC S11.85 ☑
superficial NEC S10.87 ☑
insect S10.86 ☑
superficial NEC S10.97 ☑
insect S10.96 ☑
throat S11.85 ☑
superficial NEC S10.17 ☑
insect S10.16 ☑
nose (septum) (sinus) S01.25 ☑
superficial NEC S00.37 ☑
insect S00.36 ☑
occipital region — *see* Bite, scalp
oral cavity S01.552 ☑
superficial NEC S00.572 ☑
insect S00.562 ☑
orbital region — *see* Bite, eyelid
palate — *see* Bite, oral cavity
palm — *see* Bite, hand
parietal region — *see* Bite, scalp
pelvis S31.050 ☑
with penetration into retroperitoneal space S31.051
superficial NEC S30.870 ☑
insect S30.860 ☑
penis S31.25 ☑
superficial NEC S30.872 ☑
insect S30.862 ☑
perineum
female — *see* Bite, vulva
male — *see* Bite, pelvis
periocular area (with or without lacrimal passages) — *see* Bite, eyelid
phalanges
finger — *see* Bite, finger
toe — *see* Bite, toe
pharynx S11.25 ☑
superficial NEC S10.17 ☑
insect S10.16 ☑
pinna — *see* Bite, ear
poisonous — *see* Venom
popliteal space — *see* Bite, knee
prepuce — *see* Bite, penis
pubic region — *see* Bite, abdomen, wall
rectovaginal septum — *see* Bite, vulva
red bug B88.0
reptile NEC — *see also* Venom, bite, reptile
nonvenomous — *see* Bite, by site
snake — *see* Venom, bite, snake
sacral region — *see* Bite, back, lower
sacroiliac region — *see* Bite, back, lower
salivary gland — *see* Bite, oral cavity
scalp S01.05 ☑
superficial NEC S00.07 ☑
insect S00.06 ☑
scapular region — *see* Bite, shoulder
scrotum S31.35 ☑
superficial NEC S30.873 ☑
insect S30.863 ☑
sea-snake (venomous) — *see* Toxicity, venom, snake, sea snake
shin — *see* Bite, leg
shoulder S41.05- ☑
superficial NEC S40.27- ☑
insect S40.26- ☑
snake — *see also* Venom, bite, snake
nonvenomous — *see* Bite, by site
spermatic cord — *see* Bite, testis
spider (venomous) — *see* Toxicity, venom, spider
nonvenomous — *see* Bite, by site, superficial, insect
sternal region — *see* Bite, thorax, front
submaxillary region — *see* Bite, head, specified site NEC
submental region — *see* Bite, head, specified site NEC

Bite(s) — *continued*
subungual
finger(s) — *see* Bite, finger
toe — *see* Bite, toe
superficial — *see* Bite, by site, superficial
supraclavicular fossa S11.85 ☑
supraorbital — *see* Bite, head, specified site NEC
temple, temporal region — *see* Bite, head, specified site NEC
temporomandibular area — *see* Bite, cheek
testis S31.35 ☑
superficial NEC S30.873 ☑
insect S30.863 ☑
thigh S71.15- ☑
superficial NEC S70.37- ☑
insect S70.36- ☑
thorax, thoracic (wall) S21.95 ☑
back S21.25- ☑
with penetration into thoracic cavity S21.45- ☑
breast — *see* Bite, breast
front S21.15- ☑
with penetration into thoracic cavity S21.35- ☑
superficial NEC S20.97 ☑
back S20.47- ☑
front S20.37- ☑
insect S20.96 ☑
back S20.46- ☑
front S20.36- ☑
throat — *see* Bite, neck, throat
thumb S61.05- ☑
with
damage to nail S61.15- ☑
superficial NEC S60.37- ☑
insect S60.36- ☑
thyroid S11.15 ☑
superficial NEC S10.87 ☑
insect S10.86 ☑
toe(s) S91.15- ☑
with
damage to nail S91.25- ☑
great S91.15- ☑
with
damage to nail S91.25- ☑
lesser S91.15- ☑
with
damage to nail S91.25- ☑
superficial NEC S90.47- ☑
great S90.47- ☑
insect S90.46- ☑
great S90.46- ☑
tongue S01.552 ☑
trachea S11.025 ☑
superficial NEC S10.17 ☑
insect S10.16 ☑
tunica vaginalis — *see* Bite, testis
tympanum, tympanic membrane — *see* Bite, ear
umbilical region S31.155 ☑
uvula — *see* Bite, oral cavity
vagina — *see* Bite, vulva
venomous — *see* Venom
vocal cords S11.035 ☑
superficial NEC S10.17 ☑
insect S10.16 ☑
vulva S31.45 ☑
superficial NEC S30.874 ☑
insect S30.864 ☑
wrist S61.55- ☑
superficial NEC S60.87- ☑
insect S60.86- ☑
Biting, cheek or lip K13.1
Biventricular failure (heart) I50.82
Björck (-Thorson) **syndrome** (malignant carcinoid) E34.0
Black
death A20.9
eye S00.1- ☑
hairy tongue K14.3
heel (foot) S90.3- ☑
lung (disease) J60
palm (hand) S60.22- ☑
Blackfan-Diamond anemia or syndrome (congenital hypoplastic anemia) D61.01
Blackhead L70.0
Blackout R55
Bladder — *see* condition
Blast (air) (hydraulic) (immersion) (underwater)
blindness S05.8X- ☑

38

☑ Additional Character Required — Refer to the Tabular List for Character Selection   ⏷ Subterms under main terms may continue to next column or page

Bite — Blast

Blast — *continued*
  injury
    abdomen or thorax — *see* Injury, by site
    ear (acoustic nerve trauma) — *see* Injury, nerve,
      acoustic, specified type NEC
    syndrome NEC T70.8 ☑
Blastoma — *see* Neoplasm, malignant, by site
  pulmonary — *see* Neoplasm, lung, malignant
Blastomycosis, blastomycotic B40.9
  Brazilian — *see* Paracoccidioidomycosis
  cutaneous B40.3
  disseminated B40.7
  European — *see* Cryptococcosis
  generalized B40.7
  keloidal B48.0
  North American B40.9
  primary pulmonary B40.0
  pulmonary B40.2
    acute B40.0
    chronic B40.1
  skin B40.3
  South American — *see* Paracoccidioidomycosis
  specified NEC B40.89
Bleb(s) R23.8
  emphysematous (lung) (solitary) J43.9
  endophthalmitis H59.43
  filtering (vitreous), after glaucoma surgery Z98.83
  inflamed (infected), postprocedural H59.40
    stage 1 H59.41
    stage 2 H59.42
    stage 3 H59.43
  lung (ruptured) J43.9
    congenital — *see* Atelectasis
    newborn P25.8
  subpleural (emphysematous) J43.9
Blebitis, postprocedural H59.40
  stage 1 H59.41
  stage 2 H59.42
  stage 3 H59.43
Bleeder (familial) (hereditary) — *see* Hemophilia
Bleeding — *see also* Hemorrhage
  anal K62.5
  anovulatory N97.0
  atonic, following delivery O72.1
  capillary I78.8
    puerperal O72.2
  contact (postcoital) N93.0
  due to uterine subinvolution N85.3
  ear — *see* Otorrhagia
  excessive, associated with menopausal onset N92.4
  familial — *see* Defect, coagulation
  following intercourse N93.0
  gastrointestinal K92.2
  hemorrhoids — *see* Hemorrhoids
  intermenstrual (regular) N92.3
    irregular N92.1
  intraoperative — *see* Complication, intraoperative,
    hemorrhage
  irregular N92.6
  menopausal N92.4
  newborn, intraventricular — *see* Newborn, affected
    by, hemorrhage, intraventricular
  nipple N64.59
  nose R04.0
  ovulation N92.3
  perimenopausal N92.4
  postclimacteric N95.0
  postcoital N93.0
  postmenopausal N95.0
  postoperative — *see* Complication, postprocedural,
    hemorrhage
  preclimacteric N92.4
  pre-pubertal vaginal N93.1
  puberty (excessive, with onset of menstrual periods)
    N92.2
  rectum, rectal K62.5
    newborn P54.2
  tendencies — *see* Defect, coagulation
  throat R04.1
  tooth socket (post-extraction) K91.840
  umbilical stump P51.9
  uterus, uterine NEC N93.9
    climacteric N92.4
    dysfunctional or functional N93.8
    menopausal N92.4
    preclimacteric or premenopausal N92.4
    unrelated to menstrual cycle N93.9
  vagina, vaginal (abnormal) N93.9

Bleeding — *continued*
  vagina, vaginal — *continued*
    dysfunctional or functional N93.8
    newborn P54.6
    pre-pubertal N93.1
    vicarious N94.89
Blennorrhagia, blennorrhagic — *see* Gonorrhea
Blennorrhea (acute) (chronic) — *see also* Gonorrhea
  inclusion (neonatal) (newborn) P39.1
  lower genitourinary tract (gonococcal) A54.00
  neonatorum (gonococcal ophthalmia) A54.31
Blepharelosis — *see* Entropion
Blepharitis (angularis) (ciliaris) (eyelid) (marginal)
  (nonulcerative) H01.009
  herpes zoster B02.39
  left H01.006
    lower H01.005
    upper H01.004
    upper and lower H01.00B
  right H01.003
    lower H01.002
    upper H01.001
    upper and lower H01.00A
  squamous H01.029
    left H01.026
      lower H01.025
      upper H01.024
      upper and lower H01.02B
    right H01.023
      lower H01.022
      upper H01.021
      upper and lower H01.02A
  ulcerative H01.019
    left H01.016
      lower H01.015
      upper H01.014
      upper and lower H01.01B
    right H01.013
      lower H01.012
      upper H01.011
      upper and lower H01.01A
Blepharochalasis H02.30
  congenital Q10.0
  left H02.36
    lower H02.35
    upper H02.34
  right H02.33
    lower H02.32
    upper H02.31
Blepharoclonus H02.59
Blepharoconjunctivitis H10.50- ☑
  angular H10.52- ☑
  contact H10.53- ☑
  ligneous H10.51- ☑
Blepharophimosis (eyelid) H02.529
  congenital Q10.3
  left H02.526
    lower H02.525
    upper H02.524
  right H02.523
    lower H02.522
    upper H02.521
Blepharoptosis H02.40- ☑
  congenital Q10.0
  mechanical H02.41- ☑
  myogenic H02.42- ☑
  neurogenic H02.43- ☑
  paralytic H02.43- ☑
Blepharopyorrhea, gonococcal A54.39
Blepharospasm G24.5
  drug induced G24.01
Blighted ovum O02.0
Blind — *see also* Blindness
  bronchus (congenital) Q32.4
  loop syndrome K90.2
    congenital Q43.8
  sac, fallopian tube (congenital) Q50.6
  spot, enlarged — *see* Defect, visual field, localized,
    scotoma, blind spot area
  tract or tube, congenital NEC — *see* Atresia, by site
Blindness (acquired) (congenital) (both eyes) H54.0X- ☑
  blast S05.8X- ☑
  color — *see* Deficiency, color vision
  concussion S05.8X- ☑
  cortical H47.619
    left brain H47.612
    right brain H47.611
  day H53.11

Blindness — *continued*
  due to injury (current episode) S05.9- ☑
    sequelae — *code to* injury with seventh character
      S
  eclipse (total) — *see* Retinopathy, solar
  emotional (hysterical) F44.6
  face H53.16
  hysterical F44.6
  legal (both eyes) (USA definition) H54.8
  mind R48.8
  night H53.60
    abnormal dark adaptation curve H53.61
    acquired H53.62
    congenital H53.63
    specified type NEC H53.69
    vitamin A deficiency E50.5
  one eye (other eye normal) H54.40
    left (normal vision on right) H54.42- ☑
      low vision on right H54.12- ☑
    low vision, other eye H54.10
    right (normal vision on left) H54.41- ☑
      low vision on left H54.11- ☑
  psychic R48.8
  river B73.01
  snow — *see* Photokeratitis
  sun, solar — *see* Retinopathy, solar
  transient — *see* Disturbance, vision, subjective, loss,
    transient
  traumatic (current episode) S05.9- ☑
  word (developmental) F81.0
    acquired R48.0
    secondary to organic lesion R48.0
Blister (nonthermal)
  abdominal wall S30.821 ☑
  alveolar process S00.522 ☑
  ankle S90.52- ☑
  antecubital space — *see* Blister, elbow
  anus S30.827 ☑
  arm (upper) S40.82- ☑
  auditory canal — *see* Blister, ear
  auricle — *see* Blister, ear
  axilla — *see* Blister, arm
  back, lower S30.820 ☑
  beetle dermatitis L24.89
  breast S20.12- ☑
  brow S00.82 ☑
  calf — *see* Blister, leg
  canthus — *see* Blister, eyelid
  cheek S00.82 ☑
    internal S00.522 ☑
  chest wall — *see* Blister, thorax
  chin S00.82 ☑
  costal region — *see* Blister, thorax
  digit(s)
    foot — *see* Blister, toe
    hand — *see* Blister, finger
  due to burn — *see* Burn, by site, second degree
  ear S00.42- ☑
  elbow S50.32- ☑
  epiglottis S10.12 ☑
  esophagus, cervical S10.12 ☑
  eyebrow — *see* Blister, eyelid
  eyelid S00.22- ☑
  face S00.82 ☑
  fever B00.1
  finger(s) S60.429 ☑
    index S60.42- ☑
    little S60.42- ☑
    middle S60.42- ☑
    ring S60.42- ☑
  foot (except toe(s) alone) S90.82- ☑
    toe — *see* Blister, toe
  forearm S50.82- ☑
    elbow only — *see* Blister, elbow
  forehead S00.82 ☑
  fracture — *omit code*
  genital organ
    female S30.826 ☑
    male S30.825 ☑
  gum S00.522 ☑
  hand S60.52- ☑
  head S00.92 ☑
    ear — *see* Blister, ear
    eyelid — *see* Blister, eyelid
    lip S00.521 ☑
    nose S00.32 ☑

Blister — *continued*
head — *continued*
oral cavity S00.522 ☑
scalp S00.02 ☑
specified site NEC S00.82 ☑
heel — *see* Blister, foot
hip S70.22-
interscapular region S20.429 ☑
jaw S00.82 ☑
knee S80.22-
larynx S10.12 ☑
leg (lower) S80.82- ☑
knee — *see* Blister, knee
upper — *see* Blister, thigh
lip S00.521 ☑
malar region S00.82 ☑
mammary — *see* Blister, breast
mastoid region S00.82 ☑
mouth S00.522 ☑
multiple, skin, nontraumatic R23.8
nail
finger — *see* Blister, finger
toe — *see* Blister, toe
nasal S00.32 ☑
neck S10.92 ☑
specified site NEC S10.82 ☑
throat S10.12 ☑
nose S00.32 ☑
occipital region S00.02 ☑
oral cavity S00.522 ☑
orbital region — *see* Blister, eyelid
palate S00.522 ☑
palm — *see* Blister, hand
parietal region S00.02 ☑
pelvis S30.820 ☑
penis S30.822 ☑
periocular area — *see* Blister, eyelid
phalanges
finger — *see* Blister, finger
toe — *see* Blister, toe
pharynx S10.12 ☑
pinna — *see* Blister, ear
popliteal space — *see* Blister, knee
scalp S00.02 ☑
scapular region — *see* Blister, shoulder
scrotum S30.823 ☑
shin — *see* Blister, leg
shoulder S40.22-
sternal region S20.329 ☑
submaxillary region S00.82 ☑
submental region S00.82 ☑
subungual
finger(s) — *see* Blister, finger
toe(s) — *see* Blister, toe
supraclavicular fossa S10.82 ☑
supraorbital S00.82 ☑
temple S00.82 ☑
temporal region S00.82 ☑
testis S30.823 ☑
thermal — *see* Burn, second degree, by site
thigh S70.32-
thorax, thoracic (wall) S20.92 ☑
back S20.42-
front S20.32-
throat S10.12 ☑
thumb S60.32-
toe(s) S90.42- ☑
great S90.42- ☑
tongue S00.522 ☑
trachea S10.12 ☑
tympanum, tympanic membrane — *see* Blister, ear
upper arm — *see* Blister, arm (upper)
uvula S00.522 ☑
vagina S30.824 ☑
vocal cords S10.12 ☑
vulva S30.824 ☑
wrist S60.82- ☑
Bloating R14.0
Bloch-Sulzberger disease or syndrome Q82.3
Block, blocked
alveolocapillary J84.10
arborization (heart) I45.5
arrhythmic I45.9
atrioventricular (incomplete) (partial) I44.30
with atrioventricular dissociation I44.2
complete I44.2

Block, blocked — *continued*
atrioventricular — *continued*
complete — *continued*
congenital Q24.6
congenital Q24.6
first degree I44.0
second degree (types I and II) I44.1
specified NEC I44.39
third degree I44.2
types I and II I44.1
auriculoventricular — *see* Block, atrioventricular
bifascicular (cardiac) I45.2
bundle-branch (complete) (false) (incomplete) I45.4
bilateral I45.2
left I44.7
with right bundle branch block I45.2
hemiblock I44.60
anterior I44.4
posterior I44.5
incomplete I44.7
with right bundle branch block I45.2
right I45.10
with
left bundle branch block I45.2
left fascicular block I45.2
specified NEC I45.19
Wilson's type I45.19
cardiac I45.9
conduction I45.9
complete I44.2
fascicular (left) I44.60
anterior I44.4
posterior I44.5
right I45.0
specified NEC I44.69
foramen Magendie (acquired) G91.1
congenital Q03.1
with spina bifida — *see* Spina bifida, by site, with hydrocephalus
heart I45.9
bundle branch I45.4
bilateral I45.2
complete (atrioventricular) I44.2
congenital Q24.6
first degree (atrioventricular) I44.0
second degree (atrioventricular) I44.1
specified type NEC I45.5
third degree (atrioventricular) I44.2
hepatic vein I82.0
intraventricular (nonspecific) I45.4
bundle branch
bilateral I45.2
kidney N28.9
postcystoscopic or postprocedural N99.0
Mobitz (types I and II) I44.1
myocardial — *see* Block, heart
nodal I45.5
organ or site, congenital NEC — *see* Atresia, by site
portal (vein) I81
second degree (types I and II) I44.1
sinoatrial I45.5
sinoauricular I45.5
third degree I44.2
trifascicular I45.3
tubal N97.1
vein NOS I82.90
Wenckebach (types I and II) I44.1
Blockage — *see* Obstruction
Blocq's disease F44.4
Blood
constituents, abnormal R78.9
disease D75.9
donor — *see* Donor, blood
dyscrasia D75.9
with
abortion — *see* Abortion, by type, complicated by, hemorrhage
ectopic pregnancy O08.1
molar pregnancy O08.1
following ectopic or molar pregnancy O08.1
newborn P61.9
puerperal, postpartum O72.3
flukes NEC — *see* Schistosomiasis
in
feces K92.1
occult R19.5
urine — *see* Hematuria
mole O02.0

Blood — *continued*
occult in feces R19.5
pressure
decreased, due to shock following injury T79.4 ☑
examination only Z01.30
fluctuating I99.8
high — *see* Hypertension
borderline R03.0
incidental reading, without diagnosis of hypertension R03.0
low — *see also* Hypotension
incidental reading, without diagnosis of hypotension R03.1
spitting — *see* Hemoptysis
staining cornea — *see* Pigmentation, cornea, stroma
transfusion
reaction or complication — *see* Complications, transfusion
type
A (Rh positive) Z67.10
Rh negative Z67.11
AB (Rh positive) Z67.30
Rh negative Z67.31
B (Rh positive) Z67.20
Rh negative Z67.21
O (Rh positive) Z67.40
Rh negative Z67.41
Rh (positive) Z67.90
negative Z67.91
vessel rupture — *see* Hemorrhage
vomiting — *see* Hematemesis
Blood-forming organs, disease D75.9
Bloodgood's disease — *see* Mastopathy, cystic
Bloom (-Machacek)(-Torre) **syndrome** Q82.8
Blount's disease or osteochondrosis — *see* Osteochondrosis, juvenile, tibia
Blue
baby Q24.9
diaper syndrome E72.09
dome cyst (breast) — *see* Cyst, breast
dot cataract Q12.0
nevus D22.9
sclera Q13.5
with fragility of bone and deafness Q78.0
toe syndrome I75.02- ☑
Blueness — *see* Cyanosis
Blues, postpartal O90.6
baby O90.6
Blurring, visual H53.8
Blushing (abnormal) (excessive) R23.2
BMI — *see* Body, mass index
Boarder, hospital NEC Z76.4
accompanying sick person Z76.3
healthy infant or child Z76.2
foundling Z76.1
Bockhart's impetigo L01.02
Bodechtel-Guttman disease (subacute sclerosing panencephalitis) A81.1
Boder-Sedgwick syndrome (ataxia-telangiectasia) G11.3
Body, bodies
Aschoff's — *see* Myocarditis, rheumatic
asteroid, vitreous — *see* Deposit, crystalline
cytoid (retina) — *see* Occlusion, artery, retina
drusen (degenerative) (macula) (retinal) — *see also* Degeneration, macula, drusen
optic disc — *see* Drusen, optic disc
foreign — *see* Foreign body
loose
joint, except knee — *see* Loose, body, joint
knee M23.4- ☑
sheath, tendon — *see* Disorder, tendon, specified type NEC
mass index (BMI)
adult
19.9 or less Z68.1
20.0-20.9 Z68.20
21.0-21.9 Z68.21
22.0-22.9 Z68.22
23.0-23.9 Z68.23
24.0-24.9 Z68.24
25.0-25.9 Z68.25
26.0-26.9 Z68.26
27.0-27.9 Z68.27
28.0-28.9 Z68.28
29.0-29.9 Z68.29
30.0-30.9 Z68.30
31.0-31.9 Z68.31
32.0-32.9 Z68.32

☑ **Additional Character Required** — Refer to the Tabular List for Character Selection   **Subterms under main terms may continue to next column or page**

Body, bodies — *continued*
  mass index — *continued*
    adult — *continued*
      33.0-33.9 Z68.33
      34.0-34.9 Z68.34
      35.0-35.9 Z68.35
      36.0-36.9 Z68.36
      37.0-37.9 Z68.37
      38.0-38.9 Z68.38
      39.0-39.9 Z68.39
      40.0-44.9 Z68.41
      45.0-49.9 Z68.42
      50.0-59.9 Z68.43
      60.0-69.9 Z68.44
      70 and over Z68.45
    pediatric
      5th percentile to less than 85th percentile for age Z68.52
      85th percentile to less than 95th percentile for age Z68.53
      greater than or equal to ninety-fifth percentile for age Z68.54
      less than fifth percentile for age Z68.51
  Mooser's A75.2
  rice — *see also* Loose, body, joint
    knee M23.4- ☑
  rocking F98.4
Boeck's
  disease or sarcoid — *see* Sarcoidosis
  lupoid (miliary) D86.3
Boerhaave's syndrome (spontaneous esophageal rupture) K22.3
Boggy
  cervix N88.8
  uterus N85.8
Boil — *see also* Furuncle, by site
  Aleppo B55.1
  Baghdad B55.1
  Delhi B55.1
  lacrimal
    gland — *see* Dacryoadenitis
    passages (duct) (sac) — *see* Inflammation, lacrimal, passages, acute
  Natal B55.1
  orbit, orbital — *see* Abscess, orbit
  tropical B55.1
Bold hives — *see* Urticaria
Bombé, iris — *see* Membrane, pupillary
Bone — *see* condition
Bonnevie-Ullrich syndrome — *see also* Turner's syndrome Q87.19
Bonnier's syndrome H81.8 ☑
Bonvale dam fever T73.3 ☑
Bony block of joint — *see* Ankylosis
BOOP (bronchiolitis obliterans organized pneumonia) J84.89
Borderline
  diabetes mellitus R73.03
  hypertension R03.0
  osteopenia M85.8- ☑
  pelvis, with obstruction during labor O65.1
  personality F60.3
Borna disease A83.9
Bornholm disease B33.0
Boston exanthem A88.0
Botalli, ductus (patent) (persistent) Q25.0
Bothriocephalus latus infestation B70.0
Botulism (foodborne intoxication) A05.1
  infant A48.51
  non-foodborne A48.52
  wound A48.52
Bouba — *see* Yaws
Bouchard's nodes (with arthropathy) M15.2
Bouffée délirante F23
Bouillaud's disease or syndrome (rheumatic heart disease) I01.9
Bourneville's disease Q85.1
Boutonniere deformity (finger) — *see* Deformity, finger, boutonniere
Bouveret (-Hoffmann) **syndrome** (paroxysmal tachycardia) I47.9
Bovine heart — *see* Hypertrophy, cardiac
Bowel — *see* condition
Bowen's
  dermatosis (precancerous) — *see* Neoplasm, skin, in situ
  disease — *see* Neoplasm, skin, in situ

Bowen's — *continued*
  epithelioma — *see* Neoplasm, skin, in situ
  type
    epidermoid carcinoma-in-situ — *see* Neoplasm, skin, in situ
    intraepidermal squamous cell carcinoma — *see* Neoplasm, skin, in situ
Bowing
  femur — *see also* Deformity, limb, specified type NEC, thigh
    congenital Q68.3
  fibula — *see also* Deformity, limb, specified type NEC, lower leg
    congenital Q68.4
  forearm — *see* Deformity, limb, specified type NEC, forearm
  leg(s), long bones, congenital Q68.5
  radius — *see* Deformity, limb, specified type NEC, forearm
  tibia — *see also* Deformity, limb, specified type NEC, lower leg
    congenital Q68.4
Bowleg(s) (acquired) M21.16- ☑
  congenital Q68.5
  rachitic E64.3
Boyd's dysentery A03.2
Brachial — *see* condition
Brachycardia R00.1
Brachycephaly Q75.0
Bradley's disease A08.19
Bradyarrhythmia, cardiac I49.8
Bradycardia (sinoatrial) (sinus) (vagal) R00.1
  neonatal P29.12
  reflex G90.09
  tachycardia syndrome I49.5
Bradykinesia R25.8
Bradypnea R06.89
Bradytachycardia I49.5
Brailsford's disease or osteochondrosis — *see* Osteochondrosis, juvenile, radius
Brain — *see also* condition
  death G93.82
  syndrome — *see* Syndrome, brain
Branched-chain amino-acid disorder E71.2
Branchial — *see* condition
  cartilage, congenital Q18.2
Branchiogenic remnant (in neck) Q18.0
Brandt's syndrome (acrodermatitis enteropathica) E83.2
Brash (water) R12
Bravais-jacksonian epilepsy — *see* Epilepsy, localization-related, symptomatic, with simple partial seizures
Braxton Hicks contractions — *see* False, labor
Brazilian leishmaniasis B55.2
BRBPR K62.5
Break, retina (without detachment) H33.30- ☑
  with retinal detachment — *see* Detachment, retina
  horseshoe tear H33.31- ☑
  multiple H33.33- ☑
  round hole H33.32- ☑
Breakdown
  device, graft or implant — *see also* Complications, by site and type, mechanical T85.618 ☑
    arterial graft NEC — *see* Complication, cardiovascular device, mechanical, vascular
    breast (implant) T85.41 ☑
    catheter NEC T85.618 ☑
      cystostomy T83.010 ☑
      dialysis (renal) T82.41 ☑
        intraperitoneal T85.611 ☑
      Hopkins T83.018 ☑
      ileostomy T83.018 ☑
      infusion NEC T82.514 ☑
        cranial T85.610- ☑
        epidural T85.610 ☑
        intrathecal T85.610 ☑
        spinal T85.610 ☑
        subarachnoid T85.610 ☑
        subdural T85.610 ☑
      nephrostomy T83.012 ☑
      urethral indwelling T83.011 ☑
      urinary NEC T83.018 ☑
      urostomy T83.018 ☑
    electronic (electrode) (pulse generator) (stimulator)
      bone T84.310 ☑
      cardiac T82.119 ☑
        electrode T82.110 ☑

Breakdown — *continued*
  device, graft or implant — *see also* Complications, by site and type, mechanical — *continued*
    electronic — *continued*
      cardiac — *continued*
        pulse generator T82.111 ☑
        specified type NEC T82.118 ☑
      nervous system — *see* Complication, prosthetic device, mechanical, electronic nervous system stimulator
      urinary — *see* Complication, genitourinary, device, urinary, mechanical
    fixation, internal (orthopedic) NEC — *see* Complication, fixation device, mechanical
    gastrointestinal — *see* Complications, prosthetic device, mechanical, gastrointestinal device
    genital NEC T83.418 ☑
      intrauterine contraceptive device T83.31 ☑
      penile prosthesis (cylinder) (implanted) (pump) (resevoir) T83.410 ☑
      testicular prosthesis T83.411 ☑
    heart NEC — *see* Complication, cardiovascular device, mechanical
    intrathecal infusion pump T85.615 ☑
    joint prosthesis — *see* Complications..., joint prosthesis, internal, mechanical, by site
    nervous system, specified device NEC T85.615 ☑
    ocular NEC — *see* Complications, prosthetic device, mechanical, ocular device
    orthopedic NEC — *see* Complication, orthopedic, device, mechanical
    specified NEC T85.618 ☑
    subcutaneous device pocket
      nervous system prosthetic device, implant, or graft T85.890 ☑
      other internal prosthetic device, implant, or graft T85.898 ☑
    sutures, permanent T85.612 ☑
      used in bone repair — *see* Complications, fixation device, internal (orthopedic), mechanical
    urinary NEC T83.118 ☑
      graft T83.21 ☑
      sphincter, implanted T83.111 ☑
      stent (ileal conduit) (nephroureteral) T83.113 ☑
      ureteral indwelling T83.112 ☑
    vascular NEC — *see* Complication, cardiovascular device, mechanical
    ventricular intracranial shunt T85.01 ☑
  nervous F48.8
  perineum O90.1
  respirator J95.850
    specified NEC J95.859
  ventilator J95.850
    specified NEC J95.859
Breast — *see also* condition
  buds E30.1
    in newborn P96.89
  dense R92.2
  nodule — *see also* Lump, breast N63.0
Breath
  foul R19.6
  holder, child R06.89
  holding spell R06.89
  shortness R06.02
Breathing
  labored — *see* Hyperventilation
  mouth R06.5
    causing malocclusion M26.5 ☑
  periodic R06.3
    high altitude G47.32
Breathlessness R06.81
Breda's disease — *see* Yaws
Breech presentation (mother) O32.1 ☑
  causing obstructed labor O64.1 ☑
  footling O32.8 ☑
    causing obstructed labor O64.8 ☑
  incomplete O32.8 ☑
    causing obstructed labor O64.8 ☑
Breisky's disease N90.4
Brennemann's syndrome I88.0
Brenner
  tumor (benign) D27.9
    borderline malignancy D39.1- ☑
    malignant C56 ☑
    proliferating D39.1- ☑
Bretonneau's disease or angina A36.0
Breus' mole O02.0

Brevicollis Q76.49
Brickmakers' anemia B76.9 *[D63.8]*
Bridge, myocardial Q24.5
Bright red blood per rectum (BRBPR) K62.5
Bright's disease — *see also* Nephritis
  arteriosclerotic — *see* Hypertension, kidney
Brill (-Zinsser) **disease** (recrudescent typhus) A75.1
Brill-Symmers' disease C82.90
Brion-Kayser disease — *see* Fever, parathyroid
Briquet's disorder or syndrome F45.0
Brissaud's
  infantilism or dwarfism E23.0
  motor-verbal tic F95.2
Brittle
  bones disease Q78.0
  nails L60.3
    congenital Q84.6
Broad — *see also* condition
  beta disease E78.2
  ligament laceration syndrome N83.8
Broad- or floating-betalipoproteinemia E78.2
Brock's syndrome (atelectasis due to enlarged lymph
    nodes) J98.19
Brocq-Duhring disease (dermatitis herpetiformis) L13.0
Brodie's abscess or disease M86.8X- ☑
Broken
  arches — *see also* Deformity, limb, flat foot
  arm (meaning upper limb) — *see* Fracture, arm
  back — *see* Fracture, vertebra
  bone — *see* Fracture
  implant or internal device — *see* Complications, by site
    and type, mechanical
  leg (meaning lower limb) — *see* Fracture, leg
  nose S02.2 ☑
  tooth, teeth — *see* Fracture, tooth
Bromhidrosis, bromidrosis L75.0
Bromidism, bromism G92
  due to
    correct substance properly administered — *see* Ta-
      ble of Drugs and Chemicals, by drug, adverse
      effect
    overdose or wrong substance given or taken — *see*
      Table of Drugs and Chemicals, by drug, poi-
      soning
  chronic (dependence) F13.20
Bromidrosiphobia F40.298
Bronchi, bronchial — *see* condition
Bronchiectasis (cylindrical) (diffuse) (fusiform) (localized)
    (saccular) J47.9
  with
    acute
      bronchitis J47.0
      lower respiratory infection J47.0
    exacerbation (acute) J47.1
  congenital Q33.4
  tuberculous NEC — *see* Tuberculosis, pulmonary
Bronchiolectasis — *see* Bronchiectasis
Bronchiolitis (acute) (infective) (subacute) J21.9
  with
    bronchospasm or obstruction J21.9
    influenza, flu or grippe — *see* Influenza, with, respi-
      ratory manifestations NEC
  chemical (chronic) J68.4
    acute J68.0
  chronic (fibrosing) (obliterative) J44.9
  due to
    external agent — *see* Bronchitis, acute, due to
    human metapneumovirus J21.1
    respiratory syncytial virus (RSV) J21.0
    specified organism NEC J21.8
  fibrosa obliterans J44.9
  influenzal — *see* Influenza, with, respiratory manifesta-
    tions NEC
  obliterans J42
    with organizing pneumonia (BOOP) J84.89
  obliterative (chronic) (subacute) J44.9
    due to fumes or vapors J68.4
    due to chemicals, gases, fumes or vapors (inhalation)
      J68.4
  respiratory, interstitial lung disease J84.115
Bronchitis (diffuse) (fibrinous) (hypostatic) (infective)
    (membranous) J40
  with
    influenza, flu or grippe — *see* Influenza, with, respi-
      ratory manifestations NEC
    obstruction (airway) (lung) J44.9
    tracheitis (l5 years of age and above) J40

Bronchitis — *continued*
  with — *continued*
    tracheitis — *continued*
      acute or subacute J20.9
      chronic J42
      under l5 years of age J20.9
  acute or subacute (with bronchospasm or obstruction)
    J20.9
    with
      bronchiectasis J47.0
      chronic obstructive pulmonary disease J44.0
    chemical (due to gases, fumes or vapors) J68.0
    due to
      fumes or vapors J68.0
      Haemophilus influenzae J20.1
      Mycoplasma pneumoniae J20.0
      radiation J70.0
      specified organism NEC J20.8
      Streptococcus J20.2
      virus
        coxsackie J20.3
        echovirus J20.7
        parainfluenzae J20.4
        respiratory syncytial (RSV) J20.5
        rhinovirus J20.6
    viral NEC J20.8
  allergic (acute) J45.909
    with
      exacerbation (acute) J45.901
      status asthmaticus J45.902
  arachidic T17.528 ☑
  aspiration (due to fumes or vapors) J68.0
  asthmatic J45.9 ☑
    chronic J44.9
      with
        acute lower respiratory infection J44.0
        exacerbation (acute) J44.1
  capillary — *see* Pneumonia, broncho
  caseous (tuberculous) A15.5
  Castellani's A69.8
  catarrhal (l5 years of age and above) J40
    acute — *see* Bronchitis, acute
    chronic J41.0
    under l5 years of age J20.9
  chemical (acute) (subacute) J68.0
    chronic J68.4
    due to fumes or vapors J68.0
      chronic J68.4
  chronic J42
    with
      airways obstruction J44.9
      tracheitis (chronic) J42
    asthmatic (obstructive) J44.9
    catarrhal J41.0
    chemical (due to fumes or vapors) J68.4
    due to
      chemicals, gases, fumes or vapors (inhalation)
        J68.4
      radiation J70.1
      tobacco smoking J41.0
    emphysematous J44.9
    mucopurulent J41.1
    non-obstructive J41.0
    obliterans J44.9
    obstructive J44.9
    purulent J41.1
    simple J41.0
  croupous — *see* Bronchitis, acute
  due to gases, fumes or vapors (chemical) J68.0
  emphysematous (obstructive) J44.9
  exudative — *see* Bronchitis, acute
  fetid J41.1
  grippal — *see* Influenza, with, respiratory manifesta-
    tions NEC
  in those under l5 years age — *see* Bronchitis, acute
    chronic — *see* Bronchitis, chronic
  influenzal — *see* Influenza, with, respiratory manifesta-
    tions NEC
  mixed simple and mucopurulent J41.8
  moulder's J62.8
  mucopurulent (chronic) (recurrent) J41.1
    acute or subacute J20.9
    simple (mixed) J41.8
  obliterans (chronic) J44.9
  obstructive (chronic) (diffuse) J44.9
  pituitous J41.1
  pneumococcal, acute or subacute J20.2

Bronchitis — *continued*
  pseudomembranous, acute or subacute — *see* Bronch
    tis, chronic
  purulent (chronic) (recurrent) J41.1
    acute or subacute — *see* Bronchitis, acute
  putrid J41.1
  senile (chronic) J42
  simple and mucopurulent (mixed) J41.8
  smokers' J41.0
  spirochetal NEC A69.8
  subacute — *see* Bronchitis, acute
  suppurative (chronic) J41.1
    acute or subacute — *see* Bronchitis, acute
  tuberculous A15.5
  under l5 years of age — *see* Bronchitis, acute
    chronic — *see* Bronchitis, chronic
  viral NEC, acute or subacute — *see also* Bronchitis,
    acute J20.8
Bronchoalveolitis J18.0
Bronchoaspergillosis B44.1
Bronchocele meaning goiter E04.0
Broncholithiasis J98.09
  tuberculous NEC A15.5
Bronchomalacia J98.09
  congenital Q32.2
Bronchomycosis NOS B49 *[J99]*
  candidal B37.1
Bronchopleuropneumonia — *see* Pneumonia, bronch●
Bronchopneumonia — *see* Pneumonia, broncho
Bronchopneumonitis — *see* Pneumonia, broncho
Bronchopulmonary — *see* condition
Bronchopulmonitis — *see* Pneumonia, broncho
Bronchorrhagia (see Hemoptysis)
Bronchorrhea J98.09
  acute J20.9
  chronic (infective) (purulent) J42
Bronchospasm (acute) J98.01
  with
    bronchiolitis, acute J21.9
    bronchitis, acute (conditions in J20) — *see* Bronchi
      tis, acute
  due to external agent — *see* condition, respiratory,
    acute, due to
  exercise induced J45.990
Bronchospirochetosis A69.8
  Castellani A69.8
Bronchostenosis J98.09
Bronchus — *see* condition
Brontophobia F40.220
Bronze baby syndrome P83.88
Brooke's tumor — *see* Neoplasm, skin, benign
Brown enamel of teeth (hereditary) K00.5
Brown's sheath syndrome H50.61- ☑
Brown-Séquard disease, paralysis or syndrome
  G83.81
Bruce sepsis A23.0
Brucellosis (infection) A23.9
  abortus A23.1
  canis A23.3
  dermatitis A23.9
  melitensis A23.0
  mixed A23.8
  sepsis A23.9
    melitensis A23.0
    specified NEC A23.8
  suis A23.2
Bruck-de Lange disease Q87.19
Bruck's disease — *see* Deformity, limb
BRUE (brief resolved unexplained event) R68.13
Brugsch's syndrome Q82.8
Bruise (skin surface intact) — *see also* Contusion
  with
    open wound — *see* Wound, open
  internal organ — *see* Injury, by site
  newborn P54.5
  scalp, due to birth injury, newborn P12.3
  umbilical cord O69.5 ☑
Bruit (arterial) R09.89
  cardiac R01.1
Brush burn — *see* Abrasion, by site
Bruton's X-linked agammaglobulinemia D80.0
Bruxism
  psychogenic F45.8
  sleep related G47.63
Bubbly lung syndrome P27.0
Bubo I88.8
  blennorrhagic (gonococcal) A54.89

☑ **Additional Character Required** — Refer to the Tabular List for Character Selection   ▽ **Subterms under main terms may continue to next column or page**

Index

Bubo — *continued*
- chancroidal A57
- climatic A55
- due to Haemophilus ducreyi A57
- gonococcal A54.89
- indolent (nonspecific) I88.8
- inguinal (nonspecific) I88.8
  - chancroidal A57
  - climatic A55
  - due to H. ducreyi A57
  - infective I88.8
- scrofulous (tuberculous) A18.2
- soft chancre A57
- suppurating — *see* Lymphadenitis, acute
- syphilitic (primary) A51.0
  - congenital A50.07
- tropical A55
- virulent (chancroidal) A57

Bubonic plague A20.0

Bubonocele — *see* Hernia, inguinal

Buccal — *see* condition

Buchanan's disease or osteochondrosis M91.0

Buchem's syndrome (hyperostosis corticalis) M85.2

Bucket-handle fracture or tear (semilunar cartilage) — *see* Tear, meniscus

Budd-Chiari syndrome (hepatic vein thrombosis) I82.0

Budgerigar fancier's disease or lung J67.2

Buds
- breast E30.1
  - in newborn P96.89

Buerger's disease (thromboangiitis obliterans) I73.1

Bulbar — *see* condition

Bulbus cordis (left ventricle) (persistent) Q21.8

Bulimia (nervosa) F50.2
- atypical F50.9
- normal weight F50.9

Bulky
- stools R19.5
- uterus N85.2

Bulla (e) R23.8
- lung (emphysematous) (solitary) J43.9
  - newborn P25.8

Bullet wound — *see also* Wound, open
- fracture — *code as* Fracture, by site
- internal organ — *see* Injury, by site

Bundle
- branch block (complete) (false) (incomplete) — *see* Block, bundle-branch
- of His — *see* condition

Bunion M21.61- ☑
- tailor's M21.62- ☑

Bunionette M21.62- ☑

Buphthalmia, buphthalmos (congenital) Q15.0

Burdwan fever B55.0

Bürger-Grütz disease or syndrome E78.3

Buried
- penis (congenital) Q55.64
  - acquired N48.83
- roots K08.3

Burke's syndrome K86.89

Burkitt
- cell leukemia C91.0- ☑
- lymphoma (malignant) C83.7- ☑
  - small noncleaved, diffuse C83.7- ☑
  - spleen C83.77
  - undifferentiated C83.7- ☑
- tumor C83.7- ☑
- type
  - acute lymphoblastic leukemia C91.0- ☑
  - undifferentiated C83.7- ☑

Burn (electricity) (flame) (hot gas, liquid or hot object) (radiation) (steam) (thermal) T30.0
- abdomen, abdominal (muscle) (wall) T21.02 ☑
  - first degree T21.12 ☑
  - second degree T21.22 ☑
  - third degree T21.32 ☑
- above elbow T22.039 ☑
  - first degree T22.139 ☑
  - left T22.032 ☑
    - first degree T22.132 ☑
    - second degree T22.232 ☑
    - third degree T22.332 ☑
  - right T22.031 ☑
    - first degree T22.131 ☑
    - second degree T22.231 ☑
    - third degree T22.331 ☑
  - second degree T22.239 ☑

Burn — *continued*
- above elbow — *continued*
  - third degree T22.339 ☑
- acid (caustic) (external) (internal) — *see* Corrosion, by site
- alimentary tract NEC T28.2 ☑
  - esophagus T28.1 ☑
  - mouth T28.0 ☑
  - pharynx T28.0 ☑
- alkaline (caustic) (external) (internal) — *see* Corrosion, by site
- ankle T25.019 ☑
  - first degree T25.119 ☑
  - left T25.012 ☑
    - first degree T25.112 ☑
    - second degree T25.212 ☑
    - third degree T25.312 ☑
  - multiple with foot — *see* Burn, lower, limb, multiple, ankle and foot
  - right T25.011 ☑
    - first degree T25.111 ☑
    - second degree T25.211 ☑
    - third degree T25.311 ☑
  - second degree T25.219 ☑
  - third degree T25.319 ☑
- anus — *see* Burn, buttock
- arm (lower) (upper) — *see* Burn, upper, limb
- axilla T22.049 ☑
  - first degree T22.149 ☑
  - left T22.042 ☑
    - first degree T22.142 ☑
    - second degree T22.242 ☑
    - third degree T22.342 ☑
  - right T22.041 ☑
    - first degree T22.141 ☑
    - second degree T22.241 ☑
    - third degree T22.341 ☑
  - second degree T22.249 ☑
  - third degree T22.349 ☑
- back (lower) T21.04 ☑
  - first degree T21.14 ☑
  - second degree T21.24 ☑
  - third degree T21.34 ☑
  - upper T21.03 ☑
    - first degree T21.13 ☑
    - second degree T21.23 ☑
    - third degree T21.33 ☑
- blisters — *code as* Burn, second degree, by site
- breast(s) — *see* Burn, chest wall
- buttock(s) T21.05 ☑
  - first degree T21.15 ☑
  - second degree T21.25 ☑
  - third degree T21.35 ☑
- calf T24.039 ☑
  - first degree T24.139 ☑
  - left T24.032 ☑
    - first degree T24.132 ☑
    - second degree T24.232 ☑
    - third degree T24.332 ☑
  - right T24.031 ☑
    - first degree T24.131 ☑
    - second degree T24.231 ☑
    - third degree T24.331 ☑
  - second degree T24.239 ☑
  - third degree T24.339 ☑
- canthus (eye) — *see* Burn, eyelid
- caustic acid or alkaline — *see* Corrosion, by site
- cervix T28.3 ☑
- cheek T20.06 ☑
  - first degree T20.16 ☑
  - second degree T20.26 ☑
  - third degree T20.36 ☑
- chemical (acids) (alkalines) (caustics) (external) (internal) — *see* Corrosion, by site
- chest wall T21.01 ☑
  - first degree T21.11 ☑
  - second degree T21.21 ☑
  - third degree T21.31 ☑
- chin T20.03 ☑
  - first degree T20.13 ☑
  - second degree T20.23 ☑
  - third degree T20.33 ☑
- colon T28.2 ☑
- conjunctiva (and cornea) — *see* Burn, cornea
- cornea (and conjunctiva) T26.1- ☑
  - chemical — *see* Corrosion, cornea

Burn — *continued*
- corrosion (external) (internal) — *see* Corrosion, by site
- deep necrosis of underlying tissue — *code as* Burn, third degree, by site
- dorsum of hand T23.069 ☑
  - first degree T23.169 ☑
  - left T23.062 ☑
    - first degree T23.162 ☑
    - second degree T23.262 ☑
    - third degree T23.362 ☑
  - right T23.061 ☑
    - first degree T23.161 ☑
    - second degree T23.261 ☑
    - third degree T23.361 ☑
  - second degree T23.269 ☑
  - third degree T23.369 ☑
- due to ingested chemical agent — *see* Corrosion, by site
- ear (auricle) (external) (canal) T20.01 ☑
  - first degree T20.11 ☑
  - second degree T20.21 ☑
  - third degree T20.31 ☑
- elbow T22.029 ☑
  - first degree T22.129 ☑
  - left T22.022 ☑
    - first degree T22.122 ☑
    - second degree T22.222 ☑
    - third degree T22.322 ☑
  - right T22.021 ☑
    - first degree T22.121 ☑
    - second degree T22.221 ☑
    - third degree T22.321 ☑
  - second degree T22.229 ☑
  - third degree T22.329 ☑
- epidermal loss — *code as* Burn, second degree, by site
- erythema, erythematous — *code as* Burn, first degree, by site
- esophagus T28.1 ☑
- extent (percentage of body surface)
  - less than 10 percent T31.0
  - 10-19 percent T31.10
    - with 0-9 percent third degree burns T31.10
    - with 10-19 percent third degree burns T31.11
  - 20-29 percent T31.20
    - with 0-9 percent third degree burns T31.20
    - with 10-19 percent third degree burns T31.21
    - with 20-29 percent third degree burns T31.22
  - 30-39 percent T31.30
    - with 0-9 percent third degree burns T31.30
    - with 10-19 percent third degree burns T31.31
    - with 20-29 percent third degree burns T31.32
    - with 30-39 percent third degree burns T31.33
  - 40-49 percent T31.40
    - with 0-9 percent third degree burns T31.40
    - with 10-19 percent third degree burns T31.41
    - with 20-29 percent third degree burns T31.42
    - with 30-39 percent third degree burns T31.43
    - with 40-49 percent third degree burns T31.44
  - 50-59 percent T31.50
    - with 0-9 percent third degree burns T31.50
    - with 10-19 percent third degree burns T31.51
    - with 20-29 percent third degree burns T31.52
    - with 30-39 percent third degree burns T31.53
    - with 40-49 percent third degree burns T31.54
    - with 50-59 percent third degree burns T31.55
  - 60-69 percent T31.60
    - with 0-9 percent third degree burns T31.60
    - with 10-19 percent third degree burns T31.61
    - with 20-29 percent third degree burns T31.62
    - with 30-39 percent third degree burns T31.63
    - with 40-49 percent third degree burns T31.64
    - with 50-59 percent third degree burns T31.65
    - with 60-69 percent third degree burns T31.66
  - 70-79 percent T31.70
    - with 0-9 percent third degree burns T31.70
    - with 10-19 percent third degree burns T31.71
    - with 20-29 percent third degree burns T31.72
    - with 30-39 percent third degree burns T31.73
    - with 40-49 percent third degree burns T31.74
    - with 50-59 percent third degree burns T31.75
    - with 60-69 percent third degree burns T31.76
    - with 70-79 percent third degree burns T31.77
  - 80-89 percent T31.80
    - with 0-9 percent third degree burns T31.80
    - with 10-19 percent third degree burns T31.81
    - with 20-29 percent third degree burns T31.82
    - with 30-39 percent third degree burns T31.83

Bubo — Burn

Burn — *continued*
  extent — *continued*
    80-89 percent — *continued*
      with 40-49 percent third degree burns T31.84
      with 50-59 percent third degree burns T31.85
      with 60-69 percent third degree burns T31.86
      with 70-79 percent third degree burns T31.87
      with 80-89 percent third degree burns T31.88
    90 percent or more T31.90
      with 0-9 percent third degree burns T31.90
      with 10-19 percent third degree burns T31.91
      with 20-29 percent third degree burns T31.92
      with 30-39 percent third degree burns T31.93
      with 40-49 percent third degree burns T31.94
      with 50-59 percent third degree burns T31.95
      with 60-69 percent third degree burns T31.96
      with 70-79 percent third degree burns T31.97
      with 80-89 percent third degree burns T31.98
      with 90 percent or more third degree burns T31.99
  extremity — *see* Burn, limb
  eye(s) and adnexa T26.4- ☑
    with resulting rupture and destruction of eyeball T26.2- ☑
    conjunctival sac — *see* Burn, cornea
    cornea — *see* Burn, cornea
    lid — *see* Burn, eyelid
    periocular area — *see* Burn, eyelid
    specified site NEC T26.3- ☑
  eyeball — *see* Burn, eye
  eyelid(s) T26.0- ☑
    chemical — *see* Corrosion, eyelid
  face — *see* Burn, head
  finger T23.029 ☑
    first degree T23.129 ☑
    left T23.022 ☑
      first degree T23.122 ☑
      second degree T23.222 ☑
      third degree T23.322 ☑
    multiple sites (without thumb) T23.039 ☑
      with thumb T23.049 ☑
        first degree T23.149 ☑
        left T23.042 ☑
          first degree T23.142 ☑
          second degree T23.242 ☑
          third degree T23.342 ☑
        right T23.041 ☑
          first degree T23.141 ☑
          second degree T23.241 ☑
          third degree T23.341 ☑
        second degree T23.249 ☑
        third degree T23.349 ☑
      first degree T23.139 ☑
      left T23.032 ☑
        first degree T23.132 ☑
        second degree T23.232 ☑
        third degree T23.332 ☑
      right T23.031 ☑
        first degree T23.131 ☑
        second degree T23.231 ☑
        third degree T23.331 ☑
      second degree T23.239 ☑
      third degree T23.339 ☑
    right T23.021 ☑
      first degree T23.121 ☑
      second degree T23.221 ☑
      third degree T23.321 ☑
    second degree T23.229 ☑
    third degree T23.329 ☑
  flank — *see* Burn, abdominal wall
  foot T25.029 ☑
    first degree T25.129 ☑
    left T25.022 ☑
      first degree T25.122 ☑
      second degree T25.222 ☑
      third degree T25.322 ☑
    multiple with ankle — *see* Burn, lower, limb, multiple, ankle and foot
    right T25.021 ☑
      first degree T25.121 ☑
      second degree T25.221 ☑
      third degree T25.321 ☑
    second degree T25.229 ☑
    third degree T25.329 ☑
  forearm T22.019 ☑
    first degree T22.119 ☑

Burn — *continued*
  forearm — *continued*
    left T22.012 ☑
      first degree T22.112 ☑
      second degree T22.212 ☑
      third degree T22.312 ☑
    right T22.011 ☑
      first degree T22.111 ☑
      second degree T22.211 ☑
      third degree T22.311 ☑
    second degree T22.219 ☑
    third degree T22.319 ☑
  forehead T20.06 ☑
    first degree T20.16 ☑
    second degree T20.26 ☑
    third degree T20.36 ☑
  fourth degree — *code as* Burn, third degree, by site
  friction — *see* Burn, by site
  from swallowing caustic or corrosive substance NEC — *see* Corrosion, by site
  full thickness skin loss — *code as* Burn, third degree, by site
  gastrointestinal tract NEC T28.2 ☑
    from swallowing caustic or corrosive substance T28.7 ☑
  genital organs
    external
      female T21.07 ☑
        first degree T21.17 ☑
        second degree T21.27 ☑
        third degree T21.37 ☑
      male T21.06 ☑
        first degree T21.16 ☑
        second degree T21.26 ☑
        third degree T21.36 ☑
    internal T28.3 ☑
      from caustic or corrosive substance T28.8 ☑
  groin — *see* Burn, abdominal wall
  hand(s) T23.009 ☑
    back — *see* Burn, dorsum of hand
    finger — *see* Burn, finger
    first degree T23.109 ☑
    left T23.002 ☑
      first degree T23.102 ☑
      second degree T23.202 ☑
      third degree T23.302 ☑
    multiple sites with wrist T23.099 ☑
      first degree T23.199 ☑
      left T23.092 ☑
        first degree T23.192 ☑
        second degree T23.292 ☑
        third degree T23.392 ☑
      right T23.091 ☑
        first degree T23.191 ☑
        second degree T23.291 ☑
        third degree T23.391 ☑
      second degree T23.299 ☑
      third degree T23.399 ☑
    palm — *see* Burn, palm
    right T23.001 ☑
      first degree T23.101 ☑
      second degree T23.201 ☑
      third degree T23.301 ☑
    second degree T23.209 ☑
    third degree T23.309 ☑
    thumb — *see* Burn, thumb
  head (and face) (and neck) T20.00 ☑
    cheek — *see* Burn, cheek
    chin — *see* Burn, chin
    ear — *see* Burn, ear
    eye(s) only — *see* Burn, eye
    first degree T20.10 ☑
    forehead — *see* Burn, forehead
    lip — *see* Burn, lip
    multiple sites T20.09 ☑
      first degree T20.19 ☑
      second degree T20.29 ☑
      third degree T20.39 ☑
    neck — *see* Burn, neck
    nose — *see* Burn, nose
    scalp — *see* Burn, scalp
    second degree T20.20 ☑
    third degree T20.30 ☑
  hip(s) — *see* Burn, thigh
  inhalation — *see* Burn, respiratory tract

Burn — *continued*
  inhalation — *see* Burn, respiratory tract — *continued*
    caustic or corrosive substance (fumes) — *see* Corrosion, respiratory tract
  internal organ(s) T28.40 ☑
    alimentary tract T28.2 ☑
      esophagus T28.1 ☑
    eardrum T28.41 ☑
    esophagus T28.1 ☑
    from caustic or corrosive substance (swallowing) NEC — *see* Corrosion, by site
    genitourinary T28.3 ☑
    mouth T28.0 ☑
    pharynx T28.0 ☑
    respiratory tract — *see* Burn, respiratory tract
    specified organ NEC T28.49 ☑
  interscapular region — *see* Burn, back, upper
  intestine (large) (small) T28.2 ☑
  knee T24.029 ☑
    first degree T24.129 ☑
    left T24.022 ☑
      first degree T24.122 ☑
      second degree T24.222 ☑
      third degree T24.322 ☑
    right T24.021 ☑
      first degree T24.121 ☑
      second degree T24.221 ☑
      third degree T24.321 ☑
    second degree T24.229 ☑
    third degree T24.329 ☑
  labium (majus) (minus) — *see* Burn, genital organs, external, female
  lacrimal apparatus, duct, gland or sac — *see* Burn, eye specified site NEC
  larynx T27.0 ☑
    with lung T27.1 ☑
  leg(s) (lower) (upper) — *see* Burn, lower, limb
  lightning — *see* Burn, by site
  limb(s)
    lower (except ankle or foot alone) — *see* Burn, lower, limb
    upper — *see* Burn, upper limb
  lip(s) T20.02 ☑
    first degree T20.12 ☑
    second degree T20.22 ☑
    third degree T20.32 ☑
  lower
    back — *see* Burn, back
    limb T24.009 ☑
      ankle — *see* Burn, ankle
      calf — *see* Burn, calf
      first degree T24.109 ☑
      foot — *see* Burn, foot
      hip — *see* Burn, thigh
      knee — *see* Burn, knee
      left T24.002 ☑
        first degree T24.102 ☑
        second degree T24.202 ☑
        third degree T24.302 ☑
      multiple sites, except ankle and foot T24.099 ☑
        ankle and foot T25.099 ☑
          first degree T25.199 ☑
          left T25.092 ☑
            first degree T25.192 ☑
            second degree T25.292 ☑
            third degree T25.392 ☑
          right T25.091 ☑
            first degree T25.191 ☑
            second degree T25.291 ☑
            third degree T25.391 ☑
          second degree T25.299 ☑
          third degree T25.399 ☑
        first degree T24.199 ☑
        left T24.092 ☑
          first degree T24.192 ☑
          second degree T24.292 ☑
          third degree T24.392 ☑
        right T24.091 ☑
          first degree T24.191 ☑
          second degree T24.291 ☑
          third degree T24.391 ☑
        second degree T24.299 ☑
        third degree T24.399 ☑
      right T24.001 ☑
        first degree T24.101 ☑

☑ **Additional Character Required — Refer to the Tabular List for Character Selection**
▧ **Subterms under main terms may continue to next column or page**

Burn — *continued*
- lower — *continued*
  - limb — *continued*
    - right — *continued*
      - second degree T24.201 ✓
        - third degree T24.301 ✓
      - second degree T24.209 ✓
      - thigh — *see* Burn, thigh
        - third degree T24.309 ✓
      - toe — *see* Burn, toe
- lung (with larynx and trachea) T27.1 ✓
- mouth T28.0 ✓
- neck T20.07 ✓
  - first degree T20.17 ✓
  - second degree T20.27 ✓
  - third degree T20.37 ✓
- nose (septum) T20.04 ✓
  - first degree T20.14 ✓
  - second degree T20.24 ✓
  - third degree T20.34 ✓
- ocular adnexa — *see* Burn, eye
- orbit region — *see* Burn, eyelid
- palm T23.059 ✓
  - first degree T23.159 ✓
  - left T23.052 ✓
    - first degree T23.152 ✓
    - second degree T23.252 ✓
    - third degree T23.352 ✓
  - right T23.051 ✓
    - first degree T23.151 ✓
    - second degree T23.251 ✓
    - third degree T23.351 ✓
  - second degree T23.259 ✓
  - third degree T23.359 ✓
- partial thickness — *code as* Burn, degree, by site
- pelvis — *see* Burn, trunk
- penis — *see* Burn, genital organs, external, male
- perineum
  - female — *see* Burn, genital organs, external, female
  - male — *see* Burn, genital organs, external, male
- periocular area — *see* Burn, eyelid
- pharynx T28.0 ✓
- rectum T28.2 ✓
- respiratory tract T27.3 ✓
  - larynx — *see* Burn, larynx
  - specified part NEC T27.2 ✓
  - trachea — *see* Burn, trachea
- sac, lacrimal — *see* Burn, eye, specified site NEC
- scalp T20.05 ✓
  - first degree T20.15 ✓
  - second degree T20.25 ✓
  - third degree T20.35 ✓
- scapular region T22.069 ✓
  - first degree T22.169 ✓
  - left T22.062 ✓
    - first degree T22.162 ✓
    - second degree T22.262 ✓
    - third degree T22.362 ✓
  - right T22.061 ✓
    - first degree T22.161 ✓
    - second degree T22.261 ✓
    - third degree T22.361 ✓
  - second degree T22.269 ✓
  - third degree T22.369 ✓
- sclera — *see* Burn, eye, specified site NEC
- scrotum — *see* Burn, genital organs, external, male
- shoulder T22.059 ✓
  - first degree T22.159 ✓
  - left T22.052 ✓
    - first degree T22.152 ✓
    - second degree T22.252 ✓
    - third degree T22.352 ✓
  - right T22.051 ✓
    - first degree T22.151 ✓
    - second degree T22.251 ✓
    - third degree T22.351 ✓
  - second degree T22.259 ✓
  - third degree T22.359 ✓
- stomach T28.2 ✓
- temple — *see* Burn, head
- testis — *see* Burn, genital organs, external, male
- thigh T24.019 ✓
  - first degree T24.119 ✓
  - left T24.012 ✓
    - first degree T24.112 ✓
    - second degree T24.212 ✓

Burn — *continued*
- thigh — *continued*
  - left — *continued*
    - third degree T24.312 ✓
  - right T24.011 ✓
    - first degree T24.111 ✓
    - second degree T24.211 ✓
    - third degree T24.311 ✓
  - second degree T24.219 ✓
  - third degree T24.319 ✓
- thorax (external) — *see* Burn, trunk
- throat (meaning pharynx) T28.0 ✓
- thumb(s) T23.019 ✓
  - first degree T23.119 ✓
  - left T23.012 ✓
    - first degree T23.112 ✓
    - second degree T23.212 ✓
    - third degree T23.312 ✓
  - multiple sites with fingers T23.049 ✓
    - first degree T23.149 ✓
    - left T23.042 ✓
      - first degree T23.142 ✓
      - second degree T23.242 ✓
      - third degree T23.342 ✓
    - right T23.041 ✓
      - first degree T23.141 ✓
      - second degree T23.241 ✓
      - third degree T23.341 ✓
    - second degree T23.249 ✓
    - third degree T23.349 ✓
  - right T23.011 ✓
    - first degree T23.111 ✓
    - second degree T23.211 ✓
    - third degree T23.311 ✓
  - second degree T23.219 ✓
  - third degree T23.319 ✓
- toe T25.039 ✓
  - first degree T25.139 ✓
  - left T25.032 ✓
    - first degree T25.132 ✓
    - second degree T25.232 ✓
    - third degree T25.332 ✓
  - right T25.031 ✓
    - first degree T25.131 ✓
    - second degree T25.231 ✓
    - third degree T25.331 ✓
  - second degree T25.239 ✓
  - third degree T25.339 ✓
- tongue T28.0 ✓
- tonsil(s) T28.0 ✓
- trachea T27.0 ✓
  - with lung T27.1 ✓
- trunk T21.00 ✓
  - abdominal wall — *see* Burn, abdominal wall
  - anus — *see* Burn, buttock
  - axilla — *see* Burn, upper limb
  - back — *see* Burn, back
  - breast — *see* Burn, chest wall
  - buttock — *see* Burn, buttock
  - chest wall — *see* Burn, chest wall
  - first degree T21.10 ✓
  - flank — *see* Burn, abdominal wall
  - genital
    - female — *see* Burn, genital organs, external, female
    - male — *see* Burn, genital organs, external, male
  - groin — *see* Burn, abdominal wall
  - interscapular region — *see* Burn, back, upper
  - labia — *see* Burn, genital organs, external, female
  - lower back — *see* Burn, back
  - penis — *see* Burn, genital organs, external, male
  - perineum
    - female — *see* Burn, genital organs, external, female
    - male — *see* Burn, genital organs, external, male
  - scapula region — *see* Burn, scapular region
  - scrotum — *see* Burn, genital organs, external, male
  - second degree T21.20 ✓
  - specified site NEC T21.09 ✓
    - first degree T21.19 ✓
    - second degree T21.29 ✓
    - third degree T21.39 ✓
  - testes — *see* Burn, genital organs, external, male
  - third degree T21.30 ✓
  - upper back — *see* Burn, back, upper
  - vulva — *see* Burn, genital organs, external, female

Burn — *continued*
- unspecified site with extent of body surface involved specified
  - less than 10 percent T31.0
  - 10-19 percent (0-9 percent third degree) T31.10
    - with 10-19 percent third degree T31.11
  - 20-29 percent (0-9 percent third degree) T31.20
    - with
      - 10-19 percent third degree T31.21
      - 20-29 percent third degree T31.22
  - 30-39 percent (0-9 percent third degree) T31.30
    - with
      - 10-19 percent third degree T31.31
      - 20-29 percent third degree T31.32
      - 30-39 percent third degree T31.33
  - 40-49 percent (0-9 percent third degree) T31.40
    - with
      - 10-19 percent third degree T31.41
      - 20-29 percent third degree T31.42
      - 30-39 percent third degree T31.43
      - 40-49 percent third degree T31.44
  - 50-59 percent (0-9 percent third degree) T31.50
    - with
      - 10-19 percent third degree T31.51
      - 20-29 percent third degree T31.52
      - 30-39 percent third degree T31.53
      - 40-49 percent third degree T31.54
      - 50-59 percent third degree T31.55
  - 60-69 percent (0-9 percent third degree) T31.60
    - with
      - 10-19 percent third degree T31.61
      - 20-29 percent third degree T31.62
      - 30-39 percent third degree T31.63
      - 40-49 percent third degree T31.64
      - 50-59 percent third degree T31.65
      - 60-69 percent third degree T31.66
  - 70-79 percent (0-9 percent third degree) T31.70
    - with
      - 10-19 percent third degree T31.71
      - 20-29 percent third degree T31.72
      - 30-39 percent third degree T31.73
      - 40-49 percent third degree T31.74
      - 50-59 percent third degree T31.75
      - 60-69 percent third degree T31.76
      - 70-79 percent third degree T31.77
  - 80-89 percent (0-9 percent third degree) T31.80
    - with
      - 10-19 percent third degree T31.81
      - 20-29 percent third degree T31.82
      - 30-39 percent third degree T31.83
      - 40-49 percent third degree T31.84
      - 50-59 percent third degree T31.85
      - 60-69 percent third degree T31.86
      - 70-79 percent third degree T31.87
      - 80-89 percent third degree T31.88
  - 90 percent or more (0-9 percent third degree) T31.90
    - with
      - 10-19 percent third degree T31.91
      - 20-29 percent third degree T31.92
      - 30-39 percent third degree T31.93
      - 40-49 percent third degree T31.94
      - 50-59 percent third degree T31.95
      - 60-69 percent third degree T31.96
      - 70-79 percent third degree T31.97
      - 80-89 percent third degree T31.98
      - 90-99 percent third degree T31.99
- upper limb T22.00 ✓
  - above elbow — *see* Burn, above elbow
  - axilla — *see* Burn, axilla
  - elbow — *see* Burn, elbow
  - first degree T22.10 ✓
  - forearm — *see* Burn, forearm
  - hand — *see* Burn, hand
  - interscapular region — *see* Burn, back, upper
  - multiple sites T22.099 ✓
    - first degree T22.199 ✓
    - left T22.092 ✓
      - first degree T22.192 ✓
      - second degree T22.292 ✓
      - third degree T22.392 ✓
    - right T22.091 ✓
      - first degree T22.191 ✓
      - second degree T22.291 ✓
      - third degree T22.391 ✓
    - second degree T22.299 ✓
    - third degree T22.399 ✓
  - scapular region — *see* Burn, scapular region
  - second degree T22.20 ✓

Index

Burn — Burn

Burn — continued
  upper limb — continued
    shoulder — see Burn, shoulder
      third degree T22.30 ☑
    wrist — see Burn, wrist
  uterus T28.3 ☑
  vagina T28.3 ☑
  vulva — see Burn, genital organs, external, female
  wrist T23.079 ☑
    first degree T23.179 ☑
    left T23.072 ☑
      first degree T23.172 ☑
      second degree T23.272 ☑
      third degree T23.372 ☑
    multiple sites with hand T23.099 ☑
      first degree T23.199 ☑
      left T23.092 ☑
        first degree T23.192 ☑
        second degree T23.292 ☑
        third degree T23.392 ☑
      right T23.091 ☑
        first degree T23.191 ☑
        second degree T23.291 ☑
        third degree T23.391 ☑
      second degree T23.299 ☑
      third degree T23.399 ☑
    right T23.071 ☑
      first degree T23.171 ☑
      second degree T23.271 ☑
      third degree T23.371 ☑
    second degree T23.279 ☑
    third degree T23.379 ☑
Burnett's syndrome E83.52
Burning
  feet syndrome E53.9
  sensation R20.8
  tongue K14.6
Burn-out (state) Z73.0
Burns' disease or osteochondrosis — see Osteochondrosis, juvenile, ulna
Bursa — see condition
Bursitis M71.9
  Achilles — see Tendinitis, Achilles
  adhesive — see Bursitis, specified NEC
  ankle — see Enthesopathy, lower limb, ankle, specified type NEC
  calcaneal — see Enthesopathy, foot, specified type NEC
  collateral ligament, tibial — see Bursitis, tibial collateral
  due to use, overuse, pressure — see also Disorder, soft tissue, due to use, specified type NEC
    specified NEC — see Disorder, soft tissue, due to use, specified NEC
  Duplay's M75.0 ☑
  elbow NEC M70.3- ☑
    olecranon M70.2- ☑
  finger — see Disorder, soft tissue, due to use, specified type NEC, hand
  foot — see Enthesopathy, foot, specified type NEC
  gonococcal A54.49
  gouty — see Gout
  hand M70.1- ☑
  hip NEC M70.7- ☑
    trochanteric M70.6- ☑
  infective NEC M71.10
    abscess — see Abscess, bursa
    ankle M71.17- ☑
    elbow M71.12- ☑
    foot M71.17- ☑
    hand M71.14- ☑
    hip M71.15- ☑
    knee M71.16- ☑
    multiple sites M71.19
    shoulder M71.11- ☑
    specified site NEC M71.18
    wrist M71.13- ☑
  ischial — see Bursitis, hip
  knee NEC M70.5- ☑
    prepatellar M70.4- ☑
  occupational NEC — see also Disorder, soft tissue, due to, use
  olecranon — see Bursitis, elbow, olecranon
  pharyngeal J39.1
  popliteal — see Bursitis, knee
  prepatellar M70.4- ☑
  radiohumeral M77.8
  rheumatoid M06.20

Bursitis — continued
  rheumatoid — continued
    ankle M06.27- ☑
    elbow M06.22- ☑
    foot joint M06.27- ☑
    hand joint M06.24- ☑
    hip M06.25- ☑
    knee M06.26- ☑
    multiple site M06.29
    shoulder M06.21- ☑
    vertebra M06.28
    wrist M06.23- ☑
  scapulohumeral — see Bursitis, shoulder
  semimembranous muscle (knee) — see Bursitis, knee
  shoulder M75.5- ☑
    adhesive — see Capsulitis, adhesive
  specified NEC M71.50
    ankle M71.57- ☑
    due to use, overuse or pressure — see Disorder, soft tissue, due to, use
    elbow M71.52- ☑
    foot M71.57- ☑
    hand M71.54- ☑
    hip M71.55- ☑
    knee M71.56- ☑
    shoulder — see Bursitis, shoulder
    specified site NEC M71.58
    tibial collateral M76.4- ☑
    wrist M71.53- ☑
  subacromial — see Bursitis, shoulder
  subcoracoid — see Bursitis, shoulder
  subdeltoid — see Bursitis, shoulder
  syphilitic A52.78
  Thornwaldt, Tornwaldt J39.2
  tibial collateral M76.4- ☑
  toe — see Enthesopathy, foot, specified type NEC
  trochanteric (area) — see Bursitis, hip, trochanteric
  wrist — see Bursitis, hand
Bursopathy M71.9
  specified type NEC M71.80
    ankle M71.87- ☑
    elbow M71.82- ☑
    foot M71.87- ☑
    hand M71.84- ☑
    hip M71.85- ☑
    knee M71.86- ☑
    multiple sites M71.89
    shoulder M71.81- ☑
    specified site NEC M71.88
    wrist M71.83- ☑
Burst stitches or sutures (complication of surgery) T81.31 ☑
  external operation wound T81.31 ☑
  internal operation wound T81.32 ☑
Buruli ulcer A31.1
Bury's disease L95.1
Buschke's
  disease B45.3
  scleredema — see Sclerosis, systemic
Busse-Buschke disease B45.3
Buttock — see condition
Button
  Biskra B55.1
  Delhi B55.1
  oriental B55.1
Buttonhole deformity (finger) — see Deformity, finger, boutonniere
Bwamba fever A92.8
Byssinosis J66.0
Bywaters' syndrome T79.5 ☑

C

Cachexia R64
  cancerous R64
  cardiac — see Disease, heart
  dehydration E86.0
  due to malnutrition R64
  exophthalmic — see Hyperthyroidism
  heart — see Disease, heart
  hypophyseal E23.0
  hypopituitary E23.0
  lead — see Poisoning, lead
  malignant R64
  marsh — see Malaria
  nervous F48.8

Cachexia — continued
  old age R54
  paludal — see Malaria
  pituitary E23.0
  renal N28.9
  saturnine — see Poisoning, lead
  senile R54
  Simmonds' E23.0
  splenica D73.0
  strumipriva E03.4
  tuberculous NEC — see Tuberculosis
CADASIL (cerebral autosomal dominant arteriopathy with subcortical infarcts and leukoencephalopathy) I67.850
Café, au lait spots L81.3
Caffeine-induced
  anxiety disorder F15.980
  sleep disorder F15.982
Caffey's syndrome Q78.8
Caisson disease T70.3 ☑
Cake kidney Q63.1
Caked breast (puerperal, postpartum) O92.79
Calabar swelling B74.3
Calcaneal spur — see Spur, bone, calcaneal
Calcaneo-apophysitis M92.8
Calcareous — see condition
Calcicosis J62.8
Calciferol (vitamin D) deficiency E55.9
  with rickets E55.0
Calcification
  adrenal (capsule) (gland) E27.49
    tuberculous E35 [B90.8]
  aorta I70.0
  artery (annular) — see Arteriosclerosis
  auricle (ear) — see Disorder, pinna, specified type NE
  basal ganglia G23.8
  bladder N32.89
    due to Schistosoma hematobium B65.0
  brain (cortex) — see Calcification, cerebral
  bronchus J98.09
  bursa M71.40
    ankle M71.47- ☑
    elbow M71.42- ☑
    foot M71.47- ☑
    hand M71.44- ☑
    hip M71.45- ☑
    knee M71.46- ☑
    multiple sites M71.49
    shoulder M75.3- ☑
    specified site NEC M71.48
    wrist M71.43- ☑
  cardiac — see Degeneration, myocardial
  cerebral (cortex) G93.89
    artery I67.2
  cervix (uteri) N88.8
  choroid plexus G93.89
  conjunctiva — see Concretion, conjunctiva
  corpora cavernosa (penis) N48.89
  cortex (brain) — see Calcification, cerebral
  dental pulp (nodular) K04.2
  dentinal papilla K00.4
  fallopian tube N83.8
  falx cerebri G96.19
  gallbladder K82.8
  general E83.59
  heart — see also Degeneration, myocardial
    valve — see Endocarditis
  idiopathic infantile arterial (IIAC) Q28.8
  intervertebral cartilage or disc (postinfective) — see Disorder, disc, specified NEC
  intracranial — see Calcification, cerebral
  joint — see Disorder, joint, specified type NEC
  kidney N28.89
    tuberculous N29 [B90.1]
  larynx (senile) J38.7
  lens — see Cataract, specified NEC
  lung (active) (postinfectional) J98.4
    tuberculous B90.9
  lymph gland or node (postinfectional) I89.8
    tuberculous — see also Tuberculosis, lymph gland B90.8
  mammographic R92.1
  massive (paraplegic) — see Myositis, ossificans, in, quadriplegia
  medial — see Arteriosclerosis, extremities
  meninges (cerebral) (spinal) G96.19
  metastatic E83.59

☑ **Additional Character Required** — Refer to the Tabular List for Character Selection   ▽ **Subterms under main terms may continue to next column or page**

alcification — *continued*
Mönckeberg's — *see* Arteriosclerosis, extremities
muscle M61.9
    due to burns — *see* Myositis, ossificans, in, burns
    paralytic — *see* Myositis, ossificans, in, quadriplegia
    specified type NEC M61.40
        ankle M61.47- ☑
        foot M61.47- ☑
        forearm M61.43- ☑
        hand M61.44- ☑
        lower leg M61.46- ☑
        multiple sites M61.49
        pelvic region M61.45- ☑
        shoulder region M61.41- ☑
        specified site NEC M61.48
        thigh M61.45- ☑
        upper arm M61.42- ☑
myocardium, myocardial — *see* Degeneration, myocardial
ovary N83.8
pancreas K86.89
penis N48.89
periarticular — *see* Disorder, joint, specified type NEC
pericardium — *see also* Pericarditis I31.1
pineal gland E34.8
pleura J94.8
    postinfectional J94.8
    tuberculous NEC B90.9
pulpal (dental) (nodular) K04.2
sclera H15.89
spleen D73.89
subcutaneous L94.2
suprarenal (capsule) (gland) E27.49
tendon (sheath) — *see also* Tenosynovitis, specified type NEC
    with bursitis, synovitis or tenosynovitis — *see* Tendinitis, calcific
trachea J39.8
ureter N28.89
uterus N85.8
vitreous — *see* Deposit, crystalline
alcified — *see* Calcification
alcinosis (interstitial) (tumoral) (universalis) E83.59
    with Raynaud's phenomenon, esophageal dysfunction, sclerodactyly, telangiectasia (CREST syndrome) M34.1
circumscripta (skin) L94.2
cutis L94.2
alciphylaxis — *see also* Calcification, by site E83.59
alcium
deposits — *see* Calcification, by site
metabolism disorder E83.50
salts or soaps in vitreous — *see* Deposit, crystalline
alciuria R82.994
alculi — *see* Calculus
alculosis, intrahepatic — *see* Calculus, bile duct
alculus, calculi, calculous
ampulla of Vater — *see* Calculus, bile duct
anuria (impacted) (recurrent) — *see also* Calculus, urinary N20.9
appendix K38.1
bile duct (common) (hepatic) K80.50
    with
        calculus of gallbladder — *see* Calculus, gallbladder and bile duct
        cholangitis K80.30
            with
                cholecystitis — *see* Calculus, bile duct, with cholecystitis
                obstruction K80.31
            acute K80.32
                with
                    chronic cholangitis K80.36
                      with obstruction K80.37
                    obstruction K80.33
            chronic K80.34
                with
                    acute cholangitis K80.36
                      with obstruction K80.37
                    obstruction K80.35
        cholecystitis (with cholangitis) K80.40
            with obstruction K80.41
            acute K80.42
                with
                    chronic cholecystitis K80.46
                      with obstruction K80.47
                    obstruction K80.43
             chronic K80.44

Calculus, calculi, calculous — *continued*
bile duct — *continued*
    with — *continued*
        cholecystitis — *continued*
            chronic — *continued*
                with
                    acute cholecystitis K80.46
                      with obstruction K80.47
                    obstruction K80.45
biliary — *see also* Calculus, gallbladder
    specified NEC K80.80
        with obstruction K80.81
bilirubin, multiple — *see* Calculus, gallbladder
bladder (encysted) (impacted) (urinary) (diverticulum) N21.0
bronchus J98.09
calyx (kidney) (renal) — *see* Calculus, kidney
cholesterol (pure) (solitary) — *see* Calculus, gallbladder
common duct (bile) — *see* Calculus, bile duct
conjunctiva — *see* Concretion, conjunctiva
cystic N21.0
    duct — *see* Calculus, gallbladder
dental (subgingival) (supragingival) K03.6
diverticulum
    bladder N21.0
    kidney N20.0
epididymis N50.89
gallbladder K80.20
    with
        bile duct calculus — *see* Calculus, gallbladder and bile duct
        cholecystitis K80.10
            with obstruction K80.11
            acute K80.00
                with
                    chronic cholecystitis K80.12
                      with obstruction K80.13
                    obstruction K80.01
            chronic K80.10
                with
                    acute cholecystitis K80.12
                      with obstruction K80.13
                    obstruction K80.11
            specified NEC K80.18
                with obstruction K80.19
         obstruction K80.21
gallbladder and bile duct K80.70
    with
        cholecystitis K80.60
            with obstruction K80.61
            acute K80.62
                with
                    chronic cholecystitis K80.66
                      with obstruction K80.67
                    obstruction K80.63
            chronic K80.64
                with
                    acute cholecystitis K80.66
                      with obstruction K80.67
                    obstruction K80.65
        obstruction K80.71
hepatic (duct) — *see* Calculus, bile duct
ileal conduit N21.8
intestinal (impaction) (obstruction) K56.49
kidney (impacted) (multiple) (pelvis) (recurrent) (staghorn) N20.0
    with calculus, ureter N20.2
    congenital Q63.8
lacrimal passages — *see* Dacryolith
liver (impacted) — *see* Calculus, bile duct
lung J98.4
mammographic R92.1
nephritic (impacted) (recurrent) — *see* Calculus, kidney
nose J34.89
pancreas (duct) K86.89
parotid duct or gland K11.5
pelvis, encysted — *see* Calculus, kidney
prostate N42.0
pulmonary J98.4
pyelitis (impacted) (recurrent) N20.0
    with hydronephrosis N13.6
pyelonephritis (impacted) (recurrent) — *see* category N20 ☑
    with hydronephrosis N13.6
renal (impacted) (recurrent) — *see* Calculus, kidney
salivary (duct) (gland) K11.5
seminal vesicle N50.89
staghorn — *see* Calculus, kidney

Calculus, calculi, calculous — *continued*
Stensen's duct K11.5
stomach K31.89
sublingual duct or gland K11.5
    congenital Q38.4
submandibular duct, gland or region K11.5
submaxillary duct, gland or region K11.5
suburethral N21.8
tonsil J35.8
tooth, teeth (subgingival) (supragingival) K03.6
tunica vaginalis N50.89
ureter (impacted) (recurrent) N20.1
    with calculus, kidney N20.2
        with hydronephrosis N13.2
            with infection N13.6
urethra (impacted) N21.1
urinary (duct) (impacted) (passage) (tract) N20.9
    with hydronephrosis N13.2
        with infection N13.6
    in (due to)
    lower N21.9
        specified NEC N21.8
vagina N89.8
vesical (impacted) N21.0
Wharton's duct K11.5
xanthine E79.8 *[N22]*
Calicectasis N28.89
Caliectasis N28.89
California
disease B38.9
encephalitis A83.5
Caligo cornea — *see* Opacity, cornea, central
Callositas, callosity (infected) L84
Callus (infected) L84
bone — *see* Osteophyte
    excessive, following fracture — *code as* Sequelae of fracture
CALME (childhood asymmetric labium majus enlargement) N90.61
Calorie deficiency or malnutrition — *see also* Malnutrition E46
Calvé-Perthes disease — *see* Legg-Calvé-Perthes disease
Calvé's disease — *see* Osteochondrosis, juvenile, spine
Calvities — *see* Alopecia, androgenic
Cameroon fever — *see* Malaria
Camptocormia (hysterical) F44.4
Camurati-Engelmann syndrome Q78.3
Canal — *see also* condition
atrioventricular common Q21.2
Canaliculitis (lacrimal) (acute) (subacute) H04.33- ☑
Actinomyces A42.89
chronic H04.42- ☑
Canavan's disease E75.29
Canceled procedure (surgical) Z53.9
because of
    contraindication Z53.09
        smoking Z53.01
    left against medical advice (AMA) Z53.29
    patient's decision Z53.20
        for reasons of belief or group pressure Z53.1
        specified reason NEC Z53.29
    specified reason NEC Z53.8
Cancer — *see also* Neoplasm, by site, malignant
bile duct type liver C22.1
blood — *see* Leukemia
breast — *see also* Neoplasm, breast, malignant C50.91- ☑
hepatocellular C22.0
lung — *see also* Neoplasm, lung, malignant C34.90
ovarian — *see also* Neoplasm ovary, malignant C56.9
unspecified site (primary) C80.1
Cancer (o)phobia F45.29
Cancerous — *see* Neoplasm, malignant, by site
Cancrum oris A69.0
Candidiasis, candidal B37.9
balanitis B37.42
bronchitis B37.1
cheilitis B37.83
congenital P37.5
cystitis B37.41
disseminated B37.7
endocarditis B37.6
enteritis B37.82
esophagitis B37.81
intertrigo B37.2
lung B37.1
meningitis B37.5

▼ Subterms under main terms may continue to next column or page   ☑ Additional Character Required — Refer to the Tabular List for Character Selection   47

Calcification — Candidiasis, candidal

Candidiasis, candidal — *continued*
- mouth B37.0
- nails B37.2
- neonatal P37.5
- onychia B37.2
- oral B37.0
- osteomyelitis B37.89
- otitis externa B37.84
- paronychia B37.2
- perionyxis B37.2
- pneumonia B37.1
- proctitis B37.82
- pulmonary B37.1
- pyelonephritis B37.49
- sepsis B37.7
- skin B37.2
- specified site NEC B37.89
- stomatitis B37.0
- systemic B37.7
- urethritis B37.41
- urogenital site NEC B37.49
- vagina B37.3
- vulva B37.3
- vulvovaginitis B37.3

Candidid L30.2
Candidosis — *see* Candidiasis
Candiru infection or infestation B88.8
Canities (premature) L67.1
- congenital Q84.2

Canker (mouth) (sore) K12.0
- rash A38.9

Cannabinosis J66.2
Cannabis induced
- anxiety disorder F12.980
- psychotic disorder F12.959
- sleep disorder F12.988

Canton fever A75.9
Cantrell's syndrome Q87.89
Capillariasis (intestinal) B81.1
- hepatic B83.8

Capillary — *see* condition
Caplan's syndrome — *see* Rheumatoid, lung
Capsule — *see* condition
Capsulitis (joint) — *see also* Enthesopathy
- adhesive (shoulder) M75.0- ✓
- hepatic K65.8
- labyrinthine — *see* Otosclerosis, specified NEC
- thyroid E06.9

Caput
- crepitus Q75.8
- medusae I86.8
- succedaneum P12.81

Car sickness T75.3 ✓
Carapata (disease) A68.0
Carate — *see* Pinta
Carbon lung J60
Carbuncle L02.93
- abdominal wall L02.231
- anus K61.0
- auditory canal, external — *see* Abscess, ear, external
- auricle ear — *see* Abscess, ear, external
- axilla L02.43- ✓
- back (any part) L02.232
- breast N61.1
- buttock L02.33
- cheek (external) L02.03
- chest wall L02.233
- chin L02.03
- corpus cavernosum N48.21
- ear (any part) (external) (middle) — *see* Abscess, ear, external
- external auditory canal — *see* Abscess, ear, external
- eyelid — *see* Abscess, eyelid
- face NEC L02.03
- femoral (region) — *see* Carbuncle, lower limb
- finger — *see* Carbuncle, hand
- flank L02.231
- foot L02.63- ✓
- forehead L02.03
- genital — *see* Abscess, genital
- gluteal (region) L02.33
- groin L02.234
- hand L02.53- ✓
- head NEC L02.831
- heel — *see* Carbuncle, foot
- hip — *see* Carbuncle, lower limb
- kidney — *see* Abscess, kidney

Carbuncle — *continued*
- knee — *see* Carbuncle, lower limb
- labium (majus) (minus) N76.4
- lacrimal
  - gland — *see* Dacryoadenitis
  - passages (duct) (sac) — *see* Inflammation, lacrimal, passages, acute
- leg — *see* Carbuncle, lower limb
- lower limb L02.43- ✓
- malignant A22.0
- navel L02.236
- neck L02.13
- nose (external) (septum) J34.0
- orbit, orbital — *see* Abscess, orbit
- palmar (space) — *see* Carbuncle, hand
- partes posteriores L02.33
- pectoral region L02.233
- penis N48.21
- perineum L02.235
- pinna — *see* Abscess, ear, external
- popliteal — *see* Carbuncle, lower limb
- scalp L02.831
- seminal vesicle N49.0
- shoulder — *see* Carbuncle, upper limb
- specified site NEC L02.838
- temple (region) L02.03
- thumb — *see* Carbuncle, hand
- toe — *see* Carbuncle, foot
- trunk L02.239
  - abdominal wall L02.231
  - back L02.232
  - chest wall L02.233
  - groin L02.234
  - perineum L02.235
  - umbilicus L02.236
- umbilicus L02.236
- upper limb L02.43- ✓
- urethra N34.0
- vulva N76.4

Carbunculus — *see* Carbuncle
Carcinoid (tumor) — *see* Tumor, carcinoid
Carcinoidosis E34.0
Carcinoma (malignant) — *see also* Neoplasm, by site, malignant
- acidophil
  - specified site — *see* Neoplasm, malignant, by site
  - unspecified site C75.1
- acidophil-basophil, mixed
  - specified site — *see* Neoplasm, malignant, by site
  - unspecified site C75.1
- adnexal (skin) — *see* Neoplasm, skin, malignant
- adrenal cortical C74.0- ✓
- alveolar — *see* Neoplasm, lung, malignant
  - cell — *see* Neoplasm, lung, malignant
- ameloblastic C41.1
  - upper jaw (bone) C41.0
- apocrine
  - breast — *see* Neoplasm, breast, malignant
  - specified site NEC — *see* Neoplasm, skin, malignant
  - unspecified site C44.99
- basal cell (pigmented) (*see also* Neoplasm, skin, malignant) C44.91
  - fibro-epithelial — *see* Neoplasm, skin, malignant
  - morphea — *see* Neoplasm, skin, malignant
  - multicentric — *see* Neoplasm, skin, malignant
- basaloid
- basal-squamous cell, mixed — *see* Neoplasm, skin, malignant
- basophil
  - specified site — *see* Neoplasm, malignant, by site
  - unspecified site C75.1
- basophil-acidophil, mixed
  - specified site — *see* Neoplasm, malignant, by site
  - unspecified site C75.1
- basosquamous — *see* Neoplasm, skin, malignant
- bile duct
  - with hepatocellular, mixed C22.0
  - liver C22.1
  - specified site NEC — *see* Neoplasm, malignant, by site
  - unspecified site C22.1
- branchial or branchiogenic C10.4
- bronchial or bronchogenic — *see* Neoplasm, lung, malignant
- bronchiolar — *see* Neoplasm, lung, malignant
- bronchioloalveolar — *see* Neoplasm, lung, malignant

Carcinoma — *continued*
- C cell
  - specified site — *see* Neoplasm, malignant, by site
  - unspecified site C73
- ceruminous C44.29- ✓
- cervix uteri
  - in situ D06.9
    - endocervix D06.0
    - exocervix D06.1
    - specified site NEC D06.7
- chorionic
  - specified site — *see* Neoplasm, malignant, by site
  - unspecified site
    - female C58
    - male C62.90
- chromophobe
  - specified site — *see* Neoplasm, malignant, by site
  - unspecified site C75.1
- cloacogenic
  - specified site — *see* Neoplasm, malignant, by site
  - unspecified site C21.2
- diffuse type
  - specified site — *see* Neoplasm, malignant, by site
  - unspecified site C16.9
- duct (cell)
  - with Paget's disease — *see* Neoplasm, breast, malignant
  - infiltrating
    - with lobular carcinoma (in situ)
      - specified site — *see* Neoplasm, malignant, by site
      - unspecified site (female) C50.91- ✓
        - male C50.92- ✓
    - specified site — *see* Neoplasm, malignant, by site
    - unspecified site (female) C50.91- ✓
      - male C50.92- ✓
- ductal
  - with lobular
    - specified site — *see* Neoplasm, malignant, by site
    - unspecified site (female) C50.91- ✓
      - male C50.92- ✓
- ductular, infiltrating
  - specified site — *see* Neoplasm, malignant, by site
  - unspecified site (female) C50.91- ✓
    - male C50.92- ✓
- embryonal
  - liver C22.7
- endometrioid
  - specified site — *see* Neoplasm, malignant, by site
  - unspecified site
    - female C56.9
    - male C61
- eosinophil
  - specified site — *see* Neoplasm, malignant, by site
  - unspecified site C75.1
- epidermoid — *see also* Neoplasm, skin, malignant
  - in situ, Bowen's type — *see* Neoplasm, skin, in situ
- fibroepithelial, basal cell — *see* Neoplasm, skin, malignant
- follicular
  - with papillary (mixed) C73
  - moderately differentiated C73
  - pure follicle C73
  - specified site — *see* Neoplasm, malignant, by site
  - trabecular C73
  - unspecified site C73
  - well differentiated C73
- generalized, with unspecified primary site C80.0
- glycogen-rich — *see* Neoplasm, breast, malignant
- granulosa cell C56- ✓
- hepatic cell C22.0
- hepatocellular C22.0
  - with bile duct, mixed C22.0
  - fibrolamellar C22.0
- hepatocholangiolitic C22.0
- Hurthle cell C73
- in
  - adenomatous
    - polyposis coli C18.9
  - pleomorphic adenoma — *see* Neoplasm, salivary glands, malignant
  - situ — *see* Carcinoma-in-situ

✓ **Additional Character Required** — Refer to the Tabular List for Character Selection   ▽ **Subterms under main terms may continue to next column or page**

Carcinoma — continued
- infiltrating
  - duct
    - with lobular
      - specified site — see Neoplasm, malignant, by site
      - unspecified site (female) C50.91- ☑
        - male C50.92- ☑
    - with Paget's disease — see Neoplasm, breast, malignant
    - specified site — see Neoplasm, malignant
    - unspecified site (female) C50.91- ☑
      - male C50.92- ☑
  - ductular
    - specified site — see Neoplasm, malignant
    - unspecified site (female) C50.91- ☑
      - male C50.92- ☑
  - lobular
    - specified site — see Neoplasm, malignant
    - unspecified site (female) C50.91- ☑
      - male C50.92- ☑
- inflammatory
  - specified site — see Neoplasm, malignant
  - unspecified site (female) C50.91- ☑
    - male C50.92- ☑
- intestinal type
  - specified site — see Neoplasm, malignant, by site
  - unspecified site C16.9
- intracystic
  - noninfiltrating — see Neoplasm, in situ, by site
- intraductal (noninfiltrating)
  - with Paget's disease — see Neoplasm, breast, malignant
  - breast D05.1- ☑
  - papillary
    - with invasion
      - specified site — see Neoplasm, malignant, by site
      - unspecified site (female) C50.91- ☑
        - male C50.92- ☑
    - breast D05.1- ☑
    - specified site NEC — see Neoplasm, in situ, by site
    - unspecified site (female) D05.1- ☑
  - specified site NEC — see Neoplasm, in situ, by site
  - unspecified site (female) D05.1- ☑
- intraepidermal — see Neoplasm, in situ
  - squamous cell, Bowen's type — see Neoplasm, skin, in situ
- intraepithelial — see Neoplasm, in situ, by site
  - squamous cell — see Neoplasm, in situ, by site
- intraosseous C41.1
  - upper jaw (bone) C41.0
- islet cell
  - with exocrine, mixed
    - specified site — see Neoplasm, malignant, by site
    - unspecified site C25.9
  - pancreas C25.4
  - specified site NEC — see Neoplasm, malignant, by site
  - unspecified site C25.4
- juvenile, breast — see Neoplasm, breast, malignant
- large cell
  - small cell
    - specified site — see Neoplasm, malignant, by site
    - unspecified site C34.90
- Leydig cell (testis)
  - specified site — see Neoplasm, malignant, by site
  - unspecified site
    - female C56.9
    - male C62.90
- lipid-rich (female) C50.91- ☑
  - male C50.92- ☑
- liver cell C22.0
- liver NEC C22.7
- lobular (infiltrating)
  - with intraductal
    - specified site — see Neoplasm, malignant, by site
    - unspecified site (female) C50.91- ☑
      - male C50.92- ☑
  - noninfiltrating
    - breast D05.0- ☑
    - specified site NEC — see Neoplasm, in situ, by site

Carcinoma — continued
- lobular — continued
  - noninfiltrating — continued
    - unspecified site D05.0- ☑
  - specified site — see Neoplasm, malignant, by site
  - unspecified site (female) C50.91- ☑
    - male C50.92- ☑
- medullary
  - with
    - amyloid stroma
      - specified site — see Neoplasm, malignant, by site
      - unspecified site C73
    - lymphoid stroma
      - specified site — see Neoplasm, malignant, by site
      - unspecified site (female) C50.91- ☑
        - male C50.92- ☑
- Merkel cell C4A.9 (following C43)
  - anal margin C4A.51 (following C43)
  - anal skin C4A.51 (following C43)
  - canthus C4A.1- ☑ (following C43)
  - ear and external auricular canal C4A.2- ☑ (following C43)
  - external auricular canal C4A.2- ☑ (following C43)
  - eyelid, including canthus C4A.1- ☑ (following C43)
  - face C4A.30 (following C43)
    - specified NEC C4A.39 (following C43)
  - hip C4A.7- ☑ (following C43)
  - lip C4A.0 (following C43)
  - lower limb, including hip C4A.7- ☑ (following C43)
  - neck C4A.4 (following C43)
  - nodal presentation C7B.1 (following C75)
  - nose C4A.31 (following C43)
  - overlapping sites C4A.8 (following C43)
  - perianal skin C4A.51 (following C43)
  - scalp C4A.4 (following C43)
  - secondary C7B.1 (following C75)
  - shoulder C4A.6- ☑ (following C43)
  - skin of breast C4A.52 (following C43)
  - trunk NEC C4A.59 (following C43)
  - upper limb, including shoulder C4A.6- ☑ (following C43)
  - visceral metastatic C7B.1 (following C75)
- metastatic — see Neoplasm, secondary, by site
- metatypical — see Neoplasm, skin, malignant
- morphea, basal cell — see Neoplasm, skin, malignant
- mucoid
  - cell
    - specified site — see Neoplasm, malignant, by site
    - unspecified site C75.1
- neuroendocrine — see also Tumor, neuroendocrine
  - high grade, any site C7A.1 (following C75)
  - poorly differentiated, any site C7A.1 (following C75)
- nonencapsulated sclerosing C73
- noninfiltrating
  - intracystic — see Neoplasm, in situ, by site
  - intraductal
    - breast D05.1- ☑
    - papillary
      - breast D05.1- ☑
      - specified site NEC — see Neoplasm, in situ, by site
      - unspecified site D05.1- ☑
    - specified site NEC — see Neoplasm, in situ, by site
    - unspecified site D05.1- ☑
  - lobular
    - breast D05.0- ☑
    - specified site NEC — see Neoplasm, in situ, by site
    - unspecified site (female) D05.0- ☑
- oat cell
  - specified site — see Neoplasm, malignant, by site
  - unspecified site C34.90
- odontogenic C41.1
  - upper jaw (bone) C41.0
- papillary
  - with follicular (mixed) C73
  - follicular variant C73
  - intraductal (noninfiltrating)
    - with invasion
      - specified site — see Neoplasm, malignant, by site
      - unspecified site (female) C50.91- ☑
        - male C50.92- ☑
      - breast D05.1- ☑

Carcinoma — continued
- papillary — continued
  - intraductal — continued
    - specified site NEC — see Neoplasm, in situ, by site
    - unspecified site D05.1- ☑
  - serous
    - specified site — see Neoplasm, malignant, by site
    - surface
      - specified site — see Neoplasm, malignant, by site
      - unspecified site C56.9
    - unspecified site C56.9
- papillocystic
  - specified site — see Neoplasm, malignant, by site
  - unspecified site C56.9
- parafollicular cell
  - specified site — see Neoplasm, malignant, by site
  - unspecified site C73
- pilomatrix — see Neoplasm, skin, malignant
- pseudomucinous
  - specified site — see Neoplasm, malignant, by site
  - unspecified site C56.9
- renal cell C64- ☑
- Schmincke — see Neoplasm, nasopharynx, malignant
- Schneiderian
  - specified site — see Neoplasm, malignant, by site
  - unspecified site C30.0
- sebaceous — see Neoplasm, skin, malignant
- secondary — see also Neoplasm, secondary, by site
  - Merkel cell C7B.1 (following C75)
- secretory, breast — see Neoplasm, breast, malignant
- serous
  - papillary
    - specified site — see Neoplasm, malignant, by site
    - unspecified site C56.9
  - surface, papillary
    - specified site — see Neoplasm, malignant, by site
    - unspecified site C56.9
- Sertoli cell
  - specified site — see Neoplasm, malignant, by site
  - unspecified site C62.90
    - female C56.9
    - male C62.90
- skin appendage — see Neoplasm, skin, malignant
- small cell
  - fusiform cell
    - specified site — see Neoplasm, malignant, by site
    - unspecified site C34.90
  - intermediate cell
    - specified site — see Neoplasm, malignant, by site
    - unspecified site C34.90
  - large cell
    - specified site — see Neoplasm, malignant, by site
    - unspecified site C34.90
- solid
  - with amyloid stroma
    - specified site — see Neoplasm, malignant, by site
    - unspecified site C73
  - microinvasive
    - specified site — see Neoplasm, malignant, by site
    - unspecified site C53.9
- sweat gland — see Neoplasm, skin, malignant
- theca cell C56.- ☑
- thymic C37
- unspecified site (primary) C80.1
- water-clear cell C75.0

Carcinoma-in-situ — see also Neoplasm, in situ, by site
- breast NOS D05.9- ☑
  - specified type NEC D05.8- ☑
- epidermoid — see also Neoplasm, in situ, by site
  - with questionable stromal invasion
    - cervix D06.9
    - specified site NEC — see Neoplasm, in situ, by site
    - unspecified site D06.9
  - Bowen's type — see Neoplasm, skin, in situ
- intraductal
  - breast D05.1- ☑
  - specified site NEC — see Neoplasm, in situ, by site

Carcinoma-in-situ — *continued*
- intraductal — *continued*
  - unspecified site D05.1- ☑
- lobular
  - with
    - infiltrating duct
      - breast (female) C50.91- ☑
        - male C50.92- ☑
      - specified site NEC — *see* Neoplasm, malignant
      - unspecified site (female) C50.91- ☑
        - male C50.92- ☑
    - intraductal
      - breast D05.8- ☑
      - specified site NEC — *see* Neoplasm, in situ, by site
      - unspecified site (female) D05.8- ☑
  - breast D05.0- ☑
  - specified site NEC — *see* Neoplasm, in situ, by site
  - unspecified site D05.0- ☑
- squamous cell — *see also* Neoplasm, in situ, by site
  - with questionable stromal invasion
    - cervix D06.9
    - specified site NEC — *see* Neoplasm, in situ, by site
    - unspecified site D06.9

Carcinomaphobia F45.29

Carcinomatosis C80.0
- peritonei C78.6
- unspecified site (primary) (secondary) C80.0

Carcinosarcoma — *see* Neoplasm, malignant, by site
- embryonal — *see* Neoplasm, malignant, by site

Cardia, cardial — *see* condition

Cardiac — *see also* condition
- death, sudden — *see* Arrest, cardiac
- pacemaker
  - in situ Z95.0
  - management or adjustment Z45.018
- tamponade I31.4

Cardialgia — *see* Pain, precordial

Cardiectasis — *see* Hypertrophy, cardiac

Cardiochalasia K21.9

Cardiomalacia I51.5

Cardiomegalia glycogenica diffusa E74.02 *[I43]*

Cardiomegaly — *see also* Hypertrophy, cardiac
- congenital Q24.8
- glycogen E74.02 *[I43]*
- idiopathic I51.7

Cardiomyoliposis I51.5

Cardiomyopathy (familial) (idiopathic) I42.9
- alcoholic I42.6
- amyloid E85.4 *[I43]*
  - transthyretin-related (ATTR) familial E85.4 *[I43]*
- arteriosclerotic — *see* Disease, heart, ischemic, atherosclerotic
- beriberi E51.12
- cobalt-beer I42.6
- congenital I42.4
- congestive I42.0
- constrictive NOS I42.5
- dilated I42.0
- due to
  - alcohol I42.6
  - beriberi E51.12
  - cardiac glycogenosis E74.02 *[I43]*
  - drugs I42.7
  - external agents NEC I42.7
  - Friedreich's ataxia G11.1
  - myotonia atrophica G71.11 *[I43]*
  - progressive muscular dystrophy G71.09 *[I43]*
- glycogen storage E74.02 *[I43]*
- hypertensive — *see* Hypertension, heart
- hypertrophic (nonobstructive) I42.2
  - obstructive I42.1
    - congenital Q24.8
- in
  - Chagas' disease (chronic) B57.2
    - acute B57.0
  - sarcoidosis D86.85
- ischemic I25.5
- metabolic E88.9 *[I43]*
  - thyrotoxic E05.90 *[I43]*
    - with thyroid storm E05.91 *[I43]*
- newborn I42.8
  - congenital I42.4
- non-ischemic — *see also* by cause I42.8
- nutritional E63.9 *[I43]*
  - beriberi E51.12

Cardiomyopathy — *continued*
- obscure of Africa I42.8
- peripartum O90.3
- postpartum O90.3
- restrictive NEC I42.5
- rheumatic I09.0
- secondary I42.9
- specified NEC I42.8
- stress induced I51.81
- takotsubo I51.81
- thyrotoxic E05.90 *[I43]*
  - with thyroid storm E05.91 *[I43]*
- toxic NEC I42.7
- transthyretin-related (ATTR) familial amyloid E85.4
- tuberculous A18.84
- viral B33.24

Cardionephritis — *see* Hypertension, cardiorenal

Cardionephropathy — *see* Hypertension, cardiorenal

Cardionephrosis — *see* Hypertension, cardiorenal

Cardiopathia nigra I27.0

Cardiopathy — *see also* Disease, heart I51.9
- idiopathic I42.9
- mucopolysaccharidosis E76.3 *[I52]*

Cardiopericarditis — *see* Pericarditis

Cardiophobia F45.29

Cardiorenal — *see* condition

Cardiorrhexis — *see* Infarct, myocardium

Cardiosclerosis — *see* Disease, heart, ischemic, atherosclerotic

Cardiosis — *see* Disease, heart

Cardiospasm (esophagus) (reflex) (stomach) K22.0
- congenital Q39.5
  - with megaesophagus Q39.5

Cardiostenosis — *see* Disease, heart

Cardiosymphysis I31.0

Cardiovascular — *see* condition

Carditis (acute) (bacterial) (chronic) (subacute) I51.89
- meningococcal A39.50
- rheumatic — *see* Disease, heart, rheumatic
- rheumatoid — *see* Rheumatoid, carditis
- viral B33.20

Care (of) (for) (following)
- child (routine) Z76.2
- family member (handicapped) (sick)
  - creating problem for family Z63.6
  - provided away from home for holiday relief Z75.5
  - unavailable, due to
    - absence (person rendering care) (sufferer) Z74.2
    - inability (any reason) of person rendering care Z74.2
- foundling Z76.1
- holiday relief Z75.5
- improper — *see* Maltreatment
- lack of (at or after birth) (infant) — *see* Maltreatment, child, neglect
- lactating mother Z39.1
- palliative Z51.5
- postpartum
  - immediately after delivery Z39.0
  - routine follow-up Z39.2
- respite Z75.5
- unavailable, due to
  - absence of person rendering care Z74.2
  - inability (any reason) of person rendering care Z74.2
- well-baby Z76.2

Caries
- bone NEC A18.03
- dental (dentino enamel junction) (early childhood) (of dentine) (pre-eruptive) (recurrent) (to the pulp) K02.9
  - arrested (coronal) (root) K02.3
  - chewing surface
    - limited to enamel K02.51
    - penetrating into dentin K02.52
    - penetrating into pulp K02.53
  - coronal surface
    - chewing surface
      - limited to enamel K02.51
      - penetrating into dentin K02.52
      - penetrating into pulp K02.53
    - pit and fissure surface
      - limited to enamel K02.51
      - penetrating into dentin K02.52
      - penetrating into pulp K02.53
    - smooth surface
      - limited to enamel K02.61
      - penetrating into dentin K02.62
      - penetrating into pulp K02.63

Caries — *continued*
- dental — *continued*
  - pit and fissure surface
    - limited to enamel K02.51
    - penetrating into dentin K02.52
    - penetrating into pulp K02.53
  - primary, cervical origin K02.52
  - root K02.7
  - smooth surface
    - limited to enamel K02.61
    - penetrating into dentin K02.62
    - penetrating into pulp K02.63
- external meatus — *see* Disorder, ear, external, specified type NEC
- hip (tuberculous) A18.02
- initial (tooth)
  - chewing surface K02.51
  - pit and fissure surface K02.51
  - smooth surface K02.61
- knee (tuberculous) A18.02
- labyrinth H83.8 ☑
- limb NEC (tuberculous) A18.03
- mastoid process (chronic) — *see* Mastoiditis, chronic
  - tuberculous A18.03
- middle ear H74.8 ☑
- nose (tuberculous) A18.03
- orbit (tuberculous) A18.03
- ossicles, ear — *see* Abnormal, ear ossicles
- petrous bone — *see* Petrositis
- root (dental) (tooth) K02.7
- sacrum (tuberculous) A18.01
- spine, spinal (column) (tuberculous) A18.01
- syphilitic A52.77
  - congenital (early) A50.02 *[M90.80]*
- tooth, teeth — *see* Caries, dental
- tuberculous A18.03
- vertebra (column) (tuberculous) A18.01

Carious teeth — *see* Caries, dental

Carneous mole O02.0

Carnitine insufficiency E71.40

Carotenemia (dietary) E67.1

Carotenosis (cutis) (skin) E67.1

Carotid body or sinus syndrome G90.01

Carotidynia G90.01

Carpal tunnel syndrome — *see* Syndrome, carpal tunnel

Carpenter's syndrome Q87.0

Carpopedal spasm — *see* Tetany

Carr-Barr-Plunkett syndrome Q97.1

Carrier (suspected) of
- amebiasis Z22.1
- bacterial disease NEC Z22.39
  - diphtheria Z22.2
  - intestinal infectious NEC Z22.1
    - typhoid Z22.0
  - meningococcal Z22.31
  - sexually transmitted Z22.4
  - specified NEC Z22.39
  - staphylococcal (Methicillin susceptible) Z22.321
    - Methicillin resistant Z22.322
  - streptococcal Z22.338
    - group B Z22.330
      - complicating pregnancy or delivery O99.82- ☑
  - typhoid Z22.0
- cholera Z22.1
- diphtheria Z22.2
- gastrointestinal pathogens NEC Z22.1
- genetic Z14.8
  - cystic fibrosis Z14.1
  - hemophilia A (asymptomatic) Z14.01
    - symptomatic Z14.02
- gestational, pregnant Z33.1
- gonorrhea Z22.4
- HAA (hepatitis Australian-antigen) B18.8
- HB (c)(s)-AG B18.1
- hepatitis (viral) B18.9
  - Australia-antigen (HAA) B18.8
  - B surface antigen (HBsAg) B18.1
    - with acute delta- (super)infection B17.0
  - C B18.2
  - specified NEC B18.8
- human T-cell lymphotropic virus type-1 (HTLV-1) infection Z22.6
- infectious organism Z22.9
  - specified NEC Z22.8
- meningococci Z22.31
- Salmonella typhosa Z22.0
- serum hepatitis — *see* Carrier, hepatitis

☑ **Additional Character Required** — Refer to the Tabular List for Character Selection

▽ **Subterms under main terms may continue to next column or page**

arrier of — *continued*
staphylococci (Methicillin susceptible) Z22.321
　Methicillin resistant Z22.322
streptococci Z22.338
　group B Z22.330
　　complicating pregnancy or delivery O99.82- ☑
syphilis Z22.4
typhoid Z22.0
venereal disease NEC Z22.4
arrion's disease A44.0
arter's relapsing fever (Asiatic) A68.1
artilage — *see* condition
aruncle (inflamed)
conjunctiva (acute) — *see* Conjunctivitis, acute
labium (majus) (minus) N90.89
lacrimal — *see* Inflammation, lacrimal, passages
myrtiform N89.8
urethral (benign) N36.2
ascade stomach K31.2
aseation lymphatic gland (tuberculous) A18.2
assidy (-Scholte) syndrome (malignant carcinoid) E34.0
astellani's disease A69.8
astration, traumatic, male S38.231 ☑
asts in urine R82.998
at
cry syndrome Q93.4
ear Q17.3
eye syndrome Q92.8
atabolism, senile R54
atalepsy (hysterical) F44.2
schizophrenic F20.2
ataplexy (idiopathic) — *see* Narcolepsy
ataract (cortical) (immature) (incipient) H26.9
with
　neovascularization — *see* Cataract, complicated
age-related — *see* Cataract, senile
anterior
　and posterior axial embryonal Q12.0
　pyramidal Q12.0
associated with
　galactosemia E74.21 *[H28]*
　myotonic disorders G71.19 *[H28]*
blue Q12.0
central Q12.0
cerulean Q12.0
complicated H26.20
　with
　　neovascularization H26.21- ☑
　　ocular disorder H26.22- ☑
　　glaucomatous flecks H26.23- ☑
congenital Q12.0
coraliform Q12.0
coronary Q12.0
crystalline Q12.0
diabetic — *see* Diabetes, cataract
drug-induced H26.3- ☑
due to
　ocular disorder — *see* Cataract, complicated
　radiation H26.8
electric H26.8
extraction status Z98.4- ☑
glass-blower's H26.8
heat ray H26.8
heterochromic — *see* Cataract, complicated
hypermature — *see* Cataract, senile, morgagnian type
in (due to)
　chronic iridocyclitis — *see* Cataract, complicated
　diabetes — *see* Diabetes, cataract
　endocrine disease E34.9 *[H28]*
　eye disease — *see* Cataract, complicated
　hypoparathyroidism E20.9 *[H28]*
　malnutrition-dehydration E46 *[H28]*
　metabolic disease E88.9 *[H28]*
　myotonic disorders G71.19 *[H28]*
　nutritional disease E63.9 *[H28]*
infantile — *see* Cataract, presenile
irradiational — *see* Cataract, specified NEC
juvenile — *see* Cataract, presenile
malnutrition-dehydration E46 *[H28]*
morgagnian — *see* Cataract, senile, morgagnian type
myotonic G71.19 *[H28]*
myxedema E03.9 *[H28]*
nuclear
　embryonal Q12.0
　sclerosis — *see* Cataract, senile, nuclear
presenile H26.00- ☑
　combined forms H26.06- ☑

Cataract — *continued*
presenile — *continued*
　cortical H26.01- ☑
　　lamellar — *see* Cataract, presenile, cortical
　nuclear H26.03- ☑
　specified NEC H26.09
　subcapsular polar (anterior) H26.04- ☑
　　posterior H26.05- ☑
　zonular — *see* Cataract, presenile, cortical
secondary H26.40
　Soemmering's ring H26.41- ☑
　specified NEC H26.49- ☑
　to eye disease — *see* Cataract, complicated
senile H25.9
　brunescens — *see* Cataract, senile, nuclear
　combined forms H25.81- ☑
　coronary — *see* Cataract, senile, incipient
　cortical H25.01- ☑
　hypermature — *see* Cataract, senile, morgagnian
　　type
　incipient (mature) (total) H25.09- ☑
　　cortical — *see* Cataract, senile, cortical
　　subcapsular — *see* Cataract, senile, subcapsular
　morgagnian type (hypermature) H25.2- ☑
　nuclear (sclerosis) H25.1- ☑
　polar subcapsular (anterior) (posterior) — *see*
　　Cataract, senile, incipient
　punctate — *see* Cataract, senile, incipient
　specified NEC H25.89
　subcapsular polar (anterior) H25.03- ☑
　　posterior H25.04- ☑
snowflake — *see* Diabetes, cataract
specified NEC H26.8
toxic — *see* Cataract, drug-induced
traumatic H26.10- ☑
　localized H26.11- ☑
　partially resolved H26.12- ☑
　total H26.13- ☑
zonular (perinuclear) Q12.0
Cataracta — *see also* Cataract
brunescens — *see* Cataract, senile, nuclear
centralis pulverulenta Q12.0
cerulea Q12.0
complicata — *see* Cataract, complicated
congenita Q12.0
coralliformis Q12.0
coronaria Q12.0
diabetic — *see* Diabetes, cataract
membranacea
　accreta — *see* Cataract, secondary
　congenita Q12.0
nigra — *see* Cataract, senile, nuclear
sunflower — *see* Cataract, complicated
Catarrh, catarrhal (acute) (febrile) (infectious) (inflam-
　mation) — *see also* condition J00
bronchial — *see* Bronchitis
chest — *see* Bronchitis
chronic J31.0
due to congenital syphilis A50.03
enteric — *see* Enteritis
eustachian H68.009
fauces — *see* Pharyngitis
gastrointestinal — *see* Enteritis
gingivitis K05.00
　nonplaque induced K05.01
　plaque induced K05.00
hay — *see* Fever, hay
intestinal — *see* Enteritis
larynx, chronic J37.0
liver B15.9
　with hepatic coma B15.0
lung — *see* Bronchitis
middle ear, chronic — *see* Otitis, media, nonsuppura-
　tive, chronic, serous
mouth K12.1
nasal (chronic) — *see* Rhinitis
nasobronchial J31.1
nasopharyngeal (chronic) J31.1
　acute J00
pulmonary — *see* Bronchitis
spring (eye) (vernal) — *see* Conjunctivitis, acute, atopic
summer (hay) — *see* Fever, hay
throat J31.2
tubotympanal — *see also* Otitis, media, nonsuppurative
　chronic — *see* Otitis, media, nonsuppurative,
　　chronic, serous
Catatonia (schizophrenic) F20.2

Catatonic
disorder due to known physiologic condition F06.1
schizophrenia F20.2
stupor R40.1
Cat-scratch — *see also* Abrasion
disease or fever A28.1
Cauda equina — *see* condition
Cauliflower ear M95.1- ☑
Causalgia (upper limb) G56.4- ☑
lower limb G57.7- ☑
Cause
external, general effects T75.89 ☑
Caustic burn — *see* Corrosion, by site
Cavare's disease (familial periodic paralysis) G72.3
Cave-in, injury
crushing (severe) — *see* Crush
suffocation — *see* Asphyxia, traumatic, due to low
　oxygen, due to cave-in
Cavernitis (penis) N48.29
Cavernositis N48.29
Cavernous — *see* condition
Cavitation of lung — *see also* Tuberculosis, pulmonary
nontuberculous J98.4
Cavities, dental — *see* Caries, dental
Cavity
lung — *see* Cavitation of lung
optic papilla Q14.2
pulmonary — *see* Cavitation of lung
Cavovarus foot, congenital Q66.1- ☑
Cavus foot (congenital) Q66.7- ☑
acquired — *see* Deformity, limb, foot, specified NEC
Cazenave's disease L10.2
Cecitis K52.9
with perforation, peritonitis, or rupture K65.8
Cecoureterocele Q62.32
Cecum — *see* condition
Celiac
artery compression syndrome I77.4
disease (with steatorrhea) K90.0
infantilism K90.0
Cell(s), cellular — *see also* condition
in urine R82.998
Cellulitis (diffuse) (phlegmonous) (septic) (suppurative)
　L03.90
abdominal wall L03.311
anaerobic A48.0
ankle — *see* Cellulitis, lower limb
anus K61.0
arm — *see* Cellulitis, upper limb
auricle (ear) — *see* Cellulitis, ear
axilla L03.11- ☑
back (any part) L03.312
breast (acute) (nonpuerperal) (subacute) N61.0
　nipple N61.0
broad ligament
　acute N73.0
buttock L03.317
cervical (meaning neck) L03.221
cervix (uteri) — *see* Cervicitis
cheek (external) L03.211
　internal K12.2
chest wall L03.313
chronic L03.90
clostridial A48.0
corpus cavernosum N48.22
digit
　finger — *see* Cellulitis, finger
　toe — *see* Cellulitis, toe
Douglas' cul-de-sac or pouch
　acute N73.0
drainage site (following operation) T81.49 ☑
ear (external) H60.1- ☑
eosinophilic (granulomatous) L98.3
erysipelatous — *see* Erysipelas
external auditory canal — *see* Cellulitis, ear
eyelid — *see* Abscess, eyelid
face NEC L03.211
finger (intrathecal) (periosteal) (subcutaneous) (subcu-
　ticular) L03.01- ☑
foot — *see* Cellulitis, lower limb
gangrenous — *see* Gangrene
genital organ NEC
　female (external) N76.4
　male N49.9
　　multiple sites N49.8
　　specified NEC N49.8
gluteal (region) L03.317

Cellulitis — *continued*
  gonococcal A54.89
  groin L03.314
  hand — *see* Cellulitis, upper limb
  head NEC L03.811
    face (any part, except ear, eye and nose) L03.211
  heel — *see* Cellulitis, lower limb
  hip — *see* Cellulitis, lower limb
  jaw (region) L03.211
  knee — *see* Cellulitis, lower limb
  labium (majus) (minus) — *see* Vulvitis
  lacrimal passages — *see* Inflammation, lacrimal, passages
  larynx J38.7
  leg — *see* Cellulitis, lower limb
  lip K13.0
  lower limb L03.11- ☑
    toe — *see* Cellulitis, toe
  mouth (floor) K12.2
  multiple sites, so stated L03.90
  nasopharynx J39.1
  navel L03.316
    newborn P38.9
      with mild hemorrhage P38.1
      without hemorrhage P38.9
  neck (region) L03.221
  nipple (acute) (nonpuerperal) (subacute) N61.0
  nose (septum) (external) J34.0
  orbit, orbital H05.01- ☑
  palate (soft) K12.2
  pectoral (region) L03.313
  pelvis, pelvic (chronic)
    female — *see also* Disease, pelvis, inflammatory N73.2
      acute N73.0
    following ectopic or molar pregnancy O08.0
    male K65.0
  penis N48.22
  perineal, perineum L03.315
  periorbital L03.213
  perirectal K61.1
  peritonsillar J36
  periurethral N34.0
  periuterine — *see also* Disease, pelvis, inflammatory N73.2
    acute N73.0
  pharynx J39.1
  preseptal L03.213
  rectum K61.1
  retroperitoneal K68.9
  round ligament
    acute N73.0
  scalp (any part) L03.811
  scrotum N49.2
  seminal vesicle N49.0
  shoulder — *see* Cellulitis, upper limb
  specified site NEC L03.818
  submandibular (region) (space) (triangle) K12.2
    gland K11.3
  submaxillary (region) K12.2
    gland K11.3
  thigh — *see* Cellulitis, lower limb
  thumb (intrathecal) (periosteal) (subcutaneous) (subcuticular) — *see* Cellulitis, finger
  toe (intrathecal) (periosteal) (subcutaneous) (subcuticular) L03.03- ☑
  tonsil J36
  trunk L03.319
    abdominal wall L03.311
    back (any part) L03.312
    buttock L03.317
    chest wall L03.313
    groin L03.314
    perineal, perineum L03.315
    umbilicus L03.316
  tuberculous (primary) A18.4
  umbilicus L03.316
  upper limb L03.11- ☑
    axilla — *see* Cellulitis, axilla
    finger — *see* Cellulitis, finger
    thumb — *see* Cellulitis, finger
  vaccinal T88.0 ☑
  vocal cord J38.3
  vulva — *see* Vulvitis
  wrist — *see* Cellulitis, upper limb
Cementoblastoma, benign — *see* Cyst, calcifying odontogenic
Cementoma — *see* Cyst, calcifying odontogenic

Cementoperiostitis — *see* Periodontitis
Cementosis K03.4
Central auditory processing disorder H93.25
Central pain syndrome G89.0
Cephalematocele, cephal(o)hematocele
  newborn P52.8
    birth injury P10.8
  traumatic — *see* Hematoma, brain
Cephalematoma, cephalhematoma (calcified)
  newborn (birth injury) P12.0
  traumatic — *see* Hematoma, brain
Cephalgia, cephalalgia — *see also* Headache
  histamine G44.009
    intractable G44.001
    not intractable G44.009
  trigeminal autonomic (TAC) NEC G44.099
    intractable G44.091
    not intractable G44.099
Cephalic — *see* condition
Cephalitis — *see* Encephalitis
Cephalocele — *see* Encephalocele
Cephalomenia N94.89
Cephalopelvic — *see* condition
Cerclage (with cervical incompetence) in pregnancy — *see* Incompetence, cervix, in pregnancy
Cerebellitis — *see* Encephalitis
Cerebellum, cerebellar — *see* condition
Cerebral — *see* condition
Cerebritis — *see* Encephalitis
Cerebro-hepato-renal syndrome Q87.89
Cerebromalacia — *see* Softening, brain
  sequelae of cerebrovascular disease I69.398
Cerebroside lipidosis E75.22
Cerebrospasticity (congenital) G80.1
Cerebrospinal — *see* condition
Cerebrum — *see* condition
Ceroid-lipofuscinosis, neuronal E75.4
Cerumen (accumulation) (impacted) H61.2- ☑
Cervical — *see also* condition
  auricle Q18.2
  dysplasia in pregnancy — *see* Abnormal, cervix, in pregnancy or childbirth
  erosion in pregnancy — *see* Abnormal, cervix, in pregnancy or childbirth
  fibrosis in pregnancy — *see* Abnormal, cervix, in pregnancy or childbirth
  fusion syndrome Q76.1
  rib Q76.5
  shortening (complicating pregnancy) O26.87- ☑
Cervicalgia M54.2
Cervicitis (acute) (chronic) (nonvenereal) (senile (atrophic)) (subacute) (with ulceration) N72
  with
    abortion — *see* Abortion, by type complicated by genital tract and pelvic infection
    ectopic pregnancy O08.0
    molar pregnancy O08.0
  chlamydial A56.09
  gonococcal A54.03
  herpesviral A60.03
  puerperal (postpartum) O86.11
  syphilitic A52.76
  trichomonal A59.09
  tuberculous A18.16
Cervicocolpitis (emphysematosa) — *see also* Cervicitis N72
Cervix — *see* condition
Cesarean delivery, previous, affecting management of pregnancy O34.219
  classical (vertical) scar O34.212
  low transverse scar O34.211
Céstan (-Chenais) paralysis or syndrome G46.3
Céstan-Raymond syndrome I65.8
Cestode infestation B71.9
  specified type NEC B71.8
Cestodiasis B71.9
Chabert's disease A22.9
Chacaleh E53.8
Chafing L30.4
Chagas' (-Mazza) disease (chronic) B57.2
  with
    cardiovascular involvement NEC B57.2
    digestive system involvement B57.30
      megacolon B57.32
      megaesophagus B57.31
      other specified B57.39
    megacolon B57.32

Chagas' disease — *continued*
  with — *continued*
    megaesophagus B57.31
    myocarditis B57.2
    nervous system involvement B57.40
      meningitis B57.41
      meningoencephalitis B57.42
      other specified B57.49
    specified organ involvement NEC B57.5
  acute (with) B57.1
    cardiovascular NEC B57.0
    myocarditis B57.0
Chagres fever B50.9
Chairridden Z74.09
Chalasia (cardiac sphincter) K21.9
Chalazion H00.19
  left H00.16
    lower H00.15
    upper H00.14
  right H00.13
    lower H00.12
    upper H00.11
Chalcosis — *see also* Disorder, globe, degenerative, chalcosis
  cornea — *see* Deposit, cornea
  crystalline lens — *see* Cataract, complicated
  retina H35.89
Chalicosis (pulmonum) J62.8
Chancre (any genital site) (hard) (hunterian) (mixed) (primary) (seronegative) (seropositive) (syphilitic) A51.0
  congenital A50.07
  conjunctiva NEC A51.2
  Ducrey's A57
  extragenital A51.2
  eyelid A51.2
  lip A51.2
  nipple A51.2
  Nisbet's A57
  of
    carate A67.0
    pinta A67.0
    yaws A66.0
  palate, soft A51.2
  phagedenic A57
  simple A57
  soft A57
    bubo A57
    palate A51.2
  urethra A51.0
  yaws A66.0
Chancroid (anus) (genital) (penis) (perineum) (rectum) (urethra) (vulva) A57
Chandler's disease (osteochondritis dissecans, hip) — *see* Osteochondritis, dissecans, hip
Change(s) (in) (of) — *see also* Removal
  arteriosclerotic — *see* Arteriosclerosis
  bone — *see also* Disorder, bone
    diabetic — *see* Diabetes, bone change
  bowel habit R19.4
  cardiorenal (vascular) — *see* Hypertension, cardiorenal
  cardiovascular — *see* Disease, cardiovascular
  circulatory I99.9
  cognitive (mild) (organic) R41.89
  color, tooth, teeth
    during formation K00.8
    posteruptive K03.7
  contraceptive device Z30.433
  corneal membrane H18.30
    Bowman's membrane fold or rupture H18.31- ☑
    Descemet's membrane
      fold H18.32- ☑
      rupture H18.33- ☑
  coronary — *see* Disease, heart, ischemic
  degenerative, spine or vertebra — *see* Spondylosis
  dental pulp, regressive K04.2
  dressing (nonsurgical) Z48.00
    surgical Z48.01
  heart — *see* Disease, heart
  hip joint — *see* Derangement, joint, hip
  hyperplastic larynx J38.7
  hypertrophic
    nasal sinus J34.89
    turbinate, nasal J34.3
    upper respiratory tract J39.8
  indwelling catheter Z46.6
  inflammatory — *see also* Inflammation
    sacroiliac M46.1

Change(s) — *continued*
job, anxiety concerning Z56.1
joint — *see* Derangement, joint
life — *see* Menopause
mental status R41.82
minimal (glomerular) — *see also* N00-N07 with fourth
    character .0 N05.0
myocardium, myocardial — *see* Degeneration, myocar-
    dial
of life — *see* Menopause
pacemaker Z45.018
    pulse generator Z45.010
personality (enduring) F68.8
    due to (secondary to)
        general medical condition F07.0
        secondary (nonspecific) F60.89
regressive, dental pulp K04.2
renal — *see* Disease, renal
retina H35.9
    myopic — *see also* Myopia, degenerative H44.2- ☑
sacroiliac joint M53.3
senile — *see also* condition R54
sensory R20.8
skin R23.9
    acute, due to ultraviolet radiation L56.9
        specified NEC L56.8
    chronic, due to nonionizing radiation L57.9
        specified NEC L57.8
    cyanosis R23.0
    flushing R23.2
    pallor R23.1
    petechiae R23.3
    specified change NEC R23.8
    swelling — *see* Mass, localized
    texture R23.4
trophic
    arm — *see* Mononeuropathy, upper limb
    leg — *see* Mononeuropathy, lower limb
vascular I99.9
vasomotor I73.9
voice R49.9
    psychogenic F44.4
    specified NEC R49.8
Changing sleep-work schedule, affecting sleep
    G47.26
Changuinola fever A93.1
Chapping skin T69.8 ☑
Charcot-Marie-Tooth disease, paralysis or syndrome
    G60.0
Charcot's
arthropathy — *see* Arthropathy, neuropathic
cirrhosis K74.3
disease (tabetic arthropathy) A52.16
joint (disease) (tabetic) A52.16
    diabetic — *see* Diabetes, with, arthropathy
    syringomyelic G95.0
syndrome (intermittent claudication) I73.9
CHARGE association Q89.8
Charley-horse (quadriceps) M62.831
traumatic (quadriceps) S76.11- ☑
Charlouis' disease — *see* Yaws
Cheadle's disease E54
Checking (of)
cardiac pacemaker (battery) (electrode(s)) Z45.018
    pulse generator Z45.010
implantable subdermal contraceptive Z30.46
intrauterine contraceptive device Z30.431
wound Z48.0- ☑
    due to injury — code to Injury, by site, using appro-
        priate seventh character for subsequent en-
        counter
Check-up — *see* Examination
Chédiak-Higashi (-Steinbrinck) **syndrome** (congenital
    gigantism of peroxidase granules) E70.330
Cheek — *see* condition
Cheese itch B88.0
Cheese-washer's lung J67.8
Cheese-worker's lung J67.8
Cheilitis (acute) (angular) (catarrhal) (chronic) (exfoliative)
    (gangrenous) (glandular) (infectional) (suppurative)
    (ulcerative) (vesicular) K13.0
    actinic (due to sun) L56.8
        other than from sun L59.8
    candidal B37.83
Cheilodynia K13.0
Cheiloschisis — *see* Cleft, lip
Cheilosis (angular) K13.0
    with pellagra E52

Cheilosis — *continued*
due to
    vitamin B2 (riboflavin) deficiency E53.0
Cheiromegaly M79.89
Cheiropompholyx L30.1
Cheloid — *see* Keloid
Chemical burn — *see* Corrosion, by site
Chemodectoma — *see* Paraganglioma, nonchromaffin
Chemosis, conjunctiva — *see* Edema, conjunctival
Chemotherapy (session) (for)
cancer Z51.11
neoplasm Z51.11
Cherubism M27.8
Chest — *see* condition
Cheyne-Stokes breathing (respiration) R06.3
Chiari's
disease or syndrome (hepatic vein thrombosis) I82.0
malformation
    type I G93.5
    type II — *see* Spina bifida
    net Q24.8
Chicago disease B40.9
Chickenpox — *see* Varicella
Chiclero ulcer or sore B55.1
Chigger (infestation) B88.0
Chignon (disease) B36.8
newborn (from vacuum extraction) (birth injury) P12.1
Chilaiditi's syndrome (subphrenic displacement, colon)
    Q43.3
Chilblain(s) (lupus) T69.1 ☑
Child
custody dispute Z65.3
Childbirth — *see* Delivery
Childhood
cerebral X-linked adrenoleukodystrophy E71.520
period of rapid growth Z00.2
Chill(s) R68.83
with fever R50.9
congestive in malarial regions B54
without fever R68.83
Chilomastigiasis A07.8
Chimera 46,XX/46,XY Q99.0
Chin — *see* condition
Chinese dysentery A03.9
Chionophobia F40.228
Chitral fever A93.1
Chlamydia, chlamydial A74.9
cervicitis A56.09
conjunctivitis A74.0
cystitis A56.01
endometritis A56.11
epididymitis A56.19
female
    pelvic inflammatory disease A56.11
    pelviperitonitis A56.11
orchitis A56.19
peritonitis A74.81
pharyngitis A56.4
proctitis A56.3
psittaci (infection) A70
salpingitis A56.11
sexually-transmitted infection NEC A56.8
specified NEC A74.89
urethritis A56.01
vulvovaginitis A56.02
Chlamydiosis — *see* Chlamydia
Chloasma (skin) (idiopathic) (symptomatic) L81.1
eyelid H02.719
    hyperthyroid E05.90 *[H02.719]*
        with thyroid storm E05.91 *[H02.719]*
    left H02.716
        lower H02.715
        upper H02.714
    right H02.713
        lower H02.712
        upper H02.711
Chloroma C92.3- ☑
Chlorosis D50.9
Egyptian B76.9 *[D63.8]*
miner's B76.9 *[D63.8]*
Chlorotic anemia D50.8
Chocolate cyst (ovary) N80.1
Choked
disc or disk — *see* Papilledema
on food, phlegm, or vomitus NOS — *see* Foreign body,
    by site
while vomiting NOS — *see* Foreign body, by site

Chokes (resulting from bends) T70.3 ☑
Choking sensation R09.89
Cholangiectasis K83.8
Cholangiocarcinoma
with hepatocellular carcinoma, combined C22.0
liver C22.1
specified site NEC — *see* Neoplasm, malignant, by site
unspecified site C22.1
Cholangiohepatitis K83.8
due to fluke infestation B66.1
Cholangiohepatoma C22.0
Cholangiolitis (acute) (chronic) (extrahepatic) (gan-
    grenous) (intrahepatic) K83.09
paratyphoidal — *see* Fever, paratyphoid
typhoidal A01.09
Cholangioma D13.4
malignant — *see* Cholangiocarcinoma
Cholangitis (ascending) (recurrent) (secondary) (stenos-
    ing) (suppurative) K83.09
with calculus, bile duct — *see* Calculus, bile duct, with
    cholangitis
chronic nonsuppurative destructive K74.3
primary K83.09
    sclerosing K83.01
sclerosing K83.09
Cholecystectasia K82.8
Cholecystitis K81.9
with
    calculus, stones in
        bile duct (common) (hepatic) — *see* Calculus,
            bile duct, with cholecystitis
        cystic duct — *see* Calculus, gallbladder, with
            cholecystitis
        gallbladder — *see* Calculus, gallbladder, with
            cholecystitis
        choledocholithiasis — *see* Calculus, bile duct, with
            cholecystitis
        cholelithiasis — *see* Calculus, gallbladder, with
            cholecystitis
    gangrene of gallbladder K82.A1
    perforation of gallbladder K82.A2
acute (emphysematous) (gangrenous) (suppurative)
    K81.0
    with
        calculus, stones in
            cystic duct — *see* Calculus, gallbladder, with
                cholecystitis, acute
            gallbladder — *see* Calculus, gallbladder, with
                cholecystitis, acute
            choledocholithiasis — *see* Calculus, bile duct,
                with cholecystitis, acute
            cholelithiasis — *see* Calculus, gallbladder, with
                cholecystitis, acute
        chronic cholecystitis K81.2
            with gallbladder calculus K80.12
                with obstruction K80.13
chronic K81.1
    with acute cholecystitis K81.2
        with gallbladder calculus K80.12
            with obstruction K80.13
emphysematous (acute) — *see* Cholecystitis, acute
gangrenous — *see* Cholecystitis, acute
paratyphoidal, current A01.4
suppurative — *see* Cholecystitis, acute
typhoidal A01.09
Cholecystolithiasis — *see* Calculus, gallbladder
Choledochitis (suppurative) K83.09
Choledocholith — *see* Calculus, bile duct
Choledocholithiasis (common duct) (hepatic duct) —
    see Calculus, bile duct
cystic — *see* Calculus, gallbladder
typhoidal A01.09
Cholelithiasis (cystic duct) (gallbladder) (impacted)
    (multiple) — *see* Calculus, gallbladder
bile duct (common) (hepatic) — *see* Calculus, bile duct
hepatic duct — *see* Calculus, bile duct
specified NEC K80.80
    with obstruction K80.81
Cholemia — *see also* Jaundice
familial (simple) (congenital) E80.4
Gilbert's E80.4
Choleperitoneum, choleperitonitis K65.3
Cholera (Asiatic) (epidemic) (malignant) A00.9
antimonial — *see* Poisoning, antimony
classical A00.0
due to Vibrio cholerae 01 A00.9
    biovar cholerae A00.0

▽ Subterms under main terms may continue to next column or page   ☑ Additional Character Required — Refer to the Tabular List for Character Selection   53

Change — Cholera

Cholera — *continued*
  due to Vibrio cholerae Ø1 — *continued*
    biovar eltor AØØ.1
    el tor AØØ.1
  el tor AØØ.1
Cholerine — *see* Cholera
Cholestasis NEC K83.1
  with hepatocyte injury K71.Ø
  due to total parenteral nutrition (TPN) K76.89
  pure K71.Ø
Cholesteatoma (ear) (middle) (with reaction) H71.9- ☑
  attic H71.Ø- ☑
  external ear (canal) H6Ø.4- ☑
  mastoid H71.2- ☑
  postmastoidectomy cavity (recurrent) — *see* Complications, postmastoidectomy, recurrent cholesteatoma
  recurrent (postmastoidectomy) — *see* Complications, postmastoidectomy, recurrent cholesteatoma
  tympanum H71.1- ☑
Cholesteatosis, diffuse H71.3- ☑
Cholesteremia E78.ØØ
Cholesterin in vitreous — *see* Deposit, crystalline
Cholesterol
  deposit
    retina H35.89
    vitreous — *see* Deposit, crystalline
  elevated (high) E78.ØØ
    with elevated (high) triglycerides E78.2
    screening for Z13.22Ø
  imbibition of gallbladder K82.4
Cholesterolemia (essential) (pure) E78.ØØ
  familial E78.Ø1
  hereditary E78.Ø1
Cholesterolosis, cholesterosis (gallbladder) K82.4
  cerebrotendinous E75.5
Cholocolic fistula K82.3
Choluria R82.2
Chondritis M94.8X9
  aurical H61.Ø3- ☑
  costal (Tietze's) M94.Ø
  external ear H61.Ø3- ☑
  patella, posttraumatic — *see* Chondromalacia, patella
  pinna H61.Ø3- ☑
  purulent M94.8X- ☑
  tuberculous NEC A18.Ø2
    intervertebral A18.Ø1
Chondroblastoma — *see also* Neoplasm, bone, benign
  malignant — *see* Neoplasm, bone, malignant
Chondrocalcinosis M11.2Ø
  ankle M11.27- ☑
  elbow M11.22- ☑
  familial M11.1Ø
    ankle M11.17- ☑
    elbow M11.12- ☑
    foot joint M11.17- ☑
    hand joint M11.14- ☑
    hip M11.15- ☑
    knee M11.16- ☑
    multiple site M11.19
    shoulder M11.11- ☑
    vertebrae M11.18
    wrist M11.13- ☑
  foot joint M11.27- ☑
  hand joint M11.24- ☑
  hip M11.25- ☑
  knee M11.26- ☑
  multiple site M11.29
  shoulder M11.21- ☑
  specified type NEC M11.2Ø
    ankle M11.27- ☑
    elbow M11.22- ☑
    foot joint M11.27- ☑
    hand joint M11.24- ☑
    hip M11.25- ☑
    knee M11.26- ☑
    multiple site M11.29
    shoulder M11.21- ☑
    vertebrae M11.28
    wrist M11.23- ☑
  vertebrae M11.28
  wrist M11.23- ☑
Chondrodermatitis nodularis helicis or anthelicis — *see* Perichondritis, ear
Chondrodysplasia Q78.9
  with hemangioma Q78.4
  calcificans congenita Q77.3

Chondrodysplasia — *continued*
  fetalis Q77.4
  metaphyseal (Jansen's) (McKusick's) (Schmid's) Q78.8
  punctata Q77.3
Chondrodystrophy, chondrodystrophia (familial) (fetalis) (hypoplastic) Q78.9
  calcificans congenita Q77.3
  myotonic (congenital) G71.13
  punctata Q77.3
Chondroectodermal dysplasia Q77.6
Chondrogenesis imperfecta Q77.4
Chondrolysis M94.35- ☑
Chondroma — *see also* Neoplasm, cartilage, benign
  juxtacortical — *see* Neoplasm, bone, benign
  periosteal — *see* Neoplasm, bone, benign
Chondromalacia (systemic) M94.2Ø
  acromioclavicular joint M94.21- ☑
  ankle M94.27- ☑
  elbow M94.22- ☑
  foot joint M94.27- ☑
  glenohumeral joint M94.21- ☑
  hand joint M94.24- ☑
  hip M94.25- ☑
  knee M94.26- ☑
    patella M22.4- ☑
  multiple sites M94.29
  patella M22.4- ☑
  rib M94.28
  sacroiliac joint M94.259
  shoulder M94.21- ☑
  sternoclavicular joint M94.21- ☑
  vertebral joint M94.28
  wrist M94.23- ☑
Chondromatosis — *see also* Neoplasm, cartilage, uncertain behavior
  internal Q78.4
Chondromyxosarcoma — *see* Neoplasm, cartilage, malignant
Chondro-osteodysplasia (Morquio-Brailsford type) E76.219
Chondro-osteodystrophy E76.29
Chondro-osteoma — *see* Neoplasm, bone, benign
Chondropathia tuberosa M94.Ø
Chondrosarcoma — *see also* Neoplasm, cartilage, malignant
  juxtacortical — *see* Neoplasm, bone, malignant
  mesenchymal — *see* Neoplasm, connective tissue, malignant
  myxoid — *see* Neoplasm, cartilage, malignant
Chordee (nonvenereal) N48.89
  congenital Q54.4
  gonococcal A54.Ø9
Chorditis (fibrinous) (nodosa) (tuberosa) J38.2
Chordoma — *see* Neoplasm, vertebral (column), malignant
Chorea (chronic) (gravis) (posthemiplegic) (senile) (spasmodic) G25.5
  with
    heart involvement IØ2.Ø
      active or acute (conditions in IØ1-) IØ2.Ø
      rheumatic IØ2.9
        with valvular disorder IØ2.Ø
      rheumatic heart disease (chronic) (inactive)(quiescent) — *code to* rheumatic heart condition involved
  drug-induced G25.4
  habit F95.8
  hereditary G1Ø
  Huntington's G1Ø
  hysterical F44.4
  minor IØ2.9
    with heart involvement IØ2.Ø
  progressive G25.5
    hereditary G1Ø
  rheumatic (chronic) IØ2.9
    with heart involvement IØ2.Ø
  Sydenham's IØ2.9
    with heart involvement — *see* Chorea, with rheumatic heart disease
    nonrheumatic G25.5
Choreoathetosis (paroxysmal) G25.5
Chorioadenoma (destruens) D39.2
Chorioamnionitis O41.12- ☑
Chorioangioma D26.7
Choriocarcinoma — *see* Neoplasm, malignant, by site
  combined with
    embryonal carcinoma — *see* Neoplasm, malignant, by site

Choriocarcinoma — *continued*
  combined with — *continued*
    other germ cell elements — *see* Neoplasm, malignant, by site
    teratoma — *see* Neoplasm, malignant, by site
  specified site — *see* Neoplasm, malignant, by site
  unspecified site
    female C58
    male C62.9Ø
Chorioencephalitis (acute) (lymphocytic) (serous) A87.2
Chorioepithelioma — *see* Choriocarcinoma
Choriomeningitis (acute) (lymphocytic) (serous) A87.2
Chorionepithelioma — *see* Choriocarcinoma
Chorioretinitis — *see also* Inflammation, chorioretinal
  disseminated — *see also* Inflammation, chorioretinal, disseminated
    in neurosyphilis A52.19
  Egyptian B76.9 *[D63.8]*
  focal — *see also* Inflammation, chorioretinal, focal
  histoplasmic B39.9 *[H32]*
  in (due to)
    histoplasmosis B39.9 *[H32]*
    syphilis (secondary) A51.43
      late A52.71
    toxoplasmosis (acquired) B58.Ø1
      congenital (active) P37.1 *[H32]*
    tuberculosis A18.53
  juxtapapillary, juxtapapillaris — *see* Inflammation, chorioretinal, focal, juxtapapillary
  leprous A3Ø.9 *[H32]*
  miner's B76.9 *[D63.8]*
  progressive myopia (degeneration) — *see also* Myopia, degenerative H44.2- ☑
  syphilitic (secondary) A51.43
    congenital (early) A5Ø.Ø1 *[H32]*
      late A5Ø.32
    late A52.71
  tuberculous A18.53
Chorioretinopathy, central serous H35.71- ☑
Choroid — *see* condition
Choroideremia H31.21
Choroiditis — *see* Chorioretinitis
Choroidopathy — *see* Disorder, choroid
Choroidoretinitis — *see* Chorioretinitis
Choroidoretinopathy, central serous — *see* Chorioretinopathy, central serous
Christian-Weber disease M35.6
Christmas disease D67
Chromaffinoma — *see also* Neoplasm, benign, by site
  malignant — *see* Neoplasm, malignant, by site
Chromatopsia — *see* Deficiency, color vision
Chromhidrosis, chromidrosis L75.1
Chromoblastomycosis — *see* Chromomycosis
Chromoconversion R82.91
Chromomycosis B43.9
  brain abscess B43.1
  cerebral B43.1
  cutaneous B43.Ø
  skin B43.Ø
  specified NEC B43.8
  subcutaneous abscess or cyst B43.2
Chromophytosis B36.Ø
Chromosome — *see* Anomaly, by chromosome involved
  D (1) — *see* Anomaly, chromosome 13
  E (3) — *see* Anomaly, chromosome 18
  G — *see* Anomaly, chromosome 21
Chromotrichomycosis B36.8
Chronic — *see* condition
  fracture — *see* Fracture, pathological
Churg-Strauss syndrome M3Ø.1
Chyle cyst, mesentery I89.8
Chylocele (nonfilarial) I89.8
  filarial — *see also* Infestation, filarial B74.9 *[N51]*
  tunica vaginalis N5Ø.89
    filarial — *see also* Infestation, filarial B74.9 *[N51]*
Chylomicronemia (fasting) (with hyperprebetalipoproteinemia) E78.3
Chylopericardium I31.3
  acute I3Ø.9
Chylothorax (nonfilarial) I89.8
  filarial — *see also* Infestation, filarial B74.9 *[J91.8]*
Chylous — *see* condition
Chyluria (nonfilarial) R82.Ø
  due to
    bilharziasis B65.Ø
    Brugia (malayi) B74.1
      timori B74.2

Chyluria — continued
  due to — continued
      schistosomiasis (bilharziasis) B65.0
      Wuchereria (bancrofti) B74.0
    filarial — see Infestation, filarial
Cicatricial (deformity) — see Cicatrix
Cicatrix (adherent) (contracted) (painful) (vicious) — see also Scar L90.5
  adenoid (and tonsil) J35.8
  alveolar process M26.79
  anus K62.89
  auricle — see Disorder, pinna, specified type NEC
  bile duct (common) (hepatic) K83.8
  bladder N32.89
  bone — see Disorder, bone, specified type NEC
  brain G93.89
  cervix (postoperative) (postpartal) N88.1
  common duct K83.8
  cornea H17.9
    tuberculous A18.59
  duodenum (bulb), obstructive K31.5
  esophagus K22.2
  eyelid — see Disorder, eyelid function
  hypopharynx J39.2
  lacrimal passages — see Obstruction, lacrimal
  larynx J38.7
  lung J98.4
  middle ear H74.8 ☑
  mouth K13.79
  muscle M62.89
    with contracture — see Contraction, muscle NEC
  nasopharynx J39.2
  palate (soft) K13.79
  penis N48.89
  pharynx J39.2
  prostate N42.89
  rectum K62.89
  retina — see Scar, chorioretinal
  semilunar cartilage — see Derangement, meniscus
  seminal vesicle N50.89
  skin L90.5
    infected L08.89
    postinfective L90.5
    tuberculous B90.8
  specified site NEC L90.5
  throat J39.2
  tongue K14.8
  tonsil (and adenoid) J35.8
  trachea J39.8
  tuberculous NEC B90.9
  urethra N36.8
  uterus N85.8
  vagina N89.8
    postoperative N99.2
  vocal cord J38.3
  wrist, constricting (annular) L90.5
CIDP (chronic inflammatory demyelinating polyneuropathy) G61.81
CIN — see Neoplasia, intraepithelial, cervix
CINCA (chronic infantile neurological, cutaneous and articular syndrome) M04.2
Cinchonism — see Deafness, ototoxic
  correct substance properly administered — see Table of Drugs and Chemicals, by drug, adverse effect
  overdose or wrong substance given or taken — see Table of Drugs and Chemicals, by drug, poisoning
Circle of Willis — see condition
Circular — see condition
Circulating anticoagulants — see also Disorder, hemorrhagic D68.318
  due to drugs — see also Disorder, hemorrhagic D68.32
  following childbirth O72.3
Circulation
  collateral, any site I99.8
  defective (lower extremity) I99.9
    congenital Q28.9
  embryonic Q28.9
  failure (peripheral) R57.9
    newborn P29.89
  fetal, persistent P29.38
  heart, incomplete Q28.9
Circulatory system — see condition
Circulus senilis (cornea) — see Degeneration, cornea, senile
Circumcision (in absence of medical indication) (ritual) (routine) Z41.2
Circumscribed — see condition
Circumvallate placenta O43.11- ☑

Cirrhosis, cirrhotic (hepatic) (liver) K74.60
  alcoholic K70.30
    with ascites K70.31
  atrophic — see Cirrhosis, liver
  Baumgarten-Cruveilhier K74.69
  biliary (cholangiolitic) (cholangitic) (hypertrophic) (obstructive) (pericholangiolitic) K74.5
    due to
      Clonorchiasis B66.1
      flukes B66.3
    primary K74.3
    secondary K74.4
  cardiac (of liver) K76.1
  Charcot's K74.3
  cholangiolitic, cholangitic, cholostatic (primary) K74.3
  congestive K76.1
  Cruveilhier-Baumgarten K74.69
  cryptogenic (liver) K74.69
  due to
    hepatolenticular degeneration E83.01
    Wilson's disease E83.01
    xanthomatosis E78.2
  fatty K76.0
    alcoholic K70.0
  Hanot's (hypertrophic) K74.3
  hepatic — see Cirrhosis, liver
  hypertrophic K74.3
  Indian childhood K74.69
  kidney — see Sclerosis, renal
  Laennec's K70.30
    with ascites K70.31
    alcoholic K70.30
      with ascites K70.31
    nonalcoholic K74.69
  liver K74.60
    alcoholic K70.30
      with ascites K70.31
      fatty K70.0
    congenital P78.81
    syphilitic A52.74
  lung (chronic) J84.10
  macronodular K74.69
    alcoholic K70.30
      with ascites K70.31
  micronodular K74.69
    alcoholic K70.30
      with ascites K70.31
  mixed type K74.69
  monolobular K74.3
  nephritis — see Sclerosis, renal
  nutritional K74.69
    alcoholic K70.30
      with ascites K70.31
  obstructive — see Cirrhosis, biliary
  ovarian N83.8
  pancreas (duct) K86.89
  pigmentary E83.110
  portal K74.69
    alcoholic K70.30
      with ascites K70.31
  postnecrotic K74.69
    alcoholic K70.30
      with ascites K70.31
  pulmonary J84.10
  renal — see Sclerosis, renal
  spleen D73.2
  stasis K76.1
  Todd's K74.3
  unilobar K74.3
  xanthomatous (biliary) K74.5
    due to xanthomatosis (familial) (metabolic) (primary) E78.2
Cistern, subarachnoid R93.0
Citrullinemia E72.23
Citrullinuria E72.23
Civatte's disease or poikiloderma L57.3
Clam digger's itch B65.3
Clammy skin R23.1
Clap — see Gonorrhea
Clarke-Hadfield syndrome (pancreatic infantilism) K86.89
Clark's paralysis G80.9
Clastothrix L67.8
Claude Bernard-Horner syndrome G90.2
  traumatic — see Injury, nerve, cervical sympathetic
Claude's disease or syndrome G46.3
Claudicatio venosa intermittens I87.8
Claudication (intermittent) I73.9

Claudication — continued
  cerebral (artery) G45.9
  spinal cord (arteriosclerotic) G95.19
    syphilitic A52.09
  venous (axillary) I87.8
Claustrophobia F40.240
Clavus (infected) L84
Clawfoot (congenital) Q66.89
  acquired — see Deformity, limb, clawfoot
Clawhand (acquired) — see also Deformity, limb, clawhand
  congenital Q68.1
Clawtoe (congenital) Q66.89
  acquired — see Deformity, toe, specified NEC
Clay eating — see Pica
Cleansing of artificial opening — see Attention to, artificial, opening
Cleft (congenital) — see also Imperfect, closure
  alveolar process M26.79
  branchial (persistent) Q18.2
    cyst Q18.0
      fistula Q18.0
      sinus Q18.0
  cricoid cartilage, posterior Q31.8
  cyst Q18.0
    fistula Q18.0
    sinus Q18.0
  foot Q72.7 ☑
  hand Q71.6 ☑
  lip (unilateral) Q36.9
    with cleft palate Q37.9
      hard Q37.1
        with soft Q37.5
      soft Q37.3
        with hard Q37.5
    bilateral Q36.0
      with cleft palate Q37.8
        hard Q37.0
          with soft Q37.4
        soft Q37.2
          with hard Q37.4
    median Q36.1
  nose Q30.2
  palate Q35.9
    with cleft lip (unilateral) Q37.9
      bilateral Q37.8
    hard Q35.1
      with
        cleft lip (unilateral) Q37.1
          bilateral Q37.0
        soft Q35.5
          with cleft lip (unilateral) Q37.5
            bilateral Q37.4
    medial Q35.5
    soft Q35.3
      with
        cleft lip (unilateral) Q37.3
          bilateral Q37.2
        hard Q35.1
          with cleft lip (unilateral) Q37.5
            bilateral Q37.4
  penis Q55.69
  scrotum Q55.29
  thyroid cartilage Q31.8
  uvula Q35.7
Cleidocranial dysostosis Q74.0
Cleptomania F63.2
Clicking hip (newborn) R29.4
Climacteric (female) — see also Menopause
  arthritis (any site) NEC — see Arthritis, specified form NEC
  depression (single episode) F32.89
    recurrent episode F33.8
  male (symptoms) (syndrome) NEC N50.89
  melancholia (single episode) F32.89
    recurrent episode F33.8
  paranoid state F22
  polyarthritis NEC — see Arthritis, specified form NEC
  symptoms (female) N95.1
Clinical research investigation (clinical trial) (control subject) (normal comparison) (participant) Z00.6
Clitoris — see condition
Cloaca (persistent) Q43.7
Clonorchiasis, clonorchis infection (liver) B66.1
Clonus R25.8
Closed bite M26.29
Clostridium (C.) perfringens, as cause of disease classified elsewhere B96.7

Closure
- congenital, nose Q3Ø.Ø
- cranial sutures, premature Q75.Ø
- defective or imperfect NEC — see Imperfect, closure
- fistula, delayed — see Fistula
- foramen ovale, imperfect Q21.1
- hymen N89.6
- interauricular septum, defective Q21.1
- interventricular septum, defective Q21.Ø
- lacrimal duct — see also Stenosis, lacrimal, duct
  - congenital Q1Ø.5
- nose (congenital) Q3Ø.Ø
  - acquired M95.Ø
- of artificial opening — see Attention to, artificial, opening
- vagina N89.5
- valve — see Endocarditis
- vulva N9Ø.5

Clot (blood) — see also Embolism
- artery (obstruction) (occlusion) — see Embolism
- bladder N32.89
- brain (intradural or extradural) — see Occlusion, artery, cerebral
- circulation I74.9
- heart — see also Infarct, myocardium
  - not resulting in infarction I51.3
- vein — see Thrombosis

Clouded state R4Ø.1
- epileptic — see Epilepsy, specified NEC
- paroxysmal — see Epilepsy, specified NEC

Cloudy antrum, antra J32.Ø

Clouston's (hidrotic) **ectodermal dysplasia** Q82.4

Clubbed nail pachydermoperiostosis M89.4Ø [L62]

Clubbing of finger(s) (nails) R68.3

Clubfinger R68.3
- congenital Q68.1

Clubfoot (congenital) Q66.89
- acquired — see Deformity, limb, clubfoot
- equinovarus Q66.Ø- ☑
- paralytic — see Deformity, limb, clubfoot

Clubhand (congenital) (radial) Q71.4- ☑
- acquired — see Deformity, limb, clubhand

Clubnail R68.3
- congenital Q84.6

Clump, kidney Q63.1

Clumsiness, clumsy child syndrome F82

Cluttering F8Ø.81

Clutton's joints A5Ø.51 [M12.8Ø]

Coagulation, intravascular (diffuse) (disseminated) — see also Defibrination syndrome
- complicating abortion — see Abortion, by type, complicated by, intravascular coagulation
- following ectopic or molar pregnancy OØ8.1

Coagulopathy — see also Defect, coagulation
- consumption D65
- intravascular D65
  - newborn P6Ø

Coalition
- calcaneo-scaphoid Q66.89
- tarsal Q66.89

Coalminer's
- elbow — see Bursitis, elbow, olecranon
- lung or pneumoconiosis J6Ø

Coalworker's lung or pneumoconiosis J6Ø

Coarctation
- aorta (preductal) (postductal) Q25.1
- pulmonary artery Q25.71

Coated tongue K14.3

Coats' disease (exudative retinopathy) — see Retinopathy, exudative

Cocaine-induced
- anxiety disorder F14.98Ø
- bipolar and related disorder F14.94
- depressive disorder F14.94
- obsessive-compulsive and related disorder F14.988
- psychotic disorder F14.959
- sexual dysfunction F14.981
- sleep disorder F14.982

Cocainism — see Disorder, cocaine use

Coccidioidomycosis B38.9
- cutaneous B38.3
- disseminated B38.7
- generalized B38.7
- meninges B38.4
- prostate B38.81
- pulmonary B38.2
  - acute B38.Ø

Coccidioidomycosis — continued
- pulmonary — continued
  - chronic B38.1
- skin B38.3
- specified NEC B38.89

Coccidioidosis — see Coccidioidomycosis

Coccidiosis (intestinal) AØ7.3

Coccydynia, coccygodynia M53.3

Coccyx — see condition

Cochin-China diarrhea K9Ø.1

Cockayne's syndrome Q87.19

Cocked up toe — see Deformity, toe, specified NEC

Cock's peculiar tumor L72.3

Codman's tumor — see Neoplasm, bone, benign

Coenurosis B71.8

Coffee-worker's lung J67.8

Cogan's syndrome H16.32- ☑
- oculomotor apraxia H51.8

Coitus, painful (female) N94.1Ø
- male N53.12
- psychogenic F52.6

Cold JØØ
- with influenza, flu, or grippe — see Influenza, with, respiratory manifestations NEC
- agglutinin disease or hemoglobinuria (chronic) D59.1
- bronchial — see Bronchitis
- chest — see Bronchitis
- common (head) JØØ
- effects of T69.9 ☑
  - specified effect NEC T69.8 ☑
- excessive, effects of T69.9 ☑
  - specified effect NEC T69.8 ☑
- exhaustion from T69.8 ☑
- exposure to T69.9 ☑
  - specified effect NEC T69.8 ☑
- head JØØ
- injury syndrome (newborn) P8Ø.Ø
- on lung — see Bronchitis
- rose J3Ø.1
- sensitivity, auto-immune D59.1
- symptoms JØØ
- virus JØØ

Coldsore BØØ.1

Colibacillosis A49.8
- as the cause of other disease — see also Escherichia coli B96.2Ø
- generalized A41.5Ø

Colic (bilious) (infantile) (intestinal) (recurrent) (spasmodic) R1Ø.83
- abdomen R1Ø.83
  - psychogenic F45.8
- appendix, appendicular K38.8
- bile duct — see Calculus, bile duct
- biliary — see Calculus, bile duct
- common duct — see Calculus, bile duct
- cystic duct — see Calculus, gallbladder
- Devonshire NEC — see Poisoning, lead
- gallbladder — see Calculus, gallbladder
- gallstone — see Calculus, gallbladder
  - gallbladder or cystic duct — see Calculus, gallbladder
- hepatic (duct) — see Calculus, bile duct
- hysterical F45.8
- kidney N23
- lead NEC — see Poisoning, lead
- mucous K58.9
  - with diarrhea K58.Ø
  - psychogenic F54
- nephritic N23
- painter's NEC — see Poisoning, lead
- pancreas K86.89
- psychogenic F45.8
- renal N23
- saturnine NEC — see Poisoning, lead
- ureter N23
- urethral N36.8
  - due to calculus N21.1
- uterus NEC N94.89
  - menstrual — see Dysmenorrhea
- worm NOS B83.9

Colicystitis — see Cystitis

Colitis (acute) (catarrhal) (chronic) (noninfective) (hemorrhagic) — see also Enteritis K52.9
- allergic K52.29
  - with
    - food protein-induced enterocolitis syndrome K52.21

Colitis — continued
- allergic — continued
  - with — continued
    - proctocolitis K52.82
- amebic (acute) — see also Amebiasis AØ6.Ø
  - nondysenteric AØ6.2
- anthrax A22.2
- bacillary — see Infection, Shigella
- balantidial AØ7.Ø
- Clostridium difficile
  - not specified as recurrent AØ4.72
  - recurrent AØ4.71
- coccidial AØ7.3
- collagenous K52.831
- cystica superficialis K52.89
- dietary counseling and surveillance (for) Z71.3
- dietetic — see also Colitis, allergic K52.29
- drug-induced K52.1
- due to radiation K52.Ø
- eosinophilic K52.82
- food hypersensitivity — see also Colitis, allergic K52.29
- giardial AØ7.1
- granulomatous — see Enteritis, regional, large intestine
- indeterminate, so stated K52.3
- infectious — see Enteritis, infectious
- ischemic K55.9
  - acute (subacute) — see also Ischemia, intestine, acute K55.Ø39
  - chronic K55.1
  - due to mesenteric artery insufficiency K55.1
  - fulminant (acute) — see also Ischemia, intestine, acute K55.Ø39
- left sided K51.5Ø
  - with
    - abscess K51.514
    - complication K51.519
      - specified NEC K51.518
    - fistula K51.513
    - obstruction K51.512
    - rectal bleeding K51.511
- lymphocytic K52.832
- membranous
  - psychogenic F54
- microscopic K52.839
  - specified NEC K52.838
- mucous — see Syndrome, irritable, bowel
  - psychogenic F54
- noninfective K52.9
  - specified NEC K52.89
- polyposa — see Polyp, colon, inflammatory
- protozoal AØ7.9
- pseudomembranous
  - not specified as recurrent AØ4.72
  - recurrent AØ4.71
- pseudomucinous — see Syndrome, irritable, bowel
- regional — see Enteritis, regional, large intestine
  - infectious AØ9
- segmental — see Enteritis, regional, large intestine
- septic — see Enteritis, infectious
- spastic K58.9
  - with diarrhea K58.Ø
  - psychogenic F54
- staphylococcal AØ4.8
  - foodborne AØ5.Ø
- subacute ischemic — see also Ischemia, intestine, acute K55.Ø39
- thromboulcerative — see also Ischemia, intestine, acute K55.Ø39
- toxic NEC K52.1
  - due to Clostridium difficile
    - not specified as recurrent AØ4.72
    - recurrent AØ4.71
- transmural — see Enteritis, regional, large intestine
- trichomonal AØ7.8
- tuberculous (ulcerative) A18.32
- ulcerative (chronic) K51.9Ø
  - with
    - complication K51.919
      - abscess K51.914
      - fistula K51.913
      - obstruction K51.912
      - rectal bleeding K51.911
      - specified complication NEC K51.918
  - enterocolitis — see Enterocolitis, ulcerative
  - ileocolitis — see Ileocolitis, ulcerative
  - mucosal proctocolitis — see Proctocolitis, mucosal
  - proctitis — see Proctitis, ulcerative
  - pseudopolyposis — see Polyp, colon, inflammatory

☑ **Additional Character Required** — Refer to the Tabular List for Character Selection ▽ **Subterms under main terms may continue to next column or page**

Colitis — *continued*
  ulcerative — *continued*
    psychogenic F54
    rectosigmoiditis — *see* Rectosigmoiditis, ulcerative
    specified type NEC K51.80
      with
        complication K51.819
          abscess K51.814
          fistula K51.813
          obstruction K51.812
          rectal bleeding K51.811
          specified complication NEC K51.818
Collagenosis, collagen disease (nonvascular) (vascular) M35.9
  cardiovascular I42.8
  reactive perforating L87.1
  specified NEC M35.8
Collapse R55
  adrenal E27.2
  cardiorespiratory R57.0
  cardiovascular R57.0
    newborn P29.89
  circulatory (peripheral) R57.9
    during or after labor and delivery O75.1
    following ectopic or molar pregnancy O08.3
    newborn P29.89
  during or
    after labor and delivery O75.1
    resulting from a procedure, not elsewhere classified T81.10 ☑
  external ear canal — *see* Stenosis, external ear canal
  general R55
  heart — *see* Disease, heart
  heat T67.1 ☑
  hysterical F44.89
  labyrinth, membranous (congenital) Q16.5
  lung (massive) — *see also* Atelectasis J98.19
    pressure due to anesthesia (general) (local) or other sedation T88.2 ☑
      during labor and delivery O74.1
      in pregnancy O29.02- ☑
      postpartum, puerperal O89.09
  myocardial — *see* Disease, heart
  nervous F48.8
  neurocirculatory F45.8
  nose M95.0
  postoperative T81.10 ☑
  pulmonary — *see also* Atelectasis J98.19
    newborn — *see* Atelectasis
  trachea J39.8
  tracheobronchial J98.09
  valvular — *see* Endocarditis
  vascular (peripheral) R57.9
    during or after labor and delivery O75.1
    following ectopic or molar pregnancy O08.3
    newborn P29.89
  vertebra M48.50- ☑
    cervical region M48.52- ☑
    cervicothoracic region M48.53- ☑
    in (due to)
      metastasis — *see* Collapse, vertebra, in, specified disease NEC
      osteoporosis — *see also* Osteoporosis M80.88 ☑
        cervical region M80.88 ☑
        cervicothoracic region M80.88 ☑
        lumbar region M80.88 ☑
        lumbosacral region M80.88 ☑
        multiple sites M80.88 ☑
        occipito-atlanto-axial region M80.88 ☑
        sacrococcygeal region M80.88 ☑
        thoracic region M80.88 ☑
        thoracolumbar region M80.88 ☑
      specified disease NEC M48.50- ☑
        cervical region M48.52- ☑
        cervicothoracic region M48.53- ☑
        lumbar region M48.56- ☑
        lumbosacral region M48.57- ☑
        occipito-atlanto-axial region M48.51- ☑
        sacrococcygeal region M48.58- ☑
        thoracic region M48.54- ☑
        thoracolumbar region M48.55- ☑
    lumbar region M48.56- ☑
    lumbosacral region M48.57- ☑
    occipito-atlanto-axial region M48.51- ☑
    sacrococcygeal region M48.58- ☑
    thoracic region M48.54- ☑
    thoracolumbar region M48.55- ☑

Collateral — *see also* condition
  circulation (venous) I87.8
  dilation, veins I87.8
Colles' fracture S52.53- ☑
Collet (-Sicard) syndrome G52.7
Collier's asthma or lung J60
Collodion baby Q80.2
Colloid nodule (of thyroid) (cystic) E04.1
Coloboma (iris) Q13.0
  eyelid Q10.3
  fundus Q14.8
  lens Q12.2
  optic disc (congenital) Q14.2
    acquired H47.31- ☑
Coloenteritis — *see* Enteritis
Colon — *see* condition
Colonization
  MRSA (Methicillin resistant Staphylococcus aureus) Z22.322
  MSSA (Methicillin susceptible Staphylococcus aureus) Z22.321
  status — *see* Carrier (suspected) of
Coloptosis K63.4
Color blindness — *see* Deficiency, color vision
Colostomy
  attention to Z43.3
  fitting or adjustment Z46.89
  malfunctioning K94.03
  status Z93.3
Colpitis (acute) — *see* Vaginitis
Colpocele N81.5
Colpocystitis — *see* Vaginitis
Colpospasm N94.2
Column, spinal, vertebral — *see* condition
Coma R40.20
  with
    motor response (none) R40.231 ☑
      abnormal extensor posturing to pain or noxious stimuli (< 2 years of age) R40.232 ☑
      abnormal flexure posturing to pain or noxious stimuli (0-5 years of age) R40.233 ☑
      extensor posturing to pain or noxious stimuli (2-5 years of age) R40.232 ☑
      flexion/decorticate posturing (< 2 years of age) R40.233 ☑
      localizes pain (2-5 years of age) R40.235 ☑
      normal or spontaneous movement (< 2 years of age) R40.236 ☑
      obeys commands (2-5 years of age) R40.236 ☑
      score of
        1 R40.231 ☑
        2 R40.232 ☑
        3 R40.233 ☑
        4 R40.234 ☑
        5 R40.235 ☑
        6 R40.236 ☑
      withdraws from pain or noxious stimuli (0-5 years of age) R40.234 ☑
      withdraws to touch (< 2 years of age) R40.235 ☑
    opening of eyes (never) R40.211 ☑
      in response to
        pain R40.212 ☑
        sound R40.213 ☑
      score of
        1 R40.211 ☑
        2 R40.212 ☑
        3 R40.213 ☑
        4 R40.214 ☑
      spontaneous R40.214 ☑
    verbal response (none) R40.221 ☑
      confused conversation R40.224 ☑
      cooing or babbling or crying appropriately (<2 years of age) R40.225 ☑
      inappropriate crying or screaming (< 2 years of age) R40.223 ☑
      inappropriate words (2-5 years of age) R40.224 ☑
      incomprehensible sounds (2-5 years of age) R40.222 ☑
      incomprehensible words R40.222 ☑
      irritable cries (< 2 years of age) R40.224 ☑
      moans/grunts to pain; restless (< 2 years old) R40.222 ☑
      oriented R40.225 ☑
      score of
        1 R40.221 ☑
        2 R40.222 ☑

Coma — *continued*
  with — *continued*
    verbal response — *continued*
      score of — *continued*
        3 R40.223 ☑
        4 R40.224 ☑
        5 R40.225 ☑
      screaming (2-5 years of age) R40.223 ☑
      uses appropriate words (2-5 years of age) R40.225 ☑
  eclamptic — *see* Eclampsia
  epileptic — *see* Epilepsy
  Glasgow, scale score — *see* Glasgow coma scale
  hepatic — *see* Failure, hepatic, by type, with coma
  hyperglycemic (diabetic) — *see* Diabetes, by type, with hyperosmolarity, with coma
  hyperosmolar (diabetic) — *see* Diabetes, by type, with hyperosmolarity, with coma
  hypoglycemic (diabetic) — *see* Diabetes, by type, with hypoglycemia, with coma
    nondiabetic E15
  in diabetes — *see* Diabetes, coma
  insulin-induced — *see* Coma, hypoglycemic
  ketoacidotic (diabetic) — *see* Diabetes, by type, with ketoacidosis, with coma
  myxedematous E03.5
  newborn P91.5
  persistent vegetative state R40.3
  specified NEC, without documented Glasgow coma scale score, or with partial Glasgow coma scale score reported R40.244 ☑
Comatose — *see* Coma
Combat fatigue F43.0
Combined — *see* condition
Comedo, comedones (giant) L70.0
Comedocarcinoma — *see also* Neoplasm, breast, malignant
  noninfiltrating
    breast D05.8- ☑
    specified site — *see* Neoplasm, in situ, by site
    unspecified site D05.8- ☑
Comedomastitis — *see* Ectasia, mammary duct
Comminuted fracture — *code as* Fracture, closed
Common
  arterial trunk Q20.0
  atrioventricular canal Q21.2
  atrium Q21.1
  cold (head) J00
  truncus (arteriosus) Q20.0
  variable immunodeficiency — *see* Immunodeficiency, common variable
  ventricle Q20.4
Commotio, commotion (current)
  brain — *see* Injury, intracranial, concussion
  cerebri — *see* Injury, intracranial, concussion
  retinae S05.8X- ☑
  spinal cord — *see* Injury, spinal cord, by region
  spinalis — *see* Injury, spinal cord, by region
Communication
  between
    base of aorta and pulmonary artery Q21.4
    left ventricle and right atrium Q20.5
    pericardial sac and pleural sac Q34.8
    pulmonary artery and pulmonary vein, congenital Q25.72
  congenital between uterus and digestive or urinary tract Q51.7
Compartment syndrome (deep) (posterior) (traumatic) T79.A0 ☑ (*following* T79.7)
  abdomen T79.A3 ☑ (*following* T79.7)
  lower extremity (hip, buttock, thigh, leg, foot, toes) T79.A2 ☑ (*following* T79.7)
  nontraumatic
    abdomen M79.A3 (*following* M79.7)
    lower extremity (hip, buttock, thigh, leg, foot, toes) M79.A2- ☑ (*following* M79.7)
    specified site NEC M79.A9 (*following* M79.7)
    upper extremity (shoulder, arm, forearm, wrist, hand, fingers) M79.A1- ☑ (*following* M79.7)
  specified site NEC T79.A9 ☑ (*following* T79.7)
  upper extremity (shoulder, arm, forearm, wrist, hand, fingers) T79.A1- ☑ (*following* T79.7)
Compensation
  failure — *see* Disease, heart
  neurosis, psychoneurosis — *see* Disorder, factitious
Complaint — *see also* Disease
  bowel, functional K59.9

☑ Subterms under main terms may continue to next column or page   ☑ Additional Character Required — Refer to the Tabular List for Character Selection   57

Colitis — Complaint

Complaint — continued
  bowel, functional — continued
    psychogenic F45.8
  intestine, functional K59.9
    psychogenic F45.8
  kidney — see Disease, renal
  miners' J60
Complete — see condition
Complex
  Addison-Schilder E71.528
  cardiorenal — see Hypertension, cardiorenal
  Costen's M26.69
  disseminated mycobacterium avium- intracellulare
    (DMAC) A31.2
  Eisenmenger's (ventricular septal defect) I27.83
  hypersexual F52.8
  jumped process, spine — see Dislocation, vertebra
  primary, tuberculous A15.7
  Schilder-Addison E71.528
  subluxation (vertebral) M99.19
    abdomen M99.19
    acromioclavicular M99.17
    cervical region M99.11
    cervicothoracic M99.11
    costochondral M99.18
    costovertebral M99.18
    head region M99.10
    hip M99.15
    lower extremity M99.16
    lumbar region M99.13
    lumbosacral M99.13
    occipitocervical M99.10
    pelvic region M99.15
    pubic M99.15
    rib cage M99.18
    sacral region M99.14
    sacrococcygeal M99.14
    sacroiliac M99.14
    specified NEC M99.19
    sternochondral M99.18
    sternoclavicular M99.17
    thoracic region M99.12
    thoracolumbar M99.12
    upper extremity M99.17
  Taussig-Bing (transposition, aorta and overriding pulmonary artery) Q20.1
Complication(s) (from) (of)
  accidental puncture or laceration during a procedure
    (of) — see Complications, intraoperative (intraprocedural), puncture or laceration
  amputation stump (surgical) (late) NEC T87.9
    dehiscence T87.81
    infection or inflammation T87.40
      lower limb T87.4- ☑
      upper limb T87.4- ☑
    necrosis T87.50
      lower limb T87.5- ☑
      upper limb T87.5- ☑
    neuroma T87.30
      lower limb T87.3- ☑
      upper limb T87.3- ☑
    specified type NEC T87.89
  anastomosis (and bypass) — see also Complications,
    prosthetic device or implant
    intestinal (internal) NEC K91.89
      involving urinary tract N99.89
    urinary tract (involving intestinal tract) N99.89
    vascular — see Complications, cardiovascular device
      or implant
  anesthesia, anesthetic — see also Anesthesia, complication T88.59 ☑
    brain, postpartum, puerperal O89.2
    cardiac
      in
        labor and delivery O74.2
        pregnancy O29.19- ☑
      postpartum, puerperal O89.1
    central nervous system
      in
        labor and delivery O74.3
        pregnancy O29.29- ☑
      postpartum, puerperal O89.2
    difficult or failed intubation T88.4 ☑
      in pregnancy O29.6- ☑
    failed sedation (conscious) (moderate) during procedure T88.52 ☑
    general, unintended awareness during procedure
      T88.53 ☑

Complication(s) — continued
  anesthesia, anesthetic — see also Anesthesia, complication — continued
    hyperthermia, malignant T88.3 ☑
    hypothermia T88.51 ☑
    intubation failure T88.4 ☑
    malignant hyperthermia T88.3 ☑
    pulmonary
      in
        labor and delivery O74.1
        pregnancy NEC O29.09- ☑
      postpartum, puerperal O89.09
    shock T88.2 ☑
    spinal and epidural
      in
        labor and delivery NEC O74.6
          headache O74.5
        pregnancy NEC O29.5X- ☑
      postpartum, puerperal NEC O89.5
        headache O89.4
    unintended awareness under general anesthesia
      during procedure T88.53 ☑
  anti-reflux device — see Complications, esophageal
    anti-reflux device
  aortic (bifurcation) graft — see Complications, graft,
    vascular
  aortocoronary (bypass) graft — see Complications,
    coronary artery (bypass) graft
  aortofemoral (bypass) graft — see Complications, extremity artery (bypass) graft
  arteriovenous
    fistula, surgically created T82.9 ☑
      embolism T82.818 ☑
      fibrosis T82.828 ☑
      hemorrhage T82.838 ☑
      infection or inflammation T82.7 ☑
      mechanical
        breakdown T82.510 ☑
        displacement T82.520 ☑
        leakage T82.530 ☑
        malposition T82.520 ☑
        obstruction T82.590 ☑
        perforation T82.590 ☑
        protrusion T82.590 ☑
      pain T82.848 ☑
      specified type NEC T82.898 ☑
      stenosis T82.858 ☑
      thrombosis T82.868 ☑
    shunt, surgically created T82.9 ☑
      embolism T82.818 ☑
      fibrosis T82.828 ☑
      hemorrhage T82.838 ☑
      infection or inflammation T82.7 ☑
      mechanical
        breakdown T82.511 ☑
        displacement T82.521 ☑
        leakage T82.531 ☑
        malposition T82.521 ☑
        obstruction T82.591 ☑
        perforation T82.591 ☑
        protrusion T82.591 ☑
      pain T82.848 ☑
      specified type NEC T82.898 ☑
      stenosis T82.858 ☑
      thrombosis T82.868 ☑
  arthroplasty — see Complications, joint prosthesis
  artificial
    fertilization or insemination N98.9
      attempted introduction (of)
        embryo in embryo transfer N98.3
        ovum following in vitro fertilization N98.2
      hyperstimulation of ovaries N98.1
      infection N98.0
      specified NEC N98.8
    heart T82.9 ☑
      embolism T82.817 ☑
      fibrosis T82.827 ☑
      hemorrhage T82.837 ☑
      infection or inflammation T82.7 ☑
      mechanical
        breakdown T82.512 ☑
        displacement T82.522 ☑
        leakage T82.532 ☑
        malposition T82.522 ☑
        obstruction T82.592 ☑
        perforation T82.592 ☑

Complication(s) — continued
  artificial — continued
    heart — continued
      mechanical — continued
        protrusion T82.592 ☑
      pain T82.847 ☑
      specified type NEC T82.897 ☑
      stenosis T82.857 ☑
      thrombosis T82.867 ☑
    opening
      cecostomy — see Complications, colostomy
      colostomy — see Complications, colostomy
      cystostomy — see Complications, cystostomy
      enterostomy — see Complications, enterostomy
      gastrostomy — see Complications, gastrostomy
      ileostomy — see Complications, enterostomy
      jejunostomy — see Complications, enterostomy
      nephrostomy — see Complications, stoma, urinary tract
      tracheostomy — see Complications, tracheostomy
      ureterostomy — see Complications, stoma, urinary tract
      urethrostomy — see Complications, stoma, urinary tract
  balloon implant or device
    gastrointestinal T85.9 ☑
      embolism T85.818 ☑
      fibrosis T85.828 ☑
      hemorrhage T85.838 ☑
      infection and inflammation T85.79 ☑
      pain T85.848 ☑
      specified type NEC T85.898 ☑
      stenosis T85.858 ☑
      thrombosis T85.868 ☑
    vascular (counterpulsation) T82.9 ☑
      embolism T82.818 ☑
      fibrosis T82.828 ☑
      hemorrhage T82.838 ☑
      infection or inflammation T82.7 ☑
      mechanical
        breakdown T82.513 ☑
        displacement T82.523 ☑
        leakage T82.533 ☑
        malposition T82.523 ☑
        obstruction T82.593 ☑
        perforation T82.593 ☑
        protrusion T82.593 ☑
      pain T82.848 ☑
      specified type NEC T82.898 ☑
      stenosis T82.858 ☑
      thrombosis T82.868 ☑
  bariatric procedure
    gastric band procedure K95.09
      infection K95.01
    specified procedure NEC K95.89
      infection K95.81
  bile duct implant (prosthetic) T85.9 ☑
    embolism T85.818 ☑
    fibrosis T85.828 ☑
    hemorrhage T85.838 ☑
    infection and inflammation T85.79 ☑
    mechanical
      breakdown T85.510 ☑
      displacement T85.520 ☑
      malfunction T85.510 ☑
      malposition T85.520 ☑
      obstruction T85.590 ☑
      perforation T85.590 ☑
      protrusion T85.590 ☑
      specified NEC T85.590 ☑
    pain T85.848 ☑
    specified type NEC T85.898 ☑
    stenosis T85.858 ☑
    thrombosis T85.868 ☑
  bladder device (auxiliary) — see Complications, genitourinary, device or implant, urinary system
  bleeding (postoperative) — see Complication, postoperative, hemorrhage
    intraoperative — see Complication, intraoperative, hemorrhage
  blood vessel graft — see Complications, graft, vascular
  bone
    device NEC T84.9 ☑
      embolism T84.81 ☑
      fibrosis T84.82 ☑

☑ Additional Character Required — Refer to the Tabular List for Character Selection   ▽ Subterms under main terms may continue to next column or page

Complication(s) — *continued*
  bone — *continued*
    device — *continued*
      hemorrhage T84.83 ☑
      infection or inflammation T84.7 ☑
      mechanical
        breakdown T84.318 ☑
        displacement T84.328 ☑
        malposition T84.328 ☑
        obstruction T84.398 ☑
        perforation T84.398 ☑
        protrusion T84.398 ☑
      pain T84.84 ☑
      specified type NEC T84.89 ☑
      stenosis T84.85 ☑
      thrombosis T84.86 ☑
    graft — *see* Complications, graft, bone
    growth stimulator (electrode) — *see* Complications, electronic stimulator device, bone
    marrow transplant — *see* Complications, transplant, bone, marrow
  brain neurostimulator (electrode) — *see* Complications, electronic stimulator device, brain
  breast implant (prosthetic) T85.9 ☑
    capsular contracture T85.44 ☑
    embolism T85.818 ☑
    fibrosis T85.828 ☑
    hemorrhage T85.838 ☑
    infection and inflammation T85.79 ☑
    mechanical
      breakdown T85.41 ☑
      displacement T85.42 ☑
      leakage T85.43 ☑
      malposition T85.42 ☑
      obstruction T85.49 ☑
      perforation T85.49 ☑
      protrusion T85.49 ☑
      specified NEC T85.49 ☑
    pain T85.848 ☑
    specified type NEC T85.898 ☑
    stenosis T85.858 ☑
    thrombosis T85.868 ☑
  bypass — *see also* Complications, prosthetic device or implant
    aortocoronary — *see* Complications, coronary artery (bypass) graft
    arterial — *see also* Complications, graft, vascular
      extremity — *see* Complications, extremity artery (bypass) graft
  cardiac — *see also* Disease, heart
    device, implant or graft T82.9 ☑
      embolism T82.817 ☑
      fibrosis T82.827 ☑
      hemorrhage T82.837 ☑
      infection or inflammation T82.7 ☑
        valve prosthesis T82.6 ☑
      mechanical
        breakdown T82.519 ☑
          specified device NEC T82.518 ☑
        displacement T82.529 ☑
          specified device NEC T82.528 ☑
        leakage T82.539 ☑
          specified device NEC T82.538 ☑
        malposition T82.529 ☑
          specified device NEC T82.528 ☑
        obstruction T82.599 ☑
          specified device NEC T82.598 ☑
        perforation T82.599 ☑
          specified device NEC T82.598 ☑
        protrusion T82.599 ☑
          specified device NEC T82.598 ☑
      pain T82.847 ☑
      specified type NEC T82.897 ☑
      stenosis T82.857 ☑
      thrombosis T82.867 ☑
  cardiovascular device, graft or implant T82.9 ☑
    aortic graft — *see* Complications, graft, vascular
    arteriovenous
      fistula, artificial — *see* Complication, arteriovenous, fistula, surgically created
      shunt — *see* Complication, arteriovenous, shunt, surgically created
    artificial heart — *see* Complication, artificial, heart
    balloon (counterpulsation) device — *see* Complication, balloon implant, vascular

Complication(s) — *continued*
  cardiovascular device, graft or implant — *continued*
    carotid artery graft — *see* Complications, graft, vascular
    coronary bypass graft — *see* Complication, coronary artery (bypass) graft
    dialysis catheter (vascular) — *see* Complication, catheter, dialysis
    electronic T82.9 ☑
      electrode T82.9 ☑
        embolism T82.817 ☑
        fibrosis T82.827 ☑
        hemorrhage T82.837 ☑
        infection T82.7 ☑
        mechanical
          breakdown T82.110 ☑
          displacement T82.120 ☑
          leakage T82.190 ☑
          obstruction T82.190 ☑
          perforation T82.190 ☑
          protrusion T82.190 ☑
          specified type NEC T82.190 ☑
        pain T82.847 ☑
        specified NEC T82.897 ☑
        stenosis T82.857 ☑
        thrombosis T82.867 ☑
      embolism T82.817 ☑
      fibrosis T82.827 ☑
      hemorrhage T82.837 ☑
      infection T82.7 ☑
      mechanical
        breakdown T82.119 ☑
        displacement T82.129 ☑
        leakage T82.199 ☑
        obstruction T82.199 ☑
        perforation T82.199 ☑
        protrusion T82.199 ☑
        specified type NEC T82.199 ☑
      pain T82.847 ☑
      pulse generator T82.9 ☑
        embolism T82.817 ☑
        fibrosis T82.827 ☑
        hemorrhage T82.837 ☑
        infection T82.7 ☑
        mechanical
          breakdown T82.111 ☑
          displacement T82.121 ☑
          leakage T82.191 ☑
          obstruction T82.191 ☑
          perforation T82.191 ☑
          protrusion T82.191 ☑
          specified type NEC T82.191 ☑
        pain T82.847 ☑
        specified NEC T82.897 ☑
        stenosis T82.857 ☑
        thrombosis T82.867 ☑
      specified condition NEC T82.897 ☑
      specified device NEC T82.9 ☑
        embolism T82.817 ☑
        fibrosis T82.827 ☑
        hemorrhage T82.837 ☑
        infection T82.7 ☑
        mechanical
          breakdown T82.118 ☑
          displacement T82.128 ☑
          leakage T82.198 ☑
          obstruction T82.198 ☑
          perforation T82.198 ☑
          protrusion T82.198 ☑
          specified type NEC T82.198 ☑
        pain T82.847 ☑
        specified NEC T82.897 ☑
        stenosis T82.857 ☑
        thrombosis T82.867 ☑
      stenosis T82.857 ☑
      thrombosis T82.867 ☑
    extremity artery graft — *see* Complication, extremity artery (bypass) graft
    femoral artery graft — *see* Complication, extremity artery (bypass) graft
    heart
      transplant — *see* Complication, transplant, heart
      valve — *see* Complication, prosthetic device, heart valve
        graft — *see* Complication, heart, valve, graft

Complication(s) — *continued*
  cardiovascular device, graft or implant — *continued*
    heart-lung transplant — *see* Complication, transplant, heart, with lung
    infection or inflammation T82.7 ☑
    umbrella device — *see* Complication, umbrella device, vascular
    vascular graft (or anastomosis) — *see* Complication, graft, vascular
  carotid artery (bypass) graft — *see* Complications, graft, vascular
  catheter (device) NEC — *see also* Complications, prosthetic device or implant
    cranial infusion
      infection and inflammation T85.735 ☑
      mechanical
        breakdown T85.610 ☑
        displacement T85.620 ☑
        leakage T85.630 ☑
        malfunction T85.690 ☑
        malposition T85.620 ☑
        obstruction T85.690 ☑
        perforation T85.690 ☑
        protrusion T85.690 ☑
        specified NEC T85.690 ☑
    cystostomy T83.9 ☑
      embolism T83.81 ☑
      fibrosis T83.82 ☑
      hemorrhage T83.83 ☑
      infection and inflammation T83.510 ☑
      mechanical
        breakdown T83.010 ☑
        displacement T83.020 ☑
        leakage T83.030 ☑
        malposition T83.020 ☑
        obstruction T83.090 ☑
        perforation T83.090 ☑
        protrusion T83.090 ☑
        specified NEC T83.090 ☑
      pain T83.84 ☑
      specified type NEC T83.89 ☑
      stenosis T83.85 ☑
      thrombosis T83.86 ☑
    dialysis (vascular) T82.9 ☑
      embolism T82.818 ☑
      fibrosis T82.828 ☑
      hemorrhage T82.838 ☑
      infection and inflammation T82.7 ☑
      intraperitoneal — *see* Complications, catheter, intraperitoneal
      mechanical
        breakdown T82.41 ☑
        displacement T82.42 ☑
        leakage T82.43 ☑
        malposition T82.42 ☑
        obstruction T82.49 ☑
        perforation T82.49 ☑
        protrusion T82.49 ☑
      pain T82.848 ☑
      specified type NEC T82.898 ☑
      stenosis T82.858 ☑
      thrombosis T82.868 ☑
    epidural infusion T85.9 ☑
      embolism T85.810 ☑
      fibrosis T85.820 ☑
      hemorrhage T85.830 ☑
      infection and inflammation T85.735 ☑
      mechanical
        breakdown T85.610 ☑
        displacement T85.620 ☑
        leakage T85.630 ☑
        malfunction T85.610 ☑
        malposition T85.620 ☑
        obstruction T85.690 ☑
        perforation T85.690 ☑
        protrusion T85.690 ☑
        specified NEC T85.690 ☑
      pain T85.840 ☑
      specified type NEC T85.890 ☑
      stenosis T85.850 ☑
      thrombosis T85.860 ☑
    intraperitoneal dialysis T85.9 ☑
      embolism T85.818 ☑
      fibrosis T85.828 ☑
      hemorrhage T85.838 ☑
      infection and inflammation T85.71 ☑

Complication(s) — *continued*
catheter — *see also* Complications, prosthetic device
  or implant — *continued*
    intraperitoneal dialysis — *continued*
      mechanical
        breakdown T85.611 ☑
        displacement T85.621 ☑
        leakage T85.631 ☑
        malfunction T85.611 ☑
        malposition T85.621 ☑
        obstruction T85.691 ☑
        perforation T85.691 ☑
        protrusion T85.691 ☑
        specified NEC T85.691 ☑
      pain T85.848 ☑
      specified type NEC T85.898 ☑
      stenosis T85.858 ☑
      thrombosis T85.868 ☑
    intrathecal infusion
      infection and inflammation T85.735 ☑
      mechanical
        breakdown T85.610 ☑
        displacement T85.620 ☑
        leakage T85.630 ☑
        malfunction T85.690 ☑
        malposition T85.620 ☑
        obstruction T85.690 ☑
        perforation T85.690 ☑
        protrusion T85.690 ☑
        specified NEC T85.690 ☑
    intravenous infusion T82.9 ☑
      embolism T82.818 ☑
      fibrosis T82.828 ☑
      hemorrhage T82.838 ☑
      infection or inflammation T82.7 ☑
      mechanical
        breakdown T82.514 ☑
        displacement T82.524 ☑
        leakage T82.534 ☑
        malposition T82.524 ☑
        obstruction T82.594 ☑
        perforation T82.594 ☑
        protrusion T82.594 ☑
      pain T82.848 ☑
      specified type NEC T82.898 ☑
      stenosis T82.858 ☑
      thrombosis T82.868 ☑
    spinal infusion
      infection and inflammation T85.735 ☑
      mechanical
        breakdown T85.610 ☑
        displacement T85.620 ☑
        leakage T85.630 ☑
        malfunction T85.690 ☑
        malposition T85.620 ☑
        obstruction T85.690 ☑
        perforation T85.690 ☑
        protrusion T85.690 ☑
        specified NEC T85.690 ☑
    subarachnoid infusion
      infection and inflammation T85.735 ☑
      mechanical
        breakdown T85.610 ☑
        displacement T85.620 ☑
        leakage T85.630 ☑
        malfunction T85.690 ☑
        malposition T85.620 ☑
        obstruction T85.690 ☑
        perforation T85.690 ☑
        protrusion T85.690 ☑
        specified NEC T85.690 ☑
    subdural infusion T85.9 ☑
      embolism T85.810 ☑
      fibrosis T85.820 ☑
      hemorrhage T85.830 ☑
      infection and inflammation T85.735 ☑
      mechanical
        breakdown T85.610 ☑
        displacement T85.620 ☑
        leakage T85.630 ☑
        malfunction T85.610 ☑
        malposition T85.620 ☑
        obstruction T85.690 ☑
        perforation T85.690 ☑
        protrusion T85.690 ☑
        specified NEC T85.690 ☑

Complication(s) — *continued*
catheter — *see also* Complications, prosthetic device
  or implant — *continued*
    subdural infusion — *continued*
      pain T85.840 ☑
      specified type NEC T85.890 ☑
      stenosis T85.850 ☑
      thrombosis T85.860 ☑
    urethral T83.9 ☑
      displacement T83.028 ☑
      embolism T83.81 ☑
      fibrosis T83.82 ☑
      hemorrhage T83.83 ☑
      indwelling
        breakdown T83.011 ☑
        displacement T83.021 ☑
        infection and inflammation T83.511 ☑
        leakage T83.031 ☑
        specified complication NEC T83.091 ☑
      infection and inflammation T83.511 ☑
      leakage T83.038 ☑
      malposition T83.028 ☑
      mechanical
        breakdown T83.011 ☑
      obstruction (mechanical) T83.091 ☑
      pain T83.84 ☑
      perforation T83.091 ☑
      protrusion T83.091 ☑
      specified type NEC T83.091 ☑
      stenosis T83.85 ☑
      thrombosis T83.86 ☑
      urinary NEC
        breakdown T83.018 ☑
        displacement T83.028 ☑
        infection and inflammation T83.518 ☑
        leakage T83.038 ☑
        specified complication NEC T83.098 ☑
  cecostomy (stoma) — *see* Complications, colostomy
  cesarean delivery wound NEC O90.89
    disruption O90.0
    hematoma O90.2
    infection (following delivery) O86.00
  chemotherapy (antineoplastic) NEC T88.7 ☑
  chin implant (prosthetic) — *see* Complication, prosthetic device or implant, specified NEC
  circulatory system I99.8
    intraoperative I97.88
    postprocedural I97.89
      following cardiac surgery — *see also* Infarct, myocardium, associated with revascularization procedure I97.19- ☑
        postcardiotomy syndrome I97.0
      hypertension I97.3
      lymphedema after mastectomy I97.2
      postcardiotomy syndrome I97.0
      specified NEC I97.89
  colostomy (stoma) K94.00
    hemorrhage K94.01
    infection K94.02
    malfunction K94.03
    mechanical K94.03
    specified complication NEC K94.09
  contraceptive device, intrauterine — *see* Complications, intrauterine, contraceptive device
  cord (umbilical) — *see* Complications, umbilical cord
  corneal graft — *see* Complications, graft, cornea
  coronary artery (bypass) graft T82.9 ☑
    atherosclerosis — *see* Arteriosclerosis, coronary (artery),
    embolism T82.818 ☑
    fibrosis T82.828 ☑
    hemorrhage T82.838 ☑
    infection and inflammation T82.7 ☑
    mechanical
      breakdown T82.211 ☑
      displacement T82.212 ☑
      leakage T82.213 ☑
      malposition T82.212 ☑
      obstruction T82.218 ☑
      perforation T82.218 ☑
      protrusion T82.218 ☑
      specified NEC T82.218 ☑
    pain T82.848 ☑
    specified type NEC T82.898 ☑
    stenosis T82.858 ☑
    thrombosis T82.868 ☑

Complication(s) — *continued*
counterpulsation device (balloon), intra- aortic — *see* Complications, balloon implant, vascular
cystostomy (stoma) N99.518
  catheter — *see* Complications, catheter, cystostomy
  hemorrhage N99.510
  infection N99.511
  malfunction N99.512
  specified type NEC N99.518
delivery — *see also* Complications, obstetric O75.9
  procedure (instrumental) (manual) (surgical) O75.4
  specified NEC O75.89
dialysis (peritoneal) (renal) — *see also* Complications, infusion
  catheter (vascular) — *see* Complication, catheter, dialysis
    peritoneal, intraperitoneal — *see* Complications, catheter, intraperitoneal
dorsal column (spinal) neurostimulator — *see* Complications, electronic stimulator device, spinal cord
drug NEC T88.7 ☑
ear procedure — *see also* Disorder, ear
  intraoperative H95.88
    hematoma — *see* Complications, intraoperative, hemorrhage (hematoma) (of), ear
    hemorrhage — *see* Complications, intraoperative, hemorrhage (hematoma) (of), ear
    laceration — *see* Complications, intraoperative, puncture or laceration..., ear
    specified NEC H95.88
  postoperative H95.89
    external ear canal stenosis H95.81- ☑
    hematoma — *see* Complications, postprocedural, hematoma (of), ear
    hemorrhage — *see* Complications, postprocedural, hemorrhage (of), ear
    postmastoidectomy — *see* Complications, postmastoidectomy
    seroma — *see* Complications, postprocedural, seroma (of), mastoid process
    specified NEC H95.89
ectopic pregnancy O08.9
  damage to pelvic organs O08.6
  embolism O08.2
  genital infection O08.0
  hemorrhage (delayed) (excessive) O08.1
  metabolic disorder O08.5
  renal failure O08.4
  shock O08.3
  specified type NEC O08.0
  venous complication NEC O08.7
electronic stimulator device
  bladder (urinary) — *see* Complications, electronic stimulator device, urinary
  bone T84.9 ☑
    breakdown T84.310 ☑
    displacement T84.320 ☑
    embolism T84.81 ☑
    fibrosis T84.82 ☑
    hemorrhage T84.83 ☑
    infection or inflammation T84.7 ☑
    malfunction T84.310 ☑
    malposition T84.320 ☑
    mechanical NEC T84.390 ☑
    obstruction T84.390 ☑
    pain T84.84 ☑
    perforation T84.390 ☑
    protrusion T84.390 ☑
    specified type NEC T84.89 ☑
    stenosis T84.85 ☑
    thrombosis T84.86 ☑
  brain T85.9 ☑
    embolism T85.810 ☑
    fibrosis T85.820 ☑
    hemorrhage T85.830 ☑
    infection and inflammation T85.731 ☑
    mechanical
      breakdown T85.110 ☑
      displacement T85.120 ☑
      leakage T85.190 ☑
      malposition T85.120 ☑
      obstruction T85.190 ☑
      perforation T85.190 ☑
      protrusion T85.190 ☑
      specified NEC T85.190 ☑
    pain T85.840 ☑
    specified type NEC T85.890 ☑

☑ **Additional Character Required** — **Refer to the Tabular List for Character Selection** ▽ **Subterms under main terms may continue to next column or page**

Complication(s) — *continued*
  electronic stimulator device — *continued*
    brain — *continued*
      stenosis T85.850 ☑
      thrombosis T85.860 ☑
    cardiac (defibrillator) (pacemaker) — *see* Complications, cardiovascular device or implant, electronic
    generator (brain) (gastric) (peripheral) (sacral) (spinal)
      breakdown T85.113 ☑
      displacement T85.123 ☑
      leakage T85.193 ☑
      malposition T85.123 ☑
      obstruction T85.193 ☑
      perforation T85.193 ☑
      protrusion T85.193 ☑
      specified type NEC T85.193 ☑
    muscle T84.9 ☑
      breakdown T84.418 ☑
      displacement T84.428 ☑
      embolism T84.81 ☑
      fibrosis T84.82 ☑
      hemorrhage T84.83 ☑
      infection or inflammation T84.7 ☑
      mechanical NEC T84.498 ☑
      pain T84.84 ☑
      specified type NEC T84.89 ☑
      stenosis T84.85 ☑
      thrombosis T84.86 ☑
    nervous system T85.9 ☑
      brain — *see* Complications, electronic stimulator device, brain
      cranial nerve — *see* Complications, electronic stimulator device, peripheral nerve
      embolism T85.810 ☑
      fibrosis T85.820 ☑
      gastric nerve — *see* Complications, electronic stimulator device, peripheral nerve
      hemorrhage T85.830 ☑
      infection and inflammation T85.738 ☑
      mechanical
        breakdown T85.118 ☑
        displacement T85.128 ☑
        leakage T85.199 ☑
        malposition T85.128 ☑
        obstruction T85.199 ☑
        perforation T85.199 ☑
        protrusion T85.199 ☑
        specified NEC T85.199 ☑
      pain T85.840 ☑
      peripheral nerve — *see* Complications, electronic stimulator device, peripheral nerve
      sacral nerve — *see* Complications, electronic stimulator device, peripheral nerve
      specified type NEC T85.890 ☑
      spinal cord — *see* Complications, electronic stimulator device, spinal cord
      stenosis T85.850 ☑
      thrombosis T85.860 ☑
      vagal nerve — *see* Complications, electronic stimulator device, peripheral nerve
    peripheral nerve T85.9 ☑
      embolism T85.810 ☑
      fibrosis T85.820 ☑
      hemorrhage T85.830 ☑
      infection and inflammation T85.732 ☑
      mechanical
        breakdown T85.111 ☑
        displacement T85.121 ☑
        leakage T85.191 ☑
        malposition T85.121 ☑
        obstruction T85.191 ☑
        perforation T85.191 ☑
        protrusion T85.191 ☑
        specified NEC T85.191 ☑
      pain T85.840 ☑
      specified type NEC T85.890 ☑
      stenosis T85.850 ☑
      thrombosis T85.860 ☑
    spinal cord T85.9 ☑
      embolism T85.810 ☑
      fibrosis T85.820 ☑
      hemorrhage T85.830 ☑
      infection and inflammation T85.733 ☑

Complication(s) — *continued*
  electronic stimulator device — *continued*
    spinal cord — *continued*
      mechanical
        breakdown T85.112 ☑
        displacement T85.122 ☑
        leakage T85.192 ☑
        malposition T85.122 ☑
        obstruction T85.192 ☑
        perforation T85.192 ☑
        protrusion T85.192 ☑
        specified NEC T85.192 ☑
      pain T85.840 ☑
      specified type NEC T85.890 ☑
      stenosis T85.850 ☑
      thrombosis T85.860 ☑
    urinary T83.9 ☑
      embolism T83.81 ☑
      fibrosis T83.82 ☑
      hemorrhage T83.83 ☑
      infection and inflammation T83.598 ☑
      mechanical
        breakdown T83.110 ☑
        displacement T83.120 ☑
        malposition T83.120 ☑
        perforation T83.190 ☑
        protrusion T83.190 ☑
        specified NEC T83.190 ☑
      pain T83.84 ☑
      specified type NEC T83.89 ☑
      stenosis T83.85 ☑
      thrombosis T83.86 ☑
  electroshock therapy T88.9 ☑
    specified NEC T88.8 ☑
  endocrine E34.9
    postprocedural
      adrenal hypofunction E89.6
      hypoinsulinemia E89.1
      hypoparathyroidism E89.2
      hypopituitarism E89.3
      hypothyroidism E89.0
      ovarian failure E89.40
        asymptomatic E89.40
        symptomatic E89.41
      specified NEC E89.89
      testicular hypofunction E89.5
  endodontic treatment NEC M27.59
  enterostomy (stoma) K94.10
    hemorrhage K94.11
    infection K94.12
    malfunction K94.13
    mechanical K94.13
    specified complication NEC K94.19
  episiotomy, disruption O90.1
  esophageal anti-reflux device T85.9 ☑
    embolism T85.818 ☑
    fibrosis T85.828 ☑
    hemorrhage T85.838 ☑
    infection and inflammation T85.79 ☑
    mechanical
      breakdown T85.511 ☑
      displacement T85.521 ☑
      malfunction T85.511 ☑
      malposition T85.521 ☑
      obstruction T85.591 ☑
      perforation T85.591 ☑
      protrusion T85.591 ☑
      specified NEC T85.591 ☑
    pain T85.848 ☑
    specified type NEC T85.898 ☑
    stenosis T85.858 ☑
    thrombosis T85.868 ☑
  esophagostomy K94.30
    hemorrhage K94.31
    infection K94.32
    malfunction K94.33
    mechanical K94.33
    specified complication NEC K94.39
  extracorporeal circulation T80.90 ☑
  extremity artery (bypass) graft T82.9 ☑
    arteriosclerosis — *see* Arteriosclerosis, extremities, bypass graft
    embolism T82.818 ☑
    fibrosis T82.828 ☑
    hemorrhage T82.838 ☑
    infection and inflammation T82.7 ☑

Complication(s) — *continued*
  extremity artery graft — *continued*
    mechanical
      breakdown T82.318 ☑
        femoral artery T82.312 ☑
      displacement T82.328 ☑
        femoral artery T82.322 ☑
      leakage T82.338 ☑
        femoral artery T82.332 ☑
      malposition T82.328 ☑
        femoral artery T82.322 ☑
      obstruction T82.398 ☑
        femoral artery T82.392 ☑
      perforation T82.398 ☑
        femoral artery T82.392 ☑
      protrusion T82.398 ☑
        femoral artery T82.392 ☑
    pain T82.848 ☑
    specified type NEC T82.898 ☑
    stenosis T82.858 ☑
    thrombosis T82.868 ☑
  eye H57.9
    corneal graft — *see* Complications, graft, cornea
    implant (prosthetic) T85.9 ☑
      embolism T85.818 ☑
      fibrosis T85.828 ☑
      hemorrhage T85.838 ☑
      infection and inflammation T85.79 ☑
      mechanical
        breakdown T85.318 ☑
        displacement T85.328 ☑
        leakage T85.398 ☑
        malposition T85.328 ☑
        obstruction T85.398 ☑
        perforation T85.398 ☑
        protrusion T85.398 ☑
        specified NEC T85.398 ☑
      pain T85.848 ☑
      specified type NEC T85.898 ☑
      stenosis T85.858 ☑
      thrombosis T85.868 ☑
    intraocular lens — *see* Complications, intraocular lens
    orbital prosthesis — *see* Complications, orbital prosthesis
  female genital N94.9
    device, implant or graft NEC — *see* Complications, genitourinary, device or implant, genital tract
  femoral artery (bypass) graft — *see* Complication, extremity artery (bypass) graft
  fixation device, internal (orthopedic) T84.9 ☑
    infection and inflammation T84.60 ☑
      arm T84.61- ☑
        humerus T84.61- ☑
        radius T84.61- ☑
        ulna T84.61- ☑
      leg T84.629 ☑
        femur T84.62- ☑
        fibula T84.62- ☑
        tibia T84.62- ☑
      specified site NEC T84.89 ☑
      spine T84.63 ☑
    mechanical
      breakdown
        limb T84.119 ☑
          carpal T84.210 ☑
          femur T84.11- ☑
          fibula T84.11- ☑
          humerus T84.11- ☑
          metacarpal T84.210 ☑
          metatarsal T84.213 ☑
          phalanx
            foot T84.213 ☑
            hand T84.210 ☑
          radius T84.11- ☑
          tarsal T84.213 ☑
          tibia T84.11- ☑
          ulna T84.11- ☑
        specified bone NEC T84.218 ☑
        spine T84.216 ☑
      displacement
        limb T84.129 ☑
          carpal T84.220 ☑
          femur T84.12- ☑
          fibula T84.12- ☑
          humerus T84.12- ☑

▼ Subterms under main terms may continue to next column or page   ☑ Additional Character Required — Refer to the Tabular List for Character Selection   61

Complication — Complication

Complication(s) — *continued*
fixation device, internal — *continued*
mechanical — *continued*
displacement — *continued*
limb — *continued*
metacarpal T84.220 ☑
metatarsal T84.223 ☑
phalanx
foot T84.223 ☑
hand T84.220 ☑
radius T84.12- ☑
tarsal T84.223 ☑
tibia T84.12- ☑
ulna T84.12- ☑
specified bone NEC T84.228 ☑
spine T84.226 ☑
malposition — *see* Complications, fixation device, internal, mechanical, displacement
obstruction — *see* Complications, fixation device, internal, mechanical, specified type NEC
perforation — *see* Complications, fixation device, internal, mechanical, specified type NEC
protrusion — *see* Complications, fixation device, internal, mechanical, specified type NEC
specified type NEC
limb T84.199 ☑
carpal T84.290 ☑
femur T84.19- ☑
fibula T84.19- ☑
humerus T84.19- ☑
metacarpal T84.290 ☑
metatarsal T84.293 ☑
phalanx
foot T84.293 ☑
hand T84.290 ☑
radius T84.19- ☑
tarsal T84.293 ☑
tibia T84.19- ☑
ulna T84.19- ☑
specified bone NEC T84.298 ☑
vertebra T84.296 ☑
specified type NEC T84.89 ☑
embolism T84.81 ☑
fibrosis T84.82 ☑
hemorrhage T84.83 ☑
pain T84.84 ☑
specified complication NEC T84.89 ☑
stenosis T84.85 ☑
thrombosis T84.86 ☑
following
acute myocardial infarction NEC I23.8
aneurysm (false) (of cardiac wall) (of heart wall) (ruptured) I23.3
angina I23.7
atrial
septal defect I23.1
thrombosis I23.6
cardiac wall rupture I23.3
chordae tendinae rupture I23.4
defect
septal
atrial (heart) I23.1
ventricular (heart) I23.2
hemopericardium I23.0
papillary muscle rupture I23.5
rupture
cardiac wall I23.3
with hemopericardium I23.0
chordae tendineae I23.4
papillary muscle I23.5
specified NEC I23.8
thrombosis
atrium I23.6
auricular appendage I23.6
ventricle (heart) I23.6
ventricular
septal defect I23.2
thrombosis I23.6
ectopic or molar pregnancy O08.9
cardiac arrest O08.81
sepsis O08.82
specified type NEC O08.89
urinary tract infection O08.83
termination of pregnancy — *see* Abortion
gastrointestinal K92.9
bile duct prosthesis — *see* Complications, bile duct implant

Complication(s) — *continued*
gastrointestinal — *continued*
esophageal anti-reflux device — *see* Complications, esophageal anti-reflux device
postoperative
colostomy — *see* Complications, colostomy
dumping syndrome K91.1
enterostomy — *see* Complications, enterostomy
gastrostomy — *see* Complications, gastrostomy
malabsorption NEC K91.2
obstruction — *see also* Obstruction, intestine, postoperative K91.30
postcholecystectomy syndrome K91.5
specified NEC K91.89
vomiting after GI surgery K91.0
prosthetic device or implant
bile duct prosthesis — *see* Complications, bile duct implant
esophageal anti-reflux device — *see* Complications, esophageal anti-reflux device
specified type NEC
embolism T85.818 ☑
fibrosis T85.828 ☑
hemorrhage T85.838 ☑
mechanical
breakdown T85.518 ☑
displacement T85.528 ☑
malfunction T85.518 ☑
malposition T85.528 ☑
obstruction T85.598 ☑
perforation T85.598 ☑
protrusion T85.598 ☑
specified NEC T85.598 ☑
pain T85.848 ☑
specified complication NEC T85.898 ☑
stenosis T85.858 ☑
thrombosis T85.868 ☑
gastrostomy (stoma) K94.20
hemorrhage K94.21
infection K94.22
malfunction K94.23
mechanical K94.23
specified complication NEC K94.29
genitourinary
device or implant T83.9 ☑
genital tract T83.9 ☑
infection or inflammation T83.69 ☑
intrauterine contraceptive device — *see* Complications, intrauterine, contraceptive device
mechanical — *see* Complications, by device, mechanical
mesh — *see* Complications, prosthetic device or implant, mesh
penile prosthesis — *see* Complications, prosthetic device, penile
specified type NEC T83.89 ☑
embolism T83.81 ☑
fibrosis T83.82 ☑
hemorrhage T83.83 ☑
pain T83.84 ☑
specified complication NEC T83.89 ☑
stenosis T83.85 ☑
thrombosis T83.86 ☑
vaginal mesh — *see* Complications, prosthetic device or implant, mesh
urinary system T83.9 ☑
cystostomy catheter — *see* Complication, catheter, cystostomy
electronic stimulator — *see* Complications, electronic stimulator device, urinary
indwelling urethral catheter — *see* Complications, catheter, urethral, indwelling
infection or inflammation T83.598 ☑
indwelling urethral catheter T83.511 ☑
kidney transplant — *see* Complication, transplant, kidney
organ graft — *see* Complication, graft, urinary organ
specified type NEC T83.89 ☑
embolism T83.81 ☑
fibrosis T83.82 ☑
hemorrhage T83.83 ☑
mechanical T83.198 ☑
breakdown T83.118 ☑
displacement T83.128 ☑
malfunction T83.118 ☑

Complication(s) — *continued*
genitourinary — *continued*
device or implant — *continued*
urinary system — *continued*
specified type — *continued*
mechanical — *continued*
malposition T83.128 ☑
obstruction T83.198 ☑
perforation T83.198 ☑
protrusion T83.198 ☑
specified NEC T83.198 ☑
sphincter implant — *see* Complications, implant, urinary sphincter
sphincter, implanted T83.191 ☑
stent (ileal conduit) (nephroureteral) T83.193 ☑
pain T83.84 ☑
specified complication NEC T83.89 ☑
stenosis T83.85 ☑
thrombosis T83.86 ☑
ureteral indwelling T83.192 ☑
postprocedural
pelvic peritoneal adhesions N99.4
renal failure N99.0
specified NEC N99.89
stoma — *see* Complications, stoma, urinary tract
urethral stricture — *see* Stricture, urethra, postprocedural
vaginal
adhesions N99.2
vault prolapse N99.3
graft (bypass) (patch) — *see also* Complications, prosthetic device or implant
aorta — *see* Complications, graft, vascular
arterial — *see* Complication, graft, vascular
bone T86.839
failure T86.831
infection T86.832
mechanical T84.318 ☑
breakdown T84.318 ☑
displacement T84.328 ☑
protrusion T84.398 ☑
specified type NEC T84.398 ☑
rejection T86.830
specified type NEC T86.838
carotid artery — *see* Complications, graft, vascular
cornea T86.849
failure T86.841
infection T86.842
mechanical T85.398 ☑
breakdown T85.318 ☑
displacement T85.328 ☑
protrusion T85.398 ☑
specified type NEC T85.398 ☑
rejection T86.840
retroprosthetic membrane T85.398 ☑
specified type NEC T86.848
femoral artery (bypass) — *see* Complication, extremity artery (bypass) graft
genital organ or tract — *see* Complications, genitourinary, device or implant, genital tract
muscle T84.9 ☑
breakdown T84.410 ☑
displacement T84.420 ☑
embolism T84.81 ☑
fibrosis T84.82 ☑
hemorrhage T84.83 ☑
infection and inflammation T84.7 ☑
mechanical NEC T84.490 ☑
pain T84.84 ☑
specified type NEC T84.89 ☑
stenosis T84.85 ☑
thrombosis T84.86 ☑
nerve — *see* Complication, prosthetic device or implant, specified NEC
skin — *see* Complications, prosthetic device or implant, skin graft
tendon T84.9 ☑
breakdown T84.410 ☑
displacement T84.420 ☑
embolism T84.81 ☑
fibrosis T84.82 ☑
hemorrhage T84.83 ☑
infection and inflammation T84.7 ☑
mechanical NEC T84.490 ☑
pain T84.84 ☑
specified type NEC T84.89 ☑

☑ **Additional Character Required** — Refer to the Tabular List for Character Selection   ▽ **Subterms under main terms may continue to next column or page**

Complication(s) — *continued*
graft — *see also* Complications, prosthetic device or
   implant — *continued*
   tendon — *continued*
      stenosis T84.85 ☑
      thrombosis T84.86 ☑
   urinary organ T83.9 ☑
      embolism T83.81 ☑
      fibrosis T83.82 ☑
      hemorrhage T83.83 ☑
      infection and inflammation T83.598 ☑
         indwelling urethral catheter T83.511 ☑
      mechanical
         breakdown T83.21 ☑
         displacement T83.22 ☑
         erosion T83.24 ☑
         exposure T83.25 ☑
         leakage T83.23 ☑
         malposition T83.22 ☑
         obstruction T83.29 ☑
         perforation T83.29 ☑
         protrusion T83.29 ☑
         specified NEC T83.29 ☑
      pain T83.84 ☑
      specified type NEC T83.89 ☑
      stenosis T83.85 ☑
      thrombosis T83.86 ☑
   vascular T82.9 ☑
      embolism T82.818 ☑
      femoral artery — *see* Complication, extremity
         artery (bypass) graft
      fibrosis T82.828 ☑
      hemorrhage T82.838 ☑
      mechanical
         breakdown T82.319 ☑
           aorta (bifurcation) T82.310 ☑
           carotid artery T82.311 ☑
           specified vessel NEC T82.318 ☑
         displacement T82.329 ☑
           aorta (bifurcation) T82.320 ☑
           carotid artery T82.321 ☑
           specified vessel NEC T82.328 ☑
         leakage T82.339 ☑
           aorta (bifurcation) T82.330 ☑
           carotid artery T82.331 ☑
           specified vessel NEC T82.338 ☑
         malposition T82.329 ☑
           aorta (bifurcation) T82.320 ☑
           carotid artery T82.321 ☑
           specified vessel NEC T82.328 ☑
         obstruction T82.399 ☑
           aorta (bifurcation) T82.390 ☑
           carotid artery T82.391 ☑
           specified vessel NEC T82.398 ☑
         perforation T82.399 ☑
           aorta (bifurcation) T82.390 ☑
           carotid artery T82.391 ☑
           specified vessel NEC T82.398 ☑
         protrusion T82.399 ☑
           aorta (bifurcation) T82.390 ☑
           carotid artery T82.391 ☑
           specified vessel NEC T82.398 ☑
      pain T82.848 ☑
      specified complication NEC T82.898 ☑
      stenosis T82.858 ☑
      thrombosis T82.868 ☑
heart I51.9
   assist device
      infection and inflammation T82.7 ☑
   following acute myocardial infarction — *see* Com-
      plications, following, acute myocardial infarc-
      tion
   postoperative — *see* Complications, circulatory
      system
   transplant — *see* Complication, transplant, heart
      and lung(s) — *see* Complications, transplant,
      heart, with lung
   valve
      graft (biological) T82.9 ☑
         embolism T82.817 ☑
         fibrosis T82.827 ☑
         hemorrhage T82.837 ☑
         infection and inflammation T82.7 ☑
         mechanical T82.228 ☑
           breakdown T82.221 ☑
           displacement T82.222 ☑

Complication(s) — *continued*
heart — *continued*
   valve — *continued*
      graft — *continued*
         mechanical — *continued*
           leakage T82.223 ☑
           malposition T82.222 ☑
           obstruction T82.228 ☑
           perforation T82.228 ☑
           protrusion T82.228 ☑
         pain T82.847 ☑
         specified type NEC T82.897 ☑
         stenosis T82.857 ☑
         thrombosis T82.867 ☑
      prosthesis T82.9 ☑
         embolism T82.817 ☑
         fibrosis T82.827 ☑
         hemorrhage T82.837 ☑
         infection or inflammation T82.6 ☑
         mechanical T82.09 ☑
           breakdown T82.01 ☑
           displacement T82.02 ☑
           leakage T82.03 ☑
           malposition T82.02 ☑
           obstruction T82.09 ☑
           perforation T82.09 ☑
           protrusion T82.09 ☑
         pain T82.847 ☑
         specified type NEC T82.897 ☑
           mechanical T82.09 ☑
         stenosis T82.857 ☑
         thrombosis T82.867 ☑
hematoma
   intraoperative — *see* Complication, intraoperative,
      hemorrhage
   postprocedural — *see* Complication, postprocedu-
      ral, hematoma
hemodialysis — *see* Complications, dialysis
hemorrhage
   intraoperative — *see* Complication, intraoperative,
      hemorrhage
   postprocedural — *see* Complication, postprocedu-
      ral, hemorrhage
ileostomy (stoma) — *see* Complications, enterostomy
immunization (procedure) — *see* Complications, vaccination
implant — *see also* Complications, by site and type
   urinary sphincter T83.9 ☑
      embolism T83.81 ☑
      fibrosis T83.82 ☑
      hemorrhage T83.83 ☑
      infection and inflammation T83.591 ☑
      mechanical
         breakdown T83.111 ☑
         displacement T83.121 ☑
         leakage T83.191 ☑
         malposition T83.121 ☑
         obstruction T83.191 ☑
         perforation T83.191 ☑
         protrusion T83.191 ☑
         specified NEC T83.191 ☑
      pain T83.84 ☑
      specified type NEC T83.89 ☑
      stenosis T83.85 ☑
      thrombosis T83.86 ☑
infusion (procedure) T80.90 ☑
   air embolism T80.0 ☑
   blood — *see* Complications, transfusion
   catheter — *see* Complications, catheter
   infection T80.29 ☑
   pump — *see* Complications, cardiovascular, device
      or implant
   sepsis T80.29 ☑
   serum reaction — *see also* Reaction, serum
      T80.69 ☑
      anaphylactic shock — *see also* Shock, anaphylac-
         tic T80.59 ☑
      specified type NEC T80.89 ☑
inhalation therapy NEC T81.81 ☑
injection (procedure) T80.90 ☑
   drug reaction — *see* Reaction, drug
   infection T80.29 ☑
   sepsis T80.29 ☑
   serum (prophylactic) (therapeutic) — *see* Complica-
      tions, vaccination
   specified type NEC T80.89 ☑

Complication(s) — *continued*
injection — *continued*
   vaccine (any) — *see* Complications, vaccination
   inoculation (any) — *see* Complications, vaccination
insulin pump
   infection and inflammation T85.72 ☑
   mechanical
      breakdown T85.614 ☑
      displacement T85.624 ☑
      leakage T85.633 ☑
      malposition T85.624 ☑
      obstruction T85.694 ☑
      perforation T85.694 ☑
      protrusion T85.694 ☑
      specified NEC T85.694 ☑
intestinal pouch NEC K91.858 ☑
intraocular lens (prosthetic) T85.9 ☑
   embolism T85.818 ☑
   fibrosis T85.828 ☑
   hemorrhage T85.838 ☑
   infection and inflammation T85.79 ☑
   mechanical
      breakdown T85.21 ☑
      displacement T85.22 ☑
      malposition T85.22 ☑
      obstruction T85.29 ☑
      perforation T85.29 ☑
      protrusion T85.29 ☑
      specified NEC T85.29 ☑
   pain T85.848 ☑
   specified type NEC T85.898 ☑
   stenosis T85.858 ☑
   thrombosis T85.868 ☑
intraoperative (intraprocedural)
   cardiac arrest — *see also* Infarct, myocardium, asso-
      ciated with revascularization procedure
      during cardiac surgery I97.710
      during other surgery I97.711
   cardiac functional disturbance NEC — *see also* In-
      farct, myocardium, associated with revascular-
      ization procedure
      during cardiac surgery I97.790
      during other surgery I97.791
   hemorrhage (hematoma) (of)
      circulatory system organ or structure
         during cardiac bypass I97.411
         during cardiac catheterization I97.410
         during other circulatory system procedure
           I97.418
         during other procedure I97.42
      digestive system organ
         during procedure on digestive system K91.61
         during procedure on other organ K91.62
      ear
         during procedure on ear and mastoid process
           H95.21
         during procedure on other organ H95.22
      endocrine system organ or structure
         during procedure on endocrine system organ
           or structure E36.01
         during procedure on other organ E36.02
      eye and adnexa
         during ophthalmic procedure H59.11- ☑
         during other procedure H59.12- ☑
      genitourinary organ or structure
         during procedure on genitourinary organ or
           structure N99.61
         during procedure on other organ N99.62
      mastoid process
         during procedure on ear and mastoid process
           H95.21
         during procedure on other organ H95.22
      musculoskeletal structure
         during musculoskeletal surgery M96.810
         during non-orthopedic surgery M96.811
         during orthopedic surgery M96.810
      nervous system
         during a nervous system procedure G97.31
         during other procedure G97.32
      respiratory system
         during other procedure J95.62
         during procedure on respiratory system organ
           or structure J95.61
      skin and subcutaneous tissue
         during a dermatologic procedure L76.01
         during a procedure on other organ L76.02
      spleen
         during a procedure on other organ D78.02

Complication(s) — *continued*
  intraoperative — *continued*
    hemorrhage — *continued*
      spleen — *continued*
        during a procedure on the spleen D78.01
      puncture or laceration (accidental) (unintentional) (of)
        brain
          during a nervous system procedure G97.48
          during other procedure G97.49
        circulatory system organ or structure
          during circulatory system procedure I97.51
          during other procedure I97.52
        digestive system
          during procedure on digestive system K91.71
          during procedure on other organ K91.72
        ear
          during procedure on ear and mastoid process H95.31
          during procedure on other organ H95.32
        endocrine system organ or structure
          during procedure on endocrine system organ or structure E36.11
          during procedure on other organ E36.12
        eye and adnexa
          during ophthalmic procedure H59.21- ☑
          during other procedure H59.22- ☑
        genitourinary organ or structure
          during procedure on genitourinary organ or structure N99.71
          during procedure on other organ N99.72
        mastoid process
          during procedure on ear and mastoid process H95.31
          during procedure on other organ H95.32
        musculoskeletal structure
          during musculoskeletal surgery M96.820
          during non-orthopedic surgery M96.821
          during orthopedic surgery M96.820
        nervous system
          during a nervous system procedure G97.48
          during other procedure G97.49
        respiratory system
          during other procedure J95.72
          during procedure on respiratory system organ or structure J95.71
        skin and subcutaneous tissue
          during a dermatologic procedure L76.11
          during a procedure on other organ L76.12
        spleen
          during a procedure on other organ D78.12
          during a procedure on the spleen D78.11
    specified NEC
      circulatory system I97.88
      digestive system K91.81
      ear H95.88
      endocrine system E36.8
      eye and adnexa H59.88
      genitourinary system N99.81
      mastoid process H95.88
      musculoskeletal structure M96.89
      nervous system G97.81
      respiratory system J95.88
      skin and subcutaneous tissue L76.81
      spleen D78.81
  intraperitoneal catheter (dialysis) (infusion) — *see* Complications, catheter, intraperitoneal
  intrathecal infusion pump
    infection and inflammation T85.738 ☑
    mechanical
      breakdown T85.615 ☑
      displacement T85.625 ☑
      leakage T85.635 ☑
      malfunction T85.695 ☑
      malposition T85.625 ☑
      obstruction T85.695 ☑
      perforation T85.695 ☑
      protrusion T85.695 ☑
      specified NEC T85.695 ☑
  intrauterine
    contraceptive device
      embolism T83.81 ☑
      fibrosis T83.82 ☑
      hemorrhage T83.83 ☑
      infection and inflammation T83.69 ☑
      mechanical
        breakdown T83.31 ☑
        displacement T83.32 ☑

Complication(s) — *continued*
  intrauterine — *continued*
    contraceptive device — *continued*
      mechanical — *continued*
        malposition T83.32 ☑
        obstruction T83.39 ☑
        perforation T83.39 ☑
        protrusion T83.39 ☑
        specified NEC T83.39 ☑
      pain T83.84 ☑
      specified type NEC T83.89 ☑
      stenosis T83.85 ☑
      thrombosis T83.86 ☑
    procedure (fetal), to newborn P96.5
  jejunostomy (stoma) — *see* Complications, enterostomy
  joint prosthesis, internal T84.9 ☑
    breakage (fracture) T84.01- ☑
    dislocation T84.02- ☑
    fracture T84.01- ☑
    infection or inflammation T84.50 ☑
      hip T84.5- ☑
      knee T84.5- ☑
      specified joint NEC T84.59 ☑
    instability T84.02- ☑
    malposition — *see* Complications, joint prosthesis, mechanical, displacement
    mechanical
      breakage, broken T84.01- ☑
      dislocation T84.02- ☑
      fracture T84.01- ☑
      instability T84.02- ☑
      leakage — *see* Complications, joint prosthesis, mechanical, specified NEC
      loosening T84.039 ☑
        hip T84.03- ☑
        knee T84.03- ☑
        specified joint NEC T84.038 ☑
      obstruction — *see* Complications, joint prosthesis, mechanical, specified NEC
      perforation — *see* Complications, joint prosthesis, mechanical, specified NEC
        osteolysis T84.059 ☑
          hip T84.05- ☑
          knee T84.05- ☑
          other specified joint T84.058 ☑
        periprosthetic T84.059 ☑
      protrusion — *see* Complications, joint prosthesis, mechanical, specified NEC
      specified complication NEC T84.099 ☑
        hip T84.09- ☑
        knee T84.09- ☑
        other specified joint T84.098 ☑
      subluxation T84.02- ☑
      wear of articular bearing surface T84.069 ☑
        hip T84.06- ☑
        knee T84.06- ☑
        other specified joint T84.068 ☑
    specified joint NEC T84.89 ☑
    embolism T84.81 ☑
    fibrosis T84.82 ☑
    hemorrhage T84.83 ☑
    pain T84.84 ☑
    specified complication NEC T84.89 ☑
    stenosis T84.85 ☑
    thrombosis T84.86 ☑
    subluxation T84.02- ☑
  kidney transplant — *see* Complications, transplant, kidney
  labor O75.9
    specified NEC O75.89
  liver transplant (immune or nonimmune) — *see* Complications, transplant, liver
  lumbar puncture G97.1
    cerebrospinal fluid leak G97.0
    headache or reaction G97.1
  lung transplant — *see* Complications, transplant, lung and heart — *see* Complications, transplant, lung, with heart
  male genital N50.9
    device, implant or graft — *see* Complications, genitourinary, device or implant, genital tract
    postprocedural or postoperative — *see* Complications, genitourinary, postprocedural
      specified NEC N99.89

Complication(s) — *continued*
  mastoid (process) procedure
    intraoperative H95.88
      hematoma — *see* Complications, intraoperative hemorrhage (hematoma) (of), mastoid process
      hemorrhage — *see* Complications, intraoperative, hemorrhage (hematoma) (of), mastoid process
      laceration — *see* Complications, intraoperative puncture or laceration, mastoid process
      specified NEC H95.88
    postmastoidectomy — *see* Complications, postmastoidectomy
    postoperative H95.89
      external ear canal stenosis H95.81 ☑
      hematoma — *see* Complications, postprocedural hematoma (of), mastoid process
      hemorrhage — *see* Complications, postprocedural, hemorrhage (of), mastoid process
      postmastoidectomy — *see* Complications, postmastoidectomy
      seroma — *see* Complications, postprocedural, seroma (of), mastoid process
      specified NEC H95.89
  mastoidectomy cavity — *see* Complications, postmastoidectomy
  mechanical — *see* Complications, by site and type, mechanical
  medical procedures — *see also* Complication(s), intraoperative T88.9 ☑
  metabolic E88.9
    postoperative E89.89
    specified NEC E89.89
  molar pregnancy NOS O08.9
    damage to pelvic organs O08.6
    embolism O08.2
    genital infection O08.0
    hemorrhage (delayed) (excessive) O08.1
    metabolic disorder O08.5
    renal failure O08.4
    shock O08.3
    specified type NEC O08.0
    venous complication NEC O08.7
  musculoskeletal system — *see also* Complication, intraoperative (intraprocedural), by site
    device, implant or graft NEC — *see* Complications, orthopedic, device or implant
    internal fixation (nail) (plate) (rod) — *see* Complications, fixation device, internal
    joint prosthesis — *see* Complications, joint prosthesis
    post radiation M96.89
      kyphosis M96.2
      scoliosis M96.5
      specified complication NEC M96.89
    postoperative (postprocedural) M96.89
      with osteoporosis — *see* Osteoporosis
      fracture following insertion of device — *see* Fracture, following insertion of orthopedic implant, joint prosthesis or bone plate
      joint instability after prosthesis removal M96.89
      lordosis M96.4
      postlaminectomy syndrome NEC M96.1
        kyphosis M96.3
      pseudarthrosis M96.0
      specified complication NEC M96.89
  nephrostomy (stoma) — *see* Complications, stoma, urinary tract, external NEC
  nervous system G98.8
    central G96.9
    device, implant or graft — *see also* Complication, prosthetic device or implant, specified NEC
      electronic stimulator (electrode(s)) — *see* Complications, electronic stimulator device
      specified NEC
        infection and inflammation T85.738 ☑
        mechanical T85.695 ☑
          breakdown T85.615 ☑
          displacement T85.625 ☑
          leakage T85.635 ☑
          malfunction T85.695 ☑
          malposition T85.625 ☑
          obstruction T85.695 ☑
          perforation T85.695 ☑
          protrusion T85.695 ☑
          specified NEC T85.695 ☑

Complication(s) — *continued*
nervous system — *continued*
　device, implant or graft — *see also* Complication,
　　prosthetic device or implant, specified —
　　continued
　　ventricular shunt — *see* Complications, ventricu-
　　　lar shunt
　　electronic stimulator (electrode(s)) — *see* Complica-
　　　tions, electronic stimulator device
　　postprocedural G97.82
　　　intracranial hypotension G97.2
　　　specified NEC G97.82
　　　spinal fluid leak G97.0
　newborn, due to intrauterine (fetal) procedure P96.5
　nonabsorbable (permanent) sutures — *see* Complica-
　　tion, sutures, permanent
obstetric O75.9
　procedure (instrumental) (manual) (surgical) speci-
　　fied NEC O75.4
　specified NEC O75.89
　surgical wound NEC O90.89
　　hematoma O90.2
　　infection O86.00
ocular lens implant — *see* Complications, intraocular
　lens
ophthalmologic
　postprocedural bleb — *see* Blebitis
orbital prosthesis T85.9 ☑
　embolism T85.818 ☑
　fibrosis T85.828 ☑
　hemorrhage T85.838 ☑
　infection and inflammation T85.79 ☑
　mechanical
　　breakdown T85.31- ☑
　　displacement T85.32- ☑
　　malposition T85.32- ☑
　　obstruction T85.39- ☑
　　perforation T85.39- ☑
　　protrusion T85.39- ☑
　　specified NEC T85.39- ☑
　pain T85.848 ☑
　specified type NEC T85.898 ☑
　stenosis T85.858 ☑
　thrombosis T85.868 ☑
organ or tissue transplant (partial) (total) — *see* Com-
　plications, transplant
orthopedic — *see also* Disorder, soft tissue
　device or implant T84.9 ☑
　　bone
　　　device or implant — *see* Complication, bone,
　　　　device NEC
　　　graft — *see* Complication, graft, bone
　　breakdown T84.418 ☑
　　displacement T84.428 ☑
　　electronic bone stimulator — *see* Complications,
　　　electronic stimulator device, bone
　　embolism T84.81 ☑
　　fibrosis T84.82 ☑
　　fixation device — *see* Complication, fixation de-
　　　vice, internal
　　hemorrhage T84.83 ☑
　　infection or inflammation T84.7 ☑
　　joint prosthesis — *see* Complication, joint pros-
　　　thesis, internal
　　malfunction T84.418 ☑
　　malposition T84.428 ☑
　　mechanical NEC T84.498 ☑
　　muscle graft — *see* Complications, graft, muscle
　　obstruction T84.498 ☑
　　pain T84.84 ☑
　　perforation T84.498 ☑
　　protrusion T84.498 ☑
　　specified complication NEC T84.89 ☑
　　stenosis T84.85 ☑
　　tendon graft — *see* Complications, graft, tendon
　　thrombosis T84.86 ☑
　fracture (following insertion of device) — *see* Frac-
　　ture, following insertion of orthopedic im-
　　plant, joint prosthesis or bone plate
　postprocedural M96.89
　　fracture — *see* Fracture, following insertion of
　　　orthopedic implant, joint prosthesis or
　　　bone plate
　　postlaminectomy syndrome NEC M96.1
　　　kyphosis M96.3
　　　lordosis M96.4

Complication(s) — *continued*
orthopedic — *see also* Disorder, soft tissue — *contin-
　ued*
　postprocedural — *continued*
　　postradiation
　　　kyphosis M96.2
　　　scoliosis M96.5
　　　pseudarthrosis post-fusion M96.0
　　　specified type NEC M96.89
pacemaker (cardiac) — *see* Complications, cardiovas-
　cular device or implant, electronic
pancreas transplant — *see* Complications, transplant,
　pancreas
penile prosthesis (implant) — *see* Complications,
　prosthetic device, penile
perfusion NEC T80.90 ☑
perineal repair (obstetrical) NEC O90.89
　disruption O90.1
　hematoma O90.2
　infection (following delivery) O86.09
phototherapy T88.9 ☑
　specified NEC T88.8 ☑
postmastoidectomy NEC H95.19- ☑
　cyst, mucosal H95.13- ☑
　granulation H95.12- ☑
　inflammation, chronic H95.11- ☑
　recurrent cholesteatoma H95.0- ☑
postoperative — *see* Complications, postprocedural
　circulatory — *see* Complications, circulatory system
　ear — *see* Complications, ear
　endocrine — *see* Complications, endocrine
　eye — *see* Complications, eye
　lumbar puncture G97.1
　　cerebrospinal fluid leak G97.0
　nervous system (central) (peripheral) — *see* Compli-
　　cations, nervous system
　respiratory system — *see* Complications, respiratory
　　system
postprocedural — *see also* Complications, surgical
　procedure
　cardiac arrest — *see also* Infarct, myocardium, asso-
　　ciated with revascularization procedure
　　following cardiac surgery I97.120
　　following other surgery I97.121
　cardiac functional disturbance NEC — *see also* In-
　　farct, myocardium, associated with revascular-
　　ization procedure
　　following cardiac surgery I97.190
　　following other surgery I97.191
　cardiac insufficiency
　　following cardiac surgery I97.110
　　following other surgery I97.111
　chorioretinal scars following retinal surgery
　　H59.81- ☑
　following cataract surgery
　　cataract (lens) fragments H59.02- ☑
　　cystoid macular edema H59.03- ☑
　　specified NEC H59.09- ☑
　　vitreous (touch) syndrome H59.01- ☑
　heart failure
　　following cardiac surgery I97.130
　　following other surgery I97.131
　hematoma (of)
　　circulatory system organ or structure
　　　following cardiac bypass I97.631
　　　following cardiac catheterization I97.630
　　　following other circulatory system procedure
　　　　I97.638
　　　following other procedure I97.621
　　digestive system
　　　following procedure on digestive system
　　　　K91.870
　　　following procedure on other organ K91.871
　　ear
　　　following other procedure H95.52
　　　following procedure on ear and mastoid pro-
　　　　cess H95.51
　　endocrine system
　　　following endocrine system procedure
　　　　E89.820
　　　following other procedure E89.821
　　eye and adnexa
　　　following ophthalmic procedure H59.33- ☑
　　　following other procedure H59.34- ☑
　　genitourinary organ or structure
　　　following procedure on genitourinary organ
　　　　or structure N99.840
　　　following procedure on other organ N99.841

Complication(s) — *continued*
postprocedural — *see also* Complications, surgical
　procedure — *continued*
　hematoma — *continued*
　　mastoid process
　　　following other procedure H95.52
　　　following procedure on ear and mastoid pro-
　　　　cess H95.51
　　musculoskeletal structure
　　　following musculoskeletal surgery M96.840
　　　following non-orthopedic surgery M96.841
　　　following orthopedic surgery M96.840
　　nervous system
　　　following nervous system procedure G97.61
　　　following other procedure G97.62
　　respiratory system
　　　following other procedure J95.861
　　　following procedure on respiratory system
　　　　organ or structure J95.860
　　skin and subcutaneous tissue
　　　following dermatologic procedure L76.31
　　　following procedure on other organ L76.32
　　spleen
　　　following procedure on other organ D78.32
　　　following procedure on the spleen D78.31
　hemorrhage (of)
　　circulatory system organ or structure
　　　following cardiac bypass I97.611
　　　following cardiac catheterization I97.610
　　　following other circulatory system procedure
　　　　I97.618
　　　following other procedure I97.620
　　digestive system
　　　following procedure on digestive system
　　　　K91.840
　　　following procedure on other organ K91.841
　　ear
　　　following other procedure H95.42
　　　following procedure on ear and mastoid pro-
　　　　cess H95.41
　　endocrine system
　　　following endocrine system procedure
　　　　E89.810
　　　following other procedure E89.811
　　eye and adnexa
　　　following ophthalmic procedure H59.31- ☑
　　　following other procedure H59.32- ☑
　　genitourinary organ or structure
　　　following procedure on genitourinary organ
　　　　or structure N99.820
　　　following procedure on other organ N99.821
　　mastoid process
　　　following other procedure H95.42
　　　following procedure on ear and mastoid pro-
　　　　cess H95.41
　　musculoskeletal structure
　　　following musculoskeletal surgery M96.830
　　　following non-orthopedic surgery M96.831
　　　following orthopedic surgery M96.830
　　nervous system
　　　following nervous system procedure G97.51
　　　following other procedure G97.52
　　respiratory system
　　　following a respiratory system procedure
　　　　J95.830
　　　following other procedure J95.831
　　skin and subcutaneous tissue
　　　following a procedure on other organ L76.22
　　　following dermatologic procedure L76.21
　　spleen
　　　following procedure on other organ D78.22
　　　following procedure on the spleen D78.21
　seroma (of)
　　circulatory system organ or structure
　　　following cardiac bypass I97.641
　　　following cardiac catheterization I97.640
　　　following other circulatory system procedure
　　　　I97.648
　　　following other procedure I97.622
　　digestive system
　　　following procedure on digestive system
　　　　K91.872
　　　following procedure on other organ K91.873
　　ear
　　　following other procedure H95.54
　　　following procedure on ear and mastoid pro-
　　　　cess H95.53

Index

Complication(s) — *continued*
postprocedural — *see also* Complications, surgical procedure — *continued*
  seroma — *continued*
    endocrine system
      following endocrine system procedure E89.822
      following other procedure E89.823
    eye and adnexa
      following ophthalmic procedure H59.35- ☑
      following other procedure H59.36- ☑
    genitourinary organ or structure
      following procedure on genitourinary organ or structure N99.842
      following procedure on other organ N99.843
    mastoid process
      following other procedure H95.54
      following procedure on ear and mastoid process H95.53
    musculoskeletal structure
      following musculoskeletal surgery M96.842
      following non-orthopedic surgery M96.843
      following orthopedic surgery M96.842
    nervous system
      following nervous system procedure G97.63
      following other procedure G97.64
    respiratory system
      following other procedure J95.863
      following procedure on respiratory system organ or structure J95.862
    skin and subcutaneous tissue
      following dermatologic procedure L76.33
      following procedure on other organ L76.34
    spleen
      following procedure on other organ D78.34
      following procedure on the spleen D78.33
  specified NEC
    circulatory system I97.89
    digestive K91.89
    ear H95.89
    endocrine E89.89
    eye and adnexa H59.89
    genitourinary N99.89
    mastoid process H95.89
    metabolic E89.89
    musculoskeletal structure M96.89
    nervous system G97.82
    respiratory system J95.89
    skin and subcutaneous tissue L76.82
    spleen D78.89
pregnancy NEC — *see* Pregnancy, complicated by
prosthetic device or implant T85.9 ☑
  bile duct — *see* Complications, bile duct implant
  breast — *see* Complications, breast implant
  bulking agent
    ureteral
      erosion T83.714 ☑
      exposure T83.724 ☑
    urethral
      erosion T83.713 ☑
      exposure T83.723 ☑
  cardiac and vascular NEC — *see* Complications, cardiovascular device or implant
  corneal transplant — *see* Complications, graft, cornea
  electronic nervous system stimulator — *see* Complications, electronic stimulator device
  epidural infusion catheter — *see* Complications, catheter, epidural
  esophageal anti-reflux device — *see* Complications, esophageal anti-reflux device
  genital organ or tract — *see* Complications, genitourinary, device or implant, genital tract
    specified NEC T83.79- ☑
  heart valve — *see* Complications, heart, valve, prosthesis
  infection or inflammation T85.79 ☑
    intestine transplant T86.892
    liver transplant T86.43
    lung transplant T86.812
    pancreas transplant T86.892
    skin graft T86.822
  intraocular lens — *see* Complications, intraocular lens
  intraperitoneal (dialysis) catheter — *see* Complications, catheter, intraperitoneal
  joint — *see* Complications, joint prosthesis, internal
  mechanical NEC T85.698 ☑

Complication(s) — *continued*
prosthetic device or implant — *continued*
  mechanical — *continued*
    dialysis catheter (vascular) — *see also* Complication, catheter, dialysis, mechanical
      peritoneal — *see* Complication, catheter, intraperitoneal, mechanical
    gastrointestinal device T85.598 ☑
    ocular device T85.398 ☑
    subdural (infusion) catheter T85.690 ☑
    suture, permanent T85.692 ☑
      that for bone repair — *see* Complications, fixation device, internal (orthopedic), mechanical
    ventricular shunt
      breakdown T85.01 ☑
      displacement T85.02 ☑
      leakage T85.03 ☑
      malposition T85.02 ☑
      obstruction T85.09 ☑
      perforation T85.09 ☑
      protrusion T85.09 ☑
      specified NEC T85.09 ☑
  mesh
    erosion (to surrounding organ or tissue) T83.718 ☑
      urethral (into pelvic floor muscles) T83.712 ☑
      vaginal (into pelvic floor muscles) T83.711 ☑
    exposure (into surrounding organ or tissue) T83.728 ☑
      urethral (through urethral wall) T83.722 ☑
      vaginal (into vagina) (through vaginal wall) T83.721 ☑
  orbital — *see* Complications, orbital prosthesis
  penile T83.9 ☑
    embolism T83.81 ☑
    fibrosis T83.82 ☑
    hemorrhage T83.83 ☑
    infection and inflammation T83.61 ☑
    mechanical
      breakdown T83.410 ☑
      displacement T83.420 ☑
      leakage T83.490 ☑
      malposition T83.420 ☑
      obstruction T83.490 ☑
      perforation T83.490 ☑
      protrusion T83.490 ☑
      specified NEC T83.490 ☑
    pain T83.84 ☑
    specified type NEC T83.89 ☑
    stenosis T83.85 ☑
    thrombosis T83.86 ☑
  prosthetic materials NEC
    erosion (to surrounding organ or tissue) T83.718 ☑
    exposure (into surrounding organ or tissue) T83.728 ☑
  skin graft T86.829
    artificial skin or decellularized allodermis
      embolism T85.818 ☑
      fibrosis T85.828 ☑
      hemorrhage T85.838 ☑
      infection and inflammation T85.79 ☑
      mechanical
        breakdown T85.613 ☑
        displacement T85.623 ☑
        malfunction T85.613 ☑
        malposition T85.623 ☑
        obstruction T85.693 ☑
        perforation T85.693 ☑
        protrusion T85.693 ☑
        specified NEC T85.693 ☑
      pain T85.848 ☑
      specified type NEC T85.898 ☑
      stenosis T85.858 ☑
      thrombosis T85.868 ☑
    failure T86.821
    infection T86.822
    rejection T86.820
    specified NEC T86.828
  sling
    urethral (female) (male)
      erosion T83.712 ☑
      exposure T83.722 ☑
  specified NEC T85.9 ☑
    embolism T85.818 ☑

Complication(s) — *continued*
prosthetic device or implant — *continued*
  specified — *continued*
    fibrosis T85.828 ☑
    hemorrhage T85.838 ☑
    infection and inflammation T85.79 ☑
    mechanical
      breakdown T85.618 ☑
      displacement T85.628 ☑
      leakage T85.638 ☑
      malfunction T85.618 ☑
      malposition T85.628 ☑
      obstruction T85.698 ☑
      perforation T85.698 ☑
      protrusion T85.698 ☑
      specified NEC T85.698 ☑
    pain T85.848 ☑
    specified type NEC T85.898 ☑
    stenosis T85.858 ☑
    thrombosis T85.868 ☑
  subdural infusion catheter — *see* Complications, catheter, subdural
  sutures — *see* Complications, sutures
  urinary organ or tract NEC — *see* Complications, genitourinary, device or implant, urinary system
  vascular — *see* Complications, cardiovascular device or implant
  ventricular shunt — *see* Complications, ventricular shunt (device)
puerperium — *see* Puerperal
puncture, spinal G97.1
  cerebrospinal fluid leak G97.0
  headache or reaction G97.1
pyelogram N99.89
radiation
  kyphosis M96.2
  scoliosis M96.5
reattached
  extremity (infection) (rejection)
    lower T87.1X- ☑
    upper T87.0X- ☑
  specified body part NEC T87.2
reconstructed breast
  asymmetry between native and reconstructed breast N65.1
  deformity N65.0
  disproportion between native and reconstructed breast N65.1
  excess tissue N65.0
  misshappen N65.0
reimplant NEC — *see also* Complications, prosthetic device or implant
  limb (infection) (rejection) — *see* Complications, reattached, extremity
  organ (partial) (total) — *see* Complications, transplant
  prosthetic device NEC — *see* Complications, prosthetic device
renal N28.9
  allograft — *see* Complications, transplant, kidney
  dialysis — *see* Complications, dialysis
respirator
  mechanical J95.850
    specified NEC J95.859
respiratory system J98.9
  device, implant or graft — *see* Complication, prosthetic device or implant, specified NEC
  lung transplant — *see* Complications, prosthetic device or implant, lung transplant
  postoperative J95.89
    air leak J95.812
    Mendelson's syndrome (chemical pneumonitis) J95.4
    pneumothorax J95.811
    pulmonary insufficiency (acute) (after nonthoracic surgery) J95.2
      chronic J95.3
      following thoracic surgery J95.1
    respiratory failure (acute) J95.821
      acute and chronic J95.822
    specified NEC J95.89
    subglottic stenosis J95.5
    tracheostomy complication — *see* Complications, tracheostomy
  therapy T81.89 ☑
sedation during labor and delivery O74.9

Complication(s) — *continued*
  sedation during labor and delivery — *continued*
    cardiac O74.2
    central nervous system O74.3
    pulmonary NEC O74.1
  shunt — *see also* Complications, prosthetic device or
      implant
    arteriovenous — *see* Complications, arteriovenous,
        shunt
    ventricular (communicating) — *see* Complications,
        ventricular shunt
  skin
    graft T86.829
      failure T86.821
      infection T86.822
      rejection T86.820
      specified type NEC T86.828
  spinal
    anesthesia — *see* Complications, anesthesia, spinal
    catheter (epidural) (subdural) — *see* Complications,
        catheter
    puncture or tap G97.1
      cerebrospinal fluid leak G97.0
      headache or reaction G97.1
  stent
    bile duct — *see* Complications, bile duct prosthesis
    ureteral indwelling
      breakdown T83.112 ☑
      displacement T83.122 ☑
      leakage T83.192 ☑
      malposition T83.122 ☑
      obstruction T83.192 ☑
      perforation T83.192 ☑
      protrusion T83.192 ☑
      specified NEC T83.192 ☑
    urinary NEC (ileal conduit) (nephroureteral)
        T83.193 ☑
      embolism T83.81 ☑
      fibrosis T83.82 ☑
      hemorrhage T83.83 ☑
      infection and inflammation T83.593 ☑
      mechanical
        breakdown T83.113 ☑
        displacement T83.123 ☑
        leakage T83.193 ☑
        malposition T83.123 ☑
        obstruction T83.193 ☑
        perforation T83.193 ☑
        protrusion T83.193 ☑
        specified NEC T83.193 ☑
      pain T83.84 ☑
      specified type NEC T83.89 ☑
      stenosis T83.85 ☑
      thrombosis T83.86 ☑
  vascular
    end stent stenosis — *see* Restenosis, stent
    in stent stenosis — *see* Restenosis, stent
  stoma
    digestive tract
      colostomy — *see* Complications, colostomy
      enterostomy — *see* Complications, enterostomy
      esophagostomy — *see* Complications,
          esophagostomy
      gastrostomy — *see* Complications, gastrostomy
    urinary tract N99.528
      continent N99.538
        hemorrhage N99.530
        herniation N99.533
        infection N99.531
        malfunction N99.532
        specified type NEC N99.538
        stenosis N99.534
      cystostomy — *see* Complications, cystostomy
      external NOS N99.528
      hemorrhage N99.520
      herniation N99.523
      incontinent N99.528
        hemorrhage N99.520
        herniation N99.523
        infection N99.521
        malfunction N99.522
        specified type NEC N99.528
        stenosis N99.524
      infection N99.521
      malfunction N99.522
      specified type NEC N99.528
      stenosis N99.524

Complication(s) — *continued*
  stomach banding — *see* Complication(s), bariatric
      procedure
  stomach stapling — *see* Complication(s), bariatric
      procedure
  surgical material, nonabsorbable — *see* Complication,
      suture, permanent
  surgical procedure (on) T81.9 ☑
    amputation stump (late) — *see* Complications,
        amputation stump
    cardiac — *see* Complications, circulatory system
    cholesteatoma, recurrent — *see* Complications,
        postmastoidectomy, recurrent cholesteatoma
    circulatory (early) — *see* Complications, circulatory
        system
    digestive system — *see* Complications, gastrointesti-
        nal
    dumping syndrome (postgastrectomy) K91.1
    ear — *see* Complications, ear
    elephantiasis or lymphedema I97.89
      postmastectomy I97.2
    emphysema (surgical) T81.82 ☑
    endocrine — *see* Complications, endocrine
    eye — *see* Complications, eye
    fistula (persistent postoperative) T81.83 ☑
    foreign body inadvertently left in wound (sponge)
        (suture) (swab) — *see* Foreign body, acciden-
        tally left during a procedure
    gastrointestinal — *see* Complications, gastrointesti-
        nal
    genitourinary NEC N99.89
    hematoma
      intraoperative — *see* Complication, intraopera-
          tive, hemorrhage
      postprocedural — *see* Complication, postproce-
          dural, hematoma
    hemorrhage
      intraoperative — *see* Complication, intraopera-
          tive, hemorrhage
      postprocedural — *see* Complication, postproce-
          dural, hemorrhage
    hepatic failure K91.82
    hyperglycemia (postpancreatectomy) E89.1
    hypoinsulinemia (postpancreatectomy) E89.1
    hypoparathyroidism (postparathyroidectomy) E89.2
    hypopituitarism (posthypophysectomy) E89.3
    hypothyroidism (post-thyroidectomy) E89.0
    intestinal obstruction — *see also* Obstruction, intes-
        tine, postoperative K91.30
    intracranial hypotension following ventricular
        shunting (ventriculostomy) G97.2
    lymphedema I97.89
      postmastectomy I97.2
    malabsorption (postsurgical) NEC K91.2
      osteoporosis — *see* Osteoporosis, postsurgical
          malabsorption
    mastoidectomy cavity NEC — *see* Complications,
        postmastoidectomy
    metabolic E89.89
      specified NEC E89.89
    musculoskeletal — *see* Complications, musculoskele-
        tal system
    nervous system (central) (peripheral) — *see* Compli-
        cations, nervous system
    ovarian failure E89.40
      asymptomatic E89.40
      symptomatic E89.41
    peripheral vascular — *see* Complications, surgical
        procedure, vascular
    postcardiotomy syndrome I97.0
    postcholecystectomy syndrome K91.5
    postcommissurotomy syndrome I97.0
    postgastrectomy dumping syndrome K91.1
    postlaminectomy syndrome NEC M96.1
      kyphosis M96.3
    postmastectomy lymphedema syndrome I97.2
    postmastoidectomy cholesteatoma — *see* Compli-
        cations, postmastoidectomy, recurrent
        cholesteatoma
    postvagotomy syndrome K91.1
    postvalvulotomy syndrome I97.0
    pulmonary insufficiency (acute) J95.2
      chronic J95.3
      following thoracic surgery J95.1
    reattached body part — *see* Complications, reat-
        tached
    respiratory — *see* Complications, respiratory system
    shock (hypovolemic) T81.19 ☑

Complication(s) — *continued*
  surgical procedure — *continued*
    spleen (postoperative) D78.89
      intraoperative D78.81
    stitch abscess T81.41 ☑
    subglottic stenosis (postsurgical) J95.5
    testicular hypofunction E89.5
    transplant — *see* Complications, organ or tissue
        transplant
    urinary NEC N99.89
    vaginal vault prolapse (posthysterectomy) N99.3
    vascular (peripheral)
      artery T81.719 ☑
        mesenteric T81.710 ☑
        renal T81.711 ☑
        specified NEC T81.718 ☑
      vein T81.72 ☑
    wound infection T81.49 ☑
  suture, permanent (wire) NEC T85.9 ☑
    with repair of bone — *see* Complications, fixation
        device, internal
    embolism T85.818 ☑
    fibrosis T85.828 ☑
    hemorrhage T85.838 ☑
    infection and inflammation T85.79 ☑
    mechanical
      breakdown T85.612 ☑
      displacement T85.622 ☑
      malfunction T85.612 ☑
      malposition T85.622 ☑
      obstruction T85.692 ☑
      perforation T85.692 ☑
      protrusion T85.692 ☑
      specified NEC T85.692 ☑
    pain T85.848 ☑
    specified type NEC T85.898 ☑
    stenosis T85.858 ☑
    thrombosis T85.868 ☑
  tracheostomy J95.00
    granuloma J95.09
    hemorrhage J95.01
    infection J95.02
    malfunction J95.03
    mechanical J95.03
    obstruction J95.03
    specified type NEC J95.09
    tracheo-esophageal fistula J95.04
  transfusion (blood) (lymphocytes) (plasma) T80.92 ☑
    air emblism T80.0 ☑
    circulatory overload E87.71
    febrile nonhemolytic transfusion reaction R50.84
    hemochromatosis E83.111
    hemolysis T80.89 ☑
    hemolytic reaction (antigen unspecified) T80.919 ☑
    incompatibility reaction (antigen unspecified)
        T80.919 ☑
      ABO T80.30 ☑
        delayed serologic (DSTR) T80.39 ☑
        hemolytic transfusion reaction (HTR) (unspec-
            ified time after transfusion) T80.319 ☑
          acute (AHTR) (less than 24 hours after
              transfusion) T80.310 ☑
          delayed (DHTR) (24 hours or more after
              transfusion) T80.311 ☑
        specified NEC T80.39 ☑
      acute (antigen unspecified) T80.910 ☑
      delayed (antigen unspecified) T80.911 ☑
      delayed serologic (DSTR) T80.89 ☑
      non-ABO (minor antigens (Duffy) (K) (Kell) (Kidd)
          (Lewis) (M) (N) (P) (S)) T80.A0 ☑ (*following*
          T80.4)
        delayed serologic (DSTR) T80.A9 ☑ (*following*
            T80.4)
        hemolytic transfusion reaction (HTR) (unspec-
            ified time after transfusion) T80.A19 ☑
            (*following* T80.4)
          acute (AHTR) (less than 24 hours after
              transfusion) T80.A10 ☑ (*following*
              T80.4)
          delayed (DHTR) (24 hours or more after
              transfusion) T80.A11 ☑ (*following*
              T80.4)
        specified NEC T80.A9 ☑ (*following* T80.4)
      Rh (antigens (C) (c) (D) (E) (e)) (factor) T80.40 ☑
        delayed serologic (DSTR) T80.49 ☑
        hemolytic transfusion reaction (HTR) (unspec-
            ified time after transfusion) T80.419 ☑

Index

Complication — Complication

Complication(s) — *continued*
  transfusion — *continued*
    incompatibility reaction — *continued*
      Rh — *continued*
        hemolytic transfusion reaction — *continued*
          acute (AHTR) (less than 24 hours after
            transfusion) T80.410 ☑
          delayed (DHTR) (24 hours or more after
            transfusion) T80.411 ☑
          specified NEC T80.49 ☑
    infection T80.29 ☑
      acute T80.22- ☑
    reaction NEC T80.89 ☑
    sepsis T80.29 ☑
    shock T80.89 ☑
  transplant T86.90
    bone T86.839
      failure T86.831
      infection T86.832
      rejection T86.830
      specified type NEC T86.838
    bone marrow T86.00
      failure T86.02
      infection T86.03
      rejection T86.01
      specified type NEC T86.09
    cornea T86.849
      failure T86.841
      infection T86.842
      rejection T86.840
      specified type NEC T86.848
    failure T86.92
    heart T86.20
      with lung T86.30
      cardiac allograft vasculopathy T86.290
        failure T86.32
        infection T86.33
        rejection T86.31
        specified type NEC T86.39
      failure T86.22
      infection T86.23
      rejection T86.21
      specified type NEC T86.298
    infection T86.93
    intestine T86.859
      failure T86.851
      infection T86.852
      rejection T86.850
      specified type NEC T86.858
    kidney T86.10
      failure T86.12
      infection T86.13
      rejection T86.11
      specified type NEC T86.19
    liver T86.40
      failure T86.42
      infection T86.43
      rejection T86.41
      specified type NEC T86.49
    lung T86.819
      with heart T86.30
        failure T86.32
        infection T86.33
        rejection T86.31
        specified type NEC T86.39
      failure T86.811
      infection T86.812
      rejection T86.810
      specified type NEC T86.818
    malignant neoplasm C80.2
    pancreas T86.899
      failure T86.891
      infection T86.892
      rejection T86.890
      specified type NEC T86.898
    peripheral blood stem cells T86.5
    post-transplant lymphoproliferative disorder (PTLD)
      D47.Z1 (*following* D47.4)
    rejection T86.91
    skin T86.829
      failure T86.821
      infection T86.822
      rejection T86.820
      specified type NEC T86.828
    specified
      tissue T86.899
        failure T86.891

Complication(s) — *continued*
  transplant — *continued*
    specified — *continued*
      tissue — *continued*
        infection T86.892
        rejection T86.890
        specified type NEC T86.898
      type NEC T86.99
    stem cell (from peripheral blood) (from umbilical
      cord) T86.5
    umbilical cord stem cells T86.5
  trauma (early) T79.9
    specified NEC T79.8
  ultrasound therapy NEC T88.9
  umbilical cord NEC
    complicating delivery O69.9
      specified NEC O69.89 ☑
  umbrella device, vascular T82.9
    embolism T82.818 ☑
    fibrosis T82.828 ☑
    hemorrhage T82.838 ☑
    infection or inflammation T82.7 ☑
    mechanical
      breakdown T82.515 ☑
      displacement T82.525 ☑
      leakage T82.535 ☑
      malposition T82.525 ☑
      obstruction T82.595 ☑
      perforation T82.595 ☑
      protrusion T82.595 ☑
    pain T82.848 ☑
    specified type NEC T82.898 ☑
    stenosis T82.858 ☑
    thrombosis T82.868 ☑
  urethral catheter — *see* Complications, catheter, ure-
    thral, indwelling
  vaccination T88.1 ☑
    anaphylaxis NEC T80.52 ☑
    arthropathy — *see* Arthropathy, postimmunization
    cellulitis T88.0 ☑
    encephalitis or encephalomyelitis G04.02
    infection (general) (local) NEC T88.0 ☑
    meningitis G03.8
    myelitis G04.02
    protein sickness T80.62 ☑
    rash T88.1 ☑
    reaction (allergic) T88.1 ☑
      serum T80.62 ☑
    sepsis T88.0 ☑
    serum intoxication, sickness, rash, or other serum
      reaction NEC T80.62 ☑
      anaphylactic shock T80.52 ☑
    shock (allergic) (anaphylactic) T80.52 ☑
    vaccinia (generalized) (localized) T88.1 ☑
  vas deferens device or implant — *see* Complications,
    genitourinary, device or implant, genital tract
  vascular I99.9
    device or implant T82.9 ☑
      embolism T82.818 ☑
      fibrosis T82.828 ☑
      hemorrhage T82.838 ☑
      infection or inflammation T82.7 ☑
      mechanical
        breakdown T82.519 ☑
          specified device NEC T82.518 ☑
        displacement T82.529 ☑
          specified device NEC T82.528 ☑
        leakage T82.539 ☑
          specified device NEC T82.538 ☑
        malposition T82.529 ☑
          specified device NEC T82.528 ☑
        obstruction T82.599 ☑
          specified device NEC T82.598 ☑
        perforation T82.599 ☑
          specified device NEC T82.598 ☑
        protrusion T82.599 ☑
          specified device NEC T82.598 ☑
      pain T82.848 ☑
      specified type NEC T82.898 ☑
      stenosis T82.858 ☑
      thrombosis T82.868 ☑
    dialysis catheter — *see* Complication, catheter,
      dialysis
    following infusion, therapeutic injection or transfu-
      sion T80.1 ☑
    graft T82.9 ☑

Complication(s) — *continued*
  vascular — *continued*
    graft — *continued*
      embolism T82.818 ☑
      fibrosis T82.828 ☑
      hemorrhage T82.838 ☑
      mechanical
        breakdown T82.319 ☑
          aorta (bifurcation) T82.310 ☑
          carotid artery T82.311 ☑
          specified vessel NEC T82.318 ☑
        displacement T82.329 ☑
          aorta (bifurcation) T82.320 ☑
          carotid artery T82.321 ☑
          specified vessel NEC T82.328 ☑
        leakage T82.339 ☑
          aorta (bifurcation) T82.330 ☑
          carotid artery T82.331 ☑
          specified vessel NEC T82.338 ☑
        malposition T82.329 ☑
          aorta (bifurcation) T82.320 ☑
          carotid artery T82.321 ☑
          specified vessel NEC T82.328 ☑
        obstruction T82.399 ☑
          aorta (bifurcation) T82.390 ☑
          carotid artery T82.391 ☑
          specified vessel NEC T82.398 ☑
        perforation T82.399 ☑
          aorta (bifurcation) T82.390 ☑
          carotid artery T82.391 ☑
          specified vessel NEC T82.398 ☑
        protrusion T82.399 ☑
          aorta (bifurcation) T82.390 ☑
          carotid artery T82.391 ☑
          specified vessel NEC T82.398 ☑
      pain T82.848 ☑
      specified complication NEC T82.898 ☑
      stenosis T82.858 ☑
      thrombosis T82.868 ☑
    postoperative — *see* Complications, postoperative,
      circulatory
  vena cava device (filter) (sieve) (umbrella) — *see*
    Complications, umbrella device, vascular
  ventilation therapy NEC T81.81 ☑
  ventilator
    mechanical J95.850
      specified NEC J95.859
  ventricular (communicating) shunt (device) T85.9 ☑
    embolism T85.810 ☑
    fibrosis T85.820 ☑
    hemorrhage T85.830 ☑
    infection and inflammation T85.730 ☑
    mechanical
      breakdown T85.01 ☑
      displacement T85.02 ☑
      leakage T85.03 ☑
      malposition T85.02 ☑
      obstruction T85.09 ☑
      perforation T85.09 ☑
      protrusion T85.09 ☑
      specified NEC T85.09 ☑
    pain T85.840 ☑
    specified type NEC T85.890 ☑
    stenosis T85.850 ☑
    thrombosis T85.860 ☑
  wire suture, permanent (implanted) — *see* Complica-
    tions, suture, permanent
Compressed air disease T70.3 ☑
Compression
  with injury — *code by* Nature of injury
  artery I77.1
    celiac, syndrome I77.4
  brachial plexus G54.0
  brain (stem) G93.5
    due to
      contusion (diffuse) — *see* Injury, intracranial,
        diffuse
      focal — *see* Injury, intracranial, focal
      injury NEC — *see* Injury, intracranial, diffuse
      traumatic — *see* Injury, intracranial, diffuse
  bronchus J98.09
  cauda equina G83.4
  celiac (artery) (axis) I77.4
  cerebral — *see* Compression, brain
  cervical plexus G54.2

Compression — *continued*
  cord
    spinal — *see* Compression, spinal
    umbilical — *see* Compression, umbilical cord
  cranial nerve G52.9
    eighth H93.3 ☑
    eleventh G52.8
    fifth G50.8
    first G52.0
    fourth — *see* Strabismus, paralytic, fourth nerve
    ninth G52.1
    second — *see* Disorder, nerve, optic
    seventh G51.8
    sixth — *see* Strabismus, paralytic, sixth nerve
    tenth G52.2
    third — *see* Strabismus, paralytic, third nerve
    twelfth G52.3
  diver's squeeze T70.3 ☑
  during birth (newborn) P15.9
  esophagus K22.2
  eustachian tube — *see* Obstruction, eustachian tube, cartilaginous
  facies Q67.1
  fracture
    nontraumatic NOS — *see* Collapse, vertebra
    pathological — *see* Fracture, pathological
    traumatic — *see* Fracture, traumatic
  heart — *see* Disease, heart
  intestine — *see* Obstruction, intestine
  laryngeal nerve, recurrent G52.2
    with paralysis of vocal cords and larynx J38.00
      bilateral J38.02
      unilateral J38.01
  lumbosacral plexus G54.1
  lung J98.4
  lymphatic vessel I89.0
  medulla — *see* Compression, brain
  nerve — *see also* Disorder, nerve G58.9
    arm NEC — *see* Mononeuropathy, upper limb
    axillary G54.0
    cranial — *see* Compression, cranial nerve
    leg NEC — *see* Mononeuropathy, lower limb
    median (in carpal tunnel) — *see* Syndrome, carpal tunnel
    optic — *see* Disorder, nerve, optic
    plantar — *see* Lesion, nerve, plantar
    posterior tibial (in tarsal tunnel) — *see* Syndrome, tarsal tunnel
    root or plexus NOS (in) G54.9
      intervertebral disc disorder NEC — *see* Disorder, disc, with, radiculopathy
      with myelopathy — *see* Disorder, disc, with, myelopathy
      neoplastic disease — *see also* Neoplasm D49.9 *[G55]*
      spondylosis — *see* Spondylosis, with radiculopathy
    sciatic (acute) — *see* Lesion, nerve, sciatic
    sympathetic G90.8
    traumatic — *see* Injury, nerve
    ulnar — *see* Lesion, nerve, ulnar
    upper extremity NEC — *see* Mononeuropathy, upper limb
  spinal (cord) G95.20
    by displacement of intervertebral disc NEC — *see also* Disorder, disc, with, myelopathy
    nerve root NOS G54.9
      due to displacement of intervertebral disc NEC — *see* Disorder, disc, with, radiculopathy
      with myelopathy — *see* Disorder, disc, with, myelopathy
    specified NEC G95.29
    spondylogenic (cervical) (lumbar, lumbosacral) (thoracic) — *see* Spondylosis, with myelopathy NEC
    anterior — *see* Syndrome, anterior, spinal artery, compression
    traumatic — *see* Injury, spinal cord, by region
  subcostal nerve (syndrome) — *see* Mononeuropathy, upper limb, specified NEC
  sympathetic nerve NEC G90.8
  syndrome T79.5 ☑
  trachea J39.8
  ulnar nerve (by scar tissue) — *see* Lesion, nerve, ulnar
  umbilical cord
    complicating delivery O69.2 ☑
      cord around neck O69.1 ☑

Compression — *continued*
  umbilical cord — *continued*
    complicating delivery — *continued*
      prolapse O69.0 ☑
      specified NEC O69.2 ☑
  ureter N13.5
  vein I87.1
  vena cava (inferior) (superior) I87.1
Compulsion, compulsive
  gambling F63.0
  neurosis F42.8
  personality F60.5
  states F42.8
  swearing F42.8
    in Gilles de la Tourette's syndrome F95.2
  tics and spasms F95.9
Concato's disease (pericardial polyserositis) A19.9
  nontubercular I31.1
  pleural — *see* Pleurisy, with effusion
Concavity chest wall M95.4
Concealed penis Q55.64
Concern (normal) **about sick person in family** Z63.6
Concrescence (teeth) K00.2
Concretio cordis I31.1
  rheumatic I09.2
Concretion — *see also* Calculus
  appendicular K38.1
  canaliculus — *see* Dacryolith
  clitoris N90.89
  conjunctiva H11.12- ☑
  eyelid — *see* Disorder, eyelid, specified type NEC
  lacrimal passages — *see* Dacryolith
  prepuce (male) N47.8
  salivary gland (any) K11.5
  seminal vesicle N50.89
  tonsil J35.8
Concussion (brain) (cerebral) (current) S06.0X9 ☑
  with
    loss of consciousness of 30 minutes or less S06.0X1 ☑
    loss of consciousness of unspecified duration S06.0X9 ☑
  blast (air) (hydraulic) (immersion) (underwater)
    abdomen or thorax — *see* Injury, blast, by site
    ear with acoustic nerve injury — *see* Injury, nerve, acoustic, specified type NEC
  cauda equina S34.3 ☑
  conus medullaris S34.02 ☑
  ocular S05.8X- ☑
  spinal (cord)
    cervical S14.0 ☑
    lumbar S34.01 ☑
    sacral S34.02 ☑
    thoracic S24.0 ☑
  syndrome F07.81
  without loss of consciousness S06.0X0 ☑
Condition — *see* Disease
Conditions arising in the perinatal period — *see* Newborn, affected by
Conduct disorder — *see* Disorder, conduct
Condyloma A63.0
  acuminatum A63.0
  gonorrheal A54.09
  latum A51.31
  syphilitic A51.31
    congenital A50.07
  venereal, syphilitic A51.31
Conflagration — *see also* Burn
  asphyxia (by inhalation of gases, fumes or vapors) — *see also* Table of Drugs and Chemicals T59.9- ☑
Conflict (with) — *see also* Discord
  family Z73.9
  marital Z63.0
    involving divorce or estrangement Z63.5
  parent-child Z62.820
    parent-adopted child Z62.821
    parent-biological child Z62.820
    parent-foster child Z62.822
  social role NEC Z73.5
Confluent — *see* condition
Confusion, confused R41.0
  epileptic F05
  mental state (psychogenic) F44.89
  psychogenic F44.89
  reactive (from emotional stress, psychological trauma) F44.89
Confusional arousals G47.51

Congelation T69.9 ☑
Congenital — *see also* condition
  aortic septum Q25.49
  intrinsic factor deficiency D51.0
  malformation — *see* Anomaly
Congestion, congestive
  bladder N32.89
  bowel K63.89
  brain G93.89
  breast N64.59
  bronchial J98.09
  catarrhal J31.0
  chest R09.89
  chill, malarial — *see* Malaria
  circulatory NEC I99.8
  duodenum K31.89
  eye — *see* Hyperemia, conjunctiva
  facial, due to birth injury P15.4
  general R68.89
  glottis J37.0
  heart — *see* Failure, heart, congestive
  hepatic K76.1
  hypostatic (lung) — *see* Edema, lung
  intestine K63.89
  kidney N28.89
  labyrinth H83.8 ☑
  larynx J37.0
  liver K76.1
  lung R09.89
    active or acute — *see* Pneumonia
  malaria, malarial — *see* Malaria
  nasal R09.81
  nose R09.81
  orbit, orbital — *see also* Exophthalmos
    inflammatory (chronic) — *see* Inflammation, orbit
  ovary N83.8
  pancreas K86.89
  pelvic, female N94.89
  pleural J94.8
  prostate (active) N42.1
  pulmonary — *see* Congestion, lung
  renal N28.89
  retina H35.81
  seminal vesicle N50.1
  spinal cord G95.19
  spleen (chronic) D73.2
  stomach K31.89
  trachea   *see* Tracheitis
  urethra N36.8
  uterus N85.8
    with subinvolution N85.3
  venous (passive) I87.8
  viscera R68.89
Congestive — *see* Congestion
Conical
  cervix (hypertrophic elongation) N88.4
  cornea — *see* Keratoconus
  teeth K00.2
Conjoined twins Q89.4
Conjugal maladjustment Z63.0
  involving divorce or estrangement Z63.5
Conjunctiva — *see* condition
Conjunctivitis (staphylococcal) (streptococcal) NOS H10.9
  Acanthamoeba B60.12
  acute H10.3- ☑
    atopic H10.1- ☑
    chemical — *see also* Corrosion, cornea H10.21- ☑
    mucopurulent H10.02- ☑
      follicular H10.01- ☑
    pseudomembranous H10.22- ☑
    serous except viral H10.23- ☑
      viral — *see* Conjunctivitis, viral
    toxic H10.21- ☑
  adenoviral (acute) (follicular) B30.1
  allergic (acute) — *see* Conjunctivitis, acute, atopic
    chronic H10.45
      vernal H10.44
  anaphylactic — *see* Conjunctivitis, acute, atopic
  Apollo B30.3
  atopic (acute) — *see* Conjunctivitis, acute, atopic
  Béal's B30.2
  blennorrhagic (gonococcal) (neonatorum) A54.31
  chemical (acute) — *see also* Corrosion, cornea H10.21- ☑
  chlamydial A74.0
    due to trachoma A71.1
    neonatal P39.1

Conjunctivitis — continued
  chronic (nodosa) (petrificans) (phlyctenular) H10.40- ☑
    allergic H10.45
      vernal H10.44
    follicular H10.43- ☑
    giant papillary H10.41- ☑
    simple H10.42- ☑
    vernal H10.44
  coxsackievirus 24 B30.3
  diphtheritic A36.86
  due to
    dust — see Conjunctivitis, acute, atopic
    filariasis B74.9
    mucocutaneous leishmaniasis B55.2
  enterovirus type 70 (hemorrhagic) B30.3
  epidemic (viral) B30.9
    hemorrhagic B30.3
  gonococcal (neonatorum) A54.31
  granular (trachomatous) A71.1
    sequelae (late effect) B94.0
  hemorrhagic (acute) (epidemic) B30.3
  herpes zoster B02.31
  in (due to)
    Acanthamoeba B60.12
    adenovirus (acute) (follicular) B30.1
    Chlamydia A74.0
    coxsackievirus 24 B30.3
    diphtheria A36.86
    enterovirus type 70 (hemorrhagic) B30.3
    filariasis B74.9
    gonococci A54.31
    herpes (simplex) virus B00.53
      zoster B02.31
    infectious disease NEC B99 ☑
    meningococci A39.89
    mucocutaneous leishmaniasis B55.2
    rosacea H10.82- ☑
    syphilis (late) A52.71
    zoster B02.31
  inclusion A74.0
  infantile P39.1
    gonococcal A54.31
  Koch-Weeks' — see Conjunctivitis, acute, mucopurulent
  light — see Conjunctivitis, acute, atopic
  ligneous — see Blepharoconjunctivitis, ligneous
  meningococcal A39.89
  mucopurulent — see Conjunctivitis, acute, mucopurulent
  neonatal P39.1
    gonococcal A54.31
  Newcastle B30.8
  of Béal B30.2
  parasitic
    filariasis B74.9
    mucocutaneous leishmaniasis B55.2
  Parinaud's H10.89
  petrificans H10.89
  rosacea H10.82- ☑
  specified NEC H10.89
  swimming-pool B30.1
  trachomatous A71.1
    acute A71.0
    sequelae (late effect) B94.0
  traumatic NEC H10.89
  tuberculous A18.59
  tularemic A21.1
  tularensis A21.1
  viral B30.9
    due to
      adenovirus B30.1
      enterovirus B30.3
    specified NEC B30.8
Conjunctivochalasis H11.82- ☑
Connective tissue — see condition
Conn's syndrome E26.01
Conradi (-Hunermann) **disease** Q77.3
Consanguinity Z84.3
  counseling Z71.89
Conscious simulation (of illness) Z76.5
Consecutive — see condition
Consolidation lung (base) — see Pneumonia, lobar
Constipation (atonic) (neurogenic) (simple) (spastic)
    K59.00
  chronic K59.09
    idiopathic K59.04
  drug-induced K59.03
  functional K59.04
  outlet dysfunction K59.02

Constipation — continued
  psychogenic F45.8
  slow transit K59.01
  specified NEC K59.09
Constitutional — see also condition
  substandard F60.7
Constitutionally substandard F60.7
Constriction — see also Stricture
  auditory canal — see Stenosis, external ear canal
  bronchial J98.09
  duodenum K31.5
  esophagus K22.2
  external
    abdomen, abdominal (wall) S30.841 ☑
    alveolar process S00.542 ☑
    ankle S90.54- ☑
    antecubital space — see Constriction, external, forearm
    arm (upper) S40.84- ☑
    auricle — see Constriction, external, ear
    axilla — see Constriction, external, arm
    back, lower S30.840 ☑
    breast S20.14- ☑
    brow S00.84 ☑
    buttock S30.840 ☑
    calf — see Constriction, external, leg
    canthus — see Constriction, external, eyelid
    cheek S00.84 ☑
      internal S00.542 ☑
    chest wall — see Constriction, external, thorax
    chin S00.84 ☑
    clitoris S30.844 ☑
    costal region — see Constriction, external, thorax
    digit(s)
      foot — see Constriction, external, toe
      hand — see Constriction, external, finger
    ear S00.44- ☑
    elbow S50.34- ☑
    epididymis S30.843 ☑
    epigastric region S30.841 ☑
    esophagus, cervical S10.14 ☑
    eyebrow — see Constriction, external, eyelid
    eyelid S00.24- ☑
    face S00.84 ☑
    finger(s) S60.44- ☑
      index S60.44- ☑
      little S60.44- ☑
      middle S60.44- ☑
      ring S60.44- ☑
    flank S30.841 ☑
    foot (except toe(s) alone) S90.84- ☑
      toe — see Constriction, external, toe
    forearm S50.84- ☑
      elbow only — see Constriction, external, elbow
    forehead S00.84 ☑
    genital organs, external
      female S30.846 ☑
      male S30.845 ☑
    groin S30.841 ☑
    gum S00.542 ☑
    hand S60.54- ☑
    head S00.94 ☑
      ear — see Constriction, external, ear
      eyelid — see Constriction, external, eyelid
      lip S00.541 ☑
      nose S00.34 ☑
      oral cavity S00.542 ☑
      scalp S00.04 ☑
      specified site NEC S00.84 ☑
    heel — see Constriction, external, foot
    hip S70.24- ☑
    inguinal region S30.841 ☑
    interscapular region S20.449 ☑
    jaw S00.84 ☑
    knee S80.24- ☑
    labium (majus) (minus) S30.844 ☑
    larynx S10.14 ☑
    leg (lower) S80.84- ☑
      knee — see Constriction, external, knee
      upper — see Constriction, external, thigh
    lip S00.541 ☑
    lower back S30.840 ☑
    lumbar region S30.840 ☑
    malar region S00.84 ☑
    mammary — see Constriction, external, breast
    mastoid region S00.84 ☑

Constriction — continued
  external — continued
    mouth S00.542 ☑
    nail
      finger — see Constriction, external, finger
      toe — see Constriction, external, toe
    nasal S00.34 ☑
    neck S10.94 ☑
      specified site NEC S10.84 ☑
      throat S10.14 ☑
    nose S00.34 ☑
    occipital region S00.04 ☑
    oral cavity S00.542 ☑
    orbital region — see Constriction, external, eyelid
    palate S00.542 ☑
    palm — see Constriction, external, hand
    parietal region S00.04 ☑
    pelvis S30.840 ☑
    penis S30.842 ☑
    perineum
      female S30.844 ☑
      male S30.840 ☑
    periocular area — see Constriction, external, eyelid
    phalanges
      finger — see Constriction, external, finger
      toe — see Constriction, external, toe
    pharynx S10.14 ☑
    pinna — see Constriction, external, ear
    popliteal space — see Constriction, external, knee
    prepuce S30.842 ☑
    pubic region S30.840 ☑
    pudendum
      female S30.846 ☑
      male S30.845 ☑
    sacral region S30.840 ☑
    scalp S00.04 ☑
    scapular region — see Constriction, external, shoulder
    scrotum S30.843 ☑
    shin — see Constriction, external, leg
    shoulder S40.24- ☑
    sternal region S20.349 ☑
    submaxillary region S00.84 ☑
    submental region S00.84 ☑
    subungual
      finger(s) — see Constriction, external, finger
      toe(s) — see Constriction, external, toe
    supraclavicular fossa S10.84 ☑
    supraorbital S00.84 ☑
    temple S00.84 ☑
    temporal region S00.84 ☑
    testis S30.843 ☑
    thigh S70.34- ☑
    thorax, thoracic (wall) S20.94 ☑
      back S20.44- ☑
      front S20.34- ☑
    throat S10.14 ☑
    thumb S60.34- ☑
    toe(s) (lesser) S90.44- ☑
      great S90.44- ☑
    tongue S00.542 ☑
    trachea S10.14 ☑
    tunica vaginalis S30.843 ☑
    uvula S00.542 ☑
    vagina S30.844 ☑
    vulva S30.844 ☑
    wrist S60.84- ☑
  gallbladder — see Obstruction, gallbladder
  intestine — see Obstruction, intestine
  larynx J38.6
    congenital Q31.8
      specified NEC Q31.8
      subglottic Q31.1
  organ or site, congenital NEC — see Atresia, by site
  prepuce (acquired) (congenital) N47.1
  pylorus (adult hypertrophic) K31.1
    congenital or infantile Q40.0
    newborn Q40.0
  ring dystocia (uterus) O62.4
  spastic — see also Spasm
    ureter N13.5
  ureter N13.5
    with infection N13.6
  urethra — see Stricture, urethra
  visual field (peripheral) (functional) — see Defect, visual field

Constrictive — *see* condition

Consultation
  medical — *see* Counseling, medical
  religious Z71.81
  specified reason NEC Z71.89
  spiritual Z71.81
  without complaint or sickness Z71.9
    feared complaint unfounded Z71.1
      specified reason NEC Z71.89

Consumption — *see* Tuberculosis

Contact (with) — *see also* Exposure (to)
  acariasis Z20.7
  AIDS virus Z20.6
  air pollution Z77.110
  algae and algae toxins Z77.121
  algae bloom Z77.121
  anthrax Z20.810
  aromatic amines Z77.020
  aromatic (hazardous) compounds NEC Z77.028
  aromatic dyes NOS Z77.028
  arsenic Z77.010
  asbestos Z77.090
  bacterial disease NEC Z20.818
  benzene Z77.021
  blue-green algae bloom Z77.121
  body fluids (potentially hazardous) Z77.21
  brown tide Z77.121
  chemicals (chiefly nonmedicinal) (hazardous) NEC Z77.098
  cholera Z20.09
  chromium compounds Z77.018
  communicable disease Z20.9
    bacterial NEC Z20.818
    specified NEC Z20.89
    viral NEC Z20.828
    Zika virus Z20.821
  cyanobacteria bloom Z77.121
  dyes Z77.098
  Escherichia coli (E. coli) Z20.01
  fiberglass — *see* Table of Drugs and Chemicals, fiberglass
  German measles Z20.4
  gonorrhea Z20.2
  hazardous metals NEC Z77.018
  hazardous substances NEC Z77.29
  hazards in the physical environment NEC Z77.128
  hazards to health NEC Z77.9
  HIV Z20.6
  HTLV-III/LAV Z20.6
  human immunodeficiency virus (HIV) Z20.6
  infection Z20.9
    specified NEC Z20.89
  infestation (parasitic) NEC Z20.7
  intestinal infectious disease NEC Z20.09
    Escherichia coli (E. coli) Z20.01
  lead Z77.011
  meningococcus Z20.811
  mold (toxic) Z77.120
  nickel dust Z77.018
  noise Z77.122
  parasitic disease Z20.7
  pediculosis Z20.7
  pfiesteria piscicida Z77.121
  poliomyelitis Z20.89
  pollution
    air Z77.110
    environmental NEC Z77.118
    soil Z77.112
    water Z77.111
  polycyclic aromatic hydrocarbons Z77.028
  rabies Z20.3
  radiation, naturally occurring NEC Z77.123
  radon Z77.123
  red tide (Florida) Z77.121
  rubella Z20.4
  sexually-transmitted disease Z20.2
  smallpox (laboratory) Z20.89
  syphilis Z20.2
  tuberculosis Z20.1
  uranium Z77.012
  varicella Z20.820
  venereal disease Z20.2
  viral disease NEC Z20.828
  viral hepatitis Z20.5
  water pollution Z77.111
  Zika virus Z20.821

Contamination, food — *see* Intoxication, foodborne

Contraception, contraceptive
  advice Z30.09
  counseling Z30.09
  device (intrauterine) (in situ) Z97.5
    causing menorrhagia T83.83 ☑
    checking Z30.431
    complications — *see* Complications, intrauterine, contraceptive device
    in place Z97.5
    initial prescription Z30.014
    reinsertion Z30.433
    removal Z30.432
    replacement Z30.433
  emergency (postcoital) Z30.012
  initial prescription Z30.019
    barrier Z30.018
    diaphragm Z30.018
    injectable Z30.013
    intrauterine device Z30.014
    pills Z30.011
    postcoital (emergency) Z30.012
    specified type NEC Z30.018
    subdermal implantable Z30.017
    transdermal patch hormonal Z30.016
    vaginal ring hormonal Z30.015
  maintenance Z30.40
    barrier Z30.49
    diaphragm Z30.49
    examination Z30.8
    injectable Z30.42
    intrauterine device Z30.431
    pills Z30.41
    specified type NEC Z30.49
    subdermal implantable Z30.46
    transdermal patch hormonal Z30.45
    vaginal ring hormonal Z30.44
  management Z30.9
    specified NEC Z30.8
  postcoital (emergency) Z30.012
  prescription Z30.019
    repeat Z30.40
  sterilization Z30.2
  surveillance (drug) — *see* Contraception, maintenance

Contraction(s), contracture, contracted
  Achilles tendon — *see also* Short, tendon, Achilles
    congenital Q66.89
  amputation stump (surgical) (flexion) (late) (next proximal joint) T87.89
  anus K59.8
  bile duct (common) (hepatic) K83.8
  bladder N32.89
    neck or sphincter N32.0
  bowel, cecum, colon or intestine, any part — *see* Obstruction, intestine
  Braxton Hicks — *see* False, labor
  breast implant, capsular T85.44 ☑
  bronchial J98.09
  burn (old) — *see* Cicatrix
  cervix — *see* Stricture, cervix
  cicatricial — *see* Cicatrix
  conjunctiva, trachomatous, active A71.1
    sequelae (late effect) B94.0
  Dupuytren's M72.0
  eyelid — *see* Disorder, eyelid function
  fascia (lata) (postural) M72.8
    Dupuytren's M72.0
    palmar M72.0
    plantar M72.2
  finger NEC — *see also* Deformity, finger
    congenital Q68.1
    joint — *see* Contraction, joint, hand
  flaccid — *see* Contraction, paralytic
  gallbladder K82.0
  heart valve — *see* Endocarditis
  hip — *see* Contraction, joint, hip
  hourglass
    bladder N32.89
      congenital Q64.79
    gallbladder K82.0
      congenital Q44.1
    stomach K31.89
      congenital Q40.2
      psychogenic F45.8
    uterus (complicating delivery) O62.4
  hysterical F44.4
  internal os — *see* Stricture, cervix
  joint (abduction) (acquired) (adduction) (flexion) (rotation) M24.50

Contraction(s), contracture, contracted — *continued*
  joint — *continued*
    ankle M24.57- ☑
    congenital NEC Q68.8
      hip Q65.89
    elbow M24.52- ☑
    foot joint M24.57- ☑
    hand joint M24.54- ☑
    hip M24.55- ☑
      congenital Q65.89
    hysterical F44.4
    knee M24.56- ☑
    shoulder M24.51- ☑
    wrist M24.53- ☑
  kidney (granular) (secondary) N26.9
    congenital Q63.8
    hydronephritic — *see* Hydronephrosis
    Page N26.2
    pyelonephritic — *see* Pyelitis, chronic
    tuberculous A18.11
  ligament — *see also* Disorder, ligament
    congenital Q79.8
  muscle (postinfective) (postural) NEC M62.40
    with contracture of joint — *see* Contraction, joint
    ankle M62.47- ☑
    congenital Q79.8
      sternocleidomastoid Q68.0
    extraocular — *see* Strabismus
    eye (extrinsic) — *see* Strabismus
    foot M62.47- ☑
    forearm M62.43- ☑
    hand M62.44- ☑
    hysterical F44.4
    ischemic (Volkmann's) T79.6 ☑
    lower leg M62.46- ☑
    multiple sites M62.49
    pelvic region M62.45- ☑
    posttraumatic — *see* Strabismus, paralytic
    psychogenic F45.8
      conversion reaction F44.4
    shoulder region M62.41- ☑
    specified site NEC M62.48
    thigh M62.45- ☑
    upper arm M62.42- ☑
  neck — *see* Torticollis
  ocular muscle — *see* Strabismus
  organ or site, congenital NEC — *see* Atresia, by site
  outlet (pelvis) — *see* Contraction, pelvis
  palmar fascia M72.0
  paralytic
    joint — *see* Contraction, joint
    muscle — *see also* Contraction, muscle NEC
      ocular — *see* Strabismus, paralytic
  pelvis (acquired) (general) M95.5
    with disproportion (fetopelvic) O33.1
      causing obstructed labor O65.1
    inlet O33.2
    mid-cavity O33.3 ☑
    outlet O33.3 ☑
  plantar fascia M72.2
  premature
    atrium I49.1
    auriculoventricular I49.49
    heart I49.49
    junctional I49.2
    supraventricular I49.1
    ventricular I49.3
  prostate N42.89
  pylorus NEC — *see also* Pylorospasm
    psychogenic F45.8
  rectum, rectal (sphincter) K59.8
  ring (Bandl's) (complicating delivery) O62.4
  scar — *see* Cicatrix
  spine — *see* Dorsopathy, deforming
  sternocleidomastoid (muscle), congenital Q68.0
  stomach K31.89
    hourglass K31.89
      congenital Q40.2
      psychogenic F45.8
    psychogenic F45.8
  tendon (sheath) M62.40
    with contracture of joint — *see* Contraction, joint
    Achilles — *see* Short, tendon, Achilles
    ankle M62.47- ☑
      Achilles — *see* Short, tendon, Achilles
    foot M62.47- ☑

Contraction(s), contracture, contracted — *continued*
- tendon — *continued*
  - forearm M62.43- ☑
  - hand M62.44- ☑
  - lower leg M62.46- ☑
  - multiple sites M62.49
  - neck M62.48
  - pelvic region M62.45- ☑
  - shoulder region M62.41- ☑
  - specified site NEC M62.48
  - thigh M62.45- ☑
  - thorax M62.48
  - trunk M62.48
  - upper arm M62.42- ☑
- toe — *see* Deformity, toe, specified NEC
- ureterovesical orifice (postinfectional) N13.5
  - with infection N13.6
- urethra — *see also* Stricture, urethra
  - orifice N32.0
- uterus N85.8
  - abnormal NEC O62.9
  - clonic (complicating delivery) O62.4
  - dyscoordinate (complicating delivery) O62.4
  - hourglass (complicating delivery) O62.4
  - hypertonic O62.4
  - hypotonic NEC O62.2
  - inadequate
    - primary O62.0
    - secondary O62.1
  - incoordinate (complicating delivery) O62.4
  - poor O62.2
  - tetanic (complicating delivery) O62.4
- vagina (outlet) N89.5
- vesical N32.89
  - neck or urethral orifice N32.0
- visual field — *see* Defect, visual field, generalized
- Volkmann's (ischemic) T79.6

Contusion (skin surface intact) T14.8 ☑
- abdomen, abdominal (muscle) (wall) S30.1 ☑
- adnexa, eye NEC S05.8X- ☑
- adrenal gland S37.812 ☑
- alveolar process S00.532 ☑
- ankle S90.0- ☑
- antecubital space — *see* Contusion, forearm
- anus S30.3 ☑
- arm (upper) S40.02- ☑
  - lower (with elbow) — *see* Contusion, forearm
- auditory canal — *see* Contusion, ear
- auricle — *see* Contusion, ear
- axilla — *see* Contusion, arm, upper
- back — *see also* Contusion, thorax, back
  - lower S30.0 ☑
- bile duct S36.13 ☑
- bladder S37.22 ☑
- bone NEC T14.8 ☑
- brain (diffuse) — *see* Injury, intracranial, diffuse
  - focal — *see* Injury, intracranial, focal
- brainstem S06.38- ☑
- breast S20.0- ☑
- broad ligament S37.892 ☑
- brow S00.83 ☑
- buttock S30.0 ☑
- canthus, eye S00.1- ☑
- cauda equina S34.3 ☑
- cerebellar, traumatic S06.37- ☑
- cerebral S06.33- ☑
  - left side S06.32- ☑
  - right side S06.31- ☑
- cheek S00.83 ☑
  - internal S00.532 ☑
- chest (wall) — *see* Contusion, thorax
- chin S00.83 ☑
- clitoris S30.23 ☑
- colon — *see* Injury, intestine, large, contusion
- common bile duct S36.13 ☑
- conjunctiva S05.1- ☑
  - with foreign body (in conjunctival sac) — *see* Foreign body, conjunctival sac
- conus medullaris (spine) S34.139 ☑
- cornea — *see* Contusion, eyeball
  - with foreign body — *see* Foreign body, cornea
- corpus cavernosum S30.21 ☑
- cortex (brain) (cerebral) — *see* Injury, intracranial, diffuse
  - focal — *see* Injury, intracranial, focal
- costal region — *see* Contusion, thorax

Contusion — *continued*
- cystic duct S36.13 ☑
- diaphragm S27.802 ☑
- duodenum S36.420 ☑
- ear S00.43- ☑
- elbow S50.0- ☑
  - with forearm — *see* Contusion, forearm
- epididymis S30.22 ☑
- epigastric region S30.1 ☑
- epiglottis S10.0 ☑
- esophagus (thoracic) S27.812 ☑
  - cervical S10.0 ☑
- eyeball S05.1- ☑
- eyebrow S00.1- ☑
- eyelid (and periocular area) S00.1- ☑
- face NEC S00.83 ☑
- fallopian tube S37.529 ☑
  - bilateral S37.522 ☑
  - unilateral S37.521 ☑
- femoral triangle S30.1 ☑
- finger(s) S60.00 ☑
  - with damage to nail (matrix) S60.10 ☑
  - index S60.02- ☑
    - with damage to nail S60.12- ☑
  - little S60.05- ☑
    - with damage to nail S60.15- ☑
  - middle S60.03- ☑
    - with damage to nail S60.13- ☑
  - ring S60.04- ☑
    - with damage to nail S60.14- ☑
  - thumb — *see* Contusion, thumb
- flank S30.1 ☑
- foot (except toe(s) alone) S90.3- ☑
  - toe — *see* Contusion, toe
- forearm S50.1- ☑
  - elbow only — *see* Contusion, elbow
- forehead S00.83 ☑
- gallbladder S36.122 ☑
- genital organs, external
  - female S30.202 ☑
  - male S30.201 ☑
- globe (eye) — *see* Contusion, eyeball
- groin S30.1 ☑
- gum S00.532 ☑
- hand S60.22- ☑
  - finger(s) — *see* Contusion, finger
  - wrist — *see* Contusion, wrist
- head S00.93 ☑
  - ear — *see* Contusion, ear
  - eyelid — *see* Contusion, eyelid
  - lip S00.531 ☑
  - nose S00.33 ☑
  - oral cavity S00.532 ☑
  - scalp S00.03 ☑
  - specified part NEC S00.83 ☑
- heart — *see also* Injury, heart S26.91 ☑
- heel — *see* Contusion, foot
- hepatic duct S36.13 ☑
- hip S70.0- ☑
- ileum S36.428 ☑
- iliac region S30.1 ☑
- inguinal region S30.1 ☑
- interscapular region S20.229 ☑
- intra-abdominal organ S36.92 ☑
  - colon — *see* Injury, intestine, large, contusion
  - liver S36.112 ☑
  - pancreas — *see* Contusion, pancreas
  - rectum S36.62 ☑
  - small intestine — *see* Injury, intestine, small, contusion
  - specified organ NEC S36.892 ☑
  - spleen — *see* Contusion, spleen
  - stomach S36.32 ☑
- iris (eye) — *see* Contusion, eyeball
- jaw S00.83 ☑
- jejunum S36.428 ☑
- kidney S37.01- ☑
  - major (greater than 2 cm) S37.02- ☑
  - minor (less than 2 cm) S37.01- ☑
- knee S80.0- ☑
- labium (majus) (minus) S30.23 ☑
- lacrimal apparatus, gland or sac S05.8X- ☑
- larynx S10.0 ☑
- leg (lower) S80.1- ☑
  - knee — *see* Contusion, knee
- lens — *see* Contusion, eyeball

Contusion — *continued*
- lip S00.531 ☑
- liver S36.112 ☑
- lower back S30.0 ☑
- lumbar region S30.0 ☑
- lung S27.329 ☑
  - bilateral S27.322 ☑
  - unilateral S27.321 ☑
- malar region S00.83 ☑
- mastoid region S00.83 ☑
- membrane, brain — *see* Injury, intracranial, diffuse
  - focal — *see* Injury, intracranial, focal
- mesentery S36.892 ☑
- mesosalpinx S37.892 ☑
- mouth S00.532 ☑
- muscle — *see* Contusion, by site
- nail
  - finger — *see* Contusion, finger, with damage to nail
  - toe — *see* Contusion, toe, with damage to nail
- nasal S00.33 ☑
- neck S10.93 ☑
  - specified site NEC S10.83 ☑
  - throat S10.0 ☑
- nerve — *see* Injury, nerve
- newborn P54.5
- nose S00.33 ☑
- occipital
  - lobe (brain) — *see* Injury, intracranial, diffuse
    - focal — *see* Injury, intracranial, focal
  - region (scalp) S00.03 ☑
- orbit (region) (tissues) S05.1- ☑
- ovary S37.429 ☑
  - bilateral S37.422 ☑
  - unilateral S37.421 ☑
- palate S00.532 ☑
- pancreas S36.229 ☑
  - body S36.221 ☑
  - head S36.220 ☑
  - tail S36.222 ☑
- parietal
  - lobe (brain) — *see* Injury, intracranial, diffuse
    - focal — *see* Injury, intracranial, focal
  - region (scalp) S00.03 ☑
- pelvic organ S37.92 ☑
  - adrenal gland S37.812 ☑
  - bladder S37.22 ☑
  - fallopian tube — *see* Contusion, fallopian tube
  - kidney — *see* Contusion, kidney
  - ovary — *see* Contusion, ovary
  - prostate S37.822 ☑
  - specified organ NEC S37.892 ☑
  - ureter S37.12 ☑
  - urethra S37.32 ☑
  - uterus S37.62 ☑
- pelvis S30.0 ☑
- penis S30.21 ☑
- perineum
  - female S30.23 ☑
  - male S30.0 ☑
- periocular area S00.1- ☑
- peritoneum S36.81 ☑
- periurethral tissue — *see* Contusion, urethra
- pharynx S10.0 ☑
- pinna — *see* Contusion, ear
- popliteal space — *see* Contusion, knee
- prepuce S30.21 ☑
- prostate S37.822 ☑
- pubic region S30.1 ☑
- pudendum
  - female S30.202 ☑
  - male S30.201 ☑
- quadriceps femoris — *see* Contusion, thigh
- rectum S36.62 ☑
- retroperitoneum S36.892 ☑
- round ligament S37.892 ☑
- sacral region S30.0 ☑
- scalp S00.03 ☑
  - due to birth injury P12.3
- scapular region — *see* Contusion, shoulder
- sclera — *see* Contusion, eyeball
- scrotum S30.22 ☑
- seminal vesicle S37.892 ☑
- shoulder S40.01- ☑
- skin NEC T14.8 ☑
- small intestine — *see* Injury, intestine, small, contusion
- spermatic cord S30.22 ☑

Contusion — *continued*
spinal cord — *see* Injury, spinal cord, by region
　　cauda equina S34.3 ☑
　　conus medullaris S34.139 ☑
spleen S36.029 ☑
　　major S36.021 ☑
　　minor S36.020 ☑
sternal region S20.219 ☑
stomach S36.32 ☑
subconjunctival S05.1- ☑
subcutaneous NEC T14.8 ☑
submaxillary region S00.83 ☑
submental region S00.83 ☑
subperiosteal NEC T14.8 ☑
subungual
　　finger — *see* Contusion, finger, with damage to nail
　　toe — *see* Contusion, toe, with damage to nail
supraclavicular fossa S10.83 ☑
supraorbital S00.83 ☑
suprarenal gland S37.812 ☑
temple (region) S00.83 ☑
temporal
　　lobe (brain) — *see* Injury, intracranial, diffuse
　　　focal — *see* Injury, intracranial, focal
　　region S00.83 ☑
testis S30.22 ☑
thigh S70.1- ☑
thorax (wall) S20.20 ☑
　　back S20.22- ☑
　　front S20.21- ☑
throat S10.0 ☑
thumb S60.01- ☑
　　with damage to nail S60.11- ☑
toe(s) (lesser) S90.12- ☑
　　with damage to nail S90.22- ☑
　　great S90.11- ☑
　　　with damage to nail S90.21- ☑
tongue S00.532 ☑
trachea (cervical) S10.0 ☑
　　thoracic S27.52 ☑
tunica vaginalis S30.22 ☑
tympanum, tympanic membrane — *see* Contusion, ear
ureter S37.12 ☑
urethra S37.32 ☑
urinary organ NEC S37.892 ☑
uterus S37.62 ☑
uvula S00.532 ☑
vagina S30.23 ☑
vas deferens S37.892 ☑
vesical S37.22 ☑
vocal cord(s) S10.0 ☑
vulva S30.23 ☑
wrist S60.21- ☑
Conus (congenital) (any type) Q14.8
cornea — *see* Keratoconus
medullaris syndrome G95.81
Conversion hysteria, neurosis or reaction F44.9
Converter, tuberculosis (test reaction) R76.11
Conviction (legal), **anxiety concerning** Z65.0
with imprisonment Z65.1
Convulsions (idiopathic) — *see also* Seizure(s) R56.9
apoplectiform (cerebral ischemia) I67.82
dissociative F44.5
epileptic — *see* Epilepsy
epileptiform, epileptoid — *see* Seizure, epileptiform
ether (anesthetic) — *see* Table of Drugs and Chemicals, by drug
febrile R56.00
　　with status epilepticus G40.901
　　complex R56.01
　　　with status epilepticus G40.901
　　simple R56.00
hysterical F44.5
infantile P90
　　epilepsy — *see* Epilepsy
jacksonian — *see* Epilepsy, localization-related, symptomatic, with simple partial seizures
myoclonic G25.3
newborn P90
obstetrical (nephritic) (uremic) — *see* Eclampsia
paretic A52.17
post traumatic R56.1
psychomotor — *see* Epilepsy, localization-related, symptomatic, with complex partial seizures
recurrent R56.9

Convulsions — *continued*
reflex R25.8
scarlatinal A38.8
tetanus, tetanic — *see* Tetanus
thymic E32.8
Convulsive — *see also* Convulsions
Cooley's anemia D56.1
Coolie itch B76.9
Cooper's
disease — *see* Mastopathy, cystic
hernia — *see* Hernia, abdomen, specified site NEC
Copra itch B88.0
Coprophagy F50.89
Coprophobia F40.298
Coproporphyria, hereditary E80.29
Cor
biloculare Q20.8
bovis, bovinum — *see* Hypertrophy, cardiac
pulmonale (chronic) I27.81
　　acute I26.09
triatriatum, triatrium Q24.2
triloculare Q20.8
　　biatrium Q20.4
　　biventriculare Q21.1
Corbus' disease (gangrenous balanitis) N48.1
Cord — *see also* condition
around neck
　　complicating delivery O69.81 ☑
　　　with compression O69.1 ☑
bladder G95.89
　　tabetic A52.19
Cordis ectopia Q24.8
Corditis (spermatic) N49.1
Corectopia Q13.2
Cori's disease (glycogen storage) E74.03
Corkhandler's disease or lung J67.3
Corkscrew esophagus K22.4
Corkworker's disease or lung J67.3
Corn (infected) L84
Cornea — *see also* condition
donor Z52.5
plana Q13.4
Cornelia de Lange syndrome Q87.19
Cornu cutaneum L85.8
Cornual gestation or pregnancy O00.80
with intrauterine pregnancy O00.81
Coronary (artery) — *see* condition
Coronavirus, as cause of disease classified elsewhere
B97.29
SARS-associated B97.21
Corpora — *see also* condition
amylacea, prostate N42.89
cavernosa — *see* condition
Corpulence — *see* Obesity
Corpus — *see* condition
Corrected transposition Q20.5
Corrosion (injury) (acid) (caustic) (chemical) (lime) (external) (internal) T30.4
abdomen, abdominal (muscle) (wall) T21.42 ☑
　　first degree T21.52 ☑
　　second degree T21.62 ☑
　　third degree T21.72 ☑
above elbow T22.439 ☑
　　first degree T22.539 ☑
　　left T22.432 ☑
　　　first degree T22.532 ☑
　　　second degree T22.632 ☑
　　　third degree T22.732 ☑
　　right T22.431 ☑
　　　first degree T22.531 ☑
　　　second degree T22.631 ☑
　　　third degree T22.731 ☑
　　second degree T22.639 ☑
　　third degree T22.739 ☑
alimentary tract NEC T28.7 ☑
ankle T25.419 ☑
　　first degree T25.519 ☑
　　left T25.412 ☑
　　　first degree T25.512 ☑
　　　second degree T25.612 ☑
　　　third degree T25.712 ☑
　　multiple with foot — *see* Corrosion, lower, limb, multiple, ankle and foot
　　right T25.411 ☑
　　　first degree T25.511 ☑
　　　second degree T25.611 ☑

Corrosion — *continued*
ankle — *continued*
　　right — *continued*
　　　third degree T25.711 ☑
　　second degree T25.619 ☑
　　third degree T25.719 ☑
anus — *see* Corrosion, buttock
arm(s) (meaning upper limb(s)) — *see* Corrosion, upper limb
axilla T22.449 ☑
　　first degree T22.549 ☑
　　left T22.442 ☑
　　　first degree T22.542 ☑
　　　second degree T22.642 ☑
　　　third degree T22.742 ☑
　　right T22.441 ☑
　　　first degree T22.541 ☑
　　　second degree T22.641 ☑
　　　third degree T22.741 ☑
　　second degree T22.649 ☑
　　third degree T22.749 ☑
back (lower) T21.44 ☑
　　first degree T21.54 ☑
　　second degree T21.64 ☑
　　third degree T21.74 ☑
　　upper T21.43 ☑
　　　first degree T21.53 ☑
　　　second degree T21.63 ☑
　　　third degree T21.73 ☑
blisters — *code as* Corrosion, second degree, by site
breast(s) — *see* Corrosion, chest wall
buttock(s) T21.45 ☑
　　first degree T21.55 ☑
　　second degree T21.65 ☑
　　third degree T21.75 ☑
calf T24.439 ☑
　　first degree T24.539 ☑
　　left T24.432 ☑
　　　first degree T24.532 ☑
　　　second degree T24.632 ☑
　　　third degree T24.732 ☑
　　right T24.431 ☑
　　　first degree T24.531 ☑
　　　second degree T24.631 ☑
　　　third degree T24.731 ☑
　　second degree T24.639 ☑
　　third degree T24.739 ☑
canthus (eye) — *see* Corrosion, eyelid
cervix T28.8 ☑
cheek T20.46 ☑
　　first degree T20.56 ☑
　　second degree T20.66 ☑
　　third degree T20.76 ☑
chest wall T21.41 ☑
　　first degree T21.51 ☑
　　second degree T21.61 ☑
　　third degree T21.71 ☑
chin T20.43 ☑
　　first degree T20.53 ☑
　　second degree T20.63 ☑
　　third degree T20.73 ☑
colon T28.7 ☑
conjunctiva (and cornea) — *see* Corrosion, cornea
cornea (and conjunctiva) T26.6- ☑
deep necrosis of underlying tissue — *code as* Corrosion, third degree, by site
dorsum of hand T23.469 ☑
　　first degree T23.569 ☑
　　left T23.462 ☑
　　　first degree T23.562 ☑
　　　second degree T23.662 ☑
　　　third degree T23.762 ☑
　　right T23.461 ☑
　　　first degree T23.561 ☑
　　　second degree T23.661 ☑
　　　third degree T23.761 ☑
　　second degree T23.669 ☑
　　third degree T23.769 ☑
ear (auricle) (external) (canal) T20.41 ☑
　　drum T28.91 ☑
　　first degree T20.51 ☑
　　second degree T20.61 ☑
　　third degree T20.71 ☑
elbow T22.429 ☑
　　first degree T22.529 ☑
　　left T22.422 ☑

⬇ Subterms under main terms may continue to next column or page　　　☑ Additional Character Required — Refer to the Tabular List for Character Selection　　　73

Contusion — Corrosion

Corrosion — *continued*
elbow — *continued*
  left — *continued*
    first degree T22.522 ☑
    second degree T22.622 ☑
    third degree T22.722 ☑
  right T22.421 ☑
    first degree T22.521 ☑
    second degree T22.621 ☑
    third degree T22.721 ☑
  second degree T22.629 ☑
  third degree T22.729 ☑
entire body — *see* Corrosion, multiple body regions
epidermal loss — *code as* Corrosion, second degree, by site
epiglottis T27.4 ☑
erythema, erythematous — *code as* Corrosion, first degree, by site
esophagus T28.6 ☑
extent (percentage of body surface)
  less than 10 percent T32.0
  10-19 percent (0-9 percent third degree) T32.10
    with 10-19 percent third degree T32.11
  20-29 percent (0-9 percent third degree) T32.20
    with
      10-19 percent third degree T32.21
      20-29 percent third degree T32.22
  30-39 percent (0-9 percent third degree) T32.30
    with
      10-19 percent third degree T32.31
      20-29 percent third degree T32.32
      30-39 percent third degree T32.33
  40-49 percent (0-9 percent third degree) T32.40
    with
      10-19 percent third degree T32.41
      20-29 percent third degree T32.42
      30-39 percent third degree T32.43
      40-49 percent third degree T32.44
  50-59 percent (0-9 percent third degree) T32.50
    with
      10-19 percent third degree T32.51
      20-29 percent third degree T32.52
      30-39 percent third degree T32.53
      40-49 percent third degree T32.54
      50-59 percent third degree T32.55
  60-69 percent (0-9 percent third degree) T32.60
    with
      10-19 percent third degree T32.61
      20-29 percent third degree T32.62
      30-39 percent third degree T32.63
      40-49 percent third degree T32.64
      50-59 percent third degree T32.65
      60-69 percent third degree T32.66
  70-79 percent (0-9 percent third degree) T32.70
    with
      10-19 percent third degree T32.71
      20-29 percent third degree T32.72
      30-39 percent third degree T32.73
      40-49 percent third degree T32.74
      50-59 percent third degree T32.75
      60-69 percent third degree T32.76
      70-79 percent third degree T32.77
  80-89 percent (0-9 percent third degree) T32.80
    with
      10-19 percent third degree T32.81
      20-29 percent third degree T32.82
      30-39 percent third degree T32.83
      40-49 percent third degree T32.84
      50-59 percent third degree T32.85
      60-69 percent third degree T32.86
      70-79 percent third degree T32.87
      80-89 percent third degree T32.88
  90 percent or more (0-9 percent third degree) T32.90
    with
      10-19 percent third degree T32.91
      20-29 percent third degree T32.92
      30-39 percent third degree T32.93
      40-49 percent third degree T32.94
      50-59 percent third degree T32.95
      60-69 percent third degree T32.96
      70-79 percent third degree T32.97
      80-89 percent third degree T32.98
      90-99 percent third degree T32.99
extremity — *see* Corrosion, limb
eye(s) and adnexa T26.9- ☑
  with resulting rupture and destruction of eyeball T26.7- ☑
  conjunctival sac — *see* Corrosion, cornea

Corrosion — *continued*
eye(s) and adnexa — *continued*
  cornea — *see* Corrosion, cornea
  lid — *see* Corrosion, eyelid
  periocular area — *see* Corrosion eyelid
  specified site NEC T26.8- ☑
eyeball — *see* Corrosion, eye
eyelid(s) T26.5- ☑
face — *see* Corrosion, head
finger T23.429 ☑
  first degree T23.529 ☑
  left T23.422 ☑
    first degree T23.522 ☑
    second degree T23.622 ☑
    third degree T23.722 ☑
  multiple sites (without thumb) T23.439 ☑
    with thumb T23.449 ☑
      first degree T23.549 ☑
      left T23.442 ☑
        first degree T23.542 ☑
        second degree T23.642 ☑
        third degree T23.742 ☑
      right T23.441 ☑
        first degree T23.541 ☑
        second degree T23.641 ☑
        third degree T23.741 ☑
      second degree T23.649 ☑
      third degree T23.749 ☑
    first degree T23.539 ☑
    left T23.432 ☑
      first degree T23.532 ☑
      second degree T23.632 ☑
      third degree T23.732 ☑
    right T23.431 ☑
      first degree T23.531 ☑
      second degree T23.631 ☑
      third degree T23.731 ☑
    second degree T23.639 ☑
    third degree T23.739 ☑
  right T23.421 ☑
    first degree T23.521 ☑
    second degree T23.621 ☑
    third degree T23.721 ☑
  second degree T23.629 ☑
  third degree T23.729 ☑
flank — *see* Corrosion, abdomen
foot T25.429 ☑
  first degree T25.529 ☑
  left T25.422 ☑
    first degree T25.522 ☑
    second degree T25.622 ☑
    third degree T25.722 ☑
  multiple with ankle — *see* Corrosion, lower, limb, multiple, ankle and foot
  right T25.421 ☑
    first degree T25.521 ☑
    second degree T25.621 ☑
    third degree T25.721 ☑
  second degree T25.629 ☑
  third degree T25.729 ☑
forearm T22.419 ☑
  first degree T22.519 ☑
  left T22.412 ☑
    first degree T22.512 ☑
    second degree T22.612 ☑
    third degree T22.712 ☑
  right T22.411 ☑
    first degree T22.511 ☑
    second degree T22.611 ☑
    third degree T22.711 ☑
  second degree T22.619 ☑
  third degree T22.719 ☑
forehead T20.46 ☑
  first degree T20.56 ☑
  second degree T20.66 ☑
  third degree T20.76 ☑
fourth degree — *code as* Corrosion, third degree, by site
full thickness skin loss — *code as* Corrosion, third degree, by site
gastrointestinal tract NEC T28.7 ☑
genital organs
  external
    female T21.47 ☑
      first degree T21.57 ☑
      second degree T21.67 ☑

Corrosion — *continued*
genital organs — *continued*
  external — *continued*
    female — *continued*
      third degree T21.77 ☑
    male T21.46 ☑
      first degree T21.56 ☑
      second degree T21.66 ☑
      third degree T21.76 ☑
  internal T28.8 ☑
groin — *see* Corrosion, abdominal wall
hand(s) T23.409 ☑
  back — *see* Corrosion, dorsum of hand
  finger — *see* Corrosion, finger
  first degree T23.509 ☑
  left T23.402 ☑
    first degree T23.502 ☑
    second degree T23.602 ☑
    third degree T23.702 ☑
  multiple sites with wrist T23.499 ☑
    first degree T23.599 ☑
    left T23.492 ☑
      first degree T23.592 ☑
      second degree T23.692 ☑
      third degree T23.792 ☑
    right T23.491 ☑
      first degree T23.591 ☑
      second degree T23.691 ☑
      third degree T23.791 ☑
    second degree T23.699 ☑
    third degree T23.799 ☑
  palm — *see* Corrosion, palm
  right T23.401 ☑
    first degree T23.501 ☑
    second degree T23.601 ☑
    third degree T23.701 ☑
  second degree T23.609 ☑
  third degree T23.709 ☑
  thumb — *see* Corrosion, thumb
head (and face) (and neck) T20.40 ☑
  cheek — *see* Corrosion, cheek
  chin — *see* Corrosion, chin
  ear — *see* Corrosion, ear
  eye(s) only — *see* Corrosion, eye
  first degree T20.50 ☑
  forehead — *see* Corrosion, forehead
  lip — *see* Corrosion, lip
  multiple sites T20.49 ☑
    first degree T20.59 ☑
    second degree T20.69 ☑
    third degree T20.79 ☑
  neck — *see* Corrosion, neck
  nose — *see* Corrosion, nose
  scalp — *see* Corrosion, scalp
  second degree T20.60 ☑
  third degree T20.70 ☑
hip(s) — *see* Corrosion, lower, limb
inhalation — *see* Corrosion, respiratory tract
internal organ(s) — *see also* Corrosion, by site T28.90 ☑
  alimentary tract T28.7 ☑
    esophagus T28.6 ☑
  esophagus T28.6 ☑
  genitourinary T28.8 ☑
  mouth T28.5 ☑
  pharynx T28.5 ☑
  specified organ NEC T28.99 ☑
interscapular region — *see* Corrosion, back, upper
intestine (large) (small) T28.7 ☑
knee T24.429 ☑
  first degree T24.529 ☑
  left T24.422 ☑
    first degree T24.522 ☑
    second degree T24.622 ☑
    third degree T24.722 ☑
  right T24.421 ☑
    first degree T24.521 ☑
    second degree T24.621 ☑
    third degree T24.721 ☑
  second degree T24.629 ☑
  third degree T24.729 ☑
labium (majus) (minus) — *see* Corrosion, genital organs, external, female
lacrimal apparatus, duct, gland or sac — *see* Corrosion eye, specified site NEC
larynx T27.4 ☑

Corrosion — *continued*
  larynx — *continued*
    with lung T27.5 ☑
  leg(s) (meaning lower limb(s)) — *see* Corrosion, lower limb
  limb(s)
    lower — *see* Corrosion, lower, limb
    upper — *see* Corrosion, upper limb
  lip(s) T20.42 ☑
    first degree T20.52 ☑
    second degree T20.62 ☑
    third degree T20.72 ☑
  lower
    back — *see* Corrosion, back
    limb T24.409 ☑
      ankle — *see* Corrosion, ankle
      calf — *see* Corrosion, calf
      first degree T24.509 ☑
      foot — *see* Corrosion, foot
      knee — *see* Corrosion, knee
      left T24.402 ☑
        first degree T24.502 ☑
        second degree T24.602 ☑
        third degree T24.702 ☑
      multiple sites, except ankle and foot T24.499 ☑
        ankle and foot T25.499 ☑
          first degree T25.599 ☑
          left T25.492 ☑
            first degree T25.592 ☑
            second degree T25.692 ☑
            third degree T25.792 ☑
          right T25.491 ☑
            first degree T25.591 ☑
            second degree T25.691 ☑
            third degree T25.791 ☑
          second degree T25.699 ☑
          third degree T25.799 ☑
        first degree T24.599 ☑
        left T24.492 ☑
          first degree T24.592 ☑
          second degree T24.692 ☑
          third degree T24.792 ☑
        right T24.491 ☑
          first degree T24.591 ☑
          second degree T24.691 ☑
          third degree T24.791 ☑
      second degree T24.699 ☑
      third degree T24.799 ☑
      right T24.401 ☑
        first degree T24.501 ☑
        second degree T24.601 ☑
        third degree T24.701 ☑
      second degree T24.609 ☑
      thigh — *see* Corrosion, thigh
      third degree T24.709 ☑
  lung (with larynx and trachea) T27.5 ☑
  mouth T28.5 ☑
  neck T20.47 ☑
    first degree T20.57 ☑
    second degree T20.67 ☑
    third degree T20.77 ☑
  nose (septum) T20.44 ☑
    first degree T20.54 ☑
    second degree T20.64 ☑
    third degree T20.74 ☑
  ocular adnexa — *see* Corrosion, eye
  orbit region — *see* Corrosion, eyelid
  palm T23.459 ☑
    first degree T23.559 ☑
    left T23.452 ☑
      first degree T23.552 ☑
      second degree T23.652 ☑
      third degree T23.752 ☑
    right T23.451 ☑
      first degree T23.551 ☑
      second degree T23.651 ☑
      third degree T23.751 ☑
    second degree T23.659 ☑
    third degree T23.759 ☑
  partial thickness — *code as* Corrosion, unspecified degree, by site
  pelvis — *see* Corrosion, trunk
  penis — *see* Corrosion, genital organs, external, male
  perineum
    female — *see* Corrosion, genital organs, external, female

Corrosion — *continued*
  perineum — *continued*
    male — *see* Corrosion, genital organs, external, male
  periocular area — *see* Corrosion, eyelid
  pharynx T28.5 ☑
  rectum T28.7 ☑
  respiratory tract T27.7 ☑
    larynx — *see* Corrosion, larynx
    specified part NEC T27.6 ☑
    trachea — *see* Corrosion, larynx
  sac, lacrimal — *see* Corrosion, eye, specified site NEC
  scalp T20.45 ☑
    first degree T20.55 ☑
    second degree T20.65 ☑
    third degree T20.75 ☑
  scapular region T22.469 ☑
    first degree T22.569 ☑
    left T22.462 ☑
      first degree T22.562 ☑
      second degree T22.662 ☑
      third degree T22.762 ☑
    right T22.461 ☑
      first degree T22.561 ☑
      second degree T22.661 ☑
      third degree T22.761 ☑
    second degree T22.669 ☑
    third degree T22.769 ☑
  sclera — *see* Corrosion, eye, specified site NEC
  scrotum — *see* Corrosion, genital organs, external, male
  shoulder T22.459 ☑
    first degree T22.559 ☑
    left T22.452 ☑
      first degree T22.552 ☑
      second degree T22.652 ☑
      third degree T22.752 ☑
    right T22.451 ☑
      first degree T22.551 ☑
      second degree T22.651 ☑
      third degree T22.751 ☑
    second degree T22.659 ☑
    third degree T22.759 ☑
  stomach T28.7 ☑
  temple — *see* Corrosion, head
  testis — *see* Corrosion, genital organs, external, male
  thigh T24.419 ☑
    first degree T24.519 ☑
    left T24.412 ☑
      first degree T24.512 ☑
      second degree T24.612 ☑
      third degree T24.712 ☑
    right T24.411 ☑
      first degree T24.511 ☑
      second degree T24.611 ☑
      third degree T24.711 ☑
    second degree T24.619 ☑
    third degree T24.719 ☑
  thorax (external) — *see* Corrosion, trunk
  throat (meaning pharynx) T28.5 ☑
  thumb(s) T23.419 ☑
    first degree T23.519 ☑
    left T23.412 ☑
      first degree T23.512 ☑
      second degree T23.612 ☑
      third degree T23.712 ☑
    multiple sites with fingers T23.449 ☑
      first degree T23.549 ☑
      left T23.442 ☑
        first degree T23.542 ☑
        second degree T23.642 ☑
        third degree T23.742 ☑
      right T23.441 ☑
        first degree T23.541 ☑
        second degree T23.641 ☑
        third degree T23.741 ☑
      second degree T23.649 ☑
      third degree T23.749 ☑
    right T23.411 ☑
      first degree T23.511 ☑
      second degree T23.611 ☑
      third degree T23.711 ☑
    second degree T23.619 ☑
    third degree T23.719 ☑
  toe T25.439 ☑
    first degree T25.539 ☑
    left T25.432 ☑

Corrosion — *continued*
  toe — *continued*
    left — *continued*
      first degree T25.532 ☑
      second degree T25.632 ☑
      third degree T25.732 ☑
    right T25.431 ☑
      first degree T25.531 ☑
      second degree T25.631 ☑
      third degree T25.731 ☑
    second degree T25.639 ☑
    third degree T25.739 ☑
  tongue T28.5 ☑
  tonsil(s) T28.5 ☑
  total body — *see* Corrosion, multiple body regions
  trachea T27.4 ☑
    with lung T27.5 ☑
  trunk T21.40 ☑
    abdominal wall — *see* Corrosion, abdominal wall
    anus — *see* Corrosion, buttock
    axilla — *see* Corrosion, upper limb
    back — *see* Corrosion, back
    breast — *see* Corrosion, chest wall
    buttock — *see* Corrosion, buttock
    chest wall — *see* Corrosion, chest wall
    first degree T21.50 ☑
    flank — *see* Corrosion, abdominal wall
    genital
      female — *see* Corrosion, genital organs, external, female
      male — *see* Corrosion, genital organs, external, male
    groin — *see* Corrosion, abdominal wall
    interscapular region — *see* Corrosion, back, upper
    labia — *see* Corrosion, genital organs, external, female
    lower back — *see* Corrosion, back
    penis — *see* Corrosion, genital organs, external, male
    perineum
      female — *see* Corrosion, genital organs, external, female
      male — *see* Corrosion, genital organs, external, male
    scapular region — *see* Corrosion, upper limb
    scrotum — *see* Corrosion, genital organs, external, male
    second degree T21.60 ☑
    shoulder — *see* Corrosion, upper limb
    specified site NEC T21.49 ☑
      first degree T21.59 ☑
      second degree T21.69 ☑
      third degree T21.79 ☑
    testes — *see* Corrosion, genital organs, external, male
    third degree T21.70 ☑
    upper back — *see* Corrosion, back, upper
    vagina T28.8 ☑
    vulva — *see* Corrosion, genital organs, external, female
  unspecified site with extent of body surface involved specified
    less than 10 percent T32.0
    10-19 percent (0-9 percent third degree) T32.10
      with 10-19 percent third degree T32.11
    20-29 percent (0-9 percent third degree) T32.20
      with
        10-19 percent third degree T32.21
        20-29 percent third degree T32.22
    30-39 percent (0-9 percent third degree) T32.30
      with
        10-19 percent third degree T32.31
        20-29 percent third degree T32.32
        30-39 percent third degree T32.33
    40-49 percent (0-9 percent third degree) T32.40
      with
        10-19 percent third degree T32.41
        20-29 percent third degree T32.42
        30-39 percent third degree T32.43
        40-49 percent third degree T32.44
    50-59 percent (0-9 percent third degree) T32.50
      with
        10-19 percent third degree T32.51
        20-29 percent third degree T32.52
        30-39 percent third degree T32.53
        40-49 percent third degree T32.54
        50-59 percent third degree T32.55

Corrosion — *continued*
  unspecified site with extent of body surface involved
    specified — *continued*
      60-69 percent (0-9 percent third degree) T32.60
        with
          10-19 percent third degree T32.61
          20-29 percent third degree T32.62
          30-39 percent third degree T32.63
          40-49 percent third degree T32.64
          50-59 percent third degree T32.65
          60-69 percent third degree T32.66
      70-79 percent (0-9 percent third degree) T32.70
        with
          10-19 percent third degree T32.71
          20-29 percent third degree T32.72
          30-39 percent third degree T32.73
          40-49 percent third degree T32.74
          50-59 percent third degree T32.75
          60-69 percent third degree T32.76
          70-79 percent third degree T32.77
      80-89 percent (0-9 percent third degree) T32.80
        with
          10-19 percent third degree T32.81
          20-29 percent third degree T32.82
          30-39 percent third degree T32.83
          40-49 percent third degree T32.84
          50-59 percent third degree T32.85
          60-69 percent third degree T32.86
          70-79 percent third degree T32.87
          80-89 percent third degree T32.88
      90 percent or more (0-9 percent third degree) T32.90
        with
          10-19 percent third degree T32.91
          20-29 percent third degree T32.92
          30-39 percent third degree T32.93
          40-49 percent third degree T32.94
          50-59 percent third degree T32.95
          60-69 percent third degree T32.96
          70-79 percent third degree T32.97
          80-89 percent third degree T32.98
          90-99 percent third degree T32.99
  upper limb (axilla) (scapular region) T22.40 ☑
    above elbow — *see* Corrosion, above elbow
    axilla — *see* Corrosion, axilla
    elbow — *see* Corrosion, elbow
    first degree T22.50 ☑
    forearm — *see* Corrosion, forearm
    hand — *see* Corrosion, hand
    interscapular region — *see* Corrosion, back, upper
    multiple sites T22.499 ☑
      first degree T22.599 ☑
      left T22.492 ☑
        first degree T22.592 ☑
        second degree T22.692 ☑
        third degree T22.792 ☑
      right T22.491 ☑
        first degree T22.591 ☑
        second degree T22.691 ☑
        third degree T22.791 ☑
      second degree T22.699 ☑
      third degree T22.799 ☑
    scapular region — *see* Corrosion, scapular region
    second degree T22.60 ☑
    shoulder — *see* Corrosion, shoulder
    third degree T22.70 ☑
    wrist — *see* Corrosion, hand
  uterus T28.8 ☑
  vagina T28.8 ☑
  vulva — *see* Corrosion, genital organs, external, female
  wrist T23.479 ☑
    first degree T23.579 ☑
    left T23.472 ☑
      first degree T23.572 ☑
      second degree T23.672 ☑
      third degree T23.772 ☑
    multiple sites with hand T23.499 ☑
      first degree T23.599 ☑
      left T23.492 ☑
        first degree T23.592 ☑
        second degree T23.692 ☑
        third degree T23.792 ☑
      right T23.491 ☑
        first degree T23.591 ☑
        second degree T23.691 ☑
        third degree T23.791 ☑
      second degree T23.699 ☑
      third degree T23.799 ☑

Corrosion — *continued*
  wrist — *continued*
    right T23.471 ☑
      first degree T23.571 ☑
      second degree T23.671 ☑
      third degree T23.771 ☑
    second degree T23.679 ☑
    third degree T23.779 ☑
Corrosive burn — *see* Corrosion
Corsican fever — *see* Malaria
Cortical — *see* condition
Cortico-adrenal — *see* condition
Coryza (acute) J00
  with grippe or influenza — *see* Influenza, with, respiratory manifestations NEC
  syphilitic
    congenital (chronic) A50.05
Costen's syndrome or complex M26.69
Costiveness — *see* Constipation
Costochondritis M94.0
Cot death R99
Cotard's syndrome F22
Cotia virus B08.8
Cotton wool spots (retinal) H35.81
Cotungo's disease — *see* Sciatica
Cough (affected) (chronic) (epidemic) (nervous) R05
  with hemorrhage — *see* Hemoptysis
  bronchial R05
    with grippe or influenza — *see* Influenza, with, respiratory manifestations NEC
  functional F45.8
  hysterical F45.8
  laryngeal, spasmodic R05
  psychogenic F45.8
  smokers' J41.0
  tea taster's B49
Counseling (for) Z71.9
  abuse NEC
    perpetrator Z69.82
    victim Z69.81
  alcohol abuser Z71.41
    family Z71.42
  child abuse
    nonparental
      perpetrator Z69.021
      victim Z69.020
    parental
      perpetrator Z69.011
      victim Z69.010
  consanguinity Z71.89
  contraceptive Z30.09
  dietary Z71.3
  drug abuser Z71.51
    family member Z71.52
  exercise Z71.82
  family Z71.89
  fertility preservation (prior to cancer therapy) (prior to removal of gonads) Z31.62
  for non-attending third party Z71.0
    related to sexual behavior or orientation Z70.2
  genetic
    nonprocreative Z71.83
    procreative NEC Z31.5
  gestational carrier Z31.7
  health (advice) (education) (instruction) — *see* Counseling, medical
    risk for travel (international) Z71.84
  human immunodeficiency virus (HIV) Z71.7
  impotence Z70.1
  insulin pump use Z46.81
  medical (for) Z71.9
    boarding school resident Z59.3
    consanguinity Z71.89
    feared complaint and no disease found Z71.1
    human immunodeficiency virus (HIV) Z71.7
    institutional resident Z59.3
    on behalf of another Z71.0
      related to sexual behavior or orientation Z70.2
    person living alone Z60.2
    specified reason NEC Z71.89
  natural family planning
    procreative Z31.61
    to avoid pregnancy Z30.02
  perpetrator (of)
    abuse NEC Z69.82
    child abuse
      non-parental Z69.021
      parental Z69.011

Counseling — *continued*
  perpetrator — *continued*
    rape NEC Z69.82
    spousal abuse Z69.12
  procreative NEC Z31.69
    fertility preservation (prior to cancer therapy) (prior to removal of gonads) Z31.62
    using natural family planning Z31.61
  promiscuity Z70.1
  rape victim Z69.81
  religious Z71.81
  safety for travel (international) Z71.84
  sex, sexual (related to) Z70.9
    attitude(s) Z70.0
    behavior or orientation Z70.1
    combined concerns Z70.3
    non-responsiveness Z70.1
    on behalf of third party Z70.2
    specified reason NEC Z70.8
  specified reason NEC Z71.89
  spiritual Z71.81
  spousal abuse (perpetrator) Z69.12
    victim Z69.11
  substance abuse Z71.89
    alcohol Z71.41
    drug Z71.51
    tobacco Z71.6
  tobacco use Z71.6
  travel (international) Z71.84
  use (of)
    insulin pump Z46.81
  victim (of)
    abuse Z69.81
    child abuse
      by parent Z69.010
      non-parental Z69.020
    rape NEC Z69.81
Coupled rhythm R00.8
Couvelaire syndrome or uterus (complicating delivery) O45.8X- ☑
Cowperitis — *see* Urethritis
Cowper's gland — *see* condition
Cowpox B08.010
  due to vaccination T88.1 ☑
Coxa
  magna M91.4- ☑
  plana M91.2- ☑
  valga (acquired) — *see also* Deformity, limb, specifie type NEC, thigh
    congenital Q65.81
    sequelae (late effect) of rickets E64.3
  vara (acquired) — *see also* Deformity, limb, specifiec type NEC, thigh
    congenital Q65.82
    sequelae (late effect) of rickets E64.3
Coxalgia, coxalgic (nontuberculous) — *see also* Pain, joint, hip
  tuberculous A18.02
Coxitis — *see* Monoarthritis, hip
Coxsackie (virus) (infection) B34.1
  as cause of disease classified elsewhere B97.11
  carditis B33.20
  central nervous system NEC A88.8
  endocarditis B33.21
  enteritis A08.39
  meningitis (aseptic) A87.0
  myocarditis B33.22
  pericarditis B33.23
  pharyngitis B08.5
  pleurodynia B33.0
  specific disease NEC B33.8
Crabs, meaning pubic lice B85.3
Crack baby P04.41
Cracked nipple N64.0
  associated with
    lactation O92.13
    pregnancy O92.11- ☑
    puerperium O92.12
Cracked tooth K03.81
Cradle cap L21.0
Craft neurosis F48.8
Cramp(s) R25.2
  abdominal — *see* Pain, abdominal
  bathing T75.1 ☑
  colic R10.83
    psychogenic F45.8
  due to immersion T75.1 ☑
  fireman T67.2 ☑

☑ **Additional Character Required** — Refer to the Tabular List for Character Selection
🔻 Subterms under main terms may continue to next column or page

Cramp(s) — *continued*
  heat T67.2 ☑
  immersion T75.1 ☑
  intestinal — *see* Pain, abdominal
    psychogenic F45.8
  leg, sleep related G47.62
  limb (lower) (upper) NEC R25.2
    sleep related G47.62
  linotypist's F48.8
    organic G25.89
  muscle (limb) (general) R25.2
    due to immersion T75.1 ☑
    psychogenic F45.8
  occupational (hand) F48.8
    organic G25.89
  salt-depletion E87.1
  sleep related, leg G47.62
  stoker's T67.2 ☑
  swimmer's T75.1 ☑
  telegrapher's F48.8
    organic G25.89
  typist's F48.8
    organic G25.89
  uterus N94.89
    menstrual — *see* Dysmenorrhea
  writer's F48.8
    organic G25.89
Cranial — *see* condition
Craniocleidodysostosis Q74.0
Craniofenestria (skull) Q75.8
Craniolacunia (skull) Q75.8
Craniopagus Q89.4
Craniopathy, metabolic M85.2
Craniopharyngeal — *see* condition
Craniopharyngioma D44.4
Craniorachischisis (totalis) Q00.1
Cranioschisis Q75.8
Craniostenosis Q75.0
Craniosynostosis Q75.0
Craniotabes (cause unknown) M83.8
  neonatal P96.3
  rachitic E64.3
  syphilitic A50.56
Cranium — *see* condition
Craw-craw — *see* Onchocerciasis
Creaking joint — *see* Derangement, joint, specified type NEC
Creeping
  eruption B76.9
  palsy or paralysis G12.22
Crenated tongue K14.8
Creotoxism A05.9
Crepitus
  caput Q75.8
  joint — *see* Derangement, joint, specified type NEC
Crescent or conus choroid, congenital Q14.3
CREST syndrome M34.1
Cretin, cretinism (congenital) (endemic) (nongoitrous) (sporadic) E00.9
  pelvis
    with disproportion (fetopelvic) O33.0
      causing obstructed labor O65.0
  type
    hypothyroid E00.1
    mixed E00.2
    myxedematous E00.1
    neurological E00.0
Creutzfeldt-Jakob disease or syndrome (with dementia) A81.00
  familial A81.09
  iatrogenic A81.09
  specified NEC A81.09
  sporadic A81.09
  variant (vCJD) A81.01
Crib death R99
Cribriform hymen Q52.3
Cri-du-chat syndrome Q93.4
Crigler-Najjar disease or syndrome E80.5
Crime, victim of Z65.4
Criminalism F60.2
Crisis
  abdomen R10.0
  acute reaction F43.0
  addisonian E27.2
  adrenal (cortical) E27.2
  celiac K90.0

Crisis — *continued*
  Dietl's N13.8
  emotional — *see also* Disorder, adjustment
    acute reaction to stress F43.0
    specific to childhood and adolescence F93.8
  glaucomatocyclitic — *see* Glaucoma, secondary, inflammation
  heart — *see* Failure, heart
  nitritoid I95.2
    correct substance properly administered — *see* Table of Drugs and Chemicals, by drug, adverse effect
    overdose or wrong substance given or taken — *see* Table of Drugs and Chemicals, by drug, poisoning
  oculogyric H51.8
    psychogenic F45.8
  Pel's (tabetic) A52.11
  psychosexual identity F64.2
  renal N28.0
  sickle-cell D57.00
    with
      acute chest syndrome D57.01
      splenic sequestration D57.02
  state (acute reaction) F43.0
  tabetic A52.11
  thyroid — *see* Thyrotoxicosis with thyroid storm
  thyrotoxic — *see* Thyrotoxicosis with thyroid storm
Crocq's disease (acrocyanosis) I73.89
Crohn's disease — *see* Enteritis, regional
Crooked septum, nasal J34.2
Cross syndrome E70.328
Crossbite (anterior) (posterior) M26.24
Cross-eye — *see* Strabismus, convergent concomitant
Croup, croupous (catarrhal) (infectious) (inflammatory) (nondiphtheritic) J05.0
  bronchial J20.9
  diphtheritic A36.2
  false J38.5
  spasmodic J38.5
    diphtheritic A36.2
  stridulous J38.5
    diphtheritic A36.2
Crouzon's disease Q75.1
Crowding, tooth, teeth, fully erupted M26.31
CRST syndrome M34.1
Cruchet's disease A85.8
Cruelty in children — *see also* Disorder, conduct
Crural ulcer — *see* Ulcer, lower limb
Crush, crushed, crushing T14.8 ☑
  abdomen S38.1 ☑
  ankle S97.0- ☑
  arm (upper) (and shoulder) S47.- ☑
  axilla — *see* Crush, arm
  back, lower S38.1 ☑
  buttock S38.1 ☑
  cheek S07.0 ☑
  chest S28.0 ☑
  cranium S07.1 ☑
  ear S07.0 ☑
  elbow S57.0- ☑
  extremity
    lower
      ankle — *see* Crush, ankle
      below knee — *see* Crush, leg
      foot — *see* Crush, foot
      hip — *see* Crush, hip
      knee — *see* Crush, knee
      thigh — *see* Crush, thigh
      toe — *see* Crush, toe
    upper
      below elbow S67.9- ☑
      elbow — *see* Crush, elbow
      finger — *see* Crush, finger
      forearm — *see* Crush, forearm
      hand — *see* Crush, hand
      thumb — *see* Crush, thumb
      upper arm — *see* Crush, arm
      wrist — *see* Crush, wrist
  face S07.0 ☑
  finger(s) S67.1- ☑
    with hand (and wrist) — *see* Crush, hand, specified site NEC
    index S67.19- ☑
    little S67.19- ☑
    middle S67.19- ☑
    ring S67.19- ☑

Crush, crushed, crushing — *continued*
  finger(s) — *continued*
    thumb — *see* Crush, thumb
  foot S97.8- ☑
    toe — *see* Crush, toe
  forearm S57.8- ☑
  genitalia, external
    female S38.002 ☑
      vagina S38.03 ☑
      vulva S38.03 ☑
    male S38.001 ☑
      penis S38.01 ☑
      scrotum S38.02 ☑
      testis S38.02 ☑
  hand (except fingers alone) S67.2- ☑
    with wrist S67.4- ☑
  head S07.9 ☑
    specified NEC S07.8 ☑
  heel — *see* Crush, foot
  hip S77.0- ☑
    with thigh S77.2- ☑
  internal organ (abdomen, chest, or pelvis) NEC T14.8 ☑
  knee S87.0- ☑
  labium (majus) (minus) S38.03 ☑
  larynx S17.0 ☑
  leg (lower) S87.8- ☑
    knee — *see* Crush, knee
  lip S07.0 ☑
  lower
    back S38.1 ☑
    leg — *see* Crush, leg
  neck S17.9 ☑
  nerve — *see* Injury, nerve
  nose S07.0 ☑
  pelvis S38.1 ☑
  penis S38.01 ☑
  scalp S07.8 ☑
  scapular region — *see* Crush, arm
  scrotum S38.02 ☑
  severe, unspecified site T14.8 ☑
  shoulder (and upper arm) — *see* Crush, arm
  skull S07.1 ☑
  syndrome (complication of trauma) T79.5 ☑
  testis S38.02 ☑
  thigh S77.1- ☑
    with hip S77.2- ☑
  throat S17.8 ☑
  thumb S67.0- ☑
    with hand (and wrist) — *see* Crush, hand, specified site NEC
  toe(s) S97.10- ☑
    great S97.11- ☑
    lesser S97.12- ☑
  trachea S17.0 ☑
  vagina S38.03 ☑
  vulva S38.03 ☑
  wrist S67.3- ☑
    with hand S67.4- ☑
Crusta lactea L21.0
Crusts R23.4
Crutch paralysis — *see* Injury, brachial plexus
Cruveilhier-Baumgarten cirrhosis, disease or syndrome K74.69
Cruveilhier's atrophy or disease G12.8
Crying (constant) (continuous) (excessive)
  child, adolescent, or adult R45.83
  infant (baby) (newborn) R68.11
Cryofibrinogenemia D89.2
Cryoglobulinemia (essential) (idiopathic) (mixed) (primary) (purpura) (secondary) (vasculitis) D89.1
  with lung involvement D89.1 *[J99]*
Cryptitis (anal) (rectal) K62.89
Cryptococcosis, cryptococcus (infection) (neoformans) B45.9
  bone B45.3
  cerebral B45.1
  cutaneous B45.2
  disseminated B45.7
  generalized B45.7
  meningitis B45.1
  meningocerebralis B45.1
  osseous B45.3
  pulmonary B45.0
  skin B45.2
  specified NEC B45.8
Cryptopapillitis (anus) K62.89

Cryptophthalmos Q11.2
  syndrome Q87.0
Cryptorchid, cryptorchism, cryptorchidism Q53.9
  bilateral Q53.20
    abdominal Q53.211
    perineal Q53.22
  unilateral Q53.10
    abdominal Q53.111
    perineal Q53.12
Cryptosporidiosis A07.2
  hepatobiliary B88.8
  respiratory B88.8
Cryptostromosis J67.6
Crystalluria R82.998
Cubitus
  congenital Q68.8
  valgus (acquired) M21.0- ☑
    congenital Q68.8
    sequelae (late effect) of rickets E64.3
  varus (acquired) M21.1- ☑
    congenital Q68.8
    sequelae (late effect) of rickets E64.3
Cultural deprivation or shock Z60.3
Curling esophagus K22.4
Curling's ulcer — see Ulcer, peptic, acute
Curschmann (-Batten) (-Steinert) **disease or syndrome**
  G71.11
Curse, Ondine's — see Apnea, sleep
Curvature
  organ or site, congenital NEC — see Distortion
  penis (lateral) Q55.61
  Pott's (spinal) A18.01
  radius, idiopathic, progressive (congenital) Q74.0
  spine (acquired) (angular) (idiopathic) (incorrect)
    (postural) — see Dorsopathy, deforming
    congenital Q67.5
    due to or associated with
      Charcot-Marie-Tooth disease — see also subcat-
        egory M49.8 G60.0
      osteitis
        deformans M88.88
        fibrosa cystica — see also subcategory M49.8
          E21.0
      tuberculosis (Pott's curvature) A18.01
    sequelae (late effect) of rickets E64.3
    tuberculous A18.01
Cushingoid due to steroid therapy E24.2
  correct substance properly administered — see Table
    of Drugs and Chemicals, by drug, adverse effect
  overdose or wrong substance given or taken — see
    Table of Drugs and Chemicals, by drug, poisoning
Cushing's
  syndrome or disease E24.9
    drug-induced E24.2
    iatrogenic E24.2
    pituitary-dependent E24.0
    specified NEC E24.8
  ulcer — see Ulcer, peptic, acute
Cusp, Carabelli — omit code
Cut (external) — see also Laceration
  muscle — see Injury, muscle
Cutaneous — see also condition
  hemorrhage R23.3
  larva migrans B76.9
Cutis — see also condition
  hyperelastica Q82.8
    acquired L57.4
  laxa (hyperelastica) — see Dermatolysis
  marmorata R23.8
  osteosis L94.2
  pendula — see Dermatolysis
  rhomboidalis nuchae L57.2
  verticis gyrata Q82.8
    acquired L91.8
Cyanosis R23.0
  due to
    patent foramen botalli Q21.1
    persistent foramen ovale Q21.1
  enterogenous D74.8
  paroxysmal digital — see Raynaud's disease
    with gangrene I73.01
  retina, retinal H35.89
Cyanotic heart disease I24.9
  congenital Q24.9
Cycle
  anovulatory N97.0
  menstrual, irregular N92.6
Cyclencephaly Q04.9

Cyclical vomiting, in migraine — see also Vomiting,
  cyclical G43.A0 (following G43.7)
  psychogenic F50.89
Cyclitis — see also Iridocyclitis H20.9
  chronic — see Iridocyclitis, chronic
  Fuchs' heterochromic H20.81- ☑
  granulomatous — see Iridocyclitis, chronic
  lens-induced — see Iridocyclitis, lens-induced
  posterior H30.2- ☑
Cycloid personality F34.0
Cyclophoria H50.54
Cyclopia, cyclops Q87.0
Cyclopism Q87.0
Cyclosporiasis A07.4
Cyclothymia F34.0
Cyclothymic personality F34.0
Cyclotropia H50.41- ☑
Cylindroma — see also Neoplasm, malignant, by site
  eccrine dermal — see Neoplasm, skin, benign
  skin — see Neoplasm, skin, benign
Cylindruria R82.998
Cynanche
  diphtheritic A36.2
  tonsillaris J36
Cynophobia F40.218
Cynorexia R63.2
Cyphosis — see Kyphosis
Cyprus fever — see Brucellosis
Cyst (colloid) (mucous) (simple) (retention)
  adenoid (infected) J35.8
  adrenal gland E27.8
    congenital Q89.1
  air, lung J98.4
  allantoic Q64.4
  alveolar process (jaw bone) M27.40
  amnion, amniotic O41.8X- ☑
  aneurysmal M27.49
  anterior
    chamber (eye) — see Cyst, iris
    nasopalatine K09.1
  antrum J34.1
  anus K62.89
  apical (tooth) (periodontal) K04.8
  appendix K38.8
  arachnoid, brain (acquired) G93.0
    congenital Q04.6
  arytenoid J38.7
  Baker's M71.2- ☑
    ruptured M66.0
    tuberculous A18.02
  Bartholin's gland N75.0
  bile duct (common) (hepatic) K83.5
  bladder (multiple) (trigone) N32.89
  blue dome (breast) — see Cyst, breast
  bone (local) NEC M85.60
    aneurysmal M85.50
      ankle M85.57- ☑
      foot M85.57- ☑
      forearm M85.53- ☑
      hand M85.54- ☑
      jaw M27.49
      lower leg M85.56- ☑
      multiple site M85.59
      neck M85.58
      rib M85.58
      shoulder M85.51- ☑
      skull M85.58
      specified site NEC M85.58
      thigh M85.55- ☑
      toe M85.57- ☑
      upper arm M85.52- ☑
      vertebra M85.58
    solitary M85.40
      ankle M85.47- ☑
      fibula M85.46- ☑
      foot M85.47- ☑
      hand M85.44- ☑
      humerus M85.42- ☑
      jaw M27.49
      neck M85.48
      pelvis M85.45- ☑
      radius M85.43- ☑
      rib M85.48
      shoulder M85.41- ☑
      skull M85.48
      specified site NEC M85.48
      tibia M85.46- ☑

Cyst — continued
  bone — continued
    solitary — continued
      toe M85.47- ☑
      ulna M85.43- ☑
      vertebra M85.48
    specified type NEC M85.60
      ankle M85.67- ☑
      foot M85.67- ☑
      forearm M85.63- ☑
      hand M85.64- ☑
      jaw M27.40
        developmental (nonodontogenic) K09.1
          odontogenic K09.0
        latent M27.0
      lower leg M85.66- ☑
      multiple site M85.69
      neck M85.68
      rib M85.68
      shoulder M85.61- ☑
      skull M85.68
      specified site NEC M85.68
      thigh M85.65- ☑
      toe M85.67- ☑
      upper arm M85.62- ☑
      vertebra M85.68
  brain (acquired) G93.0
    congenital Q04.6
    hydatid B67.99 [G94]
    third ventricle (colloid), congenital Q04.6
  branchial (cleft) Q18.0
  branchiogenic Q18.0
  breast (benign) (blue dome) (pedunculated) (solitar
    N60.0- ☑
    involution — see Dysplasia, mammary, specified
      type NEC
    sebaceous — see Dysplasia, mammary, specified
      type NEC
  broad ligament (benign) N83.8
  bronchogenic (mediastinal) (sequestration) J98.4
    congenital Q33.0
  buccal K09.8
  bulbourethral gland N36.8
  bursa, bursal NEC M71.30
    with rupture — see Rupture, synovium
    ankle M71.37- ☑
    elbow M71.32- ☑
    foot M71.37- ☑
    hand M71.34- ☑
    hip M71.35- ☑
    multiple sites M71.39
    pharyngeal J39.2
    popliteal space — see Cyst, Baker's
    shoulder M71.31- ☑
    specified site NEC M71.38
    wrist M71.33- ☑
  calcifying odontogenic D16.5
    upper jaw (bone) (maxilla) D16.4
  canal of Nuck (female) N94.89
    congenital Q52.4
  canthus — see Cyst, conjunctiva
  carcinomatous — see Neoplasm, malignant, by site
  cauda equina G95.89
  cavum septi pellucidi — see Cyst, brain
  celomic (pericardium) Q24.8
  cerebellopontine (angle) — see Cyst, brain
  cerebellum — see Cyst, brain
  cerebral — see Cyst, brain
  cervical lateral Q18.0
  cervix NEC N88.8
    embryonic Q51.6
    nabothian N88.8
  chiasmal optic NEC — see Disorder, optic, chiasm
  chocolate (ovary) N80.1
  choledochus, congenital Q44.4
  chorion O41.8X- ☑
  choroid plexus G93.0
    congenital Q04.6
  ciliary body — see Cyst, iris
  clitoris N90.7
  colon K63.89
  common (bile) duct K83.5
  congenital NEC Q89.8
    adrenal gland Q89.1
    epiglottis Q31.8
    esophagus Q39.8
    fallopian tube Q50.4
    kidney Q61.00

☑ **Additional Character Required** — **Refer to the Tabular List for Character Selection**   ▼ Subterms under main terms may continue to next column or page

Cyst — continued
  congenital — continued
    kidney — continued
      more than one (multiple) Q61.02
        specified as polycystic Q61.3
          adult type Q61.2
          infantile type NEC Q61.19
            collecting duct dilation Q61.11
      solitary Q61.01
    larynx Q31.8
    liver Q44.6
    lung Q33.0
    mediastinum Q34.1
    ovary Q50.1
    oviduct Q50.4
    periurethral (tissue) Q64.79
    prepuce Q55.69
    salivary gland (any) Q38.4
    sublingual Q38.6
    submaxillary gland Q38.6
    thymus (gland) Q89.2
    tongue Q38.3
    ureterovesical orifice Q62.8
    vulva Q52.79
  conjunctiva H11.44- ☑
  cornea H18.89- ☑
  corpora quadrigemina G93.0
  corpus
    albicans N83.29- ☑
    luteum (hemorrhagic) (ruptured) N83.1- ☑
  Cowper's gland (benign) (infected) N36.8
  cranial meninges G93.0
  craniobuccal pouch E23.6
  craniopharyngeal pouch E23.6
  cystic duct K82.8
  Cysticercus — see Cysticercosis
  Dandy-Walker Q03.1
    with spina bifida — see Spina bifida
  dental (root) K04.8
    developmental K09.0
    eruption K09.0
    primordial K09.0
  dentigerous (mandible) (maxilla) K09.0
  dermoid — see Neoplasm, benign, by site
    with malignant transformation C56.- ☑
    implantation
      external area or site (skin) NEC L72.0
      iris — see Cyst, iris, implantation
      vagina N89.8
      vulva N90.7
    mouth K09.8
    oral soft tissue K09.8
    sacrococcygeal — see Cyst, pilonidal
  developmental K09.1
    odontogenic K09.0
    oral region (nonodontogenic) K09.1
    ovary, ovarian Q50.1
  dura (cerebral) G93.0
    spinal G96.19
  ear (external) Q18.1
  echinococcal — see Echinococcus
  embryonic
    cervix uteri Q51.6
    fallopian tube Q50.4
    vagina Q52.4
  endometrium, endometrial (uterus) N85.8
    ectopic — see Endometriosis
  enterogenous Q43.8
  epidermal, epidermoid (inclusion) (see also Cyst, skin)
    L72.0
    mouth K09.8
    oral soft tissue K09.8
  epididymis N50.3
  epiglottis J38.7
  epiphysis cerebri E34.8
  epithelial (inclusion) L72.0
  epoophoron Q50.5
  eruption K09.0
  esophagus K22.8
  ethmoid sinus J34.1
  external female genital organs NEC N90.7
  eyelid (sebaceous) H02.829
    infected — see Hordeolum
    left H02.826
      lower H02.825
      upper H02.824
    right H02.823
      lower H02.822

Cyst — continued
  eyelid — continued
    right — continued
      upper H02.821
  eye NEC H57.89
    congenital Q15.8
  fallopian tube N83.8
    congenital Q50.4
  fimbrial (twisted) Q50.4
  fissural (oral region) K09.1
  follicle (graafian) (hemorrhagic) N83.0- ☑
    nabothian N88.8
  follicular (atretic) (hemorrhagic) (ovarian) N83.0- ☑
    dentigerous K09.0
    odontogenic K09.0
    skin L72.9
      specified NEC L72.8
  frontal sinus J34.1
  gallbladder K82.8
  ganglion — see Ganglion
  Gartner's duct Q52.4
  gingiva K09.0
  gland of Moll — see Cyst, eyelid
  globulomaxillary K09.1
  graafian follicle (hemorrhagic) N83.0- ☑
  granulosal lutein (hemorrhagic) N83.1- ☑
  hemangiomatous D18.00
    intra-abdominal D18.03
    intracranial D18.02
    skin D18.01
    specified site NEC D18.09
  hemorrhagic M27.49
  hydatid — see also Echinococcus B67.90
    brain B67.99 [G94]
    liver — see also Cyst, liver, hydatid B67.8
    lung NEC B67.99 [J99]
    Morgagni
      female Q50.5
      male (epididymal) Q55.4
        testicular Q55.29
    specified site NEC B67.99
  hymen N89.8
    embryonic Q52.4
  hypopharynx J39.2
  hypophysis, hypophyseal (duct) (recurrent) E23.6
    cerebri E23.6
  implantation (dermoid)
    external area or site (skin) NEC L72.0
    iris — see Cyst, iris, implantation
    vagina N89.8
    vulva N90.7
  incisive canal K09.1
  inclusion (epidermal) (epithelial) (epidermoid) (squamous) L72.0
    not of skin — code under Cyst, by site
  intestine (large) (small) K63.89
  intracranial — see Cyst, brain
  intraligamentous — see also Disorder, ligament
    knee — see Derangement, knee
  intrasellar E23.6
  iris H21.309
    exudative H21.31- ☑
    idiopathic H21.30- ☑
    implantation H21.32- ☑
    parasitic H21.33- ☑
    pars plana (primary) H21.34- ☑
      exudative H21.35- ☑
  jaw (bone) M27.40
    aneurysmal M27.49
    developmental (odontogenic) K09.0
    fissural K09.1
    hemorrhagic M27.49
    traumatic M27.49
  joint NEC — see Disorder, joint, specified type NEC
  kidney (acquired) N28.1
    calyceal — see Hydronephrosis
    congenital Q61.00
    more than one (multiple) Q61.02
      specified as polycystic Q61.3
        adult type (autosomal dominant) Q61.2
        infantile type (autosomal recessive) NEC
          Q61.19
          collecting duct dilation Q61.11
    pyelogenic — see Hydronephrosis
    simple N28.1
    solitary (single) Q61.01
      acquired N28.1
  labium (majus) (minus) N90.7

Cyst — continued
  labium — continued
    sebaceous N90.7
  lacrimal — see also Disorder, lacrimal system, specified
    NEC
    gland H04.13- ☑
    passages or sac — see Disorder, lacrimal system,
      specified NEC
  larynx J38.7
  lateral periodontal K09.0
  lens H27.8
    congenital Q12.8
  lip (gland) K13.0
  liver (idiopathic) (simple) K76.89
    congenital Q44.6
    hydatid B67.8
      granulosus B67.0
      multilocularis B67.5
  lung J98.4
    congenital Q33.0
    giant bullous J43.9
  lutein N83.1- ☑
  lymphangiomatous D18.1
  lymphoepithelial, oral soft tissue K09.8
  macula — see Degeneration, macula, hole
  malignant — see Neoplasm, malignant, by site
  mammary gland — see Cyst, breast
  mandible M27.40
    dentigerous K09.0
    radicular K04.8
  maxilla M27.40
    dentigerous K09.0
    radicular K04.8
  medial, face and neck Q18.8
  median
    anterior maxillary K09.1
    palatal K09.1
  mediastinum, congenital Q34.1
  meibomian (gland) — see Chalazion
    infected — see Hordeolum
  membrane, brain G93.0
  meninges (cerebral) G93.0
    spinal G96.19
  meniscus, knee — see Derangement, knee, meniscus,
    cystic
  mesentery, mesenteric K66.8
    chyle I89.8
  mesonephric duct
    female Q50.5
    male Q55.4
  milk N64.89
  Morgagni (hydatid)
    female Q50.5
    male (epididymal) Q55.4
      testicular Q55.29
  mouth K09.8
  Müllerian duct Q50.4
    appendix testis Q55.29
    cervix Q51.6
    fallopian tube Q50.4
    female Q50.4
    male Q55.29
    prostatic utricle Q55.4
    vagina (embryonal) Q52.4
  multilocular (ovary) D39.10
    benign — see Neoplasm, benign, by site
  myometrium N85.8
  nabothian (follicle) (ruptured) N88.8
  nasoalveolar K09.1
  nasolabial K09.1
  nasopalatine (anterior) (duct) K09.1
  nasopharynx J39.2
  neoplastic — see Neoplasm, uncertain behavior, by
    site
    benign — see Neoplasm, benign, by site
  nervous system NEC G96.8
  neuroenteric (congenital) Q06.8
  nipple — see Cyst, breast
  nose (turbinates) J34.1
    sinus J34.1
  odontogenic, developmental K09.0
  omentum (lesser) K66.8
    congenital Q45.8
  ora serrata — see Cyst, retina, ora serrata
  oral
    region K09.9
      developmental (nonodontogenic) K09.1
      specified NEC K09.8

ᴬᴰ Subterms under main terms may continue to next column or page   ☑ Additional Character Required — Refer to the Tabular List for Character Selection   79

Cyst — Cyst

Cyst — continued
- oral — continued
  - soft tissue K09.9
    - specified NEC K09.8
- orbit H05.81- ☑
- ovary, ovarian (twisted) N83.20- ☑
  - adherent N83.20- ☑
  - chocolate N80.1
  - corpus
    - albicans N83.29- ☑
    - luteum (hemorrhagic) N83.1- ☑
  - dermoid D27.9
  - developmental Q50.1
  - due to failure of involution NEC N83.20- ☑
  - endometrial N80.1
  - follicular (graafian) (hemorrhagic) N83.0- ☑
  - hemorrhagic N83.20- ☑
  - in pregnancy or childbirth O34.8- ☑
    - with obstructed labor O65.5
  - multilocular D39.10
  - pseudomucinous D27.9
  - retention N83.29- ☑
  - serous N83.20- ☑
  - specified NEC N83.29- ☑
  - theca lutein (hemorrhagic) N83.1- ☑
  - tuberculous A18.18
- oviduct N83.8
- palate (median) (fissural) K09.1
- palatine papilla (jaw) K09.1
- pancreas, pancreatic (hemorrhagic) (true) K86.2
  - congenital Q45.2
  - false K86.3
- paralabral
  - hip M24.85- ☑
  - shoulder S43.43- ☑
- paramesonephric duct Q50.4
  - female Q50.4
  - male Q55.29
- paranephric N28.1
- paraphysis, cerebri, congenital Q04.6
- parasitic B89
- parathyroid (gland) E21.4
- paratubal N83.8
- paraurethral duct N36.8
- paroophoron Q50.5
- parotid gland K11.6
- parovarian Q50.5
- pelvis, female N94.89
  - in pregnancy or childbirth O34.8- ☑
    - causing obstructed labor O65.5
- penis (sebaceous) N48.89
- periapical K04.8
- pericardial (congenital) Q24.8
  - acquired (secondary) I31.8
- pericoronal K09.0
- periodontal K04.8
  - lateral K09.0
- peripelvic (lymphatic) N28.1
- peritoneum K66.8
  - chylous I89.8
- periventricular, acquired, newborn P91.1
- pharynx (wall) J39.2
- pilar L72.11
- pilonidal (infected) (rectum) L05.91
  - with abscess L05.01
  - malignant C44.59- ☑
- pituitary (duct) (gland) E23.6
- placenta O43.19- ☑
- pleura J94.8
- popliteal — see Cyst, Baker's
- porencephalic Q04.6
  - acquired G93.0
- postanal (infected) — see Cyst, pilonidal
- postmastoidectomy cavity (mucosal) — see Complications, postmastoidectomy, cyst
- preauricular Q18.1
- prepuce N47.4
  - congenital Q55.69
- primordial (jaw) K09.0
- prostate N42.83
- pseudomucinous (ovary) D27.9
- pupillary, miotic H21.27- ☑
- radicular (residual) K04.8
- radiculodental K04.8
- ranular K11.8
- Rathke's pouch E23.6
- rectum (epithelium) (mucous) K62.89
- renal — see Cyst, kidney

Cyst — continued
- residual (radicular) K04.8
- retention (ovary) N83.29- ☑
  - salivary gland K11.6
- retina H33.19- ☑
  - ora serrata H33.11- ☑
  - parasitic H33.12- ☑
- retroperitoneal K68.9
- sacrococcygeal (dermoid) — see Cyst, pilonidal
- salivary gland or duct (mucous extravasation or retention) K11.6
- Sampson's N80.1
- sclera H15.89
- scrotum L72.9
  - sebaceous L72.3
- sebaceous (duct) (gland) L72.3
  - breast — see Dysplasia, mammary, specified type NEC
  - eyelid — see Cyst, eyelid
  - genital organ NEC
    - female N94.89
    - male N50.89
  - scrotum L72.3
- semilunar cartilage (knee) (multiple) — see Derangement, knee, meniscus, cystic
- seminal vesicle N50.89
- serous (ovary) N83.20- ☑
- sinus (accessory) (nasal) J34.1
- Skene's gland N36.8
- skin L72.9
  - breast — see Dysplasia, mammary, specified type NEC
  - epidermal, epidermoid L72.0
  - epithelial L72.0
  - eyelid — see Cyst, eyelid
  - genital organ NEC
    - female N90.7
    - male N50.89
  - inclusion L72.0
  - scrotum L72.9
  - sebaceous L72.3
  - sweat gland or duct L74.8
- solitary
  - bone — see Cyst, bone, solitary
  - jaw M27.40
  - kidney N28.1
- spermatic cord N50.89
- sphenoid sinus J34.1
- spinal meninges G96.19
- spleen NEC D73.4
  - congenital Q89.09
  - hydatid — see also Echinococcus B67.99 [D77]
- Stafne's M27.0
- subarachnoid intrasellar R93.0
- subcutaneous, pheomycotic (chromomycotic) B43.2
- subdural (cerebral) G93.0
  - spinal cord G96.19
- sublingual gland K11.6
- submandibular gland K11.6
- submaxillary gland K11.6
- suburethral N36.8
- suprarenal gland E27.8
- suprasellar — see Cyst, brain
- sweat gland or duct L74.8
- synovial — see also Cyst, bursa
  - ruptured — see Rupture, synovium
- tarsal — see Chalazion
- tendon (sheath) — see Disorder, tendon, specified type NEC
- testis N44.2
  - tunica albuginea N44.1
- theca lutein (ovary) N83.1- ☑
- Thornwaldt's J39.2
- thymus (gland) E32.8
- thyroglossal duct (infected) (persistent) Q89.2
- thyroid (gland) E04.1
- thyrolingual duct (infected) (persistent) Q89.2
- tongue K14.8
- tonsil J35.8
- tooth — see Cyst, dental
- Tornwaldt's J39.2
- trichilemmal (proliferating) L72.12
- trichodermal L72.12
- tubal (fallopian) N83.8
  - inflammatory — see Salpingitis, chronic
- tubo-ovarian N83.8
  - inflammatory N70.13

Cyst — continued
- tunica
  - albuginea testis N44.1
  - vaginalis N50.89
- turbinate (nose) J34.1
- Tyson's gland N48.89
- urachus, congenital Q64.4
- ureter N28.89
- ureterovesical orifice N28.89
- urethra, urethral (gland) N36.8
- uterine ligament N83.8
- uterus (body) (corpus) (recurrent) N85.8
  - embryonic Q51.818
    - cervix Q51.6
- vagina, vaginal (implantation) (inclusion) (squamous cell) (wall) N89.8
  - embryonic Q52.4
- vallecula, vallecular (epiglottis) J38.7
- vesical (orifice) N32.89
- vitreous body H43.89
- vulva (implantation) (inclusion) N90.7
  - congenital Q52.79
  - sebaceous gland N90.7
- vulvovaginal gland N90.7
- wolffian
  - female Q50.5
  - male Q55.4

Cystadenocarcinoma — see Neoplasm, malignant, by site
- bile duct C22.1
- endometrioid — see Neoplasm, malignant, by site
  - specified site — see Neoplasm, malignant, by site
  - unspecified site
    - female C56.9
    - male C61
- mucinous
  - papillary
    - specified site — see Neoplasm, malignant, by site
    - unspecified site C56.9
  - specified site — see Neoplasm, malignant, by site
  - unspecified site C56.9
- papillary
  - mucinous
    - specified site — see Neoplasm, malignant, by site
    - unspecified site C56.9
  - pseudomucinous
    - specified site — see Neoplasm, malignant, by site
    - unspecified site C56.9
  - serous
    - specified site — see Neoplasm, malignant, by site
    - unspecified site C56.9
  - specified site — see Neoplasm, malignant, by site
  - unspecified site C56.9
- pseudomucinous
  - papillary
    - specified site — see Neoplasm, malignant, by site
    - unspecified site C56.9
  - specified site — see Neoplasm, malignant, by site
  - unspecified site C56.9
- serous
  - papillary
    - specified site — see Neoplasm, malignant, by site
    - unspecified site C56.9
  - specified site — see Neoplasm, malignant, by site
  - unspecified site C56.9

Cystadenofibroma
- clear cell — see Neoplasm, benign, by site
- endometrioid D27.9
  - borderline malignancy D39.1- ☑
  - malignant C56.- ☑
- mucinous
  - specified site — see Neoplasm, benign, by site
  - unspecified site D27.9
- serous
  - specified site — see Neoplasm, benign, by site
  - unspecified site D27.9
- specified site — see Neoplasm, benign, by site
- unspecified site D27.9

Cystadenoma — see also Neoplasm, benign, by site
- bile duct D13.4
- endometrioid — see Neoplasm, benign, by site

☑ **Additional Character Required** — Refer to the Tabular List for Character Selection

▽ **Subterms under main terms may continue to next column or page**

ystadenoma — *continued*
  endometrioid — *see* Neoplasm, benign, by site —
     continued
    borderline malignancy — *see* Neoplasm, uncertain
     behavior, by site
  malignant — *see* Neoplasm, malignant, by site
  mucinous
    borderline malignancy
     ovary C56.- ☑
     specified site NEC — *see* Neoplasm, uncertain
      behavior, by site
     unspecified site C56.9
    papillary
     borderline malignancy
      ovary C56.- ☑
      specified site NEC — *see* Neoplasm, uncertain
       behavior, by site
      unspecified site C56.9
     specified site — *see* Neoplasm, benign, by site
     unspecified site D27.9
    specified site — *see* Neoplasm, benign, by site
    unspecified site D27.9
  papillary
    borderline malignancy
     ovary C56.- ☑
     specified site NEC — *see* Neoplasm, uncertain
      behavior, by site
     unspecified site C56.9
    lymphomatosum
     specified site — *see* Neoplasm, benign, by site
     unspecified site D11.9
    mucinous
     borderline malignancy
      ovary C56.- ☑
      specified site NEC — *see* Neoplasm, uncertain
       behavior, by site
      unspecified site C56.9
     specified site — *see* Neoplasm, benign, by site
     unspecified site D27.9
    pseudomucinous
     borderline malignancy
      ovary C56.- ☑
      specified site NEC — *see* Neoplasm, uncertain
       behavior, by site
      unspecified site C56.9
     specified site — *see* Neoplasm, benign, by site
     unspecified site D27.9
    serous
     borderline malignancy
      ovary C56.- ☑
      specified site NEC — *see* Neoplasm, uncertain
       behavior, by site
      unspecified site C56.9
     specified site — *see* Neoplasm, benign, by site
     unspecifled slte D27.9
    specified site — *see* Neoplasm, benign, by site
    unspecified site D27.9
  pseudomucinous
    borderline malignancy
     ovary C56.- ☑
     specified site NEC — *see* Neoplasm, uncertain
      behavior, by site
     unspecified site C56.9
    papillary
     borderline malignancy
      ovary C56.- ☑
      specified site NEC — *see* Neoplasm, uncertain
       behavior, by site
      unspecified site C56.9
     specified site — *see* Neoplasm, benign, by site
     unspecified site D27.9
    specified site — *see* Neoplasm, benign, by site
    unspecified site D27.9
  serous
    borderline malignancy
     ovary C56.- ☑
     specified site NEC — *see* Neoplasm, uncertain
      behavior, by site
     unspecified site C56.9

Cystadenoma — *continued*
  serous — *continued*
    papillary
     borderline malignancy
      ovary C56.- ☑
      specified site NEC — *see* Neoplasm, uncertain
       behavior, by site
      unspecified site C56.9
     specified site — *see* Neoplasm, benign, by site
     unspecified site D27.9
    specified site — *see* Neoplasm, benign, by site
    unspecified site D27.9
Cystathionine synthase deficiency E72.11
Cystathioninemia E72.19
Cystathioninuria E72.19
Cystic — *see also* condition
  breast (chronic) — *see* Mastopathy, cystic
  corpora lutea (hemorrhagic) N83.1- ☑
  duct — *see* condition
  eyeball (congenital) Q11.0
  fibrosis — *see* Fibrosis, cystic
  kidney (congenital) Q61.9
    adult type Q61.2
    infantile type NEC Q61.19
     collecting duct dilatation Q61.11
    medullary Q61.5
  liver, congenital Q44.6
  lung disease J98.4
    congenital Q33.0
  mastitis, chronic — *see* Mastopathy, cystic
  medullary, kidney Q61.5
  meniscus — *see* Derangement, knee, meniscus, cystic
  ovary N83.20- ☑
Cysticercosis, cysticerciasis B69.9
  with
    epileptiform fits B69.0
    myositis B69.81
  brain B69.0
  central nervous system B69.0
  cerebral B69.0
  ocular B69.1
  specified NEC B69.89
Cysticercus cellulose infestation — *see* Cysticercosis
Cystinosis (malignant) E72.04
Cystinuria E72.01
Cystitis (exudative) (hemorrhagic) (septic) (suppurative)
  N30.90
  with
    fibrosis — *see* Cystitis, chronic, interstitial
    hematuria N30.91
    leukoplakia — *see* Cystitis, chronic, interstitial
    malakoplakia — *see* Cystitis, chronic, interstitial
    metaplasia — *see* Cystitis, chronic, interstitial
    prostatitis N41.3
  acute N30.00
    with hematuria N30.01
    of trigone N30.30
     with hematuria N30.31
  allergic — *see* Cystitis, specified type NEC
  amebic A06.81
  bilharzial B65.9 [N33]
  blennorrhagic (gonococcal) A54.01
  bullous — *see* Cystitis, specified type NEC
  calculous N21.0
  chlamydial A56.01
  chronic N30.20
    with hematuria N30.21
    interstitial N30.10
     with hematuria N30.11
    of trigone N30.30
     with hematuria N30.31
    specified NEC N30.20
     with hematuria N30.21
  cystic (a) — *see* Cystitis, specified type NEC
  diphtheritic A36.85
  echinococcal
    granulosus B67.39
    multilocularis B67.69
  emphysematous — *see* Cystitis, specified type NEC
  encysted — *see* Cystitis, specified type NEC

Cystitis — *continued*
  eosinophilic — *see* Cystitis, specified type NEC
  follicular — *see* Cystitis, of trigone
  gangrenous — *see* Cystitis, specified type NEC
  glandularis — *see* Cystitis, specified type NEC
  gonococcal A54.01
  incrusted — *see* Cystitis, specified type NEC
  interstitial (chronic) — *see* Cystitis, chronic, interstitial
  irradiation N30.40
    with hematuria N30.41
  irritation — *see* Cystitis, specified type NEC
  malignant — *see* Cystitis, specified type NEC
  of trigone N30.30
    with hematuria N30.31
  panmural — *see* Cystitis, chronic, interstitial
  polyposa — *see* Cystitis, specified type NEC
  prostatic N41.3
  puerperal (postpartum) O86.22
  radiation — *see* Cystitis, irradiation
  specified type NEC N30.80
    with hematuria N30.81
  subacute — *see* Cystitis, chronic
  submucous — *see* Cystitis, chronic, interstitial
  syphilitic (late) A52.76
  trichomonal A59.03
  tuberculous A18.12
  ulcerative — *see* Cystitis, chronic, interstitial
Cystocele (-urethrocele)
  female N81.10
    with prolapse of uterus — *see* Prolapse, uterus
    lateral N81.12
    midline N81.11
    paravaginal N81.12
  in pregnancy or childbirth O34.8- ☑
    causing obstructed labor O65.5
  male N32.89
Cystolithiasis N21.0
Cystoma — *see also* Neoplasm, benign, by site
  endometrial, ovary N80.1
  mucinous
    specified site — *see* Neoplasm, benign, by site
    unspecified site D27.9
  serous
    specified site — *see* Neoplasm, benign, by site
    unspecified site D27.9
  simple (ovary) N83.29- ☑
Cystoplegia N31.2
Cystoptosis N32.89
Cystopyelitis — *see* Pyelonephritis
Cystorrhagia N32.89
Cystosarcoma phyllodes D48.6- ☑
  benign D24- ☑
  malignant — *see* Neoplasm, breast, malignant
Cystostomy
  attention to Z43.5
  complication — *see* Complications, cystostomy
  status Z93.50
    appendico-vesicostomy Z93.52
    cutaneous Z93.51
    specified NEC Z93.59
Cystourethritis — *see* Urethritis
Cystourethrocele — *see also* Cystocele
  female N81.10
    with uterine prolapse — *see* Prolapse, uterus
    lateral N81.12
    midline N81.11
    paravaginal N81.12
  male N32.89
Cytomegalic inclusion disease
  congenital P35.1
Cytomegalovirus infection B25.9
Cytomycosis (reticuloendothelial) B39.4
Cytopenia D75.9
  refractory
    with multilineage dysplasia D46.A (*following* D46.2)
    and ring sideroblasts (RCMD RS) D46.B (*following* D46.2)
Czerny's disease (periodic hydrarthrosis of the knee) —
  see Effusion, joint, knee

D

Da Costa's syndrome F45.8
Daae (-Finsen) **disease** (epidemic pleurodynia) B33.0
Dabney's grip B33.0
Dacryoadenitis, dacryadenitis H04.00- ☑
  acute H04.01- ☑
  chronic H04.02- ☑
Dacryocystitis H04.30- ☑
  acute H04.32- ☑
  chronic H04.41- ☑
  neonatal P39.1
  phlegmonous H04.31- ☑
  syphilitic A52.71
    congenital (early) A50.01
  trachomatous, active A71.1
    sequelae (late effect) B94.0
Dacryocystoblenorrhea — *see* Inflammation, lacrimal, passages, chronic
Dacryocystocele — *see* Disorder, lacrimal system, changes
Dacryolith, dacryolithiasis H04.51- ☑
Dacryoma — *see* Disorder, lacrimal system, changes
Dacryopericystitis — *see* Dacryocystitis
Dacryops H04.11- ☑
Dacryostenosis — *see also* Stenosis, lacrimal
  congenital Q10.5
Dactylitis
  bone — *see* Osteomyelitis
  sickle-cell D57.00
    Hb C D57.219
    Hb SS D57.00
    specified NEC D57.819
  skin L08.9
  syphilitic A52.77
  tuberculous A18.03
Dactylolysis spontanea (ainhum) L94.6
Dactylosymphysis Q70.9
  fingers — *see* Syndactylism, complex, fingers
  toes — *see* Syndactylism, complex, toes
Damage
  arteriosclerotic — *see* Arteriosclerosis
  brain (nontraumatic) G93.9
    anoxic, hypoxic G93.1
      resulting from a procedure G97.82
    child NEC G80.9
    due to birth injury P11.2
  cardiorenal (vascular) — *see* Hypertension, cardiorenal
  cerebral NEC — *see* Damage, brain
  coccyx, complicating delivery O71.6
  coronary — *see* Disease, heart, ischemic
  deep tissue, pressure-induced — *see also* L89 with final character .6
  eye, birth injury P15.3
  liver (nontraumatic) K76.9
    alcoholic K70.9
    due to drugs — *see* Disease, liver, toxic
    toxic — *see* Disease, liver, toxic
  medication T88.7 ☑
  pelvic
    joint or ligament, during delivery O71.6
    organ NEC
      during delivery O71.5
      following ectopic or molar pregnancy O08.6
  renal — *see* Disease, renal
  subendocardium, subendocardial — *see* Degeneration, myocardial
  vascular I99.9
Dana-Putnam syndrome (subacute combined sclerosis with pernicious anemia) — *see* Degeneration, combined
Danbolt (-Cross) **syndrome** (acrodermatitis enteropathica) E83.2
Dandruff L21.0
Dandy-Walker syndrome Q03.1
  with spina bifida — *see* Spina bifida
Danlos' syndrome — *see also* Syndrome, Ehlers-Danlos Q79.60
Darier (-White) **disease** (congenital) Q82.8
  meaning erythema annulare centrifugum L53.1
Darier-Roussy sarcoid D86.3
Darling's disease or histoplasmosis B39.4
Darwin's tubercle Q17.8
Dawson's (inclusion body) **encephalitis** A81.1
De Beurmann (-Gougerot) **disease** B42.1
De la Tourette's syndrome F95.2

De Lange's syndrome Q87.19
De Morgan's spots (senile angiomas) I78.1
De Quervain's
  disease (tendon sheath) M65.4
  syndrome E34.51
  thyroiditis (subacute granulomatous thyroiditis) E06.1
De Toni-Fanconi (-Debré) **syndrome** E72.09
  with cystinosis E72.04
Dead
  fetus, retained (mother) O36.4 ☑
    early pregnancy O02.1
  labyrinth H83.2 ☑
  ovum, retained O02.0
Deaf nonspeaking NEC H91.3
Deafmutism (acquired) (congenital) NEC H91.3
  hysterical F44.6
  syphilitic, congenital — *see also* subcategory H94.8 A50.09
Deafness (acquired) (complete) (hereditary) (partial) H91.9- ☑
  with blue sclera and fragility of bone Q78.0
  auditory fatigue — *see* Deafness, specified type NEC
  aviation T70.0 ☑
    nerve injury — *see* Injury, nerve, acoustic, specified type NEC
  boilermaker's H83.3 ☑
  central — *see* Deafness, sensorineural
  conductive H90.2
    and sensorineural
      mixed H90.8
        bilateral H90.6
      bilateral H90.0
      unilateral H90.1- ☑
        with restricted hearing on the contralateral side H90.A- ☑
  congenital H90.5
    with blue sclera and fragility of bone Q78.0
  due to toxic agents — *see* Deafness, ototoxic
  emotional (hysterical) F44.6
  functional (hysterical) F44.6
  high frequency H91.9- ☑
  hysterical F44.6
  low frequency H91.9- ☑
  mental R48.8
  mixed conductive and sensorineural H90.8
    bilateral H90.6
    unilateral H90.7- ☑
  nerve — *see* Deafness, sensorineural
  neural — *see* Deafness, sensorineural
  noise-induced — *see also* subcategory H83.3
    nerve injury — *see* Injury, nerve, acoustic, specified type NEC
  nonspeaking H91.3
  ototoxic H91.0 ☑
  perceptive — *see* Deafness, sensorineural
  psychogenic (hysterical) F44.6
  sensorineural H90.5
    and conductive
      bilateral H90.6
      mixed H90.8
        bilateral H90.6
    bilateral H90.3
    unilateral H90.4- ☑
      with restricted hearing on the contralateral side H90.A- ☑
  sensory — *see* Deafness, sensorineural
  specified type NEC H91.8 ☑
  sudden (idiopathic) H91.2- ☑
  syphilitic A52.15
  transient ischemic H93.01- ☑
  traumatic — *see* Injury, nerve, acoustic, specified type NEC
  word (developmental) H93.25
Death (cause unknown) (of) (unexplained) (unspecified cause) R99
  brain G93.82
  cardiac (sudden) (with successful resuscitation) — *code to* underlying disease
    family history of Z82.41
    personal history of Z86.74
  family member (assumed) Z63.4
Debility (chronic) (general) (nervous) R53.81
  congenital or neonatal NOS P96.9
  nervous R53.81
  old age R54
  senile R54
Débove's disease (splenomegaly) R16.1

Decalcification
  bone — *see* Osteoporosis
  teeth K03.89
Decapsulation, kidney N28.89
Decay
  dental — *see* Caries, dental
  senile R54
  tooth, teeth — *see* Caries, dental
Deciduitis (acute)
  following ectopic or molar pregnancy O08.0
Decline (general) — *see* Debility
  cognitive, age-associated R41.81
Decompensation
  cardiac (acute) (chronic) — *see* Disease, heart
  cardiovascular — *see* Disease, cardiovascular
  heart — *see* Disease, heart
  hepatic — *see* Failure, hepatic
  myocardial (acute) (chronic) — *see* Disease, heart
  respiratory J98.8
Decompression sickness T70.3 ☑
Decrease (d)
  absolute neutrophil count — *see* Neutropenia
  blood
    platelets — *see* Thrombocytopenia
    pressure R03.1
      due to shock following
        injury T79.4 ☑
        operation T81.19 ☑
  estrogen E28.39
    postablative E89.40
      asymptomatic E89.40
      symptomatic E89.41
  fragility of erythrocytes D58.8
  function
    lipase (pancreatic) K90.3
    ovary in hypopituitarism E23.0
    parenchyma of pancreas K86.89
    pituitary (gland) (anterior) (lobe) E23.0
      posterior (lobe) E23.0
  functional activity R68.89
  glucose R73.09
  hematocrit R71.0
  hemoglobin R71.0
  leukocytes D72.819
    specified NEC D72.818
  libido R68.82
  lymphocytes D72.810
  platelets D69.6
  respiration, due to shock following injury T79.4 ☑
  sexual desire R68.82
  tear secretion NEC — *see* Syndrome, dry eye
  tolerance
    fat K90.49
    glucose R73.09
    pancreatic K90.3
    salt and water E87.8
  vision NEC H54.7
  white blood cell count D72.819
    specified NEC D72.818
Decubitus (ulcer) — *see* Ulcer, pressure, by site
  cervix N86
Deepening acetabulum — *see* Derangement, joint, specified type NEC, hip
Defect, defective Q89.9
  3-beta-hydroxysteroid dehydrogenase E25.0
  11-hydroxylase E25.0
  21-hydroxylase E25.0
  abdominal wall, congenital Q79.59
  antibody immunodeficiency D80.9
  aorticopulmonary septum Q21.4
  atrial septal (ostium secundum type) Q21.1
    following acute myocardial infarction (current complication) I23.1
    ostium primum type Q21.2
  atrioventricular
    canal Q21.2
    septum Q21.2
  auricular septal Q21.1
  bilirubin excretion NEC E80.6
  biosynthesis, androgen (testicular) E29.1
  bulbar septum Q21.0
  catalase E80.3
  cell membrane receptor complex (CR3) D71
  circulation I99.9
    congenital Q28.9
    newborn Q28.9
  coagulation (factor) — *see also* Deficiency, factor D68

Defect, defective — *continued*

coagulation — *see also* Deficiency, factor — *continued*
  with
    ectopic pregnancy O08.1
    molar pregnancy O08.1
  acquired D68.4
  antepartum with hemorrhage — *see* Hemorrhage, antepartum, with coagulation defect
  due to
    liver disease D68.4
    vitamin K deficiency D68.4
  hereditary NEC D68.2
  intrapartum O67.0
  newborn, transient P61.6
  postpartum O99.13
    with hemorrhage O72.3
  specified type NEC D68.8
complement system D84.1
conduction (heart) I45.9
  bone — *see* Deafness, conductive
congenital, organ or site not listed — *see* Anomaly, by site
coronary sinus Q21.1
cushion, endocardial Q21.2
degradation, glycoprotein E77.1
dental bridge, crown, fillings — *see* Defect, dental restoration
dental restoration K08.50
  specified NEC K08.59
dentin (hereditary) K00.5
Descemet's membrane, congenital Q13.89
developmental — *see also* Anomaly
  cauda equina Q06.3
diaphragm
  with elevation, eventration or hernia — *see* Hernia, diaphragm
  congenital Q79.1
    with hernia Q79.0
    gross (with hernia) Q79.0
ectodermal, congenital Q82.9
Eisenmenger's Q21.8
enzyme
  catalase E80.3
  peroxidase E80.3
esophagus, congenital Q39.9
extensor retinaculum M62.89
fibrin polymerization D68.2
filling
  bladder R93.41
  kidney R93.42- ☑
  renal pelvis R93.41
  stomach R93.3
  ureter R93.41
  urinary organs, specified NEC R93.49
GABA (gamma aminobutyric acid) metabolic E72.81
Gerbode Q21.0
glycoprotein degradation E77.1
Hageman (factor) D68.2
hearing — *see* Deafness
high grade F70
interatrial septal Q21.1
interauricular septal Q21.1
interventricular septal Q21.0
  with dextroposition of aorta, pulmonary stenosis and hypertrophy of right ventricle Q21.3
  in tetralogy of Fallot Q21.3
learning (specific) — *see* Disorder, learning
lymphocyte function antigen-1 (LFA-1) D84.0
lysosomal enzyme, post-translational modification E77.0
major osseous M89.70
  ankle M89.77- ☑
  carpus M89.74- ☑
  clavicle M89.71- ☑
  femur M89.75- ☑
  fibula M89.76- ☑
  fingers M89.74- ☑
  foot M89.77- ☑
  forearm M89.73- ☑
  hand M89.74- ☑
  humerus M89.72- ☑
  lower leg M89.76- ☑
  metacarpus M89.74- ☑
  metatarsus M89.77- ☑
  multiple sites M89.79
  pelvic region M89.75- ☑
  pelvis M89.75- ☑

Defect, defective — *continued*

major osseous — *continued*
  radius M89.73- ☑
  scapula M89.71- ☑
  shoulder region M89.71- ☑
  specified NEC M89.78
  tarsus M89.77- ☑
  thigh M89.75- ☑
  tibia M89.76- ☑
  toes M89.77- ☑
  ulna M89.73- ☑
mental — *see* Disability, intellectual
modification, lysosomal enzymes, post-translational E77.0
obstructive, congenital
  renal pelvis Q62.39
  ureter Q62.39
    atresia — *see* Atresia, ureter
    cecoureterocele Q62.32
    megaureter Q62.2
    orthotopic ureterocele Q62.31
osseous, major M89.70
  ankle M89.77- ☑
  carpus M89.74- ☑
  clavicle M89.71- ☑
  femur M89.75- ☑
  fibula M89.76- ☑
  fingers M89.74- ☑
  foot M89.77- ☑
  forearm M89.73- ☑
  hand M89.74- ☑
  humerus M89.72- ☑
  lower leg M89.76- ☑
  metacarpus M89.74- ☑
  metatarsus M89.77- ☑
  multiple sites M89.9
  pelvic region M89.75- ☑
  pelvis M89.75- ☑
  radius M89.73- ☑
  scapula M89.71- ☑
  shoulder region M89.71- ☑
  specified NEC M89.78
  tarsus M89.77- ☑
  thigh M89.75- ☑
  tibia M89.76- ☑
  toes M89.77- ☑
  ulna M89.73- ☑
osteochondral NEC — *see also* Deformity M95.8
ostium
  primum Q21.2
  secundum Q21.1
peroxidase E80.3
placental blood supply — *see* Insufficiency, placental
platelets, qualitative D69.1
  constitutional D68.0
postural NEC, spine — *see* Dorsopathy, deforming
reduction
  limb Q73.8
    lower Q72.9- ☑
      absence — *see* Agenesis, leg
        foot — *see* Agenesis, foot
      longitudinal
        femur Q72.4- ☑
        fibula Q72.6- ☑
        tibia Q72.5- ☑
      specified type NEC Q72.89- ☑
      split foot Q72.7- ☑
    specified type NEC Q73.8
    upper Q71.9- ☑
      absence — *see* Agenesis, arm
        forearm — *see* Agenesis, forearm
        hand — *see* Agenesis, hand
      lobster-claw hand Q71.6- ☑
      longitudinal
        radius Q71.4- ☑
        ulna Q71.5- ☑
      specified type NEC Q71.89- ☑
renal pelvis Q63.8
  obstructive Q62.39
respiratory system, congenital Q34.9
restoration, dental K08.50
  specified NEC K08.59
retinal nerve bundle fibers H35.89
septal (heart) NOS Q21.9
  acquired (atrial) (auricular) (ventricular) (old) I51.0
  atrial Q21.1

Defect, defective — *continued*

septal — *continued*
  atrial — *continued*
    concurrent with acute myocardial infarction — *see* Infarct, myocardium
    following acute myocardial infarction (current complication) I23.1
  ventricular — *see also* Defect, ventricular septal Q21.0
  sinus venosus Q21.1
speech R47.9
  developmental F80.9
  specified NEC R47.89
Taussig-Bing (aortic transposition and overriding pulmonary artery) Q20.1
teeth, wedge K03.1
vascular (local) I99.9
  congenital Q27.9
ventricular septal Q21.0
  concurrent with acute myocardial infarction — *see* Infarct, myocardium
  following acute myocardial infarction (current complication) I23.2
  in tetralogy of Fallot Q21.3
vision NEC H54.7
visual field H53.40
  bilateral
    heteronymous H53.47
    homonymous H53.46- ☑
  generalized contraction H53.48- ☑
  localized
    arcuate H53.43- ☑
    scotoma (central area) H53.41- ☑
      blind spot area H53.42- ☑
    sector H53.43- ☑
    specified type NEC H53.45- ☑
voice R49.9
  specified NEC R49.8
wedge, tooth, teeth (abrasion) K03.1

Deferentitis N49.1
  gonorrheal (acute) (chronic) A54.23

Defibrination (syndrome) D65
  antepartum — *see* Hemorrhage, antepartum, with coagulation defect, disseminated intravascular coagulation
  following ectopic or molar pregnancy O08.1
  intrapartum O67.0
  newborn P60
  postpartum O72.3

Deficiency, deficient
  3-beta hydroxysteroid dehydrogenase E25.0
  5-alpha reductase (with male pseudohermaphroditism) E29.1
  11-hydroxylase E25.0
  21-hydroxylase E25.0
  abdominal muscle syndrome Q79.4
  AC globulin (congenital) (hereditary) D68.2
    acquired D68.4
  accelerator globulin (Ac G) (blood) D68.2
  acid phosphatase E83.39
  activating factor (blood) D68.2
  ADA2 (adenosine deaminase 2) D81.32
  adenosine deaminase (ADA) D81.30
    with severe combined immunodeficiency (SCID) D81.31
    partial (type 1) D81.39
    specified NEC D81.39
    type 1 (without SCID) (without severe combined immunodeficiency) D81.39
    type 2 D81.32
  aldolase (hereditary) E74.19
  alpha-1-antitrypsin E88.01
  amino-acids E72.9
  anemia — *see* Anemia
  aneurin E51.9
  antibody with
    hyperimmunoglobulinemia D80.6
    near-normal immunoglobins D80.6
  antidiuretic hormone E23.2
  anti-hemophilic
    factor (A) D66
      B D67
      C D68.1
    globulin (AHG) NEC D66
  antithrombin (antithrombin III) D68.59
  ascorbic acid E54
  attention (disorder) (syndrome) F98.8

Deficiency, deficient — *continued*
attention — *continued*
with hyperactivity — *see* Disorder, attention-deficit hyperactivity
autoprothrombin
C D68.2
I D68.2
II D67
beta-glucuronidase E76.29
biotin E53.8
biotin-dependent carboxylase D81.819
biotinidase D81.810
brancher enzyme (amylopectinosis) E74.03
C1 esterase inhibitor (C1-INH) D84.1
calciferol E55.9
with
adult osteomalacia M83.8
rickets — *see* Rickets
calcium (dietary) E58
calorie, severe E43
with marasmus E41
and kwashiorkor E42
cardiac — *see* Insufficiency, myocardial
carnitine E71.40
due to
hemodialysis E71.43
inborn errors of metabolism E71.42
Valproic acid therapy E71.43
iatrogenic E71.43
muscle palmityltransferase E71.314
primary E71.41
secondary E71.448
carotene E50.9
central nervous system G96.8
ceruloplasmin (Wilson) E83.01
choline E53.8
Christmas factor D67
chromium E61.4
clotting (blood) — *see also* Deficiency, coagulation factor D68.9
clotting factor NEC (hereditary) — *see also* Deficiency, factor D68.2
coagulation NOS D68.9
with
ectopic pregnancy O08.1
molar pregnancy O08.1
acquired (any) D68.4
antepartum hemorrhage — *see* Hemorrhage, antepartum, with coagulation defect
clotting factor NEC — *see also* Deficiency, factor D68.2
due to
hyperprothrombinemia D68.4
liver disease D68.4
vitamin K deficiency D68.4
newborn, transient P61.6
postpartum O72.3
specified NEC D68.8
cognitive F09
color vision H53.50
achromatopsia H53.51
acquired H53.52
deuteranomaly H53.53
protanomaly H53.54
specified type NEC H53.59
tritanomaly H53.55
combined glucocorticoid and mineralocorticoid E27.49
contact factor D68.2
copper (nutritional) E61.0
corticoadrenal E27.40
primary E27.1
craniofacial axis Q75.0
cyanocobalamin E53.8
debrancher enzyme (limit dextrinosis) E74.03
dehydrogenase
long chain/very long chain acyl CoA E71.310
medium chain acyl CoA E71.311
short chain acyl CoA E71.312
diet E63.9
dihydropyrimidine dehydrogenase (DPD) E88.89
disaccharidase E73.9
edema — *see* Malnutrition, severe
endocrine E34.9
energy-supply — *see* Malnutrition
enzymes, circulating NEC E88.09
ergosterol E55.9
with
adult osteomalacia M83.8

Deficiency, deficient — *continued*
ergosterol — *continued*
with — *continued*
rickets — *see* Rickets
essential fatty acid (EFA) E63.0
factor — *see also* Deficiency, coagulation
Hageman D68.2
I (congenital) (hereditary) D68.2
II (congenital) (hereditary) D68.2
IX (congenital) (functional) (hereditary) (with functional defect) D67
multiple (congenital) D68.8
acquired D68.4
V (congenital) (hereditary) D68.2
VII (congenital) (hereditary) D68.2
VIII (congenital) (functional) (hereditary) (with functional defect) D66
with vascular defect D68.0
X (congenital) (hereditary) D68.2
XI (congenital) (hereditary) D68.1
XII (congenital) (hereditary) D68.2
XIII (congenital) (hereditary) D68.2
femoral, proximal focal (congenital) — *see* Defect, reduction, lower limb, longitudinal, femur
fibrinase D68.2
fibrinogen (congenital) (hereditary) D68.2
acquired D65
fibrin-stabilizing factor (congenital) (hereditary) D68.2
acquired D68.4
folate E53.8
folic acid E53.8
foreskin N47.3
fructokinase E74.11
fructose 1,6-diphosphatase E74.19
fructose-1-phosphate aldolase E74.19
GABA (gamma aminobutyric acid) transaminase E72.81
GABA-T (gamma aminobutyric acid transaminase) E72.81
galactokinase E74.29
galactose-1-phosphate uridyl transferase E74.29
gammaglobulin in blood D80.1
hereditary D80.0
glass factor D68.2
glucocorticoid E27.49
mineralocorticoid E27.49
glucose-6-phosphatase E74.01
glucose-6-phosphate dehydrogenase
anemia D55.0
without anemia D75.A
glucuronyl transferase E80.5
glycogen synthetase E74.09
gonadotropin (isolated) E23.0
growth hormone (idiopathic) (isolated) E23.0
Hageman factor D68.2
hemoglobin D64.9
hepatophosphorylase E74.09
homogentisate 1,2-dioxygenase E70.29
hormone
anterior pituitary (partial) NEC E23.0
growth E23.0
growth (isolated) E23.0
pituitary E23.0
testicular E29.1
hypoxanthine- (guanine)-phosphoribosyltransferase (HG- PRT) (total H-PRT) E79.1
immunity D84.9
cell-mediated D84.8
with thrombocytopenia and eczema D82.0
combined D81.9
humoral D80.9
IgA (secretory) D80.2
IgG D80.3
IgM D80.4
immuno — *see* Immunodeficiency
immunoglobulin, selective
A (IgA) D80.2
G (IgG) (subclasses) D80.3
M (IgM) D80.4
inositol (B complex) E53.8
intrinsic
factor (congenital) D51.0
sphincter N36.42
with urethral hypermobility N36.43
iodine E61.8
congenital syndrome — *see* Syndrome, iodine-deficiency, congenital
iron E61.1
anemia D50.9
kalium E87.6

Deficiency, deficient — *continued*
kappa-light chain D80.8
labile factor (congenital) (hereditary) D68.2
acquired D68.4
lacrimal fluid (acquired) — *see also* Syndrome, dry e
congenital Q10.6
lactase
congenital E73.0
secondary E73.1
Laki-Lorand factor D68.2
lecithin cholesterol acyltransferase E78.6
lipocaic K86.89
lipoprotein (familial) (high density) E78.6
liver phosphorylase E74.09
lysosomal alpha-1, 4 glucosidase E74.02
magnesium E61.2
major histocompatibility complex
class I D81.6
class II D81.7
manganese E61.3
menadione (vitamin K) E56.1
newborn P53
mental (familial) (hereditary) — *see* Disability, intelle
tual
methylenetetrahydrofolate reductase (MTHFR) E72.
mevalonate kinase M04.1
mineralocorticoid E27.49
with glucocorticoid E27.49
mineral NEC E61.8
molybdenum (nutritional) E61.5
moral F60.2
multiple nutrient elements E61.7
multiple sulfatase (MSD) E75.26
muscle
carnitine (palmityltransferase) E71.314
phosphofructokinase E74.09
myoadenylate deaminase E79.2
myocardial — *see* Insufficiency, myocardial
myophosphorylase E74.04
NADH diaphorase or reductase (congenital) D74.9
NADH-methemoglobin reductase (congenital) D74.
natrium E87.1
niacin (amide) (-tryptophan) E52
nicotinamide E52
nicotinic acid E52
number of teeth — *see* Anodontia
nutrient element E61.9
multiple E61.7
specified NEC E61.8
nutrition, nutritional E63.9
sequelae — *see* Sequelae, nutritional deficiency
specified NEC E63.8
of interleukin 1 receptor antagonist [DIRA] M04.8
ornithine transcarbamylase E72.4
ovarian E28.39
oxygen — *see* Anoxia
pantothenic acid E53.8
parathyroid (gland) E20.9
perineum (female) N81.89
phenylalanine hydroxylase E70.1
phosphoenolpyruvate carboxykinase E74.4
phosphofructokinase E74.19
phosphomannomutuse E74.8
phosphomannose isomerase E74.8
phosphomannosyl mutase E74.8
phosphorylase kinase, liver E74.09
pituitary hormone (isolated) E23.0
plasma thromboplastin
antecedent (PTA) D68.1
component (PTC) D67
plasminogen (type 1) (type 2) E88.02
platelet NEC D69.1
constitutional D68.0
polyglandular E31.8
autoimmune E31.0
potassium (K) E87.6
prepuce N47.3
proaccelerin (congenital) (hereditary) D68.2
acquired D68.4
proconvertin factor (congenital) (hereditary) D68.2
acquired D68.4
protein — *see also* Malnutrition E46
anemia D53.0
C D68.59
S D68.59
prothrombin (congenital) (hereditary) D68.2
acquired D68.4
Prower factor D68.2

☑ **Additional Character Required** — Refer to the Tabular List for Character Selection   ▽ **Subterms under main terms may continue to next column or pag**

Deficiency, deficient — *continued*
pseudocholinesterase E88.09
PTA (plasma thromboplastin antecedent) D68.1
PTC (plasma thromboplastin component) D67
purine nucleoside phosphorylase (PNP) D81.5
pyracin (alpha) (beta) E53.1
pyridoxal E53.1
pyridoxamine E53.1
pyridoxine (derivatives) E53.1
pyruvate
　carboxylase E74.4
　dehydrogenase E74.4
riboflavin (vitamin B2) E53.0
salt E87.1
secretion
　ovary E28.39
　salivary gland (any) K11.7
　urine R34
selenium (dietary) E59
serum antitrypsin, familial E88.01
short stature homeobox gene (SHOX)
　with
　　dyschondrosteosis Q78.8
　　short stature (idiopathic) E34.3
　　Turner's syndrome Q96.9
sodium (Na) E87.1
SPCA (factor VII) D68.2
sphincter, intrinsic N36.42
　with urethral hypermobility N36.43
stable factor (congenital) (hereditary) D68.2
　acquired D68.4
Stuart-Prower (factor X) D68.2
succinic semialdehyde dehydrogenase E72.81
sucrase E74.39
sulfatase E75.26
sulfite oxidase E72.19
thiamin, thiaminic (chloride) E51.9
　beriberi (dry) E51.11
　　wet E51.12
thrombokinase D68.2
　newborn P53
thyroid (gland) — *see* Hypothyroidism
tocopherol E56.0
tooth bud K00.0
transcobalamine II (anemia) D51.2
vanadium E61.6
vascular I99.9
vasopressin E23.2
vertical ridge K06.8
viosterol — *see* Deficiency, calciferol
vitamin (multiple) NOS E56.9
　A E50.9
　　with
　　　Bitot's spot (corneal) E50.1
　　　follicular keratosis E50.8
　　　keratomalacia E50.4
　　　manifestations NEC E50.8
　　　night blindness E50.5
　　　scar of cornea, xerophthalmic E50.6
　　　xeroderma E50.8
　　　xerophthalmia E50.7
　　　xerosis
　　　　conjunctival E50.0
　　　　　and Bitot's spot E50.1
　　　　cornea E50.2
　　　　　and ulceration E50.3
　　　sequelae E64.1
　B (complex) NOS E53.9
　　with
　　　beriberi (dry) E51.11
　　　　wet E51.12
　　　pellagra E52
　　B1 NOS E51.9
　　　beriberi (dry) E51.11
　　　　with circulatory system manifestations E51.11
　　　　wet E51.12
　　B12 E53.8
　　B2 (riboflavin) E53.0
　　B6 E53.1
　　C E54
　　　sequelae E64.2
　　D E55.9
　　　with
　　　　adult osteomalacia M83.8
　　　　rickets — *see* Rickets
　　　　25-hydroxylase E83.32
　　E E56.0
　　folic acid E53.8
　　G E53.0

Deficiency, deficient — *continued*
vitamin — *continued*
　group B E53.9
　　specified NEC E53.8
　H (biotin) E53.8
　K E56.1
　　of newborn P53
　nicotinic E52
　P E56.8
　PP (pellagra-preventing) E52
　specified NEC E56.8
　thiamin E51.9
　　beriberi — *see* Beriberi
zinc, dietary E60
Deficit — *see also* Deficiency
attention and concentration R41.840
　disorder — *see* Attention, deficit
　following
　　cerebral infarction I69.310
　　cerebrovascular disease I69.910
　　　specified disease NEC I69.810
　　nontraumatic
　　　intracerebral hemorrhage I69.110
　　　specified intracranial hemorrhage NEC I69.210
　　　subarachnoid hemorrhage I69.010
cognitive
　communication R41.841
　emotional
　　following
　　　cerebral infarction I69.315
　　　cerebrovascular disease I69.915
　　　　specified disease NEC I69.815
　　　nontraumatic
　　　　intracerebral hemorrhage I69.115
　　　　specified intracranial hemorrhage NEC I69.215
　　　　subarachnoid hemorrhage I69.015
　following
　　cerebral infarction I69.319
　　cerebrovascular disease I69.919
　　　specified disease NEC I69.819
　　nontraumatic
　　　intracerebral hemorrhage I69.119
　　　specified intracranial hemorrhage NEC I69.219
　　　subarachnoid hemorrhage I69.019
　social
　　following
　　　cerebral infarction I69.315
　　　cerebrovascular disease I69.915
　　　　specified disease NEC I69.815
　　　nontraumatic
　　　　intracerebral hemorrhage I69.115
　　　　specified intracranial hemorrhage NEC I69.215
　　　　subarachnoid hemorrhage I69.015
cognitive NEC R41.89
　following
　　cerebral infarction I69.318
　　cerebrovascular disease I69.918
　　　specified disease NEC I69.818
　　nontraumatic
　　　intracerebral hemorrhage I69.118
　　　specified intracranial hemorrhage NEC I69.218
　　　subarachnoid hemorrhage I69.018
concentration R41.840
executive function R41.844
　following
　　cerebral infarction I69.314
　　cerebrovascular disease I69.914
　　　specified disease NEC I69.814
　　nontraumatic
　　　intracerebral hemorrhage I69.114
　　　specified intracranial hemorrhage NEC I69.214
　　　subarachnoid hemorrhage I69.014
frontal lobe R41.844
　following
　　cerebral infarction I69.314
　　cerebrovascular disease I69.914
　　　specified disease NEC I69.814
　　nontraumatic
　　　intracerebral hemorrhage I69.114
　　　specified intracranial hemorrhage NEC I69.214
　　　subarachnoid hemorrhage I69.014
memory
　following
　　cerebral infarction I69.311
　　cerebrovascular disease I69.911
　　　specified disease NEC I69.811

Deficit — *continued*
memory — *continued*
　following — *continued*
　　nontraumatic
　　　intracerebral hemorrhage I69.111
　　　specified intracranial hemorrhage NEC I69.211
　　　subarachnoid hemorrhage I69.011
neurologic NEC R29.818
　ischemic
　　reversible (RIND) I63.9
　　prolonged (PRIND) I63.9
oxygen R09.02
prolonged reversible ischemic neurologic (PRIND) I63.9
psychomotor R41.843
　following
　　cerebral infarction I69.313
　　cerebrovascular disease I69.913
　　　specified disease NEC I69.813
　　nontraumatic
　　　intracerebral hemorrhage I69.113
　　　specified intracranial hemorrhage NEC I69.213
　　　subarachnoid hemorrhage I69.013
visuospatial R41.842
　following
　　cerebral infarction I69.312
　　cerebrovascular disease I69.912
　　　specified disease NEC I69.812
　　nontraumatic
　　　intracerebral hemorrhage I69.112
　　　specified intracranial hemorrhage NEC I69.212
　　　subarachnoid hemorrhage I69.012
Deflection
radius — *see* Deformity, limb, specified type NEC, forearm
septum (acquired) (nasal) (nose) J34.2
spine — *see* Curvature, spine
turbinate (nose) J34.2
Defluvium
capillorum — *see* Alopecia
ciliorum — *see* Madarosis
unguium L60.8
Deformity Q89.9
abdomen, congenital Q89.9
abdominal wall
　acquired M95.8
　congenital Q79.59
acquired (unspecified site) M95.9
adrenal gland Q89.1
alimentary tract, congenital Q45.9
　upper Q40.9
ankle (joint) (acquired) — *see also* Deformity, limb, lower leg
　abduction — *see* Contraction, joint, ankle
　congenital Q68.8
　contraction — *see* Contraction, joint, ankle
　specified type NEC — *see* Deformity, limb, foot, specified NEC
anus (acquired) K62.89
　congenital Q43.9
aorta (arch) (congenital) Q25.40
　acquired I77.89
aortic
　arch, acquired I77.89
　cusp or valve (congenital) Q23.8
　　acquired — *see also* Endocarditis, aortic I35.8
arm (acquired) (upper) — *see also* Deformity, limb, upper arm
　congenital Q68.8
　forearm — *see* Deformity, limb, forearm
artery (congenital) (peripheral) NOS Q27.9
　acquired I77.89
　coronary (acquired) I25.9
　　congenital Q24.5
　umbilical Q27.0
atrial septal Q21.1
auditory canal (external) (congenital) — *see also* Malformation, ear, external
　acquired — *see* Disorder, ear, external, specified type NEC
auricle
　ear (congenital) — *see also* Malformation, ear, external
　acquired — *see* Disorder, pinna, deformity
back — *see* Dorsopathy, deforming
bile duct (common) (congenital) (hepatic) Q44.5
　acquired K83.8
biliary duct or passage (congenital) Q44.5
　acquired K83.8

Deformity — *continued*

bladder (neck) (trigone) (sphincter) (acquired) N32.89
  congenital Q64.79
bone (acquired) NOS M95.9
  congenital Q79.9
  turbinate M95.0
brain (congenital) Q04.9
  acquired G93.89
  reduction Q04.3
breast (acquired) N64.89
  congenital Q83.9
  reconstructed N65.0
bronchus (congenital) Q32.4
  acquired NEC J98.09
bursa, congenital Q79.9
canaliculi (lacrimalis) (acquired) — *see also* Disorder, lacrimal system, changes
  congenital Q10.6
canthus, acquired — *see* Disorder, eyelid, specified type NEC
capillary (acquired) I78.8
cardiovascular system, congenital Q28.9
caruncle, lacrimal (acquired) — *see also* Disorder, lacrimal system, changes
  congenital Q10.6
cascade, stomach K31.2
cecum (congenital) Q43.9
  acquired K63.89
cerebral, acquired G93.89
  congenital Q04.9
cervix (uterus) (acquired) NEC N88.8
  congenital Q51.9
cheek (acquired) M95.2
  congenital Q18.9
chest (acquired) (wall) M95.4
  congenital Q67.8
  sequelae (late effect) of rickets E64.3
chin (acquired) M95.2
  congenital Q18.9
choroid (congenital) Q14.3
  acquired H31.8
  plexus Q07.8
   acquired G96.19
cicatricial — *see* Cicatrix
cilia, acquired — *see* Disorder, eyelid, specified type NEC
clavicle (acquired) M95.8
  congenital Q68.8
clitoris (congenital) Q52.6
  acquired N90.89
clubfoot — *see* Clubfoot
coccyx (acquired) — *see* subcategory M43.8 ☑
colon (congenital) Q43.9
  acquired K63.89
concha (ear), congenital — *see also* Malformation, ear, external
  acquired — *see* Disorder, pinna, deformity
cornea (acquired) H18.70
  congenital Q13.4
  descemetocele — *see* Descemetocele
  ectasia — *see* Ectasia, cornea
  specified NEC H18.79- ☑
  staphyloma — *see* Staphyloma, cornea
coronary artery (acquired) I25.9
  congenital Q24.5
cranium (acquired) — *see* Deformity, skull
cricoid cartilage (congenital) Q31.8
  acquired J38.7
cystic duct (congenital) Q44.5
  acquired K82.8
Dandy-Walker Q03.1
  with spina bifida — *see* Spina bifida
diaphragm (congenital) Q79.1
  acquired J98.6
digestive organ NOS Q45.9
ductus arteriosus Q25.0
duodenal bulb K31.89
duodenum (congenital) Q43.9
  acquired K31.89
dura — *see* Deformity, meninges
ear (acquired) — *see also* Disorder, pinna, deformity
  congenital (external) Q17.9
   internal Q16.5
   middle Q16.4
    ossicles Q16.3
   ossicles Q16.3
ectodermal (congenital) NEC Q84.9
ejaculatory duct (congenital) Q55.4

Deformity — *continued*

ejaculatory duct — *continued*
  acquired N50.89
elbow (joint) (acquired) — *see also* Deformity, limb, upper arm
  congenital Q68.8
  contraction — *see* Contraction, joint, elbow
endocrine gland NEC Q89.2
epididymis (congenital) Q55.4
  acquired N50.89
epiglottis (congenital) Q31.8
  acquired J38.7
esophagus (congenital) Q39.9
  acquired K22.8
eustachian tube (congenital) NEC Q17.8
eye, congenital Q15.9
eyebrow (congenital) Q18.8
eyelid (acquired) — *see also* Disorder, eyelid, specified type NEC
  congenital Q10.3
face (acquired) M95.2
  congenital Q18.9
fallopian tube, acquired N83.8
femur (acquired) — *see* Deformity, limb, specified type NEC, thigh
fetal
  with fetopelvic disproportion O33.7 ☑
  causing obstructed labor O66.3
finger (acquired) M20.00- ☑
  boutonniere M20.02- ☑
  congenital Q68.1
  flexion contracture — *see* Contraction, joint, hand
  mallet finger M20.01- ☑
  specified NEC M20.09- ☑
  swan-neck M20.03- ☑
flexion (joint) (acquired) — *see also* Deformity, limb, flexion M21.20
  congenital NOS Q74.9
  hip Q65.89
foot (acquired) — *see also* Deformity, limb, lower leg
  cavovarus (congenital) Q66.1- ☑
  congenital NOS Q66.9- ☑
   specified type NEC Q66.89
  specified type NEC — *see* Deformity, limb, foot, specified NEC
  valgus (congenital) Q66.6
   acquired — *see* Deformity, valgus, ankle
  varus (congenital) NEC Q66.3- ☑
   acquired — *see* Deformity, varus, ankle
forearm (acquired) — *see also* Deformity, limb, forearm
  congenital Q68.8
forehead (acquired) M95.2
  congenital Q75.8
frontal bone (acquired) M95.2
  congenital Q75.8
gallbladder (congenital) Q44.1
  acquired K82.8
gastrointestinal tract (congenital) NOS Q45.9
  acquired K63.89
genitalia, genital organ(s) or system NEC
  female (congenital) Q52.9
   acquired N94.89
   external Q52.70
  male (congenital) Q55.9
   acquired N50.89
globe (eye) (congenital) Q15.8
  acquired H44.89
gum, acquired NEC K06.8
hand (acquired) — *see* Deformity, limb, hand
  congenital Q68.1
head (acquired) M95.2
  congenital Q75.8
heart (congenital) Q24.9
  septum Q21.9
   auricular Q21.1
   ventricular Q21.0
  valve (congenital) NEC Q24.8
   acquired — *see* Endocarditis
heel (acquired) — *see* Deformity, foot
hepatic duct (congenital) Q44.5
  acquired K83.8
hip (joint) (acquired) (*see also* Deformity, limb, thigh)
  congenital Q65.9
  due to (previous) juvenile osteochondrosis — *see* Coxa, plana
  flexion — *see* Contraction, joint, hip
hourglass — *see* Contraction, hourglass
humerus (acquired) M21.82- ☑

Deformity — *continued*

humerus — *continued*
  congenital Q74.0
hypophyseal (congenital) Q89.2
ileocecal (coil) (valve) (acquired) K63.89
  congenital Q43.9
ileum (congenital) Q43.9
  acquired K63.89
ilium (acquired) M95.5
  congenital Q74.2
integument (congenital) Q84.9
intervertebral cartilage or disc (acquired) — *see* Disorder, disc, specified NEC
intestine (large) (small) (congenital) NOS Q43.9
  acquired K63.89
intrinsic minus or plus (hand) — *see* Deformity, limb, specified type NEC, forearm
iris (acquired) H21.89
  congenital Q13.2
ischium (acquired) M95.5
  congenital Q74.2
jaw (acquired) (congenital) M26.9
joint (acquired) NEC M21.90
  congenital Q68.8
  elbow M21.92- ☑
  hand M21.94- ☑
  hip M21.95- ☑
  knee M21.96- ☑
  shoulder M21.92- ☑
  wrist M21.93- ☑
kidney(s) (calyx) (pelvis) (congenital) Q63.9
  acquired N28.89
  artery (congenital) Q27.2
   acquired I77.89
Klippel-Feil (brevicollis) Q76.1
knee (acquired) NEC — *see also* Deformity, limb, leg
  congenital Q68.2
labium (majus) (minus) (congenital) Q52.79
  acquired N90.89
lacrimal passages or duct (congenital) NEC Q10.6
  acquired — *see* Disorder, lacrimal system, chang
larynx (muscle) (congenital) Q31.8
  acquired J38.7
  web (glottic) Q31.0
leg (upper) (acquired) NEC — *see also* Deformity, lim thigh
  congenital Q68.8
  lower leg — *see* Deformity, limb, lower leg
lens (acquired) H27.8
  congenital Q12.9
lid (fold) (acquired) — *see also* Disorder, eyelid, spe fied type NEC
  congenital Q10.3
ligament (acquired) — *see* Disorder, ligament
  congenital Q79.9
limb (acquired) M21.90
  clawfoot M21.53- ☑
  clawhand M21.51- ☑
  clubfoot M21.54- ☑
  clubhand M21.52- ☑
  congenital, except reduction deformity Q74.9
  flat foot M21.4- ☑
  flexion M21.20
   ankle M21.27- ☑
   elbow M21.22- ☑
   finger M21.24- ☑
   hip M21.25- ☑
   knee M21.26- ☑
   shoulder M21.21- ☑
   toe M21.27- ☑
   wrist M21.23- ☑
  foot
   claw — *see* Deformity, limb, clawfoot
   club — *see* Deformity, limb, clubfoot
   drop M21.37- ☑
   flat — *see* Deformity, limb, flat foot
   specified NEC M21.6X- ☑
  forearm M21.93- ☑
  hand M21.94- ☑
  lower leg M21.96- ☑
  specified type NEC M21.80
   forearm M21.83- ☑
   lower leg M21.86- ☑
   thigh M21.85- ☑
   upper arm M21.82- ☑
  thigh M21.95- ☑

eformity — *continued*
limb — *continued*
　unequal length M21.70
　　short site is
　　　femur M21.75- ☑
　　　fibula M21.76- ☑
　　　humerus M21.72- ☑
　　　radius M21.73- ☑
　　　tibia M21.76- ☑
　　　ulna M21.73- ☑
　　upper arm M21.92- ☑
　valgus — *see* Deformity, valgus
　varus — *see* Deformity, varus
　wrist drop M21.33- ☑
lip (acquired) NEC K13.0
　congenital Q38.0
liver (congenital) Q44.7
　acquired K76.89
lumbosacral (congenital) (joint) (region) Q76.49
　acquired — *see* subcategory M43.8 ☑
　kyphosis — *see* Kyphosis, congenital
　lordosis — *see* Lordosis, congenital
lung (congenital) Q33.9
　acquired J98.4
lymphatic system, congenital Q89.9
Madelung's (radius) Q74.0
mandible (acquired) (congenital) M26.9
maxilla (acquired) (congenital) M26.9
meninges or membrane (congenital) Q07.9
　cerebral Q04.8
　　acquired G96.19
　spinal cord (congenital) G96.19
　　acquired G96.19
metacarpus (acquired) — *see* Deformity, limb, forearm
　congenital Q74.0
metatarsus (acquired) — *see* Deformity, foot
　congenital Q66.9- ☑
middle ear (congenital) Q16.4
　ossicles Q16.3
mitral (leaflets) (valve) I05.8
　parachute Q23.2
　stenosis, congenital Q23.2
mouth (acquired) K13.79
　congenital Q38.6
multiple, congenital NEC Q89.7
muscle (acquired) M62.89
　congenital Q79.9
　　sternocleidomastoid Q68.0
musculoskeletal system (acquired) M95.9
　congenital Q79.9
　specified NEC M95.8
nail (acquired) L60.8
　congenital Q84.6
nasal — *see* Deformity, nose
neck (acquired) M95.3
　congenital Q18.9
　　sternocleidomastoid Q68.0
nervous system (congenital) Q07.9
nipple (congenital) Q83.9
　acquired N64.89
nose (acquired) (cartilage) M95.0
　bone (turbinate) M95.0
　congenital Q30.9
　　bent or squashed Q67.4
　saddle M95.0
　　syphilitic A50.57
　septum (acquired) J34.2
　　congenital Q30.8
　sinus (wall) (congenital) Q30.8
　　acquired M95.0
　syphilitic (congenital) A50.57
　　late A52.73
ocular muscle (congenital) Q10.3
　acquired — *see* Strabismus, mechanical
opticociliary vessels (congenital) Q13.2
orbit (eye) (acquired) H05.30
　atrophy — *see* Atrophy, orbit
　congenital Q10.7
　due to
　　bone disease NEC H05.32- ☑
　　trauma or surgery H05.33- ☑
　enlargement — *see* Enlargement, orbit
　exostosis — *see* Exostosis, orbit
organ of Corti (congenital) Q16.5
ovary (congenital) Q50.39
　acquired N83.8
oviduct, acquired N83.8
palate (congenital) Q38.5

Deformity — *continued*
palate — *continued*
　acquired M27.8
　cleft (congenital) — *see* Cleft, palate
pancreas (congenital) Q45.3
　acquired K86.89
parathyroid (gland) Q89.2
parotid (gland) (congenital) Q38.4
　acquired K11.8
patella (acquired) — *see* Disorder, patella, specified
　NEC
pelvis, pelvic (acquired) (bony) M95.5
　with disproportion (fetopelvic) O33.0
　　causing obstructed labor O65.0
　congenital Q74.2
　rachitic sequelae (late effect) E64.3
penis (glans) (congenital) Q55.69
　acquired N48.89
pericardium (congenital) Q24.8
　acquired — *see* Pericarditis
pharynx (congenital) Q38.8
　acquired J39.2
pinna, acquired — *see also* Disorder, pinna, deformity
　congenital Q17.9
pituitary (congenital) Q89.2
posture — *see* Dorsopathy, deforming
prepuce (congenital) Q55.69
　acquired N47.8
prostate (congenital) Q55.4
　acquired N42.89
pupil (congenital) Q13.2
　acquired — *see* Abnormality, pupillary
pylorus (congenital) Q40.3
　acquired K31.89
rachitic (acquired), old or healed E64.3
radius (acquired) — *see also* Deformity, limb, forearm
　congenital Q68.8
rectum (congenital) Q43.9
　acquired K62.89
reduction (extremity) (limb), congenital — *see also*
　condition and site Q73.8
　brain Q04.3
　lower — *see* Defect, reduction, lower limb
　upper — *see* Defect, reduction, upper limb
renal — *see* Deformity, kidney
respiratory system (congenital) Q34.9
rib (acquired) M95.4
　congenital Q76.6
　　cervical Q76.5
rotation (joint) (acquired) — *see* Deformity, limb,
　specified site NEC
　congenital Q74.9
　hip — *see* Deformity, limb, specified type NEC, thigh
　　congenital Q65.89
sacroiliac joint (congenital) — *see* subcategory Q74.2
　acquired — *see* subcategory M43.8 ☑
sacrum (acquired) — *see* subcategory M43.8 ☑
saddle
　back — *see* Lordosis
　nose M95.0
　　syphilitic A50.57
salivary gland or duct (congenital) Q38.4
　acquired K11.8
scapula (acquired) M95.8
　congenital Q68.8
scrotum (congenital) — *see also* Malformation, testis
　and scrotum
　acquired N50.89
seminal vesicles (congenital) Q55.4
　acquired N50.89
septum, nasal (acquired) J34.2
shoulder (joint) (acquired) — *see* Deformity, limb, up-
　per arm
　congenital Q74.0
　contraction — *see* Contraction, joint, shoulder
sigmoid (flexure) (congenital) Q43.9
　acquired K63.89
skin (congenital) Q82.9
skull (acquired) M95.2
　congenital Q75.8
　　with
　　　anencephaly Q00.0
　　　encephalocele — *see* Encephalocele
　　　hydrocephalus Q03.9
　　　　with spina bifida — *see* Spina bifida, by
　　　　　site, with hydrocephalus
　　　microcephaly Q02

Deformity — *continued*
soft parts, organs or tissues (of pelvis)
　in pregnancy or childbirth NEC O34.8- ☑
　　causing obstructed labor O65.5
spermatic cord (congenital) Q55.4
　acquired N50.89
　torsion — *see* Torsion, spermatic cord
spinal — *see* Dorsopathy, deforming
　column (acquired) — *see* Dorsopathy, deforming
　congenital Q67.5
　cord (congenital) Q06.9
　　acquired G95.89
　nerve root (congenital) Q07.9
spine (acquired) — *see also* Dorsopathy, deforming
　congenital Q67.5
　rachitic E64.3
　specified NEC — *see* Dorsopathy, deforming, speci-
　　fied NEC
spleen
　acquired D73.89
　congenital Q89.09
Sprengel's (congenital) Q74.0
sternocleidomastoid (muscle), congenital Q68.0
sternum (acquired) M95.4
　congenital NEC Q76.7
stomach (congenital) Q40.3
　acquired K31.89
submandibular gland (congenital) Q38.4
submaxillary gland (congenital) Q38.4
　acquired K11.8
talipes — *see* Talipes
testis (congenital) — *see also* Malformation, testis and
　scrotum
　acquired N44.8
　torsion — *see* Torsion, testis
thigh (acquired) — *see also* Deformity, limb, thigh
　congenital NEC Q68.8
thorax (acquired) (wall) M95.4
　congenital Q67.8
　sequelae of rickets E64.3
thumb (acquired) — *see also* Deformity, finger
　congenital NEC Q68.1
thymus (tissue) (congenital) Q89.2
thyroid (gland) (congenital) Q89.2
　cartilage Q31.8
　　acquired J38.7
tibia (acquired) — *see also* Deformity, limb, specified
　type NEC, lower leg
　congenital NEC Q68.8
　saber (syphilitic) A50.56
toe (acquired) M20.6- ☑
　congenital Q66.9- ☑
　hallux rigidus M20.2- ☑
　hallux valgus M20.1- ☑
　hallux varus M20.3 ☑
　hammer toe M20.4- ☑
　specified NEC M20.5X- ☑
tongue (congenital) Q38.3
　acquired K14.8
tooth, teeth K00.2
trachea (rings) (congenital) Q32.1
　acquired J39.8
transverse aortic arch (congenital) Q25.49
tricuspid (leaflets) (valve) I07.8
　atresia or stenosis Q22.4
　Ebstein's Q22.5
trunk (acquired) M95.8
　congenital Q89.9
ulna (acquired) — *see also* Deformity, limb, forearm
　congenital NEC Q68.8
urachus, congenital Q64.4
ureter (opening) (congenital) Q62.8
　acquired N28.89
urethra (congenital) Q64.79
　acquired N36.8
urinary tract (congenital) Q64.9
　urachus Q64.4
uterus (congenital) Q51.9
　acquired N85.8
uvula (congenital) Q38.5
vagina (acquired) N89.8
　congenital Q52.4
valgus NEC M21.00
　ankle M21.07- ☑
　elbow M21.02- ☑
　hip M21.05- ☑
　knee M21.06- ☑
valve, valvular (congenital) (heart) Q24.8

Deformity — *continued*
  valve, valvular — *continued*
    acquired — *see* Endocarditis
  varus NEC M21.10
    ankle M21.17- ☑
    elbow M21.12- ☑
    hip M21.15 ☑
    knee M21.16- ☑
    tibia — *see* Osteochondrosis, juvenile, tibia
  vas deferens (congenital) Q55.4
    acquired N50.89
  vein (congenital) Q27.9
    great Q26.9
  vertebra — *see* Dorsopathy, deforming
  vertical talus (congenital) Q66.80
    left foot Q66.82
    right foot Q66.81
  vesicourethral orifice (acquired) N32.89
    congenital NEC Q64.79
  vessels of optic papilla (congenital) Q14.2
  visual field (contraction) — *see* Defect, visual field
  vitreous body, acquired H43.89
  vulva (congenital) Q52.79
    acquired N90.89
  wrist (joint) (acquired) — *see also* Deformity, limb, forearm
    congenital Q68.8
    contraction — *see* Contraction, joint, wrist

Degeneration, degenerative
  adrenal (capsule) (fatty) (gland) (hyaline) (infectional) E27.8
  amyloid — *see also* Amyloidosis E85.9
  anterior cornua, spinal cord G12.29
  anterior labral S43.49- ☑
  aorta, aortic I70.0
    fatty I77.89
  aortic valve (heart) — *see* Endocarditis, aortic
  arteriovascular — *see* Arteriosclerosis
  artery, arterial (atheromatous) (calcareous) — *see also* Arteriosclerosis
    cerebral, amyloid E85.4 *[I68.0]*
    medial — *see* Arteriosclerosis, extremities
  articular cartilage NEC — *see* Derangement, joint, articular cartilage, by site
  atheromatous — *see* Arteriosclerosis
  basal nuclei or ganglia G23.9
    specified NEC G23.8
  bone NEC — *see* Disorder, bone, specified type NEC
  brachial plexus G54.0
  brain (cortical) (progressive) G31.9
    alcoholic G31.2
    arteriosclerotic I67.2
    childhood G31.9
      specified NEC G31.89
    cystic G31.89
      congenital Q04.6
    in
      alcoholism G31.2
      beriberi E51.2
      cerebrovascular disease I67.9
      congenital hydrocephalus Q03.9
        with spina bifida — *see also* Spina bifida
      Fabry-Anderson disease E75.21
      Gaucher's disease E75.22
      Hunter's syndrome E76.1
      lipidosis
        cerebral E75.4
        generalized E75.6
      mucopolysaccharidosis — *see* Mucopolysaccharidosis
      myxedema E03.9 *[G32.89]*
      neoplastic disease — *see also* Neoplasm D49.6 *[G32.89]*
      Niemann-Pick disease E75.249 *[G32.89]*
      sphingolipidosis E75.3 *[G32.89]*
      vitamin B12 deficiency E53.8 *[G32.89]*
    senile NEC G31.1
  breast N64.89
  Bruch's membrane — *see* Degeneration, choroid
  capillaries (fatty) I78.8
    amyloid E85.89 *[I79.8]*
  cardiac — *see also* Degeneration, myocardial
    valve, valvular — *see* Endocarditis
  cardiorenal — *see* Hypertension, cardiorenal
  cardiovascular — *see also* Disease, cardiovascular
    renal — *see* Hypertension, cardiorenal
  cerebellar NOS G31.9
    alcoholic G31.2

Degeneration, degenerative — *continued*
  cerebellar — *continued*
    primary (hereditary) (sporadic) G11.9
  cerebral — *see* Degeneration, brain
  cerebrovascular I67.9
    due to hypertension I67.4
  cervical plexus G54.2
  cervix N88.8
    due to radiation (intended effect) N88.8
      adverse effect or misadventure N99.89
  chamber angle H21.21- ☑
  changes, spine or vertebra — *see* Spondylosis
  chorioretinal — *see also* Degeneration, choroid
    hereditary H31.20
  choroid (colloid) (drusen) H31.10- ☑
    atrophy — *see* Atrophy, choroidal
    hereditary — *see* Dystrophy, choroidal, hereditary
  ciliary body H21.22- ☑
  cochlear — *see* subcategory H83.8 ☑
  combined (spinal cord) (subacute) E53.8 *[G32.0]*
    with anemia (pernicious) D51.0 *[G32.0]*
      due to dietary vitamin B12 deficiency D51.3 *[G32.0]*
    in (due to)
      vitamin B12 deficiency E53.8 *[G32.0]*
      anemia D51.9 *[G32.0]*
  conjunctiva H11.10
    concretions — *see* Concretion, conjunctiva
    deposits — *see* Deposit, conjunctiva
    pigmentations — *see* Pigmentation, conjunctiva
    pinguecula — *see* Pinguecula
    xerosis — *see* Xerosis, conjunctiva
  cornea H18.40
    calcerous H18.43
      band keratopathy H18.42- ☑
    familial, hereditary — *see* Dystrophy, cornea
    hyaline (of old scars) H18.49
    keratomalacia — *see* Keratomalacia
    nodular H18.45- ☑
    peripheral H18.46- ☑
    senile H18.41- ☑
    specified type NEC H18.49
  cortical (cerebellar) (parenchymatous) G31.89
    alcoholic G31.2
    diffuse, due to arteriopathy I67.2
  corticobasal G31.85
  cutis L98.8
    amyloid E85.4 *[L99]*
  dental pulp K04.2
  disc disease — *see* Degeneration, intervertebral disc NEC
  dorsolateral (spinal cord) — *see* Degeneration, combined
  extrapyramidal G25.9
  eye, macular — *see also* Degeneration, macula
    congenital or hereditary — *see* Dystrophy, retina
  facet joints — *see* Spondylosis
  fatty
    liver NEC K76.0
      alcoholic K70.0
  grey matter (brain) (Alpers') G31.81
  heart — *see also* Degeneration, myocardial
    amyloid E85.4 *[I43]*
    atheromatous — *see* Disease, heart, ischemic, atherosclerotic
    ischemic — *see* Disease, heart, ischemic
  hepatolenticular (Wilson's) E83.01
  hepatorenal K76.7
  hyaline (diffuse) (generalized)
    localized — *see* Degeneration, by site
  infrapatellar fat pad M79.4
  intervertebral disc NOS
    with
      myelopathy — *see* Disorder, disc, with, myelopathy
      radiculitis or radiculopathy — *see* Disorder, disc, with, radiculopathy
    cervical, cervicothoracic — *see* Disorder, disc, cervical, degeneration
      with
        myelopathy — *see* Disorder, disc, cervical, with myelopathy
        neuritis, radiculitis or radiculopathy — *see* Disorder, disc, cervical, with neuritis
    lumbar region M51.36
      with
        myelopathy M51.06

Degeneration, degenerative — *continued*
  intervertebral disc — *continued*
    lumbar region — *continued*
      with — *continued*
        neuritis, radiculitis, radiculopathy or sciati◄ M51.16
    lumbosacral region M51.37
      with
        neuritis, radiculitis, radiculopathy or sciati◄ M51.17
    sacrococcygeal region M53.3
    thoracic region M51.34
      with
        myelopathy M51.04
        neuritis, radiculitis, radiculopathy M51.14
    thoracolumbar region M51.35
      with
        myelopathy M51.05
        neuritis, radiculitis, radiculopathy M51.15
  intestine, amyloid E85.4
  iris (pigmentary) H21.23- ☑
  ischemic — *see* Ischemia
  joint disease — *see* Osteoarthritis
  kidney N28.89
    amyloid E85.4 *[N29]*
    cystic, congenital Q61.9
    fatty N28.89
    polycystic Q61.3
      adult type (autosomal dominant) Q61.2
      infantile type (autosomal recessive) NEC Q61◄
        collecting duct dilatation Q61.11
  Kuhnt-Junius — *see also* Degeneration, macula H35.32- ☑
  lens — *see* Cataract
  lenticular (familial) (progressive) (Wilson's) (with cirr◄ sis of liver) E83.01
  liver (diffuse) NEC K76.89
    amyloid E85.4 *[K77]*
    cystic K76.89
      congenital Q44.6
    fatty NEC K76.0
      alcoholic K70.0
    hypertrophic K76.89
    parenchymatous, acute or subacute K72.00
      with coma K72.01
    pigmentary K76.89
    toxic (acute) K71.9
  lung J98.4
  lymph gland I89.8
    hyaline I89.8
  macula, macular (acquired) (age-related) (senile) H35.30
    angioid streaks H35.33
    atrophic age-related H35.31- ☑
    congenital or hereditary — *see* Dystrophy, retin◄
    cystoid H35.35- ☑
    drusen H35.36- ☑
    dry age-related H35.31- ☑
    exudative H35.32- ☑
    hole H35.34- ☑
    nonexudative H35.31- ☑
    puckering H35.37- ☑
    toxic H35.38- ☑
    wet age-related H35.32- ☑
  membranous labyrinth, congenital (causing impair◄ ment of hearing) Q16.5
  meniscus — *see* Derangement, meniscus
  mitral — *see* Insufficiency, mitral
  Mönckeberg's — *see* Arteriosclerosis, extremities
  motor centers, senile G31.1
  multi-system G90.3
  mural — *see* Degeneration, myocardial
  muscle (fatty) (fibrous) (hyaline) (progressive) M62◄
    heart — *see* Degeneration, myocardial
  myelin, central nervous system G37.9
  myocardial, myocardium (fatty) (hyaline) (senile) I5◄
    with rheumatic fever (conditions in I00) I09.0
      active, acute or subacute I01.2
        with chorea I02.0
      inactive or quiescent (with chorea) I09.0
    hypertensive — *see* Hypertension, heart
    rheumatic — *see* Degeneration, myocardial, wi◄ rheumatic fever
    syphilitic A52.06
  nasal sinus (mucosa) J32.9
    frontal J32.1
    maxillary J32.0
  nerve — *see* Disorder, nerve

   ☑ **Additional Character Required** — Refer to the Tabular List for Character Selection   ▽ **Subterms under main terms may continue to next column or pa**

egeneration, degenerative — continued
nervous system G31.9
alcoholic G31.2
amyloid E85.4 [G99.8]
autonomic G90.9
fatty G31.89
specified NEC G31.89
nipple N64.89
olivopontocerebellar (hereditary) (familial) G23.8
osseous labyrinth — see subcategory H83.8 ☑
ovary N83.8
cystic N83.20- ☑
microcystic N83.20- ☑
pallidal pigmentary (progressive) G23.0
pancreas K86.89
tuberculous A18.83
penis N48.89
pigmentary (diffuse) (general)
localized — see Degeneration, by site
pallidal (progressive) G23.0
pineal gland E34.8
pituitary (gland) E23.6
popliteal fat pad M79.4
posterolateral (spinal cord) — see Degeneration,
combined
pulmonary valve (heart) I37.8
pulp (tooth) K04.2
pupillary margin H21.24- ☑
renal — see Degeneration, kidney
retina H35.9
hereditary (cerebroretinal) (congenital) (juvenile)
(macula) (peripheral) (pigmentary) — see
Dystrophy, retina
Kuhnt-Junius — see also Degeneration, macula
H35.32- ☑
macula (cystic) (exudative) (hole) (nonexudative)
(pseudohole) (senile) (toxic) — see Degeneration, macula
peripheral H35.40
lattice H35.41- ☑
microcystoid H35.42- ☑
paving stone H35.43- ☑
secondary
pigmentary H35.45- ☑
vitreoretinal H35.46- ☑
senile reticular H35.44- ☑
pigmentary (primary) — see also Dystrophy, retina
secondary — see Degeneration, retina, peripheral, secondary
posterior pole — see Degeneration, macula
saccule, congenital (causing impairment of hearing)
Q16.5
senile R54
brain G31.1
cardiac, heart or myocardium — see Degeneration,
myocardial
motor centers G31.1
vascular — see Arteriosclerosis
sinus (cystic) — see also Sinusitis
polypoid J33.1
skin L98.8
amyloid E85.4 [L99]
colloid L98.8
spinal (cord) G31.89
amyloid E85.4 [G32.89]
combined (subacute) — see Degeneration, combined
dorsolateral — see Degeneration, combined
familial NEC G31.89
fatty G31.89
funicular — see Degeneration, combined
posterolateral — see Degeneration, combined
subacute combined — see Degeneration, combined
tuberculous A17.81
spleen D73.0
amyloid E85.4 [D77]
stomach K31.89
striatonigral G23.2
suprarenal (capsule) (gland) E27.8
synovial membrane (pulpy) — see Disorder, synovium,
specified type NEC
tapetoretinal — see Dystrophy, retina
thymus (gland) E32.8
fatty E32.8
thyroid (gland) E07.89
tricuspid (heart) (valve) I07.9
tuberculous NEC — see Tuberculosis
turbinate J34.89

Degeneration, degenerative — continued
uterus (cystic) N85.8
vascular (senile) — see Arteriosclerosis
hypertensive — see Hypertension
vitreoretinal, secondary — see Degeneration, retina,
peripheral, secondary, vitreoretinal
vitreous (body) H43.81- ☑
Wallerian — see Disorder, nerve
Wilson's hepatolenticular E83.01
Deglutition
paralysis R13.0
hysterical F44.4
pneumonia J69.0
Degos' disease I77.89
Dehiscence (of)
amputation stump T87.81
cesarean wound O90.0
closure of
cornea T81.31 ☑
craniotomy T81.32 ☑
fascia (muscular) (superficial) T81.32 ☑
internal organ or tissue T81.32 ☑
laceration (external) (internal) T81.33 ☑
ligament T81.32 ☑
mucosa T81.31 ☑
muscle or muscle flap T81.32 ☑
ribs or rib cage T81.32 ☑
skin and subcutaneous tissue (full-thickness) (superficial) T81.31 ☑
skull T81.32 ☑
sternum (sternotomy) T81.32 ☑
tendon T81.32 ☑
traumatic laceration (external) (internal) T81.33 ☑
episiotomy O90.1
operation wound NEC T81.31 ☑
external operation wound (superficial) T81.31 ☑
internal operation wound (deep) T81.32 ☑
perineal wound (postpartum) O90.1
traumatic injury wound repair T81.33 ☑
wound T81.30 ☑
traumatic repair T81.33 ☑
Dehydration E86.0
newborn P74.1
Déjérine-Roussy syndrome G89.0
Déjérine-Sottas disease or neuropathy (hypertrophic)
G60.0
Déjérine-Thomas atrophy G23.8
Delay, delayed
any plane in pelvis
complicating delivery O66.9
birth or delivery NOS O63.9
closure, ductus arteriosus (Botalli) P29.38
coagulation — see Defect, coagulation
conduction (cardiac) (ventricular) I45.9
delivery, second twin, triplet, etc O63.2
development R62.50
global F88
intellectual (specific) F81.9
language F80.9
due to hearing loss F80.4
learning F81.9
pervasive F84.9
physiological R62.50
specified stage NEC R62.0
reading F81.0
sexual E30.0
speech F80.9
due to hearing loss F80.4
spelling F81.81
ejaculation F52.32
gastric emptying K30
menarche E30.0
menstruation (cause unknown) N91.0
milestone R62.0
passage of meconium (newborn) P76.0
primary respiration P28.9
puberty (constitutional) E30.0
separation of umbilical cord P96.82
sexual maturation, female E30.0
sleep phase syndrome G47.21
union, fracture — see Fracture, by site
vaccination Z28.9
Deletion(s)
autosome Q93.9
identified by fluorescence in situ hybridization (FISH)
Q93.89
identified by in situ hybridization (ISH) Q93.89

Deletion(s) — continued
chromosome
with complex rearrangements NEC Q93.7
part of NEC Q93.59
seen only at prometaphase Q93.89
short arm
22q11.2 Q93.81
4 Q93.3
5p Q93.4
specified NEC Q93.89
long arm chromosome 18 or 21 Q93.89
with complex rearrangements NEC Q93.7
microdeletions NEC Q93.88
Delhi boil or button B55.1
Delinquency (juvenile) (neurotic) F91.8
group Z72.810
Delinquent immunization status Z28.3
Delirium, delirious (acute or subacute) (not alcohol- or
drug-induced) (with dementia) R41.0
alcoholic (acute) (tremens) (withdrawal) F10.921
with intoxication F10.921
with
in
abuse F10.121
dependence F10.221
due to (secondary to)
alcohol
intoxication F10.921
in
abuse F10.121
dependence F10.221
withdrawal F10.231
amphetamine intoxication F15.921
in
abuse F15.121
dependence F15.221
anxiolytic
intoxication F13.921
in
abuse F13.121
dependence F13.221
withdrawal F13.231
cannabis intoxication (acute) F12.921
in
abuse F12.121
dependence F12.221
cocaine intoxication (acute) F14.921
in
abuse F14.121
dependence F14.221
general medical condition F05
hallucinogen intoxication F16.921
in
abuse F16.121
dependence F16.221
hypnotic
intoxication F13.921
in
abuse F13.121
dependence F13.221
withdrawal F13.231
inhalant intoxication (acute) F18.921
in
abuse F18.121
dependence F18.221
multiple etiologies F05
opioid intoxication (acute) F11.921
in
abuse F11.121
dependence F11.221
other (or unknown) substance F19.921
phencyclidine intoxication (acute) F16.921
in
abuse F16.121
dependence F16.221
psychoactive substance NEC intoxication (acute)
F19.921
in
abuse F19.121
dependence F19.221
sedative
intoxication F13.921
in
abuse F13.121
dependence F13.221
withdrawal F13.231
unknown etiology R41.0
exhaustion F43.0
hysterical F44.89
postprocedural (postoperative) F05

Index

Delirium, delirious — Delivery

Delirium, delirious — *continued*
puerperal F05
thyroid — *see* Thyrotoxicosis with thyroid storm
traumatic — *see* Injury, intracranial
tremens (alcohol-induced) F10.231
sedative-induced F13.231
Delivery (childbirth) (labor)
arrested active phase O62.1
cesarean (for)
abnormal
pelvis (bony) (deformity) (major) NEC with disproportion (fetopelvic) O33.0
with obstructed labor O65.0
presentation or position O32.9 ☑
abruptio placentae — *see also* Abruptio placentae
O45.9-
acromion presentation O32.2 ☑
atony, uterus O62.2
breech presentation O32.1 ☑
incomplete O32.8 ☑
brow presentation O32.3 ☑
cephalopelvic disproportion O33.9
cerclage O34.3- ☑
chin presentation O32.3 ☑
cicatrix of cervix O34.4- ☑
contracted pelvis (general)
inlet O33.2
outlet O33.3 ☑
cord presentation or prolapse O69.0 ☑
cystocele O34.8- ☑
deformity (acquired) (congenital)
pelvic organs or tissues NEC O34.8- ☑
pelvis (bony) NEC O33.0
disproportion NOS O33.9
eclampsia — *see* Eclampsia
face presentation O32.3 ☑
failed
forceps O66.5
induction of labor O61.9
instrumental O61.1
mechanical O61.1
medical O61.0
specified NEC O61.8
surgical O61.1
trial of labor NOS O66.40
following previous cesarean delivery O66.41
vacuum extraction O66.5
ventouse O66.5
fetal-maternal hemorrhage O43.01- ☑
hemorrhage (intrapartum) O67.9
with coagulation defect O67.0
specified cause NEC O67.8
high head at term O32.4 ☑
hydrocephalic fetus O33.6 ☑
incarceration of uterus O34.51- ☑
incoordinate uterine action O62.4
increased size, fetus O33.5 ☑
inertia, uterus O62.2
primary O62.0
secondary O62.1
lateroversion, uterus O34.59- ☑
mal lie O32.9 ☑
malposition
fetus O32.9 ☑
pelvic organs or tissues NEC O34.8- ☑
uterus NEC O34.59- ☑
malpresentation NOS O32.9 ☑
oblique presentation O32.2 ☑
occurring after 37 completed weeks of gestation
but before 39 completed weeks gestation due
to (spontaneous) onset of labor O75.82
oversize fetus O33.5 ☑
pelvic tumor NEC O34.8- ☑
placenta previa O44.0- ☑
complete O44.0- ☑
with hemorrhage O44.1- ☑
placental insufficiency O36.51- ☑
planned, occurring after 37 completed weeks of
gestation but before 39 completed weeks
gestation due to (spontaneous) onset of labor
O75.82
polyp, cervix O34.4- ☑
causing obstructed labor O65.5
poor dilatation, cervix O62.0
pre-eclampsia O14.94
mild O14.04
moderate O14.04

Delivery — *continued*
cesarean — *continued*
pre-eclampsia — *continued*
severe O14.14
with hemolysis, elevated liver enzymes and
low platelet count (HELLP) O14.24
previous
cesarean delivery O34.219
classical (vertical) scar O34.212
low transverse scar O34.211
surgery (to)
cervix O34.4- ☑
gynecological NEC O34.8- ☑
rectum O34.7- ☑
uterus O34.29
vagina O34.6- ☑
prolapse
arm or hand O32.2 ☑
uterus O34.52- ☑
prolonged labor NOS O63.9
rectocele O34.8- ☑
retroversion
uterus O34.53- ☑
rigid
cervix O34.4- ☑
pelvic floor O34.8- ☑
perineum O34.7- ☑
vagina O34.6- ☑
vulva O34.7- ☑
sacculation, pregnant uterus O34.59- ☑
scar(s)
cervix O34.4- ☑
cesarean delivery O34.219
classical (vertical) O34.212
low transverse O34.211
transmural uterine O34.29
uterus O34.29
Shirodkar suture in situ O34.3- ☑
shoulder presentation O32.2 ☑
stenosis or stricture, cervix O34.4- ☑
streptococcus group B (GBS) carrier state O99.824
transmural uterine scar O34.29
transverse presentation or lie O32.2 ☑
tumor, pelvic organs or tissues NEC O34.8- ☑
cervix O34.4- ☑
umbilical cord presentation or prolapse O69.0 ☑
without indication O82
completely normal case O80
complicated O75.9
by
abnormal, abnormality (of)
forces of labor O62.9
specified type NEC O62.8
glucose O99.814
uterine contractions NOS O62.9
abruptio placentae — *see also* Abruptio placentae O45.9- ☑
abuse
physical O9A.32 (*following* O99)
psychological O9A.52 (*following* O99)
sexual O9A.42 (*following* O99)
adherent placenta O72.0
without hemorrhage O73.0
alcohol use O99.314
anemia (pre-existing) O99.02
anesthetic death O74.8
annular detachment of cervix O71.3
atony, uterus O62.2
attempted vacuum extraction and forceps O66.5
Bandl's ring O62.4
bariatric surgery status O99.844
biliary tract disorder O26.62
bleeding — *see* Delivery, complicated by, hemorrhage
blood disorder NEC O99.12
cervical dystocia (hypotonic) O62.2
primary O62.0
secondary O62.1
circulatory system disorder O99.42
compression of cord (umbilical) NEC O69.2 ☑
condition NEC O99.89
contraction, contracted ring O62.4
cord (umbilical)
around neck
with compression O69.1 ☑
without compression O69.81 ☑
bruising O69.5 ☑
complication O69.9 ☑

Delivery — *continued*
complicated — *continued*
by — *continued*
cord — *continued*
complication — *continued*
specified NEC O69.89 ☑
compression NEC O69.2 ☑
entanglement O69.2 ☑
without compression O69.82 ☑
hematoma O69.5 ☑
presentation O69.0 ☑
prolapse O69.0 ☑
short O69.3 ☑
thrombosis (vessels) O69.5 ☑
vascular lesion O69.5 ☑
Couvelaire uterus O45.8X- ☑
damage to (injury to) NEC
perineum O71.82
periurethral tissue O71.82
vulva O71.82
delay following rupture of membranes (spon-
neous) — *see* Pregnancy, complicated
premature rupture of membranes
depressed fetal heart tones O76
diabetes O24.92
gestational O24.429
diet controlled O24.420
insulin controlled O24.424
oral drug controlled (antidiabetic) (hyp-
glycemic) O24.425
pre-existing O24.32
specified NEC O24.82
type 1 O24.02
type 2 O24.12
diastasis recti (abdominis) O71.89
dilatation
bladder O66.8
cervix incomplete, poor or slow O62.0
disease NEC O99.89
disruptio uteri — *see* Delivery, complicated
rupture, uterus
drug use O99.324
dysfunction, uterus NOS O62.9
hypertonic O62.4
hypotonic O62.2
primary O62.0
secondary O62.1
incoordinate O62.4
eclampsia O15.1
embolism (pulmonary) — *see* Embolism, obst
ric
endocrine, nutritional or metabolic disease N
O99.284
failed
attempted vaginal birth after previous ces-
an delivery O66.41
induction of labor O61.9
instrumental O61.1
mechanical O61.1
medical O61.0
specified NEC O61.8
surgical O61.1
trial of labor O66.40
female genital mutilation O65.5
fetal
abnormal acid-base balance O68
acidemia O68
acidosis O68
alkalosis O68
death, early O02.1
deformity O66.3
heart rate or rhythm (abnormal) (non-reass
ing) O76
hypoxia O77.8
stress O77.9
due to drug administration O77.1
electrocardiographic evidence of O77
specified NEC O77.8
ultrasound evidence of O77.8
fever during labor O75.2
gastric banding status O99.844
gastric bypass status O99.844
gastrointestinal disease NEC O99.62
gestational
diabetes O24.429
diet controlled O24.420
insulin (and diet) controlled O24.424

Delivery — *continued*
complicated — *continued*
  by — *continued*
    gestational — *continued*
      diabetes — *continued*
        oral drug controlled (antidiabetic) (hypo-glycemic) O24.425
      edema O12.04
        with proteinuria O12.24
      proteinuria O12.14
    gonorrhea O98.22
    hematoma O71.7
      ischial spine O71.7
      pelvic O71.7
      vagina O71.7
      vulva or perineum O71.7
    hemorrhage (uterine) O67.9
      associated with
        afibrinogenemia O67.0
        coagulation defect O67.0
        hyperfibrinolysis O67.0
        hypofibrinogenemia O67.0
      due to
        low implantation of placenta O44.5- ☑
        low-lying placenta O44.5- ☑
        placenta previa O44.1- ☑
          marginal O44.3- ☑
          partial O44.3- ☑
        premature separation of placenta (normally implanted) — *see also* Abruptio placentae O45.9- ☑
        retained placenta O72.0
        uterine leiomyoma O67.8
      placenta NEC O67.8
      postpartum NEC (atonic) (immediate) O72.1
        with retained or trapped placenta O72.0
        delayed O72.2
        secondary O72.2
        third stage O72.0
    hourglass contraction, uterus O62.4
    hypertension, hypertensive (pre-existing) — *see* Hypertension, complicated by, childbirth (labor)
    hypotension O26.5- ☑
    incomplete dilatation (cervix) O62.0
    incoordinate uterus contractions O62.4
    inertia, uterus O62.2
      during latent phase of labor O62.0
      primary O62.0
      secondary O62.1
    infection (maternal) O98.92
      carrier state NEC O99.834
      gonorrhea O98.22
      human immunodeficiency virus (HIV) O98.72
      sexually transmitted NEC O98.32
      specified NEC O98.82
      syphilis O98.12
      tuberculosis O98.02
      viral hepatitis O98.42
      viral NEC O98.52
    injury (to mother) — *see also* Delivery, complicated, by, damage to O71.9
      nonobstetric O9A.22 (*following* O99)
        caused by abuse — *see* Delivery, complicated by, abuse
    intrauterine fetal death, early O02.1
    inversion, uterus O71.2
    laceration (perineal) O70.9
      anus (sphincter) O70.4
        with third degree laceration — *see also* Delivery, complicated, by, laceration, perineum, third degree O70.20
          with mucosa O70.3
        without third degree laceration O70.2 ☑
      bladder (urinary) O71.5
      bowel O71.5
      cervix (uteri) O71.3
      fourchette O70.0
      hymen O70.0
      labia O70.0
      pelvic
        floor O70.1
        organ NEC O71.5
      perineum, perineal O70.9
        first degree O70.0
        fourth degree O70.3
        muscles O70.1

Delivery — *continued*
complicated — *continued*
  by — *continued*
    laceration — *continued*
      perineum, perineal — *continued*
        second degree O70.1
        skin O70.0
        slight O70.0
        third degree O70.20
          with
            both external anal sphincter (EAS) and internal anal sphincter (IAS) torn (IIIc) O70.23
            less than 50% of external anal sphincter (EAS) thickness torn (IIIa) O70.21
            more than 50% external anal sphincter (EAS) thickness torn (IIIb) O70.22
          IIIa O70.21
          IIIb O70.22
          IIIc O70.23
      peritoneum (pelvic) O71.5
      rectovaginal (septum) (without perineal laceration) O71.4
        with perineum — *see also* Delivery, complicated, by, laceration, perineum, third degree O70.20
          with anal or rectal mucosa O70.3
      specified NEC O71.89
      sphincter ani — *see* Delivery, complicated, by, laceration, anus (sphincter)
      urethra O71.5
      uterus O71.81
        before labor O71.81
      vagina, vaginal (deep) (high) (without perineal laceration) O71.4
        with perineum O70.0
        muscles, with perineum O70.1
      vulva O70.0
    liver disorder O26.62
    malignancy O9A.12 (*following* O99)
    malnutrition O25.2
    malposition, malpresentation
      uterus or cervix O65.5
      placenta O44.0- ☑
        with hemorrhage O44.1- ☑
      without obstruction — *see also* Delivery, complicated by, obstruction O32.9 ☑
        breech O32.1 ☑
        compound O32.6 ☑
        face (brow) (chin) O32.3 ☑
        footling O32.8 ☑
        high head O32.4 ☑
        oblique O32.2 ☑
        specified NEC O32.8 ☑
        transverse O32.2 ☑
        unstable lie O32.0 ☑
    meconium in amniotic fluid O77.0
    mental disorder NEC O99.344
    metrorrhexis — *see* Delivery, complicated by, rupture, uterus
    nervous system disorder O99.354
    obesity (pre-existing) O99.214
    obesity surgery status O99.844
    obstetric trauma O71.9
      specified NEC O71.89
    obstructed labor
      due to
        breech (complete) (frank) presentation O64.1 ☑
          incomplete O64.8 ☑
        brow presentation O64.3 ☑
        buttock presentation O64.1 ☑
        chin presentation O64.2 ☑
        compound presentation O64.5 ☑
        contracted pelvis O65.1
        deep transverse arrest O64.0 ☑
        deformed pelvis O65.0
        dystocia (fetal) O66.9
          due to
            conjoined twins O66.3
            fetal
              abnormality NEC O66.3
              ascites O66.3
              hydrops O66.3
              meningomyelocele O66.3
              sacral teratoma O66.3

Delivery — *continued*
complicated — *continued*
  by — *continued*
    obstructed labor — *continued*
      due to — *continued*
        dystocia — *continued*
          due to — *continued*
            fetal — *continued*
              tumor O66.3
            hydrocephalic fetus O66.3
            shoulder O66.0
        face presentation O64.2 ☑
        fetopelvic disproportion O65.4
        footling presentation O64.8 ☑
        impacted shoulders O66.0
        incomplete rotation of fetal head O64.0 ☑
        large fetus O66.2
        locked twins O66.1
        malposition O64.9 ☑
          specified NEC O64.8 ☑
        malpresentation O64.9 ☑
          specified NEC O64.8 ☑
        multiple fetuses NEC O66.6
        pelvic
          abnormality (maternal) O65.9
            organ O65.5
            specified NEC O65.8
          contraction
            inlet O65.2
            mid-cavity O65.3
            outlet O65.3
        persistent (position)
          occipitoiliac O64.0 ☑
          occipitoposterior O64.0 ☑
          occipitosacral O64.0 ☑
          occipitotransverse O64.0 ☑
        prolapsed arm O64.4 ☑
        shoulder presentation O64.4 ☑
      specified NEC O66.8
    pathological retraction ring, uterus O62.4
    penetration, pregnant uterus by instrument O71.1
    perforation — *see* Delivery, complicated by, laceration
    placenta, placental
      ablatio — *see also* Abruptio placentae O45.9- ☑
      abnormality O43.9- ☑
        specified NEC O43.89- ☑
      abruptio — *see also* Abruptio placentae O45.9- ☑
      accreta O43.21- ☑
      adherent (with hemorrhage) O72.0
        without hemorrhage O73.0
      detachment (premature) — *see also* Abruptio placentae O45.9- ☑
      disorder O43.9- ☑
        specified NEC O43.89- ☑
      hemorrhage NEC O67.8
      increta O43.22- ☑
      low (implantation) (lying) O44.4- ☑
        with hemorrhage O44.5- ☑
      malformation O43.10- ☑
      malposition O44.0- ☑
        without hemorrhage O44.1- ☑
      percreta O43.23- ☑
      previa (central) (complete) (lateral) (total) O44.0- ☑
        with hemorrhage O44.1- ☑
        marginal O44.2- ☑
          with hemorrhage O44.3- ☑
        partial O44.2- ☑
          with hemorrhage O44.3- ☑
      retained (with hemorrhage) O72.0
        without hemorrhage O73.0
      separation (premature) O45.9- ☑
        specified NEC O45.8X- ☑
      vicious insertion O44.1- ☑
    precipitate labor O62.3
    premature rupture, membranes — *see also* Pregnancy, complicated by, premature rupture of membranes O42.90
    prolapse
      arm or hand O32.2 ☑
      cord (umbilical) O69.0 ☑
      foot or leg O32.8 ☑

Subterms under main terms may continue to next column or page   ☑ Additional Character Required — Refer to the Tabular List for Character Selection   91

Delivery — Delivery

Delivery — *continued*
- complicated — *continued*
  - by — *continued*
    - prolapse — *continued*
      - uterus O34.52- ☑
    - prolonged labor O63.9
      - first stage O63.0
      - second stage O63.1
    - protozoal disease (maternal) O98.62
    - respiratory disease NEC O99.52
    - retained membranes or portions of placenta O72.2
      - without hemorrhage O73.1
    - retarded birth O63.9
    - retention of secundines (with hemorrhage) O72.0
      - without hemorrhage O73.0
        - partial O72.2
          - without hemorrhage O73.1
    - rupture
      - bladder (urinary) O71.5
      - cervix O71.3
      - pelvic organ NEC O71.5
      - urethra O71.5
      - uterus (during or after labor) O71.1
        - before labor O71.0- ☑
    - separation, pubic bone (symphysis pubis) O71.6
    - shock O75.1
    - shoulder presentation O64.4 ☑
    - skin disorder NEC O99.72
    - spasm, cervix O62.4
    - stenosis or stricture, cervix O65.5
    - streptococcus group B (GBS) carrier state O99.824
    - subluxation of symphysis (pubis) O26.72
    - syphilis (maternal) O98.12
    - tear — *see* Delivery, complicated by, laceration
    - tetanic uterus O62.4
    - trauma (obstetrical) — *see also* Delivery, complicated, by, damage to O71.9
      - non-obstetric O9A.22 (*following* O99)
      - periurethral O71.82
      - specified NEC O71.89
    - tuberculosis (maternal) O98.02
    - tumor, pelvic organs or tissues NEC O65.5
    - umbilical cord around neck
      - with compression O69.1 ☑
      - without compression O69.81 ☑
    - uterine inertia O62.2
      - during latent phase of labor O62.0
      - primary O62.0
      - secondary O62.1
    - vasa previa O69.4 ☑
    - velamentous insertion of cord O43.12- ☑
  - specified complication NEC O75.89
- delayed NOS O63.9
  - following rupture of membranes
    - artificial O75.5
  - second twin, triplet, etc. O63.2
- forceps, low following failed vacuum extraction O66.5
- missed (at or near term) O36.4 ☑
- normal O80
- obstructed — *see* Delivery, complicated by, obstructed labor
- precipitate O62.3
- preterm — *see also* Pregnancy, complicated by, preterm labor O60.10 ☑
- spontaneous O80
- term pregnancy NOS O80
- uncomplicated O80
- vaginal, following previous cesarean delivery O34.219
  - classical (vertical) scar O34.212
  - low transverse scar O34.211

Delusions (paranoid) — *see* Disorder, delusional

Dementia (degenerative (primary)) (old age) (persisting) F03.90
- with
  - aggressive behavior F03.91
  - behavioral disturbance F03.91
  - combative behavior F03.91
  - Lewy bodies G31.83 *[F02.80]*
    - with behavioral disturbance G31.83 *[F02.81]*
  - Parkinsonism G31.83 *[F02.80]*
    - with behavioral disturbance G31.83 *[F02.81]*
  - Parkinson's disease G20 *[F02.80]*
    - with behavioral disturbance G20 *[F02.81]*
  - violent behavior F03.91
- alcoholic F10.97
  - with dependence F10.27
- Alzheimer's type — *see* Disease, Alzheimer's

Dementia — *continued*
- arteriosclerotic — *see* Dementia, vascular
- atypical, Alzheimer's type — *see* Disease, Alzheimer's, specified NEC
- congenital — *see* Disability, intellectual
- frontal (lobe) G31.09 *[F02.80]*
  - with behavioral disturbance G31.09 *[F02.81]*
- frontotemporal G31.09 *[F02.80]*
  - with behavioral disturbance G31.09 *[F02.81]*
  - specified NEC G31.09 *[F02.80]*
    - with behavioral disturbance G31.09 *[F02.81]*
- Huntington's disease or chorea G10
  - with dementia G10 *[F02.80]*
- in (due to)
  - with behavioral disturbance G31.83 *[F02.81]*
  - alcohol F10.97
    - with dependence F10.27
  - Alzheimer's disease — *see* Disease, Alzheimer's
  - arteriosclerotic brain disease — *see* Dementia, vascular
  - cerebral lipidoses E75.- ☑ *[F02.80]*
    - with behavioral disturbance E75.- ☑ *[F02.81]*
  - Creutzfeldt-Jakob disease — *see also* Creutzfeldt-Jakob disease or syndrome (with dementia) A81.00
  - epilepsy G40.- ☑ *[F02.80]*
    - with behavioral disturbance G40.- ☑ *[F02.81]*
  - hepatolenticular degeneration E83.01 *[F02.80]*
    - with behavioral disturbance E83.01 *[F02.81]*
  - human immunodeficiency virus (HIV) disease B20 *[F02.80]*
    - with behavioral disturbance B20 *[F02.81]*
  - Huntington's disease or chorea G10 *[F02.80]*
    - with behavioral disturbance G10 *[F02.81]*
  - hypercalcemia E83.52 *[F02.80]*
    - with behavioral disturbance E83.52 *[F02.81]*
  - hypothyroidism, acquired E03.9 *[F02.80]*
    - with behavioral disturbance E03.9 *[F02.81]*
    - due to iodine deficiency E01.8 *[F02.80]*
      - with behavioral disturbance E01.8 *[F02.81]*
  - inhalants F18.97
    - with dependence F18.27
  - multiple
    - etiologies F03 ☑
    - sclerosis G35 *[F02.80]*
      - with behavioral disturbance G35 *[F02.81]*
  - neurosyphilis A52.17 *[F02.80]*
    - with behavioral disturbance A52.17 *[F02.81]*
    - juvenile A50.49 *[F02.80]*
      - with behavioral disturbance A50.49 *[F02.81]*
  - niacin deficiency E52 *[F02.80]*
    - with behavioral disturbance E52 *[F02.81]*
  - paralysis agitans G20 *[F02.80]*
    - with behavioral disturbance G20 *[F02.81]*
  - Parkinson's disease G20 *[F02.80]*
  - pellagra E52 *[F02.80]*
    - with behavioral disturbance E52 *[F02.81]*
  - Pick's G31.01 *[F02.80]*
    - with behavioral disturbance G31.01 *[F02.81]*
  - polyarteritis nodosa M30.0 *[F02.80]*
    - with behavioral disturbance M30.0 *[F02.81]*
  - psychoactive drug F19.97
    - with dependence F19.27
    - inhalants F18.97
      - with dependence F18.27
    - sedatives, hypnotics or anxiolytics F13.97
      - with dependence F13.27
  - sedatives, hypnotics or anxiolytics F13.97
    - with dependence F13.27
  - systemic lupus erythematosus M32.- ☑ *[F02.80]*
    - with behavioral disturbance M32.- ☑ *[F02.81]*
  - trypanosomiasis
    - African B56.9 *[F02.80]*
      - with behavioral disturbance B56.9 *[F02.81]*
  - unknown etiology F03 ☑
  - vitamin B12 deficiency E53.8 *[F02.80]*
    - with behavioral disturbance E53.8 *[F02.81]*
  - volatile solvents F18.97
    - with dependence F18.27
- infantile, infantilis F84.3
- Lewy body G31.83 *[F02.80]*
  - with behavioral disturbance G31.83 *[F02.81]*
- multi-infarct — *see* Dementia, vascular
- paralytica, paralytic (syphilitic) A52.17 *[F02.80]*
  - with behavioral disturbance A52.17 *[F02.81]*
  - juvenilis A50.45
- paretic A52.17

Dementia — *continued*
- praecox — *see* Schizophrenia
- presenile F03 ☑
  - Alzheimer's type — *see* Disease, Alzheimer's, ea[rly] onset
- primary degenerative F03 ☑
- progressive, syphilitic A52.17
- senile F03 ☑
  - with acute confusional state F05
  - Alzheimer's type — *see* Disease, Alzheimer's, la[te] onset
  - depressed or paranoid type F03 ☑
- vascular (acute onset) (mixed) (multi-infarct) (subco[rti]cal) F01.50
  - with behavioral disturbance F01.51

Demineralization, bone — *see* Osteoporosis

Demodex folliculorum (infestation) B88.0

Demophobia F40.248

Demoralization R45.3

Demyelination, demyelinization
- central nervous system G37.9
  - specified NEC G37.8
- corpus callosum (central) G37.1
- disseminated, acute G36.9
  - specified NEC G36.8
- global G35
- in optic neuritis G36.0

Dengue (classical) (fever) A90
- hemorrhagic A91
- sandfly A93.1

Dennie-Marfan syphilitic syndrome A50.45

Dens evaginatus, in dente or invaginatus K00.2

Dense breasts R92.2

Density
- increased, bone (disseminated) (generalized) (spott[ed]) — *see* Disorder, bone, density and structure[,] specified type NEC
- lung (nodular) J98.4

Dental — *see also* condition
- examination Z01.20
  - with abnormal findings Z01.21
- restoration
  - aesthetically inadequate or displeasing K08.56
  - defective K08.50
    - specified NEC K08.59
  - failure of marginal integrity K08.51
  - failure of periodontal anatomical integrity K08.5[?]

Dentia praecox K00.6

Denticles (pulp) K04.2

Dentigerous cyst K09.0

Dentin
- irregular (in pulp) K04.3
- opalescent K00.5
- secondary (in pulp) K04.3
- sensitive K03.89

Dentinogenesis imperfecta K00.5

Dentinoma — *see* Cyst, calcifying odontogenic

Dentition (syndrome) K00.7
- delayed K00.6
- difficult K00.7
- precocious K00.6
- premature K00.6
- retarded K00.6

Dependence (on) (syndrome) F19.20
- with remission F19.21
- alcohol (ethyl) (methyl) (without remission) F10.20
  - with
    - amnestic disorder, persisting F10.26
    - anxiety disorder F10.280
    - dementia, persisting F10.27
    - intoxication F10.229
      - with delirium F10.221
      - uncomplicated F10.220
    - mood disorder F10.24
    - psychotic disorder F10.259
      - with
        - delusions F10.250
        - hallucinations F10.251
    - remission F10.21
    - sexual dysfunction F10.281
    - sleep disorder F10.282
    - specified disorder NEC F10.288
    - withdrawal F10.239
      - with
        - delirium F10.231
        - perceptual disturbance F10.232
      - uncomplicated F10.230
  - counseling and surveillance Z71.41

pendence — *continued*
amobarbital — *see* Dependence, drug, sedative
amphetamine(s) (type) — *see* Dependence, drug, stimulant NEC
amytal (sodium) — *see* Dependence, drug, sedative
analgesic NEC F55.8
anesthetic (agent) (gas) (general) (local) NEC — *see* Dependence, drug, psychoactive NEC
anxiolytic NEC — *see* Dependence, drug, sedative
barbital(s) — *see* Dependence, drug, sedative
barbiturate(s) (compounds) (drugs classifiable to T42) — *see* Dependence, drug, sedative
benzedrine — *see* Dependence, drug, stimulant NEC
bhang — *see* Dependence, drug, cannabis
bromide(s) NEC — *see* Dependence, drug, sedative
caffeine — *see* Dependence, drug, stimulant NEC
cannabis (sativa) (indica) (resin) (derivatives) (type) — *see* Dependence, drug, cannabis
chloral (betaine) (hydrate) — *see* Dependence, drug, sedative
chlordiazepoxide — *see* Dependence, drug, sedative
coca (leaf) (derivatives) — *see* Dependence, drug, cocaine
cocaine — *see* Dependence, drug, cocaine
codeine — *see* Dependence, drug, opioid
combinations of drugs F19.20
dagga — *see* Dependence, drug, cannabis
demerol — *see* Dependence, drug, opioid
dexamphetamine — *see* Dependence, drug, stimulant NEC
dexedrine — *see* Dependence, drug, stimulant NEC
dextromethorphan — *see* Dependence, drug, opioid
dextromoramide — *see* Dependence, drug, opioid
dextro-nor-pseudo-ephedrine — *see* Dependence, drug, stimulant NEC
dextrorphan — *see* Dependence, drug, opioid
diazepam — *see* Dependence, drug, sedative
dilaudid — *see* Dependence, drug, opioid
D-lysergic acid diethylamide — *see* Dependence, drug, hallucinogen
drug NEC F19.20
 with sleep disorder F19.282
 cannabis F12.20
  with
   anxiety disorder F12.280
   intoxication F12.229
    with
     delirium F12.221
     perceptual disturbance F12.222
    uncomplicated F12.220
   other specified disorder F12.288
   psychosis F12.259
    delusions F12.250
    hallucinations F12.251
   unspecified disorder F12.29
   withdrawal F12.23
  in remission F12.21
 cocaine F14.20
  with
   anxiety disorder F14.280
   intoxication F14.229
    with
     delirium F14.221
     perceptual disturbance F14.222
    uncomplicated F14.220
   mood disorder F14.24
   other specified disorder F14.288
   psychosis F14.259
    delusions F14.250
    hallucinations F14.251
   sexual dysfunction F14.281
   sleep disorder F14.282
   unspecified disorder F14.29
   withdrawal F14.23
  in remission F14.21
  withdrawal symptoms in newborn P96.1
 counseling and surveillance Z71.51
 hallucinogen F16.20
  with
   anxiety disorder F16.280
   flashbacks F16.283
   intoxication F16.229
    with delirium F16.221
    uncomplicated F16.220
   mood disorder F16.24
   other specified disorder F16.288
   perception disorder, persisting F16.283
   psychosis F16.259

Dependence — *continued*
 drug — *continued*
  hallucinogen — *continued*
   with — *continued*
    psychosis — *continued*
     delusions F16.250
     hallucinations F16.251
    unspecified disorder F16.29
   in remission F16.21
  in remission F19.21
  inhalant F18.20
   with
    anxiety disorder F18.280
    dementia, persisting F18.27
    intoxication F18.229
     with delirium F18.221
     uncomplicated F18.220
    mood disorder F18.24
    other specified disorder F18.288
    psychosis F18.259
     delusions F18.250
     hallucinations F18.251
    unspecified disorder F18.29
   in remission F18.21
  nicotine F17.200
   with disorder F17.209
    in remission F17.201
    specified disorder NEC F17.208
    withdrawal F17.203
   chewing tobacco F17.220
    with disorder F17.229
     in remission F17.221
     specified disorder NEC F17.228
     withdrawal F17.223
   cigarettes F17.210
    with disorder F17.219
     in remission F17.211
     specified disorder NEC F17.218
     withdrawal F17.213
   specified product NEC F17.290
    with disorder F17.299
     remission F17.291
     specified disorder NEC F17.298
     withdrawal F17.293
  opioid F11.20
   with
    intoxication F11.229
     with
      delirium F11.221
      perceptual disturbance F11.222
     uncomplicated F11.220
    mood disorder F11.24
    other specified disorder F11.288
    psychosis F11.259
     delusions F11.250
     hallucinations F11.251
    sexual dysfunction F11.281
    sleep disorder F11.282
    unspecified disorder F11.29
    withdrawal F11.23
   in remission F11.21
  psychoactive NEC F19.20
   with
    amnestic disorder F19.26
    anxiety disorder F19.280
    dementia F19.27
    intoxication F19.229
     with
      delirium F19.221
      perceptual disturbance F19.222
     uncomplicated F19.220
    mood disorder F19.24
    other specified disorder F19.288
    psychosis F19.259
     delusions F19.250
     hallucinations F19.251
    sexual dysfunction F19.281
    sleep disorder F19.282
    unspecified disorder F19.29
    withdrawal F19.239
     with
      delirium F19.231
      perceptual disturbance F19.232
     uncomplicated F19.230
  sedative, hypnotic or anxiolytic F13.20
   with
    amnestic disorder F13.26
    anxiety disorder F13.280
    dementia, persisting F13.27

Dependence — *continued*
 drug — *continued*
  sedative, hypnotic or anxiolytic — *continued*
   with — *continued*
    intoxication F13.229
     with delirium F13.221
     uncomplicated F13.220
    mood disorder F13.24
    other specified disorder F13.288
    psychosis F13.259
     delusions F13.250
     hallucinations F13.251
    sexual dysfunction F13.281
    sleep disorder F13.282
    unspecified disorder F13.29
    withdrawal F13.239
     with
      delirium F13.231
      perceptual disturbance F13.232
     uncomplicated F13.230
   in remission F13.21
  stimulant NEC F15.20
   with
    anxiety disorder F15.280
    intoxication F15.229
     with
      delirium F15.221
      perceptual disturbance F15.222
     uncomplicated F15.220
    mood disorder F15.24
    other specified disorder F15.288
    psychosis F15.259
     delusions F15.250
     hallucinations F15.251
    sexual dysfunction F15.281
    sleep disorder F15.282
    unspecified disorder F15.29
    withdrawal F15.23
   in remission F15.21
 ethyl
  alcohol (without remission) F10.20
   with remission F10.21
  bromide — *see* Dependence, drug, sedative
  carbamate F19.20
  chloride F19.20
  morphine — *see* Dependence, drug, opioid
 ganja — *see* Dependence, drug, cannabis
 glue (airplane) (sniffing) — *see* Dependence, drug, inhalant
 glutethimide — *see* Dependence, drug, sedative
 hallucinogenics — *see* Dependence, drug, hallucinogen
 hashish — *see* Dependence, drug, cannabis
 hemp — *see* Dependence, drug, cannabis
 heroin (salt) (any) — *see* Dependence, drug, opioid
 hypnotic NEC — *see* Dependence, drug, sedative
 Indian hemp — *see* Dependence, drug, cannabis
 inhalants — *see* Dependence, drug, inhalant
 khat — *see* Dependence, drug, stimulant NEC
 laudanum — *see* Dependence, drug, opioid
 LSD (-25) (derivatives) — *see* Dependence, drug, hallucinogen
 luminal — *see* Dependence, drug, sedative
 lysergic acid — *see* Dependence, drug, hallucinogen
 maconha — *see* Dependence, drug, cannabis
 marihuana — *see* Dependence, drug, cannabis
 meprobamate — *see* Dependence, drug, sedative
 mescaline — *see* Dependence, drug, hallucinogen
 methadone — *see* Dependence, drug, opioid
 methamphetamine(s) — *see* Dependence, drug, stimulant NEC
 methaqualone — *see* Dependence, drug, sedative
 methyl
  alcohol (without remission) F10.20
   with remission F10.21
  bromide — *see* Dependence, drug, sedative
  morphine — *see* Dependence, drug, opioid
  phenidate — *see* Dependence, drug, stimulant NEC
  sulfonal — *see* Dependence, drug, sedative
 morphine (sulfate) (sulfite) (type) — *see* Dependence, drug, opioid
 narcotic (drug) NEC — *see* Dependence, drug, opioid
 nembutal — *see* Dependence, drug, sedative
 neraval — *see* Dependence, drug, sedative
 neravan — *see* Dependence, drug, sedative
 neurobarb — *see* Dependence, drug, sedative
 nicotine — *see* Dependence, drug, nicotine
 nitrous oxide F19.20

Dependence — continued
  nonbarbiturate sedatives and tranquilizers with similar effect — see Dependence, drug, sedative
  on
    artificial heart (fully implantable) (mechanical) Z95.812
    aspirator Z99.0
    care provider (because of) Z74.9
      impaired mobility Z74.09
      need for
        assistance with personal care Z74.1
        continuous supervision Z74.3
      no other household member able to render care Z74.2
      specified reason NEC Z74.8
    machine Z99.89
      enabling NEC Z99.89
      specified type NEC Z99.89
    renal dialysis (hemodialysis) (peritoneal) Z99.2
    respirator Z99.11
    ventilator Z99.11
    wheelchair Z99.3
  opiate — see Dependence, drug, opioid
  opioids — see Dependence, drug, opioid
  opium (alkaloids) (derivatives) (tincture) — see Dependence, drug, opioid
  oxygen (long-term) (supplemental) Z99.81
  paraldehyde — see Dependence, drug, sedative
  paregoric — see Dependence, drug, opioid
  PCP (phencyclidine) (or related substance) — see Dependence, drug, hallucinogen
  pentobarbital — see Dependence, drug, sedative
  pentobarbitone (sodium) — see Dependence, drug, sedative
  pentothal — see Dependence, drug, sedative
  peyote — see Dependence, drug, hallucinogen
  phencyclidine (PCP) (or related substance) — see Dependence, drug, hallucinogen
  phenmetrazine — see Dependence, drug, stimulant NEC
  phenobarbital — see Dependence, drug, sedative
  polysubstance F19.20
  psilocibin, psilocin, psilocyn, psilocyline — see Dependence, drug, hallucinogen
  psychostimulant NEC — see Dependence, drug, stimulant NEC
  secobarbital — see Dependence, drug, sedative
  seconal — see Dependence, drug, sedative
  sedative NEC — see Dependence, drug, sedative
  specified drug NEC — see Dependence, drug
  stimulant NEC — see Dependence, drug, stimulant NEC
  substance NEC — see Dependence, drug
  supplemental oxygen Z99.81
  tobacco — see Dependence, drug, nicotine
    counseling and surveillance Z71.6
  tranquilizer NEC — see Dependence, drug, sedative
  vitamin B6 E53.1
  volatile solvents — see Dependence, drug, inhalant

Dependency
  care-provider Z74.9
  passive F60.7
  reactions (persistent) F60.7

Depersonalization (in neurotic state) (neurotic) (syndrome) F48.1

Depletion
  extracellular fluid E86.9
  plasma E86.1
  potassium E87.6
    nephropathy N25.89
  salt or sodium E87.1
    causing heat exhaustion or prostration T67.4 ☑
    nephropathy N28.9
  volume NOS E86.9

Deployment (current) (military) status Z56.82
  in theater or in support of military war, peacekeeping and humanitarian operations Z56.82
  personal history of Z91.82
    military war, peacekeeping and humanitarian deployment (current or past conflict) Z91.82
  returned from Z91.82

Depolarization, premature I49.40
  atrial I49.1
  junctional I49.2
  specified NEC I49.49
  ventricular I49.3

Deposit
  bone in Boeck's sarcoid D86.89
  calcareous, calcium — see Calcification

Deposit — continued
  cholesterol
    retina H35.89
    vitreous (body) (humor) — see Deposit, crystalline
  conjunctiva H11.11-
  cornea H18.00- ☑
    argentous H18.02- ☑
    due to metabolic disorder H18.03- ☑
    Kayser-Fleischer ring H18.04- ☑
    pigmentation — see Pigmentation, cornea
  crystalline, vitreous (body) (humor) H43.2- ☑
  hemosiderin in old scars of cornea — see Pigmentation, cornea, stromal
  metallic in lens — see Cataract, specified NEC
  skin R23.8
  tooth, teeth (betel) (black) (green) (materia alba) (orange) (tobacco) K03.6
  urate, kidney — see Calculus, kidney

Depraved appetite — see Pica

Depressed
  HDL cholesterol E78.6

Depression (acute) (mental) F32.9
  agitated (single episode) F32.2
  anaclitic — see Disorder, adjustment
  anxiety F41.8
    persistent F34.1
  arches — see also Deformity, limb, flat foot
  atypical (single episode) F32.89
    recurrent episode F33.8
  basal metabolic rate R94.8
  bone marrow D75.89
  central nervous system R09.2
  cerebral R29.818
    newborn P91.4
  cerebrovascular I67.9
  chest wall M95.4
  climacteric (single episode) F32.89
    recurrent episode F33.8
  endogenous (without psychotic symptoms) F33.2
    with psychotic symptoms F33.3
  functional activity R68.89
  hysterical F44.89
  involutional (single episode) F32.89
    recurrent episode F33.8
  major F32.9
    with psychotic symptoms F32.3
    recurrent — see Disorder, depressive, recurrent
  manic-depressive — see Disorder, depressive, recurrent
  masked (single episode) F32.89
  medullary G93.89
  menopausal (single episode) F32.89
    recurrent episode F33.8
  metatarsus — see Depression, arches
  monopolar F33.9
  nervous F34.1
  neurotic F34.1
  nose M95.0
  postnatal (NOS) F53.0
  postpartum (NOS) F53.0
  post-psychotic of schizophrenia F32.89
  post-schizophrenic F32.89
  psychogenic (reactive) (single episode) F32.9
  psychoneurotic F34.1
  psychotic (single episode) F32.3
    recurrent F33.3
  reactive (psychogenic) (single episode) F32.9
    psychotic (single episode) F32.3
  recurrent — see Disorder, depressive, recurrent
  respiratory center G93.89
  seasonal — see Disorder, depressive, recurrent
  senile F03 ☑
  severe, single episode F32.2
  situational F43.21
  skull Q67.4
  specified NEC (single episode) F32.89
  sternum M95.4
  visual field — see Defect, visual field
  vital (recurrent) (without psychotic symptoms) F33.2
    with psychotic symptoms F33.3
    single episode F32.2

Deprivation
  cultural Z60.3
  effects NOS T73.9 ☑
    specified NEC T73.8 ☑
  emotional NEC Z65.8
    affecting infant or child — see Maltreatment, child, psychological
  food T73.0 ☑

Deprivation — continued
  protein — see Malnutrition
  sleep Z72.820
  social Z60.4
    affecting infant or child — see Maltreatment, ch psychological
  specified NEC T73.8 ☑
  vitamins — see Deficiency, vitamin
  water T73.1 ☑

Derangement
  ankle (internal) — see Derangement, joint, ankle
  cartilage (articular) NEC — see Derangement, joint, articular cartilage, by site
    recurrent — see Dislocation, recurrent
  cruciate ligament, anterior, current injury — see Sprain knee, cruciate, anterior
  elbow (internal) — see Derangement, joint, elbow
  hip (joint) (internal) (old) — see Derangement, join hip
  joint (internal) M24.9
    ankylosis — see Ankylosis
    articular cartilage M24.10
      ankle M24.17- ☑
      elbow M24.12- ☑
      foot M24.17- ☑
      hand M24.14- ☑
      hip M24.15- ☑
      knee NEC M23.9- ☑
      loose body — see Loose, body
      shoulder M24.11- ☑
      wrist M24.13- ☑
    contracture — see Contraction, joint
    current injury — see also Dislocation
      knee, meniscus or cartilage — see Tear, menisc
    dislocation
      pathological — see Dislocation, pathologica
      recurrent — see Dislocation, recurrent
    knee — see Derangement, knee
    ligament — see Disorder, ligament
    loose body — see Loose, body
    recurrent — see Dislocation, recurrent
    specified type NEC M24.80
      ankle M24.87- ☑
      elbow M24.82- ☑
      foot joint M24.87- ☑
      hand joint M24.84- ☑
      hip M24.85- ☑
      shoulder M24.81- ☑
      wrist M24.83- ☑
    temporomandibular M26.69
  knee (recurrent) M23.9- ☑
    ligament disruption, spontaneous M23.60- ☑
      anterior cruciate M23.61- ☑
      capsular M23.67- ☑
      instability, chronic M23.5- ☑
      lateral collateral M23.64- ☑
      medial collateral M23.63- ☑
      posterior cruciate M23.62- ☑
    loose body M23.4- ☑
    meniscus M23.30- ☑
      cystic M23.00- ☑
        lateral M23.002
          anterior horn M23.04- ☑
          posterior horn M23.05- ☑
          specified NEC M23.06- ☑
        medial M23.005
          anterior horn M23.01- ☑
          posterior horn M23.02- ☑
          specified NEC M23.03- ☑
      degenerate — see Derangement, knee, meniscus, specified NEC
      detached — see Derangement, knee, meniscus specified NEC
      due to old tear or injury M23.20- ☑
        lateral M23.20- ☑
          anterior horn M23.24- ☑
          posterior horn M23.25- ☑
          specified NEC M23.26- ☑
        medial M23.20- ☑
          anterior horn M23.21- ☑
          posterior horn M23.22- ☑
          specified NEC M23.23- ☑
      retained — see Derangement, knee, meniscus specified NEC
      specified NEC M23.30- ☑
        lateral M23.30- ☑

☑ **Additional Character Required** — Refer to the Tabular List for Character Selection   ▽ **Subterms under main terms may continue to next column or pa**

angement — *continued*
 knee — *continued*
  meniscus — *continued*
   specified — *continued*
    lateral — *continued*
     anterior horn M23.34- ☑
     posterior horn M23.35- ☑
     specified NEC M23.36- ☑
    medial M23.30- ☑
     anterior horn M23.31- ☑
     posterior horn M23.32- ☑
     specified NEC M23.33- ☑
  old M23.8X- ☑
  specified NEC — *see* subcategory M23.8 ☑
 ow back NEC — *see* Dorsopathy, specified NEC
 meniscus — *see* Derangement, knee, meniscus
 mental — *see* Psychosis
 patella, specified NEC — *see* Disorder, patella, derangement NEC
 emilunar cartilage (knee) — *see* Derangement, knee, meniscus, specified NEC
 houlder (internal) — *see* Derangement, joint, shoulder
cum's disease E88.2
ealization (neurotic) F48.1
mal — *see* condition
maphytid — *see* Dermatophytosis
matitis (eczematous) L30.9
 b igne L59.0
 carine B88.0
 ctinic (due to sun) L57.8
  other than from sun L59.8
 llergic — *see* Dermatitis, contact, allergic
 mbustionis, due to burn or scald — *see* Burn
 mebic A06.7
 mmonia L22
 rsenical (ingested) L27.8
 rtefacta L98.1
  psychogenic F54
 topic L20.9
  psychogenic F54
  specified NEC L20.89
 utoimmune progesterone L30.8
 erlock, berloque L56.2
 lastomycotic B40.3
 lister beetle L24.89
 ullous, bullosa L13.9
  mucosynechial, atrophic L12.1
  seasonal L30.8
  specified NEC L13.8
 alorica L59.0
  due to burn or scald — *see* Burn
 aterpillar L24.89
 ercarial B65.3
 ombustionis L59.0
  duc to burn or scald — *see* Burn
 ongelationis T69.1 ☑
 ontact (occupational) L25.9
  allergic L23.9
   due to
    adhesives L23.1
    cement L23.5
    chemical products NEC L23.5
    chromium L23.0
    cosmetics L23.2
    dander (cat) (dog) L23.81
    drugs in contact with skin L23.3
    dyes L23.4
    food in contact with skin L23.6
    hair (cat) (dog) L23.81
    insecticide L23.5
    metals L23.0
    nickel L23.0
    plants, non-food L23.7
    plastic L23.5
    rubber L23.5
    specified agent NEC L23.89
  due to
   cement L25.3
   chemical products NEC L25.3
   cosmetics L25.0
   dander (cat) (dog) L23.81
   drugs in contact with skin L25.1
   dyes L25.2
   food in contact with skin L25.4
   hair (cat) (dog) L23.81
   plants, non-food L25.5
   specified agent NEC L25.8
  irritant L24.9

Dermatitis — *continued*
 contact — *continued*
  irritant — *continued*
   due to
    cement L24.5
    chemical products NEC L24.5
    cosmetics L24.3
    detergents L24.0
    drugs in contact with skin L24.4
    food in contact with skin L24.6
    oils and greases L24.1
    plants, non-food L24.7
    solvents L24.2
    specified agent NEC L24.89
 contusiformis L52
 diabetic — *see* E08-E13 with .620
 diaper L22
 diphtheritica A36.3
 dry skin L85.3
 due to
  acetone (contact) (irritant) L24.2
  acids (contact) (irritant) L24.5
  adhesive(s) (allergic) (contact) (plaster) L23.1
   irritant L24.5
  alcohol (irritant) (skin contact) (substances in category T51) L24.2
   taken internally L27.8
  alkalis (contact) (irritant) L24.5
  arsenic (ingested) L27.8
  carbon disulfide (contact) (irritant) L24.2
  caustics (contact) (irritant) L24.5
  cement (contact) L25.3
  cereal (ingested) L27.2
  chemical(s) NEC L25.3
   taken internally L27.8
  chlorocompounds L24.2
  chromium (contact) (irritant) L24.81
  coffee (ingested) L27.2
  cold weather L30.8
  cosmetics (contact) L25.0
   allergic L23.2
   irritant L24.3
  cyclohexanes L24.2
  dander (cat) (dog) L23.81
  Demodex species B88.0
  Dermanyssus gallinae B88.0
  detergents (contact) (irritant) L24.0
  dichromate L24.81
  drugs and medicaments (generalized) (internal use) L27.0
   external — *see* Dermatitis, due to, drugs, in contact with skin
   in contact with skin L25.1
    allergic L23.3
    irritant L24.4
   localized skin eruption L27.1
   specified substance — *see* Table of Drugs and Chemicals
  dyes (contact) L25.2
   allergic L23.4
   irritant L24.89
  epidermophytosis — *see* Dermatophytosis
  esters L24.2
  external irritant NEC L24.9
  fish (ingested) L27.2
  flour (ingested) L27.2
  food (ingested) L27.2
   in contact with skin L25.4
  fruit (ingested) L27.2
  furs (allergic) (contact) L23.81
  glues — *see* Dermatitis, due to, adhesives
  glycols L24.2
  greases NEC (contact) (irritant) L24.1
  hair (cat) (dog) L23.81
  hot
   objects and materials — *see* Burn
   weather or places L59.0
  hydrocarbons L24.2
  infrared rays L59.8
  ingestion, ingested substance L27.9
   chemical NEC L27.8
   drugs and medicaments — *see* Dermatitis, due to, drugs
   food L27.2
   specified NEC L27.8
  insecticide in contact with skin L24.5
  internal agent L27.9

Dermatitis — *continued*
 due to — *continued*
  internal agent — *continued*
   drugs and medicaments (generalized) — *see* Dermatitis, due to, drugs
   food L27.2
  irradiation — *see* Dermatitis, due to, radioactive substance
  ketones L24.2
  lacquer tree (allergic) (contact) L23.7
  light (sun) NEC L57.8
   acute L56.8
   other L59.8
  Liponyssoides sanguineus B88.0
  low temperature L30.8
  meat (ingested) L27.2
  metals, metal salts (contact) (irritant) L24.81
  milk (ingested) L27.2
  nickel (contact) (irritant) L24.81
  nylon (contact) (irritant) L24.5
  oils NEC (contact) (irritant) L24.1
  paint solvent (contact) (irritant) L24.2
  petroleum products (contact) (irritant) (substances in T52.0) L24.2
  plants NEC (contact) L25.5
   allergic L23.7
   irritant L24.7
  plasters (adhesive) (any) (allergic) (contact) L23.1
   irritant L24.5
  plastic (contact) L25.3
  preservatives (contact) — *see* Dermatitis, due to, chemical, in contact with skin
  primrose (allergic) (contact) L23.7
  primula (allergic) (contact) L23.7
  radiation L59.8
   nonionizing (chronic exposure) L57.8
   sun NEC L57.8
    acute L56.8
  radioactive substance L58.9
   acute L58.0
   chronic L58.1
  radium L59.8
   acute L58.0
   chronic L58.1
  ragweed (allergic) (contact) L23.7
  Rhus (allergic) (contact) (diversiloba) (radicans) (toxicodendron) (venenata) (verniciflua) L23.7
  rubber (contact) L24.5
  Senecio jacobaea (allergic) (contact) L23.7
  solvents (contact) (irritant) (substances in category T52) L24.2
  specified agent NEC (contact) L25.8
   allergic L23.89
   irritant L24.89
  sunshine NEC L57.8
   acute L56.8
  tetrachlorethylene (contact) (irritant) L24.2
  toluene (contact) (irritant) L24.2
  turpentine (contact) L24.2
  ultraviolet rays (sun NEC) (chronic exposure) L57.8
   acute L56.8
  vaccine or vaccination L27.0
   specified substance — *see* Table of Drugs and Chemicals
  varicose veins — *see* Varix, leg, with, inflammation
  X-rays L58.9
   acute L58.0
   chronic L58.1
 dyshydrotic L30.1
 dysmenorrheica N94.6
 escharotica — *see* Burn
 exfoliative, exfoliativa (generalized) L26
  neonatorum L00
 eyelid — *see also* Dermatosis, eyelid
  allergic H01.119
   left H01.116
    lower H01.115
    upper H01.114
   right H01.113
    lower H01.112
    upper H01.111
  contact — *see* Dermatitis, eyelid, allergic
  due to
   Demodex species B88.0
   herpes (zoster) B02.39
    simplex B00.59
  eczematous H01.139
   left H01.136

Dermatitis — *continued*
eyelid — *see also* Dermatosis, eyelid — *continued*
  eczematous — *continued*
   left — *continued*
    lower H01.135
    upper H01.134
   right H01.133
    lower H01.132
    upper H01.131
facta, factitia, factitial L98.1
  psychogenic F54
flexural NEC L20.82
friction L30.4
fungus B36.9
  specified type NEC B36.8
gangrenosa, gangrenous infantum L08.0
harvest mite B88.0
heat L59.0
herpesviral, vesicular (ear) (lip) B00.1
herpetiformis (bullous) (erythematous) (pustular)
  (vesicular) L13.0
  juvenile L12.2
  senile L12.0
hiemalis L30.8
hypostatic, hypostatica — *see* Varix, leg, with, inflammation
infectious eczematoid L30.3
infective L30.3
irritant — *see* Dermatitis, contact, irritant
Jacquet's (diaper dermatitis) L22
Leptus B88.0
lichenified NEC L28.0
medicamentosa (generalized) (internal use) — *see*
  Dermatitis, due to drugs
mite B88.0
multiformis L13.0
  juvenile L12.2
napkin L22
neurotica L13.0
nummular L30.0
papillaris capillitii L73.0
pellagrous E52
perioral L71.0
photocontact L56.2
polymorpha dolorosa L13.0
pruriginosa L13.0
pruritic NEC L30.8
psychogenic F54
purulent L08.0
pustular
  contagious B08.02
  subcorneal L13.1
pyococcal L08.0
pyogenica L08.0
repens L40.2
Ritter's (exfoliativa) L00
Schamberg's L81.7
schistosome B65.3
seasonal bullous L30.8
seborrheic L21.9
  infantile L21.1
  specified NEC L21.8
sensitization NOS L23.9
septic L08.0
solare L57.8
specified NEC L30.8
stasis I87.2
  with
   varicose ulcer — *see* Varix, leg, with ulcer, with
    inflammation
   varicose veins — *see* Varix, leg, with, inflamma-
    tion
   due to postthrombotic syndrome — *see* Syndrome,
    postthrombotic
suppurative L08.0
traumatic NEC L30.4
trophoneurotica L13.0
ultraviolet (sun) (chronic exposure) L57.8
  acute L56.8
varicose — *see* Varix, leg, with, inflammation
vegetans L10.1
verrucosa B43.0
vesicular, herpesviral B00.1
Dermatoarthritis, lipoid E78.81
Dermatochalasis, eyelid H02.839
  left H02.836
   lower H02.835
   upper H02.834

Dermatochalasis, eyelid — *continued*
  right H02.833
   lower H02.832
   upper H02.831
Dermatofibroma (lenticulare) — *see* Neoplasm, skin,
  benign
  protuberans — *see* Neoplasm, skin, uncertain behavior
Dermatofibrosarcoma (pigmented) (protuberans) —
  see Neoplasm, skin, malignant
Dermatographia L50.3
Dermatolysis (exfoliativa) (congenital) Q82.8
  acquired L57.4
  eyelids — *see* Blepharochalasis
  palpebrarum — *see* Blepharochalasis
  senile L57.4
Dermatomegaly NEC Q82.8
Dermatomucosomyositis M33.10
  with
   myopathy M33.12
   respiratory involvement M33.11
   specified organ involvement NEC M33.19
Dermatomycosis B36.9
  furfuracea B36.0
  specified type NEC B36.8
Dermatomyositis (acute) (chronic) — *see also* Dermatopolymyositis
  adult — *see also* Dermatomyositis, specified NEC
   M33.10
  in (due to) neoplastic disease — *see also* Neoplasm
   D49.9 *[M36.0]*
  juvenile M33.00
   with
    myopathy M33.02
    respiratory involvement M33.01
    specified organ involvement NEC M33.09
   without myopathy M33.03
  specified NEC M33.10
   with
    myopathy M33.12
    respiratory involvement M33.11
    specified organ involvement NEC M33.19
   without myopathy M33.13
Dermatoneuritis of children — *see* Poisoning, mercury
Dermatophilosis A48.8
Dermatophytid L30.2
Dermatophytide — *see* Dermatophytosis
Dermatophytosis (epidermophyton) (infection) (Microsporum) (tinea) (Trichophyton) B35.9
  beard B35.0
  body B35.4
  capitis B35.0
  corporis B35.4
  deep-seated B35.8
  disseminated B35.8
  foot B35.3
  granulomatous B35.8
  groin B35.6
  hand B35.2
  nail B35.1
  perianal (area) B35.6
  scalp B35.0
  specified NEC B35.8
Dermatopolymyositis M33.90
  with
   myopathy M33.92
   respiratory involvement M33.91
   specified organ involvement NEC M33.99
  in neoplastic disease — *see also* Neoplasm
   D49.9 *[M36.0]*
  juvenile M33.00
   with
    myopathy M33.02
    respiratory involvement M33.01
    specified organ involvement NEC M33.09
  specified NEC M33.10
   myopathy M33.12
   respiratory involvement M33.11
   specified organ involvement NEC M33.19
  without myopathy M33.93
Dermatopolyneuritis — *see* Poisoning, mercury
Dermatorrhexis — *see also* Syndrome, Ehlers-Danlos
  Q79.60
  acquired L57.4
Dermatosclerosis — *see also* Scleroderma
  localized L94.0
Dermatosis L98.9
  Andrews' L08.89
  Bowen's — *see* Neoplasm, skin, in situ

Dermatosis — *continued*
  bullous L13.9
   specified NEC L13.8
  exfoliativa L26
  eyelid (noninfectious)
   dermatitis — *see* Dermatitis, eyelid
   discoid lupus erythematosus — *see* Lupus, eryt
    matosus, eyelid
   xeroderma — *see* Xeroderma, acquired, eyelid
  factitial L98.1
  febrile neutrophilic L98.2
  gonococcal A54.89
  herpetiformis L13.0
   juvenile L12.2
  linear IgA L13.8
  menstrual NEC L98.8
  neutrophilic, febrile L98.2
  occupational — *see* Dermatitis, contact
  papulosa nigra L82.1
  pigmentary L81.9
   progressive L81.7
   Schamberg's L81.7
  psychogenic F54
  purpuric, pigmented L81.7
  pustular, subcorneal L13.1
  transient acantholytic L11.1
Dermographia, dermographism L50.3
Dermoid (cyst) — *see also* Neoplasm, benign, by site
  with malignant transformation C56- ☑
  due to radiation (nonionizing) L57.8
Dermopathy
  infiltrative with thyrotoxicosis — *see* Thyrotoxicos
  nephrogenic fibrosing L90.8
Dermophytosis — *see* Dermatophytosis
Descemetocele H18.73- ☑
Descemet's membrane — *see* condition
Descending — *see* condition
Descensus uteri — *see* Prolapse, uterus
Desert
  rheumatism B38.0
  sore — *see* Ulcer, skin
Desertion (newborn) — *see* Maltreatment
Desmoid (extra-abdominal) (tumor) — *see* Neoplasm
  connective tissue, uncertain behavior
  abdominal D48.1
Despondency F32.9
Desquamation, skin R23.4
Destruction, destructive — *see also* Damage
  articular facet — *see also* Derangement, joint, speci
   type NEC
   knee M23.8X- ☑
   vertebra — *see* Spondylosis
  bone — *see also* Disorder, bone, specified type NE
   syphilitic A52.77
  joint — *see also* Derangement, joint, specified typ
   NEC
   sacroiliac M53.3
  rectal sphincter K62.89
  septum (nasal) J34.89
  tuberculous NEC — *see* Tuberculosis
  tympanum, tympanic membrane (nontraumatic) -
   see Disorder, tympanic membrane, specified
  vertebral disc — *see* Degeneration, intervertebral
Destructiveness — *see also* Disorder, conduct
  adjustment reaction — *see* Disorder, adjustment
Desultory labor O62.2
Detachment
  cartilage — *see* Sprain
  cervix, annular N88.8
   complicating delivery O71.3
  choroid (old) (postinfectional) (simple) (spontanee
   H31.40- ☑
   hemorrhagic H31.41- ☑
   serous H31.42- ☑
  ligament — *see* Sprain
  meniscus (knee) — *see also* Derangement, knee,
   meniscus, specified NEC
   current injury — *see* Tear, meniscus
   due to old tear or injury — *see* Derangement, kr
    meniscus, due to old tear
  retina (without retinal break) (serous) H33.2- ☑
   with retinal:
    break H33.00- ☑
     giant H33.03- ☑
     multiple H33.02- ☑
     single H33.01- ☑
    dialysis H33.04- ☑

☑ **Additional Character Required** — **Refer to the Tabular List for Character Selection**   🔻 **Subterms under main terms may continue to next column or pa**

Index

Detachment — Diabetes, diabetic

Diabetes, diabetic — *continued*
 due to drug or chemical — *continued*
  with — *continued*
   retinopathy — *continued*
    proliferative — *continued*
     with — *continued*
      stable proliferative diabetic retinopathy E09.355 ☑
      traction retinal detachment involving the macula E09.352 ☑
      traction retinal detachment not involving the macula E09.353 ☑
    skin complication NEC E09.628
    skin ulcer NEC E09.622
 due to underlying condition E08.9
  with
   amyotrophy E08.44
   arthropathy NEC E08.618
   autonomic (poly)neuropathy E08.43
   cataract E08.36
   Charcot's joints E08.610
   chronic kidney disease E08.22
   circulatory complication NEC E08.59
   complication E08.8
    specified NEC E08.69
   dermatitis E08.620
   foot ulcer E08.621
   gangrene E08.52
   gastroparalysis E08.43
   gastroparesis E08.43
   glomerulonephrosis, intracapillary E08.21
   glomerulosclerosis, intercapillary E08.21
   hyperglycemia E08.65
   hyperosmolarity E08.00
    with coma E08.01
   hypoglycemia E08.649
    with coma E08.641
   ketoacidosis E08.10
    with coma E08.11
   kidney complications NEC E08.29
   Kimmelsteil-WIlson disease E08.21
   mononeuropathy E08.41
   myasthenia E08.44
   necrobiosis lipoidica E08.620
   nephropathy E08.21
   neuralgia E08.42
   neurologic complication NEC E08.49
   neuropathic arthropathy E08.610
   neuropathy E08.40
   ophthalmic complication NEC E08.39
   oral complication NEC E08.638
   periodontal disease E08.630
   peripheral angiopathy E08.51
    with gangrene E08.52
   polyneuropathy E08.42
   renal complication NEC E08.29
   renal tubular degeneration E08.29
   retinopathy E08.319
    with macular edema E08.311
    resolved following treatment E08.37 ☑
    nonproliferative E08.329 ☑
     with macular edema E08.321 ☑
     mild E08.329 ☑
      with macular edema E08.321 ☑
     moderate E08.339 ☑
      with macular edema E08.331 ☑
     severe E08.349 ☑
      with macular edema E08.341 ☑
    proliferative E08.359 ☑
     with
      combined traction retinal detachment and rhegmatogenous retinal detachment E08.354 ☑
      macular edema E08.351 ☑
      stable proliferative diabetic retinopathy E08.355 ☑
      traction retinal detachment involving the macula E08.352 ☑
      traction retinal detachment not involving the macula E08.353 ☑
    skin complication NEC E08.628
    skin ulcer NEC E08.622
 gestational (in pregnancy) O24.419
  affecting newborn P70.0
  diet controlled O24.410
  in childbirth O24.429
   diet controlled O24.420
   insulin (and diet) controlled O24.424

Diabetes, diabetic — *continued*
 gestational — *continued*
  in childbirth — *continued*
   oral drug controlled (antidiabetic) (hypoglycemic) O24.425
  insulin (and diet) controlled O24.414
  oral drug controlled (antidiabetic) (hypoglycemic) O24.415
  puerperal O24.439
   diet controlled O24.430
   insulin (and diet) controlled O24.434
   oral drug controlled (antidiabetic) (hypoglycemic) O24.435
 hepatogenous E13.9
 idiopathic — *see* Diabetes, type 1
 inadequately controlled — *code to* Diabetes, by type, with hyperglycemia
 insipidus E23.2
  nephrogenic N25.1
  pituitary E23.2
  vasopressin resistant N25.1
 insulin dependent — *code to* type of diabetes
 juvenile-onset — *see* Diabetes, type 1
 ketosis-prone — *see* Diabetes, type 1
 latent R73.03
 neonatal (transient) P70.2
 non-insulin dependent — *code to* type of diabetes
 out of control — *code to* Diabetes, by type, with hyperglycemia
 phosphate E83.39
 poorly controlled — *code to* Diabetes, by type, with hyperglycemia
 postpancreatectomy — *see* Diabetes, specified type NEC
 postprocedural — *see* Diabetes, specified type NEC
 secondary diabetes mellitus NEC — *see* Diabetes, specified type NEC
 specified type NEC E13.9
  with
   amyotrophy E13.44
   arthropathy NEC E13.618
   autonomic (poly)neuropathy E13.43
   cataract E13.36
   Charcot's joints E13.610
   chronic kidney disease E13.22
   circulatory complication NEC E13.59
   complication E13.8
    specified NEC E13.69
   dermatitis E13.620
   foot ulcer E13.621
   gangrene E13.52
   gastroparalysis E13.43
   gastroparesis E13.43
   glomerulonephrosis, intracapillary E13.21
   glomerulosclerosis, intercapillary E13.21
   hyperglycemia E13.65
   hyperosmolarity E13.00
    with coma E13.01
   hypoglycemia E13.649
    with coma E13.641
   ketoacidosis E13.10
    with coma E13.11
   kidney complications NEC E13.29
   Kimmelsteil-Wilson disease E13.21
   mononeuropathy E13.41
   myasthenia E13.44
   necrobiosis lipoidica E13.620
   nephropathy E13.21
   neuralgia E13.42
   neurologic complication NEC E13.49
   neuropathic arthropathy E13.610
   neuropathy E13.40
   ophthalmic complication NEC E13.39
   oral complication NEC E13.638
   periodontal disease E13.630
   peripheral angiopathy E13.51
    with gangrene E13.52
   polyneuropathy E13.42
   renal complication NEC E13.29
   renal tubular degeneration E13.29
   retinopathy E13.319
    with macular edema E13.311
    resolved following treatment E13.37 ☑
    nonproliferative E13.329 ☑
     with macular edema E13.321 ☑
     mild E13.329 ☑
      with macular edema E13.321 ☑
     moderate E13.339 ☑

Diabetes, diabetic — *continued*
 specified type — *continued*
  with — *continued*
   retinopathy — *continued*
    nonproliferative — *continued*
     moderate — *continued*
      with macular edema E13.331 ☑
     severe E13.349 ☑
      with macular edema E13.341 ☑
    proliferative E13.359 ☑
     with
      combined traction retinal detachment and rhegmatogenous retinal detachment E13.354 ☑
      macular edema E13.351 ☑
      stable proliferative diabetic retinopathy E13.355 ☑
      traction retinal detachment involving the macula E13.352 ☑
      traction retinal detachment not involving the macula E13.353 ☑
    skin complication NEC E13.628
    skin ulcer NEC E13.622
 steroid-induced — *see* Diabetes, due to, drug or chemical
 type 1 E10.9
  with
   amyotrophy E10.44
   arthropathy NEC E10.618
   autonomic (poly)neuropathy E10.43
   cataract E10.36
   Charcot's joints E10.610
   chronic kidney disease E10.22
   circulatory complication NEC E10.59
   complication E10.8
    specified NEC E10.69
   dermatitis E10.620
   foot ulcer E10.621
   gangrene E10.52
   gastroparalysis E10.43
   gastroparesis E10.43
   glomerulonephrosis, intracapillary E10.21
   glomerulosclerosis, intercapillary E10.21
   hyperglycemia E10.65
   hypoglycemia E10.649
    with coma E10.641
   ketoacidosis E10.10
    with coma E10.11
   kidney complications NEC E10.29
   Kimmelsteil-Wilson disease E10.21
   mononeuropathy E10.41
   myasthenia E10.44
   necrobiosis lipoidica E10.620
   nephropathy E10.21
   neuralgia E10.42
   neurologic complication NEC E10.49
   neuropathic arthropathy E10.610
   neuropathy E10.40
   ophthalmic complication NEC E10.39
   oral complication NEC E10.638
   osteomyelitis E10.69
   periodontal disease E10.630
   peripheral angiopathy E10.51
    with gangrene E10.52
   polyneuropathy E10.42
   renal complication NEC E10.29
   renal tubular degeneration E10.29
   retinopathy E10.319
    with macular edema E10.311
    resolved following treatment E10.37 ☑
    nonproliferative E10.329 ☑
     with macular edema E10.321 ☑
     mild E10.329 ☑
      with macular edema E10.321 ☑
     moderate E10.339 ☑
      with macular edema E10.331 ☑
     severe E10.349 ☑
      with macular edema E10.341 ☑
    proliferative E10.359 ☑
     with
      combined traction retinal detachment and rhegmatogenous retinal detachment E10.354 ☑
      macular edema E10.351 ☑
      stable proliferative diabetic retinopathy E10.355 ☑
      traction retinal detachment involving the macula E10.352 ☑

☑ **Additional Character Required** — Refer to the Tabular List for Character Selection   ▽ **Subterms under main terms may continue to next column or page**

Diabetes, diabetic — *continued*
  type 1 — *continued*
    with — *continued*
      retinopathy — *continued*
        proliferative — *continued*
          with — *continued*
            traction retinal detachment not involving the macula E10.353 ☑
      skin complication NEC E10.628
      skin ulcer NEC E10.622
  type 2 E11.9
    with
      amyotrophy E11.44
      arthropathy NEC E11.618
      autonomic (poly)neuropathy E11.43
      cataract E11.36
      Charcot's joints E11.610
      chronic kidney disease E11.22
      circulatory complication NEC E11.59
      complication E11.8
        specified NEC E11.69
      dermatitis E11.620
      foot ulcer E11.621
      gangrene E11.52
      gastroparalysis E11.43
      gastroparesis E11.43
      glomerulonephrosis, intracapillary E11.21
      glomerulosclerosis, intercapillary E11.21
      hyperglycemia E11.65
      hyperosmolarity E11.00
        with coma E11.01
      hypoglycemia E11.649
        with coma E11.641
      ketoacidosis E11.10
        with coma E11.11
      kidney complications NEC E11.29
      Kimmelsteil-Wilson disease E11.21
      mononeuropathy E11.41
      myasthenia E11.44
      necrobiosis lipoidica E11.620
      nephropathy E11.21
      neuralgia E11.42
      neurologic complication NEC E11.49
      neuropathic arthropathy E11.610
      neuropathy E11.40
      ophthalmic complication NEC E11.39
      oral complication NEC E11.638
      osteomyelitis E11.69
      periodontal disease E11.630
      peripheral angiopathy E11.51
        with gangrene E11.52
      polyneuropathy E11.42
      renal complication NEC E11.29
      renal tubular degeneration E11.29
      retinopathy E11.319
        with macular edema E11.311
        resolved following treatment E11.37 ☑
        nonproliferative E11.329 ☑
          with macular edema E11.321 ☑
          mild E11.329 ☑
            with macular edema E11.321 ☑
          moderate E11.339 ☑
            with macular edema E11.331 ☑
          severe E11.349 ☑
            with macular edema E11.341 ☑
        proliferative E11.359 ☑
          with
            combined traction retinal detachment and rhegmatogenous retinal detachment E11.354 ☑
            macular edema E11.351 ☑
            stable proliferative diabetic retinopathy E11.355 ☑
            traction retinal detachment involving the macula E11.352 ☑
            traction retinal detachment not involving the macula E11.353 ☑
      skin complication NEC E11.628
      skin ulcer NEC E11.622
  uncontrolled
    meaning
      hyperglycemia — *see* Diabetes, by type, with, hyperglycemia
      hypoglycemia — *see* Diabetes, by type, with, hypoglycemia
Diacyclothrombopathia D69.1
Diagnosis deferred R69

Dialysis (intermittent) (treatment)
  noncompliance (with) Z91.15
  renal (hemodialysis) (peritoneal), status Z99.2
  retina, retinal — *see* Detachment, retina, with retinal, dialysis
Diamond-Blackfan anemia (congenital hypoplastic) D61.01
Diamond-Gardener syndrome (autoerythrocyte sensitization) D69.2
Diaper rash L22
Diaphoresis (excessive) R61
Diaphragm — *see* condition
Diaphragmalgia R07.1
Diaphragmatitis, diaphragmitis J98.6
Diaphysial aclasis Q78.6
Diaphysitis — *see* Osteomyelitis, specified type NEC
Diarrhea, diarrheal (disease) (infantile) (inflammatory) R19.7
  achlorhydric K31.83
  allergic K52.29
    due to
      colitis — *see* Colitis, allergic
      enteritis — *see* Enteritis, allergic
  amebic — *see also* Amebiasis A06.0
    with abscess — *see* Abscess, amebic
    acute A06.0
    chronic A06.1
    nondysenteric A06.2
  bacillary — *see* Dysentery, bacillary
  balantidial A07.0
  cachectic NEC K52.89
  Chilomastix A07.8
  choleriformis A00.1
  chronic (noninfectious) K52.9
  coccidial A07.3
  Cochin-China K90.1
    strongyloidiasis B78.0
  Dientamoeba A07.8
  dietetic — *see also* Diarrhea, allergic K52.29
  drug-induced K52.1
  due to
    bacteria A04.9
      specified NEC A04.8
    Campylobacter A04.5
    Capillaria philippinensis B81.1
    Clostridium difficile
      not specified as recurrent A04.72
      recurrent A04.71
    Clostridium perfringens (C) (F) A04.8
    Cryptosporidium A07.2
    drugs K52.1
    Escherichia coli A04.4
      enteroaggregative A04.4
      enterohemorrhagic A04.3
      enteroinvasive A04.2
      enteropathogenic A04.0
      enterotoxigenic A04.1
      specified NEC A04.4
    food hypersensitivity — *see also* Diarrhea, allergic K52.29
    Necator americanus B76.1
    S. japonicum B65.2
    specified organism NEC A08.8
      bacterial A04.8
      viral A08.39
    Staphylococcus A04.8
    Trichuris trichiuria B79
    virus — *see* Enteritis, viral
    Yersinia enterocolitica A04.6
  dysenteric A09
  endemic A09
  epidemic A09
  flagellate A07.9
  Flexner's (ulcerative) A03.1
  functional K59.1
    following gastrointestinal surgery K91.89
    psychogenic F45.8
  Giardia lamblia A07.1
  giardial A07.1
  hill K90.1
  infectious A09
  malarial — *see* Malaria
  mite B88.0
  mycotic NEC B49
  neonatal (noninfectious) P78.3
  nervous F45.8
  neurogenic K59.1
  noninfectious K52.9

Diarrhea, diarrheal — *continued*
  postgastrectomy K91.1
  postvagotomy K91.1
  protozoal A07.9
    specified NEC A07.8
  psychogenic F45.8
  specified
    bacterium NEC A04.8
    virus NEC A08.39
  strongyloidiasis B78.0
  toxic K52.1
  trichomonal A07.8
  tropical K90.1
  tuberculous A18.32
  viral — *see* Enteritis, viral
Diastasis
  cranial bones M84.88
    congenital NEC Q75.8
  joint (traumatic) — *see* Dislocation
  muscle M62.00
    ankle M62.07- ☑
    congenital Q79.8
    foot M62.07- ☑
    forearm M62.03- ☑
    hand M62.04- ☑
    lower leg M62.06- ☑
    pelvic region M62.05- ☑
    shoulder region M62.01- ☑
    specified site NEC M62.08
    thigh M62.05- ☑
    upper arm M62.02- ☑
  recti (abdomen)
    complicating delivery O71.89
    congenital Q79.59
Diastema, tooth, teeth, fully erupted M26.32
Diastematomyelia Q06.2
Diataxia, cerebral G80.4
Diathesis
  allergic — *see* History, allergy
  bleeding (familial) D69.9
  cystine (familial) E72.00
  gouty — *see* Gout
  hemorrhagic (familial) D69.9
    newborn NEC P53
  spasmophilic R29.0
Diaz's disease or osteochondrosis (juvenile) (talus) — *see* Osteochondrosis, juvenile, tarsus
Dibothriocephalus, dibothriocephaliasis (latus) (infection) (infestation) B70.0
  larval B70.1
Dicephalus, dicephaly Q89.4
Dichotomy, teeth K00.2
Dichromat, dichromatopsia (congenital) — *see* Deficiency, color vision
Dichuchwa A65
Dicroceliasis B66.2
Didelphia, didelphys — *see* Double uterus
Didymytis N45.1
  with orchitis N45.3
Dietary
  inadequacy or deficiency E63.9
  surveillance and counseling Z71.3
Dietl's crisis N13.8
Dieulafoy lesion (hemorrhagic)
  duodenum K31.82
  esophagus K22.8
  intestine (colon) K63.81
  stomach K31.82
Difficult, difficulty (in)
  acculturation Z60.3
  feeding R63.3
    newborn P92.9
      breast P92.5
      specified NEC P92.8
    nonorganic (infant or child) F98.29
  intubation, in anesthesia T88.4 ☑
  mechanical, gastroduodenal stoma K91.89
    causing obstruction — *see also* Obstruction, intestine, postoperative K91.30
  micturition
    need to immediately re-void R39.191
    position dependent R39.192
    specified NEC R39.198
  reading (developmental) F81.0
    secondary to emotional disorders F93.9
  spelling (specific) F81.81
    with reading disorder F81.89
    due to inadequate teaching Z55.8

▼ **Subterms under main terms may continue to next column or page**   ☑ **Additional Character Required — Refer to the Tabular List for Character Selection**   **99**

Diabetes, diabetic — Difficult, difficulty

Difficult, difficulty — *continued*
- swallowing — *see* Dysphagia
- walking R26.2
- work
  - conditions NEC Z56.5
  - schedule Z56.3

Diffuse — *see* condition

Digestive — *see* condition

Dihydropyrimidine dehydrogenase disease (DPD) E88.89

Diktyoma — *see* Neoplasm, malignant, by site

Dilaceration, tooth K00.4

Dilatation
- anus K59.8
  - venule — *see* Hemorrhoids
- aorta (focal) (general) — *see* Ectasia, aorta
  - with aneuysm — *see* Aneurysm, aorta
  - congenital Q25.44
- artery — *see* Aneurysm
- bladder (sphincter) N32.89
  - congenital Q64.79
- blood vessel I99.8
- bronchial J47.9
  - with
    - exacerbation (acute) J47.1
    - lower respiratory infection J47.0
- calyx (due to obstruction) — *see* Hydronephrosis
- capillaries I78.8
- cardiac (acute) (chronic) — *see also* Hypertrophy, cardiac
  - congenital Q24.8
    - valve NEC Q24.8
      - pulmonary Q22.3
  - valve — *see* Endocarditis
- cavum septi pellucidi Q06.8
- cervix (uteri) — *see also* Incompetency, cervix
  - incomplete, poor, slow complicating delivery O62.0
- colon K59.39
  - congenital Q43.1
  - psychogenic F45.8
  - toxic K59.31
- common duct (acquired) K83.8
  - congenital Q44.5
- cystic duct (acquired) K82.8
  - congenital Q44.5
- duct, mammary — *see* Ectasia, mammary duct
- duodenum K59.8
- esophagus K22.8
  - congenital Q39.5
  - due to achalasia K22.0
- eustachian tube, congenital Q17.8
- gallbladder K82.8
- gastric — *see* Dilatation, stomach
- heart (acute) (chronic) — *see also* Hypertrophy, cardiac
  - congenital Q24.8
  - valve — *see* Endocarditis
- ileum K59.8
  - psychogenic F45.8
- jejunum K59.8
  - psychogenic F45.8
- kidney (calyx) (collecting structures) (cystic) (parenchyma) (pelvis) (idiopathic) N28.89
- lacrimal passages or duct — *see* Disorder, lacrimal system, changes
- lymphatic vessel I89.0
- mammary duct — *see* Ectasia, mammary duct
- Meckel's diverticulum (congenital) Q43.0
  - malignant — *see* Table of Neoplasms, small intestine, malignant
- myocardium (acute) (chronic) — *see* Hypertrophy, cardiac
- organ or site, congenital NEC — *see* Distortion
- pancreatic duct K86.89
- pericardium — *see* Pericarditis
- pharynx J39.2
- prostate N42.89
- pulmonary
  - artery (idiopathic) I28.8
  - valve, congenital Q22.3
- pupil H57.04
- rectum K59.39
- saccule, congenital Q16.5
- salivary gland (duct) K11.8
- sphincter ani K62.89
- stomach K31.89
  - acute K31.0
  - psychogenic F45.8
- submaxillary duct K11.8

Dilatation — *continued*
- trachea, congenital Q32.1
- ureter (idiopathic) N28.82
  - congenital Q62.2
  - due to obstruction N13.4
- urethra (acquired) N36.8
- vasomotor I73.9
- vein I86.8
- ventricular, ventricle (acute) (chronic) — *see also* Hypertrophy, cardiac
  - cerebral, congenital Q04.8
- venule NEC I86.8
- vesical orifice N32.89

Dilated, dilation — *see* Dilatation

Diminished, diminution
- hearing (acuity) — *see* Deafness
- sense or sensation (cold) (heat) (tactile) (vibratory) R20.8
- vision NEC H54.7
- vital capacity R94.2

Diminuta taenia B71.0

Dimitri-Sturge-Weber disease Q85.8

Dimple
- congenital sacral Q82.6
- parasacral Q82.6
- pilonidal or postanal — *see* Cyst, pilonidal

Dioctophyme renalis (infection) (infestation) B83.8

Dipetalonemiasis B74.4

Diphallus Q55.69

Diphtheria, diphtheritic (gangrenous) (hemorrhagic) A36.9
- carrier (suspected) Z22.2
- cutaneous A36.3
- faucial A36.0
- infection of wound A36.3
- laryngeal A36.2
- myocarditis A36.81
- nasal, anterior A36.89
- nasopharyngeal A36.1
- neurological complication A36.89
- pharyngeal A36.0
- specified site NEC A36.89
- tonsillar A36.0

Diphyllobothriasis (intestine) B70.0
- larval B70.1

Diplacusis H93.22- ☑

Diplegia (upper limbs) G83.0
- congenital (cerebral) G80.8
- facial G51.0
- lower limbs G82.20
- spastic G80.1

Diplococcus, diplococcal — *see* condition

Diplopia H53.2

Dipsomania F10.20
- with
  - psychosis — *see* Psychosis, alcoholic
  - remission F10.21

Dipylidiasis B71.1

DIRA (deficiency of interleukin 1 receptor antagonist) M04.8

Direction, teeth, abnormal, fully erupted M26.30

Dirofilariasis B74.8

Dirt-eating child F98.3

Disability, disabilities
- heart — *see* Disease, heart
- intellectual F79
  - with
    - autistic features F84.9
  - mild (I.Q. 50-69) F70
  - moderate (I.Q. 35-49) F71
  - profound (I.Q. under 20) F73
  - severe (I.Q. 20-34) F72
  - specified level NEC F78
- knowledge acquisition F81.9
- learning F81.9
- limiting activities Z73.6
- spelling, specific F81.81

Disappearance of family member Z63.4

Disarticulation — *see* Amputation
- meaning traumatic amputation — *see* Amputation, traumatic

Discharge (from)
- abnormal finding in — *see* Abnormal, specimen
- breast (female) (male) N64.52
- diencephalic autonomic idiopathic — *see* Epilepsy, specified NEC
- ear — *see also* Otorrhea
  - blood — *see* Otorrhagia

Discharge — *continued*
- excessive urine R35.8
- nipple N64.52
- penile R36.9
- postnasal R09.82
- prison, anxiety concerning Z65.2
- urethral R36.9
  - without blood R36.0
  - hematospermia R36.1
- vaginal N89.8

Discitis, diskitis M46.40
- cervical region M46.42
- cervicothoracic region M46.43
- lumbar region M46.46
- lumbosacral region M46.47
- multiple sites M46.49
- occipito-atlanto-axial region M46.41
- pyogenic — *see* Infection, intervertebral disc, pyogen
- sacrococcygeal region M46.48
- thoracic region M46.44
- thoracolumbar region M46.45

Discoid
- meniscus (congenital) Q68.6
- semilunar cartilage (congenital) — *see* Derangemen knee, meniscus, specified NEC

Discoloration
- nails L60.8
- teeth (posteruptive) K03.7
  - during formation K00.8

Discomfort
- chest R07.89
- visual H53.14- ☑

Discontinuity, ossicles, ear H74.2- ☑

Discord (with)
- boss Z56.4
- classmates Z55.4
- counselor Z64.4
- employer Z56.4
- family Z63.8
- fellow employees Z56.4
- in-laws Z63.1
- landlord Z59.2
- lodgers Z59.2
- neighbors Z59.2
- probation officer Z64.4
- social worker Z64.4
- teachers Z55.4
- workmates Z56.4

Discordant connection
- atrioventricular (congenital) Q20.5
- ventriculoarterial Q20.3

Discrepancy
- centric occlusion maximum intercuspation M26.55
- leg length (acquired) — *see* Deformity, limb, unequ length
  - congenital — *see* Defect, reduction, lower limb
- uterine size date O26.84- ☑

Discrimination
- ethnic Z60.5
- political Z60.5
- racial Z60.5
- religious Z60.5
- sex Z60.5

Disease, diseased — *see also* Syndrome
- absorbent system I87.8
- acid-peptic K30
- Acosta's T70.29 ☑
- Adams-Stokes (-Morgagni) (syncope with heart bloc I45.9
- Addison's anemia (pernicious) D51.0
- adenoids (and tonsils) J35.9
- adrenal (capsule) (cortex) (gland) (medullary) E27.9
  - hyperfunction E27.0
  - specified NEC E27.8
- ainhum L94.6
- airway
  - obstructive, chronic J44.9
    - due to
      - cotton dust J66.0
      - specific organic dusts NEC J66.8
  - reactive — *see* Asthma
- akamushi (scrub typhus) A75.3
- Albers-Schönberg (marble bones) Q78.2
- Albert's — *see* Tendinitis, Achilles
- alimentary canal K63.9
- alligator-skin Q80.9
  - acquired L85.0
- alpha heavy chain C88.3

sease, diseased — continued
alpine T70.29 ☑
altitude T70.20 ☑
alveolar ridge
  edentulous K06.9
    specified NEC K06.8
alveoli, teeth K08.9
Alzheimer's G30.9 [F02.80]
  with behavioral disturbance G30.9 [F02.81]
  early onset G30.0 [F02.80]
    with behavioral disturbance G30.0 [F02.81]
  late onset G30.1 [F02.80]
    with behavioral disturbance G30.1 [F02.81]
  specified NEC G30.8 [F02.80]
    with behavioral disturbance G30.8 [F02.81]
amyloid — see Amyloidosis
Andersen's (glycogenosis IV) E74.09
Andes T70.29 ☑
Andrews' (bacterid) L08.89
angiospastic I73.9
  cerebral G45.9
  vein I87.8
anterior
  chamber H21.9
  horn cell G12.29
antiglomerular basement membrane (anti- GBM) antibody M31.0
  tubulo-interstitial nephritis N12
antral — see Sinusitis, maxillary
anus K62.9
  specified NEC K62.89
aorta (nonsyphilitic) I77.9
  syphilitic NEC A52.02
aortic (heart) (valve) I35.9
  rheumatic I06.9
Apollo B30.3
aponeuroses — see Enthesopathy
appendix K38.9
  specified NEC K38.8
aqueous (chamber) H21.9
Arnold-Chiari — see Arnold-Chiari disease
arterial I77.9
  occlusive — see Occlusion, by site
    due to stricture or stenosis I77.1
  peripheral I73.9
arteriocardiorenal — see Hypertension, cardiorenal
arteriolar (generalized) (obliterative) I77.9
arteriorenal — see Hypertension, kidney
arteriosclerotic — see also Arteriosclerosis
  cardiovascular — see Disease, heart, ischemic,
    atherosclerotic
  coronary (artery) — see Disease, heart, ischemic,
    atherosclerotic
  heart — see Disease, heart, ischemic, atherosclerotic
artery I77.9
  cerebral I67.9
  coronary I25.10
    with angina pectoris — see Arteriosclerosis,
      coronary (artery)
  peripheral I73.9
arthropod-borne NOS (viral) A94
  specified type NEC A93.8
atticoantral, chronic H66.20
  left H66.22
    with right H66.23
  right H66.21
    with left H66.23
auditory canal — see Disorder, ear, external
auricle, ear NEC — see Disorder, pinna
Australian X A83.4
autoimmune (systemic) NOS M35.9
  hemolytic (cold type) (warm type) D59.1
    drug-induced D59.0
  thyroid E06.3
autoinflammatory M04.9
  NOD2-associated M04.8
  specified type NEC M04.8
aviator's — see Effect, adverse, high altitude
Ayerza's (pulmonary artery sclerosis with pulmonary
  hypertension) I27.0
Babington's (familial hemorrhagic telangiectasia) I78.0
bacterial A49.9
  specified NEC A48.8
  zoonotic A28.9
    specified type NEC A28.8
Baelz's (cheilitis glandularis apostematosa) K13.0
bagasse J67.1
balloon — see Effect, adverse, high altitude

Disease, diseased — continued
Bang's (brucella abortus) A23.1
Bannister's T78.3 ☑
barometer makers' — see Poisoning, mercury
Barraquer (-Simons') (progressive lipodystrophy) E88.1
Barrett's — see Barrett's, esophagus
Bartholin's gland N75.9
basal ganglia G25.9
  degenerative G23.9
    specified NEC G23.8
  specified NEC G25.89
Basedow's (exophthalmic goiter) — see Hyperthy-
  roidism, with, goiter (diffuse)
Bateman's B08.1
Batten-Steinert G71.11
Battey A31.0
Beard's (neurasthenia) F48.8
Becker
  idiopathic mural endomyocardial I42.3
  myotonia congenita G71.12
Begbie's (exophthalmic goiter) — see Hyperthyroidism,
  with, goiter (diffuse)
behavioral, organic F07.9
Beigel's (white piedra) B36.2
Benson's — see Deposit, crystalline
Bernard-Soulier (thrombopathy) D69.1
Bernhardt (-Roth) — see Mononeuropathy, lower limb,
  meralgia paresthetica
Biermer's (pernicious anemia) D51.0
bile duct (common) (hepatic) K83.9
  with calculus, stones — see Calculus, bile duct
  specified NEC K83.8
biliary (tract) K83.9
  specified NEC K83.8
Billroth's — see Spina bifida
bird fancier's J67.2
black lung J60
bladder N32.9
  in (due to)
    schistosomiasis (bilharziasis) B65.0 [N33]
  specified NEC N32.89
bleeder's D66
blood D75.9
  forming organs D75.9
  vessel I99.9
Bloodgood's — see Mastopathy, cystic
Bodechtel-Guttmann (subacute sclerosing panencephalitis) A81.1
bone — see also Disorder, bone
  aluminum M83.4
  fibrocystic NEC
    jaw M27.49
bone-marrow D75.9
Borna A83.9
Bornholm (epidemic pleurodynia) B33.0
Bouchard's (myopathic dilatation of the stomach) K31.0
Bouillaud's (rheumatic heart disease) I01.9
Bourneville (-Brissaud) (tuberous sclerosis) Q85.1
Bouveret (-Hoffmann) (paroxysmal tachycardia) I47.9
bowel K63.9
  functional K59.9
    psychogenic F45.8
brain G93.9
  arterial, artery I67.9
  arteriosclerotic I67.2
  congenital Q04.9
  degenerative — see Degeneration, brain
  inflammatory — see Encephalitis
  organic G93.9
    arteriosclerotic I67.2
  parasitic NEC B71.9 [G94]
  senile NEC G31.1
  specified NEC G93.89
breast — see also Disorder, breast N64.9
  cystic (chronic) — see Mastopathy, cystic
  fibrocystic — see Mastopathy, cystic
  Paget's
    female, unspecified side C50.91- ☑
    male, unspecified side C50.92- ☑
  specified NEC N64.89
Breda's — see Yaws
Bretonneau's (diphtheritic malignant angina) A36.0
Bright's — see Nephritis
  arteriosclerotic — see Hypertension, kidney
Brill's (recrudescent typhus) A75.1
Brill-Zinsser (recrudescent typhus) A75.1
Brion-Kayser — see Fever, paratyphoid

Disease, diseased — continued
broad
  beta E78.2
  ligament (noninflammatory) N83.9
    inflammatory — see Disease, pelvis, inflammato-
      ry
    specified NEC N83.8
Brocq-Duhring (dermatitis herpetiformis) L13.0
Brocq's
  meaning
    dermatitis herpetiformis L13.0
    prurigo L28.2
bronchopulmonary J98.4
bronchus NEC J98.09
bronze Addison's E27.1
  tuberculous A18.7
budgerigar fancier's J67.2
Buerger's (thromboangiitis obliterans) I73.1
bullous L13.9
  chronic of childhood L12.2
  specified NEC L13.8
Bürger-Grütz (essential familial hyperlipemia) E78.3
bursa — see Bursopathy
caisson T70.3 ☑
California — see Coccidioidomycosis
capillaries I78.9
  specified NEC I78.8
Carapata A68.0
cardiac — see Disease, heart
cardiopulmonary, chronic I27.9
cardiorenal (hepatic) (hypertensive) (vascular) — see
  Hypertension, cardiorenal
cardiovascular (atherosclerotic) I25.10
  with angina pectoris — see Arteriosclerosis, coro-
    nary (artery),
  congenital Q28.9
  hypertensive — see Hypertension, heart
  newborn P29.9
    specified NEC P29.89
  renal (hypertensive) — see Hypertension, cardiore-
    nal
  syphilitic (asymptomatic) A52.00
cartilage — see Disorder, cartilage
Castellani's A69.8
Castleman (unicentric) (multicentric) D47.Z2
  HHV-8-associated — see also Herpesvirus, human,
    8 D47.Z2
cat-scratch A28.1
Cavare's (familial periodic paralysis) G72.3
cecum K63.9
celiac (adult) (infantile) (with steatorrhea) K90.0
cellular tissue L98.9
central core G71.2
cerebellar, cerebellum — see Disease, brain
cerebral — see also Disease, brain
  degenerative — see Degeneration, brain
cerebrospinal G96.9
cerebrovascular I67.9
  acute I67.89
    embolic I63.4- ☑
    thrombotic I63.3- ☑
  arteriosclerotic I67.2
  hereditary NEC I67.858
  specified NEC I67.89
cervix (uteri) (noninflammatory) N88.9
  inflammatory — see Cervicitis
  specified NEC N88.8
Chabert's A22.9
Chandler's (osteochondritis dissecans, hip) — see Osteochondritis, dissecans, hip
Charlouis — see Yaws
Chédiak-Steinbrinck (-Higashi) (congenital gigantism
  of peroxidase granules) E70.330
chest J98.9
Chiari's (hepatic vein thrombosis) I82.0
Chicago B40.9
Chignon B36.8
chigo, chigoe B88.1
childhood granulomatous D71
Chinese liver fluke B66.1
chlamydial A74.9
  specified NEC A74.89
cholecystic K82.9
choroid H31.9
  specified NEC H31.8
Christmas D67
chronic bullous of childhood L12.2
chylomicron retention E78.3

Disease, diseased — *continued*
- ciliary body H21.9
  - specified NEC H21.89
- circulatory (system) NEC I99.8
  - newborn P29.9
  - syphilitic A52.00
    - congenital A50.54
- coagulation factor deficiency (congenital) — *see* Defect, coagulation
- coccidioidal — *see* Coccidioidomycosis
- cold
  - agglutinin or hemoglobinuria D59.1
    - paroxysmal D59.6
  - hemagglutinin (chronic) D59.1
- collagen NOS (nonvascular) (vascular) M35.9
  - specified NEC M35.8
- colon K63.9
  - functional K59.9
    - congenital Q43.2
  - ischemic — *see also* Ischemia, intestine, acute K55.039
- colonic inflammatory bowel, unclassified (IBDU) K52.3
- combined system — *see* Degeneration, combined
- compressed air T70.3 ☑
- Concato's (pericardial polyserositis) A19.9
  - nontubercular I31.1
  - pleural — *see* Pleurisy, with effusion
- conjunctiva H11.9
  - chlamydial A74.0
  - specified NEC H11.89
  - viral B30.9
    - specified NEC B30.8
- connective tissue, systemic (diffuse) M35.9
  - in (due to)
    - hypogammaglobulinemia D80.1 *[M36.8]*
    - ochronosis E70.29 *[M36.8]*
  - specified NEC M35.8
- Conor and Bruch's (boutonneuse fever) A77.1
- Cooper's — *see* Mastopathy, cystic
- Cori's (glycogenosis III) E74.03
- corkhandler's or corkworker's J67.3
- cornea H18.9
  - specified NEC H18.89- ☑
- coronary (artery) — *see* Disease, heart, ischemic, atherosclerotic
  - congenital Q24.5
  - ostial, syphilitic (aortic) (mitral) (pulmonary) A52.03
- corpus cavernosum N48.9
  - specified NEC N48.89
- Cotugno's — *see* Sciatica
- coxsackie (virus) NEC B34.1
- cranial nerve NOS G52.9
- Creutzfeldt-Jakob — *see* Creutzfeldt-Jakob disease or syndrome
- Crocq's (acrocyanosis) I73.89
- Crohn's — *see* Enteritis, regional
- Curschmann G71.11
- cystic
  - breast (chronic) — *see* Mastopathy, cystic
  - kidney, congenital Q61.9
  - liver, congenital Q44.6
  - lung J98.4
    - congenital Q33.0
- cytomegalic inclusion (generalized) B25.9
  - with pneumonia B25.0
  - congenital P35.1
- cytomegaloviral B25.9
  - specified NEC B25.8
- Czerny's (periodic hydrarthrosis of the knee) — *see* Effusion, joint, knee
- Daae (-Finsen) (epidemic pleurodynia) B33.0
- Darling's — *see* Histoplasmosis capsulati
- de Quervain's (tendon sheath) M65.4
  - thyroid (subacute granulomatous thyroiditis) E06.1
- Débove's (splenomegaly) R16.1
- deer fly — *see* Tularemia
- Degos' I77.89
- demyelinating, demyelinizing (nervous system) G37.9
  - multiple sclerosis G35
  - specified NEC G37.8
- dense deposit — *see also* N00-N07 with fourth character .6 N05.6
- deposition, hydroxyapatite — *see* Disease, hydroxyapatite deposition
- Devergie's (pityriasis rubra pilaris) L44.0
- Devic's G36.0
- diaphorase deficiency D71.0
- diaphragm J98.6

Disease, diseased — *continued*
- diarrheal, infectious NEC A09
- digestive system K92.9
  - specified NEC K92.89
- disc, degenerative — *see* Degeneration, intervertebral disc
- discogenic — *see also* Displacement, intervertebral disc NEC
  - with myelopathy — *see* Disorder, disc, with, myelopathy
- diverticular — *see* Diverticula
- Dubois (thymus) A50.59 *[E35]*
- Duchenne-Griesinger G71.01
- Duchenne's
  - muscular dystrophy G71.01
  - pseudohypertrophy, muscles G71.01
- ductless glands E34.9
- duodenum K31.9
  - specified NEC K31.89
- Dupré's (meningism) R29.1
- Dupuytren's (muscle contracture) M72.0
- Durand-Nicholas-Favre (climatic bubo) A55
- Duroziez's (congenital mitral stenosis) Q23.2
- ear — *see* Disorder, ear
- Eberth's — *see* Fever, typhoid
- Ebola (virus) A98.4
- Ebstein's heart Q22.5
- Echinococcus — *see* Echinococcus
- echovirus NEC B34.1
- Eddowes' (brittle bones and blue sclera) Q78.0
- edentulous (alveolar) ridge K06.9
  - specified NEC K06.8
- Edsall's T67.2 ☑
- Eichstedt's (pityriasis versicolor) B36.0
- Eisenmenger's (irreversible) I27.83
- Ellis-van Creveld (chondroectodermal dysplasia) Q77.6
- end stage renal (ESRD) N18.6
  - due to hypertension I12.0
- endocrine glands or system NEC E34.9
- endomyocardial (eosinophilic) I42.3
- English (rickets) E55.0
- enteroviral, enterovirus NEC B34.1
  - central nervous system NEC A88.8
- epidemic B99.9
  - specified NEC B99.8
- epididymis N50.9
- Erb (-Landouzy) G71.02
- Erdheim-Chester (ECD) E88.89
- esophagus K22.9
  - functional K22.4
  - psychogenic F45.8
  - specified NEC K22.8
- Eulenburg's (congenital paramyotonia) G71.19
- eustachian tube — *see* Disorder, eustachian tube
- external
  - auditory canal — *see* Disorder, ear, external
  - ear — *see* Disorder, ear, external
- extrapyramidal G25.9
  - specified NEC G25.89
- eye H57.9
  - anterior chamber H21.9
  - inflammatory NEC H57.89
  - muscle (external) — *see* Strabismus
  - specified NEC H57.89
  - syphilitic — *see* Oculopathy, syphilitic
- eyeball H44.9
  - specified NEC H44.89
- eyelid — *see* Disorder, eyelid
  - specified NEC — *see* Disorder, eyelid, specified type NEC
- eyeworm of Africa B74.3
- facial nerve (seventh) G51.9
  - newborn (birth injury) P11.3
- Fahr (of brain) G23.8
- Fahr Volhard (of kidney) I12.- ☑
- fallopian tube (noninflammatory) N83.9
  - inflammatory — *see* Salpingo-oophoritis
  - specified NEC N83.8
- familial periodic paralysis G72.3
- Fanconi's (congenital pancytopenia) D61.09
- fascia NEC — *see also* Disorder, muscle
  - inflammatory — *see* Myositis
  - specified NEC M62.89
- Fauchard's (periodontitis) — *see* Periodontitis
- Favre-Durand-Nicolas (climatic bubo) A55
- Fede's K14.0
- Feer's — *see* Poisoning, mercury

Disease, diseased — *continued*
- female pelvic inflammatory — *see also* Disease, pelv inflammatory N73.9
  - syphilitic (secondary) A51.42
  - tuberculous A18.17
- Fernels' (aortic aneurysm) I71.9
- fibrocaseous of lung — *see* Tuberculosis, pulmonar
- fibrocystic — *see* Fibrocystic disease
- Fiedler's (leptospiral jaundice) A27.0
- fifth B08.3
- file-cutter's — *see* Poisoning, lead
- fish-skin Q80.9
  - acquired L85.0
- Flajani (-Basedow) (exophthalmic goiter) — *see* Hype thyroidism, with, goiter (diffuse)
- flax-dresser's J66.1
- fluke — *see* Infestation, fluke
- foot and mouth B08.8
- foot process N04.9
- Forbes' (glycogenosis III) E74.03
- Fordyce-Fox (apocrine miliaria) L75.2
- Fordyce's (ectopic sebaceous glands) (mouth) Q38.(
- Forestier's (rhizomelic pseudopolyarthritis) M35.3
  - meaning ankylosing hyperostosis — *see* Hyperost sis, ankylosing
- Fothergill's
  - neuralgia — *see* Neuralgia, trigeminal
  - scarlatina anginosa A38.9
- Fournier (gangrene) N49.3
  - female N76.89
- fourth B08.8
- Fox (-Fordyce) (apocrine miliaria) L75.2
- Francis' — *see* Tularemia
- Franklin C88.2
- Frei's (climatic bubo) A55
- Friedreich's
  - combined systemic or ataxia G11.1
  - myoclonia G25.3
- frontal sinus — *see* Sinusitis, frontal
- fungus NEC B49
- Gaisböck's (polycythemia hypertonica) D75.1
- gallbladder K82.9
  - calculus — *see* Calculus, gallbladder
  - cholecystitis — *see* Cholecystitis
  - cholesterolosis K82.4
  - fistula — *see* Fistula, gallbladder
  - hydrops K82.1
  - obstruction — *see* Obstruction, gallbladder
  - perforation K82.2
  - specified NEC K82.8
- gamma heavy chain C88.2
- Gamna's (siderotic splenomegaly) D73.2
- Gamstorp's (adynamia episodica hereditaria) G72.3
- Gandy-Nanta (siderotic splenomegaly) D73.2
- ganister J62.8
- gastric — *see* Disease, stomach
- gastroesophageal reflux (GERD) K21.9
  - with esophagitis K21.0
- gastrointestinal (tract) K92.9
  - amyloid E85.4
  - functional K59.9
    - psychogenic F45.8
  - specified NEC K92.89
- Gee (-Herter) (-Heubner) (-Thaysen) (nontropical spru K90.0
- genital organs
  - female N94.9
  - male N50.9
- Gerhardt's (erythromelalgia) I73.81
- Gibert's (pityriasis rosea) L42
- Gierke's (glycogenosis I) E74.01
- Gilles de la Tourette's (motor-verbal tic) F95.2
- gingiva K06.9
  - plaque induced K05.00
  - specified NEC K06.8
- gland (lymph) I89.9
- Glanzmann's (hereditary hemorrhagic thrombasthen D69.1
- glass-blower's (cataract) — *see* Cataract, specified NI
  - salivary gland hypertrophy K11.1
- Glisson's — *see* Rickets
- globe H44.9
  - specified NEC H44.89
- glomerular — *see also* Glomerulonephritis
  - with edema — *see* Nephrosis
  - acute — *see* Nephritis, acute
  - chronic — *see* Nephritis, chronic
  - minimal change N05.0

   ☑ **Additional Character Required** — Refer to the Tabular List for Character Selection   ▽ **Subterms under main terms may continue to next column or pag**

Disease, diseased — continued
glomerular — see also Glomerulonephritis — continued
  rapidly progressive N01.9
glycogen storage E74.00
  Andersen's E74.09
  Cori's E74.03
  Forbes' E74.03
  generalized E74.00
  glucose-6-phosphatase deficiency E74.01
  heart E74.02 [143]
  hepatorenal E74.09
  Hers' E74.09
  liver and kidney E74.09
  McArdle's E74.04
  muscle phosphofructokinase E74.09
  myocardium E74.02 [143]
  Pompe's E74.02
  Tauri's E74.09
  type 0 E74.09
  type I E74.01
  type II E74.02
  type III E74.03
  type IV E74.09
  type V E74.04
  type VI-XI E74.09
  Von Gierke's E74.01
Goldstein's (familial hemorrhagic telangiectasia) I78.0
gonococcal NOS A54.9
graft-versus-host (GVH) D89.813
  acute D89.810
  acute on chronic D89.812
  chronic D89.811
grainhandler's J67.8
granulomatous (childhood) (chronic) D71
Graves' (exophthalmic goiter) — see Hyperthyroidism, with, goiter (diffuse)
Griesinger's — see Ancylostomiasis
Grisel's M43.6
Gruby's (tinea tonsurans) B35.0
Guillain-Barré G61.0
Guinon's (motor-verbal tic) F95.2
gum K06.9
gynecological N94.9
H (Hartnup's) E72.02
Haff — see Poisoning, mercury
Hageman (congenital factor XII deficiency) D68.2
hair (color) (shaft) L67.9
  follicles L73.9
    specified NEC L73.8
Hamman's (spontaneous mediastinal emphysema) J98.2
hand, foot and mouth B08.4
Hansen's — see Leprosy
Hantavirus, with pulmonary manifestations B33.4
  with renal manifestations A98.5
Harada's H30.81- ☑
Hartnup (pellagra-cerebellar ataxia-renal aminoaciduria) E72.02
Hart's (pellagra-cerebellar ataxia-renal aminoaciduria) E72.02
Hashimoto's (struma lymphomatosa) E06.3
Hb — see Disease, hemoglobin
heart (organic) I51.9
  with
    pulmonary edema (acute) — see also Failure, ventricular, left I50.1
    rheumatic fever (conditions in I00)
      active I01.9
        with chorea I02.0
        specified NEC I01.8
      inactive or quiescent (with chorea) I09.9
        specified NEC I09.89
  amyloid E85.4 [143]
  aortic (valve) I35.9
  arteriosclerotic or sclerotic (senile) — see Disease, heart, ischemic, atherosclerotic
  artery, arterial — see Disease, heart, ischemic, atherosclerotic
  beer drinkers' I42.6
  beriberi (wet) E51.12
  black I27.0
  congenital Q24.9
    cyanotic Q24.9
    specified NEC Q24.8
  coronary — see Disease, heart, ischemic
  cryptogenic I51.9
  fibroid — see Myocarditis

Disease, diseased — continued
heart — continued
  functional I51.89
    psychogenic F45.8
  glycogen storage E74.02 [143]
  gonococcal A54.83
  hypertensive — see Hypertension, heart
  hyperthyroid — see also Hyperthyroidism E05.90 [143]
    with thyroid storm E05.91 [143]
  ischemic (chronic or with a stated duration of over 4 weeks) I25.9
    atherosclerotic (of) I25.10
      with angina pectoris — see Arteriosclerosis, coronary (artery)
      coronary artery bypass graft — see Arteriosclerosis, coronary (artery),
    cardiomyopathy I25.5
    diagnosed on ECG or other special investigation, but currently presenting no symptoms I25.6
    silent I25.6
    specified form NEC I25.89
  kyphoscoliotic I27.1
  meningococcal A39.50
    endocarditis A39.51
    myocarditis A39.52
    pericarditis A39.53
  mitral I05.9
    specified NEC I05.8
  muscular — see Degeneration, myocardial
  psychogenic (functional) F45.8
  pulmonary (chronic) I27.9
    in schistosomiasis B65.9 [I52]
    specified NEC I27.89
  rheumatic (chronic) (inactive) (old) (quiescent) (with chorea) I09.9
    active or acute I01.9
      with chorea (acute) (rheumatic) (Sydenham's) I02.0
    specified NEC I09.89
  senile — see Myocarditis
  syphilitic A52.06
    aortic A52.03
      aneurysm A52.01
    congenital A50.54 [I52]
  thyrotoxic — see also Thyrotoxicosis E05.90 [143]
    with thyroid storm E05.91 [143]
  valve, valvular (obstructive) (regurgitant) — see also Endocarditis
    congenital NEC Q24.8
      pulmonary Q22.3
  vascular — see Disease, cardiovascular
heavy chain NEC C88.2
  alpha C88.3
  gamma C88.2
  mu C88.2
Hebra's
  pityriasis
    maculata et circinata L42
    rubra pilaris L44.0
  prurigo L28.2
hematopoietic organs D75.9
hemoglobin or Hb
  abnormal (mixed) NEC D58.2
    with thalassemia D56.9
  AS genotype D57.3
  Bart's D56.0
  C (Hb-C) D58.2
    with other abnormal hemoglobin NEC D58.2
    elliptocytosis D58.1
    Hb-S D57.2- ☑
      sickle-cell D57.2- ☑
    thalassemia D56.8
  Constant Spring D58.2
  D (Hb-D) D58.2
  E (Hb-E) D58.2
  E-beta thalassemia D56.5
  elliptocytosis D58.1
  H (Hb-H) (thalassemia) D56.0
    with other abnormal hemoglobin NEC D56.9
    Constant Spring D56.0
  I thalassemia D56.9
  M D74.0
  S or SS D57.1
  SC D57.2- ☑
  SD D57.8- ☑
  SE D57.8- ☑

Disease, diseased — continued
hemoglobin or Hb — continued
  spherocytosis D58.0
  unstable, hemolytic D58.2
hemolytic (newborn) P55.9
  autoimmune (cold type) (warm type) D59.1
  drug-induced D59.0
  due to or with
    incompatibility
      ABO (blood group) P55.1
      blood (group) (Duffy) (K) (Kell) (Kidd) (Lewis) (M) (S) NEC P55.8
      Rh (blood group) (factor) P55.0
      Rh negative mother P55.0
  specified type NEC P55.8
  unstable hemoglobin D58.2
hemorrhagic D69.9
  newborn P53
Henoch (-Schönlein) (purpura nervosa) D69.0
hepatic — see Disease, liver
hepatolenticular E83.01
heredodegenerative NEC
  spinal cord G95.89
herpesviral, disseminated B00.7
Hers' (glycogenosis VI) E74.09
Herter (-Gee) (-Heubner) (nontropical sprue) K90.0
Heubner-Herter (nontropical sprue) K90.0
high fetal gene or hemoglobin thalassemia D56.9
Hildenbrand's — see Typhus
hip (joint) M25.9
  congenital Q65.89
  suppurative M00.9
  tuberculous A18.02
His (-Werner) (trench fever) A79.0
Hodgson's I71.2
  ruptured I71.1
Holla — see Spherocytosis
hookworm B76.9
  specified NEC B76.8
host-versus-graft D89.813
  acute D89.810
  acute on chronic D89.812
  chronic D89.811
human immunodeficiency virus (HIV) B20
Huntington's G10
  with dementia G10 [F02.80]
Hutchinson's (cheiropompholyx) — see Hutchinson's disease
hyaline (diffuse) (generalized)
  membrane (lung) (newborn) P22.0
    adult J80
hydatid — see Echinococcus
hydroxyapatite deposition M11.00
  ankle M11.07- ☑
  elbow M11.02- ☑
  foot joint M11.07- ☑
  hand joint M11.04- ☑
  hip M11.05- ☑
  knee M11.06- ☑
  multiple site M11.09
  shoulder M11.01- ☑
  vertebra M11.08
  wrist M11.03- ☑
hyperkinetic — see Hyperkinesia
hypertensive — see Hypertension
hypophysis E23.7
Iceland G93.3
I-cell E77.0
immune D89.9
immunoproliferative (malignant) C88.9
  small intestinal C88.3
  specified NEC C88.8
inclusion B25.9
  salivary gland B25.9
infectious, infective B99.9
  congenital P37.9
    specified NEC P37.8
    viral P35.9
      specified type NEC P35.8
  specified NEC B99.8
inflammatory
  penis N48.29
    abscess N48.21
    cellulitis N48.22
  prepuce N47.7
    balanoposthitis N47.6
  tubo-ovarian — see Salpingo-oophoritis
intervertebral disc — see also Disorder, disc

Disease, diseased — *continued*
  intervertebral disc — *see also* Disorder, disc — *continued*
    with myelopathy — *see* Disorder, disc, with, myelopathy
    cervical, cervicothoracic — *see* Disorder, disc, cervical
    with
      myelopathy — *see* Disorder, disc, cervical, with myelopathy
      neuritis, radiculitis or radiculopathy — *see* Disorder, disc, cervical, with neuritis
      specified NEC — *see* Disorder, disc, cervical, specified type NEC
    lumbar (with)
      myelopathy M51.06
      neuritis, radiculitis, radiculopathy or sciatica M51.16
      specified NEC M51.86
    lumbosacral (with)
      neuritis, radiculitis, radiculopathy or sciatica M51.17
      specified NEC M51.87
    specified NEC — *see* Disorder, disc, specified NEC
    thoracic (with)
      myelopathy M51.04
      neuritis, radiculitis or radiculopathy M51.14
      specified NEC M51.84
    thoracolumbar (with)
      myelopathy M51.05
      neuritis, radiculitis or radiculopathy M51.15
      specified NEC M51.85
  intestine K63.9
    functional K59.9
      psychogenic F45.8
      specified NEC K59.8
    organic K63.9
    protozoal A07.9
    specified NEC K63.89
  iris H21.9
    specified NEC H21.89
  iron metabolism or storage E83.10
  island (scrub typhus) A75.3
  itai-itai — *see* Poisoning, cadmium
  Jakob-Creutzfeldt — *see* Creutzfeldt-Jakob disease or syndrome
  jaw M27.9
    fibrocystic M27.49
    specified NEC M27.8
  jigger B88.1
  joint — *see also* Disorder, joint
    Charcot's — *see* Arthropathy, neuropathic (Charcot)
    degenerative — *see* Osteoarthritis
      multiple M15.9
      spine — *see* Spondylosis
    hypertrophic — *see* Osteoarthritis
    sacroiliac M53.3
    specified NEC — *see* Disorder, joint, specified type NEC
    spine NEC — *see* Dorsopathy
    suppurative — *see* Arthritis, pyogenic or pyemic
  Jourdain's (acute gingivitis) K05.00
    nonplaque induced K05.01
    plaque induced K05.00
  Kaschin-Beck (endemic polyarthritis) M12.10
    ankle M12.17- ☑
    elbow M12.12- ☑
    foot joint M12.17- ☑
    hand joint M12.14- ☑
    hip M12.15- ☑
    knee M12.16- ☑
    multiple site M12.19
    shoulder M12.11- ☑
    vertebra M12.18
    wrist M12.13- ☑
  Katayama B65.2
  Kedani (scrub typhus) A75.3
  Keshan E59
  kidney (functional) (pelvis) N28.9
    chronic N18.9
      hypertensive — *see* Hypertension, kidney
      stage 1 N18.1
      stage 2 (mild) N18.2
      stage 3 (moderate) N18.3
      stage 4 (severe) N18.4
      stage 5 N18.5
    complicating pregnancy — *see* Pregnancy, complicated by, renal disease

kidney — *continued*
  cystic (congenital) Q61.9
  fibrocystic (congenital) Q61.8
  hypertensive — *see* Hypertension, kidney
  in (due to)
    schistosomiasis (bilharziasis) B65.9 *[N29]*
  multicystic Q61.4
  polycystic Q61.3
    adult type Q61.2
    childhood type NEC Q61.19
      collecting duct dilatation Q61.11
Kimmelstiel (-Wilson) (intercapillary polycystic (congenital) glomerulosclerosis) — *see* E08-E13 with .21
Kinnier Wilson's (hepatolenticular degeneration) E83.01
kissing — *see* Mononucleosis, infectious
Klebs' — *see also* Glomerulonephritis N05- ☑
Klippel-Feil (brevicollis) Q76.1
Köhler-Pellegrini-Stieda (calcification, knee joint) — *see* Bursitis, tibial collateral
Kok Q89.8
König's (osteochondritis dissecans) — *see* Osteochondritis, dissecans
Korsakoff's (nonalcoholic) F04
  alcoholic F10.96
    with dependence F10.26
Kostmann's (infantile genetic agranulocytosis) D70.0
kuru A81.81
Kyasanur Forest A98.2
labyrinth, ear — *see* Disorder, ear, inner
lacrimal system — *see* Disorder, lacrimal system
Lafora's — *see* Epilepsy, generalized, idiopathic
Lancereaux-Mathieu (leptospiral jaundice) A27.0
Landry's G61.0
Larrey-Weil (leptospiral jaundice) A27.0
larynx J38.7
legionnaires' A48.1
  nonpneumonic A48.2
Lenegre's I44.2
lens H27.9
  specified NEC H27.8
Lev's (acquired complete heart block) I44.2
Lewy body (dementia) G31.83 *[F02.80]*
  with behavioral disturbance G31.83 *[F02.81]*
Lichtheim's (subacute combined sclerosis with pernicious anemia) D51.0
Lightwood's (renal tubular acidosis) N25.89
Lignac's (cystinosis) E72.04
lip K13.0
lipid-storage E75.6
  specified NEC E75.5
Lipschütz's N76.6
liver (chronic) (organic) K76.9
  alcoholic (chronic) K70.9
    acute — *see* Disease, liver, alcoholic, hepatitis
    cirrhosis K70.30
      with ascites K70.31
    failure K70.40
      with coma K70.41
    fatty liver K70.0
    fibrosis K70.2
    hepatitis K70.10
      with ascites K70.11
    sclerosis K70.2
  cystic, congenital Q44.6
  drug-induced (idiosyncratic) (toxic) (predictable) (unpredictable) — *see* Disease, liver, toxic
  end stage K72.90
    due to hepatitis — *see* Hepatitis
  fatty, nonalcoholic (NAFLD) K76.0
    alcoholic K70.0
  fibrocystic (congenital) Q44.6
  fluke
    Chinese B66.1
    oriental B66.1
    sheep B66.3
  gestational alloimmune (GALD) P78.84
  glycogen storage E74.09 *[K77]*
  in (due to)
    schistosomiasis (bilharziasis) B65.9 *[K77]*
  inflammatory K75.9
    alcoholic K70.1 ☑
    specified NEC K75.89
  polycystic (congenital) Q44.6
  toxic K71.9
    with
      cholestasis K71.0
      cirrhosis (liver) K71.7

liver — *continued*
  toxic — *continued*
    with — *continued*
      fibrosis (liver) K71.7
      focal nodular hyperplasia K71.8
      hepatic granuloma K71.8
      hepatic necrosis K71.10
        with coma K71.11
      hepatitis NEC K71.6
        acute K71.2
        chronic
          active K71.50
            with ascites K71.51
          lobular K71.4
          persistent K71.3
        lupoid K71.50
          with ascites K71.51
      peliosis hepatis K71.8
      veno-occlusive disease (VOD) of liver K71.8
  veno-occlusive K76.5
Lobo's (keloid blastomycosis) B48.0
Lobstein's (brittle bones and blue sclera) Q78.0
Ludwig's (submaxillary cellulitis) K12.2
lumbosacral region M53.87
lung J98.4
  black J60
  congenital Q33.9
  cystic J98.4
    congenital Q33.0
  fibroid (chronic) — *see* Fibrosis, lung
  fluke B66.4
    oriental B66.4
  in
    amyloidosis E85.4 *[J99]*
    sarcoidosis D86.0
    Sjögren's syndrome M35.02
    systemic
      lupus erythematosus M32.13
      sclerosis M34.81
  interstitial J84.9
    of childhood, specified NEC J84.848
    respiratory bronchiolitis J84.115
    specified NEC J84.89
  obstructive (chronic) J43.9
    with
      acute
        bronchitis J44.0
        exacerbation NEC J44.1
        lower respiratory infection J44.0
      alveolitis, allergic J67.9
      asthma J44.9
      bronchiectasis J47.9
        with
          exacerbation (acute) J47.1
          lower respiratory infection J47.0
      bronchitis J44.9
        with
          exacerbation (acute) J44.1
          lower respiratory infection J44.0
      emphysema J43.9
      hypersensitivity pneumonitis J67.9
    decompensated J44.1
      with
        exacerbation (acute) J44.1
  polycystic J98.4
    congenital Q33.0
  rheumatoid (diffuse) (interstitial) — *see* Rheumatoid, lung
Lutembacher's (atrial septal defect with mitral stenos Q21.1
Lyme A69.20
lymphatic (gland) (system) (channel) (vessel) I89.9
lymphoproliferative D47.9
  specified NEC D47.Z9 *(following* D47.4)
  T-gamma D47.Z9 *(following* D47.4)
  X-linked D82.3
Magitot's M27.2
malarial — *see* Malaria
malignant — *see also* Neoplasm, malignant, by site
Manson's B65.1
maple bark J67.6
maple-syrup-urine E71.0
Marburg (virus) A98.3
Marion's (bladder neck obstruction) N32.0
Marsh's (exophthalmic goiter) — *see* Hyperthyroidisr with, goiter (diffuse)
mastoid (process) — *see* Disorder, ear, middle
Mathieu's (leptospiral jaundice) A27.0

Disease, diseased — *continued*
- Maxcy's A75.2
- McArdle (-Schmid-Pearson) (glycogenosis V) E74.04
- mediastinum J98.59
- medullary center (idiopathic) (respiratory) G93.89
- Meige's (chronic hereditary edema) Q82.0
- meningococcal — *see* Infection, meningococcal
- mental F99
  - organic F09
- mesenchymal M35.9
- mesenteric embolic — *see also* Ischemia, intestine, acute K55.039
- metabolic, metabolism E88.9
  - bilirubin E80.7
- metal-polisher's J62.8
- metastatic — *see also* Neoplasm, secondary, by site C79.9
- microvascular - code to condition
- microvillus
  - atrophy Q43.8
  - inclusion (MVD) Q43.8
- middle ear — *see* Disorder, ear, middle
- Mikulicz' (dryness of mouth, absent or decreased lacrimation) K11.8
- Milroy's (chronic hereditary edema) Q82.0
- Minamata — *see* Poisoning, mercury
- minicore G71.2
- Minor's G95.19
- Minot's (hemorrhagic disease, newborn) P53
- Minot-von Willebrand-Jürgens (angiohemophilia) D68.0
- Mitchell's (erythromelalgia) I73.81
- mitral (valve) I05.9
  - nonrheumatic I34.9
- mixed connective tissue M35.1
- moldy hay J67.0
- Monge's T70.29 ☑
- Morgagni-Adams-Stokes (syncope with heart block) I45.9
- Morgagni's (syndrome) (hyperostosis frontalis interna) M85.2
- Morton's (with metatarsalgia) — *see* Lesion, nerve, plantar
- Morvan's G60.8
- motor neuron (bulbar) (mixed type) (spinal) G12.20
  - amyotrophic lateral sclerosis G12.21
  - familial G12.24
  - progressive bulbar palsy G12.22
  - specified NEC G12.29
- moyamoya I67.5
- mu heavy chain disease C88.2
- multicore G71.2
- muscle — *see also* Disorder, muscle
  - inflammatory — *see* Myositis
  - ocular (external) — *see* Strabismus
- musculoskeletal system, soft tissue — *see also* Disorder, soft tissue
  - specified NEC — *see* Disorder, soft tissue, specified type NEC
- mushroom workers' J67.5
- mycotic B49
- myelodysplastic, not classified C94.6
- myeloproliferative, not classified C94.6
  - chronic D47.1
- myocardium, myocardial — *see also* Degeneration, myocardial I51.5
  - primary (idiopathic) I42.9
- myoneural G70.9
- Naegeli's D69.1
- nails L60.9
  - specified NEC L60.8
- Nairobi (sheep virus) A93.8
- nasal J34.9
- nemaline body G71.2
- nerve — *see* Disorder, nerve
- nervous system G98.8
  - autonomic G90.9
  - central G96.9
    - specified NEC G96.8
  - congenital Q07.9
  - parasympathetic G90.9
  - specified NEC G98.8
  - sympathetic G90.9
  - vegetative G90.9
- neuromuscular system G70.9
- Newcastle B30.8
- Nicolas (-Durand)-Favre (climatic bubo) A55
- nipple N64.9
  - Paget's C50.01- ☑

Disease, diseased — *continued*
- nipple — *continued*
  - Paget's — *continued*
    - female C50.01- ☑
    - male C50.02- ☑
- Nishimoto (-Takeuchi) I67.5
- nonarthropod-borne NOS (viral) B34.9
  - enterovirus NEC B34.1
- nonautoimmune hemolytic D59.4
  - drug-induced D59.2
- Nonne-Milroy-Meige (chronic hereditary edema) Q82.0
- nose J34.9
- nucleus pulposus — *see* Disorder, disc
- nutritional E63.9
- oast-house-urine E72.19
  - ocular
    - herpesviral B00.50
    - zoster B02.30
- obliterative vascular I77.1
- Ohara's — *see* Tularemia
- Opitz's (congestive splenomegaly) D73.2
- Oppenheim-Urbach (necrobiosis lipoidica diabetico-rum) — *see* E08-E13 with .620
- optic nerve NEC — *see* Disorder, nerve, optic
- orbit — *see* Disorder, orbit
- Oriental liver fluke B66.1
- Oriental lung fluke B66.4
- Ormond's N13.5
- Oropouche virus A93.0
- Osler-Rendu (familial hemorrhagic telangiectasia) I78.0
- osteofibrocystic E21.0
- Otto's M24.7
- outer ear — *see* Disorder, ear, external
- ovary (noninflammatory) N83.9
  - cystic N83.20- ☑
  - inflammatory — *see* Salpingo-oophoritis
  - polycystic E28.2
  - specified NEC N83.8
- Owren's (congenital) — *see* Defect, coagulation
- pancreas K86.9
  - cystic K86.2
  - fibrocystic E84.9
  - specified NEC K86.89
- panvalvular I08.9
  - specified NEC I08.8
- parametrium (noninflammatory) N83.9
- parasitic B89
  - cerebral NEC B71.9 *[G94]*
  - intestinal NOS B82.9
  - mouth B37.0
  - skin NOS B88.9
  - specified type — *see* Infestation
  - tongue B37.0
- parathyroid (gland) E21.5
  - specified NEC E21.4
- Parkinson's G20
- parodontal K05.6
- Parrot's (syphilitic osteochondritis) A50.02
- Parry's (exophthalmic goiter) — *see* Hyperthyroidism, with, goiter (diffuse)
- Parson's (exophthalmic goiter) — *see* Hyperthyroidism, with, goiter (diffuse)
- Paxton's (white piedra) B36.2
- pearl-worker's — *see* Osteomyelitis, specified type NEC
- Pellegrini-Stieda (calcification, knee joint) — *see* Bursitis, tibial collateral
- pelvis, pelvic
  - female NOS N94.9
    - specified NEC N94.89
  - gonococcal (acute) (chronic) A54.24
  - inflammatory (female) N73.9
    - acute N73.0
    - chlamydial A56.11
    - chronic N73.1
    - specified NEC N73.8
    - syphilitic (secondary) A51.42
      - late A52.76
    - tuberculous A18.17
  - organ, female N94.9
  - peritoneum, female NEC N94.89
- penis N48.9
  - inflammatory N48.29
    - abscess N48.21
    - cellulitis N48.22
  - specified NEC N48.89
- periapical tissues NOS K04.90
- periodontal K05.6
  - specified NEC K05.5

Disease, diseased — *continued*
- periosteum — *see* Disorder, bone, specified type NEC
- peripheral
  - arterial I73.9
  - autonomic nervous system G90.9
  - nerves — *see* Polyneuropathy
  - vascular NOS I73.9
- peritoneum K66.9
  - pelvic, female NEC N94.89
  - specified NEC K66.8
- persistent mucosal (middle ear) H66.20
  - left H66.22
    - with right H66.23
  - right H66.21
    - with left H66.23
- Petit's — *see* Hernia, abdomen, specified site NEC
- pharynx J39.2
  - specified NEC J39.2
- Phocas' — *see* Mastopathy, cystic
- photochromogenic (acid-fast bacilli) (pulmonary) A31.0
  - nonpulmonary A31.9
- Pick's G31.01 *[F02.80]*
  - with behavioral disturbance G31.01 *[F02.81]*
  - brain G31.01 *[F02.80]*
    - with behavioral disturbance G31.01 *[F02.81]*
  - of pericardium (pericardial pseudocirrhosis of liver) I31.1
- pigeon fancier's J67.2
- pineal gland E34.8
- pink — *see* Poisoning, mercury
- Pinkus' (lichen nitidus) L44.1
- pinworm B80
- Piry virus A93.8
- pituitary (gland) E23.7
- pituitary-snuff-taker's J67.8
- pleura (cavity) J94.9
  - specified NEC J94.8
- pneumatic drill (hammer) T75.21 ☑
- Pollitzer's (hidradenitis suppurativa) L73.2
- polycystic
  - kidney or renal Q61.3
    - adult type Q61.2
    - childhood type NEC Q61.19
      - collecting duct dilatation Q61.11
  - liver or hepatic Q44.6
  - lung or pulmonary J98.4
    - congenital Q33.0
  - ovary, ovaries E28.2
  - spleen Q89.09
- polyethylene T84.05- ☑
- Pompe's (glycogenosis II) E74.02
- Posadas-Wernicke B38.9
- Potain's (pulmonary edema) — *see* Edema, lung
- prepuce N47.8
  - inflammatory N47.7
    - balanoposthitis N47.6
- Pringle's (tuberous sclerosis) Q85.1
- prion, central nervous system A81.9
  - specified NEC A81.89
- prostate N42.9
  - specified NEC N42.89
- protozoal B64
  - acanthamebiasis — *see* Acanthamebiasis
  - African trypanosomiasis — *see* African trypanosomiasis
  - babesiosis B60.0
  - Chagas disease — *see* Chagas disease
  - intestine, intestinal A07.9
  - leishmaniasis — *see* Leishmaniasis
  - malaria — *see* Malaria
  - naegleriasis B60.2
  - pneumocystosis B59
  - specified organism NEC B60.8
  - toxoplasmosis — *see* Toxoplasmosis
- pseudo-Hurler's E77.0
- psychiatric F99
- psychotic — *see* Psychosis
- Puente's (simple glandular cheilitis) K13.0
- puerperal — *see also* Puerperal O90.89
- pulmonary — *see also* Disease, lung
  - artery I28.9
  - chronic obstructive J44.9
    - with
      - acute bronchitis J44.0
      - exacerbation (acute) J44.1
      - lower respiratory infection (acute) J44.0
    - decompensated J44.1

Disease, diseased — *continued*
pulmonary — *see also* Disease, lung — *continued*
  chronic obstructive — *continued*
    decompensated — *continued*
      with
        exacerbation (acute) J44.1
  heart I27.9
    specified NEC I27.89
  hypertensive (vascular) — *see also* Hypertension,
    pulmonary I27.20
    NEC I27.2 ☑
      primary (idiopathic) I27.0
  valve I37.9
    rheumatic I09.89
pulp (dental) NOS K04.90
pulseless M31.4
Putnam's (subacute combined sclerosis with pernicious
  anemia) D51.0
Pyle (-Cohn) (metaphyseal dysplasia) Q78.5
ragpicker's or ragsorter's A22.1
Raynaud's — *see* Raynaud's disease
reactive airway — *see* Asthma
Reclus' (cystic) — *see* Mastopathy, cystic
rectum K62.9
  specified NEC K62.89
Refsum's (heredopathia atactica polyneuritiformis)
  G60.1
renal (functional) (pelvis) — *see also* Disease, kidney
  N28.9
  with
    edema — *see* Nephrosis
    glomerular lesion — *see* Glomerulonephritis
      with edema — *see* Nephrosis
    interstitial nephritis N12
  acute N28.9
  chronic — *see also* Disease, kidney, chronic N18.9
  cystic, congenital Q61.9
  diabetic — *see* E08-E13 with .22
  end-stage (failure) N18.6
    due to hypertension I12.0
  fibrocystic (congenital) Q61.8
  hypertensive — *see* Hypertension, kidney
  lupus M32.14
  phosphate-losing (tubular) N25.0
  polycystic (congenital) Q61.3
    adult type Q61.2
    childhood type NEC Q61.19
      collecting duct dilatation Q61.11
  rapidly progressive N01.9
  subacute N01.9
Rendu-Osler-Weber (familial hemorrhagic telangiectasia) I78.0
renovascular (arteriosclerotic) — *see* Hypertension,
  kidney
respiratory (tract) J98.9
  acute or subacute NOS J06.9
    due to
      chemicals, gases, fumes or vapors (inhalation)
        J68.3
      external agent J70.9
        specified NEC J70.8
      radiation J70.0
      smoke inhalation J70.5
    noninfectious J39.8
  chronic NOS J98.9
    due to
      chemicals, gases, fumes or vapors J68.4
      external agent J70.9
        specified NEC J70.8
      radiation J70.1
    newborn P27.9
      specified NEC P27.8
  due to
    chemicals, gases, fumes or vapors J68.9
      acute or subacute NEC J68.3
      chronic J68.4
    external agent J70.9
      specified NEC J70.8
  newborn P28.9
    specified type NEC P28.89
  upper J39.9
    acute or subacute J06.9
    noninfectious NEC J39.8
    specified NEC J39.8
    streptococcal J06.9
retina, retinal H35.9
  Batten's or Batten-Mayou E75.4 *[H36]*
  specified NEC H35.89

Disease, diseased — *continued*
rheumatoid — *see* Arthritis, rheumatoid
rickettsial NOS A79.9
  specified type NEC A79.89
Riga (-Fede) (cachectic aphthae) K14.0
Riggs' (compound periodontitis) — *see* Periodontitis
Ritter's L00
Rivalta's (cervicofacial actinomycosis) A42.2
Robles' (onchocerciasis) B73.01
Roger's (congenital interventricular septal defect) Q21.0
Rosenthal's (factor XI deficiency) D68.1
Ross River B33.1
Rossbach's (hyperchlorhydria) K31.89
  psychogenic F45.8
Rotes Quérol — *see* Hyperostosis, ankylosing
Roth (-Bernhardt) — *see* Mononeuropathy, lower limb,
  meralgia paresthetica
Runeberg's (progressive pernicious anemia) D51.0
sacroiliac NEC M53.3
salivary gland or duct K11.9
  inclusion B25.9
  specified NEC K11.8
  virus B25.9
sandworm B76.9
Schimmelbusch's — *see* Mastopathy, cystic
Schmorl's — *see* Schmorl's disease or nodes
Schönlein (-Henoch) (purpura rheumatica) D69.0
Schottmüller's — *see* Fever, paratyphoid
Schultz's (agranulocytosis) — *see* Agranulocytosis
Schwalbe-Ziehen-Oppenheim G24.1
Schwartz-Jampel G71.13
sclera H15.9
  specified NEC H15.89
scrofulous (tuberculous) A18.2
scrotum N50.9
sebaceous glands L73.9
semilunar cartilage, cystic — *see also* Derangement,
  knee, meniscus, cystic
seminal vesicle N50.9
serum NEC — *see also* Reaction, serum T80.69 ☑
sexually transmitted A64
  anogenital
    herpesviral infection — *see* Herpes, anogenital
    warts A63.0
  chancroid A57
  chlamydial infection — *see* Chlamydia
  gonorrhea — *see* Gonorrhea
  granuloma inguinale A58
  specified organism NEC A63.8
  syphilis — *see* Syphilis
  trichomoniasis — *see* Trichomoniasis
Sézary C84.1- ☑
shimamushi (scrub typhus) A75.3
shipyard B30.0
sickle-cell D57.1
  with crisis (vasoocclusive pain) D57.00
    with
      acute chest syndrome D57.01
      splenic sequestration D57.02
  elliptocytosis D57.8- ☑
  Hb-C D57.20
    with crisis (vasoocclusive pain) D57.219
      with
        acute chest syndrome D57.211
        splenic sequestration D57.212
    without crisis D57.20
  Hb-SD D57.80
    with crisis D57.819
      with
        acute chest syndrome D57.811
        splenic sequestration D57.812
  Hb-SE D57.80
    with crisis D57.819
      with
        acute chest syndrome D57.811
        splenic sequestration D57.812
  specified NEC D57.80
    with crisis D57.819
      with
        acute chest syndrome D57.811
        splenic sequestration D57.812
  spherocytosis D57.80
    with crisis D57.819
      with
        acute chest syndrome D57.811
        splenic sequestration D57.812
  thalassemia D57.40
    with crisis (vasoocclusive pain) D57.419

Disease, diseased — *continued*
sickle-cell — *continued*
  thalassemia — *continued*
    with crisis — *continued*
      with
        acute chest syndrome D57.411
        splenic sequestration D57.412
    without crisis D57.40
silo-filler's J68.8
  bronchitis J68.0
  pneumonitis J68.0
  pulmonary edema J68.1
simian B B00.4
Simons' (progressive lipodystrophy) E88.1
sin nombre virus B33.4
sinus — *see* Sinusitis
Sirkari's B55.0
sixth B08.20
  due to human herpesvirus 6 B08.21
  due to human herpesvirus 7 B08.22
skin L98.9
  due to metabolic disorder NEC E88.9 *[L99]*
  specified NEC L98.8
slim (HIV) B20
small vessel I73.9
Sneddon-Wilkinson (subcorneal pustular dermatosis)
  L13.1
South African creeping B88.0
spinal (cord) G95.9
  congenital Q06.9
  specified NEC G95.89
spine — *see also* Spondylopathy
  joint — *see* Dorsopathy
  tuberculous A18.01
spinocerebellar (hereditary) G11.9
  specified NEC G11.8
spleen D73.9
  amyloid E85.4 *[D77]*
  organic D73.9
  polycystic Q89.09
  postinfectional D73.89
sponge-diver's — *see* Toxicity, venom, marine anima
  sea anemone
Startle Q89.8
Steinert's G71.11
Sticker's (erythema infectiosum) B08.3
Stieda's (calcification, knee joint) — *see* Bursitis, tibi
  collateral
Stokes' (exophthalmic goiter) — *see* Hyperthyroidisr
  with, goiter (diffuse)
Stokes-Adams (syncope with heart block) I45.9
stomach K31.9
  functional, psychogenic F45.8
  specified NEC K31.89
stonemason's J62.8
storage
  glycogen — *see* Disease, glycogen storage
  mucopolysaccharide — *see* Mucopolysaccharidos
striatopallidal system NEC G25.89
Stuart-Prower (congenital factor X deficiency) D68.2
Stuart's (congenital factor X deficiency) D68.2
subcutaneous tissue — *see* Disease, skin
supporting structures of teeth K08.9
  specified NEC K08.89
suprarenal (capsule) (gland) E27.9
  hyperfunction E27.0
  specified NEC E27.8
sweat glands L74.9
  specified NEC L74.8
Sweeley-Klionsky E75.21
Swift (-Feer) — *see* Poisoning, mercury
swimming-pool granuloma A31.1
Sylvest's (epidemic pleurodynia) B33.0
sympathetic nervous system G90.9
synovium — *see* Disorder, synovium
syphilitic — *see* Syphilis
systemic tissue mast cell D47.02
tanapox (virus) B08.71
Tangier E78.6
Tarral-Besnier (pityriasis rubra pilaris) L44.0
Tauri's E74.09
tear duct — *see* Disorder, lacrimal system
tendon, tendinous — *see also* Disorder, tendon
  nodular — *see* Trigger finger
terminal vessel I73.9
testis N50.9
thalassemia Hb-S — *see* Disease, sickle-cell, thalassem
Thaysen-Gee (nontropical sprue) K90.0

☑ Additional Character Required — Refer to the Tabular List for Character Selection   ▽ Subterms under main terms may continue to next column or pag

Index

Disease, diseased — Disease, diseased

Disease, diseased — *continued*

Thomsen G71.12
throat J39.2
  septic J02.0
thromboembolic — *see* Embolism
thymus (gland) E32.9
  specified NEC E32.8
thyroid (gland) E07.9
  heart — *see also* Hyperthyroidism E05.90 *[I43]*
    with thyroid storm E05.91 *[I43]*
  specified NEC E07.89
Tietze's M94.0
tongue K14.9
  specified NEC K14.8
tonsils, tonsillar (and adenoids) J35.9
tooth, teeth K08.9
  hard tissues K03.9
    specified NEC K03.89
  pulp NEC K04.99
  specified NEC K08.89
Tourette's F95.2
trachea NEC J39.8
tricuspid I07.9
  nonrheumatic I36.9
triglyceride-storage E75.5
trophoblastic — *see* Mole, hydatidiform
tsutsugamushi A75.3
tube (fallopian) (noninflammatory) N83.9
  inflammatory — *see* Salpingitis
  specified NEC N83.8
tuberculous NEC — *see* Tuberculosis
tubo-ovarian (noninflammatory) N83.9
  inflammatory — *see* Salpingo-oophoritis
  specified NEC N83.8
tubotympanic, chronic — *see* Otitis, media, suppurative, chronic, tubotympanic
tubulo-interstitial N15.9
  specified NEC N15.8
tympanum — *see* Disorder, tympanic membrane
Uhl's Q24.8
Underwood's (sclerema neonatorum) P83.0
Unverricht (-Lundborg) — *see* Epilepsy, generalized, idiopathic
Urbach-Oppenheim (necrobiosis lipoidica diabeticorum) — *see* E08-E13 with .620
ureter N28.9
  in (due to)
    schistosomiasis (bilharziasis) B65.0 *[N29]*
urethra N36.9
  specified NEC N36.8
urinary (tract) N39.9
  bladder N32.9
    specified NEC N32.89
  specified NEC N39.8
uterus (noninflammatory) N85.9
  infective — *see* Endometritis
  inflammatory — *see* Endometritis
  specified NEC N85.8
uveal tract (anterior) H21.9
  posterior H31.9
vagabond's B85.1
vagina, vaginal (noninflammatory) N89.9
  inflammatory NEC N76.89
  specified NEC N89.8
valve, valvular I38
  multiple I08.9
    specified NEC I08.8
van Creveld-von Gierke (glycogenosis I) E74.01
vas deferens N50.9
vascular I99.9
  arteriosclerotic — *see* Arteriosclerosis
  ciliary body NEC — *see* Disorder, iris, vascular
  hypertensive — *see* Hypertension
  iris NEC — *see* Disorder, iris, vascular
  obliterative I77.1
    peripheral I73.9
  occlusive I99.8
  peripheral (occlusive) I73.9
    in diabetes mellitus — *see* E08-E13 with .51
vasomotor I73.9
vasospastic I73.9
vein I87.9
venereal — *see also* Disease, sexually transmitted A64
  chlamydial NEC A56.8
    anus A56.3
    genitourinary NOS A56.2
    pharynx A56.4
    rectum A56.3

Disease, diseased — *continued*

venereal — *see also* Disease, sexually transmitted — *continued*
  fifth A55
  sixth A55
  specified nature or type NEC A63.8
vertebra, vertebral — *see also* Spondylopathy
  disc — *see* Disorder, disc
vibration — *see* Vibration, adverse effects
viral, virus — *see also* Disease, by type of virus B34.9
  arbovirus NOS A94
  arthropod-borne NOS A94
  congenital P35.9
    specified NEC P35.8
  Hanta (with renal manifestations) (Dobrava) (Puumala) (Seoul) A98.5
    with pulmonary manifestations (Andes) (Bayou) (Bermejo) (Black Creek Canal) (Choclo) (Juquitiba) (Laguna negra) (Lechiguanas) (New York) (Oran) (Sin nombre) B33.4
  Hantaan (Korean hemorrhagic fever) A98.5
  human immunodeficiency (HIV) B20
  Kunjin A83.4
  nonarthropod-borne NOS B34.9
  Powassan A84.8
  Rocio (encephalitis) A83.6
  Sin nombre (Hantavirus) (cardio)-pulmonary syndrome) B33.4
  Tahyna B33.8
  vesicular stomatitis A93.8
vitreous H43.9
  specified NEC H43.89
vocal cord J38.3
Volkmann's, acquired T79.6 ✓
von Eulenburg's (congenital paramyotonia) G71.19
von Gierke's (glycogenosis I) E74.01
von Graefe's — *see* Strabismus, paralytic, ophthalmoplegia, progressive
von Willebrand (-Jürgens) (angiohemophilia) D68.0
Vrolik's (osteogenesis imperfecta) Q78.0
vulva (noninflammatory) N90.9
  inflammatory NEC N76.89
  specified NEC N90.89
Wallgren's (obstruction of splenic vein with collateral circulation) I87.8
Wassilieff's (leptospiral jaundice) A27.0
wasting NEC R64
  due to malnutrition E41
Waterhouse-Friderichsen A39.1
Wegner's (syphilitic osteochondritis) A50.02
Weil's (leptospiral jaundice of lung) A27.0
Weir Mitchell's (erythromelalgia) I73.81
Werdnig-Hoffmann G12.0
Wermer's E31.21
Werner-His (trench fever) A79.0
Werner-Schultz (neutropenic splenomegaly) D73.81
Wernicke-Posadas B38.9
whipworm B79
white blood cells D72.9
  specified NEC D72.89
white matter R90.82
white-spot, meaning lichen sclerosus et atrophicus L90.0
  penis N48.0
  vulva N90.4
Wilkie's K55.1
Wilkinson-Sneddon (subcorneal pustular dermatosis) L13.1
Willis' — *see* Diabetes
Wilson's (hepatolenticular degeneration) E83.01
woolsorter's A22.1
yaba monkey tumor B08.72
yaba pox (virus) B08.72
Zika virus A92.5
  congenital P35.4
zoonotic, bacterial A28.9
  specified type NEC A28.8
Disfigurement (due to scar) L90.5
Disgerminoma — *see* Dysgerminoma
DISH (diffuse idiopathic skeletal hyperostosis) — *see* Hyperostosis, ankylosing
Disinsertion, retina — *see* Detachment, retina
Dislocatable hip, congenital Q65.6
Dislocation (articular)
  with fracture — *see* Fracture
  acromioclavicular (joint) S43.10- ✓
    with displacement
      100%-200% S43.12- ✓

Dislocation — *continued*

acromioclavicular — *continued*
  with displacement — *continued*
    more than 200% S43.13- ✓
  inferior S43.14- ✓
  posterior S43.15- ✓
ankle S93.0- ✓
astragalus — *see* Dislocation, ankle
atlantoaxial S13.121 ✓
atlantooccipital S13.111 ✓
atloidooccipital S13.111 ✓
breast bone S23.29 ✓
capsule, joint — *code by* site under Dislocation
carpal (bone) — *see* Dislocation, wrist
carpometacarpal (joint) NEC S63.05- ✓
  thumb S63.04- ✓
cartilage (joint) — *code by* site under Dislocation
cervical spine (vertebra) — *see* Dislocation, vertebra, cervical
chronic — *see* Dislocation, recurrent
clavicle — *see* Dislocation, acromioclavicular joint
coccyx S33.2 ✓
congenital NEC Q68.8
coracoid — *see* Dislocation, shoulder
costal cartilage S23.29 ✓
costochondral S23.29 ✓
cricoarytenoid articulation S13.29 ✓
cricothyroid articulation S13.29 ✓
dorsal vertebra — *see* Dislocation, vertebra, thoracic
ear ossicle — *see* Discontinuity, ossicles, ear
elbow S53.10- ✓
  congenital Q68.8
  pathological — *see* Dislocation, pathological NEC, elbow
  radial head alone — *see* Dislocation, radial head
  recurrent — *see* Dislocation, recurrent, elbow
  traumatic S53.10- ✓
    anterior S53.11- ✓
    lateral S53.14- ✓
    medial S53.13- ✓
    posterior S53.12- ✓
    specified type NEC S53.19- ✓
eye, nontraumatic — *see* Luxation, globe
eyeball, nontraumatic — *see* Luxation, globe
femur
  distal end — *see* Dislocation, knee
  proximal end — *see* Dislocation, hip
fibula
  distal end — *see* Dislocation, ankle
  proximal end — *see* Dislocation, knee
finger S63.25- ✓
  index S63.25- ✓
  interphalangeal S63.27- ✓
    distal S63.29- ✓
      index S63.29- ✓
      little S63.29- ✓
      middle S63.29- ✓
      ring S63.29- ✓
    index S63.27- ✓
    little S63.27- ✓
    middle S63.27- ✓
    proximal S63.28- ✓
      index S63.28- ✓
      little S63.28- ✓
      middle S63.28- ✓
      ring S63.28- ✓
    ring S63.27- ✓
  little S63.25- ✓
  metacarpophalangeal S63.26- ✓
    index S63.26- ✓
    little S63.26- ✓
    middle S63.26- ✓
    ring S63.26- ✓
  middle S63.25- ✓
  recurrent — *see* Dislocation, recurrent, finger
  ring S63.25- ✓
  thumb — *see* Dislocation, thumb
foot S93.30- ✓
  recurrent — *see* Dislocation, recurrent, foot
  specified site NEC S93.33- ✓
  tarsal joint S93.31- ✓
  tarsometatarsal joint S93.32- ✓
  toe — *see* Dislocation, toe
fracture — *see* Fracture
glenohumeral (joint) — *see* Dislocation, shoulder
glenoid — *see* Dislocation, shoulder

Subterms under main terms may continue to next column or page   ✓ **Additional Character Required — Refer to the Tabular List for Character Selection**   **107**

Disease, diseased — Dislocation

Dislocation — continued

habitual — see Dislocation, recurrent
hip S73.00- ☑
　anterior S73.03- ☑
　　obturator S73.02- ☑
　central S73.04- ☑
　congenital (total) Q65.2
　　bilateral Q65.1
　　partial Q65.5
　　　bilateral Q65.4
　　　unilateral Q65.3- ☑
　　unilateral Q65.0- ☑
　developmental M24.85- ☑
　pathological — see Dislocation, pathological NEC, hip
　posterior S73.01- ☑
　recurrent — see Dislocation, recurrent, hip
humerus, proximal end — see Dislocation, shoulder
incomplete — see Subluxation, by site
incus — see Discontinuity, ossicles, ear
infracoracoid — see Dislocation, shoulder
innominate (pubic junction) (sacral junction) S33.39 ☑
　acetabulum — see Dislocation, hip
interphalangeal (joint(s))
　finger S63.279 ☑
　　distal S63.29- ☑
　　　index S63.29- ☑
　　　little S63.29- ☑
　　　middle S63.29- ☑
　　　ring S63.29- ☑
　　index S63.27- ☑
　　little S63.27- ☑
　　middle S63.27- ☑
　　proximal S63.28- ☑
　　　index S63.28- ☑
　　　little S63.28- ☑
　　　middle S63.28- ☑
　　　ring S63.28- ☑
　　ring S63.27- ☑
　foot or toe — see Dislocation, toe
　thumb S63.12- ☑
jaw (cartilage) (meniscus) S03.0- ☑
joint prosthesis — see Complications, joint prosthesis, mechanical, displacement, by site
knee S83.106 ☑
　cap — see Dislocation, patella
　congenital Q68.2
　old M23.8X- ☑
　patella — see Dislocation, patella
　pathological — see Dislocation, pathological NEC, knee
　proximal tibia
　　anteriorly S83.11- ☑
　　laterally S83.14- ☑
　　medially S83.13- ☑
　　posteriorly S83.12- ☑
　recurrent — see also Derangement, knee, specified NEC
　specified type NEC S83.19- ☑
lacrimal gland H04.16- ☑
lens (complete) H27.10
　anterior H27.12- ☑
　congenital Q12.1
　ocular implant — see Complications, intraocular lens
　partial H27.11- ☑
　posterior H27.13- ☑
　traumatic S05.8X- ☑
ligament — code by site under Dislocation
lumbar (vertebra) — see Dislocation, vertebra, lumbar
lumbosacral (vertebra) — see also Dislocation, vertebra, lumbar
　congenital Q76.49
mandible S03.0- ☑
meniscus (knee) — see Tear, meniscus
　other sites - code by site under Dislocation
metacarpal (bone)
　distal end — see Dislocation, finger
　proximal end S63.06- ☑
metacarpophalangeal (joint)
　finger S63.26- ☑
　　index S63.26- ☑
　　little S63.26- ☑
　　middle S63.26- ☑
　　ring S63.26- ☑
　thumb S63.11- ☑

Dislocation — continued

metatarsal (bone) — see Dislocation, foot
metatarsophalangeal (joint(s)) — see Dislocation, toe
midcarpal (joint) S63.03- ☑
midtarsal (joint) — see Dislocation, foot
neck S13.20 ☑
　specified site NEC S13.29 ☑
　vertebra — see Dislocation, vertebra, cervical
nose (septal cartilage) S03.1 ☑
occipitoatloid S13.111 ☑
old — see Derangement, joint, specified type NEC
ossicles, ear — see Discontinuity, ossicles, ear
partial — see Subluxation, by site
patella S83.006 ☑
　congenital Q74.1
　lateral S83.01- ☑
　recurrent (nontraumatic) M22.0- ☑
　　incomplete M22.1- ☑
　specified type NEC S83.09- ☑
pathological NEC M24.30
　ankle M24.37- ☑
　elbow M24.32- ☑
　foot joint M24.37- ☑
　hand joint M24.34- ☑
　hip M24.35- ☑
　knee M24.36- ☑
　lumbosacral joint — see subcategory M53.2 ☑
　pelvic region — see Dislocation, pathological, hip
　sacroiliac — see subcategory M53.2 ☑
　shoulder M24.31- ☑
　wrist M24.33- ☑
pelvis NEC S33.30 ☑
　specified NEC S33.39 ☑
phalanx
　finger or hand — see Dislocation, finger
　foot or toe — see Dislocation, toe
prosthesis, internal — see Complications, prosthetic device, by site, mechanical
radial head S53.006 ☑
　anterior S53.01- ☑
　posterior S53.02- ☑
　specified type NEC S53.09- ☑
radiocarpal (joint) S63.02- ☑
radiohumeral (joint) — see Dislocation, radial head
radioulnar (joint)
　distal S63.01- ☑
　proximal — see Dislocation, elbow
radius
　distal end — see Dislocation, wrist
　proximal end — see Dislocation, radial head
recurrent M24.40
　ankle M24.47- ☑
　elbow M24.42- ☑
　finger M24.44- ☑
　foot joint M24.47- ☑
　hand joint M24.44- ☑
　hip M24.45- ☑
　knee M24.46- ☑
　　patella — see Dislocation, patella, recurrent
　patella — see Dislocation, patella, recurrent
　sacroiliac — see subcategory M53.2 ☑
　shoulder M24.41- ☑
　toe M24.47- ☑
　vertebra — see also subcategory M43.5 ☑
　　atlantoaxial M43.4
　　　with myelopathy M43.3
　wrist M24.43- ☑
rib (cartilage) S23.29 ☑
sacrococcygeal S33.2 ☑
sacroiliac (joint) (ligament) S33.2 ☑
　congenital Q74.2
　recurrent — see subcategory M53.2 ☑
sacrum S33.2 ☑
scaphoid (bone) (hand) (wrist) — see Dislocation, wrist
　foot — see Dislocation, foot
scapula — see Dislocation, shoulder, girdle, scapula
semilunar cartilage, knee — see Tear, meniscus
septal cartilage (nose) S03.1 ☑
septum (nasal) (old) J34.2
sesamoid bone — code by site under Dislocation
shoulder (blade) (ligament) (joint) (traumatic) S43.006 ☑
　acromioclavicular — see Dislocation, acromioclavicular
　chronic — see Dislocation, recurrent, shoulder
　congenital Q68.8

Dislocation — continued

shoulder — continued
　girdle S43.30- ☑
　　scapula S43.31- ☑
　　specified site NEC S43.39- ☑
　humerus S43.00- ☑
　　anterior S43.01- ☑
　　inferior S43.03- ☑
　　posterior S43.02- ☑
　pathological — see Dislocation, pathological NE◄ shoulder
　recurrent — see Dislocation, recurrent, shoulder
　specified type NEC S43.08- ☑
spine
　cervical — see Dislocation, vertebra, cervical
　congenital Q76.49
　due to birth trauma P11.5
　lumbar — see Dislocation, vertebra, lumbar
　thoracic — see Dislocation, vertebra, thoracic
spontaneous — see Dislocation, pathological
sternoclavicular (joint) S43.206 ☑
　anterior S43.21- ☑
　posterior S43.22- ☑
sternum S23.29 ☑
subglenoid — see Dislocation, shoulder
symphysis pubis S33.4 ☑
talus — see Dislocation, ankle
tarsal (bone(s)) (joint(s)) — see Dislocation, foot
tarsometatarsal (joint(s)) — see Dislocation, foot
temporomandibular (joint) S03.0- ☑
thigh, proximal end — see Dislocation, hip
thorax S23.20 ☑
　specified site NEC S23.29 ☑
　vertebra — see Dislocation, vertebra
thumb S63.10- ☑
　interphalangeal joint — see Dislocation, interph. langeal (joint), thumb
　metacarpophalangeal joint — see Dislocation, metacarpophalangeal (joint), thumb
thyroid cartilage S13.29 ☑
tibia
　distal end — see Dislocation, ankle
　proximal end — see Dislocation, knee
tibiofibular (joint)
　distal — see Dislocation, ankle
　superior — see Dislocation, knee
toe(s) S93.106 ☑
　great S93.10- ☑
　　interphalangeal joint S93.11- ☑
　　metatarsophalangeal joint S93.12- ☑
　interphalangeal joint S93.119 ☑
　lesser S93.106 ☑
　　interphalangeal joint S93.11- ☑
　　metatarsophalangeal joint S93.12- ☑
　metatarsophalangeal joint S93.12- ☑
tooth S03.2 ☑
trachea S23.29 ☑
ulna
　distal end S63.07- ☑
　proximal end — see Dislocation, elbow
ulnohumeral (joint) — see Dislocation, elbow
vertebra (articular process) (body) (traumatic)
　cervical S13.101 ☑
　　atlantoaxial joint S13.121 ☑
　　atlantooccipital joint S13.111 ☑
　　atloidooccipital joint S13.111 ☑
　　joint between
　　　C0 and C1 S13.111 ☑
　　　C1 and C2 S13.121 ☑
　　　C2 and C3 S13.131 ☑
　　　C3 and C4 S13.141 ☑
　　　C4 and C5 S13.151 ☑
　　　C5 and C6 S13.161 ☑
　　　C6 and C7 S13.171 ☑
　　　C7 and T1 S13.181 ☑
　　occipitoatloid joint S13.111 ☑
　congenital Q76.49
　lumbar S33.101 ☑
　　joint between
　　　L1 and L2 S33.111 ☑
　　　L2 and L3 S33.121 ☑
　　　L3 and L4 S33.131 ☑
　　　L4 and L5 S33.141 ☑
　nontraumatic — see Displacement, intervertebra disc
　partial — see Subluxation, by site

Dislocation — continued
  vertebra — continued
    recurrent NEC — see subcategory M43.5 ☑
    thoracic S23.101 ☑
      joint between
        T1 and T2 S23.111 ☑
        T2 and T3 S23.121 ☑
        T3 and T4 S23.123 ☑
        T4 and T5 S23.131 ☑
        T5 and T6 S23.133 ☑
        T6 and T7 S23.141 ☑
        T7 and T8 S23.143 ☑
        T8 and T9 S23.151 ☑
        T9 and T10 S23.153 ☑
        T10 and T11 S23.161 ☑
        T11 and T12 S23.163 ☑
        T12 and L1 S23.171 ☑
  wrist (carpal bone) S63.006 ☑
    carpometacarpal joint — see Dislocation, car-
      pometacarpal (joint)
    distal radioulnar joint — see Dislocation, radioulnar
      (joint), distal
    metacarpal bone, proximal — see Dislocation,
      metacarpal (bone), proximal end
    midcarpal — see Dislocation, midcarpal (joint)
    radiocarpal joint — see Dislocation, radiocarpal
      (joint)
    recurrent — see Dislocation, recurrent, wrist
    specified site NEC S63.09- ☑
    ulna — see Dislocation, ulna, distal end
  xiphoid cartilage S23.29 ☑
Disorder (of) — see also Disease
  acantholytic L11.9
    specified NEC L11.8
  acute
    psychotic — see Psychosis, acute
    stress F43.0
  adjustment (grief) F43.20
    with
      anxiety F43.22
        with depressed mood F43.23
      conduct disturbance F43.24
        with emotional disturbance F43.25
      depressed mood F43.21
        with anxiety F43.23
      other specified symptom F43.29
  adrenal (capsule) (gland) (medullary) E27.9
    specified NEC E27.8
  adrenogenital E25.9
    drug-induced E25.8
    iatrogenic E25.8
    idiopathic E25.8
  adult personality (and behavior) F69
    specified NEC F68.8
  affective (mood) — see Disorder, mood
  aggressive, unsocialized F91.1
  alcohol use
    mild F10.10
      with
        alcohol intoxication F10.129
          delirium F10.121
        alcohol-induced
          anxiety disorder F10.180
          bipolar and related disorder F10.14
          depressive disorder F10.14
          psychotic disorder F10.159
          sexual dysfunction F10.181
          sleep disorder F10.182
      in remission (early) (sustained) F10.11
    moderate or severe F10.20
      with
        alcohol intoxication F10.229
          delirium F10.221
        alcohol-induced
          anxiety disorder F10.280
          bipolar and related disorder F10.24
          depressive disorder F10.24
          major neurocognitive disorder, amnestic-
            confabulatory type F10.26
          major neurocognitive disorder, non-
            amnestic-confabulatory type
            F10.27
          mild neurocognitive disorder F10.288
          psychotic disorder F10.259
          sexual dysfunction F10.281
          sleep disorder F10.282
      in remission (early) (sustained) F10.21
  alcohol-related F10.99

Disorder — continued
  alcohol-related — continued
    with
      amnestic disorder, persisting F10.96
      anxiety disorder F10.980
      dementia, persisting F10.97
      intoxication F10.929
        with delirium F10.921
        uncomplicated F10.920
      mood disorder F10.94
      other specified F10.988
      psychotic disorder F10.959
        with
          delusions F10.950
          hallucinations F10.951
      sexual dysfunction F10.981
      sleep disorder F10.982
  allergic — see Allergy
  alveolar NEC J84.09
  amino-acid
    cystathioninuria E72.19
    cystinosis E72.04
    cystinuria E72.01
    glycinuria E72.09
    homocystinuria E72.11
    metabolism — see Disturbance, metabolism, amino-
      acid
    specified NEC E72.89
    neonatal, transitory P74.8
    renal transport NEC E72.09
    transport NEC E72.09
  amnesic, amnestic
    alcohol-induced F10.96
      with dependence F10.26
    due to (secondary to) general medical condition F04
    psychoactive NEC-induced F19.96
      with
        abuse F19.16
        dependence F19.26
    sedative, hypnotic or anxiolytic-induced F13.96
      with dependence F13.26
  amphetamine (or other stimulant) use
    mild
      with
        amphetamine, cocaine, or other stimulant
          intoxication
          with perceptual disturbances F15.122
          without perceptual disturbances F15.129
        amphetamine (or other stimulant) -induced
          anxiety disorder F15.180
          bipolar and related disorder F15.14
          depressive disorder F15.14
          obsessive-compulsive and related disor-
            der F15.188
          psychotic disorder F15.159
          sexual dysfunction F15.181
        intoxication delirium F15.121
    moderate or severe
      with
        amphetamine, cocaine, or other stimulant
          intoxication
          with perceptual disturbances F15.222
          without perceptual disturbances F15.229
        amphetamine (or other stimulant) -induced
          anxiety disorder F15.280
          bipolar and related disorder F15.24
          depressive disorder F15.24
          obsessive-compulsive and related disor-
            der F15.288
          psychotic disorder F15.259
          sexual dysfunction F15.281
        intoxication delirium F15.221
  amphetamine-type substance use
    mild F15.10
      in remission (early) (sustained) F15.11
    moderate F15.20
      in remission (early) (sustained) F15.21
    severe F15.20
      in remission (early) (sustained) F15.21
  anaerobic glycolysis with anemia D55.2
  anxiety F41.9
    due to (secondary to)
      alcohol F10.980
        in
          abuse F10.180
          dependence F10.280
      amphetamine F15.980
        in
          abuse F15.180

Disorder — continued
  anxiety — continued
    due to — continued
      amphetamine — continued
        in — continued
          dependence F15.280
      anxiolytic F13.980
        in
          abuse F13.180
          dependence F13.280
      caffeine F15.980
        in
          abuse F15.180
          dependence F15.280
      cannabis F12.980
        in
          abuse F12.180
          dependence F12.280
      cocaine F14.980
        in
          abuse F14.180
          dependence F14.180
      general medical condition F06.4
      hallucinogen F16.980
        in
          abuse F16.180
          dependence F16.280
      hypnotic F13.980
        in
          abuse F13.180
          dependence F13.280
      inhalant F18.980
        in
          abuse F18.180
          dependence F18.280
      phencyclidine F16.980
        in
          abuse F16.180
          dependence F16.280
      psychoactive substance NEC F19.980
        in
          abuse F19.180
          dependence F19.280
      sedative F13.980
        in
          abuse F13.180
          dependence F13.280
      volatile solvents F18.980
        in
          abuse F18.180
          dependence F18.280
    generalized F41.1
    illness F45.21
    mixed
      with depression (mild) F41.8
      specified NEC F41.3
    organic F06.4
    phobic F40.9
      of childhood F40.8
    specified NEC F41.8
  aortic valve — see Endocarditis, aortic
  aromatic amino-acid metabolism E70.9
    specified NEC E70.8
  arteriole NEC I77.89
  artery NEC I77.89
  articulation — see Disorder, joint
  attachment (childhood)
    disinhibited F94.2
    reactive F94.1
  attention-deficit hyperactivity (adolescent) (adult)
    (child) F90.9
    combined
      presentation F90.2
      type F90.2
    hyperactive
      impulsive presentation F90.1
      type F90.1
    inattentive
      presentation F90.0
      type F90.0
    specified type NEC F90.8
  attention-deficit without hyperactivity (adolescent)
    (adult) (child) F98.8
  auditory processing (central) H93.25
  autism spectrum F84.0
  autistic F84.0
  autoimmune D89.89
  autonomic nervous system G90.9
    specified NEC G90.8

Disorder — continued
- avoidant
  - child or adolescent F40.10
  - restrictive food intake F50.82
- balance
  - acid-base E87.8
    - mixed E87.4
  - electrolyte E87.8
  - fluid NEC E87.8
- behavioral (disruptive) — see Disorder, conduct
- beta-amino-acid metabolism E72.89
- bile acid and cholesterol metabolism E78.70
  - Barth syndrome E78.71
  - other specified E78.79
  - Smith-Lemli-Opitz syndrome E78.72
- bilirubin excretion E80.6
- binge eating F50.81
- binocular
  - movement H51.9
    - convergence
      - excess H51.12
      - insufficiency H51.11
    - internuclear ophthalmoplegia — see Ophthalmoplegia, internuclear
    - palsy of conjugate gaze H51.0
    - specified type NEC H51.8
  - vision NEC — see Disorder, vision, binocular
- bipolar (I) (type I) F31.9
  - and related due to a known physiological condition
    - with
      - manic features F06.33
      - manic- or hypomanic-like episodes F06.33
      - mixed features F06.34
  - current (or most recent) episode
    - depressed F31.9
      - with psychotic features F31.5
      - without psychotic features F31.30
        - mild F31.31
        - moderate F31.32
        - severe (without psychotic features) F31.4
          - with psychotic features F31.5
    - hypomanic F31.0
    - manic F31.9
      - with psychotic features F31.2
      - without psychotic features F31.10
        - mild F31.11
        - moderate F31.12
        - severe (without psychotic features) F31.13
          - with psychotic features F31.2
    - mixed F31.60
      - mild F31.61
      - moderate F31.62
      - severe (without psychotic features) F31.63
        - with psychotic features F31.64
      - severe depression (without psychotic features) F31.4
        - with psychotic features F31.5
  - in remission (currently) F31.70
    - in full remission
      - most recent episode
        - depressed F31.76
        - hypomanic F31.72
        - manic F31.74
        - mixed F31.78
    - in partial remission
      - most recent episode
        - depressed F31.75
        - hypomanic F31.71
        - manic F31.73
        - mixed F31.77
  - organic F06.30
  - single manic episode F30.9
    - mild F30.11
    - moderate F30.12
    - severe (without psychotic symptoms) F30.13
      - with psychotic symptoms F30.2
  - specified NEC F31.89
- bipolar II (type 2) F31.81
- bladder N32.9
  - functional NEC N31.9
  - in schistosomiasis B65.0 [N33]
  - specified NEC N32.89
- bleeding D68.9
- blood D75.9
  - in congenital early syphilis A50.09 [D77]
- body dysmorphic F45.22
- bone M89.9
  - continuity M84.9

Disorder — continued
- bone — continued
  - continuity — continued
    - specified type NEC M84.80
      - ankle M84.87- ☑
      - fibula M84.86- ☑
      - foot M84.87- ☑
      - hand M84.84- ☑
      - humerus M84.82- ☑
      - neck M84.88
      - pelvis M84.859
      - radius M84.83- ☑
      - rib M84.88
      - shoulder M84.81- ☑
      - skull M84.88
      - thigh M84.85- ☑
      - tibia M84.86- ☑
      - ulna M84.83- ☑
      - vertebra M84.88
  - density and structure M85.9
    - cyst — see also Cyst, bone, specified type NEC
      - aneurysmal — see Cyst, bone, aneurysmal
      - solitary — see Cyst, bone, solitary
    - diffuse idiopathic skeletal hyperostosis — see Hyperostosis, ankylosing
    - fibrous dysplasia (monostotic) — see Dysplasia, fibrous, bone
    - fluorosis — see Fluorosis, skeletal
    - hyperostosis of skull M85.2
    - osteitis condensans — see Osteitis, condensans
    - specified type NEC M85.8- ☑
      - ankle M85.87- ☑
      - foot M85.87- ☑
      - forearm M85.83- ☑
      - hand M85.84- ☑
      - lower leg M85.86- ☑
      - multiple sites M85.89
      - neck M85.88
      - rib M85.88
      - shoulder M85.81- ☑
      - skull M85.88
      - thigh M85.85- ☑
      - upper arm M85.82- ☑
      - vertebra M85.88
  - development and growth NEC M89.20
    - carpus M89.24- ☑
    - clavicle M89.21- ☑
    - femur M89.25- ☑
    - fibula M89.26- ☑
    - finger M89.24- ☑
    - humerus M89.22- ☑
    - ilium M89.259
    - ischium M89.259
    - metacarpus M89.24- ☑
    - metatarsus M89.27- ☑
    - multiple sites M89.29
    - neck M89.28
    - radius M89.23- ☑
    - rib M89.28
    - scapula M89.21- ☑
    - skull M89.28
    - tarsus M89.27- ☑
    - tibia M89.26- ☑
    - toe M89.27- ☑
    - ulna M89.23- ☑
    - vertebra M89.28
  - specified type NEC M89.8X- ☑
- brachial plexus G54.0
- branched-chain amino-acid metabolism E71.2
  - specified NEC E71.19
- breast N64.9
  - agalactia — see Agalactia
  - associated with
    - lactation O92.70
      - specified NEC O92.79
    - pregnancy O92.20
      - specified NEC O92.29
    - puerperium O92.20
      - specified NEC O92.29
  - cracked nipple — see Cracked nipple
  - galactorrhea — see Galactorrhea
  - hypogalactia O92.4
  - lactation disorder NEC O92.79
  - mastitis — see Mastitis
  - nipple infection — see Infection, nipple
  - retracted nipple — see Retraction, nipple
  - specified type NEC N64.89

Disorder — continued
- Briquet's F45.0
- bullous, in diseases classified elsewhere L14
- caffeine use
  - mild
    - with
      - caffeine-induced
        - anxiety disorder F15.180
        - sleep disorder F15.182
  - moderate or severe
    - with
      - caffeine-induced
        - anxiety disorder F15.280
        - sleep disorder F15.282
- cannabis use
  - mild F12.10
    - with
      - cannabis intoxication delirium F12.121
        - with perceptual disturbances F12.122
        - without perceptual disturbances F12.129
      - cannabis-induced
        - anxiety disorder F12.180
        - psychotic disorder F12.159
        - sleep disorder F12.188
      - in remission (early) (sustained) F12.11
  - moderate or severe F12.20
    - with
      - cannabis intoxication
        - with perceptual disturbances F12.222
        - without perceptual disturbances F12.229
      - cannabis-induced
        - anxiety disorder F12.280
        - psychotic disorder F12.259
        - sleep disorder F12.288
      - delirium F12.221
      - in remission (early) (sustained) F12.21
- carbohydrate
  - absorption, intestinal NEC E74.39
  - metabolism (congenital) E74.9
    - specified NEC E74.8
- cardiac, functional I51.89
- carnitine metabolism E71.40
- cartilage M94.9
  - articular NEC — see Derangement, joint, articular cartilage
  - chondrocalcinosis — see Chondrocalcinosis
  - specified type NEC M94.8X- ☑
    - articular — see Derangement, joint, articular cartilage
    - multiple sites M94.8X0
- catatonia (due to known physiological condition) (with another mental disorder) F06.1
- catatonic
  - due to (secondary to) known physiological condition F06.1
  - organic F06.1
- central auditory processing H93.25
- cervical
  - region NEC M53.82
  - root (nerve) NEC G54.2
- character NOS F60.9
- childhood disintegrative NEC F84.3
- cholesterol and bile acid metabolism E78.70
  - Barth syndrome E78.71
  - other specified E78.79
  - Smith-Lemli-Opitz syndrome E78.72
- choroid H31.9
  - atrophy — see Atrophy, choroid
  - degeneration — see Degeneration, choroid
  - detachment — see Detachment, choroid
  - dystrophy — see Dystrophy, choroid
  - hemorrhage — see Hemorrhage, choroid
  - rupture — see Rupture, choroid
  - scar — see Scar, chorioretinal
  - solar retinopathy — see Retinopathy, solar
  - specified type NEC H31.8
- ciliary body — see Disorder, iris
  - degeneration — see Degeneration, ciliary body
- coagulation (factor) — see also Defect, coagulation D68.9
  - newborn, transient P61.6
- cocaine use
  - mild F14.10
    - with
      - amphetamine, cocaine, or other stimulant intoxication
        - with perceptual disturbances F14.122
        - without perceptual disturbances F14.129

☑ **Additional Character Required** — Refer to the Tabular List for Character Selection   🔼 **Subterms under main terms may continue to next column or page**

isorder — continued
  cocaine use — continued
    mild — continued
      with — continued
        cocaine intoxication delirium F14.121
        cocaine-induced
          anxiety disorder F14.180
          bipolar and related disorder F14.14
          depressive disorder F14.14
          obsessive-compulsive and related disor-
            der F14.188
          psychotic disorder F14.159
          sexual dysfunction F14.181
          sleep disorder F14.182
        in remission (early) (sustained) F14.11
    moderate or severe F14.20
      with
        amphetamine, cocaine, or other stimulant
          intoxication
          with perceptual disturbances F14.222
          without perceptual disturbances F14.229
        cocaine intoxication delirium F14.221
        cocaine-induced
          anxiety disorder F14.280
          bipolar and related disorder F14.24
          depressive disorder F14.24
          obsessive-compulsive and related disor-
            der F14.288
          psychotic disorder F14.259
          sexual dysfunction F14.281
          sleep disorder F14.282
      in remission (early) (sustained) F14.21
coccyx NEC M53.3
cognitive F09
  due to (secondary to) general medical condition F09
  persisting R41.89
    due to
      alcohol F10.97
        with dependence F10.27
      anxiolytics F13.97
        with dependence F13.27
      hypnotics F13.97
        with dependence F13.27
      sedatives F13.97
        with dependence F13.27
      specified substance NEC F19.97
        with
          abuse F19.17
          dependence F19.27
communication F80.9
  social pragmatic F80.82
conduct (childhood) F91.9
  adjustment reaction — see Disorder, adjustment
  adolescent onset type F91.2
  childhood onset type F91.1
  compulsive F63.9
  confined to family context F91.0
  depressive F91.8
  group type F91.2
  hyperkinetic — see Disorder, attention-deficit hy-
    peractivity
  oppositional defiance F91.3
  socialized F91.2
  solitary aggressive type F91.1
  specified NEC F91.8
  unsocialized (aggressive) F91.1
conduction, heart I45.9
congenital glycosylation (CDG) E74.8
conjunctiva H11.9
  infection — see Conjunctivitis
connective tissue, localized L94.9
  specified NEC L94.8
conversion (functional neurological symptom disorder)
  with
    abnormal movement F44.4
    anesthesia or sensory loss F44.6
    attacks or seizures F44.5
    mixed symptoms F44.7
    special sensory symptoms F44.6
    speech symptoms F44.4
    swallowing symptoms F44.4
    weakness or paralysis F44.4
convulsive (secondary) — see Convulsions
cornea H18.9
  deformity — see Deformity, cornea
  degeneration — see Degeneration, cornea
  deposits — see Deposit, cornea
  due to contact lens H18.82- ☑

Disorder — continued
  cornea — continued
    due to contact lens — continued
      specified as edema — see Edema, cornea
    edema — see Edema, cornea
    keratitis — see Keratitis
    keratoconjunctivitis — see Keratoconjunctivitis
    membrane change — see Change, corneal mem-
      brane
    neovascularization — see Neovascularization,
      cornea
    scar — see Opacity, cornea
    specified type NEC H18.89- ☑
    ulcer — see Ulcer, cornea
  corpus cavernosum N48.9
  cranial nerve — see Disorder, nerve, cranial
  cyclothymic F34.0
  defiant oppositional F91.3
  delusional (persistent) (systematized) F22
    induced F24
  depersonalization F48.1
  depressive F32.9
    due to known physiological condition
      with
        depressive features F06.31
        major depressive-like episode F06.32
        mixed features F06.34
    major F32.9
      with psychotic symptoms F32.3
      in remission (full) F32.5
        partial F32.4
      recurrent F33.9
        with psychotic features F33.3
      single episode F32.9
        mild F32.0
        moderate F32.1
        severe (without psychotic symptoms) F32.2
          with psychotic symptoms F32.3
    organic F06.31
    persistent F34.1
    recurrent F33.9
      current episode
        mild F33.0
        moderate F33.1
        severe (without psychotic symptoms) F33.2
          with psychotic symptoms F33.3
      in remission F33.40
        full F33.42
        partial F33.41
      specified NEC F33.8
    single episode — see Episode, depressive
    specified NEC F32.89
  developmental F89
    arithmetical skills F81.2
    coordination (motor) F82
    expressive writing F81.81
    language F80.9
      expressive F80.1
      mixed receptive and expressive F80.2
      receptive type F80.2
      specified NEC F80.89
    learning F81.9
      arithmetical F81.2
      reading F81.0
    mixed F88
    motor coordination or function F82
    pervasive F84.9
      specified NEC F84.8
    phonological F80.0
    reading F81.0
    scholastic skills — see also Disorder, learning
      mixed F81.89
    specified NEC F88
    speech F80.9
      articulation F80.0
      specified NEC F80.89
    written expression F81.81
  diaphragm J98.6
  digestive (system) K92.9
    newborn P78.9
      specified NEC P78.89
    postprocedural — see Complication, gastrointestinal
    psychogenic F45.8
  disc (intervertebral) M51.9
    with
      myelopathy
        cervical region M50.00
        cervicothoracic region M50.03

Disorder — continued
  disc — continued
    with — continued
      myelopathy — continued
        high cervical region M50.01
        lumbar region M51.06
        mid-cervical region M50.020
        sacrococcygeal region M53.3
        thoracic region M51.04
        thoracolumbar region M51.05
      radiculopathy
        cervical region M50.10
        cervicothoracic region M50.13
        high cervical region M50.11
        lumbar region M51.16
        lumbosacral region M51.17
        mid-cervical region M50.120
        sacrococcygeal region M53.3
        thoracic region M51.14
        thoracolumbar region M51.15
    cervical M50.90
      with
        myelopathy M50.00
          C2-C3 M50.01
          C3-C4 M50.01
          C4-C5 M50.021
          C5-C6 M50.022
          C6-C7 M50.023
          C7-T1 M50.03
          cervicothoracic region M50.03
          high cervical region M50.01
          mid-cervical region M50.020
        neuritis, radiculitis or radiculopathy M50.10
          C2-C3 M50.11
          C3-C4 M50.11
          C4-C5 M50.121
          C5-C6 M50.122
          C6-C7 M50.123
          C7-T1 M50.13
          cervicothoracic region M50.13
          high cervical region M50.11
          mid-cervical region M50.120
      C2-C3 M50.91
      C3-C4 M50.91
      C4-C5 M50.921
      C5-C6 M50.922
      C6-C7 M50.923
      C7-T1 M50.93
      cervicothoracic region M50.93
      degeneration M50.30
        C2-C3 M50.31
        C3-C4 M50.31
        C4-C5 M50.321
        C5-C6 M50.322
        C6-C7 M50.323
        C7-T1 M50.33
        cervicothoracic region M50.33
        high cervical region M50.31
        mid-cervical region M50.320
      displacement M50.20
        C2-C3 M50.21
        C3-C4 M50.21
        C4-C5 M50.221
        C5-C6 M50.222
        C6-C7 M50.223
        C7-T1 M50.23
        cervicothoracic region M50.23
        high cervical region M50.21
        mid-cervical region M50.220
      high cervical region M50.91
      mid-cervical region M50.920
      specified type NEC M50.80
        C2-C3 M50.81
        C3-C4 M50.81
        C4-C5 M50.821
        C5-C6 M50.822
        C6-C7 M50.823
        C7-T1 M50.83
        cervicothoracic region M50.83
        high cervical region M50.81
        mid-cervical region M50.820
    specified NEC
      lumbar region M51.86
      lumbosacral region M51.87
      sacrococcygeal region M53.3
      thoracic region M51.84
      thoracolumbar region M51.85
  disinhibited attachment (childhood) F94.2
  disintegrative, childhood NEC F84.3

▼ Subterms under main terms may continue to next column or page　　　☑ Additional Character Required — Refer to the Tabular List for Character Selection　　　111

Disorder — Disorder

Disorder — continued
  disruptive F91.9
    mood dysregulation F34.81
    specified NEC F91.8
  disruptive behavior — see Disorder, conduct
  dissocial personality F60.2
  dissociative F44.9
    affecting
      motor function F44.4
        and sensation F44.7
      sensation F44.6
        and motor function F44.7
    brief reactive F43.0
    due to (secondary to) general medical condition
      F06.8
    mixed F44.7
    organic F06.8
    other specified NEC F44.89
  double heterozygous sickling — see Disease, sickle-cell
  dream anxiety F51.5
  drug induced hemorrhagic D68.32
  drug related F19.99
    abuse — see Abuse, drug
    dependence — see Dependence, drug
  dysmorphic body F45.22
  dysthymic F34.1
  ear H93.9- ☑
    bleeding — see Otorrhagia
    deafness — see Deafness
    degenerative H93.09- ☑
    discharge — see Otorrhea
    external H61.9- ☑
      auditory canal stenosis — see Stenosis, external
        ear canal
      exostosis — see Exostosis, external ear canal
      impacted cerumen — see Impaction, cerumen
      otitis — see Otitis, externa
      perichondritis — see Perichondritis, ear
      pinna — see Disorder, pinna
      specified type NEC H61.89- ☑
    inner H83.9- ☑
      vestibular dysfunction — see Disorder, vestibular
        function
    middle H74.9- ☑
      adhesive H74.1- ☑
      ossicle — see Abnormal, ear ossicles
      polyp — see Polyp, ear (middle)
      specified NEC, in diseases classified elsewhere
        H75.8- ☑
    postprocedural — see Complications, ear, procedure
    specified NEC, in diseases classified elsewhere
      H94.8- ☑
  eating (adult) (psychogenic) F50.9
    anorexia — see Anorexia
    binge F50.81
    bulimia F50.2
    child F98.29
      pica F98.3
      rumination disorder F98.21
    pica F50.89
      childhood F98.3
  electrolyte (balance) NEC E87.8
    with
      abortion — see Abortion by type complicated
        by specified condition NEC
      ectopic pregnancy O08.5
      molar pregnancy O08.5
    acidosis (metabolic) (respiratory) E87.2
    alkalosis (metabolic) (respiratory) E87.3
  elimination, transepidermal L87.9
    specified NEC L87.8
  emotional (persistent) F34.9
    of childhood F93.9
      specified NEC F93.8
  endocrine E34.9
    postprocedural E89.89
    specified NEC E89.89
  erectile (male) (organic) — see also Dysfunction, sexual,
    male, erectile N52.9
    nonorganic F52.21
  erythematous — see Erythema
  esophagus K22.9
    functional K22.4
    psychogenic F45.8
  eustachian tube H69.9- ☑
    infection — see Salpingitis, eustachian
    obstruction — see Obstruction, eustachian tube
    patulous — see Patulous, eustachian tube

Disorder — continued
  eustachian tube — continued
    specified NEC H69.8- ☑
  exhibitionistic F65.2
  extrapyramidal G25.9
    in deseases classified elsewhere — see category
      G26
    specified type NEC G25.89
  eye H57.9
    postprocedural — see Complication, postprocedu-
      ral, eye
  eyelid H02.9
    cyst — see Cyst, eyelid
    degenerative H02.70
      chloasma — see Chloasma, eyelid
      madarosis — see Madarosis
      specified type NEC H02.79
      vitiligo — see Vitiligo, eyelid
      xanthelasma — see Xanthelasma
    dermatochalasis — see Dermatochalasis
    edema — see Edema, eyelid
    elephantiasis — see Elephantiasis, eyelid
    foreign body, retained — see Foreign body, re-
      tained, eyelid
    function H02.59
      abnormal innervation syndrome — see Syn-
        drome, abnormal innervation
      blepharochalasis — see Blepharochalasis
      blepharoclonus — see Blepharoclonus
      blepharophimosis — see Blepharophimosis
      blepharoptosis — see Blepharoptosis
      lagophthalmos — see Lagophthalmos
      lid retraction — see Retraction, lid
    hypertrichosis — see Hypertrichosis, eyelid
    specified type NEC H02.89
    vascular H02.879
      left H02.876
        lower H02.875
        upper H02.874
      right H02.873
        lower H02.872
        upper H02.871
  factitious
    by proxy F68.A
    imposed on another F68.A
    imposed on self F68.10
      with predominantly
        psychological symptoms F68.11
          with physical symptoms F68.13
        physical symptoms F68.12
          with psychological symptoms F68.13
  factor, coagulation — see Defect, coagulation
  fatty acid
    metabolism E71.30
      specified NEC E71.39
    oxidation
      LCAD E71.310
      MCAD E71.311
      SCAD E71.312
      specified deficiency NEC E71.318
  feeding (infant or child) — see also Disorder, eating
    R63.3
    or eating disorder F50.9
    specified NEC F50.9
  feigned (with obvious motivation) Z76.5
    without obvious motivation — see Disorder, facti-
      tious
  female
    hypoactive sexual desire F52.0
    orgasmic F52.31
    sexual interest/arousal F52.22
  fetishistic F65.0
  fibroblastic M72.9
    specified NEC M72.8
  fluency
    adult onset F98.5
    childhood onset F80.81
    following
      cerebral infarction I69.323
      cerebrovascular disease I69.923
        specified disease NEC I69.823
      intracerebral hemorrhage I69.123
      nontraumatic intracranial hemorrhage NEC
        I69.223
      subarachnoid hemorrhage I69.023
    in conditions classified elsewhere R47.82
  fluid balance E87.8
  follicular (skin) L73.9

Disorder — continued
  follicular — continued
    specified NEC L73.8
  frotteuristic F65.81
  fructose metabolism E74.10
    essential fructosuria E74.11
    fructokinase deficiency E74.11
    fructose-1, 6-diphosphatase deficiency E74.19
    hereditary fructose intolerance E74.12
    other specified E74.19
  functional polymorphonuclear neutrophils D71
  gallbladder, biliary tract and pancreas in diseases cla-
    sified elsewhere K87
  gambling F63.0
  gamma aminobutyric acid (GABA) metabolism E72.8
  gamma-glutamyl cycle E72.89
  gastric (functional) K31.9
    motility K30
    psychogenic F45.8
    secretion K30
  gastrointestinal (functional) NOS K92.9
    newborn P78.9
    psychogenic F45.8
  gender-identity or -role F64.9
    childhood F64.2
    effect on relationship F66
    of adolescence or adulthood F64.0
      nontranssexual F64.8
    specified NEC F64.8
    uncertainty F66
  genito-pelvic pain penetration F52.6
  genitourinary system
    female N94.9
    male N50.9
    psychogenic F45.8
  globe H44.9
    degenerated condition H44.50
      absolute glaucoma H44.51- ☑
      atrophy H44.52- ☑
      leucocoria H44.53- ☑
    degenerative H44.30
      chalcosis H44.31- ☑
      myopia — see also Myopia, degenerative
        H44.2- ☑
      siderosis H44.32- ☑
      specified type NEC H44.39- ☑
    endophthalmitis — see Endophthalmitis
    foreign body, retained — see Foreign body, intrao-
      ular, old, retained
    hemophthalmos — see Hemophthalmos
    hypotony H44.40
      due to
        ocular fistula H44.42- ☑
        specified disorder NEC H44.43- ☑
      flat anterior chamber H44.41- ☑
      primary H44.44- ☑
    luxation — see Luxation, globe
    specified type NEC H44.89
  glomerular (in) N05.9
    amyloidosis E85.4 [N08]
    cryoglobulinemia D89.1 [N08]
    disseminated intravascular coagulation D65 [N08]
    Fabry's disease E75.21 [N08]
    familial lecithin cholesterol acyltransferase deficien-
      cy E78.6 [N08]
    Goodpasture's syndrome M31.0
    hemolytic-uremic syndrome D59.3
    Henoch (-Schönlein) purpura D69.0 [N08]
    malariae malaria B52.0
    microscopic polyangiitis M31.7 [N08]
    multiple myeloma C90.0- ☑ [N08]
    mumps B26.83
    schistosomiasis B65.9 [N08]
    sepsis NEC A41.- ☑ [N08]
      streptococcal A40.- ☑ [N08]
    sickle-cell disorders D57.- ☑ [N08]
    strongyloidiasis B78.9 [N08]
    subacute bacterial endocarditis I33.0 [N08]
    syphilis A52.75
    systemic lupus erythematosus M32.14
    thrombotic thrombocytopenic purpura M31.1 [N08]
    Waldenström macroglobulinemia C88.0 [N08]
    Wegener's granulomatosis M31.31
  gluconeogenesis E74.4
  glucosaminoglycan metabolism — see Disorder,
    metabolism, glucosaminoglycan
  glycine metabolism E72.50
    d-glycericacidemia E72.59

  ☑ **Additional Character Required** — **Refer to the Tabular List for Character Selection**   ▽ **Subterms under main terms may continue to next column or page**

isorder — *continued*
- glycine metabolism — *continued*
  - hyperhydroxyprolinemia E72.59
  - hyperoxaluria R82.992
    - primary E72.53
  - hyperprolinemia E72.59
  - non-ketotic hyperglycinemia E72.51
  - oxalosis E72.53
  - oxaluria E72.53
  - sarcosinemia E72.59
  - trimethylaminuria E72.52
- glycoprotein metabolism E77.9
  - specified NEC E77.8
- habit (and impulse) F63.9
  - involving sexual behavior NEC F65.9
  - specified NEC F63.89
- hallucinogen use
  - mild F16.10
    - with
      - hallucinogen intoxication delirium F16.121
      - hallucinogen-induced
        - anxiety disorder F16.180
        - bipolar and related disorder F16.14
        - depressive disorder F16.14
        - psychotic disorder F16.159
      - other hallucinogen intoxication F16.129
    - in remission (early) (sustained) F16.11
  - moderate or severe F16.20
    - with
      - hallucinogen intoxication delirium F16.221
      - hallucinogen-induced
        - anxiety disorder F16.280
        - bipolar and related disorder F16.24
        - depressive disorder F16.24
        - psychotic disorder F16.259
      - other hallucinogen intoxication F16.229
    - in remission (early) (sustained) F16.21
- heart action I49.9
- hematological D75.9
  - newborn (transient) P61.9
    - specified NEC P61.8
- hematopoietic organs D75.9
- hemorrhagic NEC D69.9
  - drug-induced D68.32
  - due to
    - extrinsic circulating anticoagulants D68.32
    - increase in
      - anti-IIa D68.32
      - anti-Xa D68.32
    - intrinsic
      - circulating anticoagulants D68.318
      - increase in
        - anti-IXa D68.318
        - antithrombin D68.318
        - anti-VIIIa D68.318
        - anti-XIa D68.318
  - following childbirth O72.3
- hemostasis — *see* Defect, coagulation
- histidine metabolism E70.40
  - histidinemia E70.41
  - other specified E70.49
- hoarding F42.3
- hyperkinetic — *see* Disorder, attention-deficit hyperactivity
- hyperleucine-isoleucinemia E71.19
- hypervalinemia E71.19
- hypoactive sexual desire F52.0
- hypochondriacal F45.20
  - body dysmorphic F45.22
  - neurosis F45.21
  - other specified F45.29
- identity
  - dissociative F44.81
  - illness anxiety F45.21
  - of childhood F93.8
- immune mechanism (immunity) D89.9
  - specified type NEC D89.89
- impaired renal tubular function N25.9
  - specified NEC N25.89
- impulse (control) F63.9
- inflammatory
  - pelvic, in diseases classified elsewhere — *see* category N74
  - penis N48.29
    - abscess N48.21
    - cellulitis N48.22
- inhalant use
  - mild F18.10

Disorder — *continued*
- inhalant use — *continued*
  - mild — *continued*
    - with
      - inhalant intoxication F18.129
      - inhalant intoxication delirium F18.121
      - inhalant-induced
        - anxiety disorder F18.180
        - depressive disorder F18.14
        - major neurocognitive disorder F18.17
        - mild neurocognitive disorder F18.188
        - psychotic disorder F18.159
    - in remission (early) (sustained) F18.11
  - moderate or severe F18.20
    - with
      - inhalant intoxication F18.229
      - inhalant intoxication delirium F18.221
      - inhalant-induced
        - anxiety disorder F18.280
        - depressive disorder F18.24
        - major neurocognitive disorder F18.27
        - mild neurocognitive disorder F18.288
        - psychotic disorder F18.259
    - in remission (early) (sustained) F18.21
- integument, newborn P83.9
  - specified NEC P83.88
- intermittent explosive F63.81
- internal secretion pancreas — *see* Increased, secretion, pancreas, endocrine
- intestine, intestinal
  - carbohydrate absorption NEC E74.39
    - postoperative K91.2
  - functional NEC K59.9
    - postoperative K91.89
  - psychogenic F45.8
  - vascular K55.9
    - chronic K55.1
    - specified NEC K55.8
- intraoperative (intraprocedural) — *see* Complications, intraoperative
- involuntary emotional expression (IEED) F07.89
- iris H21.9
  - adhesions — *see* Adhesions, iris
  - atrophy — *see* Atrophy, iris
  - chamber angle recession — *see* Recession, chamber angle
  - cyst — *see* Cyst, iris
  - degeneration — *see* Degeneration, iris
  - in diseases classified elsewhere H22
  - iridodialysis — *see* Iridodialysis
  - iridoschisis — *see* Iridoschisis
  - miotic pupillary cyst — *see* Cyst, pupillary
  - pupillary
    - abnormality — *see* Abnormality, pupillary
    - membrane — *see* Membrane, pupillary
  - specified type NEC H21.89
  - vascular NEC H21.1X- ☑
- iron metabolism E83.10
  - specified NEC E83.19
- isovaleric acidemia E71.110
- jaw, developmental M27.0
  - temporomandibular — *see also* Anomaly, dentofacial, temporomandibular joint M26.60- ☑
- joint M25.9
  - derangement — *see* Derangement, joint
  - effusion — *see* Effusion, joint
  - fistula — *see* Fistula, joint
  - hemarthrosis — *see* Hemarthrosis
  - instability — *see* Instability, joint
  - osteophyte — *see* Osteophyte
  - pain — *see* Pain, joint
  - psychogenic F45.8
  - specified type NEC M25.80
    - ankle M25.87- ☑
    - elbow M25.82- ☑
    - foot joint M25.87- ☑
    - hand joint M25.84- ☑
    - hip M25.85- ☑
    - knee M25.86- ☑
    - shoulder M25.81- ☑
    - wrist M25.83- ☑
  - stiffness — *see* Stiffness, joint
- ketone metabolism E71.32
- kidney N28.9
  - functional (tubular) N25.9
  - in
    - schistosomiasis B65.9 *[N29]*
    - tubular function N25.9

Disorder — *continued*
- kidney — *continued*
  - tubular function — *continued*
    - specified NEC N25.89
- lacrimal system H04.9
  - changes H04.69
    - fistula — *see* Fistula, lacrimal
  - gland H04.19
    - atrophy — *see* Atrophy, lacrimal gland
    - cyst — *see* Cyst, lacrimal, gland
    - dacryops — *see* Dacryops
    - dislocation — *see* Dislocation, lacrimal gland
    - dry eye syndrome — *see* Syndrome, dry eye
    - infection — *see* Dacryoadenitis
    - granuloma — *see* Granuloma, lacrimal
    - inflammation — *see* Inflammation, lacrimal
    - obstruction — *see* Obstruction, lacrimal
    - specified NEC H04.89
- lactation NEC O92.79
- language (developmental) F80.9
  - expressive F80.1
  - mixed receptive and expressive F80.2
  - receptive F80.2
- late luteal phase dysphoric N94.89
- learning (specific) F81.9
  - acalculia R48.8
  - alexia R48.0
  - mathematics F81.2
  - reading F81.0
  - specified
    - with impairment in
      - mathematics F81.2
      - reading F81.0
      - written expression F81.81
  - specified NEC F81.89
  - spelling F81.81
  - written expression F81.81
- lens H27.9
  - aphakia — *see* Aphakia
  - cataract — *see* Cataract
  - dislocation — *see* Dislocation, lens
  - specified type NEC H27.8
- ligament M24.20
  - ankle M24.27- ☑
  - attachment, spine — *see* Enthesopathy, spinal
  - elbow M24.22- ☑
  - foot joint M24.27- ☑
  - hand joint M24.24- ☑
  - hip M24.25- ☑
  - knee — *see* Derangement, knee, specified NEC
  - shoulder M24.21- ☑
  - vertebra M24.28
  - wrist M24.23- ☑
- ligamentous attachments — *see also* Enthesopathy
  - spine — *see* Enthesopathy, spinal
- lipid
  - metabolism, congenital E78.9
  - storage E75.6
    - specified NEC E75.5
- lipoprotein
  - deficiency (familial) E78.6
  - metabolism E78.9
    - specified NEC E78.89
- liver K76.9
  - malarial B54 *[K77]*
- low back — *see also* Dorsopathy, specified NEC
- lumbosacral
  - plexus G54.1
  - root (nerve) NEC G54.4
- lung, interstitial, drug-induced J70.4
  - acute J70.2
  - chronic J70.3
- lymphoproliferative, post-transplant (PTLD) D47.Z1 (*following* D47.4)
- lysine and hydroxylysine metabolism E72.3
- major neurocognitive — *see* Dementia, in (due to)
- male
  - erectile (organic) — *see also* Dysfunction, sexual, male, erectile N52.9
    - nonorganic F52.21
  - hypoactive sexual desire F52.0
  - orgasmic F52.32
- manic F30.9
  - organic F06.33
- mast cell activation — *see* Activation, mast cell
- mastoid — *see also* Disorder, ear, middle
  - postprocedural — *see* Complications, ear, procedure
- meniscus — *see* Derangement, knee, meniscus

☞ Subterms under main terms may continue to next column or page   ☑ Additional Character Required — Refer to the Tabular List for Character Selection   **113**

Disorder — Disorder

Disorder — *continued*
menopausal N95.9
specified NEC N95.8
menstrual N92.6
psychogenic F45.8
specified NEC N92.5
mental (or behavioral) (nonpsychotic) F99
due to (secondary to)
amphetamine
due to drug abuse — *see* Abuse, drug, stimulant
due to drug dependence — *see* Dependence, drug, stimulant
brain disease, damage and dysfunction F09
caffeine use
due to drug abuse — *see* Abuse, drug, stimulant
due to drug dependence — *see* Dependence, drug, stimulant
cannabis use
due to drug abuse — *see* Abuse, drug, cannabis
due to drug dependence — *see* Dependence, drug, cannabis
general medical condition F09
sedative or hypnotic use
due to drug abuse — *see* Abuse, drug, sedative
due to drug dependence — *see* Dependence, drug, sedative
tobacco (nicotine) use — *see* Dependence, drug, nicotine
following organic brain damage F07.9
frontal lobe syndrome F07.0
personality change F07.0
postconcussional syndrome F07.81
specified NEC F07.89
infancy, childhood or adolescence F98.9
neurotic — *see* Neurosis
organic or symptomatic F09
presenile, psychotic F03 ☑
problem NEC
psychoneurotic — *see* Neurosis
psychotic — *see* Psychosis
puerperal F53.0
senile, psychotic NEC F03 ☑
metabolic, amino acid, transitory, newborn P74.8
metabolism NOS E88.9
amino-acid E72.9
aromatic E70.9
albinism — *see* Albinism
histidine E70.40
histidinemia E70.41
other specified E70.49
hyperphenylalaninemia E70.1
classical phenylketonuria E70.0
other specified E70.8
tryptophan E70.5
tyrosine E70.20
hypertyrosinemia E70.21
other specified E70.29
branched chain E71.2
3-methylglutaconic aciduria E71.111
hyperleucine-isoleucinemia E71.19
hypervalinemia E71.19
isovaleric acidemia E71.110
maple syrup urine disease E71.0
methylmalonic acidemia E71.120
organic aciduria NEC E71.118
other specified E71.19
proprionate NEC E71.128
proprionic acidemia E71.121
glycine E72.50
d-glycericacidemia E72.59
hyperhydroxyprolinemia E72.59
hyperoxaluria R82.992
primary E72.53
hyperprolinemia E72.59
non-ketotic hyperglycinemia E72.51
other specified E72.59
sarcosinemia E72.59
trimethylaminuria E72.52
hydroxylysine E72.3
lysine E72.3
ornithine E72.4
other specified E72.89
beta amino acid E72.09
gamma-glutamyl cycle E72.89

Disorder — *continued*
metabolism — *continued*
amino-acid — *continued*
straight-chain E72.89
sulfur-bearing E72.10
homocystinuria E72.11
methylenetetrahydrofolate reductase deficiency E72.12
other specified E72.19
bile acid and cholesterol metabolism E78.70
bilirubin E80.7
specified NEC E80.6
calcium E83.50
hypercalcemia E83.52
hypocalcemia E83.51
other specified E83.59
carbohydrate E74.9
specified NEC E74.8
cholesterol and bile acid metabolism E78.70
congenital E88.9
copper E83.00
specified type NEC E83.09
Wilson's disease E83.01
cystinuria E72.01
fructose E74.10
galactose E74.20
glucosaminoglycan E76.9
mucopolysaccharidosis — *see* Mucopolysaccharidosis
specified NEC E76.8
glutamine E72.89
glycine E72.50
glycogen storage (hepatorenal) E74.09
glycoprotein E77.9
specified NEC E77.8
glycosaminoglycan E76.9
specified NEC E76.8
in labor and delivery O75.89
iron E83.10
isoleucine E71.19
leucine E71.19
lipoid E78.9
lipoprotein E78.9
specified NEC E78.89
magnesium E83.40
hypermagnesemia E83.41
hypomagnesemia E83.42
other specified E83.49
mineral E83.9
specified NEC E83.89
mitochondrial E88.40
MELAS syndrome E88.41
MERRF syndrome (myoclonic epilepsy associated with ragged-red fibers) E88.42
other specified E88.49
ornithine E72.4
phosphatases E83.30
phosphorus E83.30
acid phosphatase deficiency E83.39
hypophosphatasia E83.39
hypophosphatemia E83.39
familial E83.31
other specified E83.39
pseudovitamin D deficiency E83.32
plasma protein NEC E88.09
porphyrin — *see* Porphyria
postprocedural E89.89
specified NEC E89.89
purine E79.9
specified NEC E79.8
pyrimidine E79.9
specified NEC E79.8
pyruvate E74.4
serine E72.89
sodium E87.8
specified NEC E88.89
threonine E72.89
valine E71.19
zinc E83.2
methylmalonic acidemia E71.120
micturition NEC — *see also* Difficulty, micturition R39.198
feeling of incomplete emptying R39.14
hesitancy R39.11
poor stream R39.12
psychogenic F45.8
split stream R39.13
straining R39.16
urgency R39.15

Disorder — *continued*
mild neurocognitive G31.84
mitochondrial metabolism E88.40
mitral (valve) — *see* Endocarditis, mitral
mixed
anxiety and depressive F41.8
of scholastic skills (developmental) F81.89
receptive expressive language F80.2
mood F39
bipolar — *see* Disorder, bipolar
depressive — *see* Disorder, depressive
due to (secondary to)
alcohol F10.94
amphetamine F15.94
in
abuse F15.14
dependence F15.24
anxiolytic F13.94
in
abuse F13.14
dependence F13.24
cocaine F14.94
in
abuse F14.14
dependence F14.24
general medical condition F06.30
hallucinogen F16.94
in
abuse F16.14
dependence F16.24
hypnotic F13.94
in
abuse F13.14
dependence F13.24
inhalant F18.94
in
abuse F18.14
dependence F18.24
opioid F11.94
in
abuse F11.14
dependence F11.24
phencyclidine (PCP) F16.94
in
abuse F16.14
dependence F16.24
physiological condition F06.30
with
depressive features F06.31
major depressive-like episode F06.32
manic features F06.33
mixed features F06.34
psychoactive substance NEC F19.94
in
abuse F19.14
dependence F19.24
sedative F13.94
in
abuse F13.14
dependence F13.24
volatile solvents F18.94
in
abuse F18.14
dependence F18.24
manic episode F30.9
with psychotic symptoms F30.2
in remission (full) F30.4
partial F30.3
specified type NEC F30.8
without psychotic symptoms F30.10
mild F30.11
moderate F30.12
severe F30.13
organic F06.30
right hemisphere F07.89
persistent F34.9
cyclothymia F34.0
dysthymia F34.1
specified type NEC F34.89
recurrent F39
right hemisphere organic F07.89
movement G25.9
drug-induced G25.70
akathisia G25.71
specified NEC G25.79
hysterical F44.4
in diseases classified elsewhere — *see category* G2
periodic limb G47.61
sleep related G47.61

☑ Additional Character Required — Refer to the Tabular List for Character Selection ▽ Subterms under main terms may continue to next column or page

isorder — continued
  movement — continued
    sleep related NEC G47.69
    specified NEC G25.89
    stereotyped F98.4
    treatment-induced G25.9
  multiple personality F44.81
  muscle M62.9
    attachment, spine — see Enthesopathy, spinal
    in trichinellosis — see Trichinellosis, with muscle
      disorder
    psychogenic F45.8
    specified type NEC M62.89
    tone, newborn P94.9
      specified NEC P94.8
  muscular
    attachments — see also Enthesopathy
      spine — see Enthesopathy, spinal
    urethra N36.44
  musculoskeletal system, soft tissue — see Disorder,
    soft tissue
    postprocedural M96.89
    psychogenic F45.8
  myoneural G70.9
    due to lead G70.1
    specified NEC G70.89
    toxic G70.1
  myotonic NEC G71.19
  nail, in diseases classified elsewhere L62
  neck region NEC — see Dorsopathy, specified NEC
  neonatal onset multisystemic inflammatory (NOMID)
    M04.2
  nerve G58.9
    abducent NEC — see Strabismus, paralytic, sixth
      nerve
    accessory G52.8
    acoustic — see subcategory H93.3 ☑
    auditory — see subcategory H93.3 ☑
    auriculotemporal G50.8
    axillary G54.0
    cerebral — see Disorder, nerve, cranial
    cranial G52.9
      eighth — see subcategory H93.3 ☑
      eleventh G52.8
      fifth G50.9
      first G52.0
      fourth NEC — see Strabismus, paralytic, fourth
        nerve
      multiple G52.7
      ninth G52.1
      second NEC — see Disorder, nerve, optic
      seventh NEC G51.8
      sixth NEC — see Strabismus, paralytic, sixth nerve
      specified NEC G52.8
      tenth G52.2
      third NEC — see Strabismus, paralytic, third nerve
      twelfth G52.3
    entrapment — see Neuropathy, entrapment
    facial G51.9
      specified NEC G51.8
    femoral — see Lesion, nerve, femoral
    glossopharyngeal NEC G52.1
    hypoglossal G52.3
    intercostal G58.0
    lateral
      cutaneous of thigh — see Mononeuropathy,
        lower limb, meralgia paresthetica
      popliteal — see Lesion, nerve, popliteal
    lower limb — see Mononeuropathy, lower limb
    medial popliteal — see Lesion, nerve, popliteal,
      medial
    median NEC — see Lesion, nerve, median
    multiple G58.7
    oculomotor NEC — see Strabismus, paralytic, third
      nerve
    olfactory G52.0
    optic NEC H47.09- ☑
      hemorrhage into sheath — see Hemorrhage,
        optic nerve
      ischemic H47.01- ☑
    peroneal — see Lesion, nerve, popliteal
    phrenic G58.8
    plantar — see Lesion, nerve, plantar
    pneumogastric G52.2
    posterior tibial — see Syndrome, tarsal tunnel
    radial — see Lesion, nerve, radial
    recurrent laryngeal G52.2
    root G54.9

Disorder — continued
  nerve — continued
    root — continued
      cervical G54.2
      lumbosacral G54.1
      specified NEC G54.8
      thoracic G54.3
    sciatic NEC — see Lesion, nerve, sciatic
    specified NEC G58.8
      lower limb — see Mononeuropathy, lower limb,
        specified NEC
      upper limb — see Mononeuropathy, upper limb,
        specified NEC
    sympathetic G90.9
    tibial — see Lesion, nerve, popliteal, medial
    trigeminal G50.9
      specified NEC G50.8
    trochlear NEC — see Strabismus, paralytic, fourth
      nerve
    ulnar — see Lesion, nerve, ulnar
    upper limb — see Mononeuropathy, upper limb
    vagus G52.2
  nervous system G98.8
    autonomic (peripheral) G90.9
      specified NEC G90.8
    central G96.9
      specified NEC G96.8
    parasympathetic G90.9
    specified NEC G98.8
    sympathetic G90.9
    vegetative G90.9
  neurocognitive R41.9
    major
      with
        aggressive behavior F01.51
        combative behavior F01.51
        violent behavior F01.51
      due to vascular disease, with behavioral distur-
        bance F01.51
      in (due to) (other diseases classified elsewhere)
        — see also Dementia, in (due to) F02.80
        with
          aggressive behavior F02.81
          combative behavior F02.81
          violent behavior F02.81
      without behavioral disturbance F01.50
    mild G31.84
  neurodevelopmental F89
    specified NEC F88
  neurohypophysis NEC E23.3
  neurological NEC R29.818
  neuromuscular G70.9
    hereditary NEC G71.9
    specified NEC G70.89
    toxic G70.1
  neurotic F48.9
    specified NEC F48.8
  neutrophil, polymorphonuclear D71
  nicotine use — see Dependence, drug, nicotine
  nightmare F51.5
  non-rapid eye movement sleep arousal
    sleep terror type F51.4
    sleepwalking type F51.3
  nose J34.9
    specified NEC J34.89
  obsessive-compulsive F42.9
    and related disorder due to a known physiological
      condition F06.8
  odontogenesis NOS K00.9
  opioid use
    with
      opioid-induced psychotic disorder F11.959
        with
          delusions F11.950
          hallucinations F11.951
    due to drug abuse — see Abuse, drug, opioid
    due to drug dependence — see Dependence, drug,
      opioid
    mild F11.10
      with
        opioid-induced
          anxiety disorder F11.188
          depressive disorder F11.14
          sexual dysfunction F11.181
        opioid intoxication
          with perceptual disturbances F11.122
          delirium F11.121
          without perceptual disturbances F11.129

Disorder — continued
  opioid use — continued
    mild — continued
      in remission (early) (sustained) F11.11
    moderate or severe F11.20
      with
        opioid-induced
          anxiety disorder F11.288
          anxiety disorder F11.988
          depressive disorder F11.24
          depressive disorder F11.94
          sexual dysfunction F11.281
          sexual dysfunction F11.981
        opioid intoxication
          with perceptual disturbances F11.222
          delirium F11.221
          without perceptual disturbances F11.229
      in remission (early) (sustained) F11.21
  oppositional defiant F91.3
  optic
    chiasm H47.49
      due to
        inflammatory disorder H47.41
        neoplasm H47.42
        vascular disorder H47.43
    disc H47.39- ☑
      coloboma — see Coloboma, optic disc
      drusen — see Drusen, optic disc
      pseudopapilledema — see Pseudopapilledema
    radiations — see Disorder, visual, pathway
    tracts — see Disorder, visual, pathway
  orbit H05.9
    cyst — see Cyst, orbit
    deformity — see Deformity, orbit
    edema — see Edema, orbit
    enophthalmos — see Enophthalmos
    exophthalmos — see Exophthalmos
    hemorrhage — see Hemorrhage, orbit
    inflammation — see Inflammation, orbit
    myopathy — see Myopathy, extraocular muscles
    retained foreign body — see Foreign body, orbit,
      old
    specified type NEC H05.89
  organic
    anxiety F06.4
    catatonic F06.1
    delusional F06.2
    dissociative F06.8
    emotionally labile (asthenic) F06.8
    mood (affective) F06.30
    schizophrenia-like F06.2
  orgasmic (female) F52.31
    male F52.32
  ornithine metabolism E72.4
  overanxious F41.1
    of childhood F93.8
  pain
    with related psychological factors F45.42
    exclusively related to psychological factors F45.41
    genito-pelvic penetration disorder F52.6
  pancreatic internal secretion E16.9
    specified NEC E16.8
  panic F41.0
    with agoraphobia F40.01
  papulosquamous L44.9
    in diseases classified elsewhere L45
    specified NEC L44.8
  paranoid F22
    induced F24
    shared F24
  paraphilic F65.9
    specified NEC F65.89
  parathyroid (gland) E21.5
    specified NEC E21.4
  parietoalveolar NEC J84.09
  paroxysmal, mixed R56.9
  patella M22.9- ☑
    chondromalacia — see Chondromalacia, patella
    derangement NEC M22.3X- ☑
    recurrent
      dislocation — see Dislocation, patella, recurrent
      subluxation — see Dislocation, patella, recurrent,
        incomplete
    specified NEC M22.8X- ☑
  patellofemoral M22.2X- ☑
  pedophilic F65.4
  pentose phosphate pathway with anemia D55.1
  perception, due to hallucinogens F16.983

Subterms under main terms may continue to next column or page   ☑ Additional Character Required — Refer to the Tabular List for Character Selection   115

Disorder — Disorder

Disorder — *continued*
  perception, due to hallucinogens — *continued*
    in
      abuse F16.183
      dependence F16.283
  peripheral nervous system NEC G64
  peroxisomal E71.50
    biogenesis
      neonatal adrenoleukodystrophy E71.511
      specified disorder NEC E71.518
      Zellweger syndrome E71.510
    rhizomelic chondrodysplasia punctata E71.540
    specified form NEC E71.548
      group 1 E71.518
      group 2 E71.53
      group 3 E71.542
    X-linked adrenoleukodystrophy E71.529
      adolescent E71.521
      adrenomyeloneuropathy E71.522
      childhood E71.520
      specified form NEC E71.528
    Zellweger-like syndrome E71.541
  persistent
    (somatoform) pain F45.41
    affective (mood) F34.9
  personality — *see also* Personality F60.9
    affective F34.0
    aggressive F60.3
    amoral F60.2
    anankastic F60.5
    antisocial F60.2
    anxious F60.6
    asocial F60.2
    asthenic F60.7
    avoidant F60.6
    borderline F60.3
    change (secondary) due to general medical condi-
        tion F07.0
    compulsive F60.5
    cyclothymic F34.0
    dependent (passive) F60.7
    depressive F34.1
    dissocial F60.2
    emotional instability F60.3
    expansive paranoid F60.0
    explosive F60.3
    following organic brain damage F07.9
    histrionic F60.4
    hyperthymic F34.0
    hypothymic F34.1
    hysterical F60.4
    immature F60.89
    inadequate F60.7
    labile F60.3
    mixed (nonspecific) F60.89
    moral deficiency F60.2
    narcissistic F60.81
    negativistic F60.89
    obsessional F60.5
    obsessive (-compulsive) F60.5
    organic F07.9
    overconscientious F60.5
    paranoid F60.0
    passive (-dependent) F60.7
    passive-aggressive F60.89
    pathological NEC F60.9
    pseudosocial F60.2
    psychopathic F60.2
    schizoid F60.1
    schizotypal F21
    self-defeating F60.7
    specified NEC F60.89
    type A F60.5
    unstable (emotional) F60.3
  pervasive, developmental F84.9
  phencyclidine use
    mild F16.10
      with
        phencyclidine intoxication F16.129
        phencyclidine intoxication delirium F16.121
        phencyclidine-induced
          anxiety disorder F16.180
          bipolar and related disorder F16.14
          depressive disorder F16.14
          psychotic disorder F16.159
      in remission (early) (sustained) F16.11
    moderate or severe F16.20
      with
        phencyclidine intoxication F16.229

Disorder — *continued*
  phencyclidine use — *continued*
    moderate or severe — *continued*
      with — *continued*
        phencyclidine intoxication delirium F16.221
        phencyclidine-induced
          anxiety disorder F16.280
          bipolar and related disorder F16.14
          depressive disorder F16.24
          psychotic disorder F16.259
      in remission (early) (sustained) F16.21
  phobic anxiety, childhood F40.8
  phosphate-losing tubular N25.0
  pigmentation L81.9
    choroid, congenital Q14.3
    diminished melanin formation L81.6
    iron L81.8
    specified NEC L81.8
  pinna (noninfective) H61.10- ☑
    deformity, acquired H61.11- ☑
    hematoma H61.12- ☑
    perichondritis — *see* Perichondritis, ear
    specified type NEC H61.19- ☑
  pituitary gland E23.7
    iatrogenic (postprocedural) E89.3
    specified NEC E23.6
  platelets D69.1
  plexus G54.9
    specified NEC G54.8
  polymorphonuclear neutrophils D71
  porphyrin metabolism — *see* Porphyria
  postconcussional F07.81
  posthallucinogen perception F16.983
    in
      abuse F16.183
      dependence F16.283
  postmenopausal N95.9
    specified NEC N95.8
  postprocedural (postoperative) — *see* Complications,
      postprocedural
  post-transplant lymphoproliferative D47.Z1 (*following*
      D47.4)
  post-traumatic stress (PTSD) F43.10
    acute F43.11
    chronic F43.12
  premenstrual dysphoric (PMDD) F32.81
  prepuce N47.8
  propionic acidemia E71.121
  prostate N42.9
    specified NEC N42.89
  psychogenic NOS — *see also* condition F45.9
    anxiety F41.8
    appetite F50.9
    asthenic F48.8
    cardiovascular (system) F45.8
    compulsive F42.8
    cutaneous F54
    depressive F32.9
    digestive (system) F45.8
    dysmenorrheic F45.8
    dyspneic F45.8
    endocrine (system) F54
    eye NEC F45.8
    feeding — *see* Disorder, eating
    functional NEC F45.8
    gastric F45.8
    gastrointestinal (system) F45.8
    genitourinary (system) F45.8
    heart (function) (rhythm) F45.8
    hyperventilatory F45.8
    hypochondriacal — *see* Disorder, hypochondriacal
    intestinal F45.8
    joint F45.8
    learning F81.9
    limb F45.8
    lymphatic (system) F45.8
    menstrual F45.8
    micturition F45.8
    monoplegic NEC F44.4
    motor F44.4
    muscle F45.8
    musculoskeletal F45.8
    neurocirculatory F45.8
    obsessive F42.8
    occupational F48.8
    organ or part of body NEC F45.8
    paralytic NEC F44.4
    phobic F40.9

Disorder — *continued*
  psychogenic — *see also* condition — *continued*
    physical NEC F45.8
    rectal F45.8
    respiratory (system) F45.8
    rheumatic F45.8
    sexual (function) F52.9
    skin (allergic) (eczematous) F54
    sleep F51.9
    specified part of body NEC F45.8
    stomach F45.8
  psychological F99
    associated with
      disease classified elsewhere F54
      sexual
        development F66
        relationship F66
      uncertainty about gender identity F64.9
  psychomotor NEC F44.4
    hysterical F44.4
  psychoneurotic — *see also* Neurosis
    mixed NEC F48.8
  psychophysiologic — *see* Disorder, somatoform
  psychosexual F65.9
    development F66
    identity of childhood F64.2
  psychosomatic NOS — *see* Disorder, somatoform
    multiple F45.0
    undifferentiated F45.1
  psychotic — *see* Psychosis
    transient (acute) F23
  puberty E30.9
    specified NEC E30.8
  pulmonary (valve) — *see* Endocarditis, pulmonary
  purine metabolism E79.9
  pyrimidine metabolism E79.9
  pyruvate metabolism E74.4
  reactive attachment (childhood) F94.1
  reading R48.0
    developmental (specific) F81.0
  receptive language F80.2
  receptor, hormonal, peripheral — *see also* Syndrom
      androgen insensitivity E34.50
  recurrent brief depressive F33.8
  reflex R29.2
  refraction H52.7
    aniseikonia H52.32
    anisometropia H52.31
    astigmatism — *see* Astigmatism
    hypermetropia — *see* Hypermetropia
    myopia — *see* Myopia
    presbyopia H52.4
    specified NEC H52.6
  relationship F68.8
    due to sexual orientation F66
  REM sleep behavior G47.52
  renal function, impaired (tubular) N25.9
  resonance R49.9
    specified NEC R49.8
  respiratory function, impaired — *see also* Failure, re
      piration
    postprocedural — *see* Complication, postoperativ
        respiratory system
    psychogenic F45.8
  retina H35.9
    angioid streaks H35.33
    changes in vascular appearance H35.01- ☑
    degeneration — *see* Degeneration, retina
    dystrophy (hereditary) — *see* Dystrophy, retina
    edema H35.81
    hemorrhage — *see* Hemorrhage, retina
    ischemia H35.82
    macular degeneration — *see* Degeneration, macul
    microaneurysms H35.04- ☑
    microvascular abnormality NEC H35.09
    neovascularization — *see* Neovascularization, retir
    retinopathy — *see* Retinopathy
    separation of layers H35.70
      central serous chorioretinopathy H35.71- ☑
      pigment epithelium detachment (serous)
          H35.72- ☑
      hemorrhagic H35.73- ☑
    specified type NEC H35.89
    telangiectasis — *see* Telangiectasis, retina
    vasculitis — *see* Vasculitis, retina
  retroperitoneal K68.9
  right hemisphere organic affective F07.89
  rumination (infant or child) F98.21

☑ **Additional Character Required** — Refer to the Tabular List for Character Selection   ▽ **Subterms under main terms may continue to next column or page**

Disorder — *continued*
- sacrum, sacrococcygeal NEC M53.3
- schizoaffective F25.9
  - bipolar type F25.0
  - depressive type F25.1
  - manic type F25.0
  - mixed type F25.0
  - specified NEC F25.8
- schizoid of childhood F84.5
- schizophrenia spectrum and other psychotic disorder F29
  - specified NEC F28
- schizophreniform F20.81
  - brief F23
- schizotypal (personality) F21
- secretion, thyrocalcitonin E07.0
- sedative, hypnotic, or anxiolytic use
  - mild F13.10
    - with
      - sedative, hypnotic, or anxiolytic intoxication F13.129
      - sedative, hypnotic, or anxiolytic intoxication delirium F13.121
      - sedative, hypnotic, or anxiolytic-induced
        - anxiety disorder F13.180
        - bipolar and related disorder F13.14
        - depressive disorder F13.14
        - psychotic disorder F13.159
        - sexual dysfunction F13.181
      - in remission (early) (sustained) F13.11
  - moderate or severe F13.20
    - with
      - sedative, hypnotic, or anxiolytic intoxication F13.229
      - sedative, hypnotic, or anxiolytic intoxication delirium F13.221
      - sedative, hypnotic, or anxiolytic-induced
        - anxiety disorder F13.280
        - bipolar and related disorder F13.24
        - depressive disorder F13.24
        - major neurocognitive disorder F13.27
        - mild neurocognitive disorder F13.288
        - psychotic disorder F13.259
        - sexual dysfunction F13.281
      - in remission (early) (sustained) F13.21
- seizure — *see also* Epilepsy G40.909
  - intractable G40.919
    - with status epilepticus G40.911
- semantic pragmatic F80.89
  - with autism F84.0
- sense of smell R43.1
  - psychogenic F45.8
- separation anxiety, of childhood F93.0
- sexual
  - aversion F52.1
  - function, psychogenic F52.9
  - interest/arousal, female F52.22
  - masochism F65.51
  - maturation F66
  - nonorganic F52.9
  - preference — *see also* Deviation, sexual F65.9
    - fetishistic transvestism F65.1
  - relationship F66
  - sadism F65.52
- shyness, of childhood and adolescence F40.10
- sibling rivalry F93.8
- sickle-cell (sickling) (homozygous) — *see* Disease, sickle-cell
  - heterozygous D57.3
  - specified type NEC D57.8- ☑
  - trait D57.3
- sinus (nasal) J34.9
  - specified NEC J34.89
- skin L98.9
  - atrophic L90.9
    - specified NEC L90.8
  - granulomatous L92.9
    - specified NEC L92.8
  - hypertrophic L91.9
    - specified NEC L91.8
  - infiltrative NEC L98.6
  - newborn P83.9
    - specified NEC P83.88
  - picking F42.4
  - psychogenic (allergic) (eczematous) F54
- sleep G47.9
  - breathing-related — *see* Apnea, sleep
  - circadian rhythm G47.20
    - advance sleep phase type G47.22

Disorder — *continued*
- sleep — *continued*
  - circadian rhythm — *continued*
    - delayed sleep phase type G47.21
    - due to
      - alcohol
        - abuse F10.182
        - dependence F10.282
        - use F10.982
      - amphetamines
        - abuse F15.182
        - dependence F15.282
        - use F15.982
      - caffeine
        - abuse F15.182
        - dependence F15.282
        - use F15.982
      - cocaine
        - abuse F14.182
        - dependence F14.282
        - use F14.982
      - drug NEC
        - abuse F19.182
        - dependence F19.282
        - use F19.982
      - opioid
        - abuse F11.182
        - dependence F11.282
        - use F11.982
      - psychoactive substance NEC
        - abuse F19.182
        - dependence F19.282
        - use F19.982
      - sedative, hypnotic, or anxiolytic
        - abuse F13.182
        - dependence F13.282
        - use F13.982
      - stimulant NEC
        - abuse F15.182
        - dependence F15.282
        - use F15.982
    - free running type G47.24
    - in conditions classified elsewhere G47.27
    - irregular sleep wake type G47.23
    - jet lag type G47.25
    - non 24 hour sleep wake type G47.24
    - shift work type G47.26
    - specified NEC G47.29
  - due to
    - alcohol
      - abuse F10.182
      - dependence F10.282
      - use F10.982
    - amphetamine
      - abuse F15.182
      - dependence F15.282
      - use F15.982
    - anxiolytic
      - abuse F13.182
      - dependence F13.282
      - use F13.982
    - caffeine
      - abuse F15.182
      - dependence F15.282
      - use F15.982
    - cocaine
      - abuse F14.182
      - dependence F14.282
      - use F14.982
    - drug NEC
      - abuse F19.182
      - dependence F19.282
      - use F19.982
    - hypnotic
      - abuse F13.182
      - dependence F13.282
      - use F13.982
    - opioid
      - abuse F11.182
      - dependence F11.282
      - use F11.982
    - psychoactive substance NEC
      - abuse F19.182
      - dependence F19.282
      - use F19.982
    - sedative
      - abuse F13.182
      - dependence F13.282
      - use F13.982

Disorder — *continued*
- sleep — *continued*
  - due to — *continued*
    - stimulant NEC
      - abuse F15.182
      - dependence F15.282
      - use F15.982
    - emotional F51.9
    - excessive somnolence — *see* Hypersomnia
    - hypersomnia type — *see* Hypersomnia
    - initiating or maintaining — *see* Insomnia
    - nightmares F51.5
    - nonorganic F51.9
      - specified NEC F51.8
    - parasomnia type G47.50
    - specified NEC G47.8
    - terrors F51.4
    - walking F51.3
  - sleep-wake pattern or schedule — *see also* Disorder, sleep, circadian rhythm G47.9
    - specified NEC G47.8
  - social
    - anxiety (of childhood) F40.10
      - generalized F40.11
    - functioning in childhood F94.9
      - specified NEC F94.8
    - pragmatic F80.82
  - soft tissue M79.9
    - ankle M79.9
    - due to use, overuse and pressure M70.90
      - ankle M70.97- ☑
      - bursitis — *see* Bursitis
      - foot M70.97- ☑
      - forearm M70.93- ☑
      - hand M70.94- ☑
      - lower leg M70.96- ☑
      - multiple sites M70.99
      - pelvic region M70.95- ☑
      - shoulder region M70.91- ☑
      - specified site NEC M70.98
      - specified type NEC M70.80
        - ankle M70.87- ☑
        - foot M70.87- ☑
        - forearm M70.83- ☑
        - hand M70.84- ☑
        - lower leg M70.86- ☑
        - multiple sites M70.89
        - pelvic region M70.85 ☑
        - shoulder region M70.81- ☑
        - specified site NEC M70.88
        - thigh M70.85- ☑
        - upper arm M70.82- ☑
      - thigh M70.95- ☑
      - upper arm M70.92- ☑
    - foot M79.9
    - forearm M79.9
    - hand M79.9
    - lower leg M79.9
    - multiple sites M79.9
    - occupational — *see* Disorder, soft tissue, due to use, overuse and pressure
    - pelvic region M79.9
    - shoulder region M79.9
    - specified type NEC M79.89
    - thigh M79.9
    - upper arm M79.9
  - somatic symptom F45.1
  - somatization F45.0
  - somatoform F45.9
    - pain (persistent) F45.41
    - somatization (multiple) (long-lasting) F45.0
    - specified NEC F45.8
    - undifferentiated F45.1
  - somnolence, excessive — *see* Hypersomnia
  - specific
    - arithmetical F81.2
    - developmental, of motor F82
    - reading F81.0
    - speech and language F80.9
    - spelling F81.81
    - written expression F81.81
  - speech R47.9
    - articulation (functional) (specific) F80.0
    - developmental F80.9
    - specified NEC R47.89
  - speech-sound F80.0
  - spelling (specific) F81.81
  - spine — *see also* Dorsopathy

Disorder — *continued*
  spine — *see also* Dorsopathy — *continued*
    ligamentous or muscular attachments, peripheral
      — *see* Enthesopathy, spinal
    specified NEC — *see* Dorsopathy, specified NEC
  stereotyped, habit or movement F98.4
  stimulant use (other) (unspecified)
    mild F15.10
      in remission (early) (sustained) F15.11
    moderate or severe F15.20
      in remission (early) (sustained) F15.21
  stomach (functional) — *see* Disorder, gastric
  stress F43.9
    acute F43.0
    post-traumatic F43.10
      acute F43.11
      chronic F43.12
  substance use (other) (unknown)
    mild F19.10
      with substance-induced
        anxiety disorder F19.180
        bipolar and related disorder F19.14
        depressive disorder F19.14
        major neurocognitive disorder F19.17
        mild neurocognitive disorder F19.188
        obsessive-compulsive and related disorder
          F19.188
        sexual dysfunction F19.181
      substance intoxication F19.129
      substance intoxication delirium F19.121
    moderate or severe F19.20
      with substance-induced
        anxiety disorder F19.280
        bipolar and related disorder F19.24
        depressive disorder F19.24
        major neurocognitive disorder F19.27
        mild neurocognitive disorder F19.288
        obsessive-compulsive and related disorder
          F19.288
        sexual dysfunction F19.281
      in remission (early) (sustained) F19.21
      substance intoxication F19.229
      substance intoxication delirium F19.221
  sulfur-bearing amino-acid metabolism E72.10
  sweat gland (eccrine) L74.9
    apocrine L75.9
      specified NEC L75.8
    specified NEC L74.8
  synovium M67.90
    acromioclavicular M67.91- ☑
    ankle M67.97- ☑
    elbow M67.92- ☑
    foot M67.97- ☑
    forearm M67.93- ☑
    hand M67.94- ☑
    hip M67.95- ☑
    knee M67.96- ☑
    multiple sites M67.99
    rupture — *see* Rupture, synovium
    shoulder M67.91- ☑
    specified type NEC M67.80
      acromioclavicular M67.81- ☑
      ankle M67.87- ☑
      elbow M67.82- ☑
      foot M67.87- ☑
      hand M67.84- ☑
      hip M67.85- ☑
      knee M67.86- ☑
      multiple sites M67.89
      wrist M67.83- ☑
    synovitis — *see* Synovitis
    upper arm M67.92- ☑
    wrist M67.93- ☑
  temperature regulation, newborn P81.9
    specified NEC P81.8
  temporomandibular joint M26.60- ☑
  tendon M67.90
    acromioclavicular M67.91- ☑
    ankle M67.97- ☑
    contracture — *see* Contracture, tendon
    elbow M67.92- ☑
    foot M67.97- ☑
    forearm M67.93- ☑
    hand M67.94- ☑
    hip M67.95- ☑
    knee M67.96- ☑
    multiple sites M67.99

Disorder — *continued*
  tendon — *continued*
    rupture — *see* Rupture, tendon
    shoulder M67.91- ☑
    specified type NEC M67.80
      acromioclavicular M67.81- ☑
      ankle M67.87- ☑
      elbow M67.82- ☑
      foot M67.87- ☑
      hand M67.84- ☑
      hip M67.85- ☑
      knee M67.86- ☑
      multiple sites M67.89
      trunk M67.88
      wrist M67.83- ☑
    synovitis — *see* Synovitis
    tendinitis — *see* Tendinitis
    tenosynovitis — *see* Tenosynovitis
    trunk M67.98
    upper arm M67.92- ☑
    wrist M67.93- ☑
  thoracic root (nerve) NEC G54.3
  thyrocalcitonin hypersecretion E07.0
  thyroid (gland) E07.9
    function NEC, neonatal, transitory P72.2
    iodine-deficiency related E01.8
    specified NEC E07.89
  tic — *see* Tic
  tobacco use
    chewing tobacco (mild) (moderate) (severe)
      in remission (early) (sustained) F17.221
    cigarettes (mild) (moderate) (severe)
      in remission (early) (sustained) F17.211
    mild F17.200
      in remission (early) (sustained) F17.201
    moderate F17.200
      in remission (early) (sustained) F17.201
    severe F17.200
      in remission (early) (sustained) F17.201
    specified product NEC (mild) (moderate) (severe)
      in remission (early) (sustained) F17.291
  tooth K08.9
    development K00.9
      specified NEC K00.8
    eruption K00.6
  Tourette's F95.2
  trance and possession F44.89
  transvestic F65.1
  trauma and stressor-related F43.9
    other specified F43.8
  tricuspid (valve) — *see* Endocarditis, tricuspid
  tryptophan metabolism E70.5
  tubular, phosphate-losing N25.0
  tubulo-interstitial (in)
    brucellosis A23.9 *[N16]*
    cystinosis E72.04
    diphtheria A36.84
    glycogen storage disease E74.00 *[N16]*
    leukemia NEC C95.9- ☑ *[N16]*
    lymphoma NEC C85.9- ☑ *[N16]*
    mixed cryoglobulinemia D89.1 *[N16]*
    multiple myeloma C90.0- ☑ *[N16]*
    Salmonella infection A02.25
    sarcoidosis D86.84
    sepsis A41.9 *[N16]*
      streptococcal A40.9 *[N16]*
    systemic lupus erythematosus M32.15
    toxoplasmosis B58.83
    transplant rejection T86.91 *[N16]*
    Wilson's disease E83.01 *[N16]*
  tubulo-renal function, impaired N25.9
    specified NEC N25.89
  tympanic membrane H73.9- ☑
    atrophy — *see* Atrophy, tympanic membrane
    infection — *see* Myringitis
    perforation — *see* Perforation, tympanum
    specified NEC H73.89- ☑
  unsocialized aggressive F91.1
  urea cycle metabolism E72.20
    argininemia E72.21
    arginosuccinic aciduria E72.22
    citrullinemia E72.23
    ornithine transcarbamylase deficiency E72.4
    other specified E72.29
  ureter (in) N28.9
    schistosomiasis B65.0 *[N29]*
    tuberculosis A18.11
  urethra N36.9

Disorder — *continued*
  urethra — *continued*
    specified NEC N36.8
  urinary system N39.9
    specified NEC N39.8
  valve, heart
    aortic — *see* Endocarditis, aortic
    mitral — *see* Endocarditis, mitral
    pulmonary — *see* Endocarditis, pulmonary
    rheumatic
      aortic — *see* Endocarditis, aortic, rheumatic
      mitral — *see* Endocarditis, mitral
      pulmonary — *see* Endocarditis, pulmonary,
        rheumatic
      tricuspid — *see* Endocarditis, tricuspid
    tricuspid — *see* Endocarditis, tricuspid
  vestibular function H81.9- ☑
    specified NEC — *see* subcategory H81.8 ☑
      in diseases classified elsewhere H82.- ☑
    vertigo — *see* Vertigo
  vision, binocular H53.30
    abnormal retinal correspondence H53.31
    diplopia H53.2
    fusion with defective stereopsis H53.32
    simultaneous perception H53.33
    suppression H53.34
  visual
    cortex
      blindness H47.619
        left brain H47.612
        right brain H47.611
      due to
        inflammatory disorder H47.629
          left brain H47.622
          right brain H47.621
        neoplasm H47.639
          left brain H47.632
          right brain H47.631
        vascular disorder H47.649
          left brain H47.642
          right brain H47.641
    pathway H47.9
      due to
        inflammatory disorder H47.51- ☑
        neoplasm H47.52- ☑
        vascular disorder H47.53- ☑
    optic chiasm — *see* Disorder, optic, chiasm
  vitreous body H43.9
    crystalline deposits — *see* Deposit, crystalline
    degeneration — *see* Degeneration, vitreous
    hemorrhage — *see* Hemorrhage, vitreous
    opacities — *see* Opacity, vitreous
    prolapse — *see* Prolapse, vitreous
    specified type NEC H43.89
  voice R49.9
    specified type NEC R49.8
  volatile solvent use
    due to drug abuse — *see* Abuse, drug, inhalant
    due to drug dependence — *see* Dependence, drug,
      inhalant
  voyeuristic F65.3
  white blood cells D72.9
    specified NEC D72.89
  withdrawing, child or adolescent F40.10
Disorientation R41.0
Displacement, displaced
  acquired traumatic of bone, cartilage, joint, tendon
    NEC — *see* Dislocation
  adrenal gland (congenital) Q89.1
  appendix, retrocecal (congenital) Q43.8
  auricle (congenital) Q17.4
  bladder (acquired) N32.89
    congenital Q64.19
  brachial plexus (congenital) Q07.8
  brain stem, caudal (congenital) Q04.8
  canaliculus (lacrimalis), congenital Q10.6
  cardia through esophageal hiatus (congenital) Q40.1
  cerebellum, caudal (congenital) Q04.8
  cervix — *see* Malposition, uterus
  colon (congenital) Q43.3
  device, implant or graft — *see also* Complications, by
    site and type, mechanical T85.628 ☑
    arterial graft NEC — *see* Complication, cardiovascu
      lar device, mechanical, vascular
    breast (implant) T85.42 ☑
    catheter NEC T85.628 ☑
      dialysis (renal) T82.42 ☑
        intraperitoneal T85.621 ☑

☑ Additional Character Required — Refer to the Tabular List for Character Selection   ▽ Subterms under main terms may continue to next column or page

Displacement, displaced — *continued*
- device, implant or graft — *see also* Complications, by site and type, mechanical — *continued*
  - catheter — *continued*
    - infusion NEC T82.524 ☑
      - spinal (epidural) (subdural) T85.620 ☑
    - urinary
      - cystostomy T83.020 ☑
      - Hopkins T83.028 ☑
      - ileostomy T83.028 ☑
      - indwelling T83.021 ☑
      - nephrostomy T83.022 ☑
      - specified NEC T83.028 ☑
      - urostomy T83.028 ☑
  - electronic (electrode) (pulse generator) (stimulator) — *see* Complication, electronic stimulator
  - fixation, internal (orthopedic) NEC — *see* Complication, fixation device, mechanical
  - gastrointestinal — *see* Complications, prosthetic device, mechanical, gastrointestinal device
  - genital NEC T83.428 ☑
    - intrauterine contraceptive device (string) T83.32 ☑
    - penile prosthesis (cylinder) (implanted) (pump) (reservoir) T83.420 ☑
    - testicular prosthesis T83.421 ☑
  - heart NEC — *see* Complication, cardiovascular device, mechanical
  - joint prosthesis — *see* Complications, joint prosthesis, mechanical
  - ocular — *see* Complications, prosthetic device, mechanical, ocular device
  - orthopedic NEC — *see* Complication, orthopedic, device or graft, mechanical
  - specified NEC T85.628 ☑
  - urinary NEC T83.128 ☑
    - graft T83.22 ☑
    - sphincter, implanted T83.121 ☑
    - stent (ileal conduit) (nephroureteral) T83.123 ☑
    - ureteral indwelling T83.122 ☑
  - vascular NEC — *see* Complication, cardiovascular device, mechanical
  - ventricular intracranial shunt T85.02 ☑
- electronic stimulator
  - bone T04.320 ☑
  - cardiac — *see* Complications, cardiac device, electronic
  - nervous system — *see* Complication, prosthetic device, mechanical, electronic nervous system stimulator
  - urinary — *see* Complications, electronic stimulator, urinary
- esophageal mucosa into cardia of stomach, congenital Q39.8
- esophagus (acquired) K22.8
  - congenital Q39.8
- eyeball (acquired) (lateral) (old) — *see* Displacement, globe
  - congenital Q15.8
  - current — *see* Avulsion, eye
- fallopian tube (acquired) N83.4- ☑
  - congenital Q50.6
  - opening (congenital) Q50.6
- gallbladder (congenital) Q44.1
- gastric mucosa (congenital) Q40.2
- globe (acquired) (old) (lateral) H05.21- ☑
  - current — *see* Avulsion, eye
- heart (congenital) Q24.8
  - acquired I51.89
- hymen (upward) (congenital) Q52.4
- intervertebral disc NEC
  - with myelopathy — *see* Disorder, disc, with, myelopathy
  - cervical, cervicothoracic (with) M50.20
    - myelopathy — *see* Disorder, disc, cervical, with myelopathy
    - neuritis, radiculitis or radiculopathy — *see* Disorder, disc, cervical, with neuritis
  - due to trauma — *see* Dislocation, vertebra
  - lumbar region M51.26
    - with
      - myelopathy M51.06
      - neuritis, radiculitis, radiculopathy or sciatica M51.16
  - lumbosacral region M51.27

Displacement, displaced — *continued*
- intervertebral disc — *continued*
  - lumbosacral region — *continued*
    - with
      - neuritis, radiculitis, radiculopathy or sciatica M51.17
  - sacrococcygeal region M53.3
  - thoracic region M51.24
    - with
      - myelopathy M51.04
      - neuritis, radiculitis, radiculopathy M51.14
  - thoracolumbar region M51.25
    - with
      - myelopathy M51.05
      - neuritis, radiculitis, radiculopathy M51.15
- intrauterine device (string) T83.32 ☑
- kidney (acquired) N28.83
  - congenital Q63.2
- lachrymal, lacrimal apparatus or duct (congenital) Q10.6
- lens, congenital Q12.1
- macula (congenital) Q14.1
- Meckel's diverticulum Q43.0
  - malignant — *see* Table of Neoplasms, small intestine, malignant
- nail (congenital) Q84.6
  - acquired L60.8
- opening of Wharton's duct in mouth Q38.4
- organ or site, congenital NEC — *see* Malposition, congenital
- ovary (acquired) N83.4- ☑
  - congenital Q50.39
  - free in peritoneal cavity (congenital) Q50.39
  - into hernial sac N83.4- ☑
- oviduct (acquired) N83.4- ☑
  - congenital Q50.6
- parathyroid (gland) E21.4
- parotid gland (congenital) Q38.4
- punctum lacrimale (congenital) Q10.6
- sacro-iliac (joint) (congenital) Q74.2
  - current injury S33.2 ☑
  - old — *see* subcategory M53.2 ☑
- salivary gland (any) (congenital) Q38.4
- spleen (congenital) Q89.09
- stomach, congenital Q40.2
- sublingual duct Q38.4
- tongue (downward) (congenital) Q38.3
- tooth, teeth, fully erupted M26.30
  - horizontal M26.33
  - vertical M26.34
- trachea (congenital) Q32.1
- ureter or ureteric opening or orifice (congenital) Q62.62
- uterine opening of oviducts or fallopian tubes Q50.6
- uterus, uterine — *see* Malposition, uterus
- ventricular septum Q21.0
  - with rudimentary ventricle Q20.4

Disproportion
- between native and reconstructed breast N65.1
- fiber-type G71.2

Disruptio uteri — *see* Rupture, uterus
Disruption (of)
- ciliary body NEC H21.89
- closure of
  - cornea T81.31 ☑
  - craniotomy T81.32 ☑
  - fascia (muscular) (superficial) T81.32 ☑
  - internal organ or tissue T81.32 ☑
  - laceration (external) (internal) T81.33 ☑
  - ligament T81.32 ☑
  - mucosa T81.31 ☑
  - muscle or muscle flap T81.32 ☑
  - ribs or rib cage T81.32 ☑
  - skin and subcutaneous tissue (full-thickness) (superficial) T81.31 ☑
  - skull T81.32 ☑
  - sternum (sternotomy) T81.32 ☑
  - tendon T81.32 ☑
  - traumatic laceration (external) (internal) T81.33 ☑
- family Z63.8
  - due to
    - absence of family member due to military deployment Z63.31
    - absence of family member NEC Z63.32
    - alcoholism and drug addiction in family Z63.72
    - bereavement Z63.4
    - death (assumed) or disappearance of family member Z63.4
    - divorce or separation Z63.5
    - drug addiction in family Z63.72

Disruption — *continued*
- family — *continued*
  - due to — *continued*
    - return of family member from military deployment (current or past conflict) Z63.71
    - stressful life events NEC Z63.79
- iris NEC H21.89
- ligament(s) — *see also* Sprain
  - knee
    - current injury — *see* Dislocation, knee
    - old (chronic) — *see* Derangement, knee, instability
    - spontaneous NEC — *see* Derangement, knee, disruption ligament
  - ossicular chain — *see* Discontinuity, ossicles, ear
- pelvic ring (stable) S32.810 ☑
  - unstable S32.811 ☑
- traumatic injury wound repair T81.33 ☑
- wound T81.30 ☑
  - episiotomy O90.1
  - operation T81.31 ☑
    - cesarean O90.0
    - external operation wound (superficial) T81.31 ☑
    - internal operation wound (deep) T81.32 ☑
  - perineal (obstetric) O90.1
  - traumatic injury repair T81.33 ☑

Dissatisfaction with
- employment Z56.9
- school environment Z55.4

Dissecting — *see* condition
Dissection
- aorta I71.00
  - abdominal I71.02
  - thoracic I71.01
  - thoracoabdominal I71.03
- artery I77.70
  - basilar (trunk) I77.75
  - carotid I77.71
  - cerebral (nonruptured) I67.0
    - ruptured — *see* Hemorrhage, intracranial, subarachnoid
  - coronary I25.42
  - extremity
    - lower I77.77
    - upper I77.76
  - iliac I77.72
  - precerebral
    - congenital (nonruptured) Q28.1
    - specified site NEC I77.75
  - renal I77.73
  - specified NEC I77.79
  - vertebral I77.74
- precerebral artery, congenital (nonruptured) Q28.1
  - Heartland A93.8
- traumatic — *see* Wound, open, by site
- vascular I99.8
- wound — *see* Wound, open

Disseminated — *see* condition
Dissociation
- auriculoventricular or atrioventricular (AV) (any degree) (isorhythmic) I45.89
  - with heart block I44.2
- interference I45.89

Dissociative reaction, state F44.9
Dissolution, vertebra — *see* Osteoporosis
Distension, distention
- abdomen R14.0
- bladder N32.89
- cecum K63.89
- colon K63.89
- gallbladder K82.8
- intestine K63.89
- kidney N28.89
- liver K76.89
- seminal vesicle N50.89
- stomach K31.89
  - acute K31.0
  - psychogenic F45.8
- ureter — *see* Dilatation, ureter
- uterus N85.8

Distoma hepaticum infestation B66.3
Distomiasis B66.9
- bile passages B66.3
- hemic B65.9
- hepatic B66.3
  - due to Clonorchis sinensis B66.1
- intestinal B66.5
- liver B66.3

Distomiasis — continued
  liver — continued
    due to Clonorchis sinensis B66.1
  lung B66.4
  pulmonary B66.4
Distomolar (fourth molar) K00.1
Disto-occlusion (Division I) (Division II) M26.212
Distortion(s) (congenital)
  adrenal (gland) Q89.1
  arm NEC Q68.8
  bile duct or passage Q44.5
  bladder Q64.79
  brain Q04.9
  cervix (uteri) Q51.9
  chest (wall) Q67.8
    bones Q76.8
  clavicle Q74.0
  clitoris Q52.6
  coccyx Q76.49
  common duct Q44.5
  coronary Q24.5
  cystic duct Q44.5
  ear (auricle) (external) Q17.3
    inner Q16.5
    middle Q16.4
      ossicles Q16.3
  endocrine NEC Q89.2
  eustachian tube Q17.8
  eye (adnexa) Q15.8
  face bone(s) NEC Q75.8
  fallopian tube Q50.6
  femur NEC Q68.8
  fibula NEC Q68.8
  finger(s) Q68.1
  foot Q66.9- ☑
  genitalia, genital organ(s)
    female Q52.8
      external Q52.79
      internal NEC Q52.8
  gyri Q04.8
  hand bone(s) Q68.1
  heart (auricle) (ventricle) Q24.8
    valve (cusp) Q24.8
  hepatic duct Q44.5
  humerus NEC Q68.8
  hymen Q52.4
  intrafamilial communications Z63.8
  jaw NEC M26.89
  labium (majus) (minus) Q52.79
  leg NEC Q68.8
  lens Q12.8
  liver Q44.7
  lumbar spine Q76.49
    with disproportion O33.8
      causing obstructed labor O65.0
  lumbosacral (joint) (region) Q76.49
    kyphosis — see Kyphosis, congenital
    lordosis — see Lordosis, congenital
  nerve Q07.8
  nose Q30.8
  organ
    of Corti Q16.5
    or site not listed — see Anomaly, by site
  ossicles, ear Q16.3
  oviduct Q50.6
  pancreas Q45.3
  parathyroid (gland) Q89.2
  pituitary (gland) Q89.2
  radius NEC Q68.8
  sacroiliac joint Q74.2
  sacrum Q76.49
  scapula Q74.0
  shoulder girdle Q74.0
  skull bone(s) NEC Q75.8
    with
      anencephalus Q00.0
      encephalocele — see Encephalocele
      hydrocephalus Q03.9
        with spina bifida — see Spina bifida, with hydrocephalus
      microcephaly Q02
  spinal cord Q06.8
  spine Q76.49
    kyphosis — see Kyphosis, congenital
    lordosis — see Lordosis, congenital
  spleen Q89.09
  sternum NEC Q76.7
  thorax (wall) Q67.8

Distortion(s) — continued
  thorax — continued
    bony Q76.8
  thymus (gland) Q89.2
  thyroid (gland) Q89.2
  tibia NEC Q68.8
  toe(s) Q66.9- ☑
  tongue Q38.3
  trachea (cartilage) Q32.1
  ulna NEC Q68.8
  ureter Q62.8
  urethra Q64.79
    causing obstruction Q64.39
  uterus Q51.9
  vagina Q52.4
  vertebra Q76.49
    kyphosis — see Kyphosis, congenital
    lordosis — see Lordosis, congenital
  visual — see also Disturbance, vision
    shape and size H53.15
  vulva Q52.79
  wrist (bones) (joint) Q68.8
Distress
  abdomen — see Pain, abdominal
  acute respiratory R06.03
    syndrome (adult) (child) J80
  epigastric R10.13
  fetal P84
    complicating pregnancy — see Stress, fetal
  gastrointestinal (functional) K30
    psychogenic F45.8
  intestinal (functional) NOS K59.9
    psychogenic F45.8
  maternal, during labor and delivery O75.0
  relationship, with spouse or intimate partner Z63.0
  respiratory (adult) (child) R06.03
    newborn P22.9
      specified NEC P22.8
    orthopnea R06.01
    psychogenic F45.8
    shortness of breath R06.02
    specified type NEC R06.09
Distribution vessel, atypical Q27.9
  coronary artery Q24.5
  precerebral Q28.1
Districhiasis L68.8
Disturbance(s) — see also Disease
  absorption K90.9
    calcium E58
    carbohydrate K90.49
    fat K90.49
      pancreatic K90.3
    protein K90.49
    starch K90.49
    vitamin — see Deficiency, vitamin
  acid-base equilibrium E87.8
    mixed E87.4
  activity and attention (with hyperkinesis) — see Disorder, attention-deficit hyperactivity
  amino acid transport E72.00
  assimilation, food K90.9
  auditory nerve, except deafness — see subcategory H93.3 ☑
  behavior — see Disorder, conduct
  blood clotting (mechanism) — see also Defect, coagulation D68.9
  cerebral
    nerve — see Disorder, nerve, cranial
    status, newborn P91.9
      specified NEC P91.88
  circulatory I99.9
  conduct — see also Disorder, conduct F91.9
    adjustment reaction — see Disorder, adjustment
    compulsive F63.9
    disruptive F91.9
    hyperkinetic — see Disorder, attention-deficit hyperactivity
    socialized F91.2
    specified NEC F91.8
    unsocialized F91.1
  coordination R27.8
  cranial nerve — see Disorder, nerve, cranial
  deep sensibility — see Disturbance, sensation
  digestive K30
    psychogenic F45.8
  electrolyte — see also Imbalance, electrolyte
    newborn, transitory P74.49
      hyperammonemia P74.6

Disturbance(s) — continued
  electrolyte — see also Imbalance, electrolyte — continued
    newborn, transitory — continued
      hyperchloremia P74.421
      hyperchloremic metabolic acidosis P74.421
      hypochloremia P74.422
      potassium balance
        hyperkalemia P74.31
        hypokalemia P74.32
      sodium balance
        hypernatremia P74.21
        hyponatremia P74.22
      specified type NEC P74.49
  emotions specific to childhood and adolescence F93.9
    with
      anxiety and fearfulness NEC F93.8
      elective mutism F94.0
      oppositional disorder F91.3
      sensitivity (withdrawal) F40.10
      shyness F40.10
      social withdrawal F40.10
    involving relationship problems F93.8
    mixed F93.8
    specified NEC F93.8
  endocrine (gland) E34.9
    neonatal, transitory P72.9
      specified NEC P72.8
  equilibrium R42
  fructose metabolism E74.10
  gait — see Gait
    hysterical F44.4
    psychogenic F44.4
  gastrointestinal (functional) K30
    psychogenic F45.8
  habit, child F98.9
  hearing, except deafness and tinnitus — see Abnormal, auditory perception
  heart, functional (conditions in I44-I50)
    due to presence of (cardiac) prosthesis I97.19- ☑
    postoperative I97.89
      cardiac surgery — see also Infarct, myocardium, associated with revascularization procedure I97.19- ☑
  hormones E34.9
  innervation uterus (parasympathetic) (sympathetic) N85.8
  keratinization NEC
    gingiva K05.10
      nonplaque induced K05.11
      plaque induced K05.10
    lip K13.0
    oral (mucosa) (soft tissue) K13.29
    tongue K13.29
  learning (specific) — see Disorder, learning
  memory — see Amnesia
    mild, following organic brain damage F06.8
  mental F99
    associated with diseases classified elsewhere F54
  metabolism E88.9
    with
      abortion — see Abortion, by type with other specified complication
      ectopic pregnancy O08.5
      molar pregnancy O08.5
    amino-acid E72.9
      aromatic E70.9
      branched-chain E71.2
      straight-chain E72.89
      sulfur-bearing E72.10
    ammonia E72.20
    arginine E72.21
    arginosuccinic acid E72.22
    carbohydrate E74.9
    cholesterol E78.9
    citrulline E72.23
    cystathionine E72.19
    general E88.9
    glutamine E72.89
    histidine E70.40
    homocystine E72.19
    hydroxylysine E72.3
    in labor or delivery O75.89
    iron E83.10
    lipoid E78.9
    lysine E72.3
    methionine E72.19
    neonatal, transitory P74.9

Disturbance(s) — continued
  metabolism — continued
    neonatal, transitory — continued
      calcium and magnesium P71.9
        specified type NEC P71.8
      carbohydrate metabolism P70.9
        specified type NEC P70.8
      specified NEC P74.8
    ornithine E72.4
    phosphate E83.39
    sodium NEC E87.8
    threonine E72.89
    tryptophan E70.5
    tyrosine E70.20
    urea cycle E72.20
  motor R29.2
  nervous, functional R45.0
  neuromuscular mechanism (eye), due to syphilis A52.15
  nutritional E63.9
    nail L60.3
  ocular motion H51.9
    psychogenic F45.8
  oculogyric H51.8
    psychogenic F45.8
  oculomotor H51.9
    psychogenic F45.8
  olfactory nerve R43.1
  optic nerve NEC — see Disorder, nerve, optic
  oral epithelium, including tongue NEC K13.29
  perceptual due to
    alcohol withdrawal F10.232
    amphetamine intoxication F15.922
      in
        abuse F15.122
        dependence F15.222
    anxiolytic withdrawal F13.232
    cannabis intoxication (acute) F12.922
      in
        abuse F12.122
        dependence F12.222
    cocaine intoxication (acute) F14.922
      in
        abuse F14.122
        dependence F14.222
    hypnotic withdrawal F13.232
    opioid intoxication (acute) F11.922
      in
        abuse F11.122
        dependence F11.222
    phencyclidine intoxication (acute) F16.122
    sedative withdrawal F13.232
  personality (pattern) (trait) — see also Disorder, personality F60.9
    following organic brain damage F07.9
  polyglandular E31.9
    specified NEC E31.8
  potassium balance, newborn
    hyperkalemia P74.31
    hypokalemia P74.32
  psychogenic F45.9
  psychomotor F44.4
  psychophysical visual H53.16
  pupillary — see Anomaly, pupil, function
  reflex R29.2
  rhythm, heart I49.9
  salivary secretion K11.7
  sensation (cold) (heat) (localization) (tactile discrimination) (texture) (vibratory) NEC R20.9
    hysterical F44.6
    skin R20.9
      anesthesia R20.0
      hyperesthesia R20.3
      hypoesthesia R20.1
      paresthesia R20.2
      specified type NEC R20.8
    smell R43.9
      and taste (mixed) R43.8
      anosmia R43.0
      parosmia R43.1
      specified NEC R43.8
    taste R43.9
      and smell (mixed) R43.8
      parageusia R43.2
      specified NEC R43.8
  sensory — see Disturbance, sensation
  situational (transient) — see also Disorder, adjustment
    acute F43.0
  sleep G47.9
    nonorganic origin F51.9

Disturbance(s) — continued
  smell — see Disturbance, sensation, smell
  sociopathic F60.2
  sodium balance, newborn
    hypernatremia P74.21
    hyponatremia P74.22
  speech R47.9
    developmental F80.9
    specified NEC R47.89
  stomach (functional) K31.9
  sympathetic (nerve) G90.9
  taste — see Disturbance, sensation, taste
  temperature
    regulation, newborn P81.9
      specified NEC P81.8
    sense R20.8
      hysterical F44.6
  tooth
    eruption K00.6
    formation K00.4
    structure, hereditary NEC K00.5
  touch — see Disturbance, sensation
  vascular I99.9
    arteriosclerotic — see Arteriosclerosis
  vasomotor I73.9
  vasospastic I73.9
  vision, visual H53.9
    following
      cerebral infarction I69.398
      cerebrovascular disease I69.998
        specified NEC I69.898
      intracerebral hemorrhage I69.198
      nontraumatic intracranial hemorrhage NEC I69.298
      specified disease NEC I69.898
      subarachnoid hemorrhage I69.098
    psychophysical H53.16
    specified NEC H53.8
    subjective H53.10
      day blindness H53.11
      discomfort H53.14- ☑
      distortions of shape and size H53.15
      loss
        sudden H53.13- ☑
        transient H53.12- ☑
      specified type NEC H53.19
  voice R49.9
    psychogenic F44.4
    specified NEC R49.8
Diuresis R35.8
Diver's palsy, paralysis or squeeze T70.3 ☑
Diverticulitis (acute) K57.92
  bladder — see Cystitis
  ileum — see Diverticulitis, intestine, small
  intestine K57.92
    with
      abscess, perforation or peritonitis K57.80
        with bleeding K57.81
      bleeding K57.93
    congenital Q43.8
    large K57.32
      with
        abscess, perforation or peritonitis K57.20
          with bleeding K57.21
        bleeding K57.33
        small intestine K57.52
          with
            abscess, perforation or peritonitis K57.40
              with bleeding K57.41
            bleeding K57.53
    small K57.12
      with
        abscess, perforation or peritonitis K57.00
          with bleeding K57.01
        bleeding K57.13
        large intestine K57.52
          with
            abscess, perforation or peritonitis K57.40
              with bleeding K57.41
            bleeding K57.53
Diverticulosis K57.90
  with bleeding K57.91
  large intestine K57.30
    with
      bleeding K57.31
      small intestine K57.50

Diverticulosis — continued
  large intestine — continued
    with — continued
      small intestine — continued
        with bleeding K57.51
    small intestine K57.10
      with
        bleeding K57.11
        large intestine K57.50
          with bleeding K57.51
Diverticulum, diverticula (multiple) K57.90
  appendix (noninflammatory) K38.2
  bladder (sphincter) N32.3
    congenital Q64.6
  bronchus (congenital) Q32.4
    acquired J98.09
  calyx, calyceal (kidney) N28.89
  cardia (stomach) K31.4
  cecum — see Diverticulosis, intestine, large
    congenital Q43.8
  colon — see Diverticulosis, intestine, large
    congenital Q43.8
  duodenum — see Diverticulosis, intestine, small
    congenital Q43.8
  epiphrenic (esophagus) K22.5
  esophagus (congenital) Q39.6
    acquired (epiphrenic) (pulsion) (traction) K22.5
  eustachian tube — see Disorder, eustachian tube, specified NEC
  fallopian tube N83.8
  gastric K31.4
  heart (congenital) Q24.8
  ileum — see Diverticulosis, intestine, small
  jejunum — see Diverticulosis, intestine, small
  kidney (pelvis) (calyces) N28.89
    with calculus — see Calculus, kidney
  Meckel's (displaced) (hypertrophic) Q43.0
    malignant — see Table of Neoplasms, small intestine, malignant
  midthoracic K22.5
  organ or site, congenital NEC — see Distortion
  pericardium (congenital) (cyst) Q24.8
    acquired I31.8
  pharyngoesophageal (congenital) Q39.6
    acquired K22.5
  pharynx (congenital) Q38.7
  rectosigmoid — see Diverticulosis, intestine, large
    congenital Q43.8
  rectum — see Diverticulosis, intestine, large
  Rokitansky's K22.5
  seminal vesicle N50.89
  sigmoid — see Diverticulosis, intestine, large
    congenital Q43.8
  stomach (acquired) K31.4
    congenital Q40.2
  trachea (acquired) J39.8
  ureter (acquired) N28.89
    congenital Q62.8
  ureterovesical orifice N28.89
  urethra (acquired) N36.1
    congenital Q64.79
  ventricle, left (congenital) Q24.8
  vesical N32.3
    congenital Q64.6
  Zenker's (esophagus) K22.5
Division
  cervix uteri (acquired) N88.8
  glans penis Q55.69
  labia minora (congenital) Q52.79
  ligament (partial or complete) (current) — see also Sprain
    with open wound — see Wound, open
  muscle (partial or complete) (current) — see also Injury, muscle
    with open wound — see Wound, open
  nerve (traumatic) — see Injury, nerve
  spinal cord — see Injury, spinal cord, by region
  vein I87.8
Divorce, causing family disruption Z63.5
Dix-Hallpike neurolabyrinthitis — see Neuronitis, vestibular
Dizziness R42
  hysterical F44.89
  psychogenic F45.8
DMAC (disseminated mycobacterium avium- intracellulare complex) A31.2
DNR (do not resuscitate) Z66

Doan-Wiseman syndrome (primary splenic neutropenia) — *see* Agranulocytosis
Doehle-Heller aortitis A52.02
Dog bite — *see* Bite
Dohle body panmyelopathic syndrome D72.0
Dolichocephaly Q67.2
Dolichocolon Q43.8
Dolichostenomelia — *see* Syndrome, Marfan's
Donohue's syndrome E34.8
Donor (organ or tissue) Z52.9
  blood (whole) Z52.000
    autologous Z52.010
    specified component (lymphocytes) (platelets) NEC Z52.008
      autologous Z52.018
      specified donor NEC Z52.098
    specified donor NEC Z52.090
    stem cells Z52.001
      autologous Z52.011
      specified donor NEC Z52.091
  bone Z52.20
    autologous Z52.21
    marrow Z52.3
    specified type NEC Z52.29
  cornea Z52.5
  egg (Oocyte) Z52.819
    age 35 and over Z52.812
      anonymous recipient Z52.812
      designated recipient Z52.813
    under age 35 Z52.810
      anonymous recipient Z52.810
      designated recipient Z52.811
  kidney Z52.4
  liver Z52.6
  lung Z52.89
  lymphocyte — *see* Donor, blood, specified components NEC
  Oocyte — *see* Donor, egg
  platelets Z52.008
  potential, examination of Z00.5
  semen Z52.89
  skin Z52.10
    autologous Z52.11
    specified type NEC Z52.19
  specified organ or tissue NEC Z52.89
  sperm Z52.89
Donovanosis A58
Dorsalgia M54.9
  psychogenic F45.41
  specified NEC M54.89
Dorsopathy M53.9
  deforming M43.9
    specified NEC — *see* subcategory M43.8 ☑
  specified NEC M53.80
    cervical region M53.82
    cervicothoracic region M53.83
    lumbar region M53.86
    lumbosacral region M53.87
    occipito-atlanto-axial region M53.81
    sacrococcygeal region M53.88
    thoracic region M53.84
    thoracolumbar region M53.85
Double
  albumin E88.09
  aortic arch Q25.45
  auditory canal Q17.8
  auricle (heart) Q20.8
  bladder Q64.79
  cervix Q51.820
    with doubling of uterus (and vagina) Q51.10
      with obstruction Q51.11
  inlet ventricle Q20.4
  kidney with double pelvis (renal) Q63.0
  meatus urinarius Q64.75
  monster Q89.4
  outlet
    left ventricle Q20.2
    right ventricle Q20.1
  pelvis (renal) with double ureter Q62.5
  tongue Q38.3
  ureter (one or both sides) Q62.5
    with double pelvis (renal) Q62.5
  urethra Q64.74
  urinary meatus Q64.75
  uterus Q51.20
    with
      doubling of cervix (and vagina) Q51.10
        with obstruction Q51.11

Double — *continued*
  uterus — *continued*
    complete Q51.21
    in pregnancy or childbirth O34.0- ☑
      causing obstructed labor O65.5
    partial Q51.22
    specified NEC Q51.28
  vagina Q52.10
    with doubling of uterus (and cervix) Q51.10
      with obstruction Q51.11
  vision H53.2
  vulva Q52.79
Douglas' pouch, cul-de-sac — *see* condition
Down syndrome Q90.9
  meiotic nondisjunction Q90.0
  mitotic nondisjunction Q90.1
  mosaicism Q90.1
  translocation Q90.2
DPD (dihydropyrimidine dehydrogenase deficiency) E88.89
Dracontiasis B72
Dracunculiasis, dracunculosis B72
Dream state, hysterical F44.89
Drepanocytic anemia — *see* Disease, sickle-cell
Dresbach's syndrome (elliptocytosis) D58.1
Dreschlera (hawaiiensis) (infection) B43.8
Dressler's syndrome I24.1
Drift, ulnar — *see* Deformity, limb, specified type NEC, forearm
Drinking (alcohol)
  excessive, to excess NEC (without dependence) F10.10
    habitual (continual) (without remission) F10.20
      with remission F10.21
Drip, postnasal (chronic) R09.82
  due to
    allergic rhinitis — *see* Rhinitis, allergic
    common cold J00
    gastroesophageal reflux — *see* Reflux, gastroesophageal
    nasopharyngitis — *see* Nasopharyngitis
    other known condition — *code to* condition
    sinusitis — *see* Sinusitis
Droop
  facial R29.810
    cerebrovascular disease I69.992
      cerebral infarction I69.392
      intracerebral hemorrhage I69.192
      nontraumatic intracranial hemorrhage NEC I69.292
      specified disease NEC I69.892
      subarachnoid hemorrhage I69.092
Drop (in)
  attack NEC R55
  finger — *see* Deformity, finger
  foot — *see* Deformity, limb, foot, drop
  hematocrit (precipitous) R71.0
  hemoglobin R71.0
  toe — *see* Deformity, toe, specified NEC
  wrist — *see* Deformity, limb, wrist drop
Dropped heart beats I45.9
Dropsy, dropsical — *see also* Hydrops
  abdomen R18.8
  brain — *see* Hydrocephalus
  cardiac, heart — *see* Failure, heart, congestive
  gangrenous — *see* Gangrene
  heart — *see* Failure, heart, congestive
  kidney — *see* Nephrosis
  lung — *see* Edema, lung
  newborn due to isoimmunization P56.0
  pericardium — *see* Pericarditis
Drowned, drowning (near) T75.1 ☑
Drowsiness R40.0
Drug
  abuse counseling and surveillance Z71.51
  addiction — *see* Dependence
  dependence — *see* Dependence
  habit — *see* Dependence
  harmful use — *see* Abuse, drug
  induced fever R50.2
  overdose — *see* Table of Drugs and Chemicals, by drug, poisoning
  poisoning — *see* Table of Drugs and Chemicals, by drug, poisoning
  resistant organism infection — *see also* Resistant, organism, to, drug Z16.30

Drug — *continued*
  therapy
    long term (current) (prophylactic) — *see* Therap drug long-term (current) (prophylactic)
    short term — *omit code*
    wrong substance given or taken in error — *see* Tab of Drugs and Chemicals, by drug, poisoning
Drunkenness (without dependence) F10.129
  acute in alcoholism F10.229
  chronic (without remission) F10.20
    with remission F10.21
  pathological (without dependence) F10.129
    with dependence F10.229
  sleep F51.9
Drusen
  macula (degenerative) (retina) — *see* Degeneration macula, drusen
  optic disc H47.32- ☑
Dry, dryness — *see also* condition
  larynx J38.7
  mouth R68.2
    due to dehydration E86.0
  nose J34.89
  socket (teeth) M27.3
  throat J39.2
DSAP L56.5
Duane's syndrome H50.81- ☑
Dubin-Johnson disease or syndrome E80.6
Dubois' disease (thymus gland) A50.59 *[E35]*
Dubowitz' syndrome Q87.19
Duchenne-Aran muscular atrophy G12.21
Duchenne-Griesinger disease G71.01
Duchenne's
  disease or syndrome
    motor neuron disease G12.22
    muscular dystrophy G71.01
  locomotor ataxia (syphilitic) A52.11
  paralysis
    birth injury P14.0
    due to or associated with
      motor neuron disease G12.22
      muscular dystrophy G71.01
Ducrey's chancre A57
Duct, ductus — *see* condition
Duhring's disease (dermatitis herpetiformis) L13.0
Dullness, cardiac (decreased) (increased) R01.2
Dumb ague — *see* Malaria
Dumbness — *see* Aphasia
Dumdum fever B55.0
Dumping syndrome (postgastrectomy) K91.1
Duodenitis (nonspecific) (peptic) K29.80
  with bleeding K29.81
Duodenocholangitis — *see* Cholangitis
Duodenum, duodenal — *see* condition
Duplay's bursitis or periarthritis — *see* Tendinitis, calcific, shoulder
Duplication, duplex — *see also* Accessory
  alimentary tract Q45.8
  anus Q43.4
  appendix (and cecum) Q43.4
  biliary duct (any) Q44.5
  bladder Q64.79
  cecum (and appendix) Q43.4
  cervix Q51.820
  chromosome NEC
    with complex rearrangements NEC Q92.5
    seen only at prometaphase Q92.8
  cystic duct Q44.5
  digestive organs Q45.8
  esophagus Q39.8
  frontonasal process Q75.8
  intestine (large) (small) Q43.4
  kidney Q63.0
  liver Q44.7
  pancreas Q45.3
  penis Q55.69
  respiratory organs NEC Q34.8
  salivary duct Q38.4
  spinal cord (incomplete) Q06.2
  stomach Q40.2
Dupré's disease (meningism) R29.1
Dupuytren's contraction or disease M72.0
Durand-Nicolas-Favre disease A55
Durotomy (inadvertent) (incidental) G97.41
Duroziez's disease (congenital mitral stenosis) Q23.2
Dutton's relapsing fever (West African) A68.1
Dwarfism E34.3
  achondroplastic Q77.4

☑ **Additional Character Required** — Refer to the Tabular List for Character Selection   ▽ Subterms under main terms may continue to next column or pa

Dwarfism — continued
congenital E34.3
constitutional E34.3
hypochondroplastic Q77.4
hypophyseal E23.0
infantile E34.3
Laron-type E34.3
Lorain (-Levi) type E23.0
metatropic Q77.8
nephrotic-glycosuric (with hypophosphatemic rickets) E72.09
nutritional E45
pancreatic K86.89
pituitary E23.0
renal N25.0
thanatophoric Q77.1
Dyke-Young anemia (secondary) (symptomatic) D59.1
Dysacusis — see Abnormal, auditory perception
Dysadrenocortism E27.9
hyperfunction E27.0
Dysarthria R47.1
following
cerebral infarction I69.322
cerebrovascular disease I69.922
specified disease NEC I69.822
intracerebral hemorrhage I69.122
nontraumatic intracranial hemorrhage NEC I69.222
subarachnoid hemorrhage I69.022
Dysautonomia (familial) G90.1
Dysbarism T70.3 ☑
Dysbasia R26.2
angiosclerotica intermittens I73.9
hysterical F44.4
lordotica (progressiva) G24.1
nonorganic origin F44.4
psychogenic F44.4
Dysbetalipoproteinemia (familial) E78.2
Dyscalculia R48.8
developmental F81.2
Dyschezia K59.00
Dyschondroplasia (with hemangiomata) Q78.4
Dyschromia (skin) L81.9
Dyscollagenosis M35.9
Dyscranio-pygo-phalangy Q87.0
Dyscrasia
blood (with) D75.9
antepartum hemorrhage — see Hemorrhage, antepartum, with coagulation defect
intrapartum hemorrhage O67.0
newborn P61.9
specified type NEC P61.8
puerperal, postpartum O72.3
polyglandular, pluriglandular E31.9
Dysendocrinism E34.9
Dysentery, dysenteric (catarrhal) (diarrhea) (epidemic) (hemorrhagic) (infectious) (sporadic) (tropical) A09
abscess, liver A06.4
amebic — see also Amebiasis A06.0
with abscess — see Abscess, amebic
acute A06.0
chronic A06.1
arthritis — see also category M01 A09
bacillary (see also category M01) A03.9
bacillary A03.9
arthritis — see also category M01 A03.9
Boyd A03.2
Flexner A03.1
Schmitz (-Stutzer) A03.0
Shiga (-Kruse) A03.0
Shigella A03.9
boydii A03.2
dysenteriae A03.0
flexneri A03.1
group A A03.0
group B A03.1
group C A03.2
group D A03.3
sonnei A03.3
specified type NEC A03.8
Sonne A03.3
specified type NEC A03.8
balantidial A07.0
Balantidium coli A07.0
Boyd's A03.2
candidal B37.82
Chilomastix A07.8
Chinese A03.9
coccidial A07.3

Dysentery, dysenteric — continued
Dientamoeba (fragilis) A07.8
Embadomonas A07.8
Entamoeba, entambic — see Dysentery, amebic
Flexner-Boyd A03.2
Flexner's A03.1
Giardia lamblia A07.1
Hiss-Russell A03.1
Lamblia A07.1
leishmanial B55.0
malarial — see Malaria
metazoal B82.0
monilial B37.82
protozoal A07.9
Salmonella A02.0
schistosomal B65.1
Schmitz (-Stutzer) A03.0
Shiga (-Kruse) A03.0
Shigella NOS — see Dysentery, bacillary
Sonne A03.3
strongyloidiasis B78.0
trichomonal A07.8
viral — see also Enteritis, viral A08.4
Dysequilibrium R42
Dysesthesia R20.8
hysterical F44.6
Dysfibrinogenemia (congenital) D68.2
Dysfunction
adrenal E27.9
hyperfunction E27.0
autonomic
due to alcohol G31.2
somatoform F45.8
bladder N31.9
neurogenic NOS — see Dysfunction, bladder, neuromuscular
neuromuscular NOS N31.9
atonic (motor) (sensory) N31.2
autonomous N31.2
flaccid N31.2
nonreflex N31.2
reflex N31.1
specified NEC N31.8
uninhibited N31.0
bleeding, uterus N93.8
cerebral G93.89
colon K59.9
psychogenic F45.8
colostomy K94.03
cystic duct K82.8
cystostomy (stoma) — see Complications, cystostomy
ejaculatory N53.19
anejaculatory orgasm N53.13
painful N53.12
premature F52.4
retarded N53.11
endocrine NOS E34.9
endometrium N85.8
enterostomy K94.13
erectile — see Dysfunction, sexual, male, erectile
gallbladder K82.8
gastrostomy (stoma) K94.23
gland, glandular NOS E34.9
meibomian, of eyelid — see Dysfunction, meibomian gland
heart I51.89
hemoglobin D75.89
hepatic K76.89
hypophysis E23.7
hypothalamic NEC E23.3
ileostomy (stoma) K94.13
jejunostomy (stoma) K94.13
kidney — see Disease, renal
labyrinthine — see subcategory H83.2 ☑
left ventricular, following sudden emotional stress I51.81
liver K76.89
male — see Dysfunction, sexual, male
meibomian gland, of eyelid H02.889
left H02.886
lower H02.885
upper H02.884
upper and lower eyelids H02.88B
right H02.883
lower H02.882
upper H02.881
upper and lower eyelids H02.88A
orgasmic (female) F52.31

Dysfunction — continued
orgasmic — continued
male F52.32
ovary E28.9
specified NEC E28.8
papillary muscle I51.89
parathyroid E21.4
physiological NEC R68.89
psychogenic F59
pineal gland E34.8
pituitary (gland) E23.3
platelets D69.1
polyglandular E31.9
specified NEC E31.8
psychophysiologic F59
psychosexual F52.9
with
dyspareunia F52.6
premature ejaculation F52.4
vaginismus F52.5
pylorus K31.9
rectum K59.9
psychogenic F45.8
reflex (sympathetic) — see Syndrome, pain, complex regional I
segmental — see Dysfunction, somatic
senile R54
sexual (due to) R37
alcohol F10.981
amphetamine F15.981
in
abuse F15.181
dependence F15.281
anxiolytic F13.981
in
abuse F13.181
dependence F13.281
cocaine F14.981
in
abuse F14.181
dependence F14.281
excessive sexual drive F52.8
failure of genital response (male) F52.21
female F52.22
female N94.9
aversion F52.1
dyspareunia N94.10
psychogenic F52.6
frigidity F52.22
nymphomania F52.8
orgasmic F52.31
psychogenic F52.9
aversion F52.1
dyspareunia F52.6
frigidity F52.22
nymphomania F52.8
orgasmic F52.31
vaginismus F52.5
vaginismus N94.2
psychogenic F52.5
hypnotic F13.981
in
abuse F13.181
dependence F13.281
inhibited orgasm (female) F52.31
male F52.32
lack
of sexual enjoyment F52.1
or loss of sexual desire F52.0
male N53.9
anejaculatory orgasm N53.13
ejaculatory N53.19
painful N53.12
premature F52.4
retarded N53.11
erectile N52.9
drug induced N52.2
due to
disease classified elsewhere N52.1
drug N52.2
postoperative (postprocedural) N52.39
following
cryotherapy N52.37
interstitial seed therapy N52.36
prostate ablative therapy N52.37
prostatectomy N52.34
radical N52.31
radiation therapy N52.35
radical cystectomy N52.32

Subterms under main terms may continue to next column or page   ☑ Additional Character Required — Refer to the Tabular List for Character Selection   123

Dwarfism — Dysfunction

Index

Dysfunction — continued
  sexual — continued
    male — continued
      erectile — continued
        postoperative — continued
          following — continued
            ultrasound ablative therapy N52.37
            urethral surgery N52.33
        psychogenic F52.21
        specified cause NEC N52.8
        vasculogenic
          arterial insufficiency N52.01
            with corporo-venous occlusive N52.03
          corporo-venous occlusive N52.02
            with arterial insufficiency N52.03
      impotence — see Dysfunction, sexual, male, erectile
      psychogenic F52.9
        aversion F52.1
        erectile F52.21
        orgasmic F52.32
        premature ejaculation F52.4
        satyriasis F52.8
        specified type NEC F52.8
      specified type NEC N53.8
    nonorganic F52.9
      specified NEC F52.8
    opioid F11.981
      in
        abuse F11.181
        dependence F11.281
    orgasmic dysfunction (female) F52.31
      male F52.32
    premature ejaculation F52.4
    psychoactive substances NEC F19.981
      in
        abuse F19.181
        dependence F19.281
    psychogenic F52.9
    sedative F13.981
      in
        abuse F13.181
        dependence F13.281
    sexual aversion F52.1
    vaginismus (nonorganic) (psychogenic) F52.5
  sinoatrial node I49.5
  somatic M99.09
    abdomen M99.09
    acromioclavicular M99.07
    cervical region M99.01
    cervicothoracic M99.01
    costochondral M99.08
    costovertebral M99.08
    head region M99.00
    hip M99.05
    lower extremity M99.06
    lumbar region M99.03
    lumbosacral M99.03
    occipitocervical M99.00
    pelvic region M99.05
    pubic M99.05
    rib cage M99.08
    sacral region M99.04
    sacrococcygeal M99.04
    sacroiliac M99.04
    specified NEC M99.09
    sternochondral M99.08
    sternoclavicular M99.07
    thoracic region M99.02
    thoracolumbar M99.02
    upper extremity M99.07
  somatoform autonomic F45.8
  stomach K31.89
    psychogenic F45.8
  suprarenal E27.9
    hyperfunction E27.0
  symbolic R48.9
    specified type NEC R48.8
  temporomandibular (joint) M26.69
    joint-pain syndrome M26.62- ☑
  testicular (endocrine) E29.9
    specified NEC E29.8
  thymus E32.9
  thyroid E07.9
  ureterostomy (stoma) — see Complications, stoma, urinary tract
  urethrostomy (stoma) — see Complications, stoma, urinary tract
  uterus, complicating delivery O62.9

Dysfunction — continued
  uterus, complicating delivery — continued
    hypertonic O62.4
    hypotonic O62.2
      primary O62.0
      secondary O62.1
  ventricular I51.9
    with congestive heart failure — see also Failure, heart I50.9
    left, reversible, following sudden emotional stress I51.81
Dysgenesis
  gonadal (due to chromosomal anomaly) Q96.9
    pure Q99.1
  renal Q60.5
    bilateral Q60.4
    unilateral Q60.3
  reticular D72.0
  tidal platelet D69.3
Dysgerminoma
  specified site — see Neoplasm, malignant, by site
  unspecified site
    female C56.9
    male C62.90
Dysgeusia R43.2
Dysgraphia R27.8
Dyshidrosis, dysidrosis L30.1
Dyskaryotic cervical smear R87.619
Dyskeratosis L85.8
  cervix — see Dysplasia, cervix
  congenital Q82.8
  uterus NEC N85.8
Dyskinesia G24.9
  biliary (cystic duct or gallbladder) K82.8
  drug induced
    orofacial G24.01
  esophagus K22.4
  hysterical F44.4
  intestinal K59.8
  nonorganic origin F44.4
  orofacial (idiopathic) G24.4
    drug induced G24.01
  psychogenic F44.4
  subacute, drug induced G24.01
  tardive G24.01
    neuroleptic induced G24.01
  trachea J39.8
  tracheobronchial J98.09
Dyslalia (developmental) F80.0
Dyslexia R48.0
  developmental F81.0
Dyslipidemia E78.5
  depressed HDL cholesterol E78.6
  elevated fasting triglycerides E78.1
Dysmaturity — see also Light for dates
  pulmonary (newborn) (Wilson-Mikity) P27.0
Dysmenorrhea (essential) (exfoliative) N94.6
  congestive (syndrome) N94.6
  primary N94.4
  psychogenic F45.8
  secondary N94.5
Dysmetabolic syndrome X E88.81
Dysmetria R27.8
Dysmorphism (due to)
  alcohol Q86.0
  exogenous cause NEC Q86.8
  hydantoin Q86.1
  warfarin Q86.2
Dysmorphophobia (nondelusional) F45.22
  delusional F22
Dysnomia R47.01
Dysorexia R63.0
  psychogenic F50.89
Dysostosis
  cleidocranial, cleidocranialis Q74.0
  craniofacial Q75.1
  Fairbank's (idiopathic familial generalized osteophytosis) Q78.9
  mandibulofacial (incomplete) Q75.4
  multiplex E76.01
  oculomandibular Q75.5
Dyspareunia (female) N94.10
  deep N94.12
  male N53.12
  nonorganic F52.6
  psychogenic F52.6
  secondary N94.19
  specified NEC N94.19

Dyspareunia — continued
  superficial (introital) N94.11
Dyspepsia R10.13
  atonic K30
  functional (allergic) (congenital) (gastrointestinal) (occupational) (reflex) K30
  intestinal K59.8
  nervous F45.8
  neurotic F45.8
  psychogenic F45.8
Dysphagia R13.10
  cervical R13.19
  following
    cerebral infarction I69.391
    cerebrovascular disease I69.991
      specified NEC I69.891
    intracerebral hemorrhage I69.191
    nontraumatic intracranial hemorrhage NEC I69.2
    specified disease NEC I69.891
    subarachnoid hemorrhage I69.091
  functional (hysterical) F45.8
  hysterical F45.8
  nervous (hysterical) F45.8
  neurogenic R13.19
  oral phase R13.11
  oropharyngeal phase R13.12
  pharyngeal phase R13.13
  pharyngoesophageal phase R13.14
  psychogenic F45.8
  sideropenic D50.1
  spastica K22.4
  specified NEC R13.19
Dysphagocytosis, congenital D71
Dysphasia R47.02
  developmental
    expressive type F80.1
    receptive type F80.2
  following
    cerebrovascular disease I69.921
    cerebral infarction I69.321
      intracerebral hemorrhage I69.121
      nontraumatic intracranial hemorrhage NEC I69.221
    specified disease NEC I69.821
    subarachnoid hemorrhage I69.021
Dysphonia R49.0
  functional F44.4
  hysterical F44.4
  psychogenic F44.4
  spastica J38.3
Dysphoria
  gender F64.9
    in
      adolescence and adulthood F64.0
      children F64.2
    specified NEC F64.8
  postpartal O90.6
Dyspituitarism E23.3
Dysplasia — see also Anomaly
  acetabular, congenital Q65.89
  alveolar capillary, with vein misalignment J84.843
  anus (histologically confirmed) (mild) (moderate) K62.82
    severe D01.3
  arrhythmogenic right ventricular I42.8
  arterial, fibromuscular I77.3
  asphyxiating thoracic (congenital) Q77.2
  brain Q07.9
  bronchopulmonary, perinatal P27.1
  cervix (uteri) N87.9
    mild N87.0
    moderate N87.1
    severe D06.9
  chondroectodermal Q77.6
  colon D12.6
  craniometaphyseal Q78.8
  dentinal K00.5
  diaphyseal, progressive Q78.3
  dystrophic Q77.5
  ectodermal (anhidrotic) (congenital) (hereditary) Q8.
    hydrotic Q82.8
  epithelial, uterine cervix — see Dysplasia, cervix
  eye (congenital) Q11.2
  fibrous
    bone NEC (monostotic) M85.00
      ankle M85.07- ☑
      foot M85.07- ☑
      forearm M85.03- ☑

Dysfunction — Dysplasia

ysplasia — continued
  fibrous — continued
    bone — continued
      hand M85.04- ☑
      lower leg M85.06- ☑
      multiple site M85.09
      neck M85.08
      rib M85.08
      shoulder M85.01- ☑
      skull M85.08
      specified site NEC M85.08
      thigh M85.05- ☑
      toe M85.07- ☑
      upper arm M85.02- ☑
      vertebra M85.08
    diaphyseal, progressive Q78.3
    jaw M27.8
    polyostotic Q78.1
  florid osseous — see also Cyst, calcifying odontogenic
  high grade, focal D12.6
  hip, congenital Q65.89
  joint, congenital Q74.8
  kidney Q61.4
    multicystic Q61.4
  leg Q74.2
  lung, congenital (not associated with short gestation) Q33.6
  mammary (gland) (benign) N60.9- ☑
    cyst (solitary) — see Cyst, breast
    cystic — see Mastopathy, cystic
    duct ectasia — see Ectasia, mammary duct
    fibroadenosis — see Fibroadenosis, breast
    fibrosclerosis — see Fibrosclerosis, breast
    specified type NEC N60.8- ☑
  metaphyseal Q78.5
  muscle Q79.8
  oculodentodigital Q87.0
  periapical (cemental) (cemento-osseous) — see Cyst, calcifying odontogenic
  periosteum — see Disorder, bone, specified type NEC
  polyostotic fibrous Q78.1
  prostate — see also Neoplasia, intraepithelial, prostate N42.30
    severe D07.5
    specified NEC N42.39
  renal Q61.4
    multicystic Q61.4
  retinal, congenital Q14.1
  right ventricular, arrhythmogenic I42.8
  septo-optic Q04.4
  skin L98.8
  spinal cord Q06.1
  spondyloepiphyseal Q77.7
  thymic, with immunodeficiency D82.1
  vagina N89.3
    mild N89.0
    moderate N89.1
    severe NEC D07.2
  vulva N90.3
    mild N90.0
    moderate N90.1
    severe NEC D07.1
ysplasminogenemia E88.02
yspnea (nocturnal) (paroxysmal) R06.00
  asthmatic (bronchial) J45.909
    with
      bronchitis J45.909
        with
          exacerbation (acute) J45.901
            status asthmaticus J45.902
        chronic J44.9
      exacerbation (acute) J45.901
      status asthmaticus J45.902
    cardiac — see Failure, ventricular, left
  cardiac — see Failure, ventricular, left
  functional F45.8
  hyperventilation R06.4
  hysterical F45.8
  newborn P28.89
  orthopnea R06.01
  psychogenic F45.8
  shortness of breath R06.02
  specified type NEC R06.09
yspraxia R27.8
  developmental (syndrome) F82
ysproteinemia E88.09
ysreflexia, autonomic G90.4

Dysrhythmia
  cardiac I49.9
    newborn
      bradycardia P29.12
      occurring before birth P03.819
        before onset of labor P03.810
        during labor P03.811
      tachycardia P29.11
    postoperative I97.89
  cerebral or cortical — see Epilepsy
Dyssomnia — see Disorder, sleep
Dyssynergia
  biliary K83.8
  bladder sphincter N36.44
  cerebellaris myoclonica (Hunt's ataxia) G11.1
Dysthymia F34.1
Dysthyroidism E07.9
Dystocia O66.9
  affecting newborn P03.1
  cervical (hypotonic) O62.2
    affecting newborn P03.6
    primary O62.0
    secondary O62.1
  contraction ring O62.4
  fetal O66.9
    abnormality NEC O66.3
    conjoined twins O66.3
    oversize O66.2
  maternal O66.9
  positional O64.9 ☑
  shoulder (girdle) O66.0
    causing obstructed labor O66.0
  uterine NEC O62.4
Dystonia G24.9
  cervical G24.3
  deformans progressiva G24.1
  drug induced NEC G24.09
    acute G24.02
    specified NEC G24.09
  familial G24.1
  idiopathic G24.1
    familial G24.1
    nonfamilial G24.2
    orofacial G24.4
  lenticularis G24.8
  musculorum deformans G24.1
  neuroleptic induced (acute) G24.02
  orofacial (idiopathic) G24.4
  oromandibular G24.4
    due to drug G24.01
  specified NEC G24.8
  torsion (familial) (idiopathic) G24.1
    acquired G24.8
    genetic G24.1
    symptomatic (nonfamilial) G24.2
Dystonic movements R25.8
Dystrophy, dystrophia
  adiposogenital E23.6
  autosomal recessive, childhood type, muscular dystrophy resembling Duchenne or Becker G71.01
  Becker's type G71.01
  cervical sympathetic G90.2
  choroid (hereditary) H31.20
    central areolar H31.22
    choroideremia H31.21
    gyrate atrophy H31.23
    specified type NEC H31.29
  cornea (hereditary) H18.50
    endothelial H18.51
    epithelial H18.52
    granular H18.53
    lattice H18.54
    macular H18.55
    specified type NEC H18.59
  Duchenne's type G71.01
  due to malnutrition E45
  Erb's G71.02
  Fuchs' H18.51
  Gower's muscular G71.01
  hair L67.8
  infantile neuraxonal G31.89
  Landouzy-Déjérine G71.02
  Leyden-Möbius G71.09
  muscular G71.00
    autosomal recessive, childhood type, muscular dystrophy resembling Duchenne or Becker G71.01
    benign (Becker type) G71.01

Dystrophy, dystrophia — continued
  muscular — continued
    benign — continued
      scapuloperoneal with early contractures [Emery-Dreifuss] G71.09
    congenital (hereditary) (progressive) (with specific morphological abnormalities of the muscle fiber) G71.09
      myotonic G71.11
    distal G71.09
    Duchenne type G71.01
    Emery-Dreifuss G71.09
    Erb type G71.02
    facioscapulohumeral G71.02
    Gower's G71.01
    hereditary (progressive) G71.09
    Landouzy-Déjérine type G71.02
    limb-girdle G71.09
    myotonic G71.11
    progressive (hereditary) G71.09
      Charcot-Marie (-Tooth) type G60.0
    pseudohypertrophic (infantile) G71.01
    scapulohumeral G71.02
    scapuloperoneal G71.09
    severe (Duchenne type) G71.01
    specified type NEC G71.09
  myocardium, myocardial — see Degeneration, myocardial
  nail L60.3
    congenital Q84.6
  nutritional E45
  ocular G71.09
  oculocerebrorenal E72.03
  oculopharyngeal G71.09
  ovarian N83.8
  polyglandular E31.8
  reflex (neuromuscular) (sympathetic) — see Syndrome, pain, complex regional I
  retinal (hereditary) H35.50
    in
      lipid storage disorders E75.6 [H36]
      systemic lipidoses E75.6 [H36]
    involving
      pigment epithelium H35.54
      sensory area H35.53
    pigmentary H35.52
    vitreoretinal H35.51
  Salzmann's nodular — see Degeneration, cornea, nodular
  scapuloperoneal G71.09
  skin NEC L98.8
  sympathetic (reflex) — see Syndrome, pain, complex regional I
    cervical G90.2
  tapetoretinal H35.54
  thoracic, asphyxiating Q77.2
  unguium L60.3
    congenital Q84.6
  vitreoretinal H35.51
  vulva N90.4
  yellow (liver) — see Failure, hepatic
Dysuria R30.0
  psychogenic F45.8

E

Eales' disease H35.06- ☑
Ear — see also condition
  piercing Z41.3
  tropical NEC B36.9 [H62.40]
    in
      aspergillosis B44.89
      candidiasis B37.84
      moniliasis B37.84
  wax (impacted) H61.20
    left H61.22
      with right H61.23
    right H61.21
      with left H61.23
Earache — see subcategory H92.0 ☑
Early satiety R68.81
Eaton-Lambert syndrome — see Syndrome, Lambert-Eaton
Eberth's disease (typhoid fever) A01.00
Ebola virus disease A98.4
Ebstein's anomaly or syndrome (heart) Q22.5
Eccentro-osteochondrodysplasia E76.29
Ecchondroma — see Neoplasm, bone, benign

Ecchondrosis D48.0
Ecchymosis R58
  conjunctiva — *see* Hemorrhage, conjunctiva
  eye (traumatic) — *see* Contusion, eyeball
  eyelid (traumatic) — *see* Contusion, eyelid
  newborn P54.5
  spontaneous R23.3
  traumatic — *see* Contusion
Echinocociasis — *see* Echinococcus
Echinococcosis — *see* Echinococcus
Echinococcus (infection) B67.90
  granulosus B67.4
    bone B67.2
    liver B67.0
    lung B67.1
    multiple sites B67.32
    specified site NEC B67.39
    thyroid B67.31
  liver NOS B67.8
    granulosus B67.0
    multilocularis B67.5
  lung NEC B67.99
    granulosus B67.1
    multilocularis B67.69
  multilocularis B67.7
    liver B67.5
    multiple sites B67.61
    specified site NEC B67.69
  specified site NEC B67.99
    granulosus B67.39
    multilocularis B67.69
  thyroid NEC B67.99
    granulosus B67.31
    multilocularis B67.69 *[E35]*
Echinorhynchiasis B83.8
Echinostomiasis B66.8
Echolalia R48.8
Echovirus, as cause of disease classified elsewhere B97.12
Eclampsia, eclamptic (coma) (convulsions) (delirium) (with hypertension) NEC O15.9
  complicating
    labor and delivery O15.1
    postpartum O15.2
    pregnancy O15.0- ☑
    puerperium O15.2
Economic circumstances affecting care Z59.9
Economo's disease A85.8
Ectasia, ectasis
  annuloaortic I35.8
  aorta I77.819
    with aneurysm — *see* Aneurysm, aorta
    abdominal I77.811
    thoracic I77.810
    thoracoabdominal I77.812
  breast — *see* Ectasia, mammary duct
  capillary I78.8
  cornea H18.71- ☑
  gastric antral vascular (GAVE) K31.819
    with hemorrhage K31.811
    without hemorrhage K31.819
  mammary duct N60.4- ☑
  salivary gland (duct) K11.8
  sclera — *see* Sclerectasia
Ecthyma L08.0
  contagiosum B08.02
  gangrenosum L08.0
  infectiosum B08.02
Ectocardia Q24.8
Ectodermal dysplasia (anhidrotic) Q82.4
Ectodermosis erosiva pluriorificialis L51.1
Ectopic, ectopia (congenital)
  abdominal viscera Q45.8
    due to defect in anterior abdominal wall Q79.59
  ACTH syndrome E24.3
  adrenal gland Q89.1
  anus Q43.5
  atrial beats I49.1
  beats I49.49
    atrial I49.1
    ventricular I49.3
  bladder Q64.10
  bone and cartilage in lung Q33.5
  brain Q04.8
  breast tissue Q83.8
  cardiac Q24.8
  cerebral Q04.8
  cordis Q24.8

Ectopic, ectopia — *continued*
  endometrium — *see* Endometriosis
  gastric mucosa Q40.2
  gestation — *see* Pregnancy, by site
  heart Q24.8
  hormone secretion NEC E34.2
  kidney (crossed) (pelvis) Q63.2
  lens, lentis Q12.1
  mole — *see* Pregnancy, by site
  organ or site NEC — *see* Malposition, congenital
  pancreas Q45.3
  pregnancy — *see* Pregnancy, ectopic
  pupil — *see* Abnormality, pupillary
  renal Q63.2
  sebaceous glands of mouth Q38.6
  spleen Q89.09
  testis Q53.00
    bilateral Q53.02
    unilateral Q53.01
  thyroid Q89.2
  tissue in lung Q33.5
  ureter Q62.63
  ventricular beats I49.3
  vesicae Q64.10
Ectromelia Q73.8
  lower limb — *see* Defect, reduction, limb, lower, specified type NEC
  upper limb — *see* Defect, reduction, limb, upper, specified type NEC
Ectropion H02.109
  cervix N86
    with cervicitis N72
  congenital Q10.1
  eyelid H02.109
    cicatricial H02.119
      left H02.116
        lower H02.115
        upper H02.114
      right H02.113
        lower H02.112
        upper H02.111
    congenital Q10.1
    left H02.106
      lower H02.105
      upper H02.104
    mechanical H02.129
      left H02.126
        lower H02.125
        upper H02.124
      right H02.123
        lower H02.122
        upper H02.121
    paralytic H02.159
      left H02.156
        lower H02.155
        upper H02.154
      right H02.153
        lower H02.152
        upper H02.151
    right H02.103
      lower H02.102
      upper H02.101
    senile H02.139
      left H02.136
        lower H02.135
        upper H02.134
      right H02.133
        lower H02.132
        upper H02.131
    spastic H02.149
      left H02.146
        lower H02.145
        upper H02.144
      right H02.143
        lower H02.142
        upper H02.141
  iris H21.89
  lip (acquired) K13.0
    congenital Q38.0
  urethra N36.8
  uvea H21.89
Eczema (acute) (chronic) (erythematous) (fissum) (rubrum) (squamous) — *see also* Dermatitis L30.9
  contact — *see* Dermatitis, contact
  dyshydrotic L30.1
  external ear — *see* Otitis, externa, acute, eczematoid
  flexural L20.82
  herpeticum B00.0

Eczema — *continued*
  hypertrophicum L28.0
  hypostatic — *see* Varix, leg, with, inflammation
  impetiginous L01.1
  infantile (due to any substance) L20.83
    intertriginous L21.1
    seborrheic L21.1
  intertriginous NEC L30.4
    infantile L21.1
  intrinsic (allergic) L20.84
  lichenified NEC L28.0
  marginatum (hebrae) B35.6
  pustular L30.3
  stasis I87.2
    with varicose veins — *see* Varix, leg, with, inflammation
  vaccination, vaccinatum T88.1 ☑
  varicose — *see* Varix, leg, with, inflammation
Eczematid L30.2
Eddowes (-Spurway) **syndrome** Q78.0
Edema, edematous (infectious) (pitting) (toxic) R60.*
  with nephritis — *see* Nephrosis
  allergic T78.3 ☑
  amputation stump (surgical) (sequelae (late effect)) T87.89
  angioneurotic (allergic) (any site) (with urticaria) T78.3 ☑
    hereditary D84.1
  angiospastic I73.9
  Berlin's (traumatic) S05.8X- ☑
  brain (cytotoxic) (vasogenic) G93.6
    due to birth injury P11.0
      newborn (anoxia or hypoxia) P52.4
        birth injury P11.0
    traumatic — *see* Injury, intracranial, cerebral edem
  cardiac — *see* Failure, heart, congestive
  cardiovascular — *see* Failure, heart, congestive
  cerebral — *see* Edema, brain
  cerebrospinal — *see* Edema, brain
  cervix (uteri) (acute) N88.8
    puerperal, postpartum O90.89
  chronic hereditary Q82.0
  circumscribed, acute T78.3 ☑
    hereditary D84.1
  conjunctiva H11.42- ☑
  cornea H18.2- ☑
    idiopathic H18.22- ☑
    secondary H18.23- ☑
      due to contact lens H18.21- ☑
  due to
    lymphatic obstruction I89.0
    salt retention E87.0
  epiglottis — *see* Edema, glottis
  essential, acute T78.3 ☑
    hereditary D84.1
  extremities, lower — *see* Edema, legs
  eyelid NEC H02.849
    left H02.846
      lower H02.845
      upper H02.844
    right H02.843
      lower H02.842
      upper H02.841
  familial, hereditary Q82.0
  famine — *see* Malnutrition, severe
  generalized R60.1
  glottis, glottic, glottidis (obstructive) (passive) J38.4
    allergic T78.3 ☑
      hereditary D84.1
  heart — *see* Failure, heart, congestive
  heat T67.7 ☑
  hereditary Q82.0
  inanition — *see* Malnutrition, severe
  intracranial G93.6
  iris H21.89
  joint — *see* Effusion, joint
  larynx — *see* Edema, glottis
  legs R60.0
    due to venous obstruction I87.1
    hereditary Q82.0
  localized R60.0
    due to venous obstruction I87.1
  lower limbs — *see* Edema, legs
  lung J81.9
    with heart condition or failure — *see* Failure, ventricular, left
    acute J81.0
    chemical (acute) J68.1

☑ **Additional Character Required — Refer to the Tabular List for Character Selection**   ▽ Subterms under main terms may continue to next column or pa◄

Ekman's syndrome (brittle bones and blue sclera) Q78.0
Elastic skin Q82.8
   acquired L57.4
Elastofibroma — see Neoplasm, connective tissue, benign
Elastoma (juvenile) Q82.8
   Miescher's L87.2
Elastomyofibrosis I42.4
Elastosis
   actinic, solar L57.8
   atrophicans (senile) L57.4
   perforans serpiginosa L87.2
   senilis L57.4
Elbow — see condition
Electric current, electricity, effects (concussion) (fatal) (nonfatal) (shock) T75.4 ☑
   burn — see Burn
Electric feet syndrome E53.8
Electrocution T75.4 ☑
   from electroshock gun (taser) T75.4 ☑
Electrolyte imbalance E87.8
   with
      abortion — see Abortion by type, complicated by, electrolyte imbalance
      ectopic pregnancy O08.5
      molar pregnancy O08.5
Elephantiasis (nonfilarial) I89.0
   arabicum — see Infestation, filarial
   bancroftian B74.0
   congenital (any site) (hereditary) Q82.0
   due to
      Brugia (malayi) B74.1
         timori B74.2
      mastectomy I97.2
      Wuchereria (bancrofti) B74.0
   eyelid H02.859
      left H02.856
         lower H02.855
         upper H02.854
      right H02.853
         lower H02.852
         upper H02.851
   filarial, filariensis — see Infestation, filarial
   glandular I89.0
   graecorum A30.9
   lymphangiectatic I89.0
   lymphatic vessel I89.0
      due to mastectomy I97.2
   scrotum (nonfilarial) I89.0
   streptococcal I89.0
   surgical I97.89
      postmastectomy I97.2
   telangiectodes I89.0
   vulva (nonfilarial) N90.89
Elevated, elevation
   antibody titer R76.0
   basal metabolic rate R94.8
   blood pressure — see also Hypertension
      reading (incidental) (isolated) (nonspecific), no diagnosis of hypertension R03.0
   blood sugar R73.9
   body temperature (of unknown origin) R50.9
   cancer antigen 125 [CA 125] R97.1
   carcinoembryonic antigen [CEA] R97.0
   cholesterol E78.00
      with high triglycerides E78.2
   conjugate, eye H51.0
   C-reactive protein (CRP) R79.82
   diaphragm, congenital Q79.1
   erythrocyte sedimentation rate R70.0
   fasting glucose R73.01
   fasting triglycerides E78.1
   finding on laboratory examination — see Findings, abnormal, inconclusive, without diagnosis, by type of exam
   GFR (glomerular filtration rate) — see Findings, abnormal, inconclusive, without diagnosis, by type of exam
   glucose tolerance (oral) R73.02
   immunoglobulin level R76.8
   indoleacetic acid R82.5
   lactic acid dehydrogenase (LDH) level R74.0
   leukocytes D72.829
   lipoprotein a (Lp(a)) level E78.41
   liver function
      study R94.5
      test R79.89
         alkaline phosphatase R74.8

Elevated, elevation — continued
   liver function — continued
      test — continued
         aminotransferase R74.0
         bilirubin R17
         hepatic enzyme R74.8
         lactate dehydrogenase R74.0
   Lp(a) (lipoprotein(a)) E78.41
   lymphocytes D72.820
   prostate specific antigen [PSA] R97.20
   Rh titer — see Complication(s), transfusion, incompatibility reaction, Rh (factor)
   scapula, congenital Q74.0
   sedimentation rate R70.0
   SGOT R74.0
   SGPT R74.0
   transaminase level R74.0
   triglycerides E78.1
      with high cholesterol E78.2
   tumor associated antigens [TAA] NEC R97.8
   tumor specific antigens [TSA] NEC R97.8
   urine level of
      17-ketosteroids R82.5
      catecholamine R82.5
      indoleacetic acid R82.5
      steroids R82.5
      vanillylmandelic acid (VMA) R82.5
   venous pressure I87.8
   white blood cell count D72.829
      specified NEC D72.828
Elliptocytosis (congenital) (hereditary) D58.1
   Hb C (disease) D58.1
   hemoglobin disease D58.1
   sickle-cell (disease) D57.8- ☑
      trait D57.3
Ellison-Zollinger syndrome E16.4
Ellis-van Creveld syndrome (chondroectodermal dysplasia) Q77.6
Elongated, elongation (congenital) — see also Distortion
   bone Q79.9
   cervix (uteri) Q51.828
      acquired N88.4
      hypertrophic N88.4
   colon Q43.8
   common bile duct Q44.5
   cystic duct Q44.5
   frenulum, penis Q55.69
   labia minora (acquired) N90.69
   ligamentum patellae Q74.1
   petiolus (epiglottidis) Q31.8
   tooth, teeth K00.2
   uvula Q38.6
Eltor cholera A00.1
Emaciation (due to malnutrition) E41
Embadomoniasis A07.8
Embedded tooth, teeth K01.0
   root only K08.3
Embolic — see condition
Embolism (multiple) (paradoxical) I74.9
   air (any site) (traumatic) T79.0 ☑
      following
         abortion — see Abortion by type complicated by embolism
         ectopic pregnancy O08.2
         infusion, therapeutic injection or transfusion T80.0 ☑
         molar pregnancy O08.2
         procedure NEC
            artery T81.719 ☑
               mesenteric T81.710 ☑
               renal T81.711 ☑
               specified NEC T81.718 ☑
            vein T81.72 ☑
      in pregnancy, childbirth or puerperium — see Embolism, obstetric
   amniotic fluid (pulmonary) — see also Embolism, obstetric
      following
         abortion — see Abortion by type complicated by embolism
         ectopic pregnancy O08.2
         molar pregnancy O08.2
   aorta, aortic I74.10
      abdominal I74.09
         saddle I74.01
      bifurcation I74.09
      saddle I74.01

Embolism — continued
   aorta, aortic — continued
      thoracic I74.11
   artery I74.9
      auditory, internal I65.8
      basilar — see Occlusion, artery, basilar
      carotid (common) (internal) — see Occlusion, artery, carotid
      cerebellar (anterior inferior) (posterior inferior) (perior) I66.3
      cerebral — see Occlusion, artery, cerebral
      choroidal (anterior) I65.8
      communicating posterior I65.8
      coronary — see also Infarct, myocardium
         not resulting in infarction I24.0
      extremity I74.4
         lower I74.3
         upper I74.2
      hypophyseal I65.8
      iliac I74.5
      limb I74.4
         lower I74.3
         upper I74.2
      mesenteric (with gangrene) — see also Ischemia intestine, acute K55.059
      ophthalmic — see Occlusion, artery, retina
      peripheral I74.4
      pontine I65.8
      precerebral — see Occlusion, artery, precerebra
      pulmonary — see Embolism, pulmonary
      renal N28.0
      retinal — see Occlusion, artery, retina
      septic I76
      specified NEC I74.8
      vertebral — see Occlusion, artery, vertebral
   basilar (artery) I65.1
   blood clot
      following
         abortion — see Abortion by type complicate by embolism
         ectopic or molar pregnancy O08.2
      in pregnancy, childbirth or puerperium — see Embolism, obstetric
   brain — see also Occlusion, artery, cerebral
      following
         abortion — see Abortion by type complicate by embolism
         ectopic or molar pregnancy O08.2
      puerperal, postpartum, childbirth — see Embolis obstetric
   capillary I78.8
   cardiac — see also Infarct, myocardium
      not resulting in infarction I51.3
   carotid (artery) (common) (internal) — see Occlusion artery, carotid
   cavernous sinus (venous) — see Embolism, intracran venous sinus
   cerebral — see Occlusion, artery, cerebral
   cholesterol — see Atheroembolism
   coronary (artery or vein) (systemic) — see Occlusio coronary
   due to device, implant or graft — see also Complications, by site and type, specified NEC
      arterial graft NEC T82.818 ☑
      breast (implant) T85.818 ☑
      catheter NEC T85.818 ☑
         dialysis (renal) T82.818 ☑
            intraperitoneal T85.818 ☑
         infusion NEC T82.818 ☑
            spinal (epidural) (subdural) T85.810 ☑
         urinary (indwelling) T83.81 ☑
      electronic (electrode) (pulse generator) (stimulat
         bone T84.81 ☑
         cardiac T82.817 ☑
         nervous system (brain) (peripheral nerve) (spir
            T85.810 ☑
         urinary T83.81 ☑
      fixation, internal (orthopedic) NEC T84.81 ☑
      gastrointestinal (bile duct) (esophagus) T85.818
      genital NEC T83.81 ☑
      heart (graft) (valve) T82.817 ☑
      joint prosthesis T84.81 ☑
      ocular (corneal graft) (orbital implant) T85.818 ☑
      orthopedic (bone graft) NEC T86.838
      specified NEC T85.818 ☑
      urinary (graft) NEC T83.81 ☑
      vascular NEC T82.818 ☑

☑ **Additional Character Required** — Refer to the Tabular List for Character Selection   ▽ Subterms under main terms may continue to next column or pa

mbolism — *continued*
  due to device, implant or graft — *see also* Complications, by site and type, specified — *continued*
    ventricular intracranial shunt T85.810 ☑
  extremities
    lower — *see* Embolism, vein, lower extremity
      arterial I74.3
    upper I74.2
  eye H34.9
  fat (cerebral) (pulmonary) (systemic) T79.1 ☑
    complicating delivery — *see* Embolism, obstetric
    following
      abortion — *see* Abortion by type complicated by embolism
      ectopic or molar pregnancy O08.2
  following
    abortion — *see* Abortion by type complicated by embolism
    ectopic or molar pregnancy O08.2
    infusion, therapeutic injection or transfusion
      air T80.0 ☑
  heart (fatty) — *see also* Infarct, myocardium
    not resulting in infarction I51.3
  hepatic (vein) I82.0
  in pregnancy, childbirth or puerperium — *see* Embolism, obstetric
  intestine (artery) (vein) (with gangrene) — *see also* Ischemia, intestine, acute K55.039
  intracranial — *see also* Occlusion, artery, cerebral
    venous sinus (any) G08
      nonpyogenic I67.6
  intraspinal venous sinuses or veins G08
    nonpyogenic G95.19
  kidney (artery) N28.0
  lateral sinus (venous) — *see* Embolism, intracranial, venous sinus
  leg — *see* Embolism, vein, lower extremity
    arterial I74.3
  longitudinal sinus (venous) — *see* Embolism, intracranial, venous sinus
  lung (massive) — *see* Embolism, pulmonary
  meninges I66.8
  mesenteric (artery) (vein) (with gangrene) — *see also* Ischemia, intestine, acute K55.059
  obstetric (in) (pulmonary)
    childbirth O88.22
      air O88.02
      amniotic fluid O88.12
      blood clot O88.22
      fat O88.82
      pyemic O88.32
      septic O88.32
      specified type NEC O88.82
    pregnancy O88.21- ☑
      air O88.01- ☑
      amniotic fluid O88.11- ☑
      blood clot O88.21- ☑
      fat O88.81- ☑
      pyemic O88.31- ☑
      septic O88.31- ☑
      specified type NEC O88.81- ☑
    puerperal O88.23
      air O88.03
      amniotic fluid O88.13
      blood clot O88.23
      fat O88.83
      pyemic O88.33
      septic O88.33
      specified type NEC O88.83
  ophthalmic — *see* Occlusion, artery, retina
  penis N48.81
  peripheral artery NOS I74.4
  pituitary E23.6
  popliteal (artery) I74.3
  portal (vein) I81
  postoperative, postprocedural
    artery T81.719 ☑
      mesenteric T81.710 ☑
      renal T81.711 ☑
      specified NEC T81.718 ☑
    vein T81.72 ☑
  precerebral artery — *see* Occlusion, artery, precerebral
  puerperal — *see* Embolism, obstetric
  pulmonary (acute) (artery) (vein) I26.99
    with acute cor pulmonale I26.09
    chronic I27.82

Embolism — *continued*
  pulmonary — *continued*
    following
      abortion — *see* Abortion by type complicated by embolism
      ectopic or molar pregnancy O08.2
    healed or old Z86.711
    in pregnancy, childbirth or puerperium — *see* Embolism, obstetric
    multiple subsegmental without acute cor pulmonale I26.94
    personal history of Z86.711
    saddle I26.92
      with acute cor pulmonale I26.02
    septic I26.90
      with acute cor pulmonale I26.01
    single subsegmental without acute cor pulmonale I26.93
    subsegmental NOS I26.93
  pyemic (multiple) I76
    following
      abortion — *see* Abortion by type complicated by embolism
      ectopic or molar pregnancy O08.2
    Hemophilus influenzae A41.3
    pneumococcal A40.3
      with pneumonia J13
    puerperal, postpartum, childbirth (any organism) — *see* Embolism, obstetric
    specified organism NEC A41.89
    staphylococcal A41.2
    streptococcal A40.9
  renal (artery) N28.0
    vein I82.3
  retina, retinal — *see* Occlusion, artery, retina
  saddle
    abdominal aorta I74.01
    pulmonary artery I26.92
      with acute cor pulmonale I26.02
  septic (arterial) I76
    complicating abortion — *see* Abortion, by type, complicated by, embolism
  sinus — *see* Embolism, intracranial, venous sinus
  soap complicating abortion — *see* Abortion, by type, complicated by, embolism
  spinal cord G95.19
    pyogenic origin G06.1
  spleen, splenic (artery) I74.8
  upper extremity I74.2
  vein (acute) I82.90
    antecubital I82.61- ☑
      chronic I82.71- ☑
    axillary I82.A1- ☑ (*following* I82.7)
      chronic I82.A2- ☑ (*following* I82.7)
    basilic I82.61- ☑
      chronic I82.71- ☑
    brachial I82.62- ☑
      chronic I82.72- ☑
    brachiocephalic (innominate) I82.290
      chronic I82.291
    cephalic I82.61- ☑
      chronic I82.71- ☑
    chronic I82.91
    deep (DVT) I82.40- ☑
      calf I82.4Z- ☑
        chronic I82.5Z- ☑
      lower leg I82.4Z- ☑
        chronic I82.5Z- ☑
      thigh I82.4Y- ☑
        chronic I82.5Y- ☑
      upper leg I82.4Y ☑
        chronic I82.5Y-
    femoral I82.41- ☑
      chronic I82.51- ☑
    iliac (iliofemoral) I82.42- ☑
      chronic I82.52- ☑
    innominate I82.290
      chronic I82.291
    internal jugular I82.C1- ☑ (*following* I82.7)
      chronic I82.C2- ☑ (*following* I82.7)
    lower extremity
      deep I82.40- ☑
        chronic I82.50- ☑
        specified NEC I82.49- ☑
          chronic NEC I82.59- ☑
      distal
        deep I82.4Z- ☑

Embolism — *continued*
  vein — *continued*
    lower extremity — *continued*
      proximal
        deep I82.4Y- ☑
          chronic I82.5Y- ☑
        superficial I82.81- ☑
      popliteal I82.43- ☑
        chronic I82.53- ☑
    radial I82.62- ☑
      chronic I82.72- ☑
    renal I82.3
    saphenous (greater) (lesser) I82.81- ☑
    specified NEC I82.890
      chronic NEC I82.891
    subclavian I82.B1- ☑ (*following* I82.7)
      chronic I82.B2- ☑ (*following* I82.7)
    thoracic NEC I82.290
      chronic I82.291
    tibial I82.44- ☑
      chronic I82.54- ☑
    ulnar I82.62- ☑
      chronic I82.72- ☑
    upper extremity I82.60- ☑
      chronic I82.70- ☑
      deep I82.62- ☑
        chronic I82.72- ☑
      superficial I82.61- ☑
        chronic I82.71- ☑
  vena cava
    inferior (acute) I82.220
      chronic I82.221
    superior (acute) I82.210
      chronic I82.211
  venous sinus G08
  vessels of brain — *see* Occlusion, artery, cerebral
Embolus — *see* Embolism
Embryoma — *see also* Neoplasm, uncertain behavior, by site
  benign — *see* Neoplasm, benign, by site
  kidney C64.- ☑
  liver C22.0
  malignant — *see also* Neoplasm, malignant, by site
    kidney C64.- ☑
    liver C22.0
    testis C62.9- ☑
      descended (scrotal) C62.1- ☑
      undescended C62.0- ☑
  testis C62.9- ☑
    descended (scrotal) C62.1- ☑
    undescended C62.0- ☑
Embryonic
  circulation Q28.9
  heart Q28.9
  vas deferens Q55.4
Embryopathia NOS Q89.9
Embryotoxon Q13.4
Emesis — *see* Vomiting
Emotional lability R45.86
Emotionality, pathological F60.3
Emotogenic disease — *see* Disorder, psychogenic
Emphysema (atrophic) (bullous) (chronic) (interlobular) (lung) (obstructive) (pulmonary) (senile) (vesicular) J43.9
  cellular tissue (traumatic) T79.7 ☑
    surgical T81.82 ☑
  centrilobular J43.2
  compensatory J98.3
  congenital (interstitial) P25.0
  conjunctiva H11.89
  connective tissue (traumatic) T79.7 ☑
    surgical T81.82 ☑
  due to chemicals, gases, fumes or vapors J68.4
  eyelid(s) — *see* Disorder, eyelid, specified type NEC
    surgical T81.82 ☑
    traumatic T79.7 ☑
  interstitial J98.2
    congenital P25.0
    perinatal period P25.0
  laminated tissue T79.7 ☑
    surgical T81.82 ☑
  mediastinal J98.2
    newborn P25.2
  orbit, orbital — *see* Disorder, orbit, specified type NEC
  panacinar J43.1
  panlobular J43.1
  specified NEC J43.8

Emphysema — *continued*
  subcutaneous (traumatic) T79.7 ☑
    nontraumatic J98.2
    postprocedural T81.82 ☑
    surgical T81.82 ☑
  surgical T81.82 ☑
  thymus (gland) (congenital) E32.8
  traumatic (subcutaneous) T79.7 ☑
  unilateral J43.0
Empty nest syndrome Z60.0
Empyema (acute) (chest) (double) (pleura) (supradiaphrag-
    matic) (thorax) J86.9
  with fistula J86.0
  accessory sinus (chronic) — *see* Sinusitis
  antrum (chronic) — *see* Sinusitis, maxillary
  brain (any part) — *see* Abscess, brain
  ethmoidal (chronic) (sinus) — *see* Sinusitis, ethmoidal
  extradural — *see* Abscess, extradural
  frontal (chronic) (sinus) — *see* Sinusitis, frontal
  gallbladder K81.0
  mastoid (process) (acute) — *see* Mastoiditis, acute
  maxilla, maxillary M27.2
    sinus (chronic) — *see* Sinusitis, maxillary
  nasal sinus (chronic) — *see* Sinusitis
  sinus (accessory) (chronic) (nasal) — *see* Sinusitis
  sphenoidal (sinus) (chronic) — *see* Sinusitis, sphenoidal
  subarachnoid — *see* Abscess, extradural
  subdural — *see* Abscess, subdural
  tuberculous A15.6
  ureter — *see* Ureteritis
  ventricular — *see* Abscess, brain
En coup de sabre lesion L94.1
Enamel pearls K00.2
Enameloma K00.2
Enanthema, viral B09
Encephalitis (chronic) (hemorrhagic) (idiopathic)
    (nonepidemic) (spurious) (subacute) G04.90
  acute — *see also* Encephalitis, viral A86
    disseminated G04.00
      infectious G04.01
      noninfectious G04.81
      postimmunization (postvaccination) G04.02
      postinfectious G04.01
    inclusion body A85.8
    necrotizing hemorrhagic G04.30
      postimmunization G04.32
      postinfectious G04.31
      specified NEC G04.39
  arboviral, arbovirus NEC A85.2
  arthropod-borne NEC (viral) A85.2
  Australian A83.4
  California (virus) A83.5
  Central European (tick-borne) A84.1
  Czechoslovakian A84.1
  Dawson's (inclusion body) A81.1
  diffuse sclerosing A81.1
  disseminated, acute G04.00
  due to
    cat scratch disease A28.1
    human immunodeficiency virus (HIV) disease
      B20 *[G05.3]*
    malaria — *see* Malaria
    rickettsiosis — *see* Rickettsiosis
    smallpox inoculation G04.02
    typhus — *see* Typhus
  Eastern equine A83.2
  endemic (viral) A86
  epidemic NEC (viral) A86
  equine (acute) (infectious) (viral) A83.9
    Eastern A83.2
    Venezuelan A92.2
    Western A83.1
  Far Eastern (tick-borne) A84.0
  following vaccination or other immunization procedure
    G04.02
  herpes zoster B02.0
  herpesviral B00.4
    due to herpesvirus 6 B10.01
    due to herpesvirus 7 B10.09
    specified NEC B10.09
  Ilheus (virus) A83.8
  in (due to)
    actinomycosis A42.82
    adenovirus A85.1
    African trypanosomiasis B56.9 *[G05.3]*
    Chagas' disease (chronic) B57.42
    cytomegalovirus B25.8
    enterovirus A85.0

Encephalitis — *continued*
  in — *continued*
    herpes (simplex) virus B00.4
      due to herpesvirus 6 B10.01
      due to herpesvirus 7 B10.09
      specified NEC B10.09
    infectious disease NEC B99 ☑ *[G05.3]*
    influenza — *see* Influenza, with, encephalopathy
    listeriosis A32.12
    measles B05.0
    mumps B26.2
    naegleriasis B60.2
    parasitic disease NEC B89 *[G05.3]*
    poliovirus A80.9 *[G05.3]*
    rubella B06.01
    syphilis
      congenital A50.42
      late A52.14
    systemic lupus erythematosus M32.19
    toxoplasmosis (acquired) B58.2
      congenital P37.1
    tuberculosis A17.82
    zoster B02.0
  inclusion body A81.1
  infectious (acute) (virus) NEC A86
  Japanese (B type) A83.0
  La Crosse A83.5
  lead — *see* Poisoning, lead
  lethargica (acute) (infectious) A85.8
  louping ill A84.8
  lupus erythematosus, systemic M32.19
  lymphatica A87.2
  Mengo A85.8
  meningococcal A39.81
  Murray Valley A83.4
  otitic NEC H66.40 *[G05.3]*
  parasitic NOS B71.9
  periaxial G37.0
  periaxialis (concentrica) (diffuse) G37.5
  postchickenpox B01.11
  postexanthematous NEC B09
  postimmunization G04.02
  postinfectious NEC G04.01
  postmeasles B05.0
  postvaccinal G04.02
  postvaricella B01.11
  postviral NEC A86
  Powassan A84.8
  Rasmussen G04.81
  Rio Bravo A85.8
  Russian
    autumnal A83.0
    spring-summer (taiga) A84.0
  saturnine — *see* Poisoning, lead
  specified NEC G04.81
  St. Louis A83.3
  subacute sclerosing A81.1
  summer A83.0
  suppurative G04.81
  tick-borne A84.9
  Torula, torular (cryptococcal) B45.1
  toxic NEC G92
  trichinosis B75 *[G05.3]*
  type
    B A83.0
    C A83.3
  van Bogaert's A81.1
  Venezuelan equine A92.2
  Vienna A85.8
  viral, virus A86
    arthropod-borne NEC A85.2
      mosquito-borne A83.9
        Australian X disease A83.4
        California virus A83.5
        Eastern equine A83.2
        Japanese (B type) A83.0
        Murray Valley A83.4
        specified NEC A83.8
        St. Louis A83.3
        type B A83.0
        type C A83.3
        Western equine A83.1
      tick-borne A84.9
        biundulant A84.1
        central European A84.1
        Czechoslovakian A84.1
        diphasic meningoencephalitis A84.1
        Far Eastern A84.0

Encephalitis — *continued*
  viral, virus — *continued*
    arthropod-borne — *continued*
      tick-borne — *continued*
        Russian spring-summer (taiga) A84.0
        specified NEC A84.8
      specified type NEC A85.8
    Western equine A83.1
Encephalocele Q01.9
  frontal Q01.0
  nasofrontal Q01.1
  occipital Q01.2
  specified NEC Q01.8
Encephalocystocele — *see* Encephalocele
Encephaloduroarteriomyosynangiosis (EDAMS) I6
Encephalomalacia (brain) (cerebellar) (cerebral) — *s*
  Softening, brain
Encephalomeningitis — *see* Meningoencephalitis
Encephalomeningocele — *see* Encephalocele
Encephalomeningomyelitis — *see* Meningoencepha
Encephalomyelitis — *see also* Encephalitis G04.90
  acute disseminated G04.00
    infectious G04.01
    noninfectious G04.81
    postimmunization G04.02
    postinfectious G04.01
  acute necrotizing hemorrhagic G04.30
    postimmunization G04.32
    postinfectious G04.31
    specified NEC G04.39
  benign myalgic G93.3
  equine A83.9
    Eastern A83.2
    Venezuelan A92.2
    Western A83.1
  in diseases classified elsewhere G05.3
  myalgic, benign G93.3
  postchickenpox B01.11
  postinfectious NEC G04.01
  postmeasles B05.0
  postvaccinal G04.02
  postvaricella B01.11
  rubella B06.01
  specified NEC G04.81
  Venezuelan equine A92.2
Encephalomyelocele — *see* Encephalocele
Encephalomyelomeningitis — *see* Meningoencepha
Encephalomyelopathy G96.9
Encephalomyeloradiculitis (acute) G61.0
Encephalomyeloradiculoneuritis (acute) (Guillain-
  Barré) G61.0
Encephalomyeloradiculopathy G96.9
Encephalopathia hyperbilirubinemica, newborn
  P57.9
  due to isoimmunization (conditions in P55) P57.0
Encephalopathy (acute) G93.40
  acute necrotizing hemorrhagic G04.30
    postimmunization G04.32
    postinfectious G04.31
    specified NEC G04.39
  alcoholic G31.2
  anoxic — *see* Damage, brain, anoxic
  arteriosclerotic I67.2
  centrolobar progressive (Schilder) G37.0
  congenital Q07.9
  degenerative, in specified disease NEC G32.89
  demyelinating callosal G37.1
  due to
    drugs — *see also* Table of Drugs and Chemicals G
  hepatic — *see* Failure, hepatic
  hyperbilirubinemic, newborn P57.9
    due to isoimmunization (conditions in P55) P57
  hypertensive I67.4
  hypoglycemic E16.2
  hypoxic — *see* Damage, brain, anoxic
  hypoxic ischemic P91.60
    mild P91.61
    moderate P91.62
    severe P91.63
  in (due to) (with)
    birth injury P11.1
    hyperinsulinism E16.1 *[G94]*
    influenza — *see* Influenza, with, encephalopath
    lack of vitamin — *see also* Deficiency, vitamin
      E56.9 *[G32.89]*
    neoplastic disease — *see also* Neoplasm
      D49.9 *[G13.1]*
    serum — *see also* Reaction, serum T80.69 ☑

cephalopathy — *continued*
  in — *continued*
    syphilis A52.17
    trauma (postconcussional) F07.81
      current injury — *see* Injury, intracranial
    vaccination G04.02
  lead — *see* Poisoning, lead
  metabolic G93.41
    drug induced G92
    toxic G92
  myoclonic, early, symptomatic — *see* Epilepsy, generalized, specified NEC
  necrotizing, subacute (Leigh) G31.82
  neonatal P91.819
    in diseases classified elsewhere P91.811
  pellagrous E52 *[G32.89]*
  portosystemic — *see* Failure, hepatic
  postcontusional F07.81
    current injury — *see* Injury, intracranial, diffuse
  posthypoglycemic (coma) E16.1 *[G94]*
  postradiation G93.89
  saturnine — *see* Poisoning, lead
  septic G93.41
  specified NEC G93.49
  spongiform, subacute (viral) A81.09
  toxic G92
    metabolic G92
  traumatic (postconcussional) F07.81
    current injury — *see* Injury, intracranial
  vitamin B deficiency NEC E53.9 *[G32.89]*
    vitamin B1 E51.2
  Wernicke's E51.2
cephalorrhagia — *see* Hemorrhage, intracranial, intracerebral
cephalosis, posttraumatic F07.81
chondroma — *see also* Neoplasm, bone, benign
chondromatosis (cartilaginous) (multiple) Q78.4
copresis R15.9
  functional F98.1
  nonorganic origin F98.1
  psychogenic F98.1
counter (with health service) (for) Z76.89
  adjustment and management (of)
    breast implant Z45.81 ☑
    implanted device NEC Z45.89
    myringotomy device (stent) (tube) Z45.82
    neurostimulator (brain) (gastric) (peripheral nerve) (sacral nerve) (spinal cord) (vagus nerve) Z45.42
  administrative purpose only Z02.9
    examination for
      adoption Z02.82
      armed forces Z02.3
      disability determination Z02.71
      driving license Z02.4
      employment Z02.1
      insurance Z02.6
      medical certificate NEC Z02.79
      paternity testing Z02.81
      residential institution admission Z02.2
      school admission Z02.0
      sports Z02.5
    specified reason NEC Z02.89
  aftercare — *see* Aftercare
  antenatal screening Z36.9
    cervical length Z36.86
    chromosomal anomalies Z36.0
    congenital cardiac abnormalities Z36.83
    elevated maternal serum alphafetoprotein Z36.1
    fetal growth retardation Z36.4
    fetal lung maturity Z36.84
    fetal macrosomia Z36.88
    hydrops fetalis Z36.81
    intrauterine growth restriction (IUGR) /small-for-dates Z36.4
    isoimmunization Z36.5
    large-for-dates Z36.88
    malformations Z36.3
    non-visualized anatomy on a previous scan Z36.2
    nuchal translucency Z36.82
    raised alphafetoprotein level Z36.1
    risk of pre-term labor Z36.86
    specified follow-up NEC Z36.2
    specified genetic defects NEC Z36.8A
    specified type NEC Z36.89
    Streptococcus B Z36.85
    suspected anomaly Z36.3
    uncertain dates Z36.87

Encounter — *continued*
  assisted reproductive fertility procedure cycle Z31.83
  blood typing Z01.83
    Rh typing Z01.83
  breast augmentation or reduction Z41.1
  breast implant exchange (different material) (different size) Z45.81 ☑
  breast reconstruction following mastectomy Z42.1
  check-up — *see* Examination
  chemotherapy for neoplasm Z51.11
  colonoscopy, screening Z12.11
  counseling — *see* Counseling
  delivery, full-term, uncomplicated O80
    cesarean, without indication O82
  desensitization to allergens Z51.6
  ear piercing Z41.3
  examination — *see* Examination
  expectant parent(s) (adoptive) pre-birth pediatrician visit Z76.81
  fertility preservation procedure (prior to cancer therapy) (prior to removal of gonads) Z31.84
  fitting (of) — *see* Fitting (and adjustment) (of)
  genetic
    counseling
      nonprocreative Z71.83
      procreative Z31.5
    testing — *see* Test, genetic
  hearing conservation and treatment Z01.12
  immunotherapy for neoplasm Z51.12
  in vitro fertilization cycle Z31.83
  instruction (in)
    child care (postpartal) (prenatal) Z32.3
    childbirth Z32.2
    natural family planning
      procreative Z31.61
      to avoid pregnancy Z30.02
  insulin pump titration Z46.81
  joint prosthesis insertion following prior explantation of joint prosthesis (staged procedure)
    hip Z47.32
    knee Z47.33
    shoulder Z47.31
  laboratory (as part of a general medical examination) Z00.00
    with abnormal findings Z00.01
  mental health services (for)
    abuse NEC
      perpetrator Z69.82
      victim Z69.81
    child abuse
      nonparental
        perpetrator Z69.021
        victim Z69.020
      parental
        perpetrator Z69.011
        victim Z69.010
    child neglect
      nonparental
        perpetrator Z69.021
        victim Z69.020
      parental
        perpetrator Z69.011
        victim Z69.010
    child psychological abuse
      nonparental
        perpetrator Z69.021
        victim Z69.020
      parental
        perpetrator Z69.011
        victim Z69.010
    child sexual abuse
      nonparental
        perpetrator Z69.021
        victim Z69.020
      parental
        perpetrator Z69.011
        victim Z69.010
    non-spousal adult abuse
      perpetrator Z69.82
      victim Z69.81
    spousal or partner
      abuse
        perpetrator Z69.12
        victim Z69.11
      neglect
        perpetrator Z69.12
        victim Z69.11
      psychological abuse
        perpetrator Z69.12

Encounter — *continued*
  mental health services — *continued*
    spousal or partner — *continued*
      psychological abuse — *continued*
        victim Z69.11
      violence
        perpetrator (physical) (sexual) Z69.12
        victim (physical) Z69.11
        sexual Z69.81
  observation (for) (ruled out)
    exposure to (suspected)
      anthrax Z03.810
      biological agent NEC Z03.818
  pediatrician visit, by expectant parent(s) (adoptive) Z76.81
  placental sample (taken vaginally) — *see also* Encounter, antenatal screening Z36.9
  plastic and reconstructive surgery following medical procedure or healed injury NEC Z42.8
  pregnancy
    supervision of — *see* Pregnancy, supervision of
    test Z32.00
      result negative Z32.02
      result positive Z32.01
  procreative management and counseling for gestational carrier Z31.7
  prophylactic measures Z29.9
    antivenin Z29.12
    fluoride administration Z29.3
    immunotherapy for respiratory syncytial virus (RSV) Z29.11
    rabies immune globin Z29.14
    Rho (D) immune globulin Z29.13
    specified NEC Z29.8
  radiation therapy (antineoplastic) Z51.0
  radiological (as part of a general medical examination) Z00.00
    with abnormal findings Z00.01
  reconstructive surgery following medical procedure or healed injury NEC Z42.8
  removal (of) — *see also* Removal
    artificial
      arm Z44.00- ☑
        complete Z44.01- ☑
        partial Z44.02- ☑
      eye Z44.2- ☑
      leg Z44.10- ☑
        complete Z44.11- ☑
        partial Z44.12- ☑
    breast implant Z45.81 ☑
      tissue expander (with or without synchronous insertion of permanent implant) Z45.81 ☑
    device Z46.9
      specified NEC Z46.89
    external
      fixation device — *code to* fracture with seventh character D
      prosthesis, prosthetic device Z44.9
        breast Z44.3- ☑
        specified NEC Z44.8
    implanted device NEC Z45.89
    insulin pump Z46.81
    internal fixation device Z47.2
    myringotomy device (stent) (tube) Z45.82
    nervous system device NEC Z46.2
      brain neuropacemaker Z46.2
      visual substitution device Z46.2
        implanted Z45.31
    non-vascular catheter Z46.82
    orthodontic device Z46.4
    stent
      ureteral Z46.6
    urinary device Z46.6
  repeat cervical smear to confirm findings of recent normal smear following initial abnormal smear Z01.42
  respirator [ventilator] use during power failure Z99.12
  Rh typing Z01.83
  screening — *see* Screening
  specified NEC Z76.89
  sterilization Z30.2
  suspected condition, ruled out
    amniotic cavity and membrane Z03.71
    cervical shortening Z03.75
    fetal anomaly Z03.73
    fetal growth Z03.74
    maternal and fetal conditions NEC Z03.79
    oligohydramnios Z03.71

⟡ **Subterms under main terms may continue to next column or page**   ☑ **Additional Character Required — Refer to the Tabular List for Character Selection**   **131**

Encephalopathy — Encounter

Encounter — continued
  suspected condition, ruled out — continued
    placental problem Z03.72
    polyhydramnios Z03.71
  suspected exposure (to), ruled out
    anthrax Z03.810
    biological agents NEC Z03.818
  termination of pregnancy, elective Z33.2
  testing — see Test
  therapeutic drug level monitoring Z51.81
  titration, insulin pump Z46.81
  to determine fetal viability of pregnancy O36.80 ☑
  training
    insulin pump Z46.81
  X-ray of chest (as part of a general medical examination) Z00.00
    with abnormal findings Z00.01
Encystment — see Cyst
Endarteritis (bacterial, subacute) (infective) I77.6
  brain I67.7
  cerebral or cerebrospinal I67.7
  deformans — see Arteriosclerosis
  embolic — see Embolism
  obliterans — see also Arteriosclerosis
    pulmonary I28.8
  pulmonary I28.8
  retina — see Vasculitis, retina
  senile — see Arteriosclerosis
  syphilitic A52.09
    brain or cerebral A52.04
    congenital A50.54 [I79.8]
  tuberculous A18.89
Endemic — see condition
Endocarditis (chronic) (marantic) (nonbacterial) (thrombotic) (valvular) I38
  with rheumatic fever (conditions in I00)
    active — see Endocarditis, acute, rheumatic
    inactive or quiescent (with chorea) I09.1
  acute or subacute I33.9
    infective I33.0
    rheumatic (aortic) (mitral) (pulmonary) (tricuspid) I01.1
      with chorea (acute) (rheumatic) (Sydenham's) I02.0
  aortic (heart) (nonrheumatic) (valve) I35.8
    with
      mitral disease I08.0
        with tricuspid (valve) disease I08.3
          active or acute I01.1
            with chorea (acute) (rheumatic) (Sydenham's) I02.0
        rheumatic fever (conditions in I00)
          active — see Endocarditis, acute, rheumatic
          inactive or quiescent (with chorea) I06.9
        tricuspid (valve) disease I08.2
          with mitral (valve) disease I08.3
    acute or subacute I33.9
    arteriosclerotic I35.8
    rheumatic I06.9
      with mitral disease I08.0
        with tricuspid (valve) disease I08.3
          active or acute I01.1
            with chorea (acute) (rheumatic) (Sydenham's) I02.0
      active or acute I01.1
        with chorea (acute) (rheumatic) (Sydenham's) I02.0
    specified NEC I06.8
    specified cause NEC I35.8
    syphilitic A52.03
  arteriosclerotic I38
  atypical verrucous (Libman-Sacks) M32.11
  bacterial (acute) (any valve) (subacute) I33.0
  candidal B37.6
  congenital Q24.8
  constrictive I33.0
  Coxiella burnetii A78 [I39]
  Coxsackie B33.21
  due to
    prosthetic cardiac valve T82.6 ☑
    Q fever A78 [I39]
    Serratia marcescens I33.0
    typhoid (fever) A01.02
  gonococcal A54.83
  infectious or infective (acute) (any valve) (subacute) I33.0
  lenta (acute) (any valve) (subacute) I33.0
  Libman-Sacks M32.11

Endocarditis — continued
  listerial A32.82
  Löffler's I42.3
  malignant (acute) (any valve) (subacute) I33.0
  meningococcal A39.51
  mitral (chronic) (double) (fibroid) (heart) (inactive) (valve) (with chorea) I05.9
    with
      aortic (valve) disease I08.0
        with tricuspid (valve) disease I08.3
          active or acute I01.1
            with chorea (acute) (rheumatic) (Sydenham's) I02.0
      rheumatic fever (conditions in I00)
        active — see Endocarditis, acute, rheumatic
        inactive or quiescent (with chorea) I05.9
      tricuspid (valve) disease I08.1
        with aortic (valve) disease I08.3
    active or acute I01.1
      with chorea (acute) (rheumatic) (Sydenham's) I02.0
    bacterial I33.0
    arteriosclerotic I34.8
    nonrheumatic I34.8
      acute or subacute I33.9
    specified NEC I05.8
  monilial B37.6
  multiple valves I08.9
    specified disorders I08.8
  mycotic (acute) (any valve) (subacute) I33.0
  pneumococcal (acute) (any valve) (subacute) I33.0
  pulmonary (chronic) (heart) (valve) I37.8
    with rheumatic fever (conditions in I00)
      active — see Endocarditis, acute, rheumatic
      inactive or quiescent (with chorea) I09.89
        with aortic, mitral or tricuspid disease I08.8
    acute or subacute I33.9
      rheumatic I01.1
        with chorea (acute) (rheumatic) (Sydenham's) I02.0
    arteriosclerotic I37.8
    congenital Q22.2
    rheumatic (chronic) (inactive) (with chorea) I09.89
      active or acute I01.1
        with chorea (acute) (rheumatic) (Sydenham's) I02.0
    syphilitic A52.03
  purulent (acute) (any valve) (subacute) I33.0
  Q fever A78 [I39]
  rheumatic (chronic) (inactive) (with chorea) I09.1
    active or acute (aortic) (mitral) (pulmonary) (tricuspid) I01.1
      with chorea (acute) (rheumatic) (Sydenham's) I02.0
  rheumatoid — see Rheumatoid, carditis
  septic (acute) (any valve) (subacute) I33.0
  streptococcal (acute) (any valve) (subacute) I33.0
  subacute — see Endocarditis, acute
  suppurative (acute) (any valve) (subacute) I33.0
  syphilitic A52.03
  toxic I33.9
  tricuspid (chronic) (heart) (inactive) (rheumatic) (valve) (with chorea) I07.9
    with
      aortic (valve) disease I08.2
        mitral (valve) disease I08.3
      mitral (valve) disease I08.1
        aortic (valve) disease I08.3
      rheumatic fever (conditions in I00)
        active — see Endocarditis, acute, rheumatic
        inactive or quiescent (with chorea) I07.8
    active or acute I01.1
      with chorea (acute) (rheumatic) (Sydenham's) I02.0
    arteriosclerotic I36.8
    nonrheumatic I36.8
      acute or subacute I33.9
    specified cause, except rheumatic I36.8
  tuberculous — see Tuberculosis, endocarditis
  typhoid A01.02
  ulcerative (acute) (any valve) (subacute) I33.0
  vegetative (acute) (any valve) (subacute) I33.0
  verrucous (atypical) (nonbacterial) (nonrheumatic) M32.11
Endocardium, endocardial — see also condition
  cushion defect Q21.2
Endocervicitis — see also Cervicitis
  due to intrauterine (contraceptive) device T83.69 ☑

Endocervicitis — continued
  hyperplastic N72
Endocrine — see condition
Endocrinopathy, pluriglandular E31.9
Endodontic
  overfill M27.52
  underfill M27.53
Endodontitis K04.01
  irreversible K04.02
  reversible K04.01
Endomastoiditis — see Mastoiditis
Endometrioma N80.9
Endometriosis N80.9
  appendix N80.5
  bladder N80.8
  bowel N80.5
  broad ligament N80.3
  cervix N80.0
  colon N80.5
  cul-de-sac (Douglas') N80.3
  exocervix N80.0
  fallopian tube N80.2
  female genital organ NEC N80.8
  gallbladder N80.8
  in scar of skin N80.6
  internal N80.0
  intestine N80.5
  lung N80.8
  myometrium N80.0
  ovary N80.1
  parametrium N80.3
  pelvic peritoneum N80.3
  peritoneal (pelvic) N80.3
  rectovaginal septum N80.4
  rectum N80.5
  round ligament N80.3
  skin (scar) N80.6
  specified site NEC N80.8
  stromal D39.0
  thorax N80.8
  umbilicus N80.8
  uterus (internal) N80.0
  vagina N80.4
  vulva N80.8
Endometritis (decidual) (nonspecific) (purulent) (sen◄ (atrophic) (suppurative) N71.9
  with ectopic pregnancy O08.0
  acute N71.0
  blenorrhagic (gonococcal) (acute) (chronic) A54.24
  cervix, cervical (with erosion or ectropion) — see a◄
    Cervicitis
    hyperplastic N72
  chlamydial A56.11
  chronic N71.1
  following
    abortion — see Abortion by type complicated b◄ genital infection
    ectopic or molar pregnancy O08.0
  gonococcal, gonorrheal (acute) (chronic) A54.24
  hyperplastic — see also Hyperplasia, endometrial N85.00
    cervix N72
  puerperal, postpartum, childbirth O86.12
  subacute N71.0
  tuberculous A18.17
Endometrium — see condition
Endomyocardiopathy, South African I42.3
Endomyocarditis — see Endocarditis
Endomyofibrosis I42.3
Endomyometritis — see Endometritis
Endopericarditis — see Endocarditis
Endoperineuritis — see Disorder, nerve
Endophlebitis — see Phlebitis
Endophthalmia — see Endophthalmitis, purulent
Endophthalmitis (acute) (infective) (metastatic) (sub◄ cute) H44.009
  bleb associated — see also Bleb, inflamed (infecte◄
    postprocedural H59.4 ☑
  gonorrheal A54.39
  in (due to)
    cysticercosis B69.1
    onchocerciasis B73.01
    toxocariasis B83.0
  panuveitis — see Panuveitis
  parasitic H44.12- ☑
  purulent H44.00- ☑
    panophthalmitis — see Panophthalmitis
    vitreous abscess H44.02- ☑

dophthalmitis — *continued*
specified NEC H44.19
sympathetic — *see* Uveitis, sympathetic
dosalpingioma D28.2
dosalpingiosis N94.89
dosteitis — *see* Osteomyelitis
dothelioma, bone — *see* Neoplasm, bone, malignant
dotheliosis (hemorrhagic infectional) D69.8
dotoxemia — code to condition
dotrachelitis — *see* Cervicitis
gelmann (-Camurati) **syndrome** Q78.3
glish disease — *see* Rickets
gman's disease L30.3
gorgement
breast N64.59
newborn P83.4
puerperal, postpartum O92.79
lung (passive) — *see* Edema, lung
pulmonary (passive) — *see* Edema, lung
stomach K31.89
venous, retina — *see* Occlusion, retina, vein, engorgement
largement, enlarged — *see also* Hypertrophy
adenoids J35.2
with tonsils J35.3
alveolar ridge K08.89
congenital — *see* Anomaly, alveolar
apertures of diaphragm (congenital) Q79.1
gingival K06.1
heart, cardiac — *see* Hypertrophy, cardiac
labium majus, childhood asymmetric (CALME) N90.61
lacrimal gland, chronic H04.03- ☑
liver — *see* Hypertrophy, liver
lymph gland or node R59.9
generalized R59.1
localized R59.0
orbit H05.34- ☑
organ or site, congenital NEC — *see* Anomaly, by site
parathyroid (gland) E21.0
pituitary fossa R93.0
prostate N40.0
with lower urinary tract symptoms (LUTS) N40.1
without lower urinary tract symtpoms (LUTS) N40.0
sella turcica R93.0
spleen — *see* Splenomegaly
thymus (gland) (congenital) E32.0
thyroid (gland) — *see* Goiter
tongue K14.8
tonsils J35.1
with adenoids J35.3
uterus N85.2
vestibular aqueduct Q16.5
ophthalmos H05.40- ☑
due to
orbital tissue atrophy H05.41- ☑
trauma or surgery H05.42- ☑
ostosis M27.8
tamebic, entamebiasis — *see* Amebiasis
tanglement
umbilical cord(s) O69.82 ☑
with compression O69.2 ☑
around neck (with compression) O69.81 ☑
with compression O69.1 ☑
without compression O69.81 ☑
of twins in monoamniotic sac O69.2 ☑
without compression O69.82 ☑
teralgia — *see* Pain, abdominal
teric — *see* condition
teritis (acute) (diarrheal) (hemorrhagic) (noninfective)
K52.9
adenovirus A08.2
aertrycke infection A02.0
allergic K52.29
with
eosinophilic gastritis or gastroenteritis K52.81
food protein-induced enterocolitis syndrome
K52.21
food protein-induced enteropathy K52.22
FPIES K52.21
amebic (acute) A06.0
with abscess — *see* Abscess, amebic
chronic A06.1
with abscess — *see* Abscess, amebic
nondysenteric A06.2
nondysenteric A06.2
astrovirus A08.32
bacillary NOS A03.9

Enteritis — *continued*
bacterial A04.9
specified NEC A04.8
calicivirus A08.31
candidal B37.82
Chilomastix A07.8
choleriformis A00.1
chronic (noninfectious) K52.9
ulcerative — *see* Colitis, ulcerative
cicatrizing (chronic) — *see* Enteritis, regional, small intestine
Clostridium
botulinum (food poisoning) A05.1
difficile
not specified as recurrent A04.72
recurrent A04.71
coccidial A07.3
coxsackie virus A08.39
dietetic — *see also* Enteritis, allergic K52.29
drug-induced K52.1
due to
astrovirus A08.32
calicivirus A08.31
coxsackie virus A08.39
drugs K52.1
echovirus A08.39
enterovirus NEC A08.39
food hypersensitivity — *see also* Enteritis, allergic
K52.29
infectious organism (bacterial) (viral) — *see* Enteritis,
infectious
torovirus A08.39
Yersinia enterocolitica A04.6
echovirus A08.39
eltor A00.1
enterovirus NEC A08.39
eosinophilic K52.81
epidemic (infectious) A09
fulminant — *see also* Ischemia, intestine, acute K55.019
gangrenous — *see* Enteritis, infectious
giardial A07.1
infectious NOS A09
due to
adenovirus A08.2
Aerobacter aerogenes A04.8
Arizona (bacillus) A02.0
bacteria NOS A04.9
specified NEC A04.8
Campylobacter A04.5
Clostridium difficile
not specified as recurrent A04.72
recurrent A04.71
Clostridium perfringens A04.8
Enterobacter aerogenes A04.8
enterovirus A08.39
Escherichia coli A04.4
enteroaggregative A04.4
enterohemorrhagic A04.3
enteroinvasive A04.2
enteropathogenic A04.0
enterotoxigenic A04.1
specified NEC A04.4
specified
bacteria NEC A04.8
virus NEC A08.39
Staphylococcus A04.8
virus NEC A08.4
specified type NEC A08.39
Yersinia enterocolitica A04.6
specified organism NEC A08.8
influenzal — *see* Influenza, with, digestive manifestations
ischemic K55.9
acute — *see also* Ischemia, intestine, acute K55.019
chronic K55.1
microsporidial A07.8
mucomembranous, myxomembranous — *see* Syndrome, irritable bowel
mucous — *see* Syndrome, irritable bowel
necroticans A05.2
necrotizing of newborn — *see* Enterocolitis, necrotizing, in newborn
neurogenic — *see* Syndrome, irritable bowel
newborn necrotizing — *see* Enterocolitis, necrotizing,
in newborn
noninfectious K52.9
norovirus A08.11
parasitic NEC B82.9

Enteritis — *continued*
paratyphoid (fever) — *see* Fever, paratyphoid
protozoal A07.9
specified NEC A07.8
radiation K52.0
regional (of) K50.90
with
complication K50.919
abscess K50.914
fistula K50.913
intestinal obstruction K50.912
rectal bleeding K50.911
specified complication NEC K50.918
colon — *see* Enteritis, regional, large intestine
duodenum — *see* Enteritis, regional, small intestine
ileum — *see* Enteritis, regional, small intestine
jejunum — *see* Enteritis, regional, small intestine
large bowel — *see* Enteritis, regional, large intestine
large intestine (colon) (rectum) K50.10
with
complication K50.119
abscess K50.114
fistula K50.113
intestinal obstruction K50.112
rectal bleeding K50.111
small intestine (duodenum) (ileum) (jejunum) involvement K50.80
with
complication K50.819
abscess K50.814
fistula K50.813
intestinal obstruction K50.812
rectal bleeding K50.811
specified complication NEC
K50.818
specified complication NEC K50.118
rectum — *see* Enteritis, regional, large intestine
small intestine (duodenum) (ileum) (jejunum)
K50.00
with
complication K50.019
abscess K50.014
fistula K50.013
intestinal obstruction K50.012
large intestine (colon) (rectum) involvement K50.80
with
complication K50.819
abscess K50.814
fistula K50.813
intestinal obstruction K50.812
rectal bleeding K50.811
specified complication NEC
K50.818
rectal bleeding K50.011
specified complication NEC K50.018
rotaviral A08.0
Salmonella, salmonellosis (arizonae) (cholerae-suis)
(enteritidis) (typhimurium) A02.0
segmental — *see* Enteritis, regional
septic A09
Shigella — *see* Infection, Shigella
small round structured NEC A08.19
spasmodic, spastic — *see* Syndrome, irritable bowel
staphylococcal A04.8
due to food A05.0
torovirus A08.39
toxic NEC K52.1
due to Clostridium difficile
not specified as recurrent A04.72
recurrent A04.71
trichomonal A07.8
tuberculous A18.32
typhosa A01.00
ulcerative (chronic) — *see* Colitis, ulcerative
viral A08.4
adenovirus A08.2
enterovirus A08.39
Rotavirus A08.0
small round structured NEC A08.19
specified NEC A08.39
virus specified NEC A08.39
Enterobiasis B80
Enterobius vermicularis (infection) (infestation) B80
Enterocele — *see also* Hernia, abdomen
pelvic, pelvis (acquired) (congenital) N81.5
vagina, vaginal (acquired) (congenital) NEC N81.5
Enterocolitis — *see also* Enteritis K52.9

Enterocolitis — *continued*
  due to Clostridium difficile
    not specified as recurrent A04.72
    recurrent A04.71
  fulminant ischemic — *see also* Ischemia, intestine,
    acute K55.059
  granulomatous — *see* Enteritis, regional
  hemorrhagic (acute) — *see also* Ischemia, intestine,
    acute K55.059
    chronic K55.1
  infectious NEC A09
  ischemic K55.9
  necrotizing K55.30
    with
      perforation K55.33
      pneumatosis K55.32
        and perforation K55.33
    due to Clostridium difficile
      not specified as recurrent A04.72
      recurrent A04.71
    in non-newborn K55.30
      stage 1 (without pneumatosis, without perfora-
        tion) K55.31
      stage 2 (with pneumatosis, without perforation)
        K55.32
      stage 3 (with pneumatosis, with perforation)
        K55.33
    in newborn P77.9
      stage 1 (without pneumatosis, without perfora-
        tion) P77.1
      stage 2 (with pneumatosis, without perforation)
        P77.2
      stage 3 (with pneumatosis, with perforation)
        P77.3
    without pneumatosis or perforation K55.31
  noninfectious K52.9
    newborn — *see* Enterocolitis, necrotizing, in new-
      born
  pseudomembranous (newborn)
    not specified as recurrent A04.72
    recurrent A04.71
  radiation K52.0
    newborn — *see* Enterocolitis, necrotizing, in new-
      born
  ulcerative (chronic) — *see* Pancolitis, ulcerative
    (chronic)
Enterogastritis — *see* Enteritis
Enteropathy K63.9
  celiac-gluten-sensitive K90.0
    non-celiac K90.41
  food protein-induced K52.22
  hemorrhagic, terminal — *see also* Ischemia, intestine,
    acute K55.059
  protein-losing K90.49
Enteroperitonitis — *see* Peritonitis
Enteroptosis K63.4
Enterorrhagia K92.2
Enterospasm — *see also* Syndrome, irritable, bowel
  psychogenic F45.8
Enterostenosis — *see also* Obstruction, intestine, specified NEC K56.699
Enterostomy
  complication — *see* Complication, enterostomy
  status Z93.4
Enterovirus, as cause of disease classified elsewhere
  B97.10
  coxsackievirus B97.11
  echovirus B97.12
  other specified B97.19
Enthesopathy (peripheral) M77.9
  Achilles tendinitis — *see* Tendinitis, Achilles
  ankle and tarsus M77.5- ☑
    specified type NEC — *see* Enthesopathy, foot,
      specified type NEC
  anterior tibial syndrome M76.81- ☑
  calcaneal spur — *see* Spur, bone, calcaneal
  elbow region M77.8
    lateral epicondylitis — *see* Epicondylitis, lateral
    medial epicondylitis — *see* Epicondylitis, medial
  foot NEC M77.9
    metatarsalgia — *see* Metatarsalgia
    specified type NEC M77.5- ☑
  forearm M77.9
  gluteal tendinitis — *see* Tendinitis, gluteal
  hand M77.9
  hip — *see* Enthesopathy, lower limb, specified type
    NEC
  iliac crest spur — *see* Spur, bone, iliac crest

Enthesopathy — *continued*
  iliotibial band syndrome — *see* Syndrome, iliotibial
    band
  knee — *see* Enthesopathy, lower limb, lower leg,
    specified type NEC
  lateral epicondylitis — *see* Epicondylitis, lateral
  lower limb (excluding foot) M76.9
    Achilles tendinitis — *see* Tendinitis, Achilles
    ankle and tarsus M77.5- ☑
      specified type NEC — *see* Enthesopathy, foot,
        specified type NEC
    anterior tibial syndrome M76.81- ☑
    gluteal tendinitis — *see* Tendinitis, gluteal
    iliac crest spur — *see* Spur, bone, iliac crest
    iliotibial band syndrome — *see* Syndrome, iliotibial
      band
    patellar tendinitis — *see* Tendinitis, patellar
    pelvic region — *see* Enthesopathy, lower limb,
      specified type NEC
    peroneal tendinitis — *see* Tendinitis, peroneal
    posterior tibial syndrome M76.82- ☑
    psoas tendinitis — *see* Tendinitis, psoas
    specified type NEC M76.89- ☑
    tibial collateral bursitis — *see* Bursitis, tibial collater-
      al
  medial epicondylitis — *see* Epicondylitis, medial
  metatarsalgia — *see* Metatarsalgia
  multiple sites M77.9
  patellar tendinitis — *see* Tendinitis, patellar
  pelvis M77.9
  periarthritis of wrist — *see* Periarthritis, wrist
  peroneal tendinitis — *see* Tendinitis, peroneal
  posterior tibial syndrome M76.82- ☑
  psoas tendinitis — *see* Tendinitis, psoas
  shoulder M77.9
  shoulder region — *see* Lesion, shoulder
  specified site NEC M77.9
  specified type NEC M77.8
  spinal M46.00
    cervical region M46.02
    cervicothoracic region M46.03
    lumbar region M46.06
    lumbosacral region M46.07
    multiple sites M46.09
    occipito-atlanto-axial region M46.01
    sacrococcygeal region M46.08
    thoracic region M46.04
    thoracolumbar region M46.05
  tibial collateral bursitis — *see* Bursitis, tibial collateral
  upper arm M77.9
  wrist and carpus NEC M77.8
    calcaneal spur — *see* Spur, bone, calcaneal
    periarthritis of wrist — *see* Periarthritis, wrist
Entomophobia F40.218
Entomophthoromycosis B46.8
Entrance, air into vein — *see* Embolism, air
Entrapment, nerve — *see* Neuropathy, entrapment
Entropion (eyelid) (paralytic) H02.009
  cicatricial H02.019
    left H02.016
      lower H02.015
      upper H02.014
    right H02.013
      lower H02.012
      upper H02.011
  congenital Q10.2
  left H02.006
    lower H02.005
    upper H02.004
  mechanical H02.029
    left H02.026
      lower H02.025
      upper H02.024
    right H02.023
      lower H02.022
      upper H02.021
  right H02.003
    lower H02.002
    upper H02.001
  senile H02.039
    left H02.036
      lower H02.035
      upper H02.034
    right H02.033
      lower H02.032
      upper H02.031
  spastic H02.049
    left H02.046

Entropion — *continued*
  spastic — *continued*
    left — *continued*
      lower H02.045
      upper H02.044
    right H02.043
      lower H02.042
      upper H02.041
Enucleated eye (traumatic, current) S05.7- ☑
Enuresis R32
  functional F98.0
  habit disturbance F98.0
  nocturnal N39.44
    psychogenic F98.0
  nonorganic origin F98.0
  psychogenic F98.0
Eosinopenia — *see* Agranulocytosis
Eosinophilia (allergic) (hereditary) (idiopathic) (secondary) D72.1
  with
    angiolymphoid hyperplasia (ALHE) D18.01
  infiltrative J82
  Löffler's J82
  peritoneal — *see* Peritonitis, eosinophilic
  pulmonary NEC J82
  tropical (pulmonary) J82
Eosinophilia-myalgia syndrome M35.8
Ependymitis (acute) (cerebral) (chronic) (granular) —
  see Encephalomyelitis
Ependymoblastoma
  specified site — *see* Neoplasm, malignant, by site
  unspecified site C71.9
Ependymoma (epithelial) (malignant)
  anaplastic
    specified site — *see* Neoplasm, malignant, by si
    unspecified site C71.9
  benign
    specified site — *see* Neoplasm, benign, by site
    unspecified site D33.2
  myxopapillary D43.2
    specified site — *see* Neoplasm, uncertain behav
      by site
    unspecified site D43.2
  papillary D43.2
    specified site — *see* Neoplasm, uncertain behav
      by site
    unspecified site D43.2
  specified site — *see* Neoplasm, malignant, by site
  unspecified site C71.9
Ependymopathy G93.89
Ephelis, ephelides L81.2
Epiblepharon (congenital) Q10.3
Epicanthus, epicanthic fold (eyelid) (congenital) Q1
Epicondylitis (elbow)
  lateral M77.1- ☑
  medial M77.0- ☑
Epicystitis — *see* Cystitis
Epidemic — *see* condition
Epidermidalization, cervix — *see* Dysplasia, cervix
Epidermis, epidermal — *see* condition
Epidermodysplasia verruciformis B07.8
Epidermolysis
  bullosa (congenital) Q81.9
    acquired L12.30
      drug-induced L12.31
      specified cause NEC L12.35
    dystrophica Q81.2
    letalis Q81.1
    simplex Q81.0
    specified NEC Q81.8
  necroticans combustiformis L51.2
    due to drug — *see* Table of Drugs and Chemica
      by drug
Epidermophytid — *see* Dermatophytosis
Epidermophytosis (infected) — *see* Dermatophytos
Epididymis — *see* condition
Epididymitis (acute) (nonvenereal) (recurrent) (residu
  N45.1
  with orchitis N45.3
  blennorrhagic (gonococcal) A54.23
  caseous (tuberculous) A18.15
  chlamydial A56.19
  filarial — *see also* Infestation, filarial B74.9 [N51]
  gonococcal A54.23
  syphilitic A52.76
  tuberculous A18.15
Epididymo-orchitis — *see also* Epididymitis N45.3
Epidural — *see* condition

gastrium, epigastric — *see* condition
gastrocele — *see* Hernia, ventral
glottis — *see* condition
glottitis, epiglottiditis (acute) J05.10
with obstruction J05.11
chronic J37.0
gnathus Q89.4
lepsia partialis continua — *see also* Kozhevnikof's
epilepsy G40.1- ☑
lepsy, epileptic, epilepsia (attack) (cerebral) (convulsion) (fit) (seizure) G40.909

ote: the following terms are to be considered
quivalent to intractable: pharmacoresistant
pharmacologically resistant), treatment resistant,
fractory (medically) and poorly controlled

with
complex partial seizures — *see* Epilepsy, localization-related, symptomatic, with complex partial seizures
grand mal seizures on awakening — *see* Epilepsy, generalized, specified NEC
myoclonic absences — *see* Epilepsy, generalized, specified NEC
myoclonic-astatic seizures — *see* Epilepsy, generalized, specified NEC
simple partial seizures — *see* Epilepsy, localization-related, symptomatic, with simple partial seizures
akinetic — *see* Epilepsy, generalized, specified NEC
benign childhood with centrotemporal EEG spikes — *see* Epilepsy, localization-related, idiopathic
benign myoclonic in infancy G40.80- ☑
Bravais-jacksonian — *see* Epilepsy, localization-related, symptomatic, with simple partial seizures
childhood
with occipital EEG paroxysms — *see* Epilepsy, localization-related, idiopathic
absence G40.A09 (*following* G40.3)
intractable G40.A19 (*following* G40.3)
with status epilepticus G40.A11 (*following* G40.3)
without status epilepticus G40.A19 (*following* G40.3)
not intractable G40.A09 (*following* G40.3)
with status epilepticus G40.A01 (*following* G40.3)
without status epilepticus G40.A09 (*following* G40.3)
climacteric — *see* Epilepsy, specified NEC
cysticercosis B69.0
deterioration (mental) F06.8
due to syphilis A52.19
focal — *see* Epilepsy, localization-related, symptomatic, with simple partial seizures
generalized
idiopathic G40.309
intractable G40.319
with status epilepticus G40.311
without status epilepticus G40.319
not intractable G40.309
with status epilepticus G40.301
without status epilepticus G40.309
specified NEC G40.409
intractable G40.419
with status epilepticus G40.411
without status epilepticus G40.419
not intractable G40.409
with status epilepticus G40.401
without status epilepticus G40.409
impulsive petit mal — *see* Epilepsy, juvenile myoclonic
ntractable G40.919
with status epilepticus G40.911
without status epilepticus G40.919
juvenile absence G40.A09 (*following* G40.3)
intractable G40.A19 (*following* G40.3)
with status epilepticus G40.A11 (*following* G40.3)
without status epilepticus G40.A19 (*following* G40.3)
not intractable G40.A09 (*following* G40.3)
with status epilepticus G40.A01 (*following* G40.3)
without status epilepticus G40.A09 (*following* G40.3)
juvenile myoclonic G40.B09 (*following* G40.3)
intractable G40.B19 (*following* G40.3)
with status epilepticus G40.B11 (*following* G40.3)
without status epilepticus G40.B19 (*following* G40.3)

Epilepsy, epileptic, epilepsia — *continued*
juvenile myoclonic — *continued*
not intractable G40.B09 (*following* G40.3)
with status epilepticus G40.B01 (*following* G40.3)
without status epilepticus G40.B09 (*following* G40.3)
localization-related (focal) (partial)
idiopathic G40.009
with seizures of localized onset G40.009
intractable G40.019
with status epilepticus G40.011
without status epilepticus G40.019
not intractable G40.009
with status epilepticus G40.001
without status epilepticus G40.009
symptomatic
with complex partial seizures G40.209
intractable G40.219
with status epilepticus G40.211
without status epilepticus G40.219
not intractable G40.209
with status epilepticus G40.201
without status epilepticus G40.209
with simple partial seizures G40.109
intractable G40.119
with status epilepticus G40.111
without status epilepticus G40.119
not intractable G40.109
with status epilepticus G40.101
without status epilepticus G40.109
myoclonus, myoclonic — *see* Epilepsy, generalized, specified NEC
progressive — *see* Epilepsy, generalized, idiopathic
not intractable G40.909
with status epilepticus G40.901
without status epilepticus G40.909
on awakening — *see* Epilepsy, generalized, specified NEC
parasitic NOS B71.9 *[G94]*
partialis continua — *see also* Kozhevnikof's epilepsy G40.1- ☑
peripheral — *see* Epilepsy, specified NEC
procursiva — *see* Epilepsy, localization-related, symptomatic, with simple partial seizures
progressive (familial) myoclonic — *see* Epilepsy, generalized, idiopathic
reflex — *see* Epilepsy, specified NEC
related to
alcohol G40.509
not intractable G40.509
with status epilepticus G40.501
without status epilepticus G40.509
drugs G40.509
not intractable G40.509
with status epilepticus G40.501
without status epilepticus G40.509
external causes G40.509
not intractable G40.509
with status epilepticus G40.501
without status epilepticus G40.509
hormonal changes G40.509
not intractable G40.509
with status epilepticus G40.501
without status epilepticus G40.509
sleep deprivation G40.509
not intractable G40.509
with status epilepticus G40.501
without status epilepticus G40.509
stress G40.509
not intractable G40.509
with status epilepticus G40.501
without status epilepticus G40.509
somatomotor — *see* Epilepsy, localization-related, symptomatic, with simple partial seizures
somatosensory — *see* Epilepsy, localization-related, symptomatic, with simple partial seizures
spasms G40.822
intractable G40.824
with status epilepticus G40.823
without status epilepticus G40.824
not intractable G40.822
with status epilepticus G40.821
without status epilepticus G40.822
specified NEC G40.802
intractable G40.804
with status epilepticus G40.803
without status epilepticus G40.804
not intractable G40.802

Epilepsy, epileptic, epilepsia — *continued*
specified — *continued*
not intractable — *continued*
with status epilepticus G40.801
without status epilepticus G40.802
syndromes
generalized
idiopathic G40.309
intractable G40.319
with status epilepticus G40.311
without status epilepticus G40.319
not intractable G40.309
with status epilepticus G40.301
without status epilepticus G40.309
specified NEC G40.409
intractable G40.419
with status epilepticus G40.411
without status epilepticus G40.419
not intractable G40.409
with status epilepticus G40.401
without status epilepticus G40.409
localization-related (focal) (partial)
idiopathic G40.009
with seizures of localized onset G40.009
intractable G40.019
with status epilepticus G40.011
without status epilepticus G40.019
not intractable G40.009
with status epilepticus G40.001
without status epilepticus G40.009
symptomatic
with complex partial seizures G40.209
intractable G40.219
with status epilepticus G40.211
without status epilepticus G40.219
not intractable G40.209
with status epilepticus G40.201
without status epilepticus G40.209
with simple partial seizures G40.109
intractable G40.119
with status epilepticus G40.111
without status epilepticus G40.119
not intractable G40.109
with status epilepticus G40.101
without status epilepticus G40.109
specified NEC G40.802
intractable G40.804
with status epilepticus G40.803
without status epilepticus G40.804
not intractable G40.802
with status epilepticus G40.801
without status epilepticus G40.802
tonic (-clonic) — *see* Epilepsy, generalized, specified NEC
twilight F05
uncinate (gyrus) — *see* Epilepsy, localization-related, symptomatic, with complex partial seizures
Unverricht (-Lundborg) (familial myoclonic) — *see* Epilepsy, generalized, idiopathic
visceral — *see* Epilepsy, specified NEC
visual — *see* Epilepsy, specified NEC
Epiloia Q85.1
Epimenorrhea N92.0
Epipharyngitis — *see* Nasopharyngitis
Epiphora H04.20- ☑
due to
excess lacrimation H04.21- ☑
insufficient drainage H04.22- ☑
Epiphyseal arrest — *see* Arrest, epiphyseal
Epiphyseolysis, epiphysiolysis — *see* Osteochondropathy
Epiphysitis — *see also* Osteochondropathy
juvenile M92.9
syphilitic (congenital) A50.02
Epiplocele — *see* Hernia, abdomen
Epiploitis — *see* Peritonitis
Epiplosarcomphalocele — *see* Hernia, umbilicus
Episcleritis (suppurative) H15.10- ☑
in (due to)
syphilis A52.71
tuberculosis A18.51
nodular H15.12- ☑
periodica fugax H15.11- ☑
angioneurotic — *see* Edema, angioneurotic
syphilitic (late) A52.71
tuberculous A18.51
Episode
affective, mixed F39

Episode — *continued*
  depersonalization (in neurotic state) F48.1
  depressive F32.9
    major F32.9
      mild F32.0
      moderate F32.1
      severe (without psychotic symptoms) F32.2
        with psychotic symptoms F32.3
    recurrent F33.9
      brief F33.8
    specified NEC F32.89
  hypomanic F30.8
  manic F30.9
    with
      psychotic symptoms F30.2
      remission (full) F30.4
        partial F30.3
    other specified F30.8
    recurrent F31.89
    without psychotic symptoms F30.10
      mild F30.11
      moderate F30.12
      severe (without psychotic symptoms) F30.13
        with psychotic symptoms F30.2
  psychotic F23
    organic F06.8
  schizophrenic (acute) NEC, brief F23
Epispadias (female) (male) Q64.0
Episplenitis D73.89
Epistaxis (multiple) R04.0
  hereditary I78.0
  vicarious menstruation N94.89
Epithelioma (malignant) — *see also* Neoplasm, malignant, by site
  adenoides cysticum — *see* Neoplasm, skin, benign
  basal cell — *see* Neoplasm, skin, malignant
  benign — *see* Neoplasm, benign, by site
  Bowen's — *see* Neoplasm, skin, in situ
  calcifying, of Malherbe — *see* Neoplasm, skin, benign
  external site — *see* Neoplasm, skin, malignant
  intraepidermal, Jadassohn — *see* Neoplasm, skin, benign
  squamous cell — *see* Neoplasm, malignant, by site
Epitheliomatosis pigmented Q82.1
Epitheliopathy, multifocal placoid pigment H30.14- ☑
Epithelium, epithelial — *see* condition
Epituberculosis (with atelectasis) (allergic) A15.7
Eponychia Q84.6
Epstein's
  nephrosis or syndrome — *see* Nephrosis
  pearl K09.8
Epulis (gingiva) (fibrous) (giant cell) K06.8
Equinia A24.0
Equinovarus (congenital) (talipes) Q66.0- ☑
  acquired — *see* Deformity, limb, clubfoot
Equivalent
  convulsive (abdominal) — *see* Epilepsy, specified NEC
  epileptic (psychic) — *see* Epilepsy, localization-related, symptomatic, with complex partial seizures
Erb (-Duchenne) **paralysis** (birth injury) (newborn) P14.0
Erb-Goldflam disease or syndrome G70.00
  with exacerbation (acute) G70.01
  in crisis G70.01
Erb's
  disease G71.02
  palsy, paralysis (brachial) (birth) (newborn) P14.0
    spinal (spastic) syphilitic A52.17
  pseudohypertrophic muscular dystrophy G71.02
Erdheim's syndrome (acromegalic macrospondylitis) E22.0
Erection, painful (persistent) — *see* Priapism
Ergosterol deficiency (vitamin D) E55.9
  with
    adult osteomalacia M83.8
    rickets — *see* Rickets
Ergotism — *see also* Poisoning, food, noxious, plant
  from ergot used as drug (migraine therapy) — *see* Table of Drugs and Chemicals
Erosio interdigitalis blastomycetica B37.2
Erosion
  artery I77.2
    without rupture I77.89
  bone — *see* Disorder, bone, density and structure, specified NEC
  bronchus J98.09

Erosion — *continued*
  cartilage (joint) — *see* Disorder, cartilage, specified type NEC
  cervix (uteri) (acquired) (chronic) (congenital) N86
    with cervicitis N72
  cornea (nontraumatic) — *see* Ulcer, cornea
    recurrent H18.83- ☑
    traumatic — *see* Abrasion, cornea
  dental (idiopathic) (occupational) (due to diet, drugs or vomiting) K03.2
  duodenum, postpyloric — *see* Ulcer, duodenum
  esophagus K22.10
    with bleeding K22.11
  gastric — *see* Ulcer, stomach
  gastrojejunal — *see* Ulcer, gastrojejunal
  implanted mesh — *see* Complications, prosthetic device or implant, mesh
  intestine K63.3
  lymphatic vessel I89.8
  pylorus, pyloric (ulcer) — *see* Ulcer, stomach
  spine, aneurysmal A52.09
  stomach — *see* Ulcer, stomach
  subcutaneous device pocket
    nervous system prosthetic device, implant, or graft T85.890 ☑
    other internal prosthetic device, implant, or graft T85.898 ☑
  teeth (idiopathic) (occupational) (due to diet, drugs or vomiting) K03.2
  urethra N36.8
  uterus N85.8
Erotomania F52.8
Error
  metabolism, inborn — *see* Disorder, metabolism
  refractive — *see* Disorder, refraction
Eructation R14.2
  nervous or psychogenic F45.8
Eruption
  creeping B76.9
  drug (generalized) (taken internally) L27.0
    fixed L27.1
    in contact with skin — *see* Dermatitis, due to drugs
    localized L27.1
  Hutchinson, summer L56.4
  Kaposi's varicelliform B00.0
  napkin L22
  polymorphous light (sun) L56.4
  recalcitrant pustular L13.8
  ringed R23.8
  skin (nonspecific) R21
    creeping (meaning hookworm) B76.9
    due to inoculation/vaccination (generalized) — *see also* Dermatitis, due to, vaccine L27.0
      localized L27.1
    erysipeloid A26.0
    feigned L98.1
    Kaposi's varicelliform B00.0
    lichenoid L28.0
    meaning dermatitis — *see* Dermatitis
    toxic NEC L53.0
  tooth, teeth, abnormal (incomplete) (late) (premature) (sequence) K00.6
  vesicular R23.8
Erysipelas (gangrenous) (infantile) (newborn) (phlegmonous) (suppurative) A46
  external ear A46 *[H62.40]*
  puerperal, postpartum O86.89
Erysipeloid A26.9
  cutaneous (Rosenbach's) A26.0
  disseminated A26.8
  sepsis A26.7
  specified NEC A26.8
Erythema, erythematous (infectional) (inflammation) L53.9
  ab igne L59.0
  annulare (centrifugum) (rheumaticum) L53.1
  arthriticum epidemicum A25.1
  brucellum — *see* Brucellosis
  chronic figurate NEC L53.3
  chronicum migrans (Borrelia burgdorferi) A69.20
  diaper L22
  due to
    chemical NEC L53.0
      in contact with skin L24.5
    drug (internal use) — *see* Dermatitis, due to, drugs
  elevatum diutinum L95.1
  endemic E52
  epidemic, arthritic A25.1

Erythema, erythematous — *continued*
  figuratum perstans L53.3
  gluteal L22
  heat — *code by site under* Burn, first degree
  ichthyosiforme congenitum bullous Q80.3
  in diseases classified elsewhere L54
  induratum (nontuberculous) L52
    tuberculous A18.4
  infectiosum B08.3
  intertrigo L30.4
  iris L51.9
  marginatum L53.2
    in (due to) acute rheumatic fever I00
  medicamentosum — *see* Dermatitis, due to, drugs
  migrans A26.0
    chronicum A69.20
    tongue K14.1
  multiforme (major) (minor) L51.9
    bullous, bullosum L51.1
    conjunctiva L51.1
    nonbullous L51.0
    pemphigoides L12.0
    specified NEC L51.8
  napkin L22
  neonatorum P83.88
    toxic P83.1
  nodosum L52
    tuberculous A18.4
  palmar L53.8
  pernio T69.1 ☑
  rash, newborn P83.88
  scarlatiniform (recurrent) (exfoliative) L53.8
  solare L55.0
  specified NEC L53.8
  toxic, toxicum NEC L53.0
    newborn P83.1
  tuberculous (primary) A18.4
Erythematous, erythematosus — *see* condition
Erythermalgia (primary) I73.81
Erythralgia I73.81
Erythrasma L08.1
Erythredema (polyneuropathy) — *see* Poisoning, mercury
Erythremia (acute) C94.0- ☑
  chronic D45
  secondary D75.1
Erythroblastopenia — *see also* Aplasia, red cell D6•
  congenital D61.01
Erythroblastophthisis D61.09
Erythroblastosis (fetalis) (newborn) P55.9
  due to
    ABO (antibodies) (incompatibility) (isoimmunizat P55.1
    Rh (antibodies) (incompatibility) (isoimmunizat P55.0
Erythrocyanosis (crurum) I73.89
Erythrocythemia — *see* Erythremia
Erythrocytosis (megalosplenic) (secondary) D75.1
  familial D75.0
  oval, hereditary — *see* Elliptocytosis
  secondary D75.1
  stress D75.1
Erythroderma (secondary) — *see also* Erythema L53
  bullous ichthyosiform, congenital Q80.3
  desquamativum L21.1
  ichthyosiform, congenital (bullous) Q80.3
  neonatorum P83.88
  psoriaticum L40.8
Erythrodysesthesia, palmar plantar (PPE) L27.1
Erythrogenesis imperfecta D61.09
Erythroleukemia C94.0- ☑
Erythromelalgia I73.81
Erythrophagocytosis D75.89
Erythrophobia F40.298
Erythroplakia, oral epithelium, and tongue K13.
Erythroplasia (Queyrat) D07.4
  specified site — *see* Neoplasm, skin, in situ
  unspecified site D07.4
Escherichia coli (E. coli), **as cause of disease classif elsewhere** B96.20
  non-O157 Shiga toxin-producing (with known O gr B96.22
  non-Shiga toxin-producing B96.29
  O157 with confirmation of Shiga toxin when H anti is unknown, or is not H7 B96.21
  O157:H- (nonmotile) with confirmation of Shiga t B96.21

☑ **Additional Character Required** — **Refer to the Tabular List for Character Selection**   ▽ **Subterms under main terms may continue to next column or pa**

:herichia coli (E. coli), **as cause of disease classified elsewhere** — *continued*
  O157:H7 with or without confirmation of Shiga toxin-production B96.21
    specified NEC B96.22-
  Shiga toxin-producing (with unspecified O group) (STEC) B96.23
  O157 B96.21
  specified NEC B96.29
:phagismus K22.4
:phagitis (acute) (alkaline) (chemical) (chronic) (infectional) (necrotic) (peptic) (postoperative) K20.9
  candidal B37.81
  due to gastrointestinal reflux disease K21.0
  eosinophilic K20.0
  reflux K21.0
  specified NEC K20.8
  tuberculous A18.83
  ulcerative K22.10
    with bleeding K22.11
:phagocele K22.5
:phagomalacia K22.8
:phagospasm K22.4
:phagostenosis K22.2
:phagostomiasis B81.8
:phagotracheal — *see* condition
:phagus — *see* condition
:phoria H50.51
  convergence, excess H51.12
  divergence, insufficiency H51.8
:tropia — *see* Strabismus, convergent concomitant
:undia B55.2
:ential — *see* condition
:hesioneuroblastoma C30.0
:hesioneurocytoma C30.0
:hesioneuroepithelioma C30.0
:hiomene A55
:ivo-autumnal malaria (fever) B50.9
:rangement (marital) Z63.5
  parent-child NEC Z62.890
:riasis — *see* Myiasis
:anolism — *see* Alcoholism
:erism — *see* Dependence, drug, inhalant
:moid, ethmoidal — *see* condition
:moiditis (chronic) (nonpurulent) (purulent) *see also* Sinusitis, ethmoidal
  influenzal — *see* Influenza, with, respiratory manifestations NEC
  Woakes' J33.1
:ylism — *see* Alcoholism
:lenburg's disease (congenital paramyotonia) G71.19
:mycetoma B47.0
:nuchoidism E29.1
  hypogonadotropic E23.0
:ropean blastomycosis — *see* Cryptococcosis
:stachian — *see* condition
:aluation (for) (of)
  development state
    adolescent Z00.3
    period of
      delayed growth in childhood Z00.70
        with abnormal findings Z00.71
      rapid growth in childhood Z00.2
      puberty Z00.3
  growth and developmental state (period of rapid growth) Z00.2
    delayed growth Z00.70
      with abnormal findings Z00.71
  mental health (status) Z00.8
    requested by authority Z04.6
  period of
    delayed growth in childhood Z00.70
      with abnormal findings Z00.71
    rapid growth in childhood Z00.2
  suspected condition — *see* Observation
:ans syndrome D69.41
:ent
  apparent life threatening in newborn and infant (ALTE) R68.13
  brief resolved unexplained event (BRUE) R68.13
:entration — *see also* Hernia, ventral
  colon into chest — *see* Hernia, diaphragm
  diaphragm (congenital) Q79.1
:ersion
  bladder N32.89
  cervix (uteri) N86
    with cervicitis N72

Eversion — *continued*
  foot NEC — *see also* Deformity, valgus, ankle
    congenital Q66.6
  punctum lacrimale (postinfectional) (senile) H04.52- ☑
  ureter (meatus) N28.89
  urethra (meatus) N36.8
  uterus N81.4
Evidence
  cytologic
    of malignancy on anal smear R85.614
    of malignancy on cervical smear R87.614
    of malignancy on vaginal smear R87.624
Evisceration
  birth injury P15.8
  traumatic NEC
    eye — *see* Enucleated eye
Evulsion — *see* Avulsion
Ewing's sarcoma or tumor — *see* Neoplasm, bone, malignant
Examination (for) (following) (general) (of) (routine) Z00.00
  with abnormal findings Z00.01
  abuse, physical (alleged), ruled out
    adult Z04.71
    child Z04.72
  adolescent (development state) Z00.3
  alleged rape or sexual assault (victim), ruled out
    adult Z04.41
    child Z04.42
  allergy Z01.82
  annual (adult) (periodic) (physical) Z00.00
    with abnormal findings Z00.01
    gynecological Z01.419
      with abnormal findings Z01.411
  antibody response Z01.84
  blood — *see* Examination, laboratory
  blood pressure Z01.30
    with abnormal findings Z01.31
  cancer staging — *see* Neoplasm, malignant, by site
  cervical Papanicolaou smear Z12.4
    as part of routine gynecological examination Z01.419
      with abnormal findings Z01.411
  child (over 28 days old) Z00.129
    with abnormal findings Z00.121
    under 28 days old — *see* Newborn, examination
  clinical research control or normal comparison (control) (participant) Z00.6
  contraceptive (drug) maintenance (routine) Z30.8
    device (intrauterine) Z30.431
  dental Z01.20
    with abnormal findings Z01.21
  developmental — *see* Examination, child
  donor (potential) Z00.5
  ear Z01.10
    with abnormal findings NEC Z01.118
  eye Z01.00
    with abnormal findings Z01.01
    following failed vision screening Z01.020
      with abnormal findings Z01.021
  follow-up (routine) (following) Z09
    chemotherapy NEC Z09
      malignant neoplasm Z08
    fracture Z09
    malignant neoplasm Z08
    postpartum Z39.2
    psychotherapy Z09
    radiotherapy NEC Z09
      malignant neoplasm Z08
    surgery NEC Z09
      malignant neoplasm Z08
  following
    accident NEC Z04.3
      transport Z04.1
      work Z04.2
    assault, alleged, ruled out
      adult Z04.71
      child Z04.72
    motor vehicle accident Z04.1
    treatment (for) Z09
      combined NEC Z09
        fracture Z09
        malignant neoplasm Z08
      malignant neoplasm Z08
      mental disorder Z09
      specified condition NEC Z09
  forced sexual exploitation Z04.81
  forced labor exploitation Z04.82

Examination — *continued*
  gynecological Z01.419
    with abnormal findings Z01.411
    for contraceptive maintenance Z30.8
  health — *see* Examination, medical
  hearing Z01.10
    with abnormal findings NEC Z01.118
    following failed hearing screening Z01.110
    infant or child (over 28 days old) Z00.129
      with abnormal findings Z00.121
  immunity status testing Z01.84
  laboratory (as part of a general medical examination) Z00.00
    with abnormal findings Z00.01
    preprocedural Z01.812
  lactating mother Z39.1
  medical (adult) (for) (of) Z00.00
    with abnormal findings Z00.01
    administrative purpose only Z02.9
      specified NEC Z02.89
    admission to
      armed forces Z02.3
      old age home Z02.2
      prison Z02.89
      residential institution Z02.2
      school Z02.0
        following illness or medical treatment Z02.0
      summer camp Z02.89
    adoption Z02.82
    blood alcohol or drug level Z02.83
    camp (summer) Z02.89
    clinical research, normal subject (control) (participant) Z00.6
    control subject in clinical research (normal comparison) (participant) Z00.6
    donor (potential) Z00.5
    driving license Z02.4
    general (adult) Z00.00
      with abnormal findings Z00.01
    immigration Z02.89
    insurance purposes Z02.6
    marriage Z02.89
    medicolegal reasons NEC Z04.89
    naturalization Z02.89
    participation in sport Z02.5
    paternity testing Z02.81
    population survey Z00.8
    pre-employment Z02.1
    pre-operative — *see* Examination, pre-procedural
    pre-procedural
      cardiovascular Z01.810
      respiratory Z01.811
      specified NEC Z01.818
    preschool children
      for admission to school Z02.0
    prisoners
      for entrance into prison Z02.89
    recruitment for armed forces Z02.3
    specified NEC Z00.8
    sport competition Z02.5
  medicolegal reason NEC Z04.89
    following
      forced sexual exploitation Z04.81
      forced labor exploitation Z04.82
  newborn — *see* Newborn, examination
  pelvic (annual) (periodic) Z01.419
    with abnormal findings Z01.411
  period of rapid growth in childhood Z00.2
  periodic (adult) (annual) (routine) Z00.00
    with abnormal findings Z00.01
  physical (adult) — *see also* Examination, medical Z00.00
    sports Z02.5
  postpartum
    immediately after delivery Z39.0
    routine follow-up Z39.2
  pre-chemotherapy (antineoplastic) Z01.818
  prenatal (normal pregnancy) — *see also* Pregnancy, normal Z34.9- ☑
  pre-procedural (pre-operative)
    cardiovascular Z01.810
    laboratory Z01.812
    respiratory Z01.811
    specified NEC Z01.818
  prior to chemotherapy (antineoplastic) Z01.818
  psychiatric NEC Z00.8
    follow-up not needing further care Z09
    requested by authority Z04.6
  radiological (as part of a general medical examination) Z00.00

Examination — *continued*
  radiological — *continued*
    with abnormal findings Z00.01
    repeat cervical smear to confirm findings of recent
        normal smear following initial abnormal smear
        Z01.42
  skin (hypersensitivity) Z01.82
  special — *see also* Examination, by type Z01.89
    specified type NEC Z01.89
  specified type or reason NEC Z04.89
  teeth Z01.20
    with abnormal findings Z01.21
  urine — *see* Examination, laboratory
  vision Z01.00
    with abnormal findings Z01.01
    following failed vision screening Z01.020
      with abnormal findings Z01.021
    infant or child (over 28 days old) Z00.129
      with abnormal findings Z00.121
Exanthem, exanthema — *see also* Rash
  with enteroviral vesicular stomatitis B08.4
  Boston A88.0
  epidemic with meningitis A88.0 *[G02]*
  subitum B08.20
    due to human herpesvirus 6 B08.21
    due to human herpesvirus 7 B08.22
  viral, virus B09
    specified type NEC B08.8
Excess, excessive, excessively
  alcohol level in blood R78.0
  androgen (ovarian) E28.1
  attrition, tooth, teeth K03.0
  carotene, carotin (dietary) E67.1
  cold, effects of T69.9 ☑
    specified effect NEC T69.8 ☑
  convergence H51.12
  crying
    in child, adolescent, or adult R45.83
    in infant R68.11
  development, breast N62
  divergence H51.8
  drinking (alcohol) NEC (without dependence) F10.10
    habitual (continual) (without remission) F10.20
  eating R63.2
  estrogen E28.0
  fat — *see also* Obesity
    in heart — *see* Degeneration, myocardial
    localized E65
  foreskin N47.8
  gas R14.0
  glucagon E16.3
  heat — *see* Heat
  intermaxillary vertical dimension of fully erupted teeth
      M26.37
  interocclusal distance of fully erupted teeth M26.37
  kalium E87.5
  large
    colon K59.39
      congenital Q43.8
    infant P08.0
    organ or site, congenital NEC — *see* Anomaly, by
        site
  long
    organ or site, congenital NEC — *see* Anomaly, by
        site
  menstruation (with regular cycle) N92.0
    with irregular cycle N92.1
  napping Z72.821
  natrium E87.0
  number of teeth K00.1
  nutrient (dietary) NEC R63.2
  potassium (K) E87.5
  salivation K11.7
  secretion — *see also* Hypersecretion
    milk O92.6
    sputum R09.3
    sweat R61
  sexual drive F52.8
  short
    organ or site, congenital NEC — *see* Anomaly, by
        site
    umbilical cord in labor or delivery O69.3 ☑
  skin L98.7
    and subcutaneous tissue L98.7
    eyelid (acquired) — *see* Blepharochalasis
      congenital Q10.3
  sodium (Na) E87.0
  spacing of fully erupted teeth M26.32

Excess, excessive, excessively — *continued*
  sputum R09.3
  sweating R61
  thirst R63.1
    due to deprivation of water T73.1 ☑
  tuberosity of jaw M26.07
  vitamin
    A (dietary) E67.0
      administered as drug (prolonged intake) — *see*
          Table of Drugs and Chemicals, vitamins,
          adverse effect
      overdose or wrong substance given or taken —
          see Table of Drugs and Chemicals, vita-
          mins, poisoning
    D (dietary) E67.3
      administered as drug (prolonged intake) — *see*
          Table of Drugs and Chemicals, vitamins,
          adverse effect
      overdose or wrong substance given or taken —
          see Table of Drugs and Chemicals, vita-
          mins, poisoning
  weight
    gain R63.5
    loss R63.4
Excitability, abnormal, under minor stress (personal-
    ity disorder) F60.3
Excitation
  anomalous atrioventricular I45.6
  psychogenic F30.8
  reactive (from emotional stress, psychological trauma)
      F30.8
Excitement
  hypomanic F30.8
  manic F30.9
  mental, reactive (from emotional stress, psychological
      trauma) F30.8
  state, reactive (from emotional stress, psychological
      trauma) F30.8
Excoriation (traumatic) — *see also* Abrasion
  neurotic L98.1
  skin picking disorder F42.4
Exfoliation
  due to erythematous conditions according to extent
      of body surface involved L49.0
      10-19 percent of body surface L49.1
      20-29 percent of body surface L49.2
      30-39 percent of body surface L49.3
      40-49 percent of body surface L49.4
      50-59 percent of body surface L49.5
      60-69 percent of body surface L49.6
      70-79 percent of body surface L49.7
      80-89 percent of body surface L49.8
      90-99 percent of body surface L49.9
      less than 10 percent of body surface L49.0
  teeth, due to systemic causes K08.0
Exfoliative — *see* condition
Exhaustion, exhaustive (physical NEC) R53.83
  battle F43.0
  cardiac — *see* Failure, heart
  delirium F43.0
  due to
    cold T69.8 ☑
    excessive exertion T73.3 ☑
    exposure T73.2 ☑
    neurasthenia F48.8
  heart — *see* Failure, heart
  heat — *see also* Heat, exhaustion T67.5 ☑
    due to
      salt depletion T67.4 ☑
      water depletion T67.3 ☑
  maternal, complicating delivery O75.81
  mental F48.8
  myocardium, myocardial — *see* Failure, heart
  nervous F48.8
  old age R54
  psychogenic F48.8
  psychosis F43.0
  senile R54
  vital NEC Z73.0
Exhibitionism F65.2
Exocervicitis — *see* Cervicitis
Exomphalos Q79.2
  meaning hernia — *see* Hernia, umbilicus
Exophoria H50.52
  convergence, insufficiency H51.11
  divergence, excess H51.8
Exophthalmos H05.2- ☑
  congenital Q15.8

Exophthalmos — *continued*
  constant NEC H05.24- ☑
  displacement, globe — *see* Displacement, globe
  due to thyrotoxicosis (hyperthyroidism) — *see* Hyp
      thyroidism, with, goiter (diffuse)
  dysthyroid — *see* Hyperthyroidism, with, goiter (di
      fuse)
  goiter — *see* Hyperthyroidism, with, goiter (diffuse
  intermittent NEC H05.25- ☑
  malignant — *see* Hyperthyroidism, with, goiter (diffu
  orbital
    edema — *see* Edema, orbit
    hemorrhage — *see* Hemorrhage, orbit
  pulsating NEC H05.26- ☑
  thyrotoxic, thyrotropic — *see* Hyperthyroidism, wi
      goiter (diffuse)
Exostosis — *see also* Disorder, bone
  cartilaginous — *see* Neoplasm, bone, benign
  congenital (multiple) Q78.6
  external ear canal H61.81- ☑
  gonococcal A54.49
  jaw (bone) M27.8
  multiple, congenital Q78.6
  orbit H05.35- ☑
  osteocartilaginous — *see* Neoplasm, bone, benign
  syphilitic A52.77
Exotropia — *see* Strabismus, divergent concomitan
Explanation of
  investigation finding Z71.2
  medication Z71.89
Exposure (to) — *see also* Contact, with T75.89 ☑
  acariasis Z20.7
  AIDS virus Z20.6
  air pollution Z77.110
  algae and algae toxins Z77.121
  algae bloom Z77.121
  anthrax Z20.810
  aromatic amines Z77.020
  aromatic (hazardous) compounds NEC Z77.028
  aromatic dyes NOS Z77.028
  arsenic Z77.010
  asbestos Z77.090
  bacterial disease NEC Z20.818
  benzene Z77.021
  blue-green algae bloom Z77.121
  body fluids (potentially hazardous) Z77.21
  brown tide Z77.121
  chemicals (chiefly nonmedicinal) (hazardous) NEC
      Z77.098
  cholera Z20.09
  chromium compounds Z77.018
  cold, effects of T69.9 ☑
    specified effect NEC T69.8 ☑
  communicable disease Z20.9
    bacterial NEC Z20.818
    specified NEC Z20.89
    viral NEC Z20.828
    Zika virus Z20.821
  cyanobacteria bloom Z77.121
  disaster Z65.5
  discrimination Z60.5
  dyes Z77.098
  effects of T73.9 ☑
  environmental tobacco smoke (acute) (chronic) Z77
  Escherichia coli (E. coli) Z20.01
  exhaustion due to T73.2 ☑
  fiberglass — *see* Table of Drugs and Chemicals, fib
      glass
  German measles Z20.4
  gonorrhea Z20.2
  hazardous metals NEC Z77.018
  hazardous substances NEC Z77.29
  hazards in the physical environment NEC Z77.128
  hazards to health NEC Z77.9
  human immunodeficiency virus (HIV) Z20.6
  human T-lymphotropic virus type-1 (HTLV-1) Z20.
  implanted
    mesh — *see* Complications, prosthetic devise o
        implant, mesh
    prosthetic materials NEC — *see* Complications,
        prosthetic materials NEC
  infestation (parasitic) NEC Z20.7
  intestinal infectious disease NEC Z20.09
    Escherichia coli (E. coli) Z20.01
  lead Z77.011
  meningococcus Z20.811
  mold (toxic) Z77.120
  nickel dust Z77.018

osure — continued
noise Z77.122
occupational
 air contaminants NEC Z57.39
 dust Z57.2
 environmental tobacco smoke Z57.31
 extreme temperature Z57.6
 noise Z57.0
 radiation Z57.1
 risk factors Z57.9
  specified NEC Z57.8
 toxic agents (gases) (liquids) (solids) (vapors) in
  agriculture Z57.4
 toxic agents (gases) (liquids) (solids) (vapors) in industry NEC Z57.5
 vibration Z57.7
parasitic disease NEC Z20.7
pediculosis Z20.7
persecution Z60.5
pfiesteria piscicida Z77.121
poliomyelitis Z20.89
pollution
 air Z77.110
 environmental NEC Z77.118
 soil Z77.112
 water Z77.111
polycyclic aromatic hydrocarbons Z77.028
prenatal (drugs) (toxic chemicals) — see Newborn, affected by, noxious substances transmitted via
  placenta or breast milk
rabies Z20.3
radiation, naturally occurring NEC Z77.123
radon Z77.123
red tide (Florida) Z77.121
rubella Z20.4
second hand tobacco smoke (acute) (chronic) Z77.22
 in the perinatal period P96.81
sexually-transmitted disease Z20.2
smallpox (laboratory) Z20.89
syphilis Z20.2
terrorism Z65.4
torture Z65.4
tuberculosis Z20.1
uranium Z77.012
varicella Z20.820
venereal disease Z20.2
viral disease NEC Z20.828
war Z65.5
water pollution Z77.111
Zika virus Z20.821
sanguination — see Hemorrhage
strophy
abdominal contents Q45.8
bladder Q64.10
 cloacal Q64.12
 specified type NEC Q64.19
 supravesical fissure Q64.11
tensive — see condition
ra — see also Accessory
marker chromosomes (normal individual) Q92.61
 in abnormal individual Q92.62
rib Q76.6
 cervical Q76.5
rasystoles (supraventricular) I49.49
atrial I49.1
auricular I49.1
junctional I49.2
ventricular I49.3
rauterine gestation or pregnancy — see Pregnancy,
 by site
travasation
blood R58
chyle into mesentery I89.8
pelvicalyceal N13.8
pyelosinus N13.8
urine (from ureter) R39.0
vesicant agent
 antineoplastic chemotherapy T80.810 ☑
 other agent NEC T80.818 ☑
tremity — see condition, limb
trophy — see Exstrophy
troversion
bladder Q64.19
uterus N81.4
 complicating delivery O71.2
 postpartal (old) N81.4
truded tooth (teeth) M26.34

Extrusion
 breast implant (prosthetic) T85.42 ☑
 eye implant (globe) (ball) T85.328 ☑
 intervertebral disc — see Displacement, intervertebral
  disc
 ocular lens implant (prosthetic) — see Complications,
  intraocular lens
 vitreous — see Prolapse, vitreous
Exudate
 pleural — see Effusion, pleura
 retina H35.89
Exudative — see condition
Eye, eyeball, eyelid — see condition
Eyestrain — see Disturbance, vision, subjective
Eyeworm disease of Africa B74.3

F

Faber's syndrome (achlorhydric anemia) D50.9
Fabry (-Anderson) **disease** E75.21
Faciocephalalgia, autonomic — see also Neuropathy,
  peripheral, autonomic G90.09
Factor(s)
 psychic, associated with diseases classified elsewhere
  F54
 psychological
  affecting physical conditions F54
  or behavioral
   affecting general medical condition F54
   associated with disorders or diseases classified
    elsewhere F54
Fahr disease (of brain) G23.8
Fahr Volhard disease (of kidney) I12.- ☑
Failure, failed
 abortion — see Abortion, attempted
 aortic (valve) I35.8
  rheumatic I06.8
 attempted abortion — see Abortion, attempted
 biventricular I50.82
  due to left heart failure I50.814
 bone marrow — see Anemia, aplastic
 cardiac — see Failure, heart
 cardiorenal (chronic) — see also Failure, renal, and
  Failure, heart I50.9
  hypertensive I13.2
 cardiorespiratory — see also Failure, heart R09.2
 cardiovascular (chronic) — see Failure, heart
 cerebrovascular I67.9
 cervical dilatation in labor O62.0
 circulation, circulatory (peripheral) R57.9
  newborn P29.89
 compensation — see Disease, heart
 compliance with medical treatment or regimen — see
  Noncompliance
 congestive — see Failure, heart, congestive
 dental implant (endosseous) M27.69
  due to
   failure of dental prosthesis M27.63
   lack of attached gingiva M27.62
   occlusal trauma (poor prosthetic design) M27.62
   parafunctional habits M27.62
   periodontal infection (peri-implantitis) M27.62
   poor oral hygiene M27.62
   osseointegration M27.61
    due to
     complications of systemic disease M27.61
     poor bone quality M27.61
    iatrogenic M27.61
   post-osseointegration
    biological M27.62
    due to complications of systemic disease M27.62
    iatrogenic M27.62
    mechanical M27.63
   pre-integration M27.61
   pre-osseointegration M27.61
   specified NEC M27.69
  descent of head (at term) of pregnancy (mother)
   O32.4 ☑
  endosseous dental implant — see Failure, dental implant
  engagement of head (term of pregnancy) (mother)
   O32.4 ☑
  erection (penile) — see also Dysfunction, sexual, male,
   erectile N52.9
   nonorganic F52.21
  examination(s), anxiety concerning Z55.2

Failure, failed — continued
 expansion terminal respiratory units (newborn) (primary) P28.0
 forceps NOS (with subsequent cesarean delivery) O66.5
 gain weight (child over 28 days old) R62.51
  adult R62.7
  newborn P92.6
 genital response (male) F52.21
  female F52.22
 heart (acute) (senile) (sudden) I50.9
  with
   acute pulmonary edema — see Failure, ventricu-
    lar, left
   decompensation — see also Failure, heart, by
    type as diastolic or systolic, acute and
    chronic I50.9
   dilatation — see Disease, heart
   hypertension — see Hypertension, heart
   normal ejection fraction — see Failure, heart,
    diastolic
   preserved ejection fraction — see Failure, heart,
    diastolic
   reduced ejection fraction — see Failure, heart,
    systolic
  arteriosclerotic I70.90
  biventricular I50.82
   due to left heart failure I50.814
  combined left-right sided I50.82
   due to left heart failure I50.814
  compensated — see also Failure, heart, by type as
   diastolic or systolic, chronic I50.9
  complicating
   anesthesia (general) (local) or other sedation
    in labor and delivery O74.2
    in pregnancy O29.12- ☑
    postpartum, puerperal O89.1
   delivery (cesarean) (instrumental) O75.4
  congestive I50.9
   with rheumatic fever (conditions in I00)
    active I01.8
    inactive or quiescent (with chorea) I09.81
   newborn P29.0
   rheumatic (chronic) (inactive) (with chorea)
    I09.81
    active or acute I01.8
     with chorea I02.0
  decompensated — see also Failure, heart, by type
   as diastolic or systolic, acute and chronic I50.9
  degenerative — see Degeneration, myocardial
  diastolic (congestive) (left ventricular) I50.30
   acute (congestive) I50.31
    and (on) chronic (congestive) I50.33
   chronic (congestive) I50.32
    and (on) acute (congestive) I50.33
   combined with systolic (congestive) I50.40
    acute (congestive) I50.41
     and (on) chronic (congestive) I50.43
    chronic (congestive) I50.42
     and (on) acute (congestive) I50.43
  due to presence of cardiac prosthesis I97.13- ☑
  end stage — see also Failure, heart, by type as diastolic or systolic, chronic I50.84
  following cardiac surgery I97.13- ☑
  high output NOS I50.83
  hypertensive — see Hypertension, heart
  left (ventricular) — see also Failure, ventricular, left
   combined diastolic and systolic — see Failure,
    heart, diastolic, combined with systolic
   diastolic — see Failure, heart, diastolic
   systolic — see Failure, heart, systolic
  low output (syndrome) NOS I50.9
  newborn P29.0
  organic — see Disease, heart
  peripartum O90.3
  postprocedural I97.13- ☑
  rheumatic (chronic) (inactive) I09.9
  right (isolated) (ventricular) I50.810
   acute I50.811
    and (on) chronic I50.813
   chronic I50.812
    and acute I50.813
   secondary to left heart failure I50.814

Failure, failed — *continued*
  heart — *continued*
    specified NEC I50.89

> *Note: heart failure stages A, B, C, and D are based on the American College of Cardiology and American Heart Association stages of heart failure, which complement and should not be confused with the New York Heart Association Classification of Heart Failure, into Class I, Class II, Class III, and Class IV*

      stage A Z91.89
      stage B — *see also* Failure, heart, by type as diastolic or systolic I50.9
      stage C — *see also* Failure, heart, by type as diastolic or systolic I50.9
      stage D — *see also* Failure, heart, by type as diastolic or systolic, chronic I50.84
      systolic (congestive) (left ventricular) I50.20
        acute (congestive) I50.21
          and (on) chronic (congestive) I50.23
        chronic (congestive) I50.22
          and (on) acute (congestive) I50.23
        combined with diastolic (congestive) I50.40
          acute (congestive) I50.41
            and (on) chronic (congestive) I50.43
          chronic (congestive) I50.42
            and (on) acute (congestive) I50.43
      thyrotoxic — *see also* Thyrotoxicosis E05.90 *[I43]*
        with
          high output — *see also* Thyrotoxicosis I50.83
          thyroid storm E05.91 *[I43]*
            high output — *see also* Thyrotoxicosis I50.83
      valvular — *see* Endocarditis
  hepatic K72.90
    with coma K72.91
    acute or subacute K72.00
      with coma K72.01
      due to drugs K71.10
        with coma K71.11
    alcoholic (acute) (chronic) (subacute) K70.40
      with coma K70.41
    chronic K72.10
      with coma K72.11
      due to drugs (acute) (subacute) (chronic) K71.10
        with coma K71.11
    due to drugs (acute) (subacute) (chronic) K71.10
      with coma K71.11
    postprocedural K91.82
  hepatorenal K76.7
  induction (of labor) O61.9
    abortion — *see* Abortion, attempted
    by
      oxytocic drugs O61.0
      prostaglandins O61.0
    instrumental O61.1
    mechanical O61.1
    medical O61.0
    specified NEC O61.8
    surgical O61.1
  intubation during anesthesia T88.4 ☑
    in pregnancy O29.6- ☑
    labor and delivery O74.7
    postpartum, puerperal O89.6
  involution, thymus (gland) E32.0
  kidney — *see also* Disease, kidney, chronic N19
    acute — *see also* Failure, renal, acute N17.9
  lactation (complete) O92.3
    partial O92.4
  Leydig's cell, adult E29.1
  liver — *see* Failure, hepatic
  menstruation at puberty N91.0
  mitral I05.8
  myocardial, myocardium — *see also* Failure, heart I50.9
    chronic — *see also* Failure, heart, congestive I50.9
    congestive — *see also* Failure, heart, congestive I50.9
  orgasm (female) (psychogenic) F52.31
    male F52.32
  ovarian (primary) E28.39
    iatrogenic E89.40
      asymptomatic E89.40
      symptomatic E89.41
    postprocedural (postablative) (postirradiation) (postsurgical) E89.40
      asymptomatic E89.40
      symptomatic E89.41
  ovulation causing infertility N97.0

Failure, failed — *continued*
  polyglandular, autoimmune E31.0
  prosthetic joint implant — *see* Complications, joint prosthesis, mechanical, breakdown, by site
  renal N19
    with
      tubular necrosis (acute) N17.0
    acute N17.9
      with
        cortical necrosis N17.1
        medullary necrosis N17.2
        tubular necrosis N17.0
      specified NEC N17.8
    chronic N18.9
      hypertensive — *see* Hypertension, kidney
    congenital P96.0
    end stage (chronic) N18.6
      due to hypertension I12.0
    following
      abortion — *see* Abortion by type complicated by specified condition NEC
      crushing T79.5 ☑
      ectopic or molar pregnancy O08.4
      labor and delivery (acute) O90.4
    hypertensive — *see* Hypertension, kidney
    postprocedural N99.0
  respiration, respiratory J96.90
    with
      hypercapnia J96.92
      hypercarbia J96.92
      hypoxia J96.91
    acute J96.00
      with
        hypercapnia J96.02
        hypercarbia J96.02
        hypoxia J96.01
    center G93.89
    acute and (on) chronic J96.20
      with
        hypercapnia J96.22
        hypercarbia J96.22
        hypoxia J96.21
    chronic J96.10
      with
        hypercapnia J96.12
        hypercarbia J96.12
        hypoxia J96.11
    newborn P28.5
    postprocedural (acute) J95.821
      acute and chronic J95.822
  rotation
    cecum Q43.3
    colon Q43.3
    intestine Q43.3
    kidney Q63.2
  sedation (conscious) (moderate) during procedure T88.52 ☑
    history of Z92.83
  segmentation — *see also* Fusion
    fingers — *see* Syndactylism, complex, fingers
    vertebra Q76.49
      with scoliosis Q76.3
  seminiferous tubule, adult E29.1
  senile (general) R54
  sexual arousal (male) F52.21
    female F52.22
  testicular endocrine function E29.1
  to thrive (child over 28 days old) R62.51
    adult R62.7
    newborn P92.6
  transplant T86.92
    bone T86.831
      marrow T86.02
    cornea T86.841
    heart T86.22
      with lung(s) T86.32
    intestine T86.851
    kidney T86.12
    liver T86.42
    lung(s) T86.811
      with heart T86.32
    pancreas T86.891
    skin (allograft) (autograft) T86.821
    specified organ or tissue NEC T86.891
    stem cell (peripheral blood) (umbilical cord) T86.5
  trial of labor (with subsequent cesarean delivery) O66.40
    following previous cesarean delivery O66.41

Failure, failed — *continued*
  tubal ligation N99.89
  urinary — *see* Disease, kidney, chronic
  vacuum extraction NOS (with subsequent cesarean delivery) O66.5
  vasectomy N99.89
  ventouse NOS (with subsequent cesarean delivery) O66.5
  ventricular — *see also* Failure, heart I50.9
    left — *see also* Failure, heart, left I50.1
      with rheumatic fever (conditions in I00)
        active I01.8
          with chorea I02.0
        inactive or quiescent (with chorea) I09.81
        rheumatic (chronic) (inactive) (with chorea) I09.81
          active or acute I01.8
            with chorea I02.0
    right — *see* Failure, heart, right
  vital centers, newborn P91.88
Fainting (fit) R55
Fallen arches — *see* Deformity, limb, flat foot
Falling, falls (repeated) R29.6
  any organ or part — *see* Prolapse
Fallopian
  insufflation Z31.41
  tube — *see* condition
Fallot's
  pentalogy Q21.8
  tetrad or tetralogy Q21.3
  triad or trilogy Q22.3
False — *see also* condition
  croup J38.5
  joint — *see* Nonunion, fracture
  labor (pains) O47.9
    at or after 37 completed weeks of gestation O4
    before 37 completed weeks of gestation O47.0-
  passage, urethra (prostatic) N36.5
  pregnancy F45.8
Family, familial — *see also* condition
  disruption Z63.8
    involving divorce or separation Z63.5
  Li-Fraumeni (syndrome) Z15.01
  planning advice Z30.09
  problem Z63.9
    specified NEC Z63.8
  retinoblastoma C69.2- ☑
Famine (effects of) T73.0 ☑
  edema — *see* Malnutrition, severe
Fanconi (-de Toni)(-Debré) **syndrome** E72.09
  with cystinosis E72.04
Fanconi's anemia (congenital pancytopenia) D61.09
Farber's disease or syndrome E75.29
Farcy A24.0
Farmer's
  lung J67.0
  skin L57.8
Farsightedness — *see* Hypermetropia
Fascia — *see* condition
Fasciculation R25.3
Fasciitis M72.9
  diffuse (eosinophilic) M35.4
  infective M72.8
    necrotizing M72.6
  necrotizing M72.6
  nodular M72.4
  perirenal (with ureteral obstruction) N13.5
    with infection N13.6
  plantar M72.2
  specified NEC M72.8
  traumatic (old) M72.8
    current — *code by* site under Sprain
Fascioliasis B66.3
Fasciolopsis, fasciolopsiasis (intestinal) B66.5
Fascioscapulohumeral myopathy G71.02
Fast pulse R00.0
Fat
  embolism — *see* Embolism, fat
  excessive — *see also* Obesity
    in heart — *see* Degeneration, myocardial
  in stool R19.5
  localized (pad) E65
    heart — *see* Degeneration, myocardial
    knee M79.4
    retropatellar M79.4
  necrosis
    breast N64.1
    mesentery K65.4

— continued

necrosis — continued
  omentum K65.4
 ad E65
  knee M79.4
igue R53.83
 auditory deafness — see Deafness
 chronic R53.82
 combat F43.0
 general R53.83
  psychogenic F48.8
 heat (transient) T67.6 ☑
 muscle M62.89
 myocardium — see Failure, heart
 neoplasm-related R53.0
 nervous, neurosis F48.8
 operational F48.8
 psychogenic (general) F48.8
 senile R54
 voice R49.8
ness — see Obesity
ty — see also condition
 apron E65
 degeneration — see Degeneration, fatty
 heart (enlarged) — see Degeneration, myocardial
 liver NEC K76.0
  alcoholic K70.0
  nonalcoholic K76.0
 necrosis — see Degeneration, fatty
ces — see condition
chard's disease (periodontitis) — see Periodontitis
citis J02.9
ism (anemia) D55.0
us — see Dermatophytosis
io-Londe disease or syndrome G12.1
r complex or reaction F40.9
r of — see Phobia
red complaint unfounded Z71.1
oris, febrile — see also Fever
flava — see also Fever, yellow A95.9
 melitensis A23.0
 pestis — see Plague
 recurrens — see Fever, relapsing
 rubra A38.9
al
 incontinence R15.9
 smearing R15.1
 soiling R15.1
 urgency R15.2
alith (impaction) K56.41
 appendix K38.1
 congenital P76.8
le's disease K14.0
ble rapid pulse due to shock following injury T79.4 ☑
ble-minded F70
eding
 difficulties R63.3
 problem R63.3
  newborn P92.9
   specified NEC P92.8
  nonorganic (adult) — see Disorder, eating
ling (of)
 foreign body in throat R09.89
r's disease — see Poisoning, mercury
t — see condition
gned illness Z76.5
-Klippel syndrome (brevicollis) Q76.1
nmesser's (hidrotic) **ectodermal dysplasia** Q82.4
inophobia F40.218
on — see also Cellulitis, digit
 with lymphangitis — see Lymphangitis, acute, digit
ty's syndrome M05.00
 ankle M05.07- ☑
 elbow M05.02- ☑
 foot joint M05.07- ☑
 hand joint M05.04- ☑
 hip M05.05- ☑
 knee M05.06- ☑
 multiple site M05.09
 shoulder M05.01- ☑
 vertebra — see Spondylitis, ankylosing
 wrist M05.03- ☑
male genital cutting status — see Female genital mutilation status (FGM)
male genital mutilation status (FGM) N90.810
 specified NEC N90.818

Female genital mutilation status — continued
 type I (clitorectomy status) N90.811
 type II (clitorectomy with excision of labia minora status) N90.812
 type III (infibulation status) N90.813
 type IV N90.818
Femur, femoral — see condition
Fenestration, fenestrated — see also Imperfect, closure
 aortico-pulmonary Q21.4
 cusps, heart valve NEC Q24.8
  pulmonary Q22.3
 pulmonic cusps Q22.3
Fernell's disease (aortic aneurysm) I71.9
Fertile eunuch syndrome E23.0
Fetid
 breath R19.6
 sweat L75.0
Fetishism F65.0
 transvestic F65.1
Fetus, fetal — see also condition
 alcohol syndrome (dysmorphic) Q86.0
 compressus O31.0- ☑
 hydantoin syndrome Q86.1
 lung tissue P28.0
 papyraceous O31.0- ☑
Fever (inanition) (of unknown origin) (persistent) (with chills) (with rigor) R50.9
 abortus A23.1
 Aden (dengue) A90
 African tick-borne A68.1
 American
  mountain (tick) A93.2
  spotted A77.0
 aphthous B08.8
 arbovirus, arboviral A94
  hemorrhagic A94
  specified NEC A93.8
 Argentinian hemorrhagic A96.0
 Assam B55.0
 Australian Q A78
 Bangkok hemorrhagic A91
 Barmah forest A92.8
 Bartonella A44.0
 bilious, hemoglobinuric B50.8
 blackwater B50.8
 blister B00.1
 Bolivian hemorrhagic A96.1
 Bonvale dam T73.3 ☑
 boutonneuse A77.1
 brain — see Encephalitis
 Brazilian purpuric A48.4
 breakbone A90
 Bullis A77.0
 Bunyamwera A92.8
 Burdwan B55.0
 Bwamba A92.8
 Cameroon — see Malaria
 Canton A75.9
 catarrhal (acute) J00
  chronic J31.0
 cat-scratch A28.1
 Central Asian hemorrhagic A98.0
 cerebral — see Encephalitis
 cerebrospinal meningococcal A39.0
 Chagres B50.9
 Chandipura A92.8
 Changuinola A93.1
 Charcot's (biliary) (hepatic) (intermittent) — see Calculus, bile duct
 Chikungunya (viral) (hemorrhagic) A92.0
 Chitral A93.1
 Colombo — see Fever, paratyphoid
 Colorado tick (virus) A93.2
 congestive (remittent) — see Malaria
 Congo virus A98.0
 continued malarial B50.9
 Corsican — see Malaria
 Crimean-Congo hemorrhagic A98.0
 Cyprus — see Brucellosis
 dandy A90
 deer fly — see Tularemia
 dengue (virus) A90
  hemorrhagic A91
  sandfly A93.1
 desert B38.0
 drug induced R50.2
 due to
  conditions classified elsewhere R50.81

Fever — continued
 due to — continued
  heat T67.01 ☑
 enteric A01.00
 enteroviral exanthematous (Boston exanthem) A88.0
 ephemeral (of unknown origin) R50.9
 epidemic hemorrhagic A98.5
 erysipelatous — see Erysipelas
 estivo-autumnal (malarial) B50.9
 famine A75.0
 five day A79.0
 following delivery O86.4
 Fort Bragg A27.89
 gastroenteric A01.00
 gastromalarial — see Malaria
 Gibraltar — see Brucellosis
 glandular — see Mononucleosis, infectious
 Guama (viral) A92.8
 Haverhill A25.1
 hay (allergic) J30.1
  with asthma (bronchial) J45.909
   with
    exacerbation (acute) J45.901
    status asthmaticus J45.902
  due to
   allergen other than pollen J30.89
   pollen, any plant or tree J30.1
 heat (effects) T67.01 ☑
 hematuric, bilious B50.8
 hemoglobinuric (malarial) (bilious) B50.8
 hemorrhagic (arthropod-borne) NOS A94
  with renal syndrome A98.5
  arenaviral A96.9
   specified NEC A96.8
  Argentinian A96.0
  Bangkok A91
  Bolivian A96.1
  Central Asian A98.0
  Chikungunya A92.0
  Crimean-Congo A98.0
  dengue (virus) A91
  epidemic A98.5
  Junin (virus) A96.0
  Korean A98.5
  Kyasanur forest A98.2
  Machupo (virus) A96.1
  mite-borne A93.8
  mosquito-borne A92.8
  Omsk A98.1
  Philippine A91
  Russian A98.5
  Singapore A91
  Southeast Asia A91
  Thailand A91
  tick-borne NEC A93.8
  viral A99
   specified NEC A98.8
 hepatic — see Cholecystitis
 herpetic — see Herpes
 icterohemorrhagic A27.0
 Indiana A93.8
 infective B99.9
  specified NEC B99.8
 intermittent (bilious) — see also Malaria
  of unknown origin R50.9
  pernicious B50.9
 iodide R50.2
 Japanese river A75.3
 jungle — see also Malaria
  yellow A95.0
 Junin (virus) hemorrhagic A96.0
 Katayama B65.2
 kedani A75.3
 Kenya (tick) A77.1
 Kew Garden A79.1
 Korean hemorrhagic A98.5
 Lassa A96.2
 Lone Star A77.0
 Machupo (virus) hemorrhagic A96.1
 malaria, malarial — see Malaria
 Malta A23.9
 Marseilles A77.1
 marsh — see Malaria
 Mayaro (viral) A92.8
 Mediterranean — see also Brucellosis A23.9
  familial M04.1
  tick A77.1
 meningeal — see Meningitis

Fever — continued
- Meuse A79.0
- Mexican A75.2
- mianeh A68.1
- miasmatic — see Malaria
- mosquito-borne (viral) A92.9
  - hemorrhagic A92.8
- mountain — see also Brucellosis
  - meaning Rocky Mountain spotted fever A77.0
  - tick (American) (Colorado) (viral) A93.2
- Mucambo (viral) A92.8
- mud A27.9
- Neapolitan — see Brucellosis
- neutropenic D70.9
- newborn P81.9
  - environmental P81.0
- Nine-Mile A78
- non-exanthematous tick A93.2
- North Asian tick-borne A77.2
- Omsk hemorrhagic A98.1
- O'nyong-nyong (viral) A92.1
- Oropouche (viral) A93.0
- Oroya A44.0
- paludal — see Malaria
- Panama (malarial) B50.9
- Pappataci A93.1
- paratyphoid A01.4
  - A A01.1
  - B A01.2
  - C A01.3
- parrot A70
- periodic (Mediterranean) M04.1
- persistent (of unknown origin) R50.9
- petechial A39.0
- pharyngoconjunctival B30.2
- Philippine hemorrhagic A91
- phlebotomus A93.1
- Piry (virus) A93.8
- Pixuna (viral) A92.8
- Plasmodium ovale B53.0
- polioviral (nonparalytic) A80.4
- Pontiac A48.2
- postimmunization R50.83
- postoperative R50.82
  - due to infection T81.40 ☑
- posttransfusion R50.84
- postvaccination R50.83
- presenting with conditions classified elsewhere R50.81
- pretibial A27.89
- puerperal O86.4
- Q A78
- quadrilateral A78
- quartan (malaria) B52.9
- Queensland (coastal) (tick) A77.3
- quintan A79.0
- rabbit — see Tularemia
- rat-bite A25.9
  - due to
    - Spirillum A25.0
    - Streptobacillus moniliformis A25.1
- recurrent — see Fever, relapsing
- relapsing (Borrelia) A68.9
  - Carter's (Asiatic) A68.1
  - Dutton's (West African) A68.1
  - Koch's A68.9
  - louse-borne A68.0
  - Novy's
    - louse-borne A68.0
    - tick-borne A68.1
  - Obermeyer's (European) A68.0
  - tick-borne A68.1
- remittent (bilious) (congestive) (gastric) — see Malaria
- rheumatic (active) (acute) (chronic) (subacute) I00
  - with central nervous system involvement I02.9
  - active with heart involvement — see category I01 ☑
  - inactive or quiescent with
    - cardiac hypertrophy I09.89
    - carditis I09.9
    - endocarditis I09.1
      - aortic (valve) I06.9
        - with mitral (valve) disease I08.0
      - mitral (valve) I05.9
        - with aortic (valve) disease I08.0
      - pulmonary (valve) I09.89
      - tricuspid (valve) I07.8
    - heart disease NEC I09.89
    - heart failure (congestive) (conditions in category I50.) I09.81

Fever — continued
- rheumatic — continued
  - inactive or quiescent with — continued
    - left ventricular failure (conditions in I50.1- I50.4-) I09.81
    - myocarditis, myocardial degeneration (conditions in I51.4) I09.0
    - pancarditis I09.9
    - pericarditis I09.2
- Rift Valley (viral) A92.4
- Rocky Mountain spotted A77.0
- rose J30.1
- Ross River B33.1
- Russian hemorrhagic A98.5
- San Joaquin (Valley) B38.0
- sandfly A93.1
- Sao Paulo A77.0
- scarlet A38.9
- seven day (leptospirosis) (autumnal) (Japanese) A27.89
  - dengue A90
- shin-bone A79.0
- Singapore hemorrhagic A91
- solar A90
- Songo A98.5
- sore B00.1
- South African tick-bite A68.1
- Southeast Asia hemorrhagic A91
- spinal — see Meningitis
- spirillary A25.0
- splenic — see Anthrax
- spotted A77.9
  - American A77.0
  - Brazilian A77.0
  - cerebrospinal meningitis A39.0
  - Colombian A77.0
  - due to Rickettsia
    - australis A77.3
    - conorii A77.1
    - rickettsii A77.0
    - sibirica A77.2
    - specified type NEC A77.8
  - Ehrlichiosis A77.40
    - due to
      - E. chafeensis A77.41
      - specified organism NEC A77.49
  - Rocky Mountain A77.0
- steroid R50.2
- streptobacillary A25.1
- subtertian B50.9
- Sumatran mite A75.3
- sun A90
- swamp A27.9
- swine A02.8
- sylvatic, yellow A95.0
- Tahyna B33.8
- tertian — see Malaria, tertian
- Thailand hemorrhagic A91
- thermic T67.01 ☑
- three-day A93.1
- tick
  - American mountain A93.2
  - Colorado A93.2
  - Kemerovo A93.8
  - Mediterranean A77.1
  - mountain A93.2
  - nonexanthematous A93.2
  - Quaranfil A93.8
- tick-bite NEC A93.8
- tick-borne (hemorrhagic) NEC A93.8
- trench A79.0
- tsutsugamushi A75.3
- typhogastric A01.00
- typhoid (abortive) (hemorrhagic) (intermittent) (malignant) A01.00
  - complicated by
    - arthritis A01.04
    - heart involvement A01.02
    - meningitis A01.01
    - osteomyelitis A01.05
    - pneumonia A01.03
    - specified NEC A01.09
- typhomalarial — see Malaria
- typhus — see Typhus (fever)
- undulant — see Brucellosis
- unknown origin R50.9
- uveoparotid D86.89
- valley B38.0
- Venezuelan equine A92.2

Fever — continued
- vesicular stomatitis A93.8
- viral hemorrhagic — see Fever, hemorrhagic, by t of virus
- Volhynian A79.0
- Wesselsbron (viral) A92.8
- West
  - African B50.8
  - Nile (viral) A92.30
    - with
      - complications NEC A92.39
      - cranial nerve disorders A92.32
      - encephalitis A92.31
      - encephalomyelitis A92.31
      - neurologic manifestation NEC A92.32
      - optic neuritis A92.32
      - polyradiculitis A92.32
- Whitmore's — see Melioidosis
- Wolhynian A79.0
- worm B83.9
- yellow A95.9
  - jungle A95.0
  - sylvatic A95.0
  - urban A95.1
- Zika virus A92.5

Fibrillation
- atrial or auricular (established) I48.91
  - chronic I48.20
    - persistent I48.19
  - paroxysmal I48.0
  - permanent I48.21
  - persistent (chronic) (NOS) (other) I48.19
    - longstanding I48.11
- cardiac I49.8
- heart I49.8
- muscular M62.89
- ventricular I49.01

Fibrin
- ball or bodies, pleural (sac) J94.1
- chamber, anterior (eye) (gelatinous exudate) — se Iridocyclitis, acute

Fibrinogenolysis — see Fibrinolysis
Fibrinogenopenia D68.8
- acquired D65
- congenital D68.2

Fibrinolysis (hemorrhagic) (acquired) D65
- antepartum hemorrhage — see Hemorrhage, ante tum, with coagulation defect
- following
  - abortion — see Abortion by type complicated I hemorrhage
  - ectopic or molar pregnancy O08.1
- intrapartum O67.0
- newborn, transient P60
- postpartum O72.3

Fibrinopenia (hereditary) D68.2
- acquired D68.4

Fibrinopurulent — see condition
Fibrinous — see condition
Fibroadenoma
- cellular intracanalicular D24- ☑
- giant D24- ☑
- intracanalicular
  - cellular D24- ☑
  - giant D24- ☑
  - specified site — see Neoplasm, benign, by site
  - unspecified site D24- ☑
- juvenile D24- ☑
- pericanalicular
  - specified site — see Neoplasm, benign, by site
  - unspecified site D24- ☑
- phyllodes D24- ☑
- prostate D29.1
- specified site NEC — see Neoplasm, benign, by sit
- unspecified site D24- ☑

Fibroadenosis, breast (chronic) (cystic) (diffuse) (peri ic) (segmental) N60.2- ☑
Fibroangioma — see also Neoplasm, benign, by sit◆
- juvenile
  - specified site — see Neoplasm, benign, by site
  - unspecified site D10.6

Fibrochondrosarcoma — see Neoplasm, cartilage, ◆ lignant
Fibrocystic
- disease — see also Fibrosis, cystic
  - breast — see Mastopathy, cystic
  - jaw M27.49
  - kidney (congenital) Q61.8

rocystic — *continued*
disease — *see also* Fibrosis, cystic — *continued*
  liver Q44.6
  pancreas E84.9
kidney (congenital) Q61.8
rodysplasia ossificans progressiva — *see* Myositis, ossificans, progressiva
roelastosis (cordis) (endocardial) (endomyocardial) I42.4
roid (tumor) — *see also* Neoplasm, connective tissue, benign
disease, lung (chronic) — *see* Fibrosis, lung
heart (disease) — *see* Myocarditis
in pregnancy or childbirth O34.1- ☑
  causing obstructed labor O65.5
induration, lung (chronic) — *see* Fibrosis, lung
lung — *see* Fibrosis, lung
pneumonia (chronic) — *see* Fibrosis, lung
uterus — *see also* Leiomyoma, uterus D25.9
rolipoma — *see* Lipoma
roliposarcoma — *see* Neoplasm, connective tissue, malignant
roma — *see also* Neoplasm, connective tissue, benign
ameloblastic — *see* Cyst, calcifying odontogenic
bone (nonossifying) — *see* Disorder, bone, specified type NEC
  ossifying — *see* Neoplasm, bone, benign
cementifying — *see* Neoplasm, bone, benign
chondromyxoid — *see* Neoplasm, bone, benign
desmoplastic — *see* Neoplasm, connective tissue, uncertain behavior
durum — *see* Neoplasm, connective tissue, benign
fascial — *see* Neoplasm, connective tissue, benign
invasive — *see* Neoplasm, connective tissue, uncertain behavior
molle — *see* Lipoma
myxoid — *see* Neoplasm, connective tissue, benign
nasopharynx, nasopharyngeal (juvenile) D10.6
nonosteogenic (nonossifying) — *see* Dysplasia, fibrous
odontogenic (central) — *see* Cyst, calcifying odontogenic
ossifying — *see* Neoplasm, bone, benign
periosteal — *see* Neoplasm, bone, benign
soft — *see* Lipoma
romatosis M72.9
abdominal — *see* Neoplasm, connective tissue, uncertain behavior
aggressive — *see* Neoplasm, connective tissue, uncertain behavior
congenital generalized — *see* Neoplasm, connective tissue, uncertain behavior
Dupuytren's M72.0
gingival K06.1
palmar (fascial) M72.0
plantar (fascial) M72.2
pseudosarcomatous (proliferative) (subcutaneous) M72.4
retroperitoneal D48.3
specified NEC M72.8
romyalgia M79.7
romyoma — *see also* Neoplasm, connective tissue, benign
uterus (corpus) — *see also* Leiomyoma, uterus
  in pregnancy or childbirth — *see* Fibroid, in pregnancy or childbirth
   causing obstructed labor O65.5
romyositis M79.7
romyxolipoma D17.9
romyxoma — *see* Neoplasm, connective tissue, benign
romyxosarcoma — *see* Neoplasm, connective tissue, malignant
ro-odontoma, ameloblastic — *see* Cyst, calcifying odontogenic
ro-osteoma — *see* Neoplasm, bone, benign
roplasia, retrolental H35.17- ☑
ropurulent — *see* condition
rosarcoma — *see also* Neoplasm, connective tissue, malignant
ameloblastic C41.1
  upper jaw (bone) C41.0
congenital — *see* Neoplasm, connective tissue, malignant
fascial — *see* Neoplasm, connective tissue, malignant
infantile — *see* Neoplasm, connective tissue, malignant
odontogenic C41.1
  upper jaw (bone) C41.0

Fibrosarcoma — *continued*
periosteal — *see* Neoplasm, bone, malignant
Fibrosclerosis
breast N60.3- ☑
multifocal M35.5
penis (corpora cavernosa) N48.6
Fibrosis, fibrotic
adrenal (gland) E27.8
amnion O41.8X- ☑
anal papillae K62.89
arteriocapillary — *see* Arteriosclerosis
bladder N32.89
  interstitial — *see* Cystitis, chronic, interstitial
  localized submucosal — *see* Cystitis, chronic, interstitial
  panmural — *see* Cystitis, chronic, interstitial
breast — *see* Fibrosclerosis, breast
capillary — *see also* Arteriosclerosis I70.90
  lung (chronic) — *see* Fibrosis, lung
cardiac — *see* Myocarditis
cervix N88.8
chorion O41.8X- ☑
corpus cavernosum (sclerosing) N48.6
cystic (of pancreas) E84.9
  with
   distal intestinal obstruction syndrome E84.19
   fecal impaction E84.19
   intestinal manifestations NEC E84.19
   pulmonary manifestations E84.0
   specified manifestations NEC E84.8
due to device, implant or graft — *see also* Complications, by site and type, specified NEC T85.828 ☑
  arterial graft NEC T82.828 ☑
  breast (implant) T85.828 ☑
  catheter NEC T85.828 ☑
   dialysis (renal) T82.828 ☑
    intraperitoneal T85.828 ☑
   infusion NEC T82.828 ☑
    spinal (epidural) (subdural) T85.820 ☑
   urinary (indwelling) T83.82 ☑
  electronic (electrode) (pulse generator) (stimulator)
   bone T84.82 ☑
   cardiac T82.827 ☑
   nervous system (brain) (peripheral nerve) (spinal) T85.820 ☑
   urinary T83.82 ☑
  fixation, internal (orthopedic) NEC T84.82 ☑
  gastrointestinal (bile duct) (esophagus) T85.828 ☑
  genital NEC T83.82 ☑
  heart NEC T82.827 ☑
  joint prosthesis T84.82 ☑
  ocular (corneal graft) (orbital implant) NEC T85.828 ☑
  orthopedic NEC T84.82 ☑
  specified NEC T85.828 ☑
  urinary NEC T83.82 ☑
  vascular NEC T82.828 ☑
  ventricular intracranial shunt T85.820 ☑
ejaculatory duct N50.89
endocardium — *see* Endocarditis
endomyocardial (tropical) I42.3
epididymis N50.89
eye muscle — *see* Strabismus, mechanical
heart — *see* Myocarditis
hepatic — *see* Fibrosis, liver
hepatolienal (portal hypertension) K76.6
hepatosplenic (portal hypertension) K76.6
infrapatellar fat pad M79.4
intrascrotal N50.89
kidney N26.9
liver K74.0
  with sclerosis K74.2
  alcoholic K70.2
lung (atrophic) (chronic) (confluent) (massive) (perialveolar) (peribronchial) J84.10
  with
   anthracosilicosis J60
   anthracosis J60
   asbestosis J61
   bagassosis J67.1
   bauxite J63.1
   berylliosis J63.2
   byssinosis J66.0
   calcicosis J62.8
   chalicosis J62.8
   dust reticulation J64
   farmer's lung J67.0

Fibrosis, fibrotic — *continued*
lung — *continued*
  with — *continued*
   ganister disease J62.8
   graphite J63.3
   pneumoconiosis NOS J64
   siderosis J63.4
   silicosis J62.8
  capillary J84.10
  congenital P27.8
  diffuse (idiopathic) J84.10
   chemicals, gases, fumes or vapors (inhalation) J68.4
   interstitial J84.10
    acute J84.114
   talc J62.0
  following radiation J70.1
  idiopathic J84.112
  postinflammatory J84.10
  silicotic J62.8
  tuberculous — *see* Tuberculosis, pulmonary
lymphatic gland I89.8
median bar — *see* Hyperplasia, prostate
mediastinum (idiopathic) J98.59
meninges G96.19
myocardium, myocardial — *see* Myocarditis
ovary N83.8
oviduct N83.8
pancreas K86.89
penis NEC N48.6
pericardium I31.0
perineum, in pregnancy or childbirth O34.7- ☑
  causing obstructed labor O65.5
pleura J94.1
popliteal fat pad M79.4
prostate (chronic) — *see* Hyperplasia, prostate
pulmonary — *see also* Fibrosis, lung J84.10
  congenital P27.8
  idiopathic J84.112
rectal sphincter K62.89
retroperitoneal, idiopathic (with ureteral obstruction) N13.5
  with infection N13.6
sclerosing mesenteric (idiopathic) K65.4
scrotum N50.89
seminal vesicle N50.89
senile R54
skin L90.5
spermatic cord N50.89
spleen D73.89
  in schistosomiasis (bilharziasis) B65.9 *[D77]*
subepidermal nodular — *see* Neoplasm, skin, benign
submucous (oral) (tongue) K13.5
testis N44.8
  chronic, due to syphilis A52.76
thymus (gland) E32.8
tongue, submucous K13.5
tunica vaginalis N50.89
uterus (non-neoplastic) N85.8
vagina N89.8
valve, heart — *see* Endocarditis
vas deferens N50.89
vein I87.8
Fibrositis (periarticular) M79.7
nodular, chronic (Jaccoud's) (rheumatoid) — *see* Arthropathy, postrheumatic, chronic
Fibrothorax J94.1
Fibrotic — *see* Fibrosis
Fibrous — *see* condition
Fibroxanthoma — *see also* Neoplasm, connective tissue, benign
atypical — *see* Neoplasm, connective tissue, uncertain behavior
malignant — *see* Neoplasm, connective tissue, malignant
Fibroxanthosarcoma — *see* Neoplasm, connective tissue, malignant
Fiedler's
disease (icterohemorrhagic leptospirosis) A27.0
myocarditis (acute) I40.1
Fifth disease B08.3
venereal A55
Filaria, filarial, filariasis — *see* Infestation, filarial
Filatov's disease — *see* Mononucleosis, infectious
File-cutter's disease — *see* Poisoning, lead
Filling defect
biliary tract R93.2
bladder R93.41

Filling defect — *continued*
- duodenum R93.3
- gallbladder R93.2
- gastrointestinal tract R93.3
- intestine R93.3
- kidney R93.42- ☑
- stomach R93.3
- ureter R93.41
- urinary organs, specified NEC R93.49

Fimbrial cyst Q50.4

Financial problem affecting care NOS Z59.9
- bankruptcy Z59.8
- foreclosure on loan Z59.8

Findings, abnormal, inconclusive, without diagnosis
— *see also* Abnormal
- 17-ketosteroids, elevated R82.5
- acetonuria R82.4
- alcohol in blood R78.0
- anisocytosis R71.8
- antenatal screening of mother O28.9
  - biochemical O28.1
  - chromosomal O28.5
  - cytological O28.2
  - genetic O28.5
  - hematological O28.0
  - radiological O28.4
  - specified NEC O28.8
  - ultrasonic O28.3
- antibody titer, elevated R76.0
- anticardiolipin antibody R76.0
- antiphosphatidylglycerol antibody R76.0
- antiphosphatidylinositol antibody R76.0
- antiphosphatidylserine antibody R76.0
- antiphospholipid antibody R76.0
- bacteriuria R82.71
- bicarbonate E87.8
- bile in urine R82.2
- blood sugar R73.09
  - high R73.9
  - low (transient) E16.2
- body fluid or substance, specified NEC R88.8
- casts, urine R82.998
- catecholamines R82.5
- cells, urine R82.998
- chloride E87.8
- cholesterol E78.9
  - high E78.00
    - with high triglycerides E78.2
- chyluria R82.0
- cloudy
  - dialysis effluent R88.0
  - urine R82.90
- creatinine clearance R94.4
- crystals, urine R82.998
- culture
  - blood R78.81
  - positive — *see* Positive, culture
- echocardiogram R93.1
- electrolyte level, urinary R82.998
- function study NEC R94.8
  - bladder R94.8
  - endocrine NEC R94.7
    - thyroid R94.6
  - kidney R94.4
  - liver R94.5
  - pancreas R94.8
  - placenta R94.8
  - pulmonary R94.2
  - spleen R94.8
- gallbladder, nonvisualization R93.2
- glucose (tolerance test) (non-fasting) R73.09
- glycosuria R81
- heart
  - shadow R93.1
  - sounds R01.2
- hematinuria R82.3
- hematocrit drop (precipitous) R71.0
- hemoglobinuria R82.3
- human papillomavirus (HPV) DNA test positive
  - cervix
    - high risk R87.810
    - low risk R87.820
  - vagina
    - high risk R87.811
    - low risk R87.821
- in blood (of substance not normally found in blood) R78.9
  - addictive drug NEC R78.4
  - alcohol (excessive level) R78.0

Findings, abnormal, inconclusive, without diagnosis
— *continued*
- in blood — *continued*
  - cocaine R78.2
  - hallucinogen R78.3
  - heavy metals (abnormal level) R78.79
  - lead R78.71
  - lithium (abnormal level) R78.89
  - opiate drug R78.1
  - psychotropic drug R78.5
  - specified substance NEC R78.89
  - steroid agent R78.6
- indoleacetic acid, elevated R82.5
- ketonuria R82.4
- lactic acid dehydrogenase (LDH) R74.0
- liver function test R79.89
- mammogram NEC R92.8
  - calcification (calculus) R92.1
  - inconclusive result (due to dense breasts) R92.2
  - microcalcification R92.0
- mediastinal shift R93.89
- melanin, urine R82.998
- myoglobinuria R82.1
- neonatal screening P09
- nonvisualization of gallbladder R93.2
- odor of urine NOS R82.90
- Papanicolaou cervix R87.619
  - non-atypical endometrial cells R87.618
- pneumoencephalogram R93.0
- poikilocytosis R71.8
- potassium (deficiency) E87.6
  - excess E87.5
- PPD R76.11
- radiologic (X-ray) R93.89
  - abdomen R93.5
  - biliary tract R93.2
  - breast R92.8
  - gastrointestinal tract R93.3
  - genitourinary organs R93.89
  - head R93.0
  - inconclusive due to excess body fat of patient R93.9
  - intrathoracic organs NEC R93.1
  - musculoskeletal
    - limbs R93.6
    - other than limb R93.7
  - placenta R93.89
  - retroperitoneum R93.5
  - skin R93.89
  - skull R93.0
  - subcutaneous tissue R93.89
  - testis R93.81- ☑
- red blood cell (count) (morphology) (sickling) (volume) R71.8
- scan NEC R94.8
  - bladder R94.8
  - bone R94.8
  - kidney R94.4
  - liver R93.2
  - lung R94.2
  - pancreas R94.8
  - placental R94.8
  - spleen R94.8
  - thyroid R94.6
- sedimentation rate, elevated R70.0
- SGOT R74.0
- SGPT R74.0
- sodium (deficiency) E87.1
  - excess E87.0
- specified body fluid NEC R88.8
- stress test R94.39
- testis R93.81- ☑
- thyroid (function) (metabolic rate) (scan) (uptake) R94.6
- transaminase (level) R74.0
- triglycerides E78.9
  - high E78.1
    - with high cholesterol E78.2
- tuberculin skin test (without active tuberculosis) R76.11
- urine R82.90
  - acetone R82.4
  - bacteria R82.71
  - bile R82.2
  - casts or cells R82.998
  - chyle R82.0
  - culture positive R82.79
  - glucose R81
  - hemoglobin R82.3
  - ketone R82.4
  - sugar R81
- vanillylmandelic acid (VMA), elevated R82.5

Findings, abnormal, inconclusive, without diagno
— *continued*
- vectorcardiogram (VCG) R94.39
- ventriculogram R93.0
- white blood cell (count) (differential) (morphology) D72.9
- xerography R92.8

Finger — *see* condition

Fire, Saint Anthony's — *see* Erysipelas

Fire-setting
- pathological (compulsive) F63.1

Fish hook stomach K31.89

Fishmeal-worker's lung J67.8

Fissure, fissured
- anus, anal K60.2
  - acute K60.0
  - chronic K60.1
  - congenital Q43.8
- ear, lobule, congenital Q17.8
- epiglottis (congenital) Q31.8
- larynx J38.7
  - congenital Q31.8
- lip K13.0
  - congenital — *see* Cleft, lip
- nipple N64.0
  - associated with
    - lactation O92.13
    - pregnancy O92.11- ☑
    - puerperium O92.12
- nose Q30.2
- palate (congenital) — *see* Cleft, palate
- skin R23.4
- spine (congenital) — *see also* Spina bifida
  - with hydrocephalus — *see* Spina bifida, by site, v hydrocephalus
- tongue (acquired) K14.5
  - congenital Q38.3

Fistula (cutaneous) L98.8
- abdomen (wall) K63.2
  - bladder N32.2
  - intestine NEC K63.2
  - ureter N28.89
  - uterus N82.5
- abdominorectal K63.2
- abdominosigmoidal K63.2
- abdominothoracic J86.0
- abdominouterine N82.5
  - congenital Q51.7
- abdominovesical N32.2
- accessory sinuses — *see* Sinusitis
- actinomycotic — *see* Actinomycosis
- alveolar antrum — *see* Sinusitis, maxillary
- alveolar process K04.6
- anorectal K60.5
- antrobuccal — *see* Sinusitis, maxillary
- antrum — *see* Sinusitis, maxillary
- anus, anal (recurrent) (infectional) K60.3
  - congenital Q43.6
    - with absence, atresia and stenosis Q42.2
  - tuberculous A18.32
- aorta-duodenal I77.2
- appendix, appendicular K38.3
- arteriovenous (acquired) (nonruptured) I77.0
  - brain I67.1
    - congenital Q28.2
      - ruptured — *see* Fistula, arteriovenous, br ruptured
    - ruptured I60.8
      - intracerebral I61.8
      - intraparenchymal I61.8
      - intraventricular I61.5
      - subarachnoid I60.8
  - cerebral — *see* Fistula, arteriovenous, brain
  - congenital (peripheral) — *see also* Malformatic arteriovenous
    - brain Q28.2
      - ruptured — *see* Fistula, arteriovenous, br ruptured
    - coronary Q24.5
    - pulmonary Q25.72
  - coronary I25.41
    - congenital Q24.5
  - pulmonary I28.0
    - congenital Q25.72
  - surgically created (for dialysis) Z99.2
    - complication — *see* Complication, arteriove fistula, surgically created
    - traumatic — *see* Injury, blood vessel

☑ **Additional Character Required** — Refer to the Tabular List for Character Selection   ▽ **Subterms under main terms may continue to next column or pa**

stula — *continued*
 artery I77.2
 aural (mastoid) — *see* Mastoiditis, chronic
 auricle — *see also* Disorder, pinna, specified type NEC
    congenital Q18.1
 Bartholin's gland N82.8
 bile duct (common) (hepatic) K83.3
    with calculus, stones — *see* Calculus, bile duct
 biliary (tract) — *see* Fistula, bile duct
 bladder (sphincter) NEC — *see also* Fistula, vesico-
    N32.2
    into seminal vesicle N32.2
 bone — *see also* Disorder, bone, specified type NEC
    with osteomyelitis, chronic — *see* Osteomyelitis,
       chronic, with draining sinus
 brain G93.89
    arteriovenous (acquired) — *see also* Fistula, arteri-
       ovenous, brain I67.1
    congenital Q28.2
 branchial (cleft) Q18.0
 branchiogenous Q18.0
 breast N61.0
    puerperal, postpartum or gestational, due to mastitis
       (purulent) — *see* Mastitis, obstetric, purulent
 bronchial J86.0
 bronchocutaneous, bronchomediastinal, bronchopleu-
    ral, bronchopleuromediastinal (infective) J86.0
    tuberculous NEC A15.5
 bronchoesophageal J86.0
    congenital Q39.2
       with atresia of esophagus Q39.1
 bronchovisceral J86.0
 buccal cavity (infective) K12.2
 cecosigmoidal K63.2
 cecum K63.2
 cerebrospinal (fluid) G96.0
 cervical, lateral Q18.1
 cervicoaural Q18.1
 cervicosigmoidal N82.4
 cervicovesical N82.1
 cervix N82.8
 chest (wall) J86.0
 cholecystenteric — *see* Fistula, gallbladder
 cholecystocolic — *see* Fistula, gallbladder
 cholecystocolonic — *see* Fistula, gallbladder
 cholecystoduodenal — *see* Fistula, gallbladder
 cholecystogastric — *see* Fistula, gallbladder
 cholecystointestinal — *see* Fistula, gallbladder
 choledochoduodenal — *see* Fistula, bile duct
 cholocolic K82.3
 coccyx — *see* Sinus, pilonidal
 colon K63.2
 colostomy K94.09
 colovesical N32.1
 common duct — *see* Fistula, bile duct
 congenital, site not listed — *see* Anomaly, by site
 coronary, arteriovenous I25.41
    congenital Q24.5
 costal region J86.0
 cul-de-sac, Douglas' N82.8
 cystic duct — *see also* Fistula, gallbladder
    congenital Q44.5
 dental K04.6
 diaphragm J86.0
 duodenum K31.6
 ear (external) (canal) — *see* Disorder, ear, external,
    specified type NEC
 enterocolic K63.2
 enterocutaneous K63.2
 enterouterine N82.4
    congenital Q51.7
 enterovaginal N82.4
    congenital Q52.2
    large intestine N82.3
    small intestine N82.2
 enterovesical N32.1
 epididymis N50.89
    tuberculous A18.15
 esophagobronchial J86.0
    congenital Q39.2
       with atresia of esophagus Q39.1
 esophagocutaneous K22.8
 esophagopleural-cutaneous J86.0
 esophagotracheal J86.0
    congenital Q39.2
       with atresia of esophagus Q39.1
 esophagus K22.8
    congenital Q39.2

Fistula — *continued*
 esophagus — *continued*
    congenital — *continued*
       with atresia of esophagus Q39.1
 ethmoid — *see* Sinusitis, ethmoidal
 eyeball (cornea) (sclera) — *see* Disorder, globe, hy-
    potony
 eyelid H01.8
 fallopian tube, external N82.5
 fecal K63.2
    congenital Q43.6
 from periapical abscess K04.6
 frontal sinus — *see* Sinusitis, frontal
 gallbladder K82.3
    with calculus, cholelithiasis, stones — *see* Calculus,
       gallbladder
 gastric K31.6
 gastrocolic K31.6
    congenital Q40.2
    tuberculous A18.32
 gastroenterocolic K31.6
 gastroesophageal K31.6
 gastrojejunal K31.6
 gastrojejunocolic K31.6
 genital tract (female) N82.9
    specified NEC N82.8
    to intestine NEC N82.4
    to skin N82.5
 hepatic artery-portal vein, congenital Q26.6
 hepatopleural J86.0
 hepatopulmonary J86.0
 ileorectal or ileosigmoidal K63.2
 ileovaginal N82.2
 ileovesical N32.1
 ileum K63.2
 in ano K60.3
    tuberculous A18.32
 inner ear (labyrinth) — *see* subcategory H83.1 ☑
 intestine NEC K63.2
 intestinocolonic (abdominal) K63.2
 intestinoureteral N28.89
 intestinouterine N82.4
 intestinovaginal N82.4
    large intestine N82.3
    small intestine N82.2
 intestinovesical N32.1
 ischiorectal (fossa) K61.39
 jejunum K63.2
 joint M25.10
    ankle M25.17- ☑
    elbow M25.12- ☑
    foot joint M25.17- ☑
    hand joint M25.14- ☑
    hip M25.15- ☑
    knee M25.16- ☑
    shoulder M25.11- ☑
    specified joint NEC M25.18
    tuberculous — *see* Tuberculosis, joint
    vertebrae M25.18
    wrist M25.13- ☑
 kidney N28.89
 labium (majus) (minus) N82.8
 labyrinth — *see* subcategory H83.1 ☑
 lacrimal (gland) (sac) H04.61- ☑
 lacrimonasal duct — *see* Fistula, lacrimal
 laryngotracheal, congenital Q34.8
 larynx J38.7
 lip K13.0
    congenital Q38.0
 lumbar, tuberculous A18.01
 lung J86.0
 lymphatic I89.8
 mammary (gland) N61.0
 mastoid (process) (region) — *see* Mastoiditis, chronic
 maxillary J32.0
 medial, face and neck Q18.8
 mediastinal J86.0
 mediastinobronchial J86.0
 mediastinocutaneous J86.0
 middle ear — *see* subcategory H74.8 ☑
 mouth K12.2
 nasal J34.89
    sinus — *see* Sinusitis
 nasopharynx J39.2
 nipple N64.0
 nose J34.89
 oral (cutaneous) K12.2
    maxillary J32.0

Fistula — *continued*
 oral — *continued*
    nasal (with cleft palate) — *see* Cleft, palate
 orbit, orbital — *see* Disorder, orbit, specified type NEC
 oroantral J32.0
 oviduct, external N82.5
 palate (hard) M27.8
 pancreatic K86.89
 pancreaticoduodenal K86.89
 parotid (gland) K11.4
    region K12.2
 penis N48.89
 perianal K60.3
 pericardium (pleura) (sac) — *see* Pericarditis
 pericecal K63.2
 perineorectal K60.4
 perineosigmoidal K63.2
 perineum, perineal (with urethral involvement) NEC
    N36.0
    tuberculous A18.13
    ureter N28.89
 perirectal K60.4
    tuberculous A18.32
 peritoneum K65.9
 pharyngoesophageal J39.2
 pharynx J39.2
    branchial cleft (congenital) Q18.0
 pilonidal (infected) (rectum) — *see* Sinus, pilonidal
 pleura, pleural, pleurocutaneous, pleuroperitoneal
    J86.0
    tuberculous NEC A15.6
 pleuropericardial I31.8
 portal vein-hepatic artery, congenital Q26.6
 postauricular H70.81- ☑
 postoperative, persistent T81.83 ☑
    specified site — *see* Fistula, by site
 preauricular (congenital) Q18.1
 prostate N42.89
 pulmonary J86.0
    arteriovenous I28.0
       congenital Q25.72
    tuberculous — *see* Tuberculosis, pulmonary
 pulmonoperitoneal J86.0
 rectolabial N82.4
 rectosigmoid (intercommunicating) K63.2
 rectoureteral N28.89
 rectourethral N36.0
    congenital Q64.73
 rectouterine N82.4
    congenital Q51.7
 rectovaginal N82.3
    congenital Q52.2
    tuberculous A18.18
 rectovesical N32.1
    congenital Q64.79
 rectovesicovaginal N82.3
 rectovulval N82.4
    congenital Q52.79
 rectum (to skin) K60.4
    congenital Q43.6
       with absence, atresia and stenosis Q42.0
    tuberculous A18.32
 renal N28.89
 retroauricular — *see* Fistula, postauricular
 salivary duct or gland (any) K11.4
    congenital Q38.4
 scrotum (urinary) N50.89
    tuberculous A18.15
 semicircular canals — *see* subcategory H83.1 ☑
 sigmoid K63.2
    to bladder N32.1
 sinus — *see* Sinusitis
 skin L98.8
    to genital tract (female) N82.5
 splenocolic D73.89
 stercoral K63.2
 stomach K31.6
 sublingual gland K11.4
 submandibular gland K11.4
 submaxillary (gland) K11.4
    region K12.2
 thoracic J86.0
    duct I89.8
 thoracoabdominal J86.0
 thoracogastric J86.0
 thoracointestinal J86.0
 thorax J86.0
 thyroglossal duct Q89.2

▽ Subterms under main terms may continue to next column or page   ☑ **Additional Character Required** — Refer to the Tabular List for Character Selection   **145**

Fistula — Fistula

Fistula — *continued*
thyroid E07.89
trachea, congenital (external) (internal) Q32.1
tracheoesophageal J86.0
congenital Q39.2
with atresia of esophagus Q39.1
following tracheostomy J95.04
traumatic arteriovenous — *see* Injury, blood vessel, by site
tuberculous — *code by* site under Tuberculosis
typhoid A01.09
umbilicourinary Q64.8
urachus, congenital Q64.4
ureter (persistent) N28.89
ureteroabdominal N28.89
ureterorectal N28.89
ureterosigmoido-abdominal N28.89
ureterovaginal N82.1
ureterovesical N32.2
urethra N36.0
congenital Q64.79
tuberculous A18.13
urethroperineal N36.0
urethroperineovesical N32.2
urethrorectal N36.0
congenital Q64.73
urethroscrotal N50.89
urethrovaginal N82.1
urethrovesical N32.2
urinary (tract) (persistent) (recurrent) N36.0
uteroabdominal N82.5
congenital Q51.7
uteroenteric, uterointestinal N82.4
congenital Q51.7
uterorectal N82.4
congenital Q51.7
uteroureteric N82.1
uterourethral Q51.7
uterovaginal N82.8
uterovesical N82.1
congenital Q51.7
uterus N82.8
vagina (postpartal) (wall) N82.8
vaginocutaneous (postpartal) N82.5
vaginointestinal NEC N82.4
large intestine N82.3
small intestine N82.2
vaginoperineal N82.5
vasocutaneous, congenital Q55.7
vesical NEC N32.2
vesicoabdominal N32.2
vesicocervicovaginal N82.1
vesicocolic N32.1
vesicocutaneous N32.2
vesicoenteric N32.1
vesicointestinal N32.1
vesicometrorectal N82.4
vesicoperineal N32.2
vesicorectal N32.1
congenital Q64.79
vesicosigmoidal N32.1
vesicosigmoidovaginal N82.3
vesicoureteral N32.2
vesicoureterovaginal N82.1
vesicourethral N32.2
vesicourethrorectal N32.1
vesicouterine N82.1
congenital Q51.7
vesicovaginal N82.0
vulvorectal N82.4
congenital Q52.79

Fit R56.9
epileptic — *see* Epilepsy
fainting R55
hysterical F44.5
newborn P90
Fitting (and adjustment) (of)
artificial
arm — *see* Admission, adjustment, artificial, arm
breast Z44.3 ☑
eye Z44.2 ☑
leg — *see* Admission, adjustment, artificial, leg
automatic implantable cardiac defibrillator (with synchronous cardiac pacemaker) Z45.02
brain neuropacemaker Z46.2
implanted Z45.42
cardiac defibrillator — *see* Fitting (and adjustment) (of), automatic implantable cardiac defibrillator

Fitting — *continued*
catheter, non-vascular Z46.82
colostomy belt Z46.89
contact lenses Z46.0
CRT-D (resynchronization therapy defibrillator) Z45.02
CRT-P (cardiac resynchronization therapy pacemaker) Z45.018
pulse generator Z45.010
cystostomy device Z46.6
defibrillator, cardiac — *see* Fitting (and adjustment) (of), automatic implantable cardiac defibrillator
dentures Z46.3
device NOS Z46.9
abdominal Z46.89
gastrointestinal NEC Z46.59
implanted NEC Z45.89
nervous system Z46.2
implanted — *see* Admission, adjustment, device, implanted, nervous system
orthodontic Z46.4
orthoptic Z46.0
orthotic Z46.89
prosthetic (external) Z44.9
breast Z44.3 ☑
dental Z46.3
eye Z44.2 ☑
specified NEC Z44.8
specified NEC Z46.89
substitution
auditory Z46.2
implanted — *see* Admission, adjustment, device, implanted, hearing device
nervous system Z46.2
implanted — *see* Admission, adjustment, device, implanted, nervous system
visual Z46.2
implanted Z45.31
urinary Z46.6
gastric lap band Z46.51
gastrointestinal appliance NEC Z46.59
glasses (reading) Z46.0
hearing aid Z46.1
ileostomy device Z46.89
insulin pump Z46.81
intestinal appliance NEC Z46.89
myringotomy device (stent) (tube) Z45.82
neuropacemaker Z46.2
implanted Z45.42
non-vascular catheter Z46.82
orthodontic device Z46.4
orthopedic device (brace) (cast) (corset) (shoes) Z46.89
pacemaker (cardiac) (cardiac resynchronization therapy (CRT-P)) Z45.018
nervous system (brain) (peripheral nerve) (spinal cord) Z46.2
implanted Z45.42
pulse generator Z45.010
portacath (port-a-cath) Z45.2
prosthesis (external) Z44.9
arm — *see* Admission, adjustment, artificial, arm
breast Z44.3 ☑
dental Z46.3
eye Z44.2 ☑
leg — *see* Admission, adjustment, artificial, leg
specified NEC Z44.8
spectacles Z46.0
wheelchair Z46.89
Fitzhugh-Curtis syndrome
due to
Chlamydia trachomatis A74.81
Neisseria gonorrhorea (gonococcal peritonitis) A54.85
Fitz's syndrome (acute hemorrhagic pancreatitis) — *see also* Pancreatitis, acute K85.80
Fixation
joint — *see* Ankylosis
larynx J38.7
stapes — *see* Ankylosis, ear ossicles
deafness — *see* Deafness, conductive
uterus (acquired) — *see* Malposition, uterus
vocal cord J38.3
Flabby ridge K06.8
Flaccid — *see also* condition
palate, congenital Q38.5
Flail
chest S22.5 ☑
newborn (birth injury) P13.8
joint (paralytic) M25.20

Flail — *continued*
joint — *continued*
ankle M25.27- ☑
elbow M25.22- ☑
foot joint M25.27- ☑
hand joint M25.24- ☑
hip M25.25- ☑
knee M25.26- ☑
shoulder M25.21- ☑
specified joint NEC M25.28
wrist M25.23- ☑
Flajani's disease — *see* Hyperthyroidism, with, goite (diffuse)
Flap, liver K71.3
Flashbacks (residual to hallucinogen use) F16.283
Flat
chamber (eye) — *see* Disorder, globe, hypotony, fla anterior chamber
chest, congenital Q67.8
foot (acquired) (fixed type) (painful) (postural) — *se also* Deformity, limb, flat foot
congenital (rigid) (spastic (everted)) Q66.5- ☑
rachitic sequelae (late effect) E64.3
organ or site, congenital NEC — *see* Anomaly, by si
pelvis M95.5
with disproportion (fetopelvic) O33.0
causing obstructed labor O65.0
congenital Q74.2
Flatau-Schilder disease G37.0
Flatback syndrome M40.30
lumbar region M40.36
lumbosacral region M40.37
thoracolumbar region M40.35
Flattening
head, femur M89.8X5
hip — *see* Coxa, plana
lip (congenital) Q18.8
nose (congenital) Q67.4
acquired M95.0
Flatulence R14.3
psychogenic F45.8
Flatus R14.3
vaginalis N89.8
Flax-dresser's disease J66.1
Flea bite — *see* Injury, bite, by site, superficial, insect
Flecks, glaucomatous (subcapsular) — *see* Cataract, complicated
Fleischer (-Kayser) **ring** (cornea) H18.04- ☑
Fleshy mole O02.0
Flexibilitas cerea — *see* Catalepsy
Flexion
amputation stump (surgical) T87.89
cervix — *see* Malposition, uterus
contracture, joint — *see* Contraction, joint
deformity, joint — *see also* Deformity, limb, flexion M21.20
hip, congenital Q65.89
uterus — *see also* Malposition, uterus
lateral — *see* Lateroversion, uterus
Flexner-Boyd dysentery A03.2
Flexner's dysentery A03.1
Flexure — *see* Flexion
Flint murmur (aortic insufficiency) I35.1
Floater, vitreous — *see* Opacity, vitreous
Floating
cartilage (joint) — *see also* Loose, body, joint
knee — *see* Derangement, knee, loose body
gallbladder, congenital Q44.1
kidney N28.89
congenital Q63.8
spleen D73.89
Flooding N92.0
Floor — *see* condition
Floppy
baby syndrome (nonspecific) P94.2
iris syndrome (intraoperative) (IFIS) H21.81
nonrheumatic mitral valve syndrome I34.1
Flu — *see also* Influenza
avian — *see also* Influenza, due to, identified novel i fluenza A virus J09.X2
bird — *see also* Influenza, due to, identified novel ir fluenza A virus J09.X2
intestinal NEC A08.4
swine (viruses that normally cause infections in pigs — *see also* Influenza, due to, identified novel influenza A virus J09.X2
Fluctuating blood pressure I99.8

uid
abdomen R18.8
chest J94.8
heart — *see* Failure, heart, congestive
joint — *see* Effusion, joint
loss (acute) E86.9
lung — *see* Edema, lung
overload E87.70
　　specified NEC E87.79
peritoneal cavity R18.8
pleural cavity J94.8
retention R60.9

ukes NEC — *see also* Infestation, fluke
blood NEC — *see* Schistosomiasis
liver B66.3

uor (vaginalis) N89.8
trichomonal or due to Trichomonas (vaginalis) A59.00

uorosis
dental K00.3
skeletal M85.10
　　ankle M85.17- ☑
　　foot M85.17- ☑
　　forearm M85.13- ☑
　　hand M85.14- ☑
　　lower leg M85.16- ☑
　　multiple site M85.19
　　neck M85.18
　　rib M85.18
　　shoulder M85.11- ☑
　　skull M85.18
　　specified site NEC M85.18
　　thigh M85.15- ☑
　　toe M85.17- ☑
　　upper arm M85.12- ☑
　　vertebra M85.18

lush syndrome E34.0

lushing R23.2
menopausal N95.1

lutter
atrial or auricular I48.92
　　atypical I48.4
　　type I I48.3
　　type II I48.4
　　typical I48.3
heart I49.8
　　atrial or auricular I48.92
　　　　atypical I48.4
　　　　type I I48.3
　　　　type II I48.4
　　　　typical I48.3
　　ventricular I49.02
ventricular I49.02

NHTR (febrile nonhemolytic transfusion reaction) R50.84

ochier's abscess — *code by* site under Abscess

ocus, Assmann's — *see* Tuberculosis, pulmonary

ogo selvagem L10.3

oix-Alajouanine syndrome G95.19

old, folds (anomalous) — *see also* Anomaly, by site
Descemet's membrane — *see* Change, corneal membrane, Descemet's, fold
epicanthic Q10.3
heart Q24.8

olie à deux F24

ollicle
cervix (nabothian) (ruptured) N88.8
graafian, ruptured, with hemorrhage N83.0- ☑
nabothian N88.8

ollicular — *see* condition

olliculitis (superficial) L73.9
abscedens et suffodiens L66.3
cyst N83.0- ☑
decalvans L66.2
deep — *see* Furuncle, by site
gonococcal (acute) (chronic) A54.01
keloid, keloidalis L73.0
pustular L01.02
ulerythematosa reticulata L66.4

olliculome lipidique
specified site — *see* Neoplasm, benign, by site
unspecified site
　　female D27.9
　　male D29.20

ølling's disease E70.0

ollow-up — *see* Examination, follow-up

ong's syndrome (hereditary osteo-onychodysplasia) Q87.2

Food
allergy L27.2
asphyxia (from aspiration or inhalation) — *see* Foreign body, by site
choked on — *see* Foreign body, by site
deprivation T73.0 ☑
　　specified kind of food NEC E63.8
intoxication — *see* Poisoning, food
lack of T73.0 ☑
poisoning — *see* Poisoning, food
rejection NEC — *see* Disorder, eating
strangulation or suffocation — *see* Foreign body, by site
toxemia — *see* Poisoning, food

Foot — *see* condition

Foramen ovale (nonclosure) (patent) (persistent) Q21.1

Forbes' glycogen storage disease E74.03

Fordyce-Fox disease L75.2

Fordyce's disease (mouth) Q38.6

Forearm — *see* condition

Foreign body
with
　　laceration — *see* Laceration, by site, with foreign body
　　puncture wound — *see* Puncture, by site, with foreign body
accidentally left following a procedure T81.509 ☑
　　aspiration T81.506 ☑
　　　　resulting in
　　　　　　adhesions T81.516 ☑
　　　　　　obstruction T81.526 ☑
　　　　　　perforation T81.536 ☑
　　　　　　specified complication NEC T81.596 ☑
　　cardiac catheterization T81.505 ☑
　　　　resulting in
　　　　　　acute reaction T81.60 ☑
　　　　　　　　aseptic peritonitis T81.61 ☑
　　　　　　　　specified NEC T81.69 ☑
　　　　　　adhesions T81.515 ☑
　　　　　　obstruction T81.525 ☑
　　　　　　perforation T81.535 ☑
　　　　　　specified complication NEC T81.595 ☑
　　causing
　　　　acute reaction T81.60 ☑
　　　　　　aseptic peritonitis T81.61 ☑
　　　　　　specified complication NEC T81.69 ☑
　　　　adhesions T81.519 ☑
　　　　aseptic peritonitis T81.61 ☑
　　　　obstruction T81.529 ☑
　　　　perforation T81.539 ☑
　　　　specified complication NEC T81.599 ☑
　　endoscopy T81.504 ☑
　　　　resulting in
　　　　　　adhesions T81.514 ☑
　　　　　　obstruction T81.524 ☑
　　　　　　perforation T81.534 ☑
　　　　　　specified complication NEC T81.594 ☑
　　immunization T81.503 ☑
　　　　resulting in
　　　　　　adhesions T81.513 ☑
　　　　　　obstruction T81.523 ☑
　　　　　　perforation T81.533 ☑
　　　　　　specified complication NEC T81.593 ☑
　　infusion T81.501 ☑
　　　　resulting in
　　　　　　adhesions T81.511 ☑
　　　　　　obstruction T81.521 ☑
　　　　　　perforation T81.531 ☑
　　　　　　specified complication NEC T81.591 ☑
　　injection T81.503 ☑
　　　　resulting in
　　　　　　adhesions T81.513 ☑
　　　　　　obstruction T81.523 ☑
　　　　　　perforation T81.533 ☑
　　　　　　specified complication NEC T81.593 ☑
　　kidney dialysis T81.502 ☑
　　　　resulting in
　　　　　　adhesions T81.512 ☑
　　　　　　obstruction T81.522 ☑
　　　　　　perforation T81.532 ☑
　　　　　　specified complication NEC T81.592 ☑
　　packing removal T81.507 ☑
　　　　resulting in
　　　　　　acute reaction T81.60 ☑
　　　　　　　　aseptic peritonitis T81.61 ☑
　　　　　　　　specified NEC T81.69 ☑

Foreign body — *continued*
accidentally left following a procedure — *continued*
　　packing removal — *continued*
　　　　resulting in — *continued*
　　　　　　adhesions T81.517 ☑
　　　　　　obstruction T81.527 ☑
　　　　　　perforation T81.537 ☑
　　　　　　specified complication NEC T81.597 ☑
　　puncture T81.506 ☑
　　　　resulting in
　　　　　　adhesions T81.516 ☑
　　　　　　obstruction T81.526 ☑
　　　　　　perforation T81.536 ☑
　　　　　　specified complication NEC T81.596 ☑
　　specified procedure NEC T81.508 ☑
　　　　resulting in
　　　　　　acute reaction T81.60 ☑
　　　　　　　　aseptic peritonitis T81.61 ☑
　　　　　　　　specified NEC T81.69 ☑
　　　　　　adhesions T81.518 ☑
　　　　　　obstruction T81.528 ☑
　　　　　　perforation T81.538 ☑
　　　　　　specified complication NEC T81.598 ☑
　　surgical operation T81.500 ☑
　　　　resulting in
　　　　　　acute reaction T81.60 ☑
　　　　　　　　aseptic peritonitis T81.61 ☑
　　　　　　　　specified NEC T81.69 ☑
　　　　　　adhesions T81.510 ☑
　　　　　　obstruction T81.520 ☑
　　　　　　perforation T81.530 ☑
　　　　　　specified complication NEC T81.590 ☑
　　transfusion T81.501 ☑
　　　　resulting in
　　　　　　adhesions T81.511 ☑
　　　　　　obstruction T81.521 ☑
　　　　　　perforation T81.531 ☑
　　　　　　specified complication NEC T81.591 ☑
alimentary tract T18.9 ☑
　　anus T18.5 ☑
　　colon T18.4 ☑
　　esophagus — *see* Foreign body, esophagus
　　mouth T18.0 ☑
　　multiple sites T18.8 ☑
　　rectosigmoid (junction) T18.5 ☑
　　rectum T18.5 ☑
　　small intestine T18.3 ☑
　　specified site NEC T18.8 ☑
　　stomach T18.2 ☑
anterior chamber (eye) S05.5- ☑
auditory canal — *see* Foreign body, entering through orifice, ear
bronchus T17.508 ☑
　　causing
　　　　asphyxiation T17.500 ☑
　　　　　　food (bone) (seed) T17.520 ☑
　　　　　　gastric contents (vomitus) T17.510 ☑
　　　　　　specified type NEC T17.590 ☑
　　　　injury NEC T17.508 ☑
　　　　　　food (bone) (seed) T17.528 ☑
　　　　　　gastric contents (vomitus) T17.518 ☑
　　　　　　specified type NEC T17.598 ☑
canthus — *see* Foreign body, conjunctival sac
ciliary body (eye) S05.5- ☑
conjunctival sac T15.1- ☑
cornea T15.0- ☑
entering through orifice
　　accessory sinus T17.0 ☑
　　alimentary canal T18.9 ☑
　　　　multiple parts T18.8 ☑
　　　　specified part NEC T18.8 ☑
　　alveolar process T18.0 ☑
　　antrum (Highmore's) T17.0 ☑
　　anus T18.5 ☑
　　appendix T18.4 ☑
　　auditory canal — *see* Foreign body, entering through orifice, ear
　　auricle — *see* Foreign body, entering through orifice, ear
　　bladder T19.1 ☑
　　bronchioles — *see* Foreign body, respiratory tract, specified site NEC
　　bronchus (main) — *see* Foreign body, bronchus
　　buccal cavity T18.0 ☑
　　canthus (inner) — *see* Foreign body, conjunctival sac

Fluid — Foreign body

Foreign body — *continued*
  entering through orifice — *continued*
    cecum T18.4 ☑
    cervix (canal) (uteri) T19.3 ☑
    colon T18.4 ☑
    conjunctival sac — *see* Foreign body, conjunctival sac
    cornea — *see* Foreign body, cornea
    digestive organ or tract NOS T18.9 ☑
      multiple parts T18.8 ☑
      specified part NEC T18.8 ☑
    duodenum T18.3 ☑
    ear (external) T16.- ☑
    esophagus — *see* Foreign body, esophagus
    eye (external) NOS T15.9-
      conjunctival sac — *see* Foreign body, conjunctival sac
      cornea — *see* Foreign body, cornea
      specified part NEC T15.8-
    eyeball — *see also* Foreign body, entering through orifice, eye, specified part NEC
      with penetrating wound — *see* Puncture, eyeball
    eyelid — *see also* Foreign body, conjunctival sac
      with
        laceration — *see* Laceration, eyelid, with foreign body
        puncture — *see* Puncture, eyelid, with foreign body
        superficial injury — *see* Foreign body, superficial, eyelid
    gastrointestinal tract T18.9 ☑
      multiple parts T18.8 ☑
      specified part NEC T18.8 ☑
    genitourinary tract T19.9 ☑
      multiple parts T19.8 ☑
      specified part NEC T19.8 ☑
    globe — *see* Foreign body, entering through orifice, eyeball
    gum T18.0 ☑
    Highmore's antrum T17.0 ☑
    hypopharynx — *see* Foreign body, pharynx
    ileum T18.3 ☑
    intestine (small) T18.3 ☑
      large T18.4 ☑
    lacrimal apparatus (punctum) — *see* Foreign body, entering through orifice, eye, specified part NEC
    large intestine T18.4 ☑
    larynx — *see* Foreign body, larynx
    lung — *see* Foreign body, respiratory tract, specified site NEC
    maxillary sinus T17.0 ☑
    mouth T18.0 ☑
    nasal sinus T17.0 ☑
    nasopharynx — *see* Foreign body, pharynx
    nose (passage) T17.1 ☑
    nostril T17.1 ☑
    oral cavity T18.0 ☑
    palate T18.0 ☑
    penis T19.4 ☑
    pharynx — *see* Foreign body, pharynx
    piriform sinus — *see* Foreign body, pharynx
    rectosigmoid (junction) T18.5 ☑
    rectum T18.5 ☑
    respiratory tract — *see* Foreign body, respiratory tract
    sinus (accessory) (frontal) (maxillary) (nasal) T17.0 ☑
      piriform — *see* Foreign body, pharynx
    small intestine T18.3 ☑
    stomach T18.2 ☑
    suffocation by — *see* Foreign body, by site
    tear ducts or glands — *see* Foreign body, entering through orifice, eye, specified part NEC
    throat — *see* Foreign body, pharynx
    tongue T18.0 ☑
    tonsil, tonsillar (fossa) — *see* Foreign body, pharynx
    trachea — *see* Foreign body, trachea
    ureter T19.8 ☑
    urethra T19.0 ☑
    uterus (any part) T19.3 ☑
    vagina T19.2 ☑
    vulva T19.2 ☑
  esophagus T18.108 ☑
    causing
      injury NEC T18.108 ☑
        food (bone) (seed) T18.128 ☑

Foreign body — *continued*
  esophagus — *continued*
    causing — *continued*
      injury — *continued*
        gastric contents (vomitus) T18.118 ☑
        specified type NEC T18.198 ☑
        tracheal compression T18.100 ☑
        food (bone) (seed) T18.120 ☑
        gastric contents (vomitus) T18.110 ☑
        specified type NEC T18.190 ☑
  feeling of, in throat R09.89
  fragment — *see* Retained, foreign body fragments (type of)
  genitourinary tract T19.9 ☑
    bladder T19.1 ☑
    multiple parts T19.8 ☑
    penis T19.4 ☑
    specified site NEC T19.8 ☑
    urethra T19.0 ☑
    uterus T19.3 ☑
      IUD Z97.5
    vagina T19.2 ☑
      contraceptive device Z97.5
    vulva T19.2 ☑
  granuloma (old) (soft tissue) — *see also* Granuloma, foreign body
    skin L92.3
  in
    laceration — *see* Laceration, by site, with foreign body
    puncture wound — *see* Puncture, by site, with foreign body
    soft tissue (residual) M79.5
  inadvertently left in operation wound — *see* Foreign body, accidentally left during a procedure
  ingestion, ingested NOS T18.9 ☑
  inhalation or inspiration — *see* Foreign body, by site
  internal organ, not entering through a natural orifice — code as specific injury with foreign body
  intraocular S05.5- ☑
    old, retained (nonmagnetic) H44.70- ☑
      anterior chamber H44.71- ☑
      ciliary body H44.72- ☑
      iris H44.72- ☑
      lens H44.73- ☑
      magnetic H44.60- ☑
        anterior chamber H44.61- ☑
        ciliary body H44.62- ☑
        iris H44.62- ☑
        lens H44.63- ☑
        posterior wall H44.64- ☑
        specified site NEC H44.69- ☑
        vitreous body H44.65- ☑
      posterior wall H44.74- ☑
      specified site NEC H44.79- ☑
      vitreous body H44.75- ☑
    iris — *see* Foreign body, intraocular
  lacrimal punctum — *see* Foreign body, entering through orifice, eye, specified part NEC
  larynx T17.308 ☑
    causing
      asphyxiation T17.300 ☑
        food (bone) (seed) T17.320 ☑
        gastric contents (vomitus) T17.310 ☑
        specified type NEC T17.390 ☑
      injury NEC T17.308 ☑
        food (bone) (seed) T17.328 ☑
        gastric contents (vomitus) T17.318 ☑
        specified type NEC T17.398 ☑
  lens — *see* Foreign body, intraocular
  ocular muscle S05.4- ☑
    old, retained — *see* Foreign body, orbit, old
  old or residual
    soft tissue (residual) M79.5
  operation wound, left accidentally — *see* Foreign body, accidentally left during a procedure
  orbit S05.4- ☑
    old, retained H05.5- ☑
  pharynx T17.208 ☑
    causing
      asphyxiation T17.200 ☑
        food (bone) (seed) T17.220 ☑
        gastric contents (vomitus) T17.210 ☑
        specified type NEC T17.290 ☑
      injury NEC T17.208 ☑
        food (bone) (seed) T17.228 ☑

Foreign body — *continued*
  pharynx — *continued*
    causing — *continued*
      injury — *continued*
        gastric contents (vomitus) T17.218 ☑
        specified type NEC T17.298 ☑
  respiratory tract T17.908 ☑
    bronchioles — *see* Foreign body, respiratory tract, specified site NEC
    bronchus — *see* Foreign body, bronchus
    causing
      asphyxiation T17.900 ☑
        food (bone) (seed) T17.920 ☑
        gastric contents (vomitus) T17.910 ☑
        specified type NEC T17.990 ☑
      injury NEC T17.908 ☑
        food (bone) (seed) T17.928 ☑
        gastric contents (vomitus) T17.918 ☑
        specified type NEC T17.998 ☑
    larynx — *see* Foreign body, larynx
    lung — *see* Foreign body, respiratory tract, specified site NEC
    multiple parts — *see* Foreign body, respiratory tract, specified site NEC
    nasal sinus T17.0 ☑
    nasopharynx — *see* Foreign body, pharynx
    nose T17.1 ☑
    nostril T17.1 ☑
    pharynx — *see* Foreign body, pharynx
    specified site NEC T17.808 ☑
      causing
        asphyxiation T17.800 ☑
          food (bone) (seed) T17.820 ☑
          gastric contents (vomitus) T17.810 ☑
          specified type NEC T17.890 ☑
        injury NEC T17.808 ☑
          food (bone) (seed) T17.828 ☑
          gastric contents (vomitus) T17.818 ☑
          specified type NEC T17.898 ☑
    throat — *see* Foreign body, pharynx
    trachea — *see* Foreign body, trachea
  retained (old) (nonmagnetic) (in)
    anterior chamber (eye) — *see* Foreign body, intraocular, old, retained, anterior chamber
      magnetic — *see* Foreign body, intraocular, old, retained, magnetic, anterior chamber
    ciliary body — *see* Foreign body, intraocular, old, retained, ciliary body
      magnetic — *see* Foreign body, intraocular, old, retained, magnetic, ciliary body
    eyelid H02.819
      left H02.816
        lower H02.815
        upper H02.814
      right H02.813
        lower H02.812
        upper H02.811
    fragments — *see* Retained, foreign body fragment (type of)
    globe — *see* Foreign body, intraocular, old, retained
      magnetic — *see* Foreign body, intraocular, old, retained, magnetic
    intraocular — *see* Foreign body, intraocular, old, retained
      magnetic — *see* Foreign body, intraocular, old, retained, magnetic
    iris — *see* Foreign body, intraocular, old, retained, iris
      magnetic — *see* Foreign body, intraocular, old, retained, magnetic, iris
    lens — *see* Foreign body, intraocular, old, retained, lens
      magnetic — *see* Foreign body, intraocular, old, retained, magnetic, lens
    muscle — *see* Foreign body, retained, soft tissue
    orbit — *see* Foreign body, orbit, old
    posterior wall of globe — *see* Foreign body, intraocular, old, retained, posterior wall
      magnetic — *see* Foreign body, intraocular, old, retained, magnetic, posterior wall
    retrobulbar — *see* Foreign body, orbit, old, retrobulbar
    soft tissue M79.5
    vitreous — *see* Foreign body, intraocular, old, retained, vitreous body
      magnetic — *see* Foreign body, intraocular, old, retained, magnetic, vitreous body

☑ **Additional Character Required** — **Refer to the Tabular List for Character Selection**   ▽ **Subterms under main terms may continue to next column or page**

reign body — *continued*
retina S05.5- ☑
superficial, without open wound
  abdomen, abdominal (wall) S30.851 ☑
  alveolar process S00.552 ☑
  ankle S90.55- ☑
  antecubital space — *see* Foreign body, superficial, forearm
  anus S30.857 ☑
  arm (upper) S40.85- ☑
  auditory canal — *see* Foreign body, superficial, ear
  auricle — *see* Foreign body, superficial, ear
  axilla — *see* Foreign body, superficial, arm
  back, lower S30.850 ☑
  breast S20.15- ☑
  brow S00.85 ☑
  buttock S30.850 ☑
  calf — *see* Foreign body, superficial, leg
  canthus — *see* Foreign body, superficial, eyelid
  cheek S00.85 ☑
    internal S00.552 ☑
  chest wall — *see* Foreign body, superficial, thorax
  chin S00.85 ☑
  clitoris S30.854 ☑
  costal region — *see* Foreign body, superficial, thorax
  digit(s)
    foot — *see* Foreign body, superficial, toe
    hand — *see* Foreign body, superficial, finger
  ear S00.45- ☑
  elbow S50.35- ☑
  epididymis S30.853 ☑
  epigastric region S30.851 ☑
  epiglottis S10.15 ☑
  esophagus, cervical S10.15 ☑
  eyebrow — *see* Foreign body, superficial, eyelid
  eyelid S00.25- ☑
  face S00.85 ☑
  finger(s) S60.459 ☑
    index S60.45- ☑
    little S60.45- ☑
    middle S60.45- ☑
    ring S60.45- ☑
  flank S30.851 ☑
  foot (except toe(s) alone) S90.85- ☑
    toe — *see* Foreign body, superficial, toe
  forearm S50.85- ☑
    elbow only — *see* Foreign body, superficial, elbow
  forehead S00.85 ☑
  genital organs, external
    female S30.856 ☑
    male S30.855 ☑
  groin S30.851 ☑
  gum S00.552 ☑
  hand S60.55- ☑
  head S00.95 ☑
    ear — *see* Foreign body, superficial, ear
    eyelid — *see* Foreign body, superficial, eyelid
    lip S00.551 ☑
    nose S00.35 ☑
    oral cavity S00.552 ☑
    scalp S00.05 ☑
    specified site NEC S00.85 ☑
  heel — *see* Foreign body, superficial, foot
  hip S70.25- ☑
  inguinal region S30.851 ☑
  interscapular region S20.459 ☑
  jaw S00.85 ☑
  knee S80.25- ☑
  labium (majus) (minus) S30.854 ☑
  larynx S10.15 ☑
  leg (lower) S80.85- ☑
    knee — *see* Foreign body, superficial, knee
    upper — *see* Foreign body, superficial, thigh
  lip S00.551 ☑
  lower back S30.850 ☑
  lumbar region S30.850 ☑
  malar region S00.85 ☑
  mammary — *see* Foreign body, superficial, breast
  mastoid region S00.85 ☑
  mouth S00.552 ☑
  nail
    finger — *see* Foreign body, superficial, finger
    toe — *see* Foreign body, superficial, toe
  nape S10.85 ☑
  nasal S00.35 ☑

Foreign body — *continued*
  superficial, without open wound — *continued*
  neck S10.95
    specified site NEC S10.85 ☑
    throat S10.15 ☑
  nose S00.35 ☑
  occipital region S00.05 ☑
  oral cavity S00.552 ☑
  orbital region — *see* Foreign body, superficial, eyelid
  palate S00.552 ☑
  palm — *see* Foreign body, superficial, hand
  parietal region S00.05 ☑
  pelvis S30.850 ☑
  penis S30.852 ☑
  perineum
    female S30.854 ☑
    male S30.850 ☑
  periocular area — *see* Foreign body, superficial, eyelid
  phalanges
    finger — *see* Foreign body, superficial, finger
    toe — *see* Foreign body, superficial, toe
  pharynx S10.15 ☑
  pinna — *see* Foreign body, superficial, ear
  popliteal space — *see* Foreign body, superficial, knee
  prepuce S30.852 ☑
  pubic region S30.850 ☑
  pudendum
    female S30.856 ☑
    male S30.855 ☑
  sacral region S30.850 ☑
  scalp S00.05 ☑
  scapular region — *see* Foreign body, superficial, shoulder
  scrotum S30.853 ☑
  shin — *see* Foreign body, superficial, leg
  shoulder S40.25- ☑
  sternal region S20.359 ☑
  submaxillary region S00.85 ☑
  submental region S00.85 ☑
  subungual
    finger(s) — *see* Foreign body, superficial, finger
    toe(s) — *see* Foreign body, superficial, toe
  supraclavicular fossa S10.85 ☑
  supraorbital S00.85 ☑
  temple S00.85 ☑
  temporal region S00.85 ☑
  testis S30.853 ☑
  thigh S70.35- ☑
  thorax, thoracic (wall) S20.95 ☑
    back S20.45- ☑
    front S20.35- ☑
  throat S10.15 ☑
  thumb S60.35- ☑
  toe(s) (lesser) S90.456 ☑
    great S90.45- ☑
  tongue S00.552 ☑
  trachea S10.15 ☑
  tunica vaginalis S30.853 ☑
  tympanum, tympanic membrane — *see* Foreign body, superficial, ear
  uvula S00.552 ☑
  vagina S30.854 ☑
  vocal cords S10.15 ☑
  vulva S30.854 ☑
  wrist S60.85- ☑
swallowed T18.9 ☑
trachea T17.408 ☑
  causing
    asphyxiation T17.400 ☑
      food (bone) (seed) T17.420 ☑
      gastric contents (vomitus) T17.410 ☑
      specified type NEC T17.490 ☑
    injury NEC T17.408 ☑
      food (bone) (seed) T17.428 ☑
      gastric contents (vomitus) T17.418 ☑
      specified type NEC T17.498 ☑
type of fragment — *see* Retained, foreign body fragments (type of)
vitreous (humor) S05.5- ☑
Forestier's disease (rhizomelic pseudopolyarthritis) M35.3
  meaning ankylosing hyperostosis — *see* Hyperostosis, ankylosing

Formation
  hyalin in cornea — *see* Degeneration, cornea
  sequestrum in bone (due to infection) — *see* Osteomyelitis, chronic
  valve
    colon, congenital Q43.8
    ureter (congenital) Q62.39
Formication R20.2
Fort Bragg fever A27.89
Fossa — *see also* condition
  pyriform — *see* condition
Foster-Kennedy syndrome H47.14- ☑
Fothergill's
  disease (trigeminal neuralgia) — *see also* Neuralgia, trigeminal
  scarlatina anginosa A38.9
Foul breath R19.6
Foundling Z76.1
Fournier disease or gangrene N49.3
  female N76.89
Fourth
  cranial nerve — *see* condition
  molar K00.1
Foville's (peduncular) **disease or syndrome** G46.3
Fox (-Fordyce) disease (apocrine miliaria) L75.2
FPIES (food protein-induced enterocolitis syndrome) K52.21
Fracture, burst — *see* Fracture, traumatic, by site
Fracture, chronic — *see* Fracture, pathological, by site
Fracture, insufficiency — *see* Fracture, pathological, by site
Fracture, nontraumatic, NEC
  atypical
    femur M84.750- ☑
      complete
        oblique M84.759 ☑
          left side M84.758 ☑
          right side M84.757 ☑
        transverse M84.756 ☑
          left side M84.755 ☑
          right side M84.754 ☑
      incomplete M84.753 ☑
        left side M84.752 ☑
        right side M84.751 ☑
Fracture, pathological (pathologic) *see also* Fracture, traumatic M84.40 ☑
  ankle M84.47- ☑
  carpus M84.44- ☑
  clavicle M84.41- ☑
  compression (not due to trauma) — *see also* Collapse, vertebra M48.50- ☑
  dental implant M27.63
  dental restorative material K08.539
    with loss of material K08.531
    without loss of material K08.530
  due to
    neoplastic disease NEC — *see also* Neoplasm M84.50 ☑
      ankle M84.57- ☑
      carpus M84.54- ☑
      clavicle M84.51- ☑
      femur M84.55- ☑
      fibula M84.56- ☑
      finger M84.54- ☑
      hip M84.559 ☑
      humerus M84.52- ☑
      ilium M84.550 ☑
      ischium M84.550 ☑
      metacarpus M84.54- ☑
      metatarsus M84.57- ☑
      neck M84.58 ☑
      pelvis M84.550 ☑
      radius M84.53- ☑
      rib M84.58 ☑
      scapula M84.51- ☑
      skull M84.58 ☑
      specified site NEC M84.58 ☑
      tarsus M84.57- ☑
      tibia M84.56- ☑
      toe M84.57- ☑
      ulna M84.53- ☑
      vertebra M84.58 ☑
    osteoporosis M80.00 ☑
      disuse — *see* Osteoporosis, specified type NEC, with pathological fracture

Fracture, pathological — *continued*
due to — *continued*
osteoporosis — *continued*
drug-induced — *see* Osteoporosis, drug induced, with pathological fracture
idiopathic — *see* Osteoporosis, specified type NEC, with pathological fracture
postmenopausal — *see* Osteoporosis, post-menopausal, with pathological fracture
postoophorectomy — *see* Osteoporosis, pos-toophorectomy, with pathological fracture
postsurgical malabsorption — *see* Osteoporosis, specified type NEC, with pathological fracture
specified cause NEC — *see* Osteoporosis, speci-fied type NEC, with pathological fracture
specified disease NEC M84.60 ☑
ankle M84.67- ☑
carpus M84.64- ☑
clavicle M84.61- ☑
femur M84.65- ☑
fibula M84.66- ☑
finger M84.64- ☑
hip M84.65- ☑
humerus M84.62- ☑
ilium M84.650 ☑
ischium M84.650 ☑
metacarpus M84.64- ☑
metatarsus M84.67- ☑
neck M84.68 ☑
radius M84.63- ☑
rib M84.68 ☑
scapula M84.61- ☑
skull M84.68 ☑
tarsus M84.67- ☑
tibia M84.66- ☑
toe M84.67- ☑
ulna M84.63- ☑
vertebra M84.68 ☑
femur M84.45- ☑
fibula M84.46- ☑
finger M84.44- ☑
hip M84.459 ☑
humerus M84.42- ☑
ilium M84.454 ☑
ischium M84.454 ☑
joint prosthesis — *see* Complications, joint prosthesis, mechanical, breakdown, by site
periprosthetic — *see* Fracture, pathological, periprosthetic
metacarpus M84.44- ☑
metatarsus M84.47- ☑
neck M84.48 ☑
pelvis M84.454 ☑
periprosthetic M97.9 ☑
ankle M97.2- ☑
elbow M97.4- ☑
finger M97.8 ☑
hip M97.0- ☑
knee M97.1- ☑
other specified joint M97.8 ☑
shoulder M97.3- ☑
spinal joint M97.8 ☑
toe joint M97.8 ☑
wrist joint M97.8 ☑
radius M84.43- ☑
restorative material (dental) K08.539
with loss of material K08.531
without loss of material K08.530
rib M84.48 ☑
scapula M84.41- ☑
skull M84.48 ☑
tarsus M84.47- ☑
tibia M84.46- ☑
toe M84.47- ☑
ulna M84.43- ☑
vertebra M84.48 ☑

Fracture, traumatic (abduction) (adduction) (separation) — *see also* Fracture, pathological T14.8 ☑
acetabulum S32.40- ☑
column
anterior (displaced) (iliopubic) S32.43- ☑
nondisplaced S32.436
posterior (displaced) (ilioischial) S32.443 ☑
nondisplaced S32.44- ☑
dome (displaced) S32.48- ☑

Fracture, traumatic — *continued*
acetabulum — *continued*
dome — *continued*
nondisplaced S32.48 ☑
specified NEC S32.49- ☑
transverse (displaced) S32.45- ☑
with associated posterior wall fracture (displaced) S32.46- ☑
nondisplaced S32.46- ☑
nondisplaced S32.45- ☑
wall
anterior (displaced) S32.41- ☑
nondisplaced S32.41- ☑
medial (displaced) S32.47- ☑
nondisplaced S32.47- ☑
posterior (displaced) S32.42- ☑
with associated transverse fracture (displaced) S32.46- ☑
nondisplaced S32.46- ☑
nondisplaced S32.42- ☑
acromion — *see* Fracture, scapula, acromial process
ankle S82.899 ☑
bimalleolar (displaced) S82.84- ☑
nondisplaced S82.84- ☑
lateral malleolus only (displaced) S82.6- ☑
nondisplaced S82.6- ☑
medial malleolus (displaced) S82.5- ☑
associated with Maisonneuve's fracture — *see* Fracture, Maisonneuve's
nondisplaced S82.5- ☑
talus — *see* Fracture, tarsal, talus
trimalleolar (displaced) S82.85- ☑
nondisplaced S82.85- ☑
arm (upper) — *see also* Fracture, humerus, shaft
humerus — *see* Fracture, humerus
radius — *see* Fracture, radius
ulna — *see* Fracture, ulna
astragalus — *see* Fracture, tarsal, talus
atlas — *see* Fracture, neck, cervical vertebra, first
axis — *see* Fracture, neck, cervical vertebra, second
back — *see* Fracture, vertebra
Barton's — *see* Barton's fracture
base of skull — *see* Fracture, skull, base
basicervical (basal) (femoral) S72.0 ☑
Bennett's — *see* Bennett's fracture
bimalleolar — *see* Fracture, ankle, bimalleolar
blow-out S02.3- ☑
bone NEC T14.8 ☑
birth injury P13.9
following insertion of orthopedic implant, joint prosthesis or bone plate — *see* Fracture, fol-lowing insertion of orthopedic implant, joint prosthesis or bone plate
in (due to) neoplastic disease NEC — *see* Fracture, pathological, due to, neoplastic disease
pathological (cause unknown) — *see* Fracture, pathological
breast bone — *see* Fracture, sternum
bucket handle (semilunar cartilage) — *see* Tear, meniscus
burst — *see* Fracture, traumatic, by site
calcaneus — *see* Fracture, tarsal, calcaneus
carpal bone(s) S62.10- ☑
capitate (displaced) S62.13- ☑
nondisplaced S62.13- ☑
cuneiform — *see* Fracture, carpal bone, triquetrum
hamate (body) (displaced) S62.143 ☑
hook process (displaced) S62.15- ☑
nondisplaced S62.15- ☑
nondisplaced S62.14- ☑
larger multangular — *see* Fracture, carpal bones, trapezium
lunate (displaced) S62.12- ☑
nondisplaced S62.12- ☑
navicular S62.00- ☑
distal pole (displaced) S62.01- ☑
nondisplaced S62.01- ☑
middle third (displaced) S62.02- ☑
nondisplaced S62.02- ☑
proximal third (displaced) S62.03- ☑
nondisplaced S62.03- ☑
volar tuberosity — *see* Fracture, carpal bones, navicular, distal pole
os magnum — *see* Fracture, carpal bones, capitate
pisiform (displaced) S62.16- ☑
nondisplaced S62.16- ☑

Fracture, traumatic — *continued*
carpal bone(s) — *continued*
semilunar — *see* Fracture, carpal bones, lunate
smaller multangular — *see* Fracture, carpal bone, trapezoid
trapezium (displaced) S62.17- ☑
nondisplaced S62.17- ☑
trapezoid (displaced) S62.18- ☑
nondisplaced S62.18- ☑
triquetrum (displaced) S62.11- ☑
nondisplaced S62.11- ☑
unciform — *see* Fracture, carpal bones, hamate
cervical — *see* Fracture, vertebra, cervical
clavicle S42.00- ☑
acromial end (displaced) S42.03- ☑
nondisplaced S42.03- ☑
birth injury P13.4
lateral end — *see* Fracture, clavicle, acromial end
shaft (displaced) S42.02- ☑
nondisplaced S42.02- ☑
sternal end (anterior) (displaced) S42.01- ☑
nondisplaced S42.01- ☑
posterior S42.01- ☑
coccyx S32.2 ☑
collapsed — *see* Collapse, vertebra
collar bone — *see* Fracture, clavicle
Colles' — *see* Colles' fracture
coronoid process — *see* Fracture, ulna, upper end, coronoid process
corpus cavernosum penis S39.840 ☑
costochondral cartilage S23.41
costochondral, costosternal junction — *see* Fracture, rib
cranium — *see* Fracture, skull
cricoid cartilage S12.8 ☑
cuboid (ankle) — *see* Fracture, tarsal, cuboid
cuneiform
foot — *see* Fracture, tarsal, cuneiform
wrist — *see* Fracture, carpal, triquetrum
delayed union — *see* Delay, union, fracture
dental restorative material K08.539
with loss of material K08.531
without loss of material K08.530
due to
birth injury — *see* Birth, injury, fracture
osteoporosis — *see* Osteoporosis, with fracture
Dupuytren's — *see* Fracture, ankle, lateral malleolus
elbow S42.40- ☑
ethmoid (bone) (sinus) — *see* Fracture, skull, base
face bone S02.92 ☑
fatigue — *see also* Fracture, stress
vertebra M48.40 ☑
cervical region M48.42 ☑
cervicothoracic region M48.43 ☑
lumbar region M48.46 ☑
lumbosacral region M48.47 ☑
occipito-atlanto-axial region M48.41 ☑
sacrococcygeal region M48.48 ☑
thoracic region M48.44 ☑
thoracolumbar region M48.45 ☑
femur, femoral S72.9- ☑
basicervical (basal) S72.0 ☑
birth injury P13.2
capital epiphyseal S79.01- ☑
condyles, epicondyles — *see* Fracture, femur, lower end
distal end — *see* Fracture, femur, lower end
epiphysis
head — *see* Fracture, femur, upper end, epiphysis
lower — *see* Fracture, femur, lower end, epiphysis
upper — *see* Fracture, femur, upper end, epiphysis
following insertion of implant, prosthesis or plate M96.66- ☑
head — *see* Fracture, femur, upper end, head
intertrochanteric — *see* Fracture, femur, trochanteric
intratrochanteric — *see* Fracture, femur, trochanteric
lower end S72.40- ☑
condyle (displaced) S72.41- ☑
lateral (displaced) S72.42- ☑
nondisplaced S72.42- ☑
medial (displaced) S72.43- ☑
nondisplaced S72.43- ☑

☑ **Additional Character Required** — **Refer to the Tabular List for Character Selection**   ▽ **Subterms under main terms may continue to next column or page**

Fracture, traumatic — *continued*
femur, femoral — *continued*
  lower end — *continued*
    condyle — *continued*
      nondisplaced S72.41- ☑
    epiphysis (displaced) S72.44- ☑
      nondisplaced S72.44- ☑
    physeal S79.10- ☑
      Salter-Harris
        Type I S79.11- ☑
        Type II S79.12- ☑
        Type III S79.13- ☑
        Type IV S79.14- ☑
      specified NEC S79.19- ☑
    specified NEC S72.49- ☑
    supracondylar (displaced) S72.45- ☑
      with intracondylar extension (displaced)
        S72.46- ☑
        nondisplaced S72.46- ☑
      nondisplaced S72.45- ☑
    torus S72.47- ☑
  neck — *see* Fracture, femur, upper end, neck
  pertrochanteric — *see* Fracture, femur, trochanteric
  shaft (lower third) (middle third) (upper third)
    S72.30- ☑
    comminuted (displaced) S72.35- ☑
      nondisplaced S72.35- ☑
    oblique (displaced) S72.33- ☑
      nondisplaced S72.33- ☑
    segmental (displaced) S72.36- ☑
      nondisplaced S72.36- ☑
    specified NEC S72.39- ☑
    spiral (displaced) S72.34- ☑
      nondisplaced S72.34- ☑
    transverse (displaced) S72.32- ☑
      nondisplaced S72.32- ☑
  specified site NEC — *see* subcategory S72.8 ☑
  subcapital (displaced) S72.01- ☑
  subtrochanteric (region) (section) (displaced)
    S72.2- ☑
    nondisplaced S72.2- ☑
  transcervical — *see* Fracture, femur, midcervical
  transtrochanteric — *see* Fracture, femur,
    trochanteric
  trochanteric S72.10- ☑
    apophyseal (displaced) S72.13- ☑
      nondisplaced S72.13- ☑
    greater trochanter (displaced) S72.11- ☑
      nondisplaced S72.11- ☑
    intertrochanteric (displaced) S72.14- ☑
      nondisplaced S72.14- ☑
    lesser trochanter (displaced) S72.12- ☑
      nondisplaced S72.12- ☑
  upper end S72.00- ☑
    apophyseal (displaced) S72.13- ☑
      nondisplaced S72.13- ☑
    cervicotrochanteric — *see* Fracture, femur, upper
      end, neck, base
    epiphysis (displaced) S72.02- ☑
      nondisplaced S72.02- ☑
    head S72.05- ☑
      articular (displaced) S72.06- ☑
        nondisplaced S72.06- ☑
      specified NEC S72.09- ☑
    intertrochanteric (displaced) S72.14- ☑
      nondisplaced S72.14- ☑
    intracapsular S72.01- ☑
    midcervical (displaced) S72.03- ☑
      nondisplaced S72.03- ☑
    neck S72.00- ☑
      base (displaced) S72.04- ☑
        nondisplaced S72.04- ☑
      specified NEC S72.09- ☑
    pertrochanteric — *see* Fracture, femur, upper
      end, trochanteric
    physeal S79.00- ☑
      Salter-Harris type I S79.01- ☑
      specified NEC S79.09- ☑
    subcapital (displaced) S72.01- ☑
    subtrochanteric (displaced) S72.2- ☑
      nondisplaced S72.2- ☑
    transcervical — *see* Fracture, femur, upper end,
      midcervical
    trochanteric S72.10- ☑
      greater (displaced) S72.11- ☑
        nondisplaced S72.11- ☑

Fracture, traumatic — *continued*
femur, femoral — *continued*
  upper end — *continued*
    trochanteric — *continued*
      lesser (displaced) S72.12- ☑
        nondisplaced S72.12- ☑
fibula (shaft) (styloid) S82.40- ☑
  comminuted (displaced) S82.45- ☑
    nondisplaced S82.45- ☑
  following insertion of implant, prosthesis or plate
    M96.67- ☑
  involving ankle or malleolus — *see* Fracture, fibula,
    lateral malleolus
  lateral malleolus (displaced) S82.6- ☑
    nondisplaced S82.6- ☑
  lower end
    physeal S89.30- ☑
      Salter-Harris
        Type I S89.31- ☑
        Type II S89.32- ☑
      specified NEC S89.39- ☑
    specified NEC S82.83- ☑
    torus S82.82- ☑
  oblique (displaced) S82.43- ☑
    nondisplaced S82.43- ☑
  segmental (displaced) S82.46- ☑
    nondisplaced S82.46- ☑
  specified NEC S82.49- ☑
  spiral (displaced) S82.44- ☑
    nondisplaced S82.44- ☑
  transverse (displaced) S82.42- ☑
    nondisplaced S82.42- ☑
  upper end
    physeal S89.20- ☑
      Salter-Harris
        Type I S89.21- ☑
        Type II S89.22- ☑
      specified NEC S89.29- ☑
    specified NEC S82.83- ☑
    torus S82.81- ☑
finger (except thumb) S62.60- ☑
  distal phalanx (displaced) S62.63- ☑
    nondisplaced S62.66- ☑
  index S62.60- ☑
    distal phalanx (displaced) S62.63- ☑
      nondisplaced S62.66- ☑
    middle phalanx (displaced) S62.62- ☑
      nondisplaced S62.65- ☑
    proximal phalanx (displaced) S62.61- ☑
      nondisplaced S62.64- ☑
  little S62.60- ☑
    distal phalanx (displaced) S62.63- ☑
      nondisplaced S62.66- ☑
    middle phalanx (displaced) S62.62- ☑
      nondisplaced S62.65- ☑
    proximal phalanx (displaced) S62.61- ☑
      nondisplaced S62.64- ☑
  middle S62.60- ☑
    distal phalanx (displaced) S62.63- ☑
      nondisplaced S62.66- ☑
    middle phalanx (displaced) S62.62- ☑
      nondisplaced S62.65- ☑
    proximal phalanx (displaced) S62.61- ☑
      nondisplaced S62.64- ☑
  middle phalanx (displaced) S62.62- ☑
    nondisplaced S62.65- ☑
  proximal phalanx (displaced) S62.61- ☑
    nondisplaced S62.64- ☑
  ring S62.60- ☑
    distal phalanx (displaced) S62.63- ☑
      nondisplaced S62.66- ☑
    middle phalanx (displaced) S62.62- ☑
      nondisplaced S62.65- ☑
    proximal phalanx (displaced) S62.61- ☑
      nondisplaced S62.64- ☑
  thumb — *see* Fracture, thumb
following insertion (intraoperative) (postoperative) of
  orthopedic implant, joint prosthesis or bone
  plate M96.69
  femur M96.66- ☑
  fibula M96.67- ☑
  humerus M96.62- ☑
  pelvis M96.65
  radius M96.63- ☑
  specified bone NEC M96.69
  tibia M96.67- ☑

Fracture, traumatic — *continued*
  following insertion of orthopedic implant, joint pros-
    thesis or bone plate — *continued*
    ulna M96.63- ☑
foot S92.90- ☑
  astragalus — *see* Fracture, tarsal, talus
  calcaneus — *see* Fracture, tarsal, calcaneus
  cuboid — *see* Fracture, tarsal, cuboid
  cuneiform — *see* Fracture, tarsal, cuneiform
  metatarsal — *see* Fracture, metatarsal
  navicular — *see* Fracture, tarsal, navicular
  sesamoid 92.81- ☑
  specified NEC S92.81- ☑
  talus — *see* Fracture, tarsal, talus
  tarsal — *see* Fracture, tarsal
  toe — *see* Fracture, toe
forearm S52.9- ☑
  radius — *see* Fracture, radius
  ulna — *see* Fracture, ulna
fossa (anterior) (middle) (posterior) S02.19 ☑
fragility — *see* Fracture, pathological, due to osteoporosis
frontal (bone) (skull) S02.0 ☑
  sinus S02.19 ☑
glenoid (cavity) (scapula) — *see* Fracture, scapula,
  glenoid cavity
greenstick — *see* Fracture, by site
hallux — *see* Fracture, toe, great
hand S62.9- ☑
  carpal — *see* Fracture, carpal bone
  finger (except thumb) — *see* Fracture, finger
  metacarpal — *see* Fracture, metacarpal
  navicular (scaphoid) (hand) — *see* Fracture, carpal
    bone, navicular
  thumb — *see* Fracture, thumb
healed or old
  with complications — *code by* Nature of the compli-
    cation
heel bone — *see* Fracture, tarsal, calcaneus
Hill-Sachs S42.29- ☑
hip — *see* Fracture, femur, neck
humerus S42.30- ☑
  anatomical neck — *see* Fracture, humerus, upper
    end
  articular process — *see* Fracture, humerus, lower
    end
  capitellum — *see* Fracture, humerus, lower end,
    condyle, lateral
  distal end — *see* Fracture, humerus, lower end
  epiphysis
    lower — *see* Fracture, humerus, lower end, phy-
      seal
    upper — *see* Fracture, humerus, upper end,
      physeal
  external condyle — *see* Fracture, humerus, lower
    end, condyle, lateral
  following insertion of implant, prosthesis or plate
    M96.62- ☑
  great tuberosity — *see* Fracture, humerus, upper
    end, greater tuberosity
  intercondylar — *see* Fracture, humerus, lower end
  internal epicondyle — *see* Fracture, humerus, lower
    end, epicondyle, medial
  lesser tuberosity — *see* Fracture, humerus, upper
    end, lesser tuberosity
  lower end S42.40- ☑
    condyle
      lateral (displaced) S42.45- ☑
        nondisplaced S42.45- ☑
      medial (displaced) S42.46- ☑
        nondisplaced S42.46- ☑
    epicondyle
      lateral (displaced) S42.43- ☑
        nondisplaced S42.43- ☑
      medial (displaced) S42.44- ☑
        incarcerated S42.44- ☑
        nondisplaced S42.44- ☑
    physeal S49.10- ☑
      Salter-Harris
        Type I S49.11- ☑
        Type II S49.12- ☑
        Type III S49.13- ☑
        Type IV S49.14- ☑
      specified NEC S49.19- ☑
    specified NEC (displaced) S42.49- ☑
      nondisplaced S42.49- ☑

◄ **Subterms under main terms may continue to next column or page**   ☑ **Additional Character Required — Refer to the Tabular List for Character Selection**   **151**

Fracture, traumatic — Fracture, traumatic

Fracture, traumatic — *continued*
  humerus — *continued*
    lower end — *continued*
      supracondylar (simple) (displaced) S42.41- ☑
        with intercondylar fracture — *see* Fracture,
          humerus, lower end
        comminuted (displaced) S42.42- ☑
          nondisplaced S42.42- ☑
        nondisplaced S42.41- ☑
      torus S42.48- ☑
      transcondylar (displaced) S42.47- ☑
        nondisplaced S42.47- ☑
    proximal end — *see* Fracture, humerus, upper end
    shaft S42.30- ☑
      comminuted (displaced) S42.35- ☑
        nondisplaced S42.35- ☑
      greenstick S42.31- ☑
      oblique (displaced) S42.33- ☑
        nondisplaced S42.33- ☑
      segmental (displaced) S42.36- ☑
        nondisplaced S42.36- ☑
      specified NEC S42.39- ☑
      spiral (displaced) S42.34- ☑
        nondisplaced S42.34- ☑
      transverse (displaced) S42.32- ☑
        nondisplaced S42.32- ☑
    supracondylar — *see* Fracture, humerus, lower end
    surgical neck — *see* Fracture, humerus, upper end,
      surgical neck
    trochlea — *see* Fracture, humerus, lower end,
      condyle, medial
    tuberosity — *see* Fracture, humerus, upper end
    upper end S42.20- ☑
      anatomical neck — *see* Fracture, humerus, upper
        end, specified NEC
      articular head — *see* Fracture, humerus, upper
        end, specified NEC
      epiphysis — *see* Fracture, humerus, upper end,
        physeal
      greater tuberosity (displaced) S42.25- ☑
        nondisplaced S42.25- ☑
      lesser tuberosity (displaced) S42.26- ☑
        nondisplaced S42.26- ☑
      physeal S49.00- ☑
        Salter-Harris
          Type I S49.01- ☑
          Type II S49.02- ☑
          Type III S49.03- ☑
          Type IV S49.04- ☑
        specified NEC S49.09- ☑
      specified NEC (displaced) S42.29- ☑
        nondisplaced S42.29- ☑
      surgical neck (displaced) S42.21- ☑
        four-part S42.24- ☑
        nondisplaced S42.21- ☑
        three-part S42.23- ☑
        two-part (displaced) S42.22- ☑
          nondisplaced S42.22- ☑
      torus S42.27- ☑
      transepiphyseal — *see* Fracture, humerus, upper
        end, physeal
  hyoid bone S12.8 ☑
  ilium S32.30- ☑
    with disruption of pelvic ring — *see* Disruption,
      pelvic ring
    avulsion (displaced) S32.31- ☑
      nondisplaced S32.31- ☑
    specified NEC S32.39- ☑
  impaction, impacted — *code as* Fracture, by site
  innominate bone — *see* Fracture, ilium
  instep — *see* Fracture, foot
  ischium S32.60- ☑
    with disruption of pelvic ring — *see* Disruption,
      pelvic ring
    avulsion (displaced) S32.61- ☑
      nondisplaced S32.61- ☑
    specified NEC S32.69- ☑
  jaw (bone) (lower) — *see* Fracture, mandible
    upper — *see* Fracture, maxilla
  joint prosthesis — *see* Complications, joint prosthesis,
    mechanical, breakdown, by site
    periprosthetic — *see* Fracture, traumatic, peripros-
      thetic
  knee cap — *see* Fracture, patella
  larynx S12.8 ☑
  late effects — *see* Sequelae, fracture

Fracture, traumatic — *continued*
  leg (lower) S82.9-
    ankle — *see* Fracture, ankle
    femur — *see* Fracture, femur
    fibula — *see* Fracture, fibula
    malleolus — *see* Fracture, ankle
    patella — *see* Fracture, patella
    specified site NEC S82.89-
    tibia — *see* Fracture, tibia
  lumbar spine — *see* Fracture, vertebra, lumbar
  lumbosacral spine S32.9
  Maisonneuve's (displaced) S82.86- ☑
    nondisplaced S82.86- ☑
  malar bone — *see also* Fracture, maxilla S02.400 ☑
    left side S02.40B ☑
    right side S02.40A ☑
  malleolus — *see* Fracture, ankle
  malunion — *see* Fracture, by site
  mandible (lower jaw (bone)) S02.609 ☑
    alveolus S02.67- ☑
    angle (of jaw) S02.65- ☑
    body, unspecified S02.600 ☑
      left side S02.602 ☑
      right side S02.601 ☑
    condylar process S02.61- ☑
    coronoid process S02.63- ☑
    ramus, unspecified S02.64- ☑
    specified site NEC S02.69 ☑
    subcondylar process S02.62- ☑
    symphysis S02.66 ☑
  manubrium (sterni) S22.21 ☑
    dissociation from sternum S22.23 ☑
  march — *see* Fracture, traumatic, stress, by site
  maxilla, maxillary (bone) (sinus) (superior) (upper jaw)
    S02.401 ☑
    alveolus S02.42 ☑
    inferior — *see* Fracture, mandible
    LeFort I S02.411 ☑
    LeFort II S02.412 ☑
    LeFort III S02.413 ☑
    left side S02.40D ☑
    right side S02.40C ☑
  metacarpal S62.309 ☑
    base (displaced) S62.319 ☑
      nondisplaced S62.349 ☑
    fifth S62.30- ☑
      base (displaced) S62.31- ☑
        nondisplaced S62.34- ☑
      neck (displaced) S62.33- ☑
        nondisplaced S62.36- ☑
      shaft (displaced) S62.32- ☑
        nondisplaced S62.35- ☑
      specified NEC S62.398 ☑
    first S62.20- ☑
      base NEC (displaced) S62.23- ☑
        nondisplaced S62.23- ☑
      Bennett's — *see* Bennett's fracture
      neck (displaced) S62.25- ☑
        nondisplaced S62.25- ☑
      shaft (displaced) S62.24- ☑
        nondisplaced S62.24- ☑
      specified NEC S62.29- ☑
    fourth S62.30- ☑
      base (displaced) S62.31- ☑
        nondisplaced S62.34- ☑
      neck (displaced) S62.33- ☑
        nondisplaced S62.36- ☑
      shaft (displaced) S62.32- ☑
        nondisplaced S62.35- ☑
      specified NEC S62.39- ☑
    neck (displaced) S62.33- ☑
      nondisplaced S62.36- ☑
    Rolando's — *see* Rolando's fracture
    second S62.30- ☑
      base (displaced) S62.31- ☑
        nondisplaced S62.34- ☑
      neck (displaced) S62.33- ☑
        nondisplaced S62.36- ☑
      shaft (displaced) S62.32- ☑
        nondisplaced S62.35- ☑
      specified NEC S62.39- ☑
    shaft (displaced) S62.32- ☑
      nondisplaced S62.35- ☑
    specified NEC S62.399 ☑
    third S62.30- ☑
      base (displaced) S62.31- ☑

Fracture, traumatic — *continued*
  metacarpal — *continued*
    third — *continued*
      base — *continued*
        nondisplaced S62.34- ☑
      neck (displaced) S62.33- ☑
        nondisplaced S62.36- ☑
      shaft (displaced) S62.32- ☑
        nondisplaced S62.35- ☑
      specified NEC S62.39- ☑
  metastatic — *see* Fracture, pathological, due to, nec
    plastic disease — *see also* Neoplasm
  metatarsal bone S92.30- ☑
    fifth (displaced) S92.35- ☑
      nondisplaced S92.35- ☑
    first (displaced) S92.31- ☑
      nondisplaced S92.31- ☑
    fourth (displaced) S92.34- ☑
      nondisplaced S92.34- ☑
    physeal S99.10- ☑
      Salter-Harris
        Type I S99.11- ☑
        Type II S99.12- ☑
        Type III S99.13- ☑
        Type IV S99.14- ☑
      specified NEC S99.19- ☑
    second (displaced) S92.32- ☑
      nondisplaced S92.32- ☑
    third (displaced) S92.33- ☑
      nondisplaced S92.33- ☑
  Monteggia's — *see* Monteggia's fracture
  multiple
    hand (and wrist) NEC — *see* Fracture, by site
    ribs — *see* Fracture, rib, multiple
  nasal (bone(s)) S02.2 ☑
  navicular (scaphoid) (foot) — *see also* Fracture, tars
    navicular
    hand — *see* Fracture, carpal, navicular
  neck S12.9 ☑
    cervical vertebra S12.9 ☑
      fifth (displaced) S12.400 ☑
        nondisplaced S12.401 ☑
        specified type NEC (displaced) S12.490 ☑
          nondisplaced S12.491 ☑
      first (displaced) S12.000 ☑
        burst (stable) S12.01 ☑
          unstable S12.02 ☑
        lateral mass (displaced) S12.040 ☑
          nondisplaced S12.041 ☑
        nondisplaced S12.001 ☑
        posterior arch (displaced) S12.030 ☑
          nondisplaced S12.031 ☑
        specified type NEC (displaced) S12.090 ☑
          nondisplaced S12.091 ☑
      fourth (displaced) S12.300 ☑
        nondisplaced S12.301 ☑
        specified type NEC (displaced) S12.390 ☑
          nondisplaced S12.391 ☑
      second (displaced) S12.100 ☑
        dens (anterior) (displaced) (type II) S12.110 ☑
          nondisplaced S12.112 ☑
          posterior S12.111 ☑
        specified type NEC (displaced) S12.120 ☑
          nondisplaced S12.121 ☑
        nondisplaced S12.101 ☑
        specified type NEC (displaced) S12.190 ☑
          nondisplaced S12.191 ☑
      seventh (displaced) S12.600 ☑
        nondisplaced S12.601 ☑
        specified type NEC (displaced) S12.690 ☑
          nondisplaced S12.691 ☑
      sixth (displaced) S12.500 ☑
        nondisplaced S12.501 ☑
        specified type NEC (displaced) S12.590 ☑
          nondisplaced S12.591 ☑
      third (displaced) S12.200 ☑
        nondisplaced S12.201 ☑
        specified type NEC (displaced) S12.290 ☑
          nondisplaced S12.291 ☑
    hyoid bone S12.8 ☑
    larynx S12.8 ☑
    specified site NEC S12.8 ☑
    thyroid cartilage S12.8 ☑
    trachea S12.8 ☑
  neoplastic NEC — *see* Fracture, pathological, due to
    neoplastic disease

Fracture, traumatic — *continued*
- neural arch — *see* Fracture, vertebra
- newborn — *see* Birth, injury, fracture
- nontraumatic — *see* Fracture, pathological
- nonunion — *see* Nonunion, fracture
- nose, nasal (bone) (septum) S02.2- ☑
- occiput — *see* Fracture, skull, base, occiput
- odontoid process — *see* Fracture, neck, cervical vertebra, second
- olecranon (process) (ulna) — *see* Fracture, ulna, upper end, olecranon process
- orbit, orbital (bone) (region) S02.85- ☑
  - floor (blow-out) S02.3- ☑
  - roof S02.12- ☑
  - wall S02.85- ☑
    - lateral S02.84- ☑
    - medial S02.83- ☑
- os
  - calcis — *see* Fracture, tarsal, calcaneus
  - magnum — *see* Fracture, carpal, capitate
  - pubis — *see* Fracture, pubis
- palate S02.8- ☑
- parietal bone (skull) S02.0- ☑
- patella S82.00- ☑
  - comminuted (displaced) S82.04- ☑
    - nondisplaced S82.04- ☑
  - longitudinal (displaced) S82.02- ☑
    - nondisplaced S82.02- ☑
  - osteochondral (displaced) S82.01- ☑
    - nondisplaced S82.01- ☑
  - specified NEC S82.09- ☑
  - transverse (displaced) S82.03- ☑
    - nondisplaced S82.03- ☑
- pedicle (of vertebral arch) — *see* Fracture, vertebra
- pelvis, pelvic (bone) S32.9
  - acetabulum — *see* Fracture, acetabulum
  - circle — *see* Disruption, pelvic ring
  - following insertion of implant, prosthesis or plate M96.65
  - ilium — *see* Fracture, ilium
  - ischium — *see* Fracture, ischium
  - multiple
    - with disruption of pelvic ring (circle) — *see* Disruption, pelvic ring
    - without disruption of pelvic ring (circle) S32.82 ☑
  - pubis — *see* Fracture, pubis
  - sacrum — *see* Fracture, sacrum
  - specified site NEC S32.89 ☑
- periprosthetic, around internal prosthetic joint M97.9 ☑
  - ankle M97.2- ☑
  - elbow M97.4- ☑
  - finger M97.8 ☑
  - hip M97.0- ☑
  - knee M97.1- ☑
  - shoulder M97.3- ☑
  - specified joint NEC M97.8 ☑
  - spine M97.8 ☑
  - toe M97.8 ☑
  - wrist M97.8 ☑
- phalanx
  - foot — *see* Fracture, toe
  - hand — *see* Fracture, finger
- pisiform — *see* Fracture, carpal, pisiform
- pond — *see* Fracture, skull
- prosthetic device, internal — *see* Complications, prosthetic device, by site, mechanical
- pubis S32.50- ☑
  - with disruption of pelvic ring — *see* Disruption, pelvic ring
  - specified site NEC S32.59- ☑
  - superior rim S32.51- ☑
- radius S52.9- ☑
  - distal end — *see* Fracture, radius, lower end
  - following insertion of implant, prosthesis or plate M96.63- ☑
  - head — *see* Fracture, radius, upper end, head
  - lower end S52.50- ☑
    - Barton's — *see* Barton's fracture
    - Colles' — *see* Colles' fracture
    - extraarticular NEC S52.55- ☑
    - intraarticular NEC S52.57- ☑
    - physeal S59.20- ☑
      - Salter-Harris
        - Type I S59.21- ☑

Fracture, traumatic — *continued*
- radius — *continued*
  - lower end — *continued*
    - physeal — *continued*
      - Salter-Harris — *continued*
        - Type II S59.22- ☑
        - Type III S59.23- ☑
        - Type IV S59.24- ☑
      - specified NEC S59.29- ☑
    - Smith's — *see* Smith's fracture
    - specified NEC S52.59- ☑
    - styloid process (displaced) S52.51- ☑
      - nondisplaced S52.51- ☑
    - torus S52.52- ☑
  - neck — *see* Fracture, radius, upper end
  - proximal end — *see* Fracture, radius, upper end
  - shaft S52.30- ☑
    - bent bone S52.38- ☑
    - comminuted (displaced) S52.35- ☑
      - nondisplaced S52.35- ☑
    - Galeazzi's — *see* Galeazzi's fracture
    - greenstick S52.31- ☑
    - oblique (displaced) S52.33- ☑
      - nondisplaced S52.33- ☑
    - segmental (displaced) S52.36- ☑
      - nondisplaced S52.36- ☑
    - specified NEC S52.39- ☑
    - spiral (displaced) S52.34- ☑
      - nondisplaced S52.34- ☑
    - transverse (displaced) S52.32- ☑
      - nondisplaced S52.32- ☑
  - upper end S52.10- ☑
    - head (displaced) S52.12- ☑
      - nondisplaced S52.12- ☑
    - neck (displaced) S52.13- ☑
      - nondisplaced S52.13- ☑
    - physeal S59.10- ☑
      - Salter-Harris
        - Type I S59.11- ☑
        - Type II S59.12- ☑
        - Type III S59.13- ☑
        - Type IV S59.14- ☑
      - specified NEC S59.19- ☑
    - specified NEC S52.18- ☑
    - torus S52.11- ☑
- ramus
  - inferior or superior, pubis — *see* Fracture, pubis
  - mandible — *see* Fracture, mandible
- restorative material (dental) K08.539
  - with loss of material K08.531
  - without loss of material K08.530
- rib S22.3- ☑
  - with flail chest — *see* Flail, chest
  - multiple S22.4- ☑
    - with flail chest — *see* Flail, chest
- root, tooth — *see* Fracture, tooth
- sacrum S32.10 ☑
  - specified NEC S32.19 ☑
  - Type
    - 1 S32.14 ☑
    - 2 S32.15 ☑
    - 3 S32.16 ☑
    - 4 S32.17 ☑
  - Zone
    - I S32.119 ☑
      - displaced (minimally) S32.111 ☑
        - severely S32.112 ☑
      - nondisplaced S32.110 ☑
    - II S32.129 ☑
      - displaced (minimally) S32.121 ☑
        - severely S32.122 ☑
      - nondisplaced S32.120 ☑
    - III S32.139 ☑
      - displaced (minimally) S32.131 ☑
        - severely S32.132 ☑
      - nondisplaced S32.130 ☑
- scaphoid (hand) — *see also* Fracture, carpal, navicular
  - foot — *see* Fracture, tarsal, navicular
- scapula S42.10- ☑
  - acromial process (displaced) S42.12- ☑
    - nondisplaced S42.12- ☑
  - body (displaced) S42.11- ☑
    - nondisplaced S42.11- ☑
  - coracoid process (displaced) S42.13- ☑
    - nondisplaced S42.13- ☑
  - glenoid cavity (displaced) S42.14- ☑

Fracture, traumatic — *continued*
- scapula — *continued*
  - glenoid cavity — *continued*
    - nondisplaced S42.14- ☑
  - neck (displaced) S42.15- ☑
    - nondisplaced S42.15- ☑
  - specified NEC S42.19- ☑
- semilunar bone, wrist — *see* Fracture, carpal, lunate
- sequelae — *see* Sequelae, fracture
- sesamoid bone
  - foot S92.81- ☑
  - hand — *see* Fracture, carpal
  - other — *see* Fracture, traumatic, by site
- shepherd's — *see* Fracture, tarsal, talus
- shoulder (girdle) S42.9- ☑
  - blade — *see* Fracture, scapula
- sinus (ethmoid) (frontal) S02.19 ☑
- skull S02.91 ☑
  - base S02.10- ☑
    - occiput S02.119 ☑
      - condyle S02.113 ☑
        - specified NEC S02.118 ☑
          - left side S02.11H ☑
          - right side S02.11G ☑
        - type I S02.110 ☑
          - left side S02.11B ☑
          - right side S02.11A ☑
        - type II S02.111 ☑
          - left side S02.11D ☑
          - right side S02.11C ☑
        - type III S02.112 ☑
          - left side S02.11F ☑
          - right side S02.11E ☑
      - specified NEC S02.19 ☑ ·
  - birth injury P13.0
  - frontal bone S02.0 ☑
  - parietal bone S02.0 ☑
  - specified site NEC S02.8- ☑
  - temporal bone S02.19 ☑
  - vault S02.0 ☑
- Smith's — *see* Smith's fracture
- sphenoid (bone) (sinus) S02.19 ☑
- spine — *see* Fracture, vertebra
- spinous process — *see* Fracture, vertebra
- spontaneous (cause unknown) — *see* Fracture, pathological
- stave (of thumb) — *see* Fracture, metacarpal, first
- sternum S22.20 ☑
  - with flail chest — *see* Flail, chest
  - body S22.22 ☑
  - manubrium S22.21 ☑
  - xiphoid (process) S22.24 ☑
- stress M84.30 ☑
  - ankle M84.37- ☑
  - carpus M84.34- ☑
  - clavicle M84.31- ☑
  - femoral neck M84.359 ☑
  - femur M84.35- ☑
  - fibula M84.36- ☑
  - finger M84.34- ☑
  - hip M84.359 ☑
  - humerus M84.32- ☑
  - ilium M84.350 ☑
  - ischium M84.350 ☑
  - metacarpus M84.34- ☑
  - metatarsus M84.37- ☑
  - neck — *see* Fracture, fatigue, vertebra
  - pelvis M84.350 ☑
  - radius M84.33- ☑
  - rib M84.38 ☑
  - scapula M84.31- ☑
  - skull M84.38 ☑
  - tarsus M84.37- ☑
  - tibia M84.36- ☑
  - toe M84.37- ☑
  - ulna M84.33- ☑
  - vertebra — *see* Fracture, fatigue, vertebra
- supracondylar, elbow — *see* Fracture, humerus, lower end, supracondylar
- symphysis pubis — *see* Fracture, pubis
- talus (ankle bone) — *see* Fracture, tarsal, talus
- tarsal bone(s) S92.20- ☑
  - astragalus — *see* Fracture, tarsal, talus
  - calcaneus S92.00- ☑
    - anterior process (displaced) S92.02- ☑
      - nondisplaced S92.02- ☑

Index

Fracture, traumatic — Fracture, traumatic

Fracture, traumatic   ICD-10-CM 202

Fracture, traumatic — *continued*
- tarsal bone(s) — *continued*
  - calcaneus — *continued*
    - body (displaced) S92.01- ☑
      - nondisplaced S92.01- ☑
    - extraarticular NEC (displaced) S92.05- ☑
      - nondisplaced S92.05- ☑
    - intraarticular (displaced) S92.06- ☑
      - nondisplaced S92.06- ☑
    - physeal S99.00- ☑
      - Salter-Harris
        - Type I S99.01- ☑
        - Type II S99.02- ☑
        - Type III S99.03- ☑
        - Type IV S99.04- ☑
      - specified NEC S99.09- ☑
    - tuberosity (displaced) S92.04- ☑
      - avulsion (displaced) S92.03- ☑
        - nondisplaced S92.03- ☑
      - nondisplaced S92.04- ☑
  - cuboid (displaced) S92.21- ☑
    - nondisplaced S92.21- ☑
  - cuneiform
    - intermediate (displaced) S92.23- ☑
      - nondisplaced S92.23- ☑
    - lateral (displaced) S92.22- ☑
      - nondisplaced S92.22- ☑
    - medial (displaced) S92.24- ☑
      - nondisplaced S92.24- ☑
  - navicular (displaced) S92.25- ☑
    - nondisplaced S92.25- ☑
  - scaphoid — *see* Fracture, tarsal, navicular
  - talus S92.10- ☑
    - avulsion (displaced) S92.15- ☑
      - nondisplaced S92.15- ☑
    - body (displaced) S92.12- ☑
      - nondisplaced S92.12- ☑
    - dome (displaced) S92.14- ☑
      - nondisplaced S92.14- ☑
    - head (displaced) S92.12- ☑
      - nondisplaced S92.12- ☑
    - lateral process (displaced) S92.14- ☑
      - nondisplaced S92.14- ☑
    - neck (displaced) S92.11- ☑
      - nondisplaced S92.11- ☑
    - posterior process (displaced) S92.13- ☑
      - nondisplaced S92.13- ☑
    - specified NEC S92.19- ☑
- temporal bone (styloid) S02.19 ☑
- thorax (bony) S22.9 ☑
  - with flail chest — *see* Flail, chest
  - rib S22.3- ☑
    - multiple S22.4- ☑
      - with flail chest — *see* Flail, chest
  - sternum S22.20 ☑
    - body S22.22 ☑
    - manubrium S22.21 ☑
    - xiphoid process S22.24 ☑
  - vertebra (displaced) S22.009 ☑
    - burst (stable) S22.001 ☑
      - unstable S22.002 ☑
    - eighth S22.069 ☑
      - burst (stable) S22.061 ☑
        - unstable S22.062 ☑
      - specified type NEC S22.068 ☑
      - wedge compression S22.060 ☑
    - eleventh S22.089 ☑
      - burst (stable) S22.081 ☑
        - unstable S22.082 ☑
      - specified type NEC S22.088 ☑
      - wedge compression S22.080 ☑
    - fifth S22.059 ☑
      - burst (stable) S22.051 ☑
        - unstable S22.052 ☑
      - specified type NEC S22.058 ☑
      - wedge compression S22.050 ☑
    - first S22.019 ☑
      - burst (stable) S22.011 ☑
        - unstable S22.012 ☑
      - specified type NEC S22.018 ☑
      - wedge compression S22.010 ☑
    - fourth S22.049 ☑
      - burst (stable) S22.041 ☑
        - unstable S22.042 ☑
      - specified type NEC S22.048 ☑
      - wedge compression S22.040 ☑

Fracture, traumatic — *continued*
- thorax — *continued*
  - vertebra — *continued*
    - ninth S22.079 ☑
      - burst (stable) S22.071 ☑
        - unstable S22.072 ☑
      - specified type NEC S22.078 ☑
      - wedge compression S22.070 ☑
    - nondisplaced S22.001 ☑
    - second S22.029 ☑
      - burst (stable) S22.021 ☑
        - unstable S22.022 ☑
      - specified type NEC S22.028 ☑
      - wedge compression S22.020 ☑
    - seventh S22.069 ☑
      - burst (stable) S22.061 ☑
        - unstable S22.062 ☑
      - specified type NEC S22.068 ☑
      - wedge compression S22.060 ☑
    - sixth S22.059 ☑
      - burst (stable) S22.051 ☑
        - unstable S22.052 ☑
      - specified type NEC S22.058 ☑
      - wedge compression S22.050 ☑
    - specified type NEC S22.008 ☑
    - tenth S22.079 ☑
      - burst (stable) S22.071 ☑
        - unstable S22.072 ☑
      - specified type NEC S22.078 ☑
      - wedge compression S22.070 ☑
    - third S22.039 ☑
      - burst (stable) S22.031 ☑
        - unstable S22.032 ☑
      - specified type NEC S22.038 ☑
      - wedge compression S22.030 ☑
    - twelfth S22.089 ☑
      - burst (stable) S22.081 ☑
        - unstable S22.082 ☑
      - specified type NEC S22.088 ☑
      - wedge compression S22.080 ☑
    - wedge compression S22.000 ☑
  - thumb S62.50- ☑
    - distal phalanx (displaced) S62.52- ☑
      - nondisplaced S62.52- ☑
    - proximal phalanx (displaced) S62.51- ☑
      - nondisplaced S62.51- ☑
  - thyroid cartilage S12.8 ☑
  - tibia (shaft) S82.20- ☑
    - comminuted (displaced) S82.25- ☑
      - nondisplaced S82.25- ☑
    - condyles — *see* Fracture, tibia, upper end
    - distal end — *see* Fracture, tibia, lower end
    - epiphysis
      - lower — *see* Fracture, tibia, lower end
      - upper — *see* Fracture, tibia, upper end
    - following insertion of implant, prosthesis or plate M96.67- ☑
    - head (involving knee joint) — *see* Fracture, tibia, upper end
    - intercondyloid eminence — *see* Fracture, tibia, upper end
    - involving ankle or malleolus — *see* Fracture, ankle, medial malleolus
    - lower end S82.30- ☑
      - physeal S89.10- ☑
        - Salter-Harris
          - Type I S89.11- ☑
          - Type II S89.12- ☑
          - Type III S89.13- ☑
          - Type IV S89.14- ☑
          - specified NEC S89.19- ☑
      - pilon (displaced) S82.87- ☑
        - nondisplaced S82.87- ☑
      - specified NEC S82.39- ☑
      - torus S82.31- ☑
    - malleolus — *see* Fracture, ankle, medial malleolus
    - oblique (displaced) S82.23- ☑
      - nondisplaced S82.23- ☑
    - pilon — *see* Fracture, tibia, lower end, pilon
    - proximal end — *see* Fracture, tibia, upper end
    - segmental (displaced) S82.26- ☑
      - nondisplaced S82.26- ☑
    - specified NEC S82.29- ☑
    - spine — *see* Fracture, tibia, upper end, spine
    - spiral (displaced) S82.24- ☑
      - nondisplaced S82.24- ☑

Fracture, traumatic — *continued*
- tibia — *continued*
  - transverse (displaced) S82.22- ☑
    - nondisplaced S82.22- ☑
  - tuberosity — *see* Fracture, tibia, upper end, tuberosity
  - upper end S82.10- ☑
    - bicondylar (displaced) S82.14- ☑
      - nondisplaced S82.14- ☑
    - lateral condyle (displaced) S82.12- ☑
      - nondisplaced S82.12- ☑
    - medial condyle (displaced) S82.13- ☑
      - nondisplaced S82.13- ☑
    - physeal S89.00- ☑
      - Salter-Harris
        - Type I S89.01- ☑
        - Type II S89.02- ☑
        - Type III S89.03- ☑
        - Type IV S89.04- ☑
      - specified NEC S89.09- ☑
    - plateau — *see* Fracture, tibia, upper end, bicondylar
    - specified NEC S82.19- ☑
    - spine (displaced) S82.11- ☑
      - nondisplaced S82.11- ☑
    - torus S82.16- ☑
    - tuberosity (displaced) S82.15- ☑
      - nondisplaced S82.15- ☑
  - toe S92.91- ☑
    - great (displaced) S92.40- ☑
      - distal phalanx (displaced) S92.42- ☑
        - nondisplaced S92.42- ☑
      - nondisplaced S92.40- ☑
      - proximal phalanx (displaced) S92.41- ☑
        - nondisplaced S92.41- ☑
      - specified NEC S92.49- ☑
    - lesser (displaced) S92.50- ☑
      - distal phalanx (displaced) S92.53- ☑
        - nondisplaced S92.53- ☑
      - middle phalanx (displaced) S92.52- ☑
        - nondisplaced S92.52- ☑
      - nondisplaced S92.50- ☑
      - proximal phalanx (displaced) S92.51- ☑
        - nondisplaced S92.51- ☑
      - specified NEC S92.59- ☑
    - physeal
      - phalanx S99.20- ☑
        - Salter-Harris
          - Type I S99.21- ☑
          - Type II S99.22- ☑
          - Type III S99.23- ☑
          - Type IV S99.24- ☑
          - specified NEC S99.29- ☑
  - tooth (root) S02.5 ☑
  - trachea (cartilage) S12.8 ☑
  - transverse process — *see* Fracture, vertebra
  - trapezium or trapezoid bone — *see* Fracture, carpal
  - trimalleolar — *see* Fracture, ankle, trimalleolar
  - triquetrum (cuneiform of carpus) — *see* Fracture, carpal, triquetrum
  - trochanter — *see* Fracture, femur, trochanteric
  - tuberosity (external) — *see* Fracture, traumatic, by site
  - ulna (shaft) S52.20- ☑
    - bent bone S52.28- ☑
    - coronoid process — *see* Fracture, ulna, upper end, coronoid process
    - distal end — *see* Fracture, ulna, lower end
    - following insertion of implant, prosthesis or plate M96.63- ☑
    - head S52.60- ☑
    - lower end S52.60- ☑
      - physeal S59.00- ☑
        - Salter-Harris
          - Type I S59.01- ☑
          - Type II S59.02- ☑
          - Type III S59.03- ☑
          - Type IV S59.04- ☑
          - specified NEC S59.09- ☑
      - specified NEC S52.69- ☑
      - styloid process (displaced) S52.61- ☑
        - nondisplaced S52.61- ☑
      - torus S52.62- ☑
    - proximal end — *see* Fracture, ulna, upper end
    - shaft S52.20- ☑
      - comminuted (displaced) S52.25- ☑
        - nondisplaced S52.25- ☑

  ☑ **Additional Character Required** — Refer to the Tabular List for Character Selection ▽ **Subterms under main terms may continue to next column or page**

Index

Fracture, traumatic — Fuchs'

Fucosidosis E77.1
Fugue R68.89
  dissociative F44.1
  hysterical (dissociative) F44.1
  postictal in epilepsy — *see* Epilepsy
  reaction to exceptional stress (transient) F43.0
Fulminant, fulminating — *see* condition
Functional — *see also* condition
  bleeding (uterus) N93.8
Functioning, intellectual, borderline R41.83
Fundus — *see* condition
Fungemia NOS B49
Fungus, fungous
  cerebral G93.89
  disease NOS B49
  infection — *see* Infection, fungus
Funiculitis (acute) (chronic) (endemic) N49.1
  gonococcal (acute) (chronic) A54.23
  tuberculous A18.15
Funnel
  breast (acquired) M95.4
    congenital Q67.6
    sequelae (late effect) of rickets E64.3
  chest (acquired) M95.4
    congenital Q67.6
    sequelae (late effect) of rickets E64.3
  pelvis (acquired) M95.5
    with disproportion (fetopelvic) O33.3 ☑
      causing obstructed labor O65.3
    congenital Q74.2
FUO (fever of unknown origin) R50.9
Furfur L21.0
  microsporon B36.0
Furrier's lung J67.8
Furrowed K14.5
  nail(s) (transverse) L60.4
    congenital Q84.6
  tongue K14.5
    congenital Q38.3
Furuncle L02.92
  abdominal wall L02.221
  ankle — *see* Furuncle, lower limb
  antecubital space — *see* Furuncle, upper limb
  anus K61.0
  arm — *see* Furuncle, upper limb
  auditory canal, external — *see* Abscess, ear, external
  auricle (ear) — *see* Abscess, ear, external
  axilla (region) L02.42- ☑
  back (any part) L02.222
  breast N61.1
  buttock L02.32
  cheek (external) L02.02
  chest wall L02.223
  chin L02.02
  corpus cavernosum N48.21
  ear, external — *see* Abscess, ear, external
  external auditory canal — *see* Abscess, ear, external
  eyelid — *see* Abscess, eyelid
  face L02.02
  femoral (region) — *see* Furuncle, lower limb

Furuncle — *continued*
  finger — *see* Furuncle, hand
  flank L02.221
  foot L02.62- ☑
  forehead L02.02
  gluteal (region) L02.32
  groin L02.224
  hand L02.52- ☑
  head L02.821
    face L02.02
  hip — *see* Furuncle, lower limb
  kidney — *see* Abscess, kidney
  knee — *see* Furuncle, lower limb
  labium (majus) (minus) N76.4
  lacrimal
    gland — *see* Dacryoadenitis
    passages (duct) (sac) — *see* Inflammation, lacrimal, passages, acute
  leg (any part) — *see* Furuncle, lower limb
  lower limb L02.42- ☑
  malignant A22.0
  mouth K12.2
  navel L02.226
  neck L02.12
  nose J34.0
  orbit, orbital — *see* Abscess, orbit
  palmar (space) — *see* Furuncle, hand
  partes posteriores L02.32
  pectoral region L02.223
  penis N48.21
  perineum L02.225
  pinna — *see* Abscess, ear, external
  popliteal — *see* Furuncle, lower limb
  prepatellar — *see* Furuncle, lower limb
  scalp L02.821
  seminal vesicle N49.0
  shoulder — *see* Furuncle, upper limb
  specified site NEC L02.828
  submandibular K12.2
  temple (region) L02.02
  thumb — *see* Furuncle, hand
  toe — *see* Furuncle, foot
  trunk L02.229
    abdominal wall L02.221
    back L02.222
    chest wall L02.223
    groin L02.224
    perineum L02.225
    umbilicus L02.226
  umbilicus L02.226
  upper limb L02.42- ☑
  vulva N76.4
Furunculosis — *see* Furuncle
Fused — *see* Fusion, fused
Fusion, fused (congenital)
  astragaloscaphoid Q74.2
  atria Q21.1
  auditory canal Q16.1
  auricles, heart Q21.1
  binocular with defective stereopsis H53.32

Fusion, fused — *continued*
  bone Q79.8
  cervical spine M43.22
  choanal Q30.0
  commissure, mitral valve Q23.2
  cusps, heart valve NEC Q24.8
    mitral Q23.2
    pulmonary Q22.1
    tricuspid Q22.4
  ear ossicles Q16.3
  fingers Q70.0 ☑
  hymen Q52.3
  joint (acquired) — *see also* Ankylosis
    congenital Q74.8
  kidneys (incomplete) Q63.1
  labium (majus) (minus) Q52.5
  larynx and trachea Q34.8
  limb, congenital Q74.8
    lower Q74.2
    upper Q74.0
  lobes, lung Q33.8
  lumbosacral (acquired) M43.27
    arthrodesis status Z98.1
    congenital Q76.49
    postprocedural status Z98.1
  nares, nose, nasal, nostril(s) Q30.0
  organ or site not listed — *see* Anomaly, by site
  ossicles Q79.9
    auditory Q16.3
  pulmonic cusps Q22.1
  ribs Q76.6
  sacroiliac (joint) (acquired) M43.28
    arthrodesis status Z98.1
    congenital Q74.2
    postprocedural status Z98.1
  spine (acquired) NEC M43.20
    arthrodesis status Z98.1
    cervical region M43.22
    cervicothoracic region M43.23
    congenital Q76.49
    lumbar M43.26
    lumbosacral region M43.27
    occipito-atlanto-axial region M43.21
    postoperative status Z98.1
    sacrococcygeal region M43.28
    thoracic region M43.24
    thoracolumbar region M43.25
  sublingual duct with submaxillary duct at opening mouth Q38.4
  testes Q55.1
  toes Q70.2- ☑
  tooth, teeth K00.2
  trachea and esophagus Q39.8
  twins Q89.4
  vagina Q52.4
  ventricles, heart Q21.0
  vertebra (arch) — *see* Fusion, spine
  vulva Q52.5
Fusospirillosis (mouth) (tongue) (tonsil) A69.1
Fussy baby R68.12

G

Gain in weight (abnormal) (excessive) — *see also* Weight, gain

Gaisböck's disease (polycythemia hypertonica) D75.1

Gait abnormality R26.9
ataxic R26.0
falling R29.6
hysterical (ataxic) (staggering) F44.4
paralytic R26.1
spastic R26.1
specified type NEC R26.89
staggering R26.0
unsteadiness R26.81
walking difficulty NEC R26.2

Galactocele (breast) N64.89
puerperal, postpartum O92.79

Galactokinase deficiency E74.29

Galactophoritis N61.0
gestational, puerperal, postpartum O91.2- ☑

Galactorrhea O92.6
not associated with childbirth N64.3

Galactosemia (classic) (congenital) E74.21

Galactosuria E74.29

Galacturia R82.0
schistosomiasis (bilharziasis) B65.0

GALD (gestational alloimmune liver disease) P78.84

Galeazzi's fracture S52.37- ☑

Galen's vein — *see* condition

Gall duct — *see* condition

Gallbladder — *see also* condition
acute K81.0

Gallop rhythm R00.8

Gallstone (colic) (cystic duct) (gallbladder) (impacted) (multiple) — *see also* Calculus, gallbladder
with
cholecystitis — *see* Calculus, gallbladder, with cholecystitis
bile duct (common) (hepatic) — *see* Calculus, bile duct
causing intestinal obstruction K56.3
specified NEC K80.80
with obstruction K80.81

Gambling Z72.6
pathological (compulsive) F63.0

Gammopathy (of undetermined significance [MGUS]) D47.2
associated with lymphoplasmacytic dyscrasia D47.2
monoclonal D47.2
polyclonal D89.0

Gamna's disease (siderotic splenomegaly) D73.1

Gamophobia F40.298

Gampsodactylia (congenital) Q66.7- ☑

Gamstorp's disease (adynamia episodica hereditaria) G72.3

Gandy-Nanta disease (siderotic splenomegaly) D73.1

Gang
membership offenses Z72.810

Gangliocytoma D36.10

Ganglioglioma — *see* Neoplasm, uncertain behavior, by site

Ganglion (compound) (diffuse) (joint) (tendon (sheath)) M67.40
ankle M67.47- ☑
foot M67.47- ☑
forearm M67.43- ☑
hand M67.44- ☑
lower leg M67.46- ☑
multiple sites M67.49
of yaws (early) (late) A66.6
pelvic region M67.45- ☑
periosteal — *see* Periostitis
shoulder region M67.41- ☑
specified site NEC M67.48
thigh region M67.45- ☑
tuberculous A18.09
upper arm M67.42- ☑
wrist M67.43- ☑

Ganglioneuroblastoma — *see* Neoplasm, nerve, malignant

Ganglioneuroma D36.10
malignant — *see* Neoplasm, nerve, malignant

Ganglioneuromatosis D36.10

Ganglionitis
fifth nerve — *see* Neuralgia, trigeminal
gasserian (postherpetic) (postzoster) B02.21

Ganglionitis — *continued*
geniculate G51.1
newborn (birth injury) P11.3
postherpetic, postzoster B02.21
herpes zoster B02.21
postherpetic geniculate B02.21

Gangliosidosis E75.10
GM1 E75.19
GM2 E75.00
other specified E75.09
Sandhoff disease E75.01
Tay-Sachs disease E75.02
GM3 E75.19
mucolipidosis IV E75.11

Gangosa A66.5

Gangrene, gangrenous (connective tissue) (dropsical) (dry) (moist) (skin) (ulcer) — *see also* Necrosis I96
with diabetes (mellitus) — *see* Diabetes, gangrene
abdomen (wall) I96
alveolar M27.3
appendix K35.80
with
peritonitis, localized — *see also* Appendicitis K35.31
arteriosclerotic (general) (senile) — *see* Arteriosclerosis, extremities, with, gangrene
auricle I96
Bacillus welchii A48.0
bladder (infectious) — *see* Cystitis, specified type NEC
bowel, cecum, or colon — *see* Gangrene, intestine
Clostridium perfringens or welchii A48.0
cornea H18.89- ☑
corpora cavernosa N48.29
noninfective N48.89
cutaneous, spreading I96
decubital — *see* Ulcer, pressure, by site
diabetic (any site) — *see* Diabetes, gangrene
emphysematous — *see* Gangrene, gas
epidemic — *see* Poisoning, food, noxious, plant
epididymis (infectional) N45.1
erysipelas — *see* Erysipelas
extremity (lower) (upper) I96
Fournier N49.3
female N76.89
fusospirochetal A69.0
gallbladder — *see* Cholecystitis, acute
gas (bacillus) A48.0
following
abortion — *see* Abortion by type complicated by infection
ectopic or molar pregnancy O08.0
glossitis K14.0
hernia — *see* Hernia, by site, with gangrene
intestine, intestinal (hemorrhagic) (massive) — *see also* Infarct, intestine K55.069
with
mesenteric embolism — *see also* Infarct, intestine K55.069
obstruction — *see* Obstruction, intestine
laryngitis J04.0
limb (lower) (upper) I96
lung J85.0
spirochetal A69.8
lymphangitis I89.1
Meleney's (synergistic) — *see* Ulcer, skin
mesentery — *see also* Infarct, intestine K55.069
with
embolism — *see also* Infarct, intestine K55.069
intestinal obstruction — *see* Obstruction, intestine
mouth A69.0
ovary — *see* Oophoritis
pancreas — *see* Pancreatitis, acute
penis N48.29
noninfective N48.89
perineum I96
pharynx — *see also* Pharyngitis
Vincent's A69.1
presenile I73.1
progressive synergistic — *see* Ulcer, skin
pulmonary J85.0
pulpal (dental) K04.1
quinsy J36
Raynaud's (symmetric gangrene) I73.01
retropharyngeal J39.2
scrotum N49.3
noninfective N50.89

Gangrene, gangrenous — *continued*
senile (atherosclerotic) — *see* Arteriosclerosis, extremities, with, gangrene
spermatic cord N49.1
noninfective N50.89
spine I96
spirochetal NEC A69.8
spreading cutaneous I96
stomatitis A69.0
symmetrical I73.01
testis (infectional) N45.2
noninfective N44.8
throat — *see also* Pharyngitis
diphtheritic A36.0
Vincent's A69.1
thyroid (gland) E07.89
tooth (pulp) K04.1
tuberculous NEC — *see* Tuberculosis
tunica vaginalis N49.1
noninfective N50.89
umbilicus I96
uterus — *see* Endometritis
uvulitis K12.2
vas deferens N49.1
noninfective N50.89
vulva N76.89

Ganister disease J62.8

Ganser's syndrome (hysterical) F44.89

Gardner-Diamond syndrome (autoerythrocyte sensitization) D69.2

Gargoylism E76.01

Garré's disease, osteitis (sclerosing), osteomyelitis — *see* Osteomyelitis, specified type NEC

Garrod's pad, knuckle M72.1

Gartner's duct
cyst Q52.4
persistent Q50.6

Gas R14.3
asphyxiation, inhalation, poisoning, suffocation NEC — *see* Table of Drugs and Chemicals
excessive R14.0
gangrene A48.0
following
abortion — *see* Abortion by type complicated by infection
ectopic or molar pregnancy O08.0
on stomach R14.0
pains R14.1

Gastralgia — *see also* Pain, abdominal

Gastrectasis K31.0
psychogenic F45.8

Gastric — *see* condition

Gastrinoma
malignant
pancreas C25.4
specified site NEC — *see* Neoplasm, malignant, by site
unspecified site C25.4
specified site — *see* Neoplasm, uncertain behavior
unspecified site D37.9

Gastritis (simple) K29.70
with bleeding K29.71
acute (erosive) K29.00
with bleeding K29.01
alcoholic K29.20
with bleeding K29.21
allergic K29.60
with bleeding K29.61
atrophic (chronic) K29.40
with bleeding K29.41
chronic (antral) (fundal) K29.50
with bleeding K29.51
atrophic K29.40
with bleeding K29.41
superficial K29.30
with bleeding K29.31
dietary counseling and surveillance Z71.3
due to diet deficiency E63.9
eosinophilic K52.81
giant hypertrophic K29.60
with bleeding K29.61
granulomatous K29.60
with bleeding K29.61
hypertrophic (mucosa) K29.60
with bleeding K29.61
nervous F54
spastic K29.60
with bleeding K29.61

Gastritis — *continued*
 specified NEC K29.60
  with bleeding K29.61
 superficial chronic K29.30
  with bleeding K29.31
 tuberculous A18.83
 viral NEC A08.4
Gastrocarcinoma — *see* Neoplasm, malignant, stomach
Gastrocolic — *see* condition
Gastrodisciasis, gastrodiscoidiasis B66.8
Gastroduodenitis K29.90
 with bleeding K29.91
 virus, viral A08.4
  specified type NEC A08.39
Gastrodynia — *see* Pain, abdominal
Gastroenteritis (acute) (chronic) (noninfectious) — *see also* Enteritis K52.9
 allergic K52.29
  with
   eosinophilic gastritis or gastroenteritis K52.81
   food protein-induced enterocolitis syndrome K52.21
   food protein-induced enteropathy K52.22
 dietetic — *see also* Gastroenteritis, allergic K52.29
 drug-induced K52.1
 due to
  Cryptosporidium A07.2
  drugs K52.1
  food poisoning — *see* Intoxication, foodborne
  radiation K52.0
 eosinophilic K52.81
 epidemic (infectious) A09
 food hypersensitivity — *see also* Gastroenteritis, allergic K52.29
 infectious — *see* Enteritis, infectious
 influenzal — *see* Influenza, with gastroenteritis
 noninfectious K52.9
  specified NEC K52.89
 rotaviral A08.0
 Salmonella A02.0
 toxic K52.1
 viral NEC A08.4
  acute infectious A08.39
   type Norwalk A08.11
  infantile (acute) A08.39
  Norwalk agent A08.11
  rotaviral A08.0
  severe of infants A08.39
  specified type NEC A08.39
Gastroenteropathy — *see also* Gastroenteritis K52.9
 acute, due to Norovirus A08.11
 acute, due to Norwalk agent A08.11
 infectious A09
Gastroenteroptosis K63.4
Gastroesophageal laceration- hemorrhage syndrome K22.6
Gastrointestinal — *see* condition
Gastrojejunal — *see* condition
Gastrojejunitis — *see* Enteritis K52.9
Gastrojejunocolic — *see* condition
Gastroliths K31.89
Gastromalacia K31.89
Gastroparalysis K31.84
 diabetic — *see* Diabetes, gastroparalysis
Gastroparesis K31.84
 diabetic — *see* Diabetes, by type, with gastroparesis
Gastropathy K31.9
 congestive portal K31.89
 erythematous K29.70
 exudative K90.89
 portal hypertensive K31.89
Gastroptosis K31.89
Gastrorrhagia K92.2
 psychogenic F45.8
Gastroschisis (congenital) Q79.3
Gastrospasm (neurogenic) (reflex) K31.89
 neurotic F45.8
 psychogenic F45.8
Gastrostaxis — *see* Gastritis, with bleeding
Gastrostenosis K31.89
Gastrostomy
 attention to Z43.1
 status Z93.1
Gastrosuccorrhea (continuous) (intermittent) K31.89
 neurotic F45.8
 psychogenic F45.8
Gatophobia F40.218

Gaucher's disease or splenomegaly (adult) (infantile) E75.22
Gee (-Herter)(-Thaysen) **disease** (nontropical sprue) K90.0
Gélineau's syndrome G47.419
 with cataplexy G47.411
Gemination, tooth, teeth K00.2
Gemistocytoma
 specified site — *see* Neoplasm, malignant, by site
 unspecified site C71.9
General, generalized — *see* condition
Genetic
 carrier (status)
  cystic fibrosis Z14.1
  hemophilia A (asymptomatic) Z14.01
   symptomatic Z14.02
  specified NEC Z14.8
 susceptibility to disease NEC Z15.89
  malignant neoplasm Z15.09
   breast Z15.01
   endometrium Z15.04
   ovary Z15.02
   prostate Z15.03
   specified NEC Z15.09
  multiple endocrine neoplasia Z15.81
Genital — *see* condition
Genito-anorectal syndrome A55
Genitourinary system — *see* condition
Genu
 congenital Q74.1
 extrorsum (acquired) — *see also* Deformity, varus, knee
  congenital Q74.1
  sequelae (late effect) of rickets E64.3
 introrsum (acquired) — *see also* Deformity, valgus, knee
  congenital Q74.1
  sequelae (late effect) of rickets E64.3
 rachitic (old) E64.3
 recurvatum (acquired) — *see also* Deformity, limb, specified type NEC, lower leg
  congenital Q68.2
  sequelae (late effect) of rickets E64.3
 valgum (acquired) (knock-knee) M21.06- ☑
  congenital Q74.1
  sequelae (late effect) of rickets E64.3
 varum (acquired) (bowleg) M21.16- ☑
  congenital Q74.1
  sequelae (late effect) of rickets E64.3
Geographic tongue K14.1
Geophagia — *see* Pica
Geotrichosis B48.3
 stomatitis B48.3
Gephyrophobia F40.242
Gerbode defect Q21.0
GERD (gastroesophageal reflux disease) K21.9
Gerhardt's
 disease (erythromelalgia) I73.81
 syndrome (vocal cord paralysis) J38.00
  bilateral J38.02
  unilateral J38.01
German measles — *see also* Rubella
 exposure to Z20.4
Germinoblastoma (diffuse) C85.9- ☑
 follicular C82.9- ☑
Germinoma — *see* Neoplasm, malignant, by site
Gerontoxon — *see* Degeneration, cornea, senile
Gerstmann's syndrome R48.8
 developmental F81.2
Gerstmann-Sträussler-Scheinker syndrome (GSS) A81.82
Gestation (period) — *see also* Pregnancy
 ectopic — *see* Pregnancy, by site
 multiple O30.9- ☑
  greater than quadruplets — *see* Pregnancy, multiple (gestation), specified NEC
  specified NEC — *see* Pregnancy, multiple (gestation), specified NEC
Gestational
 mammary abscess O91.11- ☑
 purulent mastitis O91.11- ☑
 subareolar abscess O91.11- ☑
Ghon tubercle, primary infection A15.7
Ghost
 teeth K00.4
 vessels (cornea) H16.41- ☑
Ghoul hand A66.3
Gianotti-Crosti disease L44.4

Giant
 cell
  epulis K06.8
  peripheral granuloma K06.8
 esophagus, congenital Q39.5
 kidney, congenital Q63.3
 urticaria T78.3 ☑
  hereditary D84.1
Giardiasis A07.1
Gibert's disease or pityriasis L42
Giddiness R42
 hysterical F44.89
 psychogenic F45.8
Gierke's disease (glycogenosis I) E74.01
Gigantism (cerebral) (hypophyseal) (pituitary) E22.0
 constitutional E34.4
Gilbert's disease or syndrome E80.4
Gilchrist's disease B40.9
Gilford-Hutchinson disease E34.8
Gilles de la Tourette's disease or syndrome (moto verbal tic) F95.2
Gingivitis K05.10
 acute (catarrhal) K05.00
  necrotizing A69.1
  nonplaque induced K05.01
  plaque induced K05.00
 chronic (desquamative) (hyperplastic) (simple margin (pregnancy associated) (ulcerative) K05.10
  nonplaque induced K05.11
  plaque induced K05.10
 expulsiva — *see* Periodontitis
 necrotizing ulcerative (acute) A69.1
 pellagrous E52
  acute necrotizing A69.1
 Vincent's A69.1
Gingivoglossitis K14.0
Gingivopericementitis — *see* Periodontitis
Gingivosis — *see* Gingivitis, chronic
Gingivostomatitis K05.10
 herpesviral B00.2
 necrotizing ulcerative (acute) A69.1
Gland, glandular — *see* condition
Glanders A24.0
Glanzmann (-Naegeli) **disease or thrombasthenia** D69.1
Glasgow coma scale
 total score
  13-15 R40.241 ☑
  3-8 R40.243 ☑
  9-12 R40.242 ☑
Glass-blower's disease (cataract) — *see* Cataract, spe ified NEC
Glaucoma H40.9
 with
  increased episcleral venous pressure H40.81- ☑
  pseudoexfoliation of lens — *see* Glaucoma, oper angle, primary, capsular
 absolute H44.51- ☑
 angle-closure (primary) H40.20- ☑
  acute (attack) (crisis) H40.21- ☑
  chronic H40.22- ☑
  intermittent H40.23- ☑
  residual stage H40.24- ☑
 borderline H40.00- ☑
 capsular (with pseudoexfoliation of lens) — *see* Gla coma, open angle, primary, capsular
 childhood Q15.0
 closed angle — *see* Glaucoma, angle-closure
 congenital Q15.0
 corticosteroid-induced — *see* Glaucoma, secondary drugs
 hypersecretion H40.82- ☑
 in (due to)
  amyloidosis E85.4 [H42]
  aniridia Q13.1 [H42]
  concussion of globe — *see* Glaucoma, secondary trauma
  dislocation of lens — *see* Glaucoma, secondary
  disorder of lens NEC — *see* Glaucoma, secondary
  drugs — *see* Glaucoma, secondary, drugs
  endocrine disease NOS E34.9 [H42]
  eye
   inflammation — *see* Glaucoma, secondary, in flammation
   trauma — *see* Glaucoma, secondary, trauma
  hypermature cataract — *see* Glaucoma, seconda

☑ Additional Character Required — Refer to the Tabular List for Character Selection
▽ Subterms under main terms may continue to next column or pag

Glaucoma — *continued*
in — *continued*
iridocyclitis — *see* Glaucoma, secondary, inflammation
lens disorder — *see* Glaucoma, secondary
Lowe's syndrome E72.03 *[H42]*
metabolic disease NOS E88.9 *[H42]*
ocular disorders NEC — *see* Glaucoma, secondary
onchocerciasis B73.02
pupillary block — *see* Glaucoma, secondary
retinal vein occlusion — *see* Glaucoma, secondary
Rieger's anomaly Q13.81 *[H42]*
rubeosis of iris — *see* Glaucoma, secondary
tumor of globe — *see* Glaucoma, secondary
infantile Q15.0
low tension — *see* Glaucoma, open angle, primary, low-tension
malignant H40.83- ☑
narrow angle — *see* Glaucoma, angle-closure
newborn Q15.0
noncongestive (chronic) — *see* Glaucoma, open angle
nonobstructive — *see* Glaucoma, open angle
obstructive — *see also* Glaucoma, angle-closure
due to lens changes — *see* Glaucoma, secondary
open angle H40.10- ☑
primary H40.11- ☑
capsular (with pseudoexfoliation of lens) H40.14- ☑
low-tension H40.12- ☑
pigmentary H40.13- ☑
residual stage H40.15- ☑
phacolytic — *see* Glaucoma, secondary
pigmentary — *see* Glaucoma, open angle, primary, pigmentary
postinfectious — *see* Glaucoma, secondary, inflammation
secondary (to) H40.5- ☑
drugs H40.6- ☑
inflammation H40.4- ☑
trauma H40.3- ☑
simple (chronic) H40.11- ☑
simplex H40.11- ☑
specified type NEC H40.89
suspect H40.00- ☑
syphilitic A52.71
traumatic — *see also* Glaucoma, secondary, trauma
newborn (birth injury) P15.3
tuberculous A18.59
Glaucomatous flecks (subcapsular) — *see* Cataract, complicated
Glazed tongue K14.4
Gleet (gonococcal) A54.01
Glénard's disease K63.4
Glioblastoma (multiforme)
with sarcomatous component
specified site — *see* Neoplasm, malignant, by site
unspecified site C71.9
giant cell
specified site — *see* Neoplasm, malignant, by site
unspecified site C71.9
specified site — *see* Neoplasm, malignant, by site
unspecified site C71.9
Glioma (malignant)
astrocytic
specified site — *see* Neoplasm, malignant, by site
unspecified site C71.9
mixed
specified site — *see* Neoplasm, malignant, by site
unspecified site C71.9
nose Q30.8
specified site NEC — *see* Neoplasm, malignant, by site
subependymal D43.2
specified site — *see* Neoplasm, uncertain behavior, by site
unspecified site D43.2
unspecified site C71.9
Gliomatosis cerebri C71.0
Glioneuroma — *see* Neoplasm, uncertain behavior, by site
Gliosarcoma
specified site — *see* Neoplasm, malignant, by site
unspecified site C71.9
Gliosis (cerebral) G93.89
spinal G95.89
Glisson's disease — *see* Rickets
Globinuria R82.3
Globus (hystericus) F45.8

Glomangioma D18.00
intra-abdominal D18.03
intracranial D18.02
skin D18.01
specified site NEC D18.09
Glomangiomyoma D18.00
intra-abdominal D18.03
intracranial D18.02
skin D18.01
specified site NEC D18.09
Glomangiosarcoma — *see* Neoplasm, connective tissue, malignant
Glomerular
disease in syphilis A52.75
nephritis — *see* Glomerulonephritis
Glomerulitis — *see* Glomerulonephritis
Glomerulonephritis — *see also* Nephritis N05.9
with
edema — *see* Nephrosis
minimal change N05.0
minor glomerular abnormality N05.0
acute N00.9
chronic N03.9
crescentic (diffuse) NEC — *see also* N00-N07 with fourth character .7 N05.7
dense deposit — *see also* N00-N07 with fourth character .6 N05.6
diffuse
crescentic — *see also* N00-N07 with fourth character .7 N05.7
endocapillary proliferative — *see also* N00-N07 with fourth character .4 N05.4
membranous — *see also* N00-N07 with fourth character .2 N05.2
mesangial proliferative — *see also* N00-N07 with fourth character .3 N05.3
mesangiocapillary — *see also* N00-N07 with fourth character .5 N05.5
sclerosing N18.9
endocapillary proliferative (diffuse) NEC — *see also* N00-N07 with fourth character .4 N05.4
extracapillary NEC — *see also* N00-N07 with fourth character .7 N05.7
focal (and segmental) — *see also* N00-N07 with fourth character .1 N05.1
hypocomplementemic — *see* Glomerulonephritis, membranoproliferative
IgA — *see* Nephropathy, IgA
immune complex (circulating) NEC N05.8
in (due to)
amyloidosis E85.4 *[N08]*
bilharziasis B65.9 *[N08]*
cryoglobulinemia D89.1 *[N08]*
defibrination syndrome D65 *[N08]*
diabetes mellitus — *see* Diabetes, glomerulosclerosis
disseminated intravascular coagulation D65 *[N08]*
Fabry (-Anderson) disease E75.21 *[N08]*
Goodpasture's syndrome M31.0
hemolytic-uremic syndrome D59.3
Henoch (-Schönlein) purpura D69.0 *[N08]*
lecithin cholesterol acyltransferase deficiency E78.6 *[N08]*
microscopic polyangiitis M31.7 *[N08]*
multiple myeloma C90.0- ☑ *[N08]*
Plasmodium malariae B52.0
schistosomiasis B65.9 *[N08]*
sepsis A41.9 *[N08]*
streptococcal A40- ☑ *[N08]*
sickle-cell disorders D57.- ☑ *[N08]*
strongyloidiasis B78.9 *[N08]*
subacute bacterial endocarditis I33.0 *[N08]*
syphilis (late) congenital A50.59 *[N08]*
systemic lupus erythematosus M32.14
thrombotic thrombocytopenic purpura M31.1 *[N08]*
typhoid fever A01.09
Waldenström macroglobulinemia C88.0 *[N08]*
Wegener's granulomatosis M31.31
latent or quiescent N03.9
lobular, lobulonodular — *see* Glomerulonephritis, membranoproliferative
membranoproliferative (diffuse)(type 1 or 3) — *see also* N00-N07 with fourth character .5 N05.5
dense deposit (type 2) NEC — *see also* N00-N07 with fourth character .6 N05.6
membranous (diffuse) NEC — *see also* N00-N07 with fourth character .2 N05.2

Glomerulonephritis — *continued*
mesangial
IgA/IgG — *see* Nephropathy, IgA
proliferative (diffuse) NEC — *see also* N00-N07 with fourth character .3 N05.3
mesangiocapillary (diffuse) NEC — *see also* N00-N07 with fourth character .5 N05.5
necrotic, necrotizing NEC — *see also* N00- N07 with fourth character .8 N05.8
nodular — *see* Glomerulonephritis, membranoproliferative
poststreptococcal NEC N05.9
acute N00.9
chronic N03.9
rapidly progressive N01.9
proliferative NEC — *see also* N00-N07 with fourth character .8 N05.8
diffuse (lupus) M32.14
rapidly progressive N01.9
sclerosing, diffuse N18.9
specified pathology NEC — *see also* N00- N07 with fourth character .8 N05.8
subacute N01.9
Glomerulopathy — *see* Glomerulonephritis
Glomerulosclerosis — *see also* Sclerosis, renal
intercapillary (nodular) (with diabetes) — *see* Diabetes, glomerulosclerosis
intracapillary — *see* Diabetes, glomerulosclerosis
Glossagra K14.6
Glossalgia K14.6
Glossitis (chronic superficial) (gangrenous) (Moeller's) K14.0
areata exfoliativa K14.1
atrophic K14.4
benign migratory K14.1
cortical superficial, sclerotic K14.0
Hunter's D51.0
interstitial, sclerous K14.0
median rhomboid K14.2
pellagrous E52
superficial, chronic K14.0
Glossocele K14.8
Glossodynia K14.6
exfoliativa K14.4
Glossoncus K14.8
Glossopathy K14.9
Glossophytia K14.3
Glossoplegia K14.8
Glossoptosis K14.8
Glossopyrosis K14.6
Glossotrichia K14.3
Glossy skin L90.8
Glottis — *see* condition
Glottitis — *see also* Laryngitis J04.0
Glucagonoma
pancreas
benign D13.7
malignant C25.4
uncertain behavior D37.8
specified site NEC
benign — *see* Neoplasm, benign, by site
malignant — *see* Neoplasm, malignant, by site
uncertain behavior — *see* Neoplasm, uncertain behavior, by site
unspecified site
benign D13.7
malignant C25.4
uncertain behavior D37.8
Glucoglycinuria E72.51
Glucose-galactose malabsorption E74.39
Glue
ear — *see* Otitis, media, nonsuppurative, chronic, mucoid
sniffing (airplane) — *see* Abuse, drug, inhalant
dependence — *see* Dependence, drug, inhalant
Glutaric aciduria E72.3
Glycinemia E72.51
Glycinuria (renal) (with ketosis) E72.09
Glycogen
infiltration — *see* Disease, glycogen storage
storage disease — *see* Disease, glycogen storage
Glycogenosis (diffuse) (generalized) — *see also* Disease, glycogen storage
cardiac E74.02 *[I43]*
diabetic, secondary — *see* Diabetes, glycogenosis, secondary
pulmonary interstitial J84.842

Glycopenia E16.2
Glycosuria R81
  renal E74.8
Gnathostoma spinigerum (infection) (infestation),
  gnathostomiasis (wandering swelling) B83.1
Goiter (plunging) (substernal) E04.9
  with
    hyperthyroidism (recurrent) — see Hyperthyroidism,
      with, goiter
    thyrotoxicosis — see Hyperthyroidism, with, goiter
  adenomatous — see Goiter, nodular
  cancerous C73
  congenital (nontoxic) E03.0
    diffuse E03.0
    parenchymatous E03.0
    transitory, with normal functioning P72.0
  cystic E04.2
    due to iodine-deficiency E01.1
  due to
    enzyme defect in synthesis of thyroid hormone
      E07.1
    iodine-deficiency (endemic) E01.2
  dyshormonogenetic (familial) E07.1
  endemic (iodine-deficiency) E01.2
    diffuse E01.0
    multinodular E01.1
  exophthalmic — see Hyperthyroidism, with, goiter
  iodine-deficiency (endemic) E01.2
    diffuse E01.0
    multinodular E01.1
    nodular E01.1
  lingual Q89.2
  lymphadenoid E06.3
  malignant C73
  multinodular (cystic) (nontoxic) E04.2
    toxic or with hyperthyroidism E05.20
      with thyroid storm E05.21
  neonatal NEC P72.0
  nodular (nontoxic) (due to) E04.9
    with
      hyperthyroidism E05.20
        with thyroid storm E05.21
      thyrotoxicosis E05.20
        with thyroid storm E05.21
    endemic E01.1
    iodine-deficiency E01.1
    sporadic E04.9
    toxic E05.20
      with thyroid storm E05.21
  nontoxic E04.9
    diffuse (colloid) E04.0
    multinodular E04.2
    simple E04.0
    specified NEC E04.8
    uninodular E04.1
  simple E04.0
  toxic — see Hyperthyroidism, with, goiter
  uninodular (nontoxic) E04.1
    toxic or with hyperthyroidism E05.10
      with thyroid storm E05.11
Goiter-deafness syndrome E07.1
Goldberg syndrome Q89.8
Goldberg-Maxwell syndrome E34.51
Goldblatt's hypertension or kidney I70.1
Goldenhar (-Gorlin) **syndrome** Q87.0
Goldflam-Erb disease or syndrome G70.00
  with exacerbation (acute) G70.01
  in crisis G70.01
Goldscheider's disease Q81.8
Goldstein's disease (familial hemorrhagic telangiectasia)
  I78.0
Golfer's elbow — see Epicondylitis, medial
Gonadoblastoma
  specified site — see Neoplasm, uncertain behavior, by
    site
  unspecified site
    female D39.10
    male D40.10
Gonecystitis — see Vesiculitis
Gongylonemiasis B83.8
Goniosynechiae — see Adhesions, iris, goniosynechiae
Gonococcemia A54.86
Gonococcus, gonococcal (disease) (infection) — see
  also condition A54.9
  anus A54.6
  bursa, bursitis A54.49
  conjunctiva, conjunctivitis (neonatorum) A54.31
  endocardium A54.83

Gonococcus, gonococcal — continued
  eye A54.30
    conjunctivitis A54.31
    iridocyclitis A54.32
    keratitis A54.33
    newborn A54.31
    other specified A54.39
  fallopian tubes (acute) (chronic) A54.24
  genitourinary (organ) (system) (tract) (acute)
    lower A54.00
      with abscess (accessory gland) (periurethral)
        A54.1
    upper — see also condition A54.29
  heart A54.83
  iridocyclitis A54.32
  joint A54.42
  lymphatic (gland) (node) A54.89
  meninges, meningitis A54.81
  musculoskeletal A54.40
    arthritis A54.42
    osteomyelitis A54.43
    other specified A54.49
    spondylopathy A54.41
  pelviperitonitis A54.24
  pelvis (acute) (chronic) A54.24
  pharynx A54.5
  proctitis A54.6
  pyosalpinx (acute) (chronic) A54.24
  rectum A54.6
  skin A54.89
  specified site NEC A54.89
  tendon sheath A54.49
  throat A54.5
  urethra (acute) (chronic) A54.01
    with abscess (accessory gland) (periurethral) A54.1
  vulva (acute) (chronic) A54.02
Gonocytoma
  specified site — see Neoplasm, uncertain behavior, by
    site
  unspecified site
    female D39.10
    male D40.10
Gonorrhea (acute) (chronic) A54.9
  Bartholin's gland (acute) (chronic) (purulent) A54.02
    with abscess (accessory gland) (periurethral) A54.1
  bladder A54.01
  cervix A54.03
  conjunctiva, conjunctivitis (neonatorum) A54.31
  contact Z20.2
  Cowper's gland (with abscess) A54.1
  exposure to Z20.2
  fallopian tube (acute) (chronic) A54.24
  kidney (acute) (chronic) A54.21
  lower genitourinary tract A54.00
    with abscess (accessory gland) (periurethral) A54.1
  ovary (acute) (chronic) A54.24
  pelvis (acute) (chronic) A54.24
    female pelvic inflammatory disease A54.24
  penis A54.09
  prostate (acute) (chronic) A54.22
  seminal vesicle (acute) (chronic) A54.23
  specified site not listed — see also Gonococcus A54.89
  spermatic cord (acute) (chronic) A54.23
  urethra A54.01
    with abscess (accessory gland) (periurethral) A54.1
  vagina A54.02
  vas deferens (acute) (chronic) A54.23
  vulva A54.02
Goodall's disease A08.19
Goodpasture's syndrome M31.0
Gopalan's syndrome (burning feet) E53.0
Gorlin-Chaudry-Moss syndrome Q87.0
Gottron's papules L94.4
Gougerot-Blum syndrome (pigmented purpuric
  lichenoid dermatitis) L81.7
Gougerot-Carteaud disease or syndrome (confluent
  reticulate papillomatosis) L83
Gougerot's syndrome (trisymptomatic) L81.7
Gouley's syndrome (constrictive pericarditis) I31.1
Goundou A66.6
Gout, chronic — see also Gout, gouty M1A.9 ☑ (following
  M08)
  drug-induced M1A.20 ☑ (following M08)
    ankle M1A.27- ☑ (following M08)
    elbow M1A.22- ☑ (following M08)
    foot joint M1A.27- ☑ (following M08)
    hand joint M1A.24- ☑ (following M08)
    hip M1A.25- ☑ (following M08)

Gout, chronic — continued
  drug-induced — continued
    knee M1A.26- ☑ (following M08)
    multiple site M1A.29- ☑ (following M08)
    shoulder M1A.21- ☑ (following M08)
    vertebrae M1A.28 ☑ (following M08)
    wrist M1A.23- ☑ (following M08)
  idiopathic M1A.00 ☑ (following M08)
    ankle M1A.07- ☑ (following M08)
    elbow M1A.02- ☑ (following M08)
    foot joint M1A.07- ☑ (following M08)
    hand joint M1A.04- ☑ (following M08)
    hip M1A.05- ☑ (following M08)
    knee M1A.06- ☑ (following M08)
    multiple site M1A.09 ☑ (following M08)
    shoulder M1A.01- ☑ (following M08)
    vertebrae M1A.08 ☑ (following M08)
    wrist M1A.03- ☑ (following M08)
  in (due to) renal impairment M1A.30 ☑ (following M08)
    ankle M1A.37- ☑ (following M08)
    elbow M1A.32- ☑ (following M08)
    foot joint M1A.37- ☑ (following M08)
    hand joint M1A.34- ☑ (following M08)
    hip M1A.35- ☑ (following M08)
    knee M1A.36- ☑ (following M08)
    multiple site M1A.39 ☑ (following M08)
    shoulder M1A.31- ☑ (following M08)
    vertebrae M1A.38 ☑ (following M08)
    wrist M1A.33- ☑ (following M08)
  lead-induced M1A.10 ☑ (following M08)
    ankle M1A.17- ☑ (following M08)
    elbow M1A.12- ☑ (following M08)
    foot joint M1A.17- ☑ (following M08)
    hand joint M1A.14- ☑ (following M08)
    hip M1A.15- ☑ (following M08)
    knee M1A.16- ☑ (following M08)
    multiple site M1A.19 ☑ (following M08)
    shoulder M1A.11- ☑ (following M08)
    vertebrae M1A.18 ☑ (following M08)
    wrist M1A.13- ☑ (following M08)
  primary — see Gout, chronic, idiopathic
  saturnine — see Gout, chronic, lead-induced
  secondary NEC M1A.40 ☑ (following M08)
    ankle M1A.47- ☑ (following M08)
    elbow M1A.42- ☑ (following M08)
    foot joint M1A.47- ☑ (following M08)
    hand joint M1A.44- ☑ (following M08)
    hip M1A.45- ☑ (following M08)
    knee M1A.46- ☑ (following M08)
    multiple site M1A.49 ☑ (following M08)
    shoulder M1A.41- ☑ (following M08)
    vertebrae M1A.48 ☑ (following M08)
    wrist M1A.43- ☑ (following M08)
  syphilitic — see also subcategory M14.8- A52.77
  tophi M1A.9 ☑ (following M08)
Gout, gouty (acute) (attack) (flare) — see also Gout,
  chronic M10.9
  drug-induced M10.20
    ankle M10.27- ☑
    elbow M10.22- ☑
    foot joint M10.27- ☑
    hand joint M10.24- ☑
    hip M10.25- ☑
    knee M10.26- ☑
    multiple site M10.29
    shoulder M10.21- ☑
    vertebrae M10.28
    wrist M10.23- ☑
  idiopathic M10.00
    ankle M10.07- ☑
    elbow M10.02- ☑
    foot joint M10.07- ☑
    hand joint M10.04- ☑
    hip M10.05- ☑
    knee M10.06- ☑
    multiple site M10.09
    shoulder M10.01- ☑
    vertebrae M10.08
    wrist M10.03- ☑
  in (due to) renal impairment M10.30
    ankle M10.37- ☑
    elbow M10.32- ☑
    foot joint M10.37- ☑
    hand joint M10.34- ☑
    hip M10.35- ☑
    knee M10.36- ☑

Gout, gouty — *continued*
  in renal impairment — *continued*
    multiple site M10.39
    shoulder M10.31- ☑
    vertebrae M10.38
    wrist M10.33- ☑
  lead-induced M10.10
    ankle M10.17- ☑
    elbow M10.12- ☑
    foot joint M10.17- ☑
    hand joint M10.14- ☑
    hip M10.15- ☑
    knee M10.16- ☑
    multiple site M10.19
    shoulder M10.11- ☑
    vertebrae M10.18
    wrist M10.13- ☑
  primary — *see* Gout, idiopathic
  saturnine — *see* Gout, lead-induced
  secondary NEC M10.40
    ankle M10.47- ☑
    elbow M10.42- ☑
    foot joint M10.47- ☑
    hand joint M10.44- ☑
    hip M10.45- ☑
    knee M10.46- ☑
    multiple site M10.49
    shoulder M10.41- ☑
    vertebrae M10.48
    wrist M10.43- ☑
  syphilitic — *see also* subcategory M14.8- A52.77
  tophi — *see* Gout, chronic
ower's
  muscular dystrophy G71.01
  syndrome (vasovagal attack) R55
radenigo's syndrome — *see* Otitis, media, suppurative, acute
raefe's disease — *see* Strabismus, paralytic, ophthalmoplegia, progressive
raft-versus-host disease D89.813
  acute D89.810
  acute on chronic D89.812
  chronic D89.811
rain mite (itch) B88.0
rainhandler's disease or lung J67.8
rand mal — *see* Epilepsy, generalized, specified NEC
rand multipara status only (not pregnant) Z64.1
  pregnant — *see* Pregnancy, complicated by, grand multiparity
ranite worker's lung J62.8
ranular — *see also* condition
  inflammation, pharynx J31.2
  kidney (contracting) — *see* Sclerosis, renal
  liver K74.69
ranulation tissue (abnormal) (excessive) L92.9
  postmastoidectomy cavity — *see* Complications, postmastoidectomy, granulation
ranulocytopenia (primary) (malignant) — *see* Agranulocytosis
ranuloma L92.9
  abdomen K66.8
    from residual foreign body L92.3
    pyogenicum L98.0
  actinic L57.5
  annulare (perforating) L92.0
  apical K04.5
  aural — *see* Otitis, externa, specified NEC
  beryllium (skin) L92.3
  bone
    eosinophilic C96.6
    from residual foreign body — *see* Osteomyelitis, specified type NEC
    lung C96.6
  brain (any site) G06.0
    schistosomiasis B65.9 [G07]
  canaliculus lacrimalis — *see* Granuloma, lacrimal
  candidal (cutaneous) B37.2
  cerebral (any site) G06.0
  coccidioidal (primary) (progressive) B38.7
    lung B38.1
    meninges B38.4
  colon K63.89
  conjunctiva H11.22- ☑
  dental K04.5
  ear, middle — *see* Cholesteatoma
  eosinophilic C96.6
    bone C96.6

Granuloma — *continued*
  eosinophilic — *continued*
    lung C96.6
    oral mucosa K13.4
    skin L92.2
  eyelid H01.8
  facial (e) L92.2
  foreign body (in soft tissue) NEC M60.20
    ankle M60.27- ☑
    foot M60.27- ☑
    forearm M60.23- ☑
    hand M60.24- ☑
    in operation wound — *see* Foreign body, accidentally left during a procedure
    lower leg M60.26- ☑
    pelvic region M60.25- ☑
    shoulder region M60.21- ☑
    skin L92.3
    specified site NEC M60.28
    subcutaneous tissue L92.3
    thigh M60.25- ☑
    upper arm M60.22- ☑
  gangraenescens M31.2
  genito-inguinale A58
  giant cell (central) (reparative) (jaw) M27.1
    gingiva (peripheral) K06.8
  gland (lymph) I88.8
  hepatic NEC K75.3
    in (due to)
      berylliosis J63.2 [K77]
      sarcoidosis D86.89
  Hodgkin C81.9 ☑
  ileum K63.89
  infectious B99.9
    specified NEC B99.8
  inguinale (Donovan) (venereal) A58
  intestine NEC K63.89
  intracranial (any site) G06.0
  intraspinal (any part) G06.1
  iridocyclitis — *see* Iridocyclitis, chronic
  jaw (bone) (central) M27.1
    reparative giant cell M27.1
  kidney — *see also* Infection, kidney N15.8
  lacrimal H04.81- ☑
  larynx J38.7
  lethal midline (faciale(e)) M31.2
  liver NEC — *see* Granuloma, hepatic
  lung (infectious) — *see also* Fibrosis, lung
    coccidioidal B38.1
    eosinophilic C96.6
  Majocchi's B35.8
  malignant (facial(e)) M31.2
  mandible (central) M27.1
  midline (lethal) M31.2
  monilial (cutaneous) B37.2
  nasal sinus — *see* Sinusitis
  operation wound T81.89 ☑
    foreign body — *see* Foreign body, accidentally left during a procedure
    stitch T81.89 ☑
    talc — *see* Foreign body, accidentally left during a procedure
  oral mucosa K13.4
  orbit, orbital H05.11- ☑
  paracoccidioidal B41.8
  penis, venereal A58
  periapical K04.5
  peritoneum K66.8
    due to ova of helminths NOS — *see also* Helminthiasis B83.9 [K67]
  postmastoidectomy cavity — *see* Complications, postmastoidectomy, recurrent cholesteatoma
  prostate N42.89
  pudendi (ulcerating) A58
  pulp, internal (tooth) K03.3
  pyogenic, pyogenicum (of) (skin) L98.0
    gingiva K06.8
    maxillary alveolar ridge K04.5
    oral mucosa K13.4
  rectum K62.89
  reticulohistiocytic D76.3
  rubrum nasi L74.8
  Schistosoma — *see* Schistosomiasis
  septic (skin) L98.0
  silica (skin) L92.3
  sinus (accessory) (infective) (nasal) — *see* Sinusitis
  skin L92.9
    from residual foreign body L92.3

Granuloma — *continued*
  skin — *continued*
    pyogenicum L98.0
  spine
    syphilitic (epidural) A52.19
    tuberculous A18.01
  stitch (postoperative) T81.89 ☑
  suppurative (skin) L98.0
  swimming pool A31.1
  talc — *see also* Granuloma, foreign body
    in operation wound — *see* Foreign body, accidentally left during a procedure
  telangiectaticum (skin) L98.0
  tracheostomy J95.09
  trichophyticum B35.8
  tropicum A66.4
  umbilical P83.81
  umbilicus P83.81
  urethra N36.8
  uveitis — *see* Iridocyclitis, chronic
  vagina A58
  venereum A58
  vocal cord J38.3
Granulomatosis L92.9
  lymphoid C83.8- ☑
  miliary (listerial) A32.89
  necrotizing, respiratory M31.30
  progressive septic D71
  specified NEC L92.8
  Wegener's M31.30
    with renal involvement M31.31
Granulomatous tissue (abnormal) (excessive) L92.9
Granulosis rubra nasi L74.8
Graphite fibrosis (of lung) J63.3
Graphospasm F48.8
  organic G25.89
Grating scapula M89.8X1
Gravel (urinary) — *see* Calculus, urinary
Graves' disease — *see* Hyperthyroidism, with, goiter
Gravis — *see* condition
Grawitz tumor C64.- ☑
Gray syndrome (newborn) P93.0
Grayness, hair (premature) L67.1
  congenital Q84.2
Green sickness D50.8
Greenfield's disease
  meaning
    concentric sclerosis (encephalitis periaxialis concentrica) G37.5
    metachromatic leukodystrophy E75.25
Greenstick fracture — *code as* Fracture, by site
Grey syndrome (newborn) P93.0
Grief F43.21
  prolonged F43.29
  reaction — *see also* Disorder, adjustment F43.20
Griesinger's disease B76.0
Grinder's lung or pneumoconiosis J62.8
Grinding, teeth
  psychogenic F45.8
  sleep related G47.63
Grip
  Dabney's B33.0
  devil's B33.0
Grippe, grippal — *see also* Influenza
  Balkan A78
  summer, of Italy A93.1
Grisel's disease M43.6
Groin — *see* condition
Grooved tongue K14.5
Ground itch B76.9
Grover's disease or syndrome L11.1
Growing pains, children R29.898
Growth (fungoid) (neoplastic) (new) — *see also* Neoplasm
  adenoid (vegetative) J35.8
  benign — *see* Neoplasm, benign, by site
  malignant — *see* Neoplasm, malignant, by site
  rapid, childhood Z00.2
  secondary — *see* Neoplasm, secondary, by site
Gruby's disease B35.0
Gubler-Millard paralysis or syndrome G46.3
Guerin-Stern syndrome Q74.3
Guidance, insufficient anterior (occlusal) M26.54
Guillain-Barré disease or syndrome G61.0
  sequelae G65.0
Guinea worms (infection) (infestation) B72
Guinon's disease (motor-verbal tic) F95.2
Gull's disease E03.4

▽ **Subterms under main terms may continue to next column or page**   ☑ **Additional Character Required — Refer to the Tabular List for Character Selection**   **161**

Gout, gouty — Gull's disease

Gum — see condition
Gumboil K04.7
  with sinus K04.6
Gumma (syphilitic) A52.79
  artery A52.09
    cerebral A52.04
  bone A52.77
    of yaws (late) A66.6
  brain A52.19
  cauda equina A52.19
  central nervous system A52.3
  ciliary body A52.71
  congenital A50.59
  eyelid A52.71
  heart A52.06
  intracranial A52.19
  iris A52.71
  kidney A52.75
  larynx A52.73
  leptomeninges A52.19
  liver A52.74
  meninges A52.19
  myocardium A52.06
  nasopharynx A52.73
  neurosyphilitic A52.3
  nose A52.73
  orbit A52.71
  palate (soft) A52.79
  penis A52.76
  pericardium A52.06
  pharynx A52.73
  pituitary A52.79
  scrofulous (tuberculous) A18.4
  skin A52.79
  specified site NEC A52.79
  spinal cord A52.19
  tongue A52.79
  tonsil A52.73
  trachea A52.73
  tuberculous A18.4
  ulcerative due to yaws A66.4
  ureter A52.75
  yaws A66.4
    bone A66.6
Gunn's syndrome Q07.8
Gunshot wound — see also Wound, open
  fracture — code as Fracture, by site
  internal organs — see Injury, by site
Gynandrism Q56.0
Gynandroblastoma
  specified site — see Neoplasm, uncertain behavior, by site
  unspecified site
    female D39.10
    male D40.10
Gynecological examination (periodic) (routine) Z01.419
  with abnormal findings Z01.411
Gynecomastia N62
Gynephobia F40.291
Gyrate scalp Q82.8

H

H (Hartnup's) **disease** E72.02
Haas' disease or osteochondrosis (juvenile) (head of humerus) — see Osteochondrosis, juvenile, humerus
Habit, habituation
  bad sleep Z72.821
  chorea F95.8
  disturbance, child F98.9
  drug — see Dependence, drug
  irregular sleep Z72.821
  laxative F55.2
  spasm — see Tic
  tic — see Tic
Haemophilus (H.) **influenzae, as cause of disease classified elsewhere** B96.3
Haff disease — see Poisoning, mercury
Hageman's factor defect, deficiency or disease D68.2
Haglund's disease or osteochondrosis (juvenile) (os tibiale externum) — see Osteochondrosis, juvenile, tarsus
Hailey-Hailey disease Q82.8
Hair — see also condition
  plucking F63.3
    in stereotyped movement disorder F98.4
  tourniquet syndrome — see also Constriction, external, by site

Hair — continued
  tourniquet syndrome — see also Constriction, external, by site — continued
    finger S60.44- ☑
    penis S30.842 ☑
    thumb S60.34- ☑
    toe S90.44- ☑
Hairball in stomach T18.2 ☑
Hair-pulling, pathological (compulsive) F63.3
Hairy black tongue K14.3
Half vertebra Q76.49
Halitosis R19.6
Hallerman-Streiff syndrome Q87.0
Hallervorden-Spatz disease G23.0
Hallopeau's acrodermatitis or disease L40.2
Hallucination R44.3
  auditory R44.0
  gustatory R44.2
  olfactory R44.2
  specified NEC R44.2
  tactile R44.2
  visual R44.1
Hallucinosis (chronic) F28
  alcoholic (acute) F10.951
    in
      abuse F10.151
      dependence F10.251
  drug-induced F19.951
    cannabis F12.951
    cocaine F14.951
    hallucinogen F16.151
    in
      abuse F19.151
        cannabis F12.151
        cocaine F14.151
        hallucinogen F16.151
        inhalant F18.151
        opioid F11.151
        sedative, anxiolytic or hypnotic F13.151
        stimulant NEC F15.151
      dependence F19.251
        cannabis F12.251
        cocaine F14.251
        hallucinogen F16.251
        inhalant F18.251
        opioid F11.251
        sedative, anxiolytic or hypnotic F13.251
        stimulant NEC F15.251
    inhalant F18.951
    opioid F11.951
    sedative, anxiolytic or hypnotic F13.951
    stimulant NEC F15.951
  organic F06.0
Hallux
  deformity (acquired) NEC M20.5X- ☑
  limitus M20.5X- ☑
  malleus (acquired) NEC M20.3- ☑
  rigidus (acquired) M20.2- ☑
    congenital Q74.2
    sequelae (late effect) of rickets E64.3
  valgus (acquired) M20.1- ☑
    congenital Q66.6
  varus (acquired) M20.3- ☑
    congenital Q66.3- ☑
Halo, visual H53.19
Hamartoma, hamartoblastoma Q85.9
  epithelial (gingival), odontogenic, central or peripheral — see Cyst, calcifying odontogenic
Hamartosis Q85.9
Hamman-Rich syndrome J84.114
Hammer toe (acquired) NEC — see also Deformity, toe, hammer toe
  congenital Q66.89
  sequelae (late effect) of rickets E64.3
Hand — see condition
Hand-foot syndrome L27.1
Handicap, handicapped
  educational Z55.9
    specified NEC Z55.8
Hand-Schüller-Christian disease or syndrome C96.5
Hanging (asphyxia) (strangulation) (suffocation) — see Asphyxia, traumatic, due to mechanical threat
Hangnail — see also Cellulitis, digit
  with lymphangitis — see Lymphangitis, acute, digit
Hangover (alcohol) F10.129
Hanhart's syndrome Q87.0
Hanot-Chauffard (-Troisier) **syndrome** E83.19

Hanot's cirrhosis or disease K74.3
Hansen's disease — see Leprosy
Hantaan virus disease (Korean hemorrhagic fever) A98
Hantavirus disease (with renal manifestations) (Dobrav (Puumala) (Seoul) A98.5
  with pulmonary manifestations (Andes) (Bayou) (Bermejo) (Black Creek Canal) (Choclo) (Juquitib (Laguna negra) (Lechiguanas) (New York) (Ora (Sin nombre) B33.4
Happy puppet syndrome Q93.51
Harada's disease or syndrome H30.81- ☑
Hardening
  artery — see Arteriosclerosis
  brain G93.89
Harelip (complete) (incomplete) — see Cleft, lip
Harlequin (newborn) Q80.4
Harley's disease D59.6
Harmful use (of)
  alcohol F10.10
  anxiolytics — see Abuse, drug, sedative
  cannabinoids — see Abuse, drug, cannabis
  cocaine — see Abuse, drug, cocaine
  drug — see Abuse, drug
  hallucinogens — see Abuse, drug, hallucinogen
  hypnotics — see Abuse, drug, sedative
  opioids — see Abuse, drug, opioid
  PCP (phencyclidine) — see Abuse, drug, hallucinoge
  sedatives — see Abuse, drug, sedative
  stimulants NEC — see Abuse, drug, stimulant
Harris' lines — see Arrest, epiphyseal
Hartnup's disease E72.02
Harvester's lung J67.0
Harvesting ovum for in vitro fertilization Z31.83
Hashimoto's disease or thyroiditis E06.3
Hashitoxicosis (transient) E06.3
Hassal-Henle bodies or warts (cornea) H18.49
Haut mal — see Epilepsy, generalized, specified NEC
Haverhill fever A25.1
Hay fever — see also Fever, hay J30.1
Hayem-Widal syndrome D59.8
Haygarth's nodes M15.8
Haymaker's lung J67.0
Hb (abnormal)
  Bart's disease D56.0
  disease — see Disease, hemoglobin
  trait — see Trait
Head — see condition
Headache R51
  allergic NEC G44.89
  associated with sexual activity G44.82
  chronic daily R51
  cluster G44.009
    chronic G44.029
      intractable G44.021
      not intractable G44.029
    episodic G44.019
      intractable G44.011
      not intractable G44.019
    intractable G44.001
    not intractable G44.009
  cough (primary) G44.83
  daily chronic R51
  drug-induced NEC G44.40
    intractable G44.41
    not intractable G44.40
  exertional (primary) G44.84
  histamine G44.009
    intractable G44.001
    not intractable G44.009
  hypnic G44.81
  lumbar puncture G97.1
  medication overuse G44.40
    intractable G44.41
    not intractable G44.40
  menstrual — see Migraine, menstrual
  migraine (type) — see also Migraine G43.909
  nasal septum R51
  neuralgiform, short lasting unilateral, with conjunctiv injection and tearing (SUNCT) G44.059
    intractable G44.051
    not intractable G44.059
  new daily persistent (NDPH) G44.52
  orgasmic G44.82
  periodic syndromes in adults and children G43.C0 (fo lowing G43.7)
    with refractory migraine G43.C1 (following G43.7
    intractable G43.C1 (following G43.7)

  ☑ **Additional Character Required** — Refer to the Tabular List for Character Selection   ▽ **Subterms under main terms may continue to next column or pag**

Headache — *continued*
  periodic syndromes in adults and children — *contin-*
    ued
    not intractable G43.C0 (*following* G43.7)
    without refractory migraine G43.C0 (*following* G43.7)
  postspinal puncture G97.1
  post-traumatic G44.309
    acute G44.319
      intractable G44.311
      not intractable G44.319
    chronic G44.329
      intractable G44.321
      not intractable G44.329
    intractable G44.301
    not intractable G44.309
  pre-menstrual — *see* Migraine, menstrual
  preorgasmic G44.82
  primary
    cough G44.83
    exertional G44.84
    stabbing G44.85
    thunderclap G44.53
  rebound G44.40
    intractable G44.41
    not intractable G44.40
  short lasting unilateral neuralgiform, with conjunctival
    injection and tearing (SUNCT) G44.059
    intractable G44.051
    not intractable G44.059
  specified syndrome NEC G44.89
  spinal and epidural anesthesia - induced T88.59 ☑
    in labor and delivery O74.5
    in pregnancy O29.4- ☑
    postpartum, puerperal O89.4
  spinal fluid loss (from puncture) G97.1
  stabbing (primary) G44.85
  tension (-type) G44.209
    chronic G44.229
      intractable G44.221
      not intractable G44.229
    episodic G44.219
      intractable G44.211
      not intractable G44.219
    intractable G44.201
    not intractable G44.209
  thunderclap (primary) G44.53
  vascular NEC G44.1
Healthy
  infant
    accompanying sick mother Z76.3
    receiving care Z76.2
  person accompanying sick person Z76.3
Hearing examination Z01.10
  with abnormal findings NEC Z01.118
  following failed hearing screening Z01.110
  for hearing conservation and treatment Z01.12
  infant or child (over 28 days old) Z00.129
    with abnormal findings Z00.121
Heart — *see* condition
Heart beat
  abnormality R00.9
    specified NEC R00.8
  awareness R00.2
  rapid R00.0
  slow R00.1
Heartburn R12
  psychogenic F45.8
Heartland virus disease A93.8
Heat (effects) T67.9 ☑
  apoplexy T67.01 ☑
  burn — *see also* Burn L55.9
  collapse T67.1 ☑
  cramps T67.2 ☑
  dermatitis or eczema L59.0
  edema T67.7 ☑
  erythema — *code by site under* Burn, first degree
  excessive T67.9 ☑
    specified effect NEC T67.8 ☑
  exhaustion T67.5 ☑
    anhydrotic T67.3 ☑
    due to
      salt (and water) depletion T67.4 ☑
      water depletion T67.3 ☑
        with salt depletion T67.4 ☑
  fatigue (transient) T67.6 ☑
  fever T67.01 ☑
  hyperpyrexia T67.01 ☑
  prickly L74.0

Heat — *continued*
  prostration — *see* Heat, exhaustion
  pyrexia T67.01 ☑
  rash L74.0
  specified effect NEC T67.8 ☑
  stroke T67.01 ☑
    exertional T67.02 ☑
    specified NEC T67.09 ☑
  sunburn — *see* Sunburn
  syncope T67.1 ☑
Heavy-for-dates NEC (infant) (4000g to 4499g) P08.1
  exceptionally (4500g or more) P08.0
Hebephrenia, hebephrenic (schizophrenia) F20.1
Heberden's disease or nodes (with arthropathy) M15.1
Hebra's
  pityriasis L26
  prurigo L28.2
Heel — *see* condition
Heerfordt's disease D86.89
Hegglin's anomaly or syndrome D72.0
Heilmeyer-Schoner disease D45
Heine-Medin disease A80.9
Heinz body anemia, congenital D58.2
Heliophobia F40.228
Heller's disease or syndrome F84.3
HELLP syndrome (hemolysis, elevated liver enzymes and
    low platelet count) O14.2- ☑
  complicating
    childbirth O14.24
    puerperium O14.25
Helminthiasis — *see also* Infestation, helminth
  Ancylostoma B76.0
  intestinal B82.0
    mixed types (types classifiable to more than one of
      the titles B65.0-B81.3 and B81.8) B81.4
    specified type NEC B81.8
  mixed types (intestinal) (types classifiable to more than
    one of the titles B65.0-B81.3 and B81.8) B81.4
  Necator (americanus) B76.1
  specified type NEC B83.8
Heloma L84
Hemangioblastoma — *see* Neoplasm, connective tissue,
  uncertain behavior
  malignant — *see* Neoplasm, connective tissue, malig-
    nant
Hemangioendothelioma — *see also* Neoplasm, uncertain behavior, by site
  benign D18.00
    intra-abdominal D18.03
    intracranial D18.02
    skin D18.01
    specified site NEC D18.09
  bone (diffuse) — *see* Neoplasm, bone, malignant
  epithelioid — *see also* Neoplasm, uncertain behavior,
    by site
    malignant — *see* Neoplasm, malignant, by site
  malignant — *see* Neoplasm, connective tissue, malig-
    nant
Hemangiofibroma — *see* Neoplasm, benign, by site
Hemangiolipoma — *see* Lipoma
Hemangioma D18.00
  arteriovenous D18.00
    intra-abdominal D18.03
    intracranial D18.02
    skin D18.01
    specified site NEC D18.09
  capillary I78.1
    intra-abdominal D18.03
    intracranial D18.02
    skin D18.01
    specified site NEC D18.09
  cavernous D18.00
    intra-abdominal D18.03
    intracranial D18.02
    skin D18.01
    specified site NEC D18.09
  epithelioid D18.00
    intra-abdominal D18.03
    intracranial D18.02
    skin D18.01
    specified site NEC D18.09
  histiocytoid D18.00
    intra-abdominal D18.03
    intracranial D18.02
    skin D18.01
    specified site NEC D18.09
  infantile D18.00
    intra-abdominal D18.03

Hemangioma — *continued*
  infantile — *continued*
    intracranial D18.02
    skin D18.01
    specified site NEC D18.09
  intra-abdominal D18.03
  intracranial D18.02
  intramuscular D18.00
    intra-abdominal D18.03
    intracranial D18.02
    skin D18.01
    specified site NEC D18.09
  intrathoracic structures D18.09
  juvenile D18.00
  malignant — *see* Neoplasm, connective tissue, malig-
    nant
  plexiform D18.00
    intra-abdominal D18.03
    intracranial D18.02
    skin D18.01
    specified site NEC D18.09
  racemose D18.00
    intra-abdominal D18.03
    intracranial D18.02
    skin D18.01
    specified site NEC D18.09
  sclerosing — *see* Neoplasm, skin, benign
  simplex D18.00
    intra-abdominal D18.03
    intracranial D18.02
    skin D18.01
    specified site NEC D18.09
  skin D18.01
  specified site NEC D18.09
  venous D18.00
    intra-abdominal D18.03
    intracranial D18.02
    skin D18.01
    specified site NEC D18.09
  verrucous keratotic D18.00
    intra-abdominal D18.03
    intracranial D18.02
    skin D18.01
    specified site NEC D18.09
Hemangiomatosis (systemic) I78.8
  involving single site — *see* Hemangioma
Hemangiopericytoma — *see also* Neoplasm, connective
  tissue, uncertain behavior
  benign — *see* Neoplasm, connective tissue, benign
  malignant — *see* Neoplasm, connective tissue, malig-
    nant
Hemangiosarcoma — *see* Neoplasm, connective tissue,
  malignant
Hemarthrosis (nontraumatic) M25.00
  ankle M25.07- ☑
  elbow M25.02- ☑
  foot joint M25.07- ☑
  hand joint M25.04- ☑
  hip M25.05- ☑
  in hemophilic arthropathy — *see* Arthropathy,
    hemophilic
  knee M25.06- ☑
  shoulder M25.01- ☑
  specified joint NEC M25.08
  traumatic — *see* Sprain, by site
  vertebrae M25.08
  wrist M25.03- ☑
Hematemesis K92.0
  with ulcer — *code by site under* Ulcer, with hemorrhage
    K27.4
  newborn, neonatal P54.0
    due to swallowed maternal blood P78.2
Hematidrosis L74.8
Hematinuria — *see also* Hemoglobinuria
  malarial B50.8
Hematobilia K83.8
Hematocele
  female NEC N94.89
    with ectopic pregnancy O00.90
      with intrauterine pregnancy O00.91
    ovary N83.8
  male N50.1
Hematochezia — *see also* Melena K92.1
Hematochyluria — *see also* Infestation, filarial
  schistosomiasis (bilharziasis) B65.0
Hematocolpos (with hematometra or hematosalpinx)
  N89.7
Hematocornea — *see* Pigmentation, cornea, stromal

▼ Subterms under main terms may continue to next column or page   ☑ Additional Character Required — Refer to the Tabular List for Character Selection   163

Headache — Hematocornea

Hematogenous — *see* condition

Hematoma (traumatic) (skin surface intact) — *see also* Contusion
- with
  - injury of internal organs — *see* Injury, by site
  - open wound — *see* Wound, open
- amputation stump (surgical) (late) T87.89
- aorta, dissecting I71.00
  - abdominal I71.02
  - thoracic I71.01
  - thoracoabdominal I71.03
- aortic intramural — *see* Dissection, aorta
- arterial (complicating trauma) — *see* Injury, blood vessel, by site
- auricle — *see* Contusion, ear
  - nontraumatic — *see* Disorder, pinna, hematoma
- birth injury NEC P15.8
- brain (traumatic)
  - with
    - cerebral laceration or contusion (diffuse) — *see* Injury, intracranial, diffuse
      - focal — *see* Injury, intracranial, focal
  - cerebellar, traumatic S06.37- ☑
  - intracerebral, traumatic — *see* Injury, intracranial, intracerebral hemorrhage
    - newborn NEC P52.4
      - birth injury P10.1
    - nontraumatic — *see* Hemorrhage, intracranial
  - subarachnoid, arachnoid, traumatic — *see* Injury, intracranial, subarachnoid hemorrhage
  - subdural, traumatic — *see* Injury, intracranial, subdural hemorrhage
- breast (nontraumatic) N64.89
- broad ligament (nontraumatic) N83.7
  - traumatic S37.892 ☑
- cerebellar, traumatic S06.37- ☑
- cerebral — *see* Hematoma, brain
- cerebrum S06.36- ☑
  - left S06.35- ☑
  - right S06.34- ☑
- cesarean delivery wound O90.2
- complicating delivery (perineal) (pelvic) (vagina) (vulva) O71.7
- corpus cavernosum (nontraumatic) N48.89
- epididymis (nontraumatic) N50.1
- epidural (traumatic) — *see* Injury, intracranial, epidural hemorrhage
  - spinal — *see* Injury, spinal cord, by region
- episiotomy O90.2
- face, birth injury P15.4
- genital organ NEC (nontraumatic)
  - female (nonobstetric) N94.89
    - traumatic S30.202 ☑
  - male N50.1
    - traumatic S30.201 ☑
- internal organs — *see* Injury, by site
- intracerebral, traumatic — *see* Injury, intracranial, intracerebral hemorrhage
- intraoperative — *see* Complications, intraoperative, hemorrhage
- labia (nontraumatic) (nonobstetric) N90.89
- liver (subcapsular) (nontraumatic) K76.89
  - birth injury P15.0
- mediastinum — *see* Injury, intrathoracic
- mesosalpinx (nontraumatic) N83.7
  - traumatic S37.898 ☑
- muscle — code by site under Contusion
- nontraumatic
  - muscle M79.81
  - soft tissue M79.81
- obstetrical surgical wound O90.2
- orbit, orbital (nontraumatic) — *see also* Hemorrhage, orbit
  - traumatic — *see* Contusion, orbit
- pelvis (female) (nontraumatic) (nonobstetric) N94.89
  - obstetric O71.7
  - traumatic — *see* Injury, by site
- penis (nontraumatic) N48.89
  - birth injury P15.5
- perianal (nontraumatic) K64.5
- perineal S30.23 ☑
  - complicating delivery O71.7
- perirenal — *see* Injury, kidney
- pinna — *see* Contusion, ear
  - nontraumatic — *see* Disorder, pinna, hematoma
- placenta O43.89- ☑

Hematoma — *continued*
- postoperative (postprocedural) — *see* Complication, postprocedural, hematoma
- retroperitoneal (nontraumatic) K66.1
  - traumatic S36.892 ☑
- scrotum, superficial S30.22 ☑
  - birth injury P15.5
- seminal vesicle (nontraumatic) N50.1
  - traumatic S37.892 ☑
- spermatic cord (traumatic) S37.892 ☑
  - nontraumatic N50.1
- spinal (cord) (meninges) — *see also* Injury, spinal cord, by region
  - newborn (birth injury) P11.5
- spleen D73.5
  - intraoperative — *see* Complications, intraoperative, hemorrhage, spleen
  - postprocedural (postoperative) — *see* Complications, postprocedural, hemorrhage, spleen
- sternocleidomastoid, birth injury P15.2
- sternomastoid, birth injury P15.2
- subarachnoid (traumatic) — *see* Injury, intracranial, subarachnoid hemorrhage
  - newborn (nontraumatic) P52.5
    - due to birth injury P10.3
  - nontraumatic — *see* Hemorrhage, intracranial, subarachnoid
- subdural (traumatic) — *see* Injury, intracranial, subdural hemorrhage
  - newborn (localized) P52.8
    - birth injury P10.0
  - nontraumatic — *see* Hemorrhage, intracranial, subdural
- superficial, newborn P54.5
- testis (nontraumatic) N50.1
  - birth injury P15.5
- tunica vaginalis (nontraumatic) N50.1
- umbilical cord, complicating delivery O69.5 ☑
- uterine ligament (broad) (nontraumatic) N83.7
  - traumatic S37.892 ☑
- vagina (ruptured) (nontraumatic) N89.8
  - complicating delivery O71.7
- vas deferens (nontraumatic) N50.1
  - traumatic S37.892 ☑
- vitreous — *see* Hemorrhage, vitreous
- vulva (nontraumatic) (nonobstetric) N90.89
  - complicating delivery O71.7
  - newborn (birth injury) P15.5

Hematometra N85.7
- with hematocolpos N89.7

Hematomyelia (central) G95.19
- newborn (birth injury) P11.5
- traumatic T14.8 ☑

Hematomyelitis G04.90

Hematoperitoneum — *see* Hemoperitoneum

Hematophobia F40.230

Hematopneumothorax (see Hemothorax)

Hematopoiesis, cyclic D70.4

Hematoporphyria — *see* Porphyria

Hematorachis, hematorrhachis G95.19
- newborn (birth injury) P11.5

Hematosalpinx N83.6
- with
  - hematocolpos N89.7
  - hematometra N85.7
    - with hematocolpos N89.7
- infectional — *see* Salpingitis

Hematospermia R36.1

Hematothorax (see Hemothorax)

Hematuria R31.9
- benign (familial) (of childhood) — *see also* Hematuria, idiopathic
  - essential microscopic R31.1
- due to sulphonamide, sulfonamide — *see* Table of Drugs and Chemicals, by drug
- endemic — *see also* Schistosomiasis B65.0
- gross R31.0
- idiopathic N02.9
  - with glomerular lesion
    - crescentic (diffuse) glomerulonephritis N02.7
    - dense deposit disease N02.6
    - endocapillary proliferative glomerulonephritis N02.4
    - focal and segmental hyalinosis or sclerosis N02.1
    - membranoproliferative (diffuse) N02.5
    - membranous (diffuse) N02.2
    - mesangial proliferative (diffuse) N02.3
    - mesangiocapillary (diffuse) N02.5

Hematuria — *continued*
- idiopathic — *continued*
  - with glomerular lesion — *continued*
    - minor abnormality N02.0
    - proliferative NEC N02.8
    - specified pathology NEC N02.8
  - intermittent — *see* Hematuria, idiopathic
- malarial B50.8
- microscopic NEC (with symptoms) R31.29
  - asymptomatic R31.21
  - benign essential R31.1
- paroxysmal — *see also* Hematuria, idiopathic
  - nocturnal D59.5
- persistent — *see* Hematuria, idiopathic
- recurrent — *see* Hematuria, idiopathic
- tropical — *see also* Schistosomiasis B65.0
- tuberculous A18.13

Hemeralopia (day blindness) H53.11
- vitamin A deficiency E50.5

Hemi-akinesia R41.4

Hemianalgesia R20.0

Hemianencephaly Q00.0

Hemianesthesia R20.0

Hemianopia, hemianopsia (heteronymous) H53.47
- homonymous H53.46- ☑
- syphilitic A52.71

Hemiathetosis R25.8

Hemiatrophy R68.89
- cerebellar G31.9
- face, facial, progressive (Romberg) G51.8
- tongue K14.8

Hemiballism (us) G25.5

Hemicardia Q24.8

Hemicephalus, hemicephaly Q00.0

Hemichorea G25.5

Hemicolitis, left — *see* Colitis, left sided

Hemicrania
- congenital malformation Q00.0
- continua G44.51
- meaning migraine — *see also* Migraine G43.909
- paroxysmal G44.039
  - chronic G44.049
    - intractable G44.041
    - not intractable G44.049
  - episodic G44.039
    - intractable G44.031
    - not intractable G44.039
  - intractable G44.031
  - not intractable G44.039

Hemidystrophy — *see* Hemiatrophy

Hemiectromelia Q73.8

Hemihypalgesia R20.8

Hemihypesthesia R20.1

Hemi-inattention R41.4

Hemimelia Q73.8
- lower limb — *see* Defect, reduction, lower limb, specified type NEC
- upper limb — *see* Defect, reduction, upper limb, specified type NEC

Hemiparalysis — *see* Hemiplegia

Hemiparesis — *see* Hemiplegia

Hemiparesthesia R20.2

Hemiparkinsonism G20

Hemiplegia G81.9- ☑
- alternans facialis G83.89
- ascending NEC G81.90
  - spinal G95.89
- congenital (cerebral) G80.8
  - spastic G80.2
- embolic (current episode) I63.4- ☑
- flaccid G81.0- ☑
- following
  - cerebrovascular disease I69.959
    - cerebral infarction I69.35- ☑
    - intracerebral hemorrhage I69.15- ☑
    - nontraumatic intracranial hemorrhage NEC I69.25- ☑
    - specified disease NEC I69.85- ☑
    - stroke NOS I69.35- ☑
    - subarachnoid hemorrhage I69.05- ☑
- hysterical F44.4
- newborn NEC P91.88
  - birth injury P11.9
- spastic G81.1- ☑
  - congenital G80.2
- thrombotic (current episode) I63.3- ☑

Hemisection, spinal cord — *see* Injury, spinal cord, by region
Hemispasm (facial) R25.2
Hemisporosis B48.8
Hemitremor R25.1
Hemivertebra Q76.49
  failure of segmentation with scoliosis Q76.3
  fusion with scoliosis Q76.3
Hemochromatosis E83.119
  with refractory anemia D46.1
  due to repeated red blood cell transfusion E83.111
  hereditary (primary) E83.110
  neonatal P78.84
  primary E83.110
  specified NEC E83.118
Hemoglobin — *see also* condition
  abnormal (disease) — *see* Disease, hemoglobin
  AS genotype D57.3
  Constant Spring D58.2
  E-beta thalassemia D56.5
  fetal, hereditary persistence (HPFH) D56.4
  H Constant Spring D56.0
  low NOS D64.9
  S (Hb S), heterozygous D57.3
Hemoglobinemia D59.9
  due to blood transfusion T80.89 ☑
  paroxysmal D59.6
    nocturnal D59.5
Hemoglobinopathy (mixed) D58.2
  with thalassemia D56.8
  sickle-cell D57.1
    with thalassemia D57.40
      with crisis (vasoocclusive pain) D57.419
        with
          acute chest syndrome D57.411
          splenic sequestration D57.412
      without crisis D57.40
Hemoglobinuria R82.3
  with anemia, hemolytic, acquired (chronic) NEC D59.6
  cold (agglutinin) (paroxysmal) (with Raynaud's syndrome) D59.6
  due to exertion or hemolysis NEC D59.6
  intermittent D59.6
  malarial B50.8
  march D59.6
  nocturnal (paroxysmal) D59.5
  paroxysmal (cold) D59.6
    nocturnal D59.5
Hemolymphangioma D18.1
Hemolysis
  intravascular
    with
      abortion — *see* Abortion, by type, complicated by, hemorrhage
      ectopic or molar pregnancy O08.1
      hemorrhage
        antepartum — *see* Hemorrhage, antepartum, with coagulation defect
        intrapartum — *see also* Hemorrhage, complicating, delivery O67.0
      postpartum O72.3
  neonatal (excessive) P58.9
    specified NEC P58.8
Hemolytic — *see* condition
Hemopericardium I31.2
  following acute myocardial infarction (current complication) I23.0
  newborn P54.8
  traumatic — *see* Injury, heart, with hemopericardium
Hemoperitoneum K66.1
  infectional K65.9
  traumatic S36.899 ☑
    with open wound — *see* Wound, open, with penetration into peritoneal cavity
Hemophilia (classical) (familial) (hereditary) D66
  A D66
    acquired D68.311
    autoimmune D68.311
  B D67
  C D68.1
  calcipriva — *see also* Defect, coagulation D68.4
  nonfamilial — *see also* Defect, coagulation D68.4
  secondary D68.311
  vascular D68.0
Hemophthalmos H44.81- ☑
Hemopneumothorax — *see also* Hemothorax
  traumatic S27.2 ☑
Hemoptysis R04.2

Hemoptysis — *continued*
  newborn P26.9
  tuberculous — *see* Tuberculosis, pulmonary
Hemorrhage, hemorrhagic (concealed) R58
  abdomen R58
  accidental antepartum — *see* Hemorrhage, antepartum
  acute idiopathic pulmonary, in infants R04.81
  adenoid J35.8
  adrenal (capsule) (gland) E27.49
    medulla E27.8
    newborn P54.4
  after delivery — *see* Hemorrhage, postpartum
  alveolar
    lung, newborn P26.8
    process K08.89
  alveolus K08.89
  amputation stump (surgical) T87.89
  anemia (chronic) D50.0
    acute D62
  antepartum (with) O46.90
    with coagulation defect O46.00- ☑
      afibrinogenemia O46.01- ☑
      disseminated intravascular coagulation O46.02- ☑
      hypofibrinogenemia O46.01- ☑
      specified defect NEC O46.09- ☑
    before 20 weeks gestation O20.9
      specified type NEC O20.8
      threatened abortion O20.0
    due to
      abruptio placenta — *see also* Abruptio placentae O45.9- ☑
      leiomyoma, uterus — *see* Hemorrhage, antepartum, specified cause NEC
      placenta previa O44.1- ☑
    specified cause NEC — *see* subcategory O46.8X- ☑
  anus (sphincter) K62.5
  apoplexy (stroke) — *see* Hemorrhage, intracranial, intracerebral
  arachnoid — *see* Hemorrhage, intracranial, subarachnoid
  artery R58
    brain — *see* Hemorrhage, intracranial, intracerebral
  basilar (ganglion) I61.0
  bladder N32.89
  bowel K92.2
    newborn P54.3
  brain (miliary) (nontraumatic) — *see* Hemorrhage, intracranial, intracerebral
    due to
      birth injury P10.1
      syphilis A52.05
    epidural or extradural (traumatic) — *see* Injury, intracranial, epidural hemorrhage
    newborn P52.4
      birth injury P10.1
    subarachnoid — *see* Hemorrhage, intracranial, subarachnoid
    subdural — *see* Hemorrhage, intracranial, subdural
  brainstem (nontraumatic) I61.3
    traumatic S06.38- ☑
  breast N64.59
  bronchial tube — *see* Hemorrhage, lung
  bronchopulmonary — *see* Hemorrhage, lung
  bronchus — *see* Hemorrhage, lung
  bulbar I61.5
  capillary I78.8
    primary D69.8
  cecum K92.2
  cerebellar, cerebellum (nontraumatic) I61.4
    newborn P52.6
    traumatic S06.37- ☑
  cerebral, cerebrum — *see also* Hemorrhage, intracranial, intracerebral
    lobe I61.1
    newborn (anoxic) P52.4
      birth injury P10.1
  cerebromeningeal I61.8
  cerebrospinal — *see* Hemorrhage, intracranial, intracerebral
  cervix (uteri) (stump) NEC N88.8
  chamber, anterior (eye) — *see* Hyphema
  childbirth — *see* Hemorrhage, complicating, delivery
  choroid H31.30- ☑
    expulsive H31.31- ☑
  ciliary body — *see* Hyphema
  cochlea — *see* subcategory H83.8 ☑
  colon K92.2

Hemorrhage, hemorrhagic — *continued*
  complicating
    abortion — *see* Abortion, by type, complicated by, hemorrhage
    delivery O67.9
      associated with coagulation defect (afibrinogenemia) (DIC) (hyperfibrinolysis) O67.0
      specified cause NEC O67.8
    surgical procedure — *see* Hemorrhage, intraoperative
  conjunctiva H11.3- ☑
    newborn P54.8
  cord, newborn (stump) P51.9
  corpus luteum (ruptured) cyst N83.1- ☑
  cortical (brain) I61.1
  cranial — *see* Hemorrhage, intracranial
  cutaneous R23.3
    due to autosensitivity, erythrocyte D69.2
    newborn P54.5
  delayed
    following ectopic or molar pregnancy O08.1
    postpartum O72.2
  diathesis (familial) D69.9
  disease D69.9
    newborn P53
    specified type NEC D69.8
  due to or associated with
    afibrinogenemia or other coagulation defect (conditions in categories D65- D69)
      antepartum — *see* Hemorrhage, antepartum, with coagulation defect
      intrapartum O67.0
  dental implant M27.61
  device, implant or graft — *see also* Complications, by site and type, specified NEC T85.838 ☑
    arterial graft NEC T82.838 ☑
    breast T85.838 ☑
    catheter NEC T85.838 ☑
      dialysis (renal) T82.838 ☑
        intraperitoneal T85.838 ☑
      infusion NEC T82.838 ☑
        spinal (epidural) (subdural) T85.830 ☑
      urinary (indwelling) T83.83 ☑
    electronic (electrode) (pulse generator) (stimulator)
      bone T84.83 ☑
      cardiac T82.837 ☑
      nervous system (brain) (peripheral nerve) (spinal) T85.830 ☑
      urinary T83.83 ☑
    fixation, internal (orthopedic) NEC T84.83 ☑
    gastrointestinal (bile duct) (esophagus) T85.838 ☑
    genital NEC T83.83 ☑
    heart NEC T82.837 ☑
    joint prosthesis T84.83 ☑
    ocular (corneal graft) (orbital implant) NEC T85.838 ☑
    orthopedic NEC T84.83 ☑
      bone graft T86.838
    specified NEC T85.838 ☑
    urinary NEC T83.83 ☑
    vascular NEC T82.838 ☑
    ventricular intracranial shunt T85.830 ☑
  duodenum, duodenal K92.2
    ulcer — *see* Ulcer, duodenum, with hemorrhage
  dura mater — *see* Hemorrhage, intracranial, subdural
  endotracheal — *see* Hemorrhage, lung
  epicranial subaponeurotic (massive), birth injury P12.2
  epidural (traumatic) — *see also* Injury, intracranial, epidural hemorrhage
    nontraumatic I62.1
  esophagus K22.8
    varix I85.01
      secondary I85.11
  excessive, following ectopic gestation (subsequent episode) O08.1
  extradural (traumatic) — *see* Injury, intracranial, epidural hemorrhage
    birth injury P10.8
    newborn (anoxic) (nontraumatic) P52.8
    nontraumatic I62.1
  eye NEC H57.89
    fundus — *see* Hemorrhage, retina
    lid — *see* Disorder, eyelid, specified type NEC
  fallopian tube N83.6
  fibrinogenolysis — *see* Fibrinolysis

Hemorrhage, hemorrhagic — *continued*
fibrinolytic (acquired) — *see* Fibrinolysis
from
  ear (nontraumatic) — *see* Otorrhagia
  tracheostomy stoma J95.01
fundus, eye — *see* Hemorrhage, retina
funis — *see* Hemorrhage, umbilicus, cord
gastric — *see* Hemorrhage, stomach
gastroenteric K92.2
  newborn P54.3
gastrointestinal (tract) K92.2
  newborn P54.3
genital organ, male N50.1
genitourinary (tract) NOS R31.9
gingiva K06.8
globe (eye) — *see* Hemophthalmos
graafian follicle cyst (ruptured) N83.0- ☑
gum K06.8
heart I51.89
hypopharyngeal (throat) R04.1
intermenstrual (regular) N92.3
  irregular N92.1
internal (organs) NEC R58
  capsule I61.0
  ear — *see* subcategory H83.8 ☑
  newborn P54.8
intestine K92.2
  newborn P54.3
intra-abdominal R58
intra-alveolar (lung), newborn P26.8
intracerebral (nontraumatic) — *see* Hemorrhage, intracranial, intracerebral
intracranial (nontraumatic) I62.9
  birth injury P10.9
  epidural, nontraumatic I62.1
  extradural, nontraumatic I62.1
  intracerebral (nontraumatic) (in) I61.9
    brain stem I61.3
    cerebellum I61.4
    hemisphere I61.2
      cortical (superficial) I61.1
      subcortical (deep) I61.0
    intraoperative
      during a nervous system procedure G97.31
      during other procedure G97.32
    intraventricular I61.5
    multiple localized I61.6
    newborn P52.4
      birth injury P10.1
    postprocedural
      following a nervous system procedure G97.51
      following other procedure G97.52
    specified NEC I61.8
    superficial I61.1
    traumatic (diffuse) — *see* Injury, intracranial, diffuse
      focal — *see* Injury, intracranial, focal
  newborn P52.9
  specified NEC P52.8
  subarachnoid (nontraumatic) (from) I60.9
    intracranial (cerebral) artery I60.7
      anterior communicating I60.2
      basilar I60.4
      carotid siphon and bifurcation I60.0- ☑
      communicating I60.7
        anterior I60.2
        posterior I60.3- ☑
      middle cerebral I60.1- ☑
      posterior communicating I60.3- ☑
      specified artery NEC I60.6
      vertebral I60.5- ☑
    newborn P52.5
      birth injury P10.3
    specified NEC I60.8
    traumatic S06.6X- ☑
  subdural (nontraumatic) I62.00
    acute I62.01
    birth injury P10.0
    chronic I62.03
    newborn (anoxic) (hypoxic) P52.8
      birth injury P10.0
    spinal G95.19
    subacute I62.02
    traumatic — *see* Injury, intracranial, subdural hemorrhage
  traumatic — *see* Injury, intracranial, focal brain injury
intramedullary NEC G95.19

Hemorrhage, hemorrhagic — *continued*
intraocular — *see* Hemophthalmos
intraoperative, intraprocedural — *see* Complication, hemorrhage (hematoma), intraoperative (intraprocedural), by site
intrapartum — *see* Hemorrhage, complicating, delivery
intrapelvic
  female N94.89
  male K66.1
intraperitoneal K66.1
intrapontine I61.3
intraprocedural — *see* Complication, hemorrhage (hematoma), intraoperative (intraprocedural), by site
intrauterine N85.7
  complicating delivery — *see also* Hemorrhage, complicating, delivery O67.9
  postpartum — *see* Hemorrhage, postpartum
intraventricular I61.5
  newborn (nontraumatic) — *see also* Newborn, affected by, hemorrhage P52.3
    due to birth injury P10.2
    grade
      1 P52.0
      2 P52.1
      3 P52.21
      4 P52.22
intravesical N32.89
iris (postinfectional) (postinflammatory) (toxic) — *see* Hyphema
joint (nontraumatic) — *see* Hemarthrosis
kidney N28.89
knee (joint) (nontraumatic) — *see* Hemarthrosis, knee
labyrinth — *see* subcategory H83.8 ☑
lenticular striate artery I61.0
ligature, vessel — *see* Hemorrhage, postoperative
liver K76.89
lung R04.89
  newborn P26.9
    massive P26.1
    specified NEC P26.8
  tuberculous — *see* Tuberculosis, pulmonary
massive umbilical, newborn P51.0
mediastinum — *see* Hemorrhage, lung
medulla I61.3
membrane (brain) I60.8
  spinal cord — *see* Hemorrhage, spinal cord
meninges, meningeal (brain) (middle) I60.8
  spinal cord — *see* Hemorrhage, spinal cord
mesentery K66.1
metritis — *see* Endometritis
mouth K13.79
mucous membrane NEC R58
  newborn P54.8
muscle M62.89
nail (subungual) L60.8
nasal turbinate R04.0
  newborn P54.8
navel, newborn P51.9
newborn P54.9
  specified NEC P54.8
nipple N64.59
nose R04.0
  newborn P54.8
omentum K66.1
optic nerve (sheath) H47.02- ☑
orbit, orbital H05.23- ☑
ovary NEC N83.8
oviduct N83.6
pancreas K86.89
parathyroid (gland) (spontaneous) E21.4
parturition — *see* Hemorrhage, complicating, delivery
penis N48.89
pericardium, pericarditis I31.2
peritoneum, peritoneal K66.1
peritonsillar tissue J35.8
  due to infection J36
petechial R23.3
  due to autosensitivity, erythrocyte D69.2
pituitary (gland) E23.6
pleura — *see* Hemorrhage, lung
polioencephalitis, superior E51.2
polymyositis — *see* Polymyositis
pons, pontine I61.3
posterior fossa (nontraumatic) I61.8
  newborn P52.6
postmenopausal N95.0
postnasal R04.0

Hemorrhage, hemorrhagic — *continued*
postoperative — *see* Complications, postprocedural hemorrhage, by site
postpartum NEC (following delivery of placenta) O72.
  delayed or secondary O72.2
  retained placenta O72.0
  third stage O72.0
pregnancy — *see* Hemorrhage, antepartum
preretinal — *see* Hemorrhage, retina
prostate N42.1
puerperal — *see* Hemorrhage, postpartum
  delayed or secondary O72.2
pulmonary R04.89
  newborn P26.9
    massive P26.1
    specified NEC P26.8
  tuberculous — *see* Tuberculosis, pulmonary
purpura (primary) D69.3
rectum (sphincter) K62.5
  newborn P54.2
recurring, following initial hemorrhage at time of injur T79.2 ☑
renal N28.89
respiratory passage or tract R04.9
  specified NEC R04.89
retina, retinal (vessels) H35.6- ☑
  diabetic — *see* Diabetes, retinal, hemorrhage
retroperitoneal R58
scalp R58
scrotum N50.1
secondary (nontraumatic) R58
  following initial hemorrhage at time of injury T79.2 ☑
seminal vesicle N50.1
skin R23.3
  newborn P54.5
slipped umbilical ligature P51.8
spermatic cord N50.1
spinal (cord) G95.19
  newborn (birth injury) P11.5
spleen D73.5
  intraoperative — *see* Complications, intraoperative hemorrhage, spleen
  postprocedural — *see* Complications, postprocedural, hemorrhage, spleen
stomach K92.2
  newborn P54.3
  ulcer — *see* Ulcer, stomach, with hemorrhage
subarachnoid (nontraumatic) — *see* Hemorrhage, intracranial, subarachnoid
subconjunctival — *see also* Hemorrhage, conjunctival
  birth injury P15.3
subcortical (brain) I61.0
subcutaneous R23.3
subdiaphragmatic R58
subdural (acute) (nontraumatic) — *see* Hemorrhage, intracranial, subdural
subependymal
  newborn P52.0
    with intraventricular extension P52.1
      and intracerebral extension P52.22
subgaleal P12.2
subhyaloid — *see* Hemorrhage, retina
subperiosteal — *see* Disorder, bone, specified type NE
subretinal — *see* Hemorrhage, retina
subtentorial — *see* Hemorrhage, intracranial, subdura
subungual L60.8
suprarenal (capsule) (gland) E27.49
  newborn P54.4
tentorium (traumatic) NEC — *see* Hemorrhage, brain
  newborn (birth injury) P10.4
testis N50.1
third stage (postpartum) O72.0
thorax — *see* Hemorrhage, lung
throat R04.1
thymus (gland) E32.8
thyroid (cyst) (gland) E07.89
tongue K14.8
tonsil J35.8
trachea — *see* Hemorrhage, lung
tracheobronchial R04.89
  newborn P26.0
traumatic — *code to* specific injury
  cerebellar — *see* Hemorrhage, brain
  intracranial — *see* Hemorrhage, brain
  recurring or secondary (following initial hemorrhage at time of injury) T79.2 ☑

☑ **Additional Character Required — Refer to the Tabular List for Character Selection**   🔺 **Subterms under main terms may continue to next column or page**

Hemorrhage, hemorrhagic — *continued*
  tuberculous NEC — *see also* Tuberculosis, pulmonary
    A15.0
  tunica vaginalis N50.1
  ulcer — *code by* site under Ulcer, with hemorrhage
    K27.4
  umbilicus, umbilical
    cord
      after birth, newborn P51.9
      complicating delivery O69.5 ☑
    newborn P51.9
      massive P51.0
      slipped ligature P51.8
    stump P51.9
  urethra (idiopathic) N36.8
  uterus, uterine (abnormal) N93.9
    climacteric N92.4
    complicating delivery — *see* Hemorrhage, compli-
      cating, delivery
    dysfunctional or functional N93.8
    intermenstrual (regular) N92.3
      irregular N92.1
    postmenopausal N95.0
    postpartum — *see* Hemorrhage, postpartum
    preclimacteric or premenopausal N92.4
    prepubertal N93.8
    pubertal N92.2
  vagina (abnormal) N93.9
    newborn P54.6
  vas deferens N50.1
  vasa previa O69.4 ☑
  ventricular I61.5
  vesical N32.89
  viscera NEC R58
    newborn P54.8
  vitreous (humor) (intraocular) H43.1- ☑
  vulva N90.89
Hemorrhoids (bleeding) (without mention of degree)
  K64.9
  1st degree (grade/stage I) (without prolapse outside
    of anal canal) K64.0
  2nd degree (grade/stage II) (that prolapse with strain-
    ing but retract spontaneously) K64.1
  3rd degree (grade/stage III) (that prolapse with strain-
    ing and require manual replacement back inside
    anal canal) K64.2
  4th degree (grade/stage IV) (with prolapsed tissue that
    cannot be manually replaced) K64.3
  complicating
    pregnancy O22.4 ☑
    puerperium O87.2
  external K64.4
    with
      thrombosis K64.5
  internal (without mention of degree) K64.8
  prolapsed K64.8
  skin tags
    anus K64.4
    residual K64.4
  specified NEC K64.8
  strangulated — *see also* Hemorrhoids, by degree K64.8
  thrombosed — *see also* Hemorrhoids, by degree K64.5
  ulcerated — *see also* Hemorrhoids, by degree K64.8
Hemosalpinx N83.6
  with
    hematocolpos N89.7
    hematometra N85.7
      with hematocolpos N89.7
Hemosiderosis (dietary) E83.19
  pulmonary, idiopathic E83.1- ☑ *[J84.03]*
  transfusion T80.89 ☑
Hemothorax (bacterial) (nontuberculous) J94.2
  newborn P54.8
  traumatic S27.1 ☑
    with pneumothorax S27.2 ☑
  tuberculous NEC A15.6
Henoch (-Schönlein) **disease or syndrome** (purpura)
  D69.0
Henpue, henpuye A66.6
Hepar lobatum (syphilitic) A52.74
Hepatalgia K76.89
Hepatitis K75.9
  acute B17.9
    with coma K72.01
    with hepatic failure — *see* Failure, hepatic
    alcoholic — *see* Hepatitis, alcoholic
    infectious B17.9
    non-viral K72.0 ☑

Hepatitis — *continued*
  acute — *continued*
    viral B17.9
  alcoholic (acute) (chronic) K70.10
    with ascites K70.11
  amebic — *see* Abscess, liver, amebic
  anicteric, (viral) — *see* Hepatitis, viral
  antigen-associated (HAA) — *see* Hepatitis, B
  Australia-antigen (positive) — *see* Hepatitis, B
  autoimmune K75.4
  B B19.10
    with hepatic coma B19.11
    acute B16.9
      with
        delta-agent (coinfection) (without hepatic
          coma) B16.1
          with hepatic coma B16.0
        hepatic coma (without delta-agent coinfec-
          tion) B16.2
    chronic B18.1
      with delta-agent B18.0
  bacterial NEC K75.89
  C (viral) B19.20
    with hepatic coma B19.21
    acute B17.10
      with hepatic coma B17.11
    chronic B18.2
  catarrhal (acute) B15.9
    with hepatic coma B15.0
  cholangiolitic K75.89
  cholestatic K75.89
  chronic K73.9
    active NEC K73.2
    lobular NEC K73.1
    persistent NEC K73.0
    specified NEC K73.8
  cytomegaloviral B25.1
  due to ethanol (acute) (chronic) — *see* Hepatitis, alco-
    holic
  epidemic B15.9
    with hepatic coma B15.0
  fulminant NEC (viral) — *see* Hepatitis, viral
  granulomatous NEC K75.3
  herpesviral B00.81
  history of
    B Z86.19
    C Z86.19
  homologous serum — *see* Hepatitis, viral, type B
  in (due to)
    mumps B26.81
    toxoplasmosis (acquired) B58.1
      congenital (active) P37.1 *[K77]*
  infectious, infective B15.9
    acute (subacute) B17.9
    chronic B18.9
  inoculation — *see* Hepatitis, viral, type B
  interstitial (chronic) K74.69
  lupoid NEC K75.4
  malignant NEC (with hepatic failure) K72.90
    with coma K72.91
  neonatal (idiopathic) (toxic) P59.29
  neonatal giant cell P59.29
  newborn P59.29
  non-viral K72.0 ☑
  postimmunization — *see* Hepatitis, viral, type B
  post-transfusion — *see* Hepatitis, viral, type B
  reactive, nonspecific K75.2
  serum — *see* Hepatitis, viral, type B
  specified type NEC
    with hepatic failure — *see* Failure, hepatic
  syphilitic (late) A52.74
    congenital (early) A50.08 *[K77]*
      late A50.59 *[K77]*
    secondary A51.45
  toxic — *see also* Disease, liver, toxic K71.6
  tuberculous A18.83
  viral, virus B19.9
    with hepatic coma B19.0
    acute B17.9
    chronic B18.9
      specified NEC B18.8
      type
        B B18.1
          with delta-agent B18.0
        C B18.2
    congenital P35.3
    coxsackie B33.8 *[K77]*
    cytomegalic inclusion B25.1

Hepatitis — *continued*
  viral, virus — *continued*
    in remission, any type — *code to* Hepatitis, chronic,
      by type
    non-A, non-B B17.8
    specified type NEC (with or without coma) B17.8
    type
      A B15.9
        with hepatic coma B15.0
      B B19.10
        with hepatic coma B19.11
        acute B16.9
          with
            delta-agent (coinfection) (without
              hepatic coma) B16.1
              with hepatic coma B16.0
            hepatic coma (without delta-agent
              coinfection) B16.2
        chronic B18.1
          with delta-agent B18.0
      C B19.20
        with hepatic coma B19.21
        acute B17.10
          with hepatic coma B17.11
        chronic B18.2
      E B17.2
    non-A, non-B B17.8
Hepatization lung (acute) — *see* Pneumonia, lobar
Hepatoblastoma C22.2
Hepatocarcinoma C22.0
Hepatocholangiocarcinoma C22.0
Hepatocholangioma, benign D13.4
Hepatocholangitis K75.89
Hepatolenticular degeneration E83.01
Hepatoma (malignant) C22.0
  benign D13.4
  embryonal C22.0
Hepatomegaly — *see also* Hypertrophy, liver
  with splenomegaly R16.2
  congenital Q44.7
  in mononucleosis
    gammaherpesviral B27.09
    infectious specified NEC B27.89
Hepatoptosis K76.89
Hepatorenal syndrome following labor and delivery
  O90.4
Hepatosis K76.89
Hepatosplenomegaly R16.2
  hyperlipemic (Bürger-Grütz type) E78.3 *[K77]*
Hereditary — *see* condition
Heredodegeneration, macular — *see* Dystrophy, retina
Heredopathia atactica polyneuritiformis G60.1
Heredosyphilis — *see* Syphilis, congenital
Herlitz' syndrome Q81.1
Hermansky-Pudlak syndrome E70.331
Hermaphrodite, hermaphroditism (true) Q56.0
  46,XX with streak gonads Q99.1
  46,XX/46,XY Q99.0
  46,XY with streak gonads Q99.1
  chimera 46,XX/46,XY Q99.0
Hernia, hernial (acquired) (recurrent) K46.9
  with
    gangrene — *see* Hernia, by site, with, gangrene
    incarceration — *see* Hernia, by site, with, obstruction
    irreducible — *see* Hernia, by site, with, obstruction
    obstruction — *see* Hernia, by site, with, obstruction
    strangulation — *see* Hernia, by site, with, obstruc-
      tion
  abdomen, abdominal K46.9
    with
      gangrene (and obstruction) K46.1
      obstruction K46.0
    femoral — *see* Hernia, femoral
    incisional — *see* Hernia, incisional
    inguinal — *see* Hernia, inguinal
    specified site NEC K45.8
      with
        gangrene (and obstruction) K45.1
        obstruction K45.0
    umbilical — *see* Hernia, umbilical
    wall — *see* Hernia, ventral
  appendix — *see* Hernia, abdomen
  bladder (mucosa) (sphincter)
    congenital (female) (male) Q79.51
    female — *see* Cystocele
    male N32.89
  brain, congenital — *see* Encephalocele

Hernia, hernial — *continued*
- cartilage, vertebra — *see* Displacement, intervertebral disc
- cerebral, congenital — *see also* Encephalocele
  - endaural Q01.8
- ciliary body (traumatic) S05.2- ☑
- colon — *see* Hernia, abdomen
- Cooper's — *see* Hernia, abdomen, specified site NEC
- crural — *see* Hernia, femoral
- diaphragm, diaphragmatic K44.9
  - with
    - gangrene (and obstruction) K44.1
    - obstruction K44.0
  - congenital Q79.0
- direct (inguinal) — *see* Hernia, inguinal
- diverticulum, intestine — *see* Hernia, abdomen
- double (inguinal) — *see* Hernia, inguinal, bilateral
- due to adhesions (with obstruction) K56.50
- epigastric — *see also* Hernia, ventral K43.9
- esophageal hiatus — *see* Hernia, hiatal
- external (inguinal) — *see* Hernia, inguinal
- fallopian tube N83.4- ☑
- fascia M62.89
- femoral K41.90
  - with
    - gangrene (and obstruction) K41.40
      - not specified as recurrent K41.40
      - recurrent K41.41
    - obstruction K41.30
      - not specified as recurrent K41.30
      - recurrent K41.31
  - not specified as recurrent K41.90
  - recurrent K41.91
  - bilateral K41.20
    - with
      - gangrene (and obstruction) K41.10
        - not specified as recurrent K41.10
        - recurrent K41.11
      - obstruction K41.00
        - not specified as recurrent K41.00
        - recurrent K41.01
    - not specified as recurrent K41.20
    - recurrent K41.21
  - unilateral K41.90
    - with
      - gangrene (and obstruction) K41.40
        - not specified as recurrent K41.40
        - recurrent K41.41
      - obstruction K41.30
        - not specified as recurrent K41.30
        - recurrent K41.31
    - not specified as recurrent K41.90
    - recurrent K41.91
- foramen magnum G93.5
  - congenital Q01.8
- funicular (umbilical) — *see also* Hernia, umbilicus
  - spermatic (cord) — *see* Hernia, inguinal
- gastrointestinal tract — *see* Hernia, abdomen
- Hesselbach's — *see* Hernia, femoral, specified site NEC
- hiatal (esophageal) (sliding) K44.9
  - with
    - gangrene (and obstruction) K44.1
    - obstruction K44.0
  - congenital Q40.1
- hypogastric — *see* Hernia, ventral
- incarcerated — *see also* Hernia, by site, with obstruction
  - with gangrene — *see* Hernia, by site, with gangrene
- incisional K43.2
  - with
    - gangrene (and obstruction) K43.1
    - obstruction K43.0
- indirect (inguinal) — *see* Hernia, inguinal
- inguinal (direct) (external) (funicular) (indirect) (internal) (oblique) (scrotal) (sliding) K40.90
  - with
    - gangrene (and obstruction) K40.40
      - not specified as recurrent K40.40
      - recurrent K40.41
    - obstruction K40.30
      - not specified as recurrent K40.30
      - recurrent K40.31
  - not specified as recurrent K40.90
  - recurrent K40.91
  - bilateral K40.20
    - with
      - gangrene (and obstruction) K40.10
        - not specified as recurrent K40.10

Hernia, hernial — *continued*
- inguinal — *continued*
  - bilateral — *continued*
    - with — *continued*
      - gangrene — *continued*
        - recurrent K40.11
      - obstruction K40.00
        - not specified as recurrent K40.00
        - recurrent K40.01
    - not specified as recurrent K40.20
    - recurrent K40.21
  - unilateral K40.90
    - with
      - gangrene (and obstruction) K40.40
        - not specified as recurrent K40.40
        - recurrent K40.41
      - obstruction K40.30
        - not specified as recurrent K40.30
        - recurrent K40.31
    - not specified as recurrent K40.90
    - recurrent K40.91
- internal — *see also* Hernia, abdomen
  - inguinal — *see* Hernia, inguinal
- interstitial — *see* Hernia, abdomen
- intervertebral cartilage or disc — *see* Displacement, intervertebral disc
- intestine, intestinal — *see* Hernia, by site
- intra-abdominal — *see* Hernia, abdomen
- iris (traumatic) S05.2- ☑
- irreducible — *see also* Hernia, by site, with obstruction
  - with gangrene — *see* Hernia, by site, with gangrene
- ischiatic — *see* Hernia, abdomen, specified site NEC
- ischiorectal — *see* Hernia, abdomen, specified site NEC
- lens (traumatic) S05.2- ☑
- linea (alba) (semilunaris) — *see* Hernia, ventral
- Littre's — *see* Hernia, abdomen
- lumbar — *see* Hernia, abdomen, specified site NEC
- lung (subcutaneous) J98.4
- mediastinum J98.59
- mesenteric (internal) — *see* Hernia, abdomen
- midline — *see* Hernia, ventral
- muscle (sheath) M62.89
- nucleus pulposus — *see* Displacement, intervertebral disc
- oblique (inguinal) — *see* Hernia, inguinal
- obstructive — *see also* Hernia, by site, with obstruction
  - with gangrene — *see* Hernia, by site, with gangrene
- obturator — *see* Hernia, abdomen, specified site NEC
- omental — *see* Hernia, abdomen
- ovary N83.4- ☑
- oviduct N83.4- ☑
- paraesophageal — *see also* Hernia, diaphragm
  - congenital Q40.1
- parastomal K43.5
  - with
    - gangrene (and obstruction) K43.4
    - obstruction K43.3
- paraumbilical — *see* Hernia, umbilicus
- perineal — *see* Hernia, abdomen, specified site NEC
- Petit's — *see* Hernia, abdomen, specified site NEC
- postoperative — *see* Hernia, incisional
- pregnant uterus — *see* Abnormal, uterus in pregnancy or childbirth
- prevesical N32.89
- properitoneal — *see* Hernia, abdomen, specified site NEC
- pudendal — *see* Hernia, abdomen, specified site NEC
- rectovaginal N81.6
- retroperitoneal — *see* Hernia, abdomen, specified site NEC
- Richter's — *see* Hernia, abdomen, with obstruction
- Rieux's, Riex's — *see* Hernia, abdomen, specified site NEC
- sac condition (adhesion) (dropsy) (inflammation) (laceration) (suppuration) — *code by site under* Hernia
- sciatic — *see* Hernia, abdomen, specified site NEC
- scrotum, scrotal — *see* Hernia, inguinal
- sliding (inguinal) — *see also* Hernia, inguinal
  - hiatus — *see* Hernia, hiatal
- spigelian — *see* Hernia, ventral
- spinal — *see* Spina bifida
- strangulated — *see also* Hernia, by site, with obstruction
  - with gangrene — *see* Hernia, by site, with gangrene
- subxiphoid — *see* Hernia, ventral
- supra-umbilicus — *see* Hernia, ventral

Hernia, hernial — *continued*
- tendon — *see* Disorder, tendon, specified type NEC
- Treitz's (fossa) — *see* Hernia, abdomen, specified site NEC
- tunica vaginalis Q55.29
- umbilicus, umbilical K42.9
  - with
    - gangrene (and obstruction) K42.1
    - obstruction K42.0
- ureter N28.89
- urethra, congenital Q64.79
- urinary meatus, congenital Q64.79
- uterus N81.4
  - pregnant — *see* Abnormal, uterus in pregnancy or childbirth
- vaginal (anterior) (wall) — *see* Cystocele
- Velpeau's — *see* Hernia, femoral
- ventral K43.9
  - with
    - gangrene (and obstruction) K43.7
    - obstruction K43.6
  - incisional K43.2
    - with
      - gangrene (and obstruction) K43.1
      - obstruction K43.0
    - recurrent — *see* Hernia, incisional
  - specified NEC K43.9
    - with
      - gangrene (and obstruction) K43.7
      - obstruction K43.6
- vesical
  - congenital (female) (male) Q79.51
  - female — *see* Cystocele
  - male N32.89
- vitreous (into wound) S05.2- ☑
  - into anterior chamber — *see* Prolapse, vitreous

Herniation — *see also* Hernia
- brain (stem) G93.5
- cerebral G93.5
- mediastinum J98.59
- nucleus pulposus — *see* Displacement, intervertebral disc

Herpangina B08.5

Herpes, herpesvirus, herpetic B00.9
- anogenital A60.9
  - perianal skin A60.1
  - rectum A60.1
  - urogenital tract A60.00
    - cervix A60.03
    - male genital organ NEC A60.02
    - penis A60.01
    - specified site NEC A60.09
    - vagina A60.04
    - vulva A60.04
- blepharitis (zoster) B02.39
  - simplex B00.59
- circinatus B35.4
  - bullosus L12.0
- conjunctivitis (simplex) B00.53
  - zoster B02.31
- cornea B02.33
- encephalitis B00.4
  - due to herpesvirus 6 B10.01
  - due to herpesvirus 7 B10.09
  - specified NEC B10.09
- eye (zoster) B02.30
  - simplex B00.50
- eyelid (zoster) B02.39
  - simplex B00.59
- facialis B00.1
- febrilis B00.1
- geniculate ganglionitis B02.21
- genital, genitalis A60.00
  - female A60.09
  - male A60.02
- gestational, gestationis O26.4- ☑
- gingivostomatitis B00.2
- human B00.9
  - 1 — *see* Herpes, simplex
  - 2 — *see* Herpes, simplex
  - 3 — *see* Varicella
  - 4 — *see* Mononucleosis, Epstein-Barr (virus)
  - 5 — *see* Disease, cytomegalic inclusion (generalized
  - 6
    - encephalitis B10.01
    - specified NEC B10.81
  - 7
    - encephalitis B10.09

☑ **Additional Character Required** — Refer to the Tabular List for Character Selection ▼ **Subterms under main terms may continue to next column or page**

Herpes, herpesvirus, herpetic — *continued*
  human — *continued*
    7 — *continued*
      specified NEC B10.82
    8 B10.89
  infection NEC B10.89
    Kaposi's sarcoma associated B10.89
  iridocyclitis (simplex) B00.51
    zoster B02.32
  iris (vesicular erythema multiforme) L51.9
  iritis (simplex) B00.51
  Kaposi's sarcoma associated B10.89
  keratitis (simplex) (dendritic) (disciform) (interstitial)
    B00.52
    zoster (interstitial) B02.33
  keratoconjunctivitis (simplex) B00.52
    zoster B02.33
  labialis B00.1
  lip B00.1
  meningitis (simplex) B00.3
    zoster B02.1
  ophthalmicus (zoster) NEC B02.30
    simplex B00.50
  penis A60.01
  perianal skin A60.1
  pharyngitis, pharyngotonsillitis B00.2
  rectum A60.1
  scrotum A60.02
  sepsis B00.7
  simplex B00.9
    complicated NEC B00.89
    congenital P35.2
    conjunctivitis B00.53
    external ear B00.1
    eyelid B00.59
    hepatitis B00.81
    keratitis (interstitial) B00.52
    myelitis B00.82
    specified complication NEC B00.89
    visceral B00.89
  stomatitis B00.2
  tonsurans B35.0
  visceral B00.89
  vulva A60.04
  whitlow B00.89
  zoster   *see also* condition B02.9
    auricularis B02.21
    complicated NEC B02.8
    conjunctivitis B02.31
    disseminated B02.7
    encephalitis B02.0
    eye (lid) B02.39
    geniculate ganglionitis B02.21
    keratitis (interstitial) B02.33
    meningitis B02.1
    myelitis B02.24
    neuritis, neuralgia B02.29
    ophthalmicus NEC B02.30
    oticus B02.21
    polyneuropathy B02.23
    specified complication NEC B02.8
    trigeminal neuralgia B02.22
Herpesvirus (human) — *see* Herpes
Herpetophobia F40.218
Herrick's anemia — *see* Disease, sickle-cell
Hers' disease E74.09
Herter-Gee syndrome K90.0
Herxheimer's reaction R68.89
Hesitancy
  of micturition R39.11
  urinary R39.11
Hesselbach's hernia — *see* Hernia, femoral, specified
    site NEC
Heterochromia (congenital) Q13.2
  cataract — *see* Cataract, complicated
  cyclitis (Fuchs) — *see* Cyclitis, Fuchs' heterochromic
  hair L67.1
  iritis — *see* Cyclitis, Fuchs' heterochromic
  retained metallic foreign body (nonmagnetic) — *see*
    Foreign body, intraocular, old, retained
    magnetic — *see* Foreign body, intraocular, old, re-
      tained, magnetic
  uveitis — *see* Cyclitis, Fuchs' heterochromic
Heterophoria — *see* Strabismus, heterophoria
Heterophyes, heterophyiasis (small intestine) B66.8
Heterotopia, heterotopic — *see also* Malposition,
    congenital
  cerebralis Q04.8

Heterotropia — *see* Strabismus
Heubner-Herter disease K90.0
Hexadactylism Q69.9
HGSIL (cytology finding) (high grade squamous intraep-
    ithelial lesion on cytologic smear) (Pap smear find-
    ing)
  anus R85.613
  cervix R87.613
    biopsy (histology) finding — *see* Neoplasia, intraep-
      ithelial, cervix, grade II or grade III
  vagina R87.623
    biopsy (histology) finding — *see* Neoplasia, intraep-
      ithelial, cervix, grade II or grade III
Hibernoma — *see* Lipoma
Hiccup, hiccough R06.6
  epidemic B33.0
  psychogenic F45.8
Hidden penis (congenital) Q55.64
  acquired N48.83
Hidradenitis (axillaris) (suppurative) L73.2
Hidradenoma (nodular) — *see also* Neoplasm, skin, be-
    nign
  clear cell — *see* Neoplasm, skin, benign
  papillary — *see* Neoplasm, skin, benign
Hidrocystoma — *see* Neoplasm, skin, benign
High
  altitude effects T70.20 ☑
    anoxia T70.29 ☑
    on
      ears T70.0 ☑
      sinuses T70.1 ☑
    polycythemia D75.1
  arch
    foot Q66.7- ☑
    palate, congenital Q38.5
  arterial tension — *see* Hypertension
  basal metabolic rate R94.8
  blood pressure — *see also* Hypertension
    borderline R03.0
    reading (incidental) (isolated) (nonspecific), without
      diagnosis of hypertension R03.0
  cholesterol E78.00
    with high triglycerides E78.2
  diaphragm (congenital) Q79.1
  expressed emotional level within family Z63.8
  head at term O32.4 ☑
  palate, congenital Q38.5
  risk
    infant NEC Z76.2
    sexual behavior (heterosexual) Z72.51
      bisexual Z72.53
      homosexual Z72.52
  scrotal testis, testes
    bilateral Q53.23
    unilateral Q53.13
  temperature (of unknown origin) R50.9
  thoracic rib Q76.6
  triglycerides E78.1
    with high cholesterol E78.2
Hildenbrand's disease A75.0
Hilum — *see* condition
Hip — *see* condition
Hippel's disease Q85.8
Hippophobia F40.218
Hippus H57.09
Hirschsprung's disease or megacolon Q43.1
Hirsutism, hirsuties L68.0
Hirudiniasis
  external B88.3
  internal B83.4
Hiss-Russell dysentery A03.1
Histidinemia, histidinuria E70.41
Histiocytoma — *see also* Neoplasm, skin, benign
  fibrous — *see also* Neoplasm, skin, benign
    atypical — *see* Neoplasm, connective tissue, uncer-
      tain behavior
    malignant — *see* Neoplasm, connective tissue, ma-
      lignant
Histiocytosis D76.3
  acute differentiated progressive C96.0
  Langerhans' cell NEC C96.6
    multifocal X
      multisystemic (disseminated) C96.0
      unisystemic C96.5
    pulmonary, adult (adult PLCH) J84.82
    unifocal (X) C96.6
  lipid, lipoid D76.3

Histiocytosis — *continued*
  lipid, lipoid — *continued*
    essential E75.29
  malignant C96.A (*following* C96.6)
  mononuclear phagocytes NEC D76.1
    Langerhans' cells C96.6
  non-Langerhans cell D76.3
  polyostotic sclerosing D76.3
  sinus, with massive lymphadenopathy D76.3
  syndrome NEC D76.3
  X NEC C96.6
    acute (progressive) C96.0
    chronic C96.6
    multifocal C96.5
    multisystemic C96.0
    unifocal C96.6
Histoplasmosis B39.9
  with pneumonia NEC B39.2
  African B39.5
  American — *see* Histoplasmosis, capsulati
  capsulati B39.4
    disseminated B39.3
    generalized B39.3
    pulmonary B39.2
      acute B39.0
      chronic B39.1
  Darling's B39.4
  duboisii B39.5
  lung NEC B39.2
History
  family (of) — *see also* History, personal (of)
    alcohol abuse Z81.1
    allergy NEC Z84.89
    anemia Z83.2
    arthritis Z82.61
    asthma Z82.5
    blindness Z82.1
    cardiac death (sudden) Z82.41
    carrier of genetic disease Z84.81
    chromosomal anomaly Z82.79
    chronic
      disabling disease NEC Z82.8
      lower respiratory disease Z82.5
    colonic polyps Z83.71
    congenital malformations and deformations Z82.79
      polycystic kidney Z82.71
    consanguinity Z84.3
    deafness Z82.2
    diabetes mellitus Z83.3
    disability NEC Z82.8
    disease or disorder (of)
      allergic NEC Z84.89
      behavioral NEC Z81.8
      blood and blood-forming organs Z83.2
      cardiovascular NEC Z82.49
      chronic disabling NEC Z82.8
      digestive Z83.79
      ear NEC Z83.52
      elevated lipoprotein (a) (Lp(a)) Z83.430
      endocrine NEC Z83.49
      eye NEC Z83.518
        glaucoma Z83.511
      familial hypercholesterolemia Z83.42
      genitourinary NEC Z84.2
      glaucoma Z83.511
      hematological Z83.2
      immune mechanism Z83.2
      infectious NEC Z83.1
      ischemic heart Z82.49
      kidney Z84.1
      lipoprotein metabolism Z83.438
      mental NEC Z81.8
      metabolic Z83.49
      musculoskeletal NEC Z82.69
      neurological NEC Z82.0
      nutritional Z83.49
      parasitic NEC Z83.1
      psychiatric NEC Z81.8
      respiratory NEC Z83.6
      skin and subcutaneous tissue NEC Z84.0
      specified NEC Z84.89
    drug abuse NEC Z81.3
    elevated lipoprotein (a) (Lp(a)) Z83.430
    epilepsy Z82.0
    familial hypercholesterolemia Z83.42
    genetic disease carrier Z84.81
    glaucoma Z83.511
    hearing loss Z82.2
    human immunodeficiency virus (HIV) infection Z83.0

History — continued
    family — see also History, personal — continued
      Huntington's chorea Z82.0
      hyperlipidemia, familial combined Z83.438
      intellectual disability Z81.0
      leukemia Z80.6
      lipidemia NEC Z83.438
      malignant neoplasm (of) NOS Z80.9
        bladder Z80.52
        breast Z80.3
        bronchus Z80.1
        digestive organ Z80.0
        gastrointestinal tract Z80.0
        genital organ Z80.49
          ovary Z80.41
          prostate Z80.42
          specified organ NEC Z80.49
          testis Z80.43
        hematopoietic NEC Z80.7
        intrathoracic organ NEC Z80.2
        kidney Z80.51
        lung Z80.1
        lymphatic NEC Z80.7
        ovary Z80.41
        prostate Z80.42
        respiratory organ NEC Z80.2
        specified site NEC Z80.8
        testis Z80.43
        trachea Z80.1
        urinary organ or tract Z80.59
          bladder Z80.52
          kidney Z80.51
      mental
        disorder NEC Z81.8
      multiple endocrine neoplasia (MEN) syndrome
        Z83.41
      osteoporosis Z82.62
      polycystic kidney Z82.71
      polyps (colon) Z83.71
      psychiatric disorder Z81.8
      psychoactive substance abuse NEC Z81.3
      respiratory condition NEC Z83.6
        asthma and other lower respiratory conditions
          Z82.5
      self-harmful behavior Z81.8
      SIDS (sudden infant death syndrome) Z84.82
      skin condition Z84.0
      specified condition NEC Z84.89
      stroke (cerebrovascular) Z82.3
      substance abuse NEC Z81.4
        alcohol Z81.1
        drug NEC Z81.3
        psychoactive NEC Z81.3
        tobacco Z81.2
      sudden
        cardiac death Z82.41
        infant death syndrome (SIDS) Z84.82
      tobacco abuse Z81.2
      violence, violent behavior Z81.8
      visual loss Z82.1
    personal (of) — see also History, family (of)
      abuse
        adult Z91.419
          forced labor or sexual exploitation Z91.42
          physical and sexual Z91.410
          psychological Z91.411
        childhood Z62.819
          forced labor or sexual exploitation in child-
            hood Z62.813
          physical Z62.810
          psychological Z62.811
          sexual Z62.810
      alcohol dependence F10.21
      allergy (to) Z88.9
        analgesic agent NEC Z88.6
        anesthetic Z88.4
        antibiotic agent NEC Z88.1
        anti-infective agent NEC Z88.3
        contrast media Z91.041
        drugs, medicaments and biological substances
          Z88.9
          specified NEC Z88.8
        food Z91.018
          additives Z91.02
          eggs Z91.012
          milk products Z91.011
          peanuts Z91.010
          seafood Z91.013
          specified food NEC Z91.018

History — continued
    personal — see also History, family — continued
      allergy — continued
        insect Z91.038
          bee Z91.030
        latex Z91.040
        medicinal agents Z88.9
          specified NEC Z88.8
        narcotic agent NEC Z88.5
        nonmedicinal agents Z91.048
        penicillin Z88.0
        serum Z88.7
        specified NEC Z91.09
        sulfonamides Z88.2
        vaccine Z88.7
      anaphylactic shock Z87.892
      anaphylaxis Z87.892
      behavioral disorders Z86.59
      benign carcinoid tumor Z86.012
      benign neoplasm Z86.018
        brain Z86.011
        carcinoid Z86.012
        colonic polyps Z86.010
      brain injury (traumatic) Z87.820
      breast implant removal Z98.86
      calculi, renal Z87.442
      cancer — see History, personal (of), malignant
        neoplasm (of)
      cardiac arrest (death), successfully resuscitated
        Z86.74
      cerebral infarction without residual deficit Z86.73
      cervical dysplasia Z87.410
      chemotherapy for neoplastic condition Z92.21
      childhood abuse — see History, personal (of), abuse
      cleft lip (corrected) Z87.730
      cleft palate (corrected) Z87.730
      collapsed vertebra (healed) Z87.311
        due to osteoporosis Z87.310
      combat and operational stress reaction Z86.51
      congenital malformation (corrected) Z87.798
        circulatory system (corrected) Z87.74
        digestive system (corrected) NEC Z87.738
        ear (corrected) Z87.721
        eye (corrected) Z87.720
        face and neck (corrected) Z87.790
        genitourinary system (corrected) NEC Z87.718
        heart (corrected) Z87.74
        integument (corrected) Z87.76
        limb(s) (corrected) Z87.76
        musculoskeletal system (corrected) Z87.76
        neck (corrected) Z87.790
        nervous system (corrected) NEC Z87.728
        respiratory system (corrected) Z87.75
        sense organs (corrected) NEC Z87.728
        specified NEC Z87.798
      contraception Z92.0
      deployment (military) Z91.82
      diabetic foot ulcer Z86.31
      disease or disorder (of) Z87.898
        anaphylaxis Z87.892
        blood and blood-forming organs Z86.2
        circulatory system Z86.79
          specified condition NEC Z86.79
        connective tissue Z87.39
        digestive system Z87.19
          colonic polyp Z86.010
          peptic ulcer disease Z87.11
          specified condition NEC Z87.19
        ear Z86.69
        endocrine Z86.39
          diabetic foot ulcer Z86.31
          gestational diabetes Z86.32
          specified type NEC Z86.39
        eye Z86.69
        genital (track) system NEC
          female Z87.42
          male Z87.438
        hematological Z86.2
        Hodgkin Z85.71
        immune mechanism Z86.2
        infectious Z86.19
          malaria Z86.13
          Methicillin resistant Staphylococcus aureus
            (MRSA) Z86.14
          poliomyelitis Z86.12
          specified NEC Z86.19
          tuberculosis Z86.11
        mental NEC Z86.59
        metabolic Z86.39

History — continued
    personal — see also History, family — continued
      disease or disorder — continued
        metabolic — continued
          diabetic foot ulcer Z86.31
          gestational diabetes Z86.32
          specified type NEC Z86.39
        musculoskeletal NEC Z87.39
        nervous system Z86.69
        nutritional Z86.39
        parasitic Z86.19
        respiratory system NEC Z87.09
        sense organs Z86.69
        skin Z87.2
        specified site or type NEC Z87.898
        subcutaneous tissue Z87.2
        trophoblastic Z87.59
        urinary system NEC Z87.448
      drug dependence — see Dependence, drug, by
        type, in remission
      drug therapy
        antineoplastic chemotherapy Z92.21
        estrogen Z92.23
        immunosupression Z92.25
        inhaled steroids Z92.240
        monoclonal drug Z92.22
        specified NEC Z92.29
        steroid Z92.241
        systemic steroids Z92.241
      dysplasia
        cervical (mild) (moderate) Z87.410
          severe (grade III) Z86.001
        prostatic Z87.430
        vaginal (mild) (moderate) Z87.411
          severe (grade III) Z86.002
        vulvar (mild) (moderate) Z87.412
          severe (grade III) Z86.002
      embolism (venous) Z86.718
        pulmonary Z86.711
      encephalitis Z86.61
      estrogen therapy Z92.23
      extracorporeal membrane oxygenation (ECMO)
        Z92.81
      failed conscious sedation Z92.83
      failed moderate sedation Z92.83
      fall, falling Z91.81
      forced labor or sexual exploitation Z91.42
        in childhood Z62.813
      fracture (healed)
        fatigue Z87.312
        fragility Z87.310
        osteoporosis Z87.310
        pathological NEC Z87.311
        stress Z87.312
        traumatic Z87.81
      gestational diabetes Z86.32
      hepatitis
        B Z86.19
        C Z86.19
      Hodgkin disease Z85.71
      hyperthermia, malignant Z88.4
      hypospadias (corrected) Z87.710
      hysterectomy Z90.710
      immunosupression therapy Z92.25
      in situ neoplasm
        breast Z86.000
        cervix uteri Z86.001
        digestive organs, specified NEC Z86.004
        esophagus Z86.003
        genital organs, specified NEC Z86.002
        melanoma Z86.006
        middle ear Z86.005
        oral cavity Z86.003
        respiratory system Z86.005
        skin Z86.007
        specified NEC Z86.008
        stomach Z86.003
      in utero procedure during pregnancy Z98.870
      in utero procedure while a fetus Z98.871
      infection NEC Z86.19
        central nervous system Z86.61
        latent tuberculosis Z86.15
        Methicillin resistant Staphylococcus aureus
          (MRSA) Z86.14
        urinary (recurrent) (tract) Z87.440
      injury NEC Z87.828
      irradiation Z92.3
      kidney stones Z87.442
      latent tuberculosis infection Z86.15

History — *continued*
personal — *see also* History, family — *continued*
  leukemia Z85.6
  lymphoma (non-Hodgkin) Z85.72
  malignant melanoma (skin) Z85.820
  malignant neoplasm (of) Z85.9
    accessory sinuses Z85.22
    anus NEC Z85.048
      carcinoid Z85.040
    bladder Z85.51
    bone Z85.830
    brain Z85.841
    breast Z85.3
    bronchus NEC Z85.118
      carcinoid Z85.110
    carcinoid — *see* History, personal (of), malignant neoplasm, by site, carcinoid
    cervix Z85.41
    colon NEC Z85.038
      carcinoid Z85.030
    digestive organ Z85.00
      specified NEC Z85.09
    endocrine gland NEC Z85.858
    epididymis Z85.48
    esophagus Z85.01
    eye Z85.840
    gastrointestinal tract — *see* History, malignant neoplasm, digestive organ
    genital organ
      female Z85.40
        specified NEC Z85.44
      male Z85.45
        specified NEC Z85.49
    hematopoietic NEC Z85.79
    intrathoracic organ Z85.20
    kidney NEC Z85.528
      carcinoid Z85.520
    large intestine NEC Z85.038
      carcinoid Z85.030
    larynx Z85.21
    liver Z85.05
    lung NEC Z85.118
      carcinoid Z85.110
    mediastinum Z85.29
    Merkel cell Z85.821
    middle ear Z85.22
    nasal cavities Z85.22
    nervous system NEC Z85.848
    oral cavity Z85.819
      specified site NEC Z85.818
    ovary Z85.43
    pancreas Z85.07
    pelvis Z85.53
    pharynx Z85.819
      specified site NEC Z85.818
    pleura Z85.29
    prostate Z85.46
    rectosigmoid junction NEC Z85.048
      carcinoid Z85.040
    rectum NEC Z85.048
      carcinoid Z85.040
    respiratory organ Z85.20
    sinuses, accessory Z85.22
    skin NEC Z85.828
      melanoma Z85.820
      Merkel cell Z85.821
    small intestine NEC Z85.068
      carcinoid Z85.060
    soft tissue Z85.831
    specified site NEC Z85.89
    stomach NEC Z85.028
      carcinoid Z85.020
    testis Z85.47
    thymus NEC Z85.238
      carcinoid Z85.230
    thyroid Z85.850
    tongue Z85.810
    trachea Z85.12
    urinary organ or tract Z85.50
      specified NEC Z85.59
    uterus Z85.42
  maltreatment Z91.89
  medical treatment NEC Z92.89
  melanoma Z85.820
    in situ Z86.006
    malignant (skin) Z85.820
  meningitis Z86.61
  mental disorder Z86.59
  Merkel cell carcinoma (skin) Z85.821

History — *continued*
personal — *see also* History, family — *continued*
  Methicillin resistant Staphylococcus aureus (MRSA) Z86.14
  military deployment Z91.82
  military war, peacekeeping and humanitarian deployment (current or past conflict) Z91.82
  myocardial infarction (old) I25.2
  neglect (in)
    adult Z91.412
    childhood Z62.812
  neoplasia
    anal intraepithelial, III [AIN III] Z86.004
    high-grade prostatic intraepithelial, III [HGPIN III] Z86.002
    vaginal intraepithelial, III [VAIN III] Z86.002
    vulvar intraepithelial, III [VIN III] Z86.002
  neoplasm
    benign Z86.018
      brain Z86.011
      colon polyp Z86.010
    in situ
      breast Z86.000
      cervix uteri Z86.001
      digestive organs, specified NEC Z86.004
      esophagus Z86.003
      genital organs, specified NEC Z86.002
      melanoma Z86.006
      middle ear Z86.005
      oral cavity Z86.003
      respiratory system Z86.005
      skin Z86.007
      specified NEC Z86.008
      stomach Z86.003
    malignant — *see* History of, malignant neoplasm
    uncertain behavior Z86.03
  nephrotic syndrome Z87.441
  nicotine dependence Z87.891
  noncompliance with medical treatment or regimen — *see* Noncompliance
  nutritional deficiency Z86.39
  obstetric complications Z87.59
    childbirth Z87.59
    pregnancy Z87.59
    pre-term labor Z87.51
    puerperium Z87.59
  osteoporosis fractures Z87.31 ☑
  parasuicide (attempt) Z91.5
  physical trauma NEC Z87.828
    self-harm or suicide attempt Z91.5
  pneumonia (recurrent) Z87.01
  poisoning NEC Z91.89
    self-harm or suicide attempt Z91.5
  poor personal hygiene Z91.89
  preterm labor Z87.51
  procedure during pregnancy Z98.870
  procedure while a fetus Z98.871
  prolonged reversible ischemic neurologic deficit (PRIND) Z86.73
  prostatic dysplasia Z87.430
  psychological
    abuse
      adult Z91.411
      child Z62.811
    trauma, specified NEC Z91.49
  radiation therapy Z92.3
  removal
    implant
      breast Z98.86
    renal calculi Z87.442
  respiratory condition NEC Z87.09
  retained foreign body fully removed Z87.821
  risk factors NEC Z91.89
  self-harm Z91.5
  self-poisoning attempt Z91.5
  sex reassignment Z87.890
  sleep-wake cycle problem Z72.821
  specified NEC Z87.898
  steroid therapy (systemic) Z92.241
    inhaled Z92.240
  stroke without residual deficits Z86.73
  substance abuse NEC F10-F19
  sudden cardiac arrest Z86.74
  sudden cardiac death successfully resuscitated Z86.74
  suicide attempt Z91.5
  surgery NEC Z98.890
    with uterine scar Z98.891
    sex reassignment Z87.890

History — *continued*
personal — *see also* History, family — *continued*
  surgery — *continued*
    transplant — *see* Transplant
    thrombophlebitis Z86.72
    thrombosis (venous) Z86.718
      pulmonary Z86.711
    tobacco dependence Z87.891
    transient ischemic attack (TIA) without residual deficits Z86.73
    trauma (physical) NEC Z87.828
      psychological NEC Z91.49
      self-harm Z91.5
    traumatic brain injury Z87.820
    tuberculosis, latent infection Z86.15
    unhealthy sleep-wake cycle Z72.821
    unintended awareness under general anesthesia Z92.84
    urinary calculi Z87.442
    urinary (recurrent) (tract) infection(s) Z87.440
    uterine scar from previous surgery Z98.891
    vaginal dysplasia Z87.411
    venous thrombosis or embolism Z86.718
      pulmonary Z86.711
    vulvar dysplasia Z87.412
His-Werner disease A79.0
HIV — *see also* Human, immunodeficiency virus B20
  laboratory evidence (nonconclusive) R75
  nonconclusive test (in infants) R75
  positive, seropositive Z21
Hives (bold) — *see* Urticaria
Hoarseness R49.0
Hobo Z59.0
Hodgkin disease — *see* Lymphoma, Hodgkin
Hodgson's disease I71.2
  ruptured I71.1
Hoffa-Kastert disease E88.89
Hoffa's disease E88.89
Hoffmann-Bouveret syndrome I47.9
Hoffmann's syndrome E03.9 *[G73.7]*
Hole (round)
  macula H35.34 ☑
  retina (without detachment) — *see* Break, retina, round hole
    with detachment — *see* Detachment, retina, with retinal, break
Holiday relief care Z75.5
Hollenhorst's plaque — *see* Occlusion, artery, retina
Hollow foot (congenital) Q66.7- ☑
  acquired — *see* Deformity, limb, foot, specified NEC
Holoprosencephaly Q04.2
Holt-Oram syndrome Q87.2
Homelessness Z59.0
Homesickness — *see* Disorder, adjustment
Homocystinemia, homocystinuria E72.11
Homogentisate 1,2-dioxygenase deficiency E70.29
Homologous serum hepatitis (prophylactic) (therapeutic) — *see* Hepatitis, viral, type B
Honeycomb lung J98.4
  congenital Q33.0
Hooded
  clitoris Q52.6
  penis Q55.69
Hookworm (disease) (infection) (infestation) B76.9
  with anemia B76.9 *[D63.8]*
  specified NEC B76.8
Hordeolum (eyelid) (externum) (recurrent) H00.019
  internum H00.029
    left H00.026
      lower H00.025
      upper H00.024
    right H00.023
      lower H00.022
      upper H00.021
  left H00.016
    lower H00.015
    upper H00.014
  right H00.013
    lower H00.012
    upper H00.011
Horn
  cutaneous L85.8
  nail L60.2
    congenital Q84.6
Horner (-Claude Bernard) **syndrome** G90.2
  traumatic — *see* Injury, nerve, cervical sympathetic
Horseshoe kidney (congenital) Q63.1

Horton's headache or neuralgia G44.099
  intractable G44.091
  not intractable G44.099
Hospital hopper syndrome — *see* Disorder, factitious
Hospitalism in children — *see* Disorder, adjustment
Hostility R45.5
  towards child Z62.3
Hot flashes
  menopausal N95.1
Hourglass (contracture) — *see also* Contraction, hourglass
  stomach K31.89
    congenital Q40.2
    stricture K31.2
Household, housing circumstance affecting care Z59.9
  specified NEC Z59.8
Housemaid's knee — *see* Bursitis, prepatellar
Hudson (-Stähli) **line** (cornea) — *see* Pigmentation, cornea, anterior
Human
  bite (open wound) — *see also* Bite
    intact skin surface — *see* Bite, superficial
  herpesvirus — *see* Herpes
  immunodeficiency virus (HIV) disease (infection) B20
    asymptomatic status Z21
    contact Z20.6
    counseling Z71.7
    dementia B20 [F02.80]
      with behavioral disturbance B20 [F02.81]
    exposure to Z20.6
    laboratory evidence R75
    type-2 (HIV 2) as cause of disease classified elsewhere B97.35
  papillomavirus (HPV)
    DNA test positive
      high risk
        cervix R87.810
        vagina R87.811
      low risk
        cervix R87.820
        vagina R87.821
    screening for Z11.51
  T-cell lymphotropic virus
    type-1 (HTLV-I) infection B33.3
      as cause of disease classified elsewhere B97.33
      carrier Z22.6
    type-2 (HTLV-II) as cause of disease classified elsewhere B97.34
Humidifier lung or pneumonitis J67.7
Humiliation (experience) **in childhood** Z62.898
Humpback (acquired) — *see* Kyphosis
Hunchback (acquired) — *see* Kyphosis
Hunger T73.0 ☑
  air, psychogenic F45.8
Hungry bone syndrome E83.81
Hunner's ulcer — *see* Cystitis, chronic, interstitial
Hunter's
  glossitis D51.0
  syndrome E76.1
Huntington's disease or chorea G10
  with dementia G10 [F02.80]
    with behavioral disturbance G10 [F02.81]
Hunt's
  disease or syndrome (herpetic geniculate ganglionitis) B02.21
    dyssynergia cerebellaris myoclonica G11.1
  neuralgia B02.21
Hurler (-Scheie) **disease or syndrome** E76.02
Hurst's disease G36.1
Hurthle cell
  adenocarcinoma C73
  adenoma D34
  carcinoma C73
  tumor D34
Hutchinson-Boeck disease or syndrome — *see* Sarcoidosis
Hutchinson-Gilford disease or syndrome E34.8
Hutchinson's
  disease, meaning
    angioma serpiginosum L81.7
    pompholyx (cheiropompholyx) L30.1
    prurigo estivalis L56.4
    summer eruption or summer prurigo L56.4
  melanotic freckle — *see* Melanoma, in situ
    malignant melanoma in — *see* Melanoma
  teeth or incisors (congenital syphilis) A50.52
  triad (congenital syphilis) A50.53

Hyalin plaque, sclera, senile H15.89
Hyaline membrane (disease) (lung) (pulmonary) (newborn) P22.0
Hyalinosis
  cutis (et mucosae) E78.89
  focal and segmental (glomerular) — *see also* N00-N07 with fourth character .1 N05.1
Hyalitis, hyalosis, asteroid — *see also* Deposit, crystalline
  syphilitic (late) A52.71
Hydatid
  cyst or tumor — *see* Echinococcus
  mole — *see* Hydatidiform mole
  Morgagni
    female Q50.5
    male (epididymal) Q55.4
    testicular Q55.29
Hydatidiform mole (benign) (complicating pregnancy) (delivered) (undelivered) O01.9
  classical O01.0
  complete O01.0
  incomplete O01.1
  invasive D39.2
  malignant D39.2
  partial O01.1
Hydatidosis — *see* Echinococcus
Hydradenitis (axillaris) (suppurative) L73.2
Hydradenoma — *see* Hidradenoma
Hydramnios O40.-
Hydrancephaly, hydranencephaly Q04.3
  with spina bifida — *see* Spina bifida, with hydrocephalus
Hydrargyrism NEC — *see* Poisoning, mercury
Hydrarthrosis — *see also* Effusion, joint
  gonococcal A54.42
  intermittent M12.40
    ankle M12.47- ☑
    elbow M12.42- ☑
    foot joint M12.47- ☑
    hand joint M12.44- ☑
    hip M12.45- ☑
    knee M12.46- ☑
    multiple site M12.49
    shoulder M12.41- ☑
    specified joint NEC M12.48
    wrist M12.43- ☑
  of yaws (early) (late) — *see also* subcategory M14.8-A66.6
  syphilitic (late) A52.77
    congenital A50.55 [M12.80]
Hydremia D64.89
Hydrencephalocele (congenital) — *see* Encephalocele
Hydrencephalomeningocele (congenital) — *see* Encephalocele
Hydroa R23.8
  aestivale L56.4
  vacciniforme L56.4
Hydroadenitis (axillaris) (suppurative) L73.2
Hydrocalycosis — *see* Hydronephrosis
Hydrocele (spermatic cord) (testis) (tunica vaginalis) N43.3
  canal of Nuck N94.89
  communicating N43.2
    congenital P83.5
  congenital P83.5
  encysted N43.0
  female NEC N94.89
  infected N43.1
  newborn P83.5
  round ligament N94.89
  specified NEC N43.2
  spinalis — *see* Spina bifida
  vulva N90.89
Hydrocephalus (acquired) (external) (internal) (malignant) (recurrent) G91.9
  aqueduct Sylvius stricture Q03.0
  causing disproportion O33.6 ☑
    with obstructed labor O66.3
  communicating G91.0
  congenital (external) (internal) Q03.9
    with spina bifida Q05.4
      cervical Q05.0
      dorsal Q05.1
      lumbar Q05.2
      lumbosacral Q05.2
      sacral Q05.3
      thoracic Q05.1

Hydrocephalus — *continued*
  congenital — *continued*
    with spina bifida — *continued*
      thoracolumbar Q05.1
    specified NEC Q03.8
  due to toxoplasmosis (congenital) P37.1
  foramen Magendie block (acquired) G91.1
    congenital — *see also* Hydrocephalus, congenital Q03.1
  in (due to)
    infectious disease NEC B89 [G91.4]
    neoplastic disease NEC — *see also* Neoplasm G91
    parasitic disease B89 [G91.4]
  newborn Q03.9
    with spina bifida — *see* Spina bifida, with hydrocephalus
  noncommunicating G91.1
  normal pressure G91.2
    secondary G91.0
  obstructive G91.1
  otitic G93.2
  post-traumatic NEC G91.3
  secondary G91.4
    post-traumatic G91.3
  specified NEC G91.8
  syphilitic, congenital A50.49
Hydrocolpos (congenital) N89.8
Hydrocystoma — *see* Neoplasm, skin, benign
Hydroencephalocele (congenital) — *see* Encephalocele
Hydroencephalomeningocele (congenital) — *see* Encephalocele
Hydrohematopneumothorax — *see* Hemothorax
Hydromeningitis — *see* Meningitis
Hydromeningocele (spinal) — *see also* Spina bifida
  cranial — *see* Encephalocele
Hydrometra N85.8
Hydrometrocolpos N89.8
Hydromicrocephaly Q02
Hydromphalos (since birth) Q45.8
Hydromyelia Q06.4
Hydromyelocele — *see* Spina bifida
Hydronephrosis (atrophic) (early) (functionless) (intermittent) (primary) (secondary) NEC N13.30
  with
    infection N13.6
    obstruction (by) (of)
      renal calculus N13.2
        with infection N13.6
      ureteral NEC N13.1
        with infection N13.6
        calculus N13.2
          with infection N13.6
      ureteropelvic junction (congenital) Q62.11
        acquired N13.0
          with infection N13.6
    ureteral stricture NEC N13.1
      with infection N13.6
  congenital Q62.0
    due to acquired occlusion of ureteropelvic junction N13.0
  specified type NEC N13.39
  tuberculous A18.11
Hydropericarditis — *see* Pericarditis
Hydropericardium — *see* Pericarditis
Hydroperitoneum R18.8
Hydrophobia — *see* Rabies
Hydrophthalmos Q15.0
Hydropneumohemothorax — *see* Hemothorax
Hydropneumopericarditis — *see* Pericarditis
Hydropneumopericardium — *see* Pericarditis
Hydropneumothorax J94.8
  traumatic — *see* Injury, intrathoracic, lung
  tuberculous NEC A15.6
Hydrops R60.9
  abdominis R18.8
  articulorum intermittens — *see* Hydrarthrosis, intermittent
  cardiac — *see* Failure, heart, congestive
  causing obstructed labor (mother) O66.3
  endolymphatic H81.0- ☑
  fetal — *see* Pregnancy, complicated by, hydrops, feta
  fetalis P83.2
    due to
      ABO isoimmunization P56.0
      alpha thalassemia D56.0
      hemolytic disease P56.90
        specified NEC P56.99
      isoimmunization (ABO) (Rh) P56.0

Hydrops — *continued*
  fetalis — *continued*
    due to — *continued*
      other specified nonhemolytic disease NEC P83.2
      Rh incompatibility P56.0
    during pregnancy — *see* Pregnancy, complicated by, hydrops, fetalis
  gallbladder K82.1
  joint — *see* Effusion, joint
  labyrinth H81.0- ☑
  newborn (idiopathic) P83.2
    due to
      ABO isoimmunization P56.0
      alpha thalassemia D56.0
      hemolytic disease P56.90
        specified NEC P56.99
      isoimmunization (ABO) (Rh) P56.0
      Rh incompatibility P56.0
  nutritional — *see* Malnutrition, severe
  pericardium — *see* Pericarditis
  pleura — *see* Hydrothorax
  spermatic cord — *see* Hydrocele
Hydropyonephrosis N13.6
Hydrorachis Q06.4
Hydrorrhea (nasal) J34.89
  pregnancy — *see* Rupture, membranes, premature
Hydrosadenitis (axillaris) (suppurative) L73.2
Hydrosalpinx (fallopian tube) (follicularis) N70.11
Hydrothorax (double) (pleura) J94.8
  chylous (nonfilarial) I89.8
    filarial — *see also* Infestation, filarial B74.9 [J91.8]
  traumatic — *see* Injury, intrathoracic
  tuberculous NEC (non primary) A15.6
Hydroureter — *see also* Hydronephrosis N13.4
  with infection N13.6
  congenital Q62.39
Hydroureteronephrosis — *see* Hydronephrosis
Hydrourethra N36.8
Hydroxykynureninuria E70.8
Hydroxylysinemia E72.3
Hydroxyprolinemia E72.59
Hygiene, sleep
  abuse Z72.821
  inadequate Z72.821
  poor Z72.821
Hygroma (congenital) (cystic) D18.1
  praepatellare, prepatellar — *see* Bursitis, prepatellar
Hymen — *see* condition
Hymenolepis, hymenolepiasis (diminuta) (infection) (infestation) (nana) B71.0
Hypalgesia R20.8
Hyperacidity (gastric) K31.89
  psychogenic F45.8
Hyperactive, hyperactivity F90.9
  basal cell, uterine cervix — *see* Dysplasia, cervix
  bowel sounds R19.12
  cervix epithelial (basal) — *see* Dysplasia, cervix
  child F90.9
    attention deficit — *see* Disorder, attention-deficit hyperactivity
  detrusor muscle N32.81
  gastrointestinal K31.89
    psychogenic F45.8
  nasal mucous membrane J34.3
  stomach K31.89
  thyroid (gland) — *see* Hyperthyroidism
Hyperacusis H93.23- ☑
Hyperadrenalism E27.5
Hyperadrenocorticism E24.9
  congenital E25.0
  iatrogenic E24.2
    correct substance properly administered — *see* Table of Drugs and Chemicals, by drug, adverse effect
    overdose or wrong substance given or taken — *see* Table of Drugs and Chemicals, by drug, poisoning
  not associated with Cushing's syndrome E27.0
  pituitary-dependent E24.0
Hyperaldosteronism E26.9
  familial (type I) E26.02
  glucocorticoid-remediable E26.02
  primary (due to (bilateral) adrenal hyperplasia) E26.09
  primary NEC E26.09
  secondary E26.1
  specified NEC E26.89
Hyperalgesia R20.8

Hyperalimentation R63.2
  carotene, carotin E67.1
  specified NEC E67.8
  vitamin
    A E67.0
    D E67.3
Hyperaminoaciduria
  arginine E72.21
  cystine E72.01
  lysine E72.3
  ornithine E72.4
Hyperammonemia (congenital) E72.20
Hyperazotemia — *see* Uremia
Hyperbetalipoproteinemia (familial) E78.00
  with prebetalipoproteinemia E78.2
Hyperbicarbonatemia P74.41
Hyperbilirubinemia
  constitutional E80.6
  familial conjugated E80.6
  neonatal (transient) — *see* Jaundice, newborn
Hypercalcemia, hypocalciuric, familial E83.52
Hypercalciuria, idiopathic R82.994
Hypercapnia R06.89
  newborn P84
Hypercarotenemia (dietary) E67.1
Hypercementosis K03.4
Hyperchloremia E87.8
Hyperchlorhydria K31.89
  neurotic F45.8
  psychogenic F45.8
Hypercholesterinemia — *see* Hypercholesterolemia
Hypercholesterolemia (essential) (primary) (pure) E78.00
  with hyperglyceridemia, endogenous E78.2
  dietary counseling and surveillance Z71.3
  familial E78.00
  hereditary E78.01
Hyperchylia gastrica, psychogenic F45.8
Hyperchylomicronemia (familial) (primary) E78.3
  with hyperbetalipoproteinemia E78.3
Hypercoagulable (state) D68.59
  activated protein C resistance D68.51
  antithrombin (III) deficiency D68.59
  factor V Leiden mutation D68.51
  primary NEC D68.59
  protein C deficiency D68.59
  protein S deficiency D68.59
  prothrombin gene mutation D68.52
  secondary D68.69
  specified NEC D68.69
Hypercoagulation (state) D68.59
Hypercorticalism, pituitary-dependent E24.0
Hypercorticosolism — *see* Cushing's, syndrome
Hypercorticosteronism E24.2
  correct substance properly administered — *see* Table of Drugs and Chemicals, by drug, adverse effect
  overdose or wrong substance given or taken — *see* Table of Drugs and Chemicals, by drug, poisoning
Hypercortisonism E24.2
  correct substance properly administered — *see* Table of Drugs and Chemicals, by drug, adverse effect
  overdose or wrong substance given or taken — *see* Table of Drugs and Chemicals, by drug, poisoning
Hyperekplexia Q89.8
Hyperelectrolytemia E87.8
Hyperemesis R11.10
  with nausea R11.2
  gravidarum (mild) O21.0
    with
      carbohydrate depletion O21.1
      dehydration O21.1
      electrolyte imbalance O21.1
      metabolic disturbance O21.1
    severe (with metabolic disturbance) O21.1
  projectile R11.12
  psychogenic F45.8
Hyperemia (acute) (passive) R68.89
  anal mucosa K62.89
  bladder N32.89
  cerebral I67.89
  conjunctiva H11.43- ☑
  ear internal, acute — *see* subcategory H83.0 ☑
  enteric K59.8
  eye — *see* Hyperemia, conjunctiva
  eyelid (active) (passive) — *see* Disorder, eyelid, specified type NEC
  intestine K59.8
  iris — *see* Disorder, iris, vascular
  kidney N28.89

Hyperemia — *continued*
  labyrinth — *see* subcategory H83.0 ☑
  liver (active) K76.89
  lung (passive) — *see* Edema, lung
  pulmonary (passive) — *see* Edema, lung
  renal N28.89
  retina H35.89
  stomach K31.89
Hyperesthesia (body surface) R20.3
  larynx (reflex) J38.7
    hysterical F44.89
  pharynx (reflex) J39.2
    hysterical F44.89
Hyperestrogenism (drug-induced) (iatrogenic) E28.0
Hyperexplexia Q89.8
Hyperfibrinolysis — *see* Fibrinolysis
Hyperfructosemia E74.19
Hyperfunction
  adrenal cortex, not associated with Cushing's syndrome E27.0
    medulla E27.5
      adrenomedullary E27.5
      virilism E25.9
        congenital E25.0
  ovarian E28.8
  pancreas K86.89
  parathyroid (gland) E21.3
  pituitary (gland) (anterior) E22.9
    specified NEC E22.8
  polyglandular E31.1
  testicular E29.0
Hypergammaglobulinemia D89.2
  polyclonal D89.0
  Waldenström D89.0
Hypergastrinemia E16.4
Hyperglobulinemia R77.1
Hyperglycemia, hyperglycemic (transient) R73.9
  coma — *see* Diabetes, by type, with coma
  postpancreatectomy E89.1
Hyperglyceridemia (endogenous) (essential) (familial) (hereditary) (pure) E78.1
  mixed E78.3
Hyperglycinemia (non-ketotic) E72.51
Hypergonadism
  ovarian E28.8
  testicular (primary) (infantile) E29.0
Hyperheparinemia D68.32
Hyperhidrosis, hyperidrosis R61
  focal
    primary L74.519
      axilla L74.510
      face L74.511
      palms L74.512
      soles L74.513
    secondary L74.52
  generalized R61
  localized
    primary L74.519
      axilla L74.510
      face L74.511
      palms L74.512
      soles L74.513
    secondary L74.52
  psychogenic F45.8
  secondary R61
    focal L74.52
Hyperhistidinemia E70.41
Hyperhomocysteinemia E72.11
Hyperhydroxyprolinemia E72.59
Hyperinsulinism (functional) E16.1
  with
    coma (hypoglycemic) E15
    encephalopathy E16.1 [G94]
  ectopic E16.1
  therapeutic misadventure (from administration of insulin) — *see* subcategory T38.3 ☑
Hyperkalemia E87.5
Hyperkeratosis — *see also* Keratosis L85.9
  cervix N88.0
  due to yaws (early) (late) (palmar or plantar) A66.3
  follicularis Q82.8
    penetrans (in cutem) L87.0
  palmoplantaris climacterica L85.1
  pinta A67.1
  senile (with pruritus) L57.0
  universalis congenita Q80.8
  vocal cord J38.3
  vulva N90.4

Hyperkinesia, hyperkinetic (disease) (reaction) (syndrome) (childhood) (adolescence) — see also Disorder, attention-deficit hyperactivity
  heart I51.89
Hyperleucine-isoleucinemia E71.19
Hyperlipemia, hyperlipidemia E78.5
  combined E78.2
    familial E78.49
  group
    A E78.00
    B E78.1
    C E78.2
    D E78.3
  mixed E78.2
  specified NEC E78.49
Hyperlipidosis E75.6
  hereditary NEC E75.5
Hyperlipoproteinemia E78.5
  Fredrickson's type
    I E78.3
    IIa E78.00
    IIb E78.2
    III E78.2
    IV E78.1
    V E78.3
  low-density-lipoprotein-type (LDL) E78.00
  very-low-density-lipoprotein-type (VLDL) E78.1
Hyperlucent lung, unilateral J43.0
Hyperlysinemia E72.3
Hypermagnesemia E83.41
  neonatal P71.8
Hypermenorrhea N92.0
Hypermethioninemia E72.19
Hypermetropia (congenital) H52.0- ☑
Hypermobility, hypermotility
  cecum — see Syndrome, irritable bowel
  coccyx — see subcategory M53.2 ☑
  colon — see Syndrome, irritable bowel
    psychogenic F45.8
  ileum K58.9
  intestine — see also Syndrome, irritable bowel K58.9
    psychogenic F45.8
  meniscus (knee) — see Derangement, knee, meniscus
  scapula — see Instability, joint, shoulder
  stomach K31.89
    psychogenic F45.8
  syndrome M35.7
  urethra N36.41
    with intrinsic sphincter deficiency N36.43
Hypernasality R49.21
Hypernatremia E87.0
Hypernephroma C64.- ☑
Hyperopia — see Hypermetropia
Hyperorexia nervosa F50.2
Hyperornithinemia E72.4
Hyperosmia R43.1
Hyperosmolality E87.0
Hyperostosis (monomelic) — see also Disorder, bone, density and structure, specified NEC
  ankylosing (spine) M48.10
    cervical region M48.12
    cervicothoracic region M48.13
    lumbar region M48.16
    lumbosacral region M48.17
    multiple sites M48.19
    occipito-atlanto-axial region M48.11
    sacrococcygeal region M48.18
    thoracic region M48.14
    thoracolumbar region M48.15
  cortical (skull) M85.2
    infantile M89.8X- ☑
  frontal, internal of skull M85.2
  interna frontalis M85.2
  skeletal, diffuse idiopathic — see Hyperostosis, ankylosing
  skull M85.2
    congenital Q75.8
  vertebral, ankylosing — see Hyperostosis, ankylosing
Hyperovarism E28.8
Hyperoxaluria R82.992
  primary E72.53
Hyperparathyroidism E21.3
  primary E21.0
  secondary (renal) N25.81
    non-renal E21.1
  specified NEC E21.2
  tertiary E21.2
Hyperpathia R20.8

Hyperperistalsis R19.2
  psychogenic F45.8
Hyperpermeability, capillary I78.8
Hyperphagia R63.2
Hyperphenylalaninemia NEC E70.1
Hyperphoria (alternating) H50.53
Hyperphosphatemia E83.39
Hyperpiesis, hyperpiesia — see Hypertension
Hyperpigmentation — see also Pigmentation
  melanin NEC L81.4
  postinflammatory L81.0
Hyperpinealism E34.8
Hyperpituitarism E22.9
Hyperplasia, hyperplastic
  adenoids J35.2
  adrenal (capsule) (cortex) (gland) E27.8
    with
      sexual precocity (male) E25.9
        congenital E25.0
      virilism, adrenal E25.9
        congenital E25.0
      virilization (female) E25.9
        congenital E25.0
    congenital E25.0
    salt-losing E25.0
  adrenomedullary E27.5
  angiolymphoid, eosinophilia (ALHE) D18.01
  appendix (lymphoid) K38.0
  artery, fibromuscular I77.3
  bone — see also Hypertrophy, bone
    marrow D75.89
  breast — see also Hypertrophy, breast
    atypical, atypia N60.9- ☑
      ductal N60.9- ☑
      lobular N60.9- ☑
  C-cell, thyroid E07.0
  cementation (tooth) (teeth) K03.4
  cervical gland R59.0
  cervix (uteri) (basal cell) (endometrium) (polypoid) — see also Dysplasia, cervix
    congenital Q51.828
  clitoris, congenital Q52.6
  denture K06.2
  endocervicitis N72
  endometrium, endometrial (adenomatous) (cystic) (glandular) (glandular-cystic) (polypoid) N85.00
    with atypia N85.02
    benign N85.01
    cervix — see Dysplasia, cervix
    complex (without atypia) N85.01
    simple (without atypia) N85.01
  epithelial L85.9
    focal, oral, including tongue K13.29
    nipple N62
    skin L85.9
    tongue K13.29
    vaginal wall N89.3
  erythroid D75.89
  fibromuscular of artery (carotid) (renal) I77.3
  genital
    female NEC N94.89
    male N50.89
  gingiva K06.1
  glandularis cystica uteri (interstitialis) — see also Hyperplasia, endometrial N85.00
  gum K06.1
  hymen, congenital Q52.4
  irritative, edentulous (alveolar) K06.2
  jaw M26.09
    alveolar M26.79
    lower M26.03
      alveolar M26.72
    upper M26.01
      alveolar M26.71
  kidney (congenital) Q63.3
  labia N90.69
    epithelial N90.3
  liver (congenital) Q44.7
    nodular, focal K76.89
  lymph gland or node R59.9
  mandible, mandibular M26.03
    alveolar M26.72
    unilateral condylar M27.8
  maxilla, maxillary M26.01
    alveolar M26.71
  myometrium, myometrial N85.2
  neuroendocrine cell, of infancy J84.841

Hyperplasia, hyperplastic — continued
  nose
    lymphoid J34.89
    polypoid J33.9
  oral mucosa (irritative) K13.6
  organ or site, congenital NEC — see Anomaly, by site
  ovary N83.8
  palate, papillary (irritative) K13.6
  pancreatic islet cells E16.9
    alpha E16.8
      with excess
        gastrin E16.4
        glucagon E16.3
    beta E16.1
  parathyroid (gland) E21.0
  pharynx (lymphoid) J39.2
  prostate (adenofibromatous) (nodular) N40.0
    with lower urinary tract symptoms (LUTS) N40.1
    without lower urinary tract symtpoms (LUTS) N40.0
  renal artery I77.89
  reticulo-endothelial (cell) D75.89
  salivary gland (any) K11.1
  Schimmelbusch's — see Mastopathy, cystic
  suprarenal capsule (gland) E27.8
  thymus (gland) (persistent) E32.0
  thyroid (gland) — see Goiter
  tonsils (faucial) (infective) (lingual) (lymphoid) J35.1
    with adenoids J35.3
  unilateral condylar M27.8
  uterus, uterine N85.2
    endometrium (glandular) — see also Hyperplasia, endometrial N85.00
  vulva N90.69
    epithelial N90.3
Hyperpnea — see Hyperventilation
Hyperpotassemia E87.5
Hyperprebetalipoproteinemia (familial) E78.1
Hyperprolactinemia E22.1
Hyperprolinemia (type I) (type II) E72.59
Hyperproteinemia E88.09
Hyperprothrombinemia, causing coagulation factor deficiency D68.4
Hyperpyrexia R50.9
  heat (effects) T67.01 ☑
  malignant, due to anesthetic T88.3 ☑
  rheumatic — see Fever, rheumatic
  unknown origin R50.9
Hyper-reflexia R29.2
Hypersalivation K11.7
Hypersecretion
  ACTH (not associated with Cushing's syndrome) E27.0
    pituitary E24.0
  adrenaline E27.5
  adrenomedullary E27.5
  androgen (testicular) E29.0
    ovarian (drug-induced) (iatrogenic) E28.1
  calcitonin E07.0
  catecholamine E27.5
  corticoadrenal E24.9
  cortisol E24.9
  epinephrine E27.5
  estrogen E28.0
  gastric K31.89
    psychogenic F45.8
  gastrin E16.4
  glucagon E16.3
  hormone(s)
    ACTH (not associated with Cushing's syndrome) E27.0
      pituitary E24.0
    antidiuretic E22.2
    growth E22.0
    intestinal NEC E34.1
    ovarian androgen E28.1
    pituitary E22.9
    testicular E29.0
    thyroid stimulating E05.80
      with thyroid storm E05.81
  insulin — see Hyperinsulinism
  lacrimal glands — see Epiphora
  medulloadrenal E27.5
  milk O92.6
  ovarian androgens E28.1
  salivary gland (any) K11.7
  thyrocalcitonin E07.0
  upper respiratory J39.8
Hypersegmentation, leukocytic, hereditary D72.0

ypersensitive, hypersensitiveness, hypersensitivity
— *see also* Allergy
  carotid sinus G90.01
  colon — *see* Irritable, colon
  drug T88.7 ☑
  gastrointestinal K52.29
    immediate K52.29
    psychogenic F45.8
  labyrinth — *see* subcategory H83.2 ☑
  pain R20.8
  pneumonitis — *see* Pneumonitis, allergic
  reaction T78.40 ☑
    upper respiratory tract NEC J39.3
ypersomnia (organic) G47.10
  due to
    alcohol
      abuse F10.182
      dependence F10.282
      use F10.982
    amphetamines
      abuse F15.182
      dependence F15.282
      use F15.982
    caffeine
      abuse F15.182
      dependence F15.282
      use F15.982
    cocaine
      abuse F14.182
      dependence F14.282
      use F14.982
    drug NEC
      abuse F19.182
      dependence F19.282
      use F19.982
    medical condition G47.14
    mental disorder F51.13
    opioid
      abuse F11.182
      dependence F11.282
      use F11.982
    psychoactive substance NEC
      abuse F19.182
      dependence F19.282
      use F19.982
    sedative, hypnotic, or anxiolytic
      abuse F13.182
      dependence F13.282
      use F13.982
    stimulant NEC
      abuse F15.182
      dependence F15.282
      use F15.982
  idiopathic G47.11
    with long sleep time G47.11
    without long sleep time G47.12
  menstrual related G47.13
  nonorganic origin F51.11
    specified NEC F51.19
  not due to a substance or known physiological condition F51.11
    specified NEC F51.19
  primary F51.11
  recurrent G47.13
  specified NEC G47.19
ypersplenia, hypersplenism D73.1
yperstimulation, ovaries (associated with induced ovulation) N98.1
ypersusceptibility — *see* Allergy
ypertelorism (ocular) (orbital) Q75.2
ypertension, hypertensive (accelerated) (benign) (essential) (idiopathic) (malignant) (systemic) I10
  with
    heart failure (congestive) I11.0
    heart involvement (conditions in I50.-, I51.4- I51.9 due to hypertension) — *see* Hypertension, heart
    kidney involvement — *see* Hypertension, kidney
  benign, intracranial G93.2
  borderline R03.0
  cardiorenal (disease) I13.10
    with heart failure I13.0
      with stage 1 through stage 4 chronic kidney disease I13.0
      with stage 5 or end stage renal disease I13.2
    without heart failure I13.10
      with stage 1 through stage 4 chronic kidney disease I13.10

Hypertension, hypertensive — *continued*
  cardiorenal — *continued*
    without heart failure — *continued*
      with stage 5 or end stage renal disease I13.11
  cardiovascular
    disease (arteriosclerotic) (sclerotic) — *see* Hypertension, heart
    renal (disease) — *see* Hypertension, cardiorenal
  chronic venous — *see* Hypertension, venous (chronic)
  complicating
    childbirth (labor) O16.4
      pre-existing O10.92
        with
          heart disease O10.12
            with renal disease O10.32
          pre-eclampsia O11.4
          renal disease O10.22
            with heart disease O10.32
          essential O10.02
      secondary O10.42
    pregnancy O16.- ☑
      with edema — *see also* Pre-eclampsia O14.9- ☑
      gestational (pregnancy induced) (without proteinuria) O13.- ☑
        with proteinuria O14.9- ☑
          mild pre-eclampsia O14.0- ☑
          moderate pre-eclampsia O14.0- ☑
          severe pre-eclampsia O14.1- ☑
            with hemolysis, elevated liver enzymes and low platelet count (HELLP) O14.2- ☑
      pre-existing O10.91- ☑
        with
          heart disease O10.11- ☑
            with renal disease O10.31- ☑
          pre-eclampsia — *see* category O11
          renal disease O10.21- ☑
            with heart disease O10.31- ☑
          essential O10.01- ☑
        secondary O10.41- ☑
      transient O13- ☑
    puerperium, pre-existing O16.5
      pre-existing
        with
          heart disease O10.13
            with renal disease O10.33
          pre-eclampsia O11.5
          renal disease O10.23
            with heart disease O10.33
          essential O10.03
      pregnancy-induced O13.9
      secondary O10.43
  crisis I16.9
  due to
    endocrine disorders I15.2
    pheochromocytoma I15.2
    renal disorders NEC I15.1
      arterial I15.0
    renovascular disorders I15.0
    specified disease NEC I15.8
  emergency I16.1
  encephalopathy I67.4
  gestational (without significant proteinuria) (pregnancy-induced) (transient) O13.- ☑
    with significant proteinuria — *see* Pre-eclampsia
    complicating
      delivery O13.4
      puerperium O13.5
  Goldblatt's I70.1
  heart (disease) (conditions in I51.4-I51.9 due to hypertension) I11.9
    with
      heart failure (congestive) I11.0
      kidney disease (chronic) — *see* Hypertension, cardiorenal
  intracranial (benign) G93.2
  kidney I12.9
    with
      heart disease — *see* Hypertension, cardiorenal
      stage 1 through stage 4 chronic kidney disease I12.9
      stage 5 chronic kidney disease (CKD) or end stage renal disease (ESRD) I12.0
  lesser circulation I27.0
  maternal O16- ☑
  newborn P29.2
    pulmonary (persistent) P29.30
  ocular H40.05- ☑

Hypertension, hypertensive — *continued*
  pancreatic duct — *code to* underlying condition
    with chronic pancreatitis K86.1
  portal (due to chronic liver disease) (idiopathic) K76.6
    gastropathy K31.89
    in (due to) schistosomiasis (bilharziasis) B65.9 *[K77]*
  postoperative I97.3
  psychogenic F45.8
  pulmonary I27.20
    with
      cor pulmonale (chronic) I27.29
        acute I26.09
      right heart ventricular strain/failure I27.29
        acute I26.09
      right to left shunt related to congenital heart disease I27.83
      unclear multifactorial mechanisms I27.29
    arterial (associated) (drug-induced) (toxin-induced) I27.21
    chronic thromboembolic I27.24
    due to
      hematologic disorders I27.29
      left heart disease I27.22
      lung diseases and hypoxia I27.23
      metabolic disorders I27.29
      specified systemic disorders I27.29
    group 1 (associated) (drug-induced) (toxin-induced) I27.21
    group 2 I27.22
    group 3 I27.23
    group 4 I27.24
    group 5 I27.29
    of newborn (persistent) P29.30
    primary (idiopathic) I27.0
    secondary
      arterial I27.21
      specified NEC I27.29
  renal — *see* Hypertension, kidney
  renovascular I15.0
  secondary NEC I15.9
    due to
      endocrine disorders I15.2
      pheochromocytoma I15.2
      renal disorders NEC I15.1
        arterial I15.0
      renovascular disorders I15.0
    specified NEC I15.8
  transient R03.0
    of pregnancy O13.- ☑
  urgency I16.0
  venous (chronic)
    due to
      deep vein thrombosis — *see* Syndrome, post-thrombotic
    idiopathic I87.309
      with
        inflammation I87.32- ☑
          with ulcer I87.33- ☑
        specified complication NEC I87.39- ☑
        ulcer I87.31- ☑
          with inflammation I87.33- ☑
        asymptomatic I87.30- ☑
Hypertensive urgency — *see* Hypertension
Hyperthecosis ovary E28.8
Hyperthermia (of unknown origin) — *see also* Hyperpyrexia
  malignant, due to anesthesia T88.3 ☑
  newborn P81.9
    environmental P81.0
Hyperthyroid (recurrent) — *see* Hyperthyroidism
Hyperthyroidism (latent) (pre-adult) (recurrent) E05.90
  with
    goiter (diffuse) E05.00
      with thyroid storm E05.01
      nodular (multinodular) E05.20
        with thyroid storm E05.21
        uninodular E05.10
          with thyroid storm E05.11
    storm E05.91
  due to ectopic thyroid tissue E05.30
    with thyroid storm E05.31
  neonatal, transitory P72.1
  specified NEC E05.80
    with thyroid storm E05.81
Hypertony, hypertonia, hypertonicity
  bladder N31.8
  congenital P94.1
  stomach K31.89

Hypertony, hypertonia, hypertonicity — *continued*
  stomach — *continued*
    psychogenic F45.8
  uterus, uterine (contractions) (complicating delivery)
    O62.4
Hypertrichosis L68.9
  congenital Q84.2
  eyelid H02.869
    left H02.866
      lower H02.865
      upper H02.864
    right H02.863
      lower H02.862
      upper H02.861
  lanuginosa Q84.2
    acquired L68.1
  localized L68.2
  specified NEC L68.8
Hypertriglyceridemia, essential E78.1
Hypertrophy, hypertrophic
  adenofibromatous, prostate — *see* Enlargement, enlarged, prostate
  adenoids (infective) J35.2
    with tonsils J35.3
  adrenal cortex E27.8
  alveolar process or ridge — *see* Anomaly, alveolar
  anal papillae K62.89
  artery I77.89
    congenital NEC Q27.8
      digestive system Q27.8
      lower limb Q27.8
      specified site NEC Q27.8
      upper limb Q27.8
  auricular — *see* Hypertrophy, cardiac
  Bartholin's gland N75.8
  bile duct (common) (hepatic) K83.8
  bladder (sphincter) (trigone) N32.89
  bone M89.30
    carpus M89.34- ☑
    clavicle M89.31- ☑
    femur M89.35- ☑
    fibula M89.36- ☑
    finger M89.34- ☑
    humerus M89.32- ☑
    ilium M89.359
    ischium M89.359
    metacarpus M89.34- ☑
    metatarsus M89.37- ☑
    multiple sites M89.39
    neck M89.38
    radius M89.33- ☑
    rib M89.38
    scapula M89.31- ☑
    skull M89.38
    tarsus M89.37- ☑
    tibia M89.36- ☑
    toe M89.37- ☑
    ulna M89.33- ☑
    vertebra M89.38
  brain G93.89
  breast N62
    cystic — *see* Mastopathy, cystic
    newborn P83.4
    pubertal, massive N62
    puerperal, postpartum — *see* Disorder, breast, specified type NEC
    senile (parenchymatous) N62
  cardiac (chronic) (idiopathic) I51.7
    with rheumatic fever (conditions in I00)
      active I01.8
      inactive or quiescent (with chorea) I09.89
    congenital NEC Q24.8
    fatty — *see* Degeneration, myocardial
    hypertensive — *see* Hypertension, heart
    rheumatic (with chorea) I09.89
      active or acute I01.8
        with chorea I02.0
    valve — *see* Endocarditis
  cartilage — *see* Disorder, cartilage, specified type NEC
  cecum — *see* Megacolon
  cervix (uteri) N88.8
    congenital Q51.828
    elongation N88.4
  clitoris (cirrhotic) N90.89
    congenital Q52.6
  colon — *see also* Megacolon
    congenital Q43.2

Hypertrophy, hypertrophic — *continued*
  conjunctiva, lymphoid H11.89
  corpora cavernosa N48.89
  cystic duct K82.8
  duodenum K31.89
  endometrium (glandular) — *see also* Hyperplasia, endometrial N85.00
    cervix N88.8
  epididymis N50.89
  esophageal hiatus (congenital) Q79.1
    with hernia — *see* Hernia, hiatal
  eyelid — *see* Disorder, eyelid, specified type NEC
  fat pad E65
    knee (infrapatellar) (popliteal) (prepatellar) (retropatellar) M79.4
  foot (congenital) Q74.2
  frenulum, frenum (tongue) K14.8
    lip K13.0
  gallbladder K82.8
  gastric mucosa K29.60
    with bleeding K29.61
  gland, glandular R59.9
    generalized R59.1
    localized R59.0
  gum (mucous membrane) K06.1
  heart (idiopathic) — *see also* Hypertrophy, cardiac
    valve — *see also* Endocarditis I38
  hemifacial Q67.4
  hepatic — *see* Hypertrophy, liver
  hiatus (esophageal) Q79.1
  hilus gland R59.0
  hymen, congenital Q52.4
  ileum K63.89
  intestine NEC K63.89
  jejunum K63.89
  kidney (compensatory) N28.81
    congenital Q63.3
  labium (majus) (minus) N90.60
  ligament — *see* Disorder, ligament
  lingual tonsil (infective) J35.1
    with adenoids J35.3
  lip K13.0
    congenital Q18.6
  liver R16.0
    acute K76.89
    cirrhotic — *see* Cirrhosis, liver
    congenital Q44.7
    fatty — *see* Fatty, liver
  lymph, lymphatic gland R59.9
    generalized R59.1
    localized R59.0
    tuberculous — *see* Tuberculosis, lymph gland
  mammary gland — *see* Hypertrophy, breast
  Meckel's diverticulum (congenital) Q43.0
    malignant — *see* Table of Neoplasms, small intestine, malignant
  median bar — *see* Hyperplasia, prostate
  meibomian gland — *see* Chalazion
  meniscus, knee, congenital Q74.1
  metatarsal head — *see* Hypertrophy, bone, metatarsus
  metatarsus — *see* Hypertrophy, bone, metatarsus
  mucous membrane
    alveolar ridge K06.2
    gum K06.1
    nose (turbinate) J34.3
  muscle M62.89
  muscular coat, artery I77.89
  myocardium — *see also* Hypertrophy, cardiac
    idiopathic I42.2
  myometrium N85.2
  nail L60.2
    congenital Q84.5
  nasal J34.89
    alae J34.89
    bone J34.89
    cartilage J34.89
    mucous membrane (septum) J34.3
    sinus J34.89
    turbinate J34.3
  nasopharynx, lymphoid (infectional) (tissue) (wall) J35.2
  nipple N62
  organ or site, congenital NEC — *see* Anomaly, by site
  ovary N83.8
  palate (hard) M27.8
    soft K13.79
  pancreas, congenital Q45.3
  parathyroid (gland) E21.0
  parotid gland K11.1

Hypertrophy, hypertrophic — *continued*
  penis N48.89
  pharyngeal tonsil J35.2
  pharynx J39.2
    lymphoid (infectional) (tissue) (wall) J35.2
  pituitary (anterior) (fossa) (gland) E23.6
  prepuce (congenital) N47.8
    female N90.89
  prostate — *see* Enlargement, enlarged, prostate
    congenital Q55.4
  pseudomuscular G71.09
  pylorus (adult) (muscle) (sphincter) K31.1
    congenital or infantile Q40.0
  rectal, rectum (sphincter) K62.89
  rhinitis (turbinate) J31.0
  salivary gland (any) K11.1
    congenital Q38.4
  scaphoid (tarsal) — *see* Hypertrophy, bone, tarsus
  scar L91.0
  scrotum N50.89
  seminal vesicle N50.89
  sigmoid — *see* Megacolon
  skin L91.9
    specified NEC L91.8
  spermatic cord N50.89
  spleen — *see* Splenomegaly
  spondylitis — *see* Spondylosis
  stomach K31.89
  sublingual gland K11.1
  submandibular gland K11.1
  suprarenal cortex (gland) E27.8
  synovial NEC M67.20
    acromioclavicular M67.21- ☑
    ankle M67.27- ☑
    elbow M67.22- ☑
    foot M67.27- ☑
    hand M67.24- ☑
    hip M67.25- ☑
    knee M67.26- ☑
    multiple sites M67.29
    specified site NEC M67.28
    wrist M67.23- ☑
  tendon — *see* Disorder, tendon, specified type NEC
  testis N44.8
    congenital Q55.29
  thymic, thymus (gland) (congenital) E32.0
  thyroid (gland) — *see* Goiter
  toe (congenital) Q74.2
    acquired — *see also* Deformity, toe, specified NEC
  tongue K14.8
    congenital Q38.2
    papillae (foliate) K14.3
  tonsils (faucial) (infective) (lingual) (lymphoid) J35.1
    with adenoids J35.3
  tunica vaginalis N50.89
  ureter N28.89
  urethra N36.8
  uterus N85.2
    neck (with elongation) N88.4
    puerperal O90.89
  uvula K13.79
  vagina N89.8
  vas deferens N50.89
  vein I87.8
  ventricle, ventricular (heart) — *see also* Hypertrophy, cardiac
    congenital Q24.8
    in tetralogy of Fallot Q21.3
  verumontanum N36.8
  vocal cord J38.3
  vulva N90.60
    stasis (nonfilarial) N90.69
Hypertropia H50.2- ☑
Hypertyrosinemia E70.21
Hyperuricemia (asymptomatic) E79.0
Hyperuricosuria R82.993
Hypervalinemia E71.19
Hyperventilation (tetany) R06.4
  hysterical F45.8
  psychogenic F45.8
  syndrome F45.8
Hypervitaminosis (dietary) NEC E67.8
  A E67.0
    administered as drug (prolonged intake) — *see* Table of Drugs and Chemicals, vitamins, adverse effect

☑ **Additional Character Required — Refer to the Tabular List for Character Selection**

▽ Subterms under main terms may continue to next column or page

ypervitaminosis — *continued*
A — *continued*
overdose or wrong substance given or taken — *see Table of Drugs and Chemicals, vitamins, poisoning*
B6 E67.2
D E67.3
administered as drug (prolonged intake) — *see Table of Drugs and Chemicals, vitamins, adverse effect*
overdose or wrong substance given or taken — *see Table of Drugs and Chemicals, vitamins, poisoning*
K E67.8
administered as drug (prolonged intake) — *see Table of Drugs and Chemicals, vitamins, adverse effect*
overdose or wrong substance given or taken — *see Table of Drugs and Chemicals, vitamins, poisoning*
ypervolemia E87.70
specified NEC E87.79
ypesthesia R20.1
cornea — *see Anesthesia, cornea*
yphema H21.0- ☑
traumatic S05.1- ☑
ypoacidity, gastric K31.89
psychogenic F45.8
ypoadrenalism, hypoadrenia E27.40
primary E27.1
tuberculous A18.7
ypoadrenocorticism E27.40
pituitary E23.0
primary E27.1
ypoalbuminemia E88.09
ypoaldosteronism E27.40
ypoalphalipoproteinemia E78.6
ypobarism T70.29 ☑
ypobaropathy T70.29 ☑
ypobetalipoproteinemia (familial) E78.6
ypocalcemia E83.51
dietary E58
neonatal P71.1
due to cow's milk P71.0
phosphate-loading (newborn) P71.1
ypochloremia E87.8
ypochlorhydria K31.89
neurotic F45.8
psychogenic F45.8
ypochondria, hypochondriac, hypochondriasis (reaction) F45.21
sleep F51.03
ypochondrogenesis Q77.0
ypochondroplasia Q77.4
ypochromasia, blood cells D50.8
ypocitraturia R82.991
ypodontia — *see Anodontia*
ypoeosinophilia D72.89
ypoesthesia R20.1
ypofibrinogenemia D68.8
acquired D65
congenital (hereditary) D68.2
ypofunction
adrenocortical E27.40
drug-induced E27.3
postprocedural E89.6
primary E27.1
adrenomedullary, postprocedural E89.6
cerebral R29.818
corticoadrenal NEC E27.40
intestinal K59.8
labyrinth — *see subcategory* H83.2 ☑
ovary E28.39
pituitary (gland) (anterior) E23.0
testicular E29.1
postprocedural (postsurgical) (postirradiation) (iatrogenic) E89.5
ypogalactia O92.4
ypogammaglobulinemia — *see also Agammaglobulinemia* D80.1
hereditary D80.0
nonfamilial D80.1
transient, of infancy D80.7
ypogenitalism (congenital) — *see Hypogonadism*
ypoglossia Q38.3
ypoglycemia (spontaneous) E16.2
coma E15

Hypoglycemia — *continued*
coma — *continued*
diabetic — *see Diabetes, by type, with hypoglycemia, with coma*
diabetic — *see Diabetes, hypoglycemia*
dietary counseling and surveillance Z71.3
drug-induced E16.0
with coma (nondiabetic) E15
due to insulin E16.0
with coma (nondiabetic) E15
therapeutic misadventure — *see subcategory* T38.3 ☑
functional, nonhyperinsulinemic E16.1
iatrogenic E16.0
with coma (nondiabetic) E15
in infant of diabetic mother P70.1
gestational diabetes P70.0
infantile E16.1
leucine-induced E71.19
neonatal (transitory) P70.4
iatrogenic P70.3
reactive (not drug-induced) E16.1
transitory neonatal P70.4
Hypogonadism
female E28.39
hypogonadotropic E23.0
male E29.1
ovarian (primary) E28.39
pituitary E23.0
testicular (primary) E29.1
Hypohidrosis, hypoidrosis L74.4
Hypoinsulinemia, postprocedural E89.1
Hypokalemia E87.6
Hypoleukocytosis — *see Agranulocytosis*
Hypolipoproteinemia (alpha) (beta) E78.6
Hypomagnesemia E83.42
neonatal P71.2
Hypomania, hypomanic reaction F30.8
Hypomenorrhea — *see Oligomenorrhea*
Hypometabolism R63.8
Hypomotility
gastrointestinal (tract) K31.89
psychogenic F45.8
intestine K59.8
psychogenic F45.8
stomach K31.89
psychogenic F45.8
Hyponasality R49.22
Hyponatremia E87.1
Hypo-osmolality E87.1
Hypo-ovarianism, hypo-ovarism E28.39
Hypoparathyroidism E20.9
familial E20.8
idiopathic E20.0
neonatal, transitory P71.4
postprocedural E89.2
specified NEC E20.8
Hypoperfusion (in)
newborn P96.89
Hypopharyngitis — *see Laryngopharyngitis*
Hypophoria H50.53
Hypophosphatemia, hypophosphatasia (acquired) (congenital) (renal) E83.39
familial E83.31
Hypophyseal, hypophysis — *see also condition*
dwarfism E23.0
gigantism E22.0
Hypopiesis — *see Hypotension*
Hypopinealism E34.8
Hypopituitarism (juvenile) E23.0
drug-induced E23.1
due to
hypophysectomy E89.3
radiotherapy E89.3
iatrogenic NEC E23.1
postirradiation E89.3
postpartum O99.285
postprocedural E89.3
Hypoplasia, hypoplastic
adrenal (gland), congenital Q89.1
alimentary tract, congenital Q45.8
upper Q40.8
anus, anal (canal) Q42.3
with fistula Q42.2
aorta, aortic Q25.42
ascending, in hypoplastic left heart syndrome Q23.4
valve Q23.1
in hypoplastic left heart syndrome Q23.4

Hypoplasia, hypoplastic — *continued*
areola, congenital Q83.8
arm (congenital) — *see Defect, reduction, upper limb*
artery (peripheral) Q27.8
brain (congenital) Q28.3
coronary Q24.5
digestive system Q27.8
lower limb Q27.8
pulmonary Q25.79
functional, unilateral J43.0
retinal (congenital) Q14.1
specified site NEC Q27.8
umbilical Q27.0
upper limb Q27.8
auditory canal Q17.8
causing impairment of hearing Q16.9
biliary duct or passage Q44.5
bone NOS Q79.9
face Q75.8
marrow D61.9
megakaryocytic D69.49
skull — *see Hypoplasia, skull*
brain Q02
gyri Q04.3
part of Q04.3
breast (areola) N64.82
bronchus Q32.4
cardiac Q24.8
carpus — *see Defect, reduction, upper limb, specified type NEC*
cartilage hair Q78.8
cecum Q42.8
cementum K00.4
cephalic Q02
cerebellum Q04.3
cervix (uteri), congenital Q51.821
clavicle (congenital) Q74.0
coccyx Q76.49
colon Q42.9
specified NEC Q42.8
corpus callosum Q04.0
cricoid cartilage Q31.2
digestive organ(s) or tract NEC Q45.8
upper (congenital) Q40.8
ear (auricle) (lobe) Q17.2
middle Q16.4
enamel of teeth (neonatal) (postnatal) (prenatal) K00.4
endocrine (gland) NEC Q89.2
endometrium N85.8
epididymis (congenital) Q55.4
epiglottis Q31.2
erythroid, congenital D61.01
esophagus (congenital) Q39.8
eustachian tube Q17.8
eye Q11.2
eyelid (congenital) Q10.3
face Q18.8
bone(s) Q75.8
femur (congenital) — *see Defect, reduction, lower limb, specified type NEC*
fibula (congenital) — *see Defect, reduction, lower limb, specified type NEC*
finger (congenital) — *see Defect, reduction, upper limb, specified type NEC*
focal dermal Q82.8
foot — *see Defect, reduction, lower limb, specified type NEC*
gallbladder Q44.0
genitalia, genital organ(s)
female, congenital Q52.8
external Q52.79
internal NEC Q52.8
in adiposogenital dystrophy E23.6
glottis Q31.2
hair Q84.2
hand (congenital) — *see Defect, reduction, upper limb, specified type NEC*
heart Q24.8
humerus (congenital) — *see Defect, reduction, upper limb, specified type NEC*
intestine (small) Q41.9
large Q42.9
specified NEC Q42.8
jaw M26.09
alveolar M26.79
lower M26.04
alveolar M26.74
upper M26.02

Hypoplasia, hypoplastic — *continued*
 jaw — *continued*
  upper — *continued*
   alveolar M26.73
 kidney(s) Q60.5
  bilateral Q60.4
  unilateral Q60.3
 labium (majus) (minus), congenital Q52.79
 larynx Q31.2
 left heart syndrome Q23.4
 leg (congenital) — *see* Defect, reduction, lower limb
 limb Q73.8
  lower (congenital) — *see* Defect, reduction, lower limb
  upper (congenital) — *see* Defect, reduction, upper limb
 liver Q44.7
 lung (lobe) (not associated with short gestation) Q33.6
  associated with immaturity, low birth weight, prematurity, or short gestation P28.0
 mammary (areola), congenital Q83.8
 mandible, mandibular M26.04
  alveolar M26.74
  unilateral condylar M27.8
 maxillary M26.02
  alveolar M26.73
 medullary D61.9
 megakaryocytic D69.49
 metacarpus — *see* Defect, reduction, upper limb, specified type NEC
 metatarsus — *see* Defect, reduction, lower limb, specified type NEC
 muscle Q79.8
 nail(s) Q84.6
 nose, nasal Q30.1
 optic nerve H47.03- ☑
 osseous meatus (ear) Q17.8
 ovary, congenital Q50.39
 pancreas Q45.0
 parathyroid (gland) Q89.2
 parotid gland Q38.4
 patella Q74.1
 pelvis, pelvic girdle Q74.2
 penis (congenital) Q55.62
 peripheral vascular system Q27.8
  digestive system Q27.8
  lower limb Q27.8
  specified site NEC Q27.8
  upper limb Q27.8
 pituitary (gland) (congenital) Q89.2
 pulmonary (not associated with short gestation) Q33.6
  artery, functional J43.0
  associated with short gestation P28.0
 radioulnar — *see* Defect, reduction, upper limb, specified type NEC
 radius — *see* Defect, reduction, upper limb
 rectum Q42.1
  with fistula Q42.0
 respiratory system NEC Q34.8
 rib Q76.6
 right heart syndrome Q22.6
 sacrum Q76.49
 scapula Q74.0
 scrotum Q55.1
 shoulder girdle Q74.0
 skin Q82.8
 skull (bone) Q75.8
  with
   anencephaly Q00.0
   encephalocele — *see* Encephalocele
   hydrocephalus Q03.9
    with spina bifida — *see* Spina bifida, by site, with hydrocephalus
   microcephaly Q02
 spinal (cord) (ventral horn cell) Q06.1
 spine Q76.49
 sternum Q76.7
 tarsus — *see* Defect, reduction, lower limb, specified type NEC
 testis Q55.1
 thymic, with immunodeficiency D82.1
 thymus (gland) Q89.2
  with immunodeficiency D82.1
 thyroid (gland) E03.1
  cartilage Q31.2
 tibiofibular (congenital) — *see* Defect, reduction, lower limb, specified type NEC

Hypoplasia, hypoplastic — *continued*
 toe — *see* Defect, reduction, lower limb, specified type NEC
 tongue Q38.3
 Turner's K00.4
 ulna (congenital) — *see* Defect, reduction, upper limb
 umbilical artery Q27.0
 unilateral condylar M27.8
 ureter Q62.8
 uterus, congenital Q51.811
 vagina Q52.4
 vascular NEC peripheral Q27.8
  brain Q28.3
  digestive system Q27.8
  lower limb Q27.8
  specified site NEC Q27.8
  upper limb Q27.8
 vein(s) (peripheral) Q27.8
  brain Q28.3
  digestive system Q27.8
  great Q26.8
  lower limb Q27.8
  specified site NEC Q27.8
  upper limb Q27.8
 vena cava (inferior) (superior) Q26.8
 vertebra Q76.49
 vulva, congenital Q52.79
 zonule (ciliary) Q12.8
Hypoplasminogenemia E88.02
Hypopnea, obstructive sleep apnea G47.33
Hypopotassemia E87.6
Hypoproconvertinemia, congenital (hereditary) D68.2
Hypoproteinemia E77.8
Hypoprothrombinemia (congenital) (hereditary) (idiopathic) D68.2
 acquired D68.4
 newborn, transient P61.6
Hypoptyalism K11.7
Hypopyon (eye) (anterior chamber) — *see* Iridocyclitis, acute, hypopyon
Hypopyrexia R68.0
Hyporeflexia R29.2
Hyposecretion
 ACTH E23.0
 antidiuretic hormone E23.2
 ovary E28.39
 salivary gland (any) K11.7
 vasopressin E23.2
Hyposegmentation, leukocytic, hereditary D72.0
Hyposiderinemia D50.9
Hypospadias Q54.9
 balanic Q54.0
 coronal Q54.0
 glandular Q54.0
 penile Q54.1
 penoscrotal Q54.2
 perineal Q54.3
 specified NEC Q54.8
Hypospermatogenesis — *see* Oligospermia
Hyposplenism D73.0
Hypostasis pulmonary, passive — *see* Edema, lung
Hypostatic — *see* condition
Hyposthenuria N28.89
Hypotension (arterial) (constitutional) I95.9
 chronic I95.89
 due to (of) hemodialysis I95.3
 drug-induced I95.2
 iatrogenic I95.89
 idiopathic (permanent) I95.0
 intracranial, following ventricular shunting (ventriculostomy) G97.2
 intra-dialytic I95.3
 maternal, syndrome (following labor and delivery) O26.5- ☑
 neurogenic, orthostatic G90.3
 orthostatic (chronic) I95.1
  due to drugs I95.2
  neurogenic G90.3
 postoperative I95.81
 postural I95.1
 specified NEC I95.89
Hypothermia (accidental) T68 ☑
 due to anesthesia, anesthetic T88.51 ☑
 low environmental temperature T68 ☑
 neonatal P80.9
  environmental (mild) NEC P80.8
  mild P80.8
  severe (chronic) (cold injury syndrome) P80.0

Hypothermia — *continued*
 neonatal — *continued*
  specified NEC P80.8
 not associated with low environmental temperature R68.0
Hypothyroidism (acquired) E03.9
 autoimmune — *see* Thyroiditis, autoimmune
 congenital (without goiter) E03.1
  with goiter (diffuse) E03.0
 due to
  exogenous substance NEC E03.2
  iodine-deficiency, acquired E01.8
   subclinical E02
  irradiation therapy E89.0
  medicament NEC E03.2
  P-aminosalicylic acid (PAS) E03.2
  phenylbutazone E03.2
  resorcinol E03.2
  sulfonamide E03.2
  surgery E89.0
  thiourea group drugs E03.2
 iatrogenic NEC E03.2
 iodine-deficiency (acquired) E01.8
  congenital — *see* Syndrome, iodine- deficiency, congenital
  subclinical E02
 neonatal, transitory P72.2
 postinfectious E03.3
 postirradiation E89.0
 postprocedural E89.0
 postsurgical E89.0
 specified NEC E03.8
 subclinical, iodine-deficiency related E02
Hypotonia, hypotonicity, hypotony
 bladder N31.2
 congenital (benign) P94.2
 eye — *see* Disorder, globe, hypotony
Hypotrichosis — *see* Alopecia
Hypotropia H50.2- ☑
Hypoventilation R06.89
 congenital central alveolar G47.35
 sleep related
  idiopathic nonobstructive alveolar G47.34
  in conditions classified elsewhere G47.36
Hypovitaminosis — *see* Deficiency, vitamin
Hypovolemia E86.1
 surgical shock T81.19 ☑
 traumatic (shock) T79.4 ☑
Hypoxemia R09.02
 newborn P84
 sleep related, in conditions classified elsewhere G47
Hypoxia — *see also* Anoxia R09.02
 cerebral, during a procedure NEC G97.81
  postprocedural NEC G97.82
 intrauterine P84
 myocardial — *see* Insufficiency, coronary
 newborn P84
 sleep-related G47.34
Hypsarrhythmia — *see* Epilepsy, generalized, specifie NEC
Hysteralgia, pregnant uterus O26.89- ☑
Hysteria, hysterical (conversion) (dissociative state) F44.9
 anxiety F41.8
 convulsions F44.5
 psychosis, acute F44.9
Hysteroepilepsy F44.5

I

IBDU (colonic inflammatory bowel dissease unclassifie K52.3
Ichthyoparasitism due to Vandellia cirrhosa B88.
Ichthyosis (congenital) Q80.9
 acquired L85.0
 fetalis Q80.4
 hystrix Q80.8
 lamellar Q80.2
 lingual K13.29
 palmaris and plantaris Q82.8
 simplex Q80.0
 vera Q80.8
 vulgaris Q80.0
 X-linked Q80.1
Ichthyotoxism — *see* Poisoning, fish
 bacterial — *see* Intoxication, foodborne
Icteroanemia, hemolytic (acquired) D59.9
 congenital — *see* Spherocytosis

...terus — *see also* Jaundice
  conjunctiva R17
  gravis, newborn P55.0
  hematogenous (acquired) D59.9
  hemolytic (acquired) D59.9
    congenital — *see* Spherocytosis
  hemorrhagic (acute) (leptospiral) (spirochetal) A27.0
    newborn P53
  infectious B15.9
    with hepatic coma B15.0
    leptospiral A27.0
    spirochetal A27.0
  neonatorum — *see* Jaundice, newborn
  newborn P59.9
  spirocheteal A27.0
...tus solaris, solis T67.01 ☑
...reaction (due to bacteria) L30.2
...eation
  homicidal R45.850
  suicidal R45.851
...entity disorder (child) F64.9
  gender role F64.2
  psychosexual F64.2
...ioglossia F80.0
...iopathic — *see* condition
...iot, idiocy (congenital) F73
  amaurotic (Bielschowsky(-Jansky)) (family) (infantile
    (late)) (juvenile (late)) (Vogt-Spielmeyer) E75.4
  microcephalic Q02
...E asthma J45.909
...AC (idiopathic infantile arterial calcification) Q28.8
...eitis (chronic) (noninfectious) — *see also* Enteritis K52.9
  backwash — *see* Pancolitis, ulcerative (chronic)
  infectious A09
  regional (ulcerative) — *see* Enteritis, regional, small
    intestine
  segmental — *see* Enteritis, regional
  terminal (ulcerative) — *see* Enteritis, regional, small
    intestine
...eocolitis — *see also* Enteritis K52.9
  infectious A09
  regional — *see* Enteritis, regional
  ulcerative K51.0- ☑
...eostomy
  attention to Z43.2
  malfunctioning K94.13
  status Z93.2
    with complication — *see* Complications, enterosto-
      my
...eotyphus — *see* Typhoid
...eum — *see* condition
...eus (bowel) (colon) (inhibitory) (intestine) K56.7
  adynamic K56.0
  due to gallstone (in intestine) K56.3
  duodenal (chronic) K31.5
  gallstone K56.3
  mechanical NEC — *see also* Obstruction, intestine,
    specified NEC K56.699
  meconium P76.0
    in cystic fibrosis E84.11
    meaning meconium plug (without cystic fibrosis)
      P76.0
  myxedema K59.8
  neurogenic K56.0
    Hirschsprung's disease or megacolon Q43.1
  newborn
    due to meconium P76.0
      in cystic fibrosis E84.11
      meaning meconium plug (without cystic fibrosis)
        P76.0
    transitory P76.1
  obstructive — *see also* Obstruction, intestine, specified
    NEC K56.699
  paralytic K56.0
  postoperative K91.89
...ac — *see* condition
...iotibial band syndrome M76.3- ☑
...literacy Z55.0
...lness — *see also* Disease R69
  manic-depressive — *see* Disorder, bipolar
...mbalance R26.89
  autonomic G90.8
  constituents of food intake E63.1
  electrolyte E87.8
    with
      abortion — *see* Abortion by type, complicated
        by, electrolyte imbalance
      molar pregnancy O08.5

Imbalance — *continued*
  electrolyte — *continued*
    due to hyperemesis gravidarum O21.1
    following ectopic or molar pregnancy O08.5
    neonatal, transitory NEC P74.49
      potassium
        hyperkalemia P74.31
        hypokalemia P74.32
      sodium
        hypernatremia P74.21
        hyponatremia P74.22
  endocrine E34.9
  eye muscle NOS H50.9
  hormone E34.9
  hysterical F44.4
  labyrinth — *see* subcategory H83.2 ☑
  posture R29.3
  protein-energy — *see* Malnutrition
  sympathetic G90.8
Imbecile, imbecility (I.Q. 35-49) F71
Imbedding, intrauterine device T83.39 ☑
Imbibition, cholesterol (gallbladder) K82.4
Imbrication, teeth,, fully erupted M26.30
Imerslund (-Gräsbeck) **syndrome** D51.1
Immature — *see also* Immaturity
  birth (less than 37 completed weeks) — *see* Preterm,
    newborn
    extremely (less than 28 completed weeks) — *see*
      Immaturity, extreme
  personality F60.89
Immaturity (less than 37 completed weeks) — *see also*
  Preterm, newborn
  extreme of newborn (less than 28 completed weeks of
    gestation) (less than 196 completed days of
    gestation) (unspecified weeks of gestation)
    P07.20
    gestational age
      23 completed weeks (23 weeks, 0 days through
        23 weeks, 6 days) P07.22
      24 completed weeks (24 weeks, 0 days through
        24 weeks, 6 days) P07.23
      25 completed weeks (25 weeks, 0 days through
        25 weeks, 6 days) P07.24
      26 completed weeks (26 weeks, 0 days through
        26 weeks, 6 days) P07.25
      27 completed weeks (27 weeks, 0 days through
        27 weeks, 6 days) P07.26
      less than 23 completed weeks P07.21
  fetus or infant light-for-dates — *see* Light-for-dates
  lung, newborn P28.0
  organ or site NEC — *see* Hypoplasia
  pulmonary, newborn P28.0
  reaction F60.89
  sexual (female) (male), after puberty E30.0
Immersion T75.1 ☑
  foot T69.02- ☑
  hand T69.01- ☑
Immobile, immobility
  complete, due to severe physical disability or frailty
    R53.2
  intestine K59.8
  syndrome (paraplegic) M62.3
Immune reconstitution (inflammatory) syndrome [IRIS]
  D89.3
Immunization — *see also* Vaccination
  ABO — *see* Incompatibility, ABO
    in newborn P55.1
  appropriate for age
    child (over 28 days old) Z00.129
      with abnormal findings Z00.121
  complication — *see* Complications, vaccination
  encounter for Z23
  not done (not carried out) Z28.9
    because (of)
      acute illness of patient Z28.01
      allergy to vaccine (or component) Z28.04
      caregiver refusal Z28.82
      chronic illness of patient Z28.02
      contraindication NEC Z28.09
      delay in delivery of vaccine Z28.83
      group pressure Z28.1
      guardian refusal Z28.82
      immune compromised state of patient Z28.03
      lack of availability of vaccine Z28.83
      manufacturer delay of vaccine Z28.83
      parent refusal Z28.82
      patient had disease being vaccinated against
        Z28.81

Immunization — *continued*
  not done — *continued*
    because — *continued*
      patient refusal Z28.21
      patient's belief Z28.1
      religious beliefs of patient Z28.1
      specified reason NEC Z28.89
        of patient Z28.29
      unavailability of vaccine Z28.83
      unspecified patient reason Z28.20
  Rh factor
    affecting management of pregnancy NEC O36.09- ☑
      anti-D antibody O36.01- ☑
    from transfusion — *see* Complication(s), transfusion,
      incompatibility reaction, Rh (factor)
Immunocytoma C83.0- ☑
Immunodeficiency D84.9
  with
    adenosine-deaminase deficiency — *see also* Defi-
      ciency, adenosine deaminase D81.30
    antibody defects D80.9
      specified type NEC D80.8
    hyperimmunoglobulinemia D80.6
    increased immunoglobulin M (IgM) D80.5
    major defect D82.9
      specified type NEC D82.8
    partial albinism D82.8
    short-limbed stature D82.2
    thrombocytopenia and eczema D82.0
  antibody with
    hyperimmunoglobulinemia D80.6
    near-normal immunoglobulins D80.6
  autosomal recessive, Swiss type D80.0
  combined D81.9
    biotin-dependent carboxylase D81.819
      biotinidase D81.810
      holocarboxylase synthetase D81.818
      specified type NEC D81.818
    severe (SCID) D81.9
      with
        low or normal B-cell numbers D81.2
        low T- and B-cell numbers D81.1
        reticular dysgenesis D81.0
    specified type NEC D81.89
  common variable D83.9
    with
      abnormalities of B-cell numbers and function
        D83.0
      autoantibodies to B- or T-cells D83.2
      immunoregulatory T-cell disorders D83.1
    specified type NEC D83.8
  following hereditary defective response to Epstein-Barr
    virus (EBV) D82.3
  selective, immunoglobulin
    A (IgA) D80.2
    G (IgG) (subclasses) D80.3
    M (IgM) D80.4
  severe combined (SCID) D81.9
    due to adenosine deaminase deficiency D81.31
  specified type NEC D84.8
  X-linked, with increased IgM D80.5
Immunotherapy (encounter for)
  antineoplastic Z51.12
Impaction, impacted
  bowel, colon, rectum — *see also* Impaction, fecal
    K56.49
    by gallstone K56.3
  calculus — *see* Calculus
  cerumen (ear) (external) H61.2- ☑
  cuspid — *see* Impaction, tooth
  dental (same or adjacent tooth) K01.1
  fecal, feces K56.41
  fracture — *see* Fracture, by site
  gallbladder — *see* Calculus, gallbladder
  gallstone(s) — *see* Calculus, gallbladder
    bile duct (common) (hepatic) — *see* Calculus, bile
      duct
    cystic duct — *see* Calculus, gallbladder
    in intestine, with obstruction (any part) K56.3
  intestine (calculous) NEC — *see also* Impaction, fecal
    K56.49
    gallstone, with ileus K56.3
  intrauterine device (IUD) T83.39 ☑
  molar — *see* Impaction, tooth
  shoulder, causing obstructed labor O66.0
  tooth, teeth K01.1
  turbinate J34.89

Impaired, impairment (function)
  auditory discrimination — *see* Abnormal, auditory perception
  cognitive, mild, so stated G31.84
  dual sensory Z73.82
  fasting glucose R73.01
  glucose tolerance (oral) R73.02
  hearing — *see* Deafness
  heart — *see* Disease, heart
  kidney N28.9
    disorder resulting from N25.9
      specified NEC N25.89
  liver K72.90
    with coma K72.91
  mastication K08.89
  mild cognitive, so stated G31.84
  mobility
    ear ossicles — *see* Ankylosis, ear ossicles
    requiring care provider Z74.09
  myocardium, myocardial — *see* Insufficiency, myocardial
  rectal sphincter R19.8
  renal (acute) (chronic) N28.9
    disorder resulting from N25.9
      specified NEC N25.89
  vision NEC H54.7
    both eyes H54.3
Impediment, speech R47.9
  psychogenic (childhood) F98.8
  slurring R47.81
  specified NEC R47.89
Impending
  coronary syndrome I20.0
  delirium tremens F10.239
  myocardial infarction I20.0
Imperception auditory (acquired) — *see also* Deafness
  congenital H93.25
Imperfect
  aeration, lung (newborn) NEC — *see* Atelectasis
  closure (congenital)
    alimentary tract NEC Q45.8
      lower Q43.8
      upper Q40.8
    atrioventricular ostium Q21.2
    atrium (secundum) Q21.1
    branchial cleft NOS Q18.2
      cyst Q18.0
      fistula Q18.0
      sinus Q18.0
    choroid Q14.3
    cricoid cartilage Q31.8
    cusps, heart valve NEC Q24.8
      pulmonary Q22.3
    ductus
      arteriosus Q25.0
      Botalli Q25.0
    ear drum (causing impairment of hearing) Q16.4
    esophagus with communication to bronchus or trachea Q39.1
    eyelid Q10.3
    foramen
      botalli Q21.1
      ovale Q21.1
    genitalia, genital organ(s) or system
      female Q52.8
        external Q52.79
        internal NEC Q52.8
      male Q55.8
    glottis Q31.8
    interatrial ostium or septum Q21.1
    interauricular ostium or septum Q21.1
    interventricular ostium or septum Q21.0
    larynx Q31.8
    lip — *see* Cleft, lip
    nasal septum Q30.3
    nose Q30.2
    omphalomesenteric duct Q43.0
    optic nerve entry Q14.2
    organ or site not listed — *see* Anomaly, by site
    ostium
      interatrial Q21.1
      interauricular Q21.1
      interventricular Q21.0
    palate — *see* Cleft, palate
    preauricular sinus Q18.1
    retina Q14.1
    roof of orbit Q75.8
    sclera Q13.5

Imperfect — *continued*
  closure — *continued*
    septum
      aorticopulmonary Q21.4
      atrial (secundum) Q21.1
      between aorta and pulmonary artery Q21.4
      heart Q21.9
      interatrial (secundum) Q21.1
      interauricular (secundum) Q21.1
      interventricular Q21.0
        in tetralogy of Fallot Q21.3
      nasal Q30.3
      ventricular Q21.0
        with pulmonary stenosis or atresia, dextraposition of aorta, and hypertrophy of right ventricle Q21.3
        in tetralogy of Fallot Q21.3
    skull Q75.0
      with
        anencephaly Q00.0
        encephalocele — *see* Encephalocele
        hydrocephalus Q03.9
          with spina bifida — *see* Spina bifida, by site, with hydrocephalus
        microcephaly Q02
    spine (with meningocele) — *see* Spina bifida
    trachea Q32.1
    tympanic membrane (causing impairment of hearing) Q16.4
    uterus Q51.818
    vitelline duct Q43.0
  erection — *see* Dysfunction, sexual, male, erectile
  fusion — *see* Imperfect, closure
  inflation, lung (newborn) — *see* Atelectasis
  posture R29.3
  rotation, intestine Q43.3
  septum, ventricular Q21.0
Imperfectly descended testis — *see* Cryptorchid
Imperforate (congenital) — *see also* Atresia
  anus Q42.3
    with fistula Q42.2
  cervix (uteri) Q51.828
  esophagus Q39.0
    with tracheoesophageal fistula Q39.1
  hymen Q52.3
  jejunum Q41.1
  pharynx Q38.8
  rectum Q42.1
    with fistula Q42.0
  urethra Q64.39
  vagina Q52.4
Impervious (congenital) — *see also* Atresia
  anus Q42.3
    with fistula Q42.2
  bile duct Q44.2
  esophagus Q39.0
    with tracheoesophageal fistula Q39.1
  intestine (small) Q41.9
    large Q42.9
      specified NEC Q42.8
  rectum Q42.1
    with fistula Q42.0
  ureter — *see* Atresia, ureter
  urethra Q64.39
Impetiginization of dermatoses L01.1
Impetigo (any organism) (any site) (circinate) (contagiosa) (simplex) (vulgaris) L01.00
  Bockhart's L01.02
  bullous, bullosa L01.03
  external ear L01.00 *[H62.40]*
  follicularis L01.02
  furfuracea L30.5
  herpetiformis L40.1
    nonobstetrical L40.1
  neonatorum L01.03
  nonbullous L01.01
  specified type NEC L01.09
  ulcerative L01.09
Impingement (on teeth)
  joint — *see* Disorder, joint, specified type NEC
  soft tissue
    anterior M26.81
    posterior M26.82
Implant, endometrial N80.9
Implantation
  anomalous — *see* Anomaly, by site
    ureter Q62.63

Implantation — *continued*
  cyst
    external area or site (skin) NEC L72.0
    iris — *see* Cyst, iris, implantation
    vagina N89.8
    vulva N90.7
  dermoid (cyst) — *see* Implantation, cyst
Impotence (sexual) N52.9
  counseling Z70.1
  organic origin — *see also* Dysfunction, sexual, male, erectile N52.9
  psychogenic F52.21
Impression, basilar Q75.8
Imprisonment, anxiety concerning Z65.1
Improper care (child) (newborn) — *see* Maltreatment
Improperly tied umbilical cord (causing hemorrhag P51.8
Impulsiveness (impulsive) R45.87
Inability to swallow — *see* Aphagia
Inaccessible, inaccessibility
  health care NEC Z75.3
    due to
      waiting period Z75.2
        for admission to facility elsewhere Z75.1
    other helping agencies Z75.4
Inactive — *see* condition
Inadequate, inadequacy
  aesthetics of dental restoration K08.56
  biologic, constitutional, functional, or social F60.7
  development
    child R62.50
    genitalia
      after puberty NEC E30.0
      congenital
        female Q52.8
          external Q52.79
          internal Q52.8
        male Q55.8
    lungs Q33.6
      associated with short gestation P28.0
    organ or site not listed — *see* Anomaly, by site
  diet (causing nutritional deficiency) E63.9
  eating habits Z72.4
  environment, household Z59.1
  family support Z63.8
  food (supply) NEC Z59.4
    hunger effects T73.0 ☑
  functional F60.7
  household care, due to
    family member
      handicapped or ill Z74.2
      on vacation Z75.5
      temporarily away from home Z74.2
    technical defects in home Z59.1
    temporary absence from home of person renderi care Z74.2
  housing (heating) (space) Z59.1
  income (financial) Z59.6
  intrafamilial communication Z63.8
  material resources Z59.9
  mental — *see* Disability, intellectual
  parental supervision or control of child Z62.0
  personality F60.7
  pulmonary
    function R06.89
      newborn P28.5
    ventilation, newborn P28.5
  sample of cytologic smear
    anus R85.615
    cervix R87.615
    vagina R87.625
  social F60.7
    insurance Z59.7
    skills NEC Z73.4
  supervision of child by parent Z62.0
  teaching affecting education Z55.8
  welfare support Z59.7
Inanition R64
  with edema — *see* Malnutrition, severe
  due to
    deprivation of food T73.0 ☑
    malnutrition — *see* Malnutrition
  fever R50.9
Inappropriate
  change in quantitative human chorionic gonadotrop (hCG) in early pregnancy O02.81
  diet or eating habits Z72.4

☑ **Additional Character Required** — Refer to the Tabular List for Character Selection   ▼ **Subterms under main terms may continue to next column or pag**

appropriate — *continued*
  level of quantitative human chorionic gonadotropin (hCG) for gestational age in early pregnancy O02.81
  secretion
    antidiuretic hormone (ADH) (excessive) E22.2
      deficiency E23.2
    pituitary (posterior) E22.2
attention at or after birth — *see* Neglect
carceration, incarcerated
  enterocele K46.0
    gangrenous K46.1
  epiplocele K46.0
    gangrenous K46.1
  exomphalos K42.0
    gangrenous K42.1
  hernia — *see also* Hernia, by site, with obstruction
    with gangrene — *see* Hernia, by site, with gangrene
  iris, in wound — *see* Injury, eye, laceration, with prolapse
  lens, in wound — *see* Injury, eye, laceration, with prolapse
  omphalocele K42.0
  prison, anxiety concerning Z65.1
  rupture — *see* Hernia, by site
  sarcoepiplocele K46.0
    gangrenous K46.1
  sarcoepiplomphalocele K42.0
    with gangrene K42.1
  uterus N85.8
    gravid O34.51- ☑
      causing obstructed labor O65.5
cised wound
  external — *see* Laceration
  internal organs — *see* Injury, by site
cision, incisional
  hernia K43.2
    with
      gangrene (and obstruction) K43.1
      obstruction K43.0
  surgical, complication — *see* Complications, surgical procedure
  traumatic
    external — *see* Laceration
    internal organs — *see* Injury, by site
clusion
  azurophilic leukocytic D72.0
  blennorrhea (neonatal) (newborn) P39.1
  gallbladder in liver (congenital) Q44.1
compatibility
  ABO
    affecting management of pregnancy O36.11- ☑
      anti-A sensitization O36.11- ☑
      anti-B sensitization O36.19- ☑
      specified NEC O36.19- ☑
    infusion or transfusion reaction — *see* Complication(s), transfusion, incompatibility reaction, ABO
    newborn P55.1
  blood (group) (Duffy) (K) (Kell) (Kidd) (Lewis) (M) (S) NEC
    affecting management of pregnancy O36.11- ☑
      anti-A sensitization O36.11- ☑
      anti-B sensitization O36.19- ☑
    infusion or transfusion reaction T80.89 ☑
    newborn P55.8
  divorce or estrangement Z63.5
  Rh (blood group) (factor) Z31.82
    affecting management of pregnancy NEC O36.09- ☑
      anti-D antibody O36.01- ☑
    infusion or transfusion reaction — *see* Complication(s), transfusion, incompatibility reaction, Rh (factor)
    newborn P55.0
  rhesus — *see* Incompatibility, Rh
competency, incompetent, incompetence
  annular
    aortic (valve) — *see* Insufficiency, aortic
    mitral (valve) I34.0
    pulmonary valve (heart) I37.1
  aortic (valve) — *see* Insufficiency, aortic
  cardiac valve — *see* Endocarditis
  cervix, cervical (os) N88.3
    in pregnancy O34.3- ☑
  chronotropic I45.89
    with
      autonomic dysfunction G90.8
      ischemic heart disease I25.89

Incompetency, incompetent, incompetence — *continued*
  chronotropic — *continued*
    with — *continued*
      left ventricular dysfunction I51.89
      sinus node dysfunction I49.8
  esophagogastric (junction) (sphincter) K22.0
  mitral (valve) — *see* Insufficiency, mitral
  pelvic fundus N81.89
  pubocervical tissue N81.82
  pulmonary valve (heart) I37.1
    congenital Q22.3
  rectovaginal tissue N81.83
  tricuspid (annular) (valve) — *see* Insufficiency, tricuspid
  valvular — *see* Endocarditis
    congenital Q24.8
  vein, venous (saphenous) (varicose) — *see* Varix, leg
Incomplete — *see also* condition
  bladder, emptying R33.9
  defecation R15.0
  expansion lungs (newborn) NEC — *see* Atelectasis
  rotation, intestine Q43.3
Inconclusive
  diagnostic imaging due to excess body fat of patient R93.9
  findings on diagnostic imaging of breast NEC R92.8
  mammogram (due to dense breasts) R92.2
Incontinence R32
  anal sphincter R15.9
  coital N39.491
  feces R15.9
    nonorganic origin F98.1
  insensible (urinary) N39.42
  overflow N39.490
  postural (urinary) N39.492
  psychogenic F45.8
  rectal R15.9
  reflex N39.498
  stress (female) (male) N39.3
    and urge N39.46
  urethral sphincter R32
  urge N39.41
    and stress (female) (male) N39.46
  urine (urinary) R32
    continuous N39.45
    due to cognitive impairment, or severe physical disability or immobility R39.81
    functional R39.81
    insensible N39.42
    mixed (stress and urge) N39.46
    nocturnal N39.44
    nonorganic origin F98.0
    overflow N39.490
    post dribbling N39.43
    postural N39.492
    reflex N39.498
    specified NEC N39.498
    stress (female) (male) N39.3
      and urge N39.46
    total N39.498
    unaware N39.42
    urge N39.41
      and stress (female) (male) N39.46
Incontinentia pigmenti Q82.3
Incoordinate, incoordination
  esophageal-pharyngeal (newborn) — *see* Dysphagia
  muscular R27.8
  uterus (action) (contractions) (complicating delivery) O62.4
Increase, increased
  abnormal, in development R63.8
  androgens (ovarian) E28.1
  anticoagulants (antithrombin) (anti-VIIIa) (anti-IXa) (anti-Xa) (anti-XIa) — *see* Circulating anticoagulants
  cold sense R20.8
  estrogen E28.0
  function
    adrenal
      cortex — *see* Cushing's, syndrome
      medulla E27.5
    pituitary (gland) (anterior) (lobe) E22.9
      posterior E22.2
  heat sense R20.8
  intracranial pressure (benign) G93.2
  permeability, capillaries I78.8
  pressure, intracranial G93.2

Increase, increased — *continued*
  secretion
    gastrin E16.4
    glucagon E16.3
    pancreas, endocrine E16.9
      growth hormone-releasing hormone E16.8
      pancreatic polypeptide E16.8
      somatostatin E16.8
      vasoactive-intestinal polypeptide E16.8
  sphericity, lens Q12.4
  splenic activity D73.1
  venous pressure I87.8
    portal K76.6
Increta placenta O43.22- ☑
Incrustation, cornea, foreign body (lead)(zinc) — *see* Foreign body, cornea
Incyclophoria H50.54
Incyclotropia — *see* Cyclotropia
Indeterminate sex Q56.4
India rubber skin Q82.8
Indigestion (acid) (bilious) (functional) K30
  catarrhal K31.89
  due to decomposed food NOS A05.9
  nervous F45.8
  psychogenic F45.8
Indirect — *see* condition
Induratio penis plastica N48.6
Induration, indurated
  brain G93.89
  breast (fibrous) N64.51
    puerperal, postpartum O92.29
  broad ligament N83.8
  chancre
    anus A51.1
    congenital A50.07
    extragenital NEC A51.2
  corpora cavernosa (penis) (plastic) N48.6
  liver (chronic) K76.89
  lung (black) (chronic) (fibroid) — *see also* Fibrosis, lung J84.10
    essential brown J84.03
  penile (plastic) N48.6
  phlebitic — *see* Phlebitis
  skin R23.4
Inebriety (without dependence) — *see* Alcohol, intoxication
Inefficiency, kidney N28.9
Inelasticity, skin R23.4
Inequality, leg (length) (acquired) — *see also* Deformity, limb, unequal length
  congenital — *see* Defect, reduction, lower limb
  lower leg — *see* Deformity, limb, unequal length
Inertia
  bladder (neurogenic) N31.2
  stomach K31.89
    psychogenic F45.8
  uterus, uterine during labor O62.2
    during latent phase of labor O62.0
    primary O62.0
    secondary O62.1
  vesical (neurogenic) N31.2
Infancy, infantile, infantilism — *see also* condition
  celiac K90.0
  genitalia, genitals (after puberty) E30.0
  Herter's (nontropical sprue) K90.0
  intestinal K90.0
  Lorain E23.0
  pancreatic K86.89
  pelvis M95.5
    with disproportion (fetopelvic) O33.1
      causing obstructed labor O65.1
  pituitary E23.0
  renal N25.0
  uterus — *see* Infantile, genitalia
Infant(s) — *see also* Infancy
  excessive crying R68.11
  irritable child R68.12
  lack of care — *see* Neglect
  liveborn (singleton) Z38.2
    born in hospital Z38.00
      by cesarean Z38.01
    born outside hospital Z38.1
    multiple NEC Z38.8
      born in hospital Z38.68
        by cesarean Z38.69
      born outside hospital Z38.7
    quadruplet Z38.8
      born in hospital Z38.63

⤶ **Subterms under main terms may continue to next column or page**   ☑ **Additional Character Required — Refer to the Tabular List for Character Selection**   **181**

Inappropriate — Infant

Infant(s) — continued
   liveborn — continued
      quadruplet — continued
         born in hospital — continued
            by cesarean Z38.64
            born outside hospital Z38.7
         quintuplet Z38.8
            born in hospital Z38.65
               by cesarean Z38.66
            born outside hospital Z38.7
         triplet Z38.8
            born in hospital Z38.61
               by cesarean Z38.62
            born outside hospital Z38.7
         twin Z38.5
            born in hospital Z38.30
               by cesarean Z38.31
            born outside hospital Z38.4
      of diabetic mother (syndrome of) P70.1
         gestational diabetes P70.0
Infantile — see also condition
   genitalia, genitals E30.0
   os, uterine E30.0
   penis E30.0
   testis E29.1
   uterus E30.0
Infantilism — see Infancy
Infarct, infarction
   adrenal (capsule) (gland) E27.49
   appendices epiploicae — see also Infarct, intestine
      K55.069
   bowel — see also Infarct, intestine K55.069
   brain (stem) — see Infarct, cerebral
   breast N64.89
   brewer's (kidney) N28.0
   cardiac — see Infarct, myocardium
   cerebellar — see Infarct, cerebral
   cerebral (acute) (chronic) — see also Occlusion, artery
      cerebral or precerebral, with infarction I63.9
      aborted I63.9
      cortical I63.9
      due to
         cerebral venous thrombosis, nonpyogenic I63.6
         embolism
            cerebral arteries I63.4- ☑
            precerebral arteries I63.1- ☑
         occlusion NEC
            cerebral arteries I63.5- ☑
            precerebral arteries I63.2- ☑
            small artery I63.81
         stenosis NEC
            cerebral arteries I63.5- ☑
            precerebral arteries I63.2- ☑
            small artery I63.81
         thrombosis
            cerebral artery I63.3- ☑
            precerebral artery I63.0- ☑
      intraoperative
         during cardiac surgery I97.810
         during other surgery I97.811
      postprocedural
         following cardiac surgery I97.820
         following other surgery I97.821
      specified NEC I63.89
   colon (acute) (agnogenic) (embolic) (hemorrhagic)
      (nonocclusive) (nonthrombotic) (occlusive)
      (segmental) (thrombotic) (with gangrene) — see
      also Infarct, intestine K55.049
   coronary artery — see Infarct, myocardium
   embolic — see Embolism
   fallopian tube N83.8
   gallbladder K82.8
   heart — see Infarct, myocardium
   hepatic K76.3
   hypophysis (anterior lobe) E23.6
   impending (myocardium) I20.0
   intestine (acute) (agnogenic) (embolic) (hemorrhagic)
      (nonocclusive) (nonthrombotic) (occlusive)
      (thrombotic) (with gangrene) K55.069
      diffuse K55.062
      focal K55.061
      large K55.049
         diffuse K55.042
         focal K55.041
      small K55.029
         diffuse K55.022
         focal K55.021
   kidney N28.0

Infarct, infarction — continued
   lacunar I63.81
   liver K76.3
   lung (embolic) (thrombotic) — see Embolism, pul-
      monary
   lymph node I89.8
   mesentery, mesenteric (embolic) (thrombotic) (with
      gangrene) — see also Infarct, intestine K55.069
   muscle (ischemic) M62.20
      ankle M62.27- ☑
      foot M62.27- ☑
      forearm M62.23- ☑
      hand M62.24- ☑
      lower leg M62.26- ☑
      pelvic region M62.25- ☑
      shoulder region M62.21- ☑
      specified site NEC M62.28
      thigh M62.25- ☑
      upper arm M62.22- ☑
   myocardium, myocardial (acute) (with stated duration
      of 4 weeks or less) I21.9
      associated with revascularization procedure I21.A9
      diagnosed on ECG, but presenting no symptoms
         I25.2
      due to
         demand ischemia I21.A1
         ischemic imbalance I21.A1
      healed or old I25.2
      intraoperative — see also Infarct, myocardium, as-
         sociated with revascularization procedure
         during cardiac surgery I97.790
         during other surgery I97.791
      non-Q wave I21.4
      non-ST elevation (NSTEMI) I21.4
         subsequent I22.2
      nontransmural I21.4
      past (diagnosed on ECG or other investigation, but
         currently presenting no symptoms) I25.2
      postprocedural — see also Infarct, myocardium,
         associated with revascularization procedure
         following cardiac surgery — see also Infarct,
            myocardium, type 4 or type 5 I97.190
         following other surgery I97.191
      Q wave (see also Infarct, myocardium, by site) I21.3
      secondary to
         demand ischemia I21.A1
         ischemic imbalance I21.A1
      ST elevation (STEMI) I21.3
         anterior (anteroapical) (anterolateral) (anterosep-
            tal) (Q wave) (wall) I21.09
            subsequent I22.0
         inferior (diaphragmatic) (inferolateral) (inferopos-
            terior) (wall) NEC I21.19
            subsequent I22.1
         inferoposterior transmural (Q wave) I21.11
         involving
            coronary artery of anterior wall NEC I21.09
            coronary artery of inferior wall NEC I21.19
            diagonal coronary artery I21.02
            left anterior descending coronary artery I21.02
            left circumflex coronary artery I21.21
            left main coronary artery I21.01
            oblique marginal coronary artery I21.21
            right coronary artery I21.11
         lateral (apical-lateral) (basal-lateral) (high) I21.29
            subsequent I22.8
         posterior (posterobasal) (posterolateral) (pos-
            teroseptal) (true) I21.29
            subsequent I22.8
         septal I21.29
            subsequent I22.8
         specified NEC I21.29
            subsequent I22.8
         subsequent I22.9
      subsequent (recurrent) (reinfarction) I22.9
         anterior (anteroapical) (anterolateral) (anterosep-
            tal) (wall) I22.0
         diaphragmatic (wall) I22.1
         inferior (diaphragmatic) (inferolateral) (inferopos-
            terior) (wall) I22.1
         lateral (apical-lateral) (basal-lateral) (high) I22.8
         non-ST elevation (NSTEMI) I22.2
         posterior (posterobasal) (posterolateral) (pos-
            teroseptal) (true) I22.8
         septal I22.8
         specified NEC I22.8
         ST elevation I22.9

Infarct, infarction — continued
   myocardium, myocardial — continued
      subsequent — continued
         ST elevation — continued
            anterior (anteroapical) (anterolateral) (an-
               teroseptal) (wall) I22.0
            inferior (diaphragmatic) (inferolateral) (infe
               oposterior) (wall) I22.1
            specified NEC I22.8
         subendocardial I22.2
         transmural I22.9
            anterior (anteroapical) (anterolateral) (an-
               teroseptal) (wall) I22.0
            diaphragmatic (wall) I22.1
            inferior (diaphragmatic) (inferolateral) (infe
               oposterior) (wall) I22.1
            lateral (apical-lateral) (basal-lateral) (high)
               I22.8
            posterior (posterobasal) (posterolateral)
               (posteroseptal) (true) I22.8
            specified NEC I22.8
         type 1 — see also Infarction, myocardial, subs
            quent, by site, or by ST elevation or nor
            ST elevation I22.9
         type 2 I21.A1
         type 3 I21.A9
         type 4 I21.A9
         type 5 I21.A9
      syphilitic A52.06
      transmural I21.9
         anterior (anteroapical) (anterolateral) (anterose
            tal) (Q wave) (wall) NEC I21.09
         inferior (diaphragmatic) (inferolateral) (inferopc
            terior) (Q wave) (wall) NEC I21.19
         inferoposterior (Q wave) I21.11
         lateral (apical-lateral) (basal-lateral) (high) NE
            I21.29
         posterior (posterobasal) (posterolateral) (pos-
            teroseptal) (true) NEC I21.29
         septal NEC I21.29
         specified NEC I21.29
         type 1 — see also Infarction, myocardial, by site,
            by ST elevation or non-ST elevation I21.9
         type 2 I21.A1
         type 3 I21.A9
         type 4 (a) (b) (c) I21.A9
         type 5 I21.A9
      nontransmural I21.4
   omentum — see also Infarct, intestine K55.069
   ovary N83.8
   pancreas K86.89
   papillary muscle — see Infarct, myocardium
   parathyroid gland E21.4
   pituitary (gland) E23.6
   placenta O43.81- ☑
   prostate N42.89
   pulmonary (artery) (vein) (hemorrhagic) — see Em-
      bolism, pulmonary
   renal (embolic) (thrombotic) N28.0
   retina, retinal (artery) — see Occlusion, artery, retin
   spinal (cord) (acute) (embolic) (nonembolic) G95.11
   spleen D73.5
      embolic or thrombotic I74.8
   subendocardial (acute) (nontransmural) I21.4
   suprarenal (capsule) (gland) E27.49
   testis N50.1
   thrombotic — see also Thrombosis
      artery, arterial — see Embolism
   thyroid (gland) E07.89
   ventricle (heart) — see Infarct, myocardium
Infecting — see condition
Infection, infected, infective (opportunistic) B99.9
   with
      drug resistant organism — see Resistance (to), dr
         — see also specific organism
      lymphangitis — see Lymphangitis
      organ dysfunction (acute) R65.20
         with septic shock R65.21
   abscess (skin) — code by site under Abscess
   Absidia — see Mucormycosis
   Acanthamoeba — see Acanthamebiasis
   Acanthocheilonema (perstans) (streptocerca) B74.4
   accessory sinus (chronic) — see Sinusitis
   achorion — see Dermatophytosis
   Acremonium falciforme B47.0
   acromioclavicular M00.9
   Actinobacillus (actinomycetem-comitans) A28.8
      mallei A24.0

Infection, infected, infective — *continued*
Actinobacillus — *continued*
  muris A25.1
Actinomadura B47.1
Actinomyces (israelii) — *see also* Actinomycosis A42.9
Actinomycetales — *see* Actinomycosis
actinomycotic NOS — *see* Actinomycosis
adenoid (and tonsil) J03.90
  chronic J35.02
adenovirus NEC
  as cause of disease classified elsewhere B97.0
  unspecified nature or site B34.0
aerogenes capsulatus A48.0
aertrycke — *see* Infection, salmonella
alimentary canal NOS — *see* Enteritis, infectious
Allescheria boydii B48.2
Alternaria B48.8
alveolus, alveolar (process) K04.7
Ameba, amebic (histolytica) — *see* Amebiasis
amniotic fluid, sac or cavity O41.10- ☑
  chorioamnionitis O41.12- ☑
  placentitis O41.14- ☑
amputation stump (surgical) — *see* Complication, amputation stump, infection
Ancylostoma (duodenalis) B76.0
Anisakiasis, Anisakis larvae B81.0
anthrax — *see* Anthrax
antrum (chronic) — *see* Sinusitis, maxillary
anus, anal (papillae) (sphincter) K62.89
arbovirus (arbor virus) A94
  specified type NEC A93.8
artificial insemination N98.0
Ascaris lumbricoides — *see* Ascariasis
Ascomycetes B47.0
Aspergillus (flavus) (fumigatus) (terreus) — *see* Aspergillosis
atypical
  acid-fast (bacilli) — *see* Mycobacterium, atypical
  mycobacteria — *see* Mycobacterium, atypical
  virus A81.9
    specified type NEC A81.89
auditory meatus (external) — *see* Otitis, externa, infective
auricle (ear) — *see* Otitis, externa, infective
axillary gland (lymph) L04.2
Bacillus A49.9
  abortus A23.1
  anthracis — *see* Anthrax
  Ducrey's (any location) A57
  Flexner's A03.1
  Friedländer's NEC A49.8
  gas (gangrene) A48.0
  mallei A24.0
  melitensis A23.0
  paratyphoid, paratyphosus A01.4
    A A01.1
    B A01.2
    C A01.3
  Shiga (-Kruse) A03.0
  suipestifer — *see* Infection, salmonella
  swimming pool A31.1
  typhosa A01.00
  welchii — *see* Gangrene, gas
bacterial NOS A49.9
  as cause of disease classified elsewhere B96.89
    Bacteroides fragilis [B. fragilis] B96.6
    Clostridium perfringens [C. perfringens] B96.7
    Enterobacter sakazakii B96.89
    Enterococcus B95.2
    Escherichia coli [E. coli] — *see also* Escherichia coli B96.20
    Helicobacter pylori [H.pylori] B96.81
    Hemophilus influenzae [H. influenzae] B96.3
    Klebsiella pneumoniae [K. pneumoniae] B96.1
    Mycoplasma pneumoniae [M. pneumoniae] B96.0
    Proteus (mirabilis) (morganii) B96.4
    Pseudomonas (aeruginosa) (mallei) (pseudomallei) B96.5
    Staphylococcus B95.8
      aureus (methicillin susceptible) (MSSA) B95.61
        methicillin resistant (MRSA) B95.62
      specified NEC B95.7
    Streptococcus B95.5
      group A B95.0
      group B B95.1
      pneumoniae B95.3
      specified NEC B95.4

Infection, infected, infective — *continued*
bacterial — *continued*
  as cause of disease classified elsewhere — *continued*
    Vibrio vulnificus B96.82
    specified NEC A48.8
Bacterium
  paratyphosum A01.4
    A A01.1
    B A01.2
    C A01.3
  typhosum A01.00
Bacteroides NEC A49.8
  fragilis, as cause of disease classified elsewhere B96.6
Balantidium coli A07.0
Bartholin's gland N75.8
Basidiobolus B46.8
bile duct (common) (hepatic) — *see* Cholangitis
bladder — *see* Cystitis
Blastomyces, blastomycotic — *see also* Blastomycosis
  brasiliensis — *see* Paracoccidioidomycosis
  dermatitidis — *see* Blastomycosis
  European — *see* Cryptococcosis
  Loboi B48.0
  North American B40.9
  South American — *see* Paracoccidioidomycosis
bleb, postprocedure — *see* Blebitis
bone — *see* Osteomyelitis
Bordetella — *see* Whooping cough
Borrelia bergdorfi A69.20
brain — *see also* Encephalitis G04.90
  membranes — *see* Meningitis
  septic G06.0
    meninges — *see* Meningitis, bacterial
branchial cyst Q18.0
breast — *see* Mastitis
bronchus — *see* Bronchitis
Brucella A23.9
  abortus A23.1
  canis A23.3
  melitensis A23.0
  mixed A23.8
  specified NEC A23.8
  suis A23.2
Brugia (malayi) B74.1
  timori B74.2
bursa — *see* Bursitis, infective
buttocks (skin) L08.9
Campylobacter, intestinal A04.5
  as cause of disease classified elsewhere B96.81
Candida (albicans) (tropicalis) — *see* Candidiasis
candiru B88.8
Capillaria (intestinal) B81.1
  hepatica B83.8
  philippinensis B81.1
cartilage — *see* Disorder, cartilage, specified type NEC
cat liver fluke B66.0
catheter-related bloodstream (CRBSI) T80.211 ☑
cellulitis — *code by* site under Cellulitis
central line-associated T80.219 ☑
  bloodstream (CLABSI) T80.211 ☑
  specified NEC T80.218 ☑
Cephalosporium falciforme B47.0
cerebrospinal — *see* Meningitis
cervical gland (lymph) L04.0
cervix — *see* Cervicitis
cesarean delivery wound (puerperal) O86.00
cestodes — *see* Infestation, cestodes
chest J22
Chilomastix (intestinal) A07.8
Chlamydia, chlamydial A74.9
  anus A56.3
  genitourinary tract A56.2
    lower A56.00
    specified NEC A56.19
  lymphogranuloma A55
  pharynx A56.4
  psittaci A70
  rectum A56.3
  sexually transmitted NEC A56.8
cholera — *see* Cholera
Cladosporium
  bantianum (brain abscess) B43.1
  carrionii B43.0
  castellanii B36.1
  trichoides (brain abscess) B43.1
  werneckii B36.1

Infection, infected, infective — *continued*
Clonorchis (sinensis) (liver) B66.1
Clostridium NEC
  bifermentans A48.0
  botulinum (food poisoning) A05.1
    infant A48.51
    wound A48.52
  difficile
    as cause of disease classified elsewhere B96.89
    foodborne (disease)
      not specified as recurrent A04.72
      recurrent A04.71
    gas gangrene A48.0
    necrotizing enterocolitis
      not specified as recurrent A04.72
      recurrent A04.71
    sepsis A41.4
  gas-forming NEC A48.0
  histolyticum A48.0
  novyi, causing gas gangrene A48.0
  oedematiens A48.0
  perfringens
    as cause of disease classified elsewhere B96.7
    due to food A05.2
    foodborne (disease) A05.2
    gas gangrene A48.0
    sepsis A41.4
  septicum, causing gas gangrene A48.0
  sordellii, causing gas gangrene A48.0
  welchii
    as cause of disease classified elsewhere B96.7
    foodborne (disease) A05.2
    gas gangrene A48.0
    necrotizing enteritis A05.2
    sepsis A41.4
Coccidioides (immitis) — *see* Coccidioidomycosis
colon — *see* Enteritis, infectious
colostomy K94.02
common duct — *see* Cholangitis
congenital P39.9
  Candida (albicans) P37.5
  cytomegalovirus P35.1
  hepatitis, viral P35.3
  herpes simplex P35.2
  infectious or parasitic disease P37.9
    specified NEC P37.8
  listeriosis (disseminated) P37.2
  malaria NEC P37.4
    falciparum P37.3
  Plasmodium falciparum P37.3
  poliomyelitis P35.8
  rubella P35.0
  skin P39.4
  toxoplasmosis (acute) (subacute) (chronic) P37.1
  tuberculosis P37.0
  urinary (tract) P39.3
  vaccinia P35.8
  virus P35.9
    specified type NEC P35.8
Conidiobolus B46.8
coronavirus NEC B34.2
  as cause of disease classified elsewhere B97.29
  severe acute respiratory syndrome (SARS associated) B97.21
corpus luteum — *see* Salpingo-oophoritis
Corynebacterium diphtheriae — *see* Diphtheria
cotia virus B08.8
Coxiella burnetii A78
coxsackie — *see* Coxsackie
Cryptococcus neoformans — *see* Cryptococcosis
Cryptosporidium A07.2
Cunninghamella — *see* Mucormycosis
cyst — *see* Cyst
cystic duct — *see also* Cholecystitis K81.9
Cysticercus cellulosae — *see* Cysticercosis
cytomegalovirus, cytomegaloviral B25.9
  congenital P35.1
  maternal, maternal care for (suspected) damage to fetus O35.3 ☑
  mononucleosis B27.10
    with
      complication NEC B27.19
      meningitis B27.12
      polyneuropathy B27.11
delta-agent (acute), in hepatitis B carrier B17.0
dental (pulpal origin) K04.7
Deuteromycetes B47.0
Dicrocoelium dendriticum B66.2

Infection, infected, infective — *continued*
  Dipetalonema (perstans) (streptocerca) B74.4
  diphtherial — *see* Diphtheria
  Diphyllobothrium (adult) (latum) (pacificum) B70.0
    larval B70.1
  Diplogonoporus (grandis) B71.8
  Dipylidium caninum B67.4
  Dirofilaria B74.8
  Dracunculus medinensis B72
  Drechslera (hawaiiensis) B43.8
  Ducrey Haemophilus (any location) A57
  due to or resulting from
    artificial insemination N98.0
    central venous catheter T80.219 ☑
      bloodstream T80.211 ☑
      exit or insertion site T80.212 ☑
      localized T80.212 ☑
      port or reservoir T80.212 ☑
      specified NEC T80.218 ☑
      tunnel T80.212 ☑
    device, implant or graft — *see also* Complications,
        by site and type, infection or inflammation
        T85.79 ☑
      arterial graft NEC T82.7 ☑
      breast (implant) T85.79 ☑
      catheter NEC T85.79 ☑
        dialysis (renal) T82.7 ☑
          intraperitoneal T85.71 ☑
        infusion NEC T82.7 ☑
          cranial T85.735 ☑
          intrathecal T85.735 ☑
          spinal (epidural) (subdural) T85.735 ☑
          subarachnoid T85.735 ☑
        urinary T83.518 ☑
          cystostomy T83.510 ☑
          Hopkins T83.518 ☑
          ileostomy T83.518 ☑
          nephrostomy T83.512 ☑
          specified NEC T83.518 ☑
          urethral indwelling T83.511 ☑
          urostomy T83.518 ☑
      electronic (electrode) (pulse generator) (stimula-
          tor)
        bone T84.7 ☑
        cardiac T82.7 ☑
        nervous system T85.738 ☑
          brain T85.731 ☑
          cranial nerve T85.732 ☑
          gastric nerve T85.732 ☑
          generator pocket T85.734 ☑
          neurostimulator generator T85.734 ☑
          peripheral nerve T85.732 ☑
          sacral nerve T85.732 ☑
          spinal cord T85.733 ☑
          vagal nerve T85.732 ☑
        urinary (indwelling) T83.51 ☑
      fixation, internal (orthopedic) NEC — *see* Compli-
          cation, fixation device, infection
      gastrointestinal (bile duct) (esophagus) T85.79 ☑
        neurostimulator electrode (lead) T85.732 ☑
      genital NEC T83.69 ☑
      heart NEC T82.7 ☑
        valve (prosthesis) T82.6 ☑
          graft T82.7 ☑
      joint prosthesis — *see* Complication, joint pros-
          thesis, infection
      ocular (corneal graft) (orbital implant) NEC
          T85.79 ☑
      orthopedic NEC T84.7 ☑
      penile (cylinder) (pump) (resevoir) T83.61 ☑
      specified NEC T85.79 ☑
      testicular T83.62 ☑
      urinary NEC T83.598 ☑
        ileal conduit stent T83.593 ☑
        implanted neurostimulation T83.590 ☑
        implanted sphincter T83.591 ☑
        indwelling ureteral stent T83.592 ☑
        nephroureteral stent T83.593 ☑
        specified stent NEC T83.593 ☑
      vascular NEC T82.7 ☑
      ventricular intracranial (communicating) shunt
          T85.730 ☑
    Hickman catheter T80.219 ☑
      bloodstream T80.211 ☑
      localized T80.212 ☑
      specified NEC T80.218 ☑

Infection, infected, infective — *continued*
  due to or resulting from — *continued*
    immunization or vaccination T88.0 ☑
    infusion, injection or transfusion NEC T80.29 ☑
    injury NEC — *code by* site under Wound, open
    peripherally inserted central catheter (PICC)
        T80.219 ☑
      bloodstream T80.211 ☑
      localized T80.212 ☑
      specified NEC T80.218 ☑
    portacath (port-a-cath) T80.219 ☑
      bloodstream T80.211 ☑
      localized T80.212 ☑
      specified NEC T80.218 ☑
    pulmonary artery catheter — *see* Infection, due to
        or resulting from, central venous catheter
    surgery T81.40 ☑
    Swan Ganz catheter — *see* Infection, due to or re-
        sulting from, central venous catheter
    triple lumen catheter T80.219 ☑
      bloodstream T80.211 ☑
      localized T80.212 ☑
      specified NEC T80.218 ☑
    umbilical venous catheter T80.219 ☑
      bloodstream T80.211 ☑
      localized T80.212 ☑
      specified NEC T80.218 ☑
  during labor NEC O75.3
  ear (middle) — *see also* Otitis media
    external — *see* Otitis, externa, infective
    inner — *see* subcategory H83.0 ☑
  Eberthella typhosa A01.00
  Echinococcus — *see* Echinococcus
  echovirus
    as cause of disease classified elsewhere B97.12
    unspecified nature or site B34.1
  endocardium I33.0
  endocervix — *see* Cervicitis
  Entamoeba — *see* Amebiasis
  enteric — *see* Enteritis, infectious
  Enterobacter sakazakii B96.89
  Enterobius vermicularis B80
  enterostomy K94.12
  enterovirus B34.1
    as cause of disease classified elsewhere B97.10
      coxsackievirus B97.11
      echovirus B97.12
      specified NEC B97.19
  Entomophthora B46.8
  Epidermophyton — *see* Dermatophytosis
  epididymis — *see* Epididymitis
  episiotomy (puerperal) O86.09
  Erysipelothrix (insidiosa) (rhusiopathiae) — *see*
      Erysipeloid
  erythema infectiosum B08.3
  Escherichia (E.) coli NEC A49.8
    as cause of disease classified elsewhere — *see also*
        Escherichia coli B96.20
    congenital P39.8
      sepsis P36.4
    generalized A41.51
    intestinal — *see* Enteritis, infectious, due to, Es-
        cherichia coli
  ethmoidal (chronic) (sinus) — *see* Sinusitis, ethmoidal
  eustachian tube (ear) — *see* Salpingitis, eustachian
  external auditory canal (meatus) NEC — *see* Otitis, ex-
      terna, infective
  eye (purulent) — *see* Endophthalmitis, purulent
  eyelid — *see* Inflammation, eyelid
  fallopian tube — *see* Salpingo-oophoritis
  Fasciola (gigantica) (hepatica) (indica) B66.3
  Fasciolopsis (buski) B66.5
  filarial — *see* Infestation, filarial
  finger (skin) L08.9
    nail L03.01-
      fungus B35.1
  fish tapeworm B70.0
    larval B70.1
  flagellate, intestinal A07.9
  fluke — *see* Infestation, fluke
  focal
    teeth (pulpal origin) K04.7
    tonsils J35.01
  Fonsecaea (compactum) (pedrosoi) B43.0
  food — *see* Intoxication, foodborne
  foot (skin) L08.9
    dermatophytic fungus B35.3

Infection, infected, infective — *continued*
  Francisella tularensis — *see* Tularemia
  frontal (sinus) (chronic) — *see* Sinusitis, frontal
  fungus NOS B49
    beard B35.0
    dermatophytic — *see* Dermatophytosis
    foot B35.3
    groin B35.6
    hand B35.2
    nail B35.1
    pathogenic to compromised host only B48.8
    perianal (area) B35.6
    scalp B35.0
    skin B36.9
      foot B35.3
      hand B35.2
      toenails B35.1
  Fusarium B48.8
  gallbladder — *see* Cholecystitis
  gas bacillus — *see* Gangrene, gas
  gastrointestinal — *see* Enteritis, infectious
  generalized NEC — *see* Sepsis
  generator pocket, implanted electronic neurostimula
      T85.734 ☑
  genital organ or tract
    female — *see* Disease, pelvis, inflammatory
    male N49.9
      multiple sites N49.8
      specified NEC N49.8
  Ghon tubercle, primary A15.7
  Giardia lamblia A07.1
  gingiva (chronic) K05.10
    acute K05.00
      nonplaque induced K05.01
      plaque induced K05.00
    nonplaque induced K05.11
    plaque induced K05.10
  glanders A24.0
  glenosporopsis B48.0
  Gnathostoma (spinigerum) B83.1
  Gongylonema B83.8
  gonococcal — *see* Gonococcus
  gram-negative bacilli NOS A49.9
  guinea worm B72
  gum (chronic) K05.10
    acute K05.00
      nonplaque induced K05.01
      plaque induced K05.00
    nonplaque induced K05.11
    plaque induced K05.10
  Haemophilus — *see* Infection, Hemophilus
  heart — *see* Carditis
  Helicobacter pylori A04.8
    as cause of disease classified elsewhere B96.81
  helminths B83.9
    intestinal B82.0
      mixed (types classifiable to more than one of
          titles B65.0-B81.3 and B81.8) B81.4
      specified type NEC B81.8
    specified type NEC B83.8
  Hemophilus
    aegyptius, systemic A48.4
    ducrey (any location) A57
    generalized A41.3
    influenzae NEC A49.2
      as cause of disease classified elsewhere B96.
  herpes (simplex) — *see also* Herpes
    congenital P35.2
    disseminated B00.7
    zoster B02.9
  herpesvirus, herpesviral — *see* Herpes
  Heterophyes (heterophyes) B66.8
  hip (joint) NEC M00.9
    due to internal joint prosthesis
      left T84.52 ☑
      right T84.51 ☑
    skin NEC L08.9
  Histoplasma — *see* Histoplasmosis
    American B39.4
    capsulatum B39.4
  hookworm B76.9
  human
    papilloma virus A63.0
    T-cell lymphotropic virus type-1 (HTLV-1) B33.3
  hydrocele N43.0
  Hymenolepis B71.0
  hypopharynx — *see* Pharyngitis
  inguinal (lymph) glands L04.1

fection, infected, infective — *continued*
  inguinal glands — *continued*
    due to soft chancre A57
  intervertebral disc, pyogenic M46.30
    cervical region M46.32
    cervicothoracic region M46.33
    lumbar region M46.36
    lumbosacral region M46.37
    multiple sites M46.39
    occipito-atlanto-axial region M46.31
    sacrococcygeal region M46.38
    thoracic region M46.34
    thoracolumbar region M46.35
  intestine, intestinal — *see* Enteritis, infectious
    specified NEC A08.8
  intra-amniotic affecting newborn NEC P39.2
  Isospora belli or hominis A07.3
  Japanese B encephalitis A83.0
  jaw (bone) (lower) (upper) M27.2
  joint NEC M00.9
    due to internal joint prosthesis T84.50 ☑
  kidney (cortex) (hematogenous) N15.9
    with calculus N20.0
      with hydronephrosis N13.6
    following ectopic gestation O08.83
    pelvis and ureter (cystic) N28.85
    puerperal (postpartum) O86.21
    specified NEC N15.8
  Klebsiella (K.) pneumoniae NEC A49.8
    as cause of disease classified elsewhere B96.1
  knee (joint) NEC M00.9
    joint M00.9
    due to internal joint prosthesis
      left T84.54 ☑
      right T84.53 ☑
    skin L08.9
  Koch's — *see* Tuberculosis
  labia (majora) (minora) (acute) — *see* Vulvitis
  lacrimal
    gland — *see* Dacryoadenitis
    passages (duct) (sac) — *see* Inflammation, lacrimal, passages
  lancet fluke B66.2
  larynx NEC J38.7
  leg (skin) NOS L08.9
  Legionella pneumophila A48.1
    nonpneumonic A48.2
  Leishmania — *see also* Leishmaniasis
    aethiopica B55.1
    braziliensis B55.2
    chagasi B55.0
    donovani B55.0
    infantum B55.0
    major B55.1
    mexicana B55.1
    tropica B55.1
  lentivirus, as cause of disease classified elsewhere B97.31
  Leptosphaeria senegalensis B47.0
  Leptospira interrogans A27.9
    autumnalis A27.89
    canicola A27.89
    hebdomadis A27.89
    icterohaemorrhagiae A27.0
    pomona A27.89
    specified type NEC A27.89
  leptospirochetal NEC — *see* Leptospirosis
  Listeria monocytogenes — *see also* Listeriosis
    congenital P37.2
  Loa loa B74.3
    with conjunctival infestation B74.3
    eyelid B74.3
  Loboa loboi B48.0
  local, skin (staphylococcal) (streptococcal) L08.9
    abscess — *code by* site under Abscess
    cellulitis — *code by* site under Cellulitis
    specified NEC L08.89
    ulcer — *see* Ulcer, skin
  Loefflerella mallei A24.0
  lung — *see also* Pneumonia J18.9
    atypical Mycobacterium A31.0
    spirochetal A69.8
    tuberculous — *see* Tuberculosis, pulmonary
    virus — *see* Pneumonia, viral
  lymph gland — *see also* Lymphadenitis, acute
    mesenteric I88.0
  lymphoid tissue, base of tongue or posterior pharynx, NEC (chronic) J35.03

Infection, infected, infective — *continued*
  Madurella (grisea) (mycetomii) B47.0
  major
    following ectopic or molar pregnancy O08.0
    puerperal, postpartum, childbirth O85
  Malassezia furfur B36.0
  Malleomyces
    mallei A24.0
    pseudomallei (whitmori) — *see* Melioidosis
  mammary gland N61.0
  Mansonella (ozzardi) (perstans) (streptocerca) B74.4
  mastoid — *see* Mastoiditis
  maxilla, maxillary M27.2
    sinus (chronic) — *see* Sinusitis, maxillary
  mediastinum J98.51
  Medina (worm) B72
  meibomian cyst or gland — *see* Hordeolum
  meninges — *see* Meningitis, bacterial
  meningococcal — *see also* condition A39.9
    adrenals A39.1
    brain A39.81
    cerebrospinal A39.0
    conjunctiva A39.89
    endocardium A39.51
    heart A39.50
      endocardium A39.51
      myocardium A39.52
      pericardium A39.53
    joint A39.83
    meninges A39.0
    meningococcemia A39.4
      acute A39.2
      chronic A39.3
    myocardium A39.52
    pericardium A39.53
    retrobulbar neuritis A39.82
    specified site NEC A39.89
  mesenteric lymph nodes or glands NEC I88.0
  Metagonimus B66.8
  metatarsophalangeal M00.9
  methicillin
    resistant Staphylococcus aureus (MRSA) A49.02
    susceptible Staphylococcus aureus (MSSA) A49.01
  Microsporum, microsporic — *see* Dermatophytosis
  mixed flora (bacterial) NEC A49.8
  Monilia — *see* Candidiasis
  Monosporium apiospermum B48.2
  mouth, parasitic B37.0
  Mucor — *see* Mucormycosis
  muscle NEC — *see* Myositis, infective
  mycelium NOS B49
  mycetoma B47.9
    actinomycotic NEC B47.1
    mycotic NEC B47.0
  Mycobacterium, mycobacterial — *see* Mycobacterium
  Mycoplasma NEC A49.3
    pneumoniae, as cause of disease classified elsewhere B96.0
  mycotic NOS B49
    pathogenic to compromised host only B48.8
    skin NOS B36.9
  myocardium NEC I40.0
  nail (chronic)
    with lymphangitis — *see* Lymphangitis, acute, digit
    finger L03.01- ☑
      fungus B35.1
      ingrowing L60.0
    toe L03.03- ☑
      fungus B35.1
  nasal sinus (chronic) — *see* Sinusitis
  nasopharynx — *see* Nasopharyngitis
  navel L08.82
  Necator americanus B76.1
  Neisseria — *see* Gonococcus
  Neotestudina rosatii B47.0
  newborn P39.9
    intra-amniotic NEC P39.2
    skin P39.4
    specified type NEC P39.8
  nipple N61.0
    associated with
      lactation O91.03
      pregnancy O91.01- ☑
      puerperium O91.02
  Nocardia — *see* Nocardiosis
  obstetrical surgical wound (puerperal) O86.00
    incisional site
      deep O86.02

Infection, infected, infective — *continued*
  obstetrical surgical wound — *continued*
    incisional site — *continued*
      superficial O86.01
    organ and space site O86.03
    surgical site specified NEC O86.09
  Oesophagostomum (apiostomum) B81.8
  Oestrus ovis — *see* Myiasis
  Oidium albicans B37.9
  Onchocerca (volvulus) — *see* Onchocerciasis
  oncovirus, as cause of disease classified elsewhere B97.32
  operation wound T81.49 ☑
  Opisthorchis (felineus) (viverrini) B66.0
  orbit, orbital — *see* Inflammation, orbit
  orthopoxvirus NEC B08.09
  ovary — *see* Salpingo-oophoritis
  Oxyuris vermicularis B80
  pancreas (acute) — *see* Pancreatitis, acute
    abscess — *see* Pancreatitis, acute
    specified NEC — *see also* Pancreatitis, acute K85.80
  papillomavirus, as cause of disease classified elsewhere B97.7
  papovavirus NEC B34.4
  Paracoccidioides brasiliensis — *see* Paracoccidioidomycosis
  Paragonimus (westermani) B66.4
  parainfluenza virus B34.8
  parameningococcus NOS A39.9
  parapoxvirus B08.60
    specified NEC B08.69
  parasitic B89
  Parastrongylus
    cantonensis B83.2
    costaricensis B81.3
    paratyphoid A01.4
      Type A A01.1
      Type B A01.2
      Type C A01.3
  paraurethral ducts N34.2
  parotid gland — *see* Sialoadenitis
  parvovirus NEC B34.3
    as cause of disease classified elsewhere B97.6
  Pasteurella NEC A28.0
    multocida A28.0
    pestis — *see* Plague
    pseudotuberculosis A28.0
    septica (cat bite) (dog bite) A28.0
    tularensis — *see* Tularemia
  pelvic, female — *see* Disease, pelvis, inflammatory
  Penicillium (marneffei) B48.4
  penis (glans) (retention) NEC N48.29
  periapical K04.5
  peridental, periodontal K05.20
    generalized — *see* Periodontitis, aggressive, generalized
    localized — *see* Periodontitis, aggressive, localized
  perinatal period P39.9
    specified type NEC P39.8
  perineal repair (puerperal) O86.09
  periorbital — *see* Inflammation, orbit
  perirectal K62.89
  perirenal — *see* Infection, kidney
  peritoneal — *see* Peritonitis
  periureteral N28.89
  Petriellidium boydii B48.2
  pharynx — *see* Pharyngitis
    coxsackievirus B08.5
    posterior, lymphoid (chronic) J35.03
  Phialophora
    gougerotii (subcutaneous abscess or cyst) B43.2
    jeanselmei (subcutaneous abscess or cyst) B43.2
    verrucosa (skin) B43.0
  Piedraia hortae B36.3
  pinta A67.9
    intermediate A67.1
    late A67.2
    mixed A67.3
    primary A67.0
  pinworm B80
  pityrosporum furfur B36.0
  pleuro-pneumonia-like organism (PPLO) NEC A49.3
    as cause of disease classified elsewhere B96.0
  pneumococcus, pneumococcal NEC A49.1
    as cause of disease classified elsewhere B95.3
    generalized (purulent) A40.3
      with pneumonia J13
  Pneumocystis carinii (pneumonia) B59

Infection, infected, infective — *continued*
Pneumocystis jiroveci (pneumonia) B59
port or reservoir T80.212 ☑
postoperative T81.40 ☑
postoperative wound T81.49 ☑
  surgical site
    deep incisional T81.42 ☑
    organ and space T81.43 ☑
    specified NEC T81.49 ☑
    superficial incisional T81.41 ☑
postprocedural T81.40 ☑
postvaccinal T88.0 ☑
prepuce NEC N47.7
  with penile inflammation N47.6
prion — *see* Disease, prion, central nervous system
prostate (capsule) — *see* Prostatitis
Proteus (mirabilis) (morganii) (vulgaris) NEC A49.8
  as cause of disease classified elsewhere B96.4
protozoal NEC B64
  intestinal A07.9
    specified NEC A07.8
  specified NEC B60.8
Pseudoallescheria boydii B48.2
Pseudomonas NEC A49.8
  as cause of disease classified elsewhere B96.5
  mallei A24.0
  pneumonia J15.1
  pseudomallei — *see* Melioidosis
puerperal O86.4
  genitourinary tract NEC O86.89
  major or generalized O85
  minor O86.4
  specified NEC O86.89
pulmonary — *see* Infection, lung
purulent — *see* Abscess
Pyrenochaeta romeroi B47.0
Q fever A78
rectum (sphincter) K62.89
renal — *see also* Infection, kidney
  pelvis and ureter (cystic) N28.85
reovirus, as cause of disease classified elsewhere B97.5
respiratory (tract) NEC J98.8
  acute J22
  chronic J98.8
  influenzal (upper) (acute) — *see* Influenza, with, respiratory manifestations NEC
  lower (acute) J22
    chronic — *see* Bronchitis, chronic
  rhinovirus J00
  syncytial virus (RSV) — *see* Infection, virus, respiratory syncytial (RSV)
  upper (acute) NOS J06.9
    chronic J39.8
    streptococcal J06.9
    viral NOS J06.9
      due to respiratory syncytial virus (RSV) J06.9 [B97.4]
resulting from
  presence of internal prosthesis, implant, graft — *see* Complications, by site and type, infection
retortamoniasis A07.8
retroperitoneal NEC K68.9
retrovirus B33.3
  as cause of disease classified elsewhere B97.30
    human
      immunodeficiency, type 2 (HIV 2) B97.35
      T-cell lymphotropic
        type I (HTLV-I) B97.33
        type II (HTLV-II) B97.34
    lentivirus B97.31
    oncovirus B97.32
    specified NEC B97.39
Rhinosporidium (seeberi) B48.1
rhinovirus
  as cause of disease classified elsewhere B97.89
  unspecified nature or site B34.8
Rhizopus — *see* Mucormycosis
rickettsial NOS A79.9
roundworm (large) NEC B82.0
  Ascariasis — *see also* Ascariasis B77.9
rubella — *see* Rubella
Saccharomyces — *see* Candidiasis
salivary duct or gland (any) — *see* Sialoadenitis
Salmonella (aertrycke) (arizonae) (callinarum) (cholerae-suis) (enteritidis) (suipestifer) (typhimurium) A02.9
  with
    (gastro)enteritis A02.0

Infection, infected, infective — *continued*
Salmonella — *continued*
  with — *continued*
    sepsis A02.1
    specified manifestation NEC A02.8
  due to food (poisoning) A02.9
  hirschfeldii A01.3
  localized A02.20
    arthritis A02.23
    meningitis A02.21
    osteomyelitis A02.24
    pneumonia A02.22
    pyelonephritis A02.25
    specified NEC A02.29
  paratyphi A01.4
    A A01.1
    B A01.2
    C A01.3
  schottmuelleri A01.2
  typhi, typhosa — *see* Typhoid
Sarcocystis A07.8
scabies B86
Schistosoma — *see* Infestation, Schistosoma
scrotum (acute) NEC N49.2
seminal vesicle — *see* Vesiculitis
septic
  localized, skin — *see* Abscess
sheep liver fluke B66.3
Shigella A03.9
  boydii A03.2
  dysenteriae A03.0
  flexneri A03.1
  group
    A A03.0
    B A03.1
    C A03.2
    D A03.3
  Schmitz (-Stutzer) A03.0
  schmitzii A03.0
  shigae A03.0
  sonnei A03.3
  specified NEC A03.8
shoulder (joint) NEC M00.9
  due to internal joint prosthesis T84.59 ☑
  skin NEC L08.9
sinus (accessory) (chronic) (nasal) — *see also* Sinusitis
  pilonidal — *see* Sinus, pilonidal
  skin NEC L08.89
Skene's duct or gland — *see* Urethritis
skin (local) (staphylococcal) (streptococcal) L08.9
  abscess — *code by* site under Abscess
  cellulitis — *code by* site under Cellulitis
  due to fungus B36.9
    specified type NEC B36.8
  mycotic B36.9
    specified type NEC B36.8
  newborn P39.4
  ulcer — *see* Ulcer, skin
slow virus A81.9
  specified NEC A81.89
Sparganum (mansoni) (proliferum) (baxteri) B70.1
specific — *see also* Syphilis
  to perinatal period — *see* Infection, congenital
specified NEC B99.8
spermatic cord NEC N49.1
sphenoidal (sinus) — *see* Sinusitis, sphenoidal
spinal cord NOS — *see also* Myelitis G04.91
  abscess G06.1
  meninges — *see* Meningitis
  streptococcal G04.89
Spirillum A25.0
spirochetal NOS A69.9
  lung A69.8
  specified NEC A69.8
Spirometra larvae B70.1
spleen D73.89
Sporotrichum, Sporothrix (schenckii) — *see* Sporotrichosis
staphylococcal, unspecified site
  as cause of disease classified elsewhere B95.8
    aureus (methicillin susceptible) (MSSA) B95.61
      methicillin resistant (MRSA) B95.62
    specified NEC B95.7
  aureus (methicillin susceptible) (MSSA) A49.01
    methicillin resistant (MRSA) A49.02
  food poisoning A05.0
  generalized (purulent) A41.2
  pneumonia — *see* Pneumonia, staphylococcal

Infection, infected, infective — *continued*
Stellantchasmus falcatus B66.8
streptobacillus moniliformis A25.1
streptococcal NEC A49.1
  as cause of disease classified elsewhere B95.5
  B genitourinary complicating
    childbirth O98.82
    pregnancy O98.81- ☑
    puerperium O98.83
  congenital
    sepsis P36.10
      group B P36.0
      specified NEC P36.19
  generalized (purulent) A40.9
Streptomyces B47.1
Strongyloides (stercoralis) — *see* Strongyloidiasis
stump (amputation) (surgical) — *see* Complication, amputation stump, infection
subcutaneous tissue, local L08.9
suipestifer — *see* Infection, salmonella
swimming pool bacillus A31.1
Taenia — *see* Infestation, Taenia
Taeniarhynchus saginatus B68.1
tapeworm — *see* Infestation, tapeworm
tendon (sheath) — *see* Tenosynovitis, infective NEC
Ternidens diminutus B81.8
testis — *see* Orchitis
threadworm B80
throat — *see* Pharyngitis
thyroglossal duct K14.8
toe (skin) L08.9
  cellulitis L03.03- ☑
    fungus B35.1
  nail L03.03- ☑
    fungus B35.1
tongue NEC K14.0
  parasitic B37.0
tonsil (and adenoid) (faucial) (lingual) (pharyngeal) — *see* Tonsillitis
tooth, teeth K04.7
  periapical K04.7
  peridental, periodontal K05.20
    generalized — *see* Periodontitis, aggressive, generalized
    localized — *see* Periodontitis, aggressive, localized
  pulp K04.01
    irreversible K04.02
    reversible K04.01
  socket M27.3
TORCH — *see* Infection, congenital
  without active infection P00.2
Torula histolytica — *see* Cryptococcosis
Toxocara (canis) (cati) (felis) B83.0
Toxoplasma gondii — *see* Toxoplasma
trachea, chronic J42
trematode NEC — *see* Infestation, fluke
trench fever A79.0
Treponema pallidum — *see* Syphilis
Trichinella (spiralis) B75
Trichomonas A59.9
  cervix A59.09
  intestine A07.8
  prostate A59.02
  specified site NEC A59.8
  urethra A59.03
  urogenitalis A59.00
  vagina A59.01
  vulva A59.01
Trichophyton, trichophytic — *see* Dermatophytosis
Trichosporon (beigelii) cutaneum B36.2
Trichostrongylus B81.2
Trichuris (trichiura) B79
Trombicula (irritans) B88.0
Trypanosoma
  brucei
    gambiense B56.0
    rhodesiense B56.1
  cruzi — *see* Chagas' disease
tubal — *see* Salpingo-oophoritis
tuberculous
  latent (LTBI) Z22.7
  NEC — *see* Tuberculosis
tubo-ovarian — *see* Salpingo-oophoritis
tunica vaginalis N49.1
tunnel T80.212 ☑
tympanic membrane NEC — *see* Myringitis
typhoid (abortive) (ambulant) (bacillus) — *see* Typho

☑ **Additional Character Required — Refer to the Tabular List for Character Selection**   ▽ **Subterms under main terms may continue to next column or pag**

Infection, infected, infective — *continued*
  typhus A75.9
    flea-borne A75.2
    mite-borne A75.3
    recrudescent A75.1
    tick-borne A77.9
      African A77.1
      North Asian A77.2
  umbilicus L08.82
  ureter — *see* Ureteritis
  urethra — *see* Urethritis
  urinary (tract) N39.0
    bladder — *see* Cystitis
    complicating
      pregnancy O23.4- ☑
      specified type NEC O23.3- ☑
    kidney — *see* Infection, kidney
    newborn P39.3
    puerperal (postpartum) O86.20
    tuberculous A18.13
    urethra — *see* Urethritis
  uterus, uterine — *see* Endometritis
  vaccination T88.0 ☑
  vaccinia not from vaccination B08.011
  vagina (acute) — *see* Vaginitis
  varicella B01.9
  varicose veins — *see* Varix
  vas deferens NEC N49.1
  vesical — *see* Cystitis
  Vibrio
    cholerae A00.0
      El Tor A00.1
    parahaemolyticus (food poisoning) A05.3
    vulnificus
      as cause of disease classified elsewhere B96.82
      foodborne intoxication A05.5
  Vincent's (gum) (mouth) (tonsil) A69.1
  virus, viral NOS B34.9
    adenovirus
      as cause of disease classified elsewhere B97.0
      unspecified nature or site B34.0
    arborvirus, arbovirus arthropod-borne A94
    as cause of disease classified elsewhere B97.89
      adenovirus B97.0
      coronavirus B97.29
        SARS-associated B97.21
      coxsackievirus B97.11
      echovirus B97.12
      enterovirus B97.10
        coxsackievirus B97.11
        echovirus B97.12
        specified NEC B97.19
      human
        immunodeficiency, type 2 (HIV 2) B97.35
        metapneumovirus B97.81
        T-cell lymphotropic,
          type I (HTLV-I) B97.33
          type II (HTLV-II) B97.34
      papillomavirus B97.7
      parvovirus B97.6
      reovirus B97.5
      respiratory syncytial (RSV) — *see* Infection, virus, respiratory syncytial (RSV)
      retrovirus B97.30
        human
          immunodeficiency, type 2 (HIV 2) B97.35
          T-cell lymphotropic,
            type I (HTLV-I) B97.33
            type II (HTLV-II) B97.34
        lentivirus B97.31
        oncovirus B97.32
        specified NEC B97.39
      specified NEC B97.89
    central nervous system A89
      atypical A81.9
        specified NEC A81.89
      enterovirus NEC A88.8
        meningitis A87.0
      slow virus A81.9
        specified NEC A81.89
      specified NEC A88.8
    chest J98.8
    cotia B08.8
    coxsackie — *see also* Infection, coxsackie B34.1
      as cause of disease classified elsewhere B97.11
    ECHO
      as cause of disease classified elsewhere B97.12
      unspecified nature or site B34.1

Infection, infected, infective — *continued*
  virus, viral — *continued*
    encephalitis, tick-borne A84.9
    enterovirus, as cause of disease classified elsewhere B97.10
      coxsackievirus B97.11
      echovirus B97.12
      specified NEC B97.19
    exanthem NOS B09
    human metapneumovirus as cause of disease classified elsewhere B97.81
    human papilloma as cause of disease classified elsewhere B97.7
    intestine — *see* Enteritis, viral
    respiratory syncytial (RSV)
      as cause of disease classified elsewhere B97.4
      bronchiolitis J21.0
      bronchitis J20.5
      bronchopneumonia J12.1
      otitis media H65- ☑ *[B97.4]*
      pneumonia J12.1
      upper respiratory infection J06.9 *[B97.4]*
    rhinovirus
      as cause of disease classified elsewhere B97.89
      unspecified nature or site B34.8
    slow A81.9
      specified NEC A81.89
    specified type NEC B33.8
      as cause of disease classified elsewhere B97.89
      unspecified nature or site B34.8
    unspecified nature or site B34.9
    West Nile — *see* Virus, West Nile
  vulva (acute) — *see* Vulvitis
  West Nile — *see* Virus, West Nile
  whipworm B79
  worms B83.9
    specified type NEC B83.8
  Wuchereria (bancrofti) B74.0
    malayi B74.1
  yatapoxvirus B08.70
    specified NEC B08.79
  yeast — *see also* Candidiasis B37.9
  yellow fever — *see* Fever, yellow
  Yersinia
    enterocolitica (intestinal) A04.6
    pestis — *see* Plague
    pseudotuberculosis A28.2
  Zeis' gland — *see* Hordeolum
  Zika virus A92.5
    congenital P35.4
  zoonotic bacterial NOS A28.9
  Zopfia senegalensis B47.0
Infective, infectious — *see* condition
Infertility
  female N97.9
    age-related N97.8
    associated with
      anovulation N97.0
      cervical (mucus) disease or anomaly N88.3
      congenital anomaly
        cervix N88.3
        fallopian tube N97.1
        uterus N97.2
        vagina N97.8
      dysmucorrhea N88.3
      fallopian tube disease or anomaly N97.1
      pituitary-hypothalamic origin E23.0
      specified origin NEC N97.8
      Stein-Leventhal syndrome E28.2
      uterine disease or anomaly N97.2
      vaginal disease or anomaly N97.8
    due to
      cervical anomaly N88.3
      fallopian tube anomaly N97.1
      ovarian failure E28.39
      Stein-Leventhal syndrome E28.2
      uterine anomaly N97.2
      vaginal anomaly N97.8
    nonimplantation N97.2
    origin
      cervical N88.3
      tubal (block) (occlusion) (stenosis) N97.1
      uterine N97.2
      vaginal N97.8
  male N46.9
    azoospermia N46.01
      extratesticular cause N46.029
        drug therapy N46.021

Infertility — *continued*
  male — *continued*
    azoospermia — *continued*
      extratesticular cause — *continued*
        efferent duct obstruction N46.023
        infection N46.022
        radiation N46.024
        specified cause NEC N46.029
        systemic disease N46.025
    oligospermia N46.11
      extratesticular cause N46.129
        drug therapy N46.121
        efferent duct obstruction N46.123
        infection N46.122
        radiation N46.124
        specified cause NEC N46.129
        systemic disease N46.125
    specified type NEC N46.8
Infestation B88.9
  Acanthocheilonema (perstans) (streptocerca) B74.4
  Acariasis B88.0
    demodex folliculorum B88.0
    sarcoptes scabiei B86
    trombiculae B88.0
  Agamofilaria streptocerca B74.4
  Ancylostoma, ankylostoma (braziliense) (caninum) (ceylanicum) (duodenale) B76.0
    americanum B76.1
    new world B76.1
  Anisakis larvae, anisakiasis B81.0
  arthropod NEC B88.2
  Ascaris lumbricoides — *see* Ascariasis
  Balantidium coli A07.0
  beef tapeworm B68.1
  Bothriocephalus (latus) B70.0
    larval B70.1
  broad tapeworm B70.0
    larval B70.1
  Brugia (malayi) B74.1
    timori B74.2
  candiru B88.8
  Capillaria
    hepatica B83.8
    philippinensis B81.1
  cat liver fluke B66.0
  cestodes B71.9
    diphyllobothrium — *see* Infestation, diphyllobothrium
    dipylidiasis B71.1
    hymenolepiasis B71.0
    specified type NEC B71.8
  chigger B88.0
  chigo, chigoe B88.1
  Clonorchis (sinensis) (liver) B66.1
  coccidial A07.3
  crab-lice B85.3
  Cysticercus cellulosae — *see* Cysticercosis
  Demodex (folliculorum) B88.0
  Dermanyssus gallinae B88.0
  Dermatobia (hominis) — *see* Myiasis
  Dicrocoelium dendriticum B66.2
  Diphyllobothrium (adult) (latum) (intestinal) (pacificum) B70.0
    larval B70.1
  Diplogonoporus (grandis) B71.8
  Dipylidium caninum B67.4
  Distoma hepaticum B66.3
  dog tapeworm B67.4
  Dracunculus medinensis B72
  dragon worm B72
  dwarf tapeworm B71.0
  Echinococcus — *see* Echinococcus
  Echinostomum ilocanum B66.8
  Entamoeba (histolytica) — *see* Infection, Ameba
  Enterobius vermicularis B80
  eyelid
    in (due to)
      leishmaniasis B55.1
      loiasis B74.3
      onchocerciasis B73.09
      phthiriasis B85.3
      parasitic NOS B89
  eyeworm B74.3
  Fasciola (gigantica) (hepatica) (indica) B66.3
  Fasciolopsis (buski) (intestine) B66.5
  filarial B74.9

Infestation — continued
filarial — continued
  bancroftian B74.0
  conjunctiva B74.9
  due to
    Acanthocheilonema (perstans) (streptocerca) B74.4
    Brugia (malayi) B74.1
      timori B74.2
    Dracunculus medinensis B72
    guinea worm B72
    loa loa B74.3
    Mansonella (ozzardi) (perstans) (streptocerca) B74.4
    Onchocerca volvulus B73.00
      eye B73.00
      eyelid B73.09
    Wuchereria (bancrofti) B74.0
  Malayan B74.1
  ozzardi B74.4
  specified type NEC B74.8
fish tapeworm B70.0
  larval B70.1
fluke B66.9
  blood NOS — see Schistosomiasis
  cat liver B66.0
  intestinal B66.5
  lancet B66.2
  liver (sheep) B66.3
    cat B66.0
    Chinese B66.1
    due to clonorchiasis B66.1
    oriental B66.1
  lung (oriental) B66.4
  sheep liver B66.3
  specified type NEC B66.8
fly larvae — see Myiasis
Gasterophilus (intestinalis) — see Myiasis
Gastrodiscoides hominis B66.8
Giardia lamblia A07.1
Gnathostoma (spinigerum) B83.1
Gongylonema B83.8
guinea worm B72
helminth B83.9
  angiostrongyliasis B83.2
    intestinal B81.3
  gnathostomiasis B83.1
  hirudiniasis, internal B83.4
  intestinal B82.0
    angiostrongyliasis B81.3
    anisakiasis B81.0
    ascariasis — see Ascariasis
    capillariasis B81.1
    cysticercosis — see Cysticercosis
    diphyllobothriasis — see Infestation, diphyllobothriasis
    dracunculiasis B72
    echinococcus — see Echinococcosis
    enterobiasis B80
    filariasis — see Infestation, filarial
    fluke — see Infestation, fluke
    hookworm — see Infestation, hookworm
    mixed (types classifiable to more than one of the titles B65.0-B81.3 and B81.8) B81.4
    onchocerciasis — see Onchocerciasis
    schistosomiasis — see Infestation, schistosoma
    specified
      cestode NEC — see Infestation, cestode
      type NEC B81.8
    strongyloidiasis — see Strongyloidiasis
    taenia — see Infestation, taenia
    trichinellosis B75
    trichostrongyliasis B81.2
    trichuriasis B79
  specified type NEC B83.8
  syngamiasis B83.3
  visceral larva migrans B83.0
Heterophyes (heterophyes) B66.8
hookworm B76.9
  ancylostomiasis B76.0
  necatoriasis B76.1
  specified type NEC B76.8
Hymenolepis (diminuta) (nana) B71.0
intestinal NEC B82.9
leeches (aquatic) (land) — see Hirudiniasis
Leishmania — see Leishmaniasis
lice, louse — see Infestation, Pediculus
Linguatula B88.8

Infestation — continued
Liponyssoides sanguineus B88.0
Loa loa B74.3
  conjunctival B74.3
  eyelid B74.3
louse — see Infestation, Pediculus
maggots — see Myiasis
Mansonella (ozzardi) (perstans) (streptocerca) B74.4
Medina (worm) B72
Metagonimus (yokogawai) B66.8
microfilaria streptocerca — see Onchocerciasis
  eye B73.00
  eyelid B73.09
mites B88.9
  scabic B86
Monilia (albicans) — see Candidiasis
mouth B37.0
Necator americanus B76.1
nematode NEC (intestinal) B82.0
  Ancylostoma B76.0
  conjunctiva NEC B83.9
  Enterobius vermicularis B80
  Gnathostoma spinigerum B83.1
  physaloptera B80
  specified NEC B81.8
  trichostrongylus B81.2
  trichuris (trichuria) B79
Oesophagostomum (apiostomum) B81.8
Oestrus ovis — see also Myiasis B87.9
Onchocerca (volvulus) — see Onchocerciasis
Opisthorchis (felineus) (viverrini) B66.0
orbit, parasitic NOS B89
Oxyuris vermicularis B80
Paragonimus (westermani) B66.4
parasite, parasitic B89
  eyelid B89
  intestinal NOS B82.9
  mouth B37.0
  skin B88.9
  tongue B37.0
Parastrongylus
  cantonensis B83.2
  costaricensis B81.3
Pediculus B85.2
  body B85.1
  capitis (humanus) (any site) B85.0
  corporis (humanus) (any site) B85.1
  head B85.0
  mixed (classifiable to more than one of the titles B85.0 - B85.3) B85.4
  pubis (any site) B85.3
Pentastoma B88.8
Phthirus (pubis) (any site) B85.3
  with any infestation classifiable to B85.0 - B85.2 B85.4
pinworm B80
pork tapeworm (adult) B68.0
protozoal NEC B64
  intestinal A07.9
    specified NEC A07.8
  specified NEC B60.8
pubic, louse B85.3
rat tapeworm B71.0
red bug B88.0
roundworm (large) NEC B82.0
  Ascariasis — see also Ascariasis B77.9
sandflea B88.1
Sarcoptes scabiei B86
scabies B86
Schistosoma B65.9
  bovis B65.8
  cercariae B65.3
  haematobium B65.0
  intercalatum B65.8
  japonicum B65.2
  mansoni B65.1
  mattheei B65.8
  mekongi B65.8
  specified type NEC B65.8
  spindale B65.8
screw worms — see Myiasis
skin NOS B88.9
Sparganum (mansoni) (proliferum) (baxteri) B70.1
  larval B70.1
specified type NEC B88.8
Spirometra larvae B70.1
Stellantchasmus falcatus B66.8
Strongyloides stercoralis — see Strongyloidiasis

Infestation — continued
Taenia B68.9
  diminuta B71.0
  echinococcus — see Echinococcus
  mediocanellata B68.1
  nana B71.0
  saginata B68.1
  solium (intestinal form) B68.0
    larval form — see Cysticercosis
Taeniarhynchus saginatus B68.1
tapeworm B71.9
  beef B68.1
  broad B70.0
    larval B70.1
  dog B67.4
  dwarf B71.0
  fish B70.0
    larval B70.1
  pork B68.0
  rat B71.0
Ternidens diminutus B81.8
Tetranychus molestissimus B88.0
threadworm B80
tongue B37.0
Toxocara (canis) (cati) (felis) B83.0
trematode(s) NEC — see Infestation, fluke
Trichinella (spiralis) B75
Trichocephalus B79
Trichomonas — see Trichomoniasis
Trichostrongylus B81.2
Trichuris (trichiura) B79
Trombicula (irritans) B88.0
Tunga penetrans B88.1
Uncinaria americana B76.1
Vandellia cirrhosa B88.8
whipworm B79
worms B83.9
  intestinal B82.0
Wuchereria (bancrofti) B74.0

Infiltrate, infiltration
amyloid (generalized) (localized) — see Amyloidos
calcareous NEC R89.7
  localized — see Degeneration, by site
calcium salt R89.7
cardiac
  fatty — see Degeneration, myocardial
  glycogenic E74.02 [I43]
corneal — see Edema, cornea
eyelid — see Inflammation, eyelid
glycogen, glycogenic — see Disease, glycogen stora
heart, cardiac
  fatty — see Degeneration, myocardial
  glycogenic E74.02 [I43]
inflammatory in vitreous H43.89
kidney N28.89
leukemic — see Leukemia
liver K76.89
  fatty — see Fatty, liver NEC
  glycogen — see also Disease, glycogen storage E74.03 [K77]
lung R91.8
  eosinophilic J82
lymphatic — see also Leukemia, lymphatic C91.9-
  gland I88.9
muscle, fatty M62.89
myocardium, myocardial
  fatty — see Degeneration, myocardial
  glycogenic E74.02 [I43]
on chest x-ray R91.8
pulmonary R91.8
  with eosinophilia J82
skin (lymphocytic) L98.6
thymus (gland) (fatty) E32.8
urine R39.0
vesicant agent
  antineoplastic chemotherapy T80.810 ☑
  other agent NEC T80.818 ☑
vitreous body H43.89

Infirmity R68.89
senile R54

Inflammation, inflamed, inflammatory (with exudation)
abducent (nerve) — see Strabismus, paralytic, sixth nerve
accessory sinus (chronic) — see Sinusitis
adrenal (gland) E27.8
alveoli, teeth M27.3
  scorbutic E54

Inflammation, inflamed, inflammatory — *continued*
- anal canal, anus K62.89
- antrum (chronic) — *see* Sinusitis, maxillary
- appendix — *see* Appendicitis
- arachnoid — *see* Meningitis
- areola N61.0
  - puerperal, postpartum or gestational — *see* Infection, nipple
- areolar tissue NOS L08.9
- artery — *see* Arteritis
- auditory meatus (external) — *see* Otitis, externa
- Bartholin's gland N75.8
- bile duct (common) (hepatic) or passage — *see* Cholangitis
- bladder — *see* Cystitis
- bone — *see* Osteomyelitis
- brain — *see also* Encephalitis
  - membrane — *see* Meningitis
- breast N61.0
  - puerperal, postpartum, gestational — *see* Mastitis, obstetric
- broad ligament — *see* Disease, pelvis, inflammatory
- bronchi — *see* Bronchitis
- catarrhal J00
- cecum — *see* Appendicitis
- cerebral — *see also* Encephalitis
  - membrane — *see* Meningitis
- cerebrospinal
  - meningococcal A39.0
- cervix (uteri) — *see* Cervicitis
- chest J98.8
- chorioretinal H30.9- ☑
  - cyclitis — *see* Cyclitis
  - disseminated H30.10- ☑
    - generalized H30.13- ☑
    - peripheral H30.12- ☑
    - posterior pole H30.11- ☑
  - epitheliopathy — *see* Epitheliopathy
  - focal H30.00- ☑
    - juxtapapillary H30.01- ☑
    - macular H30.04- ☑
    - paramacular — *see* Inflammation, chorioretinal, focal, macular
    - peripheral H30.03- ☑
    - posterior pole H30.02- ☑
  - specified type NEC H30.89- ☑
- choroid — *see* Inflammation, chorioretinal
- chronic, postmastoidectomy cavity — *see* Complications, postmastoidectomy, inflammation
- colon — *see* Enteritis
- connective tissue (diffuse) NEC — *see* Disorder, soft tissue, specified type NEC
- cornea — *see* Keratitis
- corpora cavernosa N48.29
- cranial nerve — *see* Disorder, nerve, cranial
- Douglas' cul-de-sac or pouch (chronic) N73.0
- due to device, implant or graft — *see also* Complications, by site and type, infection or inflammation
  - arterial graft T82.7 ☑
  - breast (implant) T85.79 ☑
  - catheter T85.79 ☑
    - dialysis (renal) T82.7 ☑
      - intraperitoneal T85.71 ☑
    - infusion T82.7 ☑
      - cranial T85.735 ☑
      - intrathecal T85.735 ☑
      - spinal (epidural) (subdural) T85.735 ☑
      - subarachnoid T85.735 ☑
    - urinary T83.518 ☑
      - cystostomy T83.510 ☑
      - Hopkins T83.518 ☑
      - ileostomy T83.518 ☑
      - nephrostomy T83.512 ☑
      - specified NEC T83.518 ☑
      - urethral indwelling T83.511 ☑
      - urostomy T83.518 ☑
  - electronic (electrode) (pulse generator) (stimulator)
    - bone T84.7 ☑
    - cardiac T82.7 ☑
    - nervous system T85.738 ☑
      - brain T85.731 ☑
      - cranial nerve T85.732 ☑
      - gastric nerve T85.732 ☑
      - neurostimulator generator T85.734 ☑
      - peripheral nerve T85.732 ☑

Inflammation, inflamed, inflammatory — *continued*
- due to device, implant or graft — *see also* Complications, by site and type, infection or inflammation — *continued*
  - electronic — *continued*
    - nervous system — *continued*
      - sacral nerve T85.732 ☑
      - spinal cord T85.733 ☑
      - vagal nerve T85.732 ☑
    - urinary T83.590 ☑
  - fixation, internal (orthopedic) NEC — *see* Complication, fixation device, infection
  - gastrointestinal (bile duct) (esophagus) T85.79 ☑
    - neurostimulator electrode (lead) T85.732 ☑
  - genital NEC T83.69 ☑
  - heart NEC T82.7 ☑
    - valve (prosthesis) T82.6 ☑
      - graft T82.7 ☑
  - joint prosthesis — *see* Complication, joint prosthesis, infection
  - ocular (corneal graft) (orbital implant) NEC T85.79 ☑
  - orthopedic NEC T84.7 ☑
  - penile (cylinder) (pump) (resevoir) T83.61 ☑
  - specified NEC T85.79 ☑
  - testicular T83.62 ☑
  - urinary NEC T83.598 ☑
    - ileal conduit stent T83.593 ☑
    - implanted neurostimulation T83.590 ☑
    - implanted sphincter T83.591 ☑
    - indwelling ureteral stent T83.592 ☑
    - nephroureteral stent T83.593 ☑
    - specified stent NEC T83.593 ☑
  - vascular NEC T82.7 ☑
  - ventricular intracranial (communicating) shunt T85.730 ☑
- duodenum K29.80
  - with bleeding K29.81
- dura mater — *see* Meningitis
- ear (middle) — *see also* Otitis, media
  - external — *see* Otitis, externa
  - inner — *see* subcategory H83.0 ☑
- epididymis — *see* Epididymitis
- esophagus K20.9
- ethmoidal (sinus) (chronic) — *see* Sinusitis, ethmoidal
- eustachian tube (catarrhal) — *see* Salpingitis, eustachian
- eyelid H01.9
  - abscess — *see* Abscess, eyelid
  - blepharitis — *see* Blepharitis
  - chalazion — *see* Chalazion
  - dermatosis (noninfectious) — *see* Dermatosis, eyelid
  - hordeolum — *see* Hordeolum
  - specified NEC H01.8
- fallopian tube — *see* Salpingo-oophoritis
- fascia — *see* Myositis
- follicular, pharynx J31.2
- frontal (sinus) (chronic) — *see* Sinusitis, frontal
- gallbladder — *see* Cholecystitis
- gastric — *see* Gastritis
- gastrointestinal — *see* Enteritis
- genital organ (internal) (diffuse)
  - female — *see* Disease, pelvis, inflammatory
  - male N49.9
    - multiple sites N49.8
    - specified NEC N49.8
- gland (lymph) — *see* Lymphadenitis
- glottis — *see* Laryngitis
- granular, pharynx J31.2
- gum K05.10
  - nonplaque induced K05.11
  - plaque induced K05.10
- heart — *see* Carditis
- hepatic duct — *see* Cholangitis
- ileoanal (internal) pouch K91.850
- ileum — *see also* Enteritis
  - regional or terminal — *see* Enteritis, regional
- intestinal pouch K91.850
- intestine (any part) — *see* Enteritis
- jaw (acute) (bone) (chronic) (lower) (suppurative) (upper) M27.2
- joint NEC — *see* Arthritis
  - sacroiliac M46.1
- kidney — *see* Nephritis
- knee (joint) M13.169
  - tuberculous A18.02
- labium (majus) (minus) — *see* Vulvitis

Inflammation, inflamed, inflammatory — *continued*
- lacrimal
  - gland — *see* Dacryoadenitis
  - passages (duct) (sac) — *see also* Dacryocystitis
    - canaliculitis — *see* Canaliculitis, lacrimal
- larynx — *see* Laryngitis
- leg NOS L08.9
- lip K13.0
- liver (capsule) — *see also* Hepatitis
  - chronic K73.9
  - suppurative K75.0
- lung (acute) — *see also* Pneumonia
  - chronic J98.4
- lymph gland or node — *see* Lymphadenitis
- lymphatic vessel — *see* Lymphangitis
- maxilla, maxillary M27.2
  - sinus (chronic) — *see* Sinusitis, maxillary
- membranes of brain or spinal cord — *see* Meningitis
- meninges — *see* Meningitis
- mouth K12.1
- muscle — *see* Myositis
- myocardium — *see* Myocarditis
- nasal sinus (chronic) — *see* Sinusitis
- nasopharynx — *see* Nasopharyngitis
- navel L08.82
- nerve NEC — *see* Neuralgia
- nipple N61.0
  - puerperal, postpartum or gestational — *see* Infection, nipple
- nose — *see* Rhinitis
- oculomotor (nerve) — *see* Strabismus, paralytic, third nerve
- optic nerve — *see* Neuritis, optic
- orbit (chronic) H05.10
  - acute H05.00
    - abscess — *see* Abscess, orbit
    - cellulitis — *see* Cellulitis, orbit
    - osteomyelitis — *see* Osteomyelitis, orbit
    - periostitis — *see* Periostitis, orbital
    - tenonitis — *see* Tenonitis, eye
  - granuloma — *see* Granuloma, orbit
  - myositis — *see* Myositis, orbital
- ovary — *see* Salpingo-oophoritis
- oviduct — *see* Salpingo-oophoritis
- pancreas (acute) — *see* Pancreatitis
- parametrium N73.0
- parotid region L08.9
- pelvis, female — *see* Disease, pelvis, inflammatory
- penis (corpora cavernosa) N48.29
- perianal K62.89
- pericardium — *see* Pericarditis
- perineum (female) (male) L08.9
- perirectal K62.89
- peritoneum — *see* Peritonitis
- periuterine — *see* Disease, pelvis, inflammatory
- perivesical — *see* Cystitis
- petrous bone (acute) (chronic) — *see* Petrositis
- pharynx (acute) — *see* Pharyngitis
- pia mater — *see* Meningitis
- pleura — *see* Pleurisy
- polyp, colon — *see also* Polyp, colon, inflammatory K51.40
- prostate — *see also* Prostatitis
  - specified type NEC N41.8
- rectosigmoid — *see* Rectosigmoiditis
- rectum — *see also* Proctitis K62.89
- respiratory, upper — *see also* Infection, respiratory, upper J06.9
  - acute, due to radiation J70.0
  - chronic, due to external agent — *see* condition, respiratory, chronic, due to
  - due to
    - chemicals, gases, fumes or vapors (inhalation) J68.2
    - radiation J70.1
- retina — *see* Chorioretinitis
- retrocecal — *see* Appendicitis
- retroperitoneal — *see* Peritonitis
- salivary duct or gland (any) (suppurative) — *see* Sialoadenitis
- scorbutic, alveoli, teeth E54
- scrotum N49.2
- seminal vesicle — *see* Vesiculitis
- sigmoid — *see* Enteritis
- sinus — *see* Sinusitis
- Skene's duct or gland — *see* Urethritis

Inflammation, inflamed, inflammatory — continued

skin L08.9
spermatic cord N49.1
sphenoidal (sinus) — see Sinusitis, sphenoidal
spinal
  cord — see Encephalitis
  membrane — see Meningitis
  nerve — see Disorder, nerve
spine — see Spondylopathy, inflammatory
spleen (capsule) D73.89
stomach — see Gastritis
subcutaneous tissue L08.9
suprarenal (gland) E27.8
synovial — see Tenosynovitis
tendon (sheath) NEC — see Tenosynovitis
testis — see Orchitis
throat (acute) — see Pharyngitis
thymus (gland) E32.8
thyroid (gland) — see Thyroiditis
tongue K14.0
tonsil — see Tonsillitis
trachea — see Tracheitis
trochlear (nerve) — see Strabismus, paralytic, fourth
    nerve
tubal — see Salpingo-oophoritis
tuberculous NEC — see Tuberculosis
tubo-ovarian — see Salpingo-oophoritis
tunica vaginalis N49.1
tympanic membrane — see Tympanitis
umbilicus, umbilical L08.82
uterine ligament — see Disease, pelvis, inflammatory
uterus (catarrhal) — see Endometritis
uveal tract (anterior) NOS — see also Iridocyclitis
    posterior — see Chorioretinitis
vagina — see Vaginitis
vas deferens N49.1
vein — see also Phlebitis
  intracranial or intraspinal (septic) G08
  thrombotic I80.9
    leg — see Phlebitis, leg
    lower extremity — see Phlebitis, leg
vocal cord J38.3
vulva — see Vulvitis
Wharton's duct (suppurative) — see Sialoadenitis
Inflation, lung, imperfect (newborn) — see Atelectasis
Influenza (bronchial) (epidemic) (respiratory (upper))
    (unidentified influenza virus) J11.1
  with
    digestive manifestations J11.2
    encephalopathy J11.81
    enteritis J11.2
    gastroenteritis J11.2
    gastrointestinal manifestations J11.2
    laryngitis J11.1
    myocarditis J11.82
    otitis media J11.83
    pharyngitis J11.1
    pneumonia J11.00
      specified type J11.08
    respiratory manifestations NEC J11.1
    specified manifestation NEC J11.89
  A/H5N1 — see also Influenza, due to, identified novel
      influenza A virus J09.X2
  avian — see also Influenza, due to, identified novel in-
      fluenza A virus J09.X2
  bird — see also Influenza, due to, identified novel in-
      fluenza A virus J09.X2
  novel (2009) H1N1 influenza — see also Influenza, due
      to, identified influenza virus NEC J10.1
  novel influenza A/H1N1 — see also Influenza, due to,
      identified influenza virus NEC J10.1
  due to
    avian — see also Influenza, due to, identified novel
        influenza A virus J09.X2
    identified influenza virus NEC J10.1
      with
        digestive manifestations J10.2
        encephalopathy J10.81
        enteritis J10.2
        gastroenteritis J10.2
        gastrointestinal manifestations J10.2
        laryngitis J10.1
        myocarditis J10.82
        otitis media J10.83
        pharyngitis J10.1
        pneumonia (unspecified type) J10.00

Influenza — continued
  due to — continued
    identified influenza virus — continued
      with — continued
        pneumonia — continued
          with same identified influenza virus
            J10.01
          specified type NEC J10.08
        respiratory manifestations NEC J10.1
        specified manifestation NEC J10.89
    identified novel influenza A virus J09.X2
      with
        digestive manifestations J09.X3
        encephalopathy J09.X9
        enteritis J09.X3
        gastroenteritis J09.X3
        gastrointestinal manifestations J09.X3
        laryngitis J09.X2
        myocarditis J09.X9
        otitis media J09.X9
        pharyngitis J09.X2
        pneumonia J09.X1
        respiratory manifestations NEC J09.X2
        specified manifestation NEC J09.X9
        upper respiratory symptoms J09.X2
    of other animal origin, not bird or swine — see also
        Influenza, due to, identified novel influenza A
        virus J09.X2
    swine (viruses that normally cause infections in pigs)
        — see also Influenza, due to, identified novel
        influenza A virus J09.X2
Influenzal — see Influenza
Influenza-like disease — see Influenza
Infraction, Freiberg's (metatarsal head) — see Osteo-
    chondrosis, juvenile, metatarsus
Infraeruption of tooth (teeth) M26.34
Infusion complication, misadventure, or reaction —
    see Complications, infusion
Ingestion
  chemical — see Table of Drugs and Chemicals, by
      substance, poisoning
  drug or medicament
    correct substance properly administered — see Ta-
        ble of Drugs and Chemicals, by drug, adverse
        effect
    overdose or wrong substance given or taken — see
        Table of Drugs and Chemicals, by drug, poi-
        soning
  foreign body — see Foreign body, alimentary tract
  multiple drug — see Table of Drugs and Chemicals,
      multiple
  tularemia A21.3
Ingrowing
  hair (beard) L73.1
  nail (finger) (toe) L60.0
Inguinal — see also condition
  testicle Q53.9
    bilateral Q53.212
    unilateral Q53.112
Inhalant-induced
  anxiety disorder F18.980
  depressive disorder F18.94
  major neurocognitive disorder F18.97
  mild neurocognitive disorder F18.988
  psychotic disorder F18.959
Inhalation
  anthrax A22.1
  flame T27.3 ☑
  food or foreign body — see Foreign body, by site
  gases, fumes, or vapors NEC T59.9- ☑
    specified agent — see Table of Drugs and Chemicals,
        by substance
  liquid or vomitus — see Asphyxia
  meconium (newborn) P24.00
    with
      with respiratory symptoms P24.01
      pneumonia (pneumonitis) P24.01
  mucus — see Asphyxia, mucus
  oil or gasoline (causing suffocation) — see Foreign
      body, by site
  smoke J70.5
    due to chemicals, gases, fumes and vapors J68.9
  steam — see Toxicity, vapors
  stomach contents or secretions — see Foreign body,
      by site
    due to anesthesia (general) (local) or other sedation
        T88.59 ☑
      in labor and delivery O74.0

Inhalation — continued
  stomach contents or secretions — see Foreign bod
      by site — continued
    due to anesthesia or other sedation — continue
      in pregnancy O29.01- ☑
      postpartum, puerperal O89.01
Inhibition, orgasm
  female F52.31
  male F52.32
Inhibitor, systemic lupus erythematosus (presence
    of) D68.62
Iniencephalus, iniencephaly Q00.2
Injection, traumatic jet (air) (industrial) (water) (pa
    or dye) T70.4 ☑
Injury — see also specified injury type T14.90 ☑
  abdomen, abdominal S39.91 ☑
    blood vessel — see Injury, blood vessel, abdom
    cavity — see Injury, intra-abdominal
    contusion S30.1 ☑
    internal — see Injury, intra-abdominal
    intra-abdominal organ — see Injury, intra-abdor
        nal
    nerve — see Injury, nerve, abdomen
    open — see Wound, open, abdomen
    specified NEC S39.81 ☑
    superficial — see Injury, superficial, abdomen
  Achilles tendon S86.00- ☑
    laceration S86.02- ☑
    specified type NEC S86.09- ☑
    strain S86.01- ☑
  acoustic, resulting in deafness — see Injury, nerve,
      acoustic
  adrenal (gland) S37.819 ☑
    contusion S37.812 ☑
    laceration S37.813 ☑
    specified type NEC S37.818 ☑
  alveolar (process) S09.93 ☑
  ankle S99.91- ☑
    contusion — see Contusion, ankle
    dislocation — see Dislocation, ankle
    fracture — see Fracture, ankle
    nerve — see Injury, nerve, ankle
    open — see Wound, open, ankle
    specified type NEC S99.81- ☑
    sprain — see Sprain, ankle
    superficial — see Injury, superficial, ankle
  anterior chamber, eye — see Injury, eye, specified s
      NEC
  anus — see Injury, abdomen
  aorta (thoracic) S25.00 ☑
    abdominal S35.00 ☑
      laceration (minor) (superficial) S35.01 ☑
        major S35.02 ☑
      specified type NEC S35.09 ☑
    laceration (minor) (superficial) S25.01 ☑
      major S25.02 ☑
    specified type NEC S25.09 ☑
  arm (upper) S49.9- ☑
    blood vessel — see Injury, blood vessel, arm
    contusion — see Contusion, arm, upper
    fracture — see Fracture, humerus
    lower — see Injury, forearm
    muscle — see Injury, muscle, shoulder
    nerve — see Injury, nerve, arm
    open — see Wound, open, arm
    specified type NEC S49.8- ☑
    superficial — see Injury, superficial, arm
  artery (complicating trauma) — see also Injury, blc
      vessel, by site
    cerebral or meningeal — see Injury, intracrania
  auditory canal (external) (meatus) S09.91 ☑
  auricle, auris, ear S09.91 ☑
  axilla — see Injury, shoulder
  back — see Injury, back, lower
  bile duct S36.13 ☑
  birth — see also Birth, injury P15.9
  bladder (sphincter) S37.20 ☑
    at delivery O71.5
    contusion S37.22 ☑
    laceration S37.23 ☑
    obstetrical trauma O71.5
    specified type NEC S37.29 ☑
  blast (air) (hydraulic) (immersion) (underwater) NE
      T14.8 ☑
    acoustic nerve trauma — see Injury, nerve, acou
    bladder — see Injury, bladder

☑ **Additional Character Required — Refer to the Tabular List for Character Selection**   ⬚ **Subterms under main terms may continue to next column or pa**

ury — *continued*
blast — *continued*
  brain — *see* Concussion
  colon — *see* Injury, intestine, large
  ear (primary) S09.31- ☑
    secondary S09.39- ☑
  generalized T70.8 ☑
  lung — *see* Injury, intrathoracic, lung
  multiple body organs T70.8 ☑
  peritoneum S36.81 ☑
  rectum S36.61 ☑
  retroperitoneum S36.898 ☑
  small intestine S36.419 ☑
    duodenum S36.410 ☑
    specified site NEC S36.418 ☑
  specified
    intra-abdominal organ NEC S36.898 ☑
    pelvic organ NEC S37.899 ☑
blood vessel NEC T14.8 ☑
  abdomen S35.9 ☑
    aorta — *see* Injury, aorta, abdominal
    celiac artery — *see* Injury, blood vessel, celiac artery
    iliac vessel — *see* Injury, blood vessel, iliac
    laceration S35.91 ☑
    mesenteric vessel — *see* Injury, mesenteric
    portal vein — *see* Injury, blood vessel, portal vein
    renal vessel — *see* Injury, blood vessel, renal
    specified vessel NEC S35.8X- ☑
    splenic vessel — *see* Injury, blood vessel, splenic
    vena cava — *see* Injury, vena cava, inferior
  ankle — *see* Injury, blood vessel, foot
  aorta (abdominal) (thoracic) — *see* Injury, aorta
  arm (upper) NEC S45.90- ☑
    forearm — *see* Injury, blood vessel, forearm
    laceration S45.91- ☑
    specified
      site NEC S45.80- ☑
        laceration S45.81- ☑
        specified type NEC S45.89- ☑
      type NEC S45.99- ☑
    superficial vein S45.30- ☑
      laceration S45.31- ☑
      specified type NEC S45.39- ☑
  axillary
    artery S45.00- ☑
      laceration S45.01- ☑
      specified type NEC S45.09- ☑
    vein S45.20- ☑
      laceration S45.21- ☑
      specified type NEC S45.29- ☑
  azygos vein — *see* Injury, blood vessel, thoracic, specified site NEC
  brachial
    artery S45.10- ☑
      laceration S45.11- ☑
      specified type NEC S45.19- ☑
    vein S45.20- ☑
      laceration S45.219 ☑
      specified type NEC S45.29- ☑
  carotid artery (common) (external) (internal, extracranial) S15.00- ☑
    internal, intracranial S06.8- ☑
    laceration (minor) (superficial) S15.01- ☑
      major S15.02- ☑
    specified type NEC S15.09- ☑
  celiac artery S35.219 ☑
    branch S35.299 ☑
      laceration (minor) (superficial) S35.291 ☑
        major S35.292 ☑
      specified NEC S35.298 ☑
    laceration (minor) (superficial) S35.211 ☑
      major S35.212 ☑
    specified type NEC S35.218 ☑
  cerebral — *see* Injury, intracranial
  deep plantar — *see* Injury, blood vessel, plantar artery
  digital (hand) — *see* Injury, blood vessel, finger
  dorsal
    artery (foot) S95.00- ☑
      laceration S95.01- ☑
      specified type NEC S95.09- ☑
    vein (foot) S95.20- ☑
      laceration S95.21- ☑
      specified type NEC S95.29- ☑

Injury — *continued*
  blood vessel — *continued*
    due to accidental laceration during procedure — *see* Laceration, accidental complicating surgery
    extremity — *see* Injury, blood vessel, limb
    femoral
      artery (common) (superficial) S75.00- ☑
        laceration (minor) (superficial) S75.01- ☑
          major S75.02- ☑
        specified type NEC S75.09- ☑
      vein (hip level) (thigh level) S75.10- ☑
        laceration (minor) (superficial) S75.11- ☑
          major S75.12- ☑
        specified type NEC S75.19- ☑
    finger S65.50- ☑
      index S65.50- ☑
        laceration S65.51- ☑
        specified type NEC S65.59- ☑
      laceration S65.51- ☑
      little S65.50- ☑
        laceration S65.51- ☑
        specified type NEC S65.59- ☑
      middle S65.50- ☑
        laceration S65.51- ☑
        specified type NEC S65.59- ☑
      specified type NEC S65.59- ☑
      thumb — *see* Injury, blood vessel, thumb
    foot S95.90- ☑
      dorsal
        artery — *see* Injury, blood vessel, dorsal, artery
        vein — *see* Injury, blood vessel, dorsal, vein
      laceration S95.91- ☑
      plantar artery — *see* Injury, blood vessel, plantar artery
      specified
        site NEC S95.80- ☑
          laceration S95.81- ☑
          specified type NEC S95.89- ☑
        specified type NEC S95.99- ☑
    forearm S55.90- ☑
      laceration S55.91- ☑
      radial artery — *see* Injury, blood vessel, radial artery
      specified
        site NEC S55.80- ☑
          laceration S55.81- ☑
          specified type NEC S55.89- ☑
        type NEC S55.99- ☑
      ulnar artery — *see* Injury, blood vessel, ulnar artery
      vein S55.20- ☑
        laceration S55.21- ☑
        specified type NEC S55.29- ☑
    gastric
      artery — *see* Injury, mesenteric, artery, branch
      vein — *see* Injury, blood vessel, abdomen
    gastroduodenal artery — *see* Injury, mesenteric, artery, branch
    greater saphenous vein (lower leg level) S85.30- ☑
      hip (and thigh) level S75.20- ☑
        laceration (minor) (superficial) S75.21- ☑
          major S75.22- ☑
        specified type NEC S75.29- ☑
      laceration S85.31- ☑
      specified type NEC S85.39- ☑
    hand (level) S65.90- ☑
      finger — *see* Injury, blood vessel, finger
      laceration S65.91- ☑
      palmar arch — *see* Injury, blood vessel, palmar arch
      radial artery — *see* Injury, blood vessel, radial artery, hand
      specified
        site NEC S65.80- ☑
          laceration S65.81- ☑
          specified type NEC S65.89- ☑
        type NEC S65.99- ☑
      thumb — *see* Injury, blood vessel, thumb
      ulnar artery — *see* Injury, blood vessel, ulnar artery, hand
    head S09.0 ☑
      intracranial — *see* Injury, intracranial
      multiple S09.0 ☑

Injury — *continued*
  blood vessel — *continued*
    hepatic
      artery — *see* Injury, mesenteric, artery
      vein — *see* Injury, vena cava, inferior
    hip S75.90- ☑
      femoral artery — *see* Injury, blood vessel, femoral, artery
      femoral vein — *see* Injury, blood vessel, femoral, vein
      greater saphenous vein — *see* Injury, blood vessel, greater saphenous, hip level
      laceration S75.91- ☑
      specified
        site NEC S75.80- ☑
          laceration S75.81- ☑
          specified type NEC S75.89- ☑
        type NEC S75.99- ☑
    hypogastric (artery) (vein) — *see* Injury, blood vessel, iliac
    iliac S35.5- ☑
      artery S35.51- ☑
      specified vessel NEC S35.5- ☑
      uterine vessel — *see* Injury, blood vessel, uterine
      vein S35.51- ☑
    innominate — *see* Injury, blood vessel, thoracic, innominate
    intercostal (artery) (vein) — *see* Injury, blood vessel, thoracic, intercostal
    jugular vein (external) S15.20- ☑
      internal S15.30- ☑
        laceration (minor) (superficial) S15.31- ☑
          major S15.32- ☑
        specified type NEC S15.39- ☑
      laceration (minor) (superficial) S15.21- ☑
        major S15.22- ☑
      specified type NEC S15.29- ☑
    leg (level) (lower) S85.90- ☑
      greater saphenous — *see* Injury, blood vessel, greater saphenous
      laceration S85.91- ☑
      lesser saphenous — *see* Injury, blood vessel, lesser saphenous
      peroneal artery — *see* Injury, blood vessel, peroneal artery
      popliteal
        artery — *see* Injury, blood vessel, popliteal, artery
        vein — *see* Injury, blood vessel, popliteal, vein
      specified
        site NEC S85.80- ☑
          laceration S85.81- ☑
          specified type NEC S85.89- ☑
        type NEC S85.99- ☑
      thigh — *see* Injury, blood vessel, hip
      tibial artery — *see* Injury, blood vessel, tibial artery
    lesser saphenous vein (lower leg level) S85.40- ☑
      laceration S85.41- ☑
      specified type NEC S85.49- ☑
    limb
      lower — *see* Injury, blood vessel, leg
      upper — *see* Injury, blood vessel, arm
    lower back — *see* Injury, blood vessel, abdomen
      specified NEC — *see* Injury, blood vessel, abdomen, specified, site NEC
    mammary (artery) (vein) — *see* Injury, blood vessel, thoracic, specified site NEC
    mesenteric (inferior) (superior)
      artery — *see* Injury, mesenteric, artery
      vein — *see* Injury, blood vessel, mesenteric, vein
    neck S15.9 ☑
      specified site NEC S15.8 ☑
    ovarian (artery) (vein) — *see* subcategory S35.8 ☑
    palmar arch (superficial) S65.20- ☑
      deep S65.30- ☑
        laceration S65.31- ☑
        specified type NEC S65.39- ☑
      laceration S65.21- ☑
      specified type NEC S65.29- ☑
    pelvis — *see* Injury, blood vessel, abdomen
      specified NEC — *see* Injury, blood vessel, abdomen, specified, site NEC
    peroneal artery S85.20- ☑
      laceration S85.21- ☑
      specified type NEC S85.29- ☑

Injury — *continued*
- blood vessel — *continued*
  - plantar artery (deep) (foot) S95.10- ☑
    - laceration S95.11- ☑
    - specified type NEC S95.19- ☑
  - popliteal
    - artery S85.00- ☑
      - laceration S85.01- ☑
      - specified type NEC S85.09- ☑
    - vein S85.50- ☑
      - laceration S85.51- ☑
      - specified type NEC S85.59- ☑
  - portal vein S35.319 ☑
    - laceration S35.311 ☑
    - specified type NEC S35.318 ☑
  - precerebral — *see* Injury, blood vessel, neck
  - pulmonary (artery) (vein) — *see* Injury, blood vessel, thoracic, pulmonary
  - radial artery (forearm level) S55.10- ☑
    - hand and wrist (level) S65.10- ☑
      - laceration S65.11- ☑
      - specified type NEC S65.19- ☑
    - laceration S55.11- ☑
    - specified type NEC S55.19- ☑
  - renal
    - artery S35.40- ☑
      - laceration S35.41- ☑
      - specified NEC S35.49- ☑
    - vein S35.40- ☑
      - laceration S35.41- ☑
      - specified NEC S35.49- ☑
  - saphenous vein (greater) (lower leg level) — *see* Injury, blood vessel, greater saphenous
    - hip and thigh level — *see* Injury, blood vessel, greater saphenous, hip level
    - lesser — *see* Injury, blood vessel, lesser saphenous
  - shoulder
    - specified NEC — *see* Injury, blood vessel, arm, specified site NEC
    - superficial vein — *see* Injury, blood vessel, arm, superficial vein
  - specified NEC T14.8 ☑
  - splenic
    - artery — *see* Injury, blood vessel, celiac artery, branch
    - vein S35.329 ☑
      - laceration S35.321 ☑
      - specified NEC S35.328 ☑
  - subclavian — *see* Injury, blood vessel, thoracic, innominate
  - thigh — *see* Injury, blood vessel, hip
  - thoracic S25.90 ☑
    - aorta S25.00 ☑
      - laceration (minor) (superficial) S25.01 ☑
        - major S25.02 ☑
      - specified type NEC S25.09 ☑
    - azygos vein — *see* Injury, blood vessel, thoracic, specified, site NEC
    - innominate
      - artery S25.10- ☑
        - laceration (minor) (superficial) S25.11- ☑
          - major S25.12- ☑
        - specified type NEC S25.19- ☑
      - vein S25.30- ☑
        - laceration (minor) (superficial) S25.31- ☑
          - major S25.32- ☑
        - specified type NEC S25.39- ☑
    - intercostal S25.50- ☑
      - laceration S25.51- ☑
      - specified type NEC S25.59- ☑
    - laceration S25.91 ☑
    - mammary vessel — *see* Injury, blood vessel, thoracic, specified, site NEC
    - pulmonary S25.40- ☑
      - laceration (minor) (superficial) S25.41- ☑
        - major S25.42- ☑
      - specified type NEC S25.49- ☑
    - specified
      - site NEC S25.80- ☑
        - laceration S25.81 ☑
        - specified type NEC S25.89 ☑
      - type NEC S25.99 ☑
    - subclavian — *see* Injury, blood vessel, thoracic, innominate
    - vena cava (superior) S25.20 ☑

Injury — *continued*
- blood vessel — *continued*
  - thoracic — *continued*
    - vena cava — *continued*
      - laceration (minor) (superficial) S25.21 ☑
        - major S25.22 ☑
      - specified type NEC S25.29 ☑
  - thumb S65.40- ☑
    - laceration S65.41- ☑
    - specified type NEC S65.49- ☑
  - tibial artery S85.10- ☑
    - anterior S85.13- ☑
      - laceration S85.14- ☑
      - specified injury NEC S85.15- ☑
    - laceration S85.11- ☑
    - posterior S85.16- ☑
      - laceration S85.17- ☑
      - specified injury NEC S85.18- ☑
    - specified injury NEC S85.12- ☑
  - ulnar artery (forearm level) S55.00- ☑
    - hand and wrist (level) S65.00- ☑
      - laceration S65.01- ☑
      - specified type NEC S65.09- ☑
    - laceration S55.01- ☑
    - specified type NEC S55.09- ☑
  - upper arm (level) — *see* Injury, blood vessel, arm
    - superficial vein — *see* Injury, blood vessel, arm, superficial vein
  - uterine S35.5- ☑
    - artery S35.53- ☑
    - vein S35.53- ☑
  - vena cava — *see* Injury, vena cava
  - vertebral artery S15.10- ☑
    - laceration (minor) (superficial) S15.11- ☑
      - major S15.12- ☑
    - specified type NEC S15.19- ☑
  - wrist (level) — *see* Injury, blood vessel, hand
- brachial plexus S14.3 ☑
  - newborn P14.3
- brain (traumatic) S06.9- ☑
  - diffuse (axonal) S06.2X- ☑
  - focal S06.30- ☑
- brainstem S06.38- ☑
- breast NOS S29.9 ☑
- broad ligament — *see* Injury, pelvic organ, specified site NEC
- bronchus, bronchi — *see* Injury, intrathoracic, bronchus
- brow S09.90 ☑
- buttock S39.92 ☑
- canthus, eye S05.90 ☑
- cardiac plexus — *see* Injury, nerve, thorax, sympathetic
- cauda equina S34.3 ☑
- cavernous sinus — *see* Injury, intracranial
- cecum — *see* Injury, colon
- celiac ganglion or plexus — *see* Injury, nerve, lumbosacral, sympathetic
- cerebellum — *see* Injury, intracranial
- cerebral — *see* Injury, intracranial
- cervix (uteri) — *see* Injury, uterus
- cheek (wall) S09.93 ☑
- chest — *see* Injury, thorax
- childbirth (newborn) — *see also* Birth, injury
  - maternal NEC O71.9
- chin S09.93 ☑
- choroid (eye) — *see* Injury, eye, specified site NEC
- clitoris S39.94 ☑
- coccyx — *see also* Injury, back, lower
  - complicating delivery O71.6
- colon — *see* Injury, intestine, large
- common bile duct — *see* Injury, liver
- conjunctiva (superficial) — *see* Injury, eye, conjunctiva
- conus medullaris — *see* Injury, spinal, sacral
- cord
  - spermatic (pelvic region) S37.898 ☑
    - scrotal region S39.848 ☑
  - spinal — *see* Injury, spinal cord, by region
- cornea — *see* Injury, eye, specified site NEC
  - abrasion — *see* Injury, eye, cornea, abrasion
- cortex (cerebral) — *see also* Injury, intracranial
  - visual — *see* Injury, nerve, optic
- costal region NEC S29.9 ☑
- costochondral NEC S29.9 ☑
- cranial
  - cavity — *see* Injury, intracranial
  - nerve — *see* Injury, nerve, cranial
- crushing — *see* Crush

Injury — *continued*
- cutaneous sensory nerve
- cystic duct — *see* Injury, liver
- deep tissue — *see* Contusion, by site
  - meaning pressure ulcer — *see* Ulcer, pressure, u stageable, by site
- delivery (newborn) P15.9
  - maternal NEC O71.9
- Descemet's membrane — *see* Injury, eyeball, penetrating
- diaphragm — *see* Injury, intrathoracic, diaphragm
- duodenum — *see* Injury, intestine, small, duodenu
- ear (auricle) (external) (canal) S09.91 ☑
  - abrasion — *see* Abrasion, ear
  - bite — *see* Bite, ear
  - blister — *see* Blister, ear
  - bruise — *see* Contusion, ear
  - contusion — *see* Contusion, ear
  - external constriction — *see* Constriction, externa ear
  - hematoma — *see* Hematoma, ear
  - inner — *see* Injury, ear, middle
  - laceration — *see* Laceration, ear
  - middle S09.30- ☑
    - blast — *see* Injury, blast, ear
    - specified NEC S09.39- ☑
  - puncture — *see* Puncture, ear
  - superficial — *see* Injury, superficial, ear
- eighth cranial nerve (acoustic or auditory) — *see* Inju nerve, acoustic
- elbow S59.90- ☑
  - contusion — *see* Contusion, elbow
  - dislocation — *see* Dislocation, elbow
  - fracture — *see* Fracture, ulna, upper end
  - open — *see* Wound, open, elbow
  - specified NEC S59.80- ☑
  - sprain — *see* Sprain, elbow
  - superficial — *see* Injury, superficial, elbow
- eleventh cranial nerve (accessory) — *see* Injury, ner accessory
- epididymis S39.94 ☑
- epigastric region S39.91 ☑
- epiglottis NEC S19.89 ☑
- esophageal plexus — *see* Injury, nerve, thorax, symp thetic
- esophagus (thoracic part) — *see also* Injury, intrath racic, esophagus
  - cervical NEC S19.85 ☑
- eustachian tube S09.30 ☑
- eye S05.9- ☑
  - avulsion S05.7- ☑
  - ball — *see* Injury, eyeball
  - conjunctiva S05.0- ☑
  - cornea
    - abrasion S05.0- ☑
    - laceration S05.3- ☑
      - with prolapse S05.2- ☑
  - lacrimal apparatus S05.8X- ☑
  - orbit penetration S05.4- ☑
  - specified site NEC S05.8X- ☑
- eyeball S05.8X- ☑
  - contusion S05.1- ☑
  - penetrating S05.6- ☑
    - with
      - foreign body S05.5- ☑
      - prolapse or loss of intraocular tissue S05.2-
      - without prolapse or loss of intraocular tissue S05.3- ☑
  - specified type NEC S05.8- ☑
- eyebrow S09.93 ☑
- eyelid S09.93 ☑
  - abrasion — *see* Abrasion, eyelid
  - contusion — *see* Contusion, eyelid
  - open — *see* Wound, open, eyelid
- face S09.93 ☑
- fallopian tube S37.509 ☑
  - bilateral S37.502 ☑
    - blast injury S37.512 ☑
    - contusion S37.522 ☑
    - laceration S37.532 ☑
    - specified type NEC S37.592 ☑
  - blast injury (primary) S37.519 ☑
    - bilateral S37.512 ☑
    - secondary — *see* Injury, fallopian tube, specifi type NEC
    - unilateral S37.511 ☑

ury — *continued*
fallopian tube — *continued*
 contusion S37.529 ☑
  bilateral S37.522 ☑
  unilateral S37.521 ☑
 laceration S37.539 ☑
  bilateral S37.532 ☑
  unilateral S37.531 ☑
 specified type NEC S37.599 ☑
  bilateral S37.592 ☑
  unilateral S37.591 ☑
 unilateral S37.501 ☑
  blast injury S37.511 ☑
  contusion S37.521 ☑
  laceration S37.531 ☑
  specified type NEC S37.591 ☑
fascia — *see* Injury, muscle
fifth cranial nerve (trigeminal) — *see* Injury, nerve, trigeminal
finger (nail) S69.9- ☑
 blood vessel — *see* Injury, blood vessel, finger
 contusion — *see* Contusion, finger
 dislocation — *see* Dislocation, finger
 fracture — *see* Fracture, finger
 muscle — *see* Injury, muscle, finger
 nerve — *see* Injury, nerve, digital, finger
 open — *see* Wound, open, finger
 specified NEC S69.8- ☑
 sprain — *see* Sprain, finger
 superficial — *see* Injury, superficial, finger
first cranial nerve (olfactory) — *see* Injury, nerve, olfactory
flank — *see* Injury, abdomen
foot S99.92- ☑
 blood vessel — *see* Injury, blood vessel, foot
 contusion — *see* Contusion, foot
 dislocation — *see* Dislocation, foot
 fracture — *see* Fracture, foot
 muscle — *see* Injury, muscle, foot
 open — *see* Wound, open, foot
 specified type NEC S99.82- ☑
 sprain — *see* Sprain, foot
 superficial — *see* Injury, superficial, foot
forceps NOS P15.9
forearm S59.91- ☑
 blood vessel — *see* Injury, blood vessel, forearm
 contusion — *see* Contusion, forearm
 fracture — *see* Fracture, forearm
 muscle — *see* Injury, muscle, forearm
 nerve — *see* Injury, nerve, forearm
 open — *see* Wound, open, forearm
 specified NEC S59.81- ☑
 superficial — *see* Injury, superficial, forearm
forehead S09.90 ☑
fourth cranial nerve (trochlear) — *see* Injury, nerve, trochlear
gallbladder S36.129 ☑
 contusion S36.122 ☑
 laceration S36.123 ☑
 specified NEC S36.128 ☑
ganglion
 celiac, coeliac — *see* Injury, nerve, lumbosacral, sympathetic
 gasserian — *see* Injury, nerve, trigeminal
 stellate — *see* Injury, nerve, thorax, sympathetic
 thoracic sympathetic — *see* Injury, nerve, thorax, sympathetic
gasserian ganglion — *see* Injury, nerve, trigeminal
gastric artery — *see* Injury, blood vessel, celiac artery, branch
gastroduodenal artery — *see* Injury, blood vessel, celiac artery, branch
gastrointestinal tract — *see* Injury, intra-abdominal
 with open wound into abdominal cavity — *see* Wound, open, with penetration into peritoneal cavity
 colon — *see* Injury, intestine, large
 rectum — *see* Injury, intestine, large, rectum
  with open wound into abdominal cavity S36.61 ☑
 small intestine — *see* Injury, intestine, small
 specified site NEC — *see* Injury, intra-abdominal, specified, site NEC
 stomach — *see* Injury, stomach
genital organ(s)
 external S39.94 ☑

Injury — *continued*
genital organ(s) — *continued*
 external — *continued*
  specified NEC S39.848 ☑
 internal S37.90 ☑
  fallopian tube — *see* Injury, fallopian tube
  ovary — *see* Injury, ovary
  prostate — *see* Injury, prostate
  seminal vesicle — *see* Injury, pelvis, organ, specified site NEC
  uterus — *see* Injury, uterus
  vas deferens — *see* Injury, pelvis, organ, specified site NEC
 obstetrical trauma O71.9
gland
 lacrimal laceration — *see* Injury, eye, specified site NEC
 salivary S09.93 ☑
 thyroid NEC S19.84 ☑
globe (eye) S05.90 ☑
 specified NEC S05.8X- ☑
groin — *see* Injury, abdomen
gum S09.90 ☑
hand S69.9- ☑
 blood vessel — *see* Injury, blood vessel, hand
 contusion — *see* Contusion, hand
 fracture — *see* Fracture, hand
 muscle — *see* Injury, muscle, hand
 nerve — *see* Injury, nerve, hand
 open — *see* Wound, open, hand
 specified NEC S69.8- ☑
 sprain — *see* Sprain, hand
 superficial — *see* Injury, superficial, hand
head S09.90 ☑
 with loss of consciousness S06.9- ☑
 specified NEC S09.8 ☑
heart S26.90 ☑
 with hemopericardium S26.00 ☑
  contusion S26.01 ☑
  laceration (mild) S26.020 ☑
   major S26.022 ☑
   moderate S26.021 ☑
  specified type NEC S26.09 ☑
 contusion S26.91 ☑
 laceration S26.92 ☑
 specified type NEC S26.99 ☑
 without hemopericardium S26.10 ☑
  contusion S26.11 ☑
  laceration S26.12 ☑
  specified type NEC S26.19 ☑
heel — *see* Injury, foot
hepatic
 artery — *see* Injury, blood vessel, celiac artery, branch
 duct — *see* Injury, liver
 vein — *see* Injury, vena cava, inferior
hip S79.91- ☑
 blood vessel — *see* Injury, blood vessel, hip
 contusion — *see* Contusion, hip
 dislocation — *see* Dislocation, hip
 fracture — *see* Fracture, femur, neck
 muscle — *see* Injury, muscle, hip
 nerve — *see* Injury, nerve, hip
 open — *see* Wound, open, hip
 specified NEC S79.81- ☑
 sprain — *see* Sprain, hip
 superficial — *see* Injury, superficial, hip
hymen S39.94 ☑
hypogastric
 blood vessel — *see* Injury, blood vessel, iliac
 plexus — *see* Injury, nerve, lumbosacral, sympathetic
ileum — *see* Injury, intestine, small
iliac region S39.91 ☑
instrumental (during surgery) — *see* Laceration, accidental complicating surgery
 birth injury — *see* Birth, injury
 nonsurgical — *see* Injury, by site
 obstetrical O71.9
  bladder O71.5
  cervix O71.3
  high vaginal O71.4
  perineal NOS O70.9
  urethra O71.5
  uterus O71.5
   with rupture or perforation O71.1

Injury — *continued*
internal T14.8 ☑
 aorta — *see* Injury, aorta
 bladder (sphincter) — *see* Injury, bladder
 with
  ectopic or molar pregnancy O08.6
  following ectopic or molar pregnancy O08.6
  obstetrical trauma O71.5
 bronchus, bronchi — *see* Injury, intrathoracic, bronchus
 cecum — *see* Injury, intestine, large
 cervix (uteri) — *see also* Injury, uterus
  with ectopic or molar pregnancy O08.6
  following ectopic or molar pregnancy O08.6
  obstetrical trauma O71.3
 chest — *see* Injury, intrathoracic
 gastrointestinal tract — *see* Injury, intra-abdominal
 heart — *see* Injury, heart
 intestine NEC — *see* Injury, intestine
 intrauterine — *see* Injury, uterus
 mesentery — *see* Injury, intra-abdominal, specified, site NEC
 pelvis, pelvic (organ) S37.90 ☑
  following ectopic or molar pregnancy (subsequent episode) O08.6
  obstetrical trauma NEC O71.5
   rupture or perforation O71.1
  specified NEC S39.83 ☑
 rectum — *see* Injury, intestine, large, rectum
 stomach — *see* Injury, stomach
 ureter — *see* Injury, ureter
 urethra (sphincter) following ectopic or molar pregnancy O08.6
 uterus — *see* Injury, uterus
interscapular area — *see* Injury, thorax
intestine
 large S36.509 ☑
  ascending (right) S36.500 ☑
   blast injury (primary) S36.510 ☑
    secondary S36.590 ☑
   contusion S36.520 ☑
   laceration S36.530 ☑
   specified type NEC S36.590 ☑
  blast injury (primary) S36.519 ☑
   ascending (right) S36.510 ☑
   descending (left) S36.512 ☑
   rectum S36.61 ☑
   sigmoid S36.513 ☑
   specified site NEC S36.518 ☑
   transverse S36.511 ☑
  contusion S36.529 ☑
   ascending (right) S36.520 ☑
   descending (left) S36.522 ☑
   rectum S36.62 ☑
   sigmoid S36.523 ☑
   specified site NEC S36.528 ☑
   transverse S36.521 ☑
  descending (left) S36.502 ☑
   blast injury (primary) S36.512 ☑
    secondary S36.592 ☑
   contusion S36.522 ☑
   laceration S36.532 ☑
   specified type NEC S36.592 ☑
  laceration S36.539 ☑
   ascending (right) S36.530 ☑
   descending (left) S36.532 ☑
   rectum S36.63 ☑
   sigmoid S36.533 ☑
   specified site NEC S36.538 ☑
   transverse S36.531 ☑
  rectum S36.60 ☑
   blast injury (primary) S36.61 ☑
    secondary S36.69 ☑
   contusion S36.62 ☑
   laceration S36.63 ☑
   specified type NEC S36.69 ☑
  sigmoid S36.503 ☑
   blast injury (primary) S36.513 ☑
    secondary S36.593 ☑
   contusion S36.523 ☑
   laceration S36.533 ☑
   specified type NEC S36.593 ☑
  specified
   site NEC S36.508 ☑
    blast injury (primary) S36.518 ☑
     secondary S36.598 ☑

Injury — *continued*
  intestine — *continued*
    large — *continued*
      specified — *continued*
        site — *continued*
          contusion S36.528 ☑
          laceration S36.538 ☑
          specified type NEC S36.598 ☑
        type NEC S36.599 ☑
          ascending (right) S36.590 ☑
          descending (left) S36.592 ☑
          rectum S36.69 ☑
          sigmoid S36.593 ☑
          specified site NEC S36.598 ☑
          transverse S36.591 ☑
      transverse S36.501 ☑
        blast injury (primary) S36.511 ☑
          secondary S36.591 ☑
        contusion S36.521 ☑
        laceration S36.531 ☑
        specified type NEC S36.591 ☑
    small S36.409 ☑
      blast injury (primary) S36.419 ☑
        duodenum S36.410 ☑
        secondary S36.499 ☑
          duodenum S36.490 ☑
          specified site NEC S36.498 ☑
        specified site NEC S36.418 ☑
      contusion S36.429 ☑
        duodenum S36.420 ☑
        specified site NEC S36.428 ☑
      duodenum S36.400 ☑
        blast injury (primary) S36.410 ☑
          secondary S36.490 ☑
        contusion S36.420 ☑
        laceration S36.430 ☑
        specified NEC S36.490 ☑
      laceration S36.439 ☑
        duodenum S36.430 ☑
        specified site NEC S36.438 ☑
      specified
        site NEC S36.408 ☑
        type NEC S36.499 ☑
          duodenum S36.490 ☑
          specified site NEC S36.498 ☑
  intra-abdominal S36.90 ☑
    adrenal gland — *see* Injury, adrenal gland
    bladder — *see* Injury, bladder
    colon — *see* Injury, intestine, large
    contusion S36.92 ☑
    fallopian tube — *see* Injury, fallopian tube
    gallbladder — *see* Injury, gallbladder
    intestine — *see* Injury, intestine
    kidney — *see* Injury, kidney
    laceration S36.93 ☑
    liver — *see* Injury, liver
    ovary — *see* Injury, ovary
    pancreas — *see* Injury, pancreas
    pelvic NOS S37.90 ☑
    peritoneum — *see* Injury, intra-abdominal, specified, site NEC
    prostate — *see* Injury, prostate
    rectum — *see* Injury, intestine, large, rectum
    retroperitoneum — *see* Injury, intra-abdominal, specified, site NEC
    seminal vesicle — *see* Injury, pelvis, organ, specified site NEC
    small intestine — *see* Injury, intestine, small
    specified
      pelvic S37.90 ☑
        specified
          site NEC S37.899 ☑
            specified type NEC S37.898 ☑
          type NEC S37.99 ☑
      site NEC S36.899 ☑
        contusion S36.892 ☑
        laceration S36.893 ☑
        specified type NEC S36.898 ☑
      type NEC S36.99 ☑
    spleen — *see* Injury, spleen
    stomach — *see* Injury, stomach
    ureter — *see* Injury, ureter
    urethra — *see* Injury, urethra
    uterus — *see* Injury, uterus
    vas deferens — *see* Injury, pelvis, organ, specified site NEC

Injury — *continued*
  intracranial (traumatic) S06.9- ☑
    cerebellar hemorrhage, traumatic — *see* Injury, intracranial, focal
    cerebral edema, traumatic S06.1X- ☑
      diffuse S06.1X- ☑
      focal S06.1X- ☑
    diffuse (axonal) S06.2X- ☑
    epidural hemorrhage (traumatic) S06.4X- ☑
    focal brain injury S06.30- ☑
      contusion — *see* Contusion, cerebral
      laceration — *see* Laceration, cerebral
    intracerebral hemorrhage, traumatic S06.36- ☑
      left side S06.35- ☑
      right side S06.34- ☑
    subarachnoid hemorrhage, traumatic S06.6X- ☑
    subdural hemorrhage, traumatic S06.5X- ☑
  intraocular — *see* Injury, eyeball, penetrating
  intrathoracic S27.9 ☑
    bronchus S27.409 ☑
      bilateral S27.402 ☑
      blast injury (primary) S27.419 ☑
        bilateral S27.412 ☑
        secondary — *see* Injury, intrathoracic, bronchus, specified type NEC
        unilateral S27.411 ☑
      contusion S27.429 ☑
        bilateral S27.422 ☑
        unilateral S27.421 ☑
      laceration S27.439 ☑
        bilateral S27.432 ☑
        unilateral S27.431 ☑
      specified type NEC S27.499 ☑
        bilateral S27.492 ☑
        unilateral S27.491 ☑
      unilateral S27.401 ☑
    diaphragm S27.809 ☑
      contusion S27.802 ☑
      laceration S27.803 ☑
      specified type NEC S27.808 ☑
    esophagus (thoracic) S27.819 ☑
      contusion S27.812 ☑
      laceration S27.813 ☑
      specified type NEC S27.818 ☑
    heart — *see* Injury, heart
    hemopneumothorax S27.2 ☑
    hemothorax S27.1 ☑
    lung S27.309 ☑
      aspiration J69.0
      bilateral S27.302 ☑
      blast injury (primary) S27.319 ☑
        bilateral S27.312 ☑
        secondary — *see* Injury, intrathoracic, lung, specified type NEC
        unilateral S27.311 ☑
      contusion S27.329 ☑
        bilateral S27.322 ☑
        unilateral S27.321 ☑
      laceration S27.339 ☑
        bilateral S27.332 ☑
        unilateral S27.331 ☑
      specified type NEC S27.399 ☑
        bilateral S27.392 ☑
        unilateral S27.391 ☑
      unilateral S27.301 ☑
    pleura S27.60 ☑
      laceration S27.63 ☑
      specified type NEC S27.69 ☑
    pneumothorax S27.0 ☑
    specified organ NEC S27.899 ☑
      contusion S27.892 ☑
      laceration S27.893 ☑
      specified type NEC S27.898 ☑
    thoracic duct — *see* Injury, intrathoracic, specified organ NEC
    thymus gland — *see* Injury, intrathoracic, specified organ NEC
    trachea, thoracic S27.50 ☑
      blast (primary) S27.51 ☑
      contusion S27.52 ☑
      laceration S27.53 ☑
      specified type NEC S27.59 ☑
  iris — *see* Injury, eye, specified site NEC
    penetrating — *see* Injury, eyeball, penetrating
  jaw S09.93 ☑
  jejunum — *see* Injury, intestine, small

Injury — *continued*
  joint NOS T14.8 ☑
    old or residual — *see* Disorder, joint, specified ty NEC
  kidney S37.00- ☑
    acute (nontraumatic) N17.9
    contusion — *see* Contusion, kidney
    laceration — *see* Laceration, kidney
    specified NEC S37.09- ☑
  knee S89.9- ☑
    contusion — *see* Contusion, knee
    dislocation — *see* Dislocation, knee
    meniscus (lateral) (medial) — *see* Sprain, knee, specified site NEC
      old injury or tear — *see* Derangement, knee, meniscus, due to old injury
    open — *see* Wound, open, knee
    specified NEC S89.8- ☑
    sprain — *see* Sprain, knee
    superficial — *see* Injury, superficial, knee
  labium (majus) (minus) S39.94 ☑
  labyrinth, ear S09.30- ☑
  lacrimal apparatus, duct, gland, or sac — *see* Injury eye, specified site NEC
  larynx NEC S19.81 ☑
  leg (lower) S89.9- ☑
    blood vessel — *see* Injury, blood vessel, leg
    contusion — *see* Contusion, leg
    fracture — *see* Fracture, leg
    muscle — *see* Injury, muscle, leg
    nerve — *see* Injury, nerve, leg
    open — *see* Wound, open, leg
    specified NEC S89.8- ☑
    superficial — *see* Injury, superficial, leg
  lens, eye — *see* Injury, eye, specified site NEC
    penetrating — *see* Injury, eyeball, penetrating
  limb NEC T14.8 ☑
  lip S09.93 ☑
  liver S36.119 ☑
    contusion S36.112 ☑
    laceration S36.113 ☑
      major (stellate) S36.116 ☑
      minor S36.114 ☑
      moderate S36.115 ☑
      specified NEC S36.118 ☑
  lower back S39.92 ☑
    specified NEC S39.82 ☑
  lumbar, lumbosacral (region) S39.92 ☑
    plexus — *see* Injury, lumbosacral plexus
  lumbosacral plexus S34.4 ☑
  lung — *see also* Injury, intrathoracic, lung
    aspiration J69.0
    transfusion-related (TRALI) J95.84
  lymphatic thoracic duct — *see* Injury, intrathoracic specified organ NEC
  malar region S09.93 ☑
  mastoid region S09.90 ☑
  maxilla S09.93 ☑
  mediastinum — *see* Injury, intrathoracic, specified gan NEC
  membrane, brain — *see* Injury, intracranial
  meningeal artery — *see* Injury, intracranial, subdur hemorrhage
  meninges (cerebral) — *see* Injury, intracranial
  mesenteric
    artery
      branch S35.299 ☑
        laceration (minor) (superficial) S35.291 ☑
          major S35.292 ☑
        specified NEC S35.298 ☑
      inferior S35.239 ☑
        laceration (minor) (superficial) S35.231 ☑
          major S35.232 ☑
        specified NEC S35.238 ☑
      superior S35.229 ☑
        laceration (minor) (superficial) S35.221 ☑
          major S35.222 ☑
        specified NEC S35.228 ☑
    plexus (inferior) (superior) — *see* Injury, nerve, lumbosacral, sympathetic
    vein
      inferior S35.349 ☑
        laceration S35.341 ☑
        specified NEC S35.348 ☑
      superior S35.339 ☑
        laceration S35.331 ☑

☑ **Additional Character Required — Refer to the Tabular List for Character Selection** ▽ **Subterms under main terms may continue to next column or pa**

Injury — Injury

Injury — *continued*
  muscle — *continued*
    peroneal muscle group, at leg level (lower) S86.30- ☑
      laceration S86.32- ☑
      specified type NEC S86.39- ☑
      strain S86.31- ☑
    posterior muscle (group)
      leg level (lower) S86.10- ☑
        laceration S86.12- ☑
        specified type NEC S86.19- ☑
        strain S86.11- ☑
      thigh level S76.30- ☑
        laceration S76.32- ☑
        specified type NEC S76.39- ☑
        strain S76.31- ☑
    quadriceps (thigh) S76.10- ☑
      laceration S76.12- ☑
      specified type NEC S76.19- ☑
      strain S76.11- ☑
    shoulder S46.90- ☑
      laceration S46.92- ☑
      rotator cuff — *see* Injury, rotator cuff
      specified site NEC S46.80- ☑
        laceration S46.82- ☑
        specified type NEC S46.89- ☑
        strain S46.81- ☑
      specified type NEC S46.99- ☑
      strain S46.91- ☑
    thigh NEC (level) S76.90- ☑
      adductor — *see* Injury, muscle, adductor, thigh
      laceration S76.92- ☑
      posterior muscle (group) — *see* Injury, muscle, posterior muscle, thigh level
      quadriceps — *see* Injury, muscle, quadriceps
      specified
        site NEC S76.80- ☑
          laceration S76.82- ☑
          specified type NEC S76.89- ☑
          strain S76.81- ☑
        type NEC S76.99- ☑
      strain S76.91- ☑
    thorax (level) S29.009 ☑
      back wall S29.002 ☑
      front wall S29.001 ☑
      laceration S29.029 ☑
        back wall S29.022 ☑
        front wall S29.021 ☑
      specified type NEC S29.099 ☑
        back wall S29.092 ☑
        front wall S29.091 ☑
      strain S29.019 ☑
        back wall S29.012 ☑
        front wall S29.011 ☑
    thumb
      abductor (forearm level) S56.30- ☑
        laceration S56.32- ☑
        specified type NEC S56.39- ☑
        strain S56.31- ☑
      extensor (forearm level) S56.30- ☑
        hand level S66.20- ☑
          laceration S66.22- ☑
          specified type NEC S66.29- ☑
          strain S66.21- ☑
        laceration S56.32- ☑
        specified type NEC S56.39- ☑
        strain S56.31- ☑
      flexor (forearm level) S56.00- ☑
        hand level S66.00- ☑
          laceration S66.02- ☑
          specified type NEC S66.09- ☑
          strain S66.01- ☑
        laceration S56.02- ☑
        specified type NEC S56.09- ☑
        strain S56.01- ☑
        wrist level — *see* Injury, muscle, thumb, flexor, hand level
      intrinsic S66.40- ☑
        laceration S66.42- ☑
        specified type NEC S66.49- ☑
        strain S66.41- ☑
    toe — *see also* Injury, muscle, foot
      extensor, long S96.10- ☑
        laceration S96.12- ☑
        specified type NEC S96.19- ☑
        strain S96.11- ☑

Injury — *continued*
  muscle — *continued*
    toe — *see also* Injury, muscle, foot — *continued*
      flexor, long S96.00- ☑
        laceration S96.02- ☑
        specified type NEC S96.09- ☑
        strain S96.01- ☑
      triceps S46.30- ☑
        laceration S46.32- ☑
        specified type NEC S46.39- ☑
        strain S46.31- ☑
    wrist (and hand) level — *see* Injury, muscle, hand
  musculocutaneous nerve — *see* Injury, nerve, musculocutaneous
  myocardium — *see* Injury, heart
  nape — *see* Injury, neck
  nasal (septum) (sinus) S09.92 ☑
  nasopharynx S09.92 ☑
  neck S19.9 ☑
    specified NEC S19.80 ☑
    specified site NEC S19.89 ☑
  nerve NEC T14.8 ☑
    abdomen S34.9 ☑
      peripheral S34.6 ☑
      specified site NEC S34.8 ☑
    abducens S04.4- ☑
      contusion S04.4- ☑
      laceration S04.4- ☑
      specified type NEC S04.4- ☑
    abducent — *see* Injury, nerve, abducens
    accessory S04.7- ☑
      contusion S04.7- ☑
      laceration S04.7- ☑
      specified type NEC S04.7- ☑
    acoustic S04.6- ☑
      contusion S04.6- ☑
      laceration S04.6- ☑
      specified type NEC S04.6- ☑
    ankle S94.9- ☑
      cutaneous sensory S94.3- ☑
      specified site NEC — *see* subcategory S94.8 ☑
    anterior crural, femoral — *see* Injury, nerve, femoral
    arm (upper) S44.9- ☑
      axillary — *see* Injury, nerve, axillary
      cutaneous — *see* Injury, nerve, cutaneous, arm
      median — *see* Injury, nerve, median, upper arm
      musculocutaneous — *see* Injury, nerve, musculocutaneous
      radial — *see* Injury, nerve, radial, upper arm
      specified site NEC — *see* subcategory S44.8 ☑
      ulnar — *see* Injury, nerve, ulnar, arm
    auditory — *see* Injury, nerve, acoustic
    axillary S44.3- ☑
    brachial plexus — *see* Injury, brachial plexus
    cervical sympathetic S14.5 ☑
    cranial S04.9 ☑
      contusion S04.9 ☑
      eighth (acoustic or auditory) — *see* Injury, nerve, acoustic
      eleventh (accessory) — *see* Injury, nerve, accessory
      fifth (trigeminal) — *see* Injury, nerve, trigeminal
      first (olfactory) — *see* Injury, nerve, olfactory
      fourth (trochlear) — *see* Injury, nerve, trochlear
      laceration S04.9 ☑
      ninth (glossopharyngeal) — *see* Injury, nerve, glossopharyngeal
      second (optic) — *see* Injury, nerve, optic
      seventh (facial) — *see* Injury, nerve, facial
      sixth (abducent) — *see* Injury, nerve, abducens
      specified
        nerve NEC S04.89- ☑
          contusion S04.89- ☑
          laceration S04.89- ☑
          specified type NEC S04.89- ☑
        type NEC S04.9 ☑
      tenth (pneumogastric or vagus) — *see* Injury, nerve, vagus
      third (oculomotor) — *see* Injury, nerve, oculomotor
      twelfth (hypoglossal) — *see* Injury, nerve, hypoglossal
    cutaneous sensory
      ankle (level) S94.3- ☑
      arm (upper) (level) S44.5 ☑

Injury — *continued*
  nerve — *continued*
    cutaneous sensory — *continued*
      foot (level) — *see* Injury, nerve, cutaneous sensory, ankle
      forearm (level) S54.3- ☑
      hip (level) S74.2- ☑
      leg (lower level) S84.2- ☑
      shoulder (level) — *see* Injury, nerve, cutaneous sensory, arm
      thigh (level) — *see* Injury, nerve, cutaneous sensory, hip
    deep peroneal — *see* Injury, nerve, peroneal, foot
    digital
      finger S64.4- ☑
        index S64.49- ☑
        little S64.49- ☑
        middle S64.49- ☑
        ring S64.49- ☑
      thumb S64.3- ☑
      toe — *see* Injury, nerve, ankle, specified site N
    eighth cranial (acoustic or auditory) — *see* Injury, nerve, acoustic
    eleventh cranial (accessory) — *see* Injury, nerve, accessory
    facial S04.5- ☑
      contusion S04.5- ☑
      laceration S04.5- ☑
      newborn P11.3
      specified type NEC S04.5- ☑
    femoral (hip level) (thigh level) S74.1- ☑
    fifth cranial (trigeminal) — *see* Injury, nerve, trigeminal
    finger (digital) — *see* Injury, nerve, digital, finger
    first cranial (olfactory) — *see* Injury, nerve, olfactory
    foot S94.9- ☑
      cutaneous sensory S94.3- ☑
      deep peroneal S94.2- ☑
      lateral plantar S94.0- ☑
      medial plantar S94.1- ☑
      specified site NEC — *see* subcategory S94.8
    forearm (level) S54.9- ☑
      cutaneous sensory — *see* Injury, nerve, cutaneous sensory, forearm
      median — *see* Injury, nerve, median
      radial — *see* Injury, nerve, radial
      specified site NEC — *see* subcategory S54.8
      ulnar — *see* Injury, nerve, ulnar
    fourth cranial (trochlear) — *see* Injury, nerve, trochlear
    glossopharyngeal S04.89- ☑
      specified type NEC S04.89- ☑
    hand S64.9- ☑
      median — *see* Injury, nerve, median, hand
      radial — *see* Injury, nerve, radial, hand
      specified NEC — *see* subcategory S64.8 ☑
      ulnar — *see* Injury, nerve, ulnar, hand
    hip (level) S74.9- ☑
      cutaneous sensory — *see* Injury, nerve, cutaneous sensory, hip
      femoral — *see* Injury, nerve, femoral
      sciatic — *see* Injury, nerve, sciatic
      specified site NEC — *see* subcategory S74.8
    hypoglossal S04.89- ☑
      specified type NEC S04.89- ☑
    lateral plantar S94.0- ☑
    leg (lower) S84.9- ☑
      cutaneous sensory — *see* Injury, nerve, cutaneous sensory, leg
      peroneal — *see* Injury, nerve, peroneal
      specified site NEC — *see* subcategory S84.8
      tibial — *see* Injury, nerve, tibial
      upper — *see* Injury, nerve, thigh
    lower
      back — *see* Injury, nerve, abdomen, specified site NEC
        peripheral — *see* Injury, nerve, abdomen, peripheral
      limb — *see* Injury, nerve, leg
    lumbar plexus — *see* Injury, nerve, lumbosacral sympathetic
    lumbar spinal — *see* Injury, nerve, spinal, lumba
    lumbosacral
      plexus — *see* Injury, nerve, lumbosacral, sympathetic
      sympathetic S34.5 ☑

Injury — *continued*
nerve — *continued*
  medial plantar S94.1- ☑
  median (forearm level) S54.1- ☑
    hand (level) S64.1- ☑
    upper arm (level) S44.1- ☑
    wrist (level) — *see* Injury, nerve, median, hand
  musculocutaneous S44.4- ☑
  musculospiral (upper arm level) — *see* Injury, nerve, radial, upper arm
  neck S14.9 ☑
    peripheral S14.4 ☑
    specified site NEC S14.8 ☑
    sympathetic S14.5 ☑
  ninth cranial (glossopharyngeal) — *see* Injury, nerve, glossopharyngeal
  oculomotor S04.1- ☑
    contusion S04.1- ☑
    laceration S04.1- ☑
    specified type NEC S04.1- ☑
  olfactory S04.81- ☑
    specified type NEC S04.81- ☑
  optic S04.01- ☑
    contusion S04.01- ☑
    laceration S04.01- ☑
    specified type NEC S04.01- ☑
  pelvic girdle — *see* Injury, nerve, hip
  pelvis — *see* Injury, nerve, abdomen, specified site NEC
  peripheral — *see* Injury, nerve, abdomen, peripheral
  peripheral NEC T14.8 ☑
    abdomen — *see* Injury, nerve, abdomen, peripheral
    lower back — *see* Injury, nerve, abdomen, peripheral
    neck — *see* Injury, nerve, neck, peripheral
    pelvis — *see* Injury, nerve, abdomen, peripheral
    specified NEC T14.8 ☑
  peroneal (lower leg level) S84.1- ☑
    foot S94.2- ☑
  plexus
    brachial — *see* Injury, brachial plexus
    celiac, coeliac — *see* Injury, nerve, lumbosacral, sympathetic
    mesenteric, inferior — *see* Injury, nerve, lumbosacral, sympathetic
    sacral — *see* Injury, lumbosacral plexus
    spinal
      brachial — *see* Injury, brachial plexus
      lumbosacral — *see* Injury, lumbosacral plexus
  pneumogastric — *see* Injury, nerve, vagus
  radial (forearm level) S54.2- ☑
    hand (level) S64.2- ☑
    upper arm (level) S44.2- ☑
    wrist (level) — *see* Injury, nerve, radial, hand
  root — *see* Injury, nerve, spinal, root
  sacral plexus — *see* Injury, lumbosacral plexus
  sacral spinal — *see* Injury, nerve, spinal, sacral
  sciatic (hip level) (thigh level) S74.0- ☑
  second cranial (optic) — *see* Injury, nerve, optic
  seventh cranial (facial) — *see* Injury, nerve, facial
  shoulder — *see* Injury, nerve, arm
  sixth cranial (abducent) — *see* Injury, nerve, abducens
  spinal
    plexus — *see* Injury, nerve, plexus, spinal
    root
      cervical S14.2 ☑
      dorsal S24.2 ☑
      lumbar S34.21 ☑
      sacral S34.22 ☑
      thoracic — *see* Injury, nerve, spinal, root, dorsal
  splanchnic — *see* Injury, nerve, lumbosacral, sympathetic
  sympathetic NEC — *see* Injury, nerve, lumbosacral, sympathetic
    cervical — *see* Injury, nerve, cervical sympathetic
  tenth cranial (pneumogastric or vagus) — *see* Injury, nerve, vagus
  thigh (level) — *see* Injury, nerve, hip
    cutaneous sensory — *see* Injury, nerve, cutaneous sensory, hip
    femoral — *see* Injury, nerve, femoral
    sciatic — *see* Injury, nerve, sciatic

Injury — *continued*
nerve — *continued*
  thigh — *see* Injury, nerve, hip — *continued*
    specified NEC — *see* Injury, nerve, hip
  third cranial (oculomotor) — *see* Injury, nerve, oculomotor
  thorax S24.9 ☑
    peripheral S24.3 ☑
    specified site NEC S24.8 ☑
    sympathetic S24.4 ☑
  thumb, digital — *see* Injury, nerve, digital, thumb
  tibial (lower leg level) (posterior) S84.0- ☑
  toe — *see* Injury, nerve, ankle
  trigeminal S04.3- ☑
    contusion S04.3- ☑
    laceration S04.3- ☑
    specified type NEC S04.3- ☑
  trochlear S04.2- ☑
    contusion S04.2- ☑
    laceration S04.2- ☑
    specified type NEC S04.2- ☑
  twelfth cranial (hypoglossal) — *see* Injury, nerve, hypoglossal
  ulnar (forearm level) S54.0- ☑
    arm (upper) (level) S44.0- ☑
    hand (level) S64.0- ☑
    wrist (level) — *see* Injury, nerve, ulnar, hand
  vagus S04.89- ☑
    specified type NEC S04.89- ☑
  wrist (level) — *see* Injury, nerve, hand
ninth cranial nerve (glossopharyngeal) — *see* Injury, nerve, glossopharyngeal
nose (septum) S09.92 ☑
obstetrical O71.9
  specified NEC O71.89
occipital (region) (scalp) S09.90 ☑
  lobe — *see* Injury, intracranial
optic chiasm S04.02 ☑
optic radiation S04.03- ☑
optic tract and pathways S04.03- ☑
orbit, orbital (region) — *see* Injury, eye
  penetrating (with foreign body) — *see* Injury, eye, orbit, penetrating
  specified NEC — *see* Injury, eye, specified site NEC
ovary, ovarian S37.409 ☑
  bilateral S37.402 ☑
    contusion S37.422 ☑
    laceration S37.432 ☑
    specified type NEC S37.492 ☑
  blood vessel — *see* Injury, blood vessel, ovarian
  contusion S37.429 ☑
    bilateral S37.422 ☑
    unilateral S37.421 ☑
  laceration S37.439 ☑
    bilateral S37.432 ☑
    unilateral S37.431 ☑
  specified type NEC S37.499 ☑
    bilateral S37.492 ☑
    unilateral S37.491 ☑
  unilateral S37.401 ☑
    contusion S37.421 ☑
    laceration S37.431 ☑
    specified type NEC S37.491 ☑
palate (hard) (soft) S09.93 ☑
pancreas S36.209 ☑
  body S36.201 ☑
    contusion S36.221 ☑
    laceration S36.231 ☑
      major S36.261 ☑
      minor S36.241 ☑
      moderate S36.251 ☑
    specified type NEC S36.291 ☑
  contusion S36.229 ☑
  head S36.200 ☑
    contusion S36.220 ☑
    laceration S36.230 ☑
      major S36.260 ☑
      minor S36.240 ☑
      moderate S36.250 ☑
    specified type NEC S36.290 ☑
  laceration S36.239 ☑
    major S36.269 ☑
    minor S36.249 ☑
    moderate S36.259 ☑
  specified type NEC S36.299 ☑
  tail S36.202 ☑

Injury — *continued*
pancreas — *continued*
  tail — *continued*
    contusion S36.222 ☑
    laceration S36.232 ☑
      major S36.262 ☑
      minor S36.242 ☑
      moderate S36.252 ☑
    specified type NEC S36.292 ☑
parietal (region) (scalp) S09.90 ☑
  lobe — *see* Injury, intracranial
patellar ligament (tendon) S76.10- ☑
  laceration S76.12- ☑
  specified NEC S76.19- ☑
  strain S76.11- ☑
pelvis, pelvic (floor) S39.93 ☑
  complicating delivery O70.1
  joint or ligament, complicating delivery O71.6
  organ S37.90 ☑
    with ectopic or molar pregnancy O08.6
    complication of abortion — *see* Abortion
    contusion S37.92 ☑
    following ectopic or molar pregnancy O08.6
    laceration S37.93 ☑
    obstetrical trauma NEC O71.5
    specified
      site NEC S37.899 ☑
        contusion S37.892 ☑
        laceration S37.893 ☑
        specified type NEC S37.898 ☑
      type NEC S37.99 ☑
  specified NEC S39.83 ☑
penis S39.94 ☑
perineum S39.94 ☑
peritoneum S36.81 ☑
  laceration S36.893 ☑
periurethral tissue — *see* Injury, urethra
  complicating delivery O71.82
phalanges
  foot — *see* Injury, foot
  hand — *see* Injury, hand
pharynx NEC S19.85 ☑
pleura — *see* Injury, intrathoracic, pleura
plexus
  brachial — *see* Injury, brachial plexus
  cardiac — *see* Injury, nerve, thorax, sympathetic
  celiac, coeliac — *see* Injury, nerve, lumbosacral, sympathetic
  esophageal — *see* Injury, nerve, thorax, sympathetic
  hypogastric — *see* Injury, nerve, lumbosacral, sympathetic
  lumbar, lumbosacral — *see* Injury, lumbosacral plexus
  mesenteric — *see* Injury, nerve, lumbosacral, sympathetic
  pulmonary — *see* Injury, nerve, thorax, sympathetic
postcardiac surgery (syndrome) I97.0
prepuce S39.94 ☑
pressure
  injury — *see* Ulcer, pressure, by site
prostate S37.829 ☑
  contusion S37.822 ☑
  laceration S37.823 ☑
  specified type NEC S37.828 ☑
pubic region S39.94 ☑
pudendum S39.94 ☑
pulmonary plexus — *see* Injury, nerve, thorax, sympathetic
rectovaginal septum NEC S39.83 ☑
rectum — *see* Injury, intestine, large, rectum
retina — *see* Injury, eye, specified site NEC
  penetrating — *see* Injury, eyeball, penetrating
retroperitoneal — *see* Injury, intra-abdominal, specified site NEC
rotator cuff (muscle(s)) (tendon(s)) S46.00- ☑
  laceration S46.02- ☑
  specified type NEC S46.09- ☑
  strain S46.01- ☑
round ligament — *see* Injury, pelvic organ, specified site NEC
sacral plexus — *see* Injury, lumbosacral plexus
salivary duct or gland S09.93 ☑
scalp S09.90 ☑
  newborn (birth injury) P12.9
    due to monitoring (electrode) (sampling incision) P12.4

◢ **Subterms under main terms may continue to next column or page**   ☑ **Additional Character Required** — **Refer to the Tabular List for Character Selection**   **197**

Injury — Injury

Injury — continued
scalp — continued
 newborn — continued
  specified NEC P12.89
   caput succedaneum P12.81
scapular region — see Injury, shoulder
sclera — see Injury, eye, specified site NEC
 penetrating — see Injury, eyeball, penetrating
scrotum S39.94 ☑
second cranial nerve (optic) — see Injury, nerve, optic
seminal vesicle — see Injury, pelvic organ, specified
  site NEC
seventh cranial nerve (facial) — see Injury, nerve, facial
shoulder S49.9- ☑
 blood vessel — see Injury, blood vessel, arm
 contusion — see Contusion, shoulder
 dislocation — see Dislocation, shoulder
 fracture — see Fracture, shoulder
 muscle — see Injury, muscle, shoulder
 nerve — see Injury, nerve, shoulder
 open — see Wound, open, shoulder
 specified type NEC S49.8- ☑
 sprain — see Sprain, shoulder girdle
 superficial — see Injury, superficial, shoulder
sinus
 cavernous — see Injury, intracranial
 nasal S09.92 ☑
sixth cranial nerve (abducent) — see Injury, nerve, abducens
skeleton, birth injury P13.9
 specified part NEC P13.8
skin NEC T14.8 ☑
 surface intact — see Injury, superficial
skull NEC S09.90 ☑
specified NEC T14.8 ☑
spermatic cord (pelvic region) S37.898 ☑
 scrotal region S39.848 ☑
spinal (cord)
 cervical (neck) S14.109 ☑
  anterior cord syndrome S14.139 ☑
   C1 level S14.131 ☑
   C2 level S14.132 ☑
   C3 level S14.133 ☑
   C4 level S14.134 ☑
   C5 level S14.135 ☑
   C6 level S14.136 ☑
   C7 level S14.137 ☑
   C8 level S14.138 ☑
  Brown-Séquard syndrome S14.149 ☑
   C1 level S14.141 ☑
   C2 level S14.142 ☑
   C3 level S14.143 ☑
   C4 level S14.144 ☑
   C5 level S14.145 ☑
   C6 level S14.146 ☑
   C7 level S14.147 ☑
   C8 level S14.148 ☑
  C1 level S14.101 ☑
  C2 level S14.102 ☑
  C3 level S14.103 ☑
  C4 level S14.104 ☑
  C5 level S14.105 ☑
  C6 level S14.106 ☑
  C7 level S14.107 ☑
  C8 level S14.108 ☑
  central cord syndrome S14.129 ☑
   C1 level S14.121 ☑
   C2 level S14.122 ☑
   C3 level S14.123 ☑
   C4 level S14.124 ☑
   C5 level S14.125 ☑
   C6 level S14.126 ☑
   C7 level S14.127 ☑
   C8 level S14.128 ☑
  complete lesion S14.119 ☑
   C1 level S14.111 ☑
   C2 level S14.112 ☑
   C3 level S14.113 ☑
   C4 level S14.114 ☑
   C5 level S14.115 ☑
   C6 level S14.116 ☑
   C7 level S14.117 ☑
   C8 level S14.118 ☑
  concussion S14.0 ☑
  edema S14.0 ☑
  incomplete lesion specified NEC S14.159 ☑

Injury — continued
spinal — continued
 cervical — continued
  incomplete lesion specified — continued
   C1 level S14.151 ☑
   C2 level S14.152 ☑
   C3 level S14.153 ☑
   C4 level S14.154 ☑
   C5 level S14.155 ☑
   C6 level S14.156 ☑
   C7 level S14.157 ☑
   C8 level S14.158 ☑
  posterior cord syndrome S14.159 ☑
   C1 level S14.151 ☑
   C2 level S14.152 ☑
   C3 level S14.153 ☑
   C4 level S14.154 ☑
   C5 level S14.155 ☑
   C6 level S14.156 ☑
   C7 level S14.157 ☑
   C8 level S14.158 ☑
 dorsal — see Injury, spinal, thoracic
 lumbar S34.109 ☑
  complete lesion S34.119 ☑
   L1 level S34.111 ☑
   L2 level S34.112 ☑
   L3 level S34.113 ☑
   L4 level S34.114 ☑
   L5 level S34.115 ☑
  concussion S34.01 ☑
  edema S34.01 ☑
  incomplete lesion S34.129 ☑
   L1 level S34.121 ☑
   L2 level S34.122 ☑
   L3 level S34.123 ☑
   L4 level S34.124 ☑
   L5 level S34.125 ☑
  L1 level S34.101 ☑
  L2 level S34.102 ☑
  L3 level S34.103 ☑
  L4 level S34.104 ☑
  L5 level S34.105 ☑
 nerve root NEC
  cervical — see Injury, nerve, spinal, root, cervical
  dorsal — see Injury, nerve, spinal, root, dorsal
  lumbar S34.21 ☑
  sacral S34.22 ☑
  thoracic — see Injury, nerve, spinal, root, dorsal
 plexus
  brachial — see Injury, brachial plexus
  lumbosacral — see Injury, lumbosacral plexus
 sacral S34.139 ☑
  complete lesion S34.131 ☑
  incomplete lesion S34.132 ☑
 thoracic S24.109 ☑
  anterior cord syndrome S24.139 ☑
   T1 level S24.131 ☑
   T2-T6 level S24.132 ☑
   T7-T10 level S24.133 ☑
   T11-T12 level S24.134 ☑
  Brown-Séquard syndrome S24.149 ☑
   T1 level S24.141 ☑
   T2-T6 level S24.142 ☑
   T7-T10 level S24.143 ☑
   T11-T12 level S24.144 ☑
  complete lesion S24.119 ☑
   T1 level S24.111 ☑
   T2-T6 level S24.112 ☑
   T7-T10 level S24.113 ☑
   T11-T12 level S24.114 ☑
  concussion S24.0 ☑
  edema S24.0 ☑
  incomplete lesion specified NEC S24.159 ☑
   T1 level S24.151 ☑
   T2-T6 level S24.152 ☑
   T7-T10 level S24.153 ☑
   T11-T12 level S24.154 ☑
  posterior cord syndrome S24.159 ☑
   T1 level S24.151 ☑
   T2-T6 level S24.152 ☑
   T7-T10 level S24.153 ☑
   T11-T12 level S24.154 ☑
  T1 level S24.101 ☑
  T2-T6 level S24.102 ☑
  T7-T10 level S24.103 ☑
  T11-T12 level S24.104 ☑

Injury — continued
splanchnic nerve — see Injury, nerve, lumbosacral,
  sympathetic
spleen S36.00 ☑
 contusion S36.029 ☑
  major S36.021 ☑
  minor S36.020 ☑
 laceration S36.039 ☑
  major (massive) (stellate) S36.032 ☑
  moderate S36.031 ☑
  superficial (capsular) (minor) S36.030 ☑
 specified type NEC S36.09 ☑
splenic artery — see Injury, blood vessel, celiac arte
  branch
stellate ganglion — see Injury, nerve, thorax, symp
  thetic
sternal region S29.9 ☑
stomach S36.30 ☑
 contusion S36.32 ☑
 laceration S36.33 ☑
 specified type NEC S36.39 ☑
subconjunctival — see Injury, eye, conjunctiva
subcutaneous NEC T14.8 ☑
submaxillary region S09.93 ☑
submental region S09.93 ☑
subungual
 fingers — see Injury, hand
 toes — see Injury, foot
superficial NEC T14.8 ☑
 abdomen, abdominal (wall) S30.92 ☑
  abrasion S30.811 ☑
  bite S30.871 ☑
   insect S30.861 ☑
  contusion S30.1 ☑
  external constriction S30.841 ☑
  foreign body S30.851 ☑
 abrasion — see Abrasion, by site
 adnexa, eye NEC — see Injury, eye, specified site
   NEC
 alveolar process — see Injury, superficial, oral cav
 ankle S90.91- ☑
  abrasion — see Abrasion, ankle
  bite — see Bite, ankle
  blister — see Blister, ankle
  contusion — see Contusion, ankle
  external constriction — see Constriction, ext
    nal, ankle
  foreign body — see Foreign body, superficia
    ankle
 anus S30.98 ☑
 arm (upper) S40.92- ☑
  abrasion — see Abrasion, arm
  bite — see Bite, superficial, arm
  blister — see Blister, arm (upper)
  contusion — see Contusion, arm
  external constriction — see Constriction, ext
    nal, arm
  foreign body — see Foreign body, superficia
    arm
 auditory canal (external) (meatus) — see Injury, s
   perficial, ear
 auricle — see Injury, superficial, ear
 axilla — see Injury, superficial, arm
 back — see also Injury, superficial, thorax, back
  lower S30.91 ☑
   abrasion S30.810 ☑
   contusion S30.0 ☑
   external constriction S30.840 ☑
   superficial
    bite NEC S30.870 ☑
     insect S30.860 ☑
    foreign body S30.850 ☑
 bite NEC — see Bite, superficial NEC, by site
 blister — see Blister, by site
 breast S20.10- ☑
  abrasion — see Abrasion, breast
  bite — see Bite, superficial, breast
  contusion — see Contusion, breast
  external constriction — see Constriction, ext
    nal, breast
  foreign body — see Foreign body, superficial
    breast
 brow — see Injury, superficial, head, specified N
 buttock S30.91 ☑
 calf — see Injury, superficial, leg

☑ Additional Character Required — Refer to the Tabular List for Character Selection   ▽ Subterms under main terms may continue to next column or pag

Injury — *continued*
  superficial — *continued*
    canthus, eye — *see* Injury, superficial, periocular area
    cheek (external) — *see* Injury, superficial, head, specified NEC
      internal — *see* Injury, superficial, oral cavity
    chest wall — *see* Injury, superficial, thorax
    chin — *see* Injury, superficial, head NEC
    clitoris S30.95 ☑
    conjunctiva — *see* Injury, eye, conjunctiva
      with foreign body (in conjunctival sac) — *see* Foreign body, conjunctival sac
    contusion — *see* Contusion, by site
    costal region — *see* Injury, superficial, thorax
    digit(s)
      hand — *see* Injury, superficial, finger
    ear (auricle) (canal) (external) S00.40- ☑
      abrasion — *see* Abrasion, ear
      bite — *see* Bite, superficial, ear
      contusion — *see* Contusion, ear
      external constriction — *see* Constriction, external, ear
      foreign body — *see* Foreign body, superficial, ear
    elbow S50.90- ☑
      abrasion — *see* Abrasion, elbow
      bite — *see* Bite, superficial, elbow
      blister — *see* Blister, elbow
      contusion — *see* Contusion, elbow
      external constriction — *see* Constriction, external, elbow
      foreign body — *see* Foreign body, superficial, elbow
    epididymis S30.94 ☑
    epigastric region S30.92 ☑
    epiglottis — *see* Injury, superficial, throat
    esophagus
      cervical — *see* Injury, superficial, throat
    external constriction — *see* Constriction, external, by site
    extremity NEC T14.8 ☑
    eyeball NEC — *see* Injury, eye, specified site NEC
    eyebrow — *see* Injury, superficial, periocular area
    eyelid S00.20- ☑
      abrasion — *see* Abrasion, eyelid
      bite — *see* Bite, superficial, eyelid
      contusion — *see* Contusion, eyelid
      external constriction — *see* Constriction, external, eyelid
      foreign body — *see* Foreign body, superficial, eyelid
    face NEC — *see* Injury, superficial, head, specified NEC
    finger(s) S60.949 ☑
      abrasion — *see* Abrasion, finger
      bite — *see* Bite, superficial, finger
      blister — *see* Blister, finger
      contusion — *see* Contusion, finger
      external constriction — *see* Constriction, external, finger
      foreign body — *see* Foreign body, superficial, finger
      index S60.94- ☑
      insect bite — *see* Bite, by site, superficial, insect
      little S60.94- ☑
      middle S60.94- ☑
      ring S60.94- ☑
    flank S30.92 ☑
    foot S90.92- ☑
      abrasion — *see* Abrasion, foot
      bite — *see* Bite, foot
      blister — *see* Blister, foot
      contusion — *see* Contusion, foot
      external constriction — *see* Constriction, external, foot
      foreign body — *see* Foreign body, superficial, foot
    forearm S50.91- ☑
      abrasion — *see* Abrasion, forearm
      bite — *see* Bite, forearm, superficial
      blister — *see* Blister, forearm
      contusion — *see* Contusion, forearm
      elbow only — *see* Injury, superficial, elbow
      external constriction — *see* Constriction, external, forearm

Injury — *continued*
  superficial — *continued*
    forearm — *continued*
      foreign body — *see* Foreign body, superficial, forearm
    forehead — *see* Injury, superficial, head NEC
    foreign body — *see* Foreign body, superficial
    genital organs, external
      female S30.97 ☑
      male S30.96 ☑
    globe (eye) — *see* Injury, eye, specified site NEC
    groin S30.92 ☑
    gum — *see* Injury, superficial, oral cavity
    hand S60.92- ☑
      abrasion — *see* Abrasion, hand
      bite — *see* Bite, superficial, hand
      contusion — *see* Contusion, hand
      external constriction — *see* Constriction, external, hand
      foreign body — *see* Foreign body, superficial, hand
    head S00.90 ☑
      ear — *see* Injury, superficial, ear
      eyelid — *see* Injury, superficial, eyelid
      nose S00.30 ☑
      oral cavity S00.502 ☑
      scalp S00.00 ☑
      specified site NEC S00.80 ☑
    heel — *see* Injury, superficial, foot
    hip S70.91- ☑
      abrasion — *see* Abrasion, hip
      bite — *see* Bite, superficial, hip
      blister — *see* Blister, hip
      contusion — *see* Contusion, hip
      external constriction — *see* Constriction, external, hip
      foreign body — *see* Foreign body, superficial, hip
    iliac region — *see* Injury, superficial, abdomen
    inguinal region — *see* Injury, superficial, abdomen
    insect bite — *see* Bite, by site, superficial, insect
    interscapular region — *see* Injury, superficial, thorax, back
    jaw — *see* Injury, superficial, head, specified NEC
    knee S80.91- ☑
      abrasion — *see* Abrasion, knee
      bite — *see* Bite, superficial, knee
      blister — *see* Blister, knee
      contusion — *see* Contusion, knee
      external constriction — *see* Constriction, external, knee
      foreign body — *see* Foreign body, superficial, knee
    labium (majus) (minus) S30.95 ☑
    lacrimal (apparatus) (gland) (sac) — *see* Injury, eye, specified site NEC
    larynx — *see* Injury, superficial, throat
    leg (lower) S80.92- ☑
      abrasion — *see* Abrasion, leg
      bite — *see* Bite, superficial, leg
      contusion — *see* Contusion, leg
      external constriction — *see* Constriction, external, leg
      foreign body — *see* Foreign body, superficial, leg
      knee — *see* Injury, superficial, knee
    limb NEC T14.8 ☑
    lip S00.501 ☑
    lower back S30.91 ☑
    lumbar region S30.91 ☑
    malar region — *see* Injury, superficial, head, specified NEC
    mammary — *see* Injury, superficial, breast
    mastoid region — *see* Injury, superficial, head, specified NEC
    mouth — *see* Injury, superficial, oral cavity
    muscle NEC T14.8 ☑
    nail NEC T14.8 ☑
      finger — *see* Injury, superficial, finger
      toe — *see* Injury, superficial, toe
    nasal (septum) — *see* Injury, superficial, nose
    neck S10.90 ☑
      specified site NEC S10.80 ☑
    nose (septum) S00.30 ☑
    occipital region — *see* Injury, superficial, scalp
    oral cavity S00.502 ☑

Injury — *continued*
  superficial — *continued*
    orbital region — *see* Injury, superficial, periocular area
    palate — *see* Injury, superficial, oral cavity
    palm — *see* Injury, superficial, hand
    parietal region — *see* Injury, superficial, scalp
    pelvis S30.91 ☑
      girdle — *see* Injury, superficial, hip
    penis S30.93 ☑
    perineum
      female S30.95 ☑
      male S30.91 ☑
    periocular area S00.20- ☑
      abrasion — *see* Abrasion, eyelid
      bite — *see* Bite, superficial, eyelid
      contusion — *see* Contusion, eyelid
      external constriction — *see* Constriction, external, eyelid
      foreign body — *see* Foreign body, superficial, eyelid
    phalanges
      finger — *see* Injury, superficial, finger
      toe — *see* Injury, superficial, toe
    pharynx — *see* Injury, superficial, throat
    pinna — *see* Injury, superficial, ear
    popliteal space — *see* Injury, superficial, knee
    prepuce S30.93 ☑
    pubic region S30.91 ☑
    pudendum
      female S30.97 ☑
      male S30.96 ☑
    sacral region S30.91 ☑
    scalp S00.00 ☑
    scapular region — *see* Injury, superficial, shoulder
    sclera — *see* Injury, eye, specified site NEC
    scrotum S30.94 ☑
    shin — *see* Injury, superficial, leg
    shoulder S40.91- ☑
      abrasion — *see* Abrasion, shoulder
      bite — *see* Bite, superficial, shoulder
      blister — *see* Blister, shoulder
      contusion — *see* Contusion, shoulder
      external constriction — *see* Constriction, external, shoulder
      foreign body — *see* Foreign body, superficial, shoulder
    skin NEC T14.8 ☑
    sternal region — *see* Injury, superficial, thorax, front
    subconjunctival — *see* Injury, eye, specified site NEC
    subcutaneous NEC T14.8 ☑
    submaxillary region — *see* Injury, superficial, head, specified NEC
    submental region — *see* Injury, superficial, head, specified NEC
    subungual
      finger(s) — *see* Injury, superficial, finger
      toe(s) — *see* Injury, superficial, toe
    supraclavicular fossa — *see* Injury, superficial, neck
    supraorbital — *see* Injury, superficial, head, specified NEC
    temple — *see* Injury, superficial, head, specified NEC
    temporal region — *see* Injury, superficial, head, specified NEC
    testis S30.94 ☑
    thigh S70.92- ☑
      abrasion — *see* Abrasion, thigh
      bite — *see* Bite, superficial, thigh
      blister — *see* Blister, thigh
      contusion — *see* Contusion, thigh
      external constriction — *see* Constriction, external, thigh
      foreign body — *see* Foreign body, superficial, thigh
    thorax, thoracic (wall) S20.90 ☑
      abrasion — *see* Abrasion, thorax
      back S20.40- ☑
      bite — *see* Bite, thorax, superficial
      blister — *see* Blister, thorax
      contusion — *see* Contusion, thorax
      external constriction — *see* Constriction, external, thorax
      foreign body — *see* Foreign body, superficial, thorax
      front S20.30- ☑
    throat S10.10 ☑

Injury — *continued*
  superficial — *continued*
    throat — *continued*
      abrasion S10.11 ☑
      bite S10.17 ☑
        insect S10.16 ☑
      blister S10.12 ☑
      contusion S10.0 ☑
      external constriction S10.14 ☑
      foreign body S10.15 ☑
    thumb S60.93- ☑
      abrasion — *see* Abrasion, thumb
      bite — *see* Bite, superficial, thumb
      blister — *see* Blister, thumb
      contusion — *see* Contusion, thumb
      external constriction — *see* Constriction, external, thumb
      foreign body — *see* Foreign body, superficial, thumb
      insect bite — *see* Bite, by site, superficial, insect
      specified type NEC S60.39 ☑
    toe(s) S90.93- ☑
      abrasion — *see* Abrasion, toe
      bite — *see* Bite, toe
      blister — *see* Blister, toe
      contusion — *see* Contusion, toe
      external constriction — *see* Constriction, external, toe
      foreign body — *see* Foreign body, superficial, toe
      great S90.93- ☑
    tongue — *see* Injury, superficial, oral cavity
    tooth, teeth — *see* Injury, superficial, oral cavity
    trachea S10.10 ☑
    tunica vaginalis S30.94 ☑
    tympanum, tympanic membrane — *see* Injury, superficial, ear
    uvula — *see* Injury, superficial, oral cavity
    vagina S30.95 ☑
    vocal cords — *see* Injury, superficial, throat
    vulva S30.95 ☑
    wrist S60.91- ☑
  supraclavicular region — *see* Injury, neck
  supraorbital S09.93 ☑
  suprarenal gland (multiple) — *see* Injury, adrenal
  surgical complication (external or internal site) — *see* Laceration, accidental complicating surgery
  temple S09.90 ☑
  temporal region S09.90 ☑
  tendon — *see also* Injury, muscle, by site
    abdomen — *see* Injury, muscle, abdomen
    Achilles — *see* Injury, Achilles tendon
    lower back — *see* Injury, muscle, lower back
    pelvic organs — *see* Injury, muscle, pelvis
  tenth cranial nerve (pneumogastric or vagus) — *see* Injury, nerve, vagus
  testis S39.94 ☑
  thigh S79.92- ☑
    blood vessel — *see* Injury, blood vessel, hip
    contusion — *see* Contusion, thigh
    fracture — *see* Fracture, femur
    muscle — *see* Injury, muscle, thigh
    nerve — *see* Injury, nerve, thigh
    open — *see* Wound, open, thigh
    specified NEC S79.82- ☑
    superficial — *see* Injury, superficial, thigh
  third cranial nerve (oculomotor) — *see* Injury, nerve, oculomotor
  thorax, thoracic S29.9 ☑
    blood vessel — *see* Injury, blood vessel, thorax
    cavity — *see* Injury, intrathoracic
    dislocation — *see* Dislocation, thorax
    external (wall) S29.9 ☑
      contusion — *see* Contusion, thorax
      nerve — *see* Injury, nerve, thorax
      open — *see* Wound, open, thorax
      specified NEC S29.8 ☑
      sprain — *see* Sprain, thorax
      superficial — *see* Injury, superficial, thorax
    fracture — *see* Fracture, thorax
    internal — *see* Injury, intrathoracic
    intrathoracic organ — *see* Injury, intrathoracic
    sympathetic ganglion — *see* Injury, nerve, thorax, sympathetic
  throat — *see also* Injury, neck S19.9 ☑
  thumb S69.9- ☑

Injury — *continued*
  thumb — *continued*
    blood vessel — *see* Injury, blood vessel, thumb
    contusion — *see* Contusion, thumb
    dislocation — *see* Dislocation, thumb
    fracture — *see* Fracture, thumb
    muscle — *see* Injury, muscle, thumb
    nerve — *see* Injury, nerve, digital, thumb
    open — *see* Wound, open, thumb
    specified NEC S69.8- ☑
    sprain — *see* Sprain, thumb
    superficial — *see* Injury, superficial, thumb
  thymus (gland) — *see* Injury, intrathoracic, specified organ NEC
  thyroid (gland) NEC S19.84 ☑
  toe S99.92- ☑
    contusion — *see* Contusion, toe
    dislocation — *see* Dislocation, toe
    fracture — *see* Fracture, toe
    muscle — *see* Injury, muscle, toe
    open — *see* Wound, open, toe
    specified type NEC S99.82- ☑
    sprain — *see* Sprain, toe
    superficial — *see* Injury, superficial, toe
  tongue S09.93 ☑
  tonsil S09.93 ☑
  tooth S09.93 ☑
  trachea (cervical) NEC S19.82 ☑
    thoracic — *see* Injury, intrathoracic, trachea, thoracic
  transfusion-related acute lung (TRALI) J95.84
  tunica vaginalis S39.94 ☑
  twelfth cranial nerve (hypoglossal) — *see* Injury, nerve, hypoglossal
  ureter S37.10 ☑
    contusion S37.12 ☑
    laceration S37.13 ☑
    specified type NEC S37.19 ☑
  urethra (sphincter) S37.30 ☑
    at delivery O71.5
    contusion S37.32 ☑
    laceration S37.33 ☑
    specified type NEC S37.39 ☑
  urinary organ S37.90 ☑
    contusion S37.92 ☑
    laceration S37.93 ☑
    specified
      site NEC S37.899 ☑
        contusion S37.892 ☑
        laceration S37.893 ☑
        specified type NEC S37.898 ☑
      type NEC S37.99 ☑
  uterus, uterine S37.60 ☑
    with ectopic or molar pregnancy O08.6
    blood vessel — *see* Injury, blood vessel, iliac
    contusion S37.62 ☑
    laceration S37.63 ☑
      cervix at delivery O71.3
    rupture associated with obstetrics — *see* Rupture, uterus
    specified type NEC S37.69 ☑
  uvula S09.93 ☑
  vagina S39.93 ☑
    abrasion S30.814 ☑
    bite S31.45 ☑
      insect S30.864 ☑
      superficial NEC S30.874 ☑
    contusion S30.23 ☑
    crush S38.03 ☑
    during delivery — *see* Laceration, vagina, during delivery
    external constriction S30.844 ☑
    insect bite S30.864 ☑
    laceration S31.41 ☑
      with foreign body S31.42 ☑
    open wound S31.40 ☑
    puncture S31.43 ☑
      with foreign body S31.44 ☑
    superficial S30.95 ☑
      foreign body S30.854 ☑
  vas deferens — *see* Injury, pelvic organ, specified site NEC
  vascular NEC T14.8 ☑
  vein — *see* Injury, blood vessel
  vena cava (superior) S25.20 ☑
    inferior S35.10 ☑
      laceration (minor) (superficial) S35.11 ☑

Injury — *continued*
  vena cava — *continued*
    inferior — *continued*
      laceration — *continued*
        major S35.12 ☑
        specified type NEC S35.19 ☑
    laceration (minor) (superficial) S25.21 ☑
      major S25.22 ☑
    specified type NEC S25.29 ☑
  vesical (sphincter) — *see* Injury, bladder
  visual cortex S04.04- ☑
  vitreous (humor) S05.90 ☑
    specified NEC S05.8X- ☑
  vocal cord NEC S19.83 ☑
  vulva S39.94 ☑
    abrasion S30.814 ☑
    bite S31.45 ☑
      insect S30.864 ☑
      superficial NEC S30.874 ☑
    contusion S30.23 ☑
    crush S38.03 ☑
    during delivery — *see* Laceration, perineum, female, during delivery
    external constriction S30.844 ☑
    insect bite S30.864 ☑
    laceration S31.41 ☑
      with foreign body S31.42 ☑
    open wound S31.40 ☑
    puncture S31.43 ☑
      with foreign body S31.44 ☑
    superficial S30.95 ☑
      foreign body S30.854 ☑
  whiplash (cervical spine) S13.4 ☑
  wrist S69.9- ☑
    blood vessel — *see* Injury, blood vessel, hand
    contusion — *see* Contusion, wrist
    dislocation — *see* Dislocation, wrist
    fracture — *see* Fracture, wrist
    muscle — *see* Injury, muscle, hand
    nerve — *see* Injury, nerve, hand
    open — *see* Wound, open, wrist
    specified NEC S69.8- ☑
    sprain — *see* Sprain, wrist
    superficial — *see* Injury, superficial, wrist
Inoculation — *see also* Vaccination
  complication or reaction — *see* Complications, vaccination
Insanity, insane — *see also* Psychosis
  adolescent — *see* Schizophrenia
  confusional F28
    acute or subacute F05
  delusional F22
  senile F03 ☑
Insect
  bite — *see* Bite, by site, superficial, insect
  venomous, poisoning NEC (by) — *see* Venom, arthropod
Insensitivity
  adrenocorticotropin hormone (ACTH) E27.49
  androgen E34.50
    complete E34.51
    partial E34.52
Insertion
  cord (umbilical) lateral or velamentous O43.12-
  intrauterine contraceptive device (encounter for) — *see* Intrauterine contraceptive device
Insolation (sunstroke) T67.01 ☑
Insomnia (organic) G47.00
  adjustment F51.02
  adjustment disorder F51.02
  behavioral, of childhood Z73.819
    combined type Z73.812
    limit setting type Z73.811
    sleep-onset association type Z73.810
  childhood Z73.819
  chronic F51.04
    somatized tension F51.04
  conditioned F51.04
  due to
    alcohol
      abuse F10.182
      dependence F10.282
      use F10.982
    amphetamines
      abuse F15.182
      dependence F15.282
      use F15.982

☑ **Additional Character Required** — **Refer to the Tabular List for Character Selection**
▽ **Subterms under main terms may continue to next column or page**

somnia — continued
  due to — continued
    anxiety disorder F51.05
    caffeine
      abuse F15.182
      dependence F15.282
      use F15.982
    cocaine
      abuse F14.182
      dependence F14.282
      use F14.982
    depression F51.05
    drug NEC
      abuse F19.182
      dependence F19.282
      use F19.982
    medical condition G47.01
    mental disorder NEC F51.05
    opioid
      abuse F11.182
      dependence F11.282
      use F11.982
    psychoactive substance NEC
      abuse F19.182
      dependence F19.182
      use F19.982
    sedative, hypnotic, or anxiolytic
      abuse F13.182
      dependence F13.282
      use F13.982
    stimulant NEC
      abuse F15.182
      dependence F15.282
      use F15.982
  fatal familial (FFI) A81.83
  idiopathic F51.01
  learned F51.3
  nonorganic origin F51.01
  not due to a substance or known physiological condition F51.01
    specified NEC F51.09
  paradoxical F51.03
  primary F51.01
  psychiatric F51.05
  psychophysiologic F51.04
  related to psychopathology F51.05
  short-term F51.02
  specified NEC G47.09
  stress-related F51.02
  transient F51.02
  without objective findings F51.02
spiration
  food or foreign body — see Foreign body, by site
  mucus — see Asphyxia, mucus
spissated bile syndrome (newborn) P59.1
stability
  emotional (excessive) F60.3
  joint (post-traumatic) M25.30
    ankle M25.37- ☑
    due to old ligament injury — see Disorder, ligament
    elbow M25.32- ☑
    flail — see Flail, joint
    foot M25.37- ☑
    hand M25.34- ☑
    hip M25.35- ☑
    knee M25.36- ☑
    lumbosacral — see subcategory M53.2 ☑
    prosthesis — see Complications, joint prosthesis, mechanical, displacement, by site
    sacroiliac — see subcategory M53.2 ☑
    secondary to
      old ligament injury — see Disorder, ligament
      removal of joint prosthesis M96.89
    shoulder (region) M25.31- ☑
    spine — see subcategory M53.2 ☑
    wrist M25.33- ☑
  knee (chronic) M23.5- ☑
  lumbosacral — see subcategory M53.2 ☑
  nervous F48.8
  personality (emotional) F60.3
  spine — see Instability, joint, spine
  vasomotor R55
stitutional syndrome (childhood) F94.2
stitutionalization, affecting child Z62.22
  disinhibited attachment F94.2
sufficiency, insufficient
  accommodation, old age H52.4
  adrenal (gland) E27.40

Insufficiency, insufficient — continued
  adrenal — continued
    primary E27.1
  adrenocortical E27.40
    drug-induced E27.3
    iatrogenic E27.3
    primary E27.1
  anatomic crown height K08.89
  anterior (occlusal) guidance M26.54
  anus K62.89
  aortic (valve) I35.1
    with
      mitral (valve) disease I08.0
        with tricuspid (valve) disease I08.3
      stenosis I35.2
      tricuspid (valve) disease I08.2
        with mitral (valve) disease I08.3
    congenital Q23.1
    rheumatic I06.1
      with
        mitral (valve) disease I08.0
          with tricuspid (valve) disease I08.3
        stenosis I06.2
          with mitral (valve) disease I08.0
            with tricuspid (valve) disease I08.3
        tricuspid (valve) disease I08.2
          with mitral (valve) disease I08.3
    specified cause NEC I35.1
    syphilitic A52.03
  arterial I77.1
    basilar G45.0
    carotid (hemispheric) G45.1
    cerebral I67.81
    coronary (acute or subacute) I24.8
    mesenteric K55.1
    peripheral I73.9
    precerebral (multiple) (bilateral) G45.2
    vertebral G45.0
  arteriovenous I99.8
  biliary K83.8
  cardiac — see also Insufficiency, myocardial
    due to presence of (cardiac) prosthesis I97.11- ☑
    postprocedural I97.11- ☑
  cardiorenal, hypertensive I13.2
  cardiovascular — see Disease, cardiovascular
  cerebrovascular (acute) I67.81
    with transient focal neurological signs and symptoms G45.8
  circulatory NEC I99.8
    newborn P29.89
  clinical crown length K08.89
  convergence H51.11
  coronary (acute or subacute) I24.8
    chronic or with a stated duration of over 4 weeks I25.89
  corticoadrenal E27.40
    primary E27.1
  dietary E63.9
  divergence H51.8
  food T73.0 ☑
  gastroesophageal K22.8
  gonadal
    ovary E28.39
    testis E29.1
  heart — see also Insufficiency, myocardial
    newborn P29.0
    valve — see Endocarditis
  hepatic — see Failure, hepatic
  idiopathic autonomic G90.09
  interocclusal distance of fully erupted teeth (ridge) M26.36
  kidney N28.9
    acute N28.9
    chronic N18.9
  lacrimal (secretion) H04.12- ☑
    passages — see Stenosis, lacrimal
  liver — see Failure, hepatic
  lung — see Insufficiency, pulmonary
  mental (congenital) — see Disability, intellectual
  mesenteric K55.1
  mitral (valve) I34.0
    with
      aortic valve disease I08.0
        with tricuspid (valve) disease I08.3
      obstruction or stenosis I05.2
        with aortic valve disease I08.0
      tricuspid (valve) disease I08.1
        with aortic (valve) disease I08.3

Insufficiency, insufficient — continued
  mitral — continued
    congenital Q23.3
    rheumatic I05.1
      with
        aortic valve disease I08.0
          with tricuspid (valve) disease I08.3
        obstruction or stenosis I05.2
          with aortic valve disease I08.0
            with tricuspid (valve) disease I08.3
        tricuspid (valve) disease I08.1
          with aortic (valve) disease I08.3
    active or acute I01.1
      with chorea, rheumatic (Sydenham's) I02.0
    specified cause, except rheumatic I34.0
  muscle — see also Disease, muscle
    heart — see Insufficiency, myocardial
    ocular NEC H50.9
  myocardial, myocardium (with arteriosclerosis) — see also Failure, heart I50.9
    with
      rheumatic fever (conditions in I00) I09.0
        active, acute or subacute I01.2
          with chorea I02.0
        inactive or quiescent (with chorea) I09.0
    congenital Q24.8
    hypertensive — see Hypertension, heart
    newborn P29.0
    rheumatic I09.0
      active, acute, or subacute I01.2
    syphilitic A52.06
  nourishment T73.0 ☑
  pancreatic K86.89
    exocrine K86.81
  parathyroid (gland) E20.9
  peripheral vascular (arterial) I73.9
  pituitary E23.0
  placental (mother) O36.51- ☑
  platelets D69.6
  prenatal care affecting management of pregnancy O09.3- ☑
  progressive pluriglandular E31.0
  pulmonary J98.4
    acute, following surgery (nonthoracic) J95.2
      thoracic J95.1
    chronic, following surgery J95.3
    following
      shock J98.4
      trauma J98.4
    newborn P28.89
    valve I37.1
      with stenosis I37.2
      congenital Q22.2
      rheumatic I09.89
        with aortic, mitral or tricuspid (valve) disease I08.8
  pyloric K31.89
  renal (acute) N28.9
    chronic N18.9
  respiratory R06.89
    newborn P28.5
  rotation — see Malrotation
  sleep syndrome F51.12
  social insurance Z59.7
  suprarenal E27.40
    primary E27.1
  tarso-orbital fascia, congenital Q10.3
  testis E29.1
  thyroid (gland) (acquired) E03.9
    congenital E03.1
  tricuspid (valve) (rheumatic) I07.1
    with
      aortic (valve) disease I08.2
        with mitral (valve) disease I08.3
      mitral (valve) disease I08.1
        with aortic (valve) disease I08.3
      obstruction or stenosis I07.2
        with aortic (valve) disease I08.2
          with mitral (valve) disease I08.3
    congenital Q22.8
    nonrheumatic I36.1
      with stenosis I36.2
  urethral sphincter R32
  valve, valvular (heart) I38
    aortic — see Insufficiency, aortic (valve)
    congenital Q24.8
    mitral — see Insufficiency, mitral (valve)
    pulmonary — see Insufficiency, pulmonary, valve

Insufficiency, insufficient — *continued*
  valve, valvular — *continued*
    tricuspid — *see* Insufficiency, tricuspid (valve)
  vascular I99.8
    intestine K55.9
      acute — *see also* Ischemia, intestine, acute
        K55.059
    mesenteric K55.1
    peripheral I73.9
    renal — *see* Hypertension, kidney
  velopharyngeal
    acquired K13.79
    congenital Q38.8
  venous (chronic) (peripheral) I87.2
  ventricular — *see* Insufficiency, myocardial
  welfare support Z59.7
Insufflation, fallopian Z31.41
Insular — *see* condition
Insulinoma
  pancreas
    benign D13.7
    malignant C25.4
    uncertain behavior D37.8
  specified site
    benign — *see* Neoplasm, by site, benign
    malignant — *see* Neoplasm, by site, malignant
    uncertain behavior — *see* Neoplasm, by site, uncertain behavior
  unspecified site
    benign D13.7
    malignant C25.4
    uncertain behavior D37.8
Insuloma — *see* Insulinoma
Interference
  balancing side M26.56
  non-working side M26.56
Intermenstrual — *see* condition
Intermittent — *see* condition
Internal — *see* condition
Interrogation
  cardiac defibrillator (automatic) (implantable) Z45.02
  cardiac pacemaker Z45.018
  cardiac (event) (loop) recorder Z45.09
  infusion pump (implanted) (intrathecal) Z45.1
  neurostimulator Z46.2
Interruption
  aortic arch Q25.21
  bundle of His I44.30
  phase-shift, sleep cycle — *see* Disorder, sleep, circadian rhythm
  sleep phase-shift, or 24 hour sleep-wake cycle — *see* Disorder, sleep, circadian rhythm
Interstitial — *see* condition
Intertrigo L30.4
  labialis K13.0
Intervertebral disc — *see* condition
Intestine, intestinal — *see* condition
Intolerance
  carbohydrate K90.49
  disaccharide, hereditary E73.0
  fat NEC K90.49
    pancreatic K90.3
  food K90.49
    dietary counseling and surveillance Z71.3
  fructose E74.10
    hereditary E74.12
  glucose (-galactose) E74.39
  gluten K90.41
  lactose E73.9
    specified NEC E73.8
  lysine E72.3
  milk NEC K90.49
    lactose E73.9
  protein K90.49
  starch NEC K90.49
  sucrose (-isomaltose) E74.31
Intoxicated NEC (without dependence) — *see* Alcohol, intoxication
Intoxication
  acid E87.2
  alcoholic (acute) (without dependence) — *see* Alcohol, intoxication
  alimentary canal K52.1
  amphetamine (without dependence) — *see also* Abuse, drug, stimulant, with intoxication
    with dependence — *see* Dependence, drug, stimulant, with intoxication
    stimulant NEC F15.10

Intoxication — *continued*
  amphetamine — *see also* Abuse, drug, stimulant, with intoxication — *continued*
    stimulant — *continued*
      with
        anxiety disorder F15.180
        intoxication F15.129
          with
            delirium F15.121
            perceptual disturbance F15.122
  anxiolytic (acute) (without dependence) — *see* Abuse, drug, sedative, with intoxication
    with dependence — *see* Dependence, drug, sedative, with intoxication
  caffeine F15.929
    with dependence — *see* Dependence, drug, stimulant, with intoxication
  cannabinoids (acute) (without dependence) — *see* Use, cannabis, with intoxication
    with
      abuse — *see* Abuse, drug, cannabis, with intoxication
      dependence — *see* Dependence, drug, cannabis, with intoxication
  chemical — *see* Table of Drugs and Chemicals
    via placenta or breast milk — *see* - Absorption, chemical, through placenta
  cocaine (acute) (without dependence) — *see* Abuse, drug, cocaine, with intoxication
    with dependence — *see* Dependence, drug, cocaine, with intoxication
  drug
    acute (without dependence) — *see* Abuse, drug, by type with intoxication
      with dependence — *see* Dependence, drug, by type with intoxication
    addictive
      via placenta or breast milk — *see* Absorption, drug, addictive, through placenta
    newborn P93.8
      gray baby syndrome P93.0
    overdose or wrong substance given or taken — *see* Table of Drugs and Chemicals, by drug, poisoning
  enteric K52.1
  foodborne A05.9
    bacterial A05.9
    classical (Clostridium botulinum) A05.1
    due to
      Bacillus cereus A05.4
      bacterium A05.9
        specified NEC A05.8
      Clostridium
        botulinum A05.1
        perfringens A05.2
        welchii A05.2
      Salmonella A02.9
        with
          (gastro)enteritis A02.0
          localized infection(s) A02.20
            arthritis A02.23
            meningitis A02.21
            osteomyelitis A02.24
            pneumonia A02.22
            pyelonephritis A02.25
            specified NEC A02.29
          sepsis A02.1
          specified manifestation NEC A02.8
      Staphylococcus A05.0
      Vibrio
        parahaemolyticus A05.3
        vulnificus A05.5
    enterotoxin, staphylococcal A05.0
    noxious — *see* Poisoning, food, noxious
  gastrointestinal K52.1
  hallucinogenic (without dependence) — *see* Abuse, drug, hallucinogen, with intoxication
    with dependence — *see* Dependence, drug, hallucinogen, with intoxication
  hypnotic (acute) (without dependence) — *see* Abuse, drug, sedative, with intoxication
    with dependence — *see* Dependence, drug, sedative, with intoxication
  inhalant (acute) (without dependence) — *see* Abuse, drug, inhalant, with intoxication
    with dependence — *see* Dependence, drug, inhalant, with intoxication

Intoxication — *continued*
  meaning
    inebriation — *see* category F10 ☑
    poisoning — *see* Table of Drugs and Chemicals
  methyl alcohol (acute) (without dependence) — *se* Alcohol, intoxication
  opioid (acute) (without dependence) — *see* Abuse drug, opioid, with intoxication
    with dependence — *see* Dependence, drug, opio with intoxication
  pathologic NEC (without dependence) — *see* Alcoh intoxication
  phencyclidine (without dependence) — *see* Abuse drug, hallucinogen, with intoxication
    with dependence — *see* Dependence, drug, ha cinogen, with intoxication
  potassium (K) E87.5
  psychoactive substance NEC (without dependence)
    see Abuse, drug, psychoactive NEC, with into cation
    with dependence — *see* Dependence, drug, ps choactive NEC, with intoxication
  sedative (acute) (without dependence) — *see* Abu drug, sedative, with intoxication
    with dependence — *see* Dependence, drug, se tive, with intoxication
  serum — *see also* Reaction, serum T80.69 ☑
  uremic — *see* Uremia
  volatile solvents (acute) (without dependence) — Abuse, drug, inhalant, with intoxication
    with dependence — *see* Dependence, drug, in halant, with intoxication
  water E87.79
Intraabdominal testis, testes
  bilateral Q53.211
  unilateral Q53.111
Intracranial — *see* condition
Intrahepatic gallbladder Q44.1
Intraligamentous — *see* condition
Intrathoracic — *see also* condition
  kidney Q63.2
Intrauterine contraceptive device
  checking Z30.431
  in situ Z97.5
  insertion Z30.430
    immediately following removal Z30.433
  management Z30.431
  reinsertion Z30.433
  removal Z30.432
  replacement Z30.433
  retention in pregnancy O26.3- ☑
Intraventricular — *see* condition
Intrinsic deformity — *see* Deformity
Intubation, difficult or failed T88.4 ☑
Intumescence, lens (eye) (cataract) — *see* Cataract
Intussusception (bowel) (colon) (enteric) (ileocecal) (ileocolic) (intestine) (rectum) K56.1
  appendix K38.8
  congenital Q43.8
  ureter (with obstruction) N13.5
Invagination (bowel, colon, intestine or rectum) K56
Inversion
  albumin-globulin (A-G) ratio E88.09
  bladder N32.89
  cecum — *see* Intussusception
  cervix N88.8
  chromosome in normal individual Q95.1
  circadian rhythm — *see* Disorder, sleep, circadian rhythm
  nipple N64.59
    congenital Q83.8
    gestational — *see* Retraction, nipple
    puerperal, postpartum — *see* Retraction, nipple
  nyctohemeral rhythm — *see* Disorder, sleep, circad rhythm
  optic papilla Q14.2
  organ or site, congenital NEC — *see* Anomaly, by s
  sleep rhythm — *see* Disorder, sleep, circadian rhyt
  testis (congenital) Q55.29
  uterus (chronic) (postinfectional) (postpartal, old) N8 postpartum O71.2
  vagina (posthysterectomy) N99.3
  ventricular Q20.5
Investigation — *see also* Examination Z04.9
  clinical research subject (control) (normal comparis (participant) Z00.6
Involuntary movement, abnormal R25.9

☑ **Additional Character Required** — Refer to the Tabular List for Character Selection   ▽ **Subterms under main terms may continue to next column or pa**

volution, involutional — *see also* condition
  breast, cystic — *see* Dysplasia, mammary, specified type NEC
  depression (single episode) F32.89
    recurrent episode F33.9
  melancholia (single episode) F32.89
    recurrent episode F33.8
  ovary, senile — *see* Atrophy, ovary
  thymus failure E32.8
Q.
  20-34 F72
  35-49 F71
  50-69 F70
  under 20 F73
DS (type I) P22.0
  type II P22.1
deremia Q13.1
dis rubeosis — *see* Disorder, iris, vascular
dochoroiditis (panuveitis) — *see* Panuveitis
docyclitis H20.9
  acute H20.0- ☑
    hypopyon H20.05- ☑
    primary H20.01- ☑
    recurrent H20.02- ☑
    secondary (noninfectious) H20.04- ☑
      infectious H20.03- ☑
  chronic H20.1- ☑
  due to allergy — *see* Iridocyclitis, acute, secondary
  endogenous — *see* Iridocyclitis, acute, primary
  Fuchs' — *see* Cyclitis, Fuchs' heterochromic
  gonococcal A54.32
  granulomatous — *see* Iridocyclitis, chronic
  herpes, herpetic (simplex) B00.51
    zoster B02.32
  hypopyon — *see* Iridocyclitis, acute, hypopyon
  in (due to)
    ankylosing spondylitis M45.9
    gonococcal infection A54.32
    herpes (simplex) virus B00.51
      zoster B02.32
    infectious disease NOS B99 ☑
    parasitic disease NOS B89 *[H22]*
    sarcoidosis D86.83
    syphilis A51.43
    tuberculosis A18.54
    zoster B02.32
  lens-induced H20.2- ☑
  nongranulomatous — *see* Iridocyclitis, acute
  recurrent — *see* Iridocyclitis, acute, recurrent
  rheumatic — *see* Iridocyclitis, chronic
  subacute — *see* Iridocyclitis, acute
  sympathetic — *see* Uveitis, sympathetic
  syphilitic (secondary) A51.43
  tuberculous (chronic) A18.54
  Vogt-Koyanagi H20.82- ☑
docyclochoroiditis (panuveitis) — *see* Panuveitis
dodialysis H21.53- ☑
dodonesis H21.89
doplegia (complete) (partial) (reflex) H57.09
doschisis H21.25- ☑
s — *see also* condition
  bombé — *see* Membrane, pupillary
tis — *see also* Iridocyclitis
  chronic — *see* Iridocyclitis, chronic
  diabetic — *see* E08-E13 with .39
  due to
    herpes simplex B00.51
    leprosy A30.9 *[H22]*
  gonococcal A54.32
  gouty — *see also* Gout, by type M10.9 *[H22]*
  granulomatous — *see* Iridocyclitis, chronic
  lens induced — *see* Iridocyclitis, lens-induced
  papulosa (syphilitic) A52.71
  rheumatic — *see* Iridocyclitis, chronic
  syphilitic (secondary) A51.43
    congenital (early) A50.01
    late A52.71
  tuberculous A18.54
on — *see* condition
on-miner's lung J63.4
radiated enamel (tooth, teeth) K03.89
radiation effects, adverse T66 ☑
reducible, irreducibility — *see* condition
regular, irregularity
  action, heart I49.9
  alveolar process K08.89
  bleeding N92.6

Irregular, irregularity — *continued*
  breathing R06.89
  contour of cornea (acquired) — *see* Deformity, cornea
    congenital Q13.4
  contour, reconstructed breast N65.0
  dentin (in pulp) K04.3
  eye movements H55.89
    nystagmus — *see* Nystagmus
    saccadic H55.81
  labor O62.2
  menstruation (cause unknown) N92.6
  periods N92.6
  prostate N42.9
  pupil — *see* Abnormality, pupillary
  reconstructed breast N65.0
  respiratory R06.89
  septum (nasal) J34.2
  shape, organ or site, congenital NEC — *see* Distortion
  sleep-wake pattern (rhythm) G47.23
Irritable, irritability R45.4
  bladder N32.89
  bowel (syndrome) K58.9
    with
      constipation K58.1
      diarrhea K58.0
    mixed K58.2
    psychogenic F45.8
    specified NEC K58.8
  bronchial — *see* Bronchitis
  cerebral, in newborn P91.3
  colon — *see also* Irritable, bowel K58.9
    with diarrhea K58.0
    psychogenic F45.8
  duodenum K59.8
  heart (psychogenic) F45.8
  hip — *see* Derangement, joint, specified type NEC, hip
  ileum K59.8
  infant R68.12
  jejunum K59.8
  rectum K59.8
  stomach K31.89
    psychogenic F45.8
  sympathetic G90.8
  urethra N36.8
Irritation
  anus K62.89
  axillary nerve G54.0
  bladder N32.89
  brachial plexus G54.0
  bronchial — *see* Bronchitis
  cervical plexus G54.2
  cervix — *see* Cervicitis
  choroid, sympathetic — *see* Endophthalmitis
  cranial nerve — *see* Disorder, nerve, cranial
  gastric K31.89
    psychogenic F45.8
  globe, sympathetic — *see* Uveitis, sympathetic
  labyrinth — *see* subcategory H83.2 ☑
  lumbosacral plexus G54.1
  meninges (traumatic) — *see* Injury, intracranial
    nontraumatic — *see* Meningismus
  nerve — *see* Disorder, nerve
  nervous R45.0
  penis N48.89
  perineum NEC L29.3
  peripheral autonomic nervous system G90.8
  peritoneum — *see* Peritonitis
  pharynx J39.2
  plantar nerve — *see* Lesion, nerve, plantar
  spinal (cord) (traumatic) — *see also* Injury, spinal cord, by region
    nerve G58.9
      root NEC — *see* Radiculopathy
    nontraumatic — *see* Myelopathy
  stomach K31.89
    psychogenic F45.8
  sympathetic nerve NEC G90.8
  ulnar nerve — *see* Lesion, nerve, ulnar
  vagina N89.8
Ischemia, ischemic I99.8
  bowel (transient)
    acute — *see also* Ischemia, intestine, acute K55.059
    chronic K55.1
    due to mesenteric artery insufficiency K55.1
  brain — *see* Ischemia, cerebral
  cardiac (see Disease, heart, ischemic)
  cardiomyopathy I25.5
  cerebral (chronic) (generalized) I67.82

Ischemia, ischemic — *continued*
  cerebral — *continued*
    arteriosclerotic I67.2
    intermittent G45.9
    newborn P91.0
    recurrent focal G45.8
    transient G45.9
  colon chronic (due to mesenteric artery insufficiency) K55.1
  coronary — *see* Disease, heart, ischemic
  demand (coronary) — *see also* Angina I24.8
    with myocardial infarction I21.A1
    resulting in myocardial infarction I21.A1
  heart (chronic or with a stated duration of over 4 weeks) I25.9
    acute or with a stated duration of 4 weeks or less I24.9
    subacute I24.9
  infarction, muscle — *see* Infarct, muscle
  intestine (large) (small) (transient) K55.9
    acute K55.059
      diffuse K55.052
      focal K55.051
      large K55.039
        diffuse K55.032
        focal K55.031
      small K55.019
        diffuse K55.012
        focal K55.011
    chronic K55.1
    due to mesenteric artery insufficiency K55.1
  kidney N28.0
  mesenteric, acute — *see also* Ischemia, intestine, acute K55.059
  muscle, traumatic T79.6 ☑
  myocardium, myocardial (chronic or with a stated duration of over 4 weeks) I25.9
    acute, without myocardial infarction I51.3
    silent (asymptomatic) I25.6
    transient of newborn P29.4
  renal N28.0
  retina, retinal — *see* Occlusion, artery, retina
  small bowel
    acute K55.019
      diffuse K55.012
      focal K55.011
    chronic K55.1
    due to mesenteric artery insufficiency K55.1
  spinal cord G95.11
  subendocardial — *see* Insufficiency, coronary
  supply (coronary) — *see also* Angina I25.9
    due to vasospasm I20.1
Ischial spine — *see* condition
Ischialgia — *see* Sciatica
Ischiopagus Q89.4
Ischium, ischial — *see* condition
Ischuria R34
Iselin's disease or osteochondrosis — *see* Osteochondrosis, juvenile, metatarsus
Islands of
  parotid tissue in
    lymph nodes Q38.6
    neck structures Q38.6
  submaxillary glands in
    fascia Q38.6
    lymph nodes Q38.6
    neck muscles Q38.6
Islet cell tumor, pancreas D13.7
Isoimmunization NEC — *see also* Incompatibility
  affecting management of pregnancy (ABO) (with hydrops fetalis) O36.11- ☑
    anti-A sensitization O36.11- ☑
    anti-B sensitization O36.19- ☑
    anti-c sensitization O36.09- ☑
    anti-C sensitization O36.09- ☑
    anti-e sensitization O36.09- ☑
    anti-E sensitization O36.09- ☑
    Rh NEC O36.09- ☑
      anti-D antibody O36.01- ☑
    specified NEC O36.19- ☑
  newborn P55.9
    with
      hydrops fetalis P56.0
      kernicterus P57.0
    ABO (blood groups) P55.1
    Rhesus (Rh) factor P55.0
    specified type NEC P55.8

⬇ **Subterms under main terms may continue to next column or page**   ☑ **Additional Character Required** — **Refer to the Tabular List for Character Selection**   **203**

Involution, involutional — Isoimmunization NEC

Isolation, isolated
dwelling Z59.8
family Z63.79
social Z60.4
Isoleucinosis E71.19
Isomerism atrial appendages (with asplenia or polysplenia) Q20.6
Isosporiasis, isosporosis A07.3
Isovaleric acidemia E71.110
Issue of
medical certificate Z02.79
for disability determination Z02.71
repeat prescription (appliance) (glasses) (medicinal substance, medicament, medicine) Z76.0
contraception — see Contraception
Itch, itching — see also Pruritus
baker's L23.6
barber's B35.0
bricklayer's L24.5
cheese B88.0
clam digger's B65.3
coolie B76.9
copra B88.0
dew B76.9
dhobi B35.6
filarial — see Infestation, filarial
grain B88.0
grocer's B88.0
ground B76.9
harvest B88.0
jock B35.6
Malabar B35.5
beard B35.0
foot B35.3
scalp B35.0
meaning scabies B86
Norwegian B86
perianal L29.0
poultrymen's B88.0
sarcoptic B86
scabies B86
scrub B88.0
straw B88.0
swimmer's B65.3
water B76.9
winter L29.8
Ivemark's syndrome (asplenia with congenital heart disease) Q89.01
Ivory bones Q78.2
Ixodiasis NEC B88.8

J

Jaccoud's syndrome — see Arthropathy, postrheumatic, chronic
Jackson's
membrane Q43.3
paralysis or syndrome G83.89
veil Q43.3
Jacquet's dermatitis (diaper dermatitis) L22
Jadassohn-Pellizari's disease or anetoderma L90.2
Jadassohn's
blue nevus — see Nevus
intraepidermal epithelioma — see Neoplasm, skin, benign
Jaffe-Lichtenstein (-Uehlinger) **syndrome** — see Dysplasia, fibrous, bone NEC
Jakob-Creutzfeldt disease or syndrome — see Creutzfeldt-Jakob disease or syndrome
Jaksch-Luzet disease D64.89
Jamaican
neuropathy G92
paraplegic tropical ataxic-spastic syndrome G92
Janet's disease F48.8
Janiceps Q89.4
Jansky-Bielschowsky amaurotic idiocy E75.4
Japanese
B-type encephalitis A83.0
river fever A75.3
Jaundice (yellow) R17
acholuric (familial) (splenomegalic) — see also Spherocytosis
acquired D59.8
breast-milk (inhibitor) P59.3
catarrhal (acute) B15.9
with hepatic coma B15.0
cholestatic (benign) R17

Jaundice — continued
due to or associated with
delayed conjugation P59.8
associated with (due to) preterm delivery P59.0
preterm delivery P59.0
epidemic (catarrhal) B15.9
with hepatic coma B15.0
leptospiral A27.0
spirochetal A27.0
familial nonhemolytic (congenital) (Gilbert) E80.4
Crigler-Najjar E80.5
febrile (acute) B15.9
with hepatic coma B15.0
leptospiral A27.0
spirochetal A27.0
hematogenous D59.9
hemolytic (acquired) D59.9
congenital — see Spherocytosis
hemorrhagic (acute) (leptospiral) (spirochetal) A27.0
infectious (acute) (subacute) B15.9
with hepatic coma B15.0
leptospiral A27.0
spirochetal A27.0
leptospiral (hemorrhagic) A27.0
malignant (without coma) K72.90
with coma K72.91
neonatal — see Jaundice, newborn
newborn P59.9
due to or associated with
ABO
antibodies P55.1
incompatibility, maternal/fetal P55.1
isoimmunization P55.1
absence or deficiency of enzyme system for bilirubin conjugation (congenital) P59.8
bleeding P58.1
breast milk inhibitors to conjugation P59.3
associated with preterm delivery P59.0
bruising P58.0
Crigler-Najjar syndrome E80.5
delayed conjugation P59.8
associated with preterm delivery P59.0
drugs or toxins
given to newborn P58.42
transmitted from mother P58.41
excessive hemolysis P58.9
due to
bleeding P58.1
bruising P58.0
drugs or toxins
given to newborn P58.42
transmitted from mother P58.41
infection P58.2
polycythemia P58.3
swallowed maternal blood P58.5
specified type NEC P58.8
galactosemia E74.21
Gilbert syndrome E80.4
hemolytic disease P55.9
ABO isoimmunization P55.1
Rh isoimmunization P55.0
specified NEC P55.8
hepatocellular damage P59.20
specified NEC P59.29
hereditary hemolytic anemia P58.8
hypothyroidism, congenital E03.1
incompatibility, maternal/fetal NOS P55.9
infection P58.2
inspissated bile syndrome P59.1
isoimmunization NOS P55.9
mucoviscidosis E84.9
polycythemia P58.3
preterm delivery P59.0
Rh
antibodies P55.0
incompatibility, maternal/fetal P55.0
isoimmunization P55.0
specified cause NEC P59.8
swallowed maternal blood P58.5
spherocytosis (congenital) D58.0
nonhemolytic congenital familial (Gilbert) E80.4
nuclear, newborn — see also Kernicterus of newborn P57.9
obstructive — see also Obstruction, bile duct K83.1
post-immunization — see Hepatitis, viral, type, B
post-transfusion — see Hepatitis, viral, type, B
regurgitation — see also Obstruction, bile duct K83.1

Jaundice — continued
serum (homologous) (prophylactic) (therapeutic) — see Hepatitis, viral, type, B
spirochetal (hemorrhagic) A27.0
symptomatic R17
newborn P59.9
Jaw — see condition
Jaw-winking phenomenon or syndrome Q07.8
Jealousy
alcoholic F10.988
childhood F93.8
sibling F93.8
Jejunitis — see Enteritis
Jejunostomy status Z93.4
Jejunum, jejunal — see condition
Jensen's disease — see Inflammation, chorioretinal, cal, juxtapapillary
Jerks, myoclonic G25.3
Jervell-Lange-Nielsen syndrome I45.81
Jeune's disease Q77.2
Jigger disease B88.1
Job's syndrome (chronic granulomatous disease) D7▮
Joint — see also condition
mice — see Loose, body, joint
knee M23.4- ☑
Jordan's anomaly or syndrome D72.0
Joseph-Diamond-Blackfan anemia (congenital hypoplastic) D61.01
Jungle yellow fever A95.0
Jüngling's disease — see Sarcoidosis
Juvenile — see condition

K

Kahler's disease C90.0- ☑
Kakke E51.11
Kala-azar B55.0
Kallmann's syndrome E23.0
Kanner's syndrome (autism) — see Psychosis, childho▮
Kaposi's
dermatosis (xeroderma pigmentosum) Q82.1
lichen ruber L44.0
acuminatus L44.0
sarcoma
colon C46.4
connective tissue C46.1
gastrointestinal organ C46.4
lung C46.5- ☑
lymph node (multiple) C46.3
palate (hard) (soft) C46.2
rectum C46.4
skin (multiple sites) C46.0
specified site NEC C46.7
stomach C46.4
unspecified site C46.9
varicelliform eruption B00.0
vaccinia T88.1 ☑
Kartagener's syndrome or triad (sinusitis, bronchiec▮ sis, situs inversus) Q89.3
Karyotype
with abnormality except iso (Xq) Q96.2
45,X Q96.0
46,X
iso (Xq) Q96.1
46,XX Q98.3
with streak gonads Q50.32
hermaphrodite (true) Q99.1
male Q98.3
46,XY
with streak gonads Q56.1
female Q97.3
hermaphrodite (true) Q99.1
47,XXX Q97.0
47,XXY Q98.0
47,XYY Q98.5
Kaschin-Beck disease — see Disease, Kaschin-Beck
Katayama's disease or fever B65.2
Kawasaki's syndrome M30.3
Kayser-Fleischer ring (cornea) (pseudosclerosis) H18.04- ☑
Kaznelson's syndrome (congenital hypoplastic anem▮ D61.01
Kearns-Sayre syndrome H49.81- ☑
Kedani fever A75.3
Kelis L91.0
Kelly (-Patterson) **syndrome** (sideropenic dysphagia▮ D50.1

loid, cheloid L91.0
  acne L73.0
  Addison's L94.0
  cornea — *see* Opacity, cornea
  Hawkin's L91.0
  scar L91.0
•loma L91.0
•nya fever A77.1
•ratectasia — *see also* Ectasia, cornea
  congenital Q13.4
•ratinization of alveolar ridge mucosa
  excessive K13.23
  minimal K13.22
•ratinized residual ridge mucosa
  excessive K13.23
  minimal K13.22
•ratitis (nodular) (nonulcerative) (simple) (zonular) H16.9
  with ulceration (central) (marginal) (perforated) (ring) — *see* Ulcer, cornea
  actinic — *see* Photokeratitis
  arborescens (herpes simplex) B00.52
  areolar H16.11- ☑
  bullosa H16.8
  deep H16.309
    specified type NEC H16.399
  dendritic (a) (herpes simplex) B00.52
  disciform (is) (herpes simplex) B00.52
    varicella B01.81
  filamentary H16.12- ☑
  gonococcal (congenital or prenatal) A54.33
  herpes, herpetic (simplex) B00.52
    zoster B02.33
  in (due to)
    acanthamebiasis B60.13
    adenovirus B30.0
    exanthema — *see also* Exanthem B09
    herpes (simplex) virus B00.52
    measles B05.81
    syphilis A50.31
    tuberculosis A18.52
    zoster B02.33
  interstitial (nonsyphilitic) H16.30- ☑
    diffuse H16.32- ☑
    herpes, herpetic (simplex) B00.52
      zoster B02.33
    sclerosing H16.33- ☑
    specified type NEC H16.39 ☑
    syphilitic (congenital) (late) A50.31
    tuberculous A18.52
  macular H16.11- ☑
  nummular H16.11- ☑
  oyster shuckers' H16.8
  parenchymatous — *see* Keratitis, interstitial
  petrificans H16.8
  postmeasles B05.81
  punctata
    leprosa A30.9 [H16.14-] ☑
    syphilitic (profunda) A50.31
  punctate H16.14- ☑
  purulent H16.8
  rosacea L71.8
  sclerosing H16.33- ☑
  specified type NEC H16.8
  stellate H16.11- ☑
  striate H16.11- ☑
  superficial H16.10- ☑
    with conjunctivitis — *see* Keratoconjunctivitis
    due to light — *see* Photokeratitis
  suppurative H16.8
  syphilitic (congenital) (prenatal) A50.31
  trachomatous A71.1
    sequelae B94.0
  tuberculous A18.52
  vesicular H16.8
  xerotic — *see also* Keratomalacia H16.8
    vitamin A deficiency E50.4
•ratoacanthoma L85.8
•ratocele — *see* Descemetocele
•ratoconjunctivitis H16.20- ☑
  Acanthamoeba B60.13
  adenoviral B30.0
  epidemic B30.0
  exposure H16.21- ☑
  herpes, herpetic (simplex) B00.52
    zoster B02.33
  in exanthema — *see also* Exanthem B09
  infectious B30.0

Keratoconjunctivitis — *continued*
  lagophthalmic — *see* Keratoconjunctivitis, specified type NEC
  neurotrophic H16.23- ☑
  phlyctenular H16.25- ☑
  postmeasles B05.81
  shipyard B30.0
  sicca (Sjogren's) M35.0- ☑
    not Sjogren's H16.22- ☑
  specified type NEC H16.29- ☑
  tuberculous (phlyctenular) A18.52
  vernal H16.26- ☑
Keratoconus H18.60- ☑
  congenital Q13.4
  stable H18.61- ☑
  unstable H18.62- ☑
Keratocyst (dental) (odontogenic) — *see* Cyst, calcifying odontogenic
Keratoderma, keratodermia (congenital) (palmaris et plantaris) (symmetrical) Q82.8
  acquired L85.1
    in diseases classified elsewhere L86
  climactericum L85.1
  gonococcal A54.89
  gonorrheal A54.89
  punctata L85.2
  Reiter's — *see* Reiter's disease
Keratodermatocele — *see* Descemetocele
Keratoglobus H18.79 ☑
  congenital Q15.8
    with glaucoma Q15.0
Keratohemia — *see* Pigmentation, cornea, stromal
Keratoiritis — *see also* Iridocyclitis
  syphilitic A50.39
  tuberculous A18.54
Keratoma L57.0
  palmaris and plantaris hereditarium Q82.8
  senile L57.0
Keratomalacia H18.44- ☑
  vitamin A deficiency E50.4
Keratomegaly Q13.4
Keratomycosis B49
  nigrans, nigricans (palmaris) B36.1
Keratopathy H18.9
  band H18.42- ☑
  bullous (aphakic), following cataract surgery H59.01- ☑
  bullous H18.1- ☑
Keratoscleritis, tuberculous A18.52
Keratosis L57.0
  actinic L57.0
  arsenical L85.8
  congenital, specified NEC Q80.8
  female genital NEC N94.89
  follicularis Q82.8
    acquired L11.0
    congenita Q82.8
    et parafollicularis in cutem penetrans L87.0
    spinulosa (decalvans) Q82.8
    vitamin A deficiency E50.8
  gonococcal A54.89
  male genital (external) N50.89
  nigricans L83
  obturans, external ear (canal) — *see* Cholesteatoma, external ear
  palmaris et plantaris (inherited) (symmetrical) Q82.8
    acquired L85.1
  penile N48.89
  pharynx J39.2
  pilaris, acquired L85.8
  punctata (palmaris et plantaris) L85.2
  scrotal N50.89
  seborrheic L82.1
    inflamed L82.0
  senile L57.0
  solar L57.0
  tonsillaris J35.8
  vagina N89.4
  vegetans Q82.8
  vitamin A deficiency E50.8
  vocal cord J38.3
Kerato-uveitis — *see* Iridocyclitis
Kerion (celsi) B35.0
Kernicterus of newborn (not due to isoimmunization) P57.9
  due to isoimmunization (conditions in P55.0-P55.9) P57.0
  specified type NEC P57.8
Kerunoparalysis T75.09 ☑

Keshan disease E59
Ketoacidosis E87.2
  diabetic — *see* Diabetes, by type, with ketoacidosis
Ketonuria R82.4
Ketosis NEC E88.89
  diabetic — *see* Diabetes, by type, with ketoacidosis
Kew Garden fever A79.1
Kidney — *see* condition
Kienböck's disease — *see also* Osteochondrosis, juvenile, hand, carpal lunate
  adult M93.1
Kimmelstiel (-Wilson) **disease** — *see* Diabetes, Kimmelstiel (-Wilson) disease
Kink, kinking
  artery I77.1
  hair (acquired) L67.8
  ileum or intestine — *see* Obstruction, intestine
  Lane's — *see* Obstruction, intestine
  organ or site, congenital NEC — *see* Anomaly, by site
  ureter (pelvic junction) N13.5
    with
      hydronephrosis N13.1
        with infection N13.6
      pyelonephritis (chronic) N11.1
    congenital Q62.39
  vein(s) I87.8
    caval I87.1
    peripheral I87.1
Kinnier Wilson's disease (hepatolenticular degeneration) E83.01
Kissing spine M48.20
  cervical region M48.22
  cervicothoracic region M48.23
  lumbar region M48.26
  lumbosacral region M48.27
  occipito-atlanto-axial region M48.21
  thoracic region M48.24
  thoracolumbar region M48.25
Klatskin's tumor C22.1
Klauder's disease A26.8
Klebs' disease — *see also* Glomerulonephritis N05- ☑
Klebsiella (K.) **pneumoniae, as cause of disease classified elsewhere** B96.1
Klein (e)-**Levin syndrome** G47.13
Kleptomania F63.2
Klinefelter's syndrome Q98.4
  karyotype 47,XXY Q98.0
  male with more than two X chromosomes Q98.1
Klippel-Feil deficiency, disease, or syndrome (brevicollis) Q76.1
Klippel's disease I67.2
Klippel-Trenaunay (-Weber) **syndrome** Q87.2
Klumpke (-Déjerine) **palsy, paralysis** (birth) (newborn) P14.1
Knee — *see* condition
Knock knee (acquired) M21.06- ☑
  congenital Q74.1
Knot(s)
  intestinal, syndrome (volvulus) K56.2
  surfer S89.8- ☑
  umbilical cord (true) O69.2 ☑
Knotting (of)
  hair L67.8
  intestine K56.2
Knuckle pad (Garrod's) M72.1
Koch's
  infection — *see* Tuberculosis
  relapsing fever A68.9
Koch-Weeks' conjunctivitis — *see* Conjunctivitis, acute, mucopurulent
Köebner's syndrome Q81.8
Köenig's disease (osteochondritis dissecans) — *see* Osteochondritis, dissecans
Köhler-Pellegrini-Steida disease or syndrome (calcification, knee joint) — *see* Bursitis, tibial collateral
Köhler's disease
  patellar — *see* Osteochondrosis, juvenile, patella
  tarsal navicular — *see* Osteochondrosis, juvenile, tarsus
Koilonychia L60.3
  congenital Q84.6
Kojevnikov's, epilepsy — *see* Kozhevnikof's epilepsy
Koplik's spots B05.9
Kopp's asthma E32.8
Korsakoff's (Wernicke) **disease, psychosis or syndrome** (alcoholic) F10.96
  with dependence F10.26

Korsakoff's (Wernicke) disease, psychosis or syndrome — continued
  drug-induced
    due to drug abuse — see Abuse, drug, by type, with amnestic disorder
    due to drug dependence — see Dependence, drug, by type, with amnestic disorder
    nonalcoholic F04
Korsakov's disease, psychosis or syndrome — see Korsakoff's disease
Korsakow's disease, psychosis or syndrome — see Korsakoff's disease
Kostmann's disease or syndrome (infantile genetic agranulocytosis) — see Agranulocytosis
Kozhevnikof's epilepsy G40.109
  intractable G40.119
    with status epilepticus G40.111
    without status epilepticus G40.119
  not intractable G40.109
    with status epilepticus G40.101
    without status epilepticus G40.109
Krabbe's
  disease E75.23
  syndrome, congenital muscle hypoplasia Q79.8
Kraepelin-Morel disease — see Schizophrenia
Kraft-Weber-Dimitri disease Q85.8
Kraurosis
  ani K62.89
  penis N48.0
  vagina N89.8
  vulva N90.4
Kreotoxism A05.9
Krukenberg's
  spindle — see Pigmentation, cornea, posterior
  tumor C79.6- ☑
Kufs' disease E75.4
Kugelberg-Welander disease G12.1
Kuhnt-Junius degeneration — see also Degeneration, macula H35.32- ☑
Kümmell's disease or spondylitis — see Spondylopathy, traumatic
Kupffer cell sarcoma C22.3
Kuru A81.81
Kussmaul's
  disease M30.0
  respiration E87.2
    in diabetic acidosis — see Diabetes, by type, with ketoacidosis
Kwashiorkor E40
  marasmic, marasmus type E42
Kyasanur Forest disease A98.2
Kyphoscoliosis, kyphoscoliotic (acquired) — see also Scoliosis M41.9
  congenital Q67.5
  heart (disease) I27.1
  sequelae of rickets E64.3
  tuberculous A18.01
Kyphosis, kyphotic (acquired) M40.209
  cervical region M40.202
  cervicothoracic region M40.203
  congenital Q76.419
    cervical region Q76.412
    cervicothoracic region Q76.413
    occipito-atlanto-axial region Q76.411
    thoracic region Q76.414
    thoracolumbar region Q76.415
    Morquio-Brailsford type (spinal) — see also subcategory M49.8 E76.219
  postlaminectomy M96.3
  postradiation therapy M96.2
  postural (adolescent) M40.00
    cervicothoracic region M40.03
    thoracic region M40.04
    thoracolumbar region M40.05
  secondary NEC M40.10
    cervical region M40.12
    cervicothoracic region M40.13
    thoracic region M40.14
    thoracolumbar region M40.15
  sequelae of rickets E64.3
  specified type NEC M40.299
    cervical region M40.292
    cervicothoracic region M40.293
    thoracic region M40.294
    thoracolumbar region M40.295
  syphilitic, congenital A50.56
  thoracic region M40.204
  thoracolumbar region M40.205

Kyphosis, kyphotic — continued
  tuberculous A18.01
Kyrle disease L87.0

L

Labia, labium — see condition
Labile
  blood pressure R09.89
  vasomotor system I73.9
Labioglossal paralysis G12.29
Labium leporinum — see Cleft, lip
Labor — see Delivery
Labored breathing — see Hyperventilation
Labyrinthitis (circumscribed) (destructive) (diffuse) (inner ear) (latent) (purulent) (suppurative) — see also subcategory H83.0 ☑
  syphilitic A52.79
Laceration
  with abortion — see Abortion, by type, complicated by laceration of pelvic organs
  abdomen, abdominal
    wall S31.119 ☑
      with
        foreign body S31.129 ☑
        penetration into peritoneal cavity S31.619 ☑
          with foreign body S31.629 ☑
      epigastric region S31.112 ☑
        with
          foreign body S31.122 ☑
          penetration into peritoneal cavity S31.612 ☑
            with foreign body S31.622 ☑
      left
        lower quadrant S31.114 ☑
          with
            foreign body S31.124 ☑
            penetration into peritoneal cavity S31.614 ☑
              with foreign body S31.624 ☑
        upper quadrant S31.111 ☑
          with
            foreign body S31.121 ☑
            penetration into peritoneal cavity S31.611 ☑
              with foreign body S31.621 ☑
      periumbilic region S31.115 ☑
        with
          foreign body S31.125 ☑
          penetration into peritoneal cavity S31.615 ☑
            with foreign body S31.625 ☑
      right
        lower quadrant S31.113 ☑
          with
            foreign body S31.123 ☑
            penetration into peritoneal cavity S31.613 ☑
              with foreign body S31.623 ☑
        upper quadrant S31.110 ☑
          with
            foreign body S31.120 ☑
            penetration into peritoneal cavity S31.610 ☑
              with foreign body S31.620 ☑
  accidental, complicating surgery — see Complications, surgical, accidental puncture or laceration
  Achilles tendon S86.02- ☑
  adrenal gland S37.813 ☑
  alveolar (process) — see Laceration, oral cavity
  ankle S91.01- ☑
    with
      foreign body S91.02- ☑
  antecubital space — see Laceration, elbow
  anus (sphincter) S31.831 ☑
    with
      ectopic or molar pregnancy O08.6
      foreign body S31.832 ☑
    complicating delivery — see Delivery, complicated, by, laceration, anus (sphincter)
    following ectopic or molar pregnancy O08.6
    nontraumatic, nonpuerperal — see Fissure, anus
  arm (upper) S41.11- ☑
    with foreign body S41.12- ☑
    lower — see Laceration, forearm

Laceration — continued
  auditory canal (external) (meatus) — see Laceration, ear
  auricle, ear — see Laceration, ear
  axilla — see Laceration, arm
  back — see also Laceration, thorax, back
    lower S31.010 ☑
      with
        foreign body S31.020 ☑
          with penetration into retroperitoneal space S31.021 ☑
        penetration into retroperitoneal space S31.011 ☑
  bile duct S36.13 ☑
  bladder S37.23 ☑
    with ectopic or molar pregnancy O08.6
    following ectopic or molar pregnancy O08.6
    obstetrical trauma O71.5
  blood vessel — see Injury, blood vessel
  bowel — see also Laceration, intestine
    with ectopic or molar pregnancy O08.6
    complicating abortion — see Abortion, by type, complicated by, specified condition NEC
    following ectopic or molar pregnancy O08.6
    obstetrical trauma O71.5
  brain (any part) (cortex) (diffuse) (membrane) — se also Injury, intracranial, diffuse
    during birth P10.8
      with hemorrhage P10.1
    focal — see Injury, intracranial, focal brain injury
  brainstem S06.38- ☑
  breast S21.01- ☑
    with foreign body S21.02- ☑
  broad ligament S37.893 ☑
    with ectopic or molar pregnancy O08.6
    following ectopic or molar pregnancy O08.6
    laceration syndrome N83.8
    obstetrical trauma O71.6
    syndrome (laceration) N83.8
  buttock S31.801 ☑
    with foreign body S31.802 ☑
    left S31.821 ☑
      with foreign body S31.822 ☑
    right S31.811 ☑
      with foreign body S31.812 ☑
  calf — see Laceration, leg
  canaliculus lacrimalis — see Laceration, eyelid
  canthus, eye — see Laceration, eyelid
  capsule, joint — see Sprain
  causing eversion of cervix uteri (old) N86
  central (perineal), complicating delivery O70.9
  cerebellum, traumatic S06.37- ☑
  cerebral S06.33- ☑
    during birth P10.8
      with hemorrhage P10.1
    left side S06.32- ☑
    right side S06.31- ☑
  cervix (uteri)
    with ectopic or molar pregnancy O08.6
    following ectopic or molar pregnancy O08.6
    nonpuerperal, nontraumatic N88.1
    obstetrical trauma (current) O71.3
    old (postpartal) N88.1
    traumatic S37.63 ☑
  cheek (external) S01.41- ☑
    with foreign body S01.42- ☑
    internal — see Laceration, oral cavity
  chest wall — see Laceration, thorax
  chin — see Laceration, head, specified site NEC
  chordae tendinae NEC I51.1
    concurrent with acute myocardial infarction — s Infarct, myocardium
    following acute myocardial infarction (current complication) I23.4
  clitoris — see Laceration, vulva
  colon — see Laceration, intestine, large, colon
  common bile duct S36.13 ☑
  cortex (cerebral) — see Injury, intracranial, diffuse
  costal region — see Laceration, thorax
  cystic duct S36.13 ☑
  diaphragm S27.803 ☑
  digit(s)
    foot — see Laceration, toe
    hand — see Laceration, finger
  duodenum S36.430 ☑
  ear (canal) (external) S01.31- ☑
    with foreign body S01.32- ☑

☑ **Additional Character Required** — Refer to the Tabular List for Character Selection   ▽ **Subterms under main terms may continue to next column or pa**

ceration — continued
  ear — continued
    drum S09.2- ☑
  elbow S51.01- ☑
    with
      foreign body S51.02- ☑
  epididymis — see Laceration, testis
  epigastric region — see Laceration, abdomen, wall,
    epigastric region
  esophagus K22.8
    traumatic
      cervical S11.21 ☑
        with foreign body S11.22 ☑
      thoracic S27.813 ☑
  eye (ball) S05.3- ☑
    with prolapse or loss of intraocular tissue S05.2- ☑
    penetrating S05.6- ☑
  eyebrow — see Laceration, eyelid
  eyelid S01.11- ☑
    with foreign body S01.12- ☑
  face NEC — see Laceration, head, specified site NEC
  fallopian tube S37.539 ☑
    bilateral S37.532 ☑
    unilateral S37.531 ☑
  finger(s) S61.219 ☑
    with
      damage to nail S61.319 ☑
        with
          foreign body S61.329 ☑
      foreign body S61.229 ☑
    index S61.218 ☑
      with
        damage to nail S61.318 ☑
          with
            foreign body S61.328 ☑
        foreign body S61.228 ☑
      left S61.211 ☑
        with
          damage to nail S61.311 ☑
            with
              foreign body S61.321 ☑
          foreign body S61.221 ☑
      right S61.210 ☑
        with
          damage to nail S61.310 ☑
            with
              foreign body S61.320 ☑
          foreign body S61.220 ☑
    little S61.218 ☑
      with
        damage to nail S61.318 ☑
          with
            foreign body S61.328 ☑
        foreign body S61.228 ☑
      left S61.217 ☑
        with
          damage to nail S61.317 ☑
            with
              foreign body S61.327 ☑
          foreign body S61.227 ☑
      right S61.216 ☑
        with
          damage to nail S61.316 ☑
            with
              foreign body S61.326 ☑
          foreign body S61.226 ☑
    middle S61.218 ☑
      with
        damage to nail S61.318 ☑
          with
            foreign body S61.328 ☑
        foreign body S61.228 ☑
      left S61.213 ☑
        with
          damage to nail S61.313 ☑
            with
              foreign body S61.323 ☑
          foreign body S61.223 ☑
      right S61.212 ☑
        with
          damage to nail S61.312 ☑
            with
              foreign body S61.322 ☑
          foreign body S61.222 ☑
    ring S61.218 ☑

Laceration — continued
  finger(s) — continued
    ring — continued
      with
        damage to nail S61.318 ☑
          with
            foreign body S61.328 ☑
        foreign body S61.228 ☑
      left S61.215 ☑
        with
          damage to nail S61.315 ☑
            with
              foreign body S61.325 ☑
          foreign body S61.225 ☑
      right S61.214 ☑
        with
          damage to nail S61.314 ☑
            with
              foreign body S61.324 ☑
          foreign body S61.224 ☑
  flank S31.119 ☑
    with foreign body S31.129 ☑
  foot (except toe(s) alone) S91.319 ☑
    with foreign body S91.329 ☑
    left S91.312 ☑
      with foreign body S91.322 ☑
    right S91.311 ☑
      with foreign body S91.321 ☑
    toe — see Laceration, toe
  forearm S51.819 ☑
    with
      foreign body S51.829 ☑
    elbow only — see Laceration, elbow
    left S51.812 ☑
      with
        foreign body S51.822 ☑
    right S51.811 ☑
      with
        foreign body S51.821 ☑
  forehead S01.81 ☑
    with foreign body S01.82 ☑
  fourchette O70.0
    with ectopic or molar pregnancy O08.6
    complicating delivery O70.0
    following ectopic or molar pregnancy O08.6
  gallbladder S36.123 ☑
  genital organs, external
    female S31.512 ☑
      with foreign body S31.522 ☑
      vagina — see Laceration, vagina
      vulva — see Laceration, vulva
    male S31.511 ☑
      with foreign body S31.521 ☑
      penis — see Laceration, penis
      scrotum — see Laceration, scrotum
      testis — see Laceration, testis
  groin — see Laceration, abdomen, wall
  gum — see Laceration, oral cavity
  hand S61.419 ☑
    with
      foreign body S61.429 ☑
    finger — see Laceration, finger
    left S61.412 ☑
      with
        foreign body S61.422 ☑
    right S61.411 ☑
      with
        foreign body S61.421 ☑
    thumb — see Laceration, thumb
  head S01.91 ☑
    with foreign body S01.92 ☑
    cheek — see Laceration, cheek
    ear — see Laceration, ear
    eyelid — see Laceration, eyelid
    lip — see Laceration, lip
    nose — see Laceration, nose
    oral cavity — see Laceration, oral cavity
    scalp S01.01 ☑
      with foreign body S01.02 ☑
    specified site NEC S01.81 ☑
      with foreign body S01.82 ☑
    temporomandibular area — see Laceration, cheek
  heart — see Injury, heart, laceration
  heel — see Laceration, foot
  hepatic duct S36.13 ☑
  hip S71.019 ☑

Laceration — continued
  hip — continued
    with foreign body S71.029 ☑
    left S71.012 ☑
      with foreign body S71.022 ☑
    right S71.011 ☑
      with foreign body S71.021 ☑
  hymen — see Laceration, vagina
  hypochondrium — see Laceration, abdomen, wall
  hypogastric region — see Laceration, abdomen, wall
  ileum S36.438 ☑
  inguinal region — see Laceration, abdomen, wall
  instep — see Laceration, foot
  internal organ — see Injury, by site
  interscapular region — see Laceration, thorax, back
  intestine
    large
      colon S36.539 ☑
        ascending S36.530 ☑
        descending S36.532 ☑
        sigmoid S36.533 ☑
        specified site NEC S36.538 ☑
      rectum S36.63 ☑
        transverse S36.531 ☑
    small S36.439 ☑
      duodenum S36.430 ☑
      specified site NEC S36.438 ☑
  intra-abdominal organ S36.93 ☑
    intestine — see Laceration, intestine
    liver — see Laceration, liver
    pancreas — see Laceration, pancreas
    peritoneum S36.81 ☑
    specified site NEC S36.893 ☑
    spleen — see Laceration, spleen
    stomach — see Laceration, stomach
  intracranial NEC — see also Injury, intracranial, diffuse
    birth injury P10.9
  jaw — see Laceration, head, specified site NEC
  jejunum S36.438 ☑
  joint capsule — see Sprain, by site
  kidney S37.03- ☑
    major (greater than 3 cm) (massive) (stellate)
      S37.06- ☑
    minor (less than 1 cm) S37.04- ☑
    moderate (1 to 3 cm) S37.05- ☑
    multiple S37.06- ☑
  knee S81.01- ☑
    with foreign body S81.02- ☑
  labium (majus) (minus) — see Laceration, vulva
  lacrimal duct — see Laceration, eyelid
  large intestine — see Laceration, intestine, large
  larynx S11.011 ☑
    with foreign body S11.012 ☑
  leg (lower) S81.819 ☑
    with foreign body S81.829 ☑
    foot — see Laceration, foot
    knee — see Laceration, knee
    left S81.812 ☑
      with foreign body S81.822 ☑
    right S81.811 ☑
      with foreign body S81.821 ☑
    upper — see Laceration, thigh
  ligament — see Sprain
  lip S01.511 ☑
    with foreign body S01.521 ☑
  liver S36.113 ☑
    major (stellate) S36.116 ☑
    minor S36.114 ☑
    moderate S36.115 ☑
  loin — see Laceration, abdomen, wall
  lower back — see Laceration, back, lower
  lumbar region — see Laceration, back, lower
  lung S27.339 ☑
    bilateral S27.332 ☑
    unilateral S27.331 ☑
  malar region — see Laceration, head, specified site NEC
  mammary — see Laceration, breast
  mastoid region — see Laceration, head, specified site
    NEC
  meninges — see Injury, intracranial, diffuse
  meniscus — see Tear, meniscus
  mesentery S36.893 ☑
  mesosalpinx S37.893 ☑
  mouth — see Laceration, oral cavity
  muscle — see Injury, muscle, by site, laceration

⁷ Subterms under main terms may continue to next column or page   ☑ Additional Character Required — Refer to the Tabular List for Character Selection   207

Laceration — Laceration

Laceration — *continued*
  nail
    finger — *see* Laceration, finger, with damage to nail
    toe — *see* Laceration, toe, with damage to nail
  nasal (septum) (sinus) — *see* Laceration, nose
  nasopharynx — *see* Laceration, head, specified site NEC
  neck S11.91 ☑
    with foreign body S11.92 ☑
    involving
      cervical esophagus S11.21 ☑
        with foreign body S11.22 ☑
      larynx — *see* Laceration, larynx
      pharynx — *see* Laceration, pharynx
      thyroid gland — *see* Laceration, thyroid gland
      trachea — *see* Laceration, trachea
    specified site NEC S11.81 ☑
      with foreign body S11.82 ☑
  nerve — *see* Injury, nerve
  nose (septum) (sinus) S01.21 ☑
    with foreign body S01.22 ☑
  ocular NOS S05.3- ☑
    adnexa NOS S01.11- ☑
  oral cavity S01.512 ☑
    with foreign body S01.522 ☑
  orbit (eye) — *see* Wound, open, ocular, orbit
  ovary S37.439 ☑
    bilateral S37.432 ☑
    unilateral S37.431 ☑
  palate — *see* Laceration, oral cavity
  palm — *see* Laceration, hand
  pancreas S36.239 ☑
  pelvic S31.010 ☑
    with
      foreign body S31.020 ☑
        penetration into retroperitoneal cavity S31.021 ☑
      penetration into retroperitoneal cavity S31.011 ☑
    floor — *see also* Laceration, back, lower
      with ectopic or molar pregnancy O08.6
      complicating delivery O70.1
      following ectopic or molar pregnancy O08.6
      old (postpartal) N81.89
    organ S37.93 ☑
  penis S31.21 ☑
    with foreign body S31.22 ☑
  perineum
    female S31.41 ☑
      with
        ectopic or molar pregnancy O08.6
        foreign body S31.42 ☑
      during delivery O70.9
        first degree O70.0
        fourth degree O70.3
        second degree O70.1
        third degree — *see also* Delivery, complicated, by, laceration, perineum, third degree O70.20
      old (postpartal) N81.89
      postpartal N81.89
      secondary (postpartal) O90.1
    male S31.119 ☑
      with foreign body S31.129 ☑
  periocular area (with or without lacrimal passages) — *see* Laceration, eyelid
  peritoneum S36.893 ☑
  periumbilic region — *see* Laceration, abdomen, wall, periumbilic
  periurethral tissue — *see* Laceration, urethra
  phalanges
    finger — *see* Laceration, finger
    toe — *see* Laceration, toe
  pharynx S11.21 ☑
    with foreign body S11.22 ☑
  pinna — *see* Laceration, ear
  popliteal space — *see* Laceration, knee
  prepuce — *see* Laceration, penis
  prostate S37.823 ☑
  pubic region S31.119 ☑
    with foreign body S31.129 ☑
  pudendum — *see* Laceration, genital organs, external
  rectovaginal septum — *see* Laceration, vagina
  rectum S36.63 ☑
  retroperitoneum S36.893 ☑
  round ligament S37.893 ☑
  sacral region — *see* Laceration, back, lower

Laceration — *continued*
  sacroiliac region — *see* Laceration, back, lower
  salivary gland — *see* Laceration, oral cavity
  scalp S01.01 ☑
    with foreign body S01.02 ☑
  scapular region — *see* Laceration, shoulder
  scrotum S31.31 ☑
    with foreign body S31.32 ☑
  seminal vesicle S37.893 ☑
  shin — *see* Laceration, leg
  shoulder S41.019 ☑
    with foreign body S41.029 ☑
    left S41.012 ☑
      with foreign body S41.022 ☑
    right S41.011 ☑
      with foreign body S41.021 ☑
  small intestine — *see* Laceration, intestine, small
  spermatic cord — *see* Laceration, testis
  spinal cord (meninges) — *see also* Injury, spinal cord, by region
    due to injury at birth P11.5
    newborn (birth injury) P11.5
  spleen S36.039 ☑
    major (massive) (stellate) S36.032 ☑
    moderate S36.031 ☑
    superficial (minor) S36.030 ☑
  sternal region — *see* Laceration, thorax, front
  stomach S36.33 ☑
  submaxillary region — *see* Laceration, head, specified site NEC
  submental region — *see* Laceration, head, specified site NEC
  subungual
    finger(s) — *see* Laceration, finger, with damage to nail
    toe(s) — *see* Laceration, toe, with damage to nail
  suprarenal gland — *see* Laceration, adrenal gland
  temple, temporal region — *see* Laceration, head, specified site NEC
  temporomandibular area — *see* Laceration, cheek
  tendon — *see* Injury, muscle, by site, laceration
    Achilles S86.02- ☑
  tentorium cerebelli — *see* Injury, intracranial, diffuse
  testis S31.31 ☑
    with foreign body S31.32 ☑
  thigh S71.11- ☑
    with foreign body S71.12- ☑
  thorax, thoracic (wall) S21.91 ☑
    with foreign body S21.92 ☑
    back S21.22- ☑
      with penetration into thoracic cavity S21.42- ☑
    front S21.12- ☑
      with penetration into thoracic cavity S21.32- ☑
    back S21.21- ☑
      with
        foreign body S21.22- ☑
          with penetration into thoracic cavity S21.42- ☑
        penetration into thoracic cavity S21.41- ☑
    breast — *see* Laceration, breast
    front S21.11- ☑
      with
        foreign body S21.12- ☑
          with penetration into thoracic cavity S21.32- ☑
        penetration into thoracic cavity S21.31- ☑
  thumb S61.019 ☑
    with
      damage to nail S61.119 ☑
        with
          foreign body S61.129 ☑
      foreign body S61.029 ☑
    left S61.012 ☑
      with
        damage to nail S61.112 ☑
          with
            foreign body S61.122 ☑
        foreign body S61.022 ☑
    right S61.011 ☑
      with
        damage to nail S61.111 ☑
          with
            foreign body S61.121 ☑
        foreign body S61.021 ☑

Laceration — *continued*
  thyroid gland S11.11 ☑
    with foreign body S11.12 ☑
  toe(s) S91.119 ☑
    with
      damage to nail S91.219 ☑
        with
          foreign body S91.229 ☑
      foreign body S91.129 ☑
    great S91.113 ☑
      with
        damage to nail S91.213 ☑
          with
            foreign body S91.223 ☑
        foreign body S91.123 ☑
      left S91.112 ☑
        with
          damage to nail S91.212 ☑
            with
              foreign body S91.222 ☑
          foreign body S91.122 ☑
      right S91.111 ☑
        with
          damage to nail S91.211 ☑
            with
              foreign body S91.221 ☑
          foreign body S91.121 ☑
    lesser S91.116 ☑
      with
        damage to nail S91.216 ☑
          with
            foreign body S91.226 ☑
        foreign body S91.126 ☑
      left S91.115 ☑
        with
          damage to nail S91.215 ☑
            with
              foreign body S91.225 ☑
          foreign body S91.125 ☑
      right S91.114 ☑
        with
          damage to nail S91.214 ☑
            with
              foreign body S91.224 ☑
          foreign body S91.124 ☑
  tongue — *see* Laceration, oral cavity
  trachea S11.021 ☑
    with foreign body S11.022 ☑
  tunica vaginalis — *see* Laceration, testis
  tympanum, tympanic membrane — *see* Laceration, ear, drum
  umbilical region S31.115 ☑
    with foreign body S31.125 ☑
  ureter S37.13 ☑
  urethra S37.33 ☑
    with or following ectopic or molar pregnancy O0█
    obstetrical trauma O71.5
  urinary organ NEC S37.893 ☑
  uterus S37.63 ☑
    with ectopic or molar pregnancy O08.6
    following ectopic or molar pregnancy O08.6
    nonpuerperal, nontraumatic N85.8
    obstetrical trauma NEC O71.81
    old (postpartal) N85.8
  uvula — *see* Laceration, oral cavity
  vagina S31.41 ☑
    with
      ectopic or molar pregnancy O08.6
      foreign body S31.42 ☑
    during delivery O71.4
      with perineal laceration — *see* Laceration, perineum, female, during delivery
    following ectopic or molar pregnancy O08.6
    nonpuerperal, nontraumatic N89.8
    old (postpartal) N89.8
  vas deferens S37.893 ☑
  vesical — *see* Laceration, bladder
  vocal cords S11.031 ☑
    with foreign body S11.032 ☑
  vulva S31.41 ☑
    with
      ectopic or molar pregnancy O08.6
      foreign body S31.42 ☑
    complicating delivery O70.0
    following ectopic or molar pregnancy O08.6
    nonpuerperal, nontraumatic N90.89
    old (postpartal) N90.89

ceration — *continued*
wrist S61.519 ☑
  with
    foreign body S61.529 ☑
  left S61.512 ☑
    with
      foreign body S61.522 ☑
  right S61.511 ☑
    with
      foreign body S61.521 ☑

ck of
achievement in school Z55.3
adequate
  food Z59.4
  intermaxillary vertical dimension of fully erupted
    teeth M26.36
  sleep Z72.820
appetite (see Anorexia) R63.0
awareness R41.9
care
  in home Z74.2
  of infant (at or after birth) T76.02 ☑
    confirmed T74.02 ☑
cognitive functions R41.9
coordination R27.9
  ataxia R27.0
  specified type NEC R27.8
development (physiological) R62.50
  failure to thrive (child over 28 days old) R62.51
    adult R62.7
    newborn P92.6
  short stature R62.52
  specified type NEC R62.59
energy R53.83
financial resources Z59.6
food T73.0 ☑
growth R62.52
heating Z59.1
housing (permanent) (temporary) Z59.0
  adequate Z59.1
learning experiences in childhood Z62.898
leisure time (affecting life-style) Z73.2
material resources Z59.9
memory — *see also* Amnesia
  mild, following organic brain damage F06.8
ovulation N97.0
parental supervision or control of child Z62.0
person able to render necessary care Z74.2
physical exercise Z72.3
play experience in childhood Z62.898
posterior occlusal support M26.57
relaxation (affecting life-style) Z73.2
sexual
  desire F52.0
  enjoyment F52.1
shelter Z59.0
sleep (adequate) Z72.820
supervision of child by parent Z62.0
support, posterior occlusal M26.57
water T73.1 ☑

crimal — *see* condition
crimation, abnormal — *see* Epiphora
crimonasal duct — *see* condition
ctation, lactating (breast) (puerperal, postpartum)
associated
  cracked nipple O92.13
  retracted nipple O92.03
defective O92.4
disorder NEC O92.79
excessive O92.6
failed (complete) O92.3
  partial O92.4
mastitis NEC — *see* Mastitis, obstetric
mother (care and/or examination) Z39.1
nonpuerperal N64.3
cticemia, excessive E87.2
cunar skull Q75.8
ennec's cirrhosis K70.30
  with ascites K70.31
  nonalcoholic K74.69
fora's disease — *see* Epilepsy, generalized, idiopathic
g, lid (nervous) — *see* Retraction, lid
gophthalmos (eyelid) (nervous) H02.209
bilateral, upper and lower eyelids H02.20C
cicatricial H02.219
  bilateral, upper and lower eyelids H02.21C
  left H02.216
    lower H02.215

Lagophthalmos — *continued*
cicatricial — *continued*
  left — *continued*
    upper H02.214
    upper and lower eyelids H02.21B
  right H02.213
    lower H02.212
    upper H02.211
    upper and lower eyelids H02.21A
keratoconjunctivitis — *see* Keratoconjunctivitis
left H02.206
  lower H02.205
  upper H02.204
  upper and lower eyelids H02.20B
mechanical H02.229
  bilateral, upper and lower eyelids H02.22C
  left H02.226
    lower H02.225
    upper H02.224
    upper and lower eyelids H02.22B
  right H02.223
    lower H02.222
    upper H02.221
    upper and lower eyelids H02.22A
paralytic H02.239
  bilateral, upper and lower eyelids H02.23C
  left H02.236
    lower H02.235
    upper H02.234
    upper and lower eyelids H02.23B
  right H02.233
    lower H02.232
    upper H02.231
    upper and lower eyelids H02.23A
right H02.203
  lower H02.202
  upper H02.201
  upper and lower eyelids H02.20A
Laki-Lorand factor deficiency — *see* Defect, coagulation, specified type NEC
Lalling F80.0
Lambert-Eaton syndrome — *see* Syndrome, Lambert-Eaton
Lambliasis, lambliosis A07.1
Landau-Kleffner syndrome — *see* Epilepsy, specified NEC
Landouzy-Déjérine dystrophy or facioscapulohumeral atrophy G71.02
Landouzy's disease (icterohemorrhagic leptospirosis) A27.0
Landry-Guillain-Barré, syndrome or paralysis G61.0
Landry's disease or paralysis G61.0
Lane's
band Q43.3
kink — *see* Obstruction, intestine
syndrome K90.2
Langdon Down syndrome — *see* Trisomy, 21
Lapsed immunization schedule status Z28.3
Large
baby (regardless of gestational age) (4000g to 4499g) P08.1
ear, congenital Q17.1
physiological cup Q14.2
stature R68.89
Large-for-dates NEC (infant) (4000g to 4499g) P08.1
affecting management of pregnancy O36.6- ☑
exceptionally (4500g or more) P08.0
Larsen-Johansson disease or osteochondrosis — *see* Osteochondrosis, juvenile, patella
Larsen's syndrome (flattened facies and multiple congenital dislocations) Q74.8
Larva migrans
cutaneous B76.9
  Ancylostoma B76.0
visceral B83.0
Laryngeal — *see* condition
Laryngismus (stridulus) J38.5
congenital P28.89
diphtheritic A36.2
Laryngitis (acute) (edematous) (fibrinous) (infective) (infiltrative) (malignant) (membranous) (phlegmonous) (pneumococcal) (pseudomembranous) (septic) (subglottic) (suppurative) (ulcerative) J04.0
with
  influenza, flu, or grippe — *see* Influenza, with, laryngitis
  tracheitis (acute) — *see* Laryngotracheitis
atrophic J37.0

Laryngitis — *continued*
catarrhal J37.0
chronic J37.0
  with tracheitis (chronic) J37.1
diphtheritic A36.2
due to external agent — *see* Inflammation, respiratory, upper, due to
H. influenzae J04.0
Hemophilus influenzae J04.0
hypertrophic J37.0
influenzal — *see* Influenza, with, respiratory manifestations NEC
obstructive J05.0
sicca J37.0
spasmodic J05.0
  acute J04.0
streptococcal J04.0
stridulous J05.0
syphilitic (late) A52.73
  congenital A50.59 *[J99]*
    early A50.03 *[J99]*
tuberculous A15.5
Vincent's A69.1
Laryngocele (congenital) (ventricular) Q31.3
Laryngofissure J38.7
congenital Q31.8
Laryngomalacia (congenital) Q31.5
Laryngopharyngitis (acute) J06.0
chronic J37.0
due to external agent — *see* Inflammation, respiratory, upper, due to
Laryngoplegia J38.00
bilateral J38.02
unilateral J38.01
Laryngoptosis J38.7
Laryngospasm J38.5
Laryngostenosis J38.6
Laryngotracheitis (acute) (Infectional) (infective) (viral) J04.2
atrophic J37.1
catarrhal J37.1
chronic J37.1
diphtheritic A36.2
due to external agent — *see* Inflammation, respiratory, upper, due to
Hemophilus influenzae J04.2
hypertrophic J37.1
influenzal — *see* Influenza, with, respiratory manifestations NEC
pachydermic J38.7
sicca J37.1
spasmodic J38.5
  acute J05.0
streptococcal J04.2
stridulous J38.5
syphilitic (late) A52.73
  congenital A50.59 *[J99]*
    early A50.03 *[J99]*
tuberculous A15.5
Vincent's A69.1
Laryngotracheobronchitis — *see* Bronchitis
Larynx, laryngeal — *see* condition
Lassa fever A96.2
Lassitude — *see* Weakness
Late
talker R62.0
walker R62.0
Late effect(s) — *see* Sequelae
Latent — *see* condition
Laterocession — *see* Lateroversion
Lateroflexion — *see* Lateroversion
Lateroversion
cervix — *see* Lateroversion, uterus
uterus, uterine (cervix) (postinfectional) (postpartal, old) N85.4
  congenital Q51.818
  in pregnancy or childbirth O34.59- ☑
Lathyrism — *see* Poisoning, food, noxious, plant
Launois' syndrome (pituitary gigantism) E22.0
Launois-Bensaude adenolipomatosis E88.89
Laurence-Moon (-Bardet)-**Biedl syndrome** Q87.89
Lax, laxity — *see also* Relaxation
ligament (ous) — *see also* Disorder, ligament
  familial M35.7
  knee — *see* Derangement, knee
skin (acquired) L57.4
  congenital Q82.8
Laxative habit F55.2

Lazy leukocyte syndrome D70.8
Lead miner's lung J63.6
Leak, leakage
  air NEC J93.82
    postprocedural J95.812
  amniotic fluid — *see* Rupture, membranes, premature
  blood (microscopic), fetal, into maternal circulation
    affecting management of pregnancy — *see*
    Pregnancy, complicated by
  cerebrospinal fluid G96.0
    from spinal (lumbar) puncture G97.0
  device, implant or graft — *see also* Complications, by
    site and type, mechanical
    arterial graft NEC — *see* Complication, cardiovascu-
      lar device, mechanical, vascular
    breast (implant) T85.43 ☑
    catheter NEC T85.638 ☑
      dialysis (renal) T82.43 ☑
        intraperitoneal T85.631 ☑
      infusion NEC T82.534 ☑
        spinal (epidural) (subdural) T85.630 ☑
      urinary T83.038 ☑
        cystostomy T83.030 ☑
        Hopkins T83.038 ☑
        ileostomy T83.038 ☑
        indwelling T83.031 ☑
        nephrostomy T83.032 ☑
        specified T83.038 ☑
        urostomy T83.038 ☑
    gastrointestinal — *see* Complications, prosthetic
      device, mechanical, gastrointestinal device
    genital NEC T83.498 ☑
      penile prosthesis (cylinder) (implanted) (pump)
        (reservoir) T83.490 ☑
      testicular prosthesis T83.491 ☑
    heart NEC — *see* Complication, cardiovascular de-
      vice, mechanical
    joint prosthesis — *see* Complications, joint prosthe-
      sis, mechanical, specified NEC, by site
    ocular NEC — *see* Complications, prosthetic device,
      mechanical, ocular device
    orthopedic NEC — *see* Complication, orthopedic,
      device, mechanical
    persistent air J93.82
    specified NEC T85.638 ☑
    urinary NEC — *see also* Complication, genitourinary,
      device, urinary, mechanical
      graft T83.23 ☑
    vascular NEC — *see* Complication, cardiovascular
      device, mechanical
    ventricular intracranial shunt T85.03 ☑
  urine — *see* Incontinence
Leaky heart — *see* Endocarditis
Learning defect (specific) F81.9
Leather bottle stomach C16.9
Leber's
  congenital amaurosis H35.50
  optic atrophy (hereditary) H47.22
Lederer's anemia D59.1
Leeches (external) — *see* Hirudiniasis
Leg — *see* condition
Legg (-Calvé)-**Perthes disease, syndrome or osteo-
  chondrosis** M91.1- ☑
Legionellosis A48.1
  nonpneumonic A48.2
Legionnaires'
  disease A48.1
    nonpneumonic A48.2
  pneumonia A48.1
Leigh's disease G31.82
Leiner's disease L21.1
Leiofibromyoma — *see* Leiomyoma
Leiomyoblastoma — *see* Neoplasm, connective tissue,
  benign
Leiomyofibroma — *see also* Neoplasm, connective tissue, benign
  uterus (cervix) (corpus) D25.9
Leiomyoma — *see also* Neoplasm, connective tissue,
  benign
  bizarre — *see* Neoplasm, connective tissue, benign
  cellular — *see* Neoplasm, connective tissue, benign
  epithelioid — *see* Neoplasm, connective tissue, benign
  uterus (cervix) (corpus) D25.9
    intramural D25.1
    submucous D25.0
    subserosal D25.2
  vascular — *see* Neoplasm, connective tissue, benign

Leiomyoma, leiomyomatosis (intravascular) — *see*
  Neoplasm, connective tissue, uncertain behavior
Leiomyosarcoma — *see also* Neoplasm, connective tissue, malignant
  epithelioid — *see* Neoplasm, connective tissue, malig-
    nant
  myxoid — *see* Neoplasm, connective tissue, malignant
Leishmaniasis B55.9
  American (mucocutaneous) B55.2
    cutaneous B55.1
  Asian Desert B55.1
  Brazilian B55.2
  cutaneous (any type) B55.1
  dermal — *see also* Leishmaniasis, cutaneous
    post-kala-azar B55.0
  eyelid B55.1
  infantile B55.0
  Mediterranean B55.0
  mucocutaneous (American) (New World) B55.2
  naso-oral B55.2
  nasopharyngeal B55.2
  old world B55.1
  tegumentaria diffusa B55.1
  visceral B55.0
Leishmanoid, dermal — *see also* Leishmaniasis, cutaneous
  post-kala-azar B55.0
Lenegre's disease I44.2
Lengthening, leg — *see* Deformity, limb, unequal length
Lennert's lymphoma — *see* Lymphoma, Lennert's
Lennox-Gastaut syndrome G40.812
  intractable G40.814
    with status epilepticus G40.813
    without status epilepticus G40.814
  not intractable G40.812
    with status epilepticus G40.811
    without status epilepticus G40.812
Lens — *see* condition
Lenticonus (anterior) (posterior) (congenital) Q12.8
Lenticular degeneration, progressive E83.01
Lentiglobus (posterior) (congenital) Q12.8
Lentigo (congenital) L81.4
  maligna — *see also* Melanoma, in situ
    melanoma — *see* Melanoma
Lentivirus, as cause of disease classified elsewhere
  B97.31
Leontiasis
  ossium M85.2
  syphilitic (late) A52.78
    congenital A50.59
Lepothrix A48.8
Lepra — *see* Leprosy
Leprechaunism E34.8
Leprosy A30.- ☑
  with muscle disorder A30.9 [M63.80]
    ankle A30.9 [M63.87-] ☑
    foot A30.9 [M63.87-] ☑
    forearm A30.9 [M63.83-] ☑
    hand A30.9 [M63.84-] ☑
    lower leg A30.9 [M63.86-] ☑
    multiple sites A30.9 [M63.89]
    pelvic region A30.9 [M63.85-] ☑
    shoulder region A30.9 [M63.81-] ☑
    specified site NEC A30.9 [M63.88]
    thigh A30.9 [M63.85-] ☑
    upper arm A30.9 [M63.82-] ☑
  anesthetic A30.9
  BB A30.3
  BL A30.4
  borderline (infiltrated) (neuritic) A30.3
    lepromatous A30.4
    tuberculoid A30.2
  BT A30.2
  dimorphous (infiltrated) (neuritic) A30.3
  I A30.0
  indeterminate (macular) (neuritic) A30.0
  lepromatous (diffuse) (infiltrated) (macular) (neuritic)
    (nodular) A30.5
  LL A30.5
  macular (early) (neuritic) (simple) A30.9
  maculoanesthetic A30.9
  mixed A30.3
  neural A30.9
  nodular A30.5
  primary neuritic A30.3
  specified type NEC A30.8
  TT A30.1

Leprosy — *continued*
  tuberculoid (major) (minor) A30.1
Leptocytosis, hereditary D56.9
Leptomeningitis (chronic) (circumscribed) (hemorrhag
  (nonsuppurative) — *see* Meningitis
Leptomeningopathy G96.19
Leptospiral — *see* condition
Leptospirochetal — *see* condition
Leptospirosis A27.9
  canicola A27.89
  due to Leptospira interrogans serovar icterohaemorr
    giae A27.0
  icterohemorrhagica A27.0
  pomona A27.89
  Weil's disease A27.0
Leptus dermatitis B88.0
Leriche's syndrome (aortic bifurcation occlusion) I74
Leri's pleonosteosis Q78.8
Leri-Weill syndrome Q77.8
Lermoyez' syndrome — *see* Vertigo, peripheral NEC
Lesch-Nyhan syndrome E79.1
Leser-Trélat disease L82.1
  inflamed L82.0
Lesion(s) (nontraumatic)
  abducens nerve — *see* Strabismus, paralytic, sixth ne
  alveolar process K08.9
  angiocentric immunoproliferative D47.Z9 (*followin*
    D47.4)
  anorectal K62.9
  aortic (valve) I35.9
  auditory nerve — *see* subcategory H93.3 ☑
  basal ganglion G25.9
  bile duct — *see* Disease, bile duct
  biomechanical M99.9
    specified type NEC M99.89
      abdomen M99.89
      acromioclavicular M99.87
      cervical region M99.81
      cervicothoracic M99.81
      costochondral M99.88
      costovertebral M99.88
      head region M99.80
      hip M99.85
      lower extremity M99.86
      lumbar region M99.83
      lumbosacral M99.83
      occipitocervical M99.80
      pelvic region M99.85
      pubic M99.85
      rib cage M99.88
      sacral region M99.84
      sacrococcygeal M99.84
      sacroiliac M99.84
      specified NEC M99.89
      sternochondral M99.88
      sternoclavicular M99.87
      thoracic region M99.82
      thoracolumbar M99.82
      upper extremity M99.87
  bladder N32.9
  bone — *see* Disorder, bone
  brachial plexus G54.0
  brain G93.9
    congenital Q04.9
    vascular I67.9
      degenerative I67.9
      hypertensive I67.4
  buccal cavity K13.79
  calcified — *see* Calcification
  canthus — *see* Disorder, eyelid
  carate — *see* Pinta, lesions
  cardia K31.9
  cardiac — *see also* Disease, heart I51.9
    congenital Q24.9
    valvular — *see* Endocarditis
  cauda equina G83.4
  cecum K63.9
  cerebral — *see* Lesion, brain
  cerebrovascular I67.9
    degenerative I67.9
    hypertensive I67.4
  cervical (nerve) root NEC G54.2
  chiasmal — *see* Disorder, optic, chiasm
  chorda tympani G51.8
  coin, lung R91.1
  colon K63.9
  combined periodontic - endodontic K05.5
  congenital — *see* Anomaly, by site

☑ **Additional Character Required** — Refer to the Tabular List for Character Selection   ▽ **Subterms under main terms may continue to next column or pa**

Lesion(s) — *continued*
  conjunctiva H11.9
  conus medullaris — *see* Injury, conus medullaris
  coronary artery — *see* Ischemia, heart
  cranial nerve G52.9
    eighth — *see* Disorder, ear
    eleventh G52.9
    fifth G50.9
    first G52.0
    fourth — *see* Strabismus, paralytic, fourth nerve
    seventh G51.9
    sixth — *see* Strabismus, paralytic, sixth nerve
    tenth G52.2
    twelfth G52.3
  cystic — *see* Cyst
  degenerative — *see* Degeneration
  duodenum K31.9
  edentulous (alveolar) ridge, associated with trauma, due to traumatic occlusion K06.2
  en coup de sabre L94.1
  eyelid — *see* Disorder, eyelid
  gasserian ganglion G50.8
  gastric K31.9
  gastroduodenal K31.9
  gastrointestinal K63.9
  gingiva, associated with trauma K06.2
  glomerular
    focal and segmental — *see also* N00-N07 with fourth character .1 N05.1
    minimal change — *see also* N00-N07 with fourth character .0 N05.0
  heart (organic) — *see* Disease, heart
  hyperchromic, due to pinta (carate) A67.1
  hyperkeratotic — *see* Hyperkeratosis
  hypothalamic E23.7
  ileocecal K63.9
  ileum K63.9
  iliohypogastric nerve G57.8- ☑
  inflammatory — *see* Inflammation
  intestine K63.9
  intracerebral — *see* Lesion, brain
  intrachiasmal (optic) — *see* Disorder, optic, chiasm
  intracranial, space-occupying R90.0
  joint — *see* Disorder, joint
    sacroiliac (old) M53.3
  keratotic — *see* Keratosis
  kidney — *see* Disease, renal
  laryngeal nerve (recurrent) G52.2
  lip K13.0
  liver K76.9
  lumbosacral
    plexus G54.1
    root (nerve) NEC G54.4
  lung (coin) R91.1
  maxillary sinus J32.0
  mitral I05.9
  Morel-Lavallée — *see* Hematoma, by site
  motor cortex NEC G93.89
  mouth K13.79
  nerve G58.9
    femoral G57.2- ☑
    median G56.1- ☑
      carpal tunnel syndrome — *see* Syndrome, carpal tunnel
    plantar G57.6- ☑
    popliteal (lateral) G57.3- ☑
      medial G57.4- ☑
    radial G56.3- ☑
    sciatic G57.0- ☑
    spinal — *see* Injury, nerve, spinal
    ulnar G56.2- ☑
  nervous system, congenital Q07.9
  nonallopathic — *see* Lesion, biomechanical
  nose (internal) J34.89
  obstructive — *see* Obstruction
  obturator nerve G57.8- ☑
  oral mucosa K13.70
  organ or site NEC — *see* Disease, by site
  osteolytic — *see* Osteolysis
  peptic K27.9
  periodontal, due to traumatic occlusion K05.5
  pharynx J39.2
  pigment, pigmented (skin) L81.9
  pinta — *see* Pinta, lesions
  polypoid — *see* Polyp
  prechiasmal (optic) — *see* Disorder, optic, chiasm
  primary — *see also* Syphilis, primary A51.0

Lesion(s) — *continued*
  primary — *see also* Syphilis, primary — *continued*
    carate A67.0
    pinta A67.0
    yaws A66.0
  pulmonary J98.4
    valve I37.9
  pylorus K31.9
  rectosigmoid K63.9
  retina, retinal H35.9
  sacroiliac (joint) (old) M53.3
  salivary gland K11.9
    benign lymphoepithelial K11.8
  saphenous nerve G57.8- ☑
  sciatic nerve G57.0- ☑
  secondary — *see* Syphilis, secondary
  shoulder (region) M75.9-
    specified NEC M75.8- ☑
  sigmoid K63.9
  sinus (accessory) (nasal) J34.89
  skin L98.9
    suppurative L08.0
  SLAP S43.43- ☑
  spinal cord G95.9
    congenital Q06.9
  spleen D73.89
  stomach K31.9
  superior glenoid labrum S43.43- ☑
  syphilitic — *see* Syphilis
  tertiary — *see* Syphilis, tertiary
  thoracic root (nerve) NEC G54.3
  tonsillar fossa J35.9
  tooth, teeth K08.9
    white spot
      chewing surface K02.51
      pit and fissure surface K02.51
      smooth surface K02.61
  traumatic — *see* specific type of injury by site
  tricuspid (valve) I07.9
    nonrheumatic I36.9
  trigeminal nerve G50.9
  ulcerated or ulcerative — *see* Ulcer, skin
  uterus N85.9
  vagina N89.8
  vagus nerve G52.2
  valvular — *see* Endocarditis
  vascular I99.9
    affecting central nervous system I67.9
    following trauma NEC T14.8 ☑
    umbilical cord, complicating delivery O69.5 ☑
  vulva N90.89
  warty — *see* Verruca
  white spot (tooth)
    chewing surface K02.51
    pit and fissure surface K02.51
    smooth surface K02.61
Lethargic — *see* condition
Lethargy R53.83
Letterer-Siwe's disease C96.0
Leukemia, leukemic C95.9- ☑
  acute basophilic C94.8- ☑
  acute bilineal C95.0- ☑
  acute erythroid C94.0- ☑
  acute lymphoblastic C91.0- ☑
  acute megakaryoblastic C94.2- ☑
  acute megakaryocytic C94.2- ☑
  acute mixed lineage C95.0- ☑
  acute monoblastic (monoblastic/monocytic) C93.0- ☑
  acute monocytic (monoblastic/monocytic) C93.0- ☑
  acute myeloblastic (minimal differentiation) (with maturation) C92.0- ☑
  acute myeloid, NOS C92.0- ☑
    with
      11q23-abnormality C92.6- ☑
      dysplasia of remaining hematopoesis and/or myelodysplastic disease in its history C92.A- ☑ (*following* C92.6)
      multilineage dysplasia C92.A- ☑ (*following* C92.6)
      variation of MLL-gene C92.6- ☑
    M6 (a)(b) C94.0- ☑
    M7 C94.2- ☑
  acute myelomonocytic C92.5- ☑
  acute promyelocytic C92.4- ☑
  adult T-cell (HTLV-1-associated) (acute variant) (chronic variant) (lymphomatoid variant) (smouldering variant) C91.5- ☑

Leukemia, leukemic — *continued*
  aggressive NK-cell C94.8- ☑
  AML (1/ETO) (M0) (M1) (M2) (without a FAB classification) C92.0- ☑
  AML M3 C92.4- ☑
  AML M4 (Eo with inv(16) or t(16;16)) C92.5- ☑
  AML M5 C93.0- ☑
  AML M5a C93.0- ☑
  AML M5b C93.0- ☑
  AML Me with t (15;17) and variants C92.4- ☑
  atypical chronic myeloid, BCR/ABL-negative C92.2- ☑
  biphenotypic acute C95.0- ☑
  blast cell C95.0- ☑
  Burkitt-type, mature B-cell C91.A- ☑ (*following* C91.6)
  chronic lymphocytic, of B-cell type C91.1- ☑
  chronic monocytic C93.1- ☑
  chronic myelogenous (Philadelphia chromosome (Ph1) positive) (t(9;22)) (q34;q11) (with crisis of blast cells) C92.1- ☑
  chronic myeloid, BCR/ABL-positive C92.1- ☑
    atypical, BCR/ABL-negative C92.2- ☑
  chronic myelomonocytic C93.1- ☑
  chronic neutrophilic D47.1
  CMML (-1) (-2) (with eosinophilia) C93.1- ☑
  granulocytic — *see also* Category C92 C92.9- ☑
  hairy cell C91.4- ☑
  juvenile myelomonocytic C93.3- ☑
  lymphoid C91.9- ☑
    specified NEC C91.Z- ☑ (*following* C91.6)
  mast cell C94.3- ☑
  mature B-cell, Burkitt-type C91.A- ☑ (*following* C91.6)
  monocytic (subacute) C93.9- ☑
    specified NEC C93.Z- ☑ (*following* C93.3)
  myelogenous — *see also* Category C92 C92.9- ☑
  myeloid C92.9- ☑
    specified NEC C92.Z- ☑ (*following* C92.6)
  plasma cell C90.1- ☑
  plasmacytic C90.1- ☑
  prolymphocytic
    of B-cell type C91.3- ☑
    of T-cell type C91.6- ☑
  specified NEC C94.8- ☑
  stem cell, of unclear lineage C95.0- ☑
  subacute lymphocytic C91.9- ☑
  T-cell large granular lymphocytic C91.Z- ☑ (*following* C91.6)
  unspecified cell type C95.9 ☑
    acute C95.0- ☑
    chronic C95.1- ☑
Leukemoid reaction — *see also* Reaction, leukemoid D72.823
Leukoaraiosis (hypertensive) I67.81
Leukoariosis — *see* Leukoaraiosis
Leukocoria — *see* Disorder, globe, degenerated condition, leucocoria
Leukocytopenia D72.819
Leukocytosis D72.829
  eosinophilic D72.1
Leukoderma, leukodermia NEC L81.5
  syphilitic A51.39
    late A52.79
Leukodystrophy E75.29
Leukoedema, oral epithelium K13.29
Leukoencephalitis G04.81
  acute (subacute) hemorrhagic G36.1
    postimmunization or postvaccinal G04.02
  postinfectious G04.01
  subacute sclerosing A81.1
  van Bogaert's (sclerosing) A81.1
Leukoencephalopathy — *see also* Encephalopathy G93.49
  Binswanger's I67.3
  heroin vapor G92
  metachromatic E75.25
  multifocal (progressive) A81.2
  postimmunization and postvaccinal G04.02
  progressive multifocal A81.2
  reversible, posterior G93.6
  van Bogaert's (sclerosing) A81.1
  vascular, progressive I67.3
Leukoerythroblastosis D75.9
Leukokeratosis — *see also* Leukoplakia
  mouth K13.21
  nicotina palati K13.24
  oral mucosa K13.21
  tongue K13.21
  vocal cord J38.3

Leukokraurosis vulva (e) N90.4
Leukoma (cornea) — see also Opacity, cornea
   adherent H17.0-
   interfering with central vision — see Opacity, cornea, central
Leukomalacia, cerebral, newborn P91.2
   periventricular P91.2
Leukomelanopathy, hereditary D72.0
Leukonychia (punctata) (striata) L60.8
   congenital Q84.4
Leukopathia unguium L60.8
   congenital Q84.4
Leukopenia D72.819
   basophilic D72.818
   chemotherapy (cancer) induced D70.1
   congenital D70.0
   cyclic D70.0
   drug induced NEC D70.2
      due to cytoreductive cancer chemotherapy D70.1
   eosinophilic D72.818
   familial D70.0
   infantile genetic D70.0
   malignant D70.9
   periodic D70.0
   transitory neonatal P61.5
Leukopenic — see condition
Leukoplakia
   anus K62.89
   bladder (postinfectional) N32.89
   buccal K13.21
   cervix (uteri) N88.0
   esophagus K22.8
   gingiva K13.21
   hairy (oral mucosa) (tongue) K13.3
   kidney (pelvis) N28.89
   larynx J38.7
   lip K13.21
   mouth K13.21
   oral epithelium, including tongue (mucosa) K13.21
   palate K13.21
   pelvis (kidney) N28.89
   penis (infectional) N48.0
   rectum K62.89
   syphilitic (late) A52.79
   tongue K13.21
   ureter (postinfectional) N28.89
   urethra (postinfectional) N36.8
   uterus N85.8
   vagina N89.4
   vocal cord J38.3
   vulva N90.4
Leukorrhea N89.8
   due to Trichomonas (vaginalis) A59.00
   trichomonal A59.00
Leukosarcoma C85.9- ☑
Levocardia (isolated) Q24.1
   with situs inversus Q89.3
Levotransposition Q20.5
Lev's disease or syndrome (acquired complete heart block) I44.2
Levulosuria — see Fructosuria
Levurid L30.2
Lewy body (ies) (dementia) (disease) G31.83
Leyden-Moebius dystrophy G71.09
Leydig cell
   carcinoma
      specified site — see Neoplasm, malignant, by site
      unspecified site
         female C56.9
         male C62.9- ☑
   tumor
      benign
         specified site — see Neoplasm, benign, by site
         unspecified site
            female D27.- ☑
            male D29.2- ☑
      malignant
         specified site — see Neoplasm, malignant, by site
         unspecified site
            female C56.- ☑
            male C62.9- ☑
      specified site — see Neoplasm, uncertain behavior, by site
      unspecified site
         female D39.1- ☑
         male D40.1- ☑

Leydig-Sertoli cell tumor
   specified site — see Neoplasm, benign, by site
   unspecified site
      female D27.- ☑
      male D29.2- ☑
LGSIL (Low grade squamous intraepithelial lesion on cytologic smear of)
   anus R85.612
   cervix R87.612
   vagina R87.622
Liar, pathologic F60.2
Libido
   decreased R68.82
Libman-Sacks disease M32.11
Lice (infestation) B85.2
   body (Pediculus corporis) B85.1
   crab B85.3
   head (Pediculus capitis) B85.0
   mixed (classifiable to more than one of the titles B85.0-B85.3) B85.4
   pubic (Phthirus pubis) B85.3
Lichen L28.0
   albus L90.0
      penis N48.0
      vulva N90.4
   amyloidosis E85.4 [L99]
   atrophicus L90.0
      penis N48.0
      vulva N90.4
   congenital Q82.8
   myxedematosus L98.5
   nitidus L44.1
   pilaris Q82.8
      acquired L85.8
   planopilaris L66.1
   planus (chronicus) L43.9
      annularis L43.8
      bullous L43.1
      follicular L66.1
      hypertrophic L43.0
      moniliformis L44.3
      of Wilson L43.9
      specified NEC L43.8
      subacute (active) L43.3
      tropicus L43.3
   ruber
      acuminatus L44.0
      moniliformis L44.3
      planus L43.9
   sclerosus (et atrophicus) L90.0
      penis N48.0
      vulva N90.4
   scrofulosus (primary) (tuberculous) A18.4
   simplex (chronicus) (circumscriptus) L28.0
   striatus L44.2
   urticatus L28.2
Lichenification L28.0
Lichenoides tuberculosis (primary) A18.4
Lichtheim's disease or syndrome D51.0
Lien migrans D73.89
Ligament — see condition
Light
   for gestational age — see Light for dates
   headedness R42
Light-for-dates (infant) P05.00
   with weight of
      499 grams or less P05.01
      500-749 grams P05.02
      750-999 grams P05.03
      1000-1249 grams P05.04
      1250-1499 grams P05.05
      1500-1749 grams P05.06
      1750-1999 grams P05.07
      2000-2499 grams P05.08
      2500 grams and over P05.09
   affecting management of pregnancy O36.59- ☑
   and small-for-dates — see Small for dates
   specified NEC P05.09
Lightning (effects) (stroke) (struck by) T75.00 ☑
   burn — see Burn
   foot E53.8
   shock T75.01 ☑
   specified effect NEC T75.09 ☑
Lightwood-Albright syndrome N25.89
Lightwood's disease or syndrome (renal tubular acidosis) N25.89
Lignac (-de Toni) (-Fanconi) (-Debré) **disease or syndrome** E72.09

Lignac (-de Toni) (-Fanconi) (-Debré) **disease or syndrome** — continued
   with cystinosis E72.04
Ligneous thyroiditis E06.5
Likoff's syndrome I20.8
Limb — see condition
Limbic epilepsy personality syndrome F07.0
Limitation, limited
   activities due to disability Z73.6
   cardiac reserve — see Disease, heart
   eye muscle duction, traumatic — see Strabismus, mechanical
   mandibular range of motion M26.52
Lindau (-von Hippel) **disease** Q85.8
Line(s)
   Beau's L60.4
   Harris' — see Arrest, epiphyseal
   Hudson's (cornea) — see Pigmentation, cornea, anter
   Stähli's (cornea) — see Pigmentation, cornea, anter
Linea corneae senilis — see Change, cornea, senile
Lingua
   geographica K14.1
   nigra (villosa) K14.3
   plicata K14.5
   tylosis K13.29
Lingual — see condition
Linguatulosis B88.8
Linitis (gastric) **plastica** C16.9
Lip — see condition
Lipedema — see Edema
Lipemia — see also Hyperlipidemia
   retina, retinalis E78.3
Lipidosis E75.6
   cerebral (infantile) (juvenile) (late) E75.4
   cerebroretinal E75.4
   cerebroside E75.22
   cholesterol (cerebral) E75.5
   glycolipid E75.21
   hepatosplenomegalic E78.3
   sphingomyelin — see Niemann-Pick disease or syndrome
   sulfatide E75.29
Lipoadenoma — see Neoplasm, benign, by site
Lipoblastoma — see Lipoma
Lipoblastomatosis — see Lipoma
Lipochondrodystrophy E76.01
Lipochrome histiocytosis (familial) D71
Lipodermatosclerosis — see Varix, leg, with, inflammation
   ulcerated — see Varix, leg, with, ulcer, with inflammation by site
Lipodystrophia progressiva E88.1
Lipodystrophy (progressive) E88.1
   insulin E88.1
   intestinal K90.81
   mesenteric K65.4
Lipofibroma — see Lipoma
Lipofuscinosis, neuronal (with ceroidosis) E75.4
Lipogranuloma, sclerosing L92.8
Lipogranulomatosis E78.89
Lipoid — see also condition
   histiocytosis D76.3
      essential E75.29
   nephrosis N04.9
   proteinosis of Urbach E78.89
Lipoidemia — see Hyperlipidemia
Lipoidosis — see Lipidosis
Lipoma D17.9
   fetal D17.9
      fat cell D17.9
   infiltrating D17.9
   intramuscular D17.9
   pleomorphic D17.9
   site classification
      arms (skin) (subcutaneous) D17.2- ☑
      connective tissue D17.30
         intra-abdominal D17.5
         intrathoracic D17.4
         peritoneum D17.79
         retroperitoneum D17.79
         specified site NEC D17.39
         spermatic cord D17.6
      face (skin) (subcutaneous) D17.0
      genitourinary organ NEC D17.72
      head (skin) (subcutaneous) D17.0
      intra-abdominal D17.5
      intrathoracic D17.4

ɔoma — *continued*
site classification — *continued*
  kidney D17.71
  legs (skin) (subcutaneous) D17.2- ☑
  neck (skin) (subcutaneous) D17.0
  peritoneum D17.79
  retroperitoneum D17.79
  skin D17.30
    specified site NEC D17.39
  specified site NEC D17.79
  spermatic cord D17.6
  subcutaneous D17.30
    specified site NEC D17.39
  trunk (skin) (subcutaneous) D17.1
  unspecified D17.9
spindle cell D17.9
ɔomatosis E88.2
dolorosa (Dercum) E88.2
fetal — *see* Lipoma
Launois-Bensaude E88.89
ɔomyoma — *see* Lipoma
ɔomyxoma — *see* Lipoma
ɔomyxosarcoma — *see* Neoplasm, connective tissue,
  malignant
ɔoprotein metabolism disorder E78.9
ɔoproteinemia E78.5
broad-beta E78.2
floating-beta E78.2
hyper-pre-beta E78.1
ɔosarcoma — *see also* Neoplasm, connective tissue,
  malignant
dedifferentiated — *see* Neoplasm, connective tissue,
    malignant
differentiated type — *see* Neoplasm, connective tissue,
    malignant
embryonal — *see* Neoplasm, connective tissue, malig-
    nant
mixed type — *see* Neoplasm, connective tissue, malig-
    nant
myxoid — *see* Neoplasm, connective tissue, malignant
pleomorphic — *see* Neoplasm, connective tissue, ma-
    lignant
round cell — *see* Neoplasm, connective tissue, malig-
    nant
well differentiated type — *see* Neoplasm, connective
    tissue, malignant
ɔosynovitis prepatellaris E88.89
ɔpping, cervix N86
ɔpschütz disease or ulcer N76.6
ɔpuria R82.0
schistosomiasis (bilharziasis) B65.0
sping F80.0
ssauer's paralysis A52.17
ssencephalia, lissencephaly Q04.3
steriosis, listerellosis A32.9
congenital (disseminated) P37.2
cutaneous A32.0
neonatal, newborn (disseminated) P37.2
oculoglandular A32.81
specified NEC A32.89
themia E79.0
thiasis — *see* Calculus
thosis J62.8
thuria R82.998
tigation, anxiety concerning Z65.3
ttle leaguer's elbow — *see* Epicondylitis, medial
ttle's disease G80.9
ttre's
gland — *see* condition
hernia — *see* Hernia, abdomen
ttritis — *see* Urethritis
vedo (annularis) (racemosa) (reticularis) R23.1
ver — *see* condition
ving alone (problems with) Z60.2
with handicapped person Z74.2
oyd's syndrome — *see* Adenomatosis, endocrine
a loa, loaiasis, loasis B74.3
ɔbar — *see* condition
ɔbomycosis B48.0
ɔbo's disease B48.0
ɔbotomy syndrome F07.0
ɔbstein (-Ekman) **disease or syndrome** Q78.0
ɔbster-claw hand Q71.6- ☑
ɔbulation (congenital) — *see also* Anomaly, by site
kidney, Q63.1
liver, abnormal Q44.7
spleen Q89.09

Lobule, lobular — *see* condition
Local, localized — *see* condition
Locked twins causing obstructed labor O66.1
Locked-in state G83.5
Locking
joint — *see* Derangement, joint, specified type NEC
  knee — *see* Derangement, knee
Lockjaw — *see* Tetanus
Löffler's
endocarditis I42.3
eosinophilia J82
pneumonia J82
syndrome (eosinophilic pneumonitis) J82
Loiasis (with conjunctival infestation) (eyelid) B74.3
Lone Star fever A77.0
Long
labor O63.9
  first stage O63.0
  second stage O63.1
QT syndrome I45.81
Longitudinal stripes or grooves, nails L60.8
congenital Q84.6
Long-term (current) (prophylactic) **drug therapy** (use
  of)
agents affecting estrogen receptors and estrogen levels
    NEC Z79.818
anastrozole (Arimidex) Z79.811
antibiotics Z79.2
  short-term use — *omit code*
anticoagulants Z79.01
anti-inflammatory, non-steroidal (NSAID) Z79.1
antiplatelet Z79.02
antithrombotics Z79.02
aromatase inhibitors Z79.811
aspirin Z79.82
birth control pill or patch Z79.3
bisphosphonates Z79.83
contraceptive, oral Z79.3
drug, specified NEC Z79.899
estrogen receptor downregulators Z79.818
Evista Z79.810
exemestane (Aromasin) Z79.811
Fareston Z79.810
fulvestrant (Faslodex) Z79.818
gonadotropin-releasing hormone (GnRH) agonist
    Z79.818
goserelin acetate (Zoladex) Z79.818
hormone replacement Z79.890
insulin Z79.4
letrozole (Femara) Z79.811
leuprolide acetate (leuprorelin) (Lupron) Z79.818
megestrol acetate (Megace) Z79.818
methadone for pain management Z79.891
Nolvadex Z79.810
non-steroidal anti-inflammatories (NSAID) Z79.1
opiate analgesic Z79.891
oral
  antidiabetic Z79.84
  contraceptive Z79.3
  hypoglycemic Z79.84
raloxifene (Evista) Z79.810
selective estrogen receptor modulators (SERMs)
    Z79.810
steroids
  inhaled Z79.51
  systemic Z79.52
tamoxifen (Nolvadex) Z79.810
toremifene (Fareston) Z79.810
Loop
intestine — *see* Volvulus
vascular on papilla (optic) Q14.2
Loose — *see also* condition
body
  joint M24.00
    ankle M24.07- ☑
    elbow M24.02- ☑
    hand M24.04- ☑
    hip M24.05- ☑
    knee M23.4- ☑
    shoulder (region) M24.01- ☑
    specified site NEC M24.08
    toe M24.07- ☑
    vertebra M24.08
    wrist M24.03- ☑
  knee M23.4- ☑
  sheath, tendon — *see* Disorder, tendon, specified
    type NEC
cartilage — *see* Loose, body, joint

Loose — *continued*
skin and subcutaneous tissue (following bariatric
  surgery weight loss) (following dietary weight
  loss) L98.7
tooth, teeth K08.89
Loosening
aseptic
  joint prosthesis — *see* Complications, joint prosthe-
    sis, mechanical, loosening, by site
  epiphysis — *see* Osteochondropathy
mechanical
  joint prosthesis — *see* Complications, joint prosthe-
    sis, mechanical, loosening, by site
Looser-Milkman (-Debray) **syndrome** M83.8
Lop ear (deformity) Q17.3
Lorain (-Levi) **short stature syndrome** E23.0
Lordosis M40.50
acquired — *see* Lordosis, specified type NEC
congenital Q76.429
  lumbar region Q76.426
  lumbosacral region Q76.427
  sacral region Q76.428
  sacrococcygeal region Q76.428
  thoracolumbar region Q76.425
lumbar region M40.56
lumbosacral region M40.57
postsurgical M96.4
postural — *see* Lordosis, specified type NEC
rachitic (late effect) (sequelae) E64.3
sequelae of rickets E64.3
specified type NEC M40.40
  lumbar region M40.46
  lumbosacral region M40.47
  thoracolumbar region M40.45
thoracolumbar region M40.55
tuberculous A18.01
Loss (of)
appetite — *see also* Anorexia R63.0
  hysterical F50.89
  nonorganic origin F50.89
  psychogenic F50.89
blood — *see* Hemorrhage
bone — *see* Loss, substance of, bone
consciousness, transient R55
  traumatic — *see* Injury, intracranial
control, sphincter, rectum R15.9
  nonorganic origin F98.1
elasticity, skin R23.4
family (member) in childhood Z62.898
fluid (acute) E86.9
function of labyrinth — *see* subcategory H83.2 ☑
hair, nonscarring — *see* Alopecia
hearing — *see also* Deafness
  central NOS H90.5
  conductive H90.2
    bilateral H90.0
    unilateral
      with
        restricted hearing on the contralateral
          side H90.A1- ☑
        unrestricted hearing on the contralateral
          side H90.1- ☑
  mixed conductive and sensorineural hearing loss
    H90.8
    bilateral H90.6
    unilateral
      with
        restricted hearing on the contralateral
          side H90.A3- ☑
        unrestricted hearing on the contralateral
          side H90.7- ☑
  neural NOS H90.5
  perceptive NOS H90.5
  sensorineural NOS H90.5
    bilateral H90.3
    unilateral
      with
        restricted hearing onthe contralateral
          side H90.A2- ☑
        unrestricted hearing on the contralateral
          side H90.4- ☑
  sensory NOS H90.5
height R29.890
limb or member, traumatic, current — *see* Amputation,
  traumatic
love relationship in childhood Z62.898
memory — *see also* Amnesia
  mild, following organic brain damage F06.8

Loss — *continued*
  mind — *see* Psychosis
  occlusal vertical dimension of fully erupted teeth M26.37
  organ or part — *see* Absence, by site, acquired
  ossicles, ear (partial) H74.32- ☑
  parent in childhood Z63.4
  pregnancy, recurrent N96
    care in current pregnancy O26.2- ☑
    without current pregnancy N96
  recurrent pregnancy — *see* Loss, pregnancy, recurrent
  self-esteem, in childhood Z62.898
  sense of
    smell — *see* Disturbance, sensation, smell
    taste — *see* Disturbance, sensation, taste
    touch R20.8
  sensory R44.9
    dissociative F44.6
  sexual desire F52.0
  sight (acquired) (complete) (congenital) — *see* Blindness
  substance of
    bone — *see* Disorder, bone, density and structure, specified NEC
      horizontal alveolar K06.3
    cartilage — *see* Disorder, cartilage, specified type NEC
      auricle (ear) — *see* Disorder, pinna, specified type NEC
    vitreous (humor) H15.89
  tooth, teeth — *see* Absence, teeth, acquired
  vision, visual H54.7
    both eyes H54.3
    one eye H54.60
      left (normal vision on right) H54.62
      right (normal vision on left) H54.61
    specified as blindness — *see* Blindness
    subjective
      sudden H53.13- ☑
      transient H53.12- ☑
  vitreous — *see* Prolapse, vitreous
  voice — *see* Aphonia
  weight (abnormal) (cause unknown) R63.4
Louis-Bar syndrome (ataxia-telangiectasia) G11.3
Louping ill (encephalitis) A84.8
Louse, lousiness — *see* Lice
Low
  achiever, school Z55.3
  back syndrome M54.5
  basal metabolic rate R94.8
  birthweight (2499 grams or less) P07.10
    with weight of
      1000-1249 grams P07.14
      1250-1499 grams P07.15
      1500-1749 grams P07.16
      1750-1999 grams P07.17
      2000-2499 grams P07.18
    extreme (999 grams or less) P07.00
      with weight of
        499 grams or less P07.01
        500-749 grams P07.02
        750-999 grams P07.03
    for gestational age — *see* Light for dates
  blood pressure — *see also* Hypotension
    reading (incidental) (isolated) (nonspecific) R03.1
  cardiac reserve — *see* Disease, heart
  function — *see also* Hypofunction
    kidney N28.9
  hematocrit D64.9
  hemoglobin D64.9
  income Z59.6
  level of literacy Z55.0
  lying
    kidney N28.89
    organ or site, congenital — *see* Malposition, congenital
  output syndrome (cardiac) — *see* Failure, heart
  platelets (blood) — *see* Thrombocytopenia
  reserve, kidney N28.89
  salt syndrome E87.1
  self esteem R45.81
  set ears Q17.4
  vision H54.2X- ☑
    one eye (other eye normal) H54.50
      left (normal vision on right) H54.52A- ☑
      other eye blind — *see* Blindness
      right (normal vision on left) H54.511- ☑

Low-density-lipoprotein-type (LDL) **hyperlipoproteinemia** E78.00
Lowe's syndrome E72.03
Lown-Ganong-Levine syndrome I45.6
LSD reaction (acute) (without dependence) F16.90
  with dependence F16.20
L-shaped kidney Q63.8
LTBI (latent tuberculosis infection) Z22.7
Ludwig's angina or disease K12.2
Lues (venerea), **luetic** — *see* Syphilis
Luetscher's syndrome (dehydration) E86.0
Lumbago, lumbalgia M54.5
  with sciatica M54.4- ☑
    due to intervertebral disc disorder M51.17
  due to displacement, intervertebral disc M51.27
    with sciatica M51.17
Lumbar — *see* condition
Lumbarization, vertebra, congenital Q76.49
Lumbermen's itch B88.0
Lump — *see also* Mass
  breast N63.0
    axillary tail
      left N63.32
      right N63.31
    left
      lower inner quadrant N63.24
      lower outer quadrant N63.23
      overlapping quadrants N63.25
      unspecified quadrant N63.20
      upper inner quadrant N63.22
      upper outer quadrant N63.21
    right
      lower inner quadrant N63.14
      lower outer quadrant N63.13
      overlapping quadrants N63.15
      unspecified quadrant N63.10
      upper inner quadrant N63.12
      upper outer quadrant N63.11
    subareolar
      left N63.42
      right N63.41
Lunacy — *see* Psychosis
Lung — *see* condition
Lupoid (miliary) **of Boeck** D86.3
Lupus
  anticoagulant D68.62
    with
      hemorrhagic disorder D68.312
      hypercoagulable state D68.62
    finding without diagnosis R76.0
  discoid (local) L93.0
  erythematosus (discoid) (local) L93.0
    disseminated — *see* Lupus, erythematosus, systemic
    eyelid H01.129
      left H01.126
        lower H01.125
        upper H01.124
      right H01.123
        lower H01.122
        upper H01.121
    profundus L93.2
    specified NEC L93.2
    subacute cutaneous L93.1
    systemic M32.9
      with organ or system involvement M32.10
        endocarditis M32.11
        lung M32.13
        pericarditis M32.12
        renal (glomerular) M32.14
          tubulo-interstitial M32.15
        specified organ or system NEC M32.19
    drug-induced M32.0
    inhibitor (presence of) D68.62
      with
        hemorrhagic disorder D68.312
        hypercoagulable state D68.62
      finding without diagnosis R76.0
    specified NEC M32.8
  exedens A18.4
  hydralazine M32.0
    correct substance properly administered — *see* Table of Drugs and Chemicals, by drug, adverse effect
    overdose or wrong substance given or taken — *see* Table of Drugs and Chemicals, by drug, poisoning
  nephritis (chronic) M32.14
  nontuberculous, not disseminated L93.0

Lupus — *continued*
  panniculitis L93.2
  pernio (Besnier) D86.3
  systemic — *see* Lupus, erythematosus, systemic
  tuberculous A18.4
    eyelid A18.4
  vulgaris A18.4
    eyelid A18.4
Luteinoma D27.- ☑
Lutembacher's disease or syndrome (atrial septal fect with mitral stenosis) Q21.1
Luteoma D27.- ☑
Lutz (-Splendore-de Almeida) **disease** — *see* Paracoccioidomycosis
Luxation — *see also* Dislocation
  eyeball (nontraumatic) — *see* Luxation, globe
    birth injury P15.3
  globe, nontraumatic H44.82- ☑
  lacrimal gland — *see* Dislocation, lacrimal gland
  lens (old) (partial) (spontaneous)
    congenital Q12.1
      syphilitic A50.39
Lycanthropy F22
Lyell's syndrome L51.2
  due to drug L51.2
    correct substance properly administered — *see* ble of Drugs and Chemicals, by drug, adve effect
    overdose or wrong substance given or taken — Table of Drugs and Chemicals, by drug, p⊕ soning
Lyme disease A69.20
Lymph
  gland or node — *see* condition
  scrotum — *see* Infestation, filarial
Lymphadenitis I88.9
  with ectopic or molar pregnancy O08.0
  acute L04.9
    axilla L04.2
    face L04.0
    head L04.0
    hip L04.3
    limb
      lower L04.3
      upper L04.2
    neck L04.0
    shoulder L04.2
    specified site NEC L04.8
    trunk L04.1
  anthracosis (occupational) J60
  any site, except mesenteric I88.9
    chronic I88.1
    subacute I88.1
  breast
    gestational — *see* Mastitis, obstetric
    puerperal, postpartum (nonpurulent) O91.22
  chancroidal (congenital) A57
  chronic I88.1
    mesenteric I88.0
  due to
    Brugia (malayi) B74.1
      timori B74.2
    chlamydial lymphogranuloma A55
    diphtheria (toxin) A36.89
    lymphogranuloma venereum A55
    Wuchereria bancrofti B74.0
  following ectopic or molar pregnancy O08.0
  gonorrheal A54.89
  infective — *see* Lymphadenitis, acute
  mesenteric (acute) (chronic) (nonspecific) (subacut I88.0
    due to Salmonella typhi A01.09
    tuberculous A18.39
  mycobacterial A31.8
  purulent — *see* Lymphadenitis, acute
  pyogenic — *see* Lymphadenitis, acute
  regional, nonbacterial I88.8
  septic — *see* Lymphadenitis, acute
  subacute, unspecified site I88.1
  suppurative — *see* Lymphadenitis, acute
  syphilitic (early) (secondary) A51.49
    late A52.79
  tuberculous — *see* Tuberculosis, lymph gland
  venereal (chlamydial) A55
Lymphadenoid goiter E06.3
Lymphadenopathy (generalized) R59.1
  angioimmunoblastic, with dysproteinemia (AILD) C8
  due to toxoplasmosis (acquired) B58.89

☑ **Additional Character Required** — **Refer to the Tabular List for Character Selection**
⬇ **Subterms under main terms may continue to next column or pa**

ymphadenopathy — continued
- due to toxoplasmosis — continued
  - congenital (acute) (subacute) (chronic) P37.1
- localized R59.Ø
- syphilitic (early) (secondary) A51.49

ymphadenosis R59.1

ymphangiectasis I89.Ø
- conjunctiva H11.89
- postinfectional I89.Ø
- scrotum I89.Ø

ymphangiectatic elephantiasis, nonfilarial I89.Ø

ymphangioendothelioma D18.1
- malignant — see Neoplasm, connective tissue, malignant

ymphangioleiomyomatosis J84.81

ymphangioma D18.1
- capillary D18.1
- cavernous D18.1
- cystic D18.1
- malignant — see Neoplasm, connective tissue, malignant

ymphangiomyoma D18.1

ymphangiomyomatosis J84.81

ymphangiosarcoma — see Neoplasm, connective tissue, malignant

ymphangitis I89.1
- with
  - abscess — code by site under Abscess
  - cellulitis — code by site under Cellulitis
- ectopic or molar pregnancy OØ8.Ø
- acute LØ3.91
  - abdominal wall LØ3.321
  - ankle — see Lymphangitis, acute, lower limb
  - arm — see Lymphangitis, acute, upper limb
  - auricle (ear) — see Lymphangitis, acute, ear
  - axilla LØ3.12- ☑
  - back (any part) LØ3.322
  - buttock LØ3.327
  - cervical (meaning neck) LØ3.222
  - cheek (external) LØ3.212
  - chest wall LØ3.323
  - digit
    - finger — see Lymphangitis, acute, finger
    - toe — see Lymphangitis, acute, toe
  - ear (external) H6Ø.1- ☑
  - external auditory canal — see Lymphangitis, acute, ear
  - eyelid — see Abscess, eyelid
  - face NEC LØ3.212
  - finger (intrathecal) (periosteal) (subcutaneous) (subcuticular) LØ3.Ø2- ☑
  - foot — see Lymphangitis, acute, lower limb
  - gluteal (region) LØ3.327
  - groin LØ3.324
  - hand — see Lymphangitis, acute, upper limb
  - head NEC LØ3.891
    - face (any part, except ear, eye and nose) LØ3.212
  - heel — see Lymphangitis, acute, lower limb
  - hip — see Lymphangitis, acute, lower limb
  - jaw (region) LØ3.212
  - knee — see Lymphangitis, acute, lower limb
  - leg — see Lymphangitis, acute, lower limb
  - lower limb LØ3.12- ☑
    - toe — see Lymphangitis, acute, toe
  - navel LØ3.326
  - neck (region) LØ3.222
  - orbit, orbital — see Cellulitis, orbit
  - pectoral (region) LØ3.323
  - perineal, perineum LØ3.325
  - scalp (any part) LØ3.891
  - shoulder — see Lymphangitis, acute, upper limb
  - specified site NEC LØ3.898
  - thigh — see Lymphangitis, acute, lower limb
  - thumb (intrathecal) (periosteal) (subcutaneous) (subcuticular) — see Lymphangitis, acute, finger
  - toe (intrathecal) (periosteal) (subcutaneous) (subcuticular) LØ3.Ø4- ☑
  - trunk LØ3.329
    - abdominal wall LØ3.321
    - back (any part) LØ3.322
    - buttock LØ3.327
    - chest wall LØ3.323
    - groin LØ3.324
    - perineal, perineum LØ3.325
    - umbilicus LØ3.326
  - umbilicus LØ3.326

Lymphangitis — continued
- acute — continued
  - upper limb LØ3.12- ☑
    - axilla — see Lymphangitis, acute, axilla
    - finger — see Lymphangitis, acute, finger
    - thumb — see Lymphangitis, acute, finger
    - wrist — see Lymphangitis, acute, upper limb
- breast
  - gestational — see Mastitis, obstetric
- chancroidal A57
- chronic (any site) I89.1
- due to
  - Brugia (malayi) B74.1
    - timori B74.2
  - Wuchereria bancrofti B74.Ø
- following ectopic or molar pregnancy OØ8.89
- penis
  - acute N48.29
  - gonococcal (acute) (chronic) A54.Ø9
- puerperal, postpartum, childbirth O86.89
- strumous, tuberculous A18.2
- subacute (any site) I89.1
- tuberculous — see Tuberculosis, lymph gland

Lymphatic (vessel) — see condition

Lymphatism E32.8

Lymphectasia I89.Ø

Lymphedema (acquired) — see also Elephantiasis
- congenital Q82.Ø
- hereditary (chronic) (idiopathic) Q82.Ø
- postmastectomy I97.2
- praecox I89.Ø
- secondary I89.Ø
- surgical NEC I97.89
  - postmastectomy (syndrome) I97.2

Lymphoblastic — see condition

Lymphoblastoma (diffuse) — see Lymphoma, lymphoblastic (diffuse)
- giant follicular — see Lymphoma, lymphoblastic (diffuse)
- macrofollicular — see Lymphoma, lymphoblastic (diffuse)

Lymphocele I89.8

Lymphocytic
- chorioencephalitis (acute) (serous) A87.2
- choriomeningitis (acute) (serous) A87.2
- meningoencephalitis A87.2

Lymphocytoma, benign cutis L98.8

Lymphocytopenia D72.81Ø

Lymphocytosis (symptomatic) D72.82Ø
- infectious (acute) B33.8

Lymphoepithelioma — see Neoplasm, malignant, by site

Lymphogranuloma (malignant) — see also Lymphoma, Hodgkin
- chlamydial A55
- inguinale A55
- venereum (any site) (chlamydial) (with stricture of rectum) A55

Lymphogranulomatosis (malignant) — see also Lymphoma, Hodgkin
- benign (Boeck's sarcoid) (Schaumann's) D86.1

Lymphohistiocytosis, hemophagocytic (familial) D76.1

Lymphoid — see condition

Lymphoma (of) (malignant) C85.9Ø
- adult T-cell (HTLV-1-associated) (acute variant) (chronic variant) (lymphomatoid variant) (smouldering variant) C91.5- ☑
- anaplastic large cell
  - ALK-negative C84.7- ☑
  - ALK-positive C84.6- ☑
  - CD3Ø-positive C84.6- ☑
  - primary cutaneous C86.6
- angioimmunoblastic T-cell C86.5
- BALT C88.4
- B-cell C85.1- ☑
- blastic NK-cell C86.4
- blastic plasmacytoid dendritic cell neoplasm (BPDCN) C86.4
- B-precursor C83.5- ☑
- bronchial-associated lymphoid tissue [BALT-lymphoma] C88.4
- Burkitt (atypical) C83.7- ☑
- Burkitt-like C83.7- ☑
- centrocytic C83.1- ☑
- cutaneous follicle center C82.6- ☑
- cutaneous T-cell C84.A- ☑ (following C84.7)
- diffuse follicle center C82.5- ☑

Lymphoma — continued
- diffuse large cell C83.3- ☑
  - anaplastic C83.3- ☑
  - B-cell C83.3- ☑
  - CD3Ø-positive C83.3- ☑
  - centroblastic C83.3- ☑
  - immunoblastic C83.3- ☑
  - plasmablastic C83.3- ☑
  - subtype not specified C83.3- ☑
  - T-cell rich C83.3- ☑
- enteropathy-type (associated) (intestinal) T-cell C86.2
- extranodal marginal zone B-cell lymphoma of mucosa-associated lymphoid tissue [MALT-lymphoma] C88.4
- extranodal NK/T-cell, nasal type C86.Ø
- follicular C82.9- ☑
  - grade
    - I C82.Ø- ☑
    - II C82.1- ☑
    - III C82.2- ☑
    - IIIa C82.3- ☑
    - IIIb C82.4- ☑
  - specified NEC C82.8- ☑
- hepatosplenic T-cell (alpha-beta) (gamma-delta) C86.1
- histiocytic C85.9- ☑
  - true C96.A (following C96.6)
- Hodgkin C81.9 ☑
  - lymphocyte depleted (classical) C81.3- ☑
  - lymphocyte-rich (classical) C81.4- ☑
  - mixed cellularity (classical) C81.2- ☑
  - nodular
    - lymphocyte predominant C81.Ø- ☑
    - sclerosis (classical) C81.1- ☑
  - nodular sclerosis (classical) C81.1- ☑
  - specified NEC (classical) C81.7- ☑
- intravascular large B-cell C83.8- ☑
- Lennert's C84.4- ☑
- lymphoblastic (diffuse) C83.5- ☑
- lymphoblastic B-cell C83.5- ☑
- lymphoblastic T-cell C83.5- ☑
- lymphoepithelioid C84.4- ☑
- lymphoplasmacytic C83.Ø- ☑
  - with IgM-production C88.Ø
- MALT C88.4
- mantle cell C83.1- ☑
- mature T-cell NEC C84.4- ☑
- mature T/NK-cell C84.9- ☑
  - specified NEC C84.Z- ☑ (following C84.7)
- mediastinal (thymic) large B-cell C85.2- ☑
- Mediterranean C88.3
- mucosa-associated lymphoid tissue [MALT-lymphoma] C88.4
- NK/T cell C84.9- ☑
- nodal marginal zone C83.Ø- ☑
- non-follicular (diffuse) C83.9- ☑
  - specified NEC C83.8- ☑
- non-Hodgkin — see also Lymphoma, by type C85.9- ☑
  - specified NEC C85.8- ☑
- non-leukemic variant of B-CLL C83.Ø- ☑
- peripheral T-cell, not classified C84.4- ☑
- primary cutaneous
  - anaplastic large cell C86.6
  - CD3Ø-positive large T-cell C86.6
- primary effusion B-cell C83.8- ☑
- SALT C88.4
- skin-associated lymphoid tissue [SALT-lymphoma] C88.4
- small cell B-cell C83.Ø- ☑
- splenic marginal zone C83.Ø- ☑
- subcutaneous panniculitis-like T-cell C86.3
- T-precursor C83.5- ☑
- true histiocytic C96.A (following C96.6)

Lymphomatosis — see Lymphoma

Lymphopathia venereum, veneris A55

Lymphopenia D72.81Ø

Lymphoplasmacytic leukemia — see Leukemia, chronic lymphocytic, B-cell type

Lymphoproliferation, X-linked disease D82.3

Lymphoreticulosis, benign (of inoculation) A28.1

Lymphorrhea I89.8

Lymphosarcoma (diffuse) — see also Lymphoma C85.9- ☑

Lymphostasis I89.8

Lypemania — see Melancholia

Lysine and hydroxylysine metabolism disorder E72.3

Lyssa — see Rabies

M

Macacus ear Q17.3
Maceration, wet feet, tropical (syndrome) T69.02- ☑
MacLeod's syndrome J43.0
Macrocephalia, macrocephaly Q75.3
Macrocheilia, macrochilia (congenital) Q18.6
Macrocolon — see also Megacolon Q43.1
Macrocornea Q15.8
　with glaucoma Q15.0
Macrocytic — see condition
Macrocytosis D75.89
Macrodactylia, macrodactylism (fingers) (thumbs)
　Q74.0
　toes Q74.2
Macrodontia K00.2
Macrogenia M26.05
Macrogenitosomia (adrenal) (male) (praecox) E25.9
　congenital E25.0
Macroglobulinemia (idiopathic) (primary) C88.0
　monoclonal (essential) D47.2
　Waldenström C88.0
Macroglossia (congenital) Q38.2
　acquired K14.8
Macrognathia, macrognathism (congenital)
　(mandibular) (maxillary) M26.09
Macrogyria (congenital) Q04.8
Macrohydrocephalus — see Hydrocephalus
Macromastia — see Hypertrophy, breast
Macrophthalmos Q11.3
　in congenital glaucoma Q15.0
Macropsia H53.15
Macrosigmoid K59.39
　congenital Q43.2
Macrospondylitis , acromegalic E22.0
Macrostomia (congenital) Q18.4
Macrotia (external ear) (congenital) Q17.1
Macula
　cornea, corneal — see Opacity, cornea
　degeneration (atrophic) (exudative) (senile) — see also
　　Degeneration, macula
　　hereditary — see Dystrophy, retina
Maculae ceruleae B85.1
Maculopathy, toxic — see Degeneration, macula, toxic
Madarosis (eyelid) H02.729
　left H02.726
　　lower H02.725
　　upper H02.724
　right H02.723
　　lower H02.722
　　upper H02.721
Madelung's
　deformity (radius) Q74.0
　disease
　　radial deformity Q74.0
　　symmetrical lipomas, neck E88.89
Madness — see Psychosis
Madura
　foot B47.9
　　actinomycotic B47.1
　　mycotic B47.0
Maduromycosis B47.0
Maffucci's syndrome Q78.4
Magnesium metabolism disorder — see Disorder,
　metabolism, magnesium
Main en griffe (acquired) — see also Deformity, limb,
　clawhand
　congenital Q74.0
Maintenance (encounter for)
　antineoplastic chemotherapy Z51.11
　antineoplastic radiation therapy Z51.0
　methadone F11.20
Majocchi's
　disease L81.7
　granuloma B35.8
Major — see condition
Mal de los pintos — see Pinta
Mal de mer T75.3 ☑
Malabar itch (any site) B35.5
Malabsorption K90.9
　calcium K90.89
　carbohydrate K90.49
　disaccharide E73.9
　fat K90.49
　galactose E74.20
　glucose (-galactose) E74.39

Malabsorption — continued
　intestinal K90.9
　　specified NEC K90.89
　isomaltose E74.31
　lactose E73.9
　methionine E72.19
　monosaccharide E74.39
　postgastrectomy K91.2
　postsurgical K91.2
　protein K90.49
　starch K90.49
　sucrose E74.39
　syndrome K90.9
　　postsurgical K91.2
Malacia, bone (adult) M83.9
　juvenile — see Rickets
Malacoplakia
　bladder N32.89
　pelvis (kidney) N28.89
　ureter N28.89
　urethra N36.8
Malacosteon, juvenile — see Rickets
Maladaptation — see Maladjustment
Maladie de Roger Q21.0
Maladjustment
　conjugal Z63.0
　　involving divorce or estrangement Z63.5
　educational Z55.4
　family Z63.9
　marital Z63.0
　　involving divorce or estrangement Z63.5
　occupational NEC Z56.89
　simple, adult — see Disorder, adjustment
　situational — see Disorder, adjustment
　social Z60.9
　　due to
　　　acculturation difficulty Z60.3
　　　discrimination and persecution (perceived) Z60.5
　　　exclusion and isolation Z60.4
　　　life-cycle (phase of life) transition Z60.0
　　　rejection Z60.4
　　　specified reason NEC Z60.8
Malaise R53.81
Malakoplakia — see Malacoplakia
Malaria, malarial (fever) B54
　with
　　blackwater fever B50.8
　　　hemoglobinuric (bilious) B50.8
　　hemoglobinuria B50.8
　accidentally induced (therapeutically) — code by type
　　under Malaria
　algid B50.9
　cerebral B50.0 [G94]
　clinically diagnosed (without parasitological confirma-
　　tion) B54
　congenital NEC P37.4
　　falciparum P37.3
　congestion, congestive B54
　continued (fever) B50.9
　estivo-autumnal B50.9
　falciparum B50.9
　　with complications NEC B50.8
　　　cerebral B50.0 [G94]
　　　severe B50.8
　hemorrhagic B54
　malariae B52.9
　　with
　　　complications NEC B52.8
　　　glomerular disorder B52.0
　malignant (tertian) — see Malaria, falciparum
　mixed infections — code to first listed type in B50-B53
　ovale B53.0
　parasitologically confirmed NEC B53.8
　pernicious, acute — see Malaria, falciparum
　Plasmodium (P.)
　　falciparum NEC — see Malaria, falciparum
　　malariae NEC B52.9
　　　with Plasmodium
　　　　falciparum (and or vivax) — see Malaria, falci-
　　　　　parum
　　　　vivax — see also Malaria, vivax
　　　　　and falciparum — see Malaria, falciparum
　　ovale B53.0
　　　with Plasmodium malariae — see also Malaria,
　　　　malariae
　　　　and vivax — see also Malaria, vivax
　　　　　and falciparum — see Malaria, falciparum
　　simian B53.1

Malaria, malarial — continued
　Plasmodium — continued
　　simian — continued
　　　with Plasmodium malariae — see also Malar
　　　　malariae
　　　　and vivax — see also Malaria, vivax
　　　　　and falciparum — see Malaria, falciparu
　　　vivax NEC B51.9
　　　　with Plasmodium falciparum — see Malaria,
　　　　　ciparum
　quartan — see Malaria, malariae
　quotidian — see Malaria, falciparum
　recurrent B54
　remittent B54
　specified type NEC (parasitologically confirmed) B5
　spleen B54
　subtertian (fever) — see Malaria, falciparum
　tertian (benign) — see also Malaria, vivax
　　malignant B50.9
　tropical B50.9
　typhoid B54
　vivax B51.9
　　with
　　　complications NEC B51.8
　　　ruptured spleen B51.0
Malassez's disease (cystic) N50.89
Malassimilation K90.9
Maldescent, testis Q53.9
　bilateral Q53.20
　　abdominal Q53.211
　　perineal Q53.22
　unilateral Q53.10
　　abdominal Q53.111
　　perineal Q53.12
Maldevelopment — see also Anomaly
　brain Q07.9
　colon Q43.9
　hip Q74.2
　　congenital dislocation Q65.2
　　　bilateral Q65.1
　　　unilateral Q65.0- ☑
　mastoid process Q75.8
　middle ear Q16.4
　　except ossicles Q16.4
　　ossicles Q16.3
　ossicles Q16.3
　spine Q76.49
　toe Q74.2
Male type pelvis Q74.2
　with disproportion (fetopelvic) O33.3 ☑
　　causing obstructed labor O65.3
Malformation (congenital) — see also Anomaly
　adrenal gland Q89.1
　affecting multiple systems with skeletal changes N
　　Q87.5
　alimentary tract Q45.9
　　specified type NEC Q45.8
　　upper Q40.9
　　　specified type NEC Q40.8
　aorta Q25.40
　　absence Q25.41
　　aneurysm, congenital Q25.43
　　aplasia Q25.41
　　atresia Q25.29
　　　aortic arch Q25.21
　　coarctation (preductal) (postductal) Q25.1
　　dilatation, congenital Q25.44
　　hypoplasia Q25.42
　　patent ductus arteriosus Q25.0
　　specified type NEC Q25.49
　　stenosis Q25.1
　　　supravalvular Q25.3
　aortic valve Q23.9
　　specified NEC Q23.8
　arteriovenous, aneurysmatic (congenital) Q27.30
　　brain Q28.2
　　　ruptured I60.8
　　　　intracerebral I61.8
　　　　intraparenchymal I61.8
　　　　intraventricular I61.5
　　　　subarachnoid I60.8
　　cerebral — see also Malformation, arteriovenou
　　　brain Q28.2
　　peripheral Q27.30
　　　digestive system — see Angiodysplasia
　　　　congenital Q27.33
　　　lower limb Q27.32
　　　other specified site Q27.39

Malformation — *continued*
  arteriovenous, aneurysmatic — *continued*
    peripheral — *continued*
      renal vessel Q27.34
      upper limb Q27.31
    precerebral vessels (nonruptured) Q28.0
  auricle
    ear (congenital) Q17.3
      acquired H61.119
        left H61.112
          with right H61.113
        right H61.111
          with left H61.113
  bile duct Q44.5
  bladder Q64.79
    aplasia Q64.5
    diverticulum Q64.6
    exstrophy — *see* Exstrophy, bladder
    neck obstruction Q64.31
  bone Q79.9
    face Q75.9
      specified type NEC Q75.8
    skull Q75.9
      specified type NEC Q75.8
  brain (multiple) Q04.9
    arteriovenous Q28.2
    specified type NEC Q04.8
  branchial cleft Q18.2
  breast Q83.9
    specified type NEC Q83.8
  broad ligament Q50.6
  bronchus Q32.4
  bursa Q79.9
  cardiac
    chambers Q20.9
      specified type NEC Q20.8
    septum Q21.9
      specified type NEC Q21.8
  cerebral Q04.9
    vessels Q28.3
  cervix uteri Q51.9
    specified type NEC Q51.828
  Chiari
    Type I G93.5
    Type II Q07.01
  choroid (congenital) Q14.3
    plexus Q07.8
  circulatory system Q28.9
  cochlea Q16.5
  cornea Q13.4
  coronary vessels Q24.5
  corpus callosum (congenital) Q04.0
  diaphragm Q79.1
  digestive system NEC, specified type NEC Q45.8
  dura Q07.9
    brain Q04.9
    spinal Q06.9
  ear Q17.9
    causing impairment of hearing Q16.9
    external Q17.9
      accessory auricle Q17.0
      causing impairment of hearing Q16.9
        absence of
          auditory canal Q16.1
          auricle Q16.0
      macrotia Q17.1
      microtia Q17.2
      misplacement Q17.4
      misshapen NEC Q17.3
      prominence Q17.5
      specified type NEC Q17.8
    inner Q16.5
    middle Q16.4
      absence of eustachian tube Q16.2
      ossicles (fusion) Q16.3
    ossicles Q16.3
    specified type NEC Q17.8
  epididymis Q55.4
  esophagus Q39.9
    specified type NEC Q39.8
  eye Q15.9
    lid Q10.3
    specified NEC Q15.8
  fallopian tube Q50.6
  genital organ — *see* Anomaly, genitalia
  great
    artery Q25.9
      aorta — *see* Malformation, aorta

Malformation — *continued*
  great — *continued*
    artery — *continued*
      pulmonary artery — *see* Malformation, pul-
        monary, artery
      specified type NEC Q25.8
    vein Q26.9
      anomalous
        portal venous connection Q26.5
        pulmonary venous connection Q26.4
          partial Q26.3
          total Q26.2
      persistent left superior vena cava Q26.1
      portal vein-hepatic artery fistula Q26.6
      specified type NEC Q26.8
      vena cava stenosis, congenital Q26.0
  gum Q38.6
  hair Q84.2
  heart Q24.9
    specified type NEC Q24.8
  integument Q84.9
    specified type NEC Q84.8
  internal ear Q16.5
  intestine Q43.9
    specified type NEC Q43.8
  iris Q13.2
  joint Q74.9
    ankle Q74.2
    lumbosacral Q76.49
    sacroiliac Q74.2
    specified type NEC Q74.8
  kidney Q63.9
    accessory Q63.0
    giant Q63.3
    horseshoe Q63.1
    hydronephrosis Q62.0
    malposition Q63.2
    specified type NEC Q63.8
  lacrimal apparatus Q10.6
  lingual Q38.3
  lip Q38.0
  liver Q44.7
  lung Q33.9
  meninges or membrane (congenital) Q07.9
    cerebral Q04.8
    spinal (cord) Q06.9
  middle ear Q16.4
    ossicles Q16.3
  mitral valve Q23.9
    specified NEC Q23.8
  Mondini's (congenital) (malformation, cochlea) Q16.5
  mouth (congenital) Q38.6
  multiple types NEC Q89.7
  musculoskeletal system Q79.9
  myocardium Q24.8
  nail Q84.6
  nervous system (central) Q07.9
  nose Q30.9
    specified type NEC Q30.8
  optic disc Q14.2
  orbit Q10.7
  ovary Q50.39
  palate Q38.5
  parathyroid gland Q89.2
  pelvic organs or tissues NEC
    in pregnancy or childbirth O34.8- ☑
      causing obstructed labor O65.5
  penis Q55.69
    aplasia Q55.5
    curvature (lateral) Q55.61
    hypoplasia Q55.62
  pericardium Q24.8
  peripheral vascular system Q27.9
    specified type NEC Q27.8
  pharynx Q38.8
  precerebral vessels Q28.1
  prostate Q55.4
  pulmonary
    arteriovenous Q25.72
    artery Q25.9
      atresia Q25.5
      specified type NEC Q25.79
      stenosis Q25.6
    valve Q22.3
  renal artery Q27.2
  respiratory system Q34.9
  retina Q14.1
  scrotum — *see* Malformation, testis and scrotum
  seminal vesicles Q55.4

Malformation — *continued*
  sense organs NEC Q07.9
  skin Q82.9
  specified NEC Q89.8
  spinal
    cord Q06.9
    nerve root Q07.8
  spine Q76.49
    kyphosis — *see* Kyphosis, congenital
    lordosis — *see* Lordosis, congenital
  spleen Q89.09
  stomach Q40.3
    specified type NEC Q40.2
  teeth, tooth K00.9
  tendon Q79.9
  testis and scrotum Q55.20
    aplasia Q55.0
    hypoplasia Q55.1
    polyorchism Q55.21
    retractile testis Q55.22
    scrotal transposition Q55.23
    specified NEC Q55.29
  thorax, bony Q76.9
  throat Q38.8
  thyroid gland Q89.2
  tongue (congenital) Q38.3
    hypertrophy Q38.2
    tie Q38.1
  trachea Q32.1
  tricuspid valve Q22.9
    specified type NEC Q22.8
  umbilical cord NEC (complicating delivery) O69.89 ☑
  umbilicus Q89.9
  ureter Q62.8
    agenesis Q62.4
    duplication Q62.5
    malposition — *see* Malposition, congenital, ureter
    obstructive defect — *see* Defect, obstructive, ureter
    vesico-uretero-renal reflux Q62.7
  urethra Q64.79
    aplasia Q64.5
    duplication Q64.74
    posterior valves Q64.2
    prolapse Q64.71
    stricture Q64.32
  urinary system Q64.9
  uterus Q51.9
    specified type NEC Q51.818
  vagina Q52.4
  vas deferens Q55.4
    atresia Q55.3
  vascular system, peripheral Q27.9
  venous — *see* Anomaly, vein(s)
  vulva Q52.70

Malformation — *see also* Dysfunction
  cardiac electronic device T82.119 ☑
    electrode T82.110 ☑
    pulse generator T82.111 ☑
    specified type NEC T82.118 ☑
  catheter device NEC T85.618 ☑
    cystostomy T83.010 ☑
    dialysis (renal) (vascular) T82.41 ☑
      intraperitoneal T85.611 ☑
    infusion NEC T82.514 ☑
      cranial T85.610 ☑
      epidural T85.610 ☑
      intrathecal T85.610 ☑
      spinal T85.610 ☑
      subarachnoid T85.610 ☑
      subdural T85.610 ☑
    urinary — *see also* Breakdown, device, catheter
      T83.018 ☑
  colostomy K94.03
    valve K94.03
  cystostomy (stoma) N99.512
    catheter T83.010 ☑
  enteric stoma K94.13
  enterostomy K94.13
  esophagostomy K94.33
  gastroenteric K31.89
  gastrostomy K94.23
  ileostomy K94.13
    valve K94.13
  intrathecal infusion pump T85.615 ☑
  jejunostomy K94.13
  nervous system device, implant or graft, specified NEC
    T85.615 ☑

Malfunction — *continued*
pacemaker — *see* Malfunction, cardiac electronic device
prosthetic device, internal — *see* Complications, prosthetic device, by site, mechanical
tracheostomy J95.03
urinary device NEC — *see* Complication, genitourinary, device, urinary, mechanical
valve
colostomy K94.03
heart T82.09 ☑
ileostomy K94.13
vascular graft or shunt NEC — *see* Complication, cardiovascular device, mechanical, vascular
ventricular (communicating shunt) T85.01 ☑
Malherbe's tumor — *see* Neoplasm, skin, benign
Malibu disease L98.8
Malignancy — *see also* Neoplasm, malignant, by site
unspecified site (primary) C80.1
Malignant — *see* condition
Malingerer, malingering Z76.5
Mallet finger (acquired) — *see* Deformity, finger, mallet finger
congenital Q74.0
sequelae of rickets E64.3
Malleus A24.0
Mallory's bodies R89.7
Mallory-Weiss syndrome K22.6
Malnutrition E46
degree
first E44.1
mild (protein) E44.1
moderate (protein) E44.0
second E44.0
severe (protein-energy) E43
intermediate form E42
with
kwashiorkor (and marasmus) E42
marasmus E41
third E43
following gastrointestinal surgery K91.2
intrauterine
light-for-dates — *see* Light for dates
small-for-dates — *see* Small for dates
lack of care, or neglect (child) (infant) T76.02 ☑
confirmed T74.02 ☑
malignant E40
protein E46
calorie E46
mild E44.1
moderate E44.0
severe E43
intermediate form E42
with
kwashiorkor (and marasmus) E42
marasmus E41
energy E46
mild E44.1
moderate E44.0
severe E43
intermediate form E42
with
kwashiorkor (and marasmus) E42
marasmus E41
severe (protein-energy) E43
with
kwashiorkor (and marasmus) E42
marasmus E41
Malocclusion (teeth) M26.4
Angle's M26.219
class I M26.211
class II M26.212
class III M26.213
due to
abnormal swallowing M26.59
mouth breathing M26.59
tongue, lip or finger habits M26.59
temporomandibular (joint) M26.69
Malposition
cervix — *see* Malposition, uterus
congenital
adrenal (gland) Q89.1
alimentary tract Q45.8
lower Q43.8
upper Q40.8
aorta Q25.49
appendix Q43.8
arterial trunk Q20.0

Malposition — *continued*
congenital — *continued*
artery (peripheral) Q27.8
coronary Q24.5
digestive system Q27.8
lower limb Q27.8
pulmonary Q25.79
specified site NEC Q27.8
upper limb Q27.8
auditory canal Q17.8
causing impairment of hearing Q16.9
auricle (ear) Q17.4
causing impairment of hearing Q16.9
cervical Q18.2
biliary duct or passage Q44.5
bladder (mucosa) — *see* Exstrophy, bladder
brachial plexus Q07.8
brain tissue Q04.8
breast Q83.8
bronchus Q32.4
cecum Q43.8
clavicle Q74.0
colon Q43.8
digestive organ or tract NEC Q45.8
lower Q43.8
upper Q40.8
ear (auricle) (external) Q17.4
ossicles Q16.3
endocrine (gland) NEC Q89.2
epiglottis Q31.8
eustachian tube Q17.8
eye Q15.8
facial features Q18.8
fallopian tube Q50.6
finger(s) Q68.1
supernumerary Q69.0
foot Q66.9-
gallbladder Q44.1
gastrointestinal tract Q45.8
genitalia, genital organ(s) or tract
female Q52.8
external Q52.79
internal NEC Q52.8
male Q55.8
glottis Q31.8
hand Q68.1
heart Q24.8
dextrocardia Q24.0
with complete transposition of viscera Q89.3
hepatic duct Q44.5
hip (joint) Q65.89
intestine (large) (small) Q43.8
with anomalous adhesions, fixation or malrotation Q43.3
joint NEC Q68.8
kidney Q63.2
larynx Q31.8
limb Q68.8
lower Q68.8
upper Q68.8
liver Q44.7
lung (lobe) Q33.8
nail(s) Q84.6
nerve Q07.8
nervous system NEC Q07.8
nose, nasal (septum) Q30.8
organ or site not listed — *see* Anomaly, by site
ovary Q50.39
pancreas Q45.3
parathyroid (gland) Q89.2
patella Q74.1
peripheral vascular system Q27.8
pituitary (gland) Q89.2
respiratory organ or system NEC Q34.8
rib (cage) Q76.6
supernumerary in cervical region Q76.5
scapula Q74.0
shoulder Q74.0
spinal cord Q06.8
spleen Q89.09
sternum NEC Q76.7
stomach Q40.2
symphysis pubis Q74.2
thymus (gland) Q89.2
thyroid (gland) (tissue) Q89.2
cartilage Q31.8
toe(s) Q66.9- ☑
supernumerary Q69.2
tongue Q38.3

Malposition — *continued*
congenital — *continued*
trachea Q32.1
ureter Q62.60
deviation Q62.61
displacement Q62.62
ectopia Q62.63
specified type NEC Q62.69
uterus Q51.818
vein(s) (peripheral) Q27.8
great Q26.8
vena cava (inferior) (superior) Q26.8
device, implant or graft — *see also* Complications, by site and type, mechanical T85.628 ☑
arterial graft NEC — *see* Complication, cardiovascular device, mechanical, vascular
breast (implant) T85.42 ☑
catheter NEC T85.628 ☑
cystostomy T83.020 ☑
dialysis (renal) T82.42 ☑
intraperitoneal T85.621 ☑
infusion NEC T82.524 ☑
spinal (epidural) (subdural) T85.620 ☑
urinary — *see also* Displacement, device, catheter, urinary T83.028 ☑
electronic (electrode) (pulse generator) (stimulator)
bone T84.320 ☑
cardiac T82.129 ☑
electrode T82.120 ☑
pulse generator T82.121 ☑
specified type NEC T82.128 ☑
nervous system — *see* Complication, prosthetic device, mechanical, electronic nervous system stimulator
urinary — *see* Complication, genitourinary, device, urinary, mechanical
fixation, internal (orthopedic) NEC — *see* Complication, fixation device, mechanical
gastrointestinal — *see* Complications, prosthetic device, mechanical, gastrointestinal device
genital NEC T83.428 ☑
intrauterine contraceptive device (string) T83.32 ☑
penile prosthesis (cylinder) (implanted) (pump) (reservoir) T83.420 ☑
testicular prosthesis T83.421 ☑
heart NEC — *see* Complication, cardiovascular device, mechanical
joint prosthesis — *see* Complication, joint prosthesis, mechanical
ocular NEC — *see* Complications, prosthetic device, mechanical, ocular device
orthopedic NEC — *see* Complication, orthopedic, device, mechanical
specified NEC T85.628 ☑
urinary NEC — *see also* Complication, genitourinary, device, urinary, mechanical
graft T83.22 ☑
vascular NEC — *see* Complication, cardiovascular device, mechanical
ventricular intracranial shunt T85.02 ☑
fetus — *see* Pregnancy, complicated by (management affected by), presentation, fetal
gallbladder K82.8
gastrointestinal tract, congenital Q45.8
heart, congenital NEC Q24.8
joint prosthesis — *see* Complications, joint prosthesis, mechanical, displacement, by site
stomach K31.89
congenital Q40.2
tooth, teeth, fully erupted M26.30
uterus (acute) (acquired) (adherent) (asymptomatic) (postinfectional) (postpartal, old) N85.4
anteflexion or anteversion N85.4
congenital Q51.818
flexion N85.4
lateral — *see* Lateroversion, uterus
inversion N85.5
lateral (flexion) (version) — *see* Lateroversion, uterus
in pregnancy or childbirth — *see* subcategory O34.5 ☑
retroflexion or retroversion — *see* Retroversion, uterus
Malposture R29.3
Malrotation
cecum Q43.3
colon Q43.3

Malrotation — *continued*
  intestine Q43.3
  kidney Q63.2
Malta fever — *see* Brucellosis
Maltreatment
  adult
    abandonment
      confirmed T74.01 ☑
      suspected T76.01 ☑
    bullying
      confirmed T74.31 ☑
      suspected T76.31 ☑
    confirmed T74.91 ☑
    history of Z91.419
    intimidation (through social media)
      confirmed T74.31 ☑
      suspected T76.31 ☑
    neglect
      confirmed T74.01 ☑
      suspected T76.01 ☑
    physical abuse
      confirmed T74.11 ☑
      suspected T76.11 ☑
    psychological abuse
      confirmed T74.31 ☑
      history of Z91.411
      suspected T76.31 ☑
    sexual abuse
      confirmed T74.21 ☑
      suspected T76.21 ☑
    suspected T76.91 ☑
  child
    abandonment
      confirmed T74.02 ☑
      suspected T76.02 ☑
    bullying
      confirmed T74.32 ☑
      suspected T76.32 ☑
    confirmed T74.92 ☑
    history of — *see* History, personal (of), abuse
    intimidation (through social media)
      confirmed T74.32 ☑
      suspected T76.32 ☑
    neglect
      confirmed T74.02 ☑
      history of — *see* History, personal (of), abuse
      suspected T76.02 ☑
    physical abuse
      confirmed T74.12 ☑
      history of — *see* History, personal (of), abuse
      suspected T76.12 ☑
    psychological abuse
      confirmed T74.32 ☑
      history of — *see* History, personal (of), abuse
      suspected T76.32 ☑
    sexual abuse
      confirmed T74.22 ☑
      history of — *see* History, personal (of), abuse
      suspected T76.22 ☑
    suspected T76.92 ☑
  personal history of Z91.89
Maltworker's lung J67.4
Malunion, fracture — *see* Fracture, by site
Mammillitis N61.0
  puerperal, postpartum O91.02
Mammitis — *see* Mastitis
Mammogram (examination) Z12.39
  routine Z12.31
Mammoplasia N62
Management (of)
  bone conduction hearing device (implanted) Z45.320
  cardiac pacemaker NEC Z45.018
  cerebrospinal fluid drainage device Z45.41
  cochlear device (implanted) Z45.321
  contraceptive Z30.9
    specified NEC Z30.8
  implanted device Z45.9
    specified NEC Z45.89
  infusion pump Z45.1
  procreative Z31.9
    male factor infertility in female Z31.81
    specified NEC Z31.89
  prosthesis (external) — *see also* Fitting Z44.9
    implanted Z45.9
      specified NEC Z45.89
  renal dialysis catheter Z49.01
  vascular access device Z45.2

Mangled — *see* specified injury by site
Mania (monopolar) — *see also* Disorder, mood, manic episode
  with psychotic symptoms F30.2
  without psychotic symptoms F30.10
    mild F30.11
    moderate F30.12
    severe F30.13
  Bell's F30.8
  chronic (recurrent) F31.89
  hysterical F44.89
  puerperal F30.8
  recurrent F31.89
Manic depression F31.9
Manic-depressive insanity, psychosis, or syndrome — *see* Disorder, bipolar
Mannosidosis E77.1
Mansonelliasis, mansonellosis B74.4
Manson's
  disease B65.1
  schistosomiasis B65.1
Manual — *see* condition
Maple-bark-stripper's lung (disease) J67.6
Maple-syrup-urine disease E71.0
Marable's syndrome (celiac artery compression) I77.4
Marasmus E41
  due to malnutrition E41
  intestinal E41
  nutritional E41
  senile R54
  tuberculous NEC — *see* Tuberculosis
Marble
  bones Q78.2
  skin R23.8
Marburg virus disease A98.3
March
  fracture — *see* Fracture, traumatic, stress, by site
  hemoglobinuria D59.6
Marchesani (-Weill) **syndrome** Q87.0
Marchiafava (-Bignami) **syndrome or disease** G37.1
Marchiafava-Micheli syndrome D59.5
Marcus Gunn's syndrome Q07.8
Marfan's syndrome — *see* Syndrome, Marfan's
Marie-Bamberger disease — *see* Osteoarthropathy, hypertrophic, specified NEC
Marie-Charcot-Tooth neuropathic muscular atrophy G60.0
Marie's
  cerebellar ataxia (late-onset) G11.2
  disease or syndrome (acromegaly) E22.0
Marie-Strümpell arthritis, disease or spondylitis — *see* Spondylitis, ankylosing
Marion's disease (bladder neck obstruction) N32.0
Marital conflict Z63.0
Mark
  port wine Q82.5
  raspberry Q82.5
  strawberry Q82.5
  stretch L90.6
  tattoo L81.8
Marker heterochromatin — *see* Extra, marker chromosomes
Maroteaux-Lamy syndrome (mild) (severe) E76.29
Marrow (bone)
  arrest D61.9
  poor function D75.89
Marseilles fever A77.1
Marsh fever — *see* Malaria
Marshall's (hidrotic) **ectodermal dysplasia** Q82.4
Marsh's disease (exophthalmic goiter) E05.00
  with storm E05.01
Masculinization (female) **with adrenal hyperplasia** E25.9
  congenital E25.0
Masculinovoblastoma D27.- ☑
Masochism (sexual) F65.51
Mason's lung J62.8
Mass
  abdominal R19.00
    epigastric R19.06
    generalized R19.07
    left lower quadrant R19.04
    left upper quadrant R19.02
    periumbilic R19.05
    right lower quadrant R19.03
    right upper quadrant R19.01
    specified site NEC R19.09

Mass — *continued*
  breast — *see also* Lump, breast N63.0
  chest R22.2
  cystic — *see* Cyst
  ear H93.8- ☑
  head R22.0
  intra-abdominal (diffuse) (generalized) — *see* Mass, abdominal
  kidney N28.89
  liver R16.0
  localized (skin) R22.9
    chest R22.2
    head R22.0
    limb
      lower R22.4- ☑
      upper R22.3- ☑
    neck R22.1
    trunk R22.2
  lung R91.8
  malignant — *see* Neoplasm, malignant, by site
  neck R22.1
  pelvic (diffuse) (generalized) — *see* Mass, abdominal
  specified organ NEC — *see* Disease, by site
  splenic R16.1
  substernal thyroid — *see* Goiter
  superficial (localized) R22.9
  umbilical (diffuse) (generalized) R19.09
Massive — *see* condition
Mast cell
  disease, systemic tissue D47.02
  leukemia C94.3- ☑
  neoplasm
    malignant C96.20
      specified type NEC C96.29
    of uncertain behavior NEC D47.09
  sarcoma C96.22
  tumor D47.09
Mastalgia N64.4
Masters-Allen syndrome N83.8
Mastitis (acute) (diffuse) (nonpuerperal) (subacute) N61.0
  with abscess N61.1
  chronic (cystic) — *see* Mastopathy, cystic
  cystic (Schimmelbusch's type) — *see* Mastopathy, cystic
  fibrocystic — *see* Mastopathy, cystic
  infective N61.0
    newborn P39.0
  interstitial, gestational or puerperal — *see* Mastitis, obstetric
  neonatal (noninfective) P83.4
    infective P39.0
  obstetric (interstitial) (nonpurulent)
    associated with
      lactation O91.23
      pregnancy O91.21- ☑
      puerperium O91.22
    purulent
      associated with
        lactation O91.13
        pregnancy O91.11- ☑
        puerperium O91.12
  periductal — *see* Ectasia, mammary duct
  phlegmonous — *see* Mastopathy, cystic
  plasma cell — *see* Ectasia, mammary duct
  without abscess N61.0
Mastocytoma (extracutaneous) D47.09
  malignant C96.29
  solitary D47.01
Mastocytosis D47.09
  aggressive systemic C96.21
  cutaneous (diffuse) (maculopapular) D47.01
    congenital Q82.2
    of neonatal onset Q82.2
    of newborn onset Q82.2
  indolent systemic D47.02
  isolated bone marrow D47.02
  malignant C96.29
  systemic (indolent) (smoldering)
    with an associated hematological non-mast cell lineage disease (SM-AHNMD) D47.02
Mastodynia N64.4
Mastoid — *see* condition
Mastoidalgia — *see* subcategory H92.0 ☑
Mastoiditis (coalescent) (hemorrhagic) (suppurative) H70.9- ☑
  acute, subacute H70.00- ☑
    complicated NEC H70.09- ☑
    subperiosteal H70.01- ☑

Mastoiditis — continued
  chronic (necrotic) (recurrent) H70.1- ☑
  in (due to)
    infectious disease NEC B99 ☑ *[H75.0-]* ☑
    parasitic disease NEC B89 *[H75.0-]* ☑
    tuberculosis A18.03
  petrositis — see Petrositis
  postauricular fistula — see Fistula, postauricular
  specified NEC H70.89- ☑
  tuberculous A18.03
Mastopathy, mastopathia N64.9
  chronica cystica — see Mastopathy, cystic
  cystic (chronic) (diffuse) N60.1- ☑
    with epithelial proliferation N60.3- ☑
  diffuse cystic — see Mastopathy, cystic
  estrogenic, oestrogenica N64.89
  ovarian origin N64.89
Mastoplasia, mastoplastia N62
Masturbation (excessive) F98.8
Maternal care (for) — see Pregnancy (complicated by) (management affected by)
Mathieu's disease (leptospiral jaundice) A27.0
Mauclaire's disease or osteochondrosis — see Osteochondrosis, juvenile, hand, metacarpal
Maxcy's disease A75.2
Maxilla, maxillary — see condition
May (-Hegglin) **anomaly or syndrome** D72.0
McArdle (-Schmid)(-Pearson) **disease** (glycogen storage) E74.04
McCune-Albright syndrome Q78.1
McQuarrie's syndrome (idiopathic familial hypoglycemia) E16.2
Meadow's syndrome Q86.1
Measles (black) (hemorrhagic) (suppressed) B05.9
  with
    complications NEC B05.89
    encephalitis B05.0
    intestinal complications B05.4
    keratitis (keratoconjunctivitis) B05.81
    meningitis B05.1
    otitis media B05.3
    pneumonia B05.2
  French — see Rubella
  German — see Rubella
  Liberty — see Rubella
Meatitis, urethral — see Urethritis
Meatus, meatal — see condition
Meat-wrappers' asthma J68.9
Meckel-Gruber syndrome Q61.9
Meckel's diverticulitis, diverticulum (displaced) (hypertrophic) Q43.0
  malignant — see Table of Neoplasms, small intestine, malignant
Meconium
  ileus, newborn P76.0
    in cystic fibrosis E84.11
    meaning meconium plug (without cystic fibrosis) P76.0
  obstruction, newborn P76.0
    due to fecaliths P76.0
    in mucoviscidosis E84.11
  peritonitis P78.0
  plug syndrome (newborn) NEC P76.0
Median — see also condition
  arcuate ligament syndrome I77.4
  bar (prostate) (vesical orifice) — see Hyperplasia, prostate
  rhomboid glossitis K14.2
Mediastinal shift R93.89
Mediastinitis (acute) (chronic) J98.51
  syphilitic A52.73
  tuberculous A15.8
Mediastinopericarditis — see also Pericarditis
  acute I30.9
  adhesive I31.0
  chronic I31.8
    rheumatic I09.2
Mediastinum, mediastinal — see condition
Medicine poisoning — see Table of Drugs and Chemicals, by drug, poisoning
Mediterranean
  fever — see Brucellosis
    familial M04.1
    tick A77.1
  kala-azar B55.0
  leishmaniasis B55.0
  tick fever A77.1

Medulla — see condition
Medullary cystic kidney Q61.5
Medullated fibers
  optic (nerve) Q14.8
  retina Q14.1
Medulloblastoma
  desmoplastic C71.6
  specified site — see Neoplasm, malignant, by site
  unspecified site C71.6
Medulloepithelioma — see also Neoplasm, malignant, by site
  teratoid — see Neoplasm, malignant, by site
Medullomyoblastoma
  specified site — see Neoplasm, malignant, by site
  unspecified site C71.6
Meekeren-Ehlers-Danlos syndrome — see also Syndrome, Ehlers-Danlos Q79.69
Megacolon (acquired) (functional) (not Hirschsprung's disease) (in) K59.39
  Chagas' disease B57.32
  congenital, congenital (aganglionic) Q43.1
  Hirschsprung's (disease) Q43.1
  toxic NEC K59.31
    due to Clostridium difficile
      not specified as recurrent A04.72
      recurrent A04.71
Megaesophagus (functional) K22.0
  congenital Q39.5
  in (due to) Chagas' disease B57.31
Megalencephaly Q04.5
Megalerythema (epidemic) B08.3
Megaloappendix Q43.8
Megalocephalus, megalocephaly NEC Q75.3
Megalocornea Q15.8
  with glaucoma Q15.0
Megalocytic anemia D53.1
Megalodactylia (fingers) (thumbs) (congenital) Q74.0
  toes Q74.2
Megaloduodenum Q43.8
Megaloesophagus (functional) K22.0
  congenital Q39.5
Megalogastria (acquired) K31.89
  congenital Q40.2
Megalophthalmos Q11.3
Megalopsia H53.15
Megalosplenia — see Splenomegaly
Megaloureter N28.82
  congenital Q62.2
Megarectum K62.89
Megasigmoid K59.39
  congenital Q43.2
Megaureter N28.82
  congenital Q62.2
Megavitamin-B6 syndrome E67.2
Megrim — see Migraine
Meibomian
  cyst, infected — see Hordeolum
  gland — see condition
  sty, stye — see Hordeolum
Meibomitis — see Hordeolum
Meige-Milroy disease (chronic hereditary edema) Q82.0
Meige's syndrome Q82.0
Melalgia, nutritional E53.8
Meiancholia F32.9
  climacteric (single episode) F32.89
    recurrent episode F33.8
  hypochondriac F45.29
  intermittent (single episode) F32.89
    recurrent episode F33.8
  involutional (single episode) F32.89
    recurrent episode F33.8
  menopausal (single episode) F32.89
    recurrent episode F33.8
  puerperal F32.89
  reactive (emotional stress or trauma) F32.3
  recurrent F33.9
  senile F03 ☑
  stuporous (single episode) F32.89
    recurrent episode F33.8
Melanemia R79.89
Melanoameloblastoma — see Neoplasm, bone, benign
Melanoblastoma — see Melanoma
Melanocarcinoma — see Melanoma
Melanocytoma, eyeball D31.9- ☑
Melanocytosis, neurocutaneous Q82.8
Melanoderma, melanodermia L81.4
Melanodontia, infantile K03.89

Melanodontoclasia K03.89
Melanoepithelioma — see Melanoma
Melanoma (malignant) C43.9
  acral lentiginous, malignant — see Melanoma, skin, by site
  amelanotic — see Melanoma, skin, by site
  balloon cell — see Melanoma, skin, by site
  benign — see Nevus
  desmoplastic, malignant — see Melanoma, skin, by site
  epithelioid cell — see Melanoma, skin, by site
    with spindle cell, mixed — see Melanoma, skin, by site
  in
    giant pigmented nevus — see Melanoma, skin, by site
    Hutchinson's melanotic freckle — see Melanoma, skin, by site
    junctional nevus — see Melanoma, skin, by site
    precancerous melanosis — see Melanoma, skin, by site
  in situ D03.9
    abdominal wall D03.59
    ala nasi D03.39
    ankle D03.7- ☑
    anus, anal (margin) (skin) D03.51
    arm D03.6- ☑
    auditory canal D03.2- ☑
    auricle (ear) D03.2- ☑
    auricular canal (external) D03.2- ☑
    axilla, axillary fold D03.59
    back D03.59
    breast D03.52
    brow D03.39
    buttock D03.59
    canthus (eye) D03.1- ☑
    cheek (external) D03.39
    chest wall D03.59
    chin D03.39
    choroid D03.8
    conjunctiva D03.8
    ear (external) D03.2- ☑
    external meatus (ear) D03.2- ☑
    eye D03.8
    eyebrow D03.39
    eyelid (lower) (upper) D03.1- ☑
    face D03.30
      specified NEC D03.39
    female genital organ (external) NEC D03.8
    finger D03.6- ☑
    flank D03.59
    foot D03.7- ☑
    forearm D03.6- ☑
    forehead D03.39
    foreskin D03.8
    gluteal region D03.59
    groin D03.59
    hand D03.6- ☑
    heel D03.7- ☑
    helix D03.2- ☑
    hip D03.7- ☑
    interscapular region D03.59
    iris D03.8
    jaw D03.39
    knee D03.7- ☑
    labium (majus) (minus) D03.8
    lacrimal gland D03.8
    leg D03.7- ☑
    lip (lower) (upper) D03.0
    lower limb NEC D03.7- ☑
    male genital organ (external) NEC D03.8
    nail D03.9
      finger D03.6- ☑
      toe D03.7- ☑
    neck D03.4
    nose (external) D03.39
    orbit D03.8
    penis D03.8
    perianal skin D03.51
    perineum D03.51
    pinna D03.2- ☑
    popliteal fossa or space D03.7- ☑
    prepuce D03.8
    pudendum D03.8
    retina D03.8
    retrobulbar D03.8
    scalp D03.4

☑ Additional Character Required — Refer to the Tabular List for Character Selection   ▽ Subterms under main terms may continue to next column or page

Melanoma — *continued*
  in situ — *continued*
    scrotum D03.8
    shoulder D03.6- ☑
    specified site NEC D03.8
    submammary fold D03.52
    temple D03.39
    thigh D03.7- ☑
    toe D03.7- ☑
    trunk NEC D03.59
    umbilicus D03.59
    upper limb NEC D03.6- ☑
    vulva D03.8
  juvenile — *see* Nevus
  malignant, of soft parts except skin — *see* Neoplasm, connective tissue, malignant
  metastatic
    breast C79.81
    genital organ C79.82
    specified site NEC C79.89
  neurotropic, malignant — *see* Melanoma, skin, by site
  nodular — *see* Melanoma, skin, by site
  regressing, malignant — *see* Melanoma, skin, by site
  skin C43.9
    abdominal wall C43.59
    ala nasi C43.31
    ankle C43.7- ☑
    anus, anal (skin) C43.51
    arm C43.6- ☑
    auditory canal (external) C43.2- ☑
    auricle (ear) C43.2- ☑
    auricular canal (external) C43.2- ☑
    axilla, axillary fold C43.59
    back C43.59
    breast (female) (male) C43.52
    brow C43.39
    buttock C43.59
    canthus (eye) C43.1- ☑
    cheek (external) C43.39
    chest wall C43.59
    chin C43.39
    ear (external) C43.2- ☑
    elbow C43.6- ☑
    external meatus (ear) C43.2- ☑
    eyebrow C43.39
    eyelid (lower) (upper) C43.1- ☑
    face C43.30
      specified NEC C43.39
    female genital organ (external) NEC C51.9
    finger C43.6- ☑
    flank C43.59
    foot C43.7- ☑
    forearm C43.6- ☑
    forehead C43.39
    foreskin C60.0
    glabella C43.39
    gluteal region C43.59
    groin C43.59
    hand C43.6- ☑
    heel C43.7- ☑
    helix C43.2- ☑
    hip C43.7- ☑
    interscapular region C43.59
    jaw (external) C43.39
    knee C43.7- ☑
    labium C51.9
      majus C51.0
      minus C51.1
    leg C43.7- ☑
    lip (lower) (upper) C43.0
    lower limb NEC C43.7- ☑
    male genital organ (external) NEC C63.9
    nail
      finger C43.6- ☑
      toe C43.7- ☑
    nasolabial groove C43.39
    nates C43.59
    neck C43.4
    nose (external) C43.31
    overlapping site C43.8
    palpebra C43.1- ☑
    penis C60.9
    perianal skin C43.51
    perineum C43.51
    pinna C43.2- ☑
    popliteal fossa or space C43.7- ☑
    prepuce C60.0

Melanoma — *continued*
  skin — *continued*
    pudendum C51.9
    scalp C43.4
    scrotum C63.2
    shoulder C43.6- ☑
    skin NEC C43.9
    submammary fold C43.52
    temple C43.39
    thigh C43.7- ☑
    toe C43.7- ☑
    trunk NEC C43.59
    umbilicus C43.59
    upper limb NEC C43.6- ☑
    vulva C51.9
      overlapping sites C51.8
  spindle cell
    with epithelioid, mixed — *see* Melanoma, skin, by site
    type A C69.4- ☑
    type B C69.4- ☑
  superficial spreading — *see* Melanoma, skin, by site
Melanosarcoma — *see also* Melanoma
  epithelioid cell — *see* Melanoma
Melanosis L81.4
  addisonian E27.1
    tuberculous A18.7
  adrenal E27.1
  colon K63.89
  conjunctiva — *see* Pigmentation, conjunctiva
    congenital Q13.89
  cornea (presenile) (senile) — *see also* Pigmentation, cornea
    congenital Q13.4
  eye NEC H57.89
    congenital Q15.8
  lenticularis progressiva Q82.1
  liver K76.89
  precancerous — *see also* Melanoma, in situ
    malignant melanoma in — *see* Melanoma
  Riehl's L81.4
  sclera H15.89
    congenital Q13.89
  suprarenal E27.1
  tar L81.4
  toxic L81.4
Melanuria R82.998
MELAS syndrome E88.41
Melasma L81.1
  adrenal (gland) E27.1
  suprarenal (gland) E27.1
Melena K92.1
  with ulcer — *code by* site under Ulcer, with hemorrhage K27.4
  due to swallowed maternal blood P78.2
  newborn, neonatal P54.1
    due to swallowed maternal blood P78.2
Meleney's
  gangrene (cutaneous) — *see* Ulcer, skin
  ulcer (chronic undermining) — *see* Ulcer, skin
Melioidosis A24.9
  acute A24.1
  chronic A24.2
  fulminating A24.1
  pneumonia A24.1
  pulmonary (chronic) A24.2
    acute A24.1
    subacute A24.2
  sepsis A24.1
  specified NEC A24.3
  subacute A24.2
Melitensis, febris A23.0
Melkersson (-Rosenthal) **syndrome** G51.2
Mellitus, diabetes — *see* Diabetes
Melorheostosis (bone) — *see* Disorder, bone, density and structure, specified NEC
Meloschisis Q18.4
Melotia Q17.4
Membrana
  capsularis lentis posterior Q13.89
  epipapillaris Q14.2
Membranacea placenta O43.19- ☑
Membranaceous uterus N85.8
Membrane(s), membranous — *see also* condition
  cyclitic — *see* Membrane, pupillary
  folds, congenital — *see* Web
  Jackson's Q43.3
  over face of newborn P28.9

Membrane(s), membranous — *continued*
  premature rupture — *see* Rupture, membranes, premature
  pupillary H21.4- ☑
    persistent Q13.89
  retained (with hemorrhage) (complicating delivery) O72.2
    without hemorrhage O73.1
  secondary cataract –– *see* Cataract, secondary
  unruptured (causing asphyxia) — *see* Asphyxia, newborn
  vitreous — *see* Opacity, vitreous, membranes and strands
Membranitis — *see* Chorioamnionitis
Memory disturbance, lack or loss — *see also* Amnesia
  mild, following organic brain damage F06.8
Menadione deficiency E56.1
Menarche
  delayed E30.0
  precocious E30.1
Mendacity, pathologic F60.2
Mendelson's syndrome (due to anesthesia) J95.4
  in labor and delivery O74.0
  in pregnancy O29.01- ☑
  obstetric O74.0
  postpartum, puerperal O89.01
Ménétrier's disease or syndrome K29.60
  with bleeding K29.61
Ménière's disease, syndrome or vertigo H81.0- ☑
Meninges, meningeal — *see* condition
Meningioma — *see also* Neoplasm, meninges, benign
  angioblastic — *see* Neoplasm, meninges, benign
  angiomatous — *see* Neoplasm, meninges, benign
  endotheliomatous — *see* Neoplasm, meninges, benign
  fibroblastic — *see* Neoplasm, meninges, benign
  fibrous — *see* Neoplasm, meninges, benign
  hemangioblastic — *see* Neoplasm, meninges, benign
  hemangiopericytic — *see* Neoplasm, meninges, benign
  malignant — *see* Neoplasm, meninges, malignant
  meningiothelial — *see* Neoplasm, meninges, benign
  meningotheliomatous — *see* Neoplasm, meninges, benign
  mixed — *see* Neoplasm, meninges, benign
  multiple — *see* Neoplasm, meninges, uncertain behavior
  papillary — *see* Neoplasm, meninges, uncertain behavior
  psammomatous — *see* Neoplasm, meninges, benign
  syncytial — *see* Neoplasm, meninges, benign
  transitional — *see* Neoplasm, meninges, benign
Meningiomatosis (diffuse) — *see* Neoplasm, meninges, uncertain behavior
Meningism — *see* Meningismus
Meningismus (infectional) (pneumococcal) R29.1
  due to serum or vaccine R29.1
  influenzal — *see* Influenza, with, manifestations NEC
Meningitis (basal) (basic) (brain) (cerebral) (cervical) (congestive) (diffuse) (hemorrhagic) (infantile) (membranous) (metastatic) (nonspecific) (pontine) (progressive) (simple) (spinal) (subacute) (sympathetic) (toxic) G03.9
  abacterial G03.0
  actinomycotic A42.81
  adenoviral A87.1
  arbovirus A87.8
  aseptic (acute) G03.0
  bacterial G00.9
    Escherichia coli (E. coli) G00.8
    Friedländer (bacillus) G00.8
    gram-negative G00.9
    H. influenzae G00.0
    Klebsiella G00.8
    pneumococcal G00.1
    specified organism NEC G00.8
    staphylococcal G00.3
    streptococcal (acute) G00.2
  benign recurrent (Mollaret) G03.2
  candidal B37.5
  caseous (tuberculous) A17.0
  cerebrospinal A39.0
  chronic NEC G03.1
  clear cerebrospinal fluid NEC G03.0
  coxsackievirus A87.0
  cryptococcal B45.1
  diplococcal (gram positive) A39.0
  echovirus A87.0
  enteroviral A87.0
  eosinophilic B83.2

Meningitis — continued
  epidemic NEC A39.Ø
  Escherichia coli (E. coli) GØØ.8
  fibrinopurulent GØØ.9
    specified organism NEC GØØ.8
  Friedländer (bacillus) GØØ.8
  gonococcal A54.81
  gram-negative cocci GØØ.9
  gram-positive cocci GØØ.9
  H. influenzae GØØ.Ø
  Haemophilus (influenzae) GØØ.Ø
  in (due to)
    adenovirus A87.1
    African trypanosomiasis B56.9 [GØ2]
    anthrax A22.8
    bacterial disease NEC A48.8 [GØ1]
    Chagas' disease (chronic) B57.41
    chickenpox BØ1.Ø
    coccidioidomycosis B38.4
    Diplococcus pneumoniae GØØ.1
    enterovirus A87.Ø
    herpes (simplex) virus BØØ.3
      zoster BØ2.1
    infectious mononucleosis B27.92
    leptospirosis A27.81
    Listeria monocytogenes A32.11
    Lyme disease A69.21
    measles BØ5.1
    mumps (virus) B26.1
    neurosyphilis (late) A52.13
    parasitic disease NEC B89 [GØ2]
    poliovirus A8Ø.9 [GØ2]
    preventive immunization, inoculation or vaccination
        GØ3.8
    rubella BØ6.Ø2
    Salmonella infection AØ2.21
    specified cause NEC GØ3.8
    Streptococcal pneumoniae GØØ.1
    typhoid fever AØ1.Ø1
    varicella BØ1.Ø
    viral disease NEC A87.8
    whooping cough A37.9Ø
    zoster BØ2.1
  infectious GØØ.9
  influenzal (H. influenzae) GØØ.Ø
  Klebsiella GØØ.8
  leptospiral (aseptic) A27.81
  lymphocytic (acute) (benign) (serous) A87.2
  meningococcal A39.Ø
  Mima polymorpha GØØ.8
  Mollaret (benign recurrent) GØ3.2
  monilial B37.5
  mycotic NEC B49 [GØ2]
  Neisseria A39.Ø
  nonbacterial GØ3.Ø
  nonpyogenic NEC GØ3.Ø
  ossificans G96.19
  pneumococcal streptococcus pneumoniae GØØ.1
  poliovirus A8Ø.9 [GØ2]
  postmeasles BØ5.1
  purulent GØØ.9
    specified organism NEC GØØ.8
  pyogenic GØØ.9
    specified organism NEC GØØ.8
  Salmonella (arizonae) (Cholerae-Suis) (enteritidis) (ty-
        phimurium) AØ2.21
  septic GØØ.9
    specified organism NEC GØØ.8
  serosa circumscripta NEC GØ3.Ø
  serous NEC G93.2
  specified organism NEC GØØ.8
  sporotrichosis B42.81
  staphylococcal GØØ.3
  sterile GØ3.Ø
  Streptococcal (acute) GØØ.2
    pneumoniae GØØ.1
  suppurative GØØ.9
    specified organism NEC GØØ.8
  syphilitic (late) (tertiary) A52.13
    acute A51.41
    congenital A5Ø.41
    secondary A51.41
  Torula histolytica (cryptococcal) B45.1
  traumatic (complication of injury) T79.8 ☑
  tuberculous A17.Ø
  typhoid AØ1.Ø1
  viral NEC A87.9
  Yersinia pestis A2Ø.3

Meningocele (spinal) — see also Spina bifida
  with hydrocephalus — see Spina bifida, by site, with
        hydrocephalus
  acquired (traumatic) G96.19
  cerebral — see Encephalocele
Meningocerebritis — see Meningoencephalitis
Meningococcemia A39.4
  acute A39.2
  chronic A39.3
Meningococcus, meningococcal — see also condition
    A39.9
  adrenalitis, hemorrhagic A39.1
  carrier (suspected) of Z22.31
  meningitis (cerebrospinal) A39.Ø
Meningoencephalitis — see also Encephalitis GØ4.9Ø
  acute NEC — see also Encephalitis, viral A86
  bacterial NEC GØ4.2
  California A83.5
  diphasic A84.1
  eosinophilic B83.2
  epidemic A39.81
  herpesviral, herpetic BØØ.4
    due to herpesvirus 6 B1Ø.Ø1
    due to herpesvirus 7 B1Ø.Ø9
    specified NEC B1Ø.Ø9
  in (due to)
    blastomycosis NEC B4Ø.81
    diseases classified elsewhere GØ5.3
    free-living amebae B6Ø.2
    H. influenzae GØØ.Ø
    Hemophilus influenzae (H .influenzae) GØØ.Ø
    herpes BØØ.4
      due to herpesvirus 6 B1Ø.Ø1
      due to herpesvirus 7 B1Ø.Ø9
      specified NEC B1Ø.Ø9
    Lyme disease A69.22
    mercury — see subcategory T56.1 ☑
    mumps B26.2
    Naegleria (amebae) (organisms) (fowleri) B6Ø.2
    Parastrongylus cantonensis B83.2
    toxoplasmosis (acquired) B58.2
      congenital P37.1
  infectious (acute) (viral) A86
  influenzal (H. influenzae) GØØ.Ø
  Listeria monocytogenes A32.12
  lymphocytic (serous) A87.2
  mumps B26.2
  parasitic NEC B89 [GØ5.3]
  pneumococcal GØ4.2
  primary amebic B6Ø.2
  specific (syphilitic) A52.14
  specified organism NEC GØ4.81
  staphylococcal GØ4.2
  streptococcal GØ4.2
  syphilitic A52.14
  toxic NEC G92
    due to mercury — see subcategory T56.1 ☑
  tuberculous A17.82
  virus NEC A86
Meningoencephalocele — see also Encephalocele
  syphilitic A52.19
    congenital A5Ø.49
Meningoencephalomyelitis — see also Meningoen-
    cephalitis
  acute NEC (viral) A86
    disseminated GØ4.ØØ
      postimmunization or postvaccination GØ4.Ø2
      postinfectious GØ4.Ø1
  due to
    actinomycosis A42.82
    Torula B45.1
    Toxoplasma or toxoplasmosis (acquired) B58.2
      congenital P37.1
  postimmunization or postvaccination GØ4.Ø2
Meningoencephalomyelopathy G96.9
Meningoencephalopathy G96.9
Meningomyelitis — see also Meningoencephalitis
  bacterial NEC GØ4.2
  blastomycotic NEC B4Ø.81
  cryptococcal B45.1
  in diseases classified elsewhere GØ5.4
  meningococcal A39.81
  syphilitic A52.14
  tuberculous A17.82
Meningomyelocele — see also Spina bifida
  syphilitic A52.19
Meningomyeloneuritis — see Meningoencephalitis
Meningoradiculitis — see Meningitis

Meningovascular — see condition
Menkes' disease or syndrome E83.Ø9
  meaning maple-syrup-urine disease E71.Ø
Menometrorrhagia N92.1
Menopause, menopausal (asymptomatic) (state) Z78.
  arthritis (any site) NEC — see Arthritis, specified form
    NEC
  bleeding N92.4
  depression (single episode) F32.89
    agitated (single episode) F32.2
      recurrent episode F33.9
    psychotic (single episode) F32.89
      recurrent episode F33.9
    recurrent episode F33.8
  melancholia (single episode) F32.89
    recurrent episode F33.8
  paranoid state F22
  premature E28.319
    asymptomatic E28.319
      postirradiation E89.4Ø
      postsurgical E89.4Ø
    symptomatic E28.31Ø
      postirradiation E89.41
      postsurgical E89.41
  psychosis NEC F28
  symptomatic N95.1
  toxic polyarthritis NEC — see Arthritis, specified form
    NEC
Menorrhagia (primary) N92.Ø
  climacteric N92.4
    menopausal N92.4
  menopausal N92.4
  perimenopausal N92.4
  postclimacteric N95.Ø
  postmenopausal N95.Ø
  preclimacteric or premenopausal N92.4
  pubertal (menses retained) N92.2
Menostaxis N92.Ø
Menses, retention N94.89
Menstrual — see Menstruation
Menstruation
  absent — see Amenorrhea
  anovulatory N97.Ø
  cycle, irregular N92.6
  delayed N91.Ø
  disorder N93.9
    psychogenic F45.8
  during pregnancy O2Ø.8
  excessive (with regular cycle) N92.Ø
    with irregular cycle N92.1
    at puberty N92.2
  frequent N92.Ø
  infrequent — see Oligomenorrhea
  irregular N92.6
    specified NEC N92.5
  latent N92.5
  membranous N92.5
  painful — see also Dysmenorrhea N94.6
    primary N94.4
    psychogenic F45.8
    secondary N94.5
  passage of clots N92.Ø
  precocious E3Ø.1
  protracted N92.5
  rare — see Oligomenorrhea
  retained N94.89
  retrograde N92.5
  scanty — see Oligomenorrhea
  suppression N94.89
  vicarious (nasal) N94.89
Mental — see also condition
  deficiency — see Disability, intellectual
  deterioration — see Psychosis
  disorder — see Disorder, mental
  exhaustion F48.8
  insufficiency (congenital) — see Disability, intellectu
  observation without need for further medical care
    ZØ3.89
  retardation — see Disability, intellectual
  subnormality — see Disability, intellectuall
  upset — see Disorder, mental
Meralgia paresthetica G57.1- ☑
Mercurial — see condition
Mercurialism — see subcategory T56.1 ☑
Merkel cell tumor — see Carcinoma, Merkel cell
Merocele — see Hernia, femoral
Meromelia
  lower limb — see Defect, reduction, lower limb

Migraine — continued
  with aura — continued
    persistent — continued
      with cerebral infarction — continued
        not intractable G43.609
          with status migrainosus G43.601
          without status migrainosus G43.609
        without refractory migraine G43.609
          with status migrainosus G43.601
          without status migrainosus G43.609
      without cerebral infarction G43.509
        with refractory migraine G43.519
          with status migrainosus G43.511
          without status migrainosus G43.519
        intractable G43.519
          with status migrainosus G43.511
          without status migrainosus G43.519
        not intractable G43.509
          with status migrainosus G43.501
          without status migrainosus G43.509
        without refractory migraine G43.509
          with status migrainosus G43.501
          without status migrainosus G43.509
    without mention of refractory migraine G43.109
      with status migrainosus G43.101
      without status migrainosus G43.109
  abdominal G43.D0 (following G43.7)
    with refractory migraine G43.D1 (following G43.7)
    intractable G43.D1 (following G43.7)
    not intractable G43.D0 (following G43.7)
    without refractory migraine G43.D0 (following G43.7)
  basilar — see Migraine, with aura
  classical — see Migraine, with aura
  common — see Migraine, without aura
  complicated G43.109
  equivalents — see Migraine, with aura
  familiar — see Migraine, hemiplegic
  hemiplegic G43.409
    with refractory migraine G43.419
      with status migrainosus G43.411
      without status migrainosus G43.419
    intractable G43.419
      with status migrainosus G43.411
      without status migrainosus G43.419
    not intractable G43.409
      with status migrainosus G43.401
      without status migrainosus G43.409
    without refractory migraine G43.409
      with status migrainosus G43.401
      without status migrainosus G43.409
  intractable G43.919
    with status migrainosus G43.911
    without status migrainosus G43.919
  menstrual G43.829
    with refractory migraine G43.839
      with status migrainosus G43.831
      without status migrainosus G43.839
    intractable G43.839
      with status migrainosus G43.831
      without status migrainosus G43.839
    not intractable 4G43.829
      with status migrainosus G43.821
      without status migrainosus G43.829
    without refractory migraine G43.829
      with status migrainosus G43.821
      without status migrainosus G43.829
  menstrually related — see Migraine, menstrual
  not intractable G43.909
    with status migrainosus G43.901
    without status migrainosus G43.919
  ophthalmoplegic G43.B0 (following G43.7)
    with refractory migraine G43.B1 (following G43.7)
    intractable G43.B1 (following G43.7)
    not intractable G43.B0 (following G43.7)
    without refractory migraine G43.B0 (following G43.7)
  persistent aura (with, without) cerebral infarction —
    see Migraine, with aura, persistent
  preceded or accompanied by transient focal neurolog-
    ical phenomena — see Migraine, with aura
  pre-menstrual — see Migraine, menstrual
  pure menstrual — see Migraine, menstrual
  retinal — see Migraine, with aura
  specified NEC G43.809
    intractable G43.819
      with status migrainosus G43.811
      without status migrainosus G43.819
    not intractable G43.809
      with status migrainosus G43.801

Migraine — continued
  specified — continued
    not intractable — continued
      without status migrainosus G43.809
  sporadic — see Migraine, hemiplegic
  transformed — see Migraine, without aura, chronic
  triggered seizures — see Migraine, with aura
  without aura G43.009
    with refractory migraine G43.019
      with status migrainosus G43.011
      without status migrainosus G43.019
    chronic G43.709
      with refractory migraine G43.719
        with status migrainosus G43.711
        without status migrainosus G43.719
      intractable
        with status migrainosus G43.711
        without status migrainosus G43.719
      not intractable
        with status migrainosus G43.701
        without status migrainosus G43.709
      without refractory migraine G43.709
        with status migrainosus G43.701
        without status migrainosus G43.709
    intractable
      with status migrainosus G43.011
      without status migrainosus G43.019
    not intractable
      with status migrainosus G43.001
      without status migrainosus G43.009
    without mention of refractory migraine G43.009
      with status migrainosus G43.001
      without status migrainosus G43.009
  without refractory migraine G43.909
    with status migrainosus G43.901
    without status migrainosus G43.919
Migrant, social Z59.0
Migration, anxiety concerning Z60.3
Migratory, migrating — see also condition
  person Z59.0
  testis Q55.29
Mikity-Wilson disease or syndrome P27.0
Mikulicz' disease or syndrome K11.8
Miliaria L74.3
  alba L74.1
  apocrine L75.2
  crystallina L74.1
  profunda L74.2
  rubra L74.0
  tropicalis L74.2
Miliary — see condition
Milium L72.0
  colloid L57.8
Milk
  crust L21.0
  excessive secretion O92.6
  poisoning — see Poisoning, food, noxious
  retention O92.79
  sickness — see Poisoning, food, noxious
  spots I31.0
Milk-alkali disease or syndrome E83.52
Milk-leg (deep vessels) (nonpuerperal) — see Embolism,
  vein, lower extremity
  complicating pregnancy O22.3- ☑
  puerperal, postpartum, childbirth O87.1
Milkman's disease or syndrome M83.8
Milky urine — see Chyluria
Millard-Gubler (-Foville) **paralysis or syndrome** G46.3
Millar's asthma J38.5
Miller Fisher syndrome G61.0
Mills' disease — see Hemiplegia
Millstone maker's pneumoconiosis J62.8
Milroy's disease (chronic hereditary edema) Q82.0
Minamata disease T56.1 ☑
Miners' asthma or lung J60
Minkowski-Chauffard syndrome — see Spherocytosis
Minor — see condition
Minor's disease (hematomyelia) G95.19
Minot's disease (hemorrhagic disease), newborn P53
Minot-von Willebrand-Jurgens disease or syndrome
  (angiohemophilia) D68.0
Minus (and plus) **hand** (intrinsic) — see Deformity, limb,
  specified type NEC, forearm
Miosis (pupil) H57.03
Mirizzi's syndrome (hepatic duct stenosis) K83.1
Mirror writing F81.0

Misadventure (of) (prophylactic) (therapeutic) — see
  also Complications T88.9 ☑
  administration of insulin (by accident) — see subcate-
    gory T38.3 ☑
  infusion — see Complications, infusion
  local applications (of fomentations, plasters, etc.)
    T88.9 ☑
    burn or scald — see Burn
    specified NEC T88.8 ☑
  medical care (early) (late) T88.9 ☑
    adverse effect of drugs or chemicals — see Table of
      Drugs and Chemicals
    burn or scald — see Burn
    specified NEC T88.8 ☑
  specified NEC T88.8 ☑
  surgical procedure (early) (late) — see Complication,
    surgical procedure
  transfusion — see Complications, transfusion
  vaccination or other immunological procedure — see
    Complications, vaccination
Miscarriage O03.9
Misdirection, aqueous H40.83- ☑
Misperception, sleep state F51.02
Misplaced, misplacement
  ear Q17.4
  kidney (acquired) N28.89
    congenital Q63.2
  organ or site, congenital NEC — see Malposition, con-
    genital
Missed
  abortion O02.1
  delivery O36.4 ☑
Missing — see also Absence
  string of intrauterine contraceptive device T83.32- ☑
Misuse of drugs F19.99
Mitchell's disease (erythromelalgia) I73.81
Mite(s) (infestation) B88.9
  diarrhea B88.0
  grain (itch) B88.0
  hair follicle (itch) B88.0
  in sputum B88.0
Mitral — see condition
Mittelschmerz N94.0
Mixed — see condition
MMN (multifocal motor neuropathy) G61.82
MNGIE (Mitochondrial Neurogastrointestinal Encephalopathy) **syndrome** E88.49
Mobile, mobility
  cecum Q43.3
  excessive — see Hypermobility
  gallbladder, congenital Q44.1
  kidney N28.89
  organ or site, congenital NEC — see Malposition, con-
    genital
Mobitz heart block (atrioventricular) I44.1
Moebius, Möbius
  disease (ophthalmoplegic migraine) — see Migraine,
    ophthalmoplegic
  syndrome Q87.0
    congenital oculofacial paralysis (with other anoma-
      lies) Q87.0
    ophthalmoplegic migraine — see Migraine, ophthal-
      moplegic
Moeller's glossitis K14.0
Mohr's syndrome (Types I and II) Q87.0
Mola destruens D39.2
Molar pregnancy O02.0
Molarization of premolars K00.2
Molding, head (during birth) — omit code
Mole (pigmented) — see also Nevus
  blood O02.0
  Breus' O02.0
  cancerous — see Melanoma
  carneous O02.0
  destructive D39.2
  fleshy O02.0
  hydatid, hydatidiform (benign) (complicating pregnan-
    cy) (delivered) (undelivered) O01.9
    classical O01.0
    complete O01.0
    incomplete O01.1
    invasive D39.2
    malignant D39.2
    partial O01.1
  intrauterine O02.0
  invasive (hydatidiform) D39.2

Mole — *continued*
  malignant
    meaning
      malignant hydatidiform mole D39.2
      melanoma — *see* Melanoma
    nonhydatidiform O02.0
    nonpigmented — *see* Nevus
    pregnancy NEC O02.0
    skin — *see* Nevus
    tubal O00.10- ☑
      with intrauterine pregnancy O00.11- ☑
    vesicular — *see* Mole, hydatidiform
Molimen, molimina (menstrual) N94.3
Molluscum contagiosum (epitheliale) B08.1
Mönckeberg's arteriosclerosis, disease, or sclerosis
      — *see* Arteriosclerosis, extremities
Mondini's malformation (cochlea) Q16.5
Mondor's disease I80.8
Monge's disease T70.29 ☑
Monilethrix (congenital) Q84.1
Moniliasis — *see also* Candidiasis B37.9
    neonatal P37.5
Monitoring (encounter for)
    therapeutic drug level Z51.81
Monkey malaria B53.1
Monkeypox B04
Monoarthritis M13.10
    ankle M13.17- ☑
    elbow M13.12- ☑
    foot joint M13.17- ☑
    hand joint M13.14- ☑
    hip M13.15- ☑
    knee M13.16- ☑
    shoulder M13.11- ☑
    wrist M13.13- ☑
Monoblastic — *see* condition
Monochromat (ism), monochromatopsia (acquired)
    (congenital) H53.51
Monocytic — *see* condition
Monocytopenia D72.818
Monocytosis (symptomatic) D72.821
Monomania — *see* Psychosis
Mononeuritis G58.9
    cranial nerve — *see* Disorder, nerve, cranial
    femoral nerve G57.2- ☑
    lateral
      cutaneous nerve of thigh G57.1- ☑
      popliteal nerve G57.3- ☑
    lower limb G57.9- ☑
      specified nerve NEC G57.8- ☑
    medial popliteal nerve G57.4- ☑
    median nerve G56.1- ☑
    multiplex G58.7
    plantar nerve G57.6- ☑
    posterior tibial nerve G57.5- ☑
    radial nerve G56.3- ☑
    sciatic nerve G57.0- ☑
    specified NEC G58.8
    tibial nerve G57.4- ☑
    ulnar nerve G56.2- ☑
    upper limb G56.9- ☑
      specified nerve NEC G56.8- ☑
    vestibular — *see* subcategory H93.3
Mononeuropathy G58.9
    carpal tunnel syndrome — *see* Syndrome, carpal tunnel
    diabetic NEC — *see* E08-E13 with .41
    femoral nerve — *see* Lesion, nerve, femoral
    ilioinguinal nerve G57.8- ☑
    in diseases classified elsewhere — *see* category G59
    intercostal G58.0
    lower limb G57.9- ☑
      causalgia — *see* Causalgia, lower limb
      femoral nerve — *see* Lesion, nerve, femoral
      meralgia paresthetica G57.1- ☑
      plantar nerve — *see* Lesion, nerve, plantar
      popliteal nerve — *see* Lesion, nerve, popliteal
      sciatic nerve — *see* Lesion, nerve, sciatic
      specified NEC G57.8- ☑
      tarsal tunnel syndrome — *see* Syndrome, tarsal
        tunnel
    median nerve — *see* Lesion, nerve, median
    multiplex G58.7
    obturator nerve G57.8- ☑
    popliteal nerve — *see* Lesion, nerve, popliteal
    radial nerve — *see* Lesion, nerve, radial
    saphenous nerve G57.8- ☑

Mononeuropathy — *continued*
    specified NEC G58.8
    tarsal tunnel syndrome — *see* Syndrome, tarsal tunnel
    tuberculous A17.83
    ulnar nerve — *see* Lesion, nerve, ulnar
    upper limb G56.9- ☑
      carpal tunnel syndrome — *see* Syndrome, carpal
        tunnel
      causalgia — *see* Causalgia
      median nerve — *see* Lesion, nerve, median
      radial nerve — *see* Lesion, nerve, radial
      specified site NEC G56.8- ☑
      ulnar nerve — *see* Lesion, nerve, ulnar
Mononucleosis, infectious B27.90
    with
      complication NEC B27.99
      meningitis B27.92
      polyneuropathy B27.91
    cytomegaloviral B27.10
      with
        complication NEC B27.19
        meningitis B27.12
        polyneuropathy B27.11
    Epstein-Barr (virus) B27.00
      with
        complication NEC B27.09
        meningitis B27.02
        polyneuropathy B27.01
    gammaherpesviral B27.00
      with
        complication NEC B27.09
        meningitis B27.02
        polyneuropathy B27.01
    specified NEC B27.80
      with
        complication NEC B27.89
        meningitis B27.82
        polyneuropathy B27.81
Monoplegia G83.3- ☑
    congenital (cerebral) G80.8
      spastic G80.1
    embolic (current episode) I63.4- ☑
    following
      cerebrovascular disease
        cerebral infarction
          lower limb I69.34- ☑
          upper limb I69.33- ☑
        intracerebral hemorrhage
          lower limb I69.14- ☑
          upper limb I69.13- ☑
        lower limb I69.94- ☑
        nontraumatic intracranial hemorrhage NEC
          lower limb I69.24- ☑
          upper limb I69.23- ☑
        specified disease NEC
          lower limb I69.84- ☑
          upper limb I69.83- ☑
        stroke NOS
          lower limb I69.34- ☑
          upper limb I69.33- ☑
        subarachnoid hemorrhage
          lower limb I69.04- ☑
          upper limb I69.03- ☑
        upper limb I69.93- ☑
    hysterical (transient) F44.4
    lower limb G83.1- ☑
    psychogenic (conversion reaction) F44.4
    thrombotic (current episode) I63.3- ☑
    transient R29.818
    upper limb G83.2- ☑
Monorchism, monorchidism Q55.0
Monosomy — *see also* Deletion, chromosome Q93.9
    specified NEC Q93.89
    whole chromosome
      meiotic nondisjunction Q93.0
      mitotic nondisjunction Q93.1
      mosaicism Q93.1
    X Q96.9
Monster, monstrosity (single) Q89.7
    acephalic Q00.0
    twin Q89.4
Monteggia's fracture (-dislocation) S52.27- ☑
Mooren's ulcer (cornea) — *see* Ulcer, cornea, Mooren's
Moore's syndrome — *see* Epilepsy, specified NEC
Mooser-Neill reaction A75.2
Mooser's bodies A75.2
Morbidity not stated or unknown R69

Morbilli — *see* Measles
Morbus — *see also* Disease
    angelicus, anglorum E55.0
    Beigel B36.2
    caducus — *see* Epilepsy
    celiacus K90.0
    comitialis — *see* Epilepsy
    cordis — *see also* Disease, heart I51.9
      valvulorum — *see* Endocarditis
    coxae senilis M16.9
      tuberculous A18.02
    hemorrhagicus neonatorum P53
    maculosus neonatorum P54.5
Morel (-Stewart)(-Morgagni) **syndrome** M85.2
Morel-Kraepelin disease — *see* Schizophrenia
Morel-Moore syndrome M85.2
Morgagni's
    cyst, organ, hydatid, or appendage
      female Q50.5
      male (epididymal) Q55.4
        testicular Q55.29
    syndrome M85.2
Morgagni-Stewart-Morel syndrome M85.2
Morgagni-Stokes-Adams syndrome I45.9
Morgagni-Turner (-Albright) **syndrome** Q96.9
Moria F07.0
Moron (I.Q. 50-69) F70
Morphea L94.0
Morphinism (without remission) F11.20
    with remission F11.21
Morphinomania (without remission) F11.20
    with remission F11.21
Morquio (-Ullrich)(-Brailsford) **disease or syndrome** —
      see Mucopolysaccharidosis
Mortification (dry) (moist) — *see* Gangrene
Morton's metatarsalgia (neuralgia)(neuroma) (syn-
      drome) G57.6- ☑
Morvan's disease or syndrome G60.8
Mosaicism, mosaic (autosomal) (chromosomal)
    45,X/46,XX Q96.3
    45,X/other cell lines NEC with abnormal sex chromo-
      some Q96.4
    sex chromosome
      female Q97.8
      lines with various numbers of X chromosomes Q97.2
      male Q98.7
    XY Q96.3
Moschowitz' disease M31.1
Mother yaw A66.0
Motion sickness (from travel, any vehicle) (from round-
      abouts or swings) T75.3 ☑
Mottled, mottling, teeth (enamel) (endemic) (nonen-
      demic) K00.3
Mounier-Kuhn syndrome Q32.4
    with bronchiectasis J47.9
      exacerbation (acute) J47.1
      lower respiratory infection J47.0
    acquired J98.09
      with bronchiectasis J47.9
        with
          exacerbation (acute) J47.1
          lower respiratory infection J47.0
Mountain
    sickness T70.29 ☑
      with polycythemia , acquired (acute) D75.1
    tick fever A93.2
Mouse, joint — *see* Loose, body, joint
    knee M23.4- ☑
Mouth — *see* condition
Movable
    coccyx — *see* subcategory M53.2 ☑
    kidney N28.89
      congenital Q63.8
    spleen D73.89
Movements, dystonic R25.8
Moyamoya disease I67.5
MRSA (Methicillin resistant Staphylococcus aureus)
    infection A49.02
      as the cause of diseases classified elsewhere B95.62
    sepsis A41.02
MSD (multiple sulfatase deficiency) E75.26
MSSA (Methicillin susceptible Staphylococcus aureus)
    infection A49.01
      as the cause of diseases classified elsewhere B95.61
    sepsis A41.01
Mucha-Habermann disease L41.0
Mucinosis (cutaneous) (focal) (papular) (skin) L98.5

Mucinosis — continued
  oral K13.79
Mucocele
  appendix K38.8
  buccal cavity K13.79
  gallbladder K82.1
  lacrimal sac, chronic H04.43- ☑
  nasal sinus J34.1
  nose J34.1
  salivary gland (any) K11.6
  sinus (accessory) (nasal) J34.1
  turbinate (bone) (middle) (nasal) J34.1
  uterus N85.8
Mucolipidosis
  I E77.1
  II, III E77.0
  IV E75.11
Mucopolysaccharidosis E76.3
  beta-glucuronidase deficiency E76.29
  cardiopathy E76.3 [I52]
  Hunter's syndrome E76.1
  Hurler's syndrome E76.01
  Hurler-Scheie syndrome E76.02
  Maroteaux-Lamy syndrome E76.29
  Morquio syndrome E76.219
    A E76.210
    B E76.211
    classic E76.210
  Sanfilippo syndrome E76.22
  Scheie's syndrome E76.03
  specified NEC E76.29
  type
    I
      Hurler's syndrome E76.01
      Hurler-Scheie syndrome E76.02
      Scheie's syndrome E76.03
    II E76.1
    III E76.22
    IV E76.219
    IVA E76.210
    IVB E76.211
    VI E76.29
    VII E76.29
Mucormycosis B46.5
  cutaneous B46.3
  disseminated B46.4
  gastrointestinal B46.2
  generalized B46.4
  pulmonary B46.0
  rhinocerebral B46.1
  skin B46.3
  subcutaneous B46.3
Mucositis (ulcerative) K12.30
  due to drugs NEC K12.32
  gastrointestinal K92.81
  mouth (oral) (oropharyngeal) K12.30
    due to antineoplastic therapy K12.31
    due to drugs NEC K12.32
    due to radiation K12.33
    specified NEC K12.39
    viral K12.39
  nasal J34.81
  oral cavity — see Mucositis, mouth
  oral soft tissues — see Mucositis, mouth
  vagina and vulva N76.81
Mucositis necroticans agranulocytica — see Agranulocytosis
Mucous — see also condition
  patches (syphilitic) A51.39
    congenital A50.07
Mucoviscidosis E84.9
  with meconium obstruction E84.11
Mucus
  asphyxia or suffocation — see Asphyxia, mucus
  in stool R19.5
  plug — see Asphyxia, mucus
Muguet B37.0
Mulberry molars (congenital syphilis) A50.52
Müllerian mixed tumor
  specified site — see Neoplasm, malignant, by site
  unspecified site C54.9
Multicystic kidney (development) Q61.4
Multiparity (grand) Z64.1
  affecting management of pregnancy, labor and delivery
    (supervision only) O09.4- ☑
  requiring contraceptive management — see Contraception
Multipartita placenta O43.19- ☑

Multiple, multiplex — see also condition
  digits (congenital) Q69.9
  endocrine neoplasia — see Neoplasia, endocrine, multiple (MEN)
  personality F44.81
Mumps B26.9
  arthritis B26.85
  complication NEC B26.89
  encephalitis B26.2
  hepatitis B26.81
  meningitis (aseptic) B26.1
  meningoencephalitis B26.2
  myocarditis B26.82
  oophoritis B26.89
  orchitis B26.0
  pancreatitis B26.3
  polyneuropathy B26.84
Mumu — see also Infestation, filarial B74.9 [N51]
Münchhausen's syndrome — see Disorder, factitious
Münchmeyer's syndrome — see Myositis, ossificans, progressiva
Mural — see condition
Murmur (cardiac) (heart) (organic) R01.1
  abdominal R19.15
  aortic (valve) — see Endocarditis, aortic
  benign R01.0
  diastolic — see Endocarditis
  Flint I35.1
  functional R01.0
  Graham Steell I37.1
  innocent R01.0
  mitral (valve) — see Insufficiency, mitral
  nonorganic R01.0
  presystolic, mitral — see Insufficiency, mitral
  pulmonic (valve) I37.8
  systolic R01.1
  tricuspid (valve) I07.9
  valvular — see Endocarditis
Murri's disease (intermittent hemoglobinuria) D59.6
Muscle, muscular — see also condition
  carnitine (palmityltransferase) deficiency E71.314
Musculoneuralgia — see Neuralgia
Mushrooming hip — see Derangement, joint, specified NEC, hip
Mushroom-workers' (pickers') **disease or lung** J67.5
Mutation(s)
  factor V Leiden D68.51
  prothrombin gene D68.52
  surfactant, of lung J84.83
Mutism — see also Aphasia
  deaf (acquired) (congenital) NEC H91.3
  elective (adjustment reaction) (childhood) F94.0
  hysterical F44.4
  selective (childhood) F94.0
MVD (microvillus inclusion disease) Q43.8
MVID (microvillus inclusion disease) Q43.8
Myalgia M79.10
  auxiliary muscles, head and neck M79.12
  epidemic (cervical) B33.0
  mastication muscle M79.11
  site specified NEC M79.18
  traumatic NEC T14.8 ☑
Myasthenia G70.9
  congenital G70.2
  cordis — see Failure, heart
  developmental G70.2
  gravis G70.00
    with exacerbation (acute) G70.01
    in crisis G70.01
    neonatal, transient P94.0
    pseudoparalytica G70.00
      with exacerbation (acute) G70.01
      in crisis G70.01
  stomach, psychogenic F45.8
  syndrome
    in
      diabetes mellitus — see E08-E13 with .44
      neoplastic disease — see also Neoplasm D49.9 [G73.3]
      pernicious anemia D51.0 [G73.3]
      thyrotoxicosis E05.90 [G73.3]
        with thyroid storm E05.91 [G73.3]
Myasthenic M62.81
Mycelium infection B49
Mycetismus — see Poisoning, food, noxious, mushroom
Mycetoma B47.9
  actinomycotic B47.1
  bone (mycotic) B47.9 [M90.80]

Mycetoma — continued
  eumycotic B47.0
  foot B47.9
    actinomycotic B47.1
    mycotic B47.0
  madurae NEC B47.9
    mycotic B47.0
  maduromycotic B47.0
  mycotic B47.0
  nocardial B47.1
Mycobacteriosis — see Mycobacterium
Mycobacterium, mycobacterial (infection) A31.9
  anonymous A31.9
  atypical A31.9
    cutaneous A31.1
    pulmonary A31.0
      tuberculous — see Tuberculosis, pulmonary
    specified site NEC A31.8
  avium (intracellulare complex) A31.0
  balnei A31.1
  Battey A31.0
  chelonei A31.8
  cutaneous A31.1
  extrapulmonary systemic A31.8
  fortuitum A31.8
  intracellulare (Battey bacillus) A31.0
  kakaferifu A31.8
  kansasii (yellow bacillus) A31.0
  kasongo A31.8
  leprae — see also Leprosy A30.9
  luciflavum A31.1
  marinum (M. balnei) A31.1
  nonspecific — see Mycobacterium, atypical
  pulmonary (atypical) A31.0
    tuberculous — see Tuberculosis, pulmonary
  scrofulaceum A31.8
  simiae A31.8
  systemic, extrapulmonary A31.8
  szulgai A31.8
  terrae A31.8
  triviale A31.8
  tuberculosis (human, bovine) — see Tuberculosis
  ulcerans A31.1
  xenopi A31.8
Mycoplasma (M.) **pneumoniae, as cause of disease classified elsewhere** B96.0
Mycosis, mycotic B49
  cutaneous NEC B36.9
  ear B36.9
    in
      aspergillosis B44.89
      candidiasis B37.84
      moniliasis B37.84
  fungoides (extranodal) (solid organ) C84.0- ☑
  mouth B37.0
  nails B35.1
  opportunistic B48.8
  skin NEC B36.9
  specified NEC B48.8
  stomatitis B37.0
  vagina, vaginitis (candidal) B37.3
Mydriasis (pupil) H57.04
Myelatelia Q06.1
Myelinolysis, pontine, central G37.2
Myelitis (acute) (ascending) (childhood) (chronic) (descending) (diffuse) (disseminated) (idiopathic) (pressure) (progressive) (spinal cord) (subacute) — see also Encephalitis G04.91
  herpes simplex B00.82
  herpes zoster B02.24
  in diseases classified elsewhere G05.4
  necrotizing, subacute G37.4
  optic neuritis in G36.0
  postchickenpox B01.12
  postherpetic B02.24
  postimmunization G04.02
  postinfectious NEC G04.89
  postvaccinal G04.02
  specified NEC G04.89
  syphilitic (transverse) A52.14
  toxic G92
  transverse (in demyelinating diseases of central nervou system) G37.3
  tuberculous A17.82
  varicella B01.12
Myeloblastic — see condition
Myeloblastoma
  granular cell — see also Neoplasm, connective tissu

Myeloblastoma — *continued*
  granular cell — *see also* Neoplasm, connective tissue
    — *continued*
    malignant — *see* Neoplasm, connective tissue, ma-
      lignant
      tongue D10.1
Myelocele — *see* Spina bifida
Myelocystocele — *see* Spina bifida
Myelocytic — *see* condition
Myelodysplasia D46.9
  specified NEC D46.Z (*following* D46.4)
  spinal cord (congenital) Q06.1
Myelodysplastic syndrome D46.9
  with
    5q deletion D46.C (*following* D46.2)
    isolated del (5q) chromosomal abnormality D46.C
      (*following* D46.2)
  specified NEC D46.Z (*following* D46.4)
Myeloencephalitis — *see* Encephalitis
Myelofibrosis D75.81
  with myeloid metaplasia D47.4
  acute C94.4- ☑
  idiopathic (chronic) D47.4
  primary D47.1
  secondary D75.81
    in myeloproliferative disease D47.4
Myelogenous — *see* condition
Myeloid — *see* condition
Myelokathexis D70.9
Myeloleukodystrophy E75.29
Myelolipoma — *see* Lipoma
Myeloma (multiple) C90.0- ☑
  monostotic C90.3 ☑
    plasma cell C90.0- ☑
  plasma cell C90.0- ☑
  solitary — *see also* Plasmacytoma, solitary C90.3- ☑
Myelomalacia G95.89
Myelomatosis C90.0- ☑
Myelomeningitis — *see* Meningoencephalitis
Myelomeningocele (spinal cord) — *see* Spina bifida
Myelo-osteo-musculodysplasia hereditaria Q79.8
Myelopathic
  anemia D64.89
  muscle atrophy — *see* Atrophy, muscle, spinal
  pain syndrome G89.0
Myelopathy (spinal cord) G95.9
  drug-induced G95.89
  in (due to)
    degeneration or displacement, intervertebral disc
      NEC — *see* Disorder, disc, with, myelopathy
    infection — *see* Encephalitis
    intervertebral disc disorder — *see also* Disorder,
      disc, with, myelopathy
    mercury — *see* subcategory T56.1 ☑
    neoplastic disease — *see also* Neoplasm
      D49.9 *[G99.2]*
    pernicious anemia D51.0 *[G99.2]*
    spondylosis — *see* Spondylosis, with myelopathy
      NEC
  necrotic (subacute) (vascular) G95.19
  radiation-induced G95.89
  spondylogenic NEC — *see* Spondylosis, with
    myelopathy NEC
  toxic G95.89
  transverse, acute G37.3
  vascular G95.19
  vitamin B12 E53.8 *[G32.0]*
Myelophthisis D61.82
Myeloradiculitis G04.91
Myeloradiculodysplasia (spinal) Q06.1
Myelosarcoma C92.3- ☑
Myelosclerosis D75.89
  with myeloid metaplasia D47.4
  disseminated, of nervous system G35
  megakaryocytic D47.4
    with myeloid metaplasia D47.4
Myelosis
  acute C92.0- ☑
  aleukemic C92.9- ☑
  chronic D47.1
  erythremic (acute) C94.0- ☑
  megakaryocytic C94.2- ☑
  nonleukemic D72.828
  subacute C92.9- ☑
Myiasis (cavernous) B87.9
  aural B87.4
  creeping B87.0

Myiasis — *continued*
  cutaneous B87.0
  dermal B87.0
  ear (external) (middle) B87.4
  eye B87.2
  genitourinary B87.81
  intestinal B87.82
  laryngeal B87.3
  nasopharyngeal B87.3
  ocular B87.2
  orbit B87.2
  skin B87.0
  specified site NEC B87.89
  traumatic B87.1
  wound B87.1
Myoadenoma, prostate — *see* Hyperplasia, prostate
Myoblastoma
  granular cell — *see also* Neoplasm, connective tissue,
    benign
    malignant — *see* Neoplasm, connective tissue, ma-
      lignant
  tongue D10.1
Myocardial — *see* condition
Myocardiopathy (congestive) (constrictive) (familial)
  (hypertrophic nonobstructive) (idiopathic) (infiltrative) (obstructive) (primary) (restrictive) (sporadic)
  — *see also* Cardiomyopathy I42.9
  alcoholic I42.6
  cobalt-beer I42.6
  glycogen storage E74.02 *[I43]*
  hypertrophic obstructive I42.1
  in (due to)
    beriberi E51.12
    cardiac glycogenosis E74.02 *[I43]*
    Friedreich's ataxia G11.1 *[I43]*
    myotonia atrophica G71.11 *[I43]*
    progressive muscular dystrophy G71.09 *[I43]*
  obscure (African) I42.8
  secondary I42.9
  thyrotoxic E05.90 *[I43]*
    with storm E05.91 *[I43]*
  toxic NEC I42.7
Myocarditis (with arteriosclerosis)(chronic)(fibroid) (interstitial) (old) (progressive) (senile) I51.4
  with
    rheumatic fever (conditions in I00) I09.0
      active — *see* Myocarditis, acute, rheumatic
      inactive or quiescent (with chorea) I09.0
  active I40.9
    rheumatic I01.2
      with chorea (acute) (rheumatic) (Sydenham's)
        I02.0
  acute or subacute (interstitial) I40.9
    due to
      streptococcus (beta-hemolytic) I01.2
    idiopathic I40.1
    rheumatic I01.2
      with chorea (acute) (rheumatic) (Sydenham's)
        I02.0
    specified NEC I40.8
  aseptic of newborn B33.22
  bacterial (acute) I40.0
  Coxsackie (virus) B33.22
  diphtheritic A36.81
  eosinophilic I40.1
  epidemic of newborn (Coxsackie) B33.22
  Fiedler's (acute) (isolated) I40.1
  giant cell (acute) (subacute) I40.1
  gonococcal A54.83
  granulomatous (idiopathic) (isolated) (nonspecific) I40.1
  hypertensive — *see* Hypertension, heart
  idiopathic (granulomatous) I40.1
  in (due to)
    diphtheria A36.81
    epidemic louse-borne typhus A75.0 *[I41]*
    Lyme disease A69.29
    sarcoidosis D86.85
    scarlet fever A38.1
    toxoplasmosis (acquired) B58.81
    typhoid A01.02
    typhus NEC A75.9 *[I41]*
  infective I40.0
  influenzal — *see* Influenza, with, myocarditis
  isolated (acute) I40.1
  meningococcal A39.52
  mumps B26.82
  nonrheumatic, active I40.9
  parenchymatous I40.9

Myocarditis — *continued*
  pneumococcal I40.0
  rheumatic (chronic) (inactive) (with chorea) I09.0
    active or acute I01.2
      with chorea (acute) (rheumatic) (Sydenham's)
        I02.0
  rheumatoid — *see* Rheumatoid, carditis
  septic I40.0
  staphylococcal I40.0
  suppurative I40.0
  syphilitic (chronic) A52.06
  toxic I40.8
    rheumatic — *see* Myocarditis, acute, rheumatic
  tuberculous A18.84
  typhoid A01.02
  valvular — *see* Endocarditis
  virus, viral I40.0
    of newborn (Coxsackie) B33.22
Myocardium, myocardial — *see* condition
Myocardosis — *see* Cardiomyopathy
Myoclonus, myoclonic, myoclonia (familial) (essential)
  (multifocal) (simplex) G25.3
  drug-induced G25.3
  epilepsy — *see also* Epilepsy, generalized, specified
    NEC G40.4- ☑
    familial (progressive) G25.3
  epileptica G40.409
    with status epilepticus G40.401
  facial G51.3- ☑
  familial progressive G25.3
  Friedreich's G25.3
  jerks G25.3
  massive G25.3
  palatal G25.3
  pharyngeal G25.3
Myocytolysis I51.5
Myodiastasis — *see* Diastasis, muscle
Myoendocarditis — *see* Endocarditis
Myoepithelioma — *see* Neoplasm, benign, by site
Myofasciitis (acute) — *see* Myositis
Myofibroma — *see also* Neoplasm, connective tissue,
  benign
  uterus (cervix) (corpus) — *see* Leiomyoma
Myofibromatosis D48.1
  infantile Q89.8
Myofibrosis M62.89
  heart — *see* Myocarditis
  scapulohumeral — *see* Lesion, shoulder, specified NEC
Myofibrositis M79.7
  scapulohumeral — *see* Lesion, shoulder, specified NEC
Myoglobulinuria, myoglobinuria (primary) R82.1
Myokymia, facial G51.4
Myolipoma — *see* Lipoma
Myoma — *see also* Neoplasm, connective tissue, benign
  malignant — *see* Neoplasm, connective tissue, malig-
    nant
  prostate D29.1
  uterus (cervix) (corpus) — *see* Leiomyoma
Myomalacia M62.89
Myometritis — *see* Endometritis
Myometrium — *see* condition
Myonecrosis, clostridial A48.0
Myopathy G72.9
  acute
    necrotizing G72.81
    quadriplegic G72.81
  alcoholic G72.1
  benign congenital G71.2
  central core G71.2
  centronuclear G71.2
  congenital (benign) G71.2
  critical illness G72.81
  distal G71.09
  drug-induced G72.0
  endocrine NEC E34.9 *[G73.7]*
  extraocular muscles H05.82- ☑
  facioscapulohumeral G71.02
  hereditary G71.9
    specified NEC G71.8
  immune NEC G72.49
  in (due to)
    Addison's disease E27.1 *[G73.7]*
    alcohol G72.1
    amyloidosis E85.0 *[G73.7]*
    cretinism E00.9 *[G73.7]*
    Cushing's syndrome E24.9 *[G73.7]*
    drugs G72.0

Myopathy — continued
  in — continued
    endocrine disease NEC E34.9 [G73.7]
    giant cell arteritis M31.6 [G73.7]
    glycogen storage disease E74.00 [G73.7]
    hyperadrenocorticism E24.9 [G73.7]
    hyperparathyroidism NEC E21.3 [G73.7]
    hypoparathyroidism E20.9 [G73.7]
    hypopituitarism E23.0 [G73.7]
    hypothyroidism E03.9 [G73.7]
    infectious disease NEC B99 ☑ [G73.7]
    lipid storage disease E75.6 [G73.7]
    metabolic disease NEC E88.9 [G73.7]
    myxedema E03.9 [G73.7]
    parasitic disease NEC B89 [G73.7]
    polyarteritis nodosa M30.0 [G73.7]
    rheumatoid arthritis — see Rheumatoid, myopathy
    sarcoidosis D86.87
    scleroderma M34.82
    sicca syndrome M35.03
    Sjögren's syndrome M35.03
    systemic lupus erythematosus M32.19
    thyrotoxicosis (hyperthyroidism) E05.90 [G73.7]
      with thyroid storm E05.91 [G73.7]
    toxic agent NEC G72.2
  inflammatory NEC G72.49
  intensive care (ICU) G72.81
  limb-girdle G71.09
  mitochondrial NEC G71.3
  myotubular G71.2
  mytonic, proximal (PROMM) G71.11
  nemaline G71.2
  ocular G71.09
  oculopharyngeal G71.09
  of critical illness G72.81
  primary G71.9
    specified NEC G71.8
  progressive NEC G72.89
  proximal myotonic (PROMM) G71.11
  rod G71.2
  scapulohumeral G71.02
  specified NEC G72.89
  toxic G72.2
Myopericarditis — see also Pericarditis
  chronic rheumatic I09.2
Myopia (axial) (congenital) H52.1- ☑
  degenerative (malignant) H44.20
    with
      choroidal neovascularization H44.2A- ☑
      foveoschisis H44.2D- ☑
      macular hole H44.2B- ☑
      retinal detachment H44.2C- ☑
      specified maculopathy NEC H44.2E- ☑
    bilateral H44.23
    left eye H44.22
    right eye H44.21
  malignant — see also Myopia, degenerative H44.2- ☑
  pernicious — see also Myopia, degenerative H44.2- ☑
  progressive high (degenerative) — see also Myopia,
    degenerative H44.2- ☑
Myosarcoma — see Neoplasm, connective tissue, malignant
Myosis (pupil) H57.03
  stromal (endolymphatic) D39.0
Myositis M60.9
  clostridial A48.0
  due to posture — see Myositis, specified type NEC
  epidemic B33.0
  fibrosa or fibrous (chronic), Volkmann's T79.6 ☑
  foreign body granuloma — see Granuloma, foreign
    body
  in (due to)
    bilharziasis B65.9 [M63.8-] ☑
    cysticercosis B69.81
    leprosy A30.9 [M63.8-] ☑
    mycosis B49 [M63.8-] ☑
    sarcoidosis D86.87
    schistosomiasis B65.9 [M63.8-] ☑
    syphilis
      late A52.78
      secondary A51.49
    toxoplasmosis (acquired) B58.82

Myositis — continued
  in — continued
    trichinellosis B75 [M63.8-] ☑
    tuberculosis A18.09
  inclusion body [IBM] G72.41
  infective M60.009
    arm M60.002
      left M60.001
      right M60.000
    leg M60.005
      left M60.004
      right M60.003
    lower limb M60.005
      ankle M60.07- ☑
      foot M60.07- ☑
      lower leg M60.06- ☑
      thigh M60.05- ☑
      toe M60.07- ☑
    multiple sites M60.09
    specified site NEC M60.08
    upper limb M60.002
      finger M60.04- ☑
      forearm M60.03- ☑
      hand M60.04- ☑
      shoulder region M60.01- ☑
      upper arm M60.02- ☑
  interstitial M60.10
    ankle M60.17- ☑
    foot M60.17- ☑
    forearm M60.13- ☑
    hand M60.14- ☑
    lower leg M60.16- ☑
    multiple sites M60.19
    shoulder region M60.11- ☑
    specified site NEC M60.18
    thigh M60.15- ☑
    upper arm M60.12- ☑
  mycotic B49 [M63.8-] ☑
  orbital, chronic H05.12- ☑
  ossificans or ossifying (circumscripta) — see also Ossi-
    fication, muscle, specified NEC
    in (due to)
      burns M61.30
        ankle M61.37- ☑
        foot M61.37- ☑
        forearm M61.33- ☑
        hand M61.34- ☑
        lower leg M61.36- ☑
        multiple sites M61.39
        pelvic region M61.35- ☑
        shoulder region M61.31- ☑
        specified site NEC M61.38
        thigh M61.35- ☑
        upper arm M61.32- ☑
      quadriplegia or paraplegia M61.20
        ankle M61.27- ☑
        foot M61.27- ☑
        forearm M61.23- ☑
        hand M61.24- ☑
        lower leg M61.26- ☑
        multiple sites M61.29
        pelvic region M61.25- ☑
        shoulder region M61.21- ☑
        specified site NEC M61.28
        thigh M61.25- ☑
        upper arm M61.22- ☑
    progressiva M61.10
      ankle M61.17- ☑
      finger M61.14- ☑
      foot M61.17- ☑
      forearm M61.13- ☑
      hand M61.14- ☑
      lower leg M61.16- ☑
      multiple sites M61.19
      pelvic region M61.15- ☑
      shoulder region M61.11- ☑
      specified site NEC M61.18
      thigh M61.15- ☑
      toe M61.17- ☑
      upper arm M61.12- ☑
    traumatica M61.00

Myositis — continued
  ossificans or ossifying — see also Ossification, muscl
    specified — continued
      traumatica — continued
        ankle M61.07- ☑
        foot M61.07- ☑
        forearm M61.03- ☑
        hand M61.04- ☑
        lower leg M61.06- ☑
        multiple sites M61.09
        pelvic region M61.05- ☑
        shoulder region M61.01- ☑
        specified site NEC M61.08
        thigh M61.05- ☑
        upper arm M61.02- ☑
  purulent — see Myositis, infective
  specified type NEC M60.80
    ankle M60.87- ☑
    foot M60.87- ☑
    forearm M60.83- ☑
    hand M60.84- ☑
    lower leg M60.86- ☑
    multiple sites M60.89
    pelvic region M60.85- ☑
    shoulder region M60.81- ☑
    specified site NEC M60.88
    thigh M60.85- ☑
    upper arm M60.82- ☑
  suppurative — see Myositis, infective
  traumatic (old) — see Myositis, specified type NEC
Myospasia impulsiva F95.2
Myotonia (acquisita) (intermittens) M62.89
  atrophica G71.11
  chondrodystrophic G71.13
  congenita (acetazolamide responsive) (dominant) (r
    cessive) G71.12
  drug-induced G71.14
  dystrophica G71.11
  fluctuans G71.19
  levior G71.12
  permanens G71.19
  symptomatic G71.19
Myotonic pupil — see Anomaly, pupil, function, tonic
  pupil
Myriapodiasis B88.2
Myringitis H73.2- ☑
  with otitis media — see Otitis, media
  acute H73.00- ☑
    bullous H73.01- ☑
    specified NEC H73.09- ☑
  bullous — see Myringitis, acute, bullous
  chronic H73.1- ☑
Mysophobia F40.228
Mytilotoxism — see Poisoning, fish
Myxadenitis labialis K13.0
Myxedema (adult) (idiocy) (infantile) (juvenile) — see
  also Hypothyroidism E03.9
  circumscribed E05.90
    with storm E05.91
  coma E03.5
  congenital E00.1
  cutis L98.5
  localized (pretibial) E05.90
    with storm E05.91
  papular L98.5
Myxochondrosarcoma — see Neoplasm, cartilage, m
  lignant
Myxofibroma — see Neoplasm, connective tissue, benig
  odontogenic — see Cyst, calcifying odontogenic
Myxofibrosarcoma — see Neoplasm, connective tissu
  malignant
Myxolipoma D17.9
Myxoliposarcoma — see Neoplasm, connective tissu
  malignant
Myxoma — see also Neoplasm, connective tissue, benig
  nerve sheath — see Neoplasm, nerve, benign
  odontogenic — see Cyst, calcifying odontogenic
Myxosarcoma — see Neoplasm, connective tissue, m
  lignant

☑ **Additional Character Required** — Refer to the Tabular List for Character Selection   ▽ **Subterms under main terms may continue to next column or pag**

N

Naegeli's
- disease Q82.8
- leukemia, monocytic C93.1- ☑

Naegleriasis (with meningoencephalitis) B60.2
Naffziger's syndrome G54.0
Naga sore — *see* Ulcer, skin
Nägele's pelvis M95.5
- with disproportion (fetopelvic) O33.0
  - causing obstructed labor O65.0
Nail — *see also* condition
- biting F98.8
- patella syndrome Q87.2
Nanism, nanosomia — *see* Dwarfism
Nanophyetiasis B66.8
Nanukayami A27.89
Napkin rash L22
Narcolepsy G47.419
- with cataplexy G47.411
- in conditions classified elsewhere G47.429
  - with cataplexy G47.421
Narcosis R06.89
Narcotism — *see* Dependence
NARP (Neuropathy, Ataxia and Retinitis pigmentosa) syndrome E88.49
Narrow
- anterior chamber angle H40.03- ☑
- gingival width (of periodontal soft tissue) K05.5
- pelvis — *see* Contraction, pelvis
Narrowing — *see also* Stenosis
- artery I77.1
  - auditory, internal I65.8
  - basilar — *see* Occlusion, artery, basilar
  - carotid — *see* Occlusion, artery, carotid
  - cerebellar — *see* Occlusion, artery, cerebellar
  - cerebral — *see* Occlusion artery, cerebral
  - choroidal — *see* Occlusion, artery, precerebral, specified NEC
  - communicating posterior — *see* Occlusion, artery, precerebral, specified NEC
  - coronary — *see also* Disease, heart, ischemic, atherosclerotic
    - congenital Q24.5
    - syphilitic A50.54 [I52]
    - due to syphilis NEC A52.06
  - hypophyseal — *see* Occlusion, artery, precerebral, specified NEC
  - pontine — *see* Occlusion, artery, precerebral, specified NEC
  - precerebral — *see* Occlusion, artery, precerebral
  - vertebral — *see* Occlusion, artery, vertebral
- auditory canal (external) — *see* Stenosis, external ear canal
- eustachian tube — *see* Obstruction, eustachian tube
- eyelid — *see* Disorder, eyelid function
- larynx J38.6
- mesenteric artery — *see also* Ischemia, intestine, acute K55.059
- palate M26.89
- palpebral fissure — *see* Disorder, eyelid function
- ureter N13.5
  - with infection N13.6
- urethra — *see* Stricture, urethra
Narrowness, abnormal, eyelid Q10.3
Nasal — *see* condition
Nasolachrymal, nasolacrimal — *see* condition
Nasopharyngeal — *see also* condition
- pituitary gland Q89.2
- torticollis M43.6
Nasopharyngitis (acute) (infective) (streptococcal) (subacute) J00
- chronic (suppurative) (ulcerative) J31.1
Nasopharynx, nasopharyngeal — *see* condition
Natal tooth, teeth K00.6
Nausea (without vomiting) R11.0
- with vomiting R11.2
- gravidarum — *see* Hyperemesis, gravidarum
- marina T75.3 ☑
- navalis T75.3 ☑
Navel — *see* condition
Neapolitan fever — *see* Brucellosis
Near drowning T75.1 ☑
Nearsightedness — *see* Myopia
Near-syncope R55
Nebula, cornea — *see* Opacity, cornea

Necator americanus infestation B76.1
Necatoriasis B76.1
Neck — *see* condition
Necrobiosis R68.89
- lipoidica NEC L92.1
  - with diabetes — *see* E08-E13 with .620
Necrolysis, toxic epidermal L51.2
- due to drug
  - correct substance properly administered — *see* Table of Drugs and Chemicals, by drug, adverse effect
  - overdose or wrong substance given or taken — *see* Table of Drugs and Chemicals, by drug, poisoning
Necrophilia F65.89
Necrosis, necrotic (ischemic) — *see also* Gangrene
- adrenal (capsule) (gland) E27.49
- amputation stump (surgical) (late) T87.50
  - arm T87.5- ☑
  - leg T87.5- ☑
- antrum J32.0
- aorta (hyaline) — *see also* Aneurysm, aorta
  - cystic medial — *see* Dissection, aorta
- artery I77.5
- bladder (aseptic) (sphincter) N32.89
- bone — *see also* Osteonecrosis M87.9
  - aseptic or avascular — *see* Osteonecrosis
    - idiopathic M87.00
  - ethmoid J32.2
  - jaw M27.2
  - tuberculous — *see* Tuberculosis, bone
- brain I67.89
- breast (aseptic) (fat) (segmental) N64.1
- bronchus J98.09
- central nervous system NEC I67.89
- cerebellar I67.89
- cerebral I67.89
- colon — *see also* Infarct, intestine K55.049
- cornea H18.89- ☑
- cortical (acute) (renal) N17.1
- cystic medial (aorta) — *see* Dissection, aorta
- dental pulp K04.1
- esophagus K22.8
- ethmoid (bone) J32.2
- eyelid — *see* Disorder, eyelid, degenerative
- fat, fatty (generalized) — *see also* Disorder, soft tissue, specified type NEC)
  - abdominal wall K65.4
  - breast (aseptic) (segmental) N64.1
  - localized — *see* Degeneration, by site, fatty
  - mesentery K65.4
  - omentum K65.4
  - pancreas K86.89
  - peritoneum K65.4
  - skin (subcutaneous), newborn P83.0
  - subcutaneous, due to birth injury P15.6
- gallbladder — *see* Cholecystitis, acute
- heart — *see* Infarct, myocardium
- hip, aseptic or avascular — *see* Osteonecrosis, by type, femur
- intestine (acute) (hemorrhagic) (massive) — *see also* Infarct, intestine K55.069
- jaw M27.2
- kidney (bilateral) N28.0
  - acute N17.9
  - cortical (acute) (bilateral) N17.1
    - with ectopic or molar pregnancy O08.4
  - medullary (bilateral) (in acute renal failure) (papillary) N17.2
  - papillary (bilateral) (in acute renal failure) N17.2
  - tubular N17.0
    - with ectopic or molar pregnancy O08.4
    - complicating
      - abortion — *see* Abortion, by type, complicated by, tubular necrosis
      - ectopic or molar pregnancy O08.4
      - pregnancy — *see* Pregnancy, complicated by, diseases of, specified type or system NEC
    - following ectopic or molar pregnancy O08.4
    - traumatic T79.5 ☑
- larynx J38.7
- liver (with hepatic failure) (cell) — *see* Failure, hepatic
  - hemorrhagic, central K76.2
- lung J85.0
- lymphatic gland — *see* Lymphadenitis, acute
- mammary gland (fat) (segmental) N64.1
- mastoid (chronic) — *see* Mastoiditis, chronic

Necrosis, necrotic — *continued*
- medullary (acute) (renal) N17.2
- mesentery — *see also* Infarct, intestine K55.069
  - fat K65.4
- mitral valve — *see* Insufficiency, mitral
- myocardium, myocardial — *see* Infarct, myocardium
- nose J34.0
- omentum (with mesenteric infarction) — *see also* Infarct, intestine K55.069
  - fat K65.4
- orbit, orbital — *see* Osteomyelitis, orbit
- ossicles, ear — *see* Abnormal, ear ossicles
- ovary N70.92
- pancreas (aseptic) (duct) (fat) K86.89
  - acute (infective) — *see* Pancreatitis, acute
  - infective — *see* Pancreatitis, acute
- papillary (acute) (renal) N17.2
- perineum N90.89
- peritoneum (with mesenteric infarction) — *see also* Infarct, intestine K55.069
  - fat K65.4
- pharynx J02.9
  - in granulocytopenia — *see* Neutropenia
  - Vincent's A69.1
- phosphorus — *see* subcategory T54.2 ☑
- pituitary (gland) E23.0
  - postpartum O99.285
  - Sheehan O99.285
- pressure — *see* Ulcer, pressure, by site
- pulmonary J85.0
- pulp (dental) K04.1
- radiation — *see* Necrosis, by site
- radium — *see* Necrosis, by site
- renal — *see* Necrosis, kidney
- sclera H15.89
- scrotum N50.89
- skin or subcutaneous tissue NEC I96
- spine, spinal (column) — *see also* Osteonecrosis, by type, vertebra
  - cord G95.19
- spleen D73.5
- stomach K31.89
- stomatitis (ulcerative) A69.0
- subcutaneous fat, newborn P83.88
- subendocardial (acute) I21.4
  - chronic I25.89
- suprarenal (capsule) (gland) E27.49
- testis N50.89
- thymus (gland) E32.8
- tonsil J35.8
- trachea J39.8
- tuberculous NEC — *see* Tuberculosis
- tubular (acute) (anoxic) (renal) (toxic) N17.0
  - postprocedural N99.0
- vagina N89.8
- vertebra — *see also* Osteonecrosis, by type, vertebra
  - tuberculous A18.01
- vulva N90.89
- X-ray — *see* Necrosis, by site
Necrospermia — *see* Infertility, male
Need (for)
- care provider because (of)
  - assistance with personal care Z74.1
  - continuous supervision required Z74.3
  - impaired mobility Z74.09
  - no other household member able to render care Z74.2
  - specified reason NEC Z74.8
- immunization — *see* Vaccination
- vaccination — *see* Vaccination
Neglect
- adult
  - confirmed T74.01 ☑
  - history of Z91.412
  - suspected T76.01 ☑
- child (childhood)
  - confirmed T74.02 ☑
  - history of Z62.812
  - suspected T76.02 ☑
- emotional, in childhood Z62.898
- hemispatial R41.4
- left-sided R41.4
- sensory R41.4
- visuospatial R41.4
Neisserian infection NEC — *see* Gonococcus
Nelaton's syndrome G60.8
Nelson's syndrome E24.1
Nematodiasis (intestinal) B82.0

⬧ Subterms under main terms may continue to next column or page   ☑ Additional Character Required — Refer to the Tabular List for Character Selection   **229**

Naegeli's — Nematodiasis

Nematodiasis — *continued*
  Ancylostoma B76.0
Neonatal — *see also* Newborn
  acne L70.4
  bradycardia P29.12
  screening, abnormal findings on P09
  tachycardia P29.11
  tooth, teeth K00.6
Neonatorum — *see* condition
Neoplasia
  endocrine, multiple (MEN) E31.20
    type I E31.21
    type IIA E31.22
    type IIB E31.23
  intraepithelial (histologically confirmed)
    anal (AIN) (histologically confirmed) K62.82
      grade I K62.82
      grade II K62.82
      severe D01.3
    cervical glandular (histologically confirmed) D06.9
    cervix (uteri) (CIN) (histologically confirmed) N87.9
      glandular D06.9
      grade I N87.0
      grade II N87.1
      grade III (severe dysplasia) — *see also* Carcinoma,
        cervix uteri, in situ D06.9
    prostate (histologically confirmed) (PIN) N42.31
      grade I N42.31
      grade II N42.31
      grade III (severe dysplasia) D07.5
    vagina (histologically confirmed) (VAIN) N89.3
      grade I N89.0
      grade II N89.1
      grade III (severe dysplasia) D07.2
    vulva (histologically confirmed) (VIN) N90.3
      grade I N90.0
      grade II N90.1
      grade III (severe dysplasia) D07.1
Neoplasm, neoplastic — *see also* Table of Neoplasms
  lipomatous, benign — *see* Lipoma
  malignant mast cell C96.20
    specified type NEC C96.29
  mast cell, of uncertain behavior NEC D47.09
Neovascularization
  ciliary body — *see* Disorder, iris, vascular
  cornea H16.40- ☑
    deep H16.44- ☑
    ghost vessels — *see* Ghost, vessels
    localized H16.43- ☑
    pannus — *see* Pannus
  iris — *see* Disorder, iris, vascular
  retina H35.05- ☑
Nephralgia N23
Nephritis, nephritic (albuminuric) (azotemic) (congenital) (disseminated) (epithelial) (familial) (focal) (granulomatous) (hemorrhagic) (infantile) (nonsuppurative, excretory) (uremic) N05.9
  with
    dense deposit disease N05.6
    diffuse
      crescentic glomerulonephritis N05.7
      endocapillary proliferative glomerulonephritis
        N05.4
      membranous glomerulonephritis N05.2
      mesangial proliferative glomerulonephritis N05.3
      mesangiocapillary glomerulonephritis N05.5
    edema — *see* Nephrosis
    focal and segmental glomerular lesions N05.1
    foot process disease N04.9
    glomerular lesion
      diffuse sclerosing N05.8
      hypocomplementemic — *see* Nephritis, membranoproliferative
      IgA — *see* Nephropathy, IgA
      lobular, lobulonodular — *see* Nephritis, membranoproliferative
      nodular — *see* Nephritis, membranoproliferative
    lesion of
      glomerulonephritis, proliferative N05.8
      renal necrosis N05.9
    minor glomerular abnormality N05.0
    specified morphological changes NEC N05.8
  acute N00.9
    with
      dense deposit disease N00.6
      diffuse
        crescentic glomerulonephritis N00.7

Nephritis, nephritic — *continued*
  acute — *continued*
    with — *continued*
      diffuse — *continued*
        endocapillary proliferative glomerulonephritis
          N00.4
        membranous glomerulonephritis N00.2
        mesangial proliferative glomerulonephritis
          N00.3
        mesangiocapillary glomerulonephritis N00.5
      focal and segmental glomerular lesions N00.1
      minor glomerular abnormality N00.0
      specified morphological changes NEC N00.8
  amyloid E85.4 *[N08]*
  antiglomerular basement membrane (anti-GBM) antibody NEC
    in Goodpasture's syndrome M31.0
  antitubular basement membrane (tubulo-interstitial)
    NEC N12
    toxic — *see* Nephropathy, toxic
  arteriolar — *see* Hypertension, kidney
  arteriosclerotic — *see* Hypertension, kidney
  ascending — *see* Nephritis, tubulo-interstitial
  atrophic N03.9
  Balkan (endemic) N15.0
  calculous, calculus — *see* Calculus, kidney
  cardiac — *see* Hypertension, kidney
  cardiovascular — *see* Hypertension, kidney
  chronic N03.9
    with
      dense deposit disease N03.6
      diffuse
        crescentic glomerulonephritis N03.7
        endocapillary proliferative glomerulonephritis
          N03.4
        membranous glomerulonephritis N03.2
        mesangial proliferative glomerulonephritis
          N03.3
        mesangiocapillary glomerulonephritis N03.5
      focal and segmental glomerular lesions N03.1
      minor glomerular abnormality N03.0
      specified morphological changes NEC N03.8
    arteriosclerotic — *see* Hypertension, kidney
  cirrhotic N26.9
  complicating pregnancy O26.83- ☑
  croupous N00.9
  degenerative — *see* Nephrosis
  diffuse sclerosing N05.8
  due to
    diabetes mellitus — *see* E08-E13 with .21
    subacute bacterial endocarditis I33.0
    systemic lupus erythematosus (chronic) M32.14
    typhoid fever A01.09
  gonococcal (acute) (chronic) A54.21
  hypocomplementemic — *see* Nephritis, membranoproliferative
  IgA — *see* Nephropathy, IgA
  immune complex (circulating) NEC N05.8
  infective — *see* Nephritis, tubulo-interstitial
  interstitial — *see* Nephritis, tubulo-interstitial
  lead N14.3
  membranoproliferative (diffuse) (type 1 or 3) — *see*
    also N00-N07 with fourth character .5 N05.5
    type 2 — *see also* N00-N07 with fourth character .6
      N05.6
  minimal change N05.0
  necrotic, necrotizing NEC — *see also* N00-N07 with
    fourth character .8 N05.8
  nephrotic — *see* Nephrosis
  nodular — *see* Nephritis, membranoproliferative
  polycystic Q61.3
    adult type Q61.2
    autosomal
      dominant Q61.2
      recessive NEC Q61.19
    childhood type NEC Q61.19
    infantile type NEC Q61.19
  poststreptococcal N05.9
    acute N00.9
    chronic N03.9
    rapidly progressive N01.9
  proliferative NEC — *see also* N00-N07 with fourth
    character .8 N05.8
  purulent — *see* Nephritis, tubulo-interstitial
  rapidly progressive N01.9
    with
      dense deposit disease N01.6

Nephritis, nephritic — *continued*
  rapidly progressive — *continued*
    with — *continued*
      diffuse
        crescentic glomerulonephritis N01.7
        endocapillary proliferative glomerulonephrit♦
          N01.4
        membranous glomerulonephritis N01.2
        mesangial proliferative glomerulonephritis
          N01.3
        mesangiocapillary glomerulonephritis N01
      focal and segmental glomerular lesions N01.1
      minor glomerular abnormality N01.0
      specified morphological changes NEC N01.8
  salt losing or wasting NEC N28.89
  saturnine N14.3
  sclerosing, diffuse N05.8
  septic — *see* Nephritis, tubulo-interstitial
  specified pathology NEC — *see also* N00-N07 with
    fourth character .8 N05.8
  subacute N01.9
  suppurative — *see* Nephritis, tubulo-interstitial
  syphilitic (late) A52.75
    congenital A50.59 *[N08]*
    early (secondary) A51.44
  toxic — *see* Nephropathy, toxic
  tubal, tubular — *see* Nephritis, tubulo-interstitial
  tuberculous A18.11
  tubulo-interstitial (in) N12
    acute (infectious) N10
    chronic (infectious) N11.9
      nonobstructive N11.8
        reflux-associated N11.0
      obstructive N11.1
      specified NEC N11.8
    due to
      brucellosis A23.9 *[N16]*
      cryoglobulinemia D89.1 *[N16]*
      glycogen storage disease E74.00 *[N16]*
      Sjögren's syndrome M35.04
  vascular — *see* Hypertension, kidney
  war N00.9
Nephroblastoma (epithelial) (mesenchymal) C64- ☑
Nephrocalcinosis E83.59 *[N29]*
Nephrocystitis, pustular — *see* Nephritis, tubulo-interstitial
Nephrolithiasis (congenital) (pelvis) (recurrent) — *see*
  also Calculus, kidney
Nephroma C64- ☑
  mesoblastic D41.0- ☑
Nephronephritis — *see* Nephrosis
Nephronophthisis Q61.5
Nephropathia epidemica A98.5
Nephropathy — *see also* Nephritis N28.9
  with
    edema — *see* Nephrosis
    glomerular lesion — *see* Glomerulonephritis
  amyloid, hereditary E85.0
  analgesic N14.0
    with medullary necrosis, acute N17.2
  Balkan (endemic) N15.0
  chemical — *see* Nephropathy, toxic
  diabetic — *see* E08-E13 with .21
  drug-induced N14.2
    specified NEC N14.1
  focal and segmental hyalinosis or sclerosis N02.1
  heavy metal-induced N14.3
  hereditary NEC N07.9
    with
      dense deposit disease N07.6
      diffuse
        crescentic glomerulonephritis N07.7
        endocapillary proliferative glomerulonephri♦
          N07.4
        membranous glomerulonephritis N07.2
        mesangial proliferative glomerulonephritis
          N07.3
        mesangiocapillary glomerulonephritis N07♦
      focal and segmental glomerular lesions N07.1
      minor glomerular abnormality N07.0
      specified morphological changes NEC N07.8
  hypercalcemic N25.89
  hypertensive — *see* Hypertension, kidney
  hypokalemic (vacuolar) N25.89
  IgA N02.8
    with glomerular lesion N02.9
      focal and segmental hyalinosis or sclerosis N02♦
      membranoproliferative (diffuse) N02.5

ephropathy — *continued*
  IgA — *continued*
    with glomerular lesion — *continued*
      membranous (diffuse) N02.2
      mesangial proliferative (diffuse) N02.3
      mesangiocapillary (diffuse) N02.5
      proliferative NEC N02.8
      specified pathology NEC N02.8
    lead N14.3
  membranoproliferative (diffuse) N02.5
  membranous (diffuse) N02.2
  mesangial (IgA/IgG) — *see* Nephropathy, IgA
    proliferative (diffuse) N02.3
  mesangiocapillary (diffuse) N02.5
  obstructive N13.8
  phenacetin N17.2
  phosphate-losing N25.0
  potassium depletion N25.89
  pregnancy-related O26.83- ☑
  proliferative NEC — *see also* N00-N07 with fourth
    character .8 N05.8
  protein-losing N25.89
  saturnine N14.3
  sickle-cell D57.- ☑ *[N08]*
  toxic NEC N14.4
    due to
      drugs N14.2
        analgesic N14.0
        specified NEC N14.1
      heavy metals N14.3
  vasomotor N17.0
  water-losing N25.89
Nephroptosis N28.83
Nephropyosis — *see* Abscess, kidney
Nephrorrhagia N28.89
Nephrosclerosis (arteriolar)(arteriosclerotic) (chronic)
  (hyaline) — *see also* Hypertension, kidney
  hyperplastic — *see* Hypertension, kidney
  senile N26.9
Nephrosis, nephrotic (Epstein's) (syndrome) (congenital)
  N04.9
  with
    foot process disease N04.9
    glomerular lesion N04.1
    hypocomplementemic N04.5
  acute N04.9
  anoxic — *see* Nephrosis, tubular
  chemical — *see* Nephrosis, tubular
  cholemic K76.7
  diabetic — *see* E08-E13 with .21
  Finnish type (congenital) Q89.8
  hemoglobin N10
  hemoglobinuric — *see* Nephrosis, tubular
  in
    amyloidosis E85.4 *[N08]*
    diabetes mellitus — *see* E08-E13 with .21
    epidemic hemorrhagic fever A98.5
    malaria (malariae) B52.0
  ischemic — *see* Nephrosis, tubular
  lipoid N04.9
  lower nephron — *see* Nephrosis, tubular
  malarial (malariae) B52.0
  minimal change N04.0
  myoglobin N10
  necrotizing — *see* Nephrosis, tubular
  osmotic (sucrose) N25.89
  radiation N04.9
  syphilitic (late) A52.75
  toxic — *see* Nephrosis, tubular
  tubular (acute) N17.0
    postprocedural N99.0
    radiation N04.9
Nephrosonephritis, hemorrhagic (endemic) A98.5
Nephrostomy
  attention to Z43.6
  status Z93.6
Nerve — *see also* condition
  injury — *see* Injury, nerve, by body site
Nerves R45.0
Nervous — *see also* condition R45.0
  heart F45.8
  stomach F45.8
  tension R45.0
Nervousness R45.0
Nesidioblastoma
  pancreas D13.7
  specified site NEC — *see* Neoplasm, benign, by site
  unspecified site D13.7

Nettleship's syndrome — *see* Urticaria pigmentosa
Neumann's disease or syndrome L10.1
Neuralgia, neuralgic (acute) M79.2
  accessory (nerve) G52.8
  acoustic (nerve) — *see* subcategory H93.3 ☑
  auditory (nerve) — *see* subcategory H93.3 ☑
  ciliary G44.009
    intractable G44.001
    not intractable G44.009
  cranial
    nerve — *see also* Disorder, nerve, cranial
      fifth or trigeminal — *see* Neuralgia, trigeminal
    postherpetic, postzoster B02.29
  ear — *see* subcategory H92.0 ☑
  facialis vera G51.1
  Fothergill's — *see* Neuralgia, trigeminal
  glossopharyngeal (nerve) G52.1
  Horton's G44.099
    intractable G44.091
    not intractable G44.099
  Hunt's B02.21
  hypoglossal (nerve) G52.3
  infraorbital — *see* Neuralgia, trigeminal
  malarial — *see* Malaria
  migrainous G44.009
    intractable G44.001
    not intractable G44.009
  Morton's G57.6- ☑
  nerve, cranial — *see* Disorder, nerve, cranial
  nose G52.0
  occipital M54.81
  olfactory G52.0
  penis N48.9
  perineum R10.2
  postherpetic NEC B02.29
    trigeminal B02.22
  pubic region R10.2
  scrotum R10.2
  Sluder's G44.89
  specified nerve NEC G58.8
  spermatic cord R10.2
  sphenopalatine (ganglion) G90.09
  trifacial — *see* Neuralgia, trigeminal
  trigeminal G50.0
    postherpetic, postzoster B02.22
  vagus (nerve) G52.2
  writer's F48.8
    organic G25.89
Neurapraxia — *see* Injury, nerve
Neurasthenia F48.8
  cardiac F45.8
  gastric F45.8
  heart F45.8
Neurilemmoma — *see also* Neoplasm, nerve, benign
  acoustic (nerve) D33.3
  malignant — *see also* Neoplasm, nerve, malignant
    acoustic (nerve) C72.4- ☑
Neurilemmosarcoma — *see* Neoplasm, nerve, malignant
Neurinoma — *see* Neoplasm, nerve, benign
Neurinomatosis — *see* Neoplasm, nerve, uncertain behavior
Neuritis (rheumatoid) M79.2
  abducens (nerve) — *see* Strabismus, paralytic, sixth
    nerve
  accessory (nerve) G52.8
  acoustic (nerve) — *see also* subcategory H93.3 ☑
    in (due to)
      infectious disease NEC B99 ☑ *[H94.0-]* ☑
      parasitic disease NEC B89 *[H94.0-]* ☑
    syphilitic A52.15
  alcoholic G62.1
    with psychosis — *see* Psychosis, alcoholic
  amyloid, any site E85.4 *[G63]*
  auditory (nerve) — *see* subcategory H93.3 ☑
  brachial — *see* Radiculopathy
    due to displacement, intervertebral disc — *see* Dis-
      order, disc, cervical, with neuritis
  cranial nerve
    due to Lyme disease A69.22
    eighth or acoustic or auditory — *see* subcategory
      H93.3 ☑
    eleventh or accessory G52.8
    fifth or trigeminal G51.0
    first or olfactory G52.0
    fourth or trochlear — *see* Strabismus, paralytic,
      fourth nerve
    second or optic — *see* Neuritis, optic

Neuritis — *continued*
  cranial nerve — *continued*
    seventh or facial G51.8
      newborn (birth injury) P11.3
    sixth or abducent — *see* Strabismus, paralytic, sixth
      nerve
    tenth or vagus G52.2
    third or oculomotor — *see* Strabismus, paralytic,
      third nerve
    twelfth or hypoglossal G52.3
  Déjérine-Sottas G60.0
  diabetic (mononeuropathy) — *see* E08-E13 with .41
    polyneuropathy — *see* E08-E13 with .42
  due to
    beriberi E51.11
    displacement, prolapse or rupture, intervertebral
      disc — *see* Disorder, disc, with, radiculopathy
    herniation, nucleus pulposus M51.9 *[G55]*
  endemic E51.11
  facial G51.8
    newborn (birth injury) P11.3
  general — *see* Polyneuropathy
  geniculate ganglion G51.1
    due to herpes (zoster) B02.21
  gouty — *see also* Gout, by type M10.9 *[G63]*
  hypoglossal (nerve) G52.3
  ilioinguinal (nerve) G57.9- ☑
  infectious (multiple) NEC G61.0
  interstitial hypertrophic progressive G60.0
  lumbar M54.16
  lumbosacral M54.17
  multiple — *see also* Polyneuropathy
    endemic E51.11
    infective, acute G61.0
  multiplex endemica E51.11
  nerve root — *see* Radiculopathy
  oculomotor (nerve) — *see* Strabismus, paralytic, third
    nerve
  olfactory nerve G52.0
  optic (nerve) (hereditary) (sympathetic) H46.9
    with demyelination G36.0
    in myelitis G36.0
    nutritional H46.2
    papillitis — *see* Papillitis, optic
    retrobulbar H46.1- ☑
    specified type NEC H46.8
    toxic H46.3
  peripheral (nerve) G62.9
    multiple — *see* Polyneuropathy
    single — *see* Mononeuritis
  pneumogastric (nerve) G52.2
  postherpetic, postzoster B02.29
  progressive hypertrophic interstitial G60.0
  retrobulbar — *see also* Neuritis, optic, retrobulbar
    in (due to)
      late syphilis A52.15
      meningococcal infection A39.82
    meningococcal A39.82
    syphilitic A52.15
  sciatic (nerve) — *see also* Sciatica
    due to displacement of intervertebral disc — *see*
      Disorder, disc, with, radiculopathy
  serum — *see also* Reaction, serum T80.69 ☑
  shoulder-girdle G54.5
  specified nerve NEC G58.8
  spinal (nerve) root — *see* Radiculopathy
  syphilitic A52.15
  thenar (median) G56.1- ☑
  thoracic M54.14
  toxic NEC G62.2
  trochlear (nerve) — *see* Strabismus, paralytic, fourth
    nerve
  vagus (nerve) G52.2
Neuroastrocytoma — *see* Neoplasm, uncertain behavior,
  by site
Neuroavitaminosis E56.9 *[G99.8]*
Neuroblastoma
  olfactory C30.0
  specified site — *see* Neoplasm, malignant, by site
  unspecified site C74.90
Neurochorioretinitis — *see* Chorioretinitis
Neurocirculatory asthenia F45.8
Neurocysticercosis B69.0
Neurocytoma — *see* Neoplasm, benign, by site
Neurodermatitis (circumscribed) (circumscripta) (local)
  L28.0
  atopic L20.81
  diffuse (Brocq) L20.81

Neurodermatitis — *continued*
 disseminated L20.81
Neuroencephalomyelopathy, optic G36.0
Neuroepithelioma — *see also* Neoplasm, malignant, by site
 olfactory C30.0
Neurofibroma — *see also* Neoplasm, nerve, benign
 melanotic — *see* Neoplasm, nerve, benign
 multiple — *see* Neurofibromatosis
 plexiform — *see* Neoplasm, nerve, benign
Neurofibromatosis (multiple) (nonmalignant) Q85.00
 acoustic Q85.02
 malignant — *see* Neoplasm, nerve, malignant
 specified NEC Q85.09
 type 1 (von Recklinghausen) Q85.01
 type 2 Q85.02
Neurofibrosarcoma — *see* Neoplasm, nerve, malignant
Neurogenic — *see also* condition
 bladder — *see also* Dysfunction, bladder, neuromuscular N31.9
  cauda equina syndrome G83.4
 bowel NEC K59.2
 heart F45.8
Neuroglioma — *see* Neoplasm, uncertain behavior, by site
Neurolabyrinthitis (of Dix and Hallpike) — *see* Neuronitis, vestibular
Neurolathyrism — *see* Poisoning, food, noxious, plant
Neuroleprosy A30.9
Neuroma — *see also* Neoplasm, nerve, benign
 acoustic (nerve) D33.3
 amputation (stump) (traumatic) (surgical complication) (late) T87.3- ☑
  arm T87.3- ☑
  leg T87.3- ☑
 digital (toe) G57.6- ☑
 interdigital G58.8
  lower limb (toe) G57.8- ☑
  upper limb G56.8- ☑
 intermetatarsal G57.8- ☑
 Morton's G57.6- ☑
 nonneoplastic
  arm G56.9- ☑
  leg G57.9- ☑
  lower extremity G57.9- ☑
  upper extremity G56.9- ☑
 optic (nerve) D33.3
 plantar G57.6- ☑
 plexiform — *see* Neoplasm, nerve, benign
 surgical (nonneoplastic)
  arm G56.9- ☑
  leg G57.9- ☑
  lower extremity G57.9- ☑
  upper extremity G56.9- ☑
Neuromyalgia — *see* Neuralgia
Neuromyasthenia (epidemic) (postinfectious) G93.3
Neuromyelitis G36.9
 ascending G61.0
 optica G36.0
Neuromyopathy G70.9
 paraneoplastic D49.9 *[G13.0]*
Neuromyotonia (Isaacs) G71.19
Neuronevus — *see* Nevus
Neuronitis G58.9
 ascending (acute) G57.2- ☑
 vestibular H81.2- ☑
Neuroparalytic — *see* condition
Neuropathy, neuropathic G62.9
 acute motor G62.81
 alcoholic G62.1
  with psychosis — *see* Psychosis, alcoholic
 arm G56.9- ☑
 autonomic, peripheral — *see* Neuropathy, peripheral, autonomic
 axillary G56.9- ☑
 bladder N31.9
  atonic (motor) (sensory) N31.2
  autonomous N31.2
  flaccid N31.2
  nonreflex N31.2
  reflex N31.1
  uninhibited N31.0
 brachial plexus G54.0
 cervical plexus G54.2
 chronic
  progressive segmentally demyelinating G62.89
  relapsing demyelinating G62.89

Neuropathy, neuropathic — *continued*
 Déjérine-Sottas G60.0
 diabetic — *see* E08-E13 with .40
  mononeuropathy — *see* E08-E13 with .41
  polyneuropathy — *see* E08-E13 with .42
 entrapment G58.9
  iliohypogastric nerve G57.8- ☑
  ilioinguinal nerve G57.8- ☑
  lateral cutaneous nerve of thigh G57.1- ☑
  median nerve G56.0- ☑
  obturator nerve G57.8- ☑
  peroneal nerve G57.3- ☑
  posterior tibial nerve G57.5- ☑
  saphenous nerve G57.8- ☑
  ulnar nerve G56.2- ☑
 facial nerve G51.9
 hereditary G60.9
  motor and sensory (types I-IV) G60.0
  sensory G60.8
  specified NEC G60.8
 hypertrophic G60.0
  Charcot-Marie-Tooth G60.0
  Déjérine-Sottas G60.0
  interstitial progressive G60.0
  of infancy G60.0
  Refsum G60.1
 idiopathic G60.9
  progressive G60.3
  specified NEC G60.8
 in association with hereditary ataxia G60.2
 intercostal G58.0
 ischemic — *see* Disorder, nerve
 Jamaica (ginger) G62.2
 leg NEC G57.9- ☑
 lower extremity G57.9- ☑
 lumbar plexus G54.1
 median nerve G56.1- ☑
 motor and sensory — *see also* Polyneuropathy
  hereditary (types I-IV) G60.0
 multifocal motor (MMN) G61.82
 multiple (acute) (chronic) — *see* Polyneuropathy
 optic (nerve) — *see also* Neuritis, optic
  ischemic H47.01- ☑
 paraneoplastic (sensorial) (Denny Brown) D49.9 *[G13.0]*
 peripheral (nerve) — *see also* Polyneuropathy G62.9
  autonomic G90.9
   idiopathic G90.09
   in (due to)
    amyloidosis E85.4 *[G99.0]*
    diabetes mellitus — *see* E08-E13 with .43
    endocrine disease NEC E34.9 *[G99.0]*
    gout M10.00 *[G99.0]*
    hyperthyroidism E05.90 *[G99.0]*
     with thyroid storm E05.91 *[G99.0]*
    metabolic disease NEC E88.9 *[G99.0]*
  idiopathic G60.9
   progressive G60.3
  in (due to)
   antitetanus serum G62.0
   arsenic G62.2
   drugs NEC G62.0
   lead G62.2
   organophosphate compounds G62.2
   toxic agent NEC G62.2
 plantar nerves G57.6- ☑
 progressive
  hypertrophic interstitial G60.0
  inflammatory G62.81
 radicular NEC — *see* Radiculopathy
 sacral plexus G54.1
 sciatic G57.0- ☑
 serum G61.1
 toxic NEC G62.2
 trigeminal sensory G50.8
 ulnar nerve G56.2- ☑
 uremic N18.9 *[G63]*
 vitamin B12 E53.8 *[G63]*
  with anemia (pernicious) D51.0 *[G63]*
   due to dietary deficiency D51.3 *[G63]*
Neurophthisis — *see also* Disorder, nerve
 peripheral, diabetic — *see* E08-E13 with .42
Neuroretinitis — *see* Chorioretinitis
Neuroretinopathy, hereditary optic H47.22
Neurosarcoma — *see* Neoplasm, nerve, malignant
Neurosclerosis — *see* Disorder, nerve
Neurosis, neurotic F10.9
 anankastic F42.8

Neurosis, neurotic — *continued*
 anxiety (state) F41.1
  panic type F41.0
 asthenic F48.8
 bladder F45.8
 cardiac (reflex) F45.8
 cardiovascular F45.8
 character F60.9
 colon F45.8
 compensation F68.10
 compulsive, compulsion F42.8
 conversion F44.9
 craft F48.8
 cutaneous F45.8
 depersonalization F48.1
 depressive (reaction) (type) F34.1
 environmental F48.8
 excoriation L98.1
 fatigue F48.8
 functional — *see* Disorder, somatoform
 gastric F45.8
 gastrointestinal F45.8
 heart F45.8
 hypochondriacal F45.21
 hysterical F44.9
 incoordination F45.8
  larynx F45.8
  vocal cord F45.8
 intestine F45.8
 larynx (sensory) F45.8
  hysterical F44.4
 mixed NEC F48.8
 musculoskeletal F45.8
 obsessional F42.8
 obsessive-compulsive F42.8
 occupational F48.8
 ocular NEC F45.8
 organ — *see* Disorder, somatoform
 pharynx F45.8
 phobic F40.9
 posttraumatic (situational) F43.10
  acute F43.11
  chronic F43.12
 psychasthenic (type) F48.8
 railroad F48.8
 rectum F45.8
 respiratory F45.8
 rumination F45.8
 sexual F65.9
 situational F48.8
 social F40.10
  generalized F40.11
 specified type NEC F48.8
 state F48.9
  with depersonalization episode F48.1
 stomach F45.8
 traumatic F43.10
  acute F43.11
  chronic F43.12
 vasomotor F45.8
 visceral F45.8
 war F48.8
Neurospongioblastosis diffusa Q85.1
Neurosyphilis (arrested) (early) (gumma) (late) (latent▼ (recurrent) (relapse) A52.3
 with ataxia (cerebellar) (locomotor) (spastic) (spinal) A52.19
 aneurysm (cerebral) A52.05
 arachnoid (adhesive) A52.13
 arteritis (any artery) (cerebral) A52.04
 asymptomatic A52.2
 congenital A50.40
 dura (mater) A52.13
 general paresis A52.17
 hemorrhagic A52.05
 juvenile (asymptomatic) (meningeal) A50.40
 leptomeninges (aseptic) A52.13
 meningeal, meninges (adhesive) A52.13
 meningitis A52.13
 meningovascular (diffuse) A52.13
 optic atrophy A52.15
 parenchymatous (degenerative) A52.19
 paresis, paretic A52.17
  juvenile A50.45
 remission in (sustained) A52.3
 serological (without symptoms) A52.2
 specified nature or site NEC A52.19
 tabes, tabetic (dorsalis) A52.11
  juvenile A50.45

☑ **Additional Character Required** — Refer to the Tabular List for Character Selection ▽ Subterms under main terms may continue to next column or pag

Neurosyphilis — continued
taboparesis A52.17
  juvenile A50.45
thrombosis (cerebral) A52.05
vascular (cerebral) NEC A52.05
Neurothekeoma — see Neoplasm, nerve, benign
Neurotic — see Neurosis
Neurotoxemia — see Toxemia
Neutroclusion M26.211
Neutropenia, neutropenic (chronic) (genetic) (idiopathic) (immune) (infantile) (malignant) (pernicious) (splenic) D70.9
congenital (primary) D70.0
cyclic D70.4
cytoreductive cancer chemotherapy sequela D70.1
drug-induced D70.2
  due to cytoreductive cancer chemotherapy D70.1
due to infection D70.3
fever D70.9
neonatal, transitory (isoimmune) (maternal transfer) P61.5
periodic D70.4
secondary (cyclic) (periodic) (splenic) D70.4
  drug-induced D70.2
    due to cytoreductive cancer chemotherapy D70.1
toxic D70.8
Neutrophilia, hereditary giant D72.0
Nevocarcinoma — see Melanoma
Nevus D22.9
achromic — see Neoplasm, skin, benign
amelanotic — see Neoplasm, skin, benign
angiomatous D18.00
  intra-abdominal D18.03
  intracranial D18.02
  skin D18.01
  specified site NEC D18.09
araneus I78.1
balloon cell — see Neoplasm, skin, benign
bathing trunk D48.5
blue — see Neoplasm, skin, benign
  cellular — see Neoplasm, skin, benign
  giant — see Neoplasm, skin, benign
  Jadassohn's — see Neoplasm, skin, benign
  malignant — see Melanoma
capillary D18.00
  intra-abdominal D18.03
  intracranial D18.02
  skin D18.01
  specified site NEC D18.09
cavernous D18.00
  intra-abdominal D18.03
  intracranial D18.02
  skin D18.01
  specified site NEC D18.09
cellular — see Neoplasm, skin, benign
  blue — see Neoplasm, skin, benign
choroid D31.3- ☑
comedonicus Q82.5
conjunctiva D31.0- ☑
dermal — see Neoplasm, skin, benign
  with epidermal nevus — see Neoplasm, skin, benign
dysplastic — see Neoplasm, skin, benign
eye D31.9- ☑
flammeus Q82.5
hemangiomatous D18.00
  intra-abdominal D18.03
  intracranial D18.02
  skin D18.01
  specified site NEC D18.09
iris D31.4- ☑
lacrimal gland D31.5- ☑
lymphatic D18.1
magnocellular
  specified site — see Neoplasm, benign, by site
  unspecified site D31.40
malignant — see Melanoma
meaning hemangioma D18.00
  intra-abdominal D18.03
  intracranial D18.02
  skin D18.01
  specified site NEC D18.09
mouth (mucosa) D10.30
  specified site NEC D10.39
  white sponge Q38.6
multiplex Q85.1
non-neoplastic I78.1
oral mucosa D10.30
  specified site NEC D10.39

Nevus — continued
oral mucosa — continued
  white sponge Q38.6
orbit D31.6- ☑
pigmented
  giant — see also Neoplasm, skin, uncertain behavior D48.5
  malignant melanoma in — see Melanoma
portwine Q82.5
retina D31.2- ☑
retrobulbar D31.6- ☑
sanguineous Q82.5
senile I78.1
skin D22.9
  abdominal wall D22.5
  ala nasi D22.39
  ankle D22.7- ☑
  anus, anal D22.5
  arm D22.6- ☑
  auditory canal (external) D22.2- ☑
  auricle (ear) D22.2- ☑
  auricular canal (external) D22.2- ☑
  axilla, axillary fold D22.5
  back D22.5
  breast D22.5
  brow D22.39
  buttock D22.5
  canthus (eye) D22.1- ☑
  cheek (external) D22.39
  chest wall D22.5
  chin D22.39
  ear (external) D22.2- ☑
  external meatus (ear) D22.2- ☑
  eyebrow D22.39
  eyelid (lower) (upper) D22.1- ☑
  face D22.30
    specified NEC D22.39
  female genital organ (external) NEC D28.0
  finger D22.6- ☑
  flank D22.5
  foot D22.7- ☑
  forearm D22.6- ☑
  forehead D22.39
  foreskin D29.0
  genital organ (external) NEC
    female D28.0
    male D29.9
  gluteal region D22.5
  groin D22.5
  hand D22.6- ☑
  heel D22.7- ☑
  helix D22.2- ☑
  hip D22.7- ☑
  interscapular region D22.5
  jaw D22.39
  knee D22.7- ☑
  labium (majus) (minus) D28.0
  leg D22.7- ☑
  lip (lower) (upper) D22.0
  lower limb D22.7- ☑
  male genital organ (external) D29.9
  nail D22.9
    finger D22.6- ☑
    toe D22.7- ☑
  nasolabial groove D22.39
  nates D22.5
  neck D22.4
  nose (external) D22.39
  palpebra D22.1- ☑
  penis D29.0
  perianal skin D22.5
  perineum D22.5
  pinna D22.2- ☑
  popliteal fossa or space D22.7- ☑
  prepuce D29.0
  pudendum D28.0
  scalp D22.4
  scrotum D29.4
  shoulder D22.6- ☑
  submammary fold D22.5
  temple D22.39
  thigh D22.7- ☑
  toe D22.7- ☑
  trunk NEC D22.5
  umbilicus D22.5
  upper limb D22.6- ☑
  vulva D28.0

Nevus — continued
specified site NEC — see Neoplasm, by site, benign
spider I78.1
stellar I78.1
strawberry Q82.5
Sutton's benign D22.9
unius lateris Q82.5
Unna's Q82.5
vascular Q82.5
verrucous Q82.5
Newborn (infant) (liveborn) (singleton) Z38.2
abstinence syndrome P96.1
acne L70.4
affected by
  abnormalities of membranes P02.9
    specified NEC P02.8
  abruptio placenta P02.1
  amino-acid metabolic disorder, transitory P74.8
  amniocentesis (while in utero) P00.6
  amnionitis P02.78
  apparent life threatening event (ALTE) R68.13
  bleeding (into)
    cerebral cortex P52.22
    germinal matrix P52.0
    ventricles P52.1
  breech delivery P03.0
  cardiac arrest P29.81
  cardiomyopathy I42.8
    congenital I42.4
  cerebral ischemia P91.0
  Cesarean delivery P03.4
  chemotherapy agents P04.11
  chorioamnionitis P02.78
  cocaine (crack) P04.41
  complications of labor and delivery P03.9
    specified NEC P03.89
  compression of umbilical cord NEC P02.5
  contracted pelvis P03.1
  cyanosis P28.2
  delivery P03.9
    Cesarean P03.4
    forceps P03.2
    vacuum extractor P03.3
  drugs of addiction P04.40
    cocaine P04.41
    hallucinogens P04.42
    specified drug NEC P04.49
  entanglement (knot) in umbilical cord P02.5
  environmental chemicals P04.6
  fetal (intrauterine)
    growth retardation P05.9
    inflammatory response syndrome (FIRS) P02.70
    malnutrition not light or small for gestational age P05.2
  FIRS (fetal inflammatory response syndrome) P02.70
  forceps delivery P03.2
  heart rate abnormalities
    bradycardia P29.12
    intrauterine P03.819
      before onset of labor P03.810
      during labor P03.811
    tachycardia P29.11
  hemorrhage (antepartum) P02.1
    cerebellar (nontraumatic) P52.6
    intracerebral (nontraumatic) P52.4
    intracranial (nontraumatic) P52.9
      specified NEC P52.8
    intraventricular (nontraumatic) P52.3
      grade 1 P52.0
      grade 2 P52.1
      grade 3 P52.21
      grade 4 P52.22
    posterior fossa (nontraumatic) P52.6
    subarachnoid (nontraumatic) P52.5
    subependymal P52.0
      with intracerebral extension P52.22
      with intraventricular extension P52.1
        with enlargment of ventricles P52.21
      without intraventricular extension P52.0
  hypoxic ischemic encephalopathy [HIE] P91.60
    mild P91.61
    moderate P91.62
    severe P91.63
  induction of labor P03.89
  intestinal perforation P78.0
  intrauterine (fetal) blood loss P50.9
    due to (from)
      cut end of co-twin cord P50.5

Newborn — *continued*
  affected by — *continued*
    intrauterine blood loss — *continued*
      due to — *continued*
        hemorrhage into
          co-twin P50.3
          maternal circulation P50.4
          placenta P50.2
          ruptured cord blood P50.1
          vasa previa P50.0
        specified NEC P50.8
    intrauterine (fetal) hemorrhage P50.9
    intrauterine (in utero) procedure P96.5
    malpresentation (malposition) NEC P03.1
    maternal (complication of) (use of)
      alcohol P04.3
      amphetamines P04.16
      analgesia (maternal) P04.0
      anesthesia (maternal) P04.0
      anticonvulsants P04.13
      antidepressants P04.15
      antineoplastic chemotherapy P04.11
      anxiolytics P04.1A
      blood loss P02.1
      cannabis P04.81
      circulatory disease P00.3
      condition P00.9
        specified NEC P00.89
      cytotoxic drugs P04.12
      delivery P03.9
        Cesarean P03.4
        forceps P03.2
        vacuum extractor P03.3
      diabetes mellitus (pre-existing) P70.1
      disorder P00.9
        specified NEC P00.89
      drugs (addictive) (illegal) NEC P04.49
      ectopic pregnancy P01.4
      gestational diabetes P70.0
      hemorrhage P02.1
      hypertensive disorder P00.0
      incompetent cervix P01.0
      infectious disease P00.2
      injury P00.5
      labor and delivery P03.9
      malpresentation before labor P01.7
      maternal death P01.6
      medical procedure P00.7
      medication P04.19
        specified type NEC P04.18
      multiple pregnancy P01.5
      nutritional disorder P00.4
      oligohydramnios P01.2
      opiates P04.14
        administered for procedures during pregnancy or labor and delivery P04.0
      parasitic disease P00.2
      periodontal disease P00.81
      placenta previa P02.0
      polyhydramnios P01.3
      precipitate delivery P03.5
      pregnancy P01.9
        specified P01.8
      premature rupture of membranes P01.1
      renal disease P00.1
      respiratory disease P00.3
      sedative-hypnotics P04.17
      surgical procedure P00.6
      tranquilizers administered for procedures during pregnancy or labor and delivery P04.0
      urinary tract disease P00.1
      uterine contraction (abnormal) P03.6
    meconium peritonitis P78.0
    medication (legal) (maternal use) (prescribed) P04.19
    membrane abnormalities P02.9
      specified NEC P02.8
    membranitis P02.78
    methamphetamine(s) P04.49
    mixed metabolic and respiratory acidosis P84
    neonatal abstinence syndrome P96.1
    noxious substances transmitted via placenta or breast milk P04.9
      cannabis P04.81
      specified NEC P04.89
    nutritional supplements P04.5
    placenta previa P02.0
    placental
      abnormality (functional) (morphological) P02.20

Newborn — *continued*
  affected by — *continued*
    placental — *continued*
      abnormality — *continued*
        specified NEC P02.29
      dysfunction P02.29
      infarction P02.29
      insufficiency P02.29
      separation NEC P02.1
      transfusion syndromes P02.3
    placentitis P02.78
    precipitate delivery P03.5
    prolapsed cord P02.4
    respiratory arrest P28.81
    slow intrauterine growth P05.9
    tobacco P04.2
    twin to twin transplacental transfusion P02.3
    umbilical cord (tightly) around neck P02.5
    umbilical cord condition P02.60
      short cord P02.69
      specified NEC P02.69
    uterine contractions (abnormal) P03.6
    vasa previa P02.69
      from intrauterine blood loss P50.0
  apnea P28.4
    obstructive P28.4
    primary P28.3
    sleep (central) (obstructive) (primary) P28.3
  born in hospital Z38.00
    by cesarean Z38.01
  born outside hospital Z38.1
  breast buds P96.89
  breast engorgement P83.4
  check-up — *see* Newborn, examination
  convulsion P90
  dehydration P74.1
  examination
    8 to 28 days old Z00.111
    under 8 days old Z00.110
  fever P81.9
    environmentally-induced P81.0
  hyperbilirubinemia P59.9
    of prematurity P59.0
  hypernatremia P74.21
  hyponatremia P74.22
  infection P39.9
    candidal P37.5
    specified NEC P39.8
    urinary tract P39.3
  jaundice P59.9
    due to
      breast milk inhibitor P59.3
      hepatocellular damage P59.20
        specified NEC P59.29
      preterm delivery P59.0
    of prematurity P59.0
    specified NEC P59.8
  late metabolic acidosis P74.0
  mastitis P39.0
    infective P39.0
    noninfective P83.4
  multiple born NEC Z38.8
    born in hospital Z38.68
      by cesarean Z38.69
    born outside hospital Z38.7
  omphalitis P38.9
    with mild hemorrhage P38.1
    without hemorrhage P38.9
  post-term P08.21
  prolonged gestation (over 42 completed weeks) P08.22
  quadruplet Z38.8
    born in hospital Z38.63
      by cesarean Z38.64
    born outside hospital Z38.7
  quintuplet Z38.8
    born in hospital Z38.65
      by cesarean Z38.66
    born outside hospital Z38.7
  seizure P90
  sepsis (congenital) P36.9
    due to
      anaerobes NEC P36.5
      Escherichia coli P36.4
      Staphylococcus P36.30
        aureus P36.2
        specified NEC P36.39
      Streptococcus P36.10
        group B P36.0
        specified NEC P36.19

Newborn — *continued*
  sepsis — *continued*
    specified NEC P36.8
  triplet Z38.8
    born in hospital Z38.61
      by cesarean Z38.62
    born outside hospital Z38.7
  twin Z38.5
    born in hospital Z38.30
      by cesarean Z38.31
    born outside hospital Z38.4
  vomiting P92.09
    bilious P92.01
  weight check Z00.111

Newcastle conjunctivitis or disease B30.8
Nezelof's syndrome (pure alymphocytosis) D81.4
Niacin (amide) **deficiency** E52
Nicolas (-Durand)-**Favre disease** A55
Nicotine — *see* Tobacco
Nicotinic acid deficiency E52
Niemann-Pick disease or syndrome E75.249
  specified NEC E75.248
  type
    A E75.240
    B E75.241
    C E75.242
    D E75.243
Night
  blindness — *see* Blindness, night
  sweats R61
  terrors (child) F51.4
Nightmares (REM sleep type) F51.5
NIHSS (National Institutes of Health Stroke Scale) **scor**
  R29.7- ☑
Nipple — *see* condition
Nisbet's chancre A57
Nishimoto (-Takeuchi) **disease** I67.5
Nitritoid crisis or reaction — *see* Crisis, nitritoid
Nitrosohemoglobinemia D74.8
Njovera A65
Nocardiosis, nocardiasis A43.9
  cutaneous A43.1
  lung A43.0
  pneumonia A43.0
  pulmonary A43.0
  specified site NEC A43.8
Nocturia R35.1
  psychogenic F45.8
Nocturnal — *see* condition
Nodal rhythm I49.8
Node(s) — *see also* Nodule
  Bouchard's (with arthropathy) M15.2
  Haygarth's M15.8
  Heberden's (with arthropathy) M15.1
  larynx J38.7
  lymph — *see* condition
  milker's B08.03
  Osler's I33.0
  Schmorl's — *see* Schmorl's disease
  singer's J38.2
  teacher's J38.2
  tuberculous — *see* Tuberculosis, lymph gland
  vocal cord J38.2
Nodule(s), **nodular**
  actinomycotic — *see* Actinomycosis
  breast NEC — *see also* Lump, breast N63.0
  colloid (cystic), thyroid E04.1
  cutaneous — *see* Swelling, localized
  endometrial (stromal) D26.1
  Haygarth's M15.8
  inflammatory — *see* Inflammation
  juxta-articular
    syphilitic A52.77
    yaws A66.7
  larynx J38.7
  lung, solitary (subsegmental branch of the bronchia tree) R91.1
    multiple R91.8
  milker's B08.03
  prostate N40.2
    with lower urinary tract symptoms (LUTS) N40.3
    without lower urinary tract symtpoms (LUTS) N40
  pulmonary, solitary (subsegmental branch of the bronchial tree) R91.1
  retrocardiac R09.89
  rheumatoid M06.30
    ankle M06.37- ☑
    elbow M06.32- ☑

☑ **Additional Character Required — Refer to the Tabular List for Character Selection**
    Subterms under main terms may continue to next column or pag

Nodule(s), **nodular** — *continued*
  rheumatoid — *continued*
    foot joint M06.37- ☑
    hand joint M06.34- ☑
    hip M06.35- ☑
    knee M06.36- ☑
    multiple site M06.39
    shoulder M06.31- ☑
    vertebra M06.38
    wrist M06.33- ☑
  scrotum (inflammatory) N49.2
  singer's J38.2
  solitary, lung (subsegmental branch of the bronchial tree) R91.1
    multiple R91.8
  subcutaneous — *see* Swelling, localized
  teacher's J38.2
  thyroid (cold) (gland) (nontoxic) E04.1
    with thyrotoxicosis E05.20
      with thyroid storm E05.21
    toxic or with hyperthyroidism E05.20
      with thyroid storm E05.21
  vocal cord J38.2
Noma (gangrenous) (hospital) (infective) A69.0
  auricle I96
  mouth A69.0
  pudendi N76.89
  vulvae N76.89
Nomad, nomadism Z59.0
NOMID (neonatal onset multisystemic inflammatory disorder) M04.2
Nonadherence to medical treatment Z91.19
Nonautoimmune hemolytic anemia D59.4
  drug-induced D59.2
Nonclosure — *see also* Imperfect, closure
  ductus arteriosus (Botallo's) Q25.0
  foramen
    botalli Q21.1
    ovale Q21.1
Noncompliance Z91.19
  with
    dialysis Z91.15
    dietary regimen Z91.11
    medical treatment Z91.19
    medication regimen NEC Z91.14
      underdosing — *see also* Table of Drugs and Chemicals, categories T36-T50, with final character 6 Z91.14
      intentional NEC Z91.128
        due to financial hardship of patient Z91.120
      unintentional NEC Z91.138
        due to patient's age related debility Z91.130
    renal dialysis Z91.15
Nondescent (congenital) — *see also* Malposition, congenital
  cecum Q43.3
  colon Q43.3
  testicle Q53.9
    bilateral Q53.20
      abdominal Q53.211
      perineal Q53.22
    unilateral Q53.10
      abdominal Q53.111
      perineal Q53.12
Nondevelopment
  brain Q02
    part of Q04.3
  heart Q24.8
  organ or site, congenital NEC — *see* Hypoplasia
Nonengagement
  head NEC O32.4 ☑
    in labor, causing obstructed labor O64.8 ☑
Nonexanthematous tick fever A93.2
Nonexpansion, lung (newborn) P28.0
Nonfunctioning
  cystic duct — *see also* Disease, gallbladder K82.8
  gallbladder — *see also* Disease, gallbladder K82.8
  kidney N28.9
  labyrinth — *see* subcategory H83.2 ☑
Non-Hodgkin lymphoma NEC — *see* Lymphoma, non-Hodgkin
Nonimplantation, ovum N97.2
Noninsufflation, fallopian tube N97.1
Non-ketotic hyperglycinemia E72.51
Nonne-Milroy syndrome Q82.0
Nonovulation N97.0

Non-palpable testicle(s)
  bilateral R39.84
  unilateral R39.83
Nonpatent fallopian tube N97.1
Nonpneumatization, lung NEC P28.0
Nonrotation — *see* Malrotation
Nonsecretion, urine — *see* Anuria
Nonunion
  fracture — *see* Fracture, by site
  joint, following fusion or arthrodesis M96.0
  organ or site, congenital NEC — *see* Imperfect, closure
  symphysis pubis, congenital Q74.2
Nonvisualization, gallbladder R93.2
Nonvital, nonvitalized tooth K04.99
Non-working side interference M26.56
Noonan's syndrome Q87.19
Normocytic anemia (infectional) due to blood loss (chronic) D50.0
  acute D62
Norrie's disease (congenital) Q15.8
North American blastomycosis B40.9
Norwegian itch B86
Nose, nasal — *see* condition
Nosebleed R04.0
Nose-picking F98.8
Nosomania F45.21
Nosophobia F45.22
Nostalgia F43.20
Notch of iris Q13.2
Notching nose, congenital (tip) Q30.2
Nothnagel's
  syndrome — *see* Strabismus, paralytic, third nerve
  vasomotor acroparesthesia I73.89
Novy's relapsing fever A68.9
  louse-borne A68.0
  tick-borne A68.1
Noxious
  foodstuffs, poisoning by — *see* Poisoning, food, noxious, plant
  substances transmitted through placenta or breast milk P04.9
Nucleus pulposus — *see* condition
Numbness R20.0
Nuns' knee — *see* Bursitis, prepatellar
Nursemaid's elbow S53.03- ☑
Nutcracker esophagus K22.4
Nutmeg liver K76.1
Nutrient element deficiency E61.9
  specified NEC E61.8
Nutrition deficient or insufficient — *see also* Malnutrition E46
  due to
    insufficient food T73.0 ☑
    lack of
      care (child) T76.02 ☑
        adult T76.01 ☑
      food T73.0 ☑
Nutritional stunting E45
Nyctalopia (night blindness) — *see* Blindness, night
Nycturia R35.1
  psychogenic F45.8
Nymphomania F52.8
Nystagmus H55.00
  benign paroxysmal — *see* Vertigo, benign paroxysmal
  central positional H81.4
  congenital H55.01
  dissociated H55.04
  latent H55.02
  miners' H55.09
  positional
    benign paroxysmal H81.4
    central H81.4
  specified form NEC H55.09
  visual deprivation H55.03

O

Obermeyer's relapsing fever (European) A68.0
Obesity E66.9
  with alveolar hypoventilation E66.2
  adrenal E27.8
  complicating
    childbirth O99.214
    pregnancy O99.21- ☑
    puerperium O99.215
  constitutional E66.8
  dietary counseling and surveillance Z71.3

Obesity — *continued*
  drug-induced E66.1
  due to
    drug E66.1
    excess calories E66.09
      morbid E66.01
      severe E66.01
  endocrine E66.8
  endogenous E66.8
  exogenous E66.09
  familial E66.8
  glandular E66.8
  hypothyroid — *see* Hypothyroidism
  hypoventilation syndrome (OHS) E66.2
  morbid E66.01
    with
      alveolar hypoventilation E66.2
      obesity hypoventilation syndrome (OHS) E66.2
    due to excess calories E66.01
  nutritional E66.09
  pituitary E23.6
  severe E66.01
  specified type NEC E66.8
Oblique — *see* condition
Obliteration
  appendix (lumen) K38.8
  artery I77.1
  bile duct (noncalculous) K83.1
  common duct (noncalculous) K83.1
  cystic duct — *see* Obstruction, gallbladder
  disease, arteriolar I77.1
  endometrium N85.8
  eye, anterior chamber — *see* Disorder, globe, hypotony
  fallopian tube N97.1
  lymphatic vessel I89.0
    due to mastectomy I97.2
  organ or site, congenital NEC — *see* Atresia, by site
  ureter N13.5
    with infection N13.6
  urethra — *see* Stricture, urethra
  vein I87.8
  vestibule (oral) K08.89
Observation (following) (for) (without need for further medical care) Z04.9
  accident NEC Z04.3
    at work Z04.2
    transport Z04.1
  adverse effect of drug Z03.6
  alleged rape or sexual assault (victim), ruled out
    adult Z04.41
    child Z04.42
  criminal assault Z04.89
  development state
    adolescent Z00.3
    period of rapid growth in childhood Z00.2
    puberty Z00.3
  disease, specified NEC Z03.89
  following work accident Z04.2
  forced sexual exploitation Z04.81
  forced labor exploitation Z04.82
  growth and development state — *see* Observation, development state
  injuries (accidental) NEC — *see also* Observation, accident
  newborn (for)
    suspected condition, related to exposure from the mother or birth process — *see* Newborn, affected by, maternal
    ruled out Z05.9
      cardiac Z05.0
      connective tissue Z05.73
      gastrointestinal Z05.5
      genetic Z05.41
      genitourinary Z05.6
      immunologic Z05.43
      infectious Z05.1
      metabolic Z05.42
      musculoskeletal Z05.72
      neurological Z05.2
      respiratory Z05.3
      skin and subcutaneous tissue Z05.71
      specified condition NEC Z05.8
  postpartum
    immediately after delivery Z39.0
    routine follow-up Z39.2
  pregnancy (normal) (without complication) Z34.9- ☑
    high risk O09.9- ☑
  suicide attempt, alleged NEC Z03.89

Observation — *continued*
suicide attempt, alleged — *continued*
self-poisoning Z03.6
suspected, ruled out — *see also* Suspected condition, ruled out
abuse, physical
adult Z04.71
child Z04.72
accident at work Z04.2
adult battering victim Z04.71
child battering victim Z04.72
condition NEC Z03.89
newborn — *see also* Observation, newborn (for), suspected condition, ruled out Z05.9
drug poisoning or adverse effect Z03.6
exposure (to)
anthrax Z03.810
biological agent NEC Z03.818
inflicted injury NEC Z04.89
suicide attempt, alleged Z03.89
self-poisoning Z03.6
toxic effects from ingested substance (drug) (poison) Z03.6
toxic effects from ingested substance (drug) (poison) Z03.6

Obsession, obsessional state F42.8
mixed thoughts and acts F42.2

Obsessive-compulsive neurosis or reaction F42.8

Obstetric embolism, septic — *see* Embolism, obstetric, septic

Obstetrical trauma (complicating delivery) O71.9
with or following ectopic or molar pregnancy O08.6
specified type NEC O71.89

Obstipation — *see* Constipation

Obstruction, obstructed, obstructive
airway J98.8
with
allergic alveolitis J67.9
asthma J45.909
with
exacerbation (acute) J45.901
status asthmaticus J45.902
bronchiectasis J47.9
with
exacerbation (acute) J47.1
lower respiratory infection J47.0
bronchitis (chronic) J44.9
emphysema J43.9
chronic J44.9
with
allergic alveolitis — *see* Pneumonitis, hypersensitivity
bronchiectasis J47.9
with
exacerbation (acute) J47.1
lower respiratory infection J47.0
due to
foreign body — *see* Foreign body, by site, causing asphyxia
inhalation of fumes or vapors J68.9
laryngospasm J38.5
ampulla of Vater K83.1
aortic (heart) (valve) — *see* Stenosis, aortic
aortoiliac I74.09
aqueduct of Sylvius G91.1
congenital Q03.0
with spina bifida — *see* Spina bifida, by site, with hydrocephalus
Arnold-Chiari — *see* Arnold-Chiari disease
artery — *see also* Atherosclerosis, artery I70.9 ☑
basilar (complete) (partial) — *see* Occlusion, artery, basilar
carotid (complete) (partial) — *see* Occlusion, artery, carotid
cerebellar — *see* Occlusion, artery, cerebellar
cerebral (anterior) (middle) (posterior) — *see* Occlusion, artery, cerebral
precerebral — *see* Occlusion, artery, precerebral
renal N28.0
retinal NEC — *see* Occlusion, artery, retina
stent — *see* Restenosis, stent
vertebral (complete) (partial) — *see* Occlusion, artery, vertebral
band (intestinal) — *see also* Obstruction, intestine, specified NEC K56.699
bile duct or passage (common) (hepatic) (noncalculous) K83.1
with calculus K80.51

Obstruction, obstructed, obstructive — *continued*
bile duct or passage — *continued*
congenital (causing jaundice) Q44.3
biliary (duct) (tract) K83.1
gallbladder K82.0
bladder-neck (acquired) N32.0
congenital Q64.31
due to hyperplasia (hypertrophy) of prostate — *see* Hyperplasia, prostate
bowel — *see* Obstruction, intestine
bronchus J98.09
canal, ear — *see* Stenosis, external ear canal
cardia K22.2
caval veins (inferior) (superior) I87.1
cecum — *see* Obstruction, intestine
circulatory I99.8
colon — *see* Obstruction, intestine
common duct (noncalculous) K83.1
coronary (artery) — *see* Occlusion, coronary
cystic duct — *see also* Obstruction, gallbladder
with calculus K80.21
device, implant or graft — *see also* Complications, by site and type, mechanical T85.698 ☑
arterial graft NEC — *see* Complication, cardiovascular device, mechanical, vascular
catheter NEC T85.628 ☑
cystostomy T83.090 ☑
dialysis (renal) T82.49 ☑
intraperitoneal T85.691 ☑
Hopkins T83.098 ☑
ileostomy T83.098 ☑
infusion NEC T82.594 ☑
spinal (epidural) (subdural) T85.690 ☑
nephrostomy T83.092 ☑
urethral indwelling T83.091 ☑
urinary T83.098 ☑
urostomy T83.098 ☑
due to infection T85.79 ☑
gastrointestinal — *see* Complications, prosthetic device, mechanical, gastrointestinal device
genital NEC T83.498 ☑
intrauterine contraceptive device T83.39 ☑
penile prosthesis (cylinder) (implanted) (pump) (resevoir) T83.490 ☑
testicular prosthesis T83.491 ☑
heart NEC — *see* Complication, cardiovascular device, mechanical
joint prosthesis — *see* Complications, joint prosthesis, mechanical, specified NEC, by site
orthopedic NEC — *see* Complication, orthopedic, device, mechanical
specified NEC T85.628 ☑
urinary NEC — *see also* Complication, genitourinary, device, urinary, mechanical
graft T83.29 ☑
vascular NEC — *see* Complication, cardiovascular device, mechanical
ventricular intracranial shunt T85.09 ☑
due to foreign body accidentally left in operative wound T81.529 ☑
duodenum K31.5
ejaculatory duct N50.89
esophagus K22.2
eustachian tube (complete) (partial) H68.10- ☑
cartilagenous (extrinsic) H68.13- ☑
intrinsic H68.12- ☑
osseous H68.11- ☑
fallopian tube (bilateral) N97.1
fecal K56.41
with hernia — *see* Hernia, by site, with obstruction
foramen of Monro (congenital) Q03.8
with spina bifida — *see* Spina bifida, by site, with hydrocephalus
foreign body — *see* Foreign body
gallbladder K82.0
with calculus, stones K80.21
congenital Q44.1
gastric outlet K31.1
gastrointestinal — *see* Obstruction, intestine
hepatic K76.89
duct (noncalculous) K83.1
ileum — *see* Obstruction, intestine
iliofemoral (artery) I74.5
intestine K56.609
with
adhesions (intestinal) (peritoneal) K56.50
complete K56.52

Obstruction, obstructed, obstructive — *continued*
intestine — *continued*
with — *continued*
adhesions — *continued*
incomplete K56.51
partial K56.51
adynamic K56.0
by gallstone K56.3
complete K56.601
congenital (small) Q41.9
large Q42.9
specified part NEC Q42.8
incomplete K56.600
neurogenic K56.0
Hirschsprung's disease or megacolon Q43.1
newborn P76.9
due to
fecaliths P76.8
inspissated milk P76.2
meconium (plug) P76.0
in mucoviscidosis E84.11
specified NEC P76.8
partial K56.600
postoperative K91.30
complete K91.32
incomplete K91.31
partial K91.31
reflex K56.0
specified NEC K56.699
complete K56.691
incomplete K56.690
partial K56.690
volvulus K56.2
intracardiac ball valve prosthesis T82.09 ☑
jejunum — *see* Obstruction, intestine
joint prosthesis — *see* Complications, joint prosthesis, mechanical, specified NEC, by site
kidney (calices) N28.89
labor — *see* Delivery
lacrimal (passages) (duct)
by
dacryolith — *see* Dacryolith
stenosis — *see* Stenosis, lacrimal
congenital Q10.5
neonatal H04.53- ☑
lacrimonasal duct — *see* Obstruction, lacrimal
lacteal, with steatorrhea K90.2
laryngitis — *see* Laryngitis
larynx NEC J38.6
congenital Q31.8
lung J98.4
disease, chronic J44.9
lymphatic I89.0
meconium (plug)
newborn P76.0
due to fecaliths P76.0
in mucoviscidosis E84.11
mitral — *see* Stenosis, mitral
nasal J34.89
nasolacrimal duct — *see also* Obstruction, lacrimal
congenital Q10.5
nasopharynx J39.2
nose J34.89
organ or site, congenital NEC — *see* Atresia, by site
pancreatic duct K86.89
parotid duct or gland K11.8
pelviureteral junction N13.5
with hydronephrosis N13.0
congenital Q62.39
pharynx J39.2
portal (circulation) (vein) I81
prostate — *see also* Hyperplasia, prostate
valve (urinary) N32.0
pulmonary valve (heart) I37.0
pyelonephritis (chronic) N11.1
pylorus
adult K31.1
congenital or infantile Q40.0
rectosigmoid — *see* Obstruction, intestine
rectum K62.4
renal N28.89
outflow N13.8
pelvis, congenital Q62.39
respiratory J98.8
chronic J44.9
retinal (vessels) H34.9
salivary duct (any) K11.8
with calculus K11.5

☑ **Additional Character Required — Refer to the Tabular List for Character Selection**   ▽ **Subterms under main terms may continue to next column or pag**

Obstruction, obstructed, obstructive — *continued*
sigmoid — *see* Obstruction, intestine
sinus (accessory) (nasal) J34.89
Stensen's duct K11.8
stomach NEC K31.89
  acute K31.0
  congenital Q40.2
  due to pylorospasm K31.3
submandibular duct K11.8
submaxillary gland K11.8
  with calculus K11.5
thoracic duct I89.0
thrombotic — *see* Thrombosis
trachea J39.8
tracheostomy airway J95.03
tricuspid (valve) — *see* Stenosis, tricuspid
upper respiratory, congenital Q34.8
ureter (functional) (pelvic junction) NEC N13.5
  with
    hydronephrosis N13.1
      with infection N13.6
      pyelonephritis (chronic) N11.1
  congenital Q62.39
  due to calculus — *see* Calculus, ureter
urethra NEC N36.8
  congenital Q64.39
urinary (moderate) N13.9
  due to hyperplasia (hypertrophy) of prostate — *see*
    Hyperplasia, prostate
  organ or tract (lower) N13.9
  prostatic valve N32.0
  specified NEC N13.8
uropathy N13.9
uterus N85.8
vagina N89.5
valvular — *see* Endocarditis
vein, venous I87.1
  caval (inferior) (superior) I87.1
  thrombotic — *see* Thrombosis
vena cava (inferior) (superior) I87.1
vesical NEC N32.0
vesicourethral orifice N32.0
  congenital Q64.31
vessel NEC I99.8
  stent — *see* Restenosis, stent
Obturator — *see* condition
Occlusal wear, teeth K03.0
Occlusio pupillae — *see* Membrane, pupillary
Occlusion, occluded
anus K62.4
  congenital Q42.3
    with fistula Q42.2
aortoiliac (chronic) I74.09
aqueduct of Sylvius G91.1
  congenital Q03.0
    with spina bifida — *see* Spina bifida, by site, with
      hydrocephalus
artery — *see also* Atherosclerosis, artery I70.9 ☑
  auditory, internal I65.8
  basilar I65.1
    with
      infarction I63.22
        due to
          embolism I63.12
          thrombosis I63.02
  brain or cerebral I66.9
    with infarction (due to) I63.5- ☑
      embolism I63.4- ☑
      thrombosis I63.3- ☑
  carotid I65.2- ☑
    with
      infarction I63.23- ☑
        due to
          embolism I63.13- ☑
          thrombosis I63.03- ☑
  cerebellar (anterior inferior) (posterior inferior) (superior) I66.3
    with infarction I63.54- ☑
      due to
        embolism I63.44- ☑
        thrombosis I63.34- ☑
  cerebral I66.9
    with infarction I63.50
      due to
        embolism I63.40
          specified NEC I63.49
        thrombosis I63.30
          specified NEC I63.39

Occlusion, occluded — *continued*
  artery — *see also* Atherosclerosis, artery — *continued*
    cerebral — *continued*
      anterior I66.1- ☑
        with infarction I63.52- ☑
          due to
            embolism I63.42- ☑
            thrombosis I63.32- ☑
      middle I66.0- ☑
        with infarction I63.51- ☑
          due to
            embolism I63.41- ☑
            thrombosis I63.31- ☑
      posterior I66.2- ☑
        with infarction I63.53- ☑
          due to
            embolism I63.43- ☑
            thrombosis I63.33- ☑
      specified NEC I66.8
        with infarction I63.59
          due to
            embolism I63.4- ☑
            thrombosis I63.3- ☑
    choroidal (anterior) — *see* Occlusion, artery, precerebral, specified NEC
    communicating posterior — *see* Occlusion, artery, precerebral, specified NEC
    complete
      coronary I25.82
      extremities I70.92
    coronary (acute) (thrombotic) (without myocardial infarction) I24.0
      with myocardial infarction — *see* Infarction, myocardium
      chronic total I25.82
      complete I25.82
      healed or old I25.2
      total (chronic) I25.82
    hypophyseal — *see* Occlusion, artery, precerebral, specified NEC
    iliac I74.5
    lower extremities due to stenosis or stricture I77.1
    mesenteric (embolic) (thrombotic) — *see also* Infarct, intestine K55.069
    perforating — *see* Occlusion, artery, cerebral, specified NEC
    peripheral I77.9
      thrombotic or embolic I74.4
    pontine — *see* Occlusion, artery, precerebral, specified NEC
    precerebral I65.9
      with infarction I63.20
        specified NEC I63.29
          due to
            embolism I63.10
              specified NEC I63.19
            thrombosis I63.00
              specified NEC I63.09
      basilar — *see* Occlusion, artery, basilar
      carotid — *see* Occlusion, artery, carotid
      puerperal O88.23
      specified NEC I65.8
        with infarction I63.29
          due to
            embolism I63.19
            thrombosis I63.09
      vertebral — *see* Occlusion, artery, vertebral
    renal N28.0
    retinal
      branch H34.23- ☑
      central H34.1- ☑
      partial H34.21- ☑
      transient H34.0- ☑
    spinal — *see* Occlusion, artery, precerebral, vertebral
    total (chronic)
      coronary I25.82
      extremities I70.92
    vertebral I65.0- ☑
      with
        infarction I63.21- ☑
          due to
            embolism I63.11- ☑
            thrombosis I63.01- ☑
  basilar artery — *see* Occlusion, artery, basilar
  bile duct (common) (hepatic) (noncalculous) K83.1
  bowel — *see* Obstruction, intestine

Occlusion, occluded — *continued*
  carotid (artery) (common) (internal) — *see* Occlusion, artery, carotid
  centric (of teeth) M26.59
    maximum intercuspation discrepancy M26.55
  cerebellar (artery) — *see* Occlusion, artery, cerebellar
  cerebral (artery) — *see* Occlusion, artery, cerebral
  cerebrovascular — *see also* Occlusion, artery, cerebral
    with infarction I63.5- ☑
  cervical canal — *see* Stricture, cervix
  cervix (uteri) — *see* Stricture, cervix
  choanal Q30.0
  choroidal (artery) — *see* Occlusion, artery, precerebral, specified NEC
  colon — *see* Obstruction, intestine
  communicating posterior artery — *see* Occlusion, artery, precerebral, specified NEC
  coronary (artery) (vein) (thrombotic) — *see also* Infarct, myocardium
    chronic total I25.82
    healed or old I25.2
    not resulting in infarction I24.0
    total (chronic) I25.82
  cystic duct — *see* Obstruction, gallbladder
  embolic — *see* Embolism
  fallopian tube N97.1
    congenital Q50.6
  gallbladder — *see also* Obstruction, gallbladder
    congenital (causing jaundice) Q44.1
  gingiva, traumatic K06.2
  hymen N89.6
    congenital Q52.3
  hypophyseal (artery) — *see* Occlusion, artery, precerebral, specified NEC
  iliac artery I74.5
  intestine — *see* Obstruction, intestine
  lacrimal passages — *see* Obstruction, lacrimal
  lung J98.4
  lymph or lymphatic channel I89.0
  mammary duct N64.89
  mesenteric artery (embolic) (thrombotic) — *see also* Infarct, intestine K55.069
  nose J34.89
    congenital Q30.0
  organ or site, congenital NEC — *see* Atresia, by site
  oviduct N97.1
    congenital Q50.6
  peripheral arteries
    due to stricture or stenosis I77.1
    upper extremity I74.2
  pontine (artery) — *see* Occlusion, artery, precerebral, specified NEC
  posterior lingual, of mandibular teeth M26.29
  precerebral artery — *see* Occlusion, artery, precerebral
  punctum lacrimale — *see* Obstruction, lacrimal
  pupil — *see* Membrane, pupillary
  pylorus, adult — *see also* Stricture, pylorus K31.1
  renal artery N28.0
  retina, retinal
    artery — *see* Occlusion, artery, retinal
    vein (central) H34.81- ☑
      engorgement H34.82- ☑
      tributary H34.83- ☑
    vessels H34.9
  spinal artery — *see* Occlusion, artery, precerebral, vertebral
  teeth (mandibular) (posterior lingual) M26.29
  thoracic duct I89.0
  thrombotic — *see* Thrombosis, artery
  traumatic
    edentulous (alveolar) ridge K06.2
    gingiva K06.2
    periodontal K05.5
  tubal N97.1
  ureter (complete) (partial) N13.5
    congenital Q62.10
  ureteropelvic junction N13.5
    congenital Q62.11
  ureterovesical orifice N13.5
    congenital Q62.12
  urethra — *see* Stricture, urethra
  uterus N85.8
  vagina N89.5
  vascular NEC I99.8
  vein — *see* Thrombosis
    retinal — *see* Occlusion, retinal, vein
  vena cava (inferior) (superior) — *see* Embolism, vena cava

Occlusion, occluded — continued
  ventricle (brain) NEC G91.1
  vertebral (artery) — see Occlusion, artery, vertebral
  vessel (blood) I99.8
  vulva N90.5
Occult
  blood in feces (stools) R19.5
Occupational
  problems NEC Z56.89
Ochlophobia — see Agoraphobia
Ochronosis (endogenous) E70.29
Ocular muscle — see condition
Oculogyric crisis or disturbance H51.8
  psychogenic F45.8
Oculomotor syndrome H51.9
Oculopathy
  syphilitic NEC A52.71
    congenital
      early A50.01
      late A50.30
    early (secondary) A51.43
    late A52.71
Oddi's sphincter spasm K83.4
Odontalgia K08.89
Odontoameloblastoma — see Cyst, calcifying odontogenic
Odontoclasia K03.89
Odontodysplasia, regional K00.4
Odontogenesis imperfecta K00.5
Odontoma (ameloblastic) (complex) (compound) (fibroameloblastic) — see Cyst, calcifying odontogenic
Odontomyelitis (closed) (open) K04.01
  irreversible K04.02
  reversible K04.01
Odontorrhagia K08.89
Odontosarcoma, ameloblastic C41.1
  upper jaw (bone) C41.0
Oestriasis — see Myiasis
Oguchi's disease H53.63
Ohara's disease — see Tularemia
OHS (obesity hypoventilation syndrome) E66.2
Oidiomycosis — see Candidiasis
Oidium albicans infection — see Candidiasis
Old age (without mention of debility) R54
  dementia F03 ☑
Old (previous) **myocardial infarction** I25.2
Olfactory — see condition
Oligemia — see Anemia
Oligoastrocytoma
  specified site — see Neoplasm, malignant, by site
  unspecified site C71.9
Oligocythemia D64.9
Oligodendroblastoma
  specified site — see Neoplasm, malignant, by site
  unspecified site C71.9
Oligodendroglioma
  anaplastic type
    specified site — see Neoplasm, malignant, by site
    unspecified site C71.9
  specified site — see Neoplasm, malignant, by site
  unspecified site C71.9
Oligodontia — see Anodontia
Oligoencephalon Q02
Oligohidrosis L74.4
Oligohydramnios O41.0- ☑
Oligohydrosis L74.4
Oligomenorrhea N91.5
  primary N91.3
  secondary N91.4
Oligophrenia — see also Disability, intellectual
  phenylpyruvic E70.0
Oligospermia N46.11
  due to
    drug therapy N46.121
    efferent duct obstruction N46.123
    infection N46.122
    radiation N46.124
    specified cause NEC N46.129
    systemic disease N46.125
Oligotrichia — see Alopecia
Oliguria R34
  with, complicating or following ectopic or molar pregnancy O08.4
  postprocedural N99.0
Ollier's disease Q78.4
Omenotocele — see Hernia, abdomen, specified site NEC
Omentitis — see Peritonitis

Omentum, omental — see condition
Omphalitis (congenital) (newborn) P38.9
  with mild hemorrhage P38.1
  without hemorrhage P38.9
  not of newborn L08.82
  tetanus A33
Omphalocele Q79.2
Omphalomesenteric duct, persistent Q43.0
Omphalorrhagia, newborn P51.9
Omsk hemorrhagic fever A98.1
Onanism (excessive) F98.8
Onchocerciasis, onchocercosis B73.1
  with
    eye disease B73.00
      endophthalmitis B73.01
      eyelid B73.09
      glaucoma B73.02
      specified NEC B73.09
  eyelid B73.09
  eye NEC B73.00
Oncocytoma — see Neoplasm, benign, by site
Oncovirus, as cause of disease classified elsewhere B97.32
Ondine's curse — see Apnea, sleep
Oneirophrenia F23
Onychauxis L60.2
  congenital Q84.5
Onychia — see also Cellulitis, digit
  with lymphangitis — see Lymphangitis, acute, digit
  candidal B37.2
  dermatophytic B35.1
Onychitis — see also Cellulitis, digit
  with lymphangitis — see Lymphangitis, acute, digit
Onychocryptosis L60.0
Onychodystrophy L60.3
  congenital Q84.6
Onychogryphosis, onychogryposis L60.2
Onycholysis L60.1
Onychomadesis L60.8
Onychomalacia L60.3
Onychomycosis (finger) (toe) B35.1
Onycho-osteodysplasia Q87.2
Onychophagia F98.8
Onychophosis L60.8
Onychoptosis L60.8
Onychorrhexis L60.3
  congenital Q84.6
Onychoschizia L60.3
Onyxis (finger) (toe) L60.0
Onyxitis — see also Cellulitis, digit
  with lymphangitis — see Lymphangitis, acute, digit
Oophoritis (cystic) (infectional) (interstitial) N70.92
  with salpingitis N70.93
  acute N70.02
    with salpingitis N70.03
  chronic N70.12
    with salpingitis N70.13
  complicating abortion — see Abortion, by type, complicated by, oophoritis
Oophorocele N83.4- ☑
Opacity, opacities
  cornea H17.- ☑
    central H17.1- ☑
    congenital Q13.3
    degenerative — see Degeneration, cornea
    hereditary — see Dystrophy, cornea
    inflammatory — see Keratitis
    minor H17.81- ☑
    peripheral H17.82- ☑
    sequelae of trachoma (healed) B94.0
    specified NEC H17.89
  enamel (teeth) (fluoride) (nonfluoride) K00.3
  lens — see Cataract
  snowball — see Deposit, crystalline
  vitreous (humor) NEC H43.39- ☑
    congenital Q14.0
    membranes and strands H43.31- ☑
Opalescent dentin (hereditary) K00.5
Open, opening
  abnormal, organ or site, congenital — see Imperfect, closure
  angle with
    borderline
      findings
        high risk H40.02- ☑
        low risk H40.01- ☑
      intraocular pressure H40.00- ☑

Open, opening — continued
  angle with — continued
    cupping of discs H40.01- ☑
    glaucoma (primary) — see Glaucoma, open angle
  bite
    anterior M26.220
    posterior M26.221
  false — see Imperfect, closure
  margin on tooth restoration K08.51
  restoration margins of tooth K08.51
  wound — see Wound, open
Operational fatigue F48.8
Operative — see condition
Operculitis — see Periodontitis
Operculum — see Break, retina
Ophiasis L63.2
Ophthalmia — see also Conjunctivitis H10.9
  actinic rays — see Photokeratitis
  allergic (acute) — see Conjunctivitis, acute, atopic
  blennorrhagic (gonococcal) (neonatorum) A54.31
  diphtheritic A36.86
  Egyptian A71.1
  electrica — see Photokeratitis
  gonococcal (neonatorum) A54.31
  metastatic — see Endophthalmitis, purulent
  migraine — see Migraine, ophthalmoplegic
  neonatorum, newborn P39.1
    gonococcal A54.31
  nodosa H16.24- ☑
  purulent — see Conjunctivitis, acute, mucopurulent
  spring — see Conjunctivitis, acute, atopic
  sympathetic — see Uveitis, sympathetic
Ophthalmitis — see Ophthalmia
Ophthalmocele (congenital) Q15.8
Ophthalmoneuromyelitis G36.0
Ophthalmoplegia — see also Strabismus, paralytic
  anterior internuclear — see Ophthalmoplegia, internuclear
  ataxia-areflexia G61.0
  diabetic — see E08-E13 with .39
  exophthalmic E05.00
    with thyroid storm E05.01
  external H49.88- ☑
    progressive H49.4- ☑
      with pigmentary retinopathy — see Kearns-Sayre syndrome
    total H49.3- ☑
  internal (complete) (total) H52.51- ☑
  internuclear H51.2- ☑
  migraine — see Migraine, ophthalmoplegic
  Parinaud's H49.88- ☑
  progressive external — see Ophthalmoplegia, external, progressive
  supranuclear, progressive G23.1
  total (external) — see Ophthalmoplegia, external, total
Opioid(s)
  abuse — see Abuse, drug, opioids
  dependence — see Dependence, drug, opioids
  induced, without use disorder
    anxiety disorder F11.988
    delirium F11.921
    depressive disorder F11.94
    sexual dysfunction F11.981
    sleep disorder F11.982
Opisthognathism M26.09
Opisthorchiasis (felineus) (viverrini) B66.0
Opitz' disease D73.2
Opiumism — see Dependence, drug, opioid
Oppenheim's disease G70.2
Oppenheim-Urbach disease (necrobiosis lipoidica diabeticorum) — see E08-E13 with .620
Optic nerve — see condition
Orbit — see condition
Orchioblastoma C62.9- ☑
Orchitis (gangrenous) (nonspecific) (septic) (suppurative) N45.2
  blennorrhagic (gonococcal) (acute) (chronic) A54.23
  chlamydial A56.19
  filarial — see also Infestation, filarial B74.9 [N51]
  gonococcal (acute) (chronic) A54.23
  mumps B26.0
  syphilitic A52.76
  tuberculous A18.15
Orf (virus disease) B08.02
Organic — see also condition
  brain syndrome F09
  heart — see Disease, heart

rganic — *continued*
  mental disorder F09
  psychosis F09
rgasm
  anejaculatory N53.13
riental
  bilharziasis B65.2
  schistosomiasis B65.2
rifice — *see* condition
rigin of both great vessels from right ventricle
  Q20.1
rmond's disease (with ureteral obstruction) N13.5
  with infection N13.6
rnithine metabolism disorder E72.4
rnithinemia (Type I) (Type II) E72.4
rnithosis A70
rotaciduria, oroticaciduria (congenital) (hereditary) (pyrimidine deficiency) E79.8
  anemia D53.0
rthodontics
  adjustment Z46.4
  fitting Z46.4
rthopnea R06.01
rthopoxvirus B08.09
s, uterus — *see* condition
sgood-Schlatter disease or osteochondrosis — *see* Osteochondrosis, juvenile, tibia
sler (-Weber)-**Rendu disease** I78.0
sler's nodes I33.0
smidrosis L75.0
sseous — *see* condition
ssification
  artery — *see* Arteriosclerosis
  auricle (ear) — *see* Disorder, pinna, specified type NEC
  bronchial J98.09
  cardiac — *see* Degeneration, myocardial
  cartilage (senile) — *see* Disorder, cartilage, specified type NEC
  coronary (artery) — *see* Disease, heart, ischemic, atherosclerotic
  diaphragm J98.6
  ear, middle — *see* Otosclerosis
  falx cerebri G96.19
  fontanel, premature Q75.0
  heart — *see also* Degeneration, myocardial
    valve — *see* Endocarditis
  larynx J38.7
  ligament — *see* Disorder, tendon, specified type NEC
    posterior longitudinal — *see* Spondylopathy, specified NEC
  meninges (cerebral) (spinal) G96.19
  multiple, eccentric centers — *see* Disorder, bone, development or growth
  muscle — *see also* Calcification, muscle
    due to burns — *see* Myositis, ossificans, in, burns
    paralytic — *see* Myositis, ossificans, in, quadriplegia
    progressive — *see* Myositis, ossificans, progressiva
    specified NEC M61.50
      ankle M61.57- ☑
      foot M61.57- ☑
      forearm M61.53- ☑
      hand M61.54- ☑
      lower leg M61.56- ☑
      multiple sites M61.59
      pelvic region M61.55- ☑
      shoulder region M61.51- ☑
      specified site NEC M61.58
      thigh M61.55- ☑
      upper arm M61.52- ☑
    traumatic — *see* Myositis, ossificans, traumatica
  myocardium, myocardial — *see* Degeneration, myocardial
  penis N48.89
  periarticular — *see* Disorder, joint, specified type NEC
  pinna — *see* Disorder, pinna, specified type NEC
  rider's bone — *see* Ossification, muscle, specified NEC
  sclera H15.89
  subperiosteal, post-traumatic M89.8X- ☑
  tendon — *see* Disorder, tendon, specified type NEC
  trachea J39.8
  tympanic membrane — *see* Disorder, tympanic membrane, specified NEC
  vitreous (humor) — *see* Deposit, crystalline
steitis — *see also* Osteomyelitis
  alveolar M27.3
  condensans M85.30
    ankle M85.37- ☑

Osteitis — *continued*
  condensans — *continued*
    foot M85.37- ☑
    forearm M85.33- ☑
    hand M85.34- ☑
    lower leg M85.36- ☑
    multiple site M85.39
    neck M85.38
    rib M85.38
    shoulder M85.31- ☑
    skull M85.38
    specified site NEC M85.38
    thigh M85.35- ☑
    toe M85.37- ☑
    upper arm M85.32- ☑
    vertebra M85.38
  deformans M88.9
    in (due to)
      malignant neoplasm of bone C41.9 *[M90.60]*
      neoplastic disease — *see also* Neoplasm D49.9 *[M90.60]*
        carpus D49.9 *[M90.64-]* ☑
        clavicle D49.9 *[M90.61-]* ☑
        femur D49.9 *[M90.65-]* ☑
        fibula D49.9 *[M90.66-]* ☑
        finger D49.9 *[M90.64-]* ☑
        humerus D49.9 *[M90.62-]* ☑
        ilium D49.9 *[M90.65-]* ☑
        ischium D49.9 *[M90.65-]* ☑
        metacarpus D49.9 *[M90.64-]* ☑
        metatarsus D49.9 *[M90.67-]* ☑
        multiple sites D49.9 *[M90.69]*
        neck D49.9 *[M90.68]*
        radius D49.9 *[M90.63-]* ☑
        rib D49.9 *[M90.68]*
        scapula D49.9 *[M90.61-]* ☑
        skull D49.9 *[M90.68]*
        tarsus D49.9 *[M90.67-]* ☑
        tibia D49.9 *[M90.66-]* ☑
        toe D49.9 *[M90.67-]* ☑
        ulna D49.9 *[M90.63-]* ☑
        vertebra D49.9 *[M90.68]*
      skull M88.0
      specified NEC — *see* Paget's disease, bone, by site
      vertebra M88.1
    due to yaws A66.6
    fibrosa NEC — *see* Cyst, bone, by site
      circumscripta — *see* Dysplasia, fibrous, bone NEC
      cystica (generalisata) E21.0
      disseminata Q78.1
      osteoplastica E21.0
    fragilitans Q78.0
    Garr's (sclerosing) — *see* Osteomyelitis, specified type NEC
    jaw (acute) (chronic) (lower) (suppurative) (upper) M27.2
    parathyroid E21.0
    petrous bone (acute) (chronic) — *see* Petrositis
    sclerotic, nonsuppurative — *see* Osteomyelitis, specified type NEC
    tuberculosa A18.09
      cystica D86.89
      multiplex cystoides D86.89
Osteoarthritis M19.90
  ankle M19.07- ☑
  elbow M19.02- ☑
  foot joint M19.07- ☑
  generalized M15.9
    erosive M15.4
    primary M15.0
    specified NEC M15.8
  hand joint M19.04- ☑
    first carpometacarpal joint M18.9
  hip M16.1- ☑
    bilateral M16.0
    due to hip dysplasia (unilateral) M16.3- ☑
      bilateral M16.2
  interphalangeal
    distal (Heberden) M15.1
    proximal (Bouchard) M15.2
  knee M17.1- ☑
    bilateral M17.0
  post-traumatic NEC M19.92
    ankle M19.17- ☑
    elbow M19.12- ☑
    foot joint M19.17- ☑
    hand joint M19.14- ☑

Osteoarthritis — *continued*
  post-traumatic — *continued*
    hand joint — *continued*
      first carpometacarpal joint M18.3- ☑
        bilateral M18.2
    hip M16.5- ☑
      bilateral M16.4
    knee M17.3- ☑
      bilateral M17.2
    shoulder M19.11- ☑
    wrist M19.13- ☑
  primary M19.91
    ankle M19.07- ☑
    elbow M19.02- ☑
    foot joint M19.07- ☑
    hand joint M19.04- ☑
      first carpometacarpal joint M18.1- ☑
        bilateral M18.0
    hip M16.1- ☑
      bilateral M16.0
    knee M17.1- ☑
      bilateral M17.0
    multiple sites M89.49
    shoulder M19.01- ☑
    spine — *see* Spondylosis
    wrist M19.03- ☑
  secondary M19.93
    ankle M19.27- ☑
    elbow M19.22- ☑
    foot joint M19.27- ☑
    hand joint M19.24- ☑
      first carpometacarpal joint M18.5- ☑
        bilateral M18.4
    hip M16.7
      bilateral M16.6
    knee M17.5
      bilateral M17.4
    multiple M15.3
    shoulder M19.21- ☑
    spine — *see* Spondylosis
    wrist M19.23- ☑
  shoulder M19.01- ☑
  spine — *see* Spondylosis
  wrist M19.03- ☑
Osteoarthropathy (hypertrophic) M19.90
  ankle — *see* Osteoarthritis, primary, ankle
  elbow — *see* Osteoarthritis, primary, elbow
  foot joint — *see* Osteoarthritis, primary, foot
  hand joint — *see* Osteoarthritis, primary, hand joint
  knee joint — *see* Osteoarthritis, primary, knee
  multiple site — *see* Osteoarthritis, primary, multiple joint
  pulmonary — *see also* Osteoarthropathy, specified type NEC
    hypertrophic — *see* Osteoarthropathy, hypertrophic, specified type NEC
  secondary — *see* Osteoarthropathy, specified type NEC
  secondary hypertrophic — *see* Osteoarthropathy, specified type NEC
  shoulder — *see* Osteoarthritis, primary, shoulder
  specified joint NEC — *see* Osteoarthritis, primary, specified joint NEC
  specified type NEC M89.40
    carpus M89.44- ☑
    clavicle M89.41- ☑
    femur M89.45- ☑
    fibula M89.46- ☑
    finger M89.44- ☑
    humerus M89.42- ☑
    ilium M89.459
    ischium M89.459
    metacarpus M89.44- ☑
    metatarsus M89.47- ☑
    multiple sites M89.49
    neck M89.48
    radius M89.43- ☑
    rib M89.48
    scapula M89.41- ☑
    skull M89.48
    tarsus M89.47- ☑
    tibia M89.46- ☑
    toe M89.47- ☑
    ulna M89.43- ☑
    vertebra M89.48
  spine — *see* Spondylosis
  wrist — *see* Osteoarthritis, primary, wrist

Osteoarthrosis (degenerative) (hypertrophic) (joint) —
see also Osteoarthritis
deformans alkaptonurica E70.29 *[M36.8]*
erosive M15.4
generalized M15.9
primary M15.0
polyarticular M15.9
spine — see Spondylosis
Osteoblastoma — see Neoplasm, bone, benign
aggressive — see Neoplasm, bone, uncertain behavior
Osteochondritis — see also Osteochondropathy, by site
Brailsford's — see Osteochondrosis, juvenile, radius
dissecans M93.20
ankle M93.27- ☑
elbow M93.22- ☑
foot M93.27- ☑
hand M93.24- ☑
hip M93.25- ☑
knee M93.26- ☑
multiple sites M93.29
shoulder joint M93.21- ☑
specified site NEC M93.28
wrist M93.23- ☑
juvenile M92.9
patellar — see Osteochondrosis, juvenile, patella
syphilitic (congenital) (early) A50.02 *[M90.80]*
ankle A50.02 *[M90.87-]* ☑
elbow A50.02 *[M90.82-]* ☑
foot A50.02 *[M90.87-]* ☑
forearm A50.02 *[M90.83-]* ☑
hand A50.02 *[M90.84-]* ☑
hip A50.02 *[M90.85-]* ☑
knee A50.02 *[M90.86-]* ☑
multiple sites A50.02 *[M90.89]*
shoulder joint A50.02 *[M90.81-]* ☑
specified site NEC A50.02 *[M90.88]*
Osteochondroarthrosis deformans endemica — see
Disease, Kaschin-Beck
Osteochondrodysplasia Q78.9
with defects of growth of tubular bones and spine
Q77.9
specified NEC Q77.8
specified NEC Q78.8
Osteochondrodystrophy E78.9
Osteochondrolysis — see Osteochondritis, dissecans
Osteochondroma — see Neoplasm, bone, benign
Osteochondromatosis D48.0
syndrome Q78.4
Osteochondromyxosarcoma — see Neoplasm, bone,
malignant
Osteochondropathy M93.90
ankle M93.97- ☑
elbow M93.92- ☑
foot M93.97- ☑
hand M93.94- ☑
hip M93.95- ☑
Kienböck's disease of adults M93.1
knee M93.96- ☑
multiple joints M93.99
osteochondritis dissecans — see Osteochondritis, dissecans
osteochondrosis — see Osteochondrosis
shoulder region M93.91- ☑
slipped upper femoral epiphysis — see Slipped, epiphysis, upper femoral
specified joint NEC M93.98
specified type NEC M93.80
ankle M93.87- ☑
elbow M93.82- ☑
foot M93.87- ☑
hand M93.84- ☑
hip M93.85- ☑
knee M93.86- ☑
multiple joints M93.89
shoulder region M93.81- ☑
specified joint NEC M93.88
wrist M93.83- ☑
syphilitic, congenital
early A50.02 *[M90.80]*
late A50.56 *[M90.80]*
wrist M93.93- ☑
Osteochondrosarcoma — see Neoplasm, bone, malignant
Osteochondrosis — see also Osteochondropathy, by
site
acetabulum (juvenile) M91.0

Osteochondrosis — continued
adult — see Osteochondropathy, specified type NEC,
by site
astragalus (juvenile) — see Osteochondrosis, juvenile,
tarsus
Blount's — see Osteochondrosis, juvenile, tibia
Buchanan's M91.0
Burns' — see Osteochondrosis, juvenile, ulna
calcaneus (juvenile) — see Osteochondrosis, juvenile,
tarsus
capitular epiphysis (femur) (juvenile) — see Legg-Calvé-
Perthes disease
carpal (juvenile) (lunate) (scaphoid) — see Osteochondrosis, juvenile, hand, carpal lunate
adult M93.1
coxae juvenilis — see Legg-Calvé-Perthes disease
deformans juvenilis, coxae — see Legg-Calvé-Perthes
disease
Diaz's — see Osteochondrosis, juvenile, tarsus
dissecans (knee) (shoulder) — see Osteochondritis,
dissecans
femoral capital epiphysis (juvenile) — see Legg-Calvé-
Perthes disease
femur (head), juvenile — see Legg-Calvé-Perthes disease
fibula (juvenile) — see Osteochondrosis, juvenile,
fibula
foot NEC (juvenile) M92.8
Freiberg's — see Osteochondrosis, juvenile, metatarsus
Haas' (juvenile) — see Osteochondrosis, juvenile,
humerus
Haglund's — see Osteochondrosis, juvenile, tarsus
hip (juvenile) — see Legg-Calvé-Perthes disease
humerus (capitulum) (head) (juvenile) — see Osteochondrosis, juvenile, humerus
ilium, iliac crest (juvenile) M91.0
ischiopubic synchondrosis M91.0
Iselin's — see Osteochondrosis, juvenile, metatarsus
juvenile, juvenilis M92.9
after congenital dislocation of hip reduction — see
Osteochondrosis, juvenile, hip, specified NEC
arm — see Osteochondrosis, juvenile, upper limb
NEC
capitular epiphysis (femur) — see Legg-Calvé-
Perthes disease
clavicle, sternal epiphysis — see Osteochondrosis,
juvenile, upper limb NEC
coxae — see Legg-Calvé-Perthes disease
deformans M92.9
fibula M92.5- ☑
foot NEC M92.8
hand M92.20- ☑
carpal lunate M92.21- ☑
metacarpal head M92.22- ☑
specified site NEC M92.29- ☑
head of femur — see Legg-Calvé-Perthes disease
hip and pelvis M91.9- ☑
coxa plana — see Coxa, plana
femoral head — see Legg-Calvé-Perthes disease
pelvis M91.0
pseudocoxalgia — see Pseudocoxalgia
specified NEC M91.8- ☑
humerus M92.0- ☑
limb
lower NEC M92.8
upper NEC — see Osteochondrosis, juvenile,
upper limb NEC
medial cuneiform bone — see Osteochondrosis,
juvenile, tarsus
metatarsus M92.7- ☑
patella M92.4- ☑
radius M92.1- ☑
specified site NEC M92.8
spine M42.00
cervical region M42.02
cervicothoracic region M42.03
lumbar region M42.06
lumbosacral region M42.07
multiple sites M42.09
occipito-atlanto-axial region M42.01
sacrococcygeal region M42.08
thoracic region M42.04
thoracolumbar region M42.05
tarsus M92.6- ☑
tibia M92.5- ☑
ulna M92.1- ☑
upper limb NEC M92.3- ☑

Osteochondrosis — continued
juvenile, juvenilis — continued
vertebra (body) (epiphyseal plates) (Calvé's)
(Scheuermann's) — see Osteochondrosis, ju
venile, spine
Kienböck's — see Osteochondrosis, juvenile, hand,
carpal lunate
adult M93.1
Köhler's
patellar — see Osteochondrosis, juvenile, patella
tarsal navicular — see Osteochondrosis, juvenile
tarsus
Legg-Perthes (-Calvé)(-Waldenström) — see Legg-
Calvé-Perthes disease
limb
lower NEC (juvenile) M92.8
upper NEC (juvenile) — see Osteochondrosis, juv
nile, upper limb NEC
lunate bone (carpal) (juvenile) — see also Osteocho
drosis, juvenile, hand, carpal lunate
adult M93.1
Mauclaire's — see Osteochondrosis, juvenile, hand,
metacarpal
metacarpal (head) (juvenile) — see Osteochondrosis
juvenile, hand, metacarpal
metatarsus (fifth) (head) (juvenile) (second) — see C
teochondrosis, juvenile, metatarsus
navicular (juvenile) — see Osteochondrosis, juvenil
tarsus
os
calcis (juvenile) — see Osteochondrosis, juvenile
tarsus
tibiale externum (juvenile) — see Osteochondros
juvenile, tarsus
Osgood-Schlatter — see Osteochondrosis, juvenile,
tibia
Panner's — see Osteochondrosis, juvenile, humerus
patellar center (juvenile) (primary) (secondary) — s
Osteochondrosis, juvenile, patella
pelvis (juvenile) M91.0
Pierson's M91.0
radius (head) (juvenile) — see Osteochondrosis, juv
nile, radius
Scheuermann's — see Osteochondrosis, juvenile, spi
Sever's — see Osteochondrosis, juvenile, tarsus
Sinding-Larsen — see Osteochondrosis, juvenile,
patella
spine M42.9
adult M42.10
cervical region M42.12
cervicothoracic region M42.13
lumbar region M42.16
lumbosacral region M42.17
multiple sites M42.19
occipito-atlanto-axial region M42.11
sacrococcygeal region M42.18
thoracic region M42.14
thoracolumbar region M42.15
juvenile — see Osteochondrosis, juvenile, spine
symphysis pubis (juvenile) M91.0
syphilitic (congenital) A50.02
talus (juvenile) — see Osteochondrosis, juvenile, tars
tarsus (navicular) (juvenile) — see Osteochondrosis
juvenile, tarsus
tibia (proximal) (tubercle) (juvenile) — see Osteocho
drosis, juvenile, tibia
tuberculous — see Tuberculosis, bone
ulna (lower) (juvenile) — see Osteochondrosis, juveni
ulna
van Neck's M91.0
vertebral — see Osteochondrosis, spine
Osteoclastoma D48.0
malignant — see Neoplasm, bone, malignant
Osteodynia — see Disorder, bone, specified type NEC
Osteodystrophy Q78.9
azotemic N25.0
congenital Q78.9
parathyroid, secondary E21.1
renal N25.0
Osteofibroma — see Neoplasm, bone, benign
Osteofibrosarcoma — see Neoplasm, bone, maligna
Osteogenesis imperfecta Q78.0
Osteogenic — see condition
Osteolysis M89.50
carpus M89.54- ☑
clavicle M89.51- ☑
femur M89.55- ☑

☑ **Additional Character Required** — Refer to the Tabular List for Character Selection   ▼ Subterms under main terms may continue to next column or pag

steolysis — *continued*
  fibula M89.56- ☑
  finger M89.54- ☑
  humerus M89.52- ☑
  ilium M89.559
  ischium M89.559
  joint prosthesis (periprosthetic) — *see* Complications, joint prosthesis, mechanical, periprosthetic, oste-olysis, by site
  metacarpus M89.54- ☑
  metatarsus M89.57- ☑
  multiple sites M89.59
  neck M89.58
  periprosthetic — *see* Complications, joint prosthesis, mechanical, periprosthetic, osteolysis, by site
  radius M89.53- ☑
  rib M89.58
  scapula M89.51- ☑
  skull M89.58
  tarsus M89.57- ☑
  tibia M89.56- ☑
  toe M89.57- ☑
  ulna M89.53- ☑
  vertebra M89.58

steoma — *see also* Neoplasm, bone, benign
  osteoid — *see also* Neoplasm, bone, benign
    giant — *see* Neoplasm, bone, benign

steomalacia M83.9
  adult M83.9
    drug-induced NEC M83.5
    due to
      malabsorption (postsurgical) M83.2
      malnutrition M83.3
    specified NEC M83.8
  aluminium-induced M83.4
  infantile — *see* Rickets
  juvenile — *see* Rickets
  oncogenic E83.89
  pelvis M83.8
  puerperal M83.0
  senile M83.1
  vitamin-D-resistant in adults E83.31 *[M90.8-]* ☑
    carpus E83.31 *[M90.84-]* ☑
    clavicle E83.31 *[M90.81-]* ☑
    femur E83.31 *[M90.85-]* ☑
    fibula E83.31 *[M90.86-]* ☑
    finger E83.31 *[M90.84-]* ☑
    humerus E83.31 *[M90.82-]* ☑
    ilium E83.31 *[M90.859]*
    ischium E83.31 *[M90.859]*
    metacarpus E83.31 *[M90.84-]* ☑
    metatarsus E83.31 *[M90.87-]* ☑
    multiple sites E83.31 *[M90.89]*
    neck E83.31 *[M90.88]*
    radius E83.31 *[M90.83-]* ☑
    rib E83.31 *[M90.88]*
    scapula E83.31 *[M90.819]*
    skull E83.31 *[M90.88]*
    tarsus E83.31 *[M90.879]*
    tibia E83.31 *[M90.869]*
    toe E83.31 *[M90.879]*
    ulna E83.31 *[M90.839]*
    vertebra E83.31 *[M90.88]*

steomyelitis (general) (infective) (localized) (neonatal) (purulent) (septic) (staphylococcal) (streptococcal) (suppurative) (with periostitis) M86.9
  acute M86.10
    carpus M86.14- ☑
    clavicle M86.11- ☑
    femur M86.15- ☑
    fibula M86.16- ☑
    finger M86.14- ☑
    hematogenous M86.00
      carpus M86.04- ☑
      clavicle M86.01- ☑
      femur M86.05- ☑
      fibula M86.06- ☑
      finger M86.04- ☑
      humerus M86.02- ☑
      ilium M86.059
      ischium M86.059
      mandible M27.2
      metacarpus M86.04- ☑
      metatarsus M86.07- ☑
      multiple sites M86.09
      neck M86.08
      orbit H05.02- ☑

Osteomyelitis — *continued*
  acute — *continued*
    hematogenous — *continued*
      petrous bone — *see* Petrositis
      radius M86.03- ☑
      rib M86.08
      scapula M86.01- ☑
      skull M86.08
      tarsus M86.07- ☑
      tibia M86.06- ☑
      toe M86.07- ☑
      ulna M86.03- ☑
      vertebra — *see* Osteomyelitis, vertebra
    humerus M86.12- ☑
    ilium M86.18
    ischium M86.18
    mandible M27.2
    metacarpus M86.14- ☑
    metatarsus M86.17- ☑
    multiple sites M86.19
    neck M86.18
    orbit H05.02- ☑
    petrous bone — *see* Petrositis
    radius M86.13- ☑
    rib M86.18
    scapula M86.11- ☑
    skull M86.18
    tarsus M86.17- ☑
    tibia M86.16- ☑
    toe M86.17- ☑
    ulna M86.13- ☑
    vertebra — *see* Osteomyelitis, vertebra
  chronic (or old) M86.60
    with draining sinus M86.40
      carpus M86.44- ☑
      clavicle M86.41- ☑
      femur M86.45- ☑
      fibula M86.46- ☑
      finger M86.44- ☑
      humerus M86.42- ☑
      ilium M86.459
      ischium M86.459
      mandible M27.2
      metacarpus M86.44- ☑
      metatarsus M86.47- ☑
      multiple sites M86.49
      neck M86.48
      orbit H05.02- ☑
      petrous bone — *see* Petrositis
      radius M86.43- ☑
      rib M86.48
      scapula M86.41- ☑
      skull M86.48
      tarsus M86.47- ☑
      tibia M86.46- ☑
      toe M86.47- ☑
      ulna M86.43- ☑
      vertebra — *see* Osteomyelitis, vertebra
    carpus M86.64- ☑
    clavicle M86.61- ☑
    femur M86.65- ☑
    fibula M86.66- ☑
    finger M86.64- ☑
    hematogenous NEC M86.50
      carpus M86.54- ☑
      clavicle M86.51- ☑
      femur M86.55- ☑
      fibula M86.56- ☑
      finger M86.54- ☑
      humerus M86.52- ☑
      ilium M86.559
      ischium M86.559
      mandible M27.2
      metacarpus M86.54- ☑
      metatarsus M86.57- ☑
      multifocal M86.30
        carpus M86.34- ☑
        clavicle M86.31- ☑
        femur M86.35- ☑
        fibula M86.36- ☑
        finger M86.34- ☑
        humerus M86.32- ☑
        ilium M86.359
        ischium M86.359
        metacarpus M86.34- ☑
        metatarsus M86.37- ☑

Osteomyelitis — *continued*
  chronic — *continued*
    hematogenous — *continued*
      multifocal — *continued*
        multiple sites M86.39
        neck M86.38
        radius M86.33- ☑
        rib M86.38
        scapula M86.31- ☑
        skull M86.38
        tarsus M86.37- ☑
        tibia M86.36- ☑
        toe M86.37- ☑
        ulna M86.33- ☑
        vertebra — *see* Osteomyelitis, vertebra
      multiple sites M86.59
      neck M86.58
      orbit H05.02- ☑
      petrous bone — *see* Petrositis
      radius M86.53- ☑
      rib M86.58
      scapula M86.51- ☑
      skull M86.58
      tarsus M86.57- ☑
      tibia M86.56- ☑
      toe M86.57- ☑
      ulna M86.53- ☑
      vertebra — *see* Osteomyelitis, vertebra
    humerus M86.62- ☑
    ilium M86.659
    ischium M86.659
    mandible M27.2
    metacarpus M86.64- ☑
    metatarsus M86.67- ☑
    multifocal — *see* Osteomyelitis, chronic, hematogenous, multifocal
    multiple sites M86.69
    neck M86.68
    orbit H05.02- ☑
    petrous bone — *see* Petrositis
    radius M86.63- ☑
    rib M86.68
    scapula M86.61- ☑
    skull M86.68
    tarsus M86.67- ☑
    tibia M86.66- ☑
    toe M86.67- ☑
    ulna M86.63- ☑
    vertebra — *see* Osteomyelitis, vertebra
  echinococcal B67.2
  Garr's — *see* Osteomyelitis, specified type NEC
  in diabetes mellitus — *see* E08-E13 with .69
  jaw (acute) (chronic) (lower) (neonatal) (suppurative) (upper) M27.2
  nonsuppurating — *see* Osteomyelitis, specified type NEC
  orbit H05.02- ☑
  petrous bone — *see* Petrositis
  Salmonella (arizonae) (cholerae-suis) (enteritidis) (ty-phimurium) A02.24
  sclerosing, nonsuppurative — *see* Osteomyelitis, specified type NEC
  specified type NEC — *see also* subcategory M86.8X- ☑
    mandible M27.2
    orbit H05.02- ☑
    petrous bone — *see* Petrositis
    vertebra — *see* Osteomyelitis, vertebra
  subacute M86.20
    carpus M86.24- ☑
    clavicle M86.21- ☑
    femur M86.25- ☑
    fibula M86.26- ☑
    finger M86.24- ☑
    humerus M86.22- ☑
    mandible M27.2
    metacarpus M86.24- ☑
    metatarsus M86.27- ☑
    multiple sites M86.29
    neck M86.28
    orbit H05.02- ☑
    petrous bone — *see* Petrositis
    radius M86.23- ☑
    rib M86.28
    scapula M86.21- ☑
    skull M86.28
    tarsus M86.27- ☑
    tibia M86.26- ☑

Osteomyelitis — *continued*
  subacute — *continued*
    toe M86.27- ☑
    ulna M86.23- ☑
    vertebra — *see* Osteomyelitis, vertebra
  syphilitic A52.77
    congenital (early) A50.02 *[M90.80]*
  tuberculous — *see* Tuberculosis, bone
  typhoid A01.05
  vertebra M46.20
    cervical region M46.22
    cervicothoracic region M46.23
    lumbar region M46.26
    lumbosacral region M46.27
    occipito-atlanto-axial region M46.21
    sacrococcygeal region M46.28
    thoracic region M46.24
    thoracolumbar region M46.25
Osteomyelofibrosis D47.4
Osteomyelosclerosis D75.89
Osteonecrosis M87.9
  due to
    drugs — *see* Osteonecrosis, secondary, due to, drugs
    trauma — *see* Osteonecrosis, secondary, due to, trauma
  idiopathic aseptic M87.00
    ankle M87.07- ☑
    carpus M87.03- ☑
    clavicle M87.01- ☑
    femur M87.05- ☑
    fibula M87.06- ☑
    finger M87.04- ☑
    humerus M87.02- ☑
    ilium M87.050
    ischium M87.050
    metacarpus M87.04- ☑
    metatarsus M87.07- ☑
    multiple sites M87.09
    neck M87.08
    pelvis M87.050
    radius M87.03- ☑
    rib M87.08
    scapula M87.01- ☑
    skull M87.08
    tarsus M87.07- ☑
    tibia M87.06- ☑
    toe M87.07- ☑
    ulna M87.03- ☑
    vertebra M87.08
  secondary NEC M87.30
    carpus M87.33- ☑
    clavicle M87.31- ☑
    due to
      drugs M87.10
        carpus M87.13- ☑
        clavicle M87.11- ☑
        femur M87.15- ☑
        fibula M87.16- ☑
        finger M87.14- ☑
        humerus M87.12- ☑
        ilium M87.159
        ischium M87.159
        jaw M87.180
        metacarpus M87.14- ☑
        metatarsus M87.17- ☑
        multiple sites M87.19
        neck M87.18
        radius M87.13- ☑
        rib M87.18 ☑
        scapula M87.11- ☑
        skull M87.18 ☑
        tarsus M87.17- ☑
        tibia M87.16- ☑
        toe M87.17- ☑
        ulna M87.13- ☑
        vertebra M87.18
      hemoglobinopathy NEC D58.2 *[M90.50]*
        carpus D58.2 *[M90.54-]* ☑
        clavicle D58.2 *[M90.51-]* ☑
        femur D58.2 *[M90.55-]* ☑
        fibula D58.2 *[M90.56-]* ☑
        finger D58.2 *[M90.54-]* ☑
        humerus D58.2 *[M90.52-]* ☑
        ilium D58.2 *[M90.55-]* ☑
        ischium D58.2 *[M90.55-]* ☑
        metacarpus D58.2 *[M90.54-]* ☑
        metatarsus D58.2 *[M90.57-]* ☑

Osteonecrosis — *continued*
  secondary — *continued*
    due to — *continued*
      hemoglobinopathy — *continued*
        multiple sites D58.2 *[M90.58]*
        neck D58.2 *[M90.58]*
        radius D58.2 *[M90.53-]* ☑
        rib D58.2 *[M90.58]*
        scapula D58.2 *[M90.51-]* ☑
        skull D58.2 *[M90.58]*
        tarsus D58.2 *[M90.57-]* ☑
        tibia D58.2 *[M90.56-]* ☑
        toe D58.2 *[M90.57-]* ☑
        ulna D58.2 *[M90.53-]* ☑
        vertebra D58.2 *[M90.58]*
      trauma (previous) M87.20
        carpus M87.23- ☑
        clavicle M87.21- ☑
        femur M87.25- ☑
        fibula M87.26- ☑
        finger M87.24- ☑
        humerus M87.22- ☑
        ilium M87.25- ☑
        ischium M87.25- ☑
        metacarpus M87.24- ☑
        metatarsus M87.27- ☑
        multiple sites M87.29
        neck M87.28
        radius M87.23- ☑
        rib M87.28
        scapula M87.21- ☑
        skull M87.28
        tarsus M87.27- ☑
        tibia M87.26- ☑
        toe M87.27- ☑
        ulna M87.23- ☑
        vertebra M87.28
    femur M87.35- ☑
    fibula M87.36- ☑
    finger M87.34- ☑
    humerus M87.32- ☑
    ilium M87.350
    in
      caisson disease T70.3 ☑ *[M90.50]*
        carpus T70.3 ☑ *[M90.54-]* ☑
        clavicle T70.3 ☑ *[M90.51-]* ☑
        femur T70.3 ☑ *[M90.55-]* ☑
        fibula T70.3 ☑ *[M90.56-]* ☑
        finger T70.3 ☑ *[M90.54-]* ☑
        humerus T70.3 ☑ *[M90.52-]* ☑
        ilium T70.3 ☑ *[M90.55-]* ☑
        ischium T70.3 ☑ *[M90.55-]* ☑
        metacarpus T70.3 ☑ *[M90.54-]* ☑
        metatarsus T70.3 ☑ *[M90.57-]* ☑
        multiple sites T70.3 ☑ *[M90.59]*
        neck T70.3 ☑ *[M90.58]*
        radius T70.3 ☑ *[M90.53-]* ☑
        rib T70.3 ☑ *[M90.58]*
        scapula T70.3 ☑ *[M90.51-]* ☑
        skull T70.3 ☑ *[M90.58]*
        tarsus T70.3 ☑ *[M90.57-]* ☑
        tibia T70.3 ☑ *[M90.56-]* ☑
        toe T70.3 ☑ *[M90.57-]* ☑
        ulna T70.3 ☑ *[M90.53-]* ☑
        vertebra T70.3 ☑ *[M90.58]*
    ischium M87.350
    metacarpus M87.34- ☑
    metatarsus M87.37- ☑
    multiple site M87.39
    neck M87.38
    radius M87.33- ☑
    rib M87.38
    scapula M87.319
    skull M87.38
    tarsus M87.379
    tibia M87.366
    toe M87.379
    ulna M87.33- ☑
    vertebra M87.38
  specified type NEC M87.80
    carpus M87.83- ☑
    clavicle M87.81- ☑
    femur M87.85- ☑
    fibula M87.86- ☑
    finger M87.84- ☑
    humerus M87.82- ☑

Osteonecrosis — *continued*
  specified type — *continued*
    ilium M87.85- ☑
    ischium M87.85- ☑
    metacarpus M87.84- ☑
    metatarsus M87.87- ☑
    multiple sites M87.89
    neck M87.88
    radius M87.83- ☑
    rib M87.88
    scapula M87.81- ☑
    skull M87.88
    tarsus M87.87- ☑
    tibia M87.86- ☑
    toe M87.87- ☑
    ulna M87.83- ☑
    vertebra M87.88
Osteo-onycho-arthro-dysplasia Q87.2
Osteo-onychodysplasia, hereditary Q87.2
Osteopathia condensans disseminata Q78.8
Osteopathy — *see also* Osteomyelitis, Osteonecrosis, Osteoporosis
  after poliomyelitis M89.60
    carpus M89.64- ☑
    clavicle M89.61- ☑
    femur M89.65- ☑
    fibula M89.66- ☑
    finger M89.64- ☑
    humerus M89.62- ☑
    ilium M89.659
    ischium M89.659
    metacarpus M89.64- ☑
    metatarsus M89.67- ☑
    multiple sites M89.69
    neck M89.68
    radius M89.63- ☑
    rib M89.68
    scapula M89.61- ☑
    skull M89.68
    tarsus M89.67- ☑
    tibia M89.66- ☑
    toe M89.67- ☑
    ulna M89.63- ☑
    vertebra M89.68
  in (due to)
    renal osteodystrophy N25.0
    specified diseases classified elsewhere — *see* subcategory M90.8
Osteopenia M85.8- ☑
  borderline M85.8- ☑
Osteoperiostitis — *see* Osteomyelitis, specified type NEC
Osteopetrosis (familial) Q78.2
Osteophyte M25.70
  ankle M25.77- ☑
  elbow M25.72- ☑
  foot joint M25.77- ☑
  hand joint M25.74- ☑
  hip M25.75- ☑
  knee M25.76- ☑
  shoulder M25.71- ☑
  spine M25.78
  vertebrae M25.78
  wrist M25.73- ☑
Osteopoikilosis Q78.8
Osteoporosis (female) (male) M81.0
  with current pathological fracture M80.00 ☑
  age-related M81.0
    with current pathologic fracture M80.00 ☑
      carpus M80.04- ☑
      clavicle M80.01- ☑
      fibula M80.06- ☑
      finger M80.04- ☑
      humerus M80.02- ☑
      ilium M80.05- ☑
      ischium M80.05- ☑
      metacarpus M80.04- ☑
      metatarsus M80.07- ☑
      pelvis M80.05- ☑
      radius M80.03- ☑
      scapula M80.01- ☑
      tarsus M80.07- ☑
      tibia M80.06- ☑
      toe M80.07- ☑
      ulna M80.03- ☑
      vertebra M80.08

☑ **Additional Character Required** — Refer to the Tabular List for Character Selection
▽ Subterms under main terms may continue to next column or page

Osteoporosis — *continued*
- disuse M81.8
  - with current pathological fracture M80.80 ☑
    - carpus M80.84- ☑
    - clavicle M80.81- ☑
    - fibula M80.86- ☑
    - finger M80.84- ☑
    - humerus M80.82- ☑
    - ilium M80.85- ☑
    - ischium M80.85- ☑
    - metacarpus M80.84- ☑
    - metatarsus M80.87- ☑
    - pelvis M80.85- ☑
    - radius M80.83- ☑
    - scapula M80.81- ☑
    - tarsus M80.87- ☑
    - tibia M80.86- ☑
    - toe M80.87- ☑
    - ulna M80.83- ☑
    - vertebra M80.88 ☑
- drug-induced — *see* Osteoporosis, specified type NEC
- idiopathic — *see* Osteoporosis, specified type NEC
- involutional — *see* Osteoporosis, age-related
- Lequesne M81.6
- localized M81.6
- postmenopausal M81.0
  - with pathological fracture M80.00 ☑
    - carpus M80.04- ☑
    - clavicle M80.01- ☑
    - fibula M80.06- ☑
    - finger M80.04- ☑
    - humerus M80.02- ☑
    - ilium M80.05- ☑
    - ischium M80.05- ☑
    - metacarpus M80.04- ☑
    - metatarsus M80.07- ☑
    - pelvis M80.05- ☑
    - radius M80.03- ☑
    - scapula M80.01- ☑
    - tarsus M80.07- ☑
    - tibia M80.06- ☑
    - toe M80.07- ☑
    - ulna M80.03- ☑
    - vertebra M80.08 ☑
- postoophorectomy — *see* Osteoporosis, specified type NEC
- postsurgical malabsorption — *see* Osteoporosis, specified type NEC
- post-traumatic — *see* Osteoporosis, specified type NEC
- senile — *see* Osteoporosis, age-related
- specified type NEC M81.8
  - with pathological fracture M80.80 ☑
    - carpus M80.84- ☑
    - clavicle M80.81- ☑
    - fibula M80.86- ☑
    - finger M80.84- ☑
    - humerus M80.82- ☑
    - ilium M80.85- ☑
    - ischium M80.85- ☑
    - metacarpus M80.84- ☑
    - metatarsus M80.87- ☑
    - pelvis M80.85- ☑
    - radius M80.83- ☑
    - scapula M80.81- ☑
    - tarsus M80.87- ☑
    - tibia M80.86- ☑
    - toe M80.87- ☑
    - ulna M80.83- ☑
    - vertebra M80.88 ☑

Osteopsathyrosis (idiopathica) Q78.0
Osteoradionecrosis, jaw (acute) (chronic) (lower) (suppurative) (upper) M27.2
Osteosarcoma (any form) — *see* Neoplasm, bone, malignant
Osteosclerosis Q78.2
- acquired M85.8- ☑
- congenita Q77.4
- fragilitas (generalisata) Q78.2
- myelofibrosis D75.81
Osteosclerotic anemia D64.89
Osteosis
- cutis L94.2
- renal fibrocystic N25.0
Osterreicher-Turner syndrome Q87.2
Ostium
- atrioventriculare commune Q21.2

Ostium — *continued*
- primum (arteriosum) (defect) (persistent) Q21.2
- secundum (arteriosum) (defect) (patent) (persistent) Q21.1
Ostrum-Furst syndrome Q75.8
Otalgia H92.0 ☑
Otitis (acute) H66.90
- with effusion — *see also* Otitis, media, nonsuppurative
  - purulent — *see* Otitis, media, suppurative
- adhesive — *see* subcategory H74.1 ☑
- chronic — *see also* Otitis, media, chronic
  - with effusion — *see also* Otitis, media, nonsuppurative, chronic
- externa H60.9- ☑
  - abscess — *see* Abscess, ear, external
  - acute (noninfective) H60.50- ☑
    - actinic H60.51- ☑
    - chemical H60.52- ☑
    - contact H60.53- ☑
    - eczematoid H60.54- ☑
    - infective — *see* Otitis, externa, infective
    - reactive H60.55- ☑
    - specified NEC H60.59- ☑
  - cellulitis — *see* Cellulitis, ear
  - chronic H60.6- ☑
  - diffuse — *see* Otitis, externa, infective, diffuse
  - hemorrhagic — *see* Otitis, externa, infective, hemorrhagic
  - in (due to)
    - aspergillosis B44.89
    - candidiasis B37.84
    - erysipelas A46 *[H62.40]*
    - herpes (simplex) virus infection B00.1
      - zoster B02.8
    - impetigo L01.00 *[H62.40]*
    - infectious disease NEC B99 ☑ *[H62.4-]* ☑
    - mycosis NEC B36.9 *[H62.40]*
    - parasitic disease NEC B89 *[H62.40]*
    - viral disease NEC B34.9 *[H62.40]*
    - zoster B02.8
  - infective NEC H60.39- ☑
    - abscess — *see* Abscess, ear, external
    - cellulitis — *see* Cellulitis, ear
    - diffuse H60.31- ☑
    - hemorrhagic H60.32- ☑
    - swimmer's ear — *see* Swimmer's, ear
  - malignant H60.2- ☑
  - mycotic NEC B36.9 *[H62.40]*
    - in
      - aspergillosis B44.89
      - candidiasis B37.84
      - moniliasis B37.84
  - necrotizing — *see* Otitis, externa, malignant
  - Pseudomonas aeruginosa — *see* Otitis, externa, malignant
  - reactive — *see* Otitis, externa, acute, reactive
  - specified NEC — *see* subcategory H60.8 ☑
  - tropical NEC B36.9 *[H62.40]*
    - in
      - aspergillosis B44.89
      - candidiasis B37.84
      - moniliasis B37.84
- insidiosa — *see* Otosclerosis
- interna H83.0 ☑
- media (hemorrhagic) (staphylococcal) (streptococcal) H66.9- ☑
  - with effusion (nonpurulent) — *see* Otitis, media, nonsuppurative
  - acute, subacute H66.90
    - allergic — *see* Otitis, media, nonsuppurative, acute, allergic
    - exudative — *see* Otitis, media, suppurative, acute
    - mucoid — *see* Otitis, media, nonsuppurative, acute
    - necrotizing — *see also* Otitis, media, suppurative, acute
      - in
        - measles B05.3
        - scarlet fever A38.0
    - nonsuppurative NEC — *see* Otitis, media, nonsuppurative, acute
    - purulent — *see* Otitis, media, suppurative, acute
    - sanguinous — *see* Otitis, media, nonsuppurative, acute
    - secretory — *see* Otitis, media, nonsuppurative, acute, serous

Otitis — *continued*
- media — *continued*
  - acute, subacute — *continued*
    - seromucinous — *see* Otitis, media, nonsuppurative, acute
    - serous — *see* Otitis, media, nonsuppurative, acute, serous
    - suppurative — *see* Otitis, media, suppurative, acute
  - allergic — *see* Otitis, media, nonsuppurative
  - catarrhal — *see* Otitis, media, nonsuppurative
  - chronic H66.90
    - with effusion (nonpurulent) — *see* Otitis, media, nonsuppurative, chronic
    - allergic — *see* Otitis, media, nonsuppurative, chronic, allergic
    - benign suppurative — *see* Otitis, media, suppurative, chronic, tubotympanic
    - catarrhal — *see* Otitis, media, nonsuppurative, chronic, serous
    - exudative — *see* Otitis, media, nonsuppurative, chronic
    - mucinous — *see* Otitis, media, nonsuppurative, chronic, mucoid
    - mucoid — *see* Otitis, media, nonsuppurative, chronic, mucoid
    - nonsuppurative NEC — *see* Otitis, media, nonsuppurative, chronic
    - purulent — *see* Otitis, media, suppurative, chronic
    - secretory — *see* Otitis, media, nonsuppurative, chronic, mucoid
    - seromucinous — *see* Otitis, media, nonsuppurative, chronic
    - serous — *see* Otitis, media, nonsuppurative, chronic, serous
    - suppurative — *see* Otitis, media, suppurative, chronic
    - transudative — *see* Otitis, media, nonsuppurative, chronic, mucoid
  - exudative — *see* Otitis, media, suppurative
  - in (due to) (with)
    - influenza — *see* Influenza, with, otitis media
    - measles B05.3
    - scarlet fever A38.0
    - tuberculosis A18.6
    - viral disease NEC B34.- ☑ *[H67.-]* ☑
  - mucoid — *see* Otitis, media, nonsuppurative
  - nonsuppurative H65.9- ☑
    - acute or subacute NEC H65.19- ☑
      - allergic H65.11- ☑
        - recurrent H65.11- ☑
      - recurrent H65.19- ☑
      - secretory — *see* Otitis, media, nonsuppurative, serous
      - serous H65.0- ☑
        - recurrent H65.0- ☑
    - chronic H65.49- ☑
      - allergic H65.41- ☑
      - mucoid H65.3- ☑
      - serous H65.2- ☑
    - postmeasles B05.3
    - purulent — *see* Otitis, media, suppurative
    - secretory — *see* Otitis, media, nonsuppurative
    - seromucinous — *see* Otitis, media, nonsuppurative
    - serous — *see* Otitis, media, nonsuppurative
  - suppurative H66.4- ☑
    - acute H66.00- ☑
      - with rupture of ear drum H66.01- ☑
      - recurrent H66.00- ☑
        - with rupture of ear drum H66.01- ☑
    - chronic — *see also* subcategory H66.3 ☑
      - atticoantral H66.2- ☑
      - benign — *see* Otitis, media, suppurative, chronic, tubotympanic
      - tubotympanic H66.1- ☑
  - transudative — *see* Otitis, media, nonsuppurative
  - tuberculous A18.6
Otocephaly Q18.2
Otolith syndrome — *see* subcategory H81.8 ☑
Otomycosis (diffuse) **NEC** B36.9 *[H62.40]*
- in
  - aspergillosis B44.89
  - candidiasis B37.84
  - moniliasis B37.84
Otoporosis — *see* Otosclerosis
Otorrhagia (nontraumatic) H92.2- ☑

☑ **Additional Character Required** — Refer to the Tabular List for Character Selection   ▽ **Subterms under main terms may continue to next column or page**

ain(s) — *continued*
  due to device, implant or graft — *see also* Complica-
    tions, by site and type, specified — *continued*
    catheter — *continued*
      dialysis — *continued*
        intraperitoneal T85.848 ☑
        infusion NEC T82.848 ☑
        spinal (epidural) (subdural) T85.840 ☑
        urinary (indwelling) T83.84 ☑
    electronic (electrode) (pulse generator) (stimulator)
      bone T85.840 ☑
      cardiac T82.847 ☑
      nervous system (brain) (peripheral nerve) (spinal)
        T85.84 ☑
      urinary T83.84 ☑
    fixation, internal (orthopedic) NEC T84.84 ☑
    gastrointestinal (bile duct) (esophagus) T85.848 ☑
    genital NEC T83.84 ☑
    heart NEC T82.847 ☑
    infusion NEC T85.848 ☑
    joint prosthesis T84.84 ☑
    ocular (corneal graft) (orbital implant) NEC
      T85.848 ☑
    orthopedic NEC T84.84 ☑
    specified NEC T85.848 ☑
    urinary NEC T83.84 ☑
    vascular NEC T82.848 ☑
    ventricular intracranial shunt T85.840 ☑
  due to malignancy (primary) (secondary) G89.3
  ear — *see* subcategory H92.0 ☑
  epigastric, epigastrium R10.13
  eye — *see* Pain, ocular
  face, facial R51
    atypical G50.1
  female genital organs NEC N94.89
  finger — *see* Pain, limb, upper
  flank — *see* Pain, abdominal
  foot — *see* Pain, limb, lower
  gallbladder K82.9
  gas (intestinal) R14.1
  gastric — *see* Pain, abdominal
  generalized NOS R52
  genital organ
    female N94.89
    male N50.89
  groin — *see* Pain, abdominal, lower
  hand — *see* Pain, limb, upper
  head — *see* Headache
  heart — *see* Pain, precordial
  infra-orbital — *see* Neuralgia, trigeminal
  intercostal R07.82
  intermenstrual N94.0
  jaw R68.84
  joint M25.50
    ankle M25.57- ☑
    elbow M25.52- ☑
    finger M25.54- ☑
    foot M25.57- ☑
    hand M25.54- ☑
    hip M25.55- ☑
    knee M25.56- ☑
    shoulder M25.51- ☑
    toe M25.57- ☑
    wrist M25.53- ☑
  kidney N23
  laryngeal R07.0
  leg — *see* Pain, limb, lower
  limb M79.609
    lower M79.60- ☑
      foot M79.67- ☑
      lower leg M79.66- ☑
      thigh M79.65- ☑
      toe M79.67- ☑
    upper M79.60- ☑
      axilla M79.62- ☑
      finger M79.64- ☑
      forearm M79.63- ☑
      hand M79.64- ☑
      upper arm M79.62- ☑
  loin M54.5
  low back M54.5
  lumbar region M54.5
  mandibular R68.84
  mastoid — *see* subcategory H92.0 ☑
  maxilla R68.84
  menstrual — *see also* Dysmenorrhea N94.6
  metacarpophalangeal (joint) — *see* Pain, joint, hand

Pain(s) — *continued*
  metatarsophalangeal (joint) — *see* Pain, joint, foot
  mouth K13.79
  muscle — *see* Myalgia
  musculoskeletal — *see also* Pain, by site M79.18
  myofascial M79.18
  nasal J34.89
  nasopharynx J39.2
  neck NEC M54.2
  nerve NEC — *see* Neuralgia
  neuromuscular — *see* Neuralgia
  nose J34.89
  ocular H57.1- ☑
  ophthalmic — *see* Pain, ocular
  orbital region — *see* Pain, ocular
  ovary N94.89
  over heart — *see* Pain, precordial
  ovulation N94.0
  pelvic (female) R10.2
  penis N48.89
  pericardial — *see* Pain, precordial
  perineal, perineum R10.2
  pharynx J39.2
  pleura, pleural, pleuritic R07.81
  postoperative NOS G89.18
  postprocedural NOS G89.18
  post-thoracotomy G89.12
  precordial (region) R07.2
  premenstrual N94.3
  psychogenic (persistent) (any site) F45.41
  radicular (spinal) — *see* Radiculopathy
  rectum K62.89
  respiration R07.1
  retrosternal R07.2
  rheumatoid, muscular — *see* Myalgia
  rib R07.81
  root (spinal) — *see* Radiculopathy
  round ligament (stretch) R10.2
  sacroiliac M53.3
  sciatic — *see* Sciatica
  scrotum N50.82
  seminal vesicle N50.89
  shoulder M25.51- ☑
  spermatic cord N50.89
  spinal root — *see* Radiculopathy
  spine M54.9
    cervical M54.2
    low back M54.5
      with sciatica M54.4- ☑
    thoracic M54.6
  stomach — *see* Pain, abdominal
  substernal R07.2
  temporomandibular (joint) M26.62- ☑
  testis N50.81- ☑
  thoracic spine M54.6
    with radicular and visceral pain M54.14
  throat R07.0
  tibia — *see* Pain, limb, lower
  toe — *see* Pain, limb, lower
  tongue K14.6
  tooth K08.89
  trigeminal — *see* Neuralgia, trigeminal
  tumor associated G89.3
  ureter N23
  urinary (organ) (system) N23
  uterus NEC N94.89
  vagina R10.2
  vertebrogenic (syndrome) M54.89
  vesical R39.89
    associated with micturition — *see* Micturition,
      painful
  vulva R10.2
Painful — *see also* Pain
  coitus
    female N94.10
    male N53.12
    psychogenic F52.6
  ejaculation (semen) N53.12
    psychogenic F52.6
  erection — *see* Priapism
  feet syndrome E53.8
  joint replacement (hip) (knee) T84.84 ☑
  menstruation — *see* Dysmenorrhea
    psychogenic F45.8
  micturition — *see* Micturition, painful
  respiration R07.1
  scar NEC L90.5
  wire sutures T81.89 ☑

Painter's colic — *see* subcategory T56.0 ☑
Palate — *see* condition
Palatoplegia K13.79
Palatoschisis — *see* Cleft, palate
Palilalia R48.8
Palliative care Z51.5
Pallor R23.1
  optic disc, temporal — *see* Atrophy, optic
Palmar — *see also* condition
  fascia — *see* condition
Palpable
  cecum K63.89
  kidney N28.89
  ovary N83.8
  prostate N42.9
  spleen — *see* Splenomegaly
Palpitations (heart) R00.2
  psychogenic F45.8
Palsy — *see also* Paralysis G83.9
  atrophic diffuse (progressive) G12.22
  Bell's — *see also* Palsy, facial
    newborn P11.3
  brachial plexus NEC G54.0
    newborn (birth injury) P14.3
  brain — *see* Palsy, cerebral
  bulbar (progressive) (chronic) G12.22
    of childhood (Fazio-Londe) G12.1
    pseudo NEC G12.29
    supranuclear (progressive) G23.1
  cerebral (congenital) G80.9
    ataxic G80.4
    athetoid G80.3
    choreathetoid G80.3
    diplegic G80.8
      spastic G80.1
    dyskinetic G80.3
      athetoid G80.3
      choreathetoid G80.3
      distonic G80.3
    dystonic G80.3
    hemiplegic G80.8
      spastic G80.2
    mixed G80.8
    monoplegic G80.8
      spastic G80.1
    paraplegic G80.8
      spastic G80.1
    quadriplegic G80.8
      spastic G80.0
    spastic G80.1
      diplegic G80.1
      hemiplegic G80.2
      monoplegic G80.1
      quadriplegic G80.0
      specified NEC G80.1
      tetrapelgic G80.0
    specified NEC G80.8
    syphilitic A52.12
      congenital A50.49
    tetraplegic G80.8
      spastic G80.0
  cranial nerve — *see also* Disorder, nerve, cranial
    multiple G52.7
      in
        infectious disease B99 ☑ *[G53]*
        neoplastic disease — *see also* Neoplasm
          D49.9 *[G53]*
        parasitic disease B89 *[G53]*
        sarcoidosis D86.82
  creeping G12.22
  diver's T70.3 ☑
  Erb's P14.0
  facial G51.0
    newborn (birth injury) P11.3
  glossopharyngeal G52.1
  Klumpke (-Déjérine) P14.1
  lead — *see* subcategory T56.0 ☑
  median nerve (tardy) G56.1- ☑
  nerve G58.9
    specified NEC G58.8
  peroneal nerve (acute) (tardy) G57.3- ☑
  progressive supranuclear G23.1
  pseudobulbar NEC G12.29
  radial nerve (acute) G56.3- ☑
  seventh nerve — *see also* Palsy, facial
    newborn P11.3
  shaking — *see* Parkinsonism
  spastic (cerebral) (spinal) G80.1

⚐ Subterms under main terms may continue to next column or page   ☑ Additional Character Required — Refer to the Tabular List for Character Selection   **245**

Pain — Palsy

Palsy — *continued*
  ulnar nerve (tardy) G56.2- ☑
  wasting G12.29
Paludism — *see* Malaria
Panangiitis M30.0
Panaris, panaritium — *see also* Cellulitis, digit
  with lymphangitis — *see* Lymphangitis, acute, digit
Panarteritis nodosa M30.0
  brain or cerebral I67.7
Pancake heart R93.1
  with cor pulmonale (chronic) I27.81
Pancarditis (acute) (chronic) I51.89
  rheumatic I09.89
    active or acute I01.8
Pancoast's syndrome or tumor C34.1- ☑
Pancolitis, ulcerative (chronic) K51.00
  with
    abscess K51.014
    complication K51.019
    fistula K51.013
    obstruction K51.012
    rectal bleeding K51.011
    specified complication NEC K51.018
Pancreas, pancreatic — *see* condition
Pancreatitis (annular) (apoplectic) (calcareous) (edematous) (hemorrhagic) (malignant) (recurrent) (subacute) (suppurative) K85.90
  with necrosis (uninfected) K85.91
    infected K85.92
  acute (without necrosis or infection) K85.90
    with necrosis (uninfected) K85.91
      infected K85.92
    alcohol induced (without necrosis or infection) K85.20
      with necrosis (uninfected) K85.21
        infected K85.22
    biliary (without necrosis or infection) K85.10
      with necrosis (uninfected) K85.11
        infected K85.12
    drug induced (without necrosis or infection) K85.30
      with necrosis (uninfected) K85.31
        infected K85.32
    gallstone (without necrosis or infection) K85.10
      with necrosis (uninfected) K85.11
        infected K85.12
    idiopathic (without necrosis or infection) K85.00
      with necrosis (uninfected) K85.01
        infected K85.02
    specified NEC (without necrosis or infection) K85.80
      with necrosis (uninfected) K85.81
        infected K85.82
  chronic (infectious) K86.1
    alcohol-induced K86.0
    recurrent K86.1
    relapsing K86.1
  cystic (chronic) K86.1
  cytomegaloviral B25.2
  fibrous (chronic) K86.1
  gallstone (without necrosis or infection) K85.10
    with necrosis (uninfected) K85.11
      infected K85.12
  gangrenous — *see* Pancreatitis, acute
  interstitial (chronic) K86.1
    acute — *see also* Pancreatitis, acute K85.80
  mumps B26.3
  recurrent (chronic) K86.1
  relapsing, chronic K86.1
  syphilitic A52.74
Pancreatoblastoma — *see* Neoplasm, pancreas, malignant
Pancreolithiasis K86.89
Pancytolysis D75.89
Pancytopenia (acquired) D61.818
  with
    malformations D61.09
    myelodysplastic syndrome — *see* Syndrome, myelodysplastic
  antineoplastic chemotherapy induced D61.810
  congenital D61.09
  drug-induced NEC D61.811
PANDAS (pediatric autoimmune neuropsychiatric disorders associated with streptococcal infections syndrome) D89.89
Panencephalitis, subacute, sclerosing A81.1
Panhematopenia D61.9
  congenital D61.09
  constitutional D61.09
  splenic, primary D73.1

Panhemocytopenia D61.9
  congenital D61.09
  constitutional D61.09
Panhypogonadism E29.1
Panhypopituitarism E23.0
  prepubertal E23.0
Panic (attack) (state) F41.0
  reaction to exceptional stress (transient) F43.0
Panmyelopathy, familial, constitutional D61.09
Panmyelophthisis D61.82
  congenital D61.09
Panmyelosis (acute) (with myelofibrosis) C94.4- ☑
Panner's disease — *see* Osteochondrosis, juvenile, humerus
Panneuritis endemica E51.11
Panniculitis (nodular) (nonsuppurative) M79.3
  back M54.06
    cervical region M54.02
    cervicothoracic region M54.03
    lumbar region M54.06
    lumbosacral region M54.07
    multiple sites M54.09
    occipito-atlanto-axial region M54.01
    sacrococcygeal region M54.08
    thoracic region M54.04
    thoracolumbar region M54.05
  lupus L93.2
  mesenteric K65.4
  neck M54.02
    cervicothoracic region M54.03
    occipito-atlanto-axial region M54.01
  relapsing M35.6
Panniculus adiposus (abdominal) E65
Pannus (allergic) (cornea) (degenerativus) (keratic) H16.42- ☑
  abdominal (symptomatic) E65
  trachomatosus, trachomatous (active) A71.1
Panophthalmitis H44.01- ☑
Pansinusitis (chronic) (hyperplastic) (nonpurulent) (purulent) J32.4
  acute J01.40
    recurrent J01.41
  tuberculous A15.8
Panuveitis (sympathetic) H44.11- ☑
Panvalvular disease I08.9
  specified NEC I08.8
PAPA (pyogenic arthritis, pyoderma gangrenosum, and acne syndrome) M04.8
Papanicolaou smear, cervix Z12.4
  as part of routine gynecological examination Z01.419
    with abnormal findings Z01.411
  for suspected neoplasm Z12.4
  nonspecific abnormal finding R87.619
  routine Z01.419
    with abnormal findings Z01.411
Papilledema (choked disc) H47.10
  associated with
    decreased ocular pressure H47.12
    increased intracranial pressure H47.11
    retinal disorder H47.13
  Foster-Kennedy syndrome H47.14- ☑
Papillitis H46.00
  anus K62.89
  chronic lingual K14.4
  necrotizing, kidney N17.2
  optic H46.0- ☑
  rectum K62.89
  renal, necrotizing N17.2
  tongue K14.0
Papilloma — *see also* Neoplasm, benign, by site
  acuminatum (female) (male) (anogenital) A63.0
  basal cell L82.1
    inflamed L82.0
  benign pinta (primary) A67.0
  bladder (urinary) (transitional cell) D41.4
  choroid plexus (lateral ventricle) (third ventricle) D33.0
    anaplastic C71.5
    fourth ventricle D33.1
    malignant C71.5
  renal pelvis (transitional cell) D41.1- ☑
    benign D30.1- ☑
  Schneiderian
    specified site — *see* Neoplasm, benign, by site
    unspecified site D14.0
  serous surface
    borderline malignancy
      specified site — *see* Neoplasm, uncertain behavior, by site

Papilloma — *continued*
  serous surface — *continued*
    borderline malignancy — *continued*
      unspecified site D39.10
    specified site — *see* Neoplasm, benign, by site
    unspecified site D27.9
  transitional (cell)
    bladder (urinary) D41.4
    inverted type — *see* Neoplasm, uncertain behavior, by site
    renal pelvis D41.1- ☑
    ureter D41.2- ☑
  ureter (transitional cell) D41.2- ☑
    benign D30.2- ☑
  urothelial — *see* Neoplasm, uncertain behavior, by site
  villous — *see* Neoplasm, uncertain behavior, by site
    adenocarcinoma in — *see* Neoplasm, malignant, by site
    in situ — *see* Neoplasm, in situ
  yaws, plantar or palmar A66.1
Papillomata, multiple, of yaws A66.1
Papillomatosis — *see also* Neoplasm, benign, by site
  confluent and reticulated L83
  cystic, breast — *see* Mastopathy, cystic
  ductal, breast — *see* Mastopathy, cystic
  intraductal (diffuse) — *see* Neoplasm, benign, by site
  subareolar duct D24- ☑
Papillomavirus, as cause of disease classified elsewhere B97.7
Papillon-Léage and Psaume syndrome Q87.0
Papule(s) R23.8
  carate (primary) A67.0
  fibrous, of nose D22.39
  Gottron's L94.4
  pinta (primary) A67.0
Papulosis
  lymphomatoid C86.6
  malignant I77.89
Papyraceous fetus O31.0- ☑
Para-albuminemia E88.09
Paracephalus Q89.7
Parachute mitral valve Q23.2
Paracoccidioidomycosis B41.9
  disseminated B41.7
  generalized B41.7
  mucocutaneous-lymphangitic B41.8
  pulmonary B41.0
  specified NEC B41.8
  visceral B41.8
Paradentosis K05.4
Paraffinoma T88.8 ☑
Paraganglioma D44.7
  adrenal D35.0- ☑
    malignant C74.1- ☑
  aortic body D44.7
    malignant C75.5
  carotid body D44.6
    malignant C75.4
  chromaffin — *see also* Neoplasm, benign, by site
    malignant — *see* Neoplasm, malignant, by site
  extra-adrenal D44.7
    malignant C75.5
      specified site — *see* Neoplasm, malignant, by site
      unspecified site C75.5
    specified site — *see* Neoplasm, uncertain behavior, by site
    unspecified site D44.7
  gangliocytic D13.2
    specified site — *see* Neoplasm, benign, by site
    unspecified site D13.2
  glomus jugulare D44.7
    malignant C75.5
  jugular D44.7
  malignant C75.5
    specified site — *see* Neoplasm, malignant, by site
    unspecified site C75.5
  nonchromaffin D44.7
    malignant C75.5
      specified site — *see* Neoplasm, malignant, by site
      unspecified site C75.5
    specified site — *see* Neoplasm, uncertain behavior, by site
    unspecified site D44.7
  parasympathetic D44.7

araganglioma — *continued*
  parasympathetic — *continued*
    specified site — *see* Neoplasm, uncertain behavior, by site
    unspecified site D44.7
  specified site — *see* Neoplasm, uncertain behavior, by site
  sympathetic D44.7
    specified site — *see* Neoplasm, uncertain behavior, by site
    unspecified site D44.7
  unspecified site D44.7
arageusia R43.2
  psychogenic F45.8
aragonimiasis B66.4
aragranuloma, Hodgkin — *see* Lymphoma, Hodgkin, specified NEC
arahemophilia — *see also* Defect, coagulation D68.2
arakeratosis R23.4
  variegata L41.0
Paralysis, paralytic (complete) (incomplete) G83.9
  with
    syphilis A52.17
  abducens, abducent (nerve) — *see* Strabismus, paralytic, sixth nerve
  abductor, lower extremity G57.9- ☑
  accessory nerve G52.8
  accommodation — *see also* Paresis, of accommodation
    hysterical F44.89
  acoustic nerve (except Deafness) H93.3 ☑
  agitans — *see also* Parkinsonism G20
    arteriosclerotic G21.4
  alternating (oculomotor) G83.89
  amyotrophic G12.21
  ankle G57.9- ☑
  anus (sphincter) K62.89
  arm — *see* Monoplegia, upper limb
  ascending (spinal), acute G61.0
  association G12.29
  asthenic bulbar G70.00
    with exacerbation (acute) G70.01
    in crisis G70.01
  ataxic (hereditary) G11.9
    general (syphilitic) A52.17
  atrophic G58.9
    infantile, acute — *see* Poliomyelitis, paralytic
    progressive G12.22
    spinal (acute) — *see* Poliomyelitis, paralytic
  axillary G54.0
  Babinski-Nageotte's G83.89
  Bell's G51.0
    newborn P11.3
  Benedikt's G46.3
  birth injury P14.9
    spinal cord P11.5
  bladder (neurogenic) (sphincter) N31.2
  bowel, colon or intestine K56.0
  brachial plexus G54.0
    birth injury P14.3
    newborn (birth injury) P14.3
  brain G83.9
    diplegia G83.0
    triplegia G83.89
  bronchial J98.09
  Brown-Séquard G83.81
  bulbar (chronic) (progressive) G12.22
    infantile — *see* Poliomyelitis, paralytic
    poliomyelitic — *see* Poliomyelitis, paralytic
    pseudo G12.29
  bulbospinal G70.00
    with exacerbation (acute) G70.01
    in crisis G70.01
  cardiac — *see also* Failure, heart I50.9
  cerebrocerebellar, diplegic G80.1
  cervical
    plexus G54.2
    sympathetic G90.09
  Céstan-Chenais G46.3
  Charcot-Marie-Tooth type G60.0
  Clark's G80.9
  colon K56.0
  compressed air T70.3 ☑
  compression
    arm G56.9- ☑
    leg G57.9- ☑
    lower extremity G57.9- ☑
    upper extremity G56.9- ☑
  congenital (cerebral) — *see* Palsy, cerebral

Paralysis, paralytic — *continued*
  conjugate movement (gaze) (of eye) H51.0
    cortical (nuclear) (supranuclear) H51.0
  cordis — *see* Failure, heart
  cranial or cerebral nerve G52.9
  creeping G12.22
  crossed leg G83.89
  crutch — *see* Injury, brachial plexus
  deglutition R13.0
    hysterical F44.4
  dementia A52.17
  descending (spinal) NEC G12.29
  diaphragm (flaccid) J98.6
    due to accidental dissection of phrenic nerve during procedure — *see* Puncture, accidental complicating surgery
  digestive organs NEC K59.8
  diplegic — *see* Diplegia
  divergence (nuclear) H51.8
  diver's T70.3 ☑
  Duchenne's
    birth injury P14.0
    due to or associated with
      motor neuron disease G12.22
      muscular dystrophy G71.01
  due to intracranial or spinal birth injury — *see* Palsy, cerebral
  embolic (current episode) I63.4- ☑
  Erb (-Duchenne) (birth) (newborn) P14.0
  Erb's syphilitic spastic spinal A52.17
  esophagus K22.8
  eye muscle (extrinsic) H49.9
    intrinsic — *see also* Paresis, of accommodation
  facial (nerve) G51.0
    birth injury P11.3
    congenital P11.3
    following operation NEC — *see* Puncture, accidental complicating surgery
    newborn (birth injury) P11.3
  familial (recurrent) (periodic) G72.3
    spastic G11.4
  fauces J39.2
  finger G56.9- ☑
  gait R26.1
  gastric nerve (nondiabetic) G52.2
  gaze, conjugate H51.0
  general (progressive) (syphilitic) A52.17
    juvenile A50.45
  glottis J38.00
    bilateral J38.02
    unilateral J38.01
  gluteal G54.1
  Gubler (-Millard) G46.3
  hand — *see* Monoplegia, upper limb
  heart — *see* Arrest, cardiac
  hemiplegic — *see* Hemiplegia
  hyperkalemic periodic (familial) G72.3
  hypoglossal (nerve) G52.3
  hypokalemic periodic G72.3
  hysterical F44.4
  ileus K56.0
  infantile — *see also* Poliomyelitis, paralytic A80.30
    bulbar — *see* Poliomyelitis, paralytic
    cerebral — *see* Palsy, cerebral
    spastic — *see* Palsy, cerebral, spastic
  infective — *see* Poliomyelitis, paralytic
  inferior nuclear G83.9
  internuclear — *see* Ophthalmoplegia, internuclear
  intestine K56.0
  iris H57.09
    due to diphtheria (toxin) A36.89
  ischemic, Volkmann's (complicating trauma) T79.6 ☑
  Jackson's G83.89
  jake — *see* Poisoning, food, noxious, plant
  Jamaica ginger (jake) G62.2
  juvenile general A50.45
  Klumpke (-Déjérine) (birth) (newborn) P14.1
  labioglossal (laryngeal) (pharyngeal) G12.29
  Landry's G61.0
  laryngeal nerve (recurrent) (superior) (unilateral) J38.00
    bilateral J38.02
    unilateral J38.01
  larynx J38.00
    bilateral J38.02
    due to diphtheria (toxin) A36.2
    unilateral J38.01
  lateral G12.23
  lead T56.0 ☑

Paralysis, paralytic — *continued*
  left side — *see* Hemiplegia
  leg G83.1- ☑
    both — *see* Paraplegia
    crossed G83.89
    hysterical F44.4
    psychogenic F44.4
    transient or transitory R29.818
    traumatic NEC — *see* Injury, nerve, leg
  levator palpebrae superioris — *see* Blepharoptosis, paralytic
  limb — *see* Monoplegia
  lip K13.0
  Lissauer's A52.17
  lower limb — *see* Monoplegia, lower limb
    both — *see* Paraplegia
  lung J98.4
  median nerve G56.1- ☑
  medullary (tegmental) G83.89
  mesencephalic NEC G83.89
    tegmental G83.89
  middle alternating G83.89
  Millard-Gubler-Foville G46.3
  monoplegic — *see* Monoplegia
  motor G83.9
  muscle, muscular NEC G72.89
    due to nerve lesion G58.9
    eye (extrinsic) H49.9
      intrinsic — *see* Paresis, of accommodation
      oblique — *see* Strabismus, paralytic, fourth nerve
    iris sphincter H21.9
    ischemic (Volkmann's) (complicating trauma) T79.6 ☑
    progressive G12.21
    progressive, spinal G12.25
    pseudohypertrophic G71.02
    spinal progressive G12.25
  musculocutaneous nerve G56.9- ☑
  musculospiral G56.9- ☑
  nerve — *see also* Disorder, nerve
    abducent — *see* Strabismus, paralytic, sixth nerve
    accessory G52.8
    auditory (except Deafness) H93.3 ☑
    birth injury P14.9
    cranial or cerebral G52.9
    facial G51.0
      birth injury P11.3
      congenital P11.3
      newborn (birth injury) P11.3
    fourth or trochlear — *see* Strabismus, paralytic, fourth nerve
    newborn (birth injury) P14.9
    oculomotor — *see* Strabismus, paralytic, third nerve
    phrenic (birth injury) P14.2
    radial G56.3- ☑
    seventh or facial G51.0
      newborn (birth injury) P11.3
    sixth or abducent — *see* Strabismus, paralytic, sixth nerve
    syphilitic A52.15
    third or oculomotor — *see* Strabismus, paralytic, third nerve
    trigeminal G50.9
    trochlear — *see* Strabismus, paralytic, fourth nerve
    ulnar G56.2- ☑
  normokalemic periodic G72.3
  ocular H49.9
    alternating G83.89
  oculofacial, congenital (Moebius) Q87.0
  oculomotor (external bilateral) (nerve) — *see* Strabismus, paralytic, third nerve
  palate (soft) K13.79
  paratrigeminal G50.9
  periodic (familial) (hyperkalemic) (hypokalemic) (myotonic) (normokalemic) (potassium sensitive) (secondary) G72.3
  peripheral autonomic nervous system — *see* Neuropathy, peripheral, autonomic
  peroneal (nerve) G57.3- ☑
  pharynx J39.2
  phrenic nerve G56.8- ☑
  plantar nerve(s) G57.6- ☑
  pneumogastric nerve G52.2
  poliomyelitis (current) — *see* Poliomyelitis, paralytic
  popliteal nerve G57.3- ☑
  postepileptic transitory G83.84
  progressive (atrophic) (bulbar) (spinal) G12.22
    general A52.17

Paralysis, paralytic — *continued*
  progressive — *continued*
    infantile acute — *see* Poliomyelitis, paralytic
      supranuclear G23.1
  pseudobulbar G12.29
  pseudohypertrophic (muscle) G71.09
  psychogenic F44.4
  quadriceps G57.9-
  quadriplegic — *see* Tetraplegia
  radial nerve G56.3-
  rectus muscle (eye) H49.9
  recurrent isolated sleep G47.53
  respiratory (muscle) (system) (tract) R06.81
    center NEC G93.89
    congenital P28.89
    newborn P28.89
  right side — *see* Hemiplegia
  saturnine T56.0
  sciatic nerve G57.0-
  senile G83.9
  shaking — *see* Parkinsonism
  shoulder G56.9-
  sleep, recurrent isolated G47.53
  spastic G83.9
    cerebral — *see* Palsy, cerebral, spastic
    congenital (cerebral) — *see* Palsy, cerebral, spastic
    familial G11.4
    hereditary G11.4
    quadriplegic G80.0
    syphilitic (spinal) A52.17
  sphincter, bladder — *see* Paralysis, bladder
  spinal (cord) G83.9
    accessory nerve G52.8
    acute — *see* Poliomyelitis, paralytic
    ascending acute G61.0
    atrophic (acute) — *see also* Poliomyelitis, paralytic
      spastic, syphilitic A52.17
    congenital NEC — *see* Palsy, cerebral
    hereditary G95.89
    infantile — *see* Poliomyelitis, paralytic
    progressive G12.21
      muscle G12.25
    sequelae NEC G83.89
  sternomastoid G52.8
  stomach K31.84
    diabetic — *see* Diabetes, by type, with gastroparesis
    nerve G52.2
      diabetic — *see* Diabetes, by type, with gastro-
        paresis
  stroke — *see* Infarct, brain
  subcapsularis G56.8-
  supranuclear (progressive) G23.1
  sympathetic G90.8
    cervical G90.09
    nervous system — *see* Neuropathy, peripheral, au-
      tonomic
  syndrome G83.9
    specified NEC G83.89
  syphilitic spastic spinal (Erb's) A52.17
  thigh G57.9-
  throat J39.2
    diphtheritic A36.0
    muscle J39.2
  thrombotic (current episode) I63.3-
  thumb G56.9-
  tick — *see* Toxicity, venom, arthropod, specified NEC
  Todd's (postepileptic transitory paralysis) G83.84
  toe G57.6-
  tongue K14.8
  transient R29.5
    arm or leg NEC R29.818
    traumatic NEC — *see* Injury, nerve
  trapezius G52.8
  traumatic, transient NEC — *see* Injury, nerve
  trembling — *see* Parkinsonism
  triceps brachii G56.9-
  trigeminal nerve G50.9
  trochlear (nerve) — *see* Strabismus, paralytic, fourth
    nerve
  ulnar nerve G56.2-
  upper limb — *see* Monoplegia, upper limb
  uremic N18.9 *[G99.8]*
  uveoparotitic D86.89
  uvula K13.79
    postdiphtheritic A36.0
  vagus nerve G52.2
  vasomotor NEC G90.8
  velum palati K13.79

Paralysis, paralytic — *continued*
  vesical — *see* Paralysis, bladder
  vestibular nerve (except Vertigo) H93.3
  vocal cords J38.00
    bilateral J38.02
    unilateral J38.01
  Volkmann's (complicating trauma) T79.6
  wasting G12.29
  Weber's G46.3
  wrist G56.9-
Paramedial urethrovesical orifice Q64.79
Paramenia N92.6
Parametritis — *see also* Disease, pelvis, inflammatory
    N73.2
  acute N73.0
  complicating abortion — *see* Abortion, by type, com-
    plicated by, parametritis
Parametrium, parametric — *see* condition
Paramnesia — *see* Amnesia
Paramolar K00.1
Paramyloidosis E85.89
Paramyoclonus multiplex G25.3
Paramyotonia (congenita) G71.19
Parangi — *see* Yaws
Paranoia (querulans) F22
  senile F03
Paranoid
  dementia (senile) F03
    praecox — *see* Schizophrenia
  personality F60.0
  psychosis (climacteric) (involutional) (menopausal) F22
    psychogenic (acute) F23
    senile F03
  reaction (acute) F23
    chronic F22
  schizophrenia F20.0
  state (climacteric) (involutional) (menopausal) (simple)
    F22
    senile F03
  tendencies F60.0
  traits F60.0
  trends F60.0
  type, psychopathic personality F60.0
Paraparesis — *see* Paraplegia
Paraphasia R47.02
Paraphilia F65.9
Paraphimosis (congenital) N47.2
  chancroidal A57
Paraphrenia, paraphrenic (late) F22
  schizophrenia F20.0
Paraplegia (lower) G82.20
  ataxic — *see* Degeneration, combined, spinal cord
  complete G82.21
  congenital (cerebral) G80.8
    spastic G80.1
  familial spastic G11.4
  functional (hysterical) F44.4
  hereditary, spastic G11.4
  hysterical F44.4
  incomplete G82.22
  Pott's A18.01
  psychogenic F44.4
  spastic
    Erb's spinal, syphilitic A52.17
    hereditary G11.4
    tropical G04.1
  syphilitic (spastic) A52.17
  traumatic
    current injury — code to injury with seventh char-
      acter A
    sequela of previous injury — code to injury with
      seventh character S
  tropical spastic G04.1
Parapoxvirus B08.60
  specified NEC B08.69
Paraproteinemia D89.2
  benign (familial) D89.2
  monoclonal D47.2
  secondary to malignant disease D47.2
Parapsoriasis L41.9
  en plaques L41.4
  guttata L41.1
  large plaque L41.4
  retiform, retiformis L41.5
  small plaque L41.3
  specified NEC L41.8
  varioliformis (acuta) L41.0
Parasitic — *see also* condition

Parasitic — *continued*
  disease NEC B89
  stomatitis B37.0
  sycosis (beard) (scalp) B35.0
  twin Q89.4
Parasitism B89
  intestinal B82.9
  skin B88.9
  specified — *see* Infestation
Parasitophobia F40.218
Parasomnia G47.50
  due to
    alcohol
      abuse F10.182
      dependence F10.282
      use F10.982
    amphetamines
      abuse F15.182
      dependence F15.282
      use F15.982
    caffeine
      abuse F15.182
      dependence F15.282
      use F15.982
    cocaine
      abuse F14.182
      dependence F14.282
      use F14.982
    drug NEC
      abuse F19.182
      dependence F19.282
      use F19.982
    opioid
      abuse F11.182
      dependence F11.282
      use F11.982
    psychoactive substance NEC
      abuse F19.182
      dependence F19.282
      use F19.982
    sedative, hypnotic, or anxiolytic
      abuse F13.182
      dependence F13.282
      use F13.982
    stimulant NEC
      abuse F15.182
      dependence F15.282
      use F15.982
  in conditions classified elsewhere G47.54
  nonorganic origin F51.8
  organic G47.50
  specified NEC G47.59
Paraspadias Q54.9
Paraspasmus facialis G51.8
Parasuicide (attempt)
  history of (personal) Z91.5
    in family Z81.8
Parathyroid gland — *see* condition
Parathyroid tetany E20.9
Paratrachoma A74.0
Paratyphilitis — *see* Appendicitis
Paratyphoid (fever) — *see* Fever, paratyphoid
Paratyphus — *see* Fever, paratyphoid
Paraurethral duct Q64.79
Paraurethritis — *see also* Urethritis
  gonococcal (acute) (with abscess) A54.1
Paravaccinia NEC B08.04
Paravaginitis — *see* Vaginitis
Parencephalitis — *see also* Encephalitis
  sequelae G09
Parent-child conflict — *see* Conflict, parent-child
  estrangement NEC Z62.890
Paresis — *see also* Paralysis
  accommodation — *see* Paresis, of accommodation
  Bernhardt's G57.1-
  bladder (sphincter) — *see also* Paralysis, bladder
    tabetic A52.17
  bowel, colon or intestine K56.0
  extrinsic muscle, eye H49.9
  general (progressive) (syphilitic) A52.17
    juvenile A50.45
  heart — *see* Failure, heart
  insane (syphilitic) A52.17
  juvenile (general) A50.45
  of accommodation H52.52-
  peripheral progressive (idiopathic) G60.3
  pseudohypertrophic G71.09
  senile G83.9

☑ **Additional Character Required** — Refer to the Tabular List for Character Selection   ▽ Subterms under main terms may continue to next column or page

aresis — *continued*
  syphilitic (general) A52.17
    congenital A50.45
  vesical NEC N31.2
aresthesia — *see also* Disturbance, sensation, skin R20.2
  Bernhardt G57.1- ☑
aretic — *see* condition
arinaud's
  conjunctivitis H10.89
  oculoglandular syndrome H10.89
  ophthalmoplegia H49.88- ☑
arkinsonism (idiopathic) (primary) G20
  with neurogenic orthostatic hypotension (symptomatic) G90.3
  arteriosclerotic G21.4
  dementia G31.83 *[F02.80]*
    with behavioral disturbance G31.83 *[F02.81]*
  due to
    drugs NEC G21.19
      neuroleptic G21.11
  medication-induced NEC G21.19
  neuroleptic induced G21.11
  postencephalitic G21.3
  secondary G21.9
    due to
      arteriosclerosis G21.4
      drugs NEC G21.19
        neuroleptic G21.11
      encephalitis G21.3
      external agents NEC G21.2
      syphilis A52.19
    specified NEC G21.8
  syphilitic A52.19
  treatment-induced NEC G21.19
  vascular G21.4
arkinson's disease, syndrome or tremor — *see*
  Parkinsonism
arodontitis — *see* Periodontitis
arodontosis K05.4
aronychia — *see also* Cellulitis, digit
  with lymphangitis — *see* Lymphangitis, acute, digit
  candidal (chronic) B37.2
  tuberculous (primary) A18.4
arorexia (psychogenic) F50.89
arosmia R43.1
  psychogenic F45.8
arotid gland — *see* condition
arotitis, parotiditis (allergic)(nonspecific toxic) (purulent) (septic) (suppurative) — *see also* Sialoadenitis
  epidemic — *see* Mumps
  infectious — *see* Mumps
  postoperative K91.89
  surgical K91.89
arrot fever A70
arrot's disease (early congenital syphilitic pseudoparalysis) A50.02
arry-Romberg syndrome G51.8
arry's disease or syndrome E05.00
  with thyroid storm E05.01
ars planitis — *see* Cyclitis
arsonage (-Aldren)-**Turner syndrome** G54.5
arson's disease (exophthalmic goiter) E05.00
  with thyroid storm E05.01
articolored infant Q82.8
arturition — *see* Delivery
arulis K04.7
  with sinus K04.6
arvovirus, as cause of disease classified elsewhere B97.6
asini and Pierini's atrophoderma L90.3
assage
  false, urethra N36.5
  meconium (newborn) during delivery P03.82
  of sounds or bougies — *see* Attention to, artificial, opening
assive — *see* condition
  smoking Z77.22
asteurella septica A28.0
asteurellosis — *see* Infection, Pasteurella
AT (paroxysmal atrial tachycardia) I47.1
atau's syndrome — *see* Trisomy, 13
atches
  mucous (syphilitic) A51.39
    congenital A50.07
  smokers' (mouth) K13.24
atellar — *see* condition
atent — *see also* Imperfect, closure

Patent — *continued*
  canal of Nuck Q52.4
  cervix N88.3
  ductus arteriosus or Botallo's Q25.0
  foramen
    botalli Q21.1
    ovale Q21.1
  interauricular septum Q21.1
  interventricular septum Q21.0
  omphalomesenteric duct Q43.0
  os (uteri) — *see* Patent, cervix
  ostium secundum Q21.1
  urachus Q64.4
  vitelline duct Q43.0
Paterson (-Brown)(-Kelly) **syndrome or web** D50.1
Pathologic, pathological — *see also* condition
  asphyxia R09.01
  fire-setting F63.1
  gambling F63.0
  ovum O02.0
  resorption, tooth K03.3
  stealing F63.2
Pathology (of) — *see* Disease
  periradicular, associated with previous endodontic treatment M27.59
Pattern, sleep-wake, irregular G47.23
Patulous — *see also* Imperfect, closure (congenital)
  alimentary tract Q45.8
    lower Q43.8
    upper Q40.8
  eustachian tube H69.0- ☑
Pause, sinoatrial I49.5
Paxton's disease B36.2
Pearl(s)
  enamel K00.2
  Epstein's K09.8
Pearl-worker's disease — *see* Osteomyelitis, specified type NEC
Pectenosis K62.4
Pectoral — *see* condition
Pectus
  carinatum (congenital) Q67.7
    acquired M95.4
    rachitic sequelae (late effect) E64.3
  excavatum (congenital) Q67.6
    acquired M95.4
    rachitic sequelae (late effect) E64.3
  recurvatum (congenital) Q67.6
Pedatrophia E41
Pederosis F65.4
Pediculosis (infestation) B85.2
  capitis (head-louse) (any site) B85.0
  corporis (body-louse) (any site) B85.1
  eyelid B85.0
  mixed (classifiable to more than one of the titles B85.0-B85.3) B85.4
  pubis (pubic louse) (any site) B85.3
  vestimenti B85.1
  vulvae B85.3
Pediculus (infestation) — *see* Pediculosis
Pedophilia F65.4
Peg-shaped teeth K00.2
Pelade — *see* Alopecia, areata
Pelger-Huët anomaly or syndrome D72.0
Peliosis (rheumatica) D69.0
  hepatis K76.4
    with toxic liver disease K71.8
Pelizaeus-Merzbacher disease E75.29
Pellagra (alcoholic) (with polyneuropathy) E52
Pellagra-cerebellar-ataxia-renal aminoaciduria syndrome E72.02
Pellegrini (-Stieda) **disease or syndrome** — *see* Bursitis, tibial collateral
Pellizzi's syndrome E34.8
Pel's crisis A52.11
Pelvic — *see also* condition
  examination (periodic) (routine) Z01.419
    with abnormal findings Z01.411
  kidney, congenital Q63.2
Pelviolithiasis — *see* Calculus, kidney
Pelviperitonitis — *see also* Peritonitis, pelvic
  gonococcal A54.24
  puerperal O85
Pelvis — *see* condition or type
Pemphigoid L12.9
  benign, mucous membrane L12.1
  bullous L12.0
  cicatricial L12.1

Pemphigoid — *continued*
  juvenile L12.2
  ocular L12.1
  specified NEC L12.8
Pemphigus L10.9
  benign familial (chronic) Q82.8
  Brazilian L10.3
  circinatus L13.0
  conjunctiva L12.1
  drug-induced L10.5
  erythematosus L10.4
  foliaceous L10.2
  gangrenous — *see* Gangrene
  neonatorum L01.03
  ocular L12.1
  paraneoplastic L10.81
  specified NEC L10.89
  syphilitic (congenital) A50.06
  vegetans L10.1
  vulgaris L10.0
  wildfire L10.3
Pendred's syndrome E07.1
Pendulous
  abdomen, in pregnancy — *see* Pregnancy, complicated by, abnormal, pelvic organs or tissues NEC
  breast N64.89
Penetrating wound — *see also* Puncture
  with internal injury — *see* Injury, by site
  eyeball — *see* Puncture, eyeball
  orbit (with or without foreign body) — *see* Puncture, orbit
  uterus by instrument with or following ectopic or molar pregnancy O08.6
Penicillosis B48.4
Penis — *see* condition
Penitis N48.29
Pentalogy of Fallot Q21.8
Pentasomy X syndrome Q97.1
Pentosuria (essential) E74.8
Percreta placenta - O43.23 ☑
Peregrinating patient — *see* Disorder, factitious
Perforation, perforated (nontraumatic) (of)
  accidental during procedure (blood vessel) (nerve) (organ) — *see* Complication, accidental puncture or laceration
  antrum — *see* Sinusitis, maxillary
  appendix K35.32
    with localized peritonitis K35.32
  atrial septum, multiple Q21.1
  attic, ear — *see* Perforation, tympanum, attic
  bile duct (common) (hepatic) K83.2
    cystic K82.2
  bladder (urinary)
    with or following ectopic or molar pregnancy O08.6
    obstetrical trauma O71.5
      traumatic S37.29 ☑
        at delivery O71.5
  bowel K63.1
    with or following ectopic or molar pregnancy O08.6
    newborn P78.0
    obstetrical trauma O71.5
    traumatic — *see* Laceration, intestine
  broad ligament N83.8
    with or following ectopic or molar pregnancy O08.6
    obstetrical trauma O71.6
  by
    device, implant or graft — *see also* Complications, by site and type, mechanical T85.628 ☑
      arterial graft NEC — *see* Complication, cardiovascular device, mechanical, vascular
      breast (implant) T85.49 ☑
      catheter NEC T85.698 ☑
        cystostomy T83.090 ☑
        dialysis (renal) T82.49 ☑
          intraperitoneal T85.691 ☑
        infusion NEC T82.594 ☑
          spinal (epidural) (subdural) T85.690 ☑
        urinary — *see also* Complications, catheter, urinary T83.098 ☑
      electronic (electrode) (pulse generator) (stimulator)
        bone T84.390 ☑
        cardiac T82.199 ☑
          electrode T82.190 ☑
          pulse generator T82.191 ☑
          specified type NEC T82.198 ☑

Perforation, perforated — *continued*

Perforation, perforated — *continued*
  by — *continued*
    device, implant or graft — *see also* Complications,
      by site and type, mechanical — *continued*
      electronic — *continued*
        nervous system — *see* Complication, prosthet-
          ic device, mechanical, electronic ner-
          vous system stimulator
        urinary — *see* Complication, genitourinary,
          device, urinary, mechanical
      fixation, internal (orthopedic) NEC — *see* Compli-
        cation, fixation device, mechanical
      gastrointestinal — *see* Complications, prosthetic
        device, mechanical, gastrointestinal device
      genital NEC T83.498 ☑
        intrauterine contraceptive device T83.39 ☑
        penile prosthesis T83.490 ☑
      heart NEC — *see* Complication, cardiovascular
        device, mechanical
      joint prosthesis — *see* Complications, joint
        prosthesis, mechanical, specified NEC, by
        site
      ocular NEC — *see* Complications, prosthetic de-
        vice, mechanical, ocular device
      orthopedic NEC — *see* Complication, orthopedic,
        device, mechanical
      specified NEC T85.628 ☑
      urinary NEC — *see also* Complication, genitouri-
        nary, device, urinary, mechanical
        graft T83.29 ☑
      vascular NEC — *see* Complication, cardiovascular
        device, mechanical
      ventricular intracranial shunt T85.09 ☑
    foreign body left accidentally in operative wound
      T81.539 ☑
    instrument (any) during a procedure, accidental —
      see Puncture, accidental complicating surgery
  cecum K35.32
    with localized peritonitis K35.32
  cervix (uteri) N88.8
    with or following ectopic or molar pregnancy O08.6
    obstetrical trauma O71.3
  colon K63.1
    newborn P78.0
    obstetrical trauma O71.5
    traumatic — *see* Laceration, intestine, large
  common duct (bile) K83.2
  cornea (due to ulceration) — *see* Ulcer, cornea, perfo-
    rated
  cystic duct K82.2
  diverticulum (intestine) K57.80
    with bleeding K57.81
    large intestine K57.20
      with
        bleeding K57.21
        small intestine K57.40
          with bleeding K57.41
      small intestine K57.00
        with
          bleeding K57.01
          large intestine K57.40
            with bleeding K57.41
  ear drum — *see* Perforation, tympanum
  esophagus K22.3
  ethmoidal sinus — *see* Sinusitis, ethmoidal
  frontal sinus — *see* Sinusitis, frontal
  gallbladder K82.2
  heart valve — *see* Endocarditis
  ileum K63.1
    newborn P78.0
    obstetrical trauma O71.5
    traumatic — *see* Laceration, intestine, small
  instrumental, surgical (accidental) (blood vessel) (nerve)
    (organ) — *see* Puncture, accidental complicating
    surgery
  intestine NEC K63.1
    with ectopic or molar pregnancy O08.6
    newborn P78.0
    obstetrical trauma O71.5
    traumatic — *see* Laceration, intestine
    ulcerative NEC K63.1
      newborn P78.0
  jejunum, jejunal K63.1
    obstetrical trauma O71.5
    traumatic — *see* Laceration, intestine, small
    ulcer — *see* Ulcer, gastrojejunal, with perforation
  joint prosthesis — *see* Complications, joint prosthesis,
    mechanical, specified NEC, by site

Perforation, perforated — *continued*
  mastoid (antrum) (cell) — *see* Disorder, mastoid,
    specified NEC
  maxillary sinus — *see* Sinusitis, maxillary
  membrana tympani — *see* Perforation, tympanum
  nasal
    septum J34.89
      congenital Q30.3
      syphilitic A52.73
    sinus J34.89
      congenital Q30.8
      due to sinusitis — *see* Sinusitis
  palate — *see also* Cleft, palate Q35.9
    syphilitic A52.79
  palatine vault — *see also* Cleft, palate, hard Q35.1
    syphilitic A52.79
    congenital A50.59
  pars flaccida (ear drum) — *see* Perforation, tympanum,
    attic
  pelvic
    floor S31.030 ☑
      with
        ectopic or molar pregnancy O08.6
        penetration into retroperitoneal space
          S31.031 ☑
        retained foreign body S31.040 ☑
          with penetration into retroperitoneal
            space S31.041 ☑
      following ectopic or molar pregnancy O08.6
      obstetrical trauma O70.1
    organ S37.99 ☑
      adrenal gland S37.818 ☑
      bladder — *see* Perforation, bladder
      fallopian tube S37.599 ☑
        bilateral S37.592 ☑
        unilateral S37.591 ☑
      kidney S37.09- ☑
      obstetrical trauma O71.5
      ovary S37.499 ☑
        bilateral S37.492 ☑
        unilateral S37.491 ☑
      prostate S37.828 ☑
      specified organ NEC S37.898 ☑
      ureter — *see* Perforation, ureter
      urethra — *see* Perforation, urethra
      uterus — *see* Perforation, uterus
  perineum — *see* Laceration, perineum
  pharynx J39.2
  rectum K63.1
    newborn P78.0
    obstetrical trauma O71.5
    traumatic S36.63 ☑
  root canal space due to endodontic treatment M27.51
  sigmoid K63.1
    newborn P78.0
    obstetrical trauma O71.5
    traumatic S36.533 ☑
  sinus (accessory) (chronic) (nasal) J34.89
  sphenoidal sinus — *see* Sinusitis, sphenoidal
  surgical (accidental) (by instrument) (blood vessel)
    (nerve) (organ) — *see* Puncture, accidental
    complicating surgery
  traumatic
    external — *see* Puncture
    eye — *see* Puncture, eyeball
    internal organ — *see* Injury, by site
  tympanum, tympanic (membrane) (persistent post-
    traumatic) (postinflammatory) H72.9- ☑
    attic H72.1- ☑
      multiple — *see* Perforation, tympanum, multiple
      total — *see* Perforation, tympanum, total
    central H72.0- ☑
      multiple — *see* Perforation, tympanum, multiple
      total — *see* Perforation, tympanum, total
    marginal NEC — *see* subcategory H72.2 ☑
    multiple H72.81- ☑
    pars flaccida — *see* Perforation, tympanum, attic
    total H72.82- ☑
    traumatic, current episode S09.2- ☑
  typhoid, gastrointestinal — *see* Typhoid
  ulcer — *see* Ulcer, by site, with perforation
  ureter N28.89
    traumatic S37.19 ☑
  urethra N36.8
    with ectopic or molar pregnancy O08.6
    following ectopic or molar pregnancy O08.6
    obstetrical trauma O71.5

Perforation, perforated — *continued*
  urethra — *continued*
    traumatic S37.39 ☑
    at delivery O71.5
  uterus
    with ectopic or molar pregnancy O08.6
    by intrauterine contraceptive device T83.39 ☑
    following ectopic or molar pregnancy O08.6
    obstetrical trauma O71.1
    traumatic S37.69 ☑
      obstetric O71.1
  uvula K13.79
    syphilitic A52.79
  vagina O71.4
    obstetrical trauma O71.4
    other trauma — *see* Puncture, vagina
Periadenitis mucosa necrotica recurrens K12.0
Periappendicitis (acute) — *see* Appendicitis
Periarteritis nodosa (disseminated) (infectious) (necrotizing) M30.0
Periarthritis (joint) — *see also* Enthesopathy
  Duplay's M75.0- ☑
  gonococcal A54.42
  humeroscapularis — *see* Capsulitis, adhesive
  scapulohumeral — *see* Capsulitis, adhesive
  shoulder — *see* Capsulitis, adhesive
  wrist M77.2- ☑
Periarthrosis (angioneural) — *see* Enthesopathy
Pericapsulitis, adhesive (shoulder) — *see* Capsulitis,
  adhesive
Pericarditis (with decompensation) (with effusion) I31.
  with rheumatic fever (conditions in I00)
    active — *see* Pericarditis, rheumatic
    inactive or quiescent I09.2
  acute (hemorrhagic) (nonrheumatic) (Sicca) I30.9
    with chorea (acute) (rheumatic) (Sydenham's) I02.
    benign I30.8
    nonspecific I30.0
    rheumatic I01.0
      with chorea (acute) (Sydenham's) I02.0
  adhesive or adherent (chronic) (external) (internal) I31.
    acute — *see* Pericarditis, acute
    rheumatic I09.2
  bacterial (acute) (subacute) (with serous or seropuru-
    lent effusion) I30.1
  calcareous I31.1
  cholesterol (chronic) I31.8
    acute I30.9
  chronic (nonrheumatic) I31.9
    rheumatic I09.2
  constrictive (chronic) I31.1
  coxsackie B33.23
  fibrinocaseous (tuberculous) A18.84
  fibrinopurulent I30.1
  fibrinous I30.8
  fibrous I31.0
  gonococcal A54.83
  idiopathic I30.0
  in systemic lupus erythematosus M32.12
  infective I30.1
  meningococcal A39.53
  neoplastic (chronic) I31.8
    acute I30.9
  obliterans, obliterating I31.0
  plastic I31.0
  pneumococcal I30.1
  postinfarction I24.1
  purulent I30.1
  rheumatic (active) (acute) (with effusion) (with pneu-
    monia) I01.0
    with chorea (acute) (rheumatic) (Sydenham's) I02.
    chronic or inactive (with chorea) I09.2
  rheumatoid — *see* Rheumatoid, carditis
  septic I30.1
  serofibrinous I30.8
  staphylococcal I30.1
  streptococcal I30.1
  suppurative I30.1
  syphilitic A52.06
  tuberculous A18.84
  uremic N18.9 [*I32*]
  viral I30.1
Pericardium, pericardial — *see* condition
Pericellulitis — *see* Cellulitis
Pericementitis (chronic) (suppurative) — *see also* Periodontitis
  acute K05.20

☑ **Additional Character Required** — Refer to the Tabular List for Character Selection   ▽ Subterms under main terms may continue to next column or page

ericementitis — *continued*
  acute — *continued*
    generalized — *see* Periodontitis, aggressive, generalized
    localized — *see* Periodontitis, aggressive, localized
erichondritis
  auricle — *see* Perichondritis, ear
  bronchus J98.09
  ear (external) H61.00- ☑
    acute H61.01- ☑
    chronic H61.02- ☑
  external auditory canal — *see* Perichondritis, ear
  larynx J38.7
    syphilitic A52.73
    typhoid A01.09
  nose J34.89
  pinna — *see* Perichondritis, ear
  trachea J39.8
ericlasia K05.4
ericoronitis — *see* Periodontitis
ericystitis N30.90
  with hematuria N30.91
eridiverticulitis (intestine) K57.92
  cecum — *see* Diverticulitis, intestine, large
  colon — *see* Diverticulitis, intestine, large
  duodenum — *see* Diverticulitis, intestine, small
  intestine — *see* Diverticulitis, intestine, large
  jejunum — *see* Diverticulitis, intestine, small
  rectosigmoid — *see* Diverticulitis, intestine, large
  rectum — *see* Diverticulitis, intestine, large
  sigmoid — *see* Diverticulitis, intestine, large
eriendocarditis — *see* Endocarditis
eriepididymitis N45.1
erifolliculitis L01.02
  abscedens, caput, scalp L66.3
  capitis, abscedens (et suffodiens) L66.3
  superficial pustular L01.02
erihepatitis K65.8
erilabyrinthitis (acute) — *see* subcategory H83.0 ☑
erimeningitis — *see* Meningitis
erimetritis — *see* Endometritis
erimetrosalpingitis — *see* Salpingo-oophoritis
erineocele N81.81
erinephric, perinephritic — *see* condition
erinephritis — *see also* Infection, kidney
  purulent — *see* Abscess, kidney
erineum, perineal — *see* condition
erineuritis NEC — *see* Neuralgia
eriodic — *see* condition
eriodontitis (chronic) (complex) (compound) (local) (simplex) K05.30
  acute K05.20
    generalized K05.229
      moderate K05.222
      severe K05.223
      slight K05.221
    localized K05.219
      moderate K05.212
      severe K05.213
      slight K05.211
  apical K04.5
    acute (pulpal origin) K04.4
  generalized K05.329
    moderate K05.322
    severe K05.323
    slight K05.321
  localized K05.319
    moderate K05.312
    severe K05.313
    slight K05.311
eriodontoclasia K05.4
eriodontosis (juvenile) K05.4
eriods — *see also* Menstruation
  heavy N92.0
  irregular N92.6
  shortened intervals (irregular) N92.1
erionychia — *see also* Cellulitis, digit
  with lymphangitis — *see* Lymphangitis, acute, digit
eriooophoritis — *see* Salpingo-oophoritis
eriorchitis N45.2
eriosteum, periosteal — *see* condition
eriostitis (albuminosa) (circumscribed) (diffuse) (infective) (monomelic) — *see also* Osteomyelitis
  alveolar M27.3
  alveolodental M27.3
  dental M27.3
  gonorrheal A54.43

Periostitis — *continued*
  jaw (lower) (upper) M27.2
  orbit H05.03- ☑
  syphilitic A52.77
    congenital (early) A50.02 [M90.80]
    secondary A51.46
  tuberculous — *see* Tuberculosis, bone
  yaws (hypertrophic) (early) (late) A66.6 [M90.80]
Periostosis (hyperplastic) — *see also* Disorder, bone, specified type NEC
  with osteomyelitis — *see* Osteomyelitis, specified type NEC
Peripartum
  cardiomyopathy O90.3
Periphlebitis — *see* Phlebitis
Periproctitis K62.89
Periprostatitis — *see* Prostatitis
Perirectal — *see* condition
Perirenal — *see* condition
Perisalpingitis — *see* Salpingo-oophoritis
Perisplenitis (infectional) D73.89
Peristalsis, visible or reversed R19.2
Peritendinitis — *see* Enthesopathy
Peritoneum, peritoneal — *see* condition
Peritonitis (adhesive) (bacterial) (fibrinous) (hemorrhagic) (idiopathic) (localized) (perforative) (primary) (with adhesions) (with effusion) K65.9
  with or following
    abscess K65.1
    appendicitis
      with perforation or rupture K35.32
      generalized — *see also* Appendicitis K35.20
      localized — *see also* Appendicitis K35.30
    diverticular disease (intestine) K57.80
      with bleeding K57.81
      ectopic or molar pregnancy O08.0
      large intestine K57.20
        with
          bleeding K57.21
          small intestine K57.40
            with bleeding K57.41
      small intestine K57.00
        with
          bleeding K57.01
          large intestine K57.40
            with bleeding K57.41
  acute (generalized) K65.0
  aseptic T81.61 ☑
  bile, biliary K65.3
  chemical T81.61 ☑
  chlamydial A74.81
  chronic proliferative K65.8
  complicating abortion — *see* Abortion, by type, complicated by, pelvic peritonitis
  congenital P78.1
  diaphragmatic K65.0
  diffuse K65.0
  diphtheritic A36.89
  disseminated K65.0
  due to
    bile K65.3
    foreign
      body or object accidentally left during a procedure (instrument) (sponge) (swab) T81.599 ☑
      substance accidentally left during a procedure (chemical) (powder) (talc) T81.61 ☑
    talc T81.61 ☑
    urine K65.8
  eosinophilic K65.8
    acute K65.0
  fibrocaseous (tuberculous) A18.31
  fibropurulent K65.0
  following ectopic or molar pregnancy O08.0
  general (ized) K65.0
  gonococcal A54.85
  meconium (newborn) P78.0
  neonatal P78.1
    meconium P78.0
  pancreatic K65.0
  paroxysmal, familial E85.0
    benign E85.0
  pelvic
    female N73.5
      acute N73.3
      chronic N73.4
        with adhesions N73.6
    male K65.0

Peritonitis — *continued*
  periodic, familial E85.0
  proliferative, chronic K65.8
  puerperal, postpartum, childbirth O85
  purulent K65.0
  septic K65.0
  specified NEC K65.8
  spontaneous bacterial K65.2
  subdiaphragmatic K65.0
  subphrenic K65.0
  suppurative K65.0
  syphilitic A52.74
    congenital (early) A50.08 [K67]
  talc T81.61 ☑
  tuberculous A18.31
  urine K65.8
Peritonsillar — *see* condition
Peritonsillitis J36
Perityphlitis K37
Periureteritis N28.89
Periurethral — *see* condition
Periurethritis (gangrenous) — *see* Urethritis
Periuterine — *see* condition
Perivaginitis — *see* Vaginitis
Perivasculitis, retinal H35.06- ☑
Perivasitis (chronic) N49.1
Perivesiculitis (seminal) — *see* Vesiculitis
Perlèche NEC K13.0
  due to
    candidiasis B37.83
    moniliasis B37.83
    riboflavin deficiency E53.0
    vitamin B2 (riboflavin) deficiency E53.0
Pernicious — *see* condition
Pernio, perniosis T69.1 ☑
Perpetrator (of abuse) — *see* Index to External Causes of Injury, Perpetrator
Persecution
  delusion F22
  social Z60.5
Perseveration (tonic) R48.8
Persistence, persistent (congenital)
  anal membrane Q42.3
    with fistula Q42.2
  arteria stapedia Q16.3
  atrioventricular canal Q21.2
  branchial cleft NOS Q18.2
    cyst Q18.0
    fistula Q18.0
    sinus Q18.0
  bulbus cordis in left ventricle Q21.8
  canal of Cloquet Q14.0
  capsule (opaque) Q12.8
  cilioretinal artery or vein Q14.8
  cloaca Q43.7
  communication — *see* Fistula, congenital
  convolutions
    aortic arch Q25.46
    fallopian tube Q50.6
    oviduct Q50.6
    uterine tube Q50.6
  double aortic arch Q25.45
  ductus arteriosus (Botalli) Q25.0
  fetal
    circulation P29.38
    form of cervix (uteri) Q51.828
    hemoglobin, hereditary (HPFH) D56.4
  foramen
    Botalli Q21.1
    ovale Q21.1
  Gartner's duct Q52.4
  hemoglobin, fetal (hereditary) (HPFH) D56.4
  hyaloid
    artery (generally Incomplete) Q14.0
    system Q14.8
  hymen, in pregnancy or childbirth — *see* Pregnancy, complicated by, abnormal, vulva
  lanugo Q84.2
  left
    posterior cardinal vein Q26.8
    root with right arch of aorta Q25.49
    superior vena cava Q26.1
  Meckel's diverticulum Q43.0
    malignant — *see* Table of Neoplasms, small intestine, malignant
  mucosal disease (middle ear) — *see* Otitis, media, suppurative, chronic, tubotympanic
  nail(s), anomalous Q84.6

▽ **Subterms under main terms may continue to next column or page**   ☑ **Additional Character Required — Refer to the Tabular List for Character Selection**   **251**

Pericementitis — Persistence, persistent

Persistence, persistent — *continued*
omphalomesenteric duct Q43.0
organ or site not listed — *see* Anomaly, by site
ostium
atrioventriculare commune Q21.2
primum Q21.2
secundum Q21.1
ovarian rests in fallopian tube Q50.6
pancreatic tissue in intestinal tract Q43.8
primary (deciduous)
teeth K00.6
vitreous hyperplasia Q14.0
pupillary membrane Q13.89
rhesus (Rh) titer — *see* Complication(s), transfusion, incompatibility reaction, Rh (factor)
right aortic arch Q25.47
sinus
urogenitalis
female Q52.8
male Q55.8
venosus with imperfect incorporation in right auricle Q26.8
thymus (gland) (hyperplasia) E32.0
thyroglossal duct Q89.2
thyrolingual duct Q89.2
truncus arteriosus or communis Q20.0
tunica vasculosa lentis Q12.2
umbilical sinus Q64.4
urachus Q64.4
vitelline duct Q43.0
Person (with)
admitted for clinical research, as a control subject (normal comparison) (participant) Z00.6
awaiting admission to adequate facility elsewhere Z75.1
concern (normal) about sick person in family Z63.6
consulting on behalf of another Z71.0
feigning illness Z76.5
living (in)
alone Z60.2
boarding school Z59.3
residential institution Z59.3
without
adequate housing (heating) (space) Z59.1
housing (permanent) (temporary) Z59.0
person able to render necessary care Z74.2
shelter Z59.0
on waiting list Z75.1
sick or handicapped in family Z63.6
Personality (disorder) F60.9
accentuation of traits (type A pattern) Z73.1
affective F34.0
aggressive F60.3
amoral F60.2
anacastic, anankastic F60.5
antisocial F60.2
anxious F60.6
asocial F60.2
asthenic F60.7
avoidant F60.6
borderline F60.3
change due to organic condition (enduring) F07.0
compulsive F60.5
cycloid F34.0
cyclothymic F34.0
dependent F60.7
depressive F34.1
dissocial F60.2
dual F44.81
eccentric F60.89
emotionally unstable F60.3
expansive paranoid F60.0
explosive F60.3
fanatic F60.0
haltose type F60.89
histrionic F60.4
hyperthymic F34.0
hypothymic F34.1
hysterical F60.4
immature F60.89
inadequate F60.7
labile (emotional) F60.3
mixed (nonspecific) F60.89
morally defective F60.2
multiple F44.81
narcissistic F60.81
obsessional F60.5
obsessive (-compulsive) F60.5
organic F07.0

Personality — *continued*
overconscientious F60.5
paranoid F60.0
passive (-dependent) F60.7
passive-aggressive F60.89
pathologic F60.9
pattern defect or disturbance F60.9
pseudopsychopathic (organic) F07.0
pseudoretarded (organic) F07.0
psychoinfantile F60.4
psychoneurotic NEC F60.89
psychopathic F60.2
querulant F60.0
sadistic F60.89
schizoid F60.1
self-defeating F60.89
sensitive paranoid F60.0
sociopathic (amoral) (antisocial) (asocial) (dissocial) F60.2
specified NEC F60.89
type A Z73.1
unstable (emotional) F60.3
Perthes' disease — *see* Legg-Calvé-Perthes disease
Pertussis — *see also* Whooping cough A37.90
Perversion, perverted
appetite F50.89
psychogenic F50.89
function
pituitary gland E23.2
posterior lobe E22.2
sense of smell and taste R43.8
psychogenic F45.8
sexual — *see* Deviation, sexual
Pervious, congenital — *see also* Imperfect, closure
ductus arteriosus Q25.0
Pes (congenital) — *see also* Talipes
acquired — *see also* Deformity, limb, foot, specified NEC
planus — *see* Deformity, limb, flat foot
adductus Q66.89
cavus Q66.7- ☑
deformity NEC, acquired — *see* Deformity, limb, foot, specified NEC
planus (acquired) (any degree) — *see also* Deformity, limb, flat foot
rachitic sequelae (late effect) E64.3
valgus Q66.6
Pest, pestis — *see* Plague
Petechia, petechiae R23.3
newborn P54.5
Petechial typhus A75.9
Peter's anomaly Q13.4
Petit mal seizure — *see* Epilepsy, childhood, absence
Petit's hernia — *see* Hernia, abdomen, specified site NEC
Petrellidosis B48.2
Petrositis H70.20- ☑
acute H70.21- ☑
chronic H70.22- ☑
Peutz-Jeghers disease or syndrome Q85.8
Peyronie's disease N48.6
PFAPA (periodic fever, aphthous stomatitis, pharyngitis, and adenopathy syndrome) M04.8
Pfeiffer's disease — *see* Mononucleosis, infectious
Phagedena (dry) (moist) (sloughing) — *see also* Gangrene
geometric L88
penis N48.29
tropical — *see* Ulcer, skin
vulva N76.6
Phagedenic — *see* condition
Phakoma H35.89
Phakomatosis — *see also* specific eponymous syndromes Q85.9
Bourneville's Q85.1
specified NEC Q85.8
Phantom limb syndrome (without pain) G54.7
with pain G54.6
Pharyngeal pouch syndrome D82.1
Pharyngitis (acute) (catarrhal) (gangrenous) (infective) (malignant) (membranous) (phlegmonous) (pseudomembranous) (simple) (subacute) (suppurative) (ulcerative) (viral) J02.9
with influenza, flu, or grippe — *see* Influenza, with, pharyngitis
aphthous B08.5
atrophic J31.2
chlamydial A56.4
chronic (atrophic) (granular) (hypertrophic) J31.2

Pharyngitis — *continued*
coxsackievirus B08.5
diphtheritic A36.0
enteroviral vesicular B08.5
follicular (chronic) J31.2
fusospirochetal A69.1
gonococcal A54.5
granular (chronic) J31.2
herpesviral B00.2
hypertrophic J31.2
infectional, chronic J31.2
influenzal — *see* Influenza, with, respiratory manifestations NEC
lymphonodular, acute (enteroviral) B08.8
pneumococcal J02.8
purulent J02.9
putrid J02.9
septic J02.0
sicca J31.2
specified organism NEC J02.8
staphylococcal J02.8
streptococcal J02.0
syphilitic, congenital (early) A50.03
tuberculous A15.8
vesicular, enteroviral B08.5
viral NEC J02.8
Pharyngoconjunctivitis, viral B30.2
Pharyngolaryngitis (acute) J06.0
chronic J37.0
Pharyngoplegia J39.2
Pharyngotonsillitis, herpesviral B00.2
Pharyngotracheitis, chronic J42
Pharynx, pharyngeal — *see* condition
Phencyclidine-induced
anxiety disorder F16.980
bipolar and related disorder F16.94
depressive disorder F16.94
psychotic disorder F16.959
Phenomenon
Arthus' — *see* Arthus' phenomenon
jaw-winking Q07.8
lupus erythematosus (LE) cell M32.9
Raynaud's (secondary) I73.00
with gangrene I73.01
vasomotor R55
vasospastic I73.9
vasovagal R55
Wenckebach's I44.1
Phenylketonuria E70.1
classical E70.0
maternal E70.1
Pheochromoblastoma
specified site — *see* Neoplasm, malignant, by site
unspecified site C74.10
Pheochromocytoma
malignant
specified site — *see* Neoplasm, malignant, by site
unspecified site C74.10
specified site — *see* Neoplasm, benign, by site
unspecified site D35.00
Pheohyphomycosis — *see* Chromomycosis
Pheomycosis — *see* Chromomycosis
Phimosis (congenital) (due to infection) N47.1
chancroidal A57
Phlebectasia — *see also* Varix
congenital Q27.4
Phlebitis (infective) (pyemic) (septic) (suppurative) I80.
antepartum — *see* Thrombophlebitis, antepartum
blue — *see* Phlebitis, leg, deep
breast, superficial I80.8
calf muscular vein (NOS) I80.25- ☑
cavernous (venous) sinus — *see* Phlebitis, intracranial (venous) sinus
cerebral (venous) sinus — *see* Phlebitis, intracranial (venous) sinus
chest wall, superficial I80.8
cranial (venous) sinus — *see* Phlebitis, intracranial (venous) sinus
deep (vessels) — *see* Phlebitis, leg, deep
due to implanted device — *see* Complications, by site and type, specified NEC
during or resulting from a procedure T81.72 ☑
femoral vein (superficial) I80.1- ☑
femoropopliteal vein I80.0- ☑
gastrocnemial vein I80.25- ☑
gestational — *see* Phlebopathy, gestational
hepatic veins I80.8
iliac vein (common) (external) (internal) I80.21- ☑

☑ **Additional Character Required** — Refer to the Tabular List for Character Selection   ▽ Subterms under main terms may continue to next column or page

Phlebitis — *continued*
iliofemoral — *see* Phlebitis, femoral vein
intracranial (venous) sinus (any) G08
  nonpyogenic I67.6
intraspinal venous sinuses and veins G08
  nonpyogenic G95.19
lateral (venous) sinus — *see* Phlebitis, intracranial (venous) sinus
leg I80.3
  antepartum — *see* Thrombophlebitis, antepartum
  deep (vessels) NEC I80.20- ☑
    iliac I80.21- ☑
    popliteal vein I80.22- ☑
    specified vessel NEC I80.29- ☑
    tibial vein (anterior) (posterior) I80.23- ☑
  femoral vein (superficial) I80.1- ☑
  superficial (vessels) I80.0- ☑
longitudinal sinus — *see* Phlebitis, intracranial (venous) sinus
lower limb — *see* Phlebitis, leg
migrans, migrating (superficial) I82.1
pelvic
  with ectopic or molar pregnancy O08.0
  following ectopic or molar pregnancy O08.0
  puerperal, postpartum O87.1
peroneal vein I80.24- ☑
popliteal vein — *see* Phlebitis, leg, deep, popliteal
portal (vein) K75.1
postoperative T81.72 ☑
pregnancy — *see* Thrombophlebitis, antepartum
puerperal, postpartum, childbirth O87.0
  deep O87.1
  pelvic O87.1
  superficial O87.0
retina — *see* Vasculitis, retina
saphenous (accessory) (great) (long) (small) — *see* Phlebitis, leg, superficial
sinus (meninges) — *see* Phlebitis, intracranial (venous) sinus
soleal vein I80.25- ☑
specified site NEC I80.8
syphilitic A52.09
tibial vein — *see* Phlebitis, leg, deep, tibial
ulcerative I80.9
  leg — *see* Phlebitis, leg
umbilicus I80.8
uterus (septic) — *see* Endometritis
varicose (leg) (lower limb) — *see* Varix, leg, with, inflammation
Phlebofibrosis I87.8
Phleboliths I87.8
Phlebopathy,
  gestational O22.9- ☑
  puerperal O87.9
Phlebosclerosis I87.8
Phlebothrombosis — *see also* Thrombosis
antepartum — *see* Thrombophlebitis, antepartum
pregnancy — *see* Thrombophlebitis, antepartum
puerperal — *see* Thrombophlebitis, puerperal
Phlebotomus fever A93.1
Phlegmasia
  alba dolens O87.1
    nonpuerperal — *see* Phlebitis, femoral vein
  cerulea dolens — *see* Phlebitis, leg, deep
Phlegmon — *see* Abscess
Phlegmonous — *see* condition
Phlyctenulosis (allergic) (keratoconjunctivitis) (nontuberculous) — *see also* Keratoconjunctivitis
  cornea — *see* Keratoconjunctivitis
  tuberculous A18.52
Phobia, phobic F40.9
animal F40.218
  spiders F40.210
examination F40.298
reaction F40.9
simple F40.298
social F40.10
  generalized F40.11
specific (isolated) F40.298
  animal F40.218
    spiders F40.210
  blood F40.230
  injection F40.231
  injury F40.233
  men F40.290
  natural environment F40.228
    thunderstorms F40.220

Phobia, phobic — *continued*
specific — *continued*
  situational F40.248
    bridges F40.242
    closed in spaces F40.240
    flying F40.243
    heights F40.241
  specified focus NEC F40.298
  transfusion F40.231
  women F40.291
specified NEC F40.8
  medical care NEC F40.232
state F40.9
Phocas' disease — *see* Mastopathy, cystic
Phocomelia Q73.1
lower limb — *see* Agenesis, leg, with foot present
upper limb — *see* Agenesis, arm, with hand present
Phoria H50.50
Phosphate-losing tubular disorder N25.0
Phosphatemia E83.39
Phosphaturia E83.39
Photodermatitis (sun) L56.8
chronic L57.8
due to drug L56.8
light other than sun L59.8
Photokeratitis H16.13- ☑
Photophobia H53.14- ☑
Photophthalmia — *see* Photokeratitis
Photopsia H53.19
Photoretinitis — *see* Retinopathy, solar
Photosensitivity, photosensitization (sun) skin L56.8
light other than sun L59.8
Phrenitis — *see* Encephalitis
Phrynoderma (vitamin A deficiency) E50.8
Phthiriasis (pubis) B85.3
with any infestation classifiable to B85.0-B85.2 B85.4
Phthirus infestation — *see* Phthiriasis
Phthisis — *see also* Tuberculosis
bulbi (infectional) — *see* Disorder, globe, degenerated condition, atrophy
eyeball (due to infection) — *see* Disorder, globe, degenerated condition, atrophy
Phycomycosis — *see* Zygomycosis
Physalopteriasis B81.8
Physical restraint status Z78.1
Phytobezoar T18.9 ☑
intestine T18.3 ☑
stomach T18.2 ☑
Pian — *see* Yaws
Pianoma A66.1
Pica F50.89
in adults F50.89
infant or child F98.3
Picking, nose F98.8
Pick-Niemann disease — *see* Niemann-Pick disease or syndrome
Pick's
cerebral atrophy G31.01 *[F02.80]*
  with behavioral disturbance G31.01 *[F02.81]*
disease or syndrome (brain) G31.01 *[F02.80]*
  with behavioral disturbance G31.01 *[F02.81]*
  brain G31.01 *[F02.80]*
    with behavioral disturbance G31.01 *[F02.81]*
  pericardium (pericardial pseudocirrhosis of liver) I31.1
syndrome
  brain G31.01 *[F02.80]*
    with behavioral disturbance G31.01 *[F02.81]*
  of heart (pericardial pseudocirrhosis of liver) I31.1
Pickwickian syndrome E66.2
Piebaldism E70.39
Piedra (beard) (scalp) B36.8
black B36.3
white B36.2
Pierre Robin deformity or syndrome Q87.0
Pierson's disease or osteochondrosis M91.0
Pig-bel A05.2
Pigeon
breast or chest (acquired) M95.4
  congenital Q67.7
    rachitic sequelae (late effect) E64.3
breeder's disease or lung J67.2
fancier's disease or lung J67.2
toe — *see* Deformity, toe, specified NEC
Pigmentation (abnormal) (anomaly) L81.9
conjunctiva H11.13- ☑
cornea (anterior) H18.01- ☑

Pigmentation — *continued*
cornea — *continued*
  posterior H18.05- ☑
  stromal H18.06- ☑
diminished melanin formation NEC L81.6
iron L81.8
lids, congenital Q82.8
limbus corneae — *see* Pigmentation, cornea
metals L81.8
optic papilla, congenital Q14.2
retina, congenital (grouped) (nevoid) Q14.1
scrotum, congenital Q82.8
tattoo L81.8
Piles — *see also* Hemorrhoids K64.9
Pili
annulati or torti (congenital) Q84.1
incarnati L73.1
Pill roller hand (intrinsic) — *see* Parkinsonism
Pilomatrixoma — *see* Neoplasm, skin, benign
malignant — *see* Neoplasm, skin, malignant
Pilonidal — *see* condition
Pimple R23.8
PIN — *see* Neoplasia, intraepithelial, prostate
Pinched nerve — *see* Neuropathy, entrapment
Pindborg tumor — *see* Cyst, calcifying odontogenic
Pineal body or gland — *see* condition
Pinealoblastoma C75.3
Pinealoma D44.5
malignant C75.3
Pineoblastoma C75.3
Pineocytoma D44.5
Pinguecula H11.15- ☑
Pingueculitis H10.81- ☑
Pinhole meatus — *see also* Stricture, urethra N35.919
Pink
disease — *see* subcategory T56.1 ☑
eye — *see* Conjunctivitis, acute, mucopurulent
Pinkus' disease (lichen nitidus) L44.1
Pinpoint
meatus — *see* Stricture, urethra
os (uteri) — *see* Stricture, cervix
Pins and needles R20.2
Pinta A67.9
cardiovascular lesions A67.2
chancre (primary) A67.0
erythematous plaques A67.1
hyperchromic lesions A67.1
hyperkeratosis A67.1
lesions A67.9
  cardiovascular A67.2
  hyperchromic A67.1
  intermediate A67.1
  late A67.2
  mixed A67.3
  primary A67.0
  skin (achromic) (cicatricial) (dyschromic) A67.2
    hyperchromic A67.1
    mixed (achromic and hyperchromic) A67.3
papule (primary) A67.0
skin lesions (achromic) (cicatricial) (dyschromic) A67.2
  hyperchromic A67.1
  mixed (achromic and hyperchromic) A67.3
vitiligo A67.2
Pintids A67.1
Pinworm (disease) (infection) (infestation) B80
Piroplasmosis B60.0
Pistol wound — *see* Gunshot wound
Pitchers' elbow — *see* Derangement, joint, specified type NEC, elbow
Pithecoid pelvis Q74.2
with disproportion (fetopelvic) O33.0
  causing obstructed labor O65.0
Pithiatism F48.8
Pitted — *see* Pitting
Pitting — *see also* Edema R60.9
lip R60.0
nail L60.8
teeth K00.4
Pituitary gland — *see* condition
Pituitary-snuff-taker's disease J67.8
Pityriasis (capitis) L21.0
alba L30.5
circinata (et maculata) L42
furfuracea L21.0
Hebra's L26
lichenoides L41.0
  chronica L41.1

Pneumonia — *continued*
- broncho-, bronchial — *continued*
  - streptococcal — *continued*
    - group B J15.3
    - pneumoniae J13
  - viral, virus — *see* Pneumonia, viral
- Butyrivibrio (fibriosolvens) J15.8
- Candida B37.1
- caseous — *see* Tuberculosis, pulmonary
- catarrhal — *see* Pneumonia, broncho
- chlamydial J16.0
  - congenital P23.1
- cholesterol J84.89
- cirrhotic (chronic) — *see* Fibrosis, lung
- Clostridium (haemolyticum) (novyi) J15.8
- confluent — *see* Pneumonia, broncho
- congenital (infective) P23.9
  - due to
    - bacterium NEC P23.6
    - Chlamydia P23.1
    - Escherichia coli P23.4
    - Haemophilus influenzae P23.6
    - infective organism NEC P23.8
    - Klebsiella pneumoniae P23.6
    - Mycoplasma P23.6
    - Pseudomonas P23.5
    - Staphylococcus P23.2
    - Streptococcus (except group B) P23.6
      - group B P23.3
    - viral agent P23.0
  - specified NEC P23.8
- croupous — *see* Pneumonia, lobar
- cryptogenic organizing J84.116
- cytomegalic inclusion B25.0
- cytomegaloviral B25.0
- deglutition — *see* Pneumonia, aspiration
- desquamative interstitial J84.117
- diffuse — *see* Pneumonia, broncho
- diplococcal, diplococcus (broncho-) (lobar) J13
- disseminated (focal) — *see* Pneumonia, broncho
- Eaton's agent J15.7
- embolic, embolism — *see* Embolism, pulmonary
- Enterobacter J15.6
- eosinophilic J82
- Escherichia coli (E. coli) J15.5
- Eubacterium J15.8
- fibrinous — *see* Pneumonia, lobar
- fibroid, fibrous (chronic) — *see* Fibrosis, lung
- Friedländer's bacillus J15.0
- Fusobacterium (nucleatum) J15.8
- gangrenous J85.0
- giant cell (measles) B05.2
- gonococcal A54.84
- gram-negative bacteria NEC J15.6
  - anaerobic J15.8
- Hemophilus influenzae (broncho) (lobar) J14
- human metapneumovirus J12.3
- hypostatic (broncho) (lobar) J18.2
- in (due to)
  - actinomycosis A42.0
  - adenovirus J12.0
  - anthrax A22.1
  - ascariasis B77.81
  - aspergillosis B44.9
  - Bacillus anthracis A22.1
  - Bacterium anitratum J15.6
  - candidiasis B37.1
  - chickenpox B01.2
  - Chlamydia J16.0
    - neonatal P23.1
  - coccidioidomycosis B38.2
    - acute B38.0
    - chronic B38.1
  - cytomegalovirus disease B25.0
  - Diplococcus (pneumoniae) J13
  - Eaton's agent J15.7
  - Enterobacter J15.6
  - Escherichia coli (E. coli) J15.5
  - Friedländer's bacillus J15.0
  - fumes and vapors (chemical) (inhalation) J68.0
  - gonorrhea A54.84
  - Hemophilus influenzae (H. influenzae) J14
  - Herellea J15.6
  - histoplasmosis B39.2
    - acute B39.0
    - chronic B39.1
  - human metapneumovirus J12.3
  - Klebsiella (pneumoniae) J15.0

Pneumonia — *continued*
- in — *continued*
  - measles B05.2
  - Mycoplasma (pneumoniae) J15.7
  - nocardiosis, nocardiasis A43.0
  - ornithosis A70
  - parainfluenza virus J12.2
  - pleuro-pneumonia-like-organism (PPLO) J15.7
  - pneumococcus J13
  - pneumocystosis (Pneumocystis carinii) (Pneumocystis jiroveci) B59
  - Proteus J15.6
  - Pseudomonas NEC J15.1
    - pseudomallei A24.1
  - psittacosis A70
  - Q fever A78
  - respiratory syncytial virus (RSV) J12.1
  - rheumatic fever I00 *[J17]*
  - rubella B06.81
  - Salmonella (infection) A02.22
    - typhi A01.03
  - schistosomiasis B65.9 *[J17]*
  - Serratia marcescens J15.6
  - specified
    - bacterium NEC J15.8
    - organism NEC J16.8
  - spirochetal NEC A69.8
  - Staphylococcus J15.20
    - aureus (methicillin susceptible) (MSSA) J15.211
      - methicillin resistant (MRSA) J15.212
    - specified NEC J15.29
  - Streptococcus J15.4
    - group B J15.3
    - pneumoniae J13
    - specified NEC J15.4
  - toxoplasmosis B58.3
  - tularemia A21.2
  - typhoid (fever) A01.03
  - varicella B01.2
  - virus — *see* Pneumonia, viral
  - whooping cough A37.91
    - due to
      - Bordetella parapertussis A37.11
      - Bordetella pertussis A37.01
      - specified NEC A37.81
  - Yersinia pestis A20.2
- inhalation of food or vomit — *see* Pneumonia, aspiration
- interstitial J84.9
  - chronic J84.111
  - desquamative J84.117
  - due to
    - collagen vascular disease J84.17
    - known underlying cause J84.17
  - idiopathic NOS J84.111
  - in disease classified elsewhere J84.17
  - lymphocytic (due to collagen vascular disease) (in diseases classified elsewhere) J84.17
  - lymphoid J84.2
  - non-specific J84.89
    - due to
      - collagen vascular disease J84.17
      - known underlying cause J84.17
    - idiopathic J84.113
    - in diseases classified elsewhere J84.17
  - plasma cell B59
  - pseudomonas J15.1
  - usual J84.112
    - due to collagen vascular disease J84.17
    - idiopathic J84.112
    - in diseases classified elsewhere J84.17
- Klebsiella (pneumoniae) J15.0
- lipid, lipoid (exogenous) J69.1
  - endogenous J84.89
- lobar (disseminated) (double) (interstitial) J18.1
  - bacterial J15.9
    - specified NEC J15.8
  - chronic — *see* Fibrosis, lung
  - Escherichia coli (E. coli) J15.5
  - Friedländer's bacillus J15.0
  - Hemophilus influenzae J14
  - hypostatic J18.2
  - Klebsiella (pneumoniae) J15.0
  - pneumococcal J13
  - Proteus J15.6
  - Pseudomonas J15.1
  - specified organism NEC J16.8
  - staphylococcal — *see* Pneumonia, staphylococcal
  - streptococcal NEC J15.4

Pneumonia — *continued*
- lobar — *continued*
  - Streptococcus pneumoniae J13
  - viral, virus — *see* Pneumonia, viral
- lobular — *see* Pneumonia, broncho
- Löffler's J82
- lymphoid interstitial J84.2
- massive — *see* Pneumonia, lobar
- meconium P24.01
- MRSA (methicillin resistant Staphylococcus aureus) J15.212
- MSSA (methicillin susceptible Staphylococcus aureus) J15.211
- multilobar — *see* Pneumonia, by type
- Mycoplasma (pneumoniae) J15.7
- necrotic J85.0
- neonatal P23.9
  - aspiration — *see* Aspiration, by substance, with pneumonia
- nitrogen dioxide J68.0
- organizing J84.89
  - due to
    - collagen vascular disease J84.17
    - known underlying cause J84.17
  - in diseases classified elsewhere J84.17
- orthostatic J18.2
- parainfluenza virus J12.2
- parenchymatous — *see* Fibrosis, lung
- passive J18.2
- patchy — *see* Pneumonia, broncho
- Peptococcus J15.8
- Peptostreptococcus J15.8
- plasma cell (of infants) B59
- pleurolobar — *see* Pneumonia, lobar
- pleuro-pneumonia-like organism (PPLO) J15.7
- pneumococcal (broncho) (lobar) J13
- Pneumocystis (carinii) (jiroveci) B59
- postinfectional NEC B99 ☑ *[J17]*
- postmeasles B05.2
- Proteus J15.6
- Pseudomonas J15.1
- psittacosis A70
- radiation J70.0
- respiratory syncytial virus (RSV) J12.1
- resulting from a procedure J95.89
- rheumatic I00 *[J17]*
- Salmonella (arizonae) (cholerae-suis) (enteritidis) (typhimurium) A02.22
  - typhi A01.03
  - typhoid fever A01.03
- SARS-associated coronavirus J12.81
- segmented, segmental — *see* Pneumonia, broncho-
- Serratia marcescens J15.6
- specified NEC J18.8
  - bacterium NEC J15.8
  - organism NEC J16.8
  - virus NEC J12.89
- spirochetal NEC A69.8
- staphylococcal (broncho) (lobar) J15.20
  - aureus (methicillin susceptible) (MSSA) J15.211
    - methicillin resistant (MRSA) J15.212
  - specified NEC J15.29
- static, stasis J18.2
- streptococcal NEC (broncho) (lobar) J15.4
  - group
    - A J15.4
    - B J15.3
    - specified NEC J15.4
  - Streptococcus pneumoniae J13
- syphilitic, congenital (early) A50.04
- traumatic (complication) (early) (secondary) T79.8 ☑
- tuberculous (any) — *see* Tuberculosis, pulmonary
- tularemic A21.2
- varicella B01.2
- Veillonella J15.8
- ventilator associated J95.851
- viral, virus (broncho) (interstitial) (lobar) J12.9
  - adenoviral J12.0
  - congenital P23.0
  - human metapneumovirus J12.3
  - parainfluenza J12.2
  - respiratory syncytial (RSV) J12.1
  - SARS-associated coronavirus J12.81
  - specified NEC J12.89
  - white (congenital) A50.04

Pneumonic — *see* condition

Pneumonitis (acute) (primary) — *see also* Pneumonia
- air-conditioner J67.7

▥ Subterms under main terms may continue to next column or page   ☑ Additional Character Required — Refer to the Tabular List for Character Selection   **255**

Pneumonia — Pneumonitis

Pneumonitis — continued
  allergic (due to) J67.9
    organic dust NEC J67.8
    red cedar dust J67.8
    sequoiosis J67.8
    wood dust J67.8
  aspiration J69.0
    due to
      anesthesia J95.4
        during
          labor and delivery O74.0
          pregnancy O29.01- ☑
          puerperium O89.01
      fumes or gases J68.0
    obstetric O74.0
  chemical (due to gases, fumes or vapors) (inhalation) J68.0
    due to anesthesia J95.4
  cholesterol J84.89
  chronic — see Fibrosis, lung
  congenital rubella P35.0
  crack (cocaine) J68.0
  due to
    beryllium J68.0
    cadmium J68.0
    crack (cocaine) J68.0
    detergent J69.8
    fluorocarbon-polymer J68.0
    food, vomit (aspiration) J69.0
    fumes or vapors J68.0
    gases, fumes or vapors (inhalation) J68.0
    inhalation
      blood J69.8
      essences J69.1
      food (regurgitated), milk, vomit J69.0
      oils, essences J69.1
      saliva J69.0
      solids, liquids NEC J69.8
    manganese J68.0
    nitrogen dioxide J68.0
    oils, essences J69.1
    solids, liquids NEC J69.8
    toxoplasmosis (acquired) B58.3
      congenital P37.1
    vanadium J68.0
    ventilator J95.851
  eosinophilic J82
  hypersensitivity J67.9
    air conditioner lung J67.7
    bagassosis J67.1
    bird fancier's lung J67.2
    farmer's lung J67.0
    maltworker's lung J67.4
    maple bark-stripper's lung J67.6
    mushroom worker's lung J67.5
    specified organic dust NEC J67.8
    suberosis J67.3
  interstitial (chronic) J84.89
    acute J84.114
    lymphoid J84.2
    non-specific J84.89
      idiopathic J84.113
  lymphoid, interstitial J84.2
  meconium P24.01
  postanesthetic J95.4
    correct substance properly administered — see Table of Drugs and Chemicals, by drug, adverse effect
    in labor and delivery O74.0
    in pregnancy O29.01- ☑
    obstetric O74.0
    overdose or wrong substance given or taken (by accident) — see Table of Drugs and Chemicals, by drug, poisoning
    postpartum, puerperal O89.01
  postoperative J95.4
    obstetric O74.0
  radiation J70.0
  rubella, congenital P35.0
  ventilation (air-conditioning) J67.7
  ventilator associated J95.851
  wood-dust J67.8
Pneumoconiosis — see Pneumoconiosis
Pneumoparotid K11.8
Pneumopathy NEC J98.4
  alveolar J84.09
  due to organic dust NEC J66.8
  parietoalveolar J84.09

Pneumopericarditis — see also Pericarditis
  acute I30.9
Pneumopericardium — see also Pericarditis
  congenital P25.3
  newborn P25.3
  traumatic (post) — see Injury, heart
Pneumophagia (psychogenic) F45.8
Pneumopleurisy, pneumopleuritis — see also Pneumonia J18.8
Pneumopyopericardium I30.1
Pneumopyothorax — see Pyopneumothorax
  with fistula J86.0
Pneumorrhagia — see also Hemorrhage, lung
  tuberculous — see Tuberculosis, pulmonary
Pneumothorax NOS J93.9
  acute J93.83
  chronic J93.81
  congenital P25.1
  perinatal period P25.1
  postprocedural J95.811
  specified NEC J93.83
  spontaneous NOS J93.83
    newborn P25.1
    primary J93.11
    secondary J93.12
    tension J93.0
  tense valvular, infectional J93.0
  tension (spontaneous) J93.0
  traumatic S27.0 ☑
    with hemothorax S27.2 ☑
  tuberculous — see Tuberculosis, pulmonary
Podagra — see also Gout M10.9
Podencephalus Q01.9
Poikilocytosis R71.8
Poikiloderma L81.6
  Civatte's L57.3
  congenital Q82.8
  vasculare atrophicans L94.5
Poikilodermatomyositis M33.10
  with
    myopathy M33.12
    respiratory involvement M33.11
    specified organ involvement NEC M33.19
Pointed ear (congenital) Q17.3
Poison ivy, oak, sumac or other plant dermatitis (allergic) (contact) L23.7
Poisoning (acute) — see also Table of Drugs and Chemicals
  algae and toxins T65.82- ☑
  Bacillus B (aertrycke) (cholerae (suis)) (paratyphosus) (suipestifer) A02.9
    botulinus A05.1
  bacterial toxins A05.9
  berries, noxious — see Poisoning, food, noxious, berries
  botulism A05.1
  ciguatera fish T61.0- ☑
  Clostridium botulinum A05.1
  death-cap (Amanita phalloides) (Amanita verna) — see Poisoning, food, noxious, mushrooms
  drug — see Table of Drugs and Chemicals, by drug, poisoning
  epidemic, fish (noxious) — see Poisoning, seafood
    bacterial A05.9
  fava bean D55.0
  fish (noxious) T61.9- ☑
    bacterial — see Intoxication, foodborne, by agent
    ciguatera fish — see Poisoning, ciguatera fish
    scombroid fish — see Poisoning, scombroid fish
    specified type NEC T61.77- ☑
  food NEC A05.9
    bacterial — see Intoxication, foodborne, by agent
    due to
      Bacillus (aertrycke) (choleraesuis) (paratyphosus) (suipestifer) A02.9
        botulinus A05.1
      Clostridium (perfringens) (Welchii) A05.2
      salmonella (aertrycke) (callinarum) (choleraesuis) (enteritidis) (paratyphi) (suipestifer) A02.9
        with
          gastroenteritis A02.0
          sepsis A02.1
      staphylococcus A05.0
      Vibrio
        parahaemolyticus A05.3
        vulnificus A05.5
    noxious or naturally toxic T62.9- ☑
      berries — see subcategory T62.1 ☑
      fish — see Poisoning, seafood

Poisoning — continued
  food — continued
    noxious or naturally toxic — continued
      mushrooms — see subcategory T62.0X ☑
      plants NEC — see subcategory T62.2X ☑
      seafood — see Poisoning, seafood
      specified NEC — see subcategory T62.8X ☑
  ichthyotoxism — see Poisoning, seafood
  kreotoxism, food A05.9
  latex T65.81- ☑
  lead T56.0- ☑
  mushroom — see Poisoning, food, noxious, mushroom
  mussels — see also Poisoning, shellfish
    bacterial — see Intoxication, foodborne, by agent
  nicotine (tobacco) T65.2- ☑
  noxious foodstuffs — see Poisoning, food, noxious
  plants, noxious — see Poisoning, food, noxious, plant NEC
  ptomaine — see Poisoning, food
  radiation J70.0
  Salmonella (arizonae) (cholerae-suis) (enteritidis) (typhimurium) A02.9
  scombroid fish T61.1- ☑
  seafood (noxious) T61.9- ☑
    bacterial — see Intoxication, foodborne, by agent
    fish — see Poisoning, fish
    shellfish — see Poisoning, shellfish
    specified NEC — see subcategory T61.8X ☑
  shellfish (amnesic) (azaspiracid) (diarrheic) (neurotoxic) (noxious) (paralytic) T61.78- ☑
    bacterial — see Intoxication, foodborne, by agent
    ciguatera mollusk — see Poisoning, ciguatera fish
  specified substance NEC T65.891 ☑
  Staphylococcus, food A05.0
  tobacco (nicotine) T65.2- ☑
  water E87.79
Poker spine — see Spondylitis, ankylosing
Poland syndrome Q79.8
Polioencephalitis (acute) (bulbar) A80.9
  inferior G12.22
  influenzal — see Influenza, with, encephalopathy
  superior hemorrhagic (acute) (Wernicke's) E51.2
  Wernicke's E51.2
Polioencephalomyelitis (acute) (anterior) A80.9
  with beriberi E51.2
Polioencephalopathy, superior hemorrhagic E51.2
  with
    beriberi E51.11
    pellagra E52
Poliomeningoencephalitis — see Meningoencephalitis
Poliomyelitis (acute) (anterior) (epidemic) A80.9
  with paralysis (bulbar) — see Poliomyelitis, paralytic
  abortive A80.4
  ascending (progressive) — see Poliomyelitis, paralytic
  bulbar (paralytic) — see Poliomyelitis, paralytic
  congenital P35.8
  nonepidemic A80.9
  nonparalytic A80.4
  paralytic A80.30
    specified NEC A80.39
    vaccine-associated A80.0
    wild virus
      imported A80.1
      indigenous A80.2
  spinal, acute A80.9
Poliosis (eyebrow) (eyelashes) L67.1
  circumscripta, acquired L67.1
Pollakiuria R35.0
  psychogenic F45.8
Pollinosis J30.1
Pollitzer's disease L73.2
Polyadenitis — see also Lymphadenitis
  malignant A20.0
Polyalgia M79.89
Polyangiitis M30.0
  microscopic M31.7
  overlap syndrome M30.8
Polyarteritis
  microscopic M31.7
  nodosa M30.0
    with lung involvement M30.1
    juvenile M30.2
    related condition NEC M30.8
Polyarthralgia — see Pain, joint
Polyarthritis, polyarthropathy — see also Arthritis M13.0

   ☑ **Additional Character Required** — Refer to the Tabular List for Character Selection   ▽ **Subterms under main terms may continue to next column or page**

olyarthritis, polyarthropathy — *continued*
  due to or associated with other specified conditions — *see* Arthritis
  epidemic (Australian) (with exanthema) B33.1
  infective — *see* Arthritis, pyogenic or pyemic
  inflammatory M06.4
  juvenile (chronic) (seronegative) M08.3
  migratory M13.8- ☑
  rheumatic, acute — *see* Fever, rheumatic

olyarthrosis M15.9
  post-traumatic M15.3
  primary M15.0
  specified NEC M15.8

olycarential syndrome of infancy E40

olychondritis (atrophic) (chronic) — *see also* Disorder, cartilage, specified type NEC
  relapsing M94.1

olycoria Q13.2

olycystic (disease)
  degeneration, kidney Q61.3
    autosomal dominant (adult type) Q61.2
    autosomal recessive (infantile type) NEC Q61.19
  kidney Q61.3
    autosomal
      dominant Q61.2
      recessive NEC Q61.19
    autosomal dominant (adult type) Q61.2
    autosomal recessive (childhood type) NEC Q61.19
    infantile type NEC Q61.19
  liver Q44.6
  lung J98.4
    congenital Q33.0
  ovary, ovaries E28.2
  spleen Q89.09

olycythemia (secondary) D75.1
  acquired D75.1
  benign (familial) D75.0
  due to
    donor twin P61.1
    erythropoietin D75.1
    fall in plasma volume D75.1
    high altitude D75.1
    maternal-fetal transfusion P61.1
    stress D75.1
  emotional D75.1
  erythropoietin D75.1
  familial (benign) D75.0
  Gaisböck's (hypertonica) D75.1
  high altitude D75.1
  hypertonica D75.1
  hypoxemic D75.1
  neonatorum P61.1
  nephrogenous D75.1
  relative D75.1
  secondary D75.1
  spurious D75.1
  stress D75.1
  vera D45

olycytosis cryptogenica D75.1

olydactylism, polydactyly Q69.9
  toes Q69.2

olydipsia R63.1

olydystrophy, pseudo-Hurler E77.0

olyembryoma — *see* Neoplasm, malignant, by site

olyglandular
  deficiency E31.0
  dyscrasia E31.9
  dysfunction E31.9
  syndrome E31.8

Polyhydramnios O40.- ☑

Polymastia Q83.1

Polymenorrhea N92.0

Polymyalgia M35.3
  arteritica, giant cell M31.5
  rheumatica M35.3
    with giant cell arteritis M31.5

Polymyositis (acute) (chronic) (hemorrhagic) M33.20
  with
    myopathy M33.22
    respiratory involvement M33.21
    skin involvement — *see* Dermatopolymyositis
    specified organ involvement NEC M33.29
  ossificans (generalisata) (progressiva) — *see* Myositis, ossificans, progressiva

Polyneuritis, polyneuritic — *see also* Polyneuropathy
  acute (post-)infective G61.0
  alcoholic G62.1
  cranialis G52.7

Polyneuritis, polyneuritic — *continued*
  demyelinating, chronic inflammatory (CIDP) G61.81
  diabetic — *see* Diabetes, polyneuropathy
  diphtheritic A36.83
  due to lack of vitamin NEC E56.9 *[G63]*
  endemic E51.11
  erythredema — *see* subcategory T56.1 ☑
  febrile, acute G61.0
  hereditary ataxic G60.1
  idiopathic, acute G61.0
  infective (acute) G61.0
  inflammatory, chronic demyelinating (CIDP) G61.81
  nutritional E63.9 *[G63]*
  postinfective (acute) G61.0
  specified NEC G62.89

Polyneuropathy (peripheral) G62.9
  alcoholic G62.1
  amyloid (Portuguese) E85.1 *[G63]*
    transthyretin-related (ATTR) familial E85.1 *[G63]*
  arsenical G62.2
  critical illness G62.81
  demyelinating, chronic inflammatory (CIDP) G61.81
  diabetic — *see* Diabetes, polyneuropathy
  drug-induced G62.0
  hereditary G60.9
    specified NEC G60.8
  idiopathic G60.9
    progressive G60.3
  in (due to)
    alcohol G62.1
      sequelae G65.2
    amyloidosis, familial (Portuguese) E85.1 *[G63]*
    antitetanus serum G61.1
    arsenic G62.2
      sequelae G65.2
    avitaminosis NEC E56.9 *[G63]*
    beriberi E51.11
    collagen vascular disease NEC M35.9 *[G63]*
    deficiency (of)
      B (-complex) vitamins E53.9 *[G63]*
      vitamin B6 E53.1 *[G63]*
    diabetes — *see* Diabetes, polyneuropathy
    diphtheria A36.83
    drug or medicament G62.0
      correct substance properly administered — *see* Table of Drugs and Chemicals, by drug, adverse effect
      overdose or wrong substance given or taken — *see* Table of Drugs and Chemicals, by drug, poisoning
    endocrine disease NEC E34.9 *[G63]*
    herpes zoster B02.23
    hypoglycemia E16.2 *[G63]*
    infectious
      disease NEC B99 ☑ *[G63]*
      mononucleosis B27.91
    lack of vitamin NEC E56.9 *[G63]*
    lead G62.2
      sequelae G65.2
    leprosy A30.9 *[G63]*
    Lyme disease A69.22
    metabolic disease NEC E88.9 *[G63]*
    microscopic polyangiitis M31.7 *[G63]*
    mumps B26.84
    neoplastic disease — *see also* Neoplasm D49.9 *[G63]*
    nutritional deficiency NEC E63.9 *[G63]*
    organophosphate compounds G62.2
      sequelae G65.2
    parasitic disease NEC B89 *[G63]*
    pellagra E52 *[G63]*
    polyarteritis nodosa M30.0
    porphyria E80.20 *[G63]*
    radiation G62.82
    rheumatoid arthritis — *see* Rheumatoid, polyneuropathy
    sarcoidosis D86.89
    serum G61.1
    syphilis (late) A52.15
      congenital A50.43
    systemic
      connective tissue disorder M35.9 *[G63]*
      lupus erythematosus M32.19
    toxic agent NEC G62.2
      sequelae G65.2
  inflammatory G61.9
    chronic demyelinating (CIDP) G61.81
    sequelae G65.1
    specified NEC G61.89

Polyneuropathy — *continued*
  lead G62.2
    sequelae G65.2
  nutritional NEC E63.9 *[G63]*
  postherpetic (zoster) B02.23
  progressive G60.3
  radiation-induced G62.82
  sensory (hereditary) (idiopathic) G60.8
  specified NEC G62.89
  syphilitic (late) A52.15
    congenital A50.43
  transthyretin-related (ATTR) familial amyloid E85.1
    triorthocresyl phosphate G62.2
      sequelae G65.2
    tuberculosis A17.89
    uremia N18.9 *[G63]*
    vitamin B12 deficiency E53.8 *[G63]*
      with anemia (pernicious) D51.0 *[G63]*
        due to dietary deficiency D51.3 *[G63]*
    zoster B02.23

Polyopia H53.8

Polyorchism, polyorchidism Q55.21

Polyosteoarthritis — *see also* Osteoarthritis, generalized M15.9
  post-traumatic M15.3
  specified NEC M15.8

Polyostotic fibrous dysplasia Q78.1

Polyotia Q17.0

Polyp, polypus
  accessory sinus J33.8
  adenocarcinoma in — *see* Neoplasm, malignant, by site
  adenocarcinoma in situ in — *see* Neoplasm, in situ, by site
  adenoid tissue J33.0
  adenomatous — *see also* Neoplasm, benign, by site
    adenocarcinoma in — *see* Neoplasm, malignant, by site
    adenocarcinoma in situ in — *see* Neoplasm, in situ, by site
    carcinoma in — *see* Neoplasm, malignant, by site
    carcinoma in situ in — *see* Neoplasm, in situ, by site
    multiple — *see* Neoplasm, benign
      adenocarcinoma in — *see* Neoplasm, malignant, by site
      adenocarcinoma in situ in — *see* Neoplasm, in situ, by site
  antrum J33.0
  anus, anal (canal) K62.0
  Bartholin's gland N84.3
  bladder D41.4
  carcinoma in — *see* Neoplasm, malignant, by site
  carcinoma in situ in — *see* Neoplasm, in situ, by site
  cecum D12.0
  cervix (uteri) N84.1
    in pregnancy or childbirth — *see* Pregnancy, complicated by, abnormal, cervix
    mucous N84.1
    nonneoplastic N84.1
  choanal J33.0
  cholesterol K82.4
  clitoris N84.3
  colon K63.5
    adenomatous D12.6
      ascending D12.2
      cecum D12.0
      descending D12.4
    hyperplastic, (any site) K63.5
    inflammatory K51.40
      with
        abscess K51.414
        complication K51.419
          specified NEC K51.418
        fistula K51.413
        intestinal obstruction K51.412
        rectal bleeding K51.411
    sigmoid D12.5
    transverse D12.3
  corpus uteri N84.0
  dental K04.01
    irreversible K04.02
    reversible K04.01
  duodenum K31.7
  ear (middle) H74.4- ☑
  endometrium N84.0
  ethmoidal (sinus) J33.8
  fallopian tube N84.8
  female genital tract N84.9

▼ Subterms under main terms may continue to next column or page   ☑ Additional Character Required — Refer to the Tabular List for Character Selection   257

Polyarthritis, polyarthropathy — Polyp, polypus

Polyp, polypus — *continued*
  female genital tract — *continued*
    specified NEC N84.8
  frontal (sinus) J33.8
  gallbladder K82.4
  gingiva, gum K06.8
  labia, labium (majus) (minus) N84.3
  larynx (mucous) J38.1
    adenomatous D14.1
  malignant — *see* Neoplasm, malignant, by site
  maxillary (sinus) J33.8
  middle ear — *see* Polyp, ear (middle)
  myometrium N84.0
  nares
    anterior J33.9
    posterior J33.0
  nasal (mucous) J33.9
    cavity J33.0
    septum J33.0
  nasopharyngeal J33.0
  nose (mucous) J33.9
  oviduct N84.8
  pharynx J39.2
  placenta O90.89
  prostate — *see* Enlargement, enlarged, prostate
  pudenda, pudendum N84.3
  pulpal (dental) K04.01
    irreversible K04.02
    reversible K04.01
  rectum (nonadenomatous) K62.1
    adenomatous — *see* Polyp, adenomatous
  septum (nasal) J33.0
  sinus (accessory) (ethmoidal) (frontal) (maxillary)
    (sphenoidal) J33.8
  sphenoidal (sinus) J33.8
  stomach K31.7
    adenomatous D13.1
  tube, fallopian N84.8
  turbinate, mucous membrane J33.8
  umbilical, newborn P83.6
  ureter N28.89
  urethra N36.2
  uterus (body) (corpus) (mucous) N84.0
    cervix N84.1
    in pregnancy or childbirth — *see* Pregnancy, com-
      plicated by, tumor, uterus
  vagina N84.2
  vocal cord (mucous) J38.1
  vulva N84.3
Polyphagia R63.2
Polyploidy Q92.7
Polypoid — *see* condition
Polyposis — *see also* Polyp
  coli (adenomatous) D12.6
    adenocarcinoma in C18.9
    adenocarcinoma in situ in — *see* Neoplasm, in situ,
      by site
    carcinoma in C18.9
  colon (adenomatous) D12.6
  familial D12.6
    adenocarcinoma in situ in — *see* Neoplasm, in situ,
      by site
  intestinal (adenomatous) D12.6
  malignant lymphomatous C83.1- ☑
  multiple, adenomatous — *see also* Neoplasm, benign
    D36.9
Polyradiculitis — *see* Polyneuropathy
Polyradiculoneuropathy (acute) (postinfective) (seg-
    mentally demyelinating) G61.0
Polyserositis
  due to pericarditis I31.1
  pericardial I31.1
  periodic, familial E85.0
  tuberculous A19.9
    acute A19.1
    chronic A19.8
Polysplenia syndrome Q89.09
Polysyndactyly — *see also* Syndactylism, syndactyly
    Q70.4
Polytrichia L68.3
Polyunguia Q84.6
Polyuria R35.8
  nocturnal R35.1
  psychogenic F45.8
Pompe's disease (glycogen storage) E74.02
Pompholyx L30.1
Poncet's disease (tuberculous rheumatism) A18.09
Pond fracture — *see* Fracture, skull

Ponos B55.0
Pons, pontine — *see* condition
Poor
  aesthetic of existing restoration of tooth K08.56
  contractions, labor O62.2
  gingival margin to tooth restoration K08.51
  personal hygiene R46.0
  prenatal care, affecting management of pregnancy —
    see Pregnancy, complicated by, insufficient,
    prenatal care
  sucking reflex (newborn) R29.2
  urinary stream R39.12
  vision NEC H54.7
Poradenitis, nostras inguinalis or venerea A55
Porencephaly (congenital) (developmental) (true) Q04.6
  acquired G93.0
  nondevelopmental G93.0
  traumatic (post) F07.89
Porocephaliasis B88.8
Porokeratosis Q82.8
Poroma, eccrine — *see* Neoplasm, skin, benign
Porphyria (South African) E80.20
  acquired E80.20
  acute intermittent (hepatic) (Swedish) E80.21
  cutanea tarda (hereditary) (symptomatic) E80.1
  due to drugs E80.20
    correct substance properly administered — *see* Ta-
      ble of Drugs and Chemicals, by drug, adverse
      effect
    overdose or wrong substance given or taken — *see*
      Table of Drugs and Chemicals, by drug, poi-
      soning
  erythropoietic (congenital) (hereditary) E80.0
  hepatocutaneous type E80.1
  secondary E80.20
  toxic NEC E80.20
  variegata E80.20
Porphyrinuria — *see* Porphyria
Porphyruria — *see* Porphyria
Port wine nevus, mark, or stain Q82.5
Portal — *see* condition
Posadas-Wernicke disease B38.9
Positive
  culture (nonspecific)
    blood R78.81
    bronchial washings R84.5
    cerebrospinal fluid R83.5
    cervix uteri R87.5
    nasal secretions R84.5
    nipple discharge R89.5
    nose R84.5
      staphylococcus (Methicillin susceptible) Z22.321
        Methicillin resistant Z22.322
    peritoneal fluid R85.5
    pleural fluid R84.5
    prostatic secretions R86.5
    saliva R85.5
    seminal fluid R86.5
    sputum R84.5
    synovial fluid R89.5
    throat scrapings R84.5
    urine R82.79
    vagina R87.5
    vulva R87.5
    wound secretions R89.5
  PPD (skin test) R76.11
  serology for syphilis A53.0
    false R76.8
    with signs or symptoms — *code as* Syphilis, by site
      and stage
  skin test, tuberculin (without active tuberculosis) R76.11
  test, human immunodeficiency virus (HIV) R75
  VDRL A53.0
    with signs or symptoms — *code by* site and stage
      under Syphilis A53.9
  Wassermann reaction A53.0
Postcardiotomy syndrome I97.0
Postcaval ureter Q62.62
Postcholecystectomy syndrome K91.5
Postclimacteric bleeding N95.0
Postcommissurotomy syndrome I97.0
Postconcussional syndrome F07.81
Postcontusion syndrome F07.81
Postcricoid region — *see* condition
Post-dates (40-42 weeks) (pregnancy) (mother) O48.0
  more than 42 weeks gestation O48.1
Postencephalitic syndrome F07.89
Posterior — *see* condition

Posterolateral sclerosis (spinal cord) — *see* Degenera●
    tion, combined
Postexanthematous — *see* condition
Postfebrile — *see* condition
Postgastrectomy dumping syndrome K91.1
Posthemiplegic chorea — *see* Monoplegia
Posthemorrhagic anemia (chronic) D50.0
  acute D62
  newborn P61.3
Postherpetic neuralgia (zoster) B02.29
  trigeminal B02.22
Posthitis N47.7
Postimmunization complication or reaction — *see*
    Complications, vaccination
Postinfectious — *see* condition
Postlaminectomy syndrome NEC M96.1
Postleukotomy syndrome F07.0
Postmastectomy lymphedema (syndrome) I97.2
Postmaturity, postmature (over 42 weeks)
  maternal (over 42 weeks gestation) O48.1
  newborn P08.22
Postmeasles complication NEC — *see also* condition
    B05.89
Postmenopausal
  endometrium (atrophic) N95.8
    suppurative — *see also* Endometritis N71.9
  osteoporosis — *see* Osteoporosis, postmenopausal
Postnasal drip R09.82
  due to
    allergic rhinitis — *see* Rhinitis, allergic
    common cold J00
    gastroesophageal reflux — *see* Reflux, gastroe-
      sophageal
    nasopharyngitis — *see* Nasopharyngitis
    other known condition — *code to* condition
    sinusitis — *see* Sinusitis
Postnatal — *see* condition
Postoperative (postprocedural) — *see* Complication,
    postoperative
  pneumothorax, therapeutic Z98.3
  state NEC Z98.890
Postpancreatectomy hyperglycemia E89.1
Postpartum — *see* Puerperal
Postphlebitic syndrome — *see* Syndrome, postthrom●
    botic
Postpolio (myelitic) **syndrome** G14
Postpoliomyelitic — *see also* condition
  osteopathy — *see* Osteopathy, after poliomyelitis
Postprocedural — *see also* Postoperative
  hypoinsulinemia E89.1
Postschizophrenic depression F32.89
Postsurgery status — *see also* Status (post)
  pneumothorax, therapeutic Z98.3
Post-term (40-42 weeks) (pregnancy) (mother) O48.0
  infant P08.21
  more than 42 weeks gestation (mother) O48.1
Post-traumatic brain syndrome, nonpsychotic F07.8●
Post-typhoid abscess A01.09
Postures, hysterical F44.2
Postvaccinal reaction or complication — *see* Compli●
    cations, vaccination
Postvalvulotomy syndrome I97.0
Potain's
  disease (pulmonary edema) — *see* Edema, lung
  syndrome (gastrectasis with dyspepsia) K31.0
Potter's
  asthma J62.8
  facies Q60.6
  lung J62.8
  syndrome (with renal agenesis) Q60.6
Pott's
  curvature (spinal) A18.01
  disease or paraplegia A18.01
  spinal curvature A18.01
  tumor, puffy — *see* Osteomyelitis, specified type NE●
Pouch
  bronchus Q32.4
  Douglas' — *see* condition
  esophagus, esophageal, congenital Q39.6
    acquired K22.5
  gastric K31.4
  Hartmann's K82.8
  pharynx, pharyngeal (congenital) Q38.7
Pouchitis K91.850
Poultrymen's itch B88.0
Poverty NEC Z59.6
  extreme Z59.5

oxvirus NEC B08.8
rader-Willi syndrome Q87.11
rader-Willi-like syndrome Q87.19
reauricular appendage or tag Q17.0
rebetalipoproteinemia (acquired) (essential) (familial)
    (hereditary) (primary) (secondary) E78.1
    with chylomicronemia E78.3
recipitate labor or delivery O62.3
reclimacteric bleeding (menorrhagia) N92.4
recocious
    adrenarche E30.1
    menarche E30.1
    menstruation E30.1
    pubarche E30.1
    puberty E30.1
        central E22.8
    sexual development NEC E30.1
    thelarche E30.8
recocity, sexual (constitutional) (cryptogenic) (female)
    (idiopathic) (male) E30.1
    with adrenal hyperplasia E25.9
        congenital E25.0
recordial pain R07.2
redeciduous teeth K00.2
rediabetes, prediabetic R73.03
    complicating
        pregnancy — *see* Pregnancy, complicated by, dis-
            eases of, specified type or system NEC
        puerperium O99.89
redislocation status of hip at birth Q65.6
re-eclampsia O14.9- ☑
    with pre-existing hypertension — *see* Hypertension,
        complicating pregnancy, pre-existing, with, pre-
        eclampsia
    complicating
        childbirth O14.94
        puerperium O14.95
    mild O14.0- ☑
        complicating
            childbirth O14.04
            puerperium O14.05
    moderate O14.0- ☑
        complicating
            childbirth O14.04
            puerperium O14.05
    severe O14.1- ☑
        with hemolysis, elevated liver enzymes and low
            platelet count (HELLP) O14.2- ☑
            complicating
                childbirth O14.24
                puerperium O14.25
        complicating
            childbirth O14.14
            puerperium O14.15
re-eruptive color change, teeth, tooth K00.8
re-excitation atrioventricular conduction I45.6
reglaucoma H40.00- ☑
regnancy (single) (uterine) — *see also* Delivery and
    Puerperal

*Note: The Tabular must be reviewed for assign-
ment of appropriate seventh character for multiple gestation codes in Chapter 15*

*Note: The Tabular must be reviewed for assign-
ment of the appropriate character indicating the
trimester of the pregnancy*

    abdominal (ectopic) O00.00
        with intrauterine pregnancy O00.01
        with viable fetus O36.7- ☑
    ampullar O00.10- ☑
        with intrauterine pregnancy O00.11- ☑
    biochemical O02.81
    broad ligament O00.80
        with intrauterine pregnancy O00.81
    cervical O00.8
        with intrauterine pregnancy O00.81
    chemical O02.81
    complicated by (care of) (management affected by)
        abnormal, abnormality
            cervix O34.4- ☑
                causing obstructed labor O65.5
            cord (umbilical) O69.9 ☑
            fetal heart rate or rhythm O36.83- ☑
            findings on antenatal screening of mother O28.9
                biochemical O28.1
                chromosomal O28.5

Pregnancy — *continued*
    complicated by — *continued*
        abnormal, abnormality — *continued*
            findings on antenatal screening of mother —
                continued
                cytological O28.2
                genetic O28.5
                hematological O28.0
                radiological O28.4
                specified NEC O28.8
                ultrasonic O28.3
            glucose (tolerance) NEC O99.810
            pelvic organs O34.9- ☑
                specified NEC O34.8- ☑
                    causing obstructed labor O65.5
            pelvis (bony) (major) NEC O33.0
            perineum O34.7- ☑
            position
                placenta O44.0- ☑
                    with hemorrhage O44.1- ☑
                uterus O34.59- ☑
            uterus O34.59-
                causing obstructed labor O65.5
                congenital O34.0- ☑
            vagina O34.6- ☑
                causing obstructed labor O65.5
            vulva O34.7- ☑
                causing obstructed labor O65.5
        abruptio placentae — *see* Abruptio placentae
        abscess or cellulitis
            bladder O23.1- ☑
            breast O91.11- ☑
            genital organ or tract O23.9- ☑
        abuse
            physical O9A.31 ☑ (*following* O99)
            psychological O9A.51 ☑ (*following* O99)
            sexual O9A.41 ☑ (*following* O99)
        adverse effect anesthesia O29.9- ☑
            aspiration pneumonitis O29.01- ☑
            cardiac arrest O29.11- ☑
            cardiac complication NEC O29.19- ☑
            cardiac failure O29.12- ☑
            central nervous system complication NEC
                O29.29- ☑
            cerebral anoxia O29.21- ☑
            failed or difficult intubation O29.6- ☑
            inhalation of stomach contents or secretions NOS
                O29.01- ☑
            local, toxic reaction O29.3X
            Mendelson's syndrome O29.01- ☑
            pressure collapse of lung O29.02- ☑
            pulmonary complications NEC O29.09- ☑
            specified NEC O29.8X- ☑
            spinal and epidural type NEC O29.5X ☑
                induced headache O29.4- ☑
        albuminuria — *see also* Proteinuria, gestational
            O12.1- ☑
        alcohol use O99.31- ☑
        amnionitis O41.12- ☑
        anaphylactoid syndrome of pregnancy O88.01- ☑
        anemia (conditions in D50-D64) (pre-existing)
            O99.01- ☑
            complicating the puerperium O99.03
        antepartum hemorrhage O46.9- ☑
            with coagulation defect — *see* Hemorrhage,
                antepartum, with coagulation defect
            specified NEC O46.8X- ☑
        appendicitis O99.61- ☑
        atrophy (yellow) (acute) liver (subacute) O26.61- ☑
        bariatric surgery status O99.84- ☑
        bicornis or bicornuate uterus O34.0- ☑
        biliary tract problems O26.61- ☑
        breech presentation O32.1
        cardiovascular diseases (conditions in I00-I09, I20-
            I52, I70-I99) O99.41- ☑
        cerebrovascular disorders (conditions in I60-I69)
            O99.41- ☑
        cervical shortening O26.87- ☑
        cervicitis O23.51- ☑
        chloasma (gravidarum) O26.89- ☑
        cholecystitis O99.61- ☑
        cholestasis (intrahepatic) O26.61- ☑
        chorioamnionitis O41.12- ☑
        circulatory system disorder (conditions in I00-I09,
            I20-I99, O99.41-)
        compound presentation O32.6 ☑

Pregnancy — *continued*
    complicated by — *continued*
        conjoined twins O30.02- ☑
        connective system disorders (conditions in M00-
            M99) O99.89
        contracted pelvis (general) O33.1
            inlet O33.2
            outlet O33.3
        convulsions (eclamptic) (uremic) — *see also*
            Eclampsia O15.9
        cracked nipple O92.11- ☑
        cystitis O23.1- ☑
        cystocele O34.8- ☑
        death of fetus (near term) O36.4 ☑
            early pregnancy O02.1
            of one fetus or more in multiple gestation
                O31.2- ☑
        deciduitis O41.14- ☑
        decreased fetal movement O36.81- ☑
        dental problems O99.61- ☑
        diabetes (mellitus) O24.91- ☑
            gestational (pregnancy induced) — *see* Diabetes,
                gestational
            pre-existing O24.31- ☑
                specified NEC O24.81- ☑
                type 1 O24.01- ☑
                type 2 O24.11- ☑
        digestive system disorders (conditions in K00-K93)
            O99.61- ☑
        diseases of — *see* Pregnancy, complicated by,
            specified body system disease
            biliary tract O26.61- ☑
            blood NEC (conditions in D65-D77) O99.11- ☑
            liver O26.61- ☑
            specified NEC O99.89
        disorders of — *see* Pregnancy, complicated by,
            specified body system disorder
            amniotic fluid and membranes O41.9- ☑
                specified NEC O41.8X- ☑
            biliary tract O26.61- ☑
            ear and mastoid process (conditions in H60-H95)
                O99.89
            eye and adnexa (conditions in H00-H59) O99.89
            liver O26.61- ☑
            skin (conditions in L00-L99) O99.71- ☑
            specified NEC O99.89
        displacement, uterus NEC O34.59- ☑
            causing obstructed labor O65.5
        disproportion (due to) O33.9
            fetal (ascites) (hydrops) (meningomyelocele)
                (sacral teratoma) (tumor) deformities NEC
                O33.7
            generally contracted pelvis O33.1
            hydrocephalic fetus O33.6
            inlet contraction of pelvis O33.2
            mixed maternal and fetal origin O33.4 ☑
            specified NEC O33.8
        double uterus O34.0- ☑
            causing obstructed labor O65.5
        drug use (conditions in F11-F19) O99.32- ☑
        eclampsia, eclamptic (coma) (convulsions) (delirium)
            (nephritis) (uremia) — *see also* Eclampsia
            O15.- ☑
        ectopic pregnancy — *see* Pregnancy, ectopic
        edema O12.0- ☑
            with
                gestational hypertension, mild — *see also*
                    Pre-eclampsia O14.0- ☑
                proteinuria O12.2- ☑
        effusion, amniotic fluid — *see* Pregnancy, compli-
            cated by, premature rupture of membranes
        elderly
            multigravida O09.52- ☑
            primigravida O09.51- ☑
        embolism — *see also* Embolism, obstetric, pregnan-
            cy O88.- ☑
        endocrine diseases NEC O99.28- ☑
        endometritis O86.12
        excessive weight gain O26.0- ☑
        exhaustion O26.81- ☑
            during labor and delivery O75.81
        face presentation O32.3
        failed induction of labor O61.9
            instrumental O61.1
            mechanical O61.1
            medical O61.0
            specified NEC O61.8

Pregnancy — *continued*
  complicated by — *continued*
    failed induction of labor — *continued*
      surgical O61.1
    failed or difficult intubation for anesthesia O29.6- ☑
    false labor (pains) O47.9
      at or after 37 completed weeks of pregnancy O47.1
      before 37 completed weeks of pregnancy O47.0- ☑
    fatigue O26.81-
      during labor and delivery O75.81
    fatty metamorphosis of liver O26.61- ☑
    female genital mutilation O34.8- ☑ *[N90.81-]* ☑
    fetal (maternal care for)
      abnormality or damage O35.9 ☑
        acid-base balance O68
        specified type NEC O35.8 ☑
      acidemia O68
      acidosis O68
      alkalosis O68
      anemia and thrombocytopenia O36.82- ☑
      anencephaly O35.0 ☑
      bradycardia O36.83- ☑
      chromosomal abnormality (conditions in Q90-Q99) O35.1 ☑
      conjoined twins O30.02- ☑
      damage from
        amniocentesis O35.7 ☑
        biopsy procedures O35.7 ☑
        drug addiction O35.5 ☑
        hematological investigation O35.7 ☑
        intrauterine contraceptive device O35.7 ☑
        maternal
          alcohol addiction O35.4 ☑
          cytomegalovirus infection O35.3 ☑
          disease NEC O35.8 ☑
          drug addiction O35.5 ☑
          listeriosis O35.8 ☑
          rubella O35.3 ☑
          toxoplasmosis O35.8 ☑
          viral infection O35.3 ☑
        medical procedure NEC O35.7 ☑
        radiation O35.6 ☑
      death (near term) O36.4 ☑
        early pregnancy O02.1
      decreased movement O36.81- ☑
      depressed heart rate tones O36.83- ☑
      disproportion due to deformity (fetal) O33.7 ☑
      excessive growth (large for dates) O36.6- ☑
      growth retardation O36.59- ☑
        light for dates O36.59- ☑
        small for dates O36.59- ☑
      heart rate irregularity (abnormal variability) (bradycardia) (decelerations) (tachycardia) O36.83- ☑
      hereditary disease O35.2 ☑
      hydrocephalus O35.0 ☑
      intrauterine death O36.4 ☑
      non-reassuring heart rate or rhythm O36.83- ☑
      poor growth O36.59- ☑
        light for dates O36.59- ☑
        small for dates O36.59- ☑
      problem O36.9- ☑
        specified NEC O36.89- ☑
      reduction (elective) O31.3- ☑
      selective termination O31.3- ☑
      spina bifida O35.0 ☑
      thrombocytopenia O36.82- ☑
    fibroid (tumor) (uterus) O34.1- ☑
    fissure of nipple O92.11- ☑
    gallstones O99.61- ☑
    gastric banding status O99.84- ☑
    gastric bypass status O99.84- ☑
    genital herpes (asymptomatic) (history of) (inactive) O98.3- ☑
    genital tract infection O23.9- ☑
    glomerular diseases (conditions in N00-N07) O26.83- ☑
      with hypertension, pre-existing — *see* Hypertension, complicating, pregnancy, pre-existing, with, renal disease
    gonorrhea O98.21- ☑
    grand multiparity O09.4 ☑
    habitual aborter — *see* Pregnancy, complicated by, recurrent pregnancy loss

Pregnancy — *continued*
  complicated by — *continued*
    HELLP syndrome (hemolysis, elevated liver enzymes and low platelet count) O14.2- ☑
    hemorrhage
      antepartum — *see* Hemorrhage, antepartum
      before 20 completed weeks gestation O20.9
        specified NEC O20.8
      due to premature separation, placenta — *see also* Abruptio placentae O45.9- ☑
      early O20.9
        specified NEC O20.8
      threatened abortion O20.0
    hemorrhoids O22.4- ☑
    hepatitis (viral) O98.41- ☑
    herniation of uterus O34.59- ☑
    high
      head at term O32.4 ☑
      risk — *see* Supervision (of) (for), high-risk
    history of in utero procedure during previous pregnancy O09.82- ☑
    HIV O98.71- ☑
    human immunodeficiency virus (HIV) disease O98.71- ☑
    hydatidiform mole — *see also* Mole, hydatidiform O01.9
    hydramnios O40.- ☑
    hydrocephalic fetus (disproportion) O33.6 ☑
    hydrops
      amnii O40.- ☑
      fetalis O36.2- ☑
        associated with isoimmunization — *see also* Pregnancy, complicated by, isoimmunization O36.11- ☑
    hydrorrhea O42.90
    hyperemesis (gravidarum) (mild) — *see also* Hyperemesis, gravidarum O21.0
    hypertension — *see* Hypertension, complicating pregnancy
    hypertensive
      heart and renal disease, pre-existing — *see* Hypertension, complicating, pregnancy, pre-existing, with, heart disease, with renal disease
      heart disease, pre-existing — *see* Hypertension, complicating, pregnancy, pre-existing, with, heart disease
      renal disease, pre-existing — *see* Hypertension, complicating, pregnancy, pre-existing, with, renal disease
    hypotension O26.5- ☑
    immune disorders NEC (conditions in D80-D89) O99.11- ☑
    incarceration, uterus O34.51- ☑
    incompetent cervix O34.3- ☑
    inconclusive fetal viability O36.80 ☑
    infection(s) O98.91- ☑
      amniotic fluid or sac O41.10- ☑
      bladder O23.1- ☑
      carrier state NEC O99.830
        streptococcus B O99.820
      genital organ or tract O23.9- ☑
        specified NEC O23.59- ☑
      genitourinary tract O23.9- ☑
      gonorrhea O98.21- ☑
      hepatitis (viral) O98.41- ☑
      HIV O98.71- ☑
      human immunodeficiency virus (HIV) O98.71- ☑
      kidney O23.0- ☑
      nipple O91.01- ☑
      parasitic disease O98.91- ☑
        specified NEC O98.81- ☑
      protozoal disease O98.61- ☑
      sexually transmitted NEC O98.31- ☑
      specified type NEC O98.81- ☑
      syphilis O98.11- ☑
      tuberculosis O98.01- ☑
      urethra O23.2- ☑
      urinary (tract) O23.4- ☑
        specified NEC O23.3- ☑
      viral disease O98.51- ☑
    injury or poisoning (conditions in S00-T88) O9A.21- ☑ (*following* O99)
      due to abuse
        physical O9A.31- ☑ (*following* O99)
        psychological O9A.51- ☑ (*following* O99)
        sexual O9A.41- ☑ (*following* O99)

Pregnancy — *continued*
  complicated by — *continued*
    insufficient
      prenatal care O09.3- ☑
      weight gain O26.1- ☑
    insulin resistance O26.89 ☑
    intrauterine fetal death (near term) O36.4 ☑
      early pregnancy O02.1
      multiple gestation (one fetus or more) O31.2- ▶
    isoimmunization O36.11- ☑
      anti-A sensitization O36.11- ☑
      anti-B sensitization O36.19- ☑
      Rh O36.09- ☑
        anti-D antibody O36.01- ☑
      specified NEC O36.19- ☑
    laceration of uterus NEC O71.81
    malformation
      placenta, placental (vessel) O43.10- ☑
        specified NEC O43.19- ☑
      uterus (congenital) O34.0- ☑
    malnutrition (conditions in E40-E46) O25.1- ☑
    maternal hypotension syndrome O26.5- ☑
    mental disorders (conditions in F01-F09, F20-F99) O99.34- ☑
      alcohol use O99.31- ☑
      drug use O99.32- ☑
      smoking O99.33- ☑
    mentum presentation O32.3 ☑
    metabolic disorders O99.28- ☑
    missed
      abortion O02.1
      delivery O36.4 ☑
    multiple gestations O30.9- ☑
      conjoined twins O30.02- ☑
      quadruplet — *see* Pregnancy, quadruplet
      specified complication NEC O31.8X- ☑
      specified number of multiples NEC — *see* Pregnancy, multiple (gestation), specified NE
      triplet — *see* Pregnancy, triplet
      twin — *see* Pregnancy, twin
    musculoskeletal condition (conditions is M00-M99 O99.89
    necrosis, liver (conditions in K72) O26.61- ☑
    neoplasm
      benign
        cervix O34.4- ☑
        corpus uteri O34.1- ☑
        uterus O34.1- ☑
      malignant O9A.11- ☑ (*following* O99)
    nephropathy NEC O26.83- ☑
    nervous system condition (conditions in G00-G99 O99.35- ☑
    nutritional diseases NEC O99.28- ☑
    obesity (pre-existing) O99.21- ☑
    obesity surgery status O99.84- ☑
    oblique lie or presentation O32.2 ☑
    older mother — *see* Pregnancy, complicated by, elderly
    oligohydramnios O41.0- ☑
      with premature rupture of membranes — *see also* Pregnancy, complicated by, premature rupture of membranes O42.- ☑
    onset (spontaneous) of labor after 37 completed weeks of gestation but before 39 completed weeks gestation, with delivery by (planned) cesarean section O75.82
    oophoritis O23.52- ☑
    overdose, drug — *see also* Table of Drugs and Chemicals, by drug, poisoning O9A.21- ☑ (*following* O99)
    oversize fetus O33.5 ☑
    papyraceous fetus O31.0- ☑
    pelvic inflammatory disease O99.89
    periodontal disease O99.61- ☑
    peripheral neuritis O26.82- ☑
    peritoneal (pelvic) adhesions O99.89
    phlebitis O22.9- ☑
    phlebopathy O22.9- ☑
    phlebothrombosis (superficial) O22.2- ☑
      deep O22.3- ☑
    placenta accreta O43.21- ☑
    placenta increta O43.22- ☑
    placenta percreta O43.23- ☑
    placenta previa O44.0- ☑
      complete O44.0 ☑
        with hemorrhage O44.1- ☑

Pregnancy — *continued*
  complicated by — *continued*
    placenta previa — *continued*
      marginal O44.2- ☑
        with hemorrhage O44.3- ☑
      partial O44.2- ☑
        with hemorrhage O44.3- ☑
    placental disorder O43.9- ☑
      specified NEC O43.89- ☑
    placental dysfunction O43.89- ☑
    placental infarction O43.81- ☑
    placental insufficiency O36.51- ☑
    placental transfusion syndromes
      fetomaternal O43.01- ☑
      fetus to fetus O43.02- ☑
      maternofetal O43.01- ☑
    placentitis O41.14- ☑
    pneumonia O99.51- ☑
    poisoning — *see also* Table of Drugs and Chemicals
      O9A.21 ☑ (*following* O99)
    polyhydramnios O40- ☑
    polymorphic eruption of pregnancy O26.86
    poor obstetric history NEC O09.29- ☑
    postmaturity (post-term) (40 to 42 weeks) O48.0
      more than 42 completed weeks gestation (prolonged) O48.1
    pre-eclampsia O14.9- ☑
      mild O14.0- ☑
      moderate O14.0- ☑
      severe O14.1- ☑
        with hemolysis, elevated liver enzymes and low platelet count (HELLP) O14.2- ☑
    premature labor — *see* Pregnancy, complicated by, preterm labor
    premature rupture of membranes O42.90
      with onset of labor
        within 24 hours O42.00
          at or after 37 weeks gestation, onset of labor within 24 hours of rupture O42.02
          pre-term (before 37 completed weeks of gestation) O42.01- ☑
        after 24 hours O42.10
          at or after 37 weeks gestation, onset of labor more than 24 hours following rupture O42.12
          pre-term (before 37 completed weeks of gestation) O42.11- ☑
      at or after 37 weeks gestation, unspecified as to length of time between rupture and onset of labor O42.92
      full-term, unspecified as to length of time between rupture and onset of labor O42.92
      pre-term (before 37 completed weeks of gestation) O42.91- ☑
    premature separation of placenta — *see also* Abruptio placentae O45.9- ☑
    presentation, fetal — *see* Delivery, complicated by, malposition
    preterm delivery O60.10 ☑
    preterm labor
      with delivery O60.10 ☑
        preterm O60.10 ☑
        term O60.20 ☑
      second trimester
        with term delivery O60.22 ☑
        without delivery O60.02
        with preterm delivery
          second trimester O60.12 ☑
          third trimester O60.13 ☑
      third trimester
        with term delivery O60.23 ☑
        without delivery O60.03
        with third trimester preterm delivery O60.14 ☑
      without delivery O60.00
        second trimester O60.02
        third trimester O60.03
    previous history of — *see* Pregnancy, supervision of, high-risk
    prolapse, uterus O34.52- ☑
    proteinuria (gestational) — *see also* Proteinuria, gestational O12.1- ☑
      with edema O12.2- ☑
    pruritic urticarial papules and plaques of pregnancy (PUPPP) O26.86
    pruritus (neurogenic) O26.89- ☑

Pregnancy — *continued*
  complicated by — *continued*
    psychosis or psychoneurosis (puerperal) F53.1
    ptyalism O26.89- ☑
    PUPPP (pruritic urticarial papules and plaques of pregnancy) O26.86
    pyelitis O23.0- ☑
    recurrent pregnancy loss O26.2- ☑
    renal disease or failure NEC O26.83- ☑
      with secondary hypertension, pre-existing — *see* Hypertension, complicating, pregnancy, pre-existing, secondary
      hypertensive, pre-existing — *see* Hypertension, complicating, pregnancy, pre-existing, with, renal disease
    respiratory condition (conditions in J00-J99) O99.51- ☑
    retained, retention
      dead ovum O02.0
      intrauterine contraceptive device O26.3- ☑
    retroversion, uterus O34.53- ☑
    Rh immunization, incompatibility or sensitization NEC O36.09- ☑
      anti-D antibody O36.01- ☑
    rupture
      amnion (premature) — *see also* Pregnancy, complicated by, premature rupture of membranes O42- ☑
      membranes (premature) — *see also* Pregnancy, complicated by, premature rupture of membranes O42- ☑
      uterus (during labor) O71.1
        before onset of labor O71.0- ☑
    salivation (excessive) O26.89- ☑
    salpingitis O23.52- ☑
    salpingo-oophoritis O23.52- ☑
    sepsis (conditions in A40, A41) O98.81- ☑
    size date discrepancy (uterine) O26.84- ☑
    skin condition (conditions in L00-L99) O99.71- ☑
    smoking (tobacco) O99.33- ☑
    social problem O09.7- ☑
    specified condition NEC O26.89- ☑
    spotting O26.85- ☑
    streptococcus group B (GBS) carrier state O99.820
    subluxation of symphysis (pubis) O26.71- ☑
    syphilis (conditions in A50-A53) O98.11- ☑
    threatened
      abortion O20.0
      labor O47.9
        at or after 37 completed weeks of gestation O47.1
        before 37 completed weeks of gestation O47.0- ☑
    thrombophlebitis (superficial) O22.2- ☑
    thrombosis O22.9- ☑
      cerebral venous O22.5- ☑
      cerebrovenous sinus O22.5- ☑
      deep O22.3- ☑
    tobacco use disorder (smoking) O99.33- ☑
    torsion of uterus O34.59- ☑
    toxemia O14.9- ☑
    transverse lie or presentation O32.2
    tuberculosis (conditions in A15-A19) O98.01- ☑
    tumor (benign)
      cervix O34.4- ☑
      malignant O9A.11- ☑ (*following* O99)
      uterus O34.1- ☑
    unstable lie O32.0 ☑
    upper respiratory infection O99.51- ☑
    urethritis O23.2- ☑
    uterine size date discrepancy O26.84- ☑
    vaginitis or vulvitis O23.59- ☑
    varicose veins (lower extremities) O22.0- ☑
      genitals O22.1- ☑
      legs O22.0- ☑
      perineal O22.1- ☑
      vaginal or vulval O22.1- ☑
    venereal disease NEC (conditions in A63.8) O98.31- ☑
    venous disorders O22.9- ☑
      specified NEC O22.8X- ☑
    very young mother — *see* Pregnancy, complicated by, young mother
    viral diseases (conditions in A80-B09, B25-B34) O98.51- ☑
    vomiting O21.9
      due to diseases classified elsewhere O21.8

Pregnancy — *continued*
  complicated by — *continued*
    vomiting — *continued*
      hyperemesis gravidarum (mild) — *see also* Hyperemesis, gravidarum O21.0
      late (occurring after 20 weeks of gestation) O21.2
    young mother
      multigravida O09.62- ☑
      primigravida O09.61- ☑
  complicated NOS O26.9- ☑
  concealed O09.3- ☑
  continuing following
    elective fetal reduction of one or more fetus O31.3- ☑
    intrauterine death of one or more fetus O31.2- ☑
    spontaneous abortion of one or more fetus O31.1- ☑
  cornual O00.80
    with intrauterine pregnancy O00.81
  ectopic (ruptured) O00.90
    with intrauterine pregnancy O00.91
    abdominal O00.00
      with
        intrauterine pregnancy O00.01
        viable fetus O36.7- ☑
    cervical O00.80
      with intrauterine pregnancy O00.81
    complicated (by) O08.9
      afibrinogenemia O08.1
      cardiac arrest O08.81
      chemical damage of pelvic organ(s) O08.6
      circulatory collapse O08.3
      defibrination syndrome O08.1
      electrolyte imbalance O08.5
      embolism (amniotic fluid) (blood clot) (pulmonary) (septic) O08.2
      endometritis O08.0
      genital tract and pelvic infection O08.0
      hemorrhage (delayed) (excessive) O08.1
      infection
        genital tract or pelvic O08.0
        kidney O08.83
        urinary tract O08.3
      intravascular coagulation O08.1
      laceration of pelvic organ(s) O08.6
      metabolic disorder O08.5
      oliguria O08.4
      oophoritis O08.0
      parametritis O08.0
      pelvic peritonitis O08.0
      perforation of pelvic organ(s) O08.6
      renal failure or shutdown O08.4
      salpingitis or salpingo-oophoritis O08.0
      sepsis O08.82
      shock O08.83
        septic O08.82
      specified condition NEC O08.89
      tubular necrosis (renal) O08.4
      uremia O08.4
      urinary infection O08.83
      venous complication NEC O08.7
        embolism O08.2
    cornual O00.80
      with intrauterine pregnancy O00.81
    intraligamentous O00.80
      with intrauterine pregnancy O00.81
    mural O00.80
      with intrauterine pregnancy O00.81
    ovarian O00.20- ☑
      with intrauterine pregnancy O00.21- ☑
    specified site NEC O00.80
      with intrauterine pregnancy O00.81
    tubal (ruptured) O00.10- ☑
      with intrauterine pregnancy O00.11- ☑
  examination (normal) Z34.9- ☑
    first Z34.0- ☑
    high-risk — *see* Pregnancy, supervision of, high-risk
    specified Z34.8- ☑
  extrauterine — *see* Pregnancy, ectopic
  fallopian O00.10- ☑
    with intrauterine pregnancy O00.11- ☑
  false F45.8
  gestational carrier Z33.3
  heptachorionic, hepta-amniotic (septuplets) O30.83- ☑
  hexachorionic, hexa-amniotic (sextuplets) O30.83- ☑
  hidden O09.3- ☑
  high-risk — *see* Pregnancy, supervision of, high-risk
  incidental finding Z33.1

Pregnancy — *continued*
  interstitial O00.80
    with intrauterine pregnancy O00.81
  intraligamentous O00.80
    with intrauterine pregnancy O00.81
  intramural O00.80
    with intrauterine pregnancy O00.81
  intraperitoneal O00.00
    with intrauterine pregnancy O00.01
  isthmian O00.10- ☑
    with intrauterine pregnancy O00.11- ☑
  mesometric (mural) O00.80
    with intrauterine pregnancy O00.81
  molar NEC O02.0
    complicated (by) O08.9
      afibrinogenemia O08.1
      cardiac arrest O08.81
      chemical damage of pelvic organ(s) O08.6
      circulatory collapse O08.3
      defibrination syndrome O08.1
      electrolyte imbalance O08.5
      embolism (amniotic fluid) (blood clot) (pulmonary) (septic) O08.2
      endometritis O08.0
      genital tract and pelvic infection O08.0
      hemorrhage (delayed) (excessive) O08.1
      infection
        genital tract or pelvic O08.0
        kidney O08.83
        urinary tract O08.83
      intravascular coagulation O08.1
      laceration of pelvic organ(s) O08.6
      metabolic disorder O08.5
      oliguria O08.4
      oophoritis O08.0
      parametritis O08.0
      pelvic peritonitis O08.0
      perforation of pelvic organ(s) O08.6
      renal failure or shutdown O08.4
      salpingitis or salpingo-oophoritis O08.0
      sepsis O08.82
      shock O08.3
        septic O08.82
      specified condition NEC O08.89
      tubular necrosis (renal) O08.4
      uremia O08.4
      urinary infection O08.83
      venous complication NEC O08.7
        embolism O08.2
  hydatidiform — *see also* Mole, hydatidiform O01.9
  multiple (gestation) O30.9- ☑
    greater than quadruplets — *see* Pregnancy, multiple (gestation), specified NEC
    specified NEC O30.80- ☑
      with
        two or more monoamniotic fetuses O30.82- ☑
        two or more monochorionic fetuses O30.81- ☑
        number of chorions and amnions are both equal to the number of fetuses O30.83- ☑
        two or more monoamniotic fetuses O30.82- ☑
        two or more monochorionic fetuses O30.81- ☑
        unable to determine number of placenta and number of amniotic sacs O30.89- ☑
        unspecified number of placenta and unspecified number of amniotic sacs O30.80- ☑
  mural O00.80
    with intrauterine pregnancy O00.81
  normal (supervision of) Z34.9- ☑
    first Z34.0- ☑
    high-risk — *see* Pregnancy, supervision of, high-risk
    specified Z34.8- ☑
  ovarian O00.20- ☑
    with intrauterine pregnancy O00.21- ☑
  pentachorionic, penta-amniotic (quintuplets) O30.83- ☑
  postmature (40 to 42 weeks) O48.0
    more than 42 weeks gestation O48.1
  post-term (40 to 42 weeks) O48.0
  prenatal care only Z34.9- ☑
    first Z34.0- ☑
    high-risk — *see* Pregnancy, supervision of, high-risk
    specified Z34.8- ☑
  prolonged (more than 42 weeks gestation) O48.1
  quadruplet O30.20- ☑
    with
      two or more monoamniotic fetuses O30.22- ☑

Pregnancy — *continued*
  quadruplet — *continued*
    with — *continued*
      two or more monochorionic fetuses O30.21- ☑
      quadrachorionic/quadra-amniotic O30.23- ☑
      two or more monoamniotic fetuses O30.22- ☑
      two or more monochorionic fetuses O30.21- ☑
      unable to determine number of placenta and number of amniotic sacs O30.29- ☑
      unspecified number of placenta and unspecified number of amniotic sacs O30.20- ☑
  quintuplet — *see* Pregnancy, multiple (gestation), specified NEC
  sextuplet — *see* Pregnancy, multiple (gestation), specified NEC
  supervision of
    concealed pregnancy O09.3- ☑
    elderly mother
      multigravida O09.52- ☑
      primigravida O09.51- ☑
    hidden pregnancy O09.3- ☑
    high-risk O09.9- ☑
      due to (history of)
        ectopic pregnancy O09.1- ☑
        elderly — *see* Pregnancy, supervision, elderly mother
        grand multiparity O09.4 ☑
        in utero procedure during previous pregnancy O09.82- ☑
        in vitro fertilization O09.81- ☑
        infertility O09.0- ☑
        insufficient prenatal care O09.3- ☑
        molar pregnancy O09.A- ☑
        multiple previous pregnancies O09.4- ☑
        older mother — *see* Pregnancy, supervision of, elderly mother
        poor reproductive or obstetric history NEC O09.29- ☑
        pre-term labor O09.21- ☑
        previous
          neonatal death O09.29- ☑
        social problems O09.7- ☑
        specified NEC O09.89- ☑
        very young mother — *see* Pregnancy, supervision, young mother
      resulting from in vitro fertilization O09.81- ☑
    normal Z34.9- ☑
      first Z34.0- ☑
      specified NEC Z34.8- ☑
    young mother
      multigravida O09.62- ☑
      primigravida O09.61- ☑
  triplet O30.10- ☑
    with
      two or more monoamniotic fetuses O30.12- ☑
      two or more monochorionic fetuses O30.11- ☑
      trichorionic/triamniotic O30.13- ☑
      two or more monoamniotic fetuses O30.12- ☑
      two or more monochorionic fetuses O30.11- ☑
      unable to determine number of placenta and number of amniotic sacs O30.19- ☑
      unspecified number of placenta and unspecified number of amniotic sacs O30.10- ☑
  tubal (with abortion) (with rupture) O00.10- ☑
    with intrauterine pregnancy O00.11- ☑
  twin O30.00- ☑
    conjoined O30.02- ☑
    dichorionic/diamniotic (two placenta, two amniotic sacs) O30.04- ☑
    monochorionic/diamniotic (one placenta, two amniotic sacs) O30.03- ☑
    monochorionic/monoamniotic (one placenta, one amniotic sac) O30.01- ☑
    unable to determine number of placenta and number of amniotic sacs O30.09- ☑
    unspecified number of placenta and unspecified number of amniotic sacs O30.00- ☑
  unwanted Z64.0
  weeks of gestation
    8 weeks Z3A.08 (*following* Z36)
    9 weeks Z3A.09 (*following* Z36)
    10 weeks Z3A.10 (*following* Z36)
    11 weeks Z3A.11 (*following* Z36)
    12 weeks Z3A.12 (*following* Z36)
    13 weeks Z3A.13 (*following* Z36)
    14 weeks Z3A.14 (*following* Z36)
    15 weeks Z3A.15 (*following* Z36)

Pregnancy — *continued*
  weeks of gestation — *continued*
    16 weeks Z3A.16 (*following* Z36)
    17 weeks Z3A.17 (*following* Z36)
    18 weeks Z3A.18 (*following* Z36)
    19 weeks Z3A.19 (*following* Z36)
    20 weeks Z3A.20 (*following* Z36)
    21 weeks Z3A.21 (*following* Z36)
    22 weeks Z3A.22 (*following* Z36)
    23 weeks Z3A.23 (*following* Z36)
    24 weeks Z3A.24 (*following* Z36)
    25 weeks Z3A.25 (*following* Z36)
    26 weeks Z3A.26 (*following* Z36)
    27 weeks Z3A.27 (*following* Z36)
    28 weeks Z3A.28 (*following* Z36)
    29 weeks Z3A.29 (*following* Z36)
    30 weeks Z3A.30 (*following* Z36)
    31 weeks Z3A.31 (*following* Z36)
    32 weeks Z3A.32 (*following* Z36)
    33 weeks Z3A.33 (*following* Z36)
    34 weeks Z3A.34 (*following* Z36)
    35 weeks Z3A.35 (*following* Z36)
    36 weeks Z3A.36 (*following* Z36)
    37 weeks Z3A.37 (*following* Z36)
    38 weeks Z3A.38 (*following* Z36)
    39 weeks Z3A.39 (*following* Z36)
    40 weeks Z3A.40 (*following* Z36)
    41 weeks Z3A.41 (*following* Z36)
    42 weeks Z3A.42 (*following* Z36)
    greater than 42 weeks Z3A.49 (*following* Z36)
    less than 8 weeks Z3A.01 (*following* Z36)
    not specified Z3A.00 (*following* Z36)
Preiser's disease — *see* Osteonecrosis, secondary, due to, trauma, metacarpus
Pre-kwashiorkor — *see* Malnutrition, severe
Preleukemia (syndrome) D46.9
Preluxation, hip, congenital Q65.6
Premature — *see also* condition
  adrenarche E27.0
  aging E34.8
  beats I49.40
    atrial I49.1
    auricular I49.1
    supraventricular I49.1
  birth NEC — *see* Preterm, newborn
  closure, foramen ovale Q21.8
  contraction
    atrial I49.1
    atrioventricular I49.2
    auricular I49.1
    auriculoventricular I49.49
    heart (extrasystole) I49.49
    junctional I49.2
    ventricular I49.3
  delivery — *see also* Pregnancy, complicated by, preterm labor O60.10 ☑
  ejaculation F52.4
  infant NEC — *see* Preterm, newborn
    light-for-dates — *see* Light for dates
  labor — *see* Pregnancy, complicated by, preterm labor
  lungs P28.0
  menopause E28.319
    asymptomatic E28.319
    symptomatic E28.310
  newborn
    extreme (less than 28 completed weeks) — *see* Immaturity, extreme
    less than 37 completed weeks — *see* Preterm, newborn
  puberty E30.1
  rupture membranes or amnion — *see* Pregnancy, complicated by, premature rupture of membranes
  senility E34.8
  thelarche E30.8
  ventricular systole I49.3
Prematurity NEC (less than 37 completed weeks) — *see* Preterm, newborn
  extreme (less than 28 completed weeks) — *see* Immaturity, extreme
Premenstrual
  dysphoric disorder (PMDD) F32.81
  tension (syndrome) N94.3
Premolarization, cuspids K00.2
Prenatal
  care, normal pregnancy — *see* Pregnancy, normal
  screening of mother — *see also* Encounter, antenatal screening Z36.9

☑ **Additional Character Required** — Refer to the Tabular List for Character Selection
▽ **Subterms under main terms may continue to next column or page**

renatal — *continued*
   teeth K00.6
reparatory care for subsequent treatment NEC
   for dialysis Z49.01
      peritoneal Z49.02
repartum — *see* condition
reponderance, left or right ventricular I51.7
repuce — *see* condition
RES (posterior reversible encephalopathy syndrome)
   I67.83
resbycardia R54
resbycusis, presbyacusia H91.1- ☑
resbyesophagus K22.8
resbyophrenia F03 ☑
resbyopia H52.4
rescription of contraceptives (initial) Z30.019
   barrier Z30.018
   diaphragm Z30.018
   emergency (postcoital) Z30.012
   implantable subdermal Z30.017
   injectable Z30.013
   intrauterine contraceptive device Z30.014
   pills Z30.011
   postcoital (emergency) Z30.012
   repeat Z30.40
      barrier Z30.49
      diaphragm Z30.49
      implantable subdermal Z30.46
      injectable Z30.42
      pills Z30.41
      specified type NEC Z30.49
      transdermal patch hormonal Z30.45
      vaginal ring hormonal Z30.44
   specified type NEC Z30.018
      transdermal patch hormonal Z30.016
      vaginal ring hormonal Z30.015
Presence (of)
   ankle-joint implant (functional) (prosthesis) Z96.66- ☑
   aortocoronary (bypass) graft Z95.1
   arterial-venous shunt (dialysis) Z99.2
   artificial
      eye (globe) Z97.0
      heart (fully implantable) (mechanical) Z95.812
         valve Z95.2
      larynx Z96.3
      lens (intraocular) Z96.1
      limb (complete) (partial) Z97.1- ☑
         arm Z97.1- ☑
            bilateral Z97.15
         leg Z97.1- ☑
            bilateral Z97.16
   audiological implant (functional) Z96.29
   bladder implant (functional) Z96.0
   bone
      conduction hearing device Z96.29
      implant (functional) NEC Z96.7
      joint (prosthesis) — *see* Presence, joint implant
   cardiac
      defibrillator (functional) (with synchronous cardiac
         pacemaker) Z95.810
      implant or graft Z95.9
         specified type NEC Z95.818
      pacemaker Z95.0
      resynchronization therapy
         defibrillator Z95.810
         pacemaker Z95.0
   cardioverter-defibrillator (ICD) Z95.810
   cerebrospinal fluid drainage device Z98.2
   cochlear implant (functional) Z96.21
   contact lens (es) Z97.3
   coronary artery graft or prosthesis Z95.5
   CRT-D (cardiac resynchronization therapy defibrillator)
      Z95.810
   CRT P (cardiac resynchronization therapy pacemaker)
      Z95.0
   CSF shunt Z98.2
   dental prosthesis device Z97.2
   dentures Z97.2
   device (external) NEC Z97.8
      cardiac NEC Z95.818
      heart assist Z95.811
      implanted (functional) Z96.9
         specified NEC Z96.89
      prosthetic Z97.8
   ear implant Z96.20
      cochlear implant Z96.21
      myringotomy tube Z96.22
      specified type NEC Z96.29

Presence — *continued*
   elbow-joint implant (functional) (prosthesis) Z96.62- ☑
   endocrine implant (functional) NEC Z96.49
   eustachian tube stent or device (functional) Z96.29
   external hearing-aid or device Z97.4
   finger-joint implant (functional) (prosthetic) Z96.69- ☑
   functional implant Z96.9
      specified NEC Z96.89
   graft
      cardiac NEC Z95.818
      vascular NEC Z95.828
   hearing-aid or device (external) Z97.4
      implant (bone) (cochlear) (functional) Z96.21
   heart assist device Z95.811
   heart valve implant (functional) Z95.2
      prosthetic Z95.2
      specified type NEC Z95.4
      xenogenic Z95.3
   hip-joint implant (functional) (prosthesis) Z96.64- ☑
   ICD (cardioverter-defibrillator) Z95.810
   implanted device (artificial) (functional) (prosthetic)
      Z96.9
      automatic cardiac defibrillator (with synchronous
         cardiac pacemaker) Z95.810
      cardiac pacemaker Z95.0
      cochlear Z96.21
      dental Z96.5
      heart Z95.812
      heart valve Z95.2
         prosthetic Z95.2
         specified NEC Z95.4
         xenogenic Z95.3
      insulin pump Z96.41
      intraocular lens Z96.1
      joint Z96.60
         ankle Z96.66- ☑
         elbow Z96.62- ☑
         finger Z96.69- ☑
         hip Z96.64- ☑
         knee Z96.65- ☑
         shoulder Z96.61- ☑
         specified NEC Z96.698
         wrist Z96.63- ☑
      larynx Z96.3
      myringotomy tube Z96.22
      otological Z96.20
         cochlear Z96.21
         eustachian stent Z96.29
         myringotomy Z96.22
         specified NEC Z96.29
         stapes Z96.29
      skin Z96.81
      skull plate Z96.7
      specified NEC Z96.89
      urogenital Z96.0
   insulin pump (functional) Z96.41
   intestinal bypass or anastomosis Z98.0
   intraocular lens (functional) Z96.1
   intrauterine contraceptive device (IUD) Z97.5
   intravascular implant (functional) (prosthetic) NEC
      Z95.9
      coronary artery Z95.5
      defibrillator (with synchronous cardiac pacemaker)
         Z95.810
      peripheral vessel (with angioplasty) Z95.820
   joint implant (prosthetic) (any) Z96.60
      ankle — *see* Presence, ankle joint implant
      elbow — *see* Presence, elbow joint implant
      finger — *see* Presence, finger joint implant
      hip — *see* Presence, hip joint implant
      knee — *see* Presence, knee joint implant
      shoulder — *see* Presence, shoulder joint implant
      specified joint NEC Z96.698
      wrist   *see* Presence, wrist joint implant
   knee-joint implant (functional) (prosthesis) Z96.65- ☑
   laryngeal implant (functional) Z96.3
   mandibular implant (dental) Z96.5
   myringotomy tube(s) Z96.22
   neurostimulator (brain) (gastric) (peripheral nerve)
      (sacral nerve) (spinal cord) (vagus nerve) Z96.82
   orthopedic-joint implant (prosthetic) (any) — *see*
      Presence, joint implant
   otological implant (functional) Z96.29
   shoulder-joint implant (functional) (prosthesis)
      Z96.61- ☑
   skull-plate implant Z96.7
   spectacles Z97.3
   stapes implant (functional) Z96.29

Presence — *continued*
   systemic lupus erythematosus [SLE] inhibitor D68.62
   tendon implant (functional) (graft) Z96.7
   tooth root(s) implant Z96.5
   ureteral stent Z96.0
   urethral stent Z96.0
   urogenital implant (functional) Z96.0
   vascular implant or device Z95.9
      access port device Z95.828
      specified type NEC Z95.828
   wrist-joint implant (functional) (prosthesis) Z96.63- ☑
Presenile — *see also* condition
   dementia F03 ☑
   premature aging E34.8
Presentation, fetal — *see* Delivery, complicated by,
   malposition
Prespondylolisthesis (congenital) Q76.2
Pressure
   area, skin — *see* Ulcer, pressure, by site
   brachial plexus G54.0
   brain G93.5
      injury at birth NEC P11.1
   cerebral — *see* Pressure, brain
   chest R07.89
   cone, tentorial G93.5
   hyposystolic — *see also* Hypotension
      incidental reading, without diagnosis of hypoten-
         sion R03.1
   increased
      intracranial (benign) G93.2
         injury at birth P11.0
      intraocular H40.05- ☑
   injury — *see* Ulcer, pressure, by site
   lumbosacral plexus G54.1
   mediastinum J98.59
   necrosis (chronic) — *see* Ulcer, pressure, by site
   parental, inappropriate (excessive) Z62.6
   sore (chronic) — *see* Ulcer, pressure, by site
   spinal cord G95.20
   ulcer (chronic) — *see* Ulcer, pressure, by site
   venous, increased I87.8
Pre-syncope R55
Preterm
   delivery — *see also* Pregnancy, complicated by,
      preterm labor O60.10 ☑
   labor — *see* Pregnancy, complicated by, preterm labor
   newborn (infant) P07.30
      gestational age
         28 completed weeks (28 weeks, 0 days through
            28 weeks, 6 days) P07.31
         29 completed weeks (29 weeks, 0 days through
            29 weeks, 6 days) P07.32
         30 completed weeks (30 weeks, 0 days through
            30 weeks, 6 days) P07.33
         31 completed weeks (31 weeks, 0 days through
            31 weeks, 6 days) P07.34
         32 completed weeks (32 weeks, 0 days through
            32 weeks, 6 days) P07.35
         33 completed weeks (33 weeks, 0 days through
            33 weeks, 6 days) P07.36
         34 completed weeks (34 weeks, 0 days through
            34 weeks, 6 days) P07.37
         35 completed weeks (35 weeks, 0 days through
            35 weeks, 6 days) P07.38
         36 completed weeks (36 weeks, 0 days through
            36 weeks, 6 days) P07.39
Previa
   placenta (total) (without hemorrhage) O44.0- ☑
      with hemorrhage O44.1- ☑
      complete O44.0- ☑
         with hemorrhage O44.1- ☑
      low — *see also* Delivery, complicated, by, placenta,
         low O44.4- ☑
         with hemorrhage O44.5- ☑
      marginal O44.2- ☑
         with hemorrhage O44.3- ☑
      partial O44.2- ☑
         with hemorrhage O44.3- ☑
   vasa O69.4 ☑
Priapism N48.30
   due to
      disease classified elsewhere N48.32
      drug N48.33
      specified cause NEC N48.39
      trauma N48.31
Prickling sensation (skin) R20.2
Prickly heat L74.0

Primary — *see* condition
Primigravida
    elderly, affecting management of pregnancy, labor and delivery (supervision only) — *see* Pregnancy, complicated by, elderly, primigravida
    older, affecting management of pregnancy, labor and delivery (supervision only) — *see* Pregnancy, complicated by, elderly, primigravida
    very young, affecting management of pregnancy, labor and delivery (supervision only) — *see* Pregnancy, complicated by, young mother, primigravida
Primipara
    elderly, affecting management of pregnancy, labor and delivery (supervision only) — *see* Pregnancy, complicated by, elderly, primigravida
    older, affecting management of pregnancy, labor and delivery (supervision only) — *see* Pregnancy, complicated by, elderly, primigravida
    very young, affecting management of pregnancy, labor and delivery (supervision only) — *see* Pregnancy, complicated by, young mother, primigravida
Primus varus Q66.21- ☑
PRIND (Prolonged reversible ischemic neurologic deficit) I63.9
Pringle's disease (tuberous sclerosis) Q85.1
Prinzmetal angina I20.1
Prizefighter ear — *see* Cauliflower ear
Problem (with) (related to)
    academic Z55.8
    acculturation Z60.3
    adjustment (to)
        change of job Z56.1
        life-cycle transition Z60.0
        pension Z60.0
        retirement Z60.0
    adopted child Z62.821
    alcoholism in family Z63.72
    atypical parenting situation Z62.9
    bankruptcy Z59.8
    behavioral (adult) F69
        drug seeking Z76.5
    birth of sibling affecting child Z62.898
    care (of)
        provider dependency Z74.9
            specified NEC Z74.8
        sick or handicapped person in family or household Z63.6
    child
        abuse (affecting the child) — *see* Maltreatment, child
        custody or support proceedings Z65.3
        in care of non-parental family member Z62.21
        in foster care Z62.21
        in welfare custody Z62.21
        living in orphanage or group home Z62.22
    child-rearing Z62.9
        specified NEC Z62.898
    communication (developmental) F80.9
    conflict or discord (with)
        boss Z56.4
        classmates Z55.4
        counselor Z64.4
        employer Z56.4
        family Z63.9
            specified NEC Z63.8
        probation officer Z64.4
        social worker Z64.4
        teachers Z55.4
        workmates Z56.4
    conviction in legal proceedings Z65.0
        with imprisonment Z65.1
    counselor Z64.4
    creditors Z59.8
    digestive K92.9
    drug addict in family Z63.72
    ear — *see* Disorder, ear
    economic Z59.9
        affecting care Z59.9
        specified NEC Z59.8
    education Z55.9
        specified NEC Z55.8
    employment Z56.9
        change of job Z56.1
        discord Z56.4
        environment Z56.5
        sexual harassment Z56.81
        specified NEC Z56.89
        stressful schedule Z56.3

Problem — *continued*
    employment — *continued*
        stress NEC Z56.6
        threat of job loss Z56.2
        unemployment Z56.0
    enuresis, child F98.0
    eye H57.9
    failed examinations (school) Z55.2
    falling Z91.81
    family — *see also* Disruption, family Z63.9
        specified NEC Z63.8
    feeding (elderly) (infant) R63.3
        newborn P92.9
            breast P92.5
            overfeeding P92.4
            slow P92.2
            specified NEC P92.8
            underfeeding P92.3
        nonorganic F50.89
    finance Z59.9
        specified NEC Z59.8
    foreclosure on loan Z59.8
    foster child Z62.822
    frightening experience(s) in childhood Z62.898
    genital NEC
        female N94.9
        male N50.9
    health care Z75.9
        specified NEC Z75.8
    hearing — *see* Deafness
    homelessness Z59.0
    housing Z59.9
        inadequate Z59.1
        isolated Z59.8
        specified NEC Z59.8
    identity (of childhood) F93.8
    illegitimate pregnancy (unwanted) Z64.0
    illiteracy Z55.0
    impaired mobility Z74.09
    imprisonment or incarceration Z65.1
    inadequate teaching affecting education Z55.8
    inappropriate (excessive) parental pressure Z62.6
    influencing health status NEC Z78.9
    in-law Z63.1
    institutionalization, affecting child Z62.22
    intrafamilial communication Z63.8
    jealousy, child F93.8
    landlord Z59.2
    language (developmental) F80.9
    learning (developmental) F81.9
    legal Z65.3
        conviction without imprisonment Z65.0
        imprisonment Z65.1
        release from prison Z65.2
    life-management Z73.9
        specified NEC Z73.89
    life-style Z72.9
        gambling Z72.6
        high-risk sexual behavior (heterosexual) Z72.51
            bisexual Z72.53
            homosexual Z72.52
        inappropriate eating habits Z72.4
        self-damaging behavior NEC Z72.89
        specified NEC Z72.89
        tobacco use Z72.0
    literacy Z55.9
        low level Z55.0
        specified NEC Z55.8
    living alone Z60.2
    lodgers Z59.2
    loss of love relationship in childhood Z62.898
    marital Z63.0
        involving
            divorce Z63.5
            estrangement Z63.5
            gender identity F66
    mastication K08.89
    medical
        care, within family Z63.6
        facilities Z75.9
            specified NEC Z75.8
    mental F48.9
    multiparity Z64.1
    negative life events in childhood Z62.9
        altered pattern of family relationships Z62.898
        frightening experience Z62.898
        loss of
            love relationship Z62.898
            self-esteem Z62.898

Problem — *continued*
    negative life events in childhood — *continued*
        physical abuse (alleged) — *see* Maltreatment, chil
        removal from home Z62.29
        specified event NEC Z62.898
    neighbor Z59.2
    neurological NEC R29.818
    new step-parent affecting child Z62.898
    none (feared complaint unfounded) Z71.1
    occupational NEC Z56.89
    parent-child — *see* Conflict, parent-child
    personal hygiene Z91.89
    personality F69
    phase-of-life transition, adjustment Z60.0
    presence of sick or disabled person in family or house hold Z63.79
        needing care Z63.6
    primary support group (family) Z63.9
        specified NEC Z63.8
    probation officer Z64.4
    psychiatric F99
    psychosexual (development) F66
    psychosocial Z65.9
        religious or spiritual Z65.8
        specified NEC Z65.8
    relationship Z63.9
        childhood F93.8
    release from prison Z65.2
        religious or spiritual Z65.8
    removal from home affecting child Z62.29
    seeking and accepting known hazardous and harmfu
        behavioral or psychological interventions Z65.8
        chemical, nutritional or physical interventions Z65.
    sexual function (nonorganic) F52.9
    sight H54.7
    sleep disorder, child F51.9
    smell — *see* Disturbance, sensation, smell
    social
        environment Z60.9
            specified NEC Z60.8
        exclusion and rejection Z60.4
        worker Z64.4
    speech R47.9
        developmental F80.9
        specified NEC R47.89
    swallowing — *see* Dysphagia
    taste — *see* Disturbance, sensation, taste
    tic, child F95.0
    underachievement in school Z55.3
    unemployment Z56.0
        threatened Z56.2
    unwanted pregnancy Z64.0
    upbringing Z62.9
        specified NEC Z62.898
    urinary N39.9
    voice production R47.89
    work schedule (stressful) Z56.3
Procedure (surgical)
    converted
        arthroscopic to open Z53.33
        laparoscopic to open Z53.31
        specified procedure NEC to open Z53.39
        thoracoscopic to open Z53.32
    for purpose other than remedying health state Z41.9
        specified NEC Z41.8
    not done Z53.9
        because of
            administrative reasons Z53.8
            contraindication Z53.09
                smoking Z53.01
            patient's decision Z53.20
                for reasons of belief or group pressure Z53.1
                left against medical advice (AMA) Z53.21
                specified reason NEC Z53.29
            specified reason NEC Z53.8
Procidentia (uteri) N81.3
Proctalgia K62.89
    fugax K59.4
    spasmodic K59.4
Proctitis K62.89
    amebic (acute) A06.0
    chlamydial A56.3
    gonococcal A54.6
    granulomatous — *see* Enteritis, regional, large intestine
    herpetic A60.1
    radiation K62.7
    tuberculous A18.32
    ulcerative (chronic) K51.20

Proctitis — *continued*
  ulcerative — *continued*
    with
      complication K51.219
        abscess K51.214
        fistula K51.213
        obstruction K51.212
        rectal bleeding K51.211
        specified NEC K51.218
Proctocele
  female (without uterine prolapse) N81.6
    with uterine prolapse N81.2
      complete N81.3
  male K62.3
Proctocolitis
  food protein-induced K52.82
  food-induced eosinophilic K52.82
  milk protein-induced K52.82
  mucosal — *see* Rectosigmoiditis, ulcerative
Proctoptosis K62.3
Proctorrhagia K62.5
Proctosigmoiditis K63.89
  ulcerative (chronic) — *see* Rectosigmoiditis, ulcerative
Proctospasm K59.4
  psychogenic F45.8
Profichet's disease — *see* Disorder, soft tissue, specified type NEC
Progeria E34.8
Prognathism (mandibular) (maxillary) M26.19
Progonoma (melanotic) — *see* Neoplasm, benign, by site
Progressive — *see* condition
Prolactinoma
  specified site — *see* Neoplasm, benign, by site
  unspecified site D35.2
Prolapse, prolapsed
  anus, anal (canal) (sphincter) K62.2
  arm or hand O32.2 ☑
    causing obstructed labor O64.4 ☑
  bladder (mucosa) (sphincter) (acquired)
    congenital Q79.4
    female — *see* Cystocele
    male N32.89
  breast implant (prosthetic) T85.49 ☑
  cecostomy K94.09
  cecum K63.4
  cervix, cervical (hypertrophied) N81.2
    anterior lip, obstructing labor O65.5
    congenital Q51.828
    postpartal, old N81.2
    stump N81.85
  ciliary body (traumatic) — *see* Laceration, eye(ball), with prolapse or loss of interocular tissue
  colon (pedunculated) K63.4
  colostomy K94.09
  disc (intervertebral) — *see* Displacement, intervertebral disc
  eye implant (orbital) T85.398 ☑
    lens (ocular) — *see* Complications, intraocular lens
  fallopian tube N83.4- ☑
  gastric (mucosa) K31.89
  genital, female N81.9
    specified NEC N81.89
  globe, nontraumatic — *see* Luxation, globe
  ileostomy bud K94.19
  intervertebral disc — *see* Displacement, intervertebral disc
  intestine (small) K63.4
  iris (traumatic) — *see* Laceration, eye(ball), with prolapse or loss of interocular tissue
    nontraumatic H21.89
  kidney N28.83
    congenital Q63.2
  laryngeal muscles or ventricle J38.7
  liver K76.89
  meatus urinarius N36.8
  mitral (valve) I34.1
  ocular lens implant — *see* Complications, intraocular lens
  organ or site, congenital NEC — *see* Malposition, congenital
  ovary N83.4- ☑
  pelvic floor, female N81.89
  perineum, female N81.89
  rectum (mucosa) (sphincter) K62.3
    due to trichuris trichuria B79
  spleen D73.89
  stomach K31.89

Prolapse, prolapsed — *continued*
  umbilical cord
    complicating delivery O69.0 ☑
  urachus, congenital Q64.4
  ureter N28.89
    with obstruction N13.5
      with infection N13.6
  ureterovesical orifice N28.89
  urethra (acquired) (infected) (mucosa) N36.8
    congenital Q64.71
  urinary meatus N36.8
    congenital Q64.72
  uterovaginal N81.4
    complete N81.3
    incomplete N81.2
  uterus (with prolapse of vagina) N81.4
    complete N81.3
    congenital Q51.818
    first degree N81.2
    in pregnancy or childbirth — *see* Pregnancy, complicated by, abnormal, uterus
    incomplete N81.2
    postpartal (old) N81.4
    second degree N81.2
    third degree N81.3
  uveal (traumatic) — *see* Laceration, eye(ball), with prolapse or loss of interocular tissue
  vagina (anterior) (wall) — *see* Cystocele
    with prolapse of uterus N81.4
      complete N81.3
      incomplete N81.2
    posterior wall N81.6
    posthysterectomy N99.3
  vitreous (humor) H43.0- ☑
    in wound — *see* Laceration, eye(ball), with prolapse or loss of interocular tissue
  womb — *see* Prolapse, uterus
Prolapsus, female N81.9
  specified NEC N81.89
Proliferation(s)
  primary cutaneous CD30-positive large T-cell C86.6
  prostate, atypical small acinar N42.32
Proliferative — *see* condition
Prolonged, prolongation (of)
  bleeding (time) (idiopathic) R79.1
  coagulation (time) R79.1
  gestation (over 42 completed weeks)
    mother O48.1
    newborn P08.22
  interval I44.0
  labor O63.9
    first stage O63.0
    second stage O63.1
  partial thromboplastin time (PTT) R79.1
  pregnancy (more than 42 weeks gestation) O48.1
  prothrombin time R79.1
  QT interval R94.31
  uterine contractions in labor O62.4
Prominence, prominent
  auricle (congenital) (ear) Q17.5
  ischial spine or sacral promontory with disproportion (fetopelvic)
    with disproportion (fetopelvic) O33.0
      causing obstructed labor O65.0
  nose (congenital) acquired M95.0
Promiscuity — *see* High, risk, sexual behavior
Pronation
  ankle — *see* Deformity, limb, foot, specified NEC
  foot — *see also* Deformity, limb, foot, specified NEC
    congenital Q74.2
Prophylactic
  administration of
    antibiotics, long-term Z79.2
      short-term use — *omit code*
    drug — *see also* Long-term (current) drug therapy (use of) Z79.899
    medication Z79.899
    organ removal (for neoplasia management) Z40.00
      breast Z40.01
      fallopian tube(s) Z40.03
        with ovary(s) Z40.02
      ovary(s) Z40.02
      specified site NEC Z40.09
    surgery Z40.9
      for risk factors related to malignant neoplasm — *see* Prophylactic, organ removal
      specified NEC Z40.8
  vaccination Z23

Propionic acidemia E71.121
Proptosis (ocular) — *see also* Exophthalmos
  thyroid — *see* Hyperthyroidism, with goiter
Prosecution, anxiety concerning Z65.3
Prosopagnosia R48.3
Prostadynia N42.81
Prostate, prostatic — *see* condition
Prostatism — *see* Hyperplasia, prostate
Prostatitis (congestive) (suppurative) (with cystitis) N41.9
  acute N41.0
  cavitary N41.8
  chronic N41.1
  diverticular N41.8
  due to Trichomonas (vaginalis) A59.02
  fibrous N41.1
  gonococcal (acute) (chronic) A54.22
  granulomatous N41.4
  hypertrophic N41.1
  subacute N41.1
  trichomonal A59.02
  tuberculous A18.14
Prostatocystitis N41.3
Prostatorrhea N42.89
Prostatosis N42.82
Prostration R53.83
  heat — *see also* Heat, exhaustion
    anhydrotic T67.3 ☑
    due to
      salt (and water) depletion T67.4 ☑
      water depletion T67.3 ☑
  nervous F48.8
  senile R54
Protanomaly (anomalous trichromat) H53.54
Protanopia (complete) (incomplete) H53.54
Protection (against) (from) — *see* Prophylactic
Protein
  deficiency NEC — *see* Malnutrition
  malnutrition — *see* Malnutrition
  sickness — *see also* Reaction, serum T80.69 ☑
Proteinemia R77.9
Proteinosis
  alveolar (pulmonary) J84.01
  lipid or lipoid (of Urbach) E78.89
Proteinuria R80.9
  Bence Jones R80.3
  complicating pregnancy — *see* Proteinuria, gestational
  gestational
    complicating
      childbirth O12.14
      pregnancy O12.1- ☑
        with edema O12.2- ☑
      puerperium O12.15
  idiopathic R80.0
  isolated R80.0
    with glomerular lesion N06.9
      dense deposit disease N06.6
      diffuse
        crescentic glomerulonephritis N06.7
        endocapillary proliferative glomerulonephritis N06.4
        mesangiocapillary glomerulonephritis N06.5
      focal and segmental hyalinosis or sclerosis N06.1
      membranous (diffuse) N06.2
      mesangial proliferative (diffuse) N06.3
      minimal change N06.0
      specified pathology NEC N06.8
  orthostatic R80.2
    with glomerular lesion — *see* Proteinuria, isolated, with glomerular lesion
  persistent R80.1
    with glomerular lesion — *see* Proteinuria, isolated, with glomerular lesion
  postural R80.2
    with glomerular lesion — *see* Proteinuria, isolated, with glomerular lesion
  pre-eclamptic — *see* Pre-eclampsia
  puerperal O12.15
  specified type NEC R80.8
Proteolysis, pathologic D65
Proteus (mirabilis) (morganii), **as cause of disease classified elsewhere** B96.4
Prothrombin gene mutation D68.52
Protoporphyria, erythropoietic E80.0
Protozoal — *see also* condition
  disease B64
    specified NEC B60.8

Protrusion, protrusio
  acetabuli M24.7
  acetabulum (into pelvis) M24.7
  device, implant or graft — *see also* Complications, by
      site and type, mechanical T85.698 ☑
    arterial graft NEC — *see* Complication, cardiovascu-
        lar device, mechanical, vascular
    breast (implant) T85.49 ☑
    catheter NEC T85.698 ☑
      cystostomy T83.090 ☑
      dialysis (renal) T82.49 ☑
        intraperitoneal T85.691 ☑
      infusion NEC T82.594 ☑
        spinal (epidural) (subdural) T85.690 ☑
      urinary — *see also* Complications, catheter, uri-
          nary T83.098 ☑
    electronic (electrode) (pulse generator) (stimulator)
        bone T84.390 ☑
      nervous system — *see* Complication, prosthetic
          device, mechanical, electronic nervous
          system stimulator
    fixation, internal (orthopedic) NEC — *see* Complica-
        tion, fixation device, mechanical
    gastrointestinal — *see* Complications, prosthetic
        device, mechanical, gastrointestinal device
    genital NEC T83.498 ☑
      intrauterine contraceptive device T83.39 ☑
      penile prosthesis (cylinder) (implanted) (pump)
          (resevoir) T83.490 ☑
      testicular prosthesis T83.491 ☑
    heart NEC — *see* Complication, cardiovascular de-
        vice, mechanical
    joint prosthesis — *see* Complications, joint prosthe-
        sis, mechanical, specified NEC, by site
    ocular NEC — *see* Complications, prosthetic device,
        mechanical, ocular device
    orthopedic NEC — *see* Complication, orthopedic,
        device, mechanical
    specified NEC T85.628 ☑
    urinary NEC — *see also* Complication, genitourinary,
        device, urinary, mechanical
      graft T83.29 ☑
    vascular NEC — *see* Complication, cardiovascular
        device, mechanical
    ventricular intracranial shunt T85.09 ☑
  intervertebral disc — *see* Displacement, intervertebral
      disc
  joint prosthesis — *see* Complications, joint prosthesis,
      mechanical, specified NEC, by site
  nucleus pulposus — *see* Displacement, intervertebral
      disc
Prune belly (syndrome) Q79.4
Prurigo (ferox) (gravis) (Hebrae) (Hebra's) (mitis) (simplex)
    L28.2
  Besnier's L20.0
  estivalis L56.4
  nodularis L28.1
  psychogenic F45.8
Pruritus, pruritic (essential) L29.9
  ani, anus L29.0
    psychogenic F45.8
  anogenital L29.3
    psychogenic F45.8
  due to onchocerca volvulus B73.1
  gravidarum — *see* Pregnancy, complicated by, speci-
      fied pregnancy-related condition NEC
  hiemalis L29.8
  neurogenic (any site) F45.8
  perianal L29.0
  psychogenic (any site) F45.8
  scroti, scrotum L29.1
    psychogenic F45.8
  senile, senilis L29.8
  specified NEC L29.8
    psychogenic F45.8
  Trichomonas A59.9
  vulva, vulvae L29.2
    psychogenic F45.8
Pseudarthrosis, pseudoarthrosis (bone) — *see*
    Nonunion, fracture
  clavicle, congenital Q74.0
  joint, following fusion or arthrodesis M96.0
Pseudoaneurysm — *see* Aneurysm
Pseudoangina (pectoris) — *see* Angina
Pseudoangioma I81
Pseudoarteriosus Q28.8
Pseudoarthrosis — *see* Pseudarthrosis

Pseudobulbar affect (PBA) F48.2
Pseudochromhidrosis L67.8
Pseudocirrhosis, liver, pericardial I31.1
Pseudocowpox B08.03
Pseudocoxalgia M91.3- ☑
Pseudocroup J38.5
Pseudo-Cushing's syndrome, alcohol-induced E24.4
Pseudocyesis F45.8
Pseudocyst
  lung J98.4
  pancreas K86.3
  retina — *see* Cyst, retina
Pseudoelephantiasis neuroarthritica Q82.0
Pseudoexfoliation, capsule (lens) — *see* Cataract,
    specified NEC
Pseudofolliculitis barbae L73.1
Pseudoglioma H44.89
Pseudohemophilia (Bernuth's) (hereditary) (type B)
    D68.0
  Type A D69.8
  vascular D69.8
Pseudohermaphroditism Q56.3
  adrenal E25.8
  female Q56.2
    with adrenocortical disorder E25.8
    without adrenocortical disorder Q56.2
      adrenal (congenital) E25.0
    unspecified E25.9
  male Q56.1
    with
      5-alpha-reductase deficiency E29.1
      adrenocortical disorder E25.8
      androgen resistance E34.51
      cleft scrotum Q56.1
      feminizing testis E34.51
    without gonadal disorder Q56.1
      adrenal E25.8
    unspecified E25.9
Pseudo-Hurler's polydystrophy E77.0
Pseudohydrocephalus G93.2
Pseudohypertrophic muscular dystrophy (Erb's)
    G71.02
Pseudohypertrophy, muscle G71.09
Pseudohypoparathyroidism E20.1
Pseudoinsomnia F51.03
Pseudoleukemia, infantile D64.89
Pseudomembranous — *see* condition
Pseudomeningocele (cerebral) (infective) (post-traumat-
    ic) G96.19
  postprocedural (spinal) G97.82
Pseudomenses (newborn) P54.6
Pseudomenstruation (newborn) P54.6
Pseudomonas
  aeruginosa, as cause of disease classified elsewhere
      B96.5
  mallei infection A24.0
    as cause of disease classified elsewhere B96.5
    pseudomallei, as cause of disease classified elsewhere
        B96.5
Pseudomyotonia G71.19
Pseudomyxoma peritonei C78.6
Pseudoneuritis, optic (nerve) (disc) (papilla), **congenital**
    Q14.2
Pseudo-obstruction intestine (acute) (chronic) (idio-
    pathic) (intermittent secondary) (primary) K59.8
Pseudopapilledema H47.33- ☑
  congenital Q14.2
Pseudoparalysis
  arm or leg R29.818
  atonic, congenital P94.2
Pseudopelade L66.0
Pseudophakia Z96.1
Pseudopolyarthritis, rhizomelic M35.3
Pseudopolycythemia D75.1
Pseudopseudohypoparathyroidism E20.1
Pseudopterygium H11.81- ☑
Pseudoptosis (eyelid) — *see* Blepharochalasis
Pseudopuberty, precocious
  female heterosexual E25.8
  male isosexual E25.8
Pseudorickets (renal) N25.0
Pseudorubella B08.20
Pseudosclerema, newborn P83.88
Pseudosclerosis (brain)
  Jakob's — *see* Creutzfeldt-Jakob disease or syndrome
    of Westphal (Strümpell) E83.01
  spastic — *see* Creutzfeldt-Jakob disease or syndrome

Pseudotetanus — *see* Convulsions
Pseudotetany R29.0
  hysterical F44.5
Pseudotruncus arteriosus Q25.49
Pseudotuberculosis A28.2
  enterocolitis A04.8
  pasteurella (infection) A28.0
Pseudotumor
  cerebri G93.2
  orbital H05.11 ☑
Pseudoxanthoma elasticum Q82.8
Psilosis (sprue) (tropical) K90.1
  nontropical K90.0
Psittacosis A70
Psoitis M60.88
Psoriasis L40.9
  arthropathic L40.50
    arthritis mutilans L40.52
    distal interphalangeal L40.51
    juvenile L40.54
    other specified L40.59
    spondylitis L40.53
  buccal K13.29
  flexural L40.8
  guttate L40.4
  mouth K13.29
  nummular L40.0
  plaque L40.0
  psychogenic F54
  pustular (generalized) L40.1
    palmaris et plantaris L40.3
  specified NEC L40.8
  vulgaris L40.0
Psychasthenia F48.8
Psychiatric disorder or problem F99
Psychogenic — *see also* condition
  factors associated with physical conditions F54
**Psychological and behavioral factors affecting
    medical condition** F59
Psychoneurosis, psychoneurotic — *see also* Neuros
  anxiety (state) F41.1
  depersonalization F48.1
  hypochondriacal F45.21
  hysteria F44.9
  neurasthenic F48.8
  personality NEC F60.89
Psychopathy, psychopathic
  affectionless F94.2
  autistic F84.5
  constitution, post-traumatic F07.81
  personality — *see* Disorder, personality
  sexual — *see* Deviation, sexual
  state F60.2
Psychosexual identity disorder of childhood F64.2
Psychosis, psychotic F29
  acute (transient) F23
    hysterical F44.9
  affective — *see* Disorder, mood
  alcoholic F10.959
    with
      abuse F10.159
      anxiety disorder F10.980
        with
          abuse F10.180
          dependence F10.280
      delirium tremens F10.231
      delusions F10.950
        with
          abuse F10.150
          dependence F10.250
      dementia F10.97
        with dependence F10.27
      dependence F10.259
      hallucinosis F10.951
        with
          abuse F10.151
          dependence F10.251
      mood disorder F10.94
        with
          abuse F10.14
          dependence F10.24
      paranoia F10.950
        with
          abuse F10.150
          dependence F10.250
      persisting amnesia F10.96
        with dependence F10.26
      amnestic confabulatory F10.96

☑ **Additional Character Required** — Refer to the Tabular List for Character Selection   ▽ **Subterms under main terms may continue to next column or page**

sychosis, psychotic — *continued*
alcoholic — *continued*
amnestic confabulatory — *continued*
with dependence F10.26
delirium tremens F10.231
Korsakoff's, Korsakov's, Korsakow's F10.26
paranoid type F10.950
with
abuse F10.150
dependence F10.250
anergastic — *see* Psychosis, organic
arteriosclerotic (simple type) (uncomplicated) F01.50
with behavioral disturbance F01.51
childhood F84.0
atypical F84.8
climacteric — *see* Psychosis, involutional
confusional F29
acute or subacute F05
reactive F23
cycloid F23
depressive — *see* Disorder, depressive
disintegrative (childhood) F84.3
drug-induced — *see* F11-F19 with .X59
paranoid and hallucinatory states — *see* F11-F19
with .X50 or .X51
due to or associated with
addiction, drug — *see* F11-F19 with .X59
dependence
alcohol F10.259
drug — *see* F11-F19 with .X59
epilepsy F06.8
Huntington's chorea F06.8
ischemia, cerebrovascular (generalized) F06.8
multiple sclerosis F06.8
physical disease F06.8
presenile dementia F03 ☑
senile dementia F03 ☑
vascular disease (arteriosclerotic) (cerebral) F01.50
with behavioral disturbance F01.51
epileptic F06.8
episode F23
due to or associated with physical condition F06.8
exhaustive F43.0
hallucinatory, chronic F28
hypomanic F30.8
hysterical (acute) F44.9
induced F24
infantile F84.0
atypical F84.8
infective (acute) (subacute) F05
involutional F28
depressive — *see* Disorder, depressive
melancholic — *see* Disorder, depressive
paranoid (state) F22
Korsakoff's, Korsakov's, Korsakow's (nonalcoholic) F04
alcoholic F10.96
in dependence F10.26
induced by other psychoactive substance — *see*
categories F11-F19 with .X5X
mania, manic (single episode) F30.2
recurrent type F31.89
manic-depressive — *see* Disorder, bipolar
menopausal — *see* Psychosis, involutional
mixed schizophrenic and affective F25.8
multi-infarct (cerebrovascular) F01.50
with behavioral disturbance F01.51
nonorganic F29
specified NEC F28
organic F09
due to or associated with
arteriosclerosis (cerebral) — *see* Psychosis, arteriosclerotic
cerebrovascular disease, arteriosclerotic — *see*
Psychosis, arteriosclerotic
childbirth — *see* Psychosis, puerperal
Creutzfeldt-Jakob disease or syndrome — *see*
Creutzfeldt-Jakob disease or syndrome
dependence, alcohol F10.259
disease
alcoholic liver F10.259
brain, arteriosclerotic — *see* Psychosis, arteriosclerotic
cerebrovascular F01.50
with behavioral disturbance F01.51
Creutzfeldt-Jakob — *see* Creutzfeldt-Jakob
disease or syndrome
endocrine or metabolic F06.8
acute or subacute F05

Psychosis, psychotic — *continued*
organic — *continued*
due to or associated with — *continued*
disease — *continued*
liver, alcoholic F10.259
epilepsy transient (acute) F05
infection
brain (intracranial) F06.8
acute or subacute F05
intoxication
alcoholic (acute) F10.259
drug F11-F19 with .x59
ischemia, cerebrovascular (generalized) — *see*
Psychosis, arteriosclerotic
puerperium — *see* Psychosis, puerperal
trauma, brain (birth) (from electric current) (surgical) F06.8
acute or subacute F05
infective F06.8
acute or subacute F05
post-traumatic F06.8
acute or subacute F05
paranoiac F22
paranoid (climacteric) (involutional) (menopausal) F22
psychogenic (acute) F23
schizophrenic F20.0
senile F03 ☑
postpartum (NOS) F53.1
presbyophrenic (type) F03 ☑
presenile F03 ☑
psychogenic (paranoid) F23
depressive F32.3
puerperal (NOS) F53.1
specified type — *see* Psychosis, by type
reactive (brief) (transient) (emotional stress) (psychological trauma) F23
depressive F32.3
recurrent F33.3
excitative type F30.8
schizoaffective F25.9
depressive type F25.1
manic type F25.0
schizophrenia, schizophrenic — *see* Schizophrenia
schizophrenia-like, in epilepsy F06.2
schizophreniform F20.81
affective type F25.9
brief F23
confusional type F23
mixed type F25.0
senile NEC F03 ☑
depressed or paranoid type F03 ☑
simple deterioration F03 ☑
specified type — *code to* condition
shared F24
situational (reactive) F23
symbiotic (childhood) F84.3
symptomatic F09
Psychosomatic — *see* Disorder, psychosomatic
Psychosyndrome, organic F07.9
Psychotic episode due to or associated with physical
condition F06.8
Pterygium (eye) H11.00- ☑
amyloid H11.01- ☑
central H11.02- ☑
colli Q18.3
double H11.03- ☑
peripheral
progressive H11.05- ☑
stationary H11.04- ☑
recurrent H11.06- ☑
Ptilosis (eyelid) — *see* Madarosis
Ptomaine (poisoning) — *see* Poisoning, food
Ptosis — *see also* Blepharoptosis
adiposa (false) — *see* Blepharoptosis
breast N64.81-
brow H57.81- ☑
cecum K63.4
colon K63.4
congenital (eyelid) Q10.0
specified site NEC — *see* Anomaly, by site
eyebrow H57.81- ☑
eyelid — *see* Blepharoptosis
congenital Q10.0
gastric K31.89
intestine K63.4
kidney N28.83
liver K76.89
renal N28.83

Ptosis — *continued*
splanchnic K63.4
spleen D73.89
stomach K31.89
viscera K63.4
PTP D69.51
Ptyalism (periodic) K11.7
hysterical F45.8
pregnancy — *see* Pregnancy, complicated by, specified
pregnancy-related condition NEC
psychogenic F45.8
Ptyalolithiasis K11.5
Pubarche, precocious E30.1
Pubertas praecox E30.1
Puberty (development state) Z00.3
bleeding (excessive) N92.2
delayed E30.0
precocious (constitutional) (cryptogenic) (idiopathic)
E30.1
central E22.8
due to
ovarian hyperfunction E28.1
estrogen E28.0
testicular hyperfunction E29.0
premature E30.1
due to
adrenal cortical hyperfunction E25.8
pineal tumor E34.8
pituitary (anterior) hyperfunction E22.8
Puckering, macula — *see* Degeneration, macula, puckering
Pudenda, pudendum — *see* condition
Puente's disease (simple glandular cheilitis) K13.0
Puerperal, puerperium (complicated by, complications)
abnormal glucose (tolerance test) O99.815
abscess
areola O91.02
associated with lactation O91.03
Bartholin's gland O86.19
breast O91.12
associated with lactation O91.13
cervix (uteri) O86.11
genital organ NEC O86.19
kidney O86.21
mammary O91.12
associated with lactation O91.13
nipple O91.02
associated with lactation O91.03
peritoneum O85
subareolar O91.12
associated with lactation O91.13
urinary tract — *see* Puerperal, infection, urinary
uterus O86.12
vagina (wall) O86.13
vaginorectal O86.13
vulvovaginal gland O86.13
adnexitis O86.19
afibrinogenemia, or other coagulation defect O72.3
albuminuria (acute) (subacute) — *see* Proteinuria,
gestational
alcohol use O99.315
anemia O90.81
pre-existing (pre-pregnancy) O99.03
anesthetic death O89.8
apoplexy O99.43
bariatric surgery status O99.845
blood disorder NEC O99.13
blood dyscrasia O72.3
cardiomyopathy O90.3
cerebrovascular disorder (conditions in I60-I69) O99.43
cervicitis O86.11
circulatory system disorder O99.43
coagulopathy (any) O99.13
with hemorrhage O72.3
complications O90.9
specified NEC O90.89
convulsions — *see* Eclampsia
cystitis O86.22
cystopyelitis O86.29
delirium NEC F05
diabetes O24.93
gestational — *see* Puerperal, gestational diabetes
pre-existing O24.33
specified NEC O24.83
type 1 O24.03
type 2 O24.13
digestive system disorder O99.63
disease O90.9

Puerperal, puerperium — *continued*
  disease — *continued*
    breast NEC O92.29
    cerebrovascular (acute) O99.43
    nonobstetric NEC O99.89
    tubo-ovarian O86.19
    Valsuani's O99.03
  disorder O90.9
    biliary tract O26.63
    lactation O92.70
    liver O26.63
    nonobstetric NEC O99.89
  disruption
    cesarean wound O90.0
    episiotomy wound O90.1
    perineal laceration wound O90.1
  drug use O99.325
  eclampsia (with pre-existing hypertension) O15.2
  embolism (pulmonary) (blood clot) — *see* Embolism, obstetric, puerperal
  endocrine, nutritional or metabolic disease NEC O99.285
  endophlebitis — *see* Puerperal, phlebitis
  endotrachelitis O86.11
  failure
    lactation (complete) O92.3
      partial O92.4
    renal, acute O90.4
  fever (of unknown origin) O86.4
    septic O85
  fissure, nipple O92.12
    associated with lactation O92.13
  fistula
    breast (due to mastitis) O91.12
      associated with lactation O91.13
    nipple O91.02
      associated with lactation O91.03
  galactophoritis O91.22
    associated with lactation O91.23
  galactorrhea O92.6
  gastric banding status O99.845
  gastric bypass status O99.845
  gastrointestinal disease NEC O99.63
  gestational
    diabetes O24.439
      diet controlled O24.430
      insulin (and diet) controlled O24.434
      oral drug controlled (antidiabetic) (hypo-glycemic) O24.435
    edema O12.05
      with proteinuria O12.25
    proteinuria O12.15
  gonorrhea O98.23
  hematoma, subdural O99.43
  hemiplegia, cerebral O99.355
    due to cerbrovascular disorder O99.43
  hemorrhage O72.1
    brain O99.43
    bulbar O99.43
    cerebellar O99.43
    cerebral O99.43
    cortical O99.43
    delayed or secondary O72.2
    extradural O99.43
    internal capsule O99.43
    intracranial O99.43
    intrapontine O99.43
    meningeal O99.43
    pontine O99.43
    retained placenta O72.0
    subarachnoid O99.43
    subcortical O99.43
    subdural O99.43
    third stage O72.0
    uterine, delayed O72.2
    ventricular O99.43
  hemorrhoids O87.2
  hepatorenal syndrome O90.4
  hypertension — *see* Hypertension, complicating, puerperium
  hypertrophy, breast O92.29
  induration breast (fibrous) O92.29
  infection O86.4
    cervix O86.11
    generalized O85
    genital tract NEC O86.19
      obstetric surgical wound O86.09
    kidney (bacillus coli) O86.21
    maternal O98.93

Puerperal, puerperium — *continued*
  infection — *continued*
    maternal — *continued*
      carrier state NEC O99.835
      gonorrhea O98.23
      human immunodeficiency virus (HIV) O98.73
      protozoal O98.63
      sexually transmitted NEC O98.33
      specified NEC O98.83
      streptococcus group B (GBS) carrier state O99.825
      syphilis O98.13
      tuberculosis O98.03
      viral hepatitis O98.43
      viral NEC O98.53
    nipple O91.02
      associated with lactation O91.03
    peritoneum O85
    renal O86.21
    specified NEC O86.89
    urinary (asymptomatic) (tract) NEC O86.20
      bladder O86.22
      kidney O86.21
      specified site NEC O86.29
      urethra O86.22
    vagina O86.13
    vein — *see* Puerperal, phlebitis
  ischemia, cerebral O99.43
  lymphangitis O86.89
    breast O91.22
      associated with lactation O91.23
  malignancy O9A.13 (*following* O99)
  malnutrition O25.3
  mammillitis O91.02
    associated with lactation O91.03
  mammitis O91.22
    associated with lactation O91.23
  mania F30.8
  mastitis O91.22
    associated with lactation O91.23
    purulent O91.12
      associated with lactation O91.13
  melancholia — *see* Disorder, depressive
  mental disorder NEC O99.345
  metroperitonitis O85
  metrorrhagia — *see* Hemorrhage, postpartum
  metrosalpingitis O86.19
  metrovaginitis O86.13
  milk leg O87.1
  monoplegia, cerebral O99.43
  mood disturbance O90.6
  necrosis, liver (acute) (subacute) (conditions in subcategory K72.0) O26.63
    with renal failure O90.4
  nervous system disorder O99.355
  obesity (pre-existing prior to pregnancy) O99.215
  obesity surgery status O99.845
  occlusion, precerebral artery O99.43
  paralysis
    bladder (sphincter) O90.89
    cerebral O99.43
  paralytic stroke O99.43
  parametritis O85
  paravaginitis O86.13
  pelviperitonitis O85
  perimetritis O86.12
  perimetrosalpingitis O86.19
  perinephritis O86.21
  periphlebitis — *see* Puerperal phlebitis
  peritoneal infection O85
  peritonitis (pelvic) O85
  perivaginitis O86.13
  phlebitis O87.0
    deep O87.1
    pelvic O87.1
    superficial O87.0
  phlebothrombosis, deep O87.1
  phlegmasia alba dolens O87.1
  placental polyp O90.89
  pneumonia, embolic — *see* Embolism, obstetric, puerperal
  pre-eclampsia — *see* Pre-eclampsia
  psychosis (NOS) F53.1
  pyelitis O86.21
  pyelocystitis O86.29
  pyelonephritis O86.21
  pyelonephrosis O86.21
  pyemia O95
  pyocystitis O86.29
  pyohemia O85

Puerperal, puerperium — *continued*
  pyometra O86.12
  pyonephritis O86.21
  pyosalpingitis O86.19
  pyrexia (of unknown origin) O86.4
  renal
    disease NEC O90.89
    failure O90.4
  respiratory disease NEC O99.53
  retention
    decidua — *see* Retention, decidua
    placenta O72.0
    secundines — *see* Retention, secundines
  retrated nipple O92.02
  salpingo-ovaritis O86.19
  salpingoperitonitis O85
  secondary perineal tear O90.1
  sepsis (pelvic) O85
  sepsis O85
  septic thrombophlebitis O86.81
  skin disorder NEC O99.73
  specified condition NEC O99.89
  stroke O99.43
  subinvolution (uterus) O90.89
  subluxation of symphysis (pubis) O26.73
  suppuration — *see* Puerperal, abscess
  tetanus A34
  thelitis O91.02
    associated with lactation O91.03
  thrombocytopenia O72.3
  thrombophlebitis (superficial) O87.0
    deep O87.1
    pelvic O87.1
    septic O86.81
  thrombosis (venous) — *see* Thrombosis, puerperal
  thyroiditis O90.5
  toxemia (eclamptic) (pre-eclamptic) (with convulsion) O15.2
  trauma, non-obstetric O9A.23 (*following* O99)
    caused by abuse (physical) (suspected) O9A.33 (*following* O99)
      confirmed O9A.33 (*following* O99)
      psychological (suspected) O9A.53 (*following* O99)
        confirmed O9A.53 (*following* O99)
      sexual (suspected) O9A.43 (*following* O99)
        confirmed O9A.43 (*following* O99)
  uremia (due to renal failure) O90.4
  urethritis O86.22
  vaginitis O86.13
  varicose veins (legs) O87.4
    vulva or perineum O87.8
  venous O87.9
  vulvitis O86.19
  vulvovaginitis O86.13
  white leg O87.1
Puerperium — *see* Puerperal
Pulmolithiasis J98.4
Pulmonary — *see* condition
Pulpitis (acute) (anachoretic) (chronic) (hyperplastic) (putrescent) (suppurative) (ulcerative) K04.01
  irreversible K04.02
  reversible K04.01
Pulpless tooth K04.99
Pulse
  alternating R00.8
  bigeminal R00.8
  fast R00.0
  feeble, rapid due to shock following injury T79.4 ☑
  rapid R00.0
  weak R09.89
Pulsus alternans or trigeminus R00.8
Punch drunk F07.81
Punctum lacrimale occlusion — *see* Obstruction, lacrimal
Puncture
  abdomen, abdominal
    wall S31.139 ☑
      with
        foreign body S31.149 ☑
        penetration into peritoneal cavity S31.639 ☑
          with foreign body S31.649 ☑
        epigastric region S31.132 ☑
          with
            foreign body S31.142 ☑
            penetration into peritoneal cavity S31.632 ☑
              with foreign body S31.642 ☑

☑ **Additional Character Required** — **Refer to the Tabular List for Character Selection**   ▽ Subterms under main terms may continue to next column or page

Puncture — *continued*
  abdomen, abdominal — *continued*
    wall — *continued*
      left
        lower quadrant S31.134 ☑
          with
            foreign body S31.144 ☑
            penetration into peritoneal cavity
              S31.634 ☑
              with foreign body S31.644 ☑
        upper quadrant S31.131 ☑
          with
            foreign body S31.141 ☑
            penetration into peritoneal cavity
              S31.631 ☑
              with foreign body S31.641 ☑
      periumbilic region S31.135 ☑
        with
          foreign body S31.145 ☑
          penetration into peritoneal cavity
            S31.635 ☑
            with foreign body S31.645 ☑
      right
        lower quadrant S31.133 ☑
          with
            foreign body S31.143 ☑
            penetration into peritoneal cavity
              S31.633 ☑
              with foreign body S31.643 ☑
        upper quadrant S31.130 ☑
          with
            foreign body S31.140 ☑
            penetration into peritoneal cavity
              S31.630 ☑
              with foreign body S31.640 ☑
  accidental, complicating surgery — *see* Complication, accidental puncture or laceration
  alveolar (process) — *see* Puncture, oral cavity
  ankle S91.039 ☑
    with
      foreign body S91.049 ☑
    left S91.032 ☑
      with
        foreign body S91.042 ☑
    right S91.031 ☑
      with
        foreign body S91.041 ☑
  anus S31.833 ☑
    with foreign body S31.834 ☑
  arm (upper) S41.139 ☑
    with foreign body S41.149 ☑
    left S41.132 ☑
      with foreign body S41.142 ☑
    lower — *see* Puncture, forearm
    right S41.131 ☑
      with foreign body S41.141 ☑
  auditory canal (external) (meatus) — *see* Puncture, ear
  auricle, ear — *see* Puncture, ear
  axilla — *see* Puncture, arm
  back — *see also* Puncture, thorax, back
    lower S31.030 ☑
      with
        foreign body S31.040 ☑
          with penetration into retroperitoneal space S31.041 ☑
        penetration into retroperitoneal space S31.031 ☑
  bladder (traumatic) S37.29 ☑
    nontraumatic N32.89
  breast S21.039 ☑
    with foreign body S21.049 ☑
    left S21.032 ☑
      with foreign body S21.042 ☑
    right S21.031 ☑
      with foreign body S21.041 ☑
  buttock S31.803 ☑
    with foreign body S31.804 ☑
    left S31.823 ☑
      with foreign body S31.824 ☑
    right S31.813 ☑
      with foreign body S31.814 ☑
  by
    device, implant or graft — *see* Complications, by site and type, mechanical
    foreign body left accidentally in operative wound T81.539 ☑

Puncture — *continued*
  by — *continued*
    instrument (any) during a procedure, accidental — *see* Puncture, accidental complicating surgery
  calf — *see* Puncture, leg
  canaliculus lacrimalis — *see* Puncture, eyelid
  canthus, eye — *see* Puncture, eyelid
  cervical esophagus S11.23 ☑
    with foreign body S11.24 ☑
  cheek (external) S01.439 ☑
    with foreign body S01.449 ☑
    internal — *see* Puncture, oral cavity
    left S01.432 ☑
      with foreign body S01.442 ☑
    right S01.431 ☑
      with foreign body S01.441 ☑
  chest wall — *see* Puncture, thorax
  chin — *see* Puncture, head, specified site NEC
  clitoris — *see* Puncture, vulva
  costal region — *see* Puncture, thorax
  digit(s)
    foot — *see* Puncture, toe
    hand — *see* Puncture, finger
  ear (canal) (external) S01.339 ☑
    with foreign body S01.349 ☑
    drum S09.2- ☑
    left S01.332 ☑
      with foreign body S01.342 ☑
    right S01.331 ☑
      with foreign body S01.341 ☑
  elbow S51.039 ☑
    with
      foreign body S51.049 ☑
    left S51.032 ☑
      with
        foreign body S51.042 ☑
    right S51.031 ☑
      with
        foreign body S51.041 ☑
  epididymis — *see* Puncture, testis
  epigastric region — *see* Puncture, abdomen, wall, epigastric
  epiglottis S11.83 ☑
    with foreign body S11.84 ☑
  esophagus
    cervical S11.23 ☑
      with foreign body S11.24 ☑
    thoracic S27.818 ☑
  eyeball S05.6- ☑
    with foreign body S05.5- ☑
  eyebrow — *see* Puncture, eyelid
  eyelid S01.13- ☑
    with foreign body S01.14- ☑
    left S01.132 ☑
      with foreign body S01.142 ☑
    right S01.131 ☑
      with foreign body S01.141 ☑
  face NEC — *see* Puncture, head, specified site NEC
  finger(s) S61.239 ☑
    with
      damage to nail S61.339 ☑
        with
          foreign body S61.349 ☑
      foreign body S61.249 ☑
    index S61.238 ☑
      with
        damage to nail S61.338 ☑
          with
            foreign body S61.348 ☑
        foreign body S61.248 ☑
      left S61.231 ☑
        with
          damage to nail S61.331 ☑
            with
              foreign body S61.341 ☑
          foreign body S61.241 ☑
      right S61.230 ☑
        with
          damage to nail S61.330 ☑
            with
              foreign body S61.340 ☑
          foreign body S61.240 ☑
    little S61.238 ☑
      with
        damage to nail S61.338 ☑

Puncture — *continued*
  finger(s) — *continued*
    little — *continued*
      with — *continued*
        damage to nail — *continued*
          with
            foreign body S61.348 ☑
        foreign body S61.248 ☑
      left S61.237 ☑
        with
          damage to nail S61.337 ☑
            with
              foreign body S61.347 ☑
          foreign body S61.247 ☑
      right S61.236 ☑
        with
          damage to nail S61.336 ☑
            with
              foreign body S61.346 ☑
          foreign body S61.246 ☑
    middle S61.238 ☑
      with
        damage to nail S61.338 ☑
          with
            foreign body S61.348 ☑
        foreign body S61.248 ☑
      left S61.233 ☑
        with
          damage to nail S61.333 ☑
            with
              foreign body S61.343 ☑
          foreign body S61.243 ☑
      right S61.232 ☑
        with
          damage to nail S61.332 ☑
            with
              foreign body S61.342 ☑
          foreign body S61.242 ☑
    ring S61.238 ☑
      with
        damage to nail S61.338 ☑
          with
            foreign body S61.348 ☑
        foreign body S61.248 ☑
      left S61.235 ☑
        with
          damage to nail S61.335 ☑
            with
              foreign body S61.345 ☑
          foreign body S61.245 ☑
      right S61.234 ☑
        with
          damage to nail S61.334 ☑
            with
              foreign body S61.344 ☑
          foreign body S61.244 ☑
  flank S31.139 ☑
    with foreign body S31.149 ☑
  foot (except toe(s) alone) S91.339 ☑
    with foreign body S91.349 ☑
    left S91.332 ☑
      with foreign body S91.342 ☑
    right S91.331 ☑
      with foreign body S91.341 ☑
    toe — *see* Puncture, toe
  forearm S51.839 ☑
    with
      foreign body S51.849 ☑
    elbow only — *see* Puncture, elbow
    left S51.832 ☑
      with
        foreign body S51.842 ☑
    right S51.831 ☑
      with
        foreign body S51.841 ☑
  forehead — *see* Puncture, head, specified site NEC
  genital organs, external
    female S31.532 ☑
      with foreign body S31.542 ☑
      vagina — *see* Puncture, vagina
      vulva — *see* Puncture, vulva
    male S31.531 ☑
      with foreign body S31.541 ☑
      penis — *see* Puncture, penis
      scrotum — *see* Puncture, scrotum
      testis — *see* Puncture, testis

Puncture — *continued*
  groin — *see* Puncture, abdomen, wall
  gum — *see* Puncture, oral cavity
  hand S61.439 ☑
    with
        foreign body S61.449 ☑
      finger — *see* Puncture, finger
      left S61.432 ☑
        with
            foreign body S61.442 ☑
      right S61.431 ☑
        with
            foreign body S61.441 ☑
      thumb — *see* Puncture, thumb
  head S01.93 ☑
    with foreign body S01.94 ☑
      cheek — *see* Puncture, cheek
      ear — *see* Puncture, ear
      eyelid — *see* Puncture, eyelid
      lip — *see* Puncture, oral cavity
      nose — *see* Puncture, nose
      oral cavity — *see* Puncture, oral cavity
      scalp S01.03 ☑
        with foreign body S01.04 ☑
      specified site NEC S01.83 ☑
        with foreign body S01.84 ☑
      temporomandibular area — *see* Puncture, cheek
  heart S26.99 ☑
    with hemopericardium S26.09 ☑
    without hemopericardium S26.19 ☑
  heel — *see* Puncture, foot
  hip S71.039 ☑
    with foreign body S71.049 ☑
      left S71.032 ☑
        with foreign body S71.042 ☑
      right S71.031 ☑
        with foreign body S71.041 ☑
  hymen — *see* Puncture, vagina
  hypochondrium — *see* Puncture, abdomen, wall
  hypogastric region — *see* Puncture, abdomen, wall
  inguinal region — *see* Puncture, abdomen, wall
  instep — *see* Puncture, foot
  internal organs — *see* Injury, by site
  interscapular region — *see* Puncture, thorax, back
  intestine
    large
      colon S36.599 ☑
        ascending S36.590 ☑
        descending S36.592 ☑
        sigmoid S36.593 ☑
        specified site NEC S36.598 ☑
        transverse S36.591 ☑
      rectum S36.69 ☑
    small S36.499 ☑
      duodenum S36.490 ☑
      specified site NEC S36.498 ☑
  intra-abdominal organ S36.99 ☑
    gallbladder S36.128 ☑
    intestine — *see* Puncture, intestine
    liver S36.118 ☑
    pancreas — *see* Puncture, pancreas
    peritoneum S36.81 ☑
    specified site NEC S36.898 ☑
    spleen S36.09 ☑
    stomach S36.39 ☑
  jaw — *see* Puncture, head, specified site NEC
  knee S81.039 ☑
    with foreign body S81.049 ☑
      left S81.032 ☑
        with foreign body S81.042 ☑
      right S81.031 ☑
        with foreign body S81.041 ☑
  labium (majus) (minus) — *see* Puncture, vulva
  lacrimal duct — *see* Puncture, eyelid
  larynx S11.013 ☑
    with foreign body S11.014 ☑
  leg (lower) S81.839 ☑
    with foreign body S81.849 ☑
    foot — *see* Puncture, foot
    knee — *see* Puncture, knee
    left S81.832 ☑
      with foreign body S81.842 ☑
    right S81.831 ☑
      with foreign body S81.841 ☑
    upper — *see* Puncture, thigh
  lip S01.531 ☑

Puncture — *continued*
  lip — *continued*
    with foreign body S01.541 ☑
  loin — *see* Puncture, abdomen, wall
  lower back — *see* Puncture, back, lower
  lumbar region — *see* Puncture, back, lower
  malar region — *see* Puncture, head, specified site NEC
  mammary — *see* Puncture, breast
  mastoid region — *see* Puncture, head, specified site NEC
  mouth — *see* Puncture, oral cavity
  nail
    finger — *see* Puncture, finger, with damage to nail
    toe — *see* Puncture, toe, with damage to nail
  nasal (septum) (sinus) — *see* Puncture, nose
  nasopharynx — *see* Puncture, head, specified site NEC
  neck S11.93 ☑
    with foreign body S11.94 ☑
    involving
        cervical esophagus — *see* Puncture, cervical esophagus
        larynx — *see* Puncture, larynx
        pharynx — *see* Puncture, pharynx
        thyroid gland — *see* Puncture, thyroid gland
        trachea — *see* Puncture, trachea
    specified site NEC S11.83 ☑
      with foreign body S11.84 ☑
  nose (septum) (sinus) S01.23 ☑
    with foreign body S01.24 ☑
  ocular — *see* Puncture, eyeball
  oral cavity S01.532 ☑
    with foreign body S01.542 ☑
  orbit S05.4- ☑
  palate — *see* Puncture, oral cavity
  palm — *see* Puncture, hand
  pancreas S36.299 ☑
    body S36.291 ☑
    head S36.290 ☑
    tail S36.292 ☑
  pelvis — *see* Puncture, back, lower
  penis S31.23 ☑
    with foreign body S31.24 ☑
  perineum
    female S31.43 ☑
      with foreign body S31.44 ☑
    male S31.139 ☑
      with foreign body S31.149 ☑
  periocular area (with or without lacrimal passages) — *see* Puncture, eyelid
  phalanges
    finger — *see* Puncture, finger
    toe — *see* Puncture, toe
  pharynx S11.23 ☑
    with foreign body S11.24 ☑
  pinna — *see* Puncture, ear
  popliteal space — *see* Puncture, knee
  prepuce — *see* Puncture, penis
  pubic region S31.139 ☑
    with foreign body S31.149 ☑
  pudendum — *see* Puncture, genital organs, external
  rectovaginal septum — *see* Puncture, vagina
  sacral region — *see* Puncture, back, lower
  sacroiliac region — *see* Puncture, back, lower
  salivary gland — *see* Puncture, oral cavity
  scalp S01.03 ☑
    with foreign body S01.04 ☑
  scapular region — *see* Puncture, shoulder
  scrotum S31.33 ☑
    with foreign body S31.34 ☑
  shin — *see* Puncture, leg
  shoulder S41.039 ☑
    with foreign body S41.049 ☑
    left S41.032 ☑
      with foreign body S41.042 ☑
    right S41.031 ☑
      with foreign body S41.041 ☑
  spermatic cord — *see* Puncture, testis
  sternal region — *see* Puncture, thorax, front
  submaxillary region — *see* Puncture, head, specified site NEC
  submental region — *see* Puncture, head, specified site NEC
  subungual
    finger(s) — *see* Puncture, finger, with damage to nail
    toe — *see* Puncture, toe, with damage to nail

Puncture — *continued*
  supraclavicular fossa — *see* Puncture, neck, specified site NEC
  temple, temporal region — *see* Puncture, head, specified site NEC
  temporomandibular area — *see* Puncture, cheek
  testis S31.33 ☑
    with foreign body S31.34 ☑
  thigh S71.139 ☑
    with foreign body S71.149 ☑
    left S71.132 ☑
      with foreign body S71.142 ☑
    right S71.131 ☑
      with foreign body S71.141 ☑
  thorax, thoracic (wall) S21.93 ☑
    with foreign body S21.94 ☑
    back S21.23- ☑
      with
          foreign body S21.24- ☑
            with penetration S21.44 ☑
          penetration S21.43 ☑
    breast — *see* Puncture, breast
    front S21.13- ☑
      with
          foreign body S21.14- ☑
            with penetration S21.34 ☑
          penetration S21.33 ☑
  throat — *see* Puncture, neck
  thumb S61.039 ☑
    with
        damage to nail S61.139 ☑
          with
              foreign body S61.149 ☑
        foreign body S61.049 ☑
    left S61.032 ☑
      with
          damage to nail S61.132 ☑
            with
                foreign body S61.142 ☑
          foreign body S61.042 ☑
    right S61.031 ☑
      with
          damage to nail S61.131 ☑
            with
                foreign body S61.141 ☑
          foreign body S61.041 ☑
  thyroid gland S11.13 ☑
    with foreign body S11.14 ☑
  toe(s) S91.139 ☑
    with
        damage to nail S91.239 ☑
          with
              foreign body S91.249 ☑
        foreign body S91.149 ☑
    great S91.133 ☑
      with
          damage to nail S91.233 ☑
            with
                foreign body S91.243 ☑
          foreign body S91.143 ☑
      left S91.132 ☑
        with
            damage to nail S91.232 ☑
              with
                  foreign body S91.242 ☑
            foreign body S91.142 ☑
      right S91.131 ☑
        with
            damage to nail S91.231 ☑
              with
                  foreign body S91.241 ☑
            foreign body S91.141 ☑
    lesser S91.136 ☑
      with
          damage to nail S91.236 ☑
            with
                foreign body S91.246 ☑
          foreign body S91.146 ☑
      left S91.135 ☑
        with
            damage to nail S91.235 ☑
              with
                  foreign body S91.245 ☑
            foreign body S91.145 ☑
      right S91.134 ☑

uncture — *continued*
  toe(s) — *continued*
    lesser — *continued*
      right — *continued*
        with
          damage to nail S91.234 ☑
            with
              foreign body S91.244 ☑
          foreign body S91.144 ☑
  tongue — *see* Puncture, oral cavity
  trachea S11.023 ☑
    with foreign body S11.024 ☑
  tunica vaginalis — *see* Puncture, testis
  tympanum, tympanic membrane S09.2- ☑
  umbilical region S31.135 ☑
    with foreign body S31.145 ☑
  uvula — *see* Puncture, oral cavity
  vagina S31.43 ☑
    with foreign body S31.44 ☑
  vocal cords S11.033 ☑
    with foreign body S11.034 ☑
  vulva S31.43 ☑
    with foreign body S31.44 ☑
  wrist S61.539 ☑
    with
      foreign body S61.549 ☑
    left S61.532 ☑
      with
        foreign body S61.542 ☑
    right S61.531 ☑
      with
        foreign body S61.541 ☑
UO (pyrexia of unknown origin) R50.9
upillary membrane (persistent) Q13.89
upillotonia — *see* Anomaly, pupil, function, tonic pupil
urpura D69.2
  abdominal D69.0
  allergic D69.0
  anaphylactoid D69.0
  annularis telangiectodes L81.7
  arthritic D69.0
  autoerythrocyte sensitization D69.2
  autoimmune D69.0
  bacterial D69.0
  Bateman's (senile) D69.2
  capillary fragility (hereditary) (idiopathic) D69.8
  cryoglobulinemic D89.1
  Devil's pinches D69.2
  fibrinolytic — *see* Fibrinolysis
  fulminans, fulminous D65
  gangrenous D65
  hemorrhagic, hemorrhagica D69.3
    not due to thrombocytopenia D69.0
  Henoch (-Schönlein) (allergic) D69.0
  hypergammaglobulinemic (benign) (Waldenström) D89.0
  idiopathic (thrombocytopenic) D69.3
    nonthrombocytopenic D69.0
  immune thrombocytopenic D69.3
  infectious D69.0
  malignant D69.0
  neonatorum P54.5
  nervosa D69.0
  newborn P54.5
  nonthrombocytopenic D69.2
    hemorrhagic D69.0
    idiopathic D69.0
  nonthrombopenic D69.2
  peliosis rheumatica D69.0
  posttransfusion (post-transfusion) (from (fresh) whole blood or blood products) D69.51
  primary D69.49
  red cell membrane sensitivity D69.2
  rheumatica D69.0
  Schönlein (-Henoch) (allergic) D69.0
  scorbutic E54 *[D77]*
  senile D69.2
  simplex D69.2
  symptomatica D69.0
  telangiectasia annularis L81.7
  thrombocytopenic D69.49
    congenital D69.42
    hemorrhagic D69.3
    hereditary D69.42
    idiopathic D69.3
    immune D69.3
    neonatal, transitory P61.0
    thrombotic M31.1

Purpura — *continued*
  thrombohemolytic — *see* Fibrinolysis
  thrombolytic — *see* Fibrinolysis
  thrombopenic D69.49
  thrombotic, thrombocytopenic M31.1
  toxic D69.0
  vascular D69.0
  visceral symptoms D69.0
Purpuric spots R23.3
Purulent — *see* condition
Pus
  in
    stool R19.5
    urine N39.0
  tube (rupture) — *see* Salpingo-oophoritis
Pustular rash L08.9
Pustule (nonmalignant) L08.9
  malignant A22.0
Pustulosis palmaris et plantaris L40.3
Putnam (-Dana) **disease or syndrome** — *see* Degeneration, combined
Putrescent pulp (dental) K04.1
Pyarthritis, pyarthrosis — *see* Arthritis, pyogenic or pyemic
  tuberculous — *see* Tuberculosis, joint
Pyelectasis — *see* Hydronephrosis
Pyelitis (congenital) (uremic) — *see also* Pyelonephritis
  with
    calculus — *see* category N20 ☑
      with hydronephrosis N13.6
    contracted kidney N11.9
  acute N10
  chronic N11.9
    with calculus — *see* category N20 ☑
      with hydronephrosis N13.6
  cystica N28.84
  puerperal (postpartum) O86.21
  tuberculous A18.11
Pyelocystitis — *see* Pyelonephritis
Pyelonephritis — *see also* Nephritis, tubulo-interstitial
  with
    calculus — *see* category N20 ☑
      with hydronephrosis N13.6
    contracted kidney N11.9
  acute N10
  calculous — *see* category N20 ☑
    with hydronephrosis N13.6
  chronic N11.9
    with calculus — *see* category N20 ☑
      with hydronephrosis N13.6
    associated with ureteral obstruction or stricture N11.1
    nonobstructive N11.8
      with reflux (vesicoureteral) N11.0
    obstructive N11.1
    specified NEC N11.8
  in (due to)
    brucellosis A23.9 *[N16]*
    cryoglobulinemia (mixed) D89.1 *[N16]*
    cystinosis E72.04
    diphtheria A36.84
    glycogen storage disease E74.09 *[N16]*
    leukemia NEC C95.9- ☑ *[N16]*
    lymphoma NEC C85.90 *[N16]*
    multiple myeloma C90.0- ☑ *[N16]*
    obstruction N11.1
    Salmonella infection A02.25
    sarcoidosis D86.84
    sepsis A41.9 *[N16]*
    Sjögren's disease M35.04
    toxoplasmosis B58.83
    transplant rejection T86.91 *[N16]*
    Wilson's disease E83.01 *[N16]*
  nonobstructive N12
    with reflux (vesicoureteral) N11.0
    chronic N11.8
  syphilitic A52.75
Pyelonephrosis (obstructive) N11.1
  chronic N11.9
Pyelophlebitis I80.8
Pyeloureteritis cystica N28.85
Pyemia, pyemic (fever) (infection) (purulent) — *see also* Sepsis
  joint — *see* Arthritis, pyogenic or pyemic
  liver K75.1
  pneumococcal A40.3
  portal K75.1

Pyemia, pyemic — *continued*
  postvaccinal T88.0 ☑
  puerperal, postpartum, childbirth O85
  specified organism NEC A41.89
  tuberculous — *see* Tuberculosis, miliary
Pygopagus Q89.4
Pyknoepilepsy (idiopathic) — *see* Pyknolepsy
Pyknolepsy G40.A09 (*following* G40.3)
  intractable G40.A19 (*following* G40.3)
    with status epilepticus G40.A11 (*following* G40.3)
    without status epilepticus G40.A19 (*following* G40.3)
  not intractable G40.A09 (*following* G40.3)
    with status epilepticus G40.A01 (*following* G40.3)
    without status epilepticus G40.A09 (*following* G40.3)
Pylephlebitis K75.1
Pyle's syndrome Q78.5
Pylethrombophlebitis K75.1
Pylethrombosis K75.1
Pyloritis K29.90
  with bleeding K29.91
Pylorospasm (reflex) **NEC** K31.3
  congenital or infantile Q40.0
  neurotic F45.8
  newborn Q40.0
  psychogenic F45.8
Pylorus, pyloric — *see* condition
Pyoarthrosis — *see* Arthritis, pyogenic or pyemic
Pyocele
  mastoid — *see* Mastoiditis, acute
  sinus (accessory) — *see* Sinusitis
  turbinate (bone) J32.9
  urethra — *see also* Urethritis N34.0
Pyocolpos — *see* Vaginitis
Pyocystitis N30.80
  with hematuria N30.81
Pyoderma, pyodermia L08.0
  gangrenosum L88
  newborn P39.4
  phagedenic L88
  vegetans L08.81
Pyodermatitis L08.0
  vegetans L08.81
Pyogenic — *see* condition
Pyohydronephrosis N13.6
Pyometra, pyometrium, pyometritis — *see* Endometritis
Pyomyositis (tropical) — *see* Myositis, infective
Pyonephritis N12
Pyonephrosis N13.6
  tuberculous A18.11
Pyo-oophoritis — *see* Salpingo-oophoritis
Pyo-ovarium — *see* Salpingo-oophoritis
Pyopericarditis, pyopericardium I30.1
Pyophlebitis — *see* Phlebitis
Pyopneumopericardium I30.1
Pyopneumothorax (infective) J86.9
  with fistula J86.0
  tuberculous NEC A15.6
Pyosalpinx, pyosalpingitis — *see also* Salpingo-oophoritis
Pyothorax J86.9
  with fistula J86.0
  tuberculous NEC A15.6
Pyoureter N28.89
  tuberculous A18.11
Pyramidopallidonigral syndrome G20
Pyrexia (of unknown origin) R50.9
  atmospheric T67.01 ☑
  during labor NEC O75.2
  heat T67.01 ☑
  newborn P81.9
    environmentally-induced P81.0
  persistent R50.9
  puerperal O86.4
Pyroglobulinemia NEC E88.09
Pyromania F63.1
Pyrosis R12
Pyuria (bacterial) (sterile) R82.81

Q

Q fever A78
  with pneumonia A78
Quadricuspid aortic valve Q23.8
Quadrilateral fever A78
Quadriparesis — *see* Quadriplegia
  meaning muscle weakness M62.81

Quadriplegia G82.50
- complete
  - C1-C4 level G82.51
  - C5-C7 level G82.53
- congenital (cerebral) (spinal) G80.8
  - spastic G80.0
- embolic (current episode) I63.4- ☑
- functional R53.2
- incomplete
  - C1-C4 level G82.52
  - C5-C7 level G82.54
- thrombotic (current episode) I63.3- ☑
- traumatic — code to injury with seventh character S
  - current episode — see Injury, spinal (cord), cervical

Quadruplet, pregnancy — see Pregnancy, quadruplet

Quarrelsomeness F60.3

Queensland fever A77.3

Quervain's disease M65.4
- thyroid E06.1

Queyrat's erythroplasia D07.4
- penis D07.4
- specified site — see Neoplasm, skin, in situ
- unspecified site D07.4

Quincke's disease or edema T78.3 ☑
- hereditary D84.1

Quinsy (gangrenous) J36

Quintan fever A79.0

Quintuplet, pregnancy — see Pregnancy, quintuplet

R

Rabbit fever — see Tularemia

Rabies A82.9
- contact Z20.3
- exposure to Z20.3
- inoculation reaction — see Complications, vaccination
- sylvatic A82.0
- urban A82.1

Rachischisis — see Spina bifida

Rachitic — see also condition
- deformities of spine (late effect) (sequelae) E64.3
- pelvis (late effect) (sequelae) E64.3
  - with disproportion (fetopelvic) O33.0
    - causing obstructed labor O65.0

Rachitis, rachitism (acute) (tarda) — see also Rickets
- renalis N25.0
- sequelae E64.3

Radial nerve — see condition

Radiation
- burn — see Burn
- effects NOS T66 ☑
- sickness NOS T66 ☑
- therapy, encounter for Z51.0

Radiculitis (pressure) (vertebrogenic) — see Radiculopathy

Radiculomyelitis — see also Encephalitis
- toxic, due to
  - Clostridium tetani A35
  - Corynebacterium diphtheriae A36.82

Radiculopathy M54.10
- cervical region M54.12
- cervicothoracic region M54.13
- due to
  - disc disorder
    - C3 M50.11
    - C4 M50.11
    - C5 M50.121
    - C6 M50.122
    - C7 M50.123
  - displacement of intervertebral disc — see Disorder, disc, with, radiculopathy
- leg M54.1- ☑
- lumbar region M54.16
- lumbosacral region M54.17
- occipito-atlanto-axial region M54.11
- postherpetic B02.29
- sacrococcygeal region M54.18
- syphilitic A52.11
- thoracic region (with visceral pain) M54.14
- thoracolumbar region M54.15

Radiodermal burns (acute, chronic, or occupational) — see Burn

Radiodermatitis L58.9
- acute L58.0
- chronic L58.1

Radiotherapy session Z51.0

RAEB (refractory anemia with excess blasts) D46.2- ☑

Rage, meaning rabies — see Rabies

Ragpicker's disease A22.1

Ragsorter's disease A22.1

Raillietiniasis B71.8

Railroad neurosis F48.8

Railway spine F48.8

Raised — see also Elevated
- antibody titer R76.0

Rake teeth, tooth M26.39

Rales R09.89

Ramifying renal pelvis Q63.8

Ramsay-Hunt disease or syndrome — see also Hunt's disease B02.21
- meaning dyssynergia cerebellaris myoclonica G11.1

Ranula K11.6
- congenital Q38.4

Rape
- adult
  - confirmed T74.21 ☑
  - suspected T76.21 ☑
- alleged, observation or examination, ruled out
  - adult Z04.41
  - child Z04.42
- child
  - confirmed T74.22 ☑
  - suspected T76.22 ☑

Rapid
- feeble pulse, due to shock, following injury T79.4 ☑
- heart (beat) R00.0
  - psychogenic F45.8
- second stage (delivery) O62.3
- time-zone change syndrome G47.25

Rarefaction, bone — see Disorder, bone, density and structure, specified NEC

Rash (toxic) R21
- canker A38.9
- diaper L22
- drug (internal use) L27.0
  - contact — see also Dermatitis, due to, drugs, external L25.1
- following immunization T88.1 ☑
- food — see Dermatitis, due to, food
- heat L74.0
- napkin (psoriasiform) L22
- nettle — see Urticaria
- pustular L08.0
- rose R21
  - epidemic B06.9
- scarlet A38.9
- serum — see also Reaction, serum T80.69 ☑
- wandering tongue K14.1

Rasmussen aneurysm — see Tuberculosis, pulmonary

Rasmussen encephalitis G04.81

Rat-bite fever A25.9
- due to Streptobacillus moniliformis A25.1
- spirochetal (morsus muris) A25.0

Rathke's pouch tumor D44.3

Raymond (-Céstan) **syndrome** I65.8

Raynaud's disease, phenomenon or syndrome (secondary) I73.00
- with gangrene (symmetric) I73.01

RDS (newborn) (type I) P22.0
- type II P22.1

Reaction — see also Disorder
- withdrawing, child or adolescent F93.8
- adaptation — see Disorder, adjustment
- adjustment (anxiety) (conduct disorder) (depressiveness) (distress) — see Disorder, adjustment
  - with
    - mutism, elective (child) (adolescent) F94.0
- adverse
  - food (any) (ingested) NEC T78.1 ☑
    - anaphylactic — see Shock, anaphylactic, due to food
- affective — see Disorder, mood
- allergic — see Allergy
- anaphylactic — see Shock, anaphylactic
- anaphylactoid — see Shock, anaphylactic
- anesthesia — see Anesthesia, complication
- antitoxin (prophylactic) (therapeutic) — see Complications, vaccination
- anxiety F41.1
- Arthus — see Arthus' phenomenon
- asthenic F48.8
- combat and operational stress F43.0
- compulsive F42.8
- conversion F44.9

Reaction — continued
- crisis, acute F43.0
- deoxyribonuclease (DNA) (DNase) hypersensitivity D69.2
- depressive (single episode) F32.9
  - affective (single episode) F31.4
    - recurrent episode F33.9
  - neurotic F34.1
  - psychoneurotic F34.1
  - psychotic F32.3
  - recurrent — see Disorder, depressive, recurrent
- dissociative F44.9
- drug NEC T88.7 ☑
  - addictive — see Dependence, drug
    - transmitted via placenta or breast milk — see Absorption, drug, addictive, through placenta
  - allergic — see Allergy, drug
  - lichenoid L43.2
  - newborn P93.8
    - gray baby syndrome P93.0
  - overdose or poisoning (by accident) — see Table Drugs and Chemicals, by drug, poisoning
  - photoallergic L56.1
  - phototoxic L56.0
  - withdrawal — see Dependence, by drug, with, withdrawal
    - infant of dependent mother P96.1
    - newborn P96.1
  - wrong substance given or taken (by accident) — see Table of Drugs and Chemicals, by drug, poisoning
- fear F40.9
  - child (abnormal) F93.8
- febrile nonhemolytic transfusion (FNHTR) R50.84
- fluid loss, cerebrospinal G97.1
- foreign
  - body NEC — see Granuloma, foreign body
    - in operative wound (inadvertently left) — see Foreign body, accidentally left during a procedure
  - substance accidentally left during a procedure (chemical) (powder) (talc) T81.60 ☑
    - aseptic peritonitis T81.61 ☑
    - body or object (instrument) (sponge) (swab) — see Foreign body, accidentally left during a procedure
  - specified reaction NEC T81.69 ☑
- grief — see Disorder, adjustment
- Herxheimer's R68.89
- hyperkinetic — see Hyperkinesia
- hypochondriacal F45.20
- hypoglycemic, due to insulin E16.0
  - with coma (diabetic) — see Diabetes, coma
    - nondiabetic E15
  - therapeutic misadventure — see subcategory T38.3 ☑
- hypomanic F30.8
- hysterical F44.9
- immunization — see Complications, vaccination
- incompatibility
  - ABO blood group (infusion) (transfusion) — see Complication(s), transfusion, incompatibility reaction, ABO
    - delayed serologic T80.39 ☑
  - minor blood group (Duffy) (E) (K) (Kell) (Kidd) (Lewis) (M) (N) (P) (S) T80.89 ☑
  - Rh (factor) (infusion) (transfusion) — see Complication(s), transfusion, incompatibility reaction, Rh (factor)
- inflammatory — see Infection
- infusion — see Complications, infusion
- inoculation (immune serum) — see Complications, vaccination
- insulin T38.3- ☑
- involutional psychotic — see Disorder, depressive
- leukemoid D72.823
  - basophilic D72.823
  - lymphocytic D72.823
  - monocytic D72.823
  - myelocytic D72.823
  - neutrophilic D72.823
- LSD (acute)
  - due to drug abuse — see Abuse, drug, hallucinogen
  - due to drug dependence — see Dependence, drug, hallucinogen
- lumbar puncture G97.1
- manic-depressive — see Disorder, bipolar

...action — *continued*
neurasthenic F48.8
neurogenic — *see* Neurosis
neurotic F48.9
neurotic-depressive F34.1
nitritoid — *see* Crisis, nitritoid
nonspecific
  to
    cell mediated immunity measurement of gamma interferon antigen response without active tuberculosis R76.12
    QuantiFERON-TB test (QFT) without active tuberculosis R76.12
    tuberculin test — *see also* Reaction, tuberculin skin test R76.11
obsessive-compulsive F42.8
organic, acute or subacute — *see* Delirium
paranoid (acute) F23
  chronic F22
  senile F03 ☑
passive dependency F60.7
phobic F40.9
post-traumatic stress, uncomplicated Z73.3
psychogenic F99
psychoneurotic — *see also* Neurosis
  compulsive F42.8
  depersonalization F48.1
  depressive F34.1
  hypochondriacal F45.20
  neurasthenic F48.8
  obsessive F42.8
psychophysiologic — *see* Disorder, somatoform
psychosomatic — *see* Disorder, somatoform
psychotic — *see* Psychosis
scarlet fever toxin — *see* Complications, vaccination
schizophrenic F23
  acute (brief) (undifferentiated) F23
  latent F21
  undifferentiated (acute) (brief) F23
serological for syphilis — *see* Serology for syphilis
serum T80.69 ☑
  anaphylactic (immediate) — *see also* Shock, anaphylactic T80.59 ☑
  specified reaction NEC
    due to
      administration of blood and blood products T80.61 ☑
      immunization T80.62 ☑
      serum specified NEC T80.69 ☑
      vaccination T80.62 ☑
situational — *see* Disorder, adjustment
somatization — *see* Disorder, somatoform
spinal puncture G97.1
stress (severe) F43.9
  acute (agitation) ("daze") (disorientation) (disturbance of consciousness) (flight reaction) (fugue) F43.0
  specified NEC F43.8
surgical procedure — *see* Complications, surgical procedure
tetanus antitoxin — *see* Complications, vaccination
toxic, to local anesthesia T88.59 ☑
  in labor and delivery O74.4
  in pregnancy O29.3X- ☑
  postpartum, puerperal O89.3
toxin-antitoxin — *see* Complications, vaccination
transfusion (blood) (bone marrow) (lymphocytes) (allergic) — *see* Complications, transfusion
tuberculin skin test, abnormal R76.11
vaccination (any) — *see* Complications, vaccination
...active airway disease — *see* Asthma
...active depression — *see* Reaction, depressive
...arrangement
chromosomal
  balanced (in) Q95.9
    abnormal individual (autosomal) Q95.2
      non-sex (autosomal) chromosomes Q95.2
      sex/non-sex chromosomes Q95.3
    specified NEC Q95.8
...calcitrant patient — *see* Noncompliance
...canalization, thrombus — *see* Thrombosis
...cession, receding
chamber angle (eye) H21.55- ☑
chin M26.09
gingival (postinfective) (postoperative)
  generalized K06.020
    minimal K06.021
    moderate K06.022

Recession, receding — *continued*
gingival — *continued*
  generalized — *continued*
    severe K06.023
  localized K06.010
    minimal K06.011
    moderate K06.012
    severe K06.013
Recklinghausen disease Q85.01
bones E21.0
Reclus' disease (cystic) — *see* Mastopathy, cystic
Recrudescent typhus (fever) A75.1
Recruitment, auditory H93.21- ☑
Rectalgia K62.89
Rectitis K62.89
Rectocele
female (without uterine prolapse) N81.6
  with uterine prolapse N81.4
    incomplete N81.2
in pregnancy — *see* Pregnancy, complicated by, abnormal, pelvic organs or tissues NEC
male K62.3
Rectosigmoid junction — *see* condition
Rectosigmoiditis K63.89
ulcerative (chronic) K51.30
  with
    complication K51.319
      abscess K51.314
      fistula K51.313
      obstruction K51.312
      rectal bleeding K51.311
      specified NEC K51.318
Rectourethral — *see* condition
Rectovaginal — *see* condition
Rectovesical — *see* condition
Rectum, rectal — *see* condition
Recurrent — *see* condition
pregnancy loss — *see* Loss (of), pregnancy, recurrent
Red bugs B88.0
Red tide — *see also* Table of Drugs and Chemicals T65.82- ☑
Red-cedar lung or pneumonitis J67.8
Reduced
mobility Z74.09
ventilatory or vital capacity R94.2
Redundant, redundancy
anus (congenital) Q43.8
clitoris N90.89
colon (congenital) Q43.8
foreskin (congenital) N47.8
intestine (congenital) Q43.8
labia N90.69
organ or site, congenital NEC — *see* Accessory
panniculus (abdominal) E65
prepuce (congenital) N47.8
pylorus K31.89
rectum (congenital) Q43.8
scrotum N50.89
sigmoid (congenital) Q43.8
skin L98.7
  and subcutaneous tissue L98.7
  of face L57.4
    eyelids — *see* Blepharochalasis
stomach K31.89
Reduplication — *see* Duplication
Reflex R29.2
hyperactive gag J39.2
pupillary, abnormal — *see* Anomaly, pupil, function
vasoconstriction I73.9
vasovagal R55
Reflux K21.9
acid K21.9
esophageal K21.9
  with esophagitis K21.0
  newborn P78.83
gastroesophageal K21.9
  with esophagitis K21.0
mitral — *see* Insufficiency, mitral
ureteral — *see* Reflux, vesicoureteral
vesicoureteral (with scarring) N13.70
  with
    nephropathy N13.729
      with hydroureter N13.739
        bilateral N13.732
        unilateral N13.731
      bilateral N13.722
      unilateral N13.721
      without hydroureter N13.729

Reflux — *continued*
vesicoureteral — *continued*
  with — *continued*
    nephropathy — *continued*
      without hydroureter — *continued*
        bilateral N13.722
        unilateral N13.721
    pyelonephritis (chronic) N11.0
  congenital Q62.7
  without nephropathy N13.71
Reforming, artificial openings — *see* Attention to, artificial, opening
Refractive error — *see* Disorder, refraction
Refsum's disease or syndrome G60.1
Refusal of
food, psychogenic F50.89
treatment (because of) Z53.20
  left against medical advice (AMA) Z53.21
  patient's decision NEC Z53.29
  reasons of belief or group pressure Z53.1
Regional — *see* condition
Regurgitation R11.10
aortic (valve) — *see* Insufficiency, aortic
food — *see also* Vomiting
  with reswallowing — *see* Rumination
  newborn P92.1
gastric contents — *see* Vomiting
heart — *see* Endocarditis
mitral (valve) — *see* Insufficiency, mitral
  congenital Q23.3
myocardial — *see* Endocarditis
pulmonary (valve) (heart) I37.1
  congenital Q22.2
  syphilitic A52.03
tricuspid — *see* Insufficiency, tricuspid
valve, valvular — *see* Endocarditis
  congenital Q24.8
vesicoureteral — *see* Reflux, vesicoureteral
Reichmann's disease or syndrome K31.89
Reifenstein syndrome E34.52
Reinsertion
implantable subdermal contraceptive Z30.46
intrauterine contraceptive device Z30.433
Reiter's disease, syndrome, or urethritis M02.30
ankle M02.37- ☑
elbow M02.32- ☑
foot joint M02.37- ☑
hand joint M02.34- ☑
hip M02.35- ☑
knee M02.36- ☑
multiple site M02.39
shoulder M02.31- ☑
vertebra M02.38
wrist M02.33- ☑
Rejection
food, psychogenic F50.89
transplant T86.91
  bone T86.830
    marrow T86.01
  cornea T86.840
  heart T86.21
    with lung(s) T86.31
  intestine T86.850
  kidney T86.11
  liver T86.41
  lung(s) T86.810
    with heart T86.31
  organ (immune or nonimmune cause) T86.91
  pancreas T86.890
  skin (allograft) (autograft) T86.820
  specified NEC T86.890
  stem cell (peripheral blood) (umbilical cord) T86.5
Relapsing fever A68.9
Carter's (Asiatic) A68.1
Dutton's (West African) A68.1
Koch's A68.9
louse-borne (epidemic) A68.0
Novy's (American) A68.1
Obermeyers's (European) A68.0
Spirillum A68.9
tick-borne (endemic) A68.1
Relationship
occlusal
  open anterior M26.220
  open posterior M26.221
Relaxation
anus (sphincter) K62.89
  psychogenic F45.8

Relaxation — *continued*
 arch (foot) — *see also* Deformity, limb, flat foot
 back ligaments — *see* Instability, joint, spine
 bladder (sphincter) N31.2
 cardioesophageal K21.9
 cervix — *see* Incompetency, cervix
 diaphragm J98.6
 joint (capsule) (ligament) (paralytic) — *see* Flail, joint
  congenital NEC Q74.8
 lumbosacral (joint) — *see* subcategory M53.2 ☑
 pelvic floor N81.89
 perineum N81.89
 posture R29.3
 rectum (sphincter) K62.89
 sacroiliac (joint) — *see* subcategory M53.2 ☑
 scrotum N50.89
 urethra (sphincter) N36.44
 vesical N31.2
Release from prison, anxiety concerning Z65.2
Remains
 canal of Cloquet Q14.0
 capsule (opaque) Q14.8
Remittent fever (malarial) B54
Remnant
 canal of Cloquet Q14.0
 capsule (opaque) Q14.8
 cervix, cervical stump (acquired) (postoperative) N88.8
 cystic duct, postcholecystectomy K91.5
 fingernail L60.8
  congenital Q84.6
 meniscus, knee — *see* Derangement, knee, meniscus,
  specified NEC
 thyroglossal duct Q89.2
 tonsil J35.8
  infected (chronic) J35.01
 urachus Q64.4
Removal (from) (of)
 artificial
  arm Z44.00- ☑
   complete Z44.01- ☑
   partial Z44.02- ☑
  eye Z44.2- ☑
  leg Z44.10- ☑
   complete Z44.11- ☑
   partial Z44.12- ☑
 breast implant Z45.81 ☑
 cardiac pulse generator (battery) (end-of-life) Z45.010
 catheter (urinary) (indwelling) Z46.6
  from artificial opening — *see* Attention to, artificial,
   opening
  non-vascular Z46.82
  vascular NEC Z45.2
 device Z46.9
  contraceptive Z30.432
   implantable subdermal Z30.46
  implanted NEC Z45.89
  specified NEC Z46.89
 drains Z48.03
 dressing (nonsurgical) Z48.00
  surgical Z48.01
 external
  fixation device — *code to* fracture with seventh
   character D
  prosthesis, prosthetic device Z44.9
   breast Z44.3- ☑
   specified NEC Z44.8
 home in childhood (to foster home or institution)
  Z62.29
 ileostomy Z43.2
 insulin pump Z46.81
 myringotomy device (stent) (tube) Z45.82
 nervous system device NEC Z46.2
  brain neuropacemaker Z46.2
  visual substitution device Z46.2
   implanted Z45.31
 non-vascular catheter Z46.82
 organ, prophylactic (for neoplasia management) —
  see Prophylactic, organ removal
 orthodontic device Z46.4
 staples Z48.02
 stent
  ureteral Z46.6
 suture Z48.02
 urinary device Z46.6
 vascular access device or catheter Z45.2
Ren
 arcuatus Q63.1
 mobile, mobilis N28.89

Ren — *continued*
 mobile, mobilis — *continued*
  congenital Q63.8
  unguliformis Q63.1
Renal — *see* condition
Rendu-Osler-Weber disease or syndrome I78.0
Reninoma D41.0- ☑
Renon-Delille syndrome E23.3
Reovirus, as cause of disease classified elsewhere
  B97.5
Repeated falls NEC R29.6
Replaced chromosome by dicentric ring Q93.2
Replacement by artificial or mechanical device or
  prosthesis of
 bladder Z96.0
 blood vessel NEC Z95.828
 bone NEC Z96.7
 cochlea Z96.21
 coronary artery Z95.5
 eustachian tube Z96.29
 eye globe Z97.0
 heart Z95.812
  valve Z95.2
   prosthetic Z95.2
   specified NEC Z95.4
   xenogenic Z95.3
 intestine Z96.89
 joint Z96.60
  hip — *see* Presence, hip joint implant
  knee — *see* Presence, knee joint implant
  specified site NEC Z96.698
 larynx Z96.3
 lens Z96.1
 limb(s) — *see* Presence, artificial, limb
 mandible NEC (for tooth root implant(s)) Z96.5
 organ NEC Z96.89
 peripheral vessel NEC Z95.828
 stapes Z96.29
 teeth Z97.2
 tendon Z96.7
 tissue NEC Z96.89
 tooth root(s) Z96.5
 vessel NEC Z95.828
  coronary (artery) Z95.5
Request for expert evidence Z04.89
Reserve, decreased or low
 cardiac — *see* Disease, heart
 kidney N28.89
Residual — *see also* condition
 ovary syndrome N99.83
 state, schizophrenic F20.5
 urine R39.198
Resistance, resistant (to)
 activated protein C D68.51
 complicating pregnancy O26.89 ☑
 insulin E88.81
 organism(s)
  to
   drug Z16.30
    aminoglycosides Z16.29
    amoxicillin Z16.11
    ampicillin Z16.11
    antibiotic(s) Z16.20
     multiple Z16.24
     specified NEC Z16.29
    antifungal Z16.32
    antimicrobial (single) Z16.30
     multiple Z16.35
     specified NEC Z16.39
    antimycobacterial (single) Z16.341
     multiple Z16.342
    antiparasitic Z16.31
    antiviral Z16.33
    beta lactam antibiotics Z16.10
     specified NEC Z16.19
    cephalosporins Z16.19
    extended beta lactamase (ESBL) Z16.12
    fluoroquinolones Z16.23
    macrolides Z16.29
    methicillin — *see* MRSA
    multiple drugs (MDRO)
     antibiotics Z16.24
     antimicrobial Z16.35
     antimycobacterials Z16.342
    penicillins Z16.11
    quinine (and related compounds) Z16.31
    quinolones Z16.23
    sulfonamides Z16.29

Resistance, resistant — *continued*
 organism(s) — *continued*
  to — *continued*
   drug — *continued*
    tetracyclines Z16.29
    tuberculostatics (single) Z16.341
     multiple Z16.342
    vancomycin Z16.21
     related antibiotics Z16.22
 thyroid hormone E07.89
Resorption
 dental (roots) K03.3
  alveoli M26.79
 teeth (external) (internal) (pathological) (roots) K03☐
Respiration
 Cheyne-Stokes R06.3
 decreased due to shock, following injury T79.4 ☑
 disorder of, psychogenic F45.8
 insufficient, or poor R06.89
  newborn P28.5
 painful R07.1
 sighing, psychogenic F45.8
Respiratory — *see also* condition
 distress syndrome (newborn) (type I) P22.0
  type II P22.1
 syncytial virus, as cause of disease classified elsewh☐
  — *see also* Virus, respiratory syncytial (RSV) B9☐
Respite care Z75.5
Response (drug)
 photoallergic L56.1
 phototoxic L56.0
Restenosis
 stent
  vascular
   end stent
    adjacent to stent — *see* Arteriosclerosis
     within the stent
      coronary T82.855 ☑
      peripheral T82.856 ☑
   in stent
    coronary vessel T82.855 ☑
    peripheral vessel T82.856 ☑
Restless legs (syndrome) G25.81
Restlessness R45.1
Restoration (of)
 dental
  aesthetically inadequate or displeasing K08.56
  defective K08.50
   specified NEC K08.59
  failure of marginal integrity K08.51
  failure of periodontal anatomical intergrity K08.☐
 organ continuity from previous sterilization (tubopl☐
  ty) (vasoplasty) Z31.0
  aftercare Z31.42
 tooth (existing)
  contours biologically incompatible with oral hea☐
   K08.54
  open margins K08.51
  overhanging K08.52
  poor aesthetic K08.56
  poor gingival margins K08.51
 unsatisfactory, of tooth K08.50
  specified NEC K08.59
Restorative material (dental)
 allergy to K08.55
 fractured K08.539
  with loss of material K08.531
  without loss of material K08.530
 unrepairable overhanging of K08.52
Restriction of housing space Z59.1
Rests, ovarian, in fallopian tube Q50.6
Restzustand (schizophrenic) F20.5
Retained — *see also* Retention
 cholelithiasis following cholecystectomy K91.86
 foreign body fragments (type of) Z18.9
  acrylics Z18.2
  animal quill(s) or spines Z18.31
  cement Z18.83
  concrete Z18.83
  crystalline Z18.83
  depleted isotope Z18.09
  depleted uranium Z18.01
  diethylhexyl phthalates Z18.2
  glass Z18.81
  isocyanate Z18.2
  magnetic metal Z18.11
  metal Z18.10
  nonmagnectic metal Z18.12

☑ **Additional Character Required — Refer to the Tabular List for Character Selection** ▽ Subterms under main terms may continue to next column or pag☐

etained — *continued*
  foreign body fragments — *continued*
    nontherapeutic radioactive Z18.09
    organic NEC Z18.39
    plastic Z18.2
    quill(s) (animal) Z18.31
    radioactive (nontherapeutic) NEC Z18.09
    specified NEC Z18.89
    spine(s) (animal) Z18.31
    stone Z18.83
    tooth (teeth) Z18.32
    wood Z18.33
  fragments (type of) Z18.9
    acrylics Z18.2
    animal quill(s) or spines Z18.31
    cement Z18.83
    concrete Z18.83
    crystalline Z18.83
    depleted isotope Z18.09
    depleted uranium Z18.01
    diethylhexyl phthalates Z18.2
    glass Z18.81
    isocyanate Z18.2
    magnetic metal Z18.11
    metal Z18.10
    nonmagnectic metal Z18.12
    nontherapeutic radioactive Z18.09
    organic NEC Z18.39
    plastic Z18.2
    quill(s) (animal) Z18.31
    radioactive (nontherapeutic) NEC Z18.09
    specified NEC Z18.89
    spine(s) (animal) Z18.31
    stone Z18.83
    tooth (teeth) Z18.32
    wood Z18.33
  gallstones, following cholecystectomy K91.86

etardation
  development, developmental, specific — *see* Disorder, developmental
  endochondral bone growth — *see* Disorder, bone, development or growth
  growth R62.50
    due to malnutrition E45
  mental — *see* Disability, intellectual
  motor function, specific F82
  physical (child) R62.52
    due to malnutrition E45
  reading (specific) F81.0
  spelling (specific) (without reading disorder) F81.81

etching — *see* Vomiting

etention — *see also* Retained
  bladder — *see* Retention, urine
  carbon dioxide E87.2
  cholelithiasis following cholecystectomy K91.86
  cyst — *see* Cyst
  dead
    fetus (at or near term) (mother) O36.4 ☑
      early fetal death O02.1
    ovum O02.0
  decidua (fragments) (following delivery) (with hemorrhage) O72.2
    without hemorrhage O73.1
  deciduous tooth K00.6
  dental root K08.3
  fecal — *see* Constipation
  fetus
    dead O36.4 ☑
      early O02.1
  fluid R60.9
  foreign body — *see also* Foreign body, retained
    current trauma — *code as* Foreign body, by site or type
  gallstones, following cholecystectomy K91.86
  gastric K31.89
  intrauterine contraceptive device, in pregnancy — *see* Pregnancy, complicated by, retention, intrauterine device
  membranes (complicating delivery) (with hemorrhage) O72.2
    with abortion — *see* Abortion, by type
    without hemorrhage O73.1
  meniscus — *see* Derangement, meniscus
  menses N94.89
  milk (puerperal, postpartum) O92.79
  nitrogen, extrarenal R39.2
  ovary syndrome N99.83
  placenta (total) (with hemorrhage) O72.0

Retention — *continued*
  placenta — *continued*
    without hemorrhage O73.0
    portions or fragments (with hemorrhage) O72.2
      without hemorrhage O73.1
  products of conception
    early pregnancy (dead fetus) O02.1
    following
      delivery (with hemorrhage) O72.2
        without hemorrhage O73.1
    secundines (following delivery) (with hemorrhage) O72.0
      without hemorrhage O73.0
    complicating puerperium (delayed hemorrhage) O72.2
    partial O72.2
      without hemorrhage O73.1
  smegma, clitoris N90.89
  urine R33.9
    due to hyperplasia (hypertrophy) of prostate — *see* Hyperplasia, prostate
    drug-induced R33.0
    organic R33.8
      drug-induced R33.0
    psychogenic F45.8
    specified NEC R33.8
  water (in tissues) — *see* Edema
Reticulation, dust — *see* Pneumoconiosis
Reticulocytosis R70.1
Reticuloendotheliosis
  acute infantile C96.0
  leukemic C91.4- ☑
  nonlipid C96.0
Reticulohistiocytoma (giant-cell) D76.3
Reticuloid, actinic L57.1
Reticulosis (skin)
  acute of infancy C96.0
  hemophagocytic, familial D76.1
  histiocytic medullary C96.A (*following* C96.6)
  lipomelanotic I89.8
  malignant (midline) C86.0
  polymorphic C83.8- ☑
  Sézary — *see* Sézary disease
Retina, retinal — *see also* condition
  dark area D49.81
Retinitis — *see also* Inflammation, chorioretinal
  albuminurica N18.9 *[H32]*
  diabetic   *see* Diabetes, retinitis
  disciformis — *see* Degeneration, macula
  focal — *see* Inflammation, chorioretinal, focal
  gravidarum — *see* Pregnancy, complicated by, specified pregnancy-related condition NEC
  juxtapapillaris — *see* Inflammation, chorioretinal, focal, juxtapapillary
  luetic — *see* Retinitis, syphilitic
  pigmentosa H35.52
  proliferans — *see* Disorder, globe, degenerative, specified type NEC
  proliferating — *see* Disorder, globe, degenerative, specified type NEC
  renal N18.9 *[H32]*
  syphilitic (early) (secondary) A51.43
    central, recurrent A52.71
    congenital (early) A50.01 *[H32]*
    late A52.71
  tuberculous A18.53
Retinoblastoma C69.2- ☑
  differentiated C69.2- ☑
  undifferentiated C69.2- ☑
Retinochoroiditis — *see also* Inflammation, chorioretinal
  disseminated — *see* Inflammation, chorioretinal, disseminated
    syphilitic A52.71
  focal — *see* Inflammation, chorioretinal
  juxtapapillaris — *see* Inflammation, chorioretinal, focal, juxtapapillary
Retinopathy (background) H35.00
  arteriosclerotic I70.8 *[H35.0-]* ☑
  atherosclerotic I70.8 *[H35.0-]* ☑
  central serous — *see* Chorioretinopathy, central serous
  Coats H35.02- ☑
  diabetic — *see* Diabetes, retinopathy
  exudative H35.02- ☑
  hypertensive H35.03- ☑
  in (due to)
    diabetes — *see* Diabetes, retinopathy
    sickle-cell disorders D57.- ☑ *[H36]*

Retinopathy — *continued*
  of prematurity H35.10- ☑
    stage 0 H35.11- ☑
    stage 1 H35.12- ☑
    stage 2 H35.13- ☑
    stage 3 H35.14- ☑
    stage 4 H35.15- ☑
    stage 5 H35.16- ☑
  pigmentary, congenital — *see* Dystrophy, retina
  proliferative NEC H35.2- ☑
    diabetic — *see* Diabetes, retinopathy, proliferative
    sickle-cell D57.- ☑ *[H36]*
  solar H31.02- ☑
Retinoschisis H33.10- ☑
  congenital Q14.1
  specified type NEC H33.19- ☑
Retortamoniasis A07.8
Retractile testis Q55.22
Retraction
  cervix — *see* Retroversion, uterus
  drum (membrane) — *see* Disorder, tympanic membrane, specified NEC
  finger — *see* Deformity, finger
  lid H02.539
    left H02.536
      lower H02.535
      upper H02.534
    right H02.533
      lower H02.532
      upper H02.531
  lung J98.4
  mediastinum J98.59
  nipple N64.53
    associated with
      lactation O92.03
      pregnancy O92.01- ☑
      puerperium O92.02
    congenital Q83.8
  palmar fascia M72.0
  pleura — *see* Pleurisy
  ring, uterus (Bandl's) (pathological) O62.4
  sternum (congenital) Q76.7
    acquired M95.4
  uterus — *see* Retroversion, uterus
  valve (heart) — *see* Endocarditis
Retrobulbar — *see* condition
Retrocecal — *see* condition
Retrocession — *see* Retroversion
Retrodisplacement — *see* Retroversion
Retroflection, retroflexion — *see* Retroversion
Retrognathia, retrognathism (mandibular) (maxillary) M26.19
Retrograde menstruation N92.5
Retroperineal — *see* condition
Retroperitoneal — *see* condition
Retroperitonitis K68.9
Retropharyngeal — *see* condition
Retroplacental — *see* condition
Retroposition — *see* Retroversion
Retroprosthetic membrane T85.398 ☑
Retrosternal thyroid (congenital) Q89.2
Retroversion, retroverted
  cervix — *see* Retroversion, uterus
  female NEC — *see* Retroversion, uterus
  iris H21.89
  testis (congenital) Q55.29
  uterus (acquired) (acute) (any degree) (asymptomatic) (cervix) (postinfectional) (postpartal, old) N85.4
    congenital Q51.818
    in pregnancy O34.53- ☑
Retrovirus, as cause of disease classified elsewhere B97.30
  human
    immunodeficiency, type 2 (HIV 2) B97.35
    T-cell lymphotropic
      type I (HTLV-I) B97.33
      type II (HTLV-II) B97.34
  lentivirus B97.31
  oncovirus B97.32
  specified NEC B97.39
Retrusion, premaxilla (developmental) M26.09
Rett's disease or syndrome F84.2
Reverse peristalsis R19.2
Reye's syndrome G93.7
Rh (factor)
  hemolytic disease (newborn) P55.0

Rh — *continued*
  incompatibility, immunization or sensitization
    affecting management of pregnancy NEC O36.09- ☑
      anti-D antibody O36.01- ☑
    newborn P55.0
    transfusion reaction — *see* Complication(s), transfusion, incompatibility reaction, Rh (factor)
  negative mother affecting newborn P55.0
  titer elevated — *see* Complication(s), transfusion, incompatibility reaction, Rh (factor)
  transfusion reaction — *see* Complication(s), transfusion, incompatibility reaction, Rh (factor)
Rhabdomyolysis (idiopathic) NEC M62.82
  traumatic T79.6 ☑
Rhabdomyoma — *see also* Neoplasm, connective tissue, benign
  adult — *see* Neoplasm, connective tissue, benign
  fetal — *see* Neoplasm, connective tissue, benign
  glycogenic — *see* Neoplasm, connective tissue, benign
Rhabdomyosarcoma (any type) — *see* Neoplasm, connective tissue, malignant
Rhabdosarcoma — *see* Rhabdomyosarcoma
Rhesus (factor) **incompatibility** — *see* Rh, incompatibility
Rheumatic (acute) (subacute)
  adherent pericardium I09.2
  chronic I09.89
  coronary arteritis I01.8
  degeneration, myocardium I09.0
  fever (acute) — *see* Fever, rheumatic
  heart — *see* Disease, heart, rheumatic
  myocardial degeneration — *see* Degeneration, myocardium
  myocarditis (chronic) (inactive) (with chorea) I09.0
    active or acute I01.2
    with chorea (acute) (rheumatic) (Sydenham's) I02.0
  pancarditis, acute I01.8
    with chorea (acute (rheumatic) Sydenham's) I02.0
  pericarditis (active) (acute) (with effusion) (with pneumonia) I01.0
    with chorea (acute) (rheumatic) (Sydenham's) I02.0
    chronic or inactive I09.2
  pneumonia I00 *[J17]*
  torticollis M43.6
  typhoid fever A01.09
Rheumatism (articular) (neuralgic) (nonarticular) M79.0
  gout — *see* Arthritis, rheumatoid
  intercostal, meaning Tietze's disease M94.0
  palindromic (any site) M12.30
    ankle M12.37- ☑
    elbow M12.32- ☑
    foot joint M12.37- ☑
    hand joint M12.34- ☑
    hip M12.35- ☑
    knee M12.36- ☑
    multiple site M12.39
    shoulder M12.31- ☑
    specified joint NEC M12.38
    vertebrae M12.38
    wrist M12.33- ☑
  sciatic M54.4- ☑
Rheumatoid — *see also* condition
  arthritis — *see also* Arthritis, rheumatoid
    with involvement of organs NEC M05.60
      ankle M05.67- ☑
      elbow M05.62- ☑
      foot joint M05.67- ☑
      hand joint M05.64- ☑
      hip M05.65- ☑
      knee M05.66- ☑
      multiple site M05.69
      shoulder M05.61- ☑
      vertebra — *see* Spondylitis, ankylosing
      wrist M05.63- ☑
    seronegative — *see* Arthritis, rheumatoid, seronegative
    seropositive — *see* Arthritis, rheumatoid, seropositive
  carditis M05.30
    ankle M05.37- ☑
    elbow M05.32- ☑
    foot joint M05.37- ☑
    hand joint M05.34- ☑
    hip M05.35- ☑
    knee M05.36- ☑
    multiple site M05.39
    shoulder M05.31- ☑

Rheumatoid — *continued*
  carditis — *continued*
    vertebra — *see* Spondylitis, ankylosing
    wrist M05.33- ☑
  endocarditis — *see* Rheumatoid, carditis
  lung (disease) M05.10
    ankle M05.17- ☑
    elbow M05.12- ☑
    foot joint M05.17- ☑
    hand joint M05.14- ☑
    hip M05.15- ☑
    knee M05.16- ☑
    multiple site M05.19
    shoulder M05.11- ☑
    vertebra — *see* Spondylitis, ankylosing
    wrist M05.13- ☑
  myocarditis — *see* Rheumatoid, carditis
  myopathy M05.40
    ankle M05.47- ☑
    elbow M05.42- ☑
    foot joint M05.47- ☑
    hand joint M05.44- ☑
    hip M05.45- ☑
    knee M05.46- ☑
    multiple site M05.49
    shoulder M05.41- ☑
    vertebra — *see* Spondylitis, ankylosing
    wrist M05.43- ☑
  pericarditis — *see* Rheumatoid, carditis
  polyarthritis — *see* Arthritis, rheumatoid
  polyneuropathy M05.50
    ankle M05.57- ☑
    elbow M05.52- ☑
    foot joint M05.57- ☑
    hand joint M05.54- ☑
    hip M05.55- ☑
    knee M05.56- ☑
    multiple site M05.59
    shoulder M05.51- ☑
    vertebra — *see* Spondylitis, ankylosing
    wrist M05.53- ☑
  vasculitis M05.20
    ankle M05.27- ☑
    elbow M05.22- ☑
    foot joint M05.27- ☑
    hand joint M05.24- ☑
    hip M05.25- ☑
    knee M05.26- ☑
    multiple site M05.29
    shoulder M05.21- ☑
    vertebra — *see* Spondylitis, ankylosing
    wrist M05.23- ☑
Rhinitis (atrophic) (catarrhal) (chronic) (croupous) (fibrinous) (granulomatous) (hyperplastic) (hypertrophic) (membranous) (obstructive) (purulent) (suppurative) (ulcerative) J31.0
  with
    sore throat — *see* Nasopharyngitis
  acute J00
  allergic J30.9
    with asthma J45.909
      with
        exacerbation (acute) J45.901
        status asthmaticus J45.902
    due to
      food J30.5
      pollen J30.1
    nonseasonal J30.89
    perennial J30.89
    seasonal NEC J30.2
    specified NEC J30.89
  infective J00
  pneumococcal J00
  syphilitic A52.73
    congenital A50.05 *[J99]*
  tuberculous A15.8
  vasomotor J30.0
Rhinoantritis (chronic) — *see* Sinusitis, maxillary
Rhinodacryolith — *see* Dacryolith
Rhinolith (nasal sinus) J34.89
Rhinomegaly J34.89
Rhinopharyngitis (acute) (subacute) — *see also* Nasopharyngitis
  chronic J31.1
  destructive ulcerating A66.5
  mutilans A66.5
Rhinophyma L71.1

Rhinorrhea J34.89
  cerebrospinal (fluid) G96.0
  paroxysmal — *see* Rhinitis, allergic
  spasmodic — *see* Rhinitis, allergic
Rhinosalpingitis — *see* Salpingitis, eustachian
Rhinoscleroma A48.8
Rhinosporidiosis B48.1
Rhinovirus infection NEC B34.8
Rhizomelic chondrodysplasia punctata E71.540
Rhythm
  atrioventricular nodal I49.8
  disorder I49.9
    coronary sinus I49.8
    ectopic I49.8
    nodal I49.8
  escape I49.9
  heart, abnormal I49.9
  idioventricular I44.2
  nodal I49.8
  sleep, inversion G47.2- ☑
    nonorganic origin — *see* Disorder, sleep, circadia rhythm, psychogenic
Rhytidosis facialis L98.8
Rib — *see also* condition
  cervical Q76.5
Riboflavin deficiency E53.0
Rice bodies — *see also* Loose, body, joint
  knee M23.4- ☑
Richter syndrome — *see* Leukemia, chronic lymphocyt B-cell type
Richter's hernia — *see* Hernia, abdomen, with obstru tion
Ricinism — *see* Poisoning, food, noxious, plant
Rickets (active) (acute) (adolescent) (chest wall) (conge ital) (current) (infantile) (intestinal) E55.0
  adult — *see* Osteomalacia
  celiac K90.0
  hypophosphatemic with nephrotic-glycosuric dwarfis E72.09
  inactive E64.3
  kidney N25.0
  renal N25.0
  sequelae, any E64.3
  vitamin-D-resistant E83.31 *[M90.80]*
Rickettsial disease A79.9
  specified type NEC A79.89
Rickettsialpox (Rickettsia akari) A79.1
Rickettsiosis A79.9
  due to
    Ehrlichia sennetsu A79.81
    Rickettsia akari (rickettsialpox) A79.1
  specified type NEC A79.89
  tick-borne A77.9
  vesicular A79.1
Rider's bone — *see* Ossification, muscle, specified NEC
Ridge, alveolus — *see also* condition
  flabby K06.8
Ridged ear, congenital Q17.3
Riedel's
  lobe, liver Q44.7
  struma, thyroiditis or disease E06.5
Rieger's anomaly or syndrome Q13.81
Riehl's melanosis L81.4
Rietti-Greppi-Micheli anemia D56.9
Rieux's hernia — *see* Hernia, abdomen, specified site NEC
Riga (-Fede) **disease** K14.0
Riggs' disease — *see* Periodontitis
Right aortic arch Q25.47
Right middle lobe syndrome J98.11
Rigid, rigidity — *see also* condition
  abdominal R19.30
    with severe abdominal pain R10.0
    epigastric R19.36
    generalized R19.37
    left lower quadrant R19.34
    left upper quadrant R19.32
    periumbilic R19.35
    right lower quadrant R19.33
    right upper quadrant R19.31
  articular, multiple, congenital Q68.8
  cervix (uteri) in pregnancy — *see* Pregnancy, compli cated by, abnormal, cervix
  hymen (acquired) (congenital) N89.6
  nuchal R29.1
  pelvic floor in pregnancy — *see* Pregnancy, complica ed by, abnormal, pelvic organs or tissues NEC

☑ **Additional Character Required** — **Refer to the Tabular List for Character Selection**   **Subterms under main terms may continue to next column or pag**

gid, rigidity — *continued*
　perineum or vulva in pregnancy — *see* Pregnancy,
　　complicated by, abnormal, vulva
　spine — *see* Dorsopathy, specified NEC
　vagina in pregnancy — *see* Pregnancy, complicated
　　by, abnormal, vagina
gors R68.89
　with fever R50.9
ey-Day syndrome G90.1
ND (reversible ischemic neurologic deficit) I63.9
ng(s)
　aorta (vascular) Q25.45
　Bandl's O62.4
　contraction, complicating delivery O62.4
　esophageal, lower (muscular) K22.2
　Fleischer's (cornea) H18.04- ☑
　hymenal, tight (acquired) (congenital) N89.6
　Kayser-Fleischer (cornea) H18.04- ☑
　retraction, uterus, pathological O62.4
　Schatzki's (esophagus) (lower) K22.2
　　congenital Q39.3
　Soemmerring's — *see* Cataract, secondary
　vascular (congenital) Q25.8
　　aorta Q25.45
nged hair (congenital) Q84.1
ngworm B35.9
　beard B35.0
　black dot B35.0
　body B35.4
　Burmese B35.5
　corporeal B35.4
　foot B35.3
　groin B35.6
　hand B35.2
　honeycomb B35.0
　nails B35.1
　perianal (area) B35.6
　scalp B35.0
　specified NEC B35.8
　Tokelau B35.5
se, venous pressure I87.8
**sing, PSA following treatment for malignant neo-
　plasm of prostate** R97.21
sk
　for
　　dental caries Z91.849
　　　high Z91.843
　　　low Z91.841
　　　moderate Z91.842
　suicidal
　　meaning personal history of attempted suicide Z91.5
　　meaning suicidal ideation — *see* Ideation, suicidal
tter's disease L00
valry, sibling Z62.891
valta's disease A42.2
ver blindness B73.01
bert's pelvis Q74.2
　with disproportion (fetopelvic) O33.0
　　causing obstructed labor O65.0
bin (-Pierre) **syndrome** Q87.0
binow-Silvermann-Smith syndrome Q87.19
binson's (hidrotic) **ectodermal dysplasia or syn-
　drome** Q82.4
bles' disease B73.01
cky Mountain (spotted) **fever** A77.0
etheln — *see* Rubella
ger's disease Q21.0
kitansky-Aschoff sinuses (gallbladder) K82.8
lando's fracture (displaced) S62.22- ☑
　nondisplaced S62.22- ☑
mano-Ward (prolonged QT interval) **syndrome** I45.81
mberg's disease or syndrome G51.8
of, mouth — *see* condition
sacea L71.9
　acne L71.9
　keratitis L71.8
　specified NEC L71.8
sary, rachitic E55.0
se
　cold J30.1
　fever J30.1
　rash R21
　　epidemic B06.9
senbach's erysipeloid A26.0
senthal's disease or syndrome D68.1
seola B09
　infantum B08.20

Roseola — *continued*
　infantum — *continued*
　　due to human herpesvirus 6 B08.21
　　due to human herpesvirus 7 B08.22
Ross River disease or fever B33.1
Rossbach's disease K31.89
　psychogenic F45.8
Rostan's asthma (cardiac) — *see* Failure, ventricular, left
Rotation
　anomalous, incomplete or insufficient, intestine Q43.3
　cecum (congenital) Q43.3
　colon (congenital) Q43.3
　spine, incomplete or insufficient — *see* Dorsopathy,
　　deforming, specified NEC
　tooth, teeth, fully erupted M26.35
　vertebra, incomplete or insufficient — *see* Dorsopathy,
　　deforming, specified NEC
Rotes Quérol disease or syndrome — *see* Hyperostosis,
　ankylosing
Roth (-Bernhardt) **disease or syndrome** — *see* Meralgia
　paraesthetica
Rothmund (-Thomson) **syndrome** Q82.8
Rotor's disease or syndrome E80.6
Round
　back (with wedging of vertebrae) — *see* Kyphosis
　　sequelae (late effect) of rickets E64.3
　worms (large) (infestation) NEC B82.0
　　Ascariasis — *see also* Ascariasis B77.9
Roussy-Lévy syndrome G60.0
Rubella (German measles) B06.9
　complication NEC B06.09
　　neurological B06.00
　congenital P35.0
　contact Z20.4
　exposure to Z20.4
　maternal
　　care for (suspected) damage to fetus O35.3 ☑
　　manifest rubella in infant P35.0
　　suspected damage to fetus affecting management
　　　of pregnancy O35.3 ☑
　specified complications NEC B06.89
Rubeola (meaning measles) — *see* Measles
　meaning rubella — *see* Rubella
Rubeosis, iris — *see* Disorder, iris, vascular
Rubinstein-Taybi syndrome Q87.2
Rudimentary (congenital) — *see also* Agenesis
　arm — *see* Defect, reduction, upper limb
　bone Q79.9
　cervix uteri Q51.828
　eye Q11.2
　lobule of ear Q17.3
　patella Q74.1
　respiratory organs in thoracopagus Q89.4
　tracheal bronchus Q32.4
　uterus Q51.818
　　in male Q56.1
　vagina Q52.0
Ruled out condition — *see* Observation, suspected
Rumination R11.10
　with nausea R11.2
　disorder of infancy F98.21
　neurotic F42.8
　newborn P92.1
　obsessional F42.8
　psychogenic F42.8
Runeberg's disease D51.0
Runny nose R09.89
Rupia (syphilitic) A51.39
　congenital A50.06
　tertiary A52.79
Rupture, ruptured
　abscess (spontaneous) — *code by* site under Abscess
　aneurysm — *see* Aneurysm
　anus (sphincter) — *see* Laceration, anus
　aorta, aortic I71.8
　　abdominal I71.3
　　arch I71.1
　　ascending I71.1
　　descending I71.8
　　　abdominal I71.3
　　　thoracic I71.1
　　syphilitic A52.01
　　thoracoabdominal I71.5
　　thorax, thoracic I71.1
　　transverse I71.1
　　traumatic — *see* Injury, aorta, laceration, major
　　valve or cusp — *see also* Endocarditis, aortic I35.8

Rupture, ruptured — *continued*
　appendix (with peritonitis) — *see also* Appendicitis
　　K35.32
　　with localized peritonitis — *see also* Appendicitis
　　　K35.32
　arteriovenous fistula, brain — *see* Fistula, arteriove-
　　nous, brain, ruptured
　artery I77.2
　　brain — *see* Hemorrhage, intracranial, intracerebral
　　coronary — *see* Infarct, myocardium
　　heart — *see* Infarct, myocardium
　　pulmonary I28.8
　　traumatic (complication) — *see* Injury, blood vessel
　bile duct (common) (hepatic) K83.2
　　cystic K82.2
　bladder (sphincter) (nontraumatic) (spontaneous)
　　N32.89
　　following ectopic or molar pregnancy O08.6
　　obstetrical trauma O71.5
　　traumatic S37.29 ☑
　blood vessel — *see also* Hemorrhage
　　brain — *see* Hemorrhage, intracranial, intracerebral
　　heart — *see* Infarct, myocardium
　　traumatic (complication) — *see* Injury, blood vessel,
　　　laceration, major, by site
　bone — *see* Fracture
　bowel (nontraumatic) K63.1
　brain
　　aneurysm (congenital) — *see also* Hemorrhage, in-
　　　tracranial, subarachnoid
　　　syphilitic A52.05
　　hemorrhagic — *see* Hemorrhage, intracranial, intrac-
　　　erebral
　capillaries I78.8
　cardiac (auricle) (ventricle) (wall) I23.3
　　with hemopericardium I23.0
　　infectional I40.9
　　traumatic — *see* Injury, heart
　cartilage (articular) (current) — *see also* Sprain
　　knee S83.3- ☑
　　semilunar — *see* Tear, meniscus
　cecum (with peritonitis) K65.0
　　with peritoneal abscess K35.33
　　traumatic S36.598 ☑
　celiac artery, traumatic — *see* Injury, blood vessel,
　　celiac artery, laceration, major
　cerebral aneurysm (congenital) (see Hemorrhage, in-
　　tracranial, subarachnoid)
　cervix (uteri)
　　with ectopic or molar pregnancy O08.6
　　following ectopic or molar pregnancy O08.6
　　obstetrical trauma O71.3
　　traumatic S37.69 ☑
　chordae tendineae NEC I51.1
　　concurrent with acute myocardial infarction — *see*
　　　Infarct, myocardium
　　following acute myocardial infarction (current
　　　complication) I23.4
　choroid (direct) (indirect) (traumatic) H31.32- ☑
　circle of Willis I60.6
　colon (nontraumatic) K63.1
　　traumatic — *see* Injury, intestine, large
　cornea (traumatic) — *see* Injury, eye, laceration
　coronary (artery) (thrombotic) — *see* Infarct, myocardi-
　　um
　corpus luteum (infected) (ovary) N83.1- ☑
　cyst — *see* Cyst
　cystic duct K82.2
　Descemet's membrane — *see* Change, corneal mem-
　　brane, Descemet's, rupture
　　traumatic — *see* Injury, eye, laceration
　diaphragm, traumatic — *see* Injury, intrathoracic, di-
　　aphragm
　disc — *see* Rupture, intervertebral disc
　diverticulum (intestine) K57.80
　　with bleeding K57.81
　　bladder N32.3
　　large intestine K57.20
　　　with
　　　　bleeding K57.21
　　　　small intestine K57.40
　　　　　with bleeding K57.41
　　small intestine K57.00
　　　with
　　　　bleeding K57.01
　　　　large intestine K57.40
　　　　　with bleeding K57.41
　duodenal stump K31.89

☑ Subterms under main terms may continue to next column or page　　　☑ Additional Character Required — Refer to the Tabular List for Character Selection　　　277

Rigid, rigidity — Rupture, ruptured

Rupture, ruptured — *continued*

ear drum (nontraumatic) — *see also* Perforation, tympanum
  traumatic S09.2- ☑
    due to blast injury — *see* Injury, blast, ear
esophagus K22.3
eye (without prolapse or loss of intraocular tissue) — *see* Injury, eye, laceration
fallopian tube NEC (nonobstetric) (nontraumatic) N83.8
  due to pregnancy O00.10- ☑
    with intrauterine pregnancy O00.11- ☑
fontanel P13.1
gallbladder K82.2
  traumatic S36.128 ☑
gastric — *see also* Rupture, stomach
  vessel K92.2
globe (eye) (traumatic) — *see* Injury, eye, laceration
graafian follicle (hematoma) N83.0- ☑
heart — *see* Rupture, cardiac
hymen (nontraumatic) (nonintentional) N89.8
internal organ, traumatic — *see* Injury, by site
intervertebral disc — *see* Displacement, intervertebral disc
  traumatic — *see* Rupture, traumatic, intervertebral disc
intestine NEC (nontraumatic) K63.1
  traumatic — *see* Injury, intestine
iris — *see also* Abnormality, pupillary
  traumatic — *see* Injury, eye, laceration
joint capsule, traumatic — *see* Sprain
kidney (traumatic) S37.06- ☑
  birth injury P15.8
  nontraumatic N28.89
lacrimal duct (traumatic) — *see* Injury, eye, specified site NEC
lens (cataract) (traumatic) — *see* Cataract, traumatic
ligament, traumatic — *see* Rupture, traumatic, ligament, by site
liver S36.116 ☑
  birth injury P15.0
lymphatic vessel I89.8
marginal sinus (placental) (with hemorrhage) — *see* Hemorrhage, antepartum, specified cause NEC
membrana tympani (nontraumatic) — *see* Perforation, tympanum
membranes (spontaneous)
  artificial
    delayed delivery following O75.5
  delayed delivery following — *see* Pregnancy, complicated by, premature rupture of membranes
meningeal artery I60.8
meniscus (knee) — *see also* Tear, meniscus
  old — *see* Derangement, meniscus
  site other than knee — *code as* Sprain
mesenteric artery, traumatic — *see* Injury, mesenteric, artery, laceration, major
mesentery (nontraumatic) K66.8
  traumatic — *see* Injury, intra-abdominal, specified, site NEC
mitral (valve) I34.8
muscle (traumatic) — *see also* Strain
  diastasis — *see* Diastasis, muscle
  nontraumatic M62.10
    ankle M62.17- ☑
    foot M62.17- ☑
    forearm M62.13- ☑
    hand M62.14- ☑
    lower leg M62.16- ☑
    pelvic region M62.15- ☑
    shoulder region M62.11- ☑
    specified site NEC M62.18
    thigh M62.15- ☑
    upper arm M62.12- ☑
  traumatic — *see* Strain, by site
musculotendinous junction NEC, nontraumatic — *see* Rupture, tendon, spontaneous
mycotic aneurysm causing cerebral hemorrhage — *see* Hemorrhage, intracranial, subarachnoid
myocardium, myocardial — *see* Rupture, cardiac
  traumatic — *see* Injury, heart
nontraumatic, meaning hernia — *see* Hernia
obstructed — *see* Hernia, by site, obstructed
operation wound — *see* Disruption, wound, operation
ovary, ovarian N83.8
  corpus luteum cyst N83.1- ☑
  follicle (graafian) N83.0- ☑
oviduct (nonobstetric) (nontraumatic) N83.8

Rupture, ruptured — *continued*

oviduct — *continued*
  due to pregnancy O00.10- ☑
    with intrauterine pregnancy O00.11- ☑
pancreas (nontraumatic) K86.89
  traumatic S36.299 ☑
papillary muscle NEC I51.2
  following acute myocardial infarction (current complication) I23.5
pelvic
  floor, complicating delivery O70.1
  organ NEC, obstetrical trauma O71.5
perineum (nonobstetric) (nontraumatic) N90.89
  complicating delivery — *see* Delivery, complicated, by, laceration, anus (sphincter)
postoperative wound — *see* Disruption, wound, operation
prostate (traumatic) S37.828 ☑
pulmonary
  artery I28.8
  valve (heart) I37.8
  vein I28.8
  vessel I28.8
pus tube — *see* Salpingitis
pyosalpinx — *see* Salpingitis
rectum (nontraumatic) K63.1
  traumatic S36.69
retina, retinal (traumatic) (without detachment) — *see also* Break, retina
  with detachment — *see* Detachment, retina, with retinal, break
rotator cuff (nontraumatic) M75.10- ☑
  complete M75.12- ☑
  incomplete M75.11- ☑
sclera — *see* Injury, eye, laceration
sigmoid (nontraumatic) K63.1
  traumatic S36.593 ☑
spinal cord — *see also* Injury, spinal cord, by region
  due to injury at birth P11.5
  newborn (birth injury) P11.5
spleen (traumatic) S36.09 ☑
  birth injury P15.1
  congenital (birth injury) P15.1
  due to P. vivax malaria B51.0
  nontraumatic D73.5
  spontaneous D73.5
splenic vein R58
  traumatic — *see* Injury, blood vessel, splenic vein
stomach (nontraumatic) (spontaneous) K31.89
  traumatic S36.39 ☑
supraspinatus (complete) (incomplete) (nontraumatic) — *see* Tear, rotator cuff
symphysis pubis
  obstetric O71.6
  traumatic S33.4 ☑
synovium (cyst) M66.10
  ankle M66.17- ☑
  elbow M66.12- ☑
  finger M66.14- ☑
  foot M66.17- ☑
  forearm M66.13- ☑
  hand M66.14- ☑
  pelvic region M66.15- ☑
  shoulder region M66.11- ☑
  specified site NEC M66.18
  thigh M66.15- ☑
  toe M66.17- ☑
  upper arm M66.12- ☑
  wrist M66.13- ☑
tendon (traumatic) — *see* Strain
  nontraumatic (spontaneous) M66.9
    ankle M66.87- ☑
    extensor M66.20
      ankle M66.27- ☑
      foot M66.27- ☑
      forearm M66.23- ☑
      hand M66.24- ☑
      lower leg M66.26- ☑
      multiple sites M66.29
      pelvic region M66.25- ☑
      shoulder region M66.21- ☑
      specified site NEC M66.28
      thigh M66.25- ☑
      upper arm M66.22- ☑
    flexor M66.30
      ankle M66.37- ☑
      foot M66.37- ☑

Rupture, ruptured — *continued*

tendon — *see* Strain — *continued*
  nontraumatic — *continued*
    flexor — *continued*
      forearm M66.33- ☑
      hand M66.34- ☑
      lower leg M66.36- ☑
      multiple sites M66.39
      pelvic region M66.35- ☑
      shoulder region M66.31- ☑
      specified site NEC M66.38
      thigh M66.35- ☑
      upper arm M66.32- ☑
    foot M66.87- ☑
    forearm M66.83- ☑
    hand M66.84- ☑
    lower leg M66.86- ☑
    multiple sites M66.89
    pelvic region M66.85- ☑
    shoulder region M66.81- ☑
    specified
      site NEC M66.88
      tendon M66.80
    thigh M66.85- ☑
    upper arm M66.82- ☑
thoracic duct I89.8
tonsil J35.8
traumatic
  aorta — *see* Injury, aorta, laceration, major
  diaphragm — *see* Injury, intrathoracic, diaphrag
  external site — *see* Wound, open, by site
  eye — *see* Injury, eye, laceration
  internal organ — *see* Injury, by site
  intervertebral disc
    cervical S13.0 ☑
    lumbar S33.0 ☑
    thoracic S23.0 ☑
  kidney S37.06- ☑
  ligament — *see also* Sprain
    ankle — *see* Sprain, ankle
    carpus — *see* Rupture, traumatic, ligament, wr
    collateral (hand) — *see* Rupture, traumatic, ligament, finger, collateral
    finger (metacarpophalangeal) (interphalange S63.40- ☑
      collateral S63.41- ☑
        index S63.41- ☑
        little S63.41- ☑
        middle S63.41- ☑
        ring S63.41- ☑
      index S63.40- ☑
      little S63.40- ☑
      middle S63.40- ☑
      palmar S63.42- ☑
        index S63.42- ☑
        little S63.42- ☑
        middle S63.42- ☑
        ring S63.42- ☑
      ring S63.40- ☑
      specified site NEC S63.499 ☑
        index S63.49- ☑
        little S63.49- ☑
        middle S63.49- ☑
        ring S63.49- ☑
      volar plate S63.43- ☑
        index S63.43- ☑
        little S63.43- ☑
        middle S63.43- ☑
        ring S63.43- ☑
    foot — *see* Sprain, foot
    radial collateral S53.2- ☑
    radiocarpal — *see* Rupture, traumatic, ligament, wrist, radiocarpal
    ulnar collateral S53.3- ☑
    ulnocarpal — *see* Rupture, traumatic, ligament, wrist, ulnocarpal
    wrist S63.30- ☑
      collateral S63.31- ☑
      radiocarpal S63.32- ☑
      specified site NEC S63.39- ☑
      ulnocarpal (palmar) S63.33- ☑
  liver S36.116 ☑
  membrana tympani — *see* Rupture, ear drum, traumatic
  muscle or tendon — *see* Strain
  myocardium — *see* Injury, heart

Sarcoma — continued

lymphoblastic — *see* Lymphoma, lymphoblastic (diffuse)
lymphocytic — *see* Lymphoma, small cell B-cell
mast cell C96.22
melanotic — *see* Melanoma
meningeal — *see* Neoplasm, meninges, malignant
meningothelial — *see* Neoplasm, meninges, malignant
mesenchymal — *see also* Neoplasm, connective tissue, malignant
  mixed — *see* Neoplasm, connective tissue, malignant
mesothelial — *see* Mesothelioma
monstrocellular
  specified site — *see* Neoplasm, malignant, by site
  unspecified site C71.9
myeloid C92.3- ☑
neurogenic — *see* Neoplasm, nerve, malignant
odontogenic C41.1
  upper jaw (bone) C41.0
osteoblastic — *see* Neoplasm, bone, malignant
osteogenic — *see also* Neoplasm, bone, malignant
  juxtacortical — *see* Neoplasm, bone, malignant
  periosteal — *see* Neoplasm, bone, malignant
periosteal — *see also* Neoplasm, bone, malignant
  osteogenic — *see* Neoplasm, bone, malignant
pleomorphic cell — *see* Neoplasm, connective tissue, malignant
reticulum cell (diffuse) — *see* Lymphoma, diffuse large cell
  nodular — *see* Lymphoma, follicular
  pleomorphic cell type — *see* Lymphoma, diffuse large cell
rhabdoid — *see* Neoplasm, malignant, by site
round cell — *see* Neoplasm, connective tissue, malignant
small cell — *see* Neoplasm, connective tissue, malignant
soft tissue — *see* Neoplasm, connective tissue, malignant
spindle cell — *see* Neoplasm, connective tissue, malignant
stromal (endometrial) C54.1
  isthmus C54.0
synovial — *see also* Neoplasm, connective tissue, malignant
  biphasic — *see* Neoplasm, connective tissue, malignant
  epithelioid cell — *see* Neoplasm, connective tissue, malignant
  spindle cell — *see* Neoplasm, connective tissue, malignant

Sarcomatosis

meningeal — *see* Neoplasm, meninges, malignant
specified site NEC — *see* Neoplasm, connective tissue, malignant
unspecified site C80.1
Sarcopenia (age-related) M62.84
Sarcosinemia E72.59
Sarcosporidiosis (intestinal) A07.8
Satiety, early R68.81
Saturnine — *see* condition
Saturnism
overdose or wrong substance given or taken — *see* Table of Drugs and Chemicals, by drug, poisoning
Satyriasis F52.8
Sauriasis — *see* Ichthyosis
SBE (subacute bacterial endocarditis) I33.0
Scabies (any site) B86
Scabs R23.4
Scaglietti-Dagnini syndrome E22.0
Scald — *see* Burn
Scalenus anticus (anterior) **syndrome** G54.0
Scales R23.4
Scaling, skin R23.4
Scalp — *see* condition
Scapegoating affecting child Z62.3
Scaphocephaly Q75.0
Scapulalgia M89.8X1
Scapulohumeral myopathy G71.02
Scar, scarring — *see also* Cicatrix L90.5
adherent L90.5
atrophic L90.5
cervix
  in pregnancy or childbirth — *see* Pregnancy, complicated by, abnormal cervix
cheloid L91.0

Scar, scarring — continued

chorioretinal H31.00- ☑
  posterior pole macula H31.01- ☑
  postsurgical H59.81- ☑
  solar retinopathy H31.02- ☑
  specified type NEC H31.09- ☑
choroid — *see* Scar, chorioretinal
conjunctiva H11.24- ☑
cornea H17.9
  xerophthalmic — *see also* Opacity, cornea
    vitamin A deficiency E50.6
duodenum, obstructive K31.5
hypertrophic L91.0
keloid L91.0
labia N90.89
lung (base) J98.4
macula — *see* Scar, chorioretinal, posterior pole
muscle M62.89
myocardium, myocardial I25.2
painful L90.5
posterior pole (eye) — *see* Scar, chorioretinal, posterior pole
retina — *see* Scar, chorioretinal
trachea J39.8
transmural uterine, in pregnancy O34.29
uterus N85.8
  in pregnancy O34.29
vagina N89.8
  postoperative N99.2
vulva N90.89
Scarabiasis B88.2
Scarlatina (anginosa) (maligna) A38.9
myocarditis (acute) A38.1
  old — *see* Myocarditis
otitis media A38.0
ulcerosa A38.8
Scarlet fever (albuminuria) (angina) A38.9
Schamberg's disease (progressive pigmentary dermatosis) L81.7
Schatzki's ring (acquired) (esophagus) (lower) K22.2
congenital Q39.3
Schaufenster krankheit I20.8
Schaumann's
benign lymphogranulomatosis D86.1
disease or syndrome — *see* Sarcoidosis
Scheie's syndrome E76.03
Schenck's disease B42.1
Scheuermann's disease or osteochondrosis — *see* Osteochondrosis, juvenile, spine
Schilder (-Flatau) **disease** G37.0
Schilling-type monocytic leukemia C93.0- ☑
Schimmelbusch's disease, cystic mastitis, or hyperplasia — *see* Mastopathy, cystic
Schistosoma infestation — *see* Infestation, Schistosoma
Schistosomiasis B65.9
with muscle disorder B65.9 [M63.80]
  ankle B65.9 [M63.87-] ☑
  foot B65.9 [M63.87-] ☑
  forearm B65.9 [M63.83-] ☑
  hand B65.9 [M63.84-] ☑
  lower leg B65.9 [M63.86-] ☑
  multiple sites B65.9 [M63.89]
  pelvic region B65.9 [M63.85-] ☑
  shoulder region B65.9 [M63.81-] ☑
  specified site NEC B65.9 [M63.88]
  thigh B65.9 [M63.85-] ☑
  upper arm B65.9 [M63.82-] ☑
Asiatic B65.2
bladder B65.0
chestermani B65.8
colon B65.1
cutaneous B65.3
due to
  S. haematobium B65.0
  S. japonicum B65.2
  S. mansoni B65.1
  S. mattheii B65.8
Eastern B65.2
genitourinary tract B65.0
intestinal B65.1
lung NEC B65.9 [J99]
  pneumonia B65.9 [J17]
Manson's (intestinal) B65.1
oriental B65.2
pulmonary NEC B65.9 [J99]
  pneumonia B65.9

Schistosomiasis — continued

Schistosoma
  haematobium B65.0
  japonicum B65.2
  mansoni B65.1
specified type NEC B65.8
urinary B65.0
vesical B65.0
Schizencephaly Q04.6
Schizoaffective psychosis F25.9
Schizodontia K00.2
Schizoid personality F60.1
Schizophrenia, schizophrenic F20.9
acute (brief) (undifferentiated) F23
atypical (form) F20.3
borderline F21
catalepsy F20.2
catatonic (type) (excited) (withdrawn) F20.2
cenesthopathic, cenesthesiopathic F20.89
childhood type F84.5
chronic undifferentiated F20.5
cyclic F25.0
disorganized (type) F20.1
flexibilitas cerea F20.2
hebephrenic (type) F20.1
incipient F21
latent F21
negative type F20.5
paranoid (type) F20.0
paraphrenic F20.0
post-psychotic depression F32.89
prepsychotic F21
prodromal F21
pseudoneurotic F21
pseudopsychopathic F21
reaction F23
residual (state) (type) F20.5
restzustand F20.5
schizoaffective (type) — *see* Psychosis, schizoaffect
simple (type) F20.89
simplex F20.89
specified type NEC F20.89
spectrum and other psychotic disorder F29
  specified NEC F28
stupor F20.2
syndrome of childhood F84.5
undifferentiated (type) F20.3
  chronic F20.5
Schizothymia (persistent) F60.1
Schlatter-Osgood disease or osteochondrosis — *s* Osteochondrosis, juvenile, tibia
Schlatter's tibia — *see* Osteochondrosis, juvenile, tib
Schmidt's syndrome (polyglandular, autoimmune) E3
Schmincke's carcinoma or tumor — *see* Neoplasm nasopharynx, malignant
Schmitz (-Stutzer) **dysentery** A03.0
Schmorl's disease or nodes
lumbar region M51.46
lumbosacral region M51.47
sacrococcygeal region M53.3
thoracic region M51.44
thoracolumbar region M51.45
Schneiderian
papilloma — *see* Neoplasm, nasopharynx, benign
  specified site — *see* Neoplasm, benign, by site
  unspecified site D14.0
specified site — *see* Neoplasm, malignant, by site
  unspecified site C30.0
Scholte's syndrome (malignant carcinoid) E34.0
Scholz (-Bielchowsky-Henneberg) **disease or syndrom** E75.25
Schönlein (-Henoch) disease or purpura (primary) (rheumatic) D69.0
Schottmuller's disease A01.4
Schroeder's syndrome (endocrine hypertensive) E2?
Schüller-Christian disease or syndrome C96.5
Schultze's type acroparesthesia, simple I73.89
Schultz's disease or syndrome — *see* Agranulocyto
Schwalbe-Ziehen-Oppenheim disease G24.1
Schwannoma — *see also* Neoplasm, nerve, benign
malignant — *see also* Neoplasm, nerve, malignant
  with rhabdomyoblastic differentiation — *see* Ne plasm, nerve, malignant
melanocytic — *see* Neoplasm, nerve, benign
pigmented — *see* Neoplasm, nerve, benign
Schwannomatosis Q85.03
Schwartz (-Jampel) **syndrome** G71.13
Schwartz-Bartter syndrome E22.2

☑ **Additional Character Required — Refer to the Tabular List for Character Selection**   ▽ **Subterms under main terms may continue to next column or pag**

hweniger-Buzzi anetoderma L90.1
:iatic — *see* condition
iatica (infective)
  with lumbago M54.4- ☑
    due to intervertebral disc disorder — *see* Disorder, disc, with, radiculopathy
  due to displacement of intervertebral disc (with lumbago) — *see* Disorder, disc, with, radiculopathy
  wallet M54.3- ☑
imitar syndrome Q26.8
:lera — *see* condition
lerectasia H15.84- ☑
leredema
  adultorum — *see* Sclerosis, systemic
  Buschke's — *see* Sclerosis, systemic
  newborn P83.0
lerema (adiposum) (edematosum) (neonatorum) (newborn) P83.0
  adultorum — *see* Sclerosis, systemic
:leriasis — *see* Scleroderma
leritis H15.00- ☑
  with corneal involvement H15.04- ☑
  anterior H15.01- ☑
  brawny H15.02- ☑
  in (due to) zoster B02.34
  posterior H15.03- ☑
  specified type NEC H15.09- ☑
  syphilitic A52.71
  tuberculous (nodular) A18.51
lerochoroiditis H31.8
:leroconjunctivitis — *see* Scleritis
:lerocystic ovary syndrome E28.2
:lerodactyly, sclerodactylia L94.3
:leroderma, sclerodermia (acrosclerotic) (diffuse) (generalized) (progressive) (pulmonary) — *see also* Sclerosis, systemic M34.9
  circumscribed L94.0
  linear L94.1
  localized L94.0
  newborn P83.88
  systemic M34.9
:lerokeratitis H16.8
  tuberculous A18.52
leroma nasi A48.8
:leromalacia (perforans) H15.05- ☑
:leromyxedema L98.5
:lérose en plaques G35
:lerosis, sclerotic
  adrenal (gland) E27.8
  Alzheimer's — *see* Disease, Alzheimer's
  amyotrophic (lateral) G12.21
  aorta, aortic I70.0
    valve — *see* Endocarditis, aortic
  artery, arterial, arteriolar, arteriovascular — *see* Arteriosclerosis
  ascending multiple G35
  brain (generalized) (lobular) G37.9
    artery, arterial I67.2
    diffuse G37.0
    disseminated G35
    insular G35
    Krabbe's E75.23
    miliary G35
    multiple G35
    presenile (Alzheimer's) — *see* Disease, Alzheimer's, early onset
    senile (arteriosclerotic) I67.2
    stem, multiple G35
    tuberous Q85.1
  bulbar, multiple G35
  bundle of His I44.39
  cardiac — *see* Disease, heart, ischemic, atherosclerotic
  cardiorenal — *see* Hypertension, cardiorenal
  cardiovascular — *see also* Disease, cardiovascular
    renal — *see* Hypertension, cardiorenal
  cerebellar — *see* Sclerosis, brain
  cerebral — *see* Sclerosis, brain
  cerebrospinal (disseminated) (multiple) G35
  cerebrovascular I67.2
  choroid — *see* Degeneration, choroid
  combined (spinal cord) — *see also* Degeneration, combined
    multiple G35
  concentric (Balo) G37.5
  cornea — *see* Opacity, cornea
  coronary (artery) I25.10

Sclerosis, sclerotic — *continued*
  coronary — *continued*
    with angina pectoris — *see* Arteriosclerosis, coronary (artery),
  corpus cavernosum
    female N90.89
    male N48.6
  diffuse (brain) (spinal cord) G37.0
  disseminated G35
  dorsal G35
  dorsolateral (spinal cord) — *see* Degeneration, combined
  endometrium N85.5
  extrapyramidal G25.9
  eye, nuclear (senile) — *see* Cataract, senile, nuclear
  focal and segmental (glomerular) — *see also* N00-N07
    with fourth character .1 N05.1
  Friedreich's (spinal cord) G11.1
  funicular (spermatic cord) N50.89
  general (vascular) — *see* Arteriosclerosis
  gland (lymphatic) I89.8
  hepatic K74.1
    alcoholic K70.2
  hereditary
    cerebellar G11.9
    spinal (Friedreich's ataxia) G11.1
  hippocampal G93.81
  insular G35
  kidney — *see* Sclerosis, renal
  larynx J38.7
  lateral (amyotrophic) (descending) (spinal) G12.21
    primary G12.23
  lens, senile nuclear — *see* Cataract, senile, nuclear
  liver K74.1
    with fibrosis K74.2
      alcoholic K70.2
    alcoholic K70.2
    cardiac K76.1
  lung — *see* Fibrosis, lung
  mastoid — *see* Mastoiditis, chronic
  mesial temporal G93.81
  mitral I05.8
  Mönckeberg's (medial) — *see* Arteriosclerosis, extremities
  multiple (brain stem) (cerebral) (generalized) (spinal cord) G35
  myocardium, myocardial — *see* Disease, heart, ischemic, atherosclerotic
  nuclear (senile), eye — *see* Cataract, senile, nuclear
  ovary N83.8
  pancreas K86.89
  penis N48.6
  peripheral arteries — *see* Arteriosclerosis, extremities
  plaques G35
  pluriglandular E31.8
  polyglandular E31.8
  posterolateral (spinal cord) — *see* Degeneration, combined
  presenile (Alzheimer's) — *see* Disease, Alzheimer's, early onset
  primary, lateral G12.23
  progressive, systemic M34.0
  pulmonary — *see* Fibrosis, lung
    artery I27.0
    valve (heart) — *see* Endocarditis, pulmonary
  renal N26.9
    with
      cystine storage disease E72.09
      hypertensive heart disease (conditions in I11) — *see* Hypertension, cardiorenal
    arteriolar (hyaline) (hyperplastic) — *see* Hypertension, kidney
  retina (senile) (vascular) H35.00
  senile (vascular) — *see* Arteriosclerosis
  spinal (cord) (progressive) G95.89
    ascending G61.0
    combined — *see also* Degeneration, combined
      multiple G35
      syphilitic A52.11
    disseminated G35
    dorsolateral — *see* Degeneration, combined
    hereditary (Friedreich's) (mixed form) G11.1
    lateral (amyotrophic) G12.21
      progressive G12.23
    multiple G35
    posterior (syphilitic) A52.11
  stomach K31.89
  subendocardial, congenital I42.4

Sclerosis, sclerotic — *continued*
  systemic M34.9
    with
      lung involvement M34.81
      myopathy M34.82
      polyneuropathy M34.83
    drug-induced M34.2
    due to chemicals NEC M34.2
    progressive M34.0
    specified NEC M34.89
  temporal (mesial) G93.81
  tricuspid (heart) (valve) I07.8
  tuberous (brain) Q85.1
  tympanic membrane — *see* Disorder, tympanic membrane, specified NEC
  valve, valvular (heart) — *see* Endocarditis
  vascular — *see* Arteriosclerosis
  vein I87.8
Scoliosis (acquired) (postural) M41.9
  adolescent (idiopathic) — *see* Scoliosis, idiopathic, adolescent
  congenital Q67.5
    due to bony malformation Q76.3
    failure of segmentation (hemivertebra) Q76.3
    hemivertebra fusion Q76.3
    postural Q67.5
  idiopathic M41.20
    adolescent M41.129
      cervical region M41.122
      cervicothoracic region M41.123
      lumbar region M41.126
      lumbosacral region M41.127
      thoracic region M41.124
      thoracolumbar region M41.125
    cervical region M41.22
    cervicothoracic region M41.23
    infantile M41.00
      cervical region M41.02
      cervicothoracic region M41.03
      lumbar region M41.06
      lumbosacral region M41.07
      sacrococcygeal region M41.08
      thoracic region M41.04
      thoracolumbar region M41.05
    juvenile M41.119
      cervical region M41.112
      cervicothoracic region M41.113
      lumbar region M41.116
      lumbosacral region M41.117
      thoracic region M41.114
      thoracolumbar region M41.115
    lumbar region M41.26
    lumbosacral region M41.27
    thoracic region M41.24
    thoracolumbar region M41.25
  infantile — *see* Scoliosis, idiopathic, infantile
  neuromuscular M41.40
    cervical region M41.42
    cervicothoracic region M41.43
    lumbar region M41.46
    lumbosacral region M41.47
    occipito-atlanto-axial region M41.41
    thoracic region M41.44
    thoracolumbar region M41.45
  paralytic — *see* Scoliosis, neuromuscular
  postradiation therapy M96.5
  rachitic (late effect or sequelae) E64.3 *[M49.80]*
    cervical region E64.3 *[M49.82]*
    cervicothoracic region E64.3 *[M49.83]*
    lumbar region E64.3 *[M49.86]*
    lumbosacral region E64.3 *[M49.87]*
    multiple sites E64.3 *[M49.89]*
    occipito-atlanto-axial region E64.3 *[M49.81]*
    sacrococcygeal region E64.3 *[M49.88]*
    thoracic region E64.3 *[M49.84]*
    thoracolumbar region E64.3 *[M49.85]*
  sciatic M54.4- ☑
  secondary (to) NEC M41.50
    cerebral palsy, Friedreich's ataxia, poliomyelitis, neuromuscular disorders — *see* Scoliosis, neuromuscular
    cervical region M41.52
    cervicothoracic region M41.53
    lumbar region M41.56
    lumbosacral region M41.57
    thoracic region M41.54
    thoracolumbar region M41.55
  specified form NEC M41.80

𝄐 Subterms under main terms may continue to next column or page   ☑ Additional Character Required — Refer to the Tabular List for Character Selection   281

Schweniger-Buzzi anetoderma — Scoliosis

Scoliosis — *continued*
  specified form — *continued*
    cervical region M41.82
    cervicothoracic region M41.83
    lumbar region M41.86
    lumbosacral region M41.87
    thoracic region M41.84
    thoracolumbar region M41.85
  thoracogenic M41.30
    thoracic region M41.34
    thoracolumbar region M41.35
  tuberculous A18.01
Scoliotic pelvis
  with disproportion (fetopelvic) O33.0
    causing obstructed labor O65.0
Scorbutus, scorbutic — *see also* Scurvy
  anemia D53.2
Score, NIHSS (National Institutes of Health Stroke Scale)
  R29.7- ☑
Scotoma (arcuate) (Bjerrum) (central) (ring) — *see also*
  Defect, visual field, localized, scotoma
  scintillating H53.19
Scratch — *see* Abrasion
Scratchy throat R09.89
Screening (for) Z13.9
  alcoholism Z13.39
  anemia Z13.0
  anomaly, congenital Z13.89
  antenatal, of mother — *see also* Encounter, antenatal
    screening Z36.9
  arterial hypertension Z13.6
  arthropod-borne viral disease NEC Z11.59
  autism Z13.41
  bacteriuria, asymptomatic Z13.89
  behavioral disorder Z13.30
    specified NEC Z13.39
  brain injury, traumatic Z13.850
  bronchitis, chronic Z13.83
  brucellosis Z11.2
  cardiovascular disorder Z13.6
  cataract Z13.5
  chlamydial diseases Z11.8
  cholera Z11.0
  chromosomal abnormalities (nonprocreative) NEC
    Z13.79
  colonoscopy Z12.11
  congenital
    dislocation of hip Z13.89
    eye disorder Z13.5
    malformation or deformation Z13.89
  contamination NEC Z13.88
  cystic fibrosis Z13.228
  dengue fever Z11.59
  dental disorder Z13.84
  depression (adult) (adolescent) (child) Z13.31
    maternal Z13.32
    perinatal Z13.32
  developmental
    delays Z13.40
      global (milestones) Z13.42
      specified NEC Z13.49
    handicap Z13.42
      in early childhood Z13.42
  diabetes mellitus Z13.1
  diphtheria Z11.2
  disability, intellectual Z13.39
  disease or disorder Z13.9
    bacterial NEC Z11.2
      intestinal infectious Z11.0
      respiratory tuberculosis Z11.1
    behavioral Z13.30
      specified NEC Z13.39
    blood or blood-forming organ Z13.0
    cardiovascular Z13.6
    Chagas' Z11.6
    chlamydial Z11.8
    dental Z13.89
    developmental delays Z13.40
      global (milestones) Z13.42
      specified NEC Z13.49
    digestive tract NEC Z13.818
      lower GI Z13.811
      upper GI Z13.810
    ear Z13.5
    endocrine Z13.29
    eye Z13.5
    genitourinary Z13.89
    heart Z13.6

Screening — *continued*
  disease or disorder — *continued*
    human immunodeficiency virus (HIV) infection Z11.4
    immunity Z13.0
    infection
      intestinal Z11.0
        specified NEC Z11.6
    infectious Z11.9
    mental health and behavioral Z13.30
      specified NEC Z13.39
    metabolic Z13.228
    neurological Z13.89
    nutritional Z13.21
      metabolic Z13.228
        lipoid disorders Z13.220
    protozoal Z11.6
      intestinal Z11.0
    respiratory Z13.83
    rheumatic Z13.828
    rickettsial Z11.8
    sexually-transmitted NEC Z11.3
      human immunodeficiency virus (HIV) Z11.4
    sickle-cell (trait) Z13.0
    skin Z13.89
    specified NEC Z13.89
    spirochetal Z11.8
    thyroid Z13.29
    vascular Z13.6
    venereal Z11.3
    viral NEC Z11.59
      human immunodeficiency virus (HIV) Z11.4
      intestinal Z11.0
  elevated titer Z13.89
  emphysema Z13.83
  encephalitis, viral (mosquito- or tick-borne) Z11.59
  exposure to contaminants (toxic) Z13.88
  fever
    dengue Z11.59
    hemorrhagic Z11.59
    yellow Z11.59
  filariasis Z11.6
  galactosemia Z13.228
  gastrointestinal condition Z13.818
  genetic (nonprocreative) - for procreative management
    — *see* Testing, genetic, for procreative manage-
    ment
    disease carrier status (nonprocreative) Z13.71
    specified NEC (nonprocreative) Z13.79
  genitourinary condition Z13.89
  glaucoma Z13.5
  gonorrhea Z11.3
  gout Z13.89
  helminthiasis (intestinal) Z11.6
  hematopoietic malignancy Z12.89
  hemoglobinopathies NEC Z13.0
  hemorrhagic fever Z11.59
  Hodgkin disease Z12.89
  human immunodeficiency virus (HIV) Z11.4
  human papillomavirus Z11.51
  hypertension Z13.6
  immunity disorders Z13.0
  infant or child (over 28 days old) Z00.129
    with abnormal findings Z00.121
  infection
    mycotic Z11.8
    parasitic Z11.8
  ingestion of radioactive substance Z13.88
  intellectual disability Z13.39
  intestinal
    helminthiasis Z11.6
    infectious disease Z11.0
  leishmaniasis Z11.6
  leprosy Z11.2
  leptospirosis Z11.8
  leukemia Z12.89
  lymphoma Z12.89
  malaria Z11.6
  malnutrition Z13.29
    metabolic Z13.228
    nutritional Z13.21
  measles Z11.59
  mental health disorder Z13.30
    specified NEC Z13.39
  metabolic errors, inborn Z13.228
  multiphasic Z13.228
  musculoskeletal disorder Z13.828
    osteoporosis Z13.820
  mycoses Z11.8
  myocardial infarction (acute) Z13.6

Screening — *continued*
  neoplasm (malignant) (of) Z12.9
    bladder Z12.6
    blood Z12.89
    breast Z12.39
      routine mammogram Z12.31
    cervix Z12.4
    colon Z12.11
    genitourinary organs NEC Z12.79
      bladder Z12.6
      cervix Z12.4
      ovary Z12.73
      prostate Z12.5
      testis Z12.71
      vagina Z12.72
    hematopoietic system Z12.89
    intestinal tract Z12.10
      colon Z12.11
      rectum Z12.12
      small intestine Z12.13
    lung Z12.2
    lymph (glands) Z12.89
    nervous system Z12.82
    oral cavity Z12.81
    prostate Z12.5
    rectum Z12.12
    respiratory organs Z12.2
    skin Z12.83
    small intestine Z12.13
    specified site NEC Z12.89
    stomach Z12.0
  nephropathy Z13.89
  nervous system disorders NEC Z13.858
  neurological condition Z13.89
  osteoporosis Z13.820
  parasitic infestation Z11.9
    specified NEC Z11.8
  phenylketonuria Z13.228
  plague Z11.2
  poisoning (chemical) (heavy metal) Z13.88
  poliomyelitis Z11.59
  postnatal, chromosomal abnormalities Z13.89
  prenatal, of mother — *see also* Encounter, antenata
    screening Z36.9
  protozoal disease Z11.6
    intestinal Z11.0
  pulmonary tuberculosis Z11.1
  radiation exposure Z13.88
  respiratory condition Z13.83
  respiratory tuberculosis Z11.1
  rheumatoid arthritis Z13.828
  rubella Z11.59
  schistosomiasis Z11.6
  sexually-transmitted disease NEC Z11.3
    human immunodeficiency virus (HIV) Z11.4
  sickle-cell disease or trait Z13.0
  skin condition Z13.89
  sleeping sickness Z11.6
  special Z13.9
    specified NEC Z13.89
  syphilis Z11.3
  tetanus Z11.2
  trachoma Z11.8
  traumatic brain injury Z13.850
  trypanosomiasis Z11.6
  tuberculosis, respiratory Z11.1
    active Z11.1
    latent Z11.7
  venereal disease Z11.3
  viral encephalitis (mosquito- or tick-borne) Z11.59
  whooping cough Z11.2
  worms, intestinal Z11.6
  yaws Z11.8
  yellow fever Z11.59
Scrofula, scrofulosis (tuberculosis of cervical lymph
  glands) A18.2
Scrofulide (primary) (tuberculous) A18.4
Scrofuloderma, scrofulodermia (any site) (primary)
  A18.4
Scrofulosus lichen (primary) (tuberculous) A18.4
Scrofulous — *see* condition
Scrotal tongue K14.5
Scrotum — *see* condition
Scurvy, scorbutic E54
  anemia D53.2
  gum E54
  infantile E54
  rickets E55.0 *[M90.80]*

☑ **Additional Character Required** — Refer to the Tabular List for Character Selection   ▽ Subterms under main terms may continue to next column or pag

alpox B08.62
asickness T75.3 ☑
atworm (infection) (infestation) B80
baceous — see also condition
cyst — see Cyst, sebaceous
borrhea, seborrheic L21.9
capillitii R23.8
capitis L21.9
dermatitis L21.9
infantile L21.1
eczema L21.9
infantile L21.1
sicca L21.0
ckel's syndrome Q87.19
clusion, pupil — see Membrane, pupillary
cond hand tobacco smoke exposure (acute)
(chronic) Z77.22
in the perinatal period P96.81
condary
dentin (in pulp) K04.3
neoplasm, secondaries — see Table of Neoplasms,
secondary
cretion
antidiuretic hormone, inappropriate E22.2
catecholamine, by pheochromocytoma E27.5
hormone
antidiuretic, inappropriate (syndrome) E22.2
by
carcinoid tumor E34.0
pheochromocytoma E27.5
ectopic NEC E34.2
urinary
excessive R35.8
suppression R34
ction
nerve, traumatic — see Injury, nerve
dative, hypnotic, or anxiolytic-induced
anxiety disorder F13.980
bipolar and related disorder F13.94
delirium F13.921
depressive disorder F13.94
major neurocognitive disorder F13.97
mild neurocognitive disorder F13.988
psychotic disorder F13.959
sexual dysfunction F13.981
sleep disorder F13.982
gmentation, incomplete (congenital) — see also
Fusion
bone NEC Q78.8
lumbosacral (joint) (vertebra) Q76.49
itelberger's syndrome (infantile neuraxonal dystrophy) G31.89
izure(s) — see also Convulsions R56.9
absence G40.A- ☑ (following G40.3)
akinetic — see Epilepsy, generalized, specified NEC
atonic — see Epilepsy, generalized, specified NEC
autonomic (hysterical) F44.5
convulsive — see Convulsions
cortical (focal) (motor) — see Epilepsy, localization-related, symptomatic, with simple partial seizures
disorder — see also Epilepsy G40.909
due to stroke — see Sequelae (of), disease, cerebrovascular, by type, specified NEC
epileptic — see Epilepsy
febrile (simple) R56.00
with status epilepticus G40.901
complex (atypical) (complicated) R56.01
with status epilepticus G40.901
grand mal G40.409
intractable G40.419
with status epilepticus G40.411
without status epilepticus G40.419
not intractable G40.409
with status epilepticus G40.401
without status epilepticus G40.409
heart — see Disease, heart
hysterical F44.5
intractable G40.919
with status epilepticus G40.911
Jacksonian (focal) (motor type) (sensory type) — see
Epilepsy, localization-related, symptomatic, with
simple partial seizures
newborn P90
nonspecific epileptic
atonic — see Epilepsy, generalized, specified NEC
clonic — see Epilepsy, generalized, specified NEC
myoclonic — see Epilepsy, generalized, specified
NEC

Seizure(s) — continued
nonspecific epileptic — continued
tonic — see Epilepsy, generalized, specified NEC
tonic-clonic — see Epilepsy, generalized, specified
NEC
partial, developing into secondarily generalized
seizures
complex — see Epilepsy, localization-related,
symptomatic, with complex partial seizures
simple — see Epilepsy, localization-related, symptomatic, with simple partial seizures
petit mal G40.A- ☑ (following G40.3)
intractable G40.419
with status epilepticus G40.411
without status epilepticus G40.419
not intractable G40.409
with status epilepticus G40.401
without status epilepticus G40.409
post traumatic R56.1
recurrent G40.909
specified NEC G40.89
uncinate — see Epilepsy, localization-related, symptomatic, with complex partial seizures
Selenium deficiency, dietary E59
Self-damaging behavior (life-style) Z72.89
Self-harm (attempted)
history (personal) Z91.5
in family Z81.8
Self-mutilation (attempted)
history (personal) Z91.5
in family Z81.8
Self-poisoning
history (personal) Z91.5
in family Z81.8
observation following (alleged) attempt Z03.6
Semicoma R40.1
Seminal vesiculitis N49.0
Seminoma C62.9- ☑
specified site — see Neoplasm, malignant, by site
Senear-Usher disease or syndrome L10.4
Senectus R54
Senescence (without mention of psychosis) R54
Senile, senility — see also condition R41.81
with
acute confusional state F05
mental changes NOS F03 ☑
psychosis NEC — see Psychosis, senile
asthenia R54
cervix (atrophic) N88.8
debility R54
endometrium (atrophic) N85.8
fallopian tube (atrophic) — see Atrophy, fallopian tube
heart (failure) R54
ovary (atrophic) — see Atrophy, ovary
premature E34.8
vagina, vaginitis (atrophic) N95.2
wart L82.1
Sensation
burning (skin) R20.8
tongue K14.6
loss of R20.8
prickling (skin) R20.2
tingling (skin) R20.2
Sense loss
smell — see Disturbance, sensation, smell
taste — see Disturbance, sensation, taste
touch R20.8
Sensibility disturbance (cortical) (deep) (vibratory) R20.9
Sensitive, sensitivity — see also Allergy
carotid sinus G90.01
child (excessive) F93.8
cold, autoimmune D59.1
dentin K03.89
gluten (non-celiac) K90.41
latex Z91.040
methemoglobin D74.8
tuberculin, without clinical or radiological symptoms
R76.11
visual
glare H53.71
impaired contrast H53.72
Sensitiver Beziehungswahn F22
Sensitization, auto-erythrocytic D69.2
Separation
anxiety, abnormal (of childhood) F93.0
apophysis, traumatic — code as Fracture, by site
choroid — see Detachment, choroid

Separation — continued
epiphysis, epiphyseal
nontraumatic — see also Osteochondropathy,
specified type NEC
upper femoral — see Slipped, epiphysis, upper
femoral
traumatic — code as Fracture, by site
fracture — see Fracture
infundibulum cardiac from right ventricle by a partition
Q24.3
joint (traumatic) (current) — code by site under Dislocation
muscle (nontraumatic) — see Diastasis, muscle
pubic bone, obstetrical trauma O71.6
retina, retinal — see Detachment, retina
symphysis pubis, obstetrical trauma O71.6
tracheal ring, incomplete, congenital Q32.1
Sepsis (generalized) (unspecified organism) A41.9
with
organ dysfunction (acute) (multiple) R65.20
with septic shock R65.21
actinomycotic A42.7
adrenal hemorrhage syndrome (meningococcal) A39.1
anaerobic A41.4
Bacillus anthracis A22.7
Brucella — see also Brucellosis A23.9
candidal B37.7
cryptogenic A41.9
due to device, implant or graft T85.79 ☑
arterial graft NEC T82.7 ☑
breast (implant) T85.79 ☑
catheter NEC T85.79 ☑
dialysis (renal) T82.7 ☑
intraperitoneal T85.71 ☑
infusion NEC T82.7 ☑
spinal (cranial) (epidural) (intrathecal) (spinal)
(subarachnoid) (subdural) T85.735 ☑
urethral indwelling T83.511 ☑
urinary T83.518 ☑
ectopic or molar pregnancy O08.82
electronic (electrode) (pulse generator) (stimulator)
bone T84.7 ☑
cardiac T82.7 ☑
nervous system T85.738 ☑
brain T85.731 ☑
neurostimulator generator T85.734 ☑
peripheral nerve T85.732 ☑
spinal cord T85.733 ☑
urinary T83.590 ☑
fixation, internal (orthopedic) — see Complication,
fixation device, infection
gastrointestinal (bile duct) (esophagus) T85.79 ☑
neurostimulator electrode (lead) T85.732 ☑
genital T83.69 ☑
heart NEC T82.7 ☑
valve (prosthesis) T82.6 ☑
graft T82.7 ☑
joint prosthesis — see Complication, joint prosthesis, infection
ocular (corneal graft) (orbital implant) T85.79 ☑
orthopedic NEC T84.7 ☑
fixation device, internal — see Complication,
fixation device, infection
specified NEC T85.79 ☑
vascular T82.7 ☑
ventricular intracranial (communicating) shunt
T85.730 ☑
during labor O75.3
Enterococcus A41.81
Erysipelothrix (rhusiopathiae) (erysipeloid) A26.7
Escherichia coli (E. coli) A41.5 ☑
extraintestinal yersiniosis A28.2
following
abortion (subsequent episode) O08.0
current episode — see Abortion
ectopic or molar pregnancy O08.82
immunization T88.0 ☑
infusion, therapeutic injection or transfusion NEC
T80.29 ☑
obstetrical procedure O86.04
gangrenous A41.9
gonococcal A54.86
Gram-negative (organism) A41.5 ☑
anaerobic A41.4
Haemophilus influenzae A41.3
herpesviral B00.7
intra-abdominal K65.1

Sepsis — *continued*
  intraocular — *see* Endophthalmitis, purulent
  Listeria monocytogenes A32.7
  localized — *code to* specific localized infection
    in operation wound T81.49 ☑
    skin — *see* Abscess
  malleus A24.Ø
  melioidosis A24.1
  meningeal — *see* Meningitis
  meningococcal A39.4
    acute A39.2
    chronic A39.3
  MSSA (Methicillin susceptible Staphylococcus aureus)
    A41.Ø1
  newborn P36.9
    due to
      anaerobes NEC P36.5
      Escherichia coli P36.4
      Staphylococcus P36.3Ø
        aureus P36.2
        specified NEC P36.39
      Streptococcus P36.1Ø
        group B P36.Ø
        specified NEC P36.19
    specified NEC P36.8
  Pasteurella multocida A28.Ø
  pelvic, puerperal, postpartum, childbirth O85
  pneumococcal A4Ø.3
  postprocedural T81.44 ☑
  puerperal, postpartum, childbirth (pelvic) O85
  Salmonella (arizonae) (cholerae-suis) (enteritidis) (ty-
    phimurium) AØ2.1
  severe R65.2Ø
    with septic shock R65.21
  Shigella — *see also* Dysentery, bacillary AØ3.9
  skin, localized — *see* Abscess
  specified organism NEC A41.89
  Staphylococcus, staphylococcal A41.2
    aureus (methicillin susceptible) (MSSA) A41.Ø1
      methicillin resistant (MRSA) A41.Ø2
    coagulase-negative A41.1
    specified NEC A41.1
  Streptococcus, streptococcal A4Ø.9
    agalactiae A4Ø.1
    group
      A A4Ø.Ø
      B A4Ø.1
      D A41.81
    neonatal P36.1Ø
      group B P36.Ø
      specified NEC P36.19
    pneumoniae A4Ø.3
    pyogenes A4Ø.Ø
    specified NEC A4Ø.8
  tracheostomy stoma J95.Ø2
  tularemic A21.7
  umbilical, umbilical cord (newborn) — *see* Sepsis,
    newborn
  Yersinia pestis A2Ø.7
Septate — *see* Septum
Septic — *see* condition
  arm — *see* Cellulitis, upper limb
    with lymphangitis — *see* Lymphangitis, acute, upper
      limb
  embolus — *see* Embolism
  finger — *see* Cellulitis, digit
    with lymphangitis — *see* Lymphangitis, acute, digit
  foot — *see* Cellulitis, lower limb
    with lymphangitis — *see* Lymphangitis, acute,
      lower limb
  gallbladder (acute) K81.Ø
  hand — *see* Cellulitis, upper limb
    with lymphangitis — *see* Lymphangitis, acute, upper
      limb
  joint — *see* Arthritis, pyogenic or pyemic
  leg — *see* Cellulitis, lower limb
    with lymphangitis — *see* Lymphangitis, acute,
      lower limb
  nail — *see also* Cellulitis, digit
    with lymphangitis — *see* Lymphangitis, acute, digit
  sore — *see also* Abscess
    throat JØ2.Ø
      streptococcal JØ2.Ø
  spleen (acute) D73.89
  teeth, tooth (pulpal origin) KØ4.4
  throat — *see* Pharyngitis
  thrombus — *see* Thrombosis
  toe — *see* Cellulitis, digit

Septic — *continued*
  toe — *see* Cellulitis, digit — *continued*
    with lymphangitis — *see* Lymphangitis, acute, digit
  tonsils, chronic J35.Ø1
    with adenoiditis J35.Ø3
  uterus — *see* Endometritis
Septicemia A41.9
  meaning sepsis — *see* Sepsis
Septum, septate (congenital) — *see also* Anomaly, by
  site
  anal Q42.3
    with fistula Q42.2
  aqueduct of Sylvius QØ3.Ø
    with spina bifida — *see* Spina bifida, by site, with
      hydrocephalus
  uterus Q51.2Ø
    complete Q51.21
    partial Q51.22
    specified NEC Q51.28
  vagina Q52.1Ø
    in pregnancy — *see* Pregnancy, complicated by,
      abnormal vagina
      causing obstructed labor O65.5
    longitudinal Q52.129
      microperforate
        left side Q52.124
        right side Q52.123
      nonobstruction Q52.12Ø
      obstructing Q52.129
        left side Q52.122
        right side Q52.121
    transverse Q52.11
Sequelae (of) — *see also* condition
  abscess, intracranial or intraspinal (conditions in GØ6)
    GØ9
  amputation — *code to* injury with seventh character
    S
  burn and corrosion — *code to* injury with seventh
    character S
  calcium deficiency E64.8
  cerebrovascular disease — *see* Sequelae, disease,
    cerebrovascular
  childbirth O94
  contusion — *code to* injury with seventh character S
  corrosion — *see* Sequelae, burn and corrosion
  crushing injury — *code to* injury with seventh character
    S
  disease
    cerebrovascular I69.9Ø
      alteration of sensation I69.998
      aphasia I69.92Ø
      apraxia I69.99Ø
      ataxia I69.993
      cognitive deficits I69.91 ☑
      disturbance of vision I69.998
      dysarthria I69.922
      dysphagia I69.991
      dysphasia I69.921
      facial droop I69.992
      facial weakness I69.992
      fluency disorder I69.923
      hemiplegia I69.95- ☑
      hemorrhage
        intracerebral — *see* Sequelae, hemorrhage,
          intracerebral
        intracranial, nontraumatic NEC — *see* Seque-
          lae, hemorrhage, intracranial, nontrau-
          matic
        subarachnoid — *see* Sequelae, hemorrhage,
          subarachnoid
      language deficit I69.928
      monoplegia
        lower limb I69.94- ☑
        upper limb I69.93- ☑
      paralytic syndrome I69.96- ☑
      specified effect NEC I69.998
      specified type NEC I69.8Ø
        alteration of sensation I69.898
        aphasia I69.82Ø
        apraxia I69.89Ø
        ataxia I69.893
        cognitive deficits I69.81 ☑
        disturbance of vision I69.898
        dysarthria I69.822
        dysphagia I69.891
        dysphasia I69.821
        facial droop I69.892
        facial weakness I69.892

Sequelae — *continued*
  disease — *continued*
    cerebrovascular — *continued*
      specified type — *continued*
        fluency disorder I69.823
        hemiplegia I69.85- ☑
        language deficit I69.828
        monoplegia
          lower limb I69.84- ☑
          upper limb I69.83- ☑
        paralytic syndrome I69.86- ☑
        specified effect NEC I69.898
      speech deficit I69.928
        speech deficit I69.828
      stroke NOS — *see* Sequelae, stroke NOS
    dislocation — *code to* injury with seventh characte
    encephalitis or encephalomyelitis (conditions in GØ
      GØ9
      in infectious disease NEC B94.8
      viral B94.1
    external cause — *code to* injury with seventh charac
      S
    foreign body entering natural orifice — *code to* inju
      with seventh character S
    fracture — *code to* injury with seventh character S
    frostbite — *code to* injury with seventh character S
    Hansen's disease B92
    hemorrhage
      intracerebral I69.1Ø
        alteration of sensation I69.198
        aphasia I69.12Ø
        apraxia I69.19Ø
        ataxia I69.193
        cognitive deficits I69.11 ☑
        disturbance of vision I69.198
        dysarthria I69.122
        dysphagia I69.191
        dysphasia I69.121
        facial droop I69.192
        facial weakness I69.192
        fluency disorder I69.123
        hemiplegia I69.15- ☑
        language deficit NEC I69.128
        monoplegia
          lower limb I69.14- ☑
          upper limb I69.13- ☑
        paralytic syndrome I69.16- ☑
        specified effect NEC I69.198
        speech deficit NEC I69.128
      intracranial, nontraumatic NEC I69.2Ø
        alteration of sensation I69.298
        aphasia I69.22Ø
        apraxia I69.29Ø
        ataxia I69.293
        cognitive deficits I69.21 ☑
        disturbance of vision I69.298
        dysarthria I69.222
        dysphagia I69.291
        dysphasia I69.221
        facial droop I69.292
        facial weakness I69.292
        fluency disorder I69.223
        hemiplegia I69.25- ☑
        language deficit NEC I69.228
        monoplegia
          lower limb I69.24- ☑
          upper limb I69.23- ☑
        paralytic syndrome I69.26- ☑
        specified effect NEC I69.298
        speech deficit NEC I69.228
      subarachnoid I69.ØØ
        alteration of sensation I69.Ø98
        aphasia I69.Ø2Ø
        apraxia I69.Ø9Ø
        ataxia I69.Ø93
        cognitive deficits — *see* subcategory I69.Ø1-
        disturbance of vision I69.Ø98
        dysarthria I69.Ø22
        dysphagia I69.Ø91
        dysphasia I69.Ø21
        facial droop I69.Ø92
        facial weakness I69.Ø92
        fluency disorder I69.Ø23
        hemiplegia I69.Ø5- ☑
        language deficit NEC I69.Ø28
        monoplegia
          lower limb I69.Ø4- ☑
          upper limb I69.Ø3- ☑

quelae — *continued*
hemorrhage — *continued*
  subarachnoid — *continued*
    paralytic syndrome I69.06- ☑
    specified effect NEC I69.098
    speech deficit NEC I69.028
hepatitis, viral B94.2
hyperalimentation E68
infarction
  cerebral I69.30
    alteration of sensation I69.398
    aphasia I69.320
    apraxia I69.390
    ataxia I69.393
    cognitive deficits I69.31 ☑
    disturbance of vision I69.398
    dysarthria I69.322
    dysphagia I69.391
    dysphasia I69.321
    facial droop I69.392
    facial weakness I69.392
    fluency disorder I69.323
    hemiplegia I69.35- ☑
    language deficit NEC I69.328
    monoplegia
      lower limb I69.34- ☑
      upper limb I69.33- ☑
    paralytic syndrome I69.36- ☑
    specified effect NEC I69.398
    speech deficit NEC I69.328
infection, pyogenic, intracranial or intraspinal G09
infectious disease B94.9
  specified NEC B94.8
injury — *code to* injury with seventh character S
leprosy B92
meningitis
  bacterial (conditions in G00) G09
  other or unspecified cause (conditions in G03) G09
muscle (and tendon) injury — *code to* injury with seventh character S
myelitis — *see* Sequelae, encephalitis
niacin deficiency E64.8
nutritional deficiency E64.9
  specified NEC E64.8
obstetrical condition O94
parasitic disease B94.9
phlebitis or thrombophlebitis of intracranial or intraspinal venous sinuses and veins (conditions in G08) G09
poisoning — *code to* poisoning with seventh character S
  nonmedicinal substance — *see* Sequelae, toxic effect, nonmedicinal substance
poliomyelitis (acute) B91
pregnancy O94
protein-energy malnutrition E64.0
puerperium O94
rickets E64.3
selenium deficiency E64.8
sprain and strain — *code to* injury with seventh character S
stroke NOS I69.30
  alteration in sensation I69.398
  aphasia I69.320
  apraxia I69.390
  ataxia I69.393
  cognitive deficits I69.31 ☑
  disturbance of vision I69.398
  dysarthria I69.322
  dysphagia I69.391
  dysphasia I69.321
  facial droop I69.392
  facial weakness I69.392
  hemiplegia I69.35 ☑
  language deficit NEC I69.328
  monoplegia
    lower limb I69.34- ☑
    upper limb I69.33- ☑
  paralytic syndrome I69.36- ☑
  specified effect NEC I69.398
  speech deficit NEC I69.328
tendon and muscle injury — *code to* injury with seventh character S
thiamine deficiency E64.8
trachoma B94.0
tuberculosis B90.9
  bones and joints B90.2
  central nervous system B90.0

Sequelae — *continued*
tuberculosis — *continued*
  genitourinary B90.1
  pulmonary (respiratory) B90.9
  specified organs NEC B90.8
viral
  encephalitis B94.1
  hepatitis B94.2
vitamin deficiency NEC E64.8
  A E64.1
  B E64.8
  C E64.2
wound, open — *code to* injury with seventh character S
Sequestration — *see also* Sequestrum
disk — *see* Displacement, intervertebral disk
lung, congenital Q33.2
Sequestrum
bone — *see* Osteomyelitis, chronic
dental M27.2
jaw bone M27.2
orbit — *see* Osteomyelitis, orbit
sinus (accessory) (nasal) — *see* Sinusitis
Sequoiosis lung or pneumonitis J67.8
Serology for syphilis
doubtful
  with signs or symptoms — *code by* site and stage under Syphilis
  follow-up of latent syphilis — *see* Syphilis, latent
negative, with signs or symptoms — *code by* site and stage under Syphilis
positive A53.0
  with signs or symptoms — *code by* site and stage under Syphilis
reactivated A53.0
Seroma — *see also* Hematoma
postprocedural — *see* Complication, postprocedural, seroma
traumatic, secondary and recurrent T79.2 ☑
Seropurulent — *see* condition
Serositis, multiple K65.8
pericardial I31.1
peritoneal K65.8
Serous — *see* condition
Sertoli cell
adenoma
  specified site — *see* Neoplasm, benign, by site
  unspecified site
    female D27.9
    male D29.20
carcinoma
  specified site — *see* Neoplasm, malignant, by site
  unspecified site (male) C62.9- ☑
    female C56.9
tumor
  with lipid storage
    specified site — *see* Neoplasm, benign, by site
    unspecified site
      female D27.9
      male D29.20
  specified site — *see* Neoplasm, benign, by site
  unspecified site
    female D27.9
    male D29.20
Sertoli-Leydig cell tumor — *see* Neoplasm, benign, by site
specified site — *see* Neoplasm, benign, by site
unspecified site
  female D27.9
  male D29.20
Serum
allergy, allergic reaction — *see also* Reaction, serum T80.69 ☑
  shock — *see also* Shock, anaphylactic T80.59 ☑
arthritis — *see also* Reaction, serum T80.69 ☑
complication or reaction NEC — *see also* Reaction, serum T80.69 ☑
disease NEC — *see also* Reaction, serum T80.69 ☑
hepatitis — *see also* Hepatitis, viral, type B
  carrier (suspected) of B18.1
intoxication — *see also* Reaction, serum T80.69 ☑
neuritis — *see also* Reaction, serum T80.69 ☑
neuropathy G61.1
poisoning NEC — *see also* Reaction, serum T80.69 ☑
rash NEC — *see also* Reaction, serum T80.69 ☑
reaction NEC — *see also* Reaction, serum T80.69 ☑
sickness NEC — *see also* Reaction, serum T80.69 ☑

Serum — *continued*
urticaria — *see also* Reaction, serum T80.69 ☑
Sesamoiditis M25.8- ☑
Severe sepsis R65.20
with septic shock R65.21
Sever's disease or osteochondrosis — *see* Osteochondrosis, juvenile, tarsus
Sex
chromosome mosaics Q97.8
  lines with various numbers of X chromosomes Q97.2
education Z70.8
reassignment surgery status Z87.890
Sextuplet pregnancy — *see* Pregnancy, sextuplet
Sexual
function, disorder of (psychogenic) F52.9
immaturity (female) (male) E30.0
impotence (psychogenic) organic origin NEC — *see* Dysfunction, sexual, male
precocity (constitutional) (cryptogenic)(female) (idiopathic) (male) E30.1
Sexuality, pathologic — *see* Deviation, sexual
Sézary disease C84.1- ☑
Shadow, lung R91.8
Shaking palsy or paralysis — *see* Parkinsonism
Shallowness, acetabulum — *see* Derangement, joint, specified type NEC, hip
Shaver's disease J63.1
Sheath (tendon) — *see* condition
Sheathing, retinal vessels H35.01- ☑
Shedding
nail L60.8
premature, primary (deciduous) teeth K00.6
Sheehan's disease or syndrome E23.0
Shelf, rectal K62.89
Shell teeth K00.5
Shellshock (current) F43.0
lasting state — *see* Disorder, post-traumatic stress
Shield kidney Q63.1
Shift
auditory threshold (temporary) H93.24- ☑
mediastinal R93.89
Shifting sleep-work schedule (affecting sleep) G47.26
Shiga (-Kruse) **dysentery** A03.0
Shiga's bacillus A03.0
Shigella (dysentery) — *see* Dysentery, bacillary
Shigellosis A03.9
Group A A03.0
Group B A03.1
Group C A03.2
Group D A03.3
Shin splints S86.89- ☑
Shingles — *see* Herpes, zoster
Shipyard disease or eye B30.0
Shirodkar suture, in pregnancy — *see* Pregnancy, complicated by, incompetent cervix
Shock R57.9
with ectopic or molar pregnancy O08.3
adrenal (cortical) (Addisonian) E27.2
adverse food reaction (anaphylactic) — *see* Shock, anaphylactic, due to food
allergic — *see* Shock, anaphylactic
anaphylactic T78.2 ☑
  chemical — *see* Table of Drugs and Chemicals
  due to drug or medicinal substance
    correct substance properly administered T88.6 ☑
    overdose or wrong substance given or taken (by accident) — *see* Table of Drugs and Chemicals, by drug, poisoning
  due to food (nonpoisonous) T78.00 ☑
    additives T78.06 ☑
    dairy products T78.07 ☑
    eggs T78.08 ☑
    fish T78.03 ☑
      shellfish T78.02 ☑
    fruit T78.04 ☑
    milk T78.07 ☑
    nuts T78.05 ☑
      multiple types T78.05 ☑
      peanuts T78.01 ☑
    peanuts T78.01 ☑
    seeds T78.05 ☑
    specified type NEC T78.09 ☑
    vegetable T78.04 ☑
  following sting(s) — *see* Venom
  immunization T80.52 ☑
  serum T80.59 ☑
    blood and blood products T80.51 ☑

Subterms under main terms may continue to next column or page   ☑ **Additional Character Required** — Refer to the Tabular List for Character Selection   **285**

Sequelae — Shock

Shock — *continued*
    anaphylactic — *continued*
        serum — *continued*
            immunization T80.52 ☑
            specified NEC T80.59 ☑
            vaccination T80.52 ☑
    anaphylactoid — *see* Shock, anaphylactic
    anesthetic
        correct substance properly administered T88.2 ☑
        overdose or wrong substance given or taken — *see* Table of Drugs and Chemicals, by drug, poisoning
        specified anesthetic — *see* Table of Drugs and Chemicals, by drug, poisoning
    cardiogenic R57.0
    chemical substance — *see* Table of Drugs and Chemicals
    complicating ectopic or molar pregnancy O08.3
    culture — *see* Disorder, adjustment
    drug
        due to correct substance properly administered T88.6 ☑
        overdose or wrong substance given or taken (by accident) — *see* Table of Drugs and Chemicals, by drug, poisoning
    during or after labor and delivery O75.1
    electric T75.4 ☑
        (taser) T75.4 ☑
    endotoxic R65.21
        postprocedural (resulting from a procedure, not elsewhere classified) T81.12 ☑
    following
        ectopic or molar pregnancy O08.3
        injury (immediate) (delayed) T79.4 ☑
        labor and delivery O75.1
    food (anaphylactic) — *see* Shock, anaphylactic, due to food
    from electroshock gun (taser) T75.4 ☑
    gram-negative R65.21
        postprocedural (resulting from a procedure, not elsewhere classified) T81.12 ☑
    hematologic R57.8
    hemorrhagic R57.8
        surgery (intraoperative) (postoperative) T81.19 ☑
        trauma T79.4 ☑
    hypovolemic R57.1
        surgical T81.19 ☑
        traumatic T79.4 ☑
    insulin E15
        therapeutic misadventure — *see* subcategory T38.3 ☑
    kidney N17.0
        traumatic (following crushing) T79.5 ☑
    lightning T75.01 ☑
    liver K72.00
    lung J80
    obstetric O75.1
        with ectopic or molar pregnancy O08.3
        following ectopic or molar pregnancy O08.3
    pleural (surgical) T81.19 ☑
        due to trauma T79.4 ☑
    postprocedural (postoperative) T81.10 ☑
        with ectopic or molar pregnancy O08.3
        cardiogenic T81.11 ☑
        endotoxic T81.12 ☑
        following ectopic or molar pregnancy O08.3
        gram-negative T81.12 ☑
        hypovolemic T81.19 ☑
        septic T81.12 ☑
        specified type NEC T81.19 ☑
    psychic F43.0
    septic (due to severe sepsis) R65.21
    specified NEC R57.8
    surgical T81.10 ☑
    taser gun (taser) T75.4 ☑
    therapeutic misadventure NEC T81.10 ☑
    thyroxin
        overdose or wrong substance given or taken — *see* Table of Drugs and Chemicals, by drug, poisoning
    toxic, syndrome A48.3
    transfusion — *see* Complications, transfusion
    traumatic (immediate) (delayed) T79.4 ☑
Shoemaker's chest M95.4
Short, shortening, shortness
    arm (acquired) — *see also* Deformity, limb, unequal length

Short, shortening, shortness — *continued*
    arm — *see also* Deformity, limb, unequal length — *continued*
        congenital Q71.81- ☑
        forearm — *see* Deformity, limb, unequal length
    bowel syndrome K91.2
    breath R06.02
    cervical (complicating pregnancy) O26.87- ☑
        non-gravid uterus N88.3
    common bile duct, congenital Q44.5
    cord (umbilical), complicating delivery O69.3 ☑
    cystic duct, congenital Q44.5
    esophagus (congenital) Q39.8
    femur (acquired) — *see* Deformity, limb, unequal length, femur
        congenital — *see* Defect, reduction, lower limb, longitudinal, femur
    frenum, frenulum, linguae (congenital) Q38.1
    hip (acquired) — *see also* Deformity, limb, unequal length
        congenital Q65.89
    leg (acquired) — *see also* Deformity, limb, unequal length
        congenital Q72.81- ☑
        lower leg — *see also* Deformity, limb, unequal length
    limbed stature, with immunodeficiency D82.2
    lower limb (acquired) — *see also* Deformity, limb, unequal length
        congenital Q72.81- ☑
    organ or site, congenital NEC — *see* Distortion
    palate, congenital Q38.5
    radius (acquired) — *see also* Deformity, limb, unequal length
        congenital — *see* Defect, reduction, upper limb, longitudinal, radius
    rib syndrome Q77.2
    stature (child) (hereditary) (idiopathic) NEC R62.52
        constitutional E34.3
        due to endocrine disorder E34.3
        Laron-type E34.3
    tendon — *see also* Contraction, tendon
        with contracture of joint — *see* Contraction, joint
        Achilles (acquired) M67.0- ☑
            congenital Q66.89
        congenital Q79.8
    thigh (acquired) — *see also* Deformity, limb, unequal length, femur
        congenital — *see* Defect, reduction, lower limb, longitudinal, femur
    tibialis anterior (tendon) — *see* Contraction, tendon
    umbilical cord
        complicating delivery O69.3 ☑
    upper limb, congenital — *see* Defect, reduction, upper limb, specified type NEC
    urethra N36.8
    uvula, congenital Q38.5
    vagina (congenital) Q52.4
Shortsightedness — *see* Myopia
Shoshin (acute fulminating beriberi) E51.11
Shoulder — *see* condition
Shovel-shaped incisors K00.2
Shower, thromboembolic — *see* Embolism
Shunt
    arterial-venous (dialysis) Z99.2
    arteriovenous, pulmonary (acquired) I28.0
        congenital Q25.72
    cerebral ventricle (communicating) in situ Z98.2
    surgical, prosthetic, with complications — *see* Complications, cardiovascular, device or implant
Shutdown, renal N28.9
Shy-Drager syndrome G90.3
Sialadenitis, sialadenosis (any gland) (chronic) (periodic) (suppurative) — *see* Sialoadenitis
Sialectasia K11.8
Sialidosis E77.1
Sialitis, silitis (any gland) (chronic) (suppurative) — *see* Sialoadenitis
Sialoadenitis (any gland) (periodic) (suppurative) K11.20
    acute K11.21
        recurrent K11.22
    chronic K11.23
Sialoadenopathy K11.9
Sialoangitis — *see* Sialoadenitis
Sialodochitis (fibrinosa) — *see* Sialoadenitis
Sialodocholithiasis K11.5
Sialolithiasis K11.5

Sialometaplasia, necrotizing K11.8
Sialorrhea — *see also* Ptyalism
    periodic — *see* Sialoadenitis
Sialosis K11.7
Siamese twin Q89.4
Sibling rivalry Z62.891
Sicard's syndrome G52.7
Sicca syndrome M35.00
    with
        keratoconjunctivitis M35.01
        lung involvement M35.02
        myopathy M35.03
        renal tubulo-interstitial disorders M35.04
    specified organ involvement NEC M35.09
Sick R69
    or handicapped person in family Z63.79
        needing care at home Z63.6
    sinus (syndrome) I49.5
Sick-euthyroid syndrome E07.81
Sickle-cell
    anemia — *see* Disease, sickle-cell
    trait D57.3
Sicklemia — *see also* Disease, sickle-cell
    trait D57.3
Sickness
    air (travel) T75.3 ☑
    airplane T75.3 ☑
    alpine T70.29 ☑
    altitude T70.20 ☑
    Andes T70.29 ☑
    aviator's T70.29 ☑
    balloon T70.29 ☑
    car T75.3 ☑
    compressed air T70.3 ☑
    decompression T70.3 ☑
    green D50.8
    milk — *see* Poisoning, food, noxious
    motion T75.3 ☑
    mountain T70.29 ☑
        acute D75.1
    protein — *see also* Reaction, serum T80.69 ☑
    radiation T66 ☑
    roundabout (motion) T75.3 ☑
    sea T75.3 ☑
    serum NEC — *see also* Reaction, serum T80.69 ☑
    sleeping (African) B56.9
        by Trypanosoma B56.9
            brucei
                gambiense B56.0
                rhodesiense B56.1
        East African B56.1
        Gambian B56.0
        Rhodesian B56.1
        West African B56.0
    swing (motion) T75.3 ☑
    train (railway) (travel) T75.3 ☑
    travel (any vehicle) T75.3 ☑
Sideropenia — *see* Anemia, iron deficiency
Siderosilicosis J62.8
Siderosis (lung) J63.4
    eye (globe) — *see* Disorder, globe, degenerative, siderosis
Siemens' syndrome (ectodermal dysplasia) Q82.8
Sighing R06.89
    psychogenic F45.8
Sigmoid — *see also* condition
    flexure — *see* condition
    kidney Q63.1
Sigmoiditis — *see also* Enteritis K52.9
    infectious A09
    noninfectious K52.9
Silfversköld's syndrome Q78.9
Silicosiderosis J62.8
Silicosis, silicotic (simple) (complicated) J62.8
    with tuberculosis J65
Silicotuberculosis J65
Silo-fillers' disease J68.8
    bronchitis J68.0
    pneumonitis J68.0
    pulmonary edema J68.1
Silver's syndrome Q87.19
Simian malaria B53.1
Simmonds' cachexia or disease E23.0
Simons' disease or syndrome (progressive lipodystrophy) E88.1
Simple, simplex — *see* condition
Simulation, conscious (of illness) Z76.5

☑ Additional Character Required — Refer to the Tabular List for Character Selection   🔻 Subterms under main terms may continue to next column or pa▮

multanagnosia (asimultagnosia) R48.3
n Nombre virus disease (Hantavirus) (cardio)-pulmonary syndrome B33.4
nding-Larsen disease or osteochondrosis — see Osteochondrosis, juvenile, patella
ngapore hemorrhagic fever A91
nger's node or nodule J38.2
ngle
  atrium Q21.2
  coronary artery Q24.5
  umbilical artery Q27.0
  ventricle Q20.4
ngultus R06.6
  epidemicus B33.0
nus — see also Fistula
  abdominal K63.89
  arrest I45.5
  arrhythmia I49.8
  bradycardia R00.1
  branchial cleft (internal) (external) Q18.0
  coccygeal — see Sinus, pilonidal
  dental K04.6
  dermal (congenital) Q06.8
    with abscess Q06.8
    coccygeal, pilonidal — see Sinus, coccygeal
  infected, skin NEC L08.89
  marginal, ruptured or bleeding — see Hemorrhage, antepartum, specified cause NEC
  medial, face and neck Q18.8
  pause I45.5
  pericranii Q01.9
  pilonidal (infected) (rectum) L05.92
    with abscess L05.02
  preauricular Q18.1
  rectovaginal N82.3
  Rokitansky-Aschoff (gallbladder) K82.8
  sacrococcygeal (dermoid) (infected) — see Sinus, pilonidal
  tachycardia R00.0
    paroxysmal I47.1
  tarsi syndrome M25.57- ☑
  testis N50.89
  tract (postinfective) — see Fistula
  urachus Q64.4
nusitis (accessory) (chronic) (hyperplastic) (nasal) (nonpurulent) (purulent) J32.9
  acute J01.90
    ethmoidal J01.20
      recurrent J01.21
    frontal J01.10
      recurrent J01.11
    involving more than one sinus, other than pansinusitis J01.80
      recurrent J01.81
    maxillary J01.00
      recurrent J01.01
    pansinusitis J01.40
      recurrent J01.41
    recurrent J01.91
    specified NEC J01.80
      recurrent J01.81
    sphenoidal J01.30
      recurrent J01.31
  allergic — see Rhinitis, allergic
  due to high altitude T70.1 ☑
  ethmoidal J32.2
    acute J01.20
      recurrent J01.21
  frontal J32.1
    acute J01.10
      recurrent J01.11
  influenzal — see Influenza, with, respiratory manifestations NEC
  involving more than one sinus but not pansinusitis J32.8
    acute J01.80
      recurrent J01.81
  maxillary J32.0
    acute J01.00
      recurrent J01.01
  sphenoidal J32.3
    acute J01.30
      recurrent J01.31
  tuberculous, any sinus A15.8
nusitis-bronchiectasis-situs inversus (syndrome) (triad) Q89.3
pple's syndrome E31.22
renomelia (syndrome) Q87.2

Siriasis T67.01 ☑
Sirkari's disease B55.0
Siti A65
Situation, psychiatric F99
Situational
  disturbance (transient) — see Disorder, adjustment
    acute F43.0
  maladjustment — see Disorder, adjustment
  reaction — see Disorder, adjustment
    acute F43.0
Situs inversus or transversus (abdominalis) (thoracis) Q89.3
Sixth disease B08.20
  due to human herpesvirus 6 B08.21
  due to human herpesvirus 7 B08.22
Sjögren-Larsson syndrome Q87.19
Sjögren's syndrome or disease — see Sicca syndrome
Skeletal — see condition
Skene's gland — see condition
Skenitis — see Urethritis
Skerljevo A65
Skevas-Zerfus disease — see Toxicity, venom, marine animal, sea anemone
Skin — see also condition
  clammy R23.1
  donor — see Donor, skin
  hidebound M35.9
Slate-dressers' or slate-miners' lung J62.8
Sleep
  apnea — see Apnea, sleep
  deprivation Z72.820
  disorder or disturbance G47.9
    child F51.9
    nonorganic origin F51.9
    specified NEC G47.8
  disturbance G47.9
    nonorganic origin F51.9
  drunkenness F51.9
  rhythm inversion G47.2- ☑
  terrors F51.4
  walking F51.3
    hysterical F44.89
Sleep hygiene
  abuse Z72.821
  inadequate Z72.821
  poor Z72.821
Sleeping sickness — see Sickness, sleeping
Sleeplessness — see Insomnia
  menopausal N95.1
Sleep-wake schedule disorder G47.20
Slim disease (in HIV infection) B20
Slipped, slipping
  epiphysis (traumatic) — see also Osteochondropathy, specified type NEC
    capital femoral (traumatic)
      acute (on chronic) S79.01- ☑
    current traumatic — code as Fracture, by site
    upper femoral (nontraumatic) M93.00- ☑
      acute M93.01- ☑
        on chronic M93.03- ☑
      chronic M93.02- ☑
  intervertebral disc — see Displacement, intervertebral disc
  ligature, umbilical P51.8
  patella — see Disorder, patella, derangement NEC
  rib M89.8X8
  sacroiliac joint — see subcategory M53.2 ☑
  tendon — see Disorder, tendon
  ulnar nerve, nontraumatic — see Lesion, nerve, ulnar
  vertebra NEC — see Spondylolisthesis
Slocumb's syndrome E27.0
Sloughing (multiple) (phagedena) (skin) — see also Gangrene
  abscess — see Abscess
  appendix K38.8
  fascia — see Disorder, soft tissue, specified type NEC
  scrotum N50.89
  tendon — see Disorder, tendon
  transplanted organ — see Rejection, transplant
  ulcer — see Ulcer, skin
Slow
  feeding, newborn P92.2
  flow syndrome, coronary I20.8
  heart (beat) R00.1
Slowing, urinary stream R39.198
Sluder's neuralgia (syndrome) G44.89
Slurred, slurring speech R47.81

Small (ness)
  for gestational age — see Small for dates
  introitus, vagina N89.6
  kidney (unknown cause) N27.9
    bilateral N27.1
    unilateral N27.0
  ovary (congenital) Q50.39
  pelvis
    with disproportion (fetopelvic) O33.1
      causing obstructed labor O65.1
  uterus N85.8
  white kidney N03.9
Small-and-light-for-dates — see Small for dates
Small-for-dates (infant) P05.10
  with weight of
    499 grams or less P05.11
    500-749 grams P05.12
    750-999 grams P05.13
    1000-1249 grams P05.14
    1250-1499 grams P05.15
    1500-1749 grams P05.16
    1750-1999 grams P05.17
    2000-2499 grams P05.18
    2500 grams and over P05.19
  specified NEC P05.19
Smallpox B03
Smearing, fecal R15.1
Smith-Lemli-Opitz syndrome E78.72
Smith's fracture S52.54- ☑
Smoker — see Dependence, drug, nicotine
Smoker's
  bronchitis J41.0
  cough J41.0
  palate K13.24
  throat J31.2
  tongue K13.24
Smoking
  passive Z77.22
Smothering spells R06.81
Snaggle teeth, tooth M26.39
Snapping
  finger — see Trigger finger
  hip — see Derangement, joint, specified type NEC, hip
    involving the iliotibial band M76.3- ☑
  knee — see Derangement, knee
    involving the iliotibial band M76.3- ☑
Sneddon-Wilkinson disease or syndrome (sub-corneal pustular dermatosis) L13.1
Sneezing (intractable) R06.7
Sniffing
  cocaine
    abuse — see Abuse, drug, cocaine
    dependence — see Dependence, drug, cocaine
  gasoline
    abuse — see Abuse, drug, inhalant
    dependence — see Dependence, drug, inhalant
  glue (airplane)
    abuse — see Abuse, drug, inhalant
    drug dependence — see Dependence, drug, inhalant
Sniffles
  newborn P28.89
Snoring R06.83
Snow blindness — see Photokeratitis
Snuffles (non-syphilitic) R06.5
  newborn P28.89
  syphilitic (infant) A50.05 [J99]
Social
  exclusion Z60.4
    due to discrimination or persecution (perceived) Z60.5
  migrant Z59.0
    acculturation difficulty Z60.3
  rejection Z60.4
    due to discrimination or persecution Z60.5
  role conflict NEC Z73.5
  skills inadequacy NEC Z73.4
  transplantation Z60.3
Sodoku A25.0
Soemmerring's ring — see Cataract, secondary
Soft — see also condition
  nails L60.3
Softening
  bone — see Osteomalacia
  brain (necrotic) (progressive) G93.89
    congenital Q04.8
    embolic I63.4- ☑

Softening — continued
- brain — continued
  - hemorrhagic — see Hemorrhage, intracranial, intracerebral
    - occlusive I63.5- ☑
    - thrombotic I63.3- ☑
  - cartilage M94.2- ☑
    - patella M22.4- ☑
  - cerebellar — see Softening, brain
  - cerebral — see Softening, brain
  - cerebrospinal — see Softening, brain
  - myocardial, heart — see Degeneration, myocardial
  - spinal cord G95.89
  - stomach K31.89

Soldier's
- heart F45.8
- patches I31.0

Solitary
- cyst, kidney N28.1
- kidney, congenital Q60.0

Solvent abuse — see Abuse, drug, inhalant
- dependence — see Dependence, drug, inhalant

Somatization reaction, somatic reaction — see Disorder, somatoform

Somnambulism F51.3
- hysterical F44.89

Somnolence R40.0
- nonorganic origin F51.11

Sonne dysentery A03.3

Soor B37.0

Sore
- bed — see Ulcer, pressure, by site
- chiclero B55.1
- Delhi B55.1
- desert — see Ulcer, skin
- eye H57.1- ☑
- Lahore B55.1
- mouth K13.79
  - canker K12.0
- muscle M79.10
- Naga — see Ulcer, skin
- of skin — see Ulcer, skin
- oriental B55.1
- pressure — see Ulcer, pressure, by site
- skin L98.9
- soft A57
- throat (acute) — see also Pharyngitis
  - with influenza, flu, or grippe — see Influenza, with, respiratory manifestations NEC
  - chronic J31.2
  - coxsackie (virus) B08.5
  - diphtheritic A36.0
  - herpesviral B00.2
  - influenzal — see Influenza, with, respiratory manifestations NEC
  - septic J02.0
  - streptococcal (ulcerative) J02.0
  - viral NEC J02.8
    - coxsackie B08.5
- tropical — see Ulcer, skin
- veldt — see Ulcer, skin

Soto's syndrome (cerebral gigantism) Q87.3
South African cardiomyopathy syndrome I42.8
Southeast Asian hemorrhagic fever A91
Spacing
- abnormal, tooth, teeth, fully erupted M26.30
- excessive, tooth, fully erupted M26.32

Spade-like hand (congenital) Q68.1
Spading nail L60.8
- congenital Q84.6

Spanish collar N47.1
Sparganosis B70.1
Spasm(s), spastic, spasticity — see also condition R25.2
- accommodation — see Spasm, of accommodation
- ampulla of Vater K83.4
- anus, ani (sphincter) (reflex) K59.4
  - psychogenic F45.8
- artery I73.9
  - cerebral G45.9
- Bell's G51.3- ☑
- bladder (sphincter, external or internal) N32.89
  - psychogenic F45.8
- bronchus, bronchiole J98.01
- cardia K22.0
- cardiac I20.1
- carpopedal — see Tetany
- cerebral (arteries) (vascular) G45.9

Spasm(s), spastic, spasticity — continued
- cervix, complicating delivery O62.4
- ciliary body (of accommodation) — see Spasm, of accommodation
- colon — see also Irritable, bowel K58.9
  - with diarrhea K58.0
  - psychogenic F45.8
- common duct K83.8
- compulsive — see Tic
- conjugate H51.8
- coronary (artery) I20.1
- diaphragm (reflex) R06.6
  - epidemic B33.0
  - psychogenic F45.8
- duodenum K59.8
- epidemic diaphragmatic (transient) B33.0
- esophagus (diffuse) K22.4
  - psychogenic F45.8
- facial G51.3- ☑
- fallopian tube N83.8
- gastrointestinal (tract) K31.89
  - psychogenic F45.8
- glottis J38.5
  - hysterical F44.4
  - psychogenic F45.8
    - conversion reaction F44.4
  - reflex through recurrent laryngeal nerve J38.5
- habit — see Tic
- heart I20.1
- hemifacial (clonic) G51.3- ☑
- hourglass — see Contraction, hourglass
- hysterical F44.4
- infantile — see Epilepsy, spasms
- inferior oblique, eye H51.8
- intestinal — see also Syndrome, irritable bowel K58.9
  - psychogenic F45.8
- larynx, laryngeal J38.5
  - hysterical F44.4
  - psychogenic F45.8
    - conversion reaction F44.4
- levator palpebrae superioris — see Disorder, eyelid function
- muscle NEC M62.838
  - back M62.830
- nerve, trigeminal G51.0
- nervous F45.8
- nodding F98.4
- occupational F48.8
- oculogyric H51.8
  - psychogenic F45.8
- of accommodation H52.53- ☑
- ophthalmic artery — see Occlusion, artery, retina
- perineal, female N94.89
- peroneo-extensor — see also Deformity, limb, flat foot
- pharynx (reflex) J39.2
  - hysterical F45.8
  - psychogenic F45.8
- psychogenic F45.8
- pylorus NEC K31.3
  - adult hypertrophic K31.89
  - congenital or infantile Q40.0
  - psychogenic F45.8
- rectum (sphincter) K59.4
  - psychogenic F45.8
- retinal (artery) — see Occlusion, artery, retina
- sigmoid — see also Syndrome, irritable bowel K58.9
  - psychogenic F45.8
- sphincter of Oddi K83.4
- stomach K31.89
  - neurotic F45.8
- throat J39.2
  - hysterical F45.8
  - psychogenic F45.8
- tic F95.9
  - chronic F95.1
  - transient of childhood F95.0
- tongue K14.8
- torsion (progressive) G24.1
- trigeminal nerve — see Neuralgia, trigeminal
- ureter N13.5
- urethra (sphincter) N35.919
- uterus N85.8
  - complicating labor O62.4
- vagina N94.2
  - psychogenic F52.5
- vascular I73.9
- vasomotor I73.9
- vein NEC I87.8

Spasm(s), spastic, spasticity — continued
- viscera — see Pain, abdominal

Spasmodic — see condition
Spasmophilia — see Tetany
Spasmus nutans F98.4
Spastic, spasticity — see also Spasm
- child (cerebral) (congenital) (paralysis) G80.1

Speaker's throat R49.8
Specific, specified — see condition
Speech
- defect, disorder, disturbance, impediment R47.9
  - psychogenic, in childhood and adolescence F98
  - slurring R47.81
  - specified NEC R47.89

Spencer's disease A08.19
Spens' syndrome (syncope with heart block) I45.9
Sperm counts (fertility testing) Z31.41
- postvasectomy Z30.8
- reversal Z31.42

Spermatic cord — see condition
Spermatocele N43.40
- congenital Q55.4
- multiple N43.42
- single N43.41

Spermatocystitis N49.0
Spermatocytoma C62.9- ☑
- specified site — see Neoplasm, malignant, by site

Spermatorrhea N50.89
Sphacelus — see Gangrene
Sphenoidal — see condition
Sphenoiditis (chronic) — see Sinusitis, sphenoidal
Sphenopalatine ganglion neuralgia G90.09
Sphericity, increased, lens (congenital) Q12.4
Spherocytosis (congenital) (familial) (hereditary) D58
- hemoglobin disease D58.0
- sickle-cell (disease) D57.8- ☑

Spherophakia Q12.4
Sphincter — see condition
Sphincteritis, sphincter of Oddi — see Cholangitis
Sphingolipidosis E75.3
- specified NEC E75.29

Sphingomyelinosis E75.3
Spicule tooth K00.2
Spider
- bite — see Toxicity, venom, spider
- fingers — see Syndrome, Marfan's
- nevus I78.1
- toes — see Syndrome, Marfan's
- vascular I78.1

Spiegler-Fendt
- benign lymphocytoma L98.8
- sarcoid L08.89

Spielmeyer-Vogt disease E75.4
Spina bifida (aperta) Q05.9
- with hydrocephalus NEC Q05.4
- cervical Q05.5
  - with hydrocephalus Q05.0
- dorsal Q05.6
  - with hydrocephalus Q05.1
- lumbar Q05.7
  - with hydrocephalus Q05.2
- lumbosacral Q05.7
  - with hydrocephalus Q05.2
- occulta Q76.0
- sacral Q05.8
  - with hydrocephalus Q05.3
- thoracic Q05.6
  - with hydrocephalus Q05.1
- thoracolumbar Q05.6
  - with hydrocephalus Q05.1

Spindle, Krukenberg's — see Pigmentation, cornea, posterior
Spine, spinal — see condition
Spiradenoma (eccrine) — see Neoplasm, skin, benign
Spirillosis A25.0
Spirillum
- minus A25.0
- obermeieri infection A68.0

Spirochetal — see condition
Spirochetosis A69.9
- arthritic, arthritica A69.9
- bronchopulmonary A69.8
- icterohemorrhagic A27.0
- lung A69.8

Spirometrosis B70.1
Spitting blood — see Hemoptysis
Splanchnoptosis K63.4

leen, splenic — *see* condition
lenectasis — *see* Splenomegaly
lenitis (interstitial) (malignant) (nonspecific) D73.89
  malarial — *see also* Malaria B54 *[D77]*
  tuberculous A18.85
lenocele D73.89
lenomegaly, splenomegalia (Bengal) (cryptogenic)
    (idiopathic) (tropical) R16.1
  with hepatomegaly R16.2
  cirrhotic D73.2
  congenital Q89.09
  congestive, chronic D73.2
  Egyptian B65.1
  Gaucher's E75.22
  malarial — *see also* Malaria B54 *[D77]*
  neutropenic D73.81
  Niemann-Pick — *see* Niemann-Pick disease or syn-
      drome
  siderotic D73.2
  syphilitic A52.79
    congenital (early) A50.08 *[D77]*
lenopathy D73.9
lenoptosis D73.89
lenosis D73.89
linter — *see* Foreign body, superficial, by site
lit, splitting
  foot Q72.7- ☑
  hand Q71.6 ☑
  heart sounds R01.2
  lip, congenital — *see* Cleft, lip
  nails L60.3
  urinary stream R39.13
ondylarthrosis — *see* Spondylosis
ondylitis (chronic) — *see also* Spondylopathy, inflam-
    matory
  ankylopoietica — *see* Spondylitis, ankylosing
  ankylosing (chronic) M45.9
    with lung involvement M45.9 *[J99]*
    cervical region M45.2
    cervicothoracic region M45.3
    juvenile M08.1
    lumbar region M45.6
    lumbosacral region M45.7
    multiple sites M45.0
    occipito-atlanto-axial region M45.1
    sacrococcygeal region M45.8
    thoracic region M45.4
    thoracolumbar region M45.5
  atrophic (ligamentous) — *see* Spondylitis, ankylosing
  deformans (chronic) — *see* Spondylosis
  gonococcal A54.41
  gouty — *see also* Gout, by type, vertebrae M10.08
  in (due to)
    brucellosis A23.9 *[M49.80]*
      cervical region A23.9 *[M49.82]*
      cervicothoracic region A23.9 *[M49.83]*
      lumbar region A23.9 *[M49.86]*
      lumbosacral region A23.9 *[M49.87]*
      multiple sites A23.9 *[M49.89]*
      occipito-atlanto-axial region A23.9 *[M49.81]*
      sacrococcygeal region A23.9 *[M49.88]*
      thoracic region A23.9 *[M49.84]*
      thoracolumbar region A23.9 *[M49.85]*
    enterobacteria — *see also* subcategory M49.8 A04.9
    tuberculosis A18.01
  infectious NEC — *see* Spondylopathy, infective
  juvenile ankylosing (chronic) M08.1
  Kümmell's — *see* Spondylopathy, traumatic
  Marie-Strümpell — *see* Spondylitis, ankylosing
  muscularis — *see* Spondylopathy, specified NEC
  psoriatic L40.53
  rheumatoid — *see* Spondylitis, ankylosing
  rhizomelica — *see* Spondylitis, ankylosing
  sacroiliac NEC M46.1
  senescent, senile — *see* Spondylosis
  traumatic (chronic) or post-traumatic — *see* Spondy-
      lopathy, traumatic
  tuberculous A18.01
  typhosa A01.05
ondylolisthesis (acquired) (degenerative) M43.10
  with disproportion (fetopelvic) O33.0
    causing obstructed labor O65.0
  cervical region M43.12
  cervicothoracic region M43.13
  congenital Q76.2
  lumbar region M43.16
  lumbosacral region M43.17

Spondylolisthesis — *continued*
  multiple sites M43.19
  occipito-atlanto-axial region M43.11
  sacrococcygeal region M43.18
  thoracic region M43.14
  thoracolumbar region M43.15
  traumatic (old) M43.10
    acute
      fifth cervical (displaced) S12.430 ☑
        nondisplaced S12.431 ☑
        specified type NEC (displaced) S12.450 ☑
          nondisplaced S12.451 ☑
        type III S12.44 ☑
      fourth cervical (displaced) S12.330 ☑
        nondisplaced S12.331 ☑
        specified type NEC (displaced) S12.350 ☑
          nondisplaced S12.351 ☑
        type III S12.34 ☑
      second cervical (displaced) S12.130 ☑
        nondisplaced S12.131 ☑
        specified type NEC (displaced) S12.150 ☑
          nondisplaced S12.151 ☑
        type III S12.14 ☑
      seventh cervical (displaced) S12.630 ☑
        nondisplaced S12.631 ☑
        specified type NEC (displaced) S12.650 ☑
          nondisplaced S12.651 ☑
        type III S12.64 ☑
      sixth cervical (displaced) S12.530 ☑
        nondisplaced S12.531 ☑
        specified type NEC (displaced) S12.550 ☑
          nondisplaced S12.551 ☑
        type III S12.54 ☑
      third cervical (displaced) S12.230 ☑
        nondisplaced S12.231 ☑
        specified type NEC (displaced) S12.250 ☑
          nondisplaced S12.251 ☑
        type III S12.24 ☑
Spondylolysis (acquired) M43.00
  cervical region M43.02
  cervicothoracic region M43.03
  congenital Q76.2
  lumbar region M43.06
  lumbosacral region M43.07
    with disproportion (fetopelvic) O33.0
      causing obstructed labor O65.8
  multiple sites M43.09
  occipito-atlanto-axial region M43.01
  sacrococcygeal region M43.08
  thoracic region M43.04
  thoracolumbar region M43.05
Spondylopathy M48.9
  infective NEC M46.50
    cervical region M46.52
    cervicothoracic region M46.53
    lumbar region M46.56
    lumbosacral region M46.57
    multiple sites M46.59
    occipito-atlanto-axial region M46.51
    sacrococcygeal region M46.58
    thoracic region M46.54
    thoracolumbar region M46.55
  inflammatory M46.90
    cervical region M46.92
    cervicothoracic region M46.93
    lumbar region M46.96
    lumbosacral region M46.97
    multiple sites M46.99
    occipito-atlanto-axial region M46.91
    sacrococcygeal region M46.98
    specified type NEC M46.80
      cervical region M46.82
      cervicothoracic region M46.83
      lumbar region M46.86
      lumbosacral region M46.87
      multiple sites M46.89
      occipito-atlanto-axial region M46.81
      sacrococcygeal region M46.88
      thoracic region M46.84
      thoracolumbar region M46.85
    thoracic region M46.94
    thoracolumbar region M46.95
  neuropathic, in
    syringomyelia and syringobulbia G95.0
    tabes dorsalis A52.11
  specified NEC — *see* subcategory M48.8 ☑
  traumatic M48.30

Spondylopathy — *continued*
  traumatic — *continued*
    cervical region M48.32
    cervicothoracic region M48.33
    lumbar region M48.36
    lumbosacral region M48.37
    occipito-atlanto-axial region M48.31
    sacrococcygeal region M48.38
    thoracic region M48.34
    thoracolumbar region M48.35
Spondylosis M47.9
  with
    disproportion (fetopelvic) O33.0
      causing obstructed labor O65.0
    myelopathy NEC M47.10
      cervical region M47.12
      cervicothoracic region M47.13
      lumbar region M47.16
      occipito-atlanto-axial region M47.11
      thoracic region M47.14
      thoracolumbar region M47.15
    radiculopathy M47.20
      cervical region M47.22
      cervicothoracic region M47.23
      lumbar region M47.26
      lumbosacral region M47.27
      occipito-atlanto-axial region M47.21
      sacrococcygeal region M47.28
      thoracic region M47.24
      thoracolumbar region M47.25
  specified NEC M47.899
    cervical region M47.892
    cervicothoracic region M47.893
    lumbar region M47.896
    lumbosacral region M47.897
    occipito-atlanto-axial region M47.891
    sacrococcygeal region M47.898
    thoracic region M47.894
    thoracolumbar region M47.895
  traumatic — *see* Spondylopathy, traumatic
  without myelopathy or radiculopathy M47.819
    cervical region M47.812
    cervicothoracic region M47.813
    lumbar region M47.816
    lumbosacral region M47.817
    occipito-atlanto-axial region M47.811
    sacrococcygeal region M47.818
    thoracic region M47.814
    thoracolumbar region M47.815
Sponge
  inadvertently left in operation wound — *see* Foreign
    body, accidentally left during a procedure
  kidney (medullary) Q61.5
Sponge-diver's disease — *see* Toxicity, venom, marine
    animal, sea anemone
Spongioblastoma (any type) — *see* Neoplasm, malig-
    nant, by site
  specified site — *see* Neoplasm, malignant, by site
  unspecified site C71.9
Spongioneuroblastoma — *see* Neoplasm, malignant,
    by site
Spontaneous — *see also* condition
  fracture (cause unknown) — *see* Fracture, pathological
Spoon nail L60.3
  congenital Q84.6
Sporadic — *see* condition
Sporothrix schenckii infection — *see* Sporotrichosis
Sporotrichosis B42.9
  arthritis B42.82
  disseminated B42.7
  generalized B42.7
  lymphocutaneous (fixed) (progressive) B42.1
  pulmonary B42.0
  specified NEC B42.89
Spots, spotting (in) (of)
  Bitot's — *see also* Pigmentation, conjunctiva
    in the young child E50.1
    vitamin A deficiency E50.1
  café, au lait L81.3
  Cayenne pepper I78.1
  cotton wool, retina — *see* Occlusion, artery, retina
  de Morgan's (senile angiomas) I78.1
  Fuchs' black (myopic) — *see also* Myopia, degenerative
    H44.2- ☑
  intermenstrual (regular) N92.0
    irregular N92.1
  Koplik's B05.9
  liver L81.4

☞ Subterms under main terms may continue to next column or page   ☑ Additional Character Required — Refer to the Tabular List for Character Selection   **289**

Spleen, splenic — Spots, spotting

Spots, spotting — continued
  pregnancy O26.85- ✓
  purpuric R23.3
  ruby I78.1
Spotted fever — see Fever, spotted N92.3
Sprain (joint) (ligament)
  acromioclavicular joint or ligament S43.5- ✓
  ankle S93.40- ✓
    calcaneofibular ligament S93.41- ✓
    deltoid ligament S93.42- ✓
    internal collateral ligament — see Sprain, ankle,
      specified ligament NEC
    specified ligament NEC S93.49- ✓
    talofibular ligament — see Sprain, ankle, specified
      ligament NEC
    tibiofibular ligament S93.43- ✓
  anterior longitudinal, cervical S13.4 ✓
  atlas, atlanto-axial, atlanto-occipital S13.4 ✓
  breast bone — see Sprain, sternum
  calcaneofibular — see Sprain, ankle
  carpal — see Sprain, wrist
  carpometacarpal — see Sprain, hand, specified site
    NEC
  cartilage
    costal S23.41 ✓
    semilunar (knee) — see Sprain, knee, specified site
      NEC
      with current tear — see Tear, meniscus
    thyroid region S13.5 ✓
    xiphoid — see Sprain, sternum
  cervical, cervicodorsal, cervicothoracic S13.4 ✓
  chondrosternal S23.421 ✓
  coracoclavicular S43.8- ✓
  coracohumeral S43.41- ✓
  coronary, knee — see Sprain, knee, specified site NEC
  costal cartilage S23.41 ✓
  cricoarytenoid articulation or ligament S13.5 ✓
  cricothyroid articulation S13.5 ✓
  cruciate, knee — see Sprain, knee, cruciate
  deltoid, ankle — see Sprain, ankle
  dorsal (spine) S23.3 ✓
  elbow S53.40- ✓
    radial collateral ligament S53.43- ✓
    radiohumeral S53.41- ✓
    rupture
      radial collateral ligament — see Rupture, trau-
        matic, ligament, radial collateral
      ulnar collateral ligament — see Rupture, traumat-
        ic, ligament, ulnar collateral
    specified type NEC S53.49- ✓
    ulnar collateral ligament S53.44- ✓
    ulnohumeral S53.42- ✓
  femur, head — see Sprain, hip
  fibular collateral, knee — see Sprain, knee, collateral
  fibulocalcaneal — see Sprain, ankle
  finger(s) S63.61- ✓
    index S63.61- ✓
    interphalangeal (joint) S63.63- ✓
      index S63.63- ✓
      little S63.63- ✓
      middle S63.63- ✓
      ring S63.63- ✓
    little S63.61- ✓
    metacarpophalangeal (joint) S63.65- ✓
    middle S63.61- ✓
    ring S63.61- ✓
    specified site NEC S63.69- ✓
      index S63.69- ✓
      little S63.69- ✓
      middle S63.69- ✓
      ring S63.69- ✓
  foot S93.60- ✓
    specified ligament NEC S93.69- ✓
    tarsal ligament S93.61- ✓
    tarsometatarsal ligament S93.62- ✓
    toe — see Sprain, toe
  hand S63.9- ✓
    finger — see Sprain, finger
    specified site NEC — see subcategory S63.8 ✓
    thumb — see Sprain, thumb
  head S03.9 ✓
  hip S73.10- ✓
    iliofemoral ligament S73.11- ✓
    ischiocapsular (ligament) S73.12- ✓
    specified NEC S73.19- ✓
  iliofemoral — see Sprain, hip

Sprain — continued
  innominate
    acetabulum — see Sprain, hip
    sacral junction S33.6 ✓
  internal
    collateral, ankle — see Sprain, ankle
    semilunar cartilage — see Sprain, knee, specified
      site NEC
  interphalangeal
    finger — see Sprain, finger, interphalangeal (joint)
    toe — see Sprain, toe, interphalangeal joint
  ischiocapsular — see Sprain, hip
  ischiofemoral — see Sprain, hip
  jaw (articular disc) (cartilage) (meniscus) S03.4- ✓
    old M26.69
  knee S83.9- ✓
    collateral ligament S83.40- ✓
      lateral (fibular) S83.42- ✓
      medial (tibial) S83.41- ✓
    cruciate ligament S83.50- ✓
      anterior S83.51- ✓
      posterior S83.52- ✓
    lateral (fibular) collateral ligament S83.42- ✓
    medial (tibial) collateral ligament S83.41- ✓
    patellar ligament S76.11- ✓
    specified site NEC S83.8X- ✓
    superior tibiofibular joint (ligament) S83.6- ✓
  lateral collateral, knee — see Sprain, knee, collateral
  lumbar (spine) S33.5 ✓
  lumbosacral S33.9 ✓
  mandible (articular disc) S03.4- ✓
    old M26.69
  medial collateral, knee — see Sprain, knee, collateral
  meniscus
    jaw S03.4- ✓
      old M26.69
    knee — see Sprain, knee, specified site NEC
      with current tear — see Tear, meniscus
        old — see Derangement, knee, meniscus, due
          to old tear
    mandible S03.4- ✓
      old M26.69
  metacarpal (distal) (proximal) — see Sprain, hand,
    specified site NEC
  metacarpophalangeal — see Sprain, finger, metacar-
    pophalangeal (joint)
  metatarsophalangeal — see Sprain, toe, metatarsopha-
    langeal joint
  midcarpal — see Sprain, hand, specified site NEC
  midtarsal — see Sprain, foot, specified site NEC
  neck S13.9 ✓
    anterior longitudinal cervical ligament S13.4 ✓
    atlanto-axial joint S13.4 ✓
    atlanto-occipital joint S13.4 ✓
    cervical spine S13.4 ✓
    cricoarytenoid ligament S13.5 ✓
    cricothyroid ligament S13.5 ✓
    specified site NEC S13.8 ✓
    thyroid region (cartilage) S13.5 ✓
  nose S03.8 ✓
  orbicular, hip — see Sprain, hip
  patella — see Sprain, knee, specified site NEC
  patellar ligament S76.11- ✓
  pelvis NEC S33.8 ✓
  phalanx
    finger — see Sprain, finger
    toe — see Sprain, toe
  pubofemoral — see Sprain, hip
  radiocarpal — see Sprain, wrist
  radiohumeral — see Sprain, elbow
  radius, collateral — see Rupture, traumatic, ligament,
    radial collateral
  rib (cage) S23.41 ✓
  rotator cuff (capsule) S43.42- ✓
  sacroiliac (region)
    chronic or old — see subcategory M53.2 ✓
    joint S33.6 ✓
  scaphoid (hand) — see Sprain, hand, specified site NEC
  scapula (r) — see Sprain, shoulder girdle, specified site
    NEC
  semilunar cartilage (knee) — see Sprain, knee, specified
    site NEC
    with current tear — see Tear, meniscus
      old — see Derangement, knee, meniscus, due to
        old tear
  shoulder joint S43.40- ✓

Sprain — continued
  shoulder joint — continued
    acromioclavicular joint (ligament) — see Sprain,
      acromioclavicular joint
    blade — see Sprain, shoulder, girdle, specified s
      NEC
    coracoclavicular joint (ligament) — see Sprain,
      coracoclavicular joint
    coracohumeral ligament — see Sprain, coracohum
      al joint
    girdle S43.9- ✓
      specified site NEC S43.8- ✓
    rotator cuff — see Sprain, rotator cuff
    specified site NEC S43.49- ✓
    sternoclavicular joint (ligament) — see Sprain,
      sternoclavicular joint
  spine
    cervical S13.4 ✓
    lumbar S33.5 ✓
    thoracic S23.3 ✓
  sternoclavicular joint S43.6- ✓
  sternum S23.429 ✓
    chondrosternal joint S23.421 ✓
    specified site NEC S23.428 ✓
    sternoclavicular (joint) (ligament) S23.420 ✓
  symphysis
    jaw S03.4- ✓
      old M26.69
    mandibular S03.4- ✓
      old M26.69
  talofibular — see Sprain, ankle
  tarsal — see Sprain, foot, specified site NEC
  tarsometatarsal — see Sprain, foot, specified site N
  temporomandibular S03.4- ✓
    old M26.69
  thorax S23.9 ✓
    ribs S23.41 ✓
    specified site NEC S23.8 ✓
    spine S23.3 ✓
    sternum — see Sprain, sternum
  thumb S63.60- ✓
    interphalangeal (joint) S63.62- ✓
    metacarpophalangeal (joint) S63.64- ✓
    specified site NEC S63.68- ✓
  thyroid cartilage or region S13.5 ✓
  tibia (proximal end) — see Sprain, knee, specified s
    NEC
  tibial collateral, knee — see Sprain, knee, collateral
  tibiofibular
    distal — see Sprain, ankle
    superior — see Sprain, knee, specified site NEC
  toe(s) S93.50- ✓
    great S93.50- ✓
    interphalangeal joint S93.51- ✓
      great S93.51- ✓
      lesser S93.51- ✓
    lesser S93.50- ✓
    metatarsophalangeal joint S93.52- ✓
      great S93.52- ✓
      lesser S93.52- ✓
  ulna, collateral — see Rupture, traumatic, ligament
    ulnar collateral
  ulnohumeral — see Sprain, elbow
  wrist S63.50- ✓
    carpal S63.51- ✓
    radiocarpal S63.52- ✓
    specified site NEC S63.59- ✓
  xiphoid cartilage — see Sprain, sternum
Sprengel's deformity (congenital) Q74.0
Sprue (tropical) K90.1
  celiac K90.0
  idiopathic K90.49
  meaning thrush B37.0
  nontropical K90.0
Spur, bone — see also Enthesopathy
  calcaneal M77.3- ✓
  iliac crest M76.2- ✓
  nose (septum) J34.89
Spurway's syndrome Q78.0
Sputum
  abnormal (amount) (color) (odor) (purulent) R09.3
  blood-stained R04.2
  excessive (cause unknown) R09.3
Squamous — see also condition
  epithelium in
    cervical canal (congenital) Q51.828

Squamous — *continued*
  epithelium in — *continued*
    uterine mucosa (congenital) Q51.818
Squashed nose M95.0
  congenital Q67.4
Squeeze, diver's T70.3 ☑
Squint — *see also* Strabismus
  accommodative — *see* Strabismus, convergent concomitant
SSADH (succinic semialdehyde dehydrogenase deficiency) E72.81
St. Hubert's disease A82.9
Stab — *see also* Laceration
  internal organs — *see* Injury, by site
Stafne's cyst or cavity M27.0
Staggering gait R26.0
  hysterical F44.4
Staghorn calculus — *see* Calculus, kidney
Stähli's line (cornea) (pigment) — *see* Pigmentation, cornea, anterior
Stain, staining
  meconium (newborn) P96.83
  port wine Q82.5
  tooth, teeth (hard tissues) (extrinsic) K03.6
    due to
      accretions K03.6
      deposits (betel) (black) (green) (materia alba) (orange) (soft) (tobacco) K03.6
      metals (copper) (silver) K03.7
      nicotine K03.6
      pulpal bleeding K03.7
      tobacco K03.6
    intrinsic K00.8
Stammering — *see also* Disorder, fluency F80.81
Standstill
  auricular I45.5
  cardiac — *see* Arrest, cardiac
  sinoatrial I45.5
  ventricular — *see* Arrest, cardiac
Stannosis J63.5
Stanton's disease — *see* Melioidosis
Staphylitis (acute) (catarrhal) (chronic) (gangrenous) (membranous) (suppurative) (ulcerative) K12.2
Staphylococcal scalded skin syndrome L00
Staphylococcemia A41.2
Staphylococcus, staphylococcal — *see also* condition
  as cause of disease classified elsewhere B95.8
    aureus (methicillin susceptible) (MSSA) B95.61
      methicillin resistant (MRSA) B95.62
    specified NEC, as cause of disease classified elsewhere B95.7
Staphyloma (sclera)
  cornea H18.72- ☑
  equatorial H15.81- ☑
  localized (anterior) H15.82- ☑
  posticum H15.83- ☑
  ring H15.85- ☑
Stargardt's disease — *see* Dystrophy, retina
Starvation (inanition) (due to lack of food) T73.0 ☑
  edema — *see* Malnutrition, severe
Stasis
  bile (noncalculous) K83.1
  bronchus J98.09
    with infection — *see* Bronchitis
  cardiac — *see* Failure, heart, congestive
  cecum K59.8
  colon K59.8
  dermatitis I87.2
    with
      varicose ulcer — *see* Varix, leg, with ulcer, with inflammation
      varicose veins — *see* Varix, leg, with, inflammation
      due to postthrombotic syndrome — *see* Syndrome, postthrombotic
  duodenal K31.5
  eczema — *see* Varix, leg, with, inflammation
  edema — *see* Hypertension, venous (chronic), idiopathic
  foot T69.0- ☑
  ileocecal coil K59.8
  ileum K59.8
  intestinal K59.8
  jejunum K59.8
  kidney N19
  liver (cirrhotic) K76.1
  lymphatic I89.8

Stasis — *continued*
  pneumonia J18.2
  pulmonary — *see* Edema, lung
  rectal K59.8
  renal N19
    tubular N17.0
  ulcer — *see* Varix, leg, with, ulcer
    without varicose veins I87.2
  urine — *see* Retention, urine
  venous I87.8
State (of)
  affective and paranoid, mixed, organic psychotic F06.8
  agitated R45.1
    acute reaction to stress F43.0
  anxiety (neurotic) F41.1
  apprehension F41.1
  burn-out Z73.0
  climacteric, female Z78.0
    symptomatic N95.1
  compulsive F42.8
    mixed with obsessional thoughts F42.2
  confusional (psychogenic) F44.89
    acute — *see also* Delirium
      with
        arteriosclerotic dementia F01.50
          with behavioral disturbance F01.51
        senility or dementia F05
      alcoholic F10.231
      epileptic F05
    reactive (from emotional stress, psychological trauma) F44.89
    subacute — *see* Delirium
  convulsive — *see* Convulsions
  crisis F43.0
  depressive F32.9
    neurotic F34.1
  dissociative F44.9
  emotional shock (stress) R45.7
  hypercoagulation — *see* Hypercoagulable
  locked-in G83.5
  menopausal Z78.0
    symptomatic N95.1
  neurotic F48.9
    with depersonalization F48.1
  obsessional F42.8
  oneiroid (schizophrenia-like) F23
  organic
    hallucinatory (nonalcoholic) F06.0
    paranoid (-hallucinatory) F06.2
  panic F41.0
  paranoid F22
    climacteric F22
    involutional F22
    menopausal F22
    organic F06.2
    senile F03 ☑
    simple F22
  persistent vegetative R40.3
  phobic F40.9
  postleukotomy F07.0
  pregnant
    gestational carrier Z33.3
    incidental Z33.1
  psychogenic, twilight F44.89
  psychopathic (constitutional) F60.2
  psychotic, organic — *see also* Psychosis, organic
    mixed paranoid and affective F06.8
    senile or presenile F03 ☑
    transient NEC F06.8
      with
        depression F06.31
        hallucinations F06.0
  residual schizophrenic F20.5
  restlessness R45.1
  stress (emotional) R45.7
  tension (mental) F48.9
    specified NEC F48.8
  transient organic psychotic NEC F06.8
    depressive type F06.31
    hallucinatory type F06.0
  twilight
    epileptic F05
    psychogenic F44.89
  vegetative, persistent R40.3
  vital exhaustion Z73.0
  withdrawal, — *see* Withdrawal, state
Status (post) — *see also* Presence (of)

Status — *continued*
  absence, epileptic — *see* Epilepsy, by type, with status epilepticus
  administration of tPA (rtPA) in a different facility within the last 24 hours prior to admission to current facility Z92.82
  adrenalectomy (unilateral) (bilateral) E89.6
  anastomosis Z98.0
  anginosus I20.9
  angioplasty (peripheral) Z98.62
    with implant Z95.820
    coronary artery Z98.61
      with implant Z95.5
  aortocoronary bypass Z95.1
  arthrodesis Z98.1
  artificial opening (of) Z93.9
    gastrointestinal tract Z93.4
    specified NEC Z93.8
    urinary tract Z93.6
    vagina Z93.8
  asthmaticus — *see* Asthma, by type, with status asthmaticus
  awaiting organ transplant Z76.82
  bariatric surgery Z98.84
  bed confinement Z74.01
  bleb, filtering (vitreous), after glaucoma surgery Z98.83
  breast implant Z98.82
    removal Z98.86
  cataract extraction Z98.4- ☑
  cholecystectomy Z90.49
  clitorectomy N90.811
    with excision of labia minora N90.812
  colectomy (complete) (partial) Z90.49
  colonization — *see* Carrier (suspected) of
  colostomy Z93.3
  convulsivus idiopathicus — *see* Epilepsy, by type, with status epilepticus
  coronary artery angioplasty — *see* Status, angioplasty, coronary artery
  coronary artery bypass graft Z95.1
  cystectomy (urinary bladder) Z90.6
  cystostomy Z93.50
    appendico-vesicostomy Z93.52
    cutaneous Z93.51
    specified NEC Z93.59
  delinquent immunization Z28.3
  dental Z98.818
    crown Z98.811
    fillings Z98.811
    restoration Z98.811
    sealant Z98.810
    specified NEC Z98.818
  deployment (current) (military) Z56.82
  dialysis (hemodialysis) (peritoneal) Z99.2
  do not resuscitate (DNR) Z66
  donor — *see* Donor
  embedded fragments — *see* Retained, foreign body fragments (type of)
  embedded splinter — *see* Retained, foreign body fragments (type of)
  enterostomy Z93.4
  epileptic, epilepticus — *see also* Epilepsy, by type, with status epilepticus G40.901
  estrogen receptor
    negative Z17.1
    positive Z17.0
  female genital cutting — *see* Female genital mutilation status
  female genital mutilation — *see* Female genital mutilation status
  filtering (vitreous) bleb after glaucoma surgery Z98.83
  gastrectomy (complete) (partial) Z90.3
  gastric banding Z98.84
  gastric bypass for obesity Z98.84
  gastrostomy Z93.1
  human immunodeficiency virus (HIV) infection, asymptomatic Z21
  hysterectomy (complete) (total) Z90.710
    partial (with remaining cervial stump) Z90.711
  ileostomy Z93.2
  implant
    breast Z98.82
  infibulation N90.813
  intestinal bypass Z98.0
  jejunostomy Z93.4
  lapsed immunization schedule Z28.3
  laryngectomy Z90.02
  lymphaticus E32.8

Status — continued
- malignancy
  - castrate resistant prostate Z19.2
  - hormone resistant Z19.2
  - hormone sensitive Z19.1
- marmoratus G80.3
- mastectomy (unilateral) (bilateral) Z90.1- ☑
- military deployment status (current) Z56.82
  - in theater or in support of military war, peacekeeping and humanitarian operations Z56.82
- nephrectomy (unilateral) (bilateral) Z90.5
- nephrostomy Z93.6
- obesity surgery Z98.84
- oophorectomy
  - bilateral Z90.722
  - unilateral Z90.721
- organ replacement
  - by artificial or mechanical device or prosthesis of
    - artery Z95.828
    - bladder Z96.0
    - blood vessel Z95.828
    - breast Z97.8
    - eye globe Z97.0
    - heart Z95.812
      - valve Z95.2
    - intestine Z97.8
    - joint Z96.60
      - hip — see Presence, hip joint implant
      - knee — see Presence, knee joint implant
      - specified site NEC Z96.698
    - kidney Z97.8
    - larynx Z96.3
    - lens Z96.1
    - limbs — see Presence, artificial, limb
    - liver Z97.8
    - lung Z97.8
    - pancreas Z97.8
  - by organ transplant (heterologous)(homologous) — see Transplant
- pacemaker
  - brain Z96.89
  - cardiac Z95.0
  - specified NEC Z96.89
- pancreatectomy Z90.410
  - complete Z90.410
  - partial Z90.411
  - total Z90.410
- physical restraint Z78.1
- pneumonectomy (complete) (partial) Z90.2
- pneumothorax, therapeutic Z98.3
- postcommotio cerebri F07.81
- postoperative (postprocedural) NEC Z98.890
  - breast implant Z98.82
  - dental Z98.818
    - crown Z98.811
    - fillings Z98.811
    - restoration Z98.811
    - sealant Z98.810
    - specified NEC Z98.818
  - pneumothorax, therapeutic Z98.3
  - uterine scar Z98.891
- postpartum (routine follow-up) Z39.2
  - care immediately after delivery Z39.0
- postsurgical (postprocedural) NEC Z98.890
  - pneumothorax, therapeutic Z98.3
- pregnancy, incidental Z33.1
- prosthesis coronary angioplasty Z95.5
- pseudophakia Z96.1
- renal dialysis (hemodialysis) (peritoneal) Z99.2
- retained foreign body — see Retained, foreign body fragments (type of)
- reversed jejunal transposition (for bypass) Z98.0
- salpingo-oophorectomy
  - bilateral Z90.722
  - unilateral Z90.721
- sex reassignment surgery status Z87.890
- shunt
  - arteriovenous (for dialysis) Z99.2
  - cerebrospinal fluid Z98.2
  - ventricular (communicating) (for drainage) Z98.2
- splenectomy Z90.81
- thymicolymphaticus E32.8
- thymicus E32.8
- thymolymphaticus E32.8
- thyroidectomy (hypothyroidism) E89.0
- tooth (teeth) extraction — see also Absence, teeth, acquired K08.409

Status — continued
- tPA (rtPA) administration in a different facility within the last 24 hours prior to admission to current facility Z92.82
- tracheostomy Z93.0
- transplant — see Transplant
  - organ removed Z98.85
- tubal ligation Z98.51
- underimmunization Z28.3
- ureterostomy Z93.6
- urethrostomy Z93.6
- vagina, artificial Z93.8
- vasectomy Z98.52
- wheelchair confinement Z99.3

Stealing
- child problem F91.8
  - in company with others Z72.810
- pathological (compulsive) F63.2

Steam burn — see Burn

Steatocystoma multiplex L72.2

Steatohepatitis (nonalcoholic) (NASH) K75.81

Steatoma L72.3
- eyelid (cystic) — see Dermatosis, eyelid
  - infected — see Hordeolum

Steatorrhea (chronic) K90.9
- with lacteal obstruction K90.2
- idiopathic (adult) (infantile) K90.9
- pancreatic K90.3
- primary K90.0
- tropical K90.1

Steatosis E88.89
- heart — see Degeneration, myocardial
- kidney N28.89
- liver NEC K76.0

Steele-Richardson-Olszewski disease or syndrome G23.1

Steinbrocker's syndrome G90.8

Steinert's disease G71.11

Stein-Leventhal syndrome E28.2

Stein's syndrome E28.2

STEMI — see also Infarct, myocardium, ST elevation I21.3

Stenocardia I20.8

Stenocephaly Q75.8

Stenosis, stenotic (cicatricial) — see also Stricture
- ampulla of Vater K83.1
- anus, anal (canal) (sphincter) K62.4
  - and rectum K62.4
  - congenital Q42.3
    - with fistula Q42.2
- aorta (ascending) (supraventricular) (congenital) Q25.1
  - arteriosclerotic I70.0
  - calcified I70.0
  - supravalvular Q25.3
- aortic (valve) I35.0
  - with insufficiency I35.2
  - congenital Q23.0
  - rheumatic I06.0
    - with
      - incompetency, insufficiency or regurgitation I06.2
        - with mitral (valve) disease I08.0
          - with tricuspid (valve) disease I08.3
        - mitral (valve) disease I08.0
          - with tricuspid (valve) disease I08.3
        - tricuspid (valve) disease I08.2
          - with mitral (valve) disease I08.3
  - specified cause NEC I35.0
  - syphilitic A52.03
- aqueduct of Sylvius (congenital) Q03.0
  - with spina bifida — see Spina bifida, by site, with hydrocephalus
  - acquired G91.1
- artery NEC — see also Arteriosclerosis I77.1
  - celiac I77.4
  - cerebral — see Occlusion, artery, cerebral
  - extremities — see Arteriosclerosis, extremities
  - precerebral — see Occlusion, artery, precerebral
  - pulmonary (congenital) Q25.6
    - acquired I28.8
  - renal I70.1
  - stent
    - coronary T82.855 ☑
    - peripheral T82.856 ☑
- bile duct (common) (hepatic) K83.1
  - congenital Q44.3
- bladder-neck (acquired) N32.0
  - congenital Q64.31
- brain G93.89

Stenosis, stenotic — continued
- bronchus J98.09
  - congenital Q32.3
  - syphilitic A52.72
- cardia (stomach) K22.2
  - congenital Q39.3
- cardiovascular — see Disease, cardiovascular
- caudal M48.08
- cervix, cervical (canal) N88.2
  - congenital Q51.828
  - in pregnancy or childbirth — see Pregnancy, complicated by, abnormal cervix
- colon — see also Obstruction, intestine
  - congenital Q42.9
    - specified NEC Q42.8
- colostomy K94.03
- common (bile) duct K83.1
  - congenital Q44.3
- coronary (artery) — see Disease, heart, ischemic, atherosclerotic
- cystic duct — see Obstruction, gallbladder
- due to presence of device, implant or graft — see also Complications, by site and type, specified NEC T85.858 ☑
  - arterial graft NEC T82.858 ☑
  - breast (implant) T85.858 ☑
  - catheter T85.858 ☑
    - dialysis (renal) T82.858 ☑
      - intraperitoneal T85.858 ☑
    - infusion NEC T82.858 ☑
      - spinal (epidural) (subdural) T85.850 ☑
    - urinary (indwelling) T83.85 ☑
  - fixation, internal (orthopedic) NEC T84.85 ☑
  - gastrointestinal (bile duct) (esophagus) T85.858
  - genital NEC T83.85 ☑
  - heart NEC T82.857 ☑
  - joint prosthesis T84.85 ☑
  - ocular (corneal graft) (orbital implant) NEC T85.858 ☑
  - orthopedic NEC T84.85 ☑
  - specified NEC T85.858 ☑
  - urinary NEC T83.85 ☑
  - vascular NEC T82.858 ☑
  - ventricular intracranial shunt T85.850 ☑
- duodenum K31.5
  - congenital Q41.0
- ejaculatory duct NEC N50.89
  - stent
    - vascular
      - end stent
        - adjacent to stent — see Arteriosclerosis
        - within the stent
          - coronary T82.855 ☑
          - peripheral T82.856 ☑
      - in stent
        - coronary vessel T82.855 ☑
        - peripheral vessel T82.856 ☑
- endocervical os — see Stenosis, cervix
- enterostomy K94.13
- esophagus K22.2
  - congenital Q39.3
  - syphilitic A52.79
    - congenital A50.59 [K23]
- eustachian tube — see Obstruction, eustachian tube
- external ear canal (acquired) H61.30- ☑
  - congenital Q16.1
  - due to
    - inflammation H61.32- ☑
    - trauma H61.31- ☑
  - postprocedural H95.81- ☑
  - specified cause NEC H61.39- ☑
- gallbladder — see Obstruction, gallbladder
- glottis J38.6
- heart valve (congenital) Q24.8
  - aortic Q23.0
  - mitral Q23.2
  - pulmonary Q22.1
  - tricuspid Q22.4
- hepatic duct K83.1
- hymen N89.6
- hypertrophic subaortic (idiopathic) I42.1
- ileum — see also Obstruction, intestine, specified NE K56.699
  - congenital Q41.2
- infundibulum cardia Q24.3
- intervertebral foramina — see also Lesion, biomechanical, specified NEC

☑ **Additional Character Required** — Refer to the Tabular List for Character Selection ▽ Subterms under main terms may continue to next column or page

enosis, stenotic — *continued*
  intervertebral foramina — *see also* Lesion, biomechan-
    ical, specified — *continued*
    connective tissue M99.79
      abdomen M99.79
      cervical region M99.71
      cervicothoracic M99.71
      head region M99.70
      lumbar region M99.73
      lumbosacral M99.73
      occipitocervical M99.70
      sacral region M99.74
      sacrococcygeal M99.74
      sacroiliac M99.74
      specified NEC M99.79
      thoracic region M99.72
      thoracolumbar M99.72
    disc M99.79
      abdomen M99.79
      cervical region M99.71
      cervicothoracic M99.71
      head region M99.70
      lower extremity M99.76
      lumbar region M99.73
      lumbosacral M99.73
      occipitocervical M99.70
      pelvic M99.75
      rib cage M99.78
      sacral region M99.74
      sacrococcygeal M99.74
      sacroiliac M99.74
      specified NEC M99.79
      thoracic region M99.72
      thoracolumbar M99.72
      upper extremity M99.77
    osseous M99.69
      abdomen M99.69
      cervical region M99.61
      cervicothoracic M99.61
      head region M99.60
      lower extremity M99.66
      lumbar region M99.63
      lumbosacral M99.63
      occipitocervical M99.60
      pelvic M99.65
      rib cage M99.68
      sacral region M99.64
      sacrococcygeal M99.64
      sacroiliac M99.64
      specified NEC M99.69
      thoracic region M99.62
      thoracolumbar M99.62
      upper extremity M99.67
    subluxation — *see* Stenosis, intervertebral foramina,
      osseous
  intestine — *see also* Obstruction, intestine
    congenital (small) Q41.9
      large Q42.9
        specified NEC Q42.8
      specified NEC Q41.8
  jejunum — *see also* Obstruction, intestine, specified
    NEC K56.699
    congenital Q41.1
  lacrimal (passage)
    canaliculi H04.54- ☑
    congenital Q10.5
    duct H04.55- ☑
    punctum H04.56- ☑
    sac H04.57- ☑
  lacrimonasal duct — *see* Stenosis, lacrimal, duct
    congenital Q10.5
  larynx J38.6
    congenital NEC Q31.8
      subglottic Q31.1
    syphilitic A52.73
      congenital A50.59 [J99]
  mitral (chronic) (inactive) (valve) I05.0
    with
      aortic valve disease I08.0
      incompetency, insufficiency or regurgitation
        I05.2
    active or acute I01.1
      with rheumatic or Sydenham's chorea I02.0
    congenital Q23.2
    specified cause, except rheumatic I34.2
    syphilitic A52.03
  myocardium, myocardial — *see also* Degeneration,
    myocardial

Stenosis, stenotic — *continued*
  myocardium, myocardial — *see also* Degeneration,
    myocardial — *continued*
    hypertrophic subaortic (idiopathic) I42.1
  nares (anterior) (posterior) J34.89
    congenital Q30.0
  nasal duct — *see also* Stenosis, lacrimal, duct
    congenital Q10.5
  nasolacrimal duct — *see also* Stenosis, lacrimal, duct
    congenital Q10.5
  neural canal — *see also* Lesion, biomechanical, speci-
    fied NEC
    connective tissue M99.49
      abdomen M99.49
      cervical region M99.41
      cervicothoracic M99.41
      head region M99.40
      lower extremity M99.46
      lumbar region M99.43
      lumbosacral M99.43
      occipitocervical M99.40
      pelvic M99.45
      rib cage M99.48
      sacral region M99.44
      sacrococcygeal M99.44
      sacroiliac M99.44
      specified NEC M99.49
      thoracic region M99.42
      thoracolumbar M99.42
      upper extremity M99.47
    intervertebral disc M99.59
      abdomen M99.59
      cervical region M99.51
      cervicothoracic M99.51
      head region M99.50
      lower extremity M99.56
      lumbar region M99.53
      lumbosacral M99.53
      occipitocervical M99.50
      pelvic M99.55
      rib cage M99.58
      sacral region M99.54
      sacrococcygeal M99.54
      sacroiliac M99.54
      specified NEC M99.59
      thoracic region M99.52
      thoracolumbar M99.52
      upper extremity M99.57
    osseous M99.39
      abdomen M99.39
      cervical region M99.31
      cervicothoracic M99.31
      head region M99.30
      lower extremity M99.36
      lumbar region M99.33
      lumbosacral M99.33
      occipitocervical M99.30
      pelvic M99.35
      rib cage M99.38
      sacral region M99.34
      sacrococcygeal M99.34
      sacroiliac M99.34
      specified NEC M99.39
      thoracic region M99.32
      thoracolumbar M99.32
      upper extremity M99.37
    subluxation M99.29
      cervical region M99.21
      cervicothoracic M99.21
      head region M99.20
      lower extremity M99.26
      lumbar region M99.23
      lumbosacral M99.23
      occipitocervical M99.20
      pelvic M99.25
      rib cage M99.28
      sacral region M99.24
      sacrococcygeal M99.24
      sacroiliac M99.24
      specified NEC M99.29
      thoracic region M99.22
      thoracolumbar M99.22
      upper extremity M99.27
  organ or site, congenital NEC — *see* Atresia, by site
  papilla of Vater K83.1
  pulmonary (artery) (congenital) Q25.6
    with ventricular septal defect, transposition of aorta,
      and hypertrophy of right ventricle Q21.3
    acquired I28.8

Stenosis, stenotic — *continued*
  pulmonary — *continued*
    in tetralogy of Fallot Q21.3
    infundibular Q24.3
    subvalvular Q24.3
    supravalvular Q25.6
    valve I37.0
      with insufficiency I37.2
      congenital Q22.1
      rheumatic I09.89
        with aortic, mitral or tricuspid (valve) disease
          I08.8
    vein, acquired I28.8
    vessel NEC I28.8
  pulmonic (congenital) Q22.1
    infundibular Q24.3
    subvalvular Q24.3
  pylorus (hypertrophic) (acquired) K31.1
    adult K31.1
    congenital Q40.0
    infantile Q40.0
  rectum (sphincter) — *see* Stricture, rectum
  renal artery I70.1
    congenital Q27.1
  salivary duct (any) K11.8
  sphincter of Oddi K83.1
  spinal M48.00
    cervical region M48.02
    cervicothoracic region M48.03
    lumbar region (NOS) (without neurogenic claudica-
      tion) M48.061
      with neurogenic claudication M48.062
    lumbosacral region M48.07
    occipito-atlanto-axial region M48.01
    sacrococcygeal region M48.08
    thoracic region M48.04
    thoracolumbar region M48.05
  stomach, hourglass K31.2
  subaortic (congenital) Q24.4
    hypertrophic (idiopathic) I42.1
  subglottic J38.6
    congenital Q31.1
    postprocedural J95.5
  trachea J39.8
    congenital Q32.1
    syphilitic A52.73
    tuberculous NEC A15.5
  tracheostomy J95.03
  tricuspid (valve) I07.0
    with
      aortic (valve) disease I08.2
      incompetency, insufficiency or regurgitation
        I07.2
        with aortic (valve) disease I08.2
          with mitral (valve) disease I08.3
      mitral (valve) disease I08.1
        with aortic (valve) disease I08.3
    congenital Q22.4
    nonrheumatic I36.0
      with insufficiency I36.2
  tubal N97.1
  ureter — *see* Atresia, ureter
  ureteropelvic junction, congenital Q62.11
  ureterovesical orifice, congenital Q62.12
  urethra (valve) *see also* Stricture, urethra
    congenital Q64.32
  urinary meatus, congenital Q64.33
  vagina N89.5
    congenital Q52.4
    in pregnancy — *see* Pregnancy, complicated by,
      abnormal vagina
      causing obstructed labor O65.5
  valve (cardiac) (heart) — *see also* Endocarditis I38
    congenital Q24.8
      aortic Q23.0
      mitral Q23.2
      pulmonary Q22.1
      tricuspid Q22.4
  vena cava (inferior) (superior) I87.1
    congenital Q26.0
  vesicourethral orifice Q64.31
  vulva N90.5
Stent jail T82.897 ☑
Stercolith (impaction) K56.41
  appendix K38.1
Stercoraceous, stercoral ulcer K63.3
  anus or rectum K62.6
Stereotypies NEC F98.4

Sterility — see Infertility
Sterilization — see Encounter (for), sterilization
Sternalgia — see Angina
Sternopagus Q89.4
Sternum bifidum Q76.7
Steroid
  effects (adverse) (adrenocortical) (iatrogenic)
    cushingoid E24.2
      correct substance properly administered — see
        Table of Drugs and Chemicals, by drug,
        adverse effect
      overdose or wrong substance given or taken —
        see Table of Drugs and Chemicals, by drug,
        poisoning
    diabetes — see subcategory E09 ☑
      correct substance properly administered — see
        Table of Drugs and Chemicals, by drug,
        adverse effect
      overdose or wrong substance given or taken —
        see Table of Drugs and Chemicals, by drug,
        poisoning
    fever R50.2
    insufficiency E27.3
      correct substance properly administered — see
        Table of Drugs and Chemicals, by drug,
        adverse effect
      overdose or wrong substance given or taken —
        see Table of Drugs and Chemicals, by drug,
        poisoning
  responder H40.04- ☑
Stevens-Johnson disease or syndrome L51.1
  toxic epidermal necrolysis overlap L51.3
Stewart-Morel syndrome M85.2
Sticker's disease B08.3
Sticky eye — see Conjunctivitis, acute, mucopurulent
Stieda's disease — see Bursitis, tibial collateral
Stiff neck — see Torticollis
Stiff-man syndrome G25.82
Stiffness, joint NEC M25.60
  ankle M25.67- ☑
  ankylosis — see Ankylosis, joint
  contracture — see Contraction, joint
  elbow M25.62- ☑
  foot M25.67- ☑
  hand M25.64- ☑
  hip M25.65- ☑
  knee M25.66- ☑
  shoulder M25.61- ☑
  wrist M25.63- ☑
Stigmata congenital syphilis A50.59
Stillbirth P95
Still-Felty syndrome — see Felty's syndrome
Still's disease or syndrome (juvenile) M08.20
  adult-onset M06.1
  ankle M08.27- ☑
  elbow M08.22- ☑
  foot joint M08.27- ☑
  hand joint M08.24- ☑
  hip M08.25- ☑
  knee M08.26- ☑
  multiple site M08.29
  shoulder M08.21- ☑
  vertebra M08.28
  wrist M08.23- ☑
Stimulation, ovary E28.1
Sting (venomous) (with allergic or anaphylactic shock)
  — see Table of Drugs and Chemicals, by animal or
  substance, poisoning
Stippled epiphyses Q78.8
Stitch
  abscess T81.41 ☑
  burst (in operation wound) — see Disruption, wound,
    operation
Stokes' disease E05.00
  with thyroid storm E05.01
Stokes-Adams disease or syndrome I45.9
Stokvis (-Talma) **disease** D74.8
Stoma malfunction
  colostomy K94.03
  enterostomy K94.13
  gastrostomy K94.23
  ileostomy K94.13
  tracheostomy J95.03
Stomach — see condition
Stomatitis (denture) (ulcerative) K12.1
  angular K13.0
    due to dietary or vitamin deficiency E53.0

Stomatitis — continued
  aphthous K12.0
  bovine B08.61
  candidal B37.0
  catarrhal K12.1
  diphtheritic A36.89
  due to
    dietary deficiency E53.0
    thrush B37.0
    vitamin deficiency
      B group NEC E53.9
      B2 (riboflavin) E53.0
  epidemic B08.8
  epizootic B08.8
  follicular K12.1
  gangrenous A69.0
  Geotrichum B48.3
  herpesviral, herpetic B00.2
  herpetiformis K12.0
  malignant K12.1
  membranous acute K12.1
  monilial B37.0
  mycotic B37.0
  necrotizing ulcerative A69.0
  parasitic B37.0
  septic K12.1
  spirochetal A69.1
  suppurative (acute) K12.2
  ulceromembranous A69.1
  vesicular K12.1
    with exanthem (enteroviral) B08.4
    virus disease A93.8
  Vincent's A69.1
Stomatocytosis D58.8
Stomatomycosis B37.0
Stomatorrhagia K13.79
Stone(s) — see also Calculus
  bladder (diverticulum) N21.0
  cystine E72.09
  heart syndrome I50.1
  kidney N20.0
  prostate N42.0
  pulpal (dental) K04.2
  renal N20.0
  salivary gland or duct (any) K11.5
  urethra (impacted) N21.1
  urinary (duct) (impacted) (passage) N20.9
    bladder (diverticulum) N21.0
    lower tract N21.9
    specified NEC N21.8
  xanthine E79.8 [N22]
Stonecutter's lung J62.8
Stonemason's asthma, disease, lung or pneumoco-
  niosis J62.8
Stoppage
  heart — see Arrest, cardiac
  urine — see Retention, urine
Storm, thyroid — see Thyrotoxicosis
Strabismus (congenital) (nonparalytic) H50.9
  concomitant H50.40
    convergent — see Strabismus, convergent concomi-
      tant
    divergent — see Strabismus, divergent concomitant
  convergent concomitant H50.00
    accommodative component H50.43
    alternating H50.05
      with
        A pattern H50.06
        specified nonconcomitances NEC H50.08
        V pattern H50.07
    monocular H50.01- ☑
      with
        A pattern H50.02- ☑
        specified nonconcomitances NEC H50.04- ☑
        V pattern H50.03- ☑
      intermittent H50.31- ☑
        alternating H50.32
  cyclotropia H50.41 ☑
  divergent concomitant H50.10
    alternating H50.15
      with
        A pattern H50.16
        specified nonconcomitances NEC H50.18
        V pattern H50.17
    monocular H50.11- ☑
      with
        A pattern H50.12- ☑
        specified nonconcomitances NEC H50.14- ☑

Strabismus — continued
  divergent concomitant — continued
    monocular — continued
      with — continued
        V pattern H50.13- ☑
      intermittent H50.33 ☑
        alternating H50.34
  Duane's syndrome H50.81- ☑
  due to adhesions, scars H50.69
  heterophoria H50.50
    alternating H50.55
    cyclophoria H50.54
    esophoria H50.51
    exophoria H50.52
    vertical H50.53
  heterotropia H50.40
    intermittent H50.30
  hypertropia H50.2- ☑
  hypotropia — see Hypertropia
  latent H50.50
  mechanical H50.60
    Brown's sheath syndrome H50.61- ☑
    specified type NEC H50.69
  monofixation syndrome H50.42
  paralytic H49.9
    abducens nerve H49.2- ☑
    fourth nerve H49.1- ☑
    Kearns-Sayre syndrome H49.81- ☑
    ophthalmoplegia (external)
      progressive H49.4- ☑
        with pigmentary retinopathy H49.81- ☑
      total H49.3- ☑
    sixth nerve H49.2- ☑
    specified type NEC H49.88- ☑
    third nerve H49.0- ☑
    trochlear nerve H49.1- ☑
  specified type NEC H50.89
  vertical H50.2- ☑
Strain
  back S39.012 ☑
  cervical S16.1 ☑
  eye NEC — see Disturbance, vision, subjective
  heart — see Disease, heart
  low back S39.012 ☑
  mental NOS Z73.3
    work-related Z56.6
  muscle (tendon) — see Injury, muscle, by site, strain
  neck S16.1 ☑
  physical NOS Z73.3
    work-related Z56.6
  postural — see also Disorder, soft tissue, due to use
  psychological NEC Z73.3
  tendon — see Injury, muscle, by site, strain
Straining, on urination R39.16
Strand, vitreous — see Opacity, vitreous, membranes
  and strands
Strangulation, strangulated — see also Asphyxia,
  traumatic
  appendix K38.8
  bladder-neck N32.0
  bowel or colon K56.2
  food or foreign body — see Foreign body, by site
  hemorrhoids — see Hemorrhoids, with complication
  hernia — see also Hernia, by site, with obstruction
    with gangrene — see Hernia, by site, with gangren
  intestine (large) (small) K56.2
    with hernia — see also Hernia, by site, with obstru
      tion
      with gangrene — see Hernia, by site, with gan
        grene
  mesentery K56.2
  mucus — see Asphyxia, mucus
  omentum K56.2
  organ or site, congenital NEC — see Atresia, by site
  ovary — see Torsion, ovary
  penis N48.89
    foreign body T19.4 ☑
  rupture — see Hernia, by site, with obstruction
  stomach due to hernia — see also Hernia, by site, wit
    obstruction
    with gangrene — see Hernia, by site, with gangren
  vesicourethral orifice N32.0
Strangury R30.0
Straw itch B88.0
Strawberry
  gallbladder K82.4
  mark Q82.5

☑ Additional Character Required — Refer to the Tabular List for Character Selection   ▽ Subterms under main terms may continue to next column or page

rawberry — continued
tongue (red) (white) K14.3
eak(s)
macula, angioid H35.33
ovarian Q50.32
ephosymbolia F81.0
secondary to organic lesion R48.8
eptobacillary fever A25.1
eptobacillosis A25.1
eptobacillus moniliformis A25.1
eptococcus, streptococcal — see also condition
as cause of disease classified elsewhere B95.5
group
    A, as cause of disease classified elsewhere B95.0
    B, as cause of disease classified elsewhere B95.1
    D, as cause of disease classified elsewhere B95.2
pneumoniae, as cause of disease classified elsewhere
    B95.3
specified NEC, as cause of disease classified elsewhere
    B95.4
eptomycosis B47.1
eptotrichosis A48.8
ress F43.9
family — see Disruption, family
fetal P84
    complicating pregnancy O77.9
        due to drug administration O77.1
mental NEC Z73.3
    work-related Z56.6
physical NEC Z73.3
    work-related Z56.6
polycythemia D75.1
reaction — see also Reaction, stress F43.9
work schedule Z56.3
retching, nerve — see Injury, nerve
iae albicantes, atrophicae or distensae (cutis) L90.6
ricture — see also Stenosis
ampulla of Vater K83.1
anus (sphincter) K62.4
    congenital Q42.3
        with fistula Q42.2
    infantile Q42.3
        with fistula Q42.2
aorta (ascending) (congenital) Q25.1
    arteriosclerotic I70.0
    calcified I70.0
    supravalvular, congenital Q25.3
aortic (valve) — see Stenosis, aortic
aqueduct of Sylvius (congenital) Q03.0
    with spina bifida — see Spina bifida, by site, with
        hydrocephalus
    acquired G91.1
artery I77.1
    basilar — see Occlusion, artery, basilar
    carotid — see Occlusion, artery, carotid
    celiac I77.4
    congenital (peripheral) Q27.8
        cerebral Q28.3
        coronary Q24.5
        digestive system Q27.8
        lower limb Q27.8
        retinal Q14.1
        specified site NEC Q27.8
        umbilical Q27.0
        upper limb Q27.8
    coronary — see Disease, heart, ischemic,
        atherosclerotic
        congenital Q24.5
    precerebral — see Occlusion, artery, precerebral
    pulmonary (congenital) Q25.6
        acquired I28.8
    renal I70.1
    vertebral — see Occlusion, artery, vertebral
auditory canal (external) (congenital)
    acquired — see Stenosis, external ear canal
bile duct (common) (hepatic) K83.1
    congenital Q44.3
    postoperative K91.89
bladder N32.89
    neck N32.0
bowel — see Obstruction, intestine
brain G93.89
bronchus J98.09
    congenital Q32.3
    syphilitic A52.72
cardia (stomach) K22.2
    congenital Q39.3
cardiac — see also Disease, heart

Stricture — continued
cardiac — see also Disease, heart — continued
    orifice (stomach) K22.2
cecum — see Obstruction, intestine
cervix, cervical (canal) N88.2
    congenital Q51.828
    in pregnancy — see Pregnancy, complicated by,
        abnormal cervix
        causing obstructed labor O65.5
colon — see also Obstruction, intestine
    congenital Q42.9
    specified NEC Q42.8
colostomy K94.03
common (bile) duct K83.1
coronary (artery) — see Disease, heart, ischemic,
    atherosclerotic
cystic duct — see Obstruction, gallbladder
digestive organs NEC, congenital Q45.8
duodenum K31.5
    congenital Q41.0
ear canal (external) (congenital) Q16.1
    acquired — see Stricture, auditory canal, acquired
ejaculatory duct N50.89
enterostomy K94.13
esophagus K22.2
    congenital Q39.3
    syphilitic A52.79
        congenital A50.59 [K23]
eustachian tube — see also Obstruction, eustachian
    tube
    congenital Q17.8
fallopian tube N97.1
    gonococcal A54.24
    tuberculous A18.17
gallbladder — see Obstruction, gallbladder
glottis J38.6
heart — see also Disease, heart
    valve — see also Endocarditis I38
        aortic Q23.0
        mitral Q23.2
        pulmonary Q22.1
        tricuspid Q22.4
hepatic duct K83.1
hourglass, of stomach K31.2
hymen N89.6
hypopharynx J39.2
ileum — see also Obstruction, intestine, specified NEC
    K56.699
    congenital Q41.2
intestine — see also Obstruction, intestine
    congenital (small) Q41.9
        large Q42.9
            specified NEC Q42.8
        specified NEC Q41.8
    ischemic K55.1
jejunum — see also Obstruction, intestine, specified
    NEC K56.699
    congenital Q41.1
lacrimal passages — see also Stenosis, lacrimal
    congenital Q10.5
larynx J38.6
    congenital NEC Q31.8
        subglottic Q31.1
    syphilitic A52.73
        congenital A50.59 [J99]
meatus
    ear (congenital) Q16.1
        acquired — see Stricture, auditory canal, ac-
            quired
    osseous (ear) (congenital) Q16.1
        acquired — see Stricture, auditory canal, ac-
            quired
    urinarius — see also Stricture, urethra
        congenital Q64.33
mitral (valve) — see Stenosis, mitral
myocardium, myocardial I51.5
    hypertrophic subaortic (idiopathic) I42.1
nares (anterior) (posterior) J34.89
    congenital Q30.0
nasal duct — see also Stenosis, lacrimal, duct
    congenital Q10.5
nasolacrimal duct — see also Stenosis, lacrimal, duct
    congenital Q10.5
nasopharynx J39.2
    syphilitic A52.73
nose J34.89
    congenital Q30.0
nostril (anterior) (posterior) J34.89

Stricture — continued
nostril — continued
    congenital Q30.0
    syphilitic A52.73
        congenital A50.59 [J99]
organ or site, congenital NEC — see Atresia, by site
os uteri — see Stricture, cervix
osseous meatus (ear) (congenital) Q16.1
    acquired — see Stricture, auditory canal, acquired
oviduct — see Stricture, fallopian tube
pelviureteric junction (congenital) Q62.11
    acquired, with hydronephrosis N13.0
penis, by foreign body T19.4 ☑
pharynx J39.2
prostate N42.89
pulmonary, pulmonic
    artery (congenital) Q25.6
        acquired I28.8
        noncongenital I28.8
    infundibulum (congenital) Q24.3
    valve I37.0
        congenital Q22.1
    vein, acquired I28.8
    vessel NEC I28.8
punctum lacrimale — see also Stenosis, lacrimal,
    punctum
    congenital Q10.5
pylorus (hypertrophic) K31.1
    adult K31.1
    congenital Q40.0
    infantile Q40.0
rectosigmoid — see also Obstruction, intestine, speci-
    fied NEC K56.699
rectum (sphincter) K62.4
    congenital Q42.1
        with fistula Q42.0
    due to
        chlamydial lymphogranuloma A55
        irradiation K91.89
        lymphogranuloma venereum A55
        gonococcal A54.6
        inflammatory (chlamydial) A55
        syphilitic A52.74
        tuberculous A18.32
renal artery I70.1
    congenital Q27.1
salivary duct or gland (any) K11.8
sigmoid (flexure) — see Obstruction, intestine
spermatic cord N50.89
stoma (following) (of)
    colostomy K94.03
    enterostomy K94.13
    gastrostomy K94.23
    ileostomy K94.13
    tracheostomy J95.03
stomach K31.89
    congenital Q40.2
    hourglass K31.2
subaortic Q24.4
    hypertrophic (acquired) (idiopathic) I42.1
subglottic J38.6
syphilitic NEC A52.79
trachea J39.8
    congenital Q32.1
    syphilitic A52.73
    tuberculous NEC A15.5
tracheostomy J95.03
tricuspid (valve) — see Stenosis, tricuspid
tunica vaginalis N50.89
ureter (postoperative) N13.5
    with
        hydronephrosis N13.1
            with infection N13.6
        pyelonephritis (chronic) N11.1
    congenital — see Atresia, ureter
    tuberculous A18.11
ureteropelvic junction (congenital) Q62.11
    acquired, with hydronephrosis N13.0
ureterovesical orifice N13.5
    with infection N13.6
urethra (organic) (spasmodic) — see also Stricture,
    urethra, male N35.919
    associated with schistosomiasis B65.0 [N37]
    congenital Q64.39
        valvular (posterior) Q64.2
    due to
        infection — see Stricture, urethra, postinfective
        trauma — see Stricture, urethra, post-traumatic

Stricture — *continued*
  urethra — *see also* Stricture, urethra, male — *continued*
    female N35.92
    gonococcal, gonorrheal A54.01
    infective NEC — *see* Stricture, urethra, postinfective
    late effect (sequelae) of injury — *see* Stricture, urethra, post-traumatic
    male N35.919
      anterior urethra N35.914
      bulbous urethra N35.912
      meatal N35.911
      membranous urethra N35.913
      overlapping sites N35.916
    postcatheterization — *see* Stricture, urethra, postprocedural
    postinfective NEC
      female N35.12
      male N35.119
        anterior urethra N35.114
        bulbous urethra N35.112
        meatal N35.111
        membranous urethra N35.113
        overlapping sites N35.116
    postobstetric N35.021
    postoperative — *see* Stricture, urethra, postprocedural
    postprocedural
      female N99.12
      male N99.114
        anterior bulbous urethra N99.113
        bulbous urethra N99.111
        fossa navicularis N99.115
        meatal N99.110
        membranous urethra N99.112
        overlapping sites N99.116
    post-traumatic
      female N35.028
        due to childbirth N35.021
      male N35.014
        anterior urethra N35.013
        bulbous urethra N35.011
        meatal N35.010
        membranous urethra N35.012
        overlapping sites N35.016
    sequela (late effect) of
      childbirth N35.021
      injury — *see* Stricture, urethra, post-traumatic
    specified cause NEC
      female N35.82
      male N35.819
        anterior urethra N35.814
        bulbous urethra N35.812
        meatal N35.811
        membranous urethra N35.813
        overlapping sites N35.816
    syphilitic A52.76
    traumatic — *see* Stricture, urethra, post-traumatic
    valvular (posterior), congenital Q64.2
  urinary meatus — *see* Stricture, urethra
  uterus, uterine (synechiae) N85.6
    os (external) (internal) — *see* Stricture, cervix
  vagina (outlet) — *see* Stenosis, vagina
  valve (cardiac) (heart) — *see also* Endocarditis
    congenital
      aortic Q23.0
      mitral Q23.2
      pulmonary Q22.1
      tricuspid Q22.4
  vas deferens N50.89
    congenital Q55.4
  vein I87.1
  vena cava (inferior) (superior) NEC I87.1
    congenital Q26.0
  vesicourethral orifice N32.0
    congenital Q64.31
  vulva (acquired) N90.5
Stridor R06.1
  congenital (larynx) P28.89
Stridulous — *see* condition
Stroke (apoplectic) (brain) (embolic) (ischemic) (paralytic) (thrombotic) I63.9
  cryptogenic — *see also* infarction, cerebral I63.9
  epileptic — *see* Epilepsy
  heat T67.01 ☑
    exertional T67.02 ☑
    specified NEC T67.09 ☑
  in evolution I63.9

Stroke — *continued*
  intraoperative
    during cardiac surgery I97.810
    during other surgery I97.811
  lightning — *see* Lightning
  meaning
    cerebral hemorrhage — *code to* Hemorrhage, intracranial
    cerebral infarction — *code to* Infarction, cerebral
  postprocedural
    following cardiac surgery I97.820
    following other surgery I97.821
  sun T67.01 ☑
    specified NEC T67.09 ☑
  unspecified (NOS) I63.9
Stromatosis, endometrial D39.0
Strongyloidiasis, strongyloidosis B78.9
  cutaneous B78.1
  disseminated B78.7
  intestinal B78.0
Strophulus pruriginosus L28.2
Struck by lightning — *see* Lightning
Struma — *see also* Goiter
  Hashimoto E06.3
  lymphomatosa E06.3
  nodosa (simplex) E04.9
    endemic E01.2
      multinodular E01.1
    multinodular E04.2
      iodine-deficiency related E01.1
    toxic or with hyperthyroidism E05.20
      with thyroid storm E05.21
      multinodular E05.20
        with thyroid storm E05.21
      uninodular E05.10
        with thyroid storm E05.11
    toxicosa E05.20
      with thyroid storm E05.21
      multinodular E05.20
        with thyroid storm E05.21
      uninodular E05.10
        with thyroid storm E05.11
    uninodular E04.1
  ovarii D27.- ☑
  Riedel's E06.5
Strumipriva cachexia E03.4
Strümpell-Marie spine — *see* Spondylitis, ankylosing
Strümpell-Westphal pseudosclerosis E83.01
Stuart deficiency disease (factor X) D68.2
Stuart-Prower factor deficiency (factor X) D68.2
Student's elbow — *see* Bursitis, elbow, olecranon
Stump — *see* Amputation
Stunting, nutritional E45
Stupor (catatonic) R40.1
  depressive (single episode) F32.89
    recurrent episode F33.8
  dissociative F44.2
  manic F30.2
  manic-depressive F31.89
  psychogenic (anergic) F44.2
  reaction to exceptional stress (transient) F43.0
Sturge (-Weber) (-Dimitri) (-Kalischer) **disease or syndrome** Q85.8
Stuttering F80.81
  adult onset F98.5
  childhood onset F80.81
  following cerebrovascular disease — *see* Disorder, fluency. following cerebrovascular disease
  in conditions classified elsewhere R47.82
Sty, stye (external) (internal) (meibomian) (zeisian) — *see* Hordeolum
Subacidity, gastric K31.89
  psychogenic F45.8
Subacute — *see* condition
Subarachnoid — *see* condition
Subcortical — *see* condition
Subcostal syndrome, nerve compression — *see* Mononeuropathy, upper limb, specified site NEC
Subcutaneous, subcuticular — *see* condition
Subdural — *see* condition
Subendocardium — *see* condition
Subependymoma
  specified site — *see* Neoplasm, uncertain behavior, by site
  unspecified site D43.2
Suberosis J67.3
Subglossitis — *see* Glossitis

Subhemophilia D66
Subinvolution
  breast (postlactational) (postpuerperal) N64.89
    puerperal O90.89
  uterus (chronic) (nonpuerperal) N85.3
    puerperal O90.89
Sublingual — *see* condition
Sublinguitis — *see* Sialoadenitis
Subluxatable hip Q65.6
Subluxation — *see also* Dislocation
  acromioclavicular S43.11- ☑
  ankle S93.0- ☑
  atlantoaxial, recurrent M43.4
    with myelopathy M43.3
  carpometacarpal (joint) NEC S63.05- ☑
    thumb S63.04- ☑
  complex, vertebral — *see* Complex, subluxation
  congenital — *see also* Malposition, congenital
    hip — *see* Dislocation, hip, congenital, partial
    joint (excluding hip)
      lower limb Q68.8
      shoulder Q68.8
      upper limb Q68.8
  elbow (traumatic) S53.10- ☑
    anterior S53.11- ☑
    lateral S53.14- ☑
    medial S53.13- ☑
    posterior S53.12- ☑
    specified type NEC S53.19- ☑
  finger S63.20- ☑
    index S63.20- ☑
    interphalangeal S63.22- ☑
      distal S63.24- ☑
        index S63.24- ☑
        little S63.24- ☑
        middle S63.24- ☑
        ring S63.24- ☑
      index S63.22- ☑
      little S63.22- ☑
      middle S63.22- ☑
      proximal S63.23- ☑
        index S63.23- ☑
        little S63.23- ☑
        middle S63.23- ☑
        ring S63.23- ☑
      ring S63.22- ☑
    little S63.20- ☑
    metacarpophalangeal S63.21- ☑
      index S63.21- ☑
      little S63.21- ☑
      middle S63.21- ☑
      ring S63.21- ☑
    middle S63.20- ☑
    ring S63.20- ☑
  foot S93.30- ☑
    specified site NEC S93.33- ☑
    tarsal joint S93.31- ☑
    tarsometatarsal joint S93.32- ☑
    toe — *see* Subluxation, toe
  hip S73.00- ☑
    anterior S73.03- ☑
      obturator S73.02- ☑
    central S73.04- ☑
    posterior S73.01- ☑
  interphalangeal (joint)
    finger S63.22- ☑
      distal joint S63.24- ☑
        index S63.24- ☑
        little S63.24- ☑
        middle S63.24- ☑
        ring S63.24- ☑
      index S63.22- ☑
      little S63.22- ☑
      middle S63.22- ☑
      proximal joint S63.23- ☑
        index S63.23- ☑
        little S63.23- ☑
        middle S63.23- ☑
        ring S63.23- ☑
      ring S63.22- ☑
    thumb S63.12- ☑
    toe S93.13- ☑
      great S93.13- ☑
      lesser S93.13- ☑
  joint prosthesis — *see* Complications, joint prosthes
    mechanical, displacement, by site

☑ **Additional Character Required — Refer to the Tabular List for Character Selection**   ▽ **Subterms under main terms may continue to next column or pag**

bluxation — *continued*
- knee S83.10- ☑
  - cap — *see* Subluxation, patella
  - patella — *see* Subluxation, patella
  - proximal tibia
    - anteriorly S83.11- ☑
    - laterally S83.14- ☑
    - medially S83.13- ☑
    - posteriorly S83.12- ☑
  - specified type NEC S83.19- ☑
- lens — *see* Dislocation, lens, partial
- ligament, traumatic — *see* Sprain, by site
- metacarpal (bone)
  - proximal end S63.06- ☑
- metacarpophalangeal (joint)
  - finger S63.21- ☑
    - index S63.21- ☑
    - little S63.21- ☑
    - middle S63.21- ☑
    - ring S63.21- ☑
  - thumb S63.11- ☑
- metatarsophalangeal joint S93.14- ☑
  - great toe S93.14- ☑
  - lesser toe S93.14- ☑
- midcarpal (joint) S63.03- ☑
- patella S83.00- ☑
  - lateral S83.01- ☑
  - recurrent (nontraumatic) — *see* Dislocation, patella, recurrent, incomplete
  - specified type NEC S83.09- ☑
- pathological — *see* Dislocation, pathological
- radial head S53.00- ☑
  - anterior S53.01- ☑
  - nursemaid's elbow S53.03- ☑
  - posterior S53.02- ☑
  - specified type NEC S53.09- ☑
- radiocarpal (joint) S63.02- ☑
- radioulnar (joint)
  - distal S63.01- ☑
  - proximal — *see* Subluxation, elbow
- shoulder
  - congenital Q68.8
  - girdle S43.30- ☑
    - scapula S43.31- ☑
    - specified site NEC S43.39- ☑
  - traumatic S43.00- ☑
    - anterior S43.01- ☑
    - inferior S43.03- ☑
    - posterior S43.02- ☑
    - specified type NEC S43.08- ☑
- sternoclavicular (joint) S43.20- ☑
  - anterior S43.21- ☑
  - posterior S43.22- ☑
- symphysis (pubis)
- thumb S63.103 ☑
  - interphalangeal joint — *see* Subluxation, interphalangeal (joint), thumb
  - metacarpophalangeal joint — *see* Subluxation, metacarpophalangeal (joint), thumb
- toe(s) S93.10- ☑
  - great S93.10- ☑
    - interphalangeal joint S93.13- ☑
    - metatarsophalangeal joint S93.14- ☑
  - interphalangeal joint S93.13- ☑
  - lesser S93.10- ☑
    - interphalangeal joint S93.13- ☑
    - metatarsophalangeal joint S93.14- ☑
  - metatarsophalangeal joint S93.149 ☑
- ulna
  - distal end S63.07- ☑
  - proximal end — *see* Subluxation, elbow
- ulnohumeral joint — *see* Subluxation, elbow
- vertebral
  - recurrent NEC — *see* subcategory M43.5 ☑
  - traumatic
    - cervical S13.100 ☑
      - atlantoaxial joint S13.120 ☑
      - atlantooccipital joint S13.110 ☑
      - atloidooccipital joint S13.110 ☑
      - joint between
        - C0 and C1 S13.110 ☑
        - C1 and C2 S13.120 ☑
        - C2 and C3 S13.130 ☑
        - C3 and C4 S13.140 ☑
        - C4 and C5 S13.150 ☑
        - C5 and C6 S13.160 ☑

Subluxation — *continued*
- vertebral — *continued*
  - traumatic — *continued*
    - cervical — *continued*
      - joint between — *continued*
        - C6 and C7 S13.170 ☑
        - C7 and T1 S13.180 ☑
      - occipitoatloid joint S13.110 ☑
    - lumbar S33.100 ☑
      - joint between
        - L1 and L2 S33.110 ☑
        - L2 and L3 S33.120 ☑
        - L3 and L4 S33.130 ☑
        - L4 and L5 S33.140 ☑
    - thoracic S23.100 ☑
      - joint between
        - T1 and T2 S23.110 ☑
        - T2 and T3 S23.120 ☑
        - T3 and T4 S23.122 ☑
        - T4 and T5 S23.130 ☑
        - T5 and T6 S23.132 ☑
        - T6 and T7 S23.140 ☑
        - T7 and T8 S23.142 ☑
        - T8 and T9 S23.150 ☑
        - T9 and T10 S23.152 ☑
        - T10 and T11 S23.160 ☑
        - T11 and T12 S23.162 ☑
        - T12 and L1 S23.170 ☑
  - wrist (carpal bone) S63.00- ☑
    - carpometacarpal joint — *see* Subluxation, carpometacarpal (joint)
    - distal radioulnar joint — *see* Subluxation, radioulnar (joint), distal
    - metacarpal bone, proximal — *see* Subluxation, metacarpal (bone), proximal end
    - midcarpal — *see* Subluxation, midcarpal (joint)
    - radiocarpal joint — *see* Subluxation, radiocarpal (joint)
    - recurrent — *see* Dislocation, recurrent, wrist
    - specified site NEC S63.09- ☑
    - ulna — *see* Subluxation, ulna, distal end

Submaxillary — *see* condition
Submersion (fatal) (nonfatal) T75.1 ☑
Submucous — *see* condition
Subnormal, subnormality
- accommodation (old age) H52.4
- mental — *see* Disability, intellectual
- temperature (accidental) T68 ☑

Subphrenic — *see* condition
Subscapular nerve — *see* condition
Subseptus uterus Q51.28
Subsiding appendicitis K36
Substance (other psychoactive) **-induced**
- anxiety disorder F19.980
- bipolar and related disorder F19.94
- delirium F19.921
- depressive disorder F19.94
- major neurocognitive disorder F19.97
- mild neurocognitive disorder F19.988
- obsessive-compulsive and related disorder F19.988
- psychotic disorder F19.959
- sexual dysfunction F19.981
- sleep disorder F19.982

Substernal thyroid E04.9
- congenital Q89.2
Substitution disorder F44.9
Subtentorial — *see* condition
Subthyroidism (acquired) — *see also* Hypothyroidism
- congenital E03.1
Succenturiate placenta O43.19- ☑
Sucking thumb, child (excessive) F98.8
Sudamen, sudamina L74.1
Sudanese kala-azar B55.0
Sudden
- hearing loss — *see* Deafness, sudden
- heart failure — *see* Failure, heart
Sudeck's atrophy, disease, or syndrome — *see* Algoneurodystrophy
Suffocation — *see* Asphyxia, traumatic
Sugar
- blood
  - high (transient) R73.9
  - low (transient) E16.2
- in urine R81
Suicide, suicidal (attempted) T14.91 ☑
- by poisoning — *see* Table of Drugs and Chemicals
- history of (personal) Z91.5

Suicide, suicidal — *continued*
- history of — *continued*
  - in family Z81.8
- ideation — *see* Ideation, suicidal
- risk
  - meaning personal history of attempted suicide Z91.5
  - meaning suicidal ideation — *see* Ideation, suicidal
- tendencies
  - meaning personal history of attempted suicide Z91.5
  - meaning suicidal ideation — *see* Ideation, suicidal
- trauma — *see* nature of injury by site
Suipestifer infection — *see* Infection, salmonella
Sulfhemoglobinemia, sulphemoglobinemia (acquired) (with methemoglobinemia) D74.8
Sumatran mite fever A75.3
Summer — *see* condition
Sunburn L55.9
- due to
  - tanning bed (acute) L56.8
    - chronic L57.8
  - ultraviolet radiation (acute) L56.8
    - chronic L57.8
- first degree L55.0
- second degree L55.1
- third degree L55.2
SUNCT (short lasting unilateral neuralgiform headache with conjunctival injection and tearing) G44.059
- intractable G44.051
- not intractable G44.059
Sundowning F05
Sunken acetabulum — *see* Derangement, joint, specified type NEC, hip
Sunstroke T67.01 ☑
- specified NEC T67.09 ☑
Superfecundation — *see* Pregnancy, multiple
Superfetation — *see* Pregnancy, multiple
Superinvolution (uterus) N85.8
Supernumerary (congenital)
- aortic cusps Q23.8
- auditory ossicles Q16.3
- bone Q79.8
- breast Q83.1
- carpal bones Q74.0
- cusps, heart valve NEC Q24.8
  - aortic Q23.8
  - mitral Q23.2
  - pulmonary Q22.3
- digit(s) Q69.9
- ear (lobule) Q17.0
- fallopian tube Q50.6
- finger Q69.0
- hymen Q52.4
- kidney Q63.0
- lacrimonasal duct Q10.6
- lobule (ear) Q17.0
- mitral cusps Q23.2
- muscle Q79.8
- nipple(s) Q83.3
- organ or site not listed — *see* Accessory
- ossicles, auditory Q16.3
- ovary Q50.31
- oviduct Q50.6
- pulmonary, pulmonic cusps Q22.3
- rib Q76.6
  - cervical or first (syndrome) Q76.5
- roots (of teeth) K00.2
- spleen Q89.09
- tarsal bones Q74.2
- teeth K00.1
- testis Q55.29
- thumb Q69.1
- toe Q69.2
- uterus Q51.28
- vagina Q52.1 ☑
- vertebra Q76.49
Supervision (of)
- contraceptive — *see* Prescription, contraceptives
- dietary (for) Z71.3
  - allergy (food) Z71.3
  - colitis Z71.3
  - diabetes mellitus Z71.3
  - food allergy or intolerance Z71.3
  - gastritis Z71.3
  - hypercholesterolemia Z71.3
  - hypoglycemia Z71.3
  - intolerance (food) Z71.3
  - obesity Z71.3
  - specified NEC Z71.3

▼ Subterms under main terms may continue to next column or page   ☑ Additional Character Required — Refer to the Tabular List for Character Selection   **297**

Subluxation — Supervision

Supervision — *continued*
  healthy infant or child Z76.2
    foundling Z76.1
  high-risk pregnancy — *see* Pregnancy, complicated
    by, high, risk
  lactation Z39.1
  pregnancy — *see* Pregnancy, supervision of
Supplemental teeth K00.1
Suppression
  binocular vision H53.34
  lactation O92.5
  menstruation N94.89
  ovarian secretion E28.39
  renal N28.9
  urine, urinary secretion R34
Suppuration, suppurative — *see also* condition
  accessory sinus (chronic) — *see* Sinusitis
  adrenal gland
  antrum (chronic) — *see* Sinusitis, maxillary
  bladder — *see* Cystitis
  brain G06.0
    sequelae G09
  breast N61.1
    puerperal, postpartum or gestational — *see* Mastitis,
      obstetric, purulent
  dental periosteum M27.3
  ear (middle) — *see also* Otitis, media
    external NEC — *see* Otitis, externa, infective
    internal — *see* subcategory H83.0 ☑
  ethmoidal (chronic) (sinus) — *see* Sinusitis, ethmoidal
  fallopian tube — *see* Salpingo-oophoritis
  frontal (chronic) (sinus) — *see* Sinusitis, frontal
  gallbladder (acute) K81.0
  gum K05.20
    generalized — *see* Periodontitis, aggressive, gener-
      alized
    localized — *see* Periodontitis, aggressive, localized
  intracranial G06.0
  joint — *see* Arthritis, pyogenic or pyemic
  labyrinthine — *see* subcategory H83.0 ☑
  lung — *see* Abscess, lung
  mammary gland N61.1
    puerperal, postpartum O91.12
      associated with lactation O91.13
  maxilla, maxillary M27.2
    sinus (chronic) — *see* Sinusitis, maxillary
  muscle — *see* Myositis, infective
  nasal sinus (chronic) — *see* Sinusitis
  pancreas, acute — *see also* Pancreatitis, acute K85.80
  parotid gland — *see* Sialoadenitis
  pelvis, pelvic
    female — *see* Disease, pelvis, inflammatory
    male K65.0
  pericranial — *see* Osteomyelitis
  salivary duct or gland (any) — *see* Sialoadenitis
  sinus (accessory) (chronic) (nasal) — *see* Sinusitis
  sphenoidal sinus (chronic) — *see* Sinusitis, sphenoidal
  thymus (gland) E32.1
  thyroid (gland) E06.0
  tonsil — *see* Tonsillitis
  uterus — *see* Endometritis
Supraeruption of tooth (teeth) M26.34
Supraglottitis J04.30
  with obstruction J04.31
Suprarenal (gland) — *see* condition
Suprascapular nerve — *see* condition
Suprasellar — *see* condition
Surfer's knots or nodules S89.8- ☑
Surgical
  emphysema T81.82 ☑
  procedures, complication or misadventure — *see*
    Complications, surgical procedures
  shock T81.10 ☑
Surveillance (of) (for) — *see also* Observation
  alcohol abuse Z71.41
  contraceptive — *see* Prescription, contraceptives
  dietary Z71.3
  drug abuse Z71.51
Susceptibility to disease, genetic Z15.89
  malignant neoplasm Z15.09
    breast Z15.01
    endometrium Z15.04
    ovary Z15.02
    prostate Z15.03
    specified NEC Z15.09
  multiple endocrine neoplasia Z15.81

Suspected condition, ruled out — *see also* Observation,
  suspected
  amniotic cavity and membrane Z03.71
  cervical shortening Z03.75
  fetal anomaly Z03.73
  fetal growth Z03.74
  maternal and fetal conditions NEC Z03.79
  newborn — *see also* Observation, newborn, suspected
    condition ruled out Z05.9
  oligohydramnios Z03.71
  placental problem Z03.72
  polyhydramnios Z03.71
Suspended uterus
  in pregnancy or childbirth — *see* Pregnancy, compli-
    cated by, abnormal uterus
Sutton's nevus D22.9
Suture
  burst (in operation wound) T81.31 ☑
    external operation wound T81.31 ☑
    internal operation wound T81.32 ☑
  inadvertently left in operation wound — *see* Foreign
    body, accidentally left during a procedure
  removal Z48.02
Swab inadvertently left in operation wound — *see*
  Foreign body, accidentally left during a procedure
Swallowed, swallowing
  difficulty — *see* Dysphagia
  foreign body — *see* Foreign body, alimentary tract
Swan-neck deformity (finger) — *see* Deformity, finger,
  swan-neck
Swearing, compulsive F42.8
  in Gilles de la Tourette's syndrome F95.2
Sweat, sweats
  fetid L75.0
  night R61
Sweating, excessive R61
Sweeley-Klionsky disease E75.21
Sweet's disease or dermatosis L98.2
Swelling (of) R60.9
  abdomen, abdominal (not referable to any particular
    organ) — *see* Mass, abdominal
  ankle — *see* Effusion, joint, ankle
  arm M79.89
    forearm M79.89
  breast — *see also* Lump, breast N63.0
  Calabar B74.3
  cervical gland R59.9
  chest, localized R22.2
  ear H93.8- ☑
  extremity (lower) (upper) — *see* Disorder, soft tissue,
    specified type NEC
  finger M79.89
  foot M79.89
  glands R59.9
    generalized R59.1
    localized R59.0
  hand M79.89
  head (localized) R22.0
  inflammatory — *see* Inflammation
  intra-abdominal — *see* Mass, abdominal
  joint — *see* Effusion, joint
  leg M79.89
    lower M79.89
  limb — *see* Disorder, soft tissue, specified type NEC
  localized (skin) R22.9
    chest R22.2
    head R22.0
    limb
      lower — *see* Mass, localized, limb, lower
      upper — *see* Mass, localized, limb, upper
    neck R22.1
    trunk R22.2
  neck (localized) R22.1
  pelvic — *see* Mass, abdominal
  scrotum N50.89
  splenic — *see* Splenomegaly
  testis N50.89
  toe M79.89
  umbilical R19.09
  wandering, due to Gnathostoma (spinigerum) B83.1
  white — *see* Tuberculosis, arthritis
Swift (-Feer) **disease**
  overdose or wrong substance given or taken — *see*
    Table of Drugs and Chemicals, by drug, poisoning
Swimmer's
  cramp T75.1 ☑
  ear H60.33- ☑

Swimmer's — *continued*
  itch B65.3
Swimming in the head R42
Swollen — *see* Swelling
Swyer syndrome Q99.1
Sycosis L73.8
  barbae (not parasitic) L73.8
  contagiosa (mycotic) B35.0
  lupoides L73.8
  mycotic B35.0
  parasitic B35.0
  vulgaris L73.8
Sydenham's chorea — *see* Chorea, Sydenham's
Sylvatic yellow fever A95.0
Sylvest's disease B33.0
Symblepharon H11.23- ☑
  congenital Q10.3
Symond's syndrome G93.2
Sympathetic — *see* condition
Sympatheticotonia G90.8
Sympathicoblastoma
  specified site — *see* Neoplasm, malignant, by site
  unspecified site C74.90
Sympathogonioma — *see* Sympathicoblastoma
Symphalangy (fingers) (toes) Q70.9
Symptoms NEC R68.89
  breast NEC N64.59
  cold J00
  development NEC R63.8
  factitious, self-induced — *see* Disorder, factitious
  genital organs, female R10.2
  involving
    abdomen NEC R19.8
    appearance NEC R46.89
    awareness R41.9
      altered mental status R41.82
      amnesia — *see* Amnesia
      borderline intellectual functioning R41.83
      coma — *see* Coma
      disorientation R41.0
      neurologic neglect syndrome R41.4
      senile cognitive decline R41.81
      specified symptom NEC R41.89
    behavior NEC R46.89
    cardiovascular system NEC R09.89
    chest NEC R09.89
    circulatory system NEC R09.89
    cognitive functions R41.9
      altered mental status R41.82
      amnesia — *see* Amnesia
      borderline intellectual functioning R41.83
      coma — *see* Coma
      disorientation R41.0
      neurologic neglect syndrome R41.4
      senile cognitive decline R41.81
      specified symptom NEC R41.89
    development NEC R62.50
    digestive system NEC R19.8
    emotional state NEC R45.89
      emotional lability R45.86
    food and fluid intake R63.8
    general perceptions and sensations R44.9
      specified NEC R44.8
    musculoskeletal system R29.91
      specified NEC R29.898
    nervous system R29.90
      specified NEC R29.818
    pelvis NEC R19.8
    respiratory system NEC R09.89
    skin and integument R23.9
    urinary system R39.9
  menopausal N95.1
  metabolism NEC R63.8
  neurotic F48.8
  of infancy R68.19
  pelvis NEC, female R10.2
  skin and integument NEC R23.9
  subcutaneous tissue NEC R23.9
  viral cold J00
Sympus Q74.2
Syncephalus Q89.4
Synchondrosis
  abnormal (congenital) Q78.8
  ischiopubic M91.0
Synchysis (scintillans) (senile) (vitreous body) H43.89
Syncope (near) (pre-) R55
  anginosa I20.8
  bradycardia R00.1

☑ **Additional Character Required** — Refer to the Tabular List for Character Selection   ▽ **Subterms under main terms may continue to next column or pag**

ncope — *continued*
cardiac R55
carotid sinus G90.01
due to spinal (lumbar) puncture G97.1
heart R55
heat T67.1 ☑
laryngeal R05
psychogenic F48.8
tussive R05
vasoconstriction R55
vasodepressor R55
vasomotor R55
vasovagal R55

ndactylism, syndactyly Q70.9
complex (with synostosis)
fingers Q70.0- ☑
toes Q70.2- ☑
simple (without synostosis)
fingers Q70.1- ☑
toes Q70.3- ☑

ndrome — *see also* Disease
5q minus NOS D46.C (*following* D46.2)
48,XXXX Q97.1
49,XXXXX Q97.1
abdominal
acute R10.0
muscle deficiency Q79.4
abnormal innervation H02.519
left H02.516
lower H02.515
upper H02.514
right H02.513
lower H02.512
upper H02.511
abstinence, neonatal P96.1
acid pulmonary aspiration, obstetric O74.0
acquired immunodeficiency — *see* Human, immunodeficiency virus (HIV) disease
acute abdominal R10.0
acute respiratory distress (adult) (child) J80
idiopathic J84.114
Adair-Dighton Q78.0
Adams-Stokes (-Morgagni) I45.9
adiposogenital E23.6
adrenal
hemorrhage (meningococcal) A39.1
meningococcic A39.1
adrenocortical — *see* Cushing's, syndrome
adrenogenital E25.9
congenital, associated with enzyme deficiency E25.0
afferent loop NEC K91.89
Alagille's Q44.7
alcohol withdrawal (without convulsions) — *see* Dependence, alcohol, with, withdrawal
Alder's D72.0
Aldrich (-Wiskott) D82.0
alien hand R41.4
Alport Q87.81
alveolar hypoventilation E66.2
alveolocapillary block J84.10
amnesic, amnestic (confabulatory) (due to) — *see* Disorder, amnesic
amyostatic (Wilson's disease) E83.01
androgen insensitivity E34.50
complete E34.51
partial E34.52
androgen resistance — *see also* Syndrome, androgen
insensitivity E34.50
Angelman Q93.51
anginal — *see* Angina
ankyloglossia superior Q38.1
anterior
chest wall R07.89
cord G83.82
spinal artery G95.19
compression M47.019
cervical region M47.012
cervicothoracic region M47.013
lumbar region M47.016
occipito-atlanto-axial region M47.011
thoracic region M47.014
thoracolumbar region M47.015
tibial M76.81- ☑
antibody deficiency D80.9
agammaglobulinemic D80.1
hereditary D80.0
congenital D80.0
hypogammaglobulinemic D80.1

Syndrome — *continued*
antibody deficiency — *continued*
hypogammaglobulinemic — *continued*
hereditary D80.0
anticardiolipin (-antibody) D68.61
antidepressant discontinuation T43.205 ☑
antiphospholipid (-antibody) D68.61
aortic
arch M31.4
bifurcation I74.09
aortomesenteric duodenum occlusion K31.5
apical ballooning (transient left ventricular) I51.81
arcuate ligament I77.4
argentaffin, argintaffinoma E34.0
Arnold-Chiari — *see* Arnold-Chiari disease
Arrillaga-Ayerza I27.0
arterial tortuosity Q87.82
arteriovenous steal T82.898- ☑
Asherman's N85.6
aspiration, of newborn — *see* Aspiration, by substance,
with pneumonia
meconium P24.01
ataxia-telangiectasia G11.3
auriculotemporal G50.8
autoerythrocyte sensitization (Gardner-Diamond) D69.2
autoimmune lymphoproliferative [ALPS] D89.82
autoimmune polyglandular E31.0
autoinflammatory M04.9
specified type NEC M04.8
autosomal — *see* Abnormal, autosomes
Avellis' G46.8
Ayerza (-Arrillaga) I27.0
Babinski-Nageotte G83.89
Bakwin-Krida Q78.5
bare lymphocyte D81.6
Barré-Guillain G61.0
Barré-Liéou M53.0
Barrett's — *see* Barrett's, esophagus
Barsony-Polgar K22.4
Bársony-Teschendorf K22.4
Barth E78.71
Bartter's E26.81
basal cell nevus Q87.89
Basedow's E05.00
with thyroid storm E05.01
basilar artery G45.0
Batten-Steinert G71.11
battered
baby or child — *see* Maltreatment, child, physical
abuse
spouse — *see* Maltreatment, adult, physical abuse
Beals Q87.40
Beau's I51.5
Beck's I65.8
Benedikt's G46.3
Béquez César (-Steinbrinck-Chédiak-Higashi) E70.330
Bernhardt-Roth — *see* Meralgia paresthetica
Bernheim's — *see* Failure, heart, right
big spleen D73.1
bilateral polycystic ovarian E28.2
Bing-Horton's — *see* Horton's headache
Birt-Hogg-Dube syndrome Q87.89
Björck (-Thorsen) E34.0
black
lung J60
widow spider bite — *see* Toxicity, venom, spider,
black widow
Blackfan-Diamond D61.01
Blau M04.8
blind loop K90.2
congenital Q43.8
postsurgical K91.2
blue sclera Q78.0
blue toe I75.02- ☑
Boder-Sedgewick G11.3
Boerhaave's K22.3
Borjeson Forssman Lehmann Q89.8
Bouillaud's I01.9
Bourneville (-Pringle) Q85.1
Bouveret (-Hoffman) I47.9
brachial plexus G54.0
bradycardia-tachycardia I49.5
brain (nonpsychotic) F09
with psychosis, psychotic reaction F09
acute or subacute — *see* Delirium
congenital — *see* Disability, intellectual
organic F09
post-traumatic (nonpsychotic) F07.81

Syndrome — *continued*
brain — *continued*
organic — *continued*
post-traumatic — *continued*
psychotic F09
personality change F07.0
postcontusional F07.81
post-traumatic, nonpsychotic F07.81
psycho-organic F09
psychotic F06.8
brain stem stroke G46.3
Brandt's (acrodermatitis enteropathica) E83.2
broad ligament laceration N83.8
Brock's J98.11
bronze baby P83.88
Brown-Sequard G83.81
Brugada I49.8
bubbly lung P27.0
Buchem's M85.2
Budd-Chiari I82.0
bulbar (progressive) G12.22
Bürger-Grütz E78.3
Burke's K86.89
Burnett's (milk-alkali) E83.52
burning feet E53.9
Bywaters' T79.5 ☑
Call-Fleming I67.841
carbohydrate-deficient glycoprotein (CDGS) E77.8
carcinogenic thrombophlebitis I82.1
carcinoid E34.0
cardiac asthma I50.1
cardiacos negros I27.0
cardiofaciocutaneous Q87.89
cardiopulmonary-obesity E66.2
cardiorenal — *see* Hypertension, cardiorenal
cardiorespiratory distress (idiopathic), newborn P22.0
cardiovascular renal — *see* Hypertension, cardiorenal
carotid
artery (hemispheric) (internal) G45.1
body G90.01
sinus G90.01
carpal tunnel G56.0- ☑
Cassidy (-Scholte) E34.0
cat cry Q93.4
cat eye Q92.8
cauda equina G83.4
causalgia — *see* Causalgia
celiac K90.0
artery compression I77.4
axis I77.4
central pain G89.0
cerebellar
hereditary G11.9
stroke G46.4
cerebellomedullary malformation — *see* Spina bifida
cerebral
artery
anterior G46.1
middle G46.0
posterior G46.2
gigantism E22.0
cervical (root) M53.1
disc — *see* Disorder, disc, cervical, with neuritis
fusion Q76.1
posterior, sympathicus M53.0
rib Q76.5
sympathetic paralysis G90.2
cervicobrachial (diffuse) M53.1
cervicocranial M53.0
cervicodorsal outlet G54.2
cervicothoracic outlet G54.2
Céstan (-Raymond) I65.8
Charcot's (angina cruris) (intermittent claudication)
I73.9
Charcot-Weiss-Baker G90.09
CHARGE Q89.8
Chédiak-Higashi (-Steinbrinck) E70.330
chest wall R07.1
Chiari's (hepatic vein thrombosis) I82.0
Chilaiditi's Q43.3
child maltreatment — *see* Maltreatment, child
chondrocostal junction M94.0
chondroectodermal dysplasia Q77.6
chromosome 4 short arm deletion Q93.3
chromosome 5 short arm deletion Q93.4
chronic
infantile neurological, cutaneous and articular
(CINCA) M04.2

▽ Subterms under main terms may continue to next column or page   ☑ Additional Character Required — Refer to the Tabular List for Character Selection   299

Syncope — Syndrome

Syndrome — *continued*
chronic — *continued*
pain G89.4
personality F68.8
Churg-Strauss M30.1
Clarke-Hadfield K86.89
Clerambault's automatism G93.89
Clouston's (hidrotic ectodermal dysplasia) Q82.4
clumsiness, clumsy child F82
cluster headache G44.009
intractable G44.001
not intractable G44.009
Coffin-Lowry Q89.8
cold injury (newborn) P80.0
combined immunity deficiency D81.9
compartment (deep) (posterior) (traumatic) T79.A0 ☑
(*following* T79.7)
abdomen T79.A3 ☑ (*following* T79.7)
lower extremity (hip, buttock, thigh, leg, foot, toes)
T79.A2 ☑ (*following* T79.7)
nontraumatic
abdomen M79.A3 (*following* M79.7)
lower extremity (hip, buttock, thigh, leg, foot,
toes) M79.A2- ☑ (*following* M79.7)
specified site NEC M79.A9 (*following* M79.7)
upper extremity (shoulder, arm, forearm, wrist,
hand, fingers) M79.A1- ☑ (*following*
M79.7)
postprocedural — *see* Syndrome, compartment,
nontraumatic
specified site NEC T79.A9 ☑ (*following* T79.7)
upper extremity (shoulder, arm, forearm, wrist,
hand, fingers) T79.A1 ☑ (*following* T79.7)
complex regional pain — *see* Syndrome, pain, complex
regional
compression T79.5 ☑
anterior spinal — *see* Syndrome, anterior, spinal
artery, compression
cauda equina G83.4
celiac artery I77.4
vertebral artery M47.029
cervical region M47.022
occipito-atlanto-axial region M47.021
concussion F07.81
congenital
affecting multiple systems NEC Q87.89
central alveolar hypoventilation G47.35
facial diplegia Q87.0
muscular hypertrophy-cerebral Q87.89
oculo-auriculovertebral Q87.0
oculofacial diplegia (Moebius) Q87.0
rubella (manifest) P35.0
congestion-fibrosis (pelvic), female N94.89
congestive dysmenorrhea N94.6
connective tissue M35.9
overlap NEC M35.1
Conn's E26.01
conus medullaris G95.81
cord
anterior G83.82
posterior G83.83
coronary
acute NEC I24.9
insufficiency or intermediate I20.0
slow flow I20.8
Costen's (complex) M26.69
costochondral junction M94.0
costoclavicular G54.0
costovertebral E22.0
Cowden Q85.8
craniovertebral M53.0
Creutzfeldt-Jakob — *see* Creutzfeldt-Jakob disease or
syndrome
crib death R99
cricopharyngeal — *see* Dysphagia
cri-du-chat Q93.4
croup J05.0
CRPS I — *see* Syndrome, pain, complex regional I
crush T79.5 ☑
cryopyrin-associated perodic M04.2
cryptophthalmos Q87.0
cubital tunnel — *see* Lesion, nerve, ulnar
Curschmann (-Batten) (-Steinert) G71.11
Cushing's E24.9
alcohol-induced E24.4
due to
alcohol
drugs E24.2

Syndrome — *continued*
Cushing's — *continued*
due to — *continued*
ectopic ACTH E24.3
overproduction of pituitary ACTH E24.0
drug-induced E24.2
overdose or wrong substance given or taken — *see*
Table of Drugs and Chemicals, by drug, poisoning
pituitary-dependent E24.0
specified type NEC E24.8
cystic duct stump K91.5
Dana-Putnam D51.0
Danbolt (-Cross) (acrodermatitis enteropathica) E83.2
Dandy-Walker Q03.1
with spina bifida Q07.01
Danlos' — *see also* Syndrome, Ehlers-Danlos Q79.60
De Quervain E34.51
de Toni-Fanconi (-Debré) E72.09
with cystinosis E72.04
defibrination — *see also* Fibrinolysis
with
antepartum hemorrhage — *see* Hemorrhage,
antepartum, with coagulation defect
intrapartum hemorrhage — *see* Hemorrhage,
complicating, delivery
newborn P60
postpartum O72.3
Degos' I77.89
Déjérine-Roussy G89.0
delayed sleep phase G47.21
demyelinating G37.9
dependence — *see* F10-F19 with fourth character .2
depersonalization (-derealization) F48.1
di George's D82.1
diabetes mellitus in newborn infant P70.2
diabetes mellitus-hypertension-nephrosis — *see* Diabetes, nephrosis
diabetes-nephrosis — *see* Diabetes, nephrosis
diabetic amyotrophy — *see* Diabetes, amyotrophy
dialysis associated steal T82.898- ☑
Diamond-Blackfan D61.01
Diamond-Gardener D69.2
DIC (diffuse or disseminated intravascular coagulopathy) D65
Dighton's Q78.0
disequilibrium E87.8
Döhle body-panmyelopathic D72.0
dorsolateral medullary G46.4
double athetosis G80.3
Down — *see also* Down syndrome Q90.9
Dresbach's (elliptocytosis) D58.1
Dressler's (postmyocardial infarction) I24.1
postcardiotomy I97.0
drug withdrawal, infant of dependent mother P96.1
dry eye H04.12- ☑
due to abnormality
chromosomal Q99.9
sex
female phenotype Q97.9
male phenotype Q98.9
specified NEC Q99.8
dumping (postgastrectomy) K91.1
nonsurgical K31.89
Dupré's (meningism) R29.1
dysmetabolic X E88.81
dyspraxia, developmental F82
Eagle-Barrett Q79.4
Eaton-Lambert — *see* Syndrome, Lambert-Eaton
Ebstein's Q22.5
ectopic ACTH E24.3
eczema-thrombocytopenia D82.0
Eddowes' Q78.0
effort (psychogenic) F45.8
Ehlers-Danlos Q79.60
classical (cEDS) (classical EDS) Q79.61
hypermobile (hEDS) (hypermobile EDS) Q79.62
specified NEC Q79.69
vascular (vascular EDS) (vEDS) Q79.63
Eisenmenger's I27.83
Ekman's Q78.0
electric feet E53.8
Ellis-van Creveld Q77.6
empty nest Z60.0
endocrine-hypertensive E27.0
entrapment — *see* Neuropathy, entrapment
eosinophilia-myalgia M35.8
epileptic — *see also* Epilepsy, by type

Syndrome — *continued*
epileptic — *see also* Epilepsy, by type — *continued*
absence G40.A09 (*following* G40.3)
intractable G40.A19 (*following* G40.3)
with status epilepticus G40.A11 (*following*
G40.3)
without status epilepticus G40.A19 (*followin*
G40.3)
not intractable G40.A09 (*following* G40.3)
with status epilepticus G40.A01 (*following*
G40.3)
without status epilepticus G40.A09 (*followin*
G40.3)
Erdheim-Chester (ECD) E88.89
Erdheim's E22.0
erythrocyte fragmentation D59.4
Evans D69.41
exhaustion F48.8
extrapyramidal G25.9
specified NEC G25.89
eye retraction — *see* Strabismus
eyelid-malar-mandible Q87.0
Faber's D50.9
facial pain, paroxysmal G50.0
Fallot's Q21.3
familial cold autoinflammatory M04.2
familial eczema-thrombocytopenia (Wiskott-Aldrich
D82.0
Fanconi (-de Toni) (-Debré) E72.09
with cystinosis E72.04
Fanconi's (anemia) (congenital pancytopenia) D61.0
fatigue
chronic R53.82
psychogenic F48.8
faulty bowel habit K59.39
Feil-Klippel (brevicollis) Q76.1
Felty's — *see* Felty's syndrome
fertile eunuch E23.0
fetal
alcohol (dysmorphic) Q86.0
hydantoin Q86.1
Fiedler's I40.1
first arch Q87.0
fish odor E72.89
Fisher's G61.0
Fitzhugh-Curtis
due to
Chlamydia trachomatis A74.81
Neisseria gonorrhorea (gonococcal peritonitis
A54.85
Fitz's — *see also* Pancreatitis, acute K85.80
Flajani (-Basedow) E05.00
with thyroid storm E05.01
flatback — *see* Flatback syndrome
floppy
baby P94.2
iris (intraoperative) (IFIS) H21.81
mitral valve I34.1
flush E34.0
Foix-Alajouanine G95.19
Fong's Q87.2
food protein-induced enterocolitis (FPIES) K52.21
foramen magnum G93.5
Foster-Kennedy H47.14- ☑
Foville's (peduncular) G46.3
fragile X Q99.2
Franceschetti Q75.4
Frey's
auriculotemporal G50.8
hyperhidrosis L74.52
Friderichsen-Waterhouse A39.1
Froin's G95.89
frontal lobe F07.0
Fukuhara E88.49
functional
bowel K59.9
prepubertal castrate E29.1
Gaisböck's D75.1
ganglion (basal ganglia brain) G25.9
geniculi G51.1
Gardner-Diamond D69.2
gastroesophageal
junction K22.0
laceration-hemorrhage K22.6
gastrojejunal loop obstruction K91.89
Gee-Herter-Heubner K90.0
Gelineau's G47.419
with cataplexy G47.411
genito-anorectal A55

☑ **Additional Character Required** — Refer to the Tabular List for Character Selection

▽ **Subterms under main terms may continue to next column or page**

Syndrome — *continued*
Gerstmann-Sträussler-Scheinker (GSS) A81.82
Gianotti-Crosti L44.4
giant platelet (Bernard-Soulier) D69.1
Gilles de la Tourette's F95.2
Glass Q87.89
goiter-deafness E07.1
Goldberg Q89.8
Goldberg-Maxwell E34.51
Good's D83.8
Gopalan' (burning feet) E53.8
Gorlin's Q87.89
Gougerot-Blum L81.7
Gouley's I31.1
Gower's R55
gray or grey (newborn) P93.0
    platelet D69.1
Gubler-Millard G46.3
Guillain-Barré (-Strohl) G61.0
gustatory sweating G50.8
Hadfield-Clarke K86.89
hair tourniquet — *see* Constriction, external, by site
Hamman's J98.19
hand-foot L27.1
hand-shoulder G90.8
hantavirus (cardio)-pulmonary (HPS) (HCPS) B33.4
happy puppet Q93.51
Harada's H30.81- ☑
Hayem-Faber D50.9
headache NEC G44.89
    complicated NEC G44.59
Heberden's I20.8
Hedinger's E34.0
Hegglin's D72.0
HELLP (hemolysis, elevated liver enzymes and low
        platelet count) O14.2- ☑
    complicating
        childbirth O14.24
        puerperium O14.25
hemolytic-uremic D59.3
hemophagocytic, infection-associated D76.2
Henoch-Schönlein D69.0
hepatic flexure K59.8
hepatopulmonary K76.81
hepatorenal K76.7
    following delivery O90.4
    postoperative or postprocedural K91.83
    postpartum, puerperal O90.4
Herter (-Gee) (nontropical sprue) K90.0
Heubner-Herter K90.0
Heyd's K76.7
Hilger's G90.09
histamine-like (fish poisoning) — *see* Poisoning, fish
histiocytic D76.3
histiocytosis NEC D76.3
HIV infection, acute B20
Hoffmann-Werdnig G12.0
Hollander-Simons E88.1
Hoppe-Goldflam G70.00
    with exacerbation (acute) G70.01
    in crisis G70.01
Horner's G90.2
hungry bone E83.81
hunterian glossitis D51.0
Hutchinson's triad A50.53
hyperabduction G54.0
hyperammonemia-hyperornithinemia-homocitrial-line-
        mia E72.4
hypereosinophilic (idiopathic) D72.1
hyperimmunoglobulin D M04.1
hyperimmunoglobulin E (IgE) D82.4
hyperkalemic E87.5
hyperkinetic — *see* Hyperkinesia
hypermobility M35.7
hypernatremia E87.0
hyperosmolarity E87.0
hyperperfusion G97.82
hypersplenic D73.1
hypertransfusion, newborn P61.1
hyperventilation F45.8
hyperviscosity (of serum)
    polycythemic D75.1
    sclerothymic D58.8
hypoglycemic (familial) (neonatal) E16.2
hypokalemic E87.6
hyponatremic E87.1
hypopituitarism E23.0
hypoplastic left-heart Q23.4

Syndrome — *continued*
hypopotassemia E87.6
hyposmolality E87.1
hypotension, maternal O26.5- ☑
hypothenar hammer I73.89
hypoventilation, obesity (OHS) E66.2
ICF (intravascular coagulation-fibrinolysis) D65
idiopathic
    cardiorespiratory distress, newborn P22.0
    nephrotic (infantile) N04.9
iliotibial band M76.3- ☑
immobility, immobilization (paraplegic) M62.3
immune reconstitution D89.3
immune reconstitution inflammatory [IRIS] D89.3
immunity deficiency, combined D81.9
immunodeficiency
    acquired — *see* Human, immunodeficiency virus
            (HIV) disease
    combined D81.9
impending coronary I20.0
impingement, shoulder M75.4- ☑
inappropriate secretion of antidiuretic hormone E22.2
infant
    gestational diabetes P70.0
    of diabetic mother P70.1
infantilism (pituitary) E23.0
inferior vena cava I87.1
inspissated bile (newborn) P59.1
institutional (childhood) F94.2
insufficient sleep F51.12
intermediate coronary (artery) I20.0
interspinous ligament — *see* Spondylopathy, specified
        NEC
intestinal
    carcinoid E34.0
    knot K56.2
intravascular coagulation-fibrinolysis (ICF) D65
iodine-deficiency, congenital E00.9
    type
        mixed E00.2
        myxedematous E00.1
        neurological E00.0
IRDS (idiopathic respiratory distress, newborn) P22.0
irritable
    bowel K58.9
        with
            constipation K58.1
            diarrhea K58.0
        mixed K58.2
        psychogenic F45.8
        specified NEC K58.8
    heart (psychogenic) F45.8
    weakness F48.8
ischemic
    bowel (transient) K55.9
        chronic K55.1
        due to mesenteric artery insufficiency K55.1
    steal T82.898 ☑
IVC (intravascular coagulopathy) D65
Ivemark's Q89.01
Jaccoud's — *see* Arthropathy, postrheumatic, chronic
Jackson's G83.89
Jakob-Creutzfeldt — *see* Creutzfeldt-Jakob disease or
        syndrome
jaw-winking Q07.8
Jervell-Lange-Nielsen I45.81
jet lag G47.25
Job's D71
Joseph-Diamond-Blackfan D61.01
jugular foramen G52.7
Kabuki Q89.8
Kanner's (autism) F84.0
Kartagener's Q89.3
Kelly's D50.1
Kimmelstiel-Wilson — *see* Diabetes, specified type,
        with Kimmelstiel-Wilson disease
Klein (e)-Levine G47.13
Klippel-Feil (brevicollis) Q76.1
Köhler-Pellegrini-Steida — *see* Bursitis, tibial collateral
König's K59.8
Korsakoff (-Wernicke) (nonalcoholic) F04
    alcoholic F10.26
Kostmann's D70.0
Krabbe's congenital muscle hypoplasia Q79.8
labyrinthine — *see* subcategory H83.2 ☑
lacunar NEC G46.7
Lambert-Eaton G70.80

Syndrome — *continued*
Lambert-Eaton — *continued*
    in
        neoplastic disease G73.1
        specified disease NEC G70.81
Landau-Kleffner — *see* Epilepsy, specified NEC
Larsen's Q74.8
lateral
    cutaneous nerve of thigh G57.1- ☑
    medullary G46.4
Launois' E22.0
lazy
    leukocyte D70.8
    posture M62.3
Lemiere I80.8
Lennox-Gastaut G40.812
    intractable G40.814
        with status epilepticus G40.813
        without status epilepticus G40.814
    not intractable G40.812
        with status epilepticus G40.811
        without status epilepticus G40.812
lenticular, progressive E83.01
Leopold-Levi's E05.90
Lev's I44.2
Lichtheim's D51.0
Li-Fraumeni Z15.01
Lightwood's N25.89
Lignac (de Toni) (-Fanconi) (-Debré) E72.09
    with cystinosis E72.04
Likoff's I20.8
limbic epilepsy personality F07.0
liver-kidney K76.7
lobotomy F07.0
Loffler's J82
long arm 18 or 21 deletion Q93.89
long QT I45.81
Louis-Barré G11.3
low
    atmospheric pressure T70.29 ☑
    back M54.5
    output (cardiac) I50.9
lower radicular, newborn (birth injury) P14.8
Luetscher's (dehydration) E86.0
Lupus anticoagulant D68.62
Lutembacher's Q21.1
macrophage activation D76.1
    due to infection D76.2
magnesium-deficiency R29.0
Majeed M04.8
Mal de Debarquement R42
malabsorption K90.9
    postsurgical K91.2
malformation, congenital, due to
    alcohol Q86.0
    exogenous cause NEC Q86.8
    hydantoin Q86.1
    warfarin Q86.2
malignant
    carcinoid E34.0
    neuroleptic G21.0
Mallory-Weiss K22.6
mandibulofacial dysostosis Q75.4
manic-depressive — *see* Disorder, bipolar
maple-syrup-urine E71.0
Marable's I77.4
Marfan's Q87.40
    with
        cardiovascular manifestations Q87.418
            aortic dilation Q87.410
        ocular manifestations Q87.42
        skeletal manifestations Q87.43
Marie's (acromegaly) E22.0
mast cell activation — *see* Activation, mast cell
maternal hypotension — *see* Syndrome, hypotension,
        maternal
May (-Hegglin) D72.0
McArdle (-Schmidt) (-Pearson) E74.04
McQuarrie's E16.2
meconium plug (newborn) P76.0
median arcuate ligament I77.4
Meekeren-Ehlers-Danlos Q79.6 ☑
megavitamin-B6 E67.2
Meige G24.4
MELAS E88.41
Mendelson's O74.0
MERRF (myoclonic epilepsy associated with ragged-
        red fibers) E88.42

Syndrome — *continued*
  mesenteric
    artery (superior) K55.1
    vascular insufficiency K55.1
  metabolic E88.81
  metastatic carcinoid E34.0
  micrognathia-glossoptosis Q87.0
  midbrain NEC G93.89
  middle lobe (lung) J98.19
  middle radicular G54.0
  migraine — *see also* Migraine G43.909
  Mikulicz' K11.8
  milk-alkali E83.52
  Millard-Gubler G46.3
  Miller-Dieker Q93.88
  Miller-Fisher G61.0
  Minkowski-Chauffard D58.0
  Mirizzi's K83.1
  MNGIE (Mitochondrial Neurogastrointestinal En-
      cephalopathy) E88.49
  Möbius, ophthalmoplegic migraine — *see* Migraine,
      ophthalmoplegic
  monofixation H50.42
  Morel-Moore M85.2
  Morel-Morgagni M85.2
  Morgagni (-Morel) (-Stewart) M85.2
  Morgagni-Adams-Stokes I45.9
  Mounier-Kuhn Q32.4
    with bronchiectasis J47.9
      with
        exacerbation (acute) J47.1
        lower respiratory infection J47.0
    acquired J98.09
      with bronchiectasis J47.9
        with
          exacerbation (acute) J47.1
          lower respiratory infection J47.0
  Muckle-Wells M04.2
  mucocutaneous lymph node (acute febrile) (MCLS)
      M30.3
  multiple endocrine neoplasia (MEN) — *see* Neoplasia,
      endocrine, multiple (MEN)
  multiple operations — *see* Disorder, factitious
  myasthenic G70.9
    in
      diabetes mellitus — *see* Diabetes, amyotrophy
      endocrine disease NEC E34.9 *[G73.3]*
      neoplastic disease — *see also* Neoplasm
          D49.9 *[G73.3]*
      thyrotoxicosis (hyperthyroidism) E05.90 *[G73.3]*
        with thyroid storm E05.91 *[G73.3]*
  myelodysplastic D46.9
    with
      5q deletion D46.C *(following D46.2)*
      isolated del (5q) chromosomal abnormality D46.C
          (following D46.2)
      lesions, low grade D46.20
      specified NEC D46.Z *(following D46.4)*
  myelopathic pain G89.0
  myeloproliferative (chronic) D47.1
  myofascial pain M79.18
  Naffziger's G54.0
  nail patella Q87.2
  NARP (Neuropathy, Ataxia and Retinitis pigmentosa)
      E88.49
  neonatal abstinence P96.1
  nephritic — *see also* Nephritis
    with edema — *see* Nephrosis
    acute N00.9
    chronic N03.9
    rapidly progressive N01.9
  nephrotic (congenital) — *see also* Nephrosis N04.9
    with
      dense deposit disease N04.6
      diffuse
        crescentic glomerulonephritis N04.7
        endocapillary proliferative glomerulonephritis
            N04.4
        membranous glomerulonephritis N04.2
        mesangial proliferative glomerulonephritis
            N04.3
        mesangiocapillary glomerulonephritis N04.5
      focal and segmental glomerular lesions N04.1
      minor glomerular abnormality N04.0
      specified morphological changes NEC N04.8
    diabetic — *see* Diabetes, nephrosis
  neurologic neglect R41.4
  Nezelof's D81.4

Syndrome — *continued*
  Nonne-Milroy-Meige Q82.0
  Nothnagel's vasomotor acroparesthesia I73.89
  obesity hypoventilation (OHS) E66.2
  oculomotor H51.9
  ophthalmoplegia-cerebellar ataxia — *see* Strabismus,
      paralytic, third nerve
  oral allergy T78.1 ☑
  oral-facial-digital Q87.0
  organic
    affective F06.30
    amnesic (not alcohol- or drug-induced) F04
    brain F09
    depressive F06.31
    hallucinosis F06.0
    personality F07.0
  Ormond's N13.5
  oro-facial-digital Q87.0
  os trigonum Q68.8
  Osler-Weber-Rendu I78.0
  osteoporosis-osteomalacia M83.8
  Osterreicher-Turner Q87.2
  otolith — *see* subcategory H81.8 ☑
  oto-palatal-digital Q87.0
  outlet (thoracic) G54.0
  ovary
    polycystic E28.2
    resistant E28.39
    sclerocystic E28.2
  Owren's D68.2
  Paget-Schroetter I82.890
  pain — *see also* Pain
    complex regional I G90.50
      lower limb G90.52- ☑
      specified site NEC G90.59
      upper limb G90.51- ☑
    complex regional II — *see* Causalgia
  painful
    bruising D69.2
    feet E53.8
    prostate N42.81
  paralysis agitans — *see* Parkinsonism
  paralytic G83.9
    specified NEC G83.89
  Parinaud's H51.0
  parkinsonian — *see* Parkinsonism
  Parkinson's — *see* Parkinsonism
  paroxysmal facial pain G50.0
  Parry's E05.00
    with thyroid storm E05.01
  Parsonage (-Aldren)-Turner G54.5
  patella clunk M25.86- ☑
  Paterson (-Brown) (-Kelly) D50.1
  pectoral girdle I77.89
  pectoralis minor I77.89
  pediatric autoimmune neuropsychiatric disorders asso-
      ciated with streptococcal infections (PANDAS)
      D89.89
  Pelger-Huet D72.0
  pellagra-cerebellar ataxia-renal aminoaciduria E72.02
  pellagroid E52
  Pellegrini-Stieda — *see* Bursitis, tibial collateral
  pelvic congestion-fibrosis, female N94.89
  penta X Q97.1
  peptic ulcer — *see* Ulcer, peptic
  perabduction I77.89
  periodic fever M04.1
  periodic fever, aphthous stomatitis, pharyngitis, and
      adenopathy [PFAPA] M04.8
  periodic headache, in adults and children — *see*
      Headache, periodic syndromes in adults and
      children
  periurethral fibrosis N13.5
  phantom limb (without pain) G54.7
    with pain G54.6
  pharyngeal pouch D82.1
  Pick's — *see* Disease, Pick's
  Pickwickian E66.2
  PIE (pulmonary infiltration with eosinophilia) J82
  pigmentary pallidal degeneration (progressive) G23.0
  pineal E34.8
  pituitary E22.0
  placental transfusion — *see* Pregnancy, complicated
      by, placental transfusion syndromes
  plantar fascia M72.2
  plateau iris (post-iridectomy) (postprocedural) H21.82
  Plummer-Vinson D50.1
  pluricarential of infancy E40

Syndrome — *continued*
  plurideficiency E40
  pluriglandular (compensatory) E31.8
    autoimmune E31.0
  pneumatic hammer T75.21 ☑
  polyangiitis overlap M30.8
  polycarential of infancy E40
  polyglandular E31.8
    autoimmune E31.0
  polysplenia Q89.09
  pontine NEC G93.89
  popliteal
    artery entrapment I77.89
    post endometrial ablation N99.85
    web Q87.89
  post chemoembolization — *code to* associated cor
      tions
  postcardiac injury
    postcardiotomy I97.0
    postmyocardial infarction I24.1
  postcardiotomy I97.0
  postcholecystectomy K91.5
  postcommissurotomy I97.0
  postconcussional F07.81
  postcontusional F07.81
  postencephalitic F07.89
  posterior
    cervical sympathetic M53.0
    cord G83.83
    fossa compression G93.5
    reversible encephalopathy (PRES) I67.83
  postgastrectomy (dumping) K91.1
  postgastric surgery K91.1
  postinfarction I24.1
  postlaminectomy NEC M96.1
  postleukotomy F07.0
  postmastectomy lymphedema I97.2
  postmyocardial infarction I24.1
  postoperative NEC T81.9 ☑
    blind loop K90.2
  postpartum panhypopituitary (Sheehan) E23.0
  postpolio (myelitic) G14
  postthrombotic I87.009
    with
      inflammation I87.02- ☑
        with ulcer I87.03- ☑
      specified complication NEC I87.09- ☑
      ulcer I87.01- ☑
        with inflammation I87.03- ☑
    asymptomatic I87.00- ☑
  postvagotomy K91.1
  postvalvulotomy I97.0
  postviral NEC G93.3
    fatigue G93.3
  Potain's K31.0
  potassium intoxication E87.5
  Prader-Willi Q87.11
  Prader-Willi-like Q87.19
  precerebral artery (multiple) (bilateral) G45.2
  preinfarction I20.0
  preleukemic D46.9
  premature senility E34.8
  premenstrual dysphoric F32.81
  premenstrual tension N94.3
  Prinzmetal-Massumi R07.1
  prune belly Q79.4
  pseudo -Turner's Q87.19
  pseudocarpal tunnel (sublimis) — *see* Syndrome, carp
      tunnel
  pseudoparalytica G70.00
    with exacerbation (acute) G70.01
    in crisis G70.01
  psycho-organic (nonpsychotic severity) F07.9
    acute or subacute F05
    depressive type F06.31
    hallucinatory type F06.0
    nonpsychotic severity F07.0
    specified NEC F07.89
  pulmonary
    arteriosclerosis I27.0
    dysmaturity (Wilson-Mikity) P27.0
    hypoperfusion (idiopathic) P22.0
    renal (hemorrhagic) (Goodpasture's) M31.0
  pure
    motor lacunar G46.5
    sensory lacunar G46.6
  Putnam-Dana D51.0

Syndrome — *continued*
pyogenic arthritis, pyoderma gangrenosum, and acne
[PAPA] M04.8
pyramidopallidonigral G20
pyriformis — *see* Lesion, nerve, sciatic
QT interval prolongation I45.81
radicular NEC — *see* Radiculopathy
upper limbs, newborn (birth injury) P14.3
rapid time-zone change G47.25
Rasmussen G04.81
Raymond (-Céstan) I65.8
Raynaud's I73.00
with gangrene I73.01
RDS (respiratory distress syndrome, newborn) P22.0
reactive airways dysfunction J68.3
Refsum's G60.1
Reifenstein E34.52
renal glomerulohyalinosis-diabetic — *see* Diabetes,
nephrosis
Rendu-Osler-Weber I78.0
residual ovary N99.83
resistant ovary E28.39
respiratory
distress
acute J80
adult J80
child J80
idiopathic J84.114
newborn (idiopathic) (type I) P22.0
type II P22.1
restless legs G25.81
retinoblastoma (familial) C69.2 ☑
retroperitoneal fibrosis N13.5
retroviral seroconversion (acute) Z21
Reye's G93.7
Richter — *see* Leukemia, chronic lymphocytic, B-cell
type
Ridley's I50.1
right
heart, hypoplastic Q22.6
ventricular obstruction — *see* Failure, heart, right
Romano-Ward (prolonged QT interval) I45.81
rotator cuff, shoulder — *see also* Tear, rotator cuff
M75.10- ☑
Rotes Quérol — *see* Hyperostosis, ankylosing
Roth — *see* Meralgia paresthetica
rubella (congenital) P35.0
Ruvalcaba-Myhre-Smith E71.440
Rytand-Lipsitch I44.2
salt
depletion E87.1
due to heat NEC T67.8 ☑
causing heat exhaustion or prostration
T67.4 ☑
low E87.1
salt-losing N28.89
SATB2-associated Q87.89
Scaglietti-Dagnini E22.0
scalenus anticus (anterior) G54.0
scapulocostal — *see* Mononeuropathy, upper limb,
specified site NEC
scapuloperoneal G71.09
schizophrenic, of childhood NEC F84.5
Schnitzler D47.2
Scholte's E34.0
Schroeder's E27.0
Schüller-Christian C96.5
Schwachman's — *see* Syndrome, Shwachman's
Schwartz (-Jampel) G71.13
Schwartz-Bartter E22.2
scimitar Q26.8
sclerocystic ovary E28.2
Seitelberger's G31.89
septicemic adrenal hemorrhage A39.1
seroconversion, retroviral (acute) Z21
serous meningitis G93.2
severe acute respiratory (SARS) J12.81
shaken infant T74.4 ☑
shock (traumatic) T79.4 ☑
kidney N17.0
following crush injury T79.5 ☑
toxic A48.3
shock-lung J80
Shone's — *code to* specific anomalies
short
bowel K91.2
rib Q77.2
shoulder-hand — *see* Algoneurodystrophy

Syndrome — *continued*
Shwachman's D70.4
sicca — *see* Sicca syndrome
sick
cell E87.1
sinus I49.5
sick-euthyroid E07.81
sideropenic D50.1
Siemens' ectodermal dysplasia Q82.4
Silfversköld's Q78.9
Simons' E88.1
sinus tarsi M25.57- ☑
sinusitis-bronchiectasis-situs inversus Q89.3
Sipple's E31.22
sirenomelia Q87.2
Slocumb's E27.0
slow flow, coronary I20.8
Sluder's G44.89
Smith-Magenis Q93.88
Sneddon-Wilkinson L13.1
Sotos' Q87.3
South African cardiomyopathy I42.8
spasmodic
upward movement, eyes H51.8
winking F95.8
Spen's I45.9
splenic
agenesis Q89.01
flexure K59.8
neutropenia D73.81
Spurway's Q78.0
staphylococcal scalded skin L00
steal
arteriovenous T82.898- ☑
ischemic T82.898- ☑
subclavian G45.8
Stein-Leventhal E28.2
Stein's E28.2
Stevens-Johnson syndrome L51.1
toxic epidermal necrolysis overlap L51.3
Stewart-Morel M85.2
Stickler Q89.8
stiff baby Q89.8
stiff man G25.82
Still-Felty — *see* Felty's syndrome
Stokes (-Adams) I45.9
stone heart I50.1
straight back, congenital Q76.49
subclavian steal G45.8
subcoracoid-pectoralis minor G54.0
subcostal nerve compression I77.89
subphrenic interposition Q43.3
superior
cerebellar artery I63.89
mesenteric artery K55.1
semi-circular canal dehiscence H83.8X- ☑
vena cava I87.1
supine hypotensive (maternal) — *see* Syndrome, hypotension, maternal
suprarenal cortical E27.0
supraspinatus — *see also* Tear, rotator cuff M75.10- ☑
Susac G93.49
swallowed blood P78.2
sweat retention L74.0
Swyer Q99.1
Symond's G93.2
sympathetic
cervical paralysis G90.2
pelvic, female N94.89
systemic inflammatory response (SIRS), of non-infectious origin (without organ dysfunction) R65.10
with acute organ dysfunction R65.11
tachycardia-bradycardia I49.5
takotsubo I51.81
TAR (thrombocytopenia with absent radius) Q87.2
tarsal tunnel G57.5- ☑
teething K00.7
tegmental G93.89
telangiectasic-pigmentation-cataract Q82.8
temporal pyramidal apex — *see* Otitis, media, suppurative, acute
temporomandibular joint-pain-dysfunction M26.62- ☑
Terry's — *see also* Myopia, degenerative H44.2- ☑
testicular feminization — *see also* Syndrome, androgen
insensitivity E34.51
thalamic pain (hyperesthetic) G89.0
thoracic outlet (compression) G54.0
Thorson-Björck E34.0

Syndrome — *continued*
thrombocytopenia with absent radius (TAR) Q87.2
thyroid-adrenocortical insufficiency E31.0
tibial
anterior M76.81- ☑
posterior M76.82- ☑
Tietze's M94.0
time-zone (rapid) G47.25
Toni-Fanconi E72.09
with cystinosis E72.04
Touraine's Q79.8
tourniquet — *see* Constriction, external, by site
toxic shock A48.3
transient left ventricular apical ballooning I51.81
traumatic vasospastic T75.22 ☑
Treacher Collins Q75.4
triple X, female Q97.0
trisomy Q92.9
13 Q91.7
meiotic nondisjunction Q91.4
mitotic nondisjunction Q91.5
mosaicism Q91.5
translocation Q91.6
18 Q91.3
meiotic nondisjunction Q91.0
mitotic nondisjunction Q91.1
mosaicism Q91.1
translocation Q91.2
20 (q)(p) Q92.8
21 Q90.9
meiotic nondisjunction Q90.0
mitotic nondisjunction Q90.1
mosaicism Q90.1
translocation Q90.2
22 Q92.8
tropical wet feet T69.0- ☑
Trousseau's I82.1
tumor lysis (following antineoplastic chemotherapy)
(spontaneous) NEC E88.3
tumor necrosis factor receptor associated periodic
(TRAPS) M04.1
Twiddler's (due to)
automatic implantable defibrillator T82.198 ☑
cardiac pacemaker T82.198 ☑
Unverricht (-Lundborg) — *see* Epilepsy, generalized,
idiopathic
upward gaze H51.8
uremia, chronic — *see also* Disease, kidney, chronic
N18.9
urethral N34.3
urethro-oculo-articular — *see* Reiter's disease
urohepatic K76.7
vago-hypoglossal G52.7
van Buchem's M85.2
van der Hoeve's Q78.0
vascular NEC in cerebrovascular disease G46.8
vasoconstriction, reversible cerebrovascular I67.841
vasomotor I73.9
vasospastic (traumatic) T75.22 ☑
vasovagal R55
VATER Q87.2
velo-cardio-facial Q93.81
vena cava (inferior) (superior) (obstruction) I87.1
vertebral
artery G45.0
compression — *see* Syndrome, anterior, spinal
artery, compression
steal G45.0
vertebro-basilar artery G45.0
vertebrogenic (pain) M54.89
vertiginous — *see* Disorder, vestibular function
Vinson-Plummer D50.1
virus B34.9
visceral larva migrans B83.0
visual disorientation H53.8
vitamin B6 deficiency E53.1
vitreal corneal H59.01- ☑
vitreous (touch) H59.01- ☑
Vogt-Koyanagi H20.82- ☑
Volkmann's T79.6 ☑
von Schroetter's I82.890
von Willebrand (-Jürgen) D68.0
Waldenström-Kjellberg D50.1
Wallenberg's G46.3
water retention E87.79
Waterhouse (-Friderichsen) A39.1
Weber-Gubler G46.3
Weber-Leyden G46.3

Syndrome — *continued*
Weber's G46.3
Wegener's M31.30
with
kidney involvement M31.31
lung involvement M31.30
with kidney involvement M31.31
Weingarten's (tropical eosinophilia) J82
Weiss-Baker G90.09
Werdnig-Hoffman G12.0
Wermer's E31.21
Werner's E34.8
Wernicke-Korsakoff (nonalcoholic) F04
alcoholic F10.26
Westphal-Strümpell E83.01
West's — *see* Epilepsy, spasms
wet
feet (maceration) (tropical) T69.0- ☑
lung, newborn P22.1
whiplash S13.4 ☑
whistling face Q87.0
Wilkie's K55.1
Wilkinson-Sneddon L13.1
Willebrand (-Jürgens) D68.0
Williams Q93.82
Wilson's (hepatolenticular degeneration) E83.01
Wiskott-Aldrich D82.0
withdrawal — *see* Withdrawal, state
drug
infant of dependent mother P96.1
therapeutic use, newborn P96.2
Woakes' (ethmoiditis) J33.1
Wright's (hyperabduction) G54.0
X I20.9
XXXX Q97.1
XXXXX Q97.1
XXXXY Q98.1
XXY Q98.0
Yao M04.8
yellow nail L60.5
Zahorsky's B08.5
Zellweger syndrome E71.510
Zellweger-like syndrome E71.541
Synechia (anterior) (iris) (posterior) (pupil) — *see also*
Adhesions, iris
intra-uterine (traumatic) N85.6
Synesthesia R20.8
Syngamiasis, syngamosis B83.3
Synodontia K00.2
Synorchidism, synorchism Q55.1
Synostosis (congenital) Q78.8
astragalo-scaphoid Q74.2
radioulnar Q74.0
Synovial sarcoma — *see* Neoplasm, connective tissue,
malignant
Synovioma (malignant) — *see also* Neoplasm, connective
tissue, malignant
benign — *see* Neoplasm, connective tissue, benign
Synoviosarcoma — *see* Neoplasm, connective tissue,
malignant
Synovitis — *see also* Tenosynovitis M65.9
crepitant
hand M70.0- ☑
wrist M70.03- ☑
gonococcal A54.49
gouty — *see* Gout
in (due to)
crystals M65.8- ☑
gonorrhea A54.49
syphilis (late) A52.78
use, overuse, pressure — *see* Disorder, soft tissue,
due to use
infective NEC — *see* Tenosynovitis, infective NEC
specified NEC — *see* Tenosynovitis, specified type NEC
syphilitic A52.78
congenital (early) A50.02
toxic — *see* Synovitis, transient
transient M67.3- ☑
ankle M67.37- ☑
elbow M67.32- ☑
foot joint M67.37- ☑
hand joint M67.34- ☑
hip M67.35- ☑
knee M67.36- ☑
multiple site M67.39
pelvic region M67.35- ☑
shoulder M67.31- ☑
specified joint NEC M67.38

Synovitis — *continued*
transient — *continued*
wrist M67.33- ☑
traumatic, current — *see* Sprain
tuberculous — *see* Tuberculosis, synovitis
villonodular (pigmented) M12.2- ☑
ankle M12.27- ☑
elbow M12.22- ☑
foot joint M12.27- ☑
hand joint M12.24- ☑
hip M12.25- ☑
knee M12.26- ☑
multiple site M12.29
pelvic region M12.25- ☑
shoulder M12.21- ☑
specified joint NEC M12.28
vertebrae M12.28
wrist M12.23- ☑
Syphilid A51.39
congenital A50.06
newborn A50.06
tubercular (late) A52.79
Syphilis, syphilitic (acquired) A53.9
abdomen (late) A52.79
acoustic nerve A52.15
adenopathy (secondary) A51.49
adrenal (gland) (with cortical hypofunction) A52.79
age under 2 years NOS — *see also* Syphilis, congenital,
early
acquired A51.9
alopecia (secondary) A51.32
anemia (late) A52.79 [D63.8]
aneurysm (aorta) (ruptured) A52.01
central nervous system A52.05
congenital A50.54 [I79.0]
anus (late) A52.74
primary A51.1
secondary A51.39
aorta (arch) (abdominal) (thoracic) A52.02
aneurysm A52.01
aortic (insufficiency) (regurgitation) (stenosis) A52.03
aneurysm A52.01
arachnoid (adhesive) (cerebral) (spinal) A52.13
asymptomatic — *see* Syphilis, latent
ataxia (locomotor) A52.11
atrophoderma maculatum A51.39
auricular fibrillation A52.06
bladder (late) A52.76
bone A52.77
secondary A51.46
brain A52.17
breast (late) A52.79
bronchus (late) A52.72
bubo (primary) A51.0
bulbar palsy A52.19
bursa (late) A52.78
cardiac decompensation A52.06
cardiovascular A52.00
central nervous system (late) (recurrent) (relapse) (tertiary) A52.3
with
ataxia A52.11
general paralysis A52.17
juvenile A50.45
paresis (general) A52.17
juvenile A50.45
tabes (dorsalis) A52.11
juvenile A50.45
taboparesis A52.17
juvenile A50.45
aneurysm A52.05
congenital A50.40
juvenile A50.40
remission in (sustained) A52.3
serology doubtful, negative, or positive A52.3
specified nature or site NEC A52.19
vascular A52.05
cerebral A52.17
meningovascular A52.13
nerves (multiple palsies) A52.15
sclerosis A52.17
thrombosis A52.05
cerebrospinal (tabetic type) A52.12
cerebrovascular A52.05
cervix (late) A52.76
chancre (multiple) A51.0
extragenital A51.2
Rollet's A51.0

Syphilis, syphilitic — *continued*
Charcot's joint A52.16
chorioretinitis A51.43
congenital A50.01
late A52.71
prenatal A50.01
choroiditis — *see* Syphilitic chorioretinitis
choroidoretinitis — *see* Syphilitic chorioretinitis
ciliary body (secondary) A51.43
late A52.71
colon (late) A52.74
combined spinal sclerosis A52.11
condyloma (latum) A51.31
congenital A50.9
with
paresis (general) A50.45
tabes (dorsalis) A50.45
taboparesis A50.45
chorioretinitis, choroiditis A50.01 [H32]
early, or less than 2 years after birth NEC A50.2
with manifestations — *see* Syphilis, congenita
early, symptomatic
latent (without manifestations) A50.1
negative spinal fluid test A50.1
serology positive A50.1
symptomatic A50.09
cutaneous A50.06
mucocutaneous A50.07
oculopathy A50.01
osteochondropathy A50.02
pharyngitis A50.03
pneumonia A50.04
rhinitis A50.05
visceral A50.08
interstitial keratitis A50.31
juvenile neurosyphilis A50.45
late, or 2 years or more after birth NEC A50.7
chorioretinitis, choroiditis A50.32
interstitial keratitis A50.31
juvenile neurosyphilis A50.45
latent (without manifestations) A50.6
negative spinal fluid test A50.6
serology positive A50.6
symptomatic or with manifestations NEC A50.5
arthropathy A50.55
cardiovascular A50.54
Clutton's joints A50.51
Hutchinson's teeth A50.52
Hutchinson's triad A50.53
osteochondropathy A50.56
saddle nose A50.57
conjugal A53.9
tabes A52.11
conjunctiva (late) A52.71
contact Z20.2
cord bladder A52.19
cornea, late A52.71
coronary (artery) (sclerosis) A52.06
coryza, congenital A50.05
cranial nerve A52.15
multiple palsies A52.15
cutaneous — *see* Syphilis, skin
dacryocystitis (late) A52.71
degeneration, spinal cord A52.12
dementia paralytica A52.17
juvenilis A50.45
destruction of bone A52.77
dilatation, aorta A52.01
due to blood transfusion A53.9
dura mater A52.13
ear A52.79
inner A52.79
nerve (eighth) A52.15
neurorecurrence A52.15
early A51.9
cardiovascular A52.00
central nervous system A52.3
latent (without manifestations) (less than 2 years
after infection) A51.5
negative spinal fluid test A51.5
serological relapse after treatment A51.5
serology positive A51.5
relapse (treated, untreated) A51.9
skin A51.39
symptomatic A51.9
extragenital chancre A51.2
primary, except extragenital chancre A51.0
secondary — *see also* Syphilis, secondary A51.3
relapse (treated, untreated) A51.49

☑ **Additional Character Required** — Refer to the Tabular List for Character Selection   ▽ **Subterms under main terms may continue to next column or page**

Index

Syphilis, syphilitic — Syphilis, syphilitic

Syphilis, syphilitic — *continued*
thorax A52.73
throat A52.73
thymus (gland) (late) A52.79
thyroid (late) A52.79
tongue (late) A52.79
tonsil (lingual) (late) A52.73
primary A51.2
secondary A51.39
trachea (late) A52.73
tunica vaginalis (late) A52.76
ulcer (any site) (early) (secondary) A51.39
late A52.79
perforating A52.79
foot A52.11
urethra (late) A52.76
urogenital (late) A52.76
uterus (late) A52.76
uveal tract (secondary) A51.43
late A52.71
uveitis (secondary) A51.43
late A52.71

Syphilis, syphilitic — *continued*
uvula (late) (perforated) A52.79
vagina A51.0
late A52.76
valvulitis NEC A52.03
vascular A52.00
brain (cerebral) A52.05
ventriculi A52.74
vesicae urinariae (late) A52.76
viscera (abdominal) (late) A52.74
secondary A51.49
vitreous (opacities) (late) A52.71
hemorrhage A52.71
vulva A51.0
late A52.76
secondary A51.39
Syphiloma A52.79
cardiovascular system A52.00
central nervous system A52.3
circulatory system A52.00
congenital A50.59
Syphilophobia F45.29

Syringadenoma — *see also* Neoplasm, skin, benign
papillary — *see* Neoplasm, skin, benign
Syringobulbia G95.0
Syringocystadenoma — *see* Neoplasm, skin, benign
papillary — *see* Neoplasm, skin, benign
Syringoma — *see also* Neoplasm, skin, benign
chondroid — *see* Neoplasm, skin, benign
Syringomyelia G95.0
Syringomyelitis — *see* Encephalitis
Syringomyelocele — *see* Spina bifida
Syringopontia G95.0
System, systemic — *see also* condition
disease, combined — *see* Degeneration, combined
inflammatory response syndrome (SIRS) of non-infe
tious origin (without organ dysfunction) R65.
with acute organ dysfunction R65.11
lupus erythematosus M32.9
inhibitor present D68.62

☑ Additional Character Required — Refer to the Tabular List for Character Selection   ▽ Subterms under main terms may continue to next column or page

T

Tabacism, tabacosis, tabagism — *see also* Poisoning, tobacco
meaning dependence (without remission) F17.200
  with
    disorder F17.299
      in remission F17.211
      specified disorder NEC F17.298
      withdrawal F17.203
Tabardillo A75.9
flea-borne A75.2
louse-borne A75.0
Tabes, tabetic A52.10
with
  central nervous system syphilis A52.10
  Charcot's joint A52.16
  cord bladder A52.19
  crisis, viscera (any) A52.19
  paralysis, general A52.17
  paresis (general) A52.17
  perforating ulcer (foot) A52.19
arthropathy (Charcot) A52.16
bladder A52.19
bone A52.11
cerebrospinal A52.12
congenital A50.45
conjugal A52.10
dorsalis A52.11
  juvenile A50.49
juvenile A50.49
latent A52.19
mesenterica A18.39
paralysis, insane, general A52.17
spasmodic A52.17
syphilis (cerebrospinal) A52.12
Taboparalysis A52.17
Taboparesis (remission) A52.17
juvenile A50.45
TAC (trigeminal autonomic cephalgia) **NEC** G44.099
intractable G44.091
not intractable G44.099
Tache noir S60.22- ☑
Tachyalimentation K91.2
Tachyarrhythmia, tachyrhythmia — *see* Tachycardia
Tachycardia R00.0
atrial (paroxysmal) I47.1
auricular I47.1
AV nodal re-entry (re-entrant) I47.1
junctional (paroxysmal) I47.1
newborn P29.11
nodal (paroxysmal) I47.1
non-paroxysmal AV nodal I45.89
paroxysmal (sustained) (nonsustained) I47.9
  with sinus bradycardia I49.5
  atrial (PAT) I47.1
  atrioventricular (AV) (re-entrant) I47.1
    psychogenic F54
  junctional I47.1
    ectopic I47.1
  nodal I47.1
  psychogenic (atrial) (supraventricular) (ventricular) F54
  supraventricular (sustained) I47.1
    psychogenic F54
  ventricular I47.2
    psychogenic F54
psychogenic F45.8
sick sinus I49.5
sinoauricular NOS R00.0
  paroxysmal I47.1
sinus [sinusal] NOS R00.0
  paroxysmal I47.1
supraventricular I47.1
ventricular (paroxysmal) (sustained) I47.2
  psychogenic F54
Tachygastria K31.89
Tachypnea R06.82
hysterical F45.8
newborn (idiopathic) (transitory) P22.1
psychogenic F45.8
transitory, of newborn P22.1
TACO (transfusion associated circulatory overload) E87.71
Taenia (infection) (infestation) B68.9
diminuta B71.0
echinococcal infestation B67.90
mediocanellata B68.1

Taenia — *continued*
nana B71.0
saginata B68.1
solium (intestinal form) B68.0
  larval form — *see* Cysticercosis
Taeniasis (intestine) — *see* Taenia
Tag (hypertrophied skin) (infected) L91.8
adenoid J35.8
anus K64.4
hemorrhoidal K64.4
hymen N89.8
perineal N90.89
preauricular Q17.0
sentinel K64.4
skin L91.8
  accessory (congenital) Q82.8
  anus K64.4
  congenital Q82.8
  preauricular Q17.0
tonsil J35.8
urethra, urethral N36.8
vulva N90.89
Tahyna fever B33.8
Takahara's disease E80.3
Takayasu's disease or syndrome M31.4
Talcosis (pulmonary) J62.0
Talipes (congenital) Q66.89
acquired, planus — *see* Deformity, limb, flat foot
asymmetric Q66.89
calcaneovalgus Q66.4- ☑
calcaneovarus Q66.1- ☑
calcaneus Q66.89
cavus Q66.7- ☑
equinovalgus Q66.6
equinovarus Q66.0- ☑
equinus Q66.89
percavus Q66.7- ☑
planovalgus Q66.6
planus (acquired) (any degree) — *see also* Deformity, limb, flat foot
  congenital Q66.5- ☑
  due to rickets (sequelae) E64.3
valgus Q66.6
varus Q66.3- ☑
Tall stature, constitutional E34.4
Talma's disease M62.89
Talon noir S90.3- ☑
hand S60.22- ☑
heel S90.3- ☑
toe S90.1- ☑
Tamponade, heart I31.4
Tanapox (virus disease) B08.71
Tangier disease E78.6
Tantrum, child problem F91.8
Tapeworm (infection) (infestation) — *see* Infestation, tapeworm
Tapia's syndrome G52.7
TAR (thrombocytopenia with absent radius) **syndrome** Q87.2
Tarral-Besnier disease L44.0
Tarsal tunnel syndrome — *see* Syndrome, tarsal tunnel
Tarsalgia — *see* Pain, limb, lower
Tarsitis (eyelid) H01.8
syphilitic A52.71
tuberculous A18.4
Tartar (teeth) (dental calculus) K03.6
Tattoo (mark) L81.8
Tauri's disease E74.09
Taurodontism K00.2
Taussig-Bing syndrome Q20.1
Taybi's syndrome Q87.2
Tay-Sachs amaurotic familial idiocy or disease E75.02
TBI (traumatic brain injury) S06.9 ☑
Teacher's node or nodule J38.2
Tear, torn (traumatic) — *see also* Laceration
with abortion — *see* Abortion
annular fibrosis M51.35
anus, anal (sphincter) S31.831 ☑
  complicating delivery
    with third degree perineal laceration — *see also* Delivery, complicated, by, laceration, perineum, third degree O70.20
      with mucosa O70.3
    without third degree perineal laceration O70.4
  nontraumatic (healed) (old) K62.81
articular cartilage, old — *see* Derangement, joint, articular cartilage, by site

Tear, torn — *continued*
bladder
  with ectopic or molar pregnancy O08.6
  following ectopic or molar pregnancy O08.6
  obstetrical O71.5
  traumatic — *see* Injury, bladder
bowel
  with ectopic or molar pregnancy O08.6
  following ectopic or molar pregnancy O08.6
  obstetrical trauma O71.5
broad ligament
  with ectopic or molar pregnancy O08.6
  following ectopic or molar pregnancy O08.6
  obstetrical trauma O71.6
bucket handle (knee) (meniscus) — *see* Tear, meniscus
capsule, joint — *see* Sprain
cartilage — *see also* Sprain
  articular, old — *see* Derangement, joint, articular cartilage, by site
cervix
  with ectopic or molar pregnancy O08.6
  following ectopic or molar pregnancy O08.6
  obstetrical trauma (current) O71.3
  old N88.1
  traumatic — *see* Injury, uterus
dural G97.41
  nontraumatic G96.11
internal organ — *see* Injury, by site
knee cartilage
  articular (current) S83.3- ☑
  old — *see* Derangement, knee, meniscus, due to old tear
ligament — *see* Sprain
meniscus (knee) (current injury) S83.209 ☑
  bucket-handle S83.20- ☑
  lateral
    bucket-handle S83.25- ☑
    complex S83.27- ☑
    peripheral S83.26- ☑
    specified type NEC S83.28- ☑
  medial
    bucket-handle S83.21- ☑
    complex S83.23- ☑
    peripheral S83.22- ☑
    specified type NEC S83.24- ☑
  old — *see* Derangement, knee, meniscus, due to old tear
  site other than knee — *code as* Sprain
  specified type NEC S83.20- ☑
muscle — *see* Strain
pelvic
  floor, complicating delivery O70.1
  organ NEC, obstetrical trauma O71.5
    with ectopic or molar pregnancy O08.6
    following ectopic or molar pregnancy O08.6
perineal, secondary O90.1
periurethral tissue, obstetrical trauma O71.82
  with ectopic or molar pregnancy O08.6
  following ectopic or molar pregnancy O08.6
rectovaginal septum — *see* Laceration, vagina
retina, retinal (without detachment) (horseshoe) — *see also* Break, retina, horseshoe
  with detachment — *see* Detachment, retina, with retinal break
rotator cuff (nontraumatic) M75.10- ☑
  complete M75.12- ☑
  incomplete M75.11- ☑
  traumatic S46.01- ☑
    capsule S43.42- ☑
semilunar cartilage, knee — *see* Tear, meniscus
supraspinatus (complete) (incomplete) (nontraumatic) — *see also* Tear, rotator cuff M75.10- ☑
tendon — *see* Strain
tentorial, at birth P10.4
umbilical cord
  complicating delivery O69.89 ☑
urethra
  with ectopic or molar pregnancy O08.6
  following ectopic or molar pregnancy O08.6
  obstetrical trauma O71.5
uterus — *see* Injury, uterus
vagina — *see* Laceration, vagina
vessel, from catheter — *see* Puncture, accidental complicating surgery
vulva, complicating delivery O70.0
Tear-stone — *see* Dacryolith
Teeth — *see also* condition

Teeth — *continued*
  grinding
    psychogenic F45.8
    sleep related G47.63
Teething (syndrome) K00.7
Telangiectasia, telangiectasis (verrucous) I78.1
  ataxic (cerebellar) (Louis-Bar) G11.3
  familial I78.0
  hemorrhagic, hereditary (congenital) (senile) I78.0
  hereditary, hemorrhagic (congenital) (senile) I78.0
  juxtafoveal H35.07- ☑
  macular H35.07- ☑
  macularis eruptiva perstans D47.01
  parafoveal H35.07- ☑
  retinal (idiopathic) (juxtafoveal) (macular) (parafoveal) H35.07- ☑
  spider I78.1
Telephone scatologia F65.89
Telescoped bowel or intestine K56.1
  congenital Q43.8
Temperature
  body, high (of unknown origin) R50.9
  cold, trauma from T69.9 ☑
    newborn P80.0
    specified effect NEC T69.8 ☑
Temple — *see* condition
Temporal — *see* condition
Temporomandibular joint pain-dysfunction syndrome M26.62- ☑
Temporosphenoidal — *see* condition
Tendency
  bleeding — *see* Defect, coagulation
  suicide
    meaning personal history of attempted suicide Z91.5
    meaning suicidal ideation — *see* Ideation, suicidal
  to fall R29.6
Tenderness, abdominal R10.819
  epigastric R10.816
  generalized R10.817
  left lower quadrant R10.814
  left upper quadrant R10.812
  periumbilic R10.815
  rebound R10.829
    epigastric R10.826
    generalized R10.827
    left lower quadrant R10.824
    left upper quadrant R10.822
    periumbilic R10.825
    right lower quadrant R10.823
    right upper quadrant R10.821
  right lower quadrant R10.813
  right upper quadrant R10.811
Tendinitis, tendonitis — *see also* Enthesopathy
  Achilles M76.6- ☑
  adhesive — *see* Tenosynovitis, specified type NEC
    shoulder — *see* Capsulitis, adhesive
  bicipital M75.2- ☑
  calcific M65.2- ☑
    ankle M65.27- ☑
    foot M65.27- ☑
    forearm M65.23- ☑
    hand M65.24- ☑
    lower leg M65.26- ☑
    multiple sites M65.29
    pelvic region M65.25- ☑
    shoulder M75.3- ☑
    specified site NEC M65.28
    thigh M65.25- ☑
    upper arm M65.22- ☑
  due to use, overuse, pressure — *see also* Disorder, soft tissue, due to use
    specified NEC — *see* Disorder, soft tissue, due to use, specified NEC
  gluteal M76.0- ☑
  patellar M76.5- ☑
  peroneal M76.7- ☑
  psoas M76.1- ☑
  tibial (posterior) M76.82- ☑
    anterior M76.81- ☑
  trochanteric — *see* Bursitis, hip, trochanteric
Tendon — *see* condition
Tendosynovitis — *see* Tenosynovitis
Tenesmus (rectal) R19.8
  vesical R30.1
Tennis elbow — *see* Epicondylitis, lateral
Tenonitis — *see also* Tenosynovitis
  eye (capsule) H05.04- ☑

Tenontosynovitis — *see* Tenosynovitis
Tenontothecitis — *see* Tenosynovitis
Tenophyte — *see* Disorder, synovium, specified type NEC
Tenosynovitis — *see also* Synovitis M65.9
  adhesive — *see* Tenosynovitis, specified type NEC
    shoulder — *see* Capsulitis, adhesive
  bicipital (calcifying) — *see* Tendinitis, bicipital
  gonococcal A54.49
  in (due to)
    crystals M65.8- ☑
    gonorrhea A54.49
    syphilis (late) A52.78
    use, overuse, pressure — *see also* Disorder, soft tissue, due to use
      specified NEC — *see* Disorder, soft tissue, due to use, specified NEC
  infective NEC M65.1- ☑
    ankle M65.17- ☑
    foot M65.17- ☑
    forearm M65.13- ☑
    hand M65.14- ☑
    lower leg M65.16- ☑
    multiple sites M65.19
    pelvic region M65.15- ☑
    shoulder region M65.11- ☑
    specified site NEC M65.18
    thigh M65.15- ☑
    upper arm M65.12- ☑
  radial styloid M65.4
  shoulder region M65.81- ☑
    adhesive — *see* Capsulitis, adhesive
  specified type NEC M65.88
    ankle M65.87- ☑
    foot M65.87- ☑
    forearm M65.83- ☑
    hand M65.84- ☑
    lower leg M65.86- ☑
    multiple sites M65.89
    pelvic region M65.85- ☑
    shoulder region M65.81- ☑
    specified site NEC M65.88
    thigh M65.85- ☑
    upper arm M65.82- ☑
  tuberculous — *see* Tuberculosis, tenosynovitis
Tenovaginitis — *see* Tenosynovitis
Tension
  arterial, high — *see also* Hypertension
    without diagnosis of hypertension R03.0
  headache G44.209
    intractable G44.201
    not intractable G44.209
  nervous R45.0
  pneumothorax J93.0
  premenstrual N94.3
  state (mental) F48.9
Tentorium — *see* condition
Teratencephalus Q89.8
Teratism Q89.7
Teratoblastoma (malignant) — *see* Neoplasm, malignant, by site
Teratocarcinoma — *see also* Neoplasm, malignant, by site
  liver C22.7
Teratoma (solid) — *see also* Neoplasm, uncertain behavior, by site
  with embryonal carcinoma, mixed — *see* Neoplasm, malignant, by site
  with malignant transformation — *see* Neoplasm, malignant, by site
  adult (cystic) — *see* Neoplasm, benign, by site
  benign — *see* Neoplasm, benign, by site
  combined with choriocarcinoma — *see* Neoplasm, malignant, by site
  cystic (adult) — *see* Neoplasm, benign, by site
  differentiated — *see* Neoplasm, benign, by site
  embryonal — *see also* Neoplasm, malignant, by site
    liver C22.7
  immature — *see* Neoplasm, malignant, by site
  liver C22.7
    adult, benign, cystic, differentiated type or mature D13.4
  malignant — *see also* Neoplasm, malignant, by site
    anaplastic — *see* Neoplasm, malignant, by site
    intermediate — *see* Neoplasm, malignant, by site
    specified site — *see* Neoplasm, malignant, by site
    unspecified site C62.90

Teratoma — *continued*
  malignant — *see also* Neoplasm, malignant, by site
    continued
    undifferentiated — *see* Neoplasm, malignant, b
      site
  mature — *see* Neoplasm, uncertain behavior, by si
    malignant — *see* Neoplasm, by site, malignant,
      site
  ovary D27.- ☑
    embryonal, immature or malignant C56- ☑
  solid — *see* Neoplasm, uncertain behavior, by site
  testis C62.9- ☑
    adult, benign, cystic, differentiated type or matu
      D29.2- ☑
    scrotal C62.1- ☑
    undescended C62.0- ☑
Termination
  anomalous — *see also* Malposition, congenital
    right pulmonary vein Q26.3
  pregnancy, elective Z33.2
Ternidens diminutus infestation B81.8
Ternidensiasis B81.8
Terror(s) night (child) F51.4
Terrorism, victim of Z65.4
Terry's syndrome — *see also* Myopia, degenerative H44.2- ☑
Tertiary — *see* condition
Test, tests, testing (for)
  adequacy (for dialysis)
    hemodialysis Z49.31
    peritoneal Z49.32
  blood pressure Z01.30
    abnormal reading — *see* Blood, pressure
  blood typing Z01.83
    Rh typing Z01.83
  blood-alcohol Z04.89
    positive — *see* Findings, abnormal, in blood
  blood-drug Z04.89
    positive — *see* Findings, abnormal, in blood
  cardiac pulse generator (battery) Z45.010
  fertility Z31.41
  genetic
    disease carrier status for procreative manageme
      female Z31.430
      male Z31.440
    male partner of patient with recurrent pregnan
      loss Z31.441
    procreative management NEC
      female Z31.438
      male Z31.448
  hearing Z01.10
    with abnormal findings NEC Z01.118
    infant or child (over 28 days old) Z00.129
      with abnormal findings Z00.121
  HIV (human immunodeficiency virus)
    nonconclusive (in infants) R75
    positive Z21
    seropositive Z21
  immunity status Z01.84
  intelligence NEC Z01.89
  laboratory (as part of a general medical examinatio
    Z00.00
    with abnormal finding Z00.01
    for medicolegal reason NEC Z04.89
  male partner of patient with recurrent pregnancy lc
    Z31.441
  Mantoux (for tuberculosis) Z11.1
    abnormal result R76.11
  pregnancy, positive first pregnancy — *see* Pregnanc
    normal, first
  procreative Z31.49
    fertility Z31.41
  skin, diagnostic
    allergy Z01.82
      special screening examination — *see* Screenin
        by name of disease
    Mantoux Z11.1
    tuberculin Z11.1
  specified NEC Z01.89
  tuberculin Z11.1
    abnormal result R76.11
  vision Z01.00
    with abnormal findings Z01.01
    following failed vision screening Z01.020
      with abnormal findings Z01.021
    infant or child (over 28 days old) Z00.129
      with abnormal findings Z00.121
  Wassermann Z11.3

Thrombophlebitis — *continued*
- leg — *continued*
  - superficial I80.0- ☑
- longitudinal (venous) sinus G08
  - nonpyogenic I67.6
- lower extremity I80.299
- migrans, migrating I82.1
- pelvic
  - with ectopic or molar pregnancy O08.0
  - following ectopic or molar pregnancy O08.0
  - puerperal O87.1
- peroneal vein I80.24- ☑
- popliteal vein — *see* Phlebitis, leg, deep, popliteal
- portal (vein) K75.1
- postoperative T81.72 ☑
- pregnancy — *see* Thrombophlebitis, antepartum
- puerperal, postpartum, childbirth O87.0
  - deep O87.1
  - pelvic O87.1
  - septic O86.81
  - superficial O87.0
- saphenous (greater) (lesser) I80.0- ☑
- sinus (intracranial) G08
  - nonpyogenic I67.6
- soleal vein I80.25- ☑
- specified site NEC I80.8
- tibial vein (anterior) (posterior) I80.23- ☑

Thrombosis, thrombotic (bland) (multiple) (progressive) (silent) (vessel) I82.90
- anal K64.5
- antepartum — *see* Thrombophlebitis, antepartum
- aorta, aortic I74.10
  - abdominal I74.09
    - saddle I74.01
  - bifurcation I74.09
  - saddle I74.01
  - specified site NEC I74.19
  - terminal I74.09
  - thoracic I74.11
  - valve — *see* Endocarditis, aortic
- apoplexy I63.3- ☑
- artery, arteries (postinfectional) I74.9
  - auditory, internal — *see* Occlusion, artery, precerebral, specified NEC
  - basilar — *see* Occlusion, artery, basilar
  - carotid (common) (internal) — *see* Occlusion, artery, carotid
  - cerebellar (anterior inferior) (posterior inferior) (superior) — *see* Occlusion, artery, cerebellar
  - cerebral — *see* Occlusion, artery, cerebral
  - choroidal (anterior) — *see* Occlusion, artery, precerebral, specified NEC
  - communicating, posterior — *see* Occlusion, artery, precerebral, specified NEC
  - coronary — *see also* Infarct, myocardium
    - not resulting in infarction I24.0
  - hepatic I74.8
  - hypophyseal — *see* Occlusion, artery, precerebral, specified NEC
  - iliac I74.5
  - limb I74.4
    - lower I74.3
    - upper I74.2
  - meningeal, anterior or posterior — *see* Occlusion, artery, cerebral, specified NEC
  - mesenteric (with gangrene) — *see also* Infarct, intestine K55.069
  - ophthalmic — *see* Occlusion, artery, retina
  - pontine — *see* Occlusion, artery, precerebral, specified NEC
  - precerebral — *see* Occlusion, artery, precerebral
  - pulmonary (iatrogenic) — *see* Embolism, pulmonary
  - renal N28.0
  - retinal — *see* Occlusion, artery, retina
  - spinal, anterior or posterior G95.11
  - traumatic NEC T14.8 ☑
  - vertebral — *see* Occlusion, artery, vertebral
- atrium, auricular — *see also* Infarct, myocardium
  - following acute myocardial infarction (current complication) I23.6
  - not resulting in infarction I51.3
  - old I51.3
- basilar (artery) — *see* Occlusion, artery, basilar
- brain (artery) (stem) — *see also* Occlusion, artery, cerebral
  - due to syphilis A52.05
  - puerperal O99.43
  - sinus — *see* Thrombosis, intracranial venous sinus

Thrombosis, thrombotic — *continued*
- capillary I78.8
- cardiac — *see also* Infarct, myocardium
  - not resulting in infarction I51.3
  - old I51.3
  - valve — *see* Endocarditis
- carotid (artery) (common) (internal) — *see* Occlusion, artery, carotid
- cavernous (venous) sinus — *see* Thrombosis, intracranial venous sinus
- cerebellar artery (anterior inferior) (posterior inferior) (superior) I66.3
- cerebral (artery) — *see* Occlusion, artery, cerebral
- cerebrovenous sinus — *see also* Thrombosis, intracranial venous sinus
  - puerperium O87.3
- chronic I82.91
- coronary (artery) (vein) — *see also* Infarct, myocardium
  - not resulting in infarction I24.0
- corpus cavernosum N48.89
- cortical I66.9
- deep — *see* Embolism, vein, lower extremity
- due to device, implant or graft — *see also* Complications, by site and type, specified NEC T85.868 ☑
  - arterial graft NEC T82.868 ☑
  - breast (implant) T85.868 ☑
  - catheter NEC T85.868 ☑
    - dialysis (renal) T82.868 ☑
      - intraperitoneal T85.868 ☑
    - infusion NEC T82.868 ☑
      - spinal (epidural) (subdural) T85.860 ☑
    - urinary (indwelling) T83.86 ☑
  - electronic (electrode) (pulse generator) (stimulator)
    - bone T84.86 ☑
    - cardiac T82.867 ☑
    - nervous system (brain) (peripheral nerve) (spinal) T85.860 ☑
    - urinary T83.86 ☑
  - fixation, internal (orthopedic) NEC T84.86 ☑
  - gastrointestinal (bile duct) (esophagus) T85.868 ☑
  - genital NEC T83.86 ☑
  - heart T82.867 ☑
  - joint prosthesis T84.86 ☑
  - ocular (corneal graft) (orbital implant) NEC T85.868 ☑
  - orthopedic NEC T84.86 ☑
  - specified NEC T85.868 ☑
  - urinary NEC T83.86 ☑
  - vascular NEC T82.868 ☑
  - ventricular intracranial shunt T85.860 ☑
- during the puerperium — *see* Thrombosis, puerperal
- endocardial — *see also* Infarct, myocardium
  - not resulting in infarction I51.3
- eye — *see* Occlusion, retina
- genital organ
  - female NEC N94.89
    - pregnancy — *see* Thrombophlebitis, antepartum
  - male N50.1
- gestational — *see* Phlebopathy, gestational
- heart (chamber) — *see also* Infarct, myocardium
  - not resulting in infarction I51.3
  - old I51.3
- hepatic (vein) I82.0
  - artery I74.8
- history (of) Z86.718
- intestine (with gangrene) — *see also* Infarct, intestine K55.069
- intracardiac NEC (apical) (atrial) (auricular) (ventricular) (old) I51.3
- intracranial (arterial) I66.9
  - venous sinus (any) G08
    - nonpyogenic origin I67.6
    - puerperium O87.3
- intramural — *see also* Infarct, myocardium
  - not resulting in infarction I51.3
  - old I51.3
- intraspinal venous sinuses and veins G08
  - nonpyogenic G95.19
- kidney (artery) N28.0
- lateral (venous) sinus — *see* Thrombosis, intracranial venous sinus
- leg — *see* Thrombosis, vein, lower extremity
  - arterial I74.3
- liver (venous) I82.0
  - artery I74.8
  - portal vein I81

Thrombosis, thrombotic — *continued*
- longitudinal (venous) sinus — *see* Thrombosis, intracranial venous sinus
- lower limb — *see* Thrombosis, vein, lower extremity
- lung (iatrogenic) (postoperative) — *see* Embolism, pulmonary
- meninges (brain) (arterial) I66.8
- mesenteric (artery) (with gangrene) — *see also* Infarct, intestine K55.069
  - vein (inferior) (superior) K55.0 ☑
- mitral I34.8
- mural — *see also* Infarct, myocardium
  - due to syphilis A52.06
  - not resulting in infarction I51.3
  - old I51.3
- omentum (with gangrene) — *see also* Infarct, intestine K55.069
- ophthalmic — *see* Occlusion, retina
- pampiniform plexus (male) N50.1
- parietal — *see also* Infarct, myocardium
  - not resulting in infarction I24.0
- penis, superficial vein N48.81
- perianal venous K64.5
- peripheral arteries I74.4
  - upper I74.2
- personal history (of) Z86.718
- portal I81
  - due to syphilis A52.09
- precerebral artery — *see* Occlusion, artery, precerebral
- puerperal, postpartum O87.0
  - brain (artery) O99.43
    - venous (sinus) O87.3
  - cardiac O99.43
  - cerebral (artery) O99.43
    - venous (sinus) O87.3
  - superficial O87.0
- pulmonary (artery) (iatrogenic) (postoperative) (vein) — *see* Embolism, pulmonary
- renal (artery) N28.0
  - vein I82.3
- resulting from presence of device, implant or graft — *see* Complications, by site and type, specified NEC
- retina, retinal — *see* Occlusion, retina
- scrotum N50.1
- seminal vesicle N50.1
- sigmoid (venous) sinus — *see* Thrombosis, intracranial venous sinus
- sinus, intracranial (any) — *see* Thrombosis, intracranial venous sinus
- specified site NEC I82.890
  - chronic I82.891
- spermatic cord N50.1
- spinal cord (arterial) G95.11
  - due to syphilis A52.09
  - pyogenic origin G06.1
- spleen, splenic D73.5
  - artery I74.8
- testis N50.1
- traumatic NEC T14.8 ☑
- tricuspid I07.8
- tumor — *see* Neoplasm, unspecified behavior, by site
- tunica vaginalis N50.1
- umbilical cord (vessels), complicating delivery O69.5 ☑
- vas deferens N50.1
- vein (acute) I82.90
  - antecubital I82.61- ☑
    - chronic I82.71- ☑
  - axillary I82.A1- ☑ (*following* ☑ I82.7)
    - chronic I82.A2- ☑ (*following* I82.7)
  - basilic I82.61- ☑
    - chronic I82.71- ☑
  - brachial I82.62- ☑
    - chronic I82.72- ☑
  - brachiocephalic (innominate) I82.290
    - chronic I82.291
  - cephalic I82.61- ☑
    - chronic I82.71- ☑
  - cerebral, nonpyogenic I67.6
  - chronic I82.91
  - deep (DVT) I82.40- ☑
    - calf I82.4Z- ☑
      - chronic I82.5Z- ☑
    - lower leg I82.4Z- ☑
      - chronic I82.5Z- ☑
    - thigh I82.4Y- ☑
      - chronic I82.5Y- ☑

☑ **Additional Character Required** — Refer to the Tabular List for Character Selection ▽ **Subterms under main terms may continue to next column or page**

Thrombosis, thrombotic — *continued*
vein — *continued*
  deep — *continued*
    upper leg I82.4Y ☑
      chronic I82.5Y- ☑
    femoral I82.41- ☑
      chronic I82.51- ☑
    iliac (iliofemoral) I82.42- ☑
      chronic I82.52- ☑
    innominate I82.290
      chronic I82.291
    internal jugular I82.C1- ☑ (*following* I82.7)
      chronic I82.C2- ☑ (*following* I82.7)
    lower extremity
      deep I82.40- ☑
        chronic I82.50- ☑
        specified NEC I82.49- ☑
          chronic NEC I82.59- ☑
      distal
        deep I82.4Z- ☑
      proximal
        deep I82.4Y- ☑
          chronic I82.5Y- ☑
    superficial I82.81- ☑
  perianal K64.5
  popliteal I82.43- ☑
    chronic I82.53- ☑
  radial I82.62- ☑
    chronic I82.72- ☑
  renal I82.3
  saphenous (greater) (lesser) I82.81- ☑
  specified NEC I82.890
    chronic NEC I82.891
  subclavian I82.B1- ☑ (*following* I82.7)
    chronic I82.B2- ☑ (*following* I82.7)
  thoracic NEC I82.290
    chronic I82.291
  tibial I82.44- ☑
    chronic I82.54- ☑
  ulnar I82.62- ☑
    chronic I82.72- ☑
  upper extremity I82.60- ☑
    chronic I82.70- ☑
    deep I82.62- ☑
      chronic I82.72- ☑
    superficial I82.61- ☑
      chronic I82.71- ☑
 vena cava
  inferior I82.220
    chronic I82.221
  superior I82.210
    chronic I82.211
 venous, perianal K64.5
 ventricle — *see also* Infarct, myocardium
  following acute myocardial infarction (current complication) I23.6
  not resulting in infarction I24.0
  old I51.3
Thrombus — *see* Thrombosis
Thrush — *see also* Candidiasis
 newborn P37.5
 oral B37.0
 vaginal B37.3
Thumb — *see also* condition
 sucking (child problem) F98.8
Thymitis E32.8
Thymoma (benign) D15.0
 malignant C37
Thymus, thymic (gland) — *see* condition
Thyrocele — *see* Goiter
Thyroglossal — *see also* condition
 cyst Q89.2
 duct, persistent Q89.2
Thyroid (gland) (body) — *see also* condition
 hormone resistance E07.89
 lingual Q89.2
 nodule (cystic) (nontoxic) (single) E04.1
Thyroiditis E06.9
 acute (nonsuppurative) (pyogenic) (suppurative) E06.0
 autoimmune E06.3
 chronic (nonspecific) (sclerosing) E06.5
  with thyrotoxicosis, transient E06.2
  fibrous E06.5
  lymphadenoid E06.3
  lymphocytic E06.3
  lymphoid E06.3
  de Quervain's E06.1

Thyroiditis — *continued*
 drug-induced E06.4
 fibrous (chronic) E06.5
 giant-cell (follicular) E06.1
 granulomatous (de Quervain) (subacute) E06.1
 Hashimoto's (struma lymphomatosa) E06.3
 iatrogenic E06.4
 ligneous E06.5
 lymphocytic (chronic) E06.3
 lymphoid E06.3
 lymphomatous E06.3
 nonsuppurative E06.1
 postpartum, puerperal O90.5
 pseudotuberculous E06.1
 pyogenic E06.0
 radiation E06.4
 Riedel's E06.5
 subacute (granulomatous) E06.1
 suppurative E06.0
 tuberculous A18.81
 viral E06.1
 woody E06.5
Thyrolingual duct, persistent Q89.2
Thyromegaly E01.0
Thyrotoxic
 crisis — *see* Thyrotoxicosis
 heart disease or failure — *see also* Thyrotoxicosis E05.90 [*I43*]
  with thyroid storm E05.91 [*I43*]
 storm — *see* Thyrotoxicosis
Thyrotoxicosis (recurrent) E05.90
 with
  goiter (diffuse) E05.00
    with thyroid storm E05.01
    adenomatous uninodular E05.10
      with thyroid storm E05.11
    multinodular E05.20
      with thyroid storm E05.21
    nodular E05.20
      with thyroid storm E05.21
    uninodular E05.10
      with thyroid storm E05.11
  infiltrative
    dermopathy E05.00
      with thyroid storm E05.01
    ophthalmopathy E05.00
      with thyroid storm E05.01
  single thyroid nodule E05.10
    with thyroid storm E05.11
  thyroid storm E05.91
 due to
  ectopic thyroid nodule or tissue E05.30
    with thyroid storm E05.31
  ingestion of (excessive) thyroid material E05.40
    with thyroid storm E05.41
  overproduction of thyroid-stimulating hormone E05.80
    with thyroid storm E05.81
  specified cause NEC E05.80
    with thyroid storm E05.81
 factitia E05.40
  with thyroid storm E05.41
 heart — *see also* Failure, heart, high-output E05.90 [*I43*]
  with thyroid storm — *see also* Failure, heart, high-output E05.91 [*I43*]
  failure — *see also* Failure, heart, high-output E05.90 [*I43*]
 neonatal (transient) P72.1
 transient with chronic thyroiditis E06.2
Tibia vara — *see* Osteochondrosis, juvenile, tibia
Tic (disorder) F95.9
 breathing F95.8
 child problem F95.0
 compulsive F95.1
 de la Tourette F95.2
 degenerative (generalized) (localized) G25.69
  facial G25.69
 disorder
  chronic
    motor F95.1
    vocal F95.1
  combined vocal and multiple motor F95.2
  transient F95.0
 douloureux G50.0
  atypical G50.1
  postherpetic, postzoster B02.22
 drug-induced G25.61
 eyelid F95.8

Tic — *continued*
 habit F95.9
  chronic F95.1
  transient of childhood F95.0
 lid, transient of childhood F95.0
 motor-verbal F95.2
 occupational F48.8
 orbicularis F95.8
  transient of childhood F95.0
 organic origin G25.69
 postchoreic G25.69
 provisional F95.0
 psychogenic, compulsive F95.1
 salaam R25.8
 spasm (motor or vocal) F95.9
  chronic F95.1
  transient of childhood F95.0
 specified NEC F95.8
Tick-borne — *see* condition
Tietze's disease or syndrome M94.0
Tight, tightness
 anus K62.89
 chest R07.89
 fascia (lata) M62.89
 foreskin (congenital) N47.1
 hymen, hymenal ring N89.6
 introitus (acquired) (congenital) N89.6
 rectal sphincter K62.89
 tendon — *see* Short, tendon
 urethral sphincter N35.919
Tilting vertebra — *see* Dorsopathy, deforming, specified NEC
Timidity, child F93.8
Tinea (intersecta) (tarsi) B35.9
 amiantacea L44.8
 asbestina B35.0
 barbae B35.0
 beard B35.0
 black dot B35.0
 blanca B36.2
 capitis B35.0
 corporis B35.4
 cruris B35.6
 flava B36.0
 foot B35.3
 furfuracea B36.0
 imbricata (Tokelau) B35.5
 kerion B35.0
 manuum B35.2
 microsporic — *see* Dermatophytosis
 nigra B36.1
 nodosa — *see* Piedra
 pedis B35.3
 scalp B35.0
 specified NEC B35.8
 sycosis B35.0
 tonsurans B35.0
 trichophytic — *see* Dermatophytosis
 unguium B35.1
 versicolor B36.0
Tingling sensation (skin) R20.2
Tin-miner's lung J63.5
Tinnitus NOS H93.1- ☑
 audible H93.1- ☑
 aurium H93.1- ☑
 pulsatile H93.A- ☑
 subjective H93.1- ☑
Tipped tooth (teeth) M26.33
Tipping
 pelvis M95.5
  with disproportion (fetopelvic) O33.0
    causing obstructed labor O65.0
 tooth (teeth), fully erupted M26.33
Tiredness R53.83
Tissue — *see* condition
Tobacco (nicotine)
 abuse — *see* Tobacco, use
 dependence — *see* Dependence, drug, nicotine
 harmful use Z72.0
 heart — *see* Tobacco, toxic effect
 maternal use, affecting newborn P04.2
 toxic effect — *see* Table of Drugs and Chemicals, by substance, poisoning
  chewing tobacco — *see* Table of Drugs and Chemicals, by substance, poisoning
  cigarettes — *see* Table of Drugs and Chemicals, by substance, poisoning
 use Z72.0

☡ Subterms under main terms may continue to next column or page   ☑ Additional Character Required — Refer to the Tabular List for Character Selection   311

Thrombosis, thrombotic — Tobacco

Tobacco — *continued*
use — *continued*
complicating
childbirth O99.334
pregnancy O99.33- ☑
puerperium O99.335
counseling and surveillance Z71.6
history Z87.891
withdrawal state — *see also* Dependence, drug, nicotine F17.203
Tocopherol deficiency E56.0
Todd's
cirrhosis K74.3
paralysis (postepileptic) (transitory) G83.84
Toe — *see* condition
Toilet, artificial opening — *see* Attention to, artificial, opening
Tokelau (ringworm) B35.5
Tollwut — *see* Rabies
Tommaselli's disease R31.9
correct substance properly administered — *see* Table of Drugs and Chemicals, by drug, adverse effect
overdose or wrong substance given or taken — *see* Table of Drugs and Chemicals, by drug, poisoning
Tongue — *see also* condition
tie Q38.1
Tonic pupil — *see* Anomaly, pupil, function, tonic pupil
Toni-Fanconi syndrome (cystinosis) E72.09
with cystinosis E72.04
Tonsil — *see* condition
Tonsillitis (acute) (catarrhal) (croupous) (follicular) (gangrenous) (infective) (lacunar) (lingual) (malignant) (membranous) (parenchymatous) (phlegmonous) (pseudomembranous) (purulent) (septic) (subacute) (suppurative) (toxic) (ulcerative) (vesicular) (viral) J03.90
chronic J35.01
with adenoiditis J35.03
diphtheritic A36.0
hypertrophic J35.01
with adenoiditis J35.03
recurrent J03.91
specified organism NEC J03.80
recurrent J03.81
staphylococcal J03.80
recurrent J03.81
streptococcal J03.00
recurrent J03.01
tuberculous A15.8
Vincent's A69.1
Tooth, teeth — *see* condition
Toothache K08.89
Topagnosis R20.8
Tophi — *see* Gout, chronic
TORCH infection — *see* Infection, congenital
without active infection P00.2
Torn — *see* Tear
Tornwaldt's cyst or disease J39.2
Torsion
accessory tube — *see* Torsion, fallopian tube
adnexa (female) — *see* Torsion, fallopian tube
aorta, acquired I77.1
appendix epididymis N44.04
appendix testis N44.03
bile duct (common) (hepatic) K83.8
congenital Q44.5
bowel, colon or intestine K56.2
cervix — *see* Malposition, uterus
cystic duct K82.8
dystonia — *see* Dystonia, torsion
epididymis (appendix) N44.04
fallopian tube N83.52- ☑
with ovary N83.53
gallbladder K82.8
congenital Q44.1
hydatid of Morgagni
female N83.52- ☑
male N44.03
kidney (pedicle) (leading to infarction) N28.0
Meckel's diverticulum (congenital) Q43.0
malignant — *see* Table of Neoplasms, small intestine, malignant
mesentery K56.2
omentum K56.2
organ or site, congenital NEC — *see* Anomaly, by site
ovary (pedicle) N83.51- ☑
with fallopian tube N83.53
congenital Q50.2

Torsion — *continued*
oviduct — *see* Torsion, fallopian tube
penis (acquired) N48.82
congenital Q55.63
spasm — *see* Dystonia, torsion
spermatic cord N44.02
extravaginal N44.01
intravaginal N44.02
spleen D73.5
testis, testicle N44.00
appendix N44.03
tibia — *see* Deformity, limb, specified type NEC, lower leg
uterus — *see* Malposition, uterus
Torticollis (intermittent) (spastic) M43.6
congenital (sternomastoid) Q68.0
due to birth injury P15.8
hysterical F44.4
ocular R29.891
psychogenic F45.8
conversion reaction F44.4
rheumatic M43.6
rheumatoid M06.88
spasmodic G24.3
traumatic, current S13.4 ☑
Tortipelvis G24.1
Tortuous
aortic arch Q25.46
artery I77.1
organ or site, congenital NEC — *see* Distortion
retinal vessel, congenital Q14.1
ureter N13.8
urethra N36.8
vein — *see* Varix
Torture, victim of Z65.4
Torula, torular (histolytica) (infection) — *see* Cryptococcosis
Torulosis — *see* Cryptococcosis
Torus (mandibularis) (palatinus) M27.0
fracture — *see* Fracture, by site, torus
Touraine's syndrome Q79.8
Tourette's syndrome F95.2
Tourniquet syndrome — *see* Constriction, external, by site
Tower skull Q75.0
with exophthalmos Q87.0
Toxemia R68.89
bacterial — *see* Sepsis
burn — *see* Burn
eclamptic (with pre-existing hypertension) — *see* Eclampsia
erysipelatous — *see* Erysipelas
fatigue R68.89
food — *see* Poisoning, food
gastrointestinal K52.1
intestinal K52.1
kidney — *see* Uremia
malarial — *see* Malaria
myocardial — *see* Myocarditis, toxic
of pregnancy — *see* Pre-eclampsia
pre-eclamptic — *see* Pre-eclampsia
small intestine K52.1
staphylococcal, due to food A05.0
stasis R68.89
uremic — *see* Uremia
urinary — *see* Uremia
Toxemica cerebropathia psychica (nonalcoholic) F04
alcoholic — *see* Alcohol, amnestic disorder
Toxic (poisoning) — *see also* condition T65.91 ☑
effect — *see* Table of Drugs and Chemicals, by substance, poisoning
shock syndrome A48.3
thyroid (gland) — *see* Thyrotoxicosis
Toxicemia — *see* Toxemia
Toxicity — *see* Table of Drugs and Chemicals, by substance, poisoning
fava bean D55.0
food, noxious — *see* Poisoning, food
from drug or nonmedicinal substance — *see* Table of Drugs and Chemicals, by drug
Toxicosis — *see also* Toxemia
capillary, hemorrhagic D69.0
Toxinfection, gastrointestinal K52.1
Toxocariasis B83.0
Toxoplasma, toxoplasmosis (acquired) B58.9
with
hepatitis B58.1

Toxoplasma, toxoplasmosis — *continued*
with — *continued*
meningoencephalitis B58.2
ocular involvement B58.00
other organ involvement B58.89
pneumonia, pneumonitis B58.3
congenital (acute) (subacute) (chronic) P37.1
maternal, manifest toxoplasmosis in infant (acute) (subacute) (chronic) P37.1
tPA (rtPA) administration in a different facility within the last 24 hours prior to admission to current facility Z92.82
Trabeculation, bladder N32.89
Trachea — *see* condition
Tracheitis (catarrhal) (infantile) (membranous) (plastic) (septal) (suppurative) (viral) J04.10
with
bronchitis (15 years of age and above) J40
acute or subacute — *see* Bronchitis, acute
chronic J42
tuberculous NEC A15.5
under 15 years of age J20.9
laryngitis (acute) J04.2
chronic J37.1
tuberculous NEC A15.5
acute J04.10
with obstruction J04.11
chronic J42
with
bronchitis (chronic) J42
laryngitis (chronic) J37.1
diphtheritic (membranous) A36.89
due to external agent — *see* Inflammation, respiratory, upper, due to
syphilitic A52.73
tuberculous A15.5
Trachelitis (nonvenereal) — *see* Cervicitis
Tracheobronchial — *see* condition
Tracheobronchitis (15 years of age and above) — *see also* Bronchitis
due to
Bordetella bronchiseptica A37.80
with pneumonia A37.81
Francisella tularensis A21.8
Tracheobronchomegaly Q32.4
with bronchiectasis J47.9
with
exacerbation (acute) J47.1
lower respiratory infection J47.0
acquired J98.09
with bronchiectasis J47.9
with
exacerbation (acute) J47.1
lower respiratory infection J47.0
Tracheobronchopneumonitis — *see* Pneumonia, broncho-
Tracheocele (external) (internal) J39.8
congenital Q32.1
Tracheomalacia J39.8
congenital Q32.0
Tracheopharyngitis (acute) J06.9
chronic J42
due to external agent — *see* Inflammation, respiratory, upper, due to
Tracheostenosis J39.8
Tracheostomy
complication — *see* Complication, tracheostomy
status Z93.0
attention to Z43.0
malfunctioning J95.03
Trachoma, trachomatous A71.9
active (stage) A71.1
contraction of conjunctiva A71.1
dubium A71.0
healed or sequelae B94.0
initial (stage) A71.0
pannus A71.1
Türck's J37.0
Traction, vitreomacular H43.82- ☑
Train sickness T75.3 ☑
Trait(s)
Hb-S D57.3
hemoglobin
abnormal NEC D58.2
with thalassemia D56.3
C — *see* Disease, hemoglobin C
S (Hb-S) D57.3
Lepore D56.3

☑ **Additional Character Required** — Refer to the Tabular List for Character Selection
▽ **Subterms under main terms may continue to next column or page**

rait(s) — *continued*
  personality, accentuated Z73.1
  sickle-cell D57.3
    with elliptocytosis or spherocytosis D57.3
  type A personality Z73.1
ramp Z59.0
rance R41.89
  hysterical F44.89
ransaminasemia R74.0
ransection
  abdomen (partial) S38.3 ☑
  aorta (incomplete) — *see also* Injury, aorta
    complete — *see* Injury, aorta, laceration, major
  carotid artery (incomplete) — *see also* Injury, blood
    vessel, carotid, laceration
    complete — *see* Injury, blood vessel, carotid, lacer-
      ation, major
  celiac artery (incomplete) S35.211 ☑
    branch (incomplete) S35.291 ☑
      complete S35.292 ☑
    complete S35.212 ☑
  innominate
    artery (incomplete) — *see also* Injury, blood vessel,
      thoracic, innominate, artery, laceration
      complete — *see* Injury, blood vessel, thoracic,
        innominate, artery, laceration, major
    vein (incomplete) — *see also* Injury, blood vessel,
      thoracic, innominate, vein, laceration
      complete — *see* Injury, blood vessel, thoracic,
        innominate, vein, laceration, major
  jugular vein (external) (incomplete) — *see also* Injury,
    blood vessel, jugular vein, laceration
    complete — *see* Injury, blood vessel, jugular vein,
      laceration, major
    internal (incomplete) — *see also* Injury, blood vessel,
      jugular vein, internal, laceration
      complete — *see* Injury, blood vessel, jugular vein,
        internal, laceration, major
  mesenteric artery (incomplete) — *see also* Injury,
    mesenteric, artery, laceration
    complete — *see* Injury, mesenteric artery, laceration,
      major
  pulmonary vessel (incomplete) — *see also* Injury, blood
    vessel, thoracic, pulmonary, laceration
    complete — *see* Injury, blood vessel, thoracic, pul-
      monary, laceration, major
  subclavian — *see* Transection, innominate
  vena cava (incomplete) — *see also* Injury, vena cava
    complete — *see* Injury, vena cava, laceration, major
  vertebral artery (incomplete) — *see also* Injury, blood
    vessel, vertebral, laceration
    complete — *see* Injury, blood vessel, vertebral, lac-
      eration, major
ransfusion
  associated (red blood cell) hemochromatosis E83.111
  blood
    ABO incompatible — *see* Complication(s), transfu-
      sion, incompatibility reaction, ABO
    minor blood group (Duffy) (E) (K) (Kell) (Kidd) (Lewis)
      (M) (N) (P) (S) T80.89 ☑
    reaction or complication — *see* Complications,
      transfusion
  fetomaternal (mother) — *see* Pregnancy, complicated
    by, placenta, transfusion syndrome
  maternofetal (mother) — *see* Pregnancy, complicated
    by, placenta, transfusion syndrome
  placental (syndrome) (mother) — *see* Pregnancy,
    complicated by, placenta, transfusion syndrome
  reaction (adverse) — *see* Complications, transfusion
  related acute lung injury (TRALI) J95.84
  twin-to-twin — *see* Pregnancy, complicated by, placen-
    ta, transfusion syndrome, fetus to fetus
Transient (meaning homeless) — *see also* condition Z59.0
Translocation
  balanced autosomal Q95.9
    in normal individual Q95.0
  chromosomes NEC Q99.8
    balanced and insertion in normal individual Q95.0
  Down syndrome Q90.2
  trisomy
    13 Q91.6
    18 Q91.2
    21 Q90.2
Translucency, iris — *see Degeneration, iris*
Transmission of chemical substances through the
  placenta — *see* Absorption, chemical, through
  placenta

Transparency, lung, unilateral J43.0
Transplant (ed) (status) Z94.9
  awaiting organ Z76.82
  bone Z94.6
    marrow Z94.81
  candidate Z76.82
  complication — *see* Complication, transplant
  cornea Z94.7
  heart Z94.1
    and lung(s) Z94.3
    valve Z95.2
      prosthetic Z95.2
      specified NEC Z95.4
      xenogenic Z95.3
  intestine Z94.82
  kidney Z94.0
  liver Z94.4
  lung(s) Z94.2
    and heart Z94.3
  organ (failure) (infection) (rejection) Z94.9
    removal status Z98.85
  pancreas Z94.83
  skin Z94.5
  social Z60.3
  specified organ or tissue NEC Z94.89
  stem cells Z94.84
  tissue Z94.9
Transplants, ovarian, endometrial N80.1
Transposed — *see* Transposition
Transposition (congenital) — *see also* Malposition,
  congenital
  abdominal viscera Q89.3
  aorta (dextra) Q20.3
  appendix Q43.8
  colon Q43.8
  corrected Q20.5
  great vessels (complete) (partial) Q20.3
  heart Q24.0
    with complete transposition of viscera Q89.3
  intestine (large) (small) Q43.8
  reversed jejunal (for bypass) (status) Z98.0
  scrotum Q55.23
  stomach Q40.2
    with general transposition of viscera Q89.3
  tooth, teeth, fully erupted M26.30
  vessels, great (complete) (partial) Q20.3
  viscera (abdominal) (thoracic) Q89.3
Transsexualism F64.0
Transverse — *see also* condition
  arrest (deep), in labor O64.0 ☑
  lie (mother) O32.2 ☑
    causing obstructed labor O64.8 ☑
Transvestism, transvestitism (dual-role) F64.1
  fetishistic F65.1
Trapped placenta (with hemorrhage) O72.0
  without hemorrhage O73.0
TRAPS (tumor necrosis factor receptor associated periodic
  syndrome) M04.1
Trauma, traumatism — *see also* Injury
  acoustic — *see* subcategory H83.3 ☑
  birth — *see* Birth, injury
  complicating ectopic or molar pregnancy O08.6
  during delivery O71.9
  following ectopic or molar pregnancy O08.6
  obstetric O71.9
    specified NEC O71.89
  occusal
    primary K08.81
    secondary K08.82
Traumatic — *see also* condition
  brain injury S06.9 ☑
Treacher Collins syndrome Q75.4
Treitz's hernia — *see* Hernia, abdomen, specified site
  NEC
Trematode infestation — *see* Infestation, fluke
Trematodiasis — *see* Infestation, fluke
Trembling paralysis — *see* Parkinsonism
Tremor(s) R25.1
  drug induced G25.1
  essential (benign) G25.0
  familial G25.0
  hereditary G25.0
  hysterical F44.4
  intention G25.2
  medication induced postural G25.1
  mercurial — *see* subcategory T56.1 ☑
  Parkinson's — *see* Parkinsonism
  psychogenic (conversion reaction) F44.4

Tremor(s) — *continued*
  senilis R54
  specified type NEC G25.2
Trench
  fever A79.0
  foot — *see* Immersion, foot
  mouth A69.1
Treponema pallidum infection — *see* Syphilis
Treponematosis
  due to
    T. pallidum — *see* Syphilis
    T. pertenue — *see* Yaws
Triad
  Hutchinson's (congenital syphilis) A50.53
  Kartagener's Q89.3
  Saint's — *see* Hernia, diaphragm
Trichiasis (eyelid) H02.059
  with entropion — *see* Entropion
  left H02.056
    lower H02.055
    upper H02.054
  right H02.053
    lower H02.052
    upper H02.051
Trichinella spiralis (infection) (infestation) B75
Trichinellosis, trichiniasis, trichinelliasis, trichinosis
  B75
  with muscle disorder B75 *[M63.80]*
    ankle B75 *[M63.87-]* ☑
    foot B75 *[M63.87-]* ☑
    forearm B75 *[M63.83-]* ☑
    hand B75 *[M63.84-]* ☑
    lower leg B75 *[M63.86-]* ☑
    multiple sites B75 *[M63.89]*
    pelvic region B75 *[M63.85-]* ☑
    shoulder region B75 *[M63.81-]* ☑
    specified site NEC B75 *[M63.88]*
    thigh B75 *[M63.85-]* ☑
    upper arm B75 *[M63.82-]* ☑
Trichobezoar T18.9 ☑
  intestine T18.3 ☑
  stomach T18.2 ☑
Trichocephaliasis, trichocephalosis B79
Trichocephalus infestation B79
Trichoclasis L67.8
Trichoepithelioma — *see also* Neoplasm, skin, benign
  malignant — *see* Neoplasm, skin, malignant
Trichofolliculoma — *see* Neoplasm, skin, benign
Tricholemmoma — *see* Neoplasm, skin, benign
Trichomoniasis A59.9
  bladder A59.03
  cervix A59.09
  intestinal A07.8
  prostate A59.02
  seminal vesicles A59.09
  specified site NEC A59.8
  urethra A59.03
  urogenitalis A59.00
  vagina A59.01
  vulva A59.01
Trichomycosis
  axillaris A48.8
  nodosa, nodularis B36.8
Trichonodosis L67.8
Trichophytid, trichophyton infection — *see* Dermato-
  phytosis
Trichophytobezoar T18.9 ☑
  intestine T18.3 ☑
  stomach T18.2 ☑
Trichophytosis — *see* Dermatophytosis
Trichoptilosis L67.8
Trichorrhexis (nodosa) (invaginata) L67.0
Trichosis axillaris A48.8
Trichosporosis nodosa B36.2
Trichostasis spinulosa (congenital) Q84.1
Trichostrongyliasis, trichostrongylosis (small intes-
  tine) B81.2
Trichostrongylus infection B81.2
Trichotillomania F63.3
Trichromat, trichromatopsia, anomalous (congenital)
  H53.55
Trichuriasis B79
Trichuris trichiura (infection) (infestation) (any site) B79
Tricuspid (valve) — *see* condition
Trifid — *see also* Accessory
  kidney (pelvis) Q63.8
  tongue Q38.3

Tuberculosis, tubercular, tuberculous — *continued*
cul-de-sac of Douglas A18.17
curvature, spine A18.01
cutis (colliquativa) (primary) A18.4
cyst, ovary A18.18
cystitis A18.12
dactylitis A18.03
diarrhea A18.32
diffuse — *see* Tuberculosis, miliary
digestive tract A18.32
disseminated — *see* Tuberculosis, miliary
duodenum A18.32
dura (mater) (cerebral) (spinal) A17.0
   abscess (cerebral) (spinal) A17.81
dysentery A18.32
ear (inner) (middle) A18.6
   bone A18.03
   external (primary) A18.4
   skin (primary) A18.4
elbow A18.02
emphysema — *see* Tuberculosis, pulmonary
empyema A15.6
encephalitis A17.82
endarteritis A18.89
endocarditis A18.84
   aortic A18.84
   mitral A18.84
   pulmonary A18.84
   tricuspid A18.84
endocrine glands NEC A18.82
endometrium A18.17
enteric, enterica, enteritis A18.32
enterocolitis A18.32
epididymis, epididymitis A18.15
epidural abscess (cerebral) (spinal) A17.81
epiglottis A15.5
episcleritis A18.51
erythema (induratum) (nodosum) (primary) A18.4
esophagus A18.83
eustachian tube A18.6
exposure (to) Z20.1
exudative — *see* Tuberculosis, pulmonary
eye A18.50
eyelid (primary) (lupus) A18.4
fallopian tube (acute) (chronic) A18.17
fascia A18.09
fauces A15.8
female pelvic inflammatory disease A18.17
finger A18.03
first infection A15.7
gallbladder A18.83
ganglion A18.09
gastritis A18.83
gastrocolic fistula A18.32
gastroenteritis A18.32
gastrointestinal tract A18.32
general, generalized — *see* Tuberculosis, miliary
genital organs A18.10
genitourinary A18.10
genu A18.02
glandula suprarenalis A18.7
glandular, general A18.2
glottis A15.5
grinder's J65
gum A18.83
hand A18.03
heart A18.84
hematogenous — *see* Tuberculosis, miliary
hemoptysis — *see* Tuberculosis, pulmonary
hemorrhage NEC — *see* Tuberculosis, pulmonary
hemothorax A15.6
hepatitis A18.83
hilar lymph nodes A15.4
   primary (progressive) A15.7
hip (joint) (disease) (bone) A18.02
hydropneumothorax A15.6
hydrothorax A15.6
hypoadrenalism A18.7
hypopharynx A15.8
ileocecal (hyperplastic) A18.32
ileocolitis A18.32
ileum A18.32
iliac spine (superior) A18.03
immunological findings only A15.7
indurativa (primary) A18.4
infantile A15.7
infection A15.9
   without clinical manifestations A15.7

Tuberculosis, tubercular, tuberculous — *continued*
infraclavicular gland A18.2
inguinal gland A18.2
inguinalis A18.2
intestine (any part) A18.32
iridocyclitis A18.54
iris, iritis A18.54
ischiorectal A18.32
jaw A18.03
jejunum A18.32
joint A18.02
   vertebral A18.01
keratitis (interstitial) A18.52
keratoconjunctivitis A18.52
kidney A18.11
knee (joint) A18.02
kyphosis, kyphoscoliosis A18.01
laryngitis A15.5
larynx A15.5
latent Z22.7
leptomeninges, leptomeningitis (cerebral) (spinal) A17.0
lichenoides (primary) A18.4
linguae A18.83
lip A18.83
liver A18.83
lordosis A18.01
lung — *see* Tuberculosis, pulmonary
lupus vulgaris A18.4
lymph gland or node (peripheral) A18.2
   abdomen A18.39
   bronchial A15.4
      primary (progressive) A15.7
   cervical A18.2
   hilar A15.4
      primary (progressive) A15.7
   intrathoracic A15.4
      primary (progressive) A15.7
   mediastinal A15.4
      primary (progressive) A15.7
   mesenteric A18.39
   retroperitoneal A18.39
   tracheobronchial A15.4
      primary (progressive) A15.7
lymphadenitis — *see* Tuberculosis, lymph gland
lymphangitis — *see* Tuberculosis, lymph gland
lymphatic (gland) (vessel) — *see* Tuberculosis, lymph gland
mammary gland A18.89
marasmus A15.9
mastoiditis A18.03
mediastinal lymph gland or node A15.4
   primary (progressive) A15.7
mediastinitis A15.8
   primary (progressive) A15.7
mediastinum A15.8
   primary (progressive) A15.7
medulla A17.81
melanosis, Addisonian A18.7
meninges, meningitis (basilar) (cerebral) (cerebrospinal) (spinal) A17.0
meningoencephalitis A17.82
mesentery, mesenteric (gland or node) A18.39
miliary A19.9
   acute A19.2
      multiple sites A19.1
      single specified site A19.0
   chronic A19.8
   specified NEC A19.8
millstone makers' J65
miner's J65
molder's J65
mouth A18.83
multiple A19.9
   acute A19.1
   chronic A19.8
muscle A18.09
myelitis A17.82
myocardium, myocarditis A18.84
nasal (passage) (sinus) A15.8
nasopharynx A15.8
neck gland A18.2
nephritis A18.11
nerve (mononeuropathy) A17.83
nervous system A17.9
nose (septum) A15.8
ocular A18.50
omentum A18.31
oophoritis (acute) (chronic) A18.17

Tuberculosis, tubercular, tuberculous — *continued*
optic (nerve trunk) (papilla) A18.59
orbit A18.59
orchitis A18.15
organ, specified NEC A18.89
osseous — *see* Tuberculosis, bone
osteitis — *see* Tuberculosis, bone
osteomyelitis — *see* Tuberculosis, bone
otitis media A18.6
ovary, ovaritis (acute) (chronic) A18.17
oviduct (acute) (chronic) A18.17
pachymeningitis A17.0
palate (soft) A18.83
pancreas A18.83
papulonecrotic (a) (primary) A18.4
parathyroid glands A18.82
paronychia (primary) A18.4
parotid gland or region A18.83
pelvis (bony) A18.03
penis A18.15
peribronchitis A15.5
pericardium, pericarditis A18.84
perichondritis, larynx A15.5
periostitis — *see* Tuberculosis, bone
perirectal fistula A18.32
peritoneum NEC A18.31
peritonitis A18.31
pharynx, pharyngitis A15.8
phlyctenulosis (keratoconjunctivitis) A18.52
phthisis NEC — *see* Tuberculosis, pulmonary
pituitary gland A18.82
pleura, pleural, pleurisy, pleuritis (fibrinous) (obliterative) (purulent) (simple plastic) (with effusion) A15.6
   primary (progressive) A15.7
pneumonia, pneumonic — *see* Tuberculosis, pulmonary
pneumothorax (spontaneous) (tense valvular) — *see* Tuberculosis, pulmonary
polyneuropathy A17.89
polyserositis A19.9
   acute A19.1
   chronic A19.8
potter's J65
prepuce A18.15
primary (complex) A15.7
proctitis A18.32
prostate, prostatitis A18.14
pulmonalis — *see* Tuberculosis, pulmonary
pulmonary (cavitated) (fibrotic) (infiltrative) (nodular) A15.0
   childhood type or first infection A15.7
   primary (complex) A15.7
pyelitis A18.11
pyelonephritis A18.11
pyemia — *see* Tuberculosis, miliary
pyonephrosis A18.11
pyopneumothorax A15.6
pyothorax A15.6
rectum (fistula) (with abscess) A18.32
reinfection stage — *see* Tuberculosis, pulmonary
renal A18.11
renis A18.11
respiratory A15.9
   primary A15.7
   specified site NEC A15.8
retina, retinitis A18.53
retroperitoneal (lymph gland or node) A18.39
rheumatism NEC A18.09
rhinitis A15.8
sacroiliac (joint) A18.01
sacrum A18.01
salivary gland A18.83
salpingitis (acute) (chronic) A18.17
sandblaster's J65
sclera A18.51
scoliosis A18.01
scrofulous A18.2
scrotum A18.15
seminal tract or vesicle A18.15
senile A15.9
septic — *see* Tuberculosis, miliary
shoulder (joint) A18.02
   blade A18.03
sigmoid A18.32
sinus (any nasal) A15.8
   bone A18.03
   epididymis A18.15

Tuberculosis, tubercular, tuberculous — *continued*
skeletal NEC A18.03
skin (any site) (primary) A18.4
small intestine A18.32
soft palate A18.83
spermatic cord A18.15
spine, spinal (column) A18.01
   cord A17.81
   medulla A17.81
   membrane A17.0
   meninges A17.0
spleen, splenitis A18.85
spondylitis A18.01
sternoclavicular joint A18.02
stomach A18.83
stonemason's J65
subcutaneous tissue (cellular) (primary) A18.4
subcutis (primary) A18.4
subdeltoid bursa A18.83
submaxillary (region) A18.83
supraclavicular gland A18.2
suprarenal (capsule) (gland) A18.7
swelling, joint (*see also* category M01) — *see also* Tuberculosis, joint A18.02
symphysis pubis A18.02
synovitis A18.09
   articular A18.02
   spine or vertebra A18.01
systemic — *see* Tuberculosis, miliary
tarsitis A18.4
tendon (sheath) — *see* Tuberculosis, tenosynovitis
tenosynovitis A18.09
   spine or vertebra A18.01
testis A18.15
throat A15.8
thymus gland A18.82
thyroid gland A18.81
tongue A18.83
tonsil, tonsillitis A15.8
trachea, tracheal A15.5
   lymph gland or node A15.4
      primary (progressive) A15.7
tracheobronchial A15.5
   lymph gland or node A15.4
      primary (progressive) A15.7
tubal (acute) (chronic) A18.17
tunica vaginalis A18.15
ulcer (skin) (primary) A18.4
   bowel or intestine A18.32
   specified NEC — *see* Tuberculosis, by site
unspecified site A15.9
ureter A18.11
urethra, urethral (gland) A18.13
urinary organ or tract A18.13
uterus A18.17
uveal tract A18.54
uvula A18.83
vagina A18.18
vas deferens A18.15
verruca, verrucosa (cutis) (primary) A18.4
vertebra (column) A18.01
vesiculitis A18.15
vulva A18.18
wrist (joint) A18.02
Tuberculum
Carabelli — *see* Excludes Note at K00.2
occlusal — *see* Excludes Note at K00.2
paramolare K00.2
Tuberosity, enitre maxillary M26.07
Tuberous sclerosis (brain) Q85.1
Tubo-ovarian — *see* condition
Tuboplasty, after previous sterilization Z31.0
aftercare Z31.42
Tubotympanitis, catarrhal (chronic) — *see* Otitis, media,
   nonsuppurative, chronic, serous
Tularemia A21.9
with
   conjunctivitis A21.1
   pneumonia A21.2
abdominal A21.3
bronchopneumonic A21.2
conjunctivitis A21.1
cryptogenic A21.3
enteric A21.3
gastrointestinal A21.3
generalized A21.7
ingestion A21.3
intestinal A21.3

Tularemia — *continued*
oculoglandular A21.1
ophthalmic A21.1
pneumonia (any), pneumonic A21.2
pulmonary A21.2
sepsis A21.7
specified NEC A21.8
typhoidal A21.7
ulceroglandular A21.0
Tularensis conjunctivitis A21.1
Tumefaction — *see also* Swelling
liver — *see* Hypertrophy, liver
Tumor — *see also* Neoplasm, unspecified behavior, by
   site
acinar cell — *see* Neoplasm, uncertain behavior, by site
acinic cell — *see* Neoplasm, uncertain behavior, by site
adenocarcinoid — *see* Neoplasm, malignant, by site
adenomatoid — *see also* Neoplasm, benign, by site
   odontogenic — *see* Cyst, calcifying odontogenic
adnexal (skin) — *see* Neoplasm, skin, benign, by site
adrenal
   cortical (benign) D35.0- ☑
      malignant C74.0- ☑
   rest — *see* Neoplasm, benign, by site
alpha-cell
   malignant
      pancreas C25.4
      specified site NEC — *see* Neoplasm, malignant,
         by site
      unspecified site C25.4
   pancreas D13.7
   specified site NEC — *see* Neoplasm, benign, by site
   unspecified site D13.7
aneurysmal — *see* Aneurysm
aortic body D44.7
   malignant C75.5
Askin's — *see* Neoplasm, connective tissue, malignant
basal cell — *see also* Neoplasm, skin, uncertain behavior D48.5
Bednar — *see* Neoplasm, skin, malignant
benign (unclassified) — *see* Neoplasm, benign, by site
beta-cell
   malignant
      pancreas C25.4
      specified site NEC — *see* Neoplasm, malignant,
         by site
      unspecified site C25.4
   pancreas D13.7
   specified site NEC — *see* Neoplasm, benign, by site
   unspecified site D13.7
Brenner D27.9
   borderline malignancy D39.1- ☑
   malignant C56- ☑
   proliferating D39.1- ☑
bronchial alveolar, intravascular D38.1
Brooke's — *see* Neoplasm, skin, benign
brown fat — *see* Lipoma
Burkitt — *see* Lymphoma, Burkitt
calcifying epithelial odontogenic — *see* Cyst, calcifying
   odontogenic
carcinoid D3A.00 (*following* D36)
   benign D3A.00 (*following* D36)
      appendix D3A.020 (*following* D36)
      ascending colon D3A.022 (*following* D36)
      bronchus (lung) D3A.090 (*following* D36)
      cecum D3A.021 (*following* D36)
      colon D3A.029 (*following* D36)
      descending colon D3A.024 (*following* D36)
      duodenum D3A.010 (*following* D36)
      foregut NOS D3A.094 (*following* D36)
      hindgut NOS D3A.096 (*following* D36)
      ileum D3A.012 (*following* D36)
      jejunum D3A.011 (*following* D36)
      kidney D3A.093 (*following* D36)
      large intestine D3A.029 (*following* D36)
      lung (bronchus) D3A.090 (*following* D36)
      midgut NOS D3A.095 (*following* D36)
      rectum D3A.026 (*following* D36)
      sigmoid colon D3A.025 (*following* D36)
      small intestine D3A.019 (*following* D36)
      specified NEC D3A.098 (*following* D36)
      stomach D3A.092 (*following* D36)
      thymus D3A.091 (*following* D36)
      transverse colon D3A.023 (*following* D36)
   malignant C7A.00 (*following* C75)
      appendix C7A.020 (*following* C75)
      ascending colon C7A.022 (*following* C75)
      bronchus (lung) C7A.090 (*following* C75)

Tumor — *continued*
carcinoid — *continued*
   malignant — *continued*
      cecum C7A.021 (*following* C75)
      colon C7A.029 (*following* C75)
      descending colon C7A.024 (*following* C75)
      duodenum C7A.010 (*following* C75)
      foregut NOS C7A.094 (*following* C75)
      hindgut NOS C7A.096 (*following* C75)
      ileum C7A.012 (*following* C75)
      jejunum C7A.011 (*following* C75)
      kidney C7A.093 (*following* C75)
      large intestine C7A.029 (*following* C75)
      lung (bronchus) C7A.090 (*following* C75)
      midgut NOS C7A.095 (*following* C75)
      rectum C7A.026 (*following* C75)
      sigmoid colon C7A.025 (*following* C75)
      small intestine C7A.019 (*following* C75)
      specified NEC C7A.098 (*following* C75)
      stomach C7A.092 (*following* C75)
      thymus C7A.091 (*following* C75)
      transverse colon C7A.023 (*following* C75)
      mesentary metastasis C7B.04 (*following* C75)
      secondary C7B.00 (*following* C75)
         bone C7B.03 (*following* C75)
         distant lymph nodes C7B.01 (*following* C75)
         liver C7B.02 (*following* C75)
         peritoneum C7B.04 (*following* C75)
         specified NEC C7B.09 (*following* C75)
carotid body D44.6
   malignant C75.4
cells — *see also* Neoplasm, unspecified behavior, by
   site
   benign — *see* Neoplasm, benign, by site
   malignant — *see* Neoplasm, malignant, by site
   uncertain whether benign or malignant — *see*
      Neoplasm, uncertain behavior, by site
cervix, in pregnancy or childbirth — *see* Pregnancy,
   complicated by, tumor, cervix
chondromatous giant cell — *see* Neoplasm, bone, b
   nign
chromaffin — *see also* Neoplasm, benign, by site
   malignant — *see* Neoplasm, malignant, by site
Cock's peculiar L72.3
Codman's — *see* Neoplasm, bone, benign
dentigerous, mixed — *see* Cyst, calcifying odontogen
dermoid — *see* Neoplasm, benign, by site
   with malignant transformation C56- ☑
desmoid (extra-abdominal) — *see also* Neoplasm,
   connective tissue, uncertain behavior
   abdominal — *see* Neoplasm, connective tissue, ur
      certain behavior
embolus — *see* Neoplasm, secondary, by site
embryonal (mixed) — *see also* Neoplasm, uncertain
   behavior, by site
   liver C22.7
endodermal sinus
   specified site — *see* Neoplasm, malignant, by site
   unspecified site
      female C56.- ☑
      male C62.90
epithelial
   benign — *see* Neoplasm, benign, by site
   malignant — *see* Neoplasm, malignant, by site
Ewing's — *see* Neoplasm, bone, malignant, by site
fatty — *see* Lipoma
fibroid — *see* Leiomyoma
G cell
   malignant
      pancreas C25.4
      specified site NEC — *see* Neoplasm, malignant
         by site
      unspecified site C25.4
   specified site — *see* Neoplasm, uncertain behavio
      by site
   unspecified site D37.8
germ cell — *see also* Neoplasm, malignant, by site
   mixed — *see* Neoplasm, malignant, by site
ghost cell, odontogenic — *see* Cyst, calcifying odonto
   genic
giant cell — *see also* Neoplasm, uncertain behavior,
   by site
   bone D48.0
      malignant — *see* Neoplasm, bone, malignant
   chondromatous — *see* Neoplasm, bone, benign
   malignant — *see* Neoplasm, malignant, by site
   soft parts — *see* Neoplasm, connective tissue, un
      certain behavior

☑ **Additional Character Required** — Refer to the Tabular List for Character Selection   ▽ **Subterms under main terms may continue to next column or page**

Tumor — continued
- turban D23.4
- uterus (body), in pregnancy or childbirth — see Pregnancy, complicated by, tumor, uterus
- vagina, in pregnancy or childbirth — see Pregnancy, complicated by
- varicose — see Varix
- von Recklinghausen's — see Neurofibromatosis
- vulva or perineum, in pregnancy or childbirth — see Pregnancy, complicated by
  - causing obstructed labor O65.5
- Warthin's — see Neoplasm, salivary gland, benign
- Wilms' C64- ☑
- yolk sac — see Neoplasm, malignant, by site
  - specified site — see Neoplasm, malignant, by site
  - unspecified site
    - female C56.9
    - male C62.90

Tumor lysis syndrome (following antineoplastic chemotherapy) (spontaneous) NEC E88.3

Tumorlet — see Neoplasm, uncertain behavior, by site

Tungiasis B88.1

Tunica vasculosa lentis Q12.2

Turban tumor D23.4

Türck's trachoma J37.0

Turner-Kieser syndrome Q87.2

Turner-like syndrome Q87.19

Turner's
- hypoplasia (tooth) K00.4
- syndrome Q96.9
  - specified NEC Q96.8
- tooth K00.4

Turner-Ullrich syndrome Q96.9

Tussis convulsiva — see Whooping cough

Twiddler's syndrome (due to)
- automatic implantable defibrillator T82.198
- cardiac pacemaker T82.198 ☑

Twilight state
- epileptic F05
- psychogenic F44.89

Twin (newborn) — see also Newborn, twin
- conjoined Q89.4
- pregnancy — see Pregnancy, twin

Twinning, teeth K00.2

Twist, twisted
- bowel, colon or intestine K56.2
- hair (congenital) Q84.1
- mesentery K56.2
- omentum K56.2
- organ or site, congenital NEC — see Anomaly, by site
- ovarian pedicle — see Torsion, ovary

Twitching R25.3

Tylosis (acquired) L84
- buccalis K13.29
- linguae K13.29
- palmaris et plantaris (congenital) (inherited) Q82.8
  - acquired L85.1

Tympanism R14.0

Tympanites (abdominal) (intestinal) R14.0

Tympanitis — see Myringitis

Tympanosclerosis H74.0 ☑

Tympanum — see condition

Tympany
- abdomen R14.0
- chest R09.89

Type A behavior pattern Z73.1

Typhlitis — see Appendicitis

Typhoenteritis — see Typhoid

Typhoid (abortive) (ambulant) (any site) (clinical) (fever) (hemorrhagic) (infection) (intermittent) (malignant) (rheumatic) (Widal negative) A01.00
- with pneumonia A01.03
- abdominal A01.09
- arthritis A01.04
- carrier (suspected) of Z22.0
- cholecystitis (current) A01.09
- endocarditis A01.02
- heart involvement A01.02
- inoculation reaction — see Complications, vaccination
- meningitis A01.01
- mesenteric lymph nodes A01.09
- myocarditis A01.02
- osteomyelitis A01.05
- perichondritis, larynx A01.09
- pneumonia A01.03
- specified NEC A01.09
- spine A01.05

Typhoid — continued
- ulcer (perforating) A01.09

Typhomalaria (fever) — see Malaria

Typhomania A01.00

Typhoperitonitis A01.09

Typhus (fever) A75.9
- abdominal, abdominalis — see Typhoid
- African tick A77.1
- amarillic A95.9
- brain A75.9 [G94]
- cerebral A75.9 [G94]
- classical A75.0
- due to Rickettsia
  - prowazekii A75.0
    - recrudescent A75.1
  - tsutsugamushi A75.3
  - typhi A75.2
- endemic (flea-borne) A75.2
- epidemic (louse-borne) A75.0
- exanthematicus SAI A75.0
  - brillii SAI A75.1
  - mexicanus SAI A75.2
  - typhus murinus A75.2
- exanthematic NEC A75.0
- flea-borne A75.2
- India tick A77.1
- Kenya (tick) A77.1
- louse-borne A75.0
- Mexican A75.2
- mite-borne A75.3
- murine A75.2
- North Asian tick-borne A77.2
- petechial A75.9
- Queensland tick A77.3
- rat A75.2
- recrudescent A75.1
- recurrens — see Fever, relapsing
- Sao Paulo A77.0
- scrub (China) (India) (Malaysia) (New Guinea) A75.3
- shop (of Malaysia) A75.2
- Siberian tick A77.2
- tick-borne A77.9
- tropical (mite-borne) A75.3

Tyrosinemia E70.21
- newborn, transitory P74.5

Tyrosinosis E70.21

Tyrosinuria E70.29

U

Uhl's anomaly or disease Q24.8

Ulcer, ulcerated, ulcerating, ulceration, ulcerative
- alveolar process M27.3
- amebic (intestine) A06.1
  - skin A06.7
- anastomotic — see Ulcer, gastrojejunal
- anorectal K62.6
- antral — see Ulcer, stomach
- anus (sphincter) (solitary) K62.6
- aorta — see Aneurysm
- aphthous (oral) (recurrent) K12.0
  - genital organ(s)
    - female N76.6
    - male N50.89
- artery I77.2
- atrophic — see Ulcer, skin
  - decubitus — see Ulcer, pressure, by site
- back L98.429
  - with
    - bone involvement without evidence of necrosis L98.426
    - bone necrosis L98.424
    - exposed fat layer L98.422
    - muscle involvement without evidence of necrosis L98.425
    - muscle necrosis L98.423
    - skin breakdown only L98.421
    - specified severity NEC L98.428
- Barrett's (esophagus) K22.10
  - with bleeding K22.11
- bile duct (common) (hepatic) K83.8
- bladder (solitary) (sphincter) NEC N32.89
  - bilharzial B65.9 [N33]
  - in schistosomiasis (bilharzial) B65.9 [N33]
  - submucosal — see Cystitis, interstitial
  - tuberculous A18.12
- bleeding K27.4
- bone — see Osteomyelitis, specified type NEC

Ulcer, ulcerated, ulcerating, ulceration, ulcerative — continued
- bowel — see Ulcer, intestine
- breast N61.1
- bronchus J98.09
- buccal (cavity) (traumatic) K12.1
- Buruli A31.1
- buttock L98.419
  - with
    - bone involvement without evidence of necrosis L98.416
    - bone necrosis L98.414
    - exposed fat layer L98.412
    - muscle involvement without evidence of necrosis L98.415
    - muscle necrosis L98.413
    - skin breakdown only L98.411
    - specified severity NEC L98.418
- cancerous — see Neoplasm, malignant, by site
- cardia K22.10
  - with bleeding K22.11
- cardioesophageal (peptic) K22.10
  - with bleeding K22.11
- cecum — see Ulcer, intestine
- cervix (uteri) (decubitus) (trophic) N86
  - with cervicitis N72
- chancroidal A57
- chiclero B55.1
- chronic (cause unknown) — see Ulcer, skin
- Cochin-China B55.1
- colon — see Ulcer, intestine
- conjunctiva H10.89
- cornea H16.00- ☑
  - with hypopyon H16.03- ☑
  - central H16.01- ☑
  - dendritic (herpes simplex) B00.52
  - marginal H16.04- ☑
  - Mooren's H16.05- ☑
  - mycotic H16.06- ☑
  - perforated H16.07- ☑
  - ring H16.02- ☑
  - tuberculous (phlyctenular) A18.52
- corpus cavernosum (chronic) N48.5
- crural — see Ulcer, lower limb
- Curling's — see Ulcer, peptic, acute
- Cushing's — see Ulcer, peptic, acute
- cystic duct K82.8
- cystitis (interstitial) — see Cystitis, interstitial
- decubitus — see Ulcer, pressure, by site
- dendritic, cornea (herpes simplex) B00.52
- diabetes, diabetic — see Diabetes, ulcer
- Dieulafoy's K25.0
- due to
  - infection NEC — see Ulcer, skin
  - radiation NEC L59.8
  - trophic disturbance (any region) — see Ulcer, skin
  - X-ray L58.1
- duodenum, duodenal (eroded) (peptic) K26.9
  - with
    - hemorrhage K26.4
      - and perforation K26.6
    - perforation K26.5
  - acute K26.3
    - with
      - hemorrhage K26.0
        - and perforation K26.2
      - perforation K26.1
  - chronic K26.7
    - with
      - hemorrhage K26.4
        - and perforation K26.6
      - perforation K26.5
- dysenteric A09
- elusive — see Cystitis, interstitial
- endocarditis (acute) (chronic) (subacute) I28.8
- epiglottis J38.7
- esophagus (peptic) K22.10
  - with bleeding K22.11
  - due to
    - aspirin K22.10
      - with bleeding K22.11
    - gastrointestinal reflux disease K21.0
    - ingestion of chemical or medicament K22.10
      - with bleeding K22.11
  - fungal K22.10
    - with bleeding K22.11
  - infective K22.10
    - with bleeding K22.11

☑ **Additional Character Required** — Refer to the Tabular List for Character Selection   ▿ **Subterms under main terms may continue to next column or page**

Ulcer, ulcerated, ulcerating, ulceration, ulcerative — continued
- esophagus — continued
  - varicose — see Varix, esophagus
- eyelid (region) H01.8
- fauces J39.2
- Fenwick (-Hunner) (solitary) — see Cystitis, interstitial
- fistulous — see Ulcer, skin
- foot (indolent) (trophic) — see Ulcer, lower limb
- frambesial, initial A66.0
- frenum (tongue) K14.0
- gallbladder or duct K82.8
- gangrenous — see Gangrene
- gastric — see Ulcer, stomach
- gastrocolic — see Ulcer, gastrojejunal
- gastroduodenal — see Ulcer, peptic
- gastroesophageal — see Ulcer, stomach
- gastrointestinal — see Ulcer, gastrojejunal
- gastrojejunal (peptic) K28.9
  - with
    - hemorrhage K28.4
      - and perforation K28.6
    - perforation K28.5
  - acute K28.3
    - with
      - hemorrhage K28.0
        - and perforation K28.2
      - perforation K28.1
  - chronic K28.7
    - with
      - hemorrhage K28.4
        - and perforation K28.6
      - perforation K28.5
- gastrojejunocolic — see Ulcer, gastrojejunal
- gingiva K06.8
- gingivitis K05.10
  - nonplaque induced K05.11
  - plaque induced K05.10
- glottis J38.7
- granuloma of pudenda A58
- gum K06.8
- gumma, due to yaws A66.4
- heel — see Ulcer, lower limb
- hemorrhoid — see also Hemorrhoids, by degree K64.8
- Hunner's — see Cystitis, interstitial
- hypopharynx J39.2
- hypopyon (chronic) (subacute) — see Ulcer, cornea, with hypopyon
- hypostaticum — see Ulcer, varicose
- ileum — see Ulcer, intestine
- intestine, intestinal K63.3
  - with perforation K63.1
  - amebic A06.1
  - duodenal — see Ulcer, duodenum
  - granulocytopenic (with hemorrhage) — see Neutropenia
  - marginal — see Ulcer, gastrojejunal
  - perforating K63.1
    - newborn P78.0
  - primary, small intestine K63.3
  - rectum K62.6
  - stercoraceous, stercoral K63.3
  - tuberculous A18.32
  - typhoid (fever) — see Typhoid
  - varicose I86.8
- jejunum, jejunal — see Ulcer, gastrojejunal
- keratitis — see Ulcer, cornea
- knee — see Ulcer, lower limb
- labium (majus) (minus) N76.6
- laryngitis — see Laryngitis
- larynx (aphthous) (contact) J38.7
  - diphtheritic A36.2
- leg — see Ulcer, lower limb
- lip K13.0
- Lipschütz's N76.6
- lower limb (atrophic) (chronic) (neurogenic) (perforating) (pyogenic) (trophic) (tropical) L97.909
  - with
    - bone involvement without evidence of necrosis L97.906
    - bone necrosis L97.904
    - exposed fat layer L97.902
    - muscle involvement without evidence of necrosis L97.905
    - muscle necrosis L97.903
    - skin breakdown only L97.901
    - specified severity NEC L97.908
  - ankle L97.309

Ulcer, ulcerated, ulcerating, ulceration, ulcerative — continued
- lower limb — continued
  - ankle — continued
    - with
      - bone involvement without evidence of necrosis L97.306
      - bone necrosis L97.304
      - exposed fat layer L97.302
      - muscle involvement without evidence of necrosis L97.305
      - muscle necrosis L97.303
      - skin breakdown only L97.301
      - specified severity NEC L97.308
    - left L97.329
      - with
        - bone involvement without evidence of necrosis L97.326
        - bone necrosis L97.324
        - exposed fat layer L97.322
        - muscle involvement without evidence of necrosis L97.325
        - muscle necrosis L97.323
        - skin breakdown only L97.321
        - specified severity NEC L97.328
    - right L97.319
      - with
        - bone involvement without evidence of necrosis L97.316
        - bone necrosis L97.314
        - exposed fat layer L97.312
        - muscle involvement without evidence of necrosis L97.315
        - muscle necrosis L97.313
        - skin breakdown only L97.311
        - specified severity NEC L97.318
  - calf L97.209
    - with
      - bone involvement without evidence of necrosis L97.206
      - bone necrosis L97.204
      - exposed fat layer L97.202
      - muscle involvement without evidence of necrosis L97.205
      - muscle necrosis L97.203
      - skin breakdown only L97.201
      - specified severity NEC L97.208
    - left L97.229
      - with
        - bone involvement without evidence of necrosis L97.226
        - bone necrosis L97.224
        - exposed fat layer L97.222
        - muscle involvement without evidence of necrosis L97.225
        - muscle necrosis L97.223
        - skin breakdown only L97.221
        - specified severity NEC L97.228
    - right L97.219
      - with
        - bone involvement without evidence of necrosis L97.216
        - bone necrosis L97.214
        - exposed fat layer L97.212
        - muscle involvement without evidence of necrosis L97.215
        - muscle necrosis L97.213
        - skin breakdown only L97.211
        - specified severity NEC L97.218
  - decubitus — see Ulcer, pressure, by site
  - foot specified NEC L97.509
    - with
      - bone involvement without evidence of necrosis L97.506
      - bone necrosis L97.504
      - exposed fat layer L97.502
      - muscle involvement without evidence of necrosis L97.505
      - muscle necrosis L97.503
      - skin breakdown only L97.501
      - specified severity NEC L97.508
    - left L97.529
      - with
        - bone involvement without evidence of necrosis L97.526
        - bone necrosis L97.524
        - exposed fat layer L97.522
        - muscle involvement without evidence of necrosis L97.525

Ulcer, ulcerated, ulcerating, ulceration, ulcerative — continued
- lower limb — continued
  - foot specified — continued
    - left — continued
      - with — continued
        - muscle necrosis L97.523
        - skin breakdown only L97.521
        - specified severity NEC L97.528
    - right L97.519
      - with
        - bone involvement without evidence of necrosis L97.516
        - bone necrosis L97.514
        - exposed fat layer L97.512
        - muscle involvement without evidence of necrosis L97.515
        - muscle necrosis L97.513
        - skin breakdown only L97.511
        - specified severity NEC L97.518
  - heel L97.409
    - with
      - bone involvement without evidence of necrosis L97.406
      - bone necrosis L97.404
      - exposed fat layer L97.402
      - muscle involvement without evidence of necrosis L97.405
      - muscle necrosis L97.403
      - skin breakdown only L97.401
      - specified severity NEC L97.408
    - left L97.429
      - with
        - bone involvement without evidence of necrosis L97.426
        - bone necrosis L97.424
        - exposed fat layer L97.422
        - muscle involvement without evidence of necrosis L97.425
        - muscle necrosis L97.423
        - skin breakdown only L97.421
        - specified severity NEC L97.428
    - right L97.419
      - with
        - bone involvement without evidence of necrosis L97.416
        - bone necrosis L97.414
        - exposed fat layer L97.412
        - muscle involvement without evidence of necrosis L97.415
        - muscle necrosis L97.413
        - skin breakdown only L97.411
        - specified severity NEC L97.418
  - left L97.929
    - with
      - bone involvement without evidence of necrosis L97.926
      - bone necrosis L97.924
      - exposed fat layer L97.922
      - muscle involvement without evidence of necrosis L97.925
      - muscle necrosis L97.923
      - skin breakdown only L97.921
      - specified severity NEC L97.928
  - leprous A30.1
  - lower leg NOS L97.909
    - with
      - bone involvement without evidence of necrosis L97.906
      - bone necrosis L97.904
      - exposed fat layer L97.902
      - muscle involvement without evidence of necrosis L97.905
      - muscle necrosis L97.903
      - skin breakdown only L97.901
      - specified severity NEC L97.908
    - left L97.929
      - with
        - bone involvement without evidence of necrosis L97.926
        - bone necrosis L97.924
        - exposed fat layer L97.922
        - muscle involvement without evidence of necrosis L97.925
        - muscle necrosis L97.923
        - skin breakdown only L97.921
        - specified severity NEC L97.928
    - right L97.919

Ulcer, ulcerated, ulcerating, ulceration, ulcerative
— *continued*
  lower limb — *continued*
    lower leg — *continued*
      right — *continued*
        with
          bone involvement without evidence of necrosis L97.916
          bone necrosis L97.914
          exposed fat layer L97.912
          muscle involvement without evidence of necrosis L97.915
          muscle necrosis L97.913
          skin breakdown only L97.911
          specified severity NEC L97.918
    specified site NEC L97.809
      with
        bone involvement without evidence of necrosis L97.806
        bone necrosis L97.804
        exposed fat layer L97.802
        muscle involvement without evidence of necrosis L97.805
        muscle necrosis L97.803
        skin breakdown only L97.801
        specified severity NEC L97.808
      left L97.829
        with
          bone involvement without evidence of necrosis L97.826
          bone necrosis L97.824
          exposed fat layer L97.822
          muscle involvement without evidence of necrosis L97.825
          muscle necrosis L97.823
          skin breakdown only L97.821
          specified severity NEC L97.828
      right L97.819
        with
          bone involvement without evidence of necrosis L97.816
          bone necrosis L97.814
          exposed fat layer L97.812
          muscle involvement without evidence of necrosis L97.815
          muscle necrosis L97.813
          skin breakdown only L97.811
          specified severity NEC L97.818
  midfoot L97.409
    with
      bone involvement without evidence of necrosis L97.406
      bone necrosis L97.404
      exposed fat layer L97.402
      muscle involvement without evidence of necrosis L97.405
      muscle necrosis L97.403
      skin breakdown only L97.401
      specified severity NEC L97.408
    left L97.429
      with
        bone involvement without evidence of necrosis L97.426
        bone necrosis L97.424
        exposed fat layer L97.422
        muscle involvement without evidence of necrosis L97.425
        muscle necrosis L97.423
        skin breakdown only L97.421
        specified severity NEC L97.428
    right L97.419
      with
        bone involvement without evidence of necrosis L97.416
        bone necrosis L97.414
        exposed fat layer L97.412
        muscle involvement without evidence of necrosis L97.415
        muscle necrosis L97.413
        skin breakdown only L97.411
        specified severity NEC L97.418
  right L97.919
    with
      bone involvement without evidence of necrosis L97.916
      bone necrosis L97.914
      exposed fat layer L97.912
      muscle involvement without evidence of necrosis L97.915

Ulcer, ulcerated, ulcerating, ulceration, ulcerative
— *continued*
  lower limb — *continued*
    right — *continued*
      with — *continued*
        muscle necrosis L97.913
        skin breakdown only L97.911
        specified severity NEC L97.918
    syphilitic A52.19
    thigh L97.109
      with
        bone involvement without evidence of necrosis L97.106
        bone necrosis L97.104
        exposed fat layer L97.102
        muscle involvement without evidence of necrosis L97.105
        muscle necrosis L97.103
        skin breakdown only L97.101
        specified severity NEC L97.108
      left L97.129
        with
          bone involvement without evidence of necrosis L97.126
          bone necrosis L97.124
          exposed fat layer L97.122
          muscle involvement without evidence of necrosis L97.125
          muscle necrosis L97.123
          skin breakdown only L97.121
          specified severity NEC L97.128
      right L97.119
        with
          bone involvement without evidence of necrosis L97.116
          bone necrosis L97.114
          exposed fat layer L97.112
          muscle involvement without evidence of necrosis L97.115
          muscle necrosis L97.113
          skin breakdown only L97.111
          specified severity NEC L97.118
    toe L97.509
      with
        bone involvement without evidence of necrosis L97.506
        bone necrosis L97.504
        exposed fat layer L97.502
        muscle involvement without evidence of necrosis L97.505
        muscle necrosis L97.503
        skin breakdown only L97.501
        specified severity NEC L97.508
      left L97.529
        with
          bone involvement without evidence of necrosis L97.526
          bone necrosis L97.524
          exposed fat layer L97.522
          muscle involvement without evidence of necrosis L97.525
          muscle necrosis L97.523
          skin breakdown only L97.521
          specified severity NEC L97.528
      right L97.519
        with
          bone involvement without evidence of necrosis L97.516
          bone necrosis L97.514
          exposed fat layer L97.512
          muscle involvement without evidence of necrosis L97.515
          muscle necrosis L97.513
          skin breakdown only L97.511
          specified severity NEC L97.518
    varicose — *see* Varix, leg, with, ulcer
  luetic — *see* Ulcer, syphilitic
  lung J98.4
    tuberculous — *see* Tuberculosis, pulmonary
  malignant — *see* Neoplasm, malignant, by site
  marginal NEC — *see* Ulcer, gastrojejunal
  meatus (urinarius) N34.2
  Meckel's diverticulum Q43.0
    malignant — *see* Table of Neoplasms, small intestine, malignant
  Meleney's (chronic undermining) — *see* Ulcer, skin
  Mooren's (cornea) — *see* Ulcer, cornea, Mooren's
  mycobacterial (skin) A31.1

Ulcer, ulcerated, ulcerating, ulceration, ulcerativ
— *continued*
  nasopharynx J39.2
  neck, uterus N86
  neurogenic NEC — *see* Ulcer, skin
  nose, nasal (passage) (infective) (septum) J34.0
    skin — *see* Ulcer, skin
    spirochetal A69.8
    varicose (bleeding) I86.8
  oral mucosa (traumatic) K12.1
  palate (soft) K12.1
  penis (chronic) N48.5
  peptic (site unspecified) K27.9
    with
      hemorrhage K27.4
        and perforation K27.6
      perforation K27.5
    acute K27.3
      with
        hemorrhage K27.0
          and perforation K27.2
        perforation K27.1
    chronic K27.7
      with
        hemorrhage K27.4
          and perforation K27.6
        perforation K27.5
    esophagus K22.10
      with bleeding K22.11
    newborn P78.82
  perforating K27.5
    skin — *see* Ulcer, skin
  peritonsillar J35.8
  phagedenic (tropical) — *see* Ulcer, skin
  pharynx J39.2
  phlebitis — *see* Phlebitis
  plaster — *see* Ulcer, pressure, by site
  popliteal space — *see* Ulcer, lower limb
  postpyloric — *see* Ulcer, duodenum
  prepuce N47.7
  prepyloric — *see* Ulcer, stomach
  pressure (pressure area) L89.9- ☑
    ankle L89.5- ☑
    back L89.1- ☑
    buttock L89.3- ☑
    coccyx L89.15- ☑
    contiguous site of back, buttock, hip L89.4- ☑
    elbow L89.0- ☑
    face L89.81- ☑
    head L89.81- ☑
    heel L89.6- ☑
    hip L89.2- ☑
    sacral region (tailbone) L89.15- ☑
    specified site NEC L89.89- ☑
    stage 1 (healing) (pre-ulcer skin changes limited persistent focal edema)
      ankle L89.5- ☑
      back L89.1- ☑
      buttock L89.3- ☑
      coccyx L89.15- ☑
      contiguous site of back, buttock, hip L89.4- ☑
      elbow L89.0- ☑
      face L89.81- ☑
      head L89.81- ☑
      heel L89.6- ☑
      hip L89.2- ☑
      sacral region (tailbone) L89.15- ☑
      specified site NEC L89.89- ☑
    stage 2 (healing) (abrasion, blister, partial thickne skin loss involving epidermis and/or dermi
      ankle L89.5- ☑
      back L89.1- ☑
      buttock L89.3- ☑
      coccyx L89.15- ☑
      contiguous site of back, buttock, hip L89.4- ☑
      elbow L89.0- ☑
      face L89.81- ☑
      head L89.81- ☑
      heel L89.6- ☑
      hip L89.2- ☑
      sacral region (tailbone) L89.15- ☑
      specified site NEC L89.89- ☑
    stage 3 (healing) (full thickness skin loss involvin damage or necrosis of subcutaneous tissue
      ankle L89.5- ☑
      back L89.1- ☑
      buttock L89.3- ☑

☑ **Additional Character Required** — Refer to the Tabular List for Character Selection   ▽ Subterms under main terms may continue to next column or pag

cer, ulcerated, ulcerating, ulceration, ulcerative
— *continued*
  pressure — *continued*
    stage 3 — *continued*
      coccyx L89.15- ☑
      contiguous site of back, buttock, hip L89.4- ☑
      elbow L89.0- ☑
      face L89.81- ☑
      head L89.81- ☑
      heel L89.6- ☑
      hip L89.2- ☑
      sacral region (tailbone) L89.15- ☑
      specified site NEC L89.89- ☑
    stage 4 (healing) (necrosis of soft tissues through
      to underlying muscle, tendon, or bone)
      ankle L89.5- ☑
      back L89.1- ☑
      buttock L89.3- ☑
      coccyx L89.15- ☑
      contiguous site of back, buttock, hip L89.4- ☑
      elbow L89.0- ☑
      face L89.81- ☑
      head L89.81- ☑
      heel L89.6- ☑
      hip L89.2- ☑
      sacral region (tailbone) L89.15- ☑
      specified site NEC L89.89- ☑
    unspecified stage
      ankle L89.5- ☑
      back L89.1- ☑
      buttock L89.3- ☑
      coccyx L89.15- ☑
      contiguous site of back, buttock, hip L89.4- ☑
      elbow L89.0- ☑
      face L89.81- ☑
      head L89.81- ☑
      heel L89.6- ☑
      hip L89.2- ☑
      sacral region (tailbone) L89.15- ☑
      specified site NEC L89.89- ☑
    unstageable
      ankle L89.5- ☑
      back L89.1- ☑
      buttock L89.3- ☑
      coccyx L89.15- ☑
      contiguous site of back, buttock, hip L89.4- ☑
      elbow L89.0- ☑
      face L89.81- ☑
      head L89.81- ☑
      heel L89.6- ☑
      hip L89.2- ☑
      sacral region (tailbone) L89.15- ☑
      specified site NEC L89.89- ☑
  primary of intestine K63.3
    with perforation K63.1
  prostate N41.9
  pyloric — *see* Ulcer, stomach
  rectosigmoid K63.3
    with perforation K63.1
  rectum (sphincter) (solitary) K62.6
    stercoraceous, stercoral K62.6
  retina — *see* Inflammation, chorioretinal
  rodent — *see also* Neoplasm, skin, malignant
  sclera — *see* Scleritis
  scrofulous (tuberculous) A18.2
  scrotum N50.89
    tuberculous A18.15
    varicose I86.1
  seminal vesicle N50.89
  sigmoid — *see* Ulcer, intestine
  skin (atrophic) (chronic) (neurogenic) (non-healing)
    (perforating) (pyogenic) (trophic) (tropical)
    L98.499
    with gangrene — *see* Gangrene
    amebic A06.7
    back — *see* Ulcer, back
    buttock — *see* Ulcer, buttock
    decubitus — *see* Ulcer, pressure
    lower limb — *see* Ulcer, lower limb
    mycobacterial A31.1
    specified site NEC L98.499
      with
        bone involvement without evidence of
          necrosis L98.496
        bone necrosis L98.494
        exposed fat layer L98.492

Ulcer, ulcerated, ulcerating, ulceration, ulcerative
— *continued*
  skin — *continued*
    specified site — *continued*
      with — *continued*
        muscle involvement without evidence of
          necrosis L98.495
        muscle necrosis L98.493
        skin breakdown only L98.491
        specified severity NEC L98.498
    tuberculous (primary) A18.4
    varicose — *see* Ulcer, varicose
  sloughing — *see* Ulcer, skin
  solitary, anus or rectum (sphincter) K62.6
  sore throat J02.9
    streptococcal J02.0
  spermatic cord N50.89
  spine (tuberculous) A18.01
  stasis (venous) — *see* Varix, leg, with, ulcer
    without varicose veins I87.2
  stercoraceous, stercoral K63.3
    with perforation K63.1
    anus or rectum K62.6
  stoma, stomal — *see* Ulcer, gastrojejunal
  stomach (eroded) (peptic) (round) K25.9
    with
      hemorrhage K25.4
        and perforation K25.6
      perforation K25.5
    acute K25.3
      with
        hemorrhage K25.0
          and perforation K25.2
        perforation K25.1
    chronic K25.7
      with
        hemorrhage K25.4
          and perforation K25.6
        perforation K25.5
  stomal — *see* Ulcer, gastrojejunal
  stomatitis K12.1
  stress — *see* Ulcer, peptic
  strumous (tuberculous) A18.2
  submucosal, bladder — *see* Cystitis, interstitial
  syphilitic (any site) (early) (secondary) A51.39
    late A52.79
    perforating A52.79
      foot A52.11
  testis N50.89
  thigh — *see* Ulcer, lower limb
  throat J39.2
    diphtheritic A36.0
  toe — *see* Ulcer, lower limb
  tongue (traumatic) K14.0
  tonsil J35.8
    diphtheritic A36.0
  trachea J39.8
  trophic — *see* Ulcer, skin
  tropical — *see* Ulcer, skin
  tuberculous — *see* Tuberculosis, ulcer
  tunica vaginalis N50.89
  turbinate J34.89
  typhoid (perforating) — *see* Typhoid
  unspecified site — *see* Ulcer, skin
  urethra (meatus) — *see* Urethritis
  uterus N85.8
    cervix N86
      with cervicitis N72
    neck N86
      with cervicitis N72
  vagina N76.5
    in Behçet's disease M35.2 *[N77.0]*
    pessary N89.8
  valve, heart I33.0
  varicose (lower limb, any part) — *see also* Varix, leg,
    with, ulcer
    broad ligament I86.2
    esophagus — *see* Varix, esophagus
    inflamed or infected — *see* Varix, leg, with ulcer,
      with inflammation
    nasal septum I86.8
    perineum I86.3
    scrotum I86.1
    specified site NEC I86.8
    sublingual I86.0
    vulva I86.3
  vas deferens N50.89
  vulva (acute) (infectional) N76.6

Ulcer, ulcerated, ulcerating, ulceration, ulcerative
— *continued*
  vulva — *continued*
    in (due to)
      Behçet's disease M35.2 *[N77.0]*
      herpesviral (herpes simplex) infection A60.04
      tuberculosis A18.18
  vulvobuccal, recurring N76.6
  X-ray L58.1
  yaws A66.4
Ulcerosa scarlatina A38.8
Ulcus — *see also* Ulcer
  cutis tuberculosum A18.4
  duodeni — *see* Ulcer, duodenum
  durum (syphilitic) A51.0
    extragenital A51.2
  gastrojejunale — *see* Ulcer, gastrojejunal
  hypostaticum — *see* Ulcer, varicose
  molle (cutis) (skin) A57
  serpens corneae — *see* Ulcer, cornea, central
  ventriculi — *see* Ulcer, stomach
Ulegyria Q04.8
Ulerythema
  ophryogenes, congenital Q84.2
  sycosiforme L73.8
Ullrich (-Bonnevie)(-Turner) **syndrome** — *see also*
  Turner's syndrome Q87.19
Ullrich-Feichtiger syndrome Q87.0
Ulnar — *see* condition
Ulorrhagia, ulorrhea K06.8
Umbilicus, umbilical — *see* condition
Unacceptable
  contours of tooth K08.54
  morphology of tooth K08.54
Unavailability (of)
  bed at medical facility Z75.1
  health service-related agencies Z75.4
  medical facilities (at) Z75.3
    due to
      investigation by social service agency Z75.2
      lack of services at home Z75.0
      remoteness from facility Z75.3
      waiting list Z75.1
    home Z75.0
    outpatient clinic Z75.3
  schooling Z55.1
  social service agencies Z75.4
Uncinaria americana infestation B76.1
Uncinariasis B76.9
Uncongenial work Z56.5
Unconscious (ness) — *see* Coma
Under observation — *see* Observation
Underachievement in school Z55.3
Underdevelopment — *see also* Undeveloped
  nose Q30.1
  sexual E30.0
Underdosing — *see also* Table of Drugs and Chemicals,
  categories T36-T50, with final character 6 Z91.14
  intentional NEC Z91.128
    due to financial hardship of patient Z91.120
  unintentional NEC Z91.138
    due to patient's age related debility Z91.130
Underfeeding, newborn P92.3
Underfill, endodontic M27.53
Underimmunization status Z28.3
Undernourishment — *see* Malnutrition
Undernutrition — *see* Malnutrition
Underweight R63.6
  for gestational age — *see* Light for dates
Underwood's disease P83.0
Undescended — *see also* Malposition, congenital
  cecum Q43.3
  colon Q43.3
  testicle — *see* Cryptorchid
Undeveloped, undevelopment — *see also* Hypoplasia
  brain (congenital) Q02
  cerebral (congenital) Q02
  heart Q24.8
  lung Q33.6
  testis E29.1
  uterus E30.0
Undiagnosed (disease) R69
Undulant fever — *see* Brucellosis
Unemployment, anxiety concerning Z56.0
  threatened Z56.2
Unequal length (acquired) (limb) — *see also* Deformity,
  limb, unequal length

Unequal length — *continued*
   leg — *see also* Deformity, limb, unequal length
     congenital Q72.9- ☑
Unextracted dental root K08.3
Unguis incarnatus L60.0
Unhappiness R45.2
Unicornate uterus Q51.4
   in pregnancy or childbirth O34.00
Unilateral — *see also* condition
   development, breast N64.89
   organ or site, congenital NEC — *see* Agenesis, by site
Unilocular heart Q20.8
Union, abnormal — *see also* Fusion
   larynx and trachea Q34.8
Universal mesentery Q43.3
**Unrepairable overhanging of dental restorative
   materials** K08.52
Unsatisfactory
   restoration of tooth K08.50
     specified NEC K08.59
   sample of cytologic smear
     anus R85.615
     cervix R87.615
     vagina R87.625
   surroundings Z59.1
   work Z56.5
Unsoundness of mind — *see* Psychosis
Unstable
   back NEC — *see* Instability, joint, spine
   hip (congenital) Q65.6
     acquired — *see* Derangement, joint, specified type
       NEC, hip
   joint — *see* Instability, joint
     secondary to removal of joint prosthesis M96.89
   lie (mother) O32.0 ☑
   lumbosacral joint (congenital) — *see* subcategory
     M53.2
   sacroiliac — *see* subcategory M53.2 ☑
   spine NEC — *see* Instability, joint, spine
Unsteadiness on feet R26.81
Untruthfulness, child problem F91.8
Unverricht (-Lundborg) **disease or epilepsy** — *see*
   Epilepsy, generalized, idiopathic
Unwanted pregnancy Z64.0
Upbringing, institutional Z62.22
   away from parents NEC Z62.29
   in care of non-parental family member Z62.21
   in foster care Z62.21
   in orphanage or group home Z62.22
   in welfare custody Z62.21
Upper respiratory — *see* condition
Upset
   gastric K30
   gastrointestinal K30
     psychogenic F45.8
   intestinal (large) (small) K59.9
     psychogenic F45.8
   menstruation N93.9
   mental F48.9
   stomach K30
     psychogenic F45.8
Urachus — *see also* condition
   patent or persistent Q64.4
Urbach-Oppenheim disease (necrobiosis lipoidica diabeticorum) — *see* E08-E13 with .620
Urbach's lipoid proteinosis E78.89
Urbach-Wiethe disease E78.89
Urban yellow fever A95.1
Urea
   blood, high — *see* Uremia
   cycle metabolism disorder — *see* Disorder, urea cycle
     metabolism
Uremia, uremic N19
   with
     ectopic or molar pregnancy O08.4
     polyneuropathy N18.9 [G63]
   chronic NOS — *see also* Disease, kidney, chronic N18.9
     due to hypertension — *see* Hypertensive, kidney
   complicating
     ectopic or molar pregnancy O08.4
   congenital P96.0
   extrarenal R39.2
   following ectopic or molar pregnancy O08.4
   newborn P96.0
   prerenal R39.2
Ureter, ureteral — *see* condition
Ureteralgia N23

Ureterectasis — *see* Hydroureter
Ureteritis N28.89
   cystica N28.86
   due to calculus N20.1
     with calculus, kidney N20.2
       with hydronephrosis N13.2
   gonococcal (acute) (chronic) A54.21
   nonspecific N28.89
Ureterocele N28.89
   congenital (orthotopic) Q62.31
   ectopic Q62.32
Ureterolith, ureterolithiasis — *see* Calculus, ureter
Ureterostomy
   attention to Z43.6
   status Z93.6
Urethra, urethral — *see* condition
Urethralgia R39.89
Urethritis (anterior) (posterior) N34.2
   calculous N21.1
   candidal B37.41
   chlamydial A56.01
   diplococcal (gonococcal) A54.01
     with abscess (accessory gland) (periurethral) A54.1
   gonococcal A54.01
     with abscess (accessory gland) (periurethral) A54.1
   nongonococcal N34.1
     Reiter's — *see* Reiter's disease
   nonspecific N34.1
   nonvenereal N34.1
   postmenopausal N34.2
   puerperal O86.22
   Reiter's — *see* Reiter's disease
   specified NEC N34.2
   trichomonal or due to Trichomonas (vaginalis) A59.03
Urethrocele N81.0
   with
     cystocele — *see* Cystocele
     prolapse of uterus — *see* Prolapse, uterus
Urethrolithiasis (with colic or infection) N21.1
Urethrorectal — *see* condition
Urethrorrhagia N36.8
Urethrorrhea R36.9
Urethrostomy
   attention to Z43.6
   status Z93.6
Urethrotrigonitis — *see* Trigonitis
Urethrovaginal — *see* condition
Urgency
   fecal R15.2
   hypertensive — *see* Hypertension
   urinary R39.15
Urhidrosis, uridrosis L74.8
Uric acid in blood (increased) E79.0
Uricacidemia (asymptomatic) E79.0
Uricemia (asymptomatic) E79.0
Uricosuria R82.998
Urinary — *see* condition
Urination
   frequent R35.0
   painful R30.9
Urine
   blood in — *see* Hematuria
   discharge, excessive R35.8
   enuresis, nonorganic origin F98.0
   extravasation R39.0
   frequency R35.0
   incontinence R32
     nonorganic origin F98.0
   intermittent stream R39.198
   pus in N39.0
   retention or stasis R33.9
     organic R33.8
       drug-induced R33.0
     psychogenic F45.8
   secretion
     deficient R34
     excessive R35.8
     frequency R35.0
   stream
     intermittent R39.198
     slowing R39.198
     splitting R39.13
     weak R39.12
Urinemia — *see* Uremia
Urinoma, urethra N36.8
Uroarthritis, infectious (Reiter's) — *see* Reiter's disease
Urodialysis R34
Urolithiasis — *see* Calculus, urinary

Uronephrosis — *see* Hydronephrosis
Uropathy N39.9
   obstructive N13.9
     specified NEC N13.8
   reflux N13.9
     specified NEC N13.8
   vesicoureteral reflux-associated — *see* Reflux, vesi-
     coureteral
Urosepsis — *code to* condition
Urticaria L50.9
   with angioneurotic edema T78.3 ☑
     hereditary D84.1
   allergic L50.0
   cholinergic L50.5
   chronic L50.8
   cold, familial L50.2
   contact L50.6
   dermatographic L50.3
   due to
     cold or heat L50.2
     drugs L50.0
     food L50.0
     inhalants L50.0
     plants L50.6
     serum — *see also* Reaction, serum T80.69 ☑
   factitial L50.3
   familial cold M04.2
   giant T78.3 ☑
     hereditary D84.1
   gigantea T78.3 ☑
   idiopathic L50.1
   larynx T78.3 ☑
     hereditary D84.1
   neonatorum P83.88
   nonallergic L50.1
   papulosa (Hebra) L28.2
   pigmentosa D47.01
     congenital Q82.2
     of neonatal onset Q82.2
     of newborn onset Q82.2
   recurrent periodic L50.8
   serum — *see also* Reaction, serum T80.69 ☑
   solar L56.3
   specified type NEC L50.8
   thermal (cold) (heat) L50.2
   vibratory L50.4
   xanthelasmoidea — *see* Urticaria pigmentosa
Use (of)
   alcohol Z72.89
     with
       intoxication F10.929
       sleep disorder F10.982
     harmful — *see* Abuse, alcohol
   amphetamines — *see* Use, stimulant NEC
   caffeine — *see* Use, stimulant NEC
   cannabis F12.90
     with
       anxiety disorder F12.980
       intoxication F12.929
         with
           delirium F12.921
           perceptual disturbance F12.922
         uncomplicated F12.920
       other specified disorder F12.988
       psychosis F12.959
         delusions F12.950
         hallucinations F12.951
       unspecified disorder F12.99
       withdrawal F12.93
   cocaine F14.90
     with
       anxiety disorder F14.980
       intoxication F14.929
         with
           delirium F14.921
           perceptual disturbance F14.922
         uncomplicated F14.920
       other specified disorder F14.988
       psychosis F14.959
         delusions F14.950
         hallucinations F14.951
       sexual dysfunction F14.981
       sleep disorder F14.982
       unspecified disorder F14.99
     harmful — *see* Abuse, drug, cocaine
   drug(s) NEC F19.90
     with sleep disorder F19.982
     harmful — *see* Abuse, drug, by type

Use — *continued*
 hallucinogen NEC F16.90
  with
   anxiety disorder F16.980
   intoxication F16.929
    with
     delirium F16.921
    uncomplicated F16.920
   mood disorder F16.94
   other specified disorder F16.988
   perception disorder (flashbacks) F16.983
   psychosis F16.959
    delusions F16.950
    hallucinations F16.951
   unspecified disorder F16.99
  harmful — *see* Abuse, drug, hallucinogen NEC
 inhalants F18.90
  with
   anxiety disorder F18.980
   intoxication F18.929
    with delirium F18.921
    uncomplicated F18.920
   mood disorder F18.94
   other specified disorder F18.988
   persisting dementia F18.97
   psychosis F18.959
    delusions F18.950
    hallucinations F18.951
   unspecified disorder F18.99
  harmful — *see* Abuse, drug, inhalant
 methadone — *see* Use, opioid
 nonprescribed drugs F19.90
  harmful — *see* Abuse, non-psychoactive substance
 opioid F11.90
  with
   disorder F11.99
    mood F11.94
    sleep F11.982
    specified type NEC F11.988
   intoxication F11.929
    with
     delirium F11.921
     perceptual disturbance F11.922
    uncomplicated F11.920
   withdrawal F11.93
  harmful — *see* Abuse, drug, opioid
 patent medicines F19.90
  harmful — *see* Abuse, non-psychoactive substance
 psychoactive drug NEC F19.90
  with
   anxiety disorder F19.980
   intoxication F19.929
    with
     delirium F19.921
     perceptual disturbance F19.922
    uncomplicated F19.920
   mood disorder F19.94
   other specified disorder F19.988
   persisting
    amnestic disorder F19.96
    dementia F19.97
   psychosis F19.959
    delusions F19.950
    hallucinations F19.951
   sexual dysfunction F19.981
   sleep disorder F19.982
   unspecified disorder F19.99
   withdrawal F19.939
    with
     delirium F19.931
     perceptual disturbance F19.932
    uncomplicated F19.930
  harmful — *see* Abuse, drug NEC, psychoactive NEC
 sedative, hypnotic, or anxiolytic F13.90
  with
   anxiety disorder F13.980
   intoxication F13.929
    with
     delirium F13.921
    uncomplicated F13.920
   other specified disorder F13.988
   persisting
    amnestic disorder F13.96
    dementia F13.97
   psychosis F13.959
    delusions F13.950
    hallucinations F13.951
   sexual dysfunction F13.981

Use — *continued*
 sedative, hypnotic, or anxiolytic — *continued*
  with — *continued*
   sleep disorder F13.982
   unspecified disorder F13.99
  harmful — *see* Abuse, drug, sedative, hypnotic, or anxiolytic
 stimulant NEC F15.90
  with
   anxiety disorder F15.980
   intoxication F15.929
    with
     delirium F15.921
     perceptual disturbance F15.922
    uncomplicated F15.920
   mood disorder F15.94
   other specified disorder F15.988
   psychosis F15.959
    delusions F15.950
    hallucinations F15.951
   sexual dysfunction F15.981
   sleep disorder F15.982
   unspecified disorder F15.99
   withdrawal F15.93
  harmful — *see* Abuse, drug, stimulant NEC
 tobacco Z72.0
  with dependence — *see* Dependence, drug, nicotine
 volatile solvents — *see also* Use, inhalant F18.90
  harmful — *see* Abuse, drug, inhalant
Usher-Senear disease or syndrome L10.4
Uta B55.1
Uteromegaly N85.2
Uterovaginal — *see* condition
Uterovesical — *see* condition
Uveal — *see* condition
Uveitis (anterior) — *see also* Iridocyclitis
 acute — *see* Iridocyclitis, acute
 chronic — *see* Iridocyclitis, chronic
 due to toxoplasmosis (acquired) B58.09
  congenital P37.1
 granulomatous — *see* Iridocyclitis, chronic
 heterochromic — *see* Cyclitis, Fuchs' heterochromic
 lens-induced — *see* Iridocyclitis, lens-induced
 posterior — *see* Chorioretinitis
 sympathetic H44.13- ☑
 syphilitic (secondary) A51.43
  congenital (early) A50.01
  late A52.71
 tuberculous A18.54
Uveoencephalitis — *see* Inflammation, chorioretinal
Uveokeratitis — *see* Iridocyclitis
Uveoparotitis D86.89
Uvula — *see* condition
Uvulitis (acute) (catarrhal) (chronic) (membranous) (suppurative) (ulcerative) K12.2

V

Vaccination (prophylactic)
 complication or reaction — *see* Complications, vaccination
 delayed Z28.9
 encounter for Z23
 not done — *see* Immunization, not done, because (of)
Vaccinia (generalized) (localized) T88.1 ☑
 congenital P35.8
 without vaccination B08.011
Vacuum, in sinus (accessory) (nasal) J34.89
Vagabond, vagabondage Z59.0
Vagabond's disease B85.1
Vagina, vaginal — *see* condition
Vaginalitis (tunica) (testis) N49.1
Vaginismus (reflex) N94.2
 functional F52.5
 nonorganic F52.5
 psychogenic F52.5
 secondary N94.2
Vaginitis (acute) (circumscribed) (diffuse) (emphysematous) (nonvenereal) (ulcerative) N76.0
 with ectopic or molar pregnancy O08.0
 amebic A06.82
 atrophic, postmenopausal N95.2
 bacterial N76.0
 blennorrhagic (gonococcal) A54.02
 candidal B37.3
 chlamydial A56.02
 chronic N76.1

Vaginitis — *continued*
 due to Trichomonas (vaginalis) A59.01
 following ectopic or molar pregnancy O08.0
 gonococcal A54.02
  with abscess (accessory gland) (periurethral) A54.1
 granuloma A58
 in (due to)
  candidiasis B37.3
  herpesviral (herpes simplex) infection A60.04
  pinworm infection B80 *[N77.1]*
 monilial B37.3
 mycotic (candidal) B37.3
 postmenopausal atrophic N95.2
 puerperal (postpartum) O86.13
 senile (atrophic) N95.2
 subacute or chronic N76.1
 syphilitic (early) A51.0
  late A52.76
 trichomonal A59.01
 tuberculous A18.18
Vaginosis — *see* Vaginitis
Vagotonia G52.2
Vagrancy Z59.0
VAIN — *see* Neoplasia, intraepithelial, vagina
Vallecula — *see* condition
Valley fever B38.0
Valsuani's disease — *see* Anemia, obstetric
Valve, valvular (formation) — *see also* condition
 cerebral ventricle (communicating) in situ Z98.2
 cervix, internal os Q51.828
 congenital NEC — *see* Atresia, by site
 ureter (pelvic junction) (vesical orifice) Q62.39
 urethra (congenital) (posterior) Q64.2
Valvulitis (chronic) — *see* Endocarditis
Valvulopathy — *see* Endocarditis
Van Bogaert's leukoencephalopathy (sclerosing) (subacute) A81.1
Van Bogaert-Scherer-Epstein disease or syndrome E75.5
Van Buchem's syndrome M85.2
Van Creveld-von Gierke disease E74.01
Van der Hoeve (-de Kleyn) **syndrome** Q78.0
Van der Woude's syndrome Q38.0
Van Neck's disease or osteochondrosis M91.0
Vanishing lung J44.9
Vapor asphyxia or suffocation T59.9 ☑
 specified agent — *see* Table of Drugs and Chemicals
Variance, lethal ball, prosthetic heart valve T82.09 ☑
Variants, thalassemic D56.8
Variations in hair color L67.1
Varicella B01.9
 with
  complications NEC B01.89
  encephalitis B01.11
  encephalomyelitis B01.11
  meningitis B01.0
  myelitis B01.12
  pneumonia B01.2
 congenital P35.8
Varices — *see* Varix
Varicocele (scrotum) (thrombosed) I86.1
 ovary I86.2
 perineum I86.3
 spermatic cord (ulcerated) I86.1
Varicose
 aneurysm (ruptured) I77.0
 dermatitis — *see* Varix, leg, with, inflammation
 eczema — *see* Varix, leg, with, inflammation
 phlebitis — *see* Varix, with, inflammation
 tumor — *see* Varix
 ulcer (lower limb, any part) — *see also* Varix, leg, with, ulcer
  anus — *see also* Hemorrhoids K64.8
  esophagus — *see* Varix, esophagus
  inflamed or infected — *see* Varix, leg, with ulcer, with inflammation
  nasal septum I86.8
  perineum I86.3
  scrotum I86.1
  specified site NEC I86.8
 vein — *see* Varix
 vessel — *see* Varix, leg
Varicosis, varicosities, varicosity — *see* Varix
Variola (major) (minor) B03
Varioloid B03
Varix (lower limb) I83.90

Varix — *continued*
  with
    bleeding I83.899
    edema I83.899
    inflammation I83.10
      with ulcer (venous) I83.209
    pain I83.819
    rupture I83.899
    specified complication NEC I83.899
    stasis dermatitis I83.10
      with ulcer (venous) I83.209
    swelling I83.899
    ulcer I83.009
      with inflammation I83.209
  aneurysmal I77.0
  asymptomatic I83.9- ☑
  bladder I86.2
  broad ligament I86.2
  complicating
    childbirth (lower extremity) O87.4
      anus or rectum O87.2
      genital (vagina, vulva or perineum) O87.8
    pregnancy (lower extremity) O22.0- ☑
      anus or rectum O22.4- ☑
      genital (vagina, vulva or perineum) O22.1- ☑
    puerperium (lower extremity) O87.4
      anus or rectum O87.2
      genital (vagina, vulva, perineum) O87.8
  congenital (any site) Q27.8
  esophagus (idiopathic) (primary) (ulcerated) I85.00
    bleeding I85.01
    congenital Q27.8
    in (due to)
      alcoholic liver disease I85.10
        bleeding I85.11
      cirrhosis of liver I85.10
        bleeding I85.11
      portal hypertension I85.10
        bleeding I85.11
      schistosomiasis I85.10
        bleeding I85.11
      toxic liver disease I85.10
        bleeding I85.11
    secondary I85.10
      bleeding I85.11
  gastric I86.4
  inflamed or infected I83.10
    ulcerated I83.209
  labia (majora) I86.3
  leg (asymptomatic) I83.90
    with
      edema I83.899
      inflammation I83.10
        with ulcer — *see* Varix, leg, with, ulcer, with inflammation by site
      pain I83.819
      specified complication NEC I83.899
      swelling I83.899
      ulcer I83.009
        with inflammation I83.209
        ankle I83.003
          with inflammation I83.203
        calf I83.002
          with inflammation I83.202
        foot NEC I83.005
          with inflammation I83.205
        heel I83.004
          with inflammation I83.204
        lower leg NEC I83.008
          with inflammation I83.208
        midfoot I83.004
          with inflammation I83.204
        thigh I83.001
          with inflammation I83.201
    bilateral (asymptomatic) I83.93
      with
        edema I83.893
        pain I83.813
        specified complication NEC I83.893
        swelling I83.893
        ulcer I83.0- ☑
          with inflammation I83.209
    left (asymptomatic) I83.92
      with
        edema I83.892
        inflammation I83.12
          with ulcer — *see* Varix, leg, with, ulcer, with inflammation by site

Varix — *continued*
  leg — *continued*
    left — *continued*
      with — *continued*
        pain I83.812
        specified complication NEC I83.892
        swelling I83.892
        ulcer I83.029
          with inflammation I83.229
          ankle I83.023
            with inflammation I83.223
          calf I83.022
            with inflammation I83.222
          foot NEC I83.025
            with inflammation I83.225
          heel I83.024
            with inflammation I83.224
          lower leg NEC I83.028
            with inflammation I83.228
          midfoot I83.024
            with inflammation I83.224
          thigh I83.021
            with inflammation I83.221
      right (asymptomatic) I83.91
        with
          edema I83.891
          inflammation I83.11
            with ulcer — *see* Varix, leg, with, ulcer, with inflammation by site
          pain I83.811
          specified complication NEC I83.891
          swelling I83.891
          ulcer I83.019
            with inflammation I83.219
            ankle I83.013
              with inflammation I83.213
            calf I83.012
              with inflammation I83.212
            foot NEC I83.015
              with inflammation I83.215
            heel I83.014
              with inflammation I83.214
            lower leg NEC I83.018
              with inflammation I83.218
            midfoot I83.014
              with inflammation I83.214
            thigh I83.011
              with inflammation I83.211
  nasal septum I86.8
  orbit I86.8
    congenital Q27.8
  ovary I86.2
  papillary I78.1
  pelvis I86.2
  perineum I86.3
  pharynx I86.8
  placenta O43.89- ☑
  renal papilla I86.8
  retina H35.09
  scrotum (ulcerated) I86.1
  sigmoid colon I86.8
  specified site NEC I86.8
  spinal (cord) (vessels) I86.8
  spleen, splenic (vein) (with phlebolith) I86.8
  stomach I86.4
  sublingual I86.0
  ulcerated I83.009
    inflamed or infected I83.209
  uterine ligament I86.2
  vagina I86.8
  vocal cord I86.8
  vulva I86.3
Vas deferens — *see* condition
Vas deferentitis N49.1
Vasa previa O69.4 ☑
  hemorrhage from, affecting newborn P50.0
Vascular — *see also* condition
  loop on optic papilla Q14.2
  spasm I73.9
  spider I78.1
Vascularization, cornea — *see* Neovascularization, cornea
Vasculitis I77.6
  allergic D69.0
  cryoglobulinemic D89.1
  disseminated I77.6
  hypocomplementemic M31.8
  kidney I77.89

Vasculitis — *continued*
  livedoid L95.0
  nodular L95.8
  retina H35.06- ☑
  rheumatic — *see* Fever, rheumatic
  rheumatoid — *see* Rheumatoid, vasculitis
  skin (limited to) L95.9
    specified NEC L95.8
  systemic M31.8
Vasculopathy, necrotizing M31.9
  cardiac allograft T86.290
  specified NEC M31.8
Vasitis (nodosa) N49.1
  tuberculous A18.15
Vasodilation I73.9
Vasomotor — *see* condition
Vasoplasty, after previous sterilization Z31.0
  aftercare Z31.42
Vasospasm (vasoconstriction) I73.9
  cerebral (cerebrovascular) (artery) I67.848
    reversible I67.841
  coronary I20.1
  nerve
    arm — *see* Mononeuropathy, upper limb
    brachial plexus G54.0
    cervical plexus G54.2
    leg — *see* Mononeuropathy, lower limb
  peripheral NOS I73.9
  retina (artery) — *see* Occlusion, artery, retina
Vasospastic — *see* condition
Vasovagal attack (paroxysmal) R55
  psychogenic F45.8
VATER syndrome Q87.2
Vater's ampulla — *see* condition
Vegetation, vegetative
  adenoid (nasal fossa) J35.8
  endocarditis (acute) (any valve) (subacute) I33.0
  heart (mycotic) (valve) I33.0
Veil
  Jackson's Q43.3
Vein, venous — *see* condition
Veldt sore — *see* Ulcer, skin
Velpeau's hernia — *see* Hernia, femoral
Venereal
  bubo A55
  disease A64
  granuloma inguinale A58
  lymphogranuloma (Durand-Nicolas-Favre) A55
Venofibrosis I87.8
Venom, venomous — *see* Table of Drugs and Chemical, by animal or substance, poisoning
Venous — *see* condition
Ventilator lung, newborn P27.8
Ventral — *see* condition
Ventricle, ventricular — *see also* condition
  escape I49.3
  inversion Q20.5
Ventriculitis (cerebral) — *see also* Encephalitis G04.90
Ventriculostomy status Z98.2
Vernet's syndrome G52.7
Verneuil's disease (syphilitic bursitis) A52.78
Verruca (due to HPV) (filiformis) (simplex) (viral) (vulgaris) B07.9
  acuminata A63.0
  necrogenica (primary) (tuberculosa) A18.4
  plana B07.8
  plantaris B07.0
  seborrheica L82.1
    inflamed L82.0
  senile (seborrheic) L82.1
    inflamed L82.0
  tuberculosa (primary) A18.4
  venereal A63.0
Verrucosities — *see* Verruca
Verruga peruana, peruviana A44.1
Version
  with extraction
  cervix — *see* Malposition, uterus
  uterus (postinfectional) (postpartal, old) — *see* Malposition, uterus
Vertebra, vertebral — *see* condition
Vertical talus (congenital) Q66.80
  left foot Q66.82
  right foot Q66.81
Vertigo R42
  auditory — *see* Vertigo, aural
  aural H81.31- ☑

☑ **Additional Character Required** — **Refer to the Tabular List for Character Selection**   ▽ **Subterms under main terms may continue to next column or page**

rtigo — *continued*
  benign paroxysmal (positional) H81.1- ☑
  central (origin) H81.4
  cerebral H81.4
  Dix and Hallpike (epidemic) — *see* Neuronitis, vestibular
  due to infrasound T75.23 ☑
  epidemic A88.1
    Dix and Hallpike — *see* Neuronitis, vestibular
    Pedersen's — *see* Neuronitis, vestibular
    vestibular neuronitis — *see* Neuronitis, vestibular
  hysterical F44.89
  infrasound T75.23 ☑
  labyrinthine — *see* subcategory H81.0 ☑
  laryngeal R05
  malignant positional H81.4
  Ménière's — *see* subcategory H81.0 ☑
  menopausal N95.1
  otogenic — *see* Vertigo, aural
  paroxysmal positional, benign — *see* Vertigo, benign paroxysmal
  Pedersen's (epidemic) — *see* Neuronitis, vestibular
  peripheral NEC H81.39- ☑
  positional
    benign paroxysmal — *see* Vertigo, benign paroxysmal
    malignant H81.4
ry-low-density-lipoprotein-type (VLDL) **hyperlipoproteinemia** E78.1
sania — *see* Psychosis
sical — *see* condition
sicle
  cutaneous R23.8
  seminal — *see* condition
  skin R23.8
sicocolic — *see* condition
sicoperineal — *see* condition
sicorectal — *see* condition
sicourethrorectal — *see* condition
sicovaginal — *see* condition
sicular — *see* condition
siculitis (seminal) N49.0
  amebic A06.82
  gonorrheal (acute) (chronic) A54.23
  trichomonal A59.09
  tuberculous A18.15
stibulitis (ear) — *see also* subcategory H83.0 ☑
  nose (external) J34.89
  vulvar N94.810
stibulopathy , acute peripheral (recurrent) — *see* Neuronitis, vestibular
stige, vestigial — *see also* Persistence
  branchial Q18.0
  structures in vitreous Q14.0
bration
  adverse effects T75.20 ☑
    pneumatic hammer syndrome T75.21 ☑
    specified effect NEC T75.29 ☑
    vasospastic syndrome T75.22 ☑
    vertigo from infrasound T75.23 ☑
  exposure (occupational) Z57.7
  vertigo T75.23 ☑
briosis A28.9
ctim (of)
  crime Z65.4
  disaster Z65.5
  terrorism Z65.4
  torture Z65.4
  war Z65.5
dal's disease L28.0
illaret's syndrome G52.7
illous — *see* condition
IN — *see* Neoplasia, intraepithelial, vulva
incent's infection (angina) (gingivitis) A69.1
  stomatitis NEC A69.1
inson-Plummer syndrome D50.1
iolence, physical R45.6
iosterol deficiency — *see* Deficiency, calciferol
ipoma — *see* Neoplasm, malignant, by site
iremia B34.9
irilism (adrenal) E25.9
  congenital E25.0
irilization (female) (suprarenal) E25.9
  congenital E25.0
  isosexual E28.2
irulent bubo A57
irus, viral — *see also* condition

Virus, viral — *continued*
  as cause of disease classified elsewhere B97.89
    respiratory syncytial virus (RSV) — *see* Virus, infection, respiratory syncytial (RSV)
  cytomegalovirus B25.9
  human immunodeficiency (HIV) — *see* Human, immunodeficiency virus (HIV) disease
  infection — *see* Infection, virus
  respiratory syncytial (RSV)
    as cause of disease classified elsewhere B97.4
    bronchiolitis J21.0
    bronchitis J20.5
    bronchopneumonia J12.1
    otitis media H65.- ☑ *[B97.4]*
    pneumonia J12.1
    upper respiratory infection J06.9 *[B97.4]*
  specified NEC B34.8
  swine influenza (viruses that normally cause infections in pigs) — *see also* Influenza, due to, identified novel influenza A virus J09.X2
  West Nile (fever) A92.30
    with
      complications NEC A92.39
      cranial nerve disorders A92.32
      encephalitis A92.31
      encephalomyelitis A92.31
      neurologic manifestation NEC A92.32
      optic neuritis A92.32
      polyradiculitis A92.32
Viscera, visceral — *see* condition
Visceroptosis K63.4
Visible peristalsis R19.2
Vision, visual
  binocular, suppression H53.34
  blurred, blurring H53.8
    hysterical F44.6
  defect, defective NEC H54.7
  disorientation (syndrome) H53.8
  disturbance H53.9
    hysterical F44.6
  double H53.2
  examination Z01.00
    with abnormal findings Z01.01
    following failed vision screening Z01.020
      with abnormal findings Z01.021
  field, limitation (defect) — *see* Defect, visual field
  hallucinations R44.1
  halos H53.19
  loss — *see* Loss, vision
    sudden — *see* Disturbance, vision, subjective, loss, sudden
  low (both eyes) — *see* Low, vision
  perception, simultaneous without fusion H53.33
Vitality, lack or want of R53.83
  newborn P96.89
Vitamin deficiency — *see* Deficiency, vitamin
Vitelline duct, persistent Q43.0
Vitiligo L80
  eyelid H02.739
    left H02.736
      lower H02.735
      upper H02.734
    right H02.733
      lower H02.732
      upper H02.731
  pinta A67.2
  vulva N90.89
Vitreal corneal syndrome H59.01- ☑
Vitreoretinopathy, proliferative — *see also* Retinopathy, proliferative
  with retinal detachment — *see* Detachment, retina, traction
Vitreous — *see also* condition
  touch syndrome — *see* Complication, postprocedural, following cataract surgery
Vocal cord — *see* condition
Vogt-Koyanagi syndrome H20.82- ☑
Vogt's disease or syndrome G80.3
Vogt-Spielmeyer amaurotic idiocy or disease E75.4
Voice
  change R49.9
    specified NEC R49.8
  loss — *see* Aphonia
Volhynian fever A79.0
Volkmann's ischemic contracture or paralysis (complicating trauma) T79.6 ☑
Volvulus (bowel) (colon) (intestine) K56.2
  with perforation K56.2

Volvulus — *continued*
  congenital Q43.8
  duodenum K31.5
  fallopian tube — *see* Torsion, fallopian tube
  oviduct — *see* Torsion, fallopian tube
  stomach (due to absence of gastrocolic ligament) K31.89
Vomiting R11.10
  with nausea R11.2
  asphyxia — *see* Foreign body, by site, causing asphyxia, gastric contents
  bilious (cause unknown) R11.14
    following gastro-intestinal surgery K91.0
    in newborn P92.01
  blood — *see* Hematemesis
  causing asphyxia, choking, or suffocation — *see* Foreign body, by site
  cyclical, in migraine G43.A0 (*following* G43.7)
    with refractory migraine G43.A1 (*following* G43.7)
    intractable G43.A1 (*following* G43.7)
    not intractable G43.A0 (*following* G43.7)
    psychogenic F50.89
    without refractory migraine G43.A0 (*following* G43.7)
  cyclical syndrome NOS (unrelated to migraine) R11.15
  fecal mater R11.13
  following gastrointestinal surgery K91.0
    psychogenic F50.89
  functional K31.89
  hysterical F50.89
  nervous F50.89
  neurotic F50.89
  newborn NEC P92.09
    bilious P92.01
  periodic R11.10
    psychogenic F50.89
  persistent R11.15
  projectile R11.12
  psychogenic F50.89
  uremic — *see* Uremia
  without nausea R11.11
Vomito negro — *see* Fever, yellow
Von Bezold's abscess — *see* Mastoiditis, acute
Von Economo-Cruchet disease A85.8
Von Eulenburg's disease G71.19
Von Gierke's disease E74.01
Von Hippel (-Lindau) **disease or syndrome** Q85.8
Von Jaksch's anemia or disease D64.89
Von Recklinghausen
  disease (neurofibromatosis) Q85.01
  bones E21.0
Von Schroetter's syndrome I82.890
Von Willebrand (-Jurgens)(-Minot) **disease or syndrome** D68.0
Von Zumbusch's disease L40.1
Voyeurism F65.3
Vrolik's disease Q78.0
Vulva — *see* condition
Vulvismus N94.2
Vulvitis (acute) (allergic) (atrophic) (hypertrophic) (intertriginous) (senile) N76.2
  with ectopic or molar pregnancy O08.0
  adhesive, congenital Q52.79
  blennorrhagic (gonococcal) A54.02
  candidal B37.3
  chlamydial A56.02
  due to Haemophilus ducreyi A57
  following ectopic or molar pregnancy O08.0
  gonococcal A54.02
    with abscess (accessory gland) (periurethral) A54.1
  herpesviral A60.04
  leukoplakic N90.4
  monilial B37.3
  puerperal (postpartum) O86.19
  subacute or chronic N76.3
  syphilitic (early) A51.0
    late A52.76
  trichomonal A59.01
  tuberculous A18.18
Vulvodynia N94.819
  specified NEC N94.818
Vulvorectal — *see* condition
Vulvovaginitis (acute) — *see* Vaginitis

W

Waiting list, person on Z75.1
  for organ transplant Z76.82
  undergoing social agency investigation Z75.2

☑ **Additional Character Required** — Refer to the Tabular List for Character Selection   ⬙ Subterms under main terms may continue to next column or pag

Worm(s) (infection) (infestation) — *see also* Infestation, helminth
  guinea B72
  in intestine NEC B82.0
Worm-eaten soles A66.3
Worn out — *see* Exhaustion
Worn
  cardiac
    defibrillator (with synchronous cardiac pacemaker) Z45.02
    pacemaker
      battery Z45.010
      lead Z45.018
  device, implant or graft — *see* Complications, by site, mechanical
Worried well Z71.1
Worries R45.82
Wound check Z48.0- ☑
  due to injury — *code to* Injury, by site, using appropriate seventh character for subsequent encounter
Wound, open T14.8- ☑
  abdomen, abdominal
    wall S31.109 ☑
      with penetration into peritoneal cavity S31.609 ☑
      bite — *see* Bite, abdomen, wall
      epigastric region S31.102 ☑
        with penetration into peritoneal cavity S31.602 ☑
        bite — *see* Bite, abdomen, wall, epigastric region
        laceration — *see* Laceration, abdomen, wall, epigastric region
        puncture — *see* Puncture, abdomen, wall, epigastric region
      laceration — *see* Laceration, abdomen, wall
      left
        lower quadrant S31.104 ☑
          with penetration into peritoneal cavity S31.604 ☑
          bite — *see* Bite, abdomen, wall, left, lower quadrant
          laceration — *see* Laceration, abdomen, wall, left, lower quadrant
          puncture — *see* Puncture, abdomen, wall, left, lower quadrant
        upper quadrant S31.101 ☑
          with penetration into peritoneal cavity S31.601 ☑
          bite — *see* Bite, abdomen, wall, left, upper quadrant
          laceration — *see* Laceration, abdomen, wall, left, upper quadrant
          puncture — *see* Puncture, abdomen, wall, left, upper quadrant
      periumbilic region S31.105 ☑
        with penetration into peritoneal cavity S31.605 ☑
        bite — *see* Bite, abdomen, wall, periumbilic region
        laceration — *see* Laceration, abdomen, wall, periumbilic region
        puncture — *see* Puncture, abdomen, wall, periumbilic region
      puncture — *see* Puncture, abdomen, wall
      right
        lower quadrant S31.103 ☑
          with penetration into peritoneal cavity S31.603 ☑
          bite — *see* Bite, abdomen, wall, right, lower quadrant
          laceration — *see* Laceration, abdomen, wall, right, lower quadrant
          puncture — *see* Puncture, abdomen, wall, right, lower quadrant
        upper quadrant S31.100 ☑
          with penetration into peritoneal cavity S31.600 ☑
          bite — *see* Bite, abdomen, wall, right, upper quadrant
          laceration — *see* Laceration, abdomen, wall, right, upper quadrant
          puncture — *see* Puncture, abdomen, wall, right, upper quadrant
  alveolar (process) — *see* Wound, open, oral cavity
  ankle S91.00- ☑
    bite — *see* Bite, ankle
    laceration — *see* Laceration, ankle

Wound, open — *continued*
  ankle — *continued*
    puncture — *see* Puncture, ankle
  antecubital space — *see* Wound, open, elbow
  anterior chamber, eye — *see* Wound, open, ocular
  anus S31.839 ☑
    bite S31.835 ☑
    laceration — *see* Laceration, anus
    puncture — *see* Puncture, anus
  arm (upper) S41.10- ☑
    with amputation — *see* Amputation, traumatic, arm
    bite — *see* Bite, arm
    forearm — *see* Wound, open, forearm
    laceration — *see* Laceration, arm
    puncture — *see* Puncture, arm
  auditory canal (external) (meatus) — *see* Wound, open, ear
  auricle, ear — *see* Wound, open, ear
  axilla — *see* Wound, open, arm
  back — *see also* Wound, open, thorax, back
    lower S31.000 ☑
      with penetration into retroperitoneal space S31.001 ☑
      bite — *see* Bite, back, lower
      laceration — *see* Laceration, back, lower
      puncture — *see* Puncture, back, lower
  bite — *see* Bite
  blood vessel — *see* Injury, blood vessel
  breast S21.00- ☑
    with amputation — *see* Amputation, traumatic, breast
    bite — *see* Bite, breast
    laceration — *see* Laceration, breast
    puncture — *see* Puncture, breast
  buttock S31.809 ☑
    bite — *see* Bite, buttock
    laceration — *see* Laceration, buttock
    left S31.829 ☑
    puncture — *see* Puncture, buttock
    right S31.819 ☑
  calf — *see* Wound, open, leg
  canaliculus lacrimalis — *see* Wound, open, eyelid
  canthus, eye — *see* Wound, open, eyelid
  cervical esophagus S11.20 ☑
    bite S11.25 ☑
    laceration — *see* Laceration, esophagus, traumatic, cervical
    puncture — *see* Puncture, cervical esophagus
  cheek (external) S01.40- ☑
    bite — *see* Bite, cheek
    internal — *see* Wound, open, oral cavity
    laceration — *see* Laceration, cheek
    puncture — *see* Puncture, cheek
  chest wall — *see* Wound, open, thorax
  chin — *see* Wound, open, head, specified site NEC
  choroid — *see* Wound, open, ocular
  ciliary body (eye) — *see* Wound, open, ocular
  clitoris S31.40 ☑
    with amputation — *see* Amputation, traumatic, clitoris
    bite S31.45 ☑
    laceration — *see* Laceration, vulva
    puncture — *see* Puncture, vulva
  conjunctiva — *see* Wound, open, ocular
  cornea — *see* Wound, open, ocular
  costal region — *see* Wound, open, thorax
  Descemet's membrane — *see* Wound, open, ocular
  digit(s)
    foot — *see* Wound, open, toe
    hand — *see* Wound, open, finger
  ear (canal) (external) S01.30- ☑
    with amputation — *see* Amputation, traumatic, ear
    bite — *see* Bite, ear
    drum S09.2- ☑
    laceration — *see* Laceration, ear
    puncture — *see* Puncture, ear
  elbow S51.00- ☑
    bite — *see* Bite, elbow
    laceration — *see* Laceration, elbow
    puncture — *see* Puncture, elbow
  epididymis — *see* Wound, open, testis
  epigastric region S31.102 ☑
    with penetration into peritoneal cavity S31.602 ☑
    bite — *see* Bite, abdomen, wall, epigastric region
    laceration — *see* Laceration, abdomen, wall, epigastric region

Wound, open — *continued*
  epigastric region — *continued*
    puncture — *see* Puncture, abdomen, wall, epigastric region
  epiglottis — *see* Wound, open, neck, specified site NEC
  esophagus (thoracic) S27.819 ☑
    cervical — *see* Wound, open, cervical esophagus
    laceration S27.813 ☑
    specified type NEC S27.818 ☑
  eye — *see* Wound, open, ocular
  eyeball — *see* Wound, open, ocular
  eyebrow — *see* Wound, open, eyelid
  eyelid S01.10- ☑
    bite — *see* Bite, eyelid
    laceration — *see* Laceration, eyelid
    puncture — *see* Puncture, eyelid
  face NEC — *see* Wound, open, head, specified site NEC
  finger(s) S61.209 ☑
    with
      amputation — *see* Amputation, traumatic, finger
      damage to nail S61.309 ☑
    bite — *see* Bite, finger
    index S61.208 ☑
      with
        damage to nail S61.308 ☑
      left S61.201 ☑
        with
          damage to nail S61.301 ☑
      right S61.200 ☑
        with
          damage to nail S61.300 ☑
    laceration — *see* Laceration, finger
    little S61.208 ☑
      with
        damage to nail S61.308 ☑
      left S61.207 ☑
        with damage to nail S61.307 ☑
      right S61.206 ☑
        with damage to nail S61.306 ☑
    middle S61.208 ☑
      with
        damage to nail S61.308 ☑
      left S61.203 ☑
        with damage to nail S61.303 ☑
      right S61.202 ☑
        with damage to nail S61.302 ☑
    puncture — *see* Puncture, finger
    ring S61.208 ☑
      with
        damage to nail S61.308 ☑
      left S61.205 ☑
        with damage to nail S61.305 ☑
      right S61.204 ☑
        with damage to nail S61.304 ☑
  flank — *see* Wound, open, abdomen, wall
  foot (except toe(s) alone) S91.30- ☑
    with amputation — *see* Amputation, traumatic, foot
    bite — *see* Bite, foot
    laceration — *see* Laceration, foot
    puncture — *see* Puncture, foot
    toe — *see* Wound, open, toe
  forearm S51.80- ☑
    with
      amputation — *see* Amputation, traumatic, forearm
    bite — *see* Bite, forearm
    elbow only — *see* Wound, open, elbow
    laceration — *see* Laceration, forearm
    puncture — *see* Puncture, forearm
  forehead — *see* Wound, open, head, specified site NEC
  genital organs, external
    with amputation — *see* Amputation, traumatic, genital organs
    bite — *see* Bite, genital organ
    female S31.502 ☑
      vagina S31.40 ☑
      vulva S31.40 ☑
    laceration — *see* Laceration, genital organ
    male S31.501 ☑
      penis S31.20 ☑
      scrotum S31.30 ☑
      testes S31.30 ☑
    puncture — *see* Puncture, genital organ
  globe (eye) — *see* Wound, open, ocular
  groin — *see* Wound, open, abdomen, wall
  gum — *see* Wound, open, oral cavity

↳ **Subterms under main terms may continue to next column or page**   ☑ **Additional Character Required** — **Refer to the Tabular List for Character Selection**   **327**

Worm(s) — Wound, open

Wound, open — *continued*
  hand S61.40- ☑
    with
      amputation — *see* Amputation, traumatic, hand
    bite — *see* Bite, hand
    finger(s) — *see* Wound, open, finger
    laceration — *see* Laceration, hand
    puncture — *see* Puncture, hand
    thumb — *see* Wound, open, thumb
  head S01.90 ☑
    bite — *see* Bite, head
    cheek — *see* Wound, open, cheek
    ear — *see* Wound, open, ear
    eyelid — *see* Wound, open, eyelid
    laceration — *see* Laceration, head
    lip — *see* Wound, open, lip
    nose S01.20 ☑
    oral cavity — *see* Wound, open, oral cavity
    puncture — *see* Puncture, head
    scalp — *see* Wound, open, scalp
    specified site NEC S01.80 ☑
    temporomandibular area — *see* Wound, open, cheek
  heel — *see* Wound, open, foot
  hip S71.00- ☑
    with amputation — *see* Amputation, traumatic, hip
    bite — *see* Bite, hip
    laceration — *see* Laceration, hip
    puncture — *see* Puncture, hip
  hymen S31.40 ☑
    bite — *see* Bite, vulva
    laceration — *see* Laceration, vagina
    puncture — *see* Puncture, vagina
  hypochondrium S31.109 ☑
    bite — *see* Bite, hypochondrium
    laceration — *see* Laceration, hypochondrium
    puncture — *see* Puncture, hypochondrium
  hypogastric region S31.109 ☑
    bite — *see* Bite, hypogastric region
    laceration — *see* Laceration, hypogastric region
    puncture — *see* Puncture, hypogastric region
  iliac (region) — *see* Wound, open, inguinal region
  inguinal region S31.109 ☑
    bite — *see* Bite, abdomen, wall, lower quadrant
    laceration — *see* Laceration, inguinal region
    puncture — *see* Puncture, inguinal region
  instep — *see* Wound, open, foot
  interscapular region — *see* Wound, open, thorax, back
  intraocular — *see* Wound, open, ocular
  iris — *see* Wound, open, ocular
  jaw — *see* Wound, open, head, specified site NEC
  knee S81.00- ☑
    bite — *see* Bite, knee
    laceration — *see* Laceration, knee
    puncture — *see* Puncture, knee
  labium (majus) (minus) — *see* Wound, open, vulva
  laceration — *see* Laceration, by site
  lacrimal duct — *see* Wound, open, eyelid
  larynx S11.019 ☑
    bite — *see* Bite, larynx
    laceration — *see* Laceration, larynx
    puncture — *see* Puncture, larynx
  left
    lower quadrant S31.104 ☑
      with penetration into peritoneal cavity
        S31.604 ☑
      bite — *see* Bite, abdomen, wall, left, lower
        quadrant
      laceration — *see* Laceration, abdomen, wall, left,
        lower quadrant
      puncture — *see* Puncture, abdomen, wall, left,
        lower quadrant
    upper quadrant S31.101 ☑
      with penetration into peritoneal cavity
        S31.601 ☑
      bite — *see* Bite, abdomen, wall, left, upper
        quadrant
      laceration — *see* Laceration, abdomen, wall, left,
        upper quadrant
      puncture — *see* Puncture, abdomen, wall, left,
        upper quadrant
  leg (lower) S81.80- ☑
    with amputation — *see* Amputation, traumatic, leg
    ankle — *see* Wound, open, ankle
    bite — *see* Bite, leg
    foot — *see* Wound, open, foot

Wound, open — *continued*
  leg — *continued*
    knee — *see* Wound, open, knee
    laceration — *see* Laceration, leg
    puncture — *see* Puncture, leg
    toe — *see* Wound, open, toe
    upper — *see* Wound, open, thigh
  lip S01.501 ☑
    bite — *see* Bite, lip
    laceration — *see* Laceration, lip
    puncture — *see* Puncture, lip
  loin S31.109 ☑
    bite — *see* Bite, abdomen, wall
    laceration — *see* Laceration, loin
    puncture — *see* Puncture, loin
  lower back — *see* Wound, open, back, lower
  lumbar region — *see* Wound, open, back, lower
  malar region — *see* Wound, open, head, specified site
    NEC
  mammary — *see* Wound, open, breast
  mastoid region — *see* Wound, open, head, specified
    site NEC
  mouth — *see* Wound, open, oral cavity
  nail
    finger — *see* Wound, open, finger, with damage to
      nail
    toe — *see* Wound, open, toe, with damage to nail
  nape (neck) — *see* Wound, open, neck
  nasal (septum) (sinus) — *see* Wound, open, nose
  nasopharynx — *see* Wound, open, head, specified site
    NEC
  neck S11.90 ☑
    bite — *see* Bite, neck
    involving
      cervical esophagus S11.20 ☑
      larynx — *see* Wound, open, larynx
      pharynx S11.20 ☑
      thyroid S11.10 ☑
      trachea (cervical) S11.029 ☑
        bite — *see* Bite, trachea
        laceration S11.021 ☑
          with foreign body S11.022 ☑
        puncture S11.023 ☑
          with foreign body S11.024 ☑
    laceration — *see* Laceration, neck
    puncture — *see* Puncture, neck
    specified site NEC S11.80 ☑
      specified type NEC S11.89 ☑
  nose (septum) (sinus) S01.20 ☑
    with amputation — *see* Amputation, traumatic,
      nose
    bite — *see* Bite, nose
    laceration — *see* Laceration, nose
    puncture — *see* Puncture, nose
  ocular S05.90 ☑
    avulsion (traumatic enucleation) S05.7- ☑
    eyeball S05.6- ☑
      with foreign body S05.5- ☑
    eyelid — *see* Wound, open, eyelid
    laceration and rupture S05.3- ☑
      with prolapse or loss of intraocular tissue
        S05.2- ☑
    orbit (penetrating) (with or without foreign body)
      S05.4- ☑
    periocular area — *see* Wound, open, eyelid
    specified NEC S05.8X- ☑
  oral cavity S01.502 ☑
    bite S01.552 ☑
    laceration — *see* Laceration, oral cavity
    puncture — *see* Puncture, oral cavity
  orbit — *see* Wound, open, ocular, orbit
  palate — *see* Wound, open, oral cavity
  palm — *see* Wound, open, hand
  pelvis, pelvic — *see also* Wound, open, back, lower
    girdle — *see* Wound, open, hip
  penetrating — *see* Puncture, by site
  penis S31.20 ☑
    with amputation — *see* Amputation, traumatic,
      penis
    bite S31.25 ☑
    laceration — *see* Laceration, penis
    puncture — *see* Puncture, penis
  perineum
    bite — *see* Bite, perineum
    female S31.502 ☑
    laceration — *see* Laceration, perineum

Wound, open — *continued*
  perineum — *continued*
    male S31.501 ☑
    puncture — *see* Puncture, perineum
  periocular area (with or without lacrimal passages) —
    see Wound, open, eyelid
  periumbilic region S31.105 ☑
    with penetration into peritoneal cavity S31.605 ☑
    bite — *see* Bite, abdomen, wall, periumbilic regi
    laceration — *see* Laceration, abdomen, wall, pe
      umbilic region
    puncture — *see* Puncture, abdomen, wall, periu
      bilic region
  phalanges
    finger — *see* Wound, open, finger
    toe — *see* Wound, open, toe
  pharynx S11.20 ☑
  pinna — *see* Wound, open, ear
  popliteal space — *see* Wound, open, knee
  prepuce — *see* Wound, open, penis
  pubic region — *see* Wound, open, back, lower
  pudendum — *see* Wound, open, genital organs, ext
    nal
  puncture wound — *see* Puncture
  rectovaginal septum — *see* Wound, open, vagina
  right
    lower quadrant S31.103 ☑
      with penetration into peritoneal cavity
        S31.603 ☑
      bite — *see* Bite, abdomen, wall, right, lower
        quadrant
      laceration — *see* Laceration, abdomen, wall,
        right, lower quadrant
      puncture — *see* Puncture, abdomen, wall, rig
        lower quadrant
    upper quadrant S31.100 ☑
      with penetration into peritoneal cavity
        S31.600 ☑
      bite — *see* Bite, abdomen, wall, right, upper
        quadrant
      laceration — *see* Laceration, abdomen, wall,
        right, upper quadrant
      puncture — *see* Puncture, abdomen, wall, rig
        upper quadrant
  sacral region — *see* Wound, open, back, lower
  sacroiliac region — *see* Wound, open, back, lower
  salivary gland — *see* Wound, open, oral cavity
  scalp S01.00 ☑
    bite S01.05 ☑
    laceration — *see* Laceration, scalp
    puncture — *see* Puncture, scalp
  scalpel, newborn (birth injury) P15.8
  scapular region — *see* Wound, open, shoulder
  sclera — *see* Wound, open, ocular
  scrotum S31.30 ☑
    with amputation — *see* Amputation, traumatic,
      scrotum
    bite S31.35 ☑
    laceration — *see* Laceration, scrotum
    puncture — *see* Puncture, scrotum
  shin — *see* Wound, open, leg
  shoulder S41.00- ☑
    with amputation — *see* Amputation, traumatic, a
    bite — *see* Bite, shoulder
    laceration — *see* Laceration, shoulder
    puncture — *see* Puncture, shoulder
  skin NOS T14.8 ☑
  spermatic cord — *see* Wound, open, testis
  sternal region — *see* Wound, open, thorax, front wa
  submaxillary region — *see* Wound, open, head, spe
    fied site NEC
  submental region — *see* Wound, open, head, specifi
    site NEC
  subungual
    finger(s) — *see* Wound, open, finger
    toe(s) — *see* Wound, open, toe
  supraclavicular region — *see* Wound, open, neck,
    specified site NEC
  temple, temporal region — *see* Wound, open, head
    specified site NEC
  temporomandibular area — *see* Wound, open, chee
  testis S31.30 ☑
    with amputation — *see* Amputation, traumatic,
      testes
    bite S31.35 ☑
    laceration — *see* Laceration, testis
    puncture — *see* Puncture, testis

☑ **Additional Character Required — Refer to the Tabular List for Character Selection**   ▽ **Subterms under main terms may continue to next column or pag**

Wound, open — *continued*
thigh S71.10- ☑
  with amputation — *see* Amputation, traumatic, hip
  bite — *see* Bite, thigh
  laceration — *see* Laceration, thigh
  puncture — *see* Puncture, thigh
thorax, thoracic (wall) S21.90 ☑
  back S21.20- ☑
    with penetration S21.40 ☑
  bite — *see* Bite, thorax
  breast — *see* Wound, open, breast
  front S21.10- ☑
    with penetration S21.30 ☑
  laceration — *see* Laceration, thorax
  puncture — *see* Puncture, thorax
  throat — *see* Wound, open, neck
thumb S61.009 ☑
  with
    amputation — *see* Amputation, traumatic, thumb
    damage to nail S61.109 ☑
  bite — *see* Bite, thumb
  laceration — *see* Laceration, thumb
  left S61.002 ☑
    with
      damage to nail S61.102 ☑
  puncture — *see* Puncture, thumb
  right S61.001 ☑
    with
      damage to nail S61.101 ☑
thyroid (gland) — *see* Wound, open, neck, thyroid
toe(s) S91.109 ☑
  with
    amputation — *see* Amputation, traumatic, toe
    damage to nail S91.209 ☑
  bite — *see* Bite, toe
  great S91.103 ☑
    with
      damage to nail S91.203 ☑
    left S91.102 ☑
      with
        damage to nail S91.202 ☑
    right S91.101 ☑
      with
        damage to nail S91.201 ☑
  laceration — *see* Laceration, toe
  lesser S91.106 ☑
    with
      damage to nail S91.206 ☑
    left S91.105 ☑
      with
        damage to nail S91.205 ☑
    right S91.104 ☑
      with
        damage to nail S91.204 ☑
  puncture — *see* Puncture, toe
tongue — *see* Wound, open, oral cavity
trachea (cervical region) — *see* Wound, open, neck, trachea
tunica vaginalis — *see* Wound, open, testis
tympanum, tympanic membrane S09.2- ☑
  laceration — *see* Laceration, ear, drum
  puncture — *see* Puncture, tympanum
umbilical region — *see* Wound, open, abdomen, wall, periumbilic region
uvula — *see* Wound, open, oral cavity
vagina S31.40 ☑
  bite S31.45 ☑
  laceration — *see* Laceration, vagina
  puncture — *see* Puncture, vagina
vitreous (humor) — *see* Wound, open, ocular
vocal cord S11.039 ☑
  bite — *see* Bite, vocal cord
  laceration S11.031 ☑
    with foreign body S11.032 ☑
  puncture S11.033 ☑
    with foreign body S11.034 ☑
vulva S31.40 ☑
  with amputation — *see* Amputation, traumatic, vulva
  bite S31.45 ☑
  laceration — *see* Laceration, vulva
  puncture — *see* Puncture, vulva
wrist S61.50- ☑
  bite — *see* Bite, wrist

Wound, open — *continued*
wrist — *continued*
  laceration — *see* Laceration, wrist
  puncture — *see* Puncture, wrist
Wound, superficial — *see* Injury — *see also* specified injury type
Wright's syndrome G54.0
Wrist — *see* condition
Wrong drug (by accident) (given in error) — *see* Table of Drugs and Chemicals, by drug, poisoning
Wry neck — *see* Torticollis
Wuchereria (bancrofti) **infestation** B74.0
Wuchereriasis B74.0
Wuchernde Struma Langhans C73

X

Xanthelasma (eyelid) (palpebrarum) H02.60
  left H02.66
    lower H02.65
    upper H02.64
  right H02.63
    lower H02.62
    upper H02.61
Xanthelasmatosis (essential) E78.2
Xanthinuria, hereditary E79.8
Xanthoastrocytoma
  specified site — *see* Neoplasm, malignant, by site
  unspecified site C71.9
Xanthofibroma — *see* Neoplasm, connective tissue, benign
Xanthogranuloma D76.3
Xanthoma(s), xanthomatosis (primary) (familial) (hereditary) E75.5
  with
    hyperlipoproteinemia
      Type I E78.3
      Type III E78.2
      Type IV E78.1
      Type V E78.3
  bone (generalisata) C96.5
  cerebrotendinous E75.5
  cutaneotendinous E75.5
  disseminatum (skin) E78.2
  eruptive E78.2
  hypercholesterinemic E78.00
  hypercholesterolemic E78.00
  hyperlipidemic E78.5
  joint E75.5
  multiple (skin) E78.2
  tendon (sheath) E75.5
  tuberosum E78.2
  tuberous E78.2
  tubo-eruptive E78.2
  verrucous, oral mucosa K13.4
Xanthosis R23.8
Xenophobia F40.10
Xeroderma — *see also* Ichthyosis
  acquired L85.0
  eyelid H01.149
    left H01.146
      lower H01.145
      upper H01.144
    right H01.143
      lower H01.142
      upper H01.141
  pigmentosum Q82.1
  vitamin A deficiency E50.8
Xerophthalmia (vitamin A deficiency) E50.7
  unrelated to vitamin A deficiency — *see* Keratoconjunctivitis
Xerosis
  conjunctiva H11.14- ☑
    with Bitot's spots — *see also* Pigmentation, conjunctiva
      vitamin A deficiency E50.1
    vitamin A deficiency E50.0
  cornea H18.89- ☑
    with ulceration — *see* Ulcer, cornea
      vitamin A deficiency E50.3
    vitamin A deficiency E50.2
  cutis L85.3
  skin L85.3
Xerostomia K11.7
Xiphopagus Q89.4
XO syndrome Q96.9

X-ray (of)
  abnormal findings — *see* Abnormal, diagnostic imaging
  breast (mammogram) (routine) Z12.31
  chest
    routine (as part of a general medical examination) Z00.00
      with abnormal findings Z00.01
  routine (as part of a general medical examination) Z00.00
    with abnormal findings Z00.01
XXXXY syndrome Q98.1
XXY syndrome Q98.0

Y

Yaba pox (virus disease) B08.72
Yatapoxvirus B08.70
  specified NEC B08.79
Yawning R06.89
  psychogenic F45.8
Yaws A66.9
  bone lesions A66.6
  butter A66.1
  chancre A66.0
  cutaneous, less than five years after infection A66.2
  early (cutaneous) (macular) (maculopapular) (micropapular) (papular) A66.2
    frambeside A66.2
    skin lesions NEC A66.2
  eyelid A66.2
  ganglion A66.6
  gangosis, gangosa A66.5
  gumma, gummata A66.4
    bone A66.6
  gummatous
    frambeside A66.4
    osteitis A66.6
    periostitis A66.6
  hydrarthrosis — *see also* subcategory M14.8- A66.6
  hyperkeratosis (early) (late) A66.3
  initial lesions A66.0
  joint lesions — *see also* subcategory M14.8- A66.6
  juxta-articular nodules A66.7
  late nodular (ulcerated) A66.4
  latent (without clinical manifestations) (with positive serology) A66.8
  mother A66.0
  mucosal A66.7
  multiple papillomata A66.1
  nodular, late (ulcerated) A66.4
  osteitis A66.6
  papilloma, plantar or palmar A66.1
  periostitis (hypertrophic) A66.6
  specified NEC A66.7
  ulcers A66.4
  wet crab A66.1
Yeast infection — *see also* Candidiasis B37.9
Yellow
  atrophy (liver) — *see* Failure, hepatic
  fever — *see* Fever, yellow
  jack — *see* Fever, yellow
  jaundice — *see* Jaundice
  nail syndrome L60.5
Yersiniosis — *see also* Infection, Yersinia
  extraintestinal A28.2
  intestinal A04.6

Z

Zahorsky's syndrome (herpangina) B08.5
Zellweger's syndrome E71.510
Zenker's diverticulum (esophagus) K22.5
Ziehen-Oppenheim disease G24.1
Zieve's syndrome K70.0
Zika NOS A92.5
  congenital P35.4
Zinc
  deficiency, dietary E60
  metabolism disorder E83.2
Zollinger-Ellison syndrome E16.4
Zona — *see* Herpes, zoster
Zoophobia F40.218
Zoster (herpes) — *see* Herpes, zoster
Zygomycosis B46.9
  specified NEC B46.8
Zymotic — *see* condition

Note: The list below gives the code number for neoplasms by anatomical site. For each site there are six possible code numbers according to whether the neoplasm in question is malignant, benign, in situ, of uncertain behavior, or of unspecified nature. The description of the neoplasm will often indicate which of the six columns is appropriate; e.g., malignant melanoma of skin, benign fibroadenoma of breast, carcinoma in situ of cervix uteri. Where such descriptors are not present, the remainder of the Index should be consulted where guidance is given to the appropriate column for each morphological (histological) variety listed; e.g., Mesonephroma – see Neoplasm, malignant; Embryoma — see also Neoplasm, uncertain behavior; Disease, Bowen's – see Neoplasm, skin, in situ. However, the guidance in the Index can be overridden if one of the descriptors mentioned above is present; e.g., malignant adenoma of colon is coded to C18.9 and not to D12.6 as the adjective "malignant" overrides the Index entry "Adenoma — see also Neoplasm, benign, by site." Codes listed with a dash -, following the code have a required additional character for laterality. The tabular list must be reviewed for the complete code.

	Malignant Primary	Malignant Secondary	Ca in situ	Benign	Uncertain Behavior	Unspecified Behavior
Neoplasm, neoplastic	C80.1	C79.9	D09.9	D36.9	D48.9	D49.9
abdomen, abdominal	C76.2	C79.8-✓	D09.8	D36.7	D48.7	D49.89
cavity	C76.2	C79.8-✓	D09.8	D36.7	D48.7	D49.89
organ	C76.2	C79.8-✓	D09.8	D36.7	D48.7	D49.89
viscera	C76.2	C79.8-✓	D09.8	D36.7	D48.7	D49.89
wall — see also Neoplasm, abdomen, wall, skin	C44.509	C79.2	D04.5	D23.5	D48.5	D49.2
connective tissue	C49.4	C79.8-✓	—	D21.4	D48.1	D49.2
skin	C44.509	—	—	—	—	—
basal cell carcinoma	C44.519	—	—	—	—	—
specified type NEC	C44.599	—	—	—	—	—
squamous cell carcinoma	C44.529	—	—	—	—	—
abdominopelvic	C76.8	C79.8-✓		D36.7	D48.7	D49.89
accessory sinus — see Neoplasm, sinus						
acoustic nerve	C72.4-✓	C79.49		D33.3	D43.3	D49.7
adenoid (pharynx) (tissue)	C11.1	C79.89	D00.08	D10.6	D37.05	D49.0
adipose tissue — see also Neoplasm, connective tissue	C49.4	C79.89	—	D21.9	D48.1	D49.2
adnexa (uterine)	C57.4	C79.89	D07.39	D28.7	D39.8	D49.59
adrenal	C74.9-✓	C79.7-✓	D09.3	D35.0-✓	D44.1-✓	D49.7
capsule	C74.9-✓	C79.7-✓	D09.3	D35.0-✓	D44.1-✓	D49.7
cortex	C74.0-✓	C79.7-✓	D09.3	D35.0-✓	D44.1-✓	D49.7
gland	C74.9-✓	C79.7-✓	D09.3	D35.0-✓	D44.1-✓	D49.7
medulla	C74.1-✓	C79.7-✓	D09.3	D35.0-✓	D44.1-✓	D49.7
ala nasi (external) — see also Neoplasm, skin, nose	C44.301	C79.2	D04.39	D23.39	D48.5	D49.2
alimentary canal or tract NEC	C26.9	C78.80	D01.9	D13.9	D37.9	D49.0
alveolar	C03.9	C79.89	D00.03	D10.39	D37.09	D49.0
mucosa	C03.9	C79.89	D00.03	D10.39	D37.09	D49.0
lower	C03.1	C79.89	D00.03	D10.39	D37.09	D49.0
upper	C03.0	C79.89	D00.03	D10.39	D37.09	D49.0
ridge or process	C41.1	C79.51	—	D16.5	D48.0	D49.2
carcinoma	C03.9	C79.8-✓	—	—	—	—
lower	C03.1	C79.8-✓	—	—	—	—
upper	C03.0	C79.8-✓	—	—	—	—
lower	C41.1	C79.51	—	D16.5	D48.0	D49.2
mucosa	C03.9	C79.89	D00.03	D10.39	D37.09	D49.0
lower	C03.1	C79.89	D00.03	D10.39	D37.09	D49.0
upper	C03.0	C79.89	D00.03	D10.39	D37.09	D49.0
upper	C41.0	C79.51	—	D16.4	D48.0	D49.2
sulcus	C06.1	C79.89	D00.02	D10.39	D37.09	D49.0
alveolus	C03.9	C79.89	D00.03	D10.39	D37.09	D49.0
lower	C03.1	C79.89	D00.03	D10.39	D37.09	D49.0
upper	C03.0	C79.89	D00.03	D10.39	D37.09	D49.0
ampulla of Vater	C24.1	C78.89	D01.5	D13.5	D37.6	D49.0
ankle NEC	C76.5-✓	C79.89	D04.7-✓	D36.7	D48.7	D49.89
anorectum, anorectal (junction)	C21.8	C78.5	D01.3	D12.9	D37.8	D49.0
antecubital fossa or space	C76.4-✓	C79.89	D04.6-✓	D36.7	D48.7	D49.89

	Malignant Primary	Malignant Secondary	Ca in situ	Benign	Uncertain Behavior	Unspecified Behavior
Neoplasm, neoplastic — continued						
antrum (Highmore) (maxillary)	C31.0	C78.39	D02.3	D14.0	D38.5	D49.1
pyloric	C16.3	C78.89	D00.2	D13.1	D37.1	D49.0
tympanicum	C30.1	C78.39	D02.3	D14.0	D38.5	D49.1
anus, anal	C21.0	C78.5	D01.3	D12.9	D37.8	D49.0
canal	C21.1	C78.5	D01.3	D12.9	D37.8	D49.0
cloacogenic zone	C21.2	C78.5	D01.3	D12.9	D37.8	D49.0
margin — see also Neoplasm, anus, skin	C44.500	C79.2	D04.5	D23.5	D48.5	D49.2
overlapping lesion with rectosigmoid junction or rectum	C21.8	—	—	—	—	—
skin	C44.500	C79.2	D04.5	D23.5	D48.5	D49.2
basal cell carcinoma	C44.510	—	—	—	—	—
specified type NEC	C44.590	—	—	—	—	—
squamous cell carcinoma	C44.520	—	—	—	—	—
sphincter	C21.1	C78.5	D01.3	D12.9	D37.8	D49.0
aorta (thoracic)	C49.3	C79.89	—	D21.3	D48.1	D49.2
abdominal	C49.4	C79.89	—	D21.4	D48.1	D49.2
aortic body	C75.5	C79.89	—	D35.6	D44.7	D49.7
aponeurosis	C49.9	C79.89	—	D21.9	D48.1	D49.2
palmar	C49.1-✓	C79.89	—	D21.1-✓	D48.1	D49.2
plantar	C49.2-✓	C79.89	—	D21.2-✓	D48.1	D49.2
appendix	C18.1	C78.5	D01.0	D12.1	D37.3	D49.0
arachnoid	C70.9	C79.49	—	D32.9	D42.9	D49.7
cerebral	C70.0	C79.32	—	D32.0	D42.0	D49.7
spinal	C70.1	C79.49	—	D32.1	D42.1	D49.7
areola	C50.0-✓	C79.81	D05-✓	D24-✓	D48.6-✓	D49.3
arm NEC	C76.4-✓	C79.89	D04.6-✓	D36.7	D48.7	D49.89
artery — see Neoplasm, connective tissue						
aryepiglottic fold	C13.1	C79.89	D00.08	D10.7	D37.05	D49.0
hypopharyngeal aspect	C13.1	C79.89	D00.08	D10.7	D37.05	D49.0
laryngeal aspect	C32.1	C78.39	D02.0	D14.1	D38.0	D49.1
marginal zone	C13.1	C79.89	D00.08	D10.7	D37.05	D49.0
arytenoid (cartilage)	C32.3	C78.39	D02.0	D14.1	D38.0	D49.1
fold — see Neoplasm, aryepiglottic						
associated with transplanted organ	C80.2	—	—	—	—	—
atlas	C41.2	C79.51	—	D16.6	D48.0	D49.2
atrium, cardiac	C38.0	C79.89	—	D15.1	D48.7	D49.89
auditory						
canal (external) (skin)	C44.20-✓	C79.2	D04.2-✓	D23.2-✓	D48.5	D49.2
internal	C30.1	C78.39	D02.3	D14.0	D38.5	D49.1
nerve	C72.4-✓	C79.49	—	D33.3	D43.3	D49.7
tube	C30.1	C78.39	D02.3	D14.0	D38.5	D49.1
opening	C11.2	C79.89	D00.08	D10.6	D37.05	D49.0
auricle, ear — see also Neoplasm, skin, ear	C44.20-✓	C79.2	D04.2-✓	D23.2-✓	D48.5	D49.2
auricular canal (external) — see also Neoplasm, skin, ear	C44.20-✓	C79.2	D04.2-✓	D23.2-✓	D48.5	D49.2
internal	C30.1	C78.39	D02.3	D14.0	D38.5	D49.2
autonomic nerve or nervous system NEC (see Neoplasm, nerve, peripheral)						
axilla, axillary	C76.1	C79.89	D09.8	D36.7	D48.7	D49.89
fold — see also Neoplasm, skin, trunk	C44.509	C79.2	D04.5	D23.5	D48.5	D49.2
back NEC	C76.8	C79.89	D04.5	D36.7	D48.7	D49.89
Bartholin's gland	C51.0	C79.82	D07.1	D28.0	D39.8	D49.59
basal ganglia	C71.0	C79.31	—	D33.0	D43.0	D49.6
basis pedunculi	C71.7	C79.31	—	D33.1	D43.1	D49.6
bile or biliary (tract)	C24.9	C78.89	D01.5	D13.5	D37.6	D49.0

☑ **Additional Character Required — Refer to the Tabular List for Character Selection**   ▽ **Subterms under main terms may continue to next column or page**

	Malignant Primary	Malignant Secondary	Ca in situ	Benign	Uncertain Behavior	Unspecified Behavior
Neoplasm, neoplastic						
— *continued*						
bile or biliary —						
continued						
canaliculi (biliferi) (intrahepatic)	C22.1	C78.7	D01.5	D13.4	D37.6	D49.0
canals, interlobular	C22.1	C78.89	D01.5	D13.4	D37.6	D49.0
duct or passage (common) (cystic) (extrahepatic)	C24.0	C78.89	D01.5	D13.5	D37.6	D49.0
interlobular	C22.1	C78.89	D01.5	D13.4	D37.6	D49.0
intrahepatic	C22.1	C78.7	D01.5	D13.4	D37.6	D49.0
and extrahepatic	C24.8	C78.89	D01.5	D13.5	D37.6	D49.0
bladder (urinary)	C67.9	C79.11	D09.0	D30.3	D41.4	D49.4
dome	C67.1	C79.11	D09.0	D30.3	D41.4	D49.4
neck	C67.5	C79.11	D09.0	D30.3	D41.4	D49.4
orifice	C67.9	C79.11	D09.0	D30.3	D41.4	D49.4
ureteric	C67.6	C79.11	D09.0	D30.3	D41.4	D49.4
urethral	C67.5	C79.11	D09.0	D30.3	D41.4	D49.4
overlapping lesion	C67.8	—	—	—	—	—
sphincter	C67.8	C79.11	D09.0	D30.3	D41.4	D49.4
trigone	C67.0	C79.11	D09.0	D30.3	D41.4	D49.4
urachus	C67.7	C79.11	D09.0	D30.3	D41.4	D49.4
wall	C67.9	C79.11	D09.0	D30.3	D41.4	D49.4
anterior	C67.3	C79.11	D09.0	D30.3	D41.4	D49.4
lateral	C67.2	C79.11	D09.0	D30.3	D41.4	D49.4
posterior	C67.4	C79.11	D09.0	D30.3	D41.4	D49.4
blood vessel — *see* Neoplasm, connective tissue						
bone (periosteum)	C41.9	C79.51	—	D16.9-	D48.0	D49.2
acetabulum						
ankle	C40.3-☑	C79.51	—	D16.3-☑	—	—
arm NEC	C40.0-☑	C79.51	—	D16.0-☑	—	—
astragalus	C40.3-☑	C79.51	—	D16.3-☑	—	—
atlas	C41.2	C79.51	—	D16.6	D48.0	D49.2
axis	C41.2	C79.51	—	D16.6	D48.0	D49.2
back NEC	C41.2	C79.51	—	D16.6	D48.0	D49.2
calcaneus	C40.3-☑	C79.51	—	D16.3-☑	—	—
calvarium	C41.0	C79.51	—	D16.4	D48.0	D49.2
carpus (any)	C40.1-☑	C79.51	—	D16.1-☑	—	—
cartilage NEC	C41.9	C79.51	—	D16.9	D48.0	D49.2
clavicle	C41.3	C79.51	—	D16.7	D48.0	D49.2
clivus	C41.0	C79.51	—	D16.4	D48.0	D49.2
coccygeal vertebra	C41.4	C79.51	—	D16.8	D48.0	D49.2
coccyx	C41.4	C79.51	—	D16.8	D48.0	D49.2
costal cartilage	C41.3	C79.51	—	D16.7	D48.0	D49.2
costovertebral joint	C41.3	C79.51	—	D16.7	D48.0	D49.2
cranial	C41.0	C79.51	—	D16.4	D48.0	D49.2
cuboid	C40.3-☑	C79.51	—	D16.3-☑	—	—
cuneiform	C41.9	C79.51	—	D16.9	D48.0	D49.2
elbow	C40.0-☑	C79.51	—	D16.0-☑	—	—
ethmoid (labyrinth)	C41.0	C79.51	—	D16.4	D48.0	D49.2
face	C41.0	C79.51	—	D16.4	D48.0	D49.2
femur (any part)	C40.2-☑	C79.51	—	D16.2-☑	—	—
fibula (any part)	C40.2-☑	C79.51	—	D16.2-☑	—	—
finger (any)	C40.1-☑	C79.51	—	D16.1-☑	—	—
foot	C40.3-☑	C79.51	—	D16.3-☑	—	—
forearm	C40.0-☑	C79.51	—	D16.0-☑	—	—
frontal	C41.0	C79.51	—	D16.4	D48.0	D49.2
hand	C40.1-☑	C79.51	—	D16.1-☑	—	—
heel	C40.3-☑	C79.51	—	D16.3-☑	—	—
hip	C41.4	C79.51	—	D16.8	D48.0	D49.2
humerus (any part)	C40.0-☑	C79.51	—	D16.0-☑	—	—
hyoid	C41.0	C79.51	—	D16.4	D48.0	D49.2
ilium	C41.4	C79.51	—	D16.8	D48.0	D49.2
innominate	C41.4	C79.51	—	D16.8	D48.0	D49.2
intervertebral cartilage or disc	C41.2	C79.51	—	D16.6	D48.0	D49.2
ischium	C41.4	C79.51	—	D16.8	D48.0	D49.2
jaw (lower)	C41.1	C79.51	—	D16.5	D48.0	D49.2
knee	C40.2-☑	C79.51	—	D16.2-☑	—	—
leg NEC	C40.2-☑	C79.51	—	D16.2-☑	—	—
limb NEC	C40.9 ☑	C79.51	—	D16.9	—	—

	Malignant Primary	Malignant Secondary	Ca in situ	Benign	Uncertain Behavior	Unspecified Behavior
Neoplasm, neoplastic						
— *continued*						
bone — *continued*						
limb — *continued*						
lower (long bones)	C40.2-☑	C79.51	—	D16.2-☑	—	—
short bones	C40.3-☑	C79.51	—	D16.3-☑	—	—
upper (long bones)	C40.0-☑	C79.51	—	D16.0-☑	—	—
short bones	C40.1-☑	C79.51	—	D16.1-☑	—	—
malar	C41.0	C79.51	—	D16.4	D48.0	D49.2
mandible	C41.1	C79.51	—	D16.5	D48.0	D49.2
marrow NEC (any bone)	C96.9	C79.52	—	—	D47.9	D49.89
mastoid	C41.0	C79.51	—	D16.4	D48.0	D49.2
maxilla, maxillary (superior)	C41.0	C79.51	—	D16.4	D48.0	D49.2
inferior	C41.1	C79.51	—	D16.5	D48.0	D49.2
metacarpus (any)	C40.1-☑	C79.51	—	D16.1-☑	—	—
metatarsus (any)	C40.3-☑	C79.51	—	D16.3-☑	—	—
navicular						
ankle	C40.3-☑	C79.51	—	—	—	—
hand	C40.1-☑	C79.51	—	—	—	—
nose, nasal	C41.0	C79.51	—	D16.4	D48.0	D49.2
occipital	C41.0	C79.51	—	D16.4	D48.0	D49.2
orbit	C41.0	C79.51	—	D16.4	D48.0	D49.2
overlapping sites	C40.8-☑	—	—	—	—	—
parietal	C41.0	C79.51	—	D16.4	D48.0	D49.2
patella	C40.2-☑	C79.51	—	—	—	—
pelvic	C41.4	C79.51	—	D16.8	D48.0	D49.2
phalanges						
foot	C40.3-☑	C79.51	—	—	—	—
hand	C40.1-☑	C79.51	—	—	—	—
pubic	C41.4	C79.51	—	D16.8	D48.0	D49.2
radius (any part)	C40.0-☑	C79.51	—	D16.0-☑	—	—
rib	C41.3	C79.51	—	D16.7	D48.0	D49.2
sacral vertebra	C41.4	C79.51	—	D16.8	D48.0	D49.2
sacrum	C41.4	C79.51	—	D16.8	D48.0	D49.2
scaphoid						
of ankle	C40.3-☑	C79.51	—	—	—	—
of hand	C40.1-☑	C79.51	—	—	—	—
scapula (any part)	C40.0-☑	C79.51	—	D16.0-☑	—	—
sella turcica	C41.0	C79.51	—	D16.4	D48.0	D49.2
shoulder	C40.0-☑	C79.51	—	D16.0-☑	—	—
skull	C41.0	C79.51	—	D16.4	D48.0	D49.2
sphenoid	C41.0	C79.51	—	D16.4	D48.0	D49.2
spine, spinal (column)	C41.2	C79.51	—	D16.6	D48.0	D49.2
coccyx	C41.4	C79.51	—	D16.8	D48.0	D49.2
sacrum	C41.4	C79.51	—	D16.8	D48.0	D49.2
sternum	C41.3	C79.51	—	D16.7	D48.0	D49.2
tarsus (any)	C40.3-☑	C79.51	—	—	—	—
temporal	C41.0	C79.51	—	D16.4	D48.0	D49.2
thumb	C40.1-☑	C79.51	—	—	—	—
tibia (any part)	C40.2-☑	C79.51	—	—	—	—
toe (any)	C40.3-☑	C79.51	—	—	—	—
trapezium	C40.1-☑	C79.51	—	—	—	—
trapezoid	C40.1-☑	C79.51	—	—	—	—
turbinate	C41.0	C79.51	—	D16.4	D48.0	D49.2
ulna (any part)	C40.0-☑	C79.51	—	D16.0-☑	—	—
unciform	C40.1-☑	C79.51	—	—	—	—
vertebra (column)	C41.2	C79.51	—	D16.6	D48.0	D49.2
coccyx	C41.4	C79.51	—	D16.8	D48.0	D49.2
sacrum	C41.4	C79.51	—	D16.8	D48.0	D49.2
vomer	C41.0	C79.51	—	D16.4	D48.0	D49.2
wrist	C40.1-☑	C79.51	—	—	—	—
xiphoid process	C41.3	C79.51	—	D16.7	D48.0	D49.2
zygomatic	C41.0	C79.51	—	D16.4	D48.0	D49.2
book-leaf (mouth) — *ventral surface of tongue and floor of mouth*	C06.89	C79.89	D00.00	D10.39	D37.09	D49.0
bowel — *see* Neoplasm, intestine						
brachial plexus	C47.1-☑	C79.89	—	D36.12	D48.2	D49.2
brain NEC	C71.9	C79.31	—	D33.2	D43.2	D49.6

Neoplasm, neoplastic	Malignant Primary	Malignant Secondary	Ca in situ	Benign	Uncertain Behavior	Unspecified Behavior
— continued						
brain — continued						
basal ganglia	C71.0	C79.31	—	D33.0	D43.0	D49.6
cerebellopontine angle	C71.6	C79.31	—	D33.1	D43.1	D49.6
cerebellum NOS	C71.6	C79.31	—	D33.1	D43.1	D49.6
cerebrum	C71.0	C79.31	—	D33.0	D43.0	D49.6
choroid plexus	C71.7	C79.31	—	D33.1	D43.1	D49.6
corpus callosum	C71.8	C79.31	—	D33.2	D43.2	D49.6
corpus striatum	C71.0	C79.31	—	D33.0	D43.0	D49.6
cortex (cerebral)	C71.0	C79.31	—	D33.0	D43.0	D49.6
frontal lobe	C71.1	C79.31	—	D33.0	D43.0	D49.6
globus pallidus	C71.0	C79.31	—	D33.0	D43.0	D49.6
hippocampus	C71.2	C79.31	—	D33.0	D43.0	D49.6
hypothalamus	C71.0	C79.31	—	D33.0	D43.0	D49.6
internal capsule	C71.0	C79.31	—	D33.0	D43.0	D49.6
medulla oblongata	C71.7	C79.31	—	D33.1	D43.1	D49.6
meninges	C70.0	C79.32	—	D32.0	D42.0	D49.7
midbrain	C71.7	C79.31	—	D33.1	D43.1	D49.6
occipital lobe	C71.4	C79.31	—	D33.0	D43.0	D49.6
overlapping lesion	C71.8	C79.31	—	—	—	—
parietal lobe	C71.3	C79.31	—	D33.0	D43.0	D49.6
peduncle	C71.7	C79.31	—	D33.1	D43.1	D49.6
pons	C71.7	C79.31	—	D33.1	D43.1	D49.6
stem	C71.7	C79.31	—	D33.1	D43.1	D49.6
tapetum	C71.8	C79.31	—	D33.2	D43.2	D49.6
temporal lobe	C71.2	C79.31	—	D33.0	D43.0	D49.6
thalamus	C71.0	C79.31	—	D33.0	D43.0	D49.6
uncus	C71.2	C79.31	—	D33.0	D43.0	D49.6
ventricle (floor)	C71.5	C79.31	—	D33.0	D43.0	D49.6
fourth	C71.7	C79.31	—	D33.1	D43.1	D49.6
branchial (cleft) (cyst) (vestiges)	C10.4	C79.89	D00.08	D10.5	D37.05	D49.0
breast (connective tissue) (glandular tissue) (soft parts)	C50.9-☑	C79.81	D05.-☑	D24.-☑	D48.6-☑	D49.3
areola	C50.0-☑	C79.81	D05.-☑	D24.-☑	D48.6-☑	D49.3
axillary tail	C50.6-☑	C79.81	D05.-☑	D24.-☑	D48.6-☑	D49.3
central portion	C50.1-☑	C79.81	D05.-☑	D24.-☑	D48.6-☑	D49.3
inner	C50.8-☑	C79.81	D05.-☑	D24.-☑	D48.6-☑	D49.3
lower	C50.8-☑	C79.81	D05.-☑	D24.-☑	D48.6-☑	D49.3
lower-inner quadrant	C50.3-☑	C79.81	D05.-☑	D24.-☑	D48.6-☑	D49.3
lower-outer quadrant	C50.5-☑	C79.81	D05.-☑	D24.-☑	D48.6-☑	D49.3
mastectomy site (skin) — see also Neoplasm, breast, skin	C44.501	C79.2	—	—	—	—
specified as breast tissue	C50.8-☑	C79.81	—	—	—	—
midline	C50.8-☑	C79.81	D05.-☑	D24.-☑	D48.6-☑	D49.3
nipple	C50.0-☑	C79.81	D05.-☑	D24.-☑	D48.6-☑	D49.3
outer	C50.8-☑	C79.81	D05.-☑	D24.-☑	D48.6-☑	D49.3
overlapping lesion	C50.8-☑	—	—	—	—	—
skin	C44.501	C79.2	D04.5	D23.5	D48.5	D49.2
basal cell carcinoma	C44.511	—	—	—	—	—
specified type NEC	C44.591	—	—	—	—	—
squamous cell carcinoma	C44.521	—	—	—	—	—
tail (axillary)	C50.6-☑	C79.81	D05.-☑	D24.-☑	D48.6-☑	D49.3
upper	C50.8-☑	C79.81	D05.-☑	D24.-☑	D48.6-☑	D49.3
upper-inner quadrant	C50.2-☑	C79.81	D05.-☑	D24.-☑	D48.6-☑	D49.3
upper-outer quadrant	C50.4-☑	C79.81	D05.-☑	D24.-☑	D48.6-☑	D49.3
broad ligament	C57.1-☑	C79.82	D07.39	D28.2	D39.8	D49.59
bronchiogenic, bronchogenic (lung)	C34.9-☑	C78.0-☑	D02.2-☑	D14.3-☑	D38.1	D49.1
bronchiole	C34.9-☑	C78.0-☑	D02.2-☑	D14.3-☑	D38.1	D49.1
bronchus	C34.9-☑	C78.0-☑	D02.2-☑	D14.3-☑	D38.1	D49.1
carina	C34.0-☑	C78.0-☑	D02.2-☑	D14.3-☑	D38.1	D49.1
lower lobe of lung	C34.3-☑	C78.0-☑	D02.2-☑	D14.3-☑	D38.1	D49.1

Neoplasm, neoplastic	Malignant Primary	Malignant Secondary	Ca in situ	Benign	Uncertain Behavior	Unspecified Behavior
— continued						
bronchus — continued						
main	C34.0-☑	C78.0-☑	D02.2-☑	D14.3-☑	D38.1	D49.1
middle lobe of lung	C34.2	C78.0-☑	D02.21	D14.31	D38.1	D49.1
overlapping lesion	C34.8-☑	—	—	—	—	—
upper lobe of lung	C34.1-☑	C78.0-☑	D02.2-☑	D14.3-☑	D38.1	D49.1
brow	C44.309	C79.2	D04.39	D23.39	D48.5	D49.2
basal cell carcinoma	C44.319	—	—	—	—	—
specified type NEC	C44.399	—	—	—	—	—
squamous cell carcinoma	C44.329	—	—	—	—	—
buccal (cavity)	C06.9	C79.89	D00.00	D10.39	D37.09	D49.0
commissure	C06.0	C79.89	D00.02	D10.39	D37.09	D49.0
groove (lower) (upper)	C06.1	C79.89	D00.02	D10.39	D37.09	D49.0
mucosa	C06.0	C79.89	D00.02	D10.39	D37.09	D49.0
sulcus (lower) (upper)	C06.1	C79.89	D00.02	D10.39	D37.09	D49.0
bulbourethral gland	C68.0	C79.19	D09.19	D30.4	D41.3	D49.59
bursa — see Neoplasm, connective tissue						
buttock NEC	C76.3	C79.89	D04.5	D36.7	D48.7	D49.89
calf	C76.5-☑	C79.89	D04.7-☑	D36.7	D48.7	D49.89
calvarium	C41.0	C79.51	—	D16.4	D48.0	D49.2
calyx, renal	C65.-☑	C79.0-☑	D09.19	D30.1-☑	D41.1-☑	D49.51-☑
canal						
anal	C21.1	C78.5	D01.3	D12.9	D37.8	D49.0
auditory (external) — see also Neoplasm, skin, ear	C44.20-☑	C79.2	D04.2-☑	D23.2-☑	D48.5	D49.2
auricular (external) — see also Neoplasm, skin, ear	C44.20-☑	C79.2	D04.2-☑	D23.2-☑	D48.5	D49.2
canaliculi, biliary (biliferi) (intrahepatic)	C22.1	C78.7	D01.5	D13.4	D37.6	D49.0
canthus (eye) (inner) (outer)	C44.10-☑	C79.2	D04.1-☑	D23.1-☑	D48.5	D49.2
basal cell carcinoma	C44.11-☑	—	—	—	—	—
sebaceous cell	C44.13-☑	—	—	—	—	—
specified type NEC	C44.19-☑	—	—	—	—	—
squamous cell carcinoma	C44.12-☑	—	—	—	—	—
capillary — see Neoplasm, connective tissue						
caput coli	C18.0	C78.5	D01.0	D12.0	D37.4	D49.0
carcinoid — see Tumor, carcinoid						
cardia (gastric)	C16.0	C78.89	D00.2	D13.1	D37.1	D49.0
cardiac orifice (stomach)	C16.0	C78.89	D00.2	D13.1	D37.1	D49.0
cardio-esophageal junction	C16.0	C78.89	D00.2	D13.1	D37.1	D49.0
cardio-esophagus	C16.0	C78.89	D00.2	D13.1	D37.1	D49.0
carina (bronchus)	C34.0-☑	C78.0-☑	D02.2-☑	D14.3-☑	D38.1	D49.1
carotid (artery)	C49.0	C79.89	—	D21.0	D48.1	D49.2
body	C75.4	C79.89	—	D35.5	D44.6	D49.7
carpus (any bone)	C40.1-☑	C79.51	—	D16.1-☑	—	—
cartilage (articular) (joint) NEC — see also Neoplasm, bone						
arytenoid	C32.3	C78.39	D02.0	D14.1	D38.0	D49.1
auricular	C49.0	C79.89	—	D21.0	D48.1	D49.2
bronchi	C34.0-☑	C78.39	—	D14.3-☑	D38.1	D49.1
costal	C41.3	C79.51	—	D16.7	D48.0	D49.2
cricoid	C32.3	C78.39	D02.0	D14.1	D38.0	D49.1
cuneiform	C32.3	C78.39	D02.0	D14.1	D38.0	D49.1
ear (external)	C49.0	C79.89	—	D21.0	D48.1	D49.2
ensiform	C41.3	C79.51	—	D16.7	D48.0	D49.2
epiglottis	C32.1	C78.39	D02.0	D14.1	D38.0	D49.1

☑ Additional Character Required — Refer to the Tabular List for Character Selection · Subterms under main terms may continue to next column or page

	Malignant Primary	Malignant Secondary	Ca in situ	Benign	Uncertain Behavior	Unspecified Behavior
Neoplasm, neoplastic						
— *continued*						
cartilage — *see also*						
Neoplasm, bone —						
continued						
epiglottis —						
continued						
anterior						
surface	C10.1	C79.89	D00.08	D10.5	D37.05	D49.0
eyelid	C49.0	C79.89	—	D21.0	D48.1	D49.2
intervertebral	C41.2	C79.51		D16.6	D48.0	D49.2
larynx, laryngeal	C32.3	C78.39	D02.0	D14.1	D38.0	D49.1
nose, nasal	C30.0	C78.39	D02.3	D14.0	D38.5	D49.1
pinna	C49.0	C79.89	—	D21.0	D48.1	D49.2
rib	C41.3	C79.51		D16.7	D48.0	D49.2
semilunar						
(knee)	C40.2-☑	C79.51	—	D16.2-☑	D48.0	D49.2
thyroid	C32.3	C78.39	D02.0	D14.1	D38.0	D49.1
trachea	C33	C78.39	D02.1	D14.2	D38.1	D49.1
cauda equina	C72.1	C79.49	—	D33.4	D43.4	D49.7
cavity						
buccal	C06.9	C79.89	D00.00	D10.30	D37.09	D49.0
nasal	C30.0	C78.39	D02.3	D14.0	D38.5	D49.1
oral	C06.9	C79.89	D00.00	D10.30	D37.09	D49.0
peritoneal	C48.2	C78.6	—	D20.1	D48.4	D49.0
tympanic	C30.1	C78.39	D02.3	D14.0	D38.5	D49.1
cecum	C18.0	C78.5	D01.0	D12.0	D37.4	D49.0
central nervous						
system	C72.9	C79.40		—	—	—
cerebellopontine						
(angle)	C71.6	C79.31		D33.1	D43.1	D49.6
cerebellum,						
cerebellar	C71.6	C79.31	—	D33.1	D43.1	D49.6
cerebrum, cerebra						
(cortex)						
(hemisphere)						
(white matter)	C71.0	C79.31	—	D33.0	D43.0	D49.6
meninges	C70.0	C79.32	—	D32.0	D42.0	D49.7
peduncle	C71.7	C79.31	—	D33.1	D43.1	D49.6
ventricle	C71.5	C79.31	—	D33.0	D43.0	D49.6
fourth	C71.7	C79.31	—	D33.1	D43.1	D49.6
cervical region	C76.0	C79.89	D09.8	D36.7	D48.7	D49.89
cervix (cervical) (uteri)						
(uterus)	C53.9	C79.82	D06.9	D26.0	D39.0	D49.59
canal	C53.0	C79.82	D06.0	D26.0	D39.0	D49.59
endocervix (canal)						
(gland)	C53.0	C79.82	D06.0	D26.0	D39.0	D49.59
exocervix	C53.1	C79.82	D06.1	D26.0	D39.0	D49.59
external os	C53.1	C79.82	D06.1	D26.0	D39.0	D49.59
internal os	C53.0	C79.82	D06.0	D26.0	D39.0	D49.59
nabothian gland	C53.0	C79.82	D06.0	D26.0	D39.0	D49.59
overlapping						
lesion	C53.8	—		—	—	—
squamocolumnar						
junction	C53.8	C79.82	D06.7	D26.0	D39.0	D49.59
stump	C53.8	C79.82	D06.7	D26.0	D39.0	D49.59
cheek	C76.0	C79.89	D09.8	D36.7	D48.7	D49.89
external	C44.309	C79.2	D04.39	D23.39	D48.5	D49.2
basal cell						
carcinoma	C44.319	—	—	—	—	—
specified type						
NEC	C44.399	—	—	—	—	—
squamous cell						
carcinoma	C44.329	—	—	—	—	—
inner aspect	C06.0	C79.89	D00.02	D10.39	D37.09	D49.0
internal	C06.0	C79.89	D00.02	D10.39	D37.09	D49.0
mucosa	C06.0	C79.89	D00.02	D10.39	D37.09	D49.0
chest (wall) NEC	C76.1	C79.89	D09.8	D36.7	D48.7	D49.89
chiasma opticum	C72.3-☑	C79.49	—	D33.3	D43.3	D49.7
chin	C44.309	C79.2	D04.39	D23.39	D48.5	D49.2
basal cell						
carcinoma	C44.319	—	—	—	—	—
specified type						
NEC	C44.399	—	—	—	—	—
squamous cell						
carcinoma	C44.329	—	—	—	—	—
choana	C11.3	C79.89	D00.08	D10.6	D37.05	D49.0
cholangiole	C22.1	C78.89	D01.5	D13.4	D37.6	D49.0
choledochal duct	C24.0	C78.89	D01.5	D13.5	D37.6	D49.0
choroid	C69.3-☑	C79.49	D09.2-☑	D31.3-☑	D48.7	D49.81
plexus	C71.5	C79.31	—	D33.0	D43.0	D49.6
ciliary body	C69.4-☑	C79.49	D09.2-☑	D31.4-☑	D48.7	D49.89
clavicle	C41.3	C79.51	—	D16.7	D48.0	D49.2

	Malignant Primary	Malignant Secondary	Ca in situ	Benign	Uncertain Behavior	Unspecified Behavior
Neoplasm, neoplastic						
— *continued*						
clitoris	C51.2	C79.82	D07.1	D28.0	D39.8	D49.59
clivus	C41.0	C79.51	—	D16.4	D48.0	D49.2
cloacogenic zone	C21.2	C78.5	D01.3	D12.9	D37.8	D49.0
coccygeal						
body or glomus	C49.5	C79.89	—	D21.5	D48.1	D49.2
vertebra	C41.4	C79.51	—	D16.8	D48.0	D49.2
coccyx	C41.4	C79.51	—	D16.8	D48.0	D49.2
colon — *see also*						
Neoplasm,						
intestine,						
large	C18.9	C78.5		—	—	—
with rectum	C19	C78.5	D01.1	D12.7	D37.5	D49.0
columnella — *see also*						
Neoplasm, skin,						
face	C44.390	C79.2	D04.39	D23.39	D48.5	D49.2
column, spinal — *see*						
Neoplasm, spine						
commissure						
labial, lip	C00.6	C79.89	D00.01	D10.39	D37.01	D49.0
laryngeal	C32.0	C78.39	D02.0	D14.1	D38.0	D49.1
common (bile)						
duct	C24.0	C78.89	D01.5	D13.5	D37.6	D49.0
concha — *see also*						
Neoplasm, skin,						
ear	C44.20-☑	C79.2	D04.2-☑	D23.2-☑	D48.5	D49.2
nose	C30.0	C78.39	D02.3	D14.0	D38.5	D49.1
conjunctiva	C69.0-☑	C79.49	D09.2-☑	D31.0-☑	D48.7	D49.89
connective tissue						
NEC	C49.9	C79.89	—	D21.9	D48.1	D49.2

> Note: For neoplasms of connective tissue (blood vessel, bursa, fascia, ligament, muscle, peripheral nerves, sympathetic and parasympathetic nerves and ganglia, synovia, tendon, etc.) or of morphological types that indicate connective tissue, code according to the list under "Neoplasm, connective tissue". For sites that do not appear in this list, code to neoplasm of that site; e.g., fibrosarcoma, pancreas (C25.9)

> Note: Morphological types that indicate connective tissue appear in their proper place in the alphabetic index with the instruction "see Neoplasm, connective tissue ...."

	Malignant Primary	Malignant Secondary	Ca in situ	Benign	Uncertain Behavior	Unspecified Behavior
abdomen	C49.4	C79.89	—	D21.4	D48.1	D49.2
abdominal wall	C49.4	C79.89	—	D21.4	D48.1	D49.2
ankle	C49.2-☑	C79.89	—	D21.2-☑	D48.1	D49.2
antecubital fossa or						
space	C49.1-☑	C79.89	—	D21.1-☑	D48.1	D49.2
arm	C49.1-☑	C79.89	—	D21.1-☑	D48.1	D49.2
auricle (ear)	C49.0	C79.89	—	D21.0	D48.1	D49.2
axilla	C49.3	C79.89	—	D21.3	D48.1	D49.2
back	C49.6	C79.89	—	D21.6	D48.1	D49.2
breast — *see*						
Neoplasm,						
breast						
buttock	C49.5	C79.89	—	D21.5	D48.1	D49.2
calf	C49.2-☑	C79.89	—	D21.2-☑	D48.1	D49.2
cervical region	C49.0	C79.89	—	D21.0	D48.1	D49.2
cheek	C49.0	C79.89	—	D21.0	D48.1	D49.2
chest (wall)	C49.3	C79.89	—	D21.3	D48.1	D49.2
chin	C49.0	C79.89	—	D21.0	D48.1	D49.2
diaphragm	C49.3	C79.89	—	D21.3	D48.1	D49.2
ear (external)	C49.0	C79.89	—	D21.0	D48.1	D49.2
elbow	C49.1-☑	C79.89	—	D21.1-☑	D48.1	D49.2
extrarectal	C49.5	C79.89	—	D21.5	D48.1	D49.2
extremity	C49.9	C79.89	—	D21.9	D48.1	D49.2
lower	C49.2-☑	C79.89	—	D21.2-☑	D48.1	D49.2
upper	C49.1-☑	C79.89	—	D21.1-☑	D48.1	D49.2
eyelid	C49.0	C79.89	—	D21.0	D48.1	D49.2
face	C49.0	C79.89	—	D21.0	D48.1	D49.2
finger	C49.1-☑	C79.89	—	D21.1-☑	D48.1	D49.2
flank	C49.6	C79.89	—	D21.6	D48.1	D49.2
foot	C49.2-☑	C79.89	—	D21.2-☑	D48.1	D49.2
forearm	C49.1-☑	C79.89	—	D21.1-☑	D48.1	D49.2
forehead	C49.0	C79.89	—	D21.0	D48.1	D49.2
gastric	C49.4	C79.89	—	D21.4	D48.1	D49.2
gastrointestinal	C49.4	C79.89	—	D21.4	D48.1	D49.2
gluteal region	C49.5	C79.89	—	D21.5	D48.1	D49.2
great vessels						
NEC	C49.3	C79.89	—	D21.3	D48.1	D49.2
groin	C49.5	C79.89	—	D21.5	D48.1	D49.2
hand	C49.1-☑	C79.89	—	D21.1-☑	D48.1	D49.2
head	C49.0	C79.89	—	D21.0	D48.1	D49.2

Neoplasm, neoplastic — continued
connective tissue — continued

	Malignant Primary	Malignant Secondary	Ca in situ	Benign	Uncertain Behavior	Unspecified Behavior
heel	C49.2-☑	C79.89	—	D21.2-☑	D48.1	D49.2
hip	C49.2-☑	C79.89	—	D21.2-☑	D48.1	D49.2
hypochondrium	C49.4	C79.89	—	D21.4	D48.1	D49.2
iliopsoas muscle	C49.5	C79.89	—	D21.5	D48.1	D49.2
infraclavicular region	C49.3	C79.89	—	D21.3	D48.1	D49.2
inguinal (canal) (region)	C49.5	C79.89	—	D21.5	D48.1	D49.2
intestinal	C49.4	C79.89	—	D21.4	D48.1	D49.2
intrathoracic	C49.3	C79.89	—	D21.3	D48.1	D49.2
ischiorectal fossa	C49.5	C79.89	—	D21.5	D48.1	D49.2
jaw	C03.9	C79.89	D00.03	D10.39	D48.1	D49.0
knee	C49.2-☑	C79.89	—	D21.2-☑	D48.1	D49.2
leg	C49.2-☑	C79.89	—	D21.2-☑	D48.1	D49.2
limb NEC	C49.9	C79.89	—	D21.9	D48.1	D49.2
lower	C49.2-☑	C79.89	—	D21.2-☑	D48.1	D49.2
upper	C49.1-☑	C79.89	—	D21.1-☑	D48.1	D49.2
nates	C49.5	C79.89	—	D21.5	D48.1	D49.2
neck	C49.0	C79.89	—	D21.0	D48.1	D49.2
orbit	C69.6-☑	C79.49	D09.2-☑	D31.6-☑	D48.1	D49.89
overlapping lesion	C49.8	—	—	—	—	—
pararectal	C49.5	C79.89	—	D21.5	D48.1	D49.2
para-urethral	C49.5	C79.89	—	D21.5	D48.1	D49.2
paravaginal	C49.5	C79.89	—	D21.5	D48.1	D49.2
pelvis (floor)	C49.5	C79.89	—	D21.5	D48.1	D49.2
pelvo-abdominal	C49.8	C79.89	—	D21.6	D48.1	D49.2
perineum	C49.5	C79.89	—	D21.5	D48.1	D49.2
perirectal (tissue)	C49.5	C79.89	—	D21.5	D48.1	D49.2
periurethral (tissue)	C49.5	C79.89	—	D21.5	D48.1	D49.2
popliteal fossa or space	C49.2-☑	C79.89	—	D21.2-☑	D48.1	D49.2
presacral	C49.5	C79.89	—	D21.5	D48.1	D49.2
psoas muscle	C49.4	C79.89	—	D21.4	D48.1	D49.2
pterygoid fossa	C49.0	C79.89	—	D21.0	D48.1	D49.2
rectovaginal septum or wall	C49.5	C79.89	—	D21.5	D48.1	D49.2
rectovesical	C49.5	C79.89	—	D21.5	D48.1	D49.2
retroperitoneum	C48.0	C78.6	—	D20.0	D48.3	D49.0
sacrococcygeal region	C49.5	C79.89	—	D21.5	D48.1	D49.2
scalp	C49.0	C79.89	—	D21.0	D48.1	D49.2
scapular region	C49.3	C79.89	—	D21.3	D48.1	D49.2
shoulder	C49.1-☑	C79.89	—	D21.1-☑	D48.1	D49.2
skin (dermis) NEC — see also Neoplasm, skin, by site	C44.90	C79.2	D04.9	D23.9	D48.5	D49.2
stomach	C49.4	C79.89	—	D21.4	D48.1	D49.2
submental	C49.0	C79.89	—	D21.0	D48.1	D49.2
supraclavicular region	C49.0	C79.89	—	D21.0	D48.1	D49.2
temple	C49.0	C79.89	—	D21.0	D48.1	D49.2
temporal region	C49.0	C79.89	—	D21.0	D48.1	D49.2
thigh	C49.2-☑	C79.89	—	D21.2-☑	D48.1	D49.2
thoracic (duct) (wall)	C49.3	C79.89	—	D21.3	D48.1	D49.2
thorax	C49.3	C79.89	—	D21.3	D48.1	D49.2
thumb	C49.1-☑	C79.89	—	D21.1-☑	D48.1	D49.2
toe	C49.2-☑	C79.89	—	D21.2-☑	D48.1	D49.2
trunk	C49.6	C79.89	—	D21.6	D48.1	D49.2
umbilicus	C49.4	C79.89	—	D21.4	D48.1	D49.2
vesicorectal	C49.5	C79.89	—	D21.5	D48.1	D49.2
wrist	C49.1-☑	C79.89	—	D21.1-☑	D48.1	D49.2
conus medullaris	C72.0	C79.49	—	D33.4	D43.4	D49.7
cord (true) (vocal)	C32.0	C78.39	D02.0	D14.1	D38.0	D49.1
false	C32.1	C78.39	D02.0	D14.1	D38.0	D49.1
spermatic	C63.1-☑	C79.82	D07.69	D29.8	D40.8	D49.59
spinal (cervical) (lumbar) (thoracic)	C72.0	C79.49	—	D33.4	D43.4	D49.7
cornea (limbus)	C69.1-☑	C79.49	D09.2-☑	D31.1-☑	D48.7	D49.89
corpus						
albicans	C56.-☑	C79.6-☑	D07.39	D27.-☑	D39.1-☑	D49.59
callosum, brain	C71.0	C79.31	—	D33.2	D43.2	D49.6

Neoplasm, neoplastic — continued
corpus — continued

	Malignant Primary	Malignant Secondary	Ca in situ	Benign	Uncertain Behavior	Unspecified Behavior
cavernosum	C60.2	C79.82	D07.4	D29.0	D40.8	D49.59
gastric	C16.2	C78.89	D00.2	D13.1	D37.1	D49.0
overlapping sites	C54.8	—	—	—	—	—
penis	C60.2	C79.82	D07.4	D29.0	D40.8	D49.59
striatum, cerebrum	C71.0	C79.31	—	D33.0	D43.0	D49.6
uteri	C54.9	C79.82	D07.0	D26.1	D39.0	D49.59
isthmus	C54.0	C79.82	D07.0	D26.1	D39.0	D49.59
cortex						
adrenal	C74.0-☑	C79.7-☑	D09.3	D35.0-☑	D44.1-☑	D49.7
cerebral	C71.0	C79.31	—	D33.0	D43.0	D49.6
costal cartilage	C41.3	C79.51	—	D16.7	D48.0	D49.2
costovertebral joint	C41.3	C79.51	—	D16.7	D48.0	D49.2
Cowper's gland	C68.0	C79.19	D09.19	D30.4	D41.3	D49.59
cranial (fossa, any)	C71.9	C79.31	—	D33.2	D43.2	D49.6
meninges	C70.0	C79.32	—	D32.0	D42.0	D49.7
nerve	C72.50	C79.49	—	D33.3	D43.3	D49.7
specified NEC	C72.59	C79.49	—	D33.3	D43.3	D49.7
craniobuccal pouch	C75.2	C79.89	D09.3	D35.2	D44.3	D49.7
craniopharyngeal (duct) (pouch)	C75.2	C79.89	D09.3	D35.3	D44.4	D49.7
cricoid	C13.0	C79.89	D00.08	D10.7	D37.05	D49.0
cartilage	C32.3	C78.39	D02.0	D14.1	D38.0	D49.1
cricopharynx	C13.0	C79.89	D00.08	D10.7	D37.05	D49.0
crypt of Morgagni	C21.8	C78.5	D01.3	D12.9	D37.8	D49.0
crystalline lens	C69.4-☑	C79.49	D09.2-☑	D31.4-☑	D48.7	D49.89
cul-de-sac (Douglas')	C48.1	C78.6	—	D20.1	D48.4	D49.0
cuneiform cartilage	C32.3	C78.39	D02.0	D14.1	D38.0	D49.1
cutaneous — see Neoplasm, skin						
cutis — see Neoplasm, skin						
cystic (bile) duct (common)	C24.0	C78.89	D01.5	D13.5	D37.6	D49.0
dermis — see Neoplasm, skin						
diaphragm	C49.3	C79.89	—	D21.3	D48.1	D49.2
digestive organs, system, tube, or tract NEC	C26.9	C78.89	D01.9	D13.9	D37.9	D49.0
disc, intervertebral	C41.2	C79.51	—	D16.6	D48.0	D49.2
disease, generalized	C80.0	—	—	—	—	—
disseminated	C80.0	—	—	—	—	—
Douglas' cul-de-sac or pouch	C48.1	C78.6	—	D20.1	D48.4	D49.0
duodenojejunal junction	C17.8	C78.4	D01.49	D13.39	D37.2	D49.0
duodenum	C17.0	C78.4	D01.49	D13.2	D37.2	D49.0
dura (cranial) (mater)	C70.9	C79.49	—	D32.9	D42.9	D49.7
cerebral	C70.0	C79.32	—	D32.0	D42.0	D49.7
spinal	C70.1	C79.49	—	D32.1	D42.1	D49.7
ear (external) — see also Neoplasm, skin, ear	C44.20-☑	C79.2	D04.2-☑	D23.2-☑	D48.5	D49.2
auricle or auris — see also Neoplasm, skin, ear	C44.20-☑	C79.2	D04.2-☑	D23.2-☑	D48.5	D49.2
canal, external — see also Neoplasm, skin, ear	C44.20-☑	C79.2	D04.2-☑	D23.2-☑	D48.5	D49.2
cartilage	C49.0	C79.89	—	D21.0	D48.1	D49.2
external meatus — see also Neoplasm, skin, ear	C44.20-☑	C79.2	D04.2-☑	D23.2-☑	D48.5	D49.2
inner	C30.1	C78.39	D02.3	D14.0	D38.5	D49.1
lobule — see also Neoplasm, skin, ear	C44.20-☑	C79.2	D04.2-☑	D23.2-☑	D48.5	D49.2
middle	C30.1	C78.39	D02.3	D14.0	D38.5	D49.1
overlapping lesion with accessory sinuses	C31.8	—	—	—	—	—

☑ Additional Character Required — Refer to the Tabular List for Character Selection   ▽ Subterms under main terms may continue to next column or pag

	Malignant Primary	Malignant Secondary	Ca in situ	Benign	Uncertain Behavior	Unspecified Behavior
Neoplasm, neoplastic						
— *continued*						
ear — *see also*						
Neoplasm, skin, ear						
— *continued*						
skin	C44.20-☑	C79.2	D04.2-☑	D23.2-☑	D48.5	D49.2
basal cell						
carcinoma	C44.21-☑	—	—	—	—	—
specified type						
NEC	C44.29-☑	—	—	—	—	—
squamous cell						
carcinoma	C44.22-☑	—	—	—	—	—
earlobe	C44.20-☑	C79.2	D04.2-☑	D23.2-☑	D48.5	D49.2
basal cell						
carcinoma	C44.21-☑	—	—	—	—	—
specified type						
NEC	C44.29-☑	—	—	—	—	—
squamous cell						
carcinoma	C44.22-☑	—	—	—	—	—
ejaculatory duct	C63.7	C79.82	D07.69	D29.8	D40.8	D49.59
elbow NEC	C76.4-☑	C79.89	D04.6-☑	D36.7	D48.7	D49.89
endocardium	C38.0	C79.89	—	D15.1	D48.7	D49.89
endocervix (canal)						
(gland)	C53.0	C79.82	D06.0	D26.0	D39.0	D49.59
endocrine gland						
NEC	C75.9	C79.89	D09.3	D35.9	D44.9	D49.7
pluriglandular	C75.8	C79.89	D09.3	D35.7	D44.9	D49.7
endometrium (gland)						
(stroma)	C54.1	C79.82	D07.0	D26.1	D39.0	D49.59
ensiform cartilage	C41.3	C79.51	—	D16.7	D48.0	D49.2
enteric — *see*						
Neoplasm,						
intestine						
ependyma (brain)	C71.5	C79.31	—	D33.0	D43.0	D49.6
fourth ventricle	C71.7	C79.31	—	D33.1	D43.1	D49.6
epicardium	C38.0	C79.89	—	D15.1	D48.7	D49.89
epididymis	C63.0-☑	C79.82	D07.69	D29.3-☑	D40.8	D49.59
epidural	C72.9	C79.49	—	D33.9	D43.9	D49.7
epiglottis	C32.1	C78.39	D02.0	D14.1	D38.0	D49.1
anterior aspect or						
surface	C10.1	C79.89	D00.08	D10.5	D37.05	D49.0
cartilage	C32.3	C78.39	D02.0	D14.1	D38.0	D49.1
free border						
(margin)	C10.1	C79.89	D00.08	D10.5	D37.05	D49.0
junctional						
region	C10.8	C79.89	D00.08	D10.5	D37.05	D49.0
posterior (laryngeal)						
surface	C32.1	C78.39	D02.0	D14.1	D38.0	D49.1
suprahyoid						
portion	C32.1	C78.39	D02.0	D14.1	D38.0	D49.1
esophagogastric						
junction	C16.0	C78.89	D00.2	D13.1	D37.1	D49.0
esophagus	C15.9	C78.89	D00.1	D13.0	D37.8	D49.0
abdominal	C15.5	C78.89	D00.1	D13.0	D37.8	D49.0
cervical	C15.3	C78.89	D00.1	D13.0	D37.8	D49.0
distal (third)	C15.5	C78.89	D00.1	D13.0	D37.8	D49.0
lower (third)	C15.5	C78.89	D00.1	D13.0	D37.8	D49.0
middle (third)	C15.4	C78.89	D00.1	D13.0	D37.8	D49.0
overlapping						
lesion	C15.8	—	—	—	—	—
proximal (third)	C15.3	C78.89	D00.1	D13.0	D37.8	D49.0
thoracic	C15.4	C78.89	D00.1	D13.0	D37.8	D49.0
upper (third)	C15.3	C78.89	D00.1	D13.0	D37.8	D49.0
ethmoid (sinus)	C31.1	C78.39	D02.3	D14.0	D38.5	D49.1
bone or						
labyrinth	C41.0	C79.51	—	D16.4	D48.0	D49.2
eustachian tube	C30.1	C78.39	D02.3	D14.0	D38.5	D49.1
exocervix	C53.1	C79.82	D06.1	D26.0	D39.0	D49.59
external						
meatus (ear) — *see*						
also Neoplasm,						
skin, ear	C44.20-☑	C79.2	D04.2-☑	D23.2-☑	D48.5	D49.2
os, cervix uteri	C53.1	C79.82	D06.1	D26.0	D39.0	D49.59
extradural	C72.9	C79.49	—	D33.9	D43.9	D49.7
extrahepatic (bile)						
duct	C24.0	C78.89	D01.5	D13.5	D37.6	D49.0
overlapping lesion						
with						
gallbladder	C24.8	—	—	—	—	—
extraocular						
muscle	C69.6-☑	C79.49	D09.2-☑	D31.6-☑	D48.7	D49.89
extrarectal	C76.3	C79.89	D09.8	D36.7	D48.7	D49.89
extremity	C76.8	C79.89	D04.8	D36.7	D48.7	D49.89

	Malignant Primary	Malignant Secondary	Ca in situ	Benign	Uncertain Behavior	Unspecified Behavior
Neoplasm, neoplastic						
— *continued*						
extremity — *continued*						
lower	C76.5-☑	C79.89	D04.7-☑	D36.7	D48.7	D49.89
upper	C76.4-☑	C79.89	D04.6-☑	D36.7	D48.7	D49.89
eyeball	C69.9-☑	C79.49	D09.2-☑	D31.9-☑	D48.7	D49.89
eyebrow	C44.309	C79.2	D04.39	D23.39	D48.5	D49.2
basal cell						
carcinoma	C44.319	—	—	—	—	—
specified type						
NEC	C44.399	—	—	—	—	—
squamous cell						
carcinoma	C44.329	—	—	—	—	—
eyelid (lower) (skin)						
(upper)	C44.10-☑	—	—	—	—	—
basal cell						
carcinoma	C44.11-☑	—	—	—	—	—
cartilage	C49.0	C79.89	—	D21.0	D48.1	D49.2
sebaceous cell	C44.13-☑	—	—	—	—	—
specified type						
NEC	C44.19-☑	—	—	—	—	—
squamous cell						
carcinoma	C44.12-☑	—	—	—	—	—
eye NEC	C69.9-☑	C79.49	D09.2-☑	D31.9-☑	D48.7	D49.89
overlapping						
sites	C69.8-☑	—	—	—	—	—
face NEC	C76.0	C79.89	D04.39	D36.7	D48.7	D49.89
fallopian tube						
(accessory)	C57.0-☑	C79.82	D07.39	D28.2	D39.8	D49.59
falx (cerebella)						
(cerebri)	C70.0	C79.32	—	D32.0	D42.0	D49.7
fascia — *see also*						
Neoplasm,						
connective tissue						
palmar	C49.1-☑	C79.89	—	D21.1-☑	D48.1	D49.2
plantar	C49.2-☑	C79.89	—	D21.2-☑	D48.1	D49.2
fatty tissue — *see*						
Neoplasm,						
connective tissue						
fauces, faucial NEC	C10.9	C79.89	D00.08	D10.5	D37.05	D49.0
pillars	C09.1	C79.89	D00.08	D10.5	D37.05	D49.0
tonsil	C09.9	C79.89	D00.08	D10.4	D37.05	D49.0
femur (any part)	C40.2-☑	—	—	D16.2-☑	—	—
fetal membrane	C58	C79.82	D07.0	D26.7	D39.2	D49.59
fibrous tissue — *see*						
Neoplasm,						
connective tissue						
fibula (any part)	C40.2-☑	C79.51	—	D16.2-☑	—	—
filum terminale	C72.0	C79.49	—	D33.4	D43.4	D49.7
finger NEC	C76.4-☑	C79.89	D04.6-☑	D36.7	D48.7	D49.89
flank NEC	C76.8	C79.89	D04.5	D36.7	D48.7	D49.89
follicle, nabothian	C53.0	C79.82	D06.0	D26.0	D39.0	D49.59
foot NEC	C76.5-☑	C79.89	D04.7-☑	D36.7	D48.7	D49.89
forearm NEC	C76.4-☑	C79.89	D04.6-☑	D36.7	D48.7	D49.89
forehead (skin)	C44.309	C79.2	D04.39	D23.39	D48.5	D49.2
basal cell						
carcinoma	C44.319	—	—	—	—	—
specified type						
NEC	C44.399	—	—	—	—	—
squamous cell						
carcinoma	C44.329	—	—	—	—	—
foreskin	C60.0	C79.82	D07.4	D29.0	D40.8	D49.59
fornix						
pharyngeal	C11.3	C79.89	D00.08	D10.6	D37.05	D49.0
vagina	C52	C79.82	D07.2	D28.1	D39.8	D49.59
fossa (of)						
anterior (cranial)	C71.9	C79.31	—	D33.2	D43.2	D49.6
cranial	C71.9	C79.31	—	D33.2	D43.2	D49.6
Ischiorectal	C76.3	C79.89	D09.8	D36.7	D48.7	D49.89
middle (cranial)	C71.9	C79.31	—	D33.2	D43.2	D49.6
piriform	C12	C79.89	D00.08	D10.7	D37.05	D49.0
pituitary	C75.1	C79.89	D09.3	D35.2	D44.3	D49.7
posterior						
(cranial)	C71.9	C79.31	—	D33.2	D43.2	D49.6
pterygoid	C49.0	C79.89	—	D21.0	D48.1	D49.2
pyriform	C12	C79.89	D00.08	D10.7	D37.05	D49.0
Rosenmuller	C11.2	C79.89	D00.08	D10.6	D37.05	D49.0
tonsillar	C09.0	C79.89	D00.08	D10.5	D37.05	D49.0
fourchette	C51.9	C79.82	D07.1	D28.0	D39.8	D49.59
frenulum						
labii — *see*						
Neoplasm, lip,						
internal						

Neoplasm, neoplastic	Malignant Primary	Malignant Secondary	Ca in situ	Benign	Uncertain Behavior	Unspecified Behavior
— continued						
frenulum — continued						
linguae	C02.2	C79.89	D00.07	D10.1	D37.02	D49.0
frontal						
bone	C41.0	C79.51	—	D16.4	D48.0	D49.2
lobe, brain	C71.1	C79.31	—	D33.0	D43.0	D49.6
pole	C71.1	C79.31	—	D33.0	D43.0	D49.6
sinus	C31.2	C78.39	D02.3	D14.0	D38.5	D49.1
fundus						
stomach	C16.1	C78.89	D00.2	D13.1	D37.1	D49.0
uterus	C54.3	C79.82	D07.0	D26.1	D39.0	D49.59
gallbladder	C23	C78.89	D01.5	D13.5	D37.6	D49.0
overlapping lesion with extrahepatic bile ducts	C24.8	—	—	—	—	—
gall duct						
(extrahepatic)	C24.0	C78.89	D01.5	D13.5	D37.6	D49.0
intrahepatic	C22.1	C78.7	D01.5	D13.4	D37.6	D49.0
ganglia — see also Neoplasm, nerve, peripheral	C47.9	C79.89	—	D36.10	D48.2	D49.2
basal	C71.0	C79.31	—	D33.0	D43.0	D49.6
cranial nerve	C72.50	C79.49	—	D33.3	D43.3	D49.7
Gartner's duct	C52	C79.82	D07.2	D28.1	D39.8	D49.59
gastric — see Neoplasm, stomach						
gastrocolic	C26.9	C78.89	D01.9	D13.9	D37.9	D49.0
gastroesophageal junction	C16.0	C78.89	D00.2	D13.1	D37.1	D49.0
gastrointestinal (tract) NEC	C26.9	C78.89	D01.9	D13.9	D37.9	D49.0
generalized	C80.0	—	—	—	—	—
genital organ or tract						
female	C57.9	C79.82	D07.30	D28.9	D39.9	D49.59
overlapping lesion	C57.8	—	—	—	—	—
specified site NEC	C57.7	C79.82	D07.39	D28.7	D39.8	D49.59
male NEC	C63.9	C79.82	D07.60	D29.9	D40.9	D49.59
overlapping lesion	C63.8	—	—	—	—	—
specified site NEC	C63.7	C79.82	D07.69	D29.8	D40.8	D49.59
genitourinary tract						
female	C57.9	C79.82	D07.30	D28.9	D39.9	D49.59
male	C63.9	C79.82	D07.60	D29.9	D40.9	D49.59
gingiva (alveolar) (marginal)	C03.9	C79.89	D00.03	D10.39	D37.09	D49.0
lower	C03.1	C79.89	D00.03	D10.39	D37.09	D49.0
mandibular	C03.1	C79.89	D00.03	D10.39	D37.09	D49.0
maxillary	C03.0	C79.89	D00.03	D10.39	D37.09	D49.0
upper	C03.0	C79.89	D00.03	D10.39	D37.09	D49.0
gland, glandular (lymphatic) (system) — see also Neoplasm, lymph gland						
endocrine NEC	C75.9	C79.89	D09.3	D35.9	D44.9	D49.7
salivary — see Neoplasm, salivary gland						
glans penis	C60.1	C79.82	D07.4	D29.0	D40.8	D49.59
globus pallidus	C71.0	C79.31	—	D33.0	D43.0	D49.6
glomus						
coccygeal	C49.5	C79.89	—	D21.5	D48.1	D49.2
jugularis	C75.5	C79.89	—	D35.6	D44.7	D49.7
glosso-epiglottic fold(s)	C10.1	C79.89	D00.08	D10.5	D37.05	D49.0
glossopalatine fold	C09.1	C79.89	D00.08	D10.5	D37.05	D49.0
glossopharyngeal sulcus	C09.0	C79.89	D00.08	D10.5	D37.05	D49.0
glottis	C32.0	C78.39	D02.0	D14.1	D38.0	D49.1
gluteal region	C76.3	C79.89	D04.5	D36.7	D48.7	D49.89
great vessels NEC	C49.3	C79.89	—	D21.3	D48.1	D49.2
groin NEC	C76.3	C79.89	D04.5	D36.7	D48.7	D49.89
gum	C03.9	C79.89	D00.03	D10.39	D37.09	D49.0
lower	C03.1	C79.89	D00.03	D10.39	D37.09	D49.0
upper	C03.0	C79.89	D00.03	D10.39	D37.09	D49.0
hand NEC	C76.4-☑	C79.89	D04.6-☑	D36.7	D48.7	D49.89
head NEC	C76.0	C79.89	D04.4	D36.7	D48.7	D49.89
heart	C38.0	C79.89	—	D15.1	D48.7	D49.89

Neoplasm, neoplastic	Malignant Primary	Malignant Secondary	Ca in situ	Benign	Uncertain Behavior	Unspecified Behavior
— continued						
heel NEC	C76.5-☑	C79.89	D04.7-☑	D36.7	D48.7	D49.89
helix — see also Neoplasm, skin, ear	C44.20-☑	C79.2	D04.2-☑	D23.2-☑	D48.5	D49.2
hematopoietic, hemopoietic tissue NEC	C96.9	—	—	—	—	—
specified NEC	C96.Z	—	—	—	—	—
hemisphere, cerebral	C71.0	C79.31	—	D33.0	D43.0	D49.6
hemorrhoidal zone	C21.1	C78.5	D01.3	D12.9	D37.8	D49.0
hepatic — see also Index to disease, by histology	C22.9	C78.7	D01.5	D13.4	D37.6	D49.0
duct (bile)	C24.0	C78.89	D01.5	D13.5	D37.6	D49.0
flexure (colon)	C18.3	C78.5	D01.0	D12.3	D37.4	D49.0
primary	C22.8	C78.7	D01.5	D13.4	D37.6	D49.0
hepatobiliary	C24.9	C78.89	D01.5	D13.5	D37.6	D49.0
hepatoblastoma	C22.2	C78.7	D01.5	D13.4	D37.6	D49.0
hepatoma	C22.0	C78.7	D01.5	D13.4	D37.6	D49.0
hilus of lung	C34.0-☑	C78.0-☑	D02.2-☑	D14.3-☑	D38.1	D49.1
hippocampus, brain	C71.2	C79.31	—	D33.0	D43.0	D49.6
hip NEC	C76.5-☑	C79.89	D04.7-☑	D36.7	D48.7	D49.89
humerus (any part)	C40.0-☑	C79.51	—	D16.0-☑	—	—
hymen	C52	C79.82	D07.2	D28.1	D39.8	D49.59
hypopharynx, hypopharyngeal NEC	C13.9	C79.89	D00.08	D10.7	D37.05	D49.0
overlapping lesion	C13.8	—	—	—	—	—
postcricoid region	C13.0	C79.89	D00.08	D10.7	D37.05	D49.0
posterior wall	C13.2	C79.89	D00.08	D10.7	D37.05	D49.0
pyriform fossa (sinus)	C12	C79.89	D00.08	D10.7	D37.05	D49.0
hypophysis	C75.1	C79.89	D09.3	D35.2	D44.3	D49.7
hypothalamus	C71.0	C79.31	—	D33.0	D43.0	D49.6
ileocecum, ileocecal (coil) (junction) (valve)	C18.0	C78.5	D01.0	D12.0	D37.4	D49.0
ileum	C17.2	C78.4	D01.49	D13.39	D37.2	D49.0
ilium	C41.4	C79.51	—	D16.8	D48.0	D49.2
immunoproliferative NEC	C88.9	—	—	—	—	—
infraclavicular (region)	C76.1	C79.89	D04.5	D36.7	D48.7	D49.89
inguinal (region)	C76.3	C79.89	D04.5	D36.7	D48.7	D49.89
insula	C71.0	C79.31	—	D33.0	D43.0	D49.6
insular tissue (pancreas)	C25.4	C78.89	D01.7	D13.7	D37.8	D49.0
brain	C71.0	C79.31	—	D33.0	D43.0	D49.6
interarytenoid fold	C13.1	C78.39	D00.08	D10.7	D37.05	D49.0
hypopharyngeal aspect	C13.1	C79.89	D00.08	D10.7	D37.05	D49.0
laryngeal aspect	C32.1	C78.39	D02.0	D14.1	D38.0	D49.1
marginal zone	C13.1	C79.89	D00.08	D10.7	D37.05	D49.0
interdental papillae	C03.9	C79.89	D00.03	D10.39	D37.09	D49.0
lower	C03.1	C79.89	D00.03	D10.39	D37.09	D49.0
upper	C03.0	C79.89	D00.03	D10.39	D37.09	D49.0
internal						
capsule	C71.0	C79.31	—	D33.0	D43.0	D49.6
os (cervix)	C53.0	C79.82	D06.0	D26.0	D39.0	D49.59
intervertebral cartilage or disc	C41.2	C79.51	—	D16.6	D48.0	D49.2
intestine, intestinal	C26.0	C78.80	D01.40	D13.9	D37.8	D49.0
large	C18.9	C78.5	D01.0	D12.6	D37.4	D49.0
appendix	C18.1	C78.5	D01.0	D12.1	D37.3	D49.0
caput coli	C18.0	C78.5	D01.0	D12.0	D37.4	D49.0
cecum	C18.0	C78.5	D01.0	D12.0	D37.4	D49.0
colon	C18.9	C78.5	D01.0	D12.6	D37.4	D49.0
and rectum	C19	C78.5	D01.1	D12.7	D37.5	D49.0
ascending	C18.2	C78.5	D01.0	D12.2	D37.4	D49.0
caput	C18.0	C78.5	D01.0	D12.0	D37.4	D49.0
descending	C18.6	C78.5	D01.0	D12.4	D37.4	D49.0
distal	C18.6	C78.5	D01.0	D12.4	D37.4	D49.0

☑ Additional Character Required — Refer to the Tabular List for Character Selection ▽ Subterms under main terms may continue to next column or page

Neoplasm Table

Neoplasm, frenulum — Neoplasm, intestine, intestinal

Neoplasm, neoplastic — continued	Malignant Primary	Malignant Secondary	Ca in situ	Benign	Uncertain Behavior	Unspecified Behavior
intestine, intestinal — continued						
large — continued						
colon — continued						
left	C18.6	C78.5	D01.0	D12.4	D37.4	D49.0
overlapping lesion	C18.8	—	—	—	—	—
pelvic	C18.7	C78.5	D01.0	D12.5	D37.4	D49.0
right	C18.2	C78.5	D01.0	D12.2	D37.4	D49.0
sigmoid (flexure)	C18.7	C78.5	D01.0	D12.5	D37.4	D49.0
transverse	C18.4	C78.5	D01.0	D12.3	D37.4	D49.0
hepatic flexure	C18.3	C78.5	D01.0	D12.3	D37.4	D49.0
ileocecum, ileocecal (coil) (valve)	C18.0	C78.5	D01.0	D12.0	D37.4	D49.0
overlapping lesion	C18.8	—	—	—	—	—
sigmoid flexure (lower)						
(upper)	C18.7	C78.5	D01.0	D12.5	D37.4	D49.0
splenic flexure	C18.5	C78.5	D01.0	D12.3	D37.4	D49.0
small	C17.9	C78.4	D01.40	D13.30	D37.2	D49.0
duodenum	C17.0	C78.4	D01.49	D13.2	D37.2	D49.0
ileum	C17.2	C78.4	D01.49	D13.39	D37.2	D49.0
jejunum	C17.1	C78.4	D01.49	D13.39	D37.2	D49.0
overlapping lesion	C17.8	—	—	—	—	—
tract NEC	C26.0	C78.89	D01.40	D13.9	D37.8	D49.0
intra-abdominal	C76.2	C79.89	D09.8	D36.7	D48.7	D49.89
intracranial NEC	C71.9	C79.31	—	D33.2	D43.2	D49.6
intrahepatic (bile) duct	C22.1	C78.7	D01.5	D13.4	D37.6	D49.0
intraocular	C69.9-☑	C79.49	D09.2-☑	D31.9-☑	D48.7	D49.89
intraorbital	C69.6-☑	C79.49	D09.2-☑	D31.6-☑	D48.7	D49.89
intrasellar	C75.1	C79.89	D09.3	D35.2	D44.3	D49.7
intrathoracic (cavity) (organs)	C76.1	C79.89	D09.8	D15.9	D48.7	D49.89
specified NEC	C76.1	C79.89	D09.8	D15.7	—	—
iris	C69.4-☑	C79.49	D09.2-☑	D31.4-☑	D48.7	D49.89
ischiorectal (fossa)	C76.3	C79.89	D09.8	D36.7	D48.7	D49.89
ischium	C41.4	C79.51	—	D16.8	D48.0	D49.2
island of Reil	C71.0	C79.31	—	D33.0	D43.0	D49.6
islands or islets of Langerhans	C25.4	C78.89	D01.7	D13.7	D37.8	D49.0
isthmus uteri	C54.0	C79.82	D07.0	D26.1	D39.0	D49.59
jaw	C76.0	C79.89	D09.8	D36.7	D48.7	D49.89
bone	C41.1	C79.51	—	D16.5	D48.0	D49.2
lower	C41.1	C79.51	—	D16.5	—	—
upper	C41.0	C79.51	—	D16.4	—	—
carcinoma (any type) (lower) (upper)	C76.0	C79.89	—	—	—	—
skin — see also Neoplasm, skin, face	C44.309	C79.2	D04.39	D23.39	D48.5	D49.2
soft tissues	C03.9	C79.89	D00.03	D10.39	D37.09	D49.0
lower	C03.1	C79.89	D00.03	D10.39	D37.09	D49.0
upper	C03.0	C79.89	D00.03	D10.39	D37.09	D49.0
jejunum	C17.1	C78.4	D01.49	D13.39	D37.2	D49.0
joint NEC — see also Neoplasm, bone	C41.9	C79.51	—	D16.9	D48.0	D49.2
acromioclavicular	C40.0-☑	C79.51	—	D16.0-☑	—	—
bursa or synovial membrane — see Neoplasm, connective tissue						
costovertebral	C41.3	C79.51	—	D16.7	D48.0	D49.2
sternocostal	C41.3	C79.51	—	D16.7	D48.0	D49.2
temporomandibular	C41.1	C79.51	—	D16.5	D48.0	D49.2
junction						
anorectal	C21.8	C78.5	D01.3	D12.9	D37.8	D49.0
cardioesophageal	C16.0	C78.89	D00.2	D13.1	D37.1	D49.0
esophagogastric	C16.0	C78.89	D00.2	D13.1	D37.1	D49.0
gastroesophageal	C16.0	C78.89	D00.2	D13.1	D37.1	D49.0
hard and soft palate	C05.9	C79.89	D00.00	D10.39	D37.09	D49.0
ileocecal	C18.0	C78.5	D01.0	D12.0	D37.4	D49.0

Neoplasm, neoplastic — continued	Malignant Primary	Malignant Secondary	Ca in situ	Benign	Uncertain Behavior	Unspecified Behavior
junction — continued						
pelvirectal	C19	C78.5	D01.1	D12.7	D37.5	D49.0
pelviureteric	C65.-☑	C79.0-☑	D09.19	D30.1-☑	D41.1-☑	D49.59
rectosigmoid	C19	C78.5	D01.1	D12.7	D37.5	D49.0
squamocolumnar, of cervix	C53.8	C79.82	D06.7	D26.0	D39.0	D49.59
Kaposi's sarcoma — see Kaposi's, sarcoma						
kidney (parenchymal)	C64.-☑	C79.0-☑	D09.19	D30.0-☑	D41.0-☑	D49.51-☑
calyx	C65.-☑	C79.0-☑	D09.19	D30.1-☑	D41.1-☑	D49.51-☑
hilus	C65.-☑	C79.0-☑	D09.19	D30.1-☑	D41.1-☑	D49.51-☑
pelvis	C65.-☑	C79.0-☑	D09.19	D30.1-☑	D41.1-☑	D49.51-☑
knee NEC	C76.5-☑	C79.89	D04.7-☑	D36.7	D48.7	D49.89
labia (skin)	C51.9	C79.82	D07.1	D28.0	D39.8	D49.59
majora	C51.0	C79.82	D07.1	D28.0	D39.8	D49.59
minora	C51.1	C79.82	D07.1	D28.0	D39.8	D49.59
labial — see also Neoplasm, lip	C00.9	C79.89	D00.01	D10.0	D37.01	D49.0
sulcus (lower) (upper)	C06.1	C79.89	D00.02	D10.39	D37.09	D49.0
labium (skin)	C51.9	C79.82	D07.1	D28.0	D39.8	D49.59
majus	C51.0	C79.82	D07.1	D28.0	D39.8	D49.59
minus	C51.1	C79.82	D07.1	D28.0	D39.8	D49.59
lacrimal						
canaliculi	C69.5-☑	C79.49	D09.2-☑	D31.5-☑	D48.7	D49.89
duct (nasal)	C69.5-☑	C79.49	D09.2-☑	D31.5-☑	D48.7	D49.89
gland	C69.5-☑	C79.49	D09.2-☑	D31.5-☑	D48.7	D49.89
punctum	C69.5-☑	C79.49	D09.2-☑	D31.5-☑	D48.7	D49.89
sac	C69.5-☑	C79.49	D09.2-☑	D31.5-☑	D48.7	D49.89
Langerhans, islands or islets	C25.4	C78.89	D01.7	D13.7	D37.8	D49.0
laryngopharynx	C13.9	C79.89	D00.08	D10.7	D37.05	D49.0
larynx, laryngeal NEC	C32.9	C78.39	D02.0	D14.1	D38.0	D49.1
aryepiglottic fold	C32.1	C78.39	D02.0	D14.1	D38.0	D49.1
cartilage (arytenoid) (cricoid) (cuneiform) (thyroid)	C32.3	C78.39	D02.0	D14.1	D38.0	D49.1
commissure (anterior) (posterior)	C32.0	C78.39	D02.0	D14.1	D38.0	D49.1
extrinsic NEC	C32.1	C78.39	D02.0	D14.1	D38.0	D49.1
meaning hypopharynx	C13.9	C79.89	D00.08	D10.7	D37.05	D49.0
interarytenoid fold	C32.1	C78.39	D02.0	D14.1	D38.0	D49.1
intrinsic	C32.0	C78.39	D02.0	D14.1	D38.0	D49.1
overlapping lesion	C32.8	—	—	—	—	—
ventricular band	C32.1	C78.39	D02.0	D14.1	D38.0	D49.1
leg NEC	C76.5-☑	C79.89	D04.7-☑	D36.7	D48.7	D49.89
lens, crystalline	C69.4-☑	C79.49	D09.2-☑	D31.4-☑	D48.7	D49.89
lid (lower) (upper)	C44.10-☑	C79.2	D04.1-☑	D23.1-☑	D48.5	D49.2
basal cell carcinoma	C44.11-☑	—	—	—	—	—
sebaceous cell	C44.13-☑	—	—	—	—	—
specified type NEC	C44.19-☑	—	—	—	—	—
squamous cell carcinoma	C44.12-☑	—	—	—	—	—
ligament — see also Neoplasm, connective tissue						
broad	C57.1-☑	C79.82	D07.39	D28.2	D39.8	D49.59
Mackenrodt's	C57.7	C79.82	D07.39	D28.7	D39.8	D49.59
non-uterine — see Neoplasm, connective tissue						
round	C57.2-☑	C79.82	—	D28.2	D39.8	D49.59
sacro-uterine	C57.3	C79.82	—	D28.2	D39.8	D49.59
uterine	C57.3	C79.82	—	D28.2	D39.8	D49.59
utero-ovarian	C57.7	C79.82	D07.39	D28.2	D39.8	D49.59
uterosacral	C57.3	C79.82	—	D28.2	D39.8	D49.59
limb	C76.8	C79.89	D04.8	D36.7	D48.7	D49.89
lower	C76.5-☑	C79.89	D04.7-☑	D36.7	D48.7	D49.89
upper	C76.4-☑	C79.89	D04.6-☑	D36.7	D48.7	D49.89
limbus of cornea	C69.1-☑	C79.49	D09.2-☑	D31.1-☑	D48.7	D49.89

Neoplasm, neoplastic — continued

	Malignant Primary	Malignant Secondary	Ca in situ	Benign	Uncertain Behavior	Unspecified Behavior
lingual NEC — see also Neoplasm, tongue	C02.9	C79.89	D00.07	D10.1	D37.02	D49.0
lingula, lung	C34.1-☑	C78.0-☑	D02.2-☑	D14.3-☑	D38.1	D49.1
lip	C00.9	C79.89	D00.01	D10.0	D37.01	D49.0
buccal aspect — see Neoplasm, lip, internal						
commissure	C00.6	C79.89	D00.01	D10.0	D37.01	D49.0
external	C00.2	C79.89	D00.01	D10.0	D37.01	D49.0
lower	C00.1	C79.89	D00.01	D10.0	D37.01	D49.0
upper	C00.0	C79.89	D00.01	D10.0	D37.01	D49.0
frenulum — see Neoplasm, lip, internal						
inner aspect — see Neoplasm, lip, internal						
internal	C00.5	C79.89	D00.01	D10.0	D37.01	D49.0
lower	C00.4	C79.89	D00.01	D10.0	D37.01	D49.0
upper	C00.3	C79.89	D00.01	D10.0	D37.01	D49.0
lipstick area	C00.2	C79.89	D00.01	D10.0	D37.01	D49.0
lower	C00.1	C79.89	D00.01	D10.0	D37.01	D49.0
upper	C00.0	C79.89	D00.01	D10.0	D37.01	D49.0
lower	C00.1	C79.89	D00.01	D10.0	D37.01	D49.0
internal	C00.4	C79.89	D00.01	D10.0	D37.01	D49.0
mucosa — see Neoplasm, lip, internal						
oral aspect — see Neoplasm, lip, internal						
overlapping lesion	C00.8	—	—	—	—	—
with oral cavity or pharynx	C14.8	—	—	—	—	—
skin (commissure) (lower) (upper)	C44.00	C79.2	D04.0	D23.0	D48.5	D49.2
basal cell carcinoma	C44.01	—	—	—	—	—
specified type NEC	C44.09	—	—	—	—	—
squamous cell carcinoma	C44.02	—	—	—	—	—
upper	C00.0	C79.89	D00.01	D10.0	D37.01	D49.0
internal	C00.3	C79.89	D00.01	D10.0	D37.01	D49.0
vermilion border	C00.2	C79.89	D00.01	D10.0	D37.01	D49.0
lower	C00.1	C79.89	D00.01	D10.0	D37.01	D49.0
upper	C00.0	C79.89	D00.01	D10.0	D37.01	D49.0
lipomatous — see Lipoma, by site						
liver — see also Index to disease, by histology	C22.9	C78.7	D01.5	D13.4	D37.6	D49.0
primary	C22.8	C78.7	D01.5	D13.4	D37.6	D49.0
lumbosacral plexus	C47.5	C79.89	—	D36.16	D48.2	D49.2
lung	C34.9-☑	C78.0-☑	D02.2-☑	D14.3-☑	D38.1	D49.1
azygos lobe	C34.1-☑	C78.0-☑	D02.2-☑	D14.3-☑	D38.1	D49.1
carina	C34.0-☑	C78.0-☑	D02.2-☑	D14.3-☑	D38.1	D49.1
hilus	C34.0-☑	C78.0-☑	D02.2-☑	D14.3-☑	D38.1	D49.1
lingula	C34.1-☑	C78.0-☑	D02.2-☑	D14.3-☑	D38.1	D49.1
lobe NEC	C34.9-☑	C78.0-☑	D02.2-☑	D14.3-☑	D38.1	D49.1
lower lobe	C34.3-☑	C78.0-☑	D02.2-☑	D14.3-☑	D38.1	D49.1
main bronchus	C34.0-☑	C78.0-☑	D02.2-☑	D14.3-☑	D38.1	D49.1
mesothelioma — see Mesothelioma						
middle lobe	C34.2	C78.0-☑	D02.21	D14.31	D38.1	D49.1
overlapping lesion	C34.8-☑	—	—	—	—	—
upper lobe	C34.1-☑	C78.0-☑	D02.2-☑	D14.3-☑	D38.1	D49.1
lymph, lymphatic channel NEC	C49.9	C79.89	—	D21.9	D48.1	D49.2
gland						
(secondary)	—	C77.9	—	D36.0	D48.7	D49.89
abdominal	—	C77.2	—	D36.0	D48.7	D49.89
aortic	—	C77.2	—	D36.0	D48.7	D49.89
arm	—	C77.3	—	D36.0	D48.7	D49.89

Neoplasm, neoplastic — continued
lymph, lymphatic channel — continued
gland — continued

	Malignant Primary	Malignant Secondary	Ca in situ	Benign	Uncertain Behavior	Unspecified Behavior
auricular (anterior) (posterior)	—	C77.0	—	D36.0	D48.7	D49.89
axilla, axillary	—	C77.3	—	D36.0	D48.7	D49.89
brachial	—	C77.3	—	D36.0	D48.7	D49.89
bronchial	—	C77.1	—	D36.0	D48.7	D49.89
bronchopulmonary	—	C77.1	—	D36.0	D48.7	D49.89
celiac	—	C77.2	—	D36.0	D48.7	D49.89
cervical	—	C77.0	—	D36.0	D48.7	D49.89
cervicofacial	—	C77.0	—	D36.0	D48.7	D49.89
Cloquet	—	C77.4	—	D36.0	D48.7	D49.89
colic	—	C77.2	—	D36.0	D48.7	D49.89
common duct	—	C77.2	—	D36.0	D48.7	D49.89
cubital	—	C77.3	—	D36.0	D48.7	D49.89
diaphragmatic	—	C77.1	—	D36.0	D48.7	D49.89
epigastric, inferior	—	C77.1	—	D36.0	D48.7	D49.89
epitrochlear	—	C77.3	—	D36.0	D48.7	D49.89
esophageal	—	C77.1	—	D36.0	D48.7	D49.89
face	—	C77.0	—	D36.0	D48.7	D49.89
femoral	—	C77.4	—	D36.0	D48.7	D49.89
gastric	—	C77.2	—	D36.0	D48.7	D49.89
groin	—	C77.4	—	D36.0	D48.7	D49.89
head	—	C77.0	—	D36.0	D48.7	D49.89
hepatic	—	C77.2	—	D36.0	D48.7	D49.89
hilar (pulmonary)	—	C77.1	—	D36.0	D48.7	D49.89
splenic	—	C77.2	—	D36.0	D48.7	D49.89
hypogastric	—	C77.5	—	D36.0	D48.7	D49.89
ileocolic	—	C77.2	—	D36.0	D48.7	D49.89
iliac	—	C77.5	—	D36.0	D48.7	D49.89
infraclavicular	—	C77.3	—	D36.0	D48.7	D49.89
inguina, inguinal	—	C77.4	—	D36.0	D48.7	D49.89
innominate	—	C77.1	—	D36.0	D48.7	D49.89
intercostal	—	C77.1	—	D36.0	D48.7	D49.89
intestinal	—	C77.2	—	D36.0	D48.7	D49.89
intrabdominal	—	C77.2	—	D36.0	D48.7	D49.89
intrapelvic	—	C77.5	—	D36.0	D48.7	D49.89
intrathoracic	—	C77.1	—	D36.0	D48.7	D49.89
jugular	—	C77.0	—	D36.0	D48.7	D49.89
leg	—	C77.4	—	D36.0	D48.7	D49.89
limb						
lower	—	C77.4	—	D36.0	D48.7	D49.89
upper	—	C77.3	—	D36.0	D48.7	D49.89
lower limb	—	C77.4	—	D36.0	D48.7	D49.89
lumbar	—	C77.2	—	D36.0	D48.7	D49.89
mandibular	—	C77.0	—	D36.0	D48.7	D49.89
mediastinal	—	C77.1	—	D36.0	D48.7	D49.89
mesenteric (inferior) (superior)	—	C77.2	—	D36.0	D48.7	D49.89
midcolic	—	C77.2	—	D36.0	D48.7	D49.89
multiple sites in categories C77.0 - C77.5	—	C77.8	—	D36.0	D48.7	D49.89
neck	—	C77.0	—	D36.0	D48.7	D49.89
obturator	—	C77.5	—	D36.0	D48.7	D49.89
occipital	—	C77.0	—	D36.0	D48.7	D49.89
pancreatic	—	C77.2	—	D36.0	D48.7	D49.89
para-aortic	—	C77.2	—	D36.0	D48.7	D49.89
paracervical	—	C77.5	—	D36.0	D48.7	D49.89
parametrial	—	C77.5	—	D36.0	D48.7	D49.89
parasternal	—	C77.1	—	D36.0	D48.7	D49.89
parotid	—	C77.0	—	D36.0	D48.7	D49.89
pectoral	—	C77.3	—	D36.0	D48.7	D49.89
pelvic	—	C77.5	—	D36.0	D48.7	D49.89
peri-aortic	—	C77.2	—	D36.0	D48.7	D49.89
peripancreatic	—	C77.2	—	D36.0	D48.7	D49.89
popliteal	—	C77.4	—	D36.0	D48.7	D49.89
porta hepatis	—	C77.2	—	D36.0	D48.7	D49.89
portal	—	C77.2	—	D36.0	D48.7	D49.89
preauricular	—	C77.0	—	D36.0	D48.7	D49.89
prelaryngeal	—	C77.0	—	D36.0	D48.7	D49.89
presymphysial	—	C77.5	—	D36.0	D48.7	D49.89
pretracheal	—	C77.0	—	D36.0	D48.7	D49.89
primary (any site) NEC	C96.9	—	—	—	—	—

☑ **Additional Character Required — Refer to the Tabular List for Character Selection**

▽ **Subterms under main terms may continue to next column or page**

Neoplasm, neoplastic — continued	Malignant Primary	Malignant Secondary	Ca in situ	Benign	Uncertain Behavior	Unspecified Behavior
lymph, lymphatic channel — continued						
gland — continued						
pulmonary (hiler)	—	C77.1	—	D36.0	D48.7	D49.89
pyloric	—	C77.2	—	D36.0	D48.7	D49.89
retroperitoneal	—	C77.2	—	D36.0	D48.7	D49.89
retropharyngeal	—	C77.0	—	D36.0	D48.7	D49.89
Rosenmuller's	—	C77.4	—	D36.0	D48.7	D49.89
sacral	—	C77.5	—	D36.0	D48.7	D49.89
scalene	—	C77.0	—	D36.0	D48.7	D49.89
site NEC	—	C77.9	—	D36.0	D48.7	D49.89
splenic (hilar)	—	C77.2	—	D36.0	D48.7	D49.89
subclavicular	—	C77.3	—	D36.0	D48.7	D49.89
subinguinal	—	C77.4	—	D36.0	D48.7	D49.89
sublingual	—	C77.0	—	D36.0	D48.7	D49.89
submandibular	—	C77.0	—	D36.0	D48.7	D49.89
submaxillary	—	C77.0	—	D36.0	D48.7	D49.89
submental	—	C77.0	—	D36.0	D48.7	D49.89
subscapular	—	C77.3	—	D36.0	D48.7	D49.89
supraclavicular	—	C77.0	—	D36.0	D48.7	D49.89
thoracic	—	C77.1	—	D36.0	D48.7	D49.89
tibial	—	C77.4	—	D36.0	D48.7	D49.89
tracheal	—	C77.1	—	D36.0	D48.7	D49.89
tracheobronchial	—	C77.1	—	D36.0	D48.7	D49.89
upper limb	—	C77.3	—	D36.0	D48.7	D49.89
Virchow's	—	C77.0	—	D36.0	D48.7	D49.89
node — see also Neoplasm, lymph gland						
primary NEC	C96.9	—	—	—	—	—
vessel — see also Neoplasm, connective tissue	C49.9	C79.89	—	D21.9	D48.1	D49.2
Mackenrodt's ligament	C57.7	C79.82	D07.39	D28.7	D39.8	D49.59
malar	C41.0	C79.51	—	D16.4	D48.0	D49.2
region — see Neoplasm, cheek						
mammary gland — see Neoplasm, breast						
mandible	C41.1	C79.51	—	D16.5	D48.0	D49.2
alveolar mucosa (carcinoma)	C03.1	C79.89	D00.03	D10.39	D37.09	D49.0
ridge or process	C41.1	C79.51	—	D16.5	D48.0	D49.2
marrow (bone) NEC	C96.9	C79.52	—	—	D47.9	D49.89
mastectomy site (skin) — see also Neoplasm, breast, skin	C44.501	C79.2	—	—	—	—
specified as breast tissue	C50.8-☑	C79.81	—	—	—	—
mastoid (air cells) (antrum) (cavity)	C30.1	C78.39	D02.3	D14.0	D38.5	D49.1
bone or process	C41.0	C79.51	—	D16.4	D48.0	D49.2
maxilla, maxillary (superior)	C41.0	C79.51	—	D16.4	D48.0	D49.2
alveolar mucosa	C03.0	C79.89	D00.03	D10.39	D37.09	D49.0
ridge or process (carcinoma)	C41.0	C79.51	—	D16.4	D48.0	D49.2
antrum	C31.0	C78.39	D02.3	D14.0	D38.5	D49.1
carcinoma	C03.0	C79.51	—	—	—	—
inferior — see Neoplasm, mandible						
sinus	C31.0	C78.39	D02.3	D14.0	D38.5	D49.1
meatus external (ear) — see also Neoplasm, skin, ear	C44.20-☑	C79.2	D04.2-☑	D23.2-☑	D48.5	D49.2
Meckel diverticulum, malignant	C17.3	C78.4	D01.49	D13.39	D37.2	D49.0
mediastinum, mediastinal	C38.3	C78.1	—	D15.2	D38.3	D49.89
anterior	C38.1	C78.1	—	D15.2	D38.3	D49.89

Neoplasm, neoplastic — continued	Malignant Primary	Malignant Secondary	Ca in situ	Benign	Uncertain Behavior	Unspecified Behavior
mediastinum, mediastinal — continued						
posterior	C38.2	C78.1	—	D15.2	D38.3	D49.89
medulla						
adrenal	C74.1-☑	C79.7-☑	D09.3	D35.0-☑	D44.1-☑	D49.7
oblongata	C71.7	C79.31	—	D33.1	D43.1	D49.6
meibomian gland	C44.10-☑	C79.2	D04.1-☑	D23.1-☑	D48.5	D49.2
basal cell carcinoma	C44.11-☑	—	—	—	—	—
sebaceous cell	C44.13-☑	—	—	—	—	—
specified type NEC	C44.19-☑	—	—	—	—	—
squamous cell carcinoma	C44.12-☑	—	—	—	—	—
melanoma — see Melanoma						
meninges	C70.9	C79.49	—	D32.9	D42.9	D49.7
brain	C70.0	C79.32	—	D32.0	D42.0	D49.7
cerebral	C70.0	C79.32	—	D32.0	D42.0	D49.7
crainial	C70.0	C79.32	—	D32.0	D42.0	D49.7
intracranial	C70.0	C79.32	—	D32.0	D42.0	D49.7
spinal (cord)	C70.1	C79.49	—	D32.1	D42.1	D49.7
meniscus, knee joint (lateral) (medial)	C40.2-☑	C79.51	—	D16.2-☑	D48.0	D49.2
Merkel cell — see Carcinoma, Merkel cell						
mesentery, mesenteric	C48.1	C78.6	—	D20.1	D48.4	D49.0
mesoappendix	C48.1	C78.6	—	D20.1	D48.4	D49.0
mesocolon	C48.1	C78.6	—	D20.1	D48.4	D49.0
mesopharynx — see Neoplasm, oropharynx						
mesosalpinx	C57.1-☑	C79.82	D07.39	D28.2	D39.8	D49.59
mesothelial tissue — see Mesothelioma						
mesothelioma — see Mesothelioma						
mesovarium	C57.1-☑	C79.82	D07.39	D28.2	D39.8	D49.59
metacarpus (any bone)	C40.1-☑	C79.51	—	D16.1-☑		
metastatic NEC — see also Neoplasm, by site, secondary	—	C79.9	—	—	—	—
metatarsus (any bone)	C40.3-☑	C79.51	—	D16.3-☑	—	—
midbrain	C71.7	C79.31	—	D33.1	D43.1	D49.6
milk duct — see Neoplasm, breast						
mons						
pubis	C51.9	C79.82	D07.1	D28.0	D39.8	D49.59
veneris	C51.9	C79.82	D07.1	D28.0	D39.8	D49.59
motor tract	C72.9	C79.49	—	D33.9	D43.9	D49.7
brain	C71.9	C79.31	—	D33.2	D43.2	D49.6
cauda equina	C72.1	C79.49	—	D33.4	D43.4	D49.7
spinal	C72.0	C79.49	—	D33.4	D43.4	D49.7
mouth	C06.9	C79.89	D00.00	D10.30	D37.09	D49.0
book-leaf	C06.89	C79.89	—	—	—	—
floor	C04.9	C79.89	D00.06	D10.2	D37.09	D49.0
anterior portion	C04.0	C79.89	D00.06	D10.2	D37.09	D49.0
lateral portion	C04.1	C79.89	D00.06	D10.2	D37.09	D49.0
overlapping lesion	C04.8	—	—	—	—	—
overlapping NEC	C06.80	—	—	—	—	—
roof	C05.9	C79.89	D00.00	D10.39	D37.09	D49.0
specified part NEC	C06.89	C79.89	D00.00	D10.39	D37.09	D49.0
vestibule	C06.1	C79.89	D00.00	D10.39	D37.09	D49.0
mucosa						
alveolar (ridge or process)	C03.9	C79.89	D00.03	D10.39	D37.09	D49.0
lower	C03.1	C79.89	D00.03	D10.39	D37.09	D49.0
upper	C03.0	C79.89	D00.03	D10.39	D37.09	D49.0
buccal	C06.0	C79.89	D00.02	D10.39	D37.09	D49.0
cheek	C06.0	C79.89	D00.02	D10.39	D37.09	D49.0

▼ Subterms under main terms may continue to next column or page   ☑ Additional Character Required — Refer to the Tabular List for Character Selection   **339**

Neoplasm, lymph, lymphatic channel NEC — Neoplasm, mucosa

Neoplasm Table

	Malignant Primary	Malignant Secondary	Ca in situ	Benign	Uncertain Behavior	Unspecified Behavior
Neoplasm, neoplastic						
— *continued*						
mucosa — *continued*						
lip — *see* Neoplasm, lip, internal						
nasal	C30.0	C78.39	D02.3	D14.0	D38.5	D49.1
oral	C06.0	C79.89	D00.02	D10.39	D37.09	D49.0
Mullerian duct						
female	C57.7	C79.82	D07.39	D28.7	D39.8	D49.59
male	C63.7	C79.82	D07.69	D29.8	D40.8	D49.59
muscle — *see also* Neoplasm, connective tissue						
extraocular	C69.6-✓	C79.49	D09.2-✓	D31.6-✓	D48.7	D49.89
myocardium	C38.0	C79.89	—	D15.1	D48.7	D49.89
myometrium	C54.2	C79.82	D07	D26.1	D39.0	D49.59
myopericardium	C38.0	C79.89	—	D15.1	D48.7	D49.89
nabothian gland (follicle)	C53.0	C79.82	D06.0	D26.0	D39.0	D49.59
nail — *see also* Neoplasm, skin, limb	C44.90	C79.2	D04.9	D23.9	D48.5	D49.2
finger — *see also* Neoplasm, skin, limb, upper	C44.60-✓	C79.2	D04.6-✓	D23.6-✓	D48.5	D49.2
toe — *see also* Neoplasm, skin, limb, lower	C44.70-✓	C79.2	D04.7-✓	D23.7-✓	D48.5	D49.2
nares, naris (anterior) (posterior)	C30.0	C78.39	D02.3	D14.0	D38.5	D49.1
nasal — *see* Neoplasm, nose						
nasolabial groove — *see also* Neoplasm, skin, face	C44.309	C79.2	D04.39	D23.39	D48.5	D49.2
nasolacrimal duct	C69.5-✓	C79.49	D09.2-✓	D31.5-✓	D48.7	D49.89
nasopharynx, nasopharyngeal	C11.9	C79.89	D00.08	D10.6	D37.05	D49.0
floor	C11.3	C79.89	D00.08	D10.6	D37.05	D49.0
overlapping lesion	C11.8	—	—	—	—	—
roof	C11.0	C79.89	D00.08	D10.6	D37.05	D49.0
wall	C11.9	C79.89	D00.08	D10.6	D37.05	D49.0
anterior	C11.3	C79.89	D00.08	D10.6	D37.05	D49.0
lateral	C11.2	C79.89	D00.08	D10.6	D37.05	D49.0
posterior	C11.1	C79.89	D00.08	D10.6	D37.05	D49.0
superior	C11.0	C79.89	D00.08	D10.6	D37.05	D49.0
nates — *see also* Neoplasm, skin, trunk	C44.509	C79.2	D04.5	D23.5	D48.5	D49.2
neck NEC	C76.0	C79.89	D09.8	D36.7	D48.7	D49.89
skin	C44.40	—	—	—	—	—
basal cell carcinoma	C44.41	—	—	—	—	—
specified type NEC	C44.49	—	—	—	—	—
squamous cell carcinoma	C44.42	—	—	—	—	—
nerve (ganglion)	C47.9	C79.89	—	D36.10	D48.2	D49.2
abducens	C72.59	C79.49	—	D33.3	D43.3	D49.7
accessory (spinal)	C72.59	C79.49	—	D33.3	D43.3	D49.7
acoustic	C72.4-✓	C79.49	—	D33.3	D43.3	D49.7
auditory	C72.4-✓	C79.49	—	D33.3	D43.3	D49.7
autonomic NEC — *see also* Neoplasm, nerve, peripheral	C47.9	C79.89	—	D36.10	D48.2	D49.2
brachial	C47.1-✓	C79.89	—	D36.12	D48.2	D49.2
cranial	C72.50	C79.49	—	D33.3	D43.3	D49.7
specified NEC	C72.59	C79.49	—	D33.3	D43.3	D49.7
facial	C72.59	C79.49	—	D33.3	D43.3	D49.7
femoral	C47.2-✓	C79.89	—	D36.13	D48.2	D49.2
ganglion NEC — *see also* Neoplasm, nerve, peripheral	C47.9	C79.89	—	D36.10	D48.2	D49.2
glossopharyngeal	C72.59	C79.49	—	D33.3	D43.3	D49.7
hypoglossal	C72.59	C79.49	—	D33.3	D43.3	D49.7
intercostal	C47.3	C79.89	—	D36.14	D48.2	D49.2
lumbar	C47.6	C79.89	—	D36.17	D48.2	D49.2
median	C47.1-✓	C79.89	—	D36.12	D48.2	D49.2
obturator	C47.2-✓	C79.89	—	D36.13	D48.2	D49.2

	Malignant Primary	Malignant Secondary	Ca in situ	Benign	Uncertain Behavior	Unspecified Behavior
Neoplasm, neoplastic						
— *continued*						
nerve — *continued*						
oculomotor	C72.59	C79.49	—	D33.3	D43.3	D49.7
olfactory	C47.2-✓	C79.49	—	D33.3	D43.3	D49.7
optic	C72.3-✓	C79.49	—	D33.3	D43.3	D49.7
parasympathetic NEC	C47.9	C79.89	—	D36.10	D48.2	D49.2
peripheral NEC	C47.9	C79.89	—	D36.10	D48.2	D49.2
abdomen	C47.4	C79.89	—	D36.15	D48.2	D49.2
abdominal wall	C47.4	C79.89	—	D36.15	D48.2	D49.2
ankle	C47.2-✓	C79.89	—	D36.13	D48.2	D49.2
antecubital fossa or space	C47.1-✓	C79.89	—	D36.12	D48.2	D49.2
arm	C47.1-✓	C79.89	—	D36.12	D48.2	D49.2
auricle (ear)	C47.0	C79.89	—	D36.11	D48.2	D49.2
axilla	C47.3	C79.89	—	D36.12	D48.2	D49.2
back	C47.6	C79.89	—	D36.17	D48.2	D49.2
buttock	C47.5	C79.89	—	D36.16	D48.2	D49.2
calf	C47.2-✓	C79.89	—	D36.13	D48.2	D49.2
cervical region	C47.0	C79.89	—	D36.11	D48.2	D49.2
cheek	C47.0	C79.89	—	D36.11	D48.2	D49.2
chest (wall)	C47.3	C79.89	—	D36.14	D48.2	D49.2
chin	C47.0	C79.89	—	D36.11	D48.2	D49.2
ear (external)	C47.0	C79.89	—	D36.11	D48.2	D49.2
elbow	C47.1-✓	C79.89	—	D36.12	D48.2	D49.2
extrarectal	C47.5	C79.89	—	D36.16	D48.2	D49.2
extremity	C47.9	C79.89	—	D36.10	D48.2	D49.2
lower	C47.2-✓	C79.89	—	D36.13	D48.2	D49.2
upper	C47.1-✓	C79.89	—	D36.12	D48.2	D49.2
eyelid	C47.0	C79.89	—	D36.11	D48.2	D49.2
face	C47.0	C79.89	—	D36.11	D48.2	D49.2
finger	C47.1-✓	C79.89	—	D36.12	D48.2	D49.2
flank	C47.6	C79.89	—	D36.17	D48.2	D49.2
foot	C47.2-✓	C79.89	—	D36.13	D48.2	D49.2
forearm	C47.1-✓	C79.89	—	D36.12	D48.2	D49.2
forehead	C47.0	C79.89	—	D36.11	D48.2	D49.2
gluteal region	C47.5	C79.89	—	D36.16	D48.2	D49.2
groin	C47.5	C79.89	—	D36.16	D48.2	D49.2
hand	C47.1-✓	C79.89	—	D36.12	D48.2	D49.2
head	C47.0	C79.89	—	D36.11	D48.2	D49.2
heel	C47.2-✓	C79.89	—	D36.13	D48.2	D49.2
hip	C47.2-✓	C79.89	—	D36.13	D48.2	D49.2
infraclavicular region	C47.3	C79.89	—	D36.14	D48.2	D49.2
inguinal (canal) (region)	C47.5	C79.89	—	D36.16	D48.2	D49.2
intrathoracic	C47.3	C79.89	—	D36.14	D48.2	D49.2
ischiorectal fossa	C47.5	C79.89	—	D36.16	D48.2	D49.2
knee	C47.2-✓	C79.89	—	D36.13	D48.2	D49.2
leg	C47.2-✓	C79.89	—	D36.13	D48.2	D49.2
limb NEC	C47.9	C79.89	—	D36.10	D48.2	D49.2
lower	C47.2-✓	C79.89	—	D36.13	D48.2	D49.2
upper	C47.1-✓	C79.89	—	D36.12	D48.2	D49.2
nates	C47.5	C79.89	—	D36.16	D48.2	D49.2
neck	C47.0	C79.89	—	D36.11	D48.2	D49.2
orbit	C69.6-✓	C79.49	—	D31.6-✓	D48.7	D49.2
pararectal	C47.5	C79.89	—	D36.16	D48.2	D49.2
paraurethral	C47.5	C79.89	—	D36.16	D48.2	D49.2
paravaginal	C47.5	C79.89	—	D36.16	D48.2	D49.2
pelvis (floor)	C47.5	C79.89	—	D36.16	D48.2	D49.2
pelvoabdominal	C47.8	C79.89	—	D36.17	D48.2	D49.2
perineum	C47.5	C79.89	—	D36.16	D48.2	D49.2
perirectal (tissue)	C47.5	C79.89	—	D36.16	D48.2	D49.2
periurethral (tissue)	C47.5	C79.89	—	D36.16	D48.2	D49.2
popliteal fossa or space	C47.2-✓	C79.89	—	D36.13	D48.2	D49.2
presacral	C47.5	C79.89	—	D36.16	D48.2	D49.2
pterygoid fossa	C47.0	C79.89	—	D36.11	D48.2	D49.2
rectovaginal septum or wall	C47.5	C79.89	—	D36.16	D48.2	D49.2
rectovesical	C47.5	C79.89	—	D36.16	D48.2	D49.2
sacrococcygeal region	C47.5	C79.89	—	D36.16	D48.2	D49.2
scalp	C47.0	C79.89	—	D36.11	D48.2	D49.2

Neoplasm, mucosa — Neoplasm, nerve

	Malignant Primary	Malignant Secondary	Ca in situ	Benign	Uncertain Behavior	Unspecified Behavior
Neoplasm, neoplastic						
— *continued*						
nerve — *continued*						
peripheral —						
continued						
scapular						
region	C47.3	C79.89	—	D36.14	D48.2	D49.2
shoulder	C47.1-☑	C79.89	—	D36.12	D48.2	D49.2
submental	C47.0	C79.89	—	D36.11	D48.2	D49.2
supraclavicular						
region	C47.0	C79.89	—	D36.11	D48.2	D49.2
temple	C47.0	C79.89	—	D36.11	D48.2	D49.2
temporal						
region	C47.0	C79.89	—	D36.11	D48.2	D49.2
thigh	C47.2-☑	C79.89	—	D36.13	D48.2	D49.2
thoracic (duct)						
(wall)	C47.3	C79.89	—	D36.14	D48.2	D49.2
thorax	C47.3	C79.89	—	D36.14	D48.2	D49.2
thumb	C47.1-☑	C79.89	—	D36.12	D48.2	D49.2
toe	C47.2-☑	C79.89	—	D36.13	D48.2	D49.2
trunk	C47.6	C79.89	—	D36.17	D48.2	D49.2
umbilicus	C47.4	C79.89	—	D36.15	D48.2	D49.2
vesicorectal	C47.5	C79.89	—	D36.16	D48.2	D49.2
wrist	C47.1-☑	C79.89	—	D36.12	D48.2	D49.2
radial	C47.1-☑	C79.89	—	D36.12	D48.2	D49.2
sacral	C47.5	C79.89	—	D36.16	D48.2	D49.2
sciatic	C47.2-☑	C79.89	—	D36.13	D48.2	D49.2
spinal NEC	C47.9	C79.89	—	D36.10	D48.2	D49.2
accessory	C72.59	C79.49	—	D33.3	D43.3	D49.7
sympathetic NEC —						
see also						
Neoplasm, nerve,						
peripheral	C47.9	C79.89	—	D36.10	D48.2	D49.2
trigeminal	C72.59	C79.49	—	D33.3	D43.3	D49.7
trochlear	C72.59	C79.49	—	D33.3	D43.3	D49.7
ulnar	C47.1-☑	C79.89	—	D36.12	D48.2	D49.2
vagus	C72.59	C79.49	—	D33.3	D43.3	D49.7
nervous system						
(central)	C72.9	C79.40	—	D33.9	D43.9	D49.7
autonomic — *see*						
Neoplasm, nerve,						
peripheral						
parasympathetic						
— *see* Neoplasm,						
nerve, peripheral						
specified site						
NEC	—	C79.49	—	D33.7	D43.8	—
sympathetic — *see*						
Neoplasm, nerve,						
peripheral						
nevus — *see* Nevus						
nipple	C50.0-☑	C79.81	D05.-☑	D24.-☑	—	—
nose, nasal	C76.0	C79.89	D09.8	D36.7	D48.7	D49.89
ala (external) (nasi)						
— *see also*						
Neoplasm, nose,						
skin	C44.301	C79.2	D04.39	D23.39	D48.5	D49.2
bone	C41.0	C79.51	—	D16.4	D48.0	D49.2
cartilage	C30.0	C78.39	D02.3	D14.0	D38.5	D49.1
cavity	C30.0	C78.39	D02.3	D14.0	D38.5	D49.1
choana	C11.3	C79.89	D00.08	D10.6	D37.05	D49.0
external (skin) — *see*						
also Neoplasm,						
nose, skin	C44.301	C79.2	D04.39	D23.39	D48.5	D49.2
fossa	C30.0	C78.39	D02.3	D14.0	D38.5	D49.1
internal	C30.0	C78.39	D02.3	D14.0	D38.5	D49.1
mucosa	C30.0	C78.39	D02.3	D14.0	D38.5	D49.1
septum	C30.0	C78.39	D02.3	D14.0	D38.5	D49.1
posterior						
margin	C11.3	C79.89	D00.08	D10.6	D37.05	D49.0
sinus — *see*						
Neoplasm, sinus						
skin	C44.301	C79.2	D04.39	D23.39	D48.5	D49.2
basal cell						
carcinoma	C44.311	—	—	—	—	—
specified type						
NEC	C44.391	—	—	—	—	—
squamous cell						
carcinoma	C44.321	—	—	—	—	—
turbinate						
(mucosa)	C30.0	C78.39	D02.3	D14.0	D38.5	D49.1
bone	C41.0	C79.51	—	D16.4	D48.0	D49.2
vestibule	C30.0	C78.39	D02.3	D14.0	D38.5	D49.1

	Malignant Primary	Malignant Secondary	Ca in situ	Benign	Uncertain Behavior	Unspecified Behavior
Neoplasm, neoplastic						
— *continued*						
nostril	C30.0	C78.39	D02.3	D14.0	D38.5	D49.1
nucleus pulposus	C41.2	C79.51	—	D16.6	D48.0	D49.2
occipital						
bone	C41.0	C79.51	—	D16.4	D48.0	D49.2
lobe or pole,						
brain	C71.4	C79.31	—	D33.0	D43.0	D49.6
odontogenic — *see*						
Neoplasm, jaw						
bone						
olfactory nerve or						
bulb	C72.2-☑	C79.49	—	D33.3	D43.3	D49.7
olive (brain)	C71.7	C79.31	—	D33.1	D43.1	D49.6
omentum	C48.1	C78.6	—	D20.1	D48.4	D49.0
operculum (brain)	C71.0	C79.31	—	D33.0	D43.0	D49.6
optic nerve, chiasm, or						
tract	C72.3-☑	C79.49	—	D33.3	D43.3	D49.7
oral (cavity)	C06.9	C79.89	D00.00	D10.30	D37.09	D49.0
ill-defined	C14.8	C79.89	D00.00	D10.30	D37.09	D49.0
mucosa	C06.0	C79.89	D00.02	D10.39	D37.09	D49.0
orbit	C69.6-☑	C79.49	D09.2-☑	D31.6-☑	D48.7	D49.89
autonomic						
nerve	C69.6-☑	C79.49	—	D31.6-☑	D48.7	D49.2
bone	C41.0	C79.51	—	D16.4	D48.0	D49.2
eye	C69.6-☑	C79.49	D09.2-☑	D31.6-☑	D48.7	D49.89
peripheral						
nerves	C69.6-☑	C79.49	—	D31.6-☑	D48.7	D49.2
soft parts	C69.6-☑	C79.49	D09.2-☑	D31.6-☑	D48.7	D49.89
organ of						
Zuckerkandl	C75.5	C79.89	—	D35.6	D44.7	D49.7
oropharynx	C10.9	C79.89	D00.08	D10.5	D37.05	D49.0
branchial cleft						
(vestige)	C10.4	C79.89	D00.08	D10.5	D37.05	D49.0
junctional						
region	C10.8	C79.89	D00.08	D10.5	D37.05	D49.0
lateral wall	C10.2	C79.89	D00.08	D10.5	D37.05	D49.0
overlapping						
lesion	C10.8	—	—	—	—	—
pillars or fauces	C09.1	C79.89	D00.08	D10.5	D37.05	D49.0
posterior wall	C10.3	C79.89	D00.08	D10.5	D37.05	D49.0
vallecula	C10.0	C79.89	D00.08	D10.5	D37.05	D49.0
os						
external	C53.1	C79.82	D06.1	D26.0	D39.0	D49.59
internal	C53.0	C79.82	D06.0	D26.0	D39.0	D49.59
ovary	C56.-☑	C79.6-☑	D07.39	D27.-☑	D39.1-☑	D49.59
oviduct	C57.0-☑	C79.82	D07.39	D28.2	D39.8	D49.59
palate	C05.9	C79.89	D00.00	D10.39	D37.09	D49.0
hard	C05.0	C79.89	D00.05	D10.39	D37.09	D49.0
junction of hard and						
soft palate	C05.9	C79.89	D00.00	D10.39	D37.09	D49.0
overlapping						
lesions	C05.8	—	—	—	—	—
soft	C05.1	C79.89	D00.04	D10.39	D37.09	D49.0
nasopharyngeal						
surface	C11.3	C79.89	D00.08	D10.6	D37.05	D49.0
posterior						
surface	C11.3	C79.89	D00.08	D10.6	D37.05	D49.0
superior						
surface	C11.3	C79.89	D00.08	D10.6	D37.05	D49.0
palatoglossal arch	C09.1	C79.89	D00.00	D10.5	D37.09	D49.0
palatopharyngeal						
arch	C09.1	C79.89	D00.00	D10.5	D37.09	D49.0
pallium	C71.0	C79.31	—	D33.0	D43.0	D49.6
palpebra	C44.10-☑	C79.2	D04.1-☑	D23.1-☑	D48.5	D49.2
basal cell						
carcinoma	C44.11-☑	—	—	—	—	—
sebaceous cell	C44.13-☑	—	—	—	—	—
specified type						
NEC	C44.19-☑	—	—	—	—	—
squamous cell						
carcinoma	C44.12-☑	—	—	—	—	—
pancreas	C25.9	C78.89	D01.7	D13.6	D37.8	D49.0
body	C25.1	C78.89	D01.7	D13.6	D37.8	D49.0
duct (of Santorini) (of						
Wirsung)	C25.3	C78.89	D01.7	D13.6	D37.8	D49.0
ectopic tissue	C25.7	C78.89	—	D13.6	D37.8	D49.0
head	C25.0	C78.89	D01.7	D13.6	D37.8	D49.0
islet cells	C25.4	C78.89	D01.7	D13.7	D37.8	D49.0
neck	C25.7	C78.89	D01.7	D13.6	D37.8	D49.0
overlapping						
lesion	C25.8	—	—	—	—	—
tail	C25.2	C78.89	D01.7	D13.6	D37.8	D49.0

	Malignant Primary	Malignant Secondary	Ca in situ	Benign	Uncertain Behavior	Unspecified Behavior
Neoplasm, neoplastic						
— continued						
para-aortic body	C75.5	C79.89	—	D35.6	D44.7	D49.7
paraganglion NEC	C75.5	C79.89	—	D35.6	D44.7	D49.7
parametrium	C57.3	C79.82	—	D28.2	D39.8	D49.59
paranephric	C48.0	C78.6	—	D20.0	D48.3	D49.0
pararectal	C76.3	C79.89	—	D36.7	D48.7	D49.89
parasagittal						
(region)	C76.0	C79.89	D09.8	D36.7	D48.7	D49.89
parasellar	C72.9	C79.49	—	D33.9	D43.8	D49.7
parathyroid						
(gland)	C75.0	C79.89	D09.3	D35.1	D44.2	D49.7
paraurethral	C76.3	C79.89	—	D36.7	D48.7	D49.89
gland	C68.1	C79.19	D09.19	D30.8	D41.8	D49.59
paravaginal	C76.3	C79.89	—	D36.7	D48.7	D49.89
parenchyma,						
kidney	C64.-☑	C79.0-☑	D09.19	D30.0-☑	D41.0-☑	D49.51-☑
parietal						
bone	C41.0	C79.51	—	D16.4	D48.0	D49.2
lobe, brain	C71.3	C79.31	—	D33.0	D43.0	D49.6
paroophoron	C57.1-☑	C79.82	D07.39	D28.2	D39.8	D49.59
parotid (duct)						
(gland)	C07	C79.89	D00.00	D11.0	D37.030	D49.0
parovarium	C57.1-☑	C79.82	D07.39	D28.2	D39.8	D49.59
patella	C40.20	C79.51	—			
peduncle, cerebral	C71.7	C79.31	—	D33.1	D43.1	D49.6
pelvirectal						
junction	C19	C78.5	D01.1	D12.7	D37.5	D49.0
pelvis, pelvic	C76.3	C79.89	D09.8	D36.7	D48.7	D49.89
bone	C41.4	C79.51	—	D16.8	D48.0	D49.2
floor	C76.3	C79.89	D09.8	D36.7	D48.7	D49.89
renal	C65.-☑	C79.0-☑	D09.19	D30.1-☑	D41.1-☑	D49.51-☑
viscera	C76.3	C79.89	D09.8	D36.7	D48.7	D49.89
wall	C76.3	C79.89	D09.8	D36.7	D48.7	D49.89
pelvo-abdominal	C76.8	C79.89	D09.8	D36.7	D48.7	D49.89
penis	C60.9	C79.82	D07.4	D29.0	D40.8	D49.59
body	C60.2	C79.82	D07.4	D29.0	D40.8	D49.59
corpus						
(cavernosum)	C60.2	C79.82	D07.4	D29.0	D40.8	D49.59
glans	C60.1	C79.82	D07.4	D29.0	D40.8	D49.59
overlapping						
sites	C60.8	—	—	—	—	—
skin NEC	C60.9	C79.82	D07.4	D29.0	D40.8	D49.59
periadrenal						
(tissue)	C48.0	C78.6	—	D20.0	D48.3	D49.0
perianal (skin) — *see also* Neoplasm,						
anus, skin	C44.500	C79.2	D04.5	D23.5	D48.5	D49.2
pericardium	C38.0	C79.89	—	D15.1	D48.7	D49.89
perinephric	C48.0	C78.6	—	D20.0	D48.3	D49.0
perineum	C76.3	C79.89	D09.8	D36.7	D48.7	D49.89
periodontal tissue						
NEC	C03.9	C79.89	D00.03	D10.39	D37.09	D49.0
periosteum — *see* Neoplasm, bone						
peripancreatic	C48.0	C78.6	—	D20.0	D48.3	D49.0
peripheral nerve						
NEC	C47.9	C79.89	—	D36.10	D48.2	D49.2
perirectal (tissue)	C76.3	C79.89	—	D36.7	D48.7	D49.89
perirenal (tissue)	C48.0	C78.6	—	D20.0	D48.3	D49.0
peritoneum, peritoneal						
(cavity)	C48.2	C78.6	—	D20.1	D48.4	D49.0
benign mesothelial tissue — *see* Mesothelioma, benign						
overlapping lesion						
with digestive						
organs	C48.8	—	—	—	—	—
	C26.9	—	—	—	—	—
parietal	C48.1	C78.6	—	D20.1	D48.4	D49.0
pelvic	C48.1	C78.6	—	D20.1	D48.4	D49.0
specified part						
NEC	C48.1	C78.6	—	D20.1	D48.4	D49.0
peritonsillar						
(tissue)	C76.0	C79.89	D09.8	D36.7	D48.7	D49.89
periurethral tissue	C76.3	C79.89	—	D36.7	D48.7	D49.89
phalanges						
foot	C40.3-☑	C79.51	—	D16.3-☑	—	—
hand	C40.1-☑	C79.51	—	D16.1-☑	—	—
pharynx,						
pharyngeal	C14.0	C79.89	D00.08	D10.9	D37.05	D49.0
bursa	C11.1	C79.89	D00.08	D10.6	D37.05	D49.0
Neoplasm, neoplastic						
— continued						
pharynx, pharyngeal						
— continued						
fornix	C11.3	C79.89	D00.08	D10.6	D37.05	D49.0
recess	C11.2	C79.89	D00.08	D10.6	D37.05	D49.0
region	C14.0	C79.89	D00.08	D10.9	D37.05	D49.0
tonsil	C11.1	C79.89	D00.08	D10.6	D37.05	D49.0
wall (lateral)						
(posterior)	C14.0	C79.89	D00.08	D10.9	D37.05	D49.0
pia mater	C70.9	C79.40	—	D32.9	D42.9	D49.7
cerebral	C70.0	C79.32	—	D32.0	D42.0	D49.7
cranial	C70.0	C79.32	—	D32.0	D42.0	D49.7
spinal	C70.1	C79.49	—	D32.1	D42.1	D49.7
pillars of fauces	C09.1	C79.89	D00.08	D10.5	D37.05	D49.0
pineal (body)						
(gland)	C75.3	C79.89	D09.3	D35.4	D44.5	D49.7
pinna (ear) NEC — *see also* Neoplasm, skin,						
ear	C44.20-☑	C79.2	D04.2-☑	D23.2-☑	D48.5	D49.2
piriform fossa or						
sinus	C12	C79.89	D00.08	D10.7	D37.05	D49.0
pituitary (body) (fossa)						
(gland) (lobe)	C75.1	C79.89	D09.3	D35.2	D44.3	D49.7
placenta	C58	C79.82	D07.0	D26.7	D39.2	D49.59
pleura, pleural						
(cavity)	C38.4	C78.2	—	D19.0	D38.2	D49.1
overlapping lesion with heart or						
mediastinum	C38.8	—	—	—	—	—
parietal	C38.4	C78.2	—	D19.0	D38.2	D49.1
visceral	C38.4	C78.2	—	D19.0	D38.2	D49.1
plexus						
brachial	C47.1-☑	C79.89	—	D36.12	D48.2	D49.2
cervical	C47.0	C79.89	—	D36.11	D48.2	D49.2
choroid	C71.5	C79.31	—	D33.0	D43.0	D49.6
lumbosacral	C47.5	C79.89	—	D36.16	D48.2	D49.2
sacral	C47.5	C79.89	—	D36.16	D48.2	D49.2
pluriendocrine	C75.8	C79.89	D09.3	D35.7	D44.9	D49.7
pole						
frontal	C71.1	C79.31	—	D33.0	D43.0	D49.6
occipital	C71.4	C79.31	—	D33.0	D43.0	D49.6
pons (varolii)	C71.7	C79.31	—	D33.1	D43.1	D49.6
popliteal fossa or						
space	C76.5-☑	C79.89	D04.7-☑	D36.7	D48.7	D49.89
postcricoid						
(region)	C13.0	C79.89	D00.08	D10.7	D37.05	D49.0
posterior fossa						
(cranial)	C71.9	C79.31	—	D33.2	D43.2	D49.6
postnasal space	C11.9	C79.89	D00.08	D10.6	D37.05	D49.0
prepuce	C60.0	C79.82	D07.4	D29.0	D40.8	D49.59
prepylorus	C16.4	C78.89	D00.2	D13.1	D37.1	D49.0
presacral (region)	C76.3	C79.89	—	D36.7	D48.7	D49.89
prostate (gland)	C61	C79.82	D07.5	D29.1	D40.0	D49.59
utricle	C68.0	C79.19	D09.19	D30.4	D41.3	D49.59
pterygoid fossa	C49.0	C79.89	—	D21.0	D48.1	D49.2
pubic bone	C41.4	C79.51	—	D16.8	D48.0	D49.2
pudenda, pudendum						
(femaie)	C51.9	C79.82	D07.1	D28.0	D39.8	D49.59
pulmonary — *see also* Neoplasm,						
lung	C34.9-☑	C78.0-☑	D02.2-☑	D14.3-☑	D38.1	D49.1
putamen	C71.0	C79.31	—	D33.0	D43.0	D49.6
pyloric						
antrum	C16.3	C78.89	D00.2	D13.1	D37.1	D49.0
canal	C16.4	C78.89	D00.2	D13.1	D37.1	D49.0
pylorus	C16.4	C78.89	D00.2	D13.1	D37.1	D49.0
pyramid (brain)	C71.7	C79.31	—	D33.1	D43.1	D49.6
pyriform fossa or						
sinus	C12	C79.89	D00.08	D10.7	D37.05	D49.0
radius (any part)	C40.0-☑	C79.51	—	D16.0-☑	—	—
Rathke's pouch	C75.1	C79.89	D09.3	D35.2	D44.3	D49.7
rectosigmoid						
(junction)	C19	C78.5	D01.1	D12.7	D37.5	D49.0
overlapping lesion with anus or						
rectum	C21.8	—	—	—	—	—
rectouterine						
pouch	C48.1	C78.6	—	D20.1	D48.4	D49.0
rectovaginal septum or						
wall	C76.3	C79.89	D09.8	D36.7	D48.7	D49.89
rectovesical						
septum	C76.3	C79.89	D09.8	D36.7	D48.7	D49.89
rectum (ampulla)	C20	C78.5	D01.2	D12.8	D37.5	D49.0

☑ **Additional Character Required** — Refer to the Tabular List for Character Selection ▽ **Subterms under main terms may continue to next column or page**

Neoplasm, neoplastic	Malignant Primary	Malignant Secondary	Ca in situ	Benign	Uncertain Behavior	Unspecified Behavior
— continued						
rectum — continued						
and colon	C19	C78.5	D01.1	D12.7	D37.5	D49.0
overlapping lesion with anus or rectosigmoid junction	C21.8	—	—	—	—	—
renal	C64.-☑	C79.0-☑	D09.19	D30.0-☑	D41.0-☑	D49.51-☑
calyx	C65.-☑	C79.0-☑	D09.19	D30.1-☑	D41.1-☑	D49.51-☑
hilus	C65.-☑	C79.0-☑	D09.19	D30.1-☑	D41.1-☑	D49.51-☑
parenchyma	C64.-☑	C79.0-☑	D09.19	D30.0-☑	D41.0-☑	D49.51-☑
pelvis	C65.-☑	C79.0-☑	D09.19	D30.1-☑	D41.1-☑	D49.51-☑
respiratory						
organs or system NEC	C39.9	C78.30	D02.4	D14.4	D38.6	D49.1
tract NEC	C39.9	C78.30	D02.4	D14.4	D38.5	D49.1
upper	C39.0	C78.30	D02.4	D14.4	D38.5	D49.1
retina	C69.2-☑	C79.49	D09.2-☑	D31.2-☑	D48.7	D49.81
retrobulbar	C69.6-☑	C79.49	—	D31.6-☑	D48.7	D49.89
retrocecal	C48.0	C78.6	—	D20.0	D48.3	D49.0
retromolar (area) (triangle) (trigone)	C06.2	C79.89	D00.00	D10.39	D37.09	D49.0
retro-orbital	C76.0	C79.89	D09.8	D36.7	D48.7	D49.89
retroperitoneal (space) (tissue)	C48.0	C78.6	—	D20.0	D48.3	D49.0
retroperitoneum	C48.0	C78.6	—	D20.0	D48.3	D49.0
retropharyngeal	C14.0	C79.89	D00.08	D10.9	D37.05	D49.0
retrovesical (septum)	C76.3	C79.89	D09.8	D36.7	D48.7	D49.89
rhinencephalon	C71.0	C79.31	—	D33.0	D43.0	D49.6
rib	C41.3	C79.51	—	D16.7	D48.0	D49.2
Rosenmuller's fossa	C11.2	C79.89	D00.08	D10.6	D37.05	D49.0
round ligament	C57.2-☑	C79.82	—	D28.2	D39.8	D49.59
sacrococcyx, sacrococcygeal	C41.4	C79.51	—	D16.8	D48.0	D49.2
region	C76.3	C79.89	D09.8	D36.7	D48.7	D49.89
sacrouterine ligament	C57.3	C79.82	—	D28.2	D39.8	D49.59
sacrum, sacral (vertebra)	C41.4	C79.51	—	D16.0	D48.0	D49.2
salivary gland or duct (major)	C08.9	C79.89	D00.00	D11.9	D37.039	D49.0
minor NEC	C06.9	C79.89	D00.00	D10.39	D37.04	D49.0
overlapping lesion	C08.9	—	—	—	—	—
parotid	C07	C79.89	D00.00	D11.0	D37.030	D49.0
pluriglandular	C08.9	C79.89	D00.00	D11.9	D37.039	D49.0
sublingual	C08.1	C79.89	D00.00	D11.7	D37.031	D49.0
submandibular	C08.0	C79.89	D00.00	D11.7	D37.032	D49.0
submaxillary	C08.0	C79.89	D00.00	D11.7	D37.032	D49.0
salpinx (uterine)	C57.0-☑	C79.82	D07.39	D28.2	D39.8	D49.59
Santorini's duct	C25.3	C78.89	D01.7	D13.6	D37.8	D49.0
scalp	C44.40	C79.2	D04.4	D23.4	D48.5	D49.2
basal cell carcinoma	C44.41	—	—	—	—	—
specified type NEC	C44.49	—	—	—	—	—
squamous cell carcinoma	C44.42	—	—	—	—	—
scapula (any part)	C40.0-☑	C79.51	—	D16.0-☑	—	—
scapular region	C76.1	C79.89	D09.8	D36.7	D48.7	D49.89
scar NEC — see also Neoplasm, skin, by site	C44.90	C79.2	D04.9	D23.9	D48.5	D49.2
sciatic nerve	C47.2-☑	C79.89	—	D36.13	D48.2	D49.2
sclera	C69.4-☑	C79.49	D09.2-☑	D31.4-☑	D48.7	D49.89
scrotum (skin)	C63.2	C79.82	D07.61	D29.4	D40.8	D49.59
sebaceous gland — see Neoplasm, skin						
sella turcica	C75.1	C79.89	D09.3	D35.2	D44.3	D49.7
bone	C41.0	C79.51	—	D16.4	D48.0	D49.2
semilunar cartilage (knee)	C40.2-☑	C79.51	—	D16.2-☑	D48.0	D49.2
seminal vesicle	C63.7	C79.82	D07.69	D29.8	D40.8	D49.59
septum						
nasal	C30.0	C78.39	D02.3	D14.0	D38.5	D49.1
posterior margin	C11.3	C79.89	D00.08	D10.6	D37.05	D49.0
rectovaginal	C76.3	C79.89	D09.8	D36.7	D48.7	D49.89
rectovesical	C76.3	C79.89	D09.8	D36.7	D48.7	D49.89

Neoplasm, neoplastic	Malignant Primary	Malignant Secondary	Ca in situ	Benign	Uncertain Behavior	Unspecified Behavior
— continued						
septum — continued						
urethrovaginal	C57.9	C79.82	D07.30	D28.9	D39.9	D49.59
vesicovaginal	C57.9	C79.82	D07.30	D28.9	D39.9	D49.59
shoulder NEC	C76.4-☑	C79.89	D04.6-☑	D36.7	D48.7	D49.89
sigmoid flexure (lower) (upper)	C18.7	C78.5	D01.0	D12.5	D37.4	D49.0
sinus (accessory)	C31.9	C78.39	D02.3	D14.0	D38.5	D49.1
bone (any)	C41.0	C79.51	—	D16.4	D48.0	D49.2
ethmoidal	C31.1	C78.39	D02.3	D14.0	D38.5	D49.1
frontal	C31.2	C78.39	D02.3	D14.0	D38.5	D49.1
maxillary	C31.0	C78.39	D02.3	D14.0	D38.5	D49.1
nasal, paranasal NEC	C31.9	C78.39	D02.3	D14.0	D38.5	D49.1
overlapping lesion	C31.8	—	—	—	—	—
pyriform	C12	C79.89	D00.08	D10.7	D37.05	D49.0
sphenoid	C31.3	C78.39	D02.3	D14.0	D38.5	D49.1
skeleton, skeletal NEC	C41.9	C79.51	—	D16.9	D48.0	D49.2
Skene's gland	C68.1	C79.19	D09.19	D30.8	D41.8	D49.59
skin NOS	C44.90	C79.2	D04.9	D23.9	D48.5	D49.2
abdominal wall	C44.509	C79.2	D04.5	D23.5	D48.5	D49.2
basal cell carcinoma	C44.519	—	—	—	—	—
specified type NEC	C44.599	—	—	—	—	—
squamous cell carcinoma	C44.529	—	—	—	—	—
ala nasi — see also Neoplasm, nose, skin	C44.301	C79.2	D04.39	D23.39	D48.5	D49.2
ankle — see also Neoplasm, skin, limb, lower	C44.70-☑	C79.2	D04.7-☑	D23.7-☑	D48.5	D49.2
antecubital space — see also Neoplasm, skin, limb, upper	C44.60-☑	C79.2	D04.6-☑	D23.6-☑	D48.5	D49.2
anus	C44.500	C79.2	D04.5	D23.5	D48.5	D49.2
basal cell carcinoma	C44.510	—	—	—	—	—
specified type NEC	C44.590	—	—	—	—	—
squamous cell carcinoma	C44.520	—	—	—	—	—
arm — see also Neoplasm, skin, limb, upper	C44.60-☑	C79.2	D04.6-☑	D23.6-☑	D48.5	D49.2
auditory canal (external) — see also Neoplasm, skin, ear	C44.20-☑	C79.2	D04.2-☑	D23.2-☑	D48.5	D49.2
auricle (ear) — see also Neoplasm, skin, ear	C44.20-☑	C79.2	D04.2-☑	D23.2-☑	D48.5	D49.2
auricular canal (external) — see also Neoplasm, skin, ear	C44.20-☑	C79.2	D04.2-☑	D23.2-☑	D48.5	D49.2
axilla, axillary fold — see also Neoplasm, skin, trunk	C44.509	C79.2	D04.5	D23.5	D48.5	D49.2
back — see also Neoplasm, skin, trunk	C44.509	C79.2	D04.5	D23.5	D48.5	D49.2
basal cell carcinoma	C44.91	—	—	—	—	—
breast	C44.501	C79.2	D04.5	D23.5	D48.5	D49.2
basal cell carcinoma	C44.511	—	—	—	—	—
specified type NEC	C44.591	—	—	—	—	—
squamous cell carcinoma	C44.521	—	—	—	—	—
brow — see also Neoplasm, skin, face	C44.309	C79.2	D04.39	D23.39	D48.5	D49.2
buttock — see also Neoplasm, skin, trunk	C44.509	C79.2	D04.5	D23.5	D48.5	D49.2

Neoplasm, neoplastic — continued — skin — continued

	Malignant Primary	Malignant Secondary	Ca in situ	Benign	Uncertain Behavior	Unspecified Behavior
calf — see also Neoplasm, skin, limb, lower	C44.70-✓	C79.2	D04.7-✓	D23.7-✓	D48.5	D49.2
canthus (eye) (inner) (outer)	C44.10-✓	C79.2	D04.1-✓	D23.1-✓	D48.5	D49.2
basal cell carcinoma	C44.11-✓	—	—	—	—	—
sebaceous cell	C44.13-✓	—	—	—	—	—
specified type NEC	C44.19-✓	—	—	—	—	—
squamous cell carcinoma	C44.12-✓	—	—	—	—	—
cervical region — see also Neoplasm, skin, neck	C44.40	C79.2	D04.4	D23.4	D48.5	D49.2
cheek (external) — see also Neoplasm, skin, face	C44.309	C79.2	D04.39	D23.39	D48.5	D49.2
chest (wall) — see also Neoplasm, skin, trunk	C44.509	C79.2	D04.5	D23.5	D48.5	D49.2
chin — see also Neoplasm, skin, face	C44.309	C79.2	D04.39	D23.39	D48.5	D49.2
clavicular area — see also Neoplasm, skin, trunk	C44.509	C79.2	D04.5	D23.5	D48.5	D49.2
clitoris	C51.2	C79.82	D07.1	D28.0	D39.8	D49.59
columnella — see also Neoplasm, skin, face	C44.309	C79.2	D04.39	D23.39	D48.5	D49.2
concha — see also Neoplasm, skin, ear	C44.20-✓	C79.2	D04.2-✓	D23.2-✓	D48.5	D49.2
ear (external)	C44.20-✓	C79.2	D04.2-✓	D23.2-✓	D48.5	D49.2
basal cell carcinoma	C44.21-✓	—	—	—	—	—
specified type NEC	C44.29-✓	—	—	—	—	—
squamous cell carcinoma	C44.22-✓	—	—	—	—	—
elbow — see also Neoplasm, skin, limb, upper	C44.60-✓	C79.2	D04.6-✓	D23.6-✓	D48.5	D49.2
eyebrow — see also Neoplasm, skin, face	C44.309	C79.2	D04.39	D23.39	D48.5	D49.2
eyelid	C44.10-✓	C79.2	D04.1-✓	D23.1-✓	D48.5	D49.2
basal cell carcinoma	C44.11-✓	—	—	—	—	—
sebaceous cell	C44.13-✓	—	—	—	—	—
specified type NEC	C44.19-✓	—	—	—	—	—
squamous cell carcinoma	C44.12-✓	—	—	—	—	—
face NOS	C44.300	C79.2	D04.30	D23.30	D48.5	D49.2
basal cell carcinoma	C44.310	—	—	—	—	—
specified type NEC	C44.390	—	—	—	—	—
squamous cell carcinoma	C44.320	—	—	—	—	—
female genital organs (external)	C51.9	C79.82	D07.1	D28.0	D39.8	D49.59
clitoris	C51.2	C79.82	D07.1	D28.0	D39.8	D49.59
labium NEC	C51.9	C79.82	D07.1	D28.0	D39.8	D49.59
majus	C51.0	C79.82	D07.1	D28.0	D39.8	D49.59
minus	C51.1	C79.82	D07.1	D28.0	D39.8	D49.59
pudendum	C51.9	C79.82	D07.1	D28.0	D39.8	D49.59
vulva	C51.9	C79.82	D07.1	D28.0	D39.8	D49.59
finger — see also Neoplasm, skin, limb, upper	C44.60-✓	C79.2	D04.6-✓	D23.6-✓	D48.5	D49.2
flank — see also Neoplasm, skin, trunk	C44.509	C79.2	D04.5	D23.5	D48.5	D49.2
foot — see also Neoplasm, skin, limb, lower	C44.70-✓	C79.2	D04.7-✓	D23.7-✓	D48.5	D49.2

Neoplasm, neoplastic — continued — skin — continued

	Malignant Primary	Malignant Secondary	Ca in situ	Benign	Uncertain Behavior	Unspecified Behavior
forearm — see also Neoplasm, skin, limb, upper	C44.60-✓	C79.2	D04.6-✓	D23.6-✓	D48.5	D49.2
forehead — see also Neoplasm, skin, face	C44.309	C79.2	D04.39	D23.39	D48.5	D49.2
glabella — see also Neoplasm, skin, face	C44.309	C79.2	D04.39	D23.39	D48.5	D49.2
gluteal region — see also Neoplasm, skin, trunk	C44.509	C79.2	D04.5	D23.5	D48.5	D49.2
groin — see also Neoplasm, skin, trunk	C44.509	C79.2	D04.5	D23.5	D48.5	D49.2
hand — see also Neoplasm, skin, limb, upper	C44.60-✓	C79.2	D04.6-✓	D23.6-✓	D48.5	D49.2
head NEC — see also Neoplasm, skin, scalp	C44.40	C79.2	D04.4	D23.4	D48.5	D49.2
heel — see also Neoplasm, skin, limb, lower	C44.70-✓	C79.2	D04.7-✓	D23.7-✓	D48.5	D49.2
helix — see also Neoplasm, skin, ear	C44.20-✓	C79.2	D04.2-✓	D23.2-✓	D48.5	D49.2
hip — see also Neoplasm, skin, limb, lower	C44.70-✓	C79.2	D04.7-✓	D23.7-✓	D48.5	D49.2
infraclavicular region — see also Neoplasm, skin, trunk	C44.509	C79.2	D04.5	D23.5	D48.5	D49.2
inguinal region — see also Neoplasm, skin, trunk	C44.509	C79.2	D04.5	D23.5	D48.5	D49.2
jaw — see also Neoplasm, skin, face	C44.309	C79.2	D04.39	D23.39	D48.5	D49.2
Kaposi's sarcoma — see Kaposi's, sarcoma, skin						
knee — see also Neoplasm, skin, limb, lower	C44.70-✓	C79.2	D04.7-✓	D23.7-✓	D48.5	D49.2
labia						
majora	C51.0	C79.82	D07.1	D28.0	D39.8	D49.59
minora	C51.1	C79.82	D07.1	D28.0	D39.8	D49.59
leg — see also Neoplasm, skin, limb, lower	C44.70-✓	C79.2	D04.7-✓	D23.7-✓	D48.5	D49.2
lid (lower) (upper)	C44.10-✓	C79.2	D04.1-✓	D23.1-✓	D48.5	D49.2
basal cell carcinoma	C44.11-✓	—	—	—	—	—
sebaceous cell	C44.13-✓	—	—	—	—	—
specified type NEC	C44.19-✓	—	—	—	—	—
squamous cell carcinoma	C44.12-✓	—	—	—	—	—
limb NEC	C44.90	C79.2	D04.9	D23.9	D48.5	D49.2
basal cell carcinoma	C44.91	—	—	—	—	—
lower	C44.70-✓	C79.2	D04.7-✓	D23.7-✓	D48.5	D49.2
basal cell carcinoma	C44.71-✓	—	—	—	—	—
specified type NEC	C44.79-✓	—	—	—	—	—
squamous cell carcinoma	C44.72-✓	—	—	—	—	—
upper	C44.60-✓	C79.2	D04.6-✓	D23.6-✓	D48.5	D49.2
basal cell carcinoma	C44.61-✓	—	—	—	—	—
specified type NEC	C44.69-✓	—	—	—	—	—
squamous cell carcinoma	C44.62-✓	—	—	—	—	—
lip (lower) (upper)	C44.00	C79.2	D04.0	D23.0	D48.5	D49.2

☑ Additional Character Required — Refer to the Tabular List for Character Selection   ▽ Subterms under main terms may continue to next column or page

Neoplasm, neoplastic — continued
skin — continued
lip — continued

	Malignant Primary	Malignant Secondary	Ca in situ	Benign	Uncertain Behavior	Unspecified Behavior
basal cell carcinoma	C44.01	—	—	—	—	—
specified type NEC	C44.09	—	—	—	—	—
squamous cell carcinoma	C44.02	—	—	—	—	—
male genital organs	C63.9	C79.82	D07.60	D29.9	D40.8	D49.59
penis	C60.9	C79.82	D07.4	D29.0	D40.8	D49.59
prepuce	C60.0	C79.82	D07.4	D29.0	D40.8	D49.59
scrotum	C63.2	C79.82	D07.61	D29.4	D40.8	D49.59
mastectomy site (skin) — see also Neoplasm, skin, breast	C44.501	C79.2				
specified as breast tissue	C50.8-✓	C79.81				
meatus, acoustic (external) — see also Neoplasm, skin, ear	C44.20-✓	C79.2	D04.2-✓	D23.2-✓	D48.5	D49.2
melanotic — see Melanoma						
Merkel cell — see Carcinoma, Merkel cell						
nates — see also Neoplasm, skin, trunk	C44.509	C79.2	D04.5	D23.5	D48.5	D49.2
neck	C44.40	C79.2	D04.4	D23.4	D48.5	D49.2
basal cell carcinoma	C44.41	—	—	—	—	—
specified type NEC	C44.49	—	—	—	—	—
squamous cell carcinoma	C44.42	—	—	—	—	—
nevus — see Nevus, skin						
nose (external) — see also Neoplasm, nose, skin	C44.301	C79.2	D04.39	D23.39	D48.5	D49.2
overlapping lesion	C44.80	—	—	—	—	—
basal cell carcinoma	C44.81	—	—	—	—	—
specified type NEC	C44.89	—	—	—	—	—
squamous cell carcinoma	C44.82	—	—	—	—	—
palm — see also Neoplasm, skin, limb, upper	C44.60-✓	C79.2	D04.6-✓	D23.6-✓	D48.5	D49.2
palpebra	C44.10-✓	C79.2	D04.1-✓	D23.1-✓	D48.5	D49.2
basal cell carcinoma	C44.11-✓	—	—	—	—	—
sebaceous cell	C44.13-✓	—	—	—	—	—
specified type NEC	C44.19-✓	—	—	—	—	—
squamous cell carcinoma	C44.12-✓	—	—	—	—	—
penis NEC	C60.9	C79.82	D07.4	D29.0	D40.8	D49.59
perianal — see also Neoplasm, skin, anus	C44.500	C79.2	D04.5	D23.5	D48.5	D49.2
perineum — see also Neoplasm, skin, anus	C44.500	C79.2	D04.5	D23.5	D48.5	D49.2
pinna — see also Neoplasm, skin, ear	C44.20-✓	C79.2	D04.2-✓	D23.2-✓	D48.5	D49.2
plantar — see also Neoplasm, skin, limb, lower	C44.70-✓	C79.2	D04.7-✓	D23.7-✓	D48.5	D49.2
popliteal fossa or space — see also Neoplasm, skin, limb, lower	C44.70-✓	C79.2	D04.7-✓	D23.7-✓	D48.5	D49.2
prepuce	C60.0	C79.82	D07.4	D29.0	D40.8	D49.59

Neoplasm, neoplastic — continued
skin — continued

	Malignant Primary	Malignant Secondary	Ca in situ	Benign	Uncertain Behavior	Unspecified Behavior
pubes — see also Neoplasm, skin, trunk	C44.509	C79.2	D04.5	D23.5	D48.5	D49.2
sacrococcygeal region — see also Neoplasm, skin, trunk	C44.509	C79.2	D04.5	D23.5	D48.5	D49.2
scalp	C44.40	C79.2	D04.4	D23.4	D48.5	D49.2
basal cell carcinoma	C44.41	—	—	—	—	—
specified type NEC	C44.49	—	—	—	—	—
squamous cell carcinoma	C44.42	—	—	—	—	—
scapular region — see also Neoplasm, skin, trunk	C44.509	C79.2	D04.5	D23.5	D48.5	D49.2
scrotum	C63.2	C79.82	D07.61	D29.4	D40.8	D49.59
shoulder — see also Neoplasm, skin, limb, upper	C44.60-✓	C79.2	D04.6-✓	D23.6-✓	D48.5	D49.2
sole (foot) — see also Neoplasm, skin, limb, lower	C44.70-✓	C79.2	D04.7-✓	D23.7-✓	D48.5	D49.2
specified sites NEC	C44.80	C79.2	D04.8	D23.9	D48.5	D49.2
basal cell carcinoma	C44.81	—	—	—	—	—
specified type NEC	C44.89	—	—	—	—	—
squamous cell carcinoma	C44.82	—	—	—	—	—
specified type NEC	C44.99	—	—	—	—	—
squamous cell carcinoma	C44.92	—	—	—	—	—
submammary fold — see also Neoplasm, skin, trunk	C44.509	C79.2	D04.5	D23.5	D48.5	D49.2
supraclavicular region — see also Neoplasm, skin, neck	C44.40	C79.2	D04.4	D23.4	D48.5	D49.2
temple — see also Neoplasm, skin, face	C44.309	C79.2	D04.39	D23.39	D48.5	D49.2
thigh — see also Neoplasm, skin, limb, lower	C44.70-✓	C79.2	D04.7-✓	D23.7-✓	D48.5	D49.2
thoracic wall — see also Neoplasm, skin, trunk	C44.509	C79.2	D04.5	D23.5	D48.5	D49.2
thumb — see also Neoplasm, skin, limb, upper	C44.60-✓	C79.2	D04.6-✓	D23.6-✓	D48.5	D49.2
toe — see also Neoplasm, skin, limb, lower	C44.70-✓	C79.2	D04.7-✓	D23.7-✓	D48.5	D49.2
tragus — see also Neoplasm, skin, ear	C44.20-✓	C79.2	D04.2-✓	D23.2-✓	D48.5	D49.2
trunk	C44.509	C79.2	D04.5	D23.5	D48.5	D49.2
basal cell carcinoma	C44.519	—	—	—	—	—
specified type NEC	C44.599	—	—	—	—	—
squamous cell carcinoma	C44.529	—	—	—	—	—
umbilicus — see also Neoplasm, skin, trunk	C44.509	C79.2	D04.5	D23.5	D48.5	D49.2
vulva	C51.9	C79.82	D07.1	D28.0	D39.8	D49.59
overlapping lesion	C51.8	—	—	—	—	—
wrist — see also Neoplasm, skin, limb, upper	C44.60-✓	C79.2	D04.6-✓	D23.6-✓	D48.5	D49.2
skull	C41.0	C79.51	—	D16.4	D48.0	D49.2

	Malignant Primary	Malignant Secondary	Ca in situ	Benign	Uncertain Behavior	Unspecified Behavior
Neoplasm, neoplastic						
— continued						
soft parts or tissues —						
see Neoplasm,						
connective tissue						
specified site NEC	C76.8	C79.89	D09.8	D36.7	D48.7	D49.89
spermatic cord	C63.1-☑	C79.82	D07.69	D29.8	D40.8	D49.59
sphenoid	C31.3	C78.39	D02.3	D14.0	D38.5	D49.1
bone	C41.0	C79.51	—	D16.4	D48.0	D49.2
sinus	C31.3	C78.39	D02.3	D14.0	D38.5	D49.1
sphincter						
anal	C21.1	C78.5	D01.3	D12.9	D37.8	D49.0
of Oddi	C24.0	C78.89	D01.5	D13.5	D37.6	D49.0
spine, spinal						
(column)	C41.2	C79.51	—	D16.6	D48.0	D49.2
bulb	C71.7	C79.31	—	D33.1	D43.1	D49.6
coccyx	C41.4	C79.51	—	D16.8	D48.0	D49.2
cord (cervical)						
(lumbar) (sacral)						
(thoracic)	C72.0	C79.49	—	D33.4	D43.4	D49.7
dura mater	C70.1	C79.49	—	D32.1	D42.1	D49.7
lumbosacral	C41.2	C79.51	—	D16.6	D48.0	D49.2
marrow NEC	C96.9	C79.52	—	—	D47.9	D49.89
membrane	C70.1	C79.49	—	D32.1	D42.1	D49.7
meninges	C70.1	C79.49	—	D32.1	D42.1	D49.7
nerve (root)	C47.9	C79.89	—	D36.10	D48.2	D49.2
pia mater	C70.1	C79.49	—	D32.1	D42.1	D49.7
root	C47.9	C79.89	—	D36.10	D48.2	D49.2
sacrum	C41.4	C79.51	—	D16.8	D48.0	D49.2
spleen, splenic						
NEC	C26.1	C78.89	D01.7	D13.9	D37.8	D49.0
flexure (colon)	C18.5	C78.5	D01.0	D12.3	D37.4	D49.0
stem, brain	C71.7	C79.31	—	D33.1	D43.1	D49.6
Stensen's duct	C07	C79.89	D00.00	D11.0	D37.030	D49.0
sternum	C41.3	C79.51	—	D16.7	D48.0	D49.2
stomach	C16.9	C78.89	D00.2	D13.1	D37.1	D49.0
antrum (pyloric)	C16.3	C78.89	D00.2	D13.1	D37.1	D49.0
body	C16.2	C78.89	D00.2	D13.1	D37.1	D49.0
cardia	C16.0	C78.89	D00.2	D13.1	D37.1	D49.0
cardiac orifice	C16.0	C78.89	D00.2	D13.1	D37.1	D49.0
corpus	C16.2	C78.89	D00.2	D13.1	D37.1	D49.0
fundus	C16.1	C78.89	D00.2	D13.1	D37.1	D49.0
greater curvature						
NEC	C16.6	C78.89	D00.2	D13.1	D37.1	D49.0
lesser curvature						
NEC	C16.5	C78.89	D00.2	D13.1	D37.1	D49.0
overlapping						
lesion	C16.8	—	—	—	—	—
prepylorus	C16.4	C78.89	D00.2	D13.1	D37.1	D49.0
pylorus	C16.4	C78.89	D00.2	D13.1	D37.1	D49.0
wall NEC	C16.9	C78.89	D00.2	D13.1	D37.1	D49.0
anterior NEC	C16.8	C78.89	D00.2	D13.1	D37.1	D49.0
posterior NEC	C16.8	C78.89	D00.2	D13.1	D37.1	D49.0
stroma,						
endometrial	C54.1	C79.82	D07.0	D26.1	D39.0	D49.59
stump, cervical	C53.8	C79.82	D06.7	D26.0	D39.0	D49.59
subcutaneous (nodule)						
(tissue) NEC — see						
Neoplasm,						
connective tissue						
subdural	C70.9	C79.32	—	D32.9	D42.9	D49.7
subglottis,						
subglottic	C32.2	C78.39	D02.0	D14.1	D38.0	D49.1
sublingual	C04.9	C79.89	D00.06	D10.2	D37.09	D49.0
gland or duct	C08.1	C79.89	D00.00	D11.7	D37.031	D49.0
submandibular						
gland	C08.0	C79.89	D00.00	D11.7	D37.032	D49.0
submaxillary gland or						
duct	C08.0	C79.89	D00.00	D11.7	D37.032	D49.0
submental	C76.0	C79.89	D09.8	D36.7	D48.7	D49.89
subpleural	C34.9-☑	C78.0-☑	D02.2-☑	D14.3-☑	D38.1	D49.1
substernal	C38.1	C78.1	—	D15.2	D38.3	D49.89
sudoriferous,						
sudoriparous gland,						
site						
unspecified	C44.90	C79.2	D04.9	D23.9	D48.5	D49.2
specified site — see						
Neoplasm, skin						
supraclavicular						
region	C76.0	C79.89	D09.8	D36.7	D48.7	D49.89
supraglottis	C32.1	C78.39	D02.0	D14.1	D38.0	D49.1
suprarenal	C74.9-☑	C79.7-☑	D09.3	D35.0-☑	D44.1-☑	D49.7
capsule	C74.9-☑	C79.7-☑	D09.3	D35.0-☑	D44.1-☑	D49.7

	Malignant Primary	Malignant Secondary	Ca in situ	Benign	Uncertain Behavior	Unspecified Behavior
Neoplasm, neoplastic						
— continued						
suprarenal —						
continued						
cortex	C74.0-☑	C79.7-☑	D09.3	D35.0-☑	D44.1-☑	D49.7
gland	C74.9-☑	C79.7-☑	D09.3	D35.0-☑	D44.1-☑	D49.7
medulla	C74.1-☑	C79.7-☑	D09.3	D35.0-☑	D44.1-☑	D49.7
suprasellar						
(region)	C71.9	C79.31	—	D33.2	D43.2	D49.6
supratentorial (brain)						
NEC	C71.0	C79.31	—	D33.0	D43.0	D49.6
sweat gland (apocrine)						
(eccrine), site						
unspecified	C44.90	C79.2	D04.9	D23.9	D48.5	D49.2
specified site — see						
Neoplasm, skin						
sympathetic nerve or						
nervous system						
NEC	C47.9	C79.89	—	D36.10	D48.2	D49.2
symphysis pubis	C41.4	C79.51	—	D16.8	D48.0	D49.2
synovial membrane —						
see Neoplasm,						
connective tissue						
tapetum, brain	C71.8	C79.31	—	D33.2	D43.2	D49.6
tarsus (any bone)	C40.3-☑	C79.51	—	D16.3-☑	—	—
temple (skin) — see						
also Neoplasm, skin,						
face	C44.309	C79.2	D04.39	D23.39	D48.5	D49.2
temporal						
bone	C41.0	C79.51	—	D16.4	D48.0	D49.2
lobe or pole	C71.2	C79.31	—	D33.0	D43.0	D49.6
region	C76.0	C79.89	D09.8	D36.7	D48.7	D49.89
skin — see also						
Neoplasm, skin,						
face	C44.309	C79.2	D04.39	D23.39	D48.5	D49.2
tendon (sheath) — see						
Neoplasm,						
connective tissue						
tentorium						
(cerebelli)	C70.0	C79.32	—	D32.0	D42.0	D49.7
testis, testes	C62.9-☑	C79.82	D07.69	D29.2-☑	D40.1-☑	D49.59
descended	C62.1-☑	C79.82	D07.69	D29.2-☑	D40.1-☑	D49.59
ectopic	C62.0-☑	C79.82	D07.69	D29.2-☑	D40.1-☑	D49.59
retained	C62.0-☑	C79.82	D07.69	D29.2-☑	D40.1-☑	D49.59
scrotal	C62.1-☑	C79.82	D07.69	D29.2-☑	D40.1-☑	D49.59
undescended	C62.0-☑	C79.82	D07.69	D29.2-☑	D40.1-☑	D49.59
unspecified whether						
descended or						
undescended	C62.9-☑	C79.82	D07.69	D29.2-☑	D40.1-☑	D49.59
thalamus	C71.0	C79.31	—	D33.0	D43.0	D49.6
thigh NEC	C76.5-☑	C79.89	D04.7-☑	D36.7	D48.7	D49.89
thorax, thoracic (cavity)						
(organs NEC)	C76.1	C79.89	D09.8	D36.7	D48.7	D49.89
duct	C49.3	C79.89	—	D21.3	D48.1	D49.2
wall NEC	C76.1	C79.89	D09.8	D36.7	D48.7	D49.89
throat	C14.0	C79.89	D00.08	D10.9	D37.05	D49.0
thumb NEC	C76.4-☑	C79.89	D04.6-☑	D36.7	D48.7	D49.89
thymus (gland)	C37	C79.89	D09.3	D15.0	D38.4	D49.89
thyroglossal duct	C73	C79.89	D09.3	D34	D44.0	D49.7
thyroid (gland)	C73	C79.89	D09.3	D34	D44.0	D49.7
cartilage	C32.3	C78.39	D02.0	D14.1	D38.0	D49.1
tibia (any part)	C40.2-☑	C79.51	—	D16.2-☑	—	—
toe NEC	C76.5-☑	C79.89	D04.7-☑	D36.7	D48.7	D49.89
tongue	C02.9	C79.89	D00.07	D10.1	D37.02	D49.0
anterior (two-thirds)						
NEC	C02.3	C79.89	D00.07	D10.1	D37.02	D49.0
dorsal surface	C02.0	C79.89	D00.07	D10.1	D37.02	D49.0
ventral surface	C02.2	C79.89	D00.07	D10.1	D37.02	D49.0
base (dorsal						
surface)	C01	C79.89	D00.07	D10.1	D37.02	D49.0
border (lateral)	C02.1	C79.89	D00.07	D10.1	D37.02	D49.0
dorsal surface						
NEC	C02.0	C79.89	D00.07	D10.1	D37.02	D49.0
fixed part NEC	C01	C79.89	D00.07	D10.1	D37.02	D49.0
foreamen						
cecum	C02.0	C79.89	D00.07	D10.1	D37.02	D49.0
frenulum						
linguae	C02.2	C79.89	D00.07	D10.1	D37.02	D49.0
junctional zone	C02.8	C79.89	D00.07	D10.1	D37.02	D49.0
margin (lateral)	C02.1	C79.89	D00.07	D10.1	D37.02	D49.0
midline NEC	C02.0	C79.89	D00.07	D10.1	D37.02	D49.0
mobile part NEC	C02.3	C79.89	D00.07	D10.1	D37.02	D49.0

☑ **Additional Character Required — Refer to the Tabular List for Character Selection**   ▽ Subterms under main terms may continue to next column or page

	Malignant Primary	Malignant Secondary	Ca in situ	Benign	Uncertain Behavior	Unspecified Behavior
Neoplasm, neoplastic — *continued*						
tongue — *continued*						
overlapping lesion	C02.8	—	—	—	—	—
posterior (third)	C01	C79.89	D00.07	D10.1	D37.02	D49.0
root	C01	C79.89	D00.07	D10.1	D37.02	D49.0
surface (dorsal)	C02.0	C79.89	D00.07	D10.1	D37.02	D49.0
base	C01	C79.89	D00.07	D10.1	D37.02	D49.0
ventral	C02.2	C79.89	D00.07	D10.1	D37.02	D49.0
tip	C02.1	C79.89	D00.07	D10.1	D37.02	D49.0
tonsil	C02.4	C79.89	D00.07	D10.1	D37.02	D49.0
tonsil	C09.9	C79.89	D00.08	D10.4	D37.05	D49.0
fauces, faucial	C09.9	C79.89	D00.08	D10.4	D37.05	D49.0
lingual	C02.4	C79.89	D00.07	D10.1	D37.02	D49.0
overlapping sites	C09.8	—	—	—	—	—
palatine	C09.9	C79.89	D00.08	D10.4	D37.05	D49.0
pharyngeal	C11.1	C79.89	D00.08	D10.6	D37.05	D49.0
pillar (anterior) (posterior)	C09.1	C79.89	D00.08	D10.5	D37.05	D49.0
tonsillar fossa	C09.0	C79.89	D00.08	D10.5	D37.05	D49.0
tooth socket NEC	C03.9	C79.89	D00.03	D10.39	D37.09	D49.0
trachea (cartilage) (mucosa)	C33	C78.39	D02.1	D14.2	D38.1	D49.1
overlapping lesion with bronchus or lung	C34.8-☑	—				
tracheobronchial	C34.8-☑	C78.39	D02.1	D14.2	D38.1	D49.1
overlapping lesion with lung	C34.8-☑	—	—	—	—	—
tragus — *see also* Neoplasm, skin, ear	C44.20-☑	C79.2	D04.2-☑	D23.2-☑	D48.5	D49.2
trunk NEC	C76.8	C79.89	D04.5	D36.7	D48.7	D49.89
tubo-ovarian	C57.8	C79.82	D07.39	D28.7	D39.8	D49.59
tunica vaginalis	C63.7	C79.82	D07.69	D29.8	D40.8	D49.59
turbinate (bone)	C41.0	C79.51		D16.4	D48.0	D49.2
nasal	C30.0	C78.39	D02.3	D14.0	D38.5	D49.1
tympanic cavity	C30.1	C78.39	D02.3	D14.0	D38.5	D49.1
ulna (any part)	C40.0-☑	C79.51		D16.0-☑	—	—
umbilicus, umbilical — *see also* Neoplasm, skin, trunk	C44.509	C79.2	D04.5	D23.5	D48.5	D49.2
uncus, brain	C71.2	C79.31	—	D33.0	D43.0	D49.6
unknown site or unspecified	C80.1	C79.9	D09.9	D36.9	D48.9	D49.9
urachus	C67.7	C79.11	D09.0	D30.3	D41.4	D49.4
ureter-bladder (junction)	C67.6	C79.11	D09.0	D30.3	D41.4	D49.4
ureter, ureteral	C66.-☑	C79.19	D09.19	D30.2-☑	D41.2-☑	D49.59
orifice (bladder)	C67.6	C79.11	D09.0	D30.3	D41.4	D49.4
urethra, urethral (gland)	C68.0	C79.19	D09.19	D30.4	D41.3	D49.59
orifice, internal	C67.5	C79.11	D09.0	D30.3	D41.4	D49.4
urethrovaginal (septum)	C57.9	C79.82	D07.30	D28.9	D39.8	D49.59
urinary organ or system	C68.9	C79.10	D09.10	D30.9	D41.9	D49.59
bladder — *see* Neoplasm, bladder						
overlapping lesion	C68.8	—		—	—	—
specified sites NEC	C68.8	C79.19	D09.19	D30.8	D41.8	D49.59
utero-ovarian	C57.8	C79.82	D07.39	D28.7	D39.8	D49.59
ligament	C57.1-☑	C79.82	D07.39	D28.2	D39.8	D49.59
uterosacral ligament	C57.3	C79.82	—	D28.2	D39.8	D49.59
uterus, uteri, uterine	C55	C79.82	D07.0	D26.9	D39.0	D49.59
adnexa NEC	C57.4	C79.82	D07.39	D28.7	D39.8	D49.59
body	C54.9	C79.82	D07.0	D26.1	D39.0	D49.59
cervix	C53.9	C79.82	D06.9	D26.0	D39.0	D49.59
cornu	C54.9	C79.82	D07.0	D26.1	D39.0	D49.59
corpus	C54.9	C79.82	D07.0	D26.1	D39.0	D49.59
endocervix (canal) (gland)	C53.0	C79.82	D06.0	D26.0	D39.0	D49.59
endometrium	C54.1	C79.82	D07.0	D26.1	D39.0	D49.59
exocervix	C53.1	C79.82	D06.1	D26.0	D39.0	D49.59
external os	C53.1	C79.82	D06.1	D26.0	D39.0	D49.59
fundus	C54.3	C79.82	D07.0	D26.1	D39.0	D49.59

	Malignant Primary	Malignant Secondary	Ca in situ	Benign	Uncertain Behavior	Unspecified Behavior
Neoplasm, neoplastic — *continued*						
uterus, uteri, uterine — *continued*						
internal os	C53.0	C79.82	D06.0	D26.0	D39.0	D49.59
isthmus	C54.0	C79.82	D07.0	D26.1	D39.0	D49.59
ligament	C57.3	C79.82	—	D28.2	D39.8	D49.59
broad	C57.1-☑	C79.82	D07.39	D28.2	D39.8	D49.59
round	C57.2-☑	C79.82	—	D28.2	D39.8	D49.59
lower segment	C54.0	C79.82	D07.0	D26.1	D39.0	D49.59
myometrium	C54.2	C79.82	D07.0	D26.1	D39.0	D49.59
overlapping sites	C54.8	—	—	—	—	—
squamocolumnar junction	C53.8	C79.82	D06.7	D26.0	D39.0	D49.59
tube	C57.0-☑	C79.82	D07.39	D28.2	D39.8	D49.59
utricle, prostatic	C68.0	C79.19	D09.19	D30.4	D41.3	D49.59
uveal tract	C69.4-☑	C79.49	D09.2-☑	D31.4-☑	D48.7	D49.89
uvula	C05.2	C79.89	D00.04	D10.39	D37.09	D49.0
vagina, vaginal (fornix) (vault) (wall)	C52	C79.82	D07.2	D28.1	D39.8	D49.59
vaginovesical	C57.9	C79.82	D07.30	D28.9	D39.9	D49.59
septum	C57.9	C79.82	D07.30	D28.9	D39.9	D49.59
vallecula (epigiottis)	C10.0	C79.89	D00.08	D10.5	D37.05	D49.0
vascular — *see* Neoplasm, connective tissue						
vas deferens	C63.1-☑	C79.82	D07.69	D29.8	D40.8	D49.59
Vater's ampulla	C24.1	C78.89	D01.5	D13.5	D37.6	D49.0
vein, venous — *see* Neoplasm, connective tissue						
vena cava (abdominal) (inferior)	C49.4	C79.89	—	D21.4	D48.1	D49.2
superior	C49.3	C79.89	—	D21.3	D48.1	D49.2
ventricle (cerebral) (floor) (lateral) (third)	C71.5	C79.31		D33.0	D43.0	D49.6
cardiac (left) (right)	C38.0	C79.89		D15.1	D48.7	D49.89
fourth	C71.7	C79.31		D33.1	D43.1	D49.6
ventricular band of larynx	C32.1	C78.39	D02.0	D14.1	D38.0	D49.1
ventriculus — *see* Neoplasm, stomach						
vermillion border — *see* Neoplasm, lip						
vermis, cerebellum	C71.6	C79.31	—	D33.1	D43.1	D49.6
vertebra (column)	C41.2	C79.51	—	D16.6	D48.0	D49.2
coccyx	C41.4	C79.51	—	D16.8	D48.0	D49.2
marrow NEC	C96.9	C79.52	—	—	D47.9	D49.89
sacrum	C41.4	C79.51	—	D16.8	D48.0	D49.2
vesical — *see* Neoplasm, bladder						
vesicle, seminal	C63.7	C79.82	D07.69	D29.8	D40.8	D49.59
vesicocervical tissue	C57.9	C79.82	D07.30	D28.9	D39.9	D49.59
vesicorectal	C76.3	C79.82	D09.8	D36.7	D48.7	D49.89
vesicovaginal	C57.9	C79.82	D07.30	D28.9	D39.9	D49.59
septum	C57.9	C79.82	D07.30	D28.9	D39.8	D49.59
vessel (blood) — *see* Neoplasm, connective tissue						
vestibular gland, greater	C51.0	C79.82	D07.1	D28.0	D39.8	D49.59
vestibule						
mouth	C06.1	C79.89	D00.00	D10.39	D37.09	D49.0
nose	C30.0	C78.39	D02.3	D14.0	D38.5	D49.1
Virchow's gland	C77.0	C77.0	—	D36.0	D48.7	D49.89
viscera NEC	C76.8	C79.89	D09.8	D36.7	D48.7	D49.89
vocal cords (true)	C32.0	C78.39	D02.0	D14.1	D38.0	D49.1
false	C32.1	C78.39	D02.0	D14.1	D38.0	D49.1
vomer	C41.0	C79.51	—	D16.4	D48.0	D49.2
vulva	C51.9	C79.82	D07.1	D28.0	D39.8	D49.59
vulvovaginal gland	C51.0	C79.82	D07.1	D28.0	D39.8	D49.59
Waldeyer's ring	C14.2	C79.89	D00.08	D10.9	D37.05	D49.0
Wharton's duct	C08.0	C79.89	D00.00	D11.7	D37.032	D49.0
white matter (central) (cerebral)	C71.0	C79.31	—	D33.0	D43.0	D49.6

	Malignant Primary	Malignant Secondary	Ca in situ	Benign	Uncertain Behavior	Unspecified Behavior
Neoplasm, neoplastic _— continued_						
windpipe	C33	C78.39	D02.1	D14.2	D38.1	D49.1
Wirsung's duct	C25.3	C78.89	D01.7	D13.6	D37.8	D49.0
wolffian (body) (duct)						
female	C57.7	C79.82	D07.39	D28.7	D39.8	D49.59
male	C63.7	C79.82	D07.69	D29.8	D40.8	D49.59
womb — _see_ Neoplasm, uterus						
wrist NEC	C76.4-☑	C79.89	D04.6-☑	D36.7	D48.7	D49.89
xiphoid process	C41.3	C79.51	—	D16.7	D48.0	D49.2
Zuckerkandl organ	C75.5	C79.89	—	D35.6	D44.7	D49.7

☑ **Additional Character Required — Refer to the Tabular List for Character Selection**   ▽ **Subterms under main terms may continue to next column or page**

Substance	Poisoning, Accidental (unintentional)	Poisoning, Intentional Self-harm	Poisoning, Assault	Poisoning, Undetermined	Adverse Effect	Under-dosing
14-Hydroxydihydromorphinone	T40.2X1	T40.2X2	T40.2X3	T40.2X4	T40.2X5	T40.2X6
1-Propanol	T51.3X1	T51.3X2	T51.3X3	T51.3X4	—	—
2,3,7,8-Tetrachlorodibenzo-p-dioxin	T53.7X1	T53.7X2	T53.7X3	T53.7X4	—	—
2,4,5-T (trichlorophenoxyacetic acid)	T60.1X1	T60.1X2	T60.1X3	T60.1X4	—	—
2,4,5-Trichlorophenoxyacetic acid	T60.3X1	T60.3X2	T60.3X3	T60.3X4	—	—
2,4-D (dichlorophenoxyacetic acid)	T60.3X1	T60.3X2	T60.3X3	T60.3X4	—	—
2,4-Toluene diisocyanate	T65.0X1	T65.0X2	T65.0X3	T65.0X4	—	—
2-Deoxy-5-fluorouridine	T45.1X1	T45.1X2	T45.1X3	T45.1X4	T45.1X5	T45.1X6
2-Ethoxyethanol	T52.3X1	T52.3X2	T52.3X3	T52.3X4	—	—
2-Methoxyethanol	T52.3X1	T52.3X2	T52.3X3	T52.3X4	—	—
2-Propanol	T51.2X1	T51.2X2	T51.2X3	T51.2X4	—	—
3,4-methylenedioxymeth-amphetamine	T43.641	T43.642	T43.643	T43.644	—	—
4-Aminobutyric acid	T43.8X1	T43.8X2	T43.8X3	T43.8X4	T43.8X5	T43.8X6
4-Aminophenol derivatives	T39.1X1	T39.1X2	T39.1X3	T39.1X4	T39.1X5	T39.1X6
5-Deoxy-5-fluorouridine	T45.1X1	T45.1X2	T45.1X3	T45.1X4	T45.1X5	T45.1X6
5-Methoxypsoralen (5-MOP)	T50.991	T50.992	T50.993	T50.994	T50.995	T50.996
8-Aminoquinoline drugs	T37.2X1	T37.2X2	T37.2X3	T37.2X4	T37.2X5	T37.2X6
8-Methoxypsoralen (8-MOP)	T50.991	T50.992	T50.993	T50.994	T50.995	T50.996
ABOB	T37.5X1	T37.5X2	T37.5X3	T37.5X4	T37.5X5	T37.5X6
Abrine	T62.2X1	T62.2X2	T62.2X3	T62.2X4	—	—
Abrus (seed)	T62.2X1	T62.2X2	T62.2X3	T62.2X4	—	—
Absinthe	T51.0X1	T51.0X2	T51.0X3	T51.0X4	—	—
beverage	T51.0X1	T51.0X2	T51.0X3	T51.0X4	—	—
Acaricide	T60.8X1	T60.8X2	T60.8X3	T60.8X4	—	—
Acebutolol	T44.7X1	T44.7X2	T44.7X3	T44.7X4	T44.7X5	T44.7X6
Acecarbromal	T42.6X1	T42.6X2	T42.6X3	T42.6X4	T42.6X5	T42.6X6
Aceclidine	T44.1X1	T44.1X2	T44.1X3	T44.1X4	T44.1X5	T44.1X6
Acedapsone	T37.0X1	T37.0X2	T37.0X3	T37.0X4	T37.0X5	T37.0X6
Acefylline piperazine	T48.6X1	T48.6X2	T48.6X3	T48.6X4	T48.6X5	T48.6X6
Acemorphan	T40.2X1	T40.2X2	T40.2X3	T40.2X4	T40.2X5	T40.2X6
Acenocoumarin	T45.511	T45.512	T45.513	T45.514	T45.515	T45.516
Acenocoumarol	T45.511	T45.512	T45.513	T45.514	T45.515	T45.516
Acepifylline	T48.6X1	T48.6X2	T48.6X3	T48.6X4	T48.6X5	T48.6X6
Acepromazine	T43.3X1	T43.3X2	T43.3X3	T43.3X4	T43.3X5	T43.3X6
Acesulfamethoxypyridazine	T37.0X1	T37.0X2	T37.0X3	T37.0X4	T37.0X5	T37.0X6
Acetal	T52.8X1	T52.8X2	T52.8X3	T52.8X4	—	—
Acetaldehyde (vapor)	T52.8X1	T52.8X2	T52.8X3	T52.8X4	—	—
liquid	T65.891	T65.892	T65.893	T65.894	—	—
Acetaminophen	T39.1X1	T39.1X2	T39.1X3	T39.1X4	T39.1X5	T39.1X6
Acetaminosalol	T39.1X1	T39.1X2	T39.1X3	T39.1X4	T39.1X5	T39.1X6
Acetanilide	T39.1X1	T39.1X2	T39.1X3	T39.1X4	T39.1X5	T39.1X6
Acetarsol	T37.3X1	T37.3X2	T37.3X3	T37.3X4	T37.3X5	T37.3X6
Acetazolamide	T50.2X1	T50.2X2	T50.2X3	T50.2X4	T50.2X5	T50.2X6
Acetiamine	T45.2X1	T45.2X2	T45.2X3	T45.2X4	T45.2X5	T45.2X6
Acetic						
acid	T54.2X1	T54.2X2	T54.2X3	T54.2X4	—	—
with sodium acetate (ointment)	T49.3X1	T49.3X2	T49.3X3	T49.3X4	T49.3X5	T49.3X6
ester (solvent)(vapor)	T52.8X1	T52.8X2	T52.8X3	T52.8X4	—	—
irrigating solution	T50.3X1	T50.3X2	T50.3X3	T50.3X4	T50.3X5	T50.3X6
medicinal (lotion)	T49.2X1	T49.2X2	T49.2X3	T49.2X4	T49.2X5	T49.2X6
anhydride	T65.891	T65.892	T65.893	T65.894	—	—
ether (vapor)	T52.8X1	T52.8X2	T52.8X3	T52.8X4	—	—
Acetohexamide	T38.3X1	T38.3X2	T38.3X3	T38.3X4	T38.3X5	T38.3X6
Acetohydroxamic acid	T50.991	T50.992	T50.993	T50.994	T50.995	T50.996
Acetomenaphthone	T45.7X1	T45.7X2	T45.7X3	T45.7X4	T45.7X5	T45.7X6
Acetomorphine	T40.1X1	T40.1X2	T40.1X3	T40.1X4	—	—
Acetone (oils)	T52.4X1	T52.4X2	T52.4X3	T52.4X4	—	—
chlorinated	T52.4X1	T52.4X2	T52.4X3	T52.4X4	—	—
vapor	T52.4X1	T52.4X2	T52.4X3	T52.4X4	—	—
Acetonitrile	T52.8X1	T52.8X2	T52.8X3	T52.8X4	—	—
Acetophenazine	T43.3X1	T43.3X2	T43.3X3	T43.3X4	T43.3X5	T43.3X6
Acetophenetedin	T39.1X1	T39.1X2	T39.1X3	T39.1X4	T39.1X5	T39.1X6
Acetophenone	T52.4X1	T52.4X2	T52.4X3	T52.4X4	—	—
Acetorphine	T40.2X1	T40.2X2	T40.2X3	T40.2X4	—	—
Acetosulfone (sodium)	T37.1X1	T37.1X2	T37.1X3	T37.1X4	T37.1X5	T37.1X6
Acetrizoate (sodium)	T50.8X1	T50.8X2	T50.8X3	T50.8X4	T50.8X5	T50.8X6
Acetrizoic acid	T50.8X1	T50.8X2	T50.8X3	T50.8X4	T50.8X5	T50.8X6
Acetyl						
bromide	T53.6X1	T53.6X2	T53.6X3	T53.6X4	—	—
chloride	T53.6X1	T53.6X2	T53.6X3	T53.6X4	—	—
Acetylcarbromal	T42.6X1	T42.6X2	T42.6X3	T42.6X4	T42.6X5	T42.6X6
Acetylcholine						
chloride	T44.1X1	T44.1X2	T44.1X3	T44.1X4	T44.1X5	T44.1X6
derivative	T44.1X1	T44.1X2	T44.1X3	T44.1X4	T44.1X5	T44.1X6

Substance	Poisoning, Accidental (unintentional)	Poisoning, Intentional Self-harm	Poisoning, Assault	Poisoning, Undetermined	Adverse Effect	Under-dosing
Acetylcysteine	T48.4X1	T48.4X2	T48.4X3	T48.4X4	T48.4X5	T48.4X6
Acetyldigitoxin	T46.0X1	T46.0X2	T46.0X3	T46.0X4	T46.0X5	T46.0X6
Acetyldigoxin	T46.0X1	T46.0X2	T46.0X3	T46.0X4	T46.0X5	T46.0X6
Acetyldihydrocodeine	T40.2X1	T40.2X2	T40.2X3	T40.2X4	—	—
Acetyldihydrocodeinone	T40.2X1	T40.2X2	T40.2X3	T40.2X4	—	—
Acetylene (gas)	T59.891	T59.892	T59.893	T59.894	—	—
dichloride	T53.6X1	T53.6X2	T53.6X3	T53.6X4	—	—
incomplete combustion of	T58.11	T58.12	T58.13	T58.14	—	—
industrial	T59.891	T59.892	T59.893	T59.894	—	—
tetrachloride	T53.6X1	T53.6X2	T53.6X3	T53.6X4	—	—
vapor	T53.6X1	T53.6X2	T53.6X3	T53.6X4	—	—
Acetylpheneturide	T42.6X1	T42.6X2	T42.6X3	T42.6X4	T42.6X5	T42.6X6
Acetylphenylhydrazine	T39.8X1	T39.8X2	T39.8X3	T39.8X4	T39.8X5	T39.8X6
Acetylsalicylic acid (salts)	T39.011	T39.012	T39.013	T39.014	T39.015	T39.016
enteric coated	T39.011	T39.012	T39.013	T39.014	T39.015	T39.016
Acetylsulfamethoxypyridazine	T37.0X1	T37.0X2	T37.0X3	T37.0X4	T37.0X5	T37.0X6
Achromycin	T36.4X1	T36.4X2	T36.4X3	T36.4X4	T36.4X5	T36.4X6
ophthalmic preparation	T49.5X1	T49.5X2	T49.5X3	T49.5X4	T49.5X5	T49.5X6
topical NEC	T49.0X1	T49.0X2	T49.0X3	T49.0X4	T49.0X5	T49.0X6
Aciclovir	T37.5X1	T37.5X2	T37.5X3	T37.5X4	T37.5X5	T37.5X6
Acidifying agent NEC	T50.901	T50.902	T50.903	T50.904	T50.905	T50.906
Acid (corrosive) NEC	T54.2X1	T54.2X2	T54.2X3	T54.2X4	—	—
Acipimox	T46.6X1	T46.6X2	T46.6X3	T46.6X4	T46.6X5	T46.6X6
Acitretin	T50.991	T50.992	T50.993	T50.994	T50.995	T50.996
Aclarubicin	T45.1X1	T45.1X2	T45.1X3	T45.1X4	T45.1X5	T45.1X6
Aclatonium napadisilate	T48.1X1	T48.1X2	T48.1X3	T48.1X4	T48.1X5	T48.1X6
Aconite (wild)	T46.991	T46.992	T46.993	T46.994	T46.995	T46.996
Aconitine	T46.991	T46.992	T46.993	T46.994	T46.995	T46.996
Aconitum ferox	T46.991	T46.992	T46.993	T46.994	T46.995	T46.996
Acridine	T65.6X1	T65.6X2	T65.6X3	T65.6X4	—	—
vapor	T59.891	T59.892	T59.893	T59.894	—	—
Acriflavine	T37.91	T37.92	T37.93	T37.94	T37.95	T37.96
Acriflavinium chloride	T49.0X1	T49.0X2	T49.0X3	T49.0X4	T49.0X5	T49.0X6
Acrinol	T49.0X1	T49.0X2	T49.0X3	T49.0X4	T49.0X5	T49.0X6
Acrisorcin	T49.0X1	T49.0X2	T49.0X3	T49.0X4	T49.0X5	T49.0X6
Acrivastine	T45.0X1	T45.0X2	T45.0X3	T45.0X4	T45.0X5	T45.0X6
Acrolein (gas)	T59.891	T59.892	T59.893	T59.894	—	—
liquid	T54.1X1	T54.1X2	T54.1X3	T54.1X4	—	—
Acrylamide	T65.891	T65.892	T65.893	T65.894	—	—
Acrylic resin	T49.3X1	T49.3X2	T49.3X3	T49.3X4	T49.3X5	T49.3X6
Acrylonitrile	T65.891	T65.892	T65.893	T65.894	—	—
Actaea spicata	T62.2X1	T62.2X2	T62.2X3	T62.2X4	—	—
berry	T62.1X1	T62.1X2	T62.1X3	T62.1X4	—	—
Acterol	T37.3X1	T37.3X2	T37.3X3	T37.3X4	T37.3X5	T37.3X6
ACTH	T38.811	T38.812	T38.813	T38.814	T38.815	T38.816
Actinomycin C	T45.1X1	T45.1X2	T45.1X3	T45.1X4	T45.1X5	T45.1X6
Actinomycin D	T45.1X1	T45.1X2	T45.1X3	T45.1X4	T45.1X5	T45.1X6
Activated charcoal — see also Charcoal, medicinal	T47.6X1	T47.6X2	T47.6X3	T47.6X4	T47.6X5	T47.6X6
Acyclovir	T37.5X1	T37.5X2	T37.5X3	T37.5X4	T37.5X5	T37.5X6
Adenine	T45.2X1	T45.2X2	T45.2X3	T45.2X4	T45.2X5	T45.2X6
arabinoside	T37.5X1	T37.5X2	T37.5X3	T37.5X4	T37.5X5	T37.5X6
Adenosine (phosphate)	T46.2X1	T46.2X2	T46.2X3	T46.2X4	T46.2X5	T46.2X6
ADH	T38.891	T38.892	T38.893	T38.894	T38.895	T38.896
Adhesive NEC	T65.891	T65.892	T65.893	T65.894	—	—
Adicillin	T36.0X1	T36.0X2	T36.0X3	T36.0X4	T36.0X5	T36.0X6
Adiphenine	T44.3X1	T44.3X2	T44.3X3	T44.3X4	T44.3X5	T44.3X6
Adipiodone	T50.8X1	T50.8X2	T50.8X3	T50.8X4	T50.8X5	T50.8X6
Adjunct, pharmaceutical	T50.901	T50.902	T50.903	T50.904	T50.905	T50.906
Adrenal (extract, cortex or medulla) (glucocorticoids) (hormones) (mineralocorticoids)	T38.0X1	T38.0X2	T38.0X3	T38.0X4	T38.0X5	T38.0X6
ENT agent	T49.6X1	T49.6X2	T49.6X3	T49.6X4	T49.6X5	T49.6X6
ophthalmic preparation	T49.5X1	T49.5X2	T49.5X3	T49.5X4	T49.5X5	T49.5X6
topical NEC	T49.0X1	T49.0X2	T49.0X3	T49.0X4	T49.0X5	T49.0X6
Adrenalin — see Adrenaline						
Adrenaline	T44.5X1	T44.5X2	T44.5X3	T44.5X4	T44.5X5	T44.5X6
Adrenergic NEC	T44.901	T44.902	T44.903	T44.904	T44.905	T44.906
blocking agent NEC	T44.8X1	T44.8X2	T44.8X3	T44.8X4	T44.8X5	T44.8X6
beta, heart	T44.7X1	T44.7X2	T44.7X3	T44.7X4	T44.7X5	T44.7X6
specified NEC	T44.991	T44.992	T44.993	T44.994	T44.995	T44.996
Adrenochrome						
derivative	T46.991	T46.992	T46.993	T46.994	T46.995	T46.996
(mono) semicarbazone	T46.991	T46.992	T46.993	T46.994	T46.995	T46.996
Adrenocorticotrophic hormone	T38.811	T38.812	T38.813	T38.814	T38.815	T38.816
Adrenocorticotrophin	T38.811	T38.812	T38.813	T38.814	T38.815	T38.816
Adriamycin	T45.1X1	T45.1X2	T45.1X3	T45.1X4	T45.1X5	T45.1X6
Aerosol spray NEC	T65.91	T65.92	T65.93	T65.94	—	—
Aerosporin	T36.8X1	T36.8X2	T36.8X3	T36.8X4	T36.8X5	T36.8X6
ENT agent	T49.6X1	T49.6X2	T49.6X3	T49.6X4	T49.6X5	T49.6X6
ophthalmic preparation	T49.5X1	T49.5X2	T49.5X3	T49.5X4	T49.5X5	T49.5X6

Substance	Poisoning, Accidental (unintentional)	Poisoning, Intentional Self-harm	Poisoning, Assault	Poisoning, Undetermined	Adverse Effect	Under-dosing
Aerosporin — *continued*						
topical NEC	T49.0X1	T49.0X2	T49.0X3	T49.0X4	T49.0X5	T49.0X6
Aethusa cynapium	T62.2X1	T62.2X2	T62.2X3	T62.2X4	—	—
Afghanistan black	T40.7X1	T40.7X2	T40.7X3	T40.7X4	T40.7X5	T40.7X6
Aflatoxin	T64.01	T64.02	T64.03	T64.04	—	—
Afloqualone	T42.8X1	T42.8X2	T42.8X3	T42.8X4	T42.8X5	T42.8X6
African boxwood	T62.2X1	T62.2X2	T62.2X3	T62.2X4	—	—
Agar	T47.4X1	T47.4X2	T47.4X3	T47.4X4	T47.4X5	T47.4X6
Agonist						
predominantly						
alpha-adrenoreceptor	T44.4X1	T44.4X2	T44.4X3	T44.4X4	T44.4X5	T44.4X6
beta-adrenoreceptor	T44.5X1	T44.5X2	T44.5X3	T44.5X4	T44.5X5	T44.5X6
Agricultural agent NEC	T65.91	T65.92	T65.93	T65.94	—	—
Agrypnal	T42.3X1	T42.3X2	T42.3X3	T42.3X4	T42.3X5	T42.3X6
AHLG	T50.Z11	T50.Z12	T50.Z13	T50.Z14	T50.Z15	T50.Z16
Air contaminant(s), source/type NOS	T65.91	T65.92	T65.93	T65.94	—	—
Ajmaline	T46.2X1	T46.2X2	T46.2X3	T46.2X4	T46.2X5	T46.2X6
Akee	T62.1X1	T62.1X2	T62.1X3	T62.1X4	—	—
Akrinol	T49.0X1	T49.0X2	T49.0X3	T49.0X4	T49.0X5	T49.0X6
Akritoin	T37.8X1	T37.8X2	T37.8X3	T37.8X4	T37.8X5	T37.8X6
Alacepril	T46.4X1	T46.4X2	T46.4X3	T46.4X4	T46.4X5	T46.4X6
Alantolactone	T37.4X1	T37.4X2	T37.4X3	T37.4X4	T37.4X5	T37.4X6
Albamycin	T36.8X1	T36.8X2	T36.8X3	T36.8X4	T36.8X5	T36.8X6
Albendazole	T37.4X1	T37.4X2	T37.4X3	T37.4X4	T37.4X5	T37.4X6
Albumin						
bovine	T45.8X1	T45.8X2	T45.8X3	T45.8X4	T45.8X5	T45.8X6
human serum	T45.8X1	T45.8X2	T45.8X3	T45.8X4	T45.8X5	T45.8X6
salt-poor	T45.8X1	T45.8X2	T45.8X3	T45.8X4	T45.8X5	T45.8X6
normal human serum	T45.8X1	T45.8X2	T45.8X3	T45.8X4	T45.8X5	T45.8X6
Albuterol	T48.6X1	T48.6X2	T48.6X3	T48.6X4	T48.6X5	T48.6X6
Albutoin	T42.0X1	T42.0X2	T42.0X3	T42.0X4	T42.0X5	T42.0X6
Alclometasone	T49.0X1	T49.0X2	T49.0X3	T49.0X4	T49.0X5	T49.0X6
Alcohol	T51.91	T51.92	T51.93	T51.94	—	—
absolute	T51.0X1	T51.0X2	T51.0X3	T51.0X4	—	—
beverage	T51.0X1	T51.0X2	T51.0X3	T51.0X4	—	—
allyl	T51.8X1	T51.8X2	T51.8X3	T51.8X4	—	—
amyl	T51.3X1	T51.3X2	T51.3X3	T51.3X4	—	—
antifreeze	T51.1X1	T51.1X2	T51.1X3	T51.1X4	—	—
beverage	T51.0X1	T51.0X2	T51.0X3	T51.0X4	—	—
butyl	T51.3X1	T51.3X2	T51.3X3	T51.3X4	—	—
dehydrated	T51.0X1	T51.0X2	T51.0X3	T51.0X4	—	—
beverage	T51.0X1	T51.0X2	T51.0X3	T51.0X4	—	—
denatured	T51.0X1	T51.0X2	T51.0X3	T51.0X4	—	—
deterrent NEC	T50.6X1	T50.6X2	T50.6X3	T50.6X4	T50.6X5	T50.6X6
diagnostic (gastric function)	T50.8X1	T50.8X2	T50.8X3	T50.8X4	T50.8X5	T50.8X6
ethyl	T51.0X1	T51.0X2	T51.0X3	T51.0X4	—	—
beverage	T51.0X1	T51.0X2	T51.0X3	T51.0X4	—	—
grain	T51.0X1	T51.0X2	T51.0X3	T51.0X4	—	—
beverage	T51.0X1	T51.0X2	T51.0X3	T51.0X4	—	—
industrial	T51.0X1	T51.0X2	T51.0X3	T51.0X4	—	—
isopropyl	T51.2X1	T51.2X2	T51.2X3	T51.2X4	—	—
methyl	T51.1X1	T51.1X2	T51.1X3	T51.1X4	—	—
preparation for consumption	T51.0X1	T51.0X2	T51.0X3	T51.0X4	—	—
propyl	T51.3X1	T51.3X2	T51.3X3	T51.3X4	—	—
secondary	T51.2X1	T51.2X2	T51.2X3	T51.2X4	—	—
radiator	T51.1X1	T51.1X2	T51.1X3	T51.1X4	—	—
rubbing	T51.2X1	T51.2X2	T51.2X3	T51.2X4	—	—
specified type NEC	T51.8X1	T51.8X2	T51.8X3	T51.8X4	—	—
surgical	T51.0X1	T51.0X2	T51.0X3	T51.0X4	—	—
vapor (from any type of Alcohol)	T59.891	T59.892	T59.893	T59.894	—	—
wood	T51.1X1	T51.1X2	T51.1X3	T51.1X4	—	—
Alcuronium (chloride)	T48.1X1	T48.1X2	T48.1X3	T48.1X4	T48.1X5	T48.1X6
Aldactone	T50.0X1	T50.0X2	T50.0X3	T50.0X4	T50.0X5	T50.0X6
Aldesulfone sodium	T37.1X1	T37.1X2	T37.1X3	T37.1X4	T37.1X5	T37.1X6
Aldicarb	T60.0X1	T60.0X2	T60.0X3	T60.0X4	—	—
Aldomet	T46.5X1	T46.5X2	T46.5X3	T46.5X4	T46.5X5	T46.5X6
Aldosterone	T50.0X1	T50.0X2	T50.0X3	T50.0X4	T50.0X5	T50.0X6
Aldrin (dust)	T60.1X1	T60.1X2	T60.1X3	T60.1X4	—	—
Aleve — *see* Naproxen						
Alexitol sodium	T47.1X1	T47.1X2	T47.1X3	T47.1X4	T47.1X5	T47.1X6
Alfacalcidol	T45.2X1	T45.2X2	T45.2X3	T45.2X4	T45.2X5	T45.2X6
Alfadolone	T41.1X1	T41.1X2	T41.1X3	T41.1X4	T41.1X5	T41.1X6
Alfaxalone	T41.1X1	T41.1X2	T41.1X3	T41.1X4	T41.1X5	T41.1X6
Alfentanil	T40.4X1	T40.4X2	T40.4X3	T40.4X4	T40.4X5	T40.4X6
Alfuzosin (hydrochloride)	T44.8X1	T44.8X2	T44.8X3	T44.8X4	T44.8X5	T44.8X6
Algae (harmful) (toxin)	T65.821	T65.822	T65.823	T65.824	—	—
Algeldrate	T47.1X1	T47.1X2	T47.1X3	T47.1X4	T47.1X5	T47.1X6
Algin	T47.8X1	T47.8X2	T47.8X3	T47.8X4	T47.8X5	T47.8X6
Alglucerase	T45.3X1	T45.3X2	T45.3X3	T45.3X4	T45.3X5	T45.3X6

Substance	Poisoning, Accidental (unintentional)	Poisoning, Intentional Self-harm	Poisoning, Assault	Poisoning, Undetermined	Adverse Effect	Under-dosing
Alidase	T45.3X1	T45.3X2	T45.3X3	T45.3X4	T45.3X5	T45...
Alimemazine	T43.3X1	T43.3X2	T43.3X3	T43.3X4	T43.3X5	T43.3...
Aliphatic thiocyanates	T65.0X1	T65.0X2	T65.0X3	T65.0X4	—	—
Alizapride	T45.0X1	T45.0X2	T45.0X3	T45.0X4	T45.0X5	T45.0...
Alkali (caustic)	T54.3X1	T54.3X2	T54.3X3	T54.3X4	—	—
Alkaline antiseptic solution (aromatic)	T49.6X1	T49.6X2	T49.6X3	T49.6X4	T49.6X5	T49.6...
Alkalinizing agents (medicinal)	T50.901	T50.902	T50.903	T50.904	T50.905	T50...
Alkalizing agent NEC	T50.901	T50.902	T50.903	T50.904	T50.905	T50.9...
Alka-seltzer	T39.011	T39.012	T39.013	T39.014	T39.015	T39...
Alkavervir	T46.5X1	T46.5X2	T46.5X3	T46.5X4	T46.5X5	T46.5...
Alkonium (bromide)	T49.0X1	T49.0X2	T49.0X3	T49.0X4	T49.0X5	T49.0...
Alkylating drug NEC	T45.1X1	T45.1X2	T45.1X3	T45.1X4	T45.1X5	T45.1...
antimyeloproliferative	T45.1X1	T45.1X2	T45.1X3	T45.1X4	T45.1X5	T45.1...
lymphatic	T45.1X1	T45.1X2	T45.1X3	T45.1X4	T45.1X5	T45.1...
Alkylisocyanate	T65.0X1	T65.0X2	T65.0X3	T65.0X4	—	—
Allantoin	T49.4X1	T49.4X2	T49.4X3	T49.4X4	T49.4X5	T49...
Allegron	T43.011	T43.012	T43.013	T43.014	T43.015	T43.0...
Allethrin	T49.0X1	T49.0X2	T49.0X3	T49.0X4	T49.0X5	T49...
Allobarbital	T42.3X1	T42.3X2	T42.3X3	T42.3X4	T42.3X5	T42.3...
Allopurinol	T50.4X1	T50.4X2	T50.4X3	T50.4X4	T50.4X5	T50.4...
Allyl						
alcohol	T51.8X1	T51.8X2	T51.8X3	T51.8X4	—	—
disulfide	T46.6X1	T46.6X2	T46.6X3	T46.6X4	T46.6X5	T46.6...
Allylestrenol	T38.5X1	T38.5X2	T38.5X3	T38.5X4	T38.5X5	T38.5...
Allylisopropylacetylurea	T42.6X1	T42.6X2	T42.6X3	T42.6X4	T42.6X5	T42.6...
Allylisopropylmalonylurea	T42.3X1	T42.3X2	T42.3X3	T42.3X4	T42.3X5	T42.3...
Allylthiourea	T49.3X1	T49.3X2	T49.3X3	T49.3X4	T49.3X5	T49.3...
Allyltribromide	T42.6X1	T42.6X2	T42.6X3	T42.6X4	T42.6X5	T42.6...
Allypropymal	T42.3X1	T42.3X2	T42.3X3	T42.3X4	T42.3X5	T42.3...
Almagate	T47.1X1	T47.1X2	T47.1X3	T47.1X4	T47.1X5	T47.1...
Almasilate	T47.1X1	T47.1X2	T47.1X3	T47.1X4	T47.1X5	T47.1...
Almitrine	T50.7X1	T50.7X2	T50.7X3	T50.7X4	T50.7X5	T50.7...
Aloes	T47.2X1	T47.2X2	T47.2X3	T47.2X4	T47.2X5	T47.2...
Aloglutamol	T47.1X1	T47.1X2	T47.1X3	T47.1X4	T47.1X5	T47.1...
Aloin	T47.2X1	T47.2X2	T47.2X3	T47.2X4	T47.2X5	T47.2...
Aloxidone	T42.2X1	T42.2X2	T42.2X3	T42.2X4	T42.2X5	T42.2...
Alpha						
acetyldigoxin	T46.0X1	T46.0X2	T46.0X3	T46.0X4	T46.0X5	T46.0...
adrenergic blocking drug	T44.6X1	T44.6X2	T44.6X3	T44.6X4	T44.6X5	T44.6...
amylase	T45.3X1	T45.3X2	T45.3X3	T45.3X4	T45.3X5	T45.3...
tocoferol (acetate)	T45.2X1	T45.2X2	T45.2X3	T45.2X4	T45.2X5	T45.2...
tocopherol	T45.2X1	T45.2X2	T45.2X3	T45.2X4	T45.2X5	T45.2...
Alphadolone	T41.1X1	T41.1X2	T41.1X3	T41.1X4	T41.1X5	T41.1...
Alphaprodine	T40.4X1	T40.4X2	T40.4X3	T40.4X4	T40.4X5	T40.4...
Alphaxalone	T41.1X1	T41.1X2	T41.1X3	T41.1X4	T41.1X5	T41.1...
Alprazolam	T42.4X1	T42.4X2	T42.4X3	T42.4X4	T42.4X5	T42.4...
Alprenolol	T44.7X1	T44.7X2	T44.7X3	T44.7X4	T44.7X5	T44.7...
Alprostadil	T46.7X1	T46.7X2	T46.7X3	T46.7X4	T46.7X5	T46.7...
Alsactide	T38.811	T38.812	T38.813	T38.814	T38.815	T38.8...
Alseroxylon	T46.5X1	T46.5X2	T46.5X3	T46.5X4	T46.5X5	T46.5...
Alteplase	T45.611	T45.612	T45.613	T45.614	T45.615	T45.6...
Altizide	T50.2X1	T50.2X2	T50.2X3	T50.2X4	T50.2X5	T50.2...
Altretamine	T45.1X1	T45.1X2	T45.1X3	T45.1X4	T45.1X5	T45.1...
Alum (medicinal)	T49.4X1	T49.4X2	T49.4X3	T49.4X4	T49.4X5	T49.4...
nonmedicinal (ammonium) (potassium)	T56.891	T56.892	T56.893	T56.894		
Aluminium, aluminum						
acetate	T49.2X1	T49.2X2	T49.2X3	T49.2X4	T49.2X5	T49.2
solution	T49.0X1	T49.0X2	T49.0X3	T49.0X4	T49.0X5	T49.0
aspirin	T39.011	T39.012	T39.013	T39.014	T39.015	T39.0
bis (acetylsalicylate)	T39.011	T39.012	T39.013	T39.014	T39.015	T39.0
carbonate (gel, basic)	T47.1X1	T47.1X2	T47.1X3	T47.1X4	T47.1X5	T47.1
chlorhydroxide-complex	T47.1X1	T47.1X2	T47.1X3	T47.1X4	T47.1X5	T47.1
chloride	T49.2X1	T49.2X2	T49.2X3	T49.2X4	T49.2X5	T49.2
clofibrate	T46.6X1	T46.6X2	T46.6X3	T46.6X4	T46.6X5	T46.6
diacetate	T49.2X1	T49.2X2	T49.2X3	T49.2X4	T49.2X5	T49.2
glycinate	T47.1X1	T47.1X2	T47.1X3	T47.1X4	T47.1X5	T47.1
hydroxide (gel)	T47.1X1	T47.1X2	T47.1X3	T47.1X4	T47.1X5	T47.1
hydroxide-magnesium carb. gel	T47.1X1	T47.1X2	T47.1X3	T47.1X4	T47.1X5	T47.1
magnesium silicate	T47.1X1	T47.1X2	T47.1X3	T47.1X4	T47.1X5	T47.1
nicotinate	T46.7X1	T46.7X2	T46.7X3	T46.7X4	T46.7X5	T46.7
ointment (surgical) (topical)	T49.3X1	T49.3X2	T49.3X3	T49.3X4	T49.3X5	T49.3
phosphate	T47.1X1	T47.1X2	T47.1X3	T47.1X4	T47.1X5	T47.1
salicylate	T39.091	T39.092	T39.093	T39.094	T39.095	T39.0
silicate	T47.1X1	T47.1X2	T47.1X3	T47.1X4	T47.1X5	T47.1
sodium silicate	T47.1X1	T47.1X2	T47.1X3	T47.1X4	T47.1X5	T47.1
subacetate	T49.2X1	T49.2X2	T49.2X3	T49.2X4	T49.2X5	T49.2
sulfate	T49.0X1	T49.0X2	T49.0X3	T49.0X4	T49.0X5	T49.0
tannate	T47.6X1	T47.6X2	T47.6X3	T47.6X4	T47.6X5	T47.6

Additional Character May Be Required — Refer to the Tabular List for Character Selection ▽ Subterms under main terms may continue to next column or page

Substance	Poisoning, Accidental (unintentional)	Poisoning, Intentional Self-harm	Poisoning, Assault	Poisoning, Undetermined	Adverse Effect	Under-dosing
Aluminium, aluminum — *continued*						
topical NEC	T49.3X1	T49.3X2	T49.3X3	T49.3X4	T49.3X5	T49.3X6
Alurate	T42.3X1	T42.3X2	T42.3X3	T42.3X4	T42.3X5	T42.3X6
Alverine	T44.3X1	T44.3X2	T44.3X3	T44.3X4	T44.3X5	T44.3X6
Alvodine	T40.2X1	T40.2X2	T40.2X3	T40.2X4	T40.2X5	T40.2X6
Amanita phalloides	T62.0X1	T62.0X2	T62.0X3	T62.0X4	—	—
Amanitine	T62.0X1	T62.0X2	T62.0X3	T62.0X4	—	—
Amantadine	T42.8X1	T42.8X2	T42.8X3	T42.8X4	T42.8X5	T42.8X6
Ambazone	T49.6X1	T49.6X2	T49.6X3	T49.6X4	T49.6X5	T49.6X6
Ambenonium (chloride)	T44.0X1	T44.0X2	T44.0X3	T44.0X4	T44.0X5	T44.0X6
Ambroxol	T48.4X1	T48.4X2	T48.4X3	T48.4X4	T48.4X5	T48.4X6
Ambuphylline	T48.6X1	T48.6X2	T48.6X3	T48.6X4	T48.6X5	T48.6X6
Ambutonium bromide	T44.3X1	T44.3X2	T44.3X3	T44.3X4	T44.3X5	T44.3X6
Amcinonide	T49.0X1	T49.0X2	T49.0X3	T49.0X4	T49.0X5	T49.0X6
Amdinocilline	T36.0X1	T36.0X2	T36.0X3	T36.0X4	T36.0X5	T36.0X6
Ametazole	T50.8X1	T50.8X2	T50.8X3	T50.8X4	T50.8X5	T50.8X6
Amethocaine	T41.3X1	T41.3X2	T41.3X3	T41.3X4	T41.3X5	T41.3X6
regional	T41.3X1	T41.3X2	T41.3X3	T41.3X4	T41.3X5	T41.3X6
spinal	T41.3X1	T41.3X2	T41.3X3	T41.3X4	T41.3X5	T41.3X6
Amethopterin	T45.1X1	T45.1X2	T45.1X3	T45.1X4	T45.1X5	T45.1X6
Amezinium metilsulfate	T44.991	T44.992	T44.993	T44.994	T44.995	T44.996
Amfebutamone	T43.291	T43.292	T43.293	T43.294	T43.295	T43.296
Amfepramone	T50.5X1	T50.5X2	T50.5X3	T50.5X4	T50.5X5	T50.5X6
Amfetamine	T43.621	T43.622	T43.623	T43.624	T43.625	T43.626
Amfetaminil	T43.621	T43.622	T43.623	T43.624	T43.625	T43.626
Amfomycin	T36.8X1	T36.8X2	T36.8X3	T36.8X4	T36.8X5	T36.8X6
Amidefrine mesilate	T48.5X1	T48.5X2	T48.5X3	T48.5X4	T48.5X5	T48.5X6
Amidone	T40.3X1	T40.3X2	T40.3X3	T40.3X4	T40.3X5	T40.3X6
Amidopyrine	T39.2X1	T39.2X2	T39.2X3	T39.2X4	T39.2X5	T39.2X6
Amidotrizoate	T50.8X1	T50.8X2	T50.8X3	T50.8X4	T50.8X5	T50.8X6
Amiflamine	T43.1X1	T43.1X2	T43.1X3	T43.1X4	T43.1X5	T43.1X6
Amikacin	T36.5X1	T36.5X2	T36.5X3	T36.5X4	T36.5X5	T36.5X6
Amikhelline	T46.3X1	T46.3X2	T46.3X3	T46.3X4	T46.3X5	T46.3X6
Amiloride	T50.2X1	T50.2X2	T50.2X3	T50.2X4	T50.2X5	T50.2X6
Aminacrine	T49.0X1	T49.0X2	T49.0X4	T49.0X5	T49.0X6	
Amineptine	T43.011	T43.012	T43.013	T43.014	T43.015	T43.016
Aminitrozole	T37.3X1	T37.3X2	T37.3X3	T37.3X4	T37.3X5	T37.3X6
Aminoacetic acid (derivatives)	T50.3X1	T50.3X2	T50.3X3	T50.3X4	T50.3X5	T50.3X6
Amino acids	T50.3X1	T50.3X2	T50.3X3	T50.3X4	T50.3X5	T50.3X6
Aminoacridine	T49.0X1	T49.0X2	T49.0X3	T49.0X4	T49.0X5	T49.0X6
Aminobenzoic acid (-p)	T49.3X1	T49.3X2	T49.3X3	T49.3X4	T49.3X5	T49.3X6
Aminocaproic acid	T45.621	T45.622	T45.623	T45.624	T45.625	T45.626
Aminoethylisothiourium	T45.8X1	T45.8X2	T45.8X3	T45.8X4	T45.8X5	T45.8X6
Aminofenazone	T39.2X1	T39.2X2	T39.2X3	T39.2X4	T39.2X5	T39.2X6
Aminoglutethimide	T45.1X1	T45.1X2	T45.1X3	T45.1X4	T45.1X5	T45.1X6
Aminohippuric acid	T50.8X1	T50.8X2	T50.8X3	T50.8X4	T50.8X5	T50.8X6
Aminomethylbenzoic acid	T45.691	T45.692	T45.693	T45.694	T45.695	T45.696
Aminometradine	T50.2X1	T50.2X2	T50.2X3	T50.2X4	T50.2X5	T50.2X6
Aminopentamide	T44.3X1	T44.3X2	T44.3X3	T44.3X4	T44.3X5	T44.3X6
Aminophenazone	T39.2X1	T39.2X2	T39.2X3	T39.2X4	T39.2X5	T39.2X6
Aminophenol	T54.0X1	T54.0X2	T54.0X3	T54.0X4	—	—
Aminophenylpyridone	T43.591	T43.592	T43.593	T43.594	T43.595	T43.596
Aminophylline	T48.6X1	T48.6X2	T48.6X3	T48.6X4	T48.6X5	T48.6X6
Aminopterin sodium	T45.1X1	T45.1X2	T45.1X3	T45.1X4	T45.1X5	T45.1X6
Aminopyrine	T39.2X1	T39.2X2	T39.2X3	T39.2X4	T39.2X5	T39.2X6
Aminorex	T50.5X1	T50.5X2	T50.5X3	T50.5X4	T50.5X5	T50.5X6
Aminosalicylic acid	T37.1X1	T37.1X2	T37.1X3	T37.1X4	T37.1X5	T37.1X6
Aminosalylum	T37.1X1	T37.1X2	T37.1X3	T37.1X4	T37.1X5	T37.1X6
Amiodarone	T46.2X1	T46.2X2	T46.2X3	T46.2X4	T46.2X5	T46.2X6
Amiphenazole	T50.7X1	T50.7X2	T50.7X3	T50.7X4	T50.7X5	T50.7X6
Amiquinsin	T46.5X1	T46.5X2	T46.5X3	T46.5X4	T46.5X5	T46.5X6
Amisometradine	T50.2X1	T50.2X2	T50.2X3	T50.2X4	T50.2X5	T50.2X6
Amisulpride	T43.591	T43.592	T43.593	T43.594	T43.595	T43.596
Amitriptyline	T43.011	T43.012	T43.013	T43.014	T43.015	T43.016
Amitriptylinoxide	T43.011	T43.012	T43.013	T43.014	T43.015	T43.016
Amlexanox	T48.6X1	T48.6X2	T48.6X3	T48.6X4	T48.6X5	T48.6X6
Ammonia (fumes) (gas)	T59.891	T59.892	T59.893	T59.894	—	—
(vapor)						
aromatic spirit	T48.991	T48.992	T48.993	T48.994	T48.995	T48.996
liquid (household)	T54.3X1	T54.3X2	T54.3X3	T54.3X4	—	—
Ammoniated mercury	T49.0X1	T49.0X2	T49.0X3	T49.0X4	T49.0X5	T49.0X6
Ammonium						
acid tartrate	T49.5X1	T49.5X2	T49.5X3	T49.5X4	T49.5X5	T49.5X6
bromide	T42.6X1	T42.6X2	T42.6X3	T42.6X4	T42.6X5	T42.6X6
carbonate	T54.3X1	T54.3X2	T54.3X3	T54.3X4	—	—
chloride	T50.991	T50.992	T50.993	T50.994	T50.995	T50.996
expectorant	T48.4X1	T48.4X2	T48.4X3	T48.4X4	T48.4X5	T48.4X6
compounds (household) NEC	T54.3X1	T54.3X2	T54.3X3	T54.3X4	—	—
fumes (any usage)	T59.891	T59.892	T59.893	T59.894	—	—
industrial	T54.3X1	T54.3X2	T54.3X3	T54.3X4	—	—

Substance	Poisoning, Accidental (unintentional)	Poisoning, Intentional Self-harm	Poisoning, Assault	Poisoning, Undetermined	Adverse Effect	Under-dosing
Ammonium — *continued*						
ichthyosulronate	T49.4X1	T49.4X2	T49.4X3	T49.4X4	T49.4X5	T49.4X6
mandelate	T37.91	T37.92	T37.93	T37.94	T37.95	T37.96
sulfamate	T60.3X1	T60.3X2	T60.3X3	T60.3X4	—	—
sulfonate resin	T47.8X1	T47.8X2	T47.8X3	T47.8X4	T47.8X5	T47.8X6
Amobarbital (sodium)	T42.3X1	T42.3X2	T42.3X3	T42.3X4	T42.3X5	T42.3X6
Amodiaquine	T37.2X1	T37.2X2	T37.2X3	T37.2X4	T37.2X5	T37.2X6
Amopyroquin (e)	T37.2X1	T37.2X2	T37.2X3	T37.2X4	T37.2X5	T37.2X6
Amoxapine	T43.011	T43.012	T43.013	T43.014	T43.015	T43.016
Amoxicillin	T36.0X1	T36.0X2	T36.0X3	T36.0X4	T36.0X5	T36.0X6
Amperozide	T43.591	T43.592	T43.593	T43.594	T43.595	T43.596
Amphenidone	T43.591	T43.592	T43.593	T43.594	T43.595	T43.596
Amphetamine NEC	T43.621	T43.622	T43.623	T43.624	T43.625	T43.626
Amphomycin	T36.8X1	T36.8X2	T36.8X3	T36.8X4	T36.8X5	T36.8X6
Amphotalide	T37.4X1	T37.4X2	T37.4X3	T37.4X4	T37.4X5	T37.4X6
Amphotericin B	T36.7X1	T36.7X2	T36.7X3	T36.7X4	T36.7X5	T36.7X6
topical	T49.0X1	T49.0X2	T49.0X3	T49.0X4	T49.0X5	T49.0X6
Ampicillin	T36.0X1	T36.0X2	T36.0X3	T36.0X4	T36.0X5	T36.0X6
Amprotropine	T44.3X1	T44.3X2	T44.3X3	T44.3X4	T44.3X5	T44.3X6
Amsacrine	T45.1X1	T45.1X2	T45.1X3	T45.1X4	T45.1X5	T45.1X6
Amygdaline	T62.2X1	T62.2X2	T62.2X3	T62.2X4	—	—
Amyl						
acetate	T52.8X1	T52.8X2	T52.8X3	T52.8X4	—	—
vapor	T59.891	T59.892	T59.893	T59.894	—	—
alcohol	T51.3X1	T51.3X2	T51.3X3	T51.3X4	—	—
chloride	T53.6X1	T53.6X2	T53.6X3	T53.6X4	—	—
formate	T52.8X1	T52.8X2	T52.8X3	T52.8X4	—	—
nitrite	T46.3X1	T46.3X2	T46.3X3	T46.3X4	T46.3X5	T46.3X6
propionate	T65.891	T65.892	T65.893	T65.894	—	—
Amylase	T47.5X1	T47.5X2	T47.5X3	T47.5X4	T47.5X5	T47.5X6
Amyleine, regional	T41.3X1	T41.3X2	T41.3X3	T41.3X4	T41.3X5	T41.3X6
Amylene						
dichloride	T53.6X1	T53.6X2	T53.6X3	T53.6X4	—	—
hydrate	T51.3X1	T51.3X2	T51.3X3	T51.3X4	—	—
Amylmetacresol	T49.6X1	T49.6X2	T49.6X3	T49.6X4	T49.6X5	T49.6X6
Amylobarbitone	T42.3X1	T42.3X2	T42.3X3	T42.3X4	T42.3X5	T42.3X6
Amylocaine, regional	T41.3X1	T41.3X2	T41.3X3	T41.3X4	T41.3X5	T41.3X6
infiltration (subcutaneous)	T41.3X1	T41.3X2	T41.3X3	T41.3X4	T41.3X5	T41.3X6
nerve block (peripheral) (plexus)	T41.3X1	T41.3X2	T41.3X3	T41.3X4	T41.3X5	T41.3X6
spinal	T41.3X1	T41.3X2	T41.3X3	T41.3X4	T41.3X5	T41.3X6
topical (surface)	T41.3X1	T41.3X2	T41.3X3	T41.3X4	T41.3X5	T41.3X6
Amylopectin	T47.6X1	T47.6X2	T47.6X3	T47.6X4	T47.6X5	T47.6X6
Amytal (sodium)	T42.3X1	T42.3X2	T42.3X3	T42.3X4	T42.3X5	T42.3X6
Anabolic steroid	T38.7X1	T38.7X2	T38.7X3	T38.7X4	T38.7X5	T38.7X6
Analeptic NEC	T50.7X1	T50.7X2	T50.7X3	T50.7X4	T50.7X5	T50.7X6
Analgesic	T39.91	T39.92	T39.93	T39.94	T39.95	T39.96
anti-inflammatory NEC	T39.91	T39.92	T39.93	T39.94	T39.95	T39.96
propionic acid derivative	T39.311	T39.312	T39.313	T39.314	T39.315	T39.316
antirheumatic NEC	T39.4X1	T39.4X2	T39.4X3	T39.4X4	T39.4X5	T39.4X6
aromatic NEC	T39.1X1	T39.1X2	T39.1X3	T39.1X4	T39.1X5	T39.1X6
narcotic NEC	T40.601	T40.602	T40.603	T40.604	T40.605	T40.606
combination	T40.601	T40.602	T40.603	T40.604	T40.605	T40.606
obstetric	T40.601	T40.602	T40.603	T40.604	T40.605	T40.606
non-narcotic NEC	T39.91	T39.92	T39.93	T39.94	T39.95	T39.96
combination	T39.91	T39.92	T39.93	T39.94	T39.95	T39.96
pyrazole	T39.2X1	T39.2X2	T39.2X3	T39.2X4	T39.2X5	T39.2X6
specified NEC	T39.8X1	T39.8X2	T39.8X3	T39.8X4	T39.8X5	T39.8X6
Analgin	T39.2X1	T39.2X2	T39.2X3	T39.2X4	T39.2X5	T39.2X6
Anamirta cocculus	T62.1X1	T62.1X2	T62.1X3	T62.1X4	—	—
Ancillin	T36.0X1	T36.0X2	T36.0X3	T36.0X4	T36.0X5	T36.0X6
Ancrod	T45.691	T45.692	T45.693	T45.694	T45.695	T45.696
Androgen	T38.7X1	T38.7X2	T38.7X3	T38.7X4	T38.7X5	T38.7X6
Androgen-estrogen mixture	T38.7X1	T38.7X2	T38.7X3	T38.7X4	T38.7X5	T38.7X6
Androstalone	T38.7X1	T38.7X2	T38.7X3	T38.7X4	T38.7X5	T38.7X6
Androstanolone	T38.7X1	T38.7X2	T38.7X3	T38.7X4	T38.7X5	T38.7X6
Androsterone	T38.7X1	T38.7X2	T38.7X3	T38.7X4	T38.7X5	T38.7X6
Anemone pulsatilla	T62.2X1	T62.2X2	T62.2X3	T62.2X4	—	—
Anesthesia						
caudal	T41.3X1	T41.3X2	T41.3X3	T41.3X4	T41.3X5	T41.3X6
endotracheal	T41.0X1	T41.0X2	T41.0X3	T41.0X4	T41.0X5	T41.0X6
epidural	T41.3X1	T41.3X2	T41.3X3	T41.3X4	T41.3X5	T41.3X6
inhalation	T41.0X1	T41.0X2	T41.0X3	T41.0X4	T41.0X5	T41.0X6
local	T41.3X1	T41.3X2	T41.3X3	T41.3X4	T41.3X5	T41.3X6
mucosal	T41.3X1	T41.3X2	T41.3X3	T41.3X4	T41.3X5	T41.3X6
muscle relaxation	T48.1X1	T48.1X2	T48.1X3	T48.1X4	T48.1X5	T48.1X6
nerve blocking	T41.3X1	T41.3X2	T41.3X3	T41.3X4	T41.3X5	T41.3X6
plexus blocking	T41.3X1	T41.3X2	T41.3X3	T41.3X4	T41.3X5	T41.3X6
potentiated	T41.201	T41.202	T41.203	T41.204	T41.205	T41.206
rectal	T41.201	T41.202	T41.203	T41.204	T41.205	T41.206
general	T41.201	T41.202	T41.203	T41.204	T41.205	T41.206
local	T41.3X1	T41.3X2	T41.3X3	T41.3X4	T41.3X5	T41.3X6

Substance	Poisoning, Accidental (unintentional)	Poisoning, Intentional Self-harm	Poisoning, Assault	Poisoning, Undetermined	Adverse Effect	Under-dosing
Anesthesia — continued						
regional	T41.3X1	T41.3X2	T41.3X3	T41.3X4	T41.3X5	T41.3X6
surface	T41.3X1	T41.3X2	T41.3X3	T41.3X4	T41.3X5	T41.3X6
Anesthetic NEC — see also	T41.41	T41.42	T41.43	T41.44	T41.45	T41.46
Anesthesia						
with muscle relaxant	T41.201	T41.202	T41.203	T41.204	T41.205	T41.206
general	T41.201	T41.202	T41.203	T41.204	T41.205	T41.206
local	T41.3X1	T41.3X2	T41.3X3	T41.3X4	T41.3X5	T41.3X6
gaseous NEC	T41.0X1	T41.0X2	T41.0X3	T41.0X4	T41.0X5	T41.0X6
general NEC	T41.201	T41.202	T41.203	T41.204	T41.205	T41.206
halogenated hydrocarbon derivatives NEC	T41.0X1	T41.0X2	T41.0X3	T41.0X4	T41.0X5	T41.0X6
infiltration NEC	T41.3X1	T41.3X2	T41.3X3	T41.3X4	T41.3X5	T41.3X6
intravenous NEC	T41.1X1	T41.1X2	T41.1X3	T41.1X4	T41.1X5	T41.1X6
local NEC	T41.3X1	T41.3X2	T41.3X3	T41.3X4	T41.3X5	T41.3X6
rectal	T41.201	T41.202	T41.203	T41.204	T41.205	T41.206
general	T41.201	T41.202	T41.203	T41.204	T41.205	T41.206
local	T41.3X1	T41.3X2	T41.3X3	T41.3X4	T41.3X5	T41.3X6
regional NEC	T41.3X1	T41.3X2	T41.3X3	T41.3X4	T41.3X5	T41.3X6
spinal NEC	T41.3X1	T41.3X2	T41.3X3	T41.3X4	T41.3X5	T41.3X6
thiobarbiturate	T41.1X1	T41.1X2	T41.1X3	T41.1X4	T41.1X5	T41.1X6
topical	T41.3X1	T41.3X2	T41.3X3	T41.3X4	T41.3X5	T41.3X6
Aneurine	T45.2X1	T45.2X2	T45.2X3	T45.2X4	T45.2X5	T45.2X6
Angio-Conray	T50.8X1	T50.8X2	T50.8X3	T50.8X4	T50.8X5	T50.8X6
Angiotensin	T44.5X1	T44.5X2	T44.5X3	T44.5X4	T44.5X5	T44.5X6
Angiotensinamide	T44.991	T44.992	T44.993	T44.994	T44.995	T44.996
Anhydrohydroxy-progesterone	T38.5X1	T38.5X2	T38.5X3	T38.5X4	T38.5X5	T38.5X6
Anhydron	T50.2X1	T50.2X2	T50.2X3	T50.2X4	T50.2X5	T50.2X6
Anileridine	T40.4X1	T40.4X2	T40.4X3	T40.4X4	T40.4X5	T40.4X6
Aniline (dye) (liquid)	T65.3X1	T65.3X2	T65.3X3	T65.3X4	—	—
analgesic	T39.1X1	T39.1X2	T39.1X3	T39.1X4	T39.1X5	T39.1X6
derivatives, therapeutic NEC	T39.1X1	T39.1X2	T39.1X3	T39.1X4	T39.1X5	T39.1X6
vapor	T65.3X1	T65.3X2	T65.3X3	T65.3X4	—	—
Aniscoropine	T44.3X1	T44.3X2	T44.3X3	T44.3X4	T44.3X5	T44.3X6
Anise oil	T47.5X1	T47.5X2	T47.5X3	T47.5X4	T47.5X5	T47.5X6
Anisidine	T65.3X1	T65.3X2	T65.3X3	T65.3X4	—	—
Anisindione	T45.511	T45.512	T45.513	T45.514	T45.515	T45.516
Anisotropine methyl-bromide	T44.3X1	T44.3X2	T44.3X3	T44.3X4	T44.3X5	T44.3X6
Anistreplase	T45.611	T45.612	T45.613	T45.614	T45.615	T45.616
Anorexiant (central)	T50.5X1	T50.5X2	T50.5X3	T50.5X4	T50.5X5	T50.5X6
Anorexic agents	T50.5X1	T50.5X2	T50.5X3	T50.5X4	T50.5X5	T50.5X6
Ansamycin	T36.6X1	T36.6X2	T36.6X3	T36.6X4	T36.6X5	T36.6X6
Ant (bite) (sting)	T63.421	T63.422	T63.423	T63.424	—	—
Antabuse	T50.6X1	T50.6X2	T50.6X3	T50.6X4	T50.6X5	T50.6X6
Antacid NEC	T47.1X1	T47.1X2	T47.1X3	T47.1X4	T47.1X5	T47.1X6
Antagonist						
Aldosterone	T50.0X1	T50.0X2	T50.0X3	T50.0X4	T50.0X5	T50.0X6
alpha-adrenoreceptor	T44.6X1	T44.6X2	T44.6X3	T44.6X4	T44.6X5	T44.6X6
anticoagulant	T45.7X1	T45.7X2	T45.7X3	T45.7X4	T45.7X5	T45.7X6
beta-adrenoreceptor	T44.7X1	T44.7X2	T44.7X3	T44.7X4	T44.7X5	T44.7X6
extrapyramidal NEC	T44.3X1	T44.3X2	T44.3X3	T44.3X4	T44.3X5	T44.3X6
folic acid	T45.1X1	T45.1X2	T45.1X3	T45.1X4	T45.1X5	T45.1X6
H2 receptor	T47.0X1	T47.0X2	T47.0X3	T47.0X4	T47.0X5	T47.0X6
heavy metal	T45.8X1	T45.8X2	T45.8X3	T45.8X4	T45.8X5	T45.8X6
narcotic analgesic	T50.7X1	T50.7X2	T50.7X3	T50.7X4	T50.7X5	T50.7X6
opiate	T50.7X1	T50.7X2	T50.7X3	T50.7X4	T50.7X5	T50.7X6
pyrimidine	T45.1X1	T45.1X2	T45.1X3	T45.1X4	T45.1X5	T45.1X6
serotonin	T46.5X1	T46.5X2	T46.5X3	T46.5X4	T46.5X5	T46.5X6
Antazolin (e)	T45.0X1	T45.0X2	T45.0X3	T45.0X4	T45.0X5	T45.0X6
Anterior pituitary hormone NEC	T38.811	T38.812	T38.813	T38.814	T38.815	T38.816
Anthelmintic NEC	T37.4X1	T37.4X2	T37.4X3	T37.4X4	T37.4X5	T37.4X6
Anthiolimine	T37.4X1	T37.4X2	T37.4X3	T37.4X4	T37.4X5	T37.4X6
Anthralin	T49.4X1	T49.4X2	T49.4X3	T49.4X4	T49.4X5	T49.4X6
Anthramycin	T45.1X1	T45.1X2	T45.1X3	T45.1X4	T45.1X5	T45.1X6
Antiadrenergic NEC	T44.8X1	T44.8X2	T44.8X3	T44.8X4	T44.8X5	T44.8X6
Antiallergic NEC	T45.0X1	T45.0X2	T45.0X3	T45.0X4	T45.0X5	T45.0X6
Antiandrogen NEC	T38.6X1	T38.6X2	T38.6X3	T38.6X4	T38.6X5	T38.6X6
Anti-anemic (drug) (preparation)	T45.8X1	T45.8X2	T45.8X3	T45.8X4	T45.8X5	T45.8X6
Antianxiety drug NEC	T43.501	T43.502	T43.503	T43.504	T43.505	T43.506
Antiaris toxicaria	T65.891	T65.892	T65.893	T65.894	—	—
Antiarteriosclerotic drug	T46.6X1	T46.6X2	T46.6X3	T46.6X4	T46.6X5	T46.6X6
Antiasthmatic drug NEC	T48.6X1	T48.6X2	T48.6X3	T48.6X4	T48.6X5	T48.6X6
Antibiotic NEC	T36.91	T36.92	T36.93	T36.94	T36.95	T36.96
aminoglycoside	T36.5X1	T36.5X2	T36.5X3	T36.5X4	T36.5X5	T36.5X6
anticancer	T45.1X1	T45.1X2	T45.1X3	T45.1X4	T45.1X5	T45.1X6
antifungal	T36.7X1	T36.7X2	T36.7X3	T36.7X4	T36.7X5	T36.7X6
antimycobacterial	T36.5X1	T36.5X2	T36.5X3	T36.5X4	T36.5X5	T36.5X6
antineoplastic	T45.1X1	T45.1X2	T45.1X3	T45.1X4	T45.1X5	T45.1X6
b-lactam NEC	T36.1X1	T36.1X2	T36.1X3	T36.1X4	T36.1X5	T36.1X6

Substance	Poisoning, Accidental (unintentional)	Poisoning, Intentional Self-harm	Poisoning, Assault	Poisoning, Undetermined	Adverse Effect	Under-dosing
Antibiotic — continued						
cephalosporin (group)	T36.1X1	T36.1X2	T36.1X3	T36.1X4	T36.1X5	T36.1
chloramphenicol (group)	T36.2X1	T36.2X2	T36.2X3	T36.2X4	T36.2X5	T36.2
ENT	T49.6X1	T49.6X2	T49.6X3	T49.6X4	T49.6X5	T49.6
eye	T49.5X1	T49.5X2	T49.5X3	T49.5X4	T49.5X5	T49.5
fungicidal (local)	T49.0X1	T49.0X2	T49.0X3	T49.0X4	T49.0X5	T49.0
intestinal	T36.8X1	T36.8X2	T36.8X3	T36.8X4	T36.8X5	T36.8
local	T49.0X1	T49.0X2	T49.0X3	T49.0X4	T49.0X5	T49.0
macrolides	T36.3X1	T36.3X2	T36.3X3	T36.3X4	T36.3X5	T36.3
polypeptide	T36.8X1	T36.8X2	T36.8X3	T36.8X4	T36.8X5	T36.8
specified NEC	T36.8X1	T36.8X2	T36.8X3	T36.8X4	T36.8X5	T36.8
tetracycline (group)	T36.4X1	T36.4X2	T36.4X3	T36.4X4	T36.4X5	T36.4
throat	T49.6X1	T49.6X2	T49.6X3	T49.6X4	T49.6X5	T49.6
Anticancer agents NEC	T45.1X1	T45.1X2	T45.1X3	T45.1X4	T45.1X5	T45.1
Anticholesterolemic drug NEC	T46.6X1	T46.6X2	T46.6X3	T46.6X4	T46.6X5	T46.6
Anticholinergic NEC	T44.3X1	T44.3X2	T44.3X3	T44.3X4	T44.3X5	T44.3
Anticholinesterase	T44.0X1	T44.0X2	T44.0X3	T44.0X4	T44.0X5	T44.0
organophosphorus	T44.0X1	T44.0X2	T44.0X3	T44.0X4	T44.0X5	T44.0
insecticide	T60.0X1	T60.0X2	T60.0X3	T60.0X4	—	—
nerve gas	T59.891	T59.892	T59.893	T59.894	—	—
reversible	T44.0X1	T44.0X2	T44.0X3	T44.0X4	T44.0X5	T44.0
ophthalmological	T49.5X1	T49.5X2	T49.5X3	T49.5X4	T49.5X5	T49.5
Anticoagulant NEC	T45.511	T45.512	T45.513	T45.514	T45.515	T45.5
Antagonist	T45.7X1	T45.7X2	T45.7X3	T45.7X4	T45.7X5	T45.7
Anti-common-cold drug NEC	T48.5X1	T48.5X2	T48.5X3	T48.5X4	T48.5X5	T48.5
Anticonvulsant	T42.71	T42.72	T42.73	T42.74	T42.75	T42.7
barbiturate	T42.3X1	T42.3X2	T42.3X3	T42.3X4	T42.3X5	T42.3
combination (with barbiturate)	T42.3X1	T42.3X2	T42.3X3	T42.3X4	T42.3X5	T42.3
hydantoin	T42.0X1	T42.0X2	T42.0X3	T42.0X4	T42.0X5	T42.0
hypnotic NEC	T42.6X1	T42.6X2	T42.6X3	T42.6X4	T42.6X5	T42.6
oxazolidinedione	T42.2X1	T42.2X2	T42.2X3	T42.2X4	T42.2X5	T42.2
pyrimidinedione	T42.6X1	T42.6X2	T42.6X3	T42.6X4	T42.6X5	T42.6
specified NEC	T42.6X1	T42.6X2	T42.6X3	T42.6X4	T42.6X5	T42.6
succinimide	T42.2X1	T42.2X2	T42.2X3	T42.2X4	T42.2X5	T42.2
Antidepressant	T43.201	T43.202	T43.203	T43.204	T43.205	T43.2
monoamine oxidase inhibitor	T43.1X1	T43.1X2	T43.1X3	T43.1X4	T43.1X5	T43.1
selective serotonin norepinephrine reuptake inhibitor	T43.211	T43.212	T43.213	T43.214	T43.215	T43.2
selective serotonin reuptake inhibitor	T43.221	T43.222	T43.223	T43.224	T43.225	T43.2
specified NEC	T43.291	T43.292	T43.293	T43.294	T43.295	T43.2
tetracyclic	T43.021	T43.022	T43.023	T43.024	T43.025	T43.0
triazolopyridine	T43.211	T43.212	T43.213	T43.214	T43.215	T43.2
tricyclic	T43.011	T43.012	T43.013	T43.014	T43.015	T43.0
Antidiabetic NEC	T38.3X1	T38.3X2	T38.3X3	T38.3X4	T38.3X5	T38.3
biguanide	T38.3X1	T38.3X2	T38.3X3	T38.3X4	T38.3X5	T38.3
and sulfonyl combined	T38.3X1	T38.3X2	T38.3X3	T38.3X4	T38.3X5	T38.3
combined	T38.3X1	T38.3X2	T38.3X3	T38.3X4	T38.3X5	T38.3
sulfonylurea	T38.3X1	T38.3X2	T38.3X3	T38.3X4	T38.3X5	T38.3
Antidiarrheal drug NEC	T47.6X1	T47.6X2	T47.6X3	T47.6X4	T47.6X5	T47.6
absorbent	T47.6X1	T47.6X2	T47.6X3	T47.6X4	T47.6X5	T47.6
Anti-D immunoglobulin (human)	T50.Z11	T50.Z12	T50.Z13	T50.Z14	T50.Z15	T50.Z
Antidiphtheria serum	T50.Z11	T50.Z12	T50.Z13	T50.Z14	T50.Z15	T50.Z
Antidiuretic hormone	T38.891	T38.892	T38.893	T38.894	T38.895	T38.8
Antidote NEC	T50.6X1	T50.6X2	T50.6X3	T50.6X4	T50.6X5	T50.6
heavy metal	T45.8X1	T45.8X2	T45.8X3	T45.8X4	T45.8X5	T45.8
Antidysrhythmic NEC	T46.2X1	T46.2X2	T46.2X3	T46.2X4	T46.2X5	T46.2
Antiemetic drug	T45.0X1	T45.0X2	T45.0X3	T45.0X4	T45.0X5	T45.0
Antiepilepsy agent	T42.71	T42.72	T42.73	T42.74	T42.75	T42.7
combination	T42.5X1	T42.5X2	T42.5X3	T42.5X4	T42.5X5	T42.5
mixed	T42.5X1	T42.5X2	T42.5X3	T42.5X4	T42.5X5	T42.5
specified, NEC	T42.6X1	T42.6X2	T42.6X3	T42.6X4	T42.6X5	T42.6
Antiestrogen NEC	T38.6X1	T38.6X2	T38.6X3	T38.6X4	T38.6X5	T38.6
Antifertility pill	T38.4X1	T38.4X2	T38.4X3	T38.4X4	T38.4X5	T38.4
Antifibrinolytic drug	T45.621	T45.622	T45.623	T45.624	T45.625	T45.62
Antifilarial drug	T37.4X1	T37.4X2	T37.4X3	T37.4X4	T37.4X5	T37.4
Antiflatulent	T47.5X1	T47.5X2	T47.5X3	T47.5X4	T47.5X5	T47.5
Antifreeze	T65.91	T65.92	T65.93	T65.94	—	—
alcohol	T51.1X1	T51.1X2	T51.1X3	T51.1X4	—	—
ethylene glycol	T51.8X1	T51.8X2	T51.8X3	T51.8X4	—	—
Antifungal						
antibiotic (systemic)	T36.7X1	T36.7X2	T36.7X3	T36.7X4	T36.7X5	T36.7
anti-infective NEC	T37.91	T37.92	T37.93	T37.94	T37.95	T37.9
disinfectant, local	T49.0X1	T49.0X2	T49.0X3	T49.0X4	T49.0X5	T49.0
nonmedicinal (spray)	T60.3X1	T60.3X2	T60.3X3	T60.3X4	—	—
topical	T49.0X1	T49.0X2	T49.0X3	T49.0X4	T49.0X5	T49.0

Additional Character May Be Required — Refer to the Tabular List for Character Selection   ▽ Subterms under main terms may continue to next column or page

Substance	Poisoning, Accidental (unintentional)	Poisoning, Intentional Self-harm	Poisoning, Assault	Poisoning, Undetermined	Adverse Effect	Under-dosing
Anti-gastric-secretion drug NEC	T47.1X1	T47.1X2	T47.1X3	T47.1X4	T47.1X5	T47.1X6
Antigonadotrophin NEC	T38.6X1	T38.6X2	T38.6X3	T38.6X4	T38.6X5	T38.6X6
Antihallucinogen	T43.501	T43.502	T43.503	T43.504	T43.505	T43.506
Antihelmintics	T37.4X1	T37.4X2	T37.4X3	T37.4X4	T37.4X5	T37.4X6
Antihemophilic						
factor	T45.8X1	T45.8X2	T45.8X3	T45.8X4	T45.8X5	T45.8X6
fraction	T45.8X1	T45.8X2	T45.8X3	T45.8X4	T45.8X5	T45.8X6
globulin concentrate	T45.7X1	T45.7X2	T45.7X3	T45.7X4	T45.7X5	T45.7X6
human plasma	T45.8X1	T45.8X2	T45.8X3	T45.8X4	T45.8X5	T45.8X6
plasma, dried	T45.7X1	T45.7X2	T45.7X3	T45.7X4	T45.7X5	T45.7X6
Antihemorrhoidal preparation	T49.2X1	T49.2X2	T49.2X3	T49.2X4	T49.2X5	T49.2X6
Antiheparin drug	T45.7X1	T45.7X2	T45.7X3	T45.7X4	T45.7X5	T45.7X6
Antihistamine	T45.0X1	T45.0X2	T45.0X3	T45.0X4	T45.0X5	T45.0X6
Antihookworm drug	T37.4X1	T37.4X2	T37.4X3	T37.4X4	T37.4X5	T37.4X6
Anti-human lymphocytic globulin	T50.Z11	T50.Z12	T50.Z13	T50.Z14	T50.Z15	T50.Z16
Antihyperlipidemic drug	T46.6X1	T46.6X2	T46.6X3	T46.6X4	T46.6X5	T46.6X6
Antihypertensive drug NEC	T46.5X1	T46.5X2	T46.5X3	T46.5X4	T46.5X5	T46.5X6
Anti-infective NEC	T37.91	T37.92	T37.93	T37.94	T37.95	T37.96
anthelmintic	T37.4X1	T37.4X2	T37.4X3	T37.4X4	T37.4X5	T37.4X6
antibiotics	T36.91	T36.92	T36.93	T36.94	T36.95	T36.96
specified NEC	T36.8X1	T36.8X2	T36.8X3	T36.8X4	T36.8X5	T36.8X6
antimalarial	T37.2X1	T37.2X2	T37.2X3	T37.2X4	T37.2X5	T37.2X6
antimycobacterial NEC	T37.1X1	T37.1X2	T37.1X3	T37.1X4	T37.1X5	T37.1X6
antibiotics	T36.5X1	T36.5X2	T36.5X3	T36.5X4	T36.5X5	T36.5X6
antiprotozoal NEC	T37.3X1	T37.3X2	T37.3X3	T37.3X4	T37.3X5	T37.3X6
blood	T37.2X1	T37.2X2	T37.2X3	T37.2X4	T37.2X5	T37.2X6
antiviral	T37.5X1	T37.5X2	T37.5X3	T37.5X4	T37.5X5	T37.5X6
arsenical	T37.8X1	T37.8X2	T37.8X3	T37.8X4	T37.8X5	T37.8X6
bismuth, local	T49.0X1	T49.0X2	T49.0X3	T49.0X4	T49.0X5	T49.0X6
ENT	T49.6X1	T49.6X2	T49.6X3	T49.6X4	T49.6X5	T49.6X6
eye NEC	T49.5X1	T49.5X2	T49.5X3	T49.5X4	T49.5X5	T49.5X6
heavy metals NEC	T37.8X1	T37.8X2	T37.8X3	T37.8X4	T37.8X5	T37.8X6
local NEC	T49.0X1	T49.0X2	T49.0X3	T49.0X4	T49.0X5	T49.0X6
specified NEC	T49.0X1	T49.0X2	T49.0X3	T49.0X4	T49.0X5	T49.0X6
mixed	T37.91	T37.92	T37.93	T37.94	T37.95	T37.96
ophthalmic preparation	T49.5X1	T49.5X2	T49.5X3	T49.5X4	T49.5X5	T49.5X6
topical NEC	T49.0X1	T49.0X2	T49.0X3	T49.0X4	T49.0X5	T49.0X6
Anti-inflammatory drug NEC	T39.391	T39.392	T39.393	T39.394	T39.395	T39.396
local	T49.0X1	T49.0X2	T49.0X3	T49.0X4	T49.0X5	T49.0X6
nonsteroidal NEC	T39.391	T39.392	T39.393	T39.394	T39.395	T39.396
propionic acid derivative	T39.311	T39.312	T39.313	T39.314	T39.315	T39.316
specified NEC	T39.391	T39.392	T39.393	T39.394	T39.395	T39.396
Antikaluretic	T50.3X1	T50.3X2	T50.3X3	T50.3X4	T50.3X5	T50.3X6
Antiknock (tetraethyl lead)	T56.0X1	T56.0X2	T56.0X3	T56.0X4	—	—
Antilipemic drug NEC	T46.6X1	T46.6X2	T46.6X3	T46.6X4	T46.6X5	T46.6X6
Antimalarial	T37.2X1	T37.2X2	T37.2X3	T37.2X4	T37.2X5	T37.2X6
prophylactic NEC	T37.2X1	T37.2X2	T37.2X3	T37.2X4	T37.2X5	T37.2X6
pyrimidine derivative	T37.2X1	T37.2X2	T37.2X3	T37.2X4	T37.2X5	T37.2X6
Antimetabolite	T45.1X1	T45.1X2	T45.1X3	T45.1X4	T45.1X5	T45.1X6
Antimitotic agent	T45.1X1	T45.1X2	T45.1X3	T45.1X4	T45.1X5	T45.1X6
Antimony (compounds) (vapor) NEC	T56.891	T56.892	T56.893	T56.894	—	—
anti-infectives	T37.8X1	T37.8X2	T37.8X3	T37.8X4	T37.8X5	T37.8X6
dimercaptosuccinate	T37.3X1	T37.3X2	T37.3X3	T37.3X4	T37.3X5	T37.3X6
hydride	T56.891	T56.892	T56.893	T56.894	—	—
pesticide (vapor)	T60.8X1	T60.8X2	T60.8X3	T60.8X4	—	—
potassium (sodium) tartrate	T37.8X1	T37.8X2	T37.8X3	T37.8X4	T37.8X5	T37.8X6
sodium dimercaptosuccinate	T37.3X1	T37.3X2	T37.3X3	T37.3X4	T37.3X5	T37.3X6
tartrated	T37.8X1	T37.8X2	T37.8X3	T37.8X4	T37.8X5	T37.8X6
Antimuscarinic NEC	T44.3X1	T44.3X2	T44.3X3	T44.3X4	T44.3X5	T44.3X6
Antimycobacterial drug NEC	T37.1X1	T37.1X2	T37.1X3	T37.1X4	T37.1X5	T37.1X6
antibiotics	T36.5X1	T36.5X2	T36.5X3	T36.5X4	T36.5X5	T36.5X6
combination	T37.1X1	T37.1X2	T37.1X3	T37.1X4	T37.1X5	T37.1X6
Antinausea drug	T45.0X1	T45.0X2	T45.0X3	T45.0X4	T45.0X5	T45.0X6
Antinematode drug	T37.4X1	T37.4X2	T37.4X3	T37.4X4	T37.4X5	T37.4X6
Antineoplastic NEC	T45.1X1	T45.1X2	T45.1X3	T45.1X4	T45.1X5	T45.1X6
alkaloidal	T45.1X1	T45.1X2	T45.1X3	T45.1X4	T45.1X5	T45.1X6
antibiotics	T45.1X1	T45.1X2	T45.1X3	T45.1X4	T45.1X5	T45.1X6
combination	T45.1X1	T45.1X2	T45.1X3	T45.1X4	T45.1X5	T45.1X6
estrogen	T38.5X1	T38.5X2	T38.5X3	T38.5X4	T38.5X5	T38.5X6
steroid	T38.7X1	T38.7X2	T38.7X3	T38.7X4	T38.7X5	T38.7X6
Antiparasitic drug (systemic)	T37.91	T37.92	T37.93	T37.94	T37.95	T37.96
local	T49.0X1	T49.0X2	T49.0X3	T49.0X4	T49.0X5	T49.0X6
specified NEC	T37.8X1	T37.8X2	T37.8X3	T37.8X4	T37.8X5	T37.8X6

Substance	Poisoning, Accidental (unintentional)	Poisoning, Intentional Self-harm	Poisoning, Assault	Poisoning, Undetermined	Adverse Effect	Under-dosing
Antiparkinsonism drug NEC	T42.8X1	T42.8X2	T42.8X3	T42.8X4	T42.8X5	T42.8X6
Antiperspirant NEC	T49.2X1	T49.2X2	T49.2X3	T49.2X4	T49.2X5	T49.2X6
Antiphlogistic NEC	T39.4X1	T39.4X2	T39.4X3	T39.4X4	T39.4X5	T39.4X6
Antiplatyhelmintic drug	T37.4X1	T37.4X2	T37.4X3	T37.4X4	T37.4X5	T37.4X6
Antiprotozoal drug NEC	T37.3X1	T37.3X2	T37.3X3	T37.3X4	T37.3X5	T37.3X6
blood	T37.2X1	T37.2X2	T37.2X3	T37.2X4	T37.2X5	T37.2X6
local	T49.0X1	T49.0X2	T49.0X3	T49.0X4	T49.0X5	T49.0X6
Antipruritic drug NEC	T49.1X1	T49.1X2	T49.1X3	T49.1X4	T49.1X5	T49.1X6
Antipsychotic drug	T43.501	T43.502	T43.503	T43.504	T43.505	T43.506
specified NEC	T43.591	T43.592	T43.593	T43.594	T43.595	T43.596
Antipyretic	T39.91	T39.92	T39.93	T39.94	T39.95	T39.96
specified NEC	T39.8X1	T39.8X2	T39.8X3	T39.8X4	T39.8X5	T39.8X6
Antipyrine	T39.2X1	T39.2X2	T39.2X3	T39.2X4	T39.2X5	T39.2X6
Antirabies hyperimmune serum	T50.Z11	T50.Z12	T50.Z13	T50.Z14	T50.Z15	T50.Z16
Antirheumatic NEC	T39.4X1	T39.4X2	T39.4X3	T39.4X4	T39.4X5	T39.4X6
Antirigidity drug NEC	T42.8X1	T42.8X2	T42.8X3	T42.8X4	T42.8X5	T42.8X6
Antischistosomal drug	T37.4X1	T37.4X2	T37.4X3	T37.4X4	T37.4X5	T37.4X6
Antiscorpion sera	T50.Z11	T50.Z12	T50.Z13	T50.Z14	T50.Z15	T50.Z16
Antiseborrheics	T49.4X1	T49.4X2	T49.4X3	T49.4X4	T49.4X5	T49.4X6
Antiseptics (external) (medicinal)	T49.0X1	T49.0X2	T49.0X3	T49.0X4	T49.0X5	T49.0X6
Antistine	T45.0X1	T45.0X2	T45.0X3	T45.0X4	T45.0X5	T45.0X6
Antitapeworm drug	T37.4X1	T37.4X2	T37.4X3	T37.4X4	T37.4X5	T37.4X6
Antitetanus immunoglobulin	T50.Z11	T50.Z12	T50.Z13	T50.Z14	T50.Z15	T50.Z16
Antithrombotic	T45.521	T45.522	T45.523	T45.524	T45.525	T45.526
Antithyroid drug NEC	T38.2X1	T38.2X2	T38.2X3	T38.2X4	T38.2X5	T38.2X6
Antitoxin	T50.Z11	T50.Z12	T50.Z13	T50.Z14	T50.Z15	T50.Z16
diphtheria	T50.Z11	T50.Z12	T50.Z13	T50.Z14	T50.Z15	T50.Z16
gas gangrene	T50.Z11	T50.Z12	T50.Z13	T50.Z14	T50.Z15	T50.Z16
tetanus	T50.Z11	T50.Z12	T50.Z13	T50.Z14	T50.Z15	T50.Z16
Antitrichomonal drug	T37.3X1	T37.3X2	T37.3X3	T37.3X4	T37.3X5	T37.3X6
Antituberculars	T37.1X1	T37.1X2	T37.1X3	T37.1X4	T37.1X5	T37.1X6
antibiotics	T36.5X1	T36.5X2	T36.5X3	T36.5X4	T36.5X5	T36.5X6
Antitussive NEC	T48.3X1	T48.3X2	T48.3X3	T48.3X4	T48.3X5	T48.3X6
codeine mixture	T40.2X1	T40.2X2	T40.2X3	T40.2X4	T40.2X5	T40.2X6
opiate	T40.2X1	T40.2X2	T40.2X3	T40.2X4	T40.2X5	T40.2X6
Antivaricose drug	T46.8X1	T46.8X2	T46.8X3	T46.8X4	T46.8X5	T46.8X6
Antivenin, antivenom (sera)	T50.Z11	T50.Z12	T50.Z13	T50.Z14	T50.Z15	T50.Z16
crotaline	T50.Z11	T50.Z12	T50.Z13	T50.Z14	T50.Z15	T50.Z16
spider bite	T50.Z11	T50.Z12	T50.Z13	T50.Z14	T50.Z15	T50.Z16
Antivertigo drug	T45.0X1	T45.0X2	T45.0X3	T45.0X4	T45.0X5	T45.0X6
Antiviral drug NEC	T37.5X1	T37.5X2	T37.5X3	T37.5X4	T37.5X5	T37.5X6
eye	T49.5X1	T49.5X2	T49.5X3	T49.5X4	T49.5X5	T49.5X6
Antiwhipworm drug	T37.4X1	T37.4X2	T37.4X3	T37.4X4	T37.4X5	T37.4X6
Ant poison — see Insecticide						
Antrol — see also by specific chemical substance	T60.91	T60.92	T60.93	T60.94	—	—
fungicide	T60.91	T60.92	T60.93	T60.94	—	—
ANTU (alpha naphthylthiourea)	T60.4X1	T60.4X2	T60.4X3	T60.4X4	—	—
Apalcillin	T36.0X1	T36.0X2	T36.0X3	T36.0X4	T36.0X5	T36.0X6
APC	T48.5X1	T48.5X2	T48.5X3	T48.5X4	T48.5X5	T48.5X6
Aplonidine	T44.4X1	T44.4X2	T44.4X3	T44.4X4	T44.4X5	T44.4X6
Apomorphine	T47.7X1	T47.7X2	T47.7X3	T47.7X4	T47.7X5	T47.7X6
Appetite depressants, central	T50.5X1	T50.5X2	T50.5X3	T50.5X4	T50.5X5	T50.5X6
Apraclonidine (hydrochloride)	T44.4X1	T44.4X2	T44.4X3	T44.4X4	T44.4X5	T44.4X6
Apresoline	T46.5X1	T46.5X2	T46.5X3	T46.5X4	T46.5X5	T46.5X6
Aprindine	T46.2X1	T46.2X2	T46.2X3	T46.2X4	T46.2X5	T46.2X6
Aprobarbital	T42.3X1	T42.3X2	T42.3X3	T42.3X4	T42.3X5	T42.3X6
Apronalide	T42.6X1	T42.6X2	T42.6X3	T42.6X4	T42.6X5	T42.6X6
Aprotinin	T45.621	T45.622	T45.623	T45.624	T45.625	T45.626
Aptocaine	T41.3X1	T41.3X2	T41.3X3	T41.3X4	T41.3X5	T41.3X6
Aqua fortis	T54.2X1	T54.2X2	T54.2X3	T54.2X4	—	—
Ara-A	T37.5X1	T37.5X2	T37.5X3	T37.5X4	T37.5X5	T37.5X6
Ara-C	T45.1X1	T45.1X2	T45.1X3	T45.1X4	T45.1X5	T45.1X6
Arachis oil	T49.3X1	T49.3X2	T49.3X3	T49.3X4	T49.3X5	T49.3X6
cathartic	T47.4X1	T47.4X2	T47.4X3	T47.4X4	T47.4X5	T47.4X6
Aralen	T37.2X1	T37.2X2	T37.2X3	T37.2X4	T37.2X5	T37.2X6
Arecoline	T44.1X1	T44.1X2	T44.1X3	T44.1X4	T44.1X5	T44.1X6
Arginine	T50.991	T50.992	T50.993	T50.994	T50.995	T50.996
glutamate	T50.991	T50.992	T50.993	T50.994	T50.995	T50.996
Argyrol	T49.0X1	T49.0X2	T49.0X3	T49.0X4	T49.0X5	T49.0X6
ENT agent	T49.6X1	T49.6X2	T49.6X3	T49.6X4	T49.6X5	T49.6X6
ophthalmic preparation	T49.5X1	T49.5X2	T49.5X3	T49.5X4	T49.5X5	T49.5X6
Aristocort	T38.0X1	T38.0X2	T38.0X3	T38.0X4	T38.0X5	T38.0X6
ENT agent	T49.6X1	T49.6X2	T49.6X3	T49.6X4	T49.6X5	T49.6X6
ophthalmic preparation	T49.5X1	T49.5X2	T49.5X3	T49.5X4	T49.5X5	T49.5X6

Substance	Poisoning, Accidental (unintentional)	Poisoning, Intentional Self-harm	Poisoning, Assault	Poisoning, Undetermined	Adverse Effect	Under-dosing
Aristocort — continued						
topical NEC	T49.0X1	T49.0X2	T49.0X3	T49.0X4	T49.0X5	T49.0X6
Aromatics, corrosive	T54.1X1	T54.1X2	T54.1X3	T54.1X4	—	—
disinfectants	T54.1X1	T54.1X2	T54.1X3	T54.1X4	—	—
Arsenate of lead	T57.0X1	T57.0X2	T57.0X3	T57.0X4	—	—
herbicide	T57.0X1	T57.0X2	T57.0X3	T57.0X4	—	—
Arsenic, arsenicals (compounds) (dust) (vapor) NEC	T57.0X1	T57.0X2	T57.0X3	T57.0X4	—	—
anti-infectives	T37.8X1	T37.8X2	T37.8X3	T37.8X4	T37.8X5	T37.8X6
pesticide (dust) (fumes)	T57.0X1	T57.0X2	T57.0X3	T57.0X4	—	—
Arsine (gas)	T57.0X1	T57.0X2	T57.0X3	T57.0X4	—	—
Arsphenamine (silver)	T37.8X1	T37.8X2	T37.8X3	T37.8X4	T37.8X5	T37.8X6
Arsthinol	T37.3X1	T37.3X2	T37.3X3	T37.3X4	T37.3X5	T37.3X6
Artane	T44.3X1	T44.3X2	T44.3X3	T44.3X4	T44.3X5	T44.3X6
Arthropod (venomous) NEC	T63.481	T63.482	T63.483	T63.484	—	—
Articaine	T41.3X1	T41.3X2	T41.3X3	T41.3X4	T41.3X5	T41.3X6
Asbestos	T57.8X1	T57.8X2	T57.8X3	T57.8X4	—	—
Ascaridole	T37.4X1	T37.4X2	T37.4X3	T37.4X4	T37.4X5	T37.4X6
Ascorbic acid	T45.2X1	T45.2X2	T45.2X3	T45.2X4	T45.2X5	T45.2X6
Asiaticoside	T49.0X1	T49.0X2	T49.0X3	T49.0X4	T49.0X5	T49.0X6
Asparaginase	T45.1X1	T45.1X2	T45.1X3	T45.1X4	T45.1X5	T45.1X6
Aspidium (oleoresin)	T37.4X1	T37.4X2	T37.4X3	T37.4X4	T37.4X5	T37.4X6
Aspirin (aluminum)	T39.011	T39.012	T39.013	T39.014	T39.015	T39.016
(soluble)						
Aspoxicillin	T36.0X1	T36.0X2	T36.0X3	T36.0X4	T36.0X5	T36.0X6
Astemizole	T45.0X1	T45.0X2	T45.0X3	T45.0X4	T45.0X5	T45.0X6
Astringent (local)	T49.2X1	T49.2X2	T49.2X3	T49.2X4	T49.2X5	T49.2X6
specified NEC	T49.2X1	T49.2X2	T49.2X3	T49.2X4	T49.2X5	T49.2X6
Astromicin	T36.5X1	T36.5X2	T36.5X3	T36.5X4	T36.5X5	T36.5X6
Ataractic drug NEC	T43.501	T43.502	T43.503	T43.504	T43.505	T43.506
Atenolol	T44.7X1	T44.7X2	T44.7X3	T44.7X4	T44.7X5	T44.7X6
Atonia drug, intestinal	T47.4X1	T47.4X2	T47.4X3	T47.4X4	T47.4X5	T47.4X6
Atophan	T50.4X1	T50.4X2	T50.4X3	T50.4X4	T50.4X5	T50.4X6
Atracurium besilate	T48.1X1	T48.1X2	T48.1X3	T48.1X4	T48.1X5	T48.1X6
Atropine	T44.3X1	T44.3X2	T44.3X3	T44.3X4	T44.3X5	T44.3X6
derivative	T44.3X1	T44.3X2	T44.3X3	T44.3X4	T44.3X5	T44.3X6
methonitrate	T44.3X1	T44.3X2	T44.3X3	T44.3X4	T44.3X5	T44.3X6
Attapulgite	T47.6X1	T47.6X2	T47.6X3	T47.6X4	T47.6X5	T47.6X6
Auramine	T65.891	T65.892	T65.893	T65.894	—	—
dye	T65.6X1	T65.6X2	T65.6X3	T65.6X4	—	—
fungicide	T60.3X1	T60.3X2	T60.3X3	T60.3X4	—	—
Auranofin	T39.4X1	T39.4X2	T39.4X3	T39.4X4	T39.4X5	T39.4X6
Aurantiin	T46.991	T46.992	T46.993	T46.994	T46.995	T46.996
Aureomycin	T36.4X1	T36.4X2	T36.4X3	T36.4X4	T36.4X5	T36.4X6
ophthalmic preparation	T49.5X1	T49.5X2	T49.5X3	T49.5X4	T49.5X5	T49.5X6
topical NEC	T49.0X1	T49.0X2	T49.0X3	T49.0X4	T49.0X5	T49.0X6
Aurothioglucose	T39.4X1	T39.4X2	T39.4X3	T39.4X4	T39.4X5	T39.4X6
Aurothioglycanide	T39.4X1	T39.4X2	T39.4X3	T39.4X4	T39.4X5	T39.4X6
Aurothiomalate sodium	T39.4X1	T39.4X2	T39.4X3	T39.4X4	T39.4X5	T39.4X6
Aurotioprol	T39.4X1	T39.4X2	T39.4X3	T39.4X4	T39.4X5	T39.4X6
Automobile fuel	T52.0X1	T52.0X2	T52.0X3	T52.0X4	—	—
Autonomic nervous system agent NEC	T44.901	T44.902	T44.903	T44.904	T44.905	T44.906
Avlosulfon	T37.1X1	T37.1X2	T37.1X3	T37.1X4	T37.1X5	T37.1X6
Avomine	T42.6X1	T42.6X2	T42.6X3	T42.6X4	T42.6X5	T42.6X6
Axerophthol	T45.2X1	T45.2X2	T45.2X3	T45.2X4	T45.2X5	T45.2X6
Azacitidine	T45.1X1	T45.1X2	T45.1X3	T45.1X4	T45.1X5	T45.1X6
Azacyclonol	T43.591	T43.592	T43.593	T43.594	T43.595	T43.596
Azadirachta	T60.2X1	T60.2X2	T60.2X3	T60.2X4	—	—
Azanidazole	T37.3X1	T37.3X2	T37.3X3	T37.3X4	T37.3X5	T37.3X6
Azapetine	T46.7X1	T46.7X2	T46.7X3	T46.7X4	T46.7X5	T46.7X6
Azapropazone	T39.2X1	T39.2X2	T39.2X3	T39.2X4	T39.2X5	T39.2X6
Azaribine	T45.1X1	T45.1X2	T45.1X3	T45.1X4	T45.1X5	T45.1X6
Azaserine	T45.1X1	T45.1X2	T45.1X3	T45.1X4	T45.1X5	T45.1X6
Azatadine	T45.0X1	T45.0X2	T45.0X3	T45.0X4	T45.0X5	T45.0X6
Azatepa	T45.1X1	T45.1X2	T45.1X3	T45.1X4	T45.1X5	T45.1X6
Azathioprine	T45.1X1	T45.1X2	T45.1X3	T45.1X4	T45.1X5	T45.1X6
Azelaic acid	T49.0X1	T49.0X2	T49.0X3	T49.0X4	T49.0X5	T49.0X6
Azelastine	T45.0X1	T45.0X2	T45.0X3	T45.0X4	T45.0X5	T45.0X6
Azidocillin	T36.0X1	T36.0X2	T36.0X3	T36.0X4	T36.0X5	T36.0X6
Azidothymidine	T37.5X1	T37.5X2	T37.5X3	T37.5X4	T37.5X5	T37.5X6
Azinphos (ethyl) (methyl)	T60.0X1	T60.0X2	T60.0X3	T60.0X4	—	—
Aziridine (chelating)	T54.1X1	T54.1X2	T54.1X3	T54.1X4	—	—
Azithromycin	T36.3X1	T36.3X2	T36.3X3	T36.3X4	T36.3X5	T36.3X6
Azlocillin	T36.0X1	T36.0X2	T36.0X3	T36.0X4	T36.0X5	T36.0X6
Azobenzene smoke	T65.3X1	T65.3X2	T65.3X3	T65.3X4	—	—
acaricide	T60.8X1	T60.8X2	T60.8X3	T60.8X4	—	—
Azosulfamide	T37.0X1	T37.0X2	T37.0X3	T37.0X4	T37.0X5	T37.0X6
AZT	T37.5X1	T37.5X2	T37.5X3	T37.5X4	T37.5X5	T37.5X6
Aztreonam	T36.1X1	T36.1X2	T36.1X3	T36.1X4	T36.1X5	T36.1X6
Azulfidine	T37.0X1	T37.0X2	T37.0X3	T37.0X4	T37.0X5	T37.0X6
Azuresin	T50.8X1	T50.8X2	T50.8X3	T50.8X4	T50.8X5	T50.8X6
b-acetyldigoxin	T46.0X1	T46.0X2	T46.0X3	T46.0X4	T46.0X5	T46.0X6

Substance	Poisoning, Accidental (unintentional)	Poisoning, Intentional Self-harm	Poisoning, Assault	Poisoning, Undetermined	Adverse Effect	Under-dosing
P-Acetamidophenol	T39.1X1	T39.1X2	T39.1X3	T39.1X4	T39.1X5	T39.1
Bacampicillin	T36.0X1	T36.0X2	T36.0X3	T36.0X4	T36.0X5	T36.0
Bacillus						
lactobacillus	T47.8X1	T47.8X2	T47.8X3	T47.8X4	T47.8X5	T47.8
subtilis	T47.6X1	T47.6X2	T47.6X3	T47.6X4	T47.6X5	T47.6
Bacimycin	T49.0X1	T49.0X2	T49.0X3	T49.0X4	T49.0X5	T49.0
ophthalmic preparation	T49.5X1	T49.5X2	T49.5X3	T49.5X4	T49.5X5	T49.5
Bacitracin zinc	T49.0X1	T49.0X2	T49.0X3	T49.0X4	T49.0X5	T49.0
with neomycin	T49.0X1	T49.0X2	T49.0X3	T49.0X4	T49.0X5	T49.0
ENT agent	T49.6X1	T49.6X2	T49.6X3	T49.6X4	T49.6X5	T49.6
ophthalmic preparation	T49.5X1	T49.5X2	T49.5X3	T49.5X4	T49.5X5	T49.5
topical NEC	T49.0X1	T49.0X2	T49.0X3	T49.0X4	T49.0X5	T49.0
Baclofen	T42.8X1	T42.8X2	T42.8X3	T42.8X4	T42.8X5	T42.8
Baking soda	T50.991	T50.992	T50.993	T50.994	T50.995	T50.9
BAL	T45.8X1	T45.8X2	T45.8X3	T45.8X4	T45.8X5	T45.8
Bambuterol	T48.6X1	T48.6X2	T48.6X3	T48.6X4	T48.6X5	T48.6
Bamethan (sulfate)	T46.7X1	T46.7X2	T46.7X3	T46.7X4	T46.7X5	T46.7
Bamifylline	T48.6X1	T48.6X2	T48.6X3	T48.6X4	T48.6X5	T48.6
Bamipine	T45.0X1	T45.0X2	T45.0X3	T45.0X4	T45.0X5	T45.0
Baneberry — see Actaea spicata						
Banewort — see Belladonna						
Barbenyl	T42.3X1	T42.3X2	T42.3X3	T42.3X4	T42.3X5	T42.3
Barbexaclone	T42.6X1	T42.6X2	T42.6X3	T42.6X4	T42.6X5	T42.6
Barbital	T42.3X1	T42.3X2	T42.3X3	T42.3X4	T42.3X5	T42.3
sodium	T42.3X1	T42.3X2	T42.3X3	T42.3X4	T42.3X5	T42.3
Barbitone	T42.3X1	T42.3X2	T42.3X3	T42.3X4	T42.3X5	T42.3
Barbiturate NEC	T42.3X1	T42.3X2	T42.3X3	T42.3X4	T42.3X5	T42.3
with tranquilizer	T42.3X1	T42.3X2	T42.3X3	T42.3X4	T42.3X5	T42.3
anesthetic (intravenous)	T41.1X1	T41.1X2	T41.1X3	T41.1X4	T41.1X5	T41.1
Barium (carbonate) (chloride) (sulfite)	T57.8X1	T57.8X2	T57.8X3	T57.8X4	—	—
diagnostic agent	T50.8X1	T50.8X2	T50.8X3	T50.8X4	T50.8X5	T50.8
pesticide	T60.4X1	T60.4X2	T60.4X3	T60.4X4	—	—
rodenticide	T60.4X1	T60.4X2	T60.4X3	T60.4X4	—	—
sulfate (medicinal)	T50.8X1	T50.8X2	T50.8X3	T50.8X4	T50.8X5	T50.8
Barrier cream	T49.3X1	T49.3X2	T49.3X3	T49.3X4	T49.3X5	T49.3
Basic fuchsin	T49.0X1	T49.0X2	T49.0X3	T49.0X4	T49.0X5	T49.0
Battery acid or fluid	T54.2X1	T54.2X2	T54.2X3	T54.2X4	—	—
Bay rum	T51.8X1	T51.8X2	T51.8X3	T51.8X4	—	—
b-benzalbutyramide	T46.6X1	T46.6X2	T46.6X3	T46.6X4	T46.6X5	T46.6
BCG (vaccine)	T50.A91	T50.A92	T50.A93	T50.A94	T50.A95	T50.A
BCNU	T45.1X1	T45.1X2	T45.1X3	T45.1X4	T45.1X5	T45.1
Bearsfoot	T62.2X1	T62.2X2	T62.2X3	T62.2X4	—	—
Beclamide	T42.6X1	T42.6X2	T42.6X3	T42.6X4	T42.6X5	T42.6
Beclomethasone	T44.5X1	T44.5X2	T44.5X3	T44.5X4	T44.5X5	T44.5
Bee (sting) (venom)	T63.441	T63.442	T63.443	T63.444	—	—
Befunolol	T49.5X1	T49.5X2	T49.5X3	T49.5X4	T49.5X5	T49.5
Bekanamycin	T36.5X1	T36.5X2	T36.5X3	T36.5X4	T36.5X5	T36.5
Belladonna — see also Nightshade						
alkaloids	T44.3X1	T44.3X2	T44.3X3	T44.3X4	T44.3X5	T44.3
extract	T44.3X1	T44.3X2	T44.3X3	T44.3X4	T44.3X5	T44.3
herb	T44.3X1	T44.3X2	T44.3X3	T44.3X4	T44.3X5	T44.3
Bemegride	T50.7X1	T50.7X2	T50.7X3	T50.7X4	T50.7X5	T50.7
Benactyzine	T44.3X1	T44.3X2	T44.3X3	T44.3X4	T44.3X5	T44.3
Benadryl	T45.0X1	T45.0X2	T45.0X3	T45.0X4	T45.0X5	T45.0
Benaprizine	T44.3X1	T44.3X2	T44.3X3	T44.3X4	T44.3X5	T44.3
Benazepril	T46.4X1	T46.4X2	T46.4X3	T46.4X4	T46.4X5	T46.4
Bencyclane	T46.7X1	T46.7X2	T46.7X3	T46.7X4	T46.7X5	T46.7
Bendazol	T46.3X1	T46.3X2	T46.3X3	T46.3X4	T46.3X5	T46.3
Bendrofluazide	T50.2X1	T50.2X2	T50.2X3	T50.2X4	T50.2X5	T50.2
Bendroflumethiazide	T50.2X1	T50.2X2	T50.2X3	T50.2X4	T50.2X5	T50.2
Benemid	T50.4X1	T50.4X2	T50.4X3	T50.4X4	T50.4X5	T50.4
Benethamine penicillin	T36.0X1	T36.0X2	T36.0X3	T36.0X4	T36.0X5	T36.0
Benexate	T47.1X1	T47.1X2	T47.1X3	T47.1X4	T47.1X5	T47.1
Benfluorex	T46.6X1	T46.6X2	T46.6X3	T46.6X4	T46.6X5	T46.6
Benfotiamine	T45.2X1	T45.2X2	T45.2X3	T45.2X4	T45.2X5	T45.2
Benisone	T49.0X1	T49.0X2	T49.0X3	T49.0X4	T49.0X5	T49.0
Benomyl	T60.0X1	T60.0X2	T60.0X3	T60.0X4	—	—
Benoquin	T49.8X1	T49.8X2	T49.8X3	T49.8X4	T49.8X5	T49.8
Benoxinate	T41.3X1	T41.3X2	T41.3X3	T41.3X4	T41.3X5	T41.3
Benperidol	T43.4X1	T43.4X2	T43.4X3	T43.4X4	T43.4X5	T43.4
Benproperine	T48.3X1	T48.3X2	T48.3X3	T48.3X4	T48.3X5	T48.3
Benserazide	T42.8X1	T42.8X2	T42.8X3	T42.8X4	T42.8X5	T42.8
Bentazepam	T42.4X1	T42.4X2	T42.4X3	T42.4X4	T42.4X5	T42.4
Bentiromide	T50.8X1	T50.8X2	T50.8X3	T50.8X4	T50.8X5	T50.8
Bentonite	T49.3X1	T49.3X2	T49.3X3	T49.3X4	T49.3X5	T49.3
Benzalbutyramide	T46.6X1	T46.6X2	T46.6X3	T46.6X4	T46.6X5	T46.6
Benzalkonium (chloride)	T49.0X1	T49.0X2	T49.0X3	T49.0X4	T49.0X5	T49.0
ophthalmic preparation	T49.5X1	T49.5X2	T49.5X3	T49.5X4	T49.5X5	T49.5
Benzamidosalicylate (calcium)	T37.1X1	T37.1X2	T37.1X3	T37.1X4	T37.1X5	T37.1
Benzamine	T41.3X1	T41.3X2	T41.3X3	T41.3X4	T41.3X5	T41.3

Additional Character May Be Required — Refer to the Tabular List for Character Selection   ▽ Subterms under main terms may continue to next column or page

Substance	Poisoning, Accidental (unintentional)	Poisoning, Intentional Self-harm	Poisoning, Assault	Poisoning, Undetermined	Adverse Effect	Underdosing
Benzamine — continued						
lactate	T49.1X1	T49.1X2	T49.1X3	T49.1X4	T49.1X5	T49.1X6
Benzamphetamine	T50.5X1	T50.5X2	T50.5X3	T50.5X4	T50.5X5	T50.5X6
Benzapril hydrochloride	T46.5X1	T46.5X2	T46.5X3	T46.5X4	T46.5X5	T46.5X6
Benzathine benzylpenicillin	T36.0X1	T36.0X2	T36.0X3	T36.0X4	T36.0X5	T36.0X6
Benzathine penicillin	T36.0X1	T36.0X2	T36.0X3	T36.0X4	T36.0X5	T36.0X6
Benzatropine	T42.8X1	T42.8X2	T42.8X3	T42.8X4	T42.8X5	T42.8X6
Benzbromarone	T50.4X1	T50.4X2	T50.4X3	T50.4X4	T50.4X5	T50.4X6
Benzcarbimine	T45.1X1	T45.1X2	T45.1X3	T45.1X4	T45.1X5	T45.1X6
Benzedrex	T44.991	T44.992	T44.993	T44.994	T44.995	T44.996
Benzedrine (amphetamine)	T43.621	T43.622	T43.623	T43.624	T43.625	T43.626
Benzenamine	T65.3X1	T65.3X2	T65.3X3	T65.3X4	—	—
Benzene	T52.1X1	T52.1X2	T52.1X3	T52.1X4	—	—
homologues (acetyl) (dimethyl) (methyl) (solvent)	T52.2X1	T52.2X2	T52.2X3	T52.2X4	—	—
Benzethonium (chloride)	T49.0X1	T49.0X2	T49.0X3	T49.0X4	T49.0X5	T49.0X6
Benzfetamine	T50.5X1	T50.5X2	T50.5X3	T50.5X4	T50.5X5	T50.5X6
Benzhexol	T44.3X1	T44.3X2	T44.3X3	T44.3X4	T44.3X5	T44.3X6
Benzhydramine (chloride)	T45.0X1	T45.0X2	T45.0X3	T45.0X4	T45.0X5	T45.0X6
Benzidine	T65.891	T65.892	T65.893	T65.894	—	—
Benzilonium bromide	T44.3X1	T44.3X2	T44.3X3	T44.3X4	T44.3X5	T44.3X6
Benzimidazole	T60.3X1	T60.3X2	T60.3X3	T60.3X4	—	—
Benzin (e) — *see* Ligroin						
Benziodarone	T46.3X1	T46.3X2	T46.3X3	T46.3X4	T46.3X5	T46.3X6
Benznidazole	T37.3X1	T37.3X2	T37.3X3	T37.3X4	T37.3X5	T37.3X6
Benzocaine	T41.3X1	T41.3X2	T41.3X3	T41.3X4	T41.3X5	T41.3X6
Benzodiapin	T42.4X1	T42.4X2	T42.4X3	T42.4X4	T42.4X5	T42.4X6
Benzodiazepine NEC	T42.4X1	T42.4X2	T42.4X3	T42.4X4	T42.4X5	T42.4X6
Benzoic acid	T49.0X1	T49.0X2	T49.0X3	T49.0X4	T49.0X5	T49.0X6
with salicylic acid	T49.0X1	T49.0X2	T49.0X3	T49.0X4	T49.0X5	T49.0X6
Benzoin (tincture)	T48.5X1	T48.5X2	T48.5X3	T48.5X4	T48.5X5	T48.5X6
Benzol (benzene)	T52.1X1	T52.1X2	T52.1X3	T52.1X4	—	—
vapor	T52.0X1	T52.0X2	T52.0X3	T52.0X4	—	—
Benzomorphan	T40.2X1	T40.2X2	T40.2X3	T40.2X4	T40.2X5	T40.2X6
Benzonatate	T48.3X1	T48.3X2	T48.3X3	T48.3X4	T48.3X5	T48.3X6
Benzophenones	T49.3X1	T49.3X2	T49.3X3	T49.3X4	T49.3X5	T49.3X6
Benzopyrone	T46.991	T46.992	T46.993	T46.994	T46.995	T46.996
Benzothiadiazides	T50.2X1	T50.2X2	T50.2X3	T50.2X4	T50.2X5	T50.2X6
Benzoxonium chloride	T49.0X1	T49.0X2	T49.0X3	T49.0X4	T49.0X5	T49.0X6
Benzoylpas calcium	T37.1X1	T37.1X2	T37.1X3	T37.1X4	T37.1X5	T37.1X6
Benzoyl peroxide	T49.0X1	T49.0X2	T49.0X3	T49.0X4	T49.0X5	T49.0X6
Benzperidin	T43.591	T43.592	T43.593	T43.594	T43.595	T43.596
Benzperidol	T43.591	T43.592	T43.593	T43.594	T43.595	T43.596
Benzphetamine	T50.5X1	T50.5X2	T50.5X3	T50.5X4	T50.5X5	T50.5X6
Benzpyrinium bromide	T44.1X1	T44.1X2	T44.1X3	T44.1X4	T44.1X5	T44.1X6
Benzquinamide	T45.0X1	T45.0X2	T45.0X3	T45.0X4	T45.0X5	T45.0X6
Benzthiazide	T50.2X1	T50.2X2	T50.2X3	T50.2X4	T50.2X5	T50.2X6
Benztropine						
anticholinergic	T44.3X1	T44.3X2	T44.3X3	T44.3X4	T44.3X5	T44.3X6
antiparkinson	T42.8X1	T42.8X2	T42.8X3	T42.8X4	T42.8X5	T42.8X6
Benzydamine	T49.0X1	T49.0X2	T49.0X3	T49.0X4	T49.0X5	T49.0X6
Benzyl						
acetate	T52.8X1	T52.8X2	T52.8X3	T52.8X4	—	—
alcohol	T49.0X1	T49.0X2	T49.0X3	T49.0X4	T49.0X5	T49.0X6
benzoate	T49.0X1	T49.0X2	T49.0X3	T49.0X4	T49.0X5	T49.0X6
Benzoic acid	T49.0X1	T49.0X2	T49.0X3	T49.0X4	T49.0X5	T49.0X6
morphine	T40.2X1	T40.2X2	T40.2X3	T40.2X4	—	—
nicotinate	T46.6X1	T46.6X2	T46.6X3	T46.6X4	T46.6X5	T46.6X6
penicillin	T36.0X1	T36.0X2	T36.0X3	T36.0X4	T36.0X5	T36.0X6
Benzylhydrochlorthiazide	T50.2X1	T50.2X2	T50.2X3	T50.2X4	T50.2X5	T50.2X6
Benzylpenicillin	T36.0X1	T36.0X2	T36.0X3	T36.0X4	T36.0X5	T36.0X6
Benzylthiouracil	T38.2X1	T38.2X2	T38.2X3	T38.2X4	T38.2X5	T38.2X6
Bephenium hydroxynaphthoate	T37.4X1	T37.4X2	T37.4X3	T37.4X4	T37.4X5	T37.4X6
Bepridil	T46.1X1	T46.1X2	T46.1X3	T46.1X4	T46.1X5	T46.1X6
Bergamot oil	T65.891	T65.892	T65.893	T65.894	—	—
Bergapten	T50.991	T50.992	T50.993	T50.994	T50.995	T50.996
Berries, poisonous	T62.1X1	T62.1X2	T62.1X3	T62.1X4	—	—
Beryllium (compounds)	T56.7X1	T56.7X2	T56.7X3	T56.7X4	—	—
beta adrenergic blocking agent, heart	T44.7X1	T44.7X2	T44.7X3	T44.7X4	T44.7X5	T44.7X6
Betacarotene	T45.2X1	T45.2X2	T45.2X3	T45.2X4	T45.2X5	T45.2X6
Beta-Chlor	T42.6X1	T42.6X2	T42.6X3	T42.6X4	T42.6X5	T42.6X6
Betahistine	T46.7X1	T46.7X2	T46.7X3	T46.7X4	T46.7X5	T46.7X6
Betaine	T47.5X1	T47.5X2	T47.5X3	T47.5X4	T47.5X5	T47.5X6
Betamethasone	T49.0X1	T49.0X2	T49.0X3	T49.0X4	T49.0X5	T49.0X6
topical	T49.0X1	T49.0X2	T49.0X3	T49.0X4	T49.0X5	T49.0X6
Betamicin	T36.8X1	T36.8X2	T36.8X3	T36.8X4	T36.8X5	T36.8X6
Betanidine	T46.5X1	T46.5X2	T46.5X3	T46.5X4	T46.5X5	T46.5X6
Betaxolol	T44.7X1	T44.7X2	T44.7X3	T44.7X4	T44.7X5	T44.7X6
Betazole	T50.8X1	T50.8X2	T50.8X3	T50.8X4	T50.8X5	T50.8X6
Bethanechol	T44.1X1	T44.1X2	T44.1X3	T44.1X4	T44.1X5	T44.1X6
Bethanechol — continued						
chloride	T44.1X1	T44.1X2	T44.1X3	T44.1X4	T44.1X5	T44.1X6
Bethanidine	T46.5X1	T46.5X2	T46.5X3	T46.5X4	T46.5X5	T46.5X6
Betoxycaine	T41.3X1	T41.3X2	T41.3X3	T41.3X4	T41.3X5	T41.3X6
Betula oil	T49.3X1	T49.3X2	T49.3X3	T49.3X4	T49.3X5	T49.3X6
Bevantolol	T44.7X1	T44.7X2	T44.7X3	T44.7X4	T44.7X5	T44.7X6
Bevonium metilsulfate	T44.3X1	T44.3X2	T44.3X3	T44.3X4	T44.3X5	T44.3X6
Bezafibrate	T46.6X1	T46.6X2	T46.6X3	T46.6X4	T46.6X5	T46.6X6
Bezitramide	T40.4X1	T40.4X2	T40.4X3	T40.4X4	T40.4X5	T40.4X6
BHA	T50.991	T50.992	T50.993	T50.994	T50.995	T50.996
Bhang	T40.7X1	T40.7X2	T40.7X3	T40.7X4	T40.7X5	T40.7X6
BHC (medicinal)	T49.0X1	T49.0X2	T49.0X3	T49.0X4	T49.0X5	T49.0X6
nonmedicinal (vapor)	T53.6X1	T53.6X2	T53.6X3	T53.6X4	—	—
Bialamicol	T37.3X1	T37.3X2	T37.3X3	T37.3X4	T37.3X5	T37.3X6
Bibenzonium bromide	T48.3X1	T48.3X2	T48.3X3	T48.3X4	T48.3X5	T48.3X6
Bibrocathol	T49.5X1	T49.5X2	T49.5X3	T49.5X4	T49.5X5	T49.5X6
Bichloride of mercury — *see* Mercury, chloride						
Bichromates (calcium) (potassium)(sodium) (crystals)	T57.8X1	T57.8X2	T57.8X3	T57.8X4	—	—
fumes	T56.2X1	T56.2X2	T56.2X3	T56.2X4	—	—
Biclotymol	T49.6X1	T49.6X2	T49.6X3	T49.6X4	T49.6X5	T49.6X6
Bicucculine	T50.7X1	T50.7X2	T50.7X3	T50.7X4	T50.7X5	T50.7X6
Bifemelane	T43.291	T43.292	T43.293	T43.294	T43.295	T43.296
Biguanide derivatives, oral	T38.3X1	T38.3X2	T38.3X3	T38.3X4	T38.3X5	T38.3X6
Bile salts	T47.5X1	T47.5X2	T47.5X3	T47.5X4	T47.5X5	T47.5X6
Biligrafin	T50.8X1	T50.8X2	T50.8X3	T50.8X4	T50.8X5	T50.8X6
Bilopaque	T50.8X1	T50.8X2	T50.8X3	T50.8X4	T50.8X5	T50.8X6
Binifibrate	T46.6X1	T46.6X2	T46.6X3	T46.6X4	T46.6X5	T46.6X6
Binitrobenzol	T65.3X1	T65.3X2	T65.3X3	T65.3X4	—	—
Bioflavonoid(s)	T46.991	T46.992	T46.993	T46.994	T46.995	T46.996
Biological substance NEC	T50.901	T50.902	T50.903	T50.904	T50.905	T50.906
Biotin	T45.2X1	T45.2X2	T45.2X3	T45.2X4	T45.2X5	T45.2X6
Biperiden	T44.3X1	T44.3X2	T44.3X3	T44.3X4	T44.3X5	T44.3X6
Bisacodyl	T47.2X1	T47.2X2	T47.2X3	T47.2X4	T47.2X5	T47.2X6
Bisbentiamine	T45.2X1	T45.2X2	T45.2X3	T45.2X4	T45.2X5	T45.2X6
Bisbutiamine	T45.2X1	T45.2X2	T45.2X3	T45.2X4	T45.2X5	T45.2X6
Bisdequalinium (salts) (diacetate)	T49.6X1	T49.6X2	T49.6X3	T49.6X4	T49.6X5	T49.6X6
Bishydroxycoumarin	T45.511	T45.512	T45.513	T45.514	T45.515	T45.516
Bismarsen	T37.8X1	T37.8X2	T37.8X3	T37.8X4	T37.8X5	T37.8X6
Bismuth salts	T47.6X1	T47.6X2	T47.6X3	T47.6X4	T47.6X5	T47.6X6
aluminate	T47.1X1	T47.1X2	T47.1X3	T47.1X4	T47.1X5	T47.1X6
anti-infectives	T37.8X1	T37.8X2	T37.8X3	T37.8X4	T37.8X5	T37.8X6
formic iodide	T49.0X1	T49.0X2	T49.0X3	T49.0X4	T49.0X5	T49.0X6
glycolylarsenate	T49.0X1	T49.0X2	T49.0X3	T49.0X4	T49.0X5	T49.0X6
nonmedicinal (compounds) NEC	T65.91	T65.92	T65.93	T65.94	—	—
subcarbonate	T47.6X1	T47.6X2	T47.6X3	T47.6X4	T47.6X5	T47.6X6
subsalicylate	T37.8X1	T37.8X2	T37.8X3	T37.8X4	T37.8X5	T37.8X6
sulfarsphenamine	T37.8X1	T37.8X2	T37.8X3	T37.8X4	T37.8X5	T37.8X6
Bisoprolol	T44.7X1	T44.7X2	T44.7X3	T44.7X4	T44.7X5	T44.7X6
Bisoxatin	T47.2X1	T47.2X2	T47.2X3	T47.2X4	T47.2X5	T47.2X6
Bisulepin (hydrochloride)	T45.0X1	T45.0X2	T45.0X3	T45.0X4	T45.0X5	T45.0X6
Bithionol	T37.8X1	T37.8X2	T37.8X3	T37.8X4	T37.8X5	T37.8X6
anthelminthic	T37.4X1	T37.4X2	T37.4X3	T37.4X4	T37.4X5	T37.4X6
Bitolterol	T48.6X1	T48.6X2	T48.6X3	T48.6X4	T48.6X5	T48.6X6
Bitoscanate	T37.4X1	T37.4X2	T37.4X3	T37.4X4	T37.4X5	T37.4X6
Bitter almond oil	T62.8X1	T62.8X2	T62.8X3	T62.8X4	—	—
Bittersweet	T62.2X1	T62.2X2	T62.2X3	T62.2X4	—	—
Black						
flag	T60.91	T60.92	T60.93	T60.94	—	—
henbane	T62.2X1	T62.2X2	T62.2X3	T62.2X4	—	—
leaf (40)	T60.91	T60.92	T60.93	T60.94	—	—
widow spider (bite)	T63.311	T63.312	T63.313	T63.314	—	—
antivenin	T50.Z11	T50.Z12	T50.Z13	T50.Z14	T50.Z15	T50.Z16
Blast furnace gas (carbon monoxide from)	T58.8X1	T58.8X2	T58.8X3	T58.8X4	—	—
Bleach	T54.91	T54.92	T54.93	T54.94	—	—
Bleaching agent (medicinal)	T49.4X1	T49.4X2	T49.4X3	T49.4X4	T49.4X5	T49.4X6
Bleomycin	T45.1X1	T45.1X2	T45.1X3	T45.1X4	T45.1X5	T45.1X6
Blockain	T41.3X1	T41.3X2	T41.3X3	T41.3X4	T41.3X5	T41.3X6
infiltration (subcutaneous)	T41.3X1	T41.3X2	T41.3X3	T41.3X4	T41.3X5	T41.3X6
nerve block (peripheral) (plexus)	T41.3X1	T41.3X2	T41.3X3	T41.3X4	T41.3X5	T41.3X6
topical (surface)	T41.3X1	T41.3X2	T41.3X3	T41.3X4	T41.3X5	T41.3X6
Blockers, calcium channel	T46.1X1	T46.1X2	T46.1X3	T46.1X4	T46.1X5	T46.1X6
Blood (derivatives) (natural) (plasma) (whole)	T45.8X1	T45.8X2	T45.8X3	T45.8X4	T45.8X5	T45.8X6
dried	T45.8X1	T45.8X2	T45.8X3	T45.8X4	T45.8X5	T45.8X6

Substance	Poisoning, Accidental (unintentional)	Poisoning, Intentional Self-harm	Poisoning, Assault	Poisoning, Undetermined	Adverse Effect	Under-dosing
Blood — *continued*						
drug affecting NEC	T45.91	T45.92	T45.93	T45.94	T45.95	T45.96
expander NEC	T45.8X1	T45.8X2	T45.8X3	T45.8X4	T45.8X5	T45.8X6
fraction NEC	T45.8X1	T45.8X2	T45.8X3	T45.8X4	T45.8X5	T45.8X6
substitute (macromolecular)	T45.8X1	T45.8X2	T45.8X3	T45.8X4	T45.8X5	T45.8X6
Blue velvet	T40.2X1	T40.2X2	T40.2X3	T40.2X4	—	—
Bone meal	T62.8X1	T62.8X2	T62.8X3	T62.8X4	—	—
Bonine	T45.0X1	T45.0X2	T45.0X3	T45.0X4	T45.0X5	T45.0X6
Bopindolol	T44.7X1	T44.7X2	T44.7X3	T44.7X4	T44.7X5	T44.7X6
Boracic acid	T49.0X1	T49.0X2	T49.0X3	T49.0X4	T49.0X5	T49.0X6
ENT agent	T49.6X1	T49.6X2	T49.6X3	T49.6X4	T49.6X5	T49.6X6
ophthalmic preparation	T49.5X1	T49.5X2	T49.5X3	T49.5X4	T49.5X5	T49.5X6
Borane complex	T57.8X1	T57.8X2	T57.8X3	T57.8X4	—	—
Borate(s)	T57.8X1	T57.8X2	T57.8X3	T57.8X4	—	—
buffer	T50.991	T50.992	T50.993	T50.994	T50.995	T50.996
cleanser	T54.91	T54.92	T54.93	T54.94	—	—
sodium	T57.8X1	T57.8X2	T57.8X3	T57.8X4	—	—
Borax (cleanser)	T54.91	T54.92	T54.93	T54.94	—	—
Bordeaux mixture	T60.3X1	T60.3X2	T60.3X3	T60.3X4	—	—
Boric acid	T49.0X1	T49.0X2	T49.0X3	T49.0X4	T49.0X5	T49.0X6
ENT agent	T49.6X1	T49.6X2	T49.6X3	T49.6X4	T49.6X5	T49.6X6
ophthalmic preparation	T49.5X1	T49.5X2	T49.5X3	T49.5X4	T49.5X5	T49.5X6
Bornaprine	T44.3X1	T44.3X2	T44.3X3	T44.3X4	T44.3X5	T44.3X6
Boron	T57.8X1	T57.8X2	T57.8X3	T57.8X4	—	—
hydride NEC	T57.8X1	T57.8X2	T57.8X3	T57.8X4	—	—
fumes or gas	T57.8X1	T57.8X2	T57.8X3	T57.8X4	—	—
trifluoride	T59.891	T59.892	T59.893	T59.894	—	—
Botox	T48.291	T48.292	T48.293	T48.294	T48.295	T48.296
Botulinus anti-toxin (type A, B)	T50.Z11	T50.Z12	T50.Z13	T50.Z14	T50.Z15	T50.Z16
Brake fluid vapor	T59.891	T59.892	T59.893	T59.894	—	—
Brallobarbital	T42.3X1	T42.3X2	T42.3X3	T42.3X4	T42.3X5	T42.3X6
Bran (wheat)	T47.4X1	T47.4X2	T47.4X3	T47.4X4	T47.4X5	T47.4X6
Brass (fumes)	T56.891	T56.892	T56.893	T56.894	—	—
Brasso	T52.0X1	T52.0X2	T52.0X3	T52.0X4	—	—
Bretylium tosilate	T46.2X1	T46.2X2	T46.2X3	T46.2X4	T46.2X5	T46.2X6
Brevital (sodium)	T41.1X1	T41.1X2	T41.1X3	T41.1X4	T41.1X5	T41.1X6
Brinase	T45.3X1	T45.3X2	T45.3X3	T45.3X4	T45.3X5	T45.3X6
British antilewisite	T45.8X1	T45.8X2	T45.8X3	T45.8X4	T45.8X5	T45.8X6
Brodifacoum	T60.4X1	T60.4X2	T60.4X3	T60.4X4	—	—
Bromal (hydrate)	T42.6X1	T42.6X2	T42.6X3	T42.6X4	T42.6X5	T42.6X6
Bromazepam	T42.4X1	T42.4X2	T42.4X3	T42.4X4	T42.4X5	T42.4X6
Bromazine	T45.0X1	T45.0X2	T45.0X3	T45.0X4	T45.0X5	T45.0X6
Brombenzylcyanide	T59.3X1	T59.3X2	T59.3X3	T59.3X4	—	—
Bromelains	T45.3X1	T45.3X2	T45.3X3	T45.3X4	T45.3X5	T45.3X6
Bromethalin	T60.4X1	T60.4X2	T60.4X3	T60.4X4	—	—
Bromhexine	T48.4X1	T48.4X2	T48.4X3	T48.4X4	T48.4X5	T48.4X6
Bromide salts	T42.6X1	T42.6X2	T42.6X3	T42.6X4	T42.6X5	T42.6X6
Bromindione	T45.511	T45.512	T45.513	T45.514	T45.515	T45.516
Bromine						
compounds (medicinal)	T42.6X1	T42.6X2	T42.6X3	T42.6X4	T42.6X5	T42.6X6
sedative	T42.6X1	T42.6X2	T42.6X3	T42.6X4	T42.6X5	T42.6X6
vapor	T59.891	T59.892	T59.893	T59.894	—	—
Bromisoval	T42.6X1	T42.6X2	T42.6X3	T42.6X4	T42.6X5	T42.6X6
Bromisovalum	T42.6X1	T42.6X2	T42.6X3	T42.6X4	T42.6X5	T42.6X6
Bromobenzylcyanide	T59.3X1	T59.3X2	T59.3X3	T59.3X4	—	—
Bromochlorosalicylani-lide	T49.0X1	T49.0X2	T49.0X3	T49.0X4	T49.0X5	T49.0X6
Bromocriptine	T42.8X1	T42.8X2	T42.8X3	T42.8X4	T42.8X5	T42.8X6
Bromodiphenhydramine	T45.0X1	T45.0X2	T45.0X3	T45.0X4	T45.0X5	T45.0X6
Bromoform	T42.6X1	T42.6X2	T42.6X3	T42.6X4	T42.6X5	T42.6X6
Bromophenol blue reagent	T50.991	T50.992	T50.993	T50.994	T50.995	T50.996
Bromopride	T47.8X1	T47.8X2	T47.8X3	T47.8X4	T47.8X5	T47.8X6
Bromosalicylchloranitide	T49.0X1	T49.0X2	T49.0X3	T49.0X4	T49.0X5	T49.0X6
Bromosalicylhydroxamic acid	T37.1X1	T37.1X2	T37.1X3	T37.1X4	T37.1X5	T37.1X6
Bromo-seltzer	T39.1X1	T39.1X2	T39.1X3	T39.1X4	T39.1X5	T39.1X6
Bromoxynil	T60.3X1	T60.3X2	T60.3X3	T60.3X4	—	—
Bromperidol	T43.4X1	T43.4X2	T43.4X3	T43.4X4	T43.4X5	T43.4X6
Brompheniramine	T45.0X1	T45.0X2	T45.0X3	T45.0X4	T45.0X5	T45.0X6
Bromsulfophthalein	T50.8X1	T50.8X2	T50.8X3	T50.8X4	T50.8X5	T50.8X6
Bromural	T42.6X1	T42.6X2	T42.6X3	T42.6X4	T42.6X5	T42.6X6
Bromvaletone	T42.6X1	T42.6X2	T42.6X3	T42.6X4	T42.6X5	T42.6X6
Bronchodilator NEC	T48.6X1	T48.6X2	T48.6X3	T48.6X4	T48.6X5	T48.6X6
Brotizolam	T42.4X1	T42.4X2	T42.4X3	T42.4X4	T42.4X5	T42.4X6
Brovincamine	T46.7X1	T46.7X2	T46.7X3	T46.7X4	T46.7X5	T46.7X6
Brown recluse spider (bite) (venom)	T63.331	T63.332	T63.333	T63.334		
Brown spider (bite) (venom)	T63.391	T63.392	T63.393	T63.394	—	—
Broxaterol	T48.6X1	T48.6X2	T48.6X3	T48.6X4	T48.6X5	T48.6X6
Broxuridine	T45.1X1	T45.1X2	T45.1X3	T45.1X4	T45.1X5	T45.1X6
Broxyquinoline	T37.8X1	T37.8X2	T37.8X3	T37.8X4	T37.8X5	T37.8
Bruceine	T48.291	T48.292	T48.293	T48.294	T48.295	T48.2
Brucia	T62.2X1	T62.2X2	T62.2X3	T62.2X4	—	—
Brucine	T65.1X1	T65.1X2	T65.1X3	T65.1X4	—	—
Brunswick green — *see* Copper						
Bruten — *see* Ibuprofen						
Bryonia	T47.2X1	T47.2X2	T47.2X3	T47.2X4	T47.2X5	T47.2
Buclizine	T45.0X1	T45.0X2	T45.0X3	T45.0X4	T45.0X5	T45.0
Buclosamide	T49.0X1	T49.0X2	T49.0X3	T49.0X4	T49.0X5	T49.0
Budesonide	T44.5X1	T44.5X2	T44.5X3	T44.5X4	T44.5X5	T44.5
Budralazine	T46.5X1	T46.5X2	T46.5X3	T46.5X4	T46.5X5	T46.5
Bufferin	T39.011	T39.012	T39.013	T39.014	T39.015	T39.0
Buflomedil	T46.7X1	T46.7X2	T46.7X3	T46.7X4	T46.7X5	T46.7
Buformin	T38.3X1	T38.3X2	T38.3X3	T38.3X4	T38.3X5	T38.3
Bufotenine	T40.991	T40.992	T40.993	T40.994	—	—
Bufrolin	T48.6X1	T48.6X2	T48.6X3	T48.6X4	T48.6X5	T48.6
Bufylline	T48.6X1	T48.6X2	T48.6X3	T48.6X4	T48.6X5	T48.6
Bulk filler	T50.5X1	T50.5X2	T50.5X3	T50.5X4	T50.5X5	T50.5
cathartic	T47.4X1	T47.4X2	T47.4X3	T47.4X4	T47.4X5	T47.4
Bumetanide	T50.1X1	T50.1X2	T50.1X3	T50.1X4	T50.1X5	T50.1
Bunaftine	T46.2X1	T46.2X2	T46.2X3	T46.2X4	T46.2X5	T46.2
Bunamiodyl	T50.8X1	T50.8X2	T50.8X3	T50.8X4	T50.8X5	T50.8
Bunazosin	T44.6X1	T44.6X2	T44.6X3	T44.6X4	T44.6X5	T44.6
Bunitrolol	T44.7X1	T44.7X2	T44.7X3	T44.7X4	T44.7X5	T44.7
Buphenine	T46.7X1	T46.7X2	T46.7X3	T46.7X4	T46.7X5	T46.7
Bupivacaine	T41.3X1	T41.3X2	T41.3X3	T41.3X4	T41.3X5	T41.3
infiltration (subcutaneous)	T41.3X1	T41.3X2	T41.3X3	T41.3X4	T41.3X5	T41.3
nerve block (peripheral) (plexus)	T41.3X1	T41.3X2	T41.3X3	T41.3X4	T41.3X5	T41.3
spinal	T41.3X1	T41.3X2	T41.3X3	T41.3X4	T41.3X5	T41.3
Bupranolol	T44.7X1	T44.7X2	T44.7X3	T44.7X4	T44.7X5	T44.7
Buprenorphine	T40.4X1	T40.4X2	T40.4X3	T40.4X4	T40.4X5	T40.4
Bupropion	T43.291	T43.292	T43.293	T43.294	T43.295	T43.2
Burimamide	T47.1X1	T47.1X2	T47.1X3	T47.1X4	T47.1X5	T47.1
Buserelin	T38.891	T38.892	T38.893	T38.894	T38.895	T38.8
Buspirone	T43.591	T43.592	T43.593	T43.594	T43.595	T43.5
Busulfan, busulphan	T45.1X1	T45.1X2	T45.1X3	T45.1X4	T45.1X5	T45.1
Butabarbital (sodium)	T42.3X1	T42.3X2	T42.3X3	T42.3X4	T42.3X5	T42.3
Butabarbitone	T42.3X1	T42.3X2	T42.3X3	T42.3X4	T42.3X5	T42.3
Butabarpal	T42.3X1	T42.3X2	T42.3X3	T42.3X4	T42.3X5	T42.3
Butacaine	T41.3X1	T41.3X2	T41.3X3	T41.3X4	T41.3X5	T41.3
Butalamine	T46.7X1	T46.7X2	T46.7X3	T46.7X4	T46.7X5	T46.7
Butalbital	T42.3X1	T42.3X2	T42.3X3	T42.3X4	T42.3X5	T42.3
Butallylonal	T42.3X1	T42.3X2	T42.3X3	T42.3X4	T42.3X5	T42.3
Butamben	T41.3X1	T41.3X2	T41.3X3	T41.3X4	T41.3X5	T41.3
Butamirate	T48.3X1	T48.3X2	T48.3X3	T48.3X4	T48.3X5	T48.3
Butane (distributed in mobile container)	T59.891	T59.892	T59.893	T59.894		
distributed through pipes	T59.891	T59.892	T59.893	T59.894	—	—
incomplete combustion	T58.11	T58.12	T58.13	T58.14		
Butanilicaine	T41.3X1	T41.3X2	T41.3X3	T41.3X4	T41.3X5	T41.3
Butanol	T51.3X1	T51.3X2	T51.3X3	T51.3X4	—	—
Butanone, 2-butanone	T52.4X1	T52.4X2	T52.4X3	T52.4X4	—	—
Butantrone	T49.4X1	T49.4X2	T49.4X3	T49.4X4	T49.4X5	T49.4
Butaperazine	T43.3X1	T43.3X2	T43.3X3	T43.3X4	T43.3X5	T43.3
Butazolidin	T39.2X1	T39.2X2	T39.2X3	T39.2X4	T39.2X5	T39.2
Butetamate	T48.6X1	T48.6X2	T48.6X3	T48.6X4	T48.6X5	T48.6
Butethal	T42.3X1	T42.3X2	T42.3X3	T42.3X4	T42.3X5	T42.3
Butethamate	T44.3X1	T44.3X2	T44.3X3	T44.3X4	T44.3X5	T44.3
Buthalitone (sodium)	T41.1X1	T41.1X2	T41.1X3	T41.1X4	T41.1X5	T41.1
Butisol (sodium)	T42.3X1	T42.3X2	T42.3X3	T42.3X4	T42.3X5	T42.3
Butizide	T50.2X1	T50.2X2	T50.2X3	T50.2X4	T50.2X5	T50.2
Butobarbital	T42.3X1	T42.3X2	T42.3X3	T42.3X4	T42.3X5	T42.3
sodium	T42.3X1	T42.3X2	T42.3X3	T42.3X4	T42.3X5	T42.3
Butobarbitone	T42.3X1	T42.3X2	T42.3X3	T42.3X4	T42.3X5	T42.3
Butoconazole (nitrate)	T49.0X1	T49.0X2	T49.0X3	T49.0X4	T49.0X5	T49.0
Butorphanol	T40.4X1	T40.4X2	T40.4X3	T40.4X4	T40.4X5	T40.4
Butriptyline	T43.011	T43.012	T43.013	T43.014	T43.015	T43.01
Butropium bromide	T44.3X1	T44.3X2	T44.3X3	T44.3X4	T44.3X5	T44.3
Buttercups	T62.2X1	T62.2X2	T62.2X3	T62.2X4		
Butter of antimony — *see* Antimony						
Butyl						
acetate (secondary)	T52.8X1	T52.8X2	T52.8X3	T52.8X4	—	—
alcohol	T51.3X1	T51.3X2	T51.3X3	T51.3X4	—	—
aminobenzoate	T41.3X1	T41.3X2	T41.3X3	T41.3X4	T41.3X5	T41.3
butyrate	T52.8X1	T52.8X2	T52.8X3	T52.8X4	—	—
carbinol	T51.3X1	T51.3X2	T51.3X3	T51.3X4	—	—
carbitol	T52.3X1	T52.3X2	T52.3X3	T52.3X4	—	—
cellosolve	T52.3X1	T52.3X2	T52.3X3	T52.3X4	—	—
chloral (hydrate)	T42.6X1	T42.6X2	T42.6X3	T42.6X4	T42.6X5	T42.6
formate	T52.8X1	T52.8X2	T52.8X3	T52.8X4	—	—
lactate	T52.8X1	T52.8X2	T52.8X3	T52.8X4	—	—

356

Additional Character May Be Required — Refer to the Tabular List for Character Selection   Subterms under main terms may continue to next column or page

Substance	Poisoning, Accidental (unintentional)	Poisoning, Intentional Self-harm	Poisoning, Assault	Poisoning, Undetermined	Adverse Effect	Under-dosing
Butyl — continued						
propionate	T52.8X1	T52.8X2	T52.8X3	T52.8X4	—	—
scopolamine bromide	T44.3X1	T44.3X2	T44.3X3	T44.3X4	T44.3X5	T44.3X6
thiobarbital sodium	T41.1X1	T41.1X2	T41.1X3	T41.1X4	T41.1X5	T41.1X6
Butylated hydroxyanisole	T50.991	T50.992	T50.993	T50.994	T50.995	T50.996
Butylchloral hydrate	T42.6X1	T42.6X2	T42.6X3	T42.6X4	T42.6X5	T42.6X6
Butyltoluene	T52.2X1	T52.2X2	T52.2X3	T52.2X4	—	—
Butyn	T41.3X1	T41.3X2	T41.3X3	T41.3X4	T41.3X5	T41.3X6
Butyrophenone (-based tranquilizers)	T43.4X1	T43.4X2	T43.4X3	T43.4X4	T43.4X5	T43.4X6
Cabergoline	T42.8X1	T42.8X2	T42.8X3	T42.8X4	T42.8X5	T42.8X6
Cacodyl, cacodylic acid	T57.0X1	T57.0X2	T57.0X3	T57.0X4	—	—
Cactinomycin	T45.1X1	T45.1X2	T45.1X3	T45.1X4	T45.1X5	T45.1X6
Cade oil	T49.4X1	T49.4X2	T49.4X3	T49.4X4	T49.4X5	T49.4X6
Cadexomer iodine	T49.0X1	T49.0X2	T49.0X3	T49.0X4	T49.0X5	T49.0X6
Cadmium (chloride) (fumes) (oxide)	T56.3X1	T56.3X2	T56.3X3	T56.3X4	—	—
sulfide (medicinal) NEC	T49.4X1	T49.4X2	T49.4X3	T49.4X4	T49.4X5	T49.4X6
Cadralazine	T46.5X1	T46.5X2	T46.5X3	T46.5X4	T46.5X5	T46.5X6
Caffeine	T43.611	T43.612	T43.613	T43.614	T43.615	T43.616
Calabar bean	T62.2X1	T62.2X2	T62.2X3	T62.2X4	—	—
Caladium seguinum	T62.2X1	T62.2X2	T62.2X3	T62.2X4	—	—
Calamine (lotion)	T49.3X1	T49.3X2	T49.3X3	T49.3X4	T49.3X5	T49.3X6
Calcifediol	T45.2X1	T45.2X2	T45.2X3	T45.2X4	T45.2X5	T45.2X6
Calciferol	T45.2X1	T45.2X2	T45.2X3	T45.2X4	T45.2X5	T45.2X6
Calcitonin	T50.991	T50.992	T50.993	T50.994	T50.995	T50.996
Calcitriol	T45.2X1	T45.2X2	T45.2X3	T45.2X4	T45.2X5	T45.2X6
Calcium	T50.3X1	T50.3X2	T50.3X3	T50.3X5	T50.3X5	T50.3X6
actylsalicylate	T39.011	T39.012	T39.013	T39.014	T39.015	T39.016
benzamidosalicylate	T37.1X1	T37.1X2	T37.1X3	T37.1X4	T37.1X5	T37.1X6
bromide	T42.6X1	T42.6X2	T42.6X3	T42.6X4	T42.6X5	T42.6X6
bromolactobionate	T42.6X1	T42.6X2	T42.6X3	T42.6X4	T42.6X5	T42.6X6
carbaspirin	T39.011	T39.012	T39.013	T39.014	T39.015	T39.016
carbimide	T50.6X1	T50.6X2	T50.6X3	T50.6X4	T50.6X5	T50.6X6
carbonate	T47.1X1	T47.1X2	T47.1X3	T47.1X4	T47.1X5	T47.1X6
chloride	T50.991	T50.992	T50.993	T50.994	T50.995	T50.996
anhydrous	T50.991	T50.992	T50.993	T50.994	T50.995	T50.996
cyanide	T57.8X1	T57.8X2	T57.8X3	T57.8X4	—	—
dioctyl sulfosuccinate	T47.4X1	T47.4X2	T47.4X3	T47.4X4	T47.4X5	T47.4X6
disodium edathamil	T45.8X1	T45.8X2	T45.8X3	T45.8X4	T45.8X5	T45.8X6
disodium edetate	T45.8X1	T45.8X2	T45.8X3	T45.8X4	T45.8X5	T45.8X6
dobesilate	T46.991	T46.992	T46.993	T46.994	T46.995	T46.996
EDTA	T45.8X1	T45.8X2	T45.8X3	T45.8X4	T45.8X5	T45.8X6
ferrous citrate	T45.4X1	T45.4X2	T45.4X3	T45.4X4	T45.4X5	T45.4X6
folinate	T45.8X1	T45.8X2	T45.8X3	T45.8X4	T45.8X5	T45.8X6
glubionate	T50.3X1	T50.3X2	T50.3X3	T50.3X4	T50.3X5	T50.3X6
gluconate	T50.3X1	T50.3X2	T50.3X3	T50.3X4	T50.3X5	T50.3X6
gluconogalactogluconate	T50.3X1	T50.3X2	T50.3X3	T50.3X4	T50.3X5	T50.3X6
hydrate, hydroxide	T54.3X1	T54.3X2	T54.3X3	T54.3X4	—	—
hypochlorite	T54.3X1	T54.3X2	T54.3X3	T54.3X4	—	—
iodide	T48.4X1	T48.4X2	T48.4X3	T48.4X4	T48.4X5	T48.4X6
ipodate	T50.8X1	T50.8X2	T50.8X3	T50.8X4	T50.8X5	T50.8X6
lactate	T50.3X1	T50.3X2	T50.3X3	T50.3X4	T50.3X5	T50.3X6
leucovorin	T45.8X1	T45.8X2	T45.8X3	T45.8X4	T45.8X5	T45.8X6
mandelate	T37.91	T37.92	T37.93	T37.94	T37.95	T37.96
oxide	T54.3X1	T54.3X2	T54.3X3	T54.3X4	—	—
pantothenate	T45.2X1	T45.2X2	T45.2X3	T45.2X4	T45.2X5	T45.2X6
phosphate	T50.3X1	T50.3X2	T50.3X3	T50.3X4	T50.3X5	T50.3X6
salicylate	T39.091	T39.092	T39.093	T39.094	T39.095	T39.096
salts	T50.3X1	T50.3X2	T50.3X3	T50.3X4	T50.3X5	T50.3X6
Calculus-dissolving drug	T50.991	T50.992	T50.993	T50.994	T50.995	T50.996
Calomel	T49.0X1	T49.0X2	T49.0X3	T49.0X4	T49.0X5	T49.0X6
Caloric agent	T50.3X1	T50.3X2	T50.3X3	T50.3X4	T50.3X5	T50.3X6
Calusterone	T38.7X1	T38.7X2	T38.7X3	T38.7X4	T38.7X5	T38.7X6
Camazepam	T42.4X1	T42.4X2	T42.4X3	T42.4X4	T42.4X5	T42.4X6
Camomile	T49.0X1	T49.0X2	T49.0X3	T49.0X4	T49.0X5	T49.0X6
Camoquin	T37.2X1	T37.2X2	T37.2X3	T37.2X4	T37.2X5	T37.2X6
Camphor						
insecticide	T60.2X1	T60.2X2	T60.2X3	T60.2X4	—	—
medicinal	T49.8X1	T49.8X2	T49.8X3	T49.8X4	T49.8X5	T49.8X6
Camylofin	T44.3X1	T44.3X2	T44.3X3	T44.3X4	T44.3X5	T44.3X6
Cancer chemotherapy drug regimen	T45.1X1	T45.1X2	T45.1X3	T45.1X4	T45.1X5	T45.1X6
Candeptin	T49.0X1	T49.0X2	T49.0X3	T49.0X4	T49.0X5	T49.0X6
Candicidin	T49.0X1	T49.0X2	T49.0X3	T49.0X4	T49.0X5	T49.0X6
Cannabinol	T40.7X1	T40.7X2	T40.7X3	T40.7X4	T40.7X5	T40.7X6
Cannabis (derivatives)	T40.7X1	T40.7X2	T40.7X3	T40.7X4	T40.7X5	T40.7X6
Canned heat	T51.1X1	T51.1X2	T51.1X3	T51.1X4	—	—
Canrenoic acid	T50.0X1	T50.0X2	T50.0X3	T50.0X4	T50.0X5	T50.0X6
Canrenone	T50.0X1	T50.0X2	T50.0X3	T50.0X4	T50.0X5	T50.0X6
Cantharides, cantharidin, cantharis	T49.8X1	T49.8X2	T49.8X3	T49.8X4	T49.8X5	T49.8X6
Canthaxanthin	T50.991	T50.992	T50.993	T50.994	T50.995	T50.996

Substance	Poisoning, Accidental (unintentional)	Poisoning, Intentional Self-harm	Poisoning, Assault	Poisoning, Undetermined	Adverse Effect	Under-dosing
Capillary-active drug NEC	T46.901	T46.902	T46.903	T46.904	T46.905	T46.906
Capreomycin	T36.8X1	T36.8X2	T36.8X3	T36.8X4	T36.8X5	T36.8X6
Capsicum	T49.4X1	T49.4X2	T49.4X3	T49.4X4	T49.4X5	T49.4X6
Captafol	T60.3X1	T60.3X2	T60.3X3	T60.3X4	—	—
Captan	T60.3X1	T60.3X2	T60.3X3	T60.3X4	—	—
Captodiame, captodiamine	T43.591	T43.592	T43.593	T43.594	T43.595	T43.596
Captopril	T46.4X1	T46.4X2	T46.4X3	T46.4X4	T46.4X5	T46.4X6
Caramiphen	T44.3X1	T44.3X2	T44.3X3	T44.3X4	T44.3X5	T44.3X6
Carazolol	T44.7X1	T44.7X2	T44.7X3	T44.7X4	T44.7X5	T44.7X6
Carbachol	T44.1X1	T44.1X2	T44.1X3	T44.1X4	T44.1X5	T44.1X6
Carbacrylamine (resin)	T50.3X1	T50.3X2	T50.3X3	T50.3X4	T50.3X5	T50.3X6
Carbamate (insecticide)	T60.0X1	T60.0X2	T60.0X3	T60.0X4	—	—
Carbamate (sedative)	T42.6X1	T42.6X2	T42.6X3	T42.6X4	T42.6X5	T42.6X6
herbicide	T60.0X1	T60.0X2	T60.0X3	T60.0X4	—	—
insecticide	T60.0X1	T60.0X2	T60.0X3	T60.0X4	—	—
Carbamazepine	T42.1X1	T42.1X2	T42.1X3	T42.1X4	T42.1X5	T42.1X6
Carbamide	T47.3X1	T47.3X2	T47.3X3	T47.3X4	T47.3X5	T47.3X6
peroxide	T49.0X1	T49.0X2	T49.0X3	T49.0X4	T49.0X5	T49.0X6
topical	T49.8X1	T49.8X2	T49.8X3	T49.8X4	T49.8X5	T49.8X6
Carbamylcholine chloride	T44.1X1	T44.1X2	T44.1X3	T44.1X4	T44.1X5	T44.1X6
Carbaril	T60.0X1	T60.0X2	T60.0X3	T60.0X4	—	—
Carbarsone	T37.3X1	T37.3X2	T37.3X3	T37.3X4	T37.3X5	T37.3X6
Carbaryl	T60.0X1	T60.0X2	T60.0X3	T60.0X4	—	—
Carbaspirin	T39.011	T39.012	T39.013	T39.014	T39.015	T39.016
Carbazochrome (salicylate) (sodium sulfonate)	T49.4X1	T49.4X2	T49.4X3	T49.4X4	T49.4X5	T49.4X6
Carbenicillin	T36.0X1	T36.0X2	T36.0X3	T36.0X4	T36.0X5	T36.0X6
Carbenoxolone	T47.1X1	T47.1X2	T47.1X3	T47.1X4	T47.1X5	T47.1X6
Carbetapentane	T48.3X1	T48.3X2	T48.3X3	T48.3X4	T48.3X5	T48.3X6
Carbethyl salicylate	T39.091	T39.092	T39.093	T39.094	T39.095	T39.096
Carbidopa (with levodopa)	T42.8X1	T42.8X2	T42.8X3	T42.8X4	T42.8X5	T42.8X6
Carbimazole	T38.2X1	T38.2X2	T38.2X3	T38.2X4	T38.2X5	T38.2X6
Carbinol	T51.1X1	T51.1X2	T51.1X3	T51.1X4	—	—
Carbinoxamine	T45.0X1	T45.0X2	T45.0X3	T45.0X4	T45.0X5	T45.0X6
Carbiphene	T39.8X1	T39.8X2	T39.8X3	T39.8X4	T39.8X5	T39.8X6
Carbitol	T52.3X1	T52.3X2	T52.3X3	T52.3X4	—	—
Carbocaine	T41.3X1	T41.3X2	T41.3X3	T41.3X4	T41.3X5	T41.3X6
infiltration (subcutaneous)	T41.3X1	T41.3X2	T41.3X3	T41.3X4	T41.3X5	T41.3X6
nerve block (peripheral) (plexus)	T41.3X1	T41.3X2	T41.3X3	T41.3X4	T41.3X5	T41.3X6
topical (surface)	T41.3X1	T41.3X2	T41.3X3	T41.3X4	T41.3X5	T41.3X6
Carbocisteine	T48.4X1	T48.4X2	T48.4X3	T48.4X4	T48.4X5	T48.4X6
Carbocromen	T46.3X1	T46.3X2	T46.3X3	T46.3X4	T46.3X5	T46.3X6
Carbol fuchsin	T49.0X1	T49.0X2	T49.0X3	T49.0X4	T49.0X5	T49.0X6
Carbolic acid — see also Phenol	T54.0X1	T54.0X2	T54.0X3	T54.0X4	—	—
Carbolonium (bromide)	T48.1X1	T48.1X2	T48.1X3	T48.1X4	T48.1X5	T48.1X6
Carbo medicinalis	T47.6X1	T47.6X2	T47.6X3	T47.6X4	T47.6X5	T47.6X6
Carbomycin	T36.8X1	T36.8X2	T36.8X3	T36.8X4	T36.8X5	T36.8X6
Carbon						
bisulfide (liquid)	T65.4X1	T65.4X2	T65.4X3	T65.4X4	—	—
vapor	T65.4X1	T65.4X2	T65.4X3	T65.4X4	—	—
dioxide (gas)	T59.7X1	T59.7X2	T59.7X3	T59.7X4	—	—
medicinal	T41.5X1	T41.5X2	T41.5X3	T41.5X4	T41.5X5	T41.5X6
nonmedicinal	T59.7X1	T59.7X2	T59.7X3	T59.7X4	—	—
snow	T49.4X1	T49.4X2	T49.4X3	T49.4X4	T49.4X5	T49.4X6
disulfide (liquid)	T65.4X1	T65.4X2	T65.4X3	T65.4X4	—	—
vapor	T65.4X1	T65.4X2	T65.4X3	T65.4X4	—	—
monoxide (from incomplete combustion)	T58.91	T58.92	T58.93	T58.94	—	—
blast furnace gas	T58.8X1	T58.8X2	T58.8X3	T58.8X4	—	—
butane (distributed in mobile container)	T58.11	T58.12	T58.13	T58.14	—	—
distributed through pipes	T58.11	T58.12	T58.13	T58.14	—	—
charcoal fumes	T58.2X1	T58.2X2	T58.2X3	T58.2X4	—	—
coal	T58.2X1	T58.2X2	T58.2X3	T58.2X4	—	—
coke (in domestic stoves, fireplaces)	T58.2X1	T58.2X2	T58.2X3	T58.2X4	—	—
exhaust gas (motor) not in transit	T58.01	T58.02	T58.03	T58.04	—	—
combustion engine, any not in watercraft	T58.01	T58.02	T58.03	T58.04	—	—
farm tractor, not in transit	T58.01	T58.02	T58.03	T58.04	—	—
gas engine	T58.01	T58.02	T58.03	T58.04	—	—
motor pump	T58.01	T58.02	T58.03	T58.04	—	—
motor vehicle, not in transit	T58.01	T58.02	T58.03	T58.04	—	—
fuel (in domestic use)	T58.2X1	T58.2X2	T58.2X3	T58.2X4	—	—
gas (piped)	T58.11	T58.12	T58.13	T58.14	—	—
in mobile container	T58.11	T58.12	T58.13	T58.14	—	—

Table of Drugs and Chemicals

Carbon — Central nervous system · Central nervous system

Substance	Poisoning, Accidental (unintentional)	Poisoning, Intentional Self-harm	Poisoning, Assault	Poisoning, Undetermined	Adverse Effect	Under-dosing
Carbon — *continued*						
monoxide — *continued*						
fuel — *continued*						
piped (natural)	T58.11	T58.12	T58.13	T58.14	—	—
utility	T58.11	T58.12	T58.13	T58.14	—	—
in mobile container	T58.11	T58.12	T58.13	T58.14	—	—
gas (piped)	T58.11	T58.12	T58.13	T58.14	—	—
illuminating gas	T58.11	T58.12	T58.13	T58.14	—	—
industrial fuels or gases, any	T58.8X1	T58.8X2	T58.8X3	T58.8X4	—	—
kerosene (in domestic stoves, fireplaces)	T58.2X1	T58.2X2	T58.2X3	T58.2X4	—	—
kiln gas or vapor	T58.8X1	T58.8X2	T58.8X3	T58.8X4	—	—
motor exhaust gas, not in transit	T58.01	T58.02	T58.03	T58.04	—	—
piped gas (manufactured) (natural)	T58.11	T58.12	T58.13	T58.14	—	—
producer gas	T58.8X1	T58.8X2	T58.8X3	T58.8X4	—	—
propane (distributed in mobile container)	T58.11	T58.12	T58.13	T58.14	—	—
distributed through pipes	T58.11	T58.12	T58.13	T58.14	—	—
solid (in domestic stoves, fireplaces)	T58.2X1	T58.2X2	T58.2X3	T58.2X4	—	—
specified source NEC	T58.8X1	T58.8X2	T58.8X3	T58.8X4	—	—
stove gas	T58.11	T58.12	T58.13	T58.14	—	—
piped	T58.11	T58.12	T58.13	T58.14	—	—
utility gas	T58.11	T58.12	T58.13	T58.14	—	—
piped	T58.11	T58.12	T58.13	T58.14	—	—
water gas	T58.11	T58.12	T58.13	T58.14	—	—
wood (in domestic stoves, fireplaces)	T58.2X1	T58.2X2	T58.2X3	T58.2X4	—	—
tetrachloride (vapor) NEC	T53.0X1	T53.0X2	T53.0X3	T53.0X4	—	—
liquid (cleansing agent) NEC	T53.0X1	T53.0X2	T53.0X3	T53.0X4	—	—
solvent	T53.0X1	T53.0X2	T53.0X3	T53.0X4	—	—
Carbonic acid gas	T59.7X1	T59.7X2	T59.7X3	T59.7X4	—	—
anhydrase inhibitor NEC	T50.2X1	T50.2X2	T50.2X3	T50.2X4	T50.2X5	T50.2X6
Carbophenothion	T60.0X1	T60.0X2	T60.0X3	T60.0X4	—	—
Carboplatin	T45.1X1	T45.1X2	T45.1X3	T45.1X4	T45.1X5	T45.1X6
Carboprost	T48.0X1	T48.0X2	T48.0X3	T48.0X4	T48.0X5	T48.0X6
Carboquone	T45.1X1	T45.1X2	T45.1X3	T45.1X4	T45.1X5	T45.1X6
Carbowax	T49.3X1	T49.3X2	T49.3X3	T49.3X4	T49.3X5	T49.3X6
Carboxymethylcellulose	T47.4X1	T47.4X2	T47.4X3	T47.4X4	T47.4X5	T47.4X6
Carbrital	T42.3X1	T42.3X2	T42.3X3	T42.3X4	T42.3X5	T42.3X6
Carbromal	T42.6X1	T42.6X2	T42.6X3	T42.6X4	T42.6X5	T42.6X6
Carbutamide	T38.3X1	T38.3X2	T38.3X3	T38.3X4	T38.3X5	T38.3X6
Carbuterol	T48.6X1	T48.6X2	T48.6X3	T48.6X4	T48.6X5	T48.6X6
Cardiac						
depressants	T46.2X1	T46.2X2	T46.2X3	T46.2X4	T46.2X5	T46.2X6
rhythm regulator	T46.2X1	T46.2X2	T46.2X3	T46.2X4	T46.2X5	T46.2X6
specified NEC	T46.2X1	T46.2X2	T46.2X3	T46.2X4	T46.2X5	T46.2X6
Cardiografin	T50.8X1	T50.8X2	T50.8X3	T50.8X4	T50.8X5	T50.8X6
Cardiogreen	T50.8X1	T50.8X2	T50.8X3	T50.8X4	T50.8X5	T50.8X6
Cardiotonic (glycoside) **NEC**	T46.0X1	T46.0X2	T46.0X3	T46.0X4	T46.0X5	T46.0X6
Cardiovascular drug NEC	T46.901	T46.902	T46.903	T46.904	T46.905	T46.906
Cardrase	T50.2X1	T50.2X2	T50.2X3	T50.2X4	T50.2X5	T50.2X6
Carfecillin	T36.0X1	T36.0X2	T36.0X3	T36.0X4	T36.0X5	T36.0X6
Carfenazine	T43.3X1	T43.3X2	T43.3X3	T43.3X4	T43.3X5	T43.3X6
Carfusin	T49.0X1	T49.0X2	T49.0X3	T49.0X4	T49.0X5	T49.0X6
Carindacillin	T36.0X1	T36.0X2	T36.0X3	T36.0X4	T36.0X5	T36.0X6
Carisoprodol	T42.8X1	T42.8X2	T42.8X3	T42.8X4	T42.8X5	T42.8X6
Carmellose	T47.4X1	T47.4X2	T47.4X3	T47.4X4	T47.4X5	T47.4X6
Carminative	T47.5X1	T47.5X2	T47.5X3	T47.5X4	T47.5X5	T47.5X6
Carmofur	T45.1X1	T45.1X2	T45.1X3	T45.1X4	T45.1X5	T45.1X6
Carmustine	T45.1X1	T45.1X2	T45.1X3	T45.1X4	T45.1X5	T45.1X6
Carotene	T45.2X1	T45.2X2	T45.2X3	T45.2X4	T45.2X5	T45.2X6
Carphenazine	T43.3X1	T43.3X2	T43.3X3	T43.3X4	T43.3X5	T43.3X6
Carpipramine	T42.4X1	T42.4X2	T42.4X3	T42.4X4	T42.4X5	T42.4X6
Carprofen	T39.311	T39.312	T39.313	T39.314	T39.315	T39.316
Carpronium chloride	T44.3X1	T44.3X2	T44.3X3	T44.3X4	T44.3X5	T44.3X6
Carrageenan	T47.8X1	T47.8X2	T47.8X3	T47.8X4	T47.8X5	T47.8X6
Carteolol	T44.7X1	T44.7X2	T44.7X3	T44.7X4	T44.7X5	T44.7X6
Carter's Little Pills	T47.2X1	T47.2X2	T47.2X3	T47.2X4	T47.2X5	T47.2X6
Cascara (sagrada)	T47.2X1	T47.2X2	T47.2X3	T47.2X4	T47.2X5	T47.2X6
Cassava	T62.2X1	T62.2X2	T62.2X3	T62.2X4	—	—
Castellani's paint	T49.0X1	T49.0X2	T49.0X3	T49.0X4	T49.0X5	T49.0X6
Castor						
bean	T62.2X1	T62.2X2	T62.2X3	T62.2X4	—	—
oil	T47.2X1	T47.2X2	T47.2X3	T47.2X4	T47.2X5	T47.2X6
Catalase	T45.3X1	T45.3X2	T45.3X3	T45.3X4	T45.3X5	T45.3X6
Caterpillar (sting)	T63.431	T63.432	T63.433	T63.434		
Catha (edulis) (tea)	T43.691	T43.692	T43.693	T43.694	—	—
Cathartic NEC	T47.4X1	T47.4X2	T47.4X3	T47.4X4	T47.4X5	T47.4
anthacene derivative	T47.2X1	T47.2X2	T47.2X3	T47.2X4	T47.2X5	T47.2
bulk	T47.4X1	T47.4X2	T47.4X3	T47.4X4	T47.4X5	T47.4
contact	T47.2X1	T47.2X2	T47.2X3	T47.2X4	T47.2X5	T47.2
emollient NEC	T47.4X1	T47.4X2	T47.4X3	T47.4X4	T47.4X5	T47.4
irritant NEC	T47.2X1	T47.2X2	T47.2X3	T47.2X4	T47.2X5	T47.2
mucilage	T47.4X1	T47.4X2	T47.4X3	T47.4X4	T47.4X5	T47.4
saline	T47.3X1	T47.3X2	T47.3X3	T47.3X4	T47.3X5	T47.3
vegetable	T47.2X1	T47.2X2	T47.2X3	T47.2X4	T47.2X5	T47.2
Cathine	T50.5X1	T50.5X2	T50.5X3	T50.5X4	T50.5X5	T50.5
Cathomycin	T36.8X1	T36.8X2	T36.8X3	T36.8X4	T36.8X5	T36.8
Cation exchange resin	T50.3X1	T50.3X2	T50.3X3	T50.3X4	T50.3X5	T50.3
Caustic(s) NEC	T54.91	T54.92	T54.93	T54.94	—	—
alkali	T54.3X1	T54.3X2	T54.3X3	T54.3X4	—	—
hydroxide	T54.3X1	T54.3X2	T54.3X3	T54.3X4	—	—
potash	T54.3X1	T54.3X2	T54.3X3	T54.3X4	—	—
soda	T54.3X1	T54.3X2	T54.3X3	T54.3X4	—	—
specified NEC	T54.91	T54.92	T54.93	T54.94	—	—
Ceepryn	T49.0X1	T49.0X2	T49.0X3	T49.0X4	T49.0X5	T49.0
ENT agent	T49.6X1	T49.6X2	T49.6X3	T49.6X4	T49.6X5	T49.6
lozenges	T49.6X1	T49.6X2	T49.6X3	T49.6X4	T49.6X5	T49.6
Cefacetrile	T36.1X1	T36.1X2	T36.1X3	T36.1X4	T36.1X5	T36.1
Cefaclor	T36.1X1	T36.1X2	T36.1X3	T36.1X4	T36.1X5	T36.1
Cefadroxil	T36.1X1	T36.1X2	T36.1X3	T36.1X4	T36.1X5	T36.1
Cefalexin	T36.1X1	T36.1X2	T36.1X3	T36.1X4	T36.1X5	T36.1
Cefaloglycin	T36.1X1	T36.1X2	T36.1X3	T36.1X4	T36.1X5	T36.1
Cefaloridine	T36.1X1	T36.1X2	T36.1X3	T36.1X4	T36.1X5	T36.1
Cefalosporins	T36.1X1	T36.1X2	T36.1X3	T36.1X4	T36.1X5	T36.1
Cefalotin	T36.1X1	T36.1X2	T36.1X3	T36.1X4	T36.1X5	T36.1
Cefamandole	T36.1X1	T36.1X2	T36.1X3	T36.1X4	T36.1X5	T36.1
Cefamycin antibiotic	T36.1X1	T36.1X2	T36.1X3	T36.1X4	T36.1X5	T36.1
Cefapirin	T36.1X1	T36.1X2	T36.1X3	T36.1X4	T36.1X5	T36.1
Cefatrizine	T36.1X1	T36.1X2	T36.1X3	T36.1X4	T36.1X5	T36.1
Cefazedone	T36.1X1	T36.1X2	T36.1X3	T36.1X4	T36.1X5	T36.1
Cefazolin	T36.1X1	T36.1X2	T36.1X3	T36.1X4	T36.1X5	T36.1
Cefbuperazone	T36.1X1	T36.1X2	T36.1X3	T36.1X4	T36.1X5	T36.1
Cefetamet	T36.1X1	T36.1X2	T36.1X3	T36.1X4	T36.1X5	T36.1
Cefixime	T36.1X1	T36.1X2	T36.1X3	T36.1X4	T36.1X5	T36.1
Cefmenoxime	T36.1X1	T36.1X2	T36.1X3	T36.1X4	T36.1X5	T36.1
Cefmetazole	T36.1X1	T36.1X2	T36.1X3	T36.1X4	T36.1X5	T36.1
Cefminox	T36.1X1	T36.1X2	T36.1X3	T36.1X4	T36.1X5	T36.1
Cefonicid	T36.1X1	T36.1X2	T36.1X3	T36.1X4	T36.1X5	T36.1
Cefoperazone	T36.1X1	T36.1X2	T36.1X3	T36.1X4	T36.1X5	T36.1
Ceforanide	T36.1X1	T36.1X2	T36.1X3	T36.1X4	T36.1X5	T36.1
Cefotaxime	T36.1X1	T36.1X2	T36.1X3	T36.1X4	T36.1X5	T36.1
Cefotetan	T36.1X1	T36.1X2	T36.1X3	T36.1X4	T36.1X5	T36.1
Cefotiam	T36.1X1	T36.1X2	T36.1X3	T36.1X4	T36.1X5	T36.1
Cefoxitin	T36.1X1	T36.1X2	T36.1X3	T36.1X4	T36.1X5	T36.1
Cefpimizole	T36.1X1	T36.1X2	T36.1X3	T36.1X4	T36.1X5	T36.1
Cefpiramide	T36.1X1	T36.1X2	T36.1X3	T36.1X4	T36.1X5	T36.1
Cefradine	T36.1X1	T36.1X2	T36.1X3	T36.1X4	T36.1X5	T36.1
Cefroxadine	T36.1X1	T36.1X2	T36.1X3	T36.1X4	T36.1X5	T36.1
Cefsulodin	T36.1X1	T36.1X2	T36.1X3	T36.1X4	T36.1X5	T36.1
Ceftazidime	T36.1X1	T36.1X2	T36.1X3	T36.1X4	T36.1X5	T36.1
Cefteram	T36.1X1	T36.1X2	T36.1X3	T36.1X4	T36.1X5	T36.1
Ceftezole	T36.1X1	T36.1X2	T36.1X3	T36.1X4	T36.1X5	T36.1
Ceftizoxime	T36.1X1	T36.1X2	T36.1X3	T36.1X4	T36.1X5	T36.1
Ceftriaxone	T36.1X1	T36.1X2	T36.1X3	T36.1X4	T36.1X5	T36.1
Cefuroxime	T36.1X1	T36.1X2	T36.1X3	T36.1X4	T36.1X5	T36.1
Cefuzonam	T36.1X1	T36.1X2	T36.1X3	T36.1X4	T36.1X5	T36.1
Celestone	T38.0X1	T38.0X2	T38.0X3	T38.0X4	T38.0X5	T38.0
topical	T49.0X1	T49.0X2	T49.0X3	T49.0X4	T49.0X5	T49.0
Celiprolol	T44.7X1	T44.7X2	T44.7X3	T44.7X4	T44.7X5	T44.7
Cellosolve	T52.91	T52.92	T52.93	T52.94	—	—
Cell stimulants and proliferants	T49.8X1	T49.8X2	T49.8X3	T49.8X4		T49.8
Cellulose						
cathartic	T47.4X1	T47.4X2	T47.4X3	T47.4X4	T47.4X5	T47.4
hydroxyethyl	T47.4X1	T47.4X2	T47.4X3	T47.4X4	T47.4X5	T47.4
nitrates (topical)	T49.3X1	T49.3X2	T49.3X3	T49.3X4	T49.3X5	T49.3
oxidized	T49.4X1	T49.4X2	T49.4X3	T49.4X4	T49.4X5	T49.4
Centipede (bite)	T63.411	T63.412	T63.413	T63.414		
Central nervous system						
depressants	T42.71	T42.72	T42.73	T42.74	T42.75	T42.76
anesthetic (general) NEC	T41.201	T41.202	T41.203	T41.204	T41.205	T41.20
gases NEC	T41.0X1	T41.0X2	T41.0X3	T41.0X4	T41.0X5	T41.0
intravenous	T41.1X1	T41.1X2	T41.1X3	T41.1X4	T41.1X5	T41.1
barbiturates	T42.3X1	T42.3X2	T42.3X3	T42.3X4	T42.3X5	T42.3
benzodiazepines	T42.4X1	T42.4X2	T42.4X3	T42.4X4	T42.4X5	T42.4
bromides	T42.6X1	T42.6X2	T42.6X3	T42.6X4	T42.6X5	T42.6
cannabis sativa	T40.7X1	T40.7X2	T40.7X3	T40.7X4	T40.7X5	T40.7
chloral hydrate	T42.6X1	T42.6X2	T42.6X3	T42.6X4	T42.6X5	T42.6
ethanol	T51.0X1	T51.0X2	T51.0X3	T51.0X4	—	—

Substance	Poisoning, Accidental (unintentional)	Poisoning, Intentional Self-harm	Poisoning, Assault	Poisoning, Undetermined	Adverse Effect	Under-dosing
Central nervous system — *continued*						
depressants — *continued*						
hallucinogenics	T40.901	T40.902	T40.903	T40.904	T40.905	T40.906
hypnotics	T42.71	T42.72	T42.73	T42.74	T42.75	T42.76
specified NEC	T42.6X1	T42.6X2	T42.6X3	T42.6X4	T42.6X5	T42.6X6
muscle relaxants	T42.8X1	T42.8X2	T42.8X3	T42.8X4	T42.8X5	T42.8X6
paraldehyde	T42.6X1	T42.6X2	T42.6X3	T42.6X4	T42.6X5	T42.6X6
sedatives;	T42.71	T42.72	T42.73	T42.74	T42.75	T42.76
sedative-hypnotics						
mixed NEC	T42.6X1	T42.6X2	T42.6X3	T42.6X4	T42.6X5	T42.6X6
specified NEC	T42.6X1	T42.6X2	T42.6X3	T42.6X4	T42.6X5	T42.6X6
muscle-tone depressants	T42.8X1	T42.8X2	T42.8X3	T42.8X4	T42.8X5	T42.8X6
stimulants	T43.601	T43.602	T43.603	T43.604	T43.605	T43.606
amphetamines	T43.621	T43.622	T43.623	T43.624	T43.625	T43.626
analeptics	T50.7X1	T50.7X2	T50.7X3	T50.7X4	T50.7X5	T50.7X6
antidepressants	T43.201	T43.202	T43.203	T43.204	T43.205	T43.206
opiate antagonists	T50.7X1	T50.7X2	T50.7X3	T50.7X4	T50.7X5	T50.7X6
specified NEC	T43.691	T43.692	T43.693	T43.694	T43.695	T43.696
Cephalexin	T36.1X1	T36.1X2	T36.1X3	T36.1X4	T36.1X5	T36.1X6
Cephaloglycin	T36.1X1	T36.1X2	T36.1X3	T36.1X4	T36.1X5	T36.1X6
Cephaloridine	T36.1X1	T36.1X2	T36.1X3	T36.1X4	T36.1X5	T36.1X6
Cephalosporins	T36.1X1	T36.1X2	T36.1X3	T36.1X4	T36.1X5	T36.1X6
N (adicillin)	T36.0X1	T36.0X2	T36.0X3	T36.0X4	T36.0X5	T36.0X6
Cephalothin	T36.1X1	T36.1X2	T36.1X3	T36.1X4	T36.1X5	T36.1X6
Cephalotin	T36.1X1	T36.1X2	T36.1X3	T36.1X4	T36.1X5	T36.1X6
Cephradine	T36.1X1	T36.1X2	T36.1X3	T36.1X4	T36.1X5	T36.1X6
Cerbera (odallam)	T62.2X1	T62.2X2	T62.2X3	T62.2X4	—	—
Cerberin	T46.0X1	T46.0X2	T46.0X3	T46.0X4	T46.0X5	T46.0X6
Cerebral stimulants	T43.601	T43.602	T43.603	T43.604	T43.605	T43.606
psychotherapeutic	T43.601	T43.602	T43.603	T43.604	T43.605	T43.606
specified NEC	T43.691	T43.692	T43.693	T43.694	T43.695	T43.696
Cerium oxalate	T45.0X1	T45.0X2	T45.0X3	T45.0X4	T45.0X5	T45.0X6
Cerous oxalate	T45.0X1	T45.0X2	T45.0X3	T45.0X4	T45.0X5	T45.0X6
Ceruletide	T50.8X1	T50.8X2	T50.8X3	T50.8X4	T50.8X5	T50.8X6
Cetalkonium (chloride)	T49.0X1	T49.0X2	T49.0X3	T49.0X4	T49.0X5	T49.0X6
Cethexonium chloride	T49.0X1	T49.0X2	T49.0X3	T49.0X4	T49.0X5	T49.0X6
Cetiedil	T46.7X1	T46.7X2	T46.7X3	T46.7X4	T46.7X5	T46.7X6
Cetirizine	T45.0X1	T45.0X2	T45.0X3	T45.0X4	T45.0X5	T45.0X6
Cetomacrogol	T50.991	T50.992	T50.993	T50.994	T50.995	T50.996
Cetotiamine	T45.2X1	T45.2X2	T45.2X3	T45.2X4	T45.2X5	T45.2X6
Cetoxime	T45.0X1	T45.0X2	T45.0X3	T45.0X4	T45.0X5	T45.0X6
Cetraxate	T47.1X1	T47.1X2	T47.1X3	T47.1X4	T47.1X5	T47.1X6
Cetrimide	T49.0X1	T49.0X2	T49.0X3	T49.0X4	T49.0X5	T49.0X6
Cetrimonium (bromide)	T49.0X1	T49.0X2	T49.0X3	T49.0X4	T49.0X5	T49.0X6
Cetylpyridinium chloride	T49.0X1	T49.0X2	T49.0X3	T49.0X4	T49.0X5	T49.0X6
ENT agent	T49.6X1	T49.6X2	T49.6X3	T49.6X4	T49.6X5	T49.6X6
lozenges	T49.6X1	T49.6X2	T49.6X3	T49.6X4	T49.6X5	T49.6X6
Cevadilla — *see* Sabadilla						
Cevitamic acid	T45.2X1	T45.2X2	T45.2X3	T45.2X4	T45.2X5	T45.2X6
Chalk, precipitated	T47.1X1	T47.1X2	T47.1X3	T47.1X4	T47.1X5	T47.1X6
Chamomile	T49.0X1	T49.0X2	T49.0X3	T49.0X4	T49.0X5	T49.0X6
Ch'an su	T46.0X1	T46.0X2	T46.0X3	T46.0X4	T46.0X5	T46.0X6
Charcoal	T47.6X1	T47.6X2	T47.6X3	T47.6X4	T47.6X5	T47.6X6
activated — *see also* Charcoal,	T47.6X1	T47.6X2	T47.6X3	T47.6X4	T47.6X5	T47.6X6
medicinal						
fumes (Carbon monoxide)	T58.2X1	T58.2X2	T58.2X3	T58.2X4	—	—
industrial	T58.8X1	T58.8X2	T58.8X3	T58.8X4	—	—
medicinal (activated)	T47.6X1	T47.6X2	T47.6X3	T47.6X4	T47.6X5	T47.6X6
antidiarrheal	T47.6X1	T47.6X2	T47.6X3	T47.6X4	T47.6X5	T47.6X6
poison control	T47.8X1	T47.8X2	T47.8X3	T47.8X4	T47.8X5	T47.8X6
specified use other than for diarrhea	T47.8X1	T47.8X2	T47.8X3	T47.8X4	T47.8X5	T47.8X6
topical	T49.8X1	T49.8X2	T49.8X3	T49.8X4	T49.8X5	T49.8X6
Chaulmosulfone	T37.1X1	T37.1X2	T37.1X3	T37.1X4	T37.1X5	T37.1X6
Chelating agent NEC	T50.6X1	T50.6X2	T50.6X3	T50.6X4	T50.6X5	T50.6X6
Chelidonium majus	T62.2X1	T62.2X2	T62.2X3	T62.2X4	—	—
Chemical substance NEC	T65.91	T65.92	T65.93	T65.94	—	—
Chenodeoxycholic acid	T47.5X1	T47.5X2	T47.5X3	T47.5X4	T47.5X5	T47.5X6
Chenodiol	T47.5X1	T47.5X2	T47.5X3	T47.5X4	T47.5X5	T47.5X6
Chenopodium	T37.4X1	T37.4X2	T37.4X3	T37.4X4	T37.4X5	T37.4X6
Cherry laurel	T62.2X1	T62.2X2	T62.2X3	T62.2X4	—	—
Chinidin (e)	T46.2X1	T46.2X2	T46.2X3	T46.2X4	T46.2X5	T46.2X6
Chiniofon	T37.8X1	T37.8X2	T37.8X3	T37.8X4	T37.8X5	T37.8X6
Chlophedianol	T48.3X1	T48.3X2	T48.3X3	T48.3X4	T48.3X5	T48.3X6
Chloral	T42.6X1	T42.6X2	T42.6X3	T42.6X4	T42.6X5	T42.6X6
derivative	T42.6X1	T42.6X2	T42.6X3	T42.6X4	T42.6X5	T42.6X6
hydrate	T42.6X1	T42.6X2	T42.6X3	T42.6X4	T42.6X5	T42.6X6
Chloralamide	T42.6X1	T42.6X2	T42.6X3	T42.6X4	T42.6X5	T42.6X6
Chloralodol	T42.6X1	T42.6X2	T42.6X3	T42.6X4	T42.6X5	T42.6X6
Chloralose	T60.4X1	T60.4X2	T60.4X3	T60.4X4	—	—
Chlorambucil	T45.1X1	T45.1X2	T45.1X3	T45.1X4	T45.1X5	T45.1X6
Chloramine	T57.8X1	T57.8X2	T57.8X3	T57.8X4	—	—

Substance	Poisoning, Accidental (unintentional)	Poisoning, Intentional Self-harm	Poisoning, Assault	Poisoning, Undetermined	Adverse Effect	Under-dosing
Chloramine — *continued*						
T	T49.0X1	T49.0X2	T49.0X3	T49.0X4	T49.0X5	T49.0X6
topical	T49.0X1	T49.0X2	T49.0X3	T49.0X4	T49.0X5	T49.0X6
Chloramphenicol	T36.2X1	T36.2X2	T36.2X3	T36.2X4	T36.2X5	T36.2X6
ENT agent	T49.6X1	T49.6X2	T49.6X3	T49.6X4	T49.6X5	T49.6X6
ophthalmic preparation	T49.5X1	T49.5X2	T49.5X3	T49.5X4	T49.5X5	T49.5X6
topical NEC	T49.0X1	T49.0X2	T49.0X3	T49.0X4	T49.0X5	T49.0X6
Chlorate (potassium) (sodium) **NEC**	T60.3X1	T60.3X2	T60.3X3	T60.3X4	—	—
herbicide	T60.3X1	T60.3X2	T60.3X3	T60.3X4	—	—
Chlorazanil	T50.2X1	T50.2X2	T50.2X3	T50.2X4	T50.2X5	T50.2X6
Chlorbenzene, chlorbenzol	T53.7X1	T53.7X2	T53.7X3	T53.7X4		
Chlorbenzoxamine	T44.3X1	T44.3X2	T44.3X3	T44.3X4	T44.3X5	T44.3X6
Chlorbutol	T42.6X1	T42.6X2	T42.6X3	T42.6X4	T42.6X5	T42.6X6
Chlorcyclizine	T45.0X1	T45.0X2	T45.0X3	T45.0X4	T45.0X5	T45.0X6
Chlordan (e) (dust)	T60.1X1	T60.1X2	T60.1X3	T60.1X4		
Chlordantoin	T49.0X1	T49.0X2	T49.0X3	T49.0X4	T49.0X5	T49.0X6
Chlordiazepoxide	T42.4X1	T42.4X2	T42.4X3	T42.4X4	T42.4X5	T42.4X6
Chlordiethyl benzamide	T49.3X1	T49.3X2	T49.3X3	T49.3X4	T49.3X5	T49.3X6
Chloresium	T49.8X1	T49.8X2	T49.8X3	T49.8X4	T49.8X5	T49.8X6
Chlorethiazol	T42.6X1	T42.6X2	T42.6X3	T42.6X4	T42.6X5	T42.6X6
Chlorethyl — *see* Ethyl chloride						
Chloretone	T42.6X1	T42.6X2	T42.6X3	T42.6X4	T42.6X5	T42.6X6
Chlorex	T53.6X1	T53.6X2	T53.6X3	T53.6X4		
insecticide	T60.1X1	T60.1X2	T60.1X3	T60.1X4		
Chlorfenvinphos	T60.0X1	T60.0X2	T60.0X3	T60.0X4		
Chlorhexadol	T42.6X1	T42.6X2	T42.6X3	T42.6X4	T42.6X5	T42.6X6
Chlorhexamide	T45.1X1	T45.1X2	T45.1X3	T45.1X4	T45.1X5	T45.1X6
Chlorhexidine	T49.0X1	T49.0X2	T49.0X3	T49.0X4	T49.0X5	T49.0X6
Chlorhydroxyquinolin	T49.0X1	T49.0X2	T49.0X3	T49.0X4	T49.0X5	T49.0X6
Chloride of lime (bleach)	T54.3X1	T54.3X2	T54.3X3	T54.3X4		
Chlorimipramine	T43.011	T43.012	T43.013	T43.014	T43.015	T43.016
Chlorinated						
camphene	T53.6X1	T53.6X2	T53.6X3	T53.6X4		
diphenyl	T53.7X1	T53.7X2	T53.7X3	T53.7X4		
hydrocarbons NEC	T53.91	T53.92	T53.93	T53.94		
solvents	T53.91	T53.92	T53.93	T53.94		
lime (bleach)	T54.3X1	T54.3X2	T54.3X3	T54.3X4		
and boric acid solution	T49.0X1	T49.0X2	T49.0X3	T49.0X4	T49.0X5	T49.0X6
naphthalene (insecticide)	T60.1X1	T60.1X2	T60.1X3	T60.1X4		
industrial (non-pesticide)	T53.7X1	T53.7X2	T53.7X3	T53.7X4		
pesticide NEC	T60.8X1	T60.8X2	T60.8X3	T60.8X4		
soda — *see also* sodium hypochlorite						
solution	T49.0X1	T49.0X2	T49.0X3	T49.0X4	T49.0X5	T49.0X6
Chlorine (fumes) (gas)	T59.4X1	T59.4X2	T59.4X3	T59.4X4		
bleach	T54.3X1	T54.3X2	T54.3X3	T54.3X4		
compound gas NEC	T59.4X1	T59.4X2	T59.4X3	T59.4X4		
disinfectant	T59.4X1	T59.4X2	T59.4X3	T59.4X4		
releasing agents NEC	T59.4X1	T59.4X2	T59.4X3	T59.4X4		
Chlorisondamine chloride	T46.991	T46.992	T46.993	T46.994	T46.995	T46.996
Chlormadinone	T38.5X1	T38.5X2	T38.5X3	T38.5X4	T38.5X5	T38.5X6
Chlormephos	T60.0X1	T60.0X2	T60.0X3	T60.0X4		
Chlormerodrin	T50.2X1	T50.2X2	T50.2X3	T50.2X4	T50.2X5	T50.2X6
Chlormethiazole	T42.6X1	T42.6X2	T42.6X3	T42.6X4	T42.6X5	T42.6X6
Chlormethine	T45.1X1	T45.1X2	T45.1X3	T45.1X4	T45.1X5	T45.1X6
Chlormethylenecycline	T36.4X1	T36.4X2	T36.4X3	T36.4X4	T36.4X5	T36.4X6
Chlormezanone	T42.6X1	T42.6X2	T42.6X3	T42.6X4	T42.6X5	T42.6X6
Chloroacetic acid	T60.3X1	T60.3X2	T60.3X3	T60.3X4		
Chloroacetone	T59.3X1	T59.3X2	T59.3X3	T59.3X4		
Chloroacetophenone	T59.3X1	T59.3X2	T59.3X3	T59.3X4		
Chloroaniline	T53.7X1	T53.7X2	T53.7X3	T53.7X4		
Chlorobenzene, chlorobenzol	T53.7X1	T53.7X2	T53.7X3	T53.7X4		
Chlorobromomethane (fire extinguisher)	T53.6X1	T53.6X2	T53.6X3	T53.6X4		
Chlorobutanol	T49.0X1	T49.0X2	T49.0X3	T49.0X4	T49.0X5	T49.0X6
Chlorocresol	T49.0X1	T49.0X2	T49.0X3	T49.0X4	T49.0X5	T49.0X6
Chlorodehydromethyltestosterone	T38.7X1	T38.7X2	T38.7X3	T38.7X4	T38.7X5	T38.7X6
Chlorodinitrobenzene	T53.7X1	T53.7X2	T53.7X3	T53.7X4		
dust or vapor	T53.7X1	T53.7X2	T53.7X3	T53.7X4		
Chlorodiphenyl	T53.7X1	T53.7X2	T53.7X3	T53.7X4		
Chloroethane — *see* Ethyl chloride						
Chloroethylene	T53.6X1	T53.6X2	T53.6X3	T53.6X4		
Chlorofluorocarbons	T53.5X1	T53.5X2	T53.5X3	T53.5X4		
Chloroform (fumes) (vapor)	T53.1X1	T53.1X2	T53.1X3	T53.1X4		
anesthetic	T41.0X1	T41.0X2	T41.0X3	T41.0X4	T41.0X5	T41.0X6
solvent	T53.1X1	T53.1X2	T53.1X3	T53.1X4		
water, concentrated	T41.0X1	T41.0X2	T41.0X3	T41.0X4	T41.0X5	T41.0X6
Chloroguanide	T37.2X1	T37.2X2	T37.2X3	T37.2X4	T37.2X5	T37.2X6

Table of Drugs and Chemicals

Substance	Poisoning, Accidental (unintentional)	Poisoning, Intentional Self-harm	Poisoning, Assault	Poisoning, Undetermined	Adverse Effect	Under-dosing
Chloromycetin	T36.2X1	T36.2X2	T36.2X3	T36.2X4	T36.2X5	T36.2X6
ENT agent	T49.6X1	T49.6X2	T49.6X3	T49.6X4	T49.6X5	T49.6X6
ophthalmic preparation	T49.5X1	T49.5X2	T49.5X3	T49.5X4	T49.5X5	T49.5X6
otic solution	T49.6X1	T49.6X2	T49.6X3	T49.6X4	T49.6X5	T49.6X6
topical NEC	T49.0X1	T49.0X2	T49.0X3	T49.0X4	T49.0X5	T49.0X6
Chloronitrobenzene	T53.7X1	T53.7X2	T53.7X3	T53.7X4	—	—
dust or vapor	T53.7X1	T53.7X2	T53.7X3	T53.7X4	—	—
Chlorophacinone	T60.4X1	T60.4X2	T60.4X3	T60.4X4	—	—
Chlorophenol	T53.7X1	T53.7X2	T53.7X3	T53.7X4	—	—
Chlorophenothane	T60.1X1	T60.1X2	T60.1X3	T60.1X4	—	—
Chlorophyll	T50.991	T50.992	T50.993	T50.994	T50.995	T50.996
Chloropicrin (fumes)	T53.6X1	T53.6X2	T53.6X3	T53.6X4	—	—
fumigant	T60.8X1	T60.8X2	T60.8X3	T60.8X4	—	—
fungicide	T60.3X1	T60.3X2	T60.3X3	T60.3X4	—	—
pesticide	T60.8X1	T60.8X2	T60.8X3	T60.8X4	—	—
Chloroprocaine	T41.3X1	T41.3X2	T41.3X3	T41.3X4	T41.3X5	T41.3X6
infiltration (subcutaneous)	T41.3X1	T41.3X2	T41.3X3	T41.3X4	T41.3X5	T41.3X6
nerve block (peripheral) (plexus)	T41.3X1	T41.3X2	T41.3X3	T41.3X4	T41.3X5	T41.3X6
spinal	T41.3X1	T41.3X2	T41.3X3	T41.3X4	T41.3X5	T41.3X6
Chloroptic	T49.5X1	T49.5X2	T49.5X3	T49.5X4	T49.5X5	T49.5X6
Chloropurine	T45.1X1	T45.1X2	T45.1X3	T45.1X4	T45.1X5	T45.1X6
Chloropyramine	T45.0X1	T45.0X2	T45.0X3	T45.0X4	T45.0X5	T45.0X6
Chloropyrifos	T60.0X1	T60.0X2	T60.0X3	T60.0X4	—	—
Chloropyrilene	T45.0X1	T45.0X2	T45.0X3	T45.0X4	T45.0X5	T45.0X6
Chloroquine	T37.2X1	T37.2X2	T37.2X3	T37.2X4	T37.2X5	T37.2X6
Chlorothalonil	T60.3X1	T60.3X2	T60.3X3	T60.3X4	—	—
Chlorothen	T45.0X1	T45.0X2	T45.0X3	T45.0X4	T45.0X5	T45.0X6
Chlorothiazide	T50.2X1	T50.2X2	T50.2X3	T50.2X4	T50.2X5	T50.2X6
Chlorothymol	T49.4X1	T49.4X2	T49.4X3	T49.4X4	T49.4X5	T49.4X6
Chlorotrianisene	T38.5X1	T38.5X2	T38.5X3	T38.5X4	T38.5X5	T38.5X6
Chlorovinyldichloroarsine, not in war	T57.0X1	T57.0X2	T57.0X3	T57.0X4	—	—
Chloroxine	T49.4X1	T49.4X2	T49.4X3	T49.4X4	T49.4X5	T49.4X6
Chloroxylenol	T49.0X1	T49.0X2	T49.0X3	T49.0X4	T49.0X5	T49.0X6
Chlorphenamine	T45.0X1	T45.0X2	T45.0X3	T45.0X4	T45.0X5	T45.0X6
Chlorphenesin	T42.8X1	T42.8X2	T42.8X3	T42.8X4	T42.8X5	T42.8X6
topical (antifungal)	T49.0X1	T49.0X2	T49.0X3	T49.0X4	T49.0X5	T49.0X6
Chlorpheniramine	T45.0X1	T45.0X2	T45.0X3	T45.0X4	T45.0X5	T45.0X6
Chlorphenoxamine	T45.0X1	T45.0X2	T45.0X3	T45.0X4	T45.0X5	T45.0X6
Chlorphentermine	T50.5X1	T50.5X2	T50.5X3	T50.5X4	T50.5X5	T50.5X6
Chlorprocaine — see Chloroprocaine						
Chlorproguanil	T37.2X1	T37.2X2	T37.2X3	T37.2X4	T37.2X5	T37.2X6
Chlorpromazine	T43.3X1	T43.3X2	T43.3X3	T43.3X4	T43.3X5	T43.3X6
Chlorpropamide	T38.3X1	T38.3X2	T38.3X3	T38.3X4	T38.3X5	T38.3X6
Chlorprothixene	T43.4X1	T43.4X2	T43.4X3	T43.4X4	T43.4X5	T43.4X6
Chlorquinaldol	T49.0X1	T49.0X2	T49.0X3	T49.0X4	T49.0X5	T49.0X6
Chlorquinol	T49.0X1	T49.0X2	T49.0X3	T49.0X4	T49.0X5	T49.0X6
Chlortalidone	T50.2X1	T50.2X2	T50.2X3	T50.2X4	T50.2X5	T50.2X6
Chlortetracycline	T36.4X1	T36.4X2	T36.4X3	T36.4X4	T36.4X5	T36.4X6
Chlorthalidone	T50.2X1	T50.2X2	T50.2X3	T50.2X4	T50.2X5	T50.2X6
Chlorthion	T60.0X1	T60.0X2	T60.0X3	T60.0X4	—	—
Chlorthiophos	T60.0X1	T60.0X2	T60.0X3	T60.0X4	—	—
Chlortrianisene	T38.5X1	T38.5X2	T38.5X3	T38.5X4	T38.5X5	T38.5X6
Chlor-Trimeton	T45.0X1	T45.0X2	T45.0X3	T45.0X4	T45.0X5	T45.0X6
Chlorzoxazone	T42.8X1	T42.8X2	T42.8X3	T42.8X4	T42.8X5	T42.8X6
Choke damp	T59.7X1	T59.7X2	T59.7X3	T59.7X4	—	—
Cholagogues	T47.5X1	T47.5X2	T47.5X3	T47.5X4	T47.5X5	T47.5X6
Cholebrine	T50.8X1	T50.8X2	T50.8X3	T50.8X4	T50.8X5	T50.8X6
Cholecalciferol	T45.2X1	T45.2X2	T45.2X3	T45.2X4	T45.2X5	T45.2X6
Cholecystokinin	T50.8X1	T50.8X2	T50.8X3	T50.8X4	T50.8X5	T50.8X6
Cholera vaccine	T50.A91	T50.A92	T50.A93	T50.A94	T50.A95	T50.A96
Choleretic	T47.5X1	T47.5X2	T47.5X3	T47.5X4	T47.5X5	T47.5X6
Cholesterol-lowering agents	T46.6X1	T46.6X2	T46.6X3	T46.6X4	T46.6X5	T46.6X6
Cholestyramine (resin)	T46.6X1	T46.6X2	T46.6X3	T46.6X4	T46.6X5	T46.6X6
Cholic acid	T47.5X1	T47.5X2	T47.5X3	T47.5X4	T47.5X5	T47.5X6
Choline	T48.6X1	T48.6X2	T48.6X3	T48.6X4	T48.6X5	T48.6X6
chloride	T50.991	T50.992	T50.993	T50.994	T50.995	T50.996
dihydrogen citrate	T50.991	T50.992	T50.993	T50.994	T50.995	T50.996
salicylate	T39.091	T39.092	T39.093	T39.094	T39.095	T39.096
theophyllinate	T48.6X1	T48.6X2	T48.6X3	T48.6X4	T48.6X5	T48.6X6
Cholinergic (drug) NEC	T44.1X1	T44.1X2	T44.1X3	T44.1X4	T44.1X5	T44.1X6
muscle tone enhancer	T44.1X1	T44.1X2	T44.1X3	T44.1X4	T44.1X5	T44.1X6
organophosphorus	T44.0X1	T44.0X2	T44.0X3	T44.0X4	T44.0X5	T44.0X6
insecticide	T60.0X1	T60.0X2	T60.0X3	T60.0X4	—	—
nerve gas	T59.891	T59.892	T59.893	T59.894	—	—
trimethyl ammonium propanediol	T44.1X1	T44.1X2	T44.1X3	T44.1X4	T44.1X5	T44.1X6
Cholinesterase reactivator	T50.6X1	T50.6X2	T50.6X3	T50.6X4	T50.6X5	T50.6X6
Cholografin	T50.8X1	T50.8X2	T50.8X3	T50.8X4	T50.8X5	T50.8X6
Chorionic gonadotropin	T38.891	T38.892	T38.893	T38.894	T38.895	T38.896

Substance	Poisoning, Accidental (unintentional)	Poisoning, Intentional Self-harm	Poisoning, Assault	Poisoning, Undetermined	Adverse Effect	Under-dosing
Chromate	T56.2X1	T56.2X2	T56.2X3	T56.2X4	—	—
dust or mist	T56.2X1	T56.2X2	T56.2X3	T56.2X4	—	—
lead — see also lead	T56.0X1	T56.0X2	T56.0X3	T56.0X4	—	—
paint	T56.0X1	T56.0X2	T56.0X3	T56.0X4	—	—
Chromic						
acid	T56.2X1	T56.2X2	T56.2X3	T56.2X4	—	—
dust or mist	T56.2X1	T56.2X2	T56.2X3	T56.2X4	—	—
phosphate 32P	T45.1X1	T45.1X2	T45.1X3	T45.1X4	T45.1X5	T45.1X6
Chromium	T56.2X1	T56.2X2	T56.2X3	T56.2X4	—	—
compounds — see Chromate						
sesquioxide	T50.8X1	T50.8X2	T50.8X3	T50.8X4	T50.8X5	T50.8X6
Chromomycin A3	T45.1X1	T45.1X2	T45.1X3	T45.1X4	T45.1X5	T45.1X6
Chromonar	T46.3X1	T46.3X2	T46.3X3	T46.3X4	T46.3X5	T46.3X6
Chromyl chloride	T56.2X1	T56.2X2	T56.2X3	T56.2X4	—	—
Chrysarobin	T49.4X1	T49.4X2	T49.4X3	T49.4X4	T49.4X5	T49.4X6
Chrysazin	T47.2X1	T47.2X2	T47.2X3	T47.2X4	T47.2X5	T47.2X6
Chymar	T45.3X1	T45.3X2	T45.3X3	T45.3X4	T45.3X5	T45.3X6
ophthalmic preparation	T49.5X1	T49.5X2	T49.5X3	T49.5X4	T49.5X5	T49.5X6
Chymopapain	T45.3X1	T45.3X2	T45.3X3	T45.3X4	T45.3X5	T45.3X6
Chymotrypsin	T45.3X1	T45.3X2	T45.3X3	T45.3X4	T45.3X5	T45.3X6
ophthalmic preparation	T49.5X1	T49.5X2	T49.5X3	T49.5X4	T49.5X5	T49.5X6
Cianidanol	T50.991	T50.992	T50.993	T50.994	T50.995	T50.996
Cianopramine	T43.011	T43.012	T43.013	T43.014	T43.015	T43.016
Cibenzoline	T46.2X1	T46.2X2	T46.2X3	T46.2X4	T46.2X5	T46.2X6
Ciclacillin	T36.0X1	T36.0X2	T36.0X3	T36.0X4	T36.0X5	T36.0X6
Ciclobarbital — see Hexobarbital						
Ciclonicate	T46.7X1	T46.7X2	T46.7X3	T46.7X4	T46.7X5	T46.7X6
Ciclopirox (olamine)	T49.0X1	T49.0X2	T49.0X3	T49.0X4	T49.0X5	T49.0X6
Ciclosporin	T45.1X1	T45.1X2	T45.1X3	T45.1X4	T45.1X5	T45.1X6
Cicuta maculata or virosa	T62.2X1	T62.2X2	T62.2X3	T62.2X4	—	—
Cicutoxin	T62.2X1	T62.2X2	T62.2X3	T62.2X4	—	—
Cigarette lighter fluid	T52.0X1	T52.0X2	T52.0X3	T52.0X4	—	—
Cigarettes (tobacco)	T65.221	T65.222	T65.223	T65.224	—	—
Ciguatoxin	T61.01	T61.02	T61.03	T61.04	—	—
Cilazapril	T46.4X1	T46.4X2	T46.4X3	T46.4X4	T46.4X5	T46.4X6
Cimetidine	T47.0X1	T47.0X2	T47.0X3	T47.0X4	T47.0X5	T47.0X6
Cimetropium bromide	T44.3X1	T44.3X2	T44.3X3	T44.3X4	T44.3X5	T44.3X6
Cinchocaine	T41.3X1	T41.3X2	T41.3X3	T41.3X4	T41.3X5	T41.3X6
topical (surface)	T41.3X1	T41.3X2	T41.3X3	T41.3X4	T41.3X5	T41.3X6
Cinchona	T37.2X1	T37.2X2	T37.2X3	T37.2X4	T37.2X5	T37.2X6
Cinchonine alkaloids	T37.2X1	T37.2X2	T37.2X3	T37.2X4	T37.2X5	T37.2X6
Cinchophen	T50.4X1	T50.4X2	T50.4X3	T50.4X4	T50.4X5	T50.4X6
Cinepazide	T46.7X1	T46.7X2	T46.7X3	T46.7X4	T46.7X5	T46.7X6
Cinnamedrine	T48.5X1	T48.5X2	T48.5X3	T48.5X4	T48.5X5	T48.5X6
Cinnarizine	T45.0X1	T45.0X2	T45.0X3	T45.0X4	T45.0X5	T45.0X6
Cinoxacin	T37.8X1	T37.8X2	T37.8X3	T37.8X4	T37.8X5	T37.8X6
Ciprofibrate	T46.6X1	T46.6X2	T46.6X3	T46.6X4	T46.6X5	T46.6X6
Ciprofloxacin	T36.8X1	T36.8X2	T36.8X3	T36.8X4	T36.8X5	T36.8X6
Cisapride	T47.8X1	T47.8X2	T47.8X3	T47.8X4	T47.8X5	T47.8X6
Cisplatin	T45.1X1	T45.1X2	T45.1X3	T45.1X4	T45.1X5	T45.1X6
Citalopram	T43.221	T43.222	T43.223	T43.224	T43.225	T43.226
Citanest	T41.3X1	T41.3X2	T41.3X3	T41.3X4	T41.3X5	T41.3X6
infiltration (subcutaneous)	T41.3X1	T41.3X2	T41.3X3	T41.3X4	T41.3X5	T41.3X6
nerve block (peripheral) (plexus)	T41.3X1	T41.3X2	T41.3X3	T41.3X4	T41.3X5	T41.3X6
Citric acid	T47.5X1	T47.5X2	T47.5X3	T47.5X4	T47.5X5	T47.5X6
Citrovorum (factor)	T45.8X1	T45.8X2	T45.8X3	T45.8X4	T45.8X5	T45.8X6
Claviceps purpurea	T62.2X1	T62.2X2	T62.2X3	T62.2X4	—	—
Clavulanic acid	T36.1X1	T36.1X2	T36.1X3	T36.1X4	T36.1X5	T36.1X6
Cleaner, cleansing agent, type not specified	T65.891	T65.892	T65.893	T65.894	—	—
of paint or varnish	T52.91	T52.92	T52.93	T52.94	—	—
specified type NEC	T65.891	T65.892	T65.893	T65.894	—	—
Clebopride	T47.8X1	T47.8X2	T47.8X3	T47.8X4	T47.8X5	T47.8X6
Clefamide	T37.3X1	T37.3X2	T37.3X3	T37.3X4	T37.3X5	T37.3X6
Clemastine	T45.0X1	T45.0X2	T45.0X3	T45.0X4	T45.0X5	T45.0X6
Clematis vitalba	T62.2X1	T62.2X2	T62.2X3	T62.2X4	—	—
Clemizole	T45.0X1	T45.0X2	T45.0X3	T45.0X4	T45.0X5	T45.0X6
penicillin	T36.0X1	T36.0X2	T36.0X3	T36.0X4	T36.0X5	T36.0X6
Clenbuterol	T48.6X1	T48.6X2	T48.6X3	T48.6X4	T48.6X5	T48.6X6
Clidinium bromide	T44.3X1	T44.3X2	T44.3X3	T44.3X4	T44.3X5	T44.3X6
Clindamycin	T36.8X1	T36.8X2	T36.8X3	T36.8X4	T36.8X5	T36.8X6
Clinofibrate	T46.6X1	T46.6X2	T46.6X3	T46.6X4	T46.6X5	T46.6X6
Clioquinol	T37.8X1	T37.8X2	T37.8X3	T37.8X4	T37.8X5	T37.8X6
Cliradon	T40.2X1	T40.2X2	T40.2X3	T40.2X4		
Clobazam	T42.4X1	T42.4X2	T42.4X3	T42.4X4	T42.4X5	T42.4X6
Clobenzorex	T50.5X1	T50.5X2	T50.5X3	T50.5X4	T50.5X5	T50.5X6
Clobetasol	T49.0X1	T49.0X2	T49.0X3	T49.0X4	T49.0X5	T49.0X6
Clobetasone	T49.0X1	T49.0X2	T49.0X3	T49.0X4	T49.0X5	T49.0X6
Clobutinol	T48.3X1	T48.3X2	T48.3X3	T48.3X4	T48.3X5	T48.3X6
Clocortolone	T38.0X1	T38.0X2	T38.0X3	T38.0X4	T38.0X5	T38.0X6
Clodantoin	T49.0X1	T49.0X2	T49.0X3	T49.0X4	T49.0X5	T49.0X6

Chloromycetin — Clodantoin

Additional Character May Be Required — Refer to the Tabular List for Character Selection

▽ Subterms under main terms may continue to next column or page

Substance	Poisoning, Accidental (unintentional)	Poisoning, Intentional Self-harm	Poisoning, Assault	Poisoning, Undetermined	Adverse Effect	Under-dosing
Clodronic acid	T50.991	T50.992	T50.993	T50.994	T50.995	T50.996
Clofazimine	T37.1X1	T37.1X2	T37.1X3	T37.1X4	T37.1X5	T37.1X6
Clofedanol	T48.3X1	T48.3X2	T48.3X3	T48.3X4	T48.3X5	T48.3X6
Clofenamide	T50.2X1	T50.2X2	T50.2X3	T50.2X4	T50.2X5	T50.2X6
Clofenotane	T49.0X1	T49.0X2	T49.0X3	T49.0X4	T49.0X5	T49.0X6
Clofezone	T39.2X1	T39.2X2	T39.2X3	T39.2X4	T39.2X5	T39.2X6
Clofibrate	T46.6X1	T46.6X2	T46.6X3	T46.6X4	T46.6X5	T46.6X6
Clofibride	T46.6X1	T46.6X2	T46.6X3	T46.6X4	T46.6X5	T46.6X6
Cloforex	T50.5X1	T50.5X2	T50.5X3	T50.5X4	T50.5X5	T50.5X6
Clomethiazole	T42.6X1	T42.6X2	T42.6X3	T42.6X4	T42.6X5	T42.6X6
Clometocillin	T36.0X1	T36.0X2	T36.0X3	T36.0X4	T36.0X5	T36.0X6
Clomifene	T38.5X1	T38.5X2	T38.5X3	T38.5X4	T38.5X5	T38.5X6
Clomiphene	T38.5X1	T38.5X2	T38.5X3	T38.5X4	T38.5X5	T38.5X6
Clomipramine	T43.011	T43.012	T43.013	T43.014	T43.015	T43.016
Clomocycline	T36.4X1	T36.4X2	T36.4X3	T36.4X4	T36.4X5	T36.4X6
Clonazepam	T42.4X1	T42.4X2	T42.4X3	T42.4X4	T42.4X5	T42.4X6
Clonidine	T46.5X1	T46.5X2	T46.5X3	T46.5X4	T46.5X5	T46.5X6
Clonixin	T39.8X1	T39.8X2	T39.8X3	T39.8X4	T39.8X5	T39.8X6
Clopamide	T50.2X1	T50.2X2	T50.2X3	T50.2X4	T50.2X5	T50.2X6
Clopenthixol	T43.4X1	T43.4X2	T43.4X3	T43.4X4	T43.4X5	T43.4X6
Cloperastine	T48.3X1	T48.3X2	T48.3X3	T48.3X4	T48.3X5	T48.3X6
Clophedianol	T48.3X1	T48.3X2	T48.3X3	T48.3X4	T48.3X5	T48.3X6
Cloponone	T36.2X1	T36.2X2	T36.2X3	T36.2X4	T36.2X5	T36.2X6
Cloprednol	T38.0X1	T38.0X2	T38.0X3	T38.0X4	T38.0X5	T38.0X6
Cloral betaine	T42.6X1	T42.6X2	T42.6X3	T42.6X4	T42.6X5	T42.6X6
Cloramfenicol	T36.2X1	T36.2X2	T36.2X3	T36.2X4	T36.2X5	T36.2X6
Clorazepate (dipotassium)	T42.4X1	T42.4X2	T42.4X3	T42.4X4	T42.4X5	T42.4X6
Clorexolone	T50.2X1	T50.2X2	T50.2X3	T50.2X4	T50.2X5	T50.2X6
Clorfenamine	T45.0X1	T45.0X2	T45.0X3	T45.0X4	T45.0X5	T45.0X6
Clorgiline	T43.1X1	T43.1X2	T43.1X3	T43.1X4	T43.1X5	T43.1X6
Clorotepine	T44.3X1	T44.3X2	T44.3X3	T44.3X4	T44.3X5	T44.3X6
Clorox (bleach)	T54.91	T54.92	T54.93	T54.94	—	—
Clorprenaline	T48.6X1	T48.6X2	T48.6X3	T48.6X4	T48.6X5	T48.6X6
Clortermine	T50.5X1	T50.5X2	T50.5X3	T50.5X4	T50.5X5	T50.5X6
Clotiapine	T43.591	T43.592	T43.593	T43.594	T43.595	T43.596
Clotiazepam	T42.4X1	T42.4X2	T42.4X3	T42.4X4	T42.4X5	T42.4X6
Clotibric acid	T46.6X1	T46.6X2	T46.6X3	T46.6X4	T46.6X5	T46.6X6
Clotrimazole	T49.0X1	T49.0X2	T49.0X3	T49.0X4	T49.0X5	T49.0X6
Cloxacillin	T36.0X1	T36.0X2	T36.0X3	T36.0X4	T36.0X5	T36.0X6
Cloxazolam	T42.4X1	T42.4X2	T42.4X3	T42.4X4	T42.4X5	T42.4X6
Cloxiquine	T49.0X1	T49.0X2	T49.0X3	T49.0X4	T49.0X5	T49.0X6
Clozapine	T42.4X1	T42.4X2	T42.4X3	T42.4X4	T42.4X5	T42.4X6
Coagulant NEC	T45.7X1	T45.7X2	T45.7X3	T45.7X1	T45.7X5	T45.7X6
Coal (carbon monoxide from) — see also Carbon, monoxide, coal	T58.2X1	T58.2X2	T58.2X3	T58.2X4	—	—
oil — see Kerosene						
tar	T49.1X1	T49.1X2	T49.1X3	T49.1X4	T49.1X5	T49.1X6
fumes	T59.891	T59.892	T59.893	T59.894	—	—
medicinal (ointment)	T49.4X1	T49.4X2	T49.4X3	T49.4X4	T49.4X5	T49.4X6
analgesics NEC	T39.2X1	T39.2X2	T39.2X3	T39.2X4	T39.2X5	T39.2X6
naphtha (solvent)	T52.0X1	T52.0X2	T52.0X3	T52.0X4	—	—
Cobalamine	T45.2X1	T45.2X2	T45.2X3	T45.2X4	T45.2X5	T45.2X6
Cobalt (nonmedicinal) (fumes) (industrial)	T56.891	T56.892	T56.893	T56.894	—	—
medicinal (trace) (chloride)	T45.8X1	T45.8X2	T45.8X3	T45.8X4	T45.8X5	T45.8X6
Cobra (venom)	T63.041	T63.042	T63.043	T63.044	—	—
Coca (leaf)	T40.5X1	T40.5X2	T40.5X3	T40.5X4	T40.5X5	T40.5X6
Cocaine	T40.5X1	T40.5X2	T40.5X3	T40.5X4	T40.5X5	T40.5X6
topical anesthetic	T41.3X1	T41.3X2	T41.3X3	T41.3X4	T41.3X5	T41.3X6
Cocarboxylase	T45.3X1	T45.3X2	T45.3X3	T45.3X4	T45.3X5	T45.3X6
Coccidioidin	T50.8X1	T50.8X2	T50.8X3	T50.8X4	T50.8X5	T50.8X6
Cocculus indicus	T62.1X1	T62.1X2	T62.1X3	T62.1X4	—	—
Cochineal	T65.6X1	T65.6X2	T65.6X3	T65.6X4	—	—
medicinal products	T50.991	T50.992	T50.993	T50.994	T50.995	T50.996
Codeine	T40.2X1	T40.2X2	T40.2X3	T40.2X4	T40.2X5	T40.2X6
Cod-liver oil	T45.2X1	T45.2X2	T45.2X3	T45.2X4	T45.2X5	T45.2X6
Coenzyme A	T50.991	T50.992	T50.993	T50.994	T50.995	T50.996
Coffee	T62.8X1	T62.8X2	T62.8X3	T62.8X4	—	—
Cogalactoisomerase	T50.991	T50.992	T50.993	T50.994	T50.995	T50.996
Cogentin	T44.3X1	T44.3X2	T44.3X3	T44.3X4	T44.3X5	T44.3X6
Coke fumes or gas (carbon monoxide)	T58.2X1	T58.2X2	T58.2X3	T58.2X4	—	—
industrial use	T58.8X1	T58.8X2	T58.8X3	T58.8X4	—	—
Colace	T47.4X1	T47.4X2	T47.4X3	T47.4X4	T47.4X5	T47.4X6
Colaspase	T45.1X1	T45.1X2	T45.1X3	T45.1X4	T45.1X5	T45.1X6
Colchicine	T50.4X1	T50.4X2	T50.4X3	T50.4X4	T50.4X5	T50.4X6
Colchicum	T62.2X1	T62.2X2	T62.2X3	T62.2X4	—	—
Cold cream	T49.3X1	T49.3X2	T49.3X3	T49.3X4	T49.3X5	T49.3X6
Colecalciferol	T45.2X1	T45.2X2	T45.2X3	T45.2X4	T45.2X5	T45.2X6
Colestipol	T46.6X1	T46.6X2	T46.6X3	T46.6X4	T46.6X5	T46.6X6
Colestyramine	T46.6X1	T46.6X2	T46.6X3	T46.6X4	T46.6X5	T46.6X6
Colimycin	T36.8X1	T36.8X2	T36.8X3	T36.8X4	T36.8X5	T36.8X6

Substance	Poisoning, Accidental (unintentional)	Poisoning, Intentional Self-harm	Poisoning, Assault	Poisoning, Undetermined	Adverse Effect	Under-dosing
Colistimethate	T36.8X1	T36.8X2	T36.8X3	T36.8X4	T36.8X5	T36.8X6
Colistin	T36.8X1	T36.8X2	T36.8X3	T36.8X4	T36.8X5	T36.8X6
sulfate (eye preparation)	T49.5X1	T49.5X2	T49.5X3	T49.5X4	T49.5X5	T49.5X6
Collagen	T50.991	T50.992	T50.993	T50.994	T50.995	T50.996
Collagenase	T49.4X1	T49.4X2	T49.4X3	T49.4X4	T49.4X5	T49.4X6
Collodion	T49.3X1	T49.3X2	T49.3X3	T49.3X4	T49.3X5	T49.3X6
Colocynth	T47.2X1	T47.2X2	T47.2X3	T47.2X4	T47.2X5	T47.2X6
Colophony adhesive	T49.3X1	T49.3X2	T49.3X3	T49.3X4	T49.3X5	T49.3X6
Colorant — see also Dye	T50.991	T50.992	T50.993	T50.994	T50.995	T50.996
Coloring matter — see Dye(s)						
Combustion gas (after combustion) — see Carbon, monoxide						
prior to combustion	T59.891	T59.892	T59.893	T59.894	—	—
Compazine	T43.3X1	T43.3X2	T43.3X3	T43.3X4	T43.3X5	T43.3X6
Compound						
1080 (sodium fluoroacetate)	T60.4X1	T60.4X2	T60.4X3	T60.4X4	—	—
269 (endrin)	T60.1X1	T60.1X2	T60.1X3	T60.1X4	—	—
3422 (parathion)	T60.0X1	T60.0X2	T60.0X3	T60.0X4	—	—
3911 (phorate)	T60.0X1	T60.0X2	T60.0X3	T60.0X4	—	—
3956 (toxaphene)	T60.1X1	T60.1X2	T60.1X3	T60.1X4	—	—
4049 (malathion)	T60.0X1	T60.0X2	T60.0X3	T60.0X4	—	—
4069 (malathion)	T60.0X1	T60.0X2	T60.0X3	T60.0X4	—	—
4124 (dicapthon)	T60.0X1	T60.0X2	T60.0X3	T60.0X4	—	—
42 (warfarin)	T60.4X1	T60.4X2	T60.4X3	T60.4X4	—	—
497 (dieldrin)	T60.1X1	T60.1X2	T60.1X3	T60.1X4	—	—
E (cortisone)	T38.0X1	T38.0X2	T38.0X3	T38.0X4	T38.0X5	T38.0X6
F (hydrocortisone)	T38.0X1	T38.0X2	T38.0X3	T38.0X4	T38.0X5	T38.0X6
Congener, anabolic	T38.7X1	T38.7X2	T38.7X3	T38.7X4	T38.7X5	T38.7X6
Congo red	T50.8X1	T50.8X2	T50.8X3	T50.8X4	T50.8X5	T50.8X6
Coniine, conine	T62.2X1	T62.2X2	T62.2X3	T62.2X4	—	—
Conium (maculatum)	T62.2X1	T62.2X2	T62.2X3	T62.2X4	—	—
Conjugated estrogenic substances	T38.5X1	T38.5X2	T38.5X3	T38.5X4	T38.5X5	T38.5X6
Contac	T48.5X1	T48.5X2	T48.5X3	T48.5X4	T48.5X5	T48.5X6
Contact lens solution	T49.5X1	T49.5X2	T49.5X3	T49.5X4	T49.5X5	T49.5X6
Contraceptive (oral)	T38.4X1	T38.4X2	T38.4X3	T38.4X4	T38.4X5	T38.4X6
vaginal	T49.8X1	T49.8X2	T49.8X3	T49.8X4	T49.8X5	T49.8X6
Contrast medium, radiography	T50.8X1	T50.8X2	T50.8X3	T50.8X4	T50.8X5	T50.8X6
Convallaria glycosides	T46.0X1	T46.0X2	T46.0X3	T46.0X4	T46.0X5	T46.0X6
Convallaria majalis	T62.2X1	T62.2X2	T62.2X3	T62.2X4	—	—
berry	T62.1X1	T62.1X2	T62.1X3	T62.1X4	—	—
Copperhead snake (bite) (venom)	T63.061	T63.062	T63.063	T63.064	—	—
Copper (dust) (fumes) (nonmedicinal) NEC	T56.4X1	T56.4X2	T56.4X3	T56.4X4	—	—
arsenate, arsenite	T57.0X1	T57.0X2	T57.0X3	T57.0X4	—	—
insecticide	T60.2X1	T60.2X2	T60.2X3	T60.2X4	—	—
emetic	T47.7X1	T47.7X2	T47.7X3	T47.7X4	T47.7X5	T47.7X6
fungicide	T60.3X1	T60.3X2	T60.3X3	T60.3X4	—	—
gluconate	T49.0X1	T49.0X2	T49.0X3	T49.0X4	T49.0X5	T49.0X6
insecticide	T60.2X1	T60.2X2	T60.2X3	T60.2X4	—	—
medicinal (trace)	T45.8X1	T45.8X2	T45.8X3	T45.8X4	T45.8X5	T45.8X6
oleate	T49.0X1	T49.0X2	T49.0X3	T49.0X4	T49.0X5	T49.0X6
sulfate	T56.4X1	T56.4X2	T56.4X3	T56.4X4	—	—
cupric	T56.4X1	T56.4X2	T56.4X3	T56.4X4	—	—
fungicide	T60.3X1	T60.3X2	T60.3X3	T60.3X4	—	—
medicinal						
ear	T49.6X1	T49.6X2	T49.6X3	T49.6X4	T49.6X5	T49.6X6
emetic	T47.7X1	T47.7X2	T47.7X3	T47.7X4	T47.7X5	T47.7X6
eye	T49.5X1	T49.5X2	T49.5X3	T49.5X4	T49.5X5	T49.5X6
cuprous	T56.4X1	T56.4X2	T56.4X3	T56.4X4	—	—
fungicide	T60.3X1	T60.3X2	T60.3X3	T60.3X4	—	—
medicinal						
ear	T49.6X1	T49.6X2	T49.6X3	T49.6X4	T49.6X5	T49.6X6
emetic	T47.7X1	T47.7X2	T47.7X3	T47.7X4	T47.7X5	T47.7X6
eye	T49.5X1	T49.5X2	T49.5X3	T49.5X4	T49.5X5	T49.5X6
Coral (sting)	T63.691	T63.692	T63.693	T63.694		
snake (bite) (venom)	T63.021	T63.022	T63.023	T63.024		
Corbadrine	T49.6X1	T49.6X2	T49.6X3	T49.6X4	T49.6X5	T49.6X6
Cordite	T65.891	T65.892	T65.893	T65.894	—	—
vapor	T59.891	T59.892	T59.893	T59.894	—	—
Cordran	T49.0X1	T49.0X2	T49.0X3	T49.0X4	T49.0X5	T49.0X6
Corn cures	T49.4X1	T49.4X2	T49.4X3	T49.4X4	T49.4X5	T49.4X6
Cornhusker's lotion	T49.3X1	T49.3X2	T49.3X3	T49.3X4	T49.3X5	T49.3X6
Corn starch	T49.3X1	T49.3X2	T49.3X3	T49.3X4	T49.3X5	T49.3X6
Coronary vasodilator NEC	T46.3X1	T46.3X2	T46.3X3	T46.3X4	T46.3X5	T46.3X6
Corrosive NEC	T54.91	T54.92	T54.93	T54.94	—	—
acid NEC	T54.2X1	T54.2X2	T54.2X3	T54.2X4	—	—
aromatics	T54.1X1	T54.1X2	T54.1X3	T54.1X4	—	—
disinfectant	T54.1X1	T54.1X2	T54.1X3	T54.1X4	—	—

▽ Subterms under main terms may continue to next column or page   Additional Character May Be Required — Refer to the Tabular List for Character Selection   361

Clodronic acid — Corrosive NEC

Substance	Poisoning, Accidental (unintentional)	Poisoning, Intentional Self-harm	Poisoning, Assault	Poisoning, Undetermined	Adverse Effect	Under-dosing
Corrosive — *continued*						
fumes NEC	T54.91	T54.92	T54.93	T54.94	—	—
specified NEC	T54.91	T54.92	T54.93	T54.94	—	—
sublimate	T56.1X1	T56.1X2	T56.1X3	T56.1X4	—	—
Cortate	T38.0X1	T38.0X2	T38.0X3	T38.0X4	T38.0X5	T38.0X6
Cort-Dome	T38.0X1	T38.0X2	T38.0X3	T38.0X4	T38.0X5	T38.0X6
ENT agent	T49.6X1	T49.6X2	T49.6X3	T49.6X4	T49.6X5	T49.6X6
ophthalmic preparation	T49.5X1	T49.5X2	T49.5X3	T49.5X4	T49.5X5	T49.5X6
topical NEC	T49.0X1	T49.0X2	T49.0X3	T49.0X4	T49.0X5	T49.0X6
Cortef	T38.0X1	T38.0X2	T38.0X3	T38.0X4	T38.0X5	T38.0X6
ENT agent	T49.6X1	T49.6X2	T49.6X3	T49.6X4	T49.6X5	T49.6X6
ophthalmic preparation	T49.5X1	T49.5X2	T49.5X3	T49.5X4	T49.5X5	T49.5X6
topical NEC	T49.0X1	T49.0X2	T49.0X3	T49.0X4	T49.0X5	T49.0X6
Corticosteroid	T38.0X1	T38.0X2	T38.0X3	T38.0X4	T38.0X5	T38.0X6
ENT agent	T49.6X1	T49.6X2	T49.6X3	T49.6X4	T49.6X5	T49.6X6
mineral	T50.0X1	T50.0X2	T50.0X3	T50.0X4	T50.0X5	T50.0X6
ophthalmic	T49.5X1	T49.5X2	T49.5X3	T49.5X4	T49.5X5	T49.5X6
topical NEC	T49.0X1	T49.0X2	T49.0X3	T49.0X4	T49.0X5	T49.0X6
Corticotropin	T38.811	T38.812	T38.813	T38.814	T38.815	T38.816
Cortisol	T38.0X1	T38.0X2	T38.0X3	T38.0X4	T38.0X5	T38.0X6
ENT agent	T49.6X1	T49.6X2	T49.6X3	T49.6X4	T49.6X5	T49.6X6
ophthalmic preparation	T49.5X1	T49.5X2	T49.5X3	T49.5X4	T49.5X5	T49.5X6
topical NEC	T49.0X1	T49.0X2	T49.0X3	T49.0X4	T49.0X5	T49.0X6
Cortisone (acetate)	T38.0X1	T38.0X2	T38.0X3	T38.0X4	T38.0X5	T38.0X6
ENT agent	T49.6X1	T49.6X2	T49.6X3	T49.6X4	T49.6X5	T49.6X6
ophthalmic preparation	T49.5X1	T49.5X2	T49.5X3	T49.5X4	T49.5X5	T49.5X6
topical NEC	T49.0X1	T49.0X2	T49.0X3	T49.0X4	T49.0X5	T49.0X6
Cortivazol	T38.0X1	T38.0X2	T38.0X3	T38.0X4	T38.0X5	T38.0X6
Cortogen	T38.0X1	T38.0X2	T38.0X3	T38.0X4	T38.0X5	T38.0X6
ENT agent	T49.6X1	T49.6X2	T49.6X3	T49.6X4	T49.6X5	T49.6X6
ophthalmic preparation	T49.5X1	T49.5X2	T49.5X3	T49.5X4	T49.5X5	T49.5X6
Cortone	T38.0X1	T38.0X2	T38.0X3	T38.0X4	T38.0X5	T38.0X6
ENT agent	T49.6X1	T49.6X2	T49.6X3	T49.6X4	T49.6X5	T49.6X6
ophthalmic preparation	T49.5X1	T49.5X2	T49.5X3	T49.5X4	T49.5X5	T49.5X6
Cortril	T38.0X1	T38.0X2	T38.0X3	T38.0X4	T38.0X5	T38.0X6
ENT agent	T49.6X1	T49.6X2	T49.6X3	T49.6X4	T49.6X5	T49.6X6
ophthalmic preparation	T49.5X1	T49.5X2	T49.5X3	T49.5X4	T49.5X5	T49.5X6
topical NEC	T49.0X1	T49.0X2	T49.0X3	T49.0X4	T49.0X5	T49.0X6
Corynebacterium parvum	T45.1X1	T45.1X2	T45.1X3	T45.1X4	T45.1X5	T45.1X6
Cosmetic preparation	T49.8X1	T49.8X2	T49.8X3	T49.8X4	T49.8X5	T49.8X6
Cosmetics	T49.8X1	T49.8X2	T49.8X3	T49.8X4	T49.8X5	T49.8X6
Cosyntropin	T38.811	T38.812	T38.813	T38.814	T38.815	T38.816
Cotarnine	T45.7X1	T45.7X2	T45.7X3	T45.7X4	T45.7X5	T45.7X6
Co-trimoxazole	T36.8X1	T36.8X2	T36.8X3	T36.8X4	T36.8X5	T36.8X6
Cottonseed oil	T49.3X1	T49.3X2	T49.3X3	T49.3X4	T49.3X5	T49.3X6
Cough mixture (syrup)	T48.4X1	T48.4X2	T48.4X3	T48.4X4	T48.4X5	T48.4X6
containing opiates	T40.2X1	T40.2X2	T40.2X3	T40.2X4	T40.2X5	T40.2X6
expectorants	T48.4X1	T48.4X2	T48.4X3	T48.4X4	T48.4X5	T48.4X6
Coumadin	T45.511	T45.512	T45.513	T45.514	T45.515	T45.516
rodenticide	T60.4X1	T60.4X2	T60.4X3	T60.4X4	—	—
Coumaphos	T60.0X1	T60.0X2	T60.0X3	T60.0X4	—	—
Coumarin	T45.511	T45.512	T45.513	T45.514	T45.515	T45.516
Coumetarol	T45.511	T45.512	T45.513	T45.514	T45.515	T45.516
Cowbane	T62.2X1	T62.2X2	T62.2X3	T62.2X4	—	—
Cozyme	T45.2X1	T45.2X2	T45.2X3	T45.2X4	T45.2X5	T45.2X6
Crack	T40.5X1	T40.5X2	T40.5X3	T40.5X4	—	—
Crataegus extract	T46.0X1	T46.0X2	T46.0X3	T46.0X4	T46.0X5	T46.0X6
Creolin	T54.1X1	T54.1X2	T54.1X3	T54.1X4	—	—
disinfectant	T54.1X1	T54.1X2	T54.1X3	T54.1X4	—	—
Creosol (compound)	T49.0X1	T49.0X2	T49.0X3	T49.0X4	T49.0X5	T49.0X6
Creosote (coal tar) (beechwood)	T49.0X1	T49.0X2	T49.0X3	T49.0X4	T49.0X5	T49.0X6
medicinal (expectorant)	T48.4X1	T48.4X2	T48.4X3	T48.4X4	T48.4X5	T48.4X6
syrup	T48.4X1	T48.4X2	T48.4X3	T48.4X4	T48.4X5	T48.4X6
Cresol(s)	T49.0X1	T49.0X2	T49.0X3	T49.0X4	T49.0X5	T49.0X6
and soap solution	T49.0X1	T49.0X2	T49.0X3	T49.0X4	T49.0X5	T49.0X6
Cresyl acetate	T49.0X1	T49.0X2	T49.0X3	T49.0X4	T49.0X5	T49.0X6
Cresylic acid	T49.0X1	T49.0X2	T49.0X3	T49.0X4	T49.0X5	T49.0X6
Crimidine	T60.4X1	T60.4X2	T60.4X3	T60.4X4	—	—
Croconazole	T37.8X1	T37.8X2	T37.8X3	T37.8X4	T37.8X5	T37.8X6
Cromoglicic acid	T48.6X1	T48.6X2	T48.6X3	T48.6X4	T48.6X5	T48.6X6
Cromolyn	T48.6X1	T48.6X2	T48.6X3	T48.6X4	T48.6X5	T48.6X6
Cromonar	T46.3X1	T46.3X2	T46.3X3	T46.3X4	T46.3X5	T46.3X6
Cropropamide	T39.8X1	T39.8X2	T39.8X3	T39.8X4	T39.8X5	T39.8X6
with crotethamide	T50.7X1	T50.7X2	T50.7X3	T50.7X4	T50.7X5	T50.7X6
Crotamiton	T49.0X1	T49.0X2	T49.0X3	T49.0X4	T49.0X5	T49.0X6
Crotethamide	T39.8X1	T39.8X2	T39.8X3	T39.8X4	T39.8X5	T39.8X6
with cropropamide	T50.7X1	T50.7X2	T50.7X3	T50.7X4	T50.7X5	T50.7X6
Croton (oil)	T47.2X1	T47.2X2	T47.2X3	T47.2X4	T47.2X5	T47.2X6
chloral	T42.6X1	T42.6X2	T42.6X3	T42.6X4	T42.6X5	T42.6X6
Crude oil	T52.0X1	T52.0X2	T52.0X3	T52.0X4	—	—
Cryogenine	T39.8X1	T39.8X2	T39.8X3	T39.8X4	T39.8X5	T39.8X6
Cryolite (vapor)	T60.1X1	T60.1X2	T60.1X3	T60.1X4	—	—

Substance	Poisoning, Accidental (unintentional)	Poisoning, Intentional Self-harm	Poisoning, Assault	Poisoning, Undetermined	Adverse Effect	Under-dosing
Cryolite — *continued*						
insecticide	T60.1X1	T60.1X2	T60.1X3	T60.1X4	—	—
Cryptenamine (tannates)	T46.5X1	T46.5X2	T46.5X3	T46.5X4	T46.5X5	T46.5…
Crystal violet	T49.0X1	T49.0X2	T49.0X3	T49.0X4	T49.0X5	T49.0…
Cuckoopint	T62.2X1	T62.2X2	T62.2X3	T62.2X4	—	—
Cumetharol	T45.511	T45.512	T45.513	T45.514	T45.515	T45.5…
Cupric						
acetate	T60.3X1	T60.3X2	T60.3X3	T60.3X4	—	—
acetoarsenite	T57.0X1	T57.0X2	T57.0X3	T57.0X4	—	—
arsenate	T57.0X1	T57.0X2	T57.0X3	T57.0X4	—	—
gluconate	T49.0X1	T49.0X2	T49.0X3	T49.0X4	T49.0X5	T49.0…
oleate	T49.0X1	T49.0X2	T49.0X3	T49.0X4	T49.0X5	T49.0…
sulfate	T56.4X1	T56.4X2	T56.4X3	T56.4X4	—	—
Cuprous sulfate — *see also* Copper sulfate	T56.4X1	T56.4X2	T56.4X3	T56.4X4	—	—
Curare, curarine	T48.1X1	T48.1X2	T48.1X3	T48.1X4	T48.1X5	T48.1…
Cyamemazine	T43.3X1	T43.3X2	T43.3X3	T43.3X4	T43.3X5	T43.3…
Cyamopsis tetragonoloba	T46.6X1	T46.6X2	T46.6X3	T46.6X4	T46.6X5	T46.6…
Cyanacetyl hydrazide	T37.1X1	T37.1X2	T37.1X3	T37.1X4	T37.1X5	T37.1…
Cyanic acid (gas)	T59.891	T59.892	T59.893	T59.894		
Cyanide(s) (compounds) (potassium) (sodium) NEC	T65.0X1	T65.0X2	T65.0X3	T65.0X4	—	—
dust or gas (inhalation) NEC	T57.3X1	T57.3X2	T57.3X3	T57.3X4	—	—
fumigant	T65.0X1	T65.0X2	T65.0X3	T65.0X4	—	—
hydrogen	T57.3X1	T57.3X2	T57.3X3	T57.3X4	—	—
mercuric — *see* Mercury						
pesticide (dust) (fumes)	T65.0X1	T65.0X2	T65.0X3	T65.0X4	—	—
Cyanoacrylate adhesive	T49.3X1	T49.3X2	T49.3X3	T49.3X4	T49.3X5	T49.3…
Cyanocobalamin	T45.8X1	T45.8X2	T45.8X3	T45.8X4	T45.8X5	T45.8…
Cyanogen (chloride) (gas) NEC	T59.891	T59.892	T59.893	T59.894		
Cyclacillin	T36.0X1	T36.0X2	T36.0X3	T36.0X4	T36.0X5	T36.0…
Cyclaine	T41.3X1	T41.3X2	T41.3X3	T41.3X4	T41.3X5	T41.3…
Cyclamate	T50.991	T50.992	T50.993	T50.994	T50.995	T50.9…
Cyclamen europaeum	T62.2X1	T62.2X2	T62.2X3	T62.2X4	—	—
Cyclandelate	T46.7X1	T46.7X2	T46.7X3	T46.7X4	T46.7X5	T46.7…
Cyclazocine	T50.7X1	T50.7X2	T50.7X3	T50.7X4	T50.7X5	T50.7…
Cyclizine	T45.0X1	T45.0X2	T45.0X3	T45.0X4	T45.0X5	T45.0…
Cyclobarbital	T42.3X1	T42.3X2	T42.3X3	T42.3X4	T42.3X5	T42.3…
Cyclobarbitone	T42.3X1	T42.3X2	T42.3X3	T42.3X4	T42.3X5	T42.3…
Cyclobenzaprine	T48.1X1	T48.1X2	T48.1X3	T48.1X4	T48.1X5	T48.1…
Cyclodrine	T44.3X1	T44.3X2	T44.3X3	T44.3X4	T44.3X5	T44.3…
Cycloguanil embonate	T37.2X1	T37.2X2	T37.2X3	T37.2X4	T37.2X5	T37.2…
Cyclohexane	T52.8X1	T52.8X2	T52.8X3	T52.8X4	—	—
Cyclohexanol	T51.8X1	T51.8X2	T51.8X3	T51.8X4	—	—
Cyclohexanone	T52.4X1	T52.4X2	T52.4X3	T52.4X4	—	—
Cycloheximide	T60.3X1	T60.3X2	T60.3X3	T60.3X4	—	—
Cyclohexyl acetate	T52.8X1	T52.8X2	T52.8X3	T52.8X4	—	—
Cycloleucin	T45.1X1	T45.1X2	T45.1X3	T45.1X4	T45.1X5	T45.1…
Cyclomethycaine	T41.3X1	T41.3X2	T41.3X3	T41.3X4	T41.3X5	T41.3…
Cyclopentamine	T44.4X1	T44.4X2	T44.4X3	T44.4X4	T44.4X5	T44.4…
Cyclopenthiazide	T50.2X1	T50.2X2	T50.2X3	T50.2X4	T50.2X5	T50.2…
Cyclopentolate	T44.3X1	T44.3X2	T44.3X3	T44.3X4	T44.3X5	T44.3…
Cyclophosphamide	T45.1X1	T45.1X2	T45.1X3	T45.1X4	T45.1X5	T45.1…
Cycloplegic drug	T49.5X1	T49.5X2	T49.5X3	T49.5X4	T49.5X5	T49.5…
Cyclopropane	T41.291	T41.292	T41.293	T41.294	T41.295	T41.2…
Cyclopyrabital	T39.8X1	T39.8X2	T39.8X3	T39.8X4	T39.8X5	T39.8…
Cycloserine	T37.1X1	T37.1X2	T37.1X3	T37.1X4	T37.1X5	T37.1…
Cyclosporin	T45.1X1	T45.1X2	T45.1X3	T45.1X4	T45.1X5	T45.1…
Cyclothiazide	T50.2X1	T50.2X2	T50.2X3	T50.2X4	T50.2X5	T50.2…
Cycrimine	T44.3X1	T44.3X2	T44.3X3	T44.3X4	T44.3X5	T44.3…
Cyhalothrin	T60.1X1	T60.1X2	T60.1X3	T60.1X4	—	—
Cymarin	T46.0X1	T46.0X2	T46.0X3	T46.0X4	T46.0X5	T46.0…
Cypermethrin	T60.1X1	T60.1X2	T60.1X3	T60.1X4	—	—
Cyphenothrin	T60.2X1	T60.2X2	T60.2X3	T60.2X4	—	—
Cyproheptadine	T45.0X1	T45.0X2	T45.0X3	T45.0X4	T45.0X5	T45.0…
Cyproterone	T38.6X1	T38.6X2	T38.6X3	T38.6X4	T38.6X5	T38.6…
Cysteamine	T50.6X1	T50.6X2	T50.6X3	T50.6X4	T50.6X5	T50.6…
Cytarabine	T45.1X1	T45.1X2	T45.1X3	T45.1X4	T45.1X5	T45.1…
Cytisus						
laburnum	T62.2X1	T62.2X2	T62.2X3	T62.2X4	—	—
scoparius	T62.2X1	T62.2X2	T62.2X3	T62.2X4	—	—
Cytochrome C	T47.5X1	T47.5X2	T47.5X3	T47.5X4	T47.5X5	T47.5…
Cytomel	T38.1X1	T38.1X2	T38.1X3	T38.1X4	T38.1X5	T38.1…
Cytosine arabinoside	T45.1X1	T45.1X2	T45.1X3	T45.1X4	T45.1X5	T45.1…
Cytoxan	T45.1X1	T45.1X2	T45.1X3	T45.1X4	T45.1X5	T45.1…
Cytozyme	T45.7X1	T45.7X2	T45.7X3	T45.7X4	T45.7X5	T45.7…
S-Carboxymethylcysteine	T48.4X1	T48.4X2	T48.4X3	T48.4X4	T48.4X5	T48.4…
Dacarbazine	T45.1X1	T45.1X2	T45.1X3	T45.1X4	T45.1X5	T45.1…
Dactinomycin	T45.1X1	T45.1X2	T45.1X3	T45.1X4	T45.1X5	T45.1…
DADPS	T37.1X1	T37.1X2	T37.1X3	T37.1X4	T37.1X5	T37.1…

Substance	Poisoning, Accidental (unintentional)	Poisoning, Intentional Self-harm	Poisoning, Assault	Poisoning, Undetermined	Adverse Effect	Under-dosing
Dakin's solution	T49.0X1	T49.0X2	T49.0X3	T49.0X4	T49.0X5	T49.0X6
Dalapon (sodium)	T60.3X1	T60.3X2	T60.3X3	T60.3X4	—	—
Dalmane	T42.4X1	T42.4X2	T42.4X3	T42.4X4	T42.4X5	T42.4X6
Danazol	T38.6X1	T38.6X2	T38.6X3	T38.6X4	T38.6X5	T38.6X6
Danilone	T45.511	T45.512	T45.513	T45.514	T45.515	T45.516
Danthron	T47.2X1	T47.2X2	T47.2X3	T47.2X4	T47.2X5	T47.2X6
Dantrolene	T42.8X1	T42.8X2	T42.8X3	T42.8X4	T42.8X5	T42.8X6
Dantron	T47.2X1	T47.2X2	T47.2X3	T47.2X4	T47.2X5	T47.2X6
Daphne (gnidium) (mezereum)	T62.2X1	T62.2X2	T62.2X3	T62.2X4	—	—
berry	T62.1X1	T62.1X2	T62.1X3	T62.1X4	—	—
Dapsone	T37.1X1	T37.1X2	T37.1X3	T37.1X4	T37.1X5	T37.1X6
Daraprim	T37.2X1	T37.2X2	T37.2X3	T37.2X4	T37.2X5	T37.2X6
Darnel	T62.2X1	T62.2X2	T62.2X3	T62.2X4	—	—
Darvon	T39.8X1	T39.8X2	T39.8X3	T39.8X4	T39.8X5	T39.8X6
Daunomycin	T45.1X1	T45.1X2	T45.1X3	T45.1X4	T45.1X5	T45.1X6
Daunorubicin	T45.1X1	T45.1X2	T45.1X3	T45.1X4	T45.1X5	T45.1X6
DBI	T38.3X1	T38.3X2	T38.3X3	T38.3X4	T38.3X5	T38.3X6
D-Con	T60.91	T60.92	T60.93	T60.94	—	—
insecticide	T60.2X1	T60.2X2	T60.2X3	T60.2X4	—	—
rodenticide	T60.4X1	T60.4X2	T60.4X3	T60.4X4	—	—
DDAVP	T38.891	T38.892	T38.893	T38.894	T38.895	T38.896
DDE (bis(chlorophenyl)-dichloroethylene)	T60.2X1	T60.2X2	T60.2X3	T60.2X4	—	—
DDS	T37.1X1	T37.1X2	T37.1X3	T37.1X4	T37.1X5	T37.1X6
DDT (dust)	T60.1X1	T60.1X2	T60.1X3	T60.1X4	—	—
Deadly nightshade — see also Belladonna	T62.2X1	T62.2X2	T62.2X3	T62.2X4	—	—
berry	T62.1X1	T62.1X2	T62.1X3	T62.1X4	—	—
Deamino-D-arginine vasopressin	T38.891	T38.892	T38.893	T38.894	T38.895	T38.896
Deanol (aceglumate)	T50.991	T50.992	T50.993	T50.994	T50.995	T50.996
Debrisoquine	T46.5X1	T46.5X2	T46.5X3	T46.5X4	T46.5X5	T46.5X6
Decaborane	T57.8X1	T57.8X2	T57.8X3	T57.8X4	—	—
fumes	T59.891	T59.892	T59.893	T59.894	—	—
Decadron	T38.0X1	T38.0X2	T38.0X3	T38.0X4	T38.0X5	T38.0X6
ENT agent	T49.6X1	T49.6X2	T49.6X3	T49.6X4	T49.6X5	T49.6X6
ophthalmic preparation	T49.5X1	T49.5X2	T49.5X3	T49.5X4	T49.5X5	T49.5X6
topical NEC	T49.0X1	T49.0X2	T49.0X3	T49.0X4	T49.0X5	T49.0X6
Decahydronaphthalene	T52.8X1	T52.8X2	T52.8X3	T52.8X4	—	—
Decalin	T52.8X1	T52.8X2	T52.8X3	T52.8X4	—	—
Decamethonium (bromide)	T48.1X1	T48.1X2	T48.1X3	T48.1X4	T48.1X5	T48.1X6
Dccholin	T47.5X1	T47.5X2	T47.5X3	T47.5X4	T47.5X5	T47.5X6
Declomycin	T36.4X1	T36.4X2	T36.4X3	T36.4X4	T36.4X5	T36.4X6
Decongestant, nasal (mucosa)	T48.5X1	T48.5X2	T48.5X3	T48.5X4	T48.5X5	T48.5X6
combination	T48.5X1	T48.5X2	T48.5X3	T48.5X4	T48.5X5	T48.5X6
Deet	T60.8X1	T60.8X2	T60.8X3	T60.8X4	—	—
Deferoxamine	T45.8X1	T45.8X2	T45.8X3	T45.8X4	T45.8X5	T45.8X6
Deflazacort	T38.0X1	T38.0X2	T38.0X3	T38.0X4	T38.0X5	T38.0X6
Deglycyrrhizinized extract of licorice	T48.4X1	T48.4X2	T48.4X3	T48.4X4	T48.4X5	T48.4X6
Dehydrocholic acid	T47.5X1	T47.5X2	T47.5X3	T47.5X4	T47.5X5	T47.5X6
Dehydroemetine	T37.3X1	T37.3X2	T37.3X3	T37.3X4	T37.3X5	T37.3X6
Dekalin	T52.8X1	T52.8X2	T52.8X3	T52.8X4	—	—
Delalutin	T38.5X1	T38.5X2	T38.5X3	T38.5X4	T38.5X5	T38.5X6
Delorazepam	T42.4X1	T42.4X2	T42.4X3	T42.4X4	T42.4X5	T42.4X6
Delphinium	T62.2X1	T62.2X2	T62.2X3	T62.2X4	—	—
Deltamethrin	T60.1X1	T60.1X2	T60.1X3	T60.1X4	—	—
Deltasone	T38.0X1	T38.0X2	T38.0X3	T38.0X4	T38.0X5	T38.0X6
Deltra	T38.0X1	T38.0X2	T38.0X3	T38.0X4	T38.0X5	T38.0X6
Delvinal	T42.3X1	T42.3X2	T42.3X3	T42.3X4	T42.3X5	T42.3X6
Demecarium (bromide)	T49.5X1	T49.5X2	T49.5X3	T49.5X4	T49.5X5	T49.5X6
Demeclocycline	T36.4X1	T36.4X2	T36.4X3	T36.4X4	T36.4X5	T36.4X6
Demecolcine	T45.1X1	T45.1X2	T45.1X3	T45.1X4	T45.1X5	T45.1X6
Demegestone	T38.5X1	T38.5X2	T38.5X3	T38.5X4	T38.5X5	T38.5X6
Demelanizing agents	T49.8X1	T49.8X2	T49.8X3	T49.8X4	T49.8X5	T49.8X6
Demephion -O and -S	T60.0X1	T60.0X2	T60.0X3	T60.0X4	—	—
Demerol	T40.2X1	T40.2X2	T40.2X3	T40.2X4	T40.2X5	T40.2X6
Demethylchlortetracycline	T36.4X1	T36.4X2	T36.4X3	T36.4X4	T36.4X5	T36.4X6
Demethyltetracycline	T36.4X1	T36.4X2	T36.4X3	T36.4X4	T36.4X5	T36.4X6
Demeton -O and -S	T60.0X1	T60.0X2	T60.0X3	T60.0X4	—	—
Demulcent (external)	T49.3X1	T49.3X2	T49.3X3	T49.3X4	T49.3X5	T49.3X6
specified NEC	T49.3X1	T49.3X2	T49.3X3	T49.3X4	T49.3X5	T49.3X6
Demulen	T38.4X1	T38.4X2	T38.4X3	T38.4X4	T38.4X5	T38.4X6
Denatured alcohol	T51.0X1	T51.0X2	T51.0X3	T51.0X4	—	—
Dendrid	T49.5X1	T49.5X2	T49.5X3	T49.5X4	T49.5X5	T49.5X6
Dental drug, topical application NEC	T49.7X1	T49.7X2	T49.7X3	T49.7X4	T49.7X5	T49.7X6
Dentifrice	T49.7X1	T49.7X2	T49.7X3	T49.7X4	T49.7X5	T49.7X6
Deodorant spray (feminine hygiene)	T49.8X1	T49.8X2	T49.8X3	T49.8X4	T49.8X5	T49.8X6
Deoxycortone	T50.0X1	T50.0X2	T50.0X3	T50.0X4	T50.0X5	T50.0X6

Substance	Poisoning, Accidental (unintentional)	Poisoning, Intentional Self-harm	Poisoning, Assault	Poisoning, Undetermined	Adverse Effect	Under-dosing
Deoxyribonuclease (pancreatic)	T45.3X1	T45.3X2	T45.3X3	T45.3X4	T45.3X5	T45.3X6
Depilatory	T49.4X1	T49.4X2	T49.4X3	T49.4X4	T49.4X5	T49.4X6
Deprenalin	T42.8X1	T42.8X2	T42.8X3	T42.8X4	T42.8X5	T42.8X6
Deprenyl	T42.8X1	T42.8X2	T42.8X3	T42.8X4	T42.8X5	T42.8X6
Depressant						
appetite (central)	T50.5X1	T50.5X2	T50.5X3	T50.5X4	T50.5X5	T50.5X6
cardiac	T46.2X1	T46.2X2	T46.2X3	T46.2X4	T46.2X5	T46.2X6
central nervous system (anesthetic) — see also Central nervous system, depressants	T42.71	T42.72	T42.73	T42.74	T42.75	T42.76
general anesthetic	T41.201	T41.202	T41.203	T41.204	T41.205	T41.206
muscle tone	T42.8X1	T42.8X2	T42.8X3	T42.8X4	T42.8X5	T42.8X6
muscle tone, central	T42.8X1	T42.8X2	T42.8X3	T42.8X4	T42.8X5	T42.8X6
psychotherapeutic	T43.501	T43.502	T43.503	T43.504	T43.505	T43.506
Depressant, appetite	T50.5X1	T50.5X2	T50.5X3	T50.5X4	T50.5X5	T50.5X6
Deptropine	T45.0X1	T45.0X2	T45.0X3	T45.0X4	T45.0X5	T45.0X6
Dequalinium (chloride)	T49.0X1	T49.0X2	T49.0X3	T49.0X4	T49.0X5	T49.0X6
Derris root	T60.2X1	T60.2X2	T60.2X3	T60.2X4	—	—
Deserpidine	T46.5X1	T46.5X2	T46.5X3	T46.5X4	T46.5X5	T46.5X6
Desferrioxamine	T45.8X1	T45.8X2	T45.8X3	T45.8X4	T45.8X5	T45.8X6
Desipramine	T43.011	T43.012	T43.013	T43.014	T43.015	T43.016
Deslanoside	T46.0X1	T46.0X2	T46.0X3	T46.0X4	T46.0X5	T46.0X6
Desloughing agent	T49.4X1	T49.4X2	T49.4X3	T49.4X4	T49.4X5	T49.4X6
Desmethylimipramine	T43.011	T43.012	T43.013	T43.014	T43.015	T43.016
Desmopressin	T38.891	T38.892	T38.893	T38.894	T38.895	T38.896
Desocodeine	T40.2X1	T40.2X2	T40.2X3	T40.2X4	T40.2X5	T40.2X6
Desogestrel	T38.5X1	T38.5X2	T38.5X3	T38.5X4	T38.5X5	T38.5X6
Desomorphine	T40.2X1	T40.2X2	T40.2X3	T40.2X4	—	—
Desonide	T49.0X1	T49.0X2	T49.0X3	T49.0X4	T49.0X5	T49.0X6
Desoximetasone	T49.0X1	T49.0X2	T49.0X3	T49.0X4	T49.0X5	T49.0X6
Desoxycorticosteroid	T50.0X1	T50.0X2	T50.0X3	T50.0X4	T50.0X5	T50.0X6
Desoxycortone	T50.0X1	T50.0X2	T50.0X3	T50.0X4	T50.0X5	T50.0X6
Desoxyephedrine	T43.621	T43.622	T43.623	T43.624	T43.625	T43.626
Detaxtran	T46.6X1	T46.6X2	T46.6X3	T46.6X4	T46.6X5	T46.6X6
Detergent	T49.2X1	T49.2X2	T49.2X3	T49.2X4	T49.2X5	T49.2X6
external medication	T49.2X1	T49.2X2	T49.2X3	T49.2X4	T49.2X5	T49.2X6
local	T49.2X1	T49.2X2	T49.2X3	T49.2X4	T49.2X5	T49.2X6
medicinal	T49.2X1	T49.2X2	T49.2X3	T49.2X4	T49.2X5	T49.2X6
nonmedicinal	T55.1X1	T55.1X2	T55.1X3	T55.1X4	—	—
specified NEC	T55.1X1	T55.1X2	T55.1X3	T55.1X4	—	—
Deterrent, alcohol	T50.6X1	T50.6X2	T50.6X3	T50.6X4	T50.6X5	T50.6X6
Detoxifying agent	T50.6X1	T50.6X2	T50.6X3	T50.6X4	T50.6X5	T50.6X6
Detrothyronine	T38.1X1	T38.1X2	T38.1X3	T38.1X4	T38.1X5	T38.1X6
Dettol (external medication)	T49.0X1	T49.0X2	T49.0X3	T49.0X4	T49.0X5	T49.0X6
Dexamethasone	T38.0X1	T38.0X2	T38.0X3	T38.0X4	T38.0X5	T38.0X6
ENT agent	T49.6X1	T49.6X2	T49.6X3	T49.6X4	T49.6X5	T49.6X6
ophthalmic preparation	T49.5X1	T49.5X2	T49.5X3	T49.5X4	T49.5X5	T49.5X6
topical NEC	T49.0X1	T49.0X2	T49.0X3	T49.0X4	T49.0X5	T49.0X6
Dexamfetamine	T43.621	T43.622	T43.623	T43.624	T43.625	T43.626
Dexamphetamine	T43.621	T43.622	T43.623	T43.624	T43.625	T43.626
Dexbrompheniramine	T45.0X1	T45.0X2	T45.0X3	T45.0X4	T45.0X5	T45.0X6
Dexchlorpheniramine	T45.0X1	T45.0X2	T45.0X3	T45.0X4	T45.0X5	T45.0X6
Dexedrine	T43.621	T43.622	T43.623	T43.624	T43.625	T43.626
Dexetimide	T44.3X1	T44.3X2	T44.3X3	T44.3X4	T44.3X5	T44.3X6
Dexfenfluramine	T50.5X1	T50.5X2	T50.5X3	T50.5X4	T50.5X5	T50.5X6
Dexpanthenol	T45.2X1	T45.2X2	T45.2X3	T45.2X4	T45.2X5	T45.2X6
Dextran (40) (70) (150)	T45.8X1	T45.8X2	T45.8X3	T45.8X4	T45.8X5	T45.8X6
Dextriferron	T45.4X1	T45.4X2	T45.4X3	T45.4X4	T45.4X5	T45.4X6
Dextroamphetamine	T43.621	T43.622	T43.623	T43.624	T43.625	T43.626
Dextro calcium pantothenate	T45.2X1	T45.2X2	T45.2X3	T45.2X4	T45.2X5	T45.2X6
Dextromethorphan	T48.3X1	T48.3X2	T48.3X3	T48.3X4	T48.3X5	T48.3X6
Dextromoramide	T40.4X1	T40.4X2	T40.4X3	T40.4X4	—	—
topical	T49.8X1	T49.8X2	T49.8X3	T49.8X4	T49.8X5	T49.8X6
Dextro pantothenyl alcohol	T45.2X1	T45.2X2	T45.2X3	T45.2X4	T45.2X5	T45.2X6
Dextropropoxyphene	T40.4X1	T40.4X2	T40.4X3	T40.4X4	T40.4X5	T40.4X6
Dextrorphan	T40.2X1	T40.2X2	T40.2X3	T40.2X4	T40.2X5	T40.2X6
Dextrose	T50.3X1	T50.3X2	T50.3X3	T50.3X4	T50.3X5	T50.3X6
concentrated solution, intravenous	T46.8X1	T46.8X2	T46.8X3	T46.8X4	T46.8X5	T46.8X6
Dextrothyroxin	T38.1X1	T38.1X2	T38.1X3	T38.1X4	T38.1X5	T38.1X6
Dextrothyroxine sodium	T38.1X1	T38.1X2	T38.1X3	T38.1X4	T38.1X5	T38.1X6
DFP	T44.0X1	T44.0X2	T44.0X3	T44.0X4	T44.0X5	T44.0X6
DHE	T37.3X1	T37.3X2	T37.3X3	T37.3X4	T37.3X5	T37.3X6
45	T46.5X1	T46.5X2	T46.5X3	T46.5X4	T46.5X5	T46.5X6
Diabinese	T38.3X1	T38.3X2	T38.3X3	T38.3X4	T38.3X5	T38.3X6
Diacetone alcohol	T52.4X1	T52.4X2	T52.4X3	T52.4X4	—	—
Diacetyl monoxime	T50.991	T50.992	T50.993	T50.994	—	—
Diacetylmorphine	T40.1X1	T40.1X2	T40.1X3	T40.1X4	—	—
Diachylon plaster	T49.4X1	T49.4X2	T49.4X3	T49.4X4	T49.4X5	T49.4X6

Substance	Poisoning, Accidental (unintentional)	Poisoning, Intentional Self-harm	Poisoning, Assault	Poisoning, Undetermined	Adverse Effect	Under-dosing
Diaethylstilboestrolum	T38.5X1	T38.5X2	T38.5X3	T38.5X4	T38.5X5	T38.5X6
Diagnostic agent NEC	T50.8X1	T50.8X2	T50.8X3	T50.8X4	T50.8X5	T50.8X6
Dial (soap)	T49.2X1	T49.2X2	T49.2X3	T49.2X4	T49.2X5	T49.2X6
sedative	T42.3X1	T42.3X2	T42.3X3	T42.3X4	T42.3X5	T42.3X6
Dialkyl carbonate	T52.91	T52.92	T52.93	T52.94	—	—
Diallylbarbituric acid	T42.3X1	T42.3X2	T42.3X3	T42.3X4	T42.3X5	T42.3X6
Diallymal	T42.3X1	T42.3X2	T42.3X3	T42.3X4	T42.3X5	T42.3X6
Dialysis solution (intraperitoneal)	T50.3X1	T50.3X2	T50.3X3	T50.3X4	T50.3X5	T50.3X6
Diaminodiphenylsulfone	T37.1X1	T37.1X2	T37.1X3	T37.1X4	T37.1X5	T37.1X6
Diamorphine	T40.1X1	T40.1X2	T40.1X3	T40.1X4	—	—
Diamox	T50.2X1	T50.2X2	T50.2X3	T50.2X4	T50.2X5	T50.2X6
Diamthazole	T49.0X1	T49.0X2	T49.0X3	T49.0X4	T49.0X5	T49.0X6
Dianthone	T47.2X1	T47.2X2	T47.2X3	T47.2X4	T47.2X5	T47.2X6
Diaphenylsulfone	T37.0X1	T37.0X2	T37.0X3	T37.0X4	T37.0X5	T37.0X6
Diasone (sodium)	T37.1X1	T37.1X2	T37.1X3	T37.1X4	T37.1X5	T37.1X6
Diastase	T47.5X1	T47.5X2	T47.5X3	T47.5X4	T47.5X5	T47.5X6
Diatrizoate	T50.8X1	T50.8X2	T50.8X3	T50.8X4	T50.8X5	T50.8X6
Diazepam	T42.4X1	T42.4X2	T42.4X3	T42.4X4	T42.4X5	T42.4X6
Diazinon	T60.0X1	T60.0X2	T60.0X3	T60.0X4	—	—
Diazomethane (gas)	T59.891	T59.892	T59.893	T59.894	—	—
Diazoxide	T46.5X1	T46.5X2	T46.5X3	T46.5X4	T46.5X5	T46.5X6
Dibekacin	T36.5X1	T36.5X2	T36.5X3	T36.5X4	T36.5X5	T36.5X6
Dibenamine	T44.6X1	T44.6X2	T44.6X3	T44.6X4	T44.6X5	T44.6X6
Dibenzepin	T43.011	T43.012	T43.013	T43.014	T43.015	T43.016
Dibenzheptropine	T45.0X1	T45.0X2	T45.0X3	T45.0X4	T45.0X5	T45.0X6
Dibenzyline	T44.6X1	T44.6X2	T44.6X3	T44.6X4	T44.6X5	T44.6X6
Diborane (gas)	T59.891	T59.892	T59.893	T59.894	—	—
Dibromochloropropane	T60.8X1	T60.8X2	T60.8X3	T60.8X4	—	—
Dibromodulcitol	T45.1X1	T45.1X2	T45.1X3	T45.1X4	T45.1X5	T45.1X6
Dibromoethane	T53.6X1	T53.6X2	T53.6X3	T53.6X4	—	—
Dibromomannitol	T45.1X1	T45.1X2	T45.1X3	T45.1X4	T45.1X5	T45.1X6
Dibromopropamidine isethionate	T49.0X1	T49.0X2	T49.0X3	T49.0X4	T49.0X5	T49.0X6
Dibrompropamidine	T49.0X1	T49.0X2	T49.0X3	T49.0X4	T49.0X5	T49.0X6
Dibucaine	T41.3X1	T41.3X2	T41.3X3	T41.3X4	T41.3X5	T41.3X6
topical (surface)	T41.3X1	T41.3X2	T41.3X3	T41.3X4	T41.3X5	T41.3X6
Dibunate sodium	T48.3X1	T48.3X2	T48.3X3	T48.3X4	T48.3X5	T48.3X6
Dibutoline sulfate	T44.3X1	T44.3X2	T44.3X3	T44.3X4	T44.3X5	T44.3X6
Dicamba	T60.3X1	T60.3X2	T60.3X3	T60.3X4	—	—
Dicapthon	T60.0X1	T60.0X2	T60.0X3	T60.0X4	—	—
Dichlobenil	T60.3X1	T60.3X2	T60.3X3	T60.3X4	—	—
Dichlone	T60.3X1	T60.3X2	T60.3X3	T60.3X4	—	—
Dichloralphenozone	T42.6X1	T42.6X2	T42.6X3	T42.6X4	T42.6X5	T42.6X6
Dichlorbenzidine	T65.3X1	T65.3X2	T65.3X3	T65.3X4	—	—
Dichlorhydrin	T52.8X1	T52.8X2	T52.8X3	T52.8X4	—	—
Dichlorhydroxyquinoline	T37.8X1	T37.8X2	T37.8X3	T37.8X4	T37.8X5	T37.8X6
Dichlorobenzene	T53.7X1	T53.7X2	T53.7X3	T53.7X4	—	—
Dichlorobenzyl alcohol	T49.6X1	T49.6X2	T49.6X3	T49.6X4	T49.6X5	T49.6X6
Dichlorodifluoromethane	T53.5X1	T53.5X2	T53.5X3	T53.5X4	—	—
Dichloroethane	T52.8X1	T52.8X2	T52.8X3	T52.8X4	—	—
Dichloroethylene	T53.6X1	T53.6X2	T53.6X3	T53.6X4	—	—
Dichloroethyl sulfide, not in war	T59.891	T59.892	T59.893	T59.894		
Dichloroformoxine, not in war	T59.891	T59.892	T59.893	T59.894		
Dichlorohydrin, alpha-dichlorohydrin	T52.8X1	T52.8X2	T52.8X3	T52.8X4		
Dichloromethane (solvent)	T53.4X1	T53.4X2	T53.4X3	T53.4X4	—	—
vapor	T53.4X1	T53.4X2	T53.4X3	T53.4X4	—	—
Dichloronaphthoquinone	T60.3X1	T60.3X2	T60.3X3	T60.3X4	—	—
Dichlorophen	T37.4X1	T37.4X2	T37.4X3	T37.4X4	T37.4X5	T37.4X6
Dichloropropene	T60.3X1	T60.3X2	T60.3X3	T60.3X4	—	—
Dichloropropionic acid	T60.3X1	T60.3X2	T60.3X3	T60.3X4	—	—
Dichlorphenamide	T50.2X1	T50.2X2	T50.2X3	T50.2X4	T50.2X5	T50.2X6
Dichlorvos	T60.0X1	T60.0X2	T60.0X3	T60.0X4	—	—
Diclofenac	T39.391	T39.392	T39.393	T39.394	T39.395	T39.396
Diclofenamide	T50.2X1	T50.2X2	T50.2X3	T50.2X4	T50.2X5	T50.2X6
Diclofensine	T43.291	T43.292	T43.293	T43.294	T43.295	T43.296
Diclonixine	T39.8X1	T39.8X2	T39.8X3	T39.8X4	T39.8X5	T39.8X6
Dicloxacillin	T36.0X1	T36.0X2	T36.0X3	T36.0X4	T36.0X5	T36.0X6
Dicophane	T49.0X1	T49.0X2	T49.0X3	T49.0X4	T49.0X5	T49.0X6
Dicoumarol, dicoumarin, dicumarol	T45.511	T45.512	T45.513	T45.514	T45.515	T45.516
Dicrotophos	T60.0X1	T60.0X2	T60.0X3	T60.0X4	—	—
Dicyanogen (gas)	T65.0X1	T65.0X2	T65.0X3	T65.0X4	—	—
Dicyclomine	T44.3X1	T44.3X2	T44.3X3	T44.3X4	T44.3X5	T44.3X6
Dicycloverine	T44.3X1	T44.3X2	T44.3X3	T44.3X4	T44.3X5	T44.3X6
Dideoxycytidine	T37.5X1	T37.5X2	T37.5X3	T37.5X4	T37.5X5	T37.5X6
Dideoxyinosine	T37.5X1	T37.5X2	T37.5X3	T37.5X4	T37.5X5	T37.5X6
Dieldrin (vapor)	T60.1X1	T60.1X2	T60.1X3	T60.1X4	—	—
Diemal	T42.3X1	T42.3X2	T42.3X3	T42.3X4	T42.3X5	T42.3X6
Dienestrol	T38.5X1	T38.5X2	T38.5X3	T38.5X4	T38.5X5	T38.5X6

Substance	Poisoning, Accidental (unintentional)	Poisoning, Intentional Self-harm	Poisoning, Assault	Poisoning, Undetermined	Adverse Effect	Under-dosing
Dienoestrol	T38.5X1	T38.5X2	T38.5X3	T38.5X4	T38.5X5	T38.5X6
Dietetic drug NEC	T50.901	T50.902	T50.903	T50.904	T50.905	T50.9
Diethazine	T42.8X1	T42.8X2	T42.8X3	T42.8X4	T42.8X5	T42.8
Diethyl						
barbituric acid	T42.3X1	T42.3X2	T42.3X3	T42.3X4	T42.3X5	T42.3
carbamazine	T37.4X1	T37.4X2	T37.4X3	T37.4X4	T37.4X5	T37.4
carbinol	T51.3X1	T51.3X2	T51.3X3	T51.3X4	—	—
carbonate	T52.8X1	T52.8X2	T52.8X3	T52.8X4	—	—
ether (vapor) — see also ether	T41.0X1	T41.0X2	T41.0X3	T41.0X4	T41.0X5	T41.0
oxide	T52.8X1	T52.8X2	T52.8X3	T52.8X4	—	—
propion	T50.5X1	T50.5X2	T50.5X3	T50.5X4	T50.5X5	T50.5
stilbestrol	T38.5X1	T38.5X2	T38.5X3	T38.5X4	T38.5X5	T38.5
toluamide (nonmedicinal)	T60.8X1	T60.8X2	T60.8X3	T60.8X4	—	—
medicinal	T49.3X1	T49.3X2	T49.3X3	T49.3X4	T49.3X5	T49.3
Diethylcarbamazine	T37.4X1	T37.4X2	T37.4X3	T37.4X4	T37.4X5	T37.4
Diethylene						
dioxide	T52.8X1	T52.8X2	T52.8X3	T52.8X4	—	—
glycol (monoacetate) (monobutyl ether) (monoethyl ether)	T52.3X1	T52.3X2	T52.3X3	T52.3X4	—	—
Diethylhexylphthalate	T65.891	T65.892	T65.893	T65.894	—	—
Diethylpropion	T50.5X1	T50.5X2	T50.5X3	T50.5X4	T50.5X5	T50.5
Diethylstilbestrol	T38.5X1	T38.5X2	T38.5X3	T38.5X4	T38.5X5	T38.5
Diethylstilboestrol	T38.5X1	T38.5X2	T38.5X3	T38.5X4	T38.5X5	T38.5
Diethylsulfone-diethylmethane	T42.6X1	T42.6X2	T42.6X3	T42.6X4	T42.6X5	T42.6
Diethyltoluamide	T49.0X1	T49.0X2	T49.0X3	T49.0X4	T49.0X5	T49.0
Diethyltryptamine (DET)	T40.991	T40.992	T40.993	T40.994	—	—
Difebarbamate	T42.3X1	T42.3X2	T42.3X3	T42.3X4	T42.3X5	T42.3
Difencloxazine	T40.2X1	T40.2X2	T40.2X3	T40.2X4	T40.2X5	T40.2
Difenidol	T45.0X1	T45.0X2	T45.0X3	T45.0X4	T45.0X5	T45.0
Difenoxin	T47.6X1	T47.6X2	T47.6X3	T47.6X4	T47.6X5	T47.6
Difetarsone	T37.3X1	T37.3X2	T37.3X3	T37.3X4	T37.3X5	T37.3
Diffusin	T45.3X1	T45.3X2	T45.3X3	T45.3X4	T45.3X5	T45.3
Diflorasone	T49.0X1	T49.0X2	T49.0X3	T49.0X4	T49.0X5	T49.0
Diflos	T44.0X1	T44.0X2	T44.0X3	T44.0X4	T44.0X5	T44.0
Diflubenzuron	T60.1X1	T60.1X2	T60.1X3	T60.1X4	—	—
Diflucortolone	T49.0X1	T49.0X2	T49.0X3	T49.0X4	T49.0X5	T49.0
Diflunisal	T39.091	T39.092	T39.093	T39.094	T39.095	T39.0
Difluoromethyldopa	T42.8X1	T42.8X2	T42.8X3	T42.8X4	T42.8X5	T42.8
Difluorophate	T44.0X1	T44.0X2	T44.0X3	T44.0X4	T44.0X5	T44.0
Digestant NEC	T47.5X1	T47.5X2	T47.5X3	T47.5X4	T47.5X5	T47.5
Digitalin (e)	T46.0X1	T46.0X2	T46.0X3	T46.0X4	T46.0X5	T46.0
Digitalis (leaf)(glycoside)	T46.0X1	T46.0X2	T46.0X3	T46.0X4	T46.0X5	T46.0
lanata	T46.0X1	T46.0X2	T46.0X3	T46.0X4	T46.0X5	T46.0
purpurea	T46.0X1	T46.0X2	T46.0X3	T46.0X4	T46.0X5	T46.0
Digitoxin	T46.0X1	T46.0X2	T46.0X3	T46.0X4	T46.0X5	T46.0
Digitoxose	T46.0X1	T46.0X2	T46.0X3	T46.0X4	T46.0X5	T46.0
Digoxin	T46.0X1	T46.0X2	T46.0X3	T46.0X4	T46.0X5	T46.0
Digoxine	T46.0X1	T46.0X2	T46.0X3	T46.0X4	T46.0X5	T46.0
Dihydralazine	T46.5X1	T46.5X2	T46.5X3	T46.5X4	T46.5X5	T46.5
Dihydrazine	T46.5X1	T46.5X2	T46.5X3	T46.5X4	T46.5X5	T46.5
Dihydrocodeine	T40.2X1	T40.2X2	T40.2X3	T40.2X4	T40.2X5	T40.2
Dihydrocodeinone	T40.2X1	T40.2X2	T40.2X3	T40.2X4	T40.2X5	T40.2
Dihydroergocornine	T46.7X1	T46.7X2	T46.7X3	T46.7X4	T46.7X5	T46.7
Dihydroergocristine (mesilate)	T46.7X1	T46.7X2	T46.7X3	T46.7X4	T46.7X5	T46.7
Dihydroergokryptine	T46.7X1	T46.7X2	T46.7X3	T46.7X4	T46.7X5	T46.7
Dihydroergotamine	T46.5X1	T46.5X2	T46.5X3	T46.5X4	T46.5X5	T46.5
Dihydroergotoxine	T46.7X1	T46.7X2	T46.7X3	T46.7X4	T46.7X5	T46.7
mesilate	T46.7X1	T46.7X2	T46.7X3	T46.7X4	T46.7X5	T46.7
Dihydrohydroxycodeinone	T40.2X1	T40.2X2	T40.2X3	T40.2X4	T40.2X5	T40.2
Dihydrohydroxymorphinone	T40.2X1	T40.2X2	T40.2X3	T40.2X4	T40.2X5	T40.2
Dihydroisocodeine	T40.2X1	T40.2X2	T40.2X3	T40.2X4	T40.2X5	T40.2
Dihydromorphine	T40.2X1	T40.2X2	T40.2X3	T40.2X4		
Dihydromorphinone	T40.2X1	T40.2X2	T40.2X3	T40.2X4	T40.2X5	T40.2
Dihydrostreptomycin	T36.5X1	T36.5X2	T36.5X3	T36.5X4	T36.5X5	T36.5
Dihydrotachysterol	T45.2X1	T45.2X2	T45.2X3	T45.2X4	T45.2X5	T45.2
Dihydroxyaluminum aminoacetate	T47.1X1	T47.1X2	T47.1X3	T47.1X4	T47.1X5	T47.1
Dihydroxyaluminum sodium carbonate	T47.1X1	T47.1X2	T47.1X3	T47.1X4	T47.1X5	T47.12
Dihydroxyanthraquinone	T47.2X1	T47.2X2	T47.2X3	T47.2X4	T47.2X5	T47.2
Dihydroxycodeinone	T40.2X1	T40.2X2	T40.2X3	T40.2X4	T40.2X5	T40.2
Dihydroxypropyl theophylline	T50.2X1	T50.2X2	T50.2X3	T50.2X4	T50.2X5	T50.2
Diiodohydroxyquin	T37.8X1	T37.8X2	T37.8X3	T37.8X4	T37.8X5	T37.8
topical	T49.0X1	T49.0X2	T49.0X3	T49.0X4	T49.0X5	T49.0
Diiodohydroxyquinoline	T37.8X1	T37.8X2	T37.8X3	T37.8X4	T37.8X5	T37.8
Diiodotyrosine	T38.2X1	T38.2X2	T38.2X3	T38.2X4	T38.2X5	T38.2
Diisopromine	T44.3X1	T44.3X2	T44.3X3	T44.3X4	T44.3X5	T44.3
Diisopropylamine	T46.3X1	T46.3X2	T46.3X3	T46.3X4	T46.3X5	T46.3
Diisopropylfluorophosphonate	T44.0X1	T44.0X2	T44.0X3	T44.0X4	T44.0X5	T44.0

Substance	Poisoning, Accidental (unintentional)	Poisoning, Intentional Self-harm	Poisoning, Assault	Poisoning, Undetermined	Adverse Effect	Under-dosing
Dilantin	T42.0X1	T42.0X2	T42.0X3	T42.0X4	T42.0X5	T42.0X6
Dilaudid	T40.2X1	T40.2X2	T40.2X3	T40.2X4	T40.2X5	T40.2X6
Dilazep	T46.3X1	T46.3X2	T46.3X3	T46.3X4	T46.3X5	T46.3X6
Dill	T47.5X1	T47.5X2	T47.5X3	T47.5X4	T47.5X5	T47.5X6
Diloxanide	T37.3X1	T37.3X2	T37.3X3	T37.3X4	T37.3X5	T37.3X6
Diltiazem	T46.1X1	T46.1X2	T46.1X3	T46.1X4	T46.1X5	T46.1X6
Dimazole	T49.0X1	T49.0X2	T49.0X3	T49.0X4	T49.0X5	T49.0X6
Dimefline	T50.7X1	T50.7X2	T50.7X3	T50.7X4	T50.7X5	T50.7X6
Dimefox	T60.0X1	T60.0X2	T60.0X3	T60.0X4	—	—
Dimemorfan	T48.3X1	T48.3X2	T48.3X3	T48.3X4	T48.3X5	T48.3X6
Dimenhydrinate	T45.0X1	T45.0X2	T45.0X3	T45.0X4	T45.0X5	T45.0X6
Dimercaprol (British anti-lewisite)	T45.8X1	T45.8X2	T45.8X3	T45.8X4	T45.8X5	T45.8X6
Dimercaptopropanol	T45.8X1	T45.8X2	T45.8X3	T45.8X4	T45.8X5	T45.8X6
Dimestrol	T38.5X1	T38.5X2	T38.5X3	T38.5X4	T38.5X5	T38.5X6
Dimetane	T45.0X1	T45.0X2	T45.0X3	T45.0X4	T45.0X5	T45.0X6
Dimethicone	T47.1X1	T47.1X2	T47.1X3	T47.1X4	T47.1X5	T47.1X6
Dimethindene	T45.0X1	T45.0X2	T45.0X3	T45.0X4	T45.0X5	T45.0X6
Dimethisoquin	T49.1X1	T49.1X2	T49.1X3	T49.1X4	T49.1X5	T49.1X6
Dimethisterone	T38.5X1	T38.5X2	T38.5X3	T38.5X4	T38.5X5	T38.5X6
Dimethoate	T60.0X1	T60.0X2	T60.0X3	T60.0X4	—	—
Dimethocaine	T41.3X1	T41.3X2	T41.3X3	T41.3X4	T41.3X5	T41.3X6
Dimethoxanate	T48.3X1	T48.3X2	T48.3X3	T48.3X4	T48.3X5	T48.3X6
Dimethyl						
arsine, arsinic acid	T57.0X1	T57.0X2	T57.0X3	T57.0X4	—	—
carbinol	T51.2X1	T51.2X2	T51.2X3	T51.2X4	—	—
carbonate	T52.8X1	T52.8X2	T52.8X3	T52.8X4	—	—
diguanide	T38.3X1	T38.3X2	T38.3X3	T38.3X4	T38.3X5	T38.3X6
ketone	T52.4X1	T52.4X2	T52.4X3	T52.4X4	—	—
vapor	T52.4X1	T52.4X2	T52.4X3	T52.4X4	—	—
meperidine	T40.2X1	T40.2X2	T40.2X3	T40.2X4	T40.2X5	T40.2X6
parathion	T60.0X1	T60.0X2	T60.0X3	T60.0X4	—	—
phthlate	T49.3X1	T49.3X2	T49.3X3	T49.3X4	T49.3X5	T49.3X6
polysiloxane	T47.8X1	T47.8X2	T47.8X3	T47.8X4	T47.8X5	T47.8X6
sulfate (fumes)	T59.891	T59.892	T59.893	T59.894	—	—
liquid	T65.891	T65.892	T65.893	T65.894	—	—
sulfoxide (nonmedicinal)	T52.8X1	T52.8X2	T52.8X3	T52.8X4	—	—
medicinal	T49.4X1	T49.4X2	T49.4X3	T49.4X4	T49.4X5	T49.4X6
tryptamine	T40.991	T40.992	T40.993	T40.994	—	—
tubocurarine	T48.1X1	T48.1X2	T48.1X3	T48.1X4	T48.1X5	T48.1X6
Dimethylamine sulfate	T49.4X1	T49.4X2	T49.4X3	T49.4X4	T49.4X5	T49.4X6
Dimethylformamide	T52.8X1	T52.8X2	T52.8X3	T52.8X4	—	—
Dimethyltubocurarinium chloride	T48.1X1	T48.1X2	T48.1X3	T48.1X4	T48.1X5	T48.1X6
Dimeticone	T47.1X1	T47.1X2	T47.1X3	T47.1X4	T47.1X5	T47.1X6
Dimetilan	T60.0X1	T60.0X2	T60.0X3	T60.0X4	—	—
Dimetindene	T45.0X1	T45.0X2	T45.0X3	T45.0X4	T45.0X5	T45.0X6
Dimetotiazine	T43.3X1	T43.3X2	T43.3X3	T43.3X4	T43.3X5	T43.3X6
Dimorpholamine	T50.7X1	T50.7X2	T50.7X3	T50.7X4	T50.7X5	T50.7X6
Dimoxyline	T46.3X1	T46.3X2	T46.3X3	T46.3X4	T46.3X5	T46.3X6
Dinitrobenzene	T65.3X1	T65.3X2	T65.3X3	T65.3X4	—	—
vapor	T59.891	T59.892	T59.893	T59.894	—	—
Dinitrobenzol	T65.3X1	T65.3X2	T65.3X3	T65.3X4	—	—
vapor	T59.891	T59.892	T59.893	T59.894	—	—
Dinitrobutylphenol	T65.3X1	T65.3X2	T65.3X3	T65.3X4	—	—
Dinitro (-ortho-)cresol (pesticide) (spray)	T65.3X1	T65.3X2	T65.3X3	T65.3X4	—	—
Dinitrocyclohexylphenol	T65.3X1	T65.3X2	T65.3X3	T65.3X4	—	—
Dinitrophenol	T65.3X1	T65.3X2	T65.3X3	T65.3X4	—	—
Dinoprost	T48.0X1	T48.0X2	T48.0X3	T48.0X4	T48.0X5	T48.0X6
Dinoprostone	T48.0X1	T48.0X2	T48.0X3	T48.0X4	T48.0X5	T48.0X6
Dinoseb	T60.3X1	T60.3X2	T60.3X3	T60.3X4	—	—
Dioctyl sulfosuccinate (calcium) (sodium)	T47.4X1	T47.4X2	T47.4X3	T47.4X4	T47.4X5	T47.4X6
Diodone	T50.8X1	T50.8X2	T50.8X3	T50.8X4	T50.8X5	T50.8X6
Diodoquin	T37.8X1	T37.8X2	T37.8X3	T37.8X4	T37.8X5	T37.8X6
Dionin	T40.2X1	T40.2X2	T40.2X3	T40.2X4	T40.2X5	T40.2X6
Diosmin	T46.991	T46.992	T46.993	T46.994	T46.995	T46.996
Dioxane	T52.8X1	T52.8X2	T52.8X3	T52.8X4	—	—
Dioxathion	T60.0X1	T60.0X2	T60.0X3	T60.0X4	—	—
Dioxin	T53.7X1	T53.7X2	T53.7X3	T53.7X4	—	—
Dioxopromethazine	T43.3X1	T43.3X2	T43.3X3	T43.3X4	T43.3X5	T43.3X6
Dioxyline	T46.3X1	T46.3X2	T46.3X3	T46.3X4	T46.3X5	T46.3X6
Dipentene	T52.8X1	T52.8X2	T52.8X3	T52.8X4	—	—
Diperodon	T41.3X1	T41.3X2	T41.3X3	T41.3X4	T41.3X5	T41.3X6
Diphacinone	T60.4X1	T60.4X2	T60.4X3	T60.4X4	—	—
Diphemanil	T44.3X1	T44.3X2	T44.3X3	T44.3X4	T44.3X5	T44.3X6
metilsulfate	T44.3X1	T44.3X2	T44.3X3	T44.3X4	T44.3X5	T44.3X6
Diphenadione	T45.511	T45.512	T45.513	T45.514	T45.515	T45.516
rodenticide	T60.4X1	T60.4X2	T60.4X3	T60.4X4	—	—
Diphenhydramine	T45.0X1	T45.0X2	T45.0X3	T45.0X4	T45.0X5	T45.0X6
Diphenidol	T45.0X1	T45.0X2	T45.0X3	T45.0X4	T45.0X5	T45.0X6
Diphenoxylate	T47.6X1	T47.6X2	T47.6X3	T47.6X4	T47.6X5	T47.6X6

Substance	Poisoning, Accidental (unintentional)	Poisoning, Intentional Self-harm	Poisoning, Assault	Poisoning, Undetermined	Adverse Effect	Under-dosing
Diphenylamine	T65.3X1	T65.3X2	T65.3X3	T65.3X4	—	—
Diphenylbutazone	T39.2X1	T39.2X2	T39.2X3	T39.2X4	T39.2X5	T39.2X6
Diphenylchloroarsine, not in war	T57.0X1	T57.0X2	T57.0X3	T57.0X4	—	—
Diphenylhydantoin	T42.0X1	T42.0X2	T42.0X3	T42.0X4	T42.0X5	T42.0X6
Diphenylmethane dye	T52.1X1	T52.1X2	T52.1X3	T52.1X4	—	—
Diphenylpyraline	T45.0X1	T45.0X2	T45.0X3	T45.0X4	T45.0X5	T45.0X6
Diphtheria						
antitoxin	T50.Z11	T50.Z12	T50.Z13	T50.Z14	T50.Z15	T50.Z16
toxoid	T50.A91	T50.A92	T50.A93	T50.A94	T50.A95	T50.A96
with tetanus toxoid	T50.A21	T50.A22	T50.A23	T50.A24	T50.A25	T50.A26
with pertussis component						
vaccine	T50.A91	T50.A92	T50.A93	T50.A94	T50.A95	T50.A96
combination						
without pertussis	T50.A21	T50.A22	T50.A23	T50.A24	T50.A25	T50.A26
including pertussis	T50.A11	T50.A12	T50.A13	T50.A14	T50.A15	T50.A16
Diphylline	T50.2X1	T50.2X2	T50.2X3	T50.2X4	T50.2X5	T50.2X6
Dipipanone	T40.4X1	T40.4X2	T40.4X3	T40.4X4	—	—
Dipivefrine	T49.5X1	T49.5X2	T49.5X3	T49.5X4	T49.5X5	T49.5X6
Diplovax	T50.B91	T50.B92	T50.B93	T50.B94	T50.B95	T50.B96
Diprophylline	T50.2X1	T50.2X2	T50.2X3	T50.2X4	T50.2X5	T50.2X6
Dipropyline	T48.291	T48.292	T48.293	T48.294	T48.295	T48.296
Dipyridamole	T46.3X1	T46.3X2	T46.3X3	T46.3X4	T46.3X5	T46.3X6
Dipyrone	T39.2X1	T39.2X2	T39.2X3	T39.2X4	T39.2X5	T39.2X6
Diquat (dibromide)	T60.3X1	T60.3X2	T60.3X3	T60.3X4	—	—
Disinfectant	T65.891	T65.892	T65.893	T65.894	—	—
alkaline	T54.3X1	T54.3X2	T54.3X3	T54.3X4	—	—
aromatic	T54.1X1	T54.1X2	T54.1X3	T54.1X4	—	—
intestinal	T37.8X1	T37.8X2	T37.8X3	T37.8X4	T37.8X5	T37.8X6
Disipal	T42.8X1	T42.8X2	T42.8X3	T42.8X4	T42.8X5	T42.8X6
Disodium edetate	T50.6X1	T50.6X2	T50.6X3	T50.6X4	T50.6X5	T50.6X6
Disoprofol	T41.291	T41.292	T41.293	T41.294	T41.295	T41.296
Disopyramide	T46.2X1	T46.2X2	T46.2X3	T46.2X4	T46.2X5	T46.2X6
Distigmine (bromide)	T44.0X1	T44.0X2	T44.0X3	T44.0X4	T44.0X5	T44.0X6
Disulfamide	T50.2X1	T50.2X2	T50.2X3	T50.2X4	T50.2X5	T50.2X6
Disulfanilamide	T37.0X1	T37.0X2	T37.0X3	T37.0X4	T37.0X5	T37.0X6
Disulfiram	T50.6X1	T50.6X2	T50.6X3	T50.6X4	T50.6X5	T50.6X6
Disulfoton	T60.0X1	T60.0X2	T60.0X3	T60.0X4	—	—
Dithiazanine iodide	T37.4X1	T37.4X2	T37.4X3	T37.4X4	T37.4X5	T37.4X6
Dithiocarbamate	T60.0X1	T60.0X2	T60.0X3	T60.0X4	—	—
Dithranol	T49.4X1	T49.4X2	T49.4X3	T49.4X4	T49.4X5	T49.4X6
Diucardin	T50.2X1	T50.2X2	T50.2X3	T50.2X4	T50.2X5	T50.2X6
Diupres	T50.2X1	T50.2X2	T50.2X3	T50.2X4	T50.2X5	T50.2X6
Diuretic NEC	T50.2X1	T50.2X2	T50.2X3	T50.2X4	T50.2X5	T50.2X6
benzothiadiazine	T50.2X1	T50.2X2	T50.2X3	T50.2X4	T50.2X5	T50.2X6
carbonic acid anhydrase inhibitors	T50.2X1	T50.2X2	T50.2X3	T50.2X4	T50.2X5	T50.2X6
furfuryl NEC	T50.2X1	T50.2X2	T50.2X3	T50.2X4	T50.2X5	T50.2X6
loop (high-ceiling)	T50.1X1	T50.1X2	T50.1X3	T50.1X4	T50.1X5	T50.1X6
mercurial NEC	T50.2X1	T50.2X2	T50.2X3	T50.2X4	T50.2X5	T50.2X6
osmotic	T50.2X1	T50.2X2	T50.2X3	T50.2X4	T50.2X5	T50.2X6
purine NEC	T50.2X1	T50.2X2	T50.2X3	T50.2X4	T50.2X5	T50.2X6
saluretic NEC	T50.2X1	T50.2X2	T50.2X3	T50.2X4	T50.2X5	T50.2X6
sulfonamide	T50.2X1	T50.2X2	T50.2X3	T50.2X4	T50.2X5	T50.2X6
thiazide NEC	T50.2X1	T50.2X2	T50.2X3	T50.2X4	T50.2X5	T50.2X6
xanthine	T50.2X1	T50.2X2	T50.2X3	T50.2X4	T50.2X5	T50.2X6
Diurgin	T50.2X1	T50.2X2	T50.2X3	T50.2X4	T50.2X5	T50.2X6
Diuril	T50.2X1	T50.2X2	T50.2X3	T50.2X4	T50.2X5	T50.2X6
Diuron	T60.3X1	T60.3X2	T60.3X3	T60.3X4	—	—
Divalproex	T42.6X1	T42.6X2	T42.6X3	T42.6X4	T42.6X5	T42.6X6
Divinyl ether	T41.0X1	T41.0X2	T41.0X3	T41.0X4	T41.0X5	T41.0X6
Dixanthogen	T49.0X1	T49.0X2	T49.0X3	T49.0X4	T49.0X5	T49.0X6
Dixyrazine	T43.3X1	T43.3X2	T43.3X3	T43.3X4	T43.3X5	T43.3X6
D-lysergic acid diethylamide	T40.8X1	T40.8X2	T40.8X3	T40.8X4	—	—
DMCT	T36.4X1	T36.4X2	T36.4X3	T36.4X4	T36.4X5	T36.4X6
DMSO — see Dimethyl sulfoxide						
DNBP	T60.3X1	T60.3X2	T60.3X3	T60.3X4	—	—
DNOC	T65.3X1	T65.3X2	T65.3X3	T65.3X4	—	—
Dobutamine	T44.5X1	T44.5X2	T44.5X3	T44.5X4	T44.5X5	T44.5X6
DOCA	T38.0X1	T38.0X2	T38.0X3	T38.0X4	T38.0X5	T38.0X6
Docusate sodium	T47.4X1	T47.4X2	T47.4X3	T47.4X4	T47.4X5	T47.4X6
Dodicin	T49.0X1	T49.0X2	T49.0X3	T49.0X4	T49.0X5	T49.0X6
Dofamium chloride	T49.0X1	T49.0X2	T49.0X3	T49.0X4	T49.0X5	T49.0X6
Dolophine	T40.3X1	T40.3X2	T40.3X3	T40.3X4	T40.3X5	T40.3X6
Doloxene	T39.8X1	T39.8X2	T39.8X3	T39.8X4	T39.8X5	T39.8X6
Domestic gas (after combustion) — see Gas, utility						
prior to combustion	T59.891	T59.892	T59.893	T59.894	—	—
Domiodol	T48.4X1	T48.4X2	T48.4X3	T48.4X4	T48.4X5	T48.4X6
Domiphen (bromide)	T49.0X1	T49.0X2	T49.0X3	T49.0X4	T49.0X5	T49.0X6
Domperidone	T45.0X1	T45.0X2	T45.0X3	T45.0X4	T45.0X5	T45.0X6

Subterms under main terms may continue to next column or page   Additional Character May Be Required — Refer to the Tabular List for Character Selection   365

Dilantin — Domperidone

Substance	Poisoning, Accidental (unintentional)	Poisoning, Intentional Self-harm	Poisoning, Assault	Poisoning, Undetermined	Adverse Effect	Under-dosing
Dopa	T42.8X1	T42.8X2	T42.8X3	T42.8X4	T42.8X5	T42.8X6
Dopamine	T44.991	T44.992	T44.993	T44.994	T44.995	T44.996
Doriden	T42.6X1	T42.6X2	T42.6X3	T42.6X4	T42.6X5	T42.6X6
Dormiral	T42.3X1	T42.3X2	T42.3X3	T42.3X4	T42.3X5	T42.3X6
Dormison	T42.6X1	T42.6X2	T42.6X3	T42.6X4	T42.6X5	T42.6X6
Dornase	T48.4X1	T48.4X2	T48.4X3	T48.4X4	T48.4X5	T48.4X6
Dorsacaine	T41.3X1	T41.3X2	T41.3X3	T41.3X4	T41.3X5	T41.3X6
Dosulepin	T43.011	T43.012	T43.013	T43.014	T43.015	T43.016
Dothiepin	T43.011	T43.012	T43.013	T43.014	T43.015	T43.016
Doxantrazole	T48.6X1	T48.6X2	T48.6X3	T48.6X4	T48.6X5	T48.6X6
Doxapram	T50.7X1	T50.7X2	T50.7X3	T50.7X4	T50.7X5	T50.7X6
Doxazosin	T44.6X1	T44.6X2	T44.6X3	T44.6X4	T44.6X5	T44.6X6
Doxepin	T43.011	T43.012	T43.013	T43.014	T43.015	T43.016
Doxifluridine	T45.1X1	T45.1X2	T45.1X3	T45.1X4	T45.1X5	T45.1X6
Doxorubicin	T45.1X1	T45.1X2	T45.1X3	T45.1X4	T45.1X5	T45.1X6
Doxycycline	T36.4X1	T36.4X2	T36.4X3	T36.4X4	T36.4X5	T36.4X6
Doxylamine	T45.0X1	T45.0X2	T45.0X3	T45.0X4	T45.0X5	T45.0X6
Dramamine	T45.0X1	T45.0X2	T45.0X3	T45.0X4	T45.0X5	T45.0X6
Drano (drain cleaner)	T54.3X1	T54.3X2	T54.3X3	T54.3X4	—	—
Dressing, live pulp	T49.7X1	T49.7X2	T49.7X3	T49.7X4	T49.7X5	T49.7X6
Drocode	T40.2X1	T40.2X2	T40.2X3	T40.2X4	T40.2X5	T40.2X6
Dromoran	T40.2X1	T40.2X2	T40.2X3	T40.2X4	T40.2X5	T40.2X6
Dromostanolone	T38.7X1	T38.7X2	T38.7X3	T38.7X4	T38.7X5	T38.7X6
Dronabinol	T40.7X1	T40.7X2	T40.7X3	T40.7X4	T40.7X5	T40.7X6
Droperidol	T43.591	T43.592	T43.593	T43.594	T43.595	T43.596
Dropropizine	T48.3X1	T48.3X2	T48.3X3	T48.3X4	T48.3X5	T48.3X6
Drostanolone	T38.7X1	T38.7X2	T38.7X3	T38.7X4	T38.7X5	T38.7X6
Drotaverine	T44.3X1	T44.3X2	T44.3X3	T44.3X4	T44.3X5	T44.3X6
Drotrecogin alfa	T45.511	T45.512	T45.513	T45.514	T45.515	T45.516
Drug NEC	T50.901	T50.902	T50.903	T50.904	T50.905	T50.906
specified NEC	T50.991	T50.992	T50.993	T50.994	T50.995	T50.996
DTIC	T45.1X1	T45.1X2	T45.1X3	T45.1X4	T45.1X5	T45.1X6
Duboisine	T44.3X1	T44.3X2	T44.3X3	T44.3X4	T44.3X5	T44.3X6
Dulcolax	T47.2X1	T47.2X2	T47.2X3	T47.2X4	T47.2X5	T47.2X6
Duponol (C) (EP)	T49.2X1	T49.2X2	T49.2X3	T49.2X4	T49.2X5	T49.2X6
Durabolin	T38.7X1	T38.7X2	T38.7X3	T38.7X4	T38.7X5	T38.7X6
Dyclone	T41.3X1	T41.3X2	T41.3X3	T41.3X4	T41.3X5	T41.3X6
Dyclonine	T41.3X1	T41.3X2	T41.3X3	T41.3X4	T41.3X5	T41.3X6
Dydrogesterone	T38.5X1	T38.5X2	T38.5X3	T38.5X4	T38.5X5	T38.5X6
Dye NEC	T65.6X1	T65.6X2	T65.6X3	T65.6X4	—	—
antiseptic	T49.0X1	T49.0X2	T49.0X3	T49.0X4	T49.0X5	T49.0X6
diagnostic agents	T50.8X1	T50.8X2	T50.8X3	T50.8X4	T50.8X5	T50.8X6
pharmaceutical NEC	T50.901	T50.902	T50.903	T50.904	T50.905	T50.906
Dyflos	T44.0X1	T44.0X2	T44.0X3	T44.0X4	T44.0X5	T44.0X6
Dymelor	T38.3X1	T38.3X2	T38.3X3	T38.3X4	T38.3X5	T38.3X6
Dynamite	T65.3X1	T65.3X2	T65.3X3	T65.3X4	—	—
fumes	T59.891	T59.892	T59.893	T59.894	—	—
Dyphylline	T44.3X1	T44.3X2	T44.3X3	T44.3X4	T44.3X5	T44.3X6
b-eucaine	T49.1X1	T49.1X2	T49.1X3	T49.1X4	T49.1X5	T49.1X6
Ear drug NEC	T49.6X1	T49.6X2	T49.6X3	T49.6X4	T49.6X5	T49.6X6
Ear preparations	T49.6X1	T49.6X2	T49.6X3	T49.6X4	T49.6X5	T49.6X6
Echothiophate, echothiopate, ecothiopate	T49.5X1	T49.5X2	T49.5X3	T49.5X4	T49.5X5	T49.5X6
Econazole	T49.0X1	T49.0X2	T49.0X3	T49.0X4	T49.0X5	T49.0X6
Ecothiopate iodide	T49.5X1	T49.5X2	T49.5X3	T49.5X4	T49.5X5	T49.5X6
Ecstasy	T43.641	T43.642	T43.643	T43.644	—	—
Ectylurea	T42.6X1	T42.6X2	T42.6X3	T42.6X4	T42.6X5	T42.6X6
Edathamil disodium	T45.8X1	T45.8X2	T45.8X3	T45.8X4	T45.8X5	T45.8X6
Edecrin	T50.1X1	T50.1X2	T50.1X3	T50.1X4	T50.1X5	T50.1X6
Edetate, disodium (calcium)	T45.8X1	T45.8X2	T45.8X3	T45.8X4	T45.8X5	T45.8X6
Edoxudine	T49.5X1	T49.5X2	T49.5X3	T49.5X4	T49.5X5	T49.5X6
Edrophonium	T44.0X1	T44.0X2	T44.0X3	T44.0X4	T44.0X5	T44.0X6
chloride	T44.0X1	T44.0X2	T44.0X3	T44.0X4	T44.0X5	T44.0X6
EDTA	T50.6X1	T50.6X2	T50.6X3	T50.6X4	T50.6X5	T50.6X6
Eflornithine	T37.2X1	T37.2X2	T37.2X3	T37.2X4	T37.2X5	T37.2X6
Efloxate	T46.3X1	T46.3X2	T46.3X3	T46.3X4	T46.3X5	T46.3X6
Elase	T49.8X1	T49.8X2	T49.8X3	T49.8X4	T49.8X5	T49.8X6
Elastase	T47.5X1	T47.5X2	T47.5X3	T47.5X4	T47.5X5	T47.5X6
Elaterium	T47.2X1	T47.2X2	T47.2X3	T47.2X4	T47.2X5	T47.2X6
Elcatonin	T50.991	T50.992	T50.993	T50.994	T50.995	T50.996
Elder	T62.2X1	T62.2X2	T62.2X3	T62.2X4	—	—
berry, (unripe)	T62.1X1	T62.1X2	T62.1X3	T62.1X4	—	—
Electrolyte balance drug	T50.3X1	T50.3X2	T50.3X3	T50.3X4	T50.3X5	T50.3X6
Electrolytes NEC	T50.3X1	T50.3X2	T50.3X3	T50.3X4	T50.3X5	T50.3X6
Electrolytic agent NEC	T50.3X1	T50.3X2	T50.3X3	T50.3X4	T50.3X5	T50.3X6
Elemental diet	T50.901	T50.902	T50.903	T50.904	T50.905	T50.906
Elliptinium acetate	T45.1X1	T45.1X2	T45.1X3	T45.1X4	T45.1X5	T45.1X6
Embramine	T45.0X1	T45.0X2	T45.0X3	T45.0X4	T45.0X5	T45.0X6
Emepronium (salts)	T44.3X1	T44.3X2	T44.3X3	T44.3X4	T44.3X5	T44.3X6
bromide	T44.3X1	T44.3X2	T44.3X3	T44.3X4	T44.3X5	T44.3X6
Emetic NEC	T47.7X1	T47.7X2	T47.7X3	T47.7X4	T47.7X5	T47.7X6
Emetine	T37.3X1	T37.3X2	T37.3X3	T37.3X4	T37.3X5	T37.3X6

Substance	Poisoning, Accidental (unintentional)	Poisoning, Intentional Self-harm	Poisoning, Assault	Poisoning, Undetermined	Adverse Effect	Under-dosing
Emollient NEC	T49.3X1	T49.3X2	T49.3X3	T49.3X4	T49.3X5	T49.3
Emorfazone	T39.8X1	T39.8X2	T39.8X3	T39.8X4	T39.8X5	T39.8
Emylcamate	T43.591	T43.592	T43.593	T43.594	T43.595	T43.5
Enalapril	T46.4X1	T46.4X2	T46.4X3	T46.4X4	T46.4X5	T46.4
Enalaprilat	T46.4X1	T46.4X2	T46.4X3	T46.4X4	T46.4X5	T46.4
Encainide	T46.2X1	T46.2X2	T46.2X3	T46.2X4	T46.2X5	T46.2
Endocaine	T41.3X1	T41.3X2	T41.3X3	T41.3X4	T41.3X5	T41.3
Endosulfan	T60.2X1	T60.2X2	T60.2X3	T60.2X4	—	—
Endothall	T60.3X1	T60.3X2	T60.3X3	T60.3X4	—	—
Endralazine	T46.5X1	T46.5X2	T46.5X3	T46.5X4	T46.5X5	T46.5
Endrin	T60.1X1	T60.1X2	T60.1X3	T60.1X4	—	—
Enflurane	T41.0X1	T41.0X2	T41.0X3	T41.0X4	T41.0X5	T41.0
Enhexymal	T42.3X1	T42.3X2	T42.3X3	T42.3X4	T42.3X5	T42.3
Enocitabine	T45.1X1	T45.1X2	T45.1X3	T45.1X4	T45.1X5	T45.1
Enovid	T38.4X1	T38.4X2	T38.4X3	T38.4X4	T38.4X5	T38.4
Enoxacin	T36.8X1	T36.8X2	T36.8X3	T36.8X4	T36.8X5	T36.8
Enoxaparin (sodium)	T45.511	T45.512	T45.513	T45.514	T45.515	T45.5
Enpiprazole	T43.591	T43.592	T43.593	T43.594	T43.595	T43.5
Enprofylline	T48.6X1	T48.6X2	T48.6X3	T48.6X4	T48.6X5	T48.6
Enprostil	T47.1X1	T47.1X2	T47.1X3	T47.1X4	T47.1X5	T47.1
Enterogastrone	T38.891	T38.892	T38.893	T38.894	T38.895	T38.8
ENT preparations (anti-infectives)	T49.6X1	T49.6X2	T49.6X3	T49.6X4	T49.6X5	T49.6
Enviomycin	T36.8X1	T36.8X2	T36.8X3	T36.8X4	T36.8X5	T36.8
Enzodase	T45.3X1	T45.3X2	T45.3X3	T45.3X4	T45.3X5	T45.3
Enzyme NEC	T45.3X1	T45.3X2	T45.3X3	T45.3X4	T45.3X5	T45.3
depolymerizing	T49.8X1	T49.8X2	T49.8X3	T49.8X4	T49.8X5	T49.8
fibrolytic	T45.3X1	T45.3X2	T45.3X3	T45.3X4	T45.3X5	T45.3
gastric	T47.5X1	T47.5X2	T47.5X3	T47.5X4	T47.5X5	T47.5
intestinal	T47.5X1	T47.5X2	T47.5X3	T47.5X4	T47.5X5	T47.5
local action	T49.4X1	T49.4X2	T49.4X3	T49.4X4	T49.4X5	T49.4
proteolytic	T49.4X1	T49.4X2	T49.4X3	T49.4X4	T49.4X5	T49.4
thrombolytic	T45.3X1	T45.3X2	T45.3X3	T45.3X4	T45.3X5	T45.3
EPAB	T41.3X1	T41.3X2	T41.3X3	T41.3X4	T41.3X5	T41.3
Epanutin	T42.0X1	T42.0X2	T42.0X3	T42.0X4	T42.0X5	T42.0
Ephedra	T44.991	T44.992	T44.993	T44.994	T44.995	T44.9
Ephedrine	T44.991	T44.992	T44.993	T44.994	T44.995	T44.9
Epichlorhydrin, epichlorohydrin	T52.8X1	T52.8X2	T52.8X3	T52.8X4	—	—
Epicillin	T36.0X1	T36.0X2	T36.0X3	T36.0X4	T36.0X5	T36.0
Epiestriol	T38.5X1	T38.5X2	T38.5X3	T38.5X4	T38.5X5	T38.5
Epilim — see Sodium valproate						
Epimestrol	T38.5X1	T38.5X2	T38.5X3	T38.5X4	T38.5X5	T38.5
Epinephrine	T44.5X1	T44.5X2	T44.5X3	T44.5X4	T44.5X5	T44.5
Epirubicin	T45.1X1	T45.1X2	T45.1X3	T45.1X4	T45.1X5	T45.1
Epitiostanol	T38.7X1	T38.7X2	T38.7X3	T38.7X4	T38.7X5	T38.7
Epitizide	T50.2X1	T50.2X2	T50.2X3	T50.2X4	T50.2X5	T50.2
EPN	T60.0X1	T60.0X2	T60.0X3	T60.0X4	—	—
EPO	T45.8X1	T45.8X2	T45.8X3	T45.8X4	T45.8X5	T45.8
Epoetin alpha	T45.8X1	T45.8X2	T45.8X3	T45.8X4	T45.8X5	T45.8
Epomediol	T50.991	T50.992	T50.993	T50.994	T50.995	T50.9
Epoprostenol	T45.521	T45.522	T45.523	T45.524	T45.525	T45.5
Epoxy resin	T65.891	T65.892	T65.893	T65.894	—	—
Eprazinone	T48.4X1	T48.4X2	T48.4X3	T48.4X4	T48.4X5	T48.4
Epsilon aminocaproic acid	T45.621	T45.622	T45.623	T45.624	T45.625	T45.6
Epsom salt	T47.3X1	T47.3X2	T47.3X3	T47.3X4	T47.3X5	T47.3
Eptazocine	T40.4X1	T40.4X2	T40.4X3	T40.4X4	T40.4X5	T40.4
Equanil	T43.591	T43.592	T43.593	T43.594	T43.595	T43.5
Equisetum	T62.2X1	T62.2X2	T62.2X3	T62.2X4	—	—
diuretic	T50.2X1	T50.2X2	T50.2X3	T50.2X4	T50.2X5	T50.2
Ergobasine	T48.0X1	T48.0X2	T48.0X3	T48.0X4	T48.0X5	T48.0
Ergocalciferol	T45.2X1	T45.2X2	T45.2X3	T45.2X4	T45.2X5	T45.2
Ergoloid mesylates	T46.7X1	T46.7X2	T46.7X3	T46.7X4	T46.7X5	T46.7
Ergometrine	T48.0X1	T48.0X2	T48.0X3	T48.0X4	T48.0X5	T48.0
Ergonovine	T48.0X1	T48.0X2	T48.0X3	T48.0X4	T48.0X5	T48.0
Ergotamine	T46.5X1	T46.5X2	T46.5X3	T46.5X4	T46.5X5	T46.5
Ergotocine	T48.0X1	T48.0X2	T48.0X3	T48.0X4	T48.0X5	T48.0
Ergotrate	T48.0X1	T48.0X2	T48.0X3	T48.0X4	T48.0X5	T48.0
Ergot NEC	T64.81	T64.82	T64.83	T64.84		
derivative	T48.0X1	T48.0X2	T48.0X3	T48.0X4	T48.0X5	T48.0×
medicinal (alkaloids)	T48.0X1	T48.0X2	T48.0X3	T48.0X4	T48.0X5	T48.0×
prepared	T48.0X1	T48.0X2	T48.0X3	T48.0X4	T48.0X5	T48.0×
Eritrityl tetranitrate	T46.3X1	T46.3X2	T46.3X3	T46.3X4	T46.3X5	T46.3×
Erythrityl tetranitrate	T46.3X1	T46.3X2	T46.3X3	T46.3X4	T46.3X5	T46.3×
Erythrol tetranitrate	T46.3X1	T46.3X2	T46.3X3	T46.3X4	T46.3X5	T46.3×
Erythromycin (salts)	T36.3X1	T36.3X2	T36.3X3	T36.3X4	T36.3X5	T36.3×
ophthalmic preparation	T49.5X1	T49.5X2	T49.5X3	T49.5X4	T49.5X5	T49.5×
topical NEC	T49.0X1	T49.0X2	T49.0X3	T49.0X4	T49.0X5	T49.0×
Erythropoietin	T45.8X1	T45.8X2	T45.8X3	T45.8X4	T45.8X5	T45.8×
human	T45.8X1	T45.8X2	T45.8X3	T45.8X4	T45.8X5	T45.8×
Escin	T46.991	T46.992	T46.993	T46.994	T46.995	T45.2×
Esculin	T45.2X1	T45.2X2	T45.2X3	T45.2X4	T45.2X5	T45.2×
Esculoside	T45.2X1	T45.2X2	T45.2X3	T45.2X4	T45.2X5	T45.2×

366

Additional Character May Be Required — Refer to the Tabular List for Character Selection · Subterms under main terms may continue to next column or page

Substance	Poisoning, Accidental (unintentional)	Poisoning, Intentional Self-harm	Poisoning, Assault	Poisoning, Undetermined	Adverse Effect	Under-dosing
ESDT (ether-soluble tar distillate)	T49.1X1	T49.1X2	T49.1X3	T49.1X4	T49.1X5	T49.1X6
Eserine	T49.5X1	T49.5X2	T49.5X3	T49.5X4	T49.5X5	T49.5X6
Esflurbiprofen	T39.311	T39.312	T39.313	T39.314	T39.315	T39.316
Eskabarb	T42.3X1	T42.3X2	T42.3X3	T42.3X4	T42.3X5	T42.3X6
Eskalith	T43.8X1	T43.8X2	T43.8X3	T43.8X4	T43.8X5	T43.8X6
Esmolol	T44.7X1	T44.7X2	T44.7X3	T44.7X4	T44.7X5	T44.7X6
Estanozolol	T38.7X1	T38.7X2	T38.7X3	T38.7X4	T38.7X5	T38.7X6
Estazolam	T42.4X1	T42.4X2	T42.4X3	T42.4X4	T42.4X5	T42.4X6
Estradiol	T38.5X1	T38.5X2	T38.5X3	T38.5X4	T38.5X5	T38.5X6
with testosterone	T38.7X1	T38.7X2	T38.7X3	T38.7X4	T38.7X5	T38.7X6
benzoate	T38.5X1	T38.5X2	T38.5X3	T38.5X4	T38.5X5	T38.5X6
Estramustine	T45.1X1	T45.1X2	T45.1X3	T45.1X4	T45.1X5	T45.1X6
Estriol	T38.5X1	T38.5X2	T38.5X3	T38.5X4	T38.5X5	T38.5X6
Estrogen	T38.5X1	T38.5X2	T38.5X3	T38.5X4	T38.5X5	T38.5X6
with progesterone	T38.5X1	T38.5X2	T38.5X3	T38.5X4	T38.5X5	T38.5X6
conjugated	T38.5X1	T38.5X2	T38.5X3	T38.5X4	T38.5X5	T38.5X6
Estrone	T38.5X1	T38.5X2	T38.5X3	T38.5X4	T38.5X5	T38.5X6
Estropipate	T38.5X1	T38.5X2	T38.5X3	T38.5X4	T38.5X5	T38.5X6
Etacrynate sodium	T50.1X1	T50.1X2	T50.1X3	T50.1X4	T50.1X5	T50.1X6
Etacrynic acid	T50.1X1	T50.1X2	T50.1X3	T50.1X4	T50.1X5	T50.1X6
Etafedrine	T48.6X1	T48.6X2	T48.6X3	T48.6X4	T48.6X5	T48.6X6
Etafenone	T46.3X1	T46.3X2	T46.3X3	T46.3X4	T46.3X5	T46.3X6
Etambutol	T37.1X1	T37.1X2	T37.1X3	T37.1X4	T37.1X5	T37.1X6
Etamiphyllin	T48.6X1	T48.6X2	T48.6X3	T48.6X4	T48.6X5	T48.6X6
Etamivan	T50.7X1	T50.7X2	T50.7X3	T50.7X4	T50.7X5	T50.7X6
Etamsylate	T45.7X1	T45.7X2	T45.7X3	T45.7X4	T45.7X5	T45.7X6
Etebenecid	T50.4X1	T50.4X2	T50.4X3	T50.4X4	T50.4X5	T50.4X6
Ethacridine	T49.0X1	T49.0X2	T49.0X3	T49.0X4	T49.0X5	T49.0X6
Ethacrynic acid	T50.1X1	T50.1X2	T50.1X3	T50.1X4	T50.1X5	T50.1X6
Ethadione	T42.2X1	T42.2X2	T42.2X3	T42.2X4	T42.2X5	T42.2X6
Ethambutol	T37.1X1	T37.1X2	T37.1X3	T37.1X4	T37.1X5	T37.1X6
Ethamide	T50.2X1	T50.2X2	T50.2X3	T50.2X4	T50.2X5	T50.2X6
Ethamivan	T50.7X1	T50.7X2	T50.7X3	T50.7X4	T50.7X5	T50.7X6
Ethamsylate	T45.7X1	T45.7X2	T45.7X3	T45.7X4	T45.7X5	T45.7X6
Ethanol	T51.0X1	T51.0X2	T51.0X3	T51.0X4	—	—
beverage	T51.0X1	T51.0X2	T51.0X3	T51.0X4	—	—
Ethanolamine oleate	T46.8X1	T46.8X2	T46.8X3	T46.8X4	T46.8X5	T46.8X6
Ethaverine	T44.3X1	T44.3X2	T44.3X3	T44.3X4	T44.3X5	T44.3X6
Ethchlorvynol	T42.6X1	T42.6X2	T42.6X3	T42.6X4	T42.6X5	T42.6X6
Ethebenecid	T50.4X1	T50.4X2	T50.4X3	T50.4X4	T50.4X5	T50.4X6
Ether (vapor)	T41.0X1	T41.0X2	T41.0X3	T41.0X4	T41.0X5	T41.0X6
anesthetic	T41.0X1	T41.0X2	T41.0X3	T41.0X4	T41.0X5	T41.0X6
divinyl	T41.0X1	T41.0X2	T41.0X3	T41.0X4	T41.0X5	T41.0X6
ethyl (medicinal)	T41.0X1	T41.0X2	T41.0X3	T41.0X4	T41.0X5	T41.0X6
nonmedicinal	T52.8X1	T52.8X2	T52.8X3	T52.8X4	—	—
petroleum — see Ligroin						
solvent	T52.8X1	T52.8X2	T52.8X3	T52.8X4	—	—
Ethiazide	T50.2X1	T50.2X2	T50.2X3	T50.2X4	T50.2X5	T50.2X6
Ethidium chloride (vapor)	T59.891	T59.892	T59.893	T59.894	—	—
Ethinamate	T42.6X1	T42.6X2	T42.6X3	T42.6X4	T42.6X5	T42.6X6
Ethinylestradiol, ethinyloestradiol	T38.5X1	T38.5X2	T38.5X3	T38.5X4	T38.5X5	T38.5X6
with						
levonorgestrel	T38.4X1	T38.4X2	T38.4X3	T38.4X4	T38.4X5	T38.4X6
norethisterone	T38.4X1	T38.4X2	T38.4X3	T38.4X4	T38.4X5	T38.4X6
Ethiodized oil (131 I)	T50.8X1	T50.8X2	T50.8X3	T50.8X4	T50.8X5	T50.8X6
Ethion	T60.0X1	T60.0X2	T60.0X3	T60.0X4	—	—
Ethionamide	T37.1X1	T37.1X2	T37.1X3	T37.1X4	T37.1X5	T37.1X6
Ethioniamide	T37.1X1	T37.1X2	T37.1X3	T37.1X4	T37.1X5	T37.1X6
Ethisterone	T38.5X1	T38.5X2	T38.5X3	T38.5X4	T38.5X5	T38.5X6
Ethobral	T42.3X1	T42.3X2	T42.3X3	T42.3X4	T42.3X5	T42.3X6
Ethocaine (infiltration) (topical)	T41.3X1	T41.3X2	T41.3X3	T41.3X4	T41.3X5	T41.3X6
nerve block (peripheral) (plexus)	T41.3X1	T41.3X2	T41.3X3	T41.3X4	T41.3X5	T41.3X6
spinal	T41.3X1	T41.3X2	T41.3X3	T41.3X4	T41.3X5	T41.3X6
Ethoheptazine	T40.4X1	T40.4X2	T40.4X3	T40.4X4	T40.4X5	T40.4X6
Ethopropazine	T44.3X1	T44.3X2	T44.3X3	T44.3X4	T44.3X5	T44.3X6
Ethosuximide	T42.2X1	T42.2X2	T42.2X3	T42.2X4	T42.2X5	T42.2X6
Ethotoin	T42.0X1	T42.0X2	T42.0X3	T42.0X4	T42.0X5	T42.0X6
Ethoxazene	T37.91	T37.92	T37.93	T37.94	T37.95	T37.96
Ethoxazorutoside	T46.991	T46.992	T46.993	T46.994	T46.995	T46.996
Ethoxzolamide	T50.2X1	T50.2X2	T50.2X3	T50.2X4	T50.2X5	T50.2X6
Ethyl						
acetate	T52.8X1	T52.8X2	T52.8X3	T52.8X4	—	—
alcohol	T51.0X1	T51.0X2	T51.0X3	T51.0X4	—	—
beverage	T51.0X1	T51.0X2	T51.0X3	T51.0X4	—	—
aldehyde (vapor)	T59.891	T59.892	T59.893	T59.894	—	—
liquid	T52.8X1	T52.8X2	T52.8X3	T52.8X4	—	—
aminobenzoate	T41.3X1	T41.3X2	T41.3X3	T41.3X4	T41.3X5	T41.3X6
aminophenothiazine	T43.3X1	T43.3X2	T43.3X3	T43.3X4	T43.3X5	T43.3X6
benzoate	T52.8X1	T52.8X2	T52.8X3	T52.8X4	—	—

Substance	Poisoning, Accidental (unintentional)	Poisoning, Intentional Self-harm	Poisoning, Assault	Poisoning, Undetermined	Adverse Effect	Under-dosing
Ethyl — continued						
biscoumacetate	T45.511	T45.512	T45.513	T45.514	T45.515	T45.516
bromide (anesthetic)	T41.0X1	T41.0X2	T41.0X3	T41.0X4	T41.0X5	T41.0X6
carbamate	T45.1X1	T45.1X2	T45.1X3	T45.1X4	T45.1X5	T45.1X6
carbinol	T51.3X1	T51.3X2	T51.3X3	T51.3X4	—	—
carbonate	T52.8X1	T52.8X2	T52.8X3	T52.8X4	—	—
chaulmoograte	T37.1X1	T37.1X2	T37.1X3	T37.1X4	T37.1X5	T37.1X6
chloride (anesthetic)	T41.0X1	T41.0X2	T41.0X3	T41.0X4	T41.0X5	T41.0X6
anesthetic (local)	T41.3X1	T41.3X2	T41.3X3	T41.3X4	T41.3X5	T41.3X6
inhaled	T41.0X1	T41.0X2	T41.0X3	T41.0X4	T41.0X5	T41.0X6
local	T49.4X1	T49.4X2	T49.4X3	T49.4X4	T49.4X5	T49.4X6
solvent	T53.6X1	T53.6X2	T53.6X3	T53.6X4	—	—
dibunate	T48.3X1	T48.3X2	T48.3X3	T48.3X4	T48.3X5	T48.3X6
dichloroarsine (vapor)	T57.0X1	T57.0X2	T57.0X3	T57.0X4	—	—
estranol	T38.7X1	T38.7X2	T38.7X3	T38.7X4	T38.7X5	T38.7X6
ether — see also ether	T52.8X1	T52.8X2	T52.8X3	T52.8X4	—	—
formate NEC (solvent)	T52.0X1	T52.0X2	T52.0X3	T52.0X4	—	—
fumarate	T49.4X1	T49.4X2	T49.4X3	T49.4X4	T49.4X5	T49.4X6
hydroxyisobutyrate NEC (solvent)	T52.8X1	T52.8X2	T52.8X3	T52.8X4	—	—
iodoacetate	T59.3X1	T59.3X2	T59.3X3	T59.3X4	—	—
lactate NEC (solvent)	T52.8X1	T52.8X2	T52.8X3	T52.8X4	—	—
loflazepate	T42.4X1	T42.4X2	T42.4X3	T42.4X4	T42.4X5	T42.4X6
mercuric chloride	T56.1X1	T56.1X2	T56.1X3	T56.1X4	—	—
methylcarbinol	T51.8X1	T51.8X2	T51.8X3	T51.8X4	—	—
morphine	T40.2X1	T40.2X2	T40.2X3	T40.2X4	T40.2X5	T40.2X6
noradrenaline	T48.6X1	T48.6X2	T48.6X3	T48.6X4	T48.6X5	T48.6X6
oxybutyrate NEC (solvent)	T52.8X1	T52.8X2	T52.8X3	T52.8X4	—	—
Ethylene (gas)	T59.891	T59.892	T59.893	T59.894	—	—
anesthetic (general)	T41.0X1	T41.0X2	T41.0X3	T41.0X4	T41.0X5	T41.0X6
chlorohydrin	T52.8X1	T52.8X2	T52.8X3	T52.8X4	—	—
vapor	T53.6X1	T53.6X2	T53.6X3	T53.6X4	—	—
dichloride	T52.8X1	T52.8X2	T52.8X3	T52.8X4	—	—
vapor	T53.6X1	T53.6X2	T53.6X3	T53.6X4	—	—
dinitrate	T52.3X1	T52.3X2	T52.3X3	T52.3X4	—	—
glycol(s)	T52.8X1	T52.8X2	T52.8X3	T52.8X4	—	—
dinitrate	T52.3X1	T52.3X2	T52.3X3	T52.3X4	—	—
monobutyl ether	T52.3X1	T52.3X2	T52.3X3	T52.3X4	—	—
imine	T54.1X1	T54.1X2	T54.1X3	T54.1X4	—	—
oxide (fumigant) (nonmedicinal)	T59.891	T59.892	T59.893	T59.894	—	—
medicinal	T49.0X1	T49.0X2		T49.0X4	T49.0X5	T49.0X6
Ethylenediaminetetra-acetic acid	T50.6X1	T50.6X2	T50.6X3	T50.6X4	T50.6X5	T50.6X6
Ethylenediamine theophylline	T48.6X1	T48.6X2	T48.6X3	T48.6X4	T48.6X5	T48.6X6
Ethylenedinitrilotetra-acetate	T50.6X1	T50.6X2	T50.6X3	T50.6X4	T50.6X5	T50.6X6
Ethylestrenol	T38.7X1	T38.7X2	T38.7X3	T38.7X4	T38.7X5	T38.7X6
Ethylhydrocellulose	T47.4X1	T47.4X2	T47.4X3	T47.4X4	T47.4X5	T47.4X6
Ethylidene						
chloride NEC	T53.6X1	T53.6X2	T53.6X3	T53.6X4	—	—
diacetate	T60.3X1	T60.3X2	T60.3X3	T60.3X4	—	—
dicoumarin	T45.511	T45.512	T45.513	T45.514	T45.515	T45.516
dicoumarol	T45.511	T45.512	T45.513	T45.514	T45.515	T45.516
diethyl ether	T52.0X1	T52.0X2	T52.0X3	T52.0X4	—	—
Ethylmorphine	T40.2X1	T40.2X2	T40.2X3	T40.2X4	T40.2X5	T40.2X6
Ethylnorepinephrine	T48.6X1	T48.6X2	T48.6X3	T48.6X4	T48.6X5	T48.6X6
Ethylparachlorophen-oxyisobutyrate	T46.6X1	T46.6X2	T46.6X3	T46.6X4	T46.6X5	T46.6X6
Ethynodiol	T38.4X1	T38.4X2	T38.4X3	T38.4X4	T38.4X5	T38.4X6
with mestranol diacetate	T38.4X1	T38.4X2	T38.4X3	T38.4X4	T38.4X5	T38.4X6
Etidocaine	T41.3X1	T41.3X2	T41.3X3	T41.3X4	T41.3X5	T41.3X6
infiltration (subcutaneous)	T41.3X1	T41.3X2	T41.3X3	T41.3X4	T41.3X5	T41.3X6
nerve (peripheral) (plexus)	T41.3X1	T41.3X2	T41.3X3	T41.3X4	T41.3X5	T41.3X6
Etidronate	T50.991	T50.992	T50.993	T50.994	T50.995	T50.996
Etidronic acid (disodium salt)	T50.991	T50.992	T50.993	T50.994	T50.995	T50.996
Etifoxine	T42.6X1	T42.6X2	T42.6X3	T42.6X4	T42.6X5	T42.6X6
Etilefrine	T44.4X1	T44.4X2	T44.4X3	T44.4X4	T44.4X5	T44.4X6
Etilfen	T42.3X1	T42.3X2	T42.3X3	T42.3X4	T42.3X5	T42.3X6
Etinodiol	T38.4X1	T38.4X2	T38.4X3	T38.4X4	T38.4X5	T38.4X6
Etiroxate	T46.6X1	T46.6X2	T46.6X3	T46.6X4	T46.6X5	T46.6X6
Etizolam	T42.4X1	T42.4X2	T42.4X3	T42.4X4	T42.4X5	T42.4X6
Etodolac	T39.391	T39.392	T39.393	T39.394	T39.395	T39.396
Etofamide	T37.3X1	T37.3X2	T37.3X3	T37.3X4	T37.3X5	T37.3X6
Etofibrate	T46.6X1	T46.6X2	T46.6X3	T46.6X4	T46.6X5	T46.6X6
Etofylline	T46.7X1	T46.7X2	T46.7X3	T46.7X4	T46.7X5	T46.7X6
clofibrate	T46.6X1	T46.6X2	T46.6X3	T46.6X4	T46.6X5	T46.6X6
Etoglucid	T45.1X1	T45.1X2	T45.1X3	T45.1X4	T45.1X5	T45.1X6
Etomidate	T41.1X1	T41.1X2	T41.1X3	T41.1X4	T41.1X5	T41.1X6
Etomide	T39.8X1	T39.8X2	T39.8X3	T39.8X4	T39.8X5	T39.8X6
Etomidoline	T44.3X1	T44.3X2	T44.3X3	T44.3X4	T44.3X5	T44.3X6
Etoposide	T45.1X1	T45.1X2	T45.1X3	T45.1X4	T45.1X5	T45.1X6

Substance	Poisoning, Accidental (unintentional)	Poisoning, Intentional Self-harm	Poisoning, Assault	Poisoning, Undetermined	Adverse Effect	Under-dosing
Etorphine	T40.2X1	T40.2X2	T40.2X3	T40.2X4	T40.2X5	T40.2X6
Etoval	T42.3X1	T42.3X2	T42.3X3	T42.3X4	T42.3X5	T42.3X6
Etozolin	T50.1X1	T50.1X2	T50.1X3	T50.1X4	T50.1X5	T50.1X6
Etretinate	T50.991	T50.992	T50.993	T50.994	T50.995	T50.996
Etryptamine	T43.691	T43.692	T43.693	T43.694	T43.695	T43.696
Etybenzatropine	T44.3X1	T44.3X2	T44.3X3	T44.3X4	T44.3X5	T44.3X6
Etynodiol	T38.4X1	T38.4X2	T38.4X3	T38.4X4	T38.4X5	T38.4X6
Eucaine	T41.3X1	T41.3X2	T41.3X3	T41.3X4	T41.3X5	T41.3X6
Eucalyptus oil	T49.7X1	T49.7X2	T49.7X3	T49.7X4	T49.7X5	T49.7X6
Eucatropine	T49.5X1	T49.5X2	T49.5X3	T49.5X4	T49.5X5	T49.5X6
Eucodal	T40.2X1	T40.2X2	T40.2X3	T40.2X4	T40.2X5	T40.2X6
Euneryl	T42.3X1	T42.3X2	T42.3X3	T42.3X4	T42.3X5	T42.3X6
Euphthalmine	T44.3X1	T44.3X2	T44.3X3	T44.3X4	T44.3X5	T44.3X6
Eurax	T49.0X1	T49.0X2	T49.0X3	T49.0X4	T49.0X5	T49.0X6
Euresol	T49.4X1	T49.4X2	T49.4X3	T49.4X4	T49.4X5	T49.4X6
Euthroid	T38.1X1	T38.1X2	T38.1X3	T38.1X4	T38.1X5	T38.1X6
Evans blue	T50.8X1	T50.8X2	T50.8X3	T50.8X4	T50.8X5	T50.8X6
Evipal	T42.3X1	T42.3X2	T42.3X3	T42.3X4	T42.3X5	T42.3X6
sodium	T41.1X1	T41.1X2	T41.1X3	T41.1X4	T41.1X5	T41.1X6
Evipan	T42.3X1	T42.3X2	T42.3X3	T42.3X4	T42.3X5	T42.3X6
sodium	T41.1X1	T41.1X2	T41.1X3	T41.1X4	T41.1X5	T41.1X6
Exalamide	T49.0X1	T49.0X2	T49.0X3	T49.0X4	T49.0X5	T49.0X6
Exalgin	T39.1X1	T39.1X2	T39.1X3	T39.1X4	T39.1X5	T39.1X6
Excipients, pharmaceutical	T50.901	T50.902	T50.903	T50.904	T50.905	T50.906
Exhaust gas (engine) (motor vehicle)	T58.01	T58.02	T58.03	T58.04	—	—
Ex-Lax (phenolphthalein)	T47.2X1	T47.2X2	T47.2X3	T47.2X4	T47.2X5	T47.2X6
Expectorant NEC	T48.4X1	T48.4X2	T48.4X3	T48.4X4	T48.4X5	T48.4X6
Extended insulin zinc suspension	T38.3X1	T38.3X2	T38.3X3	T38.3X4	T38.3X5	T38.3X6
External medications (skin) (mucous membrane)	T49.91	T49.92	T49.93	T49.94	T49.95	T49.96
dental agent	T49.7X1	T49.7X2	T49.7X3	T49.7X4	T49.7X5	T49.7X6
ENT agent	T49.6X1	T49.6X2	T49.6X3	T49.6X4	T49.6X5	T49.6X6
ophthalmic preparation	T49.5X1	T49.5X2	T49.5X3	T49.5X4	T49.5X5	T49.5X6
specified NEC	T49.8X1	T49.8X2	T49.8X3	T49.8X4	T49.8X5	T49.8X6
Extrapyramidal antagonist NEC	T44.3X1	T44.3X2	T44.3X3	T44.3X4	T44.3X5	T44.3X6
Eye agents (anti-infective)	T49.5X1	T49.5X2	T49.5X3	T49.5X4	T49.5X5	T49.5X6
Eye drug NEC	T49.5X1	T49.5X2	T49.5X3	T49.5X4	T49.5X5	T49.5X6
FAC (fluorouracil + doxorubicin + cyclophosphamide)	T45.1X1	T45.1X2	T45.1X3	T45.1X4	T45.1X5	T45.1X6
Factor						
I (fibrinogen)	T45.8X1	T45.8X2	T45.8X3	T45.8X4	T45.8X5	T45.8X6
III (thromboplastin)	T45.8X1	T45.8X2	T45.8X3	T45.8X4	T45.8X5	T45.8X6
IX complex	T45.7X1	T45.7X2	T45.7X3	T45.7X4	T45.7X5	T45.7X6
human	T45.8X1	T45.8X2	T45.8X3	T45.8X4	T45.8X5	T45.8X6
VIII (antihemophilic Factor) (concentrate)	T45.8X1	T45.8X2	T45.8X3	T45.8X4	T45.8X5	T45.8X6
Famotidine	T47.0X1	T47.0X2	T47.0X3	T47.0X4	T47.0X5	T47.0X6
Fat suspension, intravenous	T50.991	T50.992	T50.993	T50.994	T50.995	T50.996
Fazadinium bromide	T48.1X1	T48.1X2	T48.1X3	T48.1X4	T48.1X5	T48.1X6
Febarbamate	T42.3X1	T42.3X2	T42.3X3	T42.3X4	T42.3X5	T42.3X6
Fecal softener	T47.4X1	T47.4X2	T47.4X3	T47.4X4	T47.4X5	T47.4X6
Fedrilate	T48.3X1	T48.3X2	T48.3X3	T48.3X4	T48.3X5	T48.3X6
Felodipine	T46.1X1	T46.1X2	T46.1X3	T46.1X4	T46.1X5	T46.1X6
Felypressin	T38.891	T38.892	T38.893	T38.894	T38.895	T38.896
Femoxetine	T43.221	T43.222	T43.223	T43.224	T43.225	T43.226
Fenalcomine	T46.3X1	T46.3X2	T46.3X3	T46.3X4	T46.3X5	T46.3X6
Fenamisal	T37.1X1	T37.1X2	T37.1X3	T37.1X4	T37.1X5	T37.1X6
Fenazone	T39.2X1	T39.2X2	T39.2X3	T39.2X4	T39.2X5	T39.2X6
Fenbendazole	T37.4X1	T37.4X2	T37.4X3	T37.4X4	T37.4X5	T37.4X6
Fenbutrazate	T50.5X1	T50.5X2	T50.5X3	T50.5X4	T50.5X5	T50.5X6
Fencamfamine	T43.691	T43.692	T43.693	T43.694	T43.695	T43.696
Fendiline	T46.1X1	T46.1X2	T46.1X3	T46.1X4	T46.1X5	T46.1X6
Fenetylline	T43.691	T43.692	T43.693	T43.694	T43.695	T43.696
Fenflumizole	T39.391	T39.392	T39.393	T39.394	T39.395	T39.396
Fenfluramine	T50.5X1	T50.5X2	T50.5X3	T50.5X4	T50.5X5	T50.5X6
Fenobarbital	T42.3X1	T42.3X2	T42.3X3	T42.3X4	T42.3X5	T42.3X6
Fenofibrate	T46.6X1	T46.6X2	T46.6X3	T46.6X4	T46.6X5	T46.6X6
Fenoprofen	T39.311	T39.312	T39.313	T39.314	T39.315	T39.316
Fenoterol	T48.6X1	T48.6X2	T48.6X3	T48.6X4	T48.6X5	T48.6X6
Fenoverine	T44.3X1	T44.3X2	T44.3X3	T44.3X4	T44.3X5	T44.3X6
Fenoxazoline	T48.5X1	T48.5X2	T48.5X3	T48.5X4	T48.5X5	T48.5X6
Fenproporex	T50.5X1	T50.5X2	T50.5X3	T50.5X4	T50.5X5	T50.5X6
Fenquizone	T50.2X1	T50.2X2	T50.2X3	T50.2X4	T50.2X5	T50.2X6
Fentanyl	T40.4X1	T40.4X2	T40.4X3	T40.4X4	T40.4X5	T40.4X6
Fentazin	T43.3X1	T43.3X2	T43.3X3	T43.3X4	T43.3X5	T43.3X6
Fenthion	T60.0X1	T60.0X2	T60.0X3	T60.0X4	—	—
Fenticlor	T49.0X1	T49.0X2	T49.0X3	T49.0X4	T49.0X5	T49.0X6
Fenylbutazone	T39.2X1	T39.2X2	T39.2X3	T39.2X4	T39.2X5	T39.2X6

Substance	Poisoning, Accidental (unintentional)	Poisoning, Intentional Self-harm	Poisoning, Assault	Poisoning, Undetermined	Adverse Effect	Under-dosing
Feprazone	T39.2X1	T39.2X2	T39.2X3	T39.2X4	T39.2X5	T39.
Fer de lance (bite) (venom)	T63.061	T63.062	T63.063	T63.064	—	
Ferric — see also Iron						
chloride	T45.4X1	T45.4X2	T45.4X3	T45.4X4	T45.4X5	T45.
citrate	T45.4X1	T45.4X2	T45.4X3	T45.4X4	T45.4X5	T45.
hydroxide						
colloidal	T45.4X1	T45.4X2	T45.4X3	T45.4X4	T45.4X5	T45.
polymaltose	T45.4X1	T45.4X2	T45.4X3	T45.4X4	T45.4X5	T45.
pyrophosphate	T45.4X1	T45.4X2	T45.4X3	T45.4X4	T45.4X5	T45.
Ferritin	T45.4X1	T45.4X2	T45.4X3	T45.4X4	T45.4X5	T45.
Ferrocholinate	T45.4X1	T45.4X2	T45.4X3	T45.4X4	T45.4X5	T45.
Ferrodextrane	T45.4X1	T45.4X2	T45.4X3	T45.4X4	T45.4X5	T45.
Ferropolimaler	T45.4X1	T45.4X2	T45.4X3	T45.4X4	T45.4X5	T45.
Ferrous — see also Iron						
phosphate	T45.4X1	T45.4X2	T45.4X3	T45.4X4	T45.4X5	T45.
salt	T45.4X1	T45.4X2	T45.4X3	T45.4X4	T45.4X5	T45.
with folic acid	T45.4X1	T45.4X2	T45.4X3	T45.4X4	T45.4X5	T45.
Ferrous fumerate, gluconate, lactate, salt NEC, sulfate (medicinal)	T45.4X1	T45.4X2	T45.4X3	T45.4X4	T45.4X5	T45.
Ferrovanadium (fumes)	T59.891	T59.892	T59.893	T59.894	—	
Ferrum — see Iron						
Fertilizers NEC	T65.891	T65.892	T65.893	T65.894	—	
with herbicide mixture	T60.3X1	T60.3X2	T60.3X3	T60.3X4	—	
Fetoxilate	T47.6X1	T47.6X2	T47.6X3	T47.6X4	T47.6X5	T47.
Fiber, dietary	T47.4X1	T47.4X2	T47.4X3	T47.4X4	T47.4X5	T47.
Fiberglass	T65.831	T65.832	T65.833	T65.834	—	
Fibrinogen (human)	T45.8X1	T45.8X2	T45.8X3	T45.8X4	T45.8X5	T45.
Fibrinolysin (human)	T45.691	T45.692	T45.693	T45.694	T45.695	T45.
Fibrinolysis						
affecting drug	T45.601	T45.602	T45.603	T45.604	T45.605	T45.
inhibitor NEC	T45.621	T45.622	T45.623	T45.624	T45.625	T45.
Fibrinolytic drug	T45.611	T45.612	T45.613	T45.614	T45.615	T45.
Filix mas	T37.4X1	T37.4X2	T37.4X3	T37.4X4	T37.4X5	T37.
Filtering cream	T49.3X1	T49.3X2	T49.3X3	T49.3X4	T49.3X5	T49.
Fiorinal	T39.011	T39.012	T39.013	T39.014	T39.015	T39.
Firedamp	T59.891	T59.892	T59.893	T59.894	—	
Fish, noxious, nonbacterial	T61.91	T61.92	T61.93	T61.94	—	
ciguatera	T61.01	T61.02	T61.03	T61.04	—	
scombroid	T61.11	T61.12	T61.13	T61.14	—	
shell	T61.781	T61.782	T61.783	T61.784	—	
specified NEC	T61.771	T61.772	T61.773	T61.774	—	
Flagyl	T37.3X1	T37.3X2	T37.3X3	T37.3X4	T37.3X5	T37.
Flavine adenine dinucleotide	T45.2X1	T45.2X2	T45.2X3	T45.2X4	T45.2X5	T45.
Flavodic acid	T46.991	T46.992	T46.993	T46.994	T46.995	T46.
Flavoxate	T44.3X1	T44.3X2	T44.3X3	T44.3X4	T44.3X5	T44.
Flaxedil	T48.1X1	T48.1X2	T48.1X3	T48.1X4	T48.1X5	T48.
Flaxseed (medicinal)	T49.3X1	T49.3X2	T49.3X3	T49.3X4	T49.3X5	T49.
Flecainide	T46.2X1	T46.2X2	T46.2X3	T46.2X4	T46.2X5	T46.
Fleroxacin	T36.8X1	T36.8X2	T36.8X3	T36.8X4	T36.8X5	T36.
Floctafenine	T39.8X1	T39.8X2	T39.8X3	T39.8X4	T39.8X5	T39.
Flomax	T44.6X1	T44.6X2	T44.6X3	T44.6X4	T44.6X5	T44.
Flomoxef	T36.1X1	T36.1X2	T36.1X3	T36.1X4	T36.1X5	T36.
Flopropione	T44.3X1	T44.3X2	T44.3X3	T44.3X4	T44.3X5	T44.
Florantyrone	T47.5X1	T47.5X2	T47.5X3	T47.5X4	T47.5X5	T47.
Floraquin	T37.8X1	T37.8X2	T37.8X3	T37.8X4	T37.8X5	T37.
Florinef	T38.0X1	T38.0X2	T38.0X3	T38.0X4	T38.0X5	T38.
ENT agent	T49.6X1	T49.6X2	T49.6X3	T49.6X4	T49.6X5	T49.
ophthalmic preparation	T49.5X1	T49.5X2	T49.5X3	T49.5X4	T49.5X5	T49.
topical NEC	T49.0X1	T49.0X2	T49.0X3	T49.0X4	T49.0X5	T49.
Flowers of sulfur	T49.4X1	T49.4X2	T49.4X3	T49.4X4	T49.4X5	T49.
Floxuridine	T45.1X1	T45.1X2	T45.1X3	T45.1X4	T45.1X5	T45.
Fluanisone	T43.4X1	T43.4X2	T43.4X3	T43.4X4	T43.4X5	T43.
Flubendazole	T37.4X1	T37.4X2	T37.4X3	T37.4X4	T37.4X5	T37.
Fluclorolone acetonide	T49.0X1	T49.0X2	T49.0X3	T49.0X4	T49.0X5	T49.
Flucloxacillin	T36.0X1	T36.0X2	T36.0X3	T36.0X4	T36.0X5	T36.
Fluconazole	T37.8X1	T37.8X2	T37.8X3	T37.8X4	T37.8X5	T37.
Flucytosine	T37.8X1	T37.8X2	T37.8X3	T37.8X4	T37.8X5	T37.
Fludeoxyglucose (18F)	T50.8X1	T50.8X2	T50.8X3	T50.8X4	T50.8X5	T50.
Fludiazepam	T42.4X1	T42.4X2	T42.4X3	T42.4X4	T42.4X5	T42.
Fludrocortisone	T50.0X1	T50.0X2	T50.0X3	T50.0X4	T50.0X5	T50.
ENT agent	T49.6X1	T49.6X2	T49.6X3	T49.6X4	T49.6X5	T49.
ophthalmic preparation	T49.5X1	T49.5X2	T49.5X3	T49.5X4	T49.5X5	T49.
topical NEC	T49.0X1	T49.0X2	T49.0X3	T49.0X4	T49.0X5	T49.
Fludroxycortide	T49.0X1	T49.0X2	T49.0X3	T49.0X4	T49.0X5	T49.
Flufenamic acid	T39.391	T39.392	T39.393	T39.394	T39.395	T39.
Fluindione	T45.511	T45.512	T45.513	T45.514	T45.515	T45.
Flumequine	T37.8X1	T37.8X2	T37.8X3	T37.8X4	T37.8X5	T37.
Flumethasone	T49.0X1	T49.0X2	T49.0X3	T49.0X4	T49.0X5	T49.
Flumethiazide	T50.2X1	T50.2X2	T50.2X3	T50.2X4	T50.2X5	T50.
Flumidin	T37.5X1	T37.5X2	T37.5X3	T37.5X4	T37.5X5	T37.

Substance	Poisoning, Accidental (unintentional)	Poisoning, Intentional Self-harm	Poisoning, Assault	Poisoning, Undetermined	Adverse Effect	Under-dosing
Flunarizine	T46.7X1	T46.7X2	T46.7X3	T46.7X4	T46.7X5	T46.7X6
Flunidazole	T37.8X1	T37.8X2	T37.8X3	T37.8X4	T37.8X5	T37.8X6
Flunisolide	T48.6X1	T48.6X2	T48.6X3	T48.6X4	T48.6X5	T48.6X6
Flunitrazepam	T42.4X1	T42.4X2	T42.4X3	T42.4X4	T42.4X5	T42.4X6
Fluocinolone (acetonide)	T49.0X1	T49.0X2	T49.0X3	T49.0X4	T49.0X5	T49.0X6
Fluocinonide	T49.0X1	T49.0X2	T49.0X3	T49.0X4	T49.0X5	T49.0X6
Fluocortin (butyl)	T49.0X1	T49.0X2	T49.0X3	T49.0X4	T49.0X5	T49.0X6
Fluocortolone	T49.0X1	T49.0X2	T49.0X3	T49.0X4	T49.0X5	T49.0X6
Fluohydrocortisone	T38.0X1	T38.0X2	T38.0X3	T38.0X4	T38.0X5	T38.0X6
ENT agent	T49.6X1	T49.6X2	T49.6X3	T49.6X4	T49.6X5	T49.6X6
ophthalmic preparation	T49.5X1	T49.5X2	T49.5X3	T49.5X4	T49.5X5	T49.5X6
topical NEC	T49.0X1	T49.0X2	T49.0X3	T49.0X4	T49.0X5	T49.0X6
Fluonid	T49.0X1	T49.0X2	T49.0X3	T49.0X4	T49.0X5	T49.0X6
Fluopromazine	T43.3X1	T43.3X2	T43.3X3	T43.3X4	T43.3X5	T43.3X6
Fluoracetate	T60.8X1	T60.8X2	T60.8X3	T60.8X4	—	—
Fluorescein	T50.8X1	T50.8X2	T50.8X3	T50.8X4	T50.8X5	T50.8X6
Fluorhydrocortisone	T50.0X1	T50.0X2	T50.0X3	T50.0X4	T50.0X5	T50.0X6
Fluoride (nonmedicinal) (pesticide) (sodium) NEC	T60.8X1	T60.8X2	T60.8X3	T60.8X4	—	—
hydrogen — see Hydrofluoric acid						
medicinal NEC	T50.991	T50.992	T50.993	T50.994	T50.995	T50.996
dental use	T49.7X1	T49.7X2	T49.7X3	T49.7X4	T49.7X5	T49.7X6
not pesticide NEC	T54.91	T54.92	T54.93	T54.94		
stannous	T49.7X1	T49.7X2	T49.7X3	T49.7X4	T49.7X5	T49.7X6
Fluorinated corticosteroids	T38.0X1	T38.0X2	T38.0X3	T38.0X4	T38.0X5	T38.0X6
Fluorine (gas)	T59.5X1	T59.5X2	T59.5X3	T59.5X4	—	—
salt — see Fluoride(s)						
Fluoristan	T49.7X1	T49.7X2	T49.7X3	T49.7X4	T49.7X5	T49.7X6
Fluormetholone	T49.0X1	T49.0X2	T49.0X3	T49.0X4	T49.0X5	T49.0X6
Fluoroacetate	T60.8X1	T60.8X2	T60.8X3	T60.8X4	—	—
Fluorocarbon monomer	T53.6X1	T53.6X2	T53.6X3	T53.6X4	—	—
Fluorocytosine	T37.8X1	T37.8X2	T37.8X3	T37.8X4	T37.8X5	T37.8X6
Fluorodeoxyuridine	T45.1X1	T45.1X2	T45.1X3	T45.1X4	T45.1X5	T45.1X6
Fluorometholone	T49.0X1	T49.0X2	T49.0X3	T49.0X4	T49.0X5	T49.0X6
ophthalmic preparation	T49.5X1	T49.5X2	T49.5X3	T49.5X4	T49.5X5	T49.5X6
Fluorophosphate insecticide	T60.0X1	T60.0X2	T60.0X3	T60.0X4	—	—
Fluorosol	T46.3X1	T46.3X2	T46.3X3	T46.3X4	T46.3X5	T46.3X6
Fluorouracil	T45.1X1	T45.1X2	T45.1X3	T45.1X4	T45.1X5	T45.1X6
Fluorphenylalanine	T49.5X1	T49.5X2	T49.5X3	T49.5X4	T49.5X5	T49.5X6
Fluothane	T41.0X1	T41.0X2	T41.0X3	T41.0X4	T41.0X5	T41.0X6
Fluoxetine	T43.221	T43.222	T43.223	T43.224	T43.225	T43.226
Fluoxymesterone	T38.7X1	T38.7X2	T38.7X3	T38.7X4	T38.7X5	T38.7X6
Flupenthixol	T43.4X1	T43.4X2	T43.4X3	T43.4X4	T43.4X5	T43.4X6
Flupentixol	T43.4X1	T43.4X2	T43.4X3	T43.4X4	T43.4X5	T43.4X6
Fluphenazine	T43.3X1	T43.3X2	T43.3X3	T43.3X4	T43.3X5	T43.3X6
Fluprednidene	T49.0X1	T49.0X2	T49.0X3	T49.0X4	T49.0X5	T49.0X6
Fluprednisolone	T38.0X1	T38.0X2	T38.0X3	T38.0X4	T38.0X5	T38.0X6
Fluradoline	T39.8X1	T39.8X2	T39.8X3	T39.8X4	T39.8X5	T39.8X6
Flurandrenolide	T49.0X1	T49.0X2	T49.0X3	T49.0X4	T49.0X5	T49.0X6
Flurandrenolone	T49.0X1	T49.0X2	T49.0X3	T49.0X4	T49.0X5	T49.0X6
Flurazepam	T42.4X1	T42.4X2	T42.4X3	T42.4X4	T42.4X5	T42.4X6
Flurbiprofen	T39.311	T39.312	T39.313	T39.314	T39.315	T39.316
Flurobate	T49.0X1	T49.0X2	T49.0X3	T49.0X4	T49.0X5	T49.0X6
Fluroxene	T41.0X1	T41.0X2	T41.0X3	T41.0X4	T41.0X5	T41.0X6
Fluspirilene	T43.591	T43.592	T43.593	T43.594	T43.595	T43.596
Flutamide	T38.6X1	T38.6X2	T38.6X3	T38.6X4	T38.6X5	T38.6X6
Flutazolam	T38.0X1	T38.0X2	T38.0X3	T38.0X4	T38.0X5	T38.0X6
Fluticasone propionate	T38.0X1	T38.0X2	T38.0X3	T38.0X4	T38.0X5	T38.0X6
Flutoprazepam	T42.4X1	T42.4X2	T42.4X3	T42.4X4	T42.4X5	T42.4X6
Flutropium bromide	T48.6X1	T48.6X2	T48.6X3	T48.6X4	T48.6X5	T48.6X6
Fluvoxamine	T43.221	T43.222	T43.223	T43.224	T43.225	T43.226
Folacin	T45.8X1	T45.8X2	T45.8X3	T45.8X4	T45.8X5	T45.8X6
Folic acid	T45.8X1	T45.8X2	T45.8X3	T45.8X4	T45.8X5	T45.8X6
with ferrous salt	T45.2X1	T45.2X2	T45.2X3	T45.2X4	T45.2X5	T45.2X6
antagonist	T45.1X1	T45.1X2	T45.1X3	T45.1X4	T45.1X5	T45.1X6
Folinic acid	T45.8X1	T45.8X2	T45.8X3	T45.8X4	T45.8X5	T45.8X6
Folium stramoniae	T48.6X1	T48.6X2	T48.6X3	T48.6X4	T48.6X5	T48.6X6
Follicle-stimulating hormone, human	T38.811	T38.812	T38.813	T38.814	T38.815	T38.816
Folpet	T60.3X1	T60.3X2	T60.3X3	T60.3X4	—	—
Fominoben	T48.3X1	T48.3X2	T48.3X3	T48.3X4	T48.3X5	T48.3X6
Food, foodstuffs, noxious, nonbacterial, NEC	T62.91	T62.92	T62.93	T62.94	—	—
berries	T62.1X1	T62.1X2	T62.1X3	T62.1X4	—	—
fish — see also Fish	T61.91	T61.92	T61.93	T61.94	—	—
mushrooms	T62.0X1	T62.0X2	T62.0X3	T62.0X4	—	—
plants	T62.2X1	T62.2X2	T62.2X3	T62.2X4	—	—
seafood	T61.91	T61.92	T61.93	T61.94	—	—
specified NEC	T61.8X1	T61.8X2	T61.8X3	T61.8X4	—	—
seeds	T62.2X1	T62.2X2	T62.2X3	T62.2X4	—	—

Substance	Poisoning, Accidental (unintentional)	Poisoning, Intentional Self-harm	Poisoning, Assault	Poisoning, Undetermined	Adverse Effect	Under-dosing
Food, foodstuffs, noxious, nonbacterial, — continued						
shellfish	T61.781	T61.782	T61.783	T61.784	—	—
specified NEC	T62.8X1	T62.8X2	T62.8X3	T62.8X4	—	—
Fool's parsley	T62.2X1	T62.2X2	T62.2X3	T62.2X4	—	—
Formaldehyde (solution), gas or vapor	T59.2X1	T59.2X2	T59.2X3	T59.2X4	—	—
fungicide	T60.3X1	T60.3X2	T60.3X3	T60.3X4	—	—
Formalin	T59.2X1	T59.2X2	T59.2X3	T59.2X4	—	—
fungicide	T60.3X1	T60.3X2	T60.3X3	T60.3X4	—	—
vapor	T59.2X1	T59.2X2	T59.2X3	T59.2X4	—	—
Formic acid	T54.2X1	T54.2X2	T54.2X3	T54.2X4	—	—
vapor	T59.891	T59.892	T59.893	T59.894	—	—
Foscarnet sodium	T37.5X1	T37.5X2	T37.5X3	T37.5X4	T37.5X5	T37.5X6
Fosfestrol	T38.5X1	T38.5X2	T38.5X3	T38.5X4	T38.5X5	T38.5X6
Fosfomycin	T36.8X1	T36.8X2	T36.8X3	T36.8X4	T36.8X5	T36.8X6
Fosfonet sodium	T37.5X1	T37.5X2	T37.5X3	T37.5X4	T37.5X5	T37.5X6
Fosinopril	T46.4X1	T46.4X2	T46.4X3	T46.4X4	T46.4X5	T46.4X6
sodium	T46.4X1	T46.4X2	T46.4X3	T46.4X4	T46.4X5	T46.4X6
Fowler's solution	T57.0X1	T57.0X2	T57.0X3	T57.0X4	—	—
Foxglove	T62.2X1	T62.2X2	T62.2X3	T62.2X4	—	—
Framycetin	T36.5X1	T36.5X2	T36.5X3	T36.5X4	T36.5X5	T36.5X6
Frangula	T47.2X1	T47.2X2	T47.2X3	T47.2X4	T47.2X5	T47.2X6
extract	T47.2X1	T47.2X2	T47.2X3	T47.2X4	T47.2X5	T47.2X6
Frei antigen	T50.8X1	T50.8X2	T50.8X3	T50.8X4	T50.8X5	T50.8X6
Freon	T53.5X1	T53.5X2	T53.5X3	T53.5X4	—	—
Fructose	T50.3X1	T50.3X2	T50.3X3	T50.3X4	T50.3X5	T50.3X6
Frusemide	T50.1X1	T50.1X2	T50.1X3	T50.1X4	T50.1X5	T50.1X6
FSH	T38.811	T38.812	T38.813	T38.814	T38.815	T38.816
Ftorafur	T45.1X1	T45.1X2	T45.1X3	T45.1X4	T45.1X5	T45.1X6
Fuel						
automobile	T52.0X1	T52.0X2	T52.0X3	T52.0X4	—	—
exhaust gas, not in transit	T58.01	T58.02	T58.03	T58.04		
vapor NEC	T52.0X1	T52.0X2	T52.0X3	T52.0X4	—	—
gas (domestic use) — see also Carbon, monoxide, fuel, utility	T59.891	T59.892	T59.893	T59.894		
utility	T59.891	T59.892	T59.893	T59.894		
incomplete combustion of — see Carbon, monoxide, fuel, utility						
in mobile container	T59.891	T59.892	T59.893	T59.894		
piped (natural)	T59.891	T59.892	T59.893	T59.894		
industrial, incomplete combustion	T58.8X1	T58.8X2	T58.8X3	T58.8X4		
Fugillin	T36.8X1	T36.8X2	T36.8X3	T36.8X4	T36.8X5	T36.8X6
Fulminate of mercury	T56.1X1	T56.1X2	T56.1X3	T56.1X4		
Fulvicin	T36.7X1	T36.7X2	T36.7X3	T36.7X4	T36.7X5	T36.7X6
Fumadil	T36.8X1	T36.8X2	T36.8X3	T36.8X4	T36.8X5	T36.8X6
Fumagillin	T36.8X1	T36.8X2	T36.8X3	T36.8X4	T36.8X5	T36.8X6
Fumaric acid	T49.4X1	T49.4X2	T49.4X3	T49.4X4	T49.4X5	T49.4X6
Fumes (from)	T59.91	T59.92	T59.93	T59.94		
carbon monoxide — see Carbon, monoxide						
charcoal (domestic use) — see Charcoal, fumes						
chloroform — see Chloroform						
coke (in domestic stoves, fireplaces) — see Coke fumes						
corrosive NEC	T54.91	T54.92	T54.93	T54.94	—	—
ether — see ether						
freons	T53.5X1	T53.5X2	T53.5X3	T53.5X4		
hydrocarbons	T59.891	T59.892	T59.893	T59.894		
petroleum (liquefied)	T59.891	T59.892	T59.893	T59.894		
distributed through pipes (pure or mixed with air)	T59.891	T59.892	T59.893	T59.894		
lead — see lead						
metal — see Metals, or the specified metal						
nitrogen dioxide	T59.0X1	T59.0X2	T59.0X3	T59.0X4		
pesticides — see Pesticides						
petroleum (liquefied)	T59.891	T59.892	T59.893	T59.894		
distributed through pipes (pure or mixed with air)	T59.891	T59.892	T59.893	T59.894		
polyester	T59.891	T59.892	T59.893	T59.894		
specified source NEC — see also substance specified	T59.891	T59.892	T59.893	T59.894		
sulfur dioxide	T59.1X1	T59.1X2	T59.1X3	T59.1X4		
Fumigant NEC	T60.91	T60.92	T60.93	T60.94	—	—

Substance	Poisoning, Accidental (unintentional)	Poisoning, Intentional Self-harm	Poisoning, Assault	Poisoning, Undetermined	Adverse Effect	Under-dosing
Fungicide NEC (nonmedicinal)	T60.3X1	T60.3X2	T60.3X3	T60.3X4	—	—
Fungi, noxious, used as food	T62.0X1	T62.0X2	T62.0X3	T62.0X4	—	—
Fungizone	T36.7X1	T36.7X2	T36.7X3	T36.7X4	T36.7X5	T36.7X6
topical	T49.0X1	T49.0X2	T49.0X3	T49.0X4	T49.0X5	T49.0X6
Furacin	T49.0X1	T49.0X2	T49.0X3	T49.0X4	T49.0X5	T49.0X6
Furadantin	T37.91	T37.92	T37.93	T37.94	T37.95	T37.96
Furazolidone	T37.8X1	T37.8X2	T37.8X3	T37.8X4	T37.8X5	T37.8X6
Furazolium chloride	T49.0X1	T49.0X2	T49.0X3	T49.0X4	T49.0X5	T49.0X6
Furfural	T52.8X1	T52.8X2	T52.8X3	T52.8X4	—	—
Furnace (coal burning) (domestic), gas from	T58.2X1	T58.2X2	T58.2X3	T58.2X4	—	—
industrial	T58.8X1	T58.8X2	T58.8X3	T58.8X4	—	—
Furniture polish	T65.891	T65.892	T65.893	T65.894	—	—
Furosemide	T50.1X1	T50.1X2	T50.1X3	T50.1X4	T50.1X5	T50.1X6
Furoxone	T37.91	T37.92	T37.93	T37.94	T37.95	T37.96
Fursultiamine	T45.2X1	T45.2X2	T45.2X3	T45.2X4	T45.2X5	T45.2X6
Fusafungine	T36.8X1	T36.8X2	T36.8X3	T36.8X4	T36.8X5	T36.8X6
Fusel oil (any) (amyl) (butyl) (propyl), vapor	T51.3X1	T51.3X2	T51.3X3	T51.3X4	—	—
Fusidate (ethanolamine) (sodium)	T36.8X1	T36.8X2	T36.8X3	T36.8X4	T36.8X5	T36.8X6
Fusidic acid	T36.8X1	T36.8X2	T36.8X3	T36.8X4	T36.8X5	T36.8X6
Fytic acid, nonasodium	T50.6X1	T50.6X2	T50.6X3	T50.6X4	T50.6X5	T50.6X6
b-Galactosidase	T47.5X1	T47.5X2	T47.5X3	T47.5X4	T47.5X5	T47.5X6
GABA	T43.8X1	T43.8X2	T43.8X3	T43.8X4	T43.8X5	T43.8X6
Gadopentetic acid	T50.8X1	T50.8X2	T50.8X3	T50.8X4	T50.8X5	T50.8X6
Galactose	T50.3X1	T50.3X2	T50.3X3	T50.3X4	T50.3X5	T50.3X6
Galantamine	T44.0X1	T44.0X2	T44.0X3	T44.0X4	T44.0X5	T44.0X6
Gallamine (triethiodide)	T48.1X1	T48.1X2	T48.1X3	T48.1X4	T48.1X5	T48.1X6
Gallium citrate	T50.991	T50.992	T50.993	T50.994	T50.995	T50.996
Gallopamil	T46.1X1	T46.1X2	T46.1X3	T46.1X4	T46.1X5	T46.1X6
Gamboge	T47.2X1	T47.2X2	T47.2X3	T47.2X4	T47.2X5	T47.2X6
Gamimune	T50.Z11	T50.Z12	T50.Z13	T50.Z14	T50.Z15	T50.Z16
Gamma-aminobutyric acid	T43.8X1	T43.8X2	T43.8X3	T43.8X4	T43.8X5	T43.8X6
Gamma-benzene hexachloride (medicinal)	T49.0X1	T49.0X2	T49.0X3	T49.0X4	T49.0X5	T49.0X6
nonmedicinal, vapor	T53.6X1	T53.6X2	T53.6X3	T53.6X4	—	—
Gamma-BHC (medicinal) — see also Gamma-benzene hexachloride	T49.0X1	T49.0X2	T49.0X3	T49.0X4	T49.0X5	T49.0X6
Gamma globulin	T50.Z11	T50.Z12	T50.Z13	T50.Z14	T50.Z15	T50.Z16
Gamulin	T50.Z11	T50.Z12	T50.Z13	T50.Z14	T50.Z15	T50.Z16
Ganciclovir (sodium)	T37.5X1	T37.5X2	T37.5X3	T37.5X4	T37.5X5	T37.5X6
Ganglionic blocking drug NEC	T44.2X1	T44.2X2	T44.2X3	T44.2X4	T44.2X5	T44.2X6
specified NEC	T44.2X1	T44.2X2	T44.2X3	T44.2X4	T44.2X5	T44.2X6
Ganja	T40.7X1	T40.7X2	T40.7X3	T40.7X4	T40.7X5	T40.7X6
Garamycin	T36.5X1	T36.5X2	T36.5X3	T36.5X4	T36.5X5	T36.5X6
ophthalmic preparation	T49.5X1	T49.5X2	T49.5X3	T49.5X4	T49.5X5	T49.5X6
topical NEC	T49.0X1	T49.0X2	T49.0X3	T49.0X4	T49.0X5	T49.0X6
Gardenal	T42.3X1	T42.3X2	T42.3X3	T42.3X4	T42.3X5	T42.3X6
Gardepanyl	T42.3X1	T42.3X2	T42.3X3	T42.3X4	T42.3X5	T42.3X6
Gaseous substance — see Gas						
Gasoline	T52.0X1	T52.0X2	T52.0X3	T52.0X4	—	—
vapor	T52.0X1	T52.0X2	T52.0X3	T52.0X4	—	—
Gastric enzymes	T47.5X1	T47.5X2	T47.5X3	T47.5X4	T47.5X5	T47.5X6
Gastrografin	T50.8X1	T50.8X2	T50.8X3	T50.8X4	T50.8X5	T50.8X6
Gastrointestinal drug	T47.91	T47.92	T47.93	T47.94	T47.95	T47.96
biological	T47.8X1	T47.8X2	T47.8X3	T47.8X4	T47.8X5	T47.8X6
specified NEC	T47.8X1	T47.8X2	T47.8X3	T47.8X4	T47.8X5	T47.8X6
Gas NEC	T59.91	T59.92	T59.93	T59.94	—	—
acetylene	T59.891	T59.892	T59.893	T59.894	—	—
incomplete combustion of	T58.11	T58.12	T58.13	T58.14	—	—
air contaminants, source or type not specified	T59.91	T59.92	T59.93	T59.94	—	—
anesthetic	T41.0X1	T41.0X2	T41.0X3	T41.0X4	T41.0X5	T41.0X6
blast furnace	T58.8X1	T58.8X2	T58.8X3	T58.8X4	—	—
butane — see butane						
carbon monoxide — see Carbon, monoxide						
chlorine	T59.4X1	T59.4X2	T59.4X3	T59.4X4	—	—
coal	T58.2X1	T58.2X2	T58.2X3	T58.2X4	—	—
cyanide	T57.3X1	T57.3X2	T57.3X3	T57.3X4	—	—
dicyanogen	T65.0X1	T65.0X2	T65.0X3	T65.0X4	—	—
domestic — see Domestic gas						
exhaust	T58.01	T58.02	T58.03	T58.04	—	—
from utility (for cooking, heating, or lighting) (after combustion) — see Carbon, monoxide, fuel, utility						

Substance	Poisoning, Accidental (unintentional)	Poisoning, Intentional Self-harm	Poisoning, Assault	Poisoning, Undetermined	Adverse Effect	Under-dosing
Gas — continued						
from utility — see Carbon, monoxide, fuel, utility — continued						
prior to combustion	T59.891	T59.892	T59.893	T59.894		
from wood- or coal-burning stove or fireplace	T58.2X1	T58.2X2	T58.2X3	T58.2X4	—	
fuel (domestic use) (after combustion) — see also Carbon, monoxide, fuel						
industrial use	T58.8X1	T58.8X2	T58.8X3	T58.8X4	—	
prior to combustion	T59.891	T59.892	T59.893	T59.894		
utility	T59.891	T59.892	T59.893	T59.894		
incomplete combustion of — see Carbon, monoxide, fuel, utility						
in mobile container	T59.891	T59.892	T59.893	T59.894		
piped (natural)	T59.891	T59.892	T59.893	T59.894		
garage	T58.01	T58.02	T58.03	T58.04		
hydrocarbon NEC	T59.891	T59.892	T59.893	T59.894		
incomplete combustion of — see Carbon, monoxide, fuel, utility						
liquefied — see butane						
piped	T59.891	T59.892	T59.893	T59.894	—	
hydrocyanic acid	T65.0X1	T65.0X2	T65.0X3	T65.0X4	—	
illuminating (after combustion)	T58.11	T58.12	T58.13	T58.14		
prior to combustion	T59.891	T59.892	T59.893	T59.894		
incomplete combustion, any — see Carbon, monoxide						
kiln	T58.8X1	T58.8X2	T58.8X3	T58.8X4		
lacrimogenic	T59.3X1	T59.3X2	T59.3X3	T59.3X4		
liquefied petroleum — see butane						
marsh	T59.891	T59.892	T59.893	T59.894		
motor exhaust, not in transit	T58.01	T58.02	T58.03	T58.04		
mustard, not in war	T59.891	T59.892	T59.893	T59.894		
natural	T59.891	T59.892	T59.893	T59.894		
nerve, not in war	T59.91	T59.92	T59.93	T59.94		
oil	T52.0X1	T52.0X2	T52.0X3	T52.0X4		
petroleum (liquefied) (distributed in mobile containers)	T59.891	T59.892	T59.893	T59.894		
piped (pure or mixed with air)	T59.891	T59.892	T59.893	T59.894		
piped (manufactured) (natural) NEC	T59.891	T59.892	T59.893	T59.894		
producer	T58.8X1	T58.8X2	T58.8X3	T58.8X4		
propane — see propane						
refrigerant (chlorofluoro-carbon)	T53.5X1	T53.5X2	T53.5X3	T53.5X4		
not chlorofluoro-carbon	T59.891	T59.892	T59.893	T59.894		
sewer	T59.91	T59.92	T59.93	T59.94	—	
specified source NEC	T59.91	T59.92	T59.93	T59.94	—	
stove (after combustion)	T58.11	T58.12	T58.13	T58.14	—	
prior to combustion	T59.891	T59.892	T59.893	T59.894	—	
tear	T59.3X1	T59.3X2	T59.3X3	T59.3X4	—	
therapeutic	T41.5X1	T41.5X2	T41.5X3	T41.5X4	T41.5X5	T41.5
utility (for cooking, heating, or lighting) (piped) NEC	T59.891	T59.892	T59.893	T59.894	—	
incomplete combustion of — see Carbon, monoxide, fuel, utilty						
in mobile container	T59.891	T59.892	T59.893	T59.894		
piped (natural)	T59.891	T59.892	T59.893	T59.894		
water	T58.11	T58.12	T58.13	T58.14	—	
incomplete combustion of — see Carbon, monoxide, fuel, utility						
Gaultheria procumbens	T62.2X1	T62.2X2	T62.2X3	T62.2X4	—	
Gefarnate	T44.3X1	T44.3X2	T44.3X3	T44.3X4	T44.3X5	T44.3
Gelatin (intravenous)	T45.8X1	T45.8X2	T45.8X3	T45.8X4	T45.8X5	T45.8
absorbable (sponge)	T45.7X1	T45.7X2	T45.7X3	T45.7X4	T45.7X5	T45.7
Gelfilm	T49.8X1	T49.8X2	T49.8X3	T49.8X4	T49.8X5	T49.8
Gelfoam	T45.7X1	T45.7X2	T45.7X3	T45.7X4	T45.7X5	T45.7
Gelsemine	T50.991	T50.992	T50.993	T50.994	T50.995	T50.9
Gelsemium (sempervirens)	T62.2X1	T62.2X2	T62.2X3	T62.2X4		
Gemeprost	T48.0X1	T48.0X2	T48.0X3	T48.0X4	T48.0X5	T48.0
Gemfibrozil	T46.6X1	T46.6X2	T46.6X3	T46.6X4	T46.6X5	T46.6
Gemonil	T42.3X1	T42.3X2	T42.3X3	T42.3X4	T42.3X5	T42.3
Gentamicin	T36.5X1	T36.5X2	T42.3X3	T36.5X4	T36.5X5	T36.5

Substance	Poisoning, Accidental (unintentional)	Poisoning, Intentional Self-harm	Poisoning, Assault	Poisoning, Undetermined	Adverse Effect	Under-dosing
Gentamicin — *continued*						
ophthalmic preparation	T49.5X1	T49.5X2	T49.5X3	T49.5X4	T49.5X5	T49.5X6
topical NEC	T49.0X1	T49.0X2	T49.0X3	T49.0X4	T49.0X5	T49.0X6
Gentian	T47.5X1	T47.5X2	T47.5X3	T47.5X4	T47.5X5	T47.5X6
violet	T49.0X1	T49.0X2	T49.0X3	T49.0X4	T49.0X5	T49.0X6
Gepefrine	T44.4X1	T44.4X2	T44.4X3	T44.4X4	T44.4X5	T44.4X6
Gestonorone caproate	T38.5X1	T38.5X2	T38.5X3	T38.5X4	T38.5X5	T38.5X6
Gexane	T49.0X1	T49.0X2	T49.0X3	T49.0X4	T49.0X5	T49.0X6
Gila monster (venom)	T63.111	T63.112	T63.113	T63.114	—	—
Ginger	T47.5X1	T47.5X2	T47.5X3	T47.5X4	T47.5X5	T47.5X6
Jamaica — *see* Jamaica, ginger						
Gitalin	T46.0X1	T46.0X2	T46.0X3	T46.0X4	T46.0X5	T46.0X6
amorphous	T46.0X1	T46.0X2	T46.0X3	T46.0X4	T46.0X5	T46.0X6
Gitaloxin	T46.0X1	T46.0X2	T46.0X3	T46.0X4	T46.0X5	T46.0X6
Gitoxin	T46.0X1	T46.0X2	T46.0X3	T46.0X4	T46.0X5	T46.0X6
Glafenine	T39.8X1	T39.8X2	T39.8X3	T39.8X4	T39.8X5	T39.8X6
Glandular extract (medicinal) NEC	T50.Z91	T50.Z92	T50.Z93	T50.Z94	T50.Z95	T50.Z96
Glaucarubin	T37.3X1	T37.3X2	T37.3X3	T37.3X4	T37.3X5	T37.3X6
Glibenclamide	T38.3X1	T38.3X2	T38.3X3	T38.3X4	T38.3X5	T38.3X6
Glibornuride	T38.3X1	T38.3X2	T38.3X3	T38.3X4	T38.3X5	T38.3X6
Gliclazide	T38.3X1	T38.3X2	T38.3X3	T38.3X4	T38.3X5	T38.3X6
Glimidine	T38.3X1	T38.3X2	T38.3X3	T38.3X4	T38.3X5	T38.3X6
Glipizide	T38.3X1	T38.3X2	T38.3X3	T38.3X4	T38.3X5	T38.3X6
Gliquidone	T38.3X1	T38.3X2	T38.3X3	T38.3X4	T38.3X5	T38.3X6
Glisolamide	T38.3X1	T38.3X2	T38.3X3	T38.3X4	T38.3X5	T38.3X6
Glisoxepide	T38.3X1	T38.3X2	T38.3X3	T38.3X4	T38.3X5	T38.3X6
Globin zinc insulin	T38.3X1	T38.3X2	T38.3X3	T38.3X4	T38.3X5	T38.3X6
Globulin						
antilymphocytic	T50.Z11	T50.Z12	T50.Z13	T50.Z14	T50.Z15	T50.Z16
antirhesus	T50.Z11	T50.Z12	T50.Z13	T50.Z14	T50.Z15	T50.Z16
antivenin	T50.Z11	T50.Z12	T50.Z13	T50.Z14	T50.Z15	T50.Z16
antiviral	T50.Z11	T50.Z12	T50.Z13	T50.Z14	T50.Z15	T50.Z16
Glucagon	T38.3X1	T38.3X2	T38.3X3	T38.3X4	T38.3X5	T38.3X6
Glucocorticoids	T38.0X1	T38.0X2	T38.0X3	T38.0X4	T38.0X5	T38.0X6
Glucocorticosteroid	T38.0X1	T38.0X2	T38.0X3	T38.0X4	T38.0X5	T38.0X6
Gluconic acid	T50.991	T50.992	T50.993	T50.994	T50.995	T50.996
Glucosamine sulfate	T39.4X1	T39.4X2	T39.4X3	T39.4X4	T39.4X5	T39.4X6
Glucose	T50.3X1	T50.3X2	T50.3X3	T50.3X4	T50.3X5	T50.3X6
with sodium chloride	T50.3X1	T50.3X2	T50.3X3	T50.3X4	T50.3X5	T50.3X6
Glucosulfone sodium	T37.1X1	T37.1X2	T37.1X3	T37.1X4	T37.1X5	T37.1X6
Glucurolactone	T47.8X1	T47.8X2	T47.8X3	T47.8X4	T47.8X5	T47.8X6
Glue NEC	T52.8X1	T52.8X2	T52.8X3	T52.8X4	—	—
Glutamic acid	T47.5X1	T47.5X2	T47.5X3	T47.5X4	T47.5X5	T47.5X6
Glutaral (medicinal)	T49.0X1	T49.0X2	T49.0X3	T49.0X4	T49.0X5	T49.0X6
nonmedicinal	T65.891	T65.892	T65.893	T65.894	—	—
Glutaraldehyde	T65.891	T65.892	T65.893	T65.894	—	—
(nonmedicinal)						
medicinal	T49.0X1	T49.0X2	T49.0X3	T49.0X4	T49.0X5	T49.0X6
Glutathione	T50.6X1	T50.6X2	T50.6X3	T50.6X4	T50.6X5	T50.6X6
Glutethimide	T42.6X1	T42.6X2	T42.6X3	T42.6X4	T42.6X5	T42.6X6
Glyburide	T38.3X1	T38.3X2	T38.3X3	T38.3X4	T38.3X5	T38.3X6
Glycerin	T47.4X1	T47.4X2	T47.4X3	T47.4X4	T47.4X5	T47.4X6
Glycerol	T47.4X1	T47.4X2	T47.4X3	T47.4X4	T47.4X5	T47.4X6
borax	T49.6X1	T49.6X2	T49.6X3	T49.6X4	T49.6X5	T49.6X6
intravenous	T50.3X1	T50.3X2	T50.3X3	T50.3X4	T50.3X5	T50.3X6
iodinated	T48.4X1	T48.4X2	T48.4X3	T48.4X4	T48.4X5	T48.4X6
Glycerophosphate	T50.991	T50.992	T50.993	T50.994	T50.995	T50.996
Glyceryl						
gualacolate	T48.4X1	T48.4X2	T48.4X3	T48.4X4	T48.4X5	T48.4X6
nitrate	T46.3X1	T46.3X2	T46.3X3	T46.3X4	T46.3X5	T46.3X6
triacetate (topical)	T49.0X1	T49.0X2	T49.0X3	T49.0X4	T49.0X5	T49.0X6
trinitrate	T46.3X1	T46.3X2	T46.3X3	T46.3X4	T46.3X5	T46.3X6
Glycine	T50.3X1	T50.3X2	T50.3X3	T50.3X4	T50.3X5	T50.3X6
Glyclopyramide	T38.3X1	T38.3X2	T38.3X3	T38.3X4	T38.3X5	T38.3X6
Glycobiarsol	T37.3X1	T37.3X2	T37.3X3	T37.3X4	T37.3X5	T37.3X6
Glycols (ether)	T52.3X1	T52.3X2	T52.3X3	T52.3X4	—	—
Glyconiazide	T37.1X1	T37.1X2	T37.1X3	T37.1X4	T37.1X5	T37.1X6
Glycopyrrolate	T44.3X1	T44.3X2	T44.3X3	T44.3X4	T44.3X5	T44.3X6
Glycopyrronium	T44.3X1	T44.3X2	T44.3X3	T44.3X4	T44.3X5	T44.3X6
bromide	T44.3X1	T44.3X2	T44.3X3	T44.3X4	T44.3X5	T44.3X6
Glycoside, cardiac (stimulant)	T46.0X1	T46.0X2	T46.0X3	T46.0X4	T46.0X5	T46.0X6
Glycyclamide	T38.3X1	T38.3X2	T38.3X3	T38.3X4	T38.3X5	T38.3X6
Glycyrrhiza extract	T48.4X1	T48.4X2	T48.4X3	T48.4X4	T48.4X5	T48.4X6
Glycyrrhizic acid	T48.4X1	T48.4X2	T48.4X3	T48.4X4	T48.4X5	T48.4X6
Glycyrrhizinate potassium	T48.4X1	T48.4X2	T48.4X3	T48.4X4	T48.4X5	T48.4X6
Glymidine sodium	T38.3X1	T38.3X2	T38.3X3	T38.3X4	T38.3X5	T38.3X6
Glyphosate	T60.3X1	T60.3X2	T60.3X3	T60.3X4	—	—
Glyphylline	T48.6X1	T48.6X2	T48.6X3	T48.6X4	T48.6X5	T48.6X6
Gold						
colloidal (I98Au)	T45.1X1	T45.1X2	T45.1X3	T45.1X4	T45.1X5	T45.1X6
salts	T39.4X1	T39.4X2	T39.4X3	T39.4X4	T39.4X5	T39.4X6

Substance	Poisoning, Accidental (unintentional)	Poisoning, Intentional Self-harm	Poisoning, Assault	Poisoning, Undetermined	Adverse Effect	Under-dosing
Golden sulfide of antimony	T56.891	T56.892	T56.893	T56.894	—	—
Goldylocks	T62.2X1	T62.2X2	T62.2X3	T62.2X4	—	—
Gonadal tissue extract	T38.901	T38.902	T38.903	T38.904	T38.905	T38.906
female	T38.5X1	T38.5X2	T38.5X3	T38.5X4	T38.5X5	T38.5X6
male	T38.7X1	T38.7X2	T38.7X3	T38.7X4	T38.7X5	T38.7X6
Gonadorelin	T38.891	T38.892	T38.893	T38.894	T38.895	T38.896
Gonadotropin	T38.891	T38.892	T38.893	T38.894	T38.895	T38.896
chorionic	T38.891	T38.892	T38.893	T38.894	T38.895	T38.896
pituitary	T38.811	T38.812	T38.813	T38.814	T38.815	T38.816
Goserelin	T45.1X1	T45.1X2	T45.1X3	T45.1X4	T45.1X5	T45.1X6
Grain alcohol	T51.0X1	T51.0X2	T51.0X3	T51.0X4		
Gramicidin	T49.0X1	T49.0X2	T49.0X3	T49.0X4	T49.0X5	T49.0X6
Granisetron	T45.0X1	T45.0X2	T45.0X3	T45.0X4	T45.0X5	T45.0X6
Gratiola officinalis	T62.2X1	T62.2X2	T62.2X3	T62.2X4	—	—
Grease	T65.891	T65.892	T65.893	T65.894	—	—
Green hellebore	T62.2X1	T62.2X2	T62.2X3	T62.2X4	—	—
Green soap	T49.2X1	T49.2X2	T49.2X3	T49.2X4	T49.2X5	T49.2X6
Grifulvin	T36.7X1	T36.7X2	T36.7X3	T36.7X4	T36.7X5	T36.7X6
Griseofulvin	T36.7X1	T36.7X2	T36.7X3	T36.7X4	T36.7X5	T36.7X6
Growth hormone	T38.811	T38.812	T38.813	T38.814	T38.815	T38.816
Guaiacol derivatives	T48.4X1	T48.4X2	T48.4X3	T48.4X4	T48.4X5	T48.4X6
Guaiac reagent	T50.991	T50.992	T50.993	T50.994	T50.995	T50.996
Guaifenesin	T48.4X1	T48.4X2	T48.4X3	T48.4X4	T48.4X5	T48.4X6
Guaimesal	T48.4X1	T48.4X2	T48.4X3	T48.4X4	T48.4X5	T48.4X6
Guaiphenesin	T48.4X1	T48.4X2	T48.4X3	T48.4X4	T48.4X5	T48.4X6
Guamecycline	T36.4X1	T36.4X2	T36.4X3	T36.4X4	T36.4X5	T36.4X6
Guanabenz	T46.5X1	T46.5X2	T46.5X3	T46.5X4	T46.5X5	T46.5X6
Guanacline	T46.5X1	T46.5X2	T46.5X3	T46.5X4	T46.5X5	T46.5X6
Guanadrel	T46.5X1	T46.5X2	T46.5X3	T46.5X4	T46.5X5	T46.5X6
Guanatol	T37.2X1	T37.2X2	T37.2X3	T37.2X4	T37.2X5	T37.2X6
Guanethidine	T46.5X1	T46.5X2	T46.5X3	T46.5X4	T46.5X5	T46.5X6
Guanfacine	T46.5X1	T46.5X2	T46.5X3	T46.5X4	T46.5X5	T46.5X6
Guano	T65.891	T65.892	T65.893	T65.894	—	—
Guanochlor	T46.5X1	T46.5X2	T46.5X3	T46.5X4	T46.5X5	T46.5X6
Guanoclor	T46.5X1	T46.5X2	T46.5X3	T46.5X4	T46.5X5	T46.5X6
Guanoctine	T46.5X1	T46.5X2	T46.5X3	T46.5X4	T46.5X5	T46.5X6
Guanoxabenz	T46.5X1	T46.5X2	T46.5X3	T46.5X4	T46.5X5	T46.5X6
Guanoxan	T46.5X1	T46.5X2	T46.5X3	T46.5X4	T46.5X5	T46.5X6
Guar gum (medicinal)	T46.6X1	T46.6X2	T46.6X3	T46.6X4	T46.6X5	T46.6X6
Hachimycin	T36.7X1	T36.7X2	T36.7X3	T36.7X4	T36.7X5	T36.7X6
Hair						
dye	T49.4X1	T49.4X2	T49.4X3	T49.4X4	T49.4X5	T49.4X6
preparation NEC	T49.4X1	T49.4X2	T49.4X3	T49.4X4	T49.4X5	T49.4X6
Halazepam	T42.4X1	T42.4X2	T42.4X3	T42.4X4	T42.4X5	T42.4X6
Halcinolone	T49.0X1	T49.0X2	T49.0X3	T49.0X4	T49.0X5	T49.0X6
Halcinonide	T49.0X1	T49.0X2	T49.0X3	T49.0X4	T49.0X5	T49.0X6
Halethazole	T49.0X1	T49.0X2	T49.0X3	T49.0X4	T49.0X5	T49.0X6
Hallucinogen NOS	T40.901	T40.902	T40.903	T40.904	T40.905	T40.906
specified NEC	T40.991	T40.992	T40.993	T40.994	T40.995	T40.996
Halofantrine	T37.2X1	T37.2X2	T37.2X3	T37.2X4	T37.2X5	T37.2X6
Halofenate	T46.6X1	T46.6X2	T46.6X3	T46.6X4	T46.6X5	T46.6X6
Halometasone	T49.0X1	T49.0X2	T49.0X3	T49.0X4	T49.0X5	T49.0X6
Haloperidol	T43.4X1	T43.4X2	T43.4X3	T43.4X4	T43.4X5	T43.4X6
Haloprogin	T49.0X1	T49.0X2	T49.0X3	T49.0X4	T49.0X5	T49.0X6
Halotex	T49.0X1	T49.0X2	T49.0X3	T49.0X4	T49.0X5	T49.0X6
Halothane	T41.0X1	T41.0X2	T41.0X3	T41.0X4	T41.0X5	T41.0X6
Haloxazolam	T42.4X1	T42.4X2	T42.4X3	T42.4X4	T42.4X5	T42.4X6
Halquinols	T49.0X1	T49.0X2	T49.0X3	T49.0X4	T49.0X5	T49.0X6
Hamamelis	T49.2X1	T49.2X2	T49.2X3	T49.2X4	T49.2X5	T49.2X6
Haptendextran	T45.8X1	T45.8X2	T45.8X3	T45.8X4	T45.8X5	T45.8X6
Harmonyl	T46.5X1	T46.5X2	T46.5X3	T46.5X4	T46.5X5	T46.5X6
Hartmann's solution	T50.3X1	T50.3X2	T50.3X3	T50.3X4	T50.3X5	T50.3X6
Hashish	T40.7X1	T40.7X2	T40.7X3	T40.7X4	T40.7X5	T40.7X6
Hawaiian Woodrose seeds	T40.991	T40.992	T40.993	T40.994		
HCB	T60.3X1	T60.3X2	T60.3X3	T60.3X4		
HCH	T53.6X1	T53.6X2	T53.6X3	T53.6X4		
medicinal	T49.0X1	T49.0X2	T49.0X3	T49.0X4	T49.0X5	T49.0X6
HCN	T57.3X1	T57.3X2	T57.3X3	T57.3X4	—	—
Headache cures, drugs, powders NEC	T50.901	T50.902	T50.903	T50.904	T50.905	T50.906
Heavenly Blue (morning glory)	T40.991	T40.992	T40.993	T40.994		
Heavy metal antidote	T45.8X1	T45.8X2	T45.8X3	T45.8X4	T45.8X5	T45.8X6
Hedaquinium	T49.0X1	T49.0X2	T49.0X3	T49.0X4	T49.0X5	T49.0X6
Hedge hyssop	T62.2X1	T62.2X2	T62.2X3	T62.2X4	—	—
Heet	T49.8X1	T49.8X2	T49.8X3	T49.8X4	T49.8X5	T49.8X6
Helenin	T37.4X1	T37.4X2	T37.4X3	T37.4X4	T37.4X5	T37.4X6
Helium (nonmedicinal) NEC	T59.891	T59.892	T59.893	T59.894	—	—
medicinal	T48.991	T48.992	T48.993	T48.994	T48.995	T48.996
Hellebore (black) (green) (white)	T62.2X1	T62.2X2	T62.2X3	T62.2X4	—	—
Hematin	T45.8X1	T45.8X2	T45.8X3	T45.8X4	T45.8X5	T45.8X6

Table of Drugs and Chemicals

Substance	Poisoning, Accidental (unintentional)	Poisoning, Intentional Self-harm	Poisoning, Assault	Poisoning, Undetermined	Adverse Effect	Under-dosing
Hematinic preparation	T45.8X1	T45.8X2	T45.8X3	T45.8X4	T45.8X5	T45.8X6
Hematological agent	T45.91	T45.92	T45.93	T45.94	T45.95	T45.96
specified NEC	T45.8X1	T45.8X2	T45.8X3	T45.8X4	T45.8X5	T45.8X6
Hemlock	T62.2X1	T62.2X2	T62.2X3	T62.2X4	—	—
Hemostatic	T45.621	T45.622	T45.623	T45.624	T45.625	T45.626
drug, systemic	T45.621	T45.622	T45.623	T45.624	T45.625	T45.626
Hemostyptic	T49.4X1	T49.4X2	T49.4X3	T49.4X4	T49.4X5	T49.4X6
Henbane	T62.2X1	T62.2X2	T62.2X3	T62.2X4	—	—
Heparin (sodium)	T45.511	T45.512	T45.513	T45.514	T45.515	T45.516
action reverser	T45.7X1	T45.7X2	T45.7X3	T45.7X4	T45.7X5	T45.7X6
Heparin-fraction	T45.511	T45.512	T45.513	T45.514	T45.515	T45.516
Heparinoid (systemic)	T45.511	T45.512	T45.513	T45.514	T45.515	T45.516
Hepatic secretion stimulant	T47.8X1	T47.8X2	T47.8X3	T47.8X4	T47.8X5	T47.8X6
Hepatitis B						
immune globulin	T50.Z11	T50.Z12	T50.Z13	T50.Z14	T50.Z15	T50.Z16
vaccine	T50.B91	T50.B92	T50.B93	T50.B94	T50.B95	T50.B96
Hepronicate	T46.7X1	T46.7X2	T46.7X3	T46.7X4	T46.7X5	T46.7X6
Heptabarb	T42.3X1	T42.3X2	T42.3X3	T42.3X4	T42.3X5	T42.3X6
Heptabarbital	T42.3X1	T42.3X2	T42.3X3	T42.3X4	T42.3X5	T42.3X6
Heptabarbitone	T42.3X1	T42.3X2	T42.3X3	T42.3X4	T42.3X5	T42.3X6
Heptachlor	T60.1X1	T60.1X2	T60.1X3	T60.1X4	—	—
Heptalgin	T40.2X1	T40.2X2	T40.2X3	T40.2X4	T40.2X5	T40.2X6
Heptaminol	T46.3X1	T46.3X2	T46.3X3	T46.3X4	T46.3X5	T46.3X6
Herbicide NEC	T60.3X1	T60.3X2	T60.3X3	T60.3X4	—	—
Heroin	T40.1X1	T40.1X2	T40.1X3	T40.1X4	—	—
Herplex	T49.5X1	T49.5X2	T49.5X3	T49.5X4	T49.5X5	T49.5X6
HES	T45.8X1	T45.8X2	T45.8X3	T45.8X4	T45.8X5	T45.8X6
Hesperidin	T46.991	T46.992	T46.993	T46.994	T46.995	T46.996
Hetacillin	T36.0X1	T36.0X2	T36.0X3	T36.0X4	T36.0X5	T36.0X6
Hetastarch	T45.8X1	T45.8X2	T45.8X3	T45.8X4	T45.8X5	T45.8X6
HETP	T60.0X1	T60.0X2	T60.0X3	T60.0X4	—	—
Hexachlorobenzene (vapor)	T60.3X1	T60.3X2	T60.3X3	T60.3X4	—	—
Hexachlorocyclohexane	T53.6X1	T53.6X2	T53.6X3	T53.6X4	—	—
Hexachlorophene	T49.0X1	T49.0X2	T49.0X3	T49.0X4	T49.0X5	T49.0X6
Hexadiline	T46.3X1	T46.3X2	T46.3X3	T46.3X4	T46.3X5	T46.3X6
Hexadimethrine (bromide)	T45.7X1	T45.7X2	T45.7X3	T45.7X4	T45.7X5	T45.7X6
Hexadylamine	T46.3X1	T46.3X2	T46.3X3	T46.3X4	T46.3X5	T46.3X6
Hexaethyl tetraphosphate	T60.0X1	T60.0X2	T60.0X3	T60.0X4	—	—
Hexafluorenium bromide	T48.1X1	T48.1X2	T48.1X3	T48.1X4	T48.1X5	T48.1X6
Hexafluronium (bromide)	T48.1X1	T48.1X2	T48.1X3	T48.1X4	T48.1X5	T48.1X6
Hexa-germ	T49.2X1	T49.2X2	T49.2X3	T49.2X4	T49.2X5	T49.2X6
Hexahydrobenzol	T52.8X1	T52.8X2	T52.8X3	T52.8X4	—	—
Hexahydrocresol(s)	T51.8X1	T51.8X2	T51.8X3	T51.8X4	—	—
arsenide	T57.0X1	T57.0X2	T57.0X3	T57.0X4	—	—
arseniurated	T57.0X1	T57.0X2	T57.0X3	T57.0X4	—	—
cyanide	T57.3X1	T57.3X2	T57.3X3	T57.3X4	—	—
gas	T59.891	T59.892	T59.893	T59.894	—	—
Fluoride (liquid)	T57.8X1	T57.8X2	T57.8X3	T57.8X4	—	—
vapor	T59.891	T59.892	T59.893	T59.894	—	—
phophorated	T60.0X1	T60.0X2	T60.0X3	T60.0X4	—	—
sulfate	T57.8X1	T57.8X2	T57.8X3	T57.8X4	—	—
sulfide (gas)	T59.6X1	T59.6X2	T59.6X3	T59.6X4	—	—
arseniurated	T57.0X1	T57.0X2	T57.0X3	T57.0X4	—	—
sulfurated	T57.8X1	T57.8X2	T57.8X3	T57.8X4	—	—
Hexahydrophenol	T51.8X1	T51.8X2	T51.8X3	T51.8X4	—	—
Hexalen	T51.8X1	T51.8X2	T51.8X3	T51.8X4	—	—
Hexamethonium bromide	T44.2X1	T44.2X2	T44.2X3	T44.2X4	T44.2X5	T44.2X6
Hexamethylene	T52.8X1	T52.8X2	T52.8X3	T52.8X4	—	—
Hexamethylmelamine	T45.1X1	T45.1X2	T45.1X3	T45.1X4	T45.1X5	T45.1X6
Hexamidine	T49.0X1	T49.0X2	T49.0X3	T49.0X4	T49.0X5	T49.0X6
Hexamine (mandelate)	T37.8X1	T37.8X2	T37.8X3	T37.8X4	T37.8X5	T37.8X6
Hexanone, 2-hexanone	T52.4X1	T52.4X2	T52.4X3	T52.4X4	—	—
Hexanuorenium	T48.1X1	T48.1X2	T48.1X3	T48.1X4	T48.1X5	T48.1X6
Hexapropymate	T42.6X1	T42.6X2	T42.6X3	T42.6X4	T42.6X5	T42.6X6
Hexasonium iodide	T44.3X1	T44.3X2	T44.3X3	T44.3X4	T44.3X5	T44.3X6
Hexcarbacholine bromide	T48.1X1	T48.1X2	T48.1X3	T48.1X4	T48.1X5	T48.1X6
Hexemal	T42.3X1	T42.3X2	T42.3X3	T42.3X4	T42.3X5	T42.3X6
Hexestrol	T38.5X1	T38.5X2	T38.5X3	T38.5X4	T38.5X5	T38.5X6
Hexethal (sodium)	T42.3X1	T42.3X2	T42.3X3	T42.3X4	T42.3X5	T42.3X6
Hexetidine	T37.8X1	T37.8X2	T37.8X3	T37.8X4	T37.8X5	T37.8X6
Hexobarbital	T42.3X1	T42.3X2	T42.3X3	T42.3X4	T42.3X5	T42.3X6
rectal	T41.291	T41.292	T41.293	T41.294	T41.295	T41.296
sodium	T41.1X1	T41.1X2	T41.1X3	T41.1X4	T41.1X5	T41.1X6
Hexobendine	T46.3X1	T46.3X2	T46.3X3	T46.3X4	T46.3X5	T46.3X6
Hexocyclium	T44.3X1	T44.3X2	T44.3X3	T44.3X4	T44.3X5	T44.3X6
metilsulfate	T44.3X1	T44.3X2	T44.3X3	T44.3X4	T44.3X5	T44.3X6
Hexoestrol	T38.5X1	T38.5X2	T38.5X3	T38.5X4	T38.5X5	T38.5X6
Hexone	T52.4X1	T52.4X2	T52.4X3	T52.4X4	—	—
Hexoprenaline	T48.6X1	T48.6X2	T48.6X3	T48.6X4	T48.6X5	T48.6X6
Hexylcaine	T41.3X1	T41.3X2	T41.3X3	T41.3X4	T41.3X5	T41.3X6
Hexylresorcinol	T52.2X1	T52.2X2	T52.2X3	T52.2X4	—	—

Substance	Poisoning, Accidental (unintentional)	Poisoning, Intentional Self-harm	Poisoning, Assault	Poisoning, Undetermined	Adverse Effect	Under-dosing
HGH (human growth hormone)	T38.811	T38.812	T38.813	T38.814	T38.815	T38.8..
Hinkle's pills	T47.2X1	T47.2X2	T47.2X3	T47.2X4	T47.2X5	T47.2..
Histalog	T50.8X1	T50.8X2	T50.8X3	T50.8X4	T50.8X5	T50.8..
Histamine (phosphate)	T50.8X1	T50.8X2	T50.8X3	T50.8X4	T50.8X5	T50.8..
Histoplasmin	T50.8X1	T50.8X2	T50.8X3	T50.8X4	T50.8X5	T50.8..
Holly berries	T62.2X1	T62.2X2	T62.2X3	T62.2X4	—	—
Homatropine	T44.3X1	T44.3X2	T44.3X3	T44.3X4	T44.3X5	T44.3..
methylbromide	T44.3X1	T44.3X2	T44.3X3	T44.3X4	T44.3X5	T44.3..
Homochlorcyclizine	T45.0X1	T45.0X2	T45.0X3	T45.0X4	T45.0X5	T45.0..
Homosalate	T49.3X1	T49.3X2	T49.3X3	T49.3X4	T49.3X5	T49.3..
Homo-tet	T50.Z11	T50.Z12	T50.Z13	T50.Z14	T50.Z15	T50.2..
Hormone	T38.801	T38.802	T38.803	T38.804	T38.805	T38.8..
adrenal cortical steroids	T38.0X1	T38.0X2	T38.0X3	T38.0X4	T38.0X5	T38.0..
androgenic	T38.7X1	T38.7X2	T38.7X3	T38.7X4	T38.7X5	T38.7..
anterior pituitary NEC	T38.811	T38.812	T38.813	T38.814	T38.815	T38.8..
antidiabetic agents	T38.3X1	T38.3X2	T38.3X3	T38.3X4	T38.3X5	T38.3..
antidiuretic	T38.891	T38.892	T38.893	T38.894	T38.895	T38.8..
cancer therapy	T45.1X1	T45.1X2	T45.1X3	T45.1X4	T45.1X5	T45.1..
follicle stimulating	T38.811	T38.812	T38.813	T38.814	T38.815	T38.8..
gonadotropic	T38.891	T38.892	T38.893	T38.894	T38.895	T38.8..
pituitary	T38.811	T38.812	T38.813	T38.814	T38.815	T38.8..
growth	T38.811	T38.812	T38.813	T38.814	T38.815	T38.8..
luteinizing	T38.811	T38.812	T38.813	T38.814	T38.815	T38.8..
ovarian	T38.5X1	T38.5X2	T38.5X3	T38.5X4	T38.5X5	T38.5..
oxytocic	T48.0X1	T48.0X2	T48.0X3	T48.0X4	T48.0X5	T48.0..
parathyroid (derivatives)	T50.991	T50.992	T50.993	T50.994	T50.995	T50.9..
pituitary (posterior) NEC	T38.891	T38.892	T38.893	T38.894	T38.895	T38.8..
anterior	T38.811	T38.812	T38.813	T38.814	T38.815	T38.8..
specified, NEC	T38.891	T38.892	T38.893	T38.894	T38.895	T38.8..
thyroid	T38.1X1	T38.1X2	T38.1X3	T38.1X4	T38.1X5	T38.1..
Hornet (sting)	T63.451	T63.452	T63.453	T63.454	—	—
Horse anti-human lymphocytic serum	T50.Z11	T50.Z12	T50.Z13	T50.Z14	T50.Z15	T50.2..
Horticulture agent NEC	T65.91	T65.92	T65.93	T65.94	—	—
with pesticide	T60.91	T60.92	T60.93	T60.94	—	—
Human						
albumin	T45.8X1	T45.8X2	T45.8X3	T45.8X4	T45.8X5	T45.8..
growth hormone (HGH)	T38.811	T38.812	T38.813	T38.814	T38.815	T38.8..
immune serum	T50.Z11	T50.Z12	T50.Z13	T50.Z14	T50.Z15	T50.2..
Hyaluronidase	T45.3X1	T45.3X2	T45.3X3	T45.3X4	T45.3X5	T45.3..
Hyazyme	T45.3X1	T45.3X2	T45.3X3	T45.3X4	T45.3X5	T45.3..
Hycodan	T40.2X1	T40.2X2	T40.2X3	T40.2X4	T40.2X5	T40.2..
Hydantoin derivative NEC	T42.0X1	T42.0X2	T42.0X3	T42.0X4	T42.0X5	T42.0..
Hydeltra	T38.0X1	T38.0X2	T38.0X3	T38.0X4	T38.0X5	T38.0..
Hydergine	T44.6X1	T44.6X2	T44.6X3	T44.6X4	T44.6X5	T44.6..
Hydrabamine penicillin	T36.0X1	T36.0X2	T36.0X3	T36.0X4	T36.0X5	T36.0..
Hydralazine	T46.5X1	T46.5X2	T46.5X3	T46.5X4	T46.5X5	T46.5..
Hydrargaphen	T49.0X1	T49.0X2	T49.0X3	T49.0X4	T49.0X5	T49.0..
Hydrargyri aminochloridum	T49.0X1	T49.0X2	T49.0X3	T49.0X4	T49.0X5	T49.0..
Hydrastine	T48.291	T48.292	T48.293	T48.294	T48.295	T48.2..
Hydrazine	T54.1X1	T54.1X2	T54.1X3	T54.1X4	—	—
monoamine oxidase inhibitors	T43.1X1	T43.1X2	T43.1X3	T43.1X4	T43.1X5	T43.1..
Hydrazoic acid, azides	T54.2X1	T54.2X2	T54.2X3	T54.2X4	—	—
Hydriodic acid	T48.4X1	T48.4X2	T48.4X3	T48.4X4	T48.4X5	T48.4..
Hydrocarbon gas	T59.891	T59.892	T59.893	T59.894	—	—
incomplete combustion of — *see* Carbon, monoxide, fuel, utility						
liquefied (mobile container)	T59.891	T59.892	T59.893	T59.894	—	—
piped (natural)	T59.891	T59.892	T59.893	T59.894	—	—
Hydrochloric acid (liquid)	T54.2X1	T54.2X2	T54.2X3	T54.2X4	—	—
medicinal (digestant)	T47.5X1	T47.5X2	T47.5X3	T47.5X4	T47.5X5	T47.5..
vapor	T59.891	T59.892	T59.893	T59.894	—	—
Hydrochlorothiazide	T50.2X1	T50.2X2	T50.2X3	T50.2X4	T50.2X5	T50.2..
Hydrocodone	T40.2X1	T40.2X2	T40.2X3	T40.2X4	T40.2X5	T40.2..
Hydrocortisone (derivatives)	T38.0X1	T38.0X2	T38.0X3	T38.0X4	T38.0X5	T38.0..
acepontate	T49.0X1	T49.0X2	T49.0X3	T49.0X4	T49.0X5	T49.0..
ENT agent	T49.6X1	T49.6X2	T49.6X3	T49.6X4	T49.6X5	T49.6..
ophthalmic preparation	T49.5X1	T49.5X2	T49.5X3	T49.5X4	T49.5X5	T49.5..
topical NEC	T49.0X1	T49.0X2	T49.0X3	T49.0X4	T49.0X5	T49.0..
Hydrocortone	T38.0X1	T38.0X2	T38.0X3	T38.0X4	T38.0X5	T38.0..
ENT agent	T49.6X1	T49.6X2	T49.6X3	T49.6X4	T49.6X5	T49.6..
ophthalmic preparation	T49.5X1	T49.5X2	T49.5X3	T49.5X4	T49.5X5	T49.5..
topical NEC	T49.0X1	T49.0X2	T49.0X3	T49.0X4	T49.0X5	T49.0..
Hydrocyanic acid (liquid)	T57.3X1	T57.3X2	T57.3X3	T57.3X4	—	—
gas	T65.0X1	T65.0X2	T65.0X3	T65.0X4	—	—
Hydroflumethiazide	T50.2X1	T50.2X2	T50.2X3	T50.2X4	T50.2X5	T50.2..
Hydrofluoric acid (liquid)	T54.2X1	T54.2X2	T54.2X3	T54.2X4	—	—

Additional Character May Be Required — Refer to the Tabular List for Character Selection

▽ Subterms under main terms may continue to next column or page

Hematinic preparation — Hydrofluoric acid

Substance	Poisoning, Accidental (unintentional)	Poisoning, Intentional Self-harm	Poisoning, Assault	Poisoning, Undetermined	Adverse Effect	Underdosing
Hydrofluoric acid — *continued*						
vapor	T59.891	T59.892	T59.893	T59.894	—	—
Hydrogen	T59.891	T59.892	T59.893	T59.894	—	—
arsenide	T57.0X1	T57.0X2	T57.0X3	T57.0X4	—	—
arseniureted	T57.0X1	T57.0X2	T57.0X3	T57.0X4	—	—
chloride	T57.8X1	T57.8X2	T57.8X3	T57.8X4	—	—
cyanide (salts)	T57.3X1	T57.3X2	T57.3X3	T57.3X4	—	—
gas	T57.3X1	T57.3X2	T57.3X3	T57.3X4	—	—
Fluoride	T59.5X1	T59.5X2	T59.5X3	T59.5X4	—	—
vapor	T59.5X1	T59.5X2	T59.5X3	T59.5X4	—	—
peroxide	T49.0X1	T49.0X2	T49.0X3	T49.0X4	T49.0X5	T49.0X6
phosphureted	T57.1X1	T57.1X2	T57.1X3	T57.1X4	—	—
sulfide	T59.6X1	T59.6X2	T59.6X3	T59.6X4	—	—
arseniureted	T57.0X1	T57.0X2	T57.0X3	T57.0X4	—	—
sulfureted	T59.6X1	T59.6X2	T59.6X3	T59.6X4	—	—
Hydromethylpyridine	T46.7X1	T46.7X2	T46.7X3	T46.7X4	T46.7X5	T46.7X6
Hydromorphinol	T40.2X1	T40.2X2	T40.2X3	T40.2X4	—	—
Hydromorphinone	T40.2X1	T40.2X2	T40.2X3	T40.2X4	T40.2X5	T40.2X6
Hydromorphone	T40.2X1	T40.2X2	T40.2X3	T40.2X4	T40.2X5	T40.2X6
Hydromox	T50.2X1	T50.2X2	T50.2X3	T50.2X4	T50.2X5	T50.2X6
Hydrophilic lotion	T49.3X1	T49.3X2	T49.3X3	T49.3X4	T49.3X5	T49.3X6
Hydroquinidine	T46.2X1	T46.2X2	T46.2X3	T46.2X4	T46.2X5	T46.2X6
Hydroquinone	T52.2X1	T52.2X2	T52.2X3	T52.2X4	—	—
vapor	T59.891	T59.892	T59.893	T59.894	—	—
Hydrosulfuric acid (gas)	T59.6X1	T59.6X2	T59.6X3	T59.6X4	—	—
Hydrotalcite	T47.1X1	T47.1X2	T47.1X3	T47.1X4	T47.1X5	T47.1X6
Hydrous wool fat	T49.3X1	T49.3X2	T49.3X3	T49.3X4	T49.3X5	T49.3X6
Hydroxide, caustic	T54.3X1	T54.3X2	T54.3X3	T54.3X4	—	—
Hydroxocobalamin	T45.8X1	T45.8X2	T45.8X3	T45.8X4	T45.8X5	T45.8X6
Hydroxyamphetamine	T49.5X1	T49.5X2	T49.5X3	T49.5X4	T49.5X5	T49.5X6
Hydroxycarbamide	T45.1X1	T45.1X2	T45.1X3	T45.1X4	T45.1X5	T45.1X6
Hydroxychloroquine	T37.8X1	T37.8X2	T37.8X3	T37.8X4	T37.8X5	T37.8X6
Hydroxydihydrocodeinone	T40.2X1	T40.2X2	T40.2X3	T40.2X4	T40.2X5	T40.2X6
Hydroxyestrone	T38.5X1	T38.5X2	T38.5X3	T38.5X4	T38.5X5	T38.5X6
Hydroxyethyl starch	T45.8X1	T45.8X2	T45.8X3	T45.8X4	T45.8X5	T45.8X6
Hydroxymethylpentanone	T52.4X1	T52.4X2	T52.4X3	T52.4X4	—	—
Hydroxyphenamate	T43.591	T43.592	T43.593	T43.594	T43.595	T43.596
Hydroxyphenylbutazone	T39.2X1	T39.2X2	T39.2X3	T39.2X4	T39.2X5	T39.2X6
Hydroxyprogesterone	T38.5X1	T38.5X2	T38.5X3	T38.5X4	T38.5X5	T38.5X6
caproate	T38.5X1	T38.5X2	T38.5X3	T38.5X4	T38.5X5	T38.5X6
Hydroxyquinoline (derivatives) NEC	T37.8X1	T37.8X2	T37.8X3	T37.8X4	T37.8X5	T37.8X6
Hydroxystilbamidine	T37.3X1	T37.3X2	T37.3X3	T37.3X4	T37.3X5	T37.3X6
Hydroxytoluene	T54.0X1	T54.0X2	T54.0X3	T54.0X4	—	—
(nonmedicinal)						
medicinal	T49.0X1	T49.0X2	T49.0X3	T49.0X4	T49.0X5	T49.0X6
Hydroxyurea	T45.1X1	T45.1X2	T45.1X3	T45.1X4	T45.1X5	T45.1X6
Hydroxyzine	T43.591	T43.592	T43.593	T43.594	T43.595	T43.596
Hyoscine	T44.3X1	T44.3X2	T44.3X3	T44.3X4	T44.3X5	T44.3X6
Hyoscyamine	T44.3X1	T44.3X2	T44.3X3	T44.3X4	T44.3X5	T44.3X6
Hyoscyamus	T44.3X1	T44.3X2	T44.3X3	T44.3X4	T44.3X5	T44.3X6
dry extract	T44.3X1	T44.3X2	T44.3X3	T44.3X4	T44.3X5	T44.3X6
Hypaque	T50.8X1	T50.8X2	T50.8X3	T50.8X4	T50.8X5	T50.8X6
Hypertussis	T50.Z11	T50.Z12	T50.Z13	T50.Z14	T50.Z15	T50.Z16
Hypnotic	T42.71	T42.72	T42.73	T42.74	T42.75	T42.76
anticonvulsant	T42.71	T42.72	T42.73	T42.74	T42.75	T42.76
specified NEC	T42.6X1	T42.6X2	T42.6X3	T42.6X4	T42.6X5	T42.6X6
Hypochlorite	T49.0X1	T49.0X2	T49.0X3	T49.0X4	T49.0X5	T49.0X6
Hypophysis, posterior	T38.891	T38.892	T38.893	T38.894	T38.895	T38.896
Hypotensive NEC	T46.5X1	T46.5X2	T46.5X3	T46.5X4	T46.5X5	T46.5X6
Hypromellose	T49.5X1	T49.5X2	T49.5X3	T49.5X4	T49.5X5	T49.5X6
Ibacitabine	T37.5X1	T37.5X2	T37.5X3	T37.5X4	T37.5X5	T37.5X6
Ibopamine	T44.991	T44.992	T44.993	T44.994	T44.995	T44.996
Ibufenac	T39.311	T39.312	T39.313	T39.314	T39.315	T39.316
Ibuprofen	T39.311	T39.312	T39.313	T39.314	T39.315	T39.316
Ibuproxam	T39.311	T39.312	T39.313	T39.314	T39.315	T39.316
Ibuterol	T48.6X1	T48.6X2	T48.6X3	T48.6X4	T48.6X5	T48.6X6
Ichthammol	T49.0X1	T49.0X2	T49.0X3	T49.0X4	T49.0X5	T49.0X6
Ichthyol	T49.4X1	T49.4X2	T49.4X3	T49.4X4	T49.4X5	T49.4X6
Idarubicin	T45.1X1	T45.1X2	T45.1X3	T45.1X4	T45.1X5	T45.1X6
Idrocilamide	T42.8X1	T42.8X2	T42.8X3	T42.8X4	T42.8X5	T42.8X6
Ifenprodil	T46.7X1	T46.7X2	T46.7X3	T46.7X4	T46.7X5	T46.7X6
Ifosfamide	T45.1X1	T45.1X2	T45.1X3	T45.1X4	T45.1X5	T45.1X6
Iletin	T38.3X1	T38.3X2	T38.3X3	T38.3X4	T38.3X5	T38.3X6
Ilex	T62.2X1	T62.2X2	T62.2X3	T62.2X4	—	—
Illuminating gas (after combustion)	T58.11	T58.12	T58.13	T58.14	—	—
prior to combustion	T59.891	T59.892	T59.893	T59.894	—	—
Ilopan	T45.2X1	T45.2X2	T45.2X3	T45.2X4	T45.2X5	T45.2X6
Iloprost	T46.7X1	T46.7X2	T46.7X3	T46.7X4	T46.7X5	T46.7X6
Ilotycin	T36.3X1	T36.3X2	T36.3X3	T36.3X4	T36.3X5	T36.3X6
ophthalmic preparation	T49.5X1	T49.5X2	T49.5X3	T49.5X4	T49.5X5	T49.5X6
topical NEC	T49.0X1	T49.0X2	T49.0X3	T49.0X4	T49.0X5	T49.0X6
Imidazole-4-carboxamide	T45.1X1	T45.1X2	T45.1X3	T45.1X4	T45.1X5	T45.1X6
Iminostilbene	T42.1X1	T42.1X2	T42.1X3	T42.1X4	T42.1X5	T42.1X6
Imipenem	T36.0X1	T36.0X2	T36.0X3	T36.0X4	T36.0X5	T36.0X6
Imipramine	T43.011	T43.012	T43.013	T43.014	T43.015	T43.016
Immu-G	T50.Z11	T50.Z12	T50.Z13	T50.Z14	T50.Z15	T50.Z16
Immuglobin	T50.Z11	T50.Z12	T50.Z13	T50.Z14	T50.Z15	T50.Z16
Immune						
globulin	T50.Z11	T50.Z12	T50.Z13	T50.Z14	T50.Z15	T50.Z16
serum globulin	T50.Z11	T50.Z12	T50.Z13	T50.Z14	T50.Z15	T50.Z16
Immunoglobin human	T50.Z11	T50.Z12	T50.Z13	T50.Z14	T50.Z15	T50.Z16
(intravenous) (normal)						
unmodified	T50.Z11	T50.Z12	T50.Z13	T50.Z14	T50.Z15	T50.Z16
Immunosuppressive drug	T45.1X1	T45.1X2	T45.1X3	T45.1X4	T45.1X5	T45.1X6
Immu-tetanus	T50.Z11	T50.Z12	T50.Z13	T50.Z14	T50.Z15	T50.Z16
Indalpine	T43.221	T43.222	T43.223	T43.224	T43.225	T43.226
Indanazoline	T48.5X1	T48.5X2	T48.5X3	T48.5X4	T48.5X5	T48.5X6
Indandione (derivatives)	T45.511	T45.512	T45.513	T45.514	T45.515	T45.516
Indapamide	T46.5X1	T46.5X2	T46.5X3	T46.5X4	T46.5X5	T46.5X6
Indendione (derivatives)	T45.511	T45.512	T45.513	T45.514	T45.515	T45.516
Indenolol	T44.7X1	T44.7X2	T44.7X3	T44.7X4	T44.7X5	T44.7X6
Inderal	T44.7X1	T44.7X2	T44.7X3	T44.7X4	T44.7X5	T44.7X6
Indian						
hemp	T40.7X1	T40.7X2	T40.7X3	T40.7X4	T40.7X5	T40.7X6
tobacco	T62.2X1	T62.2X2	T62.2X3	T62.2X4	—	—
Indigo carmine	T50.8X1	T50.8X2	T50.8X3	T50.8X4	T50.8X5	T50.8X6
Indobufen	T45.521	T45.522	T45.523	T45.524	T45.525	T45.526
Indocin	T39.391	T39.392	T39.393	T39.394	T39.395	T39.396
Indocyanine green	T50.8X1	T50.8X2	T50.8X3	T50.8X4	T50.8X5	T50.8X6
Indometacin	T39.391	T39.392	T39.393	T39.394	T39.395	T39.396
Indomethacin	T39.391	T39.392	T39.393	T39.394	T39.395	T39.396
farnesil	T39.4X1	T39.4X2	T39.4X3	T39.4X4	T39.4X5	T39.4X6
Indoramin	T44.6X1	T44.6X2	T44.6X3	T44.6X4	T44.6X5	T44.6X6
Industrial						
alcohol	T51.0X1	T51.0X2	T51.0X3	T51.0X4	—	—
fumes	T59.891	T59.892	T59.893	T59.894	—	—
solvents (fumes) (vapors)	T52.91	T52.92	T52.93	T52.94	—	—
Influenza vaccine	T50.B91	T50.B92	T50.B93	T50.B94	T50.B95	T50.B96
Ingested substance NEC	T65.91	T65.92	T65.93	T65.94	—	—
INH	T37.1X1	T37.1X2	T37.1X3	T37.1X4	T37.1X5	T37.1X6
Inhalation, gas (noxious) — *see* Gas						
Inhibitor						
angiotensin-converting enzyme	T46.4X1	T46.4X2	T46.4X3	T46.4X4	T46.4X5	T46.4X6
carbonic anhydrase	T50.2X1	T50.2X2	T50.2X3	T50.2X4	T50.2X5	T50.2X6
fibrinolysis	T45.621	T45.622	T45.623	T45.624	T45.625	T45.626
monoamine oxidase NEC	T43.1X1	T43.1X2	T43.1X3	T43.1X4	T43.1X5	T43.1X6
hydrazine	T43.1X1	T43.1X2	T43.1X3	T43.1X4	T43.1X5	T43.1X6
postsynaptic	T43.8X1	T43.8X2	T43.8X3	T43.8X4	T43.8X5	T43.8X6
prothrombin synthesis	T45.511	T45.512	T45.513	T45.514	T45.515	T45.516
Ink	T65.891	T65.892	T65.893	T65.894	—	—
Inorganic substance NEC	T57.91	T57.92	T57.93	T57.94	—	—
Inosine pranobex	T37.5X1	T37.5X2	T37.5X3	T37.5X4	T37.5X5	T37.5X6
Inositol	T50.991	T50.992	T50.993	T50.994	T50.995	T50.996
nicotinate	T46.7X1	T46.7X2	T46.7X3	T46.7X4	T46.7X5	T46.7X6
Inproquone	T45.1X1	T45.1X2	T45.1X3	T45.1X4	T45.1X5	T45.1X6
Insecticide NEC	T60.91	T60.92	T60.93	T60.94	—	—
carbamate	T60.0X1	T60.0X2	T60.0X3	T60.0X4	—	—
chlorinated	T60.1X1	T60.1X2	T60.1X3	T60.1X4	—	—
mixed	T60.91	T60.92	T60.93	T60.94	—	—
organochlorine	T60.1X1	T60.1X2	T60.1X3	T60.1X4	—	—
organophosphorus	T60.0X1	T60.0X2	T60.0X3	T60.0X4	—	—
Insect (sting), venomous	T63.481	T63.482	T63.483	T63.484	—	—
ant	T63.421	T63.422	T63.423	T63.424	—	—
bee	T63.441	T63.442	T63.443	T63.444	—	—
caterpillar	T63.431	T63.432	T63.433	T63.434	—	—
hornet	T63.451	T63.452	T63.453	T63.454	—	—
wasp	T63.461	T63.462	T63.463	T63.464	—	—
Insular tissue extract	T38.3X1	T38.3X2	T38.3X3	T38.3X4	T38.3X5	T38.3X6
Insulin (amorphous) (globin) (isophane) (Lente) (NPH) (Semilente) (Ultralente)	T38.3X1	T38.3X2	T38.3X3	T38.3X4	T38.3X5	T38.3X6
defalan	T38.3X1	T38.3X2	T38.3X3	T38.3X4	T38.3X5	T38.3X6
human	T38.3X1	T38.3X2	T38.3X3	T38.3X4	T38.3X5	T38.3X6
injection, soluble	T38.3X1	T38.3X2	T38.3X3	T38.3X4	T38.3X5	T38.3X6
biphasic	T38.3X1	T38.3X2	T38.3X3	T38.3X4	T38.3X5	T38.3X6
intermediate acting	T38.3X1	T38.3X2	T38.3X3	T38.3X4	T38.3X5	T38.3X6
protamine zinc	T38.3X1	T38.3X2	T38.3X3	T38.3X4	T38.3X5	T38.3X6
slow acting	T38.3X1	T38.3X2	T38.3X3	T38.3X4	T38.3X5	T38.3X6
zinc						
protamine injection	T38.3X1	T38.3X2	T38.3X3	T38.3X4	T38.3X5	T38.3X6
suspension (amorphous) (crystalline)	T38.3X1	T38.3X2	T38.3X3	T38.3X4	T38.3X5	T38.3X6

Substance	Poisoning, Accidental (unintentional)	Poisoning, Intentional Self-harm	Poisoning, Assault	Poisoning, Undetermined	Adverse Effect	Under-dosing
Interferon (alpha) (beta) (gamma)	T37.5X1	T37.5X2	T37.5X3	T37.5X4	T37.5X5	T37.5X6
Intestinal motility control						
drug	T47.6X1	T47.6X2	T47.6X3	T47.6X4	T47.6X5	T47.6X6
biological	T47.8X1	T47.8X2	T47.8X3	T47.8X4	T47.8X5	T47.8X6
Intranarcon	T41.1X1	T41.1X2	T41.1X3	T41.1X4	T41.1X5	T41.1X6
Intravenous						
amino acids	T50.991	T50.992	T50.993	T50.994	T50.995	T50.996
fat suspension	T50.991	T50.992	T50.993	T50.994	T50.995	T50.996
Inulin	T50.8X1	T50.8X2	T50.8X3	T50.8X4	T50.8X5	T50.8X6
Invert sugar	T50.3X1	T50.3X2	T50.3X3	T50.3X4	T50.3X5	T50.3X6
Inza — see Naproxen						
Iobenzamic acid	T50.8X1	T50.8X2	T50.8X3	T50.8X4	T50.8X5	T50.8X6
Iocarmic acid	T50.8X1	T50.8X2	T50.8X3	T50.8X4	T50.8X5	T50.8X6
Iocetamic acid	T50.8X1	T50.8X2	T50.8X3	T50.8X4	T50.8X5	T50.8X6
Iodamide	T50.8X1	T50.8X2	T50.8X3	T50.8X4	T50.8X5	T50.8X6
Iodide NEC — see also Iodine	T49.0X1	T49.0X2	T49.0X3	T49.0X4	T49.0X5	T49.0X6
mercury (ointment)	T49.0X1	T49.0X2	T49.0X3	T49.0X4	T49.0X5	T49.0X6
methylate	T49.0X1	T49.0X2	T49.0X3	T49.0X4	T49.0X5	T49.0X6
potassium (expectorant) NEC	T48.4X1	T48.4X2	T48.4X3	T48.4X4	T48.4X5	T48.4X6
Iodinated						
contrast medium	T50.8X1	T50.8X2	T50.8X3	T50.8X4	T50.8X5	T50.8X6
glycerol	T48.4X1	T48.4X2	T48.4X3	T48.4X4	T48.4X5	T48.4X6
human serum albumin (131I)	T50.8X1	T50.8X2	T50.8X3	T50.8X4	T50.8X5	T50.8X6
Iodine (antiseptic, external) (tincture) NEC	T49.0X1	T49.0X2	T49.0X3	T49.0X4	T49.0X5	T49.0X6
125 — see also Radiation sickness, and Exposure to radioactive isotopes						
therapeutic	T50.991	T50.992	T50.993	T50.994	T50.995	T50.996
131 — see also Radiation sickness, and Exposure to radioactive isotopes						
therapeutic	T38.2X1	T38.2X2	T38.2X3	T38.2X4	T38.2X5	T38.2X6
diagnostic	T50.8X1	T50.8X2	T50.8X3	T50.8X4	T50.8X5	T50.8X6
for thyroid conditions (antithyroid)	T38.2X1	T38.2X2	T38.2X3	T38.2X4	T38.2X5	T38.2X6
solution	T49.0X1	T49.0X2	T49.0X3	T49.0X4	T49.0X5	T49.0X6
vapor	T59.891	T59.892	T59.893	T59.894	—	—
Iodipamide	T50.8X1	T50.8X2	T50.8X3	T50.8X4	T50.8X5	T50.8X6
Iodized (poppy seed) oil	T50.8X1	T50.8X2	T50.8X3	T50.8X4	T50.8X5	T50.8X6
Iodobismitol	T37.8X1	T37.8X2	T37.8X3	T37.8X4	T37.8X5	T37.8X6
Iodochlorhydroxyquin	T37.8X1	T37.8X2	T37.8X3	T37.8X4	T37.8X5	T37.8X6
topical	T49.0X1	T49.0X2	T49.0X3	T49.0X4	T49.0X5	T49.0X6
Iodochlorhydroxyquinoline	T37.8X1	T37.8X2	T37.8X3	T37.8X4	T37.8X5	T37.8X6
Iodocholesterol (131I)	T50.8X1	T50.8X2	T50.8X3	T50.8X4	T50.8X5	T50.8X6
Iodoform	T49.0X1	T49.0X2	T49.0X3	T49.0X4	T49.0X5	T49.0X6
Iodohippuric acid	T50.8X1	T50.8X2	T50.8X3	T50.8X4	T50.8X5	T50.8X6
Iodopanoic acid	T50.8X1	T50.8X2	T50.8X3	T50.8X4	T50.8X5	T50.8X6
Iodophthalein (sodium)	T50.8X1	T50.8X2	T50.8X3	T50.8X4	T50.8X5	T50.8X6
Iodopyracet	T50.8X1	T50.8X2	T50.8X3	T50.8X4	T50.8X5	T50.8X6
Iodoquinol	T37.8X1	T37.8X2	T37.8X3	T37.8X4	T37.8X5	T37.8X6
Iodoxamic acid	T50.8X1	T50.8X2	T50.8X3	T50.8X4	T50.8X5	T50.8X6
Iofendylate	T50.8X1	T50.8X2	T50.8X3	T50.8X4	T50.8X5	T50.8X6
Ioglycamic acid	T50.8X1	T50.8X2	T50.8X3	T50.8X4	T50.8X5	T50.8X6
Iohexol	T50.8X1	T50.8X2	T50.8X3	T50.8X4	T50.8X5	T50.8X6
Ion exchange resin						
anion	T47.8X1	T47.8X2	T47.8X3	T47.8X4	T47.8X5	T47.8X6
cation	T50.3X1	T50.3X2	T50.3X3	T50.3X4	T50.3X5	T50.3X6
cholestyramine	T46.6X1	T46.6X2	T46.6X3	T46.6X4	T46.6X5	T46.6X6
intestinal	T47.8X1	T47.8X2	T47.8X3	T47.8X4	T47.8X5	T47.8X6
Iopamidol	T50.8X1	T50.8X2	T50.8X3	T50.8X4	T50.8X5	T50.8X6
Iopanoic acid	T50.8X1	T50.8X2	T50.8X3	T50.8X4	T50.8X5	T50.8X6
Iophenoic acid	T50.8X1	T50.8X2	T50.8X3	T50.8X4	T50.8X5	T50.8X6
Iopodate, sodium	T50.8X1	T50.8X2	T50.8X3	T50.8X4	T50.8X5	T50.8X6
Iopodic acid	T50.8X1	T50.8X2	T50.8X3	T50.8X4	T50.8X5	T50.8X6
Iopromide	T50.8X1	T50.8X2	T50.8X3	T50.8X4	T50.8X5	T50.8X6
Iopydol	T50.8X1	T50.8X2	T50.8X3	T50.8X4	T50.8X5	T50.8X6
Iotalamic acid	T50.8X1	T50.8X2	T50.8X3	T50.8X4	T50.8X5	T50.8X6
Iothalamate	T50.8X1	T50.8X2	T50.8X3	T50.8X4	T50.8X5	T50.8X6
Iothiouracil	T38.2X1	T38.2X2	T38.2X3	T38.2X4	T38.2X5	T38.2X6
Iotrol	T50.8X1	T50.8X2	T50.8X3	T50.8X4	T50.8X5	T50.8X6
Iotrolan	T50.8X1	T50.8X2	T50.8X3	T50.8X4	T50.8X5	T50.8X6
Iotroxate	T50.8X1	T50.8X2	T50.8X3	T50.8X4	T50.8X5	T50.8X6
Iotroxic acid	T50.8X1	T50.8X2	T50.8X3	T50.8X4	T50.8X5	T50.8X6
Ioversol	T50.8X1	T50.8X2	T50.8X3	T50.8X4	T50.8X5	T50.8X6
Ioxaglate	T50.8X1	T50.8X2	T50.8X3	T50.8X4	T50.8X5	T50.8X6
Ioxaglic acid	T50.8X1	T50.8X2	T50.8X3	T50.8X4	T50.8X5	T50.8X6
Ioxitalamic acid	T50.8X1	T50.8X2	T50.8X3	T50.8X4	T50.8X5	T50.8X6
Ipecac	T47.7X1	T47.7X2	T47.7X3	T47.7X4	T47.7X5	T47.7X6

Substance	Poisoning, Accidental (unintentional)	Poisoning, Intentional Self-harm	Poisoning, Assault	Poisoning, Undetermined	Adverse Effect	Under-dosing (cut off)
Ipecacuanha	T48.4X1	T48.4X2	T48.4X3	T48.4X4	T48.4X5	T48.4…
Ipodate, calcium	T50.8X1	T50.8X2	T50.8X3	T50.8X4	T50.8X5	T50…
Ipral	T42.3X1	T42.3X2	T42.3X3	T42.3X4	T42.3X5	T42.…
Ipratropium (bromide)	T48.6X1	T48.6X2	T48.6X3	T48.6X4	T48.6X5	T48.…
Ipriflavone	T46.3X1	T46.3X2	T46.3X3	T46.3X4	T46.3X5	T46.…
Iprindole	T43.011	T43.012	T43.013	T43.014	T43.015	T43.…
Iproclozide	T43.1X1	T43.1X2	T43.1X3	T43.1X4	T43.1X5	T43.…
Iprofenin	T50.8X1	T50.8X2	T50.8X3	T50.8X4	T50.8X5	T50…
Iproheptine	T49.2X1	T49.2X2	T49.2X3	T49.2X4	T49.2X5	T49.…
Iproniazid	T43.1X1	T43.1X2	T43.1X3	T43.1X4	T43.1X5	T43.…
Iproplatin	T45.1X1	T45.1X2	T45.1X3	T45.1X4	T45.1X5	T45.…
Iproveratril	T46.1X1	T46.1X2	T46.1X3	T46.1X4	T46.1X5	T46.…
Iron (compounds) (medicinal) NEC	T45.4X1	T45.4X2	T45.4X3	T45.4X4	T45.4X5	T45…
ammonium	T45.4X1	T45.4X2	T45.4X3	T45.4X4	T45.4X5	T45.…
dextran injection	T45.4X1	T45.4X2	T45.4X3	T45.4X4	T45.4X5	T45.…
nonmedicinal	T56.891	T56.892	T56.893	T56.894	—	—
salts	T45.4X1	T45.4X2	T45.4X3	T45.4X4	T45.4X5	T45.…
sorbitex	T45.4X1	T45.4X2	T45.4X3	T45.4X4	T45.4X5	T45.…
sorbitol citric acid complex	T45.4X1	T45.4X2	T45.4X3	T45.4X4	T45.4X5	T45…
Irrigating fluid (vaginal)	T49.8X1	T49.8X2	T49.8X3	T49.8X4	T49.8X5	T49.…
eye	T49.5X1	T49.5X2	T49.5X3	T49.5X4	T49.5X5	T49.…
Isepamicin	T36.5X1	T36.5X2	T36.5X3	T36.5X4	T36.5X5	T36.…
Isoaminile (citrate)	T48.3X1	T48.3X2	T48.3X3	T48.3X4	T48.3X5	T48.…
Isoamyl nitrite	T46.3X1	T46.3X2	T46.3X3	T46.3X4	T46.3X5	T46.…
Isobenzan	T60.1X1	T60.1X2	T60.1X3	T60.1X4	—	—
Isobutyl acetate	T52.8X1	T52.8X2	T52.8X3	T52.8X4	—	—
Isocarboxazid	T43.1X1	T43.1X2	T43.1X3	T43.1X4	T43.1X5	T43.…
Isoconazole	T49.0X1	T49.0X2	T49.0X3	T49.0X4	T49.0X5	T49.…
Isocyanate	T65.0X1	T65.0X2	T65.0X3	T65.0X4	—	—
Isoephedrine	T44.991	T44.992	T44.993	T44.994	T44.995	T44.…
Isoetarine	T48.6X1	T48.6X2	T48.6X3	T48.6X4	T48.6X5	T48.…
Isoethadione	T42.2X1	T42.2X2	T42.2X3	T42.2X4	T42.2X5	T42.…
Isoetharine	T44.5X1	T44.5X2	T44.5X3	T44.5X4	T44.5X5	T44.…
Isoflurane	T41.0X1	T41.0X2	T41.0X3	T41.0X4	T41.0X5	T41.…
Isoflurophate	T44.0X1	T44.0X2	T44.0X3	T44.0X4	T44.0X5	T44.…
Isomaltose, ferric complex	T45.4X1	T45.4X2	T45.4X3	T45.4X4	T45.4X5	T45.…
Isometheptene	T44.3X1	T44.3X2	T44.3X3	T44.3X4	T44.3X5	T44.…
Isoniazid	T37.1X1	T37.1X2	T37.1X3	T37.1X4	T37.1X5	T37.…
with						
rifampicin	T36.6X1	T36.6X2	T36.6X3	T36.6X4	T36.6X5	T36.…
thioacetazone	T37.1X1	T37.1X2	T37.1X3	T37.1X4	T37.1X5	T37.…
Isonicotinic acid hydrazide	T37.1X1	T37.1X2	T37.1X3	T37.1X4	T37.1X5	T37.…
Isonipecaine	T40.4X1	T40.4X2	T40.4X3	T40.4X4	T40.4X5	T40.…
Isopentaquine	T37.2X1	T37.2X2	T37.2X3	T37.2X4	T37.2X5	T37.…
Isophane insulin	T38.3X1	T38.3X2	T38.3X3	T38.3X4	T38.3X5	T38.…
Isophorone	T65.891	T65.892	T65.893	T65.894	—	—
Isophosphamide	T45.1X1	T45.1X2	T45.1X3	T45.1X4	T45.1X5	T45.…
Isopregnenone	T38.5X1	T38.5X2	T38.5X3	T38.5X4	T38.5X5	T38.…
Isoprenaline	T48.6X1	T48.6X2	T48.6X3	T48.6X4	T48.6X5	T48.…
Isopromethazine	T43.3X1	T43.3X2	T43.3X3	T43.3X4	T43.3X5	T43.…
Isopropamide	T44.3X1	T44.3X2	T44.3X3	T44.3X4	T44.3X5	T44.…
iodide	T44.3X1	T44.3X2	T44.3X3	T44.3X4	T44.3X5	T44.…
Isopropanol	T51.2X1	T51.2X2	T51.2X3	T51.2X4	—	—
Isopropyl						
acetate	T52.8X1	T52.8X2	T52.8X3	T52.8X4	—	—
alcohol	T51.2X1	T51.2X2	T51.2X3	T51.2X4	—	—
medicinal	T49.4X1	T49.4X2	T49.4X3	T49.4X4	T49.4X5	T49.…
ether	T52.8X1	T52.8X2	T52.8X3	T52.8X4	—	—
Isopropylaminophenazone	T39.2X1	T39.2X2	T39.2X3	T39.2X4	T39.2X5	T39.…
Isoproterenol	T48.6X1	T48.6X2	T48.6X3	T48.6X4	T48.6X5	T48.…
Isosorbide dinitrate	T46.3X1	T46.3X2	T46.3X3	T46.3X4	T46.3X5	T46.…
Isothipendyl	T45.0X1	T45.0X2	T45.0X3	T45.0X4	T45.0X5	T45.…
Isotretinoin	T50.991	T50.992	T50.993	T50.994	T50.995	T50.…
Isoxazolyl penicillin	T36.0X1	T36.0X2	T36.0X3	T36.0X4	T36.0X5	T36.…
Isoxicam	T39.391	T39.392	T39.393	T39.394	T39.395	T39.…
Isoxsuprine	T46.7X1	T46.7X2	T46.7X3	T46.7X4	T46.7X5	T46.…
Ispagula	T47.4X1	T47.4X2	T47.4X3	T47.4X4	T47.4X5	T47.…
husk	T47.4X1	T47.4X2	T47.4X3	T47.4X4	T47.4X5	T47.…
Isradipine	T46.1X1	T46.1X2	T46.1X3	T46.1X4	T46.1X5	T46.…
I-thyroxine sodium	T38.1X1	T38.1X2	T38.1X3	T38.1X4	T38.1X5	T38.…
Itraconazole	T37.8X1	T37.8X2	T37.8X3	T37.8X4	T37.8X5	T37.…
Itramin tosilate	T46.3X1	T46.3X2	T46.3X3	T46.3X4	T46.3X5	T46.3…
Ivermectin	T37.4X1	T37.4X2	T37.4X3	T37.4X4	T37.4X5	T37.…
Izoniazid	T37.1X1	T37.1X2	T37.1X3	T37.1X4	T37.1X5	T37.…
with thioacetazone	T37.1X1	T37.1X2	T37.1X3	T37.1X4	T37.1X5	T37.…
Jalap	T47.2X1	T47.2X2	T47.2X3	T47.2X4	T47.2X5	T47.…
Jamaica						
dogwood (bark)	T39.8X1	T39.8X2	T39.8X3	T39.8X4	T39.8X5	T39.8…
ginger	T65.891	T65.892	T65.893	T65.894	—	—
root	T62.2X1	T62.2X2	T62.2X3	T62.2X4	—	—
Jatropha	T62.2X1	T62.2X2	T62.2X3	T62.2X4	—	—
curcas	T62.2X1	T62.2X2	T62.2X3	T62.2X4	—	—

Substance	Poisoning, Accidental (unintentional)	Poisoning, Intentional Self-harm	Poisoning, Assault	Poisoning, Undetermined	Adverse Effect	Under-dosing
Jectofer	T45.4X1	T45.4X2	T45.4X3	T45.4X4	T45.4X5	T45.4X6
Jellyfish (sting)	T63.621	T63.622	T63.623	T63.624	—	—
Jequirity (bean)	T62.2X1	T62.2X2	T62.2X3	T62.2X4	—	—
Jimson weed (stramonium)	T62.2X1	T62.2X2	T62.2X3	T62.2X4	—	—
seeds	T62.2X1	T62.2X2	T62.2X3	T62.2X4	—	—
Josamycin	T36.3X1	T36.3X2	T36.3X3	T36.3X4	T36.3X5	T36.3X6
Juniper tar	T49.1X1	T49.1X2	T49.1X3	T49.1X4	T49.1X5	T49.1X6
Kallidinogenase	T46.7X1	T46.7X2	T46.7X3	T46.7X4	T46.7X5	T46.7X6
Kallikrein	T46.7X1	T46.7X2	T46.7X3	T46.7X4	T46.7X5	T46.7X6
Kanamycin	T36.5X1	T36.5X2	T36.5X3	T36.5X4	T36.5X5	T36.5X6
Kantrex	T36.5X1	T36.5X2	T36.5X3	T36.5X4	T36.5X5	T36.5X6
Kaolin	T47.6X1	T47.6X2	T47.6X3	T47.6X4	T47.6X5	T47.6X6
light	T47.6X1	T47.6X2	T47.6X3	T47.6X4	T47.6X5	T47.6X6
Karaya (gum)	T47.4X1	T47.4X2	T47.4X3	T47.4X4	T47.4X5	T47.4X6
Kebuzone	T39.2X1	T39.2X2	T39.2X3	T39.2X4	T39.2X5	T39.2X6
Kelevan	T60.1X1	T60.1X2	T60.1X3	T60.1X4	—	—
Kemithal	T41.1X1	T41.1X2	T41.1X3	T41.1X4	T41.1X5	T41.1X6
Kenacort	T38.0X1	T38.0X2	T38.0X3	T38.0X4	T38.0X5	T38.0X6
Keratolytic drug NEC	T49.4X1	T49.4X2	T49.4X3	T49.4X4	T49.4X5	T49.4X6
anthracene	T49.4X1	T49.4X2	T49.4X3	T49.4X4	T49.4X5	T49.4X6
Keratoplastic NEC	T49.4X1	T49.4X2	T49.4X3	T49.4X4	T49.4X5	T49.4X6
Kerosene, kerosine (fuel) (solvent) NEC	T52.0X1	T52.0X2	T52.0X3	T52.0X4	—	—
insecticide	T52.0X1	T52.0X2	T52.0X3	T52.0X4	—	—
vapor	T52.0X1	T52.0X2	T52.0X3	T52.0X4	—	—
Ketamine	T41.291	T41.292	T41.293	T41.294	T41.295	T41.296
Ketazolam	T42.4X1	T42.4X2	T42.4X3	T42.4X4	T42.4X5	T42.4X6
Ketazon	T39.2X1	T39.2X2	T39.2X3	T39.2X4	T39.2X5	T39.2X6
Ketobemidone	T40.4X1	T40.4X2	T40.4X3	T40.4X4	—	—
Ketoconazole	T49.0X1	T49.0X2	T49.0X3	T49.0X4	T49.0X5	T49.0X6
Ketols	T52.4X1	T52.4X2	T52.4X3	T52.4X4	—	—
Ketone oils	T52.4X1	T52.4X2	T52.4X3	T52.4X4	—	—
Ketoprofen	T39.311	T39.312	T39.313	T39.314	T39.315	T39.316
Ketorolac	T39.8X1	T39.8X2	T39.8X3	T39.8X4	T39.8X5	T39.8X6
Ketotifen	T45.0X1	T45.0X2	T45.0X3	T45.0X4	T45.0X5	T45.0X6
Khat	T43.691	T43.692	T43.693	T43.694	—	—
Khellin	T46.3X1	T46.3X2	T46.3X3	T46.3X4	T46.3X5	T46.3X6
Khelloside	T46.3X1	T46.3X2	T46.3X3	T46.3X4	T46.3X5	T46.3X6
Kiln gas or vapor (carbon monoxide)	T58.8X1	T58.8X2	T58.8X3	T58.8X4	—	—
Kitasamycin	T36.3X1	T36.3X2	T36.3X3	T36.3X4	T36.3X5	T36.3X6
Konsyl	T47.4X1	T47.4X2	T47.4X3	T47.4X4	T47.4X5	T47.4X6
Kosam seed	T62.2X1	T62.2X2	T62.2X3	T62.2X4	—	—
Krait (venom)	T63.091	T63.092	T63.093	T63.094	—	—
Kwell (insecticide)	T60.1X1	T60.1X2	T60.1X3	T60.1X4	—	—
anti-infective (topical)	T49.0X1	T49.0X2	T49.0X3	T49.0X4	T49.0X5	T49.0X6
Labetalol	T44.8X1	T44.8X2	T44.8X3	T44.8X4	T44.8X5	T44.8X6
Laburnum (seeds)	T62.2X1	T62.2X2	T62.2X3	T62.2X4	—	—
leaves	T62.2X1	T62.2X2	T62.2X3	T62.2X4	—	—
Lachesine	T49.5X1	T49.5X2	T49.5X3	T49.5X4	T49.5X5	T49.5X6
Lacidipine	T46.5X1	T46.5X2	T46.5X3	T46.5X4	T46.5X5	T46.5X6
Lacquer	T65.6X1	T65.6X2	T65.6X3	T65.6X4	—	—
Lacrimogenic gas	T59.3X1	T59.3X2	T59.3X3	T59.3X4	—	—
Lactated potassic saline	T50.3X1	T50.3X2	T50.3X3	T50.3X4	T50.3X5	T50.3X6
Lactic acid	T49.8X1	T49.8X2	T49.8X3	T49.8X4	T49.8X5	T49.8X6
Lactobacillus						
acidophilus	T47.6X1	T47.6X2	T47.6X3	T47.6X4	T47.6X5	T47.6X6
compound	T47.6X1	T47.6X2	T47.6X3	T47.6X4	T47.6X5	T47.6X6
bifidus, lyophilized	T47.6X1	T47.6X2	T47.6X3	T47.6X4	T47.6X5	T47.6X6
bulgaricus	T47.6X1	T47.6X2	T47.6X3	T47.6X4	T47.6X5	T47.6X6
sporogenes	T47.6X1	T47.6X2	T47.6X3	T47.6X4	T47.6X5	T47.6X6
Lactoflavin	T45.2X1	T45.2X2	T45.2X3	T45.2X4	T45.2X5	T45.2X6
Lactose (as excipient)	T50.901	T50.902	T50.903	T50.904	T50.905	T50.906
Lactuca (virosa) (extract)	T42.6X1	T42.6X2	T42.6X3	T42.6X4	T42.6X5	T42.6X6
Lactucarium	T42.6X1	T42.6X2	T42.6X3	T42.6X4	T42.6X5	T42.6X6
Lactulose	T47.3X1	T47.3X2	T47.3X3	T47.3X4	T47.3X5	T47.3X6
Laevo — see Levo-						
Lanatosides	T46.0X1	T46.0X2	T46.0X3	T46.0X4	T46.0X5	T46.0X6
Lanolin	T49.3X1	T49.3X2	T49.3X3	T49.3X4	T49.3X5	T49.3X6
Largactil	T43.3X1	T43.3X2	T43.3X3	T43.3X4	T43.3X5	T43.3X6
Larkspur	T62.2X1	T62.2X2	T62.2X3	T62.2X4	—	—
Laroxyl	T43.011	T43.012	T43.013	T43.014	T43.015	T43.016
Lasix	T50.1X1	T50.1X2	T50.1X3	T50.1X4	T50.1X5	T50.1X6
Lassar's paste	T49.4X1	T49.4X2	T49.4X3	T49.4X4	T49.4X5	T49.4X6
Latamoxef	T36.1X1	T36.1X2	T36.1X3	T36.1X4	T36.1X5	T36.1X6
Latex	T65.811	T65.812	T65.813	T65.814	—	—
Lathyrus (seed)	T62.2X1	T62.2X2	T62.2X3	T62.2X4	—	—
Laudanum	T40.0X1	T40.0X2	T40.0X3	T40.0X4	T40.0X5	T40.0X6
Laudexium	T48.1X1	T48.1X2	T48.1X3	T48.1X4	T48.1X5	T48.1X6
Laughing gas	T41.0X1	T41.0X2	T41.0X3	T41.0X4	T41.0X5	T41.0X6
Laurel, black or cherry	T62.2X1	T62.2X2	T62.2X3	T62.2X4	—	—
Laurolinium	T49.0X1	T49.0X2	T49.0X3	T49.0X4	T49.0X5	T49.0X6
Lauryl sulfoacetate	T49.2X1	T49.2X2	T49.2X3	T49.2X4	T49.2X5	T49.2X6
Laxative NEC	T47.4X1	T47.4X2	T47.4X3	T47.4X4	T47.4X5	T47.4X6
osmotic	T47.3X1	T47.3X2	T47.3X3	T47.3X4	T47.3X5	T47.3X6
saline	T47.3X1	T47.3X2	T47.3X3	T47.3X4	T47.3X5	T47.3X6
stimulant	T47.2X1	T47.2X2	T47.2X3	T47.2X4	T47.2X5	T47.2X6
L-dopa	T42.8X1	T42.8X2	T42.8X3	T42.8X4	T42.8X5	T42.8X6
Lead (dust) (fumes) (vapor)	T56.0X1	T56.0X2	T56.0X3	T56.0X4	—	—
NEC						
acetate	T49.2X1	T49.2X2	T49.2X3	T49.2X4	T49.2X5	T49.2X6
alkyl (fuel additive)	T56.0X1	T56.0X2	T56.0X3	T56.0X4	—	—
anti-infectives	T37.8X1	T37.8X2	T37.8X3	T37.8X4	T37.8X5	T37.8X6
antiknock compound (tetraethyl)	T56.0X1	T56.0X2	T56.0X3	T56.0X4	—	—
arsenate, arsenite (dust)(herbicide)(insecticide)(vapor)	T57.0X1	T57.0X2	T57.0X3	T57.0X4	—	—
carbonate	T56.0X1	T56.0X2	T56.0X3	T56.0X4	—	—
paint	T56.0X1	T56.0X2	T56.0X3	T56.0X4	—	—
chromate	T56.0X1	T56.0X2	T56.0X3	T56.0X4	—	—
paint	T56.0X1	T56.0X2	T56.0X3	T56.0X4	—	—
dioxide	T56.0X1	T56.0X2	T56.0X3	T56.0X4	—	—
inorganic	T56.0X1	T56.0X2	T56.0X3	T56.0X4	—	—
iodide	T56.0X1	T56.0X2	T56.0X3	T56.0X4	—	—
pigment (paint)	T56.0X1	T56.0X2	T56.0X3	T56.0X4	—	—
monoxide (dust)	T56.0X1	T56.0X2	T56.0X3	T56.0X4	—	—
paint	T56.0X1	T56.0X2	T56.0X3	T56.0X4	—	—
organic	T56.0X1	T56.0X2	T56.0X3	T56.0X4	—	—
oxide	T56.0X1	T56.0X2	T56.0X3	T56.0X4	—	—
paint	T56.0X1	T56.0X2	T56.0X3	T56.0X4	—	—
paint	T56.0X1	T56.0X2	T56.0X3	T56.0X4	—	—
salts	T56.0X1	T56.0X2	T56.0X3	T56.0X4	—	—
specified compound NEC	T56.0X1	T56.0X2	T56.0X3	T56.0X4	—	—
tetra-ethyl	T56.0X1	T56.0X2	T56.0X3	T56.0X4	—	—
Lebanese red	T40.7X1	T40.7X2	T40.7X3	T40.7X4	T40.7X5	T40.7X6
Lefetamine	T39.8X1	T39.8X2	T39.8X3	T39.8X4	T39.8X5	T39.8X6
Lenperone	T43.4X1	T43.4X2	T43.4X3	T43.4X4	T43.4X5	T43.4X6
Lente lietin (insulin)	T38.3X1	T38.3X2	T38.3X3	T38.3X4	T38.3X5	T38.3X6
Leptazol	T50.7X1	T50.7X2	T50.7X3	T50.7X4	T50.7X5	T50.7X6
Leptophos	T60.0X1	T60.0X2	T60.0X3	T60.0X4	—	—
Leritine	T40.2X1	T40.2X2	T40.2X3	T40.2X4	T40.2X5	T40.2X6
Letosteine	T48.4X1	T48.4X2	T48.4X3	T48.4X4	T48.4X5	T48.4X6
Letter	T38.1X1	T38.1X2	T38.1X3	T38.1X4	T38.1X5	T38.1X6
Lettuce opium	T42.6X1	T42.6X2	T42.6X3	T42.6X4	T42.6X5	T42.6X6
Leucinocaine	T41.3X1	T41.3X2	T41.3X3	T41.3X4	T41.3X5	T41.3X6
Leucocianidol	T46.991	T46.992	T46.993	T46.994	T46.995	T46.996
Leucovorin (factor)	T45.8X1	T45.8X2	T45.8X3	T45.8X4	T45.8X5	T45.8X6
Leukeran	T45.1X1	T45.1X2	T45.1X3	T45.1X4	T45.1X5	T45.1X6
Leuprolide	T38.891	T38.892	T38.893	T38.894	T38.895	T38.896
Levalbuterol	T48.6X1	T48.6X2	T48.6X3	T48.6X4	T48.6X5	T48.6X6
Levallorphan	T50.7X1	T50.7X2	T50.7X3	T50.7X4	T50.7X5	T50.7X6
Levamisole	T37.4X1	T37.4X2	T37.4X3	T37.4X4	T37.4X5	T37.4X6
Levanil	T42.6X1	T42.6X2	T42.6X3	T42.6X4	T42.6X5	T42.6X6
Levarterenol	T44.4X1	T44.4X2	T44.4X3	T44.4X4	T44.4X5	T44.4X6
Levdropropizine	T48.3X1	T48.3X2	T48.3X3	T48.3X4	T48.3X5	T48.3X6
Levobunolol	T49.5X1	T49.5X2	T49.5X3	T49.5X4	T49.5X5	T49.5X6
Levocabastine (hydrochloride)	T45.0X1	T45.0X2	T45.0X3	T45.0X4	T45.0X5	T45.0X6
Levocarnitine	T50.991	T50.992	T50.993	T50.994	T50.995	T50.996
Levodopa	T42.8X1	T42.8X2	T42.8X3	T42.8X4	T42.8X5	T42.8X6
with carbidopa	T42.8X1	T42.8X2	T42.8X3	T42.8X4	T42.8X5	T42.8X6
Levo-dromoran	T40.2X1	T40.2X2	T40.2X3	T40.2X4	T40.2X5	T40.2X6
Levoglutamide	T50.991	T50.992	T50.993	T50.994	T50.995	T50.996
Levoid	T38.1X1	T38.1X2	T38.1X3	T38.1X4	T38.1X5	T38.1X6
Levo-isomethadone	T40.3X1	T40.3X2	T40.3X3	T40.3X4	T40.3X5	T40.3X6
Levomepromazine	T43.3X1	T43.3X2	T43.3X3	T43.3X4	T43.3X5	T43.3X6
Levonordefrin	T49.6X1	T49.6X2	T49.6X3	T49.6X4	T49.6X5	T49.6X6
Levonorgestrel	T38.4X1	T38.4X2	T38.4X3	T38.4X4	T38.4X5	T38.4X6
with ethinylestradiol	T38.5X1	T38.5X2	T38.5X3	T38.5X4	T38.5X5	T38.5X6
Levopromazine	T43.3X1	T43.3X2	T43.3X3	T43.3X4	T43.3X5	T43.3X6
Levoprome	T42.6X1	T42.6X2	T42.6X3	T42.6X4	T42.6X5	T42.6X6
Levopropoxyphene	T40.4X1	T40.4X2	T40.4X3	T40.4X4	T40.4X5	T40.4X6
Levopropylhexedrine	T50.5X1	T50.5X2	T50.5X3	T50.5X4	T50.5X5	T50.5X6
Levoproxyphylline	T48.6X1	T48.6X2	T48.6X3	T48.6X4	T48.6X5	T48.6X6
Levorphanol	T40.4X1	T40.4X2	T40.4X3	T40.4X4	T40.4X5	T40.4X6
Levothyroxine	T38.1X1	T38.1X2	T38.1X3	T38.1X4	T38.1X5	T38.1X6
sodium	T38.1X1	T38.1X2	T38.1X3	T38.1X4	T38.1X5	T38.1X6
Levsin	T44.3X1	T44.3X2	T44.3X3	T44.3X4	T44.3X5	T44.3X6
Levulose	T50.3X1	T50.3X2	T50.3X3	T50.3X4	T50.3X5	T50.3X6
Lewisite (gas), not in war	T57.0X1	T57.0X2	T57.0X3	T57.0X4	—	—
Librium	T42.4X1	T42.4X2	T42.4X3	T42.4X4	T42.4X5	T42.4X6
Lidex	T49.0X1	T49.0X2	T49.0X3	T49.0X4	T49.0X5	T49.0X6
Lidocaine	T41.3X1	T41.3X2	T41.3X3	T41.3X4	T41.3X5	T41.3X6
regional	T41.3X1	T41.3X2	T41.3X3	T41.3X4	T41.3X5	T41.3X6
spinal	T41.3X1	T41.3X2	T41.3X3	T41.3X4	T41.3X5	T41.3X6

Substance	Poisoning, Accidental (unintentional)	Poisoning, Intentional Self-harm	Poisoning, Assault	Poisoning, Undetermined	Adverse Effect	Under-dosing
Lidofenin	T50.8X1	T50.8X2	T50.8X3	T50.8X4	T50.8X5	T50.8X6
Lidoflazine	T46.1X1	T46.1X2	T46.1X3	T46.1X4	T46.1X5	T46.1X6
Lighter fluid	T52.0X1	T52.0X2	T52.0X3	T52.0X4	—	—
Lignin hemicellulose	T47.6X1	T47.6X2	T47.6X3	T47.6X4	T47.6X5	T47.6X6
Lignocaine	T41.3X1	T41.3X2	T41.3X3	T41.3X4	T41.3X5	T41.3X6
regional	T41.3X1	T41.3X2	T41.3X3	T41.3X4	T41.3X5	T41.3X6
spinal	T41.3X1	T41.3X2	T41.3X3	T41.3X4	T41.3X5	T41.3X6
Ligroin (e) (solvent)	T52.0X1	T52.0X2	T52.0X3	T52.0X4	—	—
vapor	T59.891	T59.892	T59.893	T59.894	—	—
Ligustrum vulgare	T62.2X1	T62.2X2	T62.2X3	T62.2X4	—	—
Lily of the valley	T62.2X1	T62.2X2	T62.2X3	T62.2X4	—	—
Lime (chloride)	T54.3X1	T54.3X2	T54.3X3	T54.3X4	—	—
Limonene	T52.8X1	T52.8X2	T52.8X3	T52.8X4	—	—
Lincomycin	T36.8X1	T36.8X2	T36.8X3	T36.8X4	T36.8X5	T36.8X6
Lindane (insecticide) (nonmedicinal) (vapor)	T53.6X1	T53.6X2	T53.6X3	T53.6X4	—	—
medicinal	T49.0X1	T49.0X2	T49.0X3	T49.0X4	T49.0X5	T49.0X6
Liniments NEC	T49.91	T49.92	T49.93	T49.94	T49.95	T49.96
Linoleic acid	T46.6X1	T46.6X2	T46.6X3	T46.6X4	T46.6X5	T46.6X6
Linolenic acid	T46.6X1	T46.6X2	T46.6X3	T46.6X4	T46.6X5	T46.6X6
Linseed	T47.4X1	T47.4X2	T47.4X3	T47.4X4	T47.4X5	T47.4X6
Liothyronine	T38.1X1	T38.1X2	T38.1X3	T38.1X4	T38.1X5	T38.1X6
Liotrix	T38.1X1	T38.1X2	T38.1X3	T38.1X4	T38.1X5	T38.1X6
Lipancreatin	T47.5X1	T47.5X2	T47.5X3	T47.5X4	T47.5X5	T47.5X6
Lipo-alprostadil	T46.7X1	T46.7X2	T46.7X3	T46.7X4	T46.7X5	T46.7X6
Lipo-Lutin	T38.5X1	T38.5X2	T38.5X3	T38.5X4	T38.5X5	T38.5X6
Lipotropic drug NEC	T50.901	T50.902	T50.903	T50.904	T50.905	T50.906
Liquefied petroleum gases	T59.891	T59.892	T59.893	T59.894	—	—
piped (pure or mixed with air)	T59.891	T59.892	T59.893	T59.894	—	—
Liquid						
paraffin	T47.4X1	T47.4X2	T47.4X3	T47.4X4	T47.4X5	T47.4X6
petrolatum	T47.4X1	T47.4X2	T47.4X3	T47.4X4	T47.4X5	T47.4X6
topical	T49.3X1	T49.3X2	T49.3X3	T49.3X4	T49.3X5	T49.3X6
specified NEC	T65.891	T65.892	T65.893	T65.894	—	—
substance	T65.91	T65.92	T65.93	T65.94	—	—
Liquor creosolis compositus	T65.891	T65.892	T65.893	T65.894	—	—
Liquorice	T48.4X1	T48.4X2	T48.4X3	T48.4X4	T48.4X5	T48.4X6
extract	T47.8X1	T47.8X2	T47.8X3	T47.8X4	T47.8X5	T47.8X6
Lisinopril	T46.4X1	T46.4X2	T46.4X3	T46.4X4	T46.4X5	T46.4X6
Lisuride	T42.8X1	T42.8X2	T42.8X3	T42.8X4	T42.8X5	T42.8X6
Lithane	T43.8X1	T43.8X2	T43.8X3	T43.8X4	T43.8X5	T43.8X6
Lithium	T56.891	T56.892	T56.893	T56.894	—	—
gluconate	T43.591	T43.592	T43.593	T43.594	T43.595	T43.596
salts (carbonate)	T43.591	T43.592	T43.593	T43.594	T43.595	T43.596
Lithonate	T43.8X1	T43.8X2	T43.8X3	T43.8X4	T43.8X5	T43.8X6
Liver						
extract	T45.8X1	T45.8X2	T45.8X3	T45.8X4	T45.8X5	T45.8X6
for parenteral use	T45.8X1	T45.8X2	T45.8X3	T45.8X4	T45.8X5	T45.8X6
fraction 1	T45.8X1	T45.8X2	T45.8X3	T45.8X4	T45.8X5	T45.8X6
hydrolysate	T45.8X1	T45.8X2	T45.8X3	T45.8X4	T45.8X5	T45.8X6
Lizard (bite) (venom)	T63.121	T63.122	T63.123	T63.124	—	—
LMD	T45.8X1	T45.8X2	T45.8X3	T45.8X4	T45.8X5	T45.8X6
Lobelia	T62.2X1	T62.2X2	T62.2X3	T62.2X4	—	—
Lobeline	T50.7X1	T50.7X2	T50.7X3	T50.7X4	T50.7X5	T50.7X6
Local action drug NEC	T49.8X1	T49.8X2	T49.8X3	T49.8X4	T49.8X5	T49.8X6
Locorten	T49.0X1	T49.0X2	T49.0X3	T49.0X4	T49.0X5	T49.0X6
Lofepramine	T43.011	T43.012	T43.013	T43.014	T43.015	T43.016
Lolium temulentum	T62.2X1	T62.2X2	T62.2X3	T62.2X4	—	—
Lomotil	T47.6X1	T47.6X2	T47.6X3	T47.6X4	T47.6X5	T47.6X6
Lomustine	T45.1X1	T45.1X2	T45.1X3	T45.1X4	T45.1X5	T45.1X6
Lonidamine	T45.1X1	T45.1X2	T45.1X3	T45.1X4	T45.1X5	T45.1X6
Loperamide	T47.6X1	T47.6X2	T47.6X3	T47.6X4	T47.6X5	T47.6X6
Loprazolam	T42.4X1	T42.4X2	T42.4X3	T42.4X4	T42.4X5	T42.4X6
Lorajmine	T46.2X1	T46.2X2	T46.2X3	T46.2X4	T46.2X5	T46.2X6
Loratidine	T45.0X1	T45.0X2	T45.0X3	T45.0X4	T45.0X5	T45.0X6
Lorazepam	T42.4X1	T42.4X2	T42.4X3	T42.4X4	T42.4X5	T42.4X6
Lorcainide	T46.2X1	T46.2X2	T46.2X3	T46.2X4	T46.2X5	T46.2X6
Lormetazepam	T42.4X1	T42.4X2	T42.4X3	T42.4X4	T42.4X5	T42.4X6
Lotions NEC	T49.91	T49.92	T49.93	T49.94	T49.95	T49.96
Lotusate	T42.3X1	T42.3X2	T42.3X3	T42.3X4	T42.3X5	T42.3X6
Lovastatin	T46.6X1	T46.6X2	T46.6X3	T46.6X4	T46.6X5	T46.6X6
Lowila	T49.2X1	T49.2X2	T49.2X3	T49.2X4	T49.2X5	T49.2X6
Loxapine	T43.591	T43.592	T43.593	T43.594	T43.595	T43.596
Lozenges (throat)	T49.6X1	T49.6X2	T49.6X3	T49.6X4	T49.6X5	T49.6X6
LSD	T40.8X1	T40.8X2	T40.8X3	T40.8X4	—	—
L-Tryptophan — see amino acid						
Lubricant, eye	T49.5X1	T49.5X2	T49.5X3	T49.5X4	T49.5X5	T49.5X6
Lubricating oil NEC	T52.0X1	T52.0X2	T52.0X3	T52.0X4	—	—
Lucanthone	T37.4X1	T37.4X2	T37.4X3	T37.4X4	T37.4X5	T37.4X6
Luminal	T42.3X1	T42.3X2	T42.3X3	T42.3X4	T42.3X5	T42.3X6
Lung irritant (gas) NEC	T59.91	T59.92	T59.93	T59.94	—	—

Substance	Poisoning, Accidental (unintentional)	Poisoning, Intentional Self-harm	Poisoning, Assault	Poisoning, Undetermined	Adverse Effect	Under-dosing
Luteinizing hormone	T38.811	T38.812	T38.813	T38.814	T38.815	T38.
Lutocylol	T38.5X1	T38.5X2	T38.5X3	T38.5X4	T38.5X5	T38.
Lutromone	T38.5X1	T38.5X2	T38.5X3	T38.5X4	T38.5X5	T38.
Lututrin	T48.291	T48.292	T48.293	T48.294	T48.295	T48.
Lye (concentrated)	T54.3X1	T54.3X2	T54.3X3	T54.3X4	—	—
Lygranum (skin test)	T50.8X1	T50.8X2	T50.8X3	T50.8X4	T50.8X5	T50.
Lymecycline	T36.4X1	T36.4X2	T36.4X3	T36.4X4	T36.4X5	T36.
Lymphogranuloma venereum antigen	T50.8X1	T50.8X2	T50.8X3	T50.8X4	T50.8X5	T50.
Lynestrenol	T38.4X1	T38.4X2	T38.4X3	T38.4X4	T38.4X5	T38
Lyovac Sodium Edecrin	T50.1X1	T50.1X2	T50.1X3	T50.1X4	T50.1X5	T50.
Lypressin	T38.891	T38.892	T38.893	T38.894	T38.895	T38
Lysergic acid diethylamide	T40.8X1	T40.8X2	T40.8X3	T40.8X4	—	—
Lysergide	T40.8X1	T40.8X2	T40.8X3	T40.8X4	—	—
Lysine vasopressin	T38.891	T38.892	T38.893	T38.894	T38.895	T38
Lysol	T54.1X1	T54.1X2	T54.1X3	T54.1X4	—	—
Lysozyme	T49.0X1	T49.0X2	T49.0X3	T49.0X4	T49.0X5	T49
Lytta (vitatta)	T49.8X1	T49.8X2	T49.8X3	T49.8X4	T49.8X5	T49.
Mace	T59.3X1	T59.3X2	T59.3X3	T59.3X4	—	—
Macrogol	T50.991	T50.992	T50.993	T50.994	T50.995	T50.
Macrolide						
anabolic drug	T38.7X1	T38.7X2	T38.7X3	T38.7X4	T38.7X5	T38.
antibiotic	T36.3X1	T36.3X2	T36.3X3	T36.3X4	T36.3X5	T36.
Mafenide	T49.0X1	T49.0X2	T49.0X3	T49.0X4	T49.0X5	T49.
Magaldrate	T47.1X1	T47.1X2	T47.1X3	T47.1X4	T47.1X5	T47.
Magic mushroom	T40.991	T40.992	T40.993	T40.994	—	—
Magnamycin	T36.8X1	T36.8X2	T36.8X3	T36.8X4	T36.8X5	T36.
Magnesia magma	T47.1X1	T47.1X2	T47.1X3	T47.1X4	T47.1X5	T47.
Magnesium NEC	T56.891	T56.892	T56.893	T56.894	—	—
carbonate	T47.1X1	T47.1X2	T47.1X3	T47.1X4	T47.1X5	T47.
citrate	T47.4X1	T47.4X2	T47.4X3	T47.4X4	T47.4X5	T47.
hydroxide	T47.1X1	T47.1X2	T47.1X3	T47.1X4	T47.1X5	T47.
oxide	T47.1X1	T47.1X2	T47.1X3	T47.1X4	T47.1X5	T47.
peroxide	T49.0X1	T49.0X2	T49.0X3	T49.0X4	T49.0X5	T49.
salicylate	T39.091	T39.092	T39.093	T39.094	T39.095	T39.
silicofluoride	T50.3X1	T50.3X2	T50.3X3	T50.3X4	T50.3X5	T50.
sulfate	T47.4X1	T47.4X2	T47.4X3	T47.4X4	T47.4X5	T47.
thiosulfate	T45.0X1	T45.0X2	T45.0X3	T45.0X4	T45.0X5	T45.
trisilicate	T47.1X1	T47.1X2	T47.1X3	T47.1X4	T47.1X5	T47.
Malathion (medicinal)	T49.0X1	T49.0X2	T49.0X3	T49.0X4	T49.0X5	T49.
insecticide	T60.0X1	T60.0X2	T60.0X3	T60.0X4	—	—
Male fern extract	T37.4X1	T37.4X2	T37.4X3	T37.4X4	T37.4X5	T37.
M-AMSA	T45.1X1	T45.1X2	T45.1X3	T45.1X4	T45.1X5	T45.
Mandelic acid	T37.8X1	T37.8X2	T37.8X3	T37.8X4	T37.8X5	T37.
Manganese (dioxide) (salts)	T57.2X1	T57.2X2	T57.2X3	T57.2X4	—	—
medicinal	T50.991	T50.992	T50.993	T50.994	T50.995	T50.
Mannitol	T47.3X1	T47.3X2	T47.3X3	T47.3X4	T47.3X5	T47.
hexanitrate	T46.3X1	T46.3X2	T46.3X3	T46.3X4	T46.3X5	T46.
Mannomustine	T45.1X1	T45.1X2	T45.1X3	T45.1X4	T45.1X5	T45.
MAO inhibitors	T43.1X1	T43.1X2	T43.1X3	T43.1X4	T43.1X5	T43.
Mapharsen	T37.8X1	T37.8X2	T37.8X3	T37.8X4	T37.8X5	T37.
Maphenide	T49.0X1	T49.0X2	T49.0X3	T49.0X4	T49.0X5	T49.
Maprotiline	T43.021	T43.022	T43.023	T43.024	T43.025	T43.
Marcaine	T41.3X1	T41.3X2	T41.3X3	T41.3X4	T41.3X5	T41.
infiltration (subcutaneous)	T41.3X1	T41.3X2	T41.3X3	T41.3X4	T41.3X5	T41.
nerve block (peripheral) (plexus)	T41.3X1	T41.3X2	T41.3X3	T41.3X4	T41.3X5	T41.
Marezine	T45.0X1	T45.0X2	T45.0X3	T45.0X4	T45.0X5	T45.
Marihuana	T40.7X1	T40.7X2	T40.7X3	T40.7X4	T40.7X5	T40.
Marijuana	T40.7X1	T40.7X2	T40.7X3	T40.7X4	T40.7X5	T40.
Marine (sting)	T63.691	T63.692	T63.693	T63.694	—	—
animals (sting)	T63.691	T63.692	T63.693	T63.694	—	—
plants (sting)	T63.711	T63.712	T63.713	T63.714	—	—
Marplan	T43.1X1	T43.1X2	T43.1X3	T43.1X4	T43.1X5	T43.
Marsh gas	T59.891	T59.892	T59.893	T59.894	—	—
Marsilid	T43.1X1	T43.1X2	T43.1X3	T43.1X4	T43.1X5	T43.
Matulane	T45.1X1	T45.1X2	T45.1X3	T45.1X4	T45.1X5	T45.
Mazindol	T50.5X1	T50.5X2	T50.5X3	T50.5X4	T50.5X5	T50.
MCPA	T60.3X1	T60.3X2	T60.3X3	T60.3X4	—	—
MDMA	T43.641	T43.642	T43.643	T43.644	—	—
Meadow saffron	T62.2X1	T62.2X2	T62.2X3	T62.2X4	—	—
Measles virus vaccine (attenuated)	T50.B91	T50.B92	T50.B93	T50.B94	T50.B95	T50.
Meat, noxious	T62.8X1	T62.8X2	T62.8X3	T62.8X4	—	—
Meballymal	T42.3X1	T42.3X2	T42.3X3	T42.3X4	T42.3X5	T42.
Mebanazine	T43.1X1	T43.1X2	T43.1X3	T43.1X4	T43.1X5	T43.
Mebaral	T42.3X1	T42.3X2	T42.3X3	T42.3X4	T42.3X5	T42.
Mebendazole	T37.4X1	T37.4X2	T37.4X3	T37.4X4	T37.4X5	T37.
Mebeverine	T44.3X1	T44.3X2	T44.3X3	T44.3X4	T44.3X5	T44.
Mebhydrolin	T45.0X1	T45.0X2	T45.0X3	T45.0X4	T45.0X5	T45.
Mebumal	T42.3X1	T42.3X2	T42.3X3	T42.3X4	T42.3X5	T42.
Mebutamate	T43.591	T43.592	T43.593	T43.594	T43.595	T43.
Mecamylamine	T44.2X1	T44.2X2	T44.2X3	T44.2X4	T44.2X5	T44.

Substance	Poisoning, Accidental (unintentional)	Poisoning, Intentional Self-harm	Poisoning, Assault	Poisoning, Undetermined	Adverse Effect	Under-dosing
Mechlorethamine	T45.1X1	T45.1X2	T45.1X3	T45.1X4	T45.1X5	T45.1X6
Mecillinam	T36.0X1	T36.0X2	T36.0X3	T36.0X4	T36.0X5	T36.0X6
Meclizine (hydrochloride)	T45.0X1	T45.0X2	T45.0X3	T45.0X4	T45.0X5	T45.0X6
Meclocycline	T36.4X1	T36.4X2	T36.4X3	T36.4X4	T36.4X5	T36.4X6
Meclofenamate	T39.391	T39.392	T39.393	T39.394	T39.395	T39.396
Meclofenamic acid	T39.391	T39.392	T39.393	T39.394	T39.395	T39.396
Meclofenoxate	T43.691	T43.692	T43.693	T43.694	T43.695	T43.696
Meclozine	T45.0X1	T45.0X2	T45.0X3	T45.0X4	T45.0X5	T45.0X6
Mecobalamin	T45.8X1	T45.8X2	T45.8X3	T45.8X4	—	T45.8X6
Mecoprop	T60.3X1	T60.3X2	T60.3X3	T60.3X4	—	—
Mecrilate	T49.3X1	T49.3X2	T49.3X3	T49.3X4	T49.3X5	T49.3X6
Mecysteine	T48.4X1	T48.4X2	T48.4X3	T48.4X4	T48.4X5	T48.4X6
Medazepam	T42.4X1	T42.4X2	T42.4X3	T42.4X4	T42.4X5	T42.4X6
Medicament NEC	T50.901	T50.902	T50.903	T50.904	T50.905	T50.906
Medinal	T42.3X1	T42.3X2	T42.3X3	T42.3X4	T42.3X5	T42.3X6
Medomin	T42.3X1	T42.3X2	T42.3X3	T42.3X4	T42.3X5	T42.3X6
Medrogestone	T38.5X1	T38.5X2	T38.5X3	T38.5X4	T38.5X5	T38.5X6
Medroxalol	T44.8X1	T44.8X2	T44.8X3	T44.8X4	T44.8X5	T44.8X6
Medroxyprogesterone acetate (depot)	T38.5X1	T38.5X2	T38.5X3	T38.5X4	T38.5X5	T38.5X6
Medrysone	T49.0X1	T49.0X2	T49.0X3	T49.0X4	T49.0X5	T49.0X6
Mefenamic acid	T39.391	T39.392	T39.393	T39.394	T39.395	T39.396
Mefenorex	T50.5X1	T50.5X2	T50.5X3	T50.5X4	T50.5X5	T50.5X6
Mefloquine	T37.2X1	T37.2X2	T37.2X3	T37.2X4	T37.2X5	T37.2X6
Mefruside	T50.2X1	T50.2X2	T50.2X3	T50.2X4	T50.2X5	T50.2X6
Megahallucinogen	T40.901	T40.902	T40.903	T40.904	T40.905	T40.906
Megestrol	T38.5X1	T38.5X2	T38.5X3	T38.5X4	T38.5X5	T38.5X6
Meglumine						
antimoniate	T37.8X1	T37.8X2	T37.8X3	T37.8X4	T37.8X5	T37.8X6
diatrizoate	T50.8X1	T50.8X2	T50.8X3	T50.8X4	T50.8X5	T50.8X6
iodipamide	T50.8X1	T50.8X2	T50.8X3	T50.8X4	T50.8X5	T50.8X6
iotroxate	T50.8X1	T50.8X2	T50.8X3	T50.8X4	T50.8X5	T50.8X6
MEK (methyl ethyl ketone)	T52.4X1	T52.4X2	T52.4X3	T52.4X4	—	—
Meladinin	T49.3X1	T49.3X2	T49.3X3	T49.3X4	T49.3X5	T49.3X6
Meladrazine	T44.3X1	T44.3X2	T44.3X3	T44.3X4	T44.3X5	T44.3X6
Melaleuca alternifolia oil	T49.0X1	T49.0X2	T49.0X3	T49.0X4	T49.0X5	T49.0X6
Melanizing agents	T49.3X1	T49.3X2	T49.3X3	T49.3X4	T49.3X5	T49.3X6
Melanocyte-stimulating hormone	T38.891	T38.892	T38.893	T38.894	T38.895	T38.896
Melarsonyl potassium	T37.3X1	T37.3X2	T37.3X3	T37.3X4	T37.3X5	T37.3X6
Melarsoprol	T37.3X1	T37.3X2	T37.3X3	T37.3X4	T37.3X5	T37.3X6
Melia azedarach	T62.2X1	T62.2X2	T62.2X3	T62.2X4	—	—
Melitracen	T43.011	T43.012	T43.013	T43.014	T43.015	T43.016
Mellaril	T43.3X1	T43.3X2	T43.3X3	T43.3X4	T43.3X5	T43.3X6
Meloxine	T49.3X1	T49.3X2	T49.3X3	T49.3X4	T49.3X5	T49.3X6
Melperone	T43.4X1	T43.4X2	T43.4X3	T43.4X4	T43.4X5	T43.4X6
Melphalan	T45.1X1	T45.1X2	T45.1X3	T45.1X4	T45.1X5	T45.1X6
Memantine	T43.8X1	T43.8X2	T43.8X3	T43.8X4	T43.8X5	T43.8X6
Menadiol	T45.7X1	T45.7X2	T45.7X3	T45.7X4	T45.7X5	T45.7X6
sodium sulfate	T45.7X1	T45.7X2	T45.7X3	T45.7X4	T45.7X5	T45.7X6
Menadione	T45.7X1	T45.7X2	T45.7X3	T45.7X4	T45.7X5	T45.7X6
sodium bisulfite	T45.7X1	T45.7X2	T45.7X3	T45.7X4	T45.7X5	T45.7X6
Menaphthone	T45.7X1	T45.7X2	T45.7X3	T45.7X4	T45.7X5	T45.7X6
Menaquinone	T45.7X1	T45.7X2	T45.7X3	T45.7X4	T45.7X5	T45.7X6
Menatetrenone	T45.7X1	T45.7X2	T45.7X3	T45.7X4	T45.7X5	T45.7X6
Meningococcal vaccine	T50.A91	T50.A92	T50.A93	T50.A94	T50.A95	T50.A96
Menningovax (-AC) (-C)	T50.A91	T50.A92	T50.A93	T50.A94	T50.A95	T50.A96
Menotropins	T38.811	T38.812	T38.813	T38.814	T38.815	T38.816
Menthol	T48.5X1	T48.5X2	T48.5X3	T48.5X4	T48.5X5	T48.5X6
Mepacrine	T37.2X1	T37.2X2	T37.2X3	T37.2X4	T37.2X5	T37.2X6
Meparfynol	T42.6X1	T42.6X2	T42.6X3	T42.6X4	T42.6X5	T42.6X6
Mepartricin	T36.7X1	T36.7X2	T36.7X3	T36.7X4	T36.7X5	T36.7X6
Mepazine	T43.3X1	T43.3X2	T43.3X3	T43.3X4	T43.3X5	T43.3X6
Mepenzolate	T44.3X1	T44.3X2	T44.3X3	T44.3X4	T44.3X5	T44.3X6
bromide	T44.3X1	T44.3X2	T44.3X3	T44.3X4	T44.3X5	T44.3X6
Meperidine	T40.4X1	T40.4X2	T40.4X3	T40.4X4	T40.4X5	T40.4X6
Mephebarbital	T42.3X1	T42.3X2	T42.3X3	T42.3X4	T42.3X5	T42.3X6
Mephenamin (e)	T42.8X1	T42.8X2	T42.8X3	T42.8X4	T42.8X5	T42.8X6
Mephenesin	T42.8X1	T42.8X2	T42.8X3	T42.8X4	T42.8X5	T42.8X6
Mephenhydramine	T45.0X1	T45.0X2	T45.0X3	T45.0X4	T45.0X5	T45.0X6
Mephenoxalone	T42.8X1	T42.8X2	T42.8X3	T42.8X4	T42.8X5	T42.8X6
Mephentermine	T44.991	T44.992	T44.993	T44.994	T44.995	T44.996
Mephenytoin	T42.0X1	T42.0X2	T42.0X3	T42.0X4	T42.0X5	T42.0X6
with phenobarbital	T42.3X1	T42.3X2	T42.3X3	T42.3X4	T42.3X5	T42.3X6
Mephobarbital	T42.3X1	T42.3X2	T42.3X3	T42.3X4	T42.3X5	T42.3X6
Mephosfolan	T60.0X1	T60.0X2	T60.0X3	T60.0X4	—	—
Mepindolol	T44.7X1	T44.7X2	T44.7X3	T44.7X4	T44.7X5	T44.7X6
Mepiperphenidol	T44.3X1	T44.3X2	T44.3X3	T44.3X4	T44.3X5	T44.3X6
Mepitiostane	T38.7X1	T38.7X2	T38.7X3	T38.7X4	T38.7X5	T38.7X6
Mepivacaine	T41.3X1	T41.3X2	T41.3X3	T41.3X4	T41.3X5	T41.3X6
epidural	T41.3X1	T41.3X2	T41.3X3	T41.3X4	T41.3X5	T41.3X6
Meprednisone	T38.0X1	T38.0X2	T38.0X3	T38.0X4	T38.0X5	T38.0X6
Meprobam	T43.591	T43.592	T43.593	T43.594	T43.595	T43.596

Substance	Poisoning, Accidental (unintentional)	Poisoning, Intentional Self-harm	Poisoning, Assault	Poisoning, Undetermined	Adverse Effect	Under-dosing
Meprobamate	T43.591	T43.592	T43.593	T43.594	T43.595	T43.596
Meproscillarin	T46.0X1	T46.0X2	T46.0X3	T46.0X4	T46.0X5	T46.0X6
Meprylcaine	T41.3X1	T41.3X2	T41.3X3	T41.3X4	T41.3X5	T41.3X6
Meptazinol	T39.8X1	T39.8X2	T39.8X3	T39.8X4	T39.8X5	T39.8X6
Mepyramine	T45.0X1	T45.0X2	T45.0X3	T45.0X4	T45.0X5	T45.0X6
Mequitazine	T43.3X1	T43.3X2	T43.3X3	T43.3X4	T43.3X5	T43.3X6
Meralluride	T50.2X1	T50.2X2	T50.2X3	T50.2X4	T50.2X5	T50.2X6
Merbaphen	T50.2X1	T50.2X2	T50.2X3	T50.2X4	T50.2X5	T50.2X6
Merbromin	T49.0X1	T49.0X2	T49.0X3	T49.0X4	T49.0X5	T49.0X6
Mercaptobenzothiazole salts	T49.0X1	T49.0X2	T49.0X3	T49.0X4	T49.0X5	T49.0X6
Mercaptomerin	T50.2X1	T50.2X2	T50.2X3	T50.2X4	T50.2X5	T50.2X6
Mercaptopurine	T45.1X1	T45.1X2	T45.1X3	T45.1X4	T45.1X5	T45.1X6
Mercumatilin	T50.2X1	T50.2X2	T50.2X3	T50.2X4	T50.2X5	T50.2X6
Mercuramide	T50.2X1	T50.2X2	T50.2X3	T50.2X4	T50.2X5	T50.2X6
Mercurochrome	T49.0X1	T49.0X2	T49.0X3	T49.0X4	T49.0X5	T49.0X6
Mercurophylline	T50.2X1	T50.2X2	T50.2X3	T50.2X4	T50.2X5	T50.2X6
Mercury, mercurial, mercuric, mercurous (compounds) (cyanide) (fumes) (nonmedicinal) (vapor) NEC	T56.1X1	T56.1X2	T56.1X3	T56.1X4	—	—
ammoniated	T49.0X1	T49.0X2	T49.0X3	T49.0X4	T49.0X5	T49.0X6
anti-infective						
local	T49.0X1	T49.0X2	T49.0X3	T49.0X4	T49.0X5	T49.0X6
systemic	T37.8X1	T37.8X2	T37.8X3	T37.8X4	T37.8X5	T37.8X6
topical	T49.0X1	T49.0X2	T49.0X3	T49.0X4	T49.0X5	T49.0X6
chloride (ammoniated)	T49.0X1	T49.0X2	T49.0X3	T49.0X4	T49.0X5	T49.0X6
fungicide	T56.1X1	T56.1X2	T56.1X3	T56.1X4	—	—
diuretic NEC	T50.2X1	T50.2X2	T50.2X3	T50.2X4	T50.2X5	T50.2X6
fungicide	T56.1X1	T56.1X2	T56.1X3	T56.1X4	—	—
organic (fungicide)	T56.1X1	T56.1X2	T56.1X3	T56.1X4	—	—
oxide, yellow	T49.0X1	T49.0X2	T49.0X3	T49.0X4	T49.0X5	T49.0X6
Mersalyl	T50.2X1	T50.2X2	T50.2X3	T50.2X4	T50.2X5	T50.2X6
Merthiolate	T49.0X1	T49.0X2	T49.0X3	T49.0X4	T49.0X5	T49.0X6
ophthalmic preparation	T49.5X1	T49.5X2	T49.5X3	T49.5X4	T49.5X5	T49.5X6
Meruvax	T50.B91	T50.B92	T50.B93	T50.B94	T50.B95	T50.B96
Mesalazine	T47.8X1	T47.8X2	T47.8X3	T47.8X4	T47.8X5	T47.8X6
Mescal buttons	T40.991	T40.992	T40.993	T40.994	—	—
Mescaline	T40.991	T40.992	T40.993	T40.994	—	—
Mesna	T48.4X1	T48.4X2	T48.4X3	T48.4X4	T48.4X5	T48.4X6
Mesoglycan	T46.6X1	T46.6X2	T46.6X3	T46.6X4	T46.6X5	T46.6X6
Mesoridazine	T43.3X1	T43.3X2	T43.3X3	T43.3X4	T43.3X5	T43.3X6
Mestanolone	T38.7X1	T38.7X2	T38.7X3	T38.7X4	T38.7X5	T38.7X6
Mesterolone	T38.7X1	T38.7X2	T38.7X3	T38.7X4	T38.7X5	T38.7X6
Mestranol	T38.5X1	T38.5X2	T38.5X3	T38.5X4	T38.5X5	T38.5X6
Mesulergine	T42.8X1	T42.8X2	T42.8X3	T42.8X4	T42.8X5	T42.8X6
Mesulfen	T49.0X1	T49.0X2	T49.0X3	T49.0X4	T49.0X5	T49.0X6
Mesuximide	T42.2X1	T42.2X2	T42.2X3	T42.2X4	T42.2X5	T42.2X6
Metabutethamine	T41.3X1	T41.3X2	T41.3X3	T41.3X4	T41.3X5	T41.3X6
Metactesylacetate	T49.0X1	T49.0X2	T49.0X3	T49.0X4	T49.0X5	T49.0X6
Metacycline	T36.4X1	T36.4X2	T36.4X3	T36.4X4	T36.4X5	T36.4X6
Metaldehyde (snail killer) NEC	T60.8X1	T60.8X2	T60.8X3	T60.8X4	—	—
Metals (heavy) (nonmedicinal)	T56.91	T56.92	T56.93	T56.94	—	—
dust, fumes, or vapor NEC	T56.91	T56.92	T56.93	T56.94	—	—
light NEC	T56.91	T56.92	T56.93	T56.94	—	—
dust, fumes, or vapor NEC	T56.91	T56.92	T56.93	T56.94	—	—
specified NEC	T56.891	T56.892	T56.893	T56.894	—	—
thallium	T56.811	T56.812	T56.813	T56.814	—	—
Metamfetamine	T43.621	T43.622	T43.623	T43.624	T43.625	T43.626
Metamizole sodium	T39.2X1	T39.2X2	T39.2X3	T39.2X4	T39.2X5	T39.2X6
Metampicillin	T36.0X1	T36.0X2	T36.0X3	T36.0X4	T36.0X5	T36.0X6
Metamucil	T47.4X1	T47.4X2	T47.4X3	T47.4X4	T47.4X5	T47.4X6
Metandienone	T38.7X1	T38.7X2	T38.7X3	T38.7X4	T38.7X5	T38.7X6
Metandrostenolone	T38.7X1	T38.7X2	T38.7X3	T38.7X4	T38.7X5	T38.7X6
Metaphen	T49.0X1	T49.0X2	T49.0X3	T49.0X4	T49.0X5	T49.0X6
Metaphos	T60.0X1	T60.0X2	T60.0X3	T60.0X4	—	—
Metapramine	T43.011	T43.012	T43.013	T43.014	T43.015	T43.016
Metaproterenol	T48.291	T48.292	T48.293	T48.294	T48.295	T48.296
Metaraminol	T44.4X1	T44.4X2	T44.4X3	T44.4X4	T44.4X5	T44.4X6
Metaxalone	T42.8X1	T42.8X2	T42.8X3	T42.8X4	T42.8X5	T42.8X6
Metenolone	T38.7X1	T38.7X2	T38.7X3	T38.7X4	T38.7X5	T38.7X6
Metergoline	T42.8X1	T42.8X2	T42.8X3	T42.8X4	T42.8X5	T42.8X6
Metescufylline	T46.991	T46.992	T46.993	T46.994	T46.995	T46.996
Metetoin	T42.0X1	T42.0X2	T42.0X3	T42.0X4	T42.0X5	T42.0X6
Metformin	T38.3X1	T38.3X2	T38.3X3	T38.3X4	T38.3X5	T38.3X6
Methacholine	T44.1X1	T44.1X2	T44.1X3	T44.1X4	T44.1X5	T44.1X6
Methacycline	T36.4X1	T36.4X2	T36.4X3	T36.4X4	T36.4X5	T36.4X6
Methadone	T40.3X1	T40.3X2	T40.3X3	T40.3X4	T40.3X5	T40.3X6
Methallenestril	T38.5X1	T38.5X2	T38.5X3	T38.5X4	T38.5X5	T38.5X6

Substance	Poisoning, Accidental (unintentional)	Poisoning, Intentional Self-harm	Poisoning, Assault	Poisoning, Undetermined	Adverse Effect	Under-dosing
Methallenoestril	T38.5X1	T38.5X2	T38.5X3	T38.5X4	T38.5X5	T38.5X6
Methamphetamine	T43.621	T43.622	T43.623	T43.624	T43.625	T43.626
Methampyrone	T39.2X1	T39.2X2	T39.2X3	T39.2X4	T39.2X5	T39.2X6
Methandienone	T38.7X1	T38.7X2	T38.7X3	T38.7X4	T38.7X5	T38.7X6
Methandriol	T38.7X1	T38.7X2	T38.7X3	T38.7X4	T38.7X5	T38.7X6
Methandrostenolone	T38.7X1	T38.7X2	T38.7X3	T38.7X4	T38.7X5	T38.7X6
Methane	T59.891	T59.892	T59.893	T59.894	—	—
Methanethiol	T59.891	T59.892	T59.893	T59.894	—	—
Methaniazide	T37.1X1	T37.1X2	T37.1X3	T37.1X4	T37.1X5	T37.1X6
Methanol (vapor)	T51.1X1	T51.1X2	T51.1X3	T51.1X4	—	—
Methantheline	T44.3X1	T44.3X2	T44.3X3	T44.3X4	T44.3X5	T44.3X6
Methanthelinium bromide	T44.3X1	T44.3X2	T44.3X3	T44.3X4	T44.3X5	T44.3X6
Methaphenilene	T45.0X1	T45.0X2	T45.0X3	T45.0X4	T45.0X5	T45.0X6
Methapyrilene	T45.0X1	T45.0X2	T45.0X3	T45.0X4	T45.0X5	T45.0X6
Methaqualone (compound)	T42.6X1	T42.6X2	T42.6X3	T42.6X4	T42.6X5	T42.6X6
Metharbital	T42.3X1	T42.3X2	T42.3X3	T42.3X4	T42.3X5	T42.3X6
Methazolamide	T50.2X1	T50.2X2	T50.2X3	T50.2X4	T50.2X5	T50.2X6
Methdilazine	T43.3X1	T43.3X2	T43.3X3	T43.3X4	T43.3X5	T43.3X6
Methedrine	T43.621	T43.622	T43.623	T43.624	T43.625	T43.626
Methenamine (mandelate)	T37.8X1	T37.8X2	T37.8X3	T37.8X4	T37.8X5	T37.8X6
Methenolone	T38.7X1	T38.7X2	T38.7X3	T38.7X4	T38.7X5	T38.7X6
Methergine	T48.0X1	T48.0X2	T48.0X3	T48.0X4	T48.0X5	T48.0X6
Methetoin	T42.0X1	T42.0X2	T42.0X3	T42.0X4	T42.0X5	T42.0X6
Methiacil	T38.2X1	T38.2X2	T38.2X3	T38.2X4	T38.2X5	T38.2X6
Methicillin	T36.0X1	T36.0X2	T36.0X3	T36.0X4	T36.0X5	T36.0X6
Methimazole	T38.2X1	T38.2X2	T38.2X3	T38.2X4	T38.2X5	T38.2X6
Methiodal sodium	T50.8X1	T50.8X2	T50.8X3	T50.8X4	T50.8X5	T50.8X6
Methionine	T50.991	T50.992	T50.993	T50.994	T50.995	T50.996
Methisazone	T37.5X1	T37.5X2	T37.5X3	T37.5X4	T37.5X5	T37.5X6
Methisoprinol	T37.5X1	T37.5X2	T37.5X3	T37.5X4	T37.5X5	T37.5X6
Methitural	T42.3X1	T42.3X2	T42.3X3	T42.3X4	T42.3X5	T42.3X6
Methixene	T44.3X1	T44.3X2	T44.3X3	T44.3X4	T44.3X5	T44.3X6
Methobarbital, methobarbitone	T42.3X1	T42.3X2	T42.3X3	T42.3X4	T42.3X5	T42.3X6
Methocarbamol	T42.8X1	T42.8X2	T42.8X3	T42.8X4	T42.8X5	T42.8X6
skeletal muscle relaxant	T48.1X1	T48.1X2	T48.1X3	T48.1X4	T48.1X5	T48.1X6
Methohexital	T41.1X1	T41.1X2	T41.1X3	T41.1X4	T41.1X5	T41.1X6
Methohexitone	T41.1X1	T41.1X2	T41.1X3	T41.1X4	T41.1X5	T41.1X6
Methoin	T42.0X1	T42.0X2	T42.0X3	T42.0X4	T42.0X5	T42.0X6
Methopholine	T39.8X1	T39.8X2	T39.8X3	T39.8X4	T39.8X5	T39.8X6
Methopromazine	T43.3X1	T43.3X2	T43.3X3	T43.3X4	T43.3X5	T43.3X6
Methorate	T48.3X1	T48.3X2	T48.3X3	T48.3X4	T48.3X5	T48.3X6
Methoserpidine	T46.5X1	T46.5X2	T46.5X3	T46.5X4	T46.5X5	T46.5X6
Methotrexate	T45.1X1	T45.1X2	T45.1X3	T45.1X4	T45.1X5	T45.1X6
Methotrimeprazine	T43.3X1	T43.3X2	T43.3X3	T43.3X4	T43.3X5	T43.3X6
Methoxa-Dome	T49.3X1	T49.3X2	T49.3X3	T49.3X4	T49.3X5	T49.3X6
Methoxamine	T44.4X1	T44.4X2	T44.4X3	T44.4X4	T44.4X5	T44.4X6
Methoxsalen	T50.991	T50.992	T50.993	T50.994	T50.995	T50.996
Methoxyaniline	T65.3X1	T65.3X2	T65.3X3	T65.3X4	—	—
Methoxybenzyl penicillin	T36.0X1	T36.0X2	T36.0X3	T36.0X4	T36.0X5	T36.0X6
Methoxychlor	T53.7X1	T53.7X2	T53.7X3	T53.7X4	—	—
Methoxy-DDT	T53.7X1	T53.7X2	T53.7X3	T53.7X4	—	—
Methoxyflurane	T41.0X1	T41.0X2	T41.0X3	T41.0X4	T41.0X5	T41.0X6
Methoxyphenamine	T48.6X1	T48.6X2	T48.6X3	T48.6X4	T48.6X5	T48.6X6
Methoxypromazine	T43.3X1	T43.3X2	T43.3X3	T43.3X4	T43.3X5	T43.3X6
Methscopolamine bromide	T44.3X1	T44.3X2	T44.3X3	T44.3X4	T44.3X5	T44.3X6
Methsuximide	T42.2X1	T42.2X2	T42.2X3	T42.2X4	T42.2X5	T42.2X6
Methyclothiazide	T50.2X1	T50.2X2	T50.2X3	T50.2X4	T50.2X5	T50.2X6
Methyl						
acetate	T52.4X1	T52.4X2	T52.4X3	T52.4X4	—	—
acetone	T52.4X1	T52.4X2	T52.4X3	T52.4X4	—	—
acrylate	T65.891	T65.892	T65.893	T65.894	—	—
alcohol	T51.1X1	T51.1X2	T51.1X3	T51.1X4	—	—
aminophenol	T65.3X1	T65.3X2	T65.3X3	T65.3X4	—	—
amphetamine	T43.621	T43.622	T43.623	T43.624	T43.625	T43.626
androstanolone	T38.7X1	T38.7X2	T38.7X3	T38.7X4	T38.7X5	T38.7X6
atropine	T44.3X1	T44.3X2	T44.3X3	T44.3X4	T44.3X5	T44.3X6
benzene	T52.2X1	T52.2X2	T52.2X3	T52.2X4	—	—
benzoate	T52.8X1	T52.8X2	T52.8X3	T52.8X4	—	—
benzol	T52.2X1	T52.2X2	T52.2X3	T52.2X4	—	—
bromide (gas)	T59.891	T59.892	T59.893	T59.894	—	—
fumigant	T60.8X1	T60.8X2	T60.8X3	T60.8X4	—	—
butanol	T51.3X1	T51.3X2	T51.3X3	T51.3X4	—	—
carbinol	T51.1X1	T51.1X2	T51.1X3	T51.1X4	—	—
carbonate	T52.8X1	T52.8X2	T52.8X3	T52.8X4	—	—
CCNU	T45.1X1	T45.1X2	T45.1X3	T45.1X4	T45.1X5	T45.1X6
cellosolve	T52.91	T52.92	T52.93	T52.94	—	—
cellulose	T47.4X1	T47.4X2	T47.4X3	T47.4X4	T47.4X5	T47.4X6
chloride (gas)	T59.891	T59.892	T59.893	T59.894	—	—
chloroformate	T59.3X1	T59.3X2	T59.3X3	T59.3X4	—	—
cyclohexane	T52.8X1	T52.8X2	T52.8X3	T52.8X4	—	—
cyclohexanol	T51.8X1	T51.8X2	T51.8X3	T51.8X4	—	—

Substance	Poisoning, Accidental (unintentional)	Poisoning, Intentional Self-harm	Poisoning, Assault	Poisoning, Undetermined	Adverse Effect	Under-dosing
Methyl — continued						
cyclohexanone	T52.8X1	T52.8X2	T52.8X3	T52.8X4	—	—
cyclohexyl acetate	T52.8X1	T52.8X2	T52.8X3	T52.8X4	—	—
demeton	T60.0X1	T60.0X2	T60.0X3	T60.0X4	—	—
dihydromorphinone	T40.2X1	T40.2X2	T40.2X3	T40.2X4	T40.2X5	T40.
ergometrine	T48.0X1	T48.0X2	T48.0X3	T48.0X4	T48.0X5	T48.
ergonovine	T48.0X1	T48.0X2	T48.0X3	T48.0X4	T48.0X5	T48.
ethyl ketone	T52.4X1	T52.4X2	T52.4X3	T52.4X4	—	—
glucamine antimonate	T37.8X1	T37.8X2	T37.8X3	T37.8X4	T37.8X5	T37.
hydrazine	T65.891	T65.892	T65.893	T65.894	—	—
iodide	T65.891	T65.892	T65.893	T65.894	—	—
isobutyl ketone	T52.4X1	T52.4X2	T52.4X3	T52.4X4	—	—
isothiocyanate	T60.3X1	T60.3X2	T60.3X3	T60.3X4	—	—
mercaptan	T59.891	T59.892	T59.893	T59.894	—	—
morphine NEC	T40.2X1	T40.2X2	T40.2X3	T40.2X4	T40.2X5	T40.
nicotinate	T49.4X1	T49.4X2	T49.4X3	T49.4X4	T49.4X5	T49.
paraben	T49.0X1	T49.0X2	T49.0X3	T49.0X4	T49.0X5	T49.
parafynol	T42.6X1	T42.6X2	T42.6X3	T42.6X4	T42.6X5	T42.
parathion	T60.0X1	T60.0X2	T60.0X3	T60.0X4	—	—
peridol	T43.4X1	T43.4X2	T43.4X3	T43.4X4	T43.4X5	T43.
phenidate	T43.631	T43.632	T43.633	T43.634	T43.635	T43.
prednisolone	T38.0X1	T38.0X2	T38.0X3	T38.0X4	T38.0X5	T38.
ENT agent	T49.6X1	T49.6X2	T49.6X3	T49.6X4	T49.6X5	T49.
ophthalmic preparation	T49.5X1	T49.5X2	T49.5X3	T49.5X4	T49.5X5	T49.
topical NEC	T49.0X1	T49.0X2	T49.0X3	T49.0X4	T49.0X5	T49.
propylcarbinol	T51.3X1	T51.3X2	T51.3X3	T51.3X4	—	—
rosaniline NEC	T49.0X1	T49.0X2	T49.0X3	T49.0X4	T49.0X5	T49.
salicylate	T49.2X1	T49.2X2	T49.2X3	T49.2X4	T49.2X5	T49.
sulfate (fumes)	T59.891	T59.892	T59.893	T59.894	—	—
liquid	T52.8X1	T52.8X2	T52.8X3	T52.8X4	—	—
sulfonal	T42.6X1	T42.6X2	T42.6X3	T42.6X4	T42.6X5	T42.
testosterone	T38.7X1	T38.7X2	T38.7X3	T38.7X4	T38.7X5	T38.
thiouracil	T38.2X1	T38.2X2	T38.2X3	T38.2X4	T38.2X5	T38.
Methylamphetamine	T43.621	T43.622	T43.623	T43.624	T43.625	T43.
Methylated spirit	T51.1X1	T51.1X2	T51.1X3	T51.1X4	—	—
Methylatropine nitrate	T44.3X1	T44.3X2	T44.3X3	T44.3X4	T44.3X5	T44.
Methylbenactyzium bromide	T44.3X1	T44.3X2	T44.3X3	T44.3X4	T44.3X5	T44.
Methylbenzethonium chloride	T49.0X1	T49.0X2	T49.0X3	T49.0X4	T49.0X5	T49.
Methylcellulose	T47.4X1	T47.4X2	T47.4X3	T47.4X4	T47.4X5	T47.
laxative	T47.4X1	T47.4X2	T47.4X3	T47.4X4	T47.4X5	T47.
Methylchlorophenoxyacetic acid	T60.3X1	T60.3X2	T60.3X3	T60.3X4	—	—
Methyldopa	T46.5X1	T46.5X2	T46.5X3	T46.5X4	T46.5X5	T46.
Methyldopate	T46.5X1	T46.5X2	T46.5X3	T46.5X4	T46.5X5	T46.
Methylene						
blue	T50.6X1	T50.6X2	T50.6X3	T50.6X4	T50.6X5	T50.
chloride or dichloride (solvent) NEC	T53.4X1	T53.4X2	T53.4X3	T53.4X4	—	—
Methylenedioxyamphetamine	T43.621	T43.622	T43.623	T43.624	T43.625	T43.
Methylenedioxymeth-amphetamine	T43.641	T43.642	T43.643	T43.644	—	—
Methylergometrine	T48.0X1	T48.0X2	T48.0X3	T48.0X4	T48.0X5	T48.
Methylergonovine	T48.0X1	T48.0X2	T48.0X3	T48.0X4	T48.0X5	T48.
Methylestrenolone	T38.5X1	T38.5X2	T38.5X3	T38.5X4	T38.5X5	T38.
Methylethyl cellulose	T50.991	T50.992	T50.993	T50.994	T50.995	T50.9
Methylhexabital	T42.3X1	T42.3X2	T42.3X3	T42.3X4	T42.3X5	T42.
Methylmorphine	T40.2X1	T40.2X2	T40.2X3	T40.2X4	T40.2X5	T40.
Methylparaben (ophthalmic)	T49.5X1	T49.5X2	T49.5X3	T49.5X4	T49.5X5	T49.
Methylparafynol	T42.6X1	T42.6X2	T42.6X3	T42.6X4	T42.6X5	T42.
Methylpentynol, methylpenthynol	T42.6X1	T42.6X2	T42.6X3	T42.6X4	T42.6X5	T42.
Methylphenidate	T43.631	T43.632	T43.633	T43.634	T43.635	T43.
Methylphenobarbital	T42.3X1	T42.3X2	T42.3X3	T42.3X4	T42.3X5	T42.
Methylpolysiloxane	T47.1X1	T47.1X2	T47.1X3	T47.1X4	T47.1X5	T47.
Methylprednisolone — see Methyl, prednisolone						
Methylrosaniline	T49.0X1	T49.0X2	T49.0X3	T49.0X4	T49.0X5	T49.
Methylrosanilinium chloride	T49.0X1	T49.0X2	T49.0X3	T49.0X4	T49.0X5	T49.
Methyltestosterone	T38.7X1	T38.7X2	T38.7X3	T38.7X4	T38.7X5	T38.
Methylthionine chloride	T50.6X1	T50.6X2	T50.6X3	T50.6X4	T50.6X5	T50.
Methylthioninium chloride	T50.6X1	T50.6X2	T50.6X3	T50.6X4	T50.6X5	T50.
Methylthiouracil	T38.2X1	T38.2X2	T38.2X3	T38.2X4	T38.2X5	T38.
Methyprylon	T42.6X1	T42.6X2	T42.6X3	T42.6X4	T42.6X5	T42.
Methysergide	T46.5X1	T46.5X2	T46.5X3	T46.5X4	T46.5X5	T46.
Metiamide	T47.1X1	T47.1X2	T47.1X3	T47.1X4	T47.1X5	T47.
Meticillin	T36.0X1	T36.0X2	T36.0X3	T36.0X4	T36.0X5	T36.
Meticrane	T50.2X1	T50.2X2	T50.2X3	T50.2X4	T50.2X5	T50.2
Metildigoxin	T46.0X1	T46.0X2	T46.0X3	T46.0X4	T46.0X5	T46.

Additional Character May Be Required — Refer to the Tabular List for Character Selection ▽ Subterms under main terms may continue to next column or pag

Substance	Poisoning, Accidental (unintentional)	Poisoning, Intentional Self-harm	Poisoning, Assault	Poisoning, Undetermined	Adverse Effect	Under-dosing
Metipranolol	T49.5X1	T49.5X2	T49.5X3	T49.5X4	T49.5X5	T49.5X6
Metirosine	T46.5X1	T46.5X2	T46.5X3	T46.5X4	T46.5X5	T46.5X6
Metisazone	T37.5X1	T37.5X2	T37.5X3	T37.5X4	T37.5X5	T37.5X6
Metixene	T44.3X1	T44.3X2	T44.3X3	T44.3X4	T44.3X5	T44.3X6
Metizoline	T48.5X1	T48.5X2	T48.5X3	T48.5X4	T48.5X5	T48.5X6
Metoclopramide	T45.0X1	T45.0X2	T45.0X3	T45.0X4	T45.0X5	T45.0X6
Metofenazate	T43.3X1	T43.3X2	T43.3X3	T43.3X4	T43.3X5	T43.3X6
Metofoline	T39.8X1	T39.8X2	T39.8X3	T39.8X4	T39.8X5	T39.8X6
Metolazone	T50.2X1	T50.2X2	T50.2X3	T50.2X4	T50.2X5	T50.2X6
Metopon	T40.2X1	T40.2X2	T40.2X3	T40.2X4	T40.2X5	T40.2X6
Metoprine	T45.1X1	T45.1X2	T45.1X3	T45.1X4	T45.1X5	T45.1X6
Metoprolol	T44.7X1	T44.7X2	T44.7X3	T44.7X4	T44.7X5	T44.7X6
Metrifonate	T60.0X1	T60.0X2	T60.0X3	T60.0X4	—	—
Metrizamide	T50.8X1	T50.8X2	T50.8X3	T50.8X4	T50.8X5	T50.8X6
Metrizoic acid	T50.8X1	T50.8X2	T50.8X3	T50.8X4	T50.8X5	T50.8X6
Metronidazole	T37.8X1	T37.8X2	T37.8X3	T37.8X4	T37.8X5	T37.8X6
Metycaine	T41.3X1	T41.3X2	T41.3X3	T41.3X4	T41.3X5	T41.3X6
infiltration (subcutaneous)	T41.3X1	T41.3X2	T41.3X3	T41.3X4	T41.3X5	T41.3X6
nerve block (peripheral) (plexus)	T41.3X1	T41.3X2	T41.3X3	T41.3X4	T41.3X5	T41.3X6
topical (surface)	T41.3X1	T41.3X2	T41.3X3	T41.3X4	T41.3X5	T41.3X6
Metyrapone	T50.8X1	T50.8X2	T50.8X3	T50.8X4	T50.8X5	T50.8X6
Mevinphos	T60.0X1	T60.0X2	T60.0X3	T60.0X4	—	—
Mexazolam	T42.4X1	T42.4X2	T42.4X3	T42.4X4	T42.4X5	T42.4X6
Mexenone	T49.3X1	T49.3X2	T49.3X3	T49.3X4	T49.3X5	T49.3X6
Mexiletine	T46.2X1	T46.2X2	T46.2X3	T46.2X4	T46.2X5	T46.2X6
Mezereon	T62.2X1	T62.2X2	T62.2X3	T62.2X4	—	—
berries	T62.1X1	T62.1X2	T62.1X3	T62.1X4	—	—
Mezlocillin	T36.0X1	T36.0X2	T36.0X3	T36.0X4	T36.0X5	T36.0X6
Mianserin	T43.021	T43.022	T43.023	T43.024	T43.025	T43.026
Micatin	T49.0X1	T49.0X2	T49.0X3	T49.0X4	T49.0X5	T49.0X6
Miconazole	T49.0X1	T49.0X2	T49.0X3	T49.0X4	T49.0X5	T49.0X6
Micronomicin	T36.5X1	T36.5X2	T36.5X3	T36.5X4	T36.5X5	T36.5X6
Midazolam	T42.4X1	T42.4X2	T42.4X3	T42.4X4	T42.4X5	T42.4X6
Midecamycin	T36.3X1	T36.3X2	T36.3X3	T36.3X4	T36.3X5	T36.3X6
Mifepristone	T38.6X1	T38.6X2	T38.6X3	T38.6X4	T38.6X5	T38.6X6
Milk of magnesia	T47.1X1	T47.1X2	T47.1X3	T47.1X4	T47.1X5	T47.1X6
Millipede (tropical) (venomous)	T63.411	T63.412	T63.413	T63.414	—	—
Miltown	T43.591	T43.592	T43.593	T43.594	T43.595	T43.596
Milverine	T44.3X1	T44.3X2	T44.3X3	T44.3X4	T44.3X5	T44.3X6
Minaprine	T43.291	T43.292	T43.293	T43.294	T43.295	T43.296
Minaxolone	T41.291	T41.292	T41.293	T41.294	T41.295	T41.296
Mineral						
acids	T54.2X1	T54.2X2	T54.2X3	T54.2X4	—	—
oil (laxative)(medicinal)	T47.4X1	T47.4X2	T47.4X3	T47.4X4	T47.4X5	T47.4X6
emulsion	T47.2X1	T47.2X2	T47.2X3	T47.2X4	T47.2X5	T47.2X6
nonmedicinal	T52.0X1	T52.0X2	T52.0X3	T52.0X4	—	—
topical	T49.3X1	T49.3X2	T49.3X3	T49.3X4	T49.3X5	T49.3X6
salt NEC	T50.3X1	T50.3X2	T50.3X3	T50.3X4	T50.3X5	T50.3X6
spirits	T52.0X1	T52.0X2	T52.0X3	T52.0X4	—	—
Mineralocorticosteroid	T50.0X1	T50.0X2	T50.0X3	T50.0X4	T50.0X5	T50.0X6
Minocycline	T36.4X1	T36.4X2	T36.4X3	T36.4X4	T36.4X5	T36.4X6
Minoxidil	T46.7X1	T46.7X2	T46.7X3	T46.7X4	T46.7X5	T46.7X6
Miokamycin	T36.3X1	T36.3X2	T36.3X3	T36.3X4	T36.3X5	T36.3X6
Miotic drug	T49.5X1	T49.5X2	T49.5X3	T49.5X4	T49.5X5	T49.5X6
Mipafox	T60.0X1	T60.0X2	T60.0X3	T60.0X4	—	—
Mirex	T60.1X1	T60.1X2	T60.1X3	T60.1X4	—	—
Mirtazapine	T43.021	T43.022	T43.023	T43.024	T43.025	T43.026
Misonidazole	T37.3X1	T37.3X2	T37.3X3	T37.3X4	T37.3X5	T37.3X6
Misoprostol	T47.1X1	T47.1X2	T47.1X3	T47.1X4	T47.1X5	T47.1X6
Mithramycin	T45.1X1	T45.1X2	T45.1X3	T45.1X4	T45.1X5	T45.1X6
Mitobronitol	T45.1X1	T45.1X2	T45.1X3	T45.1X4	T45.1X5	T45.1X6
Mitoguazone	T45.1X1	T45.1X2	T45.1X3	T45.1X4	T45.1X5	T45.1X6
Mitolactol	T45.1X1	T45.1X2	T45.1X3	T45.1X4	T45.1X5	T45.1X6
Mitomycin	T45.1X1	T45.1X2	T45.1X3	T45.1X4	T45.1X5	T45.1X6
Mitopodozide	T45.1X1	T45.1X2	T45.1X3	T45.1X4	T45.1X5	T45.1X6
Mitotane	T45.1X1	T45.1X2	T45.1X3	T45.1X4	T45.1X5	T45.1X6
Mitoxantrone	T45.1X1	T45.1X2	T45.1X3	T45.1X5	T45.1X5	T45.1X6
Mivacurium chloride	T48.1X1	T48.1X2	T48.1X3	T48.1X4	T48.1X5	T48.1X6
Miyari bacteria	T47.6X1	T47.6X2	T47.6X3	T47.6X4	T47.6X5	T47.6X6
Moclobemide	T43.1X1	T43.1X2	T43.1X3	T43.1X4	T43.1X5	T43.1X6
Moderil	T46.5X1	T46.5X2	T46.5X3	T46.5X4	T46.5X5	T46.5X6
Mofebutazone	T39.2X1	T39.2X2	T39.2X3	T39.2X4	T39.2X5	T39.2X6
Mogadon — see Nitrazepam						
Molindone	T43.591	T43.592	T43.593	T43.594	T43.595	T43.596
Molsidomine	T46.3X1	T46.3X2	T46.3X3	T46.3X4	T46.3X5	T46.3X6
Mometasone	T49.0X1	T49.0X2	T49.0X3	T49.0X4	T49.0X5	T49.0X6
Monistat	T49.0X1	T49.0X2	T49.0X3	T49.0X4	T49.0X5	T49.0X6
Monkshood	T62.2X1	T62.2X2	T62.2X3	T62.2X4	—	—
Monoamine oxidase inhibitor NEC	T43.1X1	T43.1X2	T43.1X3	T43.1X4	T43.1X5	T43.1X6
hydrazine	T43.1X1	T43.1X2	T43.1X3	T43.1X4	T43.1X5	T43.1X6

Substance	Poisoning, Accidental (unintentional)	Poisoning, Intentional Self-harm	Poisoning, Assault	Poisoning, Undetermined	Adverse Effect	Under-dosing
Monobenzone	T49.4X1	T49.4X2	T49.4X3	T49.4X4	T49.4X5	T49.4X6
Monochloroacetic acid	T60.3X1	T60.3X2	T60.3X3	T60.3X4	—	—
Monochlorobenzene	T53.7X1	T53.7X2	T53.7X3	T53.7X4	—	—
Monoethanolamine	T46.8X1	T46.8X2	T46.8X3	T46.8X4	T46.8X5	T46.8X6
oleate	T46.8X1	T46.8X2	T46.8X3	T46.8X4	T46.8X5	T46.8X6
Monooctanoin	T50.991	T50.992	T50.993	T50.994	T50.995	T50.996
Monophenylbutazone	T39.2X1	T39.2X2	T39.2X3	T39.2X4	T39.2X5	T39.2X6
Monosodium glutamate	T65.891	T65.892	T65.893	T65.894	—	—
Monosulfiram	T49.0X1	T49.0X2	T49.0X3	T49.0X4	T49.0X5	T49.0X6
Monoxide, carbon — see Carbon, monoxide						
Monoxidine hydrochloride	T46.1X1	T46.1X2	T46.1X3	T46.1X4	T46.1X5	T46.1X6
Monuron	T60.3X1	T60.3X2	T60.3X3	T60.3X4	—	—
Moperone	T43.4X1	T43.4X2	T43.4X3	T43.4X4	T43.4X5	T43.4X6
Mopidamol	T45.1X1	T45.1X2	T45.1X3	T45.1X4	T45.1X5	T45.1X6
MOPP (mechloreth-amine + vincristine + prednisone + procarba-zine)	T45.1X1	T45.1X2	T45.1X3	T45.1X4	T45.1X5	T45.1X6
Morfin	T40.2X1	T40.2X2	T40.2X3	T40.2X4	T40.2X5	T40.2X6
Morinamide	T37.1X1	T37.1X2	T37.1X3	T37.1X4	T37.1X5	T37.1X6
Morning glory seeds	T40.991	T40.992	T40.993	T40.994	—	—
Moroxydine	T37.5X1	T37.5X2	T37.5X3	T37.5X4	T37.5X5	T37.5X6
Morphazinamide	T37.1X1	T37.1X2	T37.1X3	T37.1X4	T37.1X5	T37.1X6
Morphine	T40.2X1	T40.2X2	T40.2X3	T40.2X4	T40.2X5	T40.2X6
antagonist	T50.7X1	T50.7X2	T50.7X3	T50.7X4	T50.7X5	T50.7X6
Morpholinylethylmorphine	T40.2X1	T40.2X2	T40.2X3	T40.2X4	T40.2X5	T40.2X6
Morsuximide	T42.2X1	T42.2X2	T42.2X3	T42.2X4	T42.2X5	T42.2X6
Mosapramine	T43.591	T43.592	T43.593	T43.594	T43.595	T43.596
Moth balls — see also	T60.2X1	T60.2X2	T60.2X3	T60.2X4	—	—
Pesticides						
naphthalene	T60.2X1	T60.2X2	T60.2X3	T60.2X4	—	—
paradichlorobenzene	T60.1X1	T60.1X2	T60.1X3	T60.1X4	—	—
Motor exhaust gas	T58.01	T58.02	T58.03	T58.04	—	—
Mouthwash (antiseptic) (zinc chloride)	T49.6X1	T49.6X2	T49.6X3	T49.6X4	T49.6X5	T49.6X6
Moxastine	T45.0X1	T45.0X2	T45.0X3	T45.0X4	T45.0X5	T45.0X6
Moxaverine	T44.3X1	T44.3X2	T44.3X3	T44.3X4	T44.3X5	T44.3X6
Moxisylyte	T46.7X1	T46.7X2	T46.7X3	T46.7X4	T46.7X5	T46.7X6
Mucilage, plant	T47.4X1	T47.4X2	T47.4X3	T47.4X4	T47.4X5	T47.4X6
Mucolytic drug	T48.4X1	T48.4X2	T48.4X3	T48.4X4	T48.4X5	T48.4X6
Mucomyst	T48.4X1	T48.4X2	T48.4X3	T48.4X4	T48.4X5	T48.4X6
Mucous membrane agents (external)	T49.91	T49.92	T49.93	T49.94	T49.95	T49.96
specified NEC	T49.8X1	T49.8X2	T49.8X3	T49.8X4	T49.8X5	T49.8X6
Multiple unspecified drugs, medicaments and biological substances	T50.911	T50.912	T50.913	T50.914	T50.915	T50.916
Mumps						
immune globulin (human)	T50.Z11	T50.Z12	T50.Z13	T50.Z14	T50.Z15	T50.Z16
skin test antigen	T50.8X1	T50.8X2	T50.8X3	T50.8X4	T50.8X5	T50.8X6
vaccine	T50.B91	T50.B92	T50.B93	T50.B94	T50.B95	T50.B96
Mumpsvax	T50.B91	T50.B92	T50.B93	T50.B94	T50.B95	T50.B96
Mupirocin	T49.0X1	T49.0X2	T49.0X3	T49.0X4	T49.0X5	T49.0X6
Muriatic acid — see Hydrochloric acid						
Muromonab-CD3	T45.1X1	T45.1X2	T45.1X3	T45.1X4	T45.1X5	T45.1X6
Muscle-action drug NEC	T48.201	T48.202	T48.203	T48.204	T48.205	T48.206
Muscle affecting agents NEC	T48.201	T48.202	T48.203	T48.204	T48.205	T48.206
oxytocic	T48.0X1	T48.0X2	T48.0X3	T48.0X4	T48.0X5	T48.0X6
relaxants	T48.201	T48.202	T48.203	T48.204	T48.205	T48.206
central nervous system	T42.8X1	T42.8X2	T42.8X3	T42.8X4	T42.8X5	T42.8X6
skeletal	T48.1X1	T48.1X2	T48.1X3	T48.1X4	T48.1X5	T48.1X6
smooth	T44.3X1	T44.3X2	T44.3X3	T44.3X4	T44.3X5	T44.3X6
Muscle relaxant — see Relaxant, muscle						
Muscle-tone depressant, central NEC	T42.8X1	T42.8X2	T42.8X3	T42.8X4	T42.8X5	T42.8X6
specified NEC	T42.8X1	T42.8X2	T42.8X3	T42.8X4	T42.8X5	T42.8X6
Mushroom, noxious	T62.0X1	T62.0X2	T62.0X3	T62.0X4	—	—
Mussel, noxious	T61.781	T61.782	T61.783	T61.784	—	—
Mustard (emetic)	T47.7X1	T47.7X2	T47.7X3	T47.7X4	T47.7X5	T47.7X6
black	T47.7X1	T47.7X2	T47.7X3	T47.7X4	T47.7X5	T47.7X6
gas, not in war	T59.91	T59.92	T59.93	T59.94	—	—
nitrogen	T45.1X1	T45.1X2	T45.1X3	T45.1X4	T45.1X5	T45.1X6
Mustine	T45.1X1	T45.1X2	T45.1X3	T45.1X4	T45.1X5	T45.1X6
M-vac	T45.1X1	T45.1X2	T45.1X3	T45.1X4	T45.1X5	T45.1X6
Mycifradin	T36.5X1	T36.5X2	T36.5X3	T36.5X4	T36.5X5	T36.5X6
topical	T49.0X1	T49.0X2	T49.0X3	T49.0X4	T49.0X5	T49.0X6
Mycitracin	T36.8X1	T36.8X2	T36.8X3	T36.8X4	T36.8X5	T36.8X6
ophthalmic preparation	T49.5X1	T49.5X2	T49.5X3	T49.5X4	T49.5X5	T49.5X6
Mycostatin	T36.7X1	T36.7X2	T36.7X3	T36.7X4	T36.7X5	T36.7X6
topical	T49.0X1	T49.0X2	T49.0X3	T49.0X4	T49.0X5	T49.0X6

Substance	Poisoning, Accidental (unintentional)	Poisoning, Intentional Self-harm	Poisoning, Assault	Poisoning, Undetermined	Adverse Effect	Under-dosing
Mycotoxins	T64.81	T64.82	T64.83	T64.84	—	—
aflatoxin	T64.01	T64.02	T64.03	T64.04	—	—
specified NEC	T64.81	T64.82	T64.83	T64.84	—	—
Mydriacyl	T44.3X1	T44.3X2	T44.3X3	T44.3X4	T44.3X5	T44.3X6
Mydriatic drug	T49.5X1	T49.5X2	T49.5X3	T49.5X4	T49.5X5	T49.5X6
Myelobromal	T45.1X1	T45.1X2	T45.1X3	T45.1X4	T45.1X5	T45.1X6
Myleran	T45.1X1	T45.1X2	T45.1X3	T45.1X4	T45.1X5	T45.1X6
Myochrysin (e)	T39.2X1	T39.2X2	T39.2X3	T39.2X4	T39.2X5	T39.2X6
Myoneural blocking agents	T48.1X1	T48.1X2	T48.1X3	T48.1X4	T48.1X5	T48.1X6
Myralact	T49.0X1	T49.0X2	T49.0X3	T49.0X4	T49.0X5	T49.0X6
Myristica fragrans	T62.2X1	T62.2X2	T62.2X3	T62.2X4	—	—
Myristicin	T65.891	T65.892	T65.893	T65.894	—	—
Mysoline	T42.3X1	T42.3X2	T42.3X3	T42.3X4	T42.3X5	T42.3X6
Nabilone	T40.7X1	T40.7X2	T40.7X3	T40.7X4	T40.7X5	T40.7X6
Nabumetone	T39.391	T39.392	T39.393	T39.394	T39.395	T39.396
Nadolol	T44.7X1	T44.7X2	T44.7X3	T44.7X4	T44.7X5	T44.7X6
Nafcillin	T36.0X1	T36.0X2	T36.0X3	T36.0X4	T36.0X5	T36.0X6
Nafoxidine	T38.6X1	T38.6X2	T38.6X3	T38.6X4	T38.6X5	T38.6X6
Naftazone	T46.991	T46.992	T46.993	T46.994	T46.995	T46.996
Naftidrofuryl (oxalate)	T46.7X1	T46.7X2	T46.7X3	T46.7X4	T46.7X5	T46.7X6
Naftifine	T49.0X1	T49.0X2	T49.0X3	T49.0X4	T49.0X5	T49.0X6
Nail polish remover	T52.91	T52.92	T52.93	T52.94	—	—
Nalbuphine	T40.4X1	T40.4X2	T40.4X3	T40.4X4	T40.4X5	T40.4X6
Naled	T60.0X1	T60.0X2	T60.0X3	T60.0X4	—	—
Nalidixic acid	T37.8X1	T37.8X2	T37.8X3	T37.8X4	T37.8X5	T37.8X6
Nalorphine	T50.7X1	T50.7X2	T50.7X3	T50.7X4	T50.7X5	T50.7X6
Naloxone	T50.7X1	T50.7X2	T50.7X3	T50.7X4	T50.7X5	T50.7X6
Naltrexone	T50.7X1	T50.7X2	T50.7X3	T50.7X4	T50.7X5	T50.7X6
Namenda	T43.8X1	T43.8X2	T43.8X3	T43.8X4	T43.8X5	T43.8X6
Nandrolone	T38.7X1	T38.7X2	T38.7X3	T38.7X4	T38.7X5	T38.7X6
Naphazoline	T48.5X1	T48.5X2	T48.5X3	T48.5X4	T48.5X5	T48.5X6
Naphtha (painters') (petroleum)	T52.0X1	T52.0X2	T52.0X3	T52.0X4	—	—
solvent	T52.0X1	T52.0X2	T52.0X3	T52.0X4	—	—
vapor	T52.0X1	T52.0X2	T52.0X3	T52.0X4	—	—
Naphthalene (non-chlorinated)	T60.2X1	T60.2X2	T60.2X3	T60.2X4	—	—
chlorinated	T60.1X1	T60.1X2	T60.1X3	T60.1X4	—	—
vapor	T60.1X1	T60.1X2	T60.1X3	T60.1X4	—	—
insecticide or moth repellent	T60.2X1	T60.2X2	T60.2X3	T60.2X4	—	—
chlorinated	T60.1X1	T60.1X2	T60.1X3	T60.1X4	—	—
vapor	T60.2X1	T60.2X2	T60.2X3	T60.2X4	—	—
chlorinated	T60.1X1	T60.1X2	T60.1X3	T60.1X4	—	—
Naphthol	T65.891	T65.892	T65.893	T65.894	—	—
Naphthylamine	T65.891	T65.892	T65.893	T65.894	—	—
Naphthylthiourea (ANTU)	T60.4X1	T60.4X2	T60.4X3	T60.4X4	—	—
Naprosyn — see Naproxen						
Naproxen	T39.311	T39.312	T39.313	T39.314	T39.315	T39.316
Narcotic (drug)	T40.601	T40.602	T40.603	T40.604	T40.605	T40.606
analgesic NEC	T40.601	T40.602	T40.603	T40.604	T40.605	T40.606
antagonist	T50.7X1	T50.7X2	T50.7X3	T50.7X4	T50.7X5	T50.7X6
specified NEC	T40.691	T40.692	T40.693	T40.694	T40.695	T40.696
synthetic	T40.4X1	T40.4X2	T40.4X3	T40.4X4	T40.4X5	T40.4X6
Narcotine	T48.3X1	T48.3X2	T48.3X3	T48.3X4	T48.3X5	T48.3X6
Nardil	T43.1X1	T43.1X2	T43.1X3	T43.1X4	T43.1X5	T43.1X6
Nasal drug NEC	T49.6X1	T49.6X2	T49.6X3	T49.6X4	T49.6X5	T49.6X6
Natamycin	T49.0X1	T49.0X2	T49.0X3	T49.0X4	T49.0X5	T49.0X6
Natrium cyanide — see Cyanide(s)						
Natural						
blood (product)	T45.8X1	T45.8X2	T45.8X3	T45.8X4	T45.8X5	T45.8X6
gas (piped)	T59.891	T59.892	T59.893	T59.894	—	—
incomplete combustion	T58.11	T58.12	T58.13	T58.14	—	—
Nealbarbital	T42.3X1	T42.3X2	T42.3X3	T42.3X4	T42.3X5	T42.3X6
Nectadon	T48.3X1	T48.3X2	T48.3X3	T48.3X4	T48.3X5	T48.3X6
Nedocromil	T48.6X1	T48.6X2	T48.6X3	T48.6X4	T48.6X5	T48.6X6
Nefopam	T39.8X1	T39.8X2	T39.8X3	T39.8X4	T39.8X5	T39.8X6
Nematocyst (sting)	T63.691	T63.692	T63.693	T63.694	—	—
Nembutal	T42.3X1	T42.3X2	T42.3X3	T42.3X4	T42.3X5	T42.3X6
Nemonapride	T43.591	T43.592	T43.593	T43.594	T43.595	T43.596
Neoarsphenamine	T37.8X1	T37.8X2	T37.8X3	T37.8X4	T37.8X5	T37.8X6
Neocinchophen	T50.4X1	T50.4X2	T50.4X3	T50.4X4	T50.4X5	T50.4X6
Neomycin (derivatives)	T36.5X1	T36.5X2	T36.5X3	T36.5X4	T36.5X5	T36.5X6
with						
bacitracin	T49.0X1	T49.0X2	T49.0X3	T49.0X4	T49.0X5	T49.0X6
neostigmine	T44.0X1	T44.0X2	T44.0X3	T44.0X4	T44.0X5	T44.0X6
ENT agent	T49.6X1	T49.6X2	T49.6X3	T49.6X4	T49.6X5	T49.6X6
ophthalmic preparation	T49.5X1	T49.5X2	T49.5X3	T49.5X4	T49.5X5	T49.5X6
topical NEC	T49.0X1	T49.0X2	T49.0X3	T49.0X4	T49.0X5	T49.0X6
Neonal	T42.3X1	T42.3X2	T42.3X3	T42.3X4	T42.3X5	T42.3X6
Neoprontosil	T37.0X1	T37.0X2	T37.0X3	T37.0X4	T37.0X5	T37.0X6

Substance	Poisoning, Accidental (unintentional)	Poisoning, Intentional Self-harm	Poisoning, Assault	Poisoning, Undetermined	Adverse Effect	Under-
Neosalvarsan	T37.8X1	T37.8X2	T37.8X3	T37.8X4	T37.8X5	T37
Neosilversalvarsan	T37.8X1	T37.8X2	T37.8X3	T37.8X4	T37.8X5	T37
Neosporin	T36.8X1	T36.8X2	T36.8X3	T36.8X4	T36.8X5	T36
ENT agent	T49.6X1	T49.6X2	T49.6X3	T49.6X4	T49.6X5	T49.
opthalmic preparation	T49.5X1	T49.5X2	T49.5X3	T49.5X4	T49.5X5	T49.
topical NEC	T49.0X1	T49.0X2	T49.0X3	T49.0X4	T49.0X5	T49
Neostigmine bromide	T44.0X1	T44.0X2	T44.0X3	T44.0X4	T44.0X5	T44.
Neraval	T42.3X1	T42.3X2	T42.3X3	T42.3X4	T42.3X5	T42
Neravan	T42.3X1	T42.3X2	T42.3X3	T42.3X4	T42.3X5	T42
Nerium oleander	T62.2X1	T62.2X2	T62.2X3	T62.2X4	—	—
Nerve gas, not in war	T59.91	T59.92	T59.93	T59.94	—	—
Nesacaine	T41.3X1	T41.3X2	T41.3X3	T41.3X4	T41.3X5	T41.
infiltration (subcutaneous)	T41.3X1	T41.3X2	T41.3X3	T41.3X4	T41.3X5	T41.
nerve block (peripheral) (plexus)	T41.3X1	T41.3X2	T41.3X3	T41.3X4	T41.3X5	T41.
Netilmicin	T36.5X1	T36.5X2	T36.5X3	T36.5X4	T36.5X5	T36
Neurobarb	T42.3X1	T42.3X2	T42.3X3	T42.3X4	T42.3X5	T42
Neuroleptic drug NEC	T43.501	T43.502	T43.503	T43.504	T43.505	T43
Neuromuscular blocking drug	T48.1X1	T48.1X2	T48.1X3	T48.1X4	T48.1X5	T48
Neutral insulin injection	T38.3X1	T38.3X2	T38.3X3	T38.3X4	T38.3X5	T38.
Neutral spirits	T51.0X1	T51.0X2	T51.0X3	T51.0X4	—	—
beverage	T51.0X1	T51.0X2	T51.0X3	T51.0X4	—	—
Niacin	T46.7X1	T46.7X2	T46.7X3	T46.7X4	T46.7X5	T46.
Niacinamide	T45.2X1	T45.2X2	T45.2X3	T45.2X4	T45.2X5	T45.
Nialamide	T43.1X1	T43.1X2	T43.1X3	T43.1X4	T43.1X5	T43
Niaprazine	T42.6X1	T42.6X2	T42.6X3	T42.6X4	T42.6X5	T42
Nicametate	T46.7X1	T46.7X2	T46.7X3	T46.7X4	T46.7X5	T46.
Nicardipine	T46.1X1	T46.1X2	T46.1X3	T46.1X4	T46.1X5	T46.
Nicergoline	T46.7X1	T46.7X2	T46.7X3	T46.7X4	T46.7X5	T46.
Nickel (carbonyl) (tetra-carbonyl) (fumes) (vapor)	T56.891	T56.892	T56.893	T56.894	—	—
Nickelocene	T56.891	T56.892	T56.893	T56.894	—	—
Niclosamide	T37.4X1	T37.4X2	T37.4X3	T37.4X4	T37.4X5	T37
Nicofuranose	T46.7X1	T46.7X2	T46.7X3	T46.7X4	T46.7X5	T46.
Nicomorphine	T40.2X1	T40.2X2	T40.2X3	T40.2X4	—	—
Nicorandil	T46.3X1	T46.3X2	T46.3X3	T46.3X4	T46.3X5	T46.
Nicotiana (plant)	T62.2X1	T62.2X2	T62.2X3	T62.2X4	—	—
Nicotinamide	T45.2X1	T45.2X2	T45.2X3	T45.2X4	T45.2X5	T45.
Nicotine (insecticide) (spray) (sulfate) **NEC**	T60.2X1	T60.2X2	T60.2X3	T60.2X4	—	—
from tobacco						
cigarettes	T65.291	T65.292	T65.293	T65.294	—	—
not insecticide	T65.221	T65.222	T65.223	T65.224	—	—
Nicotinic acid	T65.291	T65.292	T65.293	T65.294	—	—
Nicotinyl alcohol	T46.7X1	T46.7X2	T46.7X3	T46.7X4	T46.7X5	T46.
Nicoumalone	T45.511	T45.512	T45.513	T45.514	T45.515	T45.
Nifedipine	T46.1X1	T46.1X2	T46.1X3	T46.1X4	T46.1X5	T46.
Nifenazone	T39.2X1	T39.2X2	T39.2X3	T39.2X4	T39.2X5	T39.
Nifuraldezone	T37.91	T37.92	T37.93	T37.94	T37.95	T37
Nifuratel	T37.8X1	T37.8X2	T37.8X3	T37.8X4	T37.8X5	T37.
Nifurfoxime	T37.3X1	T37.3X2	T37.3X3	T37.3X4	T37.3X5	T37.
Nifurtimox	T37.3X1	T37.3X2	T37.3X3	T37.3X4	T37.3X5	T37.
Nifurtoinol	T37.8X1	T37.8X2	T37.8X3	T37.8X4	T37.8X5	T37.
Nightshade, deadly (solanum) — see also Belladonna	T62.2X1	T62.2X2	T62.2X3	T62.2X4	—	—
berry	T62.1X1	T62.1X2	T62.1X3	T62.1X4	—	—
Nikethamide	T50.7X1	T50.7X2	T50.7X3	T50.7X4	T50.7X5	T50.
Nilstat	T36.7X1	T36.7X2	T36.7X3	T36.7X4	T36.7X5	T36.
topical	T49.0X1	T49.0X2	T49.0X3	T49.0X4	T49.0X5	T49.
Nilutamide	T38.6X1	T38.6X2	T38.6X3	T38.6X4	T38.6X5	T38.
Nimesulide	T39.391	T39.392	T39.393	T39.394	T39.395	T39.
Nimetazepam	T42.4X1	T42.4X2	T42.4X3	T42.4X4	T42.4X5	T42.
Nimodipine	T46.1X1	T46.1X2	T46.1X3	T46.1X4	T46.1X5	T46.
Nimorazole	T37.3X1	T37.3X2	T37.3X3	T37.3X4	T37.3X5	T37.
Nimustine	T45.1X1	T45.1X2	T45.1X3	T45.1X4	T45.1X5	T45.
Niridazole	T37.4X1	T37.4X2	T37.4X3	T37.4X4	T37.4X5	T37.
Nisentil	T40.2X1	T40.2X2	T40.2X3	T40.2X4	T40.2X5	T40.
Nisoldipine	T46.1X1	T46.1X2	T46.1X3	T46.1X4	T46.1X5	T46.
Nitramine	T65.3X1	T65.3X2	T65.3X3	T65.3X4	—	—
Nitrate, organic	T46.3X1	T46.3X2	T46.3X3	T46.3X4	T46.3X5	T46.
Nitrazepam	T42.4X1	T42.4X2	T42.4X3	T42.4X4	T42.4X5	T42.
Nitrefazole	T50.6X1	T50.6X2	T50.6X3	T50.6X4	T50.6X5	T50.
Nitrendipine	T46.1X1	T46.1X2	T46.1X3	T46.1X4	T46.1X5	T46.
Nitric						
acid (liquid)	T54.2X1	T54.2X2	T54.2X3	T54.2X4	—	—
vapor	T59.891	T59.892	T59.893	T59.894	—	—
oxide (gas)	T59.0X1	T59.0X2	T59.0X3	T59.0X4	—	—
Nitrimidazine	T37.3X1	T37.3X2	T37.3X3	T37.3X4	T37.3X5	T37.
Nitrite, amyl (medicinal) (vapor)	T46.3X1	T46.3X2	T46.3X3	T46.3X4	T46.3X5	T46.
Nitroaniline	T65.3X1	T65.3X2	T65.3X3	T65.3X4	—	—
vapor	T59.891	T59.892	T59.893	T59.894	—	—
Nitrobenzene, nitrobenzol	T65.3X1	T65.3X2	T65.3X3	T65.3X4	—	—

Additional Character May Be Required — Refer to the Tabular List for Character Selection ▽ Subterms under main terms may continue to next column or pa

Substance	Poisoning, Accidental (unintentional)	Poisoning, Intentional Self-harm	Poisoning, Assault	Poisoning, Undetermined	Adverse Effect	Under-dosing
Nitrobenzene, nitrobenzol — *continued*						
vapor	T65.3X1	T65.3X2	T65.3X3	T65.3X4	—	—
Nitrocellulose	T65.891	T65.892	T65.893	T65.894	—	—
lacquer	T65.891	T65.892	T65.893	T65.894	—	—
Nitrodiphenyl	T65.3X1	T65.3X2	T65.3X3	T65.3X4	—	—
Nitrofural	T49.0X1	T49.0X2	T49.0X3	T49.0X4	T49.0X5	T49.0X6
Nitrofurantoin	T37.8X1	T37.8X2	T37.8X3	T37.8X4	T37.8X5	T37.8X6
Nitrofurazone	T49.0X1	T49.0X2	T49.0X3	T49.0X4	T49.0X5	T49.0X6
Nitrogen	T59.0X1	T59.0X2	T59.0X3	T59.0X4	—	—
mustard	T45.1X1	T45.1X2	T45.1X3	T45.1X4	T45.1X5	T45.1X6
Nitroglycerin, nitroglycerol (medicinal)	T46.3X1	T46.3X2	T46.3X3	T46.3X4	T46.3X5	T46.3X6
nonmedicinal	T65.5X1	T65.5X2	T65.5X3	T65.5X4	—	—
fumes	T65.5X1	T65.5X2	T65.5X3	T65.5X4	—	—
Nitroglycol	T52.3X1	T52.3X2	T52.3X3	T52.3X4	—	—
Nitrohydrochloric acid	T54.2X1	T54.2X2	T54.2X3	T54.2X4	—	—
Nitromersol	T49.0X1	T49.0X2	T49.0X3	T49.0X4	T49.0X5	T49.0X6
Nitronaphthalene	T65.891	T65.892	T65.893	T65.894	—	—
Nitrophenol	T54.0X1	T54.0X2	T54.0X3	T54.0X4	—	—
Nitropropane	T52.8X1	T52.8X2	T52.8X3	T52.8X4	—	—
Nitroprusside	T46.5X1	T46.5X2	T46.5X3	T46.5X4	T46.5X5	T46.5X6
Nitrosodimethylamine	T65.3X1	T65.3X2	T65.3X3	T65.3X4	—	—
Nitrothiazol	T37.4X1	T37.4X2	T37.4X3	T37.4X4	T37.4X5	T37.4X6
Nitrotoluene, nitrotoluol	T65.3X1	T65.3X2	T65.3X3	T65.3X4	—	—
vapor	T65.3X1	T65.3X2	T65.3X3	T65.3X4	—	—
Nitrous						
acid (liquid)	T54.2X1	T54.2X2	T54.2X3	T54.2X4	—	—
fumes	T59.891	T59.892	T59.893	T59.894	—	—
ether spirit	T46.3X1	T46.3X2	T46.3X3	T46.3X4	—	—
oxide	T41.0X1	T41.0X2	T41.0X3	T41.0X4	T41.0X5	T41.0X6
Nitroxoline	T37.8X1	T37.8X2	T37.8X3	T37.8X4	T37.8X5	T37.8X6
Nitrozone	T49.0X1	T49.0X2	T49.0X3	T49.0X4	T49.0X5	T49.0X6
Nizatidine	T47.0X1	T47.0X2	T47.0X3	T47.0X4	T47.0X5	T47.0X6
Nizofenone	T43.8X1	T43.8X2	T43.8X3	T43.8X4	T43.8X5	T43.8X6
Noctec	T42.6X1	T42.6X2	T42.6X3	T42.6X4	T42.6X5	T42.6X6
Noludar	T42.6X1	T42.6X2	T42.6X3	T42.6X4	T42.6X5	T42.6X6
Nomegestrol	T38.5X1	T38.5X2	T38.5X3	T38.5X4	T38.5X5	T38.5X6
Nomifensine	T43.291	T43.292	T43.293	T43.294	T43.295	T43.296
Nonoxinol	T49.8X1	T49.8X2	T49.8X3	T49.8X4	T49.8X5	T49.8X6
Nonylphenoxy (polyethoxyethanol)	T49.8X1	T49.8X2	T49.8X3	T49.8X4	T49.8X5	T49.8X6
Noptil	T42.3X1	T42.3X2	T42.3X3	T42.3X4	T42.3X5	T42.3X6
Noradrenaline	T44.4X1	T44.4X2	T44.4X3	T44.4X4	T44.4X5	T44.4X6
Noramidopyrine	T39.2X1	T39.2X2	T39.2X3	T39.2X4	T39.2X5	T39.2X6
methanesulfonate sodium	T39.2X1	T39.2X2	T39.2X3	T39.2X4	T39.2X5	T39.2X6
Norbormide	T60.4X1	T60.4X2	T60.4X3	T60.4X4	—	—
Nordazepam	T42.4X1	T42.4X2	T42.4X3	T42.4X4	T42.4X5	T42.4X6
Norepinephrine	T44.4X1	T44.4X2	T44.4X3	T44.4X4	T44.4X5	T44.4X6
Norethandrolone	T38.7X1	T38.7X2	T38.7X3	T38.7X4	T38.7X5	T38.7X6
Norethindrone	T38.4X1	T38.4X2	T38.4X3	T38.4X4	T38.4X5	T38.4X6
Norethisterone (acetate) (enantate)	T38.4X1	T38.4X2	T38.4X3	T38.4X4	T38.4X5	T38.4X6
with ethinylestradiol	T38.5X1	T38.5X2	T38.5X3	T38.5X4	T38.5X5	T38.5X6
Noretynodrel	T38.5X1	T38.5X2	T38.5X3	T38.5X4	T38.5X5	T38.5X6
Norfenefrine	T44.4X1	T44.4X2	T44.4X3	T44.4X4	T44.4X5	T44.4X6
Norfloxacin	T36.8X1	T36.8X2	T36.8X3	T36.8X4	T36.8X5	T36.8X6
Norgestrel	T38.4X1	T38.4X2	T38.4X3	T38.4X4	T38.4X5	T38.4X6
Norgestrienone	T38.4X1	T38.4X2	T38.4X3	T38.4X4	T38.4X5	T38.4X6
Norlestrin	T38.4X1	T38.4X2	T38.4X3	T38.4X4	T38.4X5	T38.4X6
Norlutin	T38.4X1	T38.4X2	T38.4X3	T38.4X4	T38.4X5	T38.4X6
Normal serum albumin (human), salt-poor	T45.8X1	T45.8X2	T45.8X3	T45.8X4	T45.8X5	T45.8X6
Normethandrone	T38.5X1	T38.5X2	T38.5X3	T38.5X4	T38.5X5	T38.5X6
Normison — *see* Benzodiazepines						
Normorphine	T40.2X1	T40.2X2	T40.2X3	T40.2X4	—	—
Norpseudoephedrine	T50.5X1	T50.5X2	T50.5X3	T50.5X4	T50.5X5	T50.5X6
Nortestosterone (furanpropionate)	T38.7X1	T38.7X2	T38.7X3	T38.7X4	T38.7X5	T38.7X6
Nortriptyline	T43.011	T43.012	T43.013	T43.014	T43.015	T43.016
Noscapine	T48.3X1	T48.3X2	T48.3X3	T48.3X4	T48.3X5	T48.3X6
Nose preparations	T49.6X1	T49.6X2	T49.6X3	T49.6X4	T49.6X5	T49.6X6
Novobiocin	T36.5X1	T36.5X2	T36.5X3	T36.5X4	T36.5X5	T36.5X6
Novocain (infiltration) (topical)	T41.3X1	T41.3X2	T41.3X3	T41.3X4	T41.3X5	T41.3X6
nerve block (peripheral) (plexus)	T41.3X1	T41.3X2	T41.3X3	T41.3X4	T41.3X5	T41.3X6
spinal	T41.3X1	T41.3X2	T41.3X3	T41.3X4	T41.3X5	T41.3X6
Noxious foodstuff	T62.91	T62.92	T62.93	T62.94	—	—
specified NEC	T62.8X1	T62.8X2	T62.8X3	T62.8X4	—	—
Noxiptiline	T43.011	T43.012	T43.013	T43.014	T43.015	T43.016
Noxytiolin	T49.0X1	T49.0X2	T49.0X3	T49.0X4	T49.0X5	T49.0X6
NPH Iletin (insulin)	T38.3X1	T38.3X2	T38.3X3	T38.3X4	T38.3X5	T38.3X6
Numorphan	T40.2X1	T40.2X2	T40.2X3	T40.2X4	T40.2X5	T40.2X6
Nunol	T42.3X1	T42.3X2	T42.3X3	T42.3X4	T42.3X5	T42.3X6
Nupercaine (spinal anesthetic)	T41.3X1	T41.3X2	T41.3X3	T41.3X4	T41.3X5	T41.3X6
topical (surface)	T41.3X1	T41.3X2	T41.3X3	T41.3X4	T41.3X5	T41.3X6
Nutmeg oil (liniment)	T49.3X1	T49.3X2	T49.3X3	T49.3X4	T49.3X5	T49.3X6
Nutritional supplement	T50.901	T50.902	T50.903	T50.904	T50.905	T50.906
Nux vomica	T65.1X1	T65.1X2	T65.1X3	T65.1X4	—	—
Nydrazid	T37.1X1	T37.1X2	T37.1X3	T37.1X4	T37.1X5	T37.1X6
Nylidrin	T46.7X1	T46.7X2	T46.7X3	T46.7X4	T46.7X5	T46.7X6
Nystatin	T36.7X1	T36.7X2	T36.7X3	T36.7X4	T36.7X5	T36.7X6
topical	T49.0X1	T49.0X2	T49.0X3	T49.0X4	T49.0X5	T49.0X6
Nytol	T45.0X1	T45.0X2	T45.0X3	T45.0X4	T45.0X5	T45.0X6
Obidoxime chloride	T50.6X1	T50.6X2	T50.6X3	T50.6X4	T50.6X5	T50.6X6
Octafonium (chloride)	T49.3X1	T49.3X2	T49.3X3	T49.3X4	T49.3X5	T49.3X6
Octamethyl pyrophosphoramide	T60.0X1	T60.0X2	T60.0X3	T60.0X4	—	—
Octanoin	T50.991	T50.992	T50.993	T50.994	T50.995	T50.996
Octatropine methylbromide	T44.3X1	T44.3X2	T44.3X3	T44.3X4	T44.3X5	T44.3X6
Octotiamine	T45.2X1	T45.2X2	T45.2X3	T45.2X4	T45.2X5	T45.2X6
Octoxinol (9)	T49.8X1	T49.8X2	T49.8X3	T49.8X4	T49.8X5	T49.8X6
Octreotide	T38.991	T38.992	T38.993	T38.994	T38.995	T38.996
Octyl nitrite	T46.3X1	T46.3X2	T46.3X3	T46.3X4	T46.3X5	T46.3X6
Oestradiol	T38.5X1	T38.5X2	T38.5X3	T38.5X4	T38.5X5	T38.5X6
Oestriol	T38.5X1	T38.5X2	T38.5X3	T38.5X4	T38.5X5	T38.5X6
Oestrogen	T38.5X1	T38.5X2	T38.5X3	T38.5X4	T38.5X5	T38.5X6
Oestrone	T38.5X1	T38.5X2	T38.5X3	T38.5X4	T38.5X5	T38.5X6
Ofloxacin	T36.8X1	T36.8X2	T36.8X3	T36.8X4	T36.8X5	T36.8X6
Oil (of)	T65.891	T65.892	T65.893	T65.894	—	—
bitter almond	T62.8X1	T62.8X2	T62.8X3	T62.8X4	—	—
cloves	T49.7X1	T49.7X2	T49.7X3	T49.7X4	T49.7X5	T49.7X6
colors	T65.6X1	T65.6X2	T65.6X3	T65.6X4	—	—
fumes	T59.891	T59.892	T59.893	T59.894	—	—
lubricating	T52.0X1	T52.0X2	T52.0X3	T52.0X4	—	—
Niobe	T52.8X1	T52.8X2	T52.8X3	T52.8X4	—	—
vitriol (liquid)	T54.2X1	T54.2X2	T54.2X3	T54.2X4	—	—
fumes	T54.2X1	T54.2X2	T54.2X3	T54.2X4	—	—
wintergreen (bitter) NEC	T49.3X1	T49.3X2	T49.3X3	T49.3X4	T49.3X5	T49.3X6
Oily preparation (for skin)	T49.3X1	T49.3X2	T49.3X3	T49.3X4	T49.3X5	T49.3X6
Ointment NEC	T49.3X1	T49.3X2	T49.3X3	T49.3X4	T49.3X5	T49.3X6
Olanzapine	T43.591	T43.592	T43.593	T43.594	T43.595	T43.596
Oleander	T62.2X1	T62.2X2	T62.2X3	T62.2X4	—	—
Oleandomycin	T36.3X1	T36.3X2	T36.3X3	T36.3X4	T36.3X5	T36.3X6
Oleandrin	T46.0X1	T46.0X2	T46.0X3	T46.0X4	T46.0X5	T46.0X6
Oleic acid	T46.6X1	T46.6X2	T46.6X3	T46.6X4	T46.6X5	T46.6X6
Oleovitamin A	T45.2X1	T45.2X2	T45.2X3	T45.2X4	T45.2X5	T45.2X6
Oleum ricini	T47.2X1	T47.2X2	T47.2X3	T47.2X4	T47.2X5	T47.2X6
Olive oil (medicinal) NEC	T47.4X1	T47.4X2	T47.4X3	T47.4X4	T47.4X5	T47.4X6
Olivomycin	T45.1X1	T45.1X2	T45.1X3	T45.1X4	T45.1X5	T45.1X6
Oisalazine	T47.8X1	T47.8X2	T47.8X3	T47.8X4	T47.8X5	T47.8X6
Omeprazole	T47.1X1	T47.1X2	T47.1X3	T47.1X4	T47.1X5	T47.1X6
OMPA	T60.0X1	T60.0X2	T60.0X3	T60.0X4	—	—
Oncovin	T45.1X1	T45.1X2	T45.1X3	T45.1X4	T45.1X5	T45.1X6
Ondansetron	T45.0X1	T45.0X2	T45.0X3	T45.0X4	T45.0X5	T45.0X6
Ophthaine	T41.3X1	T41.3X2	T41.3X3	T41.3X4	T41.3X5	T41.3X6
Ophthetic	T41.3X1	T41.3X2	T41.3X3	T41.3X4	T41.3X5	T41.3X6
Opiate NEC	T40.601	T40.602	T40.603	T40.604	T40.605	T40.606
antagonists	T50.7X1	T50.7X2	T50.7X3	T50.7X4	T50.7X5	T50.7X6
Opioid NEC	T40.2X1	T40.2X2	T40.2X3	T40.2X4	T40.2X5	T40.2X6
Opipramol	T43.011	T43.012	T43.013	T43.014	T43.015	T43.016
Opium alkaloids (total)	T40.0X1	T40.0X2	T40.0X3	T40.0X4	T40.0X5	T40.0X6
standardized powdered	T40.0X1	T40.0X2	T40.0X3	T40.0X4	T40.0X5	T40.0X6
tincture (camphorated)	T40.0X1	T40.0X2	T40.0X3	T40.0X4	T40.0X5	T40.0X6
Oracon	T38.4X1	T38.4X2	T38.4X3	T38.4X4	T38.4X5	T38.4X6
Oragrafin	T50.8X1	T50.8X2	T50.8X3	T50.8X4	T50.8X5	T50.8X6
Oral contraceptives	T38.4X1	T38.4X2	T38.4X3	T38.4X4	T38.4X5	T38.4X6
Oral rehydration salts	T50.3X1	T50.3X2	T50.3X3	T50.3X4	T50.3X5	T50.3X6
Orazamide	T50.991	T50.992	T50.993	T50.994	T50.995	T50.996
Orciprenaline	T48.291	T48.292	T48.293	T48.294	T48.295	T48.296
Organidin	T48.4X1	T48.4X2	T48.4X3	T48.4X4	T48.4X5	T48.4X6
Organonitrate NEC	T46.3X1	T46.3X2	T46.3X3	T46.3X4	T46.3X5	T46.3X6
Organophosphates	T60.0X1	T60.0X2	T60.0X3	T60.0X4	—	—
Orimune	T50.B91	T50.B92	T50.B93	T50.B94	T50.B95	T50.B96
Orinase	T38.3X1	T38.3X2	T38.3X3	T38.3X4	T38.3X5	T38.3X6
Ormeloxifene	T38.6X1	T38.6X2	T38.6X3	T38.6X4	T38.6X5	T38.6X6
Ornidazole	T37.3X1	T37.3X2	T37.3X3	T37.3X4	T37.3X5	T37.3X6
Ornithine aspartate	T50.991	T50.992	T50.993	T50.994	T50.995	T50.996
Ornoprostil	T47.1X1	T47.1X2	T47.1X3	T47.1X4	T47.1X5	T47.1X6
Orphenadrine (hydrochloride)	T42.8X1	T42.8X2	T42.8X3	T42.8X4	T42.8X5	T42.8X6
Ortal (sodium)	T42.3X1	T42.3X2	T42.3X3	T42.3X4	T42.3X5	T42.3X6

Subterms under main terms may continue to next column or page   Additional Character May Be Required — Refer to the Tabular List for Character Selection

Substance	Poisoning, Accidental (unintentional)	Poisoning, Intentional Self-harm	Poisoning, Assault	Poisoning, Undetermined	Adverse Effect	Under-dosing
Orthoboric acid	T49.0X1	T49.0X2	T49.0X3	T49.0X4	T49.0X5	T49.0X6
ENT agent	T49.6X1	T49.6X2	T49.6X3	T49.6X4	T49.6X5	T49.6X6
ophthalmic preparation	T49.5X1	T49.5X2	T49.5X3	T49.5X4	T49.5X5	T49.5X6
Orthocaine	T41.3X1	T41.3X2	T41.3X3	T41.3X4	T41.3X5	T41.3X6
Orthodichlorobenzene	T53.7X1	T53.7X2	T53.7X3	T53.7X4	—	—
Ortho-Novum	T38.4X1	T38.4X2	T38.4X3	T38.4X4	T38.4X5	T38.4X6
Orthotolidine (reagent)	T54.2X1	T54.2X2	T54.2X3	T54.2X4	—	—
Osmic acid (liquid)	T54.2X1	T54.2X2	T54.2X3	T54.2X4	—	—
fumes	T54.2X1	T54.2X2	T54.2X3	T54.2X4	—	—
Osmotic diuretics	T50.2X1	T50.2X2	T50.2X3	T50.2X4	T50.2X5	T50.2X6
Otilonium bromide	T44.3X1	T44.3X2	T44.3X3	T44.3X4	T44.3X5	T44.3X6
Otorhinolaryngological drug NEC	T49.6X1	T49.6X2	T49.6X3	T49.6X4	T49.6X5	T49.6X6
Ouabain (e)	T46.0X1	T46.0X2	T46.0X3	T46.0X4	T46.0X5	T46.0X6
Ovarian						
hormone	T38.5X1	T38.5X2	T38.5X3	T38.5X4	T38.5X5	T38.5X6
stimulant	T38.5X1	T38.5X2	T38.5X3	T38.5X4	T38.5X5	T38.5X6
Ovral	T38.4X1	T38.4X2	T38.4X3	T38.4X4	T38.4X5	T38.4X6
Ovulen	T38.4X1	T38.4X2	T38.4X3	T38.4X4	T38.4X5	T38.4X6
Oxacillin	T36.0X1	T36.0X2	T36.0X3	T36.0X4	T36.0X5	T36.0X6
Oxalic acid	T54.2X1	T54.2X2	T54.2X3	T54.2X4	—	—
ammonium salt	T50.991	T50.992	T50.993	T50.994	T50.995	T50.996
Oxamniquine	T37.4X1	T37.4X2	T37.4X3	T37.4X4	T37.4X5	T37.4X6
Oxanamide	T43.591	T43.592	T43.593	T43.594	T43.595	T43.596
Oxandrolone	T38.7X1	T38.7X2	T38.7X3	T38.7X4	T38.7X5	T38.7X6
Oxantel	T37.4X1	T37.4X2	T37.4X3	T37.4X4	T37.4X5	T37.4X6
Oxapium iodide	T44.3X1	T44.3X2	T44.3X3	T44.3X4	T44.3X5	T44.3X6
Oxaprotiline	T43.021	T43.022	T43.023	T43.024	T43.025	T43.026
Oxaprozin	T39.311	T39.312	T39.313	T39.314	T39.315	T39.316
Oxatomide	T45.0X1	T45.0X2	T45.0X3	T45.0X4	T45.0X5	T45.0X6
Oxazepam	T42.4X1	T42.4X2	T42.4X3	T42.4X4	T42.4X5	T42.4X6
Oxazimedrine	T50.5X1	T50.5X2	T50.5X3	T50.5X4	T50.5X5	T50.5X6
Oxazolam	T42.4X1	T42.4X2	T42.4X3	T42.4X4	T42.4X5	T42.4X6
Oxazolidine derivatives	T42.2X1	T42.2X2	T42.2X3	T42.2X4	T42.2X5	T42.2X6
Oxazolidinedione (derivative)	T42.2X1	T42.2X2	T42.2X3	T42.2X4	T42.2X5	T42.2X6
Ox bile extract	T47.5X1	T47.5X2	T47.5X3	T47.5X4	T47.5X5	T47.5X6
Oxcarbazepine	T42.1X1	T42.1X2	T42.1X3	T42.1X4	T42.1X5	T42.1X6
Oxedrine	T44.4X1	T44.4X2	T44.4X3	T44.4X4	T44.4X5	T44.4X6
Oxeladin (citrate)	T48.3X1	T48.3X2	T48.3X3	T48.3X4	T48.3X5	T48.3X6
Oxendolone	T38.5X1	T38.5X2	T38.5X3	T38.5X4	T38.5X5	T38.5X6
Oxetacaine	T41.3X1	T41.3X2	T41.3X3	T41.3X4	T41.3X5	T41.3X6
Oxethazine	T41.3X1	T41.3X2	T41.3X3	T41.3X4	T41.3X5	T41.3X6
Oxetorone	T39.8X1	T39.8X2	T39.8X3	T39.8X4	T39.8X5	T39.8X6
Oxiconazole	T49.0X1	T49.0X2	T49.0X3	T49.0X4	T49.0X5	T49.0X6
Oxidizing agent NEC	T54.91	T54.92	T54.93	T54.94	—	—
Oxipurinol	T50.4X1	T50.4X2	T50.4X3	T50.4X4	T50.4X5	T50.4X6
Oxitriptan	T43.291	T43.292	T43.293	T43.294	T43.295	T43.296
Oxitropium bromide	T48.6X1	T48.6X2	T48.6X3	T48.6X4	T48.6X5	T48.6X6
Oxodipine	T46.1X1	T46.1X2	T46.1X3	T46.1X4	T46.1X5	T46.1X6
Oxolamine	T48.3X1	T48.3X2	T48.3X3	T48.3X4	T48.3X5	T48.3X6
Oxolinic acid	T37.8X1	T37.8X2	T37.8X3	T37.8X4	T37.8X5	T37.8X6
Oxomemazine	T43.3X1	T43.3X2	T43.3X3	T43.3X4	T43.3X5	T43.3X6
Oxophenarsine	T37.3X1	T37.3X2	T37.3X3	T37.3X4	T37.3X5	T37.3X6
Oxprenolol	T44.7X1	T44.7X2	T44.7X3	T44.7X4	T44.7X5	T44.7X6
Oxsoralen	T49.3X1	T49.3X2	T49.3X3	T49.3X4	T49.3X5	T49.3X6
Oxtriphylline	T48.6X1	T48.6X2	T48.6X3	T48.6X4	T48.6X5	T48.6X6
Oxybate sodium	T41.291	T41.292	T41.293	T41.294	T41.295	T41.296
Oxybuprocaine	T41.3X1	T41.3X2	T41.3X3	T41.3X4	T41.3X5	T41.3X6
Oxybutynin	T44.3X1	T44.3X2	T44.3X3	T44.3X4	T44.3X5	T44.3X6
Oxychlorosene	T49.0X1	T49.0X2	T49.0X3	T49.0X4	T49.0X5	T49.0X6
Oxycodone	T40.2X1	T40.2X2	T40.2X3	T40.2X4	T40.2X5	T40.2X6
Oxyfedrine	T46.3X1	T46.3X2	T46.3X3	T46.3X4	T46.3X5	T46.3X6
Oxygen	T41.5X1	T41.5X2	T41.5X3	T41.5X4	T41.5X5	T41.5X6
Oxylone	T49.0X1	T49.0X2	T49.0X3	T49.0X4	T49.0X5	T49.0X6
ophthalmic preparation	T49.5X1	T49.5X2	T49.5X3	T49.5X4	T49.5X5	T49.5X6
Oxymesterone	T38.7X1	T38.7X2	T38.7X3	T38.7X4	T38.7X5	T38.7X6
Oxymetazoline	T48.5X1	T48.5X2	T48.5X3	T48.5X4	T48.5X5	T48.5X6
Oxymetholone	T38.7X1	T38.7X2	T38.7X3	T38.7X4	T38.7X5	T38.7X6
Oxymorphone	T40.2X1	T40.2X2	T40.2X3	T40.2X4	T40.2X5	T40.2X6
Oxypertine	T43.591	T43.592	T43.593	T43.594	T43.595	T43.596
Oxyphenbutazone	T39.2X1	T39.2X2	T39.2X3	T39.2X4	T39.2X5	T39.2X6
Oxyphencyclimine	T44.3X1	T44.3X2	T44.3X3	T44.3X4	T44.3X5	T44.3X6
Oxyphenisatine	T47.2X1	T47.2X2	T47.2X3	T47.2X4	T47.2X5	T47.2X6
Oxyphenonium bromide	T44.3X1	T44.3X2	T44.3X3	T44.3X4	T44.3X5	T44.3X6
Oxypolygelatin	T45.8X1	T45.8X2	T45.8X3	T45.8X4	T45.8X5	T45.8X6
Oxyquinoline (derivatives)	T37.8X1	T37.8X2	T37.8X3	T37.8X4	T37.8X5	T37.8X6
Oxytetracycline	T36.4X1	T36.4X2	T36.4X3	T36.4X4	T36.4X5	T36.4X6
Oxytocic drug NEC	T48.0X1	T48.0X2	T48.0X3	T48.0X4	T48.0X5	T48.0X6
Oxytocin (synthetic)	T48.0X1	T48.0X2	T48.0X3	T48.0X4	T48.0X5	T48.0X6
Ozone	T59.891	T59.892	T59.893	T59.894	—	—
PABA	T49.3X1	T49.3X2	T49.3X3	T49.3X4	T49.3X5	T49.3X6
Packed red cells	T45.8X1	T45.8X2	T45.8X3	T45.8X4	T45.8X5	T45.8X6

Substance	Poisoning, Accidental (unintentional)	Poisoning, Intentional Self-harm	Poisoning, Assault	Poisoning, Undetermined	Adverse Effect	Under-dosing
Padimate	T49.3X1	T49.3X2	T49.3X3	T49.3X4	T49.3X5	T49.
Paint NEC	T65.6X1	T65.6X2	T65.6X3	T65.6X4	—	—
cleaner	T52.91	T52.92	T52.93	T52.94	—	—
fumes NEC	T59.891	T59.892	T59.893	T59.894	—	—
lead (fumes)	T56.0X1	T56.0X2	T56.0X3	T56.0X4	—	—
solvent NEC	T52.8X1	T52.8X2	T52.8X3	T52.8X4	—	—
stripper	T52.8X1	T52.8X2	T52.8X3	T52.8X4	—	—
Palfium	T40.2X1	T40.2X2	T40.2X3	T40.2X4	—	—
Palm kernel oil	T50.991	T50.992	T50.993	T50.994	T50.995	T50.
Paludrine	T37.2X1	T37.2X2	T37.2X3	T37.2X4	T37.2X5	T37.
PAM (pralidoxime)	T50.6X1	T50.6X2	T50.6X3	T50.6X4	T50.6X5	T50.
Pamaquine (naphthoute)	T37.2X1	T37.2X2	T37.2X3	T37.2X4	T37.2X5	T37.
Panadol	T39.1X1	T39.1X2	T39.1X3	T39.1X4	T39.1X5	T39.
Pancreatic						
digestive secretion stimulant	T47.8X1	T47.8X2	T47.8X3	T47.8X4	T47.8X5	T47
dornase	T45.3X1	T45.3X2	T45.3X3	T45.3X4	T45.3X5	T45
Pancreatin	T47.5X1	T47.5X2	T47.5X3	T47.5X4	T47.5X5	T47
Pancrelipase	T47.5X1	T47.5X2	T47.5X3	T47.5X4	T47.5X5	T47
Pancuronium (bromide)	T48.1X1	T48.1X2	T48.1X3	T48.1X4	T48.1X5	T48.
Pangamic acid	T45.2X1	T45.2X2	T45.2X3	T45.2X4	T45.2X5	T45.
Panthenol	T45.2X1	T45.2X2	T45.2X3	T45.2X4	T45.2X5	T45.
topical	T49.8X1	T49.8X2	T49.8X3	T49.8X4	T49.8X5	T49.
Pantopon	T40.0X1	T40.0X2	T40.0X3	T40.0X4	T40.0X5	T40.
Pantothenic acid	T45.2X1	T45.2X2	T45.2X3	T45.2X4	T45.2X5	T45.
Panwarfin	T45.511	T45.512	T45.513	T45.514	T45.515	T45.
Papain	T47.5X1	T47.5X2	T47.5X3	T47.5X4	T47.5X5	T47
digestant	T47.5X1	T47.5X2	T47.5X3	T47.5X4	T47.5X5	T47.
Papaveretum	T40.0X1	T40.0X2	T40.0X3	T40.0X4	T40.0X5	T40.
Papaverine	T44.3X1	T44.3X2	T44.3X3	T44.3X4	T44.3X5	T44.
Para-acetamidophenol	T39.1X1	T39.1X2	T39.1X3	T39.1X4	T39.1X5	T39.
Para-aminobenzoic acid	T49.3X1	T49.3X2	T49.3X3	T49.3X4	T49.3X5	T49.
Para-aminophenol derivatives	T39.1X1	T39.1X2	T39.1X3	T39.1X4	T39.1X5	T39.
Para-aminosalicylic acid	T37.1X1	T37.1X2	T37.1X3	T37.1X4	T37.1X5	T37
Paracetaldehyde	T42.6X1	T42.6X2	T42.6X3	T42.6X4	T42.6X5	T42
Paracetamol	T39.1X1	T39.1X2	T39.1X3	T39.1X4	T39.1X5	T39.
Parachlorophenol (camphorated)	T49.0X1	T49.0X2	T49.0X3	T49.0X4	T49.0X5	T49.
Paracodin	T40.2X1	T40.2X2	T40.2X3	T40.2X4	T40.2X5	T40.
Paradione	T42.2X1	T42.2X2	T42.2X3	T42.2X4	T42.2X5	T42.
Paraffin(s) (wax)	T52.0X1	T52.0X2	T52.0X3	T52.0X4	—	—
liquid (medicinal)	T47.4X1	T47.4X2	T47.4X3	T47.4X4	T47.4X5	T47.
nonmedicinal	T52.0X1	T52.0X2	T52.0X3	T52.0X4	—	—
Paraformaldehyde	T60.3X1	T60.3X2	T60.3X3	T60.3X4	—	—
Paraldehyde	T42.6X1	T42.6X2	T42.6X3	T42.6X4	T42.6X5	T42.
Paramethadione	T42.2X1	T42.2X2	T42.2X3	T42.2X4	T42.2X5	T42.
Paramethasone	T38.0X1	T38.0X2	T38.0X3	T38.0X4	T38.0X5	T38.
acetate	T49.0X1	T49.0X2	T49.0X3	T49.0X4	T49.0X5	T49.
Paraoxon	T60.0X1	T60.0X2	T60.0X3	T60.0X4	—	—
Paraquat	T60.3X1	T60.3X2	T60.3X3	T60.3X4	—	—
Parasympatholytic NEC	T44.3X1	T44.3X2	T44.3X3	T44.3X4	T44.3X5	T44.
Parasympathomimetic drug NEC	T44.1X1	T44.1X2	T44.1X3	T44.1X4	T44.1X5	T44.
Parathion	T60.0X1	T60.0X2	T60.0X3	T60.0X4	—	—
Parathormone	T50.991	T50.992	T50.993	T50.994	T50.995	T50.
Parathyroid extract	T50.991	T50.992	T50.993	T50.994	T50.995	T50.
Paratyphoid vaccine	T50.A91	T50.A92	T50.A93	T50.A94	T50.A95	T50.
Paredrine	T44.4X1	T44.4X2	T44.4X3	T44.4X4	T44.4X5	T44.
Paregoric	T40.0X1	T40.0X2	T40.0X3	T40.0X4	T40.0X5	T40.
Pargyline	T46.5X1	T46.5X2	T46.5X3	T46.5X4	T46.5X5	T46.
Paris green	T57.0X1	T57.0X2	T57.0X3	T57.0X4	—	—
insecticide	T57.0X1	T57.0X2	T57.0X3	T57.0X4	—	—
Parnate	T43.1X1	T43.1X2	T43.1X3	T43.1X4	T43.1X5	T43.
Paromomycin	T36.5X1	T36.5X2	T36.5X3	T36.5X4	T36.5X5	T36.
Paroxypropione	T45.1X1	T45.1X2	T45.1X3	T45.1X4	T45.1X5	T45.
Parzone	T40.2X1	T40.2X2	T40.2X3	T40.2X4	T40.2X5	T40.
PAS	T37.1X1	T37.1X2	T37.1X3	T37.1X4	T37.1X5	T37.
Pasiniazid	T37.1X1	T37.1X2	T37.1X3	T37.1X4	T37.1X5	T37.
PBB (polybrominated biphenyls)	T65.891	T65.892	T65.893	T65.894	—	—
PCB	T65.891	T65.892	T65.893	T65.894	—	—
PCP						
meaning pentachlorophenol	T60.1X1	T60.1X2	T60.1X3	T60.1X4	—	—
fungicide	T60.3X1	T60.3X2	T60.3X3	T60.3X4	—	—
herbicide	T60.3X1	T60.3X2	T60.3X3	T60.3X4	—	—
insecticide	T60.1X1	T60.1X2	T60.1X3	T60.1X4	—	—
meaning phencyclidine	T40.991	T40.992	T40.993	T40.994	—	—
Peach kernel oil (emulsion)	T47.4X1	T47.4X2	T47.4X3	T47.4X4	ICD47.4X5	T47.
Peanut oil (emulsion) NEC	T47.4X1	T47.4X2	T47.4X3	T47.4X4	T47.4X5	T47.
topical	T49.3X1	T49.3X2	T49.3X3	T49.3X4	T49.3X5	T49.

Substance	Poisoning, Accidental (unintentional)	Poisoning, Intentional Self-harm	Poisoning, Assault	Poisoning, Undetermined	Adverse Effect	Underdosing
early Gates (morning glory seeds)	T40.991	T40.992	T40.993	T40.994	—	—
Pecazine	T43.3X1	T43.3X2	T43.3X3	T43.3X4	T43.3X5	T43.3X6
Pectin	T47.6X1	T47.6X2	T47.6X3	T47.6X4	T47.6X5	T47.6X6
Pefloxacin	T37.8X1	T37.8X2	T37.8X3	T37.8X4	T37.8X5	T37.8X6
Pegademase, bovine	T50.Z91	T50.Z92	T50.Z93	T50.Z94	T50.Z95	T50.Z96
Pelletierine tannate	T37.4X1	T37.4X2	T37.4X3	T37.4X4	T37.4X5	T37.4X6
Pemirolast (potassium)	T48.6X1	T48.6X2	T48.6X3	T48.6X4	T48.6X5	T48.6X6
Pemoline	T50.7X1	T50.7X2	T50.7X3	T50.7X4	T50.7X5	T50.7X6
Pempidine	T44.2X1	T44.2X2	T44.2X3	T44.2X4	T44.2X5	T44.2X6
Penamecillin	T36.0X1	T36.0X2	T36.0X3	T36.0X4	T36.0X5	T36.0X6
Penbutolol	T44.7X1	T44.7X2	T44.7X3	T44.7X4	T44.7X5	T44.7X6
Penethamate	T36.0X1	T36.0X2	T36.0X3	T36.0X4	T36.0X5	T36.0X6
Penfluridol	T43.591	T43.592	T43.593	T43.594	T43.595	T43.596
Penflutizide	T50.2X1	T50.2X2	T50.2X3	T50.2X4	T50.2X5	T50.2X6
Pengitoxin	T46.0X1	T46.0X2	T46.0X3	T46.0X4	T46.0X5	T46.0X6
Penicillamine	T50.6X1	T50.6X2	T50.6X3	T50.6X4	T50.6X5	T50.6X6
Penicillin (any)	T36.0X1	T36.0X2	T36.0X3	T36.0X4	T36.0X5	T36.0X6
Penicillinase	T45.3X1	T45.3X2	T45.3X3	T45.3X4	T45.3X5	T45.3X6
Penicilloyl polylysine	T50.8X1	T50.8X2	T50.8X3	T50.8X4	T50.8X5	T50.8X6
Penimepicycline	T36.4X1	T36.4X2	T36.4X3	T36.4X4	T36.4X5	T36.4X6
Pentachloroethane	T53.6X1	T53.6X2	T53.6X3	T53.6X4	—	—
Pentachloronaphthalene	T53.7X1	T53.7X2	T53.7X3	T53.7X4	—	—
Pentachlorophenol (pesticide)	T60.1X1	T60.1X2	T60.1X3	T60.1X4	—	—
fungicide	T60.3X1	T60.3X2	T60.3X3	T60.3X4	—	—
herbicide	T60.3X1	T60.3X2	T60.3X3	T60.3X4	—	—
insecticide	T60.1X1	T60.1X2	T60.1X3	T60.1X4	—	—
Pentaerythritol	T46.3X1	T46.3X2	T46.3X3	T46.3X4	T46.3X5	T46.3X6
chloral	T42.6X1	T42.6X2	T42.6X3	T42.6X4	T42.6X5	T42.6X6
tetranitrate NEC	T46.3X1	T46.3X2	T46.3X3	T46.3X4	T46.3X5	T46.3X6
Pentaerythrityl tetranitrate	T46.3X1	T46.3X2	T46.3X3	T46.3X4	T46.3X5	T46.3X6
Pentagastrin	T50.8X1	T50.8X2	T50.8X3	T50.8X4	T50.8X5	T50.8X6
Pentalin	T53.6X1	T53.6X2	T53.6X3	T53.6X4	—	—
Pentamethonium bromide	T44.2X1	T44.2X2	T44.2X3	T44.2X4	T44.2X5	T44.2X6
Pentamidine	T37.3X1	T37.3X2	T37.3X3	T37.3X4	T37.3X5	T37.3X6
Pentanol	T51.3X1	T51.3X2	T51.3X3	T51.3X4	—	—
Pentapyrrolinium (bitartrate)	T44.2X1	T44.2X2	T44.2X3	T44.2X4	T44.2X5	T44.2X6
Pentaquine	T37.2X1	T37.2X2	T37.2X3	T37.2X4	T37.2X5	T37.2X6
Pentazocine	T40.4X1	T40.4X2	T40.4X3	T40.4X4	T40.4X5	T40.4X6
Pentetrazole	T50.7X1	T50.7X2	T50.7X3	T50.7X4	T50.7X5	T50.7X6
Penthienate bromide	T44.3X1	T44.3X2	T44.3X3	T44.3X4	T44.3X5	T44.3X6
Pentifylline	T46.7X1	T46.7X2	T46.7X3	T46.7X4	T46.7X5	T46.7X6
Pentobarbital	T42.3X1	T42.3X2	T42.3X3	T42.3X4	T42.3X5	T42.3X6
sodium	T42.3X1	T42.3X2	T42.3X3	T42.3X4	T42.3X5	T42.3X6
Pentobarbitone	T42.3X1	T42.3X2	T42.3X3	T42.3X4	T42.3X5	T42.3X6
Pentolonium tartrate	T44.2X1	T44.2X2	T44.2X3	T44.2X4	T44.2X5	T44.2X6
Pentosan polysulfate (sodium)	T39.8X1	T39.8X2	T39.8X3	T39.8X4	T39.8X5	T39.8X6
Pentostatin	T45.1X1	T45.1X2	T45.1X3	T45.1X4	T45.1X5	T45.1X6
Pentothal	T41.1X1	T41.1X2	T41.1X3	T41.1X4	T41.1X5	T41.1X6
Pentoxifylline	T46.7X1	T46.7X2	T46.7X3	T46.7X4	T46.7X5	T46.7X6
Pentoxyverine	T48.3X1	T48.3X2	T48.3X3	T48.3X4	T48.3X5	T48.3X6
Pentrinat	T46.3X1	T46.3X2	T46.3X3	T46.3X4	T46.3X5	T46.3X6
Pentylenetetrazole	T50.7X1	T50.7X2	T50.7X3	T50.7X4	T50.7X5	T50.7X6
Pentylsalicylamide	T37.1X1	T37.1X2	T37.1X3	T37.1X4	T37.1X5	T37.1X6
Pentymal	T42.3X1	T42.3X2	T42.3X3	T42.3X4	T42.3X5	T42.3X6
Peplomycin	T45.1X1	T45.1X2	T45.1X3	T45.1X4	T45.1X5	T45.1X6
Peppermint (oil)	T47.5X1	T47.5X2	T47.5X3	T47.5X4	T47.5X5	T47.5X6
Pepsin	T47.5X1	T47.5X2	T47.5X3	T47.5X4	T47.5X5	T47.5X6
digestant	T47.5X1	T47.5X2	T47.5X3	T47.5X4	T47.5X5	T47.5X6
Pepstatin	T47.1X1	T47.1X2	T47.1X3	T47.1X4	T47.1X5	T47.1X6
Peptavlon	T50.8X1	T50.8X2	T50.8X3	T50.8X4	T50.8X5	T50.8X6
Perazine	T43.3X1	T43.3X2	T43.3X3	T43.3X4	T43.3X5	T43.3X6
Percaine (spinal)	T41.3X1	T41.3X2	T41.3X3	T41.3X4	T41.3X5	T41.3X6
topical (surface)	T41.3X1	T41.3X2	T41.3X3	T41.3X4	T41.3X5	T41.3X6
Perchloroethylene	T53.3X1	T53.3X2	T53.3X3	T53.3X4	—	—
medicinal	T37.4X1	T37.4X2	T37.4X3	T37.4X4	T37.4X5	T37.4X6
vapor	T53.3X1	T53.3X2	T53.3X3	T53.3X4	—	—
Percodan	T40.2X1	T40.2X2	T40.2X3	T40.2X4	T40.2X5	T40.2X6
Percogesic — see also acetaminophen	T45.0X1	T45.0X2	T45.0X3	T45.0X4	T45.0X5	T45.0X6
Percorten	T38.0X1	T38.0X2	T38.0X3	T38.0X4	T38.0X5	T38.0X6
Pergolide	T42.8X1	T42.8X2	T42.8X3	T42.8X4	T42.8X5	T42.8X6
Pergonal	T38.811	T38.812	T38.813	T38.814	T38.815	T38.816
Perhexilene	T46.3X1	T46.3X2	T46.3X3	T46.3X4	T46.3X5	T46.3X6
Perhexiline (maleate)	T46.3X1	T46.3X2	T46.3X3	T46.3X4	T46.3X5	T46.3X6
Periactin	T45.0X1	T45.0X2	T45.0X3	T45.0X4	T45.0X5	T45.0X6
Periciazine	T43.3X1	T43.3X2	T43.3X3	T43.3X4	T43.3X5	T43.3X6
Periclor	T42.6X1	T42.6X2	T42.6X3	T42.6X4	T42.6X5	T42.6X6
Perindopril	T46.4X1	T46.4X2	T46.4X3	T46.4X4	T46.4X5	T46.4X6
Perisoxal	T39.8X1	T39.8X2	T39.8X3	T39.8X4	T39.8X5	T39.8X6
Peritoneal dialysis solution	T50.3X1	T50.3X2	T50.3X3	T50.3X4	T50.3X5	T50.3X6
Peritrate	T46.3X1	T46.3X2	T46.3X3	T46.3X4	T46.3X5	T46.3X6
Perlapine	T42.4X1	T42.4X2	T42.4X3	T42.4X4	T42.4X5	T42.4X6
Permanganate	T65.891	T65.892	T65.893	T65.894	—	—
Permethrin	T60.1X1	T60.1X2	T60.1X3	T60.1X4	—	—
Pernocton	T42.3X1	T42.3X2	T42.3X3	T42.3X4	T42.3X5	T42.3X6
Pernoston	T42.3X1	T42.3X2	T42.3X3	T42.3X4	T42.3X5	T42.3X6
Peronine	T40.2X1	T40.2X2	T40.2X3	T40.2X4	—	—
Perphenazine	T43.3X1	T43.3X2	T43.3X3	T43.3X4	T43.3X5	T43.3X6
Pertofrane	T43.011	T43.012	T43.013	T43.014	T43.015	T43.016
Pertussis						
immune serum (human)	T50.Z11	T50.Z12	T50.Z13	T50.Z14	T50.Z15	T50.Z16
vaccine (with diphtheria toxoid) (with tetanus toxoid)	T50.A11	T50.A12	T50.A13	T50.A14	T50.A15	T50.A16
Peruvian balsam	T49.0X1	T49.0X2	T49.0X3	T49.0X4	T49.0X5	T49.0X6
Peruvoside	T46.0X1	T46.0X2	T46.0X3	T46.0X4	T46.0X5	T46.0X6
Pesticide (dust) (fumes) (vapor) NEC	T60.91	T60.92	T60.93	T60.94	—	—
arsenic	T57.0X1	T57.0X2	T57.0X3	T57.0X4	—	—
chlorinated	T60.1X1	T60.1X2	T60.1X3	T60.1X4	—	—
cyanide	T65.0X1	T65.0X2	T65.0X3	T65.0X4	—	—
kerosene	T52.0X1	T52.0X2	T52.0X3	T52.0X4	—	—
mixture (of compounds)	T60.91	T60.92	T60.93	T60.94	—	—
naphthalene	T60.2X1	T60.2X2	T60.2X3	T60.2X4	—	—
organochlorine (compounds)	T60.1X1	T60.1X2	T60.1X3	T60.1X4	—	—
petroleum (distillate) (products) NEC	T60.8X1	T60.8X2	T60.8X3	T60.8X4	—	—
specified ingredient NEC	T60.8X1	T60.8X2	T60.8X3	T60.8X4	—	—
strychnine	T65.1X1	T65.1X2	T65.1X3	T65.1X4	—	—
thallium	T60.4X1	T60.4X2	T60.4X3	T60.4X4	—	—
Pethidine	T40.4X1	T40.4X2	T40.4X3	T40.4X4	T40.4X5	T40.4X6
Petrichloral	T42.6X1	T42.6X2	T42.6X3	T42.6X4	T42.6X5	T42.6X6
Petrol	T52.0X1	T52.0X2	T52.0X3	T52.0X4	—	—
vapor	T52.0X1	T52.0X2	T52.0X3	T52.0X4	—	—
Petrolatum	T49.3X1	T49.3X2	T49.3X3	T49.3X4	T49.3X5	T49.3X6
hydrophilic	T49.3X1	T49.3X2	T49.3X3	T49.3X4	T49.3X5	T49.3X6
liquid	T47.4X1	T47.4X2	T47.4X3	T47.4X4	T47.4X5	T47.4X6
topical	T49.3X1	T49.3X2	T49.3X3	T49.3X4	T49.3X5	T49.3X6
nonmedicinal	T52.0X1	T52.0X2	T52.0X3	T52.0X4	—	—
red veterinary	T49.3X1	T49.3X2	T49.3X3	T49.3X4	T49.3X5	T49.3X6
white	T49.3X1	T49.3X2	T49.3X3	T49.3X4	T49.3X5	T49.3X6
Petroleum (products) NEC	T52.0X1	T52.0X2	T52.0X3	T52.0X4	—	—
benzine(s) — see Ligroin						
ether — see Ligroin						
jelly — see Petrolatum						
naphtha — see Ligroin						
pesticide	T60.8X1	T60.8X2	T60.8X3	T60.8X4	—	—
solids	T52.0X1	T52.0X2	T52.0X3	T52.0X4	—	—
solvents	T52.0X1	T52.0X2	T52.0X3	T52.0X4	—	—
vapor	T52.0X1	T52.0X2	T52.0X3	T52.0X4	—	—
Peyote	T40.991	T40.992	T40.993	T40.994	—	—
Phanodorm, phanodorn	T42.3X1	T42.3X2	T42.3X3	T42.3X4	T42.3X5	T42.3X6
Phanquinone	T37.3X1	T37.3X2	T37.3X3	T37.3X4	T37.3X5	T37.3X6
Phanquone	T37.3X1	T37.3X2	T37.3X3	T37.3X4	T37.3X5	T37.3X6
Pharmaceutical						
adjunct NEC	T50.901	T50.902	T50.903	T50.904	T50.905	T50.906
excipient NEC	T50.901	T50.902	T50.903	T50.904	T50.905	T50.906
sweetener	T50.901	T50.902	T50.903	T50.904	T50.905	T50.906
viscous agent	T50.901	T50.902	T50.903	T50.904	T50.905	T50.906
Phemitone	T42.3X1	T42.3X2	T42.3X3	T42.3X4	T42.3X5	T42.3X6
Phenacaine	T41.3X1	T41.3X2	T41.3X3	T41.3X4	T41.3X5	T41.3X6
Phenacemide	T42.6X1	T42.6X2	T42.6X3	T42.6X4	T42.6X5	T42.6X6
Phenacetin	T39.1X1	T39.1X2	T39.1X3	T39.1X4	T39.1X5	T39.1X6
Phenadoxone	T40.2X1	T40.2X2	T40.2X3	T40.2X4	—	—
Phenaglycodol	T43.591	T43.592	T43.593	T43.594	T43.595	T43.596
Phenantoin	T42.0X1	T42.0X2	T42.0X3	T42.0X4	T42.0X5	T42.0X6
Phenaphthazine reagent	T50.991	T50.992	T50.993	T50.994	T50.995	T50.996
Phenazocine	T40.4X1	T40.4X2	T40.4X3	T40.4X4	T40.4X5	T40.4X6
Phenazone	T39.2X1	T39.2X2	T39.2X3	T39.2X4	T39.2X5	T39.2X6
Phenazopyridine	T39.8X1	T39.8X2	T39.8X3	T39.8X4	T39.8X5	T39.8X6
Phenbenicillin	T36.0X1	T36.0X2	T36.0X3	T36.0X4	T36.0X5	T36.0X6
Phenbutrazate	T50.5X1	T50.5X2	T50.5X3	T50.5X4	T50.5X5	T50.5X6
Phencyclidine	T40.991	T40.992	T40.993	T40.994	T40.995	T40.996
Phendimetrazine	T50.5X1	T50.5X2	T50.5X3	T50.5X4	T50.5X5	T50.5X6
Phenelzine	T43.1X1	T43.1X2	T43.1X3	T43.1X4	T43.1X5	T43.1X6
Phenemal	T42.3X1	T42.3X2	T42.3X3	T42.3X4	T42.3X5	T42.3X6
Phenergan	T42.6X1	T42.6X2	T42.6X3	T42.6X4	T42.6X5	T42.6X6
Pheneticillin	T36.0X1	T36.0X2	T36.0X3	T36.0X4	T36.0X5	T36.0X6
Pheneturide	T42.6X1	T42.6X2	T42.6X3	T42.6X4	T42.6X5	T42.6X6
Phenformin	T38.3X1	T38.3X2	T38.3X3	T38.3X4	T38.3X5	T38.3X6

Substance	Poisoning, Accidental (unintentional)	Poisoning, Intentional Self-harm	Poisoning, Assault	Poisoning, Undetermined	Adverse Effect	Under-dosing
Phenglutarimide	T44.3X1	T44.3X2	T44.3X3	T44.3X4	T44.3X5	T44.3X6
Phenicarbazide	T39.8X1	T39.8X2	T39.8X3	T39.8X4	T39.8X5	T39.8X6
Phenindamine	T45.0X1	T45.0X2	T45.0X3	T45.0X4	T45.0X5	T45.0X6
Phenindione	T45.511	T45.512	T45.513	T45.514	T45.515	T45.516
Pheniprazine	T43.1X1	T43.1X2	T43.1X3	T43.1X4	T43.1X5	T43.1X6
Pheniramine	T45.0X1	T45.0X2	T45.0X3	T45.0X4	T45.0X5	T45.0X6
Phenisatin	T47.2X1	T47.2X2	T47.2X3	T47.2X4	T47.2X5	T47.2X6
Phenmetrazine	T50.5X1	T50.5X2	T50.5X3	T50.5X4	T50.5X5	T50.5X6
Phenobal	T42.3X1	T42.3X2	T42.3X3	T42.3X4	T42.3X5	T42.3X6
Phenobarbital	T42.3X1	T42.3X2	T42.3X3	T42.3X4	T42.3X5	T42.3X6
with						
mephenytoin	T42.3X1	T42.3X2	T42.3X3	T42.3X4	T42.3X5	T42.3X6
phenytoin	T42.3X1	T42.3X2	T42.3X3	T42.3X4	T42.3X5	T42.3X6
sodium	T42.3X1	T42.3X2	T42.3X3	T42.3X4	T42.3X5	T42.3X6
Phenobarbitone	T42.3X1	T42.3X2	T42.3X3	T42.3X4	T42.3X5	T42.3X6
Phenobutiodil	T50.8X1	T50.8X2	T50.8X3	T50.8X4	T50.8X5	T50.8X6
Phenoctide	T49.0X1	T49.0X2	T49.0X3	T49.0X4	T49.0X5	T49.0X6
Phenol	T49.0X1	T49.0X2	T49.0X3	T49.0X4	T49.0X5	T49.0X6
disinfectant	T54.0X1	T54.0X2	T54.0X3	T54.0X4	—	—
in oil injection	T46.8X1	T46.8X2	T46.8X3	T46.8X4	T46.8X5	T46.8X6
medicinal	T49.1X1	T49.1X2	T49.1X3	T49.1X4	T49.1X5	T49.1X6
nonmedicinal NEC	T54.0X1	T54.0X2	T54.0X3	T54.0X4	—	—
pesticide	T60.8X1	T60.8X2	T60.8X3	T60.8X4	—	—
red	T50.8X1	T50.8X2	T50.8X3	T50.8X4	T50.8X5	T50.8X6
Phenolic preparation	T49.1X1	T49.1X2	T49.1X3	T49.1X4	T49.1X5	T49.1X6
Phenolphthalein	T47.2X1	T47.2X2	T47.2X3	T47.2X4	T47.2X5	T47.2X6
Phenolsulfonphthalein	T50.8X1	T50.8X2	T50.8X3	T50.8X4	T50.8X5	T50.8X6
Phenomorphan	T40.2X1	T40.2X2	T40.2X3	T40.2X4	—	—
Phenonyl	T42.3X1	T42.3X2	T42.3X3	T42.3X4	T42.3X5	T42.3X6
Phenoperidine	T40.4X1	T40.4X2	T40.4X3	T40.4X4	—	—
Phenopyrazone	T46.991	T46.992	T46.993	T46.994	T46.995	T46.996
Phenoquin	T50.4X1	T50.4X2	T50.4X3	T50.4X4	T50.4X5	T50.4X6
Phenothiazine (psychotropic) NEC	T43.3X1	T43.3X2	T43.3X3	T43.3X4	T43.3X5	T43.3X6
insecticide	T60.2X1	T60.2X2	T60.2X3	T60.2X4	—	—
Phenothrin	T49.0X1	T49.0X2	T49.0X3	T49.0X4	T49.0X5	T49.0X6
Phenoxybenzamine	T46.7X1	T46.7X2	T46.7X3	T46.7X4	T46.7X5	T46.7X6
Phenoxyethanol	T49.0X1	T49.0X2	T49.0X3	T49.0X4	T49.0X5	T49.0X6
Phenoxymethyl penicillin	T36.0X1	T36.0X2	T36.0X3	T36.0X4	T36.0X5	T36.0X6
Phenprobamate	T42.8X1	T42.8X2	T42.8X3	T42.8X4	T42.8X5	T42.8X6
Phenprocoumon	T45.511	T45.512	T45.513	T45.514	T45.515	T45.516
Phensuximide	T42.2X1	T42.2X2	T42.2X3	T42.2X4	T42.2X5	T42.2X6
Phentermine	T50.5X1	T50.5X2	T50.5X3	T50.5X4	T50.5X5	T50.5X6
Phenthicillin	T36.0X1	T36.0X2	T36.0X3	T36.0X4	T36.0X5	T36.0X6
Phentolamine	T46.7X1	T46.7X2	T46.7X3	T46.7X4	T46.7X5	T46.7X6
Phenyl						
butazone	T39.2X1	T39.2X2	T39.2X3	T39.2X4	T39.2X5	T39.2X6
enediamine	T65.3X1	T65.3X2	T65.3X3	T65.3X4	—	—
hydrazine	T65.3X1	T65.3X2	T65.3X3	T65.3X4	—	—
antineoplastic	T45.1X1	T45.1X2	T45.1X3	T45.1X4	T45.1X5	T45.1X6
mercuric compounds — see Mercury						
salicylate	T49.3X1	T49.3X2	T49.3X3	T49.3X4	T49.3X5	T49.3X6
Phenylalanine mustard	T45.1X1	T45.1X2	T45.1X3	T45.1X4	T45.1X5	T45.1X6
Phenylbutazone	T39.2X1	T39.2X2	T39.2X3	T39.2X4	T39.2X5	T39.2X6
Phenylenediamine	T65.3X1	T65.3X2	T65.3X3	T65.3X4	—	—
Phenylephrine	T44.4X1	T44.4X2	T44.4X3	T44.4X4	T44.4X5	T44.4X6
Phenylethylbiguanide	T38.3X1	T38.3X2	T38.3X3	T38.3X4	T38.3X5	T38.3X6
Phenylmercuric						
acetate	T49.0X1	T49.0X2	T49.0X3	T49.0X4	T49.0X5	T49.0X6
borate	T49.0X1	T49.0X2	T49.0X3	T49.0X4	T49.0X5	T49.0X6
nitrate	T49.0X1	T49.0X2	T49.0X3	T49.0X4	T49.0X5	T49.0X6
Phenylmethylbarbitone	T42.3X1	T42.3X2	T42.3X3	T42.3X4	T42.3X5	T42.3X6
Phenylpropanol	T47.5X1	T47.5X2	T47.5X3	T47.5X4	T47.5X5	T47.5X6
Phenylpropanolamine	T44.991	T44.992	T44.993	T44.994	T44.995	T44.996
Phenylsulfthion	T60.0X1	T60.0X2	T60.0X3	T60.0X4	—	—
Phenyltoloxamine	T45.0X1	T45.0X2	T45.0X3	T45.0X4	T45.0X5	T45.0X6
Phenyramidol, phenyramidon	T39.8X1	T39.8X2	T39.8X3	T39.8X4	T39.8X5	T39.8X6
Phenytoin	T42.0X1	T42.0X2	T42.0X3	T42.0X4	T42.0X5	T42.0X6
with Phenobarbital	T42.3X1	T42.3X2	T42.3X3	T42.3X4	T42.3X5	T42.3X6
pHisoHex	T49.2X1	T49.2X2	T49.2X3	T49.2X4	T49.2X5	T49.2X6
Pholcodine	T48.3X1	T48.3X2	T48.3X3	T48.3X4	T48.3X5	T48.3X6
Pholedrine	T46.991	T46.992	T46.993	T46.994	T46.995	T46.996
Phorate	T60.0X1	T60.0X2	T60.0X3	T60.0X4	—	—
Phosdrin	T60.0X1	T60.0X2	T60.0X3	T60.0X4	—	—
Phosfolan	T60.0X1	T60.0X2	T60.0X3	T60.0X4	—	—
Phosgene (gas)	T59.891	T59.892	T59.893	T59.894	—	—
Phosphamidon	T60.0X1	T60.0X2	T60.0X3	T60.0X4	—	—
Phosphate	T65.891	T65.892	T65.893	T65.894	—	—
laxative	T47.4X1	T47.4X2	T47.4X3	T47.4X4	T47.4X5	T47.4X6
organic	T60.0X1	T60.0X2	T60.0X3	T60.0X4	—	—
solvent	T52.91	T52.92	T52.93	T52.94	—	—

Substance	Poisoning, Accidental (unintentional)	Poisoning, Intentional Self-harm	Poisoning, Assault	Poisoning, Undetermined	Adverse Effect	Under-dosing
Phosphate — continued						
tricresyl	T65.891	T65.892	T65.893	T65.894	—	—
Phosphine	T57.1X1	T57.1X2	T57.1X3	T57.1X4	—	—
fumigant	T57.1X1	T57.1X2	T57.1X3	T57.1X4	—	—
Phospholine	T49.5X1	T49.5X2	T49.5X3	T49.5X4	T49.5X5	T49…
Phosphoric acid	T54.2X1	T54.2X2	T54.2X3	T54.2X4	—	—
Phosphorus (compound) NEC	T57.1X1	T57.1X2	T57.1X3	T57.1X4	—	—
pesticide	T60.0X1	T60.0X2	T60.0X3	T60.0X4	—	—
Phthalates	T65.891	T65.892	T65.893	T65.894	—	—
Phthalic anhydride	T65.891	T65.892	T65.893	T65.894	—	—
Phthalimidoglutarimide	T42.6X1	T42.6X2	T42.6X3	T42.6X4	T42.6X5	T42…
Phthalylsulfathiazole	T37.0X1	T37.0X2	T37.0X3	T37.0X4	T37.0X5	T37…
Phylloquinone	T45.7X1	T45.7X2	T45.7X3	T45.7X4	T45.7X5	T45…
Physeptone	T40.3X1	T40.3X2	T40.3X3	T40.3X4	T40.3X5	T40…
Physostigma venenosum	T62.2X1	T62.2X2	T62.2X3	T62.2X4	—	—
Physostigmine	T49.5X1	T49.5X2	T49.5X3	T49.5X4	T49.5X5	T49…
Phytolacca decandra	T62.2X1	T62.2X2	T62.2X3	T62.2X4	—	—
berries	T62.1X1	T62.1X2	T62.1X3	T62.1X4	—	—
Phytomenadione	T45.7X1	T45.7X2	T45.7X3	T45.7X4	T45.7X5	T45…
Phytonadione	T45.7X1	T45.7X2	T45.7X3	T45.7X4	T45.7X5	T45…
Picoperine	T48.3X1	T48.3X2	T48.3X3	T48.3X4	T48.3X5	T48…
Picosulfate (sodium)	T47.2X1	T47.2X2	T47.2X3	T47.2X4	T47.2X5	T47…
Picric (acid)	T54.2X1	T54.2X2	T54.2X3	T54.2X4	—	—
Picrotoxin	T50.7X1	T50.7X2	T50.7X3	T50.7X4	T50.7X5	T50…
Piketoprofen	T49.0X1	T49.0X2	T49.0X3	T49.0X4	T49.0X5	T49…
Pilocarpine	T44.1X1	T44.1X2	T44.1X3	T44.1X4	T44.1X5	T44…
Pilocarpus (jaborandi) extract	T44.1X1	T44.1X2	T44.1X3	T44.1X4	T44.1X5	T44…
Pilsicainide (hydrochloride)	T46.2X1	T46.2X2	T46.2X3	T46.2X4	T46.2X5	T46…
Pimaricin	T36.7X1	T36.7X2	T36.7X3	T36.7X4	T36.7X5	T36…
Pimeclone	T50.7X1	T50.7X2	T50.7X3	T50.7X4	T50.7X5	T50…
Pimelic ketone	T52.8X1	T52.8X2	T52.8X3	T52.8X4	—	—
Pimethixene	T45.0X1	T45.0X2	T45.0X3	T45.0X4	T45.0X5	T45…
Piminodine	T40.2X1	T40.2X2	T40.2X3	T40.2X4	T40.2X5	T40…
Pimozide	T43.591	T43.592	T43.593	T43.594	T43.595	T43…
Pinacidil	T46.5X1	T46.5X2	T46.5X3	T46.5X4	T46.5X5	T46…
Pinaverium bromide	T44.3X1	T44.3X2	T44.3X3	T44.3X4	T44.3X5	T44…
Pinazepam	T42.4X1	T42.4X2	T42.4X3	T42.4X4	T42.4X5	T42…
Pindolol	T44.7X1	T44.7X2	T44.7X3	T44.7X4	T44.7X5	T44…
Pindone	T60.4X1	T60.4X2	T60.4X3	T60.4X4	—	—
Pine oil (disinfectant)	T65.891	T65.892	T65.893	T65.894	—	—
Pinkroot	T37.4X1	T37.4X2	T37.4X3	T37.4X4	T37.4X5	T37…
Pipadone	T40.2X1	T40.2X2	T40.2X3	T40.2X4	—	—
Pipamazine	T45.0X1	T45.0X2	T45.0X3	T45.0X4	T45.0X5	T45…
Pipamperone	T43.4X1	T43.4X2	T43.4X3	T43.4X4	T43.4X5	T43…
Pipazetate	T48.3X1	T48.3X2	T48.3X3	T48.3X4	T48.3X5	T48…
Pipemidic acid	T37.8X1	T37.8X2	T37.8X3	T37.8X4	T37.8X5	T37…
Pipenzolate bromide	T44.3X1	T44.3X2	T44.3X3	T44.3X4	T44.3X5	T44…
Piperacetazine	T43.3X1	T43.3X2	T43.3X3	T43.3X4	T43.3X5	T43…
Piperacillin	T36.0X1	T36.0X2	T36.0X3	T36.0X4	T36.0X5	T36…
Piperazine	T37.4X1	T37.4X2	T37.4X3	T37.4X4	T37.4X5	T37…
estrone sulfate	T38.5X1	T38.5X2	T38.5X3	T38.5X4	T38.5X5	T38…
Piper cubeba	T62.2X1	T62.2X2	T62.2X3	T62.2X4	—	—
Piperidione	T48.3X1	T48.3X2	T48.3X3	T48.3X4	T48.3X5	T48…
Piperidolate	T44.3X1	T44.3X2	T44.3X3	T44.3X4	T44.3X5	T44…
Piperocaine	T41.3X1	T41.3X2	T41.3X3	T41.3X4	T41.3X5	T41…
infiltration (subcutaneous)	T41.3X1	T41.3X2	T41.3X3	T41.3X4	T41.3X5	T41…
nerve block (peripheral) (plexus)	T41.3X1	T41.3X2	T41.3X3	T41.3X4	T41.3X5	T41…
topical (surface)	T41.3X1	T41.3X2	T41.3X3	T41.3X4	T41.3X5	T41…
Piperonyl butoxide	T60.8X1	T60.8X2	T60.8X3	T60.8X4	—	—
Pipethanate	T44.3X1	T44.3X2	T44.3X3	T44.3X4	T44.3X5	T44…
Pipobroman	T45.1X1	T45.1X2	T45.1X3	T45.1X4	T45.1X5	T45…
Pipotiazine	T43.3X1	T43.3X2	T43.3X3	T43.3X4	T43.3X5	T43…
Pipoxizine	T45.0X1	T45.0X2	T45.0X3	T45.0X4	T45.0X5	T45…
Pipradrol	T43.691	T43.692	T43.693	T43.694	T43.695	T43…
Piprinhydrinate	T45.0X1	T45.0X2	T45.0X3	T45.0X4	T45.0X5	T45…
Pirarubicin	T45.1X1	T45.1X2	T45.1X3	T45.1X4	T45.1X5	T45…
Pirazinamide	T37.1X1	T37.1X2	T37.1X3	T37.1X4	T37.1X5	T37…
Pirbuterol	T48.6X1	T48.6X2	T48.6X3	T48.6X4	T48.6X5	T48…
Pirenzepine	T47.1X1	T47.1X2	T47.1X3	T47.1X4	T47.1X5	T47…
Piretanide	T50.1X1	T50.1X2	T50.1X3	T50.1X4	T50.1X5	T50…
Piribedil	T42.8X1	T42.8X2	T42.8X3	T42.8X4	T42.8X5	T42…
Piridoxilate	T46.3X1	T46.3X2	T46.3X3	T46.3X4	T46.3X5	T46…
Piritramide	T40.4X1	T40.4X2	T40.4X3	T40.4X4	—	—
Piromidic acid	T37.8X1	T37.8X2	T37.8X3	T37.8X4	T37.8X5	T37…
Piroxicam	T39.391	T39.392	T39.393	T39.394	T39.395	T39…
beta-cyclodextrin complex	T39.8X1	T39.8X2	T39.8X3	T39.8X4	T39.8X5	T39…
Pirozadil	T46.6X1	T46.6X2	T46.6X3	T46.6X4	T46.6X5	T46…
Piscidia (bark) (erythrina)	T39.8X1	T39.8X2	T39.8X3	T39.8X4	T39.8X5	T39…
Pitch	T65.891	T65.892	T65.893	T65.894	—	—
Pitkin's solution	T41.3X1	T41.3X2	T41.3X3	T41.3X4	T41.3X5	T41…

Substance	Poisoning, Accidental (unintentional)	Poisoning, Intentional Self-harm	Poisoning, Assault	Poisoning, Undetermined	Adverse Effect	Under-dosing
Pitocin	T48.0X1	T48.0X2	T48.0X3	T48.0X4	T48.0X5	T48.0X6
Pitressin (tannate)	T38.891	T38.892	T38.893	T38.894	T38.895	T38.896
Pituitary extracts	T38.891	T38.892	T38.893	T38.894	T38.895	T38.896
(posterior)						
anterior	T38.811	T38.812	T38.813	T38.814	T38.815	T38.816
Pituitrin	T38.891	T38.892	T38.893	T38.894	T38.895	T38.896
Pivampicillin	T36.0X1	T36.0X2	T36.0X3	T36.0X4	T36.0X5	T36.0X6
Pivmecillinam	T36.0X1	T36.0X2	T36.0X3	T36.0X4	T36.0X5	T36.0X6
Placental hormone	T38.891	T38.892	T38.893	T38.894	T38.895	T38.896
Placidyl	T42.6X1	T42.6X2	T42.6X3	T42.6X4	T42.6X5	T42.6X6
Plague vaccine	T50.A91	T50.A92	T50.A93	T50.A94	T50.A95	T50.A96
Plant						
food or fertilizer NEC	T65.891	T65.892	T65.893	T65.894	—	—
containing herbicide	T60.3X1	T60.3X2	T60.3X3	T60.3X4	—	—
noxious, used as food	T62.2X1	T62.2X2	T62.2X3	T62.2X4	—	—
berries	T62.1X1	T62.1X2	T62.1X3	T62.1X4	—	—
seeds	T62.2X1	T62.2X2	T62.2X3	T62.2X4	—	—
specified type NEC	T62.2X1	T62.2X2	T62.2X3	T62.2X4	—	—
Plasma	T45.8X1	T45.8X2	T45.8X3	T45.8X4	T45.8X5	T45.8X6
expander NEC	T45.8X1	T45.8X2	T45.8X3	T45.8X4	T45.8X5	T45.8X6
protein fraction (human)	T45.8X1	T45.8X2	T45.8X3	T45.8X4	T45.8X5	T45.8X6
Plasmanate	T45.8X1	T45.8X2	T45.8X3	T45.8X4	T45.8X5	T45.8X6
Plasminogen (tissue)	T45.611	T45.612	T45.613	T45.614	T45.615	T45.616
activator						
Plaster dressing	T49.3X1	T49.3X2	T49.3X3	T49.3X4	T49.3X5	T49.3X6
Plastic dressing	T49.3X1	T49.3X2	T49.3X3	T49.3X4	T49.3X5	T49.3X6
Plegicil	T43.3X1	T43.3X2	T43.3X3	T43.3X4	T43.3X5	T43.3X6
Plicamycin	T45.1X1	T45.1X2	T45.1X3	T45.1X4	T45.1X5	T45.1X6
Podophyllotoxin	T49.8X1	T49.8X2	T49.8X3	T49.8X4	T49.8X5	T49.8X6
Podophyllum (resin)	T49.4X1	T49.4X2	T49.4X3	T49.4X4	T49.4X5	T49.4X6
Poisonous berries	T62.1X1	T62.1X2	T62.1X3	T62.1X4	—	—
Poison NEC	T65.91	T65.92	T65.93	T65.94	—	—
Pokeweed (any part)	T62.2X1	T62.2X2	T62.2X3	T62.2X4	—	—
Poldine metilsulfate	T44.3X1	T44.3X2	T44.3X3	T44.3X4	T44.3X5	T44.3X6
Polidexide (sulfate)	T46.6X1	T46.6X2	T46.6X3	T46.6X4	T46.6X5	T46.6X6
Polidocanol	T46.8X1	T46.8X2	T46.8X3	T46.8X4	T46.8X5	T46.8X6
Poliomyelitis vaccine	T50.B91	T50.B92	T50.B93	T50.B94	T50.B95	T50.B96
Polish (car) (floor) (furniture)	T65.891	T65.892	T65.893	T65.894	—	—
(metal) (porcelain)						
(silver)						
abrasive	T65.891	T65.892	T65.893	T65.894	—	—
porcelain	T65.891	T65.892	T65.893	T65.894	—	—
Poloxalkol	T47.4X1	T47.4X2	T47.4X3	T47.4X4	T47.4X5	T47.4X6
Poloxamer	T47.4X1	T47.4X2	T47.4X3	T47.4X4	T47.4X5	T47.4X6
Polyaminostyrene resins	T50.3X1	T50.3X2	T50.3X3	T50.3X4	T50.3X5	T50.3X6
Polycarbophil	T47.4X1	T47.4X2	T47.4X3	T47.4X4	T47.4X5	T47.4X6
Polychlorinated biphenyl	T65.891	T65.892	T65.893	T65.894	—	—
Polycycline	T36.4X1	T36.4X2	T36.4X3	T36.4X4	T36.4X5	T36.4X6
Polyester fumes	T59.891	T59.892	T59.893	T59.894	—	—
Polyester resin hardener	T52.91	T52.92	T52.93	T52.94	—	—
fumes	T59.891	T59.892	T59.893	T59.894	—	—
Polyestradiol phosphate	T38.5X1	T38.5X2	T38.5X3	T38.5X4	T38.5X5	T38.5X6
Polyethanolamine alkyl	T49.2X1	T49.2X2	T49.2X3	T49.2X4	T49.2X5	T49.2X6
sulfate						
Polyethylene adhesive	T49.3X1	T49.3X2	T49.3X3	T49.3X4	T49.3X5	T49.3X6
Polyferose	T45.4X1	T45.4X2	T45.4X3	T45.4X4	T45.4X5	T45.4X6
Polygeline	T45.8X1	T45.8X2	T45.8X3	T45.8X4	T45.8X5	T45.8X6
Polymyxin	T36.8X1	T36.8X2	T36.8X3	T36.8X4	T36.8X5	T36.8X6
B	T36.8X1	T36.8X2	T36.8X3	T36.8X4	T36.8X5	T36.8X6
ENT agent	T49.6X1	T49.6X2	T49.6X3	T49.6X4	T49.6X5	T49.6X6
ophthalmic preparation	T49.5X1	T49.5X2	T49.5X3	T49.5X4	T49.5X5	T49.5X6
topical NEC	T49.0X1	T49.0X2	T49.0X3	T49.0X4	T49.0X5	T49.0X6
E sulfate (eye preparation)	T49.5X1	T49.5X2	T49.5X3	T49.5X4	T49.5X5	T49.5X6
Polynoxylin	T49.0X1	T49.0X2	T49.0X3	T49.0X4	T49.0X5	T49.0X6
Polyoestradiol phosphate	T38.5X1	T38.5X2	T38.5X3	T38.5X4	T38.5X5	T38.5X6
Polyoxymethyleneurea	T49.0X1	T49.0X2	T49.0X3	T49.0X4	T49.0X5	T49.0X6
Polysilane	T47.8X1	T47.8X2	T47.8X3	T47.8X4	T47.8X5	T47.8X6
Polytetrafluoroethylene	T59.891	T59.892	T59.893	T59.894	—	—
(inhaled)						
Polythiazide	T50.2X1	T50.2X2	T50.2X3	T50.2X4	T50.2X5	T50.2X6
Polyvidone	T45.8X1	T45.8X2	T45.8X3	T45.8X4	T45.8X5	T45.8X6
Polyvinylpyrrolidone	T45.8X1	T45.8X2	T45.8X3	T45.8X4	T45.8X5	T45.8X6
Pontocaine (hydrochloride)	T41.3X1	T41.3X2	T41.3X3	T41.3X4	T41.3X5	T41.3X6
(infiltration) (topical)						
nerve block (peripheral)	T41.3X1	T41.3X2	T41.3X3	T41.3X4	T41.3X5	T41.3X6
(plexus)						
spinal	T41.3X1	T41.3X2	T41.3X3	T41.3X4	T41.3X5	T41.3X6
Porfiromycin	T45.1X1	T45.1X2	T45.1X3	T45.1X4	T45.1X5	T45.1X6
Posterior pituitary hormone	T38.891	T38.892	T38.893	T38.894	T38.895	T38.896
NEC						
Pot	T40.7X1	T40.7X2	T40.7X3	T40.7X4	T40.7X5	T40.7X6
Potash (caustic)	T54.3X1	T54.3X2	T54.3X3	T54.3X4	—	—

Substance	Poisoning, Accidental (unintentional)	Poisoning, Intentional Self-harm	Poisoning, Assault	Poisoning, Undetermined	Adverse Effect	Under-dosing
Potassic saline injection	T50.3X1	T50.3X2	T50.3X3	T50.3X4	T50.3X5	T50.3X6
(lactated)						
Potassium (salts) NEC	T50.3X1	T50.3X2	T50.3X3	T50.3X4	T50.3X5	T50.3X6
aminobenzoate	T45.8X1	T45.8X2	T45.8X3	T45.8X4	T45.8X5	T45.8X6
aminosalicylate	T37.1X1	T37.1X2	T37.1X3	T37.1X4	T37.1X5	T37.1X6
antimony ' tartrate'	T37.8X1	T37.8X2	T37.8X3	T37.8X4	T37.8X5	T37.8X6
arsenite (solution)	T57.0X1	T57.0X2	T57.0X3	T57.0X4	—	—
bichromate	T56.2X1	T56.2X2	T56.2X3	T56.2X4	—	—
bisulfate	T47.3X1	T47.3X2	T47.3X3	T47.3X4	T47.3X5	T47.3X6
bromide	T42.6X1	T42.6X2	T42.6X3	T42.6X4	T42.6X5	T42.6X6
canrenoate	T50.0X1	T50.0X2	T50.0X3	T50.0X4	T50.0X5	T50.0X6
carbonate	T54.3X1	T54.3X2	T54.3X3	T54.3X4	—	—
chlorate NEC	T65.891	T65.892	T65.893	T65.894	—	—
chloride	T50.3X1	T50.3X2	T50.3X3	T50.3X4	T50.3X5	T50.3X6
citrate	T50.991	T50.992	T50.993	T50.994	T50.995	T50.996
cyanide	T65.0X1	T65.0X2	T65.0X3	T65.0X4	—	—
ferric hexacyanoferrate	T50.6X1	T50.6X2	T50.6X3	T50.6X4	T50.6X5	T50.6X6
(medicinal)						
nonmedicinal	T65.891	T65.892	T65.893	T65.894	—	—
Fluoride	T57.8X1	T57.8X2	T57.8X3	T57.8X4	—	—
glucaldrate	T47.1X1	T47.1X2	T47.1X3	T47.1X4	T47.1X5	T47.1X6
hydroxide	T54.3X1	T54.3X2	T54.3X3	T54.3X4	—	—
iodate	T49.0X1	T49.0X2	T49.0X3	T49.0X4	T49.0X5	T49.0X6
iodide	T48.4X1	T48.4X2	T48.4X3	T48.4X4	T48.4X5	T48.4X6
nitrate	T57.8X1	T57.8X2	T57.8X3	T57.8X4	—	—
oxalate	T65.891	T65.892	T65.893	T65.894	—	—
perchlorate (nonmedicinal)	T65.891	T65.892	T65.893	T65.894	—	—
NEC						
antithyroid	T38.2X1	T38.2X2	T38.2X3	T38.2X4	T38.2X5	T38.2X6
medicinal	T38.2X1	T38.2X2	T38.2X3	T38.2X4	T38.2X5	T38.2X6
Permanganate	T65.891	T65.892	T65.893	T65.894	—	—
(nonmedicinal)						
medicinal	T49.0X1	T49.0X2	T49.0X3	T49.0X4	T49.0X5	T49.0X6
sulfate	T47.2X1	T47.2X2	T47.2X3	T47.2X4	T47.2X5	T47.2X6
Potassium-removing resin	T50.3X1	T50.3X2	T50.3X3	T50.3X4	T50.3X5	T50.3X6
Potassium-retaining drug	T50.3X1	T50.3X2	T50.3X3	T50.3X4	T50.3X5	T50.3X6
Povidone	T45.8X1	T45.8X2	T45.8X3	T45.8X4	T45.8X5	T45.8X6
iodine	T49.0X1	T49.0X2	T49.0X3	T49.0X4	T49.0X5	T49.0X6
Practolol	T44.7X1	T44.7X2	T44.7X3	T44.7X4	T44.7X5	T44.7X6
Prajmalium bitartrate	T46.2X1	T46.2X2	T46.2X3	T46.2X4	T46.2X5	T46.2X6
Pralidoxime (iodide)	T50.6X1	T50.6X2	T50.6X3	T50.6X4	T50.6X5	T50.6X6
chloride	T50.6X1	T50.6X2	T50.6X3	T50.6X4	T50.6X5	T50.6X6
Pramiverine	T44.3X1	T44.3X2	T44.3X3	T44.3X4	T44.3X5	T44.3X6
Pramocaine	T49.1X1	T49.1X2	T49.1X3	T49.1X4	T49.1X5	T49.1X6
Pramoxine	T49.1X1	T49.1X2	T49.1X3	T49.1X4	T49.1X5	T49.1X6
Prasterone	T38.7X1	T38.7X2	T38.7X3	T38.7X4	T38.7X5	T38.7X6
Pravastatin	T46.6X1	T46.6X2	T46.6X3	T46.6X4	T46.6X5	T46.6X6
Prazepam	T42.4X1	T42.4X2	T42.4X3	T42.4X4	T42.4X5	T42.4X6
Praziquantel	T37.4X1	T37.4X2	T37.4X3	T37.4X4	T37.4X5	T37.4X6
Prazitone	T43.291	T43.292	T43.293	T43.294	T43.295	T43.296
Prazosin	T44.6X1	T44.6X2	T44.6X3	T44.6X4	T44.6X5	T44.6X6
Prednicarbate	T49.0X1	T49.0X2	T49.0X3	T49.0X4	T49.0X5	T49.0X6
Prednimustine	T45.1X1	T45.1X2	T45.1X3	T45.1X4	T45.1X5	T45.1X6
Prednisolone	T38.0X1	T38.0X2	T38.0X3	T38.0X4	T38.0X5	T38.0X6
ENT agent	T49.6X1	T49.6X2	T49.6X3	T49.6X4	T49.6X5	T49.6X6
ophthalmic preparation	T49.5X1	T49.5X2	T49.5X3	T49.5X4	T49.5X5	T49.5X6
steaglate	T49.0X1	T49.0X2	T49.0X3	T49.0X4	T49.0X5	T49.0X6
topical NEC	T49.0X1	T49.0X2	T49.0X3	T49.0X4	T49.0X5	T49.0X6
Prednisone	T38.0X1	T38.0X2	T38.0X3	T38.0X4	T38.0X5	T38.0X6
Prednylidene	T38.0X1	T38.0X2	T38.0X3	T38.0X4	T38.0X5	T38.0X6
Pregnandiol	T38.5X1	T38.5X2	T38.5X3	T38.5X4	T38.5X5	T38.5X6
Pregneninolone	T38.5X1	T38.5X2	T38.5X3	T38.5X4	T38.5X5	T38.5X6
Preludin	T43.691	T43.692	T43.693	T43.694	T43.695	T43.696
Premarin	T38.5X1	T38.5X2	T38.5X3	T38.5X4	T38.5X5	T38.5X6
Premedication anesthetic	T41.201	T41.202	T41.203	T41.204	T41.205	T41.206
Prenalterol	T44.5X1	T44.5X2	T44.5X3	T44.5X4	T44.5X5	T44.5X6
Prenoxdiazine	T48.3X1	T48.3X2	T48.3X3	T48.3X4	T48.3X5	T48.3X6
Prenylamine	T46.3X1	T46.3X2	T46.3X3	T46.3X4	T46.3X5	T46.3X6
Preparation H	T49.8X1	T49.8X2	T49.8X3	T49.8X4	T49.8X5	T49.8X6
Preparation, local	T49.4X1	T49.4X2	T49.4X3	T49.4X4	T49.4X5	T49.4X6
Preservative	T65.891	T65.892	T65.893	T65.894	—	—
(nonmedicinal)						
medicinal	T50.901	T50.902	T50.903	T50.904	T50.905	T50.906
wood	T60.91	T60.92	T60.93	T60.94	—	—
Prethcamide	T50.7X1	T50.7X2	T50.7X3	T50.7X4	T50.7X5	T50.7X6
Pride of China	T62.2X1	T62.2X2	T62.2X3	T62.2X4	—	—
Pridinol	T44.3X1	T44.3X2	T44.3X3	T44.3X4	T44.3X5	T44.3X6
Prifinium bromide	T44.3X1	T44.3X2	T44.3X3	T44.3X4	T44.3X5	T44.3X6
Prilocaine	T41.3X1	T41.3X2	T41.3X3	T41.3X4	T41.3X5	T41.3X6
infiltration (subcutaneous)	T41.3X1	T41.3X2	T41.3X3	T41.3X4	T41.3X5	T41.3X6
nerve block (peripheral)	T41.3X1	T41.3X2	T41.3X3	T41.3X4	T41.3X5	T41.3X6
(plexus)						
regional	T41.3X1	T41.3X2	T41.3X3	T41.3X4	T41.3X5	T41.3X6

Substance	Poisoning, Accidental (unintentional)	Poisoning, Intentional Self-harm	Poisoning, Assault	Poisoning, Undetermined	Adverse Effect	Under-dosing
Primaquine	T37.2X1	T37.2X2	T37.2X3	T37.2X4	T37.2X5	T37.2X6
Primidone	T42.6X1	T42.6X2	T42.6X3	T42.6X4	T42.6X5	T42.6X6
Primula (veris)	T62.2X1	T62.2X2	T62.2X3	T62.2X4	—	—
Prinadol	T40.2X1	T40.2X2	T40.2X3	T40.2X4	T40.2X5	T40.2X6
Priscol, Priscoline	T44.6X1	T44.6X2	T44.6X3	T44.6X4	T44.6X5	T44.6X6
Pristinamycin	T36.3X1	T36.3X2	T36.3X3	T36.3X4	T36.3X5	T36.3X6
Privet	T62.2X1	T62.2X2	T62.2X3	T62.2X4	—	—
berries	T62.1X1	T62.1X2	T62.1X3	T62.1X4	—	—
Privine	T44.4X1	T44.4X2	T44.4X3	T44.4X4	T44.4X5	T44.4X6
Pro-Banthine	T44.3X1	T44.3X2	T44.3X3	T44.3X4	T44.3X5	T44.3X6
Probarbital	T42.3X1	T42.3X2	T42.3X3	T42.3X4	T42.3X5	T42.3X6
Probenecid	T50.4X1	T50.4X2	T50.4X3	T50.4X4	T50.4X5	T50.4X6
Probucol	T46.6X1	T46.6X2	T46.6X3	T46.6X4	T46.6X5	T46.6X6
Procainamide	T46.2X1	T46.2X2	T46.2X3	T46.2X4	T46.2X5	T46.2X6
Procaine	T41.3X1	T41.3X2	T41.3X3	T41.3X4	T41.3X5	T41.3X6
benzylpenicillin	T36.0X1	T36.0X2	T36.0X3	T36.0X4	T36.0X5	T36.0X6
nerve block (periphreal) (plexus)	T41.3X1	T41.3X2	T41.3X3	T41.3X4	T41.3X5	T41.3X6
penicillin G	T36.0X1	T36.0X2	T36.0X3	T36.0X4	T36.0X5	T36.0X6
regional	T41.3X1	T41.3X2	T41.3X3	T41.3X4	T41.3X5	T41.3X6
spinal	T41.3X1	T41.3X2	T41.3X3	T41.3X4	T41.3X5	T41.3X6
Procalmidol	T43.591	T43.592	T43.593	T43.594	T43.595	T43.596
Procarbazine	T45.1X1	T45.1X2	T45.1X3	T45.1X4	T45.1X5	T45.1X6
Procaterol	T44.5X1	T44.5X2	T44.5X3	T44.5X4	T44.5X5	T44.5X6
Prochlorperazine	T43.3X1	T43.3X2	T43.3X3	T43.3X4	T43.3X5	T43.3X6
Procyclidine	T44.3X1	T44.3X2	T44.3X3	T44.3X4	T44.3X5	T44.3X6
Producer gas	T58.8X1	T58.8X2	T58.8X3	T58.8X4	—	—
Profadol	T40.4X1	T40.4X2	T40.4X3	T40.4X4	T40.4X5	T40.4X6
Profenamine	T44.3X1	T44.3X2	T44.3X3	T44.3X4	T44.3X5	T44.3X6
Profenil	T44.3X1	T44.3X2	T44.3X3	T44.3X4	T44.3X5	T44.3X6
Proflavine	T49.0X1	T49.0X2	T49.0X3	T49.0X4	T49.0X5	T49.0X6
Progabide	T42.6X1	T42.6X2	T42.6X3	T42.6X4	T42.6X5	T42.6X6
Progesterone	T38.5X1	T38.5X2	T38.5X3	T38.5X4	T38.5X5	T38.5X6
Progestin	T38.5X1	T38.5X2	T38.5X3	T38.5X4	T38.5X5	T38.5X6
oral contraceptive	T38.4X1	T38.4X2	T38.4X3	T38.4X4	T38.4X5	T38.4X6
Progestogen NEC	T38.5X1	T38.5X2	T38.5X3	T38.5X4	T38.5X5	T38.5X6
Progestone	T38.5X1	T38.5X2	T38.5X3	T38.5X4	T38.5X5	T38.5X6
Proglumide	T47.1X1	T47.1X2	T47.1X3	T47.1X4	T47.1X5	T47.1X6
Proguanil	T37.2X1	T37.2X2	T37.2X3	T37.2X4	T37.2X5	T37.2X6
Prolactin	T38.811	T38.812	T38.813	T38.814	T38.815	T38.816
Prolintane	T43.691	T43.692	T43.693	T43.694	T43.695	T43.696
Proloid	T38.1X1	T38.1X2	T38.1X3	T38.1X4	T38.1X5	T38.1X6
Proluton	T38.5X1	T38.5X2	T38.5X3	T38.5X4	T38.5X5	T38.5X6
Promacetin	T37.1X1	T37.1X2	T37.1X3	T37.1X4	T37.1X5	T37.1X6
Promazine	T43.3X1	T43.3X2	T43.3X3	T43.3X4	T43.3X5	T43.3X6
Promedol	T40.2X1	T40.2X2	T40.2X3	T40.2X4	—	—
Promegestone	T38.5X1	T38.5X2	T38.5X3	T38.5X4	T38.5X5	T38.5X6
Promethazine (teoclate)	T43.3X1	T43.3X2	T43.3X3	T43.3X4	T43.3X5	T43.3X6
Promin	T37.1X1	T37.1X2	T37.1X3	T37.1X4	T37.1X5	T37.1X6
Pronase	T45.3X1	T45.3X2	T45.3X3	T45.3X4	T45.3X5	T45.3X6
Pronestyl (hydrochloride)	T46.2X1	T46.2X2	T46.2X3	T46.2X4	T46.2X5	T46.2X6
Pronetalol	T44.7X1	T44.7X2	T44.7X3	T44.7X4	T44.7X5	T44.7X6
Prontosil	T37.0X1	T37.0X2	T37.0X3	T37.0X4	T37.0X5	T37.0X6
Propachlor	T60.3X1	T60.3X2	T60.3X3	T60.3X4	—	—
Propafenone	T46.2X1	T46.2X2	T46.2X3	T46.2X4	T46.2X5	T46.2X6
Propallylonal	T42.3X1	T42.3X2	T42.3X3	T42.3X4	T42.3X5	T42.3X6
Propamidine	T49.0X1	T49.0X2	T49.0X3	T49.0X4	T49.0X5	T49.0X6
Propane (distributed in mobile container)	T59.891	T59.892	T59.893	T59.894	—	—
distributed through pipes	T59.891	T59.892	T59.893	T59.894	—	—
incomplete combustion	T58.11	T58.12	T58.13	T58.14	—	—
Propanidid	T41.291	T41.292	T41.293	T41.294	T41.295	T41.296
Propanil	T60.3X1	T60.3X2	T60.3X3	T60.3X4	—	—
Propantheline	T44.3X1	T44.3X2	T44.3X3	T44.3X4	T44.3X5	T44.3X6
bromide	T44.3X1	T44.3X2	T44.3X3	T44.3X4	T44.3X5	T44.3X6
Proparacaine	T41.3X1	T41.3X2	T41.3X3	T41.3X4	T41.3X5	T41.3X6
Propatylnitrate	T46.3X1	T46.3X2	T46.3X3	T46.3X4	T46.3X5	T46.3X6
Propicillin	T36.0X1	T36.0X2	T36.0X3	T36.0X4	T36.0X5	T36.0X6
Propiolactone	T49.0X1	T49.0X2	T49.0X3	T49.0X4	T49.0X5	T49.0X6
Propiomazine	T45.0X1	T45.0X2	T45.0X3	T45.0X4	T45.0X5	T45.0X6
Propionaldehyde (medicinal)	T42.6X1	T42.6X2	T42.6X3	T42.6X4	T42.6X5	T42.6X6
Propionate (calcium) (sodium)	T49.0X1	T49.0X2	T49.0X3	T49.0X4	T49.0X5	T49.0X6
Propion gel	T49.0X1	T49.0X2	T49.0X3	T49.0X4	T49.0X5	T49.0X6
Propitocaine	T41.3X1	T41.3X2	T41.3X3	T41.3X4	T41.3X5	T41.3X6
infiltration (subcutaneous)	T41.3X1	T41.3X2	T41.3X3	T41.3X4	T41.3X5	T41.3X6
nerve block (peripheral) (plexus)	T41.3X1	T41.3X2	T41.3X3	T41.3X4	T41.3X5	T41.3X6
Propofol	T41.291	T41.292	T41.293	T41.294	T41.295	T41.296
Propoxur	T60.0X1	T60.0X2	T60.0X3	T60.0X4	—	—
Propoxycaine	T41.3X1	T41.3X2	T41.3X3	T41.3X4	T41.3X5	T41.3X6
infiltration (subcutaneous)	T41.3X1	T41.3X2	T41.3X3	T41.3X4	T41.3X5	T41.3X6

Substance	Poisoning, Accidental (unintentional)	Poisoning, Intentional Self-harm	Poisoning, Assault	Poisoning, Undetermined	Adverse Effect	Under-dosing
Propoxycaine — continued						
nerve block (peripheral) (plexus)	T41.3X1	T41.3X2	T41.3X3	T41.3X4	T41.3X5	T41.3
topical (surface)	T41.3X1	T41.3X2	T41.3X3	T41.3X4	T41.3X5	T41.3
Propoxyphene	T40.4X1	T40.4X2	T40.4X3	T40.4X4	T40.4X5	T40.4
Propranolol	T44.7X1	T44.7X2	T44.7X3	T44.7X4	T44.7X5	T44.7
Propyl						
alcohol	T51.3X1	T51.3X2	T51.3X3	T51.3X4	—	—
carbinol	T51.3X1	T51.3X2	T51.3X3	T51.3X4	—	—
hexadrine	T44.4X1	T44.4X2	T44.4X3	T44.4X4	T44.4X5	T44.4
iodone	T50.8X1	T50.8X2	T50.8X3	T50.8X4	T50.8X5	T50.8
thiouracil	T38.2X1	T38.2X2	T38.2X3	T38.2X4	T38.2X5	T38.2
Propylaminophenothiazine	T43.3X1	T43.3X2	T43.3X3	T43.3X4	T43.3X5	T43.3
Propylene	T59.891	T59.892	T59.893	T59.894	—	—
Propylhexedrine	T48.5X1	T48.5X2	T48.5X3	T48.5X4	T48.5X5	T48.5
Propyliodone	T50.8X1	T50.8X2	T50.8X3	T50.8X4	T50.8X5	T50.8
Propylparaben (ophthalmic)	T49.5X1	T49.5X2	T49.5X3	T49.5X4	T49.5X5	T49.5
Propylthiouracil	T38.2X1	T38.2X2	T38.2X3	T38.2X4	T38.2X5	T38.2
Propyphenazone	T39.2X1	T39.2X2	T39.2X3	T39.2X4	T39.2X5	T39.2
Proquazone	T39.391	T39.392	T39.393	T39.394	T39.395	T39.3
Proscillaridin	T46.0X1	T46.0X2	T46.0X3	T46.0X4	T46.0X5	T46.0
Prostacyclin	T45.521	T45.522	T45.523	T45.524	T45.525	T45.5
Prostaglandin (I2)	T45.521	T45.522	T45.523	T45.524	T45.525	T45.5
E1	T46.7X1	T46.7X2	T46.7X3	T46.7X4	T46.7X5	T46.7
E2	T48.0X1	T48.0X2	T48.0X3	T48.0X4	T48.0X5	T48.0
F2 alpha	T48.0X1	T48.0X2	T48.0X3	T48.0X4	T48.0X5	T48.0
Prostigmin	T44.0X1	T44.0X2	T44.0X3	T44.0X4	T44.0X5	T44.0
Prosultiamine	T45.2X1	T45.2X2	T45.2X3	T45.2X4	T45.2X5	T45.2
Protamine sulfate	T45.7X1	T45.7X2	T45.7X3	T45.7X4	T45.7X5	T45.7
zinc insulin	T38.3X1	T38.3X2	T38.3X3	T38.3X4	T38.3X5	T38.3
Protease	T47.5X1	T47.5X2	T47.5X3	T47.5X4	T47.5X5	T47.5
Protectant, skin NEC	T49.3X1	T49.3X2	T49.3X3	T49.3X4	T49.3X5	T49.3
Protein hydrolysate	T50.991	T50.992	T50.993	T50.994	T50.995	T50.9
Prothiaden — see Dothiepin hydrochloride						
Prothionamide	T37.1X1	T37.1X2	T37.1X3	T37.1X4	T37.1X5	T37.1
Prothipendyl	T43.591	T43.592	T43.593	T43.594	T43.595	T43.5
Prothoate	T60.0X1	T60.0X2	T60.0X3	T60.0X4	—	—
Prothrombin						
activator	T45.7X1	T45.7X2	T45.7X3	T45.7X4	T45.7X5	T45.7
synthesis inhibitor	T45.511	T45.512	T45.513	T45.514	T45.515	T45.5
Protionamide	T37.1X1	T37.1X2	T37.1X3	T37.1X4	T37.1X5	T37.1
Protirelin	T38.891	T38.892	T38.893	T38.894	T38.895	T38.8
Protokylol	T48.6X1	T48.6X2	T48.6X3	T48.6X4	T48.6X5	T48.6
Protopam	T50.6X1	T50.6X2	T50.6X3	T50.6X4	T50.6X5	T50.6
Protoveratrine(s) (A) (B)	T46.5X1	T46.5X2	T46.5X3	T46.5X4	T46.5X5	T46.5
Protriptyline	T43.011	T43.012	T43.013	T43.014	T43.015	T43.0
Provera	T38.5X1	T38.5X2	T38.5X3	T38.5X4	T38.5X5	T38.5
Provitamin A	T45.2X1	T45.2X2	T45.2X3	T45.2X4	T45.2X5	T45.2
Proxibarbal	T42.3X1	T42.3X2	T42.3X3	T42.3X4	T42.3X5	T42.3
Proxymetacaine	T41.3X1	T41.3X2	T41.3X3	T41.3X4	T41.3X5	T41.3
Proxyphylline	T48.6X1	T48.6X2	T48.6X3	T48.6X4	T48.6X5	T48.6
Prozac — see Fluoxetine hydrochloride						
Prunus						
laurocerasus	T62.2X1	T62.2X2	T62.2X3	T62.2X4	—	—
virginiana	T62.2X1	T62.2X2	T62.2X3	T62.2X4	—	—
Prussian blue						
commercial	T65.891	T65.892	T65.893	T65.894	—	—
therapeutic	T50.6X1	T50.6X2	T50.6X3	T50.6X4	T50.6X5	T50.6
Prussic acid	T65.0X1	T65.0X2	T65.0X3	T65.0X4	—	—
vapor	T57.3X1	T57.3X2	T57.3X3	T57.3X4	—	—
Pseudoephedrine	T44.991	T44.992	T44.993	T44.994	T44.995	T44.99
Psilocin	T40.991	T40.992	T40.993	T40.994	—	—
Psilocybin	T40.991	T40.992	T40.993	T40.994	—	—
Psilocybine	T40.991	T40.992	T40.993	T40.994	—	—
Psoralene (nonmedicinal)	T65.891	T65.892	T65.893	T65.894	—	—
Psoralens (medicinal)	T50.991	T50.992	T50.993	T50.994	T50.995	T50.9
PSP (phenolsulfonphthalein)	T50.8X1	T50.8X2	T50.8X3	T50.8X4	T50.8X5	T50.8
Psychodysleptic drug NOS	T40.901	T40.902	T40.903	T40.904	T40.905	T40.90
specified NEC	T40.991	T40.992	T40.993	T40.994	T40.995	T40.99
Psychostimulant	T43.601	T43.602	T43.603	T43.604	T43.605	T43.60
amphetamine	T43.621	T43.622	T43.623	T43.624	T43.625	T43.6
caffeine	T43.611	T43.612	T43.613	T43.614	T43.615	T43.6
methylphenidate	T43.631	T43.632	T43.633	T43.634	T43.635	T43.6
specified NEC	T43.691	T43.692	T43.693	T43.694	T43.695	T43.6
Psychotherapeutic drug NEC	T43.91	T43.92	T43.93	T43.94	T43.95	T43.9
antidepressants — see also Antidepressant	T43.201	T43.202	T43.203	T43.204	T43.205	T43.2
specified NEC	T43.8X1	T43.8X2	T43.8X3	T43.8X4	T43.8X5	T43.8

386

Additional Character May Be Required — Refer to the Tabular List for Character Selection   ▽ Subterms under main terms may continue to next column or page

Substance	Poisoning, Accidental (unintentional)	Poisoning, Intentional Self-harm	Poisoning, Assault	Poisoning, Undetermined	Adverse Effect	Under-dosing
Psychotherapeutic drug — *continued*						
tranquilizers NEC	T43.501	T43.502	T43.503	T43.504	T43.505	T43.506
Psychotomimetic agents	T40.901	T40.902	T40.903	T40.904	T40.905	T40.906
Psychotropic drug NEC	T43.91	T43.92	T43.93	T43.94	T43.95	T43.96
specified NEC	T43.8X1	T43.8X2	T43.8X3	T43.8X4	T43.8X5	T43.8X6
Psyllium hydrophilic mucilloid	T47.4X1	T47.4X2	T47.4X3	T47.4X4	T47.4X5	T47.4X6
Pteroylglutamic acid	T45.8X1	T45.8X2	T45.8X3	T45.8X4	T45.8X5	T45.8X6
Pteroyltriglutamate	T45.1X1	T45.1X2	T45.1X3	T45.1X4	T45.1X5	T45.1X6
PTFE — *see* Polytetrafluoroethylene						
Pulp						
devitalizing paste	T49.7X1	T49.7X2	T49.7X3	T49.7X4	T49.7X5	T49.7X6
dressing	T49.7X1	T49.7X2	T49.7X3	T49.7X4	T49.7X5	T49.7X6
Pulsatilla	T62.2X1	T62.2X2	T62.2X3	T62.2X4	—	—
Pumpkin seed extract	T37.4X1	T37.4X2	T37.4X3	T37.4X4	T37.4X5	T37.4X6
Purex (bleach)	T54.91	T54.92	T54.93	T54.94	—	—
Purgative NEC — *see also* Cathartic	T47.4X1	T47.4X2	T47.4X3	T47.4X4	T47.4X5	T47.4X6
Purine analogue (antineoplastic)	T45.1X1	T45.1X2	T45.1X3	T45.1X4	T45.1X5	T45.1X6
Purine diuretics	T50.2X1	T50.2X2	T50.2X3	T50.2X4	T50.2X5	T50.2X6
Purinethol	T45.1X1	T45.1X2	T45.1X3	T45.1X4	T45.1X5	T45.1X6
PVP	T45.8X1	T45.8X2	T45.8X3	T45.8X4	T45.8X5	T45.8X6
Pyrabital	T39.8X1	T39.8X2	T39.8X3	T39.8X4	T39.8X5	T39.8X6
Pyramidon	T39.2X1	T39.2X2	T39.2X3	T39.2X4	T39.2X5	T39.2X6
Pyrantel	T37.4X1	T37.4X2	T37.4X3	T37.4X4	T37.4X5	T37.4X6
Pyrathiazine	T45.0X1	T45.0X2	T45.0X3	T45.0X4	T45.0X5	T45.0X6
Pyrazinamide	T37.1X1	T37.1X2	T37.1X3	T37.1X4	T37.1X5	T37.1X6
Pyrazinoic acid (amide)	T37.1X1	T37.1X2	T37.1X3	T37.1X4	T37.1X5	T37.1X6
Pyrazole (derivatives)	T39.2X1	T39.2X2	T39.2X3	T39.2X4	T39.2X5	T39.2X6
Pyrazolone analgesic NEC	T39.2X1	T39.2X2	T39.2X3	T39.2X4	T39.2X5	T39.2X6
Pyrethrin, pyrethrum (nonmedicinal)	T60.2X1	T60.2X2	T60.2X3	T60.2X4	—	—
Pyrethrum extract	T49.0X1	T49.0X2	T49.0X3	T49.0X4	T49.0X5	T49.0X6
Pyribenzamine	T45.0X1	T45.0X2	T45.0X3	T45.0X4	T45.0X5	T45.0X6
Pyridine	T52.8X1	T52.8X2	T52.8X3	T52.8X4	—	—
aldoxime methiodide	T50.6X1	T50.6X2	T50.6X3	T50.6X4	T50.6X5	T50.6X6
aldoxime methyl chloride	T50.6X1	T50.6X2	T50.6X3	T50.6X4	T50.6X5	T50.6X6
vapor	T59.891	T59.892	T59.893	T59.894	—	—
Pyridium	T39.8X1	T39.8X2	T39.8X3	T39.8X4	T39.8X5	T39.8X6
Pyridostigmine bromide	T44.0X1	T44.0X2	T44.0X3	T44.0X4	T44.0X5	T44.0X6
Pyridoxal phosphate	T45.2X1	T45.2X2	T45.2X3	T45.2X4	T45.2X5	T45.2X6
Pyridoxine	T45.2X1	T45.2X2	T45.2X3	T45.2X4	T45.2X5	T45.2X6
Pyrilamine	T45.0X1	T45.0X2	T45.0X3	T45.0X4	T45.0X5	T45.0X6
Pyrimethamine	T37.2X1	T37.2X2	T37.2X3	T37.2X4	T37.2X5	T37.2X6
with sulfadoxine	T37.2X1	T37.2X2	T37.2X3	T37.2X4	T37.2X5	T37.2X6
Pyrimidine antagonist	T45.1X1	T45.1X2	T45.1X3	T45.1X4	T45.1X5	T45.1X6
Pyriminil	T60.4X1	T60.4X2	T60.4X3	T60.4X4	—	—
Pyrithione zinc	T49.4X1	T49.4X2	T49.4X3	T49.4X4	T49.4X5	T49.4X6
Pyrithyldione	T42.6X1	T42.6X2	T42.6X3	T42.6X4	T42.6X5	T42.6X6
Pyrogallic acid	T49.0X1	T49.0X2	T49.0X3	T49.0X4	T49.0X5	T49.0X6
Pyrogallol	T49.0X1	T49.0X2	T49.0X3	T49.0X4	T49.0X5	T49.0X6
Pyroxylin	T49.3X1	T49.3X2	T49.3X3	T49.3X4	T49.3X5	T49.3X6
Pyrrobutamine	T45.0X1	T45.0X2	T45.0X3	T45.0X4	T45.0X5	T45.0X6
Pyrrolizidine alkaloids	T62.8X1	T62.8X2	T62.8X3	T62.8X4	—	—
Pyrvinium chloride	T37.4X1	T37.4X2	T37.4X3	T37.4X4	T37.4X5	T37.4X6
PZI	T38.3X1	T38.3X2	T38.3X3	T38.3X4	T38.3X5	T38.3X6
Quaalude	T42.6X1	T42.6X2	T42.6X3	T42.6X4	T42.6X5	T42.6X6
Quarternary ammonium						
anti-infective	T49.0X1	T49.0X2	T49.0X3	T49.0X4	T49.0X5	T49.0X6
ganglion blocking	T44.2X1	T44.2X2	T44.2X3	T44.2X4	T44.2X5	T44.2X6
parasympatholytic	T44.3X1	T44.3X2	T44.3X3	T44.3X4	T44.3X5	T44.3X6
Quazepam	T42.4X1	T42.4X2	T42.4X3	T42.4X4	T42.4X5	T42.4X6
Quicklime	T54.3X1	T54.3X2	T54.3X3	T54.3X4	—	—
Quillaja extract	T48.4X1	T48.4X2	T48.4X3	T48.4X4	T48.4X5	T48.4X6
Quinacrine	T37.2X1	T37.2X2	T37.2X3	T37.2X4	T37.2X5	T37.2X6
Quinaglute	T46.2X1	T46.2X2	T46.2X3	T46.2X4	T46.2X5	T46.2X6
Quinalbarbital	T42.3X1	T42.3X2	T42.3X3	T42.3X4	T42.3X5	T42.3X6
Quinalbarbitone sodium	T42.3X1	T42.3X2	T42.3X3	T42.3X4	T42.3X5	T42.3X6
Quinalphos	T60.0X1	T60.0X2	T60.0X3	T60.0X4	—	—
Quinapril	T46.4X1	T46.4X2	T46.4X3	T46.4X4	T46.4X5	T46.4X6
Quinestradiol	T38.5X1	T38.5X2	T38.5X3	T38.5X4	T38.5X5	T38.5X6
Quinestradol	T38.5X1	T38.5X2	T38.5X3	T38.5X4	T38.5X5	T38.5X6
Quinestrol	T38.5X1	T38.5X2	T38.5X3	T38.5X4	T38.5X5	T38.5X6
Quinethazone	T50.2X1	T50.2X2	T50.2X3	T50.2X4	T50.2X5	T50.2X6
Quingestanol	T38.4X1	T38.4X2	T38.4X3	T38.4X4	T38.4X5	T38.4X6
Quinidine	T46.2X1	T46.2X2	T46.2X3	T46.2X4	T46.2X5	T46.2X6
Quinine	T37.2X1	T37.2X2	T37.2X3	T37.2X4	T37.2X5	T37.2X6
Quiniobine	T37.8X1	T37.8X2	T37.8X3	T37.8X4	T37.8X5	T37.8X6
Quinisocaine	T49.1X1	T49.1X2	T49.1X3	T49.1X4	T49.1X5	T49.1X6
Quinocide	T37.2X1	T37.2X2	T37.2X3	T37.2X4	T37.2X5	T37.2X6
Quinoline (derivatives) NEC	T37.8X1	T37.8X2	T37.8X3	T37.8X4	T37.8X5	T37.8X6
Quinupramine	T43.011	T43.012	T43.013	T43.014	T43.015	T43.016
Quotane	T41.3X1	T41.3X2	T41.3X3	T41.3X4	T41.3X5	T41.3X6
Rabies						
immune globulin (human)	T50.Z11	T50.Z12	T50.Z13	T50.Z14	T50.Z15	T50.Z16
vaccine	T50.B91	T50.B92	T50.B93	T50.B94	T50.B95	T50.B96
Racemoramide	T40.2X1	T40.2X2	T40.2X3	T40.2X4	—	—
Racemorphan	T40.2X1	T40.2X2	T40.2X3	T40.2X4	T40.2X5	T40.2X6
Racepinefrin	T44.5X1	T44.5X2	T44.5X3	T44.5X4	T44.5X5	T44.5X6
Raclopride	T43.591	T43.592	T43.593	T43.594	T43.595	T43.596
Radiator alcohol	T51.1X1	T51.1X2	T51.1X3	T51.1X4	—	—
Radioactive drug NEC	T50.8X1	T50.8X2	T50.8X3	T50.8X4	T50.8X5	T50.8X6
Radio-opaque (drugs) (materials)	T50.8X1	T50.8X2	T50.8X3	T50.8X4	T50.8X5	T50.8X6
Ramifenazone	T39.2X1	T39.2X2	T39.2X3	T39.2X4	T39.2X5	T39.2X6
Ramipril	T46.4X1	T46.4X2	T46.4X3	T46.4X4	T46.4X5	T46.4X6
Ranitidine	T47.0X1	T47.0X2	T47.0X3	T47.0X4	T47.0X5	T47.0X6
Ranunculus	T62.2X1	T62.2X2	T62.2X3	T62.2X4	—	—
Rat poison NEC	T60.4X1	T60.4X2	T60.4X3	T60.4X4	—	—
Rattlesnake (venom)	T63.011	T63.012	T63.013	T63.014	—	—
Raubasine	T46.7X1	T46.7X2	T46.7X3	T46.7X4	T46.7X5	T46.7X6
Raudixin	T46.5X1	T46.5X2	T46.5X3	T46.5X4	T46.5X5	T46.5X6
Rautensin	T46.5X1	T46.5X2	T46.5X3	T46.5X4	T46.5X5	T46.5X6
Rautina	T46.5X1	T46.5X2	T46.5X3	T46.5X4	T46.5X5	T46.5X6
Rautotal	T46.5X1	T46.5X2	T46.5X3	T46.5X4	T46.5X5	T46.5X6
Rauwiloid	T46.5X1	T46.5X2	T46.5X3	T46.5X4	T46.5X5	T46.5X6
Rauwoldin	T46.5X1	T46.5X2	T46.5X3	T46.5X4	T46.5X5	T46.5X6
Rauwolfia (alkaloids)	T46.5X1	T46.5X2	T46.5X3	T46.5X4	T46.5X5	T46.5X6
Razoxane	T45.1X1	T45.1X2	T45.1X3	T45.1X4	T45.1X5	T45.1X6
Realgar	T57.0X1	T57.0X2	T57.0X3	T57.0X4	—	—
Recombinant (R) — *see specific* protein						
Red blood cells, packed	T45.8X1	T45.8X2	T45.8X3	T45.8X4	T45.8X5	T45.8X6
Red squill (scilliroside)	T60.4X1	T60.4X2	T60.4X3	T60.4X4	—	—
Reducing agent, industrial NEC	T65.891	T65.892	T65.893	T65.894	—	—
Refrigerant gas (chlorofluorocarbon)	T53.5X1	T53.5X2	T53.5X3	T53.5X4	—	—
not chlorofluorocarbon	T59.891	T59.892	T59.893	T59.894	—	—
Regroton	T50.2X1	T50.2X2	T50.2X3	T50.2X4	T50.2X5	T50.2X6
Rehydration salts (oral)	T50.3X1	T50.3X2	T50.3X3	T50.3X4	T50.3X5	T50.3X6
Rela	T42.8X1	T42.8X2	T42.8X3	T42.8X4	T42.8X5	T42.8X6
Relaxant, muscle						
anesthetic	T48.1X1	T48.1X2	T48.1X3	T48.1X4	T48.1X5	T48.1X6
central nervous system	T42.8X1	T42.8X2	T42.8X3	T42.8X4	T42.8X5	T42.8X6
skeletal NEC	T48.1X1	T48.1X2	T48.1X3	T48.1X4	T48.1X5	T48.1X6
smooth NEC	T44.3X1	T44.3X2	T44.3X3	T44.3X4	T44.3X5	T44.3X6
Remoxipride	T43.591	T43.592	T43.593	T43.594	T43.595	T43.596
Renese	T50.2X1	T50.2X2	T50.2X3	T50.2X4	T50.2X5	T50.2X6
Renografin	T50.8X1	T50.8X2	T50.8X3	T50.8X4	T50.8X5	T50.8X6
Replacement solution	T50.3X1	T50.3X2	T50.3X3	T50.3X4	T50.3X5	T50.3X6
Reproterol	T48.6X1	T48.6X2	T48.6X3	T48.6X4	T48.6X5	T48.6X6
Rescinnamine	T46.5X1	T46.5X2	T46.5X3	T46.5X4	T46.5X5	T46.5X6
Reserpin (e)	T46.5X1	T46.5X2	T46.5X3	T46.5X4	T46.5X5	T46.5X6
Resorcin, resorcinol (nonmedicinal)	T65.891	T65.892	T65.893	T65.894	—	—
medicinal	T49.4X1	T49.4X2	T49.4X3	T49.4X4	T49.4X5	T49.4X6
Respaire	T48.4X1	T48.4X2	T48.4X3	T48.4X4	T48.4X5	T48.4X6
Respiratory drug NEC	T48.901	T48.902	T48.903	T48.904	T48.905	T48.906
antiasthmatic NEC	T48.6X1	T48.6X2	T48.6X3	T48.6X4	T48.6X5	T48.6X6
anti-common-cold NEC	T48.5X1	T48.5X2	T48.5X3	T48.5X4	T48.5X5	T48.5X6
expectorant NEC	T48.4X1	T48.4X2	T48.4X3	T48.4X4	T48.4X5	T48.4X6
stimulant	T48.901	T48.902	T48.903	T48.904	T48.905	T48.906
Retinoic acid	T49.0X1	T49.0X2	T49.0X3	T49.0X4	T49.0X5	T49.0X6
Retinol	T45.2X1	T45.2X2	T45.2X3	T45.2X4	T45.2X5	T45.2X6
Rh (D) immune globulin (human)	T50.Z11	T50.Z12	T50.Z13	T50.Z14	T50.Z15	T50.Z16
Rhodine	T39.011	T39.012	T39.013	T39.014	T39.015	T39.016
RhoGAM	T50.Z11	T50.Z12	T50.Z13	T50.Z14	T50.Z15	T50.Z16
Rhubarb						
dry extract	T47.2X1	T47.2X2	T47.2X3	T47.2X4	T47.2X5	T47.2X6
tincture, compound	T47.2X1	T47.2X2	T47.2X3	T47.2X4	T47.2X5	T47.2X6
Ribavirin	T37.5X1	T37.5X2	T37.5X3	T37.5X4	T37.5X5	T37.5X6
Riboflavin	T45.2X1	T45.2X2	T45.2X3	T45.2X4	T45.2X5	T45.2X6
Ribostamycin	T36.5X1	T36.5X2	T36.5X3	T36.5X4	T36.5X5	T36.5X6
Ricin	T62.2X1	T62.2X2	T62.2X3	T62.2X4	—	—
Ricinus communis	T62.2X1	T62.2X2	T62.2X3	T62.2X4	—	—
Rickettsial vaccine NEC	T50.A91	T50.A92	T50.A93	T50.A94	T50.A95	T50.A96
Rifabutin	T36.6X1	T36.6X2	T36.6X3	T36.6X4	T36.6X5	T36.6X6
Rifamide	T36.6X1	T36.6X2	T36.6X3	T36.6X4	T36.6X5	T36.6X6
Rifampicin	T36.6X1	T36.6X2	T36.6X3	T36.6X4	T36.6X5	T36.6X6
with isoniazid	T37.1X1	T37.1X2	T37.1X3	T37.1X4	T37.1X5	T37.1X6
Rifampin	T36.6X1	T36.6X2	T36.6X3	T36.6X4	T36.6X5	T36.6X6

Substance	Poisoning, Accidental (unintentional)	Poisoning, Intentional Self-harm	Poisoning, Assault	Poisoning, Undetermined	Adverse Effect	Under-dosing
Rifamycin	T36.6X1	T36.6X2	T36.6X3	T36.6X4	T36.6X5	T36.6X6
Rifaximin	T36.6X1	T36.6X2	T36.6X3	T36.6X4	T36.6X5	T36.6X6
Rimantadine	T37.5X1	T37.5X2	T37.5X3	T37.5X4	T37.5X5	T37.5X6
Rimazolium metilsulfate	T39.8X1	T39.8X2	T39.8X3	T39.8X4	T39.8X5	T39.8X6
Rimifon	T37.1X1	T37.1X2	T37.1X3	T37.1X4	T37.1X5	T37.1X6
Rimiterol	T48.6X1	T48.6X2	T48.6X3	T48.6X4	T48.6X5	T48.6X6
Ringer (lactate) solution	T50.3X1	T50.3X2	T50.3X3	T50.3X4	T50.3X5	T50.3X6
Ristocetin	T36.8X1	T36.8X2	T36.8X3	T36.8X4	T36.8X5	T36.8X6
Ritalin	T43.631	T43.632	T43.633	T43.634	T43.635	T43.636
Ritodrine	T44.5X1	T44.5X2	T44.5X3	T44.5X4	T44.5X5	T44.5X6
Roach killer — see Insecticide						
Rociverine	T44.3X1	T44.3X2	T44.3X3	T44.3X4	T44.3X5	T44.3X6
Rocky Mountain spotted fever vaccine	T50.A91	T50.A92	T50.A93	T50.A94	T50.A95	T50.A96
Rodenticide NEC	T60.4X1	T60.4X2	T60.4X3	T60.4X4	—	—
Rohypnol	T42.4X1	T42.4X2	T42.4X3	T42.4X4	T42.4X5	T42.4X6
Rokitamycin	T36.3X1	T36.3X2	T36.3X3	T36.3X4	T36.3X5	T36.3X6
Rolaids	T47.1X1	T47.1X2	T47.1X3	T47.1X4	T47.1X5	T47.1X6
Rolitetracycline	T36.4X1	T36.4X2	T36.4X3	T36.4X4	T36.4X5	T36.4X6
Romilar	T48.3X1	T48.3X2	T48.3X3	T48.3X4	T48.3X5	T48.3X6
Ronifibrate	T46.6X1	T46.6X2	T46.6X3	T46.6X4	T46.6X5	T46.6X6
Rosaprostol	T47.1X1	T47.1X2	T47.1X3	T47.1X4	T47.1X5	T47.1X6
Rose bengal sodium (131I)	T50.8X1	T50.8X2	T50.8X3	T50.8X4	T50.8X5	T50.8X6
Rose water ointment	T49.3X1	T49.3X2	T49.3X3	T49.3X4	T49.3X5	T49.3X6
Rosoxacin	T37.8X1	T37.8X2	T37.8X3	T37.8X4	T37.8X5	T37.8X6
Rotenone	T60.2X1	T60.2X2	T60.2X3	T60.2X4	—	—
Rotoxamine	T45.0X1	T45.0X2	T45.0X3	T45.0X4	T45.0X5	T45.0X6
Rough-on-rats	T60.4X1	T60.4X2	T60.4X3	T60.4X4	—	—
Roxatidine	T47.0X1	T47.0X2	T47.0X3	T47.0X4	T47.0X5	T47.0X6
Roxithromycin	T36.3X1	T36.3X2	T36.3X3	T36.3X4	T36.3X5	T36.3X6
Rt-PA	T45.611	T45.612	T45.613	T45.614	T45.615	T45.616
Rubbing alcohol	T51.2X1	T51.2X2	T51.2X3	T51.2X4	—	—
Rubefacient	T49.4X1	T49.4X2	T49.4X3	T49.4X4	T49.4X5	T49.4X6
Rubella vaccine	T50.B91	T50.B92	T50.B93	T50.B94	T50.B95	T50.B96
Rubeola vaccine	T50.B91	T50.B92	T50.B93	T50.B94	T50.B95	T50.B96
Rubidium chloride Rb82	T50.8X1	T50.8X2	T50.8X3	T50.8X4	T50.8X5	T50.8X6
Rubidomycin	T45.1X1	T45.1X2	T45.1X3	T45.1X4	T45.1X5	T45.1X6
Rue	T62.2X1	T62.2X2	T62.2X3	T62.2X4	—	—
Rufocromomycin	T45.1X1	T45.1X2	T45.1X3	T45.1X4	T45.1X5	T45.1X6
Russel's viper venin	T45.7X1	T45.7X2	T45.7X3	T45.7X4	T45.7X5	T45.7X6
Ruta (graveolens)	T62.2X1	T62.2X2	T62.2X3	T62.2X4	—	—
Rutinum	T46.991	T46.992	T46.993	T46.994	T46.995	T46.996
Rutoside	T46.991	T46.992	T46.993	T46.994	T46.995	T46.996
b-sitosterol(s)	T46.6X1	T46.6X2	T46.6X3	T46.6X4	T46.6X5	T46.6X6
Sabadilla (plant)	T62.2X1	T62.2X2	T62.2X3	T62.2X4	—	—
pesticide	T60.2X1	T60.2X2	T60.2X3	T60.2X4	—	—
Saccharated iron oxide	T45.8X1	T45.8X2	T45.8X3	T45.8X4	T45.8X5	T45.8X6
Saccharin	T50.901	T50.902	T50.903	T50.904	T50.905	T50.906
Saccharomyces boulardii	T47.6X1	T47.6X2	T47.6X3	T47.6X4	T47.6X5	T47.6X6
Safflower oil	T46.6X1	T46.6X2	T46.6X3	T46.6X4	T46.6X5	T46.6X6
Safrazine	T43.1X1	T43.1X2	T43.1X3	T43.1X4	T43.1X5	T43.1X6
Salazosulfapyridine	T37.0X1	T37.0X2	T37.0X3	T37.0X4	T37.0X5	T37.0X6
Salbutamol	T48.6X1	T48.6X2	T48.6X3	T48.6X4	T48.6X5	T48.6X6
Salicylamide	T39.091	T39.092	T39.093	T39.094	T39.095	T39.096
Salicylate NEC	T39.091	T39.092	T39.093	T39.094	T39.095	T39.096
methyl	T49.3X1	T49.3X2	T49.3X3	T49.3X4	T49.3X5	T49.3X6
theobromine calcium	T50.2X1	T50.2X2	T50.2X3	T50.2X4	T50.2X5	T50.2X6
Salicylazosulfapyridine	T37.0X1	T37.0X2	T37.0X3	T37.0X4	T37.0X5	T37.0X6
Salicylhydroxamic acid	T49.0X1	T49.0X2	T49.0X3	T49.0X4	T49.0X5	T49.0X6
Salicylic acid	T49.4X1	T49.4X2	T49.4X3	T49.4X4	T49.4X5	T49.4X6
with benzoic acid	T49.4X1	T49.4X2	T49.4X3	T49.4X4	T49.4X5	T49.4X6
congeners	T39.091	T39.092	T39.093	T39.094	T39.095	T39.096
derivative	T39.091	T39.092	T39.093	T39.094	T39.095	T39.096
salts	T39.091	T39.092	T39.093	T39.094	T39.095	T39.096
Salinazid	T37.1X1	T37.1X2	T37.1X3	T37.1X4	T37.1X5	T37.1X6
Salmeterol	T48.6X1	T48.6X2	T48.6X3	T48.6X4	T48.6X5	T48.6X6
Salol	T49.3X1	T49.3X2	T49.3X3	T49.3X4	T49.3X5	T49.3X6
Salsalate	T39.091	T39.092	T39.093	T39.094	T39.095	T39.096
Salt-replacing drug	T50.901	T50.902	T50.903	T50.904	T50.905	T50.906
Salt-retaining mineralocorticoid	T50.0X1	T50.0X2	T50.0X3	T50.0X4	T50.0X5	T50.0X6
Salt substitute	T50.901	T50.902	T50.903	T50.904	T50.905	T50.906
Saluretic NEC	T50.2X1	T50.2X2	T50.2X3	T50.2X4	T50.2X5	T50.2X6
Saluron	T50.2X1	T50.2X2	T50.2X3	T50.2X4	T50.2X5	T50.2X6
Salvarsan 606 (neosilver) (silver)	T37.8X1	T37.8X2	T37.8X3	T37.8X4	T37.8X5	T37.8X6
Sambucus canadensis	T62.2X1	T62.2X2	T62.2X3	T62.2X4	—	—
berry	T62.1X1	T62.1X2	T62.1X3	T62.1X4	—	—
Sandril	T46.5X1	T46.5X2	T46.5X3	T46.5X4	T46.5X5	T46.5X6
Sanguinaria canadensis	T62.2X1	T62.2X2	T62.2X3	T62.2X4	—	—
Saniflush (cleaner)	T54.2X1	T54.2X2	T54.2X3	T54.2X4	—	—
Santonin	T37.4X1	T37.4X2	T37.4X3	T37.4X4	T37.4X5	T37.4X6
Santyl	T49.8X1	T49.8X2	T49.8X3	T49.8X4	T49.8X5	T49.8X6

Substance	Poisoning, Accidental (unintentional)	Poisoning, Intentional Self-harm	Poisoning, Assault	Poisoning, Undetermined	Adverse Effect	Under-dosing
Saralasin	T46.5X1	T46.5X2	T46.5X3	T46.5X4	T46.5X5	T46.5
Sarcolysin	T45.1X1	T45.1X2	T45.1X3	T45.1X4	T45.1X5	T45.1
Sarkomycin	T45.1X1	T45.1X2	T45.1X3	T45.1X4	T45.1X5	T45.1
Saroten	T43.011	T43.012	T43.013	T43.014	T43.015	T43.0
Saturnine — see Lead						
Savin (oil)	T49.4X1	T49.4X2	T49.4X3	T49.4X4	T49.4X5	T49.4
Scammony	T47.2X1	T47.2X2	T47.2X3	T47.2X4	T47.2X5	T47.2
Scarlet red	T49.8X1	T49.8X2	T49.8X3	T49.8X4	T49.8X5	T49.8
Scheele's green	T57.0X1	T57.0X2	T57.0X3	T57.0X4	—	—
insecticide	T57.0X1	T57.0X2	T57.0X3	T57.0X4	—	—
Schizontozide (blood) (tissue)	T37.2X1	T37.2X2	T37.2X3	T37.2X4	T37.2X5	T37.2
Schradan	T60.0X1	T60.0X2	T60.0X3	T60.0X4	—	—
Schweinfurth green	T57.0X1	T57.0X2	T57.0X3	T57.0X4	—	—
insecticide	T57.0X1	T57.0X2	T57.0X3	T57.0X4	—	—
Scilla, rat poison	T60.4X1	T60.4X2	T60.4X3	T60.4X4	—	—
Scillaren	T60.4X1	T60.4X2	T60.4X3	T60.4X4	—	—
Sclerosing agent	T46.8X1	T46.8X2	T46.8X3	T46.8X4	T46.8X5	T46.8
Scombrotoxin	T61.11	T61.12	T61.13	T61.14	—	—
Scopolamine	T44.3X1	T44.3X2	T44.3X3	T44.3X4	T44.3X5	T44.3
Scopolia extract	T44.3X1	T44.3X2	T44.3X3	T44.3X4	T44.3X5	T44.3
Scouring powder	T65.891	T65.892	T65.893	T65.894	—	—
Sea						
anemone (sting)	T63.631	T63.632	T63.633	T63.634	—	—
cucumber (sting)	T63.691	T63.692	T63.693	T63.694	—	—
snake (bite) (venom)	T63.091	T63.092	T63.093	T63.094	—	—
urchin spine (puncture)	T63.691	T63.692	T63.693	T63.694	—	—
Seafood	T61.91	T61.92	T61.93	T61.94	—	—
specified NEC	T61.8X1	T61.8X2	T61.8X3	T61.8X4	—	—
Secbutabarbital	T42.3X1	T42.3X2	T42.3X3	T42.3X4	T42.3X5	T42.3
Secbutabarbitone	T42.3X1	T42.3X2	T42.3X3	T42.3X4	T42.3X5	T42.3
Secnidazole	T37.3X1	T37.3X2	T37.3X3	T37.3X4	T37.3X5	T37.3
Secobarbital	T42.3X1	T42.3X2	T42.3X3	T42.3X4	T42.3X5	T42.3
Seconal	T42.3X1	T42.3X2	T42.3X3	T42.3X4	T42.3X5	T42.3
Secretin	T50.8X1	T50.8X2	T50.8X3	T50.8X4	T50.8X5	T50.8
Sedative NEC	T42.71	T42.72	T42.73	T42.74	T42.75	T42.
mixed NEC	T42.6X1	T42.6X2	T42.6X3	T42.6X4	T42.6X5	T42.6
Sedormid	T42.6X1	T42.6X2	T42.6X3	T42.6X4	T42.6X5	T42.6
Seed disinfectant or dressing	T60.8X1	T60.8X2	T60.8X3	T60.8X4	—	—
Seeds (poisonous)	T62.2X1	T62.2X2	T62.2X3	T62.2X4	—	—
Selegiline	T42.8X1	T42.8X2	T42.8X3	T42.8X4	T42.8X5	T42.8
Selenium NEC	T56.891	T56.892	T56.893	T56.894	—	—
disulfide or sulfide	T49.4X1	T49.4X2	T49.4X3	T49.4X4	T49.4X5	T49.4
fumes	T59.891	T59.892	T59.893	T59.894	—	—
sulfide	T49.4X1	T49.4X2	T49.4X3	T49.4X4	T49.4X5	T49.4
Selenomethionine (75Se)	T50.8X1	T50.8X2	T50.8X3	T50.8X4	T50.8X5	T50.8
Selsun	T49.4X1	T49.4X2	T49.4X3	T49.4X4	T49.4X5	T49.4
Semustine	T45.1X1	T45.1X2	T45.1X3	T45.1X4	T45.1X5	T45.1
Senega syrup	T48.4X1	T48.4X2	T48.4X3	T48.4X4	T48.4X5	T48.4
Senna	T47.2X1	T47.2X2	T47.2X3	T47.2X4	T47.2X5	T47.2
Sennoside A+B	T47.2X1	T47.2X2	T47.2X3	T47.2X4	T47.2X5	T47.2
Septisol	T49.2X1	T49.2X2	T49.2X3	T49.2X4	T49.2X5	T49.2
Seractide	T38.811	T38.812	T38.813	T38.814	T38.815	T38.8
Serax	T42.4X1	T42.4X2	T42.4X3	T42.4X4	T42.4X5	T42.4
Serenesil	T42.6X1	T42.6X2	T42.6X3	T42.6X4	T42.6X5	T42.6
Serenium (hydrochloride)	T37.91	T37.92	T37.93	T37.94	T37.95	T37.9
Serepax — see Oxazepam						
Sermorelin	T38.891	T38.892	T38.893	T38.894	T38.895	T38.8
Sernyl	T41.1X1	T41.1X2	T41.1X3	T41.1X4	T41.1X5	T41.1
Serotonin	T50.991	T50.992	T50.993	T50.994	T50.995	T50.9
Serpasil	T46.5X1	T46.5X2	T46.5X3	T46.5X4	T46.5X5	T46.5
Serrapeptase	T45.3X1	T45.3X2	T45.3X3	T45.3X4	T45.3X5	T45.3
Serum						
antibotulinus	T50.Z11	T50.Z12	T50.Z13	T50.Z14	T50.Z15	T50.Z
anticytotoxic	T50.Z11	T50.Z12	T50.Z13	T50.Z14	T50.Z15	T50.Z
antidiphtheria	T50.Z11	T50.Z12	T50.Z13	T50.Z14	T50.Z15	T50.Z
antimeningococcus	T50.Z11	T50.Z12	T50.Z13	T50.Z14	T50.Z15	T50.Z
anti-Rh	T50.Z11	T50.Z12	T50.Z13	T50.Z14	T50.Z15	T50.Z
anti-snake-bite	T50.Z11	T50.Z12	T50.Z13	T50.Z14	T50.Z15	T50.Z
antitetanic	T50.Z11	T50.Z12	T50.Z13	T50.Z14	T50.Z15	T50.Z
antitoxic	T50.Z11	T50.Z12	T50.Z13	T50.Z14	T50.Z15	T50.Z
complement (inhibitor)	T45.8X1	T45.8X2	T45.8X3	T45.8X4	T45.8X5	T45.8
convalescent	T50.Z11	T50.Z12	T50.Z13	T50.Z14	T50.Z15	T50.Z
hemolytic complement	T45.8X1	T45.8X2	T45.8X3	T45.8X4	T45.8X5	T45.8
immune (human)	T50.Z11	T50.Z12	T50.Z13	T50.Z14	T50.Z15	T50.Z
protective NEC	T50.Z11	T50.Z12	T50.Z13	T50.Z14	T50.Z15	T50.Z
Setastine	T45.0X1	T45.0X2	T45.0X3	T45.0X4	T45.0X5	T45.0
Setoperone	T43.591	T43.592	T43.593	T43.594	T43.595	T43.5
Sewer gas	T59.91	T59.92	T59.93	T59.94	—	—
Shampoo	T55.0X1	T55.0X2	T55.0X3	T55.0X4	—	—
Shellfish, noxious, nonbacterial	T61.781	T61.782	T61.783	T61.784	—	—

Additional Character May Be Required — Refer to the Tabular List for Character Selection ▽ Subterms under main terms may continue to next column or page

Substance	Poisoning, Accidental (unintentional)	Poisoning, Intentional Self-harm	Poisoning, Assault	Poisoning, Undetermined	Adverse Effect	Under-dosing
Sildenafil	T46.7X1	T46.7X2	T46.7X3	T46.7X4	T46.7X5	T46.7X6
Silibinin	T50.991	T50.992	T50.993	T50.994	T50.995	T50.996
Silicone NEC	T65.891	T65.892	T65.893	T65.894	—	—
medicinal	T49.3X1	T49.3X2	T49.3X3	T49.3X4	T49.3X5	T49.3X6
Silvadene	T49.0X1	T49.0X2	T49.0X3	T49.0X4	T49.0X5	T49.0X6
Silver	T49.0X1	T49.0X2	T49.0X3	T49.0X4	T49.0X5	T49.0X6
anti-infectives	T49.0X1	T49.0X2	T49.0X3	T49.0X4	T49.0X5	T49.0X6
arsphenamine	T37.8X1	T37.8X2	T37.8X3	T37.8X4	T37.8X5	T37.8X6
colloidal	T49.0X1	T49.0X2	T49.0X3	T49.0X4	T49.0X5	T49.0X6
nitrate	T49.0X1	T49.0X2	T49.0X3	T49.0X4	T49.0X5	T49.0X6
ophthalmic preparation	T49.5X1	T49.5X2	T49.5X3	T49.5X4	T49.5X5	T49.5X6
toughened (keratolytic)	T49.4X1	T49.4X2	T49.4X3	T49.4X4	T49.4X5	T49.4X6
nonmedicinal (dust)	T56.891	T56.892	T56.893	T56.894	—	—
protein	T49.5X1	T49.5X2	T49.5X3	T49.5X4	T49.5X5	T49.5X6
salvarsan	T37.8X1	T37.8X2	T37.8X3	T37.8X4	T37.8X5	T37.8X6
sulfadiazine	T49.4X1	T49.4X2	T49.4X3	T49.4X4	T49.4X5	T49.4X6
Silymarin	T50.991	T50.992	T50.993	T50.994	T50.995	T50.996
Simaldrate	T47.1X1	T47.1X2	T47.1X3	T47.1X4	T47.1X5	T47.1X6
Simazine	T60.3X1	T60.3X2	T60.3X3	T60.3X4	—	—
Simethicone	T47.1X1	T47.1X2	T47.1X3	T47.1X4	T47.1X5	T47.1X6
Simfibrate	T46.6X1	T46.6X2	T46.6X3	T46.6X4	T46.6X5	T46.6X6
Simvastatin	T46.6X1	T46.6X2	T46.6X3	T46.6X4	T46.6X5	T46.6X6
Sincalide	T50.8X1	T50.8X2	T50.8X3	T50.8X4	T50.8X5	T50.8X6
Sinequan	T43.011	T43.012	T43.013	T43.014	T43.015	T43.016
Singoserp	T46.5X1	T46.5X2	T46.5X3	T46.5X4	T46.5X5	T46.5X6
Sintrom	T45.511	T45.512	T45.513	T45.514	T45.515	T45.516
Sisomicin	T36.5X1	T36.5X2	T36.5X3	T36.5X4	T36.5X5	T36.5X6
Sitosterols	T46.6X1	T46.6X2	T46.6X3	T46.6X4	T46.6X5	T46.6X6
Skeletal muscle relaxants	T48.1X1	T48.1X2	T48.1X3	T48.1X4	T48.1X5	T48.1X6
Skin						
agents (external)	T49.91	T49.92	T49.93	T49.94	T49.95	T49.96
specified NEC	T49.8X1	T49.8X2	T49.8X3	T49.8X4	T49.8X5	T49.8X6
test antigen	T50.8X1	T50.8X2	T50.8X3	T50.8X4	T50.8X5	T50.8X6
Sleep-eze	T45.0X1	T45.0X2	T45.0X3	T45.0X4	T45.0X5	T45.0X6
Sleeping draught, pill	T42.71	T42.72	T42.73	T42.74	T42.75	T42.76
Smallpox vaccine	T50.B11	T50.B12	T50.B13	T50.B14	T50.B15	T50.B16
Smelter fumes NEC	T56.91	T56.92	T56.93	T56.94	—	—
Smog	T59.1X1	T59.1X2	T59.1X3	T59.1X4	—	—
Smoke NEC	T59.811	T59.812	T59.813	T59.814	—	—
Smooth muscle relaxant	T44.3X1	T44.3X2	T44.3X3	T44.3X4	T44.3X5	T44.3X6
Snail killer NEC	T60.8X1	T60.8X2	T60.8X3	T60.8X4	—	—
Snake venom or bite	T63.001	T63.002	T63.003	T63.004	—	—
hemocoagulase	T45.7X1	T45.7X2	T45.7X3	T45.7X4	T45.7X5	T45.7X6
Snuff	T65.211	T65.212	T65.213	T65.214	—	—
Soap (powder) (product)	T55.0X1	T55.0X2	T55.0X3	T55.0X4	—	—
enema	T47.4X1	T47.4X2	T47.4X3	T47.4X4	T47.4X5	T47.4X6
medicinal, soft	T49.2X1	T49.2X2	T49.2X3	T49.2X4	T49.2X5	T49.2X6
superfatted	T49.2X1	T49.2X2	T49.2X3	T49.2X4	T49.2X5	T49.2X6
Sobrerol	T48.4X1	T48.4X2	T48.4X3	T48.4X4	T48.4X5	T48.4X6
Soda (caustic)	T54.3X1	T54.3X2	T54.3X3	T54.3X4	—	—
bicarb	T47.1X1	T47.1X2	T47.1X3	T47.1X4	T47.1X5	T47.1X6
chlorinated — *see* Sodium, hypochlorite						
Sodium						
acetosulfone	T37.1X1	T37.1X2	T37.1X3	T37.1X4	T37.1X5	T37.1X6
acetrizoate	T50.8X1	T50.8X2	T50.8X3	T50.8X4	T50.8X5	T50.8X6
acid phosphate	T50.3X1	T50.3X2	T50.3X3	T50.3X4	T50.3X5	T50.3X6
alginate	T47.8X1	T47.8X2	T47.8X3	T47.8X4	T47.8X5	T47.8X6
amidotrizoate	T50.8X1	T50.8X2	T50.8X3	T50.8X4	T50.8X5	T50.8X6
aminopterin	T45.1X1	T45.1X2	T45.1X3	T45.1X4	T45.1X5	T45.1X6
amylosulfate	T47.8X1	T47.8X2	T47.8X3	T47.8X4	T47.8X5	T47.8X6
amytal	T42.3X1	T42.3X2	T42.3X3	T42.3X4	T42.3X5	T42.3X6
antimony gluconate	T37.3X1	T37.3X2	T37.3X3	T37.3X4	T37.3X5	T37.3X6
arsenate	T57.0X1	T57.0X2	T57.0X3	T57.0X4	—	—
aurothiomalate	T39.4X1	T39.4X2	T39.4X3	T39.4X4	T39.4X5	T39.4X6
aurothiosulfate	T39.4X1	T39.4X2	T39.4X3	T39.4X4	T39.4X5	T39.4X6
barbiturate	T42.3X1	T42.3X2	T42.3X3	T42.3X4	T42.3X5	T42.3X6
basic phosphate	T47.4X1	T47.4X2	T47.4X3	T47.4X4	T47.4X5	T47.4X6
bicarbonate	T47.1X1	T47.1X2	T47.1X3	T47.1X4	T47.1X5	T47.1X6
bichromate	T57.8X1	T57.8X2	T57.8X3	T57.8X4	—	—
biphosphate	T50.3X1	T50.3X2	T50.3X3	T50.3X4	T50.3X5	T50.3X6
bisulfate	T65.891	T65.892	T65.893	T65.894	—	—
borate						
cleanser	T57.8X1	T57.8X2	T57.8X3	T57.8X4	—	—
eye	T49.5X1	T49.5X2	T49.5X3	T49.5X4	T49.5X5	T49.5X6
therapeutic	T49.8X1	T49.8X2	T49.8X3	T49.8X4	T49.8X5	T49.8X6
bromide	T42.6X1	T42.6X2	T42.6X3	T42.6X4	T42.6X5	T42.6X6
cacodylate (nonmedicinal) NEC	T50.8X1	T50.8X2	T50.8X3	T50.8X4	T50.8X5	T50.8X6
anti-infective	T37.8X1	T37.8X2	T37.8X3	T37.8X4	T37.8X5	T37.8X6
herbicide	T60.3X1	T60.3X2	T60.3X3	T60.3X4	—	—
calcium edetate	T45.8X1	T45.8X2	T45.8X3	T45.8X4	T45.8X5	T45.8X6
carbonate NEC	T54.3X1	T54.3X2	T54.3X3	T54.3X4	—	—

Substance	Poisoning, Accidental (unintentional)	Poisoning, Intentional Self-harm	Poisoning, Assault	Poisoning, Undetermined	Adverse Effect	Under-dosing
Sodium — *continued*						
chlorate NEC	T65.891	T65.892	T65.893	T65.894	—	—
herbicide	T54.91	T54.92	T54.93	T54.94	—	—
chloride	T50.3X1	T50.3X2	T50.3X3	T50.3X4	T50.3X5	T50.3X6
with glucose	T50.3X1	T50.3X2	T50.3X3	T50.3X4	T50.3X5	T50.3X6
chromate	T65.891	T65.892	T65.893	T65.894	—	—
citrate	T50.991	T50.992	T50.993	T50.994	T50.995	T50.996
cromoglicate	T48.6X1	T48.6X2	T48.6X3	T48.6X4	T48.6X5	T48.6X6
cyanide	T65.0X1	T65.0X2	T65.0X3	T65.0X4	—	—
cyclamate	T50.3X1	T50.3X2	T50.3X3	T50.3X4	T50.3X5	T50.3X6
dehydrocholate	T45.8X1	T45.8X2	T45.8X3	T45.8X4	T45.8X5	T45.8X6
diatrizoate	T50.8X1	T50.8X2	T50.8X3	T50.8X4	T50.8X5	T50.8X6
dibunate	T48.4X1	T48.4X2	T48.4X3	T48.4X4	T48.4X5	T48.4X6
dioctyl sulfosuccinate	T47.4X1	T47.4X2	T47.4X3	T47.4X4	T47.4X5	T47.4X6
dipantoyl ferrate	T45.8X1	T45.8X2	T45.8X3	T45.8X4	T45.8X5	T45.8X6
edetate	T45.8X1	T45.8X2	T45.8X3	T45.8X4	T45.8X5	T45.8X6
ethacrynate	T50.1X1	T50.1X2	T50.1X3	T50.1X4	T50.1X5	T50.1X6
feredetate	T45.8X1	T45.8X2	T45.8X3	T45.8X4	T45.8X5	T45.8X6
Fluoride — *see* Fluoride						
fluoroacetate (dust) (pesticide)	T60.4X1	T60.4X2	T60.4X3	T60.4X4	—	—
free salt	T50.3X1	T50.3X2	T50.3X3	T50.3X4	T50.3X5	T50.3X6
fusidate	T36.8X1	T36.8X2	T36.8X3	T36.8X4	T36.8X5	T36.8X6
glucaldrate	T47.1X1	T47.1X2	T47.1X3	T47.1X4	T47.1X5	T47.1X6
glucosulfone	T37.1X1	T37.1X2	T37.1X3	T37.1X4	T37.1X5	T37.1X6
glutamate	T45.8X1	T45.8X2	T45.8X3	T45.8X4	T45.8X5	T45.8X6
hydrogen carbonate	T50.3X1	T50.3X2	T50.3X3	T50.3X4	T50.3X5	T50.3X6
hydroxide	T54.3X1	T54.3X2	T54.3X3	T54.3X4	—	—
hypochlorite (bleach) NEC	T54.3X1	T54.3X2	T54.3X3	T54.3X4	—	—
disinfectant	T54.3X1	T54.3X2	T54.3X3	T54.3X4	—	—
medicinal (anti-infective) (external)	T49.0X1	T49.0X2	T49.0X3	T49.0X4	T49.0X5	T49.0X6
vapor	T54.3X1	T54.3X2	T54.3X3	T54.3X4	—	—
hyposulfite	T49.0X1	T49.0X2	T49.0X3	T49.0X4	T49.0X5	T49.0X6
indigotin disulfonate	T50.8X1	T50.8X2	T50.8X3	T50.8X4	T50.8X5	T50.8X6
iodide	T50.991	T50.992	T50.993	T50.994	T50.995	T50.996
I-131	T50.8X1	T50.8X2	T50.8X3	T50.8X4	T50.8X5	T50.8X6
therapeutic	T38.2X1	T38.2X2	T38.2X3	T38.2X4	T38.2X5	T38.2X6
iodohippurate (131I)	T50.8X1	T50.8X2	T50.8X3	T50.8X4	T50.8X5	T50.8X6
iopodate	T50.8X1	T50.8X2	T50.8X3	T50.8X4	T50.8X5	T50.8X6
iothalamate	T50.8X1	T50.8X2	T50.8X3	T50.8X4	T50.8X5	T50.8X6
iron edetate	T45.4X1	T45.4X2	T45.4X3	T45.4X4	T45.4X5	T45.4X6
lactate (compound solution)	T45.8X1	T45.8X2	T45.8X3	T45.8X4	T45.8X5	T45.8X6
lauryl (sulfate)	T49.2X1	T49.2X2	T49.2X3	T49.2X4	T49.2X5	T49.2X6
L-triiodothyronine	T38.1X1	T38.1X2	T38.1X3	T38.1X4	T38.1X5	T38.1X6
magnesium citrate	T50.991	T50.992	T50.993	T50.994	T50.995	T50.996
mersalate	T50.2X1	T50.2X2	T50.2X3	T50.2X4	T50.2X5	T50.2X6
metasilicate	T65.891	T65.892	T65.893	T65.894	—	—
metrizoate	T50.8X1	T50.8X2	T50.8X3	T50.8X4	T50.8X5	T50.8X6
monofluoroacetate (pesticide)	T60.1X1	T60.1X2	T60.1X3	T60.1X4	—	—
morrhuate	T46.8X1	T46.8X2	T46.8X3	T46.8X4	T46.8X5	T46.8X6
nafcillin	T36.0X1	T36.0X2	T36.0X3	T36.0X4	T36.0X5	T36.0X6
nitrate (oxidizing agent)	T65.891	T65.892	T65.893	T65.894	—	—
nitrite	T50.6X1	T50.6X2	T50.6X3	T50.6X4	T50.6X5	T50.6X6
nitroferricyanide	T46.5X1	T46.5X2	T46.5X3	T46.5X4	T46.5X5	T46.5X6
nitroprusside	T46.5X1	T46.5X2	T46.5X3	T46.5X4	T46.5X5	T46.5X6
oxalate	T65.891	T65.892	T65.893	T65.894	—	—
oxide/peroxide	T65.891	T65.892	T65.893	T65.894	—	—
oxybate	T41.291	T41.292	T41.293	T41.294	T41.295	T41.296
para-aminohippurate	T50.8X1	T50.8X2	T50.8X3	T50.8X4	T50.8X5	T50.8X6
perborate (nonmedicinal) NEC	T65.891	T65.892	T65.893	T65.894	—	—
medicinal	T49.0X1	T49.0X2	T49.0X3	T49.0X4	T49.0X5	T49.0X6
soap	T55.0X1	T55.0X2	T55.0X3	T55.0X4	—	—
percarbonate — *see* Sodium, perborate						
pertechnetate Tc99m	T50.8X1	T50.8X2	T50.8X3	T50.8X4	T50.8X5	T50.8X6
phosphate						
cellulose	T45.8X1	T45.8X2	T45.8X3	T45.8X4	T45.8X5	T45.8X6
dibasic	T47.2X1	T47.2X2	T47.2X3	T47.2X4	T47.2X5	T47.2X6
monobasic	T47.2X1	T47.2X2	T47.2X3	T47.2X4	T47.2X5	T47.2X6
phytate	T50.6X1	T50.6X2	T50.6X3	T50.6X4	T50.6X5	T50.6X6
picosulfate	T47.2X1	T47.2X2	T47.2X3	T47.2X4	T47.2X5	T47.2X6
polyhydroxyaluminium monocarbonate	T47.1X1	T47.1X2	T47.1X3	T47.1X4	T47.1X5	T47.1X6
polystyrene sulfonate	T50.3X1	T50.3X2	T50.3X3	T50.3X4	T50.3X5	T50.3X6
propionate	T49.0X1	T49.0X2	T49.0X3	T49.0X4	T49.0X5	T49.0X6
propyl hydroxybenzoate	T50.991	T50.992	T50.993	T50.994	T50.995	T50.996
psylliate	T46.8X1	T46.8X2	T46.8X3	T46.8X4	T46.8X5	T46.8X6
removing resins	T50.3X1	T50.3X2	T50.3X3	T50.3X4	T50.3X5	T50.3X6
salicylate	T39.091	T39.092	T39.093	T39.094	T39.095	T39.096

▼ Subterms under main terms may continue to next column or page   Additional Character May Be Required — Refer to the Tabular List for Character Selection   389

Sildenafil — Sodium

Substance	Poisoning, Accidental (unintentional)	Poisoning, Intentional Self-harm	Poisoning, Assault	Poisoning, Undetermined	Adverse Effect	Underdosing
Sodium — continued						
salt NEC	T50.3X1	T50.3X2	T50.3X3	T50.3X4	T50.3X5	T50.3X6
selenate	T60.2X1	T60.2X2	T60.2X3	T60.2X4	—	—
stibogluconate	T37.3X1	T37.3X2	T37.3X3	T37.3X4	T37.3X5	T37.3X6
sulfate	T47.4X1	T47.4X2	T47.4X3	T47.4X4	T47.4X5	T47.4X6
sulfoxone	T37.1X1	T37.1X2	T37.1X3	T37.1X4	T37.1X5	T37.1X6
tetradecyl sulfate	T46.8X1	T46.8X2	T46.8X3	T46.8X4	T46.8X5	T46.8X6
thiopental	T41.1X1	T41.1X2	T41.1X3	T41.1X4	T41.1X5	T41.1X6
thiosalicylate	T39.091	T39.092	T39.093	T39.094	T39.095	T39.096
thiosulfate	T50.6X1	T50.6X2	T50.6X3	T50.6X4	T50.6X5	T50.6X6
tolbutamide	T38.3X1	T38.3X2	T38.3X3	T38.3X4	T38.3X5	T38.3X6
(L)-triiodothyronine	T38.1X1	T38.1X2	T38.1X3	T38.1X4	T38.1X5	T38.1X6
tyropanoate	T50.8X1	T50.8X2	T50.8X3	T50.8X4	T50.8X5	T50.8X6
valproate	T42.6X1	T42.6X2	T42.6X3	T42.6X4	T42.6X5	T42.6X6
versenate	T50.6X1	T50.6X2	T50.6X3	T50.6X4	T50.6X5	T50.6X6
Sodium-free salt	T50.901	T50.902	T50.903	T50.904	T50.905	T50.906
Sodium-removing resin	T50.3X1	T50.3X2	T50.3X3	T50.3X4	T50.3X5	T50.3X6
Soft soap	T55.0X1	T55.0X2	T55.0X3	T55.0X4	—	—
Solanine	T62.2X1	T62.2X2	T62.2X3	T62.2X4	—	—
berries	T62.1X1	T62.1X2	T62.1X3	T62.1X4	—	—
Solanum dulcamara	T62.2X1	T62.2X2	T62.2X3	T62.2X4	—	—
berries	T62.1X1	T62.1X2	T62.1X3	T62.1X4	—	—
Solapsone	T37.1X1	T37.1X2	T37.1X3	T37.1X4	T37.1X5	T37.1X6
Solar lotion	T49.3X1	T49.3X2	T49.3X3	T49.3X4	T49.3X5	T49.3X6
Solasulfone	T37.1X1	T37.1X2	T37.1X3	T37.1X4	T37.1X5	T37.1X6
Soldering fluid	T65.891	T65.892	T65.893	T65.894	—	—
Solid substance	T65.91	T65.92	T65.93	T65.94	—	—
specified NEC	T65.891	T65.892	T65.893	T65.894	—	—
Solvent, industrial NEC	T52.91	T52.92	T52.93	T52.94	—	—
naphtha	T52.0X1	T52.0X2	T52.0X3	T52.0X4	—	—
petroleum	T52.0X1	T52.0X2	T52.0X3	T52.0X4	—	—
specified NEC	T52.8X1	T52.8X2	T52.8X3	T52.8X4	—	—
Soma	T42.8X1	T42.8X2	T42.8X3	T42.8X4	T42.8X5	T42.8X6
Somatorelin	T38.891	T38.892	T38.893	T38.894	T38.895	T38.896
Somatostatin	T38.991	T38.992	T38.993	T38.994	T38.995	T38.996
Somatotropin	T38.811	T38.812	T38.813	T38.814	T38.815	T38.816
Somatrem	T38.811	T38.812	T38.813	T38.814	T38.815	T38.816
Somatropin	T38.811	T38.812	T38.813	T38.814	T38.815	T38.816
Sominex	T45.0X1	T45.0X2	T45.0X3	T45.0X4	T45.0X5	T45.0X6
Somnos	T42.6X1	T42.6X2	T42.6X3	T42.6X4	T42.6X5	T42.6X6
Somonal	T42.3X1	T42.3X2	T42.3X3	T42.3X4	T42.3X5	T42.3X6
Soneryl	T42.3X1	T42.3X2	T42.3X3	T42.3X4	T42.3X5	T42.3X6
Soothing syrup	T50.901	T50.902	T50.903	T50.904	T50.905	T50.906
Sopor	T42.6X1	T42.6X2	T42.6X3	T42.6X4	T42.6X5	T42.6X6
Soporific	T42.71	T42.72	T42.73	T42.74	T42.75	T42.76
Soporific drug	T42.71	T42.72	T42.73	T42.74	T42.75	T42.76
specified type NEC	T42.6X1	T42.6X2	T42.6X3	T42.6X4	T42.6X5	T42.6X6
Sorbide nitrate	T46.3X1	T46.3X2	T46.3X3	T46.3X4	T46.3X5	T46.3X6
Sorbitol	T47.4X1	T47.4X2	T47.4X3	T47.4X4	T47.4X5	T47.4X6
Sotalol	T44.7X1	T44.7X2	T44.7X3	T44.7X4	T44.7X5	T44.7X6
Sotradecol	T46.8X1	T46.8X2	T46.8X3	T46.8X4	T46.8X5	T46.8X6
Soysterol	T46.6X1	T46.6X2	T46.6X3	T46.6X4	T46.6X5	T46.6X6
Spacoline	T44.3X1	T44.3X2	T44.3X3	T44.3X4	T44.3X5	T44.3X6
Spanish fly	T49.8X1	T49.8X2	T49.8X3	T49.8X4	T49.8X5	T49.8X6
Sparine	T43.3X1	T43.3X2	T43.3X3	T43.3X4	T43.3X5	T43.3X6
Sparteine	T48.0X1	T48.0X2	T48.0X3	T48.0X4	T48.0X5	T48.0X6
Spasmolytic						
anticholinergics	T44.3X1	T44.3X2	T44.3X3	T44.3X4	T44.3X5	T44.3X6
autonomic	T44.3X1	T44.3X2	T44.3X3	T44.3X4	T44.3X5	T44.3X6
bronchial NEC	T48.6X1	T48.6X2	T48.6X3	T48.6X4	T48.6X5	T48.6X6
quaternary ammonium	T44.3X1	T44.3X2	T44.3X3	T44.3X4	T44.3X5	T44.3X6
skeletal muscle NEC	T48.1X1	T48.1X2	T48.1X3	T48.1X4	T48.1X5	T48.1X6
Spectinomycin	T36.5X1	T36.5X2	T36.5X3	T36.5X4	T36.5X5	T36.5X6
Speed	T43.621	T43.622	T43.623	T43.624	T43.625	T43.626
Spermicide	T49.8X1	T49.8X2	T49.8X3	T49.8X4	T49.8X5	T49.8X6
Spider (bite) (venom)	T63.391	T63.392	T63.393	T63.394	—	—
antivenin	T50.Z11	T50.Z12	T50.Z13	T50.Z14	T50.Z15	T50.Z16
Spigelia (root)	T37.4X1	T37.4X2	T37.4X3	T37.4X4	T37.4X5	T37.4X6
Spindle inactivator	T50.4X1	T50.4X2	T50.4X3	T50.4X4	T50.4X5	T50.4X6
Spiperone	T43.4X1	T43.4X2	T43.4X3	T43.4X4	T43.4X5	T43.4X6
Spiramycin	T36.3X1	T36.3X2	T36.3X3	T36.3X4	T36.3X5	T36.3X6
Spirapril	T46.4X1	T46.4X2	T46.4X3	T46.4X4	T46.4X5	T46.4X6
Spirilene	T43.591	T43.592	T43.593	T43.594	T43.595	T43.596
Spirit(s) (neutral) **NEC**	T51.0X1	T51.0X2	T51.0X3	T51.0X4	—	—
beverage	T51.0X1	T51.0X2	T51.0X3	T51.0X4	—	—
industrial	T51.0X1	T51.0X2	T51.0X3	T51.0X4	—	—
mineral	T52.0X1	T52.0X2	T52.0X3	T52.0X4	—	—
of salt — see Hydrochloric acid						
surgical	T51.0X1	T51.0X2	T51.0X3	T51.0X4	—	—
Spironolactone	T50.0X1	T50.0X2	T50.0X3	T50.0X4	T50.0X5	T50.0X6
Spiroperidol	T43.4X1	T43.4X2	T43.4X3	T43.4X4	T43.4X5	T43.4X6
Sponge, absorbable	T45.7X1	T45.7X2	T45.7X3	T45.7X4	T45.7X5	T45.7X6
(gelatin)						

Substance	Poisoning, Accidental (unintentional)	Poisoning, Intentional Self-harm	Poisoning, Assault	Poisoning, Undetermined	Adverse Effect	Underdosing
Sporostacin	T49.0X1	T49.0X2	T49.0X3	T49.0X4	T49.0X5	T49.0
Spray (aerosol)	T65.91	T65.92	T65.93	T65.94		
cosmetic	T65.891	T65.892	T65.893	T65.894	—	—
medicinal NEC	T50.901	T50.902	T50.903	T50.904	T50.905	T50.9
pesticides — see Pesticides						
specified content — see specific substance						
Spurge flax	T62.2X1	T62.2X2	T62.2X3	T62.2X4	—	—
Spurges	T62.2X1	T62.2X2	T62.2X3	T62.2X4	—	—
Sputum viscosity-lowering drug	T48.4X1	T48.4X2	T48.4X3	T48.4X4	T48.4X5	T48.4
Squill	T46.0X1	T46.0X2	T46.0X3	T46.0X4	T46.0X5	T46.0
rat poison	T60.4X1	T60.4X2	T60.4X3	T60.4X4	—	—
Squirting cucumber (cathartic)	T47.2X1	T47.2X2	T47.2X3	T47.2X4	T47.2X5	T47.2
Stains	T65.6X1	T65.6X2	T65.6X3	T65.6X4	—	—
Stannous fluoride	T49.7X1	T49.7X2	T49.7X3	T49.7X4	T49.7X5	T49.7
Stanolone	T38.7X1	T38.7X2	T38.7X3	T38.7X4	T38.7X5	T38.7
Stanozolol	T38.7X1	T38.7X2	T38.7X3	T38.7X4	T38.7X5	T38.7
Staphisagria or stavesacre (pediculicide)	T49.0X1	T49.0X2	T49.0X3	T49.0X4	T49.0X5	T49.0
Starch	T50.901	T50.902	T50.903	T50.904	T50.905	T50.9
Stelazine	T43.3X1	T43.3X2	T43.3X3	T43.3X4	T43.3X5	T43.3
Stemetil	T43.3X1	T43.3X2	T43.3X3	T43.3X4	T43.3X5	T43.3
Stepronin	T48.4X1	T48.4X2	T48.4X3	T48.4X4	T48.4X5	T48.4
Sterculia	T47.4X1	T47.4X2	T47.4X3	T47.4X4	T47.4X5	T47.4
Sternutator gas	T59.891	T59.892	T59.893	T59.894		
Steroid	T38.0X1	T38.0X2	T38.0X3	T38.0X4	T38.0X5	T38.0
anabolic	T38.7X1	T38.7X2	T38.7X3	T38.7X4	T38.7X5	T38.7
androgenic	T38.7X1	T38.7X2	T38.7X3	T38.7X4	T38.7X5	T38.7
antineoplastic, hormone	T38.7X1	T38.7X2	T38.7X3	T38.7X4	T38.7X5	T38.7
estrogen	T38.5X1	T38.5X2	T38.5X3	T38.5X4	T38.5X5	T38.5
ENT agent	T49.6X1	T49.6X2	T49.6X3	T49.6X4	T49.6X5	T49.6
ophthalmic preparation	T49.5X1	T49.5X2	T49.5X3	T49.5X4	T49.5X5	T49.5
topical NEC	T49.0X1	T49.0X2	T49.0X3	T49.0X4	T49.0X5	T49.0
Stibine	T56.891	T56.892	T56.893	T56.894	—	—
Stibogluconate	T37.3X1	T37.3X2	T37.3X3	T37.3X4	T37.3X5	T37.3
Stibophen	T37.4X1	T37.4X2	T37.4X3	T37.4X4	T37.4X5	T37.4
Stilbamidine (isetionate)	T37.3X1	T37.3X2	T37.3X3	T37.3X4	T37.3X5	T37.3
Stilbestrol	T38.5X1	T38.5X2	T38.5X3	T38.5X4	T38.5X5	T38.5
Stilboestrol	T38.5X1	T38.5X2	T38.5X3	T38.5X4	T38.5X5	T38.5
Stimulant						
central nervous system — see also Psychostimulant	T43.601	T43.602	T43.603	T43.604	T43.605	T43.6
analeptics	T50.7X1	T50.7X2	T50.7X3	T50.7X4	T50.7X5	T50.7
opiate antagonist	T50.7X1	T50.7X2	T50.7X3	T50.7X4	T50.7X5	T50.7
psychotherapeutic NEC — see also Psychotherapeutic drug	T43.601	T43.602	T43.603	T43.604	T43.605	T43.6
specified NEC	T43.691	T43.692	T43.693	T43.694	T43.695	T43.6
respiratory	T48.901	T48.902	T48.903	T48.904	T48.905	T48.9
Stone-dissolving drug	T50.901	T50.902	T50.903	T50.904	T50.905	T50.9
Storage battery (cells) (acid)	T54.2X1	T54.2X2	T54.2X3	T54.2X4	—	—
Stovaine	T41.3X1	T41.3X2	T41.3X3	T41.3X4	T41.3X5	T41.3
infiltration (subcutaneous)	T41.3X1	T41.3X2	T41.3X3	T41.3X4	T41.3X5	T41.3
nerve block (peripheral) (plexus)	T41.3X1	T41.3X2	T41.3X3	T41.3X4	T41.3X5	T41.3
spinal	T41.3X1	T41.3X2	T41.3X3	T41.3X4	T41.3X5	T41.3
topical (surface)	T41.3X1	T41.3X2	T41.3X3	T41.3X4	T41.3X5	T41.3
Stovarsal	T37.8X1	T37.8X2	T37.8X3	T37.8X4	T37.8X5	T37.8
Stove gas — see Gas, stove						
Stoxil	T49.5X1	T49.5X2	T49.5X3	T49.5X4	T49.5X5	T49.5
Stramonium	T48.6X1	T48.6X2	T48.6X3	T48.6X4	T48.6X5	T48.6
natural state	T62.2X1	T62.2X2	T62.2X3	T62.2X4	—	—
Streptodornase	T45.3X1	T45.3X2	T45.3X3	T45.3X4	T45.3X5	T45.3
Streptoduocin	T36.5X1	T36.5X2	T36.5X3	T36.5X4	T36.5X5	T36.5
Streptokinase	T45.611	T45.612	T45.613	T45.614	T45.615	T45.61
Streptomycin (derivative)	T36.5X1	T36.5X2	T36.5X3	T36.5X4	T36.5X5	T36.5
Streptonivicin	T36.5X1	T36.5X2	T36.5X3	T36.5X4	T36.5X5	T36.5
Streptovarycin	T36.5X1	T36.5X2	T36.5X3	T36.5X4	T36.5X5	T36.5
Streptozocin	T45.1X1	T45.1X2	T45.1X3	T45.1X4	T45.1X5	T45.1
Streptozotocin	T45.1X1	T45.1X2	T45.1X3	T45.1X4	T45.1X5	T45.1
Stripper (paint) (solvent)	T52.8X1	T52.8X2	T52.8X3	T52.8X4	—	—
Strobane	T60.1X1	T60.1X2	T60.1X3	T60.1X4	—	—
Strofantina	T46.0X1	T46.0X2	T46.0X3	T46.0X4	T46.0X5	T46.0
Strophanthin (g) (k)	T46.0X1	T46.0X2	T46.0X3	T46.0X4	T46.0X5	T46.0
Strophanthus	T46.0X1	T46.0X2	T46.0X3	T46.0X4	T46.0X5	T46.0
Strophantin	T46.0X1	T46.0X2	T46.0X3	T46.0X4	T46.0X5	T46.0
Strophantin-g	T46.0X1	T46.0X2	T46.0X3	T46.0X4	T46.0X5	T46.0
Strychnine (nonmedicinal) (pesticide) (salts)	T65.1X1	T65.1X2	T65.1X3	T65.1X4	—	—
medicinal	T48.291	T48.292	T48.293	T48.294	T48.295	T48.29

Additional Character May Be Required — Refer to the Tabular List for Character Selection   ▽ Subterms under main terms may continue to next column or page

Substance	Poisoning, Accidental (unintentional)	Poisoning, Intentional Self-harm	Poisoning, Assault	Poisoning, Undetermined	Adverse Effect	Under-dosing
Strychnos (ignatii) — *see* Strychnine						
Styramate	T42.8X1	T42.8X2	T42.8X3	T42.8X4	T42.8X5	T42.8X6
Styrene	T65.891	T65.892	T65.893	T65.894	—	—
Succinimide, antiepileptic or anticonvulsant	T42.2X1	T42.2X2	T42.2X3	T42.2X4	T42.2X5	T42.2X6
mercuric — *see* Mercury						
Succinylcholine	T48.1X1	T48.1X2	T48.1X3	T48.1X4	T48.1X5	T48.1X6
Succinylsulfathiazole	T37.0X1	T37.0X2	T37.0X3	T37.0X4	T37.0X5	T37.0X6
Sucralfate	T47.1X1	T47.1X2	T47.1X3	T47.1X4	T47.1X5	T47.1X6
Sucrose	T50.3X1	T50.3X2	T50.3X3	T50.3X4	T50.3X5	T50.3X6
Sufentanil	T40.4X1	T40.4X2	T40.4X3	T40.4X4	T40.4X5	T40.4X6
Sulbactam	T36.0X1	T36.0X2	T36.0X3	T36.0X4	T36.0X5	T36.0X6
Sulbenicillin	T36.0X1	T36.0X2	T36.0X3	T36.0X4	T36.0X5	T36.0X6
Sulbentine	T49.0X1	T49.0X2	T49.0X3	T49.0X4	T49.0X5	T49.0X6
Sulfacetamide	T49.0X1	T49.0X2	T49.0X3	T49.0X4	T49.0X5	T49.0X6
ophthalmic preparation	T49.5X1	T49.5X2	T49.5X3	T49.5X4	T49.5X5	T49.5X6
Sulfachlorpyridazine	T37.0X1	T37.0X2	T37.0X3	T37.0X4	T37.0X5	T37.0X6
Sulfacitine	T37.0X1	T37.0X2	T37.0X3	T37.0X4	T37.0X5	T37.0X6
Sulfadiasulfone sodium	T37.0X1	T37.0X2	T37.0X3	T37.0X4	T37.0X5	T37.0X6
Sulfadiazine	T37.0X1	T37.0X2	T37.0X3	T37.0X4	T37.0X5	T37.0X6
silver (topical)	T49.0X1	T49.0X2	T49.0X3	T49.0X4	T49.0X5	T49.0X6
Sulfadimethoxine	T37.0X1	T37.0X2	T37.0X3	T37.0X4	T37.0X5	T37.0X6
Sulfadimidine	T37.0X1	T37.0X2	T37.0X3	T37.0X4	T37.0X5	T37.0X6
Sulfadoxine	T37.0X1	T37.0X2	T37.0X3	T37.0X4	T37.0X5	T37.0X6
with pyrimethamine	T37.2X1	T37.2X2	T37.2X3	T37.2X4	T37.2X5	T37.2X6
Sulfaethidole	T37.0X1	T37.0X2	T37.0X3	T37.0X4	T37.0X5	T37.0X6
Sulfafurazole	T37.0X1	T37.0X2	T37.0X3	T37.0X4	T37.0X5	T37.0X6
Sulfaguanidine	T37.0X1	T37.0X2	T37.0X3	T37.0X4	T37.0X5	T37.0X6
Sulfalene	T37.0X1	T37.0X2	T37.0X3	T37.0X4	T37.0X5	T37.0X6
Sulfaloxate	T37.0X1	T37.0X2	T37.0X3	T37.0X4	T37.0X5	T37.0X6
Sulfaloxic acid	T37.0X1	T37.0X2	T37.0X3	T37.0X4	T37.0X5	T37.0X6
Sulfamazone	T39.2X1	T39.2X2	T39.2X3	T39.2X4	T39.2X5	T39.2X6
Sulfamerazine	T37.0X1	T37.0X2	T37.0X3	T37.0X4	T37.0X5	T37.0X6
Sulfameter	T37.0X1	T37.0X2	T37.0X3	T37.0X4	T37.0X5	T37.0X6
Sulfamethazine	T37.0X1	T37.0X2	T37.0X3	T37.0X4	T37.0X5	T37.0X6
Sulfamethizole	T37.0X1	T37.0X2	T37.0X3	T37.0X4	T37.0X5	T37.0X6
Sulfamethoxazole	T37.0X1	T37.0X2	T37.0X3	T37.0X4	T37.0X5	T37.0X6
with trimethoprim	T36.8X1	T36.8X2	T36.8X3	T36.8X4	T36.8X5	T36.8X6
Sulfamethoxydiazine	T37.0X1	T37.0X2	T37.0X3	T37.0X4	T37.0X5	T37.0X6
Sulfamethoxypyridazine	T37.0X1	T37.0X2	T37.0X3	T37.0X4	T37.0X5	T37.0X6
Sulfamethylthiazole	T37.0X1	T37.0X2	T37.0X3	T37.0X4	T37.0X5	T37.0X6
Sulfametoxydiazine	T37.0X1	T37.0X2	T37.0X3	T37.0X4	T37.0X5	T37.0X6
Sulfamidopyrine	T39.2X1	T39.2X2	T39.2X3	T39.2X4	T39.2X5	T39.2X6
Sulfamonomethoxine	T37.0X1	T37.0X2	T37.0X3	T37.0X4	T37.0X5	T37.0X6
Sulfamoxole	T37.0X1	T37.0X2	T37.0X3	T37.0X4	T37.0X5	T37.0X6
Sulfamylon	T49.0X1	T49.0X2	T49.0X3	T49.0X4	T49.0X5	T49.0X6
Sulfan blue (diagnostic dye)	T50.8X1	T50.8X2	T50.8X3	T50.8X4	T50.8X5	T50.8X6
Sulfanilamide	T37.0X1	T37.0X2	T37.0X3	T37.0X4	T37.0X5	T37.0X6
Sulfanilylguanidine	T37.0X1	T37.0X2	T37.0X3	T37.0X4	T37.0X5	T37.0X6
Sulfaperin	T37.0X1	T37.0X2	T37.0X3	T37.0X4	T37.0X5	T37.0X6
Sulfaphenazole	T37.0X1	T37.0X2	T37.0X3	T37.0X4	T37.0X5	T37.0X6
Sulfaphenylthiazole	T37.0X1	T37.0X2	T37.0X3	T37.0X4	T37.0X5	T37.0X6
Sulfaproxyline	T37.0X1	T37.0X2	T37.0X3	T37.0X4	T37.0X5	T37.0X6
Sulfapyridine	T37.0X1	T37.0X2	T37.0X3	T37.0X4	T37.0X5	T37.0X6
Sulfapyrimidine	T37.0X1	T37.0X2	T37.0X3	T37.0X4	T37.0X5	T37.0X6
Sulfarsphenamine	T37.8X1	T37.8X2	T37.8X3	T37.8X4	T37.8X5	T37.8X6
Sulfasalazine	T37.0X1	T37.0X2	T37.0X3	T37.0X4	T37.0X5	T37.0X6
Sulfasuxidine	T37.0X1	T37.0X2	T37.0X3	T37.0X4	T37.0X5	T37.0X6
Sulfasymazine	T37.0X1	T37.0X2	T37.0X3	T37.0X4	T37.0X5	T37.0X6
Sulfated amylopectin	T47.8X1	T47.8X2	T47.8X3	T47.8X4	T47.8X5	T47.8X6
Sulfathiazole	T37.0X1	T37.0X2	T37.0X3	T37.0X4	T37.0X5	T37.0X6
Sulfatostearate	T49.2X1	T49.2X2	T49.2X3	T49.2X4	T49.2X5	T49.2X6
Sulfinpyrazone	T50.4X1	T50.4X2	T50.4X3	T50.4X4	T50.4X5	T50.4X6
Sulfiram	T49.0X1	T49.0X2	T49.0X3	T49.0X4	T49.0X5	T49.0X6
Sulfisomidine	T37.0X1	T37.0X2	T37.0X3	T37.0X4	T37.0X5	T37.0X6
Sulfisoxazole	T37.0X1	T37.0X2	T37.0X3	T37.0X4	T37.0X5	T37.0X6
ophthalmic preparation	T49.5X1	T49.5X2	T49.5X3	T49.5X4	T49.5X5	T49.5X6
Sulfobromophthalein (sodium)	T50.8X1	T50.8X2	T50.8X3	T50.8X4	T50.8X5	T50.8X6
Sulfobromphthalein	T50.8X1	T50.8X2	T50.8X3	T50.8X4	T50.8X5	T50.8X6
Sulfogaiacol	T48.4X1	T48.4X2	T48.4X3	T48.4X4	T48.4X5	T48.4X6
Sulfomyxin	T36.8X1	T36.8X2	T36.8X3	T36.8X4	T36.8X5	T36.8X6
Sulfonal	T42.6X1	T42.6X2	T42.6X3	T42.6X4	T42.6X5	T42.6X6
Sulfonamide NEC	T37.0X1	T37.0X2	T37.0X3	T37.0X4	T37.0X5	T37.0X6
eye	T49.5X1	T49.5X2	T49.5X3	T49.5X4	T49.5X5	T49.5X6
Sulfonazide	T37.1X1	T37.1X2	T37.1X3	T37.1X4	T37.1X5	T37.1X6
Sulfones	T37.1X1	T37.1X2	T37.1X3	T37.1X4	T37.1X5	T37.1X6
Sulfonethylmethane	T42.6X1	T42.6X2	T42.6X3	T42.6X4	T42.6X5	T42.6X6
Sulfonmethane	T42.6X1	T42.6X2	T42.6X3	T42.6X4	T42.6X5	T42.6X6
Sulfonphthal, sulfonphthol	T50.8X1	T50.8X2	T50.8X3	T50.8X4	T50.8X5	T50.8X6

Substance	Poisoning, Accidental (unintentional)	Poisoning, Intentional Self-harm	Poisoning, Assault	Poisoning, Undetermined	Adverse Effect	Under-dosing
Sulfonylurea derivatives, oral	T38.3X1	T38.3X2	T38.3X3	T38.3X4	T38.3X5	T38.3X6
Sulforidazine	T43.3X1	T43.3X2	T43.3X3	T43.3X4	T43.3X5	T43.3X6
Sulfoxone	T37.1X1	T37.1X2	T37.1X3	T37.1X4	T37.1X5	T37.1X6
Sulfuric acid	T54.2X1	T54.2X2	T54.2X3	T54.2X4	—	—
Sulfur, sulfurated, sulfuric, sulfurous, sulfuryl (compounds NEC) (medicinal)	T49.4X1	T49.4X2	T49.4X3	T49.4X4	T49.4X5	T49.4X6
acid	T54.2X1	T54.2X2	T54.2X3	T54.2X4	—	—
dioxide (gas)	T59.1X1	T59.1X2	T59.1X3	T59.1X4	—	—
ether — *see* Ether(s)						
hydrogen	T59.6X1	T59.6X2	T59.6X3	T59.6X4	—	—
medicinal (keratolytic) (ointment) NEC	T49.4X1	T49.4X2	T49.4X3	T49.4X4	T49.4X5	T49.4X6
ointment	T49.0X1	T49.0X2	T49.0X3	T49.0X4	T49.0X5	T49.0X6
pesticide (vapor)	T60.91	T60.92	T60.93	T60.94	—	—
vapor NEC	T59.891	T59.892	T59.893	T59.894	—	—
Sulglicotide	T47.1X1	T47.1X2	T47.1X3	T47.1X4	T47.1X5	T47.1X6
Sulindac	T39.391	T39.392	T39.393	T39.394	T39.395	T39.396
Sulisatin	T47.2X1	T47.2X2	T47.2X3	T47.2X4	T47.2X5	T47.2X6
Sulisobenzone	T49.3X1	T49.3X2	T49.3X3	T49.3X4	T49.3X5	T49.3X6
Sulkowitch's reagent	T50.8X1	T50.8X2	T50.8X3	T50.8X4	T50.8X5	T50.8X6
Sulmetozine	T44.3X1	T44.3X2	T44.3X3	T44.3X4	T44.3X5	T44.3X6
Suloctidil	T46.7X1	T46.7X2	T46.7X3	T46.7X4	T46.7X5	T46.7X6
Sulph- — *see also* Sulf-						
Sulphadiazine	T37.0X1	T37.0X2	T37.0X3	T37.0X4	T37.0X5	T37.0X6
Sulphadimethoxine	T37.0X1	T37.0X2	T37.0X3	T37.0X4	T37.0X5	T37.0X6
Sulphadimidine	T37.0X1	T37.0X2	T37.0X3	T37.0X4	T37.0X5	T37.0X6
Sulphadione	T37.1X1	T37.1X2	T37.1X3	T37.1X4	T37.1X5	T37.1X6
Sulphafurazole	T37.0X1	T37.0X2	T37.0X3	T37.0X4	T37.0X5	T37.0X6
Sulphamethizole	T37.0X1	T37.0X2	T37.0X3	T37.0X4	T37.0X5	T37.0X6
Sulphamethoxazole	T37.0X1	T37.0X2	T37.0X3	T37.0X4	T37.0X5	T37.0X6
Sulphan blue	T50.8X1	T50.8X2	T50.8X3	T50.8X4	T50.8X5	T50.8X6
Sulphaphenazole	T37.0X1	T37.0X2	T37.0X3	T37.0X4	T37.0X5	T37.0X6
Sulphapyridine	T37.0X1	T37.0X2	T37.0X3	T37.0X4	T37.0X5	T37.0X6
Sulphasalazine	T37.0X1	T37.0X2	T37.0X3	T37.0X4	T37.0X5	T37.0X6
Sulphinpyrazone	T50.4X1	T50.4X2	T50.4X3	T50.4X4	T50.4X5	T50.4X6
Sulpiride	T43.591	T43.592	T43.593	T43.594	T43.595	T43.596
Sulprostone	T48.0X1	T48.0X2	T48.0X3	T48.0X4	T48.0X5	T48.0X6
Sulpyrine	T39.2X1	T39.2X2	T39.2X3	T39.2X4	T39.2X5	T39.2X6
Sultamicillin	T36.0X1	T36.0X2	T36.0X3	T36.0X4	T36.0X5	T36.0X6
Sulthiame	T42.6X1	T42.6X2	T42.6X3	T42.6X4	T42.6X5	T42.6X6
Sultiame	T42.6X1	T42.6X2	T42.6X3	T42.6X4	T42.6X5	T42.6X6
Sultopride	T43.591	T43.592	T43.593	T43.594	T43.595	T43.596
Sumatriptan	T39.8X1	T39.8X2	T39.8X3	T39.8X4	T39.8X5	T39.8X6
Sunflower seed oil	T46.6X1	T46.6X2	T46.6X3	T46.6X4	T46.6X5	T46.6X6
Superinone	T48.4X1	T48.4X2	T48.4X3	T48.4X4	T48.4X5	T48.4X6
Suprofen	T39.311	T39.312	T39.313	T39.314	T39.315	T39.316
Suramin (sodium)	T37.4X1	T37.4X2	T37.4X3	T37.4X4	T37.4X5	T37.4X6
Surfacaine	T41.3X1	T41.3X2	T41.3X3	T41.3X4	T41.3X5	T41.3X6
Surital	T41.1X1	T41.1X2	T41.1X3	T41.1X4	T41.1X5	T41.1X6
Sutilains	T45.3X1	T45.3X2	T45.3X3	T45.3X4	T45.3X5	T45.3X6
Suxamethonium (chloride)	T48.1X1	T48.1X2	T48.1X3	T48.1X4	T48.1X5	T48.1X6
Suxethonium (chloride)	T48.1X1	T48.1X2	T48.1X3	T48.1X4	T48.1X5	T48.1X6
Suxibuzone	T39.2X1	T39.2X2	T39.2X3	T39.2X4	T39.2X5	T39.2X6
Sweetener	T50.901	T50.902	T50.903	T50.904	T50.905	T50.906
Sweet niter spirit	T46.3X1	T46.3X2	T46.3X3	T46.3X4	T46.3X5	T46.3X6
Sweet oil (birch)	T49.3X1	T49.3X2	T49.3X3	T49.3X4	T49.3X5	T49.3X6
Sym-dichloroethyl ether	T53.6X1	T53.6X2	T53.6X3	T53.6X4	—	—
Sympatholytic NEC	T44.8X1	T44.8X2	T44.8X3	T44.8X4	T44.8X5	T44.8X6
haloalkylamine	T44.8X1	T44.8X2	T44.8X3	T44.8X4	T44.8X5	T44.8X6
Sympathomimetic NEC	T44.901	T44.902	T44.903	T44.904	T44.905	T44.906
anti-common-cold	T48.5X1	T48.5X2	T48.5X3	T48.5X4	T48.5X5	T48.5X6
bronchodilator	T48.6X1	T48.6X2	T48.6X3	T48.6X4	T48.6X5	T48.6X6
specified NEC	T44.991	T44.992	T44.993	T44.994	T44.995	T44.996
Synagis	T50.B91	T50.B92	T50.B93	T50.B94	T50.B95	T50.B96
Synalar	T49.0X1	T49.0X2	T49.0X3	T49.0X4	T49.0X5	T49.0X6
Synthroid	T38.1X1	T38.1X2	T38.1X3	T38.1X4	T38.1X5	T38.1X6
Syntocinon	T48.0X1	T48.0X2	T48.0X3	T48.0X4	T48.0X5	T48.0X6
Syrosingopine	T46.5X1	T46.5X2	T46.5X3	T46.5X4	T46.5X5	T46.5X6
Systemic drug	T45.91	T45.92	T45.93	T45.94	T45.95	T45.96
specified NEC	T45.8X1	T45.8X2	T45.8X3	T45.8X4	T45.8X5	T45.8X6
Tablets — *see also* specified substance	T50.901	T50.902	T50.903	T50.904	T50.905	T50.906
Tace	T38.5X1	T38.5X2	T38.5X3	T38.5X4	T38.5X5	T38.5X6
Tacrine	T44.0X1	T44.0X2	T44.0X3	T44.0X4	T44.0X5	T44.0X6
Tadalafil	T46.7X1	T46.7X2	T46.7X3	T46.7X4	T46.7X5	T46.7X6
Talampicillin	T36.0X1	T36.0X2	T36.0X3	T36.0X4	T36.0X5	T36.0X6
Talbutal	T42.3X1	T42.3X2	T42.3X3	T42.3X4	T42.3X5	T42.3X6
Talc powder	T49.3X1	T49.3X2	T49.3X3	T49.3X4	T49.3X5	T49.3X6
Talcum	T49.3X1	T49.3X2	T49.3X3	T49.3X4	T49.3X5	T49.3X6
Taleranol	T38.6X1	T38.6X2	T38.6X3	T38.6X4	T38.6X5	T38.6X6

Substance	Poisoning, Accidental (unintentional)	Poisoning, Intentional Self-harm	Poisoning, Assault	Poisoning, Undetermined	Adverse Effect	Under-dosing
Tamoxifen	T38.6X1	T38.6X2	T38.6X3	T38.6X4	T38.6X5	T38.6X6
Tamsulosin	T44.6X1	T44.6X2	T44.6X3	T44.6X4	T44.6X5	T44.6X6
Tandearil, tanderil	T39.2X1	T39.2X2	T39.2X3	T39.2X4	T39.2X5	T39.2X6
Tannic acid	T49.2X1	T49.2X2	T49.2X3	T49.2X4	T49.2X5	T49.2X6
medicinal (astringent)	T49.2X1	T49.2X2	T49.2X3	T49.2X4	T49.2X5	T49.2X6
Tannin — see Tannic acid						
Tansy	T62.2X1	T62.2X2	T62.2X3	T62.2X4	—	—
TAO	T36.3X1	T36.3X2	T36.3X3	T36.3X4	T36.3X5	T36.3X6
Tapazole	T38.2X1	T38.2X2	T38.2X3	T38.2X4	T38.2X5	T38.2X6
Taractan	T43.591	T43.592	T43.593	T43.594	T43.595	T43.596
Tarantula (venomous)	T63.321	T63.322	T63.323	T63.324	—	—
Tartar emetic	T37.8X1	T37.8X2	T37.8X3	T37.8X4	T37.8X5	T37.8X6
Tartaric acid	T65.891	T65.892	T65.893	T65.894	—	—
Tartrated antimony (anti-infective)	T37.8X1	T37.8X2	T37.8X3	T37.8X4	T37.8X5	T37.8X6
Tartrate, laxative	T47.4X1	T47.4X2	T47.4X3	T47.4X4	T47.4X5	T47.4X6
Tar NEC	T52.0X1	T52.0X2	T52.0X3	T52.0X4	—	—
camphor	T60.1X1	T60.1X2	T60.1X3	T60.1X4	—	—
distillate	T49.1X1	T49.1X2	T49.1X3	T49.1X4	T49.1X5	T49.1X6
fumes	T59.891	T59.892	T59.893	T59.894	—	—
medicinal	T49.1X1	T49.1X2	T49.1X3	T49.1X4	T49.1X5	T49.1X6
ointment	T49.1X1	T49.1X2	T49.1X3	T49.1X4	T49.1X5	T49.1X6
Tauromustine	T45.1X1	T45.1X2	T45.1X3	T45.1X4	T45.1X5	T45.1X6
TCA — see Trichloroacetic acid						
TCDD	T53.7X1	T53.7X2	T53.7X3	T53.7X4	—	—
TDI (vapor)	T65.0X1	T65.0X2	T65.0X3	T65.0X4	—	—
Tear						
gas	T59.3X1	T59.3X2	T59.3X3	T59.3X4	—	—
solution	T49.5X1	T49.5X2	T49.5X3	T49.5X4	T49.5X5	T49.5X6
Teclothiazide	T50.2X1	T50.2X2	T50.2X3	T50.2X4	T50.2X5	T50.2X6
Teclozan	T37.3X1	T37.3X2	T37.3X3	T37.3X4	T37.3X5	T37.3X6
Tegafur	T45.1X1	T45.1X2	T45.1X3	T45.1X4	T45.1X5	T45.1X6
Tegretol	T42.1X1	T42.1X2	T42.1X3	T42.1X4	T42.1X5	T42.1X6
Teicoplanin	T36.8X1	T36.8X2	T36.8X3	T36.8X4	T36.8X5	T36.8X6
Telepaque	T50.8X1	T50.8X2	T50.8X3	T50.8X4	T50.8X5	T50.8X6
Tellurium	T56.891	T56.892	T56.893	T56.894	—	—
fumes	T56.891	T56.892	T56.893	T56.894	—	—
TEM	T45.1X1	T45.1X2	T45.1X3	T45.1X4	T45.1X5	T45.1X6
Temazepam	T42.4X1	T42.4X2	T42.4X3	T42.4X4	T42.4X5	T42.4X6
Temocillin	T36.0X1	T36.0X2	T36.0X3	T36.0X4	T36.0X5	T36.0X6
Tenamfetamine	T43.621	T43.622	T43.623	T43.624	T43.625	T43.626
Teniposide	T45.1X1	T45.1X2	T45.1X3	T45.1X4	T45.1X5	T45.1X6
Tenitramine	T46.3X1	T46.3X2	T46.3X3	T46.3X4	T46.3X5	T46.3X6
Tenoglicin	T48.4X1	T48.4X2	T48.4X3	T48.4X4	T48.4X5	T48.4X6
Tenonitrozole	T37.3X1	T37.3X2	T37.3X3	T37.3X4	T37.3X5	T37.3X6
Tenoxicam	T39.391	T39.392	T39.393	T39.394	T39.395	T39.396
TEPA	T45.1X1	T45.1X2	T45.1X3	T45.1X4	T45.1X5	T45.1X6
TEPP	T60.0X1	T60.0X2	T60.0X3	T60.0X4	—	—
Teprotide	T46.5X1	T46.5X2	T46.5X3	T46.5X4	T46.5X5	T46.5X6
Terazosin	T44.6X1	T44.6X2	T44.6X3	T44.6X4	T44.6X5	T44.6X6
Terbufos	T60.0X1	T60.0X2	T60.0X3	T60.0X4	—	—
Terbutaline	T48.6X1	T48.6X2	T48.6X3	T48.6X4	T48.6X5	T48.6X6
Terconazole	T49.0X1	T49.0X2	T49.0X3	T49.0X4	T49.0X5	T49.0X6
Terfenadine	T45.0X1	T45.0X2	T45.0X3	T45.0X4	T45.0X5	T45.0X6
Teriparatide (acetate)	T50.991	T50.992	T50.993	T50.994	T50.995	T50.996
Terizidone	T37.1X1	T37.1X2	T37.1X3	T37.1X4	T37.1X5	T37.1X6
Terlipressin	T38.891	T38.892	T38.893	T38.894	T38.895	T38.896
Terodiline	T46.3X1	T46.3X2	T46.3X3	T46.3X4	T46.3X5	T46.3X6
Teroxalene	T37.4X1	T37.4X2	T37.4X3	T37.4X4	T37.4X5	T37.4X6
Terpin (cis) hydrate	T48.4X1	T48.4X2	T48.4X3	T48.4X4	T48.4X5	T48.4X6
Terramycin	T36.4X1	T36.4X2	T36.4X3	T36.4X4	T36.4X5	T36.4X6
Tertatolol	T44.7X1	T44.7X2	T44.7X3	T44.7X4	T44.7X5	T44.7X6
Tessalon	T48.3X1	T48.3X2	T48.3X3	T48.3X4	T48.3X5	T48.3X6
Testolactone	T38.7X1	T38.7X2	T38.7X3	T38.7X4	T38.7X5	T38.7X6
Testosterone	T38.7X1	T38.7X2	T38.7X3	T38.7X4	T38.7X5	T38.7X6
Tetanus toxoid or vaccine	T50.A91	T50.A92	T50.A93	T50.A94	T50.A95	T50.A96
antitoxin	T50.Z11	T50.Z12	T50.Z13	T50.Z14	T50.Z15	T50.Z16
immune globulin (human)	T50.Z11	T50.Z12	T50.Z13	T50.Z14	T50.Z15	T50.Z16
toxoid	T50.A91	T50.A92	T50.A93	T50.A94	T50.A95	T50.A96
with diphtheria toxoid	T50.A21	T50.A22	T50.A23	T50.A24	T50.A25	T50.A26
with pertussis	T50.A11	T50.A12	T50.A13	T50.A14	T50.A15	T50.A16
Tetrabenazine	T43.591	T43.592	T43.593	T43.594	T43.595	T43.596
Tetracaine	T41.3X1	T41.3X2	T41.3X3	T41.3X4	T41.3X5	T41.3X6
nerve block (peripheral) (plexus)	T41.3X1	T41.3X2	T41.3X3	T41.3X4	T41.3X5	T41.3X6
regional	T41.3X1	T41.3X2	T41.3X3	T41.3X4	T41.3X5	T41.3X6
spinal	T41.3X1	T41.3X2	T41.3X3	T41.3X4	T41.3X5	T41.3X6
Tetrachlorethylene — see Tetrachloroethylene						
Tetrachlormethiazide	T50.2X1	T50.2X2	T50.2X3	T50.2X4	T50.2X5	T50.2X6
Tetrachloroethane	T53.6X1	T53.6X2	T53.6X3	T53.6X4	—	—
vapor	T53.6X1	T53.6X2	T53.6X3	T53.6X4	—	—
paint or varnish	T53.6X1	T53.6X2	T53.6X3	T53.6X4	—	—
Tetrachloroethylene (liquid)	T53.3X1	T53.3X2	T53.3X3	T53.3X4	—	—
medicinal	T37.4X1	T37.4X2	T37.4X3	T37.4X4	T37.4X5	T37.4
vapor	T53.3X1	T53.3X2	T53.3X3	T53.3X4	—	—
Tetrachloromethane — see Carbon tetrachloride						
Tetracosactide	T38.811	T38.812	T38.813	T38.814	T38.815	T38.8
Tetracosactrin	T38.811	T38.812	T38.813	T38.814	T38.815	T38.8
Tetracycline	T36.4X1	T36.4X2	T36.4X3	T36.4X4	T36.4X5	T36.4
ophthalmic preparation	T49.5X1	T49.5X2	T49.5X3	T49.5X4	T49.5X5	T49.5
topical NEC	T49.0X1	T49.0X2	T49.0X3	T49.0X4	T49.0X5	T49.0
Tetradifon	T60.8X1	T60.8X2	T60.8X3	T60.8X4	—	—
Tetradotoxin	T61.771	T61.772	T61.773	T61.774	—	—
Tetraethyl						
lead	T56.0X1	T56.0X2	T56.0X3	T56.0X4	—	—
pyrophosphate	T60.0X1	T60.0X2	T60.0X3	T60.0X4	—	—
Tetraethylammonium chloride	T44.2X1	T44.2X2	T44.2X3	T44.2X4	T44.2X5	T44.2
Tetraethylthiuram disulfide	T50.6X1	T50.6X2	T50.6X3	T50.6X4	T50.6X5	T50.6
Tetrahydroaminoacridine	T44.0X1	T44.0X2	T44.0X3	T44.0X4	T44.0X5	T44.0
Tetrahydrocannabinol	T40.7X1	T40.7X2	T40.7X3	T40.7X4	T40.7X5	T40.7
Tetrahydrofuran	T52.8X1	T52.8X2	T52.8X3	T52.8X4	—	—
Tetrahydronaphthalene	T52.8X1	T52.8X2	T52.8X3	T52.8X4	—	—
Tetrahydrozoline	T49.5X1	T49.5X2	T49.5X3	T49.5X4	T49.5X5	T49.5
Tetralin	T52.8X1	T52.8X2	T52.8X3	T52.8X4	—	—
Tetramethrin	T60.2X1	T60.2X2	T60.2X3	T60.2X4	—	—
Tetramethylthiuram (disulfide) NEC	T60.3X1	T60.3X2	T60.3X3	T60.3X4	—	—
medicinal	T49.0X1	T49.0X2	T49.0X3	T49.0X4	T49.0X5	T49.0
Tetramisole	T37.4X1	T37.4X2	T37.4X3	T37.4X4	T37.4X5	T37.4
Tetranicotinoyl fructose	T46.7X1	T46.7X2	T46.7X3	T46.7X4	T46.7X5	T46.7
Tetrazepam	T42.4X1	T42.4X2	T42.4X3	T42.4X4	T42.4X5	T42.4
Tetronal	T42.6X1	T42.6X2	T42.6X3	T42.6X4	T42.6X5	T42.6
Tetryl	T65.3X1	T65.3X2	T65.3X3	T65.3X4	—	—
Tetrylammonium chloride	T44.2X1	T44.2X2	T44.2X3	T44.2X4	T44.2X5	T44.2
Tetryzoline	T49.5X1	T49.5X2	T49.5X3	T49.5X4	T49.5X5	T49.5
Thalidomide	T45.1X1	T45.1X2	T45.1X3	T45.1X4	T45.1X5	T45.1
Thallium (compounds) (dust)	T56.811	T56.812	T56.813	T56.814	—	—
NEC						
pesticide	T60.4X1	T60.4X2	T60.4X3	T60.4X4	—	—
THC	T40.7X1	T40.7X2	T40.7X3	T40.7X4	T40.7X5	T40.7
Thebacon	T48.3X1	T48.3X2	T48.3X3	T48.3X4	T48.3X5	T48.3
Thebaine	T40.2X1	T40.2X2	T40.2X3	T40.2X4	T40.2X5	T40.2
Thenoic acid	T49.6X1	T49.6X2	T49.6X3	T49.6X4	T49.6X5	T49.6
Thenyldiamine	T45.0X1	T45.0X2	T45.0X3	T45.0X4	T45.0X5	T45.0
Theobromine (calcium salicylate)	T48.6X1	T48.6X2	T48.6X3	T48.6X4	T48.6X5	T48.6
sodium salicylate	T48.6X1	T48.6X2	T48.6X3	T48.6X4	T48.6X5	T48.6
Theophyllamine	T48.6X1	T48.6X2	T48.6X3	T48.6X4	T48.6X5	T48.6
Theophylline	T48.6X1	T48.6X2	T48.6X3	T48.6X4	T48.6X5	T48.6
aminobenzoic acid	T48.6X1	T48.6X2	T48.6X3	T48.6X4	T48.6X5	T48.6
ethylenediamine	T48.6X1	T48.6X2	T48.6X3	T48.6X4	T48.6X5	T48.6
piperazine	T48.6X1	T48.6X2	T48.6X3	T48.6X4	T48.6X5	T48.6
p-amino-benzoate						
Thiabendazole	T37.4X1	T37.4X2	T37.4X3	T37.4X4	T37.4X5	T37.4
Thialbarbital	T41.1X1	T41.1X2	T41.1X3	T41.1X4	T41.1X5	T41.1
Thiamazole	T38.2X1	T38.2X2	T38.2X3	T38.2X4	T38.2X5	T38.2
Thiambutosine	T37.1X1	T37.1X2	T37.1X3	T37.1X4	T37.1X5	T37.1
Thiamine	T45.2X1	T45.2X2	T45.2X3	T45.2X4	T45.2X5	T45.2
Thiamphenicol	T36.2X1	T36.2X2	T36.2X3	T36.2X4	T36.2X5	T36.2
Thiamylal	T41.1X1	T41.1X2	T41.1X3	T41.1X4	T41.1X5	T41.1
sodium	T41.1X1	T41.1X2	T41.1X3	T41.1X4	T41.1X5	T41.1
Thiazesim	T43.291	T43.292	T43.293	T43.294	T43.295	T43.2
Thiazides (diuretics)	T50.2X1	T50.2X2	T50.2X3	T50.2X4	T50.2X5	T50.2
Thiazinamium metilsulfate	T43.3X1	T43.3X2	T43.3X3	T43.3X4	T43.3X5	T43.3
Thiethylperazine	T43.3X1	T43.3X2	T43.3X3	T43.3X4	T43.3X5	T43.3
Thimerosal	T49.0X1	T49.0X2	T49.0X3	T49.0X4	T49.0X5	T49.0
ophthalmic preparation	T49.5X1	T49.5X2	T49.5X3	T49.5X4	T49.5X5	T49.5
Thioacetazone	T37.1X1	T37.1X2	T37.1X3	T37.1X4	T37.1X5	T37.1
with isoniazid	T37.1X1	T37.1X2	T37.1X3	T37.1X4	T37.1X5	T37.1
Thiobarbital sodium	T41.1X1	T41.1X2	T41.1X3	T41.1X4	T41.1X5	T41.1
Thiobarbiturate anesthetic	T41.1X1	T41.1X2	T41.1X3	T41.1X4	T41.1X5	T41.1
Thiobismol	T37.8X1	T37.8X2	T37.8X3	T37.8X4	T37.8X5	T37.8
Thiobutabarbital sodium	T41.1X1	T41.1X2	T41.1X3	T41.1X4	T41.1X5	T41.1
Thiocarbamate (insecticide)	T60.0X1	T60.0X2	T60.0X3	T60.0X4	—	—
Thiocarbamide	T38.2X1	T38.2X2	T38.2X3	T38.2X4	T38.2X5	T38.2
Thiocarbarsone	T37.8X1	T37.8X2	T37.8X3	T37.8X4	T37.8X5	T37.8
Thiocarlide	T37.1X1	T37.1X2	T37.1X3	T37.1X4	T37.1X5	T37.1
Thioctamide	T50.991	T50.992	T50.993	T50.994	T50.995	T50.99

Additional Character May Be Required — Refer to the Tabular List for Character Selection   ▽ Subterms under main terms may continue to next column or page

Substance	Poisoning, Accidental (unintentional)	Poisoning, Intentional Self-harm	Poisoning, Assault	Poisoning, Undetermined	Adverse Effect	Under-dosing
Thioctic acid	T50.991	T50.992	T50.993	T50.994	T50.995	T50.996
Thiofos	T60.0X1	T60.0X2	T60.0X3	T60.0X4	—	—
Thioglycolate	T49.4X1	T49.4X2	T49.4X3	T49.4X4	T49.4X5	T49.4X6
Thioglycolic acid	T65.891	T65.892	T65.893	T65.894	—	—
Thioguanine	T45.1X1	T45.1X2	T45.1X3	T45.1X4	T45.1X5	T45.1X6
Thiomercaptomerin	T50.2X1	T50.2X2	T50.2X3	T50.2X4	T50.2X5	T50.2X6
Thiomerin	T50.2X1	T50.2X2	T50.2X3	T50.2X4	T50.2X5	T50.2X6
Thiomersal	T49.0X1	T49.0X2	T49.0X3	T49.0X4	T49.0X5	T49.0X6
Thionazin	T60.0X1	T60.0X2	T60.0X3	T60.0X4	—	—
Thiopental (sodium)	T41.1X1	T41.1X2	T41.1X3	T41.1X4	T41.1X5	T41.1X6
Thiopentone (sodium)	T41.1X1	T41.1X2	T41.1X3	T41.1X4	T41.1X5	T41.1X6
Thiopropazate	T43.3X1	T43.3X2	T43.3X3	T43.3X4	T43.3X5	T43.3X6
Thioproperazine	T43.3X1	T43.3X2	T43.3X3	T43.3X4	T43.3X5	T43.3X6
Thioridazine	T43.3X1	T43.3X2	T43.3X3	T43.3X4	T43.3X5	T43.3X6
Thiosinamine	T49.3X1	T49.3X2	T49.3X3	T49.3X4	T49.3X5	T49.3X6
Thiotepa	T45.1X1	T45.1X2	T45.1X3	T45.1X4	T45.1X5	T45.1X6
Thiothixene	T43.4X1	T43.4X2	T43.4X3	T43.4X4	T43.4X5	T43.4X6
Thiouracil (benzyl) (methyl) (propyl)	T38.2X1	T38.2X2	T38.2X3	T38.2X4	T38.2X5	T38.2X6
Thiourea	T38.2X1	T38.2X2	T38.2X3	T38.2X4	T38.2X5	T38.2X6
Thiphenamil	T44.3X1	T44.3X2	T44.3X3	T44.3X4	T44.3X5	T44.3X6
Thiram	T60.3X1	T60.3X2	T60.3X3	T60.3X4	—	—
medicinal	T49.2X1	T49.2X2	T49.2X3	T49.2X4	T49.2X5	T49.2X6
Thonzylamine (systemic)	T45.0X1	T45.0X2	T45.0X3	T45.0X4	T45.0X5	T45.0X6
mucosal decongestant	T48.5X1	T48.5X2	T48.5X3	T48.5X4	T48.5X5	T48.5X6
Thorazine	T43.3X1	T43.3X2	T43.3X3	T43.3X4	T43.3X5	T43.3X6
Thorium dioxide suspension	T50.8X1	T50.8X2	T50.8X3	T50.8X4	T50.8X5	T50.8X6
Thornapple	T62.2X1	T62.2X2	T62.2X3	T62.2X4	—	—
Throat drug NEC	T49.6X1	T49.6X2	T49.6X3	T49.6X4	T49.6X5	T49.6X6
Thrombin	T45.7X1	T45.7X2	T45.7X3	T45.7X4	T45.7X5	T45.7X6
Thrombolysin	T45.611	T45.612	T45.613	T45.614	T45.615	T45.616
Thromboplastin	T45.7X1	T45.7X2	T45.7X3	T45.7X4	T45.7X5	T45.7X6
Thurfyl nicotinate	T46.7X1	T46.7X2	T46.7X3	T46.7X4	T46.7X5	T46.7X6
Thymol	T49.0X1	T49.0X2	T49.0X3	T49.0X4	T49.0X5	T49.0X6
Thymopentin	T37.5X1	T37.5X2	T37.5X3	T37.5X4	T37.5X5	T37.5X6
Thymoxamine	T46.7X1	T46.7X2	T46.7X3	T46.7X4	T46.7X5	T46.7X6
Thymus extract	T38.891	T38.892	T38.893	T38.894	T38.895	T38.896
Thyreotrophic hormone	T38.811	T38.812	T38.813	T38.814	T38.815	T38.816
Thyroglobulin	T38.1X1	T38.1X2	T38.1X3	T38.1X4	T38.1X5	T38.1X6
Thyroid (hormone)	T38.1X1	T38.1X2	T38.1X3	T38.1X4	T38.1X5	T38.1X6
Thyrolar	T38.1X1	T38.1X2	T38.1X3	T38.1X4	T38.1X5	T38.1X6
Thyrotrophin	T38.811	T38.812	T38.813	T38.814	T30.015	T30.016
Thyrotropic hormone	T38.811	T38.812	T38.813	T38.814	T38.815	T38.816
Thyroxine	T38.1X1	T38.1X2	T38.1X3	T38.1X4	T38.1X5	T38.1X6
Tiabendazole	T37.4X1	T37.4X2	T37.4X3	T37.4X4	T37.4X5	T37.4X6
Tiamizide	T50.2X1	T50.2X2	T50.2X3	T50.2X4	T50.2X5	T50.2X6
Tianeptine	T43.291	T43.292	T43.293	T43.294	T43.295	T43.296
Tiapamil	T46.1X1	T46.1X2	T46.1X3	T46.1X4	T46.1X5	T46.1X6
Tiapride	T43.591	T43.592	T43.593	T43.594	T43.595	T43.596
Tiaprofenic acid	T39.311	T39.312	T39.313	T39.314	T39.315	T39.316
Tiaramide	T39.8X1	T39.8X2	T39.8X3	T39.8X4	T39.8X5	T39.8X6
Ticarcillin	T36.0X1	T36.0X2	T36.0X3	T36.0X4	T36.0X5	T36.0X6
Ticlatone	T49.0X1	T49.0X2	T49.0X3	T49.0X4	T49.0X5	T49.0X6
Ticlopidine	T45.521	T45.522	T45.523	T45.524	T45.525	T45.526
Ticrynafen	T50.1X1	T50.1X2	T50.1X3	T50.1X4	T50.1X5	T50.1X6
Tidiacic	T50.991	T50.992	T50.993	T50.994	T50.995	T50.996
Tiemonium	T44.3X1	T44.3X2	T44.3X3	T44.3X4	T44.3X5	T44.3X6
iodide	T44.3X1	T44.3X2	T44.3X3	T44.3X4	T44.3X5	T44.3X6
Tienilic acid	T50.1X1	T50.1X2	T50.1X3	T50.1X4	T50.1X5	T50.1X6
Tifenamil	T44.3X1	T44.3X2	T44.3X3	T44.3X4	T44.3X5	T44.3X6
Tigan	T45.0X1	T45.0X2	T45.0X3	T45.0X4	T45.0X5	T45.0X6
Tigloidine	T44.3X1	T44.3X2	T44.3X3	T44.3X4	T44.3X5	T44.3X6
Tilactase	T47.5X1	T47.5X2	T47.5X3	T47.5X4	T47.5X5	T47.5X6
Tiletamine	T41.291	T41.292	T41.293	T41.294	T41.295	T41.296
Tilidine	T40.4X1	T40.4X2	T40.4X3	T40.4X4	—	—
Timepidium bromide	T44.3X1	T44.3X2	T44.3X3	T44.3X4	T44.3X5	T44.3X6
Timiperone	T43.4X1	T43.4X2	T43.4X3	T43.4X4	T43.4X5	T43.4X6
Timolol	T44.7X1	T44.7X2	T44.7X3	T44.7X4	T44.7X5	T44.7X6
Tincture, iodine — see Iodine						
Tindal	T43.3X1	T43.3X2	T43.3X3	T43.3X4	T43.3X5	T43.3X6
Tinidazole	T37.3X1	T37.3X2	T37.3X3	T37.3X4	T37.3X5	T37.3X6
Tin (chloride) (dust) (oxide) NEC	T56.6X1	T56.6X2	T56.6X3	T56.6X4	—	—
anti-infectives	T37.8X1	T37.8X2	T37.8X3	T37.8X4	T37.8X5	T37.8X6
Tinoridine	T39.8X1	T39.8X2	T39.8X3	T39.8X4	T39.8X5	T39.8X6
Tiocarlide	T37.1X1	T37.1X2	T37.1X3	T37.1X4	T37.1X5	T37.1X6
Tioclomarol	T45.511	T45.512	T45.513	T45.514	T45.515	T45.516
Tioconazole	T49.0X1	T49.0X2	T49.0X3	T49.0X4	T49.0X5	T49.0X6
Tioguanine	T45.1X1	T45.1X2	T45.1X3	T45.1X4	T45.1X5	T45.1X6
Tiopronin	T50.991	T50.992	T50.993	T50.994	T50.995	T50.996
Tiotixene	T43.4X1	T43.4X2	T43.4X3	T43.4X4	T43.4X5	T43.4X6
Tioxolone	T49.4X1	T49.4X2	T49.4X3	T49.4X4	T49.4X5	T49.4X6

Substance	Poisoning, Accidental (unintentional)	Poisoning, Intentional Self-harm	Poisoning, Assault	Poisoning, Undetermined	Adverse Effect	Under-dosing
Tipepidine	T48.3X1	T48.3X2	T48.3X3	T48.3X4	T48.3X5	T48.3X6
Tiquizium bromide	T44.3X1	T44.3X2	T44.3X3	T44.3X4	T44.3X5	T44.3X6
Tiratricol	T38.1X1	T38.1X2	T38.1X3	T38.1X4	T38.1X5	T38.1X6
Tisopurine	T50.4X1	T50.4X2	T50.4X3	T50.4X4	T50.4X5	T50.4X6
Titanium (compounds) (vapor)	T56.891	T56.892	T56.893	T56.894	—	—
dioxide	T49.3X1	T49.3X2	T49.3X3	T49.3X4	T49.3X5	T49.3X6
ointment	T49.3X1	T49.3X2	T49.3X3	T49.3X4	T49.3X5	T49.3X6
oxide	T49.3X1	T49.3X2	T49.3X3	T49.3X4	T49.3X5	T49.3X6
tetrachloride	T56.891	T56.892	T56.893	T56.894	—	—
Titanocene	T56.891	T56.892	T56.893	T56.894	—	—
Titroid	T38.1X1	T38.1X2	T38.1X3	T38.1X4	T38.1X5	T38.1X6
Tizanidine	T42.8X1	T42.8X2	T42.8X3	T42.8X4	T42.8X5	T42.8X6
TMTD	T60.3X1	T60.3X2	T60.3X3	T60.3X4	—	—
TNT (fumes)	T65.3X1	T65.3X2	T65.3X3	T65.3X4	—	—
Toadstool	T62.0X1	T62.0X2	T62.0X3	T62.0X4	—	—
Tobacco NEC	T65.291	T65.292	T65.293	T65.294	—	—
cigarettes	T65.221	T65.222	T65.223	T65.224	—	—
Indian	T62.2X1	T62.2X2	T62.2X3	T62.2X4	—	—
smoke, second-hand	T65.221	T65.222	T65.223	T65.224	—	—
Tobramycin	T36.5X1	T36.5X2	T36.5X3	T36.5X4	T36.5X5	T36.5X6
Tocainide	T46.2X1	T46.2X2	T46.2X3	T46.2X4	T46.2X5	T46.2X6
Tocoferol	T45.2X1	T45.2X2	T45.2X3	T45.2X4	T45.2X5	T45.2X6
Tocopherol	T45.2X1	T45.2X2	T45.2X3	T45.2X4	T45.2X5	T45.2X6
acetate	T45.2X1	T45.2X2	T45.2X3	T45.2X4	T45.2X5	T45.2X6
Tocosamine	T48.0X1	T48.0X2	T48.0X3	T48.0X4	T48.0X5	T48.0X6
Todralazine	T46.5X1	T46.5X2	T46.5X3	T46.5X4	T46.5X5	T46.5X6
Tofisopam	T42.4X1	T42.4X2	T42.4X3	T42.4X4	T42.4X5	T42.4X6
Tofranil	T43.011	T43.012	T43.013	T43.014	T43.015	T43.016
Toilet deodorizer	T65.891	T65.892	T65.893	T65.894	—	—
Tolamolol	T44.7X1	T44.7X2	T44.7X3	T44.7X4	T44.7X5	T44.7X6
Tolazamide	T38.3X1	T38.3X2	T38.3X3	T38.3X4	T38.3X5	T38.3X6
Tolazoline	T46.7X1	T46.7X2	T46.7X3	T46.7X4	T46.7X5	T46.7X6
Tolbutamide (sodium)	T38.3X1	T38.3X2	T38.3X3	T38.3X4	T38.3X5	T38.3X6
Tolciclate	T49.0X1	T49.0X2	T49.0X3	T49.0X4	T49.0X5	T49.0X6
Tolmetin	T39.391	T39.392	T39.393	T39.394	T39.395	T39.396
Tolnaftate	T49.0X1	T49.0X2	T49.0X3	T49.0X4	T49.0X5	T49.0X6
Tolonidine	T46.5X1	T46.5X2	T46.5X3	T46.5X4	T46.5X5	T46.5X6
Toloxatone	T42.6X1	T42.6X2	T42.6X3	T42.6X4	T42.6X5	T42.6X6
Tolperisone	T44.3X1	T44.3X2	T44.3X3	T44.3X4	T44.3X5	T44.3X6
Tolserol	T42.8X1	T42.8X2	T42.8X3	T42.8X4	T42.8X5	T42.8X6
Toluene (liquid)	T52.2X1	T52.2X2	T52.2X3	T52.2X4	—	—
diisocyanate	T65.0X1	T65.0X2	T65.0X3	T65.0X4	—	—
Toluidine	T65.891	T65.892	T65.893	T65.894	—	—
vapor	T59.891	T59.892	T59.893	T59.894	—	—
Toluol (liquid)	T52.2X1	T52.2X2	T52.2X3	T52.2X4	—	—
vapor	T52.2X1	T52.2X2	T52.2X3	T52.2X4	—	—
Toluylenediamine	T65.3X1	T65.3X2	T65.3X3	T65.3X4	—	—
Tolylene-2,4-diisocyanate	T65.0X1	T65.0X2	T65.0X3	T65.0X4	—	—
Tonic NEC	T50.901	T50.902	T50.903	T50.904	T50.905	T50.906
Topical action drug NEC	T49.91	T49.92	T49.93	T49.94	T49.95	T49.96
ear, nose or throat	T49.6X1	T49.6X2	T49.6X3	T49.6X4	T49.6X5	T49.6X6
eye	T49.5X1	T49.5X2	T49.5X3	T49.5X4	T49.5X5	T49.5X6
skin	T49.91	T49.92	T49.93	T49.94	T49.95	T49.96
specified NEC	T49.8X1	T49.8X2	T49.8X3	T49.8X4	T49.8X5	T49.8X6
Toquizine	T44.3X1	T44.3X2	T44.3X3	T44.3X4	T44.3X5	T44.3X6
Toremifene	T38.6X1	T38.6X2	T38.6X3	T38.6X4	T38.6X5	T38.6X6
Tosylchloramide sodium	T49.8X1	T49.8X2	T49.8X3	T49.8X4	T49.8X5	T49.8X6
Toxaphene (dust) (spray)	T60.1X1	T60.1X2	T60.1X3	T60.1X4	—	—
Toxin, diphtheria (Schick Test)	T50.8X1	T50.8X2	T50.8X3	T50.8X4	T50.8X5	T50.8X6
Toxoid						
combined	T50.A21	T50.A22	T50.A23	T50.A24	T50.A25	T50.A26
diphtheria	T50.A91	T50.A92	T50.A93	T50.A94	T50.A95	T50.A96
tetanus	T50.A91	T50.A92	T50.A93	T50.A94	T50.A95	T50.A96
Trace element NEC	T45.8X1	T45.8X2	T45.8X3	T45.8X4	T45.8X5	T45.8X6
Tractor fuel NEC	T52.0X1	T52.0X2	T52.0X3	T52.0X4	—	—
Tragacanth	T50.991	T50.992	T50.993	T50.994	T50.995	T50.996
Tramadol	T40.4X1	T40.4X2	T40.4X3	T40.4X4	T40.4X5	T40.4X6
Tramazoline	T48.5X1	T48.5X2	T48.5X3	T48.5X4	T48.5X5	T48.5X6
Tranexamic acid	T45.621	T45.622	T45.623	T45.624	T45.625	T45.626
Tranilast	T45.0X1	T45.0X2	T45.0X3	T45.0X4	T45.0X5	T45.0X6
Tranquilizer NEC	T43.501	T43.502	T43.503	T43.504	T43.505	T43.506
with hypnotic or sedative	T42.6X1	T42.6X2	T42.6X3	T42.6X4	T42.6X5	T42.6X6
benzodiazepine NEC	T42.4X1	T42.4X2	T42.4X3	T42.4X4	T42.4X5	T42.4X6
butyrophenone NEC	T43.4X1	T43.4X2	T43.4X3	T43.4X4	T43.4X5	T43.4X6
carbamate	T43.591	T43.592	T43.593	T43.594	T43.595	T43.596
dimethylamine	T43.3X1	T43.3X2	T43.3X3	T43.3X4	T43.3X5	T43.3X6
ethylamine	T43.3X1	T43.3X2	T43.3X3	T43.3X4	T43.3X5	T43.3X6
hydroxyzine	T43.591	T43.592	T43.593	T43.594	T43.595	T43.596
major NEC	T43.501	T43.502	T43.503	T43.504	T43.505	T43.506
penothiazine NEC	T43.3X1	T43.3X2	T43.3X3	T43.3X4	T43.3X5	T43.3X6
phenothiazine-based	T43.3X1	T43.3X2	T43.3X3	T43.3X4	T43.3X5	T43.3X6

Substance	Poisoning, Accidental (unintentional)	Poisoning, Intentional Self-harm	Poisoning, Assault	Poisoning, Undetermined	Adverse Effect	Underdosing
Tranquilizer — continued						
piperazine NEC	T43.3X1	T43.3X2	T43.3X3	T43.3X4	T43.3X5	T43.3X6
piperidine	T43.3X1	T43.3X2	T43.3X3	T43.3X4	T43.3X5	T43.3X6
propylamine	T43.3X1	T43.3X2	T43.3X3	T43.3X4	T43.3X5	T43.3X6
specified NEC	T43.591	T43.592	T43.593	T43.594	T43.595	T43.596
thioxanthene NEC	T43.591	T43.592	T43.593	T43.594	T43.595	T43.596
Tranxene	T42.4X1	T42.4X2	T42.4X3	T42.4X4	T42.4X5	T42.4X6
Tranylcypromine	T43.1X1	T43.1X2	T43.1X3	T43.1X4	T43.1X5	T43.1X6
Trapidil	T46.3X1	T46.3X2	T46.3X3	T46.3X4	T46.3X5	T46.3X6
Trasentine	T44.3X1	T44.3X2	T44.3X3	T44.3X4	T44.3X5	T44.3X6
Travert	T50.3X1	T50.3X2	T50.3X3	T50.3X4	T50.3X5	T50.3X6
Trazodone	T43.211	T43.212	T43.213	T43.214	T43.215	T43.216
Trecator	T37.1X1	T37.1X2	T37.1X3	T37.1X4	T37.1X5	T37.1X6
Treosulfan	T45.1X1	T45.1X2	T45.1X3	T45.1X4	T45.1X5	T45.1X6
Tretamine	T45.1X1	T45.1X2	T45.1X3	T45.1X4	T45.1X5	T45.1X6
Tretinoin	T49.0X1	T49.0X2	T49.0X3	T49.0X4	T49.0X5	T49.0X6
Tretoquinol	T48.6X1	T48.6X2	T48.6X3	T48.6X4	T48.6X5	T48.6X6
Triacetin	T49.0X1	T49.0X2	T49.0X3	T49.0X4	T49.0X5	T49.0X6
Triacetoxyanthracene	T49.4X1	T49.4X2	T49.4X3	T49.4X4	T49.4X5	T49.4X6
Triacetyloleandomycin	T36.3X1	T36.3X2	T36.3X3	T36.3X4	T36.3X5	T36.3X6
Triamcinolone	T38.0X1	T38.0X2	T38.0X3	T38.0X4	T38.0X5	T38.0X6
ENT agent	T49.6X1	T49.6X2	T49.6X3	T49.6X4	T49.6X5	T49.6X6
hexacetonide	T49.0X1	T49.0X2	T49.0X3	T49.0X4	T49.0X5	T49.0X6
ophthalmic preparation	T49.5X1	T49.5X2	T49.5X3	T49.5X4	T49.5X5	T49.5X6
topical NEC	T49.0X1	T49.0X2	T49.0X3	T49.0X4	T49.0X5	T49.0X6
Triampyzine	T44.3X1	T44.3X2	T44.3X3	T44.3X4	T44.3X5	T44.3X6
Triamterene	T50.2X1	T50.2X2	T50.2X3	T50.2X4	T50.2X5	T50.2X6
Triazine (herbicide)	T60.3X1	T60.3X2	T60.3X3	T60.3X4	—	—
Triaziquone	T45.1X1	T45.1X2	T45.1X3	T45.1X4	T45.1X5	T45.1X6
Triazolam	T42.4X1	T42.4X2	T42.4X3	T42.4X4	T42.4X5	T42.4X6
Triazole (herbicide)	T60.3X1	T60.3X2	T60.3X3	T60.3X4	—	—
Tribenoside	T46.991	T46.992	T46.993	T46.994	T46.995	T46.996
Tribromacetaldehyde	T42.6X1	T42.6X2	T42.6X3	T42.6X4	T42.6X5	T42.6X6
Tribromoethanol, rectal	T41.291	T41.292	T41.293	T41.294	T41.295	T41.296
Tribromomethane	T42.6X1	T42.6X2	T42.6X3	T42.6X4	T42.6X5	T42.6X6
Trichlorethane	T53.2X1	T53.2X2	T53.2X3	T53.2X4	—	—
Trichlorethylene	T53.2X1	T53.2X2	T53.2X3	T53.2X4	—	—
Trichlorfon	T60.0X1	T60.0X2	T60.0X3	T60.0X4	—	—
Trichlormethiazide	T50.2X1	T50.2X2	T50.2X3	T50.2X4	T50.2X5	T50.2X6
Trichlormethine	T45.1X1	T45.1X2	T45.1X3	T45.1X4	T45.1X5	T45.1X6
Trichloroacetic acid, Trichloracetic acid	T54.2X1	T54.2X2	T54.2X3	T54.2X4	—	—
medicinal	T49.4X1	T49.4X2	T49.4X3	T49.4X4	T49.4X5	T49.4X6
Trichloroethane	T53.2X1	T53.2X2	T53.2X3	T53.2X4	—	—
Trichloroethanol	T42.6X1	T42.6X2	T42.6X3	T42.6X4	T42.6X5	T42.6X6
Trichloroethylene (liquid) (vapor)	T53.2X1	T53.2X2	T53.2X3	T53.2X4	—	—
anesthetic (gas)	T41.0X1	T41.0X2	T41.0X3	T41.0X4	T41.0X5	T41.0X6
vapor NEC	T53.2X1	T53.2X2	T53.2X3	T53.2X4	—	—
Trichloroethyl phosphate	T42.6X1	T42.6X2	T42.6X3	T42.6X4	T42.6X5	T42.6X6
Trichlorofluoromethane NEC	T53.5X1	T53.5X2	T53.5X3	T53.5X4	—	—
Trichloronate	T60.0X1	T60.0X2	T60.0X3	T60.0X4	—	—
Trichloropropane	T53.6X1	T53.6X2	T53.6X3	T53.6X4	—	—
Trichlorotriethylamine	T45.1X1	T45.1X2	T45.1X3	T45.1X4	T45.1X5	T45.1X6
Trichomonacides NEC	T37.3X1	T37.3X2	T37.3X3	T37.3X4	T37.3X5	T37.3X6
Trichomycin	T36.7X1	T36.7X2	T36.7X3	T36.7X4	T36.7X5	T36.7X6
Triclobisonium chloride	T49.0X1	T49.0X2	T49.0X3	T49.0X4	T49.0X5	T49.0X6
Triclocarban	T49.0X1	T49.0X2	T49.0X3	T49.0X4	T49.0X5	T49.0X6
Triclofos	T42.6X1	T42.6X2	T42.6X3	T42.6X4	T42.6X5	T42.6X6
Triclosan	T49.0X1	T49.0X2	T49.0X3	T49.0X4	T49.0X5	T49.0X6
Tricresyl phosphate	T65.891	T65.892	T65.893	T65.894	—	—
solvent	T52.91	T52.92	T52.93	T52.94	—	—
Tricyclamol chloride	T44.3X1	T44.3X2	T44.3X3	T44.3X4	T44.3X5	T44.3X6
Tridesilon	T49.0X1	T49.0X2	T49.0X3	T49.0X4	T49.0X5	T49.0X6
Tridihexethyl iodide	T44.3X1	T44.3X2	T44.3X3	T44.3X4	T44.3X5	T44.3X6
Tridione	T42.2X1	T42.2X2	T42.2X3	T42.2X4	T42.2X5	T42.2X6
Trientine	T45.8X1	T45.8X2	T45.8X3	T45.8X4	T45.8X5	T45.8X6
Triethanolamine NEC	T54.3X1	T54.3X2	T54.3X3	T54.3X4	—	—
detergent	T54.3X1	T54.3X2	T54.3X3	T54.3X4	—	—
trinitrate (biphosphate)	T46.3X1	T46.3X2	T46.3X3	T46.3X4	T46.3X5	T46.3X6
Triethanomelamine	T45.1X1	T45.1X2	T45.1X3	T45.1X4	T45.1X5	T45.1X6
Triethylenemelamine	T45.1X1	T45.1X2	T45.1X3	T45.1X4	T45.1X5	T45.1X6
Triethylenephosphoramide	T45.1X1	T45.1X2	T45.1X3	T45.1X4	T45.1X5	T45.1X6
Triethylenethiophosphoramide	T45.1X1	T45.1X2	T45.1X3	T45.1X4	T45.1X5	T45.1X6
Trifluoperazine	T43.3X1	T43.3X2	T43.3X3	T43.3X4	T43.3X5	T43.3X6
Trifluoroethyl vinyl ether	T41.0X1	T41.0X2	T41.0X3	T41.0X4	T41.0X5	T41.0X6
Trifluperidol	T43.4X1	T43.4X2	T43.4X3	T43.4X4	T43.4X5	T43.4X6
Triflupromazine	T43.3X1	T43.3X2	T43.3X3	T43.3X4	T43.3X5	T43.3X6
Trifluridine	T37.5X1	T37.5X2	T37.5X3	T37.5X4	T37.5X5	T37.5X6
Triflusal	T45.521	T45.522	T45.523	T45.524	T45.525	T45.526
Trihexyphenidyl	T44.3X1	T44.3X2	T44.3X3	T44.3X4	T44.3X5	T44.3X6
Triiodothyronine	T38.1X1	T38.1X2	T38.1X3	T38.1X4	T38.1X5	T38.1X6

Substance	Poisoning, Accidental (unintentional)	Poisoning, Intentional Self-harm	Poisoning, Assault	Poisoning, Undetermined	Adverse Effect	Underdosing
Trilene	T41.0X1	T41.0X2	T41.0X3	T41.0X4	T41.0X5	T41.0
Trilostane	T38.991	T38.992	T38.993	T38.994	T38.995	T38.9
Trimebutine	T44.3X1	T44.3X2	T44.3X3	T44.3X4	T44.3X5	T44.3
Trimecaine	T41.3X1	T41.3X2	T41.3X3	T41.3X4	T41.3X5	T41.3
Trimeprazine (tartrate)	T44.3X1	T44.3X2	T44.3X3	T44.3X4	T44.3X5	T44.3
Trimetaphan camsilate	T44.2X1	T44.2X2	T44.2X3	T44.2X4	T44.2X5	T44.2
Trimetazidine	T46.7X1	T46.7X2	T46.7X3	T46.7X4	T46.7X5	T46.7
Trimethadione	T42.2X1	T42.2X2	T42.2X3	T42.2X4	T42.2X5	T42.2
Trimethaphan	T44.2X1	T44.2X2	T44.2X3	T44.2X4	T44.2X5	T44.2
Trimethidinium	T44.2X1	T44.2X2	T44.2X3	T44.2X4	T44.2X5	T44.2
Trimethobenzamide	T45.0X1	T45.0X2	T45.0X3	T45.0X4	T45.0X5	T45.0
Trimethoprim	T37.8X1	T37.8X2	T37.8X3	T37.8X4	T37.8X5	T37.8
with sulfamethoxazole	T36.8X1	T36.8X2	T36.8X3	T36.8X4	T36.8X5	T36.8
Trimethylcarbinol	T51.3X1	T51.3X2	T51.3X3	T51.3X4	—	—
Trimethylpsoralen	T49.3X1	T49.3X2	T49.3X3	T49.3X4	T49.3X5	T49.3
Trimeton	T45.0X1	T45.0X2	T45.0X3	T45.0X4	T45.0X5	T45.0
Trimetrexate	T45.1X1	T45.1X2	T45.1X3	T45.1X4	T45.1X5	T45.1
Trimipramine	T43.011	T43.012	T43.013	T43.014	T43.015	T43.0
Trimustine	T45.1X1	T45.1X2	T45.1X3	T45.1X4	T45.1X5	T45.1
Trinitrine	T46.3X1	T46.3X2	T46.3X3	T46.3X4	T46.3X5	T46.3
Trinitrobenzol	T65.3X1	T65.3X2	T65.3X3	T65.3X4	—	—
Trinitrophenol	T65.3X1	T65.3X2	T65.3X3	T65.3X4	—	—
Trinitrotoluene (fumes)	T65.3X1	T65.3X2	T65.3X3	T65.3X4	—	—
Trional	T42.6X1	T42.6X2	T42.6X3	T42.6X4	T42.6X5	T42.6
Triorthocresyl phosphate	T65.891	T65.892	T65.893	T65.894	—	—
Trioxide of arsenic	T57.0X1	T57.0X2	T57.0X3	T57.0X4	—	—
Trioxysalen	T49.4X1	T49.4X2	T49.4X3	T49.4X4	T49.4X5	T49.4
Tripamide	T50.2X1	T50.2X2	T50.2X3	T50.2X4	T50.2X5	T50.2
Triparanol	T46.6X1	T46.6X2	T46.6X3	T46.6X4	T46.6X5	T46.6
Tripelennamine	T45.0X1	T45.0X2	T45.0X3	T45.0X4	T45.0X5	T45.0
Triperiden	T44.3X1	T44.3X2	T44.3X3	T44.3X4	T44.3X5	T44.3
Triperidol	T43.4X1	T43.4X2	T43.4X3	T43.4X4	T43.4X5	T43.4
Triphenylphosphate	T65.891	T65.892	T65.893	T65.894	—	—
Triple						
bromides	T42.6X1	T42.6X2	T42.6X3	T42.6X4	T42.6X5	T42.6
carbonate	T47.1X1	T47.1X2	T47.1X3	T47.1X4	T47.1X5	T47.1
vaccine						
DPT	T50.A11	T50.A12	T50.A13	T50.A14	T50.A15	T50.A
including pertussis	T50.A11	T50.A12	T50.A13	T50.A14	T50.A15	T50.A
MMR	T50.B91	T50.B92	T50.B93	T50.B94	T50.B95	T50.B
Triprolidine	T45.0X1	T45.0X2	T45.0X3	T45.0X4	T45.0X5	T45.0
Trisodium hydrogen edetate	T50.6X1	T50.6X2	T50.6X3	T50.6X4	T50.6X5	T50.6
Trisoralen	T49.3X1	T49.3X2	T49.3X3	T49.3X4	T49.3X5	T49.3
Trisulfapyrimidines	T37.0X1	T37.0X2	T37.0X3	T37.0X4	T37.0X5	T37.0
Trithiozine	T44.3X1	T44.3X2	T44.3X3	T44.3X4	T44.3X5	T44.3
Tritiozine	T44.3X1	T44.3X2	T44.3X3	T44.3X4	T44.3X5	T44.3
Tritoqualine	T45.0X1	T45.0X2	T45.0X3	T45.0X4	T45.0X5	T45.0
Trofosfamide	T45.1X1	T45.1X2	T45.1X3	T45.1X4	T45.1X5	T45.1
Troleandomycin	T36.3X1	T36.3X2	T36.3X3	T36.3X4	T36.3X5	T36.3
Trolnitrate (phosphate)	T46.3X1	T46.3X2	T46.3X3	T46.3X4	T46.3X5	T46.3
Tromantadine	T37.5X1	T37.5X2	T37.5X3	T37.5X4	T37.5X5	T37.5
Trometamol	T50.2X1	T50.2X2	T50.2X3	T50.2X4	T50.2X5	T50.2
Tromethamine	T50.2X1	T50.2X2	T50.2X3	T50.2X4	T50.2X5	T50.2
Tronothane	T41.3X1	T41.3X2	T41.3X3	T41.3X4	T41.3X5	T41.3
Tropacine	T44.3X1	T44.3X2	T44.3X3	T44.3X4	T44.3X5	T44.3
Tropatepine	T44.3X1	T44.3X2	T44.3X3	T44.3X4	T44.3X5	T44.3
Tropicamide	T44.3X1	T44.3X2	T44.3X3	T44.3X4	T44.3X5	T44.3
Trospium chloride	T44.3X1	T44.3X2	T44.3X3	T44.3X4	T44.3X5	T44.3
Troxerutin	T46.991	T46.992	T46.993	T46.994	T46.995	T46.9
Troxidone	T42.2X1	T42.2X2	T42.2X3	T42.2X4	T42.2X5	T42.2
Tryparsamide	T37.3X1	T37.3X2	T37.3X3	T37.3X4	T37.3X5	T37.3
Trypsin	T45.3X1	T45.3X2	T45.3X3	T45.3X4	T45.3X5	T45.3
Tryptizol	T43.011	T43.012	T43.013	T43.014	T43.015	T43.0
TSH	T38.811	T38.812	T38.813	T38.814	T38.815	T38.8
Tuaminoheptane	T48.5X1	T48.5X2	T48.5X3	T48.5X4	T48.5X5	T48.5
Tuberculin, purified protein derivative (PPD)	T50.8X1	T50.8X2	T50.8X3	T50.8X4	T50.8X5	T50.8
Tubocurare	T48.1X1	T48.1X2	T48.1X3	T48.1X4	T48.1X5	T48.1
Tubocurarine (chloride)	T48.1X1	T48.1X2	T48.1X3	T48.1X4	T48.1X5	T48.1
Tulobuterol	T48.6X1	T48.6X2	T48.6X3	T48.6X4	T48.6X5	T48.6
Turpentine (spirits of)	T52.8X1	T52.8X2	T52.8X3	T52.8X4	—	—
vapor	T52.8X1	T52.8X2	T52.8X3	T52.8X4	—	—
Tybamate	T43.591	T43.592	T43.593	T43.594	T43.595	T43.5
Tyloxapol	T48.4X1	T48.4X2	T48.4X3	T48.4X4	T48.4X5	T48.4
Tymazoline	T48.5X1	T48.5X2	T48.5X3	T48.5X4	T48.5X5	T48.5
Typhoid-paratyphoid vaccine	T50.A91	T50.A92	T50.A93	T50.A94	T50.A95	T50.A
Typhus vaccine	T50.A91	T50.A92	T50.A93	T50.A94	T50.A95	T50.A
Tyropanoate	T50.8X1	T50.8X2	T50.8X3	T50.8X4	T50.8X5	T50.8
Tyrothricin	T49.6X1	T49.6X2	T49.6X3	T49.6X4	T49.6X5	T49.6
ENT agent	T49.6X1	T49.6X2	T49.6X3	T49.6X4	T49.6X5	T49.6
ophthalmic preparation	T49.5X1	T49.5X2	T49.5X3	T49.5X4	T49.5X5	T49.5

Substance	Poisoning, Accidental (unintentional)	Poisoning, Intentional Self-harm	Poisoning, Assault	Poisoning, Undetermined	Adverse Effect	Under-dosing
Ufenamate	T39.391	T39.392	T39.393	T39.394	T39.395	T39.396
Ultraviolet light protectant	T49.3X1	T49.3X2	T49.3X3	T49.3X4	T49.3X5	T49.3X6
Undecenoic acid	T49.0X1	T49.0X2	T49.0X3	T49.0X4	T49.0X5	T49.0X6
Undecoylium	T49.0X1	T49.0X2	T49.0X3	T49.0X4	T49.0X5	T49.0X6
Undecylenic acid	T49.0X1	T49.0X2	T49.0X3	T49.0X4	T49.0X5	T49.0X6
(derivatives)						
Unna's boot	T49.3X1	T49.3X2	T49.3X3	T49.3X4	T49.3X5	T49.3X6
Unsaturated fatty acid	T46.6X1	T46.6X2	T46.6X3	T46.6X4	T46.6X5	T46.6X6
Uracil mustard	T45.1X1	T45.1X2	T45.1X3	T45.1X4	T45.1X5	T45.1X6
Uramustine	T45.1X1	T45.1X2	T45.1X3	T45.1X4	T45.1X5	T45.1X6
Urapidil	T46.5X1	T46.5X2	T46.5X3	T46.5X4	T46.5X5	T46.5X6
Urari	T48.1X1	T48.1X2	T48.1X3	T48.1X4	T48.1X5	T48.1X6
Urate oxidase	T50.4X1	T50.4X2	T50.4X3	T50.4X4	T50.4X5	T50.4X6
Urea	T47.3X1	T47.3X2	T47.3X3	T47.3X4	T47.3X5	T47.3X6
peroxide	T49.0X1	T49.0X2	T49.0X3	T49.0X4	T49.0X5	T49.0X6
stibamine	T37.4X1	T37.4X2	T37.4X3	T37.4X4	T37.4X5	T37.4X6
topical	T49.8X1	T49.8X2	T49.8X3	T49.8X4	T49.8X5	T49.8X6
Urethane	T45.1X1	T45.1X2	T45.1X3	T45.1X4	T45.1X5	T45.1X6
Urginea (maritima) (scilla) — *see* Squill						
Uric acid metabolism drug NEC	T50.4X1	T50.4X2	T50.4X3	T50.4X4	T50.4X5	T50.4X6
Uricosuric agent	T50.4X1	T50.4X2	T50.4X3	T50.4X4	T50.4X5	T50.4X6
Urinary anti-infective	T37.8X1	T37.8X2	T37.8X3	T37.8X4	T37.8X5	T37.8X6
Urofollitropin	T38.811	T38.812	T38.813	T38.814	T38.815	T38.816
Urokinase	T45.611	T45.612	T45.613	T45.614	T45.615	T45.616
Urokon	T50.8X1	T50.8X2	T50.8X3	T50.8X4	T50.8X5	T50.8X6
Ursodeoxycholic acid	T50.991	T50.992	T50.993	T50.994	T50.995	T50.996
Ursodiol	T50.991	T50.992	T50.993	T50.994	T50.995	T50.996
Urtica	T62.2X1	T62.2X2	T62.2X3	T62.2X4	—	—
Utility gas — *see* Gas, utility						
Vaccine NEC	T50.Z91	T50.Z92	T50.Z93	T50.Z94	T50.Z95	T50.Z96
antineoplastic	T50.Z91	T50.Z92	T50.Z93	T50.Z94	T50.Z95	T50.Z96
bacterial NEC	T50.A91	T50.A92	T50.A93	T50.A94	T50.A95	T50.A96
with						
other bacterial component	T50.A21	T50.A22	T50.A23	T50.A24	T50.A25	T50.A26
pertussis component	T50.A11	T50.A12	T50.A13	T50.A14	T50.A15	T50.A16
viral-rickettsial component	T50.A21	T50.A22	T50.A23	T50.A24	T50.A25	T50.A26
mixed NEC	T50.A21	T50.A22	T50.A23	T50.A24	T50.A25	T50.A26
BCG	T50.A91	T50.A92	T50.A93	T50.A94	T50.A95	T50.A96
cholera	T50.A91	T50.A92	T50.A93	T50.A94	T50.A95	T50.A96
diphtheria	T50.A91	T50.A92	T50.A93	T50.A94	T50.A95	T50.A96
with tetanus	T50.A21	T50.A22	T50.A23	T50.A24	T50.A25	T50.A26
and pertussis	T50.A11	T50.A12	T50.A13	T50.A14	T50.A15	T50.A16
influenza	T50.B91	T50.B92	T50.B93	T50.B94	T50.B95	T50.B96
measles	T50.B91	T50.B92	T50.B93	T50.B94	T50.B95	T50.B96
with mumps and rubella	T50.B91	T50.B92	T50.B93	T50.B94	T50.B95	T50.B96
meningococcal	T50.A91	T50.A92	T50.A93	T50.A94	T50.A95	T50.A96
mumps	T50.B91	T50.B92	T50.B93	T50.B94	T50.B95	T50.B96
paratyphoid	T50.A91	T50.A92	T50.A93	T50.A94	T50.A95	T50.A96
pertussis	T50.A11	T50.A12	T50.A13	T50.A14	T50.A15	T50.A16
with diphtheria	T50.A11	T50.A12	T50.A13	T50.A14	T50.A15	T50.A16
and tetanus	T50.A11	T50.A12	T50.A13	T50.A14	T50.A15	T50.A16
with other component	T50.A11	T50.A12	T50.A13	T50.A14	T50.A15	T50.A16
plague	T50.A91	T50.A92	T50.A93	T50.A94	T50.A95	T50.A96
poliomyelitis	T50.B91	T50.B92	T50.B93	T50.B94	T50.B95	T50.B96
poliovirus	T50.B91	T50.B92	T50.B93	T50.B94	T50.B95	T50.B96
rabies	T50.B91	T50.B92	T50.B93	T50.B94	T50.B95	T50.B96
respiratory syncytial virus	T50.B91	T50.B92	T50.B93	T50.B94	T50.B95	T50.B96
rickettsial NEC	T50.A91	T50.A92	T50.A93	T50.A94	T50.A95	T50.A96
with						
bacterial component	T50.A21	T50.A22	T50.A23	T50.A24	T50.A25	T50.A26
Rocky Mountain spotted fever	T50.A91	T50.A92	T50.A93	T50.A94	T50.A95	T50.A96
rubella	T50.B91	T50.B92	T50.B93	T50.B94	T50.B95	T50.B96
sabin oral	T50.B91	T50.B92	T50.B93	T50.B94	T50.B95	T50.B96
smallpox	T50.B11	T50.B12	T50.B13	T50.B14	T50.B15	T50.B16
TAB	T50.A91	T50.A92	T50.A93	T50.A94	T50.A95	T50.A96
tetanus	T50.A91	T50.A92	T50.A93	T50.A94	T50.A95	T50.A96
typhoid	T50.A91	T50.A92	T50.A93	T50.A94	T50.A95	T50.A96
typhus	T50.A91	T50.A92	T50.A93	T50.A94	T50.A95	T50.A96
viral NEC	T50.B91	T50.B92	T50.B93	T50.B94	T50.B95	T50.B96
yellow fever	T50.B91	T50.B92	T50.B93	T50.B94	T50.B95	T50.B96
Vaccinia immune globulin	T50.Z11	T50.Z12	T50.Z13	T50.Z14	T50.Z15	T50.Z16
Vaginal contraceptives	T49.8X1	T49.8X2	T49.8X3	T49.8X4	T49.8X5	T49.8X6
Valerian						
root	T42.6X1	T42.6X2	T42.6X3	T42.6X4	T42.6X5	T42.6X6
tincture	T42.6X1	T42.6X2	T42.6X3	T42.6X4	T42.6X5	T42.6X6
Valethamate bromide	T44.3X1	T44.3X2	T44.3X3	T44.3X4	T44.3X5	T44.3X6
Valisone	T49.0X1	T49.0X2	T49.0X3	T49.0X4	T49.0X5	T49.0X6

Substance	Poisoning, Accidental (unintentional)	Poisoning, Intentional Self-harm	Poisoning, Assault	Poisoning, Undetermined	Adverse Effect	Under-dosing
Valium	T42.4X1	T42.4X2	T42.4X3	T42.4X4	T42.4X5	T42.4X6
Valmid	T42.6X1	T42.6X2	T42.6X3	T42.6X4	T42.6X5	T42.6X6
Valnoctamide	T42.6X1	T42.6X2	T42.6X3	T42.6X4	T42.6X5	T42.6X6
Valproate (sodium)	T42.6X1	T42.6X2	T42.6X3	T42.6X4	T42.6X5	T42.6X6
Valproic acid	T42.6X1	T42.6X2	T42.6X3	T42.6X4	T42.6X5	T42.6X6
Valpromide	T42.6X1	T42.6X2	T42.6X3	T42.6X4	T42.6X5	T42.6X6
Vanadium	T56.891	T56.892	T56.893	T56.894		
Vancomycin	T36.8X1	T36.8X2	T36.8X3	T36.8X4	T36.8X5	T36.8X6
Vapor — *see also* Gas	T59.91	T59.92	T59.93	T59.94		
kiln (carbon monoxide)	T58.8X1	T58.8X2	T58.8X3	T58.8X4		
lead — *see* lead						
specified source NEC	T59.891	T59.892	T59.893	T59.894	—	—
Vardenafil	T46.7X1	T46.7X2	T46.7X3	T46.7X4	T46.7X5	T46.7X6
Varicose reduction drug	T46.8X1	T46.8X2	T46.8X3	T46.8X4	T46.8X5	T46.8X6
Varnish	T65.4X1	T65.4X2	T65.4X3	T65.4X4		
cleaner	T52.91	T52.92	T52.93	T52.94		
Vaseline	T49.3X1	T49.3X2	T49.3X3	T49.3X4	T49.3X5	T49.3X6
Vasodilan	T46.7X1	T46.7X2	T46.7X3	T46.7X4	T46.7X5	T46.7X6
Vasodilator						
coronary NEC	T46.3X1	T46.3X2	T46.3X3	T46.3X4	T46.3X5	T46.3X6
peripheral NEC	T46.7X1	T46.7X2	T46.7X3	T46.7X4	T46.7X5	T46.7X6
Vasopressin	T38.891	T38.892	T38.893	T38.894	T38.895	T38.896
Vasopressor drugs	T38.891	T38.892	T38.893	T38.894	T38.895	T38.896
Vecuronium bromide	T48.1X1	T48.1X2	T48.1X3	T48.1X4	T48.1X5	T48.1X6
Vegetable extract, astringent	T49.2X1	T49.2X2	T49.2X3	T49.2X4	T49.2X5	T49.2X6
Venlafaxine	T43.211	T43.212	T43.213	T43.214	T43.215	T43.216
Venom, venomous (bite) (sting)	T63.91	T63.92	T63.93	T63.94	—	—
amphibian NEC	T63.831	T63.832	T63.833	T63.834		
animal NEC	T63.891	T63.892	T63.893	T63.894	—	—
ant	T63.421	T63.422	T63.423	T63.424		
arthropod NEC	T63.481	T63.482	T63.483	T63.484		
bee	T63.441	T63.442	T63.443	T63.444		
centipede	T63.411	T63.412	T63.413	T63.414		
fish	T63.591	T63.592	T63.593	T63.594		
frog	T63.811	T63.812	T63.813	T63.814		
hornet	T63.451	T63.452	T63.453	T63.454		
insect NEC	T63.481	T63.482	T63.483	T63.484		
lizard	T63.121	T63.122	T63.123	T63.124		
marine						
animals	T63.691	T63.692	T63.693	T63.694		
bluebottle	T63.611	T63.612	T63.613	T63.614		
jellyfish NEC	T63.621	T63.622	T63.623	T63.624		
Portugese Man-o-war	T63.611	T63.612	T63.613	T63.614		
sea anemone	T63.631	T63.632	T63.633	T63.634		
specified NEC	T63.691	T63.692	T63.693	T63.694		
fish	T63.591	T63.592	T63.593	T63.594		
plants	T63.711	T63.712	T63.713	T63.714		
sting ray	T63.511	T63.512	T63.513	T63.514		
millipede (tropical)	T63.411	T63.412	T63.413	T63.414		
plant NEC	T63.791	T63.792	T63.793	T63.794		
marine	T63.711	T63.712	T63.713	T63.714		
reptile	T63.191	T63.192	T63.193	T63.194		
gila monster	T63.111	T63.112	T63.113	T63.114		
lizard NEC	T63.121	T63.122	T63.123	T63.124		
scorpion	T63.2X1	T63.2X2	T63.2X3	T63.2X4		
snake	T63.001	T63.002	T63.003	T63.004		
African NEC	T63.081	T63.082	T63.083	T63.084		
American (North) (South) NEC	T63.061	T63.062	T63.063	T63.064		
Asian	T63.081	T63.082	T63.083	T63.084		
Australian	T63.071	T63.072	T63.073	T63.074		
cobra	T63.041	T63.042	T63.043	T63.044		
coral snake	T63.021	T63.022	T63.023	T63.024		
rattlesnake	T63.011	T63.012	T63.013	T63.014		
specified NEC	T63.091	T63.092	T63.093	T63.094		
taipan	T63.031	T63.032	T63.033	T63.034		
specified NEC	T63.891	T63.892	T63.893	T63.894		
spider	T63.301	T63.302	T63.303	T63.304		
black widow	T63.311	T63.312	T63.313	T63.314		
brown recluse	T63.331	T63.332	T63.333	T63.334		
specified NEC	T63.391	T63.392	T63.393	T63.394		
tarantula	T63.321	T63.322	T63.323	T63.324		
sting ray	T63.511	T63.512	T63.513	T63.514		
toad	T63.821	T63.822	T63.823	T63.824		
wasp	T63.461	T63.462	T63.463	T63.464	—	—
Venous sclerosing drug NEC	T46.8X1	T46.8X2	T46.8X3	T46.8X4	T46.8X5	T46.8X6
Ventolin — *see* Albuterol						
Veramon	T42.3X1	T42.3X2	T42.3X3	T42.3X4	T42.3X5	T42.3X6
Verapamil	T46.1X1	T46.1X2	T46.1X3	T46.1X4	T46.1X5	T46.1X6
Veratrine	T46.5X1	T46.5X2	T46.5X3	T46.5X4	T46.5X5	T46.5X6

Substance	Poisoning, Accidental (unintentional)	Poisoning, Intentional Self-harm	Poisoning, Assault	Poisoning, Undetermined	Adverse Effect	Under-dosing
Veratrum						
album	T62.2X1	T62.2X2	T62.2X3	T62.2X4	—	—
alkaloids	T46.5X1	T46.5X2	T46.5X3	T46.5X4	T46.5X5	T46.5X6
viride	T62.2X1	T62.2X2	T62.2X3	T62.2X4	—	—
Verdigris	T60.3X1	T60.3X2	T60.3X3	T60.3X4		
Veronal	T42.3X1	T42.3X2	T42.3X3	T42.3X4	T42.3X5	T42.3X6
Veroxil	T50.6X1	T50.6X2	T50.6X3	T50.6X4	T50.6X5	T50.6X6
Versenate	T50.6X1	T50.6X2	T50.6X3	T50.6X4	T50.6X5	T50.6X6
Versidyne	T39.8X1	T39.8X2	T39.8X3	T39.8X4	T39.8X5	T39.8X6
Vetrabutine	T48.0X1	T48.0X2	T48.0X3	T48.0X4	T48.0X5	T48.0X6
Vidarabine	T37.5X1	T37.5X2	T37.5X3	T37.5X4	T37.5X5	T37.5X6
Vienna						
green	T57.0X1	T57.0X2	T57.0X3	T57.0X4	—	—
insecticide	T60.2X1	T60.2X2	T60.2X3	T60.2X4	—	—
red	T57.0X1	T57.0X2	T57.0X3	T57.0X4	—	—
pharmaceutical dye	T50.991	T50.992	T50.993	T50.994	T50.995	T50.996
Vigabatrin	T42.6X1	T42.6X2	T42.6X3	T42.6X4	T42.6X5	T42.6X6
Viloxazine	T43.291	T43.292	T43.293	T43.294	T43.295	T43.296
Viminol	T39.8X1	T39.8X2	T39.8X3	T39.8X4	T39.8X5	T39.8X6
Vinbarbital, vinbarbitone	T42.3X1	T42.3X2	T42.3X3	T42.3X4	T42.3X5	T42.3X6
Vinblastine	T45.1X1	T45.1X2	T45.1X3	T45.1X4	T45.1X5	T45.1X6
Vinburnine	T46.7X1	T46.7X2	T46.7X3	T46.7X4	T46.7X5	T46.7X6
Vincamine	T45.1X1	T45.1X2	T45.1X3	T45.1X4	T45.1X5	T45.1X6
Vincristine	T45.1X1	T45.1X2	T45.1X3	T45.1X4	T45.1X5	T45.1X6
Vindesine	T45.1X1	T45.1X2	T45.1X3	T45.1X4	T45.1X5	T45.1X6
Vinesthene, vinethene	T41.0X1	T41.0X2	T41.0X3	T41.0X4	T41.0X5	T41.0X6
Vinorelbine tartrate	T45.1X1	T45.1X2	T45.1X3	T45.1X4	T45.1X5	T45.1X6
Vinpocetine	T46.7X1	T46.7X2	T46.7X3	T46.7X4	T46.7X5	T46.7X6
Vinyl						
acetate	T65.891	T65.892	T65.893	T65.894	—	
bital	T42.3X1	T42.3X2	T42.3X3	T42.3X4	T42.3X5	T42.3X6
bromide	T65.891	T65.892	T65.893	T65.894	—	—
chloride	T59.891	T59.892	T59.893	T59.894	—	—
ether	T41.0X1	T41.0X2	T41.0X3	T41.0X4	T41.0X5	T41.0X6
Vinylbital	T42.3X1	T42.3X2	T42.3X3	T42.3X4	T42.3X5	T42.3X6
Vinylidene chloride	T65.891	T65.892	T65.893	T65.894		
Vioform	T37.8X1	T37.8X2	T37.8X3	T37.8X4	T37.8X5	T37.8X6
topical	T49.0X1	T49.0X2	T49.0X3	T49.0X4	T49.0X5	T49.0X6
Viomycin	T36.8X1	T36.8X2	T36.8X3	T36.8X4	T36.8X5	T36.8X6
Viosterol	T45.2X1	T45.2X2	T45.2X3	T45.2X4	T45.2X5	T45.2X6
Viper (venom)	T63.091	T63.092	T63.093	T63.094	—	—
Viprynium	T37.4X1	T37.4X2	T37.4X3	T37.4X4	T37.4X5	T37.4X6
Viquidil	T46.7X1	T46.7X2	T46.7X3	T46.7X4	T46.7X5	T46.7X6
Viral vaccine NEC	T50.B91	T50.B92	T50.B93	T50.B94	T50.B95	T50.B96
Virginiamycin	T36.8X1	T36.8X2	T36.8X3	T36.8X4	T36.8X5	T36.8X6
Virugon	T37.5X1	T37.5X2	T37.5X3	T37.5X4	T37.5X5	T37.5X6
Viscous agent	T50.901	T50.902	T50.903	T50.904	T50.905	T50.906
Visine	T49.5X1	T49.5X2	T49.5X3	T49.5X4	T49.5X5	T49.5X6
Visnadine	T46.3X1	T46.3X2	T46.3X3	T46.3X4	T46.3X5	T46.3X6
Vitamin NEC	T45.2X1	T45.2X2	T45.2X3	T45.2X4	T45.2X5	T45.2X6
A	T45.2X1	T45.2X2	T45.2X3	T45.2X4	T45.2X5	T45.2X6
B1	T45.2X1	T45.2X2	T45.2X3	T45.2X4	T45.2X5	T45.2X6
B2	T45.2X1	T45.2X2	T45.2X3	T45.2X4	T45.2X5	T45.2X6
B6	T45.2X1	T45.2X2	T45.2X3	T45.2X4	T45.2X5	T45.2X6
B12	T45.2X1	T45.2X2	T45.2X3	T45.2X4	T45.2X5	T45.2X6
B15	T45.2X1	T45.2X2	T45.2X3	T45.2X4	T45.2X5	T45.2X6
B NEC	T45.2X1	T45.2X2	T45.2X3	T45.2X4	T45.2X5	T45.2X6
nicotinic acid	T46.7X1	T46.7X2	T46.7X3	T46.7X4	T46.7X5	T46.7X6
C	T45.2X1	T45.2X2	T45.2X3	T45.2X4	T45.2X5	T45.2X6
D	T45.2X1	T45.2X2	T45.2X3	T45.2X4	T45.2X5	T45.2X6
D2	T45.2X1	T45.2X2	T45.2X3	T45.2X4	T45.2X5	T45.2X6
D3	T45.2X1	T45.2X2	T45.2X3	T45.2X4	T45.2X5	T45.2X6
E	T45.2X1	T45.2X2	T45.2X3	T45.2X4	T45.2X5	T45.2X6
E acetate	T45.2X1	T45.2X2	T45.2X3	T45.2X4	T45.2X5	T45.2X6
hematopoietic	T45.8X1	T45.8X2	T45.8X3	T45.8X4	T45.8X5	T45.8X6
K1	T45.7X1	T45.7X2	T45.7X3	T45.7X4	T45.7X5	T45.7X6
K2	T45.7X1	T45.7X2	T45.7X3	T45.7X4	T45.7X5	T45.7X6
K NEC	T45.7X1	T45.7X2	T45.7X3	T45.7X4	T45.7X5	T45.7X6
PP	T45.2X1	T45.2X2	T45.2X3	T45.2X4	T45.2X5	T45.2X6
ulceroprotectant	T47.1X1	T47.1X2	T47.1X3	T47.1X4	T47.1X5	T47.1X6
Vleminckx's solution	T49.4X1	T49.4X2	T49.4X3	T49.4X4	T49.4X5	T49.4X6
Voltaren — *see* Diclofenac						
sodium						
Warfarin	T45.511	T45.512	T45.513	T45.514	T45.515	T45.516
rodenticide	T60.4X1-	T60.4X2-	T60.4X3-	T60.4X4-	—	—
sodium	T45.511	T45.512	T45.513	T45.514	T45.515	T45.516
Wasp (sting)	T63.461	T63.462	T63.463	T63.464		
Water						
balance drug	T50.3X1	T50.3X2	T50.3X3	T50.3X4	T50.3X5	T50.3X6
distilled	T50.3X1	T50.3X2	T50.3X3	T50.3X4	T50.3X5	T50.3X6
gas — *see* Gas, water						

Substance	Poisoning, Accidental (unintentional)	Poisoning, Intentional Self-harm	Poisoning, Assault	Poisoning, Undetermined	Adverse Effect	Under-dosing
Water — *continued*						
gas — *see* Gas, water — *continued*						
incomplete combustion of — *see* Carbon, monoxide, fuel, utility						
hemlock	T62.2X1	T62.2X2	T62.2X3	T62.2X4	—	—
moccasin (venom)	T63.061	T63.062	T63.063	T63.064	—	—
purified	T50.3X1	T50.3X2	T50.3X3	T50.3X4	T50.3X5	T50.3
Wax (paraffin) (petroleum)	T52.0X1	T52.0X2	T52.0X3	T52.0X4	—	—
automobile	T65.891	T65.892	T65.893	T65.894	—	—
floor	T52.0X1	T52.0X2	T52.0X3	T52.0X4	—	—
Weed killers NEC	T60.3X1	T60.3X2	T60.3X3	T60.3X4	—	—
Welldorm	T42.6X1	T42.6X2	T42.6X3	T42.6X4	T42.6X5	T42.6
White						
arsenic	T57.0X1	T57.0X2	T57.0X3	T57.0X4	—	—
hellebore	T62.2X1	T62.2X2	T62.2X3	T62.2X4	—	—
lotion (keratolytic)	T49.4X1	T49.4X2	T49.4X3	T49.4X4	T49.4X5	T49.4
spirit	T52.0X1	T52.0X2	T52.0X3	T52.0X4	—	—
Whitewash	T65.891	T65.892	T65.893	T65.894		
Whole blood (human)	T45.8X1	T45.8X2	T45.8X3	T45.8X4	T45.8X5	T45.8
Wild						
black cherry	T62.2X1	T62.2X2	T62.2X3	T62.2X4	—	—
poisonous plants NEC	T62.2X1	T62.2X2	T62.2X3	T62.2X4	—	—
Window cleaning fluid	T65.891	T65.892	T65.893	T65.894	—	—
Wintergreen (oil)	T49.3X1	T49.3X2	T49.3X3	T49.3X4	T49.3X5	T49.3
Wisterine	T62.2X1	T62.2X2	T62.2X3	T62.2X4	—	—
Witch hazel	T49.2X1	T49.2X2	T49.2X3	T49.2X4	T49.2X5	T49.2
Wood alcohol or spirit	T51.1X1	T51.1X2	T51.1X3	T51.1X4	—	—
Wool fat (hydrous)	T49.3X1	T49.3X2	T49.3X3	T49.3X4	T49.3X5	T49.3
Woorali	T48.1X1	T48.1X2	T48.1X3	T48.1X4	T48.1X5	T48.1
Wormseed, American	T37.4X1	T37.4X2	T37.4X3	T37.4X4	T37.4X5	T37.4
Xamoterol	T44.5X1	T44.5X2	T44.5X3	T44.5X4	T44.5X5	T44.5
Xanthine diuretics	T50.2X1	T50.2X2	T50.2X3	T50.2X4	T50.2X5	T50.2
Xanthinol nicotinate	T46.7X1	T46.7X2	T46.7X3	T46.7X4	T46.7X5	T46.7
Xanthotoxin	T49.3X1	T49.3X2	T49.3X3	T49.3X4	T49.3X5	T49.3
Xantinol nicotinate	T46.7X1	T46.7X2	T46.7X3	T46.7X4	T46.7X5	T46.7
Xantocillin	T36.0X1	T36.0X2	T36.0X3	T36.0X4	T36.0X5	T36.0
Xenon (127Xe) (133Xe)	T50.8X1	T50.8X2	T50.8X3	T50.8X4	T50.8X5	T50.8
Xenysalate	T49.4X1	T49.4X2	T49.4X3	T49.4X4	T49.4X5	T49.4
Xibornol	T37.8X1	T37.8X2	T37.8X3	T37.8X4	T37.8X5	T37.8
Xigris	T45.511	T45.512	T45.513	T45.514	T45.515	T45.5
Xipamide	T50.2X1	T50.2X2	T50.2X3	T50.2X4	T50.2X5	T50.2
Xylene (vapor)	T52.2X1	T52.2X2	T52.2X3	T52.2X4		
Xylocaine (infiltration) (topical)	T41.3X1	T41.3X2	T41.3X3	T41.3X4	T41.3X5	T41.3
nerve block (peripheral) (plexus)	T41.3X1	T41.3X2	T41.3X3	T41.3X4	T41.3X5	T41.3
spinal	T41.3X1	T41.3X2	T41.3X3	T41.3X4	T41.3X5	T41.3
Xylol (vapor)	T52.2X1	T52.2X2	T52.2X3	T52.2X4	—	—
Xylometazoline	T48.5X1	T48.5X2	T48.5X3	T48.5X4	T48.5X5	T48.5
Yeast	T45.2X1	T45.2X2	T45.2X3	T45.2X4	T45.2X5	T45.2
dried	T45.2X1	T45.2X2	T45.2X3	T45.2X4	T45.2X5	T45.2
Yellow						
fever vaccine	T50.B91	T50.B92	T50.B93	T50.B94	T50.B95	T50.B9
jasmine	T62.2X1	T62.2X2	T62.2X3	T62.2X4		
phenolphthalein	T47.2X1	T47.2X2	T47.2X3	T47.2X4	T47.2X5	T47.2
Yew	T62.2X1	T62.2X2	T62.2X3	T62.2X4		
Yohimbic acid	T40.991	T40.992	T40.993	T40.994	T40.995	T40.99
Zactane	T39.8X1	T39.8X2	T39.8X3	T39.8X4	T39.8X5	T39.8
Zalcitabine	T37.5X1	T37.5X2	T37.5X3	T37.5X4	T37.5X5	T37.5
Zaroxolyn	T50.2X1	T50.2X2	T50.2X3	T50.2X4	T50.2X5	T50.2
Zephiran (topical)	T49.0X1	T49.0X2	T49.0X3	T49.0X4	T49.0X5	T49.0
ophthalmic preparation	T49.5X1	T49.5X2	T49.5X3	T49.5X4	T49.5X5	T49.5
Zeranol	T38.7X1	T38.7X2	T38.7X3	T38.7X4	T38.7X5	T38.7
Zerone	T51.1X1	T51.1X2	T51.1X3	T51.1X4		
Zidovudine	T37.5X1	T37.5X2	T37.5X3	T37.5X4	T37.5X5	T37.5
Zimeldine	T43.221	T43.222	T43.223	T43.224	T43.225	T43.22
Zinc (compounds) (fumes) (vapor)	T56.5X1	T56.5X2	T56.5X3	T56.5X4		
NEC						
anti-infectives	T49.0X1	T49.0X2	T49.0X3	T49.0X4	T49.0X5	T49.0
antivaricose	T46.8X1	T46.8X2	T46.8X3	T46.8X4	T46.8X5	T46.8
bacitracin	T49.0X1	T49.0X2	T49.0X3	T49.0X4	T49.0X5	T49.0
chloride (mouthwash)	T49.6X1	T49.6X2	T49.6X3	T49.6X4	T49.6X5	T49.6
chromate	T56.5X1	T56.5X2	T56.5X3	T56.5X4		
gelatin	T49.3X1	T49.3X2	T49.3X3	T49.3X4	T49.3X5	T49.3
oxide	T49.3X1	T49.3X2	T49.3X3	T49.3X4	T49.3X5	T49.3
plaster	T49.3X1	T49.3X2	T49.3X3	T49.3X4	T49.3X5	T49.3
peroxide	T49.0X1	T49.0X2	T49.0X3	T49.0X4	T49.0X5	T49.0
pesticides	T56.5X1	T56.5X2	T56.5X3	T56.5X4		
phosphide	T60.4X1	T60.4X2	T60.4X3	T60.4X4		
pyrithionate	T49.4X1	T49.4X2	T49.4X3	T49.4X4	T49.4X5	T49.4
stearate	T49.3X1	T49.3X2	T49.3X3	T49.3X4	T49.3X5	T49.3

Additional Character May Be Required — Refer to the Tabular List for Character Selection   ▽ Subterms under main terms may continue to next column or page

Substance	Poisoning, Accidental (unintentional)	Poisoning, Intentional Self-harm	Poisoning, Assault	Poisoning, Undetermined	Adverse Effect	Under-dosing
Zinc (compounds) (fumes) (vapor)						
NEC — *continued*						
sulfate	T49.5X1	T49.5X2	T49.5X3	T49.5X4	T49.5X5	T49.5X6
ENT agent	T49.6X1	T49.6X2	T49.6X3	T49.6X4	T49.6X5	T49.6X6
ophthalmic solution	T49.5X1	T49.5X2	T49.5X3	T49.5X4	T49.5X5	T49.5X6
topical NEC	T49.0X1	T49.0X2	T49.0X3	T49.0X4	T49.0X5	T49.0X6
undecylenate	T49.0X1	T49.0X2	T49.0X3	T49.0X4	T49.0X5	T49.0X6
Zineb	T60.0X1	T60.0X2	T60.0X3	T60.0X4	—	—
Zinostatin	T45.1X1	T45.1X2	T45.1X3	T45.1X4	T45.1X5	T45.1X6
Zipeprol	T48.3X1	T48.3X2	T48.3X3	T48.3X4	T48.3X5	T48.3X6
Zofenopril	T46.4X1	T46.4X2	T46.4X3	T46.4X4	T46.4X5	T46.4X6
Zolpidem	T42.6X1	T42.6X2	T42.6X3	T42.6X4	T42.6X5	T42.6X6
Zomepirac	T39.391	T39.392	T39.393	T39.394	T39.395	T39.396
Zopiclone	T42.6X1	T42.6X2	T42.6X3	T42.6X4	T42.6X5	T42.6X6
Zorubicin	T45.1X1	T45.1X2	T45.1X3	T45.1X4	T45.1X5	T45.1X6
Zotepine	T43.591	T43.592	T43.593	T43.594	T43.595	T43.596
Zovant	T45.511	T45.512	T45.513	T45.514	T45.515	T45.516
Zoxazolamine	T42.8X1	T42.8X2	T42.8X3	T42.8X4	T42.8X5	T42.8X6
Zuclopenthixol	T43.4X1	T43.4X2	T43.4X3	T43.4X4	T43.4X5	T43.4X6
Zygadenus (venenosus)	T62.2X1	T62.2X2	T62.2X3	T62.2X4	—	—
Zyprexa	T43.591	T43.592	T43.593	T43.594	T43.595	T43.596

▽ **Subterms under main terms may continue to next column or page**   **Additional Character May Be Required — Refer to the Tabular List for Character Selection**

A

Abandonment (causing exposure to weather conditions) (with intent to injure or kill) NEC X58 ☑
Abuse (adult) (child) (mental) (physical) (sexual) X58 ☑
Accident (to) X58 ☑
  aircraft (in transit) (powered) — *see also* Accident, transport, aircraft
    due to, caused by cataclysm — *see* Forces of nature, by type
  animal-drawn vehicle — *see* Accident, transport, animal-drawn vehicle occupant
  animal-rider — *see* Accident, transport, animal-rider
  automobile — *see* Accident, transport, car occupant
  bare foot water skier V94.4 ☑
  boat, boating — *see also* Accident, watercraft
    striking swimmer
      powered V94.11 ☑
      unpowered V94.12 ☑
  bus — *see* Accident, transport, bus occupant
  cable car, not on rails V98.0 ☑
    on rails — *see* Accident, transport, streetcar occupant
  car — *see* Accident, transport, car occupant
  caused by, due to
    animal NEC W64 ☑
    chain hoist W24.0 ☑
    cold (excessive) — *see* Exposure, cold
    corrosive liquid, substance — *see* Table of Drugs and Chemicals
    cutting or piercing instrument — *see* Contact, with, by type of instrument
    drive belt W24.0 ☑
    electric
      current — *see* Exposure, electric current
      motor — *see also* Contact, with, by type of machine W31.3 ☑
        current (of) W86.8 ☑
    environmental factor NEC X58 ☑
    explosive material — *see* Explosion
    fire, flames — *see* Exposure, fire
    firearm missile — *see* Discharge, firearm by type
    heat (excessive) — *see* Heat
    hot — *see* Contact, with, hot
    ignition — *see* Ignition
    lifting device W24.0 ☑
    lightning — *see* subcategory T75.0 ☑
      causing fire — *see* Exposure, fire
    machine, machinery — *see* Contact, with, by type of machine
    natural factor NEC X58 ☑
    pulley (block) W24.0 ☑
    radiation — *see* Radiation
    steam X13.1 ☑
      inhalation X13.0 ☑
      pipe X16 ☑
    thunderbolt — *see* subcategory T75.0 ☑
      causing fire — *see* Exposure, fire
    transmission device W24.1 ☑
  coach — *see* Accident, transport, bus occupant
  coal car — *see* Accident, transport, industrial vehicle occupant
  diving — *see also* Fall, into, water
    with
      drowning or submersion — *see* Drowning
  forklift — *see* Accident, transport, industrial vehicle occupant
  heavy transport vehicle NOS — *see* Accident, transport, truck occupant
  ice yacht V98.2 ☑
  in
    medical, surgical procedure
      as, or due to misadventure — *see* Misadventure
      causing an abnormal reaction or later complication without mention of misadventure — *see also* Complication of or following, by type of procedure Y84.9
  land yacht V98.1 ☑
  late effect of — *see* W00-X58 with 7th character S
  logging car — *see* Accident, transport, industrial vehicle occupant
  machine, machinery — *see also* Contact, with, by type of machine
    on board watercraft V93.69 ☑
      explosion — *see* Explosion, in, watercraft

Accident — *continued*
  machine, machinery — *see also* Contact, with, by type of machine — *continued*
    on board watercraft — *continued*
      fire — *see* Burn, on board watercraft
      powered craft V93.63 ☑
        ferry boat V93.61 ☑
        fishing boat V93.62 ☑
        jetskis V93.63 ☑
        liner V93.61 ☑
        merchant ship V93.60 ☑
        passenger ship V93.61 ☑
        sailboat V93.64 ☑
  mine tram — *see* Accident, transport, industrial vehicle occupant
  mobility scooter (motorized) — *see* Accident, transport, pedestrian, conveyance, specified type NEC
  motor scooter — *see* Accident, transport, motorcyclist
  motor vehicle NOS (traffic) — *see also* Accident, transport V89.2 ☑
    nontraffic V89.0 ☑
    three-wheeled NOS — *see* Accident, transport, three-wheeled motor vehicle occupant
  motorcycle NOS — *see* Accident, transport, motorcyclist
  nonmotor vehicle NOS (nontraffic) — *see also* Accident, transport V89.1 ☑
    traffic NOS V89.3 ☑
  nontraffic (victim's mode of transport NOS) V88.9 ☑
    collision (between) V88.7 ☑
      bus and truck V88.5 ☑
      car and:
        bus V88.3 ☑
        pickup V88.2 ☑
        three-wheeled motor vehicle V88.0 ☑
        train V88.6 ☑
        truck V88.4 ☑
        two-wheeled motor vehicle V88.0 ☑
        van V88.2 ☑
      specified vehicle NEC and:
        three-wheeled motor vehicle V88.1 ☑
        two-wheeled motor vehicle V88.1 ☑
    known mode of transport — *see* Accident, transport, by type of vehicle
    noncollision V88.8 ☑
  on board watercraft V93.89 ☑
    powered craft V93.83 ☑
      ferry boat V93.81 ☑
      fishing boat V93.82 ☑
      jetskis V93.83 ☑
      liner V93.81 ☑
      merchant ship V93.80 ☑
      passenger ship V93.81 ☑
    unpowered craft V93.88 ☑
      canoe V93.85 ☑
      inflatable V93.86 ☑
        in tow
          recreational V94.31 ☑
          specified NEC V94.32 ☑
      kayak V93.85 ☑
      sailboat V93.84 ☑
      surf-board V93.88 ☑
      water skis V93.87 ☑
      windsurfer V93.88 ☑
  parachutist V97.29 ☑
    entangled in object V97.21 ☑
    injured on landing V97.22 ☑
  pedal cycle — *see* Accident, transport, pedal cyclist
  pedestrian (on foot)
    with
      another pedestrian W51 ☑
        on pedestrian conveyance NEC V00.09 ☑
      with fall W03 ☑
        due to ice or snow W00.0 ☑
      roller skater (in-line) V00.01 ☑
      skate boarder V00.02 ☑
      transport vehicle — *see* Accident, transport
    on pedestrian conveyance — *see* Accident, transport, pedestrian, conveyance
  pick-up truck or van — *see* Accident, transport, pickup truck occupant
  quarry truck — *see* Accident, transport, industrial vehicle occupant
  railway vehicle (any) (in motion) — *see* Accident, transport, railway vehicle occupant
    due to cataclysm — *see* Forces of nature, by type

Accident — *continued*
  scooter (non-motorized) — *see* Accident, transport, pedestrian, conveyance, scooter
  sequelae of — *see* categories W00-X58 with 7th character S
  skateboard — *see* Accident, transport, pedestrian, conveyance, skateboard
  ski(ing) — *see* Accident, transport, pedestrian, conveyance
    lift V98.3 ☑
  specified cause NEC X58 ☑
  streetcar — *see* Accident, transport, streetcar occupant
  traffic (victim's mode of transport NOS) V87.9 ☑
    collision (between) V87.7 ☑
      bus and truck V87.5 ☑
      car and:
        bus V87.3 ☑
        pickup V87.2 ☑
        three-wheeled motor vehicle V87.0 ☑
        train V87.6 ☑
        truck V87.4 ☑
        two-wheeled motor vehicle V87.0 ☑
        van V87.2 ☑
      specified vehicle NEC V86.39 ☑
        and
          three-wheeled motor vehicle V87.1 ☑
          two-wheeled motor vehicle V87.1 ☑
        driver V86.09 ☑
        passenger V86.19 ☑
        person on outside V86.29 ☑
        while boarding or alighting V86.49 ☑
    known mode of transport — *see* Accident, transport, by type of vehicle
    noncollision V87.8 ☑
  transport (involving injury to) V99 ☑
    18 wheeler — *see* Accident, transport, truck occupant
    agricultural vehicle occupant (nontraffic) V84.9 ☑
      driver V84.5 ☑
      hanger-on V84.7 ☑
      passenger V84.6 ☑
      traffic V84.3 ☑
        driver V84.0 ☑
        hanger-on V84.2 ☑
        passenger V84.1 ☑
      while boarding or alighting V84.4 ☑
    aircraft NEC V97.89 ☑
      military NEC V97.818 ☑
        civilian injured by V97.811 ☑
        with civilian aircraft V97.810 ☑
      occupant injured (in)
        nonpowered craft accident V96.9 ☑
          balloon V96.00 ☑
            collision V96.03 ☑
            crash V96.01 ☑
            explosion V96.05 ☑
            fire V96.04 ☑
            forced landing V96.02 ☑
            specified type NEC V96.09 ☑
          glider V96.20 ☑
            collision V96.23 ☑
            crash V96.21 ☑
            explosion V96.25 ☑
            fire V96.24 ☑
            forced landing V96.22 ☑
            specified type NEC V96.29 ☑
          hang glider V96.10 ☑
            collision V96.13 ☑
            crash V96.11 ☑
            explosion V96.15 ☑
            fire V96.14 ☑
            forced landing V96.12 ☑
            specified type NEC V96.19 ☑
          specified craft NEC V96.8 ☑
        powered craft accident V95.9 ☑
          fixed wing NEC
            commercial V95.30 ☑
              collision V95.33 ☑
              crash V95.31 ☑
              explosion V95.35 ☑
              fire V95.34 ☑
              forced landing V95.32 ☑
              specified type NEC V95.39 ☑
            private V95.20 ☑
              collision V95.23 ☑
              crash V95.21 ☑

Accident — *continued*
  transport — *continued*
    aircraft — *continued*
      occupant injured — *continued*
        powered craft accident — *continued*
          fixed wing — *continued*
            private — *continued*
              explosion V95.25 ☑
              fire V95.24 ☑
              forced landing V95.22 ☑
              specified type NEC V95.29 ☑
           glider V95.10 ☑
            collision V95.13 ☑
            crash V95.11 ☑
            explosion V95.15 ☑
            fire V95.14 ☑
            forced landing V95.12 ☑
            specified type NEC V95.19 ☑
           helicopter V95.00 ☑
            collision V95.03 ☑
            crash V95.01 ☑
            explosion V95.05 ☑
            fire V95.04 ☑
            forced landing V95.02 ☑
            specified type NEC V95.09 ☑
           spacecraft V95.40 ☑
            collision V95.43 ☑
            crash V95.41 ☑
            explosion V95.45 ☑
            fire V95.44 ☑
            forced landing V95.42 ☑
            specified type NEC V95.49 ☑
          specified craft NEC V95.8 ☑
          ultralight V95.10 ☑
           collision V95.13 ☑
            crash V95.11 ☑
            explosion V95.15 ☑
            fire V95.14 ☑
            forced landing V95.12 ☑
            specified type NEC V95.19 ☑
        specified accident NEC V97.0 ☑
        while boarding or alighting V97.1 ☑
      person (injured by)
        falling from, in or on aircraft V97.0 ☑
        machinery on aircraft V97.89 ☑
        on ground with aircraft involvement V97.39 ☑
        rotating propeller V97.32 ☑
        struck by object falling from aircraft V97.31 ☑
        sucked into aircraft jet V97.33 ☑
        while boarding or alighting aircraft V97.1 ☑
    airport (battery-powered) passenger vehicle — *see* Accident, transport, industrial vehicle occupant
    all-terrain vehicle occupant (nontraffic) V86.95 ☑
      driver V86.55 ☑
      dune buggy — *see* Accident, transport, dune buggy occupant
      hanger-on V86.75 ☑
      passenger V86.65 ☑
      snowmobile — *see* Accident, transport, snowmobile occupant
      specified type NEC V86.99 ☑
        driver V86.59 ☑
        passenger V86.69 ☑
        person on outside V86.79 ☑
      traffic V86.35 ☑
        driver V86.05 ☑
        hanger-on V86.25 ☑
        passenger V86.15 ☑
      while boarding or alighting V86.45 ☑
    ambulance occupant (traffic) V86.31 ☑
      driver V86.01 ☑
      hanger-on V86.21 ☑
      nontraffic V86.91 ☑
        driver V86.51 ☑
        hanger-on V86.71 ☑
        passenger V86.61 ☑
      passenger V86.11 ☑
      while boarding or alighting V86.41 ☑
    animal-drawn vehicle occupant (in) V80.929 ☑
      collision (with)
        animal V80.12 ☑
          being ridden V80.711 ☑
        animal-drawn vehicle V80.721 ☑
        bus V80.42 ☑

Accident — *continued*
  transport — *continued*
    animal-drawn vehicle occupant — *continued*
      collision — *continued*
        car V80.42 ☑
        fixed or stationary object V80.82 ☑
        military vehicle V80.920 ☑
        nonmotor vehicle V80.791 ☑
        pedal cycle V80.22 ☑
        pedestrian V80.12 ☑
        pickup V80.42 ☑
        railway train or vehicle V80.62 ☑
        specified motor vehicle NEC V80.52 ☑
        streetcar V80.731 ☑
        truck V80.42 ☑
        two- or three-wheeled motor vehicle V80.32 ☑
        van V80.42 ☑
      noncollision V80.02 ☑
      specified circumstance NEC V80.928 ☑
    animal-rider V80.919 ☑
      collision (with)
        animal V80.11 ☑
          being ridden V80.710 ☑
        animal-drawn vehicle V80.720 ☑
        bus V80.41 ☑
        car V80.41 ☑
        fixed or stationary object V80.81 ☑
        military vehicle V80.910 ☑
        nonmotor vehicle V80.790 ☑
        pedal cycle V80.21 ☑
        pedestrian V80.11 ☑
        pickup V80.41 ☑
        railway train or vehicle V80.61 ☑
        specified motor vehicle NEC V80.51 ☑
        streetcar V80.730 ☑
        truck V80.41 ☑
        two- or three-wheeled motor vehicle V80.31 ☑
        van V80.41 ☑
      noncollision V80.018 ☑
        specified as horse rider V80.010 ☑
      specified circumstance NEC V80.918 ☑
    armored car — *see* Accident, transport, truck occupant
    battery-powered truck (baggage) (mail) — *see* Accident, transport, industrial vehicle occupant
    bus occupant V79.9 ☑
      collision (with)
        animal (traffic) V70.9 ☑
          being ridden (traffic) V76.9 ☑
            nontraffic V76.3 ☑
            while boarding or alighting V76.4 ☑
          nontraffic V70.3 ☑
            while boarding or alighting V70.4 ☑
        animal-drawn vehicle (traffic) V76.9 ☑
          nontraffic V76.3 ☑
          while boarding or alighting V76.4 ☑
        bus (traffic) V74.9 ☑
          nontraffic V74.3 ☑
          while boarding or alighting V74.4 ☑
        car (traffic) V73.9 ☑
          nontraffic V73.3 ☑
          while boarding or alighting V73.4 ☑
        motor vehicle NOS (traffic) V79.60 ☑
          nontraffic V79.20 ☑
          specified type NEC (traffic) V79.69 ☑
            nontraffic V79.29 ☑
        pedal cycle (traffic) V71.9 ☑
          nontraffic V71.3 ☑
          while boarding or alighting V71.4 ☑
        pickup truck (traffic) V73.9 ☑
          nontraffic V73.3 ☑
          while boarding or alighting V73.4 ☑
        railway vehicle (traffic) V75.9 ☑
          nontraffic V75.3 ☑
          while boarding or alighting V75.4 ☑
        specified vehicle NEC (traffic) V76.9 ☑
          nontraffic V76.3 ☑
          while boarding or alighting V76.4 ☑
        stationary object (traffic) V77.9 ☑
          nontraffic V77.3 ☑
          while boarding or alighting V77.4 ☑
        streetcar (traffic) V76.9 ☑
          nontraffic V76.3 ☑
          while boarding or alighting V76.4 ☑

Accident — *continued*
  transport — *continued*
    bus occupant — *continued*
      collision — *continued*
        three wheeled motor vehicle (traffic) V72.9 ☑
          nontraffic V72.3 ☑
          while boarding or alighting V72.4 ☑
        truck (traffic) V74.9 ☑
          nontraffic V74.3 ☑
          while boarding or alighting V74.4 ☑
        two wheeled motor vehicle (traffic) V72.9 ☑
          nontraffic V72.3 ☑
          while boarding or alighting V72.4 ☑
        van (traffic) V73.9 ☑
          nontraffic V73.3 ☑
          while boarding or alighting V73.4 ☑
    driver
      collision (with)
        animal (traffic) V70.5 ☑
          being ridden (traffic) V76.5 ☑
            nontraffic V76.0 ☑
          nontraffic V70.0 ☑
        animal-drawn vehicle (traffic) V76.5 ☑
          nontraffic V76.0 ☑
        bus (traffic) V74.5 ☑
          nontraffic V74.0 ☑
        car (traffic) V73.5 ☑
          nontraffic V73.0 ☑
        motor vehicle NOS (traffic) V79.40 ☑
          nontraffic V79.00 ☑
          specified type NEC (traffic) V79.49 ☑
            nontraffic V79.09 ☑
        pedal cycle (traffic) V71.5 ☑
          nontraffic V71.0 ☑
        pickup truck (traffic) V73.5 ☑
          nontraffic V73.0 ☑
        railway vehicle (traffic) V75.5 ☑
          nontraffic V75.0 ☑
        specified vehicle NEC (traffic) V76.5 ☑
          nontraffic V76.0 ☑
        stationary object (traffic) V77.5 ☑
          nontraffic V77.0 ☑
        streetcar (traffic) V76.5 ☑
          nontraffic V76.0 ☑
        three wheeled motor vehicle (traffic) V72.5 ☑
          nontraffic V72.0 ☑
        truck (traffic) V74.5 ☑
          nontraffic V74.0 ☑
        two wheeled motor vehicle (traffic) V72.5 ☑
          nontraffic V72.0 ☑
        van (traffic) V73.5 ☑
          nontraffic V73.0 ☑
      noncollision accident (traffic) V78.5 ☑
        nontraffic V78.0 ☑
    hanger-on
      collision (with)
        animal (traffic) V70.7 ☑
          being ridden (traffic) V76.7 ☑
            nontraffic V76.2 ☑
          nontraffic V70.2 ☑
        animal-drawn vehicle (traffic) V76.7 ☑
          nontraffic V76.2 ☑
        bus (traffic) V74.7 ☑
          nontraffic V74.2 ☑
        car (traffic) V73.7 ☑
          nontraffic V73.2 ☑
        pedal cycle (traffic) V71.7 ☑
          nontraffic V71.2 ☑
        pickup truck (traffic) V73.7 ☑
          nontraffic V73.2 ☑
        railway vehicle (traffic) V75.7 ☑
          nontraffic V75.2 ☑
        specified vehicle NEC (traffic) V76.7 ☑
          nontraffic V76.2 ☑
        stationary object (traffic) V77.7 ☑
          nontraffic V77.2 ☑
        streetcar (traffic) V76.7 ☑
          nontraffic V76.2 ☑
        three wheeled motor vehicle (traffic) V72.7 ☑
          nontraffic V72.2 ☑
        truck (traffic) V74.7 ☑
          nontraffic V74.2 ☑

Accident — *continued*
  transport — *continued*
    bus occupant — *continued*
      hanger-on — *continued*
        collision — *continued*
          two wheeled motor vehicle (traffic)
            V72.7 ☑
            nontraffic V72.2 ☑
          van (traffic) V73.7 ☑
            nontraffic V73.2 ☑
        noncollision accident (traffic) V78.7 ☑
          nontraffic V78.2 ☑
      noncollision accident (traffic) V78.9 ☑
        nontraffic V78.3 ☑
      while boarding or alighting V78.4 ☑
      nontraffic V79.3 ☑
      passenger
        collision (with)
          animal (traffic) V70.6 ☑
            being ridden (traffic) V76.6 ☑
              nontraffic V76.1 ☑
            nontraffic V70.1 ☑
          animal-drawn vehicle (traffic) V76.6 ☑
            nontraffic V76.1 ☑
          bus (traffic) V74.6 ☑
            nontraffic V74.1 ☑
          car (traffic) V73.6 ☑
            nontraffic V73.1 ☑
          motor vehicle NOS (traffic) V79.50 ☑
            nontraffic V79.10 ☑
            specified type NEC (traffic) V79.59 ☑
              nontraffic V79.19 ☑
          pedal cycle (traffic) V71.6 ☑
            nontraffic V71.1 ☑
          pickup truck (traffic) V73.6 ☑
            nontraffic V73.1 ☑
          railway vehicle (traffic) V75.6 ☑
            nontraffic V75.1 ☑
          specified vehicle NEC (traffic) V76.6 ☑
            nontraffic V76.1 ☑
          stationary object (traffic) V77.6 ☑
            nontraffic V77.1 ☑
          streetcar (traffic) V76.6 ☑
            nontraffic V76.1 ☑
          three wheeled motor vehicle (traffic)
            V72.6 ☑
            nontraffic V72.1 ☑
          truck (traffic) V74.6 ☑
            nontraffic V74.1 ☑
          two wheeled motor vehicle (traffic)
            V72.6 ☑
            nontraffic V72.1 ☑
          van (traffic) V73.6 ☑
            nontraffic V73.1 ☑
        noncollision accident (traffic) V78.6 ☑
          nontraffic V78.1 ☑
      specified type NEC V79.88 ☑
      military vehicle V79.81 ☑
    cable car, not on rails V98.0 ☑
      on rails — *see* Accident, transport, streetcar oc-
        cupant
    car occupant V49.9 ☑
      ambulance occupant — *see* Accident, transport,
        ambulance occupant
      collision (with)
        animal (traffic) V40.9 ☑
          being ridden (traffic) V46.9 ☑
            nontraffic V46.3 ☑
            while boarding or alighting V46.4 ☑
          nontraffic V40.3 ☑
          while boarding or alighting V40.4 ☑
        animal-drawn vehicle (traffic) V46.9 ☑
          nontraffic V46.3 ☑
          while boarding or alighting V46.4 ☑
        bus (traffic) V44.9 ☑
          nontraffic V44.3 ☑
          while boarding or alighting V44.4 ☑
        car (traffic) V43.92 ☑
          nontraffic V43.32 ☑
          while boarding or alighting V43.42 ☑
        motor vehicle NOS (traffic) V49.60 ☑
          nontraffic V49.20 ☑
          specified type NEC (traffic) V49.69 ☑
           nontraffic V49.29 ☑
        pedal cycle (traffic) V41.9 ☑
          nontraffic V41.3 ☑

Accident — *continued*
  transport — *continued*
    car occupant — *continued*
      collision — *continued*
        pedal cycle — *continued*
          while boarding or alighting V41.4 ☑
        pickup truck (traffic) V43.93 ☑
          nontraffic V43.33 ☑
          while boarding or alighting V43.43 ☑
        railway vehicle (traffic) V45.9 ☑
          nontraffic V45.3 ☑
          while boarding or alighting V45.4 ☑
        specified vehicle NEC (traffic) V46.9 ☑
          nontraffic V46.3 ☑
          while boarding or alighting V46.4 ☑
        sport utility vehicle (traffic) V43.91 ☑
          nontraffic V43.31 ☑
          while boarding or alighting V43.41 ☑
        stationary object (traffic) V47.9 ☑
          nontraffic V47.3 ☑
          while boarding or alighting V47.4 ☑
        streetcar (traffic) V46.9 ☑
          nontraffic V46.3 ☑
          while boarding or alighting V46.4 ☑
        three wheeled motor vehicle (traffic) V42.9 ☑
          nontraffic V42.3 ☑
          while boarding or alighting V42.4 ☑
        truck (traffic) V44.9 ☑
          nontraffic V44.3 ☑
          while boarding or alighting V44.4 ☑
        two wheeled motor vehicle (traffic) V42.9 ☑
          nontraffic V42.3 ☑
          while boarding or alighting V42.4 ☑
        van (traffic) V43.94 ☑
          nontraffic V43.34 ☑
          while boarding or alighting V43.44 ☑
      driver
        collision (with)
          animal (traffic) V40.5 ☑
           being ridden (traffic) V46.5 ☑
            nontraffic V46.0 ☑
           nontraffic V40.0 ☑
          animal-drawn vehicle (traffic) V46.5 ☑
           nontraffic V46.0 ☑
          bus (traffic) V44.5 ☑
           nontraffic V44.0 ☑
          car (traffic) V43.52 ☑
           nontraffic V43.02 ☑
          motor vehicle NOS (traffic) V49.40 ☑
           nontraffic V49.00 ☑
           specified type NEC (traffic) V49.49 ☑
            nontraffic V49.09 ☑
          pedal cycle (traffic) V41.5 ☑
           nontraffic V41.0 ☑
          pickup truck (traffic) V43.53 ☑
           nontraffic V43.03 ☑
          railway vehicle (traffic) V45.5 ☑
           nontraffic V45.0 ☑
          specified vehicle NEC (traffic) V46.5 ☑
           nontraffic V46.0 ☑
          sport utility vehicle (traffic) V43.51 ☑
           nontraffic V43.01 ☑
          stationary object (traffic) V47.5 ☑
           nontraffic V47.0 ☑
          streetcar (traffic) V46.5 ☑
           nontraffic V46.0 ☑
          three wheeled motor vehicle (traffic)
            V42.5 ☑
           nontraffic V42.0 ☑
          truck (traffic) V44.5 ☑
           nontraffic V44.0 ☑
          two wheeled motor vehicle (traffic)
            V42.5 ☑
           nontraffic V42.0 ☑
          van (traffic) V43.54 ☑
           nontraffic V43.04 ☑
        noncollision accident (traffic) V48.5 ☑
          nontraffic V48.0 ☑
      hanger-on
        collision (with)
          animal (traffic) V40.7 ☑
           being ridden (traffic) V46.7 ☑
            nontraffic V46.2 ☑
           nontraffic V40.2 ☑
          animal-drawn vehicle (traffic) V46.7 ☑
           nontraffic V46.2 ☑

Accident — *continued*
  transport — *continued*
    car occupant — *continued*
      hanger-on — *continued*
        collision — *continued*
          bus (traffic) V44.7 ☑
           nontraffic V44.2 ☑
          car (traffic) V43.72 ☑
           nontraffic V43.22 ☑
          pedal cycle (traffic) V41.7 ☑
           nontraffic V41.2 ☑
          pickup truck (traffic) V43.73 ☑
           nontraffic V43.23 ☑
          railway vehicle (traffic) V45.7 ☑
           nontraffic V45.2 ☑
          specified vehicle NEC (traffic) V46.7 ☑
           nontraffic V46.2 ☑
          sport utility vehicle (traffic) V43.71 ☑
           nontraffic V43.21 ☑
          stationary object (traffic) V47.7 ☑
           nontraffic V47.2 ☑
          streetcar (traffic) V46.7 ☑
           nontraffic V46.2 ☑
          three wheeled motor vehicle (traffic)
            V42.7 ☑
           nontraffic V42.2 ☑
          truck (traffic) V44.7 ☑
           nontraffic V44.2 ☑
          two wheeled motor vehicle (traffic)
            V42.7 ☑
           nontraffic V42.2 ☑
          van (traffic) V43.74 ☑
           nontraffic V43.24 ☑
        noncollision accident (traffic) V48.7 ☑
          nontraffic V48.2 ☑
      noncollision accident (traffic) V48.9 ☑
        nontraffic V48.3 ☑
      while boarding or alighting V48.4 ☑
      nontraffic V49.3 ☑
      passenger
        collision (with)
          animal (traffic) V40.6 ☑
           being ridden (traffic) V46.6 ☑
            nontraffic V46.1 ☑
           nontraffic V40.1 ☑
          animal-drawn vehicle (traffic) V46.6 ☑
           nontraffic V46.1 ☑
          bus (traffic) V44.6 ☑
           nontraffic V44.1 ☑
          car (traffic) V43.62 ☑
           nontraffic V43.12 ☑
          motor vehicle NOS (traffic) V49.50 ☑
           nontraffic V49.10 ☑
           specified type NEC (traffic) V49.59 ☑
            nontraffic V49.19 ☑
          pedal cycle (traffic) V41.6 ☑
           nontraffic V41.1 ☑
          pickup truck (traffic) V43.63 ☑
           nontraffic V43.13 ☑
          railway vehicle (traffic) V45.6 ☑
           nontraffic V45.1 ☑
          specified vehicle NEC (traffic) V46.6 ☑
           nontraffic V46.1 ☑
          sport utility vehicle (traffic) V43.61 ☑
           nontraffic V43.11 ☑
          stationary object (traffic) V47.6 ☑
           nontraffic V47.1 ☑
          streetcar (traffic) V46.6 ☑
           nontraffic V46.1 ☑
          three wheeled motor vehicle (traffic)
            V42.6 ☑
           nontraffic V42.1 ☑
          truck (traffic) V44.6 ☑
           nontraffic V44.1 ☑
          two wheeled motor vehicle (traffic)
            V42.6 ☑
           nontraffic V42.1 ☑
          van (traffic) V43.64 ☑
           nontraffic V43.14 ☑
        noncollision accident (traffic) V48.6 ☑
          nontraffic V48.1 ☑
      specified type NEC V49.88 ☑
      military vehicle V49.81 ☑
    coal car — *see* Accident, transport, industrial vehic
      occupant
    construction vehicle occupant (nontraffic) V85.9 ☑

☑ **Additional Character Required** — Refer to the Tabular List for Character Selection   ▽ **Subterms under main terms may continue to next column or page**

Accident — *continued*
  transport — *continued*
    construction vehicle occupant — *continued*
      driver V85.5 ☑
      hanger-on V85.7 ☑
      passenger V85.6 ☑
      traffic V85.3 ☑
        driver V85.0 ☑
        hanger-on V85.2 ☑
        passenger V85.1 ☑
      while boarding or alighting V85.4 ☑
    dirt bike rider (nontraffic) V86.96 ☑
      driver V86.56
      hanger-on V86.76 ☑
      passenger V86.66 ☑
      traffic V86.36 ☑
        driver V86.06 ☑
        hanger-on V86.26 ☑
        passenger V86.16 ☑
      while boarding or alighting V86.46 ☑
    due to cataclysm — *see* Forces of nature, by type
    dune buggy occupant (nontraffic) V86.93 ☑
      driver V86.53 ☑
      hanger-on V86.73 ☑
      passenger V86.63 ☑
      traffic V86.33 ☑
        driver V86.03 ☑
        hanger-on V86.23 ☑
        passenger V86.13 ☑
      while boarding or alighting V86.43 ☑
    forklift — *see* Accident, transport, industrial vehicle occupant
    go cart — *see* Accident, transport, all-terrain vehicle occupant
    golf cart — *see* Accident, transport, all-terrain vehicle occupant
    heavy transport vehicle occupant — *see* Accident, transport, truck occupant
    ice yacht V98.2 ☑
    industrial vehicle occupant (nontraffic) V83.9 ☑
      driver V83.5 ☑
      hanger-on V83.7 ☑
      passenger V83.6 ☑
      traffic V83.3 ☑
        driver V83.0 ☑
        hanger-on V83.2 ☑
        passenger V83.1 ☑
      while boarding or alighting V83.4 ☑
    interurban electric car — *see* Accident, transport, streetcar
    land yacht V98.1 ☑
    logging car — *see* Accident, transport, industrial vehicle occupant
    military vehicle occupant (traffic) V86.34 ☑
      driver V86.04 ☑
      hanger-on V86.24 ☑
      nontraffic V86.94 ☑
        driver V86.54 ☑
        hanger-on V86.74 ☑
        passenger V86.64 ☑
      passenger V86.14 ☑
      while boarding or alighting V86.44 ☑
    mine tram — *see* Accident, transport, industrial vehicle occupant
    motor vehicle NEC occupant (traffic) V89.2 ☑
    motorcoach — *see* Accident, transport, bus occupant
    motor/cross bike rider — *see also* Accident, transport, dirt bike rider V86.96 ☑
    motorcyclist V29.9 ☑
      collision (with)
        animal (traffic) V20.9 ☑
          being ridden (traffic) V26.9 ☑
            nontraffic V26.2 ☑
            while boarding or alighting V26.3 ☑
          nontraffic V20.2 ☑
          while boarding or alighting V20.3 ☑
        animal-drawn vehicle (traffic) V26.9 ☑
          nontraffic V26.2 ☑
          while boarding or alighting V26.3 ☑
        bus (traffic) V24.9 ☑
          nontraffic V24.2 ☑
          while boarding or alighting V24.3 ☑
        car (traffic) V23.9 ☑
          nontraffic V23.2 ☑
          while boarding or alighting V23.3 ☑

Accident — *continued*
  transport — *continued*
    motorcyclist — *continued*
      collision — *continued*
        motor vehicle NOS (traffic) V29.60 ☑
          nontraffic V29.20 ☑
          specified type NEC (traffic) V29.69 ☑
            nontraffic V29.29 ☑
        pedal cycle (traffic) V21.9 ☑
          nontraffic V21.2 ☑
          while boarding or alighting V21.3 ☑
        pickup truck (traffic) V23.9 ☑
          nontraffic V23.2 ☑
          while boarding or alighting V23.3 ☑
        railway vehicle (traffic) V25.9 ☑
          nontraffic V25.2 ☑
          while boarding or alighting V25.3 ☑
        specified vehicle NEC (traffic) V26.9 ☑
          nontraffic V26.2 ☑
          while boarding or alighting V26.3 ☑
        stationary object (traffic) V27.9 ☑
          nontraffic V27.2 ☑
          while boarding or alighting V27.3 ☑
        streetcar (traffic) V26.9 ☑
          nontraffic V26.2 ☑
          while boarding or alighting V26.3 ☑
        three wheeled motor vehicle (traffic) V22.9 ☑
          nontraffic V22.2 ☑
          while boarding or alighting V22.3 ☑
        truck (traffic) V24.9 ☑
          nontraffic V24.2 ☑
          while boarding or alighting V24.3 ☑
        two wheeled motor vehicle (traffic) V22.9 ☑
          nontraffic V22.2 ☑
          while boarding or alighting V22.3 ☑
        van (traffic) V23.9 ☑
          nontraffic V23.2 ☑
          while boarding or alighting V23.3 ☑
      driver
        collision (with)
          animal (traffic) V20.4 ☑
            being ridden (traffic) V26.4 ☑
              nontraffic V26.0 ☑
            nontraffic V20.0 ☑
          animal-drawn vehicle (traffic) V26.4 ☑
            nontraffic V26.0 ☑
          bus (traffic) V24.4 ☑
            nontraffic V24.0 ☑
          car (traffic) V23.4 ☑
            nontraffic V23.0 ☑
          motor vehicle NOS (traffic) V29.40 ☑
            nontraffic V29.00 ☑
            specified type NEC (traffic) V29.49 ☑
              nontraffic V29.09 ☑
          pedal cycle (traffic) V21.4 ☑
            nontraffic V21.0 ☑
          pickup truck (traffic) V23.4 ☑
            nontraffic V23.0 ☑
          railway vehicle (traffic) V25.4 ☑
            nontraffic V25.0 ☑
          specified vehicle NEC (traffic) V26.4 ☑
            nontraffic V26.0 ☑
          stationary object (traffic) V27.4 ☑
            nontraffic V27.0 ☑
          streetcar (traffic) V26.4 ☑
            nontraffic V26.0 ☑
          three wheeled motor vehicle (traffic) V22.4 ☑
            nontraffic V22.0 ☑
          truck (traffic) V24.4 ☑
            nontraffic V24.0 ☑
          two wheeled motor vehicle (traffic) V22.4 ☑
            nontraffic V22.0 ☑
          van (traffic) V23.4 ☑
            nontraffic V23.0 ☑
        noncollision accident (traffic) V28.4 ☑
          nontraffic V28.0 ☑
      noncollision accident (traffic) V28.9 ☑
        nontraffic V28.2 ☑
        while boarding or alighting V28.3 ☑
      nontraffic V29.3 ☑
      passenger
        collision (with)
          animal (traffic) V20.5 ☑
            being ridden (traffic) V26.5 ☑

Accident — *continued*
  transport — *continued*
    motorcyclist — *continued*
      passenger — *continued*
        collision — *continued*
          animal — *continued*
            being ridden — *continued*
              nontraffic V26.1 ☑
            nontraffic V20.1 ☑
          animal-drawn vehicle (traffic) V26.5 ☑
            nontraffic V26.1 ☑
          bus (traffic) V24.5 ☑
            nontraffic V24.1 ☑
          car (traffic) V23.5 ☑
            nontraffic V23.1 ☑
          motor vehicle NOS (traffic) V29.50 ☑
            nontraffic V29.10 ☑
            specified type NEC (traffic) V29.59 ☑
              nontraffic V29.19 ☑
          pedal cycle (traffic) V21.5 ☑
            nontraffic V21.1 ☑
          pickup truck (traffic) V23.5 ☑
            nontraffic V23.1 ☑
          railway vehicle (traffic) V25.5 ☑
            nontraffic V25.1 ☑
          specified vehicle NEC (traffic) V26.5 ☑
            nontraffic V26.1 ☑
          stationary object (traffic) V27.5 ☑
            nontraffic V27.1 ☑
          streetcar (traffic) V26.5 ☑
            nontraffic V26.1 ☑
          three wheeled motor vehicle (traffic) V22.5 ☑
            nontraffic V22.1 ☑
          truck (traffic) V24.5 ☑
            nontraffic V24.1 ☑
          two wheeled motor vehicle (traffic) V22.5 ☑
            nontraffic V22.1 ☑
          van (traffic) V23.5 ☑
            nontraffic V23.1 ☑
        noncollision accident (traffic) V28.5 ☑
          nontraffic V28.1 ☑
      specified type NEC V29.88 ☑
        military vehicle V29.81 ☑
    occupant (of)
      aircraft (powered) V95.9 ☑
        fixed wing
          commercial — *see* Accident, transport, aircraft, occupant, powered, fixed wing, commercial
          private — *see* Accident, transport, aircraft, occupant, powered, fixed wing, private
        nonpowered V96.9 ☑
        specified NEC V95.8 ☑
      airport battery-powered vehicle — *see* Accident, transport, industrial vehicle occupant
      all-terrain vehicle (ATV) — *see* Accident, transport, all-terrain vehicle occupant
      animal-drawn vehicle — *see* Accident, transport, animal-drawn vehicle occupant
      automobile — *see* Accident, transport, car occupant
      balloon V96.00 ☑
      battery-powered vehicle — *see* Accident, transport, industrial vehicle occupant
      bicycle — *see* Accident, transport, pedal cyclist
        motorized — *see* Accident, transport, motorcycle rider
      boat NEC — *see* Accident, watercraft
      bulldozer — *see* Accident, transport, construction vehicle occupant
      bus — *see* Accident, transport, bus occupant
      cable car (on rails) — *see also* Accident, transport, streetcar occupant
        not on rails V98.0 ☑
      car — *see also* Accident, transport, car occupant
        cable (on rails) — *see also* Accident, transport, streetcar occupant
        not on rails V98.0 ☑
      coach — *see* Accident, transport, bus occupant
      coal-car — *see* Accident, transport, industrial vehicle occupant
      digger — *see* Accident, transport, construction vehicle occupant

Accident

ICD-10-CM 2020

External Causes Index

402   ☑ Additional Character Required — Refer to the Tabular List for Character Selection   ▽ Subterms under main terms may continue to next column or page

Accident — Accident

Accident — *continued*
   transport — *continued*
      occupant — *continued*
         dump truck — *see* Accident, transport, construction vehicle occupant
         earth-leveler — *see* Accident, transport, construction vehicle occupant
         farm machinery (self-propelled) — *see* Accident, transport, agricultural vehicle occupant
         forklift — *see* Accident, transport, industrial vehicle occupant
         glider (unpowered) V96.20 ☑
            hang V96.10 ☑
            powered (microlight) (ultralight) — *see* Accident, transport, aircraft, occupant, powered, glider
         glider (unpowered) NEC V96.20 ☑
         hang-glider V96.10 ☑
         harvester — *see* Accident, transport, agricultural vehicle occupant
         heavy (transport) vehicle — *see* Accident, transport, truck occupant
         helicopter — *see* Accident, transport, aircraft, occupant, helicopter
         ice-yacht V98.2 ☑
         kite (carrying person) V96.8 ☑
         land-yacht V98.1 ☑
         logging car — *see* Accident, transport, industrial vehicle occupant
         mechanical shovel — *see* Accident, transport, construction vehicle occupant
         microlight — *see* Accident, transport, aircraft, occupant, powered, glider
         minibus — *see* Accident, transport, pickup truck occupant
         minivan — *see* Accident, transport, pickup truck occupant
         moped — *see* Accident, transport, motorcycle
         motor scooter— *see* Accident, transport, motorcycle
         motorcycle (with sidecar) — *see* Accident, transport, motorcycle
         off-road motor-vehicle — *see also* Accident, transport, all-terrain vehicle occupant V86.99 ☑
         pedal cycle — *see also* Accident, transport, pedal cyclist
         pick-up (truck) — *see* Accident, transport, pickup truck occupant
         railway (train) (vehicle) (subterranean) (elevated) — *see* Accident, transport, railway vehicle occupant
         rickshaw — *see* Accident, transport, pedal cycle
            motorized — *see* Accident, transport, three-wheeled motor vehicle
            pedal driven — *see* Accident, transport, pedal cyclist
         road-roller — *see* Accident, transport, construction vehicle occupant
         ship NOS V94.9 ☑
         ski-lift (chair) (gondola) V98.3 ☑
         snowmobile — *see* Accident, transport, snowmobile occupant
         spacecraft, spaceship — *see* Accident, transport, aircraft, occupant, spacecraft
         sport utility vehicle — *see* Accident, transport, pickup truck occupant
         streetcar (interurban) (operating on public street or highway) — *see* Accident, transport, streetcar occupant
         SUV — *see* Accident, transport, pickup truck occupant
         téléférique V98.0 ☑
         three-wheeled vehicle (motorized) — *see also* Accident, transport, three-wheeled motor vehicle occupant
            nonmotorized — *see* Accident, transport, pedal cycle
         tractor (farm) (and trailer) — *see* Accident, transport, agricultural vehicle occupant
         train — *see* Accident, transport, railway vehicle occupant
         tram — *see* Accident, transport, streetcar occupant
            in mine or quarry — *see* Accident, transport, industrial vehicle occupant
         tricycle — *see* Accident, transport, pedal cycle

Accident — *continued*
   transport — *continued*
      occupant — *continued*
         tricycle — *see* Accident, transport, pedal cycle — *continued*
            motorized — *see* Accident, transport, three-wheeled motor vehicle
         trolley — *see* Accident, transport, streetcar occupant
            in mine or quarry — *see* Accident, transport, industrial vehicle occupant
         tub, in mine or quarry — *see* Accident, transport, industrial vehicle occupant
         ultralight — *see* Accident, transport, aircraft, occupant, powered, glider
         van — *see* Accident, transport, van occupant
         vehicle NEC V89.9 ☑
            heavy transport — *see* Accident, transport, truck occupant
            motor (traffic) NEC V89.2 ☑
               nontraffic NEC V89.0 ☑
         watercraft NOS V94.9 ☑
            causing drowning — *see* Drowning, resulting from accident to boat
      off-road motor-vehicle — *see also* Accident, transport, all-terrain vehicle occupant V86.99 ☑
      parachutist V97.29 ☑
         after accident to aircraft — *see* Accident, transport, aircraft
         entangled in object V97.21 ☑
         injured on landing V97.22 ☑
      pedal cyclist V19.9 ☑
         collision (with)
            animal (traffic) V10.9 ☑
               being ridden (traffic) V16.9 ☑
                  nontraffic V16.2 ☑
                  while boarding or alighting V16.3 ☑
               nontraffic V10.2 ☑
               while boarding or alighting V10.3 ☑
            animal-drawn vehicle (traffic) V16.9 ☑
               nontraffic V16.2 ☑
               while boarding or alighting V16.3 ☑
            bus (traffic) V14.9 ☑
               nontraffic V14.2 ☑
               while boarding or alighting V14.3 ☑
            car (traffic) V13.9 ☑
               nontraffic V13.2 ☑
               while boarding or alighting V13.3 ☑
            motor vehicle NOS (traffic) V19.60 ☑
               nontraffic V19.20 ☑
               specified type NEC (traffic) V19.69 ☑
                  nontraffic V19.29 ☑
            pedal cycle (traffic) V11.9 ☑
               nontraffic V11.2 ☑
               while boarding or alighting V11.3 ☑
            pickup truck (traffic) V13.9 ☑
               nontraffic V13.2 ☑
               while boarding or alighting V13.3 ☑
            railway vehicle (traffic) V15.9 ☑
               nontraffic V15.2 ☑
               while boarding or alighting V15.3 ☑
            specified vehicle NEC (traffic) V16.9 ☑
               nontraffic V16.2 ☑
               while boarding or alighting V16.3 ☑
            stationary object (traffic) V17.9 ☑
               nontraffic V17.2 ☑
               while boarding or alighting V17.3 ☑
            streetcar (traffic) V16.9 ☑
               nontraffic V16.2 ☑
               while boarding or alighting V16.3 ☑
            three wheeled motor vehicle (traffic) V12.9 ☑
               nontraffic V12.2 ☑
               while boarding or alighting V12.3 ☑
            truck (traffic) V14.9 ☑
               nontraffic V14.2 ☑
               while boarding or alighting V14.3 ☑
            two wheeled motor vehicle (traffic) V12.9 ☑
               nontraffic V12.2 ☑
               while boarding or alighting V12.3 ☑
            van (traffic) V13.9 ☑
               nontraffic V13.2 ☑
               while boarding or alighting V13.3 ☑
         driver
            collision (with)
               animal (traffic) V10.4 ☑
                  being ridden (traffic) V16.4 ☑

Accident — *continued*
   transport — *continued*
      pedal cyclist — *continued*
         driver — *continued*
            collision — *continued*
               animal — *continued*
                  being ridden — *continued*
                     nontraffic V16.0 ☑
                     nontraffic V10.0 ☑
               animal-drawn vehicle (traffic) V16.4 ☑
                  nontraffic V16.0 ☑
               bus (traffic) V14.4 ☑
                  nontraffic V14.0 ☑
               car (traffic) V13.4 ☑
                  nontraffic V13.0 ☑
               motor vehicle NOS (traffic) V19.40 ☑
                  nontraffic V19.00 ☑
                  specified type NEC (traffic) V19.49 ☑
                     nontraffic V19.09 ☑
               pedal cycle (traffic) V11.4 ☑
                  nontraffic V11.0 ☑
               pickup truck (traffic) V13.4 ☑
                  nontraffic V13.0 ☑
               railway vehicle (traffic) V15.4 ☑
                  nontraffic V15.0 ☑
               specified vehicle NEC (traffic) V16.4 ☑
                  nontraffic V16.0 ☑
               stationary object (traffic) V17.4 ☑
                  nontraffic V17.0 ☑
               streetcar (traffic) V16.4 ☑
                  nontraffic V16.0 ☑
               three wheeled motor vehicle (traffic) V12.4 ☑
                  nontraffic V12.0 ☑
               truck (traffic) V14.4 ☑
                  nontraffic V14.0 ☑
               two wheeled motor vehicle (traffic) V12.4 ☑
                  nontraffic V12.0 ☑
               van (traffic) V13.4 ☑
                  nontraffic V13.0 ☑
            noncollision accident (traffic) V18.4 ☑
               nontraffic V18.0 ☑
         noncollision accident (traffic) V18.9 ☑
            nontraffic V18.2 ☑
            while boarding or alighting V18.3 ☑
         nontraffic V19.3 ☑
         passenger
            collision (with)
               animal (traffic) V10.5 ☑
                  being ridden (traffic) V16.5 ☑
                     nontraffic V16.1 ☑
                  nontraffic V10.1 ☑
               animal-drawn vehicle (traffic) V16.5 ☑
                  nontraffic V16.1 ☑
               bus (traffic) V14.5 ☑
                  nontraffic V14.1 ☑
               car (traffic) V13.5 ☑
                  nontraffic V13.1 ☑
               motor vehicle NOS (traffic) V19.50 ☑
                  nontraffic V19.10 ☑
                  specified type NEC (traffic) V19.59 ☑
                     nontraffic V19.19 ☑
               pedal cycle (traffic) V11.5 ☑
                  nontraffic V11.1 ☑
               pickup truck (traffic) V13.5 ☑
                  nontraffic V13.1 ☑
               railway vehicle (traffic) V15.5 ☑
                  nontraffic V15.1 ☑
               specified vehicle NEC (traffic) V16.5 ☑
                  nontraffic V16.1 ☑
               stationary object (traffic) V17.5 ☑
                  nontraffic V17.1 ☑
               streetcar (traffic) V16.5 ☑
                  nontraffic V16.1 ☑
               three wheeled motor vehicle (traffic) V12.5 ☑
                  nontraffic V12.1 ☑
               truck (traffic) V14.5 ☑
                  nontraffic V14.1 ☑
               two wheeled motor vehicle (traffic) V12.5 ☑
                  nontraffic V12.1 ☑
               van (traffic) V13.5 ☑
                  nontraffic V13.1 ☑
            noncollision accident (traffic) V18.5 ☑

Accident — continued
 transport — continued
  pedal cyclist — continued
   passenger — continued
    noncollision accident — continued
     nontraffic V18.1 ☑
   specified type NEC V19.88 ☑
   military vehicle V19.81 ☑
  pedestrian
   conveyance (occupant) V09.9 ☑
    baby stroller V00.828 ☑
     collision (with) V09.9 ☑
      animal being ridden or animal drawn
       vehicle V06.99 ☑
       nontraffic V06.09 ☑
       traffic V06.19 ☑
      bus or heavy transport V04.99 ☑
       nontraffic V04.09 ☑
       traffic V04.19 ☑
      car V03.99 ☑
       nontraffic V03.09 ☑
       traffic V03.19 ☑
      pedal cycle V01.99 ☑
       nontraffic V01.09 ☑
       traffic V01.19 ☑
      pick-up truck or van V03.99 ☑
       nontraffic V03.09 ☑
       traffic V03.19 ☑
      railway (train) (vehicle) V05.99 ☑
       nontraffic V05.09 ☑
       traffic V05.19 ☑
      stationary object V00.822 ☑
      streetcar V06.99 ☑
       nontraffic V06.09 ☑
       traffic V06.19 ☑
      two- or three-wheeled motor vehicle
       V02.99 ☑
       nontraffic V02.09 ☑
       traffic V02.19 ☑
      vehicle V09.9 ☑
       animal-drawn V06.99 ☑
        nontraffic V06.09 ☑
        traffic V06.19 ☑
       motor
        nontraffic V09.00 ☑
        traffic V09.20 ☑
     fall V00.821 ☑
     nontraffic V09.1 ☑
      involving motor vehicle NEC V09.00 ☑
     traffic V09.3 ☑
      involving motor vehicle NEC V09.20 ☑
    flat-bottomed NEC V00.388 ☑
     collision (with) V09.9 ☑
      animal being ridden or animal drawn
       vehicle V06.99 ☑
       nontraffic V06.09 ☑
       traffic V06.19 ☑
      bus or heavy transport V04.99 ☑
       nontraffic V04.09 ☑
       traffic V04.19 ☑
      car V03.99 ☑
       nontraffic V03.09 ☑
       traffic V03.19 ☑
      pedal cycle V01.99 ☑
       nontraffic V01.09 ☑
       traffic V01.19 ☑
      pick-up truck or van V03.99 ☑
       nontraffic V03.09 ☑
       traffic V03.19 ☑
      railway (train) (vehicle) V05.99 ☑
       nontraffic V05.09 ☑
       traffic V05.19 ☑
      stationary object V00.382 ☑
      streetcar V06.99 ☑
       nontraffic V06.09 ☑
       traffic V06.19 ☑
      two- or three-wheeled motor vehicle
       V02.99 ☑
       nontraffic V02.09 ☑
       traffic V02.19 ☑
      vehicle V09.9 ☑
       animal-drawn V06.99 ☑
        nontraffic V06.09 ☑
        traffic V06.19 ☑
       motor
        nontraffic V09.00 ☑

Accident — continued
 transport — continued
  pedestrian — continued
   conveyance — continued
    flat-bottomed — continued
     collision — continued
      vehicle — continued
       motor — continued
        traffic V09.20 ☑
     fall V00.381 ☑
     nontraffic V09.1 ☑
      involving motor vehicle NEC V09.00 ☑
     snow
      board — see Accident, transport,
       pedestrian, conveyance, snow
       board
      ski — see Accident, transport, pedes-
       trian, conveyance, skis (snow)
     traffic V09.3 ☑
      involving motor vehicle NEC V09.20 ☑
    gliding type NEC V00.288 ☑
     collision (with) V09.9 ☑
      animal being ridden or animal drawn
       vehicle V06.99 ☑
       nontraffic V06.09 ☑
       traffic V06.19 ☑
      bus or heavy transport V04.99 ☑
       nontraffic V04.09 ☑
       traffic V04.19 ☑
      car V03.99 ☑
       nontraffic V03.09 ☑
       traffic V03.19 ☑
      pedal cycle V01.99 ☑
       nontraffic V01.09 ☑
       traffic V01.19 ☑
      pick-up truck or van V03.99 ☑
       nontraffic V03.09 ☑
       traffic V03.19 ☑
      railway (train) (vehicle) V05.99 ☑
       nontraffic V05.09 ☑
       traffic V05.19 ☑
      stationary object V00.282 ☑
      streetcar V06.99 ☑
       nontraffic V06.09 ☑
       traffic V02.19 ☑
      two- or three-wheeled motor vehicle
       V02.99 ☑
       nontraffic V02.09 ☑
       traffic V02.19 ☑
      vehicle V09.9 ☑
       animal-drawn V06.99 ☑
        nontraffic V06.09 ☑
        traffic V06.19 ☑
       motor
        nontraffic V09.00 ☑
        traffic V09.20 ☑
     fall V00.281 ☑
     heelies — see Accident, transport,
      pedestrian, conveyance, heelies
     ice skate — see Accident, transport,
      pedestrian, conveyance, ice skate
     nontraffic V09.1 ☑
      involving motor vehicle NEC V09.00 ☑
     sled — see Accident, transport, pedestri-
      an, conveyance, sled
     traffic V09.3 ☑
      involving motor vehicle NEC V09.20 ☑
     wheelies — see Accident, transport,
      pedestrian, conveyance, heelies
    heelies V00.158 ☑
     colliding with stationary object
      V00.152 ☑
     fall V00.151 ☑
    ice skates V00.218 ☑
     collision (with) V09.9 ☑
      animal being ridden or animal drawn
       vehicle V06.99 ☑
       nontraffic V06.09 ☑
       traffic V06.19 ☑
      bus or heavy transport V04.99 ☑
       nontraffic V04.09 ☑
       traffic V04.19 ☑
      car V03.99 ☑
       nontraffic V03.09 ☑
       traffic V03.19 ☑
      pedal cycle V01.99 ☑

Accident — continued
 transport — continued
  pedestrian — continued
   conveyance — continued
    ice skates — continued
     collision — continued
      pedal cycle — continued
       nontraffic V01.09 ☑
       traffic V01.19 ☑
      pick-up truck or van V03.99 ☑
       nontraffic V03.09 ☑
       traffic V03.19 ☑
      railway (train) (vehicle) V05.99 ☑
       nontraffic V05.09 ☑
       traffic V05.19 ☑
      stationary object V00.212 ☑
      streetcar V06.99 ☑
       nontraffic V06.09 ☑
       traffic V06.19 ☑
      two- or three-wheeled motor vehicle
       V02.99 ☑
       nontraffic V02.09 ☑
       traffic V02.19 ☑
      vehicle V09.9 ☑
       animal-drawn V06.99 ☑
        nontraffic V06.09 ☑
        traffic V06.19 ☑
       motor
        nontraffic V09.00 ☑
        traffic V09.20 ☑
     fall V00.211 ☑
     nontraffic V09.1 ☑
      involving motor vehicle NEC V09.00 ☑
     traffic V09.3 ☑
      involving motor vehicle NEC V09.20 ☑
    motorized mobility scooter V00.838 ☑
     collision with stationary object
      V00.832 ☑
     fall from V00.831 ☑
    nontraffic V09.1 ☑
     involving motor vehicle V09.00 ☑
      military V09.01 ☑
      specified type NEC V09.09 ☑
    roller skates (non in-line) V00.128 ☑
     collision (with) V09.9 ☑
      animal being ridden or animal drawn
       vehicle V06.91 ☑
       nontraffic V06.01 ☑
       traffic V06.11 ☑
      bus or heavy transport V04.91 ☑
       nontraffic V04.01 ☑
       traffic V04.11 ☑
      car V03.91 ☑
       nontraffic V03.01 ☑
       traffic V03.11 ☑
      pedal cycle V01.91 ☑
       nontraffic V01.01 ☑
       traffic V01.11 ☑
      pick-up truck or van V03.91 ☑
       nontraffic V03.01 ☑
       traffic V03.11 ☑
      railway (train) (vehicle) V05.91 ☑
       nontraffic V05.01 ☑
       traffic V05.11 ☑
      stationary object V00.122 ☑
      streetcar V06.91 ☑
       nontraffic V06.01 ☑
       traffic V06.11 ☑
      two- or three-wheeled motor vehicle
       V02.91 ☑
       nontraffic V02.01 ☑
       traffic V02.11 ☑
      vehicle V09.9 ☑
       animal-drawn V06.91 ☑
        nontraffic V06.01 ☑
        traffic V06.11 ☑
       motor
        nontraffic V09.00 ☑
        traffic V09.20 ☑
     fall V00.121 ☑
    in-line V00.118 ☑
     collision   see also Accident, trans-
      port, pedestrian, conveyance
      occupant, roller skates, collision
      with stationary object V00.112 ☑
     fall V00.111 ☑

Accident — *continued*
  transport — *continued*
    pedestrian — *continued*
      conveyance — *continued*
        roller skates — *continued*
          nontraffic V09.1 ☑
            involving motor vehicle NEC V09.00 ☑
          traffic V09.3 ☑
            involving motor vehicle NEC V09.20 ☑
        rolling shoes V00.158 ☑
          colliding with stationary object
            V00.152 ☑
          fall V00.151 ☑
        rolling type NEC V00.188 ☑
          collision (with) V09.9 ☑
            animal being ridden or animal drawn
              vehicle V06.99 ☑
              nontraffic V06.09 ☑
              traffic V06.19 ☑
            bus or heavy transport V04.99 ☑
              nontraffic V04.09 ☑
              traffic V04.19 ☑
            car V03.99 ☑
              nontraffic V03.09 ☑
              traffic V03.19 ☑
            pedal cycle V01.99 ☑
              nontraffic V01.09 ☑
              traffic V01.19 ☑
            pick-up truck or van V03.99 ☑
              nontraffic V03.09 ☑
              traffic V03.19 ☑
            railway (train) (vehicle) V05.99 ☑
              nontraffic V05.09 ☑
              traffic V05.19 ☑
            stationary object V00.182 ☑
            streetcar V06.99 ☑
              nontraffic V06.09 ☑
              traffic V06.19 ☑
            two- or three-wheeled motor vehicle
              V02.99 ☑
              nontraffic V02.09 ☑
              traffic V02.19 ☑
            vehicle V09.9 ☑
              animal-drawn V06.99 ☑
                nontraffic V06.09 ☑
                traffic V06.19 ☑
              motor
                nontraffic V09.00 ☑
                traffic V09.20 ☑
          fall V00.181 ☑
          in-line roller skate — *see* Accident,
            transport, pedestrian, conveyance,
            roller skate, in-line
          nontraffic V09.1 ☑
            involving motor vehicle NEC V09.00 ☑
          roller skate — *see* Accident, transport,
            pedestrian, conveyance, roller
            skate
          scooter (non-motorized) — *see* Accident,
            transport, pedestrian, conveyance,
            scooter
          skateboard — *see* Accident, transport,
            pedestrian, conveyance, skate-
            board
          traffic V09.3 ☑
            involving motor vehicle NEC V09.20 ☑
        scooter (non-motorized) V00.148 ☑
          collision (with) V09.9 ☑
            animal being ridden or animal drawn
              vehicle V06.99 ☑
              nontraffic V06.09 ☑
              traffic V06.19 ☑
            bus or heavy transport V04.99 ☑
              nontraffic V04.09 ☑
              traffic V04.19 ☑
            car V03.99 ☑
              nontraffic V03.09 ☑
              traffic V03.19 ☑
            pedal cycle V01.99 ☑
              nontraffic V01.09 ☑
              traffic V01.19 ☑
            pick-up truck or van V03.99 ☑
              nontraffic V03.09 ☑
              traffic V03.19 ☑
            railway (train) (vehicle) V05.99 ☑
              nontraffic V05.09 ☑

Accident — *continued*
  transport — *continued*
    pedestrian — *continued*
      conveyance — *continued*
        scooter — *continued*
          collision — *continued*
            railway — *continued*
              traffic V05.19 ☑
            stationary object V00.142 ☑
            streetcar V06.99 ☑
              nontraffic V06.09 ☑
              traffic V06.19 ☑
            two- or three-wheeled motor vehicle
              V02.99 ☑
              nontraffic V02.09 ☑
              traffic V02.19 ☑
            vehicle V09.9 ☑
              animal-drawn V06.99 ☑
                nontraffic V06.09 ☑
                traffic V06.19 ☑
              motor
                nontraffic V09.00 ☑
                traffic V09.20 ☑
          fall V00.141 ☑
          nontraffic V09.1 ☑
            involving motor vehicle NEC V09.00 ☑
          traffic V09.3 ☑
            involving motor vehicle NEC V09.20 ☑
        skate board V00.138 ☑
          collision (with) V09.9 ☑
            animal being ridden or animal drawn
              vehicle V06.92 ☑
              nontraffic V06.02 ☑
              traffic V06.12 ☑
            bus or heavy transport V04.92 ☑
              nontraffic V04.02 ☑
              traffic V04.12 ☑
            car V03.92 ☑
              nontraffic V03.02 ☑
              traffic V03.12 ☑
            pedal cycle V01.92 ☑
              nontraffic V01.02 ☑
              traffic V01.12 ☑
            pick-up truck or van V03.92 ☑
              nontraffic V03.02 ☑
              traffic V03.12 ☑
            railway (train) (vehicle) V05.92 ☑
              nontraffic V05.02 ☑
              traffic V05.12 ☑
            stationary object V00.132 ☑
            streetcar V06.92 ☑
              nontraffic V06.02 ☑
              traffic V06.12 ☑
            two- or three-wheeled motor vehicle
              V02.92 ☑
              nontraffic V02.02 ☑
              traffic V02.12 ☑
            vehicle V09.9 ☑
              animal-drawn V06.92 ☑
                nontraffic V06.02 ☑
                traffic V06.12 ☑
              motor
                nontraffic V09.00 ☑
                traffic V09.20 ☑
          fall V00.131 ☑
          nontraffic V09.1 ☑
            involving motor vehicle NEC V09.00 ☑
          traffic V09.3 ☑
            involving motor vehicle NEC V09.20 ☑
        skis (snow) V00.328 ☑
          collision (with) V09.9 ☑
            animal being ridden or animal drawn
              vehicle V06.99 ☑
              nontraffic V06.09 ☑
              traffic V06.19 ☑
            bus or heavy transport V04.99 ☑
              nontraffic V04.09 ☑
              traffic V04.19 ☑
            car V03.99 ☑
              nontraffic V03.09 ☑
              traffic V03.19 ☑
            pedal cycle V01.99 ☑
              nontraffic V01.09 ☑
              traffic V01.19 ☑
            pick-up truck or van V03.99 ☑
              nontraffic V03.09 ☑

Accident — *continued*
  transport — *continued*
    pedestrian — *continued*
      conveyance — *continued*
        skis — *continued*
          collision — *continued*
            pick-up truck or van — *continued*
              traffic V03.19 ☑
            railway (train) (vehicle) V05.99 ☑
              nontraffic V05.09 ☑
              traffic V05.19 ☑
            stationary object V00.322 ☑
            streetcar V06.99 ☑
              nontraffic V06.09 ☑
              traffic V06.19 ☑
            two- or three-wheeled motor vehicle
              V02.99 ☑
              nontraffic V02.09 ☑
              traffic V02.19 ☑
            vehicle V09.9 ☑
              animal-drawn V06.99 ☑
                nontraffic V06.09 ☑
                traffic V06.19 ☑
              motor
                nontraffic V09.00 ☑
                traffic V09.20 ☑
          fall V00.321 ☑
          nontraffic V09.1 ☑
            involving motor vehicle NEC V09.00 ☑
          traffic V09.3 ☑
            involving motor vehicle NEC V09.20 ☑
        sled V00.228 ☑
          collision (with) V09.9 ☑
            animal being ridden or animal drawn
              vehicle V06.99 ☑
              nontraffic V06.09 ☑
              traffic V06.19 ☑
            bus or heavy transport V04.99 ☑
              nontraffic V04.09 ☑
              traffic V04.19 ☑
            car V03.99 ☑
              nontraffic V03.09 ☑
              traffic V03.19 ☑
            pedal cycle V01.99 ☑
              nontraffic V01.09 ☑
              traffic V01.19 ☑
            pick-up truck or van V03.99 ☑
              nontraffic V03.09 ☑
              traffic V03.19 ☑
            railway (train) (vehicle) V05.99 ☑
              nontraffic V05.09 ☑
              traffic V05.19 ☑
            stationary object V00.222 ☑
            streetcar V06.99 ☑
              nontraffic V06.09 ☑
              traffic V06.19 ☑
            two- or three-wheeled motor vehicle
              V02.99 ☑
              nontraffic V02.09 ☑
              traffic V02.19 ☑
            vehicle V09.9 ☑
              animal-drawn V06.99 ☑
                nontraffic V06.09 ☑
                traffic V06.19 ☑
              motor
                nontraffic V09.00 ☑
                traffic V09.20 ☑
          fall V00.221 ☑
          nontraffic V09.1 ☑
            involving motor vehicle NEC V09.00 ☑
          traffic V09.3 ☑
            involving motor vehicle NEC V09.20 ☑
        snow board V00.318 ☑
          collision (with) V09.9 ☑
            animal being ridden or animal drawn
              vehicle V06.99 ☑
              nontraffic V06.09 ☑
              traffic V06.19 ☑
            bus or heavy transport V04.99 ☑
              nontraffic V04.09 ☑
              traffic V04.19 ☑
            car V03.99 ☑
              nontraffic V03.09 ☑
              traffic V03.19 ☑
            pedal cycle V01.99 ☑
              nontraffic V01.09 ☑

☑ **Additional Character Required — Refer to the Tabular List for Character Selection**   ▽ **Subterms under main terms may continue to next column or page**

Accident — *continued*
  transport — *continued*
    pedestrian — *continued*
      conveyance — *continued*
        snow board — *continued*
          collision — *continued*
            pedal cycle — *continued*
              traffic V01.19 ☑
            pick-up truck or van V03.99 ☑
              nontraffic V03.09 ☑
              traffic V03.19 ☑
            railway (train) (vehicle) V05.99 ☑
              nontraffic V05.09 ☑
              traffic V05.19 ☑
            stationary object V00.312 ☑
            streetcar V06.99 ☑
              nontraffic V06.09 ☑
              traffic V06.19 ☑
            two- or three-wheeled motor vehicle
              V02.99 ☑
              nontraffic V02.09 ☑
              traffic V02.19 ☑
            vehicle V09.9 ☑
              animal-drawn V06.99 ☑
                nontraffic V06.09 ☑
                traffic V06.19 ☑
              motor
                nontraffic V09.00 ☑
                traffic V09.20 ☑
           fall V00.311 ☑
          nontraffic V09.1 ☑
            involving motor vehicle NEC V09.00 ☑
          traffic V09.3 ☑
            involving motor vehicle NEC V09.20 ☑
        specified type NEC V00.898 ☑
          collision (with) V09.9 ☑
            animal being ridden or animal drawn
              vehicle V06.99 ☑
              nontraffic V06.09 ☑
              traffic V06.19 ☑
            bus or heavy transport V04.99 ☑
              nontraffic V04.09 ☑
              traffic V04.19 ☑
            car V03.99 ☑
              nontraffic V03.09 ☑
              traffic V03.19 ☑
            pedal cycle V01.99 ☑
              nontraffic V01.09 ☑
              traffic V01.19 ☑
            pick-up truck or van V03.99 ☑
              nontraffic V03.09 ☑
              traffic V03.19 ☑
            railway (train) (vehicle) V05.99 ☑
              nontraffic V05.09 ☑
              traffic V05.19 ☑
            stationary object V00.892 ☑
            streetcar V06.99 ☑
              nontraffic V06.09 ☑
              traffic V06.19 ☑
            two- or three-wheeled motor vehicle
              V02.99 ☑
              nontraffic V02.09 ☑
              traffic V02.19 ☑
            vehicle V09.9 ☑
              animal-drawn V06.99 ☑
                nontraffic V06.09 ☑
                traffic V06.19 ☑
              motor
                nontraffic V09.00 ☑
                traffic V09.20 ☑
           fall V00.891 ☑
          nontraffic V09.1 ☑
            involving motor vehicle NEC V09.00 ☑
          traffic V09.3 ☑
            involving motor vehicle NEC V09.20 ☑
       traffic V09.3 ☑
         involving motor vehicle V09.20 ☑
          military V09.21 ☑
          specified type NEC V09.29 ☑
      wheelchair (powered) V00.818 ☑
        collision (with) V09.9 ☑
          animal being ridden or animal drawn
            vehicle V06.99 ☑
            nontraffic V06.09 ☑
            traffic V06.19 ☑
          bus or heavy transport V04.99 ☑

Accident — *continued*
  transport — *continued*
    pedestrian — *continued*
      conveyance — *continued*
        wheelchair — *continued*
          collision — *continued*
            bus or heavy transport — *continued*
              nontraffic V04.09 ☑
              traffic V04.19 ☑
            car V03.99 ☑
              nontraffic V03.09 ☑
              traffic V03.19 ☑
            pedal cycle V01.99 ☑
              nontraffic V01.09 ☑
              traffic V01.19 ☑
            pick-up truck or van V03.99 ☑
              nontraffic V03.09 ☑
              traffic V03.19 ☑
            railway (train) (vehicle) V05.99 ☑
              nontraffic V05.09 ☑
              traffic V05.19 ☑
            stationary object V00.812 ☑
            streetcar V06.99 ☑
              nontraffic V06.09 ☑
              traffic V06.19 ☑
            two- or three-wheeled motor vehicle
              V02.99 ☑
              nontraffic V02.09 ☑
              traffic V02.19 ☑
            vehicle V09.9 ☑
              animal-drawn V06.99 ☑
                nontraffic V06.09 ☑
                traffic V06.19 ☑
              motor
                nontraffic V09.00 ☑
                traffic V09.20 ☑
           fall V00.811 ☑
          nontraffic V09.1 ☑
            involving motor vehicle NEC V09.00 ☑
          traffic V09.3 ☑
            involving motor vehicle NEC V09.20 ☑
      wheeled shoe V00.158 ☑
        colliding with stationary object
          V00.152 ☑
        fall V00.151 ☑
    on foot — *see also* Accident, pedestrian
      collision (with)
        animal being ridden or animal drawn ve-
          hicle V06.90 ☑
          nontraffic V06.00 ☑
          traffic V06.10 ☑
        bus or heavy transport V04.90 ☑
          nontraffic V04.00 ☑
          traffic V04.10 ☑
        car V03.90 ☑
          nontraffic V03.00 ☑
          traffic V03.10 ☑
        pedal cycle V01.90 ☑
          nontraffic V01.00 ☑
          traffic V01.10 ☑
        pick-up truck or van V03.90 ☑
          nontraffic V03.00 ☑
          traffic V03.10 ☑
        railway (train) (vehicle) V05.90 ☑
          nontraffic V05.00 ☑
          traffic V05.10 ☑
        streetcar V06.90 ☑
          nontraffic V06.00 ☑
          traffic V06.10 ☑
        two- or three-wheeled motor vehicle
          V02.90 ☑
          nontraffic V02.00 ☑
          traffic V02.10 ☑
        vehicle V09.9 ☑
          animal-drawn V06.90 ☑
           nontraffic V06.00 ☑
           traffic V06.10 ☑
          motor
       nontraffic V09.1 ☑
         involving motor vehicle V09.00 ☑
          military V09.01 ☑
         specified type NEC V09.09 ☑
       traffic V09.3 ☑
        involving motor vehicle V09.20 ☑
         military V09.21 ☑

Accident — *continued*
  transport — *continued*
    pedestrian — *continued*
      on foot — *see also* Accident, pedestrian — con-
        tinued
        traffic — *continued*
          involving motor vehicle — *continued*
            specified type NEC V09.29 ☑
    person NEC (unknown way or transportation) V99 ☑
      collision (between)
        bus (with)
          heavy transport vehicle (traffic) V87.5 ☑
          nontraffic V88.5 ☑
        car (with)
          bus (traffic) V87.3 ☑
          nontraffic V88.3 ☑
          heavy transport vehicle (traffic) V87.4 ☑
          nontraffic V88.4 ☑
          nontraffic V88.5 ☑
          pick-up truck or van (traffic) V87.2 ☑
          nontraffic V88.2 ☑
          train or railway vehicle (traffic) V87.6 ☑
          nontraffic V88.6 ☑
          two-or three-wheeled motor vehicle
            (traffic) V87.0 ☑
          nontraffic V88.0 ☑
        motor vehicle (traffic) NEC V87.7 ☑
          nontraffic V88.7 ☑
        two-or three-wheeled vehicle (with) (traffic)
          motor vehicle NEC V87.1 ☑
          nontraffic V88.1 ☑
      nonmotor vehicle (collision) (noncollision) (traf-
        fic) V87.9 ☑
      nontraffic V88.9 ☑
    pickup truck occupant V59.9 ☑
      collision (with)
        animal (traffic) V50.9 ☑
          being ridden (traffic) V56.9 ☑
            nontraffic V56.3 ☑
            while boarding or alighting V56.4 ☑
          nontraffic V50.3 ☑
          while boarding or alighting V50.4 ☑
        animal-drawn vehicle (traffic) V56.9 ☑
          nontraffic V56.3 ☑
          while boarding or alighting V56.4 ☑
        bus (traffic) V54.9 ☑
          nontraffic V54.3 ☑
          while boarding or alighting V54.4 ☑
        car (traffic) V53.9 ☑
          nontraffic V53.3 ☑
          while boarding or alighting V53.4 ☑
        motor vehicle NOS (traffic) V59.60 ☑
          nontraffic V59.20 ☑
          specified type NEC (traffic) V59.69 ☑
            nontraffic V59.29 ☑
        pedal cycle (traffic) V51.9 ☑
          nontraffic V51.3 ☑
          while boarding or alighting V51.4 ☑
        pickup truck (traffic) V53.9 ☑
          nontraffic V53.3 ☑
          while boarding or alighting V53.4 ☑
        railway vehicle (traffic) V55.9 ☑
          nontraffic V55.3 ☑
          while boarding or alighting V55.4 ☑
        specified vehicle NEC (traffic) V56.9 ☑
          nontraffic V56.3 ☑
          while boarding or alighting V56.4 ☑
        stationary object (traffic) V57.9 ☑
          nontraffic V57.3 ☑
          while boarding or alighting V57.4 ☑
        streetcar (traffic) V56.9 ☑
          nontraffic V56.3 ☑
          while boarding or alighting V56.4 ☑
        three wheeled motor vehicle (traffic) V52.9 ☑
          nontraffic V52.3 ☑
          while boarding or alighting V52.4 ☑
        truck (traffic) V54.9 ☑
          nontraffic V54.3 ☑
          while boarding or alighting V54.4 ☑
        two wheeled motor vehicle (traffic) V52.9 ☑
          nontraffic V52.3 ☑
          while boarding or alighting V52.4 ☑
        van (traffic) V53.9 ☑
          nontraffic V53.3 ☑
          while boarding or alighting V53.4 ☑

▽ **Subterms under main terms may continue to next column or page**   ☑ **Additional Character Required — Refer to the Tabular List for Character Selection**   **405**

Accident — Accident

Accident — *continued*
  transport — *continued*
    pickup truck occupant — *continued*
      driver
        collision (with)
          animal (traffic) V50.5 ☑
            being ridden (traffic) V56.5 ☑
              nontraffic V56.0 ☑
            nontraffic V50.0 ☑
          animal-drawn vehicle (traffic) V56.5 ☑
            nontraffic V56.0 ☑
          bus (traffic) V54.5 ☑
            nontraffic V54.0 ☑
          car (traffic) V53.5 ☑
            nontraffic V53.0 ☑
          motor vehicle NOS (traffic) V59.40 ☑
            nontraffic V59.00 ☑
            specified type NEC (traffic) V59.49 ☑
              nontraffic V59.09 ☑
          pedal cycle (traffic) V51.5 ☑
            nontraffic V51.0 ☑
          pickup truck (traffic) V53.5 ☑
            nontraffic V53.0 ☑
          railway vehicle (traffic) V55.5 ☑
            nontraffic V55.0 ☑
          specified vehicle NEC (traffic) V56.5 ☑
            nontraffic V56.0 ☑
          stationary object (traffic) V57.5 ☑
            nontraffic V57.0 ☑
          streetcar (traffic) V56.5 ☑
            nontraffic V56.0 ☑
          three wheeled motor vehicle (traffic)
            V52.5 ☑
            nontraffic V52.0 ☑
          truck (traffic) V54.5 ☑
            nontraffic V54.0 ☑
          two wheeled motor vehicle (traffic)
            V52.5 ☑
            nontraffic V52.0 ☑
          van (traffic) V53.5 ☑
            nontraffic V53.0 ☑
        noncollision accident (traffic) V58.5 ☑
          nontraffic V58.0 ☑
      hanger-on
        collision (with)
          animal (traffic) V50.7 ☑
            being ridden (traffic) V56.7 ☑
              nontraffic V56.2 ☑
            nontraffic V50.2 ☑
          animal-drawn vehicle (traffic) V56.7 ☑
            nontraffic V56.2 ☑
          bus (traffic) V54.7 ☑
            nontraffic V54.2 ☑
          car (traffic) V53.7 ☑
            nontraffic V53.2 ☑
          pedal cycle (traffic) V51.7 ☑
            nontraffic V51.2 ☑
          pickup truck (traffic) V53.7 ☑
            nontraffic V53.2 ☑
          railway vehicle (traffic) V55.7 ☑
            nontraffic V55.2 ☑
          specified vehicle NEC (traffic) V56.7 ☑
            nontraffic V56.2 ☑
          stationary object (traffic) V57.7 ☑
            nontraffic V57.2 ☑
          streetcar (traffic) V56.7 ☑
            nontraffic V56.2 ☑
          three wheeled motor vehicle (traffic)
            V52.7 ☑
            nontraffic V52.2 ☑
          truck (traffic) V54.7 ☑
            nontraffic V54.2 ☑
          two wheeled motor vehicle (traffic)
            V52.7 ☑
            nontraffic V52.2 ☑
          van (traffic) V53.7 ☑
            nontraffic V53.2 ☑
        noncollision accident (traffic) V58.7 ☑
          nontraffic V58.2 ☑
      noncollision accident (traffic) V58.9 ☑
        nontraffic V58.3 ☑
        while boarding or alighting V58.4 ☑
      nontraffic V59.3 ☑
      passenger
        collision (with)
          animal (traffic) V50.6 ☑

Accident — *continued*
  transport — *continued*
    pickup truck occupant — *continued*
      passenger — *continued*
        collision — *continued*
          animal — *continued*
            being ridden (traffic) V56.6 ☑
              nontraffic V56.1 ☑
            nontraffic V50.1 ☑
          animal-drawn vehicle (traffic) V56.6 ☑
            nontraffic V56.1 ☑
          bus (traffic) V54.6 ☑
            nontraffic V54.1 ☑
          car (traffic) V53.6 ☑
            nontraffic V53.1 ☑
          motor vehicle NOS (traffic) V59.50 ☑
            nontraffic V59.10 ☑
            specified type NEC (traffic) V59.59 ☑
              nontraffic V59.19 ☑
          pedal cycle (traffic) V51.6 ☑
            nontraffic V51.1 ☑
          pickup truck (traffic) V53.6 ☑
            nontraffic V53.1 ☑
          railway vehicle (traffic) V55.6 ☑
            nontraffic V55.1 ☑
          specified vehicle NEC (traffic) V56.6 ☑
            nontraffic V56.1 ☑
          stationary object (traffic) V57.6 ☑
            nontraffic V57.1 ☑
          streetcar (traffic) V56.6 ☑
            nontraffic V56.1 ☑
          three wheeled motor vehicle (traffic)
            V52.6 ☑
            nontraffic V52.1 ☑
          truck (traffic) V54.6 ☑
            nontraffic V54.1 ☑
          two wheeled motor vehicle (traffic)
            V52.6 ☑
            nontraffic V52.1 ☑
          van (traffic) V53.6 ☑
            nontraffic V53.1 ☑
        noncollision accident (traffic) V58.6 ☑
          nontraffic V58.1 ☑
      specified type NEC V59.88 ☑
      military vehicle V59.81 ☑
    quarry truck — *see* Accident, transport, industrial
        vehicle occupant
    race car — *see* Accident, transport, motor vehicle
        NEC occupant
    railway vehicle occupant V81.9 ☑
      collision (with) V81.3 ☑
        motor vehicle (non-military) (traffic) V81.1 ☑
          military V81.83 ☑
          nontraffic V81.0 ☑
        rolling stock V81.2 ☑
        specified object NEC V81.3 ☑
      during derailment V81.7 ☑
        with antecedent collision — *see* Accident,
          transport, railway vehicle occupant,
          collision
      explosion V81.81 ☑
      fall (in railway vehicle) V81.5 ☑
        during derailment V81.7 ☑
          with antecedent collision — *see* Accident,
            transport, railway vehicle occupant,
            collision
        from railway vehicle V81.6 ☑
          during derailment V81.7 ☑
            with antecedent collision — *see* Acci-
              dent, transport, railway vehicle
              occupant, collision
        while boarding or alighting V81.4 ☑
      fire V81.81 ☑
      object falling onto train V81.82 ☑
      specified type NEC V81.89 ☑
      while boarding or alighting V81.4 ☑
    ski lift V98.3 ☑
    snowmobile occupant (nontraffic) V86.92 ☑
      driver V86.52 ☑
      hanger-on V86.72 ☑
      passenger V86.62 ☑
      traffic V86.32 ☑
        driver V86.02 ☑
        hanger-on V86.22 ☑
        passenger V86.12 ☑
      while boarding or alighting V86.42 ☑

Accident — *continued*
  transport — *continued*
    specified NEC V98.8 ☑
    sport utility vehicle occupant — *see also* Acciden[t]
        transport, pickup truck occupant
    streetcar occupant V82.9 ☑
      collision (with) V82.3 ☑
        motor vehicle (traffic) V82.1 ☑
          nontraffic V82.0 ☑
        rolling stock V82.2 ☑
      during derailment V82.7 ☑
        with antecedent collision — *see* Accident,
          transport, streetcar occupant, collisio[n]
      fall (in streetcar) V82.5 ☑
        during derailment V82.7 ☑
          with antecedent collision — *see* Accident,
            transport, streetcar occupant, colli-
            sion
        from streetcar V82.6 ☑
          during derailment V82.7 ☑
            with antecedent collision — *see* Acci-
              dent, transport, streetcar occu-
              pant, collision
          while boarding or alighting V82.4 ☑
        while boarding or alighting V82.4 ☑
      specified type NEC V82.8 ☑
      while boarding or alighting V82.4 ☑
    three-wheeled motor vehicle occupant V39.9 ☑
      collision (with)
        animal (traffic) V30.9 ☑
          being ridden (traffic) V36.9 ☑
            nontraffic V36.3 ☑
            while boarding or alighting V36.4 ☑
          nontraffic V30.3 ☑
          while boarding or alighting V30.4 ☑
        animal-drawn vehicle (traffic) V36.9 ☑
          nontraffic V36.3 ☑
          while boarding or alighting V36.4 ☑
        bus (traffic) V34.9 ☑
          nontraffic V34.3 ☑
          while boarding or alighting V34.4 ☑
        car (traffic) V33.9 ☑
          nontraffic V33.3 ☑
          while boarding or alighting V33.4 ☑
        motor vehicle NOS (traffic) V39.60 ☑
          nontraffic V39.20 ☑
          specified type NEC (traffic) V39.69 ☑
            nontraffic V39.29 ☑
        pedal cycle (traffic) V31.9 ☑
          nontraffic V31.3 ☑
          while boarding or alighting V31.4 ☑
        pickup truck (traffic) V33.9 ☑
          nontraffic V33.3 ☑
          while boarding or alighting V33.4 ☑
        railway vehicle (traffic) V35.9 ☑
          nontraffic V35.3 ☑
          while boarding or alighting V35.4 ☑
        specified vehicle NEC (traffic) V36.9 ☑
          nontraffic V36.3 ☑
          while boarding or alighting V36.4 ☑
        stationary object (traffic) V37.9 ☑
          nontraffic V37.3 ☑
          while boarding or alighting V37.4 ☑
        streetcar (traffic) V36.9 ☑
          nontraffic V36.3 ☑
          while boarding or alighting V36.4 ☑
        three wheeled motor vehicle (traffic) V32.9 ☑
          nontraffic V32.3 ☑
          while boarding or alighting V32.4 ☑
        truck (traffic) V34.9 ☑
          nontraffic V34.3 ☑
          while boarding or alighting V34.4 ☑
        two wheeled motor vehicle (traffic) V32.9 ☑
          nontraffic V32.3 ☑
          while boarding or alighting V32.4 ☑
        van (traffic) V33.9 ☑
          nontraffic V33.3 ☑
          while boarding or alighting V33.4 ☑
      driver
        collision (with)
          animal (traffic) V30.5 ☑
            being ridden (traffic) V36.5 ☑
              nontraffic V36.0 ☑
            nontraffic V30.0 ☑
          animal-drawn vehicle (traffic) V36.5 ☑
            nontraffic V36.0 ☑

Accident — continued
  transport — continued
    three-wheeled motor vehicle occupant — continued
      driver — continued
        collision — continued
          bus (traffic) V34.5 ☑
            nontraffic V34.0 ☑
          car (traffic) V33.5 ☑
            nontraffic V33.0 ☑
          motor vehicle NOS (traffic) V39.40 ☑
            nontraffic V39.00 ☑
            specified type NEC (traffic) V39.49 ☑
              nontraffic V39.09 ☑
          pedal cycle (traffic) V31.5 ☑
            nontraffic V31.0 ☑
          pickup truck (traffic) V33.5 ☑
            nontraffic V33.0 ☑
          railway vehicle (traffic) V35.5 ☑
            nontraffic V35.0 ☑
          specified vehicle NEC (traffic) V36.5 ☑
            nontraffic V36.0 ☑
          stationary object (traffic) V37.5 ☑
            nontraffic V37.0 ☑
          streetcar (traffic) V36.5 ☑
            nontraffic V36.0 ☑
          three wheeled motor vehicle (traffic) V32.5 ☑
            nontraffic V32.0 ☑
          truck (traffic) V34.5 ☑
            nontraffic V34.0 ☑
          two wheeled motor vehicle (traffic) V32.5 ☑
            nontraffic V32.0 ☑
          van (traffic) V33.5 ☑
            nontraffic V33.0 ☑
        noncollision accident (traffic) V38.5 ☑
          nontraffic V38.0 ☑
      hanger-on
        collision (with)
          animal (traffic) V30.7 ☑
            being ridden (traffic) V36.7 ☑
              nontraffic V36.2 ☑
            nontraffic V30.2 ☑
          animal-drawn vehicle (traffic) V36.7 ☑
            nontraffic V36.2 ☑
          bus (traffic) V34.7 ☑
            nontraffic V34.2 ☑
          car (traffic) V33.7 ☑
            nontraffic V33.2 ☑
          pedal cycle (traffic) V31.7 ☑
            nontraffic V31.2 ☑
          pickup truck (traffic) V33.7 ☑
            nontraffic V33.2 ☑
          railway vehicle (traffic) V35.7 ☑
            nontraffic V35.2 ☑
          specified vehicle NEC (traffic) V36.7 ☑
            nontraffic V36.2 ☑
          stationary object (traffic) V37.7 ☑
            nontraffic V37.2 ☑
          streetcar (traffic) V36.7 ☑
            nontraffic V36.2 ☑
          three wheeled motor vehicle (traffic) V32.7 ☑
            nontraffic V32.2 ☑
          truck (traffic) V34.7 ☑
            nontraffic V34.2 ☑
          two wheeled motor vehicle (traffic) V32.7 ☑
            nontraffic V32.2 ☑
          van (traffic) V33.7 ☑
            nontraffic V33.2 ☑
        noncollision accident (traffic) V38.7 ☑
          nontraffic V38.2 ☑
      noncollision accident (traffic) V38.9 ☑
        nontraffic V38.3 ☑
        while boarding or alighting V38.4 ☑
      nontraffic V39.3 ☑
      passenger
        collision (with)
          animal (traffic) V30.6 ☑
            being ridden (traffic) V36.6 ☑
              nontraffic V36.1 ☑
            nontraffic V30.1 ☑
          animal-drawn vehicle (traffic) V36.6 ☑
            nontraffic V36.1 ☑

Accident — continued
  transport — continued
    three-wheeled motor vehicle occupant — continued
      passenger — continued
        collision — continued
          bus (traffic) V34.6 ☑
            nontraffic V34.1 ☑
          car (traffic) V33.6 ☑
            nontraffic V33.1 ☑
          motor vehicle NOS (traffic) V39.50 ☑
            nontraffic V39.10 ☑
            specified type NEC (traffic) V39.59 ☑
              nontraffic V39.19 ☑
          pedal cycle (traffic) V31.6 ☑
            nontraffic V31.1 ☑
          pickup truck (traffic) V33.6 ☑
            nontraffic V33.1 ☑
          railway vehicle (traffic) V35.6 ☑
            nontraffic V35.1 ☑
          specified vehicle NEC (traffic) V36.6 ☑
            nontraffic V36.1 ☑
          stationary object (traffic) V37.6 ☑
            nontraffic V37.1 ☑
          streetcar (traffic) V36.6 ☑
            nontraffic V36.1 ☑
          three wheeled motor vehicle (traffic) V32.6 ☑
            nontraffic V32.1 ☑
          truck (traffic) V34.6 ☑
            nontraffic V34.1 ☑
          two wheeled motor vehicle (traffic) V32.6 ☑
            nontraffic V32.1 ☑
          van (traffic) V33.6 ☑
            nontraffic V33.1 ☑
        noncollision accident (traffic) V38.6 ☑
          nontraffic V38.1 ☑
      specified type NEC V39.89 ☑
      military vehicle V39.81 ☑
    tractor (farm) (and trailer) — see Accident, transport, agricultural vehicle occupant
    tram — see Accident, transport, streetcar
      in mine or quarry — see Accident, transport, industrial vehicle occupant
    trolley — see Accident, transport, streetcar
      in mine or quarry — see Accident, transport, industrial vehicle occupant
    truck (heavy) occupant V69.9 ☑
      collision (with)
        animal (traffic) V60.9 ☑
          being ridden (traffic) V66.9 ☑
            nontraffic V66.3 ☑
            while boarding or alighting V66.4 ☑
          nontraffic V60.3 ☑
          while boarding or alighting V60.4 ☑
        animal-drawn vehicle (traffic) V66.9 ☑
          nontraffic V66.3 ☑
          while boarding or alighting V66.4 ☑
        bus (traffic) V64.9 ☑
          nontraffic V64.3 ☑
          while boarding or alighting V64.4 ☑
        car (traffic) V63.9 ☑
          nontraffic V63.3 ☑
          while boarding or alighting V63.4 ☑
        motor vehicle NOS (traffic) V69.60 ☑
          nontraffic V69.20 ☑
          specified type NEC (traffic) V69.69 ☑
            nontraffic V69.29 ☑
        pedal cycle (traffic) V61.9 ☑
          nontraffic V61.3 ☑
          while boarding or alighting V61.4 ☑
        pickup truck (traffic) V63.9 ☑
          nontraffic V63.3 ☑
          while boarding or alighting V63.4 ☑
        railway vehicle (traffic) V65.9 ☑
          nontraffic V65.3 ☑
          while boarding or alighting V65.4 ☑
        specified vehicle NEC (traffic) V66.9 ☑
          nontraffic V66.3 ☑
          while boarding or alighting V66.4 ☑
        stationary object (traffic) V67.9 ☑
          nontraffic V67.3 ☑
          while boarding or alighting V67.4 ☑
        streetcar (traffic) V66.9 ☑
          nontraffic V66.3 ☑

Accident — continued
  transport — continued
    truck occupant — continued
      collision — continued
        streetcar — continued
          while boarding or alighting V66.4 ☑
        three wheeled motor vehicle (traffic) V62.9 ☑
          nontraffic V62.3 ☑
          while boarding or alighting V62.4 ☑
        truck (traffic) V64.9 ☑
          nontraffic V64.3 ☑
          while boarding or alighting V64.4 ☑
        two wheeled motor vehicle (traffic) V62.9 ☑
          nontraffic V62.3 ☑
          while boarding or alighting V62.4 ☑
        van (traffic) V63.9 ☑
          nontraffic V63.3 ☑
          while boarding or alighting V63.4 ☑
      driver
        collision (with)
          animal (traffic) V60.5 ☑
            being ridden (traffic) V66.5 ☑
              nontraffic V66.0 ☑
            nontraffic V60.0 ☑
          animal-drawn vehicle (traffic) V66.5 ☑
            nontraffic V66.0 ☑
          bus (traffic) V64.5 ☑
            nontraffic V64.0 ☑
          car (traffic) V63.5 ☑
            nontraffic V63.0 ☑
          motor vehicle NOS (traffic) V69.40 ☑
            nontraffic V69.00 ☑
            specified type NEC (traffic) V69.49 ☑
              nontraffic V69.09 ☑
          pedal cycle (traffic) V61.5 ☑
            nontraffic V61.0 ☑
          pickup truck (traffic) V63.5 ☑
            nontraffic V63.0 ☑
          railway vehicle (traffic) V65.5 ☑
            nontraffic V65.0 ☑
          specified vehicle NEC (traffic) V66.5 ☑
            nontraffic V66.0 ☑
          stationary object (traffic) V67.5 ☑
            nontraffic V67.0 ☑
          streetcar (traffic) V66.5 ☑
            nontraffic V66.0 ☑
          three wheeled motor vehicle (traffic) V62.5 ☑
            nontraffic V62.0 ☑
          truck (traffic) V64.5 ☑
            nontraffic V64.0 ☑
          two wheeled motor vehicle (traffic) V62.5 ☑
            nontraffic V62.0 ☑
          van (traffic) V63.5 ☑
            nontraffic V63.0 ☑
        noncollision accident (traffic) V68.5 ☑
          nontraffic V68.0 ☑
      dump — see Accident, transport, construction vehicle occupant
      hanger-on
        collision (with)
          animal (traffic) V60.7 ☑
            being ridden (traffic) V66.7 ☑
              nontraffic V66.2 ☑
            nontraffic V60.2 ☑
          animal-drawn vehicle (traffic) V66.7 ☑
            nontraffic V66.2 ☑
          bus (traffic) V64.7 ☑
            nontraffic V64.2 ☑
          car (traffic) V63.7 ☑
            nontraffic V63.2 ☑
          pedal cycle (traffic) V61.7 ☑
            nontraffic V61.2 ☑
          pickup truck (traffic) V63.7 ☑
            nontraffic V63.2 ☑
          railway vehicle (traffic) V65.7 ☑
            nontraffic V65.2 ☑
          specified vehicle NEC (traffic) V66.7 ☑
            nontraffic V66.2 ☑
          stationary object (traffic) V67.7 ☑
            nontraffic V67.2 ☑
          streetcar (traffic) V66.7 ☑
            nontraffic V66.2 ☑
          three wheeled motor vehicle (traffic) V62.7 ☑

☜ Subterms under main terms may continue to next column or page   ☑ Additional Character Required — Refer to the Tabular List for Character Selection   407

Accident — Accident

Accident — *continued*
  transport — *continued*
    truck occupant — *continued*
      hanger-on — *continued*
        collision — *continued*
          three wheeled motor vehicle — *continued*
            nontraffic V62.2 ☑
          truck (traffic) V64.7 ☑
            nontraffic V64.2 ☑
          two wheeled motor vehicle (traffic) V62.7 ☑
            nontraffic V62.2 ☑
          van (traffic) V63.7 ☑
            nontraffic V63.2 ☑
        noncollision accident (traffic) V68.7 ☑
          nontraffic V68.2 ☑
      noncollision accident (traffic) V68.9 ☑
        nontraffic V68.3 ☑
        while boarding or alighting V68.4 ☑
      nontraffic V69.3 ☑
      passenger
        collision (with)
          animal (traffic) V60.6 ☑
            being ridden (traffic) V66.6 ☑
              nontraffic V66.1- ☑
            nontraffic V60.1 ☑
          animal-drawn vehicle (traffic) V66.6 ☑
            nontraffic V66.1 ☑
          bus (traffic) V64.6 ☑
            nontraffic V64.1 ☑
          car (traffic) V63.6 ☑
            nontraffic V63.1 ☑
          motor vehicle NOS (traffic) V69.50 ☑
            nontraffic V69.10 ☑
            specified type NEC (traffic) V69.59 ☑
              nontraffic V69.19 ☑
          pedal cycle (traffic) V61.6 ☑
            nontraffic V61.1 ☑
          pickup truck (traffic) V63.6 ☑
            nontraffic V63.1 ☑
          railway vehicle (traffic) V65.6 ☑
            nontraffic V65.1 ☑
          specified vehicle NEC (traffic) V66.6 ☑
            nontraffic V66.1 ☑
          stationary object (traffic) V67.6 ☑
            nontraffic V67.1 ☑
          streetcar (traffic) V66.6 ☑
            nontraffic V66.1 ☑
          three wheeled motor vehicle (traffic) V62.6 ☑
            nontraffic V62.1 ☑
          truck (traffic) V64.6 ☑
            nontraffic V64.1 ☑
          two wheeled motor vehicle (traffic) V62.6 ☑
            nontraffic V62.1 ☑
          van (traffic) V63.6 ☑
            nontraffic V63.1 ☑
        noncollision accident (traffic) V68.6 ☑
          nontraffic V68.1 ☑
      pickup — *see* Accident, transport, pickup truck occupant
      specified type NEC V69.88 ☑
        military vehicle V69.81 ☑
    van occupant V59.9 ☑
      collision (with)
        animal (traffic) V50.9 ☑
          being ridden (traffic) V56.9 ☑
            nontraffic V56.3 ☑
            while boarding or alighting V56.4 ☑
          nontraffic V50.3 ☑
          while boarding or alighting V50.4 ☑
        animal-drawn vehicle (traffic) V56.9 ☑
          nontraffic V56.3 ☑
          while boarding or alighting V56.4 ☑
        bus (traffic) V54.9 ☑
          nontraffic V54.3 ☑
          while boarding or alighting V54.4 ☑
        car (traffic) V53.9 ☑
          nontraffic V53.3 ☑
          while boarding or alighting V53.4 ☑
        motor vehicle NOS (traffic) V59.60 ☑
          nontraffic V59.20 ☑
          specified type NEC (traffic) V59.69 ☑
            nontraffic V59.29 ☑

Accident — *continued*
  transport — *continued*
    van occupant — *continued*
      collision — *continued*
        pedal cycle (traffic) V51.9 ☑
          nontraffic V51.3 ☑
          while boarding or alighting V51.4 ☑
        pickup truck (traffic) V53.9 ☑
          nontraffic V53.3 ☑
          while boarding or alighting V53.4 ☑
        railway vehicle (traffic) V55.9 ☑
          nontraffic V55.3 ☑
          while boarding or alighting V55.4 ☑
        specified vehicle NEC (traffic) V56.9 ☑
          nontraffic V56.3 ☑
          while boarding or alighting V56.4 ☑
        stationary object (traffic) V57.9 ☑
          nontraffic V57.3 ☑
          while boarding or alighting V57.4 ☑
        streetcar (traffic) V56.9 ☑
          nontraffic V56.3 ☑
          while boarding or alighting V56.4 ☑
        three wheeled motor vehicle (traffic) V52.9 ☑
          nontraffic V52.3 ☑
          while boarding or alighting V52.4 ☑
        truck (traffic) V54.9 ☑
          nontraffic V54.3 ☑
          while boarding or alighting V54.4 ☑
        two wheeled motor vehicle (traffic) V52.9 ☑
          nontraffic V52.3 ☑
          while boarding or alighting V52.4 ☑
        van (traffic) V53.9 ☑
          nontraffic V53.3 ☑
          while boarding or alighting V53.4 ☑
    driver
      collision (with)
        animal (traffic) V50.5 ☑
          being ridden (traffic) V56.5 ☑
            nontraffic V56.0 ☑
          nontraffic V50.0 ☑
        animal-drawn vehicle (traffic) V56.5 ☑
          nontraffic V56.0 ☑
        bus (traffic) V54.5 ☑
          nontraffic V54.0 ☑
        car (traffic) V53.5 ☑
          nontraffic V53.0 ☑
        motor vehicle NOS (traffic) V59.40 ☑
          nontraffic V59.00 ☑
          specified type NEC (traffic) V59.49 ☑
            nontraffic V59.09 ☑
        pedal cycle (traffic) V51.5 ☑
          nontraffic V51.0 ☑
        pickup truck (traffic) V53.5 ☑
          nontraffic V53.0 ☑
        railway vehicle (traffic) V55.5 ☑
          nontraffic V55.0 ☑
        specified vehicle NEC (traffic) V56.5 ☑
          nontraffic V56.0 ☑
        stationary object (traffic) V57.5 ☑
          nontraffic V57.0 ☑
        streetcar (traffic) V56.5 ☑
          nontraffic V56.0 ☑
        three wheeled motor vehicle (traffic) V52.5 ☑
          nontraffic V52.0 ☑
        truck (traffic) V54.5 ☑
          nontraffic V54.0 ☑
        two wheeled motor vehicle (traffic) V52.5 ☑
          nontraffic V52.0 ☑
        van (traffic) V53.5 ☑
          nontraffic V53.0 ☑
        noncollision accident (traffic) V58.5 ☑
          nontraffic V58.0 ☑
    hanger-on
      collision (with)
        animal (traffic) V50.7 ☑
          being ridden (traffic) V56.7 ☑
            nontraffic V56.2 ☑
          nontraffic V50.2 ☑
        animal-drawn vehicle (traffic) V56.7 ☑
          nontraffic V56.2 ☑
        bus (traffic) V54.7 ☑
          nontraffic V54.2 ☑
        car (traffic) V53.7 ☑
          nontraffic V53.2 ☑

Accident — *continued*
  transport — *continued*
    van occupant — *continued*
      hanger-on — *continued*
        collision — *continued*
          pedal cycle (traffic) V51.7 ☑
            nontraffic V51.2 ☑
          pickup truck (traffic) V53.7 ☑
            nontraffic V53.2 ☑
          railway vehicle (traffic) V55.7 ☑
            nontraffic V55.2 ☑
          specified vehicle NEC (traffic) V56.7 ☑
            nontraffic V56.2 ☑
          stationary object (traffic) V57.7 ☑
            nontraffic V57.2 ☑
          streetcar (traffic) V56.7 ☑
            nontraffic V56.2 ☑
          three wheeled motor vehicle (traffic) V52.7 ☑
            nontraffic V52.2 ☑
          truck (traffic) V54.7 ☑
            nontraffic V54.2 ☑
          two wheeled motor vehicle (traffic) V52.7 ☑
            nontraffic V52.2 ☑
          van (traffic) V53.7 ☑
            nontraffic V53.2 ☑
        noncollision accident (traffic) V58.7 ☑
          nontraffic V58.2 ☑
      noncollision accident (traffic) V58.9 ☑
        nontraffic V58.3 ☑
        while boarding or alighting V58.4 ☑
      nontraffic V59.3 ☑
      passenger
        collision (with)
          animal (traffic) V50.6 ☑
            being ridden (traffic) V56.6 ☑
              nontraffic V56.1 ☑
            nontraffic V50.1 ☑
          animal-drawn vehicle (traffic) V56.6 ☑
            nontraffic V56.1 ☑
          bus (traffic) V54.6 ☑
            nontraffic V54.1 ☑
          car (traffic) V53.6 ☑
            nontraffic V53.1 ☑
          motor vehicle NOS (traffic) V59.50 ☑
            nontraffic V59.10 ☑
            specified type NEC (traffic) V59.59 ☑
              nontraffic V59.19 ☑
          pedal cycle (traffic) V51.6 ☑
            nontraffic V51.1 ☑
          pickup truck (traffic) V53.6 ☑
            nontraffic V53.1 ☑
          railway vehicle (traffic) V55.6 ☑
            nontraffic V55.1 ☑
          specified vehicle NEC (traffic) V56.6 ☑
            nontraffic V56.1 ☑
          stationary object (traffic) V57.6 ☑
            nontraffic V57.1 ☑
          streetcar (traffic) V56.6 ☑
            nontraffic V56.1 ☑
          three wheeled motor vehicle (traffic) V52.6 ☑
            nontraffic V52.1 ☑
          truck (traffic) V54.6 ☑
            nontraffic V54.1 ☑
          two wheeled motor vehicle (traffic) V52.6 ☑
            nontraffic V52.1 ☑
          van (traffic) V53.6 ☑
            nontraffic V53.1 ☑
        noncollision accident (traffic) V58.6 ☑
          nontraffic V58.1 ☑
      specified type NEC V59.88 ☑
        military vehicle V59.81 ☑
    watercraft occupant — *see* Accident, watercraft
  vehicle NEC V89.9 ☑
    animal-drawn NEC — *see* Accident, transport, animal-drawn vehicle occupant
    special
      agricultural — *see* Accident, transport, agricultural vehicle occupant
      construction — *see* Accident, transport, construction vehicle occupant
      industrial — *see* Accident, transport, industrial vehicle occupant

☑ Additional Character Required — Refer to the Tabular List for Character Selection   ▽ Subterms under main terms may continue to next column or page

Accident — *continued*
  vehicle — *continued*
    three-wheeled NEC (motorized) — *see* Accident, transport, three-wheeled motor vehicle occupant
    watercraft V94.9 ☑
      causing
        drowning — *see* Drowning, due to, accident to, watercraft
        injury NEC V91.89 ☑
          crushed between craft and object V91.19 ☑
            powered craft V91.13 ☑
              ferry boat V91.11 ☑
              fishing boat V91.12 ☑
              jetskis V91.13 ☑
              liner V91.11 ☑
              merchant ship V91.10 ☑
              passenger ship V91.11 ☑
            unpowered craft V91.18 ☑
              canoe V91.15 ☑
              inflatable V91.16 ☑
              kayak V91.15 ☑
              sailboat V91.14 ☑
              surf-board V91.18 ☑
              windsurfer V91.18 ☑
          fall on board V91.29 ☑
            powered craft V91.23 ☑
              ferry boat V91.21 ☑
              fishing boat V91.22 ☑
              jetskis V91.23 ☑
              liner V91.21 ☑
              merchant ship V91.20 ☑
              passenger ship V91.21 ☑
            unpowered craft
              canoe V91.25 ☑
              inflatable V91.26 ☑
              kayak V91.25 ☑
              sailboat V91.24 ☑
          fire on board causing burn V91.09 ☑
            powered craft V91.03 ☑
              ferry boat V91.01 ☑
              fishing boat V91.02 ☑
              jetskis V91.03 ☑
              liner V91.01 ☑
              merchant ship V91.00 ☑
              passenger ship V91.01 ☑
            unpowered craft V91.08 ☑
              canoe V91.05 ☑
              inflatable V91.06 ☑
              kayak V91.05 ☑
              sailboat V91.04 ☑
              surf-board V91.08 ☑
              water skis V91.07 ☑
              windsurfer V91.08 ☑
          hit by falling object V91.39 ☑
            powered craft V91.33 ☑
              ferry boat V91.31 ☑
              fishing boat V91.32 ☑
              jetskis V91.33 ☑
              liner V91.31 ☑
              merchant ship V91.30 ☑
              passenger ship V91.31 ☑
            unpowered craft V91.38 ☑
              canoe V91.35 ☑
              inflatable V91.36 ☑
              kayak V91.35 ☑
              sailboat V91.34 ☑
              surf-board V91.38 ☑
              water skis V91.37 ☑
              windsurfer V91.38 ☑
          specified type NEC V91.89 ☑
            powered craft V91.83 ☑
              ferry boat V91.81 ☑
              fishing boat V91.82 ☑
              jetskis V91.83 ☑
              liner V91.81 ☑
              merchant ship V91.80 ☑
              passenger ship V91.81 ☑
            unpowered craft V91.88 ☑
              canoe V91.85 ☑
              inflatable V91.86 ☑
              kayak V91.85 ☑
              sailboat V91.84 ☑
              surf-board V91.88 ☑
              water skis V91.87 ☑
              windsurfer V91.88 ☑

Accident — *continued*
  watercraft — *continued*
    due to, caused by cataclysm — *see* Forces of nature, by type
    military NEC V94.818 ☑
      civilian in water injured by V94.811 ☑
      with civilian watercraft V94.810 ☑
    nonpowered, struck by
      nonpowered vessel V94.22 ☑
      powered vessel V94.21 ☑
    specified type NEC V94.89 ☑
    striking swimmer
      powered V94.11 ☑
      unpowered V94.12 ☑
Acid throwing (assault) Y08.89 ☑
Activity (involving) (of victim at time of event) Y93.9
  aerobic and step exercise (class) Y93.A3 (*following* Y93.7)
  alpine skiing Y93.23
  animal care NEC Y93.K9 (*following* Y93.7)
  arts and handcrafts NEC Y93.D9 (*following* Y93.7)
  athletics played as a team or group NEC Y93.69
  athletics played individually NEC Y93.59
  athletics NEC Y93.79
  baking Y93.G3 (*following* Y93.7)
  ballet Y93.41
  barbells Y93.B3 (*following* Y93.7)
  BASE (Building, Antenna, Span, Earth) jumping Y93.33
  baseball Y93.64
  basketball Y93.67
  bathing (personal) Y93.E1 (*following* Y93.7)
  beach volleyball Y93.68
  bike riding Y93.55
  blackout game Y93.85
  boogie boarding Y93.18
  bowling Y93.54
  boxing Y93.71
  brass instrument playing Y93.J4 (*following* Y93.7)
  building construction Y93.H3 (*following* Y93.7)
  bungee jumping Y93.34
  calisthenics Y93.A2 (*following* Y93.7)
  canoeing (in calm and turbulent water) Y93.16
  capture the flag Y93.6A
  cardiorespiratory exercise NEC Y93.A9 (*following* Y93.7)
  caregiving (providing) NEC Y93.F9 (*following* Y93.7)
    bathing Y93.F1 (*following* Y93.7)
    lifting Y93.F2 (*following* Y93.7)
  cellular
    communication device Y93.C2 (*following* Y93.7)
    telephone Y93.C2 (*following* Y93.7)
  challenge course Y93.A5 (*following* Y93.7)
  cheerleading Y93.45
  choking game Y93.85
  circuit training Y93.A4 (*following* Y93.7)
  cleaning
    floor Y93.E5 (*following* Y93.7)
  climbing NEC Y93.39
    mountain Y93.31
    rock Y93.31
    wall Y93.31
  clothing care and maintenance NEC Y93.E9 (*following* Y93.7)
  combatives Y93.75
  computer
    keyboarding Y93.C1 (*following* Y93.7)
    technology NEC Y93.C9 (*following* Y93.7)
  confidence course Y93.A5 (*following* Y93.7)
  construction (building) Y93.H3 (*following* Y93.7)
  cooking and baking Y93.G3 (*following* Y93.7)
  cool down exercises Y93.A2 (*following* Y93.7)
  cricket Y93.69
  crocheting Y93.D1 (*following* Y93.7)
  cross country skiing Y93.24
  dancing (all types) Y93.41
  digging
    dirt Y93.H1 (*following* Y93.7)
  dirt digging Y93.H1 (*following* Y93.7)
  dishwashing Y93.G1 (*following* Y93.7)
  diving (platform) (springboard) Y93.12
    underwater Y93.15
  dodge ball Y93.6A
  downhill skiing Y93.23
  drum playing Y93.J2 (*following* Y93.7)
  dumbbells Y93.B3 (*following* Y93.7)
  electronic
    devices NEC Y93.C9 (*following* Y93.7)
      hand held interactive Y93.C2 (*following* Y93.7)

Activity — *continued*
  electronic — *continued*
    game playing (using) (with)
      interactive device Y93.C2 (*following* Y93.7)
      keyboard or other stationary device Y93.C1 (*following* Y93.7)
  elliptical machine Y93.A1 (*following* Y93.7)
  exercise(s)
    machines ((primarily) for)
      cardiorespiratory conditioning Y93.A1 (*following* Y93.7)
      muscle strengthening Y93.B1 (*following* Y93.7)
    muscle strengthening (non-machine) NEC Y93.B9 (*following* Y93.7)
  external motion NEC Y93.I9 (*following* Y93.7)
    rollercoaster Y93.I1 (*following* Y93.7)
  fainting game Y93.85
  field hockey Y93.65
  figure skating (pairs) (singles) Y93.21
  flag football Y93.62
  floor mopping and cleaning Y93.E5 (*following* Y93.7)
  food preparation and clean up Y93.G1 (*following* Y93.7)
  football (American) NOS Y93.61
    flag Y93.62
    tackle Y93.61
    touch Y93.62
  four square Y93.6A
  free weights Y93.B3 (*following* Y93.7)
  frisbee (ultimate) Y93.74
  furniture
    building Y93.D3 (*following* Y93.7)
    finishing Y93.D3 (*following* Y93.7)
    repair Y93.D3 (*following* Y93.7)
  game playing (electronic)
    using interactive device Y93.C2 (*following* Y93.7)
    using keyboard or other stationary device Y93.C1 (*following* Y93.7)
  gardening Y93.H2 (*following* Y93.7)
  golf Y93.53
  grass drills Y93.A6 (*following* Y93.7)
  grilling and smoking food Y93.G2 (*following* Y93.7)
  grooming and shearing an animal Y93.K3 (*following* Y93.7)
  guerilla drills Y93.A6 (*following* Y93.7)
  gymnastics (rhythmic) Y93.43
  hand held interactive electronic device Y93.C2 (*following* Y93.7)
  handball Y93.73
  handcrafts NEC Y93.D9 (*following* Y93.7)
  hang gliding Y93.35
  hiking (on level or elevated terrain) Y93.01
  hockey (ice) Y93.22
    field Y93.65
  horseback riding Y93.52
  household (interior) maintenance NEC Y93.E9 (*following* Y93.7)
  ice NEC Y93.29
    dancing Y93.21
    hockey Y93.22
    skating Y93.21
  inline roller skating Y93.51
  ironing Y93.E4 (*following* Y93.7)
  judo Y93.75
  jumping jacks Y93.A2 (*following* Y93.7)
  jumping rope Y93.56
  jumping (off) NEC Y93.39
    BASE (Building, Antenna, Span, Earth) Y93.33
    bungee Y93.34
    jacks Y93.A2 (*following* Y93.7)
    rope Y93.56
  karate Y93.75
  kayaking (in calm and turbulent water) Y93.16
  keyboarding (computer) Y93.C1 (*following* Y93.7)
  kickball Y93.6A
  knitting Y93.D1 (*following* Y93.7)
  lacrosse Y93.65
  land maintenance NEC Y93.H9 (*following* Y93.7)
  landscaping Y93.H2 (*following* Y93.7)
  laundry Y93.E2 (*following* Y93.7)
  machines (exercise)
    primarily for cardiorespiratory conditioning Y93.A1 (*following* Y93.7)
    primarily for muscle strengthening Y93.B1 (*following* Y93.7)
  maintenance
    exterior building NEC Y93.H9 (*following* Y93.7)
    household (interior) NEC Y93.E9 (*following* Y93.7)
    land Y93.H9 (*following* Y93.7)
    property Y93.H9 (*following* Y93.7)

Activity — *continued*
marching (on level or elevated terrain) Y93.01
martial arts Y93.75
microwave oven Y93.G3 (*following* Y93.7)
milking an animal Y93.K2 (*following* Y93.7)
mopping (floor) Y93.E5 (*following* Y93.7)
mountain climbing Y93.31
muscle strengthening
    exercises (non-machine) NEC Y93.B9 (*following* Y93.7)
    machines Y93.B1 (*following* Y93.7)
musical keyboard (electronic) playing Y93.J1 (*following* Y93.7)
nordic skiing Y93.24
obstacle course Y93.A5 (*following* Y93.7)
oven (microwave) Y93.G3 (*following* Y93.7)
packing up and unpacking in moving to a new residence Y93.E6 (*following* Y93.7)
parasailing Y93.19
pass out game Y93.85
percussion instrument playing NEC Y93.J2 (*following* Y93.7)
personal
    bathing and showering Y93.E1 (*following* Y93.7)
    hygiene NEC Y93.E8 (*following* Y93.7)
    showering Y93.E1 (*following* Y93.7)
physical games generally associated with school recess, summer camp and children Y93.6A
physical training NEC Y93.A9 (*following* Y93.7)
piano playing Y93.J1 (*following* Y93.7)
pilates Y93.B4 (*following* Y93.7)
platform diving Y93.12
playing musical instrument
    brass instrument Y93.J4 (*following* Y93.7)
    drum Y93.J2 (*following* Y93.7)
    musical keyboard (electronic) Y93.J1 (*following* Y93.7)
    percussion instrument NEC Y93.J2 (*following* Y93.7)
    piano Y93.J1 (*following* Y93.7)
    string instrument Y93.J3 (*following* Y93.7)
    winds instrument Y93.J4 (*following* Y93.7)
property maintenance
    exterior NEC Y93.H9 (*following* Y93.7)
    interior NEC Y93.E9 (*following* Y93.7)
pruning (garden and lawn) Y93.H2 (*following* Y93.7)
pull-ups Y93.B2 (*following* Y93.7)
push-ups Y93.B2 (*following* Y93.7)
racquetball Y93.73
rafting (in calm and turbulent water) Y93.16
raking (leaves) Y93.H1 (*following* Y93.7)
rappelling Y93.32
refereeing a sports activity Y93.81
residential relocation Y93.E6 (*following* Y93.7)
rhythmic gymnastics Y93.43
rhythmic movement NEC Y93.49
riding
    horseback Y93.52
    rollercoaster Y93.I1 (*following* Y93.7)
rock climbing Y93.31
roller skating (inline) Y93.51
rollercoaster riding Y93.I1 (*following* Y93.7)
rough housing and horseplay Y93.83
rowing (in calm and turbulent water) Y93.16
rugby Y93.63
running Y93.02
SCUBA diving Y93.15
sewing Y93.D2 (*following* Y93.7)
shoveling Y93.H1 (*following* Y93.7)
    dirt Y93.H1 (*following* Y93.7)
    snow Y93.H1 (*following* Y93.7)
showering (personal) Y93.E1 (*following* Y93.7)
sit-ups Y93.B2 (*following* Y93.7)
skateboarding Y93.51
skating (ice) Y93.21
    roller Y93.51
skiing (alpine) (downhill) Y93.23
    cross country Y93.24
    nordic Y93.24
    water Y93.17
sledding (snow) Y93.23
sleeping (sleep) Y93.84
smoking and grilling food Y93.G2 (*following* Y93.7)
snorkeling Y93.15
snow NEC Y93.29
    boarding Y93.23
    shoveling Y93.H1 (*following* Y93.7)
    sledding Y93.23
    tubing Y93.23
soccer Y93.66

Activity — *continued*
softball Y93.64
specified NEC Y93.89
spectator at an event Y93.82
sports NEC Y93.79
    sports played as a team or group NEC Y93.69
    sports played individually NEC Y93.59
springboard diving Y93.12
squash Y93.73
stationary bike Y93.A1 (*following* Y93.7)
step (stepping) exercise (class) Y93.A3 (*following* Y93.7)
stepper machine Y93.A1 (*following* Y93.7)
stove Y93.G3 (*following* Y93.7)
string instrument playing Y93.J3 (*following* Y93.7)
surfing Y93.18
    wind Y93.18
swimming Y93.11
tackle football Y93.61
tap dancing Y93.41
tennis Y93.73
tobogganing Y93.23
touch football Y93.62
track and field events (non-running) Y93.57
    running Y93.02
trampoline Y93.44
treadmill Y93.A1 (*following* Y93.7)
trimming shrubs Y93.H2 (*following* Y93.7)
tubing (in calm and turbulent water) Y93.16
    snow Y93.23
ultimate frisbee Y93.74
underwater diving Y93.15
unpacking in moving to a new residence Y93.E6 (*following* Y93.7)
use of stove, oven and microwave oven Y93.G3 (*following* Y93.7)
vacuuming Y93.E3 (*following* Y93.7)
volleyball (beach) (court) Y93.68
wake boarding Y93.17
walking (on level or elevated terrain) Y93.01
    an animal Y93.K1 (*following* Y93.7)
walking an animal Y93.K1 (*following* Y93.7)
wall climbing Y93.31
warm up and cool down exercises Y93.A2 (*following* Y93.7)
water NEC Y93.19
    aerobics Y93.14
    craft NEC Y93.19
    exercise Y93.14
    polo Y93.13
    skiing Y93.17
    sliding Y93.18
    survival training and testing Y93.19
weeding (garden and lawn) Y93.H2 (*following* Y93.7)
wind instrument playing Y93.J4 (*following* Y93.7)
windsurfing Y93.18
wrestling Y93.72
yoga Y93.42
Adverse effect of drugs — *see* Table of Drugs and Chemicals
Aerosinusitis — *see* Air, pressure
After-effect, late — *see* Sequelae
Air
    blast in war operations — *see* War operations, air blast
    pressure
        change, rapid
            during
                ascent W94.29 ☑
                    while (in) (surfacing from)
                        aircraft W94.23 ☑
                        deep water diving W94.21 ☑
                        underground W94.22 ☑
                descent W94.39 ☑
                    in
                        aircraft W94.31 ☑
                        water W94.32 ☑
        high, prolonged W94.0 ☑
        low, prolonged W94.12 ☑
            due to residence or long visit at high altitude W94.11 ☑
Alpine sickness W94.11 ☑
Altitude sickness W94.11 ☑
Anaphylactic shock, anaphylaxis — *see* Table of Drugs and Chemicals
Andes disease W94.11 ☑
Arachnidism, arachnoidism X58 ☑
Arson (with intent to injure or kill) X97 ☑

Asphyxia, asphyxiation
by
    food (bone) (seed) — *see* categories T17 and T18
    gas — *see also* Table of Drugs and Chemicals
        legal
            execution — *see* Legal, intervention, gas
            intervention — *see* Legal, intervention, ga
    from
        fire — *see also* Exposure, fire
            in war operations — *see* War operations, fire
        ignition — *see* Ignition
        vomitus T17.81 ☑
    in war operations — *see* War operations, restriction airway
Aspiration
    food (any type) (into respiratory tract) (with asphyx
        obstruction respiratory tract, suffocation) — *s*
        categories T17 and T18 ☑
    foreign body — *see* Foreign body, aspiration
    vomitus (with asphyxia, obstruction respiratory trac
        suffocation) T17.81 ☑
Assassination (attempt) — *see* Assault
Assault (homicidal) (by) (in) Y09
    arson X97 ☑
    bite (of human being) Y04.1 ☑
    bodily force Y04.8 ☑
        bite Y04.1 ☑
        bumping into Y04.2 ☑
        sexual — *see* subcategories T74.0, T76.0 ☑
        unarmed fight Y04.0 ☑
    bomb X96.9 ☑
        antipersonnel X96.0 ☑
        fertilizer X96.3 ☑
        gasoline X96.1 ☑
        letter X96.2 ☑
        petrol X96.1 ☑
        pipe X96.3 ☑
        specified NEC X96.8 ☑
    brawl (hand) (fists) (foot) (unarmed) Y04.0 ☑
    burning, burns (by fire) NEC X97 ☑
        acid Y08.89 ☑
        caustic, corrosive substance Y08.89 ☑
        chemical from swallowing caustic, corrosive sub-stance — *see* Table of Drugs and Chemical
        cigarette(s) X97 ☑
        hot object X98.9 ☑
            fluid NEC X98.2 ☑
            household appliance X98.3 ☑
            specified NEC X98.8 ☑
            steam X98.0 ☑
            tap water X98.1 ☑
            vapors X98.0 ☑
        scalding — *see* Assault, burning
        steam X98.0 ☑
        vitriol Y08.89 ☑
    caustic, corrosive substance (gas) Y08.89 ☑
    crashing of
        aircraft Y08.81 ☑
        motor vehicle Y03.8 ☑
            pushed in front of Y02.0 ☑
            run over Y03.0 ☑
            specified NEC Y03.8 ☑
    cutting or piercing instrument X99.9 ☑
        dagger X99.2 ☑
        glass X99.0 ☑
        knife X99.1 ☑
        specified NEC X99.8 ☑
        sword X99.2 ☑
    dagger X99.2 ☑
    drowning (in) X92.9 ☑
        bathtub X92.0 ☑
        natural water X92.3 ☑
        specified NEC X92.8 ☑
        swimming pool X92.1 ☑
            following fall X92.2 ☑
    dynamite X96.8 ☑
    explosive(s) (material) X96.9 ☑
    fight (hand) (fists) (foot) (unarmed) Y04.0 ☑
        with weapon — *see* Assault, by type of weapon
    fire X97 ☑
    firearm X95.9 ☑
        airgun X95.01 ☑
        handgun X93 ☑
        hunting rifle X94.1 ☑
        larger X94.9 ☑
            specified NEC X94.8 ☑

Assault — *continued*
  firearm — *continued*
    machine gun X94.2 ☑
    shotgun X94.0 ☑
    specified NEC X95.8 ☑
  from high place Y01 ☑
  gunshot (wound) NEC — *see* Assault, firearm, by type
  incendiary device X97 ☑
  injury Y09
    to child due to criminal abortion attempt NEC
      Y08.89 ☑
  knife X99.1 ☑
  late effect of — *see* categories X92-Y08 with 7th character S
  placing before moving object NEC Y02.8 ☑
    motor vehicle Y02.0 ☑
  poisoning — *see* categories T36-T65 with 7th character S
  puncture, any part of body — *see* Assault, cutting or piercing instrument
  pushing
    before moving object NEC Y02.8 ☑
      motor vehicle Y02.0 ☑
      subway train Y02.1 ☑
      train Y02.1 ☑
    from high place Y01 ☑
  rape T74.2- ☑
  scalding — *see* Assault, burning
  sequela of — *see* categories X92-Y08 with 7th character S
  sexual (by bodily force) T74.2- ☑
  shooting — *see* Assault, firearm
  specified means NEC Y08.89 ☑
  stab, any part of body — *see* Assault, cutting or piercing instrument
  steam X98.0 ☑
  striking against
    other person Y04.2 ☑
    sports equipment Y08.09 ☑
      baseball bat Y08.02 ☑
      hockey stick Y08.01 ☑
  struck by
    sports equipment Y08.09 ☑
      baseball bat Y08.02 ☑
      hockey stick Y08.01 ☑
  submersion — *see* Assault, drowning
  violence Y09
  weapon Y09
    blunt Y00 ☑
    cutting or piercing — *see* Assault, cutting or piercing instrument
    firearm — *see* Assault, firearm
  wound Y09
    cutting — *see* Assault, cutting or piercing instrument
    gunshot — *see* Assault, firearm
    knife X99.1 ☑
    piercing — *see* Assault, cutting or piercing instrument
    puncture — *see* Assault, cutting or piercing instrument
    stab — *see* Assault, cutting or piercing instrument
Attack by mammals NEC W55.89 ☑
Avalanche — *see* Landslide
Aviator's disease — *see* Air, pressure

B

Barotitis, barodontalgia, barosinusitis, barotrauma (otitic) (sinus) — *see* Air, pressure
Battered (baby) (child) (person) (syndrome) X58 ☑
Bayonet wound W26.1 ☑
  in
    legal intervention — *see* Legal, intervention, sharp object, bayonet
    war operations — *see* War operations, combat
  stated as undetermined whether accidental or intentional Y28.8 ☑
  suicide (attempt) X78.2 ☑
Bean in nose — *see* categories T17 and T18 ☑
Bed set on fire NEC — *see* Exposure, fire, uncontrolled, building, bed
Beheading (by guillotine)
  homicide X99.9 ☑
  legal execution — *see* Legal, intervention
Bending, injury in (prolonged) (static) X50.1 ☑

Bends — *see* Air, pressure, change
Bite, bitten by
  alligator W58.01 ☑
  arthropod (nonvenomous) NEC W57 ☑
  bull W55.21 ☑
  cat W55.01 ☑
  cow W55.21 ☑
  crocodile W58.11 ☑
  dog W54.0 ☑
  goat W55.31 ☑
  hoof stock NEC W55.31 ☑
  horse W55.11 ☑
  human being (accidentally) W50.3 ☑
    with intent to injure or kill W50.3 ☑
    as, or caused by, a crowd or human stampede (with fall) W52 ☑
    assault Y04.1 ☑
    homicide (attempt) Y04.1 ☑
    in
      fight Y04.1 ☑
  insect (nonvenomous) W57 ☑
  lizard (nonvenomous) W59.01 ☑
  mammal NEC W55.81 ☑
    marine W56.31 ☑
  marine animal (nonvenomous) W56.81 ☑
  millipede W57 ☑
  moray eel W56.51 ☑
  mouse W53.01 ☑
  person(s) (accidentally) W50.3 ☑
    with intent to injure or kill Y04.1 ☑
    as, or caused by, a crowd or human stampede (with fall) W52 ☑
    assault Y04.1 ☑
    homicide (attempt) Y04.1 ☑
    in
      fight Y04.1 ☑
  pig W55.41 ☑
  raccoon W55.51 ☑
  rat W53.11 ☑
  reptile W59.81 ☑
    lizard W59.01 ☑
    snake W59.11 ☑
    turtle W59.21 ☑
      terrestrial W59.81 ☑
  rodent W53.81 ☑
    mouse W53.01 ☑
    rat W53.11 ☑
    specified NEC W53.81 ☑
    squirrel W53.21 ☑
  shark W56.41 ☑
  sheep W55.31 ☑
  snake (nonvenomous) W59.11 ☑
  spider (nonvenomous) W57 ☑
  squirrel W53.21 ☑
Blast (air) in war operations — *see* War operations, blast
Blizzard X37.2 ☑
Blood alcohol level Y90.9
  less than 20mg/100ml Y90.0
  presence in blood, level not specified Y90.9
  20-39mg/100ml Y90.1
  40-59mg/100ml Y90.2
  60-79mg/100ml Y90.3
  80-99mg/100ml Y90.4
  100-119mg/100ml Y90.5
  120-199mg/100ml Y90.6
  200-239mg/100ml Y90.7
Blow X58 ☑
  by law-enforcing agent, police (on duty) — *see* Legal, intervention, manhandling
  blunt object — *see* Legal, intervention, blunt object
Blowing up — *see* Explosion
Brawl (hand) (fists) (foot) Y04.0 ☑
Breakage (accidental) (part of)
  ladder (causing fall) W11 ☑
  scaffolding (causing fall) W12 ☑
Broken
  glass, contact with — *see* Contact, with, glass
  power line (causing electric shock) W85 ☑
Bumping against, into (accidentally)
  object NEC W22.8 ☑
    caused by crowd or human stampede (with fall) W52 ☑
    sports equipment W21.9 ☑
    with fall — *see* Fall, due to, bumping against, object
  person(s) W51 ☑
    with fall W03 ☑

Bumping against, into — *continued*
  person(s) — *continued*
    with fall — *continued*
      due to ice or snow W00.0 ☑
      assault Y04.2 ☑
    caused by, a crowd or human stampede (with fall) W52 ☑
    homicide (attempt) Y04.2 ☑
  sports equipment W21.9 ☑
Burn, burned, burning (accidental) (by) (from) (on)
  acid NEC — *see* Table of Drugs and Chemicals
  bed linen — *see* Exposure, fire, uncontrolled, in building, bed
  blowtorch X08.8 ☑
    with ignition of clothing NEC X06.2 ☑
      nightwear X05 ☑
  bonfire, campfire (controlled) — *see also* Exposure, fire, controlled, not in building
    uncontrolled — *see* Exposure, fire, uncontrolled, not in building
  candle X08.8 ☑
    with ignition of clothing NEC X06.2 ☑
      nightwear X05 ☑
  caustic liquid, substance (external) (internal) NEC — *see* Table of Drugs and Chemicals
  chemical (external) (internal) — *see also* Table of Drugs and Chemicals
    in war operations — *see* War operations. fire
  cigar(s) or cigarette(s) X08.8 ☑
    with ignition of clothing NEC X06.2 ☑
      nightwear X05 ☑
  clothes, clothing NEC (from controlled fire) X06.2 ☑
    with conflagration — *see* Exposure, fire, uncontrolled, building
      not in building or structure — *see* Exposure, fire, uncontrolled, not in building
  cooker (hot) X15.8 ☑
    stated as undetermined whether accidental or intentional Y27.3 ☑
    suicide (attempt) X77.3 ☑
  electric blanket X16 ☑
  engine (hot) X17 ☑
  fire, flames — *see* Exposure, fire
  flare, Very pistol — *see* Discharge, firearm NEC
  heat
    from appliance (electrical) (household) X15.8 ☑
      cooker X15.8 ☑
      hotplate X15.2 ☑
      kettle X15.8 ☑
      light bulb X15.8 ☑
      saucepan X15.3 ☑
      skillet X15.3 ☑
      stated as undetermined whether accidental or intentional Y27.3 ☑
      stove X15.0 ☑
      suicide (attempt) X77.3 ☑
      toaster X15.1 ☑
    in local application or packing during medical or surgical procedure Y63.5
  heating
    appliance, radiator or pipe X16 ☑
  homicide (attempt) — *see* Assault, burning
  hot
    air X14.1 ☑
    cooker X15.8 ☑
    drink X10.0 ☑
    engine X17 ☑
    fat X10.2 ☑
    fluid NEC X12 ☑
    food X10.1 ☑
    gases X14.1 ☑
    heating appliance X16 ☑
    household appliance NEC X15.8 ☑
    kettle X15.8 ☑
    liquid NEC X12 ☑
    machinery X17 ☑
    metal (molten) (liquid) NEC X18 ☑
    object (not producing fire or flames) NEC X19 ☑
    oil (cooking) X10.2 ☑
    pipe(s) X16 ☑
    radiator X16 ☑
    saucepan (glass) (metal) X15.3 ☑
    stove (kitchen) X15.0 ☑
    substance NEC X19 ☑
      caustic or corrosive NEC — *see* Table of Drugs and Chemicals

Burn, burned, burning — *continued*
hot — *continued*
toaster X15.1 ☑
tool X17 ☑
vapor X13.1 ☑
water (tap) — *see* Contact, with, hot, tap water
hotplate X15.2 ☑
suicide (attempt) X77.3 ☑
ignition — *see* Ignition
in war operations — *see* War operations, fire
inflicted by other person X97 ☑
by hot objects, hot vapor, and steam — *see* Assault, burning, hot object
internal, from swallowed caustic, corrosive liquid, substance — *see* Table of Drugs and Chemicals
iron (hot) X15.8 ☑
stated as undetermined whether accidental or intentional Y27.3 ☑
suicide (attempt) X77.3 ☑
kettle (hot) X15.8 ☑
stated as undetermined whether accidental or intentional Y27.3 ☑
suicide (attempt) X77.3 ☑
lamp (flame) X08.8 ☑
with ignition of clothing NEC X06.2 ☑
nightwear X05 ☑
lighter (cigar) (cigarette) X08.8 ☑
with ignition of clothing NEC X06.2 ☑
nightwear X05 ☑
lightning — *see* subcategory T75.0 ☑
causing fire — *see* Exposure, fire
liquid (boiling) (hot) NEC X12 ☑
stated as undetermined whether accidental or intentional Y27.2 ☑
suicide (attempt) X77.2 ☑
local application of externally applied substance in medical or surgical care Y63.5
machinery (hot) X17 ☑
matches X08.8 ☑
with ignition of clothing NEC X06.2 ☑
nightwear X05 ☑
mattress — *see* Exposure, fire, uncontrolled, building, bed
medicament, externally applied Y63.5
metal (hot) (liquid) (molten) NEC X18 ☑
nightwear (nightclothes, nightdress, gown, pajamas, robe) X05 ☑
object (hot) NEC X19 ☑
on board watercraft
due to
accident to watercraft V91.09 ☑
powered craft V91.03 ☑
ferry boat V91.01 ☑
fishing boat V91.02 ☑
jetskis V91.03 ☑
liner V91.01 ☑
merchant ship V91.00 ☑
passenger ship V91.01 ☑
unpowered craft V91.08 ☑
canoe V91.05 ☑
inflatable V91.06 ☑
kayak V91.05 ☑
sailboat V91.04 ☑
surf-board V91.08 ☑
water skis V91.07 ☑
windsurfer V91.08 ☑
fire on board V93.09 ☑
ferry boat V93.01 ☑
fishing boat V93.02 ☑
jetskis V93.03 ☑
liner V93.01 ☑
merchant ship V93.00 ☑
passenger ship V93.01 ☑
powered craft NEC V93.03 ☑
sailboat V93.04 ☑
specified heat source NEC on board V93.19 ☑
ferry boat V93.11 ☑
fishing boat V93.12 ☑
jetskis V93.13 ☑
liner V93.11 ☑
merchant ship V93.10 ☑
passenger ship V93.11 ☑
powered craft NEC V93.13 ☑
sailboat V93.14 ☑
pipe (hot) X16 ☑
smoking X08.8 ☑

Burn, burned, burning — *continued*
pipe — *continued*
smoking — *continued*
with ignition of clothing NEC X06.2 ☑
nightwear X05 ☑
powder — *see* Powder burn
radiator (hot) X16 ☑
saucepan (hot) (glass) (metal) X15.3 ☑
stated as undetermined whether accidental or intentional Y27.3 ☑
suicide (attempt) X77.3 ☑
self-inflicted X76 ☑
stated as undetermined whether accidental or intentional Y26 ☑
stated as undetermined whether accidental or intentional Y27.0 ☑
steam X13.1 ☑
pipe X16 ☑
stated as undetermined whether accidental or intentional Y27.8 ☑
stated as undetermined whether accidental or intentional Y27.0 ☑
suicide (attempt) X77.0 ☑
stove (hot) (kitchen) X15.0 ☑
stated as undetermined whether accidental or intentional Y27.3 ☑
suicide (attempt) X77.3 ☑
substance (hot) NEC X19 ☑
boiling X12 ☑
stated as undetermined whether accidental or intentional Y27.2 ☑
suicide (attempt) X77.2 ☑
molten (metal) X18 ☑
suicide (attempt) NEC X76 ☑
hot
household appliance X77.3 ☑
object X77.9 ☑
therapeutic misadventure
heat in local application or packing during medical or surgical procedure Y63.5
overdose of radiation Y63.2
toaster (hot) X15.1 ☑
stated as undetermined whether accidental or intentional Y27.3 ☑
suicide (attempt) X77.3 ☑
tool (hot) X17 ☑
torch, welding X08.8 ☑
with ignition of clothing NEC X06.2 ☑
nightwear X05 ☑
trash fire (controlled) — *see* Exposure, fire, controlled, not in building
uncontrolled — *see* Exposure, fire, uncontrolled, not in building
vapor (hot) X13.1 ☑
stated as undetermined whether accidental or intentional Y27.0 ☑
suicide (attempt) X77.0 ☑
Very pistol — *see* Discharge, firearm NEC
Butted by animal W55.82 ☑
bull W55.22 ☑
cow W55.22 ☑
goat W55.32 ☑
horse W55.12 ☑
pig W55.42 ☑
sheep W55.32 ☑

C

Caisson disease — *see* Air, pressure, change
Campfire (exposure to) (controlled) — *see also* Exposure, fire, controlled, not in building
uncontrolled — *see* Exposure, fire, uncontrolled, not in building
Capital punishment (any means) — *see* Legal, intervention
Car sickness T75.3 ☑
Casualty (not due to war) NEC X58 ☑
war — *see* War operations
Cat
bite W55.01 ☑
scratch W55.03 ☑
Cataclysm, cataclysmic (any injury) NEC — *see* Forces of nature
Catching fire — *see* Exposure, fire

Caught
between
folding object W23.0 ☑
objects (moving) (stationary and moving) W23.0 ☑
and machinery — *see* Contact, with, by type of machine
stationary W23.1 ☑
sliding door and door frame W23.0 ☑
by, in
machinery (moving parts of) — *see* Contact, with, by type of machine
washing-machine wringer W23.0 ☑
under packing crate (due to losing grip) W23.1 ☑
Cave-in caused by cataclysmic earth surface movement or eruption — *see* Landslide
Change(s) in air pressure — *see* Air, pressure, change
Choked, choking (on) (any object except food or vomitus)
food (bone) (seed) — *see* categories T17 and T18 ☑
vomitus T17.81- ☑
Civil insurrection — *see* War operations
Cloudburst (any injury) X37.8 ☑
Cold, exposure to (accidental) (excessive) (extreme) (natural) (place) NEC — *see* Exposure, cold
Collapse
building W20.1 ☑
burning (uncontrolled fire) X00.2 ☑
dam or man-made structure (causing earth movement) X36.0 ☑
machinery — *see* Contact, with, by type of machine
structure W20.1 ☑
burning (uncontrolled fire) X00.2 ☑
Collision (accidental) NEC — *see also* Accident, transport V89.9 ☑
pedestrian W51 ☑
with fall W03 ☑
due to ice or snow W00.0 ☑
involving pedestrian conveyance — *see* Accident, transport, pedestrian, conveyance
and
crowd or human stampede (with fall) W52 ☑
object W22.8 ☑
with fall — *see* Fall, due to, bumping against object
person(s) — *see* Collision, pedestrian
transport vehicle NEC V89.9 ☑
and
avalanche, fallen or not moving — *see* Accident, transport
falling or moving — *see* Landslide
landslide, fallen or not moving — *see* Accident, transport
falling or moving — *see* Landslide
due to cataclysm — *see* Forces of nature, by type
intentional, purposeful suicide (attempt) — *see* Suicide, collision
Combustion, spontaneous — *see* Ignition
Complication (delayed) **of or following** (medical or surgical procedure) Y84.9
with misadventure — *see* Misadventure
amputation of limb(s) Y83.5
anastomosis (arteriovenous) (blood vessel) (gastrojejunal) (tendon) (natural or artificial material) Y83.2
aspiration (of fluid) Y84.4
tissue Y84.8
biopsy Y84.8
blood
sampling Y84.7
transfusion
procedure Y84.8
bypass Y83.2
catheterization (urinary) Y84.6
cardiac Y84.0
colostomy Y83.3
cystostomy Y83.3
dialysis (kidney) Y84.1
drug — *see* Table of Drugs and Chemicals
due to misadventure — *see* Misadventure
duodenostomy Y83.3
electroshock therapy Y84.3
external stoma, creation of Y83.3
formation of external stoma Y83.3
gastrostomy Y83.3
graft Y83.2
hypothermia (medically-induced) Y84.8

☑ **Additional Character Required** — Refer to the Tabular List for Character Selection   ☑ **Subterms under main terms may continue to next column or page**

Complication (delayed) **of or following** —
  continued
  implant, implantation (of)
    artificial
      internal device (cardiac pacemaker) (electrodes
        in brain) (heart valve prosthesis) (orthope-
        dic) Y83.1
      material or tissue (for anastomosis or bypass)
        Y83.2
        with creation of external stoma Y83.3
      natural tissues (for anastomosis or bypass) Y83.2
        with creation of external stoma Y83.3
  infusion
    procedure Y84.8
  injection — *see* Table of Drugs and Chemicals
    procedure Y84.8
  insertion of gastric or duodenal sound Y84.5
  insulin-shock therapy Y84.3
  paracentesis (abdominal) (thoracic) (aspirative) Y84.4
  procedures other than surgical operation — *see* Com-
    plication of or following, by type of procedure
  radiological procedure or therapy Y84.2
  removal of organ (partial) (total) NEC Y83.6
  sampling
    blood Y84.7
    fluid NEC Y84.4
    tissue Y84.8
  shock therapy Y84.3
  surgical operation NEC — *see also* Complication of or
    following, by type of operation Y83.9
    reconstructive NEC Y83.4
      with
        anastomosis, bypass or graft Y83.2
        formation of external stoma Y83.3
    specified NEC Y83.8
  transfusion — *see also* Table of Drugs and Chemicals
    procedure Y84.8
  transplant, transplantation (heart) (kidney) (liver)
    (whole organ, any) Y83.0
    partial organ Y83.4
  ureterostomy Y83.3
  vaccination — *see also* Table of Drugs and Chemicals
    procedure Y84.8

Compression
  divers' squeeze — *see* Air, pressure, change
  trachea by
    food (lodged in esophagus) — *see* categories T17
      and T18 ☑
    vomitus (lodged in esophagus) T17.81- ☑

Conflagration — *see* Exposure, fire, uncontrolled

Constriction (external)
  hair W49.01 ☑
  jewelry W49.04 ☑
  ring W49.04 ☑
  rubber band W49.03 ☑
  specified item NEC W49.09 ☑
  string W49.02 ☑
  thread W49.02 ☑

Contact (accidental)
  with
    abrasive wheel (metalworking) W31.1 ☑
    alligator W58.09 ☑
      bite W58.01 ☑
      crushing W58.03 ☑
      strike W58.02 ☑
    amphibian W62.9 ☑
      frog W62.0 ☑
      toad W62.1 ☑
    animal (nonvenomous) NEC W64 ☑
      marine W56.89 ☑
        bite W56.81 ☑
        dolphin — *see* Contact, with, dolphin
        fish NEC — *see* Contact, with, fish
        mammal — *see* Contact, with, mammal, ma-
          rine
        orca — *see* Contact, with, orca
        sea lion — *see* Contact, with, sea lion
        shark — *see* Contact, with, shark
        strike W56.82 ☑
    animate mechanical force NEC W64 ☑
    arrow W21.89 ☑
      not thrown, projected or falling W45.8 ☑
    arthropods (nonvenomous) W57 ☑
    axe W27.0 ☑
    band-saw (industrial) W31.2 ☑
    bayonet — *see* Bayonet wound
    bee(s) X58 ☑

Contact — *continued*
  with — *continued*
    bench-saw (industrial) W31.2 ☑
    bird W61.99 ☑
      bite W61.91 ☑
      chicken — *see* Contact, with, chicken
      duck — *see* Contact, with, duck
      goose — *see* Contact, with, goose
      macaw — *see* Contact, with, macaw
      parrot — *see* Contact, with, parrot
      psittacine — *see* Contact, with, psittacine
      strike W61.92 ☑
      turkey — *see* Contact, with, turkey
    blender W29.0 ☑
    boiling water X12 ☑
      stated as undetermined whether accidental or
        intentional Y27.2 ☑
      suicide (attempt) X77.2 ☑
    bore, earth-drilling or mining (land) (seabed)
      W31.0 ☑
    buffalo — *see* Contact, with, hoof stock NEC
    bull W55.29 ☑
      bite W55.21 ☑
      gored W55.22 ☑
      strike W55.22 ☑
    bumper cars W31.81 ☑
    camel — *see* Contact, with, hoof stock NEC
    can
      lid W26.8 ☑
      opener W27.4 ☑
        powered W29.0 ☑
    cat W55.09 ☑
      bite W55.01 ☑
      scratch W55.03 ☑
    caterpillar (venomous) X58 ☑
    centipede (venomous) X58 ☑
    chain
      hoist W24.0 ☑
        agricultural operations W30.89 ☑
      saw W29.3 ☑
    chicken W61.39 ☑
      peck W61.33 ☑
      strike W61.32 ☑
    chisel W27.0 ☑
    circular saw W31.2 ☑
    cobra X58 ☑
    combine (harvester) W30.0 ☑
    conveyer belt W24.1 ☑
    cooker (hot) X15.8 ☑
      stated as undetermined whether accidental or
        intentional Y27.3 ☑
      suicide (attempt) X77.3 ☑
    coral X58 ☑
    cotton gin W31.82 ☑
    cow W55.29 ☑
      bite W55.21 ☑
      strike W55.22 ☑
    crane W24.0 ☑
      agricultural operations W30.89 ☑
    crocodile W58.19 ☑
      bite W58.11 ☑
      crushing W58.13 ☑
      strike W58.12 ☑
    dagger W26.1 ☑
      stated as undetermined whether accidental or
        intentional Y28.2 ☑
      suicide (attempt) X78.2 ☑
    dairy equipment W31.82 ☑
    dart W21.89 ☑
      not thrown, projected or falling W45.8 ☑
    deer — *see* Contact, with, hoof stock NEC
    derrick W24.0 ☑
      agricultural operations W30.89 ☑
        hay W30.2 ☑
    dog W54.8 ☑
      bite W54.0 ☑
      strike W54.1 ☑
    dolphin W56.09 ☑
      bite W56.01 ☑
      strike W56.02 ☑
    donkey — *see* Contact, with, hoof stock NEC
    drill (powered) W29.8 ☑
      earth (land) (seabed) W31.0 ☑
      nonpowered W27.8 ☑
    drive belt W24.0 ☑
      agricultural operations W30.89 ☑

Contact — *continued*
  with — *continued*
    dry ice — *see* Exposure, cold, man-made
    dryer (clothes) (powered) (spin) W29.2 ☑
    duck W61.69 ☑
      bite W61.61 ☑
      strike W61.62 ☑
    earth (-)
      drilling machine (industrial) W31.0 ☑
      scraping machine in stationary use W31.83 ☑
    edge of stiff paper W26.2 ☑
    electric
      beater W29.0 ☑
      blanket X16 ☑
      fan W29.2 ☑
        commercial W31.82 ☑
      knife W29.1 ☑
      mixer W29.0 ☑
    elevator (building) W24.0 ☑
      agricultural operations W30.89 ☑
        grain W30.3 ☑
    engine(s), hot NEC X17 ☑
    excavating machine W31.0 ☑
    farm machine W30.9 ☑
    feces — *see* Contact, with, by type of animal
    fer de lance X58 ☑
    fish W56.59 ☑
      bite W56.51 ☑
      shark — *see* Contact, with, shark
      strike W56.52 ☑
    flying horses W31.81 ☑
    forging (metalworking) machine W31.1 ☑
    fork W27.4 ☑
    forklift (truck) W24.0 ☑
      agricultural operations W30.89 ☑
    frog W62.0 ☑
    garden
      cultivator (powered) W29.3 ☑
        riding W30.89 ☑
      fork W27.1 ☑
    gas turbine W31.3 ☑
    Gila monster X58 ☑
    giraffe — *see* Contact, with, hoof stock NEC
    glass (sharp) (broken) W25 ☑
      assault X99.0 ☑
      due to fall — *see* Fall, by type
      stated as undetermined whether accidental or
        intentional Y28.0 ☑
      suicide (attempt) X78.0 ☑
      with subsequent fall W18.02 ☑
    goat W55.39 ☑
      bite W55.31 ☑
      strike W55.32 ☑
    goose W61.59 ☑
      bite W61.51 ☑
      strike W61.52 ☑
    hand
      saw W27.0 ☑
      tool (not powered) NEC W27.8 ☑
        powered W29.8 ☑
    harvester W30.0 ☑
    hay-derrick W30.2 ☑
    heating
      appliance (hot) X16 ☑
      pad (electric) X16 ☑
    heat NEC X19 ☑
      from appliance (electrical) (household) — *see*
        Contact, with, hot, household appliance
      heating appliance X16 ☑
    hedge-trimmer (powered) W29.3 ☑
    hoe W27.1 ☑
    hoist (chain) (shaft) NEC W24.0 ☑
      agricultural W30.89 ☑
    hoof stock NEC W55.39 ☑
      bite W55.31 ☑
      strike W55.32 ☑
    hornet(s) X58 ☑
    horse W55.19 ☑
      bite W55.11 ☑
      strike W55.12 ☑
    hot
      air X14.1 ☑
        inhalation X14.0 ☑
      cooker X15.8 ☑
      drinks X10.0 ☑
      engine X17 ☑

Contact — *continued*
  with — *continued*
    hot — *continued*
      fats X10.2 ☑
      fluids NEC X12 ☑
        assault X98.2 ☑
        suicide (attempt) X77.2 ☑
        undetermined whether accidental or intentional Y27.2 ☑
      food X10.1 ☑
      gases X14.1 ☑
        inhalation X14.0 ☑
      heating appliance X16 ☑
      household appliance X15.8 ☑
        assault X98.3 ☑
        cooker X15.8 ☑
        hotplate X15.2 ☑
        kettle X15.8 ☑
        light bulb X15.8 ☑
        object NEC X19 ☑
          assault X98.8 ☑
          stated as undetermined whether accidental or intentional Y27.9 ☑
          suicide (attempt) X77.8 ☑
        saucepan X15.3 ☑
        skillet X15.3 ☑
        stated as undetermined whether accidental or intentional Y27.3 ☑
        stove X15.0 ☑
        suicide (attempt) X77.3 ☑
        toaster X15.1 ☑
      kettle X15.8 ☑
      light bulb X15.8 ☑
      liquid NEC — *see also* Burn X12 ☑
        drinks X10.0 ☑
        stated as undetermined whether accidental or intentional Y27.2 ☑
        suicide (attempt) X77.2 ☑
        tap water X11.8 ☑
          stated as undetermined whether accidental or intentional Y27.1 ☑
          suicide (attempt) X77.1 ☑
      machinery X17 ☑
      metal (molten) (liquid) NEC X18 ☑
      object (not producing fire or flames) NEC X19 ☑
      oil (cooking) X10.2 ☑
      pipe X16 ☑
      plate X15.2 ☑
      radiator X16 ☑
      saucepan (glass) (metal) X15.3 ☑
      skillet X15.3 ☑
      stove (kitchen) X15.0 ☑
      substance NEC X19 ☑
      tap-water X11.8 ☑
        assault X98.1 ☑
        heated on stove X12 ☑
          stated as undetermined whether accidental or intentional Y27.2 ☑
          suicide (attempt) X77.2 ☑
        in bathtub X11.0 ☑
        running X11.1 ☑
        stated as undetermined whether accidental or intentional Y27.1 ☑
        suicide (attempt) X77.1 ☑
      toaster X15.1 ☑
      tool X17 ☑
      vapors X13.1 ☑
        inhalation X13.0 ☑
      water (tap) X11.8 ☑
        boiling X12 ☑
          stated as undetermined whether accidental or intentional Y27.2 ☑
          suicide (attempt) X77.2 ☑
        heated on stove X12 ☑
          stated as undetermined whether accidental or intentional Y27.2 ☑
          suicide (attempt) X77.2 ☑
        in bathtub X11.0 ☑
        running X11.1 ☑
        stated as undetermined whether accidental or intentional Y27.1 ☑
        suicide (attempt) X77.1 ☑
    hotplate X15.2 ☑
    ice-pick W27.4 ☑
    insect (nonvenomous) NEC W57 ☑
    kettle (hot) X15.8 ☑

Contact — *continued*
  with — *continued*
    knife W26.0 ☑
      assault X99.1 ☑
      electric W29.1 ☑
      stated as undetermined whether accidental or intentional Y28.1 ☑
      suicide (attempt) X78.1 ☑
    lathe (metalworking) W31.1 ☑
      turnings W45.8 ☑
      woodworking W31.2 ☑
    lawnmower (powered) (ridden) W28 ☑
      causing electrocution W86.8 ☑
        suicide (attempt) X83.1 ☑
      unpowered W27.1 ☑
    lift, lifting (devices) W24.0 ☑
      agricultural operations W30.89 ☑
      shaft W24.0 ☑
    liquefied gas — *see* Exposure, cold, man-made
    liquid air, hydrogen, nitrogen — *see* Exposure, cold, man-made
    lizard (nonvenomous) W59.09 ☑
      bite W59.01 ☑
      strike W59.02 ☑
    llama — *see* Contact, with, hoof stock NEC
    macaw W61.19 ☑
      bite W61.11 ☑
      strike W61.12 ☑
    machine, machinery W31.9 ☑
      abrasive wheel W31.1 ☑
      agricultural including animal-powered W30.9 ☑
        combine harvester W30.0 ☑
        grain storage elevator W30.3 ☑
        hay derrick W30.2 ☑
        power take-off device W30.1 ☑
        reaper W30.0 ☑
        specified NEC W30.89 ☑
        thresher W30.0 ☑
        transport vehicle, stationary W30.81 ☑
      band saw W31.2 ☑
      bench saw W31.2 ☑
      circular saw W31.2 ☑
      commercial NEC W31.82 ☑
      drilling, metal (industrial) W31.1 ☑
      earth-drilling W31.0 ☑
      earthmoving or scraping W31.89 ☑
      excavating W31.89 ☑
      forging machine W31.1 ☑
      gas turbine W31.3 ☑
      hot X17 ☑
      internal combustion engine W31.3 ☑
      land drill W31.0 ☑
      lathe W31.1 ☑
      lifting (devices) W24.0 ☑
      metal drill W31.1 ☑
      metalworking (industrial) W31.1 ☑
      milling, metal W31.1 ☑
      mining W31.0 ☑
      molding W31.2 ☑
      overhead plane W31.2 ☑
      power press, metal W31.1 ☑
      prime mover W31.3 ☑
      printing W31.89 ☑
      radial saw W31.2 ☑
      recreational W31.81 ☑
      roller-coaster W31.81 ☑
      rolling mill, metal W31.1 ☑
      sander W31.2 ☑
      seabed drill W31.0 ☑
      shaft
        hoist W31.0 ☑
        lift W31.0 ☑
      specified NEC W31.89 ☑
      spinning W31.89 ☑
      steam engine W31.3 ☑
      transmission W24.1 ☑
      undercutter W31.0 ☑
      water driven turbine W31.3 ☑
      weaving W31.89 ☑
      woodworking or forming (industrial) W31.2 ☑
    mammal (feces) (urine) W55.89 ☑
      bull — *see* Contact, with, bull
      cat — *see* Contact, with, cat
      cow — *see* Contact, with, cow
      goat — *see* Contact, with, goat
      hoof stock — *see* Contact, with, hoof stock

Contact — *continued*
  with — *continued*
    mammal — *continued*
      horse — *see* Contact, with, horse
      marine W56.39 ☑
        dolphin — *see* Contact, with, dolphin
        orca — *see* Contact, with, orca
        sea lion — *see* Contact, with, sea lion
        specified NEC W56.39 ☑
          bite W56.31 ☑
          strike W56.32 ☑
      pig — *see* Contact, with, pig
      raccoon — *see* Contact, with, raccoon
      rodent — *see* Contact, with, rodent
      sheep — *see* Contact, with, sheep
      specified NEC W55.89 ☑
        bite W55.81 ☑
        strike W55.82 ☑
    marine
      animal W56.89 ☑
        bite W56.81 ☑
        dolphin — *see* Contact, with, dolphin
        fish NEC — *see* Contact, with, fish
        mammal — *see* Contact, with, mammal, marine
        orca — *see* Contact, with, orca
        sea lion — *see* Contact, with, sea lion
        shark — *see* Contact, with, shark
        strike W56.82 ☑
    meat
      grinder (domestic) W29.0 ☑
        industrial W31.82 ☑
        nonpowered W27.4 ☑
      slicer (domestic) W29.0 ☑
        industrial W31.82 ☑
    merry go round W31.81 ☑
    metal, hot (liquid) (molten) NEC X18 ☑
    millipede W57 ☑
    nail W45.0 ☑
      gun W29.4 ☑
    needle (sewing) W27.3 ☑
      hypodermic W46.0 ☑
        contaminated W46.1 ☑
    object (blunt) NEC
      hot NEC X19 ☑
      legal intervention — *see* Legal, intervention, blunt object
      sharp NEC W45.8 ☑
        inflicted by other person NEC W45.8 ☑
          stated as
            intentional homicide (attempt) — *see* Assault, cutting or piercing instrument
        legal intervention — *see* Legal, intervention, sharp object
        self-inflicted X78.9 ☑
    orca W56.29 ☑
      bite W56.21 ☑
      strike W56.22 ☑
    overhead plane W31.2 ☑
    paper (as sharp object) W26.2 ☑
    paper-cutter W27.5 ☑
    parrot W61.09 ☑
      bite W61.01 ☑
      strike W61.02 ☑
    pig W55.49 ☑
      bite W55.41 ☑
      strike W55.42 ☑
    pipe, hot X16 ☑
    pitchfork W27.1 ☑
    plane (metal) (wood) W27.0 ☑
      overhead W31.2 ☑
    plant thorns, spines, sharp leaves or other mechanisms W60 ☑
    powered
      garden cultivator W29.3 ☑
      household appliance, implement, or machine W29.8 ☑
      saw (industrial) W31.2 ☑
        hand W29.8 ☑
    printing machine W31.89 ☑
    psittacine bird W61.29 ☑
      bite W61.21 ☑
      macaw — *see* Contact, with, macaw
      parrot — *see* Contact, with, parrot
      strike W61.22 ☑

☑ Additional Character Required — Refer to the Tabular List for Character Selection   ▽ Subterms under main terms may continue to next column or page

Contact — *continued*
  with — *continued*
    pulley (block) (transmission) W24.0 ☑
      agricultural operations W30.89 ☑
    raccoon W55.59 ☑
      bite W55.51 ☑
      strike W55.52 ☑
    radial-saw (industrial) W31.2 ☑
    radiator (hot) X16 ☑
    rake W27.1 ☑
    rattlesnake X58 ☑
    reaper W30.0 ☑
    reptile W59.89 ☑
      lizard — *see* Contact, with, lizard
      snake — *see* Contact, with, snake
      specified NEC W59.89 ☑
        bite W59.81 ☑
        crushing W59.83 ☑
        strike W59.82 ☑
      turtle — *see* Contact, with, turtle
    rivet gun (powered) W29.4 ☑
    road scraper — *see* Accident, transport, construction vehicle
    rodent (feces) (urine) W53.89 ☑
      bite W53.81 ☑
      mouse W53.09 ☑
        bite W53.01 ☑
      rat W53.19 ☑
        bite W53.11 ☑
      specified NEC W53.89 ☑
        bite W53.81 ☑
      squirrel W53.29 ☑
        bite W53.21 ☑
    roller coaster W31.81 ☑
    rope NEC W24.0 ☑
      agricultural operations W30.89 ☑
    saliva — *see* Contact, with, by type of animal
    sander W29.8 ☑
      industrial W31.2 ☑
    saucepan (hot) (glass) (metal) X15.3 ☑
    saw W27.0 ☑
      band (industrial) W31.2 ☑
      bench (industrial) W31.2 ☑
      chain W29.3 ☑
      hand W27.0 ☑
    sawing machine, metal W31.1 ☑
    scissors W27.2 ☑
    scorpion X58 ☑
    screwdriver W27.0 ☑
      powered W29.8 ☑
    sea
      anemone, cucumber or urchin (spine) X58 ☑
      lion W56.19 ☑
        bite W56.11 ☑
        strike W56.12 ☑
    serpent — *see* Contact, with, snake, by type
    sewing-machine (electric) (powered) W29.2 ☑
      not powered W27.8 ☑
    shaft (hoist) (lift) (transmission) NEC W24.0 ☑
      agricultural W30.89 ☑
    shark W56.49 ☑
      bite W56.41 ☑
      strike W56.42 ☑
    sharp object(s) W26.9 ☑
      specified NEC W26.8 ☑
    shears (hand) W27.2 ☑
      powered (industrial) W31.1 ☑
        domestic W29.2 ☑
    sheep W55.39 ☑
      bite W55.31 ☑
      strike W55.32 ☑
    shovel W27.8 ☑
      steam — *see* Accident, transport, construction vehicle
    snake (nonvenomous) W59.19 ☑
      bite W59.11 ☑
      crushing W59.13 ☑
      strike W59.12 ☑
    spade W27.1 ☑
    spider (venomous) X58 ☑
    spin-drier W29.2 ☑
    spinning machine W31.89 ☑
    splinter W45.8 ☑
    sports equipment W21.9 ☑
    staple gun (powered) W29.8 ☑
    steam X13.1 ☑

Contact — *continued*
  with — *continued*
    steam — *continued*
      engine W31.3 ☑
      inhalation X13.0 ☑
      pipe X16 ☑
      shovel W31.89 ☑
    stove (hot) (kitchen) X15.0 ☑
    substance, hot NEC X19 ☑
      molten (metal) X18 ☑
    sword W26.1 ☑
      assault X99.2 ☑
      stated as undetermined whether accidental or intentional Y28.2 ☑
      suicide (attempt) X78.2 ☑
    tarantula X58 ☑
    thresher W30.0 ☑
    tin can lid W26.8 ☑
    toad W62.1 ☑
    toaster (hot) X15.1 ☑
    tool W27.8 ☑
      hand (not powered) W27.8 ☑
        auger W27.0 ☑
        axe W27.0 ☑
        can opener W27.4 ☑
        chisel W27.0 ☑
        fork W27.4 ☑
        garden W27.1 ☑
        handsaw W27.0 ☑
        hoe W27.1 ☑
        ice-pick W27.4 ☑
        kitchen utensil W27.4 ☑
        manual
          lawn mower W27.1 ☑
          sewing machine W27.8 ☑
        meat grinder W27.4 ☑
        needle (sewing) W27.3 ☑
          hypodermic W46.0 ☑
            contaminated W46.1 ☑
        paper cutter W27.5 ☑
        pitchfork W27.1 ☑
        rake W27.1 ☑
        scissors W27.2 ☑
        screwdriver W27.0 ☑
        specified NEC W27.8 ☑
        workbench W27.0 ☑
      hot X17 ☑
      powered W29.8 ☑
        blender W29.0 ☑
          commercial W31.82 ☑
        can opener W29.0 ☑
          commercial W31.82 ☑
        chainsaw W29.3 ☑
        clothes dryer W29.2 ☑
          commercial W31.82 ☑
        dishwasher W29.2 ☑
          commercial W31.82 ☑
        edger W29.3 ☑
        electric fan W29.2 ☑
          commercial W31.82 ☑
        electric knife W29.1 ☑
        food processor W29.0 ☑
          commercial W31.82 ☑
        garbage disposal W29.0 ☑
          commercial W31.82 ☑
        garden tool W29.3 ☑
        hedge trimmer W29.3 ☑
        ice maker W29.0 ☑
          commercial W31.82 ☑
        kitchen appliance W29.0 ☑
          commercial W31.82 ☑
        lawn mower W28 ☑
        meat grinder W29.0 ☑
          commercial W31.82 ☑
        mixer W29.0 ☑
          commercial W31.82 ☑
        rototiller W29.3 ☑
        sewing machine W29.2 ☑
          commercial W31.82 ☑
        washing machine W29.2 ☑
          commercial W31.82 ☑
    transmission device (belt, cable, chain, gear, pinion, shaft) W24.1 ☑
      agricultural operations W30.89 ☑
    turbine (gas) (water-driven) W31.3 ☑
    turkey W61.49 ☑

Contact — *continued*
  with — *continued*
    turkey — *continued*
      peck W61.43 ☑
      strike W61.42 ☑
    turtle (nonvenomous) W59.29 ☑
      bite W59.21 ☑
      strike W59.22 ☑
      terrestrial W59.89 ☑
        bite W59.81 ☑
        crushing W59.83 ☑
        strike W59.82 ☑
    under-cutter W31.0 ☑
    urine — *see* Contact, with, by type of animal
    vehicle
      agricultural use (transport) — *see* Accident, transport, agricultural vehicle
        not on public highway W30.81 ☑
      industrial use (transport) — *see* Accident, transport, industrial vehicle
        not on public highway W31.83 ☑
      off-road use (transport) — *see* Accident, transport, all-terrain or off-road vehicle
        not on public highway W31.83 ☑
      special construction use (transport) — *see* Accident, transport, construction vehicle
        not on public highway W31.83 ☑
    venomous
      animal X58 ☑
      arthropods X58 ☑
      lizard X58 ☑
      marine animal NEC X58 ☑
      marine plant NEC X58 ☑
      millipedes (tropical) X58 ☑
      plant(s) X58 ☑
      snake X58 ☑
      spider X58 ☑
      viper X58 ☑
    washing-machine (powered) W29.2 ☑
    wasp X58 ☑
    weaving-machine W31.89 ☑
    winch W24.0 ☑
      agricultural operations W30.89 ☑
    wire NEC W24.0 ☑
      agricultural operations W30.89 ☑
    wood slivers W45.8 ☑
    yellow jacket X58 ☑
    zebra — *see* Contact, with, hoof stock NEC
  pressure X50.9 ☑
  stress X50.9 ☑
Coup de soleil X32 ☑
Crash
  aircraft (in transit) (powered) V95.9 ☑
    balloon V96.01 ☑
    fixed wing NEC (private) V95.21 ☑
      commercial V95.31 ☑
    glider V96.21 ☑
      hang V96.11 ☑
      powered V95.11 ☑
    helicopter V95.01 ☑
    in war operations — *see* War operations, destruction of aircraft
    microlight V95.11 ☑
    nonpowered V96.9 ☑
      specified NEC V96.8 ☑
    powered NEC V95.8 ☑
    stated as
      homicide (attempt) Y08.81 ☑
      suicide (attempt) X83.0 ☑
    ultralight V95.11 ☑
  spacecraft V95.41 ☑
  transport vehicle NEC — *see also* Accident, transport V89.9 ☑
    homicide (attempt) Y03.8 ☑
    motor NEC (traffic) V89.2 ☑
      homicide (attempt) Y03.8 ☑
      suicide (attempt) — *see* Suicide, collision
Cruelty (mental) (physical) (sexual) X58 ☑
Crushed (accidentally) X58 ☑
  between objects (moving) (stationary and moving) W23.0 ☑
    stationary W23.1 ☑
  by
    alligator W58.03 ☑
    avalanche NEC — *see* Landslide
    cave-in W20.0 ☑

Crushed — continued
  by — continued
    cave-in — continued
      caused by cataclysmic earth surface movement
        — see Landslide
    crocodile W58.13 ☑
    crowd or human stampede W52 ☑
    falling
      aircraft V97.39 ☑
        in war operations — see War operations, de-
          struction of aircraft
      earth, material W20.0 ☑
        caused by cataclysmic earth surface move-
          ment — see Landslide
      object NEC W20.8 ☑
    landslide NEC — see Landslide
    lizard (nonvenomous) W59.09 ☑
    machinery — see Contact, with, by type of machine
    reptile NEC W59.89 ☑
    snake (nonvenomous) W59.13 ☑
  in
    machinery — see Contact, with, by type of machine
Cut, cutting (any part of body) (accidental) — see also
    Contact, with, by object or machine
  during medical or surgical treatment as misadventure
    — see Index to Diseases and Injuries, Complica-
    tions
  homicide (attempt) — see Assault, cutting or piercing
    instrument
  inflicted by other person — see Assault, cutting or
    piercing instrument
  legal
    execution — see Legal, intervention
    intervention — see Legal, intervention, sharp object
  machine NEC — see also Contact, with, by type of ma-
    chine W31.9 ☑
  self-inflicted — see Suicide, cutting or piercing instru-
    ment
  suicide (attempt) — see Suicide, cutting or piercing
    instrument
Cyclone (any injury) X37.1 ☑

D

Decapitation (accidental circumstances) NEC X58 ☑
  homicide X99.9 ☑
  legal execution — see Legal, intervention
Dehydration from lack of water X58 ☑
Deprivation X58 ☑
Derailment (accidental)
  railway (rolling stock) (train) (vehicle) (without an-
    tecedent collision) V81.7 ☑
    with antecedent collision — see Accident, transport,
      railway vehicle occupant
  streetcar (without antecedent collision) V82.7 ☑
    with antecedent collision — see Accident, transport,
      streetcar occupant
Descent
  parachute (voluntary) (without accident to aircraft)
    V97.29 ☑
    due to accident to aircraft — see Accident, transport,
      aircraft
Desertion X58 ☑
Destitution X58 ☑
Disability, late effect or sequela of injury — see Se-
    quelae
Discharge (accidental)
  airgun W34.010 ☑
    assault X95.01 ☑
    homicide (attempt) X95.01 ☑
    stated as undetermined whether accidental or inten-
      tional Y24.0 ☑
    suicide (attempt) X74.01 ☑
  BB gun — see Discharge, airgun
  firearm (accidental) W34.00 ☑
    assault X95.9 ☑
    handgun (pistol) (revolver) W32.0 ☑
      assault X93 ☑
      homicide (attempt) X93 ☑
      legal intervention — see Legal, intervention,
        firearm, handgun
      stated as undetermined whether accidental or
        intentional Y22 ☑
      suicide (attempt) X72 ☑
    homicide (attempt) X95.9 ☑
    hunting rifle W33.02 ☑

Discharge — continued
  firearm — continued
    hunting rifle — continued
      assault X94.1 ☑
      homicide (attempt) X94.1 ☑
      legal intervention
        injuring
          bystander Y35.032 ☑
          law enforcement personnel Y35.031 ☑
          suspect Y35.033 ☑
          unspecified person Y35.039 ☑
      stated as undetermined whether accidental or
        intentional Y23.1 ☑
      suicide (attempt) X73.1 ☑
    larger W33.00 ☑
      assault X94.9 ☑
      homicide (attempt) X94.9 ☑
      hunting rifle — see Discharge, firearm, hunting
        rifle
      legal intervention — see Legal, intervention,
        firearm by type of firearm
      machine gun — see Discharge, firearm, machine
        gun
      shotgun — see Discharge, firearm, shotgun
      specified NEC W33.09 ☑
        assault X94.8 ☑
        homicide (attempt) X94.8 ☑
        legal intervention
          injuring
            bystander Y35.092 ☑
            law enforcement personnel
              Y35.091 ☑
            suspect Y35.093 ☑
            unspecified person Y35.099 ☑
        stated as undetermined whether accidental
          or intentional Y23.8 ☑
        suicide (attempt) X73.8 ☑
      stated as undetermined whether accidental or
        intentional Y23.9 ☑
      suicide (attempt) X73.9 ☑
    legal intervention
      injuring
        bystander Y35.002 ☑
        law enforcement personnel Y35.001 ☑
        suspect Y35.03 ☑
        unspecified person Y35.009 ☑
      using rubber bullet
        injuring
          bystander Y35.042 ☑
          law enforcement personnel Y35.041 ☑
          suspect Y35.043 ☑
          unspecified person Y35.049 ☑
    machine gun W33.03 ☑
      assault X94.2 ☑
      homicide (attempt) X94.2 ☑
      legal intervention — see Legal, intervention,
        firearm, machine gun
      stated as undetermined whether accidental or
        intentional Y23.3 ☑
      suicide (attempt) X73.2 ☑
    pellet gun — see Discharge, airgun
    shotgun W33.01 ☑
      assault X94.0 ☑
      homicide (attempt) X94.0 ☑
      legal intervention — see Legal, intervention,
        firearm, specified NEC
      stated as undetermined whether accidental or
        intentional Y23.0 ☑
      suicide (attempt) X73.0 ☑
    specified NEC W34.09 ☑
      assault X95.8 ☑
      homicide (attempt) X95.8 ☑
      legal intervention — see Legal, intervention,
        firearm, specified NEC
      stated as undetermined whether accidental or
        intentional Y24.8 ☑
      suicide (attempt) X74.8 ☑
    stated as undetermined whether accidental or inten-
      tional Y24.9 ☑
    suicide (attempt) X74.9 ☑
    Very pistol W34.09 ☑
      assault X95.8 ☑
      homicide (attempt) X95.8 ☑
      stated as undetermined whether accidental or
        intentional Y24.8 ☑
      suicide (attempt) X74.8 ☑

Discharge — continued
  firework(s) W39 ☑
    stated as undetermined whether accidental or inten-
      tional Y25 ☑
  gas-operated gun NEC W34.018 ☑
    airgun — see Discharge, airgun
    assault X95.09 ☑
    homicide (attempt) X95.09 ☑
    paintball gun — see Discharge, paintball gun
    stated as undetermined whether accidental or inten-
      tional Y24.8 ☑
    suicide (attempt) X74.09 ☑
  gun NEC — see also Discharge, firearm NEC
    air — see Discharge, airgun
    BB — see Discharge, airgun
    for single hand use — see Discharge, firearm,
      handgun
    hand — see Discharge, firearm, handgun
    machine — see Discharge, firearm, machine gun
    other specified — see Discharge, firearm NEC
    paintball — see Discharge, paintball gun
    pellet — see Discharge, airgun
  handgun — see Discharge, firearm, handgun
  machine gun — see Discharge, firearm, machine gun
  paintball gun W34.011 ☑
    assault X95.02 ☑
    homicide (attempt) X95.02 ☑
    stated as undetermined whether accidental or inten-
      tional Y24.8 ☑
    suicide (attempt) X74.02 ☑
  pistol — see Discharge, firearm, handgun
    flare — see Discharge, firearm, Very pistol
    pellet — see Discharge, airgun
    Very — see Discharge, firearm, Very pistol
  revolver — see Discharge, firearm, handgun
  rifle (hunting) — see Discharge, firearm, hunting rifle
  shotgun — see Discharge, firearm, shotgun
  spring-operated gun NEC W34.018 ☑
    assault X95.09 ☑
    homicide (attempt) X95.09 ☑
    stated as undetermined whether accidental or inten-
      tional Y24.8 ☑
    suicide (attempt) X74.09 ☑
Disease
  Andes W94.11 ☑
  aviator's — see Air, pressure
  range W94.11 ☑
Diver's disease, palsy, paralysis, squeeze — see Air,
    pressure
Diving (into water) — see Accident, diving
Dog bite W54.0 ☑
Dragged by transport vehicle NEC — see also Accident,
    transport V09.9 ☑
Drinking poison (accidental) — see Table of Drugs and
    Chemicals
Dropped (accidentally) **while being carried or support-
    ed by other person** W04 ☑
Drowning (accidental) W74 ☑
  assault X92.9 ☑
  due to
    accident (to)
      machinery — see Contact, with, by type of ma-
        chine
      watercraft V90.89 ☑
        burning V90.29 ☑
          powered V90.23 ☑
            fishing boat V90.22 ☑
            jetskis V90.23 ☑
            merchant ship V90.20 ☑
            passenger ship V90.21 ☑
          unpowered V90.28 ☑
            canoe V90.25 ☑
            inflatable V90.26 ☑
            kayak V90.25 ☑
            sailboat V90.24 ☑
            water skis V90.27 ☑
        crushed V90.39 ☑
          powered V90.33 ☑
            fishing boat V90.32 ☑
            jetskis V90.33 ☑
            merchant ship V90.30 ☑
            passenger ship V90.31 ☑
          unpowered V90.38 ☑
            canoe V90.35 ☑
            inflatable V90.36 ☑
            kayak V90.35 ☑

☑ Additional Character Required — Refer to the Tabular List for Character Selection   ▽ Subterms under main terms may continue to next column or page

Drowning — *continued*
  due to — *continued*
    accident — *continued*
      watercraft — *continued*
        crushed — *continued*
          unpowered — *continued*
            sailboat V90.34 ☑
            water skis V90.37 ☑
        overturning V90.09 ☑
          powered V90.03 ☑
            fishing boat V90.02 ☑
            jetskis V90.03 ☑
            merchant ship V90.00 ☑
            passenger ship V90.01 ☑
          unpowered V90.08 ☑
            canoe V90.05 ☑
            inflatable V90.06 ☑
            kayak V90.05 ☑
            sailboat V90.04 ☑
        sinking V90.19 ☑
          powered V90.13 ☑
            fishing boat V90.12 ☑
            jetskis V90.13 ☑
            merchant ship V90.10 ☑
            passenger ship V90.11 ☑
          unpowered V90.18 ☑
            canoe V90.15 ☑
            inflatable V90.16 ☑
            kayak V90.15 ☑
            sailboat V90.14 ☑
        specified type NEC V90.89 ☑
          powered V90.83 ☑
            fishing boat V90.82 ☑
            jetskis V90.83 ☑
            merchant ship V90.80 ☑
            passenger ship V90.81 ☑
          unpowered V90.88 ☑
            canoe V90.85 ☑
            inflatable V90.86 ☑
            kayak V90.85 ☑
            sailboat V90.84 ☑
            water skis V90.87 ☑
  avalanche — *see* Landslide
  cataclysmic
    earth surface movement NEC — *see* Forces of
      nature, earth movement
    storm — *see* Forces of nature, cataclysmic storm
  cloudburst X37.8 ☑
  cyclone X37.1 ☑
  fall overboard (from) V92.09 ☑
    powered craft V92.03 ☑
      ferry boat V92.01 ☑
      fishing boat V92.02 ☑
      jetskis V92.03 ☑
      liner V92.01 ☑
      merchant ship V92.00 ☑
      passenger ship V92.01 ☑
    resulting from
      accident to watercraft — *see* Drowning, due
        to, accident to, watercraft
      being washed overboard (from) V92.29 ☑
        powered craft V92.23 ☑
          ferry boat V92.21 ☑
          fishing boat V92.22 ☑
          jetskis V92.23 ☑
          liner V92.21 ☑
          merchant ship V92.20 ☑
          passenger ship V92.21 ☑
        unpowered craft V92.28 ☑
          canoe V92.25 ☑
          inflatable V92.26 ☑
          kayak V92.25 ☑
          sailboat V92.24 ☑
          surf-board V92.28 ☑
          water skis V92.27 ☑
          windsurfer V92.28 ☑
      motion of watercraft V92.19 ☑
        powered craft V92.13 ☑
          ferry boat V92.11 ☑
          fishing boat V92.12 ☑
          jetskis V92.13 ☑
          liner V92.11 ☑
          merchant ship V92.10 ☑
          passenger ship V92.11 ☑
        unpowered craft
          canoe V92.15 ☑

Drowning — *continued*
  due to — *continued*
    fall overboard — *continued*
      resulting from — *continued*
        motion of watercraft — *continued*
          unpowered craft — *continued*
            inflatable V92.16 ☑
            kayak V92.15 ☑
            sailboat V92.14 ☑
        unpowered craft V92.08 ☑
          canoe V92.05 ☑
          inflatable V92.06 ☑
          kayak V92.05 ☑
          sailboat V92.04 ☑
          surf-board V92.08 ☑
          water skis V92.07 ☑
          windsurfer V92.08 ☑
    hurricane X37.0 ☑
    jumping into water from watercraft (involved in
      accident) — *see also* Drowning, due to, acci-
      dent to, watercraft
      without accident to or on watercraft W16.711 ☑
    tidal wave NEC — *see* Forces of nature, tidal wave
    torrential rain X37.8 ☑
  following
    fall
      into
        bathtub W16.211 ☑
        bucket W16.221 ☑
        fountain — *see* Drowning, following, fall, into,
          water, specified NEC
        quarry — *see* Drowning, following, fall, into,
          water, specified NEC
        reservoir — *see* Drowning, following, fall, into,
          water, specified NEC
        swimming-pool W16.011 ☑
          stated as undetermined whether acciden-
            tal or intentional Y21.3 ☑
          striking
            bottom W16.021 ☑
            wall W16.031 ☑
          suicide (attempt) X71.2 ☑
        water NOS W16.41 ☑
          natural (lake) (open sea) (river) (stream)
            (pond) W16.111 ☑
            striking
              bottom W16.121 ☑
              side W16.131 ☑
          specified NEC W16.311 ☑
            striking
              bottom W16.321 ☑
              wall W16.331 ☑
      overboard NEC — *see* Drowning, due to, fall
        overboard
    jump or dive
      from boat W16.711 ☑
        striking bottom W16.721 ☑
      into
        fountain — *see* Drowning, following, jump
          or dive, into, water, specified NEC
        quarry — *see* Drowning, following, jump or
          dive, into, water, specified NEC
        reservoir — *see* Drowning, following, jump
          or dive, into, water, specified NEC
        swimming-pool W16.511 ☑
          striking
            bottom W16.521 ☑
            wall W16.531 ☑
          suicide (attempt) X71.2 ☑
        water NOS W16.91 ☑
          natural (lake) (open sea) (river) (stream)
            (pond) W16.611 ☑
          specified NEC W16.811 ☑
            bottom W16.821 ☑
            striking
              bottom W16.821 ☑
              wall W16.831 ☑
          striking
            bottom W16.821 ☑
            wall W16.831 ☑
          striking bottom W16.621 ☑
  homicide (attempt) X92.9 ☑
  in
    bathtub (accidental) W65 ☑
      assault X92.0 ☑
      following fall W16.211 ☑

Drowning — *continued*
  in — *continued*
    bathtub — *continued*
      following fall — *continued*
        stated as undetermined whether accidental
          or intentional Y21.1 ☑
      stated as undetermined whether accidental or
        intentional Y21.0 ☑
      suicide (attempt) X71.0 ☑
    lake — *see* Drowning, in, natural water
    natural water (lake) (open sea) (river) (stream)
      (pond) W69 ☑
      assault X92.3 ☑
      following
        dive or jump W16.611 ☑
          striking bottom W16.621 ☑
        fall W16.111 ☑
          striking
            bottom W16.121 ☑
            side W16.131 ☑
      stated as undetermined whether accidental or
        intentional Y21.4 ☑
      suicide (attempt) X71.3 ☑
    quarry — *see* Drowning, in, specified place NEC
    quenching tank — *see* Drowning, in, specified place
      NEC
    reservoir — *see* Drowning, in, specified place NEC
    river — *see* Drowning, in, natural water
    sea — *see* Drowning, in, natural water
    specified place NEC W73 ☑
      assault X92.8 ☑
      following
        dive or jump W16.811 ☑
          striking
            bottom W16.821 ☑
            wall W16.831 ☑
        fall W16.311 ☑
          striking
            bottom W16.321 ☑
            wall W16.331 ☑
      stated as undetermined whether accidental or
        intentional Y21.8 ☑
      suicide (attempt) X71.8 ☑
    stream — *see* Drowning, in, natural water
    swimming-pool W67 ☑
      assault X92.1 ☑
      following fall X92.2 ☑
      following
        dive or jump W16.511 ☑
          striking
            bottom W16.521 ☑
            wall W16.531 ☑
        fall W16.011 ☑
          striking
            bottom W16.021 ☑
            wall W16.031 ☑
      stated as undetermined whether accidental or
        intentional Y21.2 ☑
      following fall Y21.3 ☑
      suicide (attempt) X71.1 ☑
      following fall X71.2 ☑
    war operations — *see* War operations, restriction
      of airway
  resulting from accident to watercraft — *see* Drowning,
    due to, accident, watercraft
  self-inflicted X71.9 ☑
  stated as undetermined whether accidental or inten-
    tional Y21.9 ☑
  suicide (attempt) X71.9 ☑

E

Earth falling (on) W20.0 ☑
  caused by cataclysmic earth surface movement or
    eruption — *see* Landslide
Earth (surface) **movement NEC** — *see* Forces of nature,
  earth movement
Earthquake (any injury) X34 ☑
Effect(s) (adverse) **of**
  air pressure (any) — *see* Air, pressure
  cold, excessive (exposure to) — *see* Exposure, cold
  heat (excessive) — *see* Heat
  hot place (weather) — *see* Heat
  insolation X30 ☑
  late — *see* Sequelae
  motion — *see* Motion

▽ Subterms under main terms may continue to next column or page   ☑ Additional Character Required — Refer to the Tabular List for Character Selection

Effect — continued

Effect(s) (adverse) **of** — continued

nuclear explosion or weapon in war operations — see War operations, nuclear weapon

radiation — see Radiation

travel — see Travel

Electric shock (accidental) (by) (in) — see Exposure, electric current

Electrocution (accidental) — see Exposure, electric current

Endotracheal tube wrongly placed during anesthetic procedure

Entanglement

in

bed linen, causing suffocation T71 ☑

wheel of pedal cycle V19.88 ☑

Entry of foreign body or material — see Foreign body

Environmental pollution related condition — see category Z57

Execution, legal (any method) — see Legal, intervention

Exhaustion

cold — see Exposure, cold

due to excessive exertion — see also Overexertion X50.9 ☑

heat — see Heat

Explosion (accidental) (of) (with secondary fire) W40.9 ☑

acetylene W40.1 ☑

aerosol can W36.1 ☑

air tank (compressed) (in machinery) W36.2 ☑

aircraft (in transit) (powered) NEC V95.9 ☑

balloon V96.05 ☑

fixed wing NEC (private) V95.25 ☑

commercial V95.35 ☑

glider V96.25 ☑

hang V96.15 ☑

powered V95.15 ☑

helicopter V95.05 ☑

in war operations — see War operations, destruction of aircraft

microlight V95.15 ☑

nonpowered V96.9 ☑

specified NEC V96.8 ☑

powered NEC V95.8 ☑

stated as

homicide (attempt) Y03.8 ☑

suicide (attempt) X83.0 ☑

ultralight V95.15 ☑

anesthetic gas in operating room W40.1 ☑

antipersonnel bomb W40.8 ☑

assault X96.0 ☑

homicide (attempt) X96.0 ☑

suicide (attempt) X75 ☑

assault X96.9 ☑

bicycle tire W37.0 ☑

blasting (cap) (materials) W40.0 ☑

boiler (machinery), not on transport vehicle W35 ☑

on watercraft — see Explosion, in, watercraft

butane W40.1 ☑

caused by other person X96.9 ☑

coal gas W40.1 ☑

detonator W40.0 ☑

dump (munitions) W40.8 ☑

dynamite W40.0 ☑

in

assault X96.8 ☑

homicide (attempt) X96.8 ☑

legal intervention

injuring

bystander Y35.112 ☑

law enforcement personnel Y35.111 ☑

suspect Y35.113 ☑

unspecified person Y35.119 ☑

suicide (attempt) X75 ☑

explosive (material) W40.9 ☑

gas W40.1 ☑

in blasting operation W40.0 ☑

specified NEC W40.8 ☑

in

assault X96.8 ☑

homicide (attempt) X96.8 ☑

legal intervention

injuring

bystander Y35.192 ☑

law enforcement personnel Y35.191 ☑

suspect Y35.193 ☑

unspecified person Y35.199 ☑

Explosion — continued

explosive — continued

specified — continued

in — continued

suicide (attempt) X75 ☑

factory (munitions) W40.8 ☑

fertilizer bomb W40.8 ☑

assault X96.3 ☑

homicide (attempt) X96.3 ☑

suicide (attempt) X75 ☑

firearm (parts) NEC W34.19 ☑

airgun W34.110 ☑

BB gun W34.110 ☑

gas, air or spring-operated gun NEC W34.118 ☑

hangun W32.1 ☑

hunting rifle W33.12 ☑

larger firearm W33.10 ☑

specified NEC W33.19 ☑

machine gun W33.13 ☑

paintball gun W34.111 ☑

pellet gun W34.110 ☑

shotgun W33.11 ☑

Very pistol [flare] W34.19 ☑

fire-damp W40.1 ☑

fireworks W39 ☑

gas (coal) (explosive) W40.1 ☑

cylinder W36.9 ☑

aerosol can W36.1 ☑

air tank W36.2 ☑

pressurized W36.3 ☑

specified NEC W36.8 ☑

gasoline (fumes) (tank) not in moving motor vehicle W40.1 ☑

bomb W40.8 ☑

assault X96.1 ☑

homicide (attempt) X96.1 ☑

suicide (attempt) X75 ☑

in motor vehicle — see Accident, transport, by type of vehicle

grain store W40.8 ☑

grenade W40.8 ☑

in

assault X96.8 ☑

homicide (attempt) X96.8 ☑

legal intervention

injuring

bystander Y35.192 ☑

law enforcement personnel Y35.191 ☑

suspect Y35.193 ☑

unspecified person Y35.199 ☑

suicide (attempt) X75 ☑

handgun (parts) — see Explosion, firearm, hangun (parts)

homicide (attempt) X96.9 ☑

antipersonnel bomb — see Explosion, antipersonnel bomb

fertilizer bomb — see Explosion, fertilizer bomb

gasoline bomb — see Explosion, gasoline bomb

letter bomb — see Explosion, letter bomb

pipe bomb — see Explosion, pipe bomb

specified NEC X96.8 ☑

hose, pressurized W37.8 ☑

hot water heater, tank (in machinery) W35 ☑

on watercraft — see Explosion, in, watercraft

in, on

dump W40.8 ☑

factory W40.8 ☑

mine (of explosive gases) NEC W40.1 ☑

watercraft W93.59 ☑

powered craft V93.53 ☑

ferry boat V93.51 ☑

fishing boat V93.52 ☑

jetskis V93.53 ☑

liner V93.51 ☑

merchant ship V93.50 ☑

passenger ship V93.51 ☑

sailboat V93.54 ☑

letter bomb W40.8 ☑

assault X96.2 ☑

homicide (attempt) X96.2 ☑

suicide (attempt) X75 ☑

machinery — see also Contact, with, by type of machine

on board watercraft — see Explosion, in, watercraft

pressure vessel — see Explosion, by type of vessel

methane W40.1 ☑

Explosion — continued

mine W40.1 ☑

missile NEC W40.8 ☑

mortar bomb W40.8 ☑

in

assault X96.8 ☑

homicide (attempt) X96.8 ☑

legal intervention

injuring

bystander Y35.192 ☑

law enforcement personnel Y35.191 ☑

suspect Y35.193 ☑

unspecified person Y35.199 ☑

suicide (attempt) X75 ☑

munitions (dump) (factory) W40.8 ☑

pipe, pressurized W37.8 ☑

bomb W40.8 ☑

assault X96.4 ☑

homicide (attempt) X96.4 ☑

suicide (attempt) X75 ☑

pressure, pressurized

cooker W38 ☑

gas tank (in machinery) W36.3 ☑

hose W37.8 ☑

pipe W37.8 ☑

specified device NEC W38 ☑

tire W37.8 ☑

bicycle W37.0 ☑

vessel (in machinery) W38 ☑

propane W40.1 ☑

self-inflicted X75 ☑

shell (artillery) NEC W40.8 ☑

during war operations — see War operations, explosion

in

legal intervention

injuring

bystander Y35.122 ☑

law enforcement personnel Y35.121 ☑

suspect Y35.123 ☑

unspecified person Y35.129 ☑

war — see War operations, explosion

spacecraft V95.45 ☑

stated as undetermined whether accidental or intentional Y25 ☑

steam or water lines (in machinery) W37.8 ☑

stove W40.9 ☑

suicide (attempt) X75 ☑

tire, pressurized W37.8 ☑

bicycle W37.0 ☑

undetermined whether accidental or intentional Y25 ☑

vehicle tire NEC W37.8 ☑

bicycle W37.0 ☑

war operations — see War operations, explosion

Exposure (to) X58 ☑

air pressure change — see Air, pressure

cold (accidental) (excessive) (extreme) (natural) (place) X31 ☑

assault Y08.89 ☑

due to

man-made conditions W93.8 ☑

dry ice (contact) W93.01 ☑

inhalation W93.02 ☑

liquid air (contact) (hydrogen) (nitrogen) W93.11 ☑

inhalation W93.12 ☑

refrigeration unit (deep freeze) W93.2 ☑

suicide (attempt) X83.2 ☑

weather (conditions) X31 ☑

homicide (attempt) Y08.89 ☑

self-inflicted X83.2 ☑

due to abandonment or neglect X58 ☑

electric current W86.8 ☑

appliance (faulty) W86.8 ☑

domestic W86.0 ☑

caused by other person Y08.89 ☑

conductor (faulty) W86.1 ☑

control apparatus (faulty) W86.1 ☑

electric power generating plant, distribution station W86.1 ☑

electroshock gun — see Exposure, electric current, taser

high-voltage cable W85 ☑

homicide (attempt) Y08.89 ☑

legal execution — see Legal, intervention, specified means NEC

☑ **Additional Character Required** — Refer to the Tabular List for Character Selection ▽ **Subterms under main terms may continue to next column or page**

Exposure — *continued*
electric current — *continued*
  lightning — *see* subcategory T75.0 ☑
  live rail W86.8 ☑
  misadventure in medical or surgical procedure in
    electroshock therapy Y63.4
  motor (electric) (faulty) W86.8 ☑
    domestic W86.0 ☑
  self-inflicted X83.1 ☑
  specified NEC W86.8 ☑
    domestic W86.0 ☑
  stun gun — *see* Exposure, electric current, taser
  suicide (attempt) X83.1 ☑
  taser W86.8 ☑
    assault Y08.89 ☑
    legal intervention — *see* category Y35 ☑
    self-harm (intentional) X83.8 ☑
    undetermined intent Y33 ☑
  third rail W86.8 ☑
  transformer (faulty) W86.1 ☑
  transmission lines W85 ☑
environmental tobacco smoke X58 ☑
excessive
  cold — *see* Exposure, cold
  heat (natural) NEC X30 ☑
    man-made W92 ☑
factor(s) NOS X58 ☑
  environmental NEC X58 ☑
    man-made NEC W99 ☑
    natural NEC — *see* Forces of nature
  specified NEC X58 ☑
fire, flames (accidental) X08.8 ☑
  assault X97 ☑
  campfire — *see* Exposure, fire, controlled, not in
    building
  controlled (in)
    with ignition (of) clothing — *see also* Ignition,
      clothes X06.2 ☑
      nightwear X05 ☑
    bonfire — *see* Exposure, fire, controlled, not in
      building
    brazier (in building or structure) — *see also* Ex-
      posure, fire, controlled, building
      not in building or structure — *see* Exposure,
        fire, controlled, not in building
    building or structure X02.0 ☑
      with
        fall from building X02.3 ☑
        from building X02.5 ☑
        injury due to building collapse X02.2 ☑
        smoke inhalation X02.1 ☑
      hit by object from building X02.4 ☑
      specified mode of injury NEC X02.8 ☑
    fireplace, furnace or stove — *see* Exposure, fire,
      controlled, building
    not in building or structure X03.0 ☑
      with
        fall X03.3 ☑
        smoke inhalation X03.1 ☑
      hit by object X03.4 ☑
      specified mode of injury NEC X03.8 ☑
    trash — *see* Exposure, fire, controlled, not in
      building
  fireplace — *see* Exposure, fire, controlled, building
  fittings or furniture (in building or structure) (uncon-
    trolled) — *see* Exposure, fire, uncontrolled,
      building
  forest (uncontrolled) — *see* Exposure, fire, uncon-
    trolled, not in building
  grass (uncontrolled) — *see* Exposure, fire, uncon-
    trolled, not in building
  hay (uncontrolled) — *see* Exposure, fire, uncon-
    trolled, not in building
  homicide (attempt) X97 ☑
  ignition of highly flammable material X04 ☑
  in, of, on, starting in
    machinery — *see* Contact, with, by type of ma-
      chine
    motor vehicle (in motion) — *see also* Accident,
      transport, occupant by type of vehicle
      V87.8 ☑
      with collision — *see* Collision
    railway rolling stock, train, vehicle V81.81 ☑
      with collision — *see* Accident, transport, rail-
        way vehicle occupant
    street car (in motion) V82.8 ☑

Exposure — *continued*
fire, flames — *continued*
  in, of, on, starting in — *continued*
    street car — *continued*
      with collision — *see* Accident, transport,
        streetcar occupant
      transport vehicle NEC — *see also* Accident,
        transport
        with collision — *see* Collision
    war operations — *see also* War operations, fire
      from nuclear explosion — *see* War operations,
        nuclear weapons
    watercraft (in transit) (not in transit) V91.09 ☑
      localized — *see* Burn, on board watercraft,
        due to, fire on board
      powered craft V91.03 ☑
        ferry boat V91.01 ☑
        fishing boat V91.02 ☑
        jet skis V91.03 ☑
        liner V91.01 ☑
        merchant ship V91.00 ☑
        passenger ship V91.01 ☑
      unpowered craft V91.08 ☑
        canoe V91.05 ☑
        inflatable V91.06 ☑
        kayak V91.05 ☑
        sailboat V91.04 ☑
        surf-board V91.08 ☑
        waterskis V91.07 ☑
        windsurfer V91.08 ☑
  lumber (uncontrolled) — *see* Exposure, fire, uncon-
    trolled, not in building
  mine (uncontrolled) — *see* Exposure, fire, uncon-
    trolled, not in building
  prairie (uncontrolled) — *see* Exposure, fire, uncon-
    trolled, not in building
  resulting from
    explosion — *see* Explosion
    lightning X08.8 ☑
  self-inflicted X76 ☑
  specified NEC X08.8 ☑
  started by other person X97 ☑
  stated as undetermined whether accidental or inten-
    tional Y26 ☑
  stove — *see* Exposure, fire, controlled, building
  suicide (attempt) X76 ☑
  tunnel (uncontrolled) — *see* Exposure, fire, uncon-
    trolled, not in building
  uncontrolled
    in building or structure X00.0 ☑
      with
        fall from building X00.3 ☑
        injury due to building collapse X00.2 ☑
        jump from building X00.5 ☑
        smoke inhalation X00.1 ☑
      bed X08.00 ☑
        due to
          cigarette X08.01 ☑
          specified material NEC X08.09 ☑
      furniture NEC X08.20 ☑
        due to
          cigarette X08.21 ☑
          specified material NEC X08.29 ☑
      hit by object from building X00.4 ☑
      sofa X08.10 ☑
        due to
          cigarette X08.11 ☑
          specified material NEC X08.19 ☑
      specified mode of injury NEC X00.8 ☑
    not in building or structure (any) X01.0 ☑
      with
        fall X01.3 ☑
        smoke inhalation X01.1 ☑
      hit by object X01.4 ☑
      specified mode of injury NEC X01.8 ☑
  undetermined whether accidental or intentional
    Y26 ☑
forces of nature NEC — *see* Forces of nature
G-forces (abnormal) W49.9 ☑
gravitational forces (abnormal) W49.9 ☑
heat (natural) NEC — *see* Heat
high-pressure jet (hydraulic) (pneumatic) W49.9 ☑
hydraulic jet W49.9 ☑
inanimate mechanical force W49.9 ☑
jet, high-pressure (hydraulic) (pneumatic) W49.9 ☑
lightning — *see* subcategory T75.0 ☑

Exposure — *continued*
lightning — *see* subcategory — *continued*
  causing fire — *see* Exposure, fire
mechanical forces NEC W49.9 ☑
  animate NEC W64
  inanimate NEC W49.9 ☑
noise W42.9 ☑
  supersonic W42.0 ☑
noxious substance — *see* Table of Drugs and Chemicals
pneumatic jet W49.9 ☑
prolonged in deep-freeze unit or refrigerator W93.2 ☑
radiation — *see* Radiation
smoke — *see also* Exposure, fire
  tobacco, second hand Z77.22
specified factors NEC X58 ☑
sunlight X32 ☑
  man-made (sun lamp) W89.8 ☑
    tanning bed W89.1 ☑
supersonic waves W42.0 ☑
transmission line(s), electric W85 ☑
vibration W49.9 ☑
waves
  infrasound W49.9 ☑
  sound W42.9 ☑
  supersonic W42.0 ☑
weather NEC — *see* Forces of nature
External cause status Y99.9
child assisting in compensated work for family Y99.8
civilian activity done for financial or other compensation Y99.0
civilian activity done for income or pay Y99.0
family member assisting in compensated work for
  other family member Y99.8
hobby not done for income Y99.8
leisure activity Y99.8
military activity Y99.1
off-duty activity of military personnel Y99.8
recreation or sport not for income or while a student
  Y99.8
specified NEC Y99.8
student activity Y99.8
volunteer activity Y99.2

F

Factors, supplemental
alcohol
  blood level
    less than 20mg/100ml Y90.0
    presence in blood, level not specified Y90.9
    20-39mg/100ml Y90.1
    40-59mg/100ml Y90.2
    60-79mg/100ml Y90.3
    80-99mg/100ml Y90.4
    100-119mg/100ml Y90.5
    120-199mg/100ml Y90.6
    200-239mg/100ml Y90.7
    240mg/100ml or more Y90.8
  presence in blood, but level not specified Y90.9
environmental-pollution-related condition- *see* Z57 ☑
nosocomial condition Y95
work-related condition Y99.0
Failure
in suture or ligature during surgical procedure Y65.2
mechanical, of instrument or apparatus (any) (during
  any medical or surgical procedure) Y65.8
sterile precautions (during medical and surgical care)
  — *see* Misadventure, failure, sterile precautions,
    by type of procedure
to
  introduce tube or instrument Y65.4
    endotracheal tube during anesthesia Y65.3
  make curve (transport vehicle) NEC — *see* Accident,
    transport
  remove tube or instrument Y65.4
Fall, falling (accidental) W19 ☑
building W20.1 ☑
  burning (uncontrolled fire) X00.3 ☑
down
  embankment W17.81 ☑
  escalator W10.0 ☑
  hill W17.81 ☑
  ladder W11 ☑
  ramp W10.2 ☑
  stairs, steps W10.9 ☑

Fall, falling — *continued*
  due to
    bumping against
      object W18.00 ☑
        sharp glass W18.02 ☑
        specified NEC W18.09 ☑
        sports equipment W18.01 ☑
      person W03 ☑
        due to ice or snow W00.0 ☑
        on pedestrian conveyance — *see* Accident,
          transport, pedestrian, conveyance
    collision with another person W03 ☑
      due to ice or snow W00.0 ☑
      involving pedestrian conveyance — *see* Acci-
        dent, transport, pedestrian, conveyance
    grocery cart tipping over W17.82 ☑
    ice or snow W00.9 ☑
      from one level to another W00.2 ☑
        on stairs or steps W00.1 ☑
      involving pedestrian conveyance — *see* Acci-
        dent, transport, pedestrian, conveyance
      on same level W00.0 ☑
    slipping (on moving sidewalk) W01.0 ☑
      with subsequent striking against object
        W01.10 ☑
        furniture W01.190 ☑
        sharp object W01.119 ☑
          glass W01.110 ☑
          power tool or machine W01.111 ☑
          specified NEC W01.118 ☑
        specified NEC W01.198 ☑
    striking against
      object W18.00 ☑
        sharp glass W18.02 ☑
        specified NEC W18.09 ☑
        sports equipment W18.01 ☑
      person W03 ☑
        due to ice or snow W00.0 ☑
        on pedestrian conveyance — *see* Accident,
          transport, pedestrian, conveyance
  earth (with asphyxia or suffocation (by pressure)) —
    see Earth, falling
  from, off, out of
    aircraft NEC (with accident to aircraft NEC) V97.0 ☑
      while boarding or alighting V97.1 ☑
    balcony W13.0 ☑
    bed W06 ☑
    boat, ship, watercraft NEC (with drowning or sub-
      mersion) — *see* Drowning, due to, fall over-
      board
      with hitting bottom or object V94.0 ☑
    bridge W13.1 ☑
    building W13.9 ☑
      burning (uncontrolled fire) X00.3 ☑
    cavity W17.2 ☑
    chair W07 ☑
    cherry picker W17.89 ☑
    cliff W15 ☑
    dock W17.4 ☑
    embankment W17.81 ☑
    escalator W10.0 ☑
    flagpole W13.8 ☑
    furniture NEC W08 ☑
    grocery cart W17.82 ☑
    haystack W17.89 ☑
    high place NEC W17.89 ☑
      stated as undetermined whether accidental or
        intentional Y30 ☑
    hole W17.2 ☑
    incline W10.2 ☑
    ladder W11 ☑
    lifting device W17.89 ☑
    machine, machinery — *see also* Contact, with, by
      type of machine
      not in operation W17.89 ☑
    manhole W17.1 ☑
    mobile elevated work platform [MEWP] W17.89 ☑
    motorized mobility scooter W05.2 ☑
    one level to another NEC W17.89 ☑
      intentional, purposeful, suicide (attempt) X80 ☑
      stated as undetermined whether accidental or
        intentional Y30 ☑
    pit W17.2 ☑
    playground equipment W09.8 ☑
      jungle gym W09.2 ☑
      slide W09.0 ☑

Fall, falling — *continued*
  from, off, out of — *continued*
    playground equipment — *continued*
      swing W09.1 ☑
    quarry W17.89 ☑
    railing W13.9 ☑
    ramp W10.2 ☑
    roof W13.2 ☑
    scaffolding W12 ☑
    scooter (nonmotorized) W05.1 ☑
      motorized mobility W05.2 ☑
    sky lift W17.89 ☑
    stairs, steps W10.9 ☑
      curb W10.1 ☑
      due to ice or snow W00.1 ☑
      escalator W10.0 ☑
      incline W10.2 ☑
      ramp W10.2 ☑
      sidewalk curb W10.1 ☑
      specified NEC W10.8 ☑
    stepladder W11 ☑
    storm drain W17.1 ☑
    streetcar NEC V82.6 ☑
      while boarding or alighting V82.4 ☑
      with antecedent collision — *see* Accident,
        transport, streetcar occupant
    structure NEC W13.8 ☑
      burning (uncontrolled fire) X00.3 ☑
    table W08 ☑
    toilet W18.11 ☑
      with subsequent striking against object
        W18.12 ☑
    train NEC V81.6 ☑
      during derailment (without antecedent collision)
        V81.7 ☑
        with antecedent collision — *see* Accident,
          transport, railway vehicle occupant
      while boarding or alighting V81.4 ☑
    transport vehicle after collision — *see* Accident,
      transport, by type of vehicle, collision
    tree W14 ☑
    vehicle (in motion) NEC — *see also* Accident, trans-
      port V89.9 ☑
      motor NEC — *see also* Accident, transport, occu-
        pant, by type of vehicle V87.8 ☑
      stationary W17.89 ☑
        while boarding or alighting — *see* Accident,
          transport, by type of vehicle, while
          boarding or alighting
    viaduct W13.8 ☑
    wall W13.8 ☑
    watercraft — *see also* Drowning, due to, fall over-
      board
      with hitting bottom or object V94.0 ☑
    well W17.0 ☑
    wheelchair, non-moving W05.0 ☑
      powered — *see* Accident, transport, pedestrian,
        conveyance occupant, specified type NEC
    window W13.4 ☑
  in, on
    aircraft NEC V97.0 ☑
      while boarding or alighting V97.1 ☑
      with accident to aircraft V97.0 ☑
    bathtub (empty) W18.2 ☑
      filled W16.212 ☑
        causing drowning W16.211 ☑
    escalator W10.0 ☑
    incline W10.2 ☑
    ladder W11 ☑
    machine, machinery — *see* Contact, with, by type
      of machine
    object, edged, pointed or sharp (with cut) — *see*
      Fall, by type
    playground equipment W09.8 ☑
      jungle gym W09.2 ☑
      slide W09.0 ☑
      swing W09.1 ☑
    ramp W10.2 ☑
    scaffolding W12 ☑
    shower W18.2 ☑
      causing drowning W16.211 ☑
    staircase, stairs, steps W10.9 ☑
      curb W10.1 ☑
      due to ice or snow W00.1 ☑
      escalator W10.0 ☑
      incline W10.2 ☑

Fall, falling — *continued*
  in, on — *continued*
    staircase, stairs, steps — *continued*
      specified NEC W10.8 ☑
    streetcar (without antecedent collision) V82.5 ☑
      with antecedent collision — *see* Accident,
        transport, streetcar occupant
      while boarding or alighting V82.4 ☑
    train (without antecedent collision) V81.5 ☑
      with antecedent collision — *see* Accident,
        transport, railway vehicle occupant
      during derailment (without antecedent collision)
        V81.7 ☑
        with antecedent collision — *see* Accident,
          transport, railway vehicle occupant
      while boarding or alighting V81.4 ☑
    transport vehicle after collision — *see* Accident,
      transport, by type of vehicle, collision
    watercraft V93.39 ☑
      due to
        accident to craft V91.29 ☑
          powered craft V91.23 ☑
            ferry boat V91.21 ☑
            fishing boat V91.22 ☑
            jetskis V91.23 ☑
            liner V91.21 ☑
            merchant ship V91.20 ☑
            passenger ship V91.21 ☑
          unpowered craft
            canoe V91.25 ☑
            inflatable V91.26 ☑
            kayak V91.25 ☑
            sailboat V91.24 ☑
        powered craft V93.33 ☑
          ferry boat V93.31 ☑
          fishing boat V93.32 ☑
          jetskis V93.33 ☑
          liner V93.31 ☑
          merchant ship V93.30 ☑
          passenger ship V93.31 ☑
        unpowered craft V93.38 ☑
          canoe V93.35 ☑
          inflatable V93.36 ☑
          kayak V93.35 ☑
          sailboat V93.34 ☑
          surf-board V93.38 ☑
          windsurfer V93.38 ☑
  into
    cavity W17.2 ☑
    dock W17.4 ☑
    fire — *see* Exposure, fire, by type
    haystack W17.89 ☑
    hole W17.2 ☑
    lake — *see* Fall, into, water
    manhole W17.1 ☑
    moving part of machinery — *see* Contact, with, b
      type of machine
    ocean — *see* Fall, into, water
    opening in surface NEC W17.89 ☑
    pit W17.2 ☑
    pond — *see* Fall, into, water
    quarry W17.89 ☑
    river — *see* Fall, into, water
    shaft W17.89 ☑
    storm drain W17.1 ☑
    stream — *see* Fall, into, water
    swimming pool — *see also* Fall, into, water, in,
      swimming pool
      empty W17.3 ☑
    tank W17.89 ☑
    water W16.42 ☑
      causing drowning W16.41 ☑
      from watercraft — *see* Drowning, due to, fall
        overboard
      hitting diving board W21.4 ☑
      in
        bathtub W16.212 ☑
          causing drowning W16.211 ☑
        bucket W16.222 ☑
          causing drowning W16.221 ☑
        natural body of water W16.112 ☑
          causing drowning W16.111 ☑
          striking
            bottom W16.122 ☑
              causing drowning W16.121 ☑
            side W16.132 ☑

Fall, falling — *continued*
  into — *continued*
    water — *continued*
      in — *continued*
        natural body of water — *continued*
          striking — *continued*
            side — *continued*
              causing drowning W16.131 ☑
        specified water NEC W16.312 ☑
          causing drowning W16.311 ☑
          striking
            bottom W16.322 ☑
              causing drowning W16.321 ☑
            wall W16.332 ☑
              causing drowning W16.331 ☑
        swimming pool W16.012 ☑
          causing drowning W16.011 ☑
          striking
            bottom W16.022 ☑
              causing drowning W16.031 ☑
            wall W16.032 ☑
              causing drowning W16.021 ☑
        utility bucket W16.222 ☑
          causing drowning W16.221 ☑
    well W17.0 ☑
  involving
    bed W06 ☑
    chair W07 ☑
    furniture NEC W08 ☑
    glass — *see* Fall, by type
    playground equipment W09.8 ☑
      jungle gym W09.2 ☑
      slide W09.0 ☑
      swing W09.1 ☑
    roller blades — *see* Accident, transport, pedestrian, conveyance
    skateboard(s) — *see* Accident, transport, pedestrian, conveyance
    skates (ice) (in line) (roller) — *see* Accident, transport, pedestrian, conveyance
    skis — *see* Accident, transport, pedestrian, conveyance
    table W08 ☑
    wheelchair, non-moving W05.0 ☑
      powered — *see* Accident, transport, pedestrian, conveyance, specified type NEC
  object — *see* Struck by, object, falling
  off
    toilet W18.11 ☑
      with subsequent striking against object W18.12 ☑
  on same level W18.30 ☑
    due to
      specified NEC W18.39 ☑
      stepping on an object W18.31 ☑
  out of
    bed W06 ☑
    building NEC W13.8 ☑
    chair W07 ☑
    furniture NEC W08 ☑
    wheelchair, non-moving W05.0 ☑
      powered — *see* Accident, transport, pedestrian, conveyance, specified type NEC
    window W13.4 ☑
  over
    animal W01.0 ☑
    cliff W15 ☑
    embankment W17.81 ☑
    small object W01.0 ☑
  rock W20.8 ☑
  same level W18.30 ☑
    from
      being crushed, pushed, or stepped on by a crowd or human stampede W52 ☑
      collision, pushing, shoving, by or with other person W03 ☑
      slipping, stumbling, tripping W01.0 ☑
    involving ice or snow W00.0 ☑
      involving skates (ice) (roller), skateboard, skis — *see* Accident, transport, pedestrian, conveyance
  snowslide (avalanche) — *see* Landslide
  stone W20.8 ☑
  structure W20.1 ☑
    burning (uncontrolled fire) X00.3 ☑

Fall, falling — *continued*
  through
    bridge W13.1 ☑
    floor W13.3 ☑
    roof W13.2 ☑
    wall W13.8 ☑
    window W13.4 ☑
    timber W20.8 ☑
    tree (caused by lightning) W20.8 ☑
  while being carried or supported by other person(s) W04 ☑
Fallen on by
  animal (not being ridden) NEC W55.89 ☑
Felo-de-se — *see* Suicide
Fight (hand) (fists) (foot) — *see* Assault, fight
Fire (accidental) — *see* Exposure, fire
Firearm discharge — *see* Discharge, firearm
Fireball effects from nuclear explosion in war operations — *see* War operations, nuclear weapons
Fireworks (explosion) W39 ☑
Flash burns from explosion — *see* Explosion
Flood (any injury) (caused by) X38 ☑
  collapse of man-made structure causing earth movement X36.0 ☑
  tidal wave — *see* Forces of nature, tidal wave
Food (any type) **in**
  air passages (with asphyxia, obstruction, or suffocation) — *see* categories T17 and T18
  alimentary tract causing asphyxia (due to compression of trachea) — *see* categories T17 and T18
Forces of nature X39.8 ☑
  avalanche X36.1 ☑
    causing transport accident — *see* Accident, transport, by type of vehicle
  blizzard X37.2 ☑
  cataclysmic storm X37.9 ☑
    with flood X38 ☑
    blizzard X37.2 ☑
    cloudburst X37.8 ☑
    cyclone X37.1 ☑
    dust storm X37.3 ☑
    hurricane X37.0 ☑
    specified storm NEC X37.8 ☑
    storm surge X37.0 ☑
    tornado X37.1 ☑
    twister X37.1 ☑
    typhoon X37.0 ☑
  cloudburst X37.8 ☑
  cold (natural) X31 ☑
  cyclone X37.1 ☑
  dam collapse causing earth movement X36.0 ☑
  dust storm X37.3 ☑
  earth movement X36.1 ☑
    caused by dam or structure collapse X36.0 ☑
    earthquake X34 ☑
  earthquake X34 ☑
  flood (caused by) X38 ☑
    dam collapse X36.0 ☑
    tidal wave — *see* Forces of nature, tidal wave
  heat (natural) X30 ☑
  hurricane X37.0 ☑
  landslide X36.1 ☑
    causing transport accident — *see* Accident, transport, by type of vehicle
  lightning — *see* subcategory T75.0 ☑
    causing fire — *see* Exposure, fire
  mudslide X36.1 ☑
    causing transport accident — *see* Accident, transport, by type of vehicle
  radiation (natural) X39.08 ☑
    radon X39.01 ☑
  radon X39.01 ☑
  specified force NEC X39.8 ☑
  storm surge X37.0 ☑
  structure collapse causing earth movement X36.0 ☑
  sunlight X32 ☑
  tidal wave X37.41 ☑
    due to
      earthquake X37.41 ☑
      landslide X37.43 ☑
      storm X37.42 ☑
      volcanic eruption X37.41 ☑
  tornado X37.1 ☑
  tsunami X37.41 ☑
  twister X37.1 ☑
  typhoon X37.0 ☑

Forces of nature — *continued*
  volcanic eruption X35 ☑
Foreign body
  aspiration — *see* Index to Diseases and Injuries, Foreign body, respiratory tract
  embedded in skin W45 ☑
  entering through skin W45.8 ☑
    can lid W26.8 ☑
    nail W45.0 ☑
    paper W26.2 ☑
    specified NEC W45.8 ☑
    splinter W45.8 ☑
Forest fire (exposure to) — *see* Exposure, fire, uncontrolled, not in building
Found injured X58 ☑
  from exposure (to) — *see* Exposure
  on
    highway, road(way), street V89.9 ☑
    railway right of way V81.9 ☑
Fracture (circumstances unknown or unspecified) X58 ☑
  due to specified cause NEC X58 ☑
Freezing — *see* Exposure, cold
Frostbite X31 ☑
  due to man-made conditions — *see* Exposure, cold, man-made
Frozen — *see* Exposure, cold

G

Gored by bull W55.22 ☑
Gunshot wound W34.00 ☑

H

Hailstones, injured by X39.8 ☑
Hanged herself or himself — *see* Hanging, self-inflicted
Hanging (accidental) — *see also* category T71 ☑
  legal execution — *see* Legal, intervention, specified means NEC
Heat (effects of) (excessive) X30 ☑
  due to
    man-made conditions W92 ☑
      on board watercraft V93.29 ☑
        fishing boat V93.22 ☑
        merchant ship V93.20 ☑
        passenger ship V93.21 ☑
        sailboat V93.24 ☑
        specified powered craft NEC V93.23 ☑
    weather (conditions) X30 ☑
  from
    electric heating apparatus causing burning X16 ☑
    nuclear explosion in war operations — *see* War operations, nuclear weapons
  inappropriate in local application or packing in medical or surgical procedure Y63.5
Hemorrhage
  delayed following medical or surgical treatment without mention of misadventure — *see* Index to Diseases and Injuries, Complication(s)
  during medical or surgical treatment as misadventure — *see* Index to Diseases and Injuries, Complication(s)
High
  altitude (effects) — *see* Air, pressure, low
  level of radioactivity, effects — *see* Radiation
  pressure (effects) — *see* Air, pressure, high
  temperature, effects — *see* Heat
Hit, hitting (accidental) by — *see* Struck by
Hitting against — *see* Striking against
Homicide (attempt) (justifiable) — *see* Assault
Hot
  place, effects — *see also* Heat
  weather, effects X30 ☑
House fire (uncontrolled) — *see* Exposure, fire, uncontrolled, building
Humidity, causing problem X39.8 ☑
Hunger X58 ☑
Hurricane (any injury) X37.0 ☑
Hypobarism, hypobaropathy — *see* Air, pressure, low

I

Ictus
  caloris — *see also* Heat
  solaris X30 ☑
Ignition (accidental) — *see also* Exposure, fire X08.8 ☑

Ignition — continued
anesthetic gas in operating room W40.1 ☑
apparel X06.2 ☑
from highly flammable material X04 ☑
nightwear X05 ☑
bed linen (sheets) (spreads) (pillows) (mattress) — see
Exposure, fire, uncontrolled, building, bed
benzine X04 ☑
clothes, clothing NEC (from controlled fire) X06.2 ☑
from
highly flammable material X04 ☑
ether X04 ☑
in operating room W40.1 ☑
explosive material — see Explosion
gasoline X04 ☑
jewelry (plastic) (any) X06.0 ☑
kerosene X04 ☑
material
explosive — see Explosion
highly flammable with secondary explosion X04 ☑
nightwear X05 ☑
paraffin X04 ☑
petrol X04 ☑
Immersion (accidental) — see also Drowning
hand or foot due to cold (excessive) X31 ☑
Implantation of quills of porcupine W55.89 ☑
Inanition (from) (hunger) X58 ☑
thirst X58 ☑
Inappropriate operation performed
correct operation on wrong side or body part (wrong
side) (wrong site) Y65.53
operation intended for another patient done on wrong
patient Y65.52
wrong operation performed on correct patient Y65.51
Inattention after, at birth (homicidal intent) (infanticidal
intent) X58 ☑
Incident, adverse
device
anesthesiology Y70.8
accessory Y70.2
diagnostic Y70.0
miscellaneous Y70.8
monitoring Y70.0
prosthetic Y70.2
rehabilitative Y70.1
surgical Y70.3
therapeutic Y70.1
cardiovascular Y71.8
accessory Y71.2
diagnostic Y71.0
miscellaneous Y71.8
monitoring Y71.0
prosthetic Y71.2
rehabilitative Y71.1
surgical Y71.3
therapeutic Y71.1
gastroenterology Y73.8
accessory Y73.2
diagnostic Y73.0
miscellaneous Y73.8
monitoring Y73.0
prosthetic Y73.2
rehabilitative Y73.1
surgical Y73.3
therapeutic Y73.1
general
hospital Y74.8
accessory Y74.2
diagnostic Y74.0
miscellaneous Y74.8
monitoring Y74.0
prosthetic Y74.2
rehabilitative Y74.1
surgical Y74.3
therapeutic Y74.1
surgical Y81.8
accessory Y81.2
diagnostic Y81.0
miscellaneous Y81.8
monitoring Y81.0
prosthetic Y81.2
rehabilitative Y81.1
surgical Y81.3
therapeutic Y81.1
gynecological Y76.8
accessory Y76.2
diagnostic Y76.0
miscellaneous Y76.8

Incident, adverse — continued
device — continued
gynecological — continued
monitoring Y76.0
prosthetic Y76.2
rehabilitative Y76.1
surgical Y76.3
therapeutic Y76.1
medical Y82.9
specified type NEC Y82.8
neurological Y75.8
accessory Y75.2
diagnostic Y75.0
miscellaneous Y75.8
monitoring Y75.0
prosthetic Y75.2
rehabilitative Y75.1
surgical Y75.3
therapeutic Y75.1
obstetrical Y76.8
accessory Y76.2
diagnostic Y76.0
miscellaneous Y76.8
monitoring Y76.0
prosthetic Y76.2
rehabilitative Y76.1
surgical Y76.3
therapeutic Y76.1
ophthalmic Y77.8
accessory Y77.2
diagnostic Y77.0
miscellaneous Y77.8
monitoring Y77.0
prosthetic Y77.2
rehabilitative Y77.1
surgical Y77.3
therapeutic Y77.1
orthopedic Y79.8
accessory Y79.2
diagnostic Y79.0
miscellaneous Y79.8
monitoring Y79.0
prosthetic Y79.2
rehabilitative Y79.1
surgical Y79.3
therapeutic Y79.1
otorhinolaryngological Y72.8
accessory Y72.2
diagnostic Y72.0
miscellaneous Y72.8
monitoring Y72.0
prosthetic Y72.2
rehabilitative Y72.1
surgical Y72.3
therapeutic Y72.1
personal use Y74.8
accessory Y74.2
diagnostic Y74.0
miscellaneous Y74.8
monitoring Y74.0
prosthetic Y74.2
rehabilitative Y74.1
surgical Y74.3
therapeutic Y74.1
physical medicine Y80.8
accessory Y80.2
diagnostic Y80.0
miscellaneous Y80.8
monitoring Y80.0
prosthetic Y80.2
rehabilitative Y80.1
surgical Y80.3
therapeutic Y80.1
plastic surgical Y81.8
accessory Y81.2
diagnostic Y81.0
miscellaneous Y81.8
monitoring Y81.0
prosthetic Y81.2
rehabilitative Y81.1
surgical Y81.3
therapeutic Y81.1
radiological Y78.8
accessory Y78.2
diagnostic Y78.0
miscellaneous Y78.8
monitoring Y78.0
prosthetic Y78.2
rehabilitative Y78.1

Incident, adverse — continued
device — continued
radiological — continued
surgical Y78.3
therapeutic Y78.1
urology Y73.8
accessory Y73.2
diagnostic Y73.0
miscellaneous Y73.8
monitoring Y73.0
prosthetic Y73.2
rehabilitative Y73.1
surgical Y73.3
therapeutic Y73.1
Incineration (accidental) — see Exposure, fire
Infanticide — see Assault
Infrasound waves (causing injury) W49.9 ☑
Ingestion
foreign body (causing injury) (with obstruction) — se
Foreign body, alimentary canal
poisonous
plant(s) X58 ☑
substance NEC — see Table of Drugs and Chemica
Inhalation
excessively cold substance, man-made — see Exposur
cold, man-made
food (any type) (into respiratory tract) (with asphyxi
obstruction respiratory tract, suffocation) — se
categories T17 and T18 ☑
foreign body — see Foreign body, aspiration
gastric contents (with asphyxia, obstruction respirato
passage, suffocation) T17.81- ☑
hot air or gases X14.0 ☑
liquid air, hydrogen, nitrogen W93.12 ☑
suicide (attempt) X83.2 ☑
steam X13.0 ☑
assault X98.0 ☑
stated as undetermined whether accidental or inte
tional Y27.0 ☑
suicide (attempt) X77.0 ☑
toxic gas — see Table of Drugs and Chemicals
vomitus (with asphyxia, obstruction respiratory passage, suffocation) T17.81- ☑
Injury, injured (accidental(ly)) NOS X58 ☑
by, caused by, from
assault — see Assault
law-enforcing agent, police, in course of legal inte
vention — see Legal intervention
suicide (attempt) X83.8 ☑
due to, in
civil insurrection — see War operations
fight — see also Assault, fight Y04.0 ☑
war operations — see War operations
homicide — see also Assault Y09
inflicted (by)
in course of arrest (attempted), suppression of di
turbance, maintenance of order, by law-en
forcing agents — see Legal intervention
other person
stated as
accidental X58 ☑
intentional, homicide (attempt) — see Assau
undetermined whether accidental or inten
tional Y33 ☑
purposely (inflicted) by other person(s) — see Assau
self-inflicted X83.8 ☑
stated as accidental X58 ☑
specified cause NEC X58 ☑
undetermined whether accidental or intentional Y33
Insolation, effects X30 ☑
Insufficient nourishment X58 ☑
Interruption of respiration (by)
food (lodged in esophagus) — see categories T17 ar
T18 ☑
vomitus (lodged in esophagus) T17.81- ☑
Intervention, legal — see Legal intervention
Intoxication
drug — see Table of Drugs and Chemicals
poison — see Table of Drugs and Chemicals

J

Jammed (accidentally)
between objects (moving) (stationary and moving)
W23.0 ☑
stationary W23.1 ☑

Jumped, jumping

before moving object NEC X81.8 ☑
   motor vehicle X81.0 ☑
   subway train X81.1 ☑
   train X81.1 ☑
   undetermined whether accidental or intentional Y31 ☑
from
   boat (into water) voluntarily, without accident (to or on boat) W16.712 ☑
      striking bottom W16.722 ☑
         causing drowning W16.721 ☑
      with
         accident to or on boat — *see* Accident, watercraft
         drowning or submersion W16.711 ☑
            suicide (attempt) X71.3 ☑
   building — *see also* Jumped, from, high place W13.9 ☑
      burning (uncontrolled fire) X00.5 ☑
   high place NEC W17.89 ☑
      suicide (attempt) X80 ☑
      undetermined whether accidental or intentional Y30 ☑
   structure — *see also* Jumped, from, high place W13.9 ☑
      burning (uncontrolled fire) X00.5 ☑
into water W16.92 ☑
   causing drowning W16.91 ☑
   from, off watercraft — *see* Jumped, from, boat
   in
      natural body W16.612 ☑
         causing drowning W16.611 ☑
         striking bottom W16.622 ☑
            causing drowning W16.621 ☑
      specified place NEC W16.812 ☑
         causing drowning W16.811 ☑
         striking
            bottom W16.822 ☑
               causing drowning W16.821 ☑
            wall W16.832 ☑
               causing drowning W16.831 ☑
      swimming pool W16.512 ☑
         causing drowning W16.511 ☑
         striking
            bottom W16.522 ☑
               causing drowning W16.521 ☑
            wall W16.532 ☑
               causing drowning W16.531 ☑
   suicide (attempt) X71.3 ☑

K

Kicked by

animal NEC W55.82 ☑
person(s) (accidentally) W50.1 ☑
   with intent to injure or kill Y04.0 ☑
   as, or caused by, a crowd or human stampede (with fall) W52 ☑
   assault Y04.0 ☑
   homicide (attempt) Y04.0 ☑
   in
      fight Y04.0 ☑
      legal intervention
         injuring
            bystander Y35.812 ☑
            law enforcement personnel Y35.811 ☑
            suspect Y35.813 ☑
            unspecified person Y35.819 ☑

Kicking

against
   object W22.8 ☑
      sports equipment W21.9 ☑
      stationary W22.09 ☑
         sports equipment W21.89 ☑
   person — *see* Striking against, person
   sports equipment W21.9 ☑
carpet stretcher with knee X50.3 ☑

Killed, killing (accidentally) NOS — *see also* Injury X58 ☑

in
   action — *see* War operations
   brawl, fight (hand) (fists) (foot) Y04.0 ☑
      by weapon — *see also* Assault
         cutting, piercing — *see* Assault, cutting or piercing instrument

---

Killed, killing — *continued*

in — *continued*
   brawl, fight — *continued*
      by weapon — *see also* Assault — *continued*
         firearm — *see* Discharge, firearm, by type, homicide
self
   stated as
      accident NOS X58 ☑
      suicide — *see* Suicide
      undetermined whether accidental or intentional Y33 ☑

Kneeling (prolonged (static) X50.1 ☑

Knocked down (accidentally) (by) NOS X58 ☑

animal (not being ridden) NEC — *see also* Struck by, by type of animal
crowd or human stampede W52 ☑
person W51 ☑
   in brawl, fight Y04.0 ☑
transport vehicle NEC — *see also* Accident, transport V09.9 ☑

L

Laceration NEC — *see* Injury

Lack of

care (helpless person) (infant) (newborn) X58 ☑
food except as result of abandonment or neglect X58 ☑
   due to abandonment or neglect X58 ☑
water except as result of transport accident X58 ☑
   due to transport accident — *see* Accident, transport, by type
   helpless person, infant, newborn X58 ☑

Landslide (falling on transport vehicle) X36.1 ☑

caused by collapse of man-made structure X36.0 ☑

Late effect — *see* Sequelae

Legal

execution (any method) — *see* Legal, intervention
intervention (by)
   baton — *see* Legal, intervention, blunt object, baton
   bayonet — *see* Legal, intervention, sharp object, bayonet
   blow — *see* Legal, intervention, manhandling
   blunt object
      baton
         injuring
            bystander Y35.312 ☑
            law enforcement personnel Y35.311 ☑
            suspect Y35.313 ☑
            unspecified person Y35.319 ☑
      injuring
         bystander Y35.302 ☑
         law enforcement personnel Y35.301 ☑
         suspect Y35.303 ☑
         unspecified person Y35.309 ☑
      specified NEC
         injuring
            bystander Y35.392 ☑
            law enforcement personnel Y35.391 ☑
            suspect Y35.393 ☑
            unspecified person Y35.399 ☑
      stave
         injuring
            bystander Y35.392 ☑
            law enforcement personnel Y35.391 ☑
            suspect Y35.393 ☑
            unspecified person Y35.399 ☑
   bomb — *see* Legal, intervention, explosive
   conducted energy device
      injuring
         bystander Y35.832 ☑
         law enforcement personnel Y35.831 ☑
         suspect Y35.833 ☑
         unspecified person Y35.839 ☑
   cutting or piercing instrument — *see* Legal, intervention, sharp object
   dynamite — *see* Legal, intervention, explosive, dynamite
   electroshock device (taser)
      injuring
         bystander Y35.832 ☑
         law enforcement personnel Y35.831 ☑
         suspect Y35.833 ☑
         unspecified person Y35.839 ☑

Legal — *continued*

intervention — *continued*
   explosive(s)
      dynamite
         injuring
            bystander Y35.112 ☑
            law enforcement personnel Y35.111 ☑
            suspect Y35.113 ☑
            unspecified person Y35.119 ☑
      grenade
         injuring
            bystander Y35.192 ☑
            law enforcement personnel Y35.191 ☑
            suspect Y35.193 ☑
            unspecified person Y35.199 ☑
      injuring
         bystander Y35.102 ☑
         law enforcement personnel Y35.101 ☑
         suspect Y35.103 ☑
         unspecified person Y35.109 ☑
      mortar bomb
         injuring
            bystander Y35.192 ☑
            law enforcement personnel Y35.191 ☑
            suspect Y35.193 ☑
            unspecified person Y35.199 ☑
      shell
         injuring
            bystander Y35.122 ☑
            law enforcement personnel Y35.121 ☑
            suspect Y35.123 ☑
            unspecified person Y35.129 ☑
      specified NEC
         injuring
            bystander Y35.192 ☑
            law enforcement personnel Y35.191 ☑
            suspect Y35.193 ☑
            unspecified person Y35.199 ☑
   firearm(s) (discharge)
      handgun
         injuring
            bystander Y35.022 ☑
            law enforcement personnel Y35.021 ☑
            suspect Y35.023 ☑
            unspecified person Y35.029 ☑
      injuring
         bystander Y35.002 ☑
         law enforcement personnel Y35.001 ☑
         suspect Y35.003 ☑
         unspecified person Y35.009 ☑
      machine gun
         injuring
            bystander Y35.012 ☑
            law enforcement personnel Y35.011 ☑
            suspect Y35.013 ☑
            unspecified person Y35.019 ☑
      rifle pellet
         injuring
            bystander Y35.032 ☑
            law enforcement personnel Y35.031 ☑
            suspect Y35.033 ☑
            unspecified person Y35.039 ☑
      rubber bullet
         injuring
            bystander Y35.042 ☑
            law enforcement personnel Y35.041 ☑
            suspect Y35.043 ☑
            unspecified person Y35.049 ☑
      shotgun — *see* Legal, intervention, firearm, specified NEC
      specified NEC
         injuring
            bystander Y35.092 ☑
            law enforcement personnel Y35.091 ☑
            suspect Y35.093 ☑
            unspecified person Y35.099 ☑
   gas (asphyxiation) (poisoning)
      injuring
         bystander Y35.202 ☑
         law enforcement personnel Y35.201 ☑
         suspect Y35.203 ☑
         unspecified person Y35.209 ☑
      specified NEC
         injuring
            bystander Y35.292 ☑
            law enforcement personnel Y35.291 ☑
            suspect Y35.293 ☑

Legal — continued
  intervention — continued
    gas — continued
      specified — continued
        injuring — continued
          unspecified person Y35.299 ☑
      tear gas
        injuring
          bystander Y35.212 ☑
          law enforcement personnel Y35.211 ☑
          suspect Y35.213 ☑
          unspecified person Y35.219 ☑
    grenade — see Legal, intervention, explosive, grenade
    injuring
      bystander Y35.92 ☑
      law enforcement personnel Y35.91 ☑
      suspect Y35.93 ☑
      unspecified person Y35.99 ☑
    late effect (of) — see with 7th character S Y35 ☑
    manhandling
      injuring
        bystander Y35.812 ☑
        law enforcement personnel Y35.811 ☑
        suspect Y35.813 ☑
        unspecified person Y35.819 ☑
    sequelae (of) — see with 7th character S Y35 ☑
    sharp objects
      bayonet
        injuring
          bystander Y35.412 ☑
          law enforcement personnel Y35.411 ☑
          suspect Y35.413 ☑
          unspecified person Y35.419 ☑
      injuring
        bystander Y35.402 ☑
        law enforcement personnel Y35.401 ☑
        suspect Y35.403 ☑
        unspecified person Y35.409 ☑
      specified NEC
        injuring
          bystander Y35.492 ☑
          law enforcement personnel Y35.491 ☑
          suspect Y35.493 ☑
          unspecified person Y35.499 ☑
    specified means NEC
      injuring
        bystander Y35.892 ☑
        law enforcement personnel Y35.891 ☑
        suspect Y35.893 ☑
    stabbing — see Legal, intervention, sharp object
    stave — see Legal, intervention, blunt object, stave
    stun gun
      injuring
        bystander Y35.832 ☑
        law enforcement personnel Y35.831 ☑
        suspect Y35.833 ☑
        unspecified person Y35.839 ☑
    taser
      injuring
        bystander Y35.832 ☑
        law enforcement personnel Y35.831 ☑
        suspect Y35.833 ☑
        unspecified person Y35.839 ☑
    tear gas — see Legal, intervention, gas, tear gas
    truncheon — see Legal, intervention, blunt object, stave

Lifting — see also Overexertion
  heavy objects X50.0 ☑
  weights X50.0 ☑
Lightning (shock) (stroke) (struck by) — see subcategory T75.0 ☑
  causing fire — see Exposure, fire
Loss of control (transport vehicle) NEC — see Accident, transport
Lost at sea NOS — see Drowning, due to, fall overboard
Low
  pressure (effects) — see Air, pressure, low
  temperature (effects) — see Exposure, cold
Lying before train, vehicle or other moving object X81.8 ☑
  subway train X81.1 ☑
  train X81.1 ☑
  undetermined whether accidental or intentional Y31 ☑
Lynching — see Assault

M

Malfunction (mechanism or component) (of)
  firearm W34.10 ☑
    airgun W34.110 ☑
    BB gun W34.110 ☑
    gas, air or spring-operated gun NEC W34.118 ☑
    handgun W32.1 ☑
    hunting rifle W33.12 ☑
    larger firearm W33.10 ☑
      specified NEC W33.19 ☑
    machine gun W33.13 ☑
    paintball gun W34.111 ☑
    pellet gun W34.110 ☑
    shotgun W33.11 ☑
    specified NEC W34.19 ☑
    Very pistol [flare] W34.19 ☑
  handgun — see Malfunction, firearm, handgun
Maltreatment — see Perpetrator
Mangled (accidentally) NOS X58 ☑
Manhandling (in brawl, fight) Y04.0 ☑
  legal intervention — see Legal, intervention, manhandling
Manslaughter (nonaccidental) — see Assault
Mauled by animal NEC W55.89 ☑
Medical procedure, complication of (delayed or as an abnormal reaction without mention of misadventure) — see Complication of or following, by specified type of procedure
  due to or as a result of misadventure — see Misadventure
Melting (due to fire) — see also Exposure, fire
  apparel NEC X06.3 ☑
  clothes, clothing NEC X06.3 ☑
    nightwear X05 ☑
  fittings or furniture (burning building) (uncontrolled fire) X00.8 ☑
  nightwear X05 ☑
  plastic jewelry X06.1 ☑
Mental cruelty X58 ☑
Military operations (injuries to military and civilians occuring during peacetime on military property and during routine military exercises and operations) (by) (from) (involving) Y37.90- ☑
  air blast Y37.20- ☑
  aircraft
    destruction — see Military operations, destruction of aircraft
    airway restriction — see Military operations, restriction of airways
    asphyxiation — see Military operations, restriction of airways
  biological weapons Y37.6X- ☑
  blast Y37.20- ☑
  blast fragments Y37.20- ☑
  blast wave Y37.20- ☑
  blast wind Y37.20- ☑
  bomb Y37.20- ☑
    dirty Y37.50- ☑
    gasoline Y37.31- ☑
    incendiary Y37.31- ☑
    petrol Y37.31- ☑
  bullet Y37.43- ☑
    incendiary Y37.32- ☑
    rubber Y37.41- ☑
  chemical weapons Y37.7X- ☑
  combat
    hand to hand (unarmed) combat Y37.44- ☑
    using blunt or piercing object Y37.45- ☑
  conflagration — see Military operations, fire
  conventional warfare NEC Y37.49- ☑
  depth-charge Y37.01- ☑
  destruction of aircraft Y37.10- ☑
    due to
      air to air missile Y37.11- ☑
      collision with other aircraft Y37.12- ☑
      detonation (accidental) of onboard munitions and explosives Y37.14- ☑
      enemy fire or explosives Y37.11- ☑
      explosive placed on aircraft Y37.11- ☑
      onboard fire Y37.13- ☑
      rocket propelled grenade [RPG] Y37.11- ☑
      small arms fire Y37.11- ☑
      surface to air missile Y37.11- ☑
    specified NEC Y37.19- ☑

Military operations — continued
  detonation (accidental) of
    onboard marine weapons Y37.05- ☑
    own munitions or munitions launch device Y37.24- ☑
  dirty bomb Y37.50- ☑
  explosion (of) Y37.20- ☑
    aerial bomb Y37.21- ☑
    bomb NOS — see also Military operations, bomb(s) Y37.20- ☑
    fragments Y37.20- ☑
    grenade Y37.29- ☑
    guided missile Y37.22- ☑
    improvised explosive device [IED] (person-borne) (roadside) (vehicle-borne) Y37.23- ☑
    land mine Y37.29- ☑
    marine mine (at sea) (in harbor) Y37.02- ☑
    marine weapon Y37.00- ☑
      specified NEC Y37.09- ☑
    own munitions or munitions launch device (accidental) Y37.24- ☑
    sea-based artillery shell Y37.03- ☑
    specified NEC Y37.29- ☑
    torpedo Y37.04- ☑
  fire Y37.30- ☑
    specified NEC Y37.39- ☑
  firearms
    discharge Y37.43- ☑
    pellets Y37.42- ☑
  flamethrower Y37.33- ☑
  fragments (from) (of)
    improvised explosive device [IED] (person-borne) (roadside) (vehicle-borne) Y37.26- ☑
    munitions Y37.25- ☑
    specified NEC Y37.29- ☑
    weapons Y37.27- ☑
  friendly fire Y37.92- ☑
  hand to hand (unarmed) combat Y37.44- ☑
  hot substances — see Military operations, fire
  incendiary bullet Y37.32- ☑
  nuclear weapon (effects of) Y37.50- ☑
    acute radiation exposure Y37.54- ☑
    blast pressure Y37.51- ☑
    direct blast Y37.51- ☑
    direct heat Y37.53- ☑
    fallout exposure Y37.54- ☑
    fireball Y37.53- ☑
    indirect blast (struck or crushed by blast debris) (being thrown by blast) Y37.52- ☑
    ionizing radiation (immediate exposure) Y37.54- ☑
    nuclear radiation Y37.54- ☑
    radiation
      ionizing (immediate exposure) Y37.54- ☑
      nuclear Y37.54- ☑
      thermal Y37.53- ☑
    secondary effects Y37.54- ☑
    specified NEC Y37.59- ☑
    thermal radiation Y37.53- ☑
  restriction of air (airway)
    intentional Y37.46- ☑
    unintentional Y37.47- ☑
  rubber bullets Y37.41- ☑
  shrapnel NOS Y37.29- ☑
  suffocation — see Military operations, restriction of airways
  unconventional warfare NEC Y37.7X- ☑
  underwater blast NOS Y37.00- ☑
  warfare
    conventional NEC Y37.49- ☑
    unconventional NEC Y37.7X- ☑
  weapon of mass destruction [WMD] Y37.91- ☑
  weapons
    biological weapons Y37.6X- ☑
    chemical Y37.7X- ☑
    nuclear (effects of) Y37.50- ☑
      acute radiation exposure Y37.54- ☑
      blast pressure Y37.51- ☑
      direct blast Y37.51- ☑
      direct heat Y37.53- ☑
      fallout exposure Y37.54- ☑
      fireball Y37.53- ☑
      radiation
        ionizing (immediate exposure) Y37.54- ☑
        nuclear Y37.54- ☑
        thermal Y37.53- ☑
      secondary effects Y37.54- ☑

☑ **Additional Character Required** — Refer to the Tabular List for Character Selection

▽ **Subterms under main terms may continue to next column or page**

Military operations — *continued*
  weapons — *continued*
    nuclear — *continued*
      specified NEC Y37.59- ☑
    of mass destruction [WMD] Y37.91- ☑
Misadventure(s) to patient(s) during surgical or medical care Y69
  contaminated medical or biological substance (blood, drug, fluid) Y64.9
    administered (by) NEC Y64.9
      immunization Y64.1
      infusion Y64.0
      injection Y64.1
      specified means NEC Y64.8
      transfusion Y64.0
      vaccination Y64.1
  excessive amount of blood or other fluid during transfusion or infusion Y63.0
  failure
    in dosage Y63.9
      electroshock therapy Y63.4
      inappropriate temperature (too hot or too cold) in local application and packing Y63.5
      infusion
        excessive amount of fluid Y63.0
        incorrect dilution of fluid Y63.1
      insulin-shock therapy Y63.4
      nonadministration of necessary drug or biological substance Y63.6
      overdose — *see* Table of Drugs and Chemicals
        radiation, in therapy Y63.2
      radiation
        overdose Y63.2
      specified procedure NEC Y63.8
      transfusion
        excessive amount of blood Y63.0
  mechanical, of instrument or apparatus (any) (during any procedure) Y65.8
  sterile precautions (during procedure) Y62.9
    aspiration of fluid or tissue (by puncture or catheterization, except heart) Y62.6
    biopsy (except needle aspiration) Y62.8
      needle (aspirating) Y62.6
    blood sampling Y62.6
    catheterization Y62.6
      heart Y62.5
    dialysis (kidney) Y62.2
    endoscopic examination Y62.4
    enema Y62.8
    immunization Y62.3
    infusion Y62.1
    injection Y62.3
    needle biopsy Y62.6
    paracentesis (abdominal) (thoracic) Y62.6
    perfusion Y62.2
    puncture (lumbar) Y62.6
    removal of catheter or packing Y62.8
    specified procedure NEC Y62.8
    surgical operation Y62.0
    transfusion Y62.1
    vaccination Y62.3
  suture or ligature during surgical procedure Y65.2
  to introduce or to remove tube or instrument — *see* Failure, to
  hemorrhage — *see* Index to Diseases and Injuries, Complication(s)
  inadvertent exposure of patient to radiation Y63.3
  inappropriate
    operation performed — *see* Inappropriate operation performed
    temperature (too hot or too cold) in local application or packing Y63.5
  infusion — *see also* Misadventure, by type, infusion Y69
    excessive amount of fluid Y63.0
    incorrect dilution of fluid Y63.1
    wrong fluid Y65.1
  mismatched blood in transfusion Y65.0
  nonadministration of necessary drug or biological substance Y63.6
  overdose — *see* Table of Drugs and Chemicals
    radiation (in therapy) Y63.2
  perforation — *see* Index to Diseases and Injuries, Complication(s)
  performance of inappropriate operation — *see* Inappropriate operation performed
  puncture — *see* Index to Diseases and Injuries, Complication(s)

Misadventure(s) to patient(s) during surgical or medical care — *continued*
  specified type NEC Y65.8
    failure
      suture or ligature during surgical operation Y65.2
      to introduce or to remove tube or instrument — *see* Failure, to
    infusion of wrong fluid Y65.1
    performance of inappropriate operation — *see* Inappropriate operation performed
    transfusion of mismatched blood Y65.0
    wrong
      fluid in infusion Y65.1
      placement of endotracheal tube during anesthetic procedure Y65.3
  transfusion — *see* Misadventure, by type, transfusion
    excessive amount of blood Y63.0
    mismatched blood Y65.0
  wrong
    drug given in error — *see* Table of Drugs and Chemicals
    fluid in infusion Y65.1
    placement of endotracheal tube during anesthetic procedure Y65.3
Mismatched blood in transfusion Y65.0
Motion sickness T75.3 ☑
Mountain sickness W94.11 ☑
Mudslide (of cataclysmic nature) — *see* Landslide
Murder (attempt) — *see* Assault

N

Nail
  contact with W45.0 ☑
    gun W29.4 ☑
  embedded in skin W45.0 ☑
Neglect (criminal) (homicidal intent) X58 ☑
Noise (causing injury) (pollution) W42.9 ☑
  supersonic W42.0 ☑
Nonadministration (of)
  drug or biological substance (necessary) Y63.6
  surgical and medical care Y66
Nosocomial condition Y95

O

Object
  falling
    from, in, on, hitting
      machinery — *see* Contact, with, by type of machine
    set in motion by
      accidental explosion or rupture of pressure vessel W38 ☑
      firearm — *see* Discharge, firearm, by type
      machine(ry) — *see* Contact, with, by type of machine
Overdose (drug) — *see* Table of Drugs and Chemicals
  radiation Y63.2
Overexertion X50.9 ☑
  from
    prolonged static or awkward postures X50.1 ☑
    repetitive movements X50.3 ☑
    specified strenuous movements or postures NEC X50.9 ☑
    strenuous movement or load X50.0 ☑
Overexposure (accidental) (to)
  cold — *see also* Exposure, cold X31 ☑
    due to man-made conditions — *see* Exposure, cold, man-made
  heat — *see also* Heat X30 ☑
  radiation — *see* Radiation
  radioactivity W88.0 ☑
  sun (sunburn) X32 ☑
  weather NEC — *see* Forces of nature
  wind NEC — *see* Forces of nature
Overheated — *see* Heat
Overturning (accidental)
  machinery — *see* Contact, with, by type of machine
  transport vehicle NEC — *see also* Accident, transport V89.9 ☑
  watercraft (causing drowning, submersion) — *see also* Drowning, due to, accident to, watercraft, overturning
    causing injury except drowning or submersion — *see* Accident, watercraft, causing, injury NEC

P

Parachute descent (voluntary) (without accident to aircraft) V97.29 ☑
  due to accident to aircraft — *see* Accident, transport, aircraft
Pecked by bird W61.99 ☑
Perforation during medical or surgical treatment as misadventure — *see* Index to Diseases and Injuries, Complication(s)
Perpetrator, perpetration, of assault, maltreatment and neglect (by) Y07.9
  boyfriend Y07.03
  brother Y07.410
    stepbrother Y07.435
  coach Y07.53
  cousin
    female Y07.491
    male Y07.490
  daycare provider Y07.519
    at-home
      adult care Y07.512
      childcare Y07.510
    care center
      adult care Y07.513
      childcare Y07.511
  family member NEC Y07.499
  father Y07.11
    adoptive Y07.13
    foster Y07.420
    stepfather Y07.430
  foster father Y07.420
  foster mother Y07.421
  girl friend Y07.04
  healthcare provider Y07.529
    mental health Y07.521
    specified NEC Y07.528
  husband Y07.01
  instructor Y07.53
  mother Y07.12
    adoptive Y07.14
    foster Y07.421
    stepmother Y07.433
  multiple perpetrators Y07.6
  nonfamily member Y07.50
    specified NEC Y07.59
  nurse Y07.528
  occupational therapist Y07.528
  partner of parent
    female Y07.434
    male Y07.432
  physical therapist Y07.528
  sister Y07.411
  speech therapist Y07.528
  stepbrother Y07.435
  stepfather Y07.430
  stepmother Y07.433
  stepsister Y07.436
  teacher Y07.53
  wife Y07.02
Piercing — *see* Contact, with, by type of object or machine
Pinched
  between objects (moving) (stationary and moving) W23.0 ☑
  stationary W23.1 ☑
Pinned under machine(ry) — *see* Contact, with, by type of machine
Place of occurrence Y92.9
  abandoned house Y92.89
  airplane Y92.813
  airport Y92.520
  ambulatory health services establishment NEC Y92.538
  ambulatory surgery center Y92.530
  amusement park Y92.831
  apartment (co-op) — *see* Place of occurrence, residence, apartment
  assembly hall Y92.29
  bank Y92.510
  barn Y92.71
  baseball field Y92.320
  basketball court Y92.310
  beach Y92.832
  boarding house — *see* Place of occurrence, residence, boarding house
  boat Y92.814
  bowling alley Y92.39

Place of occurrence — *continued*
- bridge Y92.89
- building under construction Y92.61
- bus Y92.811
  - station Y92.521
- cafe Y92.511
- campsite Y92.833
- campus — *see* Place of occurrence, school
- canal Y92.89
- car Y92.810
- casino Y92.59
- children's home — *see* Place of occurrence, residence, institutional, orphanage
- church Y92.22
- cinema Y92.26
- clubhouse Y92.29
- coal pit Y92.64
- college (community) Y92.214
- condominium — *see* Place of occurrence, residence, apartment
- construction area — *see* Place of occurrence, industrial and construction area
- convalescent home — *see* Place of occurrence, residence, institutional, nursing home
- court-house Y92.240
- cricket ground Y92.328
- cultural building Y92.258
  - art gallery Y92.250
  - museum Y92.251
  - music hall Y92.252
  - opera house Y92.253
  - specified NEC Y92.258
  - theater Y92.254
- dancehall Y92.252
- day nursery Y92.210
- dentist office Y92.531
- derelict house Y92.89
- desert Y92.820
- dockyard Y92.62
- dock NOS Y92.89
- doctor's office Y92.531
- dormitory — *see* Place of occurrence, residence, institutional, school dormitory
- dry dock Y92.62
- factory (building) (premises) Y92.63
- farm (land under cultivation) (outbuildings) Y92.79
  - barn Y92.71
  - chicken coop Y92.72
  - field Y92.73
  - hen house Y92.72
  - house — *see* Place of occurrence, residence, house
  - orchard Y92.74
  - specified NEC Y92.79
- football field Y92.321
- forest Y92.821
- freeway Y92.411
- gallery Y92.250
- garage (commercial) Y92.59
  - boarding house Y92.044
  - military base Y92.135
  - mobile home Y92.025
  - nursing home Y92.124
  - orphanage Y92.114
  - private house Y92.015
  - reform school Y92.155
- gas station Y92.524
- gasworks Y92.69
- golf course Y92.39
- gravel pit Y92.64
- grocery Y92.512
- gymnasium Y92.39
- handball court Y92.318
- harbor Y92.89
- harness racing course Y92.39
- healthcare provider office Y92.531
- highway (interstate) Y92.411
- hill Y92.828
- hockey rink Y92.330
- home — *see* Place of occurrence, residence
- hospice — *see* Place of occurrence, residence, institutional, nursing home
- hospital Y92.239
  - cafeteria Y92.233
  - corridor Y92.232
  - operating room Y92.234
  - patient
    - bathroom Y92.231
    - room Y92.230

Place of occurrence — *continued*
- hospital — *continued*
  - specified NEC Y92.238
- hotel Y92.59
- house — *see also* Place of occurrence, residence
  - abandoned Y92.89
  - under construction Y92.61
- industrial and construction area (yard) Y92.69
  - building under construction Y92.61
  - dock Y92.62
  - dry dock Y92.62
  - factory Y92.63
  - gasworks Y92.69
  - mine Y92.64
  - oil rig Y92.65
  - pit Y92.64
  - power station Y92.69
  - shipyard Y92.62
  - specified NEC Y92.69
  - tunnel under construction Y92.69
  - workshop Y92.69
- kindergarten Y92.211
- lacrosse field Y92.328
- lake Y92.828
- library Y92.241
- mall Y92.59
- market Y92.512
- marsh Y92.828
- military
  - base — *see* Place of occurrence, residence, institutional, military base
  - training ground Y92.84
- mine Y92.64
- mosque Y92.22
- motel Y92.59
- motorway (interstate) Y92.411
- mountain Y92.828
- movie-house Y92.26
- museum Y92.251
- music-hall Y92.252
- not applicable Y92.9
- nuclear power station Y92.69
- nursing home — *see* Place of occurrence, residence, institutional, nursing home
- office building Y92.59
- offshore installation Y92.65
- oil rig Y92.65
- old people's home — *see* Place of occurrence, residence, institutional, specified NEC
- opera-house Y92.253
- orphanage — *see* Place of occurrence, residence, institutional, orphanage
- outpatient surgery center Y92.530
- park (public) Y92.830
  - amusement Y92.831
- parking garage Y92.89
  - lot Y92.481
- pavement Y92.480
- physician office Y92.531
- polo field Y92.328
- pond Y92.828
- post office Y92.242
- power station Y92.69
- prairie Y92.828
- prison — *see* Place of occurrence, residence, institutional, prison
- public
  - administration building Y92.248
    - city hall Y92.243
    - courthouse Y92.240
    - library Y92.241
    - post office Y92.242
    - specified NEC Y92.248
  - building NEC Y92.29
  - hall Y92.29
  - place NOS Y92.89
- race course Y92.39
- radio station Y92.59
- railway line (bridge) Y92.85
- ranch (outbuildings) — *see* Place of occurrence, farm
- recreation area Y92.838
  - amusement park Y92.831
  - beach Y92.832
  - campsite Y92.833
  - park (public) Y92.830
  - seashore Y92.832
  - specified NEC Y92.838

Place of occurrence — *continued*
- reform school - — *see* Place of occurrence, residence, institutional, reform school
- religious institution Y92.22
- residence (non-institutional) (private) Y92.009
  - apartment Y92.039
    - bathroom Y92.031
    - bedroom Y92.032
    - kitchen Y92.030
    - specified NEC Y92.038
  - bathroom Y92.002
  - bedroom Y92.003
  - boarding house Y92.049
    - bathroom Y92.041
    - bedroom Y92.042
    - driveway Y92.043
    - garage Y92.044
    - garden Y92.046
    - kitchen Y92.040
    - specified NEC Y92.048
    - swimming pool Y92.045
    - yard Y92.046
  - dining room Y92.001
  - garden Y92.007
  - home Y92.009
  - house, single family Y92.019
    - bathroom Y92.012
    - bedroom Y92.013
    - dining room Y92.011
    - driveway Y92.014
    - garage Y92.015
    - garden Y92.017
    - kitchen Y92.010
    - specified NEC Y92.018
    - swimming pool Y92.016
    - yard Y92.017
  - institutional Y92.10
    - children's home — *see* Place of occurrence, residence, institutional, orphanage
    - hospice — *see* Place of occurrence, residence, institutional, nursing home
    - military base Y92.139
      - barracks Y92.133
      - garage Y92.135
      - garden Y92.137
      - kitchen Y92.130
      - mess hall Y92.131
      - specified NEC Y92.138
      - swimming pool Y92.136
      - yard Y92.137
    - nursing home Y92.129
      - bathroom Y92.121
      - bedroom Y92.122
      - driveway Y92.123
      - garage Y92.124
      - garden Y92.126
      - kitchen Y92.120
      - specified NEC Y92.128
      - swimming pool Y92.125
      - yard Y92.126
    - orphanage Y92.119
      - bathroom Y92.111
      - bedroom Y92.112
      - driveway Y92.113
      - garage Y92.114
      - garden Y92.116
      - kitchen Y92.110
      - specified NEC Y92.118
      - swimming pool Y92.115
      - yard Y92.116
    - prison Y92.149
      - bathroom Y92.142
      - cell Y92.143
      - courtyard Y92.147
      - dining room Y92.141
      - kitchen Y92.140
      - specified NEC Y92.148
      - swimming pool Y92.146
    - reform school Y92.159
      - bathroom Y92.152
      - bedroom Y92.153
      - dining room Y92.151
      - driveway Y92.154
      - garage Y92.155
      - garden Y92.157
      - kitchen Y92.150
      - specified NEC Y92.158
      - swimming pool Y92.156
      - yard Y92.157

☑ **Additional Character Required** — Refer to the Tabular List for Character Selection   ▽ Subterms under main terms may continue to next column or page

Place of occurrence — *continued*
  residence — *continued*
    institutional — *continued*
      school dormitory Y92.169
        bathroom Y92.162
        bedroom Y92.163
        dining room Y92.161
        kitchen Y92.160
        specified NEC Y92.168
      specified NEC Y92.199
        bathroom Y92.192
        bedroom Y92.193
        dining room Y92.191
        driveway Y92.194
        garage Y92.195
        garden Y92.197
        kitchen Y92.190
        specified NEC Y92.198
        swimming pool Y92.196
        yard Y92.197
    kitchen Y92.000
    mobile home Y92.029
      bathroom Y92.022
      bedroom Y92.023
      dining room Y92.021
      driveway Y92.024
      garage Y92.025
      garden Y92.027
      kitchen Y92.020
      specified NEC Y92.028
      swimming pool Y92.026
      yard Y92.027
    specified place in residence NEC Y92.008
    specified residence type NEC Y92.099
      bathroom Y92.091
      bedroom Y92.092
      driveway Y92.093
      garage Y92.094
      garden Y92.096
      kitchen Y92.090
      specified NEC Y92.098
      swimming pool Y92.095
      yard Y92.096
  restaurant Y92.511
  riding school Y92.39
  river Y92.828
  road Y92.410
  rodeo ring Y92.39
  rugby field Y92.328
  same day surgery center Y92.530
  sand pit Y92.64
  school (private) (public) (state) Y92.219
    college Y92.214
    daycare center Y92.210
    elementary school Y92.211
    high school Y92.213
    kindergarten Y92.211
    middle school Y92.212
    specified NEC Y92.218
    trace school Y92.215
    university Y92.214
    vocational school Y92.215
  sea (shore) Y92.832
  senior citizen center Y92.29
  service area
    airport Y92.520
    bus station Y92.521
    gas station Y92.524
    highway rest stop Y92.523
    railway station Y92.522
  shipyard Y92.62
  shop (commercial) Y92.513
  sidewalk Y92.480
  silo Y92.79
  skating rink (roller) Y92.331
    ice Y92.330
  slaughter house Y92.86
  soccer field Y92.322
  specified place NEC Y92.89
  sports area Y92.39
    athletic
      court Y92.318
        basketball Y92.310
        specified NEC Y92.318
        squash Y92.311
        tennis Y92.312
      field Y92.328
        baseball Y92.320
        cricket ground Y92.328

Place of occurrence — *continued*
  sports area — *continued*
    athletic — *continued*
      field — *continued*
        football Y92.321
        hockey Y92.328
        soccer Y92.322
        specified NEC Y92.328
    golf course Y92.39
    gymnasium Y92.39
    riding school Y92.39
    skating rink (roller) Y92.331
      ice Y92.330
    stadium Y92.39
    swimming pool Y92.34
  squash court Y92.311
  stadium Y92.39
  steeplechasing course Y92.39
  store Y92.512
  stream Y92.828
  street and highway Y92.410
    bike path Y92.482
    freeway Y92.411
    highway ramp Y92.415
    interstate highway Y92.411
    local residential or business street Y92.414
    motorway Y92.411
    parking lot Y92.481
    parkway Y92.412
    sidewalk Y92.480
    specified NEC Y92.488
    state road Y92.413
  subway car Y92.816
  supermarket Y92.512
  swamp Y92.828
  swimming pool (public) Y92.34
    private (at) Y92.095
      boarding house Y92.045
      military base Y92.136
      mobile home Y92.026
      nursing home Y92.125
      orphanage Y92.115
      prison Y92.146
      reform school Y92.156
      single family residence Y92.016
  synagogue Y92.22
  television station Y92.59
  tennis court Y92.312
  theater Y92.254
  trade area Y92.59
    bank Y92.510
    cafe Y92.511
    casino Y92.59
    garage Y92.59
    hotel Y92.59
    market Y92.512
    office building Y92.59
    radio station Y92.59
    restaurant Y92.511
    shop Y92.513
    shopping mall Y92.59
    store Y92.512
    supermarket Y92.512
    television station Y92.59
    warehouse Y92.59
  trailer park, residential — *see* Place of occurrence, residence, mobile home
  trailer site NOS Y92.89
  train Y92.815
    station Y92.522
  truck Y92.812
  tunnel under construction Y92.69
  university Y92.214
  urgent (health) care center Y92.532
  vehicle (transport) Y92.818
    airplane Y92.813
    boat Y92.814
    bus Y92.811
    car Y92.810
    specified NEC Y92.818
    subway car Y92.816
    train Y92.815
    truck Y92.812
  warehouse Y92.59
  water reservoir Y92.89
  wilderness area Y92.828
    desert Y92.820
    forest Y92.821
    marsh Y92.828

Place of occurrence — *continued*
  wilderness area — *continued*
    mountain Y92.828
    prairie Y92.828
    specified NEC Y92.828
    swamp Y92.828
  workshop Y92.69
  yard, private Y92.096
    boarding house Y92.046
    mobile home Y92.027
    single family house Y92.017
  youth center Y92.29
  zoo (zoological garden) Y92.834
Plumbism — *see* Table of Drugs and Chemicals, lead
Poisoning (accidental) (by) — *see also* Table of Drugs and Chemicals
  by plant, thorns, spines, sharp leaves or other mechanisms NEC X58 ☑
  carbon monoxide
    generated by
      motor vehicle — *see* Accident, transport
      watercraft (in transit) (not in transit) V93.89 ☑
        ferry boat V93.81 ☑
        fishing boat V93.82 ☑
        jet skis V93.83 ☑
        liner V93.81 ☑
        merchant ship V93.80 ☑
        passenger ship V93.81 ☑
        powered craft NEC V93.83 ☑
  caused by injection of poisons into skin by plant thorns, spines, sharp leaves X58 ☑
    marine or sea plants (venomous) X58 ☑
  execution — *see* Legal, intervention, gas
    intervention
      by gas — *see* Legal, intervention, gas
      other specified means — *see* Legal, intervention, specified means NEC
  exhaust gas
    generated by
      motor vehicle — *see* Accident, transport
      watercraft (in transit) (not in transit) V93.89 ☑
        ferry boat V93.81 ☑
        fishing boat V93.82 ☑
        jet skis V93.83 ☑
        liner V93.81 ☑
        merchant ship V93.80 ☑
        passenger ship V93.81 ☑
        powered craft NEC V93.83 ☑
  fumes or smoke due to
    explosion — *see also* Explosion W40.9 ☑
    fire — *see* Exposure, fire
    ignition — *see* Ignition
  gas
    in legal intervention — *see* Legal, intervention, gas
    legal execution — *see* Legal, intervention, gas
  in war operations — *see* War operations
  legal
Powder burn (by) (from)
  airgun W34.110 ☑
  BB gun W34.110 ☑
  firearm NEC W34.19 ☑
  gas, air or spring-operated gun NEC W34.118 ☑
  handgun W32.1 ☑
  hunting rifle W33.12 ☑
  larger firearm W33.10 ☑
    specified NEC W33.19 ☑
  machine gun W33.13 ☑
  paintball gun W34.111 ☑
  pellet gun W34.110 ☑
  shotgun W33.11 ☑
  Very pistol [flare] W34.19 ☑
Premature cessation (of) **surgical and medical care** Y66
Privation (food) (water) X58 ☑
Procedure (operation)
  correct, on wrong side or body part (wrong side) (wrong site) Y65.53
  intended for another patient done on wrong patient Y65.52
  performed on patient not scheduled for surgery Y65.52
  performed on wrong patient Y65.52
  wrong, performed on correct patient Y65.51
Prolonged
  sitting in transport vehicle — *see* Travel, by type of vehicle

Prolonged — continued
stay in
high altitude as cause of anoxia, barodontalgia,
barotitis or hypoxia W94.11 ☑
weightless environment X52 ☑
Pulling, excessive — see also Overexertion X50.9- ☑
Puncture, puncturing — see also Contact, with, by type
of object or machine
by
plant thorns, spines, sharp leaves or other mechanisms NEC W60 ☑
during medical or surgical treatment as misadventure
— see Index to Diseases and Injuries, Complica-
tion(s)
Pushed, pushing (accidental) (injury in)
by other person(s) (accidental) W51 ☑
as, or caused by, a crowd or human stampede (with
fall) W52 ☑
before moving object NEC Y02.8 ☑
motor vehicle Y02.0 ☑
subway train Y02.1 ☑
train Y02.1 ☑
from
high place NEC
in accidental circumstances W17.89 ☑
stated as
intentional, homicide (attempt) Y01 ☑
undetermined whether accidental or intentional Y30 ☑
transport vehicle NEC — see also Accident,
transport V89.9 ☑
stated as
intentional, homicide (attempt) Y08.89 ☑
with fall W03 ☑
due to ice or snow W00.0 ☑
overexertion X50.9 ☑

R

Radiation (exposure to)
arc lamps W89.0 ☑
atomic power plant (malfunction) NEC W88.1 ☑
complication of or abnormal reaction to medical radiotherapy Y84.2
electromagnetic, ionizing W88.0 ☑
gamma rays W88.1 ☑
in
war operations (from or following nuclear explosion)
— see War operations
inadvertent exposure of patient (receiving test or
therapy) Y63.3
infrared (heaters and lamps) W90.1 ☑
excessive heat from W92 ☑
ionized, ionizing (particles, artificially accelerated)
radioisotopes W88.1 ☑
specified NEC W88.8 ☑
x-rays W88.0 ☑
isotopes, radioactive — see Radiation, radioactive isotopes
laser(s) W90.2 ☑
in war operations — see War operations
misadventure in medical care Y63.2
light sources (man-made visible and ultraviolet)
W89.9 ☑
natural X32 ☑
specified NEC W89.8 ☑
tanning bed W89.1 ☑
welding light W89.0 ☑
man-made visible light W89.9 ☑
specified NEC W89.8 ☑
tanning bed W89.1 ☑
welding light W89.0 ☑
microwave W90.8 ☑
misadventure in medical or surgical procedure Y63.2
natural NEC X39.08 ☑
radon X39.01 ☑
overdose (in medical or surgical procedure) Y63.2
radar W90.0 ☑
radioactive isotopes (any) W88.1 ☑
atomic power plant malfunction W88.1 ☑
misadventure in medical or surgical treatment Y63.2
radiofrequency W90.0 ☑
radium NEC W88.1 ☑
sun X32 ☑
ultraviolet (light) (man-made) W89.9 ☑
natural X32 ☑

Radiation — continued
ultraviolet — continued
specified NEC W89.8 ☑
tanning bed W89.1 ☑
welding light W89.0 ☑
welding arc, torch, or light W89.0 ☑
excessive heat from W92 ☑
x-rays (hard) (soft) W88.0 ☑
Range disease W94.11 ☑
Rape (attempted) T74.2- ☑
Rat bite W53.11 ☑
Reaching (prolonged) (static) X50.1 ☑
Reaction, abnormal to medical procedure — see also
Complication of or following, by type of procedure
Y84.9
biologicals — see Table of Drugs and Chemicals
drugs — see Table of Drugs and Chemicals
vaccine — see Table of Drugs and Chemicals
with misadventure — see Misadventure
Recoil
airgun W34.110 ☑
BB gun W34.110 ☑
firearm NEC W34.19 ☑
gas, air or spring-operated gun NEC W34.118 ☑
handgun W32.1 ☑
hunting rifle W33.12 ☑
larger firearm W33.10 ☑
specified NEC W33.19 ☑
machine gun W33.13 ☑
paintball gun W34.111 ☑
pellet W34.110 ☑
shotgun W33.11 ☑
Very pistol [flare] W34.19 ☑
Reduction in
atmospheric pressure — see Air, pressure, change
Rock falling on or hitting (accidentally) (person)
W20.8 ☑
in cave-in W20.0 ☑
Run over (accidentally) (by)
animal (not being ridden) NEC W55.89 ☑
machinery — see Contact, with, by specified type of
machine
transport vehicle NEC — see also Accident, transport
V09.9 ☑
intentional homicide (attempt) Y03.0 ☑
motor NEC V09.20 ☑
intentional homicide (attempt) Y03.0 ☑
Running
before moving object X81.8 ☑
motor vehicle X81.0 ☑
Running off, away
animal (being ridden) — see also Accident, transport
V80.918 ☑
not being ridden W55.89 ☑
animal-drawn vehicle NEC — see also Accident, transport V80.928 ☑
highway, road(way), street
transport vehicle NEC — see also Accident, transport
V89.9 ☑
Rupture pressurized devices — see Explosion, by type
of device

S

Saturnism — see Table of Drugs and Chemicals, lead
Scald, scalding (accidental) (by) (from) (in) X19 ☑
air (hot) X14.1 ☑
gases (hot) X14.1 ☑
homicide (attempt) — see Assault, burning, hot object
inflicted by other person
stated as intentional, homicide (attempt) — see
Assault, burning, hot object
liquid (boiling) (hot) NEC X12 ☑
stated as undetermined whether accidental or intentional Y27.2 ☑
suicide (attempt) X77.2 ☑
local application of externally applied substance in
medical or surgical care Y63.5
metal (molten) (liquid) (hot) NEC X18 ☑
self-inflicted X77.9 ☑
stated as undetermined whether accidental or intentional Y27.8 ☑
steam X13.1 ☑
assault X98.0 ☑
stated as undetermined whether accidental or intentional Y27.0 ☑

Scald, scalding — continued
steam — continued
suicide (attempt) X77.0 ☑
suicide (attempt) X77.9 ☑
vapor (hot) X13.1 ☑
assault X98.0 ☑
stated as undetermined whether accidental or inte
tional Y27.0 ☑
suicide (attempt) X77.0 ☑
Scratched by
cat W55.03 ☑
person(s) (accidentally) W50.4 ☑
with intent to injure or kill Y04.0 ☑
as, or caused by, a crowd or human stampede (wi
fall) W52 ☑
assault Y04.0 ☑
homicide (attempt) Y04.0 ☑
in
fight Y04.0 ☑
legal intervention
injuring
bystander Y35.892 ☑
law enforcement personnel Y35.891 ☑
suspect Y35.893 ☑
Seasickness T75.3 ☑
Self-harm NEC — see also External cause by type, und
termined whether accidental or intentional
intentional — see Suicide
poisoning NEC — see Table of Drugs and Chemicals
poisoning, accidental
Self-inflicted (injury) **NEC** — see also External cause b
type, undetermined whether accidental or intentio
al
intentional — see Suicide
poisoning NEC — see Table of Drugs and Chemicals
poisoning, accidental
Sequelae (of)
accident NEC — see W00-X58 with 7th character S
assault (homicidal) (any means) — see X92-Y08 wit
7th character S
homicide, attempt (any means) — see X92-Y08 with
7th character S
injury undetermined whether accidentally or purpose
inflicted — see Y21-Y33 with 7th character S
intentional self-harm (classifiable to X71-X83) — se
X71-X83 with 7th character S
legal intervention — see with 7th character S Y35 ☑
motor vehicle accident — see V00-V99 with 7th cha
acter S
suicide, attempt (any means) — see X71-X83 with 7
character S
transport accident — see V00-V99 with 7th characte
S
war operations — see War operations
Shock
electric — see Exposure, electric current
from electric appliance (any) (faulty) W86.8 ☑
domestic W86.0 ☑
suicide (attempt) X83.1 ☑
Shooting, shot (accidental(ly)) — see also Discharge,
firearm, by type
herself or himself — see Discharge, firearm by type,
self-inflicted
homicide (attempt) — see Discharge, firearm by typ
homicide
in war operations — see War operations
inflicted by other person — see Discharge, firearm b
type, homicide
accidental — see Discharge, firearm, by type of
firearm
legal
execution — see Legal, intervention, firearm
intervention — see Legal, intervention, firearm
self-inflicted — see Discharge, firearm by type, suici
accidental — see Discharge, firearm, by type of
firearm
suicide (attempt) — see Discharge, firearm by type,
suicide
Shoving (accidentally) **by other person** — see Pushe
by other person
Sickness
alpine W94.11 ☑
motion — see Motion
mountain W94.11 ☑
Sinking (accidental)
watercraft (causing drowning, submersion) — see al
Drowning, due to, accident to, watercraft, sinkin

428
☑ Additional Character Required — Refer to the Tabular List for Character Selection
▽ Subterms under main terms may continue to next column or pag

inking — *continued*
  watercraft — *see also* Drowning, due to, accident to,
    watercraft, sinking — *continued*
    causing injury except drowning or submersion —
      see Accident, watercraft, causing, injury NEC
iriasis X32 ☑
itting (prolonged) (static) X50.1 ☑
lashed wrists — *see* Cut, self-inflicted
lipping (accidental) (on same level) (with fall) W01.0 ☑
  on
    ice W00.0 ☑
      with skates — *see* Accident, transport, pedestri-
        an, conveyance
    mud W01.0 ☑
    oil W01.0 ☑
    snow W00.0 ☑
      with skis — *see* Accident, transport, pedestrian,
        conveyance
    surface (slippery) (wet) NEC W01.0 ☑
  without fall W18.40 ☑
    due to
      specified NEC W18.49 ☑
      stepping from one level to another W18.43 ☑
      stepping into hole or opening W18.42 ☑
      stepping on object W18.41 ☑
liver, wood, contact with W45.8 ☑
moldering (due to fire) — *see* Exposure, fire
odomy (attempted) **by force** T74.2 ☑
ound waves (causing injury) W42.9 ☑
  supersonic W42.0 ☑
plinter, contact with W45.8 ☑
tab, stabbing — *see* Cut
tanding (prolonged) (static) X50.1 ☑
tarvation X58 ☑
tatus of external cause Y99.9
  child assisting in compensated work for family Y99.8
  civilian activity done for financial or other compensa-
    tion Y99.0
  civilian activity done for income or pay Y99.0
  family member assisting in compensated work for
    other family member Y99.8
  hobby not done for income Y99.8
  leisure activity Y99.8
  military activity Y99.1
  off-duty activity of military personnel Y99.8
  recreation or sport not for income or while a student
    Y99.8
  specified NEC Y99.8
  student activity Y99.8
  volunteer activity Y99.2
tepped on
  by
    animal (not being ridden) NEC W55.89 ☑
    crowd or human stampede W52 ☑
    person W50.0 ☑
tepping on
  object W22.8 ☑
    sports equipment W21.9 ☑
    stationary W22.09 ☑
      sports equipment W21.89 ☑
    with fall W18.31 ☑
  person W51 ☑
    by crowd or human stampede W52 ☑
  sports equipment W21.9 ☑
ting
  arthropod, nonvenomous W57 ☑
  insect, nonvenomous W57 ☑
torm (cataclysmic) — *see* Forces of nature, cataclysmic
  storm
training, excessive — *see also* Overexertion X50.9 ☑
trangling — *see* Strangulation
trangulation (accidental) T71 ☑
trenuous movements — *see also* Overexertion
  X50.9 ☑
triking against
  airbag (automobile) W22.10 ☑
    driver side W22.11 ☑
    front passenger side W22.12 ☑
    specified NEC W22.19 ☑
  bottom when
    diving or jumping into water (in) W16.822 ☑
      causing drowning W16.821 ☑
      from boat W16.722 ☑
        causing drowning W16.721 ☑
      natural body W16.622 ☑
        causing drowning W16.821 ☑

Striking against — *continued*
  bottom when — *continued*
    diving or jumping into water — *continued*
      swimming pool W16.522 ☑
        causing drowning W16.521 ☑
    falling into water (in) W16.322 ☑
      causing drowning W16.321 ☑
      fountain — *see* Striking against, bottom when,
        falling into water, specified NEC
      natural body W16.122 ☑
        causing drowning W16.121 ☑
      reservoir — *see* Striking against, bottom when,
        falling into water, specified NEC
      specified NEC W16.322 ☑
        causing drowning W16.321 ☑
      swimming pool W16.022 ☑
        causing drowning W16.021 ☑
  diving board (swimming-pool) W21.4 ☑
  object W22.8 ☑
    caused by crowd or human stampede (with fall)
      W52 ☑
    furniture W22.03 ☑
    lamppost W22.02 ☑
    sports equipment W21.9 ☑
    stationary W22.09 ☑
      sports equipment W21.89 ☑
    wall W22.01 ☑
    with
      drowning or submersion — *see* Drowning
      fall — *see* Fall, due to, bumping against, object
  person(s) W51 ☑
    as, or caused by, a crowd or human stampede (with
      fall) W52 ☑
    assault Y04.2 ☑
    homicide (attempt) Y04.2 ☑
    with fall W03 ☑
      due to ice or snow W00.0 ☑
  sports equipment W21.9 ☑
  wall (when) W22.01 ☑
    diving or jumping into water (in) W16.832 ☑
      causing drowning W16.831 ☑
      swimming pool W16.532 ☑
        causing drowning W16.531 ☑
    falling into water (in) W16.332 ☑
      causing drowning W16.331 ☑
      fountain — *see* Striking against, wall when,
        falling into water, specified NEC
      natural body W16.132 ☑
        causing drowning W16.131 ☑
      reservoir — *see* Striking against, wall when,
        falling into water, specified NEC
      specified NEC W16.332 ☑
        causing drowning W16.331 ☑
      swimming pool W16.032 ☑
        causing drowning W16.031 ☑
    swimming pool (when) W22.042 ☑
      causing drowning W22.041 ☑
      diving or jumping into water W16.532 ☑
        causing drowning W16.531 ☑
      falling into water W16.032 ☑
        causing drowning W16.031 ☑
Struck (accidentally) **by**
  airbag (automobile) W22.10 ☑
    driver side W22.11 ☑
    front passenger side W22.12 ☑
    specified NEC W22.19 ☑
  alligator W58.02 ☑
  animal (not being ridden) NEC W55.89 ☑
  avalanche — *see* Landslide
  ball (hit) (thrown) W21.00 ☑
    assault Y08.09 ☑
    baseball W21.03 ☑
    basketball W21.05 ☑
    football W21.01 ☑
    golf ball W21.04 ☑
    soccer W21.02 ☑
    softball W21.07 ☑
    specified NEC W21.09 ☑
    volleyball W21.06 ☑
  bat or racquet
    baseball bat W21.11 ☑
      assault Y08.02 ☑
    golf club W21.13 ☑
      assault Y08.09 ☑
    specified NEC W21.19 ☑
      assault Y08.09 ☑

Struck (accidentally) **by** — *continued*
  bat or racquet — *continued*
    tennis racquet W21.12 ☑
      assault Y08.09 ☑
  bullet — *see also* Discharge, firearm by type
    in war operations — *see* War operations
  crocodile W58.12 ☑
  dog W54.1 ☑
  flare, Very pistol — *see* Discharge, firearm NEC
  hailstones X39.8 ☑
  hockey (ice)
    field
      puck W21.221 ☑
      stick W21.211 ☑
    puck W21.220 ☑
    stick W21.210 ☑
      assault Y08.01 ☑
  landslide — *see* Landslide
  law-enforcement agent (on duty) — *see* Legal, inter-
    vention, manhandling
    with blunt object — *see* Legal, intervention, blunt
      object
  lightning T75.0 ☑
    causing fire — *see* Exposure, fire
  machine — *see* Contact, with, by type of machine
  mammal NEC W55.89 ☑
    marine W56.32 ☑
  marine animal W56.82 ☑
  missile
    firearm — *see* Discharge, firearm by type
    in war operations — *see* War operations, missile
  object W22.8 ☑
    blunt W22.8 ☑
      assault Y00 ☑
      suicide (attempt) X79 ☑
      undetermined whether accidental or intentional
        Y29 ☑
    falling W20.8 ☑
      from, in, on
        building W20.1 ☑
          burning (uncontrolled fire) X00.4 ☑
        cataclysmic
          earth surface movement NEC — *see*
            Landslide
          storm — *see* Forces of nature, cataclysmic
            storm
        cave-in W20.0 ☑
        earthquake X34 ☑
        machine (in operation) — *see* Contact, with,
          by type of machine
        structure W20.1 ☑
          burning X00.4 ☑
        transport vehicle (in motion) — *see* Accident,
          transport, by type of vehicle
        watercraft W93.49 ☑
          due to
            accident to craft V91.39 ☑
              powered craft V91.33 ☑
                ferry boat V91.31 ☑
                fishing boat V91.32 ☑
                jetskis V91.33 ☑
                liner V91.31 ☑
                merchant ship V91.30 ☑
                passenger ship V91.31 ☑
             unpowered craft V91.38 ☑
                canoe V91.35 ☑
                inflatable V91.36 ☑
                kayak V91.35 ☑
                sailboat V91.34 ☑
                surf-board V91.38 ☑
                windsurfer V91.38 ☑
            powered craft V93.43 ☑
              ferry boat V93.41 ☑
              fishing boat V93.42 ☑
              jetskis V93.43 ☑
              liner V93.41 ☑
              merchant ship V93.40 ☑
              passenger ship V93.41 ☑
            unpowered craft V93.48 ☑
              sailboat V93.44 ☑
              surf-board V93.48 ☑
              windsurfer V93.48 ☑
    moving NEC W20.8 ☑
    projected W20.8 ☑
      assault Y00 ☑
      in sports W21.9 ☑

External Causes Index

Struck — Terrorism

Struck (accidentally) **by** — *continued*
  object — *continued*
    projected — *continued*
      in sports — *continued*
        assault Y08.09 ☑
        ball W21.00 ☑
          baseball W21.03 ☑
          basketball W21.05 ☑
          football W21.01 ☑
          golf ball W21.04 ☑
          soccer W21.02 ☑
          softball W21.07 ☑
          specified NEC W21.09 ☑
          volleyball W21.06 ☑
        bat or racquet
          baseball bat W21.11 ☑
            assault Y08.02 ☑
          golf club W21.13 ☑
            assault Y08.09 ☑
          specified NEC W21.19 ☑
            assault Y08.09 ☑
          tennis racquet W21.12 ☑
            assault Y08.09 ☑
        hockey (ice)
          field
            puck W21.221 ☑
            stick W21.211 ☑
          puck W21.220 ☑
          stick W21.210 ☑
            assault Y08.01 ☑
        specified NEC W21.89 ☑
    set in motion by explosion — *see* Explosion
    thrown W20.8 ☑
      assault Y00 ☑
      in sports W21.9 ☑
        assault Y08.09 ☑
        ball W21.00 ☑
          baseball W21.03 ☑
          basketball W21.05 ☑
          football W21.01 ☑
          golf ball W21.04 ☑
          soccer W21.02 ☑
          soft ball W21.07 ☑
          specified NEC W21.09 ☑
          volleyball W21.06 ☑
        bat or racquet
          baseball bat W21.11 ☑
            assault Y08.02 ☑
          golf club W21.13 ☑
            assault Y08.09 ☑
          specified NEC W21.19 ☑
            assault Y08.09 ☑
          tennis racquet W21.12 ☑
            assault Y08.09 ☑
        hockey (ice)
          field
            puck W21.221 ☑
            stick W21.211 ☑
          puck W21.220 ☑
          stick W21.210 ☑
            assault Y08.01 ☑
        specified NEC W21.89 ☑
  other person(s) W50.0 ☑
    with
      blunt object W22.8 ☑
        intentional, homicide (attempt) Y00 ☑
        sports equipment W21.9 ☑
        undetermined whether accidental or inten-
          tional Y29 ☑
      fall W03 ☑
        due to ice or snow W00.0 ☑
    as, or caused by, a crowd or human stampede (with
      fall) W52 ☑
    assault Y04.2 ☑
    homicide (attempt) Y04.2 ☑
    in legal intervention
      injuring
        bystander Y35.812 ☑
        law enforcement personnel Y35.811 ☑
        suspect Y35.813 ☑
        unspecified person Y35.819 ☑
    sports equipment W21.9 ☑
  police (on duty) — *see* Legal, intervention, manhan-
    dling
    with blunt object — *see* Legal, intervention, blunt
      object

Struck (accidentally) **by** — *continued*
  sports equipment W21.9 ☑
    assault Y08.09 ☑
    ball W21.00 ☑
      baseball W21.03 ☑
      basketball W21.05 ☑
      football W21.01 ☑
      golf ball W21.04 ☑
      soccer W21.02 ☑
      soft ball W21.07 ☑
      specified NEC W21.09 ☑
      volleyball W21.06 ☑
    bat or racquet
      baseball bat W21.11 ☑
        assault Y08.02 ☑
      golf club W21.13 ☑
        assault Y08.09 ☑
      specified NEC W21.19 ☑
        assault Y08.09 ☑
      tennis racquet W21.12 ☑
        assault Y08.09 ☑
    cleats (shoe) W21.31 ☑
    foot wear NEC W21.39 ☑
    football helmet W21.81 ☑
    hockey (ice)
      field
        puck W21.221 ☑
        stick W21.211 ☑
      puck W21.220 ☑
      stick W21.210 ☑
        assault Y08.01 ☑
    skate blades W21.32 ☑
    specified NEC W21.89 ☑
      assault Y08.09 ☑
  thunderbolt — *see* subcategory T75.0 ☑
    causing fire — *see* Exposure, fire
  transport vehicle NEC — *see also* Accident, transport
    V09.9 ☑
    intentional, homicide (attempt) Y03.0 ☑
    motor NEC — *see also* Accident, transport V09.20 ☑
      homicide Y03.0 ☑
  vehicle (transport) NEC — *see* Accident, transport, by
    type of vehicle
    stationary (falling from jack, hydraulic lift, ramp)
      W20.8 ☑

Stumbling
  over
    animal NEC W01.0 ☑
      with fall W18.09 ☑
    carpet, rug or (small) object W22.8 ☑
      with fall W18.09 ☑
    person W51 ☑
      with fall W03 ☑
        due to ice or snow W00.0 ☑
  without fall W18.40 ☑
    due to
      specified NEC W18.49 ☑
      stepping from one level to another W18.43 ☑
      stepping into hole or opening W18.42 ☑
      stepping on object W18.41 ☑
Submersion (accidental) — *see* Drowning
Suffocation (accidental) (by external means) (by pressure)
  (mechanical) — *see also* category T71 ☑
  due to, by
    avalanche — *see* Landslide
    explosion — *see* Explosion
    fire — *see* Exposure, fire
    food, any type (aspiration) (ingestion) (inhalation)
      — *see* categories T17 and T18 ☑
    ignition — *see* Ignition
    landslide — *see* Landslide
    machine(ry) — *see* Contact, with, by type of ma-
      chine
    vomitus (aspiration) (inhalation) T17.81- ☑
  in
    burning building X00.8 ☑
Suicide, suicidal (attempted) (by) X83.8 ☑
  blunt object X79 ☑
  burning, burns X76 ☑
    hot object X77.9 ☑
      fluid NEC X77.2 ☑
      household appliance X77.3 ☑
      specified NEC X77.8 ☑
      steam X77.0 ☑
      tap water X77.1 ☑
      vapors X77.0 ☑
  caustic substance — *see* Table of Drugs and Chemicals

Suicide, suicidal — *continued*
  cold, extreme X83.2 ☑
  collision of motor vehicle with
    motor vehicle X82.0 ☑
    specified NEC X82.8 ☑
    train X82.1 ☑
    tree X82.2 ☑
  crashing of aircraft X83.0 ☑
  cut (any part of body) X78.9 ☑
  cutting or piercing instrument X78.9 ☑
    dagger X78.2 ☑
    glass X78.0 ☑
    knife X78.1 ☑
    specified NEC X78.8 ☑
    sword X78.2 ☑
  drowning (in) X71.9 ☑
    bathtub X71.0 ☑
    natural water X71.3 ☑
    specified NEC X71.8 ☑
    swimming pool X71.1 ☑
      following fall X71.2 ☑
  electrocution X83.1 ☑
  explosive(s) (material) X75 ☑
  fire, flames X76 ☑
  firearm X74.9 ☑
    airgun X74.01 ☑
    handgun X72 ☑
    hunting rifle X73.1 ☑
    larger X73.9 ☑
      specified NEC X73.8 ☑
    machine gun X73.2 ☑
    shotgun X73.0 ☑
    specified NEC X74.8 ☑
  hanging X83.8 ☑
  hot object — *see* Suicide, burning, hot object
  jumping
    before moving object X81.8 ☑
      motor vehicle X81.0 ☑
      subway train X81.1 ☑
      train X81.1 ☑
    from high place X80 ☑
  late effect of attempt — *see* X71-X83 with 7th characte
    S
  lying before moving object, train, vehicle X81.8 ☑
  poisoning — *see* Table of Drugs and Chemicals
  puncture (any part of body) — *see* Suicide, cutting o
    piercing instrument
  scald — *see* Suicide, burning, hot object
  sequelae of attempt — *see* X71-X83 with 7th characte
    S
  sharp object (any) — *see* Suicide, cutting or piercing
    instrument
  shooting — *see* Suicide, firearm
  specified means NEC X83.8 ☑
  stab (any part of body) — *see* Suicide, cutting or
    piercing instrument
  steam, hot vapors X77.0 ☑
  strangulation X83.8 ☑
  submersion — *see* Suicide, drowning
  suffocation X83.8 ☑
  wound NEC X83.8 ☑
Sunstroke X32 ☑
Supersonic waves (causing injury) W42.0 ☑
Surgical procedure, complication of (delayed or as a
  abnormal reaction without mention of misadven-
    ture) — *see also* Complication of or following, by
    type of procedure
  due to or as a result of misadventure — *see* Misadver
    ture
Swallowed, swallowing
  foreign body — *see* Foreign body, alimentary canal
  poison — *see* Table of Drugs and Chemicals
  substance
    caustic or corrosive — *see* Table of Drugs and
      Chemicals
    poisonous — *see* Table of Drugs and Chemicals

T

Tackle in sport W03 ☑
Terrorism (involving) Y38.80 ☑
  biological weapons Y38.6X- ☑
  chemical weapons Y38.7X- ☑
  conflagration Y38.3X- ☑
  drowning and submersion Y38.89- ☑
  explosion Y38.2X- ☑

Terrorism — *continued*
  explosion — *continued*
    destruction of aircraft Y38.1X- ☑
    marine weapons Y38.0X- ☑
    fire Y38.3X- ☑
    firearms Y38.4X- ☑
    hot substances Y38.3X- ☑
    lasers Y38.89- ☑
    nuclear weapons Y38.5X- ☑
    piercing or stabbing instruments Y38.89- ☑
    secondary effects Y38.9X- ☑
    specified method NEC Y38.89- ☑
    suicide bomber Y38.81- ☑
Thirst X58 ☑
Threat to breathing
  aspiration — *see* Aspiration
  due to cave-in, falling earth or substance NEC T71 ☑
Thrown (accidentally)
  against part (any) of or object in transport vehicle (in motion) NEC — *see also* Accident, transport
  from
    high place, homicide (attempt) Y01 ☑
    machinery — *see* Contact, with, by type of machine
    transport vehicle NEC — *see also* Accident, transport V89.9 ☑
  off — *see* Thrown, from
Thunderbolt — *see* subcategory T75.0 ☑
  causing fire — *see* Exposure, fire
Tidal wave (any injury) **NEC** — *see* Forces of nature, tidal wave
Took
  overdose (drug) — *see* Table of Drugs and Chemicals
  poison — *see* Table of Drugs and Chemicals
Tornado (any injury) X37.1 ☑
Torrential rain (any injury) X37.8 ☑
Torture X58 ☑
Trampled by animal NEC W55.89 ☑
Trapped (accidentally)
  between objects (moving) (stationary and moving) — *see* Caught
  by part (any) of
    motorcycle V29.88 ☑
    pedal cycle V19.88 ☑
    transport vehicle NEC — *see also* Accident, transport V89.9 ☑
Travel (effects) (sickness) T75.3 ☑
Tree falling on or hitting (accidentally) (person) W20.8 ☑
Tripping
  over
    animal W01.0 ☑
      with fall W01.0 ☑
    carpet, rug or (small) object W22.8 ☑
      with fall W18.09 ☑
    person W51
      with fall W03 ☑
        due to ice or snow W00.0 ☑
  without fall W18.40 ☑
    due to
      specified NEC W18.49 ☑
      stepping from one level to another W18.43 ☑
      stepping into hole or opening W18.42 ☑
      stepping on object W18.41 ☑
Twisted by person(s) (accidentally) W50.2 ☑
  with intent to injure or kill Y04.0 ☑
  as, or caused by, a crowd or human stampede (with fall) W52 ☑
  assault Y04.0 ☑
  homicide (attempt) Y04.0 ☑
  in
    fight Y04.0 ☑
    legal intervention — *see* Legal, intervention, manhandling
Twisting (prolonged) (static) X50.1- ☑

U

Underdosing of necessary drugs, medicaments or biological substances Y63.6
Undetermined intent (contact) (exposure)
  automobile collision Y32 ☑
  blunt object Y29 ☑
  drowning (submersion) (in) Y21.9 ☑
    bathtub Y21.0 ☑
      after fall Y21.1 ☑

Undetermined intent — *continued*
  drowning — *continued*
    natural water (lake) (ocean) (pond) (river) (stream) Y21.4 ☑
    specified place NEC Y21.8 ☑
    swimming pool Y21.2 ☑
      after fall Y21.3 ☑
  explosive material Y25 ☑
  fall, jump or push from high place Y30 ☑
  falling, lying or running before moving object Y31 ☑
  fire Y26 ☑
  firearm discharge Y24.9 ☑
    airgun (BB) (pellet) Y24.0 ☑
    handgun (pistol) (revolver) Y22 ☑
    hunting rifle Y23.1 ☑
    larger Y23.9 ☑
      hunting rifle Y23.1 ☑
      machine gun Y23.3 ☑
      military Y23.2 ☑
      shotgun Y23.0 ☑
      specified type NEC Y23.8 ☑
    machine gun Y23.3 ☑
    military Y23.2 ☑
    shotgun Y23.0 ☑
    specified type NEC Y24.8 ☑
    Very pistol Y24.8 ☑
  hot object Y27.9 ☑
    fluid NEC Y27.2 ☑
    household appliance Y27.3 ☑
    specified object NEC Y27.8 ☑
    steam Y27.0 ☑
    tap water Y27.1 ☑
    vapor Y27.0 ☑
  jump, fall or push from high place Y30 ☑
  lying, falling or running before moving object Y31 ☑
  motor vehicle crash Y32 ☑
  push, fall or jump from high place Y30 ☑
  running, falling or lying before moving object Y31 ☑
  sharp object Y28.9 ☑
    dagger Y28.2 ☑
    glass Y28.0 ☑
    knife Y28.1 ☑
    specified object NEC Y28.8 ☑
    sword Y28.2 ☑
  smoke Y26 ☑
  specified event NEC Y33 ☑
Use of hand as hammer X50.3 ☑

V

Vibration (causing injury) W49.9 ☑
Victim (of)
  avalanche — *see* Landslide
  earth movements NEC — *see* Forces of nature, earth movement
  earthquake X34 ☑
  flood — *see* Flood
  landslide — *see* Landslide
  lightning — *see* subcategory T75.0 ☑
    causing fire — *see* Exposure, fire
  storm (cataclysmic) NEC — *see* Forces of nature, cataclysmic storm
  volcanic eruption X35 ☑
Volcanic eruption (any injury) X35 ☑
Vomitus, gastric contents in air passages (with asphyxia, obstruction or suffocation) T17.81- ☑

W

Walked into stationary object (any) W22.09 ☑
  furniture W22.03 ☑
  lamppost W22.02 ☑
  wall W22.01 ☑
War operations (injuries to military personnel and civilians during war, civil insurrection and peacekeeping missions) (by) (from) (involving) Y36.90 ☑
  after cessation of hostilities Y36.89- ☑
    explosion (of)
      bomb placed during war operations Y36.82- ☑
      mine placed during war operations Y36.81- ☑
    specified NEC Y36.88- ☑
  air blast Y36.20- ☑
  aircraft
    destruction — *see* War operations, destruction of aircraft

War operations — *continued*
  airway restriction — *see* War operations, restriction of airways
  asphyxiation — *see* War operations, restriction of airways
  biological weapons Y36.6X- ☑
  blast Y36.20- ☑
  blast fragments Y36.20- ☑
  blast wave Y36.20- ☑
  blast wind Y36.20- ☑
  bomb Y36.20- ☑
    dirty Y36.50- ☑
    gasoline Y36.31- ☑
    incendiary Y36.31- ☑
    petrol Y36.31- ☑
  bullet Y36.43- ☑
    incendiary Y36.32- ☑
    rubber Y36.41- ☑
  chemical weapons Y36.7X- ☑
  combat
    hand to hand (unarmed) combat Y36.44- ☑
    using blunt or piercing object Y36.45- ☑
  conflagration — *see* War operations, fire
  conventional warfare NEC Y36.49- ☑
  depth-charge Y36.01- ☑
  destruction of aircraft Y36.10- ☑
    due to
      air to air missile Y36.11- ☑
      collision with other aircraft Y36.12- ☑
      detonation (accidental) of onboard munitions and explosives Y36.14- ☑
      enemy fire or explosives Y36.11- ☑
      explosive placed on aircraft Y36.11- ☑
      onboard fire Y36.13- ☑
      rocket propelled grenade [RPG] Y36.11- ☑
      small arms fire Y36.11- ☑
      surface to air missile Y36.11- ☑
    specified NEC Y36.19- ☑
  detonation (accidental) of
    onboard marine weapons Y36.05- ☑
    own munitions or munitions launch device Y36.24- ☑
  dirty bomb Y36.50- ☑
  explosion (of) Y36.20- ☑
    aerial bomb Y36.21- ☑
    after cessation of hostilities
      bomb placed during war operations Y36.82- ☑
      mine placed during war operations Y36.81- ☑
    bomb NOS — *see also* War operations, bomb(s) Y36.20- ☑
    fragments Y36.20- ☑
    grenade Y36.29- ☑
    guided missile Y36.22- ☑
    improvised explosive device [IED] (person-borne) (roadside) (vehicle-borne) Y36.23- ☑
    land mine Y36.29- ☑
    marine mine (at sea) (in harbor) Y36.02- ☑
    marine weapon Y36.00- ☑
      specified NEC Y36.09- ☑
    own munitions or munitions launch device (accidental) Y36.24- ☑
    sea-based artillery shell Y36.03- ☑
    specified NEC Y36.29- ☑
    torpedo Y36.04- ☑
  fire Y36.30- ☑
    specified NEC Y36.39- ☑
  firearms
    discharge Y36.43- ☑
    pellets Y36.42- ☑
  flamethrower Y36.33- ☑
  fragments (from) (of)
    improvised explosive device [IED] (person-borne) (roadside) (vehicle-borne) Y36.26- ☑
    munitions Y36.25- ☑
    specified NEC Y36.29- ☑
    weapons Y36.27- ☑
  friendly fire Y36.92 ☑
  hand to hand (unarmed) combat Y36.44- ☑
  hot substances — *see* War operations, fire
  incendiary bullet Y36.32- ☑
  nuclear weapon (effects of) Y36.50- ☑
    acute radiation exposure Y36.54- ☑
    blast pressure Y36.51- ☑
    direct blast Y36.51- ☑
    direct heat Y36.53- ☑
    fallout exposure Y36.54- ☑

War operations — *continued*
  nuclear weapon — *continued*
    fireball Y36.53- ☑
    indirect blast (struck or crushed by blast debris)
      (being thrown by blast) Y36.52- ☑
    ionizing radiation (immediate exposure) Y36.54- ☑
    nuclear radiation Y36.54- ☑
    radiation
      ionizing (immediate exposure) Y36.54- ☑
      nuclear Y36.54- ☑
      thermal Y36.53- ☑
    secondary effects Y36.54- ☑
    specified NEC Y36.59- ☑
    thermal radiation Y36.53- ☑
  restriction of air (airway)
    intentional Y36.46- ☑
    unintentional Y36.47- ☑
  rubber bullets Y36.41- ☑
  shrapnel NOS Y36.29- ☑
  suffocation — *see* War operations, restriction of airways
  unconventional warfare NEC Y36.7X- ☑
  underwater blast NOS Y36.00- ☑

War operations — *continued*
  warfare
    conventional NEC Y36.49- ☑
    unconventional NEC Y36.7X- ☑
  weapon of mass destruction [WMD] Y36.91 ☑
  weapons
    biological weapons Y36.6X- ☑
    chemical Y36.7X- ☑
    nuclear (effects of) Y36.50- ☑
      acute radiation exposure Y36.54- ☑
      blast pressure Y36.51- ☑
      direct blast Y36.51- ☑
      direct heat Y36.53- ☑
      fallout exposure Y36.54- ☑
      fireball Y36.53- ☑
      radiation
        ionizing (immediate exposure) Y36.54- ☑
        nuclear Y36.54- ☑
        thermal Y36.53- ☑
      secondary effects Y36.54- ☑
      specified NEC Y36.59- ☑

War operations — *continued*
  weapons — *continued*
    of mass destruction [WMD] Y36.91 ☑
Washed
  away by flood — *see* Flood
  off road by storm (transport vehicle) — *see* Forces o
    nature, cataclysmic storm
Weather exposure NEC — *see* Forces of nature
Weightlessness (causing injury) (effects of) (in spacecra
  real or simulated) X52 ☑
Work related condition Y99.0
Wound (accidental) NEC — *see also* Injury X58 ☑
  battle — *see also* War operations Y36.90 ☑
  gunshot — *see* Discharge, firearm by type
Wreck transport vehicle NEC — *see also* Accident,
  transport V89.9 ☑
Wrong
  device implanted into correct surgical site Y65.51
  fluid in infusion Y65.1
  patient, procedure performed on Y65.52
  procedure (operation) on correct patient Y65.51

ICD-10-CM Tabular List of Diseases and Injuries

Chapter 1. Certain Infectious and Parasitic Diseases (A00–B99)

Chapter-specific Guidelines with Coding Examples

The chapter-specific guidelines from the ICD-10-CM Official Guidelines for Coding and Reporting have been provided below. Along with these guidelines are coding examples, contained in the shaded boxes, that have been developed to help illustrate the coding and/or sequencing guidance found in these guidelines.

a. Human immunodeficiency virus (HIV) infections

1) Code only confirmed cases

Code only confirmed cases of HIV infection/illness. This is an exception to the hospital inpatient guideline Section II, H.

In this context, "confirmation" does not require documentation of positive serology or culture for HIV; the provider's diagnostic statement that the patient is HIV positive, or has an HIV-related illness is sufficient.

> Patient being seen for hypothyroidism with possible HIV infection
>
> **E03.9**   **Hypothyroidism, unspecified**
>
> *Explanation:* Only the hypothyroidism is coded in this scenario because it has not been confirmed that an HIV infection is present.

2) Selection and sequencing of HIV codes

(a) Patient admitted for HIV-related condition

If a patient is admitted for an HIV-related condition, the principal diagnosis should be B20, Human immunodeficiency virus [HIV] disease followed by additional diagnosis codes for all reported HIV-related conditions.

> HIV with CMV
>
> **B20**   **Human immunodeficiency virus [HIV] disease**
>
> **B25.9**   **Cytomegaloviral disease, unspecified**
>
> *Explanation:* Cytomegaloviral infection is an HIV related condition, so the HIV diagnosis code is reported first, followed by the code for the CMV.

(b) Patient with HIV disease admitted for unrelated condition

If a patient with HIV disease is admitted for an unrelated condition (such as a traumatic injury), the code for the unrelated condition (e.g., the nature of injury code) should be the principal diagnosis. Other diagnoses would be B20 followed by additional diagnosis codes for all reported HIV-related conditions.

> Sprain of the internal collateral ligament, right ankle; HIV
>
> **S93.491A**   **Sprain of other ligament of right ankle, initial encounter**
>
> **B20**   **Human immunodeficiency virus [HIV] disease**
>
> *Explanation:* The ankle sprain is not related to HIV, so it is the first-listed diagnosis code, and HIV is reported secondarily.

(c) Whether the patient is newly diagnosed

Whether the patient is newly diagnosed or has had previous admissions/encounters for HIV conditions is irrelevant to the sequencing decision.

> Newly diagnosed multiple cutaneous Kaposi's sarcoma lesions in previously diagnosed HIV disease
>
> **B20**   **Human immunodeficiency virus [HIV] disease**
>
> **C46.0**   **Kaposi's sarcoma of skin**
>
> *Explanation:* Even though the HIV was diagnosed on a previous encounter, it is still sequenced first when coded with an HIV related condition. Kaposi's sarcoma is an HIV-related condition.

(d) Asymptomatic human immunodeficiency virus

Z21, Asymptomatic human immunodeficiency virus [HIV] infection status, is to be applied when the patient without any documentation of symptoms is listed as being "HIV positive," "known HIV," "HIV test positive," or similar terminology. Do not use this code if the term "AIDS" is used or if the patient is treated for any HIV-related illness or is described as having any condition(s) resulting from his/her HIV positive status; use B20 in these cases.

> Patient is being seen for iron deficiency anemia. Status positive HIV test on Atripla, with no prior symptoms
>
> **D50.9**   **Iron deficiency anemia, unspecified**
>
> **Z21**   **Asymptomatic human immunodeficiency virus [HIV] infection status**
>
> *Explanation:* Code Z21 is sequenced second since documentation indicates that the patient has had a positive HIV test but has been asymptomatic. Being on medication for HIV is not an indication that code B20 is used instead of Z21. Unless there has been documentation that the patient has had current or prior symptoms or HIV-related complications, code B20 is not used. The anemia is not an AIDS-related complication and is sequenced first.

(e) Patients with inconclusive HIV serology

Patients with inconclusive HIV serology, but no definitive diagnosis or manifestations of the illness, may be assigned code R75, Inconclusive laboratory evidence of human immunodeficiency virus [HIV].

(f) Previously diagnosed HIV-related illness

Patients with any known prior diagnosis of an HIV-related illness should be coded to B20. Once a patient has developed an HIV-related illness, the patient should always be assigned code B20 on every subsequent admission/encounter. Patients previously diagnosed with any HIV illness (B20) should never be assigned to R75 or Z21, Asymptomatic human immunodeficiency virus [HIV] infection status.

(g) HIV infection in pregnancy, childbirth and the puerperium

During pregnancy, childbirth or the puerperium, a patient admitted (or presenting for a health care encounter) because of an HIV-related illness should receive a principal diagnosis code of O98.7-, Human immunodeficiency [HIV] disease complicating pregnancy, childbirth and the puerperium, followed by B20 and the code(s) for the HIV-related illness(es). Codes from Chapter 15 always take sequencing priority.

Patients with asymptomatic HIV infection status admitted (or presenting for a health care encounter) during pregnancy, childbirth, or the puerperium should receive codes of O98.7- and Z21.

(h) Encounters for testing for HIV

If a patient is being seen to determine his/her HIV status, use code Z11.4, Encounter for screening for human immunodeficiency virus [HIV]. Use additional codes for any associated high risk behavior.

If a patient with signs or symptoms is being seen for HIV testing, code the signs and symptoms. An additional counseling code Z71.7, Human immunodeficiency virus [HIV] counseling, may be used if counseling is provided during the encounter for the test.

When a patient returns to be informed of his/her HIV test results and the test result is negative, use code Z71.7, Human immunodeficiency virus [HIV] counseling.

If the results are positive, see previous guidelines and assign codes as appropriate.

b. Infectious agents as the cause of diseases classified to other chapters

Certain infections are classified in chapters other than Chapter 1 and no organism is identified as part of the infection code. In these instances, it is necessary to use an additional code from Chapter 1 to identify the organism. A code from category B95, Streptococcus, Staphylococcus, and Enterococcus as the cause of diseases classified to other chapters, B96, Other bacterial agents as the cause of diseases classified to other chapters, or B97, Viral agents as the cause of diseases classified to other chapters, is to be used as an additional code to identify the organism. An instructional note will be found at the infection code advising that an additional organism code is required.

Acute *E. coli* cystitis

N30.00	**Acute cystitis without hematuria**
B96.20	**Unspecified Escherichia coli [E.coli] as the cause of diseases classified elsewhere**

Explanation: An instructional note under the category for the cystitis indicates to code also the specific organism.

c. Infections resistant to antibiotics

Many bacterial infections are resistant to current antibiotics. It is necessary to identify all infections documented as antibiotic resistant. Assign a code from category Z16, Resistance to antimicrobial drugs, following the infection code only if the infection code does not identify drug resistance.

Penicillin-resistant *Streptococcus pneumoniae* pneumonia

J13	**Pneumonia due to Streptococcus pneumoniae**
Z16.11	**Resistance to penicillins**

Explanation: Code Z16.11 is assigned as a secondary code to represent the penicillin resistance. This code includes resistance to amoxicillin and ampicillin.

d. Sepsis, severe sepsis, and septic shock

1) Coding of Sepsis and Severe Sepsis

(a) Sepsis

For a diagnosis of sepsis, assign the appropriate code for the underlying systemic infection. If the type of infection or causal organism is not further specified, assign code A41.9, Sepsis, unspecified organism.

A code from subcategory R65.2, Severe sepsis, should not be assigned unless severe sepsis or an associated acute organ dysfunction is documented.

Gram-negative sepsis

A41.50	**Gram-negative sepsis, unspecified**

Staphylococcal sepsis

A41.2	**Sepsis due to unspecified staphylococcus**

Explanation: In both examples above the organism causing the sepsis is identified, therefore A41.9 Sepsis, unspecified organism, would not be appropriate as this code would not capture the highest degree of specificity found in the documentation. Do not use an additional code for severe sepsis unless an acute organ dysfunction was also documented as "associated with" or "due to" the sepsis or the sepsis was documented as "severe."

(i) Negative or inconclusive blood cultures and sepsis

Negative or inconclusive blood cultures do not preclude a diagnosis of sepsis in patients with clinical evidence of the condition; however, the provider should be queried.

(ii) Urosepsis

The term urosepsis is a nonspecific term. It is not to be considered synonymous with sepsis. It has no default code in the Alphabetic Index. Should a provider use this term, he/she must be queried for clarification.

(iii) Sepsis with organ dysfunction

If a patient has sepsis and associated acute organ dysfunction or multiple organ dysfunction (MOD), follow the instructions for coding severe sepsis.

(iv) Acute organ dysfunction that is not clearly associated with the sepsis

If a patient has sepsis and an acute organ dysfunction, but the medical record documentation indicates that the acute organ dysfunction is related to a medical condition other than the sepsis, do not assign a code from subcategory R65.2, Severe sepsis. An acute organ dysfunction must be associated with the sepsis in order to assign the severe sepsis code. If the documentation is not clear as to whether an acute organ dysfunction is related to the sepsis or another medical condition, query the provider.

Sepsis and acute respiratory failure due to COPD exacerbation

A41.9	**Sepsis, unspecified organism**
J44.1	**Chronic obstructive pulmonary disease with (acute) exacerbation**
J96.00	**Acute respiratory failure, unspecified whether with hypoxia or hypercapnia**

Explanation: Although acute organ dysfunction is present in the form of acute respiratory failure, severe sepsis (R65.2) is not coded in this example, as the acute respiratory failure is attributed to the COPD exacerbation rather than the sepsis. Sequencing of these codes would be determined by the reason for the encounter.

(b) Severe sepsis

The coding of severe sepsis requires a minimum of 2 codes: first a code for the underlying systemic infection, followed by a code from subcategory R65.2, Severe sepsis. If the causal organism is not documented, assign code A41.9, Sepsis, unspecified organism, for the infection. Additional code(s) for the associated acute organ dysfunction are also required.

Due to the complex nature of severe sepsis, some cases may require querying the provider prior to assignment of the codes.

2) Septic shock

(a) Septic shock generally refers to circulatory failure associated with severe sepsis, and therefore, it represents a type of acute organ dysfunction.

For cases of septic shock, the code for the systemic infection should be sequenced first, followed by code R65.21, Severe sepsis with septic shock or code T81.12, Postprocedural septic shock. Any additional codes for the other acute organ dysfunctions should also be assigned. As noted in the sequencing instructions in the Tabular List, the code for septic shock cannot be assigned as a principal diagnosis.

Sepsis with septic shock

A41.9	**Sepsis, unspecified organism**
R65.21	**Severe sepsis with septic shock**

Explanation: Documentation of septic shock automatically implies severe sepsis as it is a form of acute organ dysfunction. Septic shock is not coded as the first-listed diagnosis; it is always preceded by the code for the systemic infection.

3) Sequencing of severe sepsis

If severe sepsis is present on admission, and meets the definition of principal diagnosis, the underlying systemic infection should be assigned as principal diagnosis followed by the appropriate code from subcategory R65.2 as required by the sequencing rules in the Tabular List. A code from subcategory R65.2 can never be assigned as a principal diagnosis.

When severe sepsis develops during an encounter (it was not present on admission), the underlying systemic infection and the appropriate code from subcategory R65.2 should be assigned as secondary diagnoses.

Severe sepsis may be present on admission, but the diagnosis may not be confirmed until sometime after admission. If the documentation is not clear whether severe sepsis was present on admission, the provider should be queried.

4) Sepsis *or* severe sepsis with a localized infection

If the reason for admission is sepsis or severe sepsis and a localized infection, such as pneumonia or cellulitis, a code(s) for the underlying systemic infection should be assigned first and the code for the localized infection should be assigned as a secondary diagnosis. If the patient has severe sepsis, a code from subcategory R65.2 should also be assigned as a secondary diagnosis. If the patient is admitted with a localized infection, such as pneumonia, and sepsis/severe sepsis doesn't develop until after admission, the localized infection should be assigned first, followed by the appropriate sepsis/severe sepsis codes.

Patient presents with acute renal failure due to severe sepsis from *Pseudomonas pneumonia*

A41.52	**Sepsis due to Pseudomonas**
J15.1	**Pneumonia due to Pseudomonas**
R65.20	**Severe sepsis without septic shock**
N17.9	**Acute kidney failure, unspecified**

Explanation: If all conditions are present, the systemic infection (sepsis) is sequenced first followed by the codes for the localized infection (pneumonia), severe sepsis and any organ dysfunction.

5) Sepsis due to a postprocedural infection

(a) Documentation of causal relationship

As with all postprocedural complications, code assignment is based on the provider's documentation of the relationship between the infection and the procedure.

(b) Sepsis due to a postprocedural infection

For infections following a procedure, a code from T81.40, to T81.43 Infection following a procedure, or a code from O86.00 to O86.03, Infection of obstetric surgical wound, that identifies the site of the infection should be coded first, if known. Assign an additional code for sepsis following a procedure (T81.44) or sepsis following an obstetrical procedure (O86.04). Use an additional code to identify the infectious agent. If the patient has severe sepsis, the appropriate code from subcategory R65.2 should also be assigned with the additional code(s) for any acute organ dysfunction.

For infections following infusion, transfusion, therapeutic injection, or immunization, a code from subcategory T80.2, Infections following infusion, transfusion, and therapeutic injection, or code T88.0-, Infection following immunization, should be coded first, followed by the code for the specific infection. If the patient has severe sepsis, the appropriate code from subcategory R65.2 should also be assigned, with the additional codes(s) for any acute organ dysfunction.

(c) Postprocedural infection and postprocedural septic shock

If a postprocedural infection has resulted in postprocedural septic shock, assign the codes indicated above for sepsis due to a postprocedural infection, followed by code T81.12-, Postprocedural septic shock. Do not assign code R65.21, Severe sepsis with septic shock. Additional code(s) should be assigned for any acute organ dysfunction.

6) Sepsis and severe sepsis associated with a noninfectious process (condition)

In some cases a noninfectious process (condition), such as trauma, may lead to an infection which can result in sepsis or severe sepsis. If sepsis or severe sepsis is documented as associated with a noninfectious condition, such as a burn or serious injury, and this condition meets the definition for principal diagnosis, the code for the noninfectious condition should be sequenced first, followed by the code for the resulting infection. If severe sepsis is present, a code from subcategory R65.2 should also be assigned with any associated organ dysfunction(s) codes. It is not necessary to assign a code from subcategory R65.1, Systemic inflammatory response syndrome (SIRS) of non-infectious origin, for these cases.

If the infection meets the definition of principal diagnosis, it should be sequenced before the non-infectious condition. When both the associated non-infectious condition and the infection meet the definition of principal diagnosis, either may be assigned as principal diagnosis.

Only one code from category R65, Symptoms and signs specifically associated with systemic inflammation and infection, should be assigned. Therefore, when a non-infectious condition leads to an infection resulting in severe sepsis, assign the appropriate code from subcategory R65.2, Severe sepsis. Do not additionally assign a code from subcategory R65.1, Systemic inflammatory response syndrome (SIRS) of non-infectious origin.

See Section I.C.18. SIRS due to non-infectious process

7) Sepsis and septic shock complicating abortion, pregnancy, childbirth, and the puerperium

See Section I.C.15. Sepsis and septic shock complicating abortion, pregnancy, childbirth and the puerperium

8) Newborn sepsis

See Section I.C.16. f. Bacterial sepsis of Newborn

e. Methicillin resistant *Staphylococcus aureus* (MRSA) conditions

1) Selection and sequencing of MRSA codes

(a) Combination codes for MRSA infection

When a patient is diagnosed with an infection that is due to methicillin resistant *Staphylococcus aureus* (MRSA), and that infection has a combination code that includes the causal organism (e.g., sepsis, pneumonia) assign the appropriate combination code for the condition (e.g., code A41.02, Sepsis due to Methicillin resistant Staphylococcus aureus or code J15.212, Pneumonia due to Methicillin resistant Staphylococcus aureus). Do not assign code B95.62, Methicillin resistant Staphylococcus aureus infection as the cause of diseases classified elsewhere, as an additional code, because the combination code includes the type of infection and the MRSA organism. Do not assign a code from subcategory Z16.11, Resistance to penicillins, as an additional diagnosis.

See Section C.1. for instructions on coding and sequencing of sepsis and severe sepsis.

(b) Other codes for MRSA infection

When there is documentation of a current infection (e.g., wound infection, stitch abscess, urinary tract infection) due to MRSA, and that infection does not have a combination code that includes the causal organism, assign the appropriate code to identify the condition along with code B95.62, Methicillin resistant Staphylococcus aureus infection as the cause of diseases classified elsewhere for the MRSA infection. Do not assign a code from subcategory Z16.11, Resistance to penicillins.

(c) Methicillin susceptible Staphylococcus aureus (MSSA) and MRSA colonization

The condition or state of being colonized or carrying MSSA or MRSA is called colonization or carriage, while an individual person is described as being colonized or being a carrier. Colonization means that MSSA or MSRA is present on or in the body without necessarily causing illness. A positive MRSA colonization test might be documented by the provider as "MRSA screen positive" or "MRSA nasal swab positive".

Assign code Z22.322, Carrier or suspected carrier of Methicillin resistant Staphylococcus aureus, for patients documented as having MRSA colonization. Assign code Z22.321, Carrier or suspected carrier of Methicillin susceptible Staphylococcus aureus, for patients documented as having MSSA colonization. Colonization is not necessarily indicative of a disease process or as the cause of a specific condition the patient may have unless documented as such by the provider.

(d) MRSA colonization and infection

If a patient is documented as having both MRSA colonization and infection during a hospital admission, code Z22.322, Carrier or suspected carrier of Methicillin resistant Staphylococcus aureus, and a code for the MRSA infection may both be assigned.

f. Zika virus infections

1) Code only confirmed cases

Code only a confirmed diagnosis of Zika virus (A92.5, Zika virus disease) as documented by the provider. This is an exception to the hospital inpatient guideline Section II, H. In this context, "confirmation" does not require documentation of the type of test performed; the **provider's** diagnostic statement that the condition is confirmed is sufficient. This code should be assigned regardless of the stated mode of transmission.

If the provider documents "suspected", "possible" or "probable" Zika, do not assign code A92.5. Assign a code(s) explaining the reason for encounter (such as fever, rash, or joint pain) or Z20.821, Contact with and (suspected) exposure to Zika virus.

Chapter 1. Certain Infectious and Parasitic Diseases (A00–B99)

INCLUDES   diseases generally recognized as communicable or transmissible
Use additional code to identify resistance to antimicrobial drugs (Z16.-)
EXCLUDES 1   certain localized infections — see body system-related chapters
EXCLUDES 2   carrier or suspected carrier of infectious disease (Z22.-)
infectious and parasitic diseases complicating pregnancy, childbirth and the puerperium (O98.-)
infectious and parasitic diseases specific to the perinatal period (P35-P39)
influenza and other acute respiratory infections (J00-J22)

This chapter contains the following blocks:

A00-A09   Intestinal infectious diseases
A15-A19   Tuberculosis
A20-A28   Certain zoonotic bacterial diseases
A30-A49   Other bacterial diseases
A50-A64   Infections with a predominantly sexual mode of transmission
A65-A69   Other spirochetal diseases
A70-A74   Other diseases caused by chlamydiae
A75-A79   Rickettsioses
A80-A89   Viral and prion infections of the central nervous system
A90-A99   Arthropod-borne viral fevers and viral hemorrhagic fevers
B00-B09   Viral infections characterized by skin and mucous membrane lesions
B10   Other human herpesviruses
B15-B19   Viral hepatitis
B20   Human immunodeficiency virus [HIV] disease
B25-B34   Other viral diseases
B35-B49   Mycoses
B50-B64   Protozoal diseases
B65-B83   Helminthiases
B85-B89   Pediculosis, acariasis and other infestations
B90-B94   Sequelae of infectious and parasitic diseases
B95-B97   Bacterial and viral infectious agents
B99   Other infectious diseases

Intestinal infectious diseases (A00-A09)

✓4ᵗʰ **A00 Cholera**

DEF: Acute infection of the bowel due to vibrio cholerae that presents with profuse diarrhea, cramps, and vomiting, resulting in severe dehydration, electrolyte imbalance, and death. It is spread through ingestion of food or water contaminated with feces of infected persons.

A00.0 Cholera due to Vibrio cholerae 01, biovar cholerae
Classical cholera

A00.1 Cholera due to Vibrio cholerae 01, biovar eltor
Cholera eltor

A00.9 Cholera, unspecified

✓4ᵗʰ **A01 Typhoid and paratyphoid fevers**

DEF: Typhoid fever: Acute generalized illness caused by *Salmonella typhi*. Clinical features include fever, headache, abdominal pain, cough, toxemia, leukopenia, abnormal pulse, rose spots on the skin, bacteremia, hyperplasia of intestinal lymph nodes, mesenteric lymphadenopathy, and Peyer's patches in the intestines.
DEF: Paratyphoid fever: Prolonged febrile illness, caused by *Salmonella* serotypes other than *S. typhi*, especially *S. enterica* serotypes paratyphi A, B, and C.

✓5ᵗʰ **A01.0 Typhoid fever**
Infection due to Salmonella typhi

A01.00 Typhoid fever, unspecified
A01.01 Typhoid meningitis
A01.02 Typhoid fever with heart involvement
Typhoid endocarditis
Typhoid myocarditis
A01.03 Typhoid pneumonia   HCC
A01.04 Typhoid arthritis   HCC
A01.05 Typhoid osteomyelitis   HCC
A01.09 Typhoid fever with other complications

A01.1 Paratyphoid fever A
A01.2 Paratyphoid fever B
A01.3 Paratyphoid fever C
A01.4 Paratyphoid fever, unspecified
Infection due to Salmonella paratyphi NOS

✓4ᵗʰ **A02 Other salmonella infections**

INCLUDES   infection or foodborne intoxication due to any Salmonella species other than S. typhi and S. paratyphi

A02.0 Salmonella enteritis
Salmonellosis
TIP: Dehydration (E86.0) is a complication of salmonella enteritis and may be reported separately.

A02.1 Salmonella sepsis   HCC

✓5ᵗʰ **A02.2 Localized salmonella infections**

A02.20 Localized salmonella infection, unspecified
A02.21 Salmonella meningitis
A02.22 Salmonella pneumonia   HCC
A02.23 Salmonella arthritis   HCC
A02.24 Salmonella osteomyelitis   HCC
A02.25 Salmonella pyelonephritis
Salmonella tubulo-interstitial nephropathy
A02.29 Salmonella with other localized infection

A02.8 Other specified salmonella infections
A02.9 Salmonella infection, unspecified

✓4ᵗʰ **A03 Shigellosis**

DEF: Infection caused by the genus the *Shigella*, of the family *Enterobacteriaceae* that is known to cause an acute dysenteric infection of the bowel with fever, drowsiness, anorexia, nausea, vomiting, bloody diarrhea, abdominal cramps, and distention.

A03.0 Shigellosis due to Shigella dysenteriae
Group A shigellosis [Shiga-Kruse dysentery]

A03.1 Shigellosis due to Shigella flexneri
Group B shigellosis

A03.2 Shigellosis due to Shigella boydii
Group C shigellosis

A03.3 Shigellosis due to Shigella sonnei
Group D shigellosis

A03.8 Other shigellosis
A03.9 Shigellosis, unspecified
Bacillary dysentery NOS

✓4ᵗʰ **A04 Other bacterial intestinal infections**

EXCLUDES 1   bacterial foodborne intoxications, NEC (A05.-)
tuberculous enteritis (A18.32)

DEF: Escherichia coli: Gram negative, anaerobic of the family *Enterobacteriaceae* found in the large intestine of warm-blooded animals, generally as a nonpathologic entity aiding in digestion. They become pathogenic when an opportunity to grow somewhere outside this relationship presents itself, such as ingestion of fecal contaminated food or water.

A04.0 Enteropathogenic Escherichia coli infection
A04.1 Enterotoxigenic Escherichia coli infection
A04.2 Enteroinvasive Escherichia coli infection
A04.3 Enterohemorrhagic Escherichia coli infection
DEF: *E. coli* infection penetrating the intestinal mucosa, producing microscopic ulceration and bleeding.
A04.4 Other intestinal Escherichia coli infections
Escherichia coli enteritis NOS
A04.5 Campylobacter enteritis
TIP: For Guillain-Barre syndrome occurring as a sequela of *Campylobacter enteritis*, assign code G61.0 as the first-listed diagnosis followed by B94.8 for the sequelae.
A04.6 Enteritis due to Yersinia enterocolitica
EXCLUDES 1   extraintestinal yersiniosis (A28.2)

✓5ᵗʰ **A04.7 Enterocolitis due to Clostridium difficile**
Foodborne intoxication by Clostridium difficile
Pseudomembraneous colitis
AHA: 2017,4Q,4
A04.71 Enterocolitis due to Clostridium difficile, recurrent
A04.72 Enterocolitis due to Clostridium difficile, not specified as recurrent
A04.8 Other specified bacterial intestinal infections
A04.9 Bacterial intestinal infection, unspecified
Bacterial enteritis NOS

✓4ᵗʰ **A05**   **Other bacterial foodborne intoxications, not elsewhere classified**

> _EXCLUDES 1_   Clostridium difficile foodborne intoxication and infection
> (A04.7-)
> Escherichia coli infection (A04.0-A04.4)
> listeriosis (A32.-)
> salmonella foodborne intoxication and infection (A02.-)
> toxic effect of noxious foodstuffs (T61-T62)

A05.0   **Foodborne staphylococcal intoxication**
> **TIP:** Assign code A04.8 to report a staphylococcal infection when it is caused by the ingestion of contaminated food but not caused by _S. aureus_ toxins.

A05.1   **Botulism food poisoning**
> Botulism NOS
> Classical foodborne intoxication due to Clostridium botulinum
> > _EXCLUDES 1_   infant botulism (A48.51)
> > wound botulism (A48.52)
> **DEF:** Muscle-paralyzing neurotoxic disease caused by ingesting pre-formed toxin from the bacterium _Clostridium botulinum_. It causes vomiting and diarrhea, vision problems, slurred speech, difficulty swallowing, paralysis, and death.

A05.2   **Foodborne Clostridium perfringens [Clostridium welchii] intoxication**
> Enteritis necroticans
> Pig-bel

A05.3   **Foodborne Vibrio parahaemolyticus intoxication**

A05.4   **Foodborne Bacillus cereus intoxication**

A05.5   **Foodborne Vibrio vulnificus intoxication**

A05.8   **Other specified bacterial foodborne intoxications**

A05.9   **Bacterial foodborne intoxication, unspecified**

✓4ᵗʰ **A06**   **Amebiasis**

> _INCLUDES_   infection due to Entamoeba histolytica
> _EXCLUDES 1_   other protozoal intestinal diseases (A07.-)
> _EXCLUDES 2_   acanthamebiasis (B60.1-)
> Naegleriasis (B60.2)

DEF: Infection with a single cell protozoan known as the amoeba. Transmission occurs through ingestion of feces, contaminated food or water, use of human feces as fertilizer, or person-to-person contact.

A06.0   **Acute amebic dysentery**
> Acute amebiasis
> Intestinal amebiasis NOS

A06.1   **Chronic intestinal amebiasis**

A06.2   **Amebic nondysenteric colitis**

A06.3   **Ameboma of intestine**
> Ameboma NOS

A06.4   **Amebic liver abscess**
> Hepatic amebiasis

A06.5   **Amebic lung abscess**   `HCC`
> Amebic abscess of lung (and liver)

A06.6   **Amebic brain abscess**
> Amebic abscess of brain (and liver) (and lung)

A06.7   **Cutaneous amebiasis**

✓5ᵗʰ **A06.8**   **Amebic infection of other sites**

> **A06.81**   **Amebic cystitis**

> **A06.82**   **Other amebic genitourinary infections**
> > Amebic balanitis
> > Amebic vesiculitis
> > Amebic vulvovaginitis

> **A06.89**   **Other amebic infections**
> > Amebic appendicitis
> > Amebic splenic abscess

A06.9   **Amebiasis, unspecified**

✓4ᵗʰ **A07**   **Other protozoal intestinal diseases**

> **DEF:** Protozoa: Group comprised of the simplest, single celled organisms, ranging in size from micro to macroscopic. They can live alone or in colonies, and do not show any differentiation in tissues. Most are motile and can live free in nature, but some are parasitic, causing disease in the variety of hosts they inhabit.

A07.0   **Balantidiasis**
> Balantidial dysentery

A07.1   **Giardiasis [lambliasis]**
> **DEF:** Infection caused by the flagellate protozoan _Giardia lamblia_ causing gastrointestinal problems such as vomiting, chronic diarrhea, and weight loss. The most common parasite in the US, this is usually transmitted by ingesting contaminated water while in the cyst state and latches onto the wall of the small intestine.

A07.2   **Cryptosporidiosis**   `HCC`
> **DEF:** Microscopic parasite found in water and one of the most common causes of waterborne gastrointestinal infectious disease in the United States. It is usually transmitted by ingesting contaminated drinking water or recreational water and causes profuse watery diarrhea, flatulence, abdominal pain, and cramping.

A07.3   **Isosporiasis**
> Infection due to Isospora belli and Isospora hominis
> Intestinal coccidiosis
> Isosporosis

A07.4   **Cyclosporiasis**

A07.8   **Other specified protozoal intestinal diseases**
> Intestinal microsporidiosis
> Intestinal trichomoniasis
> Sarcocystosis
> Sarcosporidiosis

A07.9   **Protozoal intestinal disease, unspecified**
> Flagellate diarrhea
> Protozoal colitis
> Protozoal diarrhea
> Protozoal dysentery

✓4ᵗʰ **A08**   **Viral and other specified intestinal infections**

> _EXCLUDES 1_   influenza with involvement of gastrointestinal tract (J09.X3, J10.2, J11.2)

A08.0   **Rotaviral enteritis**

✓5ᵗʰ **A08.1**   **Acute gastroenteropathy due to Norwalk agent and other small round viruses**

> **A08.11**   **Acute gastroenteropathy due to Norwalk agent**
> > Acute gastroenteropathy due to Norovirus
> > Acute gastroenteropathy due to Norwalk-like agent

> **A08.19**   **Acute gastroenteropathy due to other small round viruses**
> > Acute gastroenteropathy due to small round virus [SRV] NOS

A08.2   **Adenoviral enteritis**

✓5ᵗʰ **A08.3**   **Other viral enteritis**

> **A08.31**   **Calicivirus enteritis**

> **A08.32**   **Astrovirus enteritis**

> **A08.39**   **Other viral enteritis**
> > Coxsackie virus enteritis
> > Echovirus enteritis
> > Enterovirus enteritis NEC
> > Torovirus enteritis

A08.4   **Viral intestinal infection, unspecified**
> Viral enteritis NOS
> Viral gastroenteritis NOS
> Viral gastroenteropathy NOS
> **AHA:** 2016,3Q,12

A08.8   **Other specified intestinal infections**

A09   **Infectious gastroenteritis and colitis, unspecified**
> Infectious colitis NOS
> Infectious enteritis NOS
> Infectious gastroenteritis NOS
> > _EXCLUDES 1_   colitis NOS (K52.9)
> > diarrhea NOS (R19.7)
> > enteritis NOS (K52.9)
> > gastroenteritis NOS (K52.9)
> > noninfective gastroenteritis and colitis, unspecified (K52.9)
> **DEF:** Colitis: Inflammation of mucous membranes of the colon.
> **DEF:** Enteritis: Inflammation of mucous membranes of the small intestine.
> **DEF:** Gastroenteritis: Inflammation of mucous membranes of the stomach and intestines.

✓ Additional Character Required   ✓x7ᵗʰ Placeholder Alert   Manifestation   Unspecified Dx   ▶◀ Revised Text   ● New Code   ▲ Revised Code Title

Tuberculosis (A15-A19)

INCLUDES   infections due to Mycobacterium tuberculosis and Mycobacterium bovis

EXCLUDES 1   *congenital tuberculosis (P37.Ø)*
nonspecific reaction to test for tuberculosis without active tuberculosis (R76.1-)
pneumoconiosis associated with tuberculosis, any type in A15 (J65)
positive PPD (R76.11)
positive tuberculin skin test without active tuberculosis (R76.11)
sequelae of tuberculosis (B9Ø.-)
silicotuberculosis (J65)

DEF: Bacterial infection that typically spreads by inhalation of an airborne agent that usually attacks the lungs, but may also affect other organs.

✓4ᵗʰ **A15**   **Respiratory tuberculosis**

     A15.Ø   **Tuberculosis of lung**
          Tuberculous bronchiectasis
          Tuberculous fibrosis of lung
          Tuberculous pneumonia
          Tuberculous pneumothorax

Tuberculosis of Lung

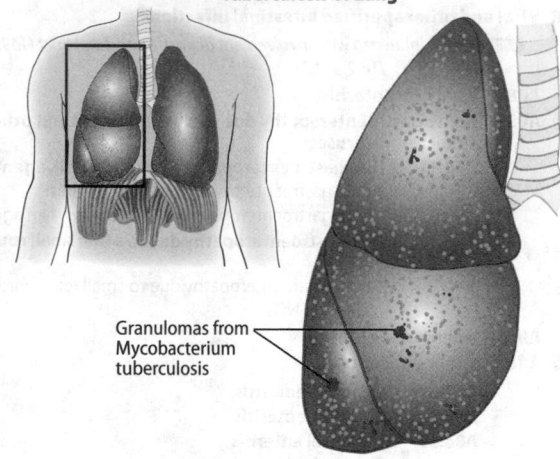

Granulomas from Mycobacterium tuberculosis

     A15.4   **Tuberculosis of intrathoracic lymph nodes**
          Tuberculosis of hilar lymph nodes
          Tuberculosis of mediastinal lymph nodes
          Tuberculosis of tracheobronchial lymph nodes
          EXCLUDES 1   *tuberculosis specified as primary (A15.7)*

     A15.5   **Tuberculosis of larynx, trachea and bronchus**
          Tuberculosis of bronchus
          Tuberculosis of glottis
          Tuberculosis of larynx
          Tuberculosis of trachea

     A15.6   **Tuberculous pleurisy**
          Tuberculosis of pleura Tuberculous empyema
          EXCLUDES 1   *primary respiratory tuberculosis (A15.7)*

     A15.7   **Primary respiratory tuberculosis**

     A15.8   **Other respiratory tuberculosis**
          Mediastinal tuberculosis
          Nasopharyngeal tuberculosis
          Tuberculosis of nose
          Tuberculosis of sinus [any nasal]

     A15.9   **Respiratory tuberculosis unspecified**

✓4ᵗʰ **A17**   **Tuberculosis of nervous system**

     A17.Ø   **Tuberculous meningitis**
          Tuberculosis of meninges (cerebral)(spinal)
          Tuberculous leptomeningitis
          EXCLUDES 1   *tuberculous meningoencephalitis (A17.82)*

     A17.1   **Meningeal tuberculoma**
          Tuberculoma of meninges (cerebral) (spinal)
          EXCLUDES 2   *tuberculoma of brain and spinal cord (A17.81)*

     ✓5ᵗʰ **A17.8**   **Other tuberculosis of nervous system**

          A17.81   **Tuberculoma of brain and spinal cord**
                   Tuberculous abscess of brain and spinal cord

          A17.82   **Tuberculous meningoencephalitis**
                   Tuberculous myelitis

          A17.83   **Tuberculous neuritis**
                   Tuberculous mononeuropathy

          A17.89   **Other tuberculosis of nervous system**
                   Tuberculous polyneuropathy

     A17.9   **Tuberculosis of nervous system, unspecified**

✓4ᵗʰ **A18**   **Tuberculosis of other organs**

     ✓5ᵗʰ **A18.Ø**   **Tuberculosis of bones and joints**

          A18.01   **Tuberculosis of spine**
                   Pott's disease or curvature of spine
                   Tuberculous arthritis
                   Tuberculous osteomyelitis of spine
                   Tuberculous spondylitis

          A18.02   **Tuberculous arthritis of other joints**
                   Tuberculosis of hip (joint)
                   Tuberculosis of knee (joint)

          A18.03   **Tuberculosis of other bones**
                   Tuberculous mastoiditis
                   Tuberculous osteomyelitis

          A18.09   **Other musculoskeletal tuberculosis**
                   Tuberculous myositis
                   Tuberculous synovitis
                   Tuberculous tenosynovitis

     ✓5ᵗʰ **A18.1**   **Tuberculosis of genitourinary system**

          A18.10   **Tuberculosis of genitourinary system, unspecified**
          A18.11   **Tuberculosis of kidney and ureter**
          A18.12   **Tuberculosis of bladder**
          A18.13   **Tuberculosis of other urinary organs**
                   Tuberculous urethritis
          A18.14   **Tuberculosis of prostate**   A ♂
          A18.15   **Tuberculosis of other male genital organs**   ♂
          A18.16   **Tuberculosis of cervix**   ♀
          A18.17   **Tuberculous female pelvic inflammatory disease**   ♀
                   Tuberculous endometritis
                   Tuberculous oophoritis and salpingitis
          A18.18   **Tuberculosis of other female genital organs**   ♀
                   Tuberculous ulceration of vulva

     A18.2   **Tuberculous peripheral lymphadenopathy**
          Tuberculous adenitis
          EXCLUDES 2   *tuberculosis of bronchial and mediastinal lymph nodes (A15.4)*
                   tuberculosis of mesenteric and retroperitoneal lymph nodes (A18.39)
                   tuberculous tracheobronchial adenopathy (A15.4)

     ✓5ᵗʰ **A18.3**   **Tuberculosis of intestines, peritoneum and mesenteric glands**

          A18.31   **Tuberculous peritonitis**
                   Tuberculous ascites
                   DEF: Tuberculous inflammation of the membrane lining the abdomen.

          A18.32   **Tuberculous enteritis**
                   Tuberculosis of anus and rectum
                   Tuberculosis of intestine (large) (small)

          A18.39   **Retroperitoneal tuberculosis**
                   Tuberculosis of mesenteric glands
                   Tuberculosis of retroperitoneal (lymph glands)

     A18.4   **Tuberculosis of skin and subcutaneous tissue**
          Erythema induratum, tuberculous
          Lupus excedens
          Lupus vulgaris NOS
          Lupus vulgaris of eyelid
          Scrofuloderma
          Tuberculosis of external ear
          EXCLUDES 2   *lupus erythematosus (L93.-)*
                   ~~*lupus NOS (M32.9)*~~
                   ▶*systemic lupus erythematosus*◀ *(M32.-)*

     ✓5ᵗʰ **A18.5**   **Tuberculosis of eye**
          EXCLUDES 2   *lupus vulgaris of eyelid (A18.4)*

          A18.50   **Tuberculosis of eye, unspecified**
          A18.51   **Tuberculous episcleritis**
          A18.52   **Tuberculous keratitis**
                   Tuberculous interstitial keratitis
                   Tuberculous keratoconjunctivitis (interstitial) (phlyctenular)
          A18.53   **Tuberculous chorioretinitis**
          A18.54   **Tuberculous iridocyclitis**

A18.59 Other tuberculosis of eye
Tuberculous conjunctivitis

A18.6 Tuberculosis of (inner) (middle) ear
Tuberculous otitis media
EXCLUDES 2   *tuberculosis of external ear (A18.4)*
tuberculous mastoiditis (A18.03)

A18.7 Tuberculosis of adrenal glands
Tuberculous Addison's disease

☑5ᵗʰ **A18.8 Tuberculosis of other specified organs**

A18.81 Tuberculosis of thyroid gland

A18.82 Tuberculosis of other endocrine glands
Tuberculosis of pituitary gland
Tuberculosis of thymus gland

A18.83 Tuberculosis of digestive tract organs, not elsewhere classified
EXCLUDES 1   *tuberculosis of intestine (A18.32)*

A18.84 Tuberculosis of heart
Tuberculous cardiomyopathy
Tuberculous endocarditis
Tuberculous myocarditis
Tuberculous pericarditis

A18.85 Tuberculosis of spleen

A18.89 Tuberculosis of other sites
Tuberculosis of muscle
Tuberculous cerebral arteritis

☑4ᵗʰ **A19 Miliary tuberculosis**
INCLUDES   disseminated tuberculosis
generalized tuberculosis
tuberculous polyserositis

A19.0 Acute miliary tuberculosis of a single specified site

A19.1 Acute miliary tuberculosis of multiple sites

A19.2 Acute miliary tuberculosis, unspecified

A19.8 Other miliary tuberculosis

A19.9 Miliary tuberculosis, unspecified

Certain zoonotic bacterial diseases (A20-A28)

☑4ᵗʰ **A20 Plague**
INCLUDES   infection due to Yersinia pestis

A20.0 Bubonic plague

A20.1 Cellulocutaneous plague

A20.2 Pneumonic plague   HCC

A20.3 Plague meningitis

A20.7 Septicemic plague   HCC

A20.8 Other forms of plague
Abortive plague
Asymptomatic plague
Pestis minor

A20.9 Plague, unspecified

☑4ᵗʰ **A21 Tularemia**
INCLUDES   deer-fly fever
infection due to Francisella tularensis
rabbit fever

DEF: Febrile disease transmitted to humans by the bites of deer flies, fleas, and ticks, by inhaling aerosolized *F. tularensis*, or by ingesting contaminated food or water. Patients quickly develop fever, chills, weakness, headache, backache, and malaise.

A21.0 Ulceroglandular tularemia

A21.1 Oculoglandular tularemia
Ophthalmic tularemia

A21.2 Pulmonary tularemia   HCC

A21.3 Gastrointestinal tularemia
Abdominal tularemia

A21.7 Generalized tularemia

A21.8 Other forms of tularemia

A21.9 Tularemia, unspecified

☑4ᵗʰ **A22 Anthrax**
INCLUDES   infection due to Bacillus anthracis

A22.0 Cutaneous anthrax
Malignant carbuncle
Malignant pustule

A22.1 Pulmonary anthrax   HCC
Inhalation anthrax
Ragpicker's disease
Woolsorter's disease

A22.2 Gastrointestinal anthrax

A22.7 Anthrax sepsis   HCC

A22.8 Other forms of anthrax
Anthrax meningitis

A22.9 Anthrax, unspecified

☑4ᵗʰ **A23 Brucellosis**
INCLUDES   Malta fever
Mediterranean fever
undulant fever

A23.0 Brucellosis due to Brucella melitensis

A23.1 Brucellosis due to Brucella abortus

A23.2 Brucellosis due to Brucella suis

A23.3 Brucellosis due to Brucella canis

A23.8 Other brucellosis

A23.9 Brucellosis, unspecified

☑4ᵗʰ **A24 Glanders and melioidosis**

A24.0 Glanders
Infection due to Pseudomonas mallei
Malleus

A24.1 Acute and fulminating melioidosis
Melioidosis pneumonia
Melioidosis sepsis

A24.2 Subacute and chronic melioidosis

A24.3 Other melioidosis

A24.9 Melioidosis, unspecified
Infection due to Pseudomonas pseudomallei NOS
Whitmore's disease

☑4ᵗʰ **A25 Rat-bite fevers**

A25.0 Spirillosis
Sodoku

A25.1 Streptobacillosis
Epidemic arthritic erythema
Haverhill fever
Streptobacillary rat-bite fever

A25.9 Rat-bite fever, unspecified

☑4ᵗʰ **A26 Erysipeloid**
DEF: Acute cutaneous infection typically caused by trauma to the skin. Presenting as cellulitis, it may become systemic affecting other organs. It is gram positive bacillus and mainly acquired by those who routinely handle meat.

A26.0 Cutaneous erysipeloid
Erythema migrans

A26.7 Erysipelothrix sepsis   HCC

A26.8 Other forms of erysipeloid

A26.9 Erysipeloid, unspecified

☑4ᵗʰ **A27 Leptospirosis**

A27.0 Leptospirosis icterohemorrhagica
Leptospiral or spirochetal jaundice (hemorrhagic)
Weil's disease

☑5ᵗʰ **A27.8 Other forms of leptospirosis**

A27.81 Aseptic meningitis in leptospirosis

A27.89 Other forms of leptospirosis

A27.9 Leptospirosis, unspecified

☑4ᵗʰ **A28 Other zoonotic bacterial diseases, not elsewhere classified**

A28.0 Pasteurellosis

A28.1 Cat-scratch disease
Cat-scratch fever

A28.2 Extraintestinal yersiniosis
EXCLUDES 1   *enteritis due to Yersinia enterocolitica (A04.6)*
plague (A20.-)

A28.8 Other specified zoonotic bacterial diseases, not elsewhere classified

A28.9 Zoonotic bacterial disease, unspecified

☑ Additional Character Required   ☑×7ᵗʰ Placeholder Alert   Manifestation   Unspecified Dx   ►◄ Revised Text   ● New Code   ▲ Revised Code Title

ICD-10-CM 2020   **439**

Chapter 1. Certain Infectious and Parasitic Diseases

Other bacterial diseases (A30-A49)

AHA: 2016,3Q,8-14

✓4th A30 Leprosy [Hansen's disease]
> INCLUDES   infection due to Mycobacterium leprae
> EXCLUDES 1   sequelae of leprosy (B92)

A30.0 Indeterminate leprosy
I leprosy

A30.1 Tuberculoid leprosy
TT leprosy

A30.2 Borderline tuberculoid leprosy
BT leprosy

A30.3 Borderline leprosy
BB leprosy

A30.4 Borderline lepromatous leprosy
BL leprosy

A30.5 Lepromatous leprosy
LL leprosy

A30.8 Other forms of leprosy

A30.9 Leprosy, unspecified

✓4th A31 Infection due to other mycobacteria
> EXCLUDES 2   leprosy (A30.-)
> tuberculosis (A15-A19)

A31.0 Pulmonary mycobacterial infection   HCC
Infection due to Mycobacterium avium
Infection due to Mycobacterium intracellulare [Battey bacillus]
Infection due to Mycobacterium kansasii

A31.1 Cutaneous mycobacterial infection
Buruli ulcer
Infection due to Mycobacterium marinum
Infection due to Mycobacterium ulcerans

A31.2 Disseminated mycobacterium avium-intracellulare complex (DMAC)   HCC
MAC sepsis

A31.8 Other mycobacterial infections

A31.9 Mycobacterial infection, unspecified
Atypical mycobacterial infection NOS
Mycobacteriosis NOS

✓4th A32 Listeriosis
> INCLUDES   listerial foodborne infection
> EXCLUDES 1   neonatal (disseminated) listeriosis (P37.2)

A32.0 Cutaneous listeriosis

✓5th A32.1 Listerial meningitis and meningoencephalitis
     A32.11 Listerial meningitis
     A32.12 Listerial meningoencephalitis

A32.7 Listerial sepsis   HCC

✓5th A32.8 Other forms of listeriosis
     A32.81 Oculoglandular listeriosis
     A32.82 Listerial endocarditis
     A32.89 Other forms of listeriosis
         Listerial cerebral arteritis

A32.9 Listeriosis, unspecified

A33 Tetanus neonatorum   N

A34 Obstetrical tetanus   M ♀

A35 Other tetanus
Tetanus NOS
> EXCLUDES 1   obstetrical tetanus (A34)
> tetanus neonatorum (A33)

DEF: Tetanus: Acute, often fatal, infectious disease caused by the anaerobic, spore-forming bacillus Clostridium tetani. The bacillus enters the body through a contaminated wound, burns, surgical wounds, or cutaneous ulcers. Symptoms include lockjaw, spasms, seizures, and paralysis.

✓4th A36 Diphtheria
A36.0 Pharyngeal diphtheria
Diphtheritic membranous angina
Tonsillar diphtheria

A36.1 Nasopharyngeal diphtheria

A36.2 Laryngeal diphtheria
Diphtheritic laryngotracheitis

A36.3 Cutaneous diphtheria
> EXCLUDES 2   erythrasma (L08.1)

✓5th A36.8 Other diphtheria
     A36.81 Diphtheritic cardiomyopathy   HCC
         Diphtheritic myocarditis
     A36.82 Diphtheritic radiculomyelitis
     A36.83 Diphtheritic polyneuritis
     A36.84 Diphtheritic tubulo-interstitial nephropathy
     A36.85 Diphtheritic cystitis
     A36.86 Diphtheritic conjunctivitis
     A36.89 Other diphtheritic complications
         Diphtheritic peritonitis

A36.9 Diphtheria, unspecified

✓4th A37 Whooping cough
DEF: Acute, highly contagious respiratory tract infection caused by Bordetella pertussis and B. bronchiseptica. Whooping cough is known by its characteristic paroxysmal cough.

✓5th A37.0 Whooping cough due to Bordetella pertussis
     A37.00 Whooping cough due to Bordetella pertussis without pneumonia
     A37.01 Whooping cough due to Bordetella pertussis with pneumonia

✓5th A37.1 Whooping cough due to Bordetella parapertussis
     A37.10 Whooping cough due to Bordetella parapertussis without pneumonia
     A37.11 Whooping cough due to Bordetella parapertussis with pneumonia

✓5th A37.8 Whooping cough due to other Bordetella species
     A37.80 Whooping cough due to other Bordetella species without pneumonia
     A37.81 Whooping cough due to other Bordetella species with pneumonia

✓5th A37.9 Whooping cough, unspecified species
     A37.90 Whooping cough, unspecified species without pneumonia
     A37.91 Whooping cough, unspecified species with pneumonia

✓4th A38 Scarlet fever
> INCLUDES   scarlatina
> EXCLUDES 2   streptococcal sore throat (J02.0)

DEF: Acute contagious disease caused by Group A bacteria, the same bacterium that causes strep throat. Individuals with strep throat can develop scarlet fever particularly if the infection is not treated with antibiotics. It is characterized by a red blush to the skin of the chest and abdomen and swelling of the nose, throat, and mouth.

A38.0 Scarlet fever with otitis media

A38.1 Scarlet fever with myocarditis

A38.8 Scarlet fever with other complications

A38.9 Scarlet fever, uncomplicated
Scarlet fever, NOS

✓4th A39 Meningococcal infection
DEF: Condition caused by Neisseria meningitidis, a bacteria that may invade the spinal cord, brain, heart, joints, optic nerve, or bloodstream.

A39.0 Meningococcal meningitis

A39.1 Waterhouse-Friderichsen syndrome   HCC
Meningococcal hemorrhagic adrenalitis
Meningococcic adrenal syndrome

A39.2 Acute meningococcemia   HCC

A39.3 Chronic meningococcemia   HCC

A39.4 Meningococcemia, unspecified   HCC

✓5th A39.5 Meningococcal heart disease
     A39.50 Meningococcal carditis, unspecified
     A39.51 Meningococcal endocarditis
     A39.52 Meningococcal myocarditis
     A39.53 Meningococcal pericarditis

✓5th A39.8 Other meningococcal infections
     A39.81 Meningococcal encephalitis
     A39.82 Meningococcal retrobulbar neuritis
     A39.83 Meningococcal arthritis   HCC
     A39.84 Postmeningococcal arthritis   HCC
     A39.89 Other meningococcal infections
         Meningococcal conjunctivitis

A39.9 Meningococcal infection, unspecified
Meningococcal disease NOS

☑️⁴ᵗʰ **A40 Streptococcal sepsis**
    Code first:
        postprocedural streptococcal sepsis (T81.4-)
        streptococcal sepsis during labor (O75.3)
        streptococcal sepsis following abortion or ectopic or molar pregnancy
          (O03-O07, O08.0)
        streptococcal sepsis following immunization (T88.0)
        streptococcal sepsis following infusion, transfusion or therapeutic
          injection (T80.2-)
      EXCLUDES 1   neonatal (P36.0-P36.1)
                  puerperal sepsis (O85)
                  sepsis due to Streptococcus, group D (A41.81)
    AHA: 2018,4Q,89; 2018,1Q,16; 2016,1Q,32

    A40.0 Sepsis due to streptococcus, group A   HCC
    A40.1 Sepsis due to streptococcus, group B   HCC
        AHA: 2019,1Q,14
    A40.3 Sepsis due to Streptococcus pneumoniae   HCC
        Pneumococcal sepsis
    A40.8 Other streptococcal sepsis   HCC
    A40.9 Streptococcal sepsis, unspecified   HCC

☑️⁴ᵗʰ **A41 Other sepsis**
    Code first:
        postprocedural sepsis (T81.4-)
        sepsis during labor (O75.3)
        sepsis following abortion, ectopic or molar pregnancy (O03-O07,
          O08.0)
        sepsis following immunization (T88.0)
        sepsis following infusion, transfusion or therapeutic injection (T80.2-)
      EXCLUDES 1   bacteremia NOS (R78.81)
                  neonatal (P36.-)
                  puerperal sepsis (O85)
                  streptococcal sepsis (A40.-)
      EXCLUDES 2   sepsis (due to) (in) actinomycotic (A42.7)
                  sepsis (due to) (in) anthrax (A22.7)
                  sepsis (due to) (in) candidal (B37.7)
                  sepsis (due to) (in) Erysipelothrix (A26.7)
                  sepsis (due to) (in) extraintestinal yersiniosis (A28.2)
                  sepsis (due to) (in) gonococcal (A54.86)
                  sepsis (due to) (in) herpesviral (B00.7)
                  sepsis (due to) (in) listerial (A32.7)
                  sepsis (due to) (in) melioidosis (A24.1)
                  sepsis (due to) (in) meningococcal (A39.2-A39.4)
                  sepsis (due to) (in) plague (A20.7)
                  sepsis (due to) (in) tularemia (A21.7)
                  toxic shock syndrome (A48.3)
    AHA: 2018,4Q,18; 2018,1Q,16; 2016,1Q,32; 2014,2Q,13

  ☑️⁵ᵗʰ **A41.0 Sepsis due to Staphylococcus aureus**
      A41.01 Sepsis due to Methicillin susceptible   HCC Q
             Staphylococcus aureus
             MSSA sepsis
             Staphylococcus aureus sepsis NOS
      A41.02 Sepsis due to Methicillin resistant   HCC
              Staphylococcus aureus
    A41.1 Sepsis due to other specified staphylococcus   HCC
        Coagulase negative staphylococcus sepsis
    A41.2 Sepsis due to unspecified staphylococcus   HCC
    A41.3 Sepsis due to Hemophilus influenzae   HCC
    A41.4 Sepsis due to anaerobes   HCC
        EXCLUDES 1   gas gangrene (A48.0)
  ☑️⁵ᵗʰ **A41.5 Sepsis due to other Gram-negative organisms**
      A41.50 Gram-negative sepsis, unspecified   HCC
             Gram-negative sepsis NOS
      A41.51 Sepsis due to Escherichia coli [E. coli]   HCC
      A41.52 Sepsis due to Pseudomonas   HCC
             Pseudomonas aeroginosa
      A41.53 Sepsis due to Serratia   HCC
      A41.59 Other Gram-negative sepsis   HCC

  ☑️⁵ᵗʰ **A41.8 Other specified sepsis**
      A41.81 Sepsis due to Enterococcus   HCC
             TIP: *E. faecium,* is a species of *Enterococcus* that is
             highly resistant to multiple antibiotics. Assign a code
             from category Z16 when resistance to antimicrobial
             drugs is documented.
      A41.89 Other specified sepsis   HCC
             AHA: 2017,1Q,51; 2016,3Q,8-14
    A41.9 Sepsis, unspecified organism   HCC
        Septicemia NOS

☑️⁴ᵗʰ **A42 Actinomycosis**
      EXCLUDES 1   actinomycetoma (B47.1)
    A42.0 Pulmonary actinomycosis   HCC
    A42.1 Abdominal actinomycosis
    A42.2 Cervicofacial actinomycosis
    A42.7 Actinomycotic sepsis   HCC
  ☑️⁵ᵗʰ **A42.8 Other forms of actinomycosis**
      A42.81 Actinomycotic meningitis
      A42.82 Actinomycotic encephalitis
      A42.89 Other forms of actinomycosis
    A42.9 Actinomycosis, unspecified

☑️⁴ᵗʰ **A43 Nocardiosis**
    DEF: Rare bacterial infection occurring most often in those with weakened
    immune systems. Can be acquired in soil, decaying plants, or standing
    water. It typically begins in the lungs and has a tendency to spread to
    other body systems.
    A43.0 Pulmonary nocardiosis   HCC
    A43.1 Cutaneous nocardiosis
    A43.8 Other forms of nocardiosis
    A43.9 Nocardiosis, unspecified

☑️⁴ᵗʰ **A44 Bartonellosis**
    A44.0 Systemic bartonellosis
        Oroya fever
    A44.1 Cutaneous and mucocutaneous bartonellosis
        Verruga peruana
    A44.8 Other forms of bartonellosis
    A44.9 Bartonellosis, unspecified

    A46 Erysipelas
      EXCLUDES 1   postpartum or puerperal erysipelas (O86.89)
    DEF: Skin infection affecting the upper dermis and superficial dermal
    lymphatics. Lesion edges are well-demarcated with distinct raised borders.
    It is often caused by group A *Streptococci.*

☑️⁴ᵗʰ **A48 Other bacterial diseases, not elsewhere classified**
      EXCLUDES 1   actinomycetoma (B47.1)
    A48.0 Gas gangrene   HCC
        Clostridial cellulitis
        Clostridial myonecrosis
        AHA: 2017,4Q,102
    A48.1 Legionnaires' disease   HCC
        DEF: Severe and often fatal infection by *Legionella pneumophila.*
        Symptoms include high fever, gastrointestinal pain, headache,
        myalgia, dry cough, and pneumonia and it is usually transmitted
        through airborne water droplets via air conditioning systems or
        hot tubs.
    A48.2 Nonpneumonic Legionnaires' disease [Pontiac fever]
    A48.3 Toxic shock syndrome   HCC
        Use additional code to identify the organism (B95, B96)
        EXCLUDES 1   endotoxic shock NOS (R57.8)
                   sepsis NOS (A41.9)
        DEF: Bacteria producing an endotoxin, such as *Staphylococci,*
        flood the body with the toxins producing a high fever, vomiting
        and diarrhea, decreasing blood pressure, a skin rash, and shock.
        Synonym(s): TSS.
    A48.4 Brazilian purpuric fever
        Systemic Hemophilus aegyptius infection
  ☑️⁵ᵗʰ **A48.5 Other specified botulism**
        Non-foodborne intoxication due to toxins of Clostridium
          botulinum [C. botulinum]
      EXCLUDES 1   food poisoning due to toxins of Clostridium
                   botulinum (A05.1)
      A48.51 Infant botulism   P

☑️ Additional Character Required   ☑️ˣ⁷ᵗʰ Placeholder Alert   Manifestation   Unspecified Dx   ▶◀ Revised Text   ● New Code   ▲ Revised Code Title

A48.52   Wound botulism
Non-foodborne botulism NOS
Use additional code for associated wound

A48.8   Other specified bacterial diseases

✓4ᵗʰ **A49   Bacterial infection of unspecified site**
EXCLUDES 1   *bacterial agents as the cause of diseases classified elsewhere (B95-B96)*
chlamydial infection NOS (A74.9)
meningococcal infection NOS (A39.9)
rickettsial infection NOS (A79.9)
spirochetal infection NOS (A69.9)

✓5ᵗʰ **A49.0   Staphylococcal infection, unspecified site**
A49.01   Methicillin susceptible Staphylococcus aureus infection, unspecified site
Methicillin susceptible Staphylococcus aureus (MSSA) infection
Staphylococcus aureus infection NOS
A49.02   Methicillin resistant Staphylococcus aureus infection, unspecified site
Methicillin resistant Staphylococcus aureus (MRSA) infection

A49.1   Streptococcal infection, unspecified site
A49.2   Hemophilus influenzae infection, unspecified site
A49.3   Mycoplasma infection, unspecified site
A49.8   Other bacterial infections of unspecified site
A49.9   Bacterial infection, unspecified
EXCLUDES 1   *bacteremia NOS (R78.81)*

Infections with a predominantly sexual mode of transmission (A50-A64)

EXCLUDES 1   *human immunodeficiency virus [HIV] disease (B20)*
nonspecific and nongonococcal urethritis (N34.1)
Reiter's disease (M02.3-)

✓4ᵗʰ **A50   Congenital syphilis**
✓5ᵗʰ **A50.0   Early congenital syphilis, symptomatic**
Any congenital syphilitic condition specified as early or manifest less than two years after birth.
A50.01   Early congenital syphilitic oculopathy
A50.02   Early congenital syphilitic osteochondropathy
A50.03   Early congenital syphilitic pharyngitis
Early congenital syphilitic laryngitis
A50.04   Early congenital syphilitic pneumonia
A50.05   Early congenital syphilitic rhinitis
A50.06   Early cutaneous congenital syphilis
A50.07   Early mucocutaneous congenital syphilis
A50.08   Early visceral congenital syphilis
A50.09   Other early congenital syphilis, symptomatic

A50.1   Early congenital syphilis, latent
Congenital syphilis without clinical manifestations, with positive serological reaction and negative spinal fluid test, less than two years after birth.

A50.2   Early congenital syphilis, unspecified
Congenital syphilis NOS less than two years after birth.

✓5ᵗʰ **A50.3   Late congenital syphilitic oculopathy**
EXCLUDES 1   *Hutchinson's triad (A50.53)*
A50.30   Late congenital syphilitic oculopathy, unspecified
A50.31   Late congenital syphilitic interstitial keratitis
A50.32   Late congenital syphilitic chorioretinitis
A50.39   Other late congenital syphilitic oculopathy

✓5ᵗʰ **A50.4   Late congenital neurosyphilis [juvenile neurosyphilis]**
Use additional code to identify any associated mental disorder
EXCLUDES 1   *Hutchinson's triad (A50.53)*
A50.40   Late congenital neurosyphilis, unspecified
Juvenile neurosyphilis NOS
A50.41   Late congenital syphilitic meningitis
A50.42   Late congenital syphilitic encephalitis
A50.43   Late congenital syphilitic polyneuropathy
A50.44   Late congenital syphilitic optic nerve atrophy
A50.45   Juvenile general paresis
Dementia paralytica juvenilis
Juvenile tabetoparetic neurosyphilis
A50.49   Other late congenital neurosyphilis
Juvenile tabes dorsalis

✓5ᵗʰ **A50.5   Other late congenital syphilis, symptomatic**
Any congenital syphilitic condition specified as late or manifest two years or more after birth.
A50.51   Clutton's joints
A50.52   Hutchinson's teeth
A50.53   Hutchinson's triad
A50.54   Late congenital cardiovascular syphilis
A50.55   Late congenital syphilitic arthropathy   HCC
A50.56   Late congenital syphilitic osteochondropathy
A50.57   Syphilitic saddle nose
A50.59   Other late congenital syphilis, symptomatic

A50.6   Late congenital syphilis, latent
Congenital syphilis without clinical manifestations, with positive serological reaction and negative spinal fluid test, two years or more after birth.

A50.7   Late congenital syphilis, unspecified
Congenital syphilis NOS two years or more after birth.

A50.9   Congenital syphilis, unspecified

✓4ᵗʰ **A51   Early syphilis**
DEF: Syphilis: Sexually transmitted disease caused by the treponema pallidum spirochete. Syphilis usually exhibits cutaneous manifestations and may exist for years without symptoms.

A51.0   Primary genital syphilis
Syphilitic chancre NOS

A51.1   Primary anal syphilis
A51.2   Primary syphilis of other sites

✓5ᵗʰ **A51.3   Secondary syphilis of skin and mucous membranes**
DEF: Transitory or chronic cutaneous eruptions that present within two to 10 weeks following an initial syphilis infection that may include nontender lymphadenopathy along with alopecia and condylomata lata.
A51.31   Condyloma latum
A51.32   Syphilitic alopecia
A51.39   Other secondary syphilis of skin
Syphilitic leukoderma
Syphilitic mucous patch
EXCLUDES 1   *late syphilitic leukoderma (A52.79)*

✓5ᵗʰ **A51.4   Other secondary syphilis**
A51.41   Secondary syphilitic meningitis
A51.42   Secondary syphilitic female pelvic disease   ♀
A51.43   Secondary syphilitic oculopathy
Secondary syphilitic chorioretinitis
Secondary syphilitic iridocyclitis, iritis
Secondary syphilitic uveitis
A51.44   Secondary syphilitic nephritis
A51.45   Secondary syphilitic hepatitis
A51.46   Secondary syphilitic osteopathy
A51.49   Other secondary syphilitic conditions
Secondary syphilitic lymphadenopathy
Secondary syphilitic myositis

A51.5   Early syphilis, latent
Syphilis (acquired) without clinical manifestations, with positive serological reaction and negative spinal fluid test, less than two years after infection.

A51.9   Early syphilis, unspecified

✓4ᵗʰ **A52   Late syphilis**
✓5ᵗʰ **A52.0   Cardiovascular and cerebrovascular syphilis**
A52.00   Cardiovascular syphilis, unspecified
A52.01   Syphilitic aneurysm of aorta
A52.02   Syphilitic aortitis
A52.03   Syphilitic endocarditis
Syphilitic aortic valve incompetence or stenosis
Syphilitic mitral valve stenosis
Syphilitic pulmonary valve regurgitation
A52.04   Syphilitic cerebral arteritis
A52.05   Other cerebrovascular syphilis
Syphilitic cerebral aneurysm (ruptured) (non-ruptured)
Syphilitic cerebral thrombosis
A52.06   Other syphilitic heart involvement
Syphilitic coronary artery disease
Syphilitic myocarditis
Syphilitic pericarditis
A52.09   Other cardiovascular syphilis

✓5ᵗʰ A52.1 Symptomatic neurosyphilis

     A52.10 Symptomatic neurosyphilis, unspecified

     A52.11 Tabes dorsalis
Locomotor ataxia (progressive)
Tabetic neurosyphilis

     A52.12 Other cerebrospinal syphilis

     A52.13 Late syphilitic meningitis

     A52.14 Late syphilitic encephalitis

     A52.15 Late syphilitic neuropathy
Late syphilitic acoustic neuritis
Late syphilitic optic (nerve) atrophy
Late syphilitic polyneuropathy
Late syphilitic retrobulbar neuritis

     A52.16 Charcôt's arthropathy (tabetic)
DEF: Progressive neurologic arthropathy in which chronic degeneration of joints in the weight-bearing areas with peripheral hypertrophy occurs as a complication of a neuropathy disorder. Supporting structures relax from a loss of sensation resulting in chronic joint instability.

     A52.17 General paresis
Dementia paralytica

     A52.19 Other symptomatic neurosyphilis
Syphilitic parkinsonism

A52.2 Asymptomatic neurosyphilis

A52.3 Neurosyphilis, unspecified
Gumma (syphilitic)
Syphilis (late)
Syphiloma

✓5ᵗʰ A52.7 Other symptomatic late syphilis

     A52.71 Late syphilitic oculopathy
Late syphilitic chorioretinitis
Late syphilitic episcleritis

     A52.72 Syphilis of lung and bronchus

     A52.73 Symptomatic late syphilis of other respiratory organs

     A52.74 Syphilis of liver and other viscera
Late syphilitic peritonitis

     A52.75 Syphilis of kidney and ureter
Syphilitic glomerular disease

     A52.76 Other genitourinary symptomatic late syphilis
Late syphilitic female pelvic inflammatory disease

     A52.77 Syphilis of bone and joint

     A52.78 Syphilis of other musculoskeletal tissue
Late syphilitic bursitis
Syphilis [stage unspecified] of bursa
Syphilis [stage unspecified] of muscle
Syphilis [stage unspecified] of synovium
Syphilis [stage unspecified] of tendon

     A52.79 Other symptomatic late syphilis
Late syphilitic leukoderma
Syphilis of adrenal gland
Syphilis of pituitary gland
Syphilis of thyroid gland
Syphilitic splenomegaly
EXCLUDES 1   syphilitic leukoderma (secondary) (A51.39)

A52.8 Late syphilis, latent
Syphilis (acquired) without clinical manifestations, with positive serological reaction and negative spinal fluid test, two years or more after infection

A52.9 Late syphilis, unspecified

✓4ᵗʰ A53 Other and unspecified syphilis

A53.0 Latent syphilis, unspecified as early or late
Latent syphilis NOS
Positive serological reaction for syphilis

A53.9 Syphilis, unspecified
Infection due to Treponema pallidum NOS
Syphilis (acquired) NOS
EXCLUDES 1   syphilis NOS under two years of age (A50.2)

✓4ᵗʰ A54 Gonococcal infection
DEF: Sexually transmitted bacterial infection caused by *Neisseria gonorrhoeae*. Women are often asymptomatic, while men tend to develop urinary symptoms quickly.

✓5ᵗʰ A54.0 Gonococcal infection of lower genitourinary tract without periurethral or accessory gland abscess
     EXCLUDES 1   gonococcal infection with genitourinary gland abscess (A54.1)
            gonococcal infection with periurethral abscess (A54.1)

     A54.00 Gonococcal infection of lower genitourinary tract, unspecified

     A54.01 Gonococcal cystitis and urethritis, unspecified

     A54.02 Gonococcal vulvovaginitis, unspecified   ♀

     A54.03 Gonococcal cervicitis, unspecified   ♀

     A54.09 Other gonococcal infection of lower genitourinary tract

A54.1 Gonococcal infection of lower genitourinary tract with periurethral and accessory gland abscess
Gonococcal Bartholin's gland abscess

✓5ᵗʰ A54.2 Gonococcal pelviperitonitis and other gonococcal genitourinary infection

     A54.21 Gonococcal infection of kidney and ureter

     A54.22 Gonococcal prostatitis   ♂

     A54.23 Gonococcal infection of other male genital organs   ♂
Gonococcal epididymitis
Gonococcal orchitis

     A54.24 Gonococcal female pelvic inflammatory disease   ♀
Gonococcal pelviperitonitis
EXCLUDES 1   gonococcal peritonitis (A54.85)

     A54.29 Other gonococcal genitourinary infections

✓5ᵗʰ A54.3 Gonococcal infection of eye

     A54.30 Gonococcal infection of eye, unspecified

     A54.31 Gonococcal conjunctivitis
Ophthalmia neonatorum due to gonococcus

     A54.32 Gonococcal iridocyclitis

     A54.33 Gonococcal keratitis

     A54.39 Other gonococcal eye infection
Gonococcal endophthalmia

✓5ᵗʰ A54.4 Gonococcal infection of musculoskeletal system

     A54.40 Gonococcal infection of musculoskeletal system, unspecified   HCC

     A54.41 Gonococcal spondylopathy   HCC

     A54.42 Gonococcal arthritis   HCC
     EXCLUDES 2   gonococcal infection of spine (A54.41)

     A54.43 Gonococcal osteomyelitis   HCC
     EXCLUDES 2   gonococcal infection of spine (A54.41)

     A54.49 Gonococcal infection of other musculoskeletal tissue   HCC
Gonococcal bursitis
Gonococcal myositis
Gonococcal synovitis
Gonococcal tenosynovitis

A54.5 Gonococcal pharyngitis

A54.6 Gonococcal infection of anus and rectum

✓5ᵗʰ A54.8 Other gonococcal infections

     A54.81 Gonococcal meningitis

     A54.82 Gonococcal brain abscess

     A54.83 Gonococcal heart infection
Gonococcal endocarditis
Gonococcal myocarditis
Gonococcal pericarditis

     A54.84 Gonococcal pneumonia   HCC

     A54.85 Gonococcal peritonitis   HCC
     EXCLUDES 1   gonococcal pelviperitonitis (A54.24)

     A54.86 Gonococcal sepsis   HCC

     A54.89 Other gonococcal infections
Gonococcal keratoderma
Gonococcal lymphadenitis

A54.9 Gonococcal infection, unspecified

Additional Character Required   ✓x7ᵗʰ Placeholder Alert   Manifestation   Unspecified Dx   ▶◀ Revised Text   ● New Code   ▲ Revised Code Title

A55 Chlamydial lymphogranuloma (venereum)
Climatic or tropical bubo
Durand-Nicolas-Favre disease
Esthiomene
Lymphogranuloma inguinale

√4ᵗʰ A56 Other sexually transmitted chlamydial diseases
> INCLUDES   sexually transmitted diseases due to Chlamydia trachomatis
> EXCLUDES 1   neonatal chlamydial conjunctivitis (P39.1)
> neonatal chlamydial pneumonia (P23.1)
> EXCLUDES 2   chlamydial lymphogranuloma (A55)
> conditions classified to A74.-

DEF: Chlamydia trachomatis: Bacterium that causes a common venereal disease. Symptoms of chlamydia are usually mild or absent, however, serious complications may cause irreversible damage, including cystitis, pelvic inflammatory disease, and infertility in women and discharge from the penis, prostatitis, and infertility in men. Genital chlamydial infection can cause arthritis, skin lesions, and inflammation of the eye and urethra.
Synonym(s): Reiter's syndrome.

√5ᵗʰ A56.0 Chlamydial infection of lower genitourinary tract

     A56.00 Chlamydial infection of lower genitourinary tract, unspecified

     A56.01 Chlamydial cystitis and urethritis

     A56.02 Chlamydial vulvovaginitis   ♀

     A56.09 Other chlamydial infection of lower genitourinary tract
     Chlamydial cervicitis

√5ᵗʰ A56.1 Chlamydial infection of pelviperitoneum and other genitourinary organs

     A56.11 Chlamydial female pelvic inflammatory disease   ♀

     A56.19 Other chlamydial genitourinary infection
     Chlamydial epididymitis
     Chlamydial orchitis

A56.2 Chlamydial infection of genitourinary tract, unspecified

A56.3 Chlamydial infection of anus and rectum

A56.4 Chlamydial infection of pharynx

A56.8 Sexually transmitted chlamydial infection of other sites

A57 Chancroid
Ulcus molle
DEF: Localized infection by *Haemophilus ducreyi*, causing genital ulcers and infecting the inguinal lymph nodes.

A58 Granuloma inguinale
Donovanosis

√4ᵗʰ A59 Trichomoniasis
> EXCLUDES 2   intestinal trichomoniasis (A07.8)

DEF: Infection with the parasitic, flagellated protozoa of the genus *Trichomonas*. This protozoon is found in the intestinal and genitourinary tracts of humans and in the mouth around tartar, cavities, and areas of periodontal disease.

√5ᵗʰ A59.0 Urogenital trichomoniasis

     A59.00 Urogenital trichomoniasis, unspecified
     Fluor (vaginalis) due to Trichomonas
     Leukorrhea (vaginalis) due to Trichomonas

     A59.01 Trichomonal vulvovaginitis   ♀

     A59.02 Trichomonal prostatitis   ♂

     A59.03 Trichomonal cystitis and urethritis

     A59.09 Other urogenital trichomoniasis
     Trichomonas cervicitis

A59.8 Trichomoniasis of other sites

A59.9 Trichomoniasis, unspecified

√4ᵗʰ A60 Anogenital herpesviral [herpes simplex] infections

√5ᵗʰ A60.0 Herpesviral infection of genitalia and urogenital tract

     A60.00 Herpesviral infection of urogenital system, unspecified

     A60.01 Herpesviral infection of penis   ♂

     A60.02 Herpesviral infection of other male genital organs   ♂

     A60.03 Herpesviral cervicitis   ♀

     A60.04 Herpesviral vulvovaginitis   ♀
     Herpesviral [herpes simplex] ulceration
     Herpesviral [herpes simplex] vaginitis
     Herpesviral [herpes simplex] vulvitis

     A60.09 Herpesviral infection of other urogenital tract

A60.1 Herpesviral infection of perianal skin and rectum

A60.9 Anogenital herpesviral infection, unspecified

√4ᵗʰ A63 Other predominantly sexually transmitted diseases, not elsewhere classified
> EXCLUDES 2   molluscum contagiosum (B08.1)
> papilloma of cervix (D26.0)

A63.0 Anogenital (venereal) warts
Anogenital warts due to (human) papillomavirus [HPV]
Condyloma acuminatum

A63.8 Other specified predominantly sexually transmitted diseases

A64 Unspecified sexually transmitted disease

Other spirochetal diseases (A65-A69)

> EXCLUDES 2   leptospirosis (A27.-)
> syphilis (A50-A53)

A65 Nonvenereal syphilis
Bejel
Endemic syphilis
Njovera

√4ᵗʰ A66 Yaws
> INCLUDES   bouba
> frambesia (tropica)
> pian

A66.0 Initial lesions of yaws
Chancre of yaws
Frambesia, initial or primary
Initial frambesial ulcer
Mother yaw

A66.1 Multiple papillomata and wet crab yaws
Frambesioma
Pianoma
Plantar or palmar papilloma of yaws

A66.2 Other early skin lesions of yaws
Cutaneous yaws, less than five years after infection
Early yaws (cutaneous) (macular) (maculopapular) (micropapular) (papular)
Frambeside of early yaws

A66.3 Hyperkeratosis of yaws
Ghoul hand
Hyperkeratosis, palmar or plantar (early) (late) due to yaws
Worm-eaten soles

A66.4 Gummata and ulcers of yaws
Gummatous frambeside
Nodular late yaws (ulcerated)

A66.5 Gangosa
Rhinopharyngitis mutilans

A66.6 Bone and joint lesions of yaws   HCC

Yaws ganglion
Yaws goundou
Yaws gumma, bone
Yaws gummatous osteitis or periostitis
Yaws hydrarthrosis
Yaws osteitis
Yaws periostitis (hypertrophic)

A66.7 Other manifestations of yaws
Juxta-articular nodules of yaws
Mucosal yaws

A66.8 Latent yaws
Yaws without clinical manifestations, with positive serology

A66.9 Yaws, unspecified

√4ᵗʰ A67 Pinta [carate]

A67.0 Primary lesions of pinta
Chancre (primary) of pinta
Papule (primary) of pinta

A67.1 Intermediate lesions of pinta
Erythematous plaques of pinta
Hyperchromic lesions of pinta
Hyperkeratosis of pinta
Pintids

A67.2 Late lesions of pinta
Achromic skin lesions of pinta
Cicatricial skin lesions of pinta
Dyschromic skin lesions of pinta

A67.3 Mixed lesions of pinta
Achromic with hyperchromic skin lesions of pinta [carate]

A67.9 Pinta, unspecified

☑4ᵗʰ **A68 Relapsing fevers**

    INCLUDES   recurrent fever

    EXCLUDES 2   *Lyme disease (A69.2-)*

   A68.0 Louse-borne relapsing fever

      Relapsing fever due to Borrelia recurrentis

   A68.1 Tick-borne relapsing fever

      Relapsing fever due to any Borrelia species other than Borrelia recurrentis

   A68.9 Relapsing fever, unspecified

☑4ᵗʰ **A69 Other spirochetal infections**

   A69.0 Necrotizing ulcerative stomatitis

      Cancrum oris

      Fusospirochetal gangrene

      Noma

      Stomatitis gangrenosa

   A69.1 Other Vincent's infections

      Fusospirochetal pharyngitis

      Necrotizing ulcerative (acute) gingivitis

      Necrotizing ulcerative (acute) gingivostomatitis

      Spirochetal stomatitis

      Trench mouth

      Vincent's angina

      Vincent's gingivitis

☑5ᵗʰ **A69.2 Lyme disease**

      Erythema chronicum migrans due to Borrelia burgdorferi

      DEF: Recurrent multisystem disorder through tick bites that begins with lesions of erythema chronicum migrans and is followed by arthritis of the large joints, myalgia, malaise, and neurological and cardiac manifestations.

    A69.20 Lyme disease, unspecified

    A69.21 Meningitis due to Lyme disease

    A69.22 Other neurologic disorders in Lyme disease

       Cranial neuritis

       Meningoencephalitis

       Polyneuropathy

    A69.23 Arthritis due to Lyme disease   HCC

    A69.29 Other conditions associated with Lyme disease

       Myopericarditis due to Lyme disease

       AHA: 2016,3Q,12

   A69.8 Other specified spirochetal infections

   A69.9 Spirochetal infection, unspecified

Other diseases caused by chlamydiae (A70-A74)

    EXCLUDES 1   *sexually transmitted chlamydial diseases (A55-A56)*

A70 Chlamydia psittaci infections

    Ornithosis

    Parrot fever

    Psittacosis

☑4ᵗʰ **A71 Trachoma**

    EXCLUDES 1   *sequelae of trachoma (B94.0)*

   A71.0 Initial stage of trachoma

      Trachoma dubium

   A71.1 Active stage of trachoma

      Granular conjunctivitis (trachomatous)

      Trachomatous follicular conjunctivitis

      Trachomatous pannus

   A71.9 Trachoma, unspecified

☑4ᵗʰ **A74 Other diseases caused by chlamydiae**

    EXCLUDES 1   *neonatal chlamydial conjunctivitis (P39.1)*

               neonatal chlamydial pneumonia (P23.1)

               Reiter's disease (M02.3-)

               sexually transmitted chlamydial diseases (A55-A56)

    EXCLUDES 2   *chlamydial pneumonia (J16.0)*

   A74.0 Chlamydial conjunctivitis

      Paratrachoma

☑5ᵗʰ **A74.8 Other chlamydial diseases**

    A74.81 Chlamydial peritonitis

    A74.89 Other chlamydial diseases

   A74.9 Chlamydial infection, unspecified

      Chlamydiosis NOS

Rickettsioses (A75-A79)

DEF: Rickettsia: Condition caused by bacteria that live in lice/ticks transmitted to humans through bites.

☑4ᵗʰ **A75 Typhus fever**

    EXCLUDES 1   *rickettsiosis due to Ehrlichia sennetsu (A79.81)*

   A75.0 Epidemic louse-borne typhus fever due to Rickettsia prowazekii

      Classical typhus (fever)

      Epidemic (louse-borne) typhus

   A75.1 Recrudescent typhus [Brill's disease]

      Brill-Zinsser disease

   A75.2 Typhus fever due to Rickettsia typhi

      Murine (flea-borne) typhus

   A75.3 Typhus fever due to Rickettsia tsutsugamushi

      Scrub (mite-borne) typhus

      Tsutsugamushi fever

   A75.9 Typhus fever, unspecified

      Typhus (fever) NOS

☑4ᵗʰ **A77 Spotted fever [tick-borne rickettsioses]**

   A77.0 Spotted fever due to Rickettsia rickettsii

      Rocky Mountain spotted fever

      Sao Paulo fever

   A77.1 Spotted fever due to Rickettsia conorii

      African tick typhus

      Boutonneuse fever

      India tick typhus

      Kenya tick typhus

      Marseilles fever

      Mediterranean tick fever

   A77.2 Spotted fever due to Rickettsia siberica

      North Asian tick fever

      Siberian tick typhus

   A77.3 Spotted fever due to Rickettsia australis

      Queensland tick typhus

☑5ᵗʰ **A77.4 Ehrlichiosis**

    EXCLUDES 1   *Rickettsiosis due to Ehrlichia sennetsu (A79.81)*

    A77.40 Ehrlichiosis, unspecified

    A77.41 Ehrlichiosis chafeensis [E. chafeensis]

    A77.49 Other ehrlichiosis

   A77.8 Other spotted fevers

   A77.9 Spotted fever, unspecified

      Tick-borne typhus NOS

A78 Q fever

    Infection due to Coxiella burnetii

    Nine Mile fever

    Quadrilateral fever

☑4ᵗʰ **A79 Other rickettsioses**

   A79.0 Trench fever

      Quintan fever

      Wolhynian fever

   A79.1 Rickettsialpox due to Rickettsia akari

      Kew Garden fever

      Vesicular rickettsiosis

☑5ᵗʰ **A79.8 Other specified rickettsioses**

    A79.81 Rickettsiosis due to Ehrlichia sennetsu

    A79.89 Other specified rickettsioses

   A79.9 Rickettsiosis, unspecified

      Rickettsial infection NOS

Viral and prion infections of the central nervous system (A80-A89)

    EXCLUDES 1   *postpolio syndrome (G14)*

               sequelae of poliomyelitis (B91)

               sequelae of viral encephalitis (B94.1)

☑4ᵗʰ **A80 Acute poliomyelitis**

   A80.0 Acute paralytic poliomyelitis, vaccine-associated

   A80.1 Acute paralytic poliomyelitis, wild virus, imported

   A80.2 Acute paralytic poliomyelitis, wild virus, indigenous

☑5ᵗʰ **A80.3 Acute paralytic poliomyelitis, other and unspecified**

    A80.30 Acute paralytic poliomyelitis, unspecified

    A80.39 Other acute paralytic poliomyelitis

   A80.4 Acute nonparalytic poliomyelitis

   A80.9 Acute poliomyelitis, unspecified

✓4ᵗʰ A81 Atypical virus infections of central nervous system

> INCLUDES   diseases of the central nervous system caused by prions

Use additional code to identify:
dementia with behavioral disturbance (F02.81)
dementia without behavioral disturbance (F02.80)

✓5ᵗʰ A81.0 Creutzfeldt-Jakob disease

> DEF: Communicable, rare spongiform encephalopathy occurring later in life with progressive destruction of the pyramidal and extrapyramidal systems eventually leading to death. Progressive dementia, wasting of muscles, tremor, and other symptoms are present.

    A81.00 Creutzfeldt-Jakob disease, unspecified   HCC
         Jakob-Creutzfeldt disease, unspecified

    A81.01 Variant Creutzfeldt-Jakob disease   HCC
         vCJD

    A81.09 Other Creutzfeldt-Jakob disease   HCC
         CJD
         Familial Creutzfeldt-Jakob disease
         Iatrogenic Creutzfeldt-Jakob disease
         Sporadic Creutzfeldt-Jakob disease
         Subacute spongiform encephalopathy (with dementia)

A81.1 Subacute sclerosing panencephalitis   HCC
     Dawson's inclusion body encephalitis
     Van Bogaert's sclerosing leukoencephalopathy

A81.2 Progressive multifocal leukoencephalopathy   HCC
     Multifocal leukoencephalopathy NOS

✓5ᵗʰ A81.8 Other atypical virus infections of central nervous system

    A81.81 Kuru   HCC

    A81.82 Gerstmann-Sträussler-Scheinker syndrome   HCC
         GSS syndrome

    A81.83 Fatal familial insomnia   HCC
         FFI

    A81.89 Other atypical virus infections of central nervous system   HCC

A81.9 Atypical virus infection of central nervous system, unspecified   HCC
     Prion diseases of the central nervous system NOS

✓4ᵗʰ A82 Rabies

A82.0 Sylvatic rabies

A82.1 Urban rabies

A82.9 Rabies, unspecified

✓4ᵗʰ A83 Mosquito-borne viral encephalitis

> INCLUDES   mosquito-borne viral meningoencephalitis
> EXCLUDES 2   Venezuelan equine encephalitis (A92.2)
>   West Nile fever (A92.3-)
>   West Nile virus (A92.3-)

A83.0 Japanese encephalitis

A83.1 Western equine encephalitis

A83.2 Eastern equine encephalitis

A83.3 St Louis encephalitis

A83.4 Australian encephalitis
     Kunjin virus disease

A83.5 California encephalitis
     California meningoencephalitis
     La Crosse encephalitis

A83.6 Rocio virus disease

A83.8 Other mosquito-borne viral encephalitis

A83.9 Mosquito-borne viral encephalitis, unspecified

✓4ᵗʰ A84 Tick-borne viral encephalitis

> INCLUDES   tick-borne viral meningoencephalitis

A84.0 Far Eastern tick-borne encephalitis [Russian spring-summer encephalitis]

A84.1 Central European tick-borne encephalitis

A84.8 Other tick-borne viral encephalitis
     Louping ill
     Powassan virus disease

A84.9 Tick-borne viral encephalitis, unspecified

✓4ᵗʰ A85 Other viral encephalitis, not elsewhere classified

> INCLUDES   specified viral encephalomyelitis NEC
>   specified viral meningoencephalitis NEC
> EXCLUDES 1   benign myalgic encephalomyelitis (G93.3)
>   encephalitis due to cytomegalovirus (B25.8)
>   encephalitis due to herpesvirus NEC (B10.0-)
>   encephalitis due to herpesvirus [herpes simplex] (B00.4)
>   encephalitis due to measles virus (B05.0)
>   encephalitis due to mumps virus (B26.2)
>   encephalitis due to poliomyelitis virus (A80.-)
>   encephalitis due to zoster (B02.0)
>   lymphocytic choriomeningitis (A87.2)

A85.0 Enteroviral encephalitis
     Enteroviral encephalomyelitis

A85.1 Adenoviral encephalitis
     Adenoviral meningoencephalitis

A85.2 Arthropod-borne viral encephalitis, unspecified
> EXCLUDES 1   West nile virus with encephalitis (A92.31)

A85.8 Other specified viral encephalitis
     Encephalitis lethargica
     Von Economo-Cruchet disease

A86 Unspecified viral encephalitis
     Viral encephalomyelitis NOS
     Viral meningoencephalitis NOS

✓4ᵗʰ A87 Viral meningitis

> EXCLUDES 1   meningitis due to herpesvirus [herpes simplex] (B00.3)
>   meningitis due to measles virus (B05.1)
>   meningitis due to mumps virus (B26.1)
>   meningitis due to poliomyelitis virus (A80.-)
>   meningitis due to zoster (B02.1)

> DEF: Meningitis: Inflammation of the meningeal layers of the brain and spine.

A87.0 Enteroviral meningitis
     Coxsackievirus meningitis
     Echovirus meningitis

A87.1 Adenoviral meningitis

A87.2 Lymphocytic choriomeningitis
     Lymphocytic meningoencephalitis

A87.8 Other viral meningitis

A87.9 Viral meningitis, unspecified

✓4ᵗʰ A88 Other viral infections of central nervous system, not elsewhere classified

> EXCLUDES 1   viral encephalitis NOS (A86)
>   viral meningitis NOS (A87.9)

A88.0 Enteroviral exanthematous fever [Boston exanthem]

A88.1 Epidemic vertigo

A88.8 Other specified viral infections of central nervous system

A89 Unspecified viral infection of central nervous system

Arthropod-borne viral fevers and viral hemorrhagic fevers (A90-A99)

A90 Dengue fever [classical dengue]
> EXCLUDES 1   dengue hemorrhagic fever (A91)

     AHA: 2016,3Q,13

A91 Dengue hemorrhagic fever

✓4ᵗʰ A92 Other mosquito-borne viral fevers
> EXCLUDES 1   Ross River disease (B33.1)

A92.0 Chikungunya virus disease
     Chikungunya (hemorrhagic) fever

A92.1 O'nyong-nyong fever

A92.2 Venezuelan equine fever
     Venezuelan equine encephalitis
     Venezuelan equine encephalomyelitis virus disease

✓5ᵗʰ A92.3 West Nile virus infection
     West Nile fever
     AHA: 2016,3Q,12

    A92.30 West Nile virus infection, unspecified
         West Nile fever NOS
         West Nile fever without complications
         West Nile virus NOS

    A92.31 West Nile virus infection with encephalitis
         West Nile encephalitis
         West Nile encephalomyelitis

A92.32   **West Nile virus infection with other neurologic manifestation**
     Use additional code to specify the neurologic manifestation

A92.39   **West Nile virus infection with other complications**
     Use additional code to specify the other conditions

A92.4   **Rift Valley fever**

A92.5   **Zika virus disease**
Zika virus fever
Zika virus infection
Zika NOS
EXCLUDES 1   *congenital Zika virus disease (P35.4)*
AHA: 2016,4Q,4-7
DEF: Virus transmitted via a bite from an infected Aedes species mosquito. Common symptoms of the virus include fever, rash, joint pain, and conjunctivitis; they are usually mild in nature and may last from several days to a week. Most people who have the Zika virus do not require medical attention; however, in pregnant women, the Zika virus can cause a serious birth defect called microcephaly, as well as other severe fetal brain defects.
TIP: Assign code Z71.1, when a patient requests testing for Zika virus but in the absence of symptoms or recent exposure to the virus.

A92.8   **Other specified mosquito-borne viral fevers**

A92.9   **Mosquito-borne viral fever, unspecified**

✓4ᵗʰ **A93**   **Other arthropod-borne viral fevers, not elsewhere classified**

A93.0   **Oropouche virus disease**
Oropouche fever

A93.1   **Sandfly fever**
Pappataci fever
Phlebotomus fever

A93.2   **Colorado tick fever**

A93.8   **Other specified arthropod-borne viral fevers**
Piry virus disease
Vesicular stomatitis virus disease [Indiana fever]

A94   **Unspecified arthropod-borne viral fever**
Arboviral fever NOS
Arbovirus infection NOS

✓4ᵗʰ **A95**   **Yellow fever**

A95.0   **Sylvatic yellow fever**
Jungle yellow fever

A95.1   **Urban yellow fever**

A95.9   **Yellow fever, unspecified**

✓4ᵗʰ **A96**   **Arenaviral hemorrhagic fever**

A96.0   **Junin hemorrhagic fever**
Argentinian hemorrhagic fever

A96.1   **Machupo hemorrhagic fever**
Bolivian hemorrhagic fever

A96.2   **Lassa fever**

A96.8   **Other arenaviral hemorrhagic fevers**

A96.9   **Arenaviral hemorrhagic fever, unspecified**

✓4ᵗʰ **A98**   **Other viral hemorrhagic fevers, not elsewhere classified**
EXCLUDES 1   *chikungunya hemorrhagic fever (A92.0)*
dengue hemorrhagic fever (A91)

A98.0   **Crimean-Congo hemorrhagic fever**
Central Asian hemorrhagic fever

A98.1   **Omsk hemorrhagic fever**

A98.2   **Kyasanur Forest disease**

A98.3   **Marburg virus disease**

A98.4   **Ebola virus disease**

A98.5   **Hemorrhagic fever with renal syndrome**
Epidemic hemorrhagic fever
Korean hemorrhagic fever
Russian hemorrhagic fever
Hantaan virus disease
Hantavirus disease with renal manifestations
Nephropathia epidemica
Songo fever
EXCLUDES 1   *hantavirus (cardio)-pulmonary syndrome (B33.4)*

A98.8   **Other specified viral hemorrhagic fevers**

A99   **Unspecified viral hemorrhagic fever**

Viral infections characterized by skin and mucous membrane lesions (B00-B09)

✓4ᵗʰ **B00**   **Herpesviral [herpes simplex] infections**
EXCLUDES 1   *congenital herpesviral infections (P35.2)*
EXCLUDES 2   *anogenital herpesviral infection (A60.-)*
gammaherpesviral mononucleosis (B27.0-)
herpangina (B08.5)

B00.0   **Eczema herpeticum**
Kaposi's varicelliform eruption

B00.1   **Herpesviral vesicular dermatitis**
Herpes simplex facialis
Herpes simplex labialis
Herpes simplex otitis externa
Vesicular dermatitis of ear
Vesicular dermatitis of lip

B00.2   **Herpesviral gingivostomatitis and pharyngotonsillitis**
Herpesviral pharyngitis

B00.3   **Herpesviral meningitis**

B00.4   **Herpesviral encephalitis**
Herpesviral meningoencephalitis
Simian B disease
EXCLUDES 1   *herpesviral encephalitis due to herpesvirus 6 and 7 (B10.01, B10.09)*
non-simplex herpesviral encephalitis (B10.0-)

✓5ᵗʰ **B00.5**   **Herpesviral ocular disease**

B00.50   **Herpesviral ocular disease, unspecified**

B00.51   **Herpesviral iridocyclitis**
Herpesviral iritis
Herpesviral uveitis, anterior

B00.52   **Herpesviral keratitis**
Herpesviral keratoconjunctivitis

B00.53   **Herpesviral conjunctivitis**

B00.59   **Other herpesviral disease of eye**
Herpesviral dermatitis of eyelid

B00.7   **Disseminated herpesviral disease**   `HCC`
Herpesviral sepsis

✓5ᵗʰ **B00.8**   **Other forms of herpesviral infections**

B00.81   **Herpesviral hepatitis**

B00.82   **Herpes simplex myelitis**   `HCC`

B00.89   **Other herpesviral infection**
Herpesviral whitlow

B00.9   **Herpesviral infection, unspecified**
Herpes simplex infection NOS

✓4ᵗʰ **B01**   **Varicella [chickenpox]**

B01.0   **Varicella meningitis**

✓5ᵗʰ **B01.1**   **Varicella encephalitis, myelitis and encephalomyelitis**
Postchickenpox encephalitis, myelitis and encephalomyelitis

B01.11   **Varicella encephalitis and encephalomyelitis**
Postchickenpox encephalitis and encephalomyelitis

B01.12   **Varicella myelitis**   `HCC`
Postchickenpox myelitis

B01.2   **Varicella pneumonia**

✓5ᵗʰ **B01.8**   **Varicella with other complications**

B01.81   **Varicella keratitis**

B01.89   **Other varicella complications**

B01.9   **Varicella without complication**
Varicella NOS

✓4ᵗʰ **B02**   **Zoster [herpes zoster]**
INCLUDES   shingles
zona

B02.0   **Zoster encephalitis**
Zoster meningoencephalitis

B02.1   **Zoster meningitis**
AHA: 2019,1Q,18

✓5ᵗʰ **B02.2**   **Zoster with other nervous system involvement**

B02.21   **Postherpetic geniculate ganglionitis**

B02.22   **Postherpetic trigeminal neuralgia**

B02.23   **Postherpetic polyneuropathy**

B02.24   **Postherpetic myelitis**   `HCC`
Herpes zoster myelitis

B02.29 **Other postherpetic nervous system involvement**
Postherpetic radiculopathy

√5ᵗʰ **B02.3** **Zoster ocular disease**

B02.30 **Zoster ocular disease, unspecified**
B02.31 **Zoster conjunctivitis**
B02.32 **Zoster iridocyclitis**
B02.33 **Zoster keratitis**
Herpes zoster keratoconjunctivitis
B02.34 **Zoster scleritis**
B02.39 **Other herpes zoster eye disease**
Zoster blepharitis

B02.7 **Disseminated zoster**

B02.8 **Zoster with other complications**
Herpes zoster otitis externa

B02.9 **Zoster without complications**
Zoster NOS

B03 **Smallpox**

> **NOTE** In 1980 the 33rd World Health Assembly declared that smallpox had been eradicated.
>
> The classification is maintained for surveillance purposes.

B04 **Monkeypox**

√4ᵗʰ **B05** **Measles**

INCLUDES morbilli

EXCLUDES 1 subacute sclerosing panencephalitis (A81.1)

B05.0 **Measles complicated by encephalitis**
Postmeasles encephalitis

B05.1 **Measles complicated by meningitis**
Postmeasles meningitis

B05.2 **Measles complicated by pneumonia**
Postmeasles pneumonia

B05.3 **Measles complicated by otitis media**
Postmeasles otitis media

B05.4 **Measles with intestinal complications**

√5ᵗʰ **B05.8** **Measles with other complications**

B05.81 **Measles keratitis and keratoconjunctivitis**
B05.89 **Other measles complications**

B05.9 **Measles without complication**
Measles NOS

√4ᵗʰ **B06** **Rubella [German measles]**

EXCLUDES 1 congenital rubella (P35.0)

DEF: Highly contagious virus in which the symptoms are mild and short-lived in most people. Rubella during pregnancy, however, can result in abortion, stillbirth, or congenital defects.

√5ᵗʰ **B06.0** **Rubella with neurological complications**

B06.00 **Rubella with neurological complication, unspecified**
B06.01 **Rubella encephalitis**
Rubella meningoencephalitis
B06.02 **Rubella meningitis**
B06.09 **Other neurological complications of rubella**

√6ᵗʰ **B06.8** **Rubella with other complications**

B06.81 **Rubella pneumonia**
B06.82 **Rubella arthritis**   HCC
B06.89 **Other rubella complications**

B06.9 **Rubella without complication**
Rubella NOS

√4ᵗʰ **B07** **Viral warts**

INCLUDES verruca simplex
verruca vulgaris
viral warts due to human papillomavirus

EXCLUDES 2 anogenital (venereal) warts (A63.0)
papilloma of bladder (D41.4)
papilloma of cervix (D26.0)
papilloma larynx (D14.1)

B07.0 **Plantar wart**
Verruca plantaris

B07.8 **Other viral warts**
Common wart
Flat wart
Verruca plana

B07.9 **Viral wart, unspecified**

√4ᵗʰ **B08** **Other viral infections characterized by skin and mucous membrane lesions, not elsewhere classified**

EXCLUDES 1 vesicular stomatitis virus disease (A93.8)

√5ᵗʰ **B08.0** **Other orthopoxvirus infections**

EXCLUDES 2 monkeypox (B04)

√6ᵗʰ **B08.01** **Cowpox and vaccinia not from vaccine**

B08.010 **Cowpox**
DEF: Disease contracted by milking infected cows. The vesicles usually appear on the fingers, hands, and adjacent areas and usually disappear without scarring. Other symptoms include local edema, lymphangitis, and regional lymphadenitis with or without fever.

B08.011 **Vaccinia not from vaccine**
EXCLUDES 1 vaccinia (from vaccination) (generalized) (T88.1)

B08.02 **Orf virus disease**
Contagious pustular dermatitis
Ecthyma contagiosum

B08.03 **Pseudocowpox [milker's node]**
B08.04 **Paravaccinia, unspecified**
B08.09 **Other orthopoxvirus infections**
Orthopoxvirus infection NOS

B08.1 **Molluscum contagiosum**
DEF: Benign poxvirus infection causing small bumps on the skin or conjunctiva and is transmitted by close contact.

√5ᵗʰ **B08.2** **Exanthema subitum [sixth disease]**

Roseola infantum

B08.20 **Exanthema subitum [sixth disease], unspecified**   P
Roseola infantum, unspecified

B08.21 **Exanthema subitum [sixth disease] due to human herpesvirus 6**   P
Roseola infantum due to human herpesvirus 6

B08.22 **Exanthema subitum [sixth disease] due to human herpesvirus 7**   P
Roseola infantum due to human herpesvirus 7

B08.3 **Erythema infectiosum [fifth disease]**
DEF: Infection with human parvovirus B19, mainly occurring in children. Symptoms include a low-grade fever, malaise, or a "cold" a few days before the appearance of a mild rash illness that presents as a "slapped-cheek" rash on the face and a lacy red rash on the trunk and limbs.

B08.4 **Enteroviral vesicular stomatitis with exanthem**
Hand, foot and mouth disease

B08.5 **Enteroviral vesicular pharyngitis**
Herpangina
DEF: Acute infectious Coxsackie virus infection causing throat lesions, fever, and vomiting that generally affects children in the summer.

√5ᵗʰ **B08.6** **Parapoxvirus infections**

B08.60 **Parapoxvirus infection, unspecified**
B08.61 **Bovine stomatitis**
B08.62 **Sealpox**
B08.69 **Other parapoxvirus infections**

√5ᵗʰ **B08.7** **Yatapoxvirus infections**

B08.70 **Yatapoxvirus infection, unspecified**
B08.71 **Tanapox virus disease**
B08.72 **Yaba pox virus disease**
Yaba monkey tumor disease
B08.79 **Other yatapoxvirus infections**

B08.8 **Other specified viral infections characterized by skin and mucous membrane lesions**
Enteroviral lymphonodular pharyngitis
Foot-and-mouth disease
Poxvirus NEC

B09 **Unspecified viral infection characterized by skin and mucous membrane lesions**
Viral enanthema NOS
Viral exanthema NOS

Other human herpesviruses (B10)

✓4ᵗʰ **B10 Other human herpesviruses**

    EXCLUDES 2 *cytomegalovirus (B25.9)*
            Epstein-Barr virus (B27.0-)
            herpes NOS (B00.9)
            herpes simplex (B00.-)
            herpes zoster (B02.-)
            human herpesvirus NOS (B00.-)
            human herpesvirus 1 and 2 (B00.-)
            human herpesvirus 3 (B01.-, B02.-)
            human herpesvirus 4 (B27.0-)
            human herpesvirus 5 (B25.-)
            varicella (B01.-)
            zoster (B02.-)

  ✓5ᵗʰ **B10.0 Other human herpesvirus encephalitis**

    EXCLUDES 2 *herpes encephalitis NOS (B00.4)*
            herpes simplex encephalitis (B00.4)
            human herpesvirus encephalitis (B00.4)
            simian B herpes virus encephalitis (B00.4)

    B10.01 Human herpesvirus 6 encephalitis

    B10.09 Other human herpesvirus encephalitis
        Human herpesvirus 7 encephalitis

  ✓5ᵗʰ **B10.8 Other human herpesvirus infection**

    B10.81 Human herpesvirus 6 infection

    B10.82 Human herpesvirus 7 infection

    B10.89 Other human herpesvirus infection
        Human herpesvirus 8 infection
        Kaposi's sarcoma-associated herpesvirus infection

Viral hepatitis (B15-B19)

  EXCLUDES 1 *sequelae of viral hepatitis (B94.2)*
  EXCLUDES 2 *cytomegaloviral hepatitis (B25.1)*
          herpesviral [herpes simplex] hepatitis (B00.81)

DEF: Hepatitis A: HAV infection that is self-limiting with flulike symptoms. Transmission is fecal-oral.
DEF: Hepatitis B: HBV infection that can be chronic and systemic. Transmission is bodily fluids.
DEF: Hepatitis C: HCV infection that can be chronic and systemic. Transmission is blood transfusion and unidentified agents.
DEF: Hepatitis D (delta): HDV that occurs only in the presence of hepatitis B virus. Transmission is contaminated blood in contact with mucous membranes.
DEF: Hepatitis E: HEV is an epidemic form. Transmission is fecal-oral, most often from contaminated water.

✓4ᵗʰ **B15 Acute hepatitis A**

  B15.0 Hepatitis A with hepatic coma

  B15.9 Hepatitis A without hepatic coma
    Hepatitis A (acute)(viral) NOS

✓4ᵗʰ **B16 Acute hepatitis B**

  AHA: 2016,3Q,13

  B16.0 Acute hepatitis B with delta-agent with hepatic coma

  B16.1 Acute hepatitis B with delta-agent without hepatic coma

  B16.2 Acute hepatitis B without delta-agent with hepatic coma

  B16.9 Acute hepatitis B without delta-agent and without hepatic coma
    Hepatitis B (acute) (viral) NOS

✓4ᵗʰ **B17 Other acute viral hepatitis**

  B17.0 Acute delta-(super) infection of hepatitis B carrier

  ✓5ᵗʰ **B17.1 Acute hepatitis C**

    B17.10 Acute hepatitis C without hepatic coma
        Acute hepatitis C NOS

    B17.11 Acute hepatitis C with hepatic coma

  B17.2 Acute hepatitis E

  B17.8 Other specified acute viral hepatitis
    Hepatitis non-A non-B (acute) (viral) NEC

  B17.9 Acute viral hepatitis, unspecified
    Acute hepatitis NOS
    Acute infectious hepatitis NOS

✓4ᵗʰ **B18 Chronic viral hepatitis**

  INCLUDES carrier of viral hepatitis
  AHA: 2017,1Q,41

  B18.0 Chronic viral hepatitis B with delta-agent HCC

  B18.1 Chronic viral hepatitis B without delta-agent HCC
    Carrier of viral hepatitis B
    Chronic (viral) hepatitis B

  B18.2 Chronic viral hepatitis C HCC
    Carrier of viral hepatitis C
    AHA: 2018,1Q,4

  B18.8 Other chronic viral hepatitis HCC
    Carrier of other viral hepatitis

  B18.9 Chronic viral hepatitis, unspecified HCC
    Carrier of unspecified viral hepatitis

✓4ᵗʰ **B19 Unspecified viral hepatitis**

  B19.0 Unspecified viral hepatitis with hepatic coma

  ✓5ᵗʰ **B19.1 Unspecified viral hepatitis B**

    B19.10 Unspecified viral hepatitis B without hepatic coma
        Unspecified viral hepatitis B NOS

    B19.11 Unspecified viral hepatitis B with hepatic coma

  ✓5ᵗʰ **B19.2 Unspecified viral hepatitis C**

    B19.20 Unspecified viral hepatitis C without hepatic coma
        Viral hepatitis C NOS

    B19.21 Unspecified viral hepatitis C with hepatic coma

  B19.9 Unspecified viral hepatitis without hepatic coma
    Viral hepatitis NOS

Human immunodeficiency virus [HIV] disease (B20)

B20 Human immunodeficiency virus [HIV] disease HCC

  INCLUDES acquired immune deficiency syndrome [AIDS]
          AIDS-related complex [ARC]
          HIV infection, symptomatic
  Code first Human immunodeficiency virus [HIV] disease complicating pregnancy, childbirth and the puerperium, if applicable (O98.7-)
  Use additional code(s) to identify all manifestations of HIV infection
  EXCLUDES 1 *asymptomatic human immunodeficiency virus [HIV] infection status (Z21)*
          exposure to HIV virus (Z20.6)
          inconclusive serologic evidence of HIV (R75)
  AHA: 2019,1Q,8-11

Other viral diseases (B25-B34)

✓4ᵗʰ **B25 Cytomegaloviral disease**

  EXCLUDES 1 *congenital cytomegalovirus infection (P35.1)*
          cytomegaloviral mononucleosis (B27.1-)

  B25.0 Cytomegaloviral pneumonitis HCC

  B25.1 Cytomegaloviral hepatitis HCC

  B25.2 Cytomegaloviral pancreatitis HCC

  B25.8 Other cytomegaloviral diseases HCC
    Cytomegaloviral encephalitis

  B25.9 Cytomegaloviral disease, unspecified HCC

✓4ᵗʰ **B26 Mumps**

  INCLUDES epidemic parotitis
          infectious parotitis

  B26.0 Mumps orchitis ♂

  B26.1 Mumps meningitis

  B26.2 Mumps encephalitis

  B26.3 Mumps pancreatitis

  ✓5ᵗʰ **B26.8 Mumps with other complications**

    B26.81 Mumps hepatitis

    B26.82 Mumps myocarditis

    B26.83 Mumps nephritis

    B26.84 Mumps polyneuropathy

    B26.85 Mumps arthritis HCC

    B26.89 Other mumps complications

  B26.9 Mumps without complication
    Mumps NOS
    Mumps parotitis NOS

✓ Additional Character Required   ✓x7ᵗʰ Placeholder Alert   Manifestation   Unspecified Dx   ▶◀ Revised Text   ● New Code   ▲ Revised Code Title

ICD-10-CM 2020   **449**

✓4ᵗʰ **B27 Infectious mononucleosis**

    INCLUDES   glandular fever
               monocytic angina
               Pfeiffer's disease

✓5ᵗʰ **B27.0 Gammaherpesviral mononucleosis**

    Mononucleosis due to Epstein-Barr virus

    B27.00 Gammaherpesviral mononucleosis without complication

    B27.01 Gammaherpesviral mononucleosis with polyneuropathy

    B27.02 Gammaherpesviral mononucleosis with meningitis

    B27.09 Gammaherpesviral mononucleosis with other complications

        Hepatomegaly in gammaherpesviral mononucleosis

✓5ᵗʰ **B27.1 Cytomegaloviral mononucleosis**

    B27.10 Cytomegaloviral mononucleosis without complications

    B27.11 Cytomegaloviral mononucleosis with polyneuropathy

    B27.12 Cytomegaloviral mononucleosis with meningitis

    B27.19 Cytomegaloviral mononucleosis with other complication

        Hepatomegaly in cytomegaloviral mononucleosis

✓5ᵗʰ **B27.8 Other infectious mononucleosis**

    B27.80 Other infectious mononucleosis without complication

    B27.81 Other infectious mononucleosis with polyneuropathy

    B27.82 Other infectious mononucleosis with meningitis

    B27.89 Other infectious mononucleosis with other complication

        Hepatomegaly in other infectious mononucleosis

✓5ᵗʰ **B27.9 Infectious mononucleosis, unspecified**

    B27.90 Infectious mononucleosis, unspecified without complication

    B27.91 Infectious mononucleosis, unspecified with polyneuropathy

    B27.92 Infectious mononucleosis, unspecified with meningitis

    B27.99 Infectious mononucleosis, unspecified with other complication

        Hepatomegaly in unspecified infectious mononucleosis

✓4ᵗʰ **B30 Viral conjunctivitis**

    EXCLUDES 1   herpesviral [herpes simplex] ocular disease (B00.5)
               ocular zoster (B02.3)

Viral Conjunctivitis

Normal conjunctiva

Inflamed conjunctiva

    B30.0 Keratoconjunctivitis due to adenovirus
        Epidemic keratoconjunctivitis
        Shipyard eye

    B30.1 Conjunctivitis due to adenovirus
        Acute adenoviral follicular conjunctivitis
        Swimming-pool conjunctivitis

    B30.2 Viral pharyngoconjunctivitis

    B30.3 Acute epidemic hemorrhagic conjunctivitis (enteroviral)
        Conjunctivitis due to coxsackievirus 24
        Conjunctivitis due to enterovirus 70
        Hemorrhagic conjunctivitis (acute)(epidemic)

    B30.8 Other viral conjunctivitis
        Newcastle conjunctivitis

    B30.9 Viral conjunctivitis, unspecified

✓4ᵗʰ **B33 Other viral diseases, not elsewhere classified**

    B33.0 Epidemic myalgia
        Bornholm disease

    B33.1 Ross River disease
        Epidemic polyarthritis and exanthema
        Ross River fever

✓5ᵗʰ **B33.2 Viral carditis**

    Coxsackie (virus) carditis

    B33.20 Viral carditis, unspecified

    B33.21 Viral endocarditis

    B33.22 Viral myocarditis

    B33.23 Viral pericarditis

    B33.24 Viral cardiomyopathy   **HCC**

    B33.3 Retrovirus infections, not elsewhere classified
        Retrovirus infection NOS

    B33.4 Hantavirus (cardio)-pulmonary syndrome [HPS] [HCPS]
        Hantavirus disease with pulmonary manifestations
        Sin nombre virus disease
        Use additional code to identify any associated acute kidney failure (N17.9)
        EXCLUDES 1   hantavirus disease with renal manifestations (A98.5)
               hemorrhagic fever with renal manifestations (A98.5)

    B33.8 Other specified viral diseases
        EXCLUDES 1   anogenital human papillomavirus infection (A63.0)
               viral warts due to human papillomavirus infection (B07)

✓4ᵗʰ **B34 Viral infection of unspecified site**

    EXCLUDES 1   anogenital human papillomavirus infection (A63.0)
               cytomegaloviral disease NOS (B25.9)
               herpesvirus [herpes simplex] infection NOS (B00.9)
               retrovirus infection NOS (B33.3)
               viral agents as the cause of diseases classified elsewhere (B97.-)
               viral warts due to human papillomavirus infection (B07)

    B34.0 Adenovirus infection, unspecified

    B34.1 Enterovirus infection, unspecified
        Coxsackievirus infection NOS
        Echovirus infection NOS

    B34.2 Coronavirus infection, unspecified
        EXCLUDES 1   pneumonia due to SARS-associated coronavirus (J12.81)

    B34.3 Parvovirus infection, unspecified

    B34.4 Papovavirus infection, unspecified

    B34.8 Other viral infections of unspecified site

    B34.9 Viral infection, unspecified
        Viremia NOS
        AHA: 2016,3Q,10

Mycoses (B35-B49)

    EXCLUDES 2   hypersensitivity pneumonitis due to organic dust (J67.-)
               mycosis fungoides (C84.0-)

✓4ᵗʰ **B35 Dermatophytosis**

    INCLUDES   favus
               infections due to species of Epidermophyton, Micro-sporum and Trichophyton
               tinea, any type except those in B36.-

    DEF: Contagious superficial fungal infection of the skin that invades and grows in dead keratin.

    B35.0 Tinea barbae and tinea capitis
        Beard ringworm
        Kerion
        Scalp ringworm
        Sycosis, mycotic

B35.1 Tinea unguium
Dermatophytic onychia
Dermatophytosis of nail
Onychomycosis
Ringworm of nails

B35.2 Tinea manuum
Dermatophytosis of hand
Hand ringworm

B35.3 Tinea pedis
Athlete's foot
Dermatophytosis of foot
Foot ringworm

B35.4 Tinea corporis
Ringworm of the body

B35.5 Tinea imbricata
Tokelau

B35.6 Tinea cruris
Dhobi itch
Groin ringworm
Jock itch

B35.8 Other dermatophytoses
Disseminated dermatophytosis
Granulomatous dermatophytosis

B35.9 Dermatophytosis, unspecified
Ringworm NOS

✓4ᵗʰ B36 Other superficial mycoses

B36.0 Pityriasis versicolor
Tinea flava
Tinea versicolor

B36.1 Tinea nigra
Keratomycosis nigricans palmaris
Microsporosis nigra
Pityriasis nigra

B36.2 White piedra
Tinea blanca

B36.3 Black piedra

B36.8 Other specified superficial mycoses

B36.9 Superficial mycosis, unspecified

✓4ᵗʰ B37 Candidiasis
INCLUDES   candidosis
moniliasis
EXCLUDES 1   neonatal candidiasis (P37.5)
DEF: Candida: Genus of yeast-like fungi that are commonly found in the mouth, skin, intestinal tract, and vagina. It may cause a white, cheesy discharge.

B37.0 Candidal stomatitis
Oral thrush

B37.1 Pulmonary candidiasis   HCC
Candidal bronchitis
Candidal pneumonia

B37.2 Candidiasis of skin and nail
Candidal onychia
Candidal paronychia
EXCLUDES 2   diaper dermatitis (L22)

B37.3 Candidiasis of vulva and vagina   ♀
Candidal vulvovaginitis
Monilial vulvovaginitis
Vaginal thrush

✓5ᵗʰ B37.4 Candidiasis of other urogenital sites

B37.41 Candidal cystitis and urethritis

B37.42 Candidal balanitis   ♂

B37.49 Other urogenital candidiasis
Candidal pyelonephritis

B37.5 Candidal meningitis

B37.6 Candidal endocarditis

B37.7 Candidal sepsis   HCC
Disseminated candidiasis
Systemic candidiasis
AHA: 2014,4Q,46
TIP: This code is assigned when sepsis is documented as due to any *Candida* type. If non-*Candida albicans* is documented, code B48.8 Other specified mycoses, is assigned.

✓5ᵗʰ B37.8 Candidiasis of other sites

B37.81 Candidal esophagitis   HCC

B37.82 Candidal enteritis
Candidal proctitis

B37.83 Candidal cheilitis

B37.84 Candidal otitis externa

B37.89 Other sites of candidiasis
Candidal osteomyelitis

B37.9 Candidiasis, unspecified
Thrush NOS

✓4ᵗʰ B38 Coccidioidomycosis

B38.0 Acute pulmonary coccidioidomycosis   HCC

B38.1 Chronic pulmonary coccidioidomycosis   HCC

B38.2 Pulmonary coccidioidomycosis, unspecified   HCC

B38.3 Cutaneous coccidioidomycosis

B38.4 Coccidioidomycosis meningitis
DEF: *Coccidioides immitis* infection of the lining of the brain and/or spinal cord.

B38.7 Disseminated coccidioidomycosis
Generalized coccidioidomycosis

✓5ᵗʰ B38.8 Other forms of coccidioidomycosis

B38.81 Prostatic coccidioidomycosis   ♂

B38.89 Other forms of coccidioidomycosis

B38.9 Coccidioidomycosis, unspecified

✓4ᵗʰ B39 Histoplasmosis
Code first associated AIDS (B20)
Use additional code for any associated manifestations, such as:
endocarditis (I39)
meningitis (G02)
pericarditis (I32)
retinitis (H32)
DEF: Type of lung infection caused by breathing in fungal spores often found in the droppings of bats and birds or soil contaminated by their droppings.

Histoplasmosis

Histoplasma capsulatum spores

Spores

B39.0 Acute pulmonary histoplasmosis capsulati   HCC

B39.1 Chronic pulmonary histoplasmosis capsulati   HCC

B39.2 Pulmonary histoplasmosis capsulati, unspecified   HCC

B39.3 Disseminated histoplasmosis capsulati
Generalized histoplasmosis capsulati

B39.4 Histoplasmosis capsulati, unspecified
American histoplasmosis

B39.5 Histoplasmosis duboisii
African histoplasmosis

B39.9 Histoplasmosis, unspecified

✓4ᵗʰ B40 Blastomycosis
EXCLUDES 1   Brazilian blastomycosis (B41.-)
keloidal blastomycosis (B48.0)

B40.0 Acute pulmonary blastomycosis   HCC

☑ Additional Character Required   ✓x7ᵗʰ Placeholder Alert   Manifestation   Unspecified Dx   ▶◀ Revised Text   ● New Code   ▲ Revised Code Title

B40.1   Chronic pulmonary **blastomycosis**   HCC

B40.2   Pulmonary **blastomycosis,** unspecified   HCC

B40.3   Cutaneous **blastomycosis**

B40.7   Disseminated **blastomycosis**
     Generalized blastomycosis

√5ᵗʰ **B40.8**   Other forms of **blastomycosis**

     B40.81   Blastomycotic **meningoencephalitis**
          Meningomyelitis due to blastomycosis

     B40.89   Other forms of blastomycosis

B40.9   Blastomycosis, unspecified

√4ᵗʰ **B41**   **Paracoccidioidomycosis**

     INCLUDES   Brazilian blastomycosis
                Lutz' disease

B41.0   Pulmonary **paracoccidioidomycosis**   HCC

B41.7   Disseminated **paracoccidioidomycosis**
     Generalized paracoccidioidomycosis

B41.8   Other forms of **paracoccidioidomycosis**

B41.9   Paracoccidioidomycosis, unspecified

√4ᵗʰ **B42**   **Sporotrichosis**

B42.0   Pulmonary **sporotrichosis**

B42.1   Lymphocutaneous **sporotrichosis**

B42.7   Disseminated **sporotrichosis**
     Generalized sporotrichosis

√5ᵗʰ **B42.8**   Other forms of **sporotrichosis**

     B42.81   Cerebral **sporotrichosis**
          Meningitis due to sporotrichosis

     B42.82   Sporotrichosis **arthritis**   HCC

     B42.89   Other forms of sporotrichosis

B42.9   Sporotrichosis, unspecified

√4ᵗʰ **B43**   **Chromomycosis and pheomycotic abscess**

B43.0   Cutaneous **chromomycosis**
     Dermatitis verrucosa

B43.1   Pheomycotic **brain abscess**
     Cerebral chromomycosis

B43.2   Subcutaneous **pheomycotic abscess** and cyst

B43.8   Other forms of chromomycosis

B43.9   Chromomycosis, unspecified

√4ᵗʰ **B44**   **Aspergillosis**

     INCLUDES   aspergilloma

B44.0   Invasive pulmonary **aspergillosis**   HCC

B44.1   Other pulmonary **aspergillosis**   HCC

B44.2   Tonsillar **aspergillosis**   HCC

B44.7   Disseminated **aspergillosis**   HCC
     Generalized aspergillosis

√5ᵗʰ **B44.8**   Other forms of **aspergillosis**

     B44.81   Allergic bronchopulmonary **aspergillosis**   HCC

     B44.89   Other forms of aspergillosis   HCC

B44.9   Aspergillosis, unspecified   HCC

√4ᵗʰ **B45**   **Cryptococcosis**

B45.0   Pulmonary **cryptococcosis**   HCC

B45.1   Cerebral **cryptococcosis**   HCC
     Cryptococcal meningitis
     Cryptococcosis meningocerebralis

B45.2   Cutaneous **cryptococcosis**   HCC

B45.3   Osseous **cryptococcosis**   HCC

B45.7   Disseminated **cryptococcosis**   HCC
     Generalized cryptococcosis

B45.8   Other forms of **cryptococcosis**   HCC

B45.9   Cryptococcosis, unspecified   HCC

√4ᵗʰ **B46**   **Zygomycosis**

B46.0   Pulmonary **mucormycosis**   HCC

B46.1   Rhinocerebral **mucormycosis**   HCC

B46.2   Gastrointestinal **mucormycosis**   HCC

B46.3   Cutaneous **mucormycosis**   HCC
     Subcutaneous mucormycosis

B46.4   Disseminated **mucormycosis**   HCC
     Generalized mucormycosis

B46.5   Mucormycosis, unspecified   HCC

B46.8   Other **zygomycoses**   HCC
     Entomophthoromycosis

B46.9   Zygomycosis, unspecified   HCC
     Phycomycosis NOS

√4ᵗʰ **B47**   **Mycetoma**

B47.0   **Eumycetoma**
     Madura foot, mycotic
     Maduromycosis

B47.1   **Actinomycetoma**

B47.9   Mycetoma, unspecified
     Madura foot NOS

√4ᵗʰ **B48**   **Other mycoses, not elsewhere classified**

B48.0   **Lobomycosis**
     Keloidal blastomycosis
     Lobo's disease

B48.1   **Rhinosporidiosis**

B48.2   **Allescheriasis**
     Infection due to Pseudallescheria boydii
     EXCLUDES 1   eumycetoma (B47.0)

B48.3   **Geotrichosis**
     Geotrichum stomatitis

B48.4   **Penicillosis**   HCC

B48.8   **Other specified mycoses**   HCC

     Adiaspiromycosis
     Infection of tissue and organs by Alternaria
     Infection of tissue and organs by Drechslera
     Infection of tissue and organs by Fusarium
     Infection of tissue and organs by saprophytic fungi NEC
     AHA: 2014,4Q,46; 2014,2Q,13
     TIP: This code is assigned when sepsis is documented as due to non-*Candida albicans*. If sepsis is due to any *Candida* type, code B37.7 Candidal sepsis, is assigned.

B49   **Unspecified mycosis**
     Fungemia NOS

Protozoal diseases (B50-B64)

     EXCLUDES 1   *amebiasis (A06.-)*
                   other protozoal intestinal diseases (A07.-)

√4ᵗʰ **B50**   **Plasmodium falciparum malaria**

     INCLUDES   mixed infections of Plasmodium falciparum with any other Plasmodium species

B50.0   Plasmodium falciparum malaria with **cerebral complications**
     Cerebral malaria NOS

B50.8   Other severe and complicated Plasmodium falciparum malaria
     Severe or complicated Plasmodium falciparum malaria NOS

B50.9   Plasmodium falciparum malaria, unspecified

√4ᵗʰ **B51**   **Plasmodium vivax malaria**

     INCLUDES   mixed infections of Plasmodium vivax with other Plasmodium species, except Plasmodium falciparum
     EXCLUDES 1   *Plasmodium vivax with Plasmodium falciparum (B50.-)*

B51.0   Plasmodium vivax malaria with **rupture of spleen**

B51.8   Plasmodium vivax malaria with **other complications**

B51.9   Plasmodium vivax malaria **without complication**
     Plasmodium vivax malaria NOS

√4ᵗʰ **B52**   **Plasmodium malariae malaria**

     INCLUDES   mixed infections of Plasmodium malariae with other Plasmodium species, except Plasmodium falciparum and Plasmodium vivax
     EXCLUDES 1   *Plasmodium falciparum (B50.-)*
                   Plasmodium vivax (B51.-)

B52.0   Plasmodium malariae malaria with **nephropathy**

B52.8   Plasmodium malariae malaria with **other complications**

B52.9   Plasmodium malariae malaria **without complication**
     Plasmodium malariae malaria NOS

√4ᵗʰ **B53**   **Other specified malaria**

B53.0   Plasmodium ovale malaria
     EXCLUDES 1   *Plasmodium ovale with Plasmodium falciparum (B50.-)*
                   Plasmodium ovale with Plasmodium malariae (B52.-)
                   Plasmodium ovale with Plasmodium vivax (B51.-)

B53.1 **Malaria due to simian plasmodia**
> EXCLUDES 1 *malaria due to simian plasmodia with Plasmodium falciparum (B50.-)*
> *malaria due to simian plasmodia with Plasmodium malariae (B52.-)*
> *malaria due to simian plasmodia with Plasmodium ovale (B53.0)*
> *malaria due to simian plasmodia with Plasmodium vivax (B51.-)*

B53.8 **Other malaria, not elsewhere classified**

B54 Unspecified malaria

√4ᵗʰ **B55 Leishmaniasis**

B55.0 **Visceral leishmaniasis**
Kala-azar
Post-kala-azar dermal leishmaniasis

B55.1 **Cutaneous leishmaniasis**

B55.2 **Mucocutaneous leishmaniasis**

B55.9 **Leishmaniasis, unspecified**

√4ᵗʰ **B56 African trypanosomiasis**

B56.0 **Gambiense trypanosomiasis**
Infection due to Trypanosoma brucei gambiense
West African sleeping sickness

B56.1 **Rhodesiense trypanosomiasis**
East African sleeping sickness
Infection due to Trypanosoma brucei rhodesiense

B56.9 **African trypanosomiasis, unspecified**
Sleeping sickness NOS

√4ᵗʰ **B57 Chagas' disease**
> INCLUDES American trypanosomiasis
> infection due to Trypanosoma cruzi

B57.0 **Acute Chagas' disease with heart involvement**
Acute Chagas' disease with myocarditis

B57.1 **Acute Chagas' disease without heart involvement**
Acute Chagas' disease NOS

B57.2 **Chagas' disease (chronic) with heart involvement**
American trypanosomiasis NOS
Chagas' disease (chronic) NOS
Chagas' disease (chronic) with myocarditis
Trypanosomiasis NOS

√5ᵗʰ B57.3 **Chagas' disease (chronic) with digestive system involvement**

B57.30 **Chagas' disease with digestive system involvement, unspecified**

B57.31 **Megaesophagus in Chagas' disease**

B57.32 **Megacolon in Chagas' disease**

B57.39 **Other digestive system involvement in Chagas' disease**

√5ᵗʰ B57.4 **Chagas' disease (chronic) with nervous system involvement**

B57.40 **Chagas' disease with nervous system involvement, unspecified**

B57.41 **Meningitis in Chagas' disease**

B57.42 **Meningoencephalitis in Chagas' disease**

B57.49 **Other nervous system involvement in Chagas' disease**

B57.5 **Chagas' disease (chronic) with other organ involvement**

√4ᵗʰ **B58 Toxoplasmosis**
> INCLUDES infection due to Toxoplasma gondii
> EXCLUDES 1 *congenital toxoplasmosis (P37.1)*

√5ᵗʰ B58.0 **Toxoplasma oculopathy**

B58.00 **Toxoplasma oculopathy, unspecified**

B58.01 **Toxoplasma chorioretinitis**

B58.09 **Other toxoplasma oculopathy**
Toxoplasma uveitis

B58.1 **Toxoplasma hepatitis**

B58.2 **Toxoplasma meningoencephalitis** HCC

B58.3 **Pulmonary toxoplasmosis** HCC

√5ᵗʰ B58.8 **Toxoplasmosis with other organ involvement**

B58.81 **Toxoplasma myocarditis**

B58.82 **Toxoplasma myositis**

B58.83 **Toxoplasma tubulo-interstitial nephropathy**
Toxoplasma pyelonephritis

B58.89 **Toxoplasmosis with other organ involvement**

B58.9 **Toxoplasmosis, unspecified**

√4ᵗʰ **B59 Pneumocystosis** HCC
Pneumonia due to Pneumocystis carinii
Pneumonia due to Pneumocystis jiroveci

√4ᵗʰ **B60 Other protozoal diseases, not elsewhere classified**
> EXCLUDES 1 *cryptosporidiosis (A07.2)*
> *intestinal microsporidiosis (A07.8)*
> *isosporiasis (A07.3)*

B60.0 **Babesiosis**
Piroplasmosis

√5ᵗʰ B60.1 **Acanthamebiasis**

B60.10 **Acanthamebiasis, unspecified**

B60.11 **Meningoencephalitis due to Acanthamoeba (culbertsoni)**

B60.12 **Conjunctivitis due to Acanthamoeba**

B60.13 **Keratoconjunctivitis due to Acanthamoeba**

B60.19 **Other acanthamebic disease**

B60.2 **Naegleriasis**
Primary amebic meningoencephalitis

B60.8 **Other specified protozoal diseases**
Microsporidiosis

B64 Unspecified protozoal disease

Helminthiases (B65-B83)

√4ᵗʰ **B65 Schistosomiasis [bilharziasis]**
> INCLUDES snail fever

B65.0 **Schistosomiasis due to Schistosoma haematobium [urinary schistosomiasis]**

B65.1 **Schistosomiasis due to Schistosoma mansoni [intestinal schistosomiasis]**

B65.2 **Schistosomiasis due to Schistosoma japonicum**
Asiatic schistosomiasis

B65.3 **Cercarial dermatitis**
Swimmer's itch

B65.8 **Other schistosomiasis**
Infection due to Schistosoma intercalatum
Infection due to Schistosoma mattheei
Infection due to Schistosoma mekongi

B65.9 **Schistosomiasis, unspecified**

√4ᵗʰ **B66 Other fluke infections**

B66.0 **Opisthorchiasis**
Infection due to cat liver fluke
Infection due to Opisthorchis (felineus)(viverrini)

B66.1 **Clonorchiasis**
Chinese liver fluke disease
Infection due to Clonorchis sinensis
Oriental liver fluke disease

B66.2 **Dicroceliasis**
Infection due to Dicrocoelium dendriticum
Lancet fluke infection

B66.3 **Fascioliasis**
Infection due to Fasciola gigantica
Infection due to Fasciola hepatica
Infection due to Fasciola indica
Sheep liver fluke disease

B66.4 **Paragonimiasis** HCC
Infection due to Paragonimus species
Lung fluke disease
Pulmonary distomiasis

B66.5 **Fasciolopsiasis**
Infection due to Fasciolopsis buski
Intestinal distomiasis

B66.8 **Other specified fluke infections**
Echinostomiasis
Heterophyiasis
Metagonimiasis
Nanophyetiasis
Watsoniasis

B66.9 **Fluke infection, unspecified**

√4ᵗʰ **B67 Echinococcosis**
> INCLUDES hydatidosis

B67.0 **Echinococcus granulosus infection of liver**

B67.1 **Echinococcus granulosus infection of lung** HCC

B67.2 **Echinococcus granulosus infection of bone**

☑ Additional Character Required | √x7ᵗʰ Placeholder Alert | Manifestation | Unspecified Dx | ▶◀ Revised Text | ● New Code | ▲ Revised Code Title

B67.3 Echinococcus granulosus infection, other and multiple sites
    B67.31 Echinococcus granulosus infection, thyroid gland
    B67.32 Echinococcus granulosus infection, multiple sites
    B67.39 Echinococcus granulosus infection, other sites
B67.4 Echinococcus granulosus infection, unspecified
    Dog tapeworm (infection)
B67.5 Echinococcus multilocularis infection of liver
B67.6 Echinococcus multilocularis infection, other and multiple sites
    B67.61 Echinococcus multilocularis infection, multiple sites
    B67.69 Echinococcus multilocularis infection, other sites
B67.7 Echinococcus multilocularis infection, unspecified
B67.8 Echinococcosis, unspecified, of liver
B67.9 Echinococcosis, other and unspecified
    B67.90 Echinococcosis, unspecified
        Echinococcosis NOS
    B67.99 Other echinococcosis

B68 Taeniasis
    EXCLUDES 1   cysticercosis (B69.-)
B68.0 Taenia solium taeniasis
    Pork tapeworm (infection)
B68.1 Taenia saginata taeniasis
    Beef tapeworm (infection)
    Infection due to adult tapeworm Taenia saginata
B68.9 Taeniasis, unspecified

B69 Cysticercosis
    INCLUDES   cysticerciasis infection due to larval form of Taenia solium
    DEF: Condition that is developed when larvae or eggs of the tapeworm *Taenia solium* are ingested, most commonly in fecally contaminated water or undercooked pork.
B69.0 Cysticercosis of central nervous system
B69.1 Cysticercosis of eye
B69.8 Cysticercosis of other sites
    B69.81 Myositis in cysticercosis
    B69.89 Cysticercosis of other sites
B69.9 Cysticercosis, unspecified

B70 Diphyllobothriasis and sparganosis
B70.0 Diphyllobothriasis
    Diphyllobothrium (adult) (latum) (pacificum) infection
    Fish tapeworm (infection)
    EXCLUDES 2   larval diphyllobothriasis (B70.1)
B70.1 Sparganosis
    Infection due to Sparganum (mansoni) (proliferum)
    Infection due to Spirometra larva
    Larval diphyllobothriasis
    Spirometrosis

B71 Other cestode infections
B71.0 Hymenolepiasis
    Dwarf tapeworm infection
    Rat tapeworm (infection)
B71.1 Dipylidiasis
B71.8 Other specified cestode infections
    Coenurosis
B71.9 Cestode infection, unspecified
    Tapeworm (infection) NOS

B72 Dracunculiasis
    INCLUDES   guinea worm infection
          infection due to Dracunculus medinensis

B73 Onchocerciasis
    INCLUDES   onchocerca volvulus infection
          onchocercosis
          river blindness
B73.0 Onchocerciasis with eye disease
    B73.00 Onchocerciasis with eye involvement, unspecified
    B73.01 Onchocerciasis with endophthalmitis
    B73.02 Onchocerciasis with glaucoma
    B73.09 Onchocerciasis with other eye involvement
        Infestation of eyelid due to onchocerciasis
B73.1 Onchocerciasis without eye disease

B74 Filariasis
    EXCLUDES 2   onchocerciasis (B73)
          tropical (pulmonary) eosinophilia NOS (J82)
B74.0 Filariasis due to Wuchereria bancrofti
    Bancroftian elephantiasis
    Bancroftian filariasis
B74.1 Filariasis due to Brugia malayi
B74.2 Filariasis due to Brugia timori
B74.3 Loiasis
    Calabar swelling
    Eyeworm disease of Africa
    Loa loa infection
B74.4 Mansonelliasis
    Infection due to Mansonella ozzardi
    Infection due to Mansonella perstans
    Infection due to Mansonella streptocerca
B74.8 Other filariases
    Dirofilariasis
B74.9 Filariasis, unspecified

B75 Trichinellosis
    INCLUDES   infection due to Trichinella species
          trichiniasis
    DEF: Infection by *Trichinella spiralis,* the smallest of the parasitic nematodes, that is transmitted by eating undercooked pork or bear meat. ***Synonym(s):*** *Trichinosis.*

B76 Hookworm diseases
    INCLUDES   uncinariasis
B76.0 Ancylostomiasis
    Infection due to Ancylostoma species
B76.1 Necatoriasis
    Infection due to Necator americanus
B76.8 Other hookworm diseases
B76.9 Hookworm disease, unspecified
    Cutaneous larva migrans NOS

B77 Ascariasis
    INCLUDES   ascaridiasis
          roundworm infection
B77.0 Ascariasis with intestinal complications
B77.8 Ascariasis with other complications
    B77.81 Ascariasis pneumonia
    B77.89 Ascariasis with other complications
B77.9 Ascariasis, unspecified

B78 Strongyloidiasis
    EXCLUDES 1   trichostrongyliasis (B81.2)
B78.0 Intestinal strongyloidiasis
B78.1 Cutaneous strongyloidiasis
B78.7 Disseminated strongyloidiasis
B78.9 Strongyloidiasis, unspecified

B79 Trichuriasis
    INCLUDES   trichocephaliasis
          whipworm (disease)(infection)

B80 Enterobiasis
    INCLUDES   oxyuriasis
          pinworm infection
          threadworm infection

B81 Other intestinal helminthiases, not elsewhere classified
    EXCLUDES 1   angiostrongyliasis due to:
          angiostrongylus cantonensis (B83.2)
          parastrongylus cantonensis (B83.2)
B81.0 Anisakiasis
    Infection due to Anisakis larva
B81.1 Intestinal capillariasis
    Capillariasis NOS
    Infection due to Capillaria philippinensis
    EXCLUDES 2   hepatic capillariasis (B83.8)
B81.2 Trichostrongyliasis
B81.3 Intestinal angiostrongyliasis
    Angiostrongyliasis due to:
    angiostrongylus costaricensis
    parastrongylus costaricensis

B81.4 Mixed intestinal helminthiases
Infection due to intestinal helminths classified to more than one of the categories B65.0-B81.3 and B81.8
Mixed helminthiasis NOS

B81.8 Other specified intestinal helminthiases
Infection due to Oesophagostomum species [esophagostomiasis]
Infection due to Ternidens diminutus [ternidensiasis]

✓4ᵗʰ **B82 Unspecified intestinal parasitism**

B82.0 Intestinal helminthiasis, unspecified

B82.9 Intestinal parasitism, unspecified

✓4ᵗʰ **B83 Other helminthiases**
EXCLUDES 1 capillariasis NOS (B81.1)
EXCLUDES 2 intestinal capillariasis (B81.1)

B83.0 Visceral larva migrans
Toxocariasis

B83.1 Gnathostomiasis
Wandering swelling

B83.2 Angiostrongyliasis due to Parastrongylus cantonensis
Eosinophilic meningoencephalitis due to Parastrongylus cantonensis
EXCLUDES 2 intestinal angiostrongyliasis (B81.3)

B83.3 Syngamiasis
Syngamosis

B83.4 Internal hirudiniasis
EXCLUDES 2 external hirudiniasis (B88.3)

B83.8 Other specified helminthiases
Acanthocephaliasis
Gongylonemiasis
Hepatic capillariasis
Metastrongyliasis
Thelaziasis

B83.9 Helminthiasis, unspecified
Worms NOS
EXCLUDES 1 intestinal helminthiasis NOS (B82.0)

Pediculosis, acariasis and other infestations (B85-B89)

✓4ᵗʰ **B85 Pediculosis and phthiriasis**

B85.0 Pediculosis due to Pediculus humanus capitis
Head-louse infestation

B85.1 Pediculosis due to Pediculus humanus corporis
Body-louse infestation

B85.2 Pediculosis, unspecified

B85.3 Phthiriasis
Infestation by crab-louse
Infestation by Phthirus pubis

B85.4 Mixed pediculosis and phthiriasis
Infestation classifiable to more than one of the categories B85.0-B85.3

B86 Scabies
Sarcoptic itch
DEF: Mite infestation that is caused by Sarcoptes scabiei. Scabies causes intense itching and sometimes secondary infection.

✓4ᵗʰ **B87 Myiasis**
INCLUDES infestation by larva of flies

B87.0 Cutaneous myiasis
Creeping myiasis

B87.1 Wound myiasis
Traumatic myiasis

B87.2 Ocular myiasis

B87.3 Nasopharyngeal myiasis
Laryngeal myiasis

B87.4 Aural myiasis

✓5ᵗʰ **B87.8 Myiasis of other sites**

B87.81 Genitourinary myiasis
B87.82 Intestinal myiasis
B87.89 Myiasis of other sites

B87.9 Myiasis, unspecified

✓4ᵗʰ **B88 Other infestations**

B88.0 Other acariasis
Acarine dermatitis
Dermatitis due to Demodex species
Dermatitis due to Dermanyssus gallinae
Dermatitis due to Liponyssoides sanguineus
Trombiculosis
EXCLUDES 2 scabies (B86)

B88.1 Tungiasis [sandflea infestation]

B88.2 Other arthropod infestations
Scarabiasis

B88.3 External hirudiniasis
Leech infestation NOS
EXCLUDES 2 internal hirudiniasis (B83.4)

B88.8 Other specified infestations
Ichthyoparasitism due to Vandellia cirrhosa
Linguatulosis
Porocephaliasis

B88.9 Infestation, unspecified
Infestation (skin) NOS
Infestation by mites NOS
Skin parasites NOS

B89 Unspecified parasitic disease

Sequelae of infectious and parasitic diseases (B90-B94)

NOTE Categories B90-B94 are to be used to indicate conditions in categories A00-B89 as the cause of sequelae, which are themselves classified elsewhere. The "sequelae" include conditions specified as such; they also include residuals of diseases classifiable to the above categories if there is evidence that the disease itself is no longer present. Codes from these categories are not to be used for chronic infections. Code chronic current infections to active infectious disease as appropriate.

Code first condition resulting from (sequela) the infectious or parasitic disease

✓4ᵗʰ **B90 Sequelae of tuberculosis**

B90.0 Sequelae of central nervous system tuberculosis

B90.1 Sequelae of genitourinary tuberculosis

B90.2 Sequelae of tuberculosis of bones and joints

B90.8 Sequelae of tuberculosis of other organs
EXCLUDES 2 sequelae of respiratory tuberculosis (B90.9)

B90.9 Sequelae of respiratory and unspecified tuberculosis
Sequelae of tuberculosis NOS

B91 Sequelae of poliomyelitis
EXCLUDES 1 postpolio syndrome (G14)

B92 Sequelae of leprosy

✓4ᵗʰ **B94 Sequelae of other and unspecified infectious and parasitic diseases**

B94.0 Sequelae of trachoma

B94.1 Sequelae of viral encephalitis

B94.2 Sequelae of viral hepatitis

B94.8 Sequelae of other specified infectious and parasitic diseases
AHA: 2017,4Q,109

B94.9 Sequelae of unspecified infectious and parasitic disease

Bacterial and viral infectious agents (B95-B97)

NOTE These categories are provided for use as supplementary or additional codes to identify the infectious agent(s) in diseases classified elsewhere.
AHA: 2018,4Q,34; 2018,1Q,16

✓4ᵗʰ **B95 Streptococcus, Staphylococcus, and Enterococcus as the cause of diseases classified elsewhere**

B95.0 Streptococcus, group A, as the cause of diseases classified elsewhere

B95.1 Streptococcus, group B, as the cause of diseases classified elsewhere
AHA: 2019,2Q,8-10

B95.2 Enterococcus as the cause of diseases classified elsewhere

B95.3 Streptococcus pneumoniae as the cause of diseases classified elsewhere

B95.4 Other streptococcus as the cause of diseases classified elsewhere

B95.5 Unspecified streptococcus as the cause of diseases classified elsewhere

☑5ᵗʰ **B95.6** Staphylococcus aureus **as the cause of diseases classified elsewhere**

B95.61 **Methicillin susceptible** Staphylococcus aureus **infection as the cause of diseases classified elsewhere**

Methicillin susceptible Staphylococcus aureus (MSSA) infection as the cause of diseases classified elsewhere

Staphylococcus aureus infection NOS as the cause of diseases classified elsewhere

B95.62 **Methicillin resistant** Staphylococcus aureus **infection as the cause of diseases classified elsewhere**

Methicillin resistant staphylococcus aureus (MRSA) infection as the cause of diseases classified elsewhere

AHA: 2016,1Q,12

B95.7 **Other staphylococcus as the cause of diseases classified elsewhere**

B95.8 **Unspecified staphylococcus as the cause of diseases classified elsewhere**

☑4ᵗʰ **B96** **Other bacterial agents as the cause of diseases classified elsewhere**

B96.0 Mycoplasma pneumoniae [M. pneumoniae] **as the cause of diseases classified elsewhere**

Pleuro-pneumonia-like-organism [PPLO]

B96.1 Klebsiella pneumoniae [K. pneumoniae] **as the cause of diseases classified elsewhere**

☑5ᵗʰ **B96.2** Escherichia coli [E. coli] **as the cause of diseases classified elsewhere**

B96.20 **Unspecified Escherichia coli [E. coli] as the cause of diseases classified elsewhere**

Escherichia coli [E. coli] NOS

▲ **B96.21** **Shiga toxin-producing** Escherichia coli [E. coli] **[STEC] O157 as the cause of diseases classified elsewhere**

E. coli O157:H- (nonmotile) with confirmation of Shiga toxin

E. coli O157 with confirmation of Shiga toxin when H antigen is unknown, or is not H7

O157:H7 Escherichia coli [E.coli] with or without confirmation of Shiga toxin-production

Shiga toxin-producing Escherichia coli [E.coli] O157:H7 with or without confirmation of Shiga toxin-production

STEC O157:H7 with or without confirmation of Shiga toxin-production

▲ **B96.22** **Other specified** Shiga toxin-producing Escherichia coli [E. coli] [STEC] **as the cause of diseases classified elsewhere**

Non-O157 Shiga toxin-producing Escherichia coli [E.coli]

Non-O157 Shiga toxin-producing Escherichia coli [E.coli] with known O group

▲ **B96.23** **Unspecified** Shiga toxin-producing Escherichia coli [E. coli] [STEC] **as the cause of diseases classified elsewhere**

Shiga toxin-producing Escherichia coli [E. coli] with unspecified O group

STEC NOS

B96.29 **Other Escherichia coli [E. coli] as the cause of diseases classified elsewhere**

Non-Shiga toxin-producing E. coli

B96.3 Hemophilus influenzae [H. influenzae] **as the cause of diseases classified elsewhere**

B96.4 Proteus (mirabilis) (morganii) **as the cause of diseases classified elsewhere**

B96.5 Pseudomonas (aeruginosa) (mallei) (pseudomallei) **as the cause of diseases classified elsewhere**

AHA: 2015,1Q,18

B96.6 Bacteroides fragilis [B. fragilis] **as the cause of diseases classified elsewhere**

B96.7 Clostridium perfringens [C. perfringens] **as the cause of diseases classified elsewhere**

☑5ᵗʰ **B96.8** **Other specified bacterial agents as the cause of diseases classified elsewhere**

B96.81 Helicobacter pylori [H. pylori] **as the cause of diseases classified elsewhere**

B96.82 Vibrio vulnificus **as the cause of diseases classified elsewhere**

B96.89 **Other specified bacterial agents as the cause of diseases classified elsewhere**

☑4ᵗʰ **B97** **Viral agents as the cause of diseases classified elsewhere**

AHA: 2016,3Q,8-10,14

B97.0 Adenovirus **as the cause of diseases classified elsewhere**

☑5ᵗʰ **B97.1** Enterovirus **as the cause of diseases classified elsewhere**

B97.10 **Unspecified enterovirus as the cause of diseases classified elsewhere**

B97.11 Coxsackievirus **as the cause of diseases classified elsewhere**

B97.12 Echovirus **as the cause of diseases classified elsewhere**

B97.19 **Other enterovirus as the cause of diseases classified elsewhere**

☑5ᵗʰ **B97.2** **Coronavirus as the cause of diseases classified elsewhere**

B97.21 **SARS-associated** coronavirus **as the cause of diseases classified elsewhere**

EXCLUDES 1 pneumonia due to SARS-associated coronavirus (J12.81)

B97.29 **Other coronavirus as the cause of diseases classified elsewhere**

☑5ᵗʰ **B97.3** **Retrovirus as the cause of diseases classified elsewhere**

EXCLUDES 1 human immunodeficiency virus [HIV] disease (B20)

B97.30 **Unspecified retrovirus as the cause of diseases classified elsewhere**

B97.31 Lentivirus **as the cause of diseases classified elsewhere**

B97.32 Oncovirus **as the cause of diseases classified elsewhere**

B97.33 **Human T-cell lymphotrophic virus, type I [HTLV-I] as the cause of diseases classified elsewhere**

B97.34 **Human T-cell lymphotrophic virus, type II [HTLV-II] as the cause of diseases classified elsewhere**

B97.35 **Human immunodeficiency virus, type 2 [HIV 2] as the cause of diseases classified elsewhere** HCC

B97.39 **Other retrovirus as the cause of diseases classified elsewhere**

B97.4 **Respiratory syncytial** virus **as the cause of diseases classified elsewhere**

▶RSV as the cause of diseases classified elsewhere◀

▶Code first related disorders, such as:◀

▶otitis media (H65.-)◀

▶upper respiratory infection (J06.9)◀

EXCLUDES 2 ▶acute bronchiolitis due to respiratory syncytial virus (RSV) (J21.0)◀

▶acute bronchitis due to respiratory syncytial virus (RSV) (J20.5)◀

▶respiratory syncytial virus (RSV) pneumonia (J12.1)◀

B97.5 Reovirus **as the cause of diseases classified elsewhere**

B97.6 Parvovirus **as the cause of diseases classified elsewhere**

B97.7 Papillomavirus **as the cause of diseases classified elsewhere**

☑5ᵗʰ **B97.8** **Other viral agents as the cause of diseases classified elsewhere**

B97.81 **Human metapneumovirus as the cause of diseases classified elsewhere**

B97.89 **Other viral agents as the cause of diseases classified elsewhere**

Other infectious diseases (B99)

☑4ᵗʰ **B99** **Other and unspecified infectious diseases**

B99.8 **Other infectious disease**

B99.9 **Unspecified infectious disease**

Chapter 2. Neoplasms (C00–D49)

Chapter-specific Guidelines with Coding Examples

The chapter-specific guidelines from the ICD-10-CM Official Guidelines for Coding and Reporting have been provided below. Along with these guidelines are coding examples, contained in the shaded boxes, that have been developed to help illustrate the coding and/or sequencing guidance found in these guidelines.

General guidelines

Chapter 2 of the ICD-10-CM contains the codes for most benign and all malignant neoplasms. Certain benign neoplasms, such as prostatic adenomas, may be found in the specific body system chapters. To properly code a neoplasm it is necessary to determine from the record if the neoplasm is benign, in-situ, malignant, or of uncertain histologic behavior. If malignant, any secondary (metastatic) sites should also be determined.

Primary malignant neoplasms overlapping site boundaries

A primary malignant neoplasm that overlaps two or more contiguous (next to each other) sites should be classified to the subcategory/code .8 ('overlapping lesion'), unless the combination is specifically indexed elsewhere. For multiple neoplasms of the same site that are not contiguous such as tumors in different quadrants of the same breast, codes for each site should be assigned.

> A 62-year-old female with a malignant lesion of the upper lip that extends from the lipstick area to the labial frenulum
>
> **C00.8**   **Malignant neoplasm of overlapping sites of lip**
>
> *Explanation*: Because this is a single lesion that overlaps two contiguous sites, a single code for overlapping sites is assigned.

> A 74-year-old male is treated for two distinct malignant lesions, one in the mucosa of the upper lip and a second in the mucosa of the lower lip.
>
> **C00.3**   **Malignant neoplasm of upper lip, inner aspect**
>
> **C00.4**   **Malignant neoplasm of lower lip, inner aspect**
>
> *Explanation*: This patient has two distinct malignant lesions of the upper and lower lips. Because the lesions are not contiguous, two codes are reported.

Malignant neoplasm of ectopic tissue

Malignant neoplasms of ectopic tissue are to be coded to the site of origin mentioned, e.g., ectopic pancreatic malignant neoplasms involving the stomach are coded to malignant neoplasm of pancreas, unspecified (C25.9).

The neoplasm table in the Alphabetic Index should be referenced first. However, if the histological term is documented, that term should be referenced first, rather than going immediately to the Neoplasm Table, in order to determine which column in the Neoplasm Table is appropriate. For example, if the documentation indicates "adenoma," refer to the term in the Alphabetic Index to review the entries under this term and the instructional note to "see also neoplasm, by site, benign." The table provides the proper code based on the type of neoplasm and the site. It is important to select the proper column in the table that corresponds to the type of neoplasm. The Tabular List should then be referenced to verify that the correct code has been selected from the table and that a more specific site code does not exist.

See Section I.C.21. Factors influencing health status and contact with health services, Status, for information regarding Z15.0, codes for genetic susceptibility to cancer.

a. Treatment directed at the malignancy

If the treatment is directed at the malignancy, designate the malignancy as the principal diagnosis.

The only exception to this guideline is if a patient admission/encounter is solely for the administration of chemotherapy, immunotherapy or external beam radiation therapy, assign the appropriate Z51.-- code as the first-listed or principal diagnosis, and the diagnosis or problem for which the service is being performed as a secondary diagnosis.

b. Treatment of secondary site

When a patient is admitted because of a primary neoplasm with metastasis and treatment is directed toward the secondary site only, the secondary neoplasm is designated as the principal diagnosis even though the primary malignancy is still present.

> Patient with primary prostate cancer with metastasis to lungs presents for wedge resection of mass in right lung
>
> **C78.01**   **Secondary malignant neoplasm of right lung**
>
> **C61**   **Malignant neoplasm of prostate**
>
> *Explanation*: Since the encounter is for treatment of the lung metastasis, the secondary lung metastasis is sequenced before the primary prostate cancer.

c. Coding and sequencing of complications

Coding and sequencing of complications associated with the malignancies or with the therapy thereof are subject to the following guidelines:

1) Anemia associated with malignancy

When admission/encounter is for management of an anemia associated with the malignancy, and the treatment is only for anemia, the appropriate code for the malignancy is sequenced as the principal or first-listed diagnosis followed by the appropriate code for the anemia (such as code D63.0, Anemia in neoplastic disease).

> Patient is seen for treatment of anemia in advanced primary liver cancer
>
> **C22.8**   **Malignant neoplasm of liver, primary, unspecified as to type**
>
> **D63.0**   **Anemia in neoplastic disease**
>
> *Explanation*: Even though the admission was solely to treat the anemia, this guideline indicates that the code for the malignancy is sequenced first.

2) Anemia associated with chemotherapy, immunotherapy and radiation therapy

When the admission/encounter is for management of an anemia associated with an adverse effect of the administration of chemotherapy or immunotherapy and the only treatment is for the anemia, the anemia code is sequenced first followed by the appropriate codes for the neoplasm and the adverse effect (T45.1X5, Adverse effect of antineoplastic and immunosuppressive drugs).

> A 56-year-old Hispanic male with grade II follicular lymphoma involving multiple lymph node sites referred for blood transfusion to treat anemia due to chemotherapy
>
> **D64.81**   **Anemia due to antineoplastic chemotherapy**
>
> **C82.18**   **Follicular lymphoma grade II, lymph nodes of multiple sites**
>
> **T45.1X5A**   **Adverse effect of antineoplastic and immunosuppressive drugs, initial encounter**
>
> *Explanation*: The code for the anemia is sequenced first followed by the code for the malignant neoplasm and lastly the code for the adverse effect.

When the admission/encounter is for management of an anemia associated with an adverse effect of radiotherapy, the anemia code should be sequenced first, followed by the appropriate neoplasm code and code Y84.2, Radiological procedure and radiotherapy as the cause of abnormal reaction of the patient, or of later complication, without mention of misadventure at the time of the procedure.

A 55-year-old male with a large malignant rectal tumor has been receiving external radiation therapy to shrink the tumor prior to planned surgery. He is referred today for a blood transfusion to treat anemia related to radiation therapy.

D64.89	**Other specified anemias**
C20	**Malignant neoplasm of rectum**
Y84.2	**Radiological procedure and radiotherapy as the cause of abnormal reaction of the patient, or of later complication, without mention of misadventure at the time of the procedure**

Explanation: The code for the anemia is sequenced first, followed by the code for the malignancy, and lastly the code for the abnormal reaction due to radiotherapy.

3) Management of dehydration due to the malignancy

When the admission/encounter is for management of dehydration due to the malignancy and only the dehydration is being treated (intravenous rehydration), the dehydration is sequenced first, followed by the code(s) for the malignancy.

4) Treatment of a complication resulting from a surgical procedure

When the admission/encounter is for treatment of a complication resulting from a surgical procedure, designate the complication as the principal or first-listed diagnosis if treatment is directed at resolving the complication.

d. Primary malignancy previously excised

When a primary malignancy has been previously excised or eradicated from its site and there is no further treatment directed to that site and there is no evidence of any existing primary malignancy at that site, a code from category Z85, Personal history of malignant neoplasm, should be used to indicate the former site of the malignancy. Any mention of extension, invasion, or metastasis to another site is coded as a secondary malignant neoplasm to that site. The secondary site may be the principal or first-listed **diagnosis** with the Z85 code used as a secondary code.

History of lung cancer, left upper lobectomy 18 months ago with no current treatment; MRI of the brain shows metastatic disease in the brain

C79.31	**Secondary malignant neoplasm of brain**
Z85.118	**Personal history of other other malignant neoplasm of bronchus and lung**

Explanation: The patient has undergone a diagnostic procedure that revealed metastatic lung cancer in the brain. The code for the secondary (metastatic) site is sequenced first, followed by a personal history code to identify the former site of the primary malignancy.

e. Admissions/encounters involving chemotherapy, immunotherapy and radiation therapy

1) Episode of care involves surgical removal of neoplasm

When an episode of care involves the surgical removal of a neoplasm, primary or secondary site, followed by adjunct chemotherapy or radiation treatment during the same episode of care, the code for the neoplasm should be assigned as principal or first-listed diagnosis.

2) Patient admission/encounter solely for administration of chemotherapy, immunotherapy and radiation therapy

If a patient admission/encounter is solely for the administration of chemotherapy, immunotherapy or external beam radiation therapy assign code Z51.0, Encounter for antineoplastic radiation therapy, or Z51.11, Encounter for antineoplastic chemotherapy, or Z51.12, Encounter for antineoplastic immunotherapy as the first-listed or principal diagnosis. If a patient receives more than one of these therapies during the same admission more than one of these codes may be assigned, in any sequence.

The malignancy for which the therapy is being administered should be assigned as a secondary diagnosis.

If a patient admission/encounter is for the insertion or implantation of radioactive elements (e.g., brachytherapy) the appropriate code for the malignancy is sequenced as the principal or first-listed diagnosis. Code Z51.0 should not be assigned.

Patient presents for second round of rituximab and fludarabine for his chronic B cell lymphocytic leukemia

Z51.11	**Encounter for antineoplastic chemotherapy**
Z51.12	**Encounter for antineoplastic immunotherapy**
C91.10	**Chronic lymphocytic leukemia of B-cell type not having achieved remission**

Explanation: Rituximab is an antineoplastic immunotherapy while fludarabine is an antineoplastic chemotherapy. The two treatments are often used together. The encounter was solely for the purpose of administering this treatment and either can be sequenced first, before the neoplastic condition.

3) Patient admitted for radiation therapy, chemotherapy or immunotherapy and develops complications

When a patient is admitted for the purpose of external beam radiotherapy, immunotherapy or chemotherapy and develops complications such as uncontrolled nausea and vomiting or dehydration, the principal or first-listed diagnosis is Z51.0, Encounter for antineoplastic radiation therapy, or Z51.11, Encounter for antineoplastic chemotherapy, or Z51.12, Encounter for antineoplastic immunotherapy followed by any codes for the complications.

When a patient is admitted for the purpose of insertion or implantation of radioactive elements (e.g., brachytherapy) and develops complications such as uncontrolled nausea and vomiting or dehydration, the principal or first-listed diagnosis is the appropriate code for the malignancy followed by any codes for the complications.

f. Admission/encounter to determine extent of malignancy

When the reason for admission/encounter is to determine the extent of the malignancy, or for a procedure such as paracentesis or thoracentesis, the primary malignancy or appropriate metastatic site is designated as the principal or first-listed diagnosis, even though chemotherapy or radiotherapy is administered.

Patient with left lung cancer with malignant pleural effusion being seen for paracentesis and initiation/administration of chemotherapy

C34.92	**Malignant neoplasm of unspecified part of left bronchus or lung**
J91.0	**Malignant pleural effusion**
Z51.11	**Encounter for antineoplastic chemotherapy**

Explanation: The lung cancer is sequenced before the chemotherapy in this instance because the paracentesis for the malignant effusion is also being performed. An instructional note under the malignant effusion instructs that the lung cancer be sequenced first.

g. Symptoms, signs, and abnormal findings listed in Chapter 18 associated with neoplasms

Symptoms, signs, and ill-defined conditions listed in Chapter 18 characteristic of, or associated with, an existing primary or secondary site malignancy cannot be used to replace the malignancy as principal or first-listed diagnosis, regardless of the number of admissions or encounters for treatment and care of the neoplasm.

See Section I.C.21. Factors influencing health status and contact with health services, Encounter for prophylactic organ removal.

h. Admission/encounter for pain control/management

See Section I.C.6. for information on coding admission/encounter for pain control/management.

i. Malignancy in two or more noncontiguous sites

A patient may have more than one malignant tumor in the same organ. These tumors may represent different primaries or metastatic disease, depending on the site. Should the documentation be unclear, the provider should be queried as to the status of each tumor so that the correct codes can be assigned.

j. Disseminated malignant neoplasm, unspecified

Code C80.0, Disseminated malignant neoplasm, unspecified, is for use only in those cases where the patient has advanced metastatic disease and no known primary or secondary sites are specified. It should not be used in place of assigning codes for the primary site and all known secondary sites.

k. Malignant neoplasm without specification of site

Code C80.1, Malignant (primary) neoplasm, unspecified, equates to Cancer, unspecified. This code should only be used when no determination can be made as to the primary site of a malignancy. This code should rarely be used in the inpatient setting.

Evaluation of painful hip leads to diagnosis of a metastatic bone lesion from an unknown primary neoplasm source

C79.51	**Secondary malignant neoplasm of bone**
C80.1	**Malignant (primary) neoplasm, unspecified**

Explanation: If only the secondary site is known, use code C80.1 for the unknown primary site.

l. Sequencing of neoplasm codes

1) Encounter for treatment of primary malignancy

If the reason for the encounter is for treatment of a primary malignancy, assign the malignancy as the principal/first-listed diagnosis. The primary site is to be sequenced first, followed by any metastatic sites.

2) Encounter for treatment of secondary malignancy

When an encounter is for a primary malignancy with metastasis and treatment is directed toward the metastatic (secondary) site(s) only, the metastatic site(s) is designated as the principal/first-listed diagnosis. The primary malignancy is coded as an additional code.

Patient has primary colon cancer with metastasis to rib and is evaluated for possible excision of portion of rib bone

C79.51	**Secondary malignant neoplasm of bone**
C18.9	**Malignant neoplasm of colon, unspecified**

Explanation: The treatment for this encounter is focused on the metastasis to the rib bone rather than the primary colon cancer, thus indicating that the bone metastasis is sequenced as the first-listed code.

3) Malignant neoplasm in a pregnant patient

When a pregnant woman has a malignant neoplasm, a code from subcategory O9A.1-, Malignant neoplasm complicating pregnancy, childbirth, and the puerperium, should be sequenced first, followed by the appropriate code from Chapter 2 to indicate the type of neoplasm.

A 30-year-old pregnant female in first trimester evaluated for pituitary gland malignancy

O9A.111	**Malignant neoplasm complicating pregnancy, first trimester**
C75.1	**Malignant neoplasm of pituitary gland**

Explanation: Codes from chapter 15 describing complications of pregnancy are sequenced as first-listed codes, further specified by codes from other chapters such as neoplastic, unless the pregnancy is documented as incidental to the condition. See also guideline 1.C.15.a.1.

4) Encounter for complication associated with a neoplasm

When an encounter is for management of a complication associated with a neoplasm, such as dehydration, and the treatment is only for the complication, the complication is coded first, followed by the appropriate code(s) for the neoplasm.

The exception to this guideline is anemia. When the admission/encounter is for management of an anemia associated with the malignancy, and the treatment is only for anemia, the appropriate code for the malignancy is sequenced as the principal or first-listed diagnosis followed by code D63.0, Anemia in neoplastic disease.

Patient with pancreatic cancer is seen for initiation of TPN for cancer-related moderate protein-calorie malnutrition

E44.0	**Moderate protein-calorie malnutrition**
C25.9	**Malignant neoplasm of pancreas, unspecified**

Explanation: The encounter is to initiate treatment for malnutrition, a common complication of many types of neoplasms, and is sequenced first.

5) Complication from surgical procedure for treatment of a neoplasm

When an encounter is for treatment of a complication resulting from a surgical procedure performed for the treatment of the neoplasm, designate the complication as the principal/first-listed diagnosis. See **the** guideline regarding the coding of a current malignancy versus personal history to determine if the code for the neoplasm should also be assigned.

6) Pathologic fracture due to a neoplasm

When an encounter is for a pathological fracture due to a neoplasm, and the focus of treatment is the fracture, a code from subcategory M84.5, Pathological fracture in neoplastic disease, should be sequenced first, followed by the code for the neoplasm.

If the focus of treatment is the neoplasm with an associated pathological fracture, the neoplasm code should be sequenced first, followed by a code from M84.5 for the pathological fracture.

m. Current malignancy versus personal history of malignancy

When a primary malignancy has been excised but further treatment, such as an additional surgery for the malignancy, radiation therapy or chemotherapy is directed to that site, the primary malignancy code should be used until treatment is completed.

Female patient with ongoing chemotherapy after right mastectomy for breast cancer

C50.911	**Malignant neoplasm of unspecified site of right female breast**
Z90.11	**Acquired absence of right breast and nipple**

Explanation: Even though the breast has been removed, the breast cancer is still being treated with chemotherapy and therefore is still coded as a current condition rather than personal history.

When a primary malignancy has been previously excised or eradicated from its site, there is no further treatment (of the malignancy) directed to that site, and there is no evidence of any existing primary malignancy at that site, a code from category Z85, Personal history of malignant neoplasm, should be used to indicate the former site of the malignancy.

Subcategories Z85.0 – Z85.7 should only be assigned for the former site of a primary malignancy, not the site of a secondary malignancy. Codes from subcategory Z85.8-, may be assigned for the former site(s) of either a primary or secondary malignancy included in this subcategory.

See Section I.C.21. Factors influencing health status and contact with health services, History (of)

n. Leukemia, multiple myeloma, and malignant plasma cell neoplasms in remission versus personal history

The categories for leukemia, and category C90, Multiple myeloma and malignant plasma cell neoplasms, have codes indicating whether or not the leukemia has achieved remission. There are also codes Z85.6, Personal history of leukemia, and Z85.79, Personal history of other malignant neoplasms of lymphoid, hematopoietic and related tissues. If the documentation is unclear as to whether the leukemia has achieved remission, the provider should be queried.

See Section I.C.21. Factors influencing health status and contact with health services, History (of)

o. Aftercare following surgery for neoplasm

See Section I.C.21. Factors influencing health status and contact with health services, Aftercare

p. Follow-up care for completed treatment of a malignancy

See Section I.C.21. Factors influencing health status and contact with health services, Follow-up

q. Prophylactic organ removal for prevention of malignancy

See Section I.C. 21, Factors influencing health status and contact with health services, Prophylactic organ removal

r. Malignant neoplasm associated with transplanted organ

A malignant neoplasm of a transplanted organ should be coded as a transplant complication. Assign first the appropriate code from category T86.-, Complications of transplanted organs and tissue, followed by code C80.2, Malignant neoplasm associated with transplanted organ. Use an additional code for the specific malignancy.

ter 2. Neoplasms (C00-D49)

NOTE

Functional activity

All neoplasms are classified in this chapter, whether they are functionally active or not. An additional code from Chapter 4 may be used, to identify functional activity associated with any neoplasm.

Morphology [Histology]

Chapter 2 classifies neoplasms primarily by site (topography), with broad groupings for behavior, malignant, in situ, benign, etc. The Table of Neoplasms should be used to identify the correct topography code. In a few cases, such as for malignant melanoma and certain neuroendocrine tumors, the morphology (histologic type) is included in the category and codes.

Primary malignant neoplasms overlapping site boundaries

A primary malignant neoplasm that overlaps two or more contiguous (next to each other) sites should be classified to the subcategory/code .8 ("overlapping lesion"), unless the combination is specifically indexed elsewhere. For multiple neoplasms of the same site that are not contiguous, such as tumors in different quadrants of the same breast, codes for each site should be assigned.

Malignant neoplasm of ectopic tissue

Malignant neoplasms of ectopic tissue are to be coded to the site mentioned, e.g., ectopic pancreatic malignant neoplasms are coded to pancreas, unspecified (C25.9).

AHA: 2017,4Q,103; 2017,1Q,4,5-6,8

This chapter contains the following blocks:

C00-C14   Malignant neoplasms of lip, oral cavity and pharynx
C15-C26   Malignant neoplasms of digestive organs
C30-C39   Malignant neoplasms of respiratory and intrathoracic organs
C40-C41   Malignant neoplasms of bone and articular cartilage
C43-C44   Melanoma and other malignant neoplasms of skin
C45-C49   Malignant neoplasms of mesothelial and soft tissue
C50   Malignant neoplasms of breast
C51-C58   Malignant neoplasms of female genital organs
C60-C63   Malignant neoplasms of male genital organs
C64-C68   Malignant neoplasms of urinary tract
C69-C72   Malignant neoplasms of eye, brain and other parts of central nervous system
C73-C75   Malignant neoplasms of thyroid and other endocrine glands
C7A   Malignant neuroendocrine tumors
C7B   Secondary neuroendocrine tumors
C76-C80   Malignant neoplasms of ill-defined, other secondary and unspecified sites
C81-C96   Malignant neoplasms of lymphoid, hematopoietic and related tissue
D00-D09   In situ neoplasms
D10-D36   Benign neoplasms, except benign neuroendocrine tumors
D3A   Benign neuroendocrine tumors
D37-D48   Neoplasms of uncertain behavior, polycythemia vera and myelodysplastic syndromes
D49   Neoplasms of unspecified behavior

MALIGNANT NEOPLASMS(C00-C96)

Malignant neoplasms, stated or presumed to be primary (of specified sites), and certain specified histologies, except neuroendocrine, and of lymphoid, hematopoietic and related tissue (C00-C75)

TIP: Codes from this code block can be assigned based on the diagnosis listed in a pathology or cytology report when authenticated by a pathologist and available at the time of code assignment.

Malignant neoplasms of lip, oral cavity and pharynx (C00-C14)

✓4ᵗʰ C00 Malignant neoplasm of lip

Use additional code to identify:
alcohol abuse and dependence (F10.-)
history of tobacco dependence (Z87.891)
tobacco dependence (F17.-)
tobacco use (Z72.0)

EXCLUDES 1   malignant melanoma of lip (C43.0)
Merkel cell carcinoma of lip (C4A.0)
other and unspecified malignant neoplasm of skin of lip (C44.0-)

C00.0 Malignant neoplasm of external upper lip
Malignant neoplasm of lipstick area of upper lip
Malignant neoplasm of upper lip NOS
Malignant neoplasm of vermilion border of upper lip

C00.1 Malignant neoplasm of external lower lip
Malignant neoplasm of lower lip NOS
Malignant neoplasm of lipstick area of lower lip
Malignant neoplasm of vermilion border of lower lip

C00.2 Malignant neoplasm of external lip, unspecified
Malignant neoplasm of vermilion border of lip NOS

C00.3 Malignant neoplasm of upper lip, inner aspect
Malignant neoplasm of buccal aspect of upper lip
Malignant neoplasm of frenulum of upper lip
Malignant neoplasm of mucosa of upper lip
Malignant neoplasm of oral aspect of upper lip

C00.4 Malignant neoplasm of lower lip, inner aspect
Malignant neoplasm of buccal aspect of lower lip
Malignant neoplasm of frenulum of lower lip
Malignant neoplasm of mucosa of lower lip
Malignant neoplasm of oral aspect of lower lip

C00.5 Malignant neoplasm of lip, unspecified, inner aspect
Malignant neoplasm of buccal aspect of lip, unspecified
Malignant neoplasm of frenulum of lip, unspecified
Malignant neoplasm of mucosa of lip, unspecified
Malignant neoplasm of oral aspect of lip, unspecified

C00.6 Malignant neoplasm of commissure of lip, unspecified

C00.8 Malignant neoplasm of overlapping sites of lip

C00.9 Malignant neoplasm of lip, unspecified

C01 Malignant neoplasm of base of tongue   HCC

Malignant neoplasm of dorsal surface of base of tongue
Malignant neoplasm of fixed part of tongue NOS
Malignant neoplasm of posterior third of tongue
Use additional code to identify:
alcohol abuse and dependence (F10.-)
history of tobacco dependence (Z87.891)
tobacco dependence (F17.-)
tobacco use (Z72.0)

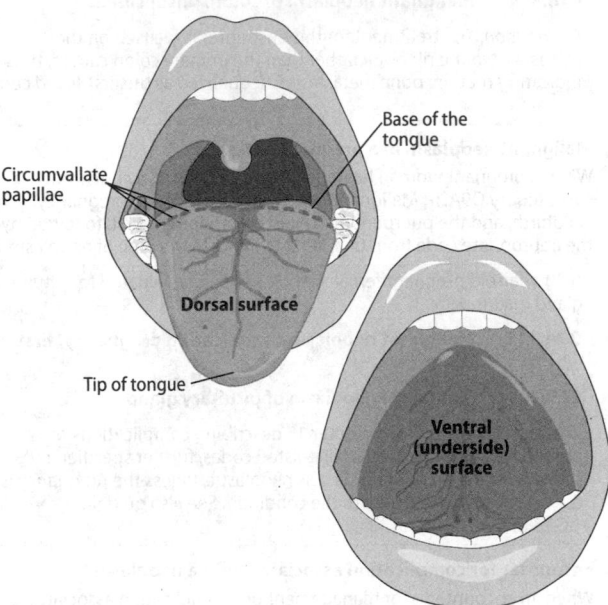

Malignant Neoplasm of Tongue

Base of the tongue
Circumvallate papillae
Dorsal surface
Tip of tongue
Ventral (underside) surface

✓4ᵗʰ C02 Malignant neoplasm of other and unspecified parts of tongue

Use additional code to identify:
alcohol abuse and dependence (F10.-)
history of tobacco dependence (Z87.891)
tobacco dependence (F17.-)
tobacco use (Z72.0)

C02.0 Malignant neoplasm of dorsal surface of tongue   HCC
Malignant neoplasm of anterior two-thirds of tongue, dorsal surface

EXCLUDES 2   malignant neoplasm of dorsal surface of base of tongue (C01)

C02.1 Malignant neoplasm of border of tongue   HCC
Malignant neoplasm of tip of tongue

C02.2 Malignant neoplasm of ventral surface of tongue   HCC
Malignant neoplasm of anterior two-thirds of tongue, ventral surface
Malignant neoplasm of frenulum linguae

C02.3   **Malignant neoplasm of anterior two-thirds of tongue, part unspecified** `HCC`

Malignant neoplasm of middle third of tongue NOS

Malignant neoplasm of mobile part of tongue NOS

C02.4   **Malignant neoplasm of lingual tonsil** `HCC`

> EXCLUDES 2   *malignant neoplasm of tonsil NOS (C09.9)*

C02.8   **Malignant neoplasm of overlapping sites of tongue** `HCC`

Malignant neoplasm of two or more contiguous sites of tongue

C02.9   **Malignant neoplasm of tongue, unspecified** `HCC`

✓4ᵗʰ **C03 Malignant neoplasm of gum**

> INCLUDES   malignant neoplasm of alveolar (ridge) mucosa
> malignant neoplasm of gingiva

Use additional code to identify:

alcohol abuse and dependence (F10.-)

history of tobacco dependence (Z87.891)

tobacco dependence (F17.-)

tobacco use (Z72.0)

> EXCLUDES 2   *malignant odontogenic neoplasms (C41.0-C41.1)*

C03.0   **Malignant neoplasm of upper gum** `HCC`

C03.1   **Malignant neoplasm of lower gum** `HCC`

C03.9   **Malignant neoplasm of gum, unspecified** `HCC`

✓4ᵗʰ **C04 Malignant neoplasm of floor of mouth**

Use additional code to identify:

alcohol abuse and dependence (F10.-)

history of tobacco dependence (Z87.891)

tobacco dependence (F17.-)

tobacco use (Z72.0)

C04.0   **Malignant neoplasm of anterior floor of mouth** `HCC`

Malignant neoplasm of anterior to the premolar-canine junction

C04.1   **Malignant neoplasm of lateral floor of mouth** `HCC`

C04.8   **Malignant neoplasm of overlapping sites of floor of mouth** `HCC`

C04.9   **Malignant neoplasm of floor of mouth, unspecified** `HCC`

✓4ᵗʰ **C05 Malignant neoplasm of palate**

Use additional code to identify:

alcohol abuse and dependence (F10.-)

history of tobacco dependence (Z87.891)

tobacco dependence (F17.-)

tobacco use (Z72.0)

> EXCLUDES 1   *Kaposi's sarcoma of palate (C46.2)*

C05.0   **Malignant neoplasm of hard palate** `HCC`

C05.1   **Malignant neoplasm of soft palate** `HCC`

> EXCLUDES 2   *malignant neoplasm of nasopharyngeal surface of soft palate (C11.3)*

C05.2   **Malignant neoplasm of uvula** `HCC`

C05.8   **Malignant neoplasm of overlapping sites of palate** `HCC`

C05.9   **Malignant neoplasm of palate, unspecified** `HCC`

Malignant neoplasm of roof of mouth

✓4ᵗʰ **C06 Malignant neoplasm of other and unspecified parts of mouth**

Use additional code to identify:

alcohol abuse and dependence (F10.-)

history of tobacco dependence (Z87.891)

tobacco dependence (F17.-)

tobacco use (Z72.0)

C06.0   **Malignant neoplasm of cheek mucosa** `HCC`

Malignant neoplasm of buccal mucosa NOS

Malignant neoplasm of internal cheek

C06.1   **Malignant neoplasm of vestibule of mouth** `HCC`

Malignant neoplasm of buccal sulcus (upper) (lower)

Malignant neoplasm of labial sulcus (upper) (lower)

C06.2   **Malignant neoplasm of retromolar area** `HCC`

✓5ᵗʰ **C06.8**   **Malignant neoplasm of overlapping sites of other and unspecified parts of mouth**

C06.80   **Malignant neoplasm of overlapping sites of unspecified parts of mouth** `HCC`

C06.89   **Malignant neoplasm of overlapping sites of other parts of mouth** `HCC`

"book leaf" neoplasm [ventral surface of tongue and floor of mouth]

C06.9   **Malignant neoplasm of mouth, unspecified** `HCC`

Malignant neoplasm of minor salivary gland, unspecified site

Malignant neoplasm of oral cavity NOS

C07 Malignant neoplasm of parotid gland `HCC`

Use additional code to identify:

alcohol abuse and dependence (F10.-)

exposure to environmental tobacco smoke (Z77.22)

exposure to tobacco smoke in the perinatal period (P96.81)

history of tobacco dependence (Z87.891)

occupational exposure to environmental tobacco smoke (Z57.31)

tobacco dependence (F17.-)

tobacco use (Z72.0)

✓4ᵗʰ **C08 Malignant neoplasm of other and unspecified major salivary glands**

> INCLUDES   malignant neoplasm of salivary ducts

Use additional code to identify:

alcohol abuse and dependence (F10.-)

exposure to environmental tobacco smoke (Z77.22)

exposure to tobacco smoke in the perinatal period (P96.81)

history of tobacco dependence (Z87.891)

occupational exposure to environmental tobacco smoke (Z57.31)

tobacco dependence (F17.-)

tobacco use (Z72.0)

> EXCLUDES 1   *malignant neoplasms of specified minor salivary glands which are classified according to their anatomical location*

> EXCLUDES 2   *malignant neoplasms of minor salivary glands NOS (C06.9)*
> *malignant neoplasm of parotid gland (C07)*

C08.0   **Malignant neoplasm of submandibular gland** `HCC`

Malignant neoplasm of submaxillary gland

C08.1   **Malignant neoplasm of sublingual gland** `HCC`

C08.9   **Malignant neoplasm of major salivary gland, unspecified** `HCC`

Malignant neoplasm of salivary gland (major) NOS

✓4ᵗʰ **C09 Malignant neoplasm of tonsil**

Use additional code to identify:

alcohol abuse and dependence (F10.-)

exposure to environmental tobacco smoke (Z77.22)

exposure to tobacco smoke in the perinatal period (P96.81)

history of tobacco dependence (Z87.891)

occupational exposure to environmental tobacco smoke (Z57.31)

tobacco dependence (F17.-)

tobacco use (Z72.0)

> EXCLUDES 2   *malignant neoplasm of lingual tonsil (C02.4)*
> *malignant neoplasm of pharyngeal tonsil (C11.1)*

C09.0   **Malignant neoplasm of tonsillar fossa** `HCC`

C09.1   **Malignant neoplasm of tonsillar pillar (anterior) (posterior)** `HCC`

C09.8   **Malignant neoplasm of overlapping sites of tonsil** `HCC`

C09.9   **Malignant neoplasm of tonsil, unspecified** `HCC`

Malignant neoplasm of tonsil NOS

Malignant neoplasm of faucial tonsils

Malignant neoplasm of palatine tonsils

✓4ᵗʰ **C10 Malignant neoplasm of oropharynx**

Use additional code to identify:

alcohol abuse and dependence (F10.-)

exposure to environmental tobacco smoke (Z77.22)

exposure to tobacco smoke in the perinatal period (P96.81)

history of tobacco dependence (Z87.891)

occupational exposure to environmental tobacco smoke (Z57.31)

tobacco dependence (F17.-)

tobacco use (Z72.0)

> EXCLUDES 2   *malignant neoplasm of tonsil (C09.-)*

DEF: Oropharynx: Middle portion of pharynx (throat); communicates with the oral cavity, nasopharynx and laryngopharynx.

C10.0   **Malignant neoplasm of vallecula** `HCC`

C10.1   **Malignant neoplasm of anterior surface of epiglottis** `HCC`

Malignant neoplasm of epiglottis, free border [margin]

Malignant neoplasm of glossoepiglottic fold(s)

> EXCLUDES 2   *malignant neoplasm of epiglottis (suprahyoid portion) NOS (C32.1)*

C10.2   **Malignant neoplasm of lateral wall of oropharynx** `HCC`

C10.3   **Malignant neoplasm of posterior wall of oropharynx** `HCC`

☑ Additional Character Required   ✓x7ᵗʰ Placeholder Alert   Manifestation   Unspecified Dx   ▶◀ Revised Text   ● New Code   ▲ Revised Code Title

ICD-10-CM 2020   461

C02.3–C10.3

C10.4   **Malignant neoplasm of** branchial cleft   `HCC`

Malignant neoplasm of branchial cyst [site of neoplasm]

C10.8   **Malignant neoplasm of** overlapping sites **of oropharynx**   `HCC`

Malignant neoplasm of junctional region of oropharynx

C10.9   **Malignant neoplasm of oropharynx, unspecified**   `HCC`

√4ᵗʰ **C11**   **Malignant neoplasm of** nasopharynx

Use additional code to identify:
exposure to environmental tobacco smoke (Z77.22)
exposure to tobacco smoke in the perinatal period (P96.81)
history of tobacco dependence (Z87.891)
occupational exposure to environmental tobacco smoke (Z57.31)
tobacco dependence (F17.-)
tobacco use (Z72.0)
DEF: Nasopharynx: Upper portion of pharynx (throat); communicates with the nasal cavities, oropharynx and tympanic cavities.

C11.0   **Malignant neoplasm of** superior wall **of nasopharynx**   `HCC`

Malignant neoplasm of roof of nasopharynx

C11.1   **Malignant neoplasm of** posterior wall **of nasopharynx**   `HCC`

Malignant neoplasm of adenoid
Malignant neoplasm of pharyngeal tonsil

C11.2   **Malignant neoplasm of** lateral wall **of nasopharynx**   `HCC`

Malignant neoplasm of fossa of Rosenmüller
Malignant neoplasm of opening of auditory tube
Malignant neoplasm of pharyngeal recess

C11.3   **Malignant neoplasm of** anterior wall **of nasopharynx**   `HCC`

Malignant neoplasm of floor of nasopharynx
Malignant neoplasm of nasopharyngeal (anterior) (posterior) surface of soft palate
Malignant neoplasm of posterior margin of nasal choana
Malignant neoplasm of posterior margin of nasal septum

C11.8   **Malignant neoplasm of** overlapping sites **of nasopharynx**   `HCC`

C11.9   **Malignant neoplasm of nasopharynx, unspecified**   `HCC`

Malignant neoplasm of nasopharyngeal wall NOS

C12   **Malignant neoplasm of** pyriform sinus   `HCC`

Malignant neoplasm of pyriform fossa
Use additional code to identify:
exposure to environmental tobacco smoke (Z77.22)
exposure to tobacco smoke in the perinatal period (P96.81)
history of tobacco dependence (Z87.891)
occupational exposure to environmental tobacco smoke (Z57.31)
tobacco dependence (F17.-)
tobacco use (Z72.0)

√4ᵗʰ **C13**   **Malignant neoplasm of** hypopharynx

Use additional code to identify:
exposure to environmental tobacco smoke (Z77.22)
exposure to tobacco smoke in the perinatal period (P96.81)
history of tobacco dependence (Z87.891)
occupational exposure to environmental tobacco smoke (Z57.31)
tobacco dependence (F17.-)
tobacco use (Z72.0)
`EXCLUDES 2`   *malignant neoplasm of pyriform sinus (C12)*
DEF: Hypopharynx: Lower portion of pharynx (throat); communicates with the oropharynx and the esophagus. **Synonyms:** *laryngopharynx.*

C13.0   **Malignant neoplasm of** postcricoid region   `HCC`

C13.1   **Malignant neoplasm of** aryepiglottic fold, hypopharyngeal aspect   `HCC`

Malignant neoplasm of aryepiglottic fold, marginal zone
Malignant neoplasm of aryepiglottic fold NOS
Malignant neoplasm of interarytenoid fold, marginal zone
Malignant neoplasm of interarytenoid fold NOS
`EXCLUDES 2`   *malignant neoplasm of aryepiglottic fold or interarytenoid fold, laryngeal aspect (C32.1)*

C13.2   **Malignant neoplasm of** posterior wall **of hypopharynx**   `HCC`

C13.8   **Malignant neoplasm of** overlapping sites **of hypopharynx**   `HCC`

C13.9   **Malignant neoplasm of hypopharynx, unspecified**   `HCC`

Malignant neoplasm of hypopharyngeal wall NOS

√4ᵗʰ **C14**   **Malignant neoplasm of** other and ill-defined sites in the lip, oral cavity and pharynx

Use additional code to identify:
alcohol abuse and dependence (F10.-)
exposure to environmental tobacco smoke (Z77.22)
exposure to tobacco smoke in the perinatal period (P96.81)
history of tobacco dependence (Z87.891)
occupational exposure to environmental tobacco smoke (Z57.31)
tobacco dependence (F17.-)
tobacco use (Z72.0)
`EXCLUDES 1`   *malignant neoplasm of oral cavity NOS (C06.9)*

C14.0   **Malignant neoplasm of pharynx, unspecified**   `HCC`

C14.2   **Malignant neoplasm of** Waldeyer's ring   `HCC`

DEF: Waldeyer's ring: Ring of lymphoid tissue that is made up of the two palatine tonsils, the pharyngeal tonsil (adenoid), and the lingual tonsil. It functions as the defense against infection and assists with the development of the immune system.

C14.8   **Malignant neoplasm of** overlapping sites **of lip, oral cavity and pharynx**   `HCC`

Primary malignant neoplasm of two or more contiguous sites of lip, oral cavity and pharynx
`EXCLUDES 1`   *"book leaf" neoplasm [ventral surface of tongue and floor of mouth] (C06.89)*

Malignant neoplasms of digestive organs (C15-C26)

`EXCLUDES 1`   *Kaposi's sarcoma of gastrointestinal sites (C46.4)*
`EXCLUDES 2`   *gastrointestinal stromal tumors (C49.A-)*

√4ᵗʰ **C15**   **Malignant neoplasm of** esophagus

Use additional code to identify:
alcohol abuse and dependence (F10.-)

C15.3   **Malignant neoplasm of** upper third **of esophagus**   `HCC`

C15.4   **Malignant neoplasm of** middle third **of esophagus**   `HCC`

C15.5   **Malignant neoplasm of** lower third **of esophagus**   `HCC`

`EXCLUDES 1`   *malignant neoplasm of cardio-esophageal junction (C16.0)*

C15.8   **Malignant neoplasm of** overlapping sites **of esophagus**   `HCC`

C15.9   **Malignant neoplasm of esophagus, unspecified**   `HCC`

√4ᵗʰ **C16**   **Malignant neoplasm of** stomach

Use additional code to identify:
alcohol abuse and dependence (F10.-)
`EXCLUDES 2`   *malignant carcinoid tumor of the stomach (C7A.092)*

C16.0   **Malignant neoplasm of** cardia   `HCC`

Malignant neoplasm of cardiac orifice
Malignant neoplasm of cardio-esophageal junction
Malignant neoplasm of esophagus and stomach
Malignant neoplasm of gastro-esophageal junction

C16.1   **Malignant neoplasm of** fundus **of stomach**   `HCC`

C16.2   **Malignant neoplasm of** body **of stomach**   `HCC`

C16.3   **Malignant neoplasm of** pyloric antrum   `HCC`

Malignant neoplasm of gastric antrum

C16.4   **Malignant neoplasm of** pylorus   `HCC`

Malignant neoplasm of prepylorus
Malignant neoplasm of pyloric canal

C16.5   **Malignant neoplasm of** lesser curvature **of stomach, unspecified**   `HCC`

Malignant neoplasm of lesser curvature of stomach, not classifiable to C16.1-C16.4

C16.6   **Malignant neoplasm of** greater curvature **of stomach, unspecified**   `HCC`

Malignant neoplasm of greater curvature of stomach, not classifiable to C16.0-C16.4

C16.8   **Malignant neoplasm of** overlapping sites **of stomach**   `HCC`

C16.9   **Malignant neoplasm of stomach, unspecified**   `HCC`

Gastric cancer NOS

√4ᵗʰ **C17**   **Malignant neoplasm of** small intestine

`EXCLUDES 1`   *malignant carcinoid tumors of the small intestine (C7A.01)*
AHA: 2016,1Q,19

C17.0   **Malignant neoplasm of** duodenum   `HCC`

C17.1   **Malignant neoplasm of** jejunum   `HCC`

C17.2   **Malignant neoplasm of** ileum   `HCC`
> `EXCLUDES 1`   *malignant neoplasm of ileocecal valve (C18.0)*

C17.3   **Meckel's diverticulum, malignant**   `HCC`
> `EXCLUDES 1`   *Meckel's diverticulum, congenital (Q43.0)*
>
> **DEF:** Congenital, abnormal remnant of embryonic digestive system development that leaves a sacculation or outpouching from the wall of the small intestine near the terminal part of the ileum made of acid-secreting tissue as in the stomach.

C17.8   **Malignant neoplasm of** overlapping sites **of small intestine**   `HCC`

C17.9   **Malignant neoplasm of small intestine, unspecified**   `HCC`

`✓4ᵗʰ` **C18**   **Malignant neoplasm of** colon
> `EXCLUDES 1`   *malignant carcinoid tumors of the colon (C7A.02-)*

Colon

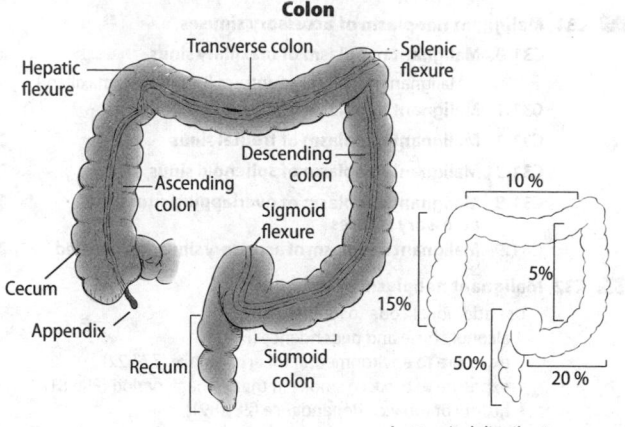

Transverse colon
Hepatic flexure
Splenic flexure
Descending colon
Ascending colon
Sigmoid flexure
Cecum
Appendix
Rectum
Sigmoid colon

10 %
5%
15%
50%
20 %

Anatomical distribution of large bowel cancers

C18.0   **Malignant neoplasm of** cecum   `HCC`
Malignant neoplasm of ileocecal valve

C18.1   **Malignant neoplasm of** appendix   `HCC`

C18.2   **Malignant neoplasm of** ascending colon   `HCC`

C18.3   **Malignant neoplasm of** hepatic flexure   `HCC`

C18.4   **Malignant neoplasm of** transverse colon   `HCC`

C18.5   **Malignant neoplasm of** splenic flexure   `HCC`

C18.6   **Malignant neoplasm of** descending colon   `HCC`

C18.7   **Malignant neoplasm of** sigmoid colon   `HCC`
Malignant neoplasm of sigmoid (flexure)
> `EXCLUDES 1`   *malignant neoplasm of rectosigmoid junction (C19)*

C18.8   **Malignant neoplasm of** overlapping sites **of colon**   `HCC`

C18.9   **Malignant neoplasm of colon, unspecified**   `HCC`
Malignant neoplasm of large intestine NOS

C19   **Malignant neoplasm of** rectosigmoid junction   `HCC`
Malignant neoplasm of colon with rectum
Malignant neoplasm of rectosigmoid (colon)
> `EXCLUDES 1`   *malignant carcinoid tumors of the colon (C7A.02-)*

C20   **Malignant neoplasm of** rectum   `HCC`
Malignant neoplasm of rectal ampulla
> `EXCLUDES 1`   *malignant carcinoid tumor of the rectum (C7A.026)*

`✓4ᵗʰ` **C21**   **Malignant neoplasm of anus and anal canal**
> `EXCLUDES 2`   *malignant carcinoid tumors of the colon (C7A.02-)*
> *malignant melanoma of anal margin (C43.51)*
> *malignant melanoma of anal skin (C43.51)*
> *malignant melanoma of perianal skin (C43.51)*
> *other and unspecified malignant neoplasm of anal margin (C44.500, C44.510, C44.520, C44.590)*
> *other and unspecified malignant neoplasm of anal skin (C44.500, C44.510, C44.520, C44.590)*
> *other and unspecified malignant neoplasm of perianal skin (C44.500, C44.510, C44.520, C44.590)*

C21.0   **Malignant neoplasm of** anus, **unspecified**   `HCC`

C21.1   **Malignant neoplasm of** anal canal   `HCC`
Malignant neoplasm of anal sphincter

C21.2   **Malignant neoplasm of** cloacogenic zone   `HCC`

C21.8   **Malignant neoplasm of** overlapping sites **of rectum, anus and anal canal**   `HCC`
Malignant neoplasm of anorectal junction
Malignant neoplasm of anorectum
Primary malignant neoplasm of two or more contiguous sites of rectum, anus and anal canal

`✓4ᵗʰ` **C22**   **Malignant neoplasm of** liver and intrahepatic bile ducts
Use additional code to identify:
alcohol abuse and dependence (F10.-)
hepatitis B (B16.-, B18.0-B18.1)
hepatitis C (B17.1-, B18.2)
> `EXCLUDES 1`   *malignant neoplasm of biliary tract NOS (C24.9)*
> *secondary malignant neoplasm of liver and intrahepatic bile duct (C78.7)*

C22.0   **Liver cell carcinoma**   `HCC`
Hepatocellular carcinoma
Hepatoma
AHA: 2016,1Q,18

C22.1   **Intrahepatic bile duct carcinoma**   `HCC`
Cholangiocarcinoma
> `EXCLUDES 1`   *malignant neoplasm of hepatic duct (C24.0)*

C22.2   **Hepatoblastoma**   `HCC`

C22.3   **Angiosarcoma of liver**   `HCC`
Kupffer cell sarcoma

C22.4   **Other sarcomas of liver**   `HCC`

C22.7   **Other specified carcinomas of liver**   `HCC`

C22.8   **Malignant neoplasm of liver, primary, unspecified as to type**   `HCC`

C22.9   **Malignant neoplasm of liver, not specified as primary or secondary**   `HCC`

C23   **Malignant neoplasm of** gallbladder   `HCC`

`✓4ᵗʰ` **C24**   **Malignant neoplasm of** other and unspecified parts of biliary tract
> `EXCLUDES 1`   *malignant neoplasm of intrahepatic bile duct (C22.1)*

C24.0   **Malignant neoplasm of** extrahepatic bile duct   `HCC`
Malignant neoplasm of biliary duct or passage NOS
Malignant neoplasm of common bile duct
Malignant neoplasm of cystic duct
Malignant neoplasm of hepatic duct

C24.1   **Malignant neoplasm of** ampulla of Vater   `HCC`
> **DEF:** Malignant neoplasm in the area of dilation at the juncture of the common bile and pancreatic ducts near the opening into the lumen of the duodenum.

C24.8   **Malignant neoplasm of** overlapping sites **of biliary tract**   `HCC`
Malignant neoplasm involving both intrahepatic and extrahepatic bile ducts
Primary malignant neoplasm of two or more contiguous sites of biliary tract

C24.9   **Malignant neoplasm of biliary tract, unspecified**   `HCC`

C25 Malignant neoplasm of pancreas

Code also exocrine pancreatic insufficiency (K86.81)
Use additional code to identify:
  alcohol abuse and dependence (F10.-)

Pancreas

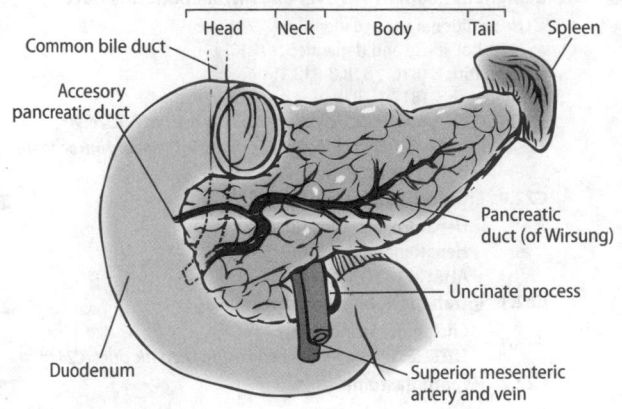

| Head | Neck | Body | Tail | Spleen |

Common bile duct
Accesory pancreatic duct
Pancreatic duct (of Wirsung)
Uncinate process
Duodenum
Superior mesenteric artery and vein

C25.0 Malignant neoplasm of head of pancreas `HCC`

C25.1 Malignant neoplasm of body of pancreas `HCC`

C25.2 Malignant neoplasm of tail of pancreas `HCC`

C25.3 Malignant neoplasm of pancreatic duct `HCC`

C25.4 Malignant neoplasm of endocrine pancreas `HCC`

Malignant neoplasm of islets of Langerhans
Use additional code to identify any functional activity

C25.7 Malignant neoplasm of other parts of pancreas `HCC`

Malignant neoplasm of neck of pancreas

C25.8 Malignant neoplasm of overlapping sites of pancreas `HCC`

C25.9 Malignant neoplasm of pancreas, unspecified `HCC`

✓4ᵗʰ C26 Malignant neoplasm of other and ill-defined digestive organs

EXCLUDES 1 malignant neoplasm of peritoneum and retroperitoneum (C48.-)

C26.0 Malignant neoplasm of intestinal tract, part unspecified `HCC`

Malignant neoplasm of intestine NOS

C26.1 Malignant neoplasm of spleen `HCC`

EXCLUDES 1 Hodgkin lymphoma (C81.-)
non-Hodgkin lymphoma (C82-C85)

C26.9 Malignant neoplasm of ill-defined sites within the digestive system `HCC`

Malignant neoplasm of alimentary canal or tract NOS
Malignant neoplasm of gastrointestinal tract NOS
EXCLUDES 1 malignant neoplasm of abdominal NOS (C76.2)
malignant neoplasm of intra-abdominal NOS (C76.2)

Malignant neoplasms of respiratory and intrathoracic organs (C30-C39)

INCLUDES malignant neoplasm of middle ear
EXCLUDES 1 mesothelioma (C45.-)

✓4ᵗʰ C30 Malignant neoplasm of nasal cavity and middle ear

C30.0 Malignant neoplasm of nasal cavity `HCC`

Malignant neoplasm of cartilage of nose
Malignant neoplasm of nasal concha
Malignant neoplasm of internal nose
Malignant neoplasm of septum of nose
Malignant neoplasm of vestibule of nose
EXCLUDES 1 malignant neoplasm of nasal bone (C41.0)
malignant neoplasm of nose NOS (C76.0)
malignant neoplasm of olfactory bulb (C72.2-)
malignant neoplasm of posterior margin of nasal septum and choana (C11.3)
malignant melanoma of skin of nose (C43.31)
malignant neoplasm of turbinates (C41.0)
other and unspecified malignant neoplasm of skin of nose (C44.301, C44.311, C44.321, C44.391)

C30.1 Malignant neoplasm of middle ear `HCC`

Malignant neoplasm of antrum tympanicum
Malignant neoplasm of auditory tube
Malignant neoplasm of eustachian tube
Malignant neoplasm of inner ear
Malignant neoplasm of mastoid air cells
Malignant neoplasm of tympanic cavity
EXCLUDES 1 malignant neoplasm of auricular canal (external) (C43.2-,C44.2-)
malignant neoplasm of bone of ear (meatus) (C41.0)
malignant neoplasm of cartilage of ear (C49.0)
malignant melanoma of skin of (external) ear (C43.2-)
other and unspecified malignant neoplasm of skin of (external) ear (C44.2-)

✓4ᵗʰ C31 Malignant neoplasm of accessory sinuses

C31.0 Malignant neoplasm of maxillary sinus `HCC`

Malignant neoplasm of antrum (Highmore) (maxillary)

C31.1 Malignant neoplasm of ethmoidal sinus `HCC`

C31.2 Malignant neoplasm of frontal sinus `HCC`

C31.3 Malignant neoplasm of sphenoid sinus `HCC`

C31.8 Malignant neoplasm of overlapping sites of accessory sinuses `HCC`

C31.9 Malignant neoplasm of accessory sinus, unspecified `HCC`

✓4ᵗʰ C32 Malignant neoplasm of larynx

Use additional code to identify:
  alcohol abuse and dependence (F10.-)
  exposure to environmental tobacco smoke (Z77.22)
  exposure to tobacco smoke in the perinatal period (P96.81)
  history of tobacco dependence (Z87.891)
  occupational exposure to environmental tobacco smoke (Z57.31)
  tobacco dependence (F17.-)
  tobacco use (Z72.0)

C32.0 Malignant neoplasm of glottis `HCC`

Malignant neoplasm of intrinsic larynx
Malignant neoplasm of laryngeal commissure (anterior)(posterior)
Malignant neoplasm of vocal cord (true) NOS

C32.1 Malignant neoplasm of supraglottis `HCC`

Malignant neoplasm of aryepiglottic fold or interarytenoid fold, laryngeal aspect
Malignant neoplasm of epiglottis (suprahyoid portion) NOS
Malignant neoplasm of extrinsic larynx
Malignant neoplasm of false vocal cord
Malignant neoplasm of posterior (laryngeal) surface of epiglottis
Malignant neoplasm of ventricular bands
EXCLUDES 2 malignant neoplasm of anterior surface of epiglottis (C10.1)
malignant neoplasm of aryepiglottic fold or interarytenoid fold, hypopharyngeal aspect (C13.1)
malignant neoplasm of aryepiglottic fold or interarytenoid fold, marginal zone (C13.1)
malignant neoplasm of aryepiglottic fold or interarytenoid fold NOS (C13.1)

C32.2 Malignant neoplasm of subglottis `HCC`

C32.3 Malignant neoplasm of laryngeal cartilage `HCC`

C32.8 Malignant neoplasm of overlapping sites of larynx `HCC`

C32.9 Malignant neoplasm of larynx, unspecified `HCC`

C33 Malignant neoplasm of trachea `HCC`

Use additional code to identify:
  exposure to environmental tobacco smoke (Z77.22)
  exposure to tobacco smoke in the perinatal period (P96.81)
  history of tobacco dependence (Z87.891)
  occupational exposure to environmental tobacco smoke (Z57.31)
  tobacco dependence (F17.-)
  tobacco use (Z72.0)

☑4ᵗʰ C34 Malignant neoplasm of bronchus and lung

Use additional code to identify:
exposure to environmental tobacco smoke (Z77.22)
exposure to tobacco smoke in the perinatal period (P96.81)
history of tobacco dependence (Z87.891)
occupational exposure to environmental tobacco smoke (Z57.31)
tobacco dependence (F17.-)
tobacco use (Z72.0)

EXCLUDES 1   Kaposi's sarcoma of lung (C46.5-)
malignant carcinoid tumor of the bronchus and lung (C7A.090)

AHA: 2019,1Q,16

TIP: When documented, assign code I31.3 for associated malignant pericardial effusion. If the sole reason for admission is to treat the effusion with no treatment of the lung malignancy rendered, code I31.3 may be sequenced first.

☑5ᵗʰ C34.0 Malignant neoplasm of main bronchus

Malignant neoplasm of carina
Malignant neoplasm of hilus (of lung)

     C34.00 Malignant neoplasm of unspecified main bronchus   HCC Q

     C34.01 Malignant neoplasm of right main bronchus   HCC Q

     C34.02 Malignant neoplasm of left main bronchus   HCC Q

☑5ᵗʰ C34.1 Malignant neoplasm of upper lobe, bronchus or lung

     C34.10 Malignant neoplasm of upper lobe, unspecified bronchus or lung   HCC Q

     C34.11 Malignant neoplasm of upper lobe, right bronchus or lung   HCC Q

     C34.12 Malignant neoplasm of upper lobe, left bronchus or lung   HCC Q

C34.2 Malignant neoplasm of middle lobe, bronchus or lung   HCC Q

☑5ᵗʰ C34.3 Malignant neoplasm of lower lobe, bronchus or lung

     C34.30 Malignant neoplasm of lower lobe, unspecified bronchus or lung   HCC Q

     C34.31 Malignant neoplasm of lower lobe, right bronchus or lung   HCC Q

     C34.32 Malignant neoplasm of lower lobe, left bronchus or lung   HCC Q

☑5ᵗʰ C34.8 Malignant neoplasm of overlapping sites of bronchus and lung

     C34.80 Malignant neoplasm of overlapping sites of unspecified bronchus and lung   HCC Q

     C34.81 Malignant neoplasm of overlapping sites of right bronchus and lung   HCC Q

     C34.82 Malignant neoplasm of overlapping sites of left bronchus and lung   HCC Q

☑5ᵗʰ C34.9 Malignant neoplasm of unspecified part of bronchus or lung

     C34.90 Malignant neoplasm of unspecified part of unspecified bronchus or lung   HCC Q

Lung cancer NOS

     C34.91 Malignant neoplasm of unspecified part of right bronchus or lung   HCC Q

     C34.92 Malignant neoplasm of unspecified part of left bronchus or lung   HCC Q

C37 Malignant neoplasm of thymus   HCC

EXCLUDES 1   malignant carcinoid tumor of the thymus (C7A.091)

☑4ᵗʰ C38 Malignant neoplasm of heart, mediastinum and pleura

EXCLUDES 1   mesothelioma (C45.-)

C38.0 Malignant neoplasm of heart   HCC

Malignant neoplasm of pericardium

EXCLUDES 1   malignant neoplasm of great vessels (C49.3)

C38.1 Malignant neoplasm of anterior mediastinum   HCC

C38.2 Malignant neoplasm of posterior mediastinum   HCC

C38.3 Malignant neoplasm of mediastinum, part unspecified   HCC

C38.4 Malignant neoplasm of pleura   HCC

C38.8 Malignant neoplasm of overlapping sites of heart, mediastinum and pleura   HCC

☑4ᵗʰ C39 Malignant neoplasm of other and ill-defined sites in the respiratory system and intrathoracic organs

Use additional code to identify:
exposure to environmental tobacco smoke (Z77.22)
exposure to tobacco smoke in the perinatal period (P96.81)
history of tobacco dependence (Z87.891)
occupational exposure to environmental tobacco smoke (Z57.31)
tobacco dependence (F17.-)
tobacco use (Z72.0)

EXCLUDES 1   intrathoracic malignant neoplasm NOS (C76.1)
thoracic malignant neoplasm NOS (C76.1)

C39.0 Malignant neoplasm of upper respiratory tract, part unspecified   HCC

C39.9 Malignant neoplasm of lower respiratory tract, part unspecified   HCC

Malignant neoplasm of respiratory tract NOS

Malignant neoplasms of bone and articular cartilage (C40-C41)

INCLUDES   malignant neoplasm of cartilage (articular) (joint)
malignant neoplasm of periosteum

EXCLUDES 1   malignant neoplasm of bone marrow NOS (C96.9)
malignant neoplasm of synovia (C49.-)

☑4ᵗʰ C40 Malignant neoplasm of bone and articular cartilage of limbs

Use additional code to identify major osseous defect, if applicable (M89.7-)

☑5ᵗʰ C40.0 Malignant neoplasm of scapula and long bones of upper limb

     C40.00 Malignant neoplasm of scapula and long bones of unspecified upper limb   HCC

     C40.01 Malignant neoplasm of scapula and long bones of right upper limb   HCC

     C40.02 Malignant neoplasm of scapula and long bones of left upper limb   HCC

☑5ᵗʰ C40.1 Malignant neoplasm of short bones of upper limb

     C40.10 Malignant neoplasm of short bones of unspecified upper limb   HCC

     C40.11 Malignant neoplasm of short bones of right upper limb   HCC

     C40.12 Malignant neoplasm of short bones of left upper limb   HCC

☑5ᵗʰ C40.2 Malignant neoplasm of long bones of lower limb

     C40.20 Malignant neoplasm of long bones of unspecified lower limb   HCC

     C40.21 Malignant neoplasm of long bones of right lower limb   HCC

     C40.22 Malignant neoplasm of long bones of left lower limb   HCC

☑5ᵗʰ C40.3 Malignant neoplasm of short bones of lower limb

     C40.30 Malignant neoplasm of short bones of unspecified lower limb   HCC

     C40.31 Malignant neoplasm of short bones of right lower limb   HCC

     C40.32 Malignant neoplasm of short bones of left lower limb   HCC

☑5ᵗʰ C40.8 Malignant neoplasm of overlapping sites of bone and articular cartilage of limb

     C40.80 Malignant neoplasm of overlapping sites of bone and articular cartilage of unspecified limb   HCC

     C40.81 Malignant neoplasm of overlapping sites of bone and articular cartilage of right limb   HCC

     C40.82 Malignant neoplasm of overlapping sites of bone and articular cartilage of left limb   HCC

☑5ᵗʰ C40.9 Malignant neoplasm of unspecified bones and articular cartilage of limb

     C40.90 Malignant neoplasm of unspecified bones and articular cartilage of unspecified limb   HCC

     C40.91 Malignant neoplasm of unspecified bones and articular cartilage of right limb   HCC

     C40.92 Malignant neoplasm of unspecified bones and articular cartilage of left limb   HCC

☑ Additional Character Required   ☑x7ᵗʰ Placeholder Alert   Manifestation   Unspecified Dx   ►◄ Revised Text   ● New Code   ▲ Revised Code Title

✓4ᵗʰ C41 Malignant neoplasm of bone and articular cartilage of other and unspecified sites

EXCLUDES 1   malignant neoplasm of bones of limbs (C4Ø.-)
malignant neoplasm of cartilage of ear (C49.Ø)
malignant neoplasm of cartilage of eyelid (C49.Ø)
malignant neoplasm of cartilage of larynx (C32.3)
malignant neoplasm of cartilage of limbs (C4Ø.-)
malignant neoplasm of cartilage of nose (C3Ø.Ø)

C41.Ø Malignant neoplasm of bones of skull and face   HCC

Malignant neoplasm of maxilla (superior)
Malignant neoplasm of orbital bone

EXCLUDES 2   carcinoma, any type except intraosseous or odontogenic of:
maxillary sinus (C31.Ø)
upper jaw (CØ3.Ø)
malignant neoplasm of jaw bone (lower) (C41.1)

C41.1 Malignant neoplasm of mandible   HCC

Malignant neoplasm of inferior maxilla
Malignant neoplasm of lower jaw bone

EXCLUDES 2   carcinoma, any type except intraosseous or odontogenic of:
jaw NOS (CØ3.9)
lower (CØ3.1)
malignant neoplasm of upper jaw bone (C41.Ø)

C41.2 Malignant neoplasm of vertebral column   HCC

EXCLUDES 1   malignant neoplasm of sacrum and coccyx (C41.4)

C41.3 Malignant neoplasm of ribs, sternum and clavicle   HCC

C41.4 Malignant neoplasm of pelvic bones, sacrum and coccyx   HCC

C41.9 Malignant neoplasm of bone and articular cartilage, unspecified   HCC

Melanoma and other malignant neoplasms of skin (C43-C44)

✓4ᵗʰ C43 Malignant melanoma of skin

EXCLUDES 1   melanoma in situ (DØ3.-)
EXCLUDES 2   malignant melanoma of skin of genital organs (C51-C52, C6Ø.-, C63.-)
Merkel cell carcinoma (C4A.-)
sites other than skin - code to malignant neoplasm of the site

C43.Ø Malignant melanoma of lip   HCC   Q

EXCLUDES 1   malignant neoplasm of vermilion border of lip (CØØ.Ø-CØØ.2)

✓5ᵗʰ C43.1 Malignant melanoma of eyelid, including canthus

AHA: 2018,4Q,4

C43.1Ø Malignant melanoma of unspecified eyelid, including canthus   HCC

✓6ᵗʰ C43.11 Malignant melanoma of right eyelid, including canthus

C43.111 Malignant melanoma of right upper eyelid, including canthus   HCC

C43.112 Malignant melanoma of right lower eyelid, including canthus   HCC

✓6ᵗʰ C43.12 Malignant melanoma of left eyelid, including canthus

C43.121 Malignant melanoma of left upper eyelid, including canthus   HCC

C43.122 Malignant melanoma of left lower eyelid, including canthus   HCC

✓5ᵗʰ C43.2 Malignant melanoma of ear and external auricular canal

C43.2Ø Malignant melanoma of unspecified ear and external auricular canal   HCC   Q

C43.21 Malignant melanoma of right ear and external auricular canal   HCC   Q

C43.22 Malignant melanoma of left ear and external auricular canal   HCC   Q

✓5ᵗʰ C43.3 Malignant melanoma of other and unspecified parts of face

C43.3Ø Malignant melanoma of unspecified part of face   HCC   Q

C43.31 Malignant melanoma of nose   HCC   Q

C43.39 Malignant melanoma of other parts of face   HCC   Q

C43.4 Malignant melanoma of scalp and neck   HCC   Q

✓5ᵗʰ C43.5 Malignant melanoma of trunk

EXCLUDES 2   malignant neoplasm of anus NOS (C21.Ø)
malignant neoplasm of scrotum (C63.2)

C43.51 Malignant melanoma of anal skin   HCC   Q

Malignant melanoma of anal margin
Malignant melanoma of perianal skin

C43.52 Malignant melanoma of skin of breast   HCC   Q

C43.59 Malignant melanoma of other part of trunk   HCC   Q

✓5ᵗʰ C43.6 Malignant melanoma of upper limb, including shoulder

C43.6Ø Malignant melanoma of unspecified upper limb, including shoulder   HCC   Q

C43.61 Malignant melanoma of right upper limb, including shoulder   HCC   Q

C43.62 Malignant melanoma of left upper limb, including shoulder   HCC   Q

✓5ᵗʰ C43.7 Malignant melanoma of lower limb, including hip

C43.7Ø Malignant melanoma of unspecified lower limb, including hip   HCC   Q

C43.71 Malignant melanoma of right lower limb, including hip   HCC   Q

C43.72 Malignant melanoma of left lower limb, including hip   HCC   Q

C43.8 Malignant melanoma of overlapping sites of skin   HCC   Q

C43.9 Malignant melanoma of skin, unspecified   HCC   Q

Malignant melanoma of unspecified site of skin
Melanoma (malignant) NOS

✓4ᵗʰ C4A Merkel cell carcinoma

DEF: Malignant cutaneous cancer predominantly found in elderly patients with sun exposure that usually presents as a flesh-colored or bluish-red lump typically seen on the neck, head, and face.

C4A.Ø Merkel cell carcinoma of lip   HCC

EXCLUDES 1   malignant neoplasm of vermilion border of lip (CØØ.Ø-CØØ.2)

✓5ᵗʰ C4A.1 Merkel cell carcinoma of eyelid, including canthus

AHA: 2018,4Q,4

C4A.1Ø Merkel cell carcinoma of unspecified eyelid, including canthus   HCC

✓6ᵗʰ C4A.11 Merkel cell carcinoma of right eyelid, including canthus

C4A.111 Merkel cell carcinoma of right upper eyelid, including canthus   HCC

C4A.112 Merkel cell carcinoma of right lower eyelid, including canthus   HCC

✓6ᵗʰ C4A.12 Merkel cell carcinoma of left eyelid, including canthus

C4A.121 Merkel cell carcinoma of left upper eyelid, including canthus   HCC

C4A.122 Merkel cell carcinoma of left lower eyelid, including canthus   HCC

✓5ᵗʰ C4A.2 Merkel cell carcinoma of ear and external auricular canal

C4A.2Ø Merkel cell carcinoma of unspecified ear and external auricular canal   HCC

C4A.21 Merkel cell carcinoma of right ear and external auricular canal   HCC

C4A.22 Merkel cell carcinoma of left ear and external auricular canal   HCC

✓5ᵗʰ C4A.3 Merkel cell carcinoma of other and unspecified parts of face

C4A.3Ø Merkel cell carcinoma of unspecified part of face   HCC

C4A.31 Merkel cell carcinoma of nose   HCC

C4A.39 Merkel cell carcinoma of other parts of face   HCC

C4A.4 Merkel cell carcinoma of scalp and neck   HCC

✓5ᵗʰ C4A.5 Merkel cell carcinoma of trunk

EXCLUDES 2   malignant neoplasm of anus NOS (C21.Ø)
malignant neoplasm of scrotum (C63.2)

C4A.51 Merkel cell carcinoma of anal skin   HCC

Merkel cell carcinoma of anal margin
Merkel cell carcinoma of perianal skin

C4A.52 Merkel cell carcinoma of skin of breast   HCC

C4A.59 Merkel cell carcinoma of other part of trunk   HCC

✓5ᵗʰ C4A.6 Merkel cell carcinoma of upper limb, including shoulder

C4A.6Ø Merkel cell carcinoma of unspecified upper limb, including shoulder   HCC

C4A.61 Merkel cell carcinoma of right upper limb, including shoulder   HCC

C4A.62 Merkel cell carcinoma of left upper limb, including shoulder   HCC

√6th **C4A.7** Merkel cell carcinoma of lower limb, including hip

  C4A.70 Merkel cell carcinoma of unspecified lower limb, including hip   HCC

  C4A.71 Merkel cell carcinoma of right lower limb, including hip   HCC

  C4A.72 Merkel cell carcinoma of left lower limb, including hip   HCC

C4A.8 Merkel cell carcinoma of overlapping sites   HCC

C4A.9 Merkel cell carcinoma, unspecified   HCC

  Merkel cell carcinoma of unspecified site

  Merkel cell carcinoma NOS

√4th **C44** Other and unspecified malignant neoplasm of skin

  INCLUDES   malignant neoplasm of sebaceous glands

          malignant neoplasm of sweat glands

  EXCLUDES 1   *Kaposi's sarcoma of skin (C46.0)*

          malignant melanoma of skin (C43.-)

          malignant neoplasm of skin of genital organs (C51-C52, C60.-, C63.2)

          Merkel cell carcinoma (C4A.-)

DEF: Basal cell carcinoma: Abnormal growth of skin cells that arises from the deepest layer of the epidermis and may present as an open sore, red patches, pink growth, or scar. Typically caused by sun exposure, it is one of the most common forms of skin cancer.

DEF: Squamous cell carcinoma: Uncontrolled growth of abnormal skin cells that arises from the outer layers of the skin (epidermis) and may present as an open sore. It is characterized by a firm, red nodule, elevated growth with a central depression, or a flat sore with a scaly crust.

√5th **C44.0** Other and unspecified malignant neoplasm of skin of lip

  EXCLUDES 1   *malignant neoplasm of lip (C00.-)*

  C44.00 Unspecified malignant neoplasm of skin of lip

  C44.01 Basal cell carcinoma of skin of lip

  C44.02 Squamous cell carcinoma of skin of lip

  C44.09 Other specified malignant neoplasm of skin of lip

√5th **C44.1** Other and unspecified malignant neoplasm of skin of eyelid, including canthus

  EXCLUDES 1   *connective tissue of eyelid (C49.0)*

  AHA: 2018,4Q,4

  √6th **C44.10** Unspecified malignant neoplasm of skin of eyelid, including canthus

    C44.101 Unspecified malignant neoplasm of skin of unspecified eyelid, including canthus

    √7th **C44.102** Unspecified malignant neoplasm of skin of right eyelid, including canthus

      C44.1021 Unspecified malignant neoplasm of skin of right upper eyelid, including canthus

      C44.1022 Unspecified malignant neoplasm of skin of right lower eyelid, including canthus

    √7th **C44.109** Unspecified malignant neoplasm of skin of left eyelid, including canthus

      C44.1091 Unspecified malignant neoplasm of skin of left upper eyelid, including canthus

      C44.1092 Unspecified malignant neoplasm of skin of left lower eyelid, including canthus

  √6th **C44.11** Basal cell carcinoma of skin of eyelid, including canthus

    C44.111 Basal cell carcinoma of skin of unspecified eyelid, including canthus

    √7th **C44.112** Basal cell carcinoma of skin of right eyelid, including canthus

      C44.1121 Basal cell carcinoma of skin of right upper eyelid, including canthus

      C44.1122 Basal cell carcinoma of skin of right lower eyelid, including canthus

    √7th **C44.119** Basal cell carcinoma of skin of left eyelid, including canthus

      C44.1191 Basal cell carcinoma of skin of left upper eyelid, including canthus

      C44.1192 Basal cell carcinoma of skin of left lower eyelid, including canthus

  √6th **C44.12** Squamous cell carcinoma of skin of eyelid, including canthus

    C44.121 Squamous cell carcinoma of skin of unspecified eyelid, including canthus

    √7th **C44.122** Squamous cell carcinoma of skin of right eyelid, including canthus

      C44.1221 Squamous cell carcinoma of skin of right upper eyelid, including canthus

      C44.1222 Squamous cell carcinoma of skin of right lower eyelid, including canthus

    √7th **C44.129** Squamous cell carcinoma of skin of left eyelid, including canthus

      C44.1291 Squamous cell carcinoma of skin of left upper eyelid, including canthus

      C44.1292 Squamous cell carcinoma of skin of left lower eyelid, including canthus

  √6th **C44.13** Sebaceous cell carcinoma of skin of eyelid, including canthus

    C44.131 Sebaceous cell carcinoma of skin of unspecified eyelid, including canthus

    √7th **C44.132** Sebaceous cell carcinoma of skin of right eyelid, including canthus

      C44.1321 Sebaceous cell carcinoma of skin of right upper eyelid, including canthus

      C44.1322 Sebaceous cell carcinoma of skin of right lower eyelid, including canthus

    √7th **C44.139** Sebaceous cell carcinoma of skin of left eyelid, including canthus

      C44.1391 Sebaceous cell carcinoma of skin of left upper eyelid, including canthus

      C44.1392 Sebaceous cell carcinoma of skin of left lower eyelid, including canthus

  √6th **C44.19** Other specified malignant neoplasm of skin of eyelid, including canthus

    C44.191 Other specified malignant neoplasm of skin of unspecified eyelid, including canthus

    √7th **C44.192** Other specified malignant neoplasm of skin of right eyelid, including canthus

      C44.1921 Other specified malignant neoplasm of skin of right upper eyelid, including canthus

      C44.1922 Other specified malignant neoplasm of skin of right lower eyelid, including canthus

    √7th **C44.199** Other specified malignant neoplasm of skin of left eyelid, including canthus

      C44.1991 Other specified malignant neoplasm of skin of left upper eyelid, including canthus

      C44.1992 Other specified malignant neoplasm of skin of left lower eyelid, including canthus

√5th **C44.2** Other and unspecified malignant neoplasm of skin of ear and external auricular canal

  EXCLUDES 1   *connective tissue of ear (C49.0)*

  √6th **C44.20** Unspecified malignant neoplasm of skin of ear and external auricular canal

    C44.201 Unspecified malignant neoplasm of skin of unspecified ear and external auricular canal

    C44.202 Unspecified malignant neoplasm of skin of right ear and external auricular canal

    C44.209 Unspecified malignant neoplasm of skin of left ear and external auricular canal

  √6th **C44.21** Basal cell carcinoma of skin of ear and external auricular canal

    C44.211 Basal cell carcinoma of skin of unspecified ear and external auricular canal

    C44.212 Basal cell carcinoma of skin of right ear and external auricular canal

    C44.219 Basal cell carcinoma of skin of left ear and external auricular canal

☑ Additional Character Required   √x7th Placeholder Alert   Manifestation   Unspecified Dx   ►◄ Revised Text   ● New Code   ▲ Revised Code Title

√6ᵗʰ **C44.22** Squamous cell carcinoma of skin of ear and external auricular canal
- **C44.221** Squamous cell carcinoma of skin of unspecified ear and external auricular canal
- **C44.222** Squamous cell carcinoma of skin of right ear and external auricular canal
- **C44.229** Squamous cell carcinoma of skin of left ear and external auricular canal

√6ᵗʰ **C44.29** Other specified malignant neoplasm of skin of ear and external auricular canal
- **C44.291** Other specified malignant neoplasm of skin of unspecified ear and external auricular canal
- **C44.292** Other specified malignant neoplasm of skin of right ear and external auricular canal
- **C44.299** Other specified malignant neoplasm of skin of left ear and external auricular canal

√5ᵗʰ **C44.3** Other and unspecified malignant neoplasm of skin of other and unspecified parts of face

√6ᵗʰ **C44.30** Unspecified malignant neoplasm of skin of other and unspecified parts of face
- **C44.300** Unspecified malignant neoplasm of skin of unspecified part of face
- **C44.301** Unspecified malignant neoplasm of skin of nose
- **C44.309** Unspecified malignant neoplasm of skin of other parts of face

√6ᵗʰ **C44.31** Basal cell carcinoma of skin of other and unspecified parts of face
- **C44.310** Basal cell carcinoma of skin of unspecified parts of face
- **C44.311** Basal cell carcinoma of skin of nose
- **C44.319** Basal cell carcinoma of skin of other parts of face

√6ᵗʰ **C44.32** Squamous cell carcinoma of skin of other and unspecified parts of face
- **C44.320** Squamous cell carcinoma of skin of unspecified parts of face
- **C44.321** Squamous cell carcinoma of skin of nose
- **C44.329** Squamous cell carcinoma of skin of other parts of face

√6ᵗʰ **C44.39** Other specified malignant neoplasm of skin of other and unspecified parts of face
- **C44.390** Other specified malignant neoplasm of skin of unspecified parts of face
- **C44.391** Other specified malignant neoplasm of skin of nose
- **C44.399** Other specified malignant neoplasm of skin of other parts of face

√5ᵗʰ **C44.4** Other and unspecified malignant neoplasm of skin of scalp and neck
- **C44.40** Unspecified malignant neoplasm of skin of scalp and neck
- **C44.41** Basal cell carcinoma of skin of scalp and neck
- **C44.42** Squamous cell carcinoma of skin of scalp and neck
- **C44.49** Other specified malignant neoplasm of skin of scalp and neck

√5ᵗʰ **C44.5** Other and unspecified malignant neoplasm of skin of trunk
- **EXCLUDES 1**   anus NOS (C21.0)
  - scrotum (C63.2)

√6ᵗʰ **C44.50** Unspecified malignant neoplasm of skin of trunk
- **C44.500** Unspecified malignant neoplasm of anal skin
  - Unspecified malignant neoplasm of anal margin
  - Unspecified malignant neoplasm of perianal skin
- **C44.501** Unspecified malignant neoplasm of skin of breast
- **C44.509** Unspecified malignant neoplasm of skin of other part of trunk

√6ᵗʰ **C44.51** Basal cell carcinoma of skin of trunk
- **C44.510** Basal cell carcinoma of anal skin
  - Basal cell carcinoma of anal margin
  - Basal cell carcinoma of perianal skin
- **C44.511** Basal cell carcinoma of skin of breast
- **C44.519** Basal cell carcinoma of skin of other part of trunk

√6ᵗʰ **C44.52** Squamous cell carcinoma of skin of trunk
- **C44.520** Squamous cell carcinoma of anal skin
  - Squamous cell carcinoma of anal margin
  - Squamous cell carcinoma of perianal skin
- **C44.521** Squamous cell carcinoma of skin of breast
- **C44.529** Squamous cell carcinoma of skin of other part of trunk

√6ᵗʰ **C44.59** Other specified malignant neoplasm of skin of trunk
- **C44.590** Other specified malignant neoplasm of anal skin
  - Other specified malignant neoplasm of anal margin
  - Other specified malignant neoplasm of perianal skin
- **C44.591** Other specified malignant neoplasm of skin of breast
- **C44.599** Other specified malignant neoplasm of skin of other part of trunk

√5ᵗʰ **C44.6** Other and unspecified malignant neoplasm of skin of upper limb, including shoulder

√6ᵗʰ **C44.60** Unspecified malignant neoplasm of skin of upper limb, including shoulder
- **C44.601** Unspecified malignant neoplasm of skin of unspecified upper limb, including shoulder
- **C44.602** Unspecified malignant neoplasm of skin of right upper limb, including shoulder
- **C44.609** Unspecified malignant neoplasm of skin of left upper limb, including shoulder

√6ᵗʰ **C44.61** Basal cell carcinoma of skin of upper limb, including shoulder
- **C44.611** Basal cell carcinoma of skin of unspecified upper limb, including shoulder
- **C44.612** Basal cell carcinoma of skin of right upper limb, including shoulder
- **C44.619** Basal cell carcinoma of skin of left upper limb, including shoulder

√6ᵗʰ **C44.62** Squamous cell carcinoma of skin of upper limb, including shoulder
- **C44.621** Squamous cell carcinoma of skin of unspecified upper limb, including shoulder
- **C44.622** Squamous cell carcinoma of skin of right upper limb, including shoulder
- **C44.629** Squamous cell carcinoma of skin of left upper limb, including shoulder

√6ᵗʰ **C44.69** Other specified malignant neoplasm of skin of upper limb, including shoulder
- **C44.691** Other specified malignant neoplasm of skin of unspecified upper limb, including shoulder
- **C44.692** Other specified malignant neoplasm of skin of right upper limb, including shoulder
- **C44.699** Other specified malignant neoplasm of skin of left upper limb, including shoulder

√5ᵗʰ **C44.7** Other and unspecified malignant neoplasm of skin of lower limb, including hip

√6ᵗʰ **C44.70** Unspecified malignant neoplasm of skin of lower limb, including hip
- **C44.701** Unspecified malignant neoplasm of skin of unspecified lower limb, including hip
- **C44.702** Unspecified malignant neoplasm of skin of right lower limb, including hip
- **C44.709** Unspecified malignant neoplasm of skin of left lower limb, including hip

√6ᵗʰ **C44.71** Basal cell carcinoma of skin of lower limb, including hip
- **C44.711** Basal cell carcinoma of skin of unspecified lower limb, including hip
- **C44.712** Basal cell carcinoma of skin of right lower limb, including hip
- **C44.719** Basal cell carcinoma of skin of left lower limb, including hip

√6ᵗʰ **C44.72** Squamous cell carcinoma of skin of lower limb, including hip
- **C44.721** Squamous cell carcinoma of skin of unspecified lower limb, including hip
- **C44.722** Squamous cell carcinoma of skin of right lower limb, including hip
- **C44.729** Squamous cell carcinoma of skin of left lower limb, including hip

☑6ᵗʰ **C44.79   Other specified malignant neoplasm of skin of lower limb, including hip**

    C44.791   Other specified malignant neoplasm of skin of unspecified lower limb, including hip

    C44.792   Other specified malignant neoplasm of skin of right lower limb, including hip

    C44.799   Other specified malignant neoplasm of skin of left lower limb, including hip

☑5ᵗʰ **C44.8   Other and unspecified malignant neoplasm of overlapping sites of skin**

    C44.80   Unspecified malignant neoplasm of overlapping sites of skin

    C44.81   Basal cell carcinoma of overlapping sites of skin

    C44.82   Squamous cell carcinoma of overlapping sites of skin

    C44.89   Other specified malignant neoplasm of overlapping sites of skin

☑6ᵗʰ **C44.9   Other and unspecified malignant neoplasm of skin, unspecified**

    C44.90   Unspecified malignant neoplasm of skin, unspecified

      Malignant neoplasm of unspecified site of skin

    C44.91   Basal cell carcinoma of skin, unspecified

    C44.92   Squamous cell carcinoma of skin, unspecified

    C44.99   Other specified malignant neoplasm of skin, unspecified

Malignant neoplasms of mesothelial and soft tissue (C45-C49)

☑4ᵗʰ **C45   Mesothelioma**

    DEF: Rare type of cancer that forms in the thin layer of protective tissue that covers the majority of internal organs (mesothelium).

    C45.0   Mesothelioma of pleura   HCC

      EXCLUDES 1   other malignant neoplasm of pleura (C38.4)

      AHA: 2017,2Q,11

      TIP: For pleural mesothelioma that has metastasized to the chest wall, assign this code for the primary site along with C79.89 for metastatic cancer in the chest wall.

    C45.1   Mesothelioma of peritoneum   HCC

      Mesothelioma of cul-de-sac
      Mesothelioma of mesentery
      Mesothelioma of mesocolon
      · Mesothelioma of omentum
      Mesothelioma of peritoneum (parietal) (pelvic)

      EXCLUDES 1   other malignant neoplasm of soft tissue of peritoneum (C48.-)

    C45.2   Mesothelioma of pericardium   HCC

      EXCLUDES 1   other malignant neoplasm of pericardium (C38.0)

    C45.7   Mesothelioma of other sites   HCC

    C45.9   Mesothelioma, unspecified   HCC

☑4ᵗʰ **C46   Kaposi's sarcoma**

    Code first any human immunodeficiency virus [HIV] disease (B20)

    DEF: Malignant neoplasm that causes patches of abnormal tissue to grow under the skin, in the lining of the mouth, nose, and throat, in lymph nodes, or in other visceral organs. Kaposi's sarcoma is caused by human herpesvirus8 (HHV8).

    C46.0   Kaposi's sarcoma of skin   HCC

    C46.1   Kaposi's sarcoma of soft tissue   HCC

      Kaposi's sarcoma of blood vessel
      Kaposi's sarcoma of connective tissue
      Kaposi's sarcoma of fascia
      Kaposi's sarcoma of ligament
      Kaposi's sarcoma of lymphatic(s) NEC
      Kaposi's sarcoma of muscle

      EXCLUDES 2   Kaposi's sarcoma of lymph glands and nodes (C46.3)

    C46.2   Kaposi's sarcoma of palate   HCC

    C46.3   Kaposi's sarcoma of lymph nodes   HCC

    C46.4   Kaposi's sarcoma of gastrointestinal sites   HCC

☑5ᵗʰ **C46.5   Kaposi's sarcoma of lung**

      AHA: 2019,1Q,16

      TIP: When associated malignant pericardial effusion is documented, assign code I31.3. If the sole reason for admission is to treat the effusion with no treatment of the lung malignancy rendered, code I31.3 may be sequenced first.

      C46.50   Kaposi's sarcoma of unspecified lung   HCC

      C46.51   Kaposi's sarcoma of right lung   HCC

      C46.52   Kaposi's sarcoma of left lung   HCC

    C46.7   Kaposi's sarcoma of other sites   HCC

    C46.9   Kaposi's sarcoma, unspecified   HCC

      Kaposi's sarcoma of unspecified site

☑4ᵗʰ **C47   Malignant neoplasm of peripheral nerves and autonomic nervous system**

    INCLUDES   malignant neoplasm of sympathetic and parasympathetic nerves and ganglia

    EXCLUDES 1   Kaposi's sarcoma of soft tissue (C46.1)

    C47.0   Malignant neoplasm of peripheral nerves of head, face and neck   HCC

      EXCLUDES 1   malignant neoplasm of peripheral nerves of orbit (C69.6-)

☑5ᵗʰ **C47.1   Malignant neoplasm of peripheral nerves of upper limb, including shoulder**

    C47.10   Malignant neoplasm of peripheral nerves of unspecified upper limb, including shoulder   HCC

    C47.11   Malignant neoplasm of peripheral nerves of right upper limb, including shoulder   HCC

    C47.12   Malignant neoplasm of peripheral nerves of left upper limb, including shoulder   HCC

☑5ᵗʰ **C47.2   Malignant neoplasm of peripheral nerves of lower limb, including hip**

    C47.20   Malignant neoplasm of peripheral nerves of unspecified lower limb, including hip   HCC

    C47.21   Malignant neoplasm of peripheral nerves of right lower limb, including hip   HCC

    C47.22   Malignant neoplasm of peripheral nerves of left lower limb, including hip   HCC

    C47.3   Malignant neoplasm of peripheral nerves of thorax   HCC

    C47.4   Malignant neoplasm of peripheral nerves of abdomen   HCC

    C47.5   Malignant neoplasm of peripheral nerves of pelvis   HCC

    C47.6   Malignant neoplasm of peripheral nerves of trunk, unspecified   HCC

      Malignant neoplasm of peripheral nerves of unspecified part of trunk

    C47.8   Malignant neoplasm of overlapping sites of peripheral nerves and autonomic nervous system   HCC

    C47.9   Malignant neoplasm of peripheral nerves and autonomic nervous system, unspecified   HCC

      Malignant neoplasm of unspecified site of peripheral nerves and autonomic nervous system

☑4ᵗʰ **C48   Malignant neoplasm of retroperitoneum and peritoneum**

    EXCLUDES 1   Kaposi's sarcoma of connective tissue (C46.1)
           mesothelioma (C45.-)

    C48.0   Malignant neoplasm of retroperitoneum   HCC

    C48.1   Malignant neoplasm of specified parts of peritoneum   HCC

      Malignant neoplasm of cul-de-sac
      Malignant neoplasm of mesentery
      Malignant neoplasm of mesocolon
      Malignant neoplasm of omentum
      Malignant neoplasm of parietal peritoneum
      Malignant neoplasm of pelvic peritoneum

    C48.2   Malignant neoplasm of peritoneum, unspecified   HCC

    C48.8   Malignant neoplasm of overlapping sites of retroperitoneum and peritoneum   HCC

☑ Additional Character Required   ☑x7ᵗʰ Placeholder Alert   Manifestation   Unspecified Dx   ▶◀ Revised Text   ● New Code   ▲ Revised Code Title

ICD-10-CM 2020   469

✓4ᵗʰ **C49　Malignant neoplasm of** other connective and soft tissue

    INCLUDES malignant neoplasm of blood vessel
        malignant neoplasm of bursa
        malignant neoplasm of cartilage
        malignant neoplasm of fascia
        malignant neoplasm of fat
        malignant neoplasm of ligament, except uterine
        malignant neoplasm of lymphatic vessel
        malignant neoplasm of muscle
        malignant neoplasm of synovia
        malignant neoplasm of tendon (sheath)

    EXCLUDES 1 *malignant neoplasm of cartilage (of):*
        articular (C40-C41)
        larynx (C32.3)
        nose (C30.0)
        malignant neoplasm of connective tissue of breast (C50.-)

    EXCLUDES 2 *Kaposi's sarcoma of soft tissue (C46.1)*
        malignant neoplasm of heart (C38.0)
        malignant neoplasm of peripheral nerves and autonomic nervous system (C47.-)
        malignant neoplasm of peritoneum (C48.2)
        malignant neoplasm of retroperitoneum (C48.0)
        malignant neoplasm of uterine ligament (C57.3)
        mesothelioma (C45.-)

C49.0　Malignant neoplasm of connective and soft tissue of head, face and neck　　HCC
    Malignant neoplasm of connective tissue of ear
    Malignant neoplasm of connective tissue of eyelid
    EXCLUDES 1 *connective tissue of orbit (C69.6-)*

✓5ᵗʰ **C49.1　Malignant neoplasm of connective and soft tissue of** upper limb, including shoulder

  C49.10　Malignant neoplasm of connective and soft tissue of unspecified upper limb, including shoulder　　HCC

  C49.11　Malignant neoplasm of connective and soft tissue of right **upper limb, including shoulder**　　HCC

  C49.12　Malignant neoplasm of connective and soft tissue of left **upper limb, including shoulder**　　HCC

✓5ᵗʰ **C49.2　Malignant neoplasm of connective and soft tissue of** lower limb, including hip

  C49.20　Malignant neoplasm of connective and soft tissue of unspecified lower limb, including hip　　HCC

  C49.21　Malignant neoplasm of connective and soft tissue of right **lower limb, including hip**　　HCC

  C49.22　Malignant neoplasm of connective and soft tissue of left **lower limb, including hip**　　HCC

C49.3　Malignant neoplasm of connective and soft tissue of thorax　　HCC
    Malignant neoplasm of axilla
    Malignant neoplasm of diaphragm
    Malignant neoplasm of great vessels
    EXCLUDES 1 *malignant neoplasm of breast (C50.-)*
        malignant neoplasm of heart (C38.0)
        malignant neoplasm of mediastinum (C38.1-C38.3)
        malignant neoplasm of thymus (C37)
    AHA: 2015,3Q,19

C49.4　Malignant neoplasm of connective and soft tissue of abdomen　　HCC
    Malignant neoplasm of abdominal wall
    Malignant neoplasm of hypochondrium

C49.5　Malignant neoplasm of connective and soft tissue of pelvis　　HCC
    Malignant neoplasm of buttock
    Malignant neoplasm of groin
    Malignant neoplasm of perineum

C49.6　Malignant neoplasm of connective and soft tissue of trunk, unspecified　　HCC
    Malignant neoplasm of back NOS

C49.8　Malignant neoplasm of overlapping sites **of connective and soft tissue**　　HCC
    Primary malignant neoplasm of two or more contiguous sites of connective and soft tissue

C49.9　Malignant neoplasm of connective and soft tissue, unspecified　　HCC

✓5ᵗʰ **C49.A　Gastrointestinal stromal tumor**

    AHA: 2016,4Q,8
    DEF: Uncommon malignant tumor found in the GI tract that originates from interstitial cells of the autonomic nervous system. Most occur in the stomach or small intestine but can originate anywhere in the GI tract.

  C49.A0　Gastrointestinal stromal tumor, unspecified site　　HCC

  C49.A1　Gastrointestinal stromal tumor of esophagus　　HCC

  C49.A2　Gastrointestinal stromal tumor of stomach　　HCC

  C49.A3　Gastrointestinal stromal tumor of small intestine　　HCC

  C49.A4　Gastrointestinal stromal tumor of large intestine　　HCC

  C49.A5　Gastrointestinal stromal tumor of rectum　　HCC

  C49.A9　Gastrointestinal stromal tumor of other sites　　HCC

Malignant neoplasms of breast (C50)

✓4ᵗʰ **C50　Malignant neoplasm of** breast

    INCLUDES connective tissue of breast
        Paget's disease of breast
        Paget's disease of nipple
    Use additional code to identify estrogen receptor status (Z17.0, Z17.1)
    EXCLUDES 1 *skin of breast (C44.501, C44.511, C44.521, C44.591)*
    AHA: 2017,4Q,19

Female Breast

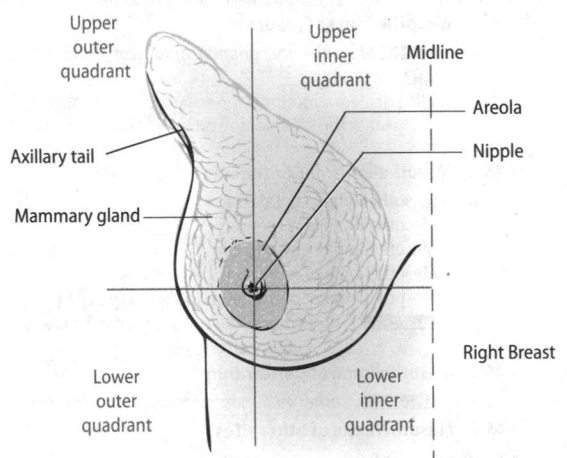

Upper outer quadrant — Upper inner quadrant — Midline — Areola — Nipple — Axillary tail — Mammary gland — Lower outer quadrant — Lower inner quadrant — Right Breast

✓5ᵗʰ **C50.0　Malignant neoplasm of** nipple and areola

  ✓6ᵗʰ **C50.01　Malignant neoplasm of nipple and areola,** female

    C50.011　Malignant neoplasm of nipple and areola, right **female breast**　　HCC ♀

    C50.012　Malignant neoplasm of nipple and areola, left **female breast**　　HCC ♀

    C50.019　Malignant neoplasm of nipple and areola, unspecified female breast　　HCC ♀

  ✓6ᵗʰ **C50.02　Malignant neoplasm of nipple and areola,** male

    C50.021　Malignant neoplasm of nipple and areola, right **male breast**　　HCC ♂

    C50.022　Malignant neoplasm of nipple and areola, left **male breast**　　HCC ♂

    C50.029　Malignant neoplasm of nipple and areola, unspecified male breast　　HCC ♂

✓5ᵗʰ **C50.1　Malignant neoplasm of** central portion **of breast**

  ✓6ᵗʰ **C50.11　Malignant neoplasm of central portion of breast, female**

    C50.111　Malignant neoplasm of central portion of right **female breast**　　HCC ♀

    C50.112　Malignant neoplasm of central portion of left **female breast**　　HCC ♀

    C50.119　Malignant neoplasm of central portion of unspecified female breast　　HCC ♀

√6ᵗʰ C50.12   **Malignant neoplasm of central portion of breast, male**

     C50.121   Malignant neoplasm of central portion of right male breast   HCC ♂

     C50.122   Malignant neoplasm of central portion of left male breast   HCC ♂

     C50.129   Malignant neoplasm of central portion of unspecified male breast   HCC ♂

√5ᵗʰ C50.2   **Malignant neoplasm of upper-inner quadrant of breast**

   √6ᵗʰ C50.21   Malignant neoplasm of upper-inner quadrant of breast, female

     C50.211   Malignant neoplasm of upper-inner quadrant of right female breast   HCC ♀

     C50.212   Malignant neoplasm of upper-inner quadrant of left female breast   HCC ♀

     C50.219   Malignant neoplasm of upper-inner quadrant of unspecified female breast   HCC ♀

   √6ᵗʰ C50.22   Malignant neoplasm of upper-inner quadrant of breast, male

     C50.221   Malignant neoplasm of upper-inner quadrant of right male breast   HCC ♂

     C50.222   Malignant neoplasm of upper-inner quadrant of left male breast   HCC ♂

     C50.229   Malignant neoplasm of upper-inner quadrant of unspecified male breast   HCC ♂

√5ᵗʰ C50.3   **Malignant neoplasm of lower-inner quadrant of breast**

   √6ᵗʰ C50.31   Malignant neoplasm of lower-inner quadrant of breast, female

     C50.311   Malignant neoplasm of lower-inner quadrant of right female breast   HCC ♀

     C50.312   Malignant neoplasm of lower-inner quadrant of left female breast   HCC ♀

     C50.319   Malignant neoplasm of lower-inner quadrant of unspecified female breast   HCC ♀

   √6ᵗʰ C50.32   Malignant neoplasm of lower-inner quadrant of breast, male

     C50.321   Malignant neoplasm of lower-inner quadrant of right male breast   HCC ♂

     C50.322   Malignant neoplasm of lower-inner quadrant of left male breast   HCC ♂

     C50.329   Malignant neoplasm of lower-inner quadrant of unspecified male breast   HCC ♂

√5ᵗʰ C50.4   **Malignant neoplasm of upper-outer quadrant of breast**

   √6ᵗʰ C50.41   Malignant neoplasm of upper-outer quadrant of breast, female

     C50.411   Malignant neoplasm of upper-outer quadrant of right female breast   HCC ♀

     C50.412   Malignant neoplasm of upper-outer quadrant of left female breast   HCC ♀

     C50.419   Malignant neoplasm of upper-outer quadrant of unspecified female breast   HCC ♀

   √6ᵗʰ C50.42   Malignant neoplasm of upper-outer quadrant of breast, male

     C50.421   Malignant neoplasm of upper-outer quadrant of right male breast   HCC ♂

     C50.422   Malignant neoplasm of upper-outer quadrant of left male breast   HCC ♂

     C50.429   Malignant neoplasm of upper-outer quadrant of unspecified male breast   HCC ♂

√5ᵗʰ C50.5   **Malignant neoplasm of lower-outer quadrant of breast**

   √6ᵗʰ C50.51   Malignant neoplasm of lower-outer quadrant of breast, female

     C50.511   Malignant neoplasm of lower-outer quadrant of right female breast   HCC ♀

     C50.512   Malignant neoplasm of lower-outer quadrant of left female breast   HCC ♀

     C50.519   Malignant neoplasm of lower-outer quadrant of unspecified female breast   HCC ♀

   √6ᵗʰ C50.52   Malignant neoplasm of lower-outer quadrant of breast, male

     C50.521   Malignant neoplasm of lower-outer quadrant of right male breast   HCC ♂

     C50.522   Malignant neoplasm of lower-outer quadrant of left male breast   HCC ♂

     C50.529   Malignant neoplasm of lower-outer quadrant of unspecified male breast   HCC ♂

√5ᵗʰ C50.6   **Malignant neoplasm of axillary tail of breast**

   √6ᵗʰ C50.61   Malignant neoplasm of axillary tail of breast, female

     C50.611   Malignant neoplasm of axillary tail of right female breast   HCC ♀

     C50.612   Malignant neoplasm of axillary tail of left female breast   HCC ♀

     C50.619   Malignant neoplasm of axillary tail of unspecified female breast   HCC ♀

   √6ᵗʰ C50.62   Malignant neoplasm of axillary tail of breast, male

     C50.621   Malignant neoplasm of axillary tail of right male breast   HCC ♂

     C50.622   Malignant neoplasm of axillary tail of left male breast   HCC ♂

     C50.629   Malignant neoplasm of axillary tail of unspecified male breast   HCC ♂

√5ᵗʰ C50.8   **Malignant neoplasm of overlapping sites of breast**

   √6ᵗʰ C50.81   Malignant neoplasm of overlapping sites of breast, female

     C50.811   Malignant neoplasm of overlapping sites of right female breast   HCC ♀

     C50.812   Malignant neoplasm of overlapping sites of left female breast   HCC ♀

     C50.819   Malignant neoplasm of overlapping sites of unspecified female breast   HCC ♀

   √6ᵗʰ C50.82   Malignant neoplasm of overlapping sites of breast, male

     C50.821   Malignant neoplasm of overlapping sites of right male breast   HCC ♂

     C50.822   Malignant neoplasm of overlapping sites of left male breast   HCC ♂

     C50.829   Malignant neoplasm of overlapping sites of unspecified male breast   HCC ♂

√5ᵗʰ C50.9   **Malignant neoplasm of breast of unspecified site**

   √6ᵗʰ C50.91   Malignant neoplasm of breast of unspecified site, female

     C50.911   Malignant neoplasm of unspecified site of right female breast   HCC ♀

     C50.912   Malignant neoplasm of unspecified site of left female breast   HCC ♀

     C50.919   Malignant neoplasm of unspecified site of unspecified female breast   HCC ♀

   √6ᵗʰ C50.92   Malignant neoplasm of breast of unspecified site, male

     C50.921   Malignant neoplasm of unspecified site of right male breast   HCC ♂

     C50.922   Malignant neoplasm of unspecified site of left male breast   HCC ♂

✅ Additional Character Required   √x7ᵗʰ Placeholder Alert   Manifestation   Unspecified Dx   ►◄ Revised Text   ● New Code   ▲ Revised Code Title

C50.929   **Malignant neoplasm of unspecified site of unspecified male breast**   HCC ♂

Malignant neoplasms of female genital organs (C51-C58)

INCLUDES   malignant neoplasm of skin of female genital organs

√4ᵗʰ **C51   Malignant neoplasm of vulva**

EXCLUDES 1   *carcinoma in situ of vulva (D07.1)*

C51.0   Malignant neoplasm of labium majus   HCC ♀

Malignant neoplasm of Bartholin's [greater vestibular] gland

C51.1   Malignant neoplasm of labium minus   HCC ♀

C51.2   Malignant neoplasm of clitoris   HCC ♀

C51.8   Malignant neoplasm of overlapping sites of vulva   HCC ♀

C51.9   Malignant neoplasm of vulva, unspecified   HCC ♀

Malignant neoplasm of external female genitalia NOS
Malignant neoplasm of pudendum

C52   Malignant neoplasm of vagina   HCC ♀

EXCLUDES 1   *carcinoma in situ of vagina (D07.2)*

√4ᵗʰ **C53   Malignant neoplasm of cervix uteri**

EXCLUDES 1   *carcinoma in situ of cervix uteri (D06.-)*

AHA: 2017,4Q,103

C53.0   Malignant neoplasm of endocervix   HCC ♀

C53.1   Malignant neoplasm of exocervix   HCC ♀

C53.8   Malignant neoplasm of overlapping sites of cervix uteri   HCC ♀

C53.9   Malignant neoplasm of cervix uteri, unspecified   HCC ♀

√4ᵗʰ **C54   Malignant neoplasm of corpus uteri**

C54.0   Malignant neoplasm of isthmus uteri   HCC ♀

Malignant neoplasm of lower uterine segment

C54.1   Malignant neoplasm of endometrium   HCC ♀

C54.2   Malignant neoplasm of myometrium   HCC ♀

C54.3   Malignant neoplasm of fundus uteri   HCC ♀

C54.8   Malignant neoplasm of overlapping sites of corpus uteri   HCC ♀

C54.9   Malignant neoplasm of corpus uteri, unspecified   HCC ♀

C55   Malignant neoplasm of uterus, part unspecified   HCC ♀

√4ᵗʰ **C56   Malignant neoplasm of ovary**

Use additional code to identify any functional activity

C56.1   Malignant neoplasm of right ovary   HCC ♀

C56.2   Malignant neoplasm of left ovary   HCC ♀

C56.9   Malignant neoplasm of unspecified ovary   HCC ♀

√4ᵗʰ **C57   Malignant neoplasm of other and unspecified female genital organs**

√5ᵗʰ **C57.0   Malignant neoplasm of fallopian tube**

Malignant neoplasm of oviduct
Malignant neoplasm of uterine tube

C57.00   Malignant neoplasm of unspecified fallopian tube   HCC ♀

C57.01   Malignant neoplasm of right fallopian tube   HCC ♀

C57.02   Malignant neoplasm of left fallopian tube   HCC ♀

√5ᵗʰ **C57.1   Malignant neoplasm of broad ligament**

C57.10   Malignant neoplasm of unspecified broad ligament   HCC ♀

C57.11   Malignant neoplasm of right broad ligament   HCC ♀

C57.12   Malignant neoplasm of left broad ligament   HCC ♀

√5ᵗʰ **C57.2   Malignant neoplasm of round ligament**

C57.20   Malignant neoplasm of unspecified round ligament   HCC ♀

C57.21   Malignant neoplasm of right round ligament   HCC ♀

C57.22   Malignant neoplasm of left round ligament   HCC ♀

C57.3   Malignant neoplasm of parametrium   HCC ♀

Malignant neoplasm of uterine ligament NOS

C57.4   Malignant neoplasm of uterine adnexa, unspecified   HCC ♀

C57.7   Malignant neoplasm of other specified female genital organs   HCC ♀

Malignant neoplasm of wolffian body or duct

C57.8   Malignant neoplasm of overlapping sites of female genital organs   HCC ♀

Primary malignant neoplasm of two or more contiguous sites of the female genital organs whose point of origin cannot be determined

Primary tubo-ovarian malignant neoplasm whose point of origin cannot be determined

Primary utero-ovarian malignant neoplasm whose point of origin cannot be determined

C57.9   Malignant neoplasm of female genital organ, unspecified   HCC ♀

Malignant neoplasm of female genitourinary tract NOS

C58   Malignant neoplasm of placenta   HCC M ♀

INCLUDES   choriocarcinoma NOS
chorionepithelioma NOS

EXCLUDES 1   *chorioadenoma (destruens) (D39.2)*
hydatidiform mole NOS (O01.9)
invasive hydatidiform mole (D39.2)
male choriocarcinoma NOS (C62.9-)
malignant hydatidiform mole (D39.2)

Malignant neoplasms of male genital organs (C60-C63)

INCLUDES   malignant neoplasm of skin of male genital organs

√4ᵗʰ **C60   Malignant neoplasm of penis**

C60.0   Malignant neoplasm of prepuce   HCC ♂

Malignant neoplasm of foreskin

C60.1   Malignant neoplasm of glans penis   HCC ♂

C60.2   Malignant neoplasm of body of penis   HCC ♂

Malignant neoplasm of corpus cavernosum

C60.8   Malignant neoplasm of overlapping sites of penis   HCC ♂

C60.9   Malignant neoplasm of penis, unspecified   HCC ♂

Malignant neoplasm of skin of penis NOS

C61   Malignant neoplasm of prostate   HCC Q ♂

Use additional code to identify:
hormone sensitivity status (Z19.1-Z19.2)
rising PSA following treatment for malignant neoplasm of prostate (R97.21)

EXCLUDES 1   *malignant neoplasm of seminal vesicle (C63.7)*

AHA: 2017,1Q,17

√4ᵗʰ **C62   Malignant neoplasm of testis**

Use additional code to identify any functional activity

√5ᵗʰ **C62.0   Malignant neoplasm of undescended testis**

Malignant neoplasm of ectopic testis
Malignant neoplasm of retained testis

C62.00   Malignant neoplasm of unspecified undescended testis   HCC ♂

C62.01   Malignant neoplasm of undescended right testis   HCC ♂

C62.02   Malignant neoplasm of undescended left testis   HCC ♂

√5ᵗʰ **C62.1   Malignant neoplasm of descended testis**

Malignant neoplasm of scrotal testis

C62.10   Malignant neoplasm of unspecified descended testis   HCC ♂

C62.11   Malignant neoplasm of descended right testis   HCC ♂

C62.12   Malignant neoplasm of descended left testis   HCC ♂

√5ᵗʰ **C62.9   Malignant neoplasm of testis, unspecified whether descended or undescended**

C62.90   Malignant neoplasm of unspecified testis, unspecified whether descended or undescended   HCC ♂

Malignant neoplasm of testis NOS

C62.91   Malignant neoplasm of right testis, unspecified whether descended or undescended   HCC ♂

C62.92   Malignant neoplasm of left testis, unspecified whether descended or undescended   HCC ♂

☑4ᵗʰ C63 Malignant neoplasm of other and unspecified male genital organs

  ☑5ᵗʰ **C63.0 Malignant neoplasm of** epididymis

    C63.00 Malignant neoplasm of unspecified epididymis   HCC ♂

    C63.01 Malignant neoplasm of right **epididymis**   HCC ♂

    C63.02 Malignant neoplasm of left **epididymis**   HCC ♂

  ☑5ᵗʰ **C63.1 Malignant neoplasm of** spermatic cord

    C63.10 Malignant neoplasm of unspecified spermatic cord   HCC ♂

    C63.11 Malignant neoplasm of right **spermatic cord**   HCC ♂

    C63.12 Malignant neoplasm of left **spermatic cord**   HCC ♂

  C63.2 Malignant neoplasm of scrotum   HCC ♂

    Malignant neoplasm of skin of scrotum

  C63.7 Malignant neoplasm of other specified male genital organs   HCC ♂

    Malignant neoplasm of seminal vesicle

    Malignant neoplasm of tunica vaginalis

  C63.8 Malignant neoplasm of overlapping sites **of male genital organs**   HCC ♂

    Primary malignant neoplasm of two or more contiguous sites of male genital organs whose point of origin cannot be determined

  C63.9 Malignant neoplasm of male genital organ, unspecified   HCC ♂

    Malignant neoplasm of male genitourinary tract NOS

Malignant neoplasms of urinary tract (C64-C68)

☑4ᵗʰ C64 Malignant neoplasm of kidney, except renal pelvis

  EXCLUDES 1   malignant carcinoid tumor of the kidney (C7A.093)

    malignant neoplasm of renal calyces (C65.-)

    malignant neoplasm of renal pelvis (C65.-)

  C64.1 Malignant neoplasm of right **kidney, except renal pelvis**   HCC

  C64.2 Malignant neoplasm of left **kidney, except renal pelvis**   HCC

  C64.9 Malignant neoplasm of unspecified kidney, except renal pelvis   HCC

☑4ᵗʰ C65 Malignant neoplasm of renal pelvis

  INCLUDES   malignant neoplasm of pelviureteric junction

    malignant neoplasm of renal calyces

  C65.1 Malignant neoplasm of right **renal pelvis**   HCC

  C65.2 Malignant neoplasm of left **renal pelvis**   HCC

  C65.9 Malignant neoplasm of unspecified renal pelvis   HCC

☑4ᵗʰ C66 Malignant neoplasm of ureter

  EXCLUDES 1   malignant neoplasm of ureteric orifice of bladder (C67.6)

  C66.1 Malignant neoplasm of right **ureter**   HCC

  C66.2 Malignant neoplasm of left **ureter**   HCC

  C66.9 Malignant neoplasm of unspecified ureter   HCC

☑4ᵗʰ C67 Malignant neoplasm of bladder

  C67.0 Malignant neoplasm of trigone **of bladder**   HCC

  C67.1 Malignant neoplasm of dome **of bladder**   HCC

  C67.2 Malignant neoplasm of lateral wall **of bladder**   HCC

  C67.3 Malignant neoplasm of anterior wall **of bladder**   HCC

  C67.4 Malignant neoplasm of posterior wall **of bladder**   HCC

  C67.5 Malignant neoplasm of bladder neck   HCC

    Malignant neoplasm of internal urethral orifice

  C67.6 Malignant neoplasm of ureteric orifice   HCC

  C67.7 Malignant neoplasm of urachus   HCC

  C67.8 Malignant neoplasm of overlapping sites **of bladder**   HCC

  C67.9 Malignant neoplasm of bladder, unspecified   HCC

    AHA: 2016,1Q,19

☑4ᵗʰ C68 Malignant neoplasm of other and unspecified urinary organs

  EXCLUDES 1   malignant neoplasm of female genitourinary tract NOS (C57.9)

    malignant neoplasm of male genitourinary tract NOS (C63.9)

  AHA: 2016,1Q,14

  C68.0 Malignant neoplasm of urethra   HCC

    EXCLUDES 1   malignant neoplasm of urethral orifice of bladder (C67.5)

  C68.1 Malignant neoplasm of paraurethral glands   HCC

  C68.8 Malignant neoplasm of overlapping sites **of urinary organs**   HCC

    Primary malignant neoplasm of two or more contiguous sites of urinary organs whose point of origin cannot be determined

  C68.9 Malignant neoplasm of urinary organ, unspecified   HCC

    Malignant neoplasm of urinary system NOS

Malignant neoplasms of eye, brain and other parts of central nervous system (C69-C72)

☑4ᵗʰ C69 Malignant neoplasm of eye and adnexa

  EXCLUDES 1   malignant neoplasm of connective tissue of eyelid (C49.0)

    malignant neoplasm of eyelid (skin) (C43.1-, C44.1-)

    malignant neoplasm of optic nerve (C72.3-)

  ☑5ᵗʰ **C69.0 Malignant neoplasm of** conjunctiva

    C69.00 Malignant neoplasm of unspecified conjunctiva   HCC

    C69.01 Malignant neoplasm of right **conjunctiva**   HCC

    C69.02 Malignant neoplasm of left **conjunctiva**   HCC

  ☑5ᵗʰ **C69.1 Malignant neoplasm of** cornea

    C69.10 Malignant neoplasm of unspecified cornea   HCC

    C69.11 Malignant neoplasm of right **cornea**   HCC

    C69.12 Malignant neoplasm of left **cornea**   HCC

  ☑5ᵗʰ **C69.2 Malignant neoplasm of** retina

    EXCLUDES 1   dark area on retina (D49.81)

      neoplasm of unspecified behavior of retina and choroid (D49.81)

      retinal freckle (D49.81)

    C69.20 Malignant neoplasm of unspecified retina   HCC

    C69.21 Malignant neoplasm of right **retina**   HCC

    C69.22 Malignant neoplasm of left **retina**   HCC

  ☑5ᵗʰ **C69.3 Malignant neoplasm of** choroid

    C69.30 Malignant neoplasm of unspecified choroid   HCC

    C69.31 Malignant neoplasm of right **choroid**   HCC

    C69.32 Malignant neoplasm of left **choroid**   HCC

  ☑5ᵗʰ **C69.4 Malignant neoplasm of** ciliary body

    C69.40 Malignant neoplasm of unspecified ciliary body   HCC

    C69.41 Malignant neoplasm of right **ciliary body**   HCC

    C69.42 Malignant neoplasm of left **ciliary body**   HCC

  ☑5ᵗʰ **C69.5 Malignant neoplasm of** lacrimal gland and duct

    Malignant neoplasm of lacrimal sac

    Malignant neoplasm of nasolacrimal duct

    C69.50 Malignant neoplasm of unspecified lacrimal gland and duct   HCC

    C69.51 Malignant neoplasm of right **lacrimal gland and duct**   HCC

    C69.52 Malignant neoplasm of left **lacrimal gland and duct**   HCC

  ☑5ᵗʰ **C69.6 Malignant neoplasm of** orbit

    Malignant neoplasm of connective tissue of orbit

    Malignant neoplasm of extraocular muscle

    Malignant neoplasm of peripheral nerves of orbit

    Malignant neoplasm of retrobulbar tissue

    Malignant neoplasm of retro-ocular tissue

    EXCLUDES 1   malignant neoplasm of orbital bone (C41.0)

    C69.60 Malignant neoplasm of unspecified orbit   HCC

    C69.61 Malignant neoplasm of right **orbit**   HCC

    C69.62 Malignant neoplasm of left **orbit**   HCC

☑ Additional Character Required   ☑x7ᵗʰ Placeholder Alert   Manifestation   Unspecified Dx   ►◄ Revised Text   ● New Code   ▲ Revised Code Title

ICD-10-CM 2020   473

Chapter 2. Neoplasms (side margin)

C69.8-C75.5 (side margin)

√5ᵗʰ **C69.8** **Malignant neoplasm of** overlapping sites **of eye and adnexa**

     C69.80 **Malignant neoplasm of overlapping sites of unspecified eye and adnexa**   HCC

     C69.81 **Malignant neoplasm of overlapping sites of** right **eye and adnexa**   HCC

     C69.82 **Malignant neoplasm of overlapping sites of** left **eye and adnexa**   HCC

√5ᵗʰ **C69.9** **Malignant neoplasm of unspecified site of eye**

     Malignant neoplasm of eyeball

     C69.90 **Malignant neoplasm of unspecified site of unspecified eye**   HCC

     C69.91 **Malignant neoplasm of unspecified site of** right **eye**   HCC

     C69.92 **Malignant neoplasm of unspecified site of** left **eye**   HCC

√4ᵗʰ **C70** **Malignant neoplasm of** meninges

     C70.0 **Malignant neoplasm of** cerebral **meninges**   HCC

     C70.1 **Malignant neoplasm of** spinal **meninges**   HCC

     C70.9 **Malignant neoplasm of meninges, unspecified**   HCC

√4ᵗʰ **C71** **Malignant neoplasm of** brain

     EXCLUDES 1   *malignant neoplasm of cranial nerves (C72.2-C72.5)*

                  retrobulbar malignant neoplasm (C69.6-)

Lobes of the Brain

Frontal lobe, Parietal lobe, Occipital lobe, Temporal lobe, Brain stem, Cerebellum

     C71.0 **Malignant neoplasm of** cerebrum, except lobes and **ventricles**   HCC

     Malignant neoplasm of supratentorial NOS

     C71.1 **Malignant neoplasm of** frontal **lobe**   HCC

     C71.2 **Malignant neoplasm of** temporal **lobe**   HCC

     C71.3 **Malignant neoplasm of** parietal **lobe**   HCC

     C71.4 **Malignant neoplasm of** occipital **lobe**   HCC

     C71.5 **Malignant neoplasm of** cerebral **ventricle**   HCC

         EXCLUDES 1   *malignant neoplasm of fourth cerebral ventricle (C71.7)*

     C71.6 **Malignant neoplasm of** cerebellum   HCC

     C71.7 **Malignant neoplasm of** brain stem   HCC

     Malignant neoplasm of fourth cerebral ventricle

     Infratentorial malignant neoplasm NOS

     C71.8 **Malignant neoplasm of** overlapping sites **of brain**   HCC

     C71.9 **Malignant neoplasm of brain, unspecified**   HCC

         AHA: 2014,3Q,3

√4ᵗʰ **C72** **Malignant neoplasm of** spinal cord, cranial nerves **and other parts of** central nervous system

     EXCLUDES 1   *malignant neoplasm of meninges (C70.-)*

                  malignant neoplasm of peripheral nerves and autonomic nervous system (C47.-)

     C72.0 **Malignant neoplasm of** spinal cord   HCC

     C72.1 **Malignant neoplasm of** cauda equina   HCC

√5ᵗʰ **C72.2** **Malignant neoplasm of** olfactory nerve

     Malignant neoplasm of olfactory bulb

     C72.20 **Malignant neoplasm of unspecified olfactory nerve**   HCC

     C72.21 **Malignant neoplasm of** right olfactory **nerve**   HCC

     C72.22 **Malignant neoplasm of** left olfactory **nerve**   HCC

√5ᵗʰ **C72.3** **Malignant neoplasm of** optic nerve

     C72.30 **Malignant neoplasm of unspecified optic nerve**   HCC

     C72.31 **Malignant neoplasm of** right optic nerve   HCC

     C72.32 **Malignant neoplasm of** left optic nerve   HCC

√5ᵗʰ **C72.4** **Malignant neoplasm of** acoustic nerve

     C72.40 **Malignant neoplasm of unspecified acoustic nerve**   HCC

     C72.41 **Malignant neoplasm of** right acoustic **nerve**   HCC

     C72.42 **Malignant neoplasm of** left acoustic nerve   HCC

√5ᵗʰ **C72.5** **Malignant neoplasm of** other and unspecified cranial nerves

     C72.50 **Malignant neoplasm of unspecified cranial nerve**   HCC

         Malignant neoplasm of cranial nerve NOS

     C72.59 **Malignant neoplasm of other cranial nerves**   HCC

     C72.9 **Malignant neoplasm of central nervous system, unspecified**   HCC

     Malignant neoplasm of unspecified site of central nervous system

     Malignant neoplasm of nervous system NOS

Malignant neoplasms of thyroid and other endocrine glands (C73-C75)

C73 **Malignant neoplasm of** thyroid gland   HCC

     Use additional code to identify any functional activity

√4ᵗʰ **C74** **Malignant neoplasm of** adrenal gland

     TIP: If an adrenal gland tumor is described as functional (producing too much of a hormone), additional codes should be assigned to report the functional activity.

√5ᵗʰ **C74.0** **Malignant neoplasm of** cortex **of adrenal gland**

     C74.00 **Malignant neoplasm of cortex of unspecified adrenal gland**   HCC

     C74.01 **Malignant neoplasm of cortex of** right **adrenal gland**   HCC

     C74.02 **Malignant neoplasm of cortex of** left **adrenal gland**   HCC

√5ᵗʰ **C74.1** **Malignant neoplasm of** medulla **of adrenal gland**

     C74.10 **Malignant neoplasm of medulla of unspecified adrenal gland**   HCC

     C74.11 **Malignant neoplasm of medulla of** right **adrenal gland**   HCC

     C74.12 **Malignant neoplasm of medulla of** left **adrenal gland**   HCC

√5ᵗʰ **C74.9** **Malignant neoplasm of unspecified part of adrenal gland**

     C74.90 **Malignant neoplasm of unspecified part of unspecified adrenal gland**   HCC

     C74.91 **Malignant neoplasm of unspecified part of** right **adrenal gland**   HCC

     C74.92 **Malignant neoplasm of unspecified part of** left **adrenal gland**   HCC

√4ᵗʰ **C75** **Malignant neoplasm of other** endocrine glands and related **structures**

     EXCLUDES 1   *malignant carcinoid tumors (C7A.0-)*

                  malignant neoplasm of adrenal gland (C74.-)

                  malignant neoplasm of endocrine pancreas (C25.4)

                  malignant neoplasm of islets of Langerhans (C25.4)

                  malignant neoplasm of ovary (C56.-)

                  malignant neoplasm of testis (C62.-)

                  malignant neoplasm of thymus (C37)

                  malignant neoplasm of thyroid gland (C73)

                  malignant neuroendocrine tumors (C7A.-)

     C75.0 **Malignant neoplasm of** parathyroid **gland**   HCC

     C75.1 **Malignant neoplasm of** pituitary **gland**   HCC

     C75.2 **Malignant neoplasm of** craniopharyngeal duct   HCC

     C75.3 **Malignant neoplasm of** pineal gland   HCC

     C75.4 **Malignant neoplasm of** carotid body   HCC

     C75.5 **Malignant neoplasm of** aortic body **and other** paraganglia   HCC

| C75.8 | Malignant neoplasm with pluriglandular involvement, unspecified | HCC |

| C75.9 | Malignant neoplasm of endocrine gland, unspecified | HCC |

Malignant neuroendocrine tumors (C7A)

✓4ᵗʰ **C7A Malignant neuroendocrine tumors**

Code also any associated multiple endocrine neoplasia [MEN] syndromes (E31.2-)

Use additional code to identify any associated endocrine syndrome, such as:

carcinoid syndrome (E34.0)

EXCLUDES 2   *malignant pancreatic islet cell tumors (C25.4)*

Merkel cell carcinoma (C4A.-)

DEF: Tumors comprised of cells that are capable of producing hormonal syndromes in which the normal hormonal balance required to support body system functions is adversely affected.

✓5ᵗʰ **C7A.0 Malignant carcinoid tumors**

DEF: Specific type of slow-growing benign or malignant neuroendocrine tumors. Carcinoid tumors occur most commonly in the hormone producing cells of the gastrointestinal tracts and can also occur in the pancreas, testes, ovaries, or lungs.

| C7A.00 | Malignant carcinoid tumor of unspecified site | HCC |

✓6ᵗʰ C7A.01 **Malignant carcinoid tumors of the small intestine**

C7A.010	Malignant carcinoid tumor of the duodenum	HCC
C7A.011	Malignant carcinoid tumor of the jejunum	HCC
C7A.012	Malignant carcinoid tumor of the ileum	HCC
C7A.019	Malignant carcinoid tumor of the small intestine, unspecified portion	HCC

✓6ᵗʰ C7A.02 **Malignant carcinoid tumors of the appendix, large intestine, and rectum**

C7A.020	Malignant carcinoid tumor of the appendix	HCC
C7A.021	Malignant carcinoid tumor of the cecum	HCC
C7A.022	Malignant carcinoid tumor of the ascending colon	HCC
C7A.023	Malignant carcinoid tumor of the transverse colon	HCC
C7A.024	Malignant carcinoid tumor of the descending colon	HCC
C7A.025	Malignant carcinoid tumor of the sigmoid colon	HCC
C7A.026	Malignant carcinoid tumor of the rectum	HCC
C7A.029	Malignant carcinoid tumor of the large intestine, unspecified portion	HCC

Malignant carcinoid tumor of the colon NOS

✓6ᵗʰ C7A.09 **Malignant carcinoid tumors of other sites**

| C7A.090 | Malignant carcinoid tumor of the bronchus and lung | HCC |

AHA: 2019,1Q,16

TIP: When associated malignant pericardial effusion is documented, assign code I31.3. If the sole reason for admission is to treat the effusion with no treatment of the lung malignancy rendered, code I31.3 may be sequenced first.

C7A.091	Malignant carcinoid tumor of the thymus	HCC
C7A.092	Malignant carcinoid tumor of the stomach	HCC
C7A.093	Malignant carcinoid tumor of the kidney	HCC
C7A.094	Malignant carcinoid tumor of the foregut, unspecified	HCC
C7A.095	Malignant carcinoid tumor of the midgut, unspecified	HCC
C7A.096	Malignant carcinoid tumor of the hindgut, unspecified	HCC
C7A.098	Malignant carcinoid tumors of other sites	HCC

| C7A.1 | Malignant poorly differentiated neuroendocrine tumors | HCC |

Malignant poorly differentiated neuroendocrine tumor NOS

High grade neuroendocrine carcinoma, any site

Malignant poorly differentiated neuroendocrine carcinoma, any site

| C7A.8 | Other malignant neuroendocrine tumors | HCC |

Secondary neuroendocrine tumors (C7B)

✓4ᵗʰ **C7B Secondary neuroendocrine tumors**

Use additional code to identify any functional activity

✓5ᵗʰ **C7B.0 Secondary carcinoid tumors**

C7B.00	Secondary carcinoid tumors, unspecified site	HCC
C7B.01	Secondary carcinoid tumors of distant lymph nodes	HCC
C7B.02	Secondary carcinoid tumors of liver	HCC
C7B.03	Secondary carcinoid tumors of bone	HCC
C7B.04	Secondary carcinoid tumors of peritoneum	HCC

Mesentary metastasis of carcinoid tumor

| C7B.09 | Secondary carcinoid tumors of other sites | HCC |

| C7B.1 | Secondary Merkel cell carcinoma | HCC |

Merkel cell carcinoma nodal presentation

Merkel cell carcinoma visceral metastatic presentation

| C7B.8 | Other secondary neuroendocrine tumors | HCC |

Malignant neoplasms of ill-defined, other secondary and unspecified sites (C76-C80)

✓4ᵗʰ **C76 Malignant neoplasm of other and ill-defined sites**

EXCLUDES 1   *malignant neoplasm of female genitourinary tract NOS (C57.9)*

malignant neoplasm of male genitourinary tract NOS (C63.9)

malignant neoplasm of lymphoid, hematopoietic and related tissue (C81-C96)

malignant neoplasm of skin (C44.-)

malignant neoplasm of unspecified site NOS (C80.1)

| C76.0 | Malignant neoplasm of head, face and neck | HCC |

Malignant neoplasm of cheek NOS

Malignant neoplasm of nose NOS

| C76.1 | Malignant neoplasm of thorax | HCC |

Intrathoracic malignant neoplasm NOS

Malignant neoplasm of axilla NOS

Thoracic malignant neoplasm NOS

| C76.2 | Malignant neoplasm of abdomen | HCC |

| C76.3 | Malignant neoplasm of pelvis | HCC |

Malignant neoplasm of groin NOS

Malignant neoplasm of sites overlapping systems within the pelvis

Rectovaginal (septum) malignant neoplasm

Rectovesical (septum) malignant neoplasm

✓5ᵗʰ **C76.4 Malignant neoplasm of upper limb**

C76.40	Malignant neoplasm of unspecified upper limb	HCC
C76.41	Malignant neoplasm of right upper limb	HCC
C76.42	Malignant neoplasm of left upper limb	HCC

✓5ᵗʰ **C76.5 Malignant neoplasm of lower limb**

C76.50	Malignant neoplasm of unspecified lower limb	HCC
C76.51	Malignant neoplasm of right lower limb	HCC
C76.52	Malignant neoplasm of left lower limb	HCC

| C76.8 | Malignant neoplasm of other specified ill-defined sites | HCC |

Malignant neoplasm of overlapping ill-defined sites

✔ Additional Character Required   ✓x7ᵗʰ Placeholder Alert   Manifestation   Unspecified Dx   ▶◀ Revised Text   ● New Code   ▲ Revised Code Title

ICD-10-CM 2020   475

Chapter 2. Neoplasms

C75.8–C76.8

√4th C77 Secondary and unspecified malignant neoplasm of lymph nodes

> EXCLUDES 1   malignant neoplasm of lymph nodes, specified as primary (C81-C86, C88, C96.-)
> mesentary metastasis of carcinoid tumor (C7B.04)
> secondary carcinoid tumors of distant lymph nodes (C7B.01)

C77.0 Secondary and unspecified malignant neoplasm of lymph nodes of head, face and neck   HCC
> Secondary and unspecified malignant neoplasm of supraclavicular lymph nodes

C77.1 Secondary and unspecified malignant neoplasm of intrathoracic lymph nodes   HCC

C77.2 Secondary and unspecified malignant neoplasm of intra-abdominal lymph nodes   HCC

C77.3 Secondary and unspecified malignant neoplasm of axilla and upper limb lymph nodes   HCC
> Secondary and unspecified malignant neoplasm of pectoral lymph nodes

C77.4 Secondary and unspecified malignant neoplasm of inguinal and lower limb lymph nodes   HCC

C77.5 Secondary and unspecified malignant neoplasm of intrapelvic lymph nodes   HCC

C77.8 Secondary and unspecified malignant neoplasm of lymph nodes of multiple regions   HCC

C77.9 Secondary and unspecified malignant neoplasm of lymph node, unspecified   HCC

√4th C78 Secondary malignant neoplasm of respiratory and digestive organs

> EXCLUDES 1   secondary carcinoid tumors of liver (C7B.02)
> secondary carcinoid tumors of peritoneum (C7B.04)
>
> EXCLUDES 2   lymph node metastases (C77.0)

√5th C78.0 Secondary malignant neoplasm of lung
> **AHA:** 2019,1Q,16

C78.00 Secondary malignant neoplasm of unspecified lung   HCC

C78.01 Secondary malignant neoplasm of right lung   HCC

C78.02 Secondary malignant neoplasm of left lung   HCC

C78.1 Secondary malignant neoplasm of mediastinum   HCC

C78.2 Secondary malignant neoplasm of pleura   HCC

√5th C78.3 Secondary malignant neoplasm of other and unspecified respiratory organs

C78.30 Secondary malignant neoplasm of unspecified respiratory organ   HCC

C78.39 Secondary malignant neoplasm of other respiratory organs   HCC

C78.4 Secondary malignant neoplasm of small intestine   HCC

C78.5 Secondary malignant neoplasm of large intestine and rectum   HCC

C78.6 Secondary malignant neoplasm of retroperitoneum and peritoneum   HCC
> **AHA:** 2017,2Q,12

C78.7 Secondary malignant neoplasm of liver and intrahepatic bile duct   HCC

√5th C78.8 Secondary malignant neoplasm of other and unspecified digestive organs

C78.80 Secondary malignant neoplasm of unspecified digestive organ   HCC

C78.89 Secondary malignant neoplasm of other digestive organs   HCC
> Code also exocrine pancreatic insufficiency (K86.81)

√4th C79 Secondary malignant neoplasm of other and unspecified sites

> EXCLUDES 1   secondary carcinoid tumors (C7B.-)
> secondary neuroendocrine tumors (C7B.-)

√5th C79.0 Secondary malignant neoplasm of kidney and renal pelvis

C79.00 Secondary malignant neoplasm of unspecified kidney and renal pelvis   HCC

C79.01 Secondary malignant neoplasm of right kidney and renal pelvis   HCC

C79.02 Secondary malignant neoplasm of left kidney and renal pelvis   HCC

√5th C79.1 Secondary malignant neoplasm of bladder and other and unspecified urinary organs

C79.10 Secondary malignant neoplasm of unspecified urinary organs   HCC

C79.11 Secondary malignant neoplasm of bladder   HCC
> EXCLUDES 2   lymph node metastases (C77.0)

C79.19 Secondary malignant neoplasm of other urinary organs   HCC

C79.2 Secondary malignant neoplasm of skin   HCC
> EXCLUDES 1   secondary Merkel cell carcinoma (C7B.1)

√5th C79.3 Secondary malignant neoplasm of brain and cerebral meninges

C79.31 Secondary malignant neoplasm of brain   HCC

C79.32 Secondary malignant neoplasm of cerebral meninges   HCC

√5th C79.4 Secondary malignant neoplasm of other and unspecified parts of nervous system

C79.40 Secondary malignant neoplasm of unspecified part of nervous system   HCC

C79.49 Secondary malignant neoplasm of other parts of nervous system   HCC

√5th C79.5 Secondary malignant neoplasm of bone and bone marrow
> EXCLUDES 1   secondary carcinoid tumors of bone (C7B.03)

C79.51 Secondary malignant neoplasm of bone   HCC
> **TIP:** Do not assign in addition to a code from subcategory C90.0 when multiple myeloma is described as metastatic to the bone; bone involvement is integral to multiple myeloma.

C79.52 Secondary malignant neoplasm of bone marrow   HCC

√5th C79.6 Secondary malignant neoplasm of ovary

C79.60 Secondary malignant neoplasm of unspecified ovary   HCC ♀

C79.61 Secondary malignant neoplasm of right ovary   HCC ♀

C79.62 Secondary malignant neoplasm of left ovary   HCC ♀

√5th C79.7 Secondary malignant neoplasm of adrenal gland

C79.70 Secondary malignant neoplasm of unspecified adrenal gland   HCC

C79.71 Secondary malignant neoplasm of right adrenal gland   HCC

C79.72 Secondary malignant neoplasm of left adrenal gland   HCC

√5th C79.8 Secondary malignant neoplasm of other specified sites

C79.81 Secondary malignant neoplasm of breast   HCC

C79.82 Secondary malignant neoplasm of genital organs   HCC

C79.89 Secondary malignant neoplasm of other specified sites   HCC
> **AHA:** 2017,2Q,11

C79.9 Secondary malignant neoplasm of unspecified site   HCC
> Metastatic cancer NOS
> Metastatic disease NOS
> EXCLUDES 1   carcinomatosis NOS (C80.0)
> generalized cancer NOS (C80.0)
> malignant (primary) neoplasm of unspecified site (C80.1)

√4th C80 Malignant neoplasm without specification of site

> EXCLUDES 1   malignant carcinoid tumor of unspecified site (C7A.00)
> malignant neoplasm of specified multiple sites — code to each site

C80.0 Disseminated malignant neoplasm, unspecified   HCC
> Carcinomatosis NOS
> Generalized cancer, unspecified site (primary) (secondary)
> Generalized malignancy, unspecified site (primary) (secondary)

C80.1 Malignant (primary) neoplasm, unspecified   HCC
> Cancer NOS
> Cancer unspecified site (primary)
> Carcinoma unspecified site (primary)
> Malignancy unspecified site (primary)
> EXCLUDES 1   secondary malignant neoplasm of unspecified site (C79.9)

C80.2 Malignant neoplasm associated with transplanted organ   HCC
> Code first complication of transplanted organ (T86.-)
> Use additional code to identify the specific malignancy

Malignant neoplasms of lymphoid, hematopoietic and related tissue (C81-C96)

> EXCLUDES 2   *Kaposi's sarcoma of lymph nodes (C46.3)*
> *secondary and unspecified neoplasm of lymph nodes (C77.-)*
> *secondary neoplasm of bone marrow (C79.52)*
> *secondary neoplasm of spleen (C78.89)*

✓4ᵗʰ C81 Hodgkin lymphoma

> EXCLUDES 1   *personal history of Hodgkin lymphoma (Z85.71)*

DEF: Malignant disorder of lymphoid cells characterized by the presence of progressively swollen lymph nodes and spleen that may also involve the liver. A diagnosis of Hodgkin's lymphoma can be confirmed by the presence of Reed-Sternberg cells. *Synonym(s): Hodgkin disease.*

✓5ᵗʰ C81.0 Nodular lymphocyte predominant Hodgkin lymphoma

- **C81.00** Nodular lymphocyte predominant Hodgkin lymphoma, unspecified site — HCC
- **C81.01** Nodular lymphocyte predominant Hodgkin lymphoma, lymph nodes of head, face, and neck — HCC
- **C81.02** Nodular lymphocyte predominant Hodgkin lymphoma, intrathoracic lymph nodes — HCC
- **C81.03** Nodular lymphocyte predominant Hodgkin lymphoma, intra-abdominal lymph nodes — HCC
- **C81.04** Nodular lymphocyte predominant Hodgkin lymphoma, lymph nodes of axilla and upper limb — HCC
- **C81.05** Nodular lymphocyte predominant Hodgkin lymphoma, lymph nodes of inguinal region and lower limb — HCC
- **C81.06** Nodular lymphocyte predominant Hodgkin lymphoma, intrapelvic lymph nodes — HCC
- **C81.07** Nodular lymphocyte predominant Hodgkin lymphoma, spleen — HCC
- **C81.08** Nodular lymphocyte predominant Hodgkin lymphoma, lymph nodes of multiple sites — HCC
- **C81.09** Nodular lymphocyte predominant Hodgkin lymphoma, extranodal and solid organ sites — HCC

✓5ᵗʰ C81.1 Nodular sclerosis Hodgkin lymphoma

Nodular sclerosis classical Hodgkin lymphoma

- **C81.10** Nodular sclerosis Hodgkin lymphoma, unspecified site — HCC
- **C81.11** Nodular sclerosis Hodgkin lymphoma, lymph nodes of head, face, and neck — HCC
- **C81.12** Nodular sclerosis Hodgkin lymphoma, intrathoracic lymph nodes — HCC
- **C81.13** Nodular sclerosis Hodgkin lymphoma, intra-abdominal lymph nodes — HCC
- **C81.14** Nodular sclerosis Hodgkin lymphoma, lymph nodes of axilla and upper limb — HCC
- **C81.15** Nodular sclerosis Hodgkin lymphoma, lymph nodes of inguinal region and lower limb — HCC
- **C81.16** Nodular sclerosis Hodgkin lymphoma, intrapelvic lymph nodes — HCC
- **C81.17** Nodular sclerosis Hodgkin lymphoma, spleen — HCC
- **C81.18** Nodular sclerosis Hodgkin lymphoma, lymph nodes of multiple sites — HCC
- **C81.19** Nodular sclerosis Hodgkin lymphoma, extranodal and solid organ sites — HCC

✓5ᵗʰ C81.2 Mixed cellularity Hodgkin lymphoma

Mixed cellularity classical Hodgkin lymphoma

- **C81.20** Mixed cellularity Hodgkin lymphoma, unspecified site — HCC
- **C81.21** Mixed cellularity Hodgkin lymphoma, lymph nodes of head, face, and neck — HCC
- **C81.22** Mixed cellularity Hodgkin lymphoma, intrathoracic lymph nodes — HCC
- **C81.23** Mixed cellularity Hodgkin lymphoma, intra-abdominal lymph nodes — HCC
- **C81.24** Mixed cellularity Hodgkin lymphoma, lymph nodes of axilla and upper limb — HCC
- **C81.25** Mixed cellularity Hodgkin lymphoma, lymph nodes of inguinal region and lower limb — HCC
- **C81.26** Mixed cellularity Hodgkin lymphoma, intrapelvic lymph nodes — HCC
- **C81.27** Mixed cellularity Hodgkin lymphoma, spleen — HCC
- **C81.28** Mixed cellularity Hodgkin lymphoma, lymph nodes of multiple sites — HCC
- **C81.29** Mixed cellularity Hodgkin lymphoma, extranodal and solid organ sites — HCC

✓5ᵗʰ C81.3 Lymphocyte depleted Hodgkin lymphoma

Lymphocyte depleted classical Hodgkin lymphoma

- **C81.30** Lymphocyte depleted Hodgkin lymphoma, unspecified site — HCC
- **C81.31** Lymphocyte depleted Hodgkin lymphoma, lymph nodes of head, face, and neck — HCC
- **C81.32** Lymphocyte depleted Hodgkin lymphoma, intrathoracic lymph nodes — HCC
- **C81.33** Lymphocyte depleted Hodgkin lymphoma, intra-abdominal lymph nodes — HCC
- **C81.34** Lymphocyte depleted Hodgkin lymphoma, lymph nodes of axilla and upper limb — HCC
- **C81.35** Lymphocyte depleted Hodgkin lymphoma, lymph nodes of inguinal region and lower limb — HCC
- **C81.36** Lymphocyte depleted Hodgkin lymphoma, intrapelvic lymph nodes — HCC
- **C81.37** Lymphocyte depleted Hodgkin lymphoma, spleen — HCC
- **C81.38** Lymphocyte depleted Hodgkin lymphoma, lymph nodes of multiple sites — HCC
- **C81.39** Lymphocyte depleted Hodgkin lymphoma, extranodal and solid organ sites — HCC

✓5ᵗʰ C81.4 Lymphocyte-rich Hodgkin lymphoma

Lymphocyte-rich classical Hodgkin lymphoma

> EXCLUDES 1   *nodular lymphocyte predominant Hodgkin lymphoma (C81.0-)*

- **C81.40** Lymphocyte-rich Hodgkin lymphoma, unspecified site — HCC
- **C81.41** Lymphocyte-rich Hodgkin lymphoma, lymph nodes of head, face, and neck — HCC
- **C81.42** Lymphocyte-rich Hodgkin lymphoma, intrathoracic lymph nodes — HCC
- **C81.43** Lymphocyte-rich Hodgkin lymphoma, intra-abdominal lymph nodes — HCC
- **C81.44** Lymphocyte-rich Hodgkin lymphoma, lymph nodes of axilla and upper limb — HCC
- **C81.45** Lymphocyte-rich Hodgkin lymphoma, lymph nodes of inguinal region and lower limb — HCC
- **C81.46** Lymphocyte-rich Hodgkin lymphoma, intrapelvic lymph nodes — HCC
- **C81.47** Lymphocyte-rich Hodgkin lymphoma, spleen — HCC
- **C81.48** Lymphocyte-rich Hodgkin lymphoma, lymph nodes of multiple sites — HCC
- **C81.49** Lymphocyte-rich Hodgkin lymphoma, extranodal and solid organ sites — HCC

✓5ᵗʰ C81.7 Other Hodgkin lymphoma

Classical Hodgkin lymphoma NOS
Other classical Hodgkin lymphoma

- **C81.70** Other Hodgkin lymphoma, unspecified site — HCC
- **C81.71** Other Hodgkin lymphoma, lymph nodes of head, face, and neck — HCC
- **C81.72** Other Hodgkin lymphoma, intrathoracic lymph nodes — HCC
- **C81.73** Other Hodgkin lymphoma, intra-abdominal lymph nodes — HCC
- **C81.74** Other Hodgkin lymphoma, lymph nodes of axilla and upper limb — HCC
- **C81.75** Other Hodgkin lymphoma, lymph nodes of inguinal region and lower limb — HCC
- **C81.76** Other Hodgkin lymphoma, intrapelvic lymph nodes — HCC
- **C81.77** Other Hodgkin lymphoma, spleen — HCC
- **C81.78** Other Hodgkin lymphoma, lymph nodes of multiple sites — HCC
- **C81.79** Other Hodgkin lymphoma, extranodal and solid organ sites — HCC

☑ Additional Character Required   ✓x7ᵗʰ Placeholder Alert   Manifestation   Unspecified Dx   ►◄ Revised Text   ● New Code   ▲ Revised Code Title

ICD-10-CM 2020   477

√5ᵗʰ **C81.9 Hodgkin lymphoma, unspecified**

    C81.90 Hodgkin lymphoma, unspecified, unspecified site `HCC`

    C81.91 Hodgkin lymphoma, unspecified, lymph nodes of head, face, and neck `HCC`

    C81.92 Hodgkin lymphoma, unspecified, intrathoracic lymph nodes `HCC`

    C81.93 Hodgkin lymphoma, unspecified, intra-abdominal lymph nodes `HCC`

    C81.94 Hodgkin lymphoma, unspecified, lymph nodes of axilla and upper limb `HCC`

    C81.95 Hodgkin lymphoma, unspecified, lymph nodes of inguinal region and lower limb `HCC`

    C81.96 Hodgkin lymphoma, unspecified, intrapelvic lymph nodes `HCC`

    C81.97 Hodgkin lymphoma, unspecified, spleen `HCC`

    C81.98 Hodgkin lymphoma, unspecified, lymph nodes of multiple sites `HCC`

    C81.99 Hodgkin lymphoma, unspecified, extranodal and solid organ sites `HCC`

√4ᵗʰ **C82 Follicular lymphoma**

    INCLUDES   follicular lymphoma with or without diffuse areas

    EXCLUDES 1   mature T/NK-cell lymphomas (C84.-)

         personal history of non-Hodgkin lymphoma (Z85.72)

    DEF: Most common subgroup of non-Hodgkin lymphomas (NHL), accounting for 20 to 30 percent of all NHLs. NHL is a B-cell lymphoma that is slow growing and characterized by the circular pattern of malignant cell growth with the cells clustered into identifiable nodules or follicles.

√5ᵗʰ **C82.0 Follicular lymphoma grade I**

    C82.00 Follicular lymphoma grade I, unspecified site `HCC`

    C82.01 Follicular lymphoma grade I, lymph nodes of head, face, and neck `HCC`

    C82.02 Follicular lymphoma grade I, intrathoracic lymph nodes `HCC`

    C82.03 Follicular lymphoma grade I, intra-abdominal lymph nodes `HCC`

    C82.04 Follicular lymphoma grade I, lymph nodes of axilla and upper limb `HCC`

    C82.05 Follicular lymphoma grade I, lymph nodes of inguinal region and lower limb `HCC`

    C82.06 Follicular lymphoma grade I, intrapelvic lymph nodes `HCC`

    C82.07 Follicular lymphoma grade I, spleen `HCC`

    C82.08 Follicular lymphoma grade I, lymph nodes of multiple sites `HCC`

    C82.09 Follicular lymphoma grade I, extranodal and solid organ sites `HCC`

√5ᵗʰ **C82.1 Follicular lymphoma grade II**

    C82.10 Follicular lymphoma grade II, unspecified site `HCC`

    C82.11 Follicular lymphoma grade II, lymph nodes of head, face, and neck `HCC`

    C82.12 Follicular lymphoma grade II, intrathoracic lymph nodes `HCC`

    C82.13 Follicular lymphoma grade II, intra-abdominal lymph nodes `HCC`

    C82.14 Follicular lymphoma grade II, lymph nodes of axilla and upper limb `HCC`

    C82.15 Follicular lymphoma grade II, lymph nodes of inguinal region and lower limb `HCC`

    C82.16 Follicular lymphoma grade II, intrapelvic lymph nodes `HCC`

    C82.17 Follicular lymphoma grade II, spleen `HCC`

    C82.18 Follicular lymphoma grade II, lymph nodes of multiple sites `HCC`

    C82.19 Follicular lymphoma grade II, extranodal and solid organ sites `HCC`

√5ᵗʰ **C82.2 Follicular lymphoma grade III, unspecified**

    C82.20 Follicular lymphoma grade III, unspecified, unspecified site `HCC`

    C82.21 Follicular lymphoma grade III, unspecified, lymph nodes of head, face, and neck `HCC`

    C82.22 Follicular lymphoma grade III, unspecified, intrathoracic lymph nodes `HCC`

    C82.23 Follicular lymphoma grade III, unspecified, intra-abdominal lymph nodes `HCC`

    C82.24 Follicular lymphoma grade III, unspecified, lymph nodes of axilla and upper limb `HCC`

    C82.25 Follicular lymphoma grade III, unspecified, lymph nodes of inguinal region and lower limb `HCC`

    C82.26 Follicular lymphoma grade III, unspecified, intrapelvic lymph nodes `HCC`

    C82.27 Follicular lymphoma grade III, unspecified, spleen `HCC`

    C82.28 Follicular lymphoma grade III, unspecified, lymph nodes of multiple sites `HCC`

    C82.29 Follicular lymphoma grade III, unspecified, extranodal and solid organ sites `HCC`

√5ᵗʰ **C82.3 Follicular lymphoma grade IIIa**

    C82.30 Follicular lymphoma grade IIIa, unspecified site `HCC`

    C82.31 Follicular lymphoma grade IIIa, lymph nodes of head, face, and neck `HCC`

    C82.32 Follicular lymphoma grade IIIa, intrathoracic lymph nodes `HCC`

    C82.33 Follicular lymphoma grade IIIa, intra-abdominal lymph nodes `HCC`

    C82.34 Follicular lymphoma grade IIIa, lymph nodes of axilla and upper limb `HCC`

    C82.35 Follicular lymphoma grade IIIa, lymph nodes of inguinal region and lower limb `HCC`

    C82.36 Follicular lymphoma grade IIIa, intrapelvic lymph nodes `HCC`

    C82.37 Follicular lymphoma grade IIIa, spleen `HCC`

    C82.38 Follicular lymphoma grade IIIa, lymph nodes of multiple sites `HCC`

    C82.39 Follicular lymphoma grade IIIa, extranodal and solid organ sites `HCC`

√5ᵗʰ **C82.4 Follicular lymphoma grade IIIb**

    C82.40 Follicular lymphoma grade IIIb, unspecified site `HCC`

    C82.41 Follicular lymphoma grade IIIb, lymph nodes of head, face, and neck `HCC`

    C82.42 Follicular lymphoma grade IIIb, intrathoracic lymph nodes `HCC`

    C82.43 Follicular lymphoma grade IIIb, intra-abdominal lymph nodes `HCC`

    C82.44 Follicular lymphoma grade IIIb, lymph nodes of axilla and upper limb `HCC`

    C82.45 Follicular lymphoma grade IIIb, lymph nodes of inguinal region and lower limb `HCC`

    C82.46 Follicular lymphoma grade IIIb, intrapelvic lymph nodes `HCC`

    C82.47 Follicular lymphoma grade IIIb, spleen `HCC`

    C82.48 Follicular lymphoma grade IIIb, lymph nodes of multiple sites `HCC`

    C82.49 Follicular lymphoma grade IIIb, extranodal and solid organ sites `HCC`

√5ᵗʰ **C82.5 Diffuse follicle center lymphoma**

    C82.50 Diffuse follicle center lymphoma, unspecified site `HCC`

    C82.51 Diffuse follicle center lymphoma, lymph nodes of head, face, and neck `HCC`

    C82.52 Diffuse follicle center lymphoma, intrathoracic lymph nodes `HCC`

    C82.53 Diffuse follicle center lymphoma, intra-abdominal lymph nodes `HCC`

    C82.54 Diffuse follicle center lymphoma, lymph nodes of axilla and upper limb `HCC`

    C82.55 Diffuse follicle center lymphoma, lymph nodes of inguinal region and lower limb `HCC`

    C82.56 Diffuse follicle center lymphoma, intrapelvic lymph nodes `HCC`

    C82.57 Diffuse follicle center lymphoma, spleen `HCC`

    C82.58 Diffuse follicle center lymphoma, lymph nodes of multiple sites `HCC`

    C82.59 Diffuse follicle center lymphoma, extranodal and solid organ sites `HCC`

√5ᵗʰ **C82.6 Cutaneous follicle center lymphoma**

    C82.60 Cutaneous follicle center lymphoma, unspecified site `HCC`

    C82.61 Cutaneous follicle center lymphoma, lymph nodes of head, face, and neck `HCC`

    C82.62   **Cutaneous follicle center lymphoma, intrathoracic lymph nodes**   HCC

    C82.63   **Cutaneous follicle center lymphoma, intra-abdominal lymph nodes**   HCC

    C82.64   **Cutaneous follicle center lymphoma, lymph nodes of axilla and upper limb**   HCC

    C82.65   **Cutaneous follicle center lymphoma, lymph nodes of inguinal region and lower limb**   HCC

    C82.66   **Cutaneous follicle center lymphoma, intrapelvic lymph nodes**   HCC

    C82.67   **Cutaneous follicle center lymphoma, spleen**   HCC

    C82.68   **Cutaneous follicle center lymphoma, lymph nodes of multiple sites**   HCC

    C82.69   **Cutaneous follicle center lymphoma, extranodal and solid organ sites**   HCC

√5th **C82.8**   **Other types of follicular lymphoma**

    C82.80   **Other types of follicular lymphoma, unspecified site**   HCC

    C82.81   **Other types of follicular lymphoma, lymph nodes of head, face, and neck**   HCC

    C82.82   **Other types of follicular lymphoma, intrathoracic lymph nodes**   HCC

    C82.83   **Other types of follicular lymphoma, intra-abdominal lymph nodes**   HCC

    C82.84   **Other types of follicular lymphoma, lymph nodes of axilla and upper limb**   HCC

    C82.85   **Other types of follicular lymphoma, lymph nodes of inguinal region and lower limb**   HCC

    C82.86   **Other types of follicular lymphoma, intrapelvic lymph nodes**   HCC

    C82.87   **Other types of follicular lymphoma, spleen**   HCC

    C82.88   **Other types of follicular lymphoma, lymph nodes of multiple sites**   HCC

    C82.89   **Other types of follicular lymphoma, extranodal and solid organ sites**   HCC

√5th **C82.9**   **Follicular lymphoma, unspecified**

    C82.90   **Follicular lymphoma, unspecified, unspecified site**   HCC

    C82.91   **Follicular lymphoma, unspecified, lymph nodes of head, face, and neck**   HCC

    C82.92   **Follicular lymphoma, unspecified, intrathoracic lymph nodes**   HCC

    C82.93   **Follicular lymphoma, unspecified, intra-abdominal lymph nodes**   HCC

    C82.94   **Follicular lymphoma, unspecified, lymph nodes of axilla and upper limb**   HCC

    C82.95   **Follicular lymphoma, unspecified, lymph nodes of inguinal region and lower limb**   HCC

    C82.96   **Follicular lymphoma, unspecified, intrapelvic lymph nodes**   HCC

    C82.97   **Follicular lymphoma, unspecified, spleen**   HCC

    C82.98   **Follicular lymphoma, unspecified, lymph nodes of multiple sites**   HCC

    C82.99   **Follicular lymphoma, unspecified, extranodal and solid organ sites**   HCC

√4th **C83**   **Non-follicular lymphoma**

    EXCLUDES 1   *personal history of non-Hodgkin lymphoma (Z85.72)*

√5th **C83.0**   **Small cell B-cell lymphoma**

    Lymphoplasmacytic lymphoma
    Nodal marginal zone lymphoma
    Non-leukemic variant of B-CLL
    Splenic marginal zone lymphoma

    EXCLUDES 1   *chronic lymphocytic leukemia (C91.1)*
               mature T/NK-cell lymphomas (C84.-)
               Waldenström macroglobulinemia (C88.0)

    DEF: Nonfollicular lymphoma that is rare, slow growing, and usually found in the older population.

    C83.00   **Small cell B-cell lymphoma, unspecified site**   HCC

    C83.01   **Small cell B-cell lymphoma, lymph nodes of head, face, and neck**   HCC

    C83.02   **Small cell B-cell lymphoma, intrathoracic lymph nodes**   HCC

    C83.03   **Small cell B-cell lymphoma, intra-abdominal lymph nodes**   HCC

    C83.04   **Small cell B-cell lymphoma, lymph nodes of axilla and upper limb**   HCC

    C83.05   **Small cell B-cell lymphoma, lymph nodes of inguinal region and lower limb**   HCC

    C83.06   **Small cell B-cell lymphoma, intrapelvic lymph nodes**   HCC

    C83.07   **Small cell B-cell lymphoma, spleen**   HCC

    C83.08   **Small cell B-cell lymphoma, lymph nodes of multiple sites**   HCC

    C83.09   **Small cell B-cell lymphoma, extranodal and solid organ sites**   HCC

√5th **C83.1**   **Mantle cell lymphoma**

    Centrocytic lymphoma
    Malignant lymphomatous polyposis
    DEF: Rare form of B-cell non-Hodgkin lymphoma named for the location of the tumor cell production, the mantle zone of the lymph nodes.

    C83.10   **Mantle cell lymphoma, unspecified site**   HCC

    C83.11   **Mantle cell lymphoma, lymph nodes of head, face, and neck**   HCC

    C83.12   **Mantle cell lymphoma, intrathoracic lymph nodes**   HCC

    C83.13   **Mantle cell lymphoma, intra-abdominal lymph nodes**   HCC

    C83.14   **Mantle cell lymphoma, lymph nodes of axilla and upper limb**   HCC

    C83.15   **Mantle cell lymphoma, lymph nodes of inguinal region and lower limb**   HCC

    C83.16   **Mantle cell lymphoma, intrapelvic lymph nodes**   HCC

    C83.17   **Mantle cell lymphoma, spleen**   HCC

    C83.18   **Mantle cell lymphoma, lymph nodes of multiple sites**   HCC

    C83.19   **Mantle cell lymphoma, extranodal and solid organ sites**   HCC

√5th **C83.3**   **Diffuse large B-cell lymphoma**

    Anaplastic diffuse large B-cell lymphoma
    CD30-positive diffuse large B-cell lymphoma
    Centroblastic diffuse large B-cell lymphoma
    Diffuse large B-cell lymphoma, subtype not specified
    Immunoblastic diffuse large B-cell lymphoma
    Plasmablastic diffuse large B-cell lymphoma
    T-cell rich diffuse large B-cell lymphoma

    EXCLUDES 1   *mediastinal (thymic) large B-cell lymphoma (C85.2-)*
               mature T/NK-cell lymphomas (C84.-)

    DEF: Nonfollicular lymphoma that is one of the more common types of lymphoma. This cancer is fast growing and affects any age but is found mostly in the older population.

    C83.30   **Diffuse large B-cell lymphoma, unspecified site**   HCC

    C83.31   **Diffuse large B-cell lymphoma, lymph nodes of head, face, and neck**   HCC

    C83.32   **Diffuse large B-cell lymphoma, intrathoracic lymph nodes**   HCC

    C83.33   **Diffuse large B-cell lymphoma, intra-abdominal lymph nodes**   HCC

    C83.34   **Diffuse large B-cell lymphoma, lymph nodes of axilla and upper limb**   HCC

    C83.35   **Diffuse large B-cell lymphoma, lymph nodes of inguinal region and lower limb**   HCC

    C83.36   **Diffuse large B-cell lymphoma, intrapelvic lymph nodes**   HCC

    C83.37   **Diffuse large B-cell lymphoma, spleen**   HCC

    C83.38   **Diffuse large B-cell lymphoma, lymph nodes of multiple sites**   HCC

    C83.39   **Diffuse large B-cell lymphoma, extranodal and solid organ sites**   HCC

√5th **C83.5**   **Lymphoblastic (diffuse) lymphoma**

    B-precursor lymphoma
    Lymphoblastic B-cell lymphoma
    Lymphoblastic lymphoma NOS
    Lymphoblastic T-cell lymphoma
    T-precursor lymphoma

    DEF: Type of non-Hodgkin lymphoma considered lymphoma or leukemia—the determination is made based on the amount of bone marrow involvement. The cells are small to medium immature T-cells that often originate in the thymus where many of the T-cells are made.

    C83.50   **Lymphoblastic (diffuse) lymphoma, unspecified site**   HCC

    C83.51   **Lymphoblastic (diffuse) lymphoma, lymph nodes of head, face, and neck**   HCC

✓ Additional Character Required   √x7th Placeholder Alert   Manifestation   Unspecified Dx   ►◄ Revised Text   ● New Code   ▲ Revised Code Title

ICD-10-CM 2020   479

C83.52 Lymphoblastic (diffuse) lymphoma, intrathoracic **lymph nodes** `HCC`

C83.53 Lymphoblastic (diffuse) lymphoma, intra-abdominal **lymph nodes** `HCC`

C83.54 Lymphoblastic (diffuse) lymphoma, lymph nodes of axilla and upper limb `HCC`

C83.55 Lymphoblastic (diffuse) lymphoma, lymph nodes of inguinal region and lower limb `HCC`

C83.56 Lymphoblastic (diffuse) lymphoma, intrapelvic **lymph nodes** `HCC`

C83.57 Lymphoblastic (diffuse) lymphoma, spleen `HCC`

C83.58 Lymphoblastic (diffuse) lymphoma, lymph nodes of multiple sites `HCC`

C83.59 Lymphoblastic (diffuse) lymphoma, extranodal and solid organ sites `HCC`

✓5ᵗʰ **C83.7** Burkitt **lymphoma**

Atypical Burkitt lymphoma

Burkitt-like lymphoma

EXCLUDES 1   *mature B-cell leukemia Burkitt type (C91.A-)*

DEF: Malignancy of the lymphatic system, most often seen as a large bone-deteriorating lesion within the jaw or as an abdominal mass. It is a form of non-Hodgkin's lymphoma and is recognized as the fastest growing human tumor.

C83.70 Burkitt lymphoma, unspecified site `HCC`

C83.71 Burkitt lymphoma, lymph nodes of head, face, and neck `HCC`

C83.72 Burkitt lymphoma, intrathoracic lymph nodes `HCC`

C83.73 Burkitt lymphoma, intra-abdominal lymph nodes `HCC`

C83.74 Burkitt lymphoma, lymph nodes of axilla and upper limb `HCC`

C83.75 Burkitt lymphoma, lymph nodes of inguinal region and lower limb `HCC`

C83.76 Burkitt lymphoma, intrapelvic lymph nodes `HCC`

C83.77 Burkitt lymphoma, spleen `HCC`

C83.78 Burkitt lymphoma, lymph nodes of multiple sites `HCC`

C83.79 Burkitt lymphoma, extranodal and solid organ sites `HCC`

✓5ᵗʰ **C83.8** Other non-follicular **lymphoma**

Intravascular large B-cell lymphoma

Lymphoid granulomatosis

Primary effusion B-cell lymphoma

EXCLUDES 1   *mediastinal (thymic) large B-cell lymphoma (C85.2-)*
          T-cell rich B-cell lymphoma (C83.3-)

C83.80 Other non-follicular lymphoma, unspecified site `HCC`

C83.81 Other non-follicular lymphoma, lymph nodes of head, face, and neck `HCC`

C83.82 Other non-follicular lymphoma, intrathoracic lymph nodes `HCC`

C83.83 Other non-follicular lymphoma, intra-abdominal lymph nodes `HCC`

C83.84 Other non-follicular lymphoma, lymph nodes of axilla and upper limb `HCC`

C83.85 Other non-follicular lymphoma, lymph nodes of inguinal region and lower limb `HCC`

C83.86 Other non-follicular lymphoma, intrapelvic lymph nodes `HCC`

C83.87 Other non-follicular lymphoma, spleen `HCC`

C83.88 Other non-follicular lymphoma, lymph nodes of multiple sites `HCC`

C83.89 Other non-follicular lymphoma, extranodal and solid organ sites `HCC`

✓5ᵗʰ **C83.9** Non-follicular (diffuse) **lymphoma, unspecified**

C83.90 Non-follicular (diffuse) lymphoma, unspecified unspecified site `HCC`

C83.91 Non-follicular (diffuse) lymphoma, unspecified, lymph nodes of head, face, and neck `HCC`

C83.92 Non-follicular (diffuse) lymphoma, unspecified, intrathoracic lymph nodes `HCC`

C83.93 Non-follicular (diffuse) lymphoma, unspecified, intra-abdominal lymph nodes `HCC`

C83.94 Non-follicular (diffuse) lymphoma, unspecified, lymph nodes of axilla and upper limb `HCC`

C83.95 Non-follicular (diffuse) lymphoma, unspecified, lymph nodes of inguinal region and lower limb `HCC`

C83.96 Non-follicular (diffuse) lymphoma, unspecified, intrapelvic lymph nodes `HCC`

C83.97 Non-follicular (diffuse) lymphoma, unspecified, spleen `HCC`

C83.98 Non-follicular (diffuse) lymphoma, unspecified, lymph nodes of multiple sites `HCC`

C83.99 Non-follicular (diffuse) lymphoma, unspecified, extranodal and solid organ sites `HCC`

✓4ᵗʰ **C84** Mature T/NK-cell lymphomas

EXCLUDES 1   *personal history of non-Hodgkin lymphoma (Z85.72)*

✓5ᵗʰ **C84.0** Mycosis fungoides

EXCLUDES 1   *peripheral T-cell lymphoma, not classified (C84.4-)*

DEF: Most common form of cutaneous T-cell lymphoma. A type of non-Hodgkin lymphoma in which white blood cells become cancerous and affect the skin and sometimes internal organs.

Synonym(s): *Alibert-Bazin syndrome.*

C84.00 Mycosis fungoides, unspecified site `HCC`

C84.01 Mycosis fungoides, lymph nodes of head, face, and neck `HCC`

C84.02 Mycosis fungoides, intrathoracic lymph nodes `HCC`

C84.03 Mycosis fungoides, intra-abdominal lymph nodes `HCC`

C84.04 Mycosis fungoides, lymph nodes of axilla and upper limb `HCC`

C84.05 Mycosis fungoides, lymph nodes of inguinal region and lower limb `HCC`

C84.06 Mycosis fungoides, intrapelvic lymph nodes `HCC`

C84.07 Mycosis fungoides, spleen `HCC`

C84.08 Mycosis fungoides, lymph nodes of multiple sites `HCC`

C84.09 Mycosis fungoides, extranodal and solid organ sites `HCC`

✓5ᵗʰ **C84.1** Sézary disease

DEF: Extension of mycosis fungoides that affects the blood and all of the skin, appearing as sunburn, rather than patches. It spreads to the lymph nodes and is often linked to a weakened immune system.

C84.10 Sézary disease, unspecified site `HCC`

C84.11 Sézary disease, lymph nodes of head, face, and neck `HCC`

C84.12 Sézary disease, intrathoracic lymph nodes `HCC`

C84.13 Sézary disease, intra-abdominal lymph nodes `HCC`

C84.14 Sézary disease, lymph nodes of axilla and upper limb `HCC`

C84.15 Sézary disease, lymph nodes of inguinal region and lower limb `HCC`

C84.16 Sézary disease, intrapelvic lymph nodes `HCC`

C84.17 Sézary disease, spleen `HCC`

C84.18 Sézary disease, lymph nodes of multiple sites `HCC`

C84.19 Sézary disease, extranodal and solid organ sites `HCC`

✓5ᵗʰ **C84.4** Peripheral T-cell lymphoma, not classified

Lennert's lymphoma

Lymphoepithelioid lymphoma

Mature T-cell lymphoma, not elsewhere classified

C84.40 Peripheral T-cell lymphoma, not classified, unspecified site `HCC`

C84.41 Peripheral T-cell lymphoma, not classified, lymph nodes of head, face, and neck `HCC`

C84.42 Peripheral T-cell lymphoma, not classified, intrathoracic lymph nodes `HCC`

C84.43 Peripheral T-cell lymphoma, not classified, intra-abdominal lymph nodes `HCC`

C84.44 Peripheral T-cell lymphoma, not classified, lymph nodes of axilla and upper limb `HCC`

C84.45 Peripheral T-cell lymphoma, not classified, lymph nodes of inguinal region and lower limb `HCC`

C84.46 Peripheral T-cell lymphoma, not classified, intrapelvic lymph nodes

C84.47 Peripheral T-cell lymphoma, not classified, spleen `HCC`

C84.48 Peripheral T-cell lymphoma, not classified, lymph nodes of multiple sites `HCC`

C84.49 Peripheral T-cell lymphoma, not classified, extranodal and solid organ sites `HCC`

√5th **C84.6** Anaplastic large cell lymphoma, ALK-positive

Anaplastic large cell lymphoma, CD30-positive

C84.60 Anaplastic large cell lymphoma, ALK-positive, unspecified site `HCC`

C84.61 Anaplastic large cell lymphoma, ALK-positive, lymph nodes of head, face, and neck `HCC`

C84.62 Anaplastic large cell lymphoma, ALK-positive, intrathoracic lymph nodes `HCC`

C84.63 Anaplastic large cell lymphoma, ALK-positive, intra-abdominal lymph nodes `HCC`

C84.64 Anaplastic large cell lymphoma, ALK-positive, lymph nodes of axilla and upper limb `HCC`

C84.65 Anaplastic large cell lymphoma, ALK-positive, lymph nodes of inguinal region and lower limb `HCC`

C84.66 Anaplastic large cell lymphoma, ALK-positive, intrapelvic lymph nodes `HCC`

C84.67 Anaplastic large cell lymphoma, ALK-positive, spleen `HCC`

C84.68 Anaplastic large cell lymphoma, ALK-positive, lymph nodes of multiple sites `HCC`

C84.69 Anaplastic large cell lymphoma, ALK-positive, extranodal and solid organ sites `HCC`

√5th **C84.7** Anaplastic large cell lymphoma, ALK-negative

EXCLUDES 1   *primary cutaneous CD30-positive T-cell proliferations (C86.6-)*

C84.70 Anaplastic large cell lymphoma, ALK-negative, unspecified site `HCC`

C84.71 Anaplastic large cell lymphoma, ALK-negative, lymph nodes of head, face, and neck `HCC`

C84.72 Anaplastic large cell lymphoma, ALK-negative, intrathoracic lymph nodes `HCC`

C84.73 Anaplastic large cell lymphoma, ALK-negative, intra-abdominal lymph nodes `HCC`

C84.74 Anaplastic large cell lymphoma, ALK-negative, lymph nodes of axilla and upper limb `HCC`

C84.75 Anaplastic large cell lymphoma, ALK-negative, lymph nodes of inguinal region and lower limb `HCC`

C84.76 Anaplastic large cell lymphoma, ALK-negative, intrapelvic lymph nodes `HCC`

C84.77 Anaplastic large cell lymphoma, ALK-negative, spleen `HCC`

C84.78 Anaplastic large cell lymphoma, ALK-negative, lymph nodes of multiple sites `HCC`

C84.79 Anaplastic large cell lymphoma, ALK-negative, extranodal and solid organ sites `HCC`

√5th **C84.A** Cutaneous T-cell lymphoma, unspecified

C84.A0 Cutaneous T-cell lymphoma, unspecified, unspecified site `HCC`

C84.A1 Cutaneous T-cell lymphoma, unspecified lymph nodes of head, face, and neck `HCC`

C84.A2 Cutaneous T-cell lymphoma, unspecified, intrathoracic lymph nodes `HCC`

C84.A3 Cutaneous T-cell lymphoma, unspecified, intra-abdominal lymph nodes `HCC`

C84.A4 Cutaneous T-cell lymphoma, unspecified, lymph nodes of axilla and upper limb `HCC`

C84.A5 Cutaneous T-cell lymphoma, unspecified, lymph nodes of inguinal region and lower limb `HCC`

C84.A6 Cutaneous T-cell lymphoma, unspecified, intrapelvic lymph nodes `HCC`

C84.A7 Cutaneous T-cell lymphoma, unspecified, spleen `HCC`

C84.A8 Cutaneous T-cell lymphoma, unspecified, lymph nodes of multiple sites `HCC`

C84.A9 Cutaneous T-cell lymphoma, unspecified, extranodal and solid organ sites `HCC`

√5th **C84.Z** Other mature T/NK-cell lymphomas

NOTE   If T-cell lineage or involvement is mentioned in conjunction with a specific lymphoma, code to the more specific description.

EXCLUDES 1   *angioimmunoblastic T-cell lymphoma (C86.5)*
blastic NK-cell lymphoma (C86.4)
enteropathy-type T-cell lymphoma (C86.2)
extranodal NK-cell lymphoma, nasal type (C86.0)
hepatosplenic T-cell lymphoma (C86.1)
primary cutaneous CD30-positive T-cell proliferations (C86.6)
subcutaneous panniculitis-like T-cell lymphoma (C86.3)
T-cell leukemia (C91.1-)

C84.Z0 Other mature T/NK-cell lymphomas, unspecified site `HCC`

C84.Z1 Other mature T/NK-cell lymphomas, lymph nodes of head, face, and neck `HCC`

C84.Z2 Other mature T/NK-cell lymphomas, intrathoracic lymph nodes `HCC`

C84.Z3 Other mature T/NK-cell lymphomas, intra-abdominal lymph nodes `HCC`

C84.Z4 Other mature T/NK-cell lymphomas, lymph nodes of axilla and upper limb `HCC`

C84.Z5 Other mature T/NK-cell lymphomas, lymph nodes of inguinal region and lower limb `HCC`

C84.Z6 Other mature T/NK-cell lymphomas, intrapelvic lymph nodes `HCC`

C84.Z7 Other mature T/NK-cell lymphomas, spleen `HCC`

C84.Z8 Other mature T/NK-cell lymphomas, lymph nodes of multiple sites `HCC`

C84.Z9 Other mature T/NK-cell lymphomas, extranodal and solid organ sites `HCC`

√5th **C84.9** Mature T/NK-cell lymphomas, unspecified

NK/T cell lymphoma NOS

EXCLUDES 1   *mature T-cell lymphoma, not elsewhere classified (C84.4-)*

C84.90 Mature T/NK-cell lymphomas, unspecified, unspecified site `HCC`

C84.91 Mature T/NK-cell lymphomas, unspecified, lymph nodes of head, face, and neck `HCC`

C84.92 Mature T/NK-cell lymphomas, unspecified, intrathoracic lymph nodes `HCC`

C84.93 Mature T/NK-cell lymphomas, unspecified, intra-abdominal lymph nodes `HCC`

C84.94 Mature T/NK-cell lymphomas, unspecified, lymph nodes of axilla and upper limb `HCC`

C84.95 Mature T/NK-cell lymphomas, unspecified, lymph nodes of inguinal region and lower limb `HCC`

C84.96 Mature T/NK-cell lymphomas, unspecified, intrapelvic lymph nodes `HCC`

C84.97 Mature T/NK-cell lymphomas, unspecified, spleen `HCC`

C84.98 Mature T/NK-cell lymphomas, unspecified, lymph nodes of multiple sites `HCC`

C84.99 Mature T/NK-cell lymphomas, unspecified, extranodal and solid organ sites `HCC`

√4th **C85** Other specified and unspecified types of non-Hodgkin lymphoma

EXCLUDES 1   *other specified types of T/NK-cell lymphoma (C86.-)*
personal history of non-Hodgkin lymphoma (Z85.72)

√5th **C85.1** Unspecified B-cell lymphoma

NOTE   If B-cell lineage or involvement is mentioned in conjunction with a specific lymphoma, code to the more specific description.

C85.10 Unspecified B-cell lymphoma, unspecified site `HCC`

C85.11 Unspecified B-cell lymphoma, lymph nodes of head, face, and neck `HCC`

C85.12 Unspecified B-cell lymphoma, intrathoracic lymph nodes `HCC`

| ☑ Additional Character Required | √x7th Placeholder Alert | Manifestation | Unspecified Dx | ►◄ Revised Text | ● New Code | ▲ Revised Code Title |

ICD-10-CM 2020   481

C85.13 Unspecified B-cell lymphoma, intra-abdominal lymph nodes `HCC`

C85.14 Unspecified B-cell lymphoma, lymph nodes of axilla and upper limb `HCC`

C85.15 Unspecified B-cell lymphoma, lymph nodes of inguinal region and lower limb `HCC`

C85.16 Unspecified B-cell lymphoma, intrapelvic lymph nodes `HCC`

C85.17 Unspecified B-cell lymphoma, spleen `HCC`

C85.18 Unspecified B-cell lymphoma, lymph nodes of multiple sites `HCC`

C85.19 Unspecified B-cell lymphoma, extranodal and solid organ sites `HCC`

✓5ᵗʰ **C85.2** Mediastinal (thymic) large B-cell lymphoma

C85.20 Mediastinal (thymic) large B-cell lymphoma, unspecified site `HCC`

C85.21 Mediastinal (thymic) large B-cell lymphoma, lymph nodes of head, face, and neck `HCC`

C85.22 Mediastinal (thymic) large B-cell lymphoma, intrathoracic lymph nodes `HCC`

C85.23 Mediastinal (thymic) large B-cell lymphoma, intra-abdominal lymph nodes `HCC`

C85.24 Mediastinal (thymic) large B-cell lymphoma, lymph nodes of axilla and upper limb `HCC`

C85.25 Mediastinal (thymic) large B-cell lymphoma, lymph nodes of inguinal region and lower limb `HCC`

C85.26 Mediastinal (thymic) large B-cell lymphoma, intrapelvic lymph nodes `HCC`

C85.27 Mediastinal (thymic) large B-cell lymphoma, spleen `HCC`

C85.28 Mediastinal (thymic) large B-cell lymphoma, lymph nodes of multiple sites `HCC`

C85.29 Mediastinal (thymic) large B-cell lymphoma, extranodal and solid organ sites `HCC`

✓5ᵗʰ **C85.8** Other specified types of non-Hodgkin lymphoma

C85.80 Other specified types of non-Hodgkin lymphoma, unspecified site `HCC`

C85.81 Other specified types of non-Hodgkin lymphoma, lymph nodes of head, face, and neck `HCC`

C85.82 Other specified types of non-Hodgkin lymphoma, intrathoracic lymph nodes `HCC`

C85.83 Other specified types of non-Hodgkin lymphoma, intra-abdominal lymph nodes `HCC`

C85.84 Other specified types of non-Hodgkin lymphoma, lymph nodes of axilla and upper limb `HCC`

C85.85 Other specified types of non-Hodgkin lymphoma, lymph nodes of inguinal region and lower limb `HCC`

C85.86 Other specified types of non-Hodgkin lymphoma, intrapelvic lymph nodes `HCC`

C85.87 Other specified types of non-Hodgkin lymphoma, spleen `HCC`

C85.88 Other specified types of non-Hodgkin lymphoma, lymph nodes of multiple sites `HCC`

C85.89 Other specified types of non-Hodgkin lymphoma, extranodal and solid organ sites `HCC`

✓5ᵗʰ **C85.9** Non-Hodgkin lymphoma, unspecified

Lymphoma NOS
Malignant lymphoma NOS
Non-Hodgkin lymphoma NOS

C85.90 Non-Hodgkin lymphoma, unspecified, unspecified site `HCC`

C85.91 Non-Hodgkin lymphoma, unspecified, lymph nodes of head, face, and neck `HCC`

C85.92 Non-Hodgkin lymphoma, unspecified, intrathoracic lymph nodes `HCC`

C85.93 Non-Hodgkin lymphoma, unspecified, intra-abdominal lymph nodes `HCC`

C85.94 Non-Hodgkin lymphoma, unspecified, lymph nodes of axilla and upper limb `HCC`

C85.95 Non-Hodgkin lymphoma, unspecified, lymph nodes of inguinal region and lower limb `HCC`

C85.96 Non-Hodgkin lymphoma, unspecified, intrapelvic lymph nodes `HCC`

C85.97 Non-Hodgkin lymphoma, unspecified, spleen `HCC`

C85.98 Non-Hodgkin lymphoma, unspecified, lymph nodes of multiple sites `HCC`

C85.99 Non-Hodgkin lymphoma, unspecified, extranodal and solid organ sites `HCC`

✓4ᵗʰ **C86** Other specified types of T/NK-cell lymphoma

EXCLUDES 1   anaplastic large cell lymphoma, ALK negative (C84.7-)
anaplastic large cell lymphoma, ALK positive (C84.6-)
mature T/NK-cell lymphomas (C84.-)
other specified types of non-Hodgkin lymphoma (C85.8-)

C86.0 Extranodal NK/T-cell lymphoma, nasal type `HCC`

C86.1 Hepatosplenic T-cell lymphoma `HCC`

Alpha-beta and gamma delta types

C86.2 Enteropathy-type (intestinal) T-cell lymphoma `HCC`

Enteropathy associated T-cell lymphoma

C86.3 Subcutaneous panniculitis-like T-cell lymphoma `HCC`

C86.4 Blastic NK-cell lymphoma `HCC`

Blastic plasmacytoid dendritic cell neoplasm (BPDCN)

C86.5 Angioimmunoblastic T-cell lymphoma `HCC`

Angioimmunoblastic lymphadenopathy with dysproteinemia (AILD)

C86.6 Primary cutaneous CD30-positive T-cell proliferations `HCC`

Lymphomatoid papulosis
Primary cutaneous anaplastic large cell lymphoma
Primary cutaneous CD30-positive large T-cell lymphoma

✓4ᵗʰ **C88** Malignant immunoproliferative diseases and certain other B-cell lymphomas

EXCLUDES 1   B-cell lymphoma, unspecified (C85.1-)
personal history of other malignant neoplasms of lymphoid, hematopoietic and related tissues (Z85.79)

C88.0 Waldenström macroglobulinemia `HCC`

Lymphoplasmacytic lymphoma with IgM-production
Macroglobulinemia (idiopathic) (primary)
EXCLUDES 1   small cell B-cell lymphoma (C83.0)

C88.2 Heavy chain disease `HCC`

Franklin disease
Gamma heavy chain disease
Mu heavy chain disease

C88.3 Immunoproliferative small intestinal disease `HCC`

Alpha heavy chain disease
Mediterranean lymphoma

C88.4 Extranodal marginal zone B-cell lymphoma of mucosa-associated lymphoid tissue [MALT-lymphoma] `HCC`

Lymphoma of skin-associated lymphoid tissue [SALT-lymphoma]
Lymphoma of bronchial-associated lymphoid tissue [BALT-lymphoma]
EXCLUDES 1   high malignant (diffuse large B-cell) lymphoma (C83.3-)

C88.8 Other malignant immunoproliferative diseases `HCC`

C88.9 Malignant immunoproliferative disease, unspecified `HCC`

Immunoproliferative disease NOS

✓4ᵗʰ **C90** Multiple myeloma and malignant plasma cell neoplasms

EXCLUDES 1   personal history of other malignant neoplasms of lymphoid, hematopoietic and related tissues (Z85.79)

AHA: 2019, 2Q, 30

✓5ᵗʰ **C90.0** Multiple myeloma

Kahler's disease
Medullary plasmacytoma
Myelomatosis
Plasma cell myeloma
EXCLUDES 1   solitary myeloma (C90.3-)
solitary plasmactyoma (C90.3-)

TIP: Do not assign an additional code for bone metastasis (C79.51) when multiple myeloma is described as metastatic to the bone; bone involvement is integral to this disease process.

C90.00 Multiple myeloma not having achieved remission `HCC`

Multiple myeloma with failed remission
Multiple myeloma NOS

C90.01   **Multiple myeloma** in remission   `HCC`

C90.02   **Multiple myeloma** in relapse   `HCC`

√5ᵗʰ **C90.1**   **Plasma cell leukemia**

    Plasmacytic leukemia

    AHA: 2019,2Q,30

    C90.10   **Plasma cell leukemia** not having achieved   `HCC`
         remission

         Plasma cell leukemia with failed remission

         Plasma cell leukemia NOS

    C90.11   **Plasma cell leukemia** in remission   `HCC`

    C90.12   **Plasma cell leukemia** in relapse   `HCC`

√5ᵗʰ **C90.2**   **Extramedullary plasmacytoma**

    C90.20   **Extramedullary plasmacytoma** not having   `HCC`
         achieved remission

         Extramedullary plasmacytoma with failed remission

         Extramedullary plasmacytoma NOS

    C90.21   **Extramedullary plasmacytoma** in   `HCC`
         remission

    C90.22   **Extramedullary plasmacytoma** in relapse   `HCC`

√5ᵗʰ **C90.3**   **Solitary plasmacytoma**

    Localized malignant plasma cell tumor NOS

    Plasmacytoma NOS

    Solitary myeloma

    C90.30   **Solitary plasmacytoma** not having   `HCC`
         achieved remission

         Solitary plasmacytoma with failed remission

         Solitary plasmacytoma NOS

    C90.31   **Solitary plasmacytoma** in remission   `HCC`

    C90.32   **Solitary plasmacytoma** in relapse   `HCC`

√4ᵗʰ **C91**   **Lymphoid leukemia**

    `EXCLUDES 1`   personal history of leukemia (Z85.6)

    DEF: Malignant proliferation of immature lymphocytes (white blood cells that make up lymphoid tissue), called lymphoblasts, that originate in the bone marrow. Can be acute (ALL) or chronic (CLL).

√5ᵗʰ **C91.0**   **Acute lymphoblastic leukemia [ALL]**

    `NOTE`   ▶Codes in subcategory C91.0- should only be used for T-cell and B-cell precursor leukemia◀

    C91.00   **Acute lymphoblastic leukemia** not having   `HCC`
         achieved remission

         Acute lymphoblastic leukemia with failed remission

         Acute lymphoblastic leukemia NOS

    C91.01   **Acute lymphoblastic leukemia,** in   `HCC`
         remission

    C91.02   **Acute lymphoblastic leukemia,** in relapse   `HCC`

√5ᵗʰ **C91.1**   **Chronic lymphocytic leukemia of B-cell type**

    Lymphoplasmacytic leukemia

    Richter syndrome

    `EXCLUDES 1`   lymphoplasmacytic lymphoma (C83.0-)

    C91.10   **Chronic lymphocytic leukemia of B-cell**   `HCC`
         type not having achieved remission

         Chronic lymphocytic leukemia of B-cell type with failed remission

         Chronic lymphocytic leukemia of B-cell type NOS

    C91.11   **Chronic lymphocytic leukemia of B-cell**   `HCC`
         type in remission

    C91.12   **Chronic lymphocytic leukemia of B-cell**   `HCC`
         type in relapse

√5ᵗʰ **C91.3**   **Prolymphocytic leukemia of B-cell type**

    C91.30   **Prolymphocytic leukemia of B-cell type**   `HCC`
         not having achieved remission

         Prolymphocytic leukemia of B-cell type with failed remission

         Prolymphocytic leukemia of B-cell type NOS

    C91.31   **Prolymphocytic leukemia of B-cell type,**   `HCC`
         in remission

    C91.32   **Prolymphocytic leukemia of B-cell type,**   `HCC`
         in relapse

√5ᵗʰ **C91.4**   **Hairy cell leukemia**

    Leukemic reticuloendotheliosis

    DEF: Rare type of leukemia that is slow growing and often also considered a type of lymphoma. The small B-cell lymphocytes appear with "hairy" projections under a microscope and are found mostly in the bone marrow, spleen, and blood.

    C91.40   **Hairy cell leukemia** not having achieved   `HCC`
         remission

         Hairy cell leukemia with failed remission

         Hairy cell leukemia NOS

    C91.41   **Hairy cell leukemia,** in remission   `HCC`

    C91.42   **Hairy cell leukemia,** in relapse   `HCC`

√5ᵗʰ **C91.5**   **Adult T-cell lymphoma/leukemia (HTLV-1-associated)**

    Acute variant of adult T-cell lymphoma/leukemia (HTLV-1-associated)

    Chronic variant of adult T-cell lymphoma/leukemia (HTLV-1-associated)

    Lymphomatoid variant of adult T-cell lymphoma/leukemia (HTLV-1-associated)

    Smouldering variant of adult T-cell lymphoma/leukemia (HTLV-1-associated)

    C91.50   **Adult T-cell lymphoma/leukemia**   `HCC` `A`
         (HTLV-1-associated) not having achieved
         remission

         Adult T-cell lymphoma/leukemia (HTLV-1-associated) with failed remission

         Adult T-cell lymphoma/leukemia (HTLV-1-associated) NOS

    C91.51   **Adult T-cell lymphoma/leukemia**   `HCC` `A`
         (HTLV-1-associated), in remission

    C91.52   **Adult T-cell lymphoma/leukemia**   `HCC` `A`
         (HTLV-1-associated), in relapse

√5ᵗʰ **C91.6**   **Prolymphocytic leukemia of T-cell type**

    C91.60   **Prolymphocytic leukemia of T-cell type**   `HCC`
         not having achieved remission

         Prolymphocytic leukemia of T-cell type with failed remission

         Prolymphocytic leukemia of T-cell type NOS

    C91.61   **Prolymphocytic leukemia of T-cell type,**   `HCC`
         in remission

    C91.62   **Prolymphocytic leukemia of T-cell type,**   `HCC`
         in relapse

√5ᵗʰ **C91.A**   **Mature B-cell leukemia Burkitt-type**

    `EXCLUDES 1`   Burkitt lymphoma (C83.7-)

    C91.A0   **Mature B-cell leukemia Burkitt-type** not   `HCC`
         having achieved remission

         Mature B-cell leukemia Burkitt-type with failed remission

         Mature B-cell leukemia Burkitt-type NOS

    C91.A1   **Mature B-cell leukemia Burkitt-type,** in   `HCC`
         remission

    C91.A2   **Mature B-cell leukemia Burkitt-type,** in   `HCC`
         relapse

√5ᵗʰ **C91.Z**   **Other lymphoid leukemia**

    T-cell large granular lymphocytic leukemia (associated with rheumatoid arthritis)

    C91.Z0   **Other lymphoid leukemia** not having   `HCC`
         achieved remission

         Other lymphoid leukemia with failed remission

         Other lymphoid leukemia NOS

    C91.Z1   **Other lymphoid leukemia,** in remission   `HCC`

    C91.Z2   **Other lymphoid leukemia,** in relapse   `HCC`

√5ᵗʰ **C91.9**   **Lymphoid leukemia, unspecified**

    C91.90   **Lymphoid leukemia, unspecified** not   `HCC`
         having achieved remission

         Lymphoid leukemia with failed remission

         Lymphoid leukemia NOS

    C91.91   **Lymphoid leukemia, unspecified,** in   `HCC`
         remission

    C91.92   **Lymphoid leukemia, unspecified,** in   `HCC`
         relapse

☑ Additional Character Required   ✓ˣ7ᵗʰ Placeholder Alert   Manifestation   Unspecified Dx   ▶◀ Revised Text   ● New Code   ▲ Revised Code Title

Chapter 2. Neoplasms

C92–C93.02

✓4ᵗʰ **C92 Myeloid leukemia**

  INCLUDES   granulocytic leukemia

                myelogenous leukemia

  EXCLUDES 1   *personal history of leukemia (Z85.6)*

  AHA: 2019,1Q,16

  DEF: Cancer that develops in immature myelocytes called myeloblasts. These are the cells that become white blood cells (except lymphocytes), red blood cells, or platelet making cells. Can be acute (AML) or chronic (CML).

  TIP: Pancytopenia, although common in some types of myeloid leukemia's, is not always inherent. When it is documented, code D61.818 can be assigned in addition to a code from this category.

  ✓5ᵗʰ **C92.0 Acute myeloblastic leukemia**

         Acute myeloblastic leukemia, minimal differentiation

         Acute myeloblastic leukemia (with maturation)

         Acute myeloblastic leukemia 1/ETO

         Acute myeloblastic leukemia MØ

         Acute myeloblastic leukemia M1

         Acute myeloblastic leukemia M2

         Acute myeloblastic leukemia with t(8;21)

         Acute myeloblastic leukemia (without a FAB classification) NOS

         Refractory anemia with excess blasts in transformation [RAEBT]

      EXCLUDES 1   *acute exacerbation of chronic myeloid leukemia (C92.10)*

                    refractory anemia with excess of blasts not in transformation (D46.2-)

      AHA: 2018,4Q,87

    C92.00 Acute myeloblastic leukemia, not having achieved remission   HCC

         Acute myeloblastic leukemia with failed remission

         Acute myeloblastic leukemia NOS

    C92.01 Acute myeloblastic leukemia, in remission   HCC

    C92.02 Acute myeloblastic leukemia, in relapse   HCC

  ✓5ᵗʰ **C92.1 Chronic myeloid leukemia, BCR/ABL-positive**

         Chronic myelogenous leukemia, Philadelphia chromosome (Ph1) positive

         Chronic myelogenous leukemia, t(9;22) (q34;q11)

         Chronic myelogenous leukemia with crisis of blast cells

      EXCLUDES 1   *atypical chronic myeloid leukemia BCR/ABL-negative (C92.2-)*

                    chronic myelomonocytic leukemia (C93.1-)

                    chronic myeloproliferative disease (D47.1)

    C92.10 Chronic myeloid leukemia, BCR/ABL-positive, not having achieved remission   HCC

         Chronic myeloid leukemia, BCR/ABL-positive with failed remission

         Chronic myeloid leukemia, BCR/ABL-positive NOS

    C92.11 Chronic myeloid leukemia, BCR/ABL-positive, in remission   HCC

    C92.12 Chronic myeloid leukemia, BCR/ABL-positive, in relapse   HCC

  ✓5ᵗʰ **C92.2 Atypical chronic myeloid leukemia, BCR/ABL-negative**

    C92.20 Atypical chronic myeloid leukemia, BCR/ABL-negative, not having achieved remission   HCC

         Atypical chronic myeloid leukemia, BCR/ABL-negative with failed remission

         Atypical chronic myeloid leukemia, BCR/ABL-negative NOS

    C92.21 Atypical chronic myeloid leukemia, BCR/ABL-negative, in remission   HCC

    C92.22 Atypical chronic myeloid leukemia, BCR/ABL-negative, in relapse   HCC

  ✓5ᵗʰ **C92.3 Myeloid sarcoma**

         A malignant tumor of immature myeloid cells

         Chloroma

         Granulocytic sarcoma

    C92.30 Myeloid sarcoma, not having achieved remission   HCC

         Myeloid sarcoma with failed remission

         Myeloid sarcoma NOS

    C92.31 Myeloid sarcoma, in remission   HCC

    C92.32 Myeloid sarcoma, in relapse   HCC

  ✓5ᵗʰ **C92.4 Acute promyelocytic leukemia**

         AML M3

         AML Me with t(15;17) and variants

    C92.40 Acute promyelocytic leukemia, not having achieved remission   HCC

         Acute promyelocytic leukemia with failed remission

         Acute promyelocytic leukemia NOS

    C92.41 Acute promyelocytic leukemia, in remission   HCC

    C92.42 Acute promyelocytic leukemia, in relapse   HCC

  ✓5ᵗʰ **C92.5 Acute myelomonocytic leukemia**

         AML M4

         AML M4 Eo with inv(16) or t(16;16)

    C92.50 Acute myelomonocytic leukemia, not having achieved remission   HCC

         Acute myelomonocytic leukemia with failed remission

         Acute myelomonocytic leukemia NOS

    C92.51 Acute myelomonocytic leukemia, in remission   HCC

    C92.52 Acute myelomonocytic leukemia, in relapse   HCC

  ✓5ᵗʰ **C92.6 Acute myeloid leukemia with 11q23-abnormality**

         Acute myeloid leukemia with variation of MLL-gene

    C92.60 Acute myeloid leukemia with 11q23-abnormality not having achieved remission   HCC

         Acute myeloid leukemia with 11q23-abnormality with failed remission

         Acute myeloid leukemia with 11q23-abnormality NOS

    C92.61 Acute myeloid leukemia with 11q23-abnormality in remission   HCC

    C92.62 Acute myeloid leukemia with 11q23-abnormality in relapse   HCC

  ✓5ᵗʰ **C92.A Acute myeloid leukemia with multilineage dysplasia**

         Acute myeloid leukemia with dysplasia of remaining hematopoesis and/or myelodysplastic disease in its history

    C92.AØ Acute myeloid leukemia with multilineage dysplasia, not having achieved remission   HCC

         Acute myeloid leukemia with multilineage dysplasia with failed remission

         Acute myeloid leukemia with multilineage dysplasia NOS

    C92.A1 Acute myeloid leukemia with multilineage dysplasia, in remission   HCC

    C92.A2 Acute myeloid leukemia with multilineage dysplasia, in relapse   HCC

  ✓5ᵗʰ **C92.Z Other myeloid leukemia**

    C92.ZØ Other myeloid leukemia not having achieved remission   HCC

         Myeloid leukemia NEC with failed remission

         Myeloid leukemia NEC

    C92.Z1 Other myeloid leukemia, in remission   HCC

    C92.Z2 Other myeloid leukemia, in relapse   HCC

  ✓5ᵗʰ **C92.9 Myeloid leukemia, unspecified**

    C92.90 Myeloid leukemia, unspecified, not having achieved remission   HCC

         Myeloid leukemia, unspecified with failed remission

         Myeloid leukemia, unspecified NOS

    C92.91 Myeloid leukemia, unspecified in remission   HCC

    C92.92 Myeloid leukemia, unspecified in relapse   HCC

✓4ᵗʰ **C93 Monocytic leukemia**

  INCLUDES   monocytoid leukemia

  EXCLUDES 1   *personal history of leukemia (Z85.6)*

  ✓5ᵗʰ **C93.0 Acute monoblastic/monocytic leukemia**

         AML M5

         AML M5a

         AML M5b

    C93.00 Acute monoblastic/monocytic leukemia, not having achieved remission   HCC

         Acute monoblastic/monocytic leukemia with failed remission

         Acute monoblastic/monocytic leukemia NOS

    C93.01 Acute monoblastic/monocytic leukemia, in remission   HCC

    C93.02 Acute monoblastic/monocytic leukemia, in relapse   HCC

√5th **C93.1** **Chronic myelomonocytic leukemia**
Chronic monocytic leukemia
CMML-1
CMML-2
CMML with eosinophilia

  C93.10 **Chronic myelomonocytic leukemia** not having achieved remission   HCC
Chronic myelomonocytic leukemia with failed remission
Chronic myelomonocytic leukemia NOS

  C93.11 **Chronic myelomonocytic leukemia, in remission**   HCC

  C93.12 **Chronic myelomonocytic leukemia, in relapse**   HCC

√5th **C93.3** **Juvenile myelomonocytic leukemia**

  C93.30 **Juvenile myelomonocytic leukemia, not having achieved remission**   HCC P
Juvenile myelomonocytic leukemia with failed remission
Juvenile myelomonocytic leukemia NOS

  C93.31 **Juvenile myelomonocytic leukemia, in remission**   HCC P

  C93.32 **Juvenile myelomonocytic leukemia, in relapse**   HCC P

√5th **C93.Z** **Other monocytic leukemia**

  C93.Z0 **Other monocytic leukemia, not having achieved remission**   HCC
Other monocytic leukemia NOS

  C93.Z1 **Other monocytic leukemia, in remission**   HCC

  C93.Z2 **Other monocytic leukemia, in relapse**   HCC

√5th **C93.9** **Monocytic leukemia, unspecified**

  C93.90 **Monocytic leukemia, unspecified, not having achieved remission**   HCC
Monocytic leukemia, unspecified with failed remission
Monocytic leukemia, unspecified NOS

  C93.91 **Monocytic leukemia, unspecified in remission**   HCC

  C93.92 **Monocytic leukemia, unspecified in relapse**   HCC

√4th **C94** **Other leukemias of specified cell type**

  EXCLUDES 1   *leukemic reticuloendotheliosis (C91.4-)*
              myelodysplastic syndromes (D46.-)
              personal history of leukemia (Z85.6)
              plasma cell leukemia (C90.1-)

√5th **C94.0** **Acute erythroid leukemia**
Acute myeloid leukemia M6(a)(b)
Erythroleukemia
DEF: Erythroleukemia: Malignant blood dyscrasia (a myeloproliferative disorder).

  C94.00 **Acute erythroid leukemia, not having achieved remission**   HCC
Acute erythroid leukemia with failed remission
Acute erythroid leukemia NOS

  C94.01 **Acute erythroid leukemia, in remission**   HCC

  C94.02 **Acute erythroid leukemia, in relapse**   HCC

√5th **C94.2** **Acute megakaryoblastic leukemia**
Acute myeloid leukemia M7
Acute megakaryocytic leukemia

  C94.20 **Acute megakaryoblastic leukemia not having achieved remission**   HCC
Acute megakaryoblastic leukemia with failed remission
Acute megakaryoblastic leukemia NOS

  C94.21 **Acute megakaryoblastic leukemia, in remission**   HCC

  C94.22 **Acute megakaryoblastic leukemia, in relapse**   HCC

√5th **C94.3** **Mast cell leukemia**
AHA: 2017,4Q,5

  C94.30 **Mast cell leukemia not having achieved remission**   HCC
Mast cell leukemia with failed remission
Mast cell leukemia NOS

  C94.31 **Mast cell leukemia, in remission**   HCC

  C94.32 **Mast cell leukemia, in relapse**   HCC

√5th **C94.4** **Acute panmyelosis with myelofibrosis**
Acute myelofibrosis
  EXCLUDES 1   *myelofibrosis NOS (D75.81)*
              secondary myelofibrosis NOS (D75.81)

  C94.40 **Acute panmyelosis with myelofibrosis not having achieved remission**   HCC
Acute myelofibrosis NOS
Acute panmyelosis with myelofibrosis with failed remission
Acute panmyelosis NOS

  C94.41 **Acute panmyelosis with myelofibrosis, in remission**   HCC

  C94.42 **Acute panmyelosis with myelofibrosis, in relapse**   HCC

C94.6 **Myelodysplastic disease, not classified**   HCC
Myeloproliferative disease, not classified

√5th **C94.8** **Other specified leukemias**
Aggressive NK-cell leukemia
Acute basophilic leukemia

  C94.80 **Other specified leukemias not having achieved remission**   HCC
Other specified leukemia with failed remission
Other specified leukemias NOS

  C94.81 **Other specified leukemias, in remission**   HCC

  C94.82 **Other specified leukemias, in relapse**   HCC

√4th **C95** **Leukemia of unspecified cell type**
  EXCLUDES 1   *personal history of leukemia (Z85.6)*

√5th **C95.0** **Acute leukemia of unspecified cell type**
Acute bilineal leukemia
Acute mixed lineage leukemia
Biphenotypic acute leukemia
Stem cell leukemia of unclear lineage
  EXCLUDES 1   *acute exacerbation of unspecified chronic leukemia (C95.10)*

  C95.00 **Acute leukemia of unspecified cell type not having achieved remission**   HCC
Acute leukemia of unspecified cell type with failed remission
Acute leukemia NOS

  C95.01 **Acute leukemia of unspecified cell type, in remission**   HCC

  C95.02 **Acute leukemia of unspecified cell type, in relapse**   HCC

√5th **C95.1** **Chronic leukemia of unspecified cell type**

  C95.10 **Chronic leukemia of unspecified cell type not having achieved remission**   HCC
Chronic leukemia of unspecified cell type with failed remission
Chronic leukemia NOS

  C95.11 **Chronic leukemia of unspecified cell type, in remission**   HCC

  C95.12 **Chronic leukemia of unspecified cell type, in relapse**   HCC

√5th **C95.9** **Leukemia, unspecified**

  C95.90 **Leukemia, unspecified not having achieved remission**   HCC
Leukemia, unspecified with failed remission
Leukemia NOS

  C95.91 **Leukemia, unspecified, in remission**   HCC

  C95.92 **Leukemia, unspecified, in relapse**   HCC

√4th **C96** **Other and unspecified malignant neoplasms of lymphoid, hematopoietic and related tissue**
  EXCLUDES 1   *personal history of other malignant neoplasms of lymphoid, hematopoietic and related tissues (Z85.79)*

C96.0 **Multifocal and multisystemic (disseminated) Langerhans-cell histiocytosis**   HCC
Histiocytosis X, multisystemic
Letterer-Siwe disease
  EXCLUDES 1   *adult pulmonary Langerhans cell histiocytosis (J84.82)*
              multifocal and unisystemic Langerhans-cell histiocytosis (C96.5)
              unifocal Langerhans-cell histiocytosis (C96.6)

✔ Additional Character Required   √x7th Placeholder Alert   Manifestation   Unspecified Dx   ►◄ Revised Text   ● New Code   ▲ Revised Code Title

C96.2 Malignant mast cell neoplasm

> EXCLUDES 1   indolent mastocytosis (D47.02)
> mast cell leukemia (C94.30)
> mastocytosis (congenital) (cutaneous) (Q82.2)

AHA: 2017,4Q,5

DEF: Mast cell: Type of white blood cell found in the loose connective tissue of blood vessels and bronchioles responsible for acute hypersensitivity reactions, including anaphylactic shock. The IgE receptors on these cells bind with allergens causing cell degranulation and diffuse, widespread histamine release that results in airway constriction and vasodilation with decreased systemic blood pressure.

   C96.20 Malignant mast cell neoplasm, unspecified HCC

   C96.21 Aggressive systemic mastocytosis HCC

   C96.22 Mast cell sarcoma HCC

   C96.29 Other malignant mast cell neoplasm HCC

C96.4 Sarcoma of dendritic cells (accessory cells) HCC

Follicular dendritic cell sarcoma
Interdigitating dendritic cell sarcoma
Langerhans cell sarcoma

C96.5 Multifocal and unisystemic Langerhans-cell histiocytosis HCC

Hand-Schüller-Christian disease
Histiocytosis X, multifocal

> EXCLUDES 1   multifocal and multisystemic (disseminated) Langerhans-cell histiocytosis (C96.0)
> unifocal Langerhans-cell histiocytosis (C96.6)

C96.6 Unifocal Langerhans-cell histiocytosis HCC

Eosinophilic granuloma
Histiocytosis X, unifocal
Histiocytosis X NOS
Langerhans-cell histiocytosis NOS

> EXCLUDES 1   multifocal and multisysemic (disseminated) Langerhans-cell histiocytosis (C96.0)
> multifocal and unisystemic Langerhans-cell histiocytosis (C96.5)

C96.A Histiocytic sarcoma HCC

Malignant histiocytosis

C96.Z Other specified malignant neoplasms of lymphoid, hematopoietic and related tissue HCC

C96.9 Malignant neoplasm of lymphoid, hematopoietic and related tissue, unspecified HCC

In situ neoplasms (D00-D09)

INCLUDES   Bowen's disease
erythroplasia
grade III intraepithelial neoplasia
Queyrat's erythroplasia

D00 Carcinoma in situ of oral cavity, esophagus and stomach

> EXCLUDES 1   melanoma in situ (D03.-)

D00.0 Carcinoma in situ of lip, oral cavity and pharynx

Use additional code to identify:
exposure to environmental tobacco smoke (Z77.22)
exposure to tobacco smoke in the perinatal period (P96.81)
history of tobacco dependence (Z87.891)
occupational exposure to environmental tobacco smoke (Z57.31)
tobacco dependence (F17.-)
tobacco use (Z72.0)

> EXCLUDES 1   carcinoma in situ of aryepiglottic fold or interarytenoid fold, laryngeal aspect (D02.0)
> carcinoma in situ of epiglottis NOS (D02.0)
> carcinoma in situ of epiglottis suprahyoid portion (D02.0)
> carcinoma in situ of skin of lip (D03.0, D04.0)

   D00.00 Carcinoma in situ of oral cavity, unspecified site

   D00.01 Carcinoma in situ of labial mucosa and vermilion border

   D00.02 Carcinoma in situ of buccal mucosa

   D00.03 Carcinoma in situ of gingiva and edentulous alveolar ridge

   D00.04 Carcinoma in situ of soft palate

   D00.05 Carcinoma in situ of hard palate

   D00.06 Carcinoma in situ of floor of mouth

   D00.07 Carcinoma in situ of tongue

   D00.08 Carcinoma in situ of pharynx

Carcinoma in situ of aryepiglottic fold NOS
Carcinoma in situ of hypopharyngeal aspect of aryepiglottic fold
Carcinoma in situ of marginal zone of aryepiglottic fold

D00.1 Carcinoma in situ of esophagus

D00.2 Carcinoma in situ of stomach

D01 Carcinoma in situ of other and unspecified digestive organs

> EXCLUDES 1   melanoma in situ (D03.-)

D01.0 Carcinoma in situ of colon

> EXCLUDES 1   carcinoma in situ of rectosigmoid junction (D01.1)

D01.1 Carcinoma in situ of rectosigmoid junction

D01.2 Carcinoma in situ of rectum

D01.3 Carcinoma in situ of anus and anal canal

Anal intraepithelial neoplasia III [AIN III]
Severe dysplasia of anus

> EXCLUDES 1   anal intraepithelial neoplasia I and II [AIN I and AIN II] (K62.82)
> carcinoma in situ of anal margin (D04.5)
> carcinoma in situ of anal skin (D04.5)
> carcinoma in situ of perianal skin (D04.5)

D01.4 Carcinoma in situ of other and unspecified parts of intestine

> EXCLUDES 1   carcinoma in situ of ampulla of Vater (D01.5)

   D01.40 Carcinoma in situ of unspecified part of intestine

   D01.49 Carcinoma in situ of other parts of intestine

D01.5 Carcinoma in situ of liver, gallbladder and bile ducts

Carcinoma in situ of ampulla of Vater

D01.7 Carcinoma in situ of other specified digestive organs

Carcinoma in situ of pancreas

D01.9 Carcinoma in situ of digestive organ, unspecified

D02 Carcinoma in situ of middle ear and respiratory system

Use additional code to identify:
exposure to environmental tobacco smoke (Z77.22)
exposure to tobacco smoke in the perinatal period (P96.81)
history of tobacco dependence (Z87.891)
occupational exposure to environmental tobacco smoke (Z57.31)
tobacco dependence (F17.-)
tobacco use (Z72.0)

> EXCLUDES 1   melanoma in situ (D03.-)

D02.0 Carcinoma in situ of larynx

Carcinoma in situ of aryepiglottic fold or interarytenoid fold, laryngeal aspect
Carcinoma in situ of epiglottis (suprahyoid portion)

> EXCLUDES 1   carcinoma in situ of aryepiglottic fold or interarytenoid fold NOS (D00.08)
> carcinoma in situ of hypopharyngeal aspect (D00.08)
> carcinoma in situ of marginal zone (D00.08)

D02.1 Carcinoma in situ of trachea

D02.2 Carcinoma in situ of bronchus and lung

   D02.20 Carcinoma in situ of unspecified bronchus and lung

   D02.21 Carcinoma in situ of right bronchus and lung

   D02.22 Carcinoma in situ of left bronchus and lung

D02.3 Carcinoma in situ of other parts of respiratory system

Carcinoma in situ of accessory sinuses
Carcinoma in situ of middle ear
Carcinoma in situ of nasal cavities

> EXCLUDES 1   carcinoma in situ of ear (external) (skin) (D04.2-)
> carcinoma in situ of nose NOS (D09.8)
> carcinoma in situ of skin of nose (D04.3)

D02.4 Carcinoma in situ of respiratory system, unspecified

D03 Melanoma in situ

D03.0 Melanoma in situ of lip HCC

D03.1 Melanoma in situ of eyelid, including canthus

AHA: 2018,4Q,4

   D03.10 Melanoma in situ of unspecified eyelid, including canthus HCC

   D03.11 Melanoma in situ of right eyelid, including canthus

      D03.111 Melanoma in situ of right upper eyelid, including canthus HCC

      D03.112 Melanoma in situ of right lower eyelid, including canthus HCC

✓6ᵗʰ D03.12   **Melanoma in situ of** left **eyelid, including canthus**

     D03.121   **Melanoma in situ of left** upper **eyelid, including canthus**   HCC

     D03.122   **Melanoma in situ of left** lower **eyelid, including canthus**   HCC

✓5ᵗʰ D03.2   **Melanoma in situ of** ear and external auricular canal

   D03.20   **Melanoma in situ of unspecified ear and external auricular canal**   HCC

   D03.21   **Melanoma in situ of** right **ear and external auricular canal**   HCC

   D03.22   **Melanoma in situ of** left **ear and external auricular canal**   HCC

✓5ᵗʰ D03.3   **Melanoma in situ of other and unspecified parts of** face

   D03.30   **Melanoma in situ of unspecified part of face**   HCC

   D03.39   **Melanoma in situ of other parts of face**   HCC

D03.4   **Melanoma in situ of** scalp and neck   HCC

✓5ᵗʰ D03.5   **Melanoma in situ of** trunk

   D03.51   **Melanoma in situ of** anal skin   HCC

     Melanoma in situ of anal margin
     Melanoma in situ of perianal skin

   D03.52   **Melanoma in situ of** breast (skin) (soft tissue)   HCC

   D03.59   **Melanoma in situ of other part of trunk**   HCC

✓5ᵗʰ D03.6   **Melanoma in situ of** upper limb, including shoulder

   D03.60   **Melanoma in situ of unspecified upper limb, including shoulder**   HCC

   D03.61   **Melanoma in situ of** right **upper limb, including shoulder**   HCC

   D03.62   **Melanoma in situ of** left **upper limb, including shoulder**   HCC

✓5ᵗʰ D03.7   **Melanoma in situ of** lower limb, including hip

   D03.70   **Melanoma in situ of unspecified lower limb, including hip**   HCC

   D03.71   **Melanoma in situ of** right **lower limb, including hip**   HCC

   D03.72   **Melanoma in situ of** left **lower limb, including hip**   HCC

D03.8   **Melanoma in situ of other sites**   HCC

     Melanoma in situ of scrotum
     EXCLUDES 1   *carcinoma in situ of scrotum (D07.61)*

D03.9   **Melanoma in situ, unspecified**   HCC

✓4ᵗʰ **D04**   **Carcinoma in situ of** skin

     EXCLUDES 1   *erythroplasia of Queyrat (penis) NOS (D07.4)*
                 melanoma in situ (D03.-)

D04.0   **Carcinoma in situ of skin of** lip

     EXCLUDES 1   *carcinoma in situ of vermilion border of lip (D00.01)*
     EXCLUDES 2   ▶*carcinoma in situ of vermilion border of lip (D00.01)*◀

✓5ᵗʰ D04.1   **Carcinoma in situ of skin of** eyelid, including canthus

     AHA: 2018,4Q,4

   D04.10   **Carcinoma in situ of skin of unspecified eyelid, including canthus**

   ✓6ᵗʰ D04.11   **Carcinoma in situ of skin of** right **eyelid, including canthus**

     D04.111   **Carcinoma in situ of skin of right** upper **eyelid, including canthus**

     D04.112   **Carcinoma in situ of skin of right** lower **eyelid, including canthus**

   ✓6ᵗʰ D04.12   **Carcinoma in situ of skin of** left **eyelid, including canthus**

     D04.121   **Carcinoma in situ of skin of left** upper **eyelid, including canthus**

     D04.122   **Carcinoma in situ of skin of left** lower **eyelid, including canthus**

✓5ᵗʰ D04.2   **Carcinoma in situ of skin of** ear and external auricular canal

   D04.20   **Carcinoma in situ of skin of unspecified ear and external auricular canal**

   D04.21   **Carcinoma in situ of skin of** right **ear and external auricular canal**

   D04.22   **Carcinoma in situ of skin of** left **ear and external auricular canal**

✓5ᵗʰ D04.3   **Carcinoma in situ of skin of other and unspecified** parts of face

   D04.30   **Carcinoma in situ of skin of unspecified part of face**

   D04.39   **Carcinoma in situ of skin of other parts of face**

D04.4   **Carcinoma in situ of skin of** scalp and neck

D04.5   **Carcinoma in situ of skin of** trunk

     Carcinoma in situ of anal margin
     Carcinoma in situ of anal skin
     Carcinoma in situ of perianal skin
     Carcinoma in situ of skin of breast

     EXCLUDES 1   *carcinoma in situ of anus NOS (D01.3)*
                 carcinoma in situ of scrotum (D07.61)
                 carcinoma in situ of skin of genital organs (D07.-)

✓5ᵗʰ D04.6   **Carcinoma in situ of skin of** upper limb, including shoulder

   D04.60   **Carcinoma in situ of skin of unspecified upper limb, including shoulder**

   D04.61   **Carcinoma in situ of skin of** right **upper limb, including shoulder**

   D04.62   **Carcinoma in situ of skin of** left **upper limb, including shoulder**

✓5ᵗʰ D04.7   **Carcinoma in situ of skin of** lower limb, including hip

   D04.70   **Carcinoma in situ of skin of unspecified lower limb, including hip**

   D04.71   **Carcinoma in situ of skin of** right **lower limb, including hip**

   D04.72   **Carcinoma in situ of skin of** left **lower limb, including hip**

D04.8   **Carcinoma in situ of skin of other sites**

D04.9   **Carcinoma in situ of skin, unspecified**

✓4ᵗʰ **D05**   **Carcinoma in situ of** breast

     EXCLUDES 1   *carcinoma in situ of skin of breast (D04.5)*
                 melanoma in situ of breast (skin) (D03.5)
                 Paget's disease of breast or nipple (C50.-)

✓5ᵗʰ D05.0   Lobular **carcinoma in situ of breast**

   D05.00   **Lobular carcinoma in situ of unspecified breast**

   D05.01   **Lobular carcinoma in situ of** right **breast**

   D05.02   **Lobular carcinoma in situ of** left **breast**

✓5ᵗʰ D05.1   Intraductal **carcinoma in situ of breast**

   D05.10   **Intraductal carcinoma in situ of unspecified breast**

   D05.11   **Intraductal carcinoma in situ of** right **breast**

   D05.12   **Intraductal carcinoma in situ of** left **breast**

✓5ᵗʰ D05.8   **Other specified type of carcinoma in situ of breast**

   D05.80   **Other specified type of carcinoma in situ of unspecified breast**

   D05.81   **Other specified type of carcinoma in situ of** right **breast**

   D05.82   **Other specified type of carcinoma in situ of** left **breast**

✓5ᵗʰ D05.9   **Unspecified type of carcinoma in situ of breast**

   D05.90   **Unspecified type of carcinoma in situ of unspecified breast**

   D05.91   **Unspecified type of carcinoma in situ of** right **breast**

   D05.92   **Unspecified type of carcinoma in situ of** left **breast**

✓4ᵗʰ **D06**   **Carcinoma in situ of** cervix uteri

     INCLUDES   cervical adenocarcinoma in situ
              cervical intraepithelial glandular neoplasia
              cervical intraepithelial neoplasia III [CIN III]
              severe dysplasia of cervix uteri

     EXCLUDES 1   *cervical intraepithelial neoplasia II [CIN II] (N87.1)*
                 cytologic evidence of malignancy of cervix without histologic confirmation (R87.614)
                 high grade squamous intraepithelial lesion (HGSIL) of cervix (R87.613)
                 melanoma in situ of cervix (D03.5)
                 moderate cervical dysplasia (N87.1)

D06.0   **Carcinoma in situ of** endocervix   ♀

D06.1   **Carcinoma in situ of** exocervix   ♀

D06.7   **Carcinoma in situ of other** parts of cervix   ♀

D06.9   **Carcinoma in situ of cervix, unspecified**   ♀

✓4ᵗʰ **D07**   **Carcinoma in situ of other and unspecified** genital organs

     EXCLUDES 1   *melanoma in situ of trunk (D03.5)*

D07.0   **Carcinoma in situ of** endometrium   ♀

D07.1   **Carcinoma in situ of** vulva   ♀

     Severe dysplasia of vulva
     Vulvar intraepithelial neoplasia III [VIN III]

     EXCLUDES 1   *moderate dysplasia of vulva (N90.1)*
                 vulvar intraepithelial neoplasia II [VIN II] (N90.1)

✓ Additional Character Required   ✓x7ᵗʰ Placeholder Alert   Manifestation   Unspecified Dx   ▶◀ Revised Text   ● New Code   ▲ Revised Code Title

ICD-10-CM 2020   487

D07.2   **Carcinoma in situ of vagina** ♀
Severe dysplasia of vagina
Vaginal intraepithelial neoplasia III [VAIN III]
> **EXCLUDES 1**   *moderate dysplasia of vagina (N89.1)*
> *vaginal intraepithelial neoplasia II [VIN II] (N89.1)*

✓5ᵗʰ **D07.3**   **Carcinoma in situ of other and unspecified female genital organs**
   D07.30   **Carcinoma in situ of unspecified female genital organs** ♀
   D07.39   **Carcinoma in situ of other female genital organs** ♀

D07.4   **Carcinoma in situ of penis** ♂
Erythroplasia of Queyrat NOS

D07.5   **Carcinoma in situ of prostate** ♂
Prostatic intraepithelial neoplasia III (PIN III)
Severe dysplasia of prostate
> **EXCLUDES 1**   *dysplasia (mild) (moderate) of prostate (N42.3-)*
> *prostatic intraepithelial neoplasia II [PIN II] (N42.3-)*

✓5ᵗʰ **D07.6**   **Carcinoma in situ of other and unspecified male genital organs**
   D07.60   **Carcinoma in situ of unspecified male genital organs** ♂
   D07.61   **Carcinoma in situ of scrotum** ♂
   D07.69   **Carcinoma in situ of other male genital organs** ♂

✓4ᵗʰ **D09**   **Carcinoma in situ of other and unspecified sites**
> **EXCLUDES 1**   *melanoma in situ (D03.-)*

D09.0   **Carcinoma in situ of bladder**

✓5ᵗʰ **D09.1**   **Carcinoma in situ of other and unspecified urinary organs**
   D09.10   **Carcinoma in situ of unspecified urinary organ**
   D09.19   **Carcinoma in situ of other urinary organs**

✓5ᵗʰ **D09.2**   **Carcinoma in situ of eye**
> **EXCLUDES 1**   *carcinoma in situ of skin of eyelid (D04.1-)*
   D09.20   **Carcinoma in situ of unspecified eye**
   D09.21   **Carcinoma in situ of right eye**
   D09.22   **Carcinoma in situ of left eye**

D09.3   **Carcinoma in situ of thyroid and other endocrine glands**
> **EXCLUDES 1**   *carcinoma in situ of endocrine pancreas (D01.7)*
> *carcinoma in situ of ovary (D07.39)*
> *carcinoma in situ of testis (D07.69)*

D09.8   **Carcinoma in situ of other specified sites**
D09.9   **Carcinoma in situ, unspecified**

Benign neoplasms, except benign neuroendocrine tumors (D10-D36)

✓4ᵗʰ **D10**   **Benign neoplasm of mouth and pharynx**

D10.0   **Benign neoplasm of lip**
Benign neoplasm of lip (frenulum) (inner aspect) (mucosa) (vermilion border)
> **EXCLUDES 1**   *benign neoplasm of skin of lip (D22.0, D23.0)*

D10.1   **Benign neoplasm of tongue**
Benign neoplasm of lingual tonsil

D10.2   **Benign neoplasm of floor of mouth**

✓5ᵗʰ **D10.3**   **Benign neoplasm of other and unspecified parts of mouth**
   D10.30   **Benign neoplasm of unspecified part of mouth**
   D10.39   **Benign neoplasm of other parts of mouth**
     Benign neoplasm of minor salivary gland NOS
> **EXCLUDES 1**   *benign odontogenic neoplasms (D16.4-D16.5)*
> *benign neoplasm of mucosa of lip (D10.0)*
> *benign neoplasm of nasopharyngeal surface of soft palate (D10.6)*

D10.4   **Benign neoplasm of tonsil**
Benign neoplasm of tonsil (faucial) (palatine)
> **EXCLUDES 1**   *benign neoplasm of lingual tonsil (D10.1)*
> *benign neoplasm of pharyngeal tonsil (D10.6)*
> *benign neoplasm of tonsillar fossa (D10.5)*
> *benign neoplasm of tonsillar pillars (D10.5)*

D10.5   **Benign neoplasm of other parts of oropharynx**
Benign neoplasm of epiglottis, anterior aspect
Benign neoplasm of tonsillar fossa
Benign neoplasm of tonsillar pillars
Benign neoplasm of vallecula
> **EXCLUDES 1**   *benign neoplasm of epiglottis NOS (D14.1)*
> *benign neoplasm of epiglottis, suprahyoid portion (D14.1)*

DEF: Oropharynx: Middle portion of pharynx (throat); communicates with the oral cavity, nasopharynx and laryngopharynx.

D10.6   **Benign neoplasm of nasopharynx**
Benign neoplasm of pharyngeal tonsil
Benign neoplasm of posterior margin of septum and choanae
DEF: Nasopharynx: Upper portion of pharynx (throat); communicates with the nasal cavities, oropharynx and tympanic cavities.

D10.7   **Benign neoplasm of hypopharynx**
DEF: Hypopharynx: Lower portion of pharynx (throat); communicates with the oropharynx and the esophagus.
Synonyms: *laryngopharynx.*

D10.9   **Benign neoplasm of pharynx, unspecified**

✓4ᵗʰ **D11**   **Benign neoplasm of major salivary glands**
> **EXCLUDES 1**   *benign neoplasms of specified minor salivary glands which are classified according to their anatomical location*
> *benign neoplasms of minor salivary glands NOS (D10.39)*

D11.0   **Benign neoplasm of parotid gland**
D11.7   **Benign neoplasm of other major salivary glands**
Benign neoplasm of sublingual salivary gland
Benign neoplasm of submandibular salivary gland
D11.9   **Benign neoplasm of major salivary gland, unspecified**

✓4ᵗʰ **D12**   **Benign neoplasm of colon, rectum, anus and anal canal**
> **EXCLUDES 1**   *benign carcinoid tumors of the large intestine, and rectum (D3A.02-)*
> ▶*polyp of colon NOS (K63.5)*◀

AHA: 2018,2Q,14; 2017,1Q,15; 2015,2Q,14
TIP: Code K63.5 Polyp of colon, is assigned when documentation states hyperplastic colon polyps, regardless of the site in the colon. Slow-growing, hyperplastic polyps are not precancerous and are classified differently from benign or adenomatous polyps.

D12.0   **Benign neoplasm of cecum**
Benign neoplasm of ileocecal valve

D12.1   **Benign neoplasm of appendix**
> **EXCLUDES 1**   *benign carcinoid tumor of the appendix (D3A.020)*

D12.2   **Benign neoplasm of ascending colon**

D12.3   **Benign neoplasm of transverse colon**
Benign neoplasm of hepatic flexure
Benign neoplasm of splenic flexure
AHA: 2017,1Q,16

D12.4   **Benign neoplasm of descending colon**

D12.5   **Benign neoplasm of sigmoid colon**

D12.6   **Benign neoplasm of colon, unspecified**
Adenomatosis of colon
Benign neoplasm of large intestine NOS
Polyposis (hereditary) of colon
> **EXCLUDES 1**   *inflammatory polyp of colon (K51.4-)*
> *polyp of colon NOS (K63.5)*

D12.7   **Benign neoplasm of rectosigmoid junction**

D12.8   **Benign neoplasm of rectum**
> **EXCLUDES 1**   *benign carcinoid tumor of the rectum (D3A.026)*
AHA: 2018,1Q,6

D12.9   **Benign neoplasm of anus and anal canal**
Benign neoplasm of anus NOS
> **EXCLUDES 1**   *benign neoplasm of anal margin (D22.5, D23.5)*
> *benign neoplasm of anal skin (D22.5, D23.5)*
> *benign neoplasm of perianal skin (D22.5, D23.5)*

✓4ᵗʰ **D13**   **Benign neoplasm of other and ill-defined parts of digestive system**
> **EXCLUDES 1**   *benign stromal tumors of digestive system (D21.4)*

D13.0   **Benign neoplasm of esophagus**
D13.1   **Benign neoplasm of stomach**
> **EXCLUDES 1**   *benign carcinoid tumor of the stomach (D3A.092)*
D13.2   **Benign neoplasm of duodenum**
> **EXCLUDES 1**   *benign carcinoid tumor of the duodenum (D3A.010)*

✓5ᵗʰ **D13.3** **Benign neoplasm of other and unspecified parts of** small intestine

     EXCLUDES 1   *benign carcinoid tumors of the small intestine (D3A.01-)*

                benign neoplasm of ileocecal valve (D12.0)

     D13.30 **Benign neoplasm of unspecified part of small intestine**

     D13.39 **Benign neoplasm of other parts of small intestine**

D13.4 **Benign neoplasm of** liver

     Benign neoplasm of intrahepatic bile ducts

D13.5 **Benign neoplasm of** extrahepatic bile ducts

D13.6 **Benign neoplasm of** pancreas

     EXCLUDES 1   *benign neoplasm of endocrine pancreas (D13.7)*

D13.7 **Benign neoplasm of** endocrine pancreas

     Benign neoplasm of islets of Langerhans

     Islet cell tumor

     Use additional code to identify any functional activity

D13.9 **Benign neoplasm of** ill-defined sites **within the digestive system**

     Benign neoplasm of digestive system NOS

     Benign neoplasm of intestine NOS

     Benign neoplasm of spleen

✓4ᵗʰ **D14** **Benign neoplasm of** middle ear and respiratory system

D14.0 **Benign neoplasm of** middle ear, nasal cavity and accessory sinuses

     Benign neoplasm of cartilage of nose

     EXCLUDES 1   *benign neoplasm of auricular canal (external) (D22.2-, D23.2-)*

                benign neoplasm of bone of ear (D16.4)

                benign neoplasm of bone of nose (D16.4)

                benign neoplasm of cartilage of ear (D21.0)

                benign neoplasm of ear (external)(skin) (D22.2-, D23.2-)

                benign neoplasm of nose NOS (D36.7)

                benign neoplasm of skin of nose (D22.39, D23.39)

                benign neoplasm of olfactory bulb (D33.3)

                benign neoplasm of posterior margin of septum and choanae (D10.6)

                polyp of accessory sinus (J33.8)

                polyp of ear (middle) (H74.4)

                polyp of nasal (cavity) (J33.-)

D14.1 **Benign neoplasm of** larynx

     Adenomatous polyp of larynx

     Benign neoplasm of epiglottis (suprahyoid portion)

     EXCLUDES 1   *benign neoplasm of epiglottis, anterior aspect (D10.5)*

                polyp (nonadenomatous) of vocal cord or larynx (J38.1)

D14.2 **Benign neoplasm of** trachea

✓5ᵗʰ **D14.3** **Benign neoplasm of** bronchus and lung

     EXCLUDES 1   *benign carcinoid tumor of the bronchus and lung (D3A.090)*

     D14.30 **Benign neoplasm of unspecified bronchus and lung**

     D14.31 **Benign neoplasm of** right **bronchus and lung**

     D14.32 **Benign neoplasm of** left **bronchus and lung**

   D14.4 **Benign neoplasm of respiratory system, unspecified**

✓4ᵗʰ **D15** **Benign neoplasm of other and unspecified** intrathoracic organs

     EXCLUDES 1   *benign neoplasm of mesothelial tissue (D19.-)*

D15.0 **Benign neoplasm of** thymus

     EXCLUDES 1   *benign carcinoid tumor of the thymus (D3A.091)*

D15.1 **Benign neoplasm of** heart

     EXCLUDES 1   *benign neoplasm of great vessels (D21.3)*

D15.2 **Benign neoplasm of** mediastinum

D15.7 **Benign neoplasm of other specified intrathoracic organs**

D15.9 **Benign neoplasm of intrathoracic organ, unspecified**

✓4ᵗʰ **D16** **Benign neoplasm of** bone and articular cartilage

     EXCLUDES 1   *benign neoplasm of connective tissue of ear (D21.0)*

                benign neoplasm of connective tissue of eyelid (D21.0)

                benign neoplasm of connective tissue of larynx (D14.1)

                benign neoplasm of connective tissue of nose (D14.0)

                benign neoplasm of synovia (D21.-)

✓6ᵗʰ **D16.0** **Benign neoplasm of** scapula and long bones of upper limb

     D16.00 **Benign neoplasm of scapula and long bones of unspecified upper limb**

     D16.01 **Benign neoplasm of scapula and long bones of** right **upper limb**

     D16.02 **Benign neoplasm of scapula and long bones of** left **upper limb**

✓5ᵗʰ **D16.1** **Benign neoplasm of** short bones of upper limb

     D16.10 **Benign neoplasm of short bones of unspecified upper limb**

     D16.11 **Benign neoplasm of short bones of** right **upper limb**

     D16.12 **Benign neoplasm of short bones of** left **upper limb**

✓5ᵗʰ **D16.2** **Benign neoplasm of** long bones of lower limb

     D16.20 **Benign neoplasm of long bones of unspecified lower limb**

     D16.21 **Benign neoplasm of long bones of** right **lower limb**

     D16.22 **Benign neoplasm of long bones of** left **lower limb**

✓5ᵗʰ **D16.3** **Benign neoplasm of** short bones of lower limb

     D16.30 **Benign neoplasm of short bones of unspecified lower limb**

     D16.31 **Benign neoplasm of short bones of** right **lower limb**

     D16.32 **Benign neoplasm of short bones of** left **lower limb**

D16.4 **Benign neoplasm of bones of** skull and face

     Benign neoplasm of maxilla (superior)

     Benign neoplasm of orbital bone

     Keratocyst of maxilla

     Keratocystic odontogenic tumor of maxilla

     EXCLUDES 2   *benign neoplasm of lower jaw bone (D16.5)*

D16.5 **Benign neoplasm of** lower jaw bone

     Keratocyst of mandible

     Keratocystic odontogenic tumor of mandible

D16.6 **Benign neoplasm of** vertebral column

     EXCLUDES 1   *benign neoplasm of sacrum and coccyx (D16.8)*

D16.7 **Benign neoplasm of** ribs, sternum and clavicle

D16.8 **Benign neoplasm of** pelvic bones, sacrum and coccyx

D16.9 **Benign neoplasm of bone and articular cartilage, unspecified**

✓4ᵗʰ **D17** **Benign** lipomatous **neoplasm**

D17.0 **Benign lipomatous neoplasm of** skin and subcutaneous tissue of head, face and neck

D17.1 **Benign lipomatous neoplasm of** skin and subcutaneous tissue of trunk

✓5ᵗʰ **D17.2** **Benign lipomatous neoplasm of** skin and subcutaneous tissue of limb

     D17.20 **Benign lipomatous neoplasm of skin and subcutaneous tissue of unspecified limb**

     D17.21 **Benign lipomatous neoplasm of skin and subcutaneous tissue of** right **arm**

     D17.22 **Benign lipomatous neoplasm of skin and subcutaneous tissue of** left **arm**

     D17.23 **Benign lipomatous neoplasm of skin and subcutaneous tissue of** right **leg**

     D17.24 **Benign lipomatous neoplasm of skin and subcutaneous tissue of** left **leg**

✓5ᵗʰ **D17.3** **Benign lipomatous neoplasm of** skin and subcutaneous tissue of other and unspecified sites

     D17.30 **Benign lipomatous neoplasm of skin and subcutaneous tissue of unspecified sites**

     D17.39 **Benign lipomatous neoplasm of skin and subcutaneous tissue of other sites**

D17.4 **Benign lipomatous neoplasm of** intrathoracic organs

D17.5 **Benign lipomatous neoplasm of** intra-abdominal organs

     EXCLUDES 1   *benign lipomatous neoplasm of peritoneum and retroperitoneum (D17.79)*

D17.6 **Benign lipomatous neoplasm of** spermatic cord   ♂

✓5ᵗʰ **D17.7** **Benign lipomatous neoplasm of** other sites

     D17.71 **Benign lipomatous neoplasm of** kidney

     D17.72 **Benign lipomatous neoplasm of other** genitourinary organ

     D17.79 **Benign lipomatous neoplasm of other sites**

        Benign lipomatous neoplasm of peritoneum

        Benign lipomatous neoplasm of retroperitoneum

D17.9 **Benign lipomatous neoplasm, unspecified**

     Lipoma NOS

☑ Additional Character Required   ✓x7ᵗʰ Placeholder Alert   Manifestation   Unspecified Dx   ▶◀ Revised Text   ● New Code   ▲ Revised Code Title

ICD-10-CM 2020   489

✓4ᵗʰ **D18 Hemangioma and lymphangioma, any site**

EXCLUDES 1   *benign neoplasm of glomus jugulare (D35.6)*
blue or pigmented nevus (D22.-)
nevus NOS (D22.-)
vascular nevus (Q82.5)

✓5ᵗʰ **D18.0 Hemangioma**

Angioma NOS
Cavernous nevus
DEF: Common benign tumor usually occurring in infancy that is composed of newly formed blood vessels due to malformation of the angioblastic tissue.

D18.00   **Hemangioma** unspecified site

D18.01   **Hemangioma of** skin and subcutaneous tissue

D18.02   **Hemangioma of** intracranial structures   HCC

D18.03   **Hemangioma of** intra-abdominal structures

D18.09   **Hemangioma of other sites**

D18.1 Lymphangioma, any site
AHA: 2018,3Q,31; 2018,2Q,13

✓4ᵗʰ **D19 Benign neoplasm of** mesothelial tissue

D19.0 Benign neoplasm of mesothelial tissue of pleura

D19.1 Benign neoplasm of mesothelial tissue of peritoneum

D19.7 Benign neoplasm of mesothelial tissue of other sites

D19.9 Benign neoplasm of mesothelial tissue, unspecified
Benign mesothelioma NOS

✓4ᵗʰ **D20 Benign neoplasm of soft tissue of** retroperitoneum and peritoneum

EXCLUDES 1   *benign lipomatous neoplasm of peritoneum and*
retroperitoneum (D17.79)
benign neoplasm of mesothelial tissue (D19.-)

D20.0 Benign neoplasm of soft tissue of retroperitoneum

D20.1 Benign neoplasm of soft tissue of peritoneum

✓4ᵗʰ **D21 Other benign neoplasms of** connective and other soft tissue

INCLUDES   benign neoplasm of blood vessel
benign neoplasm of bursa
benign neoplasm of cartilage
benign neoplasm of fascia
benign neoplasm of fat
benign neoplasm of ligament, except uterine
benign neoplasm of lymphatic channel
benign neoplasm of muscle
benign neoplasm of synovia
benign neoplasm of tendon (sheath)
benign stromal tumors

EXCLUDES 1   *benign neoplasm of articular cartilage (D16.-)*
benign neoplasm of cartilage of larynx (D14.1)
benign neoplasm of cartilage of nose (D14.0)
benign neoplasm of connective tissue of breast (D24.-)
benign neoplasm of peripheral nerves and autonomic nervous
system (D36.1-)
benign neoplasm of peritoneum (D20.1)
benign neoplasm of retroperitoneum (D20.0)
benign neoplasm of uterine ligament, any (D28.2)
benign neoplasm of vascular tissue (D18.-)
hemangioma (D18.0-)
lipomatous neoplasm (D17.-)
lymphangioma (D18.1)
uterine leiomyoma (D25.-)

D21.0 Benign neoplasm of connective and other soft tissue of head, face and neck
Benign neoplasm of connective tissue of ear
Benign neoplasm of connective tissue of eyelid

EXCLUDES 1   *benign neoplasm of connective tissue of orbit*
(D31.6-)

✓5ᵗʰ **D21.1 Benign neoplasm of connective and other soft tissue of** upper limb, including shoulder

D21.10   **Benign neoplasm of connective and other soft tissue of unspecified upper limb, including shoulder**

D21.11   **Benign neoplasm of connective and other soft tissue of** right **upper limb, including shoulder**

D21.12   **Benign neoplasm of connective and other soft tissue of** left **upper limb, including shoulder**

✓5ᵗʰ **D21.2 Benign neoplasm of connective and other soft tissue of** lower limb, including hip

D21.20   **Benign neoplasm of connective and other soft tissue of unspecified lower limb, including hip**

D21.21   **Benign neoplasm of connective and other soft tissue of** right **lower limb, including hip**

D21.22   **Benign neoplasm of connective and other soft tissue of** left **lower limb, including hip**

D21.3 Benign neoplasm of connective and other soft tissue of thorax
Benign neoplasm of axilla
Benign neoplasm of diaphragm
Benign neoplasm of great vessels

EXCLUDES 1   *benign neoplasm of heart (D15.1)*
benign neoplasm of mediastinum (D15.2)
benign neoplasm of thymus (D15.0)

D21.4 Benign neoplasm of connective and other soft tissue of abdomen
Benign stromal tumors of abdomen

D21.5 Benign neoplasm of connective and other soft tissue of pelvis

EXCLUDES 1   *benign neoplasm of any uterine ligament (D28.2)*
uterine leiomyoma (D25.-)

D21.6 Benign neoplasm of connective and other soft tissue of trunk, unspecified
▶Benign neoplasm of connective and other soft tissue back NOS◀

D21.9 Benign neoplasm of connective and other soft tissue, unspecified

✓4ᵗʰ **D22 Melanocytic nevi**

INCLUDES   atypical nevus
blue hairy pigmented nevus
nevus NOS

D22.0 Melanocytic nevi of lip

✓5ᵗʰ **D22.1 Melanocytic nevi of** eyelid, including canthus
AHA: 2018,4Q,4

D22.10   **Melanocytic nevi of unspecified eyelid, including canthus**

✓6ᵗʰ D22.11   **Melanocytic nevi of** right **eyelid, including canthus**

D22.111   **Melanocytic nevi of right** upper **eyelid, including canthus**

D22.112   **Melanocytic nevi of right** lower **eyelid, including canthus**

✓6ᵗʰ D22.12   **Melanocytic nevi of** left **eyelid, including canthus**

D22.121   **Melanocytic nevi of left** upper **eyelid, including canthus**

D22.122   **Melanocytic nevi of left** lower **eyelid, including canthus**

✓5ᵗʰ **D22.2 Melanocytic nevi of** ear and external auricular canal

D22.20   **Melanocytic nevi of unspecified ear and external auricular canal**

D22.21   **Melanocytic nevi of** right **ear and external auricular canal**

D22.22   **Melanocytic nevi of** left **ear and external auricular canal**

✓5ᵗʰ **D22.3 Melanocytic nevi of other and unspecified** parts of face

D22.30   **Melanocytic nevi of unspecified part of face**

D22.39   **Melanocytic nevi of other parts of face**

D22.4 Melanocytic nevi of scalp and neck

D22.5 Melanocytic nevi of trunk
Melanocytic nevi of anal margin
Melanocytic nevi of anal skin
Melanocytic nevi of perianal skin
Melanocytic nevi of skin of breast

✓5ᵗʰ **D22.6 Melanocytic nevi of** upper limb, including shoulder

D22.60   **Melanocytic nevi of unspecified upper limb, including shoulder**

D22.61   **Melanocytic nevi of** right **upper limb, including shoulder**

D22.62   **Melanocytic nevi of** left **upper limb, including shoulder**

✓5ᵗʰ **D22.7 Melanocytic nevi of** lower limb, including hip

D22.70   **Melanocytic nevi of unspecified lower limb, including hip**

D22.71   **Melanocytic nevi of** right **lower limb, including hip**

D22.72   **Melanocytic nevi of** left **lower limb, including hip**

D22.9 Melanocytic nevi, unspecified

☑4ᵗʰ D23   Other benign neoplasms of skin

> **INCLUDES**   benign neoplasm of hair follicles
> benign neoplasm of sebaceous glands
> benign neoplasm of sweat glands
> **EXCLUDES 1**   *benign lipomatous neoplasms of skin (D17.0-D17.3)*
> *melanocytic nevi (D22.-)*
> **EXCLUDES 2**   ▶*melanocytic nevi (D22.-)*◀

D23.0   Other benign neoplasm of skin of lip

> **EXCLUDES 1**   *benign neoplasm of vermilion border of lip (D10.0)*

☑5ᵗʰ D23.1   Other benign neoplasm of skin of eyelid, including canthus

> **AHA:** 2018,4Q,4

> **D23.10   Other benign neoplasm of skin of unspecified eyelid, including canthus**

> **☑6ᵗʰ D23.11   Other benign neoplasm of skin of right eyelid, including canthus**
>> **D23.111   Other benign neoplasm of skin of right upper eyelid, including canthus**
>> **D23.112   Other benign neoplasm of skin of right lower eyelid, including canthus**

> **☑6ᵗʰ D23.12   Other benign neoplasm of skin of left eyelid, including canthus**
>> **D23.121   Other benign neoplasm of skin of left upper eyelid, including canthus**
>> **D23.122   Other benign neoplasm of skin of left lower eyelid, including canthus**

☑5ᵗʰ D23.2   Other benign neoplasm of skin of ear and external auricular canal

> **D23.20   Other benign neoplasm of skin of unspecified ear and external auricular canal**
> **D23.21   Other benign neoplasm of skin of right ear and external auricular canal**
> **D23.22   Other benign neoplasm of skin of left ear and external auricular canal**

☑5ᵗʰ D23.3   Other benign neoplasm of skin of other and unspecified parts of face

> **D23.30   Other benign neoplasm of skin of unspecified part of face**
> **D23.39   Other benign neoplasm of skin of other parts of face**

D23.4   Other benign neoplasm of skin of scalp and neck

D23.5   Other benign neoplasm of skin of trunk
> Other benign neoplasm of anal margin
> Other benign neoplasm of anal skin
> Other benign neoplasm of perianal skin
> Other benign neoplasm of skin of breast
> **EXCLUDES 1**   *benign neoplasm of anus NOS (D12.9)*

☑5ᵗʰ D23.6   Other benign neoplasm of skin of upper limb, including shoulder

> **D23.60   Other benign neoplasm of skin of unspecified upper limb, including shoulder**
> **D23.61   Other benign neoplasm of skin of right upper limb, including shoulder**
> **D23.62   Other benign neoplasm of skin of left upper limb, including shoulder**

☑5ᵗʰ D23.7   Other benign neoplasm of skin of lower limb, including hip

> **D23.70   Other benign neoplasm of skin of unspecified lower limb, including hip**
> **D23.71   Other benign neoplasm of skin of right lower limb, including hip**
> **D23.72   Other benign neoplasm of skin of left lower limb, including hip**

D23.9   Other benign neoplasm of skin, unspecified

☑4ᵗʰ D24   Benign neoplasm of breast

> **INCLUDES**   benign neoplasm of connective tissue of breast
> benign neoplasm of soft parts of breast
> fibroadenoma of breast
> **EXCLUDES 2**   *adenofibrosis of breast (N60.2)*
> *benign cyst of breast (N60.-)*
> *benign mammary dysplasia (N60.-)*
> *benign neoplasm of skin of breast (D22.5, D23.5)*
> *fibrocystic disease of breast (N60.-)*

D24.1   Benign neoplasm of right breast
D24.2   Benign neoplasm of left breast
D24.9   Benign neoplasm of unspecified breast

☑4ᵗʰ D25   Leiomyoma of uterus

> **INCLUDES**   uterine fibroid
> uterine fibromyoma
> uterine myoma

Uterine Leiomyomas (Fibroids)

D25.0   Submucous leiomyoma of uterus   ♀
D25.1   Intramural leiomyoma of uterus   ♀
> Interstitial leiomyoma of uterus
D25.2   Subserosal leiomyoma of uterus   ♀
> Subperitoneal leiomyoma of uterus
D25.9   Leiomyoma of uterus, unspecified   ♀

☑4ᵗʰ D26   Other benign neoplasms of uterus

D26.0   Other benign neoplasm of cervix uteri   ♀
D26.1   Other benign neoplasm of corpus uteri   ♀
D26.7   Other benign neoplasm of other parts of uterus   ♀
D26.9   Other benign neoplasm of uterus, unspecified   ♀

☑4ᵗʰ D27   Benign neoplasm of ovary

> Use additional code to identify any functional activity
> **EXCLUDES 2**   *corpus albicans cyst (N83.2-)*
> *corpus luteum cyst (N83.1-)*
> *endometrial cyst (N80.1)*
> *follicular (atretic) cyst (N83.0-)*
> *graafian follicle cyst (N83.0-)*
> *ovarian cyst NEC (N83.2-)*
> *ovarian retention cyst (N83.2-)*

D27.0   Benign neoplasm of right ovary   ♀
D27.1   Benign neoplasm of left ovary   ♀
D27.9   Benign neoplasm of unspecified ovary   ♀

☑4ᵗʰ D28   Benign neoplasm of other and unspecified female genital organs

> **INCLUDES**   adenomatous polyp
> benign neoplasm of skin of female genital organs
> benign teratoma
> **EXCLUDES 1**   *epoophoron cyst (Q50.5)*
> *fimbrial cyst (Q50.4)*
> *Gartner's duct cyst (Q52.4)*
> *parovarian cyst (Q50.5)*

D28.0   Benign neoplasm of vulva   ♀
D28.1   Benign neoplasm of vagina   ♀
D28.2   Benign neoplasm of uterine tubes and ligaments   ♀
> Benign neoplasm of fallopian tube
> Benign neoplasm of uterine ligament (broad) (round)
D28.7   Benign neoplasm of other specified female genital organs   ♀
D28.9   Benign neoplasm of female genital organ, unspecified   ♀

☑4ᵗʰ D29   Benign neoplasm of male genital organs

> **INCLUDES**   benign neoplasm of skin of male genital organs
D29.0   Benign neoplasm of penis   ♂

☑ Additional Character Required   ✓ˣ7ᵗʰ Placeholder Alert   Manifestation   Unspecified Dx   ▶◀ Revised Text   ● New Code   ▲ Revised Code Title

D29.1   **Benign neoplasm of** prostate   ♂
> *EXCLUDES 1*   enlarged prostate (N40.-)

✓5ᵗʰ **D29.2**   **Benign neoplasm of** testis
> Use additional code to identify any functional activity
>> **D29.20**   **Benign neoplasm of unspecified** testis   ♂
>> **D29.21**   **Benign neoplasm of** right **testis**   ♂
>> **D29.22**   **Benign neoplasm of** left **testis**   ♂

✓5ᵗʰ **D29.3**   **Benign neoplasm of** epididymis
>> **D29.30**   **Benign neoplasm of unspecified epididymis**   ♂
>> **D29.31**   **Benign neoplasm of** right **epididymis**   ♂
>> **D29.32**   **Benign neoplasm of** left **epididymis**   ♂

D29.4   **Benign neoplasm of** scrotum   ♂
> Benign neoplasm of skin of scrotum

D29.8   **Benign neoplasm of other specified male genital organs**   ♂
> Benign neoplasm of seminal vesicle
> Benign neoplasm of spermatic cord
> Benign neoplasm of tunica vaginalis

D29.9   **Benign neoplasm of male genital organ, unspecified**   ♂

✓4ᵗʰ **D30**   **Benign neoplasm of** urinary organs

✓5ᵗʰ **D30.0**   **Benign neoplasm of** kidney
> *EXCLUDES 1*   benign carcinoid tumor of the kidney (D3A.093)
>   benign neoplasm of renal calyces (D30.1-)
>   benign neoplasm of renal pelvis (D30.1-)
>> **D30.00**   **Benign neoplasm of unspecified kidney**
>> **D30.01**   **Benign neoplasm of** right **kidney**
>> **D30.02**   **Benign neoplasm of** left **kidney**

✓5ᵗʰ **D30.1**   **Benign neoplasm of** renal pelvis
>> **D30.10**   **Benign neoplasm of unspecified renal pelvis**
>> **D30.11**   **Benign neoplasm of** right **renal pelvis**
>> **D30.12**   **Benign neoplasm of** left **renal pelvis**

✓5ᵗʰ **D30.2**   **Benign neoplasm of** ureter
> *EXCLUDES 1*   benign neoplasm of ureteric orifice of bladder (D30.3)
>> **D30.20**   **Benign neoplasm of unspecified ureter**
>> **D30.21**   **Benign neoplasm of** right **ureter**
>> **D30.22**   **Benign neoplasm of** left **ureter**

D30.3   **Benign neoplasm of** bladder
> Benign neoplasm of ureteric orifice of bladder
> Benign neoplasm of urethral orifice of bladder

D30.4   **Benign neoplasm of** urethra
> *EXCLUDES 1*   benign neoplasm of urethral orifice of bladder (D30.3)

D30.8   **Benign neoplasm of other specified urinary organs**
> Benign neoplasm of paraurethral glands

D30.9   **Benign neoplasm of urinary organ, unspecified**
> Benign neoplasm of urinary system NOS

✓4ᵗʰ **D31**   **Benign neoplasm of** eye and adnexa
> *EXCLUDES 1*   benign neoplasm of connective tissue of eyelid (D21.0)
>   benign neoplasm of optic nerve (D33.3)
>   benign neoplasm of skin of eyelid (D22.1-, D23.1-)

✓5ᵗʰ **D31.0**   **Benign neoplasm of** conjunctiva
>> **D31.00**   **Benign neoplasm of unspecified conjunctiva**
>> **D31.01**   **Benign neoplasm of** right **conjunctiva**
>> **D31.02**   **Benign neoplasm of** left **conjunctiva**

✓5ᵗʰ **D31.1**   **Benign neoplasm of** cornea
>> **D31.10**   **Benign neoplasm of unspecified cornea**
>> **D31.11**   **Benign neoplasm of** right **cornea**
>> **D31.12**   **Benign neoplasm of** left **cornea**

✓5ᵗʰ **D31.2**   **Benign neoplasm of** retina
> *EXCLUDES 1*   dark area on retina (D49.81)
>   hemangioma of retina (D49.81)
>   neoplasm of unspecified behavior of retina and choroid (D49.81)
>   retinal freckle (D49.81)
>> **D31.20**   **Benign neoplasm of unspecified retina**
>> **D31.21**   **Benign neoplasm of** right **retina**
>> **D31.22**   **Benign neoplasm of** left **retina**

✓5ᵗʰ **D31.3**   **Benign neoplasm of** choroid
>> **D31.30**   **Benign neoplasm of unspecified choroid**
>> **D31.31**   **Benign neoplasm of** right **choroid**
>> **D31.32**   **Benign neoplasm of** left **choroid**

✓5ᵗʰ **D31.4**   **Benign neoplasm of** ciliary body
>> **D31.40**   **Benign neoplasm of unspecified ciliary body**
>> **D31.41**   **Benign neoplasm of** right **ciliary body**
>> **D31.42**   **Benign neoplasm of** left **ciliary body**

✓5ᵗʰ **D31.5**   **Benign neoplasm of** lacrimal gland and duct
> Benign neoplasm of lacrimal sac
> Benign neoplasm of nasolacrimal duct
>> **D31.50**   **Benign neoplasm of unspecified lacrimal gland and duct**
>> **D31.51**   **Benign neoplasm of** right **lacrimal gland and duct**
>> **D31.52**   **Benign neoplasm of** left **lacrimal gland and duct**

✓5ᵗʰ **D31.6**   **Benign neoplasm of unspecified site of** orbit
> Benign neoplasm of connective tissue of orbit
> Benign neoplasm of extraocular muscle
> Benign neoplasm of peripheral nerves of orbit
> Benign neoplasm of retrobulbar tissue
> Benign neoplasm of retro-ocular tissue
> *EXCLUDES 1*   benign neoplasm of orbital bone (D16.4)
>> **D31.60**   **Benign neoplasm of unspecified site of unspecified orbit**
>> **D31.61**   **Benign neoplasm of unspecified site of** right **orbit**
>> **D31.62**   **Benign neoplasm of unspecified site of** left **orbit**

✓5ᵗʰ **D31.9**   **Benign neoplasm of unspecified** part of eye
> Benign neoplasm of eyeball
>> **D31.90**   **Benign neoplasm of unspecified part of unspecified eye**
>> **D31.91**   **Benign neoplasm of unspecified part of** right **eye**
>> **D31.92**   **Benign neoplasm of unspecified part of** left **eye**

✓4ᵗʰ **D32**   **Benign neoplasm of** meninges
> **D32.0**   **Benign neoplasm of** cerebral **meninges**   HCC
> **D32.1**   **Benign neoplasm of** spinal **meninges**   HCC
> **D32.9**   **Benign neoplasm of meninges, unspecified**   HCC
>> Meningioma NOS

✓4ᵗʰ **D33**   **Benign neoplasm of** brain and other parts of central nervous system
> *EXCLUDES 1*   angioma (D18.0-)
>   benign neoplasm of meninges (D32.-)
>   benign neoplasm of peripheral nerves and autonomic nervous system (D36.1-)
>   hemangioma (D18.0-)
>   neurofibromatosis (Q85.0-)
>   retro-ocular benign neoplasm (D31.6-)

> **D33.0**   **Benign neoplasm of** brain, supratentorial   HCC
>> Benign neoplasm of cerebral ventricle
>> Benign neoplasm of cerebrum
>> Benign neoplasm of frontal lobe
>> Benign neoplasm of occipital lobe
>> Benign neoplasm of parietal lobe
>> Benign neoplasm of temporal lobe
>> *EXCLUDES 1*   benign neoplasm of fourth ventricle (D33.1)

> **D33.1**   **Benign neoplasm of** brain, infratentorial   HCC
>> Benign neoplasm of brain stem
>> Benign neoplasm of cerebellum
>> Benign neoplasm of fourth ventricle

> **D33.2**   **Benign neoplasm of brain, unspecified**   HCC

> **D33.3**   **Benign neoplasm of** cranial nerves   HCC
>> Benign neoplasm of olfactory bulb

> **D33.4**   **Benign neoplasm of** spinal cord   HCC

> **D33.7**   **Benign neoplasm of other specified parts of central nervous system**   HCC

> **D33.9**   **Benign neoplasm of central nervous system, unspecified**   HCC
>> Benign neoplasm of nervous system (central) NOS

D34   **Benign neoplasm of** thyroid gland
> Use additional code to identify any functional activity

✓4ᵗʰ **D35**   **Benign neoplasm of other and unspecified** endocrine glands
> Use additional code to identify any functional activity
> *EXCLUDES 1*   benign neoplasm of endocrine pancreas (D13.7)
>   benign neoplasm of ovary (D27.-)
>   benign neoplasm of testis (D29.2.-)
>   benign neoplasm of thymus (D15.0)

✓5ᵗʰ **D35.0**   **Benign neoplasm of** adrenal gland
>> **D35.00**   **Benign neoplasm of unspecified adrenal gland**

D35.01   **Benign neoplasm of** right **adrenal gland**

D35.02   **Benign neoplasm of** left **adrenal gland**

D35.1   **Benign neoplasm of** parathyroid gland

D35.2   **Benign neoplasm of** pituitary gland   `HCC`

     AHA: 2014,3Q,22

D35.3   **Benign neoplasm of** craniopharyngeal duct   `HCC`

D35.4   **Benign neoplasm of** pineal gland   `HCC`

D35.5   **Benign neoplasm of** carotid body

D35.6   **Benign neoplasm of** aortic body and other paraganglia

     Benign tumor of glomus jugulare

D35.7   **Benign neoplasm of other specified endocrine glands**

D35.9   **Benign neoplasm of** endocrine gland, unspecified

     Benign neoplasm of unspecified endocrine gland

✓4ᵗʰ **D36   Benign neoplasm of other and unspecified sites**

D36.0   **Benign neoplasm of** lymph nodes

     EXCLUDES 1   lymphangioma (D18.1)

✓5ᵗʰ D36.1   **Benign neoplasm of** peripheral nerves and autonomic nervous system

     EXCLUDES 1   benign neoplasm of peripheral nerves of orbit (D31.6-)

                       neurofibromatosis (Q85.0-)

     D36.10   **Benign neoplasm of peripheral nerves and autonomic nervous system, unspecified**

     D36.11   **Benign neoplasm of peripheral nerves and autonomic nervous system of** face, head, and neck

     D36.12   **Benign neoplasm of peripheral nerves and autonomic nervous system,** upper limb, including shoulder

     D36.13   **Benign neoplasm of peripheral nerves and autonomic nervous system of** lower limb, including hip

     D36.14   **Benign neoplasm of peripheral nerves and autonomic nervous system of** thorax

     D36.15   **Benign neoplasm of peripheral nerves and autonomic nervous system of** abdomen

     D36.16   **Benign neoplasm of peripheral nerves and autonomic nervous system of** pelvis

     D36.17   **Benign neoplasm of peripheral nerves and autonomic nervous system of** trunk, **unspecified**

D36.7   **Benign neoplasm of other specified sites**

     ►Benign neoplasm of back NOS◄

     Benign neoplasm of nose NOS

D36.9   **Benign neoplasm, unspecified site**

Benign neuroendocrine tumors (D3A)

✓4ᵗʰ **D3A   Benign neuroendocrine tumors**

     Code also any associated multiple endocrine neoplasia [MEN] syndromes (E31.2-)

     Use additional code to identify any associated endocrine syndrome, such as:

     carcinoid syndrome (E34.0)

     EXCLUDES 2   benign pancreatic islet cell tumors (D13.7)

✓5ᵗʰ **D3A.0   Benign** carcinoid tumors

     D3A.00   **Benign carcinoid tumor of unspecified site**

                 Carcinoid tumor NOS

     ✓6ᵗʰ D3A.01   **Benign carcinoid tumors of the** small intestine

         D3A.010   **Benign carcinoid tumor of the** duodenum

         D3A.011   **Benign carcinoid tumor of the** jejunum

         D3A.012   **Benign carcinoid tumor of the** ileum

         D3A.019   **Benign carcinoid tumor of the small intestine, unspecified portion**

     ✓6ᵗʰ D3A.02   **Benign carcinoid tumors of the** appendix, large intestine, and rectum

         D3A.020   **Benign carcinoid tumor of the** appendix

         D3A.021   **Benign carcinoid tumor of the** cecum

         D3A.022   **Benign carcinoid tumor of the** ascending colon

         D3A.023   **Benign carcinoid tumor of the** transverse colon

         D3A.024   **Benign carcinoid tumor of the** descending colon

         D3A.025   **Benign carcinoid tumor of the** sigmoid colon

         D3A.026   **Benign carcinoid tumor of the** rectum

         D3A.029   **Benign carcinoid tumor of the large intestine, unspecified portion**

                 Benign carcinoid tumor of the colon NOS

     ✓6ᵗʰ D3A.09   **Benign carcinoid tumors of other sites**

         D3A.090   **Benign carcinoid tumor of the** bronchus and lung

         D3A.091   **Benign carcinoid tumor of the** thymus

         D3A.092   **Benign carcinoid tumor of the** stomach

         D3A.093   **Benign carcinoid tumor of the** kidney

         D3A.094   **Benign carcinoid tumor of the** foregut, **unspecified**

         D3A.095   **Benign carcinoid tumor of the** midgut, **unspecified**

         D3A.096   **Benign carcinoid tumor of the** hindgut, **unspecified**

         D3A.098   **Benign carcinoid tumors of other sites**

     D3A.8   **Other benign neuroendocrine tumors**

         Neuroendocrine tumor NOS

Neoplasms of uncertain behavior, polycythemia vera and myelodysplastic syndromes (D37-D48)

`NOTE`   Categories D37-D44, and D48 classify by site neoplasms of uncertain behavior, i.e., histologic confirmation whether the neoplasm is malignant or benign cannot be made.

     EXCLUDES 1   neoplasms of unspecified behavior (D49.-)

✓4ᵗʰ **D37   Neoplasm of uncertain behavior of oral cavity and digestive organs**

     EXCLUDES 1   stromal tumors of uncertain behavior of digestive system (D48.1)

✓5ᵗʰ **D37.0   Neoplasm of uncertain behavior of** lip, oral cavity and pharynx

     EXCLUDES 1   neoplasm of uncertain behavior of aryepiglottic fold or interarytenoid fold, laryngeal aspect (D38.0)

                       neoplasm of uncertain behavior of epiglottis NOS (D38.0)

                       neoplasm of uncertain behavior of skin of lip (D48.5)

                       neoplasm of uncertain behavior of suprahyoid portion of epiglottis (D38.0)

     D37.01   **Neoplasm of uncertain behavior of** lip

             Neoplasm of uncertain behavior of vermilion border of lip

     D37.02   **Neoplasm of uncertain behavior of** tongue

     ✓6ᵗʰ D37.03   **Neoplasm of uncertain behavior of the** major salivary glands

         D37.030   **Neoplasm of uncertain behavior of the** parotid **salivary glands**

         D37.031   **Neoplasm of uncertain behavior of the** sublingual **salivary glands**

         D37.032   **Neoplasm of uncertain behavior of the** submandibular **salivary glands**

         D37.039   **Neoplasm of uncertain behavior of the major salivary glands, unspecified**

     D37.04   **Neoplasm of uncertain behavior of the** minor salivary glands

         Neoplasm of uncertain behavior of submucosal salivary glands of lip

         Neoplasm of uncertain behavior of submucosal salivary glands of cheek

         Neoplasm of uncertain behavior of submucosal salivary glands of hard palate

         Neoplasm of uncertain behavior of submucosal salivary glands of soft palate

     D37.05   **Neoplasm of uncertain behavior of** pharynx

         Neoplasm of uncertain behavior of aryepiglottic fold of pharynx NOS

         Neoplasm of uncertain behavior of hypopharyngeal aspect of aryepiglottic fold of pharynx

         Neoplasm of uncertain behavior of marginal zone of aryepiglottic fold of pharynx

     D37.09   **Neoplasm of uncertain behavior of other specified sites of the oral cavity**

D37.1   **Neoplasm of uncertain behavior of** stomach

D37.2   **Neoplasm of uncertain behavior of** small intestine

D37.3   **Neoplasm of uncertain behavior of** appendix

D37.4   **Neoplasm of uncertain behavior of** colon

D37.5   **Neoplasm of uncertain behavior of** rectum

     Neoplasm of uncertain behavior of rectosigmoid junction

✔ Additional Character Required   ✓x7ᵗʰ Placeholder Alert   Manifestation   Unspecified Dx   ►◄ Revised Text   ● New Code   ▲ Revised Code Title

ICD-10-CM 2020   493

Chapter 2. Neoplasms

D37.6–D44.0

D37.6 Neoplasm of uncertain behavior of liver, gallbladder and bile ducts

Neoplasm of uncertain behavior of ampulla of Vater

D37.8 Neoplasm of uncertain behavior of other specified digestive organs

Neoplasm of uncertain behavior of anal canal

Neoplasm of uncertain behavior of anal sphincter

Neoplasm of uncertain behavior of anus NOS

Neoplasm of uncertain behavior of esophagus

Neoplasm of uncertain behavior of intestine NOS

Neoplasm of uncertain behavior of pancreas

EXCLUDES 1 *neoplasm of uncertain behavior of anal margin (D48.5)*

neoplasm of uncertain behavior of anal skin (D48.5)

neoplasm of uncertain behavior of perianal skin (D48.5)

D37.9 Neoplasm of uncertain behavior of digestive organ, unspecified

✓4ᵗʰ **D38** Neoplasm of uncertain behavior of middle ear and respiratory and intrathoracic organs

EXCLUDES 1 *neoplasm of uncertain behavior of heart (D48.7)*

D38.0 Neoplasm of uncertain behavior of larynx

Neoplasm of uncertain behavior of aryepiglottic fold or interarytenoid fold, laryngeal aspect

Neoplasm of uncertain behavior of epiglottis (suprahyoid portion)

EXCLUDES 1 *neoplasm of uncertain behavior of aryepiglottic fold or interarytenoid fold NOS (D37.05)*

neoplasm of uncertain behavior of hypopharyngeal aspect of aryepiglottic fold (D37.05)

neoplasm of uncertain behavior of marginal zone of aryepiglottic fold (D37.05)

D38.1 Neoplasm of uncertain behavior of trachea, bronchus and lung

D38.2 Neoplasm of uncertain behavior of pleura

D38.3 Neoplasm of uncertain behavior of mediastinum

D38.4 Neoplasm of uncertain behavior of thymus

D38.5 Neoplasm of uncertain behavior of other respiratory organs

Neoplasm of uncertain behavior of accessory sinuses

Neoplasm of uncertain behavior of cartilage of nose

Neoplasm of uncertain behavior of middle ear

Neoplasm of uncertain behavior of nasal cavities

EXCLUDES 1 *neoplasm of uncertain behavior of ear (external) (skin) (D48.5)*

neoplasm of uncertain behavior of nose NOS (D48.7)

neoplasm of uncertain behavior of skin of nose (D48.5)

D38.6 Neoplasm of uncertain behavior of respiratory organ, unspecified

✓4ᵗʰ **D39** Neoplasm of uncertain behavior of female genital organs

D39.0 Neoplasm of uncertain behavior of uterus   ♀

✓5ᵗʰ **D39.1** Neoplasm of uncertain behavior of ovary   ♀

Use additional code to identify any functional activity

D39.10 Neoplasm of uncertain behavior of unspecified ovary   ♀

D39.11 Neoplasm of uncertain behavior of right ovary   ♀

D39.12 Neoplasm of uncertain behavior of left ovary   ♀

D39.2 Neoplasm of uncertain behavior of placenta   M ♀

Chorioadenoma destruens

Invasive hydatidiform mole

Malignant hydatidiform mole

EXCLUDES 1 *hydatidiform mole NOS (O01.9)*

D39.8 Neoplasm of uncertain behavior of other specified female genital organs   ♀

Neoplasm of uncertain behavior of skin of female genital organs

D39.9 Neoplasm of uncertain behavior of female genital organ, unspecified   ♀

✓4ᵗʰ **D40** Neoplasm of uncertain behavior of male genital organs

D40.0 Neoplasm of uncertain behavior of prostate   ♂

✓5ᵗʰ **D40.1** Neoplasm of uncertain behavior of testis

D40.10 Neoplasm of uncertain behavior of unspecified testis   ♂

D40.11 Neoplasm of uncertain behavior of right testis   ♂

D40.12 Neoplasm of uncertain behavior of left testis   ♂

D40.8 Neoplasm of uncertain behavior of other specified male genital organs   ♂

Neoplasm of uncertain behavior of skin of male genital organs

D40.9 Neoplasm of uncertain behavior of male genital organ, unspecified   ♂

✓4ᵗʰ **D41** Neoplasm of uncertain behavior of urinary organs

✓5ᵗʰ **D41.0** Neoplasm of uncertain behavior of kidney

EXCLUDES 1 *neoplasm of uncertain behavior of renal pelvis (D41.1-)*

D41.00 Neoplasm of uncertain behavior of unspecified kidney

D41.01 Neoplasm of uncertain behavior of right kidney

D41.02 Neoplasm of uncertain behavior of left kidney

✓5ᵗʰ **D41.1** Neoplasm of uncertain behavior of renal pelvis

D41.10 Neoplasm of uncertain behavior of unspecified renal pelvis

D41.11 Neoplasm of uncertain behavior of right renal pelvis

D41.12 Neoplasm of uncertain behavior of left renal pelvis

✓5ᵗʰ **D41.2** Neoplasm of uncertain behavior of ureter

D41.20 Neoplasm of uncertain behavior of unspecified ureter

D41.21 Neoplasm of uncertain behavior of right ureter

D41.22 Neoplasm of uncertain behavior of left ureter

D41.3 Neoplasm of uncertain behavior of urethra

D41.4 Neoplasm of uncertain behavior of bladder

D41.8 Neoplasm of uncertain behavior of other specified urinary organs

D41.9 Neoplasm of uncertain behavior of unspecified urinary organ

✓4ᵗʰ **D42** Neoplasm of uncertain behavior of meninges

D42.0 Neoplasm of uncertain behavior of cerebral meninges   HCC

D42.1 Neoplasm of uncertain behavior of spinal meninges   HCC

D42.9 Neoplasm of uncertain behavior of meninges, unspecified   HCC

✓4ᵗʰ **D43** Neoplasm of uncertain behavior of brain and central nervous system

EXCLUDES 1 *neoplasm of uncertain behavior of peripheral nerves and autonomic nervous system (D48.2)*

D43.0 Neoplasm of uncertain behavior of brain, supratentorial   HCC

Neoplasm of uncertain behavior of cerebral ventricle

Neoplasm of uncertain behavior of cerebrum

Neoplasm of uncertain behavior of frontal lobe

Neoplasm of uncertain behavior of occipital lobe

Neoplasm of uncertain behavior of parietal lobe

Neoplasm of uncertain behavior of temporal lobe

EXCLUDES 1 *neoplasm of uncertain behavior of fourth ventricle (D43.1)*

D43.1 Neoplasm of uncertain behavior of brain, infratentorial   HCC

Neoplasm of uncertain behavior of brain stem

Neoplasm of uncertain behavior of cerebellum

Neoplasm of uncertain behavior of fourth ventricle

D43.2 Neoplasm of uncertain behavior of brain, unspecified   HCC

D43.3 Neoplasm of uncertain behavior of cranial nerves   HCC

D43.4 Neoplasm of uncertain behavior of spinal cord   HCC

D43.8 Neoplasm of uncertain behavior of other specified parts of central nervous system   HCC

D43.9 Neoplasm of uncertain behavior of central nervous system, unspecified   HCC

Neoplasm of uncertain behavior of nervous system (central) NOS

✓4ᵗʰ **D44** Neoplasm of uncertain behavior of endocrine glands

EXCLUDES 1 *multiple endocrine adenomatosis (E31.2-)*

multiple endocrine neoplasia (E31.2-)

neoplasm of uncertain behavior of endocrine pancreas (D37.8)

neoplasm of uncertain behavior of ovary (D39.1-)

neoplasm of uncertain behavior of testis (D40.1-)

neoplasm of uncertain behavior of thymus (D38.4)

D44.0 Neoplasm of uncertain behavior of thyroid gland

✓5ᵗʰ **D44.1** **Neoplasm of uncertain behavior of** adrenal gland

Use additional code to identify any functional activity

     D44.10 **Neoplasm of uncertain behavior of unspecified adrenal gland**

     D44.11 **Neoplasm of uncertain behavior of** right **adrenal gland**

     D44.12 **Neoplasm of uncertain behavior of** left **adrenal gland**

D44.2 **Neoplasm of uncertain behavior of** parathyroid gland

D44.3 **Neoplasm of uncertain behavior of** pituitary gland   HCC

Use additional code to identify any functional activity

D44.4 **Neoplasm of uncertain behavior of craniopharyngeal duct**   HCC

D44.5 **Neoplasm of uncertain behavior of** pineal gland   HCC

D44.6 **Neoplasm of uncertain behavior of** carotid body   HCC

D44.7 **Neoplasm of uncertain behavior of** aortic body and other paraganglia   HCC

AHA: 2016,4Q,26

D44.9 **Neoplasm of uncertain behavior of unspecified endocrine gland**

D45 **Polycythemia vera**   HCC

EXCLUDES 1   familial polycythemia (D75.0)

             secondary polycythemia (D75.1)

DEF: Abnormal proliferation of all bone marrow elements, increased red cell mass, and total blood volume. The etiology is unknown, but it is frequently associated with splenomegaly, leukocytosis, and thrombocythemia.

✓4ᵗʰ **D46** **Myelodysplastic syndromes**

Use additional code for adverse effect, if applicable, to identify drug (T36-T50 with fifth or sixth character 5)

EXCLUDES 2   drug-induced aplastic anemia (D61.1)

D46.0 **Refractory anemia** without ring sideroblasts, **so stated**   HCC

Refractory anemia without sideroblasts, without excess of blasts

D46.1 **Refractory anemia** with ring sideroblasts   HCC

RARS

✓5ᵗʰ **D46.2** **Refractory anemia** with excess of blasts [RAEB]

     D46.20 **Refractory anemia with excess of blasts, unspecified**   HCC

RAEB NOS

     D46.21 **Refractory anemia with excess of** blasts 1   HCC

RAEB 1

     D46.22 **Refractory anemia with excess of** blasts 2   HCC

RAEB 2

D46.A **Refractory** cytopenia with multilineage dysplasia   HCC

D46.B **Refractory** cytopenia with multilineage dysplasia and ring sideroblasts   HCC

RCMD RS

D46.C **Myelodysplastic syndrome** with isolated del(5q) **chromosomal abnormality**   HCC

Myelodysplastic syndrome with 5q deletion

5q minus syndrome NOS

D46.4 **Refractory anemia, unspecified**   HCC

D46.Z **Other myelodysplastic syndromes**   HCC

EXCLUDES 1   chronic myelomonocytic leukemia (C93.1-)

D46.9 **Myelodysplastic syndrome, unspecified**   HCC

Myelodysplasia NOS

✓4ᵗʰ **D47** **Other neoplasms of uncertain behavior of** lymphoid, hematopoietic and related tissue

✓5ᵗʰ **D47.0** **Mast cell neoplasms of uncertain behavior**

EXCLUDES 1   congenital cutaneous mastocytosis (Q82.2)

             histiocytic neoplasms of uncertain behavior (D47.Z9)

             malignant mast cell neoplasm (C96.2-)

AHA: 2017,4Q,5

     D47.01 **Cutaneous mastocytosis**

Diffuse cutaneous mastocytosis

Maculopapular cutaneous mastocytosis

Solitary mastocytoma

Telangiectasia macularis eruptiva perstans

Urticaria pigmentosa

EXCLUDES 1   congenital (diffuse) (maculopapular) cutaneous mastocytosis (Q82.2)

             congenital urticaria pigmentosa (Q82.2)

             extracutaneous mastocytoma (D47.09)

     D47.02 **Systemic mastocytosis**

Indolent systemic mastocytosis

Isolated bone marrow mastocytosis

Smoldering systemic mastocytosis

Systemic mastocytosis, with an associated hematological non-mast cell lineage disease (SM-AHNMD)

Code also, if applicable, any associated hematological non-mast cell lineage disease, such as:

acute myeloid leukemia (C92.6-, C92.A-)

chronic myelomonocytic leukemia (C93.1-)

essential thrombocytosis (D47.3)

hypereosinophilic syndrome (D72.1)

myelodysplastic syndrome (D46.9)

myeloproliferative syndrome (D47.1)

non-Hodgkin lymphoma (C82-C85)

plasma cell myeloma (C90.0-)

polycythemia vera (D45)

EXCLUDES 1   aggressive systemic mastocytosis (C96.21)

             mast cell leukemia (C94.3-)

     D47.09 **Other mast cell neoplasms of uncertain behavior**

Extracutaneous mastocytoma

Mast cell tumor NOS

Mastocytoma NOS

Mastocytosis NOS

D47.1 **Chronic myeloproliferative disease**   HCC

Chronic neutrophilic leukemia

Myeloproliferative disease, unspecified

EXCLUDES 1   atypical chronic myeloid leukemia BCR/ABL-negative (C92.2-)

             chronic myeloid leukemia BCR/ABL-positive (C92.1-)

             myelofibrosis NOS (D75.81)

             myelophthisic anemia (D61.82)

             myelophthisis (D61.82)

             secondary myelofibrosis NOS (D75.81)

D47.2 **Monoclonal gammopathy**

Monoclonal gammopathy of undetermined significance [MGUS]

D47.3 **Essential (hemorrhagic) thrombocythemia**   HCC

Essential thrombocytosis

Idiopathic hemorrhagic thrombocythemia

DEF: Chronic myeloproliferative neoplasm involving production of excess blood platelets that may result in abnormal clotting or hemorrhaging.

D47.4 **Osteomyelofibrosis**   HCC

Chronic idiopathic myelofibrosis

Myelofibrosis (idiopathic) (with myeloid metaplasia)

Myelosclerosis (megakaryocytic) with myeloid metaplasia

Secondary myelofibrosis in myeloproliferative disease

EXCLUDES 1   acute myelofibrosis (C94.4-)

☑ Additional Character Required   ✓x7ᵗʰ Placeholder Alert   Manifestation   Unspecified Dx   ▶◀ Revised Text   ● New Code   ▲ Revised Code Title

ICD-10-CM 2020   495

Chapter 2. Neoplasms (side margin)

D47.Z–D49.7 (side margin)

✓5ᵗʰ **D47.Z Other specified neoplasms of uncertain behavior of lymphoid, hematopoietic and related tissue**
AHA: 2016,4Q,8

D47.Z1 Post-transplant lymphoproliferative disorder (PTLD) HCC
Code first complications of transplanted organs and tissue (T86.-)
DEF: Excessive proliferation of B-cell lymphocytes following Epstein-Barr virus infection in organ transplant patients. It may progress to non-Hodgkin lymphoma.

D47.Z2 Castleman disease HCC
Code also if applicable human herpesvirus 8 infection (B10.89)
EXCLUDES 2   Kaposi's sarcoma (C46-)
DEF: Rare disease of the lymph nodes and lymphoid tissues that closely mimics lymphoma.

D47.Z9 Other specified neoplasms of uncertain behavior of lymphoid, hematopoietic and related tissue HCC
Histiocytic tumors of uncertain behavior

D47.9 Neoplasm of uncertain behavior of lymphoid, hematopoietic and related tissue, unspecified HCC
Lymphoproliferative disease NOS

✓4ᵗʰ **D48 Neoplasm of uncertain behavior of other and unspecified sites**
EXCLUDES 1   neurofibromatosis (nonmalignant) (Q85.0-)

D48.0 Neoplasm of uncertain behavior of bone and articular cartilage
EXCLUDES 1   neoplasm of uncertain behavior of cartilage of ear (D48.1)
neoplasm of uncertain behavior of cartilage of larynx (D38.0)
neoplasm of uncertain behavior of cartilage of nose (D38.5)
neoplasm of uncertain behavior of connective tissue of eyelid (D48.1)
neoplasm of uncertain behavior of synovia (D48.1)

D48.1 Neoplasm of uncertain behavior of connective and other soft tissue
Neoplasm of uncertain behavior of connective tissue of ear
Neoplasm of uncertain behavior of connective tissue of eyelid
Stromal tumors of uncertain behavior of digestive system
EXCLUDES 1   neoplasm of uncertain behavior of articular cartilage (D48.0)
neoplasm of uncertain behavior of cartilage of larynx (D38.0)
neoplasm of uncertain behavior of cartilage of nose (D38.5)
neoplasm of uncertain behavior of connective tissue of breast (D48.6-)

D48.2 Neoplasm of uncertain behavior of peripheral nerves and autonomic nervous system
EXCLUDES 1   neoplasm of uncertain behavior of peripheral nerves of orbit (D48.7)

D48.3 Neoplasm of uncertain behavior of retroperitoneum

D48.4 Neoplasm of uncertain behavior of peritoneum

D48.5 Neoplasm of uncertain behavior of skin
Neoplasm of uncertain behavior of anal margin
Neoplasm of uncertain behavior of anal skin
Neoplasm of uncertain behavior of perianal skin
Neoplasm of uncertain behavior of skin of breast
EXCLUDES 1   neoplasm of uncertain behavior of anus NOS (D37.8)
neoplasm of uncertain behavior of skin of genital organs (D39.8, D40.8)
neoplasm of uncertain behavior of vermilion border of lip (D37.0)

✓5ᵗʰ **D48.6 Neoplasm of uncertain behavior of breast**
Neoplasm of uncertain behavior of connective tissue of breast
Cystosarcoma phyllodes
EXCLUDES 1   neoplasm of uncertain behavior of skin of breast (D48.5)

D48.60 Neoplasm of uncertain behavior of unspecified breast

D48.61 Neoplasm of uncertain behavior of right breast

D48.62 Neoplasm of uncertain behavior of left breast

D48.7 Neoplasm of uncertain behavior of other specified sites
Neoplasm of uncertain behavior of eye
Neoplasm of uncertain behavior of heart
Neoplasm of uncertain behavior of peripheral nerves of orbit
EXCLUDES 1   neoplasm of uncertain behavior of connective tissue (D48.1)
neoplasm of uncertain behavior of skin of eyelid (D48.5)

D48.9 Neoplasm of uncertain behavior, unspecified

Neoplasms of unspecified behavior (D49)

✓4ᵗʰ **D49 Neoplasms of unspecified behavior**

NOTE   Category D49 classifies by site neoplasms of unspecified morphology and behavior. The term "mass", unless otherwise stated, is not to be regarded as a neoplastic growth.

INCLUDES   "growth" NOS
neoplasm NOS
new growth NOS
tumor NOS

EXCLUDES 1   neoplasms of uncertain behavior (D37-D44, D48)

D49.0 Neoplasm of unspecified behavior of digestive system
EXCLUDES 1   neoplasm of unspecified behavior of margin of anus (D49.2)
neoplasm of unspecified behavior of perianal skin (D49.2)
neoplasm of unspecified behavior of skin of anus (D49.2)

D49.1 Neoplasm of unspecified behavior of respiratory system

D49.2 Neoplasm of unspecified behavior of bone, soft tissue, and skin
EXCLUDES 1   neoplasm of unspecified behavior of anal canal (D49.0)
neoplasm of unspecified behavior of anus NOS (D49.0)
neoplasm of unspecified behavior of bone marrow (D49.89)
neoplasm of unspecified behavior of cartilage of larynx (D49.1)
neoplasm of unspecified behavior of cartilage of nose (D49.1)
neoplasm of unspecified behavior of connective tissue of breast (D49.3)
neoplasm of unspecified behavior of skin of genital organs (D49.59)
neoplasm of unspecified behavior of vermilion border of lip (D49.0)

D49.3 Neoplasm of unspecified behavior of breast
EXCLUDES 1   neoplasm of unspecified behavior of skin of breast (D49.2)

D49.4 Neoplasm of unspecified behavior of bladder

✓5ᵗʰ **D49.5 Neoplasm of unspecified behavior of other genitourinary organs**
AHA: 2016,4Q,9

✓6ᵗʰ **D49.51 Neoplasm of unspecified behavior of kidney**

D49.511 Neoplasm of unspecified behavior of right kidney

D49.512 Neoplasm of unspecified behavior of left kidney

D49.519 Neoplasm of unspecified behavior of unspecified kidney

D49.59 Neoplasm of unspecified behavior of other genitourinary organ

D49.6 Neoplasm of unspecified behavior of brain HCC
EXCLUDES 1   neoplasm of unspecified behavior of cerebral meninges (D49.7)
neoplasm of unspecified behavior of cranial nerves (D49.7)

D49.7 Neoplasm of unspecified behavior of endocrine glands and other parts of nervous system
EXCLUDES 1   neoplasm of unspecified behavior of peripheral, sympathetic, and parasympathetic nerves and ganglia (D49.2)

√5ᵗʰ **D49.8 Neoplasm of unspecified behavior of other specified sites**

EXCLUDES 1   *neoplasm of unspecified behavior of eyelid (skin) (D49.2)*

      neoplasm of unspecified behavior of eyelid cartilage (D49.2)

      neoplasm of unspecified behavior of great vessels (D49.2)

      neoplasm of unspecified behavior of optic nerve (D49.7)

D49.81 Neoplasm of unspecified behavior of retina and choroid

     Dark area on retina

     Retinal freckle

D49.89 Neoplasm of unspecified behavior of other specified sites

D49.9 Neoplasm of unspecified behavior of unspecified site

☑ Additional Character Required   √x7ᵗʰ Placeholder Alert   **Manifestation**   Unspecified Dx   ►◄ Revised Text   ● New Code   ▲ Revised Code Title

ICD-10-CM 2020   **497**

Chapter 3. Disease of the Blood and Blood-Forming Organs and Certain Disorders Involving the Immune Mechanism (D5Ø–D89)

Chapter-specific Guidelines with Coding Examples
Reserved for future guideline expansion.

Chapter 3. Diseases of the Blood and Blood-forming Organs and Certain Disorders Involving the Immune Mechanism (D50-D89)

EXCLUDES 2   autoimmune disease (systemic) NOS (M35.9)
certain conditions originating in the perinatal period (P00-P96)
complications of pregnancy, childbirth and the puerperium (O00-O9A)
congenital malformations, deformations and chromosomal abnormalities (Q00-Q99)
endocrine, nutritional and metabolic diseases (E00-E88)
human immunodeficiency virus [HIV] disease (B20)
injury, poisoning and certain other consequences of external causes (S00-T88)
neoplasms (C00-D49)
symptoms, signs and abnormal clinical and laboratory findings, not elsewhere classified (R00-R94)

This chapter contains the following blocks:

D50-D53   Nutritional anemias
D55-D59   Hemolytic anemias
D60-D64   Aplastic and other anemias and other bone marrow failure syndromes
D65-D69   Coagulation defects, purpura and other hemorrhagic conditions
D70-D77   Other disorders of blood and blood-forming organs
D78   Intraoperative and postprocedural complications of the spleen
D80-D89   Certain disorders involving the immune mechanism

Nutritional anemias (D50-D53)

DEF: Nutritional anemia: The result of inadequate intake or absorption of a vitamin or mineral that impacts the production of red blood cells or causes them to develop abnormally affecting the size and shape.
TIP: Documentation must identify a link between anemia and the nutritional deficiency; low levels of a particular nutrient may occur concurrently with anemia but not cause the anemia.

√4th **D50**   Iron **deficiency anemia**

     INCLUDES   asiderotic anemia
              hypochromic anemia

   D50.0   **Iron deficiency anemia** secondary to blood loss (chronic)
       Posthemorrhagic anemia (chronic)
       EXCLUDES 1   acute posthemorrhagic anemia (D62)
                  congenital anemia from fetal blood loss (P61.3)

   D50.1   **Sideropenic dysphagia**
       Kelly-Paterson syndrome
       Plummer-Vinson syndrome

   D50.8   **Other iron deficiency anemias**
       Iron deficiency anemia due to inadequate dietary iron intake

   D50.9   **Iron deficiency anemia, unspecified**

√4th **D51**   Vitamin B12 **deficiency anemia**

     EXCLUDES 1   vitamin B12 deficiency (E53.8)

   D51.0   **Vitamin B12 deficiency anemia due to** intrinsic factor **deficiency**
       Addison anemia
       Biermer anemia
       Pernicious (congenital) anemia
       Congenital intrinsic factor deficiency
       DEF: Chronic progressive anemia due to vitamin B12 malabsorption, caused by lack of secretion of intrinsic factor, which is produced by the gastric mucosa of the stomach.

   D51.1   **Vitamin B12 deficiency anemia due to** selective vitamin B12 **malabsorption with proteinuria**
       Imerslund (Gräsbeck) syndrome
       Megaloblastic hereditary anemia

   D51.2   **Transcobalamin II deficiency**

   D51.3   **Other dietary vitamin B12 deficiency anemia**
       Vegan anemia

   D51.8   **Other vitamin B12 deficiency anemias**

   D51.9   **Vitamin B12 deficiency anemia, unspecified**

√4th **D52**   Folate **deficiency anemia**

     EXCLUDES 1   folate deficiency without anemia (E53.8)
     DEF: Deficiency in a B complex vitamin needed for the production of healthy red blood cells. Lack of folate, or folic acid, and other absorption conditions can cause anemia resulting in large, misshapen red blood cells called megaloblasts.

   D52.0   **Dietary folate deficiency anemia**
       Nutritional megaloblastic anemia
       DEF: Result of a poor diet with inadequate intake of folate, which is needed to produce healthy red blood cells.

   D52.1   **Drug-induced folate deficiency anemia**
       Use additional code for adverse effect, if applicable, to identify drug (T36-T50 with fifth or sixth character 5)

   D52.8   **Other folate deficiency anemias**

   D52.9   **Folate deficiency anemia, unspecified**
       Folic acid deficiency anemia NOS

√4th **D53**   **Other nutritional anemias**

     INCLUDES   megaloblastic anemia unresponsive to vitamin B12 or folate therapy

   D53.0   **Protein deficiency anemia**
       Amino-acid deficiency anemia
       Orotaciduric anemia
       EXCLUDES 1   Lesch-Nyhan syndrome (E79.1)

   D53.1   **Other megaloblastic anemias, not elsewhere classified**
       Megaloblastic anemia NOS
       EXCLUDES 1   Di Guglielmo's disease (C94.0)

   D53.2   **Scorbutic anemia**
       EXCLUDES 1   scurvy (E54)

   D53.8   **Other specified nutritional anemias**
       Anemia associated with deficiency of copper
       Anemia associated with deficiency of molybdenum
       Anemia associated with deficiency of zinc
       EXCLUDES 1   nutritional deficiencies without anemia, such as:
                copper deficiency NOS (E61.0)
                molybdenum deficiency NOS (E61.5)
                zinc deficiency NOS (E60)

   D53.9   **Nutritional anemia, unspecified**
       Simple chronic anemia
       EXCLUDES 1   anemia NOS (D64.9)
       AHA: 2018,4Q,88

Hemolytic anemias (D55-D59)

√4th **D55**   **Anemia due to enzyme disorders**

     EXCLUDES 1   drug-induced enzyme deficiency anemia (D59.2)

   D55.0   **Anemia due to** glucose-6-phosphate dehydrogenase **[G6PD] deficiency**   HCC
       Favism
       G6PD deficiency anemia
       EXCLUDES 1   ▶glucose-6-phosphate dehydrogenase (G6PD) deficiency without anemia (D75.A)◀

   D55.1   **Anemia due to other disorders of** glutathione **metabolism**   HCC
       Anemia (due to) enzyme deficiencies, except G6PD, related to the hexose monophosphate [HMP] shunt pathway
       Anemia (due to) hemolytic nonspherocytic (hereditary), type I

   D55.2   **Anemia due to disorders of** glycolytic enzymes   HCC
       Hemolytic nonspherocytic (hereditary) anemia, type II
       Hexokinase deficiency anemia
       Pyruvate kinase [PK] deficiency anemia
       Triose-phosphate isomerase deficiency anemia
       EXCLUDES 1   disorders of glycolysis not associated with anemia (E74.8)

   D55.3   **Anemia due to disorders of** nucleotide metabolism   HCC

   D55.8   **Other anemias due to enzyme disorders**   HCC

   D55.9   **Anemia due to enzyme disorder, unspecified**   HCC

☑4ᵗʰ **D56 Thalassemia**

     EXCLUDES 1   *sickle-cell thalassemia (D57.4-)*

     DEF: Group of inherited disorders of hemoglobin metabolism causing mild to severe anemia. It is usually found in people of Mediterranean, African, Chinese, or Asian descent.

Thalassemia

Misshapen RBC

Misshapen RBC

Healthy RBC

    D56.Ø   Alpha thalassemia   HCC

     Alpha thalassemia major
     Hemoglobin H Constant Spring
     Hemoglobin H disease
     Hydrops fetalis due to alpha thalassemia
     Severe alpha thalassemia
     Triple gene defect alpha thalassemia
     Use additional code, if applicable, for hydrops fetalis due to alpha thalassemia (P56.99)

     EXCLUDES 1   *alpha thalassemia trait or minor (D56.3)*
                 asymptomatic alpha thalassemia (D56.3)
                 hydrops fetalis due to isoimmunization (P56.Ø)
                 hydrops fetalis not due to immune hemolysis (P83.2)

     DEF: HBA1 and HBA2 genetic variant of chromosome 16 prevalent among those of African and Southeast Asian descent. Alpha thalassemia is associated with a wide spectrum of anemic presentation and includes hemoglobin H disease subtypes.

    D56.1   Beta thalassemia   HCC

     Beta thalassemia major
     Cooley's anemia
     Homozygous beta thalassemia
     Severe beta thalassemia
     Thalassemia intermedia
     Thalassemia major

     EXCLUDES 1   *beta thalassemia minor (D56.3)*
                 beta thalassemia trait (D56.3)
                 delta-beta thalassemia (D56.2)
                 hemoglobin E-beta thalassemia (D56.5)
                 sickle-cell beta thalassemia (D57.4-)

    D56.2   Delta-beta thalassemia   HCC

     Homozygous delta-beta thalassemia
     EXCLUDES 1   *delta-beta thalassemia minor (D56.3)*
                 delta-beta thalassemia trait (D56.3)

    D56.3   Thalassemia minor

     Alpha thalassemia minor
     Alpha thalassemia silent carrier
     Alpha thalassemia trait
     Beta thalassemia minor
     Beta thalassemia trait
     Delta-beta thalassemia minor
     Delta-beta thalassemia trait
     Thalassemia trait NOS

     EXCLUDES 1   *alpha thalassemia (D56.Ø)*
                 beta thalassemia (D56.1)
                 delta-beta thalassemia (D56.2)
                 hemoglobin E-beta thalassemia (D56.5)
                 sickle-cell trait (D57.3)

     DEF: Solitary abnormal gene that identifies a carrier of the disease, yet with an absence of symptoms or a clinically mild anemic presentation.

    D56.4   Hereditary persistence of fetal hemoglobin [HPFH]   HCC

    D56.5   Hemoglobin E-beta thalassemia   HCC

     EXCLUDES 1   *beta thalassemia (D56.1)*
                 beta thalassemia minor (D56.3)
                 beta thalassemia trait (D56.3)
                 delta-beta thalassemia (D56.2)
                 delta-beta thalassemia trait (D56.3)
                 hemoglobin E disease (D58.2)
                 other hemoglobinopathies (D58.2)
                 sickle-cell beta thalassemia (D57.4-)

    D56.8   Other thalassemias   HCC

     Dominant thalassemia
     Hemoglobin C thalassemia
     Mixed thalassemia
     Thalassemia with other hemoglobinopathy

     EXCLUDES 1   *hemoglobin C disease (D58.2)*
                 hemoglobin E disease (D58.2)
                 other hemoglobinopathies (D58.2)
                 sickle-cell anemia (D57.-)
                 sickle-cell thalassemia (D57.4)

    D56.9   Thalassemia, unspecified

     Mediterranean anemia (with other hemoglobinopathy)

☑4ᵗʰ **D57 Sickle-cell disorders**

     Use additional code for any associated fever (R50.81)
     EXCLUDES 1   *other hemoglobinopathies (D58.-)*
     DEF: Severe, chronic inherited diseases caused by a genetic variation in hemoglobin protein of the red blood cell. The gene mutation causes the red blood cell to become hard, sticky, and crescent or sickle shaped making it harder for red blood cells to travel through the bloodstream disrupting blood flow and decreasing oxygen transport to tissues.

Sickle cell

Sickle cells

Normal RBCs

    ☑5ᵗʰ **D57.Ø   Hb-SS disease with crisis**

     Sickle-cell disease NOS with crisis
     Hb-SS disease with vasoocclusive pain

     D57.ØØ   Hb-SS disease with crisis, unspecified   HCC

     D57.Ø1   Hb-SS disease with acute chest syndrome   HCC

     D57.Ø2   Hb-SS disease with splenic sequestration   HCC

☑ Additional Character Required   ☑x7ᵗʰ Placeholder Alert   Manifestation   Unspecified Dx   ▶◀ Revised Text   ● New Code   ▲ Revised Code Title

Chapter 3. Diseases of the Blood and Blood-forming Organs

D57.1 Sickle-cell disease without crisis   HCC
Hb-SS disease without crisis
Sickle-cell anemia NOS
Sickle-cell disease NOS
Sickle-cell disorder NOS

✓5ᵗʰ **D57.2 Sickle-cell/Hb-C disease**
Hb-SC disease
Hb-S/Hb-C disease

     D57.20 Sickle-cell/Hb-C disease without crisis   HCC

✓6ᵗʰ   **D57.21 Sickle-cell/Hb-C disease with crisis**

         D57.211 Sickle-cell/Hb-C disease with acute chest syndrome   HCC

         D57.212 Sickle-cell/Hb-C disease with splenic sequestration   HCC

         D57.219 Sickle-cell/Hb-C disease with crisis, unspecified   HCC
Sickle-cell/Hb-C disease with crisis NOS

D57.3 Sickle-cell trait   HCC
Hb-S trait
Heterozygous hemoglobin S
DEF: Heterozygous genetic makeup characterized by one gene for normal hemoglobin and one for sickle-cell hemoglobin. The clinical disease is rarely present.

✓5ᵗʰ **D57.4 Sickle-cell thalassemia**
Sickle-cell beta thalassemia
Thalassemia Hb-S disease

     D57.40 Sickle-cell thalassemia without crisis   HCC
Microdrepanocytosis
Sickle-cell thalassemia NOS

✓6ᵗʰ   **D57.41 Sickle-cell thalassemia with crisis**
Sickle-cell thalassemia with vasoocclusive pain

         D57.411 Sickle-cell thalassemia with acute chest syndrome   HCC

         D57.412 Sickle-cell thalassemia with splenic sequestration   HCC

         D57.419 Sickle-cell thalassemia with crisis, unspecified   HCC
Sickle-cell thalassemia with crisis NOS

✓5ᵗʰ **D57.8 Other sickle-cell disorders**
Hb-SD disease
Hb-SE disease

     D57.80 Other sickle-cell disorders without crisis   HCC

✓6ᵗʰ   **D57.81 Other sickle-cell disorders with crisis**

         D57.811 Other sickle-cell disorders with acute chest syndrome   HCC

         D57.812 Other sickle-cell disorders with splenic sequestration   HCC

         D57.819 Other sickle-cell disorders with crisis, unspecified   HCC
Other sickle-cell disorders with crisis NOS

✓4ᵗʰ **D58 Other hereditary hemolytic anemias**
EXCLUDES 1   *hemolytic anemia of the newborn (P55.-)*

D58.0 Hereditary spherocytosis   HCC
Acholuric (familial) jaundice
Congenital (spherocytic) hemolytic icterus
Minkowski-Chauffard syndrome
DEF: Inherited condition caused by mutations to genes responsible for the production of proteins that form the membranes of red blood cells. The shape and flexibility of the red blood cell membrane is altered diminishing the cells ability to traverse the spleen, therefore becoming trapped and destroyed before the red blood cell has reached maturity.

D58.1 Hereditary elliptocytosis   HCC
Elliptocytosis (congenital)
Ovalocytosis (congenital) (hereditary)

D58.2 Other hemoglobinopathies   HCC
Abnormal hemoglobin NOS
Congenital Heinz body anemia
Hb-C disease
Hb-D disease
Hb-E disease
Hemoglobinopathy NOS
Unstable hemoglobin hemolytic disease
EXCLUDES 1   *familial polycythemia (D75.0)*
         Hb-M disease (D74.0)
         hemoglobin E-beta thalassemia (D56.5)
         hereditary persistence of fetal hemoglobin [HPFH] (D56.4)
         high-altitude polycythemia (D75.1)
         methemoglobinemia (D74.-)
         other hemoglobinopathies with thalassemia (D56.8)

D58.8 Other specified hereditary hemolytic anemias   HCC
Stomatocytosis

D58.9 Hereditary hemolytic anemia, unspecified   HCC

✓4ᵗʰ **D59 Acquired hemolytic anemia**
DEF: Non-hereditary anemia characterized by premature destruction of red blood cells caused by infectious organisms, poisons, and physical agents.

D59.0 Drug-induced autoimmune hemolytic anemia   HCC
Use additional code for adverse effect, if applicable, to identify drug (T36-T50 with fifth or sixth character 5)

D59.1 Other autoimmune hemolytic anemias   HCC
Autoimmune hemolytic disease (cold type) (warm type)
Chronic cold hemagglutinin disease
Cold agglutinin disease
Cold agglutinin hemoglobinuria
Cold type (secondary) (symptomatic) hemolytic anemia
Warm type (secondary) (symptomatic) hemolytic anemia
EXCLUDES 1   *Evans syndrome (D69.41)*
         hemolytic disease of newborn (P55.-)
         paroxysmal cold hemoglobinuria (D59.6)

D59.2 Drug-induced nonautoimmune hemolytic anemia   HCC
Drug-induced enzyme deficiency anemia
Use additional code for adverse effect, if applicable, to identify drug (T36-T50 with fifth or sixth character 5)

D59.3 Hemolytic-uremic syndrome   HCC
Use additional code to identify associated:
E. coli infection (B96.2-)
Pneumococcal pneumonia (J13)
Shigella dysenteriae (A03.9)
DEF: Condition typically precipitated by infection causing low platelets and destruction of red blood cells resulting in hemolytic anemia. This cell damage and blockage of renal capillaries lead to kidney failure. Mainly affects children.

D59.4 Other nonautoimmune hemolytic anemias   HCC
Mechanical hemolytic anemia
Microangiopathic hemolytic anemia
Toxic hemolytic anemia

D59.5 Paroxysmal nocturnal hemoglobinuria [Marchiafava-Micheli]   HCC
EXCLUDES 1   *hemoglobinuria NOS (R82.3)*

D59.6 Hemoglobinuria due to hemolysis from other external causes   HCC
Hemoglobinuria from exertion
March hemoglobinuria
Paroxysmal cold hemoglobinuria
Use additional code (Chapter 20) to identify external cause
EXCLUDES 1   *hemoglobinuria NOS (R82.3)*

D59.8 Other acquired hemolytic anemias   HCC

D59.9 Acquired hemolytic anemia, unspecified   HCC
Idiopathic hemolytic anemia, chronic

Aplastic and other anemias and other bone marrow failure syndromes (D60-D64)

✓4ᵗʰ D60 Acquired pure red cell aplasia [erythroblastopenia]

> **INCLUDES** red cell aplasia (acquired) (adult) (with thymoma)
> **EXCLUDES 1** congenital red cell aplasia (D61.01)
> **DEF:** Bone marrow failure characterized by underproduction of red blood cells while white blood cell and platelet production remains normal.

D60.0 Chronic acquired pure red cell aplasia   `HCC`

D60.1 Transient acquired pure red cell aplasia   `HCC`

D60.8 Other acquired pure red cell aplasias   `HCC`

D60.9 Acquired pure red cell aplasia, unspecified   `HCC`

✓4ᵗʰ D61 Other aplastic anemias and other bone marrow failure syndromes

> **EXCLUDES 1** neutropenia (D70.-)
> **AHA:** 2014,4Q,22
> **DEF:** Aplastic anemia: Bone marrow failure characterized by underproduction of red bloods cells, white blood cells and platelets.

✓5ᵗʰ D61.0 Constitutional aplastic anemia

D61.01 Constitutional (pure) red blood cell aplasia   `HCC`

Blackfan-Diamond syndrome
Congenital (pure) red cell aplasia
Familial hypoplastic anemia
Primary (pure) red cell aplasia
Red cell (pure) aplasia of infants
> **EXCLUDES 1** acquired red cell aplasia (D60.9)

D61.09 Other constitutional aplastic anemia   `HCC`

Fanconi's anemia
Pancytopenia with malformations

D61.1 Drug-induced aplastic anemia   `HCC`

Use additional code for adverse effect, if applicable, to identify drug (T36-T50 with fifth or sixth character 5)

D61.2 Aplastic anemia due to other external agents   `HCC`

Code first, if applicable, toxic effects of substances chiefly nonmedicinal as to source (T51-T65)

D61.3 Idiopathic aplastic anemia   `HCC`

✓5ᵗʰ D61.8 Other specified aplastic anemias and other bone marrow failure syndromes

✓6ᵗʰ D61.81 Pancytopenia

> **EXCLUDES 1** pancytopenia (due to) (with) aplastic anemia (D61.9)
> pancytopenia (due to) (with) bone marrow infiltration (D61.82)
> pancytopenia (due to) (with) congenital (pure) red cell aplasia (D61.01)
> pancytopenia (due to) (with) hairy cell leukemia (C91.4-)
> pancytopenia (due to) (with) human immunodeficiency virus disease (B20)
> pancytopenia (due to) (with) leukoerythroblastic anemia (D61.82)
> pancytopenia (due to) (with) myeloproliferative disease (D47.1)
> **EXCLUDES 2** pancytopenia (due to) (with) myelodysplastic syndromes (D46.-)
> **DEF:** Shortage of all three blood cells: white, red, and platelets.

D61.810 Antineoplastic chemotherapy induced pancytopenia   `HCC`

> **EXCLUDES 2** aplastic anemia due to antineoplastic chemotherapy (D61.1)

D61.811 Other drug-induced pancytopenia   `HCC`

> **EXCLUDES 2** aplastic anemia due to drugs (D61.1)

D61.818 Other pancytopenia   `HCC`

> **AHA:** 2019,1Q,16
> **TIP:** Assign this code in addition to myeloid leukemia codes (C92.-) when pancytopenia is documented. Although common in some types of myeloid leukemia, pancytopenia is not always inherent.

D61.82 Myelophthisis   `HCC`

Leukoerythroblastic anemia
Myelophthisic anemia
Panmyelophthisis
Code also the underlying disorder, such as:
  malignant neoplasm of breast (C50.-)
  tuberculosis (A15.-)
> **EXCLUDES 1** idiopathic myelofibrosis (D47.1)
> myelofibrosis NOS (D75.81)
> myelofibrosis with myeloid metaplasia (D47.4)
> primary myelofibrosis (D47.1)
> secondary myelofibrosis (D75.81)
> **DEF:** Condition that occurs when normal hematopoietic tissue in the bone marrow is replaced with abnormal tissue, such as fibrous tissue or tumors. Most commonly seen during the advanced stages of cancer.

D61.89 Other specified aplastic anemias and other bone marrow failure syndromes   `HCC`

D61.9 Aplastic anemia, unspecified   `HCC`

Hypoplastic anemia NOS
Medullary hypoplasia

D62 Acute posthemorrhagic anemia

> **EXCLUDES 1** anemia due to chronic blood loss (D50.0)
> blood loss anemia NOS (D50.0)
> congenital anemia from fetal blood loss (P61.3)

✓4ᵗʰ D63 Anemia in chronic diseases classified elsewhere

D63.0 Anemia in neoplastic disease

Code first neoplasm (C00-D49)
> **EXCLUDES 1** aplastic anemia due to antineoplastic chemotherapy (D61.1)
> **EXCLUDES 2** anemia due to antineoplastic chemotherapy (D64.81)

D63.1 Anemia in chronic kidney disease

Erythropoietin resistant anemia (EPO resistant anemia)
Code first underlying chronic kidney disease (CKD) (N18.-)

D63.8 Anemia in other chronic diseases classified elsewhere

Code first underlying disease, such as:
  diphyllobothriasis (B70.0)
  hookworm disease (B76.0-B76.9)
  hypothyroidism (E00.0-E03.9)
  malaria (B50.0-B54)
  symptomatic late syphilis (A52.79)
  tuberculosis (A18.89)

✓4ᵗʰ D64 Other anemias

> **EXCLUDES 1** refractory anemia (D46.-)
> refractory anemia with excess blasts in transformation [RAEB T] (C92.0-)
> **DEF:** Sideroblastic anemia: Hereditary or secondary disorder in which the red blood cells cannot effectively use iron, a nutrient needed to make hemoglobin. Although the iron can enter the red blood cell it is not assimilated into the hemoglobin molecule and builds up ringed sideroblasts around the cell nucleus.

D64.0 Hereditary sideroblastic anemia   `HCC`

Sex-linked hypochromic sideroblastic anemia

D64.1 Secondary sideroblastic anemia due to disease   `HCC`

Code first underlying disease

D64.2 Secondary sideroblastic anemia due to drugs and toxins   `HCC`

Code first poisoning due to drug or toxin, if applicable (T36-T65 with fifth or sixth character 1-4 or 6)
Use additional code for adverse effect, if applicable, to identify drug (T36-T50 with fifth or sixth character 5)

D64.3 Other sideroblastic anemias   `HCC`

Sideroblastic anemia NOS
Pyridoxine-responsive sideroblastic anemia NEC

D64.4 Congenital dyserythropoietic anemia

Dyshematopoietic anemia (congenital)
> **EXCLUDES 1** Blackfan-Diamond syndrome (D61.01)
> Di Guglielmo's disease (C94.0)

☑ Additional Character Required   ✓x7ᵗʰ Placeholder Alert   Manifestation   Unspecified Dx   ►◄ Revised Text   ● New Code   ▲ Revised Code Title

ICD-10-CM 2020   503

D64.8   Other specified anemias

D64.81   Anemia due to antineoplastic chemotherapy

Antineoplastic chemotherapy induced anemia

EXCLUDES 1   *aplastic anemia due to antineoplastic chemotherapy (D61.1)*

EXCLUDES 2   *anemia in neoplastic disease (D63.0)*

AHA: 2014,4Q,22

DEF: Reversible adverse effect of chemotherapy, causing inhibition of bone marrow production. A decrease in red blood cell production prevents adequate oxygenation of the tissues and organs causing fatigue, shortness of breath (SOB), and exacerbation of other medical conditions.

D64.89   Other specified anemias

Infantile pseudoleukemia

D64.9   Anemia, unspecified

AHA: 2018,4Q,88; 2017,1Q,7

Coagulation defects, purpura and other hemorrhagic conditions (D65-D69)

D65   Disseminated intravascular coagulation [defibrination syndrome]   HCC

Afibrinogenemia, acquired

Consumption coagulopathy

Diffuse or disseminated intravascular coagulation [DIC]

Fibrinolytic hemorrhage, acquired

Fibrinolytic purpura

Purpura fulminans

EXCLUDES 1   *disseminated intravascular coagulation (complicating):*

abortion or ectopic or molar pregnancy (O00-O07, O08.1)

in newborn (P60)

pregnancy, childbirth and the puerperium (O45.0, O46.0, O67.0, O72.3)

Coagulation

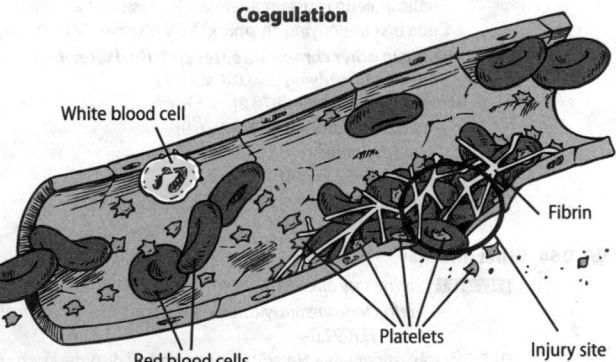

White blood cell

Fibrin

Platelets

Red blood cells

Injury site

D66   Hereditary factor VIII deficiency   HCC

Classical hemophilia

Deficiency factor VIII (with functional defect)

Hemophilia A

Hemophilia NOS

EXCLUDES 1   *factor VIII deficiency with vascular defect (D68.0)*

DEF: Hereditary, sex-linked lack of antihemophilic globulin (AHG) (factor VIII) that causes abnormal coagulation characterized by increased bleeding; large bruises of skin; bleeding in the mouth, nose, and gastrointestinal tract; and hemorrhages into joints, resulting in swelling and impaired function.

D67   Hereditary factor IX deficiency   HCC

Christmas disease

Factor IX deficiency (with functional defect)

Hemophilia B

Plasma thromboplastin component [PTC] deficiency

D68   Other coagulation defects

EXCLUDES 1   *abnormal coagulation profile (R79.1)*

coagulation defects complicating abortion or ectopic or molar pregnancy (O00-O07, O08.1)

coagulation defects complicating pregnancy, childbirth and the puerperium (O45.0, O46.0, O67.0, O72.3)

AHA: 2016,1Q,14

D68.0   Von Willebrand's disease   HCC

Angiohemophilia

Factor VIII deficiency with vascular defect

Vascular hemophilia

EXCLUDES 1   *capillary fragility (hereditary) (D69.8)*

factor VIII deficiency NOS (D66)

factor VIII deficiency with functional defect (D66)

DEF: Congenital, abnormal blood coagulation caused by deficient blood factor VII. Symptoms include excess or prolonged bleeding.

D68.1   Hereditary factor XI deficiency   HCC

Hemophilia C

Plasma thromboplastin antecedent [PTA] deficiency

Rosenthal's disease

D68.2   Hereditary deficiency of other clotting factors   HCC

AC globulin deficiency

Congenital afibrinogenemia

Deficiency of factor I [fibrinogen]

Deficiency of factor II [prothrombin]

Deficiency of factor V [labile]

Deficiency of factor VII [stable]

Deficiency of factor X [Stuart-Prower]

Deficiency of factor XII [Hageman]

Deficiency of factor XIII [fibrin stabilizing]

Dysfibrinogenemia (congenital)

Hypoproconvertinemia

Owren's disease

Proaccelerin deficiency

D68.3   Hemorrhagic disorder due to circulating anticoagulants

D68.31   Hemorrhagic disorder due to intrinsic circulating anticoagulants, antibodies, or inhibitors

D68.311   Acquired hemophilia   HCC

Autoimmune hemophilia

Autoimmune inhibitors to clotting factors

Secondary hemophilia

D68.312   Antiphospholipid antibody with hemorrhagic disorder   HCC

Lupus anticoagulant (LAC) with hemorrhagic disorder

Systemic lupus erythematosus [SLE] inhibitor with hemorrhagic disorder

EXCLUDES 1   *antiphospholipid antibody, finding without diagnosis (R76.0)*

antiphospholipid antibody syndrome (D68.61)

antiphospholipid antibody with hypercoagulable state (D68.61)

lupus anticoagulant (LAC) finding without diagnosis (R76.0)

lupus anticoagulant (LAC) with hypercoagulable state (D68.62)

systemic lupus erythematosus [SLE] inhibitor finding without diagnosis (R76.0)

systemic lupus erythematosus [SLE] inhibitor with hypercoagulable state (D68.62)

D68.318   **Other hemorrhagic disorder due to intrinsic circulating anticoagulants, antibodies, or inhibitors**   `HCC`

Antithromboplastinemia
Antithromboplastinogenemia
Hemorrhagic disorder due to intrinsic increase in antithrombin
Hemorrhagic disorder due to intrinsic increase in anti-VIIIa
Hemorrhagic disorder due to intrinsic increase in anti-IXa
Hemorrhagic disorder due to intrinsic increase in anti-XIa

D68.32   **Hemorrhagic disorder due to extrinsic circulating anticoagulants**   `HCC`

Drug-induced hemorrhagic disorder
Hemorrhagic disorder due to increase in anti-IIa
Hemorrhagic disorder due to increase in anti-Xa
Hyperheparinemia
Use additional code for adverse effect, if applicable, to identify drug (T45.515, T45.525)
AHA: 2016,1Q,14-15
TIP: Do not assign to identify routine therapeutic anticoagulation effects; assign only for documented adverse effects. An adverse effect code (T36–T50) identifying the specific therapeutic agent should also be assigned.

D68.4   **Acquired coagulation factor deficiency**   `HCC`

Deficiency of coagulation factor due to liver disease
Deficiency of coagulation factor due to vitamin K deficiency
EXCLUDES 1   *vitamin K deficiency of newborn (P53)*

✓5th **D68.5**   **Primary thrombophilia**

Primary hypercoagulable states
EXCLUDES 1   *antiphospholipid syndrome (D68.61)*
lupus anticoagulant (D68.62)
secondary activated protein C resistance (D68.69)
secondary antiphospholipid antibody syndrome (D68.69)
secondary lupus anticoagulant with hypercoagulable state (D68.69)
secondary systemic lupus erythematosus [SLE] inhibitor with hypercoagulable state (D68.69)
systemic lupus erythematosus [SLE] inhibitor finding without diagnosis (R76.0)
systemic lupus erythematosus [SLE] inhibitor with hemorrhagic disorder (D68.312)
thrombotic thrombocytopenic purpura (M31.1)
DEF: Thrombophilia: Increased tendency of the blood to clot, which can lead to thrombus or embolus formation.

D68.51   **Activated protein C resistance**   `HCC`

Factor V Leiden mutation

D68.52   **Prothrombin gene mutation**   `HCC`

D68.59   **Other primary thrombophilia**   `HCC`

Antithrombin III deficiency
Hypercoagulable state NOS
Primary hypercoagulable state NEC
Primary thrombophilia NEC
Protein C deficiency
Protein S deficiency
Thrombophilia NOS

✓5th **D68.6**   **Other thrombophilia**

Other hypercoagulable states
EXCLUDES 1   *diffuse or disseminated intravascular coagulation [DIC] (D65)*
heparin induced thrombocytopenia (HIT) (D75.82)
hyperhomocysteinemia (E72.11)

D68.61   **Antiphospholipid syndrome**   `HCC`

Anticardiolipin syndrome
Antiphospholipid antibody syndrome
EXCLUDES 1   *anti-phospholipid antibody, finding without diagnosis (R76.0)*
anti-phospholipid antibody with hemorrhagic disorder (D68.312)
lupus anticoagulant syndrome (D68.62)

D68.62   **Lupus anticoagulant syndrome**   `HCC`

Lupus anticoagulant
Presence of systemic lupus erythematosus [SLE] inhibitor
EXCLUDES 1   *anticardiolipin syndrome (D68.61)*
antiphospholipid syndrome (D68.61)
lupus anticoagulant (LAC) finding without diagnosis (R76.0)
lupus anticoagulant (LAC) with hemorrhagic disorder (D68.312)

D68.69   **Other thrombophilia**   `HCC`

Hypercoagulable states NEC
Secondary hypercoagulable state NOS

D68.8   **Other specified coagulation defects**   `HCC`

EXCLUDES 1   *hemorrhagic disease of newborn (P53)*

D68.9   **Coagulation defect, unspecified**   `HCC`

✓4th **D69**   **Purpura and other hemorrhagic conditions**

EXCLUDES 1   *benign hypergammaglobulinemic purpura (D89.0)*
cryoglobulinemic purpura (D89.1)
essential (hemorrhagic) thrombocythemia (D47.3)
hemorrhagic thrombocythemia (D47.3)
purpura fulminans (D65)
thrombotic thrombocytopenic purpura (M31.1)
Waldenström hypergammaglobulinemic purpura (D89.0)

D69.0   **Allergic purpura**   `HCC`

Allergic vasculitis
Nonthrombocytopenic hemorrhagic purpura
Nonthrombocytopenic idiopathic purpura
Purpura anaphylactoid
Purpura Henoch(-Schönlein)
Purpura rheumatica
Vascular purpura
EXCLUDES 1   *thrombocytopenic hemorrhagic purpura (D69.3)*
DEF: Any hemorrhagic condition, thrombocytic or nonthrombocytopenic in origin, caused by a presumed allergic reaction.

D69.1   **Qualitative platelet defects**   `HCC`

Bernard Soulier [giant platelet] syndrome
Glanzmann's disease
Grey platelet syndrome
Thromboasthenia (hemorrhagic) (hereditary)
Thrombocytopathy
EXCLUDES 1   *von Willebrand's disease (D68.0)*

D69.2   **Other nonthrombocytopenic purpura**   `HCC`

Purpura NOS
Purpura simplex
Senile purpura

D69.3   **Immune thrombocytopenic purpura**   `HCC`

Hemorrhagic (thrombocytopenic) purpura
Idiopathic thrombocytopenic purpura
Tidal platelet dysgenesis
DEF: Tidal platelet dysgenesis: Fluctuation of platelet counts from normal to very low within periods of 20 to 40 days and may involve autoimmune platelet destruction.

✓5th **D69.4**   **Other primary thrombocytopenia**

EXCLUDES 1   *transient neonatal thrombocytopenia (P61.0)*
Wiskott-Aldrich syndrome (D82.0)

D69.41   **Evans syndrome**   `HCC`

D69.42   **Congenital and hereditary thrombocytopenia purpura**   `HCC`

Congenital thrombocytopenia
Hereditary thrombocytopenia
Code first congenital or hereditary disorder, such as:
thrombocytopenia with absent radius (TAR syndrome) (Q87.2)

D69.49   **Other primary thrombocytopenia**   `HCC`

Megakaryocytic hypoplasia
Primary thrombocytopenia NOS

✓ Additional Character Required   ✓x7th Placeholder Alert   Manifestation   Unspecified Dx   ►◄ Revised Text   ● New Code   ▲ Revised Code Title

ICD-10-CM 2020   **505**

✓5ᵗʰ D69.5 Secondary thrombocytopenia

> EXCLUDES 1 heparin induced thrombocytopenia (HIT) (D75.82)
> transient thrombocytopenia of newborn (P61.0)

D69.51 Posttransfusion purpura
Posttransfusion purpura from whole blood (fresh) or blood products
PTP

D69.59　Other secondary thrombocytopenia
AHA: 2014,4Q,22

D69.6 Thrombocytopenia, unspecified　　HCC

D69.8 Other specified hemorrhagic conditions　　HCC
Capillary fragility (hereditary)
Vascular pseudohemophilia

D69.9 Hemorrhagic condition, unspecified　　HCC

Other disorders of blood and blood-forming organs (D70-D77)

✓4ᵗʰ D70 Neutropenia

> INCLUDES agranulocytosis
> decreased absolute neurophile count (ANC)

Use additional code for any associated:
  fever (R50.81)
  mucositis (J34.81, K12.3-, K92.81, N76.81)

> EXCLUDES 1 neutropenic splenomegaly (D73.81)
> transient neonatal neutropenia (P61.5)

DEF: Abnormally low number of neutrophils. Neutrophils are phagocytic, meaning they surround and consume harmful pathogens, primarily bacteria. When neutrophil counts decrease the risk of infection increases.

D70.0 Congenital agranulocytosis　　HCC
Congenital neutropenia
Infantile genetic agranulocytosis
Kostmann's disease

D70.1 Agranulocytosis secondary to cancer chemotherapy　　HCC
Code also underlying neoplasm
Use additional code for adverse effect, if applicable, to identify drug (T45.1X5)
AHA: 2014,4Q,22

D70.2 Other drug-induced agranulocytosis　　HCC
Use additional code for adverse effect, if applicable, to identify drug (T36-T50 with fifth or sixth character 5)

D70.3 Neutropenia due to infection　　HCC

D70.4 Cyclic neutropenia　　HCC
Cyclic hematopoiesis
Periodic neutropenia

D70.8 Other neutropenia　　HCC

D70.9 Neutropenia, unspecified　　HCC

D71 Functional disorders of polymorphonuclear neutrophils　　HCC
Cell membrane receptor complex [CR3] defect
Chronic (childhood) granulomatous disease
Congenital dysphagocytosis
Progressive septic granulomatosis

✓4ᵗʰ D72 Other disorders of white blood cells

> EXCLUDES 1 basophilia (D72.824)
> immunity disorders (D80-D89)
> neutropenia (D70)
> preleukemia (syndrome) (D46.9)

D72.0 Genetic anomalies of leukocytes　　HCC
Alder (granulation) (granulocyte) anomaly
Alder syndrome
Hereditary leukocytic hypersegmentation
Hereditary leukocytic hyposegmentation
Hereditary leukomelanopathy
May-Hegglin (granulation) (granulocyte) anomaly
May-Hegglin syndrome
Pelger-Huët (granulation) (granulocyte) anomaly
Pelger-Huët syndrome

> EXCLUDES 1 Chédiak (-Steinbrinck)-Higashi syndrome (E70.330)

D72.1 Eosinophilia
Allergic eosinophilia
Hereditary eosinophilia

> EXCLUDES 1 Löffler's syndrome (J82)
> pulmonary eosinophilia (J82)

✓5ᵗʰ D72.8 Other specified disorders of white blood cells

> EXCLUDES 1 leukemia (C91-C95)

✓6ᵗʰ D72.81 Decreased white blood cell count

> EXCLUDES 1 neutropenia (D70.-)

D72.810 Lymphocytopenia
Decreased lymphocytes

D72.818 Other decreased white blood cell count
Basophilic leukopenia
Eosinophilic leukopenia
Monocytopenia
Other decreased leukocytes
Plasmacytopenia

D72.819 Decreased white blood cell count, unspecified
Decreased leukocytes, unspecified
Leukocytopenia, unspecified
Leukopenia

> EXCLUDES 1 malignant leukopenia (D70.9)

✓6ᵗʰ D72.82 Elevated white blood cell count

> EXCLUDES 1 eosinophilia (D72.1)

D72.820 Lymphocytosis (symptomatic)
Elevated lymphocytes

D72.821 Monocytosis (symptomatic)

> EXCLUDES 1 infectious mononucleosis (B27.-)

D72.822 Plasmacytosis

D72.823 Leukemoid reaction
Basophilic leukemoid reaction
Leukemoid reaction NOS
Lymphocytic leukemoid reaction
Monocytic leukemoid reaction
Myelocytic leukemoid reaction
Neutrophilic leukemoid reaction

D72.824 Basophilia
DEF: Increase in the basophils of the blood, a type of white blood cell, often seen in conjunction with neoplastic disorders.

D72.825 Bandemia
Bandemia without diagnosis of specific infection

> EXCLUDES 1 confirmed infection — code to infection
> leukemia (C91.-, C92.-, C93.-, C94.-, C95.-)

DEF: Increase in early neutrophil cells, called band cells that may indicate infection.

D72.828 Other elevated white blood cell count

D72.829 Elevated white blood cell count, unspecified
Elevated leukocytes, unspecified
Leukocytosis, unspecified

D72.89 Other specified disorders of white blood cells
Abnormality of white blood cells NEC

D72.9 Disorder of white blood cells, unspecified
Abnormal leukocyte differential NOS

✓4ᵗʰ D73 Diseases of spleen

D73.0 Hyposplenism
Atrophy of spleen

> EXCLUDES 1 asplenia (congenital) (Q89.01)
> postsurgical absence of spleen (Z90.81)

D73.1 Hypersplenism

> EXCLUDES 1 neutropenic splenomegaly (D73.81)
> primary splenic neutropenia (D73.81)
> splenitis, splenomegaly in late syphilis (A52.79)
> splenitis, splenomegaly in tuberculosis (A18.85)
> splenomegaly NOS (R16.1)
> splenomegaly congenital (Q89.0)

D73.2 Chronic congestive splenomegaly

D73.3 Abscess of spleen

D73.4 Cyst of spleen

D73.5 Infarction of spleen
Splenic rupture, nontraumatic
Torsion of spleen

> EXCLUDES 1 rupture of spleen due to Plasmodium vivax malaria (B51.0)
> traumatic rupture of spleen (S36.03-)

☑5ᵗʰ **D73.8** **Other diseases of spleen**

    D73.81 **Neutropenic splenomegaly**
        Werner-Schultz disease

    D73.89 **Other diseases of spleen**
        Fibrosis of spleen NOS
        Perisplenitis
        Splenitis NOS

D73.9 **Disease of spleen, unspecified**

☑4ᵗʰ **D74** **Methemoglobinemia**

    D74.0 **Congenital methemoglobinemia**
        Congenital NADH-methemoglobin reductase deficiency
        Hemoglobin-M [Hb-M] disease
        Methemoglobinemia, hereditary

    D74.8 **Other methemoglobinemias**
        Acquired methemoglobinemia (with sulfhemoglobinemia)
        Toxic methemoglobinemia

    D74.9 **Methemoglobinemia, unspecified**

☑4ᵗʰ **D75** **Other and unspecified diseases of blood and blood-forming organs**

    EXCLUDES 2   *acute lymphadenitis (L04.-)*
        chronic lymphadenitis (I88.1)
        enlarged lymph nodes (R59.-)
        hypergammaglobulinemia NOS (D89.2)
        lymphadenitis NOS (I88.9)
        mesenteric lymphadenitis (acute) (chronic) (I88.0)

    D75.0 **Familial erythrocytosis**
        Benign polycythemia
        Familial polycythemia
      EXCLUDES 1 *hereditary ovalocytosis (D58.1)*

    D75.1 **Secondary polycythemia**
        Acquired polycythemia
        Emotional polycythemia
        Erythrocytosis NOS
        Hypoxemic polycythemia
        Nephrogenous polycythemia
        Polycythemia due to erythropoietin
        Polycythemia due to fall in plasma volume
        Polycythemia due to high altitude
        Polycythemia due to stress
        Polycythemia NOS
        Relative polycythemia
      EXCLUDES 1 *polycythemia neonatorum (P61.1)*
        polycythemia vera (D45)
        DEF: Elevated number of red blood cells in circulating blood as a result of reduced oxygen supply to the tissues.

☑5ᵗʰ **D75.8** **Other specified diseases of blood and blood-forming organs**

    D75.81 ***Myelofibrosis***   HCC
        Myelofibrosis NOS
        Secondary myelofibrosis NOS
        Code first the underlying disorder, such as:
          malignant neoplasm of breast (C50.-)
        Use additional code, if applicable, for associated
          therapy-related myelodysplastic syndrome
          (D46.-)
        Use additional code for adverse effect, if applicable,
          to identify drug (T45.1X5)
      EXCLUDES 1 *acute myelofibrosis (C94.4-)*
        idiopathic myelofibrosis (D47.1)
        leukoerythroblastic anemia (D61.82)
        myelofibrosis with myeloid metaplasia
          (D47.4)
        myelophthisic anemia (D61.82)
        myelophthisis (D61.82)
        primary myelofibrosis (D47.1)

    D75.82 **Heparin induced thrombocytopenia (HIT)**   HCC
        DEF: Immune-mediated reaction to heparin therapy causing an abrupt fall in platelet count and serious complications such as pulmonary embolism, stroke, AMI, or DVT.

    D75.89 **Other specified diseases of blood and blood-forming organs**

D75.9 **Disease of blood and blood-forming organs, unspecified**

● **D75.A** **Glucose-6-phosphate dehydrogenase (G6PD) deficiency without anemia**
      EXCLUDES 1 *glucose-6-phosphate dehydrogenase (G6PD)*
        deficiency with anemia (D55.0)

☑4ᵗʰ **D76** **Other specified diseases with participation of lymphoreticular and reticulohistiocytic tissue**

    EXCLUDES 1 *(Abt-) Letterer-Siwe disease (C96.0)*
        eosinophilic granuloma (C96.6)
        Hand-Schüller-Christian disease (C96.5)
        histiocytic medullary reticulosis (C96.9)
        histiocytic sarcoma (C96.A)
        histiocytosis X, multifocal (C96.5)
        histiocytosis X, unifocal (C96.6)
        Langerhans-cell histiocytosis, multifocal (C96.5)
        Langerhans-cell histiocytosis NOS (C96.6)
        Langerhans-cell histiocytosis, unifocal (C96.6)
        leukemic reticuloendotheliosis (C91.4-)
        lipomelanotic reticulosis (I89.8)
        malignant histiocytosis (C96.A)
        malignant reticulosis (C86.0)
        nonlipid reticuloendotheliosis (C96.0)

    D76.1 **Hemophagocytic lymphohistiocytosis**   HCC
        Familial hemophagocytic reticulosis
        Histiocytoses of mononuclear phagocytes

    D76.2 **Hemophagocytic syndrome, infection-associated**   HCC
        Use additional code to identify infectious agent or disease

    D76.3 **Other histiocytosis syndromes**   HCC
        Reticulohistiocytoma (giant-cell)
        Sinus histiocytosis with massive lymphadenopathy
        Xanthogranuloma

D77 ***Other disorders of blood and blood-forming organs in diseases classified elsewhere***
    Code first underlying disease, such as:
      amyloidosis (E85.-)
      congenital early syphilis (A50.0)
      echinococcosis (B67.0-B67.9)
      malaria (B50.0-B54)
      schistosomiasis [bilharziasis] (B65.0-B65.9)
      vitamin C deficiency (E54)
    EXCLUDES 1 *rupture of spleen due to Plasmodium vivax malaria (B51.0)*
        splenitis, splenomegaly in late syphilis (A52.79)
        splenitis, splenomegaly in tuberculosis (A18.85)

Intraoperative and postprocedural complications of the spleen (D78)

☑4ᵗʰ **D78** **Intraoperative and postprocedural complications of the spleen**
    AHA: 2016,4Q,9-10

  ☑5ᵗʰ **D78.0** **Intraoperative hemorrhage and hematoma of the spleen complicating a procedure**
      EXCLUDES 1 *intraoperative hemorrhage and hematoma of the*
        spleen due to accidental puncture or laceration
        during a procedure (D78.1-)

    D78.01 **Intraoperative hemorrhage and hematoma of the spleen complicating a procedure on the spleen**

    D78.02 **Intraoperative hemorrhage and hematoma of the spleen complicating other procedure**

  ☑5ᵗʰ **D78.1** **Accidental puncture and laceration of the spleen during a procedure**

    D78.11 **Accidental puncture and laceration of the spleen during a procedure on the spleen**

    D78.12 **Accidental puncture and laceration of the spleen during other procedure**

  ☑5ᵗʰ **D78.2** **Postprocedural hemorrhage of the spleen following a procedure**

    D78.21 **Postprocedural hemorrhage of the spleen following a procedure on the spleen**

    D78.22 **Postprocedural hemorrhage of the spleen following other procedure**

  ☑5ᵗʰ **D78.3** **Postprocedural hematoma and seroma of the spleen following a procedure**

    D78.31 **Postprocedural hematoma of the spleen following a procedure on the spleen**

    D78.32 **Postprocedural hematoma of the spleen following other procedure**

    D78.33 **Postprocedural seroma of the spleen following a procedure on the spleen**

    D78.34 **Postprocedural seroma of the spleen following other procedure**

☑ Additional Character Required   √x7ᵗʰ Placeholder Alert   Manifestation   Unspecified Dx   ▶◀ Revised Text   ● New Code   ▲ Revised Code Title

D78.8   **Other intraoperative and postprocedural complications of the spleen**

Use additional code, if applicable, to further specify disorder

D78.81   **Other intraoperative complications of the spleen**

D78.89   **Other postprocedural complications of the spleen**

Certain disorders involving the immune mechanism (D80-D89)

INCLUDES   defects in the complement system
immunodeficiency disorders, except human immunodeficiency virus [HIV] disease
sarcoidosis

EXCLUDES 1   *autoimmune disease (systemic) NOS (M35.9)*
functional disorders of polymorphonuclear neutrophils (D71)
human immunodeficiency virus [HIV] disease (B20)

✓4th **D80**   **Immunodeficiency with predominantly antibody defects**

D80.0   **Hereditary hypogammaglobulinemia**   HCC

Autosomal recessive agammaglobulinemia (Swiss type)
X-linked agammaglobulinemia [Bruton] (with growth hormone deficiency)

D80.1   **Nonfamilial hypogammaglobulinemia**   HCC

Agammaglobulinemia with immunoglobulin-bearing B-lymphocytes
Common variable agammaglobulinemia [CVAgamma]
Hypogammaglobulinemia NOS

D80.2   **Selective deficiency of immunoglobulin A [IgA]**   HCC

D80.3   **Selective deficiency of immunoglobulin G [IgG] subclasses**   HCC

D80.4   **Selective deficiency of immunoglobulin M [IgM]**   HCC

D80.5   **Immunodeficiency with increased immunoglobulin M [IgM]**   HCC

D80.6   **Antibody deficiency with near-normal immunoglobulins or with hyperimmunoglobulinemia**   HCC

D80.7   **Transient hypogammaglobulinemia of infancy**   HCC

D80.8   **Other immunodeficiencies with predominantly antibody defects**   HCC

Kappa light chain deficiency

D80.9   **Immunodeficiency with predominantly antibody defects, unspecified**   HCC

✓4th **D81**   **Combined immunodeficiencies**

EXCLUDES 1   *autosomal recessive agammaglobulinemia (Swiss type) (D80.0)*

D81.0   **Severe combined immunodeficiency [SCID] with reticular dysgenesis**   HCC

D81.1   **Severe combined immunodeficiency [SCID] with low T- and B-cell numbers**   HCC

D81.2   **Severe combined immunodeficiency [SCID] with low or normal B-cell numbers**   HCC

▲ ✓5th **D81.3**   **Adenosine deaminase [ADA] deficiency**

●   **D81.30**   **Adenosine deaminase deficiency, unspecified**

ADA deficiency NOS

●   **D81.31**   **Severe combined immunodeficiency due to adenosine deaminase deficiency**

ADA deficiency with SCID
Adenosine deaminase [ADA] deficiency with severe combined immunodeficiency

●   **D81.32**   **Adenosine deaminase 2 deficiency**

ADA2 deficiency
Adenosine deaminase deficiency type 2
Code also, if applicable, any associated manifestations, such as:
polyarteritis nodosa (M30.0)
stroke (I63.-)

●   **D81.39**   **Other adenosine deaminase deficiency**

Adenosine deaminase [ADA] deficiency type 1, NOS
Adenosine deaminase [ADA] deficiency type 1, without SCID
Adenosine deaminase [ADA] deficiency type 1, without severe combined immunodeficiency
Partial ADA deficiency (type 1)
Partial adenosine deaminase deficiency (type 1)

D81.4   **Nezelof's syndrome**   HCC

D81.5   **Purine nucleoside phosphorylase [PNP] deficiency**   HCC

D81.6   **Major histocompatibility complex class I deficiency**   HCC

Bare lymphocyte syndrome

D81.7   **Major histocompatibility complex class II deficiency**   HCC

✓5th **D81.8**   **Other combined immunodeficiencies**

✓6th **D81.81**   **Biotin-dependent carboxylase deficiency**

Multiple carboxylase deficiency

EXCLUDES 1   *biotin-dependent carboxylase deficiency due to dietary deficiency of biotin (E53.8)*

D81.810   **Biotinidase deficiency**

D81.818   **Other biotin-dependent carboxylase deficiency**

Holocarboxylase synthetase deficiency
Other multiple carboxylase deficiency

D81.819   **Biotin-dependent carboxylase deficiency, unspecified**

Multiple carboxylase deficiency, unspecified

D81.89   **Other combined immunodeficiencies**   HCC

D81.9   **Combined immunodeficiency, unspecified**   HCC

Severe combined immunodeficiency disorder [SCID] NOS

✓4th **D82**   **Immunodeficiency associated with other major defects**

EXCLUDES 1   *ataxia telangiectasia [Louis-Bar] (G11.3)*

D82.0   **Wiskott-Aldrich syndrome**   HCC

Immunodeficiency with thrombocytopenia and eczema

D82.1   **Di George's syndrome**   HCC

Pharyngeal pouch syndrome
Thymic alymphoplasia
Thymic aplasia or hypoplasia with immunodeficiency

D82.2   **Immunodeficiency with short-limbed stature**   HCC

D82.3   **Immunodeficiency following hereditary defective response to Epstein-Barr virus**   HCC

X-linked lymphoproliferative disease

D82.4   **Hyperimmunoglobulin E [IgE] syndrome**   HCC

D82.8   **Immunodeficiency associated with other specified major defects**   HCC

D82.9   **Immunodeficiency associated with major defect, unspecified**   HCC

✓4th **D83**   **Common variable immunodeficiency**

D83.0   **Common variable immunodeficiency with predominant abnormalities of B-cell numbers and function**   HCC

D83.1   **Common variable immunodeficiency with predominant immunoregulatory T-cell disorders**   HCC

D83.2   **Common variable immunodeficiency with autoantibodies to B- or T-cells**   HCC

D83.8   **Other common variable immunodeficiencies**   HCC

D83.9   **Common variable immunodeficiency, unspecified**   HCC

✓4th **D84**   **Other immunodeficiencies**

D84.0   **Lymphocyte function antigen-1 [LFA-1] defect**   HCC

D84.1   **Defects in the complement system**   HCC

C1 esterase inhibitor [C1-INH] deficiency

D84.8   **Other specified immunodeficiencies**   HCC

D84.9   **Immunodeficiency, unspecified**   HCC

✓4th **D86**   **Sarcoidosis**

DEF: Clustering of immune cells resulting in granuloma formation. Often affects the lungs and lymphatic system but can occur in other body sites.

D86.0   **Sarcoidosis of lung**   HCC

D86.1   **Sarcoidosis of lymph nodes**

D86.2   **Sarcoidosis of lung with sarcoidosis of lymph nodes**   HCC

D86.3   **Sarcoidosis of skin**

✓5th **D86.8**   **Sarcoidosis of other sites**

D86.81   **Sarcoid meningitis**

D86.82   **Multiple cranial nerve palsies in sarcoidosis**   HCC

D86.83   **Sarcoid iridocyclitis**

D86.84   **Sarcoid pyelonephritis**

Tubulo-interstitial nephropathy in sarcoidosis

D86.85   **Sarcoid myocarditis**

D86.86   **Sarcoid arthropathy**

Polyarthritis in sarcoidosis

D86.87   **Sarcoid myositis**

D86.89   **Sarcoidosis of other sites**

Hepatic granuloma
Uveoparotid fever [Heerfordt]

D86.9   **Sarcoidosis, unspecified**

☑4ᵗʰ **D89 Other disorders involving the immune mechanism, not elsewhere classified**

> EXCLUDES 1   hyperglobulinemia NOS (R77.1)
> monoclonal gammopathy (of undetermined significance) (D47.2)
>
> EXCLUDES 2   transplant failure and rejection (T86.-)

D89.0 Polyclonal hypergammaglobulinemia

Benign hypergammaglobulinemic purpura
Polyclonal gammopathy NOS

D89.1 Cryoglobulinemia   HCC

Cryoglobulinemic purpura
Cryoglobulinemic vasculitis
Essential cryoglobulinemia
Idiopathic cryoglobulinemia
Mixed cryoglobulinemia
Primary cryoglobulinemia
Secondary cryoglobulinemia

D89.2 Hypergammaglobulinemia, unspecified

D89.3 Immune reconstitution syndrome   HCC

Immune reconstitution inflammatory syndrome [IRIS]
Use additional code for adverse effect, if applicable, to identify drug (T36-T50 with fifth or sixth character 5)

☑5ᵗʰ **D89.4 Mast cell activation syndrome and related disorders**

> EXCLUDES 1   aggressive systemic mastocytosis (C96.21)
> congenital cutaneous mastocytosis (Q82.2)
> (non-congenital) cutaneous mastocytosis (D47.01)
> (indolent) systemic mastocytosis (D47.02)
> malignant mast cell neoplasm (C96.2-)
> malignant mastocytoma (C96.29)
> mast cell leukemia (C94.3-)
> mast cell sarcoma (C96.22)
> mastocytoma NOS (D47.09)
> other mast cell neoplasms of uncertain behavior (D47.09)
> systemic mastocytosis associated with a clonal hematologic non-mast cell lineage disease (SM-AHNMD) (D47.02)

AHA: 2016,4Q,11

D89.40 Mast cell activation, unspecified   HCC

Mast cell activation disorder, unspecified
Mast cell activation syndrome, NOS

D89.41 Monoclonal mast cell activation syndrome   HCC

D89.42 Idiopathic mast cell activation syndrome   HCC

D89.43 Secondary mast cell activation   HCC

Secondary mast cell activation syndrome
Code also underlying etiology, if known

D89.49 Other mast cell activation disorder   HCC

Other mast cell activation syndrome

☑5ᵗʰ **D89.8 Other specified disorders involving the immune mechanism, not elsewhere classified**

☑6ᵗʰ **D89.81 Graft-versus-host disease**

Code first underlying cause, such as:
> complications of transplanted organs and tissue (T86.-)
> complications of blood transfusion (T80.89)

Use additional code to identify associated manifestations, such as:
> desquamative dermatitis (L30.8)
> diarrhea (R19.7)
> elevated bilirubin (R17)
> hair loss (L65.9)

D89.810 Acute graft-versus-host disease   HCC

D89.811 Chronic graft-versus-host disease   HCC

D89.812 Acute on chronic graft-versus-host disease   HCC

D89.813 Graft-versus-host disease, unspecified   HCC

D89.82 Autoimmune lymphoproliferative syndrome [ALPS]   HCC

DEF: Rare genetic alteration of the Fas protein that impairs normal cellular apoptosis (normal cell death), causing abnormal accumulation of lymphocytes in the lymph glands, liver, and spleen. Symptoms include neutropenia, anemia, and thrombocytopenia.

D89.89 Other specified disorders involving the immune mechanism, not elsewhere classified   HCC

> EXCLUDES 1   human immunodeficiency virus disease (B20)

AHA: 2017,4Q,109

D89.9 Disorder involving the immune mechanism, unspecified   HCC

Immune disease NOS
AHA: 2015,3Q,22

☑ Additional Character Required   ☑x7ᵗʰ Placeholder Alert   Manifestation   Unspecified Dx   ▶◀ Revised Text   ● New Code   ▲ Revised Code Title

ICD-10-CM 2020   509

Chapter 4. Endocrine, Nutritional, and Metabolic Diseases (E00–E89)

Chapter-specific Guidelines with Coding Examples

The chapter-specific guidelines from the ICD-10-CM Official Guidelines for Coding and Reporting have been provided below. Along with these guidelines are coding examples, contained in the shaded boxes, that have been developed to help illustrate the coding and/or sequencing guidance found in these guidelines.

a. Diabetes mellitus

The diabetes mellitus codes are combination codes that include the type of diabetes mellitus, the body system affected, and the complications affecting that body system. As many codes within a particular category as are necessary to describe all of the complications of the disease may be used. They should be sequenced based on the reason for a particular encounter. Assign as many codes from categories E08–E13 as needed to identify all of the associated conditions that the patient has.

> Patient is seen for uncontrolled diabetes, type 2, with hyperglycemia diabetic nephropathy, and diabetic gastroparesis
>
> **E11.65**   **Type 2 diabetes mellitus with hyperglycemia**
>
> **E11.21**   **Type 2 diabetes mellitus with diabetic nephropathy**
>
> **E11.43**   **Type 2 diabetes mellitus with diabetic autonomic (poly)neuropathy**
>
> **K31.84**   **Gastroparesis**
>
> *Explanation*: Use as many codes to describe the diabetic complications as needed. Many are combination codes that describe more than one condition. Code first the reason for the encounter. The term "uncontrolled" can refer to either hyperglycemia or hypoglycemia. In this case, "uncontrolled" is described as "with hyperglycemia."

1) Type of diabetes

The age of a patient is not the sole determining factor, though most type 1 diabetics develop the condition before reaching puberty. For this reason type 1 diabetes mellitus is also referred to as juvenile diabetes.

> A 45-year-old patient is diagnosed with type 1 diabetes
>
> **E10.9**   **Type 1 diabetes mellitus without complications**
>
> *Explanation*: Although most type 1 diabetics are diagnosed in childhood or adolescence, it can also begin in adults.

2) Type of diabetes mellitus not documented

If the type of diabetes mellitus is not documented in the medical record the default is E11.-, Type 2 diabetes mellitus.

> Office visit lists diabetic retinopathy with macular edema and hypertension on patient problem list
>
> **E11.311**   **Type 2 diabetes mellitus with unspecified diabetic retinopathy with macular edema**
>
> **I10**   **Essential (primary) hypertension**
>
> *Explanation*: Since the type of diabetes was not documented, default to category E11.

3) Diabetes mellitus and the use of insulin and oral hypoglycemics

If the documentation in a medical record does not indicate the type of diabetes but does indicate that the patient uses insulin, code E11-, Type 2 diabetes mellitus, should be assigned. An additional code should be assigned from category Z79 to identify the long-term (current) use of insulin or oral hypoglycemic drugs. If the patient is treated with both oral medications and insulin, only the code for long-term (current) use of insulin should be assigned. Code Z79.4 should not be assigned if insulin is given temporarily to bring a type 2 patient's blood sugar under control during an encounter.

> Office visit lists chronic diabetes with daily insulin use on patient problem list
>
> **E11.9**   **Type 2 diabetes mellitus without complications**
>
> **Z79.4**   **Long term (current) use of insulin**
>
> *Explanation*: Do not assume that a patient on insulin must have type 1 diabetes. The default for diabetes without further specification defaults to type 2. Add the code for long term use of insulin.

4) Diabetes mellitus in pregnancy and gestational diabetes

See Section I.C.15. Diabetes mellitus in pregnancy.

See Section I.C.15. Gestational (pregnancy induced) diabetes

5) Complications due to insulin pump malfunction

(a) Underdose of insulin due to insulin pump failure

An underdose of insulin due to an insulin pump failure should be assigned to a code from subcategory T85.6, Mechanical complication of other specified internal and external prosthetic devices, implants and grafts, that specifies the type of pump malfunction, as the principal or first-listed code, followed by code T38.3X6-, Underdosing of insulin and oral hypoglycemic [antidiabetic] drugs. Additional codes for the type of diabetes mellitus and any associated complications due to the underdosing should also be assigned.

> A 24-year-old type 1 diabetic male treated in for hyperglycemia; insulin pump found to be malfunctioning and underdosing
>
> **T85.614A**   **Breakdown (mechanical) of insulin pump, initial encounter**
>
> **T38.3X6A**   **Underdosing of insulin and oral hypoglycemic [antidiabetic] drugs, initial encounter**
>
> **E10.65**   **Type 1 diabetes mellitus with hyperglycemia**
>
> *Explanation*: The complication code for the mechanical breakdown of the pump is sequenced first, followed by the underdosing code and type of diabetes with complication. Code all other diabetic complication codes necessary to describe the patient's condition.

(b) Overdose of insulin due to insulin pump failure

The principal or first-listed code for an encounter due to an insulin pump malfunction resulting in an overdose of insulin, should also be T85.6-, Mechanical complication of other specified internal and external prosthetic devices, implants and grafts, followed by code T38.3X1-, Poisoning by insulin and oral hypoglycemic [antidiabetic] drugs, accidental (unintentional).

> A 24-year-old type 1 diabetic male found down with diabetic coma, brought into ED and treated for hypoglycemia; insulin pump found to be malfunctioning and overdosing
>
> **T85.614A**   **Breakdown (mechanical) of insulin pump, initial encounter**
>
> **T38.3X1A**   **Poisoning by insulin and oral hypoglycemic [antidiabetic] drugs, accidental (unintentional), initial encounter**
>
> **E10.641**   **Type 1 diabetes mellitus with hypoglycemia with coma**
>
> *Explanation*: The complication code for the mechanical breakdown of the pump is sequenced first, followed by the poisoning code and type of diabetes with complication. All the characters in the combination code must be used to form a valid code and to fully describe the type of diabetes, the hypoglycemia, and the coma.

6) Secondary diabetes mellitus

Codes under categories E08, Diabetes mellitus due to underlying condition, E09, Drug or chemical induced diabetes mellitus, and E13, Other specified diabetes mellitus, identify complications/manifestations associated with secondary diabetes mellitus. Secondary diabetes is always caused by another condition or event (e.g., cystic fibrosis, malignant neoplasm of pancreas, pancreatectomy, adverse effect of drug, or poisoning).

(a) Secondary diabetes mellitus and the use of insulin or oral hypoglycemic drugs

For patients with secondary diabetes mellitus who routinely use insulin or oral hypoglycemic drugs, an additional code from category Z79 should be assigned to identify the long-term (current) use of insulin or oral hypoglycemic drugs. If the patient is treated with both oral medications and insulin, only the code for long-term (current) use of insulin should be assigned. Code Z79.4 should not be assigned if insulin is given temporarily to bring a secondary diabetic patient's blood sugar under control during an encounter.

Chapter 4. Endocrine, Nutritional, and Metabolic Diseases

Type 2 diabetic with no complications, normally only on oral metformin, is given insulin for three days to maintain glucose control while in the hospital recovering from surgery

E11.9   **Type 2 diabetes mellitus without complications**

Z79.84   **Long term (current) use of oral hypoglycemic drugs**

Explanation: Although the patient was given insulin for a short time during his hospital stay, the intent was only to maintain the patient's glucose levels while off his regular oral hypoglycemic medication, not for long term use. No code is needed for long term use of insulin, but a Z code for long term use of an oral hypoglycemic should be added to identify the chronic use of this drug.

Type 2 diabetic with diabetic polyneuropathy on insulin

E11.42   **Type 2 diabetes mellitus with diabetic polyneuropathy**

Z79.4   **Long term (current) use of insulin**

Explanation: Add the Z code for the long term use of insulin because the insulin is taken chronically.

(b) Assigning and sequencing secondary diabetes codes and its causes

The sequencing of the secondary diabetes codes in relationship to codes for the cause of the diabetes is based on the Tabular List instructions for categories E08, E09 and E13.

(i) Secondary diabetes mellitus due to pancreatectomy

For postpancreatectomy diabetes mellitus (lack of insulin due to the surgical removal of all or part of the pancreas), assign code E89.1, Postprocedural hypoinsulinemia. Assign a code from category E13 and a code from subcategory Z90.41-, Acquired absence of pancreas, as additional codes.

Patient with newly diagnosed diabetes after surgical removal of part of pancreas

E89.1   **Postprocedural hypoinsulinemia**

E13.9   **Other specified diabetes mellitus without complications**

Z90.411   **Acquired partial absence of pancreas**

Explanation: Sequence the postprocedural complication of the hypoinsulinemia due to the partial removal of the pancreas as the first-listed code, followed by the other specified diabetes (NEC) with or without complications and the partial or total acquired absence of the pancreas.

(ii) Secondary diabetes due to drugs

Secondary diabetes may be caused by an adverse effect of correctly administered medications, poisoning or sequela of poisoning.

See section I.C.19.e for coding of adverse effects and poisoning, and section I.C.20 for external cause code reporting.

Initial encounter for corticosteroid-induced diabetes mellitus

E09.9   **Drug or chemical induced diabetes mellitus without complications**

T38.0X5A   **Adverse effect of glucocorticoids and synthetic analogues, initial encounter**

Explanation: If the diabetes is caused by an adverse effect of a drug, the diabetic condition is coded first. If it occurs from a poisoning or overdose, the poisoning code causing the diabetes is sequenced first.

Chapter 4. Endocrine, Nutritional and Metabolic Diseases (E00-E89)

> **NOTE**   All neoplasms, whether functionally active or not, are classified in Chapter 2. Appropriate codes in this chapter (i.e. E05.8, E07.0, E16-E31, E34.-) may be used as additional codes to indicate either functional activity by neoplasms and ectopic endocrine tissue or hyperfunction and hypofunction of endocrine glands associated with neoplasms and other conditions classified elsewhere.

> *EXCLUDES 1*   *transitory endocrine and metabolic disorders specific to newborn (P70-P74)*

AHA: 2018,2Q,6

This chapter contains the following blocks:

E00-E07	Disorders of thyroid gland
E08-E13	Diabetes mellitus
E15-E16	Other disorders of glucose regulation and pancreatic internal secretion
E20-E35	Disorders of other endocrine glands
E36	Intraoperative complications of endocrine system
E40-E46	Malnutrition
E50-E64	Other nutritional deficiencies
E65-E68	Overweight, obesity and other hyperalimentation
E70-E88	Metabolic disorders
E89	Postprocedural endocrine and metabolic complications and disorders, not elsewhere classified

Disorders of thyroid gland (E00-E07)

✓4ᵗʰ E00 Congenital iodine-deficiency syndrome

Use additional code (F70-F79) to identify associated intellectual disabilities

> *EXCLUDES 1*   *subclinical iodine-deficiency hypothyroidism (E02)*

E00.0 Congenital iodine-deficiency syndrome, neurological type
Endemic cretinism, neurological type

E00.1 Congenital iodine-deficiency syndrome, myxedematous type
Endemic hypothyroid cretinism
Endemic cretinism, myxedematous type

E00.2 Congenital iodine-deficiency syndrome, mixed type
Endemic cretinism, mixed type

E00.9 Congenital iodine-deficiency syndrome, unspecified
Congenital iodine-deficiency hypothyroidism NOS
Endemic cretinism NOS

✓4ᵗʰ E01 Iodine-deficiency related thyroid disorders and allied conditions

> *EXCLUDES 1*   *congenital iodine-deficiency syndrome (E00.-)*
> *subclinical iodine-deficiency hypothyroidism (E02)*

E01.0 Iodine-deficiency related diffuse (endemic) goiter

E01.1 Iodine-deficiency related multinodular (endemic) goiter
Iodine-deficiency related nodular goiter

E01.2 Iodine-deficiency related (endemic) goiter, unspecified
Endemic goiter NOS

E01.8 Other iodine-deficiency related thyroid disorders and allied conditions
Acquired iodine-deficiency hypothyroidism NOS

E02 Subclinical iodine-deficiency hypothyroidism

✓4ᵗʰ E03 Other hypothyroidism

> *EXCLUDES 1*   *iodine-deficiency related hypothyroidism (E00-E02)*
> *postprocedural hypothyroidism (E89.0)*

DEF: Hypothyroidism: Underproduction of thyroid hormone.

E03.0 Congenital hypothyroidism with diffuse goiter
Congenital parenchymatous goiter (nontoxic)
Congenital goiter (nontoxic) NOS

> *EXCLUDES 1*   *transitory congenital goiter with normal function (P72.0)*

E03.1 Congenital hypothyroidism without goiter
Aplasia of thyroid (with myxedema)
Congenital atrophy of thyroid
Congenital hypothyroidism NOS

E03.2 Hypothyroidism due to medicaments and other exogenous substances
Code first poisoning due to drug or toxin, if applicable (T36-T65 with fifth or sixth character 1-4 or 6)
Use additional code for adverse effect, if applicable, to identify drug (T36-T50 with fifth or sixth character 5)

E03.3 Postinfectious hypothyroidism

E03.4 Atrophy of thyroid (acquired)

> *EXCLUDES 1*   *congenital atrophy of thyroid (E03.1)*

E03.5 Myxedema coma   **HCC**

E03.8 Other specified hypothyroidism

E03.9 Hypothyroidism, unspecified
Myxedema NOS

✓4ᵗʰ E04 Other nontoxic goiter

> *EXCLUDES 1*   *congenital goiter (NOS) (diffuse) (parenchymatous) (E03.0)*
> *iodine-deficiency related goiter (E00-E02)*

E04.0 Nontoxic diffuse goiter
Diffuse (colloid) nontoxic goiter
Simple nontoxic goiter

E04.1 Nontoxic single thyroid nodule
Colloid nodule (cystic) (thyroid)
Nontoxic uninodular goiter
Thyroid (cystic) nodule NOS
DEF: Enlarged thyroid, commonly due to decreased thyroid production, with a single nodule. No clinical hypothyroidism.

E04.2 Nontoxic multinodular goiter
Cystic goiter NOS
Multinodular (cystic) goiter NOS
DEF: Enlarged thyroid, commonly due to decreased thyroid production with multiple nodules. No clinical hypothyroidism.

E04.8 Other specified nontoxic goiter

E04.9 Nontoxic goiter, unspecified
Goiter NOS
Nodular goiter (nontoxic) NOS

✓4ᵗʰ E05 Thyrotoxicosis [hyperthyroidism]

> *EXCLUDES 1*   *chronic thyroiditis with transient thyrotoxicosis (E06.2)*
> *neonatal thyrotoxicosis (P72.1)*

DEF: Excessive quantities of hormones from the thyroid gland caused by overproduction or loss of storage ability.

✓5ᵗʰ E05.0 Thyrotoxicosis with diffuse goiter

Exophthalmic or toxic goiter NOS
Graves' disease
Toxic diffuse goiter
DEF: Diffuse thyroid enlargement accompanied by hyperthyroidism, bulging eyes, and dermopathy.

E05.00 Thyrotoxicosis with diffuse goiter without thyrotoxic crisis or storm

E05.01 Thyrotoxicosis with diffuse goiter with thyrotoxic crisis or storm

Goiter

✓5ᵗʰ E05.1 Thyrotoxicosis with toxic single thyroid nodule

Thyrotoxicosis with toxic uninodular goiter
DEF: Symptomatic hyperthyroidism with a single nodule on the enlarged thyroid gland. Onset of symptoms can be abrupt and include extreme nervousness, insomnia, weight loss, tremors, and psychosis or coma.

E05.10 Thyrotoxicosis with toxic single thyroid nodule without thyrotoxic crisis or storm

E05.11 Thyrotoxicosis with toxic single thyroid nodule with thyrotoxic crisis or storm

✓5ᵗʰ E05.2 Thyrotoxicosis with toxic multinodular goiter

Toxic nodular goiter NOS

E05.20 Thyrotoxicosis with toxic multinodular goiter without thyrotoxic crisis or storm

E05.21 Thyrotoxicosis with toxic multinodular goiter with thyrotoxic crisis or storm

✓5ᵗʰ E05.3 Thyrotoxicosis from ectopic thyroid tissue

E05.30 Thyrotoxicosis from ectopic thyroid tissue without thyrotoxic crisis or storm

E05.31 Thyrotoxicosis from ectopic thyroid tissue with thyrotoxic crisis or storm

---

☑ Additional Character Required   ✓ˣ⁷ᵗʰ Placeholder Alert   Manifestation   Unspecified Dx   ►◄ Revised Text   ● New Code   ▲ Revised Code Title

ICD-10-CM 2020   **513**

E05.4   Thyrotoxicosis factitia

     E05.40   **Thyrotoxicosis factitia** without thyrotoxic crisis or storm

     E05.41   **Thyrotoxicosis factitia** with thyrotoxic crisis or storm

✓5ᵗʰ **E05.8**   **Other thyrotoxicosis**

     Overproduction of thyroid-stimulating hormone

     E05.80   **Other thyrotoxicosis** without thyrotoxic crisis or storm

     E05.81   **Other thyrotoxicosis** with thyrotoxic crisis or storm

✓5ᵗʰ **E05.9**   **Thyrotoxicosis, unspecified**

     Hyperthyroidism NOS

     E05.90   **Thyrotoxicosis, unspecified** without thyrotoxic crisis or storm

     E05.91   **Thyrotoxicosis, unspecified** with thyrotoxic crisis or storm

✓4ᵗʰ **E06**   **Thyroiditis**

     EXCLUDES 1   postpartum thyroiditis (O90.5)

     DEF: Inflammation of the thyroid gland.

     E06.0   **Acute thyroiditis**

         Abscess of thyroid

         Pyogenic thyroiditis

         Suppurative thyroiditis

         Use additional code (B95-B97) to identify infectious agent

     E06.1   **Subacute thyroiditis**

         de Quervain thyroiditis

         Giant-cell thyroiditis

         Granulomatous thyroiditis

         Nonsuppurative thyroiditis

         Viral thyroiditis

         EXCLUDES 1   autoimmune thyroiditis (E06.3)

     E06.2   **Chronic thyroiditis with transient thyrotoxicosis**

         EXCLUDES 1   autoimmune thyroiditis (E06.3)

     E06.3   **Autoimmune thyroiditis**

         Hashimoto's thyroiditis

         Hashitoxicosis (transient)

         Lymphadenoid goiter

         Lymphocytic thyroiditis

         Struma lymphomatosa

     E06.4   **Drug-induced thyroiditis**

         Use additional code for adverse effect, if applicable, to identify drug (T36-T50 with fifth or sixth character 5)

     E06.5   **Other chronic thyroiditis**

         Chronic fibrous thyroiditis

         Chronic thyroiditis NOS

         Ligneous thyroiditis

         Riedel thyroiditis

     E06.9   **Thyroiditis, unspecified**

✓4ᵗʰ **E07**   **Other disorders of thyroid**

     E07.0   **Hypersecretion of calcitonin**

         C-cell hyperplasia of thyroid

         Hypersecretion of thyrocalcitonin

     E07.1   **Dyshormogenetic goiter**

         Familial dyshormogenetic goiter

         Pendred's syndrome

         EXCLUDES 1   transitory congenital goiter with normal function (P72.0)

✓5ᵗʰ **E07.8**   **Other specified disorders of thyroid**

     E07.81   **Sick-euthyroid syndrome**

         Euthyroid sick-syndrome

         DEF: Thyroid dysfunction caused by abnormal levels of thyroid hormones T3 and/or T4. This syndrome is often associated with starvation or critical illness.

     E07.89   **Other specified disorders of thyroid**

         Abnormality of thyroid-binding globulin

         Hemorrhage of thyroid

         Infarction of thyroid

     E07.9   **Disorder of thyroid, unspecified**

Diabetes mellitus (E08-E13)

AHA: 2018,4Q,88; 2018,3Q,3-4; 2018,2Q,6; 2017,4Q,6; 2017,1Q,42; 2016,4Q,11-13; 2016,2Q,36; 2016,1Q,11-13

TIP: There is no default code for diabetes mellitus documented only as uncontrolled. The provider must indicate whether the diabetic patient is hypoglycemic or hyperglycemic to determine the appropriate code.

✓4ᵗʰ **E08**   **Diabetes mellitus** due to underlying condition

     Code first the underlying condition, such as:

         congenital rubella (P35.0)

         Cushing's syndrome (E24.-)

         cystic fibrosis (E84.-)

         malignant neoplasm (C00-C96)

         malnutrition (E40-E46)

         pancreatitis and other diseases of the pancreas (K85-K86.-)

     Use additional code to identify control using:

         insulin (Z79.4)

         oral antidiabetic drugs (Z79.84)

         oral hypoglycemic drugs (Z79.84)

     EXCLUDES 1   drug or chemical induced diabetes mellitus (E09.-)

         gestational diabetes (O24.4-)

         neonatal diabetes mellitus (P70.2)

         postpancreatectomy diabetes mellitus (E13.-)

         postprocedural diabetes mellitus (E13.-)

         secondary diabetes mellitus NEC (E13.-)

         type 1 diabetes mellitus (E10.-)

         type 2 diabetes mellitus (E11.-)

     AHA: 2013,4Q,114; 2013,3Q,20

✓5ᵗʰ **E08.0**   **Diabetes mellitus due to underlying condition with hyperosmolarity**

     DEF: Diabetic hyperosmolarity: Extremely high levels of glucose in the blood without ketones.

     E08.00   *Diabetes mellitus due to underlying condition with hyperosmolarity without nonketotic hyperglycemic-hyperosmolar coma (NKHHC)*   HCC

     E08.01   *Diabetes mellitus due to underlying condition with hyperosmolarity with coma*   HCC

✓5ᵗʰ **E08.1**   **Diabetes mellitus due to underlying condition with ketoacidosis**

     DEF: Diabetic ketoacidosis: Potentially life-threatening complication due to a shortage of insulin in which the body switches to burning fatty acids and producing acidic ketone bodies.

     E08.10   *Diabetes mellitus due to underlying condition with ketoacidosis without coma*   HCC

     E08.11   *Diabetes mellitus due to underlying condition with ketoacidosis with coma*   HCC

✓5ᵗʰ **E08.2**   **Diabetes mellitus due to underlying condition with kidney complications**

     E08.21   *Diabetes mellitus due to underlying condition with diabetic nephropathy*   HCC

         Diabetes mellitus due to underlying condition with intercapillary glomerulosclerosis

         Diabetes mellitus due to underlying condition with intracapillary glomerulonephrosis

         Diabetes mellitus due to underlying condition with Kimmelstiel-Wilson disease

     E08.22   *Diabetes mellitus due to underlying condition with diabetic chronic kidney disease*   HCC

         Use additional code to identify stage of chronic kidney disease (N18.1-N18.6)

     E08.29   *Diabetes mellitus due to underlying condition with other diabetic kidney complication*   HCC

         Renal tubular degeneration in diabetes mellitus due to underlying condition

E08.3 **Diabetes mellitus due to underlying condition with ophthalmic complications**

> One of the following 7th characters is to be assigned to codes in subcategories E08.32, E08.33, E08.34, E08.35, and E08.37 to designate laterality of the disease:
> 1 right eye
> 2 left eye
> 3 bilateral
> 9 unspecified eye

E08.31 **Diabetes mellitus due to underlying condition with unspecified diabetic retinopathy**
DEF: Diabetic retinopathy: Diabetic complication from damage to the retinal vessels resulting in vision problems that can progress to blindness.

E08.311 *Diabetes mellitus due to underlying condition with unspecified diabetic retinopathy with macular edema* `HCC` `Q`

E08.319 *Diabetes mellitus due to underlying condition with unspecified diabetic retinopathy without macular edema* `HCC` `Q`

E08.32 **Diabetes mellitus due to underlying condition with mild nonproliferative diabetic retinopathy**
Diabetes mellitus due to underlying condition with nonproliferative diabetic retinopathy NOS

E08.321 *Diabetes mellitus due to underlying condition with mild nonproliferative diabetic retinopathy with macular edema* `HCC` `Q`

E08.329 *Diabetes mellitus due to underlying condition with mild nonproliferative diabetic retinopathy without macular edema* `HCC` `Q`

E08.33 **Diabetes mellitus due to underlying condition with moderate nonproliferative diabetic retinopathy**

E08.331 *Diabetes mellitus due to underlying condition with moderate nonproliferative diabetic retinopathy with macular edema* `HCC` `Q`

E08.339 *Diabetes mellitus due to underlying condition with moderate nonproliferative diabetic retinopathy without macular edema* `HCC` `Q`

E08.34 **Diabetes mellitus due to underlying condition with severe nonproliferative diabetic retinopathy**

E08.341 *Diabetes mellitus due to underlying condition with severe nonproliferative diabetic retinopathy with macular edema* `HCC` `Q`

E08.349 *Diabetes mellitus due to underlying condition with severe nonproliferative diabetic retinopathy without macular edema* `HCC` `Q`

E08.35 **Diabetes mellitus due to underlying condition with proliferative diabetic retinopathy**

E08.351 *Diabetes mellitus due to underlying condition with proliferative diabetic retinopathy with macular edema* `HCC` `Q`

E08.352 *Diabetes mellitus due to underlying condition with proliferative diabetic retinopathy with traction retinal detachment involving the macula* `HCC` `Q`

E08.353 *Diabetes mellitus due to underlying condition with proliferative diabetic retinopathy with traction retinal detachment not involving the macula* `HCC` `Q`

E08.354 *Diabetes mellitus due to underlying condition with proliferative diabetic retinopathy with combined traction retinal detachment and rhegmatogenous retinal detachment* `HCC` `Q`

E08.355 *Diabetes mellitus due to underlying condition with stable proliferative diabetic retinopathy* `HCC` `Q`

E08.359 *Diabetes mellitus due to underlying condition with proliferative diabetic retinopathy without macular edema* `HCC` `Q`

E08.36 *Diabetes mellitus due to underlying condition with diabetic cataract* `HCC`
AHA: 2019,2Q,30-31; 2016,4Q,142

E08.37 *Diabetes mellitus due to underlying condition with diabetic macular edema, resolved following treatment* `HCC`

E08.39 *Diabetes mellitus due to underlying condition with other diabetic ophthalmic complication* `HCC`
Use additional code to identify manifestation, such as:
diabetic glaucoma (H40-H42)

E08.4 **Diabetes mellitus due to underlying condition with neurological complications**

E08.40 *Diabetes mellitus due to underlying condition with diabetic neuropathy, unspecified* `HCC`

E08.41 *Diabetes mellitus due to underlying condition with diabetic mononeuropathy* `HCC`

E08.42 *Diabetes mellitus due to underlying condition with diabetic polyneuropathy* `HCC`
Diabetes mellitus due to underlying condition with diabetic neuralgia

E08.43 *Diabetes mellitus due to underlying condition with diabetic autonomic (poly)neuropathy* `HCC`
Diabetes mellitus due to underlying condition with diabetic gastroparesis
AHA: 2013,4Q,114

E08.44 *Diabetes mellitus due to underlying condition with diabetic amyotrophy* `HCC`

E08.49 *Diabetes mellitus due to underlying condition with other diabetic neurological complication* `HCC`

E08.5 **Diabetes mellitus due to underlying condition with circulatory complications**

E08.51 *Diabetes mellitus due to underlying condition with diabetic peripheral angiopathy without gangrene* `HCC`
AHA: 2018,2Q,7

E08.52 *Diabetes mellitus due to underlying condition with diabetic peripheral angiopathy with gangrene* `HCC`
Diabetes mellitus due to underlying condition with diabetic gangrene
AHA: 2018,2Q,7; 2017,4Q,102

E08.59 *Diabetes mellitus due to underlying condition with other circulatory complications* `HCC`

E08.6 **Diabetes mellitus due to underlying condition with other specified complications**

E08.61 **Diabetes mellitus due to underlying condition with diabetic arthropathy**

E08.610 *Diabetes mellitus due to underlying condition with diabetic neuropathic arthropathy* `HCC`
Diabetes mellitus due to underlying condition with Charcôt's joints
DEF: Charcot's joint: Progressive neurologic arthropathy in which chronic degeneration of joints in the weight-bearing areas with peripheral hypertrophy occurs as a complication of a neuropathy disorder. Supporting structures relax from a loss of sensation resulting in chronic joint instability.

E08.618 *Diabetes mellitus due to underlying condition with other diabetic arthropathy* `HCC`
AHA: 2018,2Q,6

E08.62 **Diabetes mellitus due to underlying condition with skin complications**

E08.620 *Diabetes mellitus due to underlying condition with diabetic dermatitis* `HCC`
Diabetes mellitus due to underlying condition with diabetic necrobiosis lipoidica

E08.621   *Diabetes mellitus due to underlying condition with foot ulcer*   HCC
>> Use additional code to identify site of ulcer (L97.4-, L97.5-)
>> **TIP:** Do not assign a code for diabetic ulcer when the ulcer is closed/resolved or to report history of diabetic ulcers; Z86.31 Personal history of diabetic foot ulcer, may be assigned.

E08.622   *Diabetes mellitus due to underlying condition with other skin ulcer*   HCC
>> Use additional code to identify site of ulcer (L97.1-L97.9, L98.41-L98.49)
>> **AHA:** 2017,4Q,17

E08.628   *Diabetes mellitus due to underlying condition with other skin complications*   HCC
>> **AHA:** 2017,4Q,100-101

√6ᵗʰ **E08.63**   **Diabetes mellitus due to underlying condition with oral complications**

E08.630   *Diabetes mellitus due to underlying condition with periodontal disease*   HCC

E08.638   *Diabetes mellitus due to underlying condition with other oral complications*   HCC

√6ᵗʰ **E08.64**   **Diabetes mellitus due to underlying condition with hypoglycemia**

E08.641   *Diabetes mellitus due to underlying condition with hypoglycemia with coma*   HCC

E08.649   *Diabetes mellitus due to underlying condition with hypoglycemia without coma*   HCC
>> **AHA:** 2016,3Q,42; 2015,3Q,21

E08.65   *Diabetes mellitus due to underlying condition with hyperglycemia*   HCC

E08.69   *Diabetes mellitus due to underlying condition with other specified complication*   HCC
>> Use additional code to identify complication
>> **AHA:** 2016,4Q,141; 2016,1Q,13

E08.8   *Diabetes mellitus due to underlying condition with unspecified complications*   HCC

E08.9   *Diabetes mellitus due to underlying condition without complications*   HCC

√4ᵗʰ **E09**   **Drug or chemical induced diabetes mellitus**
> Code first poisoning due to drug or toxin, if applicable (T36-T65 with fifth or sixth character 1-4 or 6)
> Use additional code for adverse effect, if applicable, to identify drug (T36-T50 with fifth or sixth character 5)
> Use additional code to identify control using:
> insulin (Z79.4)
> oral antidiabetic drugs (Z79.84)
> oral hypoglycemic drugs (Z79.84)
> > *EXCLUDES 1*   *diabetes mellitus due to underlying condition (E08.-)*
> > *gestational diabetes (O24.4-)*
> > *neonatal diabetes mellitus (P70.2)*
> > *postpancreatectomy diabetes mellitus (E13.-)*
> > *postprocedural diabetes mellitus (E13.-)*
> > *secondary diabetes mellitus NEC (E13.-)*
> > *type 1 diabetes mellitus (E10.-)*
> > *type 2 diabetes mellitus (E11.-)*
> **AHA:** 2013,4Q,114; 2013,3Q,20

√5ᵗʰ **E09.0**   **Drug or chemical induced diabetes mellitus with hyperosmolarity**
> **DEF:** Diabetic hyperosmolarity: Extremely high levels of glucose in the blood without ketones.

E09.00   **Drug or chemical induced diabetes mellitus with hyperosmolarity without nonketotic hyperglycemic-hyperosmolar coma (NKHHC)**   HCC

E09.01   **Drug or chemical induced diabetes mellitus with hyperosmolarity with coma**   HCC

√5ᵗʰ **E09.1**   **Drug or chemical induced diabetes mellitus with ketoacidosis**
> **DEF:** Diabetic ketoacidosis: Potentially life-threatening complication due to a shortage of insulin in which the body switches to burning fatty acids and producing acidic ketone bodies.

E09.10   **Drug or chemical induced diabetes mellitus with ketoacidosis without coma**   HCC

E09.11   **Drug or chemical induced diabetes mellitus with ketoacidosis with coma**   HCC

√5ᵗʰ **E09.2**   **Drug or chemical induced diabetes mellitus with kidney complications**

E09.21   **Drug or chemical induced diabetes mellitus with diabetic nephropathy**   HCC
>> Drug or chemical induced diabetes mellitus with intercapillary glomerulosclerosis
>> Drug or chemical induced diabetes mellitus with intracapillary glomerulonephrosis
>> Drug or chemical induced diabetes mellitus with Kimmelstiel-Wilson disease

E09.22   **Drug or chemical induced diabetes mellitus with diabetic chronic kidney disease**   HCC
>> Use additional code to identify stage of chronic kidney disease (N18.1-N18.6)

E09.29   **Drug or chemical induced diabetes mellitus with other diabetic kidney complication**   HCC
>> Drug or chemical induced diabetes mellitus with renal tubular degeneration

√5ᵗʰ **E09.3**   **Drug or chemical induced diabetes mellitus with ophthalmic complications**
> One of the following 7th characters is to be assigned to codes in subcategories E09.32, E09.33, E09.34, E09.35, and E09.37 to designate laterality of the disease:
> 1   right eye
> 2   left eye
> 3   bilateral
> 9   unspecified eye

√6ᵗʰ **E09.31**   **Drug or chemical induced diabetes mellitus with unspecified diabetic retinopathy**
>> **DEF:** Diabetic retinopathy: Diabetic complication from damage to the retinal vessels resulting in vision problems that can progress to blindness.

E09.311   **Drug or chemical induced diabetes mellitus with unspecified diabetic retinopathy with macular edema**   HCC Q

E09.319   **Drug or chemical induced diabetes mellitus with unspecified diabetic retinopathy without macular edema**   HCC Q

√6ᵗʰ **E09.32**   **Drug or chemical induced diabetes mellitus with mild nonproliferative diabetic retinopathy**
>> Drug or chemical induced diabetes mellitus with nonproliferative diabetic retinopathy NOS

√7ᵗʰ **E09.321**   **Drug or chemical induced diabetes mellitus with mild nonproliferative diabetic retinopathy with macular edema**   HCC Q

√7ᵗʰ **E09.329**   **Drug or chemical induced diabetes mellitus with mild nonproliferative diabetic retinopathy without macular edema**   HCC Q

√6ᵗʰ **E09.33**   **Drug or chemical induced diabetes mellitus with moderate nonproliferative diabetic retinopathy**

√7ᵗʰ **E09.331**   **Drug or chemical induced diabetes mellitus with moderate nonproliferative diabetic retinopathy with macular edema**   HCC Q

√7ᵗʰ **E09.339**   **Drug or chemical induced diabetes mellitus with moderate nonproliferative diabetic retinopathy without macular edema**   HCC Q

√6ᵗʰ **E09.34**   **Drug or chemical induced diabetes mellitus with severe nonproliferative diabetic retinopathy**

√7ᵗʰ **E09.341**   **Drug or chemical induced diabetes mellitus with severe nonproliferative diabetic retinopathy with macular edema**   HCC Q

✓7ᵗʰ **E09.349** **Drug or chemical induced diabetes mellitus with severe nonproliferative diabetic retinopathy** without macular edema   HCC Q

✓6ᵗʰ **E09.35** **Drug or chemical induced diabetes mellitus with** proliferative **diabetic** retinopathy

  ✓7ᵗʰ **E09.351** **Drug or chemical induced diabetes mellitus with proliferative diabetic retinopathy with** macular edema   HCC Q

  ✓7ᵗʰ **E09.352** **Drug or chemical induced diabetes mellitus with proliferative diabetic retinopathy with traction retinal detachment involving the macula**   HCC Q

  ✓7ᵗʰ **E09.353** **Drug or chemical induced diabetes mellitus with proliferative diabetic retinopathy with traction retinal detachment not involving the macula**   HCC Q

  ✓7ᵗʰ **E09.354** **Drug or chemical induced diabetes mellitus with proliferative diabetic retinopathy with combined traction retinal detachment and rhegmatogenous retinal detachment**   HCC Q

  ✓7ᵗʰ **E09.355** **Drug or chemical induced diabetes mellitus with stable proliferative diabetic retinopathy**   HCC Q

  ✓7ᵗʰ **E09.359** **Drug or chemical induced diabetes mellitus with proliferative diabetic retinopathy** without macular edema   HCC Q

E09.36 **Drug or chemical induced diabetes mellitus with diabetic** cataract   HCC
    AHA: 2019,2Q,30-31; 2016,4Q,142

✓7ᵗʰ **E09.37** **Drug or chemical induced diabetes mellitus with diabetic** macular edema, resolved following treatment   HCC

E09.39 **Drug or chemical induced diabetes mellitus with other diabetic ophthalmic complication**   HCC
    Use additional code to identify manifestation, such as:
      diabetic glaucoma (H40-H42)

✓5ᵗʰ **E09.4** **Drug or chemical induced diabetes mellitus with** neurological complications

E09.40 **Drug or chemical induced diabetes mellitus with neurological complications with diabetic** neuropathy, unspecified   HCC

E09.41 **Drug or chemical induced diabetes mellitus with neurological complications with diabetic** mononeuropathy   HCC

E09.42 **Drug or chemical induced diabetes mellitus with neurological complications with diabetic** polyneuropathy   HCC
    Drug or chemical induced diabetes mellitus with diabetic neuralgia

E09.43 **Drug or chemical induced diabetes mellitus with neurological complications with diabetic** autonomic (poly)neuropathy   HCC
    Drug or chemical induced diabetes mellitus with diabetic gastroparesis
    AHA: 2013,4Q,114

E09.44 **Drug or chemical induced diabetes mellitus with neurological complications with diabetic** amyotrophy   HCC

E09.49 **Drug or chemical induced diabetes mellitus with neurological complications with other diabetic neurological complication**   HCC

✓5ᵗʰ **E09.5** **Drug or chemical induced diabetes mellitus with** circulatory complications

E09.51 **Drug or chemical induced diabetes mellitus with diabetic** peripheral angiopathy without gangrene   HCC
    AHA: 2018,2Q,7

E09.52 **Drug or chemical induced diabetes mellitus with diabetic** peripheral angiopathy with gangrene   HCC
    Drug or chemical induced diabetes mellitus with diabetic gangrene
    AHA: 2018,2Q,7; 2017,4Q,102

E09.59 **Drug or chemical induced diabetes mellitus with other circulatory complications**   HCC

✓5ᵗʰ **E09.6** **Drug or chemical induced diabetes mellitus with other specified complications**

✓6ᵗʰ **E09.61** **Drug or chemical induced diabetes mellitus with diabetic** arthropathy

E09.610 **Drug or chemical induced diabetes mellitus with diabetic** neuropathic **arthropathy**   HCC
    Drug or chemical induced diabetes mellitus with Charcôt's joints
    DEF: Charcot's joint: Progressive neurologic arthropathy in which chronic degeneration of joints in the weight-bearing areas with peripheral hypertrophy occurs as a complication of a neuropathy disorder. Supporting structures relax from a loss of sensation resulting in chronic joint instability.

E09.618 **Drug or chemical induced diabetes mellitus with other diabetic arthropathy**   HCC
    AHA: 2018,2Q,6

✓6ᵗʰ **E09.62** **Drug or chemical induced diabetes mellitus with** skin complications

E09.620 **Drug or chemical induced diabetes mellitus with** diabetic dermatitis   HCC
    Drug or chemical induced diabetes mellitus with diabetic necrobiosis lipoidica

E09.621 **Drug or chemical induced diabetes mellitus with** foot ulcer   HCC
    Use additional code to identify site of ulcer (L97.4-, L97.5-)
    TIP: Do not assign a code for diabetic ulcer when the ulcer is closed/resolved or to report history of diabetic ulcers; Z86.31 Personal history of diabetic foot ulcer, may be assigned.

E09.622 **Drug or chemical induced diabetes mellitus with other skin ulcer**   HCC
    Use additional code to identify site of ulcer (L97.1-L97.9, L98.41-L98.49)
    AHA: 2017,4Q,17

E09.628 **Drug or chemical induced diabetes mellitus with other skin complications**   HCC
    AHA: 2017,4Q,100-101

✓6ᵗʰ **E09.63** **Drug or chemical induced diabetes mellitus with** oral complications

E09.630 **Drug or chemical induced diabetes mellitus with** periodontal disease   HCC

E09.638 **Drug or chemical induced diabetes mellitus with other oral complications**   HCC

✓6ᵗʰ **E09.64** **Drug or chemical induced diabetes mellitus with** hypoglycemia

E09.641 **Drug or chemical induced diabetes mellitus with** hypoglycemia with coma   HCC

E09.649 **Drug or chemical induced diabetes mellitus with** hypoglycemia without coma   HCC
    AHA: 2016,3Q,42; 2015,3Q,21

E09.65 **Drug or chemical induced diabetes mellitus with** hyperglycemia   HCC

E09.69 **Drug or chemical induced diabetes mellitus with other specified complication**   HCC
    Use additional code to identify complication
    AHA: 2016,4Q,141; 2016,1Q,13

E09.8 **Drug or chemical induced diabetes mellitus with unspecified complications**   HCC

E09.9 **Drug or chemical induced diabetes mellitus** without complications   HCC

✓ Additional Character Required   ✓x7ᵗʰ Placeholder Alert   Manifestation   Unspecified Dx   ▶◀ Revised Text   ● New Code   ▲ Revised Code Title

ICD-10-CM 2020   517

Type 1 diabetes mellitus

INCLUDES   brittle diabetes (mellitus)
diabetes (mellitus) due to autoimmune process
diabetes (mellitus) due to immune mediated pancreatic islet beta-cell destruction
idiopathic diabetes (mellitus)
juvenile onset diabetes (mellitus)
ketosis-prone diabetes (mellitus)

EXCLUDES 1   *diabetes mellitus due to underlying condition (E08.-)*
drug or chemical induced diabetes mellitus (E09.-)
gestational diabetes (O24.4-)
hyperglycemia NOS (R73.9)
neonatal diabetes mellitus (P70.2)
postpancreatectomy diabetes mellitus (E13.-)
postprocedural diabetes mellitus (E13.-)
secondary diabetes mellitus NEC (E13.-)
type 2 diabetes mellitus (E11.-)

AHA: 2013,4Q,114; 2013,3Q,20

√5ᵗʰ **E10.1   Type 1 diabetes mellitus with** kidney complications

     AHA: 2013,3Q,20
     DEF: Diabetic ketoacidosis: Potentially life-threatening complication due to a shortage of insulin in which the body switches to burning fatty acids and producing acidic ketone bodies.

     E10.10   Type 1 diabetes mellitus with ketoacidosis HCC Q **without coma**

     E10.11   Type 1 diabetes mellitus with ketoacidosis HCC Q **with coma**

√5ᵗʰ **E10.2   Type 1 diabetes mellitus with** kidney complications

     E10.21   Type 1 diabetes mellitus with diabetic HCC Q **nephropathy**
          Type 1 diabetes mellitus with intercapillary glomerulosclerosis
          Type 1 diabetes mellitus with intracapillary glomerulonephrosis
          Type 1 diabetes mellitus with Kimmelstiel-Wilson disease

     E10.22   Type 1 diabetes mellitus with diabetic HCC Q **chronic kidney disease**
          Use additional code to identify stage of chronic kidney disease (N18.1-N18.6)

     E10.29   Type 1 diabetes mellitus with other diabetic HCC Q **kidney complication**
          Type 1 diabetes mellitus with renal tubular degeneration
          AHA: 2016,1Q,13

√5ᵗʰ **E10.3   Type 1 diabetes mellitus with** ophthalmic complications

     One of the following 7th characters is to be assigned to codes in subcategories E10.32, E10.33, E10.34, E10.35, and E10.37 to designate laterality of the disease:
     1   right eye
     2   left eye
     3   bilateral
     9   unspecified eye

√6ᵗʰ **E10.31   Type 1 diabetes mellitus with unspecified diabetic retinopathy**
       DEF: Diabetic retinopathy: Diabetic complication from damage to the retinal vessels resulting in vision problems that can progress to blindness.

       E10.311   Type 1 diabetes mellitus with HCC Q **unspecified diabetic retinopathy with macular edema**

       E10.319   Type 1 diabetes mellitus with HCC Q **unspecified diabetic retinopathy without macular edema**

√6ᵗʰ **E10.32   Type 1 diabetes mellitus with** mild nonproliferative diabetic retinopathy
       Type 1 diabetes mellitus with nonproliferative diabetic retinopathy NOS

       √7ᵗʰ **E10.321   Type 1 diabetes mellitus with** HCC Q **mild nonproliferative diabetic retinopathy with macular edema**

       √7ᵗʰ **E10.329   Type 1 diabetes mellitus with** HCC Q **mild nonproliferative diabetic retinopathy without macular edema**

√6ᵗʰ **E10.33   Type 1 diabetes mellitus with** moderate nonproliferative **diabetic** retinopathy

     √7ᵗʰ **E10.331   Type 1 diabetes mellitus with** HCC Q **moderate nonproliferative diabetic retinopathy with macular edema**

     √7ᵗʰ **E10.339   Type 1 diabetes mellitus with** HCC Q **moderate nonproliferative diabetic retinopathy without macular edema**

√6ᵗʰ **E10.34   Type 1 diabetes mellitus with** severe nonproliferative **diabetic** retinopathy

     √7ᵗʰ **E10.341   Type 1 diabetes mellitus with** HCC Q **severe nonproliferative diabetic retinopathy with macular edema**

     √7ᵗʰ **E10.349   Type 1 diabetes mellitus with** HCC Q **severe nonproliferative diabetic retinopathy without macular edema**

√6ᵗʰ **E10.35   Type 1 diabetes mellitus with** proliferative **diabetic** retinopathy

     √7ᵗʰ **E10.351   Type 1 diabetes mellitus with** HCC Q **proliferative diabetic retinopathy with macular edema**

     √7ᵗʰ **E10.352   Type 1 diabetes mellitus with** HCC Q **proliferative diabetic retinopathy with traction retinal detachment involving the macula**

     √7ᵗʰ **E10.353   Type 1 diabetes mellitus with** HCC Q **proliferative diabetic retinopathy with traction retinal detachment not involving the macula**

     √7ᵗʰ **E10.354   Type 1 diabetes mellitus with** HCC Q **proliferative diabetic retinopathy with combined traction retinal detachment and rhegmatogenous retinal detachment**

     √7ᵗʰ **E10.355   Type 1 diabetes mellitus with** HCC Q **stable proliferative diabetic retinopathy**

     √7ᵗʰ **E10.359   Type 1 diabetes mellitus with** HCC Q **proliferative diabetic retinopathy without macular edema**

     E10.36   Type 1 diabetes mellitus with diabetic HCC Q **cataract**
       AHA: 2019,2Q,30-31; 2016,4Q,142

√x7ᵗʰ **E10.37   Type 1 diabetes mellitus with diabetic** HCC Q **macular edema, resolved following treatment**

     E10.39   Type 1 diabetes mellitus with other diabetic HCC Q **ophthalmic complication**
       Use additional code to identify manifestation, such as:
         diabetic glaucoma (H40-H42)

√5ᵗʰ **E10.4   Type 1 diabetes mellitus with** neurological complications

     E10.40   Type 1 diabetes mellitus with diabetic HCC Q **neuropathy, unspecified**

     E10.41   Type 1 diabetes mellitus with diabetic HCC Q **mononeuropathy**

     E10.42   Type 1 diabetes mellitus with diabetic HCC Q **polyneuropathy**
       Type 1 diabetes mellitus with diabetic neuralgia

     E10.43   Type 1 diabetes mellitus with diabetic HCC Q **autonomic (poly)neuropathy**
       Type 1 diabetes mellitus with diabetic gastroparesis
       AHA: 2013,4Q,114

     E10.44   Type 1 diabetes mellitus with diabetic HCC Q **amyotrophy**

     E10.49   Type 1 diabetes mellitus with other diabetic HCC Q **neurological complication**

√5ᵗʰ **E10.5   Type 1 diabetes mellitus with** circulatory complications

     E10.51   Type 1 diabetes mellitus with diabetic HCC Q **peripheral angiopathy without gangrene**
       AHA: 2018,2Q,7

     E10.52   Type 1 diabetes mellitus with diabetic HCC Q **peripheral angiopathy with gangrene**
       Type 1 diabetes mellitus with diabetic gangrene
       AHA: 2018,2Q,7; 2017,4Q,102

     E10.59   Type 1 diabetes mellitus with other HCC Q **circulatory complications**

✓5ᵗʰ **E10.6**   **Type 1 diabetes mellitus with other specified complications**

  ✓6ᵗʰ **E10.61**   **Type 1 diabetes mellitus with diabetic** arthropathy

    E10.610   **Type 1 diabetes mellitus with diabetic** neuropathic **arthropathy**   HCC Q
      Type 1 diabetes mellitus with Charcôt's joints
      DEF: Charcot's joint: Progressive neurologic arthropathy in which chronic degeneration of joints in the weight-bearing areas with peripheral hypertrophy occurs as a complication of a neuropathy disorder. Supporting structures relax from a loss of sensation resulting in chronic joint instability.

    E10.618   **Type 1 diabetes mellitus with other diabetic arthropathy**   HCC Q
      AHA: 2018,2Q,6

  ✓6ᵗʰ **E10.62**   **Type 1 diabetes mellitus with** skin complications

    E10.620   **Type 1 diabetes mellitus with diabetic** dermatitis   HCC Q
      Type 1 diabetes mellitus with diabetic necrobiosis lipoidica

    E10.621   **Type 1 diabetes mellitus with** foot HCC Q **ulcer**
      Use additional code to identify site of ulcer (L97.4-, L97.5-)
      TIP: Do not assign a code for diabetic ulcer when the ulcer is closed/resolved or to report history of diabetic ulcers; Z86.31 Personal history of diabetic foot ulcer, may be assigned.

    E10.622   **Type 1 diabetes mellitus with other skin ulcer**   HCC Q
      Use additional code to identify site of ulcer (L97.1-L97.9, L98.41-L98.49)
      AHA: 2017,4Q,17

    E10.628   **Type 1 diabetes mellitus with other skin complications**   HCC Q
      AHA: 2017,4Q,100-101

  ✓6ᵗʰ **E10.63**   **Type 1 diabetes mellitus with** oral complications

    E10.630   **Type 1 diabetes mellitus with** periodontal disease   HCC Q

    E10.638   **Type 1 diabetes mellitus with other oral complications**   HCC Q

  ✓6ᵗʰ **E10.64**   **Type 1 diabetes mellitus with** hypoglycemia

    E10.641   **Type 1 diabetes mellitus with hypoglycemia** with coma   HCC Q

    E10.649   **Type 1 diabetes mellitus with hypoglycemia** without coma   HCC Q
      AHA: 2016,3Q,42; 2016,1Q,13; 2015,3Q,21

  E10.65   **Type 1 diabetes mellitus with** hyperglycemia   HCC Q
    AHA: 2013,3Q,20

  E10.69   **Type 1 diabetes mellitus with other specified complication**   HCC Q
    Use additional code to identify complication
    AHA: 2016,4Q,141; 2016,1Q,13

E10.8   **Type 1 diabetes mellitus with unspecified complications**   HCC Q

E10.9   **Type 1 diabetes mellitus** without complications   HCC Q

✓4ᵗʰ **E11**   Type 2 **diabetes mellitus**

  INCLUDES   diabetes (mellitus) due to insulin secretory defect
    diabetes NOS
    insulin resistant diabetes (mellitus)
  Use additional code to identify control using:
    insulin (Z79.4)
    oral antidiabetic drugs (Z79.84)
    oral hypoglycemic drugs (Z79.84)
  EXCLUDES 1   diabetes mellitus due to underlying condition (E08.-)
    drug or chemical induced diabetes mellitus (E09.-)
    gestational diabetes (O24.4-)
    neonatal diabetes mellitus (P70.2)
    postpancreatectomy diabetes mellitus (E13.-)
    postprocedural diabetes mellitus (E13.-)
    secondary diabetes mellitus NEC (E13.-)
    type 1 diabetes mellitus (E10.-)
  AHA: 2016,2Q,10; 2013,4Q,114; 2013,3Q,20; 2013,1Q,26

  ✓5ᵗʰ **E11.0**   **Type 2 diabetes mellitus with** hyperosmolarity
    DEF: Diabetic hyperosmolarity: Extremely high levels of glucose in the blood without ketones.

    E11.00   **Type 2 diabetes mellitus with hyperosmolarity** without nonketotic hyperglycemic-hyperosmolar coma **(NKHHC)**   HCC Q

    E11.01   **Type 2 diabetes mellitus with hyperosmolarity** with coma   HCC Q

  ✓5ᵗʰ **E11.1**   **Type 2 diabetes mellitus with** ketoacidosis
    DEF: Diabetic ketoacidosis: Potentially life-threatening complication due to a shortage of insulin in which the body switches to burning fatty acids and producing acidic ketone bodies.

    E11.10   **Type 2 diabetes mellitus with ketoacidosis** without coma   HCC

    E11.11   **Type 2 diabetes mellitus with ketoacidosis** with coma   HCC

  ✓5ᵗʰ **E11.2**   **Type 2 diabetes mellitus with** kidney complications

    E11.21   **Type 2 diabetes mellitus with diabetic** nephropathy   HCC Q
      Type 2 diabetes mellitus with intercapillary glomerulosclerosis
      Type 2 diabetes mellitus with intracapillary glomerulonephrosis
      Type 2 diabetes mellitus with Kimmelstiel-Wilson disease

    E11.22   **Type 2 diabetes mellitus with diabetic** chronic kidney disease   HCC Q
      Use additional code to identify stage of chronic kidney disease (N18.1-N18.6)
      AHA: 2016,1Q,12

    E11.29   **Type 2 diabetes mellitus with other diabetic kidney complication**   HCC Q
      Type 2 diabetes mellitus with renal tubular degeneration

  ✓5ᵗʰ **E11.3**   **Type 2 diabetes mellitus with** ophthalmic complications

    One of the following 7th characters is to be assigned to codes in subcategories E11.32, E11.33, E11.34, E11.35, and E11.37 to designate laterality of the disease:
    1   right eye
    2   left eye
    3   bilateral
    9   unspecified eye

  ✓6ᵗʰ **E11.31**   **Type 2 diabetes mellitus with unspecified diabetic** retinopathy
    DEF: Diabetic retinopathy: Diabetic complication from damage to the retinal vessels resulting in vision problems that can progress to blindness.

    E11.311   **Type 2 diabetes mellitus with unspecified diabetic retinopathy** with macular edema   HCC Q

    E11.319   **Type 2 diabetes mellitus with unspecified diabetic retinopathy** without macular edema   HCC Q

  ✓6ᵗʰ **E11.32**   **Type 2 diabetes mellitus with** mild nonproliferative diabetic **retinopathy**
    Type 2 diabetes mellitus with nonproliferative diabetic retinopathy NOS

    ✓7ᵗʰ **E11.321**   **Type 2 diabetes mellitus with mild nonproliferative diabetic retinopathy** with macular edema   HCC Q

√7th **E11.329** **Type 2 diabetes mellitus with mild nonproliferative diabetic retinopathy** without macular edema HCC Q

√6th **E11.33** **Type 2 diabetes mellitus with** moderate nonproliferative **diabetic** retinopathy

√7th **E11.331** **Type 2 diabetes mellitus with moderate nonproliferative diabetic retinopathy with** macular edema

√7th **E11.339** **Type 2 diabetes mellitus with moderate nonproliferative diabetic retinopathy without** macular edema HCC Q

√6th **E11.34** **Type 2 diabetes mellitus with** severe nonproliferative **diabetic** retinopathy

√7th **E11.341** **Type 2 diabetes mellitus with severe nonproliferative diabetic retinopathy with macular edema** HCC Q

√7th **E11.349** **Type 2 diabetes mellitus with severe nonproliferative diabetic retinopathy without macular edema** HCC Q

√6th **E11.35** **Type 2 diabetes mellitus with** proliferative **diabetic** retinopathy

√7th **E11.351** **Type 2 diabetes mellitus with proliferative diabetic retinopathy with macular edema** HCC Q

√7th **E11.352** **Type 2 diabetes mellitus with proliferative diabetic retinopathy with traction retinal detachment involving the macula** HCC Q

√7th **E11.353** **Type 2 diabetes mellitus with proliferative diabetic retinopathy with traction retinal detachment not involving the macula** HCC Q

√7th **E11.354** **Type 2 diabetes mellitus with proliferative diabetic retinopathy with combined traction retinal detachment and rhegmatogenous retinal detachment** HCC Q

√7th **E11.355** **Type 2 diabetes mellitus with** stable **proliferative diabetic retinopathy** HCC Q

√7th **E11.359** **Type 2 diabetes mellitus with proliferative diabetic retinopathy** without macular edema HCC Q

E11.36 **Type 2 diabetes mellitus with diabetic** cataract HCC Q
AHA: 2019,2Q,30-31; 2016,4Q,142

√x7th **E11.37** **Type 2 diabetes mellitus with diabetic** macular edema, resolved following treatment HCC Q

E11.39 **Type 2 diabetes mellitus with other diabetic ophthalmic complication** HCC Q
Use additional code to identify manifestation, such as:
diabetic glaucoma (H40-H42)

√5th **E11.4** **Type 2 diabetes mellitus with** neurological complications

E11.40 **Type 2 diabetes mellitus with diabetic neuropathy, unspecified** HCC Q
AHA: 2013,4Q,129

E11.41 **Type 2 diabetes mellitus with diabetic** mononeuropathy HCC Q

E11.42 **Type 2 diabetes mellitus with diabetic** polyneuropathy HCC Q
Type 2 diabetes mellitus with diabetic neuralgia
AHA: 2016,1Q,12

E11.43 **Type 2 diabetes mellitus with diabetic autonomic (poly)neuropathy** HCC Q
Type 2 diabetes mellitus with diabetic gastroparesis
AHA: 2013,4Q,114

E11.44 **Type 2 diabetes mellitus with diabetic** amyotrophy HCC Q

E11.49 **Type 2 diabetes mellitus with other diabetic neurological complication** HCC Q

√5th **E11.5** **Type 2 diabetes mellitus with** circulatory complications

E11.51 **Type 2 diabetes mellitus with diabetic** peripheral angiopathy without gangrene HCC Q
AHA: 2018,2Q,7

E11.52 **Type 2 diabetes mellitus with diabetic peripheral angiopathy with gangrene** HCC Q
Type 2 diabetes mellitus with diabetic gangrene
AHA: 2018,2Q,7; 2017,4Q,102

E11.59 **Type 2 diabetes mellitus with other circulatory complications** HCC Q

√5th **E11.6** **Type 2 diabetes mellitus with other specified complications**

√6th **E11.61** **Type 2 diabetes mellitus with diabetic** arthropathy

E11.610 **Type 2 diabetes mellitus with diabetic** neuropathic **arthropathy** HCC Q
Type 2 diabetes mellitus with Charcôt's joints
DEF: Charcot's joint: Progressive neurologic arthropathy in which chronic degeneration of joints in the weight-bearing areas with peripheral hypertrophy occurs as a complication of a neuropathy disorder. Supporting structures relax from a loss of sensation resulting in chronic joint instability.

E11.618 **Type 2 diabetes mellitus with other diabetic arthropathy** HCC Q
AHA: 2018,2Q,6

√6th **E11.62** **Type 2 diabetes mellitus with** skin complications

E11.620 **Type 2 diabetes mellitus with diabetic dermatitis** HCC Q
Type 2 diabetes mellitus with diabetic necrobiosis lipoidica

E11.621 **Type 2 diabetes mellitus with** foot ulcer HCC Q
Use additional code to identify site of ulcer (L97.4-, L97.5-)
AHA: 2016,1Q,12
TIP: Do not assign a code for diabetic ulcer when the ulcer is closed/resolved or to report history of diabetic ulcers; Z86.31 Personal history of diabetic foot ulcer, may be assigned.

E11.622 **Type 2 diabetes mellitus with other skin ulcer** HCC Q
Use additional code to identify site of ulcer (L97.1-L97.9, L98.41-L98.49)
AHA: 2017,4Q,17

E11.628 **Type 2 diabetes mellitus with other skin complications** HCC Q
AHA: 2017,4Q,100-101

√6th **E11.63** **Type 2 diabetes mellitus with** oral complications

E11.630 **Type 2 diabetes mellitus with** periodontal disease HCC Q

E11.638 **Type 2 diabetes mellitus with other oral complications** HCC Q

√6th **E11.64** **Type 2 diabetes mellitus with** hypoglycemia

E11.641 **Type 2 diabetes mellitus with hypoglycemia** with coma HCC Q

E11.649 **Type 2 diabetes mellitus with hypoglycemia** without coma HCC Q
AHA: 2016,3Q,42; 2015,3Q,21

E11.65 **Type 2 diabetes mellitus with** hyperglycemia HCC Q
AHA: 2013,3Q,20

E11.69 **Type 2 diabetes mellitus with other specified complication** HCC Q
Use additional code to identify complication
AHA: 2016,4Q,141; 2016,1Q,13

E11.8 **Type 2 diabetes mellitus with unspecified complications** HCC Q

E11.9 **Type 2 diabetes mellitus** without complications HCC Q

✓4th **E13 Other specified diabetes mellitus**

INCLUDES   diabetes mellitus due to genetic defects of beta-cell function

diabetes mellitus due to genetic defects in insulin action

postpancreatectomy diabetes mellitus

postprocedural diabetes mellitus

secondary diabetes mellitus NEC

Use additional code to identify control using:

insulin (Z79.4)

oral antidiabetic drugs (Z79.84)

oral hypoglycemic drugs (Z79.84)

EXCLUDES 1   *diabetes (mellitus) due to autoimmune process (E10.-)*

diabetes (mellitus) due to immune mediated pancreatic islet beta-cell destruction (E10.-)

diabetes mellitus due to underlying condition (E08.-)

drug or chemical induced diabetes mellitus (E09.-)

gestational diabetes (O24.4-)

neonatal diabetes mellitus (P70.2)

type 1 diabetes mellitus (E10.-)

AHA: 2018,3Q,4; 2016,1Q,11-13; 2013,4Q,114; 2013,3Q,20

TIP: Use this category when the diabetes is documented as diabetes type 1.5. Synonymous terms used in the documentation may also include combined diabetes type 1 and type 2, latent autoimmune diabetes of adults (LADA), slow-progressing type 1 diabetes, or double diabetes.

TIP: When postprocedural or postpancreatectomy hypoinsulinemia (E89.1) is documented with postprocedural or postpancreatectomy diabetes mellitus (E13.-), code E89.1 should be sequenced first.

✓5th **E13.0 Other specified diabetes mellitus with** hyperosmolarity

DEF: Diabetic hyperosmolarity: Extremely high levels of glucose in the blood without ketones.

E13.00   Other specified diabetes mellitus with hyperosmolarity without nonketotic hyperglycemic-hyperosmolar coma (NKHHC)   HCC Q

EXCLUDES 2   *type 2 diabetes mellitus (E11.-)*

E13.01   Other specified diabetes mellitus with hyperosmolarity with coma   HCC Q

✓5th **E13.1 Other specified diabetes mellitus with** ketoacidosis

AHA: 2016,2Q,10; 2013,1Q,26

DEF: Diabetic ketoacidosis: Potentially life threatening complication due to a shortage of insulin in which the body switches to burning fatty acids and producing acidic ketone bodies.

E13.10   Other specified diabetes mellitus with ketoacidosis without coma   HCC Q

E13.11   Other specified diabetes mellitus with ketoacidosis with coma   HCC Q

✓5th **E13.2 Other specified diabetes mellitus with** kidney complications

E13.21   Other specified diabetes mellitus with diabetic nephropathy   HCC Q

Other specified diabetes mellitus with intercapillary glomerulosclerosis

Other specified diabetes mellitus with intracapillary glomerulonephrosis

Other specified diabetes mellitus with Kimmelstiel-Wilson disease

E13.22   Other specified diabetes mellitus with diabetic chronic kidney disease   HCC Q

Use additional code to identify stage of chronic kidney disease (N18.1-N18.6)

E13.29   Other specified diabetes mellitus with other diabetic kidney complication   HCC Q

Other specified diabetes mellitus with renal tubular degeneration

✓5th **E13.3 Other specified diabetes mellitus with** ophthalmic complications

One of the following 7th characters is to be assigned to codes in subcategories E13.32, E13.33, E13.34, E13.35, and E13.37 to designate laterality of the disease:

1   right eye

2   left eye

3   bilateral

9   unspecified eye

✓6th **E13.31   Other specified diabetes mellitus with unspecified diabetic** retinopathy

DEF: Diabetic retinopathy: Diabetic complication from damage to the retinal vessels resulting in vision problems that can progress to blindness.

E13.311   Other specified diabetes mellitus with unspecified diabetic retinopathy with macular edema   HCC Q

E13.319   Other specified diabetes mellitus with unspecified diabetic retinopathy without macular edema   HCC Q

✓6th **E13.32   Other specified diabetes mellitus with** mild nonproliferative **diabetic** retinopathy

Other specified diabetes mellitus with nonproliferative diabetic retinopathy NOS

E13.321   Other specified diabetes mellitus with mild nonproliferative diabetic retinopathy with macular edema   HCC Q

E13.329   Other specified diabetes mellitus with mild nonproliferative diabetic retinopathy without macular edema   HCC Q

✓6th **E13.33   Other specified diabetes mellitus with** moderate nonproliferative **diabetic** retinopathy

E13.331   Other specified diabetes mellitus with moderate nonproliferative diabetic retinopathy with macular edema   HCC Q

E13.339   Other specified diabetes mellitus with moderate nonproliferative diabetic retinopathy without macular edema   HCC Q

✓6th **E13.34   Other specified diabetes mellitus with** severe nonproliferative **diabetic** retinopathy

E13.341   Other specified diabetes mellitus with severe nonproliferative diabetic retinopathy with macular edema   HCC Q

E13.349   Other specified diabetes mellitus with severe nonproliferative diabetic retinopathy without macular edema   HCC Q

✓6th **E13.35   Other specified diabetes mellitus with** proliferative **diabetic** retinopathy

E13.351   Other specified diabetes mellitus with proliferative diabetic retinopathy with macular edema   HCC Q

E13.352   Other specified diabetes mellitus with proliferative diabetic retinopathy with traction retinal detachment involving the macula   HCC Q

E13.353   Other specified diabetes mellitus with proliferative diabetic retinopathy with traction retinal detachment not involving the macula   HCC Q

E13.354   Other specified diabetes mellitus with proliferative diabetic retinopathy with combined traction retinal detachment and rhegmatogenous retinal detachment   HCC Q

E13.355   Other specified diabetes mellitus with stable proliferative diabetic retinopathy   HCC Q

E13.359   Other specified diabetes mellitus with proliferative diabetic retinopathy without macular edema   HCC Q

E13.36   Other specified diabetes mellitus with diabetic cataract   HCC Q

AHA: 2019,2Q,30-31; 2016,4Q,142

✓ Additional Character Required   ✓x7th Placeholder Alert   Manifestation   Unspecified Dx   ▶◀ Revised Text   ● New Code   ▲ Revised Code Title

ICD-10-CM 2020   521

√x 7th **E13.37** **Other specified diabetes mellitus with** HCC Q **diabetic macular edema, resolved following treatment**

E13.39 **Other specified diabetes mellitus with other** HCC Q **diabetic ophthalmic complication**

Use additional code to identify manifestation, such as:

diabetic glaucoma (H40-H42)

√5th **E13.4** **Other specified diabetes mellitus with neurological complications**

E13.40 **Other specified diabetes mellitus with** HCC Q **diabetic neuropathy, unspecified**

E13.41 **Other specified diabetes mellitus with** HCC Q **diabetic mononeuropathy**

E13.42 **Other specified diabetes mellitus with** HCC Q **diabetic polyneuropathy**

Other specified diabetes mellitus with diabetic neuralgia

E13.43 **Other specified diabetes mellitus with** HCC Q **diabetic autonomic (poly)neuropathy**

Other specified diabetes mellitus with diabetic gastroparesis

AHA: 2013,4Q,114

E13.44 **Other specified diabetes mellitus with** HCC Q **diabetic amyotrophy**

E13.49 **Other specified diabetes mellitus with other** HCC Q **diabetic neurological complication**

√5th **E13.5** **Other specified diabetes mellitus with circulatory complications**

E13.51 **Other specified diabetes mellitus with** HCC Q **diabetic peripheral angiopathy without gangrene**

AHA: 2018,2Q,7

E13.52 **Other specified diabetes mellitus with** HCC Q **diabetic peripheral angiopathy with gangrene**

Other specified diabetes mellitus with diabetic gangrene

AHA: 2018,2Q,7; 2017,4Q,102

E13.59 **Other specified diabetes mellitus with other** HCC Q **circulatory complications**

√5th **E13.6** **Other specified diabetes mellitus with other specified complications**

√6th **E13.61** **Other specified diabetes mellitus with diabetic arthropathy**

E13.610 **Other specified diabetes mellitus** HCC Q **with diabetic neuropathic arthropathy**

Other specified diabetes mellitus with Charcôt's joints

DEF: Charcôt's joint: Progressive neurologic arthropathy in which chronic degeneration of joints in the weight-bearing areas with peripheral hypertrophy occurs as a complication of a neuropathy disorder. Supporting structures relax from a loss of sensation resulting in chronic joint instability.

E13.618 **Other specified diabetes mellitus** HCC Q **with other diabetic arthropathy**

AHA: 2018,2Q,6

√6th **E13.62** **Other specified diabetes mellitus with skin complications**

E13.620 **Other specified diabetes mellitus** HCC Q **with diabetic dermatitis**

Other specified diabetes mellitus with diabetic necrobiosis lipoidica

E13.621 **Other specified diabetes mellitus** HCC Q **with foot ulcer**

Use additional code to identify site of ulcer (L97.4-, L97.5-)

TIP: Do not assign a code for diabetic ulcer when the ulcer is closed/resolved or to report history of diabetic ulcers; Z86.31 Personal history of diabetic foot ulcer, may be assigned.

E13.622 **Other specified diabetes mellitus** HCC Q **with other skin ulcer**

Use additional code to identify site of ulcer (L97.1-L97.9, L98.41-L98.49)

AHA: 2017,4Q,17

E13.628 **Other specified diabetes mellitus** HCC Q **with other skin complications**

AHA: 2017,4Q,100-101

√6th **E13.63** **Other specified diabetes mellitus with oral complications**

E13.630 **Other specified diabetes mellitus** HCC Q **with periodontal disease**

E13.638 **Other specified diabetes mellitus** HCC Q **with other oral complications**

√6th **E13.64** **Other specified diabetes mellitus with hypoglycemia**

E13.641 **Other specified diabetes mellitus** HCC Q **with hypoglycemia with coma**

E13.649 **Other specified diabetes mellitus** HCC Q **with hypoglycemia without coma**

AHA: 2016,3Q,42; 2015,3Q,21

E13.65 **Other specified diabetes mellitus with** HCC Q **hyperglycemia**

E13.69 **Other specified diabetes mellitus with other** HCC Q **specified complication**

Use additional code to identify complication

AHA: 2016,4Q,141; 2016,1Q,13

E13.8 **Other specified diabetes mellitus with unspecified** HCC Q **complications**

E13.9 **Other specified diabetes mellitus without** HCC Q **complications**

Other disorders of glucose regulation and pancreatic internal secretion (E15-E16)

E15 Nondiabetic hypoglycemic coma HCC

INCLUDES drug-induced insulin coma in nondiabetic hyperinsulinism with hypoglycemic coma hypoglycemic coma NOS

√4th **E16 Other disorders of pancreatic internal secretion**

E16.0 **Drug-induced hypoglycemia without coma**

Use additional code for adverse effect, if applicable, to identify drug (T36-T50 with fifth or sixth character 5)

EXCLUDES 1 diabetes with hypoglycemia without coma (E09.649)

E16.1 **Other hypoglycemia**

Functional hyperinsulinism

Functional nonhyperinsulinemic hypoglycemia

Hyperinsulinism NOS

Hyperplasia of pancreatic islet beta cells NOS

EXCLUDES 1 diabetes with hypoglycemia (E08.649, E10.649, E11.649, E13.649)

hypoglycemia in infant of diabetic mother (P70.1)

neonatal hypoglycemia (P70.4)

E16.2 **Hypoglycemia, unspecified**

EXCLUDES 1 diabetes with hypoglycemia (E08.649, E10.649, E11.649, E13.649)

AHA: 2016,3Q,42

TIP: Assign for nondiabetic hypoglycemic encephalopathy not further clarified in the documentation.

E16.3 **Increased secretion of glucagon**

Hyperplasia of pancreatic endocrine cells with glucagon excess

E16.4 **Increased secretion of gastrin**

Hypergastrinemia

Hyperplasia of pancreatic endocrine cells with gastrin excess

Zollinger-Ellison syndrome

E16.8 **Other specified disorders of pancreatic internal secretion**

Increased secretion from endocrine pancreas of growth hormone-releasing hormone

Increased secretion from endocrine pancreas of pancreatic polypeptide

Increased secretion from endocrine pancreas of somatostatin

Increased secretion from endocrine pancreas of vasoactive-intestinal polypeptide

E16.9 **Disorder of pancreatic internal secretion, unspecified**

Islet-cell hyperplasia NOS

Pancreatic endocrine cell hyperplasia NOS

Disorders of other endocrine glands (E20-E35)

EXCLUDES 1   galactorrhea (N64.3)
         gynecomastia (N62)

✓4th **E20 Hypoparathyroidism**

     EXCLUDES 1   Di George's syndrome (D82.1)
            postprocedural hypoparathyroidism (E89.2)
            tetany NOS (R29.0)
            transitory neonatal hypoparathyroidism (P71.4)

E20.0 Idiopathic hypoparathyroidism   HCC

     DEF: Abnormally low secretion of parathyroid hormones, with unknown cause, which causes decreased calcium and increased phosphorus in the blood, resulting in muscle cramps, tetany, tingling, or burning in the lips, fingers, and toes, and cataracts.

E20.1 Pseudohypoparathyroidism

E20.8 Other hypoparathyroidism   HCC

E20.9 Hypoparathyroidism, unspecified   HCC

     Parathyroid tetany

✓4th **E21 Hyperparathyroidism and other disorders of parathyroid gland**

     EXCLUDES 1   adult osteomalacia (M83.-)
            ectopic hyperparathyroidism (E34.2)
            familial hypocalciuric hypercalcemia (E83.52)
            hungry bone syndrome (E83.81)
            infantile and juvenile osteomalacia (E55.0)

E21.0 Primary hyperparathyroidism   HCC

     Hyperplasia of parathyroid
     Osteitis fibrosa cystica generalisata [von Recklinghausen's disease of bone]
     DEF: Parathyroid dysfunction commonly caused by hyperplasia of two or more glands. Symptoms include hypercalcemia and increased parathyroid hormone levels.

E21.1 Secondary hyperparathyroidism, not elsewhere classified   HCC

     EXCLUDES 1   secondary hyperparathyroidism of renal origin (N25.81)

E21.2 Other hyperparathyroidism   HCC

     Tertiary hyperparathyroidism
     EXCLUDES 1   familial hypocalciuric hypercalcemia (E83.52)

E21.3 Hyperparathyroidism, unspecified   HCC

E21.4 Other specified disorders of parathyroid gland   HCC

E21.5 Disorder of parathyroid gland, unspecified   HCC

✓4th **E22 Hyperfunction of pituitary gland**

     EXCLUDES 1   Cushing's syndrome (E24.-)
            Nelson's syndrome (E24.1)
            overproduction of ACTH not associated with Cushing's disease (E27.0)
            overproduction of pituitary ACTH (E24.0)
            overproduction of thyroid-stimulating hormone (E05.8-)

E22.0 Acromegaly and pituitary gigantism   HCC

     Overproduction of growth hormone
     EXCLUDES 1   constitutional gigantism (E34.4)
            constitutional tall stature (E34.4)
            increased secretion from endocrine pancreas of growth hormone-releasing hormone (E16.8)
     DEF: Acromegaly: Chronic condition caused by overproduction of the pituitary growth hormone resulting in enlarged skeletal parts and facial features.

E22.1 Hyperprolactinemia   HCC

     Use additional code for adverse effect, if applicable, to identify drug (T36-T50 with fifth or sixth character 5)

E22.2 Syndrome of inappropriate secretion of antidiuretic hormone   HCC

E22.8 Other hyperfunction of pituitary gland   HCC

     Central precocious puberty

E22.9 Hyperfunction of pituitary gland, unspecified   HCC

✓4th **E23 Hypofunction and other disorders of the pituitary gland**

     INCLUDES   the listed conditions whether the disorder is in the pituitary or the hypothalamus

     EXCLUDES 1   postprocedural hypopituitarism (E89.3)

E23.0 Hypopituitarism   HCC

     Fertile eunuch syndrome
     Hypogonadotropic hypogonadism
     Idiopathic growth hormone deficiency
     Isolated deficiency of gonadotropin
     Isolated deficiency of growth hormone
     Isolated deficiency of pituitary hormone
     Kallmann's syndrome
     Lorain-Levi short stature
     Necrosis of pituitary gland (postpartum)
     Panhypopituitarism
     Pituitary cachexia
     Pituitary insufficiency NOS
     Pituitary short stature
     Sheehan's syndrome
     Simmonds' disease

E23.1 Drug-induced hypopituitarism   HCC

     Use additional code for adverse effect, if applicable, to identify drug (T36-T50 with fifth or sixth character 5)

E23.2 Diabetes insipidus   HCC

     EXCLUDES 1   nephrogenic diabetes insipidus (N25.1)

E23.3 Hypothalamic dysfunction, not elsewhere classified   HCC

     EXCLUDES 1   Prader-Willi syndrome ▶(Q87.11)◀
            Russell-Silver syndrome ▶(Q87.19)◀

E23.6 Other disorders of pituitary gland   HCC

     Abscess of pituitary
     Adiposogenital dystrophy

E23.7 Disorder of pituitary gland, unspecified   HCC

✓4th **E24 Cushing's syndrome**

     EXCLUDES 1   congenital adrenal hyperplasia (E25.0)

     DEF: Abdominal striae, acne, hypertension, decreased carbohydrate tolerance, moon face, obesity, protein catabolism, and psychiatric disturbances resulting from increased adrenocortical secretion of cortisol caused by ACTH-dependent adrenocortical hyperplasia or tumor, or by steroid effects.

E24.0 Pituitary-dependent Cushing's disease   HCC

     Overproduction of pituitary ACTH
     Pituitary-dependent hypercorticalism

E24.1 Nelson's syndrome   HCC

E24.2 Drug-induced Cushing's syndrome   HCC

     Use additional code for adverse effect, if applicable, to identify drug (T36-T50 with fifth or sixth character 5)

E24.3 Ectopic ACTH syndrome   HCC

E24.4 Alcohol-induced pseudo-Cushing's syndrome   HCC

E24.8 Other Cushing's syndrome   HCC

E24.9 Cushing's syndrome, unspecified   HCC

✓4th **E25 Adrenogenital disorders**

     INCLUDES   adrenogenital syndromes, virilizing or feminizing, whether acquired or due to adrenal hyperplasia consequent on inborn enzyme defects in hormone synthesis
            female adrenal pseudohermaphroditism
            female heterosexual precocious pseudopuberty
            male isosexual precocious pseudopuberty
            male macrogenitosomia praecox
            male sexual precocity with adrenal hyperplasia
            male virilization (female)

     EXCLUDES 1   indeterminate sex and pseudohermaphroditism (Q56)
            chromosomal abnormalities (Q90-Q99)

E25.0 Congenital adrenogenital disorders associated with enzyme deficiency   HCC

     Congenital adrenal hyperplasia
     21-Hydroxylase deficiency
     Salt-losing congenital adrenal hyperplasia

E25.8 Other adrenogenital disorders   HCC

     Idiopathic adrenogenital disorder
     Use additional code for adverse effect, if applicable, to identify drug (T36-T50 with fifth or sixth character 5)

✓ Additional Character Required   ✓x7th Placeholder Alert   Manifestation   Unspecified Dx   ▶◀ Revised Text   ● New Code   ▲ Revised Code Title

ICD-10-CM 2020   523

E25.9 – E31.1

Chapter 4. Endocrine, Nutritional and Metabolic Diseases

E25.9 Adrenogenital disorder, unspecified   HCC
   Adrenogenital syndrome NOS

✓4th **E26 Hyperaldosteronism**

   ✓5th **E26.0 Primary hyperaldosteronism**

      E26.01 Conn's syndrome   HCC
         Code also adrenal adenoma (D35.0-)

      E26.02 Glucocorticoid-remediable aldosteronism   HCC
         Familial aldosteronism type I
         DEF: Rare autosomal dominant familial form of primary
         aldosteronism in which the secretion of aldosterone is
         under the influence of adrenocorticotrophic hormone
         (ACTH) rather than the renin-angiotensin mechanism.
         Moderate hypersecretion of aldosterone and
         suppressed plasma renin activity that are rapidly
         reversed by administration of glucosteroids. Symptoms
         include hypertension and mild hypokalemia.

      E26.09 Other primary hyperaldosteronism   HCC
         Primary aldosteronism due to adrenal hyperplasia
         (bilateral)

   E26.1 Secondary hyperaldosteronism   HCC

   ✓5th **E26.8 Other hyperaldosteronism**

      E26.81 Bartter's syndrome   HCC

      E26.89 Other hyperaldosteronism   HCC

   E26.9 Hyperaldosteronism, unspecified   HCC
      Aldosteronism NOS
      Hyperaldosteronism NOS

✓4th **E27 Other disorders of adrenal gland**

   E27.0 Other adrenocortical overactivity   HCC
      Overproduction of ACTH, not associated with Cushing's disease
      Premature adrenarche
      EXCLUDES 1   Cushing's syndrome (E24.-)

   E27.1 Primary adrenocortical insufficiency   HCC
      Addison's disease
      Autoimmune adrenalitis
      EXCLUDES 1   Addison only phenotype adrenoleukodystrophy
                   (E71.528)
                   amyloidosis (E85.-)
                   tuberculous Addison's disease (A18.7)
                   Waterhouse-Friderichsen syndrome (A39.1)

   E27.2 Addisonian crisis   HCC
      Adrenal crisis
      Adrenocortical crisis
      DEF: Life-threatening condition that occurs when there is not
      enough cortisol excreted from the adrenal glands. This condition
      may be due to injury to the adrenal glands or to the pituitary
      gland, which controls adrenal hormone secretion, or when a
      patient stops hydrocortisone treatment too quickly or too early.

   E27.3 Drug-induced adrenocortical insufficiency   HCC
      Use additional code for adverse effect, if applicable, to identify
         drug (T36-T50 with fifth or sixth character 5)

   ✓5th **E27.4 Other and unspecified adrenocortical insufficiency**
      EXCLUDES 1   adrenoleukodystrophy [Addison-Schilder] (E71.528)
                   Waterhouse-Friderichsen syndrome (A39.1)

      E27.40 Unspecified adrenocortical insufficiency   HCC
         Adrenocortical insufficiency NOS
         Hypoaldosteronism

      E27.49 Other adrenocortical insufficiency   HCC
         Adrenal hemorrhage
         Adrenal infarction

   E27.5 Adrenomedullary hyperfunction   HCC
      Adrenomedullary hyperplasia
      Catecholamine hypersecretion

   E27.8 Other specified disorders of adrenal gland   HCC
      Abnormality of cortisol-binding globulin

   E27.9 Disorder of adrenal gland, unspecified   HCC

✓4th **E28 Ovarian dysfunction**
   EXCLUDES 1   isolated gonadotropin deficiency (E23.0)
                postprocedural ovarian failure (E89.4-)

   E28.0 Estrogen excess   ♀
      Use additional code for adverse effect, if applicable, to identify
         drug (T36-T50 with fifth or sixth character 5)

   E28.1 Androgen excess   ♀
      Hypersecretion of ovarian androgens
      Use additional code for adverse effect, if applicable, to identify
         drug (T36-T50 with fifth or sixth character 5)

   E28.2 Polycystic ovarian syndrome   ♀
      Sclerocystic ovary syndrome
      Stein-Leventhal syndrome
      DEF: Common hormonal disorder among women of reproductive
      age that involves enlarged ovaries with numerous small cysts
      located along the outer ovarian edge.

   ✓5th **E28.3 Primary ovarian failure**
      EXCLUDES 1   pure gonadal dysgenesis (Q99.1)
                   Turner's syndrome (Q96.-)

      ✓6th **E28.31 Premature menopause**

         E28.310 Symptomatic premature   A ♀
                    menopause
            Symptoms such as flushing, sleeplessness,
               headache, lack of concentration,
               associated with premature
               menopause

         E28.319 Asymptomatic premature   A ♀
                    menopause
            Premature menopause NOS

      E28.39 Other primary ovarian failure   ♀
         Decreased estrogen
         Resistant ovary syndrome

   E28.8 Other ovarian dysfunction   ♀
      Ovarian hyperfunction NOS
      EXCLUDES 1   postprocedural ovarian failure (E89.4-)

   E28.9 Ovarian dysfunction, unspecified   ♀

✓4th **E29 Testicular dysfunction**
   EXCLUDES 1   androgen insensitivity syndrome (E34.5-)
                azoospermia or oligospermia NOS (N46.0-N46.1)
                isolated gonadotropin deficiency (E23.0)
                Klinefelter's syndrome (Q98.0-Q98.1, Q98.4)

   E29.0 Testicular hyperfunction   ♂
      Hypersecretion of testicular hormones

   E29.1 Testicular hypofunction   ♂
      Defective biosynthesis of testicular androgen NOS
      5-delta-Reductase deficiency (with male
         pseudohermaphroditism)
      Testicular hypogonadism NOS
      Use additional code for adverse effect, if applicable, to identify
         drug (T36-T50 with fifth or sixth character 5)
      EXCLUDES 1   postprocedural testicular hypofunction (E89.5)

   E29.8 Other testicular dysfunction   ♂

   E29.9 Testicular dysfunction, unspecified   ♂

✓4th **E30 Disorders of puberty, not elsewhere classified**

   E30.0 Delayed puberty
      Constitutional delay of puberty
      Delayed sexual development

   E30.1 Precocious puberty   P
      Precocious menstruation
      EXCLUDES 1   Albright (-McCune) (-Sternberg) syndrome (Q78.1)
                   central precocious puberty (E22.8)
                   congenital adrenal hyperplasia (E25.0)
                   female heterosexual precocious pseudopuberty
                      (E25.-)
                   male isosexual precocious pseudopuberty (E25.-)

   E30.8 Other disorders of puberty   P
      Premature thelarche

   E30.9 Disorder of puberty, unspecified

✓4th **E31 Polyglandular dysfunction**
   EXCLUDES 1   ataxia telangiectasia [Louis-Bar] (G11.3)
                dystrophia myotonica [Steinert] (G71.11)
                pseudohypoparathyroidism (E20.1)

   E31.0 Autoimmune polyglandular failure   HCC
      Schmidt's syndrome

   E31.1 Polyglandular hyperfunction   HCC
      EXCLUDES 1   multiple endocrine adenomatosis (E31.2-)
                   multiple endocrine neoplasia (E31.2-)

√5ᵗʰ **E31.2 Multiple endocrine neoplasia [MEN] syndromes**

Multiple endocrine adenomatosis

Code also any associated malignancies and other conditions associated with the syndromes

DEF: Group of conditions in which several endocrine glands grow excessively (such as in adenomatous hyperplasia) and/or develop benign or malignant tumors. Tumors and hyperplasia associated with MEN often produce excess hormones, which impede normal physiology. There is no comprehensive cure known for MEN syndrome. Treatment is directed at the hyperplasia or tumors in each individual gland. Tumors are usually surgically removed and oral medications or hormonal injections are used to correct hormone imbalances.

E31.20 Multiple endocrine neoplasia [MEN] syndrome, unspecified   HCC

Multiple endocrine adenomatosis NOS

Multiple endocrine neoplasia [MEN] syndrome NOS

E31.21 Multiple endocrine neoplasia [MEN] type I   HCC

Wermer's syndrome

E31.22 Multiple endocrine neoplasia [MEN] type IIA   HCC

Sipple's syndrome

E31.23 Multiple endocrine neoplasia [MEN] type IIB   HCC

E31.8 Other polyglandular dysfunction   HCC

E31.9 Polyglandular dysfunction, unspecified   HCC

√4ᵗʰ **E32 Diseases of thymus**

EXCLUDES 1   aplasia or hypoplasia of thymus with immunodeficiency (D82.1)

myasthenia gravis (G70.0)

E32.0 Persistent hyperplasia of thymus   HCC

Hypertrophy of thymus

E32.1 Abscess of thymus   HCC

E32.8 Other diseases of thymus   HCC

. EXCLUDES 1   aplasia or hypoplasia with immunodeficiency (D82.1)

thymoma (D15.0)

E32.9 Disease of thymus, unspecified   HCC

√4ᵗʰ **E34 Other endocrine disorders**

EXCLUDES 1   pseudohypoparathyroidism (E20.1)

E34.0 Carcinoid syndrome   HCC

NOTE   May be used as an additional code to identify functional activity associated with a carcinoid tumor.

E34.1 Other hypersecretion of intestinal hormones

E34.2 Ectopic hormone secretion, not elsewhere classified

EXCLUDES 1   ectopic ACTH syndrome (E24.3)

E34.3 Short stature due to endocrine disorder

Constitutional short stature

Laron-type short stature

EXCLUDES 1   achondroplastic short stature (Q77.4)

hypochondroplastic short stature (Q77.4)

nutritional short stature (E45)

pituitary short stature (E23.0)

progeria (E34.8)

renal short stature (N25.0)

Russell-Silver syndrome ▶(Q87.19)◄

short-limbed stature with immunodeficiency (D82.2)

short stature in specific dysmorphic syndromes — code to syndrome — see Alphabetical Index

short stature NOS (R62.52)

E34.4 Constitutional tall stature   HCC

Constitutional gigantism

√5ᵗʰ **E34.5 Androgen insensitivity syndrome**

DEF: X-linked recessive condition in which individuals that are chromosomally male fail to develop normal male external genitalia due to an abnormality on the X chromosome that prohibits the body, completely or in part, from recognizing the androgens produced. *Synonym(s):* AIS

E34.50 Androgen insensitivity syndrome, unspecified

Androgen insensitivity NOS

E34.51 Complete androgen insensitivity syndrome

Complete androgen insensitivity

de Quervain syndrome

Goldberg-Maxwell syndrome

E34.52 Partial androgen insensitivity syndrome

Partial androgen insensitivity

Reifenstein syndrome

E34.8 Other specified endocrine disorders

Pineal gland dysfunction

Progeria

EXCLUDES 2   pseudohypoparathyroidism (E20.1)

E34.9 Endocrine disorder, unspecified

Endocrine disturbance NOS

Hormone disturbance NOS

E35   ***Disorders of endocrine glands in diseases classified elsewhere***

Code first underlying disease, such as:

late congenital syphilis of thymus gland [Dubois disease] (A50.5)

Use additional code, if applicable, to identify:

sequelae of tuberculosis of other organs (B90.8)

EXCLUDES 1   Echinococcus granulosus infection of thyroid gland (B67.3)

meningococcal hemorrhagic adrenalitis (A39.1)

syphilis of endocrine gland (A52.79)

tuberculosis of adrenal gland, except calcification (A18.7)

tuberculosis of endocrine gland NEC (A18.82)

tuberculosis of thyroid gland (A18.81)

Waterhouse-Friderichsen syndrome (A39.1)

Intraoperative complications of endocrine system (E36)

√4ᵗʰ **E36 Intraoperative complications of endocrine system**

EXCLUDES 2   postprocedural endocrine and metabolic complications and disorders, not elsewhere classified (E89.-)

√5ᵗʰ **E36.0 Intraoperative hemorrhage and hematoma of an endocrine system organ or structure complicating a procedure**

EXCLUDES 1   intraoperative hemorrhage and hematoma of an endocrine system organ or structure due to accidental puncture or laceration during a procedure (E36.1-)

E36.01 Intraoperative hemorrhage and hematoma of an endocrine system organ or structure complicating an endocrine system procedure

E36.02 Intraoperative hemorrhage and hematoma of an endocrine system organ or structure complicating other procedure

√5ᵗʰ **E36.1 Accidental puncture and laceration of an endocrine system organ or structure during a procedure**

E36.11 Accidental puncture and laceration of an endocrine system organ or structure during an endocrine system procedure

E36.12 Accidental puncture and laceration of an endocrine system organ or structure during other procedure

E36.8 Other intraoperative complications of endocrine system

Use additional code, if applicable, to further specify disorder

Malnutrition (E40-E46)

EXCLUDES 1   intestinal malabsorption (K90.-)

sequelae of protein-calorie malnutrition (E64.0)

EXCLUDES 2   nutritional anemias (D50-D53)

starvation (T73.0)

AHA: 2017,4Q,108; 2017,3Q,25

TIP: Assign additional code for BMI from category Z68, when documented. BMI can be based on documentation from clinicians who are not the patient's provider.

E40 Kwashiorkor   HCC

Severe malnutrition with nutritional edema with dyspigmentation of skin and hair

EXCLUDES 1   marasmic kwashiorkor (E42)

E41 Nutritional marasmus   HCC

Severe malnutrition with marasmus

EXCLUDES 1   marasmic kwashiorkor (E42)

AHA: 2017,3Q,24

DEF: Protein-calorie malabsorption or malnutrition in children characterized by tissue wasting, dehydration, and subcutaneous fat depletion. It may occur with infectious disease.

TIP: Assign code R64 when emaciated or emaciation is documented without documentation of malnutrition.

E42 Marasmic kwashiorkor   HCC

Intermediate form severe protein-calorie malnutrition

Severe protein-calorie malnutrition with signs of both kwashiorkor and marasmus

---

✓ Additional Character Required   ✓ˣ⁷ᵗʰ Placeholder Alert   Manifestation   Unspecified Dx   ▶◄ Revised Text   ● New Code   ▲ Revised Code Title

E43 Unspecified severe protein-calorie malnutrition `HCC`
Starvation edema
AHA: 2017,4Q,108

`√4ᵗʰ` **E44 Protein-calorie malnutrition of moderate and mild degree**

E44.0 Moderate protein-calorie malnutrition `HCC`

E44.1 Mild protein-calorie malnutrition `HCC`

E45 Retarded development following protein-calorie malnutrition `HCC`
Nutritional short stature
Nutritional stunting
Physical retardation due to malnutrition

E46 Unspecified protein-calorie malnutrition `HCC`
Malnutrition NOS
Protein-calorie imbalance NOS
`EXCLUDES 1` *nutritional deficiency NOS (E63.9)*
AHA: 2018,4Q,82

Other nutritional deficiencies (E50-E64)

`EXCLUDES 2` *nutritional anemias (D50-D53)*

`√4ᵗʰ` **E50 Vitamin A deficiency**

`EXCLUDES 1` *sequelae of vitamin A deficiency (E64.1)*

E50.0 Vitamin A deficiency with conjunctival xerosis

E50.1 Vitamin A deficiency with Bitot's spot and conjunctival xerosis
Bitot's spot in the young child
DEF: Vitamin A deficiency with conjunctival dryness and superficial spots of keratinized epithelium.

E50.2 Vitamin A deficiency with corneal xerosis

E50.3 Vitamin A deficiency with corneal ulceration and xerosis

E50.4 Vitamin A deficiency with keratomalacia
DEF: Vitamin A deficiency creating corneal dryness that progresses to corneal insensitivity, softness, and necrosis. It is usually bilateral.

E50.5 Vitamin A deficiency with night blindness

E50.6 Vitamin A deficiency with xerophthalmic scars of cornea

E50.7 Other ocular manifestations of vitamin A deficiency
Xerophthalmia NOS

E50.8 Other manifestations of vitamin A deficiency
Follicular keratosis
Xeroderma

E50.9 Vitamin A deficiency, unspecified
Hypovitaminosis A NOS

`√4ᵗʰ` **E51 Thiamine deficiency**

`EXCLUDES 1` *sequelae of thiamine deficiency (E64.8)*

`√5ᵗʰ` **E51.1 Beriberi**

E51.11 Dry beriberi
Beriberi NOS
Beriberi with polyneuropathy

E51.12 Wet beriberi
Beriberi with cardiovascular manifestations
Cardiovascular beriberi
Shoshin disease

E51.2 Wernicke's encephalopathy
DEF: Deficiency of vitamin B1 resulting in a triad of acute mental confusion, ataxia, and ophthalmoplegia. The vast majority of affected patients are alcoholics.

E51.8 Other manifestations of thiamine deficiency

E51.9 Thiamine deficiency, unspecified

E52 Niacin deficiency [pellagra]
Niacin (-tryptophan) deficiency
Nicotinamide deficiency
Pellagra (alcoholic)
`EXCLUDES 1` *sequelae of niacin deficiency (E64.8)*

`√4ᵗʰ` **E53 Deficiency of other B group vitamins**

`EXCLUDES 1` *sequelae of vitamin B deficiency (E64.8)*

E53.0 Riboflavin deficiency
Ariboflavinosis
Vitamin B2 deficiency

E53.1 Pyridoxine deficiency
Vitamin B6 deficiency
`EXCLUDES 1` *pyridoxine-responsive sideroblastic anemia (D64.3)*

E53.8 Deficiency of other specified B group vitamins
Biotin deficiency
Cyanocobalamin deficiency
Folate deficiency
Folic acid deficiency
Pantothenic acid deficiency
Vitamin B12 deficiency
`EXCLUDES 1` *folate deficiency anemia (D52.-)*
vitamin B12 deficiency anemia (D51.-)

E53.9 Vitamin B deficiency, unspecified

E54 Ascorbic acid deficiency
Deficiency of vitamin C
Scurvy
`EXCLUDES 1` *scorbutic anemia (D53.2)*
sequelae of vitamin C deficiency (E64.2)
DEF: Vitamin C deficiency causing swollen gums, myalgia, weight loss, and weakness.

`√4ᵗʰ` **E55 Vitamin D deficiency**

`EXCLUDES 1` *adult osteomalacia (M83.-)*
osteoporosis (M80.-)
sequelae of rickets (E64.3)

E55.0 Rickets, active
Infantile osteomalacia
Juvenile osteomalacia
`EXCLUDES 1` *celiac rickets (K90.0)*
Crohn's rickets (K50.-)
hereditary vitamin D-dependent rickets (E83.32)
inactive rickets (E64.3)
renal rickets (N25.0)
sequelae of rickets (E64.3)
vitamin D-resistant rickets (E83.31)
DEF: Rickets: Softening or weakening of the bones due to a lack of vitamin D, calcium, and phosphate.

E55.9 Vitamin D deficiency, unspecified
Avitaminosis D

`√4ᵗʰ` **E56 Other vitamin deficiencies**

`EXCLUDES 1` *sequelae of other vitamin deficiencies (E64.8)*

E56.0 Deficiency of vitamin E

E56.1 Deficiency of vitamin K
`EXCLUDES 1` *deficiency of coagulation factor due to vitamin K deficiency (D68.4)*
vitamin K deficiency of newborn (P53)

E56.8 Deficiency of other vitamins

E56.9 Vitamin deficiency, unspecified

E58 Dietary calcium deficiency
`EXCLUDES 1` *disorders of calcium metabolism (E83.5-)*
sequelae of calcium deficiency (E64.8)

E59 Dietary selenium deficiency
Keshan disease
`EXCLUDES 1` *sequelae of selenium deficiency (E64.8)*

E60 Dietary zinc deficiency

`√4ᵗʰ` **E61 Deficiency of other nutrient elements**
Use additional code for adverse effect, if applicable, to identify drug (T36-T50 with fifth or sixth character 5)
`EXCLUDES 1` *disorders of mineral metabolism (E83.-)*
iodine deficiency related thyroid disorders (E00-E02)
sequelae of malnutrition and other nutritional deficiencies (E64.-)

E61.0 Copper deficiency

E61.1 Iron deficiency
`EXCLUDES 1` *iron deficiency anemia (D50.-)*

E61.2 Magnesium deficiency

E61.3 Manganese deficiency

E61.4 Chromium deficiency

E61.5 Molybdenum deficiency

E61.6 Vanadium deficiency

E61.7 Deficiency of multiple nutrient elements

E61.8 Deficiency of other specified nutrient elements

E61.9 Deficiency of nutrient element, unspecified

✓4ᵗʰ **E63** **Other nutritional deficiencies**

> EXCLUDES 1   dehydration (E86.0)
> failure to thrive, adult (R62.7)
> failure to thrive, child (R62.51)
> feeding problems in newborn (P92.-)
> sequelae of malnutrition and other nutritional deficiencies
> (E64.-)

E63.0 **Essential fatty acid [EFA] deficiency**

E63.1 **Imbalance of constituents of food intake**

E63.8 **Other specified nutritional deficiencies**

E63.9 **Nutritional deficiency, unspecified**

✓4ᵗʰ **E64** **Sequelae of malnutrition and other nutritional deficiencies**

> NOTE   This category is to be used to indicate conditions in categories E43, E44, E46, E50-E63 as the cause of sequelae, which are themselves classified elsewhere. The 'sequelae' include conditions specified as such; they also include the late effects of diseases classifiable to the above categories if the disease itself is no longer present
>
> Code first condition resulting from (sequela) of malnutrition and other nutritional deficiencies

E64.0 **Sequelae of protein-calorie malnutrition**   HCC

> EXCLUDES 2   retarded development following protein-calorie malnutrition (E45)

E64.1 **Sequelae of vitamin A deficiency**

E64.2 **Sequelae of vitamin C deficiency**

E64.3 **Sequelae of rickets**

E64.8 **Sequelae of other nutritional deficiencies**

E64.9 **Sequelae of unspecified nutritional deficiency**

Overweight, obesity and other hyperalimentation (E65-E68)

E65 **Localized adiposity**

Fat pad

✓4ᵗʰ **E66** **Overweight and obesity**

> Code first obesity complicating pregnancy, childbirth and the puerperium, if applicable (O99.21-)
> Use additional code to identify body mass index (BMI), if known (Z68.-)
> EXCLUDES 1   adiposogenital dystrophy (E23.6)
> lipomatosis NOS (E88.2)
> lipomatosis dolorosa [Dercum] (E88.2)
> Prader-Willi syndrome ▶(Q87.11)◀

AHA: 2018,4Q,77,79-80

TIP: Do not assign a BMI code (Z68.-) when a pregnant patient is documented as being overweight or obese. Only a code from subcategory O99.21- and a code from this category should be assigned.

✓5ᵗʰ **E66.0** **Obesity due to excess calories**

E66.01 **Morbid (severe) obesity due to excess calories**   HCC

> EXCLUDES 1   morbid (severe) obesity with alveolar hypoventilation (E66.2)

E66.09 **Other obesity due to excess calories**

E66.1 **Drug-induced obesity**

> Use additional code for adverse effect, if applicable, to identify drug (T36-T50 with fifth or sixth character 5)

E66.2 **Morbid (severe) obesity with alveolar hypoventilation**   HCC

Obesity hypoventilation syndrome (OHS)
Pickwickian syndrome

E66.3 **Overweight**

AHA: 2018,4Q,78

E66.8 **Other obesity**

E66.9 **Obesity, unspecified**

Obesity NOS

✓4ᵗʰ **E67** **Other hyperalimentation**

> EXCLUDES 1   hyperalimentation NOS (R63.2)
> sequelae of hyperalimentation (E68)

E67.0 **Hypervitaminosis A**

E67.1 **Hypercarotenemia**

> DEF: Elevated blood carotene level as a result of excessive carotenoid ingestion or an inability to convert carotenoids to vitamin A. Characteristics often include yellow discoloration of the skin, which may follow overeating of carotenoid-rich foods such as carrots, sweet potatoes, or squash.

E67.2 **Megavitamin-B6 syndrome**

E67.3 **Hypervitaminosis D**

E67.8 **Other specified hyperalimentation**

E68 **Sequelae of hyperalimentation**

Code first condition resulting from (sequela) of hyperalimentation

Metabolic disorders (E70-E88)

> EXCLUDES 1   androgen insensitivity syndrome (E34.5-)
> congenital adrenal hyperplasia (E25.0)
> Ehlers-Danlos syndrome ▶(Q79.6-)◀
> hemolytic anemias attributable to enzyme disorders (D55.-)
> Marfan's syndrome (Q87.4)
> 5-alpha-reductase deficiency (E29.1)

AHA: 2018,2Q,6

✓4ᵗʰ **E70** **Disorders of aromatic amino-acid metabolism**

E70.0 **Classical phenylketonuria**   HCC

E70.1 **Other hyperphenylalaninemias**   HCC

✓5ᵗʰ **E70.2** **Disorders of tyrosine metabolism**

> EXCLUDES 1   transitory tyrosinemia of newborn (P74.5)

E70.20 **Disorder of tyrosine metabolism, unspecified**   HCC

E70.21 **Tyrosinemia**   HCC

Hypertyrosinemia

E70.29 **Other disorders of tyrosine metabolism**   HCC

Alkaptonuria
Ochronosis

✓5ᵗʰ **E70.3** **Albinism**

> DEF: Absence of pigment in skin, hair, and eyes. This genetic condition is often accompanied by astigmatism, photophobia, and nystagmus.

E70.30 **Albinism, unspecified**   HCC

✓6ᵗʰ **E70.31** **Ocular albinism**

E70.310 **X-linked ocular albinism**   HCC

E70.311 **Autosomal recessive ocular albinism**   HCC

E70.318 **Other ocular albinism**   HCC

E70.319 **Ocular albinism, unspecified**   HCC

✓6ᵗʰ **E70.32** **Oculocutaneous albinism**

> EXCLUDES 1   Chediak-Higashi syndrome (E70.330)
> Hermansky-Pudlak syndrome (E70.331)

E70.320 **Tyrosinase negative oculocutaneous albinism**   HCC

Albinism I
Oculocutaneous albinism ty-neg

E70.321 **Tyrosinase positive oculocutaneous albinism**   HCC

Albinism II
Oculocutaneous albinism ty-pos

E70.328 **Other oculocutaneous albinism**   HCC

Cross syndrome

E70.329 **Oculocutaneous albinism, unspecified**   HCC

✓6ᵗʰ **E70.33** **Albinism with hematologic abnormality**

E70.330 **Chediak-Higashi syndrome**   HCC

E70.331 **Hermansky-Pudlak syndrome**   HCC

E70.338 **Other albinism with hematologic abnormality**   HCC

E70.339 **Albinism with hematologic abnormality, unspecified**   HCC

E70.39 **Other specified albinism**   HCC

Piebaldism

✓5ᵗʰ **E70.4** **Disorders of histidine metabolism**

E70.40 **Disorders of histidine metabolism, unspecified**   HCC

E70.41 **Histidinemia**   HCC

E70.49 **Other disorders of histidine metabolism**   HCC

E70.5 **Disorders of tryptophan metabolism**   HCC

E70.8 **Other disorders of aromatic amino-acid metabolism**   HCC

E70.9 **Disorder of aromatic amino-acid metabolism, unspecified**   HCC

✓4ᵗʰ **E71** **Disorders of branched-chain amino-acid metabolism and fatty-acid metabolism**

E71.0 **Maple-syrup-urine disease**   HCC

✓5ᵗʰ **E71.1** **Other disorders of branched-chain amino-acid metabolism**

✓6ᵗʰ **E71.11** **Branched-chain organic acidurias**

E71.110 **Isovaleric acidemia**   HCC

✔ Additional Character Required   ✓x7ᵗʰ Placeholder Alert   Manifestation   Unspecified Dx   ▶◀ Revised Text   ● New Code   ▲ Revised Code Title

ICD-10-CM 2020   527

	E71.111	3-methylglutaconic aciduria	HCC
	E71.118	Other branched-chain organic acidurias	HCC
✓6th E71.12		**Disorders of** propionate metabolism	
	E71.120	**Methylmalonic acidemia**	HCC
	E71.121	**Propionic acidemia**	HCC
	E71.128	**Other disorders of propionate metabolism**	HCC
E71.19		**Other disorders of branched-chain amino-acid metabolism**	HCC
		Hyperleucine-isoleucinemia	
		Hypervalinemia	
E71.2		**Disorder of branched-chain amino-acid metabolism, unspecified**	HCC

✓5th E71.3 Disorders of fatty-acid metabolism

> EXCLUDES 1   peroxisomal disorders (E71.5)
> Refsum's disease (G60.1)
> Schilder's disease (G37.0)
> EXCLUDES 2   carnitine deficiency due to inborn error of metabolism (E71.42)

E71.30		**Disorder of fatty-acid metabolism, unspecified**	
✓6th E71.31		**Disorders of fatty-acid** oxidation	
	E71.310	Long chain/very long chain **acyl CoA dehydrogenase deficiency**	HCC
		LCAD	
		VLCAD	
	E71.311	**Medium chain acyl CoA dehydrogenase deficiency**	HCC
		MCAD	
	E71.312	**Short chain acyl CoA dehydrogenase deficiency**	HCC
		SCAD	
	E71.313	**Glutaric aciduria type II**	HCC
		Glutaric aciduria type II A	
		Glutaric aciduria type II B	
		Glutaric aciduria type II C	

> EXCLUDES 1   glutaric aciduria (type 1) NOS (E72.3)

	E71.314	**Muscle carnitine palmitoyltransferase deficiency**	HCC
	E71.318	**Other disorders of fatty-acid oxidation**	HCC
E71.32		**Disorders of** ketone metabolism	HCC
E71.39		**Other disorders of fatty-acid metabolism**	HCC

✓5th E71.4 Disorders of carnitine metabolism

> EXCLUDES 1   muscle carnitine palmitoyltransferase deficiency (E71.314)

E71.40		**Disorder of carnitine metabolism, unspecified**	HCC
E71.41		**Primary carnitine deficiency**	HCC
E71.42		**Carnitine deficiency due to** inborn errors of metabolism	HCC
		Code also associated inborn error or metabolism	
E71.43		**Iatrogenic carnitine deficiency**	HCC
		Carnitine deficiency due to hemodialysis	
		Carnitine deficiency due to Valproic acid therapy	
✓6th E71.44		**Other** secondary **carnitine deficiency**	
	E71.440	**Ruvalcaba-Myhre-Smith syndrome**	HCC
	E71.448	**Other secondary carnitine deficiency**	HCC

✓5th E71.5 Peroxisomal disorders

> EXCLUDES 1   Schilder's disease (G37.0)

E71.50		**Peroxisomal disorder, unspecified**	HCC
✓6th E71.51		**Disorders of peroxisome** biogenesis	
		Group 1 peroxisomal disorders	

> EXCLUDES 1   Refsum's disease (G60.1)

	E71.510	**Zellweger syndrome**	HCC
	E71.511	**Neonatal adrenoleukodystrophy**	HCC

> EXCLUDES 1   X-linked adrenoleukodystrophy (E71.42-)

	E71.518	**Other disorders of peroxisome biogenesis**	HCC

✓6th E71.52		**X-linked adrenoleukodystrophy**	
	E71.520	**Childhood cerebral X-linked adrenoleukodystrophy**	HCC
	E71.521	**Adolescent X-linked adrenoleukodystrophy**	HCC
	E71.522	**Adrenomyeloneuropathy**	HCC
	E71.528	**Other X-linked adrenoleukodystrophy**	
		Addison only phenotype adrenoleukodystrophy	
		Addison-Schilder adrenoleukodystrophy	
	E71.529	**X-linked adrenoleukodystrophy, unspecified type**	HCC
E71.53		**Other** group 2 peroxisomal disorders	HCC
✓6th E71.54		**Other peroxisomal disorders**	
	E71.540	**Rhizomelic chondrodysplasia punctata**	HCC

> EXCLUDES 1   chondrodysplasia punctata NOS (Q77.3)

	E71.541	**Zellweger-like syndrome**	HCC
	E71.542	**Other group 3 peroxisomal disorders**	HCC
	E71.548	**Other peroxisomal disorders**	HCC

✓4th E72 Other disorders of amino-acid metabolism

> EXCLUDES 1   disorders of:
> aromatic amino-acid metabolism (E70.-)
> branched-chain amino-acid metabolism (E71.0-E71.2)
> fatty-acid metabolism (E71.3)
> purine and pyrimidine metabolism (E79.-)
> gout (M1A.-, M10.-)

✓5th E72.0 Disorders of amino-acid transport

> EXCLUDES 1   disorders of tryptophan metabolism (E70.5)

E72.00		**Disorders of amino-acid transport, unspecified**	HCC
E72.01		**Cystinuria**	HCC
E72.02		**Hartnup's disease**	HCC
E72.03		**Lowe's syndrome**	HCC
		Use additional code for associated glaucoma (H42)	
E72.04		**Cystinosis**	HCC
		Fanconi (-de Toni) (-Debré) syndrome with cystinosis	

> EXCLUDES 1   Fanconi (-de Toni) (-Debré) syndrome without cystinosis (E72.09)

E72.09		**Other disorders of amino-acid transport**	HCC
		Fanconi (-de Toni) (-Debré) syndrome, unspecified	

✓5th E72.1 Disorders of sulfur-bearing **amino-acid metabolism**

> EXCLUDES 1   cystinosis (E72.04)
> cystinuria (E72.01)
> transcobalamin II deficiency (D51.2)

E72.10		**Disorders of sulfur-bearing amino-acid metabolism, unspecified**	HCC
E72.11		**Homocystinuria**	HCC
		Cystathionine synthase deficiency	
E72.12		**Methylenetetrahydrofolate reductase deficiency**	HCC
E72.19		**Other disorders of sulfur-bearing amino-acid metabolism**	HCC
		Cystathioninuria	
		Methioninemia	
		Sulfite oxidase deficiency	

✓5th E72.2 Disorders of urea cycle **metabolism**

> EXCLUDES 1   disorders of ornithine metabolism (E72.4)

E72.20		**Disorder of urea cycle metabolism, unspecified**	HCC
		Hyperammonemia	

> EXCLUDES 1   hyperammonemia- hyperornithinemia- homocitrullinemia syndrome E72.4
> transient hyperammonemia of newborn (P74.6)

E72.21		**Argininemia**	HCC
E72.22		**Arginosuccinic aciduria**	HCC
E72.23		**Citrullinemia**	HCC
E72.29		**Other disorders of urea cycle metabolism**	HCC

E72.3   **Disorders of lysine and hydroxylysine metabolism**   `HCC`

Glutaric aciduria NOS
Glutaric aciduria (type I)
Hydroxylysinemia
Hyperlysinemia
> *EXCLUDES 1*   *glutaric aciduria type II (E71.313)*
>   *Refsum's disease (G60.1)*
>   *Zellweger syndrome (E71.510)*

E72.4   **Disorders of ornithine metabolism**   `HCC`

Hyperammonemia-Hyperornithinemia-Homocitrullinemia
     syndrome
Ornithinemia (types I, II)
Ornithine transcarbamylase deficiency
> *EXCLUDES 1*   *hereditary choroidal dystrophy (H31.2-)*

☑5ᵗʰ E72.5   **Disorders of glycine metabolism**

     E72.50   **Disorder of glycine metabolism, unspecified**   `HCC`

     E72.51   **Non-ketotic hyperglycinemia**   `HCC`

     E72.52   **Trimethylaminuria**   `HCC`

     E72.53   **Primary hyperoxaluria**   `HCC`

         Oxalosis
         Oxaluria
         AHA: 2018,4Q,29

     E72.59   **Other disorders of glycine metabolism**   `HCC`

         D-glycericacidemia
         Hyperhydroxyprolinemia
         Hyperprolinemia (types I, II)
         Sarcosinemia

☑5ᵗʰ E72.8   **Other specified disorders of amino-acid metabolism**

     AHA: 2018,4Q,5

     E72.81   **Disorders of gamma aminobutyric acid metabolism**   `HCC`

         4-hydroxybutyric aciduria
         Disorders of GABA metabolism
         GABA metabolic defect
         GABA transaminase deficiency
         GABA-T deficiency
         Gamma-hydroxybutyric aciduria
         SSADHD
         Succinic semialdehyde dehydrogenase deficiency

     E72.89   **Other specified disorders of amino-acid metabolism**   `HCC`

         Disorders of beta-amino-acid metabolism
         Disorders of gamma-glutamyl cycle

     E72.9   **Disorder of amino-acid metabolism, unspecified**   `HCC`

☑4ᵗʰ E73   **Lactose intolerance**

     DEF: Inability to break down sugar in dairy products due to a deficiency in the enzyme lactase.

     E73.0   **Congenital lactase deficiency**

     E73.1   **Secondary lactase deficiency**

     E73.8   **Other lactose intolerance**

     E73.9   **Lactose intolerance, unspecified**

☑4ᵗʰ E74   **Other disorders of carbohydrate metabolism**

> *EXCLUDES 1*   *diabetes mellitus (E08-E13)*
>   *hypoglycemia NOS (E16.2)*
>   *increased secretion of glucagon (E16.3)*
>   *mucopolysaccharidosis (E76.0-E76.3)*

☑5ᵗʰ E74.0   **Glycogen storage disease**

     E74.00   **Glycogen storage disease, unspecified**   `HCC`

     E74.01   **von Gierke disease**   `HCC`

         Type I glycogen storage disease

     E74.02   **Pompe disease**   `HCC`

         Cardiac glycogenosis
         Type II glycogen storage disease

     E74.03   **Cori disease**   `HCC`

         Forbes disease
         Type III glycogen storage disease

     E74.04   **McArdle disease**   `HCC`

         Type V glycogen storage disease

     E74.09   **Other glycogen storage disease**   `HCC`

         Andersen disease
         Hers disease
         Tauri disease
         Glycogen storage disease, types 0, IV, VI-XI
         Liver phosphorylase deficiency
         Muscle phosphofructokinase deficiency

☑5ᵗʰ E74.1   **Disorders of fructose metabolism**

> *EXCLUDES 1*   *muscle phosphofructokinase deficiency (E74.09)*

     E74.10   **Disorder of fructose metabolism, unspecified**

     E74.11   **Essential fructosuria**

         Fructokinase deficiency

     E74.12   **Hereditary fructose intolerance**

         Fructosemia

     E74.19   **Other disorders of fructose metabolism**

         Fructose-1, 6-diphosphatase deficiency

☑5ᵗʰ E74.2   **Disorders of galactose metabolism**

     E74.20   **Disorders of galactose metabolism, unspecified**   `HCC`

     E74.21   **Galactosemia**   `HCC`

         DEF: Any of three genetic disorders caused by a defective galactose metabolism. Symptoms include failure to thrive in infancy, jaundice, liver and spleen damage, cataracts, and mental retardation.

     E74.29   **Other disorders of galactose metabolism**   `HCC`

         Galactokinase deficiency

☑5ᵗʰ E74.3   **Other disorders of intestinal carbohydrate absorption**

> *EXCLUDES 2*   *lactose intolerance (E73.-)*

     E74.31   **Sucrase-isomaltase deficiency**

     E74.39   **Other disorders of intestinal carbohydrate absorption**

         Disorder of intestinal carbohydrate absorption NOS
         Glucose-galactose malabsorption
         Sucrase deficiency

E74.4   **Disorders of pyruvate metabolism and gluconeogenesis**   `HCC`

Deficiency of phosphoenolpyruvate carboxykinase
Deficiency of pyruvate carboxylase
Deficiency of pyruvate dehydrogenase
> *EXCLUDES 1*   *disorders of pyruvate metabolism and gluconeogenesis with anemia (D55.-)*
>   *Leigh's syndrome (G31.82)*

E74.8   **Other specified disorders of carbohydrate metabolism**   `HCC`

Essential pentosuria
Renal glycosuria

E74.9   **Disorder of carbohydrate metabolism, unspecified**   `HCC`

☑4ᵗʰ E75   **Disorders of sphingolipid metabolism and other lipid storage disorders**

> *EXCLUDES 1*   *mucolipidosis, types I-III (E77.0-E77.1)*
>   *Refsum's disease (G60.1)*

☑5ᵗʰ E75.0   **GM2 gangliosidosis**

     E75.00   **GM2 gangliosidosis, unspecified**   `HCC`

     E75.01   **Sandhoff disease**   `HCC`

✔ Additional Character Required   ✔x7ᵗʰ Placeholder Alert   Manifestation   Unspecified Dx   ▶◀ Revised Text   ● New Code   ▲ Revised Code Title

ICD-10-CM 2020   529

Chapter 4. Endocrine, Nutritional and Metabolic Diseases

E75.Ø2   Tay-Sachs disease `HCC`

DEF: Genetic mutation of the HEXA gene that inhibits the breakdown of a toxic substance called ganglioside. The accumulation of ganglioside results in destruction of the neurons in the brain and spinal cord.

Tay-Sachs Disease

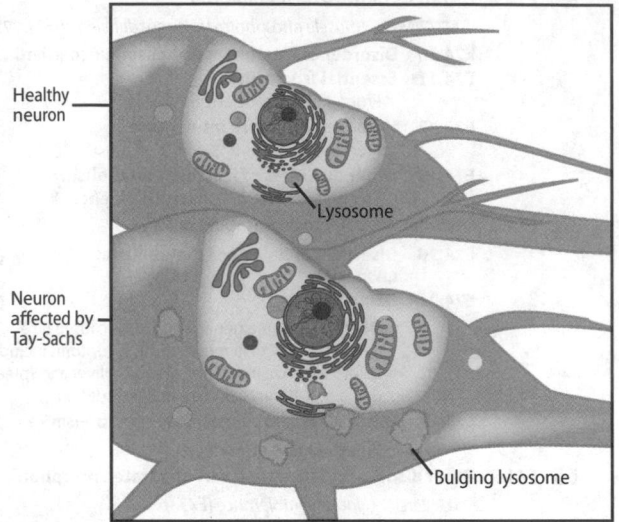

Healthy neuron

Lysosome

Neuron affected by Tay-Sachs

Bulging lysosome

E75.Ø9   Other GM2 gangliosidosis `HCC`

Adult GM2 gangliosidosis
Juvenile GM2 gangliosidosis

✓5ᵗʰ **E75.1   Other and unspecified gangliosidosis**

E75.1Ø   Unspecified gangliosidosis `HCC`

Gangliosidosis NOS

E75.11   Mucolipidosis IV `HCC`

E75.19   Other gangliosidosis `HCC`

GM1 gangliosidosis
GM3 gangliosidosis

✓5ᵗʰ **E75.2   Other sphingolipidosis**

EXCLUDES 1   adrenoleukodystrophy [Addison-Schilder] (E71.528)

E75.21   Fabry (-Anderson) disease `HCC`

E75.22   Gaucher disease `HCC`

E75.23   Krabbe disease `HCC`

✓6ᵗʰ **E75.24   Niemann-Pick disease**

E75.24Ø   Niemann-Pick disease type A `HCC`

E75.241   Niemann-Pick disease type B `HCC`

E75.242   Niemann-Pick disease type C `HCC`

E75.243   Niemann-Pick disease type D `HCC`

E75.248   Other Niemann-Pick disease `HCC`

E75.249   Niemann-Pick disease, unspecified `HCC`

E75.25   Metachromatic leukodystrophy `HCC`

E75.26   Sulfatase deficiency `HCC`

Multiple sulfatase deficiency (MSD)
AHA: 2018,4Q,5-6

E75.29   Other sphingolipidosis `HCC`

Farber's syndrome
Sulfatide lipidosis

E75.3   Sphingolipidosis, unspecified `HCC`

E75.4   Neuronal ceroid lipofuscinosis `HCC`

Batten disease
Bielschowsky-Jansky disease
Kufs disease
Spielmeyer-Vogt disease

E75.5   Other lipid storage disorders

Cerebrotendinous cholesterosis [van Bogaert-Scherer-Epstein]
Wolman's disease

E75.6   Lipid storage disorder, unspecified

✓4ᵗʰ **E76   Disorders of glycosaminoglycan metabolism**

✓5ᵗʰ **E76.Ø   Mucopolysaccharidosis, type I**

E76.Ø1   Hurler's syndrome `HCC`

E76.Ø2   Hurler-Scheie syndrome `HCC`

E76.Ø3   Scheie's syndrome `HCC`

E76.1   Mucopolysaccharidosis, type II

Hunter's syndrome

✓5ᵗʰ **E76.2   Other mucopolysaccharidoses**

✓6ᵗʰ **E76.21   Morquio mucopolysaccharidoses**

E76.21Ø   Morquio A mucopolysaccharidoses `HCC`

Classic Morquio syndrome
Morquio syndrome A
Mucopolysaccharidosis, type IVA

E76.211   Morquio B mucopolysaccharidoses `HCC`

Morquio-like mucopolysaccharidoses
Morquio-like syndrome
Morquio syndrome B
Mucopolysaccharidosis, type IVB

E76.219   Morquio mucopolysaccharidoses, unspecified `HCC`

Morquio syndrome
Mucopolysaccharidosis, type IV

E76.22   Sanfilippo mucopolysaccharidoses `HCC`

Mucopolysaccharidosis, type III (A) (B) (C) (D)
Sanfilippo A syndrome
Sanfilippo B syndrome
Sanfilippo C syndrome
Sanfilippo D syndrome

E76.29   Other mucopolysaccharidoses `HCC`

beta-Glucuronidase deficiency
Maroteaux-Lamy (mild) (severe) syndrome
Mucopolysaccharidosis, types VI, VII

E76.3   Mucopolysaccharidosis, unspecified `HCC`

E76.8   Other disorders of glucosaminoglycan metabolism `HCC`

E76.9   Glucosaminoglycan metabolism disorder, unspecified `HCC`

✓4ᵗʰ **E77   Disorders of glycoprotein metabolism**

E77.Ø   Defects in post-translational modification of lysosomal enzymes `HCC`

Mucolipidosis II [I-cell disease]
Mucolipidosis III [pseudo-Hurler polydystrophy]

E77.1   Defects in glycoprotein degradation `HCC`

Aspartylglucosaminuria
Fucosidosis
Mannosidosis
Sialidosis [mucolipidosis I]

E77.8   Other disorders of glycoprotein metabolism `HCC`

E77.9   Disorder of glycoprotein metabolism, unspecified `HCC`

✓4ᵗʰ **E78   Disorders of lipoprotein metabolism and other lipidemias**

EXCLUDES 1   sphingolipidosis (E75.Ø-E75.3)

✓5ᵗʰ **E78.Ø   Pure hypercholesterolemia**

AHA: 2016,4Q,13-14

E78.ØØ   Pure hypercholesterolemia, unspecified

Fredrickson's hyperlipoproteinemia, type IIa
Hyperbetalipoproteinemia
Low-density-lipoprotein-type [LDL] hyperlipoproteinemia
(Pure) hypercholesterolemia NOS

E78.Ø1   Familial hypercholesterolemia

E78.1   Pure hyperglyceridemia

Elevated fasting triglycerides
Endogenous hyperglyceridemia
Fredrickson's hyperlipoproteinemia, type IV
Hyperlipidemia, group B
Hyperprebetalipoproteinemia
Very-low-density-lipoprotein-type [VLDL] hyperlipoproteinemia

E78.2   **Mixed hyperlipidemia**
Broad- or floating-betalipoproteinemia
Combined hyperlipidemia NOS
Elevated cholesterol with elevated triglycerides NEC
Fredrickson's hyperlipoproteinemia, type IIb or III
Hyperbetalipoproteinemia with prebetalipoproteinemia
Hypercholesteremia with endogenous hyperglyceridemia
Hyperlipidemia, group C
Tubo-eruptive xanthoma
Xanthoma tuberosum
> EXCLUDES 1   *cerebrotendinous cholesterosis [van Bogaert-Scherer-Epstein] (E75.5)*
> *familial combined hyperlipidemia (E78.49)*

E78.3   **Hyperchylomicronemia**
Chylomicron retention disease
Fredrickson's hyperlipoproteinemia, type I or V
Hyperlipidemia, group D
Mixed hyperglyceridemia

☑5ᵗʰ E78.4   **Other hyperlipidemia**
AHA: 2018,4Q,6
  E78.41   **Elevated Lipoprotein(a)**
    Elevated Lp(a)
  E78.49   **Other hyperlipidemia**
    Familial combined hyperlipidemia

E78.5   **Hyperlipidemia, unspecified**

E78.6   **Lipoprotein deficiency**
Abetalipoproteinemia
Depressed HDL cholesterol
High-density lipoprotein deficiency
Hypoalphalipoproteinemia
Hypobetalipoproteinemia (familial)
Lecithin cholesterol acyltransferase deficiency
Tangier disease

☑5ᵗʰ E78.7   **Disorders of bile acid and cholesterol metabolism**
> EXCLUDES 1   *Niemann-Pick disease type C (E75.242)*

  E78.70   **Disorder of bile acid and cholesterol metabolism, unspecified**
  E78.71   **Barth syndrome**
  E78.72   **Smith-Lemli-Opitz syndrome**
  E78.79   **Other disorders of bile acid and cholesterol metabolism**

☑5ᵗʰ E78.8   **Other disorders of lipoprotein metabolism**
  E78.81   **Lipoid dermatoarthritis**
  E78.89   **Other lipoprotein metabolism disorders**
E78.9   **Disorder of lipoprotein metabolism, unspecified**

☑4ᵗʰ E79   **Disorders of purine and pyrimidine metabolism**
> EXCLUDES 1   *Ataxia-telangiectasia ▶(Q87.19)◄*
> *Bloom's syndrome (Q82.8)*
> *Cockayne's syndrome ▶(Q87.19)◄*
> *calculus of kidney (N20.0)*
> *combined immunodeficiency disorders (D81.-)*
> *Fanconi's anemia (D61.09)*
> *gout (M1A.-, M10.-)*
> *orotaciduric anemia (D53.0)*
> *progeria (E34.8)*
> *Werner's syndrome (E34.8)*
> *xeroderma pigmentosum (Q82.1)*

E79.0   **Hyperuricemia without signs of inflammatory arthritis and tophaceous disease**
Asymptomatic hyperuricemia

E79.1   **Lesch-Nyhan syndrome**   `HCC`
HGPRT deficiency

E79.2   **Myoadenylate deaminase deficiency**   `HCC`

E79.8   **Other disorders of purine and pyrimidine metabolism**   `HCC`
Hereditary xanthinuria

E79.9   **Disorder of purine and pyrimidine metabolism, unspecified**   `HCC`

☑4ᵗʰ E80   **Disorders of porphyrin and bilirubin metabolism**
> INCLUDES   defects of catalase and peroxidase

E80.0   **Hereditary erythropoietic porphyria**   `HCC`
Congenital erythropoietic porphyria
Erythropoietic protoporphyria

E80.1   **Porphyria cutanea tarda**   `HCC`

☑5ᵗʰ E80.2   **Other and unspecified porphyria**
  E80.20   **Unspecified porphyria**   `HCC`
    Porphyria NOS
  E80.21   **Acute intermittent (hepatic) porphyria**   `HCC`
  E80.29   **Other porphyria**   `HCC`
    Hereditary coproporphyria

E80.3   **Defects of catalase and peroxidase**   `HCC`
Acatalasia [Takahara]

E80.4   **Gilbert syndrome**

E80.5   **Crigler-Najjar syndrome**

E80.6   **Other disorders of bilirubin metabolism**
Dubin-Johnson syndrome
Rotor's syndrome

E80.7   **Disorder of bilirubin metabolism, unspecified**

☑4ᵗʰ E83   **Disorders of mineral metabolism**
> EXCLUDES 1   *dietary mineral deficiency (E58-E61)*
> *parathyroid disorders (E20-E21)*
> *vitamin D deficiency (E55.-)*

☑5ᵗʰ E83.0   **Disorders of copper metabolism**
  E83.00   **Disorder of copper metabolism, unspecified**
  E83.01   **Wilson's disease**
    Code also associated Kayser Fleischer ring (H18.04-)
  E83.09   **Other disorders of copper metabolism**
    Menkes' (kinky hair) (steely hair) disease

☑5ᵗʰ E83.1   **Disorders of iron metabolism**
> EXCLUDES 1   *iron deficiency anemia (D50.-)*
> *sideroblastic anemia (D64.0-D64.3)*

  E83.10   **Disorder of iron metabolism, unspecified**
  ☑6ᵗʰ E83.11   **Hemochromatosis**
> EXCLUDES 1   *GALD (P78.84)*
> *gestational alloimmune liver disease (P78.84)*
> *neonatal hemochromatosis (P78.84)*

    E83.110   **Hereditary hemochromatosis**   `HCC`
      Bronzed diabetes
      Pigmentary cirrhosis (of liver)
      Primary (hereditary) hemochromatosis
    E83.111   **Hemochromatosis due to repeated red blood cell transfusions**
      Iron overload due to repeated red blood cell transfusions
      Transfusion (red blood cell) associated hemochromatosis
    E83.118   **Other hemochromatosis**
    E83.119   **Hemochromatosis, unspecified**
  E83.19   **Other disorders of iron metabolism**
    Use additional code, if applicable, for idiopathic pulmonary hemosiderosis (J84.03)

E83.2   **Disorders of zinc metabolism**
Acrodermatitis enteropathica

☑5ᵗʰ E83.3   **Disorders of phosphorus metabolism and phosphatases**
> EXCLUDES 1   *adult osteomalacia (M83.-)*
> *osteoporosis (M80.-)*

  E83.30   **Disorder of phosphorus metabolism, unspecified**
  E83.31   **Familial hypophosphatemia**
    Vitamin D-resistant osteomalacia
    Vitamin D-resistant rickets
>   EXCLUDES 1   *vitamin D-deficiency rickets (E55.0)*

  E83.32   **Hereditary vitamin D-dependent rickets (type 1) (type 2)**
    25-hydroxyvitamin D 1-alpha-hydroxylase deficiency
    Pseudovitamin D deficiency
    Vitamin D receptor defect
  E83.39   **Other disorders of phosphorus metabolism**
    Acid phosphatase deficiency
    Hypophosphatasia

☑5ᵗʰ E83.4   **Disorders of magnesium metabolism**
  E83.40   **Disorders of magnesium metabolism, unspecified**
  E83.41   **Hypermagnesemia**
    AHA: 2016,4Q,54
  E83.42   **Hypomagnesemia**
  E83.49   **Other disorders of magnesium metabolism**

✓5ᵗʰ **E83.5** **Disorders of calcium metabolism**

> EXCLUDES 1　*chondrocalcinosis (M11.1-M11.2)*
> *hungry bone syndrome (E83.81)*
> *hyperparathyroidism (E21.0-E21.3)*

E83.50 **Unspecified disorder of calcium metabolism**

E83.51 **Hypocalcemia**

E83.52 **Hypercalcemia**
Familial hypocalciuric hypercalcemia

E83.59 **Other disorders of calcium metabolism**

✓5ᵗʰ **E83.8** **Other disorders of mineral metabolism**

E83.81 **Hungry bone syndrome**

E83.89 **Other disorders of mineral metabolism**

E83.9 **Disorder of mineral metabolism, unspecified**

✓4ᵗʰ **E84** **Cystic fibrosis**

> INCLUDES　mucoviscidosis

Code also exocrine pancreatic insufficiency (K86.81)
DEF: Genetic disorder affecting the respiratory, digestive, and reproductive systems in infants to young adults by disturbing exocrine gland function and causing chronic pulmonary disease with excess mucus production and pancreatic deficiency.

E84.0 **Cystic fibrosis with pulmonary manifestations**　HCC

Use additional code to identify any infectious organism present, such as:
Pseudomonas (B96.5)

✓5ᵗʰ **E84.1** **Cystic fibrosis with intestinal manifestations**

E84.11 **Meconium ileus in cystic fibrosis**　HCC N

> EXCLUDES 1　*meconium ileus not due to cystic fibrosis (P76.0)*

E84.19 **Cystic fibrosis with other intestinal manifestations**　HCC
Distal intestinal obstruction syndrome

E84.8 **Cystic fibrosis with other manifestations**　HCC

E84.9 **Cystic fibrosis, unspecified**　HCC

✓4ᵗʰ **E85** **Amyloidosis**

> EXCLUDES 2　*Alzheimer's disease (G30.0-)*

DEF: Conditions of diverse etiologies characterized by the accumulation of insoluble fibrillar proteins (amyloid) in various organs and tissues of the body, compromising vital functions.

E85.0 **Non-neuropathic heredofamilial amyloidosis**　HCC

Hereditary amyloid nephropathy
Code also associated disorders, such as:
autoinflammatory syndromes (M04.-)

> EXCLUDES 2　*transthyretin-related (ATTR) familial amyloid cardiomyopathy (E85.4)*

E85.1 **Neuropathic heredofamilial amyloidosis**　HCC

Amyloid polyneuropathy (Portuguese)
Transthyretin-related (ATTR) familial amyloid polyneuropathy
AHA: 2012,4Q,99

E85.2 **Heredofamilial amyloidosis, unspecified**　HCC

E85.3 **Secondary systemic amyloidosis**　HCC

Hemodialysis-associated amyloidosis

E85.4 **Organ-limited amyloidosis**　HCC

Localized amyloidosis
Transthyretin-related (ATTR) familial amyloid cardiomyopathy

✓5ᵗʰ **E85.8** **Other amyloidosis**

AHA: 2017,4Q,7

E85.81 **Light chain (AL) amyloidosis**　HCC

E85.82 **Wild-type transthyretin-related (ATTR) amyloidosis**　HCC
Senile systemic amyloidosis (SSA)

E85.89 **Other amyloidosis**　HCC

E85.9 **Amyloidosis, unspecified**　HCC

✓4ᵗʰ **E86** **Volume depletion**

Use additional code(s) for any associated disorders of electrolyte and acid-base balance (E87.-)

> EXCLUDES 1　*dehydration of newborn (P74.1)*
> *hypovolemic shock NOS (R57.1)*
> *postprocedural hypovolemic shock (T81.19)*
> *traumatic hypovolemic shock (T79.4)*

AHA: 2019,2Q,7; 2018,2Q,6

E86.0 **Dehydration**
AHA: 2019,2Q,7; 2019,1Q,12; 2014,1Q,7
TIP: Can be assigned in addition to hypernatremia (E87.0) or hyponatremia (E87.1), when documented.

E86.1 **Hypovolemia**
Depletion of volume of plasma

E86.9 **Volume depletion, unspecified**
DEF: Depletion of total body water (dehydration) and/or contraction of total intravascular plasma (hypovolemia).

✓4ᵗʰ **E87** **Other disorders of fluid, electrolyte and acid-base balance**

> EXCLUDES 1　*diabetes insipidus (E23.2)*
> *electrolyte imbalance associated with hyperemesis gravidarum (O21.1)*
> *electrolyte imbalance following ectopic or molar pregnancy (O08.5)*
> *familial periodic paralysis (G72.3)*

AHA: 2018,2Q,6

E87.0 **Hyperosmolality and hypernatremia**
Sodium [Na] excess
Sodium [Na] overload
AHA: 2014,1Q,7
TIP: Assign an additional code for dehydration (E86.0), when documented.

E87.1 **Hypo-osmolality and hyponatremia**
Sodium [Na] deficiency

> EXCLUDES 1　*syndrome of inappropriate secretion of antidiuretic hormone (E22.2)*

AHA: 2014,1Q,7
TIP: Assign an additional code for dehydration (E86.0), when documented.

E87.2 **Acidosis**
Acidosis NOS
Lactic acidosis
Metabolic acidosis
Respiratory acidosis

> EXCLUDES 1　*diabetic acidosis — see categories E08-E10, E13 with ketoacidosis*

DEF: Reduction of alkaline in the blood and tissues caused by an increase in acid and decrease in bicarbonate.

E87.3 **Alkalosis**
Alkalosis NOS
Metabolic alkalosis
Respiratory alkalosis

E87.4 **Mixed disorder of acid-base balance**

E87.5 **Hyperkalemia**
Potassium [K] excess
Potassium [K] overload

E87.6 **Hypokalemia**
Potassium [K] deficiency

✓5ᵗʰ **E87.7** **Fluid overload**

> EXCLUDES 1　*edema NOS (R60.9)*
> *fluid retention (R60.9)*

E87.70 **Fluid overload, unspecified**

E87.71 **Transfusion associated circulatory overload**
Fluid overload due to transfusion (blood) (blood components)
TACO

E87.79 **Other fluid overload**

E87.8 **Other disorders of electrolyte and fluid balance, not elsewhere classified**
Electrolyte imbalance NOS
Hyperchloremia
Hypochloremia

✓4ᵗʰ E88 Other and unspecified metabolic disorders

Use additional codes for associated conditions

EXCLUDES 1   histiocytosis X (chronic) (C96.6)

✓5ᵗʰ E88.Ø Disorders of plasma-protein metabolism, not elsewhere classified

EXCLUDES 1   disorder of lipoprotein metabolism (E78.-)

monoclonal gammopathy (of undetermined significance) (D47.2)

polyclonal hypergammaglobulinemia (D89.Ø)

Waldenström macroglobulinemia (C88.Ø)

E88.Ø1 Alpha-1-antitrypsin deficiency   HCC

AAT deficiency

E88.Ø2 Plasminogen deficiency

Dysplasminogenemia

Hypoplasminogenemia

Type 1 plasminogen deficiency

Type 2 plasminogen deficiency

Code also, if applicable, ligneous conjunctivitis (H1Ø.51)

Use additional code for associated findings, such as:

hydrocephalus (G91.4)

~~ligneous conjunctivitis (H1Ø.51)~~

otitis media (H67.-)

respiratory disorder related to plasminogen deficiency (J99)

AHA: 2018,4Q,6-7

E88.Ø9 Other disorders of plasma-protein metabolism, not elsewhere classified

Bisalbuminemia

E88.1 Lipodystrophy, not elsewhere classified

Lipodystrophy NOS

EXCLUDES 1   Whipple's disease (K9Ø.81)

E88.2 Lipomatosis, not elsewhere classified

Lipomatosis NOS

Lipomatosis (Check) dolorosa [Dercum]

E88.3 Tumor lysis syndrome

Tumor lysis syndrome (spontaneous)

Tumor lysis syndrome following antineoplastic drug chemotherapy

Use additional code for adverse effect, if applicable, to identify drug (T45.1X5)

AHA: 2019,2Q,24

DEF: Potentially fatal metabolic complication of tumor necrosis caused by spontaneous or treatment-related accumulation of byproducts from dying cancer cells. Symptoms include hyperkalemia, hyperphosphatemia, hypocalcemia, hyperuricemia, and hyperuricosuria.

✓5ᵗʰ E88.4 Mitochondrial metabolism disorders

EXCLUDES 1   disorders of pyruvate metabolism (E74.4)

Kearns-Sayre syndrome (H49.81)

Leber's disease (H47.22)

Leigh's encephalopathy (G31.82)

mitochondrial myopathy, NEC (G71.3)

Reye's syndrome (G93.7)

E88.4Ø Mitochondrial metabolism disorder, unspecified   HCC

E88.41 MELAS syndrome   HCC

Mitochondrial myopathy, encephalopathy, lactic acidosis and stroke-like episodes

E88.42 MERRF syndrome   HCC

Myoclonic epilepsy associated with ragged-red fibers

Code also progressive myoclonic epilepsy (G4Ø.3-)

E88.49 Other mitochondrial metabolism disorders   HCC

✓5ᵗʰ E88.8 Other specified metabolic disorders

E88.81 Metabolic syndrome

Dysmetabolic syndrome X

Use additional codes for associated manifestations, such as:

obesity (E66.-)

DEF: Group of health risks that increase the likelihood of developing heart disease, stroke, and diabetes. These risks include certain parameters for blood pressure, cholesterol, and glucose levels.

E88.89 Other specified metabolic disorders   HCC

Launois-Bensaude adenolipomatosis

EXCLUDES 1   adult pulmonary Langerhans cell histiocytosis (J84.82)

E88.9 Metabolic disorder, unspecified

Postprocedural endocrine and metabolic complications and disorders, not elsewhere classified (E89)

✓4ᵗʰ E89 Postprocedural endocrine and metabolic complications and disorders, not elsewhere classified

EXCLUDES 2   intraoperative complications of endocrine system organ or structure (E36.Ø-, E36.1-, E36.8)

E89.Ø Postprocedural hypothyroidism

Postirradiation hypothyroidism

Postsurgical hypothyroidism

E89.1 Postprocedural hypoinsulinemia

Postpancreatectomy hyperglycemia

Postsurgical hypoinsulinemia

Use additional code, if applicable, to identify:

acquired absence of pancreas (Z9Ø.41-)

diabetes mellitus (postpancreatectomy) (postprocedural) (E13.-)

insulin use (Z79.4)

EXCLUDES 1   transient postprocedural hyperglycemia (R73.9)

transient postprocedural hypoglycemia (E16.2)

E89.2 Postprocedural hypoparathyroidism   HCC

Parathyroprival tetany

E89.3 Postprocedural hypopituitarism   HCC

Postirradiation hypopituitarism

✓5ᵗʰ E89.4 Postprocedural ovarian failure

E89.4Ø Asymptomatic postprocedural ovarian failure   ♀

Postprocedural ovarian failure NOS

E89.41 Symptomatic postprocedural ovarian failure   ♀

Symptoms such as flushing, sleeplessness, headache, lack of concentration, associated with postprocedural menopause

E89.5 Postprocedural testicular hypofunction   ♂

E89.6 Postprocedural adrenocortical (-medullary) hypofunction   HCC

✓5ᵗʰ E89.8 Other postprocedural endocrine and metabolic complications and disorders

AHA: 2016,4Q,9-10

✓6ᵗʰ E89.81 Postprocedural hemorrhage of an endocrine system organ or structure following a procedure

E89.81Ø Postprocedural hemorrhage of an endocrine system organ or structure following an endocrine system procedure

E89.811 Postprocedural hemorrhage of an endocrine system organ or structure following other procedure

✓6ᵗʰ E89.82 Postprocedural hematoma and seroma of an endocrine system organ or structure

E89.82Ø Postprocedural hematoma of an endocrine system organ or structure following an endocrine system procedure

E89.821 Postprocedural hematoma of an endocrine system organ or structure following other procedure

E89.822 Postprocedural seroma of an endocrine system organ or structure following an endocrine system procedure

E89.823 Postprocedural seroma of an endocrine system organ or structure following other procedure

E89.89 Other postprocedural endocrine and metabolic complications and disorders

Use additional code, if applicable, to further specify disorder

---

✓ Additional Character Required   ✓x7ᵗʰ Placeholder Alert   Manifestation   Unspecified Dx   ►◄ Revised Text   ● New Code   ▲ Revised Code Title

Chapter 5. Mental, Behavioral and Neurodevelopmental Disorders (FØ1–F99)

Chapter-specific Guidelines with Coding Examples

The chapter-specific guidelines from the ICD-10-CM Official Guidelines for Coding and Reporting have been provided below. Along with these guidelines are coding examples, contained in the shaded boxes, that have been developed to help illustrate the coding and/or sequencing guidance found in these guidelines.

a. Pain disorders related to psychological factors

Assign code F45.41, for pain that is exclusively related to psychological disorders. As indicated by the Excludes 1 note under category G89, a code from category G89 should not be assigned with code F45.41.

> Chest pain determined to be persistent somatoform pain disorder
>
> **F45.41   Pain disorder exclusively related to psychological factors**
>
> *Explanation*: This pain was diagnosed as being exclusively psychological; therefore, no code from category G89 is added.

Code F45.42, Pain disorders with related psychological factors, should be used with a code from category G89, Pain, not elsewhere classified, if there is documentation of a psychological component for a patient with acute or chronic pain.
See Section I.C.6. Pain

b. Mental and behavioral disorders due to psychoactive substance use

1) In remission

Selection of codes for "in remission" for categories F10-F19, Mental and behavioral disorders due to psychoactive substance use (categories F1Ø-F19 with -11, -.21) requires the provider's clinical judgment. The appropriate codes for "in remission" are assigned only on the basis of provider documentation (as defined in the Official Guidelines for Coding and Reporting), unless otherwise instructed by the classification.

Mild substance use disorders in early or sustained remission are classified to the appropriate codes for substance abuse in remission, and moderate or severe substance use disorders in early or sustained remission are classified to the appropriate codes for substance dependence in remission.

> Physician documentation indicates the patient is seen to monitor progress on quitting cigarette smoking. The problem list indicates mild tobacco use disorder that is currently in remission.
>
> **F17.211   Nicotine dependence, cigarettes, in remission**
>
> *Explanation*: According to the index, Disorder, tobacco use, cigarettes (mild) (moderate) (severe), in remission (early) (sustained) is categorized to dependence (F17.211). Since the physician clearly documents mild cigarette use "disorder" and that the disorder is in remission, a code for nicotine dependence "in remission" is appropriate.

2) Psychoactive substance use, abuse and dependence

When the provider documentation refers to use, abuse and dependence of the same substance (e.g. alcohol, opioid, cannabis, etc.), only one code should be assigned to identify the pattern of use based on the following hierarchy:

- If both use and abuse are documented, assign only the code for abuse
- If both abuse and dependence are documented, assign only the code for dependence
- If use, abuse and dependence are all documented, assign only the code for dependence
- If both use and dependence are documented, assign only the code for dependence.

> History and physical notes cannabis dependence and ongoing cannabis abuse
>
> **F12.2Ø   Cannabis dependence, uncomplicated**
>
> *Explanation*: In the hierarchy, the dependence code is used if both abuse and dependence are documented.

> Current problem list indicates daily opioid use with opioid abuse.
>
> **F11.1Ø   Opioid abuse, uncomplicated**
>
> *Explanation*: In the hierarchy, the abuse code is used if both abuse and use are documented.

3) Psychoactive substance use, unspecified

As with all other unspecified diagnoses, the codes for unspecified psychoactive substance use disorders (F1Ø.9-, F11.9-, F12.9-, F13.9-, F14.9-, F15.9-, F16.9-, F18.9-, F19.9-) should only be assigned based on provider documentation and when they meet the definition of a reportable diagnosis (see Section III, Reporting Additional Diagnoses). These codes are to be used only when the psychoactive substance use is associated with a physical, mental or behavioral disorder, and such a relationship is documented by the provider.

c. Factitious disorder

Factitious disorder imposed on self or Munchausen's syndrome is a disorder in which a person falsely reports or causes his or her own physical or psychological signs or symptoms. For patients with documented factitious disorder on self or Munchausen's syndrome, assign the appropriate code from subcategory F68.1-, Factitious disorder imposed on self.

Munchausen's syndrome by proxy (MSBP) is a disorder in which a caregiver (perpetrator) falsely reports or causes an illness or injury in another person (victim) under his or her care, such as a child, an elderly adult, or a person who has a disability. The condition is also referred to as "factitious disorder imposed on another" or "factitious disorder by proxy." The perpetrator, not the victim, receives this diagnosis. Assign code F68.A, Factitious disorder imposed on another, to the perpetrator's record. For the victim of a patient suffering from MSBP, assign the appropriate code from categories T74, Adult and child abuse, neglect and other maltreatment, confirmed, or T76, Adult and child abuse, neglect and other maltreatment, suspected.
See Section I.C.19.f. Adult and child abuse, neglect and other maltreatment

r 5. Mental, Behavioral and evelopmental Disorders (F01-F99)

INCLUDES   disorders of psychological development
EXCLUDES 2   symptoms, signs and abnormal clinical laboratory findings, not elsewhere classified (R00-R99)

This chapter contains the following blocks:

F01-F09	Mental disorders due to known physiological conditions
F10-F19	Mental and behavioral disorders due to psychoactive substance use
F20-F29	Schizophrenia, schizotypal, delusional, and other non-mood psychotic disorders
F30-F39	Mood [affective] disorders
F40-F48	Anxiety, dissociative, stress-related, somatoform and other nonpsychotic mental disorders
F50-F59	Behavioral syndromes associated with physiological disturbances and physical factors
F60-F69	Disorders of adult personality and behavior
F70-F79	Intellectual disabilities
F80-F89	Pervasive and specific developmental disorders
F90-F98	Behavioral and emotional disorders with onset usually occurring in childhood and adolescence
F99	Unspecified mental disorder

Mental disorders due to known physiological conditions (F01-F09)

NOTE   This block comprises a range of mental disorders grouped together on the basis of their having in common a demonstrable etiology in cerebral disease, brain injury, or other insult leading to cerebral dysfunction. The dysfunction may be primary, as in diseases, injuries, and insults that affect the brain directly and selectively; or secondary, as in systemic diseases and disorders that attack the brain only as one of the multiple organs or systems of the body that are involved.

✓4ᵗʰ **F01   Vascular dementia**

Vascular dementia as a result of infarction of the brain due to vascular disease, including hypertensive cerebrovascular disease.
INCLUDES   arteriosclerotic dementia
Code first the underlying physiological condition or sequelae of cerebrovascular disease.

   ✓5ᵗʰ **F01.5   Vascular dementia**

     F01.50   Vascular dementia without behavioral **HCC** **A** disturbance
Major neurocognitive disorder without behavioral disturbance

     F01.51   Vascular dementia with behavioral **HCC** **Q** **A** disturbance
Major neurocognitive disorder due to vascular disease, with behavioral disturbance
Major neurocognitive disorder with aggressive behavior
Major neurocognitive disorder with combative behavior
Major neurocognitive disorder with violent behavior
Vascular dementia with aggressive behavior
Vascular dementia with combative behavior
Vascular dementia with violent behavior
Use additional code, if applicable, to identify wandering in vascular dementia (Z91.83)

✓4ᵗʰ **F02   Dementia in other diseases classified elsewhere**

INCLUDES   major neurocognitive disorder in other diseases classified elsewhere
Code first the underlying physiological condition, such as:
Alzheimer's (G30.-)
cerebral lipidosis (E75.4)
Creutzfeldt-Jakob disease (A81.0-)
dementia with Lewy bodies (G31.83)
dementia with Parkinsonism (G31.83)
epilepsy and recurrent seizures (G40.-)
frontotemporal dementia (G31.09)
hepatolenticular degeneration (E83.0)
human immunodeficiency virus [HIV] disease (B20)
Huntington's disease (G10)
hypercalcemia (E83.52)
hypothyroidism, acquired (E00-E03.-)
intoxications (T36-T65)
Jakob-Creutzfeldt disease (A81.0-)
multiple sclerosis (G35)
neurosyphilis (A52.17)
niacin deficiency [pellagra] (E52)
Parkinson's disease (G20)
Pick's disease (G31.01)
polyarteritis nodosa (M30.0)
prion disease (A81.9)
systemic lupus erythematosus (M32.-)
traumatic brain injury (S06.-)
trypanosomiasis (B56.-, B57.-)
vitamin B deficiency (E53.8)
EXCLUDES 2   dementia in alcohol and psychoactive substance disorders (F10-F19, with .17, .27, .97)
vascular dementia (F01.5-)

   ✓5ᵗʰ **F02.8   Dementia in other diseases classified elsewhere**

AHA: 2017,2Q,7; 2016,4Q,141; 2016,2Q,6
TIP: A code from this subcategory should always be assigned with a code from category G30 when Alzheimer's disease is documented, even in the absence of documented dementia.

     F02.80   Dementia in other diseases classified **HCC** **elsewhere** without behavioral disturbance
Dementia in other diseases classified elsewhere NOS
Major neurocognitive disorder in other diseases classified elsewhere

     F02.81   Dementia in other diseases classified **HCC** **elsewhere** with behavioral disturbance
Dementia in other diseases classified elsewhere with aggressive behavior
Dementia in other diseases classified elsewhere with combative behavior
Dementia in other diseases classified elsewhere with violent behavior
Major neurocognitive disorder in other diseases classified elsewhere with aggressive behavior
Major neurocognitive disorder in other diseases classified elsewhere with combative behavior
Major neurocognitive disorder in other diseases classified elsewhere with violent behavior
Use additional code, if applicable, to identify wandering in dementia in conditions classified elsewhere (Z91.83)

✓4ᵗʰ **F03   Unspecified dementia**

Presenile dementia NOS
Presenile psychosis NOS
Primary degenerative dementia NOS
Senile dementia NOS
Senile dementia depressed or paranoid type
Senile psychosis NOS
EXCLUDES 1   senility NOS (R41.81)
EXCLUDES 2   mild memory disturbance due to known physiological condition (F06.8)
senile dementia with delirium or acute confusional state (F05)

   ✓5ᵗʰ **F03.9   Unspecified dementia**

     F03.90   Unspecified dementia without behavioral **HCC** **A** disturbance
Dementia NOS
AHA: 2012,4Q,92

F03.91   **Unspecified dementia with behavioral**   `HCC` `A`
     disturbance
     Unspecified dementia with aggressive behavior
     Unspecified dementia with combative behavior
     Unspecified dementia with violent behavior
     Use additional code, if applicable, to identify
        wandering in unspecified dementia (Z91.83)

F04   **Amnestic disorder due to known physiological condition**   `HCC`
     Korsakov's psychosis or syndrome, nonalcoholic
     Code first the underlying physiological condition
     EXCLUDES 1   *amnesia NOS (R41.3)*
                  anterograde amnesia (R41.1)
                  dissociative amnesia (F44.0)
                  retrograde amnesia (R41.2)
     EXCLUDES 2   *alcohol-induced or unspecified Korsakov's syndrome (F10.26,*
                  F10.96)
                  Korsakov's syndrome induced by other psychoactive
                     substances (F13.26, F13.96, F19.16, F19.26, F19.96)

F05   **Delirium due to known physiological condition**
     Acute or subacute brain syndrome
     Acute or subacute confusional state (nonalcoholic)
     Acute or subacute infective psychosis
     Acute or subacute organic reaction
     Acute or subacute psycho-organic syndrome
     Delirium of mixed etiology
     Delirium superimposed on dementia
     Sundowning
     Code first the underlying physiological condition
     EXCLUDES 1   *delirium NOS (R41.0)*
     EXCLUDES 2   *delirium tremens alcohol-induced or unspecified (F10.231,*
                  F10.921)
     AHA: 2019,2Q,34

`✓4ᵗʰ` **F06**   **Other mental disorders due to known physiological condition**
     `INCLUDES`   mental disorders due to endocrine disorder
                  mental disorders due to exogenous hormone
                  mental disorders due to exogenous toxic substance
                  mental disorders due to primary cerebral disease
                  mental disorders due to somatic illness
                  mental disorders due to systemic disease affecting the
                     brain
     Code first the underlying physiological condition
     EXCLUDES 1   *unspecified dementia (F03)*
     EXCLUDES 2   *delirium due to known physiological condition (F05)*
                  dementia as classified in F01-F02
                  other mental disorders associated with alcohol and other
                     psychoactive substances (F10-F19)

F06.0   **Psychotic disorder with hallucinations due to known**
     physiological condition
     Organic hallucinatory state (nonalcoholic)
     EXCLUDES 2   *hallucinations and perceptual disturbance induced*
                  by alcohol and other psychoactive substances
                  (F10-F19 with .151, .251, .951)
                  schizophrenia (F20.-)

F06.1   **Catatonic disorder due to known physiological condition**
     Catatonia associated with another mental disorder
     Catatonia NOS
     EXCLUDES 1   *catatonic stupor (R40.1)*
                  stupor NOS (R40.1)
     EXCLUDES 2   *catatonic schizophrenia (F20.2)*
                  dissociative stupor (F44.2)
     DEF: Catatonic: Abnormal neuropsychiatric state characterized
     by stupor, immobility or purposeless movements, or
     unresponsiveness in a person who otherwise appears awake.

F06.2   **Psychotic disorder with delusions due to known physiological**
     condition
     Paranoid and paranoid-hallucinatory organic states
     Schizophrenia-like psychosis in epilepsy
     EXCLUDES 2   *alcohol and drug-induced psychotic disorder*
                  (F10-F19 with .150, .250, .950)
                  brief psychotic disorder (F23)
                  delusional disorder (F22)
                  schizophrenia (F20.-)

`✓5ᵗʰ` **F06.3**   **Mood disorder due to known physiological condition**
     EXCLUDES 2   *mood disorders due to alcohol and other*
                  psychoactive substances (F10-F19 with .14, .24,
                  .94)
                  mood disorders, not due to known physiological
                  condition or unspecified (F30-F39)

     F06.30   **Mood disorder due to known physiological**
           condition, unspecified
     F06.31   **Mood disorder due to known physiological**
           condition with depressive features
           Depressive disorder due to known physiological
              condition, with depressive features
     F06.32   **Mood disorder due to known physiological**
           condition with major depressive-like episode
           Depressive disorder due to known physiological
              condition, with major depressive-like episode
     F06.33   **Mood disorder due to known physiological**
           condition with manic features
           Bipolar and related disorder due to a known
              physiological condition, with manic features
           Bipolar and related disorder due to known
              physiological condition, with manic- or
              hypomanic-like episodes
     F06.34   **Mood disorder due to known physiological**
           condition with mixed features
           Bipolar and related disorder due to known
              physiological condition, with mixed features
           Depressive disorder due to known physiological
              condition, with mixed features

F06.4   **Anxiety disorder due to known physiological condition**
     EXCLUDES 2   *anxiety disorders due to alcohol and other*
                  psychoactive substances (F10-F19 with .180,
                  .280, .980)
                  anxiety disorders, not due to known physiological
                  condition or unspecified (F40.-, F41.-)

F06.8   **Other specified mental disorders due to known physiological**
     condition
     Epileptic psychosis NOS
     Obsessive-compulsive and related disorder due to a known
        physiological condition
     Organic dissociative disorder
     Organic emotionally labile [asthenic] disorder

`✓4ᵗʰ` **F07**   **Personality and behavioral disorders due to known physiological**
     condition
     Code first the underlying physiological condition

F07.0   **Personality change due to known physiological condition**
     Frontal lobe syndrome
     Limbic epilepsy personality syndrome
     Lobotomy syndrome
     Organic personality disorder
     Organic pseudopsychopathic personality
     Organic pseudoretarded personality
     Postleucotomy syndrome
     Code first underlying physiological condition
     EXCLUDES 1   *mild cognitive impairment (G31.84)*
                  postconcussional syndrome (F07.81)
                  postencephalitic syndrome (F07.89)
                  signs and symptoms involving emotional state (R45.-)
     EXCLUDES 2   *specific personality disorder (F60.-)*

`✓5ᵗʰ` **F07.8**   **Other personality and behavioral disorders due to known**
     physiological condition
     F07.81   **Postconcussional syndrome**
           Postcontusional syndrome (encephalopathy)
           Post-traumatic brain syndrome, nonpsychotic
           Use additional code to identify associated
              post-traumatic headache, if applicable (G44.3-)
              EXCLUDES 1   *current concussion (brain) (S06.0-)*
                       postencephalitic syndrome (F07.89)
           DEF: Concussion symptoms that persist for weeks or
           months after a head injury. These symptoms may
           include headache, giddiness, fatigue, insomnia, mood
           fluctuation, and a subjective feeling of impaired
           intellectual function with extreme reaction to normal
           stressors.

     F07.89   **Other personality and behavioral disorders due to**
           known physiological condition
           Postencephalitic syndrome
           Right hemispheric organic affective disorder

`✓` Additional Character Required   `✓x7ᵗʰ` Placeholder Alert   Manifestation   Unspecified Dx   ►◄ Revised Text   ● New Code   ▲ Revised Code Title

ICD-10-CM 2020   **537**

F07.9   **Unspecified personality and behavioral disorder due to known physiological condition**
Organic psychosyndrome

F09   **Unspecified mental disorder due to known physiological condition**
Mental disorder NOS due to known physiological condition
Organic brain syndrome NOS
Organic mental disorder NOS
Organic psychosis NOS
Symptomatic psychosis NOS
Code first the underlying physiological condition
EXCLUDES 1   psychosis NOS (F29)

Mental and behavioral disorders due to psychoactive substance use (F10-F19)

AHA: 2018,4Q,69-70; 2017,4Q,8; 2017,2Q,27

√4th **F10**   **Alcohol related disorders**
Use additional code for blood alcohol level, if applicable (Y90.-)

√5th **F10.1**   **Alcohol abuse**
EXCLUDES 1   alcohol dependence (F10.2-)
alcohol use, unspecified (F10.9-)
AHA: 2018,1Q,16; 2015,2Q,15
TIP: Alcohol withdrawal is classified to dependence only (F10.23-); there is no combination code for alcohol abuse with withdrawal. When alcohol abuse and alcohol withdrawal are documented for the same encounter, query the provider for clarification.
TIP: Assign when documentation indicates alcohol withdrawal without dependence; do not assign an additional code for withdrawal.

F10.10   **Alcohol abuse, uncomplicated**
Alcohol use disorder, mild

F10.11   **Alcohol abuse, in remission**
Alcohol use disorder, mild, in early remission
Alcohol use disorder, mild, in sustained remission

√6th **F10.12**   **Alcohol abuse with intoxication**
F10.120   **Alcohol abuse with intoxication, uncomplicated**   HCC
F10.121   **Alcohol abuse with intoxication delirium**   HCC
F10.129   **Alcohol abuse with intoxication, unspecified**   HCC

F10.14   **Alcohol abuse with alcohol-induced mood disorder**   HCC
Alcohol use disorder, mild, with alcohol-induced bipolar or related disorder
Alcohol use disorder, mild, with alcohol-induced depressive disorder

√6th **F10.15**   **Alcohol abuse with alcohol-induced psychotic disorder**
F10.150   **Alcohol abuse with alcohol-induced psychotic disorder with delusions**   HCC
F10.151   **Alcohol abuse with alcohol-induced psychotic disorder with hallucinations**   HCC
DEF: Psychosis lasting less than six months with slight or no clouding of consciousness in which auditory hallucinations predominate.
F10.159   **Alcohol abuse with alcohol-induced psychotic disorder, unspecified**   HCC

√6th **F10.18**   **Alcohol abuse with other alcohol-induced disorders**
F10.180   **Alcohol abuse with alcohol-induced anxiety disorder**   HCC
F10.181   **Alcohol abuse with alcohol-induced sexual dysfunction**   HCC
F10.182   **Alcohol abuse with alcohol-induced sleep disorder**   HCC
F10.188   **Alcohol abuse with other alcohol-induced disorder**   HCC
F10.19   **Alcohol abuse with unspecified alcohol-induced disorder**   HCC

√5th **F10.2**   **Alcohol dependence**
EXCLUDES 1   alcohol abuse (F10.1-)
alcohol use, unspecified (F10.9-)
EXCLUDES 2   toxic effect of alcohol (T51.0-)

F10.20   **Alcohol dependence, uncomplicated**   HCC
Alcohol use disorder, moderate
Alcohol use disorder, severe

F10.21   **Alcohol dependence, in remission**   HCC
Alcohol use disorder, moderate, in early remission
Alcohol use disorder, moderate, in sustained remission
Alcohol use disorder, severe, in early remission
Alcohol use disorder, severe, in sustained remission

√6th **F10.22**   **Alcohol dependence with intoxication**
Acute drunkenness (in alcoholism)
EXCLUDES 2   alcohol dependence with withdrawal (F10.23-)
F10.220   **Alcohol dependence with intoxication, uncomplicated**   HCC
F10.221   **Alcohol dependence with intoxication delirium**   HCC
F10.229   **Alcohol dependence with intoxication, unspecified**   HCC

√6th **F10.23**   **Alcohol dependence with withdrawal**
EXCLUDES 2   alcohol dependence with intoxication (F10.22-)
AHA: 2018,1Q,16; 2015,2Q,15
TIP: Do not assign a code from this subcategory when documentation indicates alcohol withdrawal without dependence.
F10.230   **Alcohol dependence with withdrawal, uncomplicated**   HCC
F10.231   **Alcohol dependence with withdrawal delirium**   HCC
F10.232   **Alcohol dependence with withdrawal with perceptual disturbance**   HCC
F10.239   **Alcohol dependence with withdrawal, unspecified**   HCC

F10.24   **Alcohol dependence with alcohol-induced mood disorder**   HCC
Alcohol use disorder, moderate, with alcohol-induced bipolar or related disorder
Alcohol use disorder, moderate, with alcohol-induced depressive disorder
Alcohol use disorder, severe, with alcohol-induced bipolar or related disorder
Alcohol use disorder, severe, with alcohol-induced depressive disorder

√6th **F10.25**   **Alcohol dependence with alcohol-induced psychotic disorder**
F10.250   **Alcohol dependence with alcohol-induced psychotic disorder with delusions**   HCC
F10.251   **Alcohol dependence with alcohol-induced psychotic disorder with hallucinations**   HCC
F10.259   **Alcohol dependence with alcohol-induced psychotic disorder, unspecified**   HCC

F10.26   **Alcohol dependence with alcohol-induced persisting amnestic disorder**   HCC
Alcohol use disorder, moderate, with alcohol-induced major neurocognitive disorder, amnestic-confabulatory type
Alcohol use disorder, severe, with alcohol-induced major neurocognitive disorder, amnestic-confabulatory type
DEF: Prominent and lasting reduced memory span and disordered time appreciation and confabulation that occurs in alcoholics as sequel to acute alcoholic psychosis.

F10.27   **Alcohol dependence with alcohol-induced** `HCC`
    persisting dementia
      Alcohol use disorder, moderate, with alcohol-induced
       major neurocognitive disorder,
       nonamnestic-confabulatory type
      Alcohol use disorder, severe, with alcohol-induced
       major neurocognitive disorder,
       nonamnestic-confabulatory type

✓6ᵗʰ   **F10.28**   **Alcohol dependence with other alcohol-induced**
    disorders

     F10.280   **Alcohol dependence with** `HCC`
       alcohol-induced anxiety disorder

     F10.281   **Alcohol dependence with** `HCC`
       alcohol-induced sexual
       dysfunction

     F10.282   **Alcohol dependence with** `HCC`
       alcohol-induced sleep disorder

     F10.288   **Alcohol dependence with other** `HCC`
       alcohol-induced disorder
        Alcohol use disorder, moderate, with
         alcohol-induced mild neurocognitive
         disorder
        Alcohol use disorder, severe, with
         alcohol-induced mild neurocognitive
         disorder

   F10.29   **Alcohol dependence with unspecified** `HCC`
    alcohol-induced disorder

✓5ᵗʰ   **F10.9**   **Alcohol use, unspecified**

    EXCLUDES 1   *alcohol abuse (F10.1-)*
           alcohol dependence (F10.2-)

    AHA: 2018,2Q,10-11
    TIP: Assign a substance use code only when the provider
    documents a relationship between the use and an associated
    physical, mental, or behavioral disorder. As with all diagnoses,
    substance use codes must meet the definition of a reportable
    diagnosis.

✓6ᵗʰ   **F10.92**   **Alcohol use, unspecified with** intoxication

     F10.920   **Alcohol use, unspecified with** `HCC`
       intoxication, uncomplicated
        AHA: 2018,2Q,10-11

     F10.921   **Alcohol use, unspecified with** `HCC`
       intoxication delirium

     F10.929   **Alcohol use, unspecified with** `HCC`
       intoxication, unspecified

   F10.94   **Alcohol use, unspecified with** `HCC`
    alcohol-induced mood disorder
     Alcohol induced bipolar or related disorder, without
      use disorder
     Alcohol induced depressive disorder, without use
      disorder

✓6ᵗʰ   **F10.95**   **Alcohol use, unspecified with alcohol-induced**
    psychotic disorder

     F10.950   **Alcohol use, unspecified with** `HCC`
       alcohol-induced psychotic
       disorder with delusions

     F10.951   **Alcohol use, unspecified with** `HCC`
       alcohol-induced psychotic
       disorder with hallucinations

     F10.959   **Alcohol use, unspecified with** `HCC`
       alcohol-induced psychotic
       disorder, unspecified
        Alcohol-induced psychotic disorder
         without use disorder

   F10.96   **Alcohol use, unspecified with** `HCC`
    alcohol-induced persisting amnestic
    disorder
     Alcohol-induced major neurocognitive disorder,
      amnestic-confabulatory type, without use
      disorder

   F10.97   **Alcohol use, unspecified with** `HCC`
    alcohol-induced persisting dementia
     Alcohol-induced major neurocognitive disorder,
      nonamnestic-confabulatory type, without use
      disorder

✓6ᵗʰ   **F10.98**   **Alcohol use, unspecified with other alcohol-induced**
    disorders

     F10.980   **Alcohol use, unspecified with** `HCC`
       alcohol-induced anxiety disorder
        Alcohol induced anxiety disorder, without
         use disorder

     F10.981   **Alcohol use, unspecified with** `HCC`
       alcohol-induced sexual
       dysfunction
        Alcohol induced sexual dysfunction,
         without use disorder

     F10.982   **Alcohol use, unspecified with** `HCC`
       alcohol-induced sleep disorder
        Alcohol induced sleep disorder, without
         use disorder

     F10.988   **Alcohol use, unspecified with** `HCC`
       other alcohol-induced disorder
        Alcohol induced mild neurocognitive
         disorder, without use disorder

   F10.99   **Alcohol use, unspecified with unspecified** `HCC`
    alcohol-induced disorder

✓4ᵗʰ   **F11**   **Opioid related disorders**

✓5ᵗʰ   **F11.1**   **Opioid** abuse

    EXCLUDES 1   *opioid dependence (F11.2-)*
           opioid use, unspecified (F11.9-)

   F11.10   **Opioid abuse, uncomplicated** `HCC`
     Opioid use disorder, mild

   F11.11   **Opioid abuse, in remission** `HCC`
     Opioid use disorder, mild, in early remission
     Opioid use disorder, mild, in sustained remission

✓6ᵗʰ   **F11.12**   **Opioid abuse with** intoxication

     F11.120   **Opioid abuse with intoxication,** `HCC`
       uncomplicated

     F11.121   **Opioid abuse with intoxication** `HCC`
       delirium

     F11.122   **Opioid abuse with intoxication** `HCC`
       with perceptual disturbance

     F11.129   **Opioid abuse with intoxication,** `HCC`
       unspecified

   F11.14   **Opioid abuse with opioid-induced** mood `HCC`
    disorder
     Opioid use disorder, mild, with opioid-induced
      depressive disorder

✓6ᵗʰ   **F11.15**   **Opioid abuse with opioid-induced** psychotic
    disorder

     F11.150   **Opioid abuse with opioid-induced** `HCC`
       psychotic disorder with delusions

     F11.151   **Opioid abuse with opioid-induced** `HCC`
       psychotic disorder with
       hallucinations

     F11.159   **Opioid abuse with opioid-induced** `HCC`
       psychotic disorder, unspecified

✓6ᵗʰ   **F11.18**   **Opioid abuse with other opioid-induced disorder**

     F11.181   **Opioid abuse with opioid-induced** `HCC`
       sexual dysfunction

     F11.182   **Opioid abuse with opioid-induced** `HCC`
       sleep disorder

     F11.188   **Opioid abuse with other** `HCC`
       opioid-induced disorder

   F11.19   **Opioid abuse with unspecified** `HCC`
    opioid-induced disorder

✓5ᵗʰ   **F11.2**   **Opioid** dependence

    EXCLUDES 1   *opioid abuse (F11.1-)*
           opioid use, unspecified (F11.9-)
    EXCLUDES 2   *opioid poisoning (T40.0-T40.2-)*

   F11.20   **Opioid dependence, uncomplicated** `HCC`
     Opioid use disorder, moderate
     Opioid use disorder, severe

   F11.21   **Opioid dependence, in remission** `HCC`
     Opioid use disorder, moderate, in early remission
     Opioid use disorder, moderate, in sustained remission
     Opioid use disorder, severe, in early remission
     Opioid use disorder, severe, in sustained remission

✓6ᵗʰ   **F11.22**   **Opioid dependence with** intoxication

    EXCLUDES 1   *opioid dependence with withdrawal*
           (F11.23)

     F11.220   **Opioid dependence with** `HCC`
       intoxication, uncomplicated

     F11.221   **Opioid dependence with** `HCC`
       intoxication delirium

     F11.222   **Opioid dependence with** `HCC`
       intoxication with perceptual
       disturbance

✔ Additional Character Required   ✓x7ᵗʰ Placeholder Alert   Manifestation   Unspecified Dx   ▶◀ Revised Text   ● New Code   ▲ Revised Code Title

ICD-10-CM 2020   539

        F11.229 Opioid dependence with intoxication, unspecified HCC

   F11.23 Opioid dependence with withdrawal HCC

        EXCLUDES 1   *opioid dependence with intoxication (F11.22-)*

   F11.24 Opioid dependence with opioid-induced mood disorder HCC

        Opioid use disorder, moderate, with opioid induced depressive disorder

✓6th   **F11.25 Opioid dependence with opioid-induced** psychotic disorder

        F11.250 Opioid dependence with opioid-induced psychotic disorder with delusions HCC

        F11.251 Opioid dependence with opioid-induced psychotic disorder with hallucinations HCC

        F11.259 Opioid dependence with opioid-induced psychotic disorder, unspecified HCC

✓6th   **F11.28 Opioid dependence with other opioid-induced disorder**

        F11.281 Opioid dependence with opioid-induced sexual dysfunction HCC

        F11.282 Opioid dependence with opioid-induced sleep disorder HCC

        F11.288 Opioid dependence with other opioid-induced disorder HCC

   F11.29 Opioid dependence with unspecified opioid-induced disorder HCC

✓5th **F11.9 Opioid use, unspecified**

     EXCLUDES 1   *opioid abuse (F11.1-)*

               opioid dependence (F11.2-)

     TIP: Assign a substance use code only when the provider documents a relationship between the use and an associated physical, mental, or behavioral disorder. As with all diagnoses, substance use codes must meet the definition of a reportable diagnosis.

   F11.90 Opioid use, unspecified, uncomplicated

        AHA: 2018,2Q,10-11

✓6th   **F11.92 Opioid use, unspecified with** intoxication

      EXCLUDES 1   *opioid use, unspecified with withdrawal (F11.93)*

        F11.920 Opioid use, unspecified with intoxication, uncomplicated HCC

        F11.921 Opioid use, unspecified with intoxication delirium HCC

           Opioid-induced delirium

        F11.922 Opioid use, unspecified with intoxication with perceptual disturbance HCC

        F11.929 Opioid use, unspecified with intoxication, unspecified HCC

   F11.93 Opioid use, unspecified with withdrawal HCC

      EXCLUDES 1   *opioid use, unspecified with intoxication (F11.92-)*

   F11.94 Opioid use, unspecified with opioid-induced mood disorder HCC

        Opioid induced depressive disorder, without use disorder

✓6th   **F11.95 Opioid use, unspecified with opioid-induced** psychotic disorder

        F11.950 Opioid use, unspecified with opioid-induced psychotic disorder with delusions HCC

        F11.951 Opioid use, unspecified with opioid-induced psychotic disorder with hallucinations HCC

        F11.959 Opioid use, unspecified with opioid-induced psychotic disorder, unspecified HCC

✓6th   **F11.98 Opioid use, unspecified with other specified opioid-induced disorder**

        F11.981 Opioid use, unspecified with opioid-induced sexual dysfunction HCC

           Opioid induced sexual dysfunction, without use disorder

        F11.982 Opioid use, unspecified with opioid-induced sleep disorder HCC

           Opioid induced sleep disorder, without use disorder

        F11.988 Opioid use, unspecified with other opioid-induced disorder HCC

           Opioid induced anxiety disorder, without use disorder

   F11.99 Opioid use, unspecified with unspecified opioid-induced disorder HCC

✓4th **F12 Cannabis related disorders**

     INCLUDES   marijuana

✓5th **F12.1 Cannabis** abuse

     EXCLUDES 1   *cannabis dependence (F12.2-)*

               cannabis use, unspecified (F12.9-)

   F12.10 Cannabis abuse, uncomplicated

        Cannabis use disorder, mild

   F12.11 Cannabis abuse, in remission

        Cannabis use disorder, mild, in early remission

        Cannabis use disorder, mild, in sustained remission

✓6th   **F12.12 Cannabis abuse with** intoxication

        F12.120 Cannabis abuse with intoxication, uncomplicated HCC

        F12.121 Cannabis abuse with intoxication delirium HCC

        F12.122 Cannabis abuse with intoxication with perceptual disturbance HCC

        F12.129 Cannabis abuse with intoxication, unspecified HCC

✓6th   **F12.15 Cannabis abuse with** psychotic disorder

        F12.150 Cannabis abuse with psychotic disorder with delusions HCC

        F12.151 Cannabis abuse with psychotic disorder with hallucinations HCC

        F12.159 Cannabis abuse with psychotic disorder, unspecified HCC

✓6th   **F12.18 Cannabis abuse with other cannabis-induced disorder**

        F12.180 Cannabis abuse with cannabis-induced anxiety disorder HCC

        F12.188 Cannabis abuse with other cannabis-induced disorder HCC

           Cannabis use disorder, mild, with cannabis-induced sleep disorder

   F12.19 Cannabis abuse with unspecified cannabis-induced disorder HCC

✓5th **F12.2 Cannabis** dependence

     EXCLUDES 1   *cannabis abuse (F12.1-)*

               cannabis use, unspecified (F12.9-)

     EXCLUDES 2   *cannabis poisoning (T40.7-)*

   F12.20 Cannabis dependence, uncomplicated HCC

        Cannabis use disorder, moderate

        Cannabis use disorder, severe

   F12.21 Cannabis dependence, in remission HCC

        Cannabis use disorder, moderate, in early remission

        Cannabis use disorder, moderate, in sustained remission

        Cannabis use disorder, severe, in early remission

        Cannabis use disorder, severe, in sustained remission

✓6th   **F12.22 Cannabis dependence with** intoxication

        F12.220 Cannabis dependence with intoxication, uncomplicated HCC

        F12.221 Cannabis dependence with intoxication delirium HCC

        F12.222 Cannabis dependence with intoxication with perceptual disturbance HCC

        F12.229 Cannabis dependence with intoxication, unspecified HCC

   F12.23 Cannabis dependence with withdrawal HCC

        AHA: 2018,4Q,7

✓6th   **F12.25 Cannabis dependence with** psychotic disorder

        F12.250 Cannabis dependence with psychotic disorder with delusions HCC

        F12.251 Cannabis dependence with psychotic disorder with hallucinations HCC

F12.259   Cannabis dependence with psychotic disorder, unspecified   HCC

✓6ᵗʰ **F12.28**   Cannabis dependence with other cannabis-induced disorder

F12.280   Cannabis dependence with cannabis-induced anxiety disorder   HCC

F12.288   Cannabis dependence with other cannabis-induced disorder   HCC

Cannabis use disorder, moderate, with cannabis-induced sleep disorder

Cannabis use disorder, severe, with cannabis-induced sleep disorder

F12.29   Cannabis dependence with unspecified cannabis-induced disorder   HCC

✓5ᵗʰ **F12.9**   Cannabis use, unspecified

> *EXCLUDES 1*   cannabis abuse (F12.1-)
> cannabis dependence (F12.2-)

TIP: Assign a substance use code only when the provider documents a relationship between the use and an associated physical, mental, or behavioral disorder. As with all diagnoses, substance use codes must meet the definition of a reportable diagnosis.

F12.90   Cannabis use, unspecified, uncomplicated

AHA: 2018,2Q,10-11

✓6ᵗʰ **F12.92**   Cannabis use, unspecified with intoxication

F12.920   Cannabis use, unspecified with intoxication, uncomplicated   HCC

F12.921   Cannabis use, unspecified with intoxication delirium   HCC

F12.922   Cannabis use, unspecified with intoxication with perceptual disturbance   HCC

F12.929   Cannabis use, unspecified with intoxication, unspecified   HCC

F12.93   Cannabis use, unspecified with withdrawal   HCC

AHA: 2018,4Q,7

✓6ᵗʰ **F12.95**   Cannabis use, unspecified with psychotic disorder

F12.950   Cannabis use, unspecified with psychotic disorder with delusions   HCC

F12.951   Cannabis use, unspecified with psychotic disorder with hallucinations   HCC

F12.959   Cannabis use, unspecified with psychotic disorder, unspecified   HCC

Cannabis induced psychotic disorder, without use disorder

✓6ᵗʰ **F12.98**   Cannabis use, unspecified with other cannabis-induced disorder

F12.980   Cannabis use, unspecified with anxiety disorder   HCC

Cannabis induced anxiety disorder, without use disorder

F12.988   Cannabis use, unspecified with other cannabis-induced disorder   HCC

Cannabis induced sleep disorder, without use disorder

F12.99   Cannabis use, unspecified with unspecified cannabis-induced disorder   HCC

✓4ᵗʰ **F13**   Sedative, hypnotic, or anxiolytic related disorders

✓5ᵗʰ **F13.1**   Sedative, hypnotic or anxiolytic-related abuse

> *EXCLUDES 1*   sedative, hypnotic or anxiolytic-related dependence (F13.2-)
> sedative, hypnotic, or anxiolytic use, unspecified (F13.9-)

F13.10   Sedative, hypnotic or anxiolytic abuse, uncomplicated   HCC

Sedative, hypnotic, or anxiolytic use disorder, mild

F13.11   Sedative, hypnotic or anxiolytic abuse, in remission   HCC

Sedative, hypnotic, or anxiolytic use disorder, mild, in early remission

Sedative, hypnotic, or anxiolytic use disorder, mild, in sustained remission

✓6ᵗʰ **F13.12**   Sedative, hypnotic or anxiolytic abuse with intoxication

F13.120   Sedative, hypnotic or anxiolytic abuse with intoxication, uncomplicated   HCC

F13.121   Sedative, hypnotic or anxiolytic abuse with intoxication delirium   HCC

F13.129   Sedative, hypnotic or anxiolytic abuse with intoxication, unspecified   HCC

F13.14   Sedative, hypnotic or anxiolytic abuse with sedative, hypnotic or anxiolytic-induced mood disorder   HCC

Sedative, hypnotic, or anxiolytic use disorder, mild, with sedative, hypnotic, or anxiolytic-induced bipolar or related disorder

Sedative, hypnotic, or anxiolytic use disorder, mild, with sedative, hypnotic, or anxiolytic-induced depressive disorder

✓6ᵗʰ **F13.15**   Sedative, hypnotic or anxiolytic abuse with sedative, hypnotic or anxiolytic-induced psychotic disorder

F13.150   Sedative, hypnotic or anxiolytic abuse with sedative, hypnotic or anxiolytic-induced psychotic disorder with delusions   HCC

F13.151   Sedative, hypnotic or anxiolytic abuse with sedative, hypnotic or anxiolytic-induced psychotic disorder with hallucinations   HCC

F13.159   Sedative, hypnotic or anxiolytic abuse with sedative, hypnotic or anxiolytic-induced psychotic disorder, unspecified   HCC

✓6ᵗʰ **F13.18**   Sedative, hypnotic or anxiolytic abuse with other sedative, hypnotic or anxiolytic-induced disorders

F13.180   Sedative, hypnotic or anxiolytic abuse with sedative, hypnotic or anxiolytic-induced anxiety disorder   HCC

F13.181   Sedative, hypnotic or anxiolytic abuse with sedative, hypnotic or anxiolytic-induced sexual dysfunction   HCC

F13.182   Sedative, hypnotic or anxiolytic abuse with sedative, hypnotic or anxiolytic-induced sleep disorder   HCC

F13.188   Sedative, hypnotic or anxiolytic abuse with other sedative, hypnotic or anxiolytic-induced disorder   HCC

F13.19   Sedative, hypnotic or anxiolytic abuse with unspecified sedative, hypnotic or anxiolytic-induced disorder   HCC

✓5ᵗʰ **F13.2**   Sedative, hypnotic or anxiolytic-related dependence

> *EXCLUDES 1*   sedative, hypnotic or anxiolytic-related abuse (F13.1-)
> sedative, hypnotic, or anxiolytic use, unspecified (F13.9-)
>
> *EXCLUDES 2*   sedative, hypnotic, or anxiolytic poisoning (T42.-)

F13.20   Sedative, hypnotic or anxiolytic dependence, uncomplicated   HCC

F13.21   Sedative, hypnotic or anxiolytic dependence, in remission   HCC

Sedative, hypnotic or anxiolytic use disorder, moderate, in early remission

Sedative, hypnotic or anxiolytic use disorder, moderate, in sustained remission

Sedative, hypnotic or anxiolytic use disorder, severe, in early remission

Sedative, hypnotic or anxiolytic use disorder, severe, in sustained remission

✓6ᵗʰ **F13.22**   Sedative, hypnotic or anxiolytic dependence with intoxication

> *EXCLUDES 1*   sedative, hypnotic or anxiolytic dependence with withdrawal (F13.23-)

F13.220   Sedative, hypnotic or anxiolytic dependence with intoxication, uncomplicated   HCC

F13.221   Sedative, hypnotic or anxiolytic dependence with intoxication delirium   HCC

F13.229   Sedative, hypnotic or anxiolytic dependence with intoxication, unspecified   HCC

☑ Additional Character Required   ✓×7ᵗʰ Placeholder Alert   Manifestation   Unspecified Dx   ►◄ Revised Text   ● New Code   ▲ Revised Code Title

ICD-10-CM 2020   541

Chapter 5. Mental, Behavioral and Neurodevelopmental Disorders

✓6ᵗʰ **F13.23 Sedative, hypnotic or anxiolytic dependence with withdrawal**
Sedative, hypnotic, or anxiolytic use disorder, moderate
Sedative, hypnotic, or anxiolytic use disorder, severe
> *EXCLUDES 1*   sedative, hypnotic or anxiolytic dependence with intoxication (F13.22-)

    F13.230 Sedative, hypnotic or anxiolytic dependence with withdrawal, uncomplicated HCC

    F13.231 Sedative, hypnotic or anxiolytic dependence with withdrawal delirium HCC

    F13.232 Sedative, hypnotic or anxiolytic dependence with withdrawal with perceptual disturbance HCC
Sedative, hypnotic, or anxiolytic withdrawal with perceptual disturbances

    F13.239 Sedative, hypnotic or anxiolytic dependence with withdrawal, unspecified HCC
Sedative, hypnotic, or anxiolytic withdrawal without perceptual disturbances

F13.24 Sedative, hypnotic or anxiolytic dependence with sedative, hypnotic or anxiolytic-induced mood disorder HCC
Sedative, hypnotic, or anxiolytic use disorder, moderate, with sedative, hypnotic, or anxiolytic-induced bipolar or related disorder
Sedative, hypnotic, or anxiolytic use disorder, moderate, with sedative, hypnotic, or anxiolytic-induced depressive disorder
Sedative, hypnotic, or anxiolytic use disorder, severe, with sedative, hypnotic, or anxiolytic-induced bipolar or related disorder
Sedative, hypnotic, or anxiolytic use disorder, severe, with sedative, hypnotic, or anxiolytic-induced depressive disorder

✓6ᵗʰ **F13.25 Sedative, hypnotic or anxiolytic dependence with sedative, hypnotic or anxiolytic-induced psychotic disorder**

    F13.250 Sedative, hypnotic or anxiolytic dependence with sedative, hypnotic or anxiolytic-induced psychotic disorder with delusions HCC

    F13.251 Sedative, hypnotic or anxiolytic dependence with sedative, hypnotic or anxiolytic-induced psychotic disorder with hallucinations HCC

    F13.259 Sedative, hypnotic or anxiolytic dependence with sedative, hypnotic or anxiolytic-induced psychotic disorder, unspecified HCC

F13.26 Sedative, hypnotic or anxiolytic dependence with sedative, hypnotic or anxiolytic-induced persisting amnestic disorder HCC

F13.27 Sedative, hypnotic or anxiolytic dependence with sedative, hypnotic or anxiolytic-induced persisting dementia HCC
Sedative, hypnotic, or anxiolytic use disorder, moderate, with sedative, hypnotic, or anxiolytic induced major neurocognitive disorder
Sedative, hypnotic, or anxiolytic use disorder, severe, with sedative, hypnotic, or anxiolytic-induced major neurocognitive disorder

✓6ᵗʰ **F13.28 Sedative, hypnotic or anxiolytic dependence with other sedative, hypnotic or anxiolytic-induced disorders**

    F13.280 Sedative, hypnotic or anxiolytic dependence with sedative, hypnotic or anxiolytic-induced anxiety disorder HCC

    F13.281 Sedative, hypnotic or anxiolytic dependence with sedative, hypnotic or anxiolytic-induced sexual dysfunction HCC

    F13.282 Sedative, hypnotic or anxiolytic dependence with sedative, hypnotic or anxiolytic-induced sleep disorder HCC

    F13.288 Sedative, hypnotic or anxiolytic dependence with other sedative, hypnotic or anxiolytic-induced disorder HCC
Sedative, hypnotic, or anxiolytic use disorder, moderate, with sedative, hypnotic, or anxiolytic-induced mild neurocognitive disorder
Sedative, hypnotic, or anxiolytic use disorder, severe, with sedative, hypnotic, or anxiolytic-induced mild neurocognitive disorder

F13.29 Sedative, hypnotic or anxiolytic dependence with unspecified sedative, hypnotic or anxiolytic-induced disorder HCC

✓5ᵗʰ **F13.9 Sedative, hypnotic or anxiolytic-related use, unspecified**
> *EXCLUDES 1*   sedative, hypnotic or anxiolytic-related abuse (F13.1-)
> sedative, hypnotic or anxiolytic-related dependence (F13.2-)

TIP: Assign a substance use code only when the provider documents a relationship between the use and an associated physical, mental, or behavioral disorder. As with all diagnoses, substance use codes must meet the definition of a reportable diagnosis.

F13.90 Sedative, hypnotic, or anxiolytic use, unspecified, uncomplicated
AHA: 2018,2Q,10-11

✓6ᵗʰ **F13.92 Sedative, hypnotic or anxiolytic use, unspecified with intoxication**
> *EXCLUDES 1*   sedative, hypnotic or anxiolytic use, unspecified with withdrawal (F13.93-)

    F13.920 Sedative, hypnotic or anxiolytic use, unspecified with intoxication, uncomplicated HCC

    F13.921 Sedative, hypnotic or anxiolytic use, unspecified with intoxication delirium HCC
Sedative, hypnotic, or anxiolytic-induced delirium

    F13.929 Sedative, hypnotic or anxiolytic use, unspecified with intoxication, unspecified HCC

✓6ᵗʰ **F13.93 Sedative, hypnotic or anxiolytic use, unspecified with withdrawal**
> *EXCLUDES 1*   sedative, hypnotic or anxiolytic use, unspecified with intoxication (F13.92-)

    F13.930 Sedative, hypnotic or anxiolytic use, unspecified with withdrawal, uncomplicated HCC

    F13.931 Sedative, hypnotic or anxiolytic use, unspecified with withdrawal delirium HCC

    F13.932 Sedative, hypnotic or anxiolytic use, unspecified with withdrawal with perceptual disturbances HCC

    F13.939 Sedative, hypnotic or anxiolytic use, unspecified with withdrawal, unspecified HCC

F13.94 Sedative, hypnotic or anxiolytic use, unspecified with sedative, hypnotic or anxiolytic-induced mood disorder HCC
Sedative, hypnotic, or anxiolytic-induced bipolar or related disorder, without use disorder
Sedative, hypnotic, or anxiolytic-induced depressive disorder, without use disorder

✓6ᵗʰ **F13.95 Sedative, hypnotic or anxiolytic use, unspecified with sedative, hypnotic or anxiolytic-induced psychotic disorder**

    F13.950 Sedative, hypnotic or anxiolytic use, unspecified with sedative, hypnotic or anxiolytic-induced psychotic disorder with delusions HCC

    F13.951 Sedative, hypnotic or anxiolytic use, unspecified with sedative, hypnotic or anxiolytic-induced psychotic disorder with hallucinations HCC

F13.959 Sedative, hypnotic or anxiolytic use, unspecified with sedative, hypnotic or anxiolytic-induced psychotic disorder, unspecified   HCC
> Sedative, hypnotic, or anxiolytic-induced psychotic disorder, without use disorder

F13.96 Sedative, hypnotic or anxiolytic use, unspecified with sedative, hypnotic or anxiolytic-induced persisting amnestic disorder   HCC

F13.97 Sedative, hypnotic or anxiolytic use, unspecified with sedative, hypnotic or anxiolytic-induced persisting dementia   HCC
> Sedative, hypnotic, or anxiolytic-induced major neurocognitive disorder, without use disorder

✓6ᵗʰ **F13.98** Sedative, hypnotic or anxiolytic use, unspecified with other sedative, hypnotic or anxiolytic-induced disorders

   F13.980 Sedative, hypnotic or anxiolytic use, unspecified with sedative, hypnotic or anxiolytic-induced anxiety disorder   HCC
> Sedative, hypnotic, or anxiolytic-induced anxiety disorder, without use disorder

   F13.981 Sedative, hypnotic or anxiolytic use, unspecified with sedative, hypnotic or anxiolytic-induced sexual dysfunction   HCC
> Sedative, hypnotic, or anxiolytic-induced sexual dysfunction disorder, without use disorder

   F13.982 Sedative, hypnotic or anxiolytic use, unspecified with sedative, hypnotic or anxiolytic-induced sleep disorder   HCC
> Sedative, hypnotic, or anxiolytic-induced sleep disorder, without use disorder

   F13.988 Sedative, hypnotic or anxiolytic use, unspecified with other sedative, hypnotic or anxiolytic-induced disorder   HCC
> Sedative, hypnotic, or anxiolytic-induced mild neurocognitive disorder

F13.99 Sedative, hypnotic or anxiolytic use, unspecified with unspecified sedative, hypnotic or anxiolytic-induced disorder   HCC

✓4ᵗʰ **F14** Cocaine related disorders
> EXCLUDES 2   other stimulant-related disorders (F15.-)

✓5ᵗʰ **F14.1** Cocaine abuse
> EXCLUDES 1   cocaine dependence (F14.2-)
>   cocaine use, unspecified (F14.9-)

   F14.10 Cocaine abuse, uncomplicated   HCC
> Cocaine use disorder, mild

   F14.11 Cocaine abuse, in remission   HCC
> Cocaine use disorder, mild, in early remission
> Cocaine use disorder, mild, in sustained remission

✓6ᵗʰ **F14.12** Cocaine abuse with intoxication

     F14.120 Cocaine abuse with intoxication, uncomplicated   HCC

     F14.121 Cocaine abuse with intoxication with delirium   HCC

     F14.122 Cocaine abuse with intoxication with perceptual disturbance   HCC

     F14.129 Cocaine abuse with intoxication, unspecified   HCC

   F14.14 Cocaine abuse with cocaine-induced mood disorder   HCC
> Cocaine use disorder, mild, with cocaine-induced bipolar or related disorder
> Cocaine use disorder, mild, with cocaine-induced depressive disorder

✓6ᵗʰ **F14.15** Cocaine abuse with cocaine-induced psychotic disorder

     F14.150 Cocaine abuse with cocaine-induced psychotic disorder with delusions   HCC

     F14.151 Cocaine abuse with cocaine-induced psychotic disorder with hallucinations   HCC

     F14.159 Cocaine abuse with cocaine-induced psychotic disorder, unspecified   HCC

✓6ᵗʰ **F14.18** Cocaine abuse with other cocaine-induced disorder

     F14.180 Cocaine abuse with cocaine-induced anxiety disorder   HCC

     F14.181 Cocaine abuse with cocaine-induced sexual dysfunction   HCC

     F14.182 Cocaine abuse with cocaine-induced sleep disorder   HCC

     F14.188 Cocaine abuse with other cocaine-induced disorder   HCC
> Cocaine use disorder, mild, with cocaine-induced obsessive compulsive or related disorder

   F14.19 Cocaine abuse with unspecified cocaine-induced disorder   HCC

✓5ᵗʰ **F14.2** Cocaine dependence
> EXCLUDES 1   cocaine abuse (F14.1-)
>   cocaine use, unspecified (F14.9-)
> EXCLUDES 2   cocaine poisoning (T40.5-)

   F14.20 Cocaine dependence, uncomplicated   HCC
> Cocaine use disorder, moderate
> Cocaine use disorder, severe

   F14.21 Cocaine dependence, in remission   HCC
> Cocaine use disorder, moderate, in early remission
> Cocaine use disorder, moderate, in sustained remission
> Cocaine use disorder, severe, in early remission
> Cocaine use disorder, severe, in sustained remission

✓6ᵗʰ **F14.22** Cocaine dependence with intoxication
> EXCLUDES 1   cocaine dependence with withdrawal (F14.23)

     F14.220 Cocaine dependence with intoxication, uncomplicated   HCC

     F14.221 Cocaine dependence with intoxication delirium   HCC

     F14.222 Cocaine dependence with intoxication with perceptual disturbance   HCC

     F14.229 Cocaine dependence with intoxication, unspecified   HCC

   F14.23 Cocaine dependence with withdrawal   HCC
> EXCLUDES 1   cocaine dependence with intoxication (F14.22-)

   F14.24 Cocaine dependence with cocaine-induced mood disorder   HCC
> Cocaine use disorder, moderate, with cocaine-induced bipolar or related disorder
> Cocaine use disorder, moderate, with cocaine-induced depressive disorder
> Cocaine use disorder, severe, with cocaine-induced bipolar or related disorder
> Cocaine use disorder, severe, with cocaine-induced depressive disorder

✓6ᵗʰ **F14.25** Cocaine dependence with cocaine-induced psychotic disorder

     F14.250 Cocaine dependence with cocaine-induced psychotic disorder with delusions   HCC

     F14.251 Cocaine dependence with cocaine-induced psychotic disorder with hallucinations   HCC

     F14.259 Cocaine dependence with cocaine-induced psychotic disorder, unspecified   HCC

✓6ᵗʰ **F14.28** Cocaine dependence with other cocaine-induced disorder

     F14.280 Cocaine dependence with cocaine-induced anxiety disorder   HCC

     F14.281 Cocaine dependence with cocaine-induced sexual dysfunction   HCC

     F14.282 Cocaine dependence with cocaine-induced sleep disorder   HCC

☑ Additional Character Required   ✓x7ᵗʰ Placeholder Alert   Manifestation   Unspecified Dx   ▶◀ Revised Text   ● New Code   ▲ Revised Code Title

Chapter 5. Mental, Behavioral and Neurodevelopmental Disorders

F14.288   **Cocaine dependence with other cocaine-induced disorder**   `HCC`
Cocaine use disorder, moderate, with cocaine-induced obsessive compulsive or related disorder
Cocaine use disorder, severe, with cocaine-induced obsessive compulsive or related disorder

F14.29   **Cocaine dependence with unspecified cocaine-induced disorder**   `HCC`

√5ᵗʰ **F14.9**   **Cocaine use, unspecified**

EXCLUDES 1   cocaine abuse (F14.1-)
cocaine dependence (F14.2-)

TIP: Assign a substance use code only when the provider documents a relationship between the use and an associated physical, mental, or behavioral disorder. As with all diagnoses, substance use codes must meet the definition of a reportable diagnosis.

F14.90   **Cocaine use, unspecified, uncomplicated**
AHA: 2018,2Q,10-11

√6ᵗʰ **F14.92**   **Cocaine use, unspecified with intoxication**

F14.920   **Cocaine use, unspecified with intoxication, uncomplicated**   `HCC`

F14.921   **Cocaine use, unspecified with intoxication delirium**   `HCC`

F14.922   **Cocaine use, unspecified with intoxication with perceptual disturbance**   `HCC`

F14.929   **Cocaine use, unspecified with intoxication, unspecified**   `HCC`

F14.94   **Cocaine use, unspecified with cocaine-induced mood disorder**   `HCC`
Cocaine induced bipolar or related disorder, without use disorder
Cocaine induced depressive disorder, without use disorder

√6ᵗʰ **F14.95**   **Cocaine use, unspecified with cocaine-induced psychotic disorder**

F14.950   **Cocaine use, unspecified with cocaine-induced psychotic disorder with delusions**   `HCC`

F14.951   **Cocaine use, unspecified with cocaine-induced psychotic disorder with hallucinations**   `HCC`

F14.959   **Cocaine use, unspecified with cocaine-induced psychotic disorder, unspecified**   `HCC`
Cocaine induced psychotic disorder, without use disorder

√6ᵗʰ **F14.98**   **Cocaine use, unspecified with other specified cocaine-induced disorder**

F14.980   **Cocaine use, unspecified with cocaine-induced anxiety disorder**   `HCC`
Cocaine induced anxiety disorder, without use disorder

F14.981   **Cocaine use, unspecified with cocaine-induced sexual dysfunction**   `HCC`
Cocaine induced sexual dysfunction, without use disorder

F14.982   **Cocaine use, unspecified with cocaine-induced sleep disorder**   `HCC`
Cocaine induced sleep disorder, without use disorder

F14.988   **Cocaine use, unspecified with other cocaine-induced disorder**   `HCC`
Cocaine induced obsessive compulsive or related disorder

F14.99   **Cocaine use, unspecified with unspecified cocaine-induced disorder**   `HCC`

√4ᵗʰ **F15**   **Other stimulant related disorders**

INCLUDES   amphetamine-related disorders
caffeine

EXCLUDES 2   cocaine-related disorders (F14.-)

√5ᵗʰ **F15.1**   **Other stimulant abuse**

EXCLUDES 1   other stimulant dependence (F15.2-)
other stimulant use, unspecified (F15.9-)

F15.10   **Other stimulant abuse, uncomplicated**   `HCC`
Amphetamine type substance use disorder, mild
Other or unspecified stimulant use disorder, mild

F15.11   **Other stimulant abuse, in remission**   `HCC`
Amphetamine type substance use disorder, mild, in early remission
Amphetamine type substance use disorder, mild, in sustained remission
Other or unspecified stimulant use disorder, mild, in early remission
Other or unspecified stimulant use disorder, mild, in sustained remission

√6ᵗʰ **F15.12**   **Other stimulant abuse with intoxication**

F15.120   **Other stimulant abuse with intoxication, uncomplicated**   `HCC`

F15.121   **Other stimulant abuse with intoxication delirium**   `HCC`

F15.122   **Other stimulant abuse with intoxication with perceptual disturbance**   `HCC`
Amphetamine or other stimulant use disorder, mild, with amphetamine or other stimulant intoxication, with perceptual disturbances

F15.129   **Other stimulant abuse with intoxication, unspecified**   `HCC`
Amphetamine or other stimulant use disorder, mild, with amphetamine or other stimulant intoxication, without perceptual disturbances

F15.14   **Other stimulant abuse with stimulant-induced mood disorder**   `HCC`
Amphetamine or other stimulant use disorder, mild, with amphetamine or other stimulant induced bipolar or related disorder
Amphetamine or other stimulant use disorder, mild, with amphetamine or other stimulant induced depressive disorder

√6ᵗʰ **F15.15**   **Other stimulant abuse with stimulant-induced psychotic disorder**

F15.150   **Other stimulant abuse with stimulant-induced psychotic disorder with delusions**   `HCC`

F15.151   **Other stimulant abuse with stimulant-induced psychotic disorder with hallucinations**   `HCC`

F15.159   **Other stimulant abuse with stimulant-induced psychotic disorder, unspecified**   `HCC`

√6ᵗʰ **F15.18**   **Other stimulant abuse with other stimulant-induced disorder**

F15.180   **Other stimulant abuse with stimulant-induced anxiety disorder**   `HCC`

F15.181   **Other stimulant abuse with stimulant-induced sexual dysfunction**   `HCC`

F15.182   **Other stimulant abuse with stimulant-induced sleep disorder**   `HCC`

F15.188   **Other stimulant abuse with other stimulant-induced disorder**   `HCC`
Amphetamine or other stimulant use disorder, mild, with amphetamine or other stimulant induced obsessive-compulsive or related disorder

F15.19   **Other stimulant abuse with unspecified stimulant-induced disorder**   `HCC`

☑5ᵗʰ **F15.2 Other stimulant** dependence

     EXCLUDES 1   *other stimulant abuse (F15.1-)*
                  other stimulant use, unspecified (F15.9-)

    F15.20 Other stimulant dependence,   HCC
           uncomplicated
           Amphetamine type substance use disorder, moderate
           Amphetamine type substance use disorder, severe
           Other or unspecified stimulant use disorder, moderate
           Other or unspecified stimulant use disorder, severe

    F15.21 Other stimulant dependence, in remission   HCC
           Amphetamine type substance use disorder, moderate,
              in early remission
           Amphetamine type substance use disorder, moderate,
              in sustained remission
           Amphetamine type substance use disorder, severe,
              in early remission
           Amphetamine type substance use disorder, severe,
              in sustained remission
           Other or unspecified stimulant use disorder,
              moderate, in early remission
           Other or unspecified stimulant use disorder,
              moderate, in sustained remission
           Other or unspecified stimulant use disorder, severe,
              in early remission
           Other or unspecified stimulant use disorder, severe,
              in sustained remission

☑6ᵗʰ **F15.22 Other stimulant dependence with** intoxication

     EXCLUDES 1   *other stimulant dependence with*
                  withdrawal (F15.23)

    F15.220 Other stimulant dependence with   HCC
           intoxication, uncomplicated

    F15.221 Other stimulant dependence with   HCC
           intoxication delirium

    F15.222 Other stimulant dependence with   HCC
           intoxication with perceptual
           disturbance
           Amphetamine or other stimulant use
              disorder, moderate, with
              amphetamine or other stimulant
              intoxication, with perceptual
              disturbances
           Amphetamine or other stimulant use
              disorder, severe, with amphetamine
              or other stimulant intoxication, with
              perceptual disturbances

    F15.229 Other stimulant dependence with   HCC
           intoxication, unspecified
           Amphetamine or other stimulant use
              disorder, moderate, with
              amphetamine or other stimulant
              intoxication, without perceptual
              disturbances
           Amphetamine or other stimulant use
              disorder, severe, with amphetamine
              or other stimulant intoxication,
              without perceptual disturbances

    F15.23 Other stimulant dependence with   HCC
           withdrawal
           Amphetamine or other stimulant withdrawal
      EXCLUDES 1   *other stimulant dependence with*
                  intoxication (F15.22-)

    F15.24 Other stimulant dependence with   HCC
           stimulant-induced mood disorder
           Amphetamine or other stimulant use disorder,
              moderate, with amphetamine or other
              stimulant-induced bipolar or related disorder
           Amphetamine or other stimulant use disorder,
              moderate, with amphetamine or other stimulant
              induced depressive disorder
           Amphetamine or other stimulant use disorder, severe,
              with amphetamine or other stimulant-induced
              bipolar or related disorder
           Amphetamine or other stimulant use disorder, severe,
              with amphetamine or other stimulant-induced
              depressive disorder

☑6ᵗʰ **F15.25 Other stimulant dependence with**
        stimulant-induced psychotic disorder

    F15.250 Other stimulant dependence with   HCC
           stimulant-induced psychotic
           disorder with delusions

    F15.251 Other stimulant dependence with   HCC
           stimulant-induced psychotic
           disorder with hallucinations

    F15.259 Other stimulant dependence with   HCC
           stimulant-induced psychotic
           disorder, unspecified

☑6ᵗʰ **F15.28 Other stimulant dependence with other**
        stimulant-induced disorder

    F15.280 Other stimulant dependence with   HCC
           stimulant-induced anxiety
           disorder

    F15.281 Other stimulant dependence with   HCC
           stimulant-induced sexual
           dysfunction

    F15.282 Other stimulant dependence with   HCC
           stimulant-induced sleep disorder

    F15.288 Other stimulant dependence with   HCC
           other stimulant-induced disorder
           Amphetamine or other stimulant use
              disorder, moderate, with
              amphetamine orother stimulant
              induced obsessive compulsive or
              related disorder
           Amphetamine or other stimulant use
              disorder, severe, with amphetamine
              or otherstimulant induced obsessive
              compulsive or related disorder

    F15.29 Other stimulant dependence with   HCC
           unspecified stimulant-induced disorder

☑5ᵗʰ **F15.9 Other stimulant** use, unspecified

     EXCLUDES 1   *other stimulant abuse (F15.1-)*
                  other stimulant dependence (F15.2-)

    TIP: Assign a substance use code only when the provider
    documents a relationship between the use and an associated
    physical, mental, or behavioral disorder. As with all diagnoses,
    substance use codes must meet the definition of a reportable
    diagnosis.

    F15.90 Other stimulant use, unspecified, uncomplicated
           AHA: 2018,2Q,10-11

☑6ᵗʰ **F15.92 Other stimulant use, unspecified with** intoxication

     EXCLUDES 1   *other stimulant use, unspecified with*
                  withdrawal (F15.93)

    F15.920 Other stimulant use, unspecified   HCC
           with intoxication, uncomplicated

    F15.921 Other stimulant use, unspecified   HCC
           with intoxication delirium
           Amphetamine or other stimulant-induced
              delirium

    F15.922 Other stimulant use, unspecified   HCC
           with intoxication with perceptual
           disturbance

    F15.929 Other stimulant use, unspecified   HCC
           with intoxication, unspecified
           Caffeine intoxication

    F15.93 Other stimulant use, unspecified with   HCC
           withdrawal
           Caffeine withdrawal
      EXCLUDES 1   *other stimulant use, unspecified with*
                  intoxication (F15.92-)

    F15.94 Other stimulant use, unspecified with   HCC
           stimulant-induced mood disorder
           Amphetamine or other stimulant-induced bipolar or
              related disorder, without use disorder
           Amphetamine or other stimulant-induced depressive
              disorder, without use disorder

☑6ᵗʰ **F15.95 Other stimulant use, unspecified with**
        stimulant-induced psychotic disorder

    F15.950 Other stimulant use, unspecified   HCC
           with stimulant-induced psychotic
           disorder with delusions

    F15.951 Other stimulant use, unspecified   HCC
           with stimulant-induced psychotic
           disorder with hallucinations

☑ Additional Character Required   ✓x7ᵗʰ Placeholder Alert   Manifestation   Unspecified Dx   ▶◀ Revised Text   ● New Code   ▲ Revised Code Title

ICD-10-CM 2020   545

F15.959 **Other stimulant use, unspecified with stimulant-induced psychotic disorder, unspecified** `HCC`

Amphetamine or other stimulant-induced psychotic disorder, without use disorder

✓6ᵗʰ **F15.98** **Other stimulant use, unspecified with other stimulant-induced disorder**

F15.980 **Other stimulant use, unspecified with stimulant-induced anxiety disorder** `HCC`

Amphetamine or other stimulant-induced anxiety disorder, without use disorder

Caffeine induced anxiety disorder, without use disorder

F15.981 **Other stimulant use, unspecified with stimulant-induced sexual dysfunction** `HCC`

Amphetamine or other stimulant-induced sexual dysfunction, without use disorder

F15.982 **Other stimulant use, unspecified with stimulant-induced sleep disorder** `HCC`

Amphetamine or other stimulant-induced sleep disorder, without use disorder

Caffeine induced sleep disorder, without use disorder

F15.988 **Other stimulant use, unspecified with other stimulant-induced disorder** `HCC`

Amphetamine or other stimulant-induced obsessive compulsive or related disorder, without use disorder

F15.99 **Other stimulant use, unspecified with unspecified stimulant-induced disorder** `HCC`

✓4ᵗʰ **F16** **Hallucinogen related disorders**

`INCLUDES`   ecstasy

PCP

phencyclidine

AHA: 2018,4Q,31

✓5ᵗʰ **F16.1** **Hallucinogen abuse**

EXCLUDES 1   *hallucinogen dependence (F16.2-)*

hallucinogen use, unspecified (F16.9-)

F16.10 **Hallucinogen abuse, uncomplicated** `HCC`

Other hallucinogen use disorder, mild

Phencyclidine use disorder, mild

F16.11 **Hallucinogen abuse, in remission** `HCC`

Other hallucinogen use disorder, mild, in early remission

Other hallucinogen use disorder, mild, in sustained remission

Phencyclidine use disorder, mild, in early remission

Phencyclidine use disorder, mild, in sustained remission

✓6ᵗʰ **F16.12** **Hallucinogen abuse with intoxication**

F16.120 **Hallucinogen abuse with intoxication, uncomplicated** `HCC`

F16.121 **Hallucinogen abuse with intoxication with delirium** `HCC`

F16.122 **Hallucinogen abuse with intoxication with perceptual disturbance** `HCC`

F16.129 **Hallucinogen abuse with intoxication, unspecified** `HCC`

F16.14 **Hallucinogen abuse with hallucinogen-induced mood disorder** `HCC`

Other hallucinogen use disorder, mild, with other hallucinogen induced bipolar or related disorder

Other hallucinogen use disorder, mild, with other hallucinogen induced depressive disorder

Phencyclidine use disorder, mild, with phencyclidine induced bipolar or related disorder

Phencyclidine use disorder, mild, with phencyclidine induced depressive disorder

✓6ᵗʰ **F16.15** **Hallucinogen abuse with hallucinogen-induced psychotic disorder**

F16.150 **Hallucinogen abuse with hallucinogen-induced psychotic disorder with delusions** `HCC`

F16.151 **Hallucinogen abuse with hallucinogen-induced psychotic disorder with hallucinations** `HCC`

F16.159 **Hallucinogen abuse with hallucinogen-induced psychotic disorder, unspecified** `HCC`

✓6ᵗʰ **F16.18** **Hallucinogen abuse with other hallucinogen-induced disorder**

F16.180 **Hallucinogen abuse with hallucinogen-induced anxiety disorder** `HCC`

F16.183 **Hallucinogen abuse with hallucinogen persisting perception disorder (flashbacks)**

F16.188 **Hallucinogen abuse with other hallucinogen-induced disorder** `HCC`

F16.19 **Hallucinogen abuse with unspecified hallucinogen-induced disorder** `HCC`

✓5ᵗʰ **F16.2** **Hallucinogen dependence**

EXCLUDES 1   *hallucinogen abuse (F16.1-)*

hallucinogen use, unspecified (F16.9-)

F16.20 **Hallucinogen dependence, uncomplicated** `HCC`

Other hallucinogen use disorder, moderate

Other hallucinogen use disorder, severe

Phencyclidine use disorder, moderate

Phencyclidine use disorder, severe

F16.21 **Hallucinogen dependence, in remission** `HCC`

Other hallucinogen use disorder, moderate, in early remission

Other hallucinogen use disorder, moderate, in sustained remission

Other hallucinogen use disorder, severe, in early remission

Other hallucinogen use disorder, severe, in sustained remission

Phencyclidine use disorder, moderate, in early remission

Phencyclidine use disorder, moderate, in sustained remission

Phencyclidine use disorder, severe, in early remission

Phencyclidine use disorder, severe, in sustained remission

✓6ᵗʰ **F16.22** **Hallucinogen dependence with intoxication**

F16.220 **Hallucinogen dependence with intoxication, uncomplicated** `HCC`

F16.221 **Hallucinogen dependence with intoxication with delirium** `HCC`

F16.229 **Hallucinogen dependence with intoxication, unspecified** `HCC`

F16.24 **Hallucinogen dependence with hallucinogen-induced mood disorder** `HCC`

Other hallucinogen use disorder, moderate, with other hallucinogen induced bipolar or related disorder

Other hallucinogen use disorder, moderate, with other hallucinogen induced depressive disorder

Other hallucinogen use disorder, severe, with other hallucinogen-induced bipolar or related disorder

Other hallucinogen use disorder, severe, with other hallucinogen-induced depressive disorder

Phencyclidine use disorder, moderate, with phencyclidine induced bipolar or related disorder

Phencyclidine use disorder, moderate, with phencyclidine induced depressive disorder

Phencyclidine use disorder, severe, with phencyclidine induced bipolar or related disorder

Phencyclidine use disorder, severe, with phencyclidine-induced depressive disorder

✓6ᵗʰ **F16.25** **Hallucinogen dependence with hallucinogen-induced psychotic disorder**

F16.250 **Hallucinogen dependence with hallucinogen-induced psychotic disorder with delusions** `HCC`

F16.251 Hallucinogen dependence with hallucinogen-induced psychotic disorder with **hallucinations** `HCC`

F16.259 Hallucinogen dependence with hallucinogen-induced psychotic disorder, unspecified `HCC`

√6ᵗʰ **F16.28** Hallucinogen dependence with **other** hallucinogen-induced disorder

F16.280 Hallucinogen dependence with hallucinogen-induced **anxiety** disorder `HCC`

F16.283 Hallucinogen dependence with hallucinogen **persisting perception disorder (flashbacks)** `HCC`

F16.288 Hallucinogen dependence with other hallucinogen-induced disorder `HCC`

F16.29 Hallucinogen dependence with unspecified hallucinogen-induced disorder `HCC`

√5ᵗʰ **F16.9** Hallucinogen **use, unspecified**

> EXCLUDES 1   hallucinogen abuse (F16.1-)
> hallucinogen dependence (F16.2-)

TIP: Assign a substance use code only when the provider documents a relationship between the use and an associated physical, mental, or behavioral disorder. As with all diagnoses, substance use codes must meet the definition of a reportable diagnosis.

F16.90 Hallucinogen use, unspecified, **uncomplicated**
     AHA: 2018,2Q,10-11

√6ᵗʰ **F16.92** Hallucinogen use, unspecified with **intoxication**

F16.920 Hallucinogen use, unspecified with intoxication, **uncomplicated** `HCC`

F16.921 Hallucinogen use, unspecified with intoxication with **delirium** `HCC`
     Other hallucinogen intoxication delirium

F16.929 Hallucinogen use, unspecified with intoxication, unspecified `HCC`

F16.94 Hallucinogen use, unspecified with hallucinogen-induced **mood disorder** `HCC`
     Other hallucinogen induced bipolar or related disorder, without use disorder
     Other hallucinogen induced depressive disorder, without use disorder
     Phencyclidine induced bipolar or related disorder, without use disorder
     Phencyclidine induced depressive disorder, without use disorder

√6ᵗʰ **F16.95** Hallucinogen use, unspecified with hallucinogen-induced **psychotic disorder**

F16.950 Hallucinogen use, unspecified with hallucinogen-induced psychotic disorder with **delusions** `HCC`

F16.951 Hallucinogen use, unspecified with hallucinogen-induced psychotic disorder with **hallucinations** `HCC`

F16.959 Hallucinogen use, unspecified with hallucinogen-induced psychotic disorder, unspecified `HCC`
     Other hallucinogen induced psychotic disorder, without use disorder
     Phencyclidine induced psychotic disorder, without use disorder

√6ᵗʰ **F16.98** Hallucinogen use, unspecified with other specified hallucinogen-induced disorder

F16.980 Hallucinogen use, unspecified with hallucinogen-induced **anxiety disorder** `HCC`
     Other hallucinogen-induced anxiety disorder, without use disorder
     Phencyclidine induced anxiety disorder, without use disorder

F16.983 Hallucinogen use, unspecified with hallucinogen **persisting perception disorder (flashbacks)** `HCC`

F16.988 Hallucinogen use, unspecified with other hallucinogen-induced disorder `HCC`

F16.99 Hallucinogen use, unspecified with unspecified hallucinogen-induced disorder `HCC`

√4ᵗʰ **F17** Nicotine **dependence**

> EXCLUDES 1   history of tobacco dependence (Z87.891)
> tobacco use NOS (Z72.0)
> EXCLUDES 2   tobacco use (smoking) during pregnancy, childbirth and the puerperium (O99.33-)
> toxic effect of nicotine (T65.2-)

AHA: 2013,4Q,108-109

√5ᵗʰ **F17.2** Nicotine **dependence**

√6ᵗʰ **F17.20** Nicotine dependence, unspecified

F17.200 Nicotine dependence, unspecified, **uncomplicated**
     Tobacco use disorder, mild
     Tobacco use disorder, moderate
     Tobacco use disorder, severe
     AHA: 2016,1Q,36
     TIP: Assign when provider documentation indicates "smoker" without further specification.

F17.201 Nicotine dependence, unspecified, **in remission**
     Tobacco use disorder, mild, in early remission
     Tobacco use disorder, mild, in sustained remission
     Tobacco use disorder, moderate, in early remission
     Tobacco use disorder, moderate, in sustained remission
     Tobacco use disorder, severe, in early remission
     Tobacco use disorder, severe, in sustained remission

F17.203 Nicotine dependence unspecified, **with withdrawal**
     Tobacco withdrawal

F17.208 Nicotine dependence, unspecified, with other nicotine-induced disorders

F17.209 Nicotine dependence, unspecified, with unspecified nicotine-induced disorders

√6ᵗʰ **F17.21** Nicotine dependence, **cigarettes**

F17.210 Nicotine dependence, cigarettes, **uncomplicated**
     AHA: 2017,2Q,28-29

F17.211 Nicotine dependence, cigarettes, **in remission**
     Tobacco use disorder, cigarettes, mild, in early remission
     Tobacco use disorder, cigarettes, mild, in sustained remission
     Tobacco use disorder, cigarettes, moderate, in early remission
     Tobacco use disorder, cigarettes, moderate, in sustained remission
     Tobacco use disorder, cigarettes, severe, in early remission
     Tobacco use disorder, cigarettes, severe, in sustained remission

F17.213 Nicotine dependence, cigarettes, with **withdrawal**

F17.218 Nicotine dependence, cigarettes, with other nicotine-induced disorders

F17.219 Nicotine dependence, cigarettes, with unspecified nicotine-induced disorders

√6ᵗʰ **F17.22** Nicotine dependence, **chewing tobacco**

F17.220 Nicotine dependence, chewing tobacco, **uncomplicated**

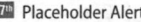 Additional Character Required   √x7ᵗʰ Placeholder Alert   Manifestation   Unspecified Dx   ▶◀ Revised Text   ● New Code   ▲ Revised Code Title

ICD-10-CM 2020   547

Chapter 5. Mental, Behavioral and Neurodevelopmental Disorders

F17.221   **Nicotine dependence, chewing tobacco, in remission**
Tobacco use disorder, chewing tobacco, mild, in early remission
Tobacco use disorder, chewing tobacco, mild, in sustained remission
Tobacco use disorder, chewing tobacco, moderate, in early remission
Tobacco use disorder, chewing tobacco, moderate, in sustained remission
Tobacco use disorder, chewing tobacco, severe, in early remission
Tobacco use disorder, chewing tobacco, severe, in sustained remission

F17.223   **Nicotine dependence, chewing tobacco, with withdrawal**

F17.228   **Nicotine dependence, chewing tobacco, with other nicotine-induced disorders**

F17.229   **Nicotine dependence, chewing tobacco, with unspecified nicotine-induced disorders**

✓6th   **F17.29**   **Nicotine dependence, other tobacco product**

F17.290   **Nicotine dependence, other tobacco product, uncomplicated**
AHA: 2017,2Q,28-29

F17.291   **Nicotine dependence, other tobacco product, in remission**
Tobacco use disorder, other tobacco product, mild, in early remission
Tobacco use disorder, other tobacco product, mild, in sustained remission
Tobacco use disorder, other tobacco product, moderate, in early remission
Tobacco use disorder, other tobacco product, moderate, in sustained remission
Tobacco use disorder, other tobacco product, severe, in early remission
Tobacco use disorder, other tobacco product, severe, in sustained remission

F17.293   **Nicotine dependence, other tobacco product, with withdrawal**

F17.298   **Nicotine dependence, other tobacco product, with other nicotine-induced disorders**

F17.299   **Nicotine dependence, other tobacco product, with unspecified nicotine-induced disorders**

✓4th   **F18**   **Inhalant related disorders**
INCLUDES   volatile solvents

✓5th   **F18.1**   **Inhalant abuse**
EXCLUDES 1   inhalant dependence (F18.2-)
inhalant use, unspecified (F18.9-)

F18.10   **Inhalant abuse, uncomplicated**   HCC
Inhalant use disorder, mild

F18.11   **Inhalant abuse, in remission**   HCC
Inhalant use disorder, mild, in early remission
Inhalant use disorder, mild, in sustained remission

✓6th   **F18.12**   **Inhalant abuse with intoxication**

F18.120   **Inhalant abuse with intoxication, uncomplicated**   HCC

F18.121   **Inhalant abuse with intoxication delirium**   HCC

F18.129   **Inhalant abuse with intoxication, unspecified**   HCC

F18.14   **Inhalant abuse with inhalant-induced mood disorder**   HCC
Inhalant use disorder, mild, with inhalant induced depressive disorder

✓6th   **F18.15**   **Inhalant abuse with inhalant-induced psychotic disorder**

F18.150   **Inhalant abuse with inhalant-induced psychotic disorder with delusions**   HCC

F18.151   **Inhalant abuse with inhalant-induced psychotic disorder with hallucinations**   HCC

F18.159   **Inhalant abuse with inhalant-induced psychotic disorder, unspecified**   HCC

F18.17   **Inhalant abuse with inhalant-induced dementia**   HCC
Inhalant use disorder, mild, with inhalant induced major neurocognitive disorder

✓6th   **F18.18**   **Inhalant abuse with other inhalant-induced disorders**

F18.180   **Inhalant abuse with inhalant-induced anxiety disorder**   HCC

F18.188   **Inhalant abuse with other inhalant-induced disorder**   HCC
Inhalant use disorder, mild, with inhalant induced mild neurocognitive disorder

F18.19   **Inhalant abuse with unspecified inhalant-induced disorder**   HCC

✓5th   **F18.2**   **Inhalant dependence**
EXCLUDES 1   inhalant abuse (F18.1-)
inhalant use, unspecified (F18.9-)

F18.20   **Inhalant dependence, uncomplicated**   HCC
Inhalant use disorder, moderate
Inhalant use disorder, severe

F18.21   **Inhalant dependence, in remission**   HCC
Inhalant use disorder, moderate, in early remission
Inhalant use disorder, moderate, in sustained remission
Inhalant use disorder, severe, in early remission
Inhalant use disorder, severe, in sustained remission

✓6th   **F18.22**   **Inhalant dependence with intoxication**

F18.220   **Inhalant dependence with intoxication, uncomplicated**   HCC

F18.221   **Inhalant dependence with intoxication delirium**   HCC

F18.229   **Inhalant dependence with intoxication, unspecified**   HCC

F18.24   **Inhalant dependence with inhalant-induced mood disorder**   HCC
Inhalant use disorder, moderate, with inhalant induced depressive disorder
Inhalant use disorder, severe, with inhalant induced depressive disorder

✓6th   **F18.25**   **Inhalant dependence with inhalant-induced psychotic disorder**

F18.250   **Inhalant dependence with inhalant-induced psychotic disorder with delusions**   HCC

F18.251   **Inhalant dependence with inhalant-induced psychotic disorder with hallucinations**   HCC

F18.259   **Inhalant dependence with inhalant-induced psychotic disorder, unspecified**   HCC

F18.27   **Inhalant dependence with inhalant-induced dementia**   HCC
Inhalant use disorder, moderate, with inhalant induced major neurocognitive disorder
Inhalant use disorder, severe, with inhalant induced major neurocognitive disorder

✓6th   **F18.28**   **Inhalant dependence with other inhalant-induced disorders**

F18.280   **Inhalant dependence with inhalant-induced anxiety disorder**   HCC

F18.288   **Inhalant dependence with other inhalant-induced disorder**   HCC
Inhalant use disorder, moderate, with inhalant-induced mild neurocognitive disorder
Inhalant use disorder, severe, with inhalant-induced mild neurocognitive disorder

F18.29   **Inhalant dependence with unspecified inhalant-induced disorder**   HCC

✓5ᵗʰ F18.9 Inhalant use, unspecified

> EXCLUDES 1   inhalant abuse (F18.1-)
> inhalant dependence (F18.2-)

  F18.90 Inhalant use, unspecified, uncomplicated
  AHA: 2018,2Q,10-11

✓6ᵗʰ F18.92 Inhalant use, unspecified with intoxication

  F18.920 Inhalant use, unspecified with intoxication, uncomplicated   HCC
  F18.921 Inhalant use, unspecified with intoxication with delirium   HCC
  F18.929 Inhalant use, unspecified with intoxication, unspecified   HCC

  F18.94 Inhalant use, unspecified with inhalant-induced mood disorder   HCC
  Inhalant induced depressive disorder

✓6ᵗʰ F18.95 Inhalant use, unspecified with inhalant-induced psychotic disorder

  F18.950 Inhalant use, unspecified with inhalant-induced psychotic disorder with delusions   HCC
  F18.951 Inhalant use, unspecified with inhalant-induced psychotic disorder with hallucinations HCC
  F18.959 Inhalant use, unspecified with inhalant-induced psychotic disorder, unspecified   HCC

  F18.97 Inhalant use, unspecified with inhalant-induced persisting dementia   HCC
  Inhalant-induced major neurocognitive disorder

✓6ᵗʰ F18.98 Inhalant use, unspecified with other inhalant-induced disorders

  F18.980 Inhalant use, unspecified with inhalant-induced anxiety disorder   HCC
  F18.988 Inhalant use, unspecified with other inhalant-induced disorder   HCC
  Inhalant-induced mild neurocognitive disorder

  F18.99 Inhalant use, unspecified with unspecified inhalant-induced disorder   HCC

✓4ᵗʰ F19 Other psychoactive substance related disorders

> INCLUDES   polysubstance drug use (indiscriminate drug use)

✓5ᵗʰ F19.1 Other psychoactive substance abuse

> EXCLUDES 1   other psychoactive substance dependence (F19.2-)
> other psychoactive substance use, unspecified (F19.9-)

  F19.10 Other psychoactive substance abuse, uncomplicated   HCC
  Other (or unknown) substance use disorder, mild

  F19.11 Other psychoactive substance abuse, in remission   HCC
  Other (or unknown) substance use disorder, mild, in early remission
  Other (or unknown) substance use disorder, mild, in sustained remission

✓6ᵗʰ F19.12 Other psychoactive substance abuse with intoxication

  F19.120 Other psychoactive substance abuse with intoxication, uncomplicated   HCC
  F19.121 Other psychoactive substance abuse with intoxication delirium   HCC
  F19.122 Other psychoactive substance abuse with intoxication with perceptual disturbances HCC
  F19.129 Other psychoactive substance abuse with intoxication, unspecified   HCC

  F19.14 Other psychoactive substance abuse with psychoactive substance-induced mood disorder   HCC
  Other (or unknown) substance use disorder, mild, with other (or unknown) substance-induced bipolar or related disorder
  Other (or unknown) substance use disorder, mild, with other (or unknown) substance-induced depressive disorder

✓6ᵗʰ F19.15 Other psychoactive substance abuse with psychoactive substance-induced psychotic disorder

  F19.150 Other psychoactive substance abuse with psychoactive substance-induced psychotic disorder with delusions   HCC
  F19.151 Other psychoactive substance abuse with psychoactive substance-induced psychotic disorder with hallucinations HCC
  F19.159 Other psychoactive substance abuse with psychoactive substance-induced psychotic disorder, unspecified   HCC

  F19.16 Other psychoactive substance abuse with psychoactive substance-induced persisting amnestic disorder   HCC
  F19.17 Other psychoactive substance abuse with psychoactive substance-induced persisting dementia   HCC
  Other (or unknown) substance use disorder, mild, with other (or unknown) substance-induced major neurocognitive disorder

✓6ᵗʰ F19.18 Other psychoactive substance abuse with other psychoactive substance-induced disorders

  F19.180 Other psychoactive substance abuse with psychoactive substance-induced anxiety disorder   HCC
  F19.181 Other psychoactive substance abuse with psychoactive substance-induced sexual dysfunction   HCC
  F19.182 Other psychoactive substance abuse with psychoactive substance-induced sleep disorder   HCC
  F19.188 Other psychoactive substance abuse with other psychoactive substance-induced disorder   HCC
  Other (or unknown) substance use disorder, mild, with other (or unknown) substance induced mild neurocognitive disorder
  Other (or unknown) substance use disorder, mild, with other (or unknown) substance induced obsessive-compulsive or related disorder

  F19.19 Other psychoactive substance abuse with unspecified psychoactive substance-induced disorder   HCC

✓5ᵗʰ F19.2 Other psychoactive substance dependence

> EXCLUDES 1   other psychoactive substance abuse (F19.1-)
> other psychoactive substance use, unspecified (F19.9-)

  F19.20 Other psychoactive substance dependence, uncomplicated   HCC
  Other (or unknown) substance use disorder, moderate
  Other (or unknown) substance use disorder, severe

  F19.21 Other psychoactive substance dependence, in remission   HCC
  Other (or unknown) substance use disorder, moderate, in early remission
  Other (or unknown) substance use disorder, moderate, in sustained remission
  Other (or unknown) substance use disorder, severe, in early remission
  Other (or unknown) substance use disorder, severe, in sustained remission

✓6ᵗʰ F19.22 Other psychoactive substance dependence with intoxication

> EXCLUDES 1   other psychoactive substance dependence with withdrawal (F19.23-)

  F19.220 Other psychoactive substance dependence with intoxication, uncomplicated   HCC
  F19.221 Other psychoactive substance dependence with intoxication delirium   HCC
  F19.222 Other psychoactive substance dependence with intoxication with perceptual disturbance HCC

✓ Additional Character Required   ✓x7ᵗʰ Placeholder Alert   Manifestation   Unspecified Dx   ▶◀ Revised Text   ● New Code   ▲ Revised Code Title

ICD-10-CM 2020   549

Chapter 5. Mental, Behavioral and Neurodevelopmental Disorders

F18.9–F19.222

F19.229 Other psychoactive substance dependence with intoxication, unspecified `HCC`

✓6th **F19.23** Other psychoactive substance dependence with withdrawal

　EXCLUDES 1　other psychoactive substance dependence with intoxication (F19.22-)

F19.230 Other psychoactive substance dependence with withdrawal, uncomplicated `HCC`

F19.231 Other psychoactive substance dependence with withdrawal delirium `HCC`

F19.232 Other psychoactive substance dependence with withdrawal with perceptual disturbance `HCC`

F19.239 Other psychoactive substance dependence with withdrawal, unspecified `HCC`

F19.24 Other psychoactive substance dependence with psychoactive substance-induced mood disorder `HCC`

Other (or unknown) substance use disorder, moderate, with other (or unknown) substance induced bipolar or related disorder

Other (or unknown) substance use disorder, moderate, with other (or unknown) substance induced depressive disorder

Other (or unknown) substance use disorder, severe, with other (or unknown) substance induced bipolar or related disorder

Other (or unknown) substance use disorder, severe, with other (or unknown) substance induced depressive disorder

✓6th **F19.25** Other psychoactive substance dependence with psychoactive substance-induced psychotic disorder

F19.250 Other psychoactive substance dependence with psychoactive substance-induced psychotic disorder with delusions `HCC`

F19.251 Other psychoactive substance dependence with psychoactive substance-induced psychotic disorder with hallucinations `HCC`

F19.259 Other psychoactive substance dependence with psychoactive substance-induced psychotic disorder, unspecified `HCC`

F19.26 Other psychoactive substance dependence with psychoactive substance-induced persisting amnestic disorder `HCC`

F19.27 Other psychoactive substance dependence with psychoactive substance-induced persisting dementia `HCC`

Other (or unknown) substance use disorder, moderate, with other (or unknown) substance induced major neurocognitive disorder

Other (or unknown) substance use disorder, severe, with other (or unknown) substance induced major neurocognitive disorder

✓6th **F19.28** Other psychoactive substance dependence with other psychoactive substance-induced disorders

F19.280 Other psychoactive substance dependence with psychoactive substance-induced anxiety disorder `HCC`

F19.281 Other psychoactive substance dependence with psychoactive substance-induced sexual dysfunction `HCC`

F19.282 Other psychoactive substance dependence with psychoactive substance-induced sleep disorder `HCC`

F19.288 Other psychoactive substance dependence with other psychoactive substance-induced disorder `HCC`

Other (or unknown) substance use disorder, moderate, with other (or unknown) substance induced mild neurocognitive disorder

Other (or unknown) substance use disorder, severe, with other (or unknown) substance induced mild neurocognitive disorder

Other (or unknown) substance use disorder, moderate, with other (or unknown) substance induced obsessive compulsive or related disorder

Other (or unknown) substance use disorder, severe, with other (or unknown) substance induced obsessive-compulsive or related disorder

F19.29 Other psychoactive substance dependence with unspecified psychoactive substance-induced disorder `HCC`

✓5th **F19.9** Other psychoactive substance use, unspecified

　EXCLUDES 1　other psychoactive substance abuse (F19.1-)
　　　　　　other psychoactive substance dependence (F19.2-)

F19.90 Other psychoactive substance use, unspecified, uncomplicated

AHA: 2018,2Q,10-11

✓6th **F19.92** Other psychoactive substance use, unspecified with intoxication

　EXCLUDES 1　other psychoactive substance use, unspecified with withdrawal (F19.93)

F19.920 Other psychoactive substance use, unspecified with intoxication, uncomplicated `HCC`

F19.921 Other psychoactive substance use, unspecified with intoxication with delirium `HCC`

Other (or unknown) substance-induced delirium

F19.922 Other psychoactive substance use, unspecified with intoxication with perceptual disturbance `HCC`

F19.929 Other psychoactive substance use, unspecified with intoxication, unspecified `HCC`

✓6th **F19.93** Other psychoactive substance use, unspecified with withdrawal

　EXCLUDES 1　other psychoactive substance use, unspecified with intoxication (F19.92-)

F19.930 Other psychoactive substance use, unspecified with withdrawal, uncomplicated `HCC`

F19.931 Other psychoactive substance use, unspecified with withdrawal delirium `HCC`

F19.932 Other psychoactive substance use, unspecified with withdrawal with perceptual disturbance `HCC`

F19.939 Other psychoactive substance use, unspecified with withdrawal, unspecified `HCC`

F19.94 Other psychoactive substance use, unspecified with psychoactive substance-induced mood disorder `HCC`

Other (or unknown) substance-induced bipolar or related disorder, without use disorder

Other (or unknown) substance-induced depressive disorder, without use disorder

✓6th **F19.95** Other psychoactive substance use, unspecified with psychoactive substance-induced psychotic disorder

F19.950 Other psychoactive substance use, unspecified with psychoactive substance-induced psychotic disorder with delusions `HCC`

F19.951 Other psychoactive substance use, unspecified with psychoactive substance-induced psychotic disorder with hallucinations   HCC

F19.959 Other psychoactive substance use, unspecified with psychoactive substance-induced psychotic disorder, unspecified   HCC

Other or unknown substance-induced psychotic disorder, without use disorder

F19.96 Other psychoactive substance use, unspecified with psychoactive substance-induced persisting amnestic disorder   HCC

F19.97 Other psychoactive substance use, unspecified with psychoactive substance-induced persisting dementia   HCC

Other (or unknown) substance-induced major neurocognitive disorder, without use disorder

√6ᵗʰ **F19.98** Other psychoactive substance use, unspecified with other psychoactive substance-induced disorders

F19.980 Other psychoactive substance use, unspecified with psychoactive substance-induced anxiety disorder   HCC

Other (or unknown) substance-induced anxiety disorder, without use disorder

F19.981 Other psychoactive substance use, unspecified with psychoactive substance-induced sexual dysfunction   HCC

Other (or unknown) substance-induced sexual dysfunction, without use disorder

F19.982 Other psychoactive substance use, unspecified with psychoactive substance-induced sleep disorder   HCC

Other (or unknown) substance-induced sleep disorder, without use disorder

F19.988 Other psychoactive substance use, unspecified with other psychoactive substance-induced disorder   HCC

Other (or unknown) substance-induced mild neurocognitive disorder, without use disorder

Other (or unknown) substance-induced obsessive-compulsive or related disorder, without use disorder

F19.99 Other psychoactive substance use, unspecified with unspecified psychoactive substance-induced disorder   HCC

Schizophrenia, schizotypal, delusional, and other non-mood psychotic disorders (F20-F29)

√4ᵗʰ **F20 Schizophrenia**

EXCLUDES 1   brief psychotic disorder (F23)
     cyclic schizophrenia (F25.0)
     mood [affective] disorders with psychotic symptoms (F30.2, F31.2, F31.5, F31.64, F32.3, F33.3)
     schizoaffective disorder (F25.-)
     schizophrenic reaction NOS (F23)

EXCLUDES 2   schizophrenic reaction in:
     alcoholism (F10.15-, F10.25-, F10.95-)
     brain disease (F06.2)
     epilepsy (F06.2)
     psychoactive drug use (F11-F19 with .15..25, .95)
     schizotypal disorder (F21)

DEF: Group of disorders with disturbances in thought (delusions, hallucinations), mood (blunted, flattened, inappropriate affect), and sense of self. Schizophrenia also includes bizarre, purposeless behavior, repetitive activity, or inactivity.

F20.0 Paranoid schizophrenia   HCC

Paraphrenic schizophrenia

EXCLUDES 1   involutional paranoid state (F22)
     paranoia (F22)

DEF: Preoccupied with delusional suspicions and auditory hallucinations related to a single theme. This type of schizophrenia is usually hostile, grandiose, threatening, persecutory, and occasionally hypochondriacal.

F20.1 Disorganized schizophrenia   HCC

Hebephrenic schizophrenia
Hebephrenia

F20.2 Catatonic schizophrenia   HCC

Schizophrenic catalepsy
Schizophrenic catatonia
Schizophrenic flexibilitas cerea

EXCLUDES 1   catatonic stupor (R40.1)

DEF: Extreme changes in motor activity. One extreme is a decreased response or reaction to the environment and the other is spontaneous activity.

F20.3 Undifferentiated schizophrenia   HCC

Atypical schizophrenia

EXCLUDES 1   acute schizophrenia-like psychotic disorder (F23)
EXCLUDES 2   post-schizophrenic depression (F32.89)

F20.5 Residual schizophrenia   HCC

Restzustand (schizophrenic)
Schizophrenic residual state

√5ᵗʰ **F20.8 Other schizophrenia**

F20.81 Schizophreniform disorder   HCC

Schizophreniform psychosis NOS

F20.89 Other schizophrenia   HCC

Cenesthopathic schizophrenia
Simple schizophrenia

F20.9 Schizophrenia, unspecified   HCC

AHA: 2019,2Q,32

F21 Schizotypal disorder   HCC

Borderline schizophrenia
Latent schizophrenia
Latent schizophrenic reaction
Prepsychotic schizophrenia
Prodromal schizophrenia
Pseudoneurotic schizophrenia
Pseudopsychopathic schizophrenia
Schizotypal personality disorder

EXCLUDES 2   Asperger's syndrome (F84.5)
     schizoid personality disorder (F60.1)

DEF: Disorder characterized by various oddities of thinking, perception, communication, and behavior that may be manifested as magical thinking, ideas of reference, paranoid ideation, recurrent illusions and derealization (depersonalization), or social isolation.

✔ Additional Character Required   √x7ᵗʰ Placeholder Alert   Manifestation   Unspecified Dx   ▶◀ Revised Text   ● New Code   ▲ Revised Code Title

ICD-10-CM 2020   551

F22 Delusional disorders `HCC`

  Delusional dysmorphophobia
  Involutional paranoid state
  Paranoia
  Paranoia querulans
  Paranoid psychosis
  Paranoid state
  Paraphrenia (late)
  Sensitiver Beziehungswahn

    EXCLUDES 1   mood [affective] disorders with psychotic symptoms (F30.2,
               F31.2, F31.5, F31.64, F32.3, F33.3)
               paranoid schizophrenia (F20.0)
    EXCLUDES 2   paranoid personality disorder (F60.0)
               paranoid psychosis, psychogenic (F23)
               paranoid reaction (F23)

F23 Brief psychotic disorder `HCC`

  Paranoid reaction
  Psychogenic paranoid psychosis

    EXCLUDES 2   mood [affective] disorders with psychotic symptoms (F30.2,
               F31.2, F31.5, F31.64, F32.3, F33.3)

  AHA: 2019,2Q,32

F24 Shared psychotic disorder `HCC`

  Folie à deux
  Induced paranoid disorder
  Induced psychotic disorder

√4ᵗʰ F25 Schizoaffective disorders

    EXCLUDES 1   mood [affective] disorders with psychotic symptoms (F30.2,
               F31.2, F31.5, F31.64, F32.3, F33.3)
               schizophrenia (F20.-)

  F25.0 Schizoaffective disorder, bipolar type `HCC`

    Cyclic schizophrenia
    Schizoaffective disorder, manic type
    Schizoaffective disorder, mixed type
    Schizoaffective psychosis, bipolar type

  F25.1 Schizoaffective disorder, depressive type `HCC`

    Schizoaffective psychosis, depressive type

  F25.8 Other schizoaffective disorders `HCC`

  F25.9 Schizoaffective disorder, unspecified `HCC`

    Schizoaffective psychosis NOS

F28 Other psychotic disorder not due to a substance or known `HCC`
physiological condition

  Chronic hallucinatory psychosis
  Other specified schizophrenia spectrum and other psychotic disorder

F29 Unspecified psychosis not due to a substance or known `HCC`
physiological condition

  Psychosis NOS
  Unspecified schizophrenia spectrum and other psychotic disorder

    EXCLUDES 1   mental disorder NOS (F99)
               unspecified mental disorder due to known physiological
               condition (F09)

Mood [affective] disorders (F30-F39)

√4ᵗʰ F30 Manic episode

    INCLUDES   bipolar disorder, single manic episode
              mixed affective episode
    EXCLUDES 1   bipolar disorder (F31.-)
               major depressive disorder, recurrent (F33.-)
               major depressive disorder, single episode (F32.-)

  DEF: Mania: Characterized by abnormal states of elation or excitement
  out of keeping with the individual's circumstances and varying from
  enhanced liveliness (hypomania) to violent, almost uncontrollable,
  excitement. Aggression and anger, flight of ideas, distractibility, impaired
  judgment, and grandiose ideas are common.

  √5ᵗʰ F30.1 Manic episode without psychotic symptoms

    F30.10 Manic episode without psychotic `HCC`
         symptoms, unspecified

    F30.11 Manic episode without psychotic `HCC`
         symptoms, mild

    F30.12 Manic episode without psychotic `HCC`
         symptoms, moderate

    F30.13 Manic episode, severe, without psychotic `HCC`
         symptoms

  F30.2 Manic episode, severe with psychotic symptoms `HCC`

    Manic stupor
    Mania with mood-congruent psychotic symptoms
    Mania with mood-incongruent psychotic symptoms

  F30.3 Manic episode in partial remission `HCC`

  F30.4 Manic episode in full remission `HCC`

  F30.8 Other manic episodes `HCC`

    Hypomania

  F30.9 Manic episode, unspecified `HCC`

    Mania NOS

√4ᵗʰ F31 Bipolar disorder

    INCLUDES   bipolar I disorder
              bipolar type I disorder
              manic-depressive illness
              manic-depressive psychosis
              manic-depressive reaction
    EXCLUDES 1   bipolar disorder, single manic episode (F30.-)
               major depressive disorder, recurrent (F33.-)
               major depressive disorder, single episode (F32.-)
    EXCLUDES 2   cyclothymia (F34.0)

  F31.0 Bipolar disorder, current episode hypomanic `HCC`

  √5ᵗʰ F31.1 Bipolar disorder, current episode manic without psychotic
  features

    F31.10 Bipolar disorder, current episode manic `HCC` `Q`
         without psychotic features, unspecified

    F31.11 Bipolar disorder, current episode manic `HCC` `Q`
         without psychotic features, mild

    F31.12 Bipolar disorder, current episode manic `HCC` `Q`
         without psychotic features, moderate

    F31.13 Bipolar disorder, current episode manic `HCC` `Q`
         without psychotic features, severe

  F31.2 Bipolar disorder, current episode manic severe with `HCC` `Q`
  psychotic features

    Bipolar disorder, current episode manic with mood-congruent
      psychotic symptoms
    Bipolar disorder, current episode manic with mood-incongruent
      psychotic symptoms
    Bipolar I disorder, current or most recent episode manic with
      psychotic features

  √5ᵗʰ F31.3 Bipolar disorder, current episode depressed, mild or
  moderate severity

    F31.30 Bipolar disorder, current episode `HCC` `Q`
         depressed, mild or moderate severity,
         unspecified

    F31.31 Bipolar disorder, current episode `HCC` `Q`
         depressed, mild

    F31.32 Bipolar disorder, current episode `HCC` `Q`
         depressed, moderate

  F31.4 Bipolar disorder, current episode depressed, severe, `HCC` `Q`
  without psychotic features

  F31.5 Bipolar disorder, current episode depressed, severe, `HCC` `Q`
  with psychotic features

    Bipolar disorder, current episode depressed with
      mood-congruent psychotic symptoms
    Bipolar disorder, current episode depressed with
      mood-incongruent psychotic symptoms
    Bipolar I disorder, current or most recent episode depressed,
      with psychotic features

  √5ᵗʰ F31.6 Bipolar disorder, current episode mixed

    F31.60 Bipolar disorder, current episode mixed, `HCC` `Q`
         unspecified

    F31.61 Bipolar disorder, current episode mixed, `HCC` `Q`
         mild

    F31.62 Bipolar disorder, current episode mixed, `HCC` `Q`
         moderate

    F31.63 Bipolar disorder, current episode mixed, `HCC` `Q`
         severe, without psychotic features

    F31.64 Bipolar disorder, current episode mixed, `HCC` `Q`
         severe, with psychotic features

      Bipolar disorder, current episode mixed with
        mood-congruent psychotic symptoms
      Bipolar disorder, current episode mixed with
        mood-incongruent psychotic symptoms

  √5ᵗʰ F31.7 Bipolar disorder, currently in remission

    F31.70 Bipolar disorder, currently in remission, `HCC` `Q`
         most recent episode unspecified

F31.71 **Bipolar disorder, in partial remission, most** HCC Q **recent episode hypomanic**

F31.72 **Bipolar disorder, in full remission, most** HCC Q **recent episode hypomanic**

F31.73 **Bipolar disorder, in partial remission, most** HCC Q **recent episode manic**

F31.74 **Bipolar disorder, in full remission, most** HCC Q **recent episode manic**

F31.75 **Bipolar disorder, in partial remission, most** HCC Q **recent episode depressed**

F31.76 **Bipolar disorder, in full remission, most** HCC Q **recent episode depressed**

F31.77 **Bipolar disorder, in partial remission, most** HCC Q **recent episode mixed**

F31.78 **Bipolar disorder, in full remission, most** HCC Q **recent episode mixed**

√5ᵗʰ **F31.8 Other bipolar disorders**

F31.81 **Bipolar II disorder** HCC Q

Bipolar disorder, type 2

F31.89 **Other bipolar disorder** HCC Q

Recurrent manic episodes NOS

F31.9 Bipolar disorder, unspecified HCC Q

Manic depression

√4ᵗʰ **F32 Major depressive disorder, single episode**

INCLUDES single episode of agitated depression
single episode of depressive reaction
single episode of major depression
single episode of psychogenic depression
single episode of reactive depression
single episode of vital depression

EXCLUDES 1 bipolar disorder (F31.-)
manic episode (F30.-)
recurrent depressive disorder (F33.-)

EXCLUDES 2 adjustment disorder (F43.2)

DEF: Mood disorder that produces depression that may exhibit as sadness, low self-esteem, or guilt feelings. Other manifestations may be withdrawal from friends and family and interrupted sleep.

F32.0 Major depressive disorder, single episode, mild HCC Q

F32.1 Major depressive disorder, single episode, moderate HCC Q

F32.2 Major depressive disorder, single episode, severe HCC Q **without psychotic features**

F32.3 Major depressive disorder, single episode, severe HCC Q **with psychotic features**

Single episode of major depression with mood-congruent psychotic symptoms
Single episode of major depression with mood-incongruent psychotic symptoms
Single episode of major depression with psychotic symptoms
Single episode of psychogenic depressive psychosis
Single episode of psychotic depression
Single episode of reactive depressive psychosis

F32.4 Major depressive disorder, single episode, in partial HCC Q **remission**

F32.5 Major depressive disorder, single episode, in full HCC Q **remission**

√5ᵗʰ **F32.8 Other depressive episodes**

AHA: 2016,4Q,14

F32.81 **Premenstrual dysphoric disorder** ♀

EXCLUDES 1 premenstrual tension syndrome (N94.3)

DEF: Severe manifestation of premenstrual syndrome (PMS) that can be disabling and destructive to day-to-day activities. It can exacerbate pre-existing emotional disorders, like depression and anxiety, and cause feelings of loss of control, fatigue, and irritability.

F32.89 **Other specified depressive episodes** Q

Atypical depression
Post-schizophrenic depression
Single episode of 'masked' depression NOS

F32.9 Major depressive disorder, single episode, unspecified Q

Depression NOS
Depressive disorder NOS
Major depression NOS
AHA: 2013,4Q,107

√4ᵗʰ **F33 Major depressive disorder, recurrent**

INCLUDES recurrent episodes of depressive reaction
recurrent episodes of endogenous depression
recurrent episodes of major depression
recurrent episodes of psychogenic depression
recurrent episodes of reactive depression
recurrent episodes of seasonal depressive disorder
recurrent episodes of vital depression

EXCLUDES 1 bipolar disorder (F31.-)
manic episode (F30.-)

DEF: Mood disorder that produces depression that may exhibit as sadness, low self-esteem, or guilt feelings. Other manifestations may be withdrawal from friends and family and interrupted sleep.

F33.0 Major depressive disorder, recurrent, mild HCC Q

F33.1 Major depressive disorder, recurrent, moderate HCC Q

F33.2 Major depressive disorder, recurrent, severe without HCC Q **psychotic features**

F33.3 Major depressive disorder, recurrent, severe with HCC Q **psychotic symptoms**

Endogenous depression with psychotic symptoms
Major depressive disorder, recurrent, with psychotic features
Recurrent severe episodes of major depression with mood-congruent psychotic symptoms
Recurrent severe episodes of major depression with mood-incongruent psychotic symptoms
Recurrent severe episodes of major depression with psychotic symptoms
Recurrent severe episodes of psychogenic depressive psychosis
Recurrent severe episodes of psychotic depression
Recurrent severe episodes of reactive depressive psychosis

√5ᵗʰ **F33.4 Major depressive disorder, recurrent, in remission**

F33.40 **Major depressive disorder, recurrent, in** HCC Q **remission, unspecified**

F33.41 **Major depressive disorder, recurrent, in** HCC Q **partial remission**

F33.42 **Major depressive disorder, recurrent, in full** HCC Q **remission**

F33.8 Other recurrent depressive disorders HCC Q

Recurrent brief depressive episodes

F33.9 Major depressive disorder, recurrent, unspecified HCC Q

Monopolar depression NOS

√4ᵗʰ **F34 Persistent mood [affective] disorders**

F34.0 Cyclothymic disorder

Affective personality disorder
Cycloid personality
Cyclothymia
Cyclothymic personality

DEF: Mood disorder characterized by fast and repeated alterations between hypomanic and depressed moods.

F34.1 Dysthymic disorder Q

Depressive neurosis
Depressive personality disorder
Dysthymia
Neurotic depression
Persistent anxiety depression
Persistent depressive disorder

EXCLUDES 2 anxiety depression (mild or not persistent) (F41.8)

DEF: Depression without psychosis. It is a less severe but persistent depression and is considered a mild to moderate chronic form of depression.

√5ᵗʰ **F34.8 Other persistent mood [affective] disorders**

AHA: 2016,4Q,14

F34.81 **Disruptive mood dysregulation disorder** HCC Q

F34.89 **Other specified persistent mood disorders** HCC Q

F34.9 Persistent mood [affective] disorder, unspecified HCC

F39 Unspecified mood [affective] disorder HCC

Affective psychosis NOS

☑ Additional Character Required   √x7ᵗʰ Placeholder Alert   Manifestation   Unspecified Dx   ►◄ Revised Text   ● New Code   ▲ Revised Code Title

Chapter 5. Mental, Behavioral and Neurodevelopmental Disorders

F40–F43.9

Anxiety, dissociative, stress-related, somatoform and other nonpsychotic mental disorders (F40-F48)

✓4ᵗʰ F40 Phobic anxiety disorders

    DEF: Phobia: Broad-range anxiety with abnormally intense dread of certain objects or specific situations that would not normally have that effect.

✓5ᵗʰ F40.0 Agoraphobia

    DEF: Profound anxiety or fear of leaving familiar settings like home, or being in unfamiliar locations or with strangers or crowds. Agoraphobia may or may not be preceded by recurrent panic attacks.

    F40.00 Agoraphobia, unspecified

    F40.01 Agoraphobia with panic disorder

        Panic disorder with agoraphobia

        EXCLUDES 1   *panic disorder without agoraphobia (F41.0)*

    F40.02 Agoraphobia without panic disorder

✓5ᵗʰ F40.1 Social phobias

    Anthropophobia

    Social anxiety disorder

    Social anxiety disorder of childhood

    Social neurosis

    F40.10 Social phobia, unspecified

    F40.11 Social phobia, generalized

✓5ᵗʰ F40.2 Specific (isolated) phobias

    EXCLUDES 2   *dysmorphophobia (nondelusional) (F45.22)*

                  nosophobia (F45.22)

    ✓6ᵗʰ F40.21 Animal type phobia

        F40.210 Arachnophobia

            Fear of spiders

        F40.218 Other animal type phobia

    ✓6ᵗʰ F40.22 Natural environment type phobia

        F40.220 Fear of thunderstorms

        F40.228 Other natural environment type phobia

    ✓6ᵗʰ F40.23 Blood, injection, injury type phobia

        F40.230 Fear of blood

        F40.231 Fear of injections and transfusions

        F40.232 Fear of other medical care

        F40.233 Fear of injury

    ✓6ᵗʰ F40.24 Situational type phobia

        F40.240 Claustrophobia

        F40.241 Acrophobia

        F40.242 Fear of bridges

        F40.243 Fear of flying

        F40.248 Other situational type phobia

    ✓6ᵗʰ F40.29 Other specified phobia

        F40.290 Androphobia

            Fear of men

        F40.291 Gynephobia

            Fear of women

        F40.298 Other specified phobia

    F40.8 Other phobic anxiety disorders

        Phobic anxiety disorder of childhood

    F40.9 Phobic anxiety disorder, unspecified

        Phobia NOS

        Phobic state NOS

✓4ᵗʰ F41 Other anxiety disorders

    EXCLUDES 2   *anxiety in:*

        acute stress reaction (F43.0)

        neurasthenia (F48.8)

        psychophysiologic disorders (F45.-)

        transient adjustment reaction (F43.2)

        separation anxiety (F93.0)

    F41.0 Panic disorder [episodic paroxysmal anxiety]

        Panic attack

        Panic state

        EXCLUDES 1   *panic disorder with agoraphobia (F40.01)*

        DEF: Neurotic disorder characterized by recurrent panic or anxiety, apprehension, fear, or terror. Symptoms include shortness of breath, palpitations, dizziness, and shakiness; fear of dying may persist.

F41.1 Generalized anxiety disorder

    Anxiety neurosis

    Anxiety reaction

    Anxiety state

    Overanxious disorder

    EXCLUDES 2   *neurasthenia (F48.8)*

F41.3 Other mixed anxiety disorders

F41.8 Other specified anxiety disorders

    Anxiety depression (mild or not persistent)

    Anxiety hysteria

    Mixed anxiety and depressive disorder

F41.9 Anxiety disorder, unspecified

    Anxiety NOS

✓4ᵗʰ F42 Obsessive-compulsive disorder

    EXCLUDES 2   *obsessive-compulsive personality (disorder) (F60.5)*

        obsessive-compulsive symptoms occurring in depression (F32-F33)

        obsessive-compulsive symptoms occurring in schizophrenia (F20.-)

    AHA: 2016,4Q,14-15

F42.2 Mixed obsessional thoughts and acts

F42.3 Hoarding disorder

F42.4 Excoriation (skin-picking) disorder

    EXCLUDES 1   *factitial dermatitis (L98.1)*

        other specified behavioral and emotional disorders with onset usually occurring in early childhood and adolescence (F98.8)

F42.8 Other obsessive-compulsive disorder

    Anancastic neurosis

    Obsessive-compulsive neurosis

F42.9 Obsessive-compulsive disorder, unspecified

✓4ᵗʰ F43 Reaction to severe stress, and adjustment disorders

    F43.0 Acute stress reaction

        Acute crisis reaction

        Acute reaction to stress

        Combat and operational stress reaction

        Combat fatigue

        Crisis state

        Psychic shock

    ✓5ᵗʰ F43.1 Post-traumatic stress disorder (PTSD)

        Traumatic neurosis

        DEF: Preoccupation with traumatic events beyond normal experience (i.e., rape, personal assault, etc.) that may also include recurring flashbacks of the trauma. Symptoms include difficulty remembering, sleeping, or concentrating, and guilt feelings for surviving.

        F43.10 Post-traumatic stress disorder, unspecified

        F43.11 Post-traumatic stress disorder, acute

        F43.12 Post-traumatic stress disorder, chronic

    ✓5ᵗʰ F43.2 Adjustment disorders

        Culture shock

        Grief reaction

        Hospitalism in children

        EXCLUDES 2   *separation anxiety disorder of childhood (F93.0)*

        F43.20 Adjustment disorder, unspecified

        F43.21 Adjustment disorder with depressed mood   **Q**

            AHA: 2014,1Q,25

        F43.22 Adjustment disorder with anxiety

        F43.23 Adjustment disorder with mixed anxiety and depressed mood   **Q**

        F43.24 Adjustment disorder with disturbance of conduct

        F43.25 Adjustment disorder with mixed disturbance of emotions and conduct

        F43.29 Adjustment disorder with other symptoms

    F43.8 Other reactions to severe stress

        Other specified trauma and stressor-related disorder

    F43.9 Reaction to severe stress, unspecified

        Trauma and stressor-related disorder, NOS

Chapter 5. Mental, Behavioral and Neurodevelopmental Disorders

✓4ᵗʰ F44 Dissociative and conversion disorders

INCLUDES   conversion hysteria
conversion reaction
hysteria
hysterical psychosis
EXCLUDES 2   *malingering [conscious simulation] (Z76.5)*

F44.0 Dissociative amnesia   HCC
EXCLUDES 1   *amnesia NOS (R41.3)*
anterograde amnesia (R41.1)
dissociative amnesia with dissociative fugue (F44.1)
retrograde amnesia (R41.2)
EXCLUDES 2   *alcohol-or other psychoactive substance-induced amnestic disorder (F10, F13, F19 with .26, .96)*
amnestic disorder due to known physiological condition (F04)
postictal amnesia in epilepsy (G40.-)

F44.1 Dissociative fugue   HCC
Dissociative amnesia with dissociative fugue
EXCLUDES 2   *postictal fugue in epilepsy (G40.-)*
DEF: Dissociative hysteria identified by memory loss and flight from familiar surroundings to a completely separate environment. Episodes may last hours or days. Conscious activity is not associated with perception of surroundings and there is no later memory of the episode.

F44.2 Dissociative stupor
EXCLUDES 1   *catatonic stupor (R40.1)*
stupor NOS (R40.1)
EXCLUDES 2   *catatonic disorder due to known physiological condition (F06.1)*
depressive stupor (F32, F33)
manic stupor (F30, F31)

F44.4 Conversion disorder with motor symptom or deficit
Conversion disorder with abnormal movement
Conversion disorder with speech symptoms
Conversion disorder with swallowing symptoms
Conversion disorder with weakness/paralysis
Dissociative motor disorders
Psychogenic aphonia
Psychogenic dysphonia

F44.5 Conversion disorder with seizures or convulsions
Conversion disorder with attacks or seizures
Dissociative convulsions
AHA: 2019,1Q,19

F44.6 Conversion disorder with sensory symptom or deficit
Conversion disorder with anesthesia or sensory loss
Conversion disorder with special sensory symptoms
Dissociative anesthesia and sensory loss
Psychogenic deafness

F44.7 Conversion disorder with mixed symptom presentation

✓5ᵗʰ F44.8 Other dissociative and conversion disorders

F44.81 Dissociative identity disorder   HCC
Multiple personality disorder

F44.89 Other dissociative and conversion disorders
Ganser's syndrome
Psychogenic confusion
Psychogenic twilight state
Trance and possession disorders

F44.9 Dissociative and conversion disorder, unspecified
Dissociative disorder NOS

✓4ᵗʰ F45 Somatoform disorders

EXCLUDES 2   *dissociative and conversion disorders (F44.-)*
factitious disorders (F68.1-, F68.A)
hair-plucking (F63.3)
lalling (F80.0)
lisping (F80.0)
malingering [conscious simulation] (Z76.5)
nail-biting (F98.8)
psychological or behavioral factors associated with disorders or diseases classified elsewhere (F54)
sexual dysfunction, not due to a substance or known physiological condition (F52.-)
thumb-sucking (F98.8)
tic disorders (in childhood and adolescence) (F95.-)
Tourette's syndrome (F95.2)
trichotillomania (F63.3)
DEF: Types of disorders causing inconsistent physical symptoms that cannot be explained.

F45.0 Somatization disorder
Briquet's disorder
Multiple psychosomatic disorder

F45.1 Undifferentiated somatoform disorder
Somatic symptom disorder
Undifferentiated psychosomatic disorder

✓5ᵗʰ F45.2 Hypochondriacal disorders
EXCLUDES 2   *delusional dysmorphophobia (F22)*
fixed delusions about bodily functions or shape (F22)

F45.20 Hypochondriacal disorder, unspecified
F45.21 Hypochondriasis
Hypochondriacal neurosis
Illness anxiety disorder
F45.22 Body dysmorphic disorder
Dysmorphophobia (nondelusional)
Nosophobia
F45.29 Other hypochondriacal disorders

✓5ᵗʰ F45.4 Pain disorders related to psychological factors
EXCLUDES 1   *pain NOS (R52)*

F45.41 Pain disorder exclusively related to psychological factors
Somatoform pain disorder (persistent)
F45.42 Pain disorder with related psychological factors
Code also associated acute or chronic pain (G89.-)

F45.8 Other somatoform disorders
Psychogenic dysmenorrhea
Psychogenic dysphagia, including 'globus hystericus'
Psychogenic pruritus
Psychogenic torticollis
Somatoform autonomic dysfunction
Teeth grinding
EXCLUDES 1   *sleep related teeth grinding (G47.63)*

F45.9 Somatoform disorder, unspecified
Psychosomatic disorder NOS

✓4ᵗʰ F48 Other nonpsychotic mental disorders

F48.1 Depersonalization-derealization syndrome   HCC

F48.2 Pseudobulbar affect
Involuntary emotional expression disorder
Code first underlying cause, if known, such as:
amyotrophic lateral sclerosis (G12.21)
multiple sclerosis (G35)
sequelae of cerebrovascular disease (I69.-)
sequelae of traumatic intracranial injury (S06.-)

F48.8 Other specified nonpsychotic mental disorders
Dhat syndrome
Neurasthenia
Occupational neurosis, including writer's cramp
Psychasthenia
Psychasthenic neurosis
Psychogenic syncope

F48.9 Nonpsychotic mental disorder, unspecified
Neurosis NOS

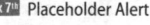 Additional Character Required   ✓x7ᵗʰ Placeholder Alert   Manifestation   Unspecified Dx   ►◄ Revised Text   ● New Code   ▲ Revised Code Title

ICD-10-CM 2020   555

F44–F48.9

Chapter 5. Mental, Behavioral and Neurodevelopmental Disorders

Behavioral syndromes associated with physiological disturbances and physical factors (F50-F59)

F50 Eating disorders

EXCLUDES 1   *anorexia NOS (R63.0)*
feeding difficulties (R63.3)
feeding problems of newborn (P92.-)
polyphagia (R63.2)

EXCLUDES 2   *feeding disorder in infancy or childhood (F98.2-)*

AHA: 2018,4Q,82

TIP: Assign additional code for BMI from category Z68, when documented. BMI can be based on documentation from clinicians who are not the patient's provider.

√5ᵗʰ **F50.0 Anorexia nervosa**

EXCLUDES 1   *loss of appetite (R63.0)*
psychogenic loss of appetite (F50.89)

DEF: Psychological eating disorder characterized by an intense fear of gaining weight and an unrealistic perception of body image that perpetuates the feeling of being fat or having too much fat. Avoidance of food and restrictive or unhealthy eating are common.

F50.00 Anorexia nervosa, unspecified
F50.01 Anorexia nervosa, restricting type
F50.02 Anorexia nervosa, binge eating/purging type
EXCLUDES 1   *bulimia nervosa (F50.2)*

F50.2 Bulimia nervosa
Bulimia NOS
Hyperorexia nervosa
EXCLUDES 1   *anorexia nervosa, binge eating/purging type (F50.02)*

DEF: Episodic pattern of overeating (binge eating) followed by purging or extreme exercise accompanied by an awareness of the abnormal eating pattern with a fear of not being able to stop eating.

√5ᵗʰ **F50.8 Other eating disorders**

EXCLUDES 2   *pica of infancy and childhood (F98.3)*

AHA: 2017,4Q,9; 2016,4Q,15-16

F50.81 Binge eating disorder
F50.82 Avoidant/restrictive food intake disorder
F50.89 Other specified eating disorder
Pica in adults
Psychogenic loss of appetite

F50.9 Eating disorder, unspecified
Atypical anorexia nervosa
Atypical bulimia nervosa
Feeding or eating disorder, unspecified
Other specified feeding disorder

√4ᵗʰ **F51 Sleep disorders not due to a substance or known physiological condition**

EXCLUDES 2   *organic sleep disorders (G47.-)*

√5ᵗʰ **F51.0 Insomnia not due to a substance or known physiological condition**

EXCLUDES 2   *alcohol related insomnia (F10.182, F10.282, F10.982)*
drug-related insomnia (F11.182, F11.282, F11.982, F13.182, F13.282, F13.982, F14.182, F14.282, F14.982, F15.182, F15.282, F15.982, F19.182, F19.282, F19.982)
insomnia NOS (G47.0-)
insomnia due to known physiological condition (G47.0-)
organic insomnia (G47.0-)
sleep deprivation (Z72.820)

F51.01 Primary insomnia
Idiopathic insomnia
F51.02 Adjustment insomnia
F51.03 Paradoxical insomnia
F51.04 Psychophysiologic insomnia
F51.05 Insomnia due to other mental disorder
Code also associated mental disorder
F51.09 Other insomnia not due to a substance or known physiological condition

√5ᵗʰ **F51.1 Hypersomnia not due to a substance or known physiological condition**

EXCLUDES 2   *alcohol related hypersomnia (F10.182, F10.282, F10.982)*
drug-related hypersomnia (F11.182, F11.282, F11.982, F13.182, F13.282, F13.982, F14.182, F14.282, F14.982, F15.182, F15.282, F15.982, F19.182, F19.282, F19.982)
hypersomnia NOS (G47.10)
hypersomnia due to known physiological condition (G47.10)
idiopathic hypersomnia (G47.11, G47.12)
narcolepsy (G47.4-)

F51.11 Primary hypersomnia
F51.12 Insufficient sleep syndrome
EXCLUDES 1   *sleep deprivation (Z72.820)*
F51.13 Hypersomnia due to other mental disorder
Code also associated mental disorder
F51.19 Other hypersomnia not due to a substance or known physiological condition

F51.3 Sleepwalking [somnambulism]
Non-rapid eye movement sleep arousal disorders, sleepwalking type

F51.4 Sleep terrors [night terrors]
Non-rapid eye movement sleep arousal disorders, sleep terror type

F51.5 Nightmare disorder
Dream anxiety disorder

F51.8 Other sleep disorders not due to a substance or known physiological condition

F51.9 Sleep disorder not due to a substance or known physiological condition, unspecified
Emotional sleep disorder NOS

√4ᵗʰ **F52 Sexual dysfunction not due to a substance or known physiological condition**

EXCLUDES 2   *Dhat syndrome (F48.8)*

F52.0 Hypoactive sexual desire disorder
Lack or loss of sexual desire
Male hypoactive sexual desire disorder
Sexual anhedonia
EXCLUDES 1   *decreased libido (R68.82)*

F52.1 Sexual aversion disorder
Sexual aversion and lack of sexual enjoyment

√5ᵗʰ **F52.2 Sexual arousal disorders**
Failure of genital response

F52.21 Male erectile disorder   ♂
Erectile disorder
Psychogenic impotence
EXCLUDES 1   *impotence of organic origin (N52.-)*
impotence NOS (N52.-)

F52.22 Female sexual arousal disorder   ♀
Female sexual interest/arousal disorder

√5ᵗʰ **F52.3 Orgasmic disorder**
Inhibited orgasm
Psychogenic anorgasmy

F52.31 Female orgasmic disorder   ♀
F52.32 Male orgasmic disorder   ♂
Delayed ejaculation

F52.4 Premature ejaculation   ♂

F52.5 Vaginismus not due to a substance or known physiological condition   ♀
Psychogenic vaginismus
EXCLUDES 2   *vaginismus (due to a known physiological condition) (N94.2)*

DEF: Psychogenic response resulting in painful contractions of the vaginal canal muscles. This condition can be severe enough to prevent sexual intercourse.

F52.6 Dyspareunia not due to a substance or known physiological condition
Genito-pelvic pain penetration disorder
Psychogenic dyspareunia
EXCLUDES 2   *dyspareunia (due to a known physiological condition) (N94.1-)*

F52.8   **Other sexual dysfunction not due to a substance or known physiological condition**

Excessive sexual drive
Nymphomania
Satyriasis

F52.9   **Unspecified sexual dysfunction not due to a substance or known physiological condition**

Sexual dysfunction NOS

✓4ᵗʰ **F53**   **Mental and behavioral disorders associated with the puerperium, not elsewhere classified**

> EXCLUDES 1   mood disorders with psychotic features (F30.2, F31.2, F31.5, F31.64, F32.3, F33.3)
> postpartum dysphoria (O90.6)
> psychosis in schizophrenia, schizotypal, delusional, and other psychotic disorders (F20-F29)

AHA: 2018,4Q,8

F53.0   **Postpartum depression**   M ♀

Postnatal depression, NOS
Postpartum depression, NOS

F53.1   **Puerperal psychosis**   HCC M ♀

Postpartum psychosis
Puerperal psychosis, NOS

F54   *Psychological and behavioral factors associated with disorders or diseases classified elsewhere*

Psychological factors affecting physical conditions
Code first the associated physical disorder, such as:
asthma (J45.-)
dermatitis (L23-L25)
gastric ulcer (K25.-)
mucous colitis (K58.-)
ulcerative colitis (K51.-)
urticaria (L50.-)

> EXCLUDES 2   tension-type headache (G44.2)

✓4ᵗʰ **F55**   **Abuse of non-psychoactive substances**

> EXCLUDES 2   abuse of psychoactive substances (F10-F19)

F55.0   **Abuse of** antacids
F55.1   **Abuse of** herbal or folk remedies
F55.2   **Abuse of** laxatives
F55.3   **Abuse of** steroids or hormones
F55.4   **Abuse of** vitamins
F55.8   **Abuse of** other non-psychoactive substances

F59   **Unspecified behavioral syndromes associated with physiological disturbances and physical factors**

Psychogenic physiological dysfunction NOS

Disorders of adult personality and behavior (F60-F69)

✓4ᵗʰ **F60**   **Specific personality disorders**

F60.0   **Paranoid** personality disorder   HCC

Expansive paranoid personality (disorder)
Fanatic personality (disorder)
Paranoid personality (disorder)
Querulant personality (disorder)
Sensitive paranoid personality (disorder)

> EXCLUDES 2   paranoia (F22)
> paranoia querulans (F22)
> paranoid psychosis (F22)
> paranoid schizophrenia (F20.0)
> paranoid state (F22)

F60.1   **Schizoid** personality disorder   HCC

> EXCLUDES 2   Asperger's syndrome (F84.5)
> delusional disorder (F22)
> schizoid disorder of childhood (F84.5)
> schizophrenia (F20.-)
> schizotypal disorder (F21)

F60.2   **Antisocial** personality disorder   HCC

Amoral personality (disorder)
Asocial personality (disorder)
Dissocial personality disorder
Psychopathic personality (disorder)
Sociopathic personality (disorder)

> EXCLUDES 1   conduct disorders (F91.-)
> EXCLUDES 2   borderline personality disorder (F60.3)

F60.3   **Borderline** personality disorder   HCC

Aggressive personality (disorder)
Emotionally unstable personality disorder
Explosive personality (disorder)

> EXCLUDES 2   antisocial personality disorder (F60.2)

F60.4   **Histrionic** personality disorder   HCC

Hysterical personality (disorder)
Psychoinfantile personality (disorder)

F60.5   **Obsessive-compulsive** personality disorder   HCC

Anankastic personality (disorder)
Compulsive personality (disorder)
Obsessional personality (disorder)

> EXCLUDES 2   obsessive-compulsive disorder (F42-)

F60.6   **Avoidant** personality disorder   HCC

Anxious personality disorder

F60.7   **Dependent** personality disorder   HCC

Asthenic personality (disorder)
Inadequate personality (disorder)
Passive personality (disorder)
DEF: Lack of self-confidence, fear of abandonment, and an obsessive need to be taken care of.

✓5ᵗʰ **F60.8**   **Other specific personality disorders**

F60.81   **Narcissistic personality disorder**   HCC

F60.89   **Other specific personality disorders**   HCC

Eccentric personality disorder
"Haltlose" type personality disorder
Immature personality disorder
Passive-aggressive personality disorder
Psychoneurotic personality disorder
Self-defeating personality disorder

F60.9   **Personality disorder, unspecified**   HCC

Character disorder NOS
Character neurosis NOS
Pathological personality NOS

✓4ᵗʰ **F63**   **Impulse disorders**

> EXCLUDES 2   habitual excessive use of alcohol or psychoactive substances (F10-F19)
> impulse disorders involving sexual behavior (F65.-)

F63.0   **Pathological gambling**

Compulsive gambling
Gambling disorder

> EXCLUDES 1   gambling and betting NOS (Z72.6)
> EXCLUDES 2   excessive gambling by manic patients (F30, F31)
> gambling in antisocial personality disorder (F60.2)

F63.1   **Pyromania**

Pathological fire-setting

> EXCLUDES 2   fire-setting (by) (in):
> adult with antisocial personality disorder (F60.2)
> alcohol or psychoactive substance intoxication (F10-F19)
> conduct disorders (F91.-)
> mental disorders due to known physiological condition (F01-F09)
> schizophrenia (F20.-)

F63.2   **Kleptomania**

Pathological stealing

> EXCLUDES 1   shoplifting as the reason for observation for suspected mental disorder (Z03.8)
> EXCLUDES 2   depressive disorder with stealing (F31-F33)
> stealing due to underlying mental condition - code to mental condition
> stealing in mental disorders due to known physiological condition (F01-F09)

F63.3   **Trichotillomania**

Hair plucking

> EXCLUDES 2   other stereotyped movement disorder (F98.4)

✓5ᵗʰ **F63.8**   **Other impulse disorders**

F63.81   **Intermittent explosive disorder**

F63.89   **Other impulse disorders**

F63.9   **Impulse disorder, unspecified**

Impulse control disorder NOS

✓ Additional Character Required   ✓x7ᵗʰ Placeholder Alert   Manifestation   Unspecified Dx   ▶◀ Revised Text   ● New Code   ▲ Revised Code Title

✓4ᵗʰ F64 Gender identity disorders
> **AHA:** 2016,4Q,16

F64.0 Transsexualism
> Gender identity disorder in adolescence and adulthood
> Gender dysphoria in adolescents and adults

F64.1 Dual role transvestism
> Use additional code to identify sex reassignment status (Z87.890)
> *EXCLUDES 1*   *gender identity disorder in childhood (F64.2)*
> *EXCLUDES 2*   *fetishistic transvestism (F65.1)*

F64.2 Gender identity disorder of childhood   P
> Gender dysphoria in children
> *EXCLUDES 1*   *gender identity disorder in adolescence and adulthood (F64.0)*
> *EXCLUDES 2*   *sexual maturation disorder (F66)*

F64.8 Other gender identity disorders
> Other specified gender dysphoria

F64.9 Gender identity disorder, unspecified
> Gender dysphoria, unspecified
> Gender-role disorder NOS

✓4ᵗʰ F65 Paraphilias

F65.0 Fetishism
> Fetishistic disorder

F65.1 Transvestic fetishism
> Fetishistic transvestism
> Transvestic disorder

F65.2 Exhibitionism
> Exhibitionistic disorder

F65.3 Voyeurism
> Voyeuristic disorder

F65.4 Pedophilia
> Pedophilic disorder

✓5ᵗʰ F65.5 Sadomasochism
> **F65.50 Sadomasochism, unspecified**
> **F65.51 Sexual masochism**
> > Sexual masochism disorder
> **F65.52 Sexual sadism**
> > Sexual sadism disorder

✓5ᵗʰ F65.8 Other paraphilias
> **F65.81 Frotteurism**
> > Frotteuristic disorder
> **F65.89 Other paraphilias**
> > Necrophilia
> > Other specified paraphilic disorder

F65.9 Paraphilia, unspecified
> Paraphilic disorder, unspecified
> Sexual deviation NOS

F66 Other sexual disorders
> Sexual maturation disorder
> Sexual relationship disorder

✓4ᵗʰ F68 Other disorders of adult personality and behavior
> **AHA:** 2018,4Q,9,65

✓5ᵗʰ F68.1 Factitious disorder imposed on self
> Compensation neurosis
> Elaboration of physical symptoms for psychological reasons
> Hospital hopper syndrome
> Münchausen's syndrome
> Peregrinating patient
> *EXCLUDES 2*   *factitial dermatitis (L98.1)*
> > *person feigning illness (with obvious motivation) (Z76.5)*
> **F68.10 Factitious disorder imposed on self, unspecified**
> **F68.11 Factitious disorder imposed on self, with predominantly psychological signs and symptoms**
> **F68.12 Factitious disorder imposed on self, with predominantly physical signs and symptoms**
> **F68.13 Factitious disorder imposed on self, with combined psychological and physical signs and symptoms**

F68.A Factitious disorder imposed on another
> Factitious disorder by proxy
> Münchausen's by proxy

F68.8 Other specified disorders of adult personality and behavior

F69 Unspecified disorder of adult personality and behavior   A

Intellectual disabilities (F70-F79)

Code first any associated physical or developmental disorders
EXCLUDES 1   *borderline intellectual functioning, IQ above 70 to 84 (R41.83)*

F70 Mild intellectual disabilities
> IQ level 50-55 to approximately 70
> Mild mental subnormality

F71 Moderate intellectual disabilities
> IQ level 35-40 to 50-55
> Moderate mental subnormality

F72 Severe intellectual disabilities
> IQ 20-25 to 35-40
> Severe mental subnormality

F73 Profound intellectual disabilities
> IQ level below 20-25
> Profound mental subnormality

F78 Other intellectual disabilities

F79 Unspecified intellectual disabilities
> Mental deficiency NOS
> Mental subnormality NOS

Pervasive and specific developmental disorders (F80-F89)

✓4ᵗʰ F80 Specific developmental disorders of speech and language

F80.0 Phonological disorder
> Dyslalia
> Functional speech articulation disorder
> Lalling
> Lisping
> Phonological developmental disorder
> Speech articulation developmental disorder
> Speech-sound disorder
> *EXCLUDES 1*   *speech articulation impairment due to aphasia NOS (R47.01)*
> > *speech articulation impairment due to apraxia (R48.2)*
> *EXCLUDES 2*   *speech articulation impairment due to hearing loss (F80.4)*
> > *speech articulation impairment due to intellectual disabilities (F70-F79)*
> > *speech articulation impairment with expressive language developmental disorder (F80.1)*
> > *speech articulation impairment with mixed receptive expressive language developmental disorder (F80.2)*

F80.1 Expressive language disorder
> Developmental dysphasia or aphasia, expressive type
> *EXCLUDES 1*   *mixed receptive-expressive language disorder (F80.2)*
> > *dysphasia and aphasia NOS (R47.-)*
> *EXCLUDES 2*   *acquired aphasia with epilepsy [Landau-Kleffner] (G40.80-)*
> > *selective mutism (F94.0)*
> > *intellectual disabilities (F70-F79)*
> > *pervasive developmental disorders (F84.-)*

F80.2 Mixed receptive-expressive language disorder
> Developmental dysphasia or aphasia, receptive type
> Developmental Wernicke's aphasia
> *EXCLUDES 1*   *central auditory processing disorder (H93.25)*
> > *dysphasia or aphasia NOS (R47.-)*
> > *expressive language disorder (F80.1)*
> > *expressive type dysphasia or aphasia (F80.1)*
> > *word deafness (H93.25)*
> *EXCLUDES 2*   *acquired aphasia with epilepsy [Landau-Kleffner] (G40.80-)*
> > *pervasive developmental disorders (F84.-)*
> > *selective mutism (F94.0)*
> > *intellectual disabilities (F70-F79)*

F80.4 Speech and language development delay due to hearing loss
> Code also type of hearing loss (H90.-, H91.-)

✓5ᵗʰ **F80.8** **Other developmental disorders of speech and language**
    AHA: 2017,1Q,27

    F80.81 **Childhood onset fluency disorder**
        Cluttering NOS
        Stuttering NOS
        EXCLUDES 1   *adult onset fluency disorder (F98.5)*
                fluency disorder in conditions classified
                    elsewhere (R47.82)
                fluency disorder (stuttering) following
                    cerebrovascular disease (I69. with
                    final characters -23)

    F80.82 **Social pragmatic communication disorder**
        EXCLUDES 1   *Asperger's syndrome (F84.5)*
                autistic disorder (F84.0)
        AHA: 2016,4Q,16

    F80.89 **Other developmental disorders of speech and language**

  F80.9 **Developmental disorder of speech and language, unspecified**
    Communication disorder NOS
    Language disorder NOS

✓4ᵗʰ **F81** **Specific developmental disorders of scholastic skills**

  F81.0 **Specific reading disorder**
    "Backward reading"
    Developmental dyslexia
    Specific learning disorder, with impairment in reading
    Specific reading retardation
    EXCLUDES 1   *alexia NOS (R48.0)*
                dyslexia NOS (R48.0)
    DEF: Serious impairment of reading skills unexplained in relation to general intelligence and teaching processes.

  F81.2 **Mathematics disorder**
    Developmental acalculia
    Developmental arithmetical disorder
    Developmental Gerstmann's syndrome
    Specific learning disorder, with impairment in mathematics
    EXCLUDES 1   *acalculia NOS (R48.8)*
    EXCLUDES 2   *arithmetical difficulties associated with a reading*
                disorder (F81.0)
                arithmetical difficulties associated with a spelling
                disorder (F81.81)
                arithmetical difficulties due to inadequate teaching
                (Z55.8)

✓5ᵗʰ **F81.8** **Other developmental disorders of scholastic skills**

    F81.81 **Disorder of written expression**
        Specific learning disorder, with impairment in written expression
        Specific spelling disorder

    F81.89 **Other developmental disorders of scholastic skills**

  F81.9 **Developmental disorder of scholastic skills, unspecified**
    Knowledge acquisition disability NOS
    Learning disability NOS
    Learning disorder NOS

F82 **Specific developmental disorder of motor function**
    Clumsy child syndrome
    Developmental coordination disorder
    Developmental dyspraxia
    EXCLUDES 1   *abnormalities of gait and mobility (R26.-)*
                lack of coordination (R27.-)
    EXCLUDES 2   *lack of coordination secondary to intellectual disabilities*
                (F70-F79)

✓4ᵗʰ **F84** **Pervasive developmental disorders**
    Use additional code to identify any associated medical condition and intellectual disabilities.

  F84.0 **Autistic disorder**
    Autism spectrum disorder
    Infantile autism
    Infantile psychosis
    Kanner's syndrome
    EXCLUDES 1   *Asperger's syndrome (F84.5)*
    AHA: 2017,1Q,27
    TIP: When the encounter is focused on treatment of conditions related to autism spectrum disorder, first assign codes to identify the problem or manifestation receiving therapeutic services.

  F84.2 **Rett's syndrome**
    EXCLUDES 1   *Asperger's syndrome (F84.5)*
                autistic disorder (F84.0)
                other childhood disintegrative disorder (F84.3)

  F84.3 **Other childhood disintegrative disorder**   ℙ
    Dementia infantilis
    Disintegrative psychosis
    Heller's syndrome
    Symbiotic psychosis
    Use additional code to identify any associated neurological condition
    EXCLUDES 1   *Asperger's syndrome (F84.5)*
                autistic disorder (F84.0)
                Rett's syndrome (F84.2)

  F84.5 **Asperger's syndrome**
    Asperger's disorder
    Autistic psychopathy
    Schizoid disorder of childhood
    DEF: High-functioning form of autism. Children with this syndrome usually develop speech on schedule, are generally very intelligent, and communicate well, but have considerable social shortcomings. *Synonym(s): AS.*

  F84.8 **Other pervasive developmental disorders**
    Overactive disorder associated with intellectual disabilities and stereotyped movements

  F84.9 **Pervasive developmental disorder, unspecified**
    Atypical autism

F88 **Other disorders of psychological development**
    Developmental agnosia
    Global developmental delay
    Other specified neurodevelopmental disorder

F89 **Unspecified disorder of psychological development**
    Developmental disorder NOS
    Neurodevelopmental disorder NOS

Behavioral and emotional disorders with onset usually occurring in childhood and adolescence (F90-F98)

NOTE   Codes within categories F90-F98 may be used regardless of the age of a patient. These disorders generally have onset within the childhood or adolescent years, but may continue throughout life or not be diagnosed until adulthood

✓4ᵗʰ **F90** **Attention-deficit hyperactivity disorders**
    INCLUDES   attention deficit disorder with hyperactivity
                attention deficit syndrome with hyperactivity
    EXCLUDES 2   *anxiety disorders (F40.-, F41.-)*
                mood [affective] disorders (F30-F39)
                pervasive developmental disorders (F84.-)
                schizophrenia (F20.-)

  F90.0 **Attention-deficit hyperactivity disorder, predominantly inattentive type**
    Attention-deficit/hyperactivity disorder, predominantly inattentive presentation

  F90.1 **Attention-deficit hyperactivity disorder, predominantly hyperactive type**
    Attention-deficit/hyperactivity disorder, predominantly hyperactive impulsive presentation

  F90.2 **Attention-deficit hyperactivity disorder, combined type**
    Attention-deficit/hyperactivity disorder, combined presentation

  F90.8 **Attention-deficit hyperactivity disorder, other type**

  F90.9 **Attention-deficit hyperactivity disorder, unspecified type**
    Attention-deficit hyperactivity disorder of childhood or adolescence NOS
    Attention-deficit hyperactivity disorder NOS

✓4ᵗʰ **F91** **Conduct disorders**
    EXCLUDES 1   *antisocial behavior (Z72.81-)*
                antisocial personality disorder (F60.2)
    EXCLUDES 2   *conduct problems associated with attention-deficit*
                hyperactivity disorder (F90.-)
                mood [affective] disorders (F30-F39)
                pervasive developmental disorders (F84.-)
                schizophrenia (F20.-)

  F91.0 **Conduct disorder confined to family context**

✔ Additional Character Required   ✔x7ᵗʰ Placeholder Alert   Manifestation   Unspecified Dx   ▶◀ Revised Text   ● New Code   ▲ Revised Code Title

ICD-10-CM 2020   **559**

F91.1 Conduct disorder, childhood-onset type
Unsocialized conduct disorder
Conduct disorder, solitary aggressive type
Unsocialized aggressive disorder

F91.2 Conduct disorder, adolescent-onset type
Socialized conduct disorder
Conduct disorder, group type

F91.3 Oppositional defiant disorder

F91.8 Other conduct disorders
Other specified conduct disorder
Other specified disruptive disorder

F91.9 Conduct disorder, unspecified
Behavioral disorder NOS
Conduct disorder NOS
Disruptive behavior disorder NOS
Disruptive disorder NOS

✓4ᵗʰ **F93 Emotional disorders with onset specific to childhood**

F93.0 Separation anxiety disorder of childhood
EXCLUDES 2   *mood [affective] disorders (F30-F39)*
nonpsychotic mental disorders (F40-F48)
phobic anxiety disorder of childhood (F40.8)
social phobia (F40.1)

F93.8 Other childhood emotional disorders
Identity disorder
EXCLUDES 2   *gender identity disorder of childhood (F64.2)*

F93.9 Childhood emotional disorder, unspecified

✓4ᵗʰ **F94 Disorders of social functioning with onset specific to childhood and adolescence**

F94.0 Selective mutism
Elective mutism
EXCLUDES 2   *pervasive developmental disorders (F84.-)*
schizophrenia (F20.-)
specific developmental disorders of speech and language (F80.-)
transient mutism as part of separation anxiety in young children (F93.0)

F94.1 Reactive attachment disorder of childhood
Use additional code to identify any associated failure to thrive or growth retardation
EXCLUDES 1   *disinhibited attachment disorder of childhood (F94.2)*
normal variation in pattern of selective attachment
EXCLUDES 2   *Asperger's syndrome (F84.5)*
maltreatment syndromes (T74.-)
sexual or physical abuse in childhood, resulting in psychosocial problems (Z62.81-)

F94.2 Disinhibited attachment disorder of childhood
Affectionless psychopathy
Institutional syndrome
EXCLUDES 1   *reactive attachment disorder of childhood (F94.1)*
EXCLUDES 2   *Asperger's syndrome (F84.5)*
attention-deficit hyperactivity disorders (F90.-)
hospitalism in children (F43.2-)

F94.8 Other childhood disorders of social functioning

F94.9 Childhood disorder of social functioning, unspecified

✓4ᵗʰ **F95 Tic disorder**

F95.0 Transient tic disorder
Provisional tic disorder

F95.1 Chronic motor or vocal tic disorder

F95.2 Tourette's disorder
Combined vocal and multiple motor tic disorder [de la Tourette]
Tourette's syndrome

F95.8 Other tic disorders

F95.9 Tic disorder, unspecified
Tic NOS

✓4ᵗʰ **F98 Other behavioral and emotional disorders with onset usually occurring in childhood and adolescence**
EXCLUDES 2   *breath-holding spells (R06.89)*
gender identity disorder of childhood (F64.2)
Kleine-Levin syndrome (G47.13)
obsessive-compulsive disorder (F42-)
sleep disorders not due to a substance or known physiological condition (F51.-)

F98.0 Enuresis not due to a substance or known physiological condition   Q
Enuresis (primary) (secondary) of nonorganic origin
Functional enuresis
Psychogenic enuresis
Urinary incontinence of nonorganic origin
EXCLUDES 1   *enuresis NOS (R32)*

F98.1 Encopresis not due to a substance or known physiological condition
Functional encopresis
Incontinence of feces of nonorganic origin
Psychogenic encopresis
Use additional code to identify the cause of any coexisting constipation
EXCLUDES 1   *encopresis NOS (R15.-)*

✓5ᵗʰ **F98.2 Other feeding disorders of infancy and childhood**
EXCLUDES 1   *feeding difficulties (R63.3)*
EXCLUDES 2   *anorexia nervosa and other eating disorders (F50.-)*
feeding problems of newborn (P92.-)
pica of infancy or childhood (F98.3)

F98.21 Rumination disorder of infancy

F98.29 Other feeding disorders of infancy and early childhood

F98.3 Pica of infancy and childhood

F98.4 Stereotyped movement disorders
Stereotype/habit disorder
EXCLUDES 1   *abnormal involuntary movements (R25.-)*
EXCLUDES 2   *compulsions in obsessive-compulsive disorder (F42-)*
hair plucking (F63.3)
movement disorders of organic origin (G20-G25)
nail-biting (F98.8)
nose-picking (F98.8)
stereotypies that are part of a broader psychiatric condition (F01-F95)
thumb-sucking (F98.8)
tic disorders (F95.-)
trichotillomania (F63.3)

F98.5 Adult onset fluency disorder
EXCLUDES 1   *childhood onset fluency disorder (F80.81)*
dysphasia (R47.02)
fluency disorder in conditions classified elsewhere (R47.82)
fluency disorder (stuttering) following cerebrovascular disease (I69. with final characters -23)
tic disorders (F95.-)

F98.8 Other specified behavioral and emotional disorders with onset usually occurring in childhood and adolescence
Excessive masturbation
Nail-biting
Nose-picking
Thumb-sucking

F98.9 Unspecified behavioral and emotional disorders with onset usually occurring in childhood and adolescence

Unspecified mental disorder (F99)

F99 Mental disorder, not otherwise specified
Mental illness NOS
EXCLUDES 1   *unspecified mental disorder due to known physiological condition (F09)*

Chapter 6. Diseases of the Nervous System (GØØ-G99)

Chapter-specific Guidelines with Coding Examples

The chapter-specific guidelines from the ICD-10-CM Official Guidelines for Coding and Reporting have been provided below. Along with these guidelines are coding examples, contained in the shaded boxes, that have been developed to help illustrate the coding and/or sequencing guidance found in these guidelines.

a. Dominant/nondominant side

Codes from category G81, Hemiplegia and hemiparesis, and subcategories G83.1, Monoplegia of lower limb, G83.2, Monoplegia of upper limb, and G83.3, Monoplegia, unspecified, identify whether the dominant or nondominant side is affected. Should the affected side be documented, but not specified as dominant or nondominant, and the classification system does not indicate a default, code selection is as follows:

- For ambidextrous patients, the default should be dominant.
- If the left side is affected, the default is non-dominant.
- If the right side is affected, the default is dominant.

> Hemiplegia affecting left side of ambidextrous patient
>
> **G81.92**   **Hemiplegia, unspecified affecting left dominant side**
>
> *Explanation*: Documentation states that the left side is affected and dominant is used for ambidextrous persons.

> Right spastic hemiplegia, unknown whether patient is right- or left-handed
>
> **G81.11**   **Spastic hemiplegia affecting right dominant side**
>
> *Explanation*: Since it is unknown whether the patient is right- or left-handed, if the right side is affected, the default is dominant.

b. Pain—Category G89

1) General coding information

Codes in category G89, Pain, not elsewhere classified, may be used in conjunction with codes from other categories and chapters to provide more detail about acute or chronic pain and neoplasm-related pain, unless otherwise indicated below.

If the pain is not specified as acute or chronic, post-thoracotomy, postprocedural, or neoplasm-related, do not assign codes from category G89.

A code from category G89 should not be assigned if the underlying (definitive) diagnosis is known, unless the reason for the encounter is pain control/ management and not management of the underlying condition.

When an admission or encounter is for a procedure aimed at treating the underlying condition (e.g., spinal fusion, kyphoplasty), a code for the underlying condition (e.g., vertebral fracture, spinal stenosis) should be assigned as the principal diagnosis. No code from category G89 should be assigned.

> Elderly patient with back pain is admitted for outpatient kyphoplasty for age-related osteopathic compression fracture at vertebra T3
>
> **M80.08XA**   **Age-related osteoporosis with current pathological fracture, vertebra(e), initial encounter for fracture**
>
> *Explanation*: No code assigned for the pain as it is inherent in the underlying condition being treated.

(a) Category G89 codes as principal or first-listed diagnosis

Category G89 codes are acceptable as principal diagnosis or the first-listed code:

- When pain control or pain management is the reason for the admission/encounter (e.g., a patient with displaced intervertebral disc, nerve impingement and severe back pain presents for injection of steroid into the spinal canal). The underlying cause of the pain should be reported as an additional diagnosis, if known.

> Patient presents for steroid injection in the right elbow due to chronic pain associated with primary degenerative joint disease.
>
> **G89.29**   **Other chronic pain**
>
> **M19.021**   **Primary osteoarthritis, right elbow**
>
> *Explanation*: Since the encounter is for control of pain, not treating the underlying condition, the pain code is sequenced first followed by the underlying condition. The M25 pain code is not necessary as the underlying condition code represents the specific site.

- When a patient is admitted for the insertion of a neurostimulator for pain control, assign the appropriate pain code as the principal or first-listed diagnosis. When an admission or encounter is for a procedure aimed at treating the underlying condition and a neurostimulator is inserted for pain control during the same admission/encounter, a code for the underlying condition should be assigned as the principal diagnosis and the appropriate pain code should be assigned as a secondary diagnosis.

(b) Use of category G89 codes in conjunction with site specific pain codes

(i) Assigning category G89 and site-specific pain codes

Codes from category G89 may be used in conjunction with codes that identify the site of pain (including codes from chapter 18) if the category G89 code provides additional information. For example, if the code describes the site of the pain, but does not fully describe whether the pain is acute or chronic, then both codes should be assigned.

> Patient is seen to evaluate chronic right knee pain
>
> **M25.561**   **Pain in right knee**
>
> **G89.29**   **Other chronic pain**
>
> *Explanation*: No underlying condition has been determined yet so the pain would be the reason for the visit. The M25 pain code in this instance does not fully describe the condition as it does not represent that the pain is chronic. The G89 chronic pain code is assigned to provide specificity.

(ii) Sequencing of category G89 codes with site-specific pain codes

The sequencing of category G89 codes with site-specific pain codes (including chapter 18 codes), is dependent on the circumstances of the encounter/admission as follows:

- If the encounter is for pain control or pain management, assign the code from category G89 followed by the code identifying the specific site of pain (e.g., encounter for pain management for acute neck pain from trauma is assigned code G89.11, Acute pain due to trauma, followed by code M54.2, Cervicalgia, to identify the site of pain).

> Management of acute, traumatic left shoulder pain
>
> **G89.11**   **Acute pain due to trauma**
>
> **M25.512**   **Pain in left shoulder**
>
> *Explanation*: The reason for the encounter is to manage or control the pain, not to treat or evaluate an underlying condition. The G89 pain code is assigned as the first-listed diagnosis but in this instance does not fully describe the condition as it does not include the site and laterality. The M25 pain code is added to provide this information.

- If the encounter is for any other reason except pain control or pain management, and a related definitive diagnosis has not been established (confirmed) by the provider, assign the code for the specific site of pain first, followed by the appropriate code from category G89.

Chapter 6. Diseases of the Nervous System

> Tests are performed to investigate the source of the patient's chronic epigastric abdominal pain
>
> **R10.13**   **Epigastric pain**
>
> **G89.29**   **Other chronic pain**
>
> *Explanation*: In this instance the patient's epigastric pain is not being treated; rather the source of the pain is being investigated. A code from chapter 18 for epigastric pain is sequenced before the additional specificity of the G89 code for the chronic pain.

2) Pain due to devices, implants and grafts

See Section I.C.19. Pain due to medical devices

3) Postoperative Pain

The provider's documentation should be used to guide the coding of postoperative pain, as well as *Section III. Reporting Additional Diagnoses* and *Section IV. Diagnostic Coding and Reporting in the Outpatient Setting*.

The default for post-thoracotomy and other postoperative pain not specified as acute or chronic is the code for the acute form.

Routine or expected postoperative pain immediately after surgery should not be coded.

> Pain pump dose is increased for the patient's unexpected, extreme pain post-thoracotomy
>
> **G89.12**   **Acute post-thoracotomy pain**
>
> *Explanation*: When acute or chronic is not documented, default to acute. The use of "unexpected, extreme" and the increase of medication dosage indicate that the pain was more than routine or expected.

(a) Postoperative pain not associated with specific postoperative complication

Postoperative pain not associated with a specific postoperative complication is assigned to the appropriate postoperative pain code in category G89.

(b) Postoperative pain associated with specific postoperative complication

Postoperative pain associated with a specific postoperative complication (such as painful wire sutures) is assigned to the appropriate code(s) found in Chapter 19, Injury, poisoning, and certain other consequences of external causes. If appropriate, use additional code(s) from category G89 to identify acute or chronic pain (G89.18 or G89.28).

4) Chronic pain

Chronic pain is classified to subcategory G89.2. There is no time frame defining when pain becomes chronic pain. The provider's documentation should be used to guide use of these codes.

5) Neoplasm related pain

Code G89.3 is assigned to pain documented as being related, associated or due to cancer, primary or secondary malignancy, or tumor. This code is assigned regardless of whether the pain is acute or chronic.

This code may be assigned as the principal or first-listed code when the stated reason for the admission/encounter is documented as pain control/pain management. The underlying neoplasm should be reported as an additional diagnosis.

> Patient referred today for pain management due to acute pain related to malignancy of the right breast.
>
> **G89.3**   **Neoplasm related pain (acute)(chronic)**
>
> **C50.911**   **Malignant neoplasm of unspecified site of right female breast**
>
> *Explanation*: Since the encounter was for pain medication management, the pain, rather than the neoplasm, was the reason for the encounter and is sequenced first. This "neoplasm-related pain" code includes both acute and chronic pain.

When the reason for the admission/encounter is management of the neoplasm and the pain associated with the neoplasm is also documented, code G89.3 may be assigned as an additional diagnosis. It is not necessary to assign an additional code for the site of the pain.

See Section I.C.2 for instructions on the sequencing of neoplasms for all other stated reasons for the admission/encounter (except for pain control/pain management).

> Patient with lung cancer presents with acute hip pain and is evaluated and found to have iliac bone metastasis
>
> **C79.51**   **Secondary malignant neoplasm of bone**
>
> **C34.90**   **Malignant neoplasm of unspecified part of unspecified bronchus or lung**
>
> **G89.3**   **Neoplasm related pain (acute)(chronic)**
>
> *Explanation*: The reason for the encounter was the evaluation and diagnosis of the bone metastasis, whose code would be assigned as first-listed, followed by codes for the primary neoplasm and the pain due to the iliac bone metastasis.

6) Chronic pain syndrome

Central pain syndrome (G89.0) and chronic pain syndrome (G89.4) are different than the term "chronic pain," and therefore codes should only be used when the provider has specifically documented this condition.

See Section I.C.5. Pain disorders related to psychological factors

Chapter 6. Diseases of the Nervous System (G00–G99)

EXCLUDES 2 certain conditions originating in the perinatal period (P04-P96)
certain infectious and parasitic diseases (A00-B99)
complications of pregnancy, childbirth and the puerperium (O00-O9A)
congenital malformations, deformations, and chromosomal abnormalities (Q00-Q99)
endocrine, nutritional and metabolic diseases (E00-E88)
injury, poisoning and certain other consequences of external causes (S00-T88)
neoplasms (C00-D49)
symptoms, signs and abnormal clinical and laboratory findings, not elsewhere classified (R00-R94)

This chapter contains the following blocks:

G00-G09 Inflammatory diseases of the central nervous system
G10-G14 Systemic atrophies primarily affecting the central nervous system
G20-G26 Extrapyramidal and movement disorders
G30-G32 Other degenerative diseases of the nervous system
G35-G37 Demyelinating diseases of the central nervous system
G40-G47 Episodic and paroxysmal disorders
G50-G59 Nerve, nerve root and plexus disorders
G60-G65 Polyneuropathies and other disorders of the peripheral nervous system
G70-G73 Diseases of myoneural junction and muscle
G80-G83 Cerebral palsy and other paralytic syndromes
G89-G99 Other disorders of the nervous system

Inflammatory diseases of the central nervous system (G00–G09)

✓4th G00 Bacterial meningitis, not elsewhere classified

INCLUDES bacterial arachnoiditis
bacterial leptomeningitis
bacterial meningitis
bacterial pachymeningitis

EXCLUDES 1 bacterial meningoencephalitis (G04.2)
bacterial meningomyelitis (G04.2)

DEF: Inflammation of meningeal layers of the brain and spinal cord due to a bacterial infection.

G00.0 **Hemophilus meningitis**
Meningitis due to Hemophilus influenzae

G00.1 **Pneumococcal meningitis**
Meningtitis due to Streptococcal pneumoniae

G00.2 **Streptococcal meningitis**
Use additional code to further identify organism (B95.0-B95.5)

G00.3 **Staphylococcal meningitis**
Use additional code to further identify organism (B95.61-B95.8)

G00.8 **Other bacterial meningitis**
Meningitis due to Escherichia coli
Meningitis due to Friedländer's bacillus
Meningitis due to Klebsiella
Use additional code to further identify organism (B96.-)

G00.9 **Bacterial meningitis, unspecified**
Meningitis due to gram-negative bacteria, unspecified
Purulent meningitis NOS
Pyogenic meningitis NOS
Suppurative meningitis NOS

G01 *Meningitis in bacterial diseases classified elsewhere*
Code first underlying disease

EXCLUDES 1 meningitis (in):
gonococcal (A54.81)
leptospirosis (A27.81)
listeriosis (A32.11)
Lyme disease (A69.21)
meningococcal (A39.0)
neurosyphilis (A52.13)
tuberculosis (A17.0)
meningoencephalitis and meningomyelitis in bacterial diseases classified elsewhere (G05)

G02 *Meningitis in other infectious and parasitic diseases classified elsewhere*
Code first underlying disease, such as:
African trypanosomiasis (B56.-)
poliovirus infection (A80.-)

EXCLUDES 1 candidal meningitis (B37.5)
coccidioidomycosis meningitis (B38.4)
cryptococcal meningitis (B45.1)
herpesviral [herpes simplex] meningitis (B00.3)
infectious mononucleosis complicated by meningitis (B27.- with fourth character 2)
measles complicated by meningitis (B05.1)
meningoencephalitis and meningomyelitis in other infectious and parasitic diseases classified elsewhere (G05)
mumps meningitis (B26.1)
rubella meningitis (B06.02)
varicella [chickenpox] meningitis (B01.0)
zoster meningitis (B02.1)

✓4th G03 Meningitis due to other and unspecified causes

INCLUDES arachnoiditis NOS
leptomeningitis NOS
meningitis NOS
pachymeningitis NOS

EXCLUDES 1 meningoencephalitis (G04.-)
meningomyelitis (G04.-)

G03.0 **Nonpyogenic meningitis**
Aseptic meningitis
Nonbacterial meningitis
DEF: Type of meningitis where no bacterial, viral, or other infectious source exists that explains the meningitis symptomology.

G03.1 **Chronic meningitis**

G03.2 **Benign recurrent meningitis [Mollaret]**
DEF: Aseptic or noninfectious inflammation of the meninges with the presence of Mollaret cells in the spinal fluid. The patient experiences recurrent bouts of inflammation, lasting anywhere from two to five days.

G03.8 **Meningitis due to other specified causes**

G03.9 **Meningitis, unspecified**
Arachnoiditis (spinal) NOS

✓4th G04 Encephalitis, myelitis and encephalomyelitis

INCLUDES acute ascending myelitis
meningoencephalitis
meningomyelitis

EXCLUDES 1 encephalopathy NOS (G93.40)

EXCLUDES 2 acute transverse myelitis (G37.3-)
alcoholic encephalopathy (G31.2)
benign myalgic encephalomyelitis (G93.3)
multiple sclerosis (G35)
subacute necrotizing myelitis (G37.4)
toxic encephalitis (G92)
toxic encephalopathy (G92)

DEF: Encephalitis: Inflammation of the brain, often caused by viral or bacterial infection.
DEF: Encephalomyelitis: Inflammatory disease, often viral in nature, that affects the brain and spinal cord.
DEF: Myelitis: Inflammation of the spinal cord.

✓5th G04.0 Acute disseminated encephalitis and encephalomyelitis (ADEM)

EXCLUDES 1 acute necrotizing hemorrhagic encephalopathy (G04.3-)
other noninfectious acute disseminated encephalomyelitis (noninfectious ADEM) (G04.81)

G04.00 **Acute disseminated encephalitis and encephalomyelitis, unspecified**

G04.01 **Postinfectious acute disseminated encephalitis and encephalomyelitis (postinfectious ADEM)**
EXCLUDES 1 post chickenpox encephalitis (B01.1)
post measles encephalitis (B05.0)
post measles myelitis (B05.1)

G04.02   **Postimmunization acute disseminated encephalitis, myelitis and encephalomyelitis**
Encephalitis, post immunization
Encephalomyelitis, post immunization
Use additional code to identify the vaccine (T50.A-, T50.B-, T50.Z-)

G04.1   **Tropical spastic paraplegia**   `HCC`

G04.2   **Bacterial meningoencephalitis and meningomyelitis, not elsewhere classified**

√5ᵗʰ G04.3   **Acute necrotizing hemorrhagic encephalopathy**
    EXCLUDES 1   *acute disseminated encephalitis and encephalomyelitis (G04.0-)*

   G04.30   **Acute necrotizing hemorrhagic encephalopathy, unspecified**

   G04.31   **Postinfectious acute necrotizing hemorrhagic encephalopathy**

   G04.32   **Postimmunization acute necrotizing hemorrhagic encephalopathy**
     Use additional code to identify the vaccine (T50.A-, T50.B-, T50.Z-)

   G04.39   **Other acute necrotizing hemorrhagic encephalopathy**
     Code also underlying etiology, if applicable

√5ᵗʰ G04.8   **Other encephalitis, myelitis and encephalomyelitis**
    Code also any associated seizure (G40.-, R56.9)

   G04.81   **Other encephalitis and encephalomyelitis**
     Noninfectious acute disseminated encephalomyelitis (noninfectious ADEM)

   G04.89   **Other myelitis**   `HCC`

√5ᵗʰ G04.9   **Encephalitis, myelitis and encephalomyelitis, unspecified**

   G04.90   **Encephalitis and encephalomyelitis, unspecified**
     Ventriculitis (cerebral) NOS

   G04.91   **Myelitis, unspecified**   `HCC`

√4ᵗʰ G05   **Encephalitis, myelitis and encephalomyelitis in diseases classified elsewhere**
    Code first underlying disease, such as:
     human immunodeficiency virus [HIV] disease (B20)
     poliovirus (A80.-)
     suppurative otitis media (H66.01-H66.4)
     trichinellosis (B75)
    EXCLUDES 1   *adenoviral encephalitis, myelitis and encephalomyelitis (A85.1)*
      congenital toxoplasmosis encephalitis, myelitis and encephalomyelitis (P37.1)
      cytomegaloviral encephalitis, myelitis and encephalomyelitis (B25.8)
      encephalitis, myelitis and encephalomyelitis (in) measles (B05.0)
      encephalitis, myelitis and encephalomyelitis (in) systemic lupus erythematosus (M32.19)
      enteroviral encephalitis, myelitis and encephalomyelitis (A85.0)
      eosinophilic meningoencephalitis (B83.2)
      herpesviral [herpes simplex] encephalitis, myelitis and encephalomyelitis (B00.4)
      listerial encephalitis, myelitis and encephalomyelitis (A32.12)
      meningococcal encephalitis, myelitis and encephalomyelitis (A39.81)
      mumps encephalitis, myelitis and encephalomyelitis (B26.2)
      postchickenpox encephalitis, myelitis and encephalomyelitis (B01.1-)
      rubella encephalitis, myelitis and encephalomyelitis (B06.01)
      toxoplasmosis encephalitis, myelitis and encephalomyelitis (B58.2)
      zoster encephalitis, myelitis and encephalomyelitis (B02.0)

G05.3   **Encephalitis and encephalomyelitis in diseases classified elsewhere**
    Meningoencephalitis in diseases classified elsewhere

G05.4   **Myelitis in diseases classified elsewhere**   `HCC`
    Meningomyelitis in diseases classified elsewhere

√4ᵗʰ G06   **Intracranial and intraspinal abscess and granuloma**
    Use additional code (B95-B97) to identify infectious agent
    DEF: Abscess: Circumscribed collection of pus resulting from bacteria, frequently associated with swelling and other signs of inflammation.
    DEF: Granuloma: Abnormal, dense collections or cells forming a mass or nodule of chronically inflamed tissue with granulations that is usually associated with an infective process.

   G06.0   **Intracranial abscess and granuloma**
     Brain [any part] abscess (embolic)
     Cerebellar abscess (embolic)
     Cerebral abscess (embolic)
     Intracranial epidural abscess or granuloma
     Intracranial extradural abscess or granuloma
     Intracranial subdural abscess or granuloma
     Otogenic abscess (embolic)
     EXCLUDES 1   *tuberculous intracranial abscess and granuloma (A17.81)*

   G06.1   **Intraspinal abscess and granuloma**
     Abscess (embolic) of spinal cord [any part]
     Intraspinal epidural abscess or granuloma
     Intraspinal extradural abscess or granuloma
     Intraspinal subdural abscess or granuloma
     EXCLUDES 1   *tuberculous intraspinal abscess and granuloma (A17.81)*

   G06.2   **Extradural and subdural abscess, unspecified**

G07   *Intracranial and intraspinal abscess and granuloma in diseases classified elsewhere*
    Code first underlying disease, such as:
     schistosomiasis granuloma of brain (B65.-)
    EXCLUDES 1   *abscess of brain:*
      amebic (A06.6)
      chromomycotic (B43.1)
      gonococcal (A54.82)
      tuberculous (A17.81)
      tuberculoma of meninges (A17.1)

G08   **Intracranial and intraspinal phlebitis and thrombophlebitis**
    Septic embolism of intracranial or intraspinal venous sinuses and veins
    Septic endophlebitis of intracranial or intraspinal venous sinuses and veins
    Septic phlebitis of intracranial or intraspinal venous sinuses and veins
    Septic thrombophlebitis of intracranial or intraspinal venous sinuses and veins
    Septic thrombosis of intracranial or intraspinal venous sinuses and veins
    EXCLUDES 1   *intracranial phlebitis and thrombophlebitis complicating:*
      abortion, ectopic or molar pregnancy (O00-O07, O08.7)
      pregnancy, childbirth and the puerperium (O22.5, O87.3)
      nonpyogenic intracranial phlebitis and thrombophlebitis (I67.6)
    EXCLUDES 2   *intracranial phlebitis and thrombophlebitis complicating nonpyogenic intraspinal phlebitis and thrombophlebitis (G95.1)*
    DEF: Inflammation and formation of a blood clot in a vein within the brain or spine, or their linings.

G09   **Sequelae of inflammatory diseases of central nervous system**
    NOTE   Category G09 is to be used to indicate conditions whose primary classification is to G00-G08 as the cause of sequelae, themselves classifiable elsewhere. The "sequelae" include conditions specified as residuals.
    Code first condition resulting from (sequela) of inflammatory diseases of central nervous system

Systemic atrophies primarily affecting the central nervous system (G10-G14)

G10   **Huntington's disease**   `HCC`
    Huntington's chorea
    Huntington's dementia
    Code also dementia in other diseases classified elsewhere without behavioral disturbance (F02.80)
    DEF: Genetic disease caused by degeneration of nerve cells in the brain, characterized by chronic progressive mental deterioration. Dementia and death occur within 15 to 20 years of onset.

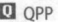

✓4th **G11   Hereditary ataxia**

    EXCLUDES 2   *cerebral palsy (G80.-)*
                hereditary and idiopathic neuropathy (G60.-)
                metabolic disorders (E70-E88)

    DEF: Ataxia: Defect in muscular control or coordination due to a central nervous system disorder, particularly when voluntary muscular movements are attempted.

    G11.0   Congenital nonprogressive ataxia   HCC

    G11.1   Early-onset cerebellar ataxia   HCC

        Early-onset cerebellar ataxia with essential tremor
        Early-onset cerebellar ataxia with myoclonus [Hunt's ataxia]
        Early-onset cerebellar ataxia with retained tendon reflexes
        Friedreich's ataxia (autosomal recessive)
        X-linked recessive spinocerebellar ataxia

    G11.2   Late-onset cerebellar ataxia   HCC   A

    G11.3   Cerebellar ataxia with defective DNA repair   HCC

        Ataxia telangiectasia [Louis-Bar]
        EXCLUDES 2   *Cockayne's syndrome ▶(Q87.19)◀*
                   other disorders of purine and pyrimidine metabolism (E79.-)
                   xeroderma pigmentosum (Q82.1)

    G11.4   Hereditary spastic paraplegia   HCC

    G11.8   Other hereditary ataxias   HCC

    G11.9   Hereditary ataxia, unspecified   HCC

        Hereditary cerebellar ataxia NOS
        Hereditary cerebellar degeneration
        Hereditary cerebellar disease
        Hereditary cerebellar syndrome

✓4th **G12   Spinal muscular atrophy and related syndromes**

    G12.0   Infantile spinal muscular atrophy, type I [Werdnig-Hoffman]   HCC

    G12.1   Other inherited spinal muscular atrophy   HCC

        Adult form spinal muscular atrophy
        Childhood form, type II spinal muscular atrophy
        Distal spinal muscular atrophy
        Juvenile form, type III spinal muscular atrophy [Kugelberg-Welander]
        Progressive bulbar palsy of childhood [Fazio-Londe]
        Scapuloperoneal form spinal muscular atrophy

    ✓5th **G12.2   Motor neuron disease**

        AHA: 2017,4Q,9-10

        G12.20   Motor neuron disease, unspecified   HCC

        G12.21   Amyotrophic lateral sclerosis   HCC   A

        G12.22   Progressive bulbar palsy   HCC

        G12.23   Primary lateral sclerosis   HCC

        G12.24   Familial motor neuron disease   HCC

        G12.25   Progressive spinal muscle atrophy   HCC

        G12.29   Other motor neuron disease   HCC

    G12.8   Other spinal muscular atrophies and related syndromes   HCC

    G12.9   Spinal muscular atrophy, unspecified   HCC

✓4th **G13   Systemic atrophies primarily affecting central nervous system in diseases classified elsewhere**

    G13.0   Paraneoplastic neuromyopathy and neuropathy   HCC

        Carcinomatous neuromyopathy
        Sensorial paraneoplastic neuropathy [Denny Brown]
        Code first underlying neoplasm (C00-D49)

    G13.1   Other systemic atrophy primarily affecting central nervous system in neoplastic disease   HCC

        Paraneoplastic limbic encephalopathy
        Code first underlying neoplasm (C00-D49)

    G13.2   Systemic atrophy primarily affecting the central nervous system in myxedema   HCC

        Code first underlying disease, such as:
          hypothyroidism (E03.-)
          myxedematous congenital iodine deficiency (E00.1)

    G13.8   Systemic atrophy primarily affecting central nervous system in other diseases classified elsewhere   HCC

        Code first underlying disease

G14   Postpolio syndrome

    INCLUDES   postpolio myelitic syndrome
    EXCLUDES 1   *sequelae of poliomyelitis (B91)*

Extrapyramidal and movement disorders (G20-G26)

G20   Parkinson's disease   HCC

    Hemiparkinsonism
    Idiopathic Parkinsonism or Parkinson's disease
    Paralysis agitans
    Parkinsonism or Parkinson's disease NOS
    Primary Parkinsonism or Parkinson's disease

    EXCLUDES 1   *dementia with Parkinsonism (G31.83)*

    AHA: 2017,2Q,7; 2016,2Q,6

    TIP: Repeated falls (R29.6) are not integral to Parkinson's disease and can be separately coded.

✓4th **G21   Secondary parkinsonism**

    EXCLUDES 1   *dementia with Parkinsonism (G31.83)*
               Huntington's disease (G10)
               Shy-Drager syndrome (G90.3)
               syphilitic Parkinsonism (A52.19)

    G21.0   Malignant neuroleptic syndrome

        Use additional code for adverse effect, if applicable, to identify drug (T43.3X5, T43.4X5, T43.5O5, T43.595)

        EXCLUDES 1   *neuroleptic induced parkinsonism (G21.11)*

    ✓5th **G21.1   Other drug-induced secondary parkinsonism**

        G21.11   Neuroleptic induced parkinsonism   HCC

            Use additional code for adverse effect, if applicable, to identify drug (T43.3X5, T43.4X5, T43.5O5, T43.595)

            EXCLUDES 1   *malignant neuroleptic syndrome (G21.0)*

        G21.19   Other drug induced secondary parkinsonism   HCC

            Other medication-induced parkinsonism
            Use additional code for adverse effect, if applicable, to identify drug (T36-T50 with fifth or sixth character 5)

    G21.2   Secondary parkinsonism due to other external agents   HCC

        Code first (T51-T65) to identify external agent

    G21.3   Postencephalitic parkinsonism   HCC

    G21.4   Vascular parkinsonism   HCC

    G21.8   Other secondary parkinsonism   HCC

    G21.9   Secondary parkinsonism, unspecified   HCC

✓4th **G23   Other degenerative diseases of basal ganglia**

    EXCLUDES 2   *multi-system degeneration of the autonomic nervous system (G90.3)*

    G23.0   Hallervorden-Spatz disease   HCC

        Pigmentary pallidal degeneration

    G23.1   Progressive supranuclear ophthalmoplegia [Steele-Richardson-Olszewski]   HCC

        Progressive supranuclear palsy

    G23.2   Striatonigral degeneration   HCC

    G23.8   Other specified degenerative diseases of basal ganglia   HCC

        Calcification of basal ganglia

    G23.9   Degenerative disease of basal ganglia, unspecified   HCC

✓4th **G24   Dystonia**

    INCLUDES   dyskinesia

    EXCLUDES 2   *athetoid cerebral palsy (G80.3)*

    DEF: Disorder of abnormal muscle tone, excessive or inadequate. Involuntary movements and prolonged muscle contractions result in tremors, abnormalities in posture, and twisting body motions that affect an isolated area or the whole body.

    ✓5th **G24.0   Drug induced dystonia**

        Use additional code for adverse effect, if applicable, to identify drug (T36-T50 with fifth or sixth character 5)

        G24.01   Drug induced subacute dyskinesia

            Drug induced blepharospasm
            Drug induced orofacial dyskinesia
            Neuroleptic induced tardive dyskinesia
            Tardive dyskinesia

        G24.02   Drug induced acute dystonia

            Acute dystonic reaction to drugs
            Neuroleptic induced acute dystonia

        G24.09   Other drug induced dystonia

✓ Additional Character Required   ✓x7th Placeholder Alert   Manifestation   Unspecified Dx   ▶◀ Revised Text   ● New Code   ▲ Revised Code Title

ICD-10-CM 2020   565

Chapter 6. Diseases of the Nervous System

G24.1   **Genetic torsion dystonia**
Dystonia deformans progressiva
Dystonia musculorum deformans
Familial torsion dystonia
Idiopathic familial dystonia
Idiopathic (torsion) dystonia NOS
(Schwalbe-) Ziehen-Oppenheim disease

G24.2   **Idiopathic nonfamilial dystonia**

G24.3   **Spasmodic torticollis**
> EXCLUDES 1   congenital torticollis (Q68.0)
> hysterical torticollis (F44.4)
> ocular torticollis (R29.891)
> psychogenic torticollis (F45.8)
> torticollis NOS (M43.6)
> traumatic recurrent torticollis (S13.4)

DEF: Twisted, unnatural position of the neck due to contracted cervical muscles that pull the head to one side or cause involuntary shaking of the head.

G24.4   **Idiopathic orofacial dystonia**
Orofacial dyskinesia
> EXCLUDES 1   drug induced orofacial dyskinesia (G24.01)

G24.5   **Blepharospasm**
> EXCLUDES 1   drug induced blepharospasm (G24.01)

DEF: Involuntary contraction of the orbicularis oculi muscle, resulting in the eyelids being completely closed.

G24.8   **Other dystonia**
Acquired torsion dystonia NOS

G24.9   **Dystonia, unspecified**
Dyskinesia NOS

✓4ᵗʰ **G25**   **Other extrapyramidal and movement disorders**
> EXCLUDES 2   sleep related movement disorders (G47.6-)

G25.0   **Essential tremor**
Familial tremor
> EXCLUDES 1   tremor NOS (R25.1)

G25.1   **Drug-induced tremor**
Use additional code for adverse effect, if applicable, to identify drug (T36-T50 with fifth or sixth character 5)

G25.2   **Other specified forms of tremor**
Intention tremor

G25.3   **Myoclonus**
Drug-induced myoclonus
Palatal myoclonus
Use additional code for adverse effect, if applicable, to identify drug (T36-T50 with fifth or sixth character 5)
> EXCLUDES 1   facial myokymia (G51.4)
> myoclonic epilepsy (G40.-)

DEF: Spasmodic, brief, involuntary muscle contractions that can be due to an undetermined etiology, drug-induced, or caused by a disease process.

G25.4   **Drug-induced chorea**
Use additional code for adverse effect, if applicable, to identify drug (T36-T50 with fifth or sixth character 5)

G25.5   **Other chorea**
Chorea NOS
> EXCLUDES 1   chorea NOS with heart involvement (I02.0)
> Huntington's chorea (G10)
> rheumatic chorea (I02.-)
> Sydenham's chorea (I02.-)

✓5ᵗʰ **G25.6**   **Drug induced tics and other tics of organic origin**

G25.61   **Drug induced tics**
Use additional code for adverse effect, if applicable, to identify drug (T36-T50 with fifth or sixth character 5)

G25.69   **Other tics of organic origin**
> EXCLUDES 1   habit spasm (F95.9)
> tic NOS (F95.9)
> Tourette's syndrome (F95.2)

✓5ᵗʰ **G25.7**   **Other and unspecified drug induced movement disorders**
Use additional code for adverse effect, if applicable, to identify drug (T36-T50 with fifth or sixth character 5)

G25.70   **Drug induced movement disorder, unspecified**

G25.71   **Drug induced akathisia**
Drug induced acathisia
Neuroleptic induced acute akathisia
Tardive akathisia

G25.79   **Other drug induced movement disorders**

✓5ᵗʰ **G25.8**   **Other specified extrapyramidal and movement disorders**

G25.81   **Restless legs syndrome**
DEF: Neurological disorder of unknown etiology creating an irresistible urge to move the legs, which may temporarily relieve the symptoms. This syndrome is accompanied by motor restlessness and sensations of pain, burning, prickling, or tingling.

G25.82   **Stiff-man syndrome**

G25.83   **Benign shuddering attacks**

G25.89   **Other specified extrapyramidal and movement disorders**

G25.9   **Extrapyramidal and movement disorder, unspecified**

G26   *Extrapyramidal and movement disorders in diseases classified elsewhere*
Code first underlying disease

Other degenerative diseases of the nervous system (G30-G32)

✓4ᵗʰ **G30**   **Alzheimer's disease**
> INCLUDES   Alzheimer's dementia senile and presenile forms

Use additional code to identify:
delirium, if applicable (F05)
dementia with behavioral disturbance (F02.81)
dementia without behavioral disturbance (F02.80)
> EXCLUDES 1   senile degeneration of brain NEC (G31.1)
> senile dementia NOS (F03)
> senility NOS (R41.81)

AHA: 2017,1Q,43
TIP: A code from subcategory F02.8 should always be assigned with a code from this category, even in the absence of documented dementia.
TIP: Functional quadriplegia (R53.2) is not integral to Alzheimer's disease and can be coded in addition to codes from category G30.

G30.0   **Alzheimer's disease with early onset**   HCC

G30.1   **Alzheimer's disease with late onset**   HCC A

G30.8   **Other Alzheimer's disease**   HCC

G30.9   **Alzheimer's disease, unspecified**   HCC
AHA: 2016,2Q,6; 2012,4Q,95

✓4ᵗʰ **G31**   **Other degenerative diseases of nervous system, not elsewhere classified**
▶For codes G31.0–G31.83, G31.85–G31.9, use additional code to identify:◄
dementia with behavioral disturbance (F02.81)
dementia without behavioral disturbance (F02.80)
> EXCLUDES 2   Reye's syndrome (G93.7)

✓5ᵗʰ **G31.0**   **Frontotemporal dementia**

G31.01   **Pick's disease**   HCC
Primary progressive aphasia
Progressive isolated aphasia
DEF: Progressive frontotemporal dementia with asymmetrical atrophy of the frontal and temporal regions of the cerebral cortex and abnormal rounded brain cells called Pick cells with the presence of abnormal staining of protein (called tau). Symptoms include prominent apathy, behavioral changes such as disinhibition and restlessness, echolalia, impairment of language, memory, and intellect, increased carelessness, poor personal hygiene, and decreased attention span.

G31.09   **Other frontotemporal dementia**   HCC
Frontal dementia

G31.1   **Senile degeneration of brain, not elsewhere classified**   HCC
> EXCLUDES 1   Alzheimer's disease (G30.-)
> senility NOS (R41.81)

G31.2   **Degeneration of nervous system due to alcohol**   HCC
Alcoholic cerebellar ataxia
Alcoholic cerebellar degeneration
Alcoholic cerebral degeneration
Alcoholic encephalopathy
Dysfunction of the autonomic nervous system due to alcohol
Code also associated alcoholism (F10.-)

✓5ᵗʰ **G31.8**   **Other specified degenerative diseases of nervous system**

G31.81   **Alpers disease**   HCC
Grey-matter degeneration

G31.82   **Leigh's disease**   HCC
Subacute necrotizing encephalopathy

G31.83   **Dementia with Lewy bodies**   `HCC`

Dementia with Parkinsonism
Lewy body dementia
Lewy body disease
AHA: 2017,2Q,7; 2016,4Q,141
DEF: Cerebral dementia with neurophysiologic changes, increased hippocampal volume, hypoperfusion in the occipital lobes, beta amyloid deposits with neurofibrillary tangles, and atrophy of the cortex and brainstem. Hallmark neuropsychological characteristics include fluctuating cognition with pronounced variation in attention and alertness, recurrent hallucinations, and Parkinsonism.

G31.84   **Mild cognitive impairment, so stated**

Mild neurocognitive disorder
> *EXCLUDES 1*   age related cognitive decline (R41.81)
> altered mental status (R41.82)
> cerebral degeneration (G31.9)
> change in mental status (R41.82)
> cognitive deficits following (sequelae of) cerebral hemorrhage or infarction (I69.01-, I69.11-, I69.21-, I69.31-, I69.81-, I69.91-)
> cognitive impairment due to intracranial or head injury (S06.-)
> dementia (F01.-, F02.-, F03)
> mild memory disturbance (F06.8)
> neurologic neglect syndrome (R41.4)
> personality change, nonpsychotic (F68.8)

G31.85   **Corticobasal degeneration**   `HCC`

G31.89   **Other specified degenerative diseases of nervous system**   `HCC`

G31.9   Degenerative disease of nervous system, unspecified   `HCC`

✓4ᵗʰ **G32**   **Other degenerative disorders of nervous system in diseases classified elsewhere**

G32.0   *Subacute combined degeneration of spinal cord in diseases classified elsewhere*   `HCC`

Dana-Putnam syndrome
Sclerosis of spinal cord (combined) (dorsolateral) (posterolateral)
Code first underlying disease, such as:
   anemia (D51.9)
   dietary (D51.3)
   pernicious (D51.0)
   vitamin B12 deficiency (E53.8)
> *EXCLUDES 1*   syphilitic combined degeneration of spinal cord (A52.11)

✓5ᵗʰ **G32.8**   **Other specified degenerative disorders of nervous system in diseases classified elsewhere**

Code first underlying disease, such as:
   amyloidosis cerebral degeneration (E85.-)
   cerebral degeneration (due to) hypothyroidism (E00.0-E03.9)
   cerebral degeneration (due to) neoplasm (C00-D49)
   cerebral degeneration (due to) vitamin B deficiency, except thiamine (E52-E53.-)
> *EXCLUDES 1*   superior hemorrhagic polioencephalitis [Wernicke's encephalopathy] (E51.2)

G32.81   *Cerebellar ataxia in diseases classified elsewhere*   `HCC`

Code first underlying disease, such as:
   celiac disease (with gluten ataxia) (K90.0)
   cerebellar ataxia (in) neoplastic disease (paraneoplastic cerebellar degeneration) (C00-D49)
   non-celiac gluten ataxia (M35.9)
> *EXCLUDES 1*   systemic atrophy primarily affecting the central nervous system in alcoholic cerebellar ataxia (G31.2)
> systemic atrophy primarily affecting the central nervous system in myxedema (G13.2)

G32.89   *Other specified degenerative disorders of nervous system in diseases classified elsewhere*

Degenerative encephalopathy in diseases classified elsewhere

Demyelinating diseases of the central nervous system (G35-G37)

G35   **Multiple sclerosis**   `HCC`

Disseminated multiple sclerosis
Generalized multiple sclerosis
Multiple sclerosis NOS
Multiple sclerosis of brain stem
Multiple sclerosis of cord

✓4ᵗʰ **G36**   **Other acute disseminated demyelination**

> *EXCLUDES 1*   postinfectious encephalitis and encephalomyelitis NOS (G04.01)

DEF: Demyelination: Abnormal loss of myelin, the protective white matter that insulates nerve endings and facilitates neuroreception and neurotransmission. When this substance is damaged, the nerve is short-circuited, resulting in impaired or loss of function.

G36.0   **Neuromyelitis optica [Devic]**   `HCC`

Demyelination in optic neuritis
> *EXCLUDES 1*   optic neuritis NOS (H46)

G36.1   **Acute and subacute hemorrhagic leukoencephalitis [Hurst]**   `HCC`

G36.8   **Other specified acute disseminated demyelination**   `HCC`

G36.9   **Acute disseminated demyelination, unspecified**   `HCC`

✓4ᵗʰ **G37**   **Other demyelinating diseases of central nervous system**

G37.0   **Diffuse sclerosis of central nervous system**   `HCC`

Periaxial encephalitis
Schilder's disease
> *EXCLUDES 1*   X linked adrenoleukodystrophy (E71.52-)

G37.1   **Central demyelination of corpus callosum**   `HCC`

G37.2   **Central pontine myelinolysis**   `HCC`

G37.3   **Acute transverse myelitis in demyelinating disease of central nervous system**   `HCC`

Acute transverse myelitis NOS
Acute transverse myelopathy
> *EXCLUDES 1*   multiple sclerosis (G35)
> neuromyelitis optica [Devic] (G36.0)

G37.4   **Subacute necrotizing myelitis of central nervous system**   `HCC`

G37.5   **Concentric sclerosis [Balo] of central nervous system**   `HCC`

G37.8   **Other specified demyelinating diseases of central nervous system**   `HCC`

G37.9   **Demyelinating disease of central nervous system, unspecified**   `HCC`

Episodic and paroxysmal disorders (G40-G47)

√4ᵗʰ G40 Epilepsy and recurrent seizures

> **NOTE** The following terms are to be considered equivalent to intractable: pharmacoresistant (pharmacologically resistant), treatment resistant, refractory (medically) and poorly controlled

> **EXCLUDES 1** conversion disorder with seizures (F44.5)
> convulsions NOS (R56.9)
> post traumatic seizures (R56.1)
> seizure (convulsive) NOS (R56.9)
> seizure of newborn (P90)

> **EXCLUDES 2** hippocampal sclerosis (G93.81)
> mesial temporal sclerosis (G93.81)
> temporal sclerosis (G93.81)
> Todd's paralysis (G83.85)

√5ᵗʰ G40.0 Localization-related (focal) (partial) idiopathic epilepsy and epileptic syndromes with seizures of localized onset
Benign childhood epilepsy with centrotemporal EEG spikes
Childhood epilepsy with occipital EEG paroxysms

> **EXCLUDES 1** adult onset localization-related epilepsy (G40.1-, G40.2-)

√6ᵗʰ G40.00 Localization-related (focal) (partial) idiopathic epilepsy and epileptic syndromes with seizures of localized onset, not intractable
Localization-related (focal) (partial) idiopathic epilepsy and epileptic syndromes with seizures of localized onset without intractability

G40.001 Localization-related (focal) (partial) idiopathic epilepsy and epileptic syndromes with seizures of localized onset, not intractable, with status epilepticus `HCC`

G40.009 Localization-related (focal) (partial) idiopathic epilepsy and epileptic syndromes with seizures of localized onset, not intractable, without status epilepticus `HCC`
Localization-related (focal) (partial) idiopathic epilepsy and epileptic syndromes with seizures of localized onset NOS

√6ᵗʰ G40.01 Localization-related (focal) (partial) idiopathic epilepsy and epileptic syndromes with seizures of localized onset, intractable

G40.011 Localization-related (focal) (partial) idiopathic epilepsy and epileptic syndromes with seizures of localized onset, intractable, with status epilepticus `HCC`

G40.019 Localization-related (focal) (partial) idiopathic epilepsy and epileptic syndromes with seizures of localized onset, intractable, without status epilepticus `HCC`

√5ᵗʰ G40.1 Localization-related (focal) (partial) symptomatic epilepsy and epileptic syndromes with simple partial seizures
Attacks without alteration of consciousness
Epilepsia partialis continua [Kozhevnikof]
Simple partial seizures developing into secondarily generalized seizures

√6ᵗʰ G40.10 Localization-related (focal) (partial) symptomatic epilepsy and epileptic syndromes with simple partial seizures, not intractable
Localization-related (focal) (partial) symptomatic epilepsy and epileptic syndromes with simple partial seizures without intractability

G40.101 Localization-related (focal) (partial) symptomatic epilepsy and epileptic syndromes with simple partial seizures, not intractable, with status epilepticus `HCC`

G40.109 Localization-related (focal) (partial) symptomatic epilepsy and epileptic syndromes with simple partial seizures, not intractable, without status epilepticus `HCC` `Q`
Localization-related (focal) (partial) symptomatic epilepsy and epileptic syndromes with simple partial seizures NOS

√6ᵗʰ G40.11 Localization-related (focal) (partial) symptomatic epilepsy and epileptic syndromes with simple partial seizures, intractable

G40.111 Localization-related (focal) (partial) symptomatic epilepsy and epileptic syndromes with simple partial seizures, intractable, with status epilepticus `HCC`

G40.119 Localization-related (focal) (partial) symptomatic epilepsy and epileptic syndromes with simple partial seizures, intractable, without status epilepticus `HCC` `Q`

√5ᵗʰ G40.2 Localization-related (focal) (partial) symptomatic epilepsy and epileptic syndromes with complex partial seizures
Attacks with alteration of consciousness, often with automatisms
Complex partial seizures developing into secondarily generalized seizures

√6ᵗʰ G40.20 Localization-related (focal) (partial) symptomatic epilepsy and epileptic syndromes with complex partial seizures, not intractable
Localization-related (focal) (partial) symptomatic epilepsy and epileptic syndromes with complex partial seizures without intractability

G40.201 Localization-related (focal) (partial) symptomatic epilepsy and epileptic syndromes with complex partial seizures, not intractable, with status epilepticus `HCC`

G40.209 Localization-related (focal) (partial) symptomatic epilepsy and epileptic syndromes with complex partial seizures, not intractable, without status epilepticus `HCC` `Q`
Localization-related (focal) (partial) symptomatic epilepsy and epileptic syndromes with complex partial seizures NOS

√6ᵗʰ G40.21 Localization-related (focal) (partial) symptomatic epilepsy and epileptic syndromes with complex partial seizures, intractable

G40.211 Localization-related (focal) (partial) symptomatic epilepsy and epileptic syndromes with complex partial seizures, intractable, with status epilepticus `HCC`

G40.219 Localization-related (focal) (partial) symptomatic epilepsy and epileptic syndromes with complex partial seizures, intractable, without status epilepticus `HCC` `Q`

√5ᵗʰ G40.3 Generalized idiopathic epilepsy and epileptic syndromes
Code also MERRF syndrome, if applicable (E88.42)

√6ᵗʰ G40.30 Generalized idiopathic epilepsy and epileptic syndromes, not intractable
Generalized idiopathic epilepsy and epileptic syndromes without intractability

G40.301 Generalized idiopathic epilepsy and epileptic syndromes, not intractable, with status epilepticus `HCC`

G40.309 **Generalized idiopathic epilepsy and epileptic syndromes, not intractable, without status epilepticus** `HCC` `Q`
     Generalized idiopathic epilepsy and epileptic syndromes NOS

✓6ᵗʰ G40.31 **Generalized idiopathic epilepsy and epileptic syndromes, intractable**
     G40.311 **Generalized idiopathic epilepsy and epileptic syndromes, intractable, with status epilepticus** `HCC`
     G40.319 **Generalized idiopathic epilepsy and epileptic syndromes, intractable, without status epilepticus** `HCC`

✓5ᵗʰ G40.A **Absence epileptic syndrome**
     Childhood absence epilepsy [pyknolepsy]
     Juvenile absence epilepsy
     Absence epileptic syndrome, NOS

✓6ᵗʰ G40.A0 **Absence epileptic syndrome, not intractable**
     G40.A01 **Absence epileptic syndrome, not intractable, with status epilepticus** `HCC`
     G40.A09 **Absence epileptic syndrome, not intractable, without status epilepticus** `HCC` `Q`

✓6ᵗʰ G40.A1 **Absence epileptic syndrome, intractable**
     G40.A11 **Absence epileptic syndrome, intractable, with status epilepticus** `HCC`
     G40.A19 **Absence epileptic syndrome, intractable, without status epilepticus** `HCC` `Q`

✓5ᵗʰ G40.B **Juvenile myoclonic epilepsy [impulsive petit mal]**

✓6ᵗʰ G40.B0 **Juvenile myoclonic epilepsy, not intractable**
     G40.B01 **Juvenile myoclonic epilepsy, not intractable, with status epilepticus** `HCC`
     G40.B09 **Juvenile myoclonic epilepsy, not intractable, without status epilepticus** `HCC`

✓6ᵗʰ G40.B1 **Juvenile myoclonic epilepsy, intractable**
     G40.B11 **Juvenile myoclonic epilepsy, intractable, with status epilepticus** `HCC`
     G40.B19 **Juvenile myoclonic epilepsy, intractable, without status epilepticus** `HCC`

✓5ᵗʰ G40.4 **Other generalized epilepsy and epileptic syndromes**
     Epilepsy with grand mal seizures on awakening
     Epilepsy with myoclonic absences
     Epilepsy with myoclonic-astatic seizures
     Grand mal seizure NOS
     Nonspecific atonic epileptic seizures
     Nonspecific clonic epileptic seizures
     Nonspecific myoclonic epileptic seizures
     Nonspecific tonic epileptic seizures
     Nonspecific tonic-clonic epileptic seizures
     Symptomatic early myoclonic encephalopathy

✓6ᵗʰ G40.40 **Other generalized epilepsy and epileptic syndromes, not intractable**
     Other generalized epilepsy and epileptic syndromes without intractability
     Other generalized epilepsy and epileptic syndromes NOS
     G40.401 **Other generalized epilepsy and epileptic syndromes, not intractable, with status epilepticus** `HCC`
     G40.409 **Other generalized epilepsy and epileptic syndromes, not intractable, without status epilepticus** `HCC` `Q`

✓6ᵗʰ G40.41 **Other generalized epilepsy and epileptic syndromes, intractable**
     G40.411 **Other generalized epilepsy and epileptic syndromes, intractable, with status epilepticus** `HCC` `Q`

G40.419 **Other generalized epilepsy and epileptic syndromes, intractable, without status epilepticus** `HCC`

✓5ᵗʰ G40.5 **Epileptic seizures related to external causes**
     Epileptic seizures related to alcohol
     Epileptic seizures related to drugs
     Epileptic seizures related to hormonal changes
     Epileptic seizures related to sleep deprivation
     Epileptic seizures related to stress
     Code also, if applicable, associated epilepsy and recurrent seizures (G40.-)
     Use additional code for adverse effect, if applicable, to identify drug (T36-T50 with fifth or sixth character 5)

✓6ᵗʰ G40.50 **Epileptic seizures related to external causes, not intractable**
     G40.501 **Epileptic seizures related to external causes, not intractable, with status epilepticus** `HCC`
     G40.509 **Epileptic seizures related to external causes, not intractable, without status epilepticus** `HCC`
     Epileptic seizures related to external causes, NOS

✓5ᵗʰ G40.8 **Other epilepsy and recurrent seizures**
     Epilepsies and epileptic syndromes undetermined as to whether they are focal or generalized
     Landau-Kleffner syndrome

✓6ᵗʰ G40.80 **Other epilepsy**
     G40.801 **Other epilepsy, not intractable, with status epilepticus** `HCC`
     Other epilepsy without intractability with status epilepticus
     G40.802 **Other epilepsy, not intractable, without status epilepticus** `HCC`
     Other epilepsy NOS
     Other epilepsy without intractability without status epilepticus
     G40.803 **Other epilepsy, intractable, with status epilepticus** `HCC`
     G40.804 **Other epilepsy, intractable, without status epilepticus** `HCC`

✓6ᵗʰ G40.81 **Lennox-Gastaut syndrome**
     DEF: Severe form of epilepsy with usual onset in early childhood. Seizures are frequent and difficult to treat, causing falls and intellectual impairment.
     G40.811 **Lennox-Gastaut syndrome, not intractable, with status epilepticus** `HCC`
     G40.812 **Lennox-Gastaut syndrome, not intractable, without status epilepticus** `HCC`
     G40.813 **Lennox-Gastaut syndrome, intractable, with status epilepticus** `HCC`
     G40.814 **Lennox-Gastaut syndrome, intractable, without status epilepticus** `HCC`

✓6ᵗʰ G40.82 **Epileptic spasms**
     Infantile spasms
     Salaam attacks
     West's syndrome
     G40.821 **Epileptic spasms, not intractable, with status epilepticus** `HCC`
     G40.822 **Epileptic spasms, not intractable, without status epilepticus** `HCC` `Q`
     G40.823 **Epileptic spasms, intractable, with status epilepticus** `HCC`
     G40.824 **Epileptic spasms, intractable, without status epilepticus** `HCC` `Q`

G40.89 **Other seizures** `HCC`
     `EXCLUDES 1` *post traumatic seizures (R56.1)*
     recurrent seizures NOS (G40.909)
     seizure NOS (R56.9)

✓5ᵗʰ G40.9 **Epilepsy, unspecified**
     AHA: 2019,1Q,19

✓6ᵗʰ G40.90 **Epilepsy, unspecified, not intractable**
     Epilepsy, unspecified, without intractability
     G40.901 **Epilepsy, unspecified, not intractable, with status epilepticus** `HCC`

G40.909   **Epilepsy, unspecified, not intractable,** without status epilepticus   HCC Q

Epilepsy NOS

Epileptic convulsions NOS

Epileptic fits NOS

Epileptic seizures NOS

Recurrent seizures NOS

Seizure disorder NOS

√6th   **G40.91**   **Epilepsy, unspecified,** intractable

Intractable seizure disorder NOS

G40.911   **Epilepsy, unspecified, intractable,** with status epilepticus   HCC

G40.919   **Epilepsy, unspecified, intractable,** without status epilepticus   HCC

√4th   **G43**   **Migraine**

> **NOTE**   The following terms are to be considered equivalent to intractable: pharmacoresistant (pharmacologically resistant), treatment resistant, refractory (medically) and poorly controlled
>
> Use additional code for adverse effect, if applicable, to identify drug (T36-T50 with fifth or sixth character 5)
>
> EXCLUDES 1   headache NOS (R51)
>
>   lower half migraine (G44.00)
>
> EXCLUDES 2   headache syndromes (G44.-)
>
> **DEF:** Headaches that occur periodically on one or both sides of the head that may be associated with nausea and vomiting, sensitivity to light and sound, dizziness, distorted vision, and cognitive disturbances.

√5th   **G43.0**   **Migraine** without aura

Common migraine

> EXCLUDES 1   chronic migraine without aura (G43.7-)

√6th   **G43.00**   **Migraine without aura,** not intractable

Migraine without aura without mention of refractory migraine

G43.001   **Migraine without aura, not intractable,** with status migrainosus   Q

G43.009   **Migraine without aura, not intractable,** without status migrainosus   Q

Migraine without aura NOS

√6th   **G43.01**   **Migraine without aura,** intractable

Migraine without aura with refractory migraine

G43.011   **Migraine without aura, intractable,** with status migrainosus   Q

G43.019   **Migraine without aura, intractable,** without status migrainosus   Q

√5th   **G43.1**   **Migraine** with aura

Basilar migraine

Classical migraine

Migraine equivalents

Migraine preceded or accompanied by transient focal neurological phenomena

Migraine triggered seizures

Migraine with acute-onset aura

Migraine with aura without headache (migraine equivalents)

Migraine with prolonged aura

Migraine with typical aura

Retinal migraine

Code also any associated seizure (G40.-, R56.9)

> EXCLUDES 1   persistent migraine aura (G43.5-, G43.6-)

√6th   **G43.10**   **Migraine with aura,** not intractable

Migraine with aura without mention of refractory migraine

G43.101   **Migraine with aura, not intractable,** with status migrainosus   Q

G43.109   **Migraine with aura, not intractable,** without status migrainosus   Q

Migraine with aura NOS

√6th   **G43.11**   **Migraine with aura,** intractable

Migraine with aura with refractory migraine

G43.111   **Migraine with aura, intractable,** with status migrainosus   Q

G43.119   **Migraine with aura, intractable,** without status migrainosus   Q

√5th   **G43.4**   **Hemiplegic migraine**

Familial migraine

Sporadic migraine

√6th   **G43.40**   **Hemiplegic migraine,** not intractable

Hemiplegic migraine without refractory migraine

G43.401   **Hemiplegic migraine, not intractable,** with status migrainosus   Q

G43.409   **Hemiplegic migraine, not intractable,** without status migrainosus   Q

Hemiplegic migraine NOS

√6th   **G43.41**   **Hemiplegic migraine,** intractable

Hemiplegic migraine with refractory migraine

G43.411   **Hemiplegic migraine, intractable,** with status migrainosus   Q

G43.419   **Hemiplegic migraine, intractable,** without status migrainosus   Q

√5th   **G43.5**   **Persistent** migraine aura without cerebral infarction

√6th   **G43.50**   **Persistent migraine aura without cerebral infarction,** not intractable

Persistent migraine aura without cerebral infarction, without refractory migraine

G43.501   **Persistent migraine aura without cerebral infarction, not intractable,** with status migrainosus   Q

G43.509   **Persistent migraine aura without cerebral infarction, not intractable,** without status migrainosus   Q

Persistent migraine aura NOS

√6th   **G43.51**   **Persistent migraine aura without cerebral infarction,** intractable

Persistent migraine aura without cerebral infarction, with refractory migraine

G43.511   **Persistent migraine aura without cerebral infarction, intractable,** with status migrainosus   Q

G43.519   **Persistent migraine aura without cerebral infarction, intractable,** without status migrainosus   Q

√5th   **G43.6**   **Persistent** migraine aura with cerebral infarction

Code also the type of cerebral infarction (I63.-)

√6th   **G43.60**   **Persistent migraine aura with cerebral infarction,** not intractable

Persistent migraine aura with cerebral infarction, without refractory migraine

G43.601   **Persistent migraine aura with cerebral infarction, not intractable,** with status migrainosus   Q

G43.609   **Persistent migraine aura with cerebral infarction, not intractable,** without status migrainosus   Q

√6th   **G43.61**   **Persistent migraine aura with cerebral infarction,** intractable

Persistent migraine aura with cerebral infarction, with refractory migraine

G43.611   **Persistent migraine aura with cerebral infarction, intractable,** with status migrainosus   Q

G43.619   **Persistent migraine aura with cerebral infarction, intractable,** without status migrainosus   Q

√5th   **G43.7**   **Chronic migraine** without aura

Transformed migraine

> EXCLUDES 1   migraine without aura (G43.0-)

√6th   **G43.70**   **Chronic migraine without aura,** not intractable

Chronic migraine without aura, without refractory migraine

G43.701   **Chronic migraine without aura, not intractable,** with status migrainosus   Q

G43.709 **Chronic migraine without aura,** **not intractable, without status migrainosus**   **Q**
     Chronic migraine without aura NOS

☑6ᵗʰ **G43.71** **Chronic migraine without aura, intractable**
     Chronic migraine without aura, with refractory migraine

G43.711 **Chronic migraine without aura, intractable, with status migrainosus**   **Q**

G43.719 **Chronic migraine without aura, intractable, without status migrainosus**   **Q**

☑5ᵗʰ **G43.A** **Cyclical vomiting**
   EXCLUDES 1 ▶cyclical vomiting syndrome unrelated to migraine (R11.15)◀

▲ **G43.A0** **Cyclical vomiting, in migraine, not intractable**
     Cyclical vomiting, without refractory migraine

▲ **G43.A1** **Cyclical vomiting, in migraine, intractable**
     Cyclical vomiting, with refractory migraine

☑5ᵗʰ **G43.B** **Ophthalmoplegic migraine**

G43.B0 **Ophthalmoplegic migraine, not intractable**
     Ophthalmoplegic migraine, without refractory migraine

G43.B1 **Ophthalmoplegic migraine, intractable**
     Ophthalmoplegic migraine, with refractory migraine

☑5ᵗʰ **G43.C** **Periodic headache syndromes in child or adult**

G43.C0 **Periodic headache syndromes in child or adult, not intractable**
     Periodic headache syndromes in child or adult, without refractory migraine

G43.C1 **Periodic headache syndromes in child or adult, intractable**
     Periodic headache syndromes in child or adult, with refractory migraine

☑5ᵗʰ **G43.D** **Abdominal migraine**

G43.D0 **Abdominal migraine, not intractable**
     Abdominal migraine, without refractory migraine

G43.D1 **Abdominal migraine, intractable**
     Abdominal migraine, with refractory migraine

☑5ᵗʰ **G43.8** **Other migraine**

☑6ᵗʰ **G43.80** **Other migraine, not intractable**
     Other migraine, without refractory migraine

G43.801 **Other migraine, not intractable, with status migrainosus**   **Q**

G43.809 **Other migraine, not intractable, without status migrainosus**   **Q**

☑6ᵗʰ **G43.81** **Other migraine, intractable**
     Other migraine, with refractory migraine

G43.811 **Other migraine, intractable, with status migrainosus**   **Q**

G43.819 **Other migraine, intractable, without status migrainosus**   **Q**

☑6ᵗʰ **G43.82** **Menstrual migraine, not intractable**
     Menstrual headache, not intractable
     Menstrual migraine, without refractory migraine
     Menstrually related migraine, not intractable
     Pre-menstrual headache, not intractable
     Pre-menstrual migraine, not intractable
     Pure menstrual migraine, not intractable
     Code also associated premenstrual tension syndrome (N94.3)

G43.821 **Menstrual migraine, not intractable, with status migrainosus**   **Q** ♀

G43.829 **Menstrual migraine, not intractable, without status migrainosus**   **Q** ♀
     Menstrual migraine NOS

☑6ᵗʰ **G43.83** **Menstrual migraine, intractable**
     Menstrual headache, intractable
     Menstrual migraine, with refractory migraine
     Menstrually related migraine, intractable
     Pre-menstrual headache, intractable
     Pre-menstrual migraine, intractable
     Pure menstrual migraine, intractable
     Code also associated premenstrual tension syndrome (N94.3)

G43.831 **Menstrual migraine, intractable, with status migrainosus**   **Q** ♀

G43.839 **Menstrual migraine, intractable, without status migrainosus**   **Q** ♀

☑5ᵗʰ **G43.9** **Migraine, unspecified**

☑6ᵗʰ **G43.90** **Migraine, unspecified, not intractable**
     Migraine, unspecified, without refractory migraine

G43.901 **Migraine, unspecified, not intractable, with status migrainosus**   **Q**
     Status migrainosus NOS

G43.909 **Migraine, unspecified, not intractable, without status migrainosus**   **Q**
     Migraine NOS

☑6ᵗʰ **G43.91** **Migraine, unspecified, intractable**
     Migraine, unspecified, with refractory migraine

G43.911 **Migraine, unspecified, intractable, with status migrainosus**   **Q**

G43.919 **Migraine, unspecified, intractable, without status migrainosus**   **Q**

☑4ᵗʰ **G44** **Other headache syndromes**
   EXCLUDES 1   headache NOS (R51)
   EXCLUDES 2   atypical facial pain (G50.1)
          headache due to lumbar puncture (G97.1)
          migraines (G43.-)
          trigeminal neuralgia (G50.0)

☑5ᵗʰ **G44.0** **Cluster headaches and other trigeminal autonomic cephalgias (TAC)**
   DEF: Cluster headache: Characteristic grouping or clustering of headaches that can last for a number of weeks or months and then completely disappear for months or years. They are typically not associated with gastrointestinal upset or light sensitivity as experienced in migraines.

☑6ᵗʰ **G44.00** **Cluster headache syndrome, unspecified**
     Ciliary neuralgia
     Cluster headache NOS
     Histamine cephalgia
     Lower half migraine
     Migrainous neuralgia

G44.001 **Cluster headache syndrome, unspecified, intractable**

G44.009 **Cluster headache syndrome, unspecified, not intractable**   **Q**
     Cluster headache syndrome NOS

☑6ᵗʰ **G44.01** **Episodic cluster headache**

G44.011 **Episodic cluster headache, intractable**

G44.019 **Episodic cluster headache, not intractable**   **Q**
     Episodic cluster headache NOS

☑6ᵗʰ **G44.02** **Chronic cluster headache**

G44.021 **Chronic cluster headache, intractable**

G44.029 **Chronic cluster headache, not intractable**   **Q**
     Chronic cluster headache NOS

☑6ᵗʰ **G44.03** **Episodic paroxysmal hemicrania**
     Paroxysmal hemicrania NOS

G44.031 **Episodic paroxysmal hemicrania, intractable**

G44.039 **Episodic paroxysmal hemicrania, not intractable**   **Q**
     Episodic paroxysmal hemicrania NOS

☑6ᵗʰ **G44.04** **Chronic paroxysmal hemicrania**

G44.041 **Chronic paroxysmal hemicrania, intractable**

☑ Additional Character Required   ☑x7ᵗʰ Placeholder Alert   Manifestation   Unspecified Dx   ▶◀ Revised Text   ● New Code   ▲ Revised Code Title

ICD-10-CM 2020   571

G44.049   **Chronic paroxysmal hemicrania,**   Ⓠ
     not intractable
       Chronic paroxysmal hemicrania NOS

✓6ᵗʰ **G44.05**   **Short lasting unilateral neuraligform headache with conjunctival injection and tearing (SUNCT)**

G44.051   **Short lasting unilateral neuraligform headache with conjunctival injection and tearing (SUNCT), intractable**

G44.059   **Short lasting unilateral neuraligform headache with conjunctival injection and tearing (SUNCT), not intractable**   Ⓠ
       Short lasting unilateral neuraligform headache with conjunctival injection and tearing (SUNCT) NOS

✓6ᵗʰ **G44.09**   **Other trigeminal autonomic cephalgias (TAC)**

G44.091   **Other trigeminal autonomic cephalgias (TAC), intractable**

G44.099   **Other trigeminal autonomic cephalgias (TAC), not intractable**   Ⓠ

G44.1   **Vascular headache, not elsewhere classified**   Ⓠ
     EXCLUDES 2   *cluster headache (G44.0)*
         complicated headache syndromes (G44.5-)
         drug-induced headache (G44.4-)
         migraine (G43.-)
         other specified headache syndromes (G44.8-)
         post-traumatic headache (G44.3-)
         tension-type headache (G44.2-)

✓5ᵗʰ **G44.2**   **Tension-type headache**

✓6ᵗʰ **G44.20**   **Tension-type headache, unspecified**

G44.201   **Tension-type headache, unspecified, intractable**

G44.209   **Tension-type headache, unspecified, not intractable**   Ⓠ
       Tension headache NOS

✓6ᵗʰ **G44.21**   **Episodic tension-type headache**

G44.211   **Episodic tension-type headache, intractable**

G44.219   **Episodic tension-type headache, not intractable**   Ⓠ
       Episodic tension-type headache NOS

✓6ᵗʰ **G44.22**   **Chronic tension-type headache**

G44.221   **Chronic tension-type headache, intractable**   Ⓠ

G44.229   **Chronic tension-type headache, not intractable**   Ⓠ
       Chronic tension-type headache NOS

✓5ᵗʰ **G44.3**   **Post-traumatic headache**

✓6ᵗʰ **G44.30**   **Post-traumatic headache, unspecified**

G44.301   **Post-traumatic headache, unspecified, intractable**

G44.309   **Post-traumatic headache, unspecified, not intractable**
       Post-traumatic headache NOS

✓6ᵗʰ **G44.31**   **Acute post-traumatic headache**

G44.311   **Acute post-traumatic headache, intractable**

G44.319   **Acute post-traumatic headache, not intractable**
       Acute post-traumatic headache NOS

✓6ᵗʰ **G44.32**   **Chronic post-traumatic headache**

G44.321   **Chronic post-traumatic headache, intractable**

G44.329   **Chronic post-traumatic headache, not intractable**
       Chronic post-traumatic headache NOS

✓5ᵗʰ **G44.4**   **Drug-induced headache, not elsewhere classified**
     Medication overuse headache
     Use additional code for adverse effect, if applicable, to identify drug (T36-T50 with fifth or sixth character 5)

G44.40   **Drug-induced headache, not elsewhere classified, not intractable**

G44.41   **Drug-induced headache, not elsewhere classified, intractable**

✓5ᵗʰ **G44.5**   **Complicated headache syndromes**

G44.51   **Hemicrania continua**   Ⓠ
     DEF: Persistent primary headache of unknown causation occurring on one side of the face and head. May last for more than three months, with daily and continuous pain of moderate intensity with severe exacerbations.

G44.52   **New daily persistent headache (NDPH)**   Ⓠ

G44.53   **Primary thunderclap headache**   Ⓠ

G44.59   **Other complicated headache syndrome**   Ⓠ

✓5ᵗʰ **G44.8**   **Other specified headache syndromes**

G44.81   **Hypnic headache**   Ⓠ

G44.82   **Headache associated with sexual activity**   Ⓠ
       Orgasmic headache
       Preorgasmic headache

G44.83   **Primary cough headache**   Ⓠ

G44.84   **Primary exertional headache**   Ⓠ

G44.85   **Primary stabbing headache**   Ⓠ

G44.89   **Other headache syndrome**   Ⓠ

✓4ᵗʰ **G45**   **Transient cerebral ischemic attacks and related syndromes**
     EXCLUDES 1   *neonatal cerebral ischemia (P91.0)*
         transient retinal artery occlusion (H34.0-)
     AHA: 2018,2Q,9
     DEF: Transient cerebral ischemic attack: Intermittent or brief cerebral dysfunction from lack of oxygenation with no persistent neurological deficits associated with occlusive vascular disease. TIA may denote an impending cerebrovascular accident.

G45.0   **Vertebro-basilar artery syndrome**

G45.1   **Carotid artery syndrome (hemispheric)**

G45.2   **Multiple and bilateral precerebral artery syndromes**

G45.3   **Amaurosis fugax**

G45.4   **Transient global amnesia**
     EXCLUDES 1   *amnesia NOS (R41.3)*

G45.8   **Other transient cerebral ischemic attacks and related syndromes**

G45.9   **Transient cerebral ischemic attack, unspecified**
     Spasm of cerebral artery
     TIA
     Transient cerebral ischemia NOS

✓4ᵗʰ **G46**   **Vascular syndromes of brain in cerebrovascular diseases**
     Code first underlying cerebrovascular disease (I60-I69)

G46.0   **Middle cerebral artery syndrome**

G46.1   **Anterior cerebral artery syndrome**

G46.2   **Posterior cerebral artery syndrome**

G46.3   **Brain stem stroke syndrome**
     Benedikt syndrome
     Claude syndrome
     Foville syndrome
     Millard-Gubler syndrome
     Wallenberg syndrome
     Weber syndrome

G46.4   **Cerebellar stroke syndrome**

G46.5   **Pure motor lacunar syndrome**

G46.6   **Pure sensory lacunar syndrome**

G46.7   **Other lacunar syndromes**

G46.8   **Other vascular syndromes of brain in cerebrovascular diseases**

✓4ᵗʰ G47 Sleep disorders

EXCLUDES 2   nightmares (F51.5)
nonorganic sleep disorders (F51.-)
sleep terrors (F51.4)
sleepwalking (F51.3)

✓5ᵗʰ G47.0 Insomnia

EXCLUDES 2   alcohol related insomnia (F10.182, F10.282, F10.982)
drug-related insomnia (F11.182, F11.282, F11.982, F13.182, F13.282, F13.982, F14.182, F14.282, F14.982, F15.182, F15.282, F15.982, F19.182, F19.282, F19.982)
idiopathic insomnia (F51.01)
insomnia due to a mental disorder (F51.05)
insomnia not due to a substance or known physiological condition (F51.0-)
nonorganic insomnia (F51.0-)
primary insomnia (F51.01)
sleep apnea (G47.3-)

G47.00   **Insomnia, unspecified**
Insomnia NOS

G47.01   **Insomnia due to medical condition**
Code also associated medical condition

G47.09   **Other insomnia**

✓5ᵗʰ G47.1 Hypersomnia

EXCLUDES 2   alcohol-related hypersomnia (F10.182, F10.282, F10.982)
drug-related hypersomnia (F11.182, F11.282, F11.982, F13.182, F13.282, F13.982, F14.182, F14.282, F14.982, F15.182, F15.282, F15.982, F19.182, F19.282, F19.982)
hypersomnia due to a mental disorder (F51.13)
hypersomnia not due to a substance or known physiological condition (F51.1-)
primary hypersomnia (F51.11)
sleep apnea (G47.3-)

G47.10   **Hypersomnia, unspecified**
Hypersomnia NOS

G47.11   **Idiopathic hypersomnia with long sleep time**
Idiopathic hypersomnia NOS

G47.12   **Idiopathic hypersomnia without long sleep time**

G47.13   **Recurrent hypersomnia**
Kleine-Levin syndrome
Menstrual related hypersomnia

G47.14   **Hypersomnia due to medical condition**
Code also associated medical condition

G47.19   **Other hypersomnia**

✓5ᵗʰ G47.2 Circadian rhythm sleep disorders

Disorders of the sleep wake schedule
Inversion of nyctohemeral rhythm
Inversion of sleep rhythm
DEF: Circadian rhythm: Daily cycle (24-hour period) of physical, mental and behavioral changes. It is largely influenced by environmental ques, such as changes in light or temperature.
Synonyms: sleep/wake cycle.

G47.20   **Circadian rhythm sleep disorder, unspecified type**
Sleep wake schedule disorder NOS

G47.21   **Circadian rhythm sleep disorder, delayed sleep phase type**
Delayed sleep phase syndrome

G47.22   **Circadian rhythm sleep disorder, advanced sleep phase type**

G47.23   **Circadian rhythm sleep disorder, irregular sleep wake type**
Irregular sleep-wake pattern

G47.24   **Circadian rhythm sleep disorder, free running type**
Circadian rhythm sleep disorder, non-24-hour sleep-wake type

G47.25   **Circadian rhythm sleep disorder, jet lag type**

G47.26   **Circadian rhythm sleep disorder, shift work type**

G47.27   **Circadian rhythm sleep disorder in conditions classified elsewhere**
Code first underlying condition

G47.29   **Other circadian rhythm sleep disorder**

✓5ᵗʰ G47.3 Sleep apnea

Code also any associated underlying condition

EXCLUDES 1   apnea NOS (R06.81)
Cheyne-Stokes breathing (R06.3)
pickwickian syndrome (E66.2)
sleep apnea of newborn (P28.3)

G47.30   **Sleep apnea, unspecified**
Sleep apnea NOS

G47.31   **Primary central sleep apnea**
Idiopathic central sleep apnea

G47.32   **High altitude periodic breathing**

G47.33   **Obstructive sleep apnea (adult) (pediatric)**
Obstructive sleep apnea hypopnea
EXCLUDES 1   obstructive sleep apnea of newborn (P28.3)

G47.34   **Idiopathic sleep related nonobstructive alveolar hypoventilation**
Sleep related hypoxia

G47.35   **Congenital central alveolar hypoventilation syndrome**

G47.36   *Sleep related hypoventilation in conditions classified elsewhere*
Sleep related hypoxemia in conditions classified elsewhere
Code first underlying condition

G47.37   *Central sleep apnea in conditions classified elsewhere*
Code first underlying condition

G47.39   **Other sleep apnea**

✓5ᵗʰ G47.4 Narcolepsy and cataplexy

✓6ᵗʰ G47.41 Narcolepsy

G47.411   **Narcolepsy with cataplexy**

G47.419   **Narcolepsy without cataplexy**
Narcolepsy NOS

✓6ᵗʰ G47.42 Narcolepsy in conditions classified elsewhere
Code first underlying condition

G47.421   *Narcolepsy in conditions classified elsewhere with cataplexy*

G47.429   *Narcolepsy in conditions classified elsewhere without cataplexy*

✓5ᵗʰ G47.5 Parasomnia

EXCLUDES 1   alcohol induced parasomnia (F10.182, F10.282, F10.982)
drug induced parasomnia (F11.182, F11.282, F11.982, F13.182, F13.282, F13.982, F14.182, F14.282, F14.982, F15.182, F15.282, F15.982, F19.182, F19.282, F19.982)
parasomnia not due to a substance or known physiological condition (F51.8)

G47.50   **Parasomnia, unspecified**
Parasomnia NOS

G47.51   **Confusional arousals**

G47.52   **REM sleep behavior disorder**

G47.53   **Recurrent isolated sleep paralysis**

G47.54   *Parasomnia in conditions classified elsewhere*
Code first underlying condition

G47.59   **Other parasomnia**

✓5ᵗʰ G47.6 Sleep related movement disorders

EXCLUDES 2   restless legs syndrome (G25.81)

G47.61   **Periodic limb movement disorder**

G47.62   **Sleep related leg cramps**

G47.63   **Sleep related bruxism**
EXCLUDES 1   psychogenic bruxism (F45.8)

G47.69   **Other sleep related movement disorders**

G47.8 Other sleep disorders
Other specified sleep-wake disorder

G47.9 Sleep disorder, unspecified
Sleep disorder NOS
Unspecified sleep-wake disorder

✔ Additional Character Required   ✓x7ᵗʰ Placeholder Alert   Manifestation   Unspecified Dx   ▶◀ Revised Text   ● New Code   ▲ Revised Code Title

Chapter 6. Diseases of the Nervous System

Nerve, nerve root and plexus disorders (G50-G59)

> EXCLUDES 1   current traumatic nerve, nerve root and plexus disorders — see Injury, nerve by body region
> neuralgia NOS (M79.2)
> neuritis NOS (M79.2)
> peripheral neuritis in pregnancy (O26.82-)
> radiculitis NOS (M54.1-)

✓4ᵗʰ G50   Disorders of trigeminal nerve

> INCLUDES   disorders of 5th cranial nerve

Trigeminal and Facial Nerve Branches

Supratrochlear nerve
Supraorbital nerve
V2 branch
Infraorbital nerve
V1 branch
Trigeminal nerve (CN V) branches in infratemporal fossa
V3 branch
Mental nerve
Mental foramen

G50.0   Trigeminal neuralgia
Syndrome of paroxysmal facial pain
Tic douloureux

G50.1   Atypical facial pain

G50.8   Other disorders of trigeminal nerve

G50.9   Disorder of trigeminal nerve, unspecified

✓4ᵗʰ G51   Facial nerve disorders

> INCLUDES   disorders of 7th cranial nerve

G51.0   Bell's palsy
Facial palsy

G51.1   Geniculate ganglionitis
> EXCLUDES 1   postherpetic geniculate ganglionitis (B02.21)

G51.2   Melkersson's syndrome
Melkersson-Rosenthal syndrome

✓5ᵗʰ **G51.3   Clonic hemifacial spasm**
> AHA: 2018,4Q,10

   G51.31   Clonic hemifacial spasm, right
   G51.32   Clonic hemifacial spasm, left
   G51.33   Clonic hemifacial spasm, bilateral
   G51.39   Clonic hemifacial spasm, unspecified

G51.4   Facial myokymia

G51.8   Other disorders of facial nerve

G51.9   Disorder of facial nerve, unspecified

✓4ᵗʰ G52   Disorders of other cranial nerves

> EXCLUDES 2   disorders of acoustic [8th] nerve (H93.3)
> disorders of optic [2nd] nerve (H46, H47.0)
> paralytic strabismus due to nerve palsy (H49.0-H49.2)

G52.0   Disorders of olfactory nerve
Disorders of 1st cranial nerve

G52.1   Disorders of glossopharyngeal nerve
Disorder of 9th cranial nerve
Glossopharyngeal neuralgia

G52.2   Disorders of vagus nerve
Disorders of pneumogastric [10th] nerve

G52.3   Disorders of hypoglossal nerve
Disorders of 12th cranial nerve

G52.7   Disorders of multiple cranial nerves
Polyneuritis cranialis

G52.8   Disorders of other specified cranial nerves

G52.9   Cranial nerve disorder, unspecified

G53   *Cranial nerve disorders in diseases classified elsewhere*

Code first underlying disease, such as:
neoplasm (C00-D49)

> EXCLUDES 1   multiple cranial nerve palsy in sarcoidosis (D86.82)
> multiple cranial nerve palsy in syphilis (A52.15)
> postherpetic geniculate ganglionitis (B02.21)
> postherpetic trigeminal neuralgia (B02.22)

✓4ᵗʰ G54   Nerve root and plexus disorders

> EXCLUDES 1   current traumatic nerve root and plexus disorders — see nerve injury by body region
> intervertebral disc disorders (M50-M51)
> neuralgia or neuritis NOS (M79.2)
> neuritis or radiculitis brachial NOS (M54.13)
> neuritis or radiculitis lumbar NOS (M54.16)
> neuritis or radiculitis lumbosacral NOS (M54.17)
> neuritis or radiculitis thoracic NOS (M54.14)
> radiculitis NOS (M54.10)
> radiculopathy NOS (M54.10)
> spondylosis (M47.-)

G54.0   Brachial plexus disorders
Thoracic outlet syndrome
DEF: Acquired disorder affecting the spinal nerves that send signals to the shoulder, arm, and hand, causing corresponding motor and sensory dysfunction. This disorder is characterized by regional paresthesia, pain, muscle weakness, and in severe cases paralysis.

G54.1   Lumbosacral plexus disorders

G54.2   Cervical root disorders, not elsewhere classified

G54.3   Thoracic root disorders, not elsewhere classified

G54.4   Lumbosacral root disorders, not elsewhere classified

G54.5   Neuralgic amyotrophy
Parsonage-Aldren-Turner syndrome
Shoulder-girdle neuritis
> EXCLUDES 1   neuralgic amyotrophy in diabetes mellitus (E08-E13 with .44)

G54.6   Phantom limb syndrome with pain   HCC

G54.7   Phantom limb syndrome without pain   HCC
Phantom limb syndrome NOS

G54.8   Other nerve root and plexus disorders

G54.9   Nerve root and plexus disorder, unspecified

G55   *Nerve root and plexus compressions in diseases classified elsewhere*

Code first underlying disease, such as:
neoplasm (C00-D49)

> EXCLUDES 1   nerve root compression (due to) (in) ankylosing spondylitis (M45.-)
> nerve root compression (due to) (in) dorsopathies (M53.-, M54.-)
> nerve root compression (due to) (in) intervertebral disc disorders (M50.1.-, M51.1.-)
> nerve root compression (due to) (in) spondylopathies (M46.-, M48.-)
> nerve root compression (due to) (in) spondylosis (M47.0-M47.2-)

✓4th **G56 Mononeuropathies of upper limb**

> EXCLUDES 1   *current traumatic nerve disorder — see nerve injury by body region*
>
> **AHA:** 2016,4Q,17-18

Nerves of Upper Limb

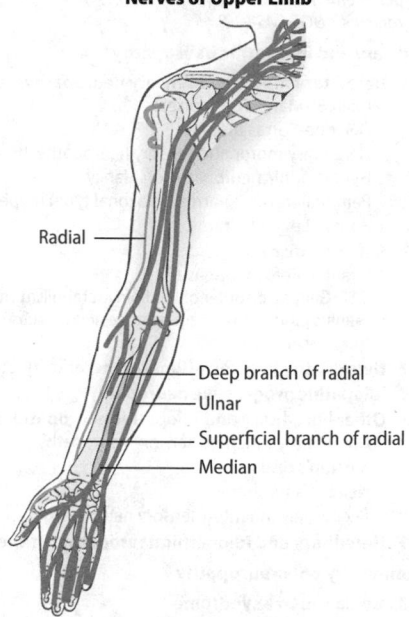

- Radial
- Deep branch of radial
- Ulnar
- Superficial branch of radial
- Median

✓5th **G56.0 Carpal tunnel syndrome**

> **DEF:** Swelling and inflammation in the tendons or bursa surrounding the median nerve caused by repetitive activity. The resulting compression on the nerve causes pain, numbness, and tingling especially to the palm, index, middle finger, and thumb.

     G56.00 Carpal tunnel syndrome, unspecified upper limb
     G56.01 Carpal tunnel syndrome, right upper limb
     G56.02 Carpal tunnel syndrome, left upper limb
     G56.03 Carpal tunnel syndrome, bilateral upper limbs

✓5th **G56.1 Other lesions of median nerve**

     G56.10 Other lesions of median nerve, unspecified upper limb
     G56.11 Other lesions of median nerve, right upper limb
     G56.12 Other lesions of median nerve, left upper limb
     G56.13 Other lesions of median nerve, bilateral upper limbs

✓5th **G56.2 Lesion of ulnar nerve**

> Tardy ulnar nerve palsy

     G56.20 Lesion of ulnar nerve, unspecified upper limb
     G56.21 Lesion of ulnar nerve, right upper limb
     G56.22 Lesion of ulnar nerve, left upper limb
     G56.23 Lesion of ulnar nerve, bilateral upper limbs

✓5th **G56.3 Lesion of radial nerve**

     G56.30 Lesion of radial nerve, unspecified upper limb
     G56.31 Lesion of radial nerve, right upper limb
     G56.32 Lesion of radial nerve, left upper limb
     G56.33 Lesion of radial nerve, bilateral upper limbs

✓5th **G56.4 Causalgia of upper limb**

> Complex regional pain syndrome II of upper limb
>
> EXCLUDES 1   *complex regional pain syndrome I of lower limb (G90.52-)*
> *complex regional pain syndrome I of upper limb (G90.51-)*
> *complex regional pain syndrome II of lower limb (G57.7-)*
> *reflex sympathetic dystrophy of lower limb (G90.52-)*
> *reflex sympathetic dystrophy of upper limb (G90.51-)*

     G56.40 Causalgia of unspecified upper limb
     G56.41 Causalgia of right upper limb
     G56.42 Causalgia of left upper limb
     G56.43 Causalgia of bilateral upper limbs

✓5th **G56.8 Other specified mononeuropathies of upper limb**

> Interdigital neuroma of upper limb

     G56.80 Other specified mononeuropathies of unspecified upper limb

     G56.81 Other specified mononeuropathies of right upper limb
     G56.82 Other specified mononeuropathies of left upper limb
     G56.83 Other specified mononeuropathies of bilateral upper limbs

✓5th **G56.9 Unspecified mononeuropathy of upper limb**

     G56.90 Unspecified mononeuropathy of unspecified upper limb
     G56.91 Unspecified mononeuropathy of right upper limb
     G56.92 Unspecified mononeuropathy of left upper limb
     G56.93 Unspecified mononeuropathy of bilateral upper limbs

✓4th **G57 Mononeuropathies of lower limb**

> EXCLUDES 1   *current traumatic nerve disorder — see nerve injury by body region*
>
> **AHA:** 2016,4Q,17-18

Nerves of Lower Limb

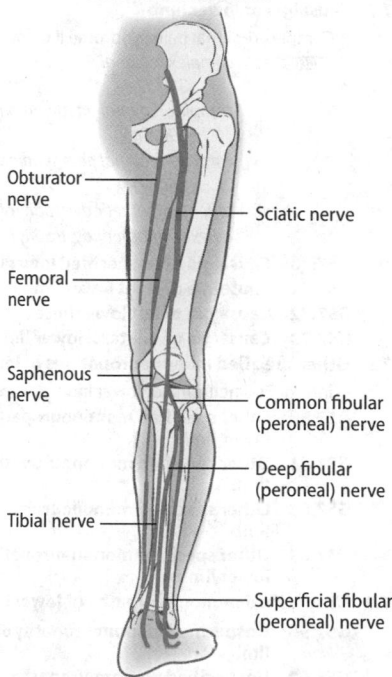

- Obturator nerve
- Sciatic nerve
- Femoral nerve
- Saphenous nerve
- Common fibular (peroneal) nerve
- Deep fibular (peroneal) nerve
- Tibial nerve
- Superficial fibular (peroneal) nerve

✓5th **G57.0 Lesion of sciatic nerve**

> EXCLUDES 1   *sciatica NOS (M54.3-)*
> EXCLUDES 2   *sciatica attributed to intervertebral disc disorder (M51.1.-)*

     G57.00 Lesion of sciatic nerve, unspecified lower limb
     G57.01 Lesion of sciatic nerve, right lower limb
     G57.02 Lesion of sciatic nerve, left lower limb
     G57.03 Lesion of sciatic nerve, bilateral lower limbs

✓5th **G57.1 Meralgia paresthetica**

> Lateral cutaneous nerve of thigh syndrome

     G57.10 Meralgia paresthetica, unspecified lower limb
     G57.11 Meralgia paresthetica, right lower limb
     G57.12 Meralgia paresthetica, left lower limb
     G57.13 Meralgia paresthetica, bilateral lower limbs

✓5th **G57.2 Lesion of femoral nerve**

     G57.20 Lesion of femoral nerve, unspecified lower limb
     G57.21 Lesion of femoral nerve, right lower limb
     G57.22 Lesion of femoral nerve, left lower limb
     G57.23 Lesion of femoral nerve, bilateral lower limbs

✓5th **G57.3 Lesion of lateral popliteal nerve**

> Peroneal nerve palsy

     G57.30 Lesion of lateral popliteal nerve, unspecified lower limb
     G57.31 Lesion of lateral popliteal nerve, right lower limb
     G57.32 Lesion of lateral popliteal nerve, left lower limb
     G57.33 Lesion of lateral popliteal nerve, bilateral lower limbs

---

✔ Additional Character Required   ✔x7th Placeholder Alert   Manifestation   Unspecified Dx   ▶◀ Revised Text   ● New Code   ▲ Revised Code Title

Chapter 6. Diseases of the Nervous System

G57.4–G62.9

√5ᵗʰ **G57.4 Lesion of medial popliteal nerve**

    G57.40 Lesion of medial popliteal nerve, unspecified lower limb

    G57.41 Lesion of medial popliteal nerve, right lower limb

    G57.42 Lesion of medial popliteal nerve, left lower limb

    G57.43 Lesion of medial popliteal nerve, bilateral lower limbs

√5ᵗʰ **G57.5 Tarsal tunnel syndrome**

    G57.50 Tarsal tunnel syndrome, unspecified lower limb

    G57.51 Tarsal tunnel syndrome, right lower limb

    G57.52 Tarsal tunnel syndrome, left lower limb

    G57.53 Tarsal tunnel syndrome, bilateral lower limbs

√5ᵗʰ **G57.6 Lesion of plantar nerve**

    Morton's metatarsalgia

    G57.60 Lesion of plantar nerve, unspecified lower limb

    G57.61 Lesion of plantar nerve, right lower limb

    G57.62 Lesion of plantar nerve, left lower limb

    G57.63 Lesion of plantar nerve, bilateral lower limbs

√5ᵗʰ **G57.7 Causalgia of lower limb**

    Complex regional pain syndrome II of lower limb

    EXCLUDES 1   *complex regional pain syndrome I of lower limb (G90.52-)*

         complex regional pain syndrome I of upper limb (G90.51-)

         complex regional pain syndrome II of upper limb (G56.4-)

         reflex sympathetic dystrophy of lower limb (G90.52-)

         reflex sympathetic dystrophy of upper limb (G90.51-)

    G57.70 Causalgia of unspecified lower limb

    G57.71 Causalgia of right lower limb

    G57.72 Causalgia of left lower limb

    G57.73 Causalgia of bilateral lower limbs

√5ᵗʰ **G57.8 Other specified mononeuropathies of lower limb**

    Interdigital neuroma of lower limb

    G57.80 Other specified mononeuropathies of unspecified lower limb

    G57.81 Other specified mononeuropathies of right lower limb

    G57.82 Other specified mononeuropathies of left lower limb

    G57.83 Other specified mononeuropathies of bilateral lower limbs

√5ᵗʰ **G57.9 Unspecified mononeuropathy of lower limb**

    G57.90 Unspecified mononeuropathy of unspecified lower limb

    G57.91 Unspecified mononeuropathy of right lower limb

    G57.92 Unspecified mononeuropathy of left lower limb

    G57.93 Unspecified mononeuropathy of bilateral lower limbs

√4ᵗʰ **G58 Other mononeuropathies**

    G58.0 Intercostal neuropathy

    G58.7 Mononeuritis multiplex

    G58.8 Other specified mononeuropathies

    G58.9 Mononeuropathy, unspecified

G59 Mononeuropathy in diseases classified elsewhere

    Code first underlying disease

    EXCLUDES 1   *diabetic mononeuropathy (E08-E13 with .41)*

         syphilitic nerve paralysis (A52.19)

         syphilitic neuritis (A52.15)

         tuberculous mononeuropathy (A17.83)

Polyneuropathies and other disorders of the peripheral nervous system (G60-G65)

EXCLUDES 1   *neuralgia NOS (M79.2)*

        neuritis NOS (M79.2)

        peripheral neuritis in pregnancy (O26.82-)

        radiculitis NOS (M54.10)

√4ᵗʰ **G60 Hereditary and idiopathic neuropathy**

    G60.0 Hereditary motor and sensory neuropathy

      Charcôt-Marie-Tooth disease

      Déjérine-Sottas disease

      Hereditary motor and sensory neuropathy, types I-IV

      Hypertrophic neuropathy of infancy

      Peroneal muscular atrophy (axonal type) (hypertrophic type)

      Roussy-Levy syndrome

    G60.1 Refsum's disease

      Infantile Refsum disease

      DEF: Genetic disorder of the lipid metabolism characterized by retinitis pigmentosa, degenerative nerve disease, ataxia, and dry, rough, scaly skin.

    G60.2 Neuropathy in association with hereditary ataxia

    G60.3 Idiopathic progressive neuropathy

    G60.8 Other hereditary and idiopathic neuropathies

      Dominantly inherited sensory neuropathy

      Morvan's disease

      Nelaton's syndrome

      Recessively inherited sensory neuropathy

    G60.9 Hereditary and idiopathic neuropathy, unspecified

√4ᵗʰ **G61 Inflammatory polyneuropathy**

    G61.0 Guillain-Barre syndrome   HCC

      Acute (post-)infective polyneuritis

      Miller Fisher syndrome

      AHA: 2014,2Q,4

      DEF: Autoimmune disorder due to an immune response to foreign antigens with paraplegia of limbs, flaccid paralysis, ophthalmoplegia, ataxia, and areflexia. In most cases, this disorder is triggered by a mild viral infection, surgery, or following an immunization.

      TIP: Guillain-Barre syndrome can occur as a sequela of *Campylobacter enteritis.* Assign code B94.8 for the sequelae as an additional diagnosis.

    G61.1 Serum neuropathy   HCC

      Use additional code for adverse effect, if applicable, to identify serum (T50.-)

    √5ᵗʰ **G61.8 Other inflammatory polyneuropathies**

      G61.81 Chronic inflammatory demyelinating polyneuritis   HCC

      G61.82 Multifocal motor neuropathy   HCC

        MMN

        AHA: 2016,4Q,18

      G61.89 Other inflammatory polyneuropathies   HCC

    G61.9 Inflammatory polyneuropathy, unspecified   HCC

√4ᵗʰ **G62 Other and unspecified polyneuropathies**

    G62.0 Drug-induced polyneuropathy   HCC

      Use additional code for adverse effect, if applicable, to identify drug (T36-T50 with fifth or sixth character 5)

    G62.1 Alcoholic polyneuropathy   HCC

    G62.2 Polyneuropathy due to other toxic agents   HCC

      Code first (T51-T65) to identify toxic agent

    √5ᵗʰ **G62.8 Other specified polyneuropathies**

      G62.81 Critical illness polyneuropathy   HCC

        Acute motor neuropathy

      G62.82 Radiation-induced polyneuropathy   HCC

        Use additional external cause code (W88-W90, X39.0-) to identify cause

      G62.89 Other specified polyneuropathies

        AHA: 2016,2Q,11

    G62.9 Polyneuropathy, unspecified

      Neuropathy NOS

G63 Polyneuropathy in diseases classified elsewhere `HCC`

Code first underlying disease, such as:

amyloidosis (E85.-)

endocrine disease, except diabetes (E00-E07, E15-E16, E20-E34)

metabolic diseases (E70-E88)

neoplasm (C00-D49)

nutritional deficiency (E40-E64)

`EXCLUDES 1`   *polyneuropathy (in):*

diabetes mellitus (E08-E13 with .42)

diphtheria (A36.83)

infectious mononucleosis (B27.0-B27.9 with 1)

Lyme disease (A69.22)

mumps (B26.84)

postherpetic (B02.23)

rheumatoid arthritis ▶(M05.5-)◀

scleroderma (M34.83)

systemic lupus erythematosus (M32.19)

AHA: 2012,4Q,99

G64 Other disorders of peripheral nervous system

Disorder of peripheral nervous system NOS

`✓4ᵗʰ` **G65 Sequelae of inflammatory and toxic polyneuropathies**

Code first condition resulting from (sequela) of inflammatory and toxic polyneuropathies

G65.0 Sequelae of Guillain-Barré syndrome `HCC`

G65.1 Sequelae of other inflammatory polyneuropathy `HCC`

G65.2 Sequelae of toxic polyneuropathy `HCC`

Diseases of myoneural junction and muscle (G70-G73)

`✓4ᵗʰ` **G70 Myasthenia gravis and other myoneural disorders**

`EXCLUDES 1`   *botulism (A05.1, A48.51-A48.52)*

transient neonatal myasthenia gravis (P94.0)

`✓6ᵗʰ` **G70.0 Myasthenia gravis**

DEF: Autoimmune neuromuscular disorder caused by antibodies to the acetylcholine receptors at the neuromuscular junction, interfering with proper binding of the neurotransmitter from the neuron to the target muscle, causing muscle weakness, fatigue, and exhaustion, without pain or atrophy.

G70.00 Myasthenia gravis without (acute) exacerbation `HCC`

Myasthenia gravis NOS

G70.01 Myasthenia gravis with (acute) exacerbation `HCC`

Myasthenia gravis in crisis

G70.1 Toxic myoneural disorders `HCC`

Code first (T51-T65) to identify toxic agent

G70.2 Congenital and developmental myasthenia `HCC`

`✓5ᵗʰ` **G70.8 Other specified myoneural disorders**

G70.80 Lambert-Eaton syndrome, unspecified `HCC`

Lambert-Eaton syndrome NOS

G70.81 *Lambert-Eaton syndrome in disease classified elsewhere* `HCC`

Code first underlying disease

`EXCLUDES 1`   *Lambert-Eaton syndrome in neoplastic disease (G73.1)*

G70.89 Other specified myoneural disorders `HCC`

G70.9 Myoneural disorder, unspecified `HCC`

`✓4ᵗʰ` **G71 Primary disorders of muscles**

`EXCLUDES 2`   *arthrogryposis multiplex congenita (Q74.3)*

metabolic disorders (E70-E88)

myositis (M60.-)

`✓5ᵗʰ` **G71.0 Muscular dystrophy**

AHA: 2018,4Q,11-12

G71.00 Muscular dystrophy, unspecified `HCC`

G71.01 Duchenne or Becker muscular dystrophy `HCC`

Autosomal recessive, childhood type, muscular dystrophy resembling Duchenne or Becker muscular dystrophy

Benign [Becker] muscular dystrophy

Severe [Duchenne] muscular dystrophy

G71.02 Facioscapulohumeral muscular dystrophy `HCC`

Scapulohumeral muscular dystrophy

G71.09 Other specified muscular dystrophies `HCC`

Benign scapuloperoneal muscular dystrophy with early contractures [Emery-Dreifuss]

Congenital muscular dystrophy NOS

Congenital muscular dystrophy with specific morphological abnormalities of the muscle fiber

Distal muscular dystrophy

Limb-girdle muscular dystrophy

Ocular muscular dystrophy

Oculopharyngeal muscular dystrophy

Scapuloperoneal muscular dystrophy

`✓5ᵗʰ` **G71.1 Myotonic disorders**

G71.11 Myotonic muscular dystrophy `HCC`

Dystrophia myotonica [Steinert]

Myotonia atrophica

Myotonic dystrophy

Proximal myotonic myopathy (PROMM)

Steinert disease

G71.12 Myotonia congenita

Acetazolamide responsive myotonia congenita

Dominant myotonia congenita [Thomsen disease]

Myotonia levior

Recessive myotonia congenita [Becker disease]

G71.13 Myotonic chondrodystrophy

Chondrodystrophic myotonia

Congenital myotonic chondrodystrophy

Schwartz-Jampel disease

G71.14 Drug induced myotonia

Use additional code for adverse effect, if applicable, to identify drug (T36-T50 with fifth or sixth character 5)

G71.19 Other specified myotonic disorders

Myotonia fluctuans

Myotonia permanens

Neuromyotonia [Isaacs]

Paramyotonia congenita (of von Eulenburg)

Pseudomyotonia

Symptomatic myotonia

G71.2 Congenital myopathies `HCC`

Central core disease

Fiber-type disproportion

Minicore disease

Multicore disease

Myotubular (centronuclear) myopathy

Nemaline myopathy

`EXCLUDES 1`   *arthrogryposis multiplex congenita (Q74.3)*

G71.3 Mitochondrial myopathy, not elsewhere classified

`EXCLUDES 1`   *Kearns-Sayre syndrome (H49.81)*

Leber's disease (H47.21)

Leigh's encephalopathy (G31.82)

mitochondrial metabolism disorders (E88.4.-)

Reye's syndrome (G93.7)

G71.8 Other primary disorders of muscles

G71.9 Primary disorder of muscle, unspecified

Hereditary myopathy NOS

`✓4ᵗʰ` **G72 Other and unspecified myopathies**

`EXCLUDES 1`   *arthrogryposis multiplex congenita (Q74.3)*

dermatopolymyositis (M33.-)

ischemic infarction of muscle (M62.2-)

myositis (M60.-)

polymyositis (M33.2.-)

G72.0 Drug-induced myopathy

Use additional code for adverse effect, if applicable, to identify drug (T36-T50 with fifth or sixth character 5)

G72.1 Alcoholic myopathy

Use additional code to identify alcoholism (F10.-)

G72.2 Myopathy due to other toxic agents

Code first (T51-T65) to identify toxic agent

☑ Additional Character Required   `✓x7ᵗʰ` Placeholder Alert   Manifestation   Unspecified Dx   ▶◀ Revised Text   ● New Code   ▲ Revised Code Title

G72.3 Periodic paralysis
Familial periodic paralysis
Hyperkalemic periodic paralysis (familial)
Hypokalemic periodic paralysis (familial)
Myotonic periodic paralysis (familial)
Normokalemic paralysis (familial)
Potassium sensitive periodic paralysis
> EXCLUDES 1   *paramyotonia congenita (of von Eulenburg) (G71.19)*

√5ᵗʰ **G72.4 Inflammatory and immune myopathies, not elsewhere classified**

G72.41 Inclusion body myositis [IBM]

G72.49 Other inflammatory and immune myopathies, not elsewhere classified
Inflammatory myopathy NOS

√5ᵗʰ **G72.8 Other specified myopathies**

G72.81 Critical illness myopathy
Acute necrotizing myopathy
Acute quadriplegic myopathy
Intensive care (ICU) myopathy
Myopathy of critical illness

G72.89 Other specified myopathies

G72.9 Myopathy, unspecified

√4ᵗʰ **G73 Disorders of myoneural junction and muscle in diseases classified elsewhere**

G73.1 *Lambert-Eaton syndrome in neoplastic disease*   HCC
Code first underlying neoplasm (C00-D49)
> EXCLUDES 1   *Lambert-Eaton syndrome not associated with neoplasm (G70.80-G70.81)*

G73.3 *Myasthenic syndromes in other diseases classified elsewhere*   HCC
Code first underlying disease, such as:
neoplasm (C00-D49)
thyrotoxicosis (E05.-)

G73.7 *Myopathy in diseases classified elsewhere*
Code first underlying disease, such as:
hyperparathyroidism (E21.0, E21.3)
hypoparathyroidism (E20.-)
glycogen storage disease (E74.0)
lipid storage disorders (E75.-)
> EXCLUDES 1   *myopathy in:*
> *rheumatoid arthritis (M05.32)*
> *sarcoidosis (D86.87)*
> *scleroderma (M34.82)*
> *sicca syndrome [Sjögren] (M35.03)*
> *systemic lupus erythematosus (M32.19)*

Cerebral palsy and other paralytic syndromes (G80-G83)

√4ᵗʰ **G80 Cerebral palsy**
> EXCLUDES 1   *hereditary spastic paraplegia (G11.4)*

G80.0 Spastic quadriplegic cerebral palsy   HCC
Congenital spastic paralysis (cerebral)

G80.1 Spastic diplegic cerebral palsy   HCC
Spastic cerebral palsy NOS

G80.2 Spastic hemiplegic cerebral palsy   HCC

G80.3 Athetoid cerebral palsy   HCC
Double athetosis (syndrome)
Dyskinetic cerebral palsy
Dystonic cerebral palsy
Vogt disease

G80.4 Ataxic cerebral palsy   HCC

G80.8 Other cerebral palsy   HCC
Mixed cerebral palsy syndromes

G80.9 Cerebral palsy, unspecified   HCC
Cerebral palsy NOS

√4ᵗʰ **G81 Hemiplegia and hemiparesis**

> **NOTE**   This category is to be used only when hemiplegia (complete)(incomplete) is reported without further specification, or is stated to be old or longstanding but of unspecified cause. The category is also for use in multiple coding to identify these types of hemiplegia resulting from any cause.

> EXCLUDES 1   *congenital cerebral palsy (G80.-)*
> *hemiplegia and hemiparesis due to sequela of cerebrovascular disease (I69.05-, I69.15-, I69.25-, I69.35-, I69.85-, I69.95-)*

AHA: 2015,1Q,25
TIP: If the documentation specifies the affected side but not whether it is the dominant or nondominant side, the default is as follows: for ambidextrous patients, the default is dominant; when the left side is affected, the default is nondominant; and when the right side is affected, the default is dominant.

√5ᵗʰ **G81.0 Flaccid hemiplegia**

G81.00 Flaccid hemiplegia affecting unspecified side   HCC

G81.01 Flaccid hemiplegia affecting right dominant side   HCC

G81.02 Flaccid hemiplegia affecting left dominant side   HCC

G81.03 Flaccid hemiplegia affecting right nondominant side   HCC

G81.04 Flaccid hemiplegia affecting left nondominant side   HCC

√5ᵗʰ **G81.1 Spastic hemiplegia**

G81.10 Spastic hemiplegia affecting unspecified side   HCC

G81.11 Spastic hemiplegia affecting right dominant side   HCC

G81.12 Spastic hemiplegia affecting left dominant side   HCC

G81.13 Spastic hemiplegia affecting right nondominant side   HCC

G81.14 Spastic hemiplegia affecting left nondominant side   HCC

√5ᵗʰ **G81.9 Hemiplegia, unspecified**
AHA: 2014,1Q,23

G81.90 Hemiplegia, unspecified affecting unspecified side   HCC

G81.91 Hemiplegia, unspecified affecting right dominant side   HCC

G81.92 Hemiplegia, unspecified affecting left dominant side   HCC

G81.93 Hemiplegia, unspecified affecting right nondominant side   HCC

G81.94 Hemiplegia, unspecified affecting left nondominant side   HCC

√4ᵗʰ **G82 Paraplegia (paraparesis) and quadriplegia (quadriparesis)**

> **NOTE**   This category is to be used only when the listed conditions are reported without further specification, or are stated to be old or longstanding but of unspecified cause. The category is also for use in multiple coding to identify these conditions resulting from any cause

> EXCLUDES 1   *congenital cerebral palsy (G80.-)*
> *functional quadriplegia (R53.2)*
> *hysterical paralysis (F44.4)*

√5ᵗʰ **G82.2 Paraplegia**
Paralysis of both lower limbs NOS
Paraparesis (lower) NOS
Paraplegia (lower) NOS
AHA: 2017,3Q,3

G82.20 Paraplegia, unspecified   HCC

G82.21 Paraplegia, complete   HCC

G82.22 Paraplegia, incomplete   HCC

√5ᵗʰ **G82.5 Quadriplegia**

G82.50 Quadriplegia, unspecified   HCC

G82.51 Quadriplegia, C1-C4 complete   HCC

G82.52 Quadriplegia, C1-C4 incomplete   HCC

G82.53 Quadriplegia, C5-C7 complete   HCC

G82.54 Quadriplegia, C5-C7 incomplete   HCC

✓⁴ᵗʰ G83 Other paralytic syndromes

> **NOTE**   This category is to be used only when the listed conditions are reported without further specification, or are stated to be old or longstanding but of unspecified cause. The category is also for use in multiple coding to identify these conditions resulting from any cause.

> **INCLUDES**   paralysis (complete) (incomplete), except as in G80-G82

G83.0 Diplegia of upper limbs   HCC

> Diplegia (upper)
> Paralysis of both upper limbs

✓⁵ᵗʰ G83.1 Monoplegia of lower limb

> Paralysis of lower limb
> **EXCLUDES 1**   monoplegia of lower limbs due to sequela of cerebrovascular disease (I69.04-, I69.14-, I69.24-, I69.34-, I69.84-, I69.94-)

> **TIP:** If the documentation specifies the affected side but not whether it is the dominant or nondominant side, the default is as follows: for ambidextrous patients, the default is dominant; when the left side is affected, the default is nondominant; and when the right side is affected, the default is dominant.

> **G83.10 Monoplegia of lower limb affecting unspecified side**   HCC
> **G83.11 Monoplegia of lower limb affecting right dominant side**   HCC
> **G83.12 Monoplegia of lower limb affecting left dominant side**   HCC
> **G83.13 Monoplegia of lower limb affecting right nondominant side**   HCC
> **G83.14 Monoplegia of lower limb affecting left nondominant side**   HCC

✓⁵ᵗʰ G83.2 Monoplegia of upper limb

> Paralysis of upper limb
> **EXCLUDES 1**   monoplegia of upper limbs due to sequela of cerebrovascular disease (I69.03-, I69.13-, I69.23-, I69.33-, I69.83-, I69.93-)

> **TIP:** If the documentation specifies the affected side but not whether it is the dominant or nondominant side, the default is as follows: for ambidextrous patients, the default is dominant; when the left side is affected, the default is nondominant; and when the right side is affected, the default is dominant.

> **G83.20 Monoplegia of upper limb affecting unspecified side**   HCC
> **G83.21 Monoplegia of upper limb affecting right dominant side**   HCC
> **G83.22 Monoplegia of upper limb affecting left dominant side**   HCC
> **G83.23 Monoplegia of upper limb affecting right nondominant side**   HCC
> **G83.24 Monoplegia of upper limb affecting left nondominant side**   HCC

✓⁵ᵗʰ G83.3 Monoplegia, unspecified

> **TIP:** If the documentation specifies the affected side but not whether it is the dominant or nondominant side, the default is as follows: for ambidextrous patients, the default is dominant; when the left side is affected, the default is nondominant; and when the right side is affected, the default is dominant.

> **G83.30 Monoplegia, unspecified affecting unspecified side**   HCC
> **G83.31 Monoplegia, unspecified affecting right dominant side**   HCC
> **G83.32 Monoplegia, unspecified affecting left dominant side**   HCC
> **G83.33 Monoplegia, unspecified affecting right nondominant side**   HCC
> **G83.34 Monoplegia, unspecified affecting left nondominant side**   HCC

G83.4 Cauda equina syndrome   HCC

> Neurogenic bladder due to cauda equina syndrome
> **EXCLUDES 1**   cord bladder NOS (G95.89)
>   neurogenic bladder NOS (N31.9)

> **DEF:** Compression of the spinal nerve roots presenting with pain and tingling radiating down the buttocks, back of the thigh and calf, and into the foot in a sciatic manner with aching in the bladder, perineum, and sacrum. Loss of bowel and bladder control may also occur.

G83.5 Locked-in state   HCC

✓⁵ᵗʰ G83.8 Other specified paralytic syndromes

> **EXCLUDES 1**   paralytic syndromes due to current spinal cord injury — code to spinal cord injury (S14, S24, S34)

> **G83.81 Brown-Séquard syndrome**   HCC
> **G83.82 Anterior cord syndrome**   HCC
> **G83.83 Posterior cord syndrome**   HCC
> **G83.84 Todd's paralysis (postepileptic)**   HCC
> **G83.89 Other specified paralytic syndromes**   HCC

G83.9 Paralytic syndrome, unspecified   HCC

Other disorders of the nervous system (G89-G99)

✓⁴ᵗʰ G89 Pain, not elsewhere classified

> Code also related psychological factors associated with pain (F45.42)
> **EXCLUDES 1**   generalized pain NOS (R52)
>   pain disorders exclusively related to psychological factors (F45.41)
>   pain NOS (R52)
> **EXCLUDES 2**   atypical face pain (G50.1)
>   headache syndromes (G44.-)
>   localized pain, unspecified type — code to pain by site, such as:
>   abdomen pain (R10.-)
>   back pain (M54.9)
>   breast pain (N64.4)
>   chest pain (R07.1-R07.9)
>   ear pain (H92.0-)
>   eye pain (H57.1)
>   headache (R51)
>   joint pain (M25.5-)
>   limb pain (M79.6-)
>   lumbar region pain (M54.5)
>   painful urination (R30.9)
>   pelvic and perineal pain (R10.2)
>   renal colic (N23)
>   shoulder pain (M25.51-)
>   spine pain (M54.-)
>   throat pain (R07.0)
>   tongue pain (K14.6)
>   tooth pain (K08.8)
>   migraines (G43.-)
>   myalgia (M79.1-)
>   pain from prosthetic devices, implants, and grafts (T82.84, T83.84, T84.84, T85.84)
>   phantom limb syndrome with pain (G54.6)
>   vulvar vestibulitis (N94.810)
>   vulvodynia (N94.81-)

G89.0 Central pain syndrome

> Déjérine-Roussy syndrome
> Myelopathic pain syndrome
> Thalamic pain syndrome (hyperesthetic)

✓⁵ᵗʰ G89.1 Acute pain, not elsewhere classified

> **G89.11 Acute pain due to trauma**
> **G89.12 Acute post-thoracotomy pain**
>   Post-thoracotomy pain NOS
> **G89.18 Other acute postprocedural pain**
>   Postoperative pain NOS
>   Postprocedural pain NOS

✓⁵ᵗʰ G89.2 Chronic pain, not elsewhere classified

> **EXCLUDES 1**   causalgia, lower limb (G57.7-)
>   causalgia, upper limb (G56.4-)
>   central pain syndrome (G89.0)
>   chronic pain syndrome (G89.4)
>   complex regional pain syndrome II, lower limb (G57.7-)
>   complex regional pain syndrome II, upper limb (G56.4-)
>   neoplasm related chronic pain (G89.3)
>   reflex sympathetic dystrophy (G90.5-)

> **G89.21 Chronic pain due to trauma**
> **G89.22 Chronic post-thoracotomy pain**
> **G89.28 Other chronic postprocedural pain**
>   Other chronic postoperative pain
> **G89.29 Other chronic pain**

☑ Additional Character Required   ✓ˣ⁷ᵗʰ Placeholder Alert   Manifestation   Unspecified Dx   ►◄ Revised Text   ● New Code   ▲ Revised Code Title

G89.3   **Neoplasm related pain (acute) (chronic)**
Cancer associated pain
Pain due to malignancy (primary) (secondary)
Tumor associated pain

G89.4   **Chronic pain syndrome**
Chronic pain associated with significant psychosocial dysfunction

✓4ᵗʰ **G90**   **Disorders of autonomic nervous system**
> EXCLUDES 1   *dysfunction of the autonomic nervous system due to alcohol (G31.2)*

✓5ᵗʰ **G90.0**   **Idiopathic peripheral autonomic neuropathy**

G90.01   **Carotid sinus syncope**
Carotid sinus syndrome
DEF: Vagal activation caused by pressure on the carotid sinus baroreceptors. Sympathetic nerve impulses may cause sinus arrest or AV block.

G90.09   **Other idiopathic peripheral autonomic neuropathy**
Idiopathic peripheral autonomic neuropathy NOS

G90.1   **Familial dysautonomia [Riley-Day]**   `HCC`

G90.2   **Horner's syndrome**
Bernard(-Horner) syndrome
Cervical sympathetic dystrophy or paralysis

G90.3   **Multi-system degeneration of the autonomic nervous system**   `HCC`
Neurogenic orthostatic hypotension [Shy-Drager]
> EXCLUDES 1   *orthostatic hypotension NOS (I95.1)*

G90.4   **Autonomic dysreflexia**
Use additional code to identify the cause, such as:
fecal impaction (K56.41)
pressure ulcer (pressure area) (L89.-)
urinary tract infection (N39.0)

✓5ᵗʰ **G90.5**   **Complex regional pain syndrome I (CRPS I)**
Reflex sympathetic dystrophy
> EXCLUDES 1   *causalgia of lower limb (G57.7-)*
> *causalgia of upper limb (G56.4-)*
> *complex regional pain syndrome II of lower limb (G57.7-)*
> *complex regional pain syndrome II of upper limb (G56.4-)*

G90.50   **Complex regional pain syndrome I, unspecified**

✓6ᵗʰ **G90.51**   **Complex regional pain syndrome I of upper limb**

G90.511   **Complex regional pain syndrome I of right upper limb**

G90.512   **Complex regional pain syndrome I of left upper limb**

G90.513   **Complex regional pain syndrome I of upper limb, bilateral**

G90.519   **Complex regional pain syndrome I of unspecified upper limb**

✓6ᵗʰ **G90.52**   **Complex regional pain syndrome I of lower limb**

G90.521   **Complex regional pain syndrome I of right lower limb**

G90.522   **Complex regional pain syndrome I of left lower limb**

G90.523   **Complex regional pain syndrome I of lower limb, bilateral**

G90.529   **Complex regional pain syndrome I of unspecified lower limb**

G90.59   **Complex regional pain syndrome I of other specified site**

G90.8   **Other disorders of autonomic nervous system**

G90.9   **Disorder of the autonomic nervous system, unspecified**

✓4ᵗʰ **G91**   **Hydrocephalus**
> INCLUDES   acquired hydrocephalus
> EXCLUDES 1   *Arnold-Chiari syndrome with hydrocephalus (Q07.-)*
> *congenital hydrocephalus (Q03.-)*
> *spina bifida with hydrocephalus (Q05.-)*

DEF: Abnormal buildup of cerebrospinal fluid in the brain causing dilation of the ventricles.

Hydrocephalus (Acquired)

Normal ventricles   Hydrocephalic ventricles

G91.0   **Communicating hydrocephalus**   `HCC`
Secondary normal pressure hydrocephalus

G91.1   **Obstructive hydrocephalus**   `HCC`
DEF: Obstruction of the cerebrospinal fluid passage from the brain into the spinal canal characterized by headaches, drowsiness, poor coordination, urinary incontinence, nausea, vomiting, and papilledema.

G91.2   **(Idiopathic) normal pressure hydrocephalus**   `HCC`
Normal pressure hydrocephalus NOS

G91.3   **Post-traumatic hydrocephalus, unspecified**   `HCC`

G91.4   *Hydrocephalus in diseases classified elsewhere*   `HCC`
Code first underlying condition, such as:
congenital syphilis (A50.4-)
neoplasm (C00-D49)
plasminogen deficiency (E88.02)
> EXCLUDES 1   *hydrocephalus due to congenital toxoplasmosis (P37.1)*

AHA: 2014,3Q,3

G91.8   **Other hydrocephalus**   `HCC`

G91.9   **Hydrocephalus, unspecified**   `HCC`

G92   **Toxic encephalopathy**
Toxic encephalitis
Toxic metabolic encephalopathy
Code first, if applicable, drug induced (T36-T50)
Code first (T51-T65) to identify toxic agent
AHA: 2017,1Q,39-40
DEF: Brain tissue degeneration due to a toxic substance.

✓4ᵗʰ **G93**   **Other disorders of brain**

G93.0   **Cerebral cysts**
Arachnoid cyst
Porencephalic cyst, acquired
> EXCLUDES 1   *acquired periventricular cysts of newborn (P91.1)*
> *congenital cerebral cysts (Q04.6)*

G93.1   **Anoxic brain damage, not elsewhere classified**   `HCC`
> EXCLUDES 1   *cerebral anoxia due to anesthesia during labor and delivery (O74.3)*
> *cerebral anoxia due to anesthesia during the puerperium (O89.2)*
> *neonatal anoxia (P84)*

DEF: Brain injury not resulting from birth trauma that is due to lack of oxygen. Brain cells, when deprived of oxygen; begin to expire after 4 minutes.

G93.2   **Benign intracranial hypertension**
> EXCLUDES 1   *hypertensive encephalopathy (I67.4)*

G93.3   **Postviral fatigue syndrome**
Benign myalgic encephalomyelitis
EXCLUDES 1   *chronic fatigue syndrome NOS (R53.82)*

✓5ᵗʰ   **G93.4**   **Other and unspecified encephalopathy**
EXCLUDES 1   *alcoholic encephalopathy (G31.2)*
encephalopathy in diseases classified elsewhere (G94)
hypertensive encephalopathy (I67.4)
toxic (metabolic) encephalopathy (G92)

    G93.40   **Encephalopathy, unspecified**
AHA: 2017,2Q,8

    G93.41   **Metabolic encephalopathy**
Septic encephalopathy
AHA: 2017,2Q,8; 2016,3Q,42; 2015,3Q,21
TIP: Assign separately when documented with diabetic hypoglycemia (E08.649, E09.649, E10.649, E11.649, E13.649).

    G93.49   **Other encephalopathy**
Encephalopathy NEC
AHA: 2018,4Q,16; 2018,2Q,22,24; 2017,2Q,9

G93.5   **Compression of brain**   HCC
Arnold-Chiari type 1 compression of brain
Compression of brain (stem)
Herniation of brain (stem)
EXCLUDES 1   *diffuse traumatic compression of brain (S06.2-)*
focal traumatic compression of brain (S06.3-)

G93.6   **Cerebral edema**   HCC
EXCLUDES 1   *cerebral edema due to birth injury (P11.0)*
traumatic cerebral edema (S06.1-)

G93.7   **Reye's syndrome**   HCC P
Code first poisoning due to salicylates, if applicable (T39.0-, with sixth character 1-4)
Use additional code for adverse effect due to salicylates, if applicable (T39.0-, with sixth character 5)
DEF: Rare childhood illness often developed after a viral upper respiratory infection. Symptoms include vomiting, elevated serum transaminase, brain swelling, disturbances of consciousness, seizures, and changes in liver and other viscera and it can be fatal.

✓5ᵗʰ   **G93.8**   **Other specified disorders of brain**

    G93.81   **Temporal sclerosis**
Hippocampal sclerosis
Mesial temporal sclerosis

    G93.82   **Brain death**

    G93.89   **Other specified disorders of brain**
Postradiation encephalopathy

    G93.9   **Disorder of brain, unspecified**

G94   *Other disorders of brain in diseases classified elsewhere*
Code first underlying disease
EXCLUDES 1   *encephalopathy in congenital syphilis (A50.49)*
encephalopathy in influenza (J09.X9, J10.81, J11.81)
encephalopathy in syphilis (A52.19)
hydrocephalus in diseases classified elsewhere (G91.4)
AHA: 2018,2Q,22; 2017,2Q,8-9

✓4ᵗʰ   **G95**   **Other and unspecified diseases of spinal cord**
EXCLUDES 2   *myelitis (G04.-)*

G95.0   **Syringomyelia and syringobulbia**   HCC

✓5ᵗʰ   **G95.1**   **Vascular myelopathies**
EXCLUDES 2   *intraspinal phlebitis and thrombophlebitis, except non-pyogenic (G08)*

    G95.11   **Acute infarction of spinal cord (embolic) (nonembolic)**   HCC
Anoxia of spinal cord
Arterial thrombosis of spinal cord

    G95.19   **Other vascular myelopathies**   HCC
Edema of spinal cord
Hematomyelia
Nonpyogenic intraspinal phlebitis and thrombophlebitis
Subacute necrotic myelopathy

✓5ᵗʰ   **G95.2**   **Other and unspecified cord compression**

    G95.20   **Unspecified cord compression**   HCC

    G95.29   **Other cord compression**   HCC

✓5ᵗʰ   **G95.8**   **Other specified diseases of spinal cord**
EXCLUDES 1   *neurogenic bladder NOS (N31.9)*
neurogenic bladder due to cauda equina syndrome (G83.4)
neuromuscular dysfunction of bladder without spinal cord lesion (N31.-)

    G95.81   **Conus medullaris syndrome**   HCC

    G95.89   **Other specified diseases of spinal cord**   HCC
Cord bladder NOS
Drug-induced myelopathy
Radiation-induced myelopathy
EXCLUDES 1   *myelopathy NOS (G95.9)*

G95.9   **Disease of spinal cord, unspecified**   HCC
Myelopathy NOS

✓4ᵗʰ   **G96**   **Other disorders of central nervous system**

G96.0   **Cerebrospinal fluid leak**
EXCLUDES 1   *cerebrospinal fluid leak from spinal puncture (G97.0)*
AHA: 2018,2Q,13
DEF: Cerebrospinal fluid discharging from the nose or the ear caused by a fracture of the frontal bone with tearing of dura mater and arachnoid. It is characterized by watery drainage usually from only one side of the nose or one ear, headache, vision changes, and hearing loss.

✓5ᵗʰ   **G96.1**   **Disorders of meninges, not elsewhere classified**

    G96.11   **Dural tear**
EXCLUDES 1   *accidental puncture or laceration of dura during a procedure (G97.41)*
AHA: 2014,4Q,24

    G96.12   **Meningeal adhesions (cerebral) (spinal)**

    G96.19   **Other disorders of meninges, not elsewhere classified**

G96.8   **Other specified disorders of central nervous system**

G96.9   **Disorder of central nervous system, unspecified**

✓4ᵗʰ   **G97**   **Intraoperative and postprocedural complications and disorders of nervous system, not elsewhere classified**
EXCLUDES 2   *intraoperative and postprocedural cerebrovascular infarction (I97.81-, I97.82-)*
AHA: 2016,4Q,9-10

G97.0   **Cerebrospinal fluid leak from spinal puncture**

Spinal Puncture

- Spinal cord
- Epidural space
- Subarachnoid space
- Vertebra
- Spinal needle

Lumbar area

G97.1   **Other reaction to spinal and lumbar puncture**
Headache due to lumbar puncture

G97.2   **Intracranial hypotension following ventricular shunting**

✓5ᵗʰ   **G97.3**   **Intraoperative hemorrhage and hematoma of a nervous system organ or structure complicating a procedure**
EXCLUDES 1   *intraoperative hemorrhage and hematoma of a nervous system organ or structure due to accidental puncture and laceration during a procedure (G97.4-)*

    G97.31   **Intraoperative hemorrhage and hematoma of a nervous system organ or structure complicating a nervous system procedure**

    G97.32   **Intraoperative hemorrhage and hematoma of a nervous system organ or structure complicating other procedure**

✓ Additional Character Required   ✓x7ᵗʰ Placeholder Alert   Manifestation   Unspecified Dx   ▶◀ Revised Text   ● New Code   ▲ Revised Code Title

ICD-10-CM 2020   581

G97.4 Accidental puncture and laceration of a nervous system organ or structure during a procedure

    G97.41 Accidental puncture or laceration of dura during a procedure

         Incidental (inadvertent) durotomy

         AHA: 2014,4Q,24

    G97.48 Accidental puncture and laceration of other nervous system organ or structure during a nervous system procedure

    G97.49 Accidental puncture and laceration of other nervous system organ or structure during other procedure

✓5ᵗʰ **G97.5 Postprocedural hemorrhage of a nervous system organ or structure following a procedure**

    G97.51 Postprocedural hemorrhage of a nervous system organ or structure following a nervous system procedure

    G97.52 Postprocedural hemorrhage of a nervous system organ or structure following other procedure

✓5ᵗʰ **G97.6 Postprocedural hematoma and seroma of a nervous system organ or structure following a procedure**

    G97.61 Postprocedural hematoma of a nervous system organ or structure following a nervous system procedure

    G97.62 Postprocedural hematoma of a nervous system organ or structure following other procedure

    G97.63 Postprocedural seroma of a nervous system organ or structure following a nervous system procedure

    G97.64 Postprocedural seroma of a nervous system organ or structure following other procedure

✓5ᵗʰ **G97.8 Other intraoperative and postprocedural complications and disorders of nervous system**

         Use additional code to further specify disorder

    G97.81 Other intraoperative complications of nervous system

    G97.82 Other postprocedural complications and disorders of nervous system

✓4ᵗʰ **G98 Other disorders of nervous system not elsewhere classified**

    INCLUDES nervous system disorder NOS

  G98.0 Neurogenic arthritis, not elsewhere classified

         Nonsyphilitic neurogenic arthropathy NEC

         Nonsyphilitic neurogenic spondylopathy NEC

         EXCLUDES 1   spondylopathy (in):

                 syringomyelia and syringobulbia (G95.0)

                 tabes dorsalis (A52.11)

  G98.8 Other disorders of nervous system

         Nervous system disorder NOS

✓4ᵗʰ **G99 Other disorders of nervous system in diseases classified elsewhere**

  G99.0 Autonomic neuropathy in diseases classified elsewhere

         Code first underlying disease, such as:

            amyloidosis (E85.-)

            gout (M1A.-, M10.-)

            hyperthyroidism (E05.-)

         EXCLUDES 1   diabetic autonomic neuropathy (E08-E13 with .43)

  G99.2 Myelopathy in diseases classified elsewhere   **HCC**

         Code first underlying disease, such as:

            neoplasm (C00-D49)

         EXCLUDES 1   myelopathy in:

                 intervertebral disease (M50.0-, M51.0-)

                 spondylosis (M47.0-, M47.1-)

         AHA: 2018,3Q,18-19

         TIP: Use this code in addition to a spondylolisthesis code (M43.1-) or a spinal stenosis code (M48.0-) when either of these disorders is documented as the cause of the myelopathy.

  G99.8 Other specified disorders of nervous system in diseases classified elsewhere

         Code first underlying disorder, such as:

            amyloidosis (E85.-)

            avitaminosis (E56.9)

         EXCLUDES 1   nervous system involvement in:

                 cysticercosis (B69.0)

                 rubella (B06.0-)

                 syphilis (A52.1-)

Chapter 7. Diseases of the Eye and Adnexa (H00–H59)

Chapter-specific Guidelines with Coding Examples

The chapter-specific guidelines from the ICD-10-CM Official Guidelines for Coding and Reporting have been provided below. Along with these guidelines are coding examples, contained in the shaded boxes, that have been developed to help illustrate the coding and/or sequencing guidance found in these guidelines.

a. Glaucoma

1) Assigning glaucoma codes

Assign as many codes from category H40, Glaucoma, as needed to identify the type of glaucoma, the affected eye, and the glaucoma stage.

2) Bilateral glaucoma with same type and stage

When a patient has bilateral glaucoma and both eyes are documented as being the same type and stage, and there is a code for bilateral glaucoma, report only the code for the type of glaucoma, bilateral, with the seventh character for the stage.

> Bilateral mild stage primary open-angle glaucoma
>
> **H40.1131** **Primary open-angle glaucoma, bilateral, mild stage**
>
> *Explanation*: In this scenario, the patient has the same type and stage of glaucoma in both eyes. As this type of glaucoma has a code for bilateral, assign only the code for the bilateral glaucoma with the seventh character for the stage.

When a patient has bilateral glaucoma and both eyes are documented as being the same type and stage, and the classification does not provide a code for bilateral glaucoma (i.e. subcategories H40.10 and H40.20) report only one code for the type of glaucoma with the appropriate seventh character for the stage.

> Bilateral open-angle glaucoma, severe stage; not specified as to type
>
> **H40.10X3** **Unspecified open-angle glaucoma, severe stage**
>
> *Explanation*: In this scenario, the patient has glaucoma of the same type and stage of both eyes, but there is no code specifically for bilateral glaucoma. Only one code is assigned with the appropriate seventh character for the stage.

3) Bilateral glaucoma stage with different types or stages

When a patient has bilateral glaucoma and each eye is documented as having a different type or stage, and the classification distinguishes laterality, assign the appropriate code for each eye rather than the code for bilateral glaucoma.

> Bilateral chronic angle-closure glaucoma; right eye is documented as mild stage and left eye as moderate stage
>
> **H40.2211** **Chronic angle-closure glaucoma, right eye, mild stage**
>
> **H40.2222** **Chronic angle-closure glaucoma, left eye, moderate stage**
>
> *Explanation*: In this scenario the patient has the same type of glaucoma in both eyes, but each eye is at a different stage. Because the subcategory for this condition identifies laterality, one code is assigned for the right eye and one code is assigned for the left eye, each with the appropriate seventh character for the stage appended.

When a patient has bilateral glaucoma and each eye is documented as having a different type, and the classification does not distinguish laterality (i.e. subcategories H40.10 and H40.20), assign one code for each type of glaucoma with the appropriate seventh character for the stage.

> Documentation relates mild, unspecified primary angle-closure glaucoma of the left eye with mild unspecified open-angle glaucoma of the right eye
>
> **H40.20X1** **Unspecified primary angle-closure glaucoma, mild stage**
>
> **H40.10X1** **Unspecified open-angle glaucoma, mild stage**
>
> *Explanation*: In this scenario the patient has a different type of glaucoma in each eye and the classification does not distinguish laterality. A code for each type of glaucoma is assigned, each with the appropriate seventh character for the stage.

When a patient has bilateral glaucoma and each eye is documented as having the same type, but different stage, and the classification does not distinguish laterality (i.e. subcategories H40.10 and H40.20), assign a code for the type of glaucoma for each eye with the seventh character for the specific glaucoma stage documented for each eye.

> Bilateral open-angle glaucoma, not specified as to type; the right eye is documented to be in mild stage and the left eye as being in moderate stage
>
> **H40.10X1** **Unspecified open-angle glaucoma, mild stage**
>
> **H40.10X2** **Unspecified open-angle glaucoma, moderate stage**
>
> *Explanation*: In this scenario the patient has the same type of glaucoma in each eye but each eye is at a different stage, and the classification does not distinguish laterality at this subcategory level. Two codes are assigned; both codes represent the same type of glaucoma but each has a different seventh character identifying the appropriate stage for each eye.

4) Patient admitted with glaucoma and stage evolves during the admission

If a patient is admitted with glaucoma and the stage progresses during the admission, assign the code for highest stage documented.

5) Indeterminate stage glaucoma

Assignment of the seventh character "4" for "indeterminate stage" should be based on the clinical documentation. The seventh character "4" is used for glaucomas whose stage cannot be clinically determined. This seventh character should not be confused with the seventh character "0", unspecified, which should be assigned when there is no documentation regarding the stage of the glaucoma.

b. Blindness

If "blindness" or "low vision" of both eyes is documented but the visual impairment category is not documented, assign code H54.3, Unqualified visual loss, both eyes. If "blindness" or "low vision" in one eye is documented but the visual impairment category is not documented, assign a code from H54.6-, Unqualified visual loss, one eye. If "blindness" or "visual loss" is documented without any information about whether one or both eyes are affected, assign code H54.7, Unspecified visual loss.

> Patient assessment indicates moderately impaired/low vision in the left eye with no visual impairments in the right eye
>
> **H54.62** **Unqualified visual loss, left eye, normal vision right eye**
>
> Report unqualified visual loss when the visual impairment category is not specified. In this case, only the left eye is impacted by visual loss with normal vision of the right eye documented.

Chapter 7. Diseases of the Eye and Adnexa (H00–H59)

NOTE   Use an external cause code following the code for the eye condition, if applicable, to identify the cause of the eye condition

EXCLUDES 2   *certain conditions originating in the perinatal period (P04-P96)*
certain infectious and parasitic diseases (A00-B99)
complications of pregnancy, childbirth and the puerperium (O00-O9A)
congenital malformations, deformations, and chromosomal abnormalities (Q00-Q99)
diabetes mellitus related eye conditions (E09.3-, E10.3-, E11.3-, E13.3-)
endocrine, nutritional and metabolic diseases (E00-E88)
injury (trauma) of eye and orbit (S05.-)
injury, poisoning and certain other consequences of external causes (S00-T88)
neoplasms (C00-D49)
symptoms, signs and abnormal clinical and laboratory findings, not elsewhere classified (R00-R94)
syphilis related eye disorders (A50.01, A50.3-, A51.43, A52.71)

This chapter contains the following blocks:

H00-H05   Disorders of eyelid, lacrimal system and orbit
H10-H11   Disorders of conjunctiva
H15-H22   Disorders of sclera, cornea, iris and ciliary body
H25-H28   Disorders of lens
H30-H36   Disorders of choroid and retina
H40-H42   Glaucoma
H43-H44   Disorders of vitreous body and globe
H46-H47   Disorders of optic nerve and visual pathways
H49-H52   Disorders of ocular muscles, binocular movement, accommodation and refraction
H53-H54   Visual disturbances and blindness
H55-H57   Other disorders of eye and adnexa
H59   Intraoperative and postprocedural complications and disorders of eye and adnexa, not elsewhere classified

Disorders of eyelid, lacrimal system and orbit (H00-H05)

EXCLUDES 2   *open wound of eyelid (S01.1-)*
superficial injury of eyelid (S00.1-, S00.2-)

✓4ᵗʰ **H00   Hordeolum and chalazion**

    ✓5ᵗʰ **H00.0   Hordeolum (externum) (internum) of eyelid**

       DEF: Acute localized infection of the gland of Zeis (external hordeolum) or Molt or of the meibomian glands (internal hordeolum) of the orbit.

      ✓6ᵗʰ **H00.01   Hordeolum externum**

        Hordeolum NOS
        Stye

        H00.011   Hordeolum externum right upper **eyelid**
        H00.012   Hordeolum externum right lower **eyelid**
        H00.013   Hordeolum externum right eye, **unspecified eyelid**
        H00.014   Hordeolum externum left upper **eyelid**
        H00.015   Hordeolum externum left lower **eyelid**
        H00.016   Hordeolum externum left eye, **unspecified eyelid**
        H00.019   Hordeolum externum unspecified eye, unspecified eyelid

      ✓6ᵗʰ **H00.02   Hordeolum internum**

        Infection of meibomian gland

        H00.021   Hordeolum internum right upper **eyelid**
        H00.022   Hordeolum internum right lower **eyelid**
        H00.023   Hordeolum internum right eye, **unspecified eyelid**
        H00.024   Hordeolum internum left upper **eyelid**
        H00.025   Hordeolum internum left lower **eyelid**
        H00.026   Hordeolum internum left eye, unspecified **eyelid**
        H00.029   Hordeolum internum unspecified eye, unspecified eyelid

      ✓6ᵗʰ **H00.03   Abscess of eyelid**

        Furuncle of eyelid

        H00.031   Abscess of right upper **eyelid**
        H00.032   Abscess of right lower **eyelid**
        H00.033   Abscess of eyelid right eye, **unspecified eyelid**
        H00.034   Abscess of left upper **eyelid**
        H00.035   Abscess of left lower **eyelid**
        H00.036   Abscess of eyelid left eye, **unspecified eyelid**
        H00.039   Abscess of eyelid unspecified eye, unspecified eyelid

✓5ᵗʰ **H00.1   Chalazion**

      Meibomian (gland) cyst

      EXCLUDES 2   *infected meibomian gland (H00.02-)*

      DEF: Noninfectious, obstructive mass in the oil gland of the eyelid that results in a small chronic lump or inflammation.

      H00.11   Chalazion right upper **eyelid**
      H00.12   Chalazion right lower **eyelid**
      H00.13   Chalazion right eye, unspecified **eyelid**
      H00.14   Chalazion left upper **eyelid**
      H00.15   Chalazion left lower **eyelid**
      H00.16   Chalazion left eye, unspecified **eyelid**
      H00.19   Chalazion unspecified eye, unspecified eyelid

✓4ᵗʰ **H01   Other inflammation of eyelid**

    ✓5ᵗʰ **H01.0   Blepharitis**

      EXCLUDES 1   *blepharoconjunctivitis (H10.5-)*

      ✓6ᵗʰ **H01.00   Unspecified blepharitis**

       AHA: 2018,4Q,13

       H01.001   Unspecified blepharitis right upper **eyelid**
       H01.002   Unspecified blepharitis right lower **eyelid**
       H01.003   Unspecified blepharitis right eye, unspecified **eyelid**
       H01.004   Unspecified blepharitis left upper **eyelid**
       H01.005   Unspecified blepharitis left lower **eyelid**
       H01.006   Unspecified blepharitis left eye, unspecified **eyelid**
       H01.009   Unspecified blepharitis unspecified eye, unspecified eyelid
       H01.00A   Unspecified blepharitis right eye, upper **and lower eyelids**
       H01.00B   Unspecified blepharitis left eye, upper **and lower eyelids**

      ✓6ᵗʰ **H01.01   Ulcerative blepharitis**

       AHA: 2018,4Q,13

       H01.011   Ulcerative blepharitis right upper **eyelid**
       H01.012   Ulcerative blepharitis right lower **eyelid**
       H01.013   Ulcerative blepharitis right eye, unspecified **eyelid**
       H01.014   Ulcerative blepharitis left upper **eyelid**
       H01.015   Ulcerative blepharitis left lower **eyelid**
       H01.016   Ulcerative blepharitis left eye, unspecified **eyelid**
       H01.019   Ulcerative blepharitis unspecified eye, unspecified eyelid
       H01.01A   Ulcerative blepharitis right eye, upper **and lower eyelids**
       H01.01B   Ulcerative blepharitis left eye, upper and **lower eyelids**

      ✓6ᵗʰ **H01.02   Squamous blepharitis**

       AHA: 2018,4Q,13

       H01.021   Squamous blepharitis right upper **eyelid**
       H01.022   Squamous blepharitis right lower **eyelid**
       H01.023   Squamous blepharitis right eye, unspecified **eyelid**
       H01.024   Squamous blepharitis left upper **eyelid**
       H01.025   Squamous blepharitis left lower **eyelid**
       H01.026   Squamous blepharitis left eye, unspecified **eyelid**
       H01.029   Squamous blepharitis unspecified eye, unspecified eyelid
       H01.02A   Squamous blepharitis right eye, upper **and lower eyelids**
       H01.02B   Squamous blepharitis left eye, upper and **lower eyelids**

    ✓5ᵗʰ **H01.1   Noninfectious dermatoses of eyelid**

      ✓6ᵗʰ **H01.11   Allergic dermatitis of eyelid**

       Contact dermatitis of eyelid

       H01.111   Allergic dermatitis of right upper **eyelid**
       H01.112   Allergic dermatitis of right lower **eyelid**
       H01.113   Allergic dermatitis of right eye, unspecified **eyelid**
       H01.114   Allergic dermatitis of left upper **eyelid**
       H01.115   Allergic dermatitis of left lower **eyelid**
       H01.116   Allergic dermatitis of left eye, unspecified **eyelid**
       H01.119   Allergic dermatitis of unspecified eye, **unspecified eyelid**

✓6ᵗʰ **H01.12** Discoid lupus erythematosus of eyelid

     H01.121 Discoid lupus erythematosus of right upper eyelid

     H01.122 Discoid lupus erythematosus of right lower eyelid

     H01.123 Discoid lupus erythematosus of right eye, unspecified eyelid

     H01.124 Discoid lupus erythematosus of left upper eyelid

     H01.125 Discoid lupus erythematosus of left lower eyelid

     H01.126 Discoid lupus erythematosus of left eye, unspecified eyelid

     H01.129 Discoid lupus erythematosus of unspecified eye, unspecified eyelid

✓6ᵗʰ **H01.13** Eczematous dermatitis of eyelid

     H01.131 Eczematous dermatitis of right upper eyelid

     H01.132 Eczematous dermatitis of right lower eyelid

     H01.133 Eczematous dermatitis of right eye, unspecified eyelid

     H01.134 Eczematous dermatitis of left upper eyelid

     H01.135 Eczematous dermatitis of left lower eyelid

     H01.136 Eczematous dermatitis of left eye, unspecified eyelid

     H01.139 Eczematous dermatitis of unspecified eye, unspecified eyelid

✓6ᵗʰ **H01.14** Xeroderma of eyelid

     H01.141 Xeroderma of right upper eyelid

     H01.142 Xeroderma of right lower eyelid

     H01.143 Xeroderma of right eye, unspecified eyelid

     H01.144 Xeroderma of left upper eyelid

     H01.145 Xeroderma of left lower eyelid

     H01.146 Xeroderma of left eye, unspecified eyelid

     H01.149 Xeroderma of unspecified eye, unspecified eyelid

H01.8 Other specified inflammations of eyelid

H01.9 Unspecified inflammation of eyelid

     Inflammation of eyelid NOS

✓4ᵗʰ **H02** Other disorders of eyelid

     EXCLUDES 1   congenital malformations of eyelid (Q10.0-Q10.3)

Entropion and Ectropion

Normal eyelid   Entropion   Ectropion

✓5ᵗʰ **H02.0** Entropion and trichiasis of eyelid

     DEF: Entropion: Inversion of the eyelid, turning the edge in toward the eyeball and causing irritation from contact of the lashes with the surface of the eye.

     DEF: Trichiasis: Condition wherein the eyelid is in a normal position but lashes are ingrown or misdirected in their growth so that they irritate the tissues of the eye.

✓6ᵗʰ **H02.00** Unspecified entropion of eyelid

     H02.001 Unspecified entropion of right upper eyelid

     H02.002 Unspecified entropion of right lower eyelid

     H02.003 Unspecified entropion of right eye, unspecified eyelid

     H02.004 Unspecified entropion of left upper eyelid

     H02.005 Unspecified entropion of left lower eyelid

     H02.006 Unspecified entropion of left eye, unspecified eyelid

     H02.009 Unspecified entropion of unspecified eye, unspecified eyelid

✓6ᵗʰ **H02.01** Cicatricial entropion of eyelid

     H02.011 Cicatricial entropion of right upper eyelid

     H02.012 Cicatricial entropion of right lower eyelid

     H02.013 Cicatricial entropion of right eye, unspecified eyelid

     H02.014 Cicatricial entropion of left upper eyelid

     H02.015 Cicatricial entropion of left lower eyelid

     H02.016 Cicatricial entropion of left eye, unspecified eyelid

     H02.019 Cicatricial entropion of unspecified eye, unspecified eyelid

✓6ᵗʰ **H02.02** Mechanical entropion of eyelid

     H02.021 Mechanical entropion of right upper eyelid

     H02.022 Mechanical entropion of right lower eyelid

     H02.023 Mechanical entropion of right eye, unspecified eyelid

     H02.024 Mechanical entropion of left upper eyelid

     H02.025 Mechanical entropion of left lower eyelid

     H02.026 Mechanical entropion of left eye, unspecified eyelid

     H02.029 Mechanical entropion of unspecified eye, unspecified eyelid

✓6ᵗʰ **H02.03** Senile entropion of eyelid

     H02.031 Senile entropion of right upper eyelid   Ⓐ

     H02.032 Senile entropion of right lower eyelid   Ⓐ

     H02.033 Senile entropion of right eye, unspecified eyelid   Ⓐ

     H02.034 Senile entropion of left upper eyelid   Ⓐ

     H02.035 Senile entropion of left lower eyelid   Ⓐ

     H02.036 Senile entropion of left eye, unspecified eyelid   Ⓐ

     H02.039 Senile entropion of unspecified eye, unspecified eyelid   Ⓐ

✓6ᵗʰ **H02.04** Spastic entropion of eyelid

     H02.041 Spastic entropion of right upper eyelid

     H02.042 Spastic entropion of right lower eyelid

     H02.043 Spastic entropion of right eye, unspecified eyelid

     H02.044 Spastic entropion of left upper eyelid

     H02.045 Spastic entropion of left lower eyelid

     H02.046 Spastic entropion of left eye, unspecified eyelid

     H02.049 Spastic entropion of unspecified eye, unspecified eyelid

✓6ᵗʰ **H02.05** Trichiasis without entropion

     H02.051 Trichiasis without entropion right upper eyelid

     H02.052 Trichiasis without entropion right lower eyelid

     H02.053 Trichiasis without entropion right eye, unspecified eyelid

     H02.054 Trichiasis without entropion left upper eyelid

     H02.055 Trichiasis without entropion left lower eyelid

     H02.056 Trichiasis without entropion left eye, unspecified eyelid

     H02.059 Trichiasis without entropion unspecified eye, unspecified eyelid

✓5ᵗʰ **H02.1** Ectropion of eyelid

     DEF: Drooping of the lower eyelid away from the eye or outward turning or eversion of the edge of the eyelid, exposing the palpebral conjunctiva and causing irritation.

✓6ᵗʰ **H02.10** Unspecified ectropion of eyelid

     H02.101 Unspecified ectropion of right upper eyelid

     H02.102 Unspecified ectropion of right lower eyelid

     H02.103 Unspecified ectropion of right eye, unspecified eyelid

     H02.104 Unspecified ectropion of left upper eyelid

     H02.105 Unspecified ectropion of left lower eyelid

☑ Additional Character Required   ✓×7ᵗʰ Placeholder Alert   Manifestation   Unspecified Dx   ►◄ Revised Text   ● New Code   ▲ Revised Code Title

H02.106 Unspecified ectropion of left eye, unspecified eyelid

H02.109 Unspecified ectropion of unspecified eye, unspecified eyelid

✓6ᵗʰ **H02.11** Cicatricial ectropion of eyelid

H02.111 Cicatricial ectropion of right upper eyelid

H02.112 Cicatricial ectropion of right lower eyelid

H02.113 Cicatricial ectropion of right eye, unspecified eyelid

H02.114 Cicatricial ectropion of left upper eyelid

H02.115 Cicatricial ectropion of left lower eyelid

H02.116 Cicatricial ectropion of left eye, unspecified eyelid

H02.119 Cicatricial ectropion of unspecified eye, unspecified eyelid

✓6ᵗʰ **H02.12** Mechanical ectropion of eyelid

H02.121 Mechanical ectropion of right upper eyelid

H02.122 Mechanical ectropion of right lower eyelid

H02.123 Mechanical ectropion of right eye, unspecified eyelid

H02.124 Mechanical ectropion of left upper eyelid

H02.125 Mechanical ectropion of left lower eyelid

H02.126 Mechanical ectropion of left eye, unspecified eyelid

H02.129 Mechanical ectropion of unspecified eye, unspecified eyelid

✓6ᵗʰ **H02.13** Senile ectropion of eyelid

H02.131 Senile ectropion of right upper eyelid 🅐

H02.132 Senile ectropion of right lower eyelid 🅐

H02.133 Senile ectropion of right eye, unspecified eyelid 🅐

H02.134 Senile ectropion of left upper eyelid 🅐

H02.135 Senile ectropion of left lower eyelid 🅐

H02.136 Senile ectropion of left eye, unspecified eyelid 🅐

H02.139 Senile ectropion of unspecified eye, unspecified eyelid 🅐

✓6ᵗʰ **H02.14** Spastic ectropion of eyelid

H02.141 Spastic ectropion of right upper eyelid

H02.142 Spastic ectropion of right lower eyelid

H02.143 Spastic ectropion of right eye, unspecified eyelid

H02.144 Spastic ectropion of left upper eyelid

H02.145 Spastic ectropion of left lower eyelid

H02.146 Spastic ectropion of left eye, unspecified eyelid

H02.149 Spastic ectropion of unspecified eye, unspecified eyelid

✓6ᵗʰ **H02.15** Paralytic ectropion of eyelid

AHA: 2018,4Q,13

H02.151 Paralytic ectropion of right upper eyelid

H02.152 Paralytic ectropion of right lower eyelid

H02.153 Paralytic ectropion of right eye, unspecified eyelid

H02.154 Paralytic ectropion of left upper eyelid

H02.155 Paralytic ectropion of left lower eyelid

H02.156 Paralytic ectropion of left eye, unspecified eyelid

H02.159 Paralytic ectropion of unspecified eye, unspecified eyelid

✓5ᵗʰ **H02.2** Lagophthalmos

AHA: 2018,4Q,14

DEF: Condition of the eye that prevents it from closing completely.

✓6ᵗʰ **H02.20** Unspecified lagophthalmos

H02.201 Unspecified lagophthalmos right upper eyelid

H02.202 Unspecified lagophthalmos right lower eyelid

H02.203 Unspecified lagophthalmos right eye, unspecified eyelid

H02.204 Unspecified lagophthalmos left upper eyelid

H02.205 Unspecified lagophthalmos left lower eyelid

H02.206 Unspecified lagophthalmos left eye, unspecified eyelid

H02.209 Unspecified lagophthalmos unspecified eye, unspecified eyelid

H02.20A Unspecified lagophthalmos right eye, upper and lower eyelids

H02.20B Unspecified lagophthalmos left eye, upper and lower eyelids

H02.20C Unspecified lagophthalmos, bilateral, upper and lower eyelids

✓6ᵗʰ **H02.21** Cicatricial lagophthalmos

H02.211 Cicatricial lagophthalmos right upper eyelid

H02.212 Cicatricial lagophthalmos right lower eyelid

H02.213 Cicatricial lagophthalmos right eye, unspecified eyelid

H02.214 Cicatricial lagophthalmos left upper eyelid

H02.215 Cicatricial lagophthalmos left lower eyelid

H02.216 Cicatricial lagophthalmos left eye, unspecified eyelid

H02.219 Cicatricial lagophthalmos unspecified eye, unspecified eyelid

H02.21A Cicatricial lagophthalmos right eye, upper and lower eyelids

H02.21B Cicatricial lagophthalmos left eye, upper and lower eyelids

H02.21C Cicatricial lagophthalmos, bilateral, upper and lower eyelids

✓6ᵗʰ **H02.22** Mechanical lagophthalmos

H02.221 Mechanical lagophthalmos right upper eyelid

H02.222 Mechanical lagophthalmos right lower eyelid

H02.223 Mechanical lagophthalmos right eye, unspecified eyelid

H02.224 Mechanical lagophthalmos left upper eyelid

H02.225 Mechanical lagophthalmos left lower eyelid

H02.226 Mechanical lagophthalmos left eye, unspecified eyelid

H02.229 Mechanical lagophthalmos unspecified eye, unspecified eyelid

H02.22A Mechanical lagophthalmos right eye, upper and lower eyelids

H02.22B Mechanical lagophthalmos left eye, upper and lower eyelids

H02.22C Mechanical lagophthalmos, bilateral, upper and lower eyelids

✓6ᵗʰ **H02.23** Paralytic lagophthalmos

H02.231 Paralytic lagophthalmos right upper eyelid

H02.232 Paralytic lagophthalmos right lower eyelid

H02.233 Paralytic lagophthalmos right eye, unspecified eyelid

H02.234 Paralytic lagophthalmos left upper eyelid

H02.235 Paralytic lagophthalmos left lower eyelid

H02.236 Paralytic lagophthalmos left eye, unspecified eyelid

H02.239 Paralytic lagophthalmos unspecified eye, unspecified eyelid

H02.23A Paralytic lagophthalmos right eye, upper and lower eyelids

H02.23B Paralytic lagophthalmos left eye, upper and lower eyelids

H02.23C Paralytic lagophthalmos, bilateral, upper and lower eyelids

✓5ᵗʰ **H02.3** Blepharochalasis

Pseudoptosis

DEF: Loss of elasticity and relaxation of skin of the eyelid, thickened or indurated skin on the eyelid associated with recurrent episodes of edema, and intracellular atrophy.

H02.30 Blepharochalasis unspecified eye, unspecified eyelid

H02.31 Blepharochalasis right upper eyelid

H02.32 Blepharochalasis right lower eyelid

H02.33 Blepharochalasis right eye, unspecified eyelid

H02.34 Blepharochalasis left upper eyelid

H02.35   **Blepharochalasis** left lower **eyelid**
H02.36   **Blepharochalasis** left eye, unspecified **eyelid**

✓5ᵗʰ **H02.4   Ptosis of eyelid**

  ✓6ᵗʰ **H02.40   Unspecified ptosis of eyelid**

    H02.401   **Unspecified ptosis of** right **eyelid**
    H02.402   **Unspecified ptosis of** left **eyelid**
    H02.403   **Unspecified ptosis of** bilateral **eyelids**
    H02.409   **Unspecified ptosis of** unspecified **eyelid**

  ✓6ᵗʰ **H02.41   Mechanical ptosis of eyelid**

    H02.411   **Mechanical ptosis of** right **eyelid**
    H02.412   **Mechanical ptosis of** left **eyelid**
    H02.413   **Mechanical ptosis of** bilateral **eyelids**
    H02.419   **Mechanical ptosis of** unspecified **eyelid**

  ✓6ᵗʰ **H02.42   Myogenic ptosis of eyelid**

    H02.421   **Myogenic ptosis of** right **eyelid**
    H02.422   **Myogenic ptosis of** left **eyelid**
    H02.423   **Myogenic ptosis of** bilateral **eyelids**
    H02.429   **Myogenic ptosis of** unspecified **eyelid**

  ✓6ᵗʰ **H02.43   Paralytic ptosis of eyelid**

    Neurogenic ptosis of eyelid
    H02.431   **Paralytic ptosis of** right **eyelid**
    H02.432   **Paralytic ptosis of** left **eyelid**
    H02.433   **Paralytic ptosis of** bilateral **eyelids**
    H02.439   **Paralytic ptosis** unspecified **eyelid**

✓5ᵗʰ **H02.5   Other disorders affecting eyelid function**

    EXCLUDES 2   *blepharospasm (G24.5)*
      organic tic (G25.69)
      psychogenic tic (F95.-)

  ✓6ᵗʰ **H02.51   Abnormal innervation syndrome**

    H02.511   **Abnormal innervation syndrome** right upper **eyelid**
    H02.512   **Abnormal innervation syndrome** right lower **eyelid**
    H02.513   **Abnormal innervation syndrome** right eye, unspecified **eyelid**
    H02.514   **Abnormal innervation syndrome** left upper **eyelid**
    H02.515   **Abnormal innervation syndrome** left lower **eyelid**
    H02.516   **Abnormal innervation syndrome** left eye, unspecified **eyelid**
    H02.519   **Abnormal innervation syndrome** unspecified eye, unspecified **eyelid**

  ✓6ᵗʰ **H02.52   Blepharophimosis**

    Ankyloblepharon
    H02.521   **Blepharophimosis** right upper **eyelid**
    H02.522   **Blepharophimosis** right lower **eyelid**
    H02.523   **Blepharophimosis** right eye, unspecified **eyelid**
    H02.524   **Blepharophimosis** left upper **eyelid**
    H02.525   **Blepharophimosis** left lower **eyelid**
    H02.526   **Blepharophimosis** left eye, unspecified **eyelid**
    H02.529   **Blepharophimosis** unspecified eye, unspecified **lid**

  ✓6ᵗʰ **H02.53   Eyelid retraction**

    Eyelid lag
    H02.531   **Eyelid retraction** right upper **eyelid**
    H02.532   **Eyelid retraction** right lower **eyelid**
    H02.533   **Eyelid retraction** right eye, unspecified **eyelid**
    H02.534   **Eyelid retraction** left upper **eyelid**
    H02.535   **Eyelid retraction** left lower **eyelid**
    H02.536   **Eyelid retraction** left eye, unspecified **eyelid**
    H02.539   **Eyelid retraction** unspecified eye, unspecified **lid**

    H02.59   **Other disorders affecting eyelid function**
      Deficient blink reflex
      Sensory disorders

✓5ᵗʰ **H02.6   Xanthelasma of eyelid**

    DEF: Condition in which there are small yellow tumors that occur on the eyelid, usually appearing near the nose.

    H02.60   **Xanthelasma of** unspecified eye, unspecified **eyelid**
    H02.61   **Xanthelasma of** right upper **eyelid**
    H02.62   **Xanthelasma of** right lower **eyelid**
    H02.63   **Xanthelasma of** right eye, unspecified **eyelid**
    H02.64   **Xanthelasma of** left upper **eyelid**

H02.65   **Xanthelasma of** left lower **eyelid**
H02.66   **Xanthelasma of** left eye, unspecified **eyelid**

✓5ᵗʰ **H02.7   Other and unspecified degenerative disorders of eyelid and periocular area**

    H02.70   **Unspecified degenerative disorders of eyelid and periocular area**

  ✓6ᵗʰ **H02.71   Chloasma of eyelid and periocular area**

    Dyspigmentation of eyelid
    Hyperpigmentation of eyelid
    H02.711   **Chloasma of** right upper **eyelid and periocular area**
    H02.712   **Chloasma of** right lower **eyelid and periocular area**
    H02.713   **Chloasma of** right eye, unspecified **eyelid and periocular area**
    H02.714   **Chloasma of** left upper **eyelid and periocular area**
    H02.715   **Chloasma of** left lower **eyelid and periocular area**
    H02.716   **Chloasma of** left eye, unspecified **eyelid and periocular area**
    H02.719   **Chloasma of** unspecified eye, unspecified **eyelid and periocular area**

  ✓6ᵗʰ **H02.72   Madarosis of eyelid and periocular area**

    Hypotrichosis of eyelid
    H02.721   **Madarosis of** right upper **eyelid and periocular area**
    H02.722   **Madarosis of** right lower **eyelid and periocular area**
    H02.723   **Madarosis of** right eye, unspecified **eyelid and periocular area**
    H02.724   **Madarosis of** left upper **eyelid and periocular area**
    H02.725   **Madarosis of** left lower **eyelid and periocular area**
    H02.726   **Madarosis of** left eye, unspecified **eyelid and periocular area**
    H02.729   **Madarosis of** unspecified eye, unspecified **eyelid and periocular area**

  ✓6ᵗʰ **H02.73   Vitiligo of eyelid and periocular area**

    Hypopigmentation of eyelid
    H02.731   **Vitiligo of** right upper **eyelid and periocular area**
    H02.732   **Vitiligo of** right lower **eyelid and periocular area**
    H02.733   **Vitiligo of** right eye, unspecified **eyelid and periocular area**
    H02.734   **Vitiligo of** left upper **eyelid and periocular area**
    H02.735   **Vitiligo of** left lower **eyelid and periocular area**
    H02.736   **Vitiligo of** left eye, unspecified **eyelid and periocular area**
    H02.739   **Vitiligo of** unspecified eye, unspecified **eyelid and periocular area**

    H02.79   **Other degenerative disorders of eyelid and periocular area**

✓5ᵗʰ **H02.8   Other specified disorders of eyelid**

  ✓6ᵗʰ **H02.81   Retained foreign body in eyelid**

    Use additional code to identify the type of retained foreign body (Z18.-)
    EXCLUDES 1   *laceration of eyelid with foreign body (S01.12-)*
      retained intraocular foreign body (H44.6-, H44.7-)
      superficial foreign body of eyelid and periocular area (S00.25-)
    H02.811   **Retained foreign body in** right upper **eyelid**
    H02.812   **Retained foreign body in** right lower **eyelid**
    H02.813   **Retained foreign body in** right eye, unspecified **eyelid**
    H02.814   **Retained foreign body in** left upper **eyelid**
    H02.815   **Retained foreign body in** left lower **eyelid**
    H02.816   **Retained foreign body in** left eye, unspecified **eyelid**
    H02.819   **Retained foreign body in** unspecified eye, unspecified **eyelid**

☑ Additional Character Required   ✓ₓ7ᵗʰ Placeholder Alert   Manifestation   Unspecified Dx   ◄► Revised Text   ● New Code   ▲ Revised Code Title

ICD-10-CM 2020   587

Chapter 7. Diseases of the Eye and Adnexa

H02.82–H04.149

✓6th **H02.82 Cysts** of eyelid

Sebaceous cyst of eyelid

H02.821 Cysts of right upper **eyelid**
H02.822 Cysts of right lower **eyelid**
H02.823 Cysts of right eye, unspecified eyelid
H02.824 Cysts of left upper **eyelid**
H02.825 Cysts of left lower **eyelid**
H02.826 Cysts of left eye, unspecified eyelid
H02.829 Cysts of unspecified eye, unspecified **eyelid**

✓6th **H02.83 Dermatochalasis** of eyelid

DEF: Acquired form of connective tissue disorder associated with decreased elastic tissue and abnormal elastin formation, resulting in loss of elasticity of the skin of the eyelid. It is generally associated with aging.

H02.831 Dermatochalasis of right upper **eyelid**
H02.832 Dermatochalasis of right lower **eyelid**
H02.833 Dermatochalasis of right eye, unspecified eyelid
H02.834 Dermatochalasis of left upper **eyelid**
H02.835 Dermatochalasis of left lower **eyelid**
H02.836 Dermatochalasis of left eye, unspecified eyelid
H02.839 Dermatochalasis of unspecified eye, unspecified eyelid

✓6th **H02.84 Edema** of eyelid

Hyperemia of eyelid

H02.841 Edema of right upper **eyelid**
H02.842 Edema of right lower **eyelid**
H02.843 Edema of right eye, unspecified eyelid
H02.844 Edema of left upper **eyelid**
H02.845 Edema of left lower **eyelid**
H02.846 Edema of left eye, unspecified eyelid
H02.849 Edema of unspecified eye, unspecified eyelid

✓6th **H02.85 Elephantiasis** of eyelid

H02.851 Elephantiasis of right upper **eyelid**
H02.852 Elephantiasis of right lower **eyelid**
H02.853 Elephantiasis of right eye, unspecified eyelid
H02.854 Elephantiasis of left upper **eyelid**
H02.855 Elephantiasis of left lower **eyelid**
H02.856 Elephantiasis of left eye, unspecified eyelid
H02.859 Elephantiasis of unspecified eye, unspecified eyelid

✓6th **H02.86 Hypertrichosis** of eyelid

H02.861 Hypertrichosis of right upper **eyelid**
H02.862 Hypertrichosis of right lower **eyelid**
H02.863 Hypertrichosis of right eye, unspecified eyelid
H02.864 Hypertrichosis of left upper **eyelid**
H02.865 Hypertrichosis of left lower **eyelid**
H02.866 Hypertrichosis of left eye, unspecified eyelid
H02.869 Hypertrichosis of unspecified eye, unspecified eyelid

✓6th **H02.87 Vascular anomalies** of eyelid

H02.871 Vascular anomalies of right upper **eyelid**
H02.872 Vascular anomalies of right lower **eyelid**
H02.873 Vascular anomalies of right eye, unspecified eyelid
H02.874 Vascular anomalies of left upper **eyelid**
H02.875 Vascular anomalies of left lower **eyelid**
H02.876 Vascular anomalies of left eye, unspecified eyelid
H02.879 Vascular anomalies of unspecified eye, unspecified eyelid

✓6th **H02.88 Meibomian gland dysfunction** of eyelid

AHA: 2018,4Q,14-15

H02.881 Meibomian gland dysfunction right upper **eyelid**
H02.882 Meibomian gland dysfunction right lower **eyelid**
H02.883 Meibomian gland dysfunction of right eye, unspecified eyelid
H02.884 Meibomian gland dysfunction left upper **eyelid**
H02.885 Meibomian gland dysfunction left lower **eyelid**

H02.886 Meibomian gland dysfunction of left eye, unspecified eyelid
H02.889 Meibomian gland dysfunction of unspecified eye, unspecified eyelid
H02.88A Meibomian gland dysfunction right eye, upper and lower **eyelids**
H02.88B Meibomian gland dysfunction left eye, upper and lower **eyelids**

H02.89 Other specified disorders of eyelid

Hemorrhage of eyelid

H02.9 Unspecified disorder of eyelid

Disorder of eyelid NOS

✓4th **H04 Disorders of lacrimal system**

EXCLUDES 1 congenital malformations of lacrimal system (Q10.4-Q10.6)

✓5th **H04.0 Dacryoadenitis**

DEF: Inflammation of the lacrimal gland.

✓6th **H04.00 Unspecified dacryoadenitis**

H04.001 Unspecified dacryoadenitis, right **lacrimal gland**
H04.002 Unspecified dacryoadenitis, left **lacrimal gland**
H04.003 Unspecified dacryoadenitis, bilateral **lacrimal glands**
H04.009 Unspecified dacryoadenitis, unspecified **lacrimal gland**

✓6th **H04.01 Acute dacryoadenitis**

H04.011 Acute dacryoadenitis, right **lacrimal gland**
H04.012 Acute dacryoadenitis, left **lacrimal gland**
H04.013 Acute dacryoadenitis, bilateral **lacrimal glands**
H04.019 Acute dacryoadenitis, unspecified **lacrimal gland**

✓6th **H04.02 Chronic dacryoadenitis**

H04.021 Chronic dacryoadenitis, right **lacrimal gland**
H04.022 Chronic dacryoadenitis, left **lacrimal gland**
H04.023 Chronic dacryoadenitis, bilateral **lacrimal gland**
H04.029 Chronic dacryoadenitis, unspecified **lacrimal gland**

✓6th **H04.03 Chronic enlargement of lacrimal gland**

H04.031 Chronic enlargement of right **lacrimal gland**
H04.032 Chronic enlargement of left **lacrimal gland**
H04.033 Chronic enlargement of bilateral **lacrimal glands**
H04.039 Chronic enlargement of unspecified **lacrimal gland**

✓5th **H04.1 Other disorders of lacrimal gland**

✓6th **H04.11 Dacryops**

H04.111 Dacryops of right **lacrimal gland**
H04.112 Dacryops of left **lacrimal gland**
H04.113 Dacryops of bilateral **lacrimal glands**
H04.119 Dacryops of unspecified **lacrimal gland**

✓6th **H04.12 Dry eye syndrome**

Tear film insufficiency, NOS

H04.121 Dry eye syndrome of right **lacrimal gland**
H04.122 Dry eye syndrome of left **lacrimal gland**
H04.123 Dry eye syndrome of bilateral **lacrimal glands**
H04.129 Dry eye syndrome of unspecified **lacrimal gland**

✓6th **H04.13 Lacrimal cyst**

Lacrimal cystic degeneration

H04.131 Lacrimal cyst, right **lacrimal gland**
H04.132 Lacrimal cyst, left **lacrimal gland**
H04.133 Lacrimal cyst, bilateral **lacrimal glands**
H04.139 Lacrimal cyst, unspecified **lacrimal gland**

✓6th **H04.14 Primary lacrimal gland atrophy**

H04.141 Primary lacrimal gland atrophy, right **lacrimal gland**
H04.142 Primary lacrimal gland atrophy, left **lacrimal gland**
H04.143 Primary lacrimal gland atrophy, bilateral **lacrimal glands**
H04.149 Primary lacrimal gland atrophy, unspecified **lacrimal gland**

✓6ᵗʰ H04.15   Secondary lacrimal gland atrophy

     H04.151   Secondary lacrimal gland atrophy, right lacrimal gland

     H04.152   Secondary lacrimal gland atrophy, left lacrimal gland

     H04.153   Secondary lacrimal gland atrophy, bilateral lacrimal glands

     H04.159   Secondary lacrimal gland atrophy, unspecified lacrimal gland

✓6ᵗʰ H04.16   Lacrimal gland dislocation

     H04.161   Lacrimal gland dislocation, right lacrimal gland

     H04.162   Lacrimal gland dislocation, left lacrimal gland

     H04.163   Lacrimal gland dislocation, bilateral lacrimal glands

     H04.169   Lacrimal gland dislocation, unspecified lacrimal gland

     H04.19   Other specified disorders of lacrimal gland

✓5ᵗʰ H04.2   Epiphora

     DEF: Excessive tearing or overflow of tears down the cheeks often due to a stricture in the lacrimal passages but can be caused by other conditions.

   ✓6ᵗʰ H04.20   Unspecified epiphora

     H04.201   Unspecified epiphora, right side

     H04.202   Unspecified epiphora, left side

     H04.203   Unspecified epiphora, bilateral

     H04.209   Unspecified epiphora, unspecified side

   ✓6ᵗʰ H04.21   Epiphora due to excess lacrimation

     H04.211   Epiphora due to excess lacrimation, right lacrimal gland

     H04.212   Epiphora due to excess lacrimation, left lacrimal gland

     H04.213   Epiphora due to excess lacrimation, bilateral lacrimal glands

     H04.219   Epiphora due to excess lacrimation, unspecified lacrimal gland

   ✓6ᵗʰ H04.22   Epiphora due to insufficient drainage

     H04.221   Epiphora due to insufficient drainage, right side

     H04.222   Epiphora due to insufficient drainage, left side

     H04.223   Epiphora due to insufficient drainage, bilateral

     H04.229   Epiphora due to insufficient drainage, unspecified side

✓5ᵗʰ H04.3   Acute and unspecified inflammation of lacrimal passages

     EXCLUDES 1   neonatal dacryocystitis (P39.1)

   ✓6ᵗʰ H04.30   Unspecified dacryocystitis

     H04.301   Unspecified dacryocystitis of right lacrimal passage

     H04.302   Unspecified dacryocystitis of left lacrimal passage

     H04.303   Unspecified dacryocystitis of bilateral lacrimal passages

     H04.309   Unspecified dacryocystitis of unspecified lacrimal passage

   ✓6ᵗʰ H04.31   Phlegmonous dacryocystitis

     H04.311   Phlegmonous dacryocystitis of right lacrimal passage

     H04.312   Phlegmonous dacryocystitis of left lacrimal passage

     H04.313   Phlegmonous dacryocystitis of bilateral lacrimal passages

     H04.319   Phlegmonous dacryocystitis of unspecified lacrimal passage

   ✓6ᵗʰ H04.32   Acute dacryocystitis

     Acute dacryopericystitis

     H04.321   Acute dacryocystitis of right lacrimal passage

     H04.322   Acute dacryocystitis of left lacrimal passage

     H04.323   Acute dacryocystitis of bilateral lacrimal passages

     H04.329   Acute dacryocystitis of unspecified lacrimal passage

   ✓6ᵗʰ H04.33   Acute lacrimal canaliculitis

     H04.331   Acute lacrimal canaliculitis of right lacrimal passage

     H04.332   Acute lacrimal canaliculitis of left lacrimal passage

     H04.333   Acute lacrimal canaliculitis of bilateral lacrimal passages

     H04.339   Acute lacrimal canaliculitis of unspecified lacrimal passage

✓5ᵗʰ H04.4   Chronic inflammation of lacrimal passages

   ✓6ᵗʰ H04.41   Chronic dacryocystitis

     H04.411   Chronic dacryocystitis of right lacrimal passage

     H04.412   Chronic dacryocystitis of left lacrimal passage

     H04.413   Chronic dacryocystitis of bilateral lacrimal passages

     H04.419   Chronic dacryocystitis of unspecified lacrimal passage

   ✓6ᵗʰ H04.42   Chronic lacrimal canaliculitis

     H04.421   Chronic lacrimal canaliculitis of right lacrimal passage

     H04.422   Chronic lacrimal canaliculitis of left lacrimal passage

     H04.423   Chronic lacrimal canaliculitis of bilateral lacrimal passages

     H04.429   Chronic lacrimal canaliculitis of unspecified lacrimal passage

   ✓6ᵗʰ H04.43   Chronic lacrimal mucocele

     H04.431   Chronic lacrimal mucocele of right lacrimal passage

     H04.432   Chronic lacrimal mucocele of left lacrimal passage

     H04.433   Chronic lacrimal mucocele of bilateral lacrimal passages

     H04.439   Chronic lacrimal mucocele of unspecified lacrimal passage

✓5ᵗʰ H04.5   Stenosis and insufficiency of lacrimal passages

   ✓6ᵗʰ H04.51   Dacryolith

     H04.511   Dacryolith of right lacrimal passage

     H04.512   Dacryolith of left lacrimal passage

     H04.513   Dacryolith of bilateral lacrimal passages

     H04.519   Dacryolith of unspecified lacrimal passage

   ✓6ᵗʰ H04.52   Eversion of lacrimal punctum

     H04.521   Eversion of right lacrimal punctum

     H04.522   Eversion of left lacrimal punctum

     H04.523   Eversion of bilateral lacrimal punctum

     H04.529   Eversion of unspecified lacrimal punctum

   ✓6ᵗʰ H04.53   Neonatal obstruction of nasolacrimal duct

     EXCLUDES 1   congenital stenosis and stricture of lacrimal duct (Q10.5)

     H04.531   Neonatal obstruction of right nasolacrimal duct   Ⓝ

     H04.532   Neonatal obstruction of left nasolacrimal duct   Ⓝ

     H04.533   Neonatal obstruction of bilateral nasolacrimal duct   Ⓝ

     H04.539   Neonatal obstruction of unspecified nasolacrimal duct   Ⓝ

   ✓6ᵗʰ H04.54   Stenosis of lacrimal canaliculi

     H04.541   Stenosis of right lacrimal canaliculi

     H04.542   Stenosis of left lacrimal canaliculi

     H04.543   Stenosis of bilateral lacrimal canaliculi

     H04.549   Stenosis of unspecified lacrimal canaliculi

   ✓6ᵗʰ H04.55   Acquired stenosis of nasolacrimal duct

     H04.551   Acquired stenosis of right nasolacrimal duct

     H04.552   Acquired stenosis of left nasolacrimal duct

     H04.553   Acquired stenosis of bilateral nasolacrimal duct

     H04.559   Acquired stenosis of unspecified nasolacrimal duct

   ✓6ᵗʰ H04.56   Stenosis of lacrimal punctum

     H04.561   Stenosis of right lacrimal punctum

     H04.562   Stenosis of left lacrimal punctum

     H04.563   Stenosis of bilateral lacrimal punctum

     H04.569   Stenosis of unspecified lacrimal punctum

   ✓6ᵗʰ H04.57   Stenosis of lacrimal sac

     H04.571   Stenosis of right lacrimal sac

     H04.572   Stenosis of left lacrimal sac

✅ Additional Character Required   ✓×7ᵗʰ Placeholder Alert   Manifestation   Unspecified Dx   ►◄ Revised Text   ● New Code   ▲ Revised Code Title

    H04.573 **Stenosis of** bilateral **lacrimal sac**
    H04.579 **Stenosis of unspecified lacrimal sac**

✓5ᵗʰ **H04.6** **Other changes of lacrimal passages**

  ✓6ᵗʰ **H04.61** **Lacrimal** fistula

    H04.611 **Lacrimal fistula** right **lacrimal passage**
    H04.612 **Lacrimal fistula** left **lacrimal passage**
    H04.613 **Lacrimal fistula** bilateral **lacrimal passages**
    H04.619 **Lacrimal fistula unspecified lacrimal passage**

  H04.69 **Other changes of lacrimal passages**

✓5ᵗʰ **H04.8** **Other disorders of lacrimal system**

  ✓6ᵗʰ **H04.81** **Granuloma of lacrimal passages**

    H04.811 **Granuloma of** right **lacrimal passage**
    H04.812 **Granuloma of** left **lacrimal passage**
    H04.813 **Granuloma of** bilateral **lacrimal passages**
    H04.819 **Granuloma of unspecified lacrimal passage**

  H04.89 **Other disorders of lacrimal system**

H04.9 **Disorder of lacrimal system, unspecified**

✓4ᵗʰ **H05** **Disorders of orbit**

  EXCLUDES 1   congenital malformation of orbit (Q10.7)

  ✓5ᵗʰ **H05.0** **Acute inflammation of orbit**

    H05.00 **Unspecified acute inflammation of orbit**

    ✓6ᵗʰ **H05.01** **Cellulitis of orbit**

      Abscess of orbit
      H05.011 **Cellulitis of** right **orbit**
      H05.012 **Cellulitis of** left **orbit**
      H05.013 **Cellulitis of** bilateral **orbits**
      H05.019 **Cellulitis of unspecified orbit**

    ✓6ᵗʰ **H05.02** **Osteomyelitis of orbit**

      H05.021 **Osteomyelitis of** right **orbit**
      H05.022 **Osteomyelitis of** left **orbit**
      H05.023 **Osteomyelitis of** bilateral **orbits**
      H05.029 **Osteomyelitis of unspecified orbit**

    ✓6ᵗʰ **H05.03** **Periostitis of orbit**

      H05.031 **Periostitis of** right **orbit**
      H05.032 **Periostitis of** left **orbit**
      H05.033 **Periostitis of** bilateral **orbits**
      H05.039 **Periostitis of unspecified orbit**

    ✓6ᵗʰ **H05.04** **Tenonitis of orbit**

      H05.041 **Tenonitis of** right **orbit**
      H05.042 **Tenonitis of** left **orbit**
      H05.043 **Tenonitis of** bilateral **orbits**
      H05.049 **Tenonitis of unspecified orbit**

  ✓5ᵗʰ **H05.1** **Chronic inflammatory disorders of orbit**

    H05.10 **Unspecified chronic inflammatory disorders of orbit**

    ✓6ᵗʰ **H05.11** **Granuloma of orbit**

      Pseudotumor (inflammatory) of orbit
      H05.111 **Granuloma of** right **orbit**
      H05.112 **Granuloma of** left **orbit**
      H05.113 **Granuloma of** bilateral **orbits**
      H05.119 **Granuloma of unspecified orbit**

    ✓6ᵗʰ **H05.12** **Orbital** myositis

      H05.121 **Orbital myositis,** right **orbit**
      H05.122 **Orbital myositis,** left **orbit**
      H05.123 **Orbital myositis,** bilateral
      H05.129 **Orbital myositis, unspecified orbit**

  ✓5ᵗʰ **H05.2** **Exophthalmic conditions**

    H05.20 **Unspecified exophthalmos**

    ✓6ᵗʰ **H05.21** **Displacement (lateral) of globe**

      H05.211 **Displacement (lateral) of globe,** right **eye**
      H05.212 **Displacement (lateral) of globe,** left **eye**
      H05.213 **Displacement (lateral) of globe,** bilateral
      H05.219 **Displacement (lateral) of globe, unspecified eye**

    ✓6ᵗʰ **H05.22** **Edema of orbit**

      Orbital congestion
      H05.221 **Edema of** right **orbit**
      H05.222 **Edema of** left **orbit**
      H05.223 **Edema of** bilateral **orbit**
      H05.229 **Edema of unspecified orbit**

    ✓6ᵗʰ **H05.23** **Hemorrhage of orbit**

      H05.231 **Hemorrhage of** right **orbit**
      H05.232 **Hemorrhage of** left **orbit**

      H05.233 **Hemorrhage of** bilateral **orbit**
      H05.239 **Hemorrhage of unspecified orbit**

    ✓6ᵗʰ **H05.24** **Constant exophthalmos**

      H05.241 **Constant exophthalmos,** right **eye**
      H05.242 **Constant exophthalmos,** left **eye**
      H05.243 **Constant exophthalmos,** bilateral
      H05.249 **Constant exophthalmos, unspecified eye**

    ✓6ᵗʰ **H05.25** **Intermittent exophthalmos**

      H05.251 **Intermittent exophthalmos,** right **eye**
      H05.252 **Intermittent exophthalmos,** left **eye**
      H05.253 **Intermittent exophthalmos,** bilateral
      H05.259 **Intermittent exophthalmos, unspecified eye**

    ✓6ᵗʰ **H05.26** **Pulsating exophthalmos**

      H05.261 **Pulsating exophthalmos,** right **eye**
      H05.262 **Pulsating exophthalmos,** left **eye**
      H05.263 **Pulsating exophthalmos,** bilateral
      H05.269 **Pulsating exophthalmos, unspecified eye**

  ✓5ᵗʰ **H05.3** **Deformity of orbit**

    EXCLUDES 1   congenital deformity of orbit (Q10.7)
                hypertelorism (Q75.2)

    H05.30 **Unspecified deformity of orbit**

    ✓6ᵗʰ **H05.31** **Atrophy of orbit**

      H05.311 **Atrophy of** right **orbit**
      H05.312 **Atrophy of** left **orbit**
      H05.313 **Atrophy of** bilateral **orbit**
      H05.319 **Atrophy of unspecified orbit**

    ✓6ᵗʰ **H05.32** **Deformity of orbit** due to bone disease

      Code also associated bone disease
      H05.321 **Deformity of** right **orbit due to bone disease**
      H05.322 **Deformity of** left **orbit due to bone disease**
      H05.323 **Deformity of** bilateral **orbits due to bone disease**
      H05.329 **Deformity of unspecified orbit due to bone disease**

    ✓6ᵗʰ **H05.33** **Deformity of orbit** due to trauma or surgery

      H05.331 **Deformity of** right **orbit due to trauma or surgery**
      H05.332 **Deformity of** left **orbit due to trauma or surgery**
      H05.333 **Deformity of** bilateral **orbits due to trauma or surgery**
      H05.339 **Deformity of unspecified orbit due to trauma or surgery**

    ✓6ᵗʰ **H05.34** **Enlargement of orbit**

      H05.341 **Enlargement of** right **orbit**
      H05.342 **Enlargement of** left **orbit**
      H05.343 **Enlargement of** bilateral **orbits**
      H05.349 **Enlargement of unspecified orbit**

    ✓6ᵗʰ **H05.35** **Exostosis of orbit**

      H05.351 **Exostosis of** right **orbit**
      H05.352 **Exostosis of** left **orbit**
      H05.353 **Exostosis of** bilateral **orbits**
      H05.359 **Exostosis of unspecified orbit**

  ✓5ᵗʰ **H05.4** **Enophthalmos**

    ✓6ᵗʰ **H05.40** **Unspecified enophthalmos**

      H05.401 **Unspecified enophthalmos,** right **eye**
      H05.402 **Unspecified enophthalmos,** left **eye**
      H05.403 **Unspecified enophthalmos,** bilateral
      H05.409 **Unspecified enophthalmos, unspecified eye**

    ✓6ᵗʰ **H05.41** **Enophthalmos** due to atrophy of orbital tissue

      H05.411 **Enophthalmos due to atrophy of orbital tissue,** right **eye**
      H05.412 **Enophthalmos due to atrophy of orbital tissue,** left **eye**
      H05.413 **Enophthalmos due to atrophy of orbital tissue,** bilateral
      H05.419 **Enophthalmos due to atrophy of orbital tissue, unspecified eye**

    ✓6ᵗʰ **H05.42** **Enophthalmos** due to trauma or surgery

      H05.421 **Enophthalmos due to trauma or surgery,** right **eye**
      H05.422 **Enophthalmos due to trauma or surgery,** left **eye**

H05.423 Enophthalmos due to trauma or surgery, bilateral

H05.429 Enophthalmos due to trauma or surgery, unspecified eye

✓5ᵗʰ **H05.5** **Retained (old) foreign body following penetrating wound of orbit**

　Retrobulbar foreign body

　Use additional code to identify the type of retained foreign body (Z18.-)

　EXCLUDES 1　*current penetrating wound of orbit (S05.4-)*

　EXCLUDES 2　*retained foreign body of eyelid (H02.81-)*

　　　　　　　retained intraocular foreign body (H44.6-, H44.7-)

　H05.50 **Retained (old) foreign body following penetrating wound of unspecified orbit**

　H05.51 **Retained (old) foreign body following penetrating wound of right orbit**

　H05.52 **Retained (old) foreign body following penetrating wound of left orbit**

　H05.53 **Retained (old) foreign body following penetrating wound of bilateral orbits**

✓5ᵗʰ **H05.8** **Other disorders of orbit**

　✓6ᵗʰ **H05.81** **Cyst of orbit**

　　Encephalocele of orbit

　　H05.811 Cyst of right orbit

　　H05.812 Cyst of left orbit

　　H05.813 Cyst of bilateral orbits

　　H05.819 Cyst of unspecified orbit

　✓6ᵗʰ **H05.82** **Myopathy of extraocular muscles**

　　H05.821 Myopathy of extraocular muscles, right orbit

　　H05.822 Myopathy of extraocular muscles, left orbit

　　H05.823 Myopathy of extraocular muscles, bilateral

　　H05.829 Myopathy of extraocular muscles, unspecified orbit

　H05.89 Other disorders of orbit

H05.9 **Unspecified disorder of orbit**

Disorders of conjunctiva (H10-H11)

✓4ᵗʰ **H10** **Conjunctivitis**

　EXCLUDES 1　*keratoconjunctivitis (H16.2-)*

✓5ᵗʰ **H10.0** **Mucopurulent conjunctivitis**

　✓6ᵗʰ **H10.01** **Acute follicular conjunctivitis**

　　H10.011 Acute follicular conjunctivitis, right eye

　　H10.012 Acute follicular conjunctivitis, left eye

　　H10.013 Acute follicular conjunctivitis, bilateral

　　H10.019 Acute follicular conjunctivitis, unspecified eye

　✓6ᵗʰ **H10.02** **Other mucopurulent conjunctivitis**

　　H10.021 Other mucopurulent conjunctivitis, right eye

　　H10.022 Other mucopurulent conjunctivitis, left eye

　　H10.023 Other mucopurulent conjunctivitis, bilateral

　　H10.029 Other mucopurulent conjunctivitis, unspecified eye

✓5ᵗʰ **H10.1** **Acute atopic conjunctivitis**

　Acute papillary conjunctivitis

　H10.10 Acute atopic conjunctivitis, unspecified eye

　H10.11 Acute atopic conjunctivitis, right eye

　H10.12 Acute atopic conjunctivitis, left eye

　H10.13 Acute atopic conjunctivitis, bilateral

✓5ᵗʰ **H10.2** **Other acute conjunctivitis**

　✓6ᵗʰ **H10.21** **Acute toxic conjunctivitis**

　　Acute chemical conjunctivitis

　　Code first (T51-T65) to identify chemical and intent

　　EXCLUDES 1　*burn and corrosion of eye and adnexa (T26.-)*

　　H10.211 Acute toxic conjunctivitis, right eye

　　H10.212 Acute toxic conjunctivitis, left eye

　　H10.213 Acute toxic conjunctivitis, bilateral

　　H10.219 Acute toxic conjunctivitis, unspecified eye

✓6ᵗʰ **H10.22** **Pseudomembranous conjunctivitis**

　H10.221 Pseudomembranous conjunctivitis, right eye

　H10.222 Pseudomembranous conjunctivitis, left eye

　H10.223 Pseudomembranous conjunctivitis, bilateral

　H10.229 Pseudomembranous conjunctivitis, unspecified eye

✓6ᵗʰ **H10.23** **Serous conjunctivitis, except viral**

　EXCLUDES 1　*viral conjunctivitis (B30.-)*

　H10.231 Serous conjunctivitis, except viral, right eye

　H10.232 Serous conjunctivitis, except viral, left eye

　H10.233 Serous conjunctivitis, except viral, bilateral

　H10.239 Serous conjunctivitis, except viral, unspecified eye

✓5ᵗʰ **H10.3** **Unspecified acute conjunctivitis**

　EXCLUDES 1　*ophthalmia neonatorum NOS (P39.1)*

　H10.30 Unspecified acute conjunctivitis, unspecified eye

　H10.31 Unspecified acute conjunctivitis, right eye

　H10.32 Unspecified acute conjunctivitis, left eye

　H10.33 Unspecified acute conjunctivitis, bilateral

✓6ᵗʰ **H10.4** **Chronic conjunctivitis**

　✓6ᵗʰ **H10.40** **Unspecified chronic conjunctivitis**

　　H10.401 Unspecified chronic conjunctivitis, right eye

　　H10.402 Unspecified chronic conjunctivitis, left eye

　　H10.403 Unspecified chronic conjunctivitis, bilateral

　　H10.409 Unspecified chronic conjunctivitis, unspecified eye

　✓6ᵗʰ **H10.41** **Chronic giant papillary conjunctivitis**

　　H10.411 Chronic giant papillary conjunctivitis, right eye

　　H10.412 Chronic giant papillary conjunctivitis, left eye

　　H10.413 Chronic giant papillary conjunctivitis, bilateral

　　H10.419 Chronic giant papillary conjunctivitis, unspecified eye

　✓6ᵗʰ **H10.42** **Simple chronic conjunctivitis**

　　H10.421 Simple chronic conjunctivitis, right eye

　　H10.422 Simple chronic conjunctivitis, left eye

　　H10.423 Simple chronic conjunctivitis, bilateral

　　H10.429 Simple chronic conjunctivitis, unspecified eye

　✓6ᵗʰ **H10.43** **Chronic follicular conjunctivitis**

　　H10.431 Chronic follicular conjunctivitis, right eye

　　H10.432 Chronic follicular conjunctivitis, left eye

　　H10.433 Chronic follicular conjunctivitis, bilateral

　　H10.439 Chronic follicular conjunctivitis, unspecified eye

　H10.44 **Vernal conjunctivitis**

　　EXCLUDES 1　*vernal keratoconjunctivitis with limbar and corneal involvement (H16.26-)*

　H10.45 Other chronic allergic conjunctivitis

✓5ᵗʰ **H10.5** **Blepharoconjunctivitis**

　✓6ᵗʰ **H10.50** **Unspecified blepharoconjunctivitis**

　　H10.501 Unspecified blepharoconjunctivitis, right eye

　　H10.502 Unspecified blepharoconjunctivitis, left eye

　　H10.503 Unspecified blepharoconjunctivitis, bilateral

　　H10.509 Unspecified blepharoconjunctivitis, unspecified eye

　✓6ᵗʰ **H10.51** **Ligneous conjunctivitis**

　　Code also underlying condition if known, such as: plasminogen deficiency (E88.02)

　　H10.511 Ligneous conjunctivitis, right eye

　　H10.512 Ligneous conjunctivitis, left eye

　　H10.513 Ligneous conjunctivitis, bilateral

　　H10.519 Ligneous conjunctivitis, unspecified eye

✓ Additional Character Required　　✓×7ᵗʰ Placeholder Alert　　Manifestation　　Unspecified Dx　　►◄ Revised Text　　● New Code　　▲ Revised Code Title

ICD-10-CM 2020　　　　　　　　　　　　　　　　　　　　　　　　　　　　　　591

√6ᵗʰ **H10.52** **Angular** blepharoconjunctivitis

  H10.521 Angular blepharoconjunctivitis, **right eye**
  H10.522 Angular blepharoconjunctivitis, **left eye**
  H10.523 Angular blepharoconjunctivitis, **bilateral**
  H10.529 Angular blepharoconjunctivitis, **unspecified eye**

√6ᵗʰ **H10.53** **Contact** blepharoconjunctivitis

  H10.531 Contact blepharoconjunctivitis, **right eye**
  H10.532 Contact blepharoconjunctivitis, **left eye**
  H10.533 Contact blepharoconjunctivitis, **bilateral**
  H10.539 Contact blepharoconjunctivitis, **unspecified eye**

√5ᵗʰ **H10.8** **Other conjunctivitis**

√6ᵗʰ **H10.81** **Pingueculitis**

  EXCLUDES 1 *pinguecula (H11.15-)*
  H10.811 Pingueculitis, **right eye**
  H10.812 Pingueculitis, **left eye**
  H10.813 Pingueculitis, **bilateral**
  H10.819 Pingueculitis, **unspecified eye**

√6ᵗʰ **H10.82** **Rosacea** conjunctivitis

  Code first underlying rosacea dermatitis (L71.-)
  AHA: 2018,4Q,15
  H10.821 Rosacea conjunctivitis, **right eye**
  H10.822 Rosacea conjunctivitis, **left eye**
  H10.823 Rosacea conjunctivitis, **bilateral**
  H10.829 Rosacea conjunctivitis, **unspecified eye**

  H10.89 **Other conjunctivitis**

H10.9 **Unspecified conjunctivitis**

✅4ᵗʰ **H11** **Other disorders of conjunctiva**

  EXCLUDES 1 *keratoconjunctivitis (H16.2-)*

√5ᵗʰ **H11.0** **Pterygium of eye**

  EXCLUDES 1 *pseudopterygium (H11.81-)*
  DEF: Benign, wedge-shaped, conjunctival thickening that advances from the inner corner of the eye toward the cornea.

Pterygium

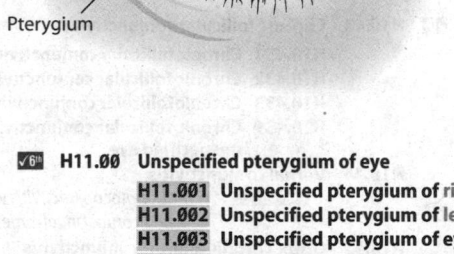

Pterygium

√6ᵗʰ **H11.00** **Unspecified pterygium of eye**

  H11.001 Unspecified pterygium of **right** eye
  H11.002 Unspecified pterygium of **left** eye
  H11.003 Unspecified pterygium of eye, **bilateral**
  H11.009 Unspecified pterygium of unspecified eye

√6ᵗʰ **H11.01** **Amyloid** pterygium

  H11.011 Amyloid pterygium of **right** eye
  H11.012 Amyloid pterygium of **left** eye
  H11.013 Amyloid pterygium of eye, **bilateral**
  H11.019 Amyloid pterygium of unspecified eye

√6ᵗʰ **H11.02** **Central** pterygium of eye

  H11.021 Central pterygium of **right** eye
  H11.022 Central pterygium of **left** eye
  H11.023 Central pterygium of eye, **bilateral**
  H11.029 Central pterygium of unspecified eye

√6ᵗʰ **H11.03** **Double** pterygium of eye

  H11.031 Double pterygium of **right** eye
  H11.032 Double pterygium of **left** eye
  H11.033 Double pterygium of eye, **bilateral**
  H11.039 Double pterygium of unspecified eye

√6ᵗʰ **H11.04** **Peripheral** pterygium of eye, **stationary**

  H11.041 Peripheral pterygium, stationary, **right eye**
  H11.042 Peripheral pterygium, stationary, **left eye**
  H11.043 Peripheral pterygium, stationary, **bilateral**
  H11.049 Peripheral pterygium, stationary, **unspecified eye**

√6ᵗʰ **H11.05** **Peripheral** pterygium of eye, **progressive**

  H11.051 Peripheral pterygium, progressive, **right eye**
  H11.052 Peripheral pterygium, progressive, **left eye**
  H11.053 Peripheral pterygium, progressive, **bilateral**
  H11.059 Peripheral pterygium, progressive, **unspecified eye**

√6ᵗʰ **H11.06** **Recurrent** pterygium of eye

  H11.061 Recurrent pterygium of **right** eye
  H11.062 Recurrent pterygium of **left** eye
  H11.063 Recurrent pterygium of eye, **bilateral**
  H11.069 Recurrent pterygium of unspecified eye

√5ᵗʰ **H11.1** **Conjunctival degenerations and deposits**

  EXCLUDES 2 *pseudopterygium (H11.81)*

  H11.10 **Unspecified conjunctival degenerations**

√6ᵗʰ **H11.11** **Conjunctival** deposits

  H11.111 Conjunctival deposits, **right eye**
  H11.112 Conjunctival deposits, **left eye**
  H11.113 Conjunctival deposits, **bilateral**
  H11.119 Conjunctival deposits, unspecified eye

√6ᵗʰ **H11.12** **Conjunctival** concretions

  H11.121 Conjunctival concretions, **right eye**
  H11.122 Conjunctival concretions, **left eye**
  H11.123 Conjunctival concretions, **bilateral**
  H11.129 Conjunctival concretions, unspecified eye

√6ᵗʰ **H11.13** **Conjunctival** pigmentations

  Conjunctival argyrosis [argyria]
  H11.131 Conjunctival pigmentations, **right eye**
  H11.132 Conjunctival pigmentations, **left eye**
  H11.133 Conjunctival pigmentations, **bilateral**
  H11.139 Conjunctival pigmentations, unspecified eye

√6ᵗʰ **H11.14** **Conjunctival xerosis, unspecified**

  EXCLUDES 1 *xerosis of conjunctiva due to vitamin A deficiency (E50.0, E50.1)*
  DEF: Abnormal dryness of the conjunctiva due to lack of insufficient tears or conjunctival secretions.
  H11.141 Conjunctival xerosis, unspecified, **right eye**
  H11.142 Conjunctival xerosis, unspecified, **left eye**
  H11.143 Conjunctival xerosis, unspecified, **bilateral**
  H11.149 Conjunctival xerosis, unspecified, **unspecified eye**

✓6ᵗʰ **H11.15 Pinguecula**

EXCLUDES 1 *pinguecultis (H10.81-)*

DEF: Proliferation on the conjunctiva near the sclerocorneal junction, usually of the side of the nose and usually in older patients.

Pinguecula

Pinguecula

H11.151 **Pinguecula, right eye**
H11.152 **Pinguecula, left eye**
H11.153 **Pinguecula, bilateral**
H11.159 **Pinguecula, unspecified eye**

✓5ᵗʰ **H11.2 Conjunctival scars**

✓6ᵗʰ **H11.21 Conjunctival adhesions and strands (localized)**

H11.211 **Conjunctival adhesions and strands (localized), right eye**
H11.212 **Conjunctival adhesions and strands (localized), left eye**
H11.213 **Conjunctival adhesions and strands (localized), bilateral**
H11.219 **Conjunctival adhesions and strands (localized), unspecified eye**

✓6ᵗʰ **H11.22 Conjunctival granuloma**

H11.221 **Conjunctival granuloma, right eye**
H11.222 **Conjunctival granuloma, left eye**
H11.223 **Conjunctival granuloma, bilateral**
H11.229 **Conjunctival granuloma, unspecified**

✓6ᵗʰ **H11.23 Symblepharon**

H11.231 **Symblepharon, right eye**
H11.232 **Symblepharon, left eye**
H11.233 **Symblepharon, bilateral**
H11.239 **Symblepharon, unspecified eye**

✓6ᵗʰ **H11.24 Scarring of conjunctiva**

H11.241 **Scarring of conjunctiva, right eye**
H11.242 **Scarring of conjunctiva, left eye**
H11.243 **Scarring of conjunctiva, bilateral**
H11.249 **Scarring of conjunctiva, unspecified eye**

✓5ᵗʰ **H11.3 Conjunctival hemorrhage**

Subconjunctival hemorrhage

H11.30 **Conjunctival hemorrhage, unspecified eye**
H11.31 **Conjunctival hemorrhage, right eye**
H11.32 **Conjunctival hemorrhage, left eye**
H11.33 **Conjunctival hemorrhage, bilateral**

✓5ᵗʰ **H11.4 Other conjunctival vascular disorders and cysts**

✓6ᵗʰ **H11.41 Vascular abnormalities of conjunctiva**

Conjunctival aneurysm

H11.411 **Vascular abnormalities of conjunctiva, right eye**
H11.412 **Vascular abnormalities of conjunctiva, left eye**
H11.413 **Vascular abnormalities of conjunctiva, bilateral**
H11.419 **Vascular abnormalities of conjunctiva, unspecified eye**

✓6ᵗʰ **H11.42 Conjunctival edema**

H11.421 **Conjunctival edema, right eye**
H11.422 **Conjunctival edema, left eye**
H11.423 **Conjunctival edema, bilateral**
H11.429 **Conjunctival edema, unspecified eye**

✓6ᵗʰ **H11.43 Conjunctival hyperemia**

H11.431 **Conjunctival hyperemia, right eye**

H11.432 **Conjunctival hyperemia, left eye**
H11.433 **Conjunctival hyperemia, bilateral**
H11.439 **Conjunctival hyperemia, unspecified eye**

✓6ᵗʰ **H11.44 Conjunctival cysts**

H11.441 **Conjunctival cysts, right eye**
H11.442 **Conjunctival cysts, left eye**
H11.443 **Conjunctival cysts, bilateral**
H11.449 **Conjunctival cysts, unspecified eye**

✓5ᵗʰ **H11.8 Other specified disorders of conjunctiva**

✓6ᵗʰ **H11.81 Pseudopterygium of conjunctiva**

H11.811 **Pseudopterygium of conjunctiva, right eye**
H11.812 **Pseudopterygium of conjunctiva, left eye**
H11.813 **Pseudopterygium of conjunctiva, bilateral**
H11.819 **Pseudopterygium of conjunctiva, unspecified eye**

✓6ᵗʰ **H11.82 Conjunctivochalasis**

H11.821 **Conjunctivochalasis, right eye**
H11.822 **Conjunctivochalasis, left eye**
H11.823 **Conjunctivochalasis, bilateral**
H11.829 **Conjunctivochalasis, unspecified eye**

H11.89 **Other specified disorders of conjunctiva**

H11.9 Unspecified disorder of conjunctiva

Disorders of sclera, cornea, iris and ciliary body (H15-H22)

✓4ᵗʰ **H15 Disorders of sclera**

✓5ᵗʰ **H15.0 Scleritis**

✓6ᵗʰ **H15.00 Unspecified scleritis**

H15.001 **Unspecified scleritis, right eye**
H15.002 **Unspecified scleritis, left eye**
H15.003 **Unspecified scleritis, bilateral**
H15.009 **Unspecified scleritis, unspecified eye**

✓6ᵗʰ **H15.01 Anterior scleritis**

H15.011 **Anterior scleritis, right eye**
H15.012 **Anterior scleritis, left eye**
H15.013 **Anterior scleritis, bilateral**
H15.019 **Anterior scleritis, unspecified eye**

✓6ᵗʰ **H15.02 Brawny scleritis**

H15.021 **Brawny scleritis, right eye**
H15.022 **Brawny scleritis, left eye**
H15.023 **Brawny scleritis, bilateral**
H15.029 **Brawny scleritis, unspecified eye**

✓6ᵗʰ **H15.03 Posterior scleritis**

Sclerotenonitis

H15.031 **Posterior scleritis, right eye**
H15.032 **Posterior scleritis, left eye**
H15.033 **Posterior scleritis, bilateral**
H15.039 **Posterior scleritis, unspecified eye**

✓6ᵗʰ **H15.04 Scleritis with corneal involvement**

H15.041 **Scleritis with corneal involvement, right eye**
H15.042 **Scleritis with corneal involvement, left eye**
H15.043 **Scleritis with corneal involvement, bilateral**
H15.049 **Scleritis with corneal involvement, unspecified eye**

✓6ᵗʰ **H15.05 Scleromalacia perforans**

H15.051 **Scleromalacia perforans, right eye**
H15.052 **Scleromalacia perforans, left eye**
H15.053 **Scleromalacia perforans, bilateral**
H15.059 **Scleromalacia perforans, unspecified eye**

✓6ᵗʰ **H15.09 Other scleritis**

Scleral abscess

H15.091 **Other scleritis, right eye**
H15.092 **Other scleritis, left eye**
H15.093 **Other scleritis, bilateral**
H15.099 **Other scleritis, unspecified eye**

✓5ᵗʰ **H15.1 Episcleritis**

✓6ᵗʰ **H15.10 Unspecified episcleritis**

H15.101 **Unspecified episcleritis, right eye**
H15.102 **Unspecified episcleritis, left eye**
H15.103 **Unspecified episcleritis, bilateral**
H15.109 **Unspecified episcleritis, unspecified eye**

☑ Additional Character Required ✓x7ᵗʰ Placeholder Alert Manifestation Unspecified Dx ▶◀ Revised Text ● New Code ▲ Revised Code Title

ICD-10-CM 2020   593

√6ᵗʰ H15.11 Episcleritis periodica fugax

H15.111 Episcleritis periodica fugax, **right eye**
H15.112 Episcleritis periodica fugax, **left eye**
H15.113 Episcleritis periodica fugax, **bilateral**
H15.119 Episcleritis periodica fugax, **unspecified eye**

√6ᵗʰ H15.12 Nodular episcleritis

H15.121 Nodular episcleritis, **right eye**
H15.122 Nodular episcleritis, **left eye**
H15.123 Nodular episcleritis, **bilateral**
H15.129 Nodular episcleritis, **unspecified eye**

√5ᵗʰ H15.8 Other disorders of sclera

EXCLUDES 2   blue sclera (Q13.5)
degenerative myopia (H44.2-)

√6ᵗʰ H15.81 Equatorial staphyloma

H15.811 Equatorial staphyloma, **right eye**
H15.812 Equatorial staphyloma, **left eye**
H15.813 Equatorial staphyloma, **bilateral**
H15.819 Equatorial staphyloma, **unspecified eye**

√6ᵗʰ H15.82 Localized anterior staphyloma

H15.821 Localized anterior staphyloma, **right eye**
H15.822 Localized anterior staphyloma, **left eye**
H15.823 Localized anterior staphyloma, **bilateral**
H15.829 Localized anterior staphyloma, **unspecified eye**

√6ᵗʰ H15.83 Staphyloma posticum

H15.831 Staphyloma posticum, **right eye**
H15.832 Staphyloma posticum, **left eye**
H15.833 Staphyloma posticum, **bilateral**
H15.839 Staphyloma posticum, **unspecified eye**

√6ᵗʰ H15.84 Scleral ectasia

H15.841 Scleral ectasia, **right eye**
H15.842 Scleral ectasia, **left eye**
H15.843 Scleral ectasia, **bilateral**
H15.849 Scleral ectasia, **unspecified eye**

√6ᵗʰ H15.85 Ring staphyloma

H15.851 Ring staphyloma, **right eye**
H15.852 Ring staphyloma, **left eye**
H15.853 Ring staphyloma, **bilateral**
H15.859 Ring staphyloma, **unspecified eye**

H15.89 **Other disorders of sclera**

H15.9 Unspecified disorder of sclera

√4ᵗʰ H16 Keratitis

DEF: Condition in which the cornea becomes inflamed and irritated.

√5ᵗʰ H16.0 Corneal ulcer

√6ᵗʰ H16.00 Unspecified corneal ulcer

H16.001 Unspecified corneal ulcer, **right eye**
H16.002 Unspecified corneal ulcer, **left eye**
H16.003 Unspecified corneal ulcer, **bilateral**
H16.009 Unspecified corneal ulcer, **unspecified eye**

√6ᵗʰ H16.01 Central corneal ulcer

H16.011 Central corneal ulcer, **right eye**
H16.012 Central corneal ulcer, **left eye**
H16.013 Central corneal ulcer, **bilateral**
H16.019 Central corneal ulcer, **unspecified eye**

√6ᵗʰ H16.02 Ring corneal ulcer

H16.021 Ring corneal ulcer, **right eye**
H16.022 Ring corneal ulcer, **left eye**
H16.023 Ring corneal ulcer, **bilateral**
H16.029 Ring corneal ulcer, **unspecified eye**

√6ᵗʰ H16.03 Corneal ulcer with hypopyon

H16.031 Corneal ulcer with hypopyon, **right eye**
H16.032 Corneal ulcer with hypopyon, **left eye**
H16.033 Corneal ulcer with hypopyon, **bilateral**
H16.039 Corneal ulcer with hypopyon, **unspecified eye**

√6ᵗʰ H16.04 Marginal corneal ulcer

H16.041 Marginal corneal ulcer, **right eye**
H16.042 Marginal corneal ulcer, **left eye**
H16.043 Marginal corneal ulcer, **bilateral**
H16.049 Marginal corneal ulcer, **unspecified eye**

√6ᵗʰ H16.05 Mooren's corneal ulcer

H16.051 Mooren's corneal ulcer, **right eye**
H16.052 Mooren's corneal ulcer, **left eye**
H16.053 Mooren's corneal ulcer, **bilateral**
H16.059 Mooren's corneal ulcer, **unspecified eye**

√6ᵗʰ H16.06 Mycotic corneal ulcer

H16.061 Mycotic corneal ulcer, **right eye**
H16.062 Mycotic corneal ulcer, **left eye**
H16.063 Mycotic corneal ulcer, **bilateral**
H16.069 Mycotic corneal ulcer, **unspecified eye**

√6ᵗʰ H16.07 Perforated corneal ulcer

H16.071 Perforated corneal ulcer, **right eye**
H16.072 Perforated corneal ulcer, **left eye**
H16.073 Perforated corneal ulcer, **bilateral**
H16.079 Perforated corneal ulcer, **unspecified eye**

√5ᵗʰ H16.1 Other and unspecified superficial keratitis without conjunctivitis

√6ᵗʰ H16.10 Unspecified superficial keratitis

H16.101 Unspecified superficial keratitis, **right eye**
H16.102 Unspecified superficial keratitis, **left eye**
H16.103 Unspecified superficial keratitis, **bilateral**
H16.109 Unspecified superficial keratitis, **unspecified eye**

√6ᵗʰ H16.11 Macular keratitis

Areolar keratitis
Nummular keratitis
Stellate keratitis
Striate keratitis

H16.111 Macular keratitis, **right eye**
H16.112 Macular keratitis, **left eye**
H16.113 Macular keratitis, **bilateral**
H16.119 Macular keratitis, **unspecified eye**

√6ᵗʰ H16.12 Filamentary keratitis

H16.121 Filamentary keratitis, **right eye**
H16.122 Filamentary keratitis, **left eye**
H16.123 Filamentary keratitis, **bilateral**
H16.129 Filamentary keratitis, **unspecified eye**

√6ᵗʰ H16.13 Photokeratitis

Snow blindness
Welders keratitis

H16.131 Photokeratitis, **right eye**
H16.132 Photokeratitis, **left eye**
H16.133 Photokeratitis, **bilateral**
H16.139 Photokeratitis, **unspecified eye**

√6ᵗʰ H16.14 Punctate keratitis

H16.141 Punctate keratitis, **right eye**
H16.142 Punctate keratitis, **left eye**
H16.143 Punctate keratitis, **bilateral**
H16.149 Punctate keratitis, **unspecified eye**

√5ᵗʰ H16.2 Keratoconjunctivitis

√6ᵗʰ H16.20 Unspecified keratoconjunctivitis

Superficial keratitis with conjunctivitis NOS

H16.201 Unspecified keratoconjunctivitis, **right eye**
H16.202 Unspecified keratoconjunctivitis, **left eye**
H16.203 Unspecified keratoconjunctivitis, **bilateral**
H16.209 Unspecified keratoconjunctivitis, **unspecified eye**

√6ᵗʰ H16.21 Exposure keratoconjunctivitis

H16.211 Exposure keratoconjunctivitis, **right eye**
H16.212 Exposure keratoconjunctivitis, **left eye**
H16.213 Exposure keratoconjunctivitis, **bilateral**
H16.219 Exposure keratoconjunctivitis, **unspecified eye**

√6ᵗʰ H16.22 Keratoconjunctivitis sicca, not specified as Sjögren's

EXCLUDES 1   Sjögren's syndrome (M35.01)

H16.221 Keratoconjunctivitis sicca, not specified as Sjögren's, **right eye**
H16.222 Keratoconjunctivitis sicca, not specified as Sjögren's, **left eye**
H16.223 Keratoconjunctivitis sicca, not specified as Sjögren's, **bilateral**
H16.229 Keratoconjunctivitis sicca, not specified as Sjögren's, **unspecified eye**

√6ᵗʰ H16.23 Neurotrophic keratoconjunctivitis

H16.231 Neurotrophic keratoconjunctivitis, **right eye**
H16.232 Neurotrophic keratoconjunctivitis, **left eye**

H16.233 **Neurotrophic keratoconjunctivitis, bilateral**

H16.239 **Neurotrophic keratoconjunctivitis, unspecified eye**

√6ᵗʰ H16.24 Ophthalmia nodosa

H16.241 **Ophthalmia nodosa, right eye**

H16.242 **Ophthalmia nodosa, left eye**

H16.243 **Ophthalmia nodosa, bilateral**

H16.249 **Ophthalmia nodosa, unspecified eye**

√6ᵗʰ H16.25 Phlyctenular keratoconjunctivitis

H16.251 **Phlyctenular keratoconjunctivitis, right eye**

H16.252 **Phlyctenular keratoconjunctivitis, left eye**

H16.253 **Phlyctenular keratoconjunctivitis, bilateral**

H16.259 **Phlyctenular keratoconjunctivitis, unspecified eye**

√6ᵗʰ H16.26 Vernal keratoconjunctivitis, with limbar and corneal involvement

     EXCLUDES 1   *vernal conjunctivitis without limbar and corneal involvement (H10.44)*

H16.261 **Vernal keratoconjunctivitis, with limbar and corneal involvement, right eye**

H16.262 **Vernal keratoconjunctivitis, with limbar and corneal involvement, left eye**

H16.263 **Vernal keratoconjunctivitis, with limbar and corneal involvement, bilateral**

H16.269 **Vernal keratoconjunctivitis, with limbar and corneal involvement, unspecified eye**

√6ᵗʰ H16.29 Other keratoconjunctivitis

H16.291 **Other keratoconjunctivitis, right eye**

H16.292 **Other keratoconjunctivitis, left eye**

H16.293 **Other keratoconjunctivitis, bilateral**

H16.299 **Other keratoconjunctivitis, unspecified eye**

√5ᵗʰ H16.3 Interstitial and deep keratitis

√6ᵗʰ H16.30 Unspecified interstitial keratitis

H16.301 **Unspecified interstitial keratitis, right eye**

H16.302 **Unspecified interstitial keratitis, left eye**

H16.303 **Unspecified interstitial keratitis, bilateral**

H16.309 **Unspecified interstitial keratitis, unspecified eye**

√6ᵗʰ H16.31 Corneal abscess

H16.311 **Corneal abscess, right eye**

H16.312 **Corneal abscess, left eye**

H16.313 **Corneal abscess, bilateral**

H16.319 **Corneal abscess, unspecified eye**

√6ᵗʰ H16.32 Diffuse interstitial keratitis

     Cogan's syndrome

H16.321 **Diffuse interstitial keratitis, right eye**

H16.322 **Diffuse interstitial keratitis, left eye**

H16.323 **Diffuse interstitial keratitis, bilateral**

H16.329 **Diffuse interstitial keratitis, unspecified eye**

√6ᵗʰ H16.33 Sclerosing keratitis

H16.331 **Sclerosing keratitis, right eye**

H16.332 **Sclerosing keratitis, left eye**

H16.333 **Sclerosing keratitis, bilateral**

H16.339 **Sclerosing keratitis, unspecified eye**

√6ᵗʰ H16.39 Other interstitial and deep keratitis

H16.391 **Other interstitial and deep keratitis, right eye**

H16.392 **Other interstitial and deep keratitis, left eye**

H16.393 **Other interstitial and deep keratitis, bilateral**

H16.399 **Other interstitial and deep keratitis, unspecified eye**

√5ᵗʰ H16.4 Corneal neovascularization

√6ᵗʰ H16.40 Unspecified corneal neovascularization

H16.401 **Unspecified corneal neovascularization, right eye**

H16.402 **Unspecified corneal neovascularization, left eye**

H16.403 **Unspecified corneal neovascularization, bilateral**

H16.409 **Unspecified corneal neovascularization, unspecified eye**

√6ᵗʰ H16.41 Ghost vessels (corneal)

H16.411 **Ghost vessels (corneal), right eye**

H16.412 **Ghost vessels (corneal), left eye**

H16.413 **Ghost vessels (corneal), bilateral**

H16.419 **Ghost vessels (corneal), unspecified eye**

√6ᵗʰ H16.42 Pannus (corneal)

H16.421 **Pannus (corneal), right eye**

H16.422 **Pannus (corneal), left eye**

H16.423 **Pannus (corneal), bilateral**

H16.429 **Pannus (corneal), unspecified eye**

√6ᵗʰ H16.43 Localized vascularization of cornea

H16.431 **Localized vascularization of cornea, right eye**

H16.432 **Localized vascularization of cornea, left eye**

H16.433 **Localized vascularization of cornea, bilateral**

H16.439 **Localized vascularization of cornea, unspecified eye**

√6ᵗʰ H16.44 Deep vascularization of cornea

H16.441 **Deep vascularization of cornea, right eye**

H16.442 **Deep vascularization of cornea, left eye**

H16.443 **Deep vascularization of cornea, bilateral**

H16.449 **Deep vascularization of cornea, unspecified eye**

H16.8 **Other keratitis**

H16.9 **Unspecified keratitis**

√4ᵗʰ **H17 Corneal scars and opacities**

√5ᵗʰ H17.0 Adherent leukoma

H17.00 **Adherent leukoma, unspecified eye**

H17.01 **Adherent leukoma, right eye**

H17.02 **Adherent leukoma, left eye**

H17.03 **Adherent leukoma, bilateral**

√5ᵗʰ H17.1 Central corneal opacity

H17.10 **Central corneal opacity, unspecified eye**

H17.11 **Central corneal opacity, right eye**

H17.12 **Central corneal opacity, left eye**

H17.13 **Central corneal opacity, bilateral**

√5ᵗʰ H17.8 Other corneal scars and opacities

√6ᵗʰ H17.81 Minor opacity of cornea

     Corneal nebula

H17.811 **Minor opacity of cornea, right eye**

H17.812 **Minor opacity of cornea, left eye**

H17.813 **Minor opacity of cornea, bilateral**

H17.819 **Minor opacity of cornea, unspecified eye**

√6ᵗʰ H17.82 Peripheral opacity of cornea

H17.821 **Peripheral opacity of cornea, right eye**

H17.822 **Peripheral opacity of cornea, left eye**

H17.823 **Peripheral opacity of cornea, bilateral**

H17.829 **Peripheral opacity of cornea, unspecified eye**

H17.89 **Other corneal scars and opacities**

H17.9 **Unspecified corneal scar and opacity**

√4ᵗʰ **H18 Other disorders of cornea**

√5ᵗʰ H18.0 Corneal pigmentations and deposits

√6ᵗʰ H18.00 Unspecified corneal deposit

H18.001 **Unspecified corneal deposit, right eye**

H18.002 **Unspecified corneal deposit, left eye**

H18.003 **Unspecified corneal deposit, bilateral**

H18.009 **Unspecified corneal deposit, unspecified eye**

√6ᵗʰ H18.01 Anterior corneal pigmentations

     Staehli's line

H18.011 **Anterior corneal pigmentations, right eye**

H18.012 **Anterior corneal pigmentations, left eye**

H18.013 **Anterior corneal pigmentations, bilateral**

H18.019 **Anterior corneal pigmentations, unspecified eye**

√6ᵗʰ H18.02 Argentous corneal deposits

H18.021 **Argentous corneal deposits, right eye**

H18.022 **Argentous corneal deposits, left eye**

H18.023 **Argentous corneal deposits, bilateral**

H18.029 **Argentous corneal deposits, unspecified eye**

☑ Additional Character Required   √x7ᵗʰ Placeholder Alert   Manifestation   Unspecified Dx   ▶◀ Revised Text   ● New Code   ▲ Revised Code Title

☑6ᵗʰ **H18.03 Corneal deposits in** metabolic disorders

Code also associated metabolic disorder

H18.031 Corneal deposits in metabolic disorders, right eye

H18.032 Corneal deposits in metabolic disorders, left eye

H18.033 Corneal deposits in metabolic disorders, bilateral

H18.039 Corneal deposits in metabolic disorders, unspecified eye

☑6ᵗʰ **H18.04 Kayser-Fleischer ring**

Code also associated Wilson's disease (E83.01)

H18.041 Kayser-Fleischer ring, right eye

H18.042 Kayser-Fleischer ring, left eye

H18.043 Kayser-Fleischer ring, bilateral

H18.049 Kayser-Fleischer ring, unspecified eye

☑6ᵗʰ **H18.05 Posterior corneal pigmentations**

Krukenberg's spindle

H18.051 Posterior corneal pigmentations, right eye

H18.052 Posterior corneal pigmentations, left eye

H18.053 Posterior corneal pigmentations, bilateral

H18.059 Posterior corneal pigmentations, unspecified eye

☑6ᵗʰ **H18.06 Stromal corneal pigmentations**

Hematocornea

H18.061 Stromal corneal pigmentations, right eye

H18.062 Stromal corneal pigmentations, left eye

H18.063 Stromal corneal pigmentations, bilateral

H18.069 Stromal corneal pigmentations, unspecified eye

☑5ᵗʰ **H18.1 Bullous keratopathy**

DEF: Corneal swelling due to a damaged corneal endothelium. Bullous keratopathy is characterized by recurring, rupturing epithelial blisters causing glaucoma, iridocyclitis, and Fuchs dystrophy.

H18.10 Bullous keratopathy, unspecified eye

H18.11 Bullous keratopathy, right eye

H18.12 Bullous keratopathy, left eye

H18.13 Bullous keratopathy, bilateral

☑5ᵗʰ **H18.2 Other and unspecified corneal edema**

H18.20 Unspecified corneal edema

☑6ᵗʰ **H18.21 Corneal edema secondary to contact lens**

EXCLUDES 2   other corneal disorders due to contact lens (H18.82-)

H18.211 Corneal edema secondary to contact lens, right eye

H18.212 Corneal edema secondary to contact lens, left eye

H18.213 Corneal edema secondary to contact lens, bilateral

H18.219 Corneal edema secondary to contact lens, unspecified eye

☑6ᵗʰ **H18.22 Idiopathic corneal edema**

H18.221 Idiopathic corneal edema, right eye

H18.222 Idiopathic corneal edema, left eye

H18.223 Idiopathic corneal edema, bilateral

H18.229 Idiopathic corneal edema, unspecified eye

☑6ᵗʰ **H18.23 Secondary corneal edema**

H18.231 Secondary corneal edema, right eye

H18.232 Secondary corneal edema, left eye

H18.233 Secondary corneal edema, bilateral

H18.239 Secondary corneal edema, unspecified eye

☑5ᵗʰ **H18.3 Changes of corneal membranes**

H18.30 Unspecified corneal membrane change

☑6ᵗʰ **H18.31 Folds and rupture in Bowman's membrane**

H18.311 Folds and rupture in Bowman's membrane, right eye

H18.312 Folds and rupture in Bowman's membrane, left eye

H18.313 Folds and rupture in Bowman's membrane, bilateral

H18.319 Folds and rupture in Bowman's membrane, unspecified eye

☑6ᵗʰ **H18.32 Folds in Descemet's membrane**

H18.321 Folds in Descemet's membrane, right eye

H18.322 Folds in Descemet's membrane, left eye

H18.323 Folds in Descemet's membrane, bilateral

H18.329 Folds in Descemet's membrane, unspecified eye

☑6ᵗʰ **H18.33 Rupture in Descemet's membrane**

H18.331 Rupture in Descemet's membrane, right eye

H18.332 Rupture in Descemet's membrane, left eye

H18.333 Rupture in Descemet's membrane, bilateral

H18.339 Rupture in Descemet's membrane, unspecified eye

☑5ᵗʰ **H18.4 Corneal degeneration**

EXCLUDES 1   Mooren's ulcer (H16.0-)

recurrent erosion of cornea (H18.83-)

H18.40 Unspecified corneal degeneration

☑6ᵗʰ **H18.41 Arcus senilis**

Senile corneal changes

H18.411 Arcus senilis, right eye

H18.412 Arcus senilis, left eye

H18.413 Arcus senilis, bilateral

H18.419 Arcus senilis, unspecified eye

☑6ᵗʰ **H18.42 Band keratopathy**

H18.421 Band keratopathy, right eye

H18.422 Band keratopathy, left eye

H18.423 Band keratopathy, bilateral

H18.429 Band keratopathy, unspecified eye

H18.43 Other calcerous corneal degeneration

☑6ᵗʰ **H18.44 Keratomalacia**

EXCLUDES 1   keratomalacia due to vitamin A deficiency (E50.4)

H18.441 Keratomalacia, right eye

H18.442 Keratomalacia, left eye

H18.443 Keratomalacia, bilateral

H18.449 Keratomalacia, unspecified eye

☑6ᵗʰ **H18.45 Nodular corneal degeneration**

H18.451 Nodular corneal degeneration, right eye

H18.452 Nodular corneal degeneration, left eye

H18.453 Nodular corneal degeneration, bilateral

H18.459 Nodular corneal degeneration, unspecified eye

☑6ᵗʰ **H18.46 Peripheral corneal degeneration**

H18.461 Peripheral corneal degeneration, right eye

H18.462 Peripheral corneal degeneration, left eye

H18.463 Peripheral corneal degeneration, bilateral

H18.469 Peripheral corneal degeneration, unspecified eye

H18.49 Other corneal degeneration

☑5ᵗʰ **H18.5 Hereditary corneal dystrophies**

H18.50 Unspecified hereditary corneal dystrophies

H18.51 Endothelial corneal dystrophy

Fuchs' dystrophy

H18.52 Epithelial (juvenile) corneal dystrophy

H18.53 Granular corneal dystrophy

H18.54 Lattice corneal dystrophy

H18.55 Macular corneal dystrophy

H18.59 Other hereditary corneal dystrophies

☑5ᵗʰ **H18.6 Keratoconus**

☑6ᵗʰ **H18.60 Keratoconus, unspecified**

H18.601 Keratoconus, unspecified, right eye

H18.602 Keratoconus, unspecified, left eye

H18.603 Keratoconus, unspecified, bilateral

H18.609 Keratoconus, unspecified, unspecified eye

☑6ᵗʰ **H18.61 Keratoconus, stable**

H18.611 Keratoconus, stable, right eye

H18.612 Keratoconus, stable, left eye

H18.613 Keratoconus, stable, bilateral

H18.619 Keratoconus, stable, unspecified eye

☑6ᵗʰ **H18.62 Keratoconus, unstable**

Acute hydrops

H18.621 Keratoconus, unstable, right eye

H18.622 Keratoconus, unstable, left eye

H18.623 Keratoconus, unstable, bilateral

H18.629 Keratoconus, unstable, unspecified eye

√5ᵗʰ **H18.7 Other and unspecified corneal deformities**
- EXCLUDES 1   *congenital malformations of cornea (Q13.3-Q13.4)*

   H18.70 Unspecified corneal deformity

√6ᵗʰ **H18.71 Corneal** ectasia
- H18.711 Corneal ectasia, **right eye**
- H18.712 Corneal ectasia, **left eye**
- H18.713 Corneal ectasia, **bilateral**
- H18.719 Corneal ectasia, **unspecified eye**

√6ᵗʰ **H18.72 Corneal** staphyloma
- H18.721 Corneal staphyloma, **right eye**
- H18.722 Corneal staphyloma, **left eye**
- H18.723 Corneal staphyloma, **bilateral**
- H18.729 Corneal staphyloma, **unspecified eye**

√6ᵗʰ **H18.73 Descemetocele**
- H18.731 Descemetocele, **right eye**
- H18.732 Descemetocele, **left eye**
- H18.733 Descemetocele, **bilateral**
- H18.739 Descemetocele, **unspecified eye**

√6ᵗʰ **H18.79 Other corneal deformities**
- H18.791 Other corneal deformities, **right eye**
- H18.792 Other corneal deformities, **left eye**
- H18.793 Other corneal deformities, **bilateral**
- H18.799 Other corneal deformities, **unspecified eye**

√5ᵗʰ **H18.8 Other specified disorders of cornea**

√6ᵗʰ **H18.81 Anesthesia and hypoesthesia of cornea**
- H18.811 Anesthesia and hypoesthesia of cornea, **right eye**
- H18.812 Anesthesia and hypoesthesia of cornea, **left eye**
- H18.813 Anesthesia and hypoesthesia of cornea, **bilateral**
- H18.819 Anesthesia and hypoesthesia of cornea, **unspecified eye**

√6ᵗʰ **H18.82 Corneal disorder due to contact lens**
- EXCLUDES 2   *corneal edema due to contact lens (H18.21-)*
- H18.821 Corneal disorder due to contact lens, **right eye**
- H18.822 Corneal disorder due to contact lens, **left eye**
- H18.823 Corneal disorder due to contact lens, **bilateral**
- H18.829 Corneal disorder due to contact lens, **unspecified eye**

√6ᵗʰ **H18.83 Recurrent erosion of cornea**
- H18.831 Recurrent erosion of cornea, **right eye**
- H18.832 Recurrent erosion of cornea, **left eye**
- H18.833 Recurrent erosion of cornea, **bilateral**
- H18.839 Recurrent erosion of cornea, **unspecified eye**

√6ᵗʰ **H18.89 Other specified disorders of cornea**
- H18.891 Other specified disorders of cornea, **right eye**
- H18.892 Other specified disorders of cornea, **left eye**
- H18.893 Other specified disorders of cornea, **bilateral**
- H18.899 Other specified disorders of cornea, **unspecified eye**

H18.9 Unspecified disorder of cornea

√4ᵗʰ **H20 Iridocyclitis**

√5ᵗʰ **H20.0 Acute and subacute iridocyclitis**
- Acute anterior uveitis
- Acute cyclitis
- Acute iritis
- Subacute anterior uveitis
- Subacute cyclitis
- Subacute iritis
- EXCLUDES 1   *iridocyclitis, iritis, uveitis (due to) (in) diabetes mellitus (E08-E13 with .39)*
  - *iridocyclitis, iritis, uveitis (due to) (in) diphtheria (A36.89)*
  - *iridocyclitis, iritis, uveitis (due to) (in) gonococcal (A54.32)*
  - *iridocyclitis, iritis, uveitis (due to) (in) herpes (simplex) (B00.51)*
  - *iridocyclitis, iritis, uveitis (due to) (in) herpes zoster (B02.32)*
  - *iridocyclitis, iritis, uveitis (due to) (in) late congenital syphilis (A50.39)*
  - *iridocyclitis, iritis, uveitis (due to) (in) late syphilis (A52.71)*
  - *iridocyclitis, iritis, uveitis (due to) (in) sarcoidosis (D86.83)*
  - *iridocyclitis, iritis, uveitis (due to) (in) syphilis (A51.43)*
  - *iridocyclitis, iritis, uveitis (due to) (in) toxoplasmosis (B58.09)*
  - *iridocyclitis, iritis, uveitis (due to) (in) tuberculosis (A18.54)*

   H20.00 Unspecified acute and subacute iridocyclitis

√6ᵗʰ **H20.01 Primary iridocyclitis**
- H20.011 Primary iridocyclitis, **right eye**
- H20.012 Primary iridocyclitis, **left eye**
- H20.013 Primary iridocyclitis, **bilateral**
- H20.019 Primary iridocyclitis, **unspecified eye**

√6ᵗʰ **H20.02 Recurrent acute iridocyclitis**
- H20.021 Recurrent acute iridocyclitis, **right eye**
- H20.022 Recurrent acute iridocyclitis, **left eye**
- H20.023 Recurrent acute iridocyclitis, **bilateral**
- H20.029 Recurrent acute iridocyclitis, **unspecified eye**

√6ᵗʰ **H20.03 Secondary infectious iridocyclitis**
- H20.031 Secondary infectious iridocyclitis, **right eye**
- H20.032 Secondary infectious iridocyclitis, **left eye**
- H20.033 Secondary infectious iridocyclitis, **bilateral**
- H20.039 Secondary infectious iridocyclitis, **unspecified eye**

√6ᵗʰ **H20.04 Secondary noninfectious iridocyclitis**
- H20.041 Secondary noninfectious iridocyclitis, **right eye**
- H20.042 Secondary noninfectious iridocyclitis, **left eye**
- H20.043 Secondary noninfectious iridocyclitis, **bilateral**
- H20.049 Secondary noninfectious iridocyclitis, **unspecified eye**

√6ᵗʰ **H20.05 Hypopyon**
- H20.051 Hypopyon, **right eye**
- H20.052 Hypopyon, **left eye**
- H20.053 Hypopyon, **bilateral**
- H20.059 Hypopyon, **unspecified eye**

√5ᵗʰ **H20.1 Chronic iridocyclitis**
- Use additional code for any associated cataract (H26.21-)
- EXCLUDES 2   *posterior cyclitis (H30.2-)*
- **H20.10 Chronic iridocyclitis, unspecified eye**
- H20.11 Chronic iridocyclitis, **right eye**
- H20.12 Chronic iridocyclitis, **left eye**
- H20.13 Chronic iridocyclitis, **bilateral**

√5ᵗʰ **H20.2 Lens-induced iridocyclitis**
- **H20.20 Lens-induced iridocyclitis, unspecified eye**
- H20.21 Lens-induced iridocyclitis, **right eye**
- H20.22 Lens-induced iridocyclitis, **left eye**
- H20.23 Lens-induced iridocyclitis, **bilateral**

☑ Additional Character Required   √x7ᵗʰ Placeholder Alert   Manifestation   Unspecified Dx   ►◄ Revised Text   ● New Code   ▲ Revised Code Title

√5ᵗʰ **H20.8 Other iridocyclitis**
     EXCLUDES 2   *glaucomatocyclitis crises (H40.4-)*
           posterior cyclitis (H30.2-)
           sympathetic uveitis (H44.13-)

√6ᵗʰ **H20.81 Fuchs' heterochromic cyclitis**
     H20.811 Fuchs' heterochromic cyclitis, right eye
     H20.812 Fuchs' heterochromic cyclitis, left eye
     H20.813 Fuchs' heterochromic cyclitis, bilateral
     H20.819 Fuchs' heterochromic cyclitis, unspecified eye

√6ᵗʰ **H20.82 Vogt-Koyanagi syndrome**
     H20.821 Vogt-Koyanagi syndrome, right eye
     H20.822 Vogt-Koyanagi syndrome, left eye
     H20.823 Vogt-Koyanagi syndrome, bilateral
     H20.829 Vogt-Koyanagi syndrome, unspecified eye

H20.9 Unspecified iridocyclitis
     Uveitis NOS

√4ᵗʰ **H21 Other disorders of iris and ciliary body**
     EXCLUDES 2   *sympathetic uveitis (H44.1-)*

√5ᵗʰ **H21.0 Hyphema**
     EXCLUDES 1   *traumatic hyphema (S05.1-)*

Hyphema

     Iris
     Cornea
     Hyphema

H21.00 Hyphema, unspecified eye
H21.01 Hyphema, right eye
H21.02 Hyphema, left eye
H21.03 Hyphema, bilateral

√5ᵗʰ **H21.1 Other vascular disorders of iris and ciliary body**
     Neovascularization of iris or ciliary body
     Rubeosis iridis
     Rubeosis of iris

√6ᵗʰ **H21.1X Other vascular disorders of iris and ciliary body**
     H21.1X1 Other vascular disorders of iris and ciliary body, right eye
     H21.1X2 Other vascular disorders of iris and ciliary body, left eye
     H21.1X3 Other vascular disorders of iris and ciliary body, bilateral
     H21.1X9 Other vascular disorders of iris and ciliary body, unspecified eye

√5ᵗʰ **H21.2 Degeneration of iris and ciliary body**

√6ᵗʰ **H21.21 Degeneration of chamber angle**
     H21.211 Degeneration of chamber angle, right eye
     H21.212 Degeneration of chamber angle, left eye
     H21.213 Degeneration of chamber angle, bilateral
     H21.219 Degeneration of chamber angle, unspecified eye

√6ᵗʰ **H21.22 Degeneration of ciliary body**
     H21.221 Degeneration of ciliary body, right eye
     H21.222 Degeneration of ciliary body, left eye
     H21.223 Degeneration of ciliary body, bilateral
     H21.229 Degeneration of ciliary body, unspecified eye

√6ᵗʰ **H21.23 Degeneration of iris (pigmentary)**
     Translucency of iris
     H21.231 Degeneration of iris (pigmentary), right eye
     H21.232 Degeneration of iris (pigmentary), left eye

H21.233 Degeneration of iris (pigmentary), bilateral
H21.239 Degeneration of iris (pigmentary), unspecified eye

√6ᵗʰ **H21.24 Degeneration of pupillary margin**
     H21.241 Degeneration of pupillary margin, right eye
     H21.242 Degeneration of pupillary margin, left eye
     H21.243 Degeneration of pupillary margin, bilateral
     H21.249 Degeneration of pupillary margin, unspecified eye

√6ᵗʰ **H21.25 Iridoschisis**
     H21.251 Iridoschisis, right eye
     H21.252 Iridoschisis, left eye
     H21.253 Iridoschisis, bilateral
     H21.259 Iridoschisis, unspecified eye

√6ᵗʰ **H21.26 Iris atrophy (essential) (progressive)**
     H21.261 Iris atrophy (essential) (progressive), right eye
     H21.262 Iris atrophy (essential) (progressive), left eye
     H21.263 Iris atrophy (essential) (progressive), bilateral
     H21.269 Iris atrophy (essential) (progressive), unspecified eye

√6ᵗʰ **H21.27 Miotic pupillary cyst**
     H21.271 Miotic pupillary cyst, right eye
     H21.272 Miotic pupillary cyst, left eye
     H21.273 Miotic pupillary cyst, bilateral
     H21.279 Miotic pupillary cyst, unspecified eye

H21.29 Other iris atrophy

√5ᵗʰ **H21.3 Cyst of iris, ciliary body and anterior chamber**
     EXCLUDES 2   *miotic pupillary cyst (H21.27-)*

√6ᵗʰ **H21.30 Idiopathic cysts of iris, ciliary body or anterior chamber**
     Cyst of iris, ciliary body or anterior chamber NOS
     H21.301 Idiopathic cysts of iris, ciliary body or anterior chamber, right eye
     H21.302 Idiopathic cysts of iris, ciliary body or anterior chamber, left eye
     H21.303 Idiopathic cysts of iris, ciliary body or anterior chamber, bilateral
     H21.309 Idiopathic cysts of iris, ciliary body or anterior chamber, unspecified eye

√6ᵗʰ **H21.31 Exudative cysts of iris or anterior chamber**
     H21.311 Exudative cysts of iris or anterior chamber, right eye
     H21.312 Exudative cysts of iris or anterior chamber, left eye
     H21.313 Exudative cysts of iris or anterior chamber, bilateral
     H21.319 Exudative cysts of iris or anterior chamber, unspecified eye

√6ᵗʰ **H21.32 Implantation cysts of iris, ciliary body or anterior chamber**
     H21.321 Implantation cysts of iris, ciliary body or anterior chamber, right eye
     H21.322 Implantation cysts of iris, ciliary body or anterior chamber, left eye
     H21.323 Implantation cysts of iris, ciliary body or anterior chamber, bilateral
     H21.329 Implantation cysts of iris, ciliary body or anterior chamber, unspecified eye

√6ᵗʰ **H21.33 Parasitic cyst of iris, ciliary body or anterior chamber**
     H21.331 Parasitic cyst of iris, ciliary body or anterior chamber, right eye
     H21.332 Parasitic cyst of iris, ciliary body or anterior chamber, left eye
     H21.333 Parasitic cyst of iris, ciliary body or anterior chamber, bilateral
     H21.339 Parasitic cyst of iris, ciliary body or anterior chamber, unspecified eye

√6ᵗʰ **H21.34 Primary cyst of pars plana**
     H21.341 Primary cyst of pars plana, right eye
     H21.342 Primary cyst of pars plana, left eye
     H21.343 Primary cyst of pars plana, bilateral

      H21.349 **Primary cyst of pars plana, unspecified eye**

  ✓6ᵗʰ **H21.35** **Exudative cyst of** pars plana

      DEF: Protein, fatty-filled bullous elevation of the nonpigmented outermost ciliary epithelium of pars plana, due to fluid leak from blood vessels.

      H21.351 **Exudative cyst of pars plana,** right eye
      H21.352 **Exudative cyst of pars plana,** left eye
      H21.353 **Exudative cyst of pars plana,** bilateral
      H21.359 **Exudative cyst of pars plana,** unspecified

✓5ᵗʰ **H21.4** **Pupillary membranes**

    Iris bombé
    Pupillary occlusion
    Pupillary seclusion
    EXCLUDES 1   *congenital pupillary membranes (Q13.8)*

    H21.4Ø **Pupillary membranes, unspecified eye**
    H21.41 **Pupillary membranes,** right eye
    H21.42 **Pupillary membranes,** left eye
    H21.43 **Pupillary membranes,** bilateral

✓5ᵗʰ **H21.5** **Other and unspecified adhesions and disruptions of iris and ciliary body**

    EXCLUDES 1   *corectopia (Q13.2)*

  ✓6ᵗʰ **H21.5Ø** **Unspecified adhesions of iris**

    Synechia (iris) NOS

      H21.5Ø1 **Unspecified adhesions of iris,** right eye
      H21.5Ø2 **Unspecified adhesions of iris,** left eye
      H21.5Ø3 **Unspecified adhesions of iris,** bilateral
      H21.5Ø9 **Unspecified adhesions of iris and ciliary body, unspecified eye**

  ✓6ᵗʰ **H21.51** **Anterior synechiae (iris)**

      H21.511 **Anterior synechiae (iris),** right eye
      H21.512 **Anterior synechiae (iris),** left eye
      H21.513 **Anterior synechiae (iris),** bilateral
      H21.519 **Anterior synechiae (iris), unspecified eye**

  ✓6ᵗʰ **H21.52** **Goniosynechiae**

      H21.521 **Goniosynechiae,** right eye
      H21.522 **Goniosynechiae,** left eye
      H21.523 **Goniosynechiae,** bilateral
      H21.529 **Goniosynechiae, unspecified eye**

  ✓6ᵗʰ **H21.53** **Iridodialysis**

      H21.531 **Iridodialysis,** right eye
      H21.532 **Iridodialysis,** left eye
      H21.533 **Iridodialysis,** bilateral
      H21.539 **Iridodialysis, unspecified eye**

  ✓6ᵗʰ **H21.54** **Posterior synechiae (iris)**

      H21.541 **Posterior synechiae (iris),** right eye
      H21.542 **Posterior synechiae (iris),** left eye
      H21.543 **Posterior synechiae (iris),** bilateral
      H21.549 **Posterior synechiae (iris), unspecified eye**

  ✓6ᵗʰ **H21.55** **Recession of chamber angle**

      H21.551 **Recession of chamber angle,** right eye
      H21.552 **Recession of chamber angle,** left eye
      H21.553 **Recession of chamber angle,** bilateral
      H21.559 **Recession of chamber angle, unspecified eye**

  ✓6ᵗʰ **H21.56** **Pupillary abnormalities**

    Deformed pupil
    Ectopic pupil
    Rupture of sphincter, pupil
    EXCLUDES 1   *congenital deformity of pupil (Q13.2-)*

      H21.561 **Pupillary abnormality,** right eye
      H21.562 **Pupillary abnormality,** left eye
      H21.563 **Pupillary abnormality,** bilateral
      H21.569 **Pupillary abnormality, unspecified eye**

✓5ᵗʰ **H21.8** **Other specified disorders of iris and ciliary body**

    H21.81 **Floppy iris syndrome**

      Intraoperative floppy iris syndrome (IFIS)
      Use additional code for adverse effect, if applicable, to identify drug (T36-T5Ø with fifth or sixth character 5)

    H21.82 **Plateau iris syndrome (post-iridectomy) (postprocedural)**

    H21.89 **Other specified disorders of iris and ciliary body**

  H21.9 **Unspecified disorder of iris and ciliary body**

H22 *Disorders of iris and ciliary body in diseases classified elsewhere*

    Code first underlying disease, such as:
    gout (M1A.-, M10.-)
    leprosy (A3Ø.-)
    parasitic disease (B89)

Disorders of lens (H25-H28)

✓4ᵗʰ **H25** **Age-related cataract**

    Senile cataract
    EXCLUDES 2   *capsular glaucoma with pseudoexfoliation of lens (H4Ø.1-)*

Cataracts

Iris, Cornea, Pupil, Lens, Vitreous, Retina

Normal lens

Clouded lens

Lens affected by cataracts

✓5ᵗʰ **H25.Ø** **Age-related** incipient **cataract**

  ✓6ᵗʰ **H25.Ø1** **Cortical** age-related **cataract**

      H25.Ø11 **Cortical age-related cataract,** right eye   Ⓐ
      H25.Ø12 **Cortical age-related cataract,** left eye   Ⓐ
      H25.Ø13 **Cortical age-related cataract,** bilateral   Ⓐ
      H25.Ø19 **Cortical age-related cataract, unspecified eye**   Ⓐ

  ✓6ᵗʰ **H25.Ø3** **Anterior subcapsular polar** age-related **cataract**

      H25.Ø31 **Anterior subcapsular polar age-related cataract,** right eye   Ⓐ
      H25.Ø32 **Anterior subcapsular polar age-related cataract,** left eye   Ⓐ
      H25.Ø33 **Anterior subcapsular polar age-related cataract,** bilateral   Ⓐ
      H25.Ø39 **Anterior subcapsular polar age-related cataract, unspecified eye**   Ⓐ

  ✓6ᵗʰ **H25.Ø4** **Posterior subcapsular polar** age-related **cataract**

      H25.Ø41 **Posterior subcapsular polar age-related cataract,** right eye   Ⓐ
      H25.Ø42 **Posterior subcapsular polar age-related cataract,** left eye   Ⓐ
      H25.Ø43 **Posterior subcapsular polar age-related cataract,** bilateral   Ⓐ
      H25.Ø49 **Posterior subcapsular polar age-related cataract, unspecified eye**   Ⓐ

  ✓6ᵗʰ **H25.Ø9** **Other age-related incipient cataract**

    Coronary age-related cataract
    Punctate age-related cataract
    Water clefts

      H25.Ø91 **Other age-related incipient cataract,** right eye   Ⓐ
      H25.Ø92 **Other age-related incipient cataract,** left eye   Ⓐ
      H25.Ø93 **Other age-related incipient cataract,** bilateral   Ⓐ
      H25.Ø99 **Other age-related incipient cataract, unspecified eye**   Ⓐ

✔ Additional Character Required   ✔x7ᵗʰ Placeholder Alert   Manifestation   Unspecified Dx   ▶◀ Revised Text   ● New Code   ▲ Revised Code Title

ICD-10-CM 2020   599

✓5ᵗʰ **H25.1 Age-related** nuclear **cataract**
Cataracta brunescens
Nuclear sclerosis cataract
AHA: 2019,2Q,31; 2016,1Q,32

   H25.10 Age-related nuclear cataract, unspecified eye   Ⓐ

   H25.11 Age-related nuclear cataract, right **eye**   Ⓐ

   H25.12 Age-related nuclear cataract, left **eye**   Ⓐ

   H25.13 Age-related nuclear cataract, bilateral   Ⓐ

✓5ᵗʰ **H25.2 Age-related cataract,** morgagnian type
Age-related hypermature cataract

   H25.20 Age-related cataract, morgagnian type, unspecified eye   Ⓐ

   H25.21 Age-related cataract, morgagnian type, right **eye**   Ⓐ

   H25.22 Age-related cataract, morgagnian type, left **eye**   Ⓐ

   H25.23 Age-related cataract, morgagnian type, bilateral   Ⓐ

✓5ᵗʰ **H25.8 Other age-related cataract**

   ✓6ᵗʰ **H25.81 Combined forms** of age-related cataract
AHA: 2019,2Q,30

     H25.811 Combined forms of age-related cataract, right **eye**   Ⓐ

     H25.812 Combined forms of age-related cataract, left **eye**   Ⓐ

     H25.813 Combined forms of age-related cataract, bilateral   Ⓐ

     H25.819 Combined forms of age-related cataract, unspecified eye   Ⓐ

   H25.89 Other age-related cataract   Ⓐ

   H25.9 Unspecified age-related cataract   Ⓐ

✓4ᵗʰ **H26 Other cataract**

   EXCLUDES 1   congenital cataract (Q12.0)

✓5ᵗʰ **H26.0 Infantile and juvenile** cataract

   ✓6ᵗʰ **H26.00 Unspecified infantile and juvenile cataract**

     H26.001 Unspecified infantile and juvenile cataract, right **eye**   Ⓟ

     H26.002 Unspecified infantile and juvenile cataract, left **eye**   Ⓟ

     H26.003 Unspecified infantile and juvenile cataract, bilateral   Ⓟ

     H26.009 Unspecified infantile and juvenile cataract, unspecified eye   Ⓟ

   ✓6ᵗʰ **H26.01 Infantile and juvenile** cortical, lamellar, or zonular cataract

     H26.011 Infantile and juvenile cortical, lamellar, or zonular cataract, right **eye**   Ⓟ

     H26.012 Infantile and juvenile cortical, lamellar, or zonular cataract, left **eye**   Ⓟ

     H26.013 Infantile and juvenile cortical, lamellar, or zonular cataract, bilateral   Ⓟ

     H26.019 Infantile and juvenile cortical, lamellar, or zonular cataract, unspecified eye   Ⓟ

   ✓6ᵗʰ **H26.03 Infantile and juvenile** nuclear **cataract**

     H26.031 Infantile and juvenile nuclear cataract, right **eye**   Ⓟ

     H26.032 Infantile and juvenile nuclear cataract, left **eye**   Ⓟ

     H26.033 Infantile and juvenile nuclear cataract, bilateral   Ⓟ

     H26.039 Infantile and juvenile nuclear cataract, unspecified eye   Ⓟ

   ✓6ᵗʰ **H26.04 Anterior** subcapsular polar **infantile and juvenile** cataract

     H26.041 Anterior subcapsular polar infantile and juvenile cataract, right **eye**   Ⓟ

     H26.042 Anterior subcapsular polar infantile and juvenile cataract, left **eye**   Ⓟ

     H26.043 Anterior subcapsular polar infantile and juvenile cataract, bilateral   Ⓟ

     H26.049 Anterior subcapsular polar infantile and juvenile cataract, unspecified eye   Ⓟ

   ✓6ᵗʰ **H26.05 Posterior** subcapsular polar **infantile and juvenile** cataract

     H26.051 Posterior subcapsular polar infantile and juvenile cataract, right **eye**   Ⓟ

     H26.052 Posterior subcapsular polar infantile and juvenile cataract, left **eye**   Ⓟ

     H26.053 Posterior subcapsular polar infantile and juvenile cataract, bilateral   Ⓟ

     H26.059 Posterior subcapsular polar infantile and juvenile cataract, unspecified eye   Ⓟ

   ✓6ᵗʰ **H26.06 Combined forms** of infantile and juvenile cataract

     H26.061 Combined forms of infantile and juvenile cataract, right **eye**   Ⓟ

     H26.062 Combined forms of infantile and juvenile cataract, left **eye**   Ⓟ

     H26.063 Combined forms of infantile and juvenile cataract, bilateral   Ⓟ

     H26.069 Combined forms of infantile and juvenile cataract, unspecified eye   Ⓟ

   H26.09 Other infantile and juvenile cataract   Ⓟ

✓5ᵗʰ **H26.1 Traumatic** cataract
Use additional code (Chapter 20) to identify external cause

   ✓6ᵗʰ **H26.10 Unspecified traumatic cataract**

     H26.101 Unspecified traumatic cataract, right **eye**

     H26.102 Unspecified traumatic cataract, left **eye**

     H26.103 Unspecified traumatic cataract, bilateral

     H26.109 Unspecified traumatic cataract, unspecified eye

   ✓6ᵗʰ **H26.11 Localized** traumatic opacities

     H26.111 Localized traumatic opacities, right **eye**

     H26.112 Localized traumatic opacities, left **eye**

     H26.113 Localized traumatic opacities, bilateral

     H26.119 Localized traumatic opacities, unspecified eye

   ✓6ᵗʰ **H26.12 Partially** resolved **traumatic cataract**

     H26.121 Partially resolved traumatic cataract, right **eye**

     H26.122 Partially resolved traumatic cataract, left **eye**

     H26.123 Partially resolved traumatic cataract, bilateral

     H26.129 Partially resolved traumatic cataract, unspecified eye

   ✓6ᵗʰ **H26.13 Total** traumatic cataract

     H26.131 Total traumatic cataract, right **eye**

     H26.132 Total traumatic cataract, left **eye**

     H26.133 Total traumatic cataract, bilateral

     H26.139 Total traumatic cataract, unspecified eye

✓5ᵗʰ **H26.2 Complicated** cataract

   H26.20 Unspecified complicated cataract
Cataracta complicata NOS

   ✓6ᵗʰ **H26.21 Cataract** with neovascularization
Code also associated condition, such as:
     chronic iridocyclitis (H20.1-)

     H26.211 Cataract with neovascularization, right **eye**

     H26.212 Cataract with neovascularization, left **eye**

     H26.213 Cataract with neovascularization, bilateral

     H26.219 Cataract with neovascularization, unspecified eye

   ✓6ᵗʰ **H26.22 Cataract** secondary to ocular disorders **(degenerative) (inflammatory)**
Code also associated ocular disorder

     H26.221 Cataract secondary to ocular disorders (degenerative) (inflammatory), right **eye**

     H26.222 Cataract secondary to ocular disorders (degenerative) (inflammatory), left **eye**

     H26.223 Cataract secondary to ocular disorders (degenerative) (inflammatory), bilateral

     H26.229 Cataract secondary to ocular disorders (degenerative) (inflammatory), unspecified eye

☑6ᵗʰ **H26.23** Glaucomatous flecks (subcapsular)

    Code first underlying glaucoma (H40-H42)

    H26.231 Glaucomatous flecks (subcapsular), right eye

    H26.232 Glaucomatous flecks (subcapsular), left eye

    H26.233 Glaucomatous flecks (subcapsular), bilateral

    H26.239 Glaucomatous flecks (subcapsular), unspecified eye

☑5ᵗʰ **H26.3** Drug-induced cataract

    Toxic cataract

    Use additional code for adverse effect, if applicable, to identify drug (T36-T50 with fifth or sixth character 5)

    H26.30 Drug-induced cataract, unspecified eye

    H26.31 Drug-induced cataract, right eye

    H26.32 Drug-induced cataract, left eye

    H26.33 Drug-induced cataract, bilateral

☑5ᵗʰ **H26.4** Secondary cataract

    H26.40 Unspecified secondary cataract

☑6ᵗʰ   **H26.41** Soemmering's ring

        H26.411 Soemmering's ring, right eye

        H26.412 Soemmering's ring, left eye

        H26.413 Soemmering's ring, bilateral

        H26.419 Soemmering's ring, unspecified eye

☑6ᵗʰ   **H26.49** Other secondary cataract

        AHA: 2018,2Q,14

        H26.491 Other secondary cataract, right eye

        H26.492 Other secondary cataract, left eye

        H26.493 Other secondary cataract, bilateral

        H26.499 Other secondary cataract, unspecified eye

    H26.8 Other specified cataract

    H26.9 Unspecified cataract

☑4ᵗʰ **H27** Other disorders of lens

    EXCLUDES 1   congenital lens malformations (Q12.-)

              mechanical complications of intraocular lens implant (T85.2)

              pseudophakia (Z96.1)

☑5ᵗʰ **H27.0** Aphakia

    Acquired absence of lens

    Acquired aphakia

    Aphakia due to trauma

    EXCLUDES 1   cataract extraction status (Z98.4-)

              congenital absence of lens (Q12.3)

              congenital aphakia (Q12.3)

    H27.00 Aphakia, unspecified eye

    H27.01 Aphakia, right eye

    H27.02 Aphakia, left eye

    H27.03 Aphakia, bilateral

☑5ᵗʰ **H27.1** Dislocation of lens

    H27.10 Unspecified dislocation of lens

☑6ᵗʰ   **H27.11** Subluxation of lens

        H27.111 Subluxation of lens, right eye

        H27.112 Subluxation of lens, left eye

        H27.113 Subluxation of lens, bilateral

        H27.119 Subluxation of lens, unspecified eye

☑6ᵗʰ   **H27.12** Anterior dislocation of lens

        H27.121 Anterior dislocation of lens, right eye

        H27.122 Anterior dislocation of lens, left eye

        H27.123 Anterior dislocation of lens, bilateral

        H27.129 Anterior dislocation of lens, unspecified eye

☑6ᵗʰ   **H27.13** Posterior dislocation of lens

        H27.131 Posterior dislocation of lens, right eye

        H27.132 Posterior dislocation of lens, left eye

        H27.133 Posterior dislocation of lens, bilateral

        H27.139 Posterior dislocation of lens, unspecified eye

    H27.8 Other specified disorders of lens

    H27.9 Unspecified disorder of lens

H28 *Cataract in diseases classified elsewhere*

    Code first underlying disease, such as:

      hypoparathyroidism (E20.-)

      myotonia (G71.1-)

      myxedema (E03.-)

      protein-calorie malnutrition (E40-E46)

    EXCLUDES 1   cataract in diabetes mellitus (E08.36, E09.36, E10.36, E11.36, E13.36)

Disorders of choroid and retina (H30-H36)

☑4ᵗʰ **H30** Chorioretinal inflammation

☑5ᵗʰ **H30.0** Focal chorioretinal inflammation

    Focal chorioretinitis

    Focal choroiditis

    Focal retinitis

    Focal retinochoroiditis

☑6ᵗʰ   **H30.00** Unspecified focal chorioretinal inflammation

        Focal chorioretinitis NOS

        Focal choroiditis NOS

        Focal retinitis NOS

        Focal retinochoroiditis NOS

        H30.001 Unspecified focal chorioretinal inflammation, right eye

        H30.002 Unspecified focal chorioretinal inflammation, left eye

        H30.003 Unspecified focal chorioretinal inflammation, bilateral

        H30.009 Unspecified focal chorioretinal inflammation, unspecified eye

☑6ᵗʰ   **H30.01** Focal chorioretinal inflammation, juxtapapillary

        H30.011 Focal chorioretinal inflammation, juxtapapillary, right eye

        H30.012 Focal chorioretinal inflammation, juxtapapillary, left eye

        H30.013 Focal chorioretinal inflammation, juxtapapillary, bilateral

        H30.019 Focal chorioretinal inflammation, juxtapapillary, unspecified eye

☑6ᵗʰ   **H30.02** Focal chorioretinal inflammation of posterior pole

        H30.021 Focal chorioretinal inflammation of posterior pole, right eye

        H30.022 Focal chorioretinal inflammation of posterior pole, left eye

        H30.023 Focal chorioretinal inflammation of posterior pole, bilateral

        H30.029 Focal chorioretinal inflammation of posterior pole, unspecified eye

☑6ᵗʰ   **H30.03** Focal chorioretinal inflammation, peripheral

        H30.031 Focal chorioretinal inflammation, peripheral, right eye

        H30.032 Focal chorioretinal inflammation, peripheral, left eye

        H30.033 Focal chorioretinal inflammation, peripheral, bilateral

        H30.039 Focal chorioretinal inflammation, peripheral, unspecified eye

☑6ᵗʰ   **H30.04** Focal chorioretinal inflammation, macular or paramacular

        H30.041 Focal chorioretinal inflammation, macular or paramacular, right eye

        H30.042 Focal chorioretinal inflammation, macular or paramacular, left eye

        H30.043 Focal chorioretinal inflammation, macular or paramacular, bilateral

        H30.049 Focal chorioretinal inflammation, macular or paramacular, unspecified eye

☑ Additional Character Required   ☑x7ᵗʰ Placeholder Alert   Manifestation   Unspecified Dx   ▶◀ Revised Text   ● New Code   ▲ Revised Code Title

ICD-10-CM 2020   601

H26.23–H30.049

Chapter 7. Diseases of the Eye and Adnexa

H30.1–H31.129

√6ᵗʰ **H30.1 Disseminated chorioretinal inflammation**
Disseminated chorioretinitis
Disseminated choroiditis
Disseminated retinitis
Disseminated retinochoroiditis
EXCLUDES 2   *exudative retinopathy (H35.02-)*

√6ᵗʰ **H30.10 Unspecified disseminated chorioretinal inflammation**
Disseminated chorioretinitis NOS
Disseminated choroiditis NOS
Disseminated retinitis NOS
Disseminated retinochoroiditis NOS

H30.101 **Unspecified disseminated chorioretinal inflammation, right eye**

H30.102 **Unspecified disseminated chorioretinal inflammation, left eye**

H30.103 **Unspecified disseminated chorioretinal inflammation, bilateral**

H30.109 **Unspecified disseminated chorioretinal inflammation, unspecified eye**

√6ᵗʰ **H30.11 Disseminated chorioretinal inflammation of posterior pole**

H30.111 **Disseminated chorioretinal inflammation of posterior pole, right eye**

H30.112 **Disseminated chorioretinal inflammation of posterior pole, left eye**

H30.113 **Disseminated chorioretinal inflammation of posterior pole, bilateral**

H30.119 **Disseminated chorioretinal inflammation of posterior pole, unspecified eye**

√6ᵗʰ **H30.12 Disseminated chorioretinal inflammation, peripheral**

H30.121 **Disseminated chorioretinal inflammation, peripheral right eye**

H30.122 **Disseminated chorioretinal inflammation, peripheral, left eye**

H30.123 **Disseminated chorioretinal inflammation, peripheral, bilateral**

H30.129 **Disseminated chorioretinal inflammation, peripheral, unspecified eye**

√6ᵗʰ **H30.13 Disseminated chorioretinal inflammation, generalized**

H30.131 **Disseminated chorioretinal inflammation, generalized, right eye**

H30.132 **Disseminated chorioretinal inflammation, generalized, left eye**

H30.133 **Disseminated chorioretinal inflammation, generalized, bilateral**

H30.139 **Disseminated chorioretinal inflammation, generalized, unspecified eye**

√6ᵗʰ **H30.14 Acute posterior multifocal placoid pigment epitheliopathy**

H30.141 **Acute posterior multifocal placoid pigment epitheliopathy, right eye**

H30.142 **Acute posterior multifocal placoid pigment epitheliopathy, left eye**

H30.143 **Acute posterior multifocal placoid pigment epitheliopathy, bilateral**

H30.149 **Acute posterior multifocal placoid pigment epitheliopathy, unspecified eye**

√5ᵗʰ **H30.2 Posterior cyclitis**
Pars planitis

H30.20 **Posterior cyclitis, unspecified eye**

H30.21 **Posterior cyclitis, right eye**

H30.22 **Posterior cyclitis, left eye**

H30.23 **Posterior cyclitis, bilateral**

√5ᵗʰ **H30.8 Other chorioretinal inflammations**

√6ᵗʰ **H30.81 Harada's disease**

H30.811 **Harada's disease, right eye**

H30.812 **Harada's disease, left eye**

H30.813 **Harada's disease, bilateral**

H30.819 **Harada's disease, unspecified eye**

√6ᵗʰ **H30.89 Other chorioretinal inflammations**

H30.891 **Other chorioretinal inflammations, right eye**

H30.892 **Other chorioretinal inflammations, left eye**

H30.893 **Other chorioretinal inflammations, bilateral**

H30.899 **Other chorioretinal inflammations, unspecified eye**

√5ᵗʰ **H30.9 Unspecified chorioretinal inflammation**
Chorioretinitis NOS
Choroiditis NOS
Neuroretinitis NOS
Retinitis NOS
Retinochoroiditis NOS

H30.90 **Unspecified chorioretinal inflammation, unspecified eye**

H30.91 **Unspecified chorioretinal inflammation, right eye**

H30.92 **Unspecified chorioretinal inflammation, left eye**

H30.93 **Unspecified chorioretinal inflammation, bilateral**

√4ᵗʰ **H31 Other disorders of choroid**

√5ᵗʰ **H31.0 Chorioretinal scars**
EXCLUDES 2   *postsurgical chorioretinal scars (H59.81-)*

√6ᵗʰ **H31.00 Unspecified chorioretinal scars**

H31.001 **Unspecified chorioretinal scars, right eye**

H31.002 **Unspecified chorioretinal scars, left eye**

H31.003 **Unspecified chorioretinal scars, bilateral**

H31.009 **Unspecified chorioretinal scars, unspecified eye**

√6ᵗʰ **H31.01 Macula scars of posterior pole (postinflammatory) (post-traumatic)**
EXCLUDES 1   *postprocedural chorioretinal scar (H59.81-)*

H31.011 **Macula scars of posterior pole (postinflammatory) (post-traumatic), right eye**

H31.012 **Macula scars of posterior pole (postinflammatory) (post-traumatic), left eye**

H31.013 **Macula scars of posterior pole (postinflammatory) (post-traumatic), bilateral**

H31.019 **Macula scars of posterior pole (postinflammatory) (post-traumatic), unspecified eye**

√6ᵗʰ **H31.02 Solar retinopathy**

H31.021 **Solar retinopathy, right eye**

H31.022 **Solar retinopathy, left eye**

H31.023 **Solar retinopathy, bilateral**

H31.029 **Solar retinopathy, unspecified eye**

√6ᵗʰ **H31.09 Other chorioretinal scars**

H31.091 **Other chorioretinal scars, right eye**

H31.092 **Other chorioretinal scars, left eye**

H31.093 **Other chorioretinal scars, bilateral**

H31.099 **Other chorioretinal scars, unspecified eye**

√5ᵗʰ **H31.1 Choroidal degeneration**
EXCLUDES 2   *angioid streaks of macula (H35.33)*

√6ᵗʰ **H31.10 Unspecified choroidal degeneration**
Choroidal sclerosis NOS

H31.101 **Choroidal degeneration, unspecified, right eye**

H31.102 **Choroidal degeneration, unspecified, left eye**

H31.103 **Choroidal degeneration, unspecified, bilateral**

H31.109 **Choroidal degeneration, unspecified, unspecified eye**

√6ᵗʰ **H31.11 Age-related choroidal atrophy**

H31.111 **Age-related choroidal atrophy, right eye**   Ⓐ

H31.112 **Age-related choroidal atrophy, left eye**   Ⓐ

H31.113 **Age-related choroidal atrophy, bilateral**   Ⓐ

H31.119 **Age-related choroidal atrophy, unspecified eye**   Ⓐ

√6ᵗʰ **H31.12 Diffuse secondary atrophy of choroid**

H31.121 **Diffuse secondary atrophy of choroid, right eye**

H31.122 **Diffuse secondary atrophy of choroid, left eye**

H31.123 **Diffuse secondary atrophy of choroid, bilateral**

H31.129 **Diffuse secondary atrophy of choroid, unspecified eye**

√5ᵗʰ **H31.2 Hereditary choroidal dystrophy**
  EXCLUDES 2   hyperornithinemia (E72.4)
            ornithinemia (E72.4)
  H31.20 Hereditary choroidal dystrophy, unspecified
  H31.21 Choroideremia
  H31.22 Choroidal dystrophy (central areolar) (generalized) (peripapillary)
  H31.23 Gyrate atrophy, choroid
  H31.29 Other hereditary choroidal dystrophy

√5ᵗʰ **H31.3 Choroidal hemorrhage and rupture**
  √6ᵗʰ **H31.30 Unspecified choroidal hemorrhage**
    H31.301 Unspecified choroidal hemorrhage, right eye
    H31.302 Unspecified choroidal hemorrhage, left eye
    H31.303 Unspecified choroidal hemorrhage, bilateral
    H31.309 Unspecified choroidal hemorrhage, unspecified eye
  √6ᵗʰ **H31.31 Expulsive choroidal hemorrhage**
    H31.311 Expulsive choroidal hemorrhage, right eye
    H31.312 Expulsive choroidal hemorrhage, left eye
    H31.313 Expulsive choroidal hemorrhage, bilateral
    H31.319 Expulsive choroidal hemorrhage, unspecified eye
  √6ᵗʰ **H31.32 Choroidal rupture**
    H31.321 Choroidal rupture, right eye
    H31.322 Choroidal rupture, left eye
    H31.323 Choroidal rupture, bilateral
    H31.329 Choroidal rupture, unspecified eye

√5ᵗʰ **H31.4 Choroidal detachment**
  √6ᵗʰ **H31.40 Unspecified choroidal detachment**
    H31.401 Unspecified choroidal detachment, right eye
    H31.402 Unspecified choroidal detachment, left eye
    H31.403 Unspecified choroidal detachment, bilateral
    H31.409 Unspecified choroidal detachment, unspecified eye
  √6ᵗʰ **H31.41 Hemorrhagic choroidal detachment**
    H31.411 Hemorrhagic choroidal detachment, right eye
    H31.412 Hemorrhagic choroidal detachment, left eye
    H31.413 Hemorrhagic choroidal detachment, bilateral
    H31.419 Hemorrhagic choroidal detachment, unspecified eye
  √6ᵗʰ **H31.42 Serous choroidal detachment**
    H31.421 Serous choroidal detachment, right eye
    H31.422 Serous choroidal detachment, left eye
    H31.423 Serous choroidal detachment, bilateral
    H31.429 Serous choroidal detachment, unspecified eye
  H31.8 Other specified disorders of choroid
  H31.9 Unspecified disorder of choroid

H32 Chorioretinal disorders in diseases classified elsewhere
  Code first underlying disease, such as:
  congenital toxoplasmosis (P37.1)
  histoplasmosis (B39.-)
  leprosy (A30.-)
  EXCLUDES 1   chorioretinitis (in):
           toxoplasmosis (acquired) (B58.01)
           tuberculosis (A18.53)

√4ᵗʰ **H33 Retinal detachments and breaks**
  EXCLUDES 1   detachment of retinal pigment epithelium (H35.72-, H35.73-)

Retinal Detachment

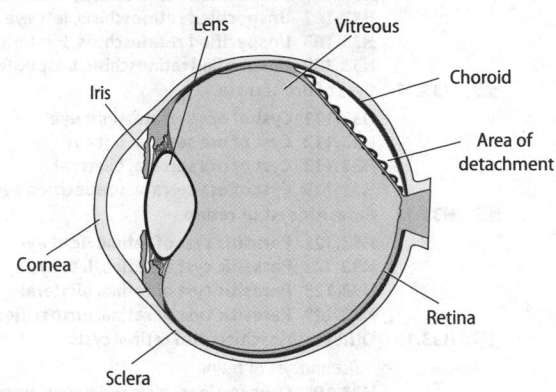

√5ᵗʰ **H33.0 Retinal detachment with retinal break**
  Rhegmatogenous retinal detachment
  EXCLUDES 1   serous retinal detachment (without retinal break) (H33.2-)
  √6ᵗʰ **H33.00 Unspecified retinal detachment with retinal break**
    H33.001 Unspecified retinal detachment with retinal break, right eye
    H33.002 Unspecified retinal detachment with retinal break, left eye
    H33.003 Unspecified retinal detachment with retinal break, bilateral
    H33.009 Unspecified retinal detachment with retinal break, unspecified eye
  √6ᵗʰ **H33.01 Retinal detachment with single break**
    H33.011 Retinal detachment with single break, right eye
    H33.012 Retinal detachment with single break, left eye
    H33.013 Retinal detachment with single break, bilateral
    H33.019 Retinal detachment with single break, unspecified eye
  √6ᵗʰ **H33.02 Retinal detachment with multiple breaks**
    H33.021 Retinal detachment with multiple breaks, right eye
    H33.022 Retinal detachment with multiple breaks, left eye
    H33.023 Retinal detachment with multiple breaks, bilateral
    H33.029 Retinal detachment with multiple breaks, unspecified eye
  √6ᵗʰ **H33.03 Retinal detachment with giant retinal tear**
    H33.031 Retinal detachment with giant retinal tear, right eye
    H33.032 Retinal detachment with giant retinal tear, left eye
    H33.033 Retinal detachment with giant retinal tear, bilateral
    H33.039 Retinal detachment with giant retinal tear, unspecified eye
  √6ᵗʰ **H33.04 Retinal detachment with retinal dialysis**
    H33.041 Retinal detachment with retinal dialysis, right eye
    H33.042 Retinal detachment with retinal dialysis, left eye
    H33.043 Retinal detachment with retinal dialysis, bilateral
    H33.049 Retinal detachment with retinal dialysis, unspecified eye
  √6ᵗʰ **H33.05 Total retinal detachment**
    H33.051 Total retinal detachment, right eye
    H33.052 Total retinal detachment, left eye
    H33.053 Total retinal detachment, bilateral
    H33.059 Total retinal detachment, unspecified eye

Chapter 7. Diseases of the Eye and Adnexa

H33.1–H35.00

✓5ᵗʰ **H33.1 Retinoschisis and retinal cysts**

     EXCLUDES 1   *congenital retinoschisis (Q14.1)*

         microcystoid degeneration of retina (H35.42-)

    ✓6ᵗʰ **H33.10 Unspecified retinoschisis**

      H33.101 Unspecified retinoschisis, right eye

      H33.102 Unspecified retinoschisis, left eye

      H33.103 Unspecified retinoschisis, bilateral

      H33.109 Unspecified retinoschisis, unspecified eye

    ✓6ᵗʰ **H33.11 Cyst of ora serrata**

      H33.111 Cyst of ora serrata, right eye

      H33.112 Cyst of ora serrata, left eye

      H33.113 Cyst of ora serrata, bilateral

      H33.119 Cyst of ora serrata, unspecified eye

    ✓6ᵗʰ **H33.12 Parasitic cyst of retina**

      H33.121 Parasitic cyst of retina, right eye

      H33.122 Parasitic cyst of retina, left eye

      H33.123 Parasitic cyst of retina, bilateral

      H33.129 Parasitic cyst of retina, unspecified eye

    ✓6ᵗʰ **H33.19 Other retinoschisis and retinal cysts**

      Pseudocyst of retina

      H33.191 Other retinoschisis and retinal cysts, right eye

      H33.192 Other retinoschisis and retinal cysts, left eye

      H33.193 Other retinoschisis and retinal cysts, bilateral

      H33.199 Other retinoschisis and retinal cysts, unspecified eye

✓5ᵗʰ **H33.2 Serous retinal detachment**

     Retinal detachment NOS

     Retinal detachment without retinal break

     EXCLUDES 1   *central serous chorioretinopathy (H35.71-)*

    H33.20 Serous retinal detachment, unspecified eye

    H33.21 Serous retinal detachment, right eye

    H33.22 Serous retinal detachment, left eye

    H33.23 Serous retinal detachment, bilateral

✓5ᵗʰ **H33.3 Retinal breaks without detachment**

     EXCLUDES 1   *chorioretinal scars after surgery for detachment (H59.81-)*

         peripheral retinal degeneration without break (H35.4-)

    ✓6ᵗʰ **H33.30 Unspecified retinal break**

      H33.301 Unspecified retinal break, right eye

      H33.302 Unspecified retinal break, left eye

      H33.303 Unspecified retinal break, bilateral

      H33.309 Unspecified retinal break, unspecified eye

    ✓6ᵗʰ **H33.31 Horseshoe tear of retina without detachment**

      Operculum of retina without detachment

      H33.311 Horseshoe tear of retina without detachment, right eye

      H33.312 Horseshoe tear of retina without detachment, left eye

      H33.313 Horseshoe tear of retina without detachment, bilateral

      H33.319 Horseshoe tear of retina without detachment, unspecified eye

    ✓6ᵗʰ **H33.32 Round hole of retina without detachment**

      H33.321 Round hole, right eye

      H33.322 Round hole, left eye

      H33.323 Round hole, bilateral

      H33.329 Round hole, unspecified eye

    ✓6ᵗʰ **H33.33 Multiple defects of retina without detachment**

      H33.331 Multiple defects of retina without detachment, right eye

      H33.332 Multiple defects of retina without detachment, left eye

      H33.333 Multiple defects of retina without detachment, bilateral

      H33.339 Multiple defects of retina without detachment, unspecified eye

✓5ᵗʰ **H33.4 Traction detachment of retina**

     Proliferative vitreo-retinopathy with retinal detachment

    H33.40 Traction detachment of retina, unspecified eye

    H33.41 Traction detachment of retina, right eye

    H33.42 Traction detachment of retina, left eye

    H33.43 Traction detachment of retina, bilateral

H33.8 Other retinal detachments

✓4ᵗʰ **H34 Retinal vascular occlusions**

     EXCLUDES 1   *amaurosis fugax (G45.3)*

    ✓5ᵗʰ **H34.0 Transient retinal artery occlusion**

      H34.00 Transient retinal artery occlusion, unspecified eye

      H34.01 Transient retinal artery occlusion, right eye

      H34.02 Transient retinal artery occlusion, left eye

      H34.03 Transient retinal artery occlusion, bilateral

    ✓5ᵗʰ **H34.1 Central retinal artery occlusion**

      H34.10 Central retinal artery occlusion, unspecified eye

      H34.11 Central retinal artery occlusion, right eye

      H34.12 Central retinal artery occlusion, left eye

      H34.13 Central retinal artery occlusion, bilateral

    ✓5ᵗʰ **H34.2 Other retinal artery occlusions**

     ✓6ᵗʰ **H34.21 Partial retinal artery occlusion**

       Hollenhorst's plaque

       Retinal microembolism

       H34.211 Partial retinal artery occlusion, right eye

       H34.212 Partial retinal artery occlusion, left eye

       H34.213 Partial retinal artery occlusion, bilateral

       H34.219 Partial retinal artery occlusion, unspecified eye

     ✓6ᵗʰ **H34.23 Retinal artery branch occlusion**

       H34.231 Retinal artery branch occlusion, right eye

       H34.232 Retinal artery branch occlusion, left eye

       H34.233 Retinal artery branch occlusion, bilateral

       H34.239 Retinal artery branch occlusion, unspecified eye

    ✓5ᵗʰ **H34.8 Other retinal vascular occlusions**

     AHA: 2016,4Q,19

     ✓6ᵗʰ **H34.81 Central retinal vein occlusion**

       One of the following 7th characters is to be assigned to codes in subcategory H34.81 to designate the severity of the occlusion:

       0   with macular edema

       1   with retinal neovascularization

       2   stable

          old central retinal vein occlusion

       ✓7ᵗʰ **H34.811 Central retinal vein occlusion, right eye**

       ✓7ᵗʰ **H34.812 Central retinal vein occlusion, left eye**

       ✓7ᵗʰ **H34.813 Central retinal vein occlusion, bilateral**

       ✓7ᵗʰ **H34.819 Central retinal vein occlusion, unspecified eye**

     ✓6ᵗʰ **H34.82 Venous engorgement**

       Incipient retinal vein occlusion

       Partial retinal vein occlusion

       H34.821 Venous engorgement, right eye

       H34.822 Venous engorgement, left eye

       H34.823 Venous engorgement, bilateral

       H34.829 Venous engorgement, unspecified eye

     ✓6ᵗʰ **H34.83 Tributary (branch) retinal vein occlusion**

       One of the following 7th characters is to be assigned to codes in subcategory H34.83 to designate the severity of the occlusion:

       0   with macular edema

       1   with retinal neovascularization

       2   stable

          old tributary (branch) retinal vein occlusion

       ✓7ᵗʰ **H34.831 Tributary (branch) retinal vein occlusion, right eye**

       ✓7ᵗʰ **H34.832 Tributary (branch) retinal vein occlusion, left eye**

       ✓7ᵗʰ **H34.833 Tributary (branch) retinal vein occlusion, bilateral**

       ✓7ᵗʰ **H34.839 Tributary (branch) retinal vein occlusion, unspecified eye**

    H34.9 Unspecified retinal vascular occlusion

✓4ᵗʰ **H35 Other retinal disorders**

     EXCLUDES 2   *diabetic retinal disorders (E08.311-E08.359, E09.311-E09.359, E10.311-E10.359, E11.311-E11.359, E13.311-E13.359)*

    ✓5ᵗʰ **H35.0 Background retinopathy and retinal vascular changes**

     Code also any associated hypertension (I10.-)

     H35.00 Unspecified background retinopathy

✓6ᵗʰ **H35.01   Changes in retinal vascular appearance**
     Retinal vascular sheathing
     H35.011   **Changes in retinal vascular appearance, right eye**
     H35.012   **Changes in retinal vascular appearance, left eye**
     H35.013   **Changes in retinal vascular appearance, bilateral**
     H35.019   **Changes in retinal vascular appearance, unspecified eye**

✓6ᵗʰ **H35.02   Exudative retinopathy**
     Coats retinopathy
     H35.021   **Exudative retinopathy, right eye**
     H35.022   **Exudative retinopathy, left eye**
     H35.023   **Exudative retinopathy, bilateral**
     H35.029   **Exudative retinopathy, unspecified eye**

✓6ᵗʰ **H35.03   Hypertensive retinopathy**
     H35.031   **Hypertensive retinopathy, right eye**
     H35.032   **Hypertensive retinopathy, left eye**
     H35.033   **Hypertensive retinopathy, bilateral**
     H35.039   **Hypertensive retinopathy, unspecified eye**

✓6ᵗʰ **H35.04   Retinal micro-aneurysms, unspecified**
     H35.041   **Retinal micro-aneurysms, unspecified, right eye**
     H35.042   **Retinal micro-aneurysms, unspecified, left eye**
     H35.043   **Retinal micro-aneurysms, unspecified, bilateral**
     H35.049   **Retinal micro-aneurysms, unspecified, unspecified eye**

✓6ᵗʰ **H35.05   Retinal neovascularization, unspecified**
     H35.051   **Retinal neovascularization, unspecified, right eye**
     H35.052   **Retinal neovascularization, unspecified, left eye**
     H35.053   **Retinal neovascularization, unspecified, bilateral**
     H35.059   **Retinal neovascularization, unspecified, unspecified eye**

✓6ᵗʰ **H35.06   Retinal vasculitis**
     Eales disease
     Retinal perivasculitis
     DEF: Sight-threatening intraocular inflammation of the retinal blood vessels that causes minimal, partial, or even complete blindness.
     H35.061   **Retinal vasculitis, right eye**
     H35.062   **Retinal vasculitis, left eye**
     H35.063   **Retinal vasculitis, bilateral**
     H35.069   **Retinal vasculitis, unspecified eye**

✓6ᵗʰ **H35.07   Retinal telangiectasis**
     H35.071   **Retinal telangiectasis, right eye**
     H35.072   **Retinal telangiectasis, left eye**
     H35.073   **Retinal telangiectasis, bilateral**
     H35.079   **Retinal telangiectasis, unspecified eye**

     H35.09   Other intraretinal microvascular abnormalities
     Retinal varices

✓5ᵗʰ **H35.1   Retinopathy of prematurity**

✓6ᵗʰ **H35.10   Retinopathy of prematurity, unspecified**
     Retinopathy of prematurity NOS
     H35.101   **Retinopathy of prematurity, unspecified, right eye**
     H35.102   **Retinopathy of prematurity, unspecified, left eye**
     H35.103   **Retinopathy of prematurity, unspecified, bilateral**
     H35.109   **Retinopathy of prematurity, unspecified, unspecified eye**

✓6ᵗʰ **H35.11   Retinopathy of prematurity, stage 0**
     H35.111   **Retinopathy of prematurity, stage 0, right eye**
     H35.112   **Retinopathy of prematurity, stage 0, left eye**
     H35.113   **Retinopathy of prematurity, stage 0, bilateral**
     H35.119   **Retinopathy of prematurity, stage 0, unspecified eye**

✓6ᵗʰ **H35.12   Retinopathy of prematurity, stage 1**
     H35.121   **Retinopathy of prematurity, stage 1, right eye**
     H35.122   **Retinopathy of prematurity, stage 1, left eye**
     H35.123   **Retinopathy of prematurity, stage 1, bilateral**
     H35.129   **Retinopathy of prematurity, stage 1, unspecified eye**

✓6ᵗʰ **H35.13   Retinopathy of prematurity, stage 2**
     H35.131   **Retinopathy of prematurity, stage 2, right eye**
     H35.132   **Retinopathy of prematurity, stage 2, left eye**
     H35.133   **Retinopathy of prematurity, stage 2, bilateral**
     H35.139   **Retinopathy of prematurity, stage 2, unspecified eye**

✓6ᵗʰ **H35.14   Retinopathy of prematurity, stage 3**
     H35.141   **Retinopathy of prematurity, stage 3, right eye**
     H35.142   **Retinopathy of prematurity, stage 3, left eye**
     H35.143   **Retinopathy of prematurity, stage 3, bilateral**
     H35.149   **Retinopathy of prematurity, stage 3, unspecified eye**

✓6ᵗʰ **H35.15   Retinopathy of prematurity, stage 4**
     H35.151   **Retinopathy of prematurity, stage 4, right eye**
     H35.152   **Retinopathy of prematurity, stage 4, left eye**
     H35.153   **Retinopathy of prematurity, stage 4, bilateral**
     H35.159   **Retinopathy of prematurity, stage 4, unspecified eye**

✓6ᵗʰ **H35.16   Retinopathy of prematurity, stage 5**
     H35.161   **Retinopathy of prematurity, stage 5, right eye**
     H35.162   **Retinopathy of prematurity, stage 5, left eye**
     H35.163   **Retinopathy of prematurity, stage 5, bilateral**
     H35.169   **Retinopathy of prematurity, stage 5, unspecified eye**

✓6ᵗʰ **H35.17   Retrolental fibroplasia**
     H35.171   **Retrolental fibroplasia, right eye**
     H35.172   **Retrolental fibroplasia, left eye**
     H35.173   **Retrolental fibroplasia, bilateral**
     H35.179   **Retrolental fibroplasia, unspecified eye**

✓5ᵗʰ **H35.2   Other non-diabetic proliferative retinopathy**
     Proliferative vitreo-retinopathy
     EXCLUDES 1   *proliferative vitreo-retinopathy with retinal detachment (H33.4-)*
     H35.20   Other non-diabetic proliferative retinopathy, unspecified eye
     H35.21   Other non-diabetic proliferative retinopathy, right eye
     H35.22   Other non-diabetic proliferative retinopathy, left eye
     H35.23   Other non-diabetic proliferative retinopathy, bilateral

✓5ᵗʰ **H35.3   Degeneration of macula and posterior pole**
     H35.30   Unspecified macular degeneration   🄠 🄰
     Age-related macular degeneration

Chapter 7. Diseases of the Eye and Adnexa

H35.31–H35.51

✓6ᵗʰ **H35.31** **Nonexudative age-related macular degeneration**

Atrophic age-related macular degeneration
Dry age-related macular degeneration
AHA: 2016,4Q,20-21

One of the following 7th characters is to be assigned to each code in subcategory H35.31 to designate the stage of the disease:
Ø   stage unspecified
1   early dry stage
2   intermediate dry stage
3   advanced atrophic without subfoveal involvement
    advanced dry stage
4   advanced atrophic with subfoveal involvement

    ✓7ᵗʰ **H35.311** **Nonexudative age-related**   Q A
                 macular degeneration, right eye
    ✓7ᵗʰ **H35.312** **Nonexudative age-related**   Q A
                 macular degeneration, left eye
    ✓7ᵗʰ **H35.313** **Nonexudative age-related**   Q A
                 macular degeneration, bilateral
    ✓7ᵗʰ **H35.319** **Nonexudative age-related**   A
                 macular degeneration, unspecified eye

✓6ᵗʰ **H35.32** **Exudative age-related macular degeneration**

Wet age-related macular degeneration
AHA: 2016,4Q,20-21

One of the following 7th characters is to be assigned to each code in subcategory H35.32 to designate the stage of the disease:
Ø   stage unspecified
1   with active choroidal neovascularization
2   with inactive choroidal neovascularization
    with involuted or regressed neovascularization
3   with inactive scar

    ✓7ᵗʰ **H35.321** **Exudative age-related macular**   HCC Q A
                 degeneration, right eye
    ✓7ᵗʰ **H35.322** **Exudative age-related macular**   HCC Q A
                 degeneration, left eye
    ✓7ᵗʰ **H35.323** **Exudative age-related macular**   HCC Q A
                 degeneration, bilateral
    ✓7ᵗʰ **H35.329** **Exudative age-related macular**   HCC A
                 degeneration, unspecified eye

H35.33 **Angioid streaks of macula**
    DEF: Degeneration of the choroid; characterized by broad, irregular, dark brown streaks radiating from optic disc; occurs with pseudoxanthoma elasticum or Paget's disease.

✓6ᵗʰ **H35.34** **Macular cyst, hole, or pseudohole**
    H35.341 **Macular cyst, hole, or pseudohole, right eye**
    H35.342 **Macular cyst, hole, or pseudohole, left eye**
    H35.343 **Macular cyst, hole, or pseudohole, bilateral**
    H35.349 **Macular cyst, hole, or pseudohole, unspecified eye**

✓6ᵗʰ **H35.35** **Cystoid macular degeneration**
    EXCLUDES 1   cystoid macular edema following cataract surgery (H59.Ø3-)
    H35.351 **Cystoid macular degeneration, right eye**
    H35.352 **Cystoid macular degeneration, left eye**
    H35.353 **Cystoid macular degeneration, bilateral**
    H35.359 **Cystoid macular degeneration, unspecified eye**

✓6ᵗʰ **H35.36** **Drusen (degenerative) of macula**
    AHA: 2017,1Q,51; 2016,4Q,21
    H35.361 **Drusen (degenerative) of macula, right eye**
    H35.362 **Drusen (degenerative) of macula, left eye**
    H35.363 **Drusen (degenerative) of macula, bilateral**
    H35.369 **Drusen (degenerative) of macula, unspecified eye**

✓6ᵗʰ **H35.37** **Puckering of macula**
    H35.371 **Puckering of macula, right eye**
    H35.372 **Puckering of macula, left eye**
    H35.373 **Puckering of macula, bilateral**
    H35.379 **Puckering of macula, unspecified eye**

✓6ᵗʰ **H35.38** **Toxic maculopathy**

Code first poisoning due to drug or toxin, if applicable (T36-T65 with fifth or sixth character 1-4 or 6)
Use additional code for adverse effect, if applicable, to identify drug (T36-T50 with fifth or sixth character 5)

    H35.381 **Toxic maculopathy, right eye**
    H35.382 **Toxic maculopathy, left eye**
    H35.383 **Toxic maculopathy, bilateral**
    H35.389 **Toxic maculopathy, unspecified eye**

✓5ᵗʰ **H35.4** **Peripheral retinal degeneration**
    EXCLUDES 1   hereditary retinal degeneration (dystrophy) (H35.5-)
                 peripheral retinal degeneration with retinal break (H33.3-)

    H35.40 **Unspecified peripheral retinal degeneration**
✓6ᵗʰ **H35.41** **Lattice degeneration of retina**
    Palisade degeneration of retina
    DEF: Degeneration of the retina, often bilateral, that is usually benign. It is characterized by lines intersecting at irregular intervals in the peripheral retina. Retinal thinning and retinal holes may occur.
    H35.411 **Lattice degeneration of retina, right eye**
    H35.412 **Lattice degeneration of retina, left eye**
    H35.413 **Lattice degeneration of retina, bilateral**
    H35.419 **Lattice degeneration of retina, unspecified eye**

✓6ᵗʰ **H35.42** **Microcystoid degeneration of retina**
    H35.421 **Microcystoid degeneration of retina, right eye**
    H35.422 **Microcystoid degeneration of retina, left eye**
    H35.423 **Microcystoid degeneration of retina, bilateral**
    H35.429 **Microcystoid degeneration of retina, unspecified eye**

✓6ᵗʰ **H35.43** **Paving stone degeneration of retina**
    H35.431 **Paving stone degeneration of retina, right eye**
    H35.432 **Paving stone degeneration of retina, left eye**
    H35.433 **Paving stone degeneration of retina, bilateral**
    H35.439 **Paving stone degeneration of retina, unspecified eye**

✓6ᵗʰ **H35.44** **Age-related reticular degeneration of retina**
    H35.441 **Age-related reticular**   A
                 degeneration of retina, right eye
    H35.442 **Age-related reticular**   A
                 degeneration of retina, left eye
    H35.443 **Age-related reticular**   A
                 degeneration of retina, bilateral
    H35.449 **Age-related reticular**   A
                 degeneration of retina, unspecified eye

✓6ᵗʰ **H35.45** **Secondary pigmentary degeneration**
    H35.451 **Secondary pigmentary degeneration, right eye**
    H35.452 **Secondary pigmentary degeneration, left eye**
    H35.453 **Secondary pigmentary degeneration, bilateral**
    H35.459 **Secondary pigmentary degeneration, unspecified eye**

✓6ᵗʰ **H35.46** **Secondary vitreoretinal degeneration**
    H35.461 **Secondary vitreoretinal degeneration, right eye**
    H35.462 **Secondary vitreoretinal degeneration, left eye**
    H35.463 **Secondary vitreoretinal degeneration, bilateral**
    H35.469 **Secondary vitreoretinal degeneration, unspecified eye**

✓5ᵗʰ **H35.5** **Hereditary retinal dystrophy**
    EXCLUDES 1   dystrophies primarily involving Bruch's membrane (H31.1-)

    H35.5Ø **Unspecified hereditary retinal dystrophy**
    H35.51 **Vitreoretinal dystrophy**

H35.52 **Pigmentary retinal dystrophy**
Albipunctate retinal dystrophy
Retinitis pigmentosa
Tapetoretinal dystrophy

H35.53 **Other dystrophies primarily involving the sensory retina**
Stargardt's disease

H35.54 **Dystrophies primarily involving the retinal pigment epithelium**
Vitelliform retinal dystrophy

✓5ᵗʰ H35.6 **Retinal hemorrhage**
H35.60 **Retinal hemorrhage, unspecified eye**
H35.61 **Retinal hemorrhage, right eye**
H35.62 **Retinal hemorrhage, left eye**
H35.63 **Retinal hemorrhage, bilateral**

✓5ᵗʰ H35.7 **Separation of retinal layers**
> EXCLUDES 1   *retinal detachment (serous) (H33.2-)*
>   *rhegmatogenous retinal detachment (H33.0-)*

H35.70 **Unspecified separation of retinal layers**
✓6ᵗʰ H35.71 **Central serous chorioretinopathy**
H35.711 **Central serous chorioretinopathy, right eye**
H35.712 **Central serous chorioretinopathy, left eye**
H35.713 **Central serous chorioretinopathy, bilateral**
H35.719 **Central serous chorioretinopathy, unspecified eye**

✓6ᵗʰ H35.72 **Serous detachment of retinal pigment epithelium**
H35.721 **Serous detachment of retinal pigment epithelium, right eye**
H35.722 **Serous detachment of retinal pigment epithelium, left eye**
H35.723 **Serous detachment of retinal pigment epithelium, bilateral**
H35.729 **Serous detachment of retinal pigment epithelium, unspecified eye**

✓6ᵗʰ H35.73 **Hemorrhagic detachment of retinal pigment epithelium**
H35.731 **Hemorrhagic detachment of retinal pigment epithelium, right eye**
H35.732 **Hemorrhagic detachment of retinal pigment epithelium, left eye**
H35.733 **Hemorrhagic detachment of retinal pigment epithelium, bilateral**
H35.739 **Hemorrhagic detachment of retinal pigment epithelium, unspecified eye**

✓5ᵗʰ H35.8 **Other specified retinal disorders**
> EXCLUDES 2   *retinal hemorrhage (H35.6-)*

H35.81 **Retinal edema**
Retinal cotton wool spots
H35.82 **Retinal ischemia**
H35.89 **Other specified retinal disorders**
H35.9 **Unspecified retinal disorder**

H36 **Retinal disorders in diseases classified elsewhere**
Code first underlying disease, such as:
    lipid storage disorders (E75.-)
    sickle-cell disorders (D57.-)
> EXCLUDES 1   *arteriosclerotic retinopathy (H35.0-)*
>   *diabetic retinopathy (E08.3-, E09.3-, E10.3-, E11.3-, E13.3-)*

Glaucoma (H40-H42)

✓4ᵗʰ **H40 Glaucoma**
> EXCLUDES 1   *absolute glaucoma (H44.51-)*
>   *congenital glaucoma (Q15.0)*
>   *traumatic glaucoma due to birth injury (P15.3)*

Open Angle/Angle Closure Glaucoma

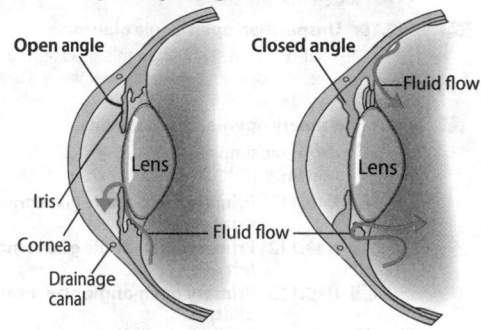

✓5ᵗʰ H40.0 **Glaucoma suspect**
✓6ᵗʰ H40.00 **Preglaucoma, unspecified**
H40.001 **Preglaucoma, unspecified, right eye**
H40.002 **Preglaucoma, unspecified, left eye**
H40.003 **Preglaucoma, unspecified, bilateral**
H40.009 **Preglaucoma, unspecified, unspecified eye**

✓6ᵗʰ H40.01 **Open angle with borderline findings, low risk**
Open angle, low risk
H40.011 **Open angle with borderline findings, low risk, right eye**
H40.012 **Open angle with borderline findings, low risk, left eye**
H40.013 **Open angle with borderline findings, low risk, bilateral**
H40.019 **Open angle with borderline findings, low risk, unspecified eye**

✓6ᵗʰ H40.02 **Open angle with borderline findings, high risk**
Open angle, high risk
H40.021 **Open angle with borderline findings, high risk, right eye**
H40.022 **Open angle with borderline findings, high risk, left eye**
H40.023 **Open angle with borderline findings, high risk, bilateral**
H40.029 **Open angle with borderline findings, high risk, unspecified eye**

✓6ᵗʰ H40.03 **Anatomical narrow angle**
Primary angle closure suspect
H40.031 **Anatomical narrow angle, right eye**
H40.032 **Anatomical narrow angle, left eye**
H40.033 **Anatomical narrow angle, bilateral**
H40.039 **Anatomical narrow angle, unspecified eye**

✓6ᵗʰ H40.04 **Steroid responder**
H40.041 **Steroid responder, right eye**
H40.042 **Steroid responder, left eye**
H40.043 **Steroid responder, bilateral**
H40.049 **Steroid responder, unspecified eye**

✓6ᵗʰ H40.05 **Ocular hypertension**
H40.051 **Ocular hypertension, right eye**
H40.052 **Ocular hypertension, left eye**
H40.053 **Ocular hypertension, bilateral**
H40.059 **Ocular hypertension, unspecified eye**

✓6ᵗʰ H40.06 **Primary angle closure without glaucoma damage**
H40.061 **Primary angle closure without glaucoma damage, right eye**
H40.062 **Primary angle closure without glaucoma damage, left eye**
H40.063 **Primary angle closure without glaucoma damage, bilateral**
H40.069 **Primary angle closure without glaucoma damage, unspecified eye**

☑ Additional Character Required   ✓x7ᵗʰ Placeholder Alert   Manifestation   Unspecified Dx   ▶◀ Revised Text   ● New Code   ▲ Revised Code Title

ICD-10-CM 2020   **607**

√5ᵗʰ H40.1 Open-angle glaucoma

> One of the following 7th characters is to be assigned to each code in subcategories H40.10, H40.11, H40.12, H40.13, and H40.14 to designate the stage of glaucoma.
> - 0   stage unspecified
> - 1   mild stage
> - 2   moderate stage
> - 3   severe stage
> - 4   indeterminate stage

   √x7ᵗʰ H40.10 Unspecified open-angle glaucoma   Q

> **TIP:** Only one code from this subcategory should be assigned when both left and right eyes are the same stage.

   √6ᵗʰ H40.11 Primary open-angle glaucoma

> Chronic simple glaucoma
> **AHA:** 2016,4Q,22

     √7ᵗʰ H40.111 Primary open-angle glaucoma, right eye   Q

     √7ᵗʰ H40.112 Primary open-angle glaucoma, left eye   Q

     √7ᵗʰ H40.113 Primary open-angle glaucoma, bilateral   Q

     √7ᵗʰ H40.119 Primary open-angle glaucoma, unspecified eye

   √6ᵗʰ H40.12 Low-tension glaucoma

     √7ᵗʰ H40.121 Low-tension glaucoma, right eye   Q

     √7ᵗʰ H40.122 Low-tension glaucoma, left eye   Q

     √7ᵗʰ H40.123 Low-tension glaucoma, bilateral   Q

     √7ᵗʰ H40.129 Low-tension glaucoma, unspecified eye

   √6ᵗʰ H40.13 Pigmentary glaucoma

     √7ᵗʰ H40.131 Pigmentary glaucoma, right eye

     √7ᵗʰ H40.132 Pigmentary glaucoma, left eye

     √7ᵗʰ H40.133 Pigmentary glaucoma, bilateral

     √7ᵗʰ H40.139 Pigmentary glaucoma, unspecified eye

   √6ᵗʰ H40.14 Capsular glaucoma with pseudoexfoliation of lens

     √7ᵗʰ H40.141 Capsular glaucoma with pseudoexfoliation of lens, right eye

     √7ᵗʰ H40.142 Capsular glaucoma with pseudoexfoliation of lens, left eye

     √7ᵗʰ H40.143 Capsular glaucoma with pseudoexfoliation of lens, bilateral

     √7ᵗʰ H40.149 Capsular glaucoma with pseudoexfoliation of lens, unspecified eye

   √6ᵗʰ H40.15 Residual stage of open-angle glaucoma

     H40.151 Residual stage of open-angle glaucoma, right eye   Q

     H40.152 Residual stage of open-angle glaucoma, left eye   Q

     H40.153 Residual stage of open-angle glaucoma, bilateral   Q

     H40.159 Residual stage of open-angle glaucoma, unspecified eye

√5ᵗʰ H40.2 Primary angle-closure glaucoma

> **EXCLUDES 1**   aqueous misdirection (H40.83-)
>   malignant glaucoma (H40.83-)

> One of the following 7th characters is to be assigned to code H40.20 and H40.22- to designate the stage of glaucoma.
> - 0   stage unspecified
> - 1   mild stage
> - 2   moderate stage
> - 3   severe stage
> - 4   indeterminate stage

   √x7ᵗʰ H40.20 Unspecified primary angle-closure glaucoma

> **TIP:** Only one code from this subcategory should be assigned when both left and right eyes are the same stage.

   √6ᵗʰ H40.21 Acute angle-closure glaucoma

> Acute angle-closure glaucoma attack
> Acute angle-closure glaucoma crisis

     H40.211 Acute angle-closure glaucoma, right eye

     H40.212 Acute angle-closure glaucoma, left eye

     H40.213 Acute angle-closure glaucoma, bilateral

     H40.219 Acute angle-closure glaucoma, unspecified eye

√6ᵗʰ H40.22 Chronic angle-closure glaucoma

> Chronic primary angle closure glaucoma

   √7ᵗʰ H40.221 Chronic angle-closure glaucoma, right eye

   √7ᵗʰ H40.222 Chronic angle-closure glaucoma, left eye

   √7ᵗʰ H40.223 Chronic angle-closure glaucoma, bilateral

   √7ᵗʰ H40.229 Chronic angle-closure glaucoma, unspecified eye

√6ᵗʰ H40.23 Intermittent angle-closure glaucoma

   H40.231 Intermittent angle-closure glaucoma, right eye

   H40.232 Intermittent angle-closure glaucoma, left eye

   H40.233 Intermittent angle-closure glaucoma, bilateral

   H40.239 Intermittent angle-closure glaucoma, unspecified eye

√6ᵗʰ H40.24 Residual stage of angle-closure glaucoma

   H40.241 Residual stage of angle-closure glaucoma, right eye

   H40.242 Residual stage of angle-closure glaucoma, left eye

   H40.243 Residual stage of angle-closure glaucoma, bilateral

   H40.249 Residual stage of angle-closure glaucoma, unspecified eye

√5ᵗʰ H40.3 Glaucoma secondary to eye trauma

> Code also underlying condition

> One of the following 7th characters is to be assigned to each code in subcategory H40.3- to designate the stage of glaucoma.
> - 0   stage unspecified
> - 1   mild stage
> - 2   moderate stage
> - 3   severe stage
> - 4   indeterminate stage

   √x7ᵗʰ H40.30 Glaucoma secondary to eye trauma, unspecified eye

   √x7ᵗʰ H40.31 Glaucoma secondary to eye trauma, right eye

   √x7ᵗʰ H40.32 Glaucoma secondary to eye trauma, left eye

   √x7ᵗʰ H40.33 Glaucoma secondary to eye trauma, bilateral

√5ᵗʰ H40.4 Glaucoma secondary to eye inflammation

> Code also underlying condition

> One of the following 7th characters is to be assigned to each code in subcategory H40.4- to designate the stage of glaucoma.
> - 0   stage unspecified
> - 1   mild stage
> - 2   moderate stage
> - 3   severe stage
> - 4   indeterminate stage

   √x7ᵗʰ H40.40 Glaucoma secondary to eye inflammation, unspecified eye

   √x7ᵗʰ H40.41 Glaucoma secondary to eye inflammation, right eye

   √x7ᵗʰ H40.42 Glaucoma secondary to eye inflammation, left eye

   √x7ᵗʰ H40.43 Glaucoma secondary to eye inflammation, bilateral

√5ᵗʰ H40.5 Glaucoma secondary to other eye disorders

> Code also underlying eye disorder

> One of the following 7th characters is to be assigned to each code in subcategory H40.5- to designate the stage of glaucoma.
> - 0   stage unspecified
> - 1   mild stage
> - 2   moderate stage
> - 3   severe stage
> - 4   indeterminate stage

   √x7ᵗʰ H40.50 Glaucoma secondary to other eye disorders, unspecified eye

   √x7ᵗʰ H40.51 Glaucoma secondary to other eye disorders, right eye

   √x7ᵗʰ H40.52 Glaucoma secondary to other eye disorders, left eye

   √x7ᵗʰ H40.53 Glaucoma secondary to other eye disorders, bilateral

✓5th H40.6 Glaucoma secondary to drugs

Use additional code for adverse effect, if applicable, to identify drug (T36-T50 with fifth or sixth character 5)

One of the following 7th characters is to be assigned to each code in subcategory H40.6- to designate the stage of glaucoma
- Ø   stage unspecified
- 1   mild stage
- 2   moderate stage
- 3   severe stage
- 4   indeterminate stage

- ✓x7th **H40.60** Glaucoma secondary to drugs, unspecified eye
- ✓x7th **H40.61** Glaucoma secondary to drugs, right eye
- ✓x7th **H40.62** Glaucoma secondary to drugs, left eye
- ✓x7th **H40.63** Glaucoma secondary to drugs, bilateral

✓5th H40.8 Other glaucoma

- ✓6th **H40.81** Glaucoma with increased episcleral venous pressure
  - **H40.811** Glaucoma with increased episcleral venous pressure, right eye
  - **H40.812** Glaucoma with increased episcleral venous pressure, left eye
  - **H40.813** Glaucoma with increased episcleral venous pressure, bilateral
  - **H40.819** Glaucoma with increased episcleral venous pressure, unspecified eye
- ✓6th **H40.82** Hypersecretion glaucoma
  - **H40.821** Hypersecretion glaucoma, right eye
  - **H40.822** Hypersecretion glaucoma, left eye
  - **H40.823** Hypersecretion glaucoma, bilateral
  - **H40.829** Hypersecretion glaucoma, unspecified eye
- ✓6th **H40.83** Aqueous misdirection
  - Malignant glaucoma
  - **H40.831** Aqueous misdirection, right eye
  - **H40.832** Aqueous misdirection, left eye
  - **H40.833** Aqueous misdirection, bilateral
  - **H40.839** Aqueous misdirection, unspecified eye
- **H40.89** Other specified glaucoma
- **H40.9** Unspecified glaucoma

H42 Glaucoma in diseases classified elsewhere

Code first underlying condition, such as:
- amyloidosis (E85.-)
- aniridia (Q13.1)
- glaucoma (in) diabetes mellitus (E08.39, E09.39, E10.39, E11.39, E13.39)
- Lowe's syndrome (E72.03)
- Reiger's anomaly (Q13.81)
- specified metabolic disorder (E70-E88)

EXCLUDES 1   *glaucoma (in) onchocerciasis (B73.02)*
          glaucoma (in) syphilis (A52.71)
          glaucoma (in) tuberculous (A18.59)

Disorders of vitreous body and globe (H43-H44)

✓4th H43 Disorders of vitreous body

✓5th H43.0 Vitreous prolapse

EXCLUDES 1   *traumatic vitreous prolapse (S05.2-)*
          vitreous syndrome following cataract surgery (H59.0-)

- **H43.00** Vitreous prolapse, unspecified eye
- **H43.01** Vitreous prolapse, right eye
- **H43.02** Vitreous prolapse, left eye
- **H43.03** Vitreous prolapse, bilateral

✓5th H43.1 Vitreous hemorrhage

- **H43.10** Vitreous hemorrhage, unspecified eye   HCC
- **H43.11** Vitreous hemorrhage, right eye   HCC
- **H43.12** Vitreous hemorrhage, left eye   HCC
- **H43.13** Vitreous hemorrhage, bilateral   HCC

✓5th H43.2 Crystalline deposits in vitreous body

- **H43.20** Crystalline deposits in vitreous body, unspecified eye
- **H43.21** Crystalline deposits in vitreous body, right eye
- **H43.22** Crystalline deposits in vitreous body, left eye
- **H43.23** Crystalline deposits in vitreous body, bilateral

✓5th H43.3 Other vitreous opacities

- ✓6th **H43.31** Vitreous membranes and strands
  - **H43.311** Vitreous membranes and strands, right eye
  - **H43.312** Vitreous membranes and strands, left eye
  - **H43.313** Vitreous membranes and strands, bilateral
  - **H43.319** Vitreous membranes and strands, unspecified eye
- ✓6th **H43.39** Other vitreous opacities
  - Vitreous floaters
  - **H43.391** Other vitreous opacities, right eye
  - **H43.392** Other vitreous opacities, left eye
  - **H43.393** Other vitreous opacities, bilateral
  - **H43.399** Other vitreous opacities, unspecified eye

✓5th H43.8 Other disorders of vitreous body

EXCLUDES 1   *proliferative vitreo-retinopathy with retinal detachment (H33.4-)*
EXCLUDES 2   *vitreous abscess (H44.02-)*

- ✓6th **H43.81** Vitreous degeneration
  - Vitreous detachment
  - **H43.811** Vitreous degeneration, right eye
  - **H43.812** Vitreous degeneration, left eye
  - **H43.813** Vitreous degeneration, bilateral
  - **H43.819** Vitreous degeneration, unspecified eye
- ✓6th **H43.82** Vitreomacular adhesion
  - Vitreomacular traction
  - **H43.821** Vitreomacular adhesion, right eye   A
  - **H43.822** Vitreomacular adhesion, left eye   A
  - **H43.823** Vitreomacular adhesion, bilateral   A
  - **H43.829** Vitreomacular adhesion, unspecified eye   A
- **H43.89** Other disorders of vitreous body
- **H43.9** Unspecified disorder of vitreous body

✓4th H44 Disorders of globe

INCLUDES   disorders affecting multiple structures of eye

✓5th H44.0 Purulent endophthalmitis

Use additional code to identify organism

EXCLUDES 1   *bleb associated endophthalmitis (H59.4-)*

- ✓6th **H44.00** Unspecified purulent endophthalmitis
  - **H44.001** Unspecified purulent endophthalmitis, right eye
  - **H44.002** Unspecified purulent endophthalmitis, left eye
  - **H44.003** Unspecified purulent endophthalmitis, bilateral
  - **H44.009** Unspecified purulent endophthalmitis, unspecified eye
- ✓6th **H44.01** Panophthalmitis (acute)
  - **H44.011** Panophthalmitis (acute), right eye
  - **H44.012** Panophthalmitis (acute), left eye
  - **H44.013** Panophthalmitis (acute), bilateral
  - **H44.019** Panophthalmitis (acute), unspecified eye
- ✓6th **H44.02** Vitreous abscess (chronic)
  - **H44.021** Vitreous abscess (chronic), right eye
  - **H44.022** Vitreous abscess (chronic), left eye
  - **H44.023** Vitreous abscess (chronic), bilateral
  - **H44.029** Vitreous abscess (chronic), unspecified eye

✓5th H44.1 Other endophthalmitis

EXCLUDES 1   *bleb associated endophthalmitis (H59.4-)*
EXCLUDES 2   *ophthalmia nodosa (H16.2-)*

- ✓6th **H44.11** Panuveitis
  - **DEF:** Inflammation of all layers of the uvea of the eye, including the choroid, iris, and ciliary body. It also typically involves the lens, retina, optic nerve, and vitreous and causes reduced vision or blindness.
  - **H44.111** Panuveitis, right eye
  - **H44.112** Panuveitis, left eye
  - **H44.113** Panuveitis, bilateral
  - **H44.119** Panuveitis, unspecified eye
- ✓6th **H44.12** Parasitic endophthalmitis, unspecified
  - **H44.121** Parasitic endophthalmitis, unspecified, right eye
  - **H44.122** Parasitic endophthalmitis, unspecified, left eye

---

✓ Additional Character Required   ✓x7th Placeholder Alert   Manifestation   Unspecified Dx   ▶◀ Revised Text   ● New Code   ▲ Revised Code Title

            H44.123   Parasitic endophthalmitis, unspecified, bilateral

            H44.129   Parasitic endophthalmitis, unspecified, unspecified eye

√6ᵗʰ   **H44.13**   **Sympathetic uveitis**

            H44.131   Sympathetic uveitis, right eye

            H44.132   Sympathetic uveitis, left eye

            H44.133   Sympathetic uveitis, bilateral

            H44.139   Sympathetic uveitis, unspecified eye

     H44.19   **Other endophthalmitis**

√5ᵗʰ   **H44.2**   **Degenerative myopia**

       Malignant myopia

       AHA: 2017,4Q,10-11

     H44.20   Degenerative myopia, unspecified eye

     H44.21   Degenerative myopia, right eye

     H44.22   Degenerative myopia, left eye

     H44.23   Degenerative myopia, bilateral

√6ᵗʰ   **H44.2A**   **Degenerative myopia with choroidal neovascularization**

       Use additional code for any associated choroid disorders (H31.-)

            H44.2A1   Degenerative myopia with choroidal neovascularization, right eye

            H44.2A2   Degenerative myopia with choroidal neovascularization, left eye

            H44.2A3   Degenerative myopia with choroidal neovascularization, bilateral eye

            H44.2A9   Degenerative myopia with choroidal neovascularization, unspecified eye

√6ᵗʰ   **H44.2B**   **Degenerative myopia with macular hole**

            H44.2B1   Degenerative myopia with macular hole, right eye

            H44.2B2   Degenerative myopia with macular hole, left eye

            H44.2B3   Degenerative myopia with macular hole, bilateral eye

            H44.2B9   Degenerative myopia with macular hole, unspecified eye

√6ᵗʰ   **H44.2C**   **Degenerative myopia with retinal detachment**

       Use additional code to identify the retinal detachment (H33.-)

            H44.2C1   Degenerative myopia with retinal detachment, right eye

            H44.2C2   Degenerative myopia with retinal detachment, left eye

            H44.2C3   Degenerative myopia with retinal detachment, bilateral eye

            H44.2C9   Degenerative myopia with retinal detachment, unspecified eye

√6ᵗʰ   **H44.2D**   **Degenerative myopia with foveoschisis**

            H44.2D1   Degenerative myopia with foveoschisis, right eye

            H44.2D2   Degenerative myopia with foveoschisis, left eye

            H44.2D3   Degenerative myopia with foveoschisis, bilateral eye

            H44.2D9   Degenerative myopia with foveoschisis, unspecified eye

√6ᵗʰ   **H44.2E**   **Degenerative myopia with other maculopathy**

            H44.2E1   Degenerative myopia with other maculopathy, right eye

            H44.2E2   Degenerative myopia with other maculopathy, left eye

            H44.2E3   Degenerative myopia with other maculopathy, bilateral eye

            H44.2E9   Degenerative myopia with other maculopathy, unspecified eye

√5ᵗʰ   **H44.3**   **Other and unspecified degenerative disorders of globe**

     H44.30   Unspecified degenerative disorder of globe

√6ᵗʰ   **H44.31**   **Chalcosis**

            H44.311   Chalcosis, right eye

            H44.312   Chalcosis, left eye

            H44.313   Chalcosis, bilateral

            H44.319   Chalcosis, unspecified eye

√6ᵗʰ   **H44.32**   **Siderosis of eye**

       DEF: Iron pigment deposits within tissue of the eyeball caused by high iron content of the blood. Symptoms include cataracts, rust-colored anterior subcapsular deposits, iris heterochromia, pupillary mydriasis, and depressed electroretinogram amplitudes.

            H44.321   Siderosis of eye, right eye

            H44.322   Siderosis of eye, left eye

            H44.323   Siderosis of eye, bilateral

            H44.329   Siderosis of eye, unspecified eye

√6ᵗʰ   **H44.39**   **Other degenerative disorders of globe**

            H44.391   Other degenerative disorders of globe, right eye

            H44.392   Other degenerative disorders of globe, left eye

            H44.393   Other degenerative disorders of globe, bilateral

            H44.399   Other degenerative disorders of globe, unspecified eye

√5ᵗʰ   **H44.4**   **Hypotony of eye**

     H44.40   Unspecified hypotony of eye

√6ᵗʰ   **H44.41**   **Flat anterior chamber hypotony of eye**

            H44.411   Flat anterior chamber hypotony of right eye

            H44.412   Flat anterior chamber hypotony of left eye

            H44.413   Flat anterior chamber hypotony of eye, bilateral

            H44.419   Flat anterior chamber hypotony of unspecified eye

√6ᵗʰ   **H44.42**   **Hypotony of eye due to ocular fistula**

            H44.421   Hypotony of right eye due to ocular fistula

            H44.422   Hypotony of left eye due to ocular fistula

            H44.423   Hypotony of eye due to ocular fistula, bilateral

            H44.429   Hypotony of unspecified eye due to ocular fistula

√6ᵗʰ   **H44.43**   **Hypotony of eye due to other ocular disorders**

            H44.431   Hypotony of eye due to other ocular disorders, right eye

            H44.432   Hypotony of eye due to other ocular disorders, left eye

            H44.433   Hypotony of eye due to other ocular disorders, bilateral

            H44.439   Hypotony of eye due to other ocular disorders, unspecified eye

√6ᵗʰ   **H44.44**   **Primary hypotony of eye**

            H44.441   Primary hypotony of right eye

            H44.442   Primary hypotony of left eye

            H44.443   Primary hypotony of eye, bilateral

            H44.449   Primary hypotony of unspecified eye

√5ᵗʰ   **H44.5**   **Degenerated conditions of globe**

     H44.50   Unspecified degenerated conditions of globe

√6ᵗʰ   **H44.51**   **Absolute glaucoma**

            H44.511   Absolute glaucoma, right eye

            H44.512   Absolute glaucoma, left eye

            H44.513   Absolute glaucoma, bilateral

            H44.519   Absolute glaucoma, unspecified eye

√6ᵗʰ   **H44.52**   **Atrophy of globe**

       Phthisis bulbi

            H44.521   Atrophy of globe, right eye

            H44.522   Atrophy of globe, left eye

            H44.523   Atrophy of globe, bilateral

            H44.529   Atrophy of globe, unspecified eye

√6ᵗʰ   **H44.53**   **Leucocoria**

            H44.531   Leucocoria, right eye

            H44.532   Leucocoria, left eye

            H44.533   Leucocoria, bilateral

            H44.539   Leucocoria, unspecified eye

√5ᵗʰ **H44.6** **Retained (old) intraocular foreign body,** magnetic

Use additional code to identify magnetic foreign body (Z18.11)

EXCLUDES 1　*current intraocular foreign body (S05.-)*

EXCLUDES 2　*retained foreign body in eyelid (H02.81-)*

retained (old) foreign body following penetrating wound of orbit (H05.5-)

retained (old) intraocular foreign body, nonmagnetic (H44.7-)

√6ᵗʰ **H44.60** **Unspecified retained (old) intraocular foreign body, magnetic**

H44.601 **Unspecified retained (old) intraocular foreign body, magnetic, right eye**

H44.602 **Unspecified retained (old) intraocular foreign body, magnetic, left eye**

H44.603 **Unspecified retained (old) intraocular foreign body, magnetic, bilateral**

H44.609 **Unspecified retained (old) intraocular foreign body, magnetic, unspecified eye**

√6ᵗʰ **H44.61** **Retained (old) magnetic foreign body in** anterior chamber

H44.611 **Retained (old) magnetic foreign body in anterior chamber, right eye**

H44.612 **Retained (old) magnetic foreign body in anterior chamber, left eye**

H44.613 **Retained (old) magnetic foreign body in anterior chamber, bilateral**

H44.619 **Retained (old) magnetic foreign body in anterior chamber, unspecified eye**

√6ᵗʰ **H44.62** **Retained (old) magnetic foreign body in** iris or ciliary body

H44.621 **Retained (old) magnetic foreign body in iris or ciliary body, right eye**

H44.622 **Retained (old) magnetic foreign body in iris or ciliary body, left eye**

H44.623 **Retained (old) magnetic foreign body in iris or ciliary body, bilateral**

H44.629 **Retained (old) magnetic foreign body in iris or ciliary body, unspecified eye**

√6ᵗʰ **H44.63** **Retained (old) magnetic foreign body in** lens

H44.631 **Retained (old) magnetic foreign body in lens, right eye**

H44.632 **Retained (old) magnetic foreign body in lens, left eye**

H44.633 **Retained (old) magnetic foreign body in lens, bilateral**

H44.639 **Retained (old) magnetic foreign body in lens, unspecified eye**

√6ᵗʰ **H44.64** **Retained (old) magnetic foreign body in** posterior wall of globe

H44.641 **Retained (old) magnetic foreign body in posterior wall of globe, right eye**

H44.642 **Retained (old) magnetic foreign body in posterior wall of globe, left eye**

H44.643 **Retained (old) magnetic foreign body in posterior wall of globe, bilateral**

H44.649 **Retained (old) magnetic foreign body in posterior wall of globe, unspecified eye**

√6ᵗʰ **H44.65** **Retained (old) magnetic foreign body in** vitreous body

H44.651 **Retained (old) magnetic foreign body in vitreous body, right eye**

H44.652 **Retained (old) magnetic foreign body in vitreous body, left eye**

H44.653 **Retained (old) magnetic foreign body in vitreous body, bilateral**

H44.659 **Retained (old) magnetic foreign body in vitreous body, unspecified eye**

√6ᵗʰ **H44.69** **Retained (old) intraocular foreign body, magnetic, in other or multiple sites**

H44.691 **Retained (old) intraocular foreign body, magnetic, in other or multiple sites, right eye**

H44.692 **Retained (old) intraocular foreign body, magnetic, in other or multiple sites, left eye**

H44.693 **Retained (old) intraocular foreign body, magnetic, in other or multiple sites, bilateral**

H44.699 **Retained (old) intraocular foreign body, magnetic, in other or multiple sites, unspecified eye**

√5ᵗʰ **H44.7** **Retained (old) intraocular foreign body,** nonmagnetic

Use additional code to identify nonmagnetic foreign body (Z18.01-Z18.10, Z18.12, Z18.2-Z18.9)

EXCLUDES 1　*current intraocular foreign body (S05.-)*

EXCLUDES 2　*retained foreign body in eyelid (H02.81-)*

retained (old) foreign body following penetrating wound of orbit (H05.5-)

retained (old) intraocular foreign body, magnetic (H44.6-)

√6ᵗʰ **H44.70** **Unspecified retained (old) intraocular foreign body, nonmagnetic**

H44.701 **Unspecified retained (old) intraocular foreign body, nonmagnetic, right eye**

H44.702 **Unspecified retained (old) intraocular foreign body, nonmagnetic, left eye**

H44.703 **Unspecified retained (old) intraocular foreign body, nonmagnetic, bilateral**

H44.709 **Unspecified retained (old) intraocular foreign body, nonmagnetic, unspecified eye**

Retained (old) intraocular foreign body NOS

√6ᵗʰ **H44.71** **Retained (nonmagnetic) (old) foreign body in** anterior chamber

H44.711 **Retained (nonmagnetic) (old) foreign body in anterior chamber, right eye**

H44.712 **Retained (nonmagnetic) (old) foreign body in anterior chamber, left eye**

H44.713 **Retained (nonmagnetic) (old) foreign body in anterior chamber, bilateral**

H44.719 **Retained (nonmagnetic) (old) foreign body in anterior chamber, unspecified eye**

√6ᵗʰ **H44.72** **Retained (nonmagnetic) (old) foreign body in** iris or ciliary body

H44.721 **Retained (nonmagnetic) (old) foreign body in iris or ciliary body, right eye**

H44.722 **Retained (nonmagnetic) (old) foreign body in iris or ciliary body, left eye**

H44.723 **Retained (nonmagnetic) (old) foreign body in iris or ciliary body, bilateral**

H44.729 **Retained (nonmagnetic) (old) foreign body in iris or ciliary body, unspecified eye**

√6ᵗʰ **H44.73** **Retained (nonmagnetic) (old) foreign body in** lens

H44.731 **Retained (nonmagnetic) (old) foreign body in lens, right eye**

H44.732 **Retained (nonmagnetic) (old) foreign body in lens, left eye**

H44.733 **Retained (nonmagnetic) (old) foreign body in lens, bilateral**

H44.739 **Retained (nonmagnetic) (old) foreign body in lens, unspecified eye**

√6ᵗʰ **H44.74** **Retained (nonmagnetic) (old) foreign body in** posterior wall of globe

H44.741 **Retained (nonmagnetic) (old) foreign body in posterior wall of globe, right eye**

H44.742 **Retained (nonmagnetic) (old) foreign body in posterior wall of globe, left eye**

H44.743 **Retained (nonmagnetic) (old) foreign body in posterior wall of globe, bilateral**

H44.749 **Retained (nonmagnetic) (old) foreign body in posterior wall of globe, unspecified eye**

√6ᵗʰ **H44.75** **Retained (nonmagnetic) (old) foreign body in** vitreous body

H44.751 **Retained (nonmagnetic) (old) foreign body in vitreous body, right eye**

H44.752 **Retained (nonmagnetic) (old) foreign body in vitreous body, left eye**

H44.753 **Retained (nonmagnetic) (old) foreign body in vitreous body, bilateral**

H44.759 **Retained (nonmagnetic) (old) foreign body in vitreous body, unspecified eye**

√6ᵗʰ **H44.79** **Retained (old) intraocular foreign body, nonmagnetic, in other or multiple sites**

H44.791 **Retained (old) intraocular foreign body, nonmagnetic, in other or multiple sites, right eye**

H44.792 **Retained (old) intraocular foreign body, nonmagnetic, in other or multiple sites, left eye**

☑ Additional Character Required　　√x7ᵗʰ Placeholder Alert　　Manifestation　　Unspecified Dx　　▶◀ Revised Text　　● New Code　　▲ Revised Code Title

Chapter 7. Diseases of the Eye and Adnexa

H44.793 Retained (old) intraocular foreign body, nonmagnetic, in other or multiple sites, bilateral

H44.799 Retained (old) intraocular foreign body, nonmagnetic, in other or multiple sites, unspecified eye

✓5ᵗʰ **H44.8 Other disorders of globe**

  ✓6ᵗʰ **H44.81 Hemophthalmos**

    DEF: Pool of blood within the eyeball, not from a current injury.

    H44.811 Hemophthalmos, right eye

    H44.812 Hemophthalmos, left eye

    H44.813 Hemophthalmos, bilateral

    H44.819 Hemophthalmos, unspecified eye

  ✓6ᵗʰ **H44.82 Luxation of globe**

    H44.821 Luxation of globe, right eye

    H44.822 Luxation of globe, left eye

    H44.823 Luxation of globe, bilateral

    H44.829 Luxation of globe, unspecified eye

  H44.89 Other disorders of globe

H44.9 Unspecified disorder of globe

Disorders of optic nerve and visual pathways (H46-H47)

✓4ᵗʰ **H46 Optic neuritis**

  EXCLUDES 2   ischemic optic neuropathy (H47.01-)
                neuromyelitis optica [Devic] (G36.0)

  ✓5ᵗʰ **H46.0 Optic papillitis**

    H46.00 Optic papillitis, unspecified eye

    H46.01 Optic papillitis, right eye

    H46.02 Optic papillitis, left eye

    H46.03 Optic papillitis, bilateral

  ✓5ᵗʰ **H46.1 Retrobulbar neuritis**

    Retrobulbar neuritis NOS

    EXCLUDES 1   syphilitic retrobulbar neuritis (A52.15)

    H46.10 Retrobulbar neuritis, unspecified eye

    H46.11 Retrobulbar neuritis, right eye

    H46.12 Retrobulbar neuritis, left eye

    H46.13 Retrobulbar neuritis, bilateral

  H46.2 Nutritional optic neuropathy

  H46.3 Toxic optic neuropathy

    Code first (T51-T65) to identify cause

  H46.8 Other optic neuritis

  H46.9 Unspecified optic neuritis

✓4ᵗʰ **H47 Other disorders of optic [2nd] nerve and visual pathways**

  ✓5ᵗʰ **H47.0 Disorders of optic nerve, not elsewhere classified**

    ✓6ᵗʰ **H47.01 Ischemic optic neuropathy**

      H47.011 Ischemic optic neuropathy, right eye

      H47.012 Ischemic optic neuropathy, left eye

      H47.013 Ischemic optic neuropathy, bilateral

      H47.019 Ischemic optic neuropathy, unspecified eye

    ✓6ᵗʰ **H47.02 Hemorrhage in optic nerve sheath**

      H47.021 Hemorrhage in optic nerve sheath, right eye

      H47.022 Hemorrhage in optic nerve sheath, left eye

      H47.023 Hemorrhage in optic nerve sheath, bilateral

      H47.029 Hemorrhage in optic nerve sheath, unspecified eye

    ✓6ᵗʰ **H47.03 Optic nerve hypoplasia**

      H47.031 Optic nerve hypoplasia, right eye

      H47.032 Optic nerve hypoplasia, left eye

      H47.033 Optic nerve hypoplasia, bilateral

      H47.039 Optic nerve hypoplasia, unspecified eye

    ✓6ᵗʰ **H47.09 Other disorders of optic nerve, not elsewhere classified**

      Compression of optic nerve

      H47.091 Other disorders of optic nerve, not elsewhere classified, right eye

      H47.092 Other disorders of optic nerve, not elsewhere classified, left eye

      H47.093 Other disorders of optic nerve, not elsewhere classified, bilateral

      H47.099 Other disorders of optic nerve, not elsewhere classified, unspecified eye

✓5ᵗʰ **H47.1 Papilledema**

  DEF: Swelling of the optic papilla, the raised area connected to the optic disk made up of nerves that enter the eyeball. It may be caused by increased intracranial pressure, decreased ocular pressure, or a retinal disorder.

  H47.10 Unspecified papilledema

  H47.11 Papilledema associated with increased intracranial pressure

  H47.12 Papilledema associated with decreased ocular pressure

  H47.13 Papilledema associated with retinal disorder

  ✓6ᵗʰ **H47.14 Foster-Kennedy syndrome**

    H47.141 Foster-Kennedy syndrome, right eye

    H47.142 Foster-Kennedy syndrome, left eye

    H47.143 Foster-Kennedy syndrome, bilateral

    H47.149 Foster-Kennedy syndrome, unspecified eye

✓5ᵗʰ **H47.2 Optic atrophy**

  H47.20 Unspecified optic atrophy

  ✓6ᵗʰ **H47.21 Primary optic atrophy**

    H47.211 Primary optic atrophy, right eye

    H47.212 Primary optic atrophy, left eye

    H47.213 Primary optic atrophy, bilateral

    H47.219 Primary optic atrophy, unspecified eye

  H47.22 Hereditary optic atrophy

    Leber's optic atrophy

  ✓6ᵗʰ **H47.23 Glaucomatous optic atrophy**

    H47.231 Glaucomatous optic atrophy, right eye

    H47.232 Glaucomatous optic atrophy, left eye

    H47.233 Glaucomatous optic atrophy, bilateral

    H47.239 Glaucomatous optic atrophy, unspecified eye

  ✓6ᵗʰ **H47.29 Other optic atrophy**

    Temporal pallor of optic disc

    H47.291 Other optic atrophy, right eye

    H47.292 Other optic atrophy, left eye

    H47.293 Other optic atrophy, bilateral

    H47.299 Other optic atrophy, unspecified eye

✓5ᵗʰ **H47.3 Other disorders of optic disc**

  ✓6ᵗʰ **H47.31 Coloboma of optic disc**

    H47.311 Coloboma of optic disc, right eye

    H47.312 Coloboma of optic disc, left eye

    H47.313 Coloboma of optic disc, bilateral

    H47.319 Coloboma of optic disc, unspecified eye

  ✓6ᵗʰ **H47.32 Drusen of optic disc**

    H47.321 Drusen of optic disc, right eye

    H47.322 Drusen of optic disc, left eye

    H47.323 Drusen of optic disc, bilateral

    H47.329 Drusen of optic disc, unspecified eye

  ✓6ᵗʰ **H47.33 Pseudopapilledema of optic disc**

    H47.331 Pseudopapilledema of optic disc, right eye

    H47.332 Pseudopapilledema of optic disc, left eye

    H47.333 Pseudopapilledema of optic disc, bilateral

    H47.339 Pseudopapilledema of optic disc, unspecified eye

  ✓6ᵗʰ **H47.39 Other disorders of optic disc**

    H47.391 Other disorders of optic disc, right eye

    H47.392 Other disorders of optic disc, left eye

    H47.393 Other disorders of optic disc, bilateral

    H47.399 Other disorders of optic disc, unspecified eye

✓5ᵗʰ **H47.4 Disorders of optic chiasm**

  Code also underlying condition

  H47.41 Disorders of optic chiasm in (due to) inflammatory disorders

  H47.42 Disorders of optic chiasm in (due to) neoplasm

  H47.43 Disorders of optic chiasm in (due to) vascular disorders

  H47.49 Disorders of optic chiasm in (due to) other disorders

✓5ᵗʰ **H47.5 Disorders of other visual pathways**

  Disorders of optic tracts, geniculate nuclei and optic radiations

  Code also underlying condition

  ✓6ᵗʰ **H47.51 Disorders of visual pathways in (due to) inflammatory disorders**

    H47.511 Disorders of visual pathways in (due to) inflammatory disorders, right side

---

H47.512 Disorders of visual pathways in (due to) inflammatory disorders, left side
H47.519 Disorders of visual pathways in (due to) inflammatory disorders, unspecified side

√6ᵗʰ H47.52 Disorders of visual pathways in (due to) neoplasm
H47.521 Disorders of visual pathways in (due to) neoplasm, right side
H47.522 Disorders of visual pathways in (due to) neoplasm, left side
H47.529 Disorders of visual pathways in (due to) neoplasm, unspecified side

√6ᵗʰ H47.53 Disorders of visual pathways in (due to) vascular disorders
H47.531 Disorders of visual pathways in (due to) vascular disorders, right side
H47.532 Disorders of visual pathways in (due to) vascular disorders, left side
H47.539 Disorders of visual pathways in (due to) vascular disorders, unspecified side

√5ᵗʰ H47.6 Disorders of visual cortex
Code also underlying condition
EXCLUDES 1 injury to visual cortex ▶S04.04-◀

√6ᵗʰ H47.61 Cortical blindness
H47.611 Cortical blindness, right side of brain
H47.612 Cortical blindness, left side of brain
H47.619 Cortical blindness, unspecified side of brain

√6ᵗʰ H47.62 Disorders of visual cortex in (due to) inflammatory disorders
H47.621 Disorders of visual cortex in (due to) inflammatory disorders, right side of brain
H47.622 Disorders of visual cortex in (due to) inflammatory disorders, left side of brain
H47.629 Disorders of visual cortex in (due to) inflammatory disorders, unspecified side of brain

√6ᵗʰ H47.63 Disorders of visual cortex in (due to) neoplasm
H47.631 Disorders of visual cortex in (due to) neoplasm, right side of brain
H47.632 Disorders of visual cortex in (due to) neoplasm, left side of brain
H47.639 Disorders of visual cortex in (due to) neoplasm, unspecified side of brain

√6ᵗʰ H47.64 Disorders of visual cortex in (due to) vascular disorders
H47.641 Disorders of visual cortex in (due to) vascular disorders, right side of brain
H47.642 Disorders of visual cortex in (due to) vascular disorders, left side of brain
H47.649 Disorders of visual cortex in (due to) vascular disorders, unspecified side of brain

H47.9 Unspecified disorder of visual pathways

Disorders of ocular muscles, binocular movement, accommodation and refraction (H49-H52)

EXCLUDES 2 nystagmus and other irregular eye movements (H55)

√4ᵗʰ H49 Paralytic strabismus
EXCLUDES 2 internal ophthalmoplegia (H52.51-)
internuclear ophthalmoplegia (H51.2-)
progressive supranuclear ophthalmoplegia (G23.1)
DEF: Strabismus: Misalignment of the eyes with the inability to move and focus in the same direction due to conditions affecting the muscles controlling them.

√5ᵗʰ H49.0 Third [oculomotor] nerve palsy
H49.00 Third [oculomotor] nerve palsy, unspecified eye
H49.01 Third [oculomotor] nerve palsy, right eye
H49.02 Third [oculomotor] nerve palsy, left eye
H49.03 Third [oculomotor] nerve palsy, bilateral

√5ᵗʰ H49.1 Fourth [trochlear] nerve palsy
H49.10 Fourth [trochlear] nerve palsy, unspecified eye
H49.11 Fourth [trochlear] nerve palsy, right eye
H49.12 Fourth [trochlear] nerve palsy, left eye
H49.13 Fourth [trochlear] nerve palsy, bilateral

√5ᵗʰ H49.2 Sixth [abducent] nerve palsy
H49.20 Sixth [abducent] nerve palsy, unspecified eye
H49.21 Sixth [abducent] nerve palsy, right eye
H49.22 Sixth [abducent] nerve palsy, left eye

H49.23 Sixth [abducent] nerve palsy, bilateral

√5ᵗʰ H49.3 Total (external) ophthalmoplegia
H49.30 Total (external) ophthalmoplegia, unspecified eye
H49.31 Total (external) ophthalmoplegia, right eye
H49.32 Total (external) ophthalmoplegia, left eye
H49.33 Total (external) ophthalmoplegia, bilateral

√5ᵗʰ H49.4 Progressive external ophthalmoplegia
EXCLUDES 1 Kearns-Sayre syndrome (H49.81-)
H49.40 Progressive external ophthalmoplegia, unspecified eye
H49.41 Progressive external ophthalmoplegia, right eye
H49.42 Progressive external ophthalmoplegia, left eye
H49.43 Progressive external ophthalmoplegia, bilateral

√5ᵗʰ H49.8 Other paralytic strabismus
√6ᵗʰ H49.81 Kearns-Sayre syndrome
Progressive external ophthalmoplegia with pigmentary retinopathy
Use additional code for other manifestation, such as: heart block (I45.9)
H49.811 Kearns-Sayre syndrome, right eye   HCC
H49.812 Kearns-Sayre syndrome, left eye   HCC
H49.813 Kearns-Sayre syndrome, bilateral   HCC
H49.819 Kearns-Sayre syndrome, unspecified eye   HCC

√6ᵗʰ H49.88 Other paralytic strabismus
External ophthalmoplegia NOS
H49.881 Other paralytic strabismus, right eye
H49.882 Other paralytic strabismus, left eye
H49.883 Other paralytic strabismus, bilateral
H49.889 Other paralytic strabismus, unspecified eye

H49.9 Unspecified paralytic strabismus

√4ᵗʰ H50 Other strabismus
DEF: Strabismus: Misalignment of the eyes with the inability to move and focus in the same direction due to conditions affecting the muscles controlling them.

√5ᵗʰ H50.0 Esotropia
Convergent concomitant strabismus
EXCLUDES 1 intermittent esotropia (H50.31-, H50.32)
H50.00 Unspecified esotropia
√6ᵗʰ H50.01 Monocular esotropia
H50.011 Monocular esotropia, right eye
H50.012 Monocular esotropia, left eye
√6ᵗʰ H50.02 Monocular esotropia with A pattern
H50.021 Monocular esotropia with A pattern, right eye
H50.022 Monocular esotropia with A pattern, left eye
√6ᵗʰ H50.03 Monocular esotropia with V pattern
H50.031 Monocular esotropia with V pattern, right eye
H50.032 Monocular esotropia with V pattern, left eye
√6ᵗʰ H50.04 Monocular esotropia with other noncomitancies
H50.041 Monocular esotropia with other noncomitancies, right eye
H50.042 Monocular esotropia with other noncomitancies, left eye
H50.05 Alternating esotropia
H50.06 Alternating esotropia with A pattern
H50.07 Alternating esotropia with V pattern

H50.08   Alternating esotropia with other noncomitancies

Eye Muscle Diseases

R.   L.
Monocular (one eye only) esotropia (inward)

Monocular exotropia (outward)

Monocular hypertropia (upward)

✓5ᵗʰ **H50.1**   **Exotropia**
    Divergent concomitant strabismus
    EXCLUDES 1   *intermittent exotropia (H50.33-, H50.34)*
    H50.10   Unspecified exotropia
   ✓6ᵗʰ **H50.11**   Monocular exotropia
      H50.111   Monocular exotropia, right eye
      H50.112   Monocular exotropia, left eye
   ✓6ᵗʰ **H50.12**   Monocular exotropia with A pattern
      H50.121   Monocular exotropia with A pattern, right eye
      H50.122   Monocular exotropia with A pattern, left eye
   ✓6ᵗʰ **H50.13**   Monocular exotropia with V pattern
      H50.131   Monocular exotropia with V pattern, right eye
      H50.132   Monocular exotropia with V pattern, left eye
   ✓6ᵗʰ **H50.14**   Monocular exotropia with other noncomitancies
      H50.141   Monocular exotropia with other noncomitancies, right eye
      H50.142   Monocular exotropia with other noncomitancies, left eye
    H50.15   Alternating exotropia
    H50.16   Alternating exotropia with A pattern
    H50.17   Alternating exotropia with V pattern
    H50.18   Alternating exotropia with other noncomitancies
✓5ᵗʰ **H50.2**   **Vertical strabismus**
    Hypertropia
    H50.21   Vertical strabismus, right eye
    H50.22   Vertical strabismus, left eye
✓5ᵗʰ **H50.3**   **Intermittent heterotropia**
    H50.30   Unspecified intermittent heterotropia
   ✓6ᵗʰ **H50.31**   Intermittent monocular esotropia
      H50.311   Intermittent monocular esotropia, right eye
      H50.312   Intermittent monocular esotropia, left eye
    H50.32   Intermittent alternating esotropia
   ✓6ᵗʰ **H50.33**   Intermittent monocular exotropia
      H50.331   Intermittent monocular exotropia, right eye
      H50.332   Intermittent monocular exotropia, left eye
    H50.34   Intermittent alternating exotropia
✓5ᵗʰ **H50.4**   **Other and unspecified heterotropia**
    H50.40   Unspecified heterotropia
   ✓6ᵗʰ **H50.41**   Cyclotropia
      H50.411   Cyclotropia, right eye
      H50.412   Cyclotropia, left eye
    H50.42   Monofixation syndrome

    H50.43   Accommodative component in esotropia
✓5ᵗʰ **H50.5**   **Heterophoria**
    H50.50   Unspecified heterophoria
    H50.51   Esophoria
    H50.52   Exophoria
    H50.53   Vertical heterophoria
    H50.54   Cyclophoria
    H50.55   Alternating heterophoria
✓5ᵗʰ **H50.6**   **Mechanical strabismus**
    H50.60   Mechanical strabismus, unspecified
   ✓6ᵗʰ **H50.61**   Brown's sheath syndrome
      H50.611   Brown's sheath syndrome, right eye
      H50.612   Brown's sheath syndrome, left eye
    H50.69   Other mechanical strabismus
      Strabismus due to adhesions
      Traumatic limitation of duction of eye muscle
✓5ᵗʰ **H50.8**   **Other specified strabismus**
   ✓6ᵗʰ **H50.81**   Duane's syndrome
      H50.811   Duane's syndrome, right eye
      H50.812   Duane's syndrome, left eye
    H50.89   Other specified strabismus
    H50.9   Unspecified strabismus
✓4ᵗʰ **H51**   **Other disorders of binocular movement**
    H51.0   Palsy (spasm) of conjugate gaze
✓5ᵗʰ **H51.1**   **Convergence insufficiency and excess**
    H51.11   Convergence insufficiency
    H51.12   Convergence excess
✓5ᵗʰ **H51.2**   **Internuclear ophthalmoplegia**
    H51.20   Internuclear ophthalmoplegia, unspecified eye
    H51.21   Internuclear ophthalmoplegia, right eye
    H51.22   Internuclear ophthalmoplegia, left eye
    H51.23   Internuclear ophthalmoplegia, bilateral
    H51.8   Other specified disorders of binocular movement
    H51.9   Unspecified disorder of binocular movement
✓4ᵗʰ **H52**   **Disorders of refraction and accommodation**
✓5ᵗʰ **H52.0**   **Hypermetropia**
    H52.00   Hypermetropia, unspecified eye
    H52.01   Hypermetropia, right eye
    H52.02   Hypermetropia, left eye
    H52.03   Hypermetropia, bilateral
✓5ᵗʰ **H52.1**   **Myopia**
    EXCLUDES 1   *degenerative myopia (H44.2-)*
    H52.10   Myopia, unspecified eye
    H52.11   Myopia, right eye
    H52.12   Myopia, left eye
    H52.13   Myopia, bilateral
✓5ᵗʰ **H52.2**   **Astigmatism**
   ✓6ᵗʰ **H52.20**   Unspecified astigmatism
      H52.201   Unspecified astigmatism, right eye
      H52.202   Unspecified astigmatism, left eye
      H52.203   Unspecified astigmatism, bilateral
      H52.209   Unspecified astigmatism, unspecified eye
   ✓6ᵗʰ **H52.21**   Irregular astigmatism
      H52.211   Irregular astigmatism, right eye
      H52.212   Irregular astigmatism, left eye
      H52.213   Irregular astigmatism, bilateral
      H52.219   Irregular astigmatism, unspecified eye
   ✓6ᵗʰ **H52.22**   Regular astigmatism
      H52.221   Regular astigmatism, right eye
      H52.222   Regular astigmatism, left eye
      H52.223   Regular astigmatism, bilateral
      H52.229   Regular astigmatism, unspecified eye
✓5ᵗʰ **H52.3**   **Anisometropia and aniseikonia**
    H52.31   Anisometropia
    H52.32   Aniseikonia
    H52.4   Presbyopia
✓5ᵗʰ **H52.5**   **Disorders of accommodation**
   ✓6ᵗʰ **H52.51**   Internal ophthalmoplegia (complete) (total)
      H52.511   Internal ophthalmoplegia (complete) (total), right eye
      H52.512   Internal ophthalmoplegia (complete) (total), left eye

H52.513   **Internal ophthalmoplegia (complete) (total), bilateral**

H52.519   **Internal ophthalmoplegia (complete) (total), unspecified eye**

✓6ᵗʰ **H52.52**   **Paresis of accommodation**

H52.521   **Paresis of accommodation, right eye**

H52.522   **Paresis of accommodation, left eye**

H52.523   **Paresis of accommodation, bilateral**

H52.529   **Paresis of accommodation, unspecified eye**

✓6ᵗʰ **H52.53**   **Spasm of accommodation**

H52.531   **Spasm of accommodation, right eye**

H52.532   **Spasm of accommodation, left eye**

H52.533   **Spasm of accommodation, bilateral**

H52.539   **Spasm of accommodation, unspecified eye**

H52.6   **Other disorders of refraction**

H52.7   **Unspecified disorder of refraction**

Visual disturbances and blindness (H53-H54)

✓4ᵗʰ **H53**   **Visual disturbances**

✓5ᵗʰ **H53.0**   **Amblyopia ex anopsia**

EXCLUDES 1   *amblyopia due to vitamin A deficiency (E50.5)*

✓6ᵗʰ **H53.00**   **Unspecified amblyopia**

H53.001   **Unspecified amblyopia, right eye**

H53.002   **Unspecified amblyopia, left eye**

H53.003   **Unspecified amblyopia, bilateral**

H53.009   **Unspecified amblyopia, unspecified eye**

✓6ᵗʰ **H53.01**   **Deprivation amblyopia**

H53.011   **Deprivation amblyopia, right eye**

H53.012   **Deprivation amblyopia, left eye**

H53.013   **Deprivation amblyopia, bilateral**

H53.019   **Deprivation amblyopia, unspecified eye**

✓6ᵗʰ **H53.02**   **Refractive amblyopia**

H53.021   **Refractive amblyopia, right eye**

H53.022   **Refractive amblyopia, left eye**

H53.023   **Refractive amblyopia, bilateral**

H53.029   **Refractive amblyopia, unspecified eye**

✓6ᵗʰ **H53.03**   **Strabismic amblyopia**

EXCLUDES 1   *strabismus (H50.-)*

H53.031   **Strabismic amblyopia, right eye**

H53.032   **Strabismic amblyopia, left eye**

H53.033   **Strabismic amblyopia, bilateral**

H53.039   **Strabismic amblyopia, unspecified eye**

✓6ᵗʰ **H53.04**   **Amblyopia suspect**

AHA: 2016,4Q,22-23

H53.041   **Amblyopia suspect, right eye**

H53.042   **Amblyopia suspect, left eye**

H53.043   **Amblyopia suspect, bilateral**

H53.049   **Amblyopia suspect, unspecified eye**

✓5ᵗʰ **H53.1**   **Subjective visual disturbances**

EXCLUDES 1   *subjective visual disturbances due to vitamin A deficiency (E50.5)*
visual hallucinations (R44.1)

H53.10   **Unspecified subjective visual disturbances**

H53.11   **Day blindness**

Hemeralopia

✓6ᵗʰ **H53.12**   **Transient visual loss**

Scintillating scotoma

EXCLUDES 1   *amaurosis fugax (G45.3-)*
transient retinal artery occlusion (H34.0-)

H53.121   **Transient visual loss, right eye**

H53.122   **Transient visual loss, left eye**

H53.123   **Transient visual loss, bilateral**

H53.129   **Transient visual loss, unspecified eye**

✓6ᵗʰ **H53.13**   **Sudden visual loss**

H53.131   **Sudden visual loss, right eye**

H53.132   **Sudden visual loss, left eye**

H53.133   **Sudden visual loss, bilateral**

H53.139   **Sudden visual loss, unspecified eye**

✓6ᵗʰ **H53.14**   **Visual discomfort**

Asthenopia

Photophobia

H53.141   **Visual discomfort, right eye**

H53.142   **Visual discomfort, left eye**

H53.143   **Visual discomfort, bilateral**

H53.149   **Visual discomfort, unspecified**

H53.15   **Visual distortions of shape and size**

Metamorphopsia

H53.16   **Psychophysical visual disturbances**

H53.19   **Other subjective visual disturbances**

Visual halos

H53.2   **Diplopia**

Double vision

✓5ᵗʰ **H53.3**   **Other and unspecified disorders of binocular vision**

H53.30   **Unspecified disorder of binocular vision**

H53.31   **Abnormal retinal correspondence**

H53.32   **Fusion with defective stereopsis**

H53.33   **Simultaneous visual perception without fusion**

H53.34   **Suppression of binocular vision**

✓5ᵗʰ **H53.4**   **Visual field defects**

H53.40   **Unspecified visual field defects**

✓6ᵗʰ **H53.41**   **Scotoma involving central area**

Central scotoma

H53.411   **Scotoma involving central area, right eye**

H53.412   **Scotoma involving central area, left eye**

H53.413   **Scotoma involving central area, bilateral**

H53.419   **Scotoma involving central area, unspecified eye**

✓6ᵗʰ **H53.42**   **Scotoma of blind spot area**

Enlarged blind spot

H53.421   **Scotoma of blind spot area, right eye**

H53.422   **Scotoma of blind spot area, left eye**

H53.423   **Scotoma of blind spot area, bilateral**

H53.429   **Scotoma of blind spot area, unspecified eye**

✓6ᵗʰ **H53.43**   **Sector or arcuate defects**

Arcuate scotoma

Bjerrum scotoma

H53.431   **Sector or arcuate defects, right eye**

H53.432   **Sector or arcuate defects, left eye**

H53.433   **Sector or arcuate defects, bilateral**

H53.439   **Sector or arcuate defects, unspecified eye**

✓6ᵗʰ **H53.45**   **Other localized visual field defect**

Peripheral visual field defect

Ring scotoma NOS

Scotoma NOS

H53.451   **Other localized visual field defect, right eye**

H53.452   **Other localized visual field defect, left eye**

H53.453   **Other localized visual field defect, bilateral**

H53.459   **Other localized visual field defect, unspecified eye**

✓6ᵗʰ **H53.46**   **Homonymous bilateral field defects**

Homonymous hemianopia

Homonymous hemianopsia

Quadrant anopia

Quadrant anopsia

H53.461   **Homonymous bilateral field defects, right side**

H53.462   **Homonymous bilateral field defects, left side**

H53.469   **Homonymous bilateral field defects, unspecified side**

Homonymous bilateral field defects NOS

H53.47   **Heteronymous bilateral field defects**

Heteronymous hemianop(s)ia

✓6ᵗʰ **H53.48**   **Generalized contraction of visual field**

H53.481   **Generalized contraction of visual field, right eye**

H53.482   **Generalized contraction of visual field, left eye**

H53.483   **Generalized contraction of visual field, bilateral**

H53.489   **Generalized contraction of visual field, unspecified eye**

✓ Additional Character Required   ✓x7ᵗʰ Placeholder Alert   Manifestation   Unspecified Dx   ▶◀ Revised Text   ● New Code   ▲ Revised Code Title

ICD-10-CM 2020   615

Chapter 7. Diseases of the Eye and Adnexa

H53.5–H54.50

✓5ᵗʰ **H53.5** **Color vision deficiencies**
Color blindness
EXCLUDES 2   day blindness (H53.11)

     H53.50 **Unspecified color vision deficiencies**
Color blindness NOS

     H53.51 **Achromatopsia**
DEF: Nonprogressive genetic visual disorder characterized by complete color blindness, decreased vision, and light sensitivity.

     H53.52 **Acquired color vision deficiency**

     H53.53 **Deuteranomaly**
Deuteranopia
DEF: Male-only genetic disorder causing difficulty in distinguishing green and red; no shortened spectrum.

     H53.54 **Protanomaly**
Protanopia

     H53.55 **Tritanomaly**
Tritanopia

     H53.59 **Other color vision deficiencies**

✓5ᵗʰ **H53.6** **Night blindness**
EXCLUDES 1   night blindness due to vitamin A deficiency (E50.5)

     H53.60 **Unspecified night blindness**

     H53.61 **Abnormal dark adaptation curve**

     H53.62 **Acquired night blindness**

     H53.63 **Congenital night blindness**

     H53.69 **Other night blindness**

✓5ᵗʰ **H53.7** **Vision sensitivity deficiencies**

     H53.71 **Glare sensitivity**

     H53.72 **Impaired contrast sensitivity**

   H53.8 **Other visual disturbances**

   H53.9 **Unspecified visual disturbance**

✓4ᵗʰ **H54** **Blindness and low vision**

     NOTE   For definition of visual impairment categories see table below

Code first any associated underlying cause of the blindness
EXCLUDES 1   amaurosis fugax (G45.3)
AHA: 2017,4Q,11-12

✓5ᵗʰ **H54.0** **Blindness, both eyes**
Visual impairment categories 3, 4, 5 in both eyes.

     ✓6ᵗʰ **H54.0X** **Blindness, both eyes, different category levels**

       ✓7ᵗʰ **H54.0X3** **Blindness right eye, category 3**

         H54.0X33 Blindness right eye category 3, blindness left eye category 3

         H54.0X34 Blindness right eye category 3, blindness left eye category 4

         H54.0X35 Blindness right eye category 3, blindness left eye category 5

       ✓7ᵗʰ **H54.0X4** **Blindness right eye, category 4**

         H54.0X43 Blindness right eye category 4, blindness left eye category 3

         H54.0X44 Blindness right eye category 4, blindness left eye category 4

         H54.0X45 Blindness right eye category 4, blindness left eye category 5

       ✓7ᵗʰ **H54.0X5** **Blindness right eye, category 5**

         H54.0X53 Blindness right eye category 5, blindness left eye category 3

         H54.0X54 Blindness right eye category 5, blindness left eye category 4

         H54.0X55 Blindness right eye category 5, blindness left eye category 5

✓5ᵗʰ **H54.1** **Blindness, one eye, low vision other eye**
Visual impairment categories 3, 4, 5 in one eye, with categories 1 or 2 in the other eye.

     H54.10 **Blindness, one eye, low vision other eye, unspecified eyes**

     ✓6ᵗʰ **H54.11** **Blindness, right eye, low vision left eye**

       ✓7ᵗʰ **H54.113** **Blindness right eye category 3, low vision left eye**

         H54.1131 Blindness right eye category 3, low vision left eye category 1

         H54.1132 Blindness right eye category 3, low vision left eye category 2

       ✓7ᵗʰ **H54.114** **Blindness right eye category 4, low vision left eye**

         H54.1141 Blindness right eye category 4, low vision left eye category 1

         H54.1142 Blindness right eye category 4, low vision left eye category 2

       ✓7ᵗʰ **H54.115** **Blindness right eye category 5, low vision left eye**

         H54.1151 Blindness right eye category 5, low vision left eye category 1

         H54.1152 Blindness right eye category 5, low vision left eye category 2

     ✓6ᵗʰ **H54.12** **Blindness, left eye, low vision right eye**

       ✓7ᵗʰ **H54.121** **Low vision right eye category 1, blindness left eye**

         H54.1213 Low vision right eye category 1, blindness left eye category 3

         H54.1214 Low vision right eye category 1, blindness left eye category 4

         H54.1215 Low vision right eye category 1, blindness left eye category 5

       ✓7ᵗʰ **H54.122** **Low vision right eye category 2, blindness left eye**

         H54.1223 Low vision right eye category 2, blindness left eye category 3

         H54.1224 Low vision right eye category 2, blindness left eye category 4

         H54.1225 Low vision right eye category 2, blindness left eye category 5

✓5ᵗʰ **H54.2** **Low vision, both eyes**
Visual impairment categories 1 or 2 in both eyes.

     ✓6ᵗʰ **H54.2X** **Low vision, both eyes, different category levels**

       ✓7ᵗʰ **H54.2X1** **Low vision, right eye, category 1**

         H54.2X11 Low vision right eye category 1, low vision left eye category 1

         H54.2X12 Low vision right eye category 1, low vision left eye category 2

       ✓7ᵗʰ **H54.2X2** **Low vision, right eye, category 2**

         H54.2X21 Low vision right eye category 2, low vision left eye category 1

         H54.2X22 Low vision right eye category 2, low vision left eye category 2

   H54.3 **Unqualified visual loss, both eyes**
Visual impairment category 9 in both eyes.
TIP: Assign only when both eyes are documented as affected by blindness or low vision but the visual impairment category is not documented.

✓5ᵗʰ **H54.4** **Blindness, one eye**
Visual impairment categories 3, 4, 5 in one eye [normal vision in other eye]

     H54.40 **Blindness, one eye, unspecified eye**

     ✓6ᵗʰ **H54.41** **Blindness, right eye, normal vision left eye**

       ✓7ᵗʰ **H54.413** **Blindness, right eye, category 3**

         H54.413A Blindness right eye category 3, normal vision left eye

       ✓7ᵗʰ **H54.414** **Blindness, right eye, category 4**

         H54.414A Blindness right eye category 4, normal vision left eye

       ✓7ᵗʰ **H54.415** **Blindness, right eye, category 5**

         H54.415A Blindness right eye category 5, normal vision left eye

     ✓6ᵗʰ **H54.42** **Blindness, left eye, normal vision right eye**

       ✓7ᵗʰ **H54.42A** **Blindness, left eye, category 3-5**

         H54.42A3 Blindness left eye category 3, normal vision right eye

         H54.42A4 Blindness left eye category 4, normal vision right eye

         H54.42A5 Blindness left eye category 5, normal vision right eye

✓5ᵗʰ **H54.5** **Low vision, one eye**
Visual impairment categories 1 or 2 in one eye [normal vision in other eye].

     H54.50 **Low vision, one eye, unspecified eye**

☑6ᵗʰ H54.51   Low vision, right eye, normal vision left eye

   ☑7ᵗʰ H54.511   Low vision, right eye, category 1-2

      H54.511A   Low vision right eye category 1, normal vision left eye

      H54.512A   Low vision right eye category 2, normal vision left eye

☑7ᵗʰ H54.52   Low vision, left eye, normal vision right eye

   ☑7ᵗʰ H54.52A   Low vision, left eye, category 1-2

      H54.52A1   Low vision left eye category 1, normal vision right eye

      H54.52A2   Low vision left eye category 2, normal vision right eye

☑5ᵗʰ H54.6   **Unqualified visual loss, one eye**

Visual impairment category 9 in one eye [normal vision in other eye].

TIP: Assign a code from this category only when one eye is documented as affected by blindness or low vision but the visual impairment category is not documented.

H54.60   **Unqualified visual loss, one eye, unspecified**

H54.61   **Unqualified visual loss, right eye, normal vision left eye**

H54.62   **Unqualified visual loss, left eye, normal vision right eye**

H54.7   **Unspecified visual loss**

Visual impairment category 9 NOS

TIP: Assign only when documentation specifies blindness, visual loss, or low vision but not whether one or both eyes are affected or the visual impairment category.

H54.8   **Legal blindness, as defined in USA**

Blindness NOS according to USA definition

EXCLUDES 1   *legal blindness with specification of impairment level (H54.0-H54.7)*

NOTE   The table below gives a classification of severity of visual impairment recommended by a WHO Study Group on the Prevention of Blindness, Geneva, 6-10 November 1972.

The term "low vision" in category H54 comprises categories 1 and 2 of the table, the term "blindness" categories 3, 4 and 5, and the term "unqualified visual loss" category 9.

If the extent of the visual field is taken into account, patients with a field no greater than 10 but greater than 5 around central fixation should be placed in category 3 and patients with a field no greater than 5 around central fixation should be placed in category 4, even if the central acuity is not impaired.

Category of visual impairment	Visual acuity with best possible correction	
	Maximum less than:	**Minimum equal to or better than:**
1	6/18 3/10 (0.3) 20/70	6/60 1/10 (0.1) 20/200
2	6/60 1/10 (0.1) 20/200	3/60 1/20 (0.05) 20/400
3	3/60 1/200 (0.05) 20/400	1/60 (finger counting at one meter) 1/50 (0.02) 5/300 (20/1200)
4	1/60 (finger counting at one meter) 1/50 (0.02) 5/300	Light perception
5	No light perception	
9	Undetermined or unspecified	

Other disorders of eye and adnexa (H55-H57)

☑4ᵗʰ H55   **Nystagmus and other irregular eye movements**

☑5ᵗʰ H55.0   **Nystagmus**

DEF: Rapid, rhythmic, involuntary movements of the eyeball in vertical, horizontal, rotational, or mixed directions.

H55.00   **Unspecified nystagmus**

H55.01   **Congenital nystagmus**

H55.02   **Latent nystagmus**

H55.03   **Visual deprivation nystagmus**

H55.04   **Dissociated nystagmus**

H55.09   **Other forms of nystagmus**

☑5ᵗʰ H55.8   **Other irregular eye movements**

H55.81   **Saccadic eye movements**

H55.89   **Other irregular eye movements**

☑4ᵗʰ H57   **Other disorders of eye and adnexa**

☑5ᵗʰ H57.0   **Anomalies of pupillary function**

H57.00   **Unspecified anomaly of pupillary function**

H57.01   **Argyll Robertson pupil, atypical**

EXCLUDES 1   *syphilitic Argyll Robertson pupil (A52.19)*

H57.02   **Anisocoria**

H57.03   **Miosis**

H57.04   **Mydriasis**

☑6ᵗʰ H57.05   **Tonic pupil**

H57.051   **Tonic pupil, right eye**

H57.052   **Tonic pupil, left eye**

H57.053   **Tonic pupil, bilateral**

H57.059   **Tonic pupil, unspecified eye**

H57.09   **Other anomalies of pupillary function**

☑5ᵗʰ H57.1   **Ocular pain**

H57.10   **Ocular pain, unspecified eye**

H57.11   **Ocular pain, right eye**

H57.12   **Ocular pain, left eye**

H57.13   **Ocular pain, bilateral**

☑5ᵗʰ H57.8   **Other specified disorders of eye and adnexa**

AHA: 2018,4Q,15-16

☑6ᵗʰ H57.81   **Brow ptosis**

H57.811   **Brow ptosis, right**

H57.812   **Brow ptosis, left**

H57.813   **Brow ptosis, bilateral**

H57.819   **Brow ptosis, unspecified**

H57.89   **Other specified disorders of eye and adnexa**

H57.9   **Unspecified disorder of eye and adnexa**

Intraoperative and postprocedural complications and disorders of eye and adnexa, not elsewhere classified (H59)

☑4ᵗʰ H59   **Intraoperative and postprocedural complications and disorders of eye and adnexa, not elsewhere classified**

EXCLUDES 1   *mechanical complication of intraocular lens (T85.2)*
mechanical complication of other ocular prosthetic devices, implants and grafts (T85.3)
pseudophakia (Z96.1)
secondary cataracts (H26.4-)

☑5ᵗʰ H59.0   **Disorders of the eye following cataract surgery**

☑6ᵗʰ H59.01   **Keratopathy (bullous aphakic) following cataract surgery**

Vitreal corneal syndrome

Vitreous (touch) syndrome

H59.011   **Keratopathy (bullous aphakic) following cataract surgery, right eye**

H59.012   **Keratopathy (bullous aphakic) following cataract surgery, left eye**

H59.013   **Keratopathy (bullous aphakic) following cataract surgery, bilateral**

H59.019   **Keratopathy (bullous aphakic) following cataract surgery, unspecified eye**

☑6ᵗʰ H59.02   **Cataract (lens) fragments in eye following cataract surgery**

H59.021   **Cataract (lens) fragments in eye following cataract surgery, right eye**

H59.022   **Cataract (lens) fragments in eye following cataract surgery, left eye**

H59.023   **Cataract (lens) fragments in eye following cataract surgery, bilateral**

☑ Additional Character Required   **☑x7ᵗʰ** Placeholder Alert   Manifestation   Unspecified Dx   ▶◀ Revised Text   ● New Code   ▲ Revised Code Title

Chapter 7. Diseases of the Eye and Adnexa

H59.029 Cataract (lens) fragments in eye following cataract surgery, unspecified eye

√6ᵗʰ **H59.03** Cystoid macular edema following cataract surgery

     H59.031 Cystoid macular edema following cataract surgery, right eye

     H59.032 Cystoid macular edema following cataract surgery, left eye

     H59.033 Cystoid macular edema following cataract surgery, bilateral

     H59.039 Cystoid macular edema following cataract surgery, unspecified eye

√6ᵗʰ **H59.09** Other disorders of the eye following cataract surgery

     H59.091 Other disorders of the right eye following cataract surgery

     H59.092 Other disorders of the left eye following cataract surgery

     H59.093 Other disorders of the eye following cataract surgery, bilateral

     H59.099 Other disorders of unspecified eye following cataract surgery

√5ᵗʰ **H59.1** Intraoperative hemorrhage and hematoma of eye and adnexa complicating a procedure

     EXCLUDES 1   *intraoperative hemorrhage and hematoma of eye and adnexa due to accidental puncture or laceration during a procedure (H59.2-)*

√6ᵗʰ **H59.11** Intraoperative hemorrhage and hematoma of eye and adnexa complicating an ophthalmic procedure

     H59.111 Intraoperative hemorrhage and hematoma of right eye and adnexa complicating an ophthalmic procedure

     H59.112 Intraoperative hemorrhage and hematoma of left eye and adnexa complicating an ophthalmic procedure

     H59.113 Intraoperative hemorrhage and hematoma of eye and adnexa complicating an ophthalmic procedure, bilateral

     H59.119 Intraoperative hemorrhage and hematoma of unspecified eye and adnexa complicating an ophthalmic procedure

√6ᵗʰ **H59.12** Intraoperative hemorrhage and hematoma of eye and adnexa complicating other procedure

     H59.121 Intraoperative hemorrhage and hematoma of right eye and adnexa complicating other procedure

     H59.122 Intraoperative hemorrhage and hematoma of left eye and adnexa complicating other procedure

     H59.123 Intraoperative hemorrhage and hematoma of eye and adnexa complicating other procedure, bilateral

     H59.129 Intraoperative hemorrhage and hematoma of unspecified eye and adnexa complicating other procedure

√5ᵗʰ **H59.2** Accidental puncture and laceration of eye and adnexa during a procedure

√6ᵗʰ **H59.21** Accidental puncture and laceration of eye and adnexa during an ophthalmic procedure

     H59.211 Accidental puncture and laceration of right eye and adnexa during an ophthalmic procedure

     H59.212 Accidental puncture and laceration of left eye and adnexa during an ophthalmic procedure

     H59.213 Accidental puncture and laceration of eye and adnexa during an ophthalmic procedure, bilateral

     H59.219 Accidental puncture and laceration of unspecified eye and adnexa during an ophthalmic procedure

√6ᵗʰ **H59.22** Accidental puncture and laceration of eye and adnexa during other procedure

     H59.221 Accidental puncture and laceration of right eye and adnexa during other procedure

     H59.222 Accidental puncture and laceration of left eye and adnexa during other procedure

     H59.223 Accidental puncture and laceration of eye and adnexa during other procedure, bilateral

     H59.229 Accidental puncture and laceration of unspecified eye and adnexa during other procedure

√5ᵗʰ **H59.3** Postprocedural hemorrhage, hematoma, and seroma of eye and adnexa following a procedure

     AHA: 2016,4Q,9-10

√6ᵗʰ **H59.31** Postprocedural hemorrhage of eye and adnexa following an ophthalmic procedure

     H59.311 Postprocedural hemorrhage of right eye and adnexa following an ophthalmic procedure

     H59.312 Postprocedural hemorrhage of left eye and adnexa following an ophthalmic procedure

     H59.313 Postprocedural hemorrhage of eye and adnexa following an ophthalmic procedure, bilateral

     H59.319 Postprocedural hemorrhage of unspecified eye and adnexa following an ophthalmic procedure

√6ᵗʰ **H59.32** Postprocedural hemorrhage of eye and adnexa following other procedure

     H59.321 Postprocedural hemorrhage of right eye and adnexa following other procedure

     H59.322 Postprocedural hemorrhage of left eye and adnexa following other procedure

     H59.323 Postprocedural hemorrhage of eye and adnexa following other procedure, bilateral

     H59.329 Postprocedural hemorrhage of unspecified eye and adnexa following other procedure

√6ᵗʰ **H59.33** Postprocedural hematoma of eye and adnexa following an ophthalmic procedure

     H59.331 Postprocedural hematoma of right eye and adnexa following an ophthalmic procedure

     H59.332 Postprocedural hematoma of left eye and adnexa following an ophthalmic procedure

     H59.333 Postprocedural hematoma of eye and adnexa following an ophthalmic procedure, bilateral

     H59.339 Postprocedural hematoma of unspecified eye and adnexa following an ophthalmic procedure

√6ᵗʰ **H59.34** Postprocedural hematoma of eye and adnexa following other procedure

     H59.341 Postprocedural hematoma of right eye and adnexa following other procedure

     H59.342 Postprocedural hematoma of left eye and adnexa following other procedure

     H59.343 Postprocedural hematoma of eye and adnexa following other procedure, bilateral

     H59.349 Postprocedural hematoma of unspecified eye and adnexa following other procedure

√6ᵗʰ **H59.35** Postprocedural seroma of eye and adnexa following an ophthalmic procedure

     H59.351 Postprocedural seroma of right eye and adnexa following an ophthalmic procedure

     H59.352 Postprocedural seroma of left eye and adnexa following an ophthalmic procedure

     H59.353 Postprocedural seroma of eye and adnexa following an ophthalmic procedure, bilateral

     H59.359 Postprocedural seroma of unspecified eye and adnexa following an ophthalmic procedure

√6ᵗʰ **H59.36** Postprocedural seroma of eye and adnexa following other procedure

     H59.361 Postprocedural seroma of right eye and adnexa following other procedure

     H59.362 Postprocedural seroma of left eye and adnexa following other procedure

     H59.363 Postprocedural seroma of eye and adnexa following other procedure, bilateral

     H59.369 Postprocedural seroma of unspecified eye and adnexa following other procedure

☑5ᵗʰ **H59.4** Inflammation **(infection) of** postprocedural bleb

    Postprocedural blebitis

       EXCLUDES 1   *filtering (vitreous) bleb after glaucoma surgery status (Z98.83)*

    H59.40   **Inflammation (infection) of postprocedural bleb, unspecified**

    H59.41   **Inflammation (infection) of postprocedural bleb, stage 1**

    H59.42   **Inflammation (infection) of postprocedural bleb, stage 2**

    H59.43   **Inflammation (infection) of postprocedural bleb, stage 3**

        Bleb endophthalmitis

☑5ᵗʰ **H59.8** **Other intraoperative and postprocedural complications and disorders of eye and adnexa, not elsewhere classified**

  ☑6ᵗʰ **H59.81**   **Chorioretinal scars after surgery for detachment**

      H59.811   **Chorioretinal scars after surgery for detachment,** right **eye**

      H59.812   **Chorioretinal scars after surgery for detachment,** left **eye**

      H59.813   **Chorioretinal scars after surgery for detachment,** bilateral

      H59.819   **Chorioretinal scars after surgery for detachment, unspecified eye**

  H59.88   **Other intraoperative complications of eye and adnexa, not elsewhere classified**

  H59.89   **Other postprocedural complications and disorders of eye and adnexa, not elsewhere classified**

☑ Additional Character Required   ☑x7ᵗʰ Placeholder Alert   Manifestation   Unspecified Dx   ▶◀ Revised Text   ● New Code   ▲ Revised Code Title

ICD-10-CM 2020   619

Chapter 8. Diseases of the Ear and Mastoid Process (H60–H95)

Chapter-specific Guidelines with Coding Examples
Reserved for future guideline expansion.

Chapter 8. Diseases of the Ear and Mastoid Process (H60-H95)

NOTE Use an external cause code following the code for the ear condition, if applicable, to identify the cause of the ear condition

EXCLUDES 2 certain conditions originating in the perinatal period (P04-P96)
certain infectious and parasitic diseases (A00-B99)
complications of pregnancy, childbirth and the puerperium (O00-O9A)
congenital malformations, deformations and chromosomal abnormalities (Q00-Q99)
endocrine, nutritional and metabolic diseases (E00-E88)
injury, poisoning and certain other consequences of external causes (S00-T88)
neoplasms (C00-D49)
symptoms, signs and abnormal clinical and laboratory findings, not elsewhere classified (R00-R94)

This chapter contains the following blocks:

H60-H62   Diseases of external ear
H65-H75   Diseases of middle ear and mastoid
H80-H83   Diseases of inner ear
H90-H94   Other disorders of ear
H95   Intraoperative and postprocedural complications and disorders of ear and mastoid process, not elsewhere classified

Diseases of external ear (H60-H62)

✓4ᵗʰ H60 Otitis externa

TIP: When the specific infectious agent is identified, a code from Chapter 1 is assigned instead of a code from this category.

✓5ᵗʰ H60.0 Abscess of external ear

Boil of external ear
Carbuncle of auricle or external auditory canal
Furuncle of external ear

H60.00 Abscess of external ear, unspecified ear
H60.01 Abscess of right external ear
H60.02 Abscess of left external ear
H60.03 Abscess of external ear, bilateral

✓5ᵗʰ H60.1 Cellulitis of external ear

Cellulitis of auricle
Cellulitis of external auditory canal

H60.10 Cellulitis of external ear, unspecified ear
H60.11 Cellulitis of right external ear
H60.12 Cellulitis of left external ear
H60.13 Cellulitis of external ear, bilateral

✓5ᵗʰ H60.2 Malignant otitis externa

H60.20 Malignant otitis externa, unspecified ear
H60.21 Malignant otitis externa, right ear
H60.22 Malignant otitis externa, left ear
H60.23 Malignant otitis externa, bilateral

✓5ᵗʰ H60.3 Other infective otitis externa

✓6ᵗʰ H60.31 Diffuse otitis externa

H60.311 Diffuse otitis externa, right ear   Q
H60.312 Diffuse otitis externa, left ear   Q
H60.313 Diffuse otitis externa, bilateral   Q
H60.319 Diffuse otitis externa, unspecified ear   Q

✓6ᵗʰ H60.32 Hemorrhagic otitis externa

H60.321 Hemorrhagic otitis externa, right ear   Q
H60.322 Hemorrhagic otitis externa, left ear   Q
H60.323 Hemorrhagic otitis externa, bilateral   Q
H60.329 Hemorrhagic otitis externa, unspecified ear   Q

✓6ᵗʰ H60.33 Swimmer's ear

DEF: Commonly occurs when water gets trapped in the ear after swimming.

H60.331 Swimmer's ear, right ear   Q
H60.332 Swimmer's ear, left ear   Q
H60.333 Swimmer's ear, bilateral   Q
H60.339 Swimmer's ear, unspecified ear   Q

✓6ᵗʰ H60.39 Other infective otitis externa

H60.391 Other infective otitis externa, right ear   Q
H60.392 Other infective otitis externa, left ear   Q

H60.393 Other infective otitis externa, bilateral   Q
H60.399 Other infective otitis externa, unspecified ear   Q

✓5ᵗʰ H60.4 Cholesteatoma of external ear

Keratosis obturans of external ear (canal)

EXCLUDES 2 cholesteatoma of middle ear (H71.-)
recurrent cholesteatoma of postmastoidectomy cavity (H95.0-)

DEF: Cholesteatoma: Noncancerous cyst-like mass of cell debris, including cholesterol and epithelial cells resulting from trauma, repeated or improperly healed infections, and congenital enclosure of epidermal cells.

H60.40 Cholesteatoma of external ear, unspecified ear
H60.41 Cholesteatoma of right external ear
H60.42 Cholesteatoma of left external ear
H60.43 Cholesteatoma of external ear, bilateral

✓5ᵗʰ H60.5 Acute noninfective otitis externa

✓6ᵗʰ H60.50 Unspecified acute noninfective otitis externa

Acute otitis externa NOS

H60.501 Unspecified acute noninfective otitis externa, right ear   Q
H60.502 Unspecified acute noninfective otitis externa, left ear   Q
H60.503 Unspecified acute noninfective otitis externa, bilateral   Q
H60.509 Unspecified acute noninfective otitis externa, unspecified ear   Q

✓6ᵗʰ H60.51 Acute actinic otitis externa

H60.511 Acute actinic otitis externa, right ear   Q
H60.512 Acute actinic otitis externa, left ear   Q
H60.513 Acute actinic otitis externa, bilateral   Q
H60.519 Acute actinic otitis externa, unspecified ear   Q

✓6ᵗʰ H60.52 Acute chemical otitis externa

H60.521 Acute chemical otitis externa, right ear   Q
H60.522 Acute chemical otitis externa, left ear   Q
H60.523 Acute chemical otitis externa, bilateral   Q
H60.529 Acute chemical otitis externa, unspecified ear   Q

✓6ᵗʰ H60.53 Acute contact otitis externa

H60.531 Acute contact otitis externa, right ear   Q
H60.532 Acute contact otitis externa, left ear   Q
H60.533 Acute contact otitis externa, bilateral   Q
H60.539 Acute contact otitis externa, unspecified ear   Q

✓6ᵗʰ H60.54 Acute eczematoid otitis externa

H60.541 Acute eczematoid otitis externa, right ear   Q
H60.542 Acute eczematoid otitis externa, left ear   Q
H60.543 Acute eczematoid otitis externa, bilateral   Q
H60.549 Acute eczematoid otitis externa, unspecified ear   Q

✓6ᵗʰ H60.55 Acute reactive otitis externa

H60.551 Acute reactive otitis externa, right ear   Q
H60.552 Acute reactive otitis externa, left ear   Q
H60.553 Acute reactive otitis externa, bilateral   Q
H60.559 Acute reactive otitis externa, unspecified ear   Q

✓6ᵗʰ H60.59 Other noninfective acute otitis externa

H60.591 Other noninfective acute otitis externa, right ear   Q
H60.592 Other noninfective acute otitis externa, left ear   Q
H60.593 Other noninfective acute otitis externa, bilateral   Q

           H60.599   Other noninfective acute otitis externa, unspecified ear   0

   ✓5ᵗʰ   **H60.6**   **Unspecified chronic otitis externa**

         H60.60   Unspecified chronic otitis externa, unspecified ear

         H60.61   Unspecified chronic otitis externa, right ear

         H60.62   Unspecified chronic otitis externa, left ear

         H60.63   Unspecified chronic otitis externa, bilateral

   ✓5ᵗʰ   **H60.8**   **Other otitis externa**

     ✓6ᵗʰ   **H60.8X**   **Other otitis externa**

         H60.8X1   Other otitis externa, right ear

         H60.8X2   Other otitis externa, left ear

         H60.8X3   Other otitis externa, bilateral   0

         H60.8X9   Other otitis externa, unspecified ear

   ✓5ᵗʰ   **H60.9**   **Unspecified otitis externa**

         H60.90   Unspecified otitis externa, unspecified ear

         H60.91   Unspecified otitis externa, right ear

         H60.92   Unspecified otitis externa, left ear

         H60.93   Unspecified otitis externa, bilateral

✓4ᵗʰ   **H61**   **Other disorders of external ear**

   ✓5ᵗʰ   **H61.0**   **Chondritis and perichondritis of external ear**

       Chondrodermatitis nodularis chronica helicis

       Perichondritis of auricle

       Perichondritis of pinna

     ✓6ᵗʰ   **H61.00**   **Unspecified perichondritis of external ear**

         H61.001   Unspecified perichondritis of right external ear

         H61.002   Unspecified perichondritis of left external ear

         H61.003   Unspecified perichondritis of external ear, bilateral

         H61.009   Unspecified perichondritis of external ear, unspecified ear

     ✓6ᵗʰ   **H61.01**   **Acute perichondritis of external ear**

         H61.011   Acute perichondritis of right external ear

         H61.012   Acute perichondritis of left external ear

         H61.013   Acute perichondritis of external ear, bilateral

         H61.019   Acute perichondritis of external ear, unspecified ear

     ✓6ᵗʰ   **H61.02**   **Chronic perichondritis of external ear**

         H61.021   Chronic perichondritis of right external ear

         H61.022   Chronic perichondritis of left external ear

         H61.023   Chronic perichondritis of external ear, bilateral

         H61.029   Chronic perichondritis of external ear, unspecified ear

     ✓6ᵗʰ   **H61.03**   **Chondritis of external ear**

         Chondritis of auricle

         Chondritis of pinna

         AHA: 2015,1Q,18

         DEF: Infection that has progressed into the cartilage and presents as indurated and edematous skin over the pinna. Vascular compromise occurs with tissue necrosis and deformity.

         H61.031   Chondritis of right external ear

         H61.032   Chondritis of left external ear

         H61.033   Chondritis of external ear, bilateral

         H61.039   Chondritis of external ear, unspecified ear

   ✓5ᵗʰ   **H61.1**   **Noninfective disorders of pinna**

       EXCLUDES 2   cauliflower ear (M95.1-)

                      gouty tophi of ear (M1A.-)

     ✓6ᵗʰ   **H61.10**   **Unspecified noninfective disorders of pinna**

         Disorder of pinna NOS

         H61.101   Unspecified noninfective disorders of pinna, right ear

         H61.102   Unspecified noninfective disorders of pinna, left ear

         H61.103   Unspecified noninfective disorders of pinna, bilateral

         H61.109   Unspecified noninfective disorders of pinna, unspecified ear

     ✓6ᵗʰ   **H61.11**   **Acquired deformity of pinna**

         Acquired deformity of auricle

         EXCLUDES 2   cauliflower ear (M95.1-)

         H61.111   Acquired deformity of pinna, right ear

         H61.112   Acquired deformity of pinna, left ear

         H61.113   Acquired deformity of pinna, bilateral

         H61.119   Acquired deformity of pinna, unspecified ear

     ✓6ᵗʰ   **H61.12**   **Hematoma of pinna**

         Hematoma of auricle

         H61.121   Hematoma of pinna, right ear

         H61.122   Hematoma of pinna, left ear

         H61.123   Hematoma of pinna, bilateral

         H61.129   Hematoma of pinna, unspecified ear

     ✓6ᵗʰ   **H61.19**   **Other noninfective disorders of pinna**

         H61.191   Noninfective disorders of pinna, right ear

         H61.192   Noninfective disorders of pinna, left ear

         H61.193   Noninfective disorders of pinna, bilateral

         H61.199   Noninfective disorders of pinna, unspecified ear

   ✓5ᵗʰ   **H61.2**   **Impacted cerumen**

       Wax in ear

         H61.20   Impacted cerumen, unspecified ear

         H61.21   Impacted cerumen, right ear

         H61.22   Impacted cerumen, left ear

         H61.23   Impacted cerumen, bilateral

   ✓5ᵗʰ   **H61.3**   **Acquired stenosis of external ear canal**

       Collapse of external ear canal

       EXCLUDES 1   postprocedural stenosis of external ear canal (H95.81-)

     ✓6ᵗʰ   **H61.30**   **Acquired stenosis of external ear canal, unspecified**

         H61.301   Acquired stenosis of right external ear canal, unspecified

         H61.302   Acquired stenosis of left external ear canal, unspecified

         H61.303   Acquired stenosis of external ear canal, unspecified, bilateral

         H61.309   Acquired stenosis of external ear canal, unspecified, unspecified ear

     ✓6ᵗʰ   **H61.31**   **Acquired stenosis of external ear canal secondary to trauma**

         H61.311   Acquired stenosis of right external ear canal secondary to trauma

         H61.312   Acquired stenosis of left external ear canal secondary to trauma

         H61.313   Acquired stenosis of external ear canal secondary to trauma, bilateral

         H61.319   Acquired stenosis of external ear canal secondary to trauma, unspecified ear

     ✓6ᵗʰ   **H61.32**   **Acquired stenosis of external ear canal secondary to inflammation and infection**

         DEF: Narrowing of the external ear canal due to chronic inflammation or infection.

         H61.321   Acquired stenosis of right external ear canal secondary to inflammation and infection

         H61.322   Acquired stenosis of left external ear canal secondary to inflammation and infection

         H61.323   Acquired stenosis of external ear canal secondary to inflammation and infection, bilateral

         H61.329   Acquired stenosis of external ear canal secondary to inflammation and infection, unspecified ear

     ✓6ᵗʰ   **H61.39**   **Other acquired stenosis of external ear canal**

         H61.391   Other acquired stenosis of right external ear canal

         H61.392   Other acquired stenosis of left external ear canal

         H61.393   Other acquired stenosis of external ear canal, bilateral

         H61.399   Other acquired stenosis of external ear canal, unspecified ear

   ✓5ᵗʰ   **H61.8**   **Other specified disorders of external ear**

     ✓6ᵗʰ   **H61.81**   **Exostosis of external canal**

         H61.811   Exostosis of right external canal

         H61.812   Exostosis of left external canal

         H61.813   Exostosis of external canal, bilateral

         H61.819   Exostosis of external canal, unspecified ear

     ✓6ᵗʰ   **H61.89**   **Other specified disorders of external ear**

         H61.891   Other specified disorders of right external ear

☑ Additional Character Required   ✓ₓ7ᵗʰ Placeholder Alert   Manifestation   Unspecified Dx   ▶◀ Revised Text   ● New Code   ▲ Revised Code Title

ICD-10-CM 2020   623

H61.892   Other specified disorders of left external ear

H61.893   Other specified disorders of external ear, bilateral

H61.899   Other specified disorders of external ear, unspecified ear

√5ᵗʰ **H61.9**   Disorder of external ear, unspecified

H61.90   Disorder of external ear, unspecified, unspecified ear

H61.91   Disorder of right external ear, unspecified

H61.92   Disorder of left external ear, unspecified

H61.93   Disorder of external ear, unspecified, bilateral

√4ᵗʰ **H62**   Disorders of external ear in diseases classified elsewhere

√5ᵗʰ **H62.4**   Otitis externa in other diseases classified elsewhere

Code first underlying disease, such as:
erysipelas (A46)
impetigo (L01.0)

EXCLUDES 1   otitis externa (in):
     candidiasis (B37.84)
     herpes viral [herpes simplex] (B00.1)
     herpes zoster (B02.8)

H62.40   *Otitis externa in other diseases classified elsewhere, unspecified ear*   Q

H62.41   *Otitis externa in other diseases classified elsewhere, right ear*   Q

H62.42   *Otitis externa in other diseases classified elsewhere, left ear*   Q

H62.43   *Otitis externa in other diseases classified elsewhere, bilateral*   Q

√5ᵗʰ **H62.8**   Other disorders of external ear in diseases classified elsewhere

Code first underlying disease, such as:
gout (M1A.-, M10.-)

√6ᵗʰ **H62.8X**   Other disorders of external ear in diseases classified elsewhere

H62.8X1   *Other disorders of right external ear in diseases classified elsewhere*

H62.8X2   *Other disorders of left external ear in diseases classified elsewhere*

H62.8X3   *Other disorders of external ear in diseases classified elsewhere, bilateral*

H62.8X9   *Other disorders of external ear in diseases classified elsewhere, unspecified ear*

Diseases of middle ear and mastoid (H65-H75)

√4ᵗʰ **H65**   Nonsuppurative otitis media

INCLUDES   nonsuppurative otitis media with myringitis

Use additional code for any associated perforated tympanic membrane (H72.-)

▶Use additional code, if applicable, to identify:◀
exposure to environmental tobacco smoke (Z77.22)
exposure to tobacco smoke in the perinatal period (P96.81)
history of tobacco dependence (Z87.891)
▶infectious agent (B95-B97)◀
occupational exposure to environmental tobacco smoke (Z57.31)
tobacco dependence (F17.-)
tobacco use (Z72.0)

√5ᵗʰ **H65.0**   Acute serous otitis media

Acute and subacute secretory otitis

H65.00   Acute serous otitis media, unspecified ear

H65.01   Acute serous otitis media, right ear

H65.02   Acute serous otitis media, left ear

H65.03   Acute serous otitis media, bilateral

H65.04   Acute serous otitis media, recurrent, right ear

H65.05   Acute serous otitis media, recurrent, left ear

H65.06   Acute serous otitis media, recurrent, bilateral

H65.07   Acute serous otitis media, recurrent, unspecified ear

√5ᵗʰ **H65.1**   Other acute nonsuppurative otitis media

EXCLUDES 1   otitic barotrauma (T70.0)
     otitis media (acute) NOS (H66.9)

√6ᵗʰ **H65.11**   Acute and subacute allergic otitis media (mucoid) (sanguinous) (serous)

H65.111   Acute and subacute allergic otitis media (mucoid) (sanguinous) (serous), right ear

H65.112   Acute and subacute allergic otitis media (mucoid) (sanguinous) (serous), left ear

H65.113   Acute and subacute allergic otitis media (mucoid) (sanguinous) (serous), bilateral

H65.114   Acute and subacute allergic otitis media (mucoid) (sanguinous) (serous), recurrent, right ear

H65.115   Acute and subacute allergic otitis media (mucoid) (sanguinous) (serous), recurrent, left ear

H65.116   Acute and subacute allergic otitis media (mucoid) (sanguinous) (serous), recurrent, bilateral

H65.117   Acute and subacute allergic otitis media (mucoid) (sanguinous) (serous), recurrent, unspecified ear

H65.119   Acute and subacute allergic otitis media (mucoid) (sanguinous) (serous), unspecified ear

√6ᵗʰ **H65.19**   Other acute nonsuppurative otitis media

Acute and subacute mucoid otitis media
Acute and subacute nonsuppurative otitis media NOS
Acute and subacute sanguinous otitis media
Acute and subacute seromucinous otitis media

H65.191   Other acute nonsuppurative otitis media, right ear

H65.192   Other acute nonsuppurative otitis media, left ear

H65.193   Other acute nonsuppurative otitis media, bilateral

H65.194   Other acute nonsuppurative otitis media, recurrent, right ear

H65.195   Other acute nonsuppurative otitis media, recurrent, left ear

H65.196   Other acute nonsuppurative otitis media, recurrent, bilateral

H65.197   Other acute nonsuppurative otitis media recurrent, unspecified ear

H65.199   Other acute nonsuppurative otitis media, unspecified ear

√5ᵗʰ **H65.2**   Chronic serous otitis media

Chronic tubotympanal catarrh

H65.20   Chronic serous otitis media, unspecified ear

H65.21   Chronic serous otitis media, right ear

H65.22   Chronic serous otitis media, left ear

H65.23   Chronic serous otitis media, bilateral

√5ᵗʰ **H65.3**   Chronic mucoid otitis media

Chronic mucinous otitis media
Chronic secretory otitis media
Chronic transudative otitis media
Glue ear

EXCLUDES 1   adhesive middle ear disease (H74.1)

H65.30   Chronic mucoid otitis media, unspecified ear

H65.31   Chronic mucoid otitis media, right ear

H65.32   Chronic mucoid otitis media, left ear

H65.33   Chronic mucoid otitis media, bilateral

√5ᵗʰ **H65.4**   Other chronic nonsuppurative otitis media

√6ᵗʰ **H65.41**   Chronic allergic otitis media

H65.411   Chronic allergic otitis media, right ear

H65.412   Chronic allergic otitis media, left ear

H65.413   Chronic allergic otitis media, bilateral

H65.419   Chronic allergic otitis media, unspecified ear

√6ᵗʰ **H65.49**   Other chronic nonsuppurative otitis media

Chronic exudative otitis media
Chronic nonsuppurative otitis media NOS
Chronic otitis media with effusion (nonpurulent)
Chronic seromucinous otitis media

H65.491   Other chronic nonsuppurative otitis media, right ear

H65.492   Other chronic nonsuppurative otitis media, left ear

H65.493   Other chronic nonsuppurative otitis media, bilateral

H65.499   Other chronic nonsuppurative otitis media, unspecified ear

✓5ᵗʰ **H65.9 Unspecified nonsuppurative otitis media**

Allergic otitis media NOS
Catarrhal otitis media NOS
Exudative otitis media NOS
Mucoid otitis media NOS
Otitis media with effusion (nonpurulent) NOS
Secretory otitis media NOS
Seromucinous otitis media NOS
Serous otitis media NOS
Transudative otitis media NOS

     H65.90 Unspecified nonsuppurative otitis media, unspecified ear
     H65.91 Unspecified nonsuppurative otitis media, right ear
     H65.92 Unspecified nonsuppurative otitis media, left ear
     H65.93 Unspecified nonsuppurative otitis media, bilateral

✓4ᵗʰ **H66 Suppurative and unspecified otitis media**

INCLUDES suppurative and unspecified otitis media with myringitis
Use additional code to identify:
    exposure to environmental tobacco smoke (Z77.22)
    exposure to tobacco smoke in the perinatal period (P96.81)
    history of tobacco dependence (Z87.891)
    occupational exposure to environmental tobacco smoke (Z57.31)
    tobacco dependence (F17.-)
    tobacco use (Z72.0)
AHA: 2016,1Q,34

✓5ᵗʰ **H66.0 Acute suppurative otitis media**

   ✓6ᵗʰ **H66.00 Acute suppurative otitis media without spontaneous rupture of ear drum**

     H66.001 Acute suppurative otitis media without spontaneous rupture of ear drum, right ear
     H66.002 Acute suppurative otitis media without spontaneous rupture of ear drum, left ear
     H66.003 Acute suppurative otitis media without spontaneous rupture of ear drum, bilateral
     H66.004 Acute suppurative otitis media without spontaneous rupture of ear drum, recurrent, right ear
     H66.005 Acute suppurative otitis media without spontaneous rupture of ear drum, recurrent, left ear
     H66.006 Acute suppurative otitis media without spontaneous rupture of ear drum, recurrent, bilateral
     H66.007 Acute suppurative otitis media without spontaneous rupture of ear drum, recurrent, unspecified ear
     H66.009 Acute suppurative otitis media without spontaneous rupture of ear drum, unspecified ear

   ✓6ᵗʰ **H66.01 Acute suppurative otitis media with spontaneous rupture of ear drum**
     DEF: Sudden, severe inflammation of the middle ear, causing pressure that perforates the ear drum tissue.

     H66.011 Acute suppurative otitis media with spontaneous rupture of ear drum, right ear
     H66.012 Acute suppurative otitis media with spontaneous rupture of ear drum, left ear
     H66.013 Acute suppurative otitis media with spontaneous rupture of ear drum, bilateral
     H66.014 Acute suppurative otitis media with spontaneous rupture of ear drum, recurrent, right ear
     H66.015 Acute suppurative otitis media with spontaneous rupture of ear drum, recurrent, left ear
     H66.016 Acute suppurative otitis media with spontaneous rupture of ear drum, recurrent, bilateral
     H66.017 Acute suppurative otitis media with spontaneous rupture of ear drum, recurrent, unspecified ear
     H66.019 Acute suppurative otitis media with spontaneous rupture of ear drum, unspecified ear

✓5ᵗʰ **H66.1 Chronic tubotympanic suppurative otitis media**

Benign chronic suppurative otitis media
Chronic tubotympanic disease
Use additional code for any associated perforated tympanic membrane (H72.-)

     H66.10 Chronic tubotympanic suppurative otitis media, unspecified
     H66.11 Chronic tubotympanic suppurative otitis media, right ear
     H66.12 Chronic tubotympanic suppurative otitis media, left ear
     H66.13 Chronic tubotympanic suppurative otitis media, bilateral

✓5ᵗʰ **H66.2 Chronic atticoantral suppurative otitis media**

Chronic atticoantral disease
Use additional code for any associated perforated tympanic membrane (H72.-)

     H66.20 Chronic atticoantral suppurative otitis media, unspecified ear
     H66.21 Chronic atticoantral suppurative otitis media, right ear
     H66.22 Chronic atticoantral suppurative otitis media, left ear
     H66.23 Chronic atticoantral suppurative otitis media, bilateral

✓5ᵗʰ **H66.3 Other chronic suppurative otitis media**

Chronic suppurative otitis media NOS
Use additional code for any associated perforated tympanic membrane (H72.-)
EXCLUDES 1 tuberculous otitis media (A18.6)

   ✓6ᵗʰ **H66.3X Other chronic suppurative otitis media**

     H66.3X1 Other chronic suppurative otitis media, right ear
     H66.3X2 Other chronic suppurative otitis media, left ear
     H66.3X3 Other chronic suppurative otitis media, bilateral
     H66.3X9 Other chronic suppurative otitis media, unspecified ear

✓5ᵗʰ **H66.4 Suppurative otitis media, unspecified**

Purulent otitis media NOS
Use additional code for any associated perforated tympanic membrane (H72.-)

     H66.40 Suppurative otitis media, unspecified, unspecified ear
     H66.41 Suppurative otitis media, unspecified, right ear
     H66.42 Suppurative otitis media, unspecified, left ear
     H66.43 Suppurative otitis media, unspecified, bilateral

✓5ᵗʰ **H66.9 Otitis media, unspecified**

Otitis media NOS
Acute otitis media NOS
Chronic otitis media NOS
Use additional code for any associated perforated tympanic membrane (H72.-)

     H66.90 Otitis media, unspecified, unspecified ear
     H66.91 Otitis media, unspecified, right ear
     H66.92 Otitis media, unspecified, left ear
     H66.93 Otitis media, unspecified, bilateral

✓4ᵗʰ **H67 Otitis media in diseases classified elsewhere**

Code first underlying disease, such as:
    plasminogen deficiency (E88.02)
    viral disease NEC (B00-B34)
Use additional code for any associated perforated tympanic membrane (H72.-)
EXCLUDES 1 otitis media in:
     influenza (J09.X9, J10.83, J11.83)
     measles (B05.3)
     scarlet fever (A38.0)
     tuberculosis (A18.6)

     H67.1 Otitis media in diseases classified elsewhere, right ear
     H67.2 Otitis media in diseases classified elsewhere, left ear
     H67.3 Otitis media in diseases classified elsewhere, bilateral
     H67.9 Otitis media in diseases classified elsewhere, unspecified ear

---

☑ Additional Character Required   ✓x7ᵗʰ Placeholder Alert   Manifestation   Unspecified Dx   ▶◀ Revised Text   ● New Code   ▲ Revised Code Title

✅4ᵗʰ **H68 Eustachian salpingitis and obstruction**

DEF: Eustachian tube: Internal channel between the tympanic cavity and the nasopharynx that equalizes internal pressure to the outside pressure and drains mucous production from the middle ear.

✅5ᵗʰ **H68.0 Eustachian salpingitis**

✅6ᵗʰ **H68.00 Unspecified Eustachian salpingitis**

H68.001 Unspecified Eustachian salpingitis, **right ear**

H68.002 Unspecified Eustachian salpingitis, **left ear**

H68.003 Unspecified Eustachian salpingitis, **bilateral**

H68.009 Unspecified Eustachian salpingitis, **unspecified ear**

✅6ᵗʰ **H68.01 Acute Eustachian salpingitis**

H68.011 Acute Eustachian salpingitis, **right** ear

H68.012 Acute Eustachian salpingitis, **left** ear

H68.013 Acute Eustachian salpingitis, **bilateral**

H68.019 Acute Eustachian salpingitis, unspecified ear

✅6ᵗʰ **H68.02 Chronic Eustachian salpingitis**

H68.021 Chronic Eustachian salpingitis, **right** ear

H68.022 Chronic Eustachian salpingitis, **left** ear

H68.023 Chronic Eustachian salpingitis, **bilateral**

H68.029 Chronic Eustachian salpingitis, **unspecified ear**

✅5ᵗʰ **H68.1 Obstruction of Eustachian tube**

Stenosis of Eustachian tube
Stricture of Eustachian tube

✅6ᵗʰ **H68.10 Unspecified obstruction of Eustachian tube**

H68.101 Unspecified obstruction of Eustachian tube, **right ear**

H68.102 Unspecified obstruction of Eustachian tube, **left ear**

H68.103 Unspecified obstruction of Eustachian tube, **bilateral**

H68.109 Unspecified obstruction of Eustachian tube, unspecified ear

✅6ᵗʰ **H68.11 Osseous obstruction of Eustachian tube**

H68.111 Osseous obstruction of Eustachian tube, **right ear**

H68.112 Osseous obstruction of Eustachian tube, **left ear**

H68.113 Osseous obstruction of Eustachian tube, **bilateral**

H68.119 Osseous obstruction of Eustachian tube, unspecified ear

✅6ᵗʰ **H68.12 Intrinsic cartilagenous obstruction of Eustachian tube**

H68.121 Intrinsic cartilagenous obstruction of Eustachian tube, **right ear**

H68.122 Intrinsic cartilagenous obstruction of Eustachian tube, **left ear**

H68.123 Intrinsic cartilagenous obstruction of Eustachian tube, **bilateral**

H68.129 Intrinsic cartilagenous obstruction of Eustachian tube, unspecified ear

✅6ᵗʰ **H68.13 Extrinsic cartilagenous obstruction of Eustachian tube**

Compression of Eustachian tube

H68.131 Extrinsic cartilagenous obstruction of Eustachian tube, **right ear**

H68.132 Extrinsic cartilagenous obstruction of Eustachian tube, **left ear**

H68.133 Extrinsic cartilagenous obstruction of Eustachian tube, **bilateral**

H68.139 Extrinsic cartilagenous obstruction of Eustachian tube, unspecified ear

✅4ᵗʰ **H69 Other and unspecified disorders of Eustachian tube**

DEF: Eustachian tube: Internal channel between the tympanic cavity and the nasopharynx that equalizes internal pressure to the outside pressure and drains mucous production from the middle ear.

✅5ᵗʰ **H69.0 Patulous Eustachian tube**

H69.00 Patulous Eustachian tube, **unspecified ear**

H69.01 Patulous Eustachian tube, **right ear**

H69.02 Patulous Eustachian tube, **left ear**

H69.03 Patulous Eustachian tube, **bilateral**

✅5ᵗʰ **H69.8 Other specified disorders of Eustachian tube**

H69.80 Other specified disorders of Eustachian tube, **unspecified ear**

H69.81 Other specified disorders of Eustachian tube, **right ear**

H69.82 Other specified disorders of Eustachian tube, **left ear**

H69.83 Other specified disorders of Eustachian tube, **bilateral**

✅5ᵗʰ **H69.9 Unspecified Eustachian tube disorder**

H69.90 Unspecified Eustachian tube disorder, **unspecified ear**

H69.91 Unspecified Eustachian tube disorder, **right ear**

H69.92 Unspecified Eustachian tube disorder, **left ear**

H69.93 Unspecified Eustachian tube disorder, **bilateral**

✅4ᵗʰ **H70 Mastoiditis and related conditions**

✅5ᵗʰ **H70.0 Acute mastoiditis**

Abscess of mastoid
Empyema of mastoid

✅6ᵗʰ **H70.00 Acute mastoiditis without complications**

H70.001 Acute mastoiditis without complications, **right ear**

H70.002 Acute mastoiditis without complications, **left ear**

H70.003 Acute mastoiditis without complications, **bilateral**

H70.009 Acute mastoiditis without complications, **unspecified ear**

✅6ᵗʰ **H70.01 Subperiosteal abscess of mastoid**

H70.011 Subperiosteal abscess of mastoid, **right ear**

H70.012 Subperiosteal abscess of mastoid, **left ear**

H70.013 Subperiosteal abscess of mastoid, **bilateral**

H70.019 Subperiosteal abscess of mastoid, **unspecified ear**

✅6ᵗʰ **H70.09 Acute mastoiditis with other complications**

H70.091 Acute mastoiditis with other complications, **right ear**

H70.092 Acute mastoiditis with other complications, **left ear**

H70.093 Acute mastoiditis with other complications, **bilateral**

H70.099 Acute mastoiditis with other complications, unspecified ear

✅5ᵗʰ **H70.1 Chronic mastoiditis**

Caries of mastoid
Fistula of mastoid

EXCLUDES 1   *tuberculous mastoiditis (A18.03)*

H70.10 Chronic mastoiditis, unspecified ear

H70.11 Chronic mastoiditis, **right ear**

H70.12 Chronic mastoiditis, **left ear**

H70.13 Chronic mastoiditis, **bilateral**

✅5ᵗʰ **H70.2 Petrositis**

Inflammation of petrous bone

✅6ᵗʰ **H70.20 Unspecified petrositis**

H70.201 Unspecified petrositis, **right ear**

H70.202 Unspecified petrositis, **left ear**

H70.203 Unspecified petrositis, **bilateral**

H70.209 Unspecified petrositis, unspecified ear

✅6ᵗʰ **H70.21 Acute petrositis**

DEF: Sudden, severe inflammation of the petrous temporal bone behind the ear, associated with a middle ear infection.

H70.211 Acute petrositis, **right ear**

H70.212 Acute petrositis, **left ear**

H70.213 Acute petrositis, **bilateral**

H70.219 Acute petrositis, **unspecified ear**

✅6ᵗʰ **H70.22 Chronic petrositis**

H70.221 Chronic petrositis, **right ear**

H70.222 Chronic petrositis, **left ear**

H70.223 Chronic petrositis, **bilateral**

H70.229 Chronic petrositis, unspecified ear

✓5ᵗʰ H70.8 Other mastoiditis and related conditions

> *EXCLUDES 1*   preauricular sinus and cyst (Q18.1)
> sinus, fistula, and cyst of branchial cleft (Q18.0)

   ✓6ᵗʰ H70.81 Postauricular fistula

     H70.811 Postauricular fistula, **right** ear
     H70.812 Postauricular fistula, **left** ear
     H70.813 Postauricular fistula, **bilateral**
     H70.819 Postauricular fistula, **unspecified** ear

   ✓6ᵗʰ H70.89 Other mastoiditis and related conditions

     H70.891 Other mastoiditis and related conditions, **right** ear
     H70.892 Other mastoiditis and related conditions, **left** ear
     H70.893 Other mastoiditis and related conditions, **bilateral**
     H70.899 Other mastoiditis and related conditions, **unspecified** ear

✓5ᵗʰ H70.9 Unspecified mastoiditis

     H70.90 Unspecified mastoiditis, **unspecified** ear
     H70.91 Unspecified mastoiditis, **right** ear
     H70.92 Unspecified mastoiditis, **left** ear
     H70.93 Unspecified mastoiditis, **bilateral**

✓4ᵗʰ H71 Cholesteatoma of middle ear

> *EXCLUDES 2*   cholesteatoma of external ear (H60.4-)
> recurrent cholesteatoma of postmastoidectomy cavity (H95.0-)

DEF: Cholesteatoma: Noncancerous cyst-like mass of cell debris, including cholesterol and epithelial cells resulting from trauma, repeated or improperly healed infections, and congenital enclosure of epidermal cells.

Cholesteatoma of Middle Ear

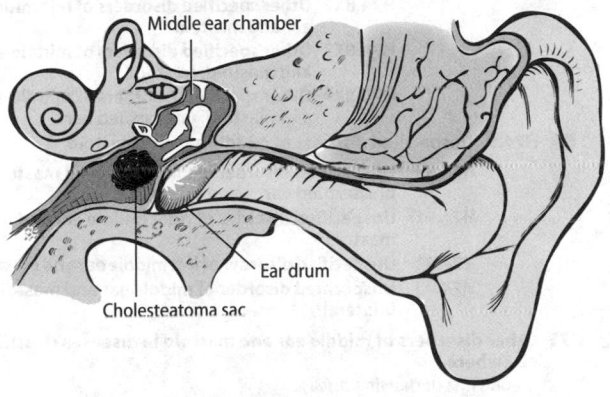

Middle ear chamber

Ear drum

Cholesteatoma sac

✓5ᵗʰ H71.0 Cholesteatoma of attic

     H71.00 Cholesteatoma of attic, **unspecified** ear
     H71.01 Cholesteatoma of attic, **right** ear
     H71.02 Cholesteatoma of attic, **left** ear
     H71.03 Cholesteatoma of attic, **bilateral**

✓5ᵗʰ H71.1 Cholesteatoma of tympanum

     H71.10 Cholesteatoma of tympanum, **unspecified** ear
     H71.11 Cholesteatoma of tympanum, **right** ear
     H71.12 Cholesteatoma of tympanum, **left** ear
     H71.13 Cholesteatoma of tympanum, **bilateral**

✓5ᵗʰ H71.2 Cholesteatoma of mastoid

     H71.20 Cholesteatoma of mastoid, **unspecified** ear
     H71.21 Cholesteatoma of mastoid, **right** ear
     H71.22 Cholesteatoma of mastoid, **left** ear
     H71.23 Cholesteatoma of mastoid, **bilateral**

✓5ᵗʰ H71.3 Diffuse cholesteatosis

     H71.30 Diffuse cholesteatosis, **unspecified** ear
     H71.31 Diffuse cholesteatosis, **right** ear
     H71.32 Diffuse cholesteatosis, **left** ear
     H71.33 Diffuse cholesteatosis, **bilateral**

✓5ᵗʰ H71.9 Unspecified cholesteatoma

     H71.90 Unspecified cholesteatoma, **unspecified** ear
     H71.91 Unspecified cholesteatoma, **right** ear
     H71.92 Unspecified cholesteatoma, **left** ear
     H71.93 Unspecified cholesteatoma, **bilateral**

✓4ᵗʰ H72 Perforation of tympanic membrane

> **INCLUDES**   persistent post-traumatic perforation of ear drum
> postinflammatory perforation of ear drum

Code first any associated otitis media (H65.-, H66.1-, H66.2-, H66.3-, H66.4-, H66.9-, H67.-)

> *EXCLUDES 1*   acute suppurative otitis media with rupture of the tympanic membrane (H66.01-)
> traumatic rupture of ear drum (S09.2-)

✓5ᵗʰ H72.0 Central perforation of tympanic membrane

     H72.00 Central perforation of tympanic membrane, **unspecified** ear
     H72.01 Central perforation of tympanic membrane, **right** ear
     H72.02 Central perforation of tympanic membrane, **left** ear
     H72.03 Central perforation of tympanic membrane, **bilateral**

✓5ᵗʰ H72.1 Attic perforation of tympanic membrane

     Perforation of pars flaccida

     H72.10 Attic perforation of tympanic membrane, **unspecified** ear
     H72.11 Attic perforation of tympanic membrane, **right** ear
     H72.12 Attic perforation of tympanic membrane, **left** ear
     H72.13 Attic perforation of tympanic membrane, **bilateral**

✓5ᵗʰ H72.2 Other marginal perforations of tympanic membrane

   ✓6ᵗʰ H72.2X Other marginal perforations of tympanic membrane

     H72.2X1 Other marginal perforations of tympanic membrane, **right** ear
     H72.2X2 Other marginal perforations of tympanic membrane, **left** ear
     H72.2X3 Other marginal perforations of tympanic membrane, **bilateral**
     H72.2X9 Other marginal perforations of tympanic membrane, **unspecified** ear

✓5ᵗʰ H72.8 Other perforations of tympanic membrane

   ✓6ᵗʰ H72.81 Multiple perforations of tympanic membrane

     H72.811 Multiple perforations of tympanic membrane, **right** ear
     H72.812 Multiple perforations of tympanic membrane, **left** ear
     H72.813 Multiple perforations of tympanic membrane, **bilateral**
     H72.819 Multiple perforations of tympanic membrane, **unspecified** ear

   ✓6ᵗʰ H72.82 Total perforations of tympanic membrane

     H72.821 Total perforations of tympanic membrane, **right** ear
     H72.822 Total perforations of tympanic membrane, **left** ear
     H72.823 Total perforations of tympanic membrane, **bilateral**
     H72.829 Total perforations of tympanic membrane, **unspecified** ear

✓5ᵗʰ H72.9 Unspecified perforation of tympanic membrane

     H72.90 Unspecified perforation of tympanic membrane, **unspecified** ear
     H72.91 Unspecified perforation of tympanic membrane, **right** ear
     H72.92 Unspecified perforation of tympanic membrane, **left** ear
     H72.93 Unspecified perforation of tympanic membrane, **bilateral**

✓4ᵗʰ H73 Other disorders of tympanic membrane

   ✓5ᵗʰ H73.0 Acute myringitis

> *EXCLUDES 1*   acute myringitis with otitis media (H65, H66)

   ✓6ᵗʰ H73.00 Unspecified acute myringitis

     Acute tympanitis NOS

     H73.001 Acute myringitis, **right** ear
     H73.002 Acute myringitis, **left** ear
     H73.003 Acute myringitis, **bilateral**
     H73.009 Acute myringitis, **unspecified** ear

   ✓6ᵗʰ H73.01 Bullous myringitis

     DEF: Bacterial or viral otitis media that is characterized by the appearance of serous or hemorrhagic blebs on the ear drum and sudden onset of severe pain in ear.

     H73.011 Bullous myringitis, **right** ear
     H73.012 Bullous myringitis, **left** ear
     H73.013 Bullous myringitis, **bilateral**

☑ Additional Character Required   ✓x7ᵗʰ Placeholder Alert   Manifestation   Unspecified Dx   ▶◀ Revised Text   ● New Code   ▲ Revised Code Title

ICD-10-CM 2020   627

Chapter 8. Diseases of the Ear and Mastoid Process

H73.019   Bullous myringitis, unspecified ear

√6ᵗʰ **H73.09**   **Other acute myringitis**

    H73.091   Other acute myringitis, right ear

    H73.092   Other acute myringitis, left ear

    H73.093   Other acute myringitis, bilateral

    H73.099   Other acute myringitis, unspecified ear

√5ᵗʰ **H73.1**   **Chronic myringitis**

    Chronic tympanitis

    EXCLUDES 1   chronic myringitis with otitis media (H65, H66)

    H73.10   **Chronic myringitis, unspecified ear**

    H73.11   **Chronic myringitis, right ear**

    H73.12   **Chronic myringitis, left ear**

    H73.13   **Chronic myringitis, bilateral**

√5ᵗʰ **H73.2**   **Unspecified myringitis**

    H73.20   **Unspecified myringitis, unspecified ear**

    H73.21   **Unspecified myringitis, right ear**

    H73.22   **Unspecified myringitis, left ear**

    H73.23   **Unspecified myringitis, bilateral**

√5ᵗʰ **H73.8**   **Other specified disorders of tympanic membrane**

√6ᵗʰ **H73.81**   Atrophic flaccid tympanic membrane

    H73.811   Atrophic flaccid tympanic membrane, right ear

    H73.812   Atrophic flaccid tympanic membrane, left ear

    H73.813   Atrophic flaccid tympanic membrane, bilateral

    H73.819   Atrophic flaccid tympanic membrane, unspecified ear

√6ᵗʰ **H73.82**   Atrophic nonflaccid tympanic membrane

    H73.821   Atrophic nonflaccid tympanic membrane, right ear

    H73.822   Atrophic nonflaccid tympanic membrane, left ear

    H73.823   Atrophic nonflaccid tympanic membrane, bilateral

    H73.829   Atrophic nonflaccid tympanic membrane, unspecified ear

√6ᵗʰ **H73.89**   Other specified disorders of tympanic membrane

    H73.891   Other specified disorders of tympanic membrane, right ear

    H73.892   Other specified disorders of tympanic membrane, left ear

    H73.893   Other specified disorders of tympanic membrane, bilateral

    H73.899   Other specified disorders of tympanic membrane, unspecified ear

√5ᵗʰ **H73.9**   **Unspecified disorder of tympanic membrane**

    H73.90   **Unspecified disorder of tympanic membrane, unspecified ear**

    H73.91   **Unspecified disorder of tympanic membrane, right ear**

    H73.92   **Unspecified disorder of tympanic membrane, left ear**

    H73.93   **Unspecified disorder of tympanic membrane, bilateral**

√4ᵗʰ **H74**   **Other disorders of middle ear mastoid**

    EXCLUDES 2   mastoiditis (H70.-)

√5ᵗʰ **H74.0**   **Tympanosclerosis**

    DEF: Calcification of tissue in the ear drum, middle ear bones, and middle ear canal.

    H74.01   **Tympanosclerosis, right ear**

    H74.02   **Tympanosclerosis, left ear**

    H74.03   **Tympanosclerosis, bilateral**

    H74.09   **Tympanosclerosis, unspecified ear**

√5ᵗʰ **H74.1**   **Adhesive middle ear disease**

    Adhesive otitis

    EXCLUDES 1   glue ear (H65.3-)

    H74.11   **Adhesive right middle ear disease**

    H74.12   **Adhesive left middle ear disease**

    H74.13   **Adhesive middle ear disease, bilateral**

    H74.19   **Adhesive middle ear disease, unspecified ear**

√5ᵗʰ **H74.2**   **Discontinuity and dislocation of ear ossicles**

    H74.20   **Discontinuity and dislocation of ear ossicles, unspecified ear**

    H74.21   **Discontinuity and dislocation of right ear ossicles**

    H74.22   **Discontinuity and dislocation of left ear ossicles**

H74.23   **Discontinuity and dislocation of ear ossicles, bilateral**

√5ᵗʰ **H74.3**   **Other acquired abnormalities of ear ossicles**

√6ᵗʰ **H74.31**   Ankylosis of ear ossicles

    H74.311   Ankylosis of ear ossicles, right ear

    H74.312   Ankylosis of ear ossicles, left ear

    H74.313   Ankylosis of ear ossicles, bilateral

    H74.319   Ankylosis of ear ossicles, unspecified ear

√6ᵗʰ **H74.32**   Partial loss of ear ossicles

    H74.321   Partial loss of ear ossicles, right ear

    H74.322   Partial loss of ear ossicles, left ear

    H74.323   Partial loss of ear ossicles, bilateral

    H74.329   Partial loss of ear ossicles, unspecified ear

√6ᵗʰ **H74.39**   Other acquired abnormalities of ear ossicles

    H74.391   Other acquired abnormalities of right ear ossicles

    H74.392   Other acquired abnormalities of left ear ossicles

    H74.393   Other acquired abnormalities of ear ossicles, bilateral

    H74.399   Other acquired abnormalities of ear ossicles, unspecified ear

√5ᵗʰ **H74.4**   **Polyp of middle ear**

    H74.40   **Polyp of middle ear, unspecified ear**

    H74.41   **Polyp of right middle ear**

    H74.42   **Polyp of left middle ear**

    H74.43   **Polyp of middle ear, bilateral**

√5ᵗʰ **H74.8**   **Other specified disorders of middle ear and mastoid**

√6ᵗʰ **H74.8X**   Other specified disorders of middle ear and mastoid

    H74.8X1   Other specified disorders of right middle ear and mastoid

    H74.8X2   Other specified disorders of left middle ear and mastoid

    H74.8X3   Other specified disorders of middle ear and mastoid, bilateral

    H74.8X9   Other specified disorders of middle ear and mastoid, unspecified ear

√5ᵗʰ **H74.9**   **Unspecified disorder of middle ear and mastoid**

    H74.90   **Unspecified disorder of middle ear and mastoid, unspecified ear**

    H74.91   **Unspecified disorder of right middle ear and mastoid**

    H74.92   **Unspecified disorder of left middle ear and mastoid**

    H74.93   **Unspecified disorder of middle ear and mastoid, bilateral**

√4ᵗʰ **H75**   **Other disorders of middle ear and mastoid in diseases classified elsewhere**

    Code first underlying disease

√5ᵗʰ **H75.0**   **Mastoiditis in infectious and parasitic diseases classified elsewhere**

    EXCLUDES 1   mastoiditis (in):

       syphilis (A52.77)

       tuberculosis (A18.03)

    H75.00   *Mastoiditis in infectious and parasitic diseases classified elsewhere, unspecified ear*

    H75.01   *Mastoiditis in infectious and parasitic diseases classified elsewhere, right ear*

    H75.02   *Mastoiditis in infectious and parasitic diseases classified elsewhere, left ear*

    H75.03   *Mastoiditis in infectious and parasitic diseases classified elsewhere, bilateral*

√5ᵗʰ **H75.8**   **Other specified disorders of middle ear and mastoid in diseases classified elsewhere**

    H75.80   *Other specified disorders of middle ear and mastoid in diseases classified elsewhere, unspecified ear*

    H75.81   *Other specified disorders of right middle ear and mastoid in diseases classified elsewhere*

    H75.82   *Other specified disorders of left middle ear and mastoid in diseases classified elsewhere*

    H75.83   *Other specified disorders of middle ear and mastoid in diseases classified elsewhere, bilateral*

Diseases of inner ear (H80-H83)

✓4ᵗʰ H80 Otosclerosis

INCLUDES   otospongiosis

✓5ᵗʰ H80.0 Otosclerosis involving oval window, nonobliterative

- **H80.00** Otosclerosis involving oval window, nonobliterative, unspecified ear
- **H80.01** Otosclerosis involving oval window, nonobliterative, right ear
- **H80.02** Otosclerosis involving oval window, nonobliterative, left ear
- **H80.03** Otosclerosis involving oval window, nonobliterative, bilateral

✓5ᵗʰ H80.1 Otosclerosis involving oval window, obliterative

- **H80.10** Otosclerosis involving oval window, obliterative, unspecified ear
- **H80.11** Otosclerosis involving oval window, obliterative, right ear
- **H80.12** Otosclerosis involving oval window, obliterative, left ear
- **H80.13** Otosclerosis involving oval window, obliterative, bilateral

✓5ᵗʰ H80.2 Cochlear otosclerosis

Otosclerosis involving otic capsule
Otosclerosis involving round window

- **H80.20** Cochlear otosclerosis, unspecified ear
- **H80.21** Cochlear otosclerosis, right ear
- **H80.22** Cochlear otosclerosis, left ear
- **H80.23** Cochlear otosclerosis, bilateral

✓5ᵗʰ H80.8 Other otosclerosis

- **H80.80** Other otosclerosis, unspecified ear
- **H80.81** Other otosclerosis, right ear
- **H80.82** Other otosclerosis, left ear
- **H80.83** Other otosclerosis, bilateral

✓5ᵗʰ H80.9 Unspecified otosclerosis

- **H80.90** Unspecified otosclerosis, unspecified ear
- **H80.91** Unspecified otosclerosis, right ear
- **H80.92** Unspecified otosclerosis, left ear
- **H80.93** Unspecified otosclerosis, bilateral

✓4ᵗʰ H81 Disorders of vestibular function

EXCLUDES 1   epidemic vertigo (A88.1)
         vertigo NOS (R42)

✓6ᵗʰ H81.0 Ménière's disease

Labyrinthine hydrops
Ménière's syndrome or vertigo
DEF: Distended membranous labyrinth of the middle ear from fluctuating pressure of fluid (hydrops) that causes vertigo, tinnitus, pressure, and hearing loss that may last on and off for several hours. Episodes may occur in clusters or may subside for weeks, months, or even years.

- **H81.01** Ménière's disease, right ear
- **H81.02** Ménière's disease, left ear
- **H81.03** Ménière's disease, bilateral
- **H81.09** Ménière's disease, unspecified ear

✓5ᵗʰ H81.1 Benign paroxysmal vertigo

- **H81.10** Benign paroxysmal vertigo, unspecified ear   Q
- **H81.11** Benign paroxysmal vertigo, right ear   Q
- **H81.12** Benign paroxysmal vertigo, left ear   Q
- **H81.13** Benign paroxysmal vertigo, bilateral   Q

✓5ᵗʰ H81.2 Vestibular neuronitis

DEF: Transient benign vertigo caused by inflammation of the vestibular nerve. It is characterized by response to caloric stimulation on one side and nystagmus with rhythmic movement of the eyes. Normal auditory function is present.

- **H81.20** Vestibular neuronitis, unspecified ear
- **H81.21** Vestibular neuronitis, right ear
- **H81.22** Vestibular neuronitis, left ear
- **H81.23** Vestibular neuronitis, bilateral

✓5ᵗʰ H81.3 Other peripheral vertigo

✓6ᵗʰ H81.31 Aural vertigo

- **H81.311** Aural vertigo, right ear
- **H81.312** Aural vertigo, left ear
- **H81.313** Aural vertigo, bilateral
- **H81.319** Aural vertigo, unspecified ear

✓6ᵗʰ H81.39 Other peripheral vertigo

Lermoyez' syndrome
Otogenic vertigo
Peripheral vertigo NOS

- **H81.391** Other peripheral vertigo, right ear
- **H81.392** Other peripheral vertigo, left ear
- **H81.393** Other peripheral vertigo, bilateral
- **H81.399** Other peripheral vertigo, unspecified ear

▲ H81.4 Vertigo of central origin

Central positional nystagmus

- ~~**H81.41** Vertigo of central origin, right ear~~
- ~~**H81.42** Vertigo of central origin, left ear~~
- ~~**H81.43** Vertigo of central origin, bilateral~~
- ~~**H81.49** Vertigo of central origin, unspecified ear~~

✓5ᵗʰ H81.8 Other disorders of vestibular function

✓6ᵗʰ H81.8X Other disorders of vestibular function

- **H81.8X1** Other disorders of vestibular function, right ear
- **H81.8X2** Other disorders of vestibular function, left ear
- **H81.8X3** Other disorders of vestibular function, bilateral
- **H81.8X9** Other disorders of vestibular function, unspecified ear

✓5ᵗʰ H81.9 Unspecified disorder of vestibular function

Vertiginous syndrome NOS

- **H81.90** Unspecified disorder of vestibular function, unspecified ear
- **H81.91** Unspecified disorder of vestibular function, right ear
- **H81.92** Unspecified disorder of vestibular function, left ear
- **H81.93** Unspecified disorder of vestibular function, bilateral

✓4ᵗʰ H82 Vertiginous syndromes in diseases classified elsewhere

Code first underlying disease
EXCLUDES 1   epidemic vertigo (A88.1)

- **H82.1** Vertiginous syndromes in diseases classified elsewhere, right ear
- **H82.2** Vertiginous syndromes in diseases classified elsewhere, left ear
- **H82.3** Vertiginous syndromes in diseases classified elsewhere, bilateral
- **H82.9** Vertiginous syndromes in diseases classified elsewhere, unspecified ear

✓4ᵗʰ H83 Other diseases of inner ear

✓5ᵗʰ H83.0 Labyrinthitis

DEF: Inflammation of the inner ear, or labyrinth, characterized by pus, vertigo, dizziness, nausea, and hearing loss.

- **H83.01** Labyrinthitis, right ear
- **H83.02** Labyrinthitis, left ear
- **H83.03** Labyrinthitis, bilateral
- **H83.09** Labyrinthitis, unspecified ear

✓5ᵗʰ H83.1 Labyrinthine fistula

- **H83.11** Labyrinthine fistula, right ear
- **H83.12** Labyrinthine fistula, left ear
- **H83.13** Labyrinthine fistula, bilateral
- **H83.19** Labyrinthine fistula, unspecified ear

✓5ᵗʰ H83.2 Labyrinthine dysfunction

Labyrinthine hypersensitivity
Labyrinthine hypofunction
Labyrinthine loss of function
DEF: Decreased function of the labyrinth sensors.

✓6ᵗʰ H83.2X Labyrinthine dysfunction

- **H83.2X1** Labyrinthine dysfunction, right ear
- **H83.2X2** Labyrinthine dysfunction, left ear
- **H83.2X3** Labyrinthine dysfunction, bilateral
- **H83.2X9** Labyrinthine dysfunction, unspecified ear

✓5ᵗʰ H83.3 Noise effects on inner ear

Acoustic trauma of inner ear
Noise-induced hearing loss of inner ear

✓6ᵗʰ H83.3X Noise effects on inner ear

- **H83.3X1** Noise effects on right inner ear
- **H83.3X2** Noise effects on left inner ear
- **H83.3X3** Noise effects on inner ear, bilateral

✔ Additional Character Required   ✓7ᵗʰ Placeholder Alert   Manifestation   Unspecified Dx   ►◄ Revised Text   ● New Code   ▲ Revised Code Title

H83.3X9 Noise effects on inner ear, unspecified ear

H83.8 Other specified diseases of inner ear

☑6th H83.8X Other specified diseases of inner ear

H83.8X1 Other specified diseases of right inner ear
H83.8X2 Other specified diseases of left inner ear
H83.8X3 Other specified diseases of inner ear, bilateral
H83.8X9 Other specified diseases of inner ear, unspecified ear

☑5th H83.9 Unspecified disease of inner ear

H83.90 Unspecified disease of inner ear, unspecified ear
H83.91 Unspecified disease of right inner ear
H83.92 Unspecified disease of left inner ear
H83.93 Unspecified disease of inner ear, bilateral

Other disorders of ear (H90-H94)

☑4th H90 Conductive and sensorineural hearing loss

EXCLUDES 1 deaf nonspeaking NEC (H91.3)
deafness NOS (H91.9-)
hearing loss NOS (H91.9-)
noise-induced hearing loss (H83.3-)
ototoxic hearing loss (H91.0-)
sudden (idiopathic) hearing loss (H91.2-)

AHA: 2015,2Q,7
DEF: Conductive hearing loss: Hearing Loss due to the inability of sound waves to move from the outer (external ear) to the inner ear.
DEF: Sensorineural hearing loss: Hearing Loss that occurs from damage to the hair cells of the inner ear or problems with the nerve pathways from the inner ear to the brain.

H90.0 Conductive hearing loss, bilateral

☑5th H90.1 Conductive hearing loss, unilateral with unrestricted hearing on the contralateral side

H90.11 Conductive hearing loss, unilateral, right ear, with unrestricted hearing on the contralateral side
H90.12 Conductive hearing loss, unilateral, left ear, with unrestricted hearing on the contralateral side

H90.2 Conductive hearing loss, unspecified
Conductive deafness NOS

H90.3 Sensorineural hearing loss, bilateral

☑5th H90.4 Sensorineural hearing loss, unilateral with unrestricted hearing on the contralateral side

H90.41 Sensorineural hearing loss, unilateral, right ear, with unrestricted hearing on the contralateral side
H90.42 Sensorineural hearing loss, unilateral, left ear, with unrestricted hearing on the contralateral side

H90.5 Unspecified sensorineural hearing loss
Central hearing loss NOS
Congenital deafness NOS
Neural hearing loss NOS
Perceptive hearing loss NOS
Sensorineural deafness NOS
Sensory hearing loss NOS

EXCLUDES 1 abnormal auditory perception (H93.2-)
psychogenic deafness (F44.6)

H90.6 Mixed conductive and sensorineural hearing loss, bilateral
AHA: 2015,2Q,7

☑5th H90.7 Mixed conductive and sensorineural hearing loss, unilateral with unrestricted hearing on the contralateral side

H90.71 Mixed conductive and sensorineural hearing loss, unilateral, right ear, with unrestricted hearing on the contralateral side
H90.72 Mixed conductive and sensorineural hearing loss, unilateral, left ear, with unrestricted hearing on the contralateral side

H90.8 Mixed conductive and sensorineural hearing loss, unspecified

☑5th H90.A Conductive and sensorineural hearing loss with restricted hearing on the contralateral side
AHA: 2016,4Q,23-25

☑6th H90.A1 Conductive hearing loss, unilateral, with restricted hearing on the contralateral side

H90.A11 Conductive hearing loss, unilateral, right ear with restricted hearing on the contralateral side
H90.A12 Conductive hearing loss, unilateral, left ear with restricted hearing on the contralateral side

☑6th H90.A2 Sensorineural hearing loss, unilateral, with restricted hearing on the contralateral side

H90.A21 Sensorineural hearing loss, unilateral, right ear, with restricted hearing on the contralateral side
H90.A22 Sensorineural hearing loss, unilateral, left ear, with restricted hearing on the contralateral side

☑6th H90.A3 Mixed conductive and sensorineural hearing loss, unilateral with restricted hearing on the contralateral side

H90.A31 Mixed conductive and sensorineural hearing loss, unilateral, right ear with restricted hearing on the contralateral side
H90.A32 Mixed conductive and sensorineural hearing, unilateral, left ear with restricted hearing on the contralateral side

☑4th H91 Other and unspecified hearing loss

EXCLUDES 1 abnormal auditory perception (H93.2-)
hearing loss as classified in H90.-
impacted cerumen (H61.2-)
noise-induced hearing loss (H83.3-)
psychogenic deafness (F44.6)
transient ischemic deafness (H93.01-)

☑5th H91.0 Ototoxic hearing loss
Code first poisoning due to drug or toxin, if applicable (T36-T65 with fifth or sixth character 1-4 or 6)
Use additional code for adverse effect, if applicable, to identify drug (T36-T50 with fifth or sixth character 5)

H91.01 Ototoxic hearing loss, right ear
H91.02 Ototoxic hearing loss, left ear
H91.03 Ototoxic hearing loss, bilateral
H91.09 Ototoxic hearing loss, unspecified ear

☑5th H91.1 Presbycusis
Presbyacusia

H91.10 Presbycusis, unspecified ear
H91.11 Presbycusis, right ear
H91.12 Presbycusis, left ear
H91.13 Presbycusis, bilateral

☑5th H91.2 Sudden idiopathic hearing loss
Sudden hearing loss NOS

H91.20 Sudden idiopathic hearing loss, unspecified ear
H91.21 Sudden idiopathic hearing loss, right ear
H91.22 Sudden idiopathic hearing loss, left ear
H91.23 Sudden idiopathic hearing loss, bilateral

H91.3 Deaf nonspeaking, not elsewhere classified

☑5th H91.8 Other specified hearing loss

☑6th H91.8X Other specified hearing loss

H91.8X1 Other specified hearing loss, right ear
H91.8X2 Other specified hearing loss, left ear
H91.8X3 Other specified hearing loss, bilateral
H91.8X9 Other specified hearing loss, unspecified ear

☑5th H91.9 Unspecified hearing loss
Deafness NOS
High frequency deafness
Low frequency deafness

H91.90 Unspecified hearing loss, unspecified ear
H91.91 Unspecified hearing loss, right ear
H91.92 Unspecified hearing loss, left ear
H91.93 Unspecified hearing loss, bilateral

☑4th H92 Otalgia and effusion of ear

☑5th H92.0 Otalgia

H92.01 Otalgia, right ear
H92.02 Otalgia, left ear
H92.03 Otalgia, bilateral
H92.09 Otalgia, unspecified ear

☑5th H92.1 Otorrhea

EXCLUDES 1 leakage of cerebrospinal fluid through ear (G96.0)

H92.10 Otorrhea, unspecified ear
H92.11 Otorrhea, right ear
H92.12 Otorrhea, left ear
H92.13 Otorrhea, bilateral

✓5ᵗʰ **H92.2** **Otorrhagia**

> EXCLUDES 1   *traumatic otorrhagia — code to injury*

     H92.20   **Otorrhagia, unspecified ear**

     H92.21   **Otorrhagia, right ear**

     H92.22   **Otorrhagia, left ear**

     H92.23   **Otorrhagia, bilateral**

✓4ᵗʰ **H93** **Other disorders of ear, not elsewhere classified**

✓5ᵗʰ   **H93.0**   **Degenerative and vascular disorders of ear**

> EXCLUDES 1   *presbycusis (H91.1)*

✓6ᵗʰ   **H93.01**   **Transient ischemic deafness**

       H93.011   **Transient ischemic deafness, right ear**

       H93.012   **Transient ischemic deafness, left ear**

       H93.013   **Transient ischemic deafness, bilateral**

       H93.019   **Transient ischemic deafness, unspecified ear**

✓6ᵗʰ   **H93.09**   **Unspecified degenerative and vascular disorders of ear**

       H93.091   **Unspecified degenerative and vascular disorders of right ear**

       H93.092   **Unspecified degenerative and vascular disorders of left ear**

       H93.093   **Unspecified degenerative and vascular disorders of ear, bilateral**

       H93.099   **Unspecified degenerative and vascular disorders of unspecified ear**

✓5ᵗʰ   **H93.1**   **Tinnitus**

     H93.11   **Tinnitus, right ear**

     H93.12   **Tinnitus, left ear**

     H93.13   **Tinnitus, bilateral**

     H93.19   **Tinnitus, unspecified ear**

✓5ᵗʰ   **H93.A**   **Pulsatile tinnitus**

     AHA: 2016,4Q,25-26

     H93.A1   **Pulsatile tinnitus, right ear**

     H93.A2   **Pulsatile tinnitus, left ear**

     H93.A3   **Pulsatile tinnitus, bilateral**

     H93.A9   **Pulsatile tinnitus, unspecified ear**

✓5ᵗʰ   **H93.2**   **Other abnormal auditory perceptions**

> EXCLUDES 2   *auditory hallucinations (R44.0)*

✓6ᵗʰ   **H93.21**   **Auditory recruitment**

       H93.211   **Auditory recruitment, right ear**

       H93.212   **Auditory recruitment, left ear**

       H93.213   **Auditory recruitment, bilateral**

       H93.219   **Auditory recruitment, unspecified ear**

✓6ᵗʰ   **H93.22**   **Diplacusis**

       H93.221   **Diplacusis, right ear**

       H93.222   **Diplacusis, left ear**

       H93.223   **Diplacusis, bilateral**

       H93.229   **Diplacusis, unspecified ear**

✓6ᵗʰ   **H93.23**   **Hyperacusis**

> **DEF:** Exceptionally acute sense of hearing caused by such conditions as Bell's palsy. This term may also refer to painful sensitivity to sounds.

       H93.231   **Hyperacusis, right ear**

       H93.232   **Hyperacusis, left ear**

       H93.233   **Hyperacusis, bilateral**

       H93.239   **Hyperacusis, unspecified ear**

✓6ᵗʰ   **H93.24**   **Temporary auditory threshold shift**

       H93.241   **Temporary auditory threshold shift, right ear**

       H93.242   **Temporary auditory threshold shift, left ear**

       H93.243   **Temporary auditory threshold shift, bilateral**

       H93.249   **Temporary auditory threshold shift, unspecified ear**

     H93.25   **Central auditory processing disorder**

       Congenital auditory imperception

       Word deafness

> EXCLUDES 1   *mixed receptive-expressive language disorder (F80.2)*

✓6ᵗʰ   **H93.29**   **Other abnormal auditory perceptions**

       H93.291   **Other abnormal auditory perceptions, right ear**

       H93.292   **Other abnormal auditory perceptions, left ear**

       H93.293   **Other abnormal auditory perceptions, bilateral**

       H93.299   **Other abnormal auditory perceptions, unspecified ear**

✓5ᵗʰ   **H93.3**   **Disorders of acoustic nerve**

     Disorder of 8th cranial nerve

> EXCLUDES 1   *acoustic neuroma (D33.3)*
>   *syphilitic acoustic neuritis (A52.15)*

✓6ᵗʰ   **H93.3X**   **Disorders of acoustic nerve**

       H93.3X1   **Disorders of right acoustic nerve**

       H93.3X2   **Disorders of left acoustic nerve**

       H93.3X3   **Disorders of bilateral acoustic nerves**

       H93.3X9   **Disorders of unspecified acoustic nerve**

✓5ᵗʰ   **H93.8**   **Other specified disorders of ear**

✓6ᵗʰ   **H93.8X**   **Other specified disorders of ear**

       H93.8X1   **Other specified disorders of right ear**

       H93.8X2   **Other specified disorders of left ear**

       H93.8X3   **Other specified disorders of ear, bilateral**

       H93.8X9   **Other specified disorders of ear, unspecified ear**

✓5ᵗʰ   **H93.9**   **Unspecified disorder of ear**

     H93.90   **Unspecified disorder of ear, unspecified ear**

     H93.91   **Unspecified disorder of right ear**

     H93.92   **Unspecified disorder of left ear**

     H93.93   **Unspecified disorder of ear, bilateral**

✓4ᵗʰ **H94** **Other disorders of ear in diseases classified elsewhere**

✓5ᵗʰ   **H94.0**   **Acoustic neuritis in infectious and parasitic diseases classified elsewhere**

     Code first underlying disease, such as:

       parasitic disease (B65-B89)

> EXCLUDES 1   *acoustic neuritis (in):*
>   *herpes zoster (B02.29)*
>   *syphilis (A52.15)*

     H94.00   *Acoustic neuritis in infectious and parasitic diseases classified elsewhere, unspecified ear*

     H94.01   *Acoustic neuritis in infectious and parasitic diseases classified elsewhere, right ear*

     H94.02   *Acoustic neuritis in infectious and parasitic diseases classified elsewhere, left ear*

     H94.03   *Acoustic neuritis in infectious and parasitic diseases classified elsewhere, bilateral*

✓5ᵗʰ   **H94.8**   **Other specified disorders of ear in diseases classified elsewhere**

     Code first underlying disease, such as:

       congenital syphilis (A50.0)

> EXCLUDES 1   *aural myiasis (B87.4)*
>   *syphilitic labyrinthitis (A52.79)*

     H94.80   *Other specified disorders of ear in diseases classified elsewhere, unspecified ear*

     H94.81   *Other specified disorders of right ear in diseases classified elsewhere*

     H94.82   *Other specified disorders of left ear in diseases classified elsewhere*

     H94.83   *Other specified disorders of ear in diseases classified elsewhere, bilateral*

Intraoperative and postprocedural complications and disorders of ear and mastoid process, not elsewhere classified (H95)

✓4ᵗʰ **H95** **Intraoperative and postprocedural complications and disorders of ear and mastoid process, not elsewhere classified**

     AHA: 2016,4Q,9-10

✓5ᵗʰ   **H95.0**   **Recurrent cholesteatoma of postmastoidectomy cavity**

     H95.00   **Recurrent cholesteatoma of postmastoidectomy cavity, unspecified ear**

     H95.01   **Recurrent cholesteatoma of postmastoidectomy cavity, right ear**

     H95.02   **Recurrent cholesteatoma of postmastoidectomy cavity, left ear**

     H95.03   **Recurrent cholesteatoma of postmastoidectomy cavity, bilateral ears**

✓5ᵗʰ   **H95.1**   **Other disorders of ear and mastoid process following mastoidectomy**

✓6ᵗʰ   **H95.11**   **Chronic inflammation of postmastoidectomy cavity**

       H95.111   **Chronic inflammation of postmastoidectomy cavity, right ear**

       H95.112   **Chronic inflammation of postmastoidectomy cavity, left ear**

✓ Additional Character Required   ✓x7ᵗʰ Placeholder Alert   Manifestation   Unspecified Dx   ▶◀ Revised Text   ● New Code   ▲ Revised Code Title

ICD-10-CM 2020   631

Chapter 8. Diseases of the Ear and Mastoid Process

H95.113   **Chronic inflammation of postmastoidectomy cavity, bilateral ears**

H95.119   **Chronic inflammation of postmastoidectomy cavity, unspecified ear**

✓6ᵗʰ   **H95.12**   **Granulation of postmastoidectomy cavity**

    H95.121   **Granulation of postmastoidectomy cavity, right ear**

    H95.122   **Granulation of postmastoidectomy cavity, left ear**

    H95.123   **Granulation of postmastoidectomy cavity, bilateral ears**

    H95.129   **Granulation of postmastoidectomy cavity, unspecified ear**

✓6ᵗʰ   **H95.13**   **Mucosal cyst of postmastoidectomy cavity**

    H95.131   **Mucosal cyst of postmastoidectomy cavity, right ear**

    H95.132   **Mucosal cyst of postmastoidectomy cavity, left ear**

    H95.133   **Mucosal cyst of postmastoidectomy cavity, bilateral ears**

    H95.139   **Mucosal cyst of postmastoidectomy cavity, unspecified ear**

✓6ᵗʰ   **H95.19**   **Other disorders following mastoidectomy**

    H95.191   **Other disorders following mastoidectomy, right ear**

    H95.192   **Other disorders following mastoidectomy, left ear**

    H95.193   **Other disorders following mastoidectomy, bilateral ears**

    H95.199   **Other disorders following mastoidectomy, unspecified ear**

✓5ᵗʰ   **H95.2**   **Intraoperative hemorrhage and hematoma of ear and mastoid process complicating a procedure**

> **EXCLUDES 1**   *intraoperative hemorrhage and hematoma of ear and mastoid process due to accidental puncture or laceration during a procedure (H95.3-)*

    H95.21   **Intraoperative hemorrhage and hematoma of ear and mastoid process complicating a procedure on the ear and mastoid process**

    H95.22   **Intraoperative hemorrhage and hematoma of ear and mastoid process complicating other procedure**

✓5ᵗʰ   **H95.3**   **Accidental puncture and laceration of ear and mastoid process during a procedure**

    H95.31   **Accidental puncture and laceration of the ear and mastoid process during a procedure on the ear and mastoid process**

    H95.32   **Accidental puncture and laceration of the ear and mastoid process during other procedure**

✓5ᵗʰ   **H95.4**   **Postprocedural hemorrhage of ear and mastoid process following a procedure**

    H95.41   **Postprocedural hemorrhage of ear and mastoid process following a procedure on the ear and mastoid process**

    H95.42   **Postprocedural hemorrhage of ear and mastoid process following other procedure**

✓5ᵗʰ   **H95.5**   **Postprocedural hematoma and seroma of ear and mastoid process following a procedure**

    H95.51   **Postprocedural hematoma of ear and mastoid process following a procedure on the ear and mastoid process**

    H95.52   **Postprocedural hematoma of ear and mastoid process following other procedure**

    H95.53   **Postprocedural seroma of ear and mastoid process following a procedure on the ear and mastoid process**

    H95.54   **Postprocedural seroma of ear and mastoid process following other procedure**

✓5ᵗʰ   **H95.8**   **Other intraoperative and postprocedural complications and disorders of the ear and mastoid process, not elsewhere classified**

> **EXCLUDES 2**   *postprocedural complications and disorders following mastoidectomy (H95.0-, H95.1-)*

✓6ᵗʰ   **H95.81**   **Postprocedural stenosis of external ear canal**

    H95.811   **Postprocedural stenosis of right external ear canal**

    H95.812   **Postprocedural stenosis of left external ear canal**

    H95.813   **Postprocedural stenosis of external ear canal, bilateral**

    H95.819   **Postprocedural stenosis of unspecified external ear canal**

H95.88   **Other intraoperative complications and disorders of the ear and mastoid process, not elsewhere classified**

> Use additional code, if applicable, to further specify disorder

H95.89   **Other postprocedural complications and disorders of the ear and mastoid process, not elsewhere classified**

> Use additional code, if applicable, to further specify disorder

Chapter 9. Diseases of the Circulatory System (I00–I99)

Chapter-specific Guidelines with Coding Examples

The chapter-specific guidelines from the ICD-10-CM Official Guidelines for Coding and Reporting have been provided below. Along with these guidelines are coding examples, contained in the shaded boxes, that have been developed to help illustrate the coding and/or sequencing guidance found in these guidelines.

a. Hypertension

The classification presumes a causal relationship between hypertension and heart involvement and between hypertension and kidney involvement, as the two conditions are linked by the term "with" in the Alphabetic Index. These conditions should be coded as related even in the absence of provider documentation explicitly linking them, unless the documentation clearly states the conditions are unrelated.

For hypertension and conditions not specifically linked by relational terms such as "with," "associated with" or "due to" in the classification, provider documentation must link the conditions in order to code them as related.

1) Hypertension with heart disease

Hypertension with heart conditions classified to I50.- or I51.4-I51.7, I51.89, I51.9, are assigned to a code from category I11, Hypertensive heart disease. Use additional code(s) from category I50, Heart failure, to identify the type(s) of heart failure in those patients with heart failure.

The same heart conditions (I50.-, I51.4-I51.7, I51.89, I51.9) with hypertension are coded separately if the provider has documented they are unrelated to the hypertension. Sequence according to the circumstances of the admission/encounter.

> Patient is treated for left heart failure. Patient also has a history of hypertension managed by medication.
>
> **I11.0**   **Hypertensive heart disease with heart failure**
>
> **I50.1**   **Left ventricular failure, unspecified**
>
> *Explanation*: Without a diagnostic statement to the contrary, hypertension and heart failure have an assumed causal relationship, and a combination code should be used. An additional code to identify the type of heart failure (I50.-) should also be provided.

2) Hypertensive chronic kidney disease

Assign codes from category I12, Hypertensive chronic kidney disease, when both hypertension and a condition classifiable to category N18, Chronic kidney disease (CKD), are present. CKD should not be coded as hypertensive if the provider indicates the CKD is not related to the hypertension.

The appropriate code from category N18 should be used as a secondary code with a code from category I12 to identify the stage of chronic kidney disease.

See Section I.C.14. Chronic kidney disease.

If a patient has hypertensive chronic kidney disease and acute renal failure, an additional code for the acute renal failure is required.

> Patient is admitted with stage IV chronic kidney disease (CKD) due to polycystic kidney disease. Patient also is on lisinopril for hypertension.
>
> **N18.4**   **Chronic kidney disease, stage 4 (severe)**
>
> **Q61.3**   **Polycystic kidney, unspecified**
>
> **I10**   **Essential (primary) hypertension**
>
> *Explanation*: A combination code describing a relationship between hypertension and CKD is not used because the physician documentation identifies the polycystic kidney disease as the cause for the CKD.

3) Hypertensive heart and chronic kidney disease

Assign codes from combination category I13, Hypertensive heart and chronic kidney disease, when there is hypertension with both heart and kidney involvement. If heart failure is present, assign an additional code from category I50 to identify the type of heart failure.

The appropriate code from category N18, Chronic kidney disease, should be used as a secondary code with a code from category I13 to identify the stage of chronic kidney disease.

See Section I.C.14. Chronic kidney disease.

The codes in category I13, Hypertensive heart and chronic kidney disease, are combination codes that include hypertension, heart disease and chronic kidney disease. The Includes note at I13 specifies that the conditions included at I11 and I12 are included together in I13. If a patient has hypertension, heart disease and chronic kidney disease, then a code from I13 should be used, not individual codes for hypertension, heart disease and chronic kidney disease, or codes from I11 or I12.

For patients with both acute renal failure and chronic kidney disease, an additional code for acute renal failure is required.

> Hypertensive heart and kidney disease with congestive heart failure and stage 2 chronic kidney disease
>
> **I13.0**   **Hypertensive heart and chronic kidney disease with heart failure and stage 1 through stage 4 chronic kidney disease, or unspecified chronic kidney disease**
>
> **I50.9**   **Heart failure, unspecified**
>
> **N18.2**   **Chronic kidney disease, stage 2 (mild)**
>
> *Explanation*: Combination codes in category I13 are used to report conditions classifiable to *both* categories I11 and I12. Do not report conditions classifiable to I11 and I12 separately. Use additional codes to report type of heart failure and stage of CKD.

4) Hypertensive cerebrovascular disease

For hypertensive cerebrovascular disease, first assign the appropriate code from categories I60-I69, followed by the appropriate hypertension code.

> Rupture of cerebral aneurysm caused by malignant hypertension
>
> **I60.7**   **Nontraumatic subarachnoid hemorrhage from unspecified introcranial artery**
>
> **I10**   **Essential (primary) hypertension**
>
> *Explanation*: Hypertensive cerebrovascular disease requires two codes: the appropriate I60–I69 code followed by the appropriate hypertension code.

5) Hypertensive retinopathy

Subcategory H35.0, Background retinopathy and retinal vascular changes, should be used with a code from category I10 – I15, Hypertensive disease to include the systemic hypertension. The sequencing is based on the reason for the encounter.

6) Hypertension, secondary

Secondary hypertension is due to an underlying condition. Two codes are required: one to identify the underlying etiology and one from category I15 to identify the hypertension. Sequencing of codes is determined by the reason for admission/encounter.

> Renovascular hypertension due to renal artery atherosclerosis
>
> **I15.0**   **Renovascular hypertension**
>
> **I70.1**   **Atherosclerosis of renal artery**
>
> *Explanation*: Secondary hypertension requires two codes: a code to identify the etiology and the appropriate I15 code.

7) Hypertension, transient

Assign code R03.0, Elevated blood pressure reading without diagnosis of hypertension, unless patient has an established diagnosis of hypertension. Assign code O13.-, Gestational [pregnancy-induced] hypertension without significant proteinuria, or O14.-, Pre-eclampsia, for transient hypertension of pregnancy.

8) Hypertension, controlled

This diagnostic statement usually refers to an existing state of hypertension under control by therapy. Assign the appropriate code from categories I10-I15, Hypertensive diseases.

9) Hypertension, uncontrolled

Uncontrolled hypertension may refer to untreated hypertension or hypertension not responding to current therapeutic regimen. In either case, assign the appropriate code from categories I10-I15, Hypertensive diseases.

10) Hypertensive crisis

Assign a code from category I16, Hypertensive crisis, for documented hypertensive urgency, hypertensive emergency or unspecified hypertensive crisis. Code also any identified hypertensive disease (I10-I15). The sequencing is based on the reason for the encounter.

11) Pulmonary hypertension

Pulmonary hypertension is classified to category I27, Other pulmonary heart diseases. For secondary pulmonary hypertension (I27.1, I27.2-), code also any associated conditions or adverse effects of drugs or toxins. The sequencing is based on the reason for the encounter, except for adverse effects of drugs (See Section I.C.19.e.).

sclerotic coronary artery disease and angina

D-10-CM has combination codes for atherosclerotic heart disease with angina pectoris. The subcategories for these codes are I25.11, Atherosclerotic heart disease of native coronary artery with angina pectoris and I25.7, Atherosclerosis of coronary artery bypass graft(s) and coronary artery of transplanted heart with angina pectoris.

When using one of these combination codes it is not necessary to use an additional code for angina pectoris. A causal relationship can be assumed in a patient with both atherosclerosis and angina pectoris, unless the documentation indicates the angina is due to something other than the atherosclerosis.

If a patient with coronary artery disease is admitted due to an acute myocardial infarction (AMI), the AMI should be sequenced before the coronary artery disease.

See Section I.C.9. Acute myocardial infarction (AMI)

> Patient is being seen for spastic angina pectoris. She also has a documented history of progressive coronary artery disease of the native vessels.
>
> **I25.111**   **Atherosclerotic heart disease of native coronary artery with angina pectoris with documented spasm**
>
> *Explanation*: Report the combination code for atherosclerotic heart disease (coronary artery disease) with angina pectoris. A causal relationship is assumed in a patient with both atherosclerosis and angina pectoris, unless the documentation indicates the angina is due to something other than the atherosclerosis. When using one of these combination codes, it is not necessary to use an additional code for angina pectoris.

c. Intraoperative and postprocedural cerebrovascular accident

Medical record documentation should clearly specify the cause- and- effect relationship between the medical intervention and the cerebrovascular accident in order to assign a code for intraoperative or postprocedural cerebrovascular accident.

Proper code assignment depends on whether it was an infarction or hemorrhage and whether it occurred intraoperatively or postoperatively. If it was a cerebral hemorrhage, code assignment depends on the type of procedure performed.

> Embolic cerebral infarction of the right middle cerebral artery that occurred during hip replacement surgery. The surgeon documented as due to the surgery.
>
> **I97.811**   **Intraoperative cerebrovascular infarction during other surgery**
>
> **I63.411**   **Cerebral infarction due to embolism of right middle cerebral artery**
>
> *Explanation*: Code assignment for intraoperative or postprocedural cerebrovascular accident is based on the provider's documentation of a cause-and-effect relationship between the condition and the procedure. Proper code assignment also depends on whether the cerebrovascular accident was an infarction or hemorrhage, occurred intraoperatively or postoperatively, and the type of procedure performed.

d. Sequelae of cerebrovascular disease

1) Category I69, Sequelae of cerebrovascular disease

Category I69 is used to indicate conditions classifiable to categories I60-I67 as the causes of sequela (neurologic deficits), themselves classified elsewhere. These "late effects" include neurologic deficits that persist after initial onset of conditions classifiable to categories I60-I67. The neurologic deficits caused by cerebrovascular disease may be present from the onset or may arise at any time after the onset of the condition classifiable to categories I60-I67.

Codes from category I69, Sequelae of cerebrovascular disease, that specify hemiplegia, hemiparesis and monoplegia identify whether the dominant or nondominant side is affected. Should the affected side be documented, but not specified as dominant or nondominant, and the classification system does not indicate a default, code selection is as follows:

- For ambidextrous patients, the default should be dominant.
- If the left side is affected, the default is non-dominant.
- If the right side is affected, the default is dominant.

2) Codes from category I69 with codes from I60–I67

Codes from category I69 may be assigned on a health care record with codes from I60-I67, if the patient has a current cerebrovascular disease and deficits from an old cerebrovascular disease.

3) Codes from category I69 and personal history of transient ischemic attack (TIA) and cerebral infarction (Z86.73)

Codes from category I69 should not be assigned if the patient does not have neurologic deficits.

See Section I.C.21. 4. History (of) for use of personal history codes

e. Acute myocardial infarction (AMI)

1) Type 1 ST elevation myocardial infarction (STEMI) and non-ST elevation myocardial infarction (NSTEMI)

The ICD-10-CM codes for type 1 acute myocardial infarction (AMI) identify the site, such as anterolateral wall or true posterior wall. Subcategories I21.0-I21.2 and code I21.3 are used for type 1 ST elevation myocardial infarction (STEMI). Code I21.4, Non-ST elevation (NSTEMI) myocardial infarction, is used for type 1 non ST elevation myocardial infarction (NSTEMI) and nontransmural MIs.

If a type 1 NSTEMI evolves to STEMI, assign the STEMI code. If a type 1 STEMI converts to NSTEMI due to thrombolytic therapy, it is still coded as STEMI.

For encounters occurring while the myocardial infarction is equal to, or less than, four weeks old, including transfers to another acute setting or a postacute setting, and the myocardial infarction meets the definition for "other diagnoses" (see Section III, Reporting Additional Diagnoses), codes from category I21 may continue to be reported. For encounters after the 4 week time frame and the patient is still receiving care related to the myocardial infarction, the appropriate aftercare code should be assigned, rather than a code from category I21. For old or healed myocardial infarctions not requiring further care, code I25.2, Old myocardial infarction, may be assigned.

2) Acute myocardial infarction, unspecified

Code I21.9, Acute myocardial infarction, unspecified, is the default for unspecified acute myocardial infarction or unspecified type. If only type 1 STEMI or transmural MI without the site is documented, assign code I21.3, ST elevation (STEMI) myocardial infarction of unspecified site.

3) AMI documented as nontransmural or subendocardial but site provided

If an AMI is documented as nontransmural or subendocardial, but the site is provided, it is still coded as a subendocardial AMI.

See Section I.C.21.3 for information on coding status post administration of tPA in a different facility within the last 24 hours.

> Acute inferior subendocardial myocardial infarction (NSTEMI)
>
> **I21.4**   **Non-ST elevation (NSTEMI) myocardial infarction**
>
> *Explanation*: An AMI documented as subendocardial or nontransmural is coded as such (I21.4, I22.2), even if the site of infarction is specified.

4) Subsequent acute myocardial infarction

A code from category I22, Subsequent ST elevation (STEMI) and non-ST elevation (NSTEMI) myocardial infarction, is to be used when a patient who has suffered a type 1 or unspecified AMI has a new AMI within the 4 week time frame of the initial AMI. A code from category I22 must be used in conjunction with a code from category I21. The sequencing of the I22 and I21 codes depends on the circumstances of the encounter.
Do not assign code I22 for subsequent myocardial infarctions other than type 1 or unspecified. For subsequent type 2 AMI assign only code I21.A1. For subsequent type 4 or type 5 AMI, assign only code I21.A9. If a subsequent myocardial infarction of one type occurs within 4 weeks of a myocardial infarction of a different type, assign the appropriate codes from category I21 to identify each type. Do not assign a code from I22. Codes from category I22 should only be assigned if both the initial and subsequent myocardial infarctions are type 1 or unspecified.

5) Other Types of Myocardial Infarction

The ICD-10-CM provides codes for different types of myocardial infarction. Type 1 myocardial infarctions are assigned to codes I21.0-I21.4.
Type 2 myocardial infarction (myocardial infarction due to demand ischemia or secondary to ischemic **im**balance) is assigned to code I21.A1, Myocardial infarction type 2 with the underlying cause **coded first**. Do not assign code I24.8, Other forms of acute ischemic heart disease, for the demand ischemia. **If** a type 2 AMI is described as NSTEMI or STEMI, only assign code I21.A1. Codes I21.01-I21.4 should only be assigned for type 1 AMIs.

Acute myocardial infarctions type 3, 4a, 4b, 4c and 5 are assigned to code I21.A9, Other myocardial infarction type.

The "Code also" and "Code first" notes should be followed related to complications, and for coding of postprocedural myocardial infarctions during or following cardiac surgery.

Chapter 9. Diseases of the Circulatory System (I00-I99)

EXCLUDES 2   *certain conditions originating in the perinatal period (P04-P96)*
certain infectious and parasitic diseases (A00-B99)
complications of pregnancy, childbirth and the puerperium (O00-O9A)
congenital malformations, deformations, and chromosomal abnormalities (Q00-Q99)
endocrine, nutritional and metabolic diseases (E00-E88)
injury, poisoning and certain other consequences of external causes (S00-T88)
neoplasms (C00-D49)
symptoms, signs and abnormal clinical and laboratory findings, not elsewhere classified (R00-R94)
systemic connective tissue disorders (M30-M36)
transient cerebral ischemic attacks and related syndromes (G45.-)

This chapter contains the following blocks:

I00-I02	Acute rheumatic fever
I05-I09	Chronic rheumatic heart diseases
I10-I16	Hypertensive diseases
I20-I25	Ischemic heart diseases
I26-I28	Pulmonary heart disease and diseases of pulmonary circulation
I30-I52	Other forms of heart disease
I60-I69	Cerebrovascular diseases
I70-I79	Diseases of arteries, arterioles and capillaries
I80-I89	Diseases of veins, lymphatic vessels and lymph nodes, not elsewhere classified
I95-I99	Other and unspecified disorders of the circulatory system

Acute rheumatic fever (I00-I02)

DEF: Inflammatory disease that can follow a throat infection by group A streptococci. Complications can involve the joints (arthritis), subcutaneous tissue (nodules), skin (erythema marginatum), heart (carditis), or brain (chorea).

I00   **Rheumatic fever without heart involvement**
    INCLUDES   arthritis, rheumatic, acute or subacute
    EXCLUDES 1   *rheumatic fever with heart involvement (I01.0-I01.9)*

√4ᵗʰ **I01**   **Rheumatic fever with heart involvement**
    EXCLUDES 1   *chronic diseases of rheumatic origin (I05-I09) unless rheumatic fever is also present or there is evidence of reactivation or activity of the rheumatic process*

    I01.0   **Acute rheumatic pericarditis**
      Any condition in I00 with pericarditis
      Rheumatic pericarditis (acute)
      EXCLUDES 1   *acute pericarditis not specified as rheumatic (I30.-)*

    I01.1   **Acute rheumatic endocarditis**
      Any condition in I00 with endocarditis or valvulitis
      Acute rheumatic valvulitis

    I01.2   **Acute rheumatic myocarditis**
      Any condition in I00 with myocarditis

    I01.8   **Other acute rheumatic heart disease**
      Any condition in I00 with other or multiple types of heart involvement
      Acute rheumatic pancarditis

    I01.9   **Acute rheumatic heart disease, unspecified**
      Any condition in I00 with unspecified type of heart involvement
      Rheumatic carditis, acute
      Rheumatic heart disease, active or acute

√4ᵗʰ **I02**   **Rheumatic chorea**
    INCLUDES   Sydenham's chorea
    EXCLUDES 1   *chorea NOS (G25.5)*
             Huntington's chorea (G10)

    I02.0   **Rheumatic chorea with heart involvement**
      Chorea NOS with heart involvement
      Rheumatic chorea with heart involvement of any type classifiable under I01.-

    I02.9   **Rheumatic chorea without heart involvement**
      Rheumatic chorea NOS

Chronic rheumatic heart diseases (I05-I09)

√4ᵗʰ **I05**   **Rheumatic mitral valve diseases**
    INCLUDES   conditions classifiable to both I05.0 and I05.2-I05.9, whether specified as rheumatic or not
    EXCLUDES 1   *mitral valve disease specified as nonrheumatic (I34.-)*
             mitral valve disease with aortic and/or tricuspid valve involvement (I08.-)

    I05.0   **Rheumatic mitral stenosis**
      Mitral (valve) obstruction (rheumatic)
      DEF: Narrowing of the mitral valve between the left atrium and left ventricle due to rheumatic fever. Symptoms include shortness of breath during or after exercise, fatigue, palpitations, chest discomfort, and swelling of feet or legs.

    I05.1   **Rheumatic mitral insufficiency**
      Rheumatic mitral incompetence
      Rheumatic mitral regurgitation
      EXCLUDES 1   *mitral insufficiency not specified as rheumatic (I34.0)*

    I05.2   **Rheumatic mitral stenosis with insufficiency**
      Rheumatic mitral stenosis with incompetence or regurgitation

    I05.8   **Other rheumatic mitral valve diseases**
      Rheumatic mitral (valve) failure

    I05.9   **Rheumatic mitral valve disease, unspecified**
      Rheumatic mitral (valve) disorder (chronic) NOS

√4ᵗʰ **I06**   **Rheumatic aortic valve diseases**
    EXCLUDES 1   *aortic valve disease not specified as rheumatic (I35.-)*
             aortic valve disease with mitral and/or tricuspid valve involvement (I08.-)

    I06.0   **Rheumatic aortic stenosis**
      Rheumatic aortic (valve) obstruction

    I06.1   **Rheumatic aortic insufficiency**
      Rheumatic aortic incompetence
      Rheumatic aortic regurgitation

    I06.2   **Rheumatic aortic stenosis with insufficiency**
      Rheumatic aortic stenosis with incompetence or regurgitation

    I06.8   **Other rheumatic aortic valve diseases**

    I06.9   **Rheumatic aortic valve disease, unspecified**
      Rheumatic aortic (valve) disease NOS

√4ᵗʰ **I07**   **Rheumatic tricuspid valve diseases**
    INCLUDES   rheumatic tricuspid valve diseases specified as rheumatic or unspecified
    EXCLUDES 1   *tricuspid valve disease specified as nonrheumatic (I36.-)*
             tricuspid valve disease with aortic and/or mitral valve involvement (I08.-)

    I07.0   **Rheumatic tricuspid stenosis**
      Tricuspid (valve) stenosis (rheumatic)

    I07.1   **Rheumatic tricuspid insufficiency**
      Tricuspid (valve) insufficiency (rheumatic)

    I07.2   **Rheumatic tricuspid stenosis and insufficiency**

    I07.8   **Other rheumatic tricuspid valve diseases**

    I07.9   **Rheumatic tricuspid valve disease, unspecified**
      Rheumatic tricuspid valve disorder NOS

√4ᵗʰ **I08**   **Multiple valve diseases**
    INCLUDES   multiple valve diseases specified as rheumatic or unspecified
    EXCLUDES 1   *endocarditis, valve unspecified (I38)*
             multiple valve disease specified a nonrheumatic (I34.-, I35.-, I36.-, I37.-, I38.-, Q22.-, Q23.-, Q24.8-)
             rheumatic valve disease NOS (I09.1)

    I08.0   **Rheumatic disorders of both mitral and aortic valves**
      Involvement of both mitral and aortic valves specified as rheumatic or unspecified
      AHA: 2019,2Q,5

    I08.1   **Rheumatic disorders of both mitral and tricuspid valves**

    I08.2   **Rheumatic disorders of both aortic and tricuspid valves**

    I08.3   **Combined rheumatic disorders of mitral, aortic and tricuspid valves**

    I08.8   **Other rheumatic multiple valve diseases**

    I08.9   **Rheumatic multiple valve disease, unspecified**

√4ᵗʰ **I09**   **Other rheumatic heart diseases**

    I09.0   **Rheumatic myocarditis**
      EXCLUDES 1   *myocarditis not specified as rheumatic (I51.4)*

☑ Additional Character Required   √x7ᵗʰ Placeholder Alert   Manifestation   Unspecified Dx   ▶◀ Revised Text   ● New Code   ▲ Revised Code Title

ICD-10-CM 2020   **635**

I09.1 **Rheumatic diseases of endocardium, valve unspecified**
Rheumatic endocarditis (chronic)
Rheumatic valvulitis (chronic)
EXCLUDES 1 endocarditis, valve unspecified (I38)

I09.2 **Chronic rheumatic pericarditis**
Adherent pericardium, rheumatic
Chronic rheumatic mediastinopericarditis
Chronic rheumatic myopericarditis
EXCLUDES 1 chronic pericarditis not specified as rheumatic (I31.-)

✓5ᵗʰ **I09.8** **Other specified rheumatic heart diseases**

I09.81 **Rheumatic heart failure** HCC
Use additional code to identify type of heart failure (I50.-)
DEF: Decreased cardiac output, edema, and hypertension due to rheumatic heart disease.

I09.89 **Other specified rheumatic heart diseases**
Rheumatic disease of pulmonary valve

I09.9 **Rheumatic heart disease, unspecified**
Rheumatic carditis
EXCLUDES 1 rheumatoid carditis (M05.31)

Hypertensive diseases (I10-I16)

Use additional code to identify:
exposure to environmental tobacco smoke (Z77.22)
history of tobacco dependence (Z87.891)
occupational exposure to environmental tobacco smoke (Z57.31)
tobacco dependence (F17.-)
tobacco use (Z72.0)
EXCLUDES 1 neonatal hypertension (P29.2)
primary pulmonary hypertension (I27.0)
EXCLUDES 2 hypertensive disease complicating pregnancy, childbirth and the puerperium (O10-O11, O13-O16)

I10 **Essential (primary) hypertension** Q
INCLUDES high blood pressure
hypertension (arterial) (benign) (essential) (malignant) (primary) (systemic)
EXCLUDES 1 hypertensive disease complicating pregnancy, childbirth and the puerperium (O10-O11, O13-O16)
EXCLUDES 2 essential (primary) hypertension involving vessels of brain (I60-I69)
essential (primary) hypertension involving vessels of eye (H35.0-)
AHA: 2018,2Q,9; 2016,4Q,27

✓4ᵗʰ **I11** **Hypertensive heart disease**
INCLUDES any condition in I50.-, I51.4-I51.9 due to hypertension
AHA: 2018,2Q,9
TIP: Do not assign a code from this category when provider documentation indicates the heart disease is attributable to another cause.

I11.0 **Hypertensive heart disease with heart failure** HCC
Hypertensive heart failure
Use additional code to identify type of heart failure (I50.-)
AHA: 2017,1Q,47

I11.9 **Hypertensive heart disease without heart failure**
Hypertensive heart disease NOS

✓4ᵗʰ **I12** **Hypertensive chronic kidney disease**
INCLUDES any condition in N18 and N26 — due to hypertension
arteriosclerosis of kidney
arteriosclerotic nephritis (chronic) (interstitial)
hypertensive nephropathy
nephrosclerosis
EXCLUDES 1 hypertension due to kidney disease (I15.0, I15.1)
renovascular hypertension (I15.0)
secondary hypertension (I15.-)
EXCLUDES 2 acute kidney failure (N17.-)
AHA: 2018,4Q,88; 2016,3Q,22
TIP: Do not assign a code from this category when provider documentation indicates the chronic kidney disease (CKD) is attributable to another cause.

I12.0 **Hypertensive chronic kidney disease with stage 5 chronic kidney disease or end stage renal disease** HCC
Use additional code to identify the stage of chronic kidney disease (N18.5, N18.6)

I12.9 **Hypertensive chronic kidney disease with stage 1 through stage 4 chronic kidney disease, or unspecified chronic kidney disease**
Hypertensive chronic kidney disease NOS
Hypertensive renal disease NOS
Use additional code to identify the stage of chronic kidney disease (N18.1-N18.4, N18.9)

✓4ᵗʰ **I13** **Hypertensive heart and chronic kidney disease**
INCLUDES any condition in I11.- with any condition in I12.-
cardiorenal disease
cardiovascular renal disease
TIP: Do not assign a code from this category when provider documentation indicates the heart and/or chronic kidney disease is attributable to another cause.

I13.0 **Hypertensive heart and chronic kidney disease with heart failure and stage 1 through stage 4 chronic kidney disease, or unspecified chronic kidney disease** HCC
Use additional code to identify type of heart failure (I50.-)
Use additional code to identify stage of chronic kidney disease (N18.1-N18.4, N18.9)

✓5ᵗʰ **I13.1** **Hypertensive heart and chronic kidney disease without heart failure**

I13.10 **Hypertensive heart and chronic kidney disease without heart failure, with stage 1 through stage 4 chronic kidney disease, or unspecified chronic kidney disease**
Hypertensive heart disease and hypertensive chronic kidney disease NOS
Use additional code to identify the stage of chronic kidney disease (N18.1-N18.4, N18.9)

I13.11 **Hypertensive heart and chronic kidney disease without heart failure, with stage 5 chronic kidney disease, or end stage renal disease** HCC
Use additional code to identify the stage of chronic kidney disease (N18.5, N18.6)

I13.2 **Hypertensive heart and chronic kidney disease with heart failure and with stage 5 chronic kidney disease, or end stage renal disease** HCC
Use additional code to identify type of heart failure (I50.-)
Use additional code to identify the stage of chronic kidney disease (N18.5, N18.6)

✓4ᵗʰ **I15** **Secondary hypertension**
Code also underlying condition
EXCLUDES 1 postprocedural hypertension (I97.3)
EXCLUDES 2 secondary hypertension involving vessels of brain (I60-I69)
secondary hypertension involving vessels of eye (H35.0-)

I15.0 **Renovascular hypertension**
I15.1 **Hypertension secondary to other renal disorders**
AHA: 2016,3Q,22
I15.2 **Hypertension secondary to endocrine disorders**
I15.8 **Other secondary hypertension**
I15.9 **Secondary hypertension, unspecified**

✓4ᵗʰ **I16** **Hypertensive crisis**
Code also any identified hypertensive disease (I10-I15)
AHA: 2016,4Q,26-28
I16.0 **Hypertensive urgency**
I16.1 **Hypertensive emergency**
I16.9 **Hypertensive crisis, unspecified**

Ischemic heart diseases (I20-I25)

Use additional code to identify presence of hypertension (I10-I16)

☑4ᵗʰ I20   Angina pectoris

Use additional code to identify:
   exposure to environmental tobacco smoke (Z77.22)
   history of tobacco dependence (Z87.891)
   occupational exposure to environmental tobacco smoke (Z57.31)
   tobacco dependence (F17.-)
   tobacco use (Z72.0)

> **EXCLUDES 1**   *angina pectoris with atherosclerotic heart disease of native coronary arteries (I25.1-)*
> *atherosclerosis of coronary artery bypass graft(s) and coronary artery of transplanted heart with angina pectoris (I25.7-)*
> *postinfarction angina (I23.7)*

DEF: Chest pain due to reduced blood flow resulting in a lack of oxygen to the heart muscles.

I20.0   Unstable angina   HCC Q

Accelerated angina
Crescendo angina
De novo effort angina
Intermediate coronary syndrome
Preinfarction syndrome
Worsening effort angina
DEF: Condition representing an intermediate stage between angina of effort and acute myocardial infarction.

I20.1   Angina pectoris with documented spasm   HCC Q

Angiospastic angina
Prinzmetal angina
Spasm-induced angina
Variant angina

I20.8   Other forms of angina pectoris   HCC Q

Angina equivalent
Angina of effort
Coronary slow flow syndrome
Stable angina
Stenocardia
Use additional code(s) for symptoms associated with angina equivalent

I20.9   Angina pectoris, unspecified   HCC Q

Angina NOS
Anginal syndrome
Cardiac angina
Ischemic chest pain

☑4ᵗʰ I21   Acute myocardial infarction

> **INCLUDES**   cardiac infarction
> coronary (artery) embolism
> coronary (artery) occlusion
> coronary (artery) rupture
> coronary (artery) thrombosis
> infarction of heart, myocardium, or ventricle
> myocardial infarction specified as acute or with a stated duration of 4 weeks (28 days) or less from onset

Use additional code, if applicable, to identify:
   exposure to environmental tobacco smoke (Z77.22)
   history of tobacco dependence (Z87.891)
   occupational exposure to environmental tobacco smoke (Z57.31)
   status post administration of tPA (rtPA) in a different facility within the last 24 hours prior to admission to current facility (Z92.82)
   tobacco dependence (F17.-)
   tobacco use (Z72.0)

> **EXCLUDES 2**   *old myocardial infarction (I25.2)*
> *postmyocardial infarction syndrome (I24.1)*
> *subsequent type 1 myocardial infarction (I22.-)*

AHA: 2019,2Q,5; 2018,4Q,68; 2018,3Q,5; 2017,4Q,12-14; 2017,1Q,44-45; 2016,4Q,140; 2015,2Q,16; 2013,1Q,25; 2012,4Q,96,102-103

TIP: When chronic total occlusion and myocardial infarction are documented as being in different vessels, assign code I25.82 Chronic total occlusion of coronary artery, in addition to the myocardial infarction code.

☑5ᵗʰ I21.0   ST elevation (STEMI) myocardial infarction of anterior wall

Type 1 ST elevation myocardial infarction of anterior wall
DEF: ST elevation myocardial infarction: Complete obstruction of one or more coronary arteries causing decreased blood flow (ischemia) and necrosis of myocardial muscle cells.

I21.01   ST elevation (STEMI) myocardial infarction involving left main coronary artery   HCC Q

I21.02   ST elevation (STEMI) myocardial infarction involving left anterior descending coronary artery   HCC Q

ST elevation (STEMI) myocardial infarction involving diagonal coronary artery
AHA: 2013,1Q,25

I21.09   ST elevation (STEMI) myocardial infarction involving other coronary artery of anterior wall   HCC Q

Acute transmural myocardial infarction of anterior wall
Anteroapical transmural (Q wave) infarction (acute)
Anterolateral transmural (Q wave) infarction (acute)
Anteroseptal transmural (O wave) infarction (acute)
Transmural (Q wave) infarction (acute) (of) anterior (wall) NOS
AHA: 2012,4Q,102-103

☑5ᵗʰ I21.1   ST elevation (STEMI) myocardial infarction of inferior wall

Type 1 ST elevation myocardial infarction of inferior wall
DEF: ST elevation myocardial infarction: Complete obstruction of one or more coronary arteries causing decreased blood flow (ischemia) and necrosis of myocardial muscle cells.

I21.11   ST elevation (STEMI) myocardial infarction involving right coronary artery   HCC Q

Inferoposterior transmural (Q wave) infarction (acute)

I21.19   ST elevation (STEMI) myocardial infarction involving other coronary artery of inferior wall   HCC Q

Acute transmural myocardial infarction of inferior wall
Inferolateral transmural (Q wave) infarction (acute)
Transmural (Q wave) infarction (acute) (of) diaphragmatic wall
Transmural (Q wave) infarction (acute) (of) inferior (wall) NOS

> **EXCLUDES 2**   *ST elevation (STEMI) myocardial infarction involving left circumflex coronary artery (I21.21)*

AHA: 2012,4Q,96

☑ **Additional Character Required**   ✓x7ᵗʰ **Placeholder Alert**   **Manifestation**   **Unspecified Dx**   ◄► **Revised Text**   ● **New Code**   ▲ **Revised Code Title**

ICD-10-CM 2020   **637**

Chapter 9. Diseases of the Circulatory System

✓5ᵗʰ **I21.2   ST elevation (STEMI) myocardial infarction of other sites**

Type 1 ST elevation myocardial infarction of other sites

DEF: ST elevation myocardial infarction: Complete obstruction of one or more coronary arteries causing decreased blood flow (ischemia) and necrosis of myocardial muscle cells.

I21.21   ST elevation (STEMI) myocardial infarction HCC Q **involving left circumflex coronary artery**

ST elevation (STEMI) myocardial infarction involving oblique marginal coronary artery

I21.29   ST elevation (STEMI) myocardial infarction HCC Q **involving other sites**

Acute transmural myocardial infarction of other sites

Apical-lateral transmural (Q wave) infarction (acute)

Basal-lateral transmural (Q wave) infarction (acute)

High lateral transmural (Q wave) infarction (acute)

Lateral (wall) NOS transmural (Q wave) infarction (acute)

Posterior (true) transmural (Q wave) infarction (acute)

Posterobasal transmural (Q wave) infarction (acute)

Posterolateral transmural (Q wave) infarction (acute)

Posteroseptal transmural (Q wave) infarction (acute)

Septal transmural (Q wave) infarction (acute) NOS

I21.3   ST elevation (STEMI) myocardial infarction of HCC Q **unspecified site**

Acute transmural myocardial infarction of unspecified site

Transmural (Q wave) myocardial infarction NOS

Type 1 ST elevation myocardial infarction of unspecified site

DEF: ST elevation myocardial infarction: Complete obstruction of one or more coronary arteries causing decreased blood flow (ischemia) and necrosis of myocardial muscle cells.

I21.4   Non-ST elevation (NSTEMI) myocardial infarction HCC Q

Acute subendocardial myocardial infarction

Non-Q wave myocardial infarction NOS

Nontransmural myocardial infarction NOS

Type 1 non-ST elevation myocardial infarction

AHA: 2019,2Q,33; 2017,1Q,44-45

DEF: Partial obstruction of one or more coronary arteries that causes decreased blood flow (ischemia) and may cause partial thickness necrosis of myocardial muscle cells.

I21.9   Acute myocardial infarction, unspecified HCC Q

Myocardial infarction (acute) NOS

✓5ᵗʰ **I21.A   Other type of myocardial infarction**

AHA: 2019,2Q,5

I21.A1   Myocardial infarction type 2 HCC Q

Myocardial infarction due to demand ischemia

Myocardial infarction secondary to ischemic imbalance

▶Code first the underlying cause, such as:◀

▶anemia (D50.0-D64.9)◀

▶chronic obstructive pulmonary disease (J44.-)◀

▶paroxysmal tachycardia (I47.0-I47.9)◀

▶shock (R57.0-R57.9)◀

~~Code also the underlying cause, if known and~~
~~applicable, such as:~~

~~anemia (D50.0-D64.9)~~

~~chronic obstructive pulmonary disease (J44.-)~~

~~heart failure (I50.-)~~

~~paroxysmal tachycardia (I47.0-I47.9)~~

~~renal failure (N17.0-N19)~~

~~shock (R57.0-R57.9)~~

AHA: 2017,4Q,13-14

DEF: Often referred to as due to demand ischemia, myocardial infarction (MI) type 2 refers to an MI due to ischemia and necrosis resulting from an oxygen imbalance to the heart. This mismatch between oxygen decreased supply and increased demand is caused by conditions other than coronary artery disease such as vasospasm, embolism, anemia, hypertension, hypotension, or arrhythmias.

I21.A9   Other myocardial infarction type HCC Q

Myocardial infarction associated with revascularization procedure

Myocardial infarction type 3

Myocardial infarction type 4a

Myocardial infarction type 4b

Myocardial infarction type 4c

Myocardial infarction type 5

Code first, if applicable, postprocedural myocardial infarction following cardiac surgery (I97.190), or postprocedural myocardial infarction during cardiac surgery (I97.790)

Code also complication, if known and applicable, such as:

(acute) stent occlusion (T82.897-)

(acute) stent stenosis ▶(T82.855-)◀

(acute) stent thrombosis (T82.867-)

cardiac arrest due to underlying cardiac condition (I46.2)

complication of percutaneous coronary intervention (PCI) (I97.89)

occlusion of coronary artery bypass graft (T82.218-)

AHA: 2019,2Q,33

✓4ᵗʰ **I22   Subsequent ST elevation (STEMI) and non-ST elevation (NSTEMI) myocardial infarction**

INCLUDES   acute myocardial infarction occurring within four weeks (28 days) of a previous acute myocardial infarction, regardless of site

cardiac infarction

coronary (artery) embolism

coronary (artery) occlusion

coronary (artery) rupture

coronary (artery) thrombosis

infarction of heart, myocardium, or ventricle

recurrent myocardial infarction

reinfarction of myocardium

rupture of heart, myocardium, or ventricle

subsequent type 1 myocardial infarction

Use additional code, if applicable, to identify:

exposure to environmental tobacco smoke (Z77.22)

history of tobacco dependence (Z87.891)

occupational exposure to environmental tobacco smoke (Z57.31)

status post administration of tPA (rtPA) in a different facility within the last 24 hours prior to admission to current facility (Z92.82)

tobacco dependence (F17.-)

tobacco use (Z72.0)

EXCLUDES 1   *subsequent myocardial infarction, type 2 (I21.A1)*

subsequent myocardial infarction of other type (type 3) (type 4) (type 5) (I21.A9)

AHA: 2018,4Q,68; 2018,3Q,5; 2017,4Q,12-13; 2017,2Q,11; 2013,1Q,25; 2012,4Q,97,102-103

DEF: Non-ST elevation myocardial infarction: Partial obstruction of one or more coronary arteries that causes decreased blood flow (ischemia) and may cause partial thickness necrosis of myocardial muscle cells.

DEF: ST elevation myocardial infarction: Complete obstruction of one or more coronary arteries causing decreased blood flow (ischemia) and necrosis of myocardial muscle cells.

TIP: When chronic total occlusion and myocardial infarction are documented as being in different vessels, assign code I25.82 Chronic total occlusion of coronary artery, in addition to the myocardial infarction code.

I22.0   Subsequent ST elevation (STEMI) myocardial HCC Q **infarction of anterior wall**

Subsequent acute transmural myocardial infarction of anterior wall

Subsequent transmural (Q wave) infarction (acute)(of) anterior (wall) NOS

Subsequent anteroapical transmural (Q wave) infarction (acute)

Subsequent anterolateral transmural (Q wave) infarction (acute)

Subsequent anteroseptal transmural (Q wave) infarction (acute)

I22.1 **Subsequent ST elevation (STEMI) myocardial** HCC Q
infarction of inferior wall
Subsequent acute transmural myocardial infarction of inferior wall
Subsequent transmural (Q wave) infarction (acute)(of) diaphragmatic wall
Subsequent transmural (Q wave) infarction (acute)(of) inferior (wall) NOS
Subsequent inferolateral transmural (Q wave) infarction (acute)
Subsequent inferoposterior transmural (Q wave) infarction (acute)
AHA: 2012,4Q,102

I22.2 **Subsequent** non-ST elevation (NSTEMI) myocardial HCC Q
infarction
Subsequent acute subendocardial myocardial infarction
Subsequent non-Q wave myocardial infarction NOS
Subsequent nontransmural myocardial infarction NOS

I22.8 **Subsequent ST elevation (STEMI) myocardial** HCC Q
infarction of other sites
Subsequent acute transmural myocardial infarction of other sites
Subsequent apical-lateral transmural (Q wave) myocardial infarction (acute)
Subsequent basal-lateral transmural (Q wave) myocardial infarction (acute)
Subsequent high lateral transmural (Q wave) myocardial infarction (acute)
Subsequent transmural (Q wave) myocardial infarction (acute)(of) lateral (wall) NOS
Subsequent posterior (true) transmural (Q wave) myocardial infarction (acute)
Subsequent posterobasal transmural (Q wave) myocardial infarction (acute)
Subsequent posterolateral transmural (Q wave) myocardial infarction (acute)
Subsequent posteroseptal transmural (Q wave) myocardial infarction (acute)
Subsequent septal NOS transmural (Q wave) myocardial infarction (acute)

I22.9 **Subsequent ST elevation (STEMI) myocardial** II88
infarction of unspecified site
Subsequent acute myocardial infarction of unspecified site
Subsequent myocardial infarction (acute) NOS

√4ᵗʰ **I23** **Certain current complications following ST elevation (STEMI) and non-ST elevation (NSTEMI) myocardial infarction (within the 28 day period)**
AHA: 2017,2Q,11
DEF: ST elevation myocardial infarction: Complete obstruction of one or more coronary arteries causing decreased blood flow (ischemia) and necrosis of myocardial muscle cells.
DEF: Non-ST elevation myocardial infarction: Partial obstruction of one or more coronary arteries that causes decreased blood flow (ischemia) and may cause partial thickness necrosis of myocardial muscle cells.

I23.0 **Hemopericardium as current complication** HCC Q A
following acute myocardial infarction
EXCLUDES 1   hemopericardium not specified as current complication following acute myocardial infarction (I31.2)

I23.1 **Atrial septal defect as current complication** HCC Q A
following acute myocardial infarction
EXCLUDES 1   acquired atrial septal defect not specified as current complication following acute myocardial infarction (I51.0)

I23.2 **Ventricular septal defect as current complication** HCC Q A
following acute myocardial infarction
EXCLUDES 1   acquired ventricular septal defect not specified as current complication following acute myocardial infarction (I51.0)

I23.3 **Rupture of cardiac wall without hemopericardium** HCC Q A
as current complication following acute myocardial infarction

I23.4 **Rupture of chordae tendineae as current** HCC Q
complication following acute myocardial infarction
EXCLUDES 1   rupture of chordae tendineae not specified as current complication following acute myocardial infarction (I51.1)

I23.5 **Rupture of papillary muscle as current complication** HCC Q
following acute myocardial infarction
EXCLUDES 1   rupture of papillary muscle not specified as current complication following acute myocardial infarction (I51.2)

I23.6 **Thrombosis of atrium, auricular appendage, and** HCC Q A
ventricle as current complications following acute myocardial infarction
EXCLUDES 1   thrombosis of atrium, auricular appendage, and ventricle not specified as current complication following acute myocardial infarction (I51.3)

I23.7 **Postinfarction angina** HCC Q A
AHA: 2015,2Q,16
TIP: When postinfarction angina occurs with atherosclerotic coronary artery disease, code both I23.7 and I25.118 for atherosclerotic disease with other forms of angina pectoris.

I23.8 **Other current complications following acute** HCC Q A
myocardial infarction

√4ᵗʰ **I24** **Other acute ischemic heart diseases**
EXCLUDES 1   angina pectoris (I20.-)
      transient myocardial ischemia in newborn (P29.4)

I24.0 **Acute coronary thrombosis not resulting in** HCC Q
myocardial infarction
Acute coronary (artery) (vein) embolism not resulting in myocardial infarction
Acute coronary (artery) (vein) occlusion not resulting in myocardial infarction
Acute coronary (artery) (vein) thromboembolism not resulting in myocardial infarction
EXCLUDES 1   atherosclerotic heart disease (I25.1-)
AHA: 2013,1Q,24

I24.1 **Dressler's syndrome** HCC Q
Postmyocardial infarction syndrome
EXCLUDES 1   postinfarction angina (I23.7)
DEF: Fever, leukocytosis, chest pain, evidence of pericarditis, pleurisy, and pneumonia occurring days or weeks after a myocardial infarction.

I24.8 **Other forms of acute ischemic heart disease** HCC Q
EXCLUDES 1   myocardial infarction due to demand ischemia (I21.A1)
AHA: 2017,4Q,13

I24.9 **Acute ischemic heart disease, unspecified** HCC Q
EXCLUDES 1   ischemic heart disease (chronic) NOS (I25.9)

Chapter 9. Diseases of the Circulatory System

I25.709

✓4ᵗʰ **I25 Chronic ischemic heart disease**

Use additional code to identify:
chronic total occlusion of coronary artery (I25.82)
exposure to environmental tobacco smoke (Z77.22)
history of tobacco dependence (Z87.891)
occupational exposure to environmental tobacco smoke (Z57.31)
tobacco dependence (F17.-)
tobacco use (Z72.0)

✓5ᵗʰ **I25.1 Atherosclerotic heart disease of native coronary artery**

Atherosclerotic cardiovascular disease
Coronary (artery) atheroma
Coronary (artery) atherosclerosis
Coronary (artery) disease
Coronary (artery) sclerosis
Use additional code, if applicable, to identify:
coronary atherosclerosis due to calcified coronary lesion
(I25.84)
coronary atherosclerosis due to lipid rich plaque (I25.83)
EXCLUDES 2   *atheroembolism (I75.-)*
*atherosclerosis of coronary artery bypass graft(s) and
transplanted heart (I25.7-)*

Atheromas

Atheromas (fatty tissue and/or plaque)   Lumen

I25.10 Atherosclerotic heart disease of native HCC Q A
coronary artery without angina pectoris
Atherosclerotic heart disease NOS
AHA: 2015,2Q,16; 2012,4Q,92

✓6ᵗʰ **I25.11 Atherosclerotic heart disease of native coronary
artery with angina pectoris**

I25.110 Atherosclerotic heart disease of HCC Q A
**native coronary artery with
unstable angina pectoris**
EXCLUDES 1   *unstable angina without
atherosclerotic heart
disease (I20.0)*

I25.111 Atherosclerotic heart disease of HCC Q A
**native coronary artery with
angina pectoris with
documented spasm**
EXCLUDES 1   *angina pectoris with
documented spasm
without atherosclerotic
heart disease (I20.1)*

I25.118 Atherosclerotic heart disease of HCC Q A
**native coronary artery with
other forms of angina pectoris**
EXCLUDES 1   *other forms of angina pectoris
without atherosclerotic
heart disease (I20.8)*
AHA: 2015,2Q,16
TIP: When postinfarction angina occurs with
atherosclerotic coronary artery disease, code
both I23.7 and I25.118 for atherosclerotic
disease with other forms of angina pectoris.

I25.119 Atherosclerotic heart disease of HCC Q A
**native coronary artery with
unspecified angina pectoris**
Atherosclerotic heart disease with angina
NOS
Atherosclerotic heart disease with ischemic
chest pain
EXCLUDES 1   *unspecified angina pectoris
without atherosclerotic
heart disease (I20.9)*

I25.2 Old myocardial infarction Q
Healed myocardial infarction
Past myocardial infarction diagnosed by ECG or other
investigation, but currently presenting no symptoms

I25.3 Aneurysm of heart Q
Mural aneurysm
Ventricular aneurysm

✓5ᵗʰ **I25.4 Coronary artery aneurysm and dissection**

I25.41 Coronary artery aneurysm
Coronary arteriovenous fistula, acquired
EXCLUDES 1   *congenital coronary (artery) aneurysm
(Q24.5)*

I25.42 Coronary artery dissection
DEF: Tear in the intimal arterial wall of a coronary artery
resulting in the sudden intrusion of blood within the
layers of the wall.

I25.5 Ischemic cardiomyopathy Q
EXCLUDES 2   *coronary atherosclerosis (I25.1-, I25.7-)*

I25.6 Silent myocardial ischemia Q

✓5ᵗʰ **I25.7 Atherosclerosis of coronary artery bypass graft(s) and
coronary artery of transplanted heart with angina pectoris**
Use additional code, if applicable, to identify:
coronary atherosclerosis due to calcified coronary lesion
(I25.84)
coronary atherosclerosis due to lipid rich plaque (I25.83)
EXCLUDES 1   *atherosclerosis of bypass graft(s) of transplanted
heart without angina pectoris (I25.812)*
*atherosclerosis of coronary artery bypass graft(s)
without angina pectoris (I25.810)*
*atherosclerosis of native coronary artery of
transplanted heart without angina pectoris
(I25.811)*

✓6ᵗʰ **I25.70 Atherosclerosis of coronary artery bypass graft(s),
unspecified, with angina pectoris**

I25.700 Atherosclerosis of coronary HCC Q A
**artery bypass graft(s),
unspecified, with unstable
angina pectoris**
EXCLUDES 1   *unstable angina pectoris
without atherosclerosis of
coronary artery bypass
graft (I20.0)*

I25.701 Atherosclerosis of coronary HCC Q A
**artery bypass graft(s),
unspecified, with angina
pectoris with documented
spasm**
EXCLUDES 1   *angina pectoris with
documented spasm
without atherosclerosis of
coronary artery bypass
graft (I20.1)*

I25.708 Atherosclerosis of coronary HCC Q A
**artery bypass graft(s),
unspecified, with other forms
of angina pectoris**
EXCLUDES 1   *other forms of angina pectoris
without atherosclerosis of
coronary artery bypass
graft (I20.8)*

I25.709 Atherosclerosis of coronary HCC Q A
**artery bypass graft(s),
unspecified, with unspecified
angina pectoris**
EXCLUDES 1   *unspecified angina pectoris
without atherosclerosis of
coronary artery bypass
graft (I20.9)*

√6ᵗʰ **I25.71** **Atherosclerosis of** autologous vein **coronary artery bypass graft(s) with angina pectoris**

I25.710 **Atherosclerosis of autologous** HCC Q A **vein coronary artery bypass graft(s) with** unstable **angina pectoris**

> EXCLUDES 1 *unstable angina without atherosclerosis of autologous vein coronary artery bypass graft(s) (I20.0)*

> EXCLUDES 2 *embolism or thrombus of coronary artery bypass graft(s) (T82.8-)*

I25.711 **Atherosclerosis of autologous** HCC Q A **vein coronary artery bypass graft(s) with angina pectoris with** documented spasm

> EXCLUDES 1 *angina pectoris with documented spasm without atherosclerosis of autologous vein coronary artery bypass graft(s) (I20.1)*

I25.718 **Atherosclerosis of autologous** HCC Q A **vein coronary artery bypass graft(s) with other forms of angina pectoris**

> EXCLUDES 1 *other forms of angina pectoris without atherosclerosis of autologous vein coronary artery bypass graft(s) (I20.8)*

I25.719 **Atherosclerosis of autologous** HCC Q A **vein coronary artery bypass graft(s) with unspecified angina pectoris**

> EXCLUDES 1 *unspecified angina pectoris without atherosclerosis of autologous vein coronary artery bypass graft(s) (I20.9)*

√6ᵗʰ **I25.72** **Atherosclerosis of** autologous artery **coronary artery bypass graft(s) with angina pectoris**

Atherosclerosis of internal mammary artery graft with angina pectoris

I25.720 **Atherosclerosis of autologous** HCC Q A **artery coronary artery bypass graft(s) with** unstable **angina pectoris**

> EXCLUDES 1 *unstable angina without atherosclerosis of autologous artery coronary artery bypass graft(s) (I20.0)*

I25.721 **Atherosclerosis of autologous** HCC Q A **artery coronary artery bypass graft(s) with angina pectoris with** documented spasm

> EXCLUDES 1 *angina pectoris with documented spasm without atherosclerosis of autologous artery coronary artery bypass graft(s) (I20.1)*

I25.728 **Atherosclerosis of autologous** HCC Q A **artery coronary artery bypass graft(s) with other forms of angina pectoris**

> EXCLUDES 1 *other forms of angina pectoris without atherosclerosis of autologous artery coronary artery bypass graft(s) (I20.8)*

I25.729 **Atherosclerosis of autologous** HCC Q A **artery coronary artery bypass graft(s) with unspecified angina pectoris**

> EXCLUDES 1 *unspecified angina pectoris without atherosclerosis of autologous artery coronary artery bypass graft(s) (I20.9)*

√6ᵗʰ **I25.73** **Atherosclerosis of** nonautologous biological **coronary artery bypass graft(s) with angina pectoris**

I25.730 **Atherosclerosis of** HCC Q A **nonautologous biological coronary artery bypass graft(s) with** unstable **angina pectoris**

> EXCLUDES 1 *unstable angina without atherosclerosis of nonautologous biological coronary artery bypass graft(s) (I20.0)*

I25.731 **Atherosclerosis of** HCC Q A **nonautologous biological coronary artery bypass graft(s) with angina pectoris with** documented spasm

> EXCLUDES 1 *angina pectoris with documented spasm without atherosclerosis of nonautologous biological coronary artery bypass graft(s) (I20.1)*

I25.738 **Atherosclerosis of** HCC Q A **nonautologous biological coronary artery bypass graft(s) with other forms of angina pectoris**

> EXCLUDES 1 *other forms of angina pectoris without atherosclerosis of nonautologous biological coronary artery bypass graft(s) (I20.8)*

I25.739 **Atherosclerosis of** HCC Q A **nonautologous biological coronary artery bypass graft(s) with unspecified angina pectoris**

> EXCLUDES 1 *unspecified angina pectoris without atherosclerosis of nonautologous biological coronary artery bypass graft(s) (I20.9)*

√6ᵗʰ **I25.75** **Atherosclerosis of** native **coronary artery of** transplanted heart **with angina pectoris**

> EXCLUDES 1 *atherosclerosis of native coronary artery of transplanted heart without angina pectoris (I25.811)*

I25.750 **Atherosclerosis of native** HCC Q **coronary artery of transplanted heart with** unstable **angina**

I25.751 **Atherosclerosis of native** HCC **coronary artery of transplanted heart with angina pectoris with** documented spasm

I25.758 **Atherosclerosis of native** HCC Q **coronary artery of transplanted heart with other forms of angina pectoris**

I25.759 **Atherosclerosis of native** HCC Q **coronary artery of transplanted heart with unspecified angina pectoris**

√6ᵗʰ **I25.76** **Atherosclerosis of** bypass graft **of coronary artery of** transplanted heart **with angina pectoris**

> EXCLUDES 1 *atherosclerosis of bypass graft of coronary artery of transplanted heart without angina pectoris (I25.812)*

I25.760 **Atherosclerosis of bypass graft** HCC Q A **of coronary artery of transplanted heart with** unstable **angina**

☑ Additional Character Required   √x7ᵗʰ Placeholder Alert   Manifestation   Unspecified Dx   ►◄ Revised Text   ● New Code   ▲ Revised Code Title

I25.761 **Atherosclerosis of bypass graft** `HCC` `Q` `A`
of coronary artery of
transplanted heart with angina
pectoris with documented
spasm

I25.768 **Atherosclerosis of bypass graft** `HCC` `Q` `A`
of coronary artery of
transplanted heart with other
forms of angina pectoris

I25.769 **Atherosclerosis of bypass graft** `HCC` `Q` `A`
of coronary artery of
transplanted heart with
unspecified angina pectoris

√6ᵗʰ **I25.79** **Atherosclerosis of other coronary artery bypass**
graft(s) with angina pectoris

I25.790 **Atherosclerosis of other** `HCC` `Q` `A`
coronary artery bypass graft(s)
with unstable **angina pectoris**
> _EXCLUDES 1_   _unstable angina without_
> _atherosclerosis of other_
> _coronary artery bypass_
> _graft(s) (I20.0)_

I25.791 **Atherosclerosis of other** `HCC` `Q` `A`
coronary artery bypass graft(s)
with angina pectoris with
documented spasm
> _EXCLUDES 1_   _angina pectoris with_
> _documented spasm_
> _without atherosclerosis of_
> _other coronary artery_
> _bypass graft(s) (I20.1)_

I25.798 **Atherosclerosis of other** `HCC` `Q` `A`
coronary artery bypass graft(s)
with other forms of angina
pectoris
> _EXCLUDES 1_   _other forms of angina pectoris_
> _without atherosclerosis of_
> _other coronary artery_
> _bypass graft(s) (I20.8)_

I25.799 **Atherosclerosis of other** `HCC` `Q` `A`
coronary artery bypass graft(s)
with unspecified angina
pectoris
> _EXCLUDES 1_   _unspecified angina pectoris_
> _without atherosclerosis of_
> _other coronary artery_
> _bypass graft(s) (I20.9)_

√5ᵗʰ **I25.8** **Other forms of chronic ischemic heart disease**

√6ᵗʰ **I25.81** **Atherosclerosis of other coronary vessels** without
angina pectoris
Use additional code, if applicable, to identify:
coronary atherosclerosis due to calcified coronary
lesion (I25.84)
coronary atherosclerosis due to lipid rich plaque
(I25.83)
> _EXCLUDES 1_   ~~_atherosclerotic heart disease of native_~~
> ~~_coronary artery without angina_~~
> ~~_pectoris (I25.10)_~~
>
> _EXCLUDES 2_   ▶_atherosclerotic heart disease of native_
> _coronary artery without angina_
> _pectoris (I25.10)_◀

I25.810 **Atherosclerosis of coronary** `Q` `A`
artery bypass graft(s) **without**
angina pectoris
Atherosclerosis of coronary artery bypass
graft NOS
> _EXCLUDES 1_   _atherosclerosis of coronary_
> _bypass graft(s) with_
> _angina pectoris_
> _(I25.70-I25.73-, I25.79-)_

I25.811 **Atherosclerosis of** native `Q`
coronary artery of transplanted
heart without angina pectoris
Atherosclerosis of native coronary artery
of transplanted heart NOS
> _EXCLUDES 1_   _atherosclerosis of native_
> _coronary artery of_
> _transplanted heart with_
> _angina pectoris (I25.75-)_

I25.812 **Atherosclerosis of** bypass graft `Q` `A`
of coronary artery of
transplanted heart **without**
angina pectoris
Atherosclerosis of bypass graft of
transplanted heart NOS
> _EXCLUDES 1_   _atherosclerosis of bypass graft_
> _of transplanted heart with_
> _angina pectoris (I25.76)_

I25.82 **Chronic total occlusion of coronary artery** `Q`
Complete occlusion of coronary artery
Total occlusion of coronary artery
Code first coronary atherosclerosis (I25.1-, I25.7-,
I25.81-)
> _EXCLUDES 1_   _acute coronary occlusion with myocardial_
> _infarction (I21.0-I21.9, I22.-)_
> _acute coronary occlusion without_
> _myocardial infarction (I24.0)_

AHA: 2018,3Q,5
DEF: Complete blockage of the coronary artery due to
plaque accumulation over an extended period of time,
resulting in substantial reduction of blood flow.
Symptoms include angina or chest pain.
TIP: Report this code in addition to a code from
category I21 or I22 when the chronic total occlusion
and the myocardial infarction are documented as being
in different vessels.

I25.83 **Coronary atherosclerosis due to** lipid rich `Q` `A`
plaque
Code first coronary atherosclerosis (I25.1-, I25.7-,
I25.81-)

I25.84 **Coronary atherosclerosis due to** calcified `Q`
coronary lesion
Coronary atherosclerosis due to severely calcified
coronary lesion
Code first coronary atherosclerosis (I25.1-, I25.7-,
I25.81-)

I25.89 **Other forms of chronic ischemic heart** `Q`
disease

I25.9 **Chronic ischemic heart disease, unspecified** `Q`
Ischemic heart disease (chronic) NOS

Pulmonary heart disease and diseases of pulmonary circulation (I26-I28)

√4ᵗʰ **I26** **Pulmonary embolism**
> `INCLUDES`   pulmonary (acute)(artery)(vein) infarction
> pulmonary (acute) (artery)(vein) thromboembolism
> pulmonary (acute)(artery)(vein) thrombosis
>
> _EXCLUDES 2_   _chronic pulmonary embolism (I27.82)_
> _personal history of pulmonary embolism (Z86.711)_
> _pulmonary embolism complicating abortion, ectopic or molar_
> _pregnancy (O00-O07, O08.2)_
> _pulmonary embolism complicating pregnancy, childbirth and_
> _the puerperium (O88.-)_
> _pulmonary embolism due to trauma (T79.0, T79.1)_
> _pulmonary embolism due to complications of surgical and_
> _medical care (T80.0, T81.7-, T82.8-)_
> _septic (non-pulmonary) arterial embolism (I76)_

√5ᵗʰ **I26.0** **Pulmonary embolism** with acute cor pulmonale
DEF: Cor pulmonale: Heart-lung disease appearing in identifiable
forms as chronic or acute. The chronic form of this heart-lung
disease is marked by dilation, hypertrophy and failure of the right
ventricle due to a disease that has affected the function of the
lungs, excluding congenital or left heart diseases and is also called
chronic cardiopulmonary disease. The acute form is an overload
of the right ventricle from a rapid onset of pulmonary
hypertension, usually arising from a pulmonary embolism.

I26.01 **Septic** **pulmonary embolism with acute** `HCC`
cor pulmonale
Code first underlying infection

I26.02 **Saddle** **embolus of pulmonary artery with** `HCC`
acute cor pulmonale

I26.09 **Other** **pulmonary embolism with acute cor** `HCC`
pulmonale
Acute cor pulmonale NOS
AHA: 2014,4Q,21

☑5th **I26.9** **Pulmonary embolism** without acute cor pulmonale

     I26.90 **Septic pulmonary embolism without acute cor pulmonale**   HCC

         Code first underlying infection

     I26.92 **Saddle embolus of pulmonary artery without acute cor pulmonale**   HCC

●   **I26.93** **Single subsegmental pulmonary embolism without acute cor pulmonale**

         Subsegmental pulmonary embolism NOS

●   **I26.94** **Multiple subsegmental pulmonary emboli without acute cor pulmonale**

     I26.99 **Other pulmonary embolism without acute cor pulmonale**   HCC

         Acute pulmonary embolism NOS

         Pulmonary embolism NOS

         AHA: 2019,2Q,22

☑4th **I27** **Other pulmonary heart diseases**

     I27.0 **Primary pulmonary hypertension**   HCC

         Heritable pulmonary arterial hypertension

         Idiopathic pulmonary arterial hypertension

         Primary group 1 pulmonary hypertension

         Primary pulmonary arterial hypertension

         EXCLUDES 1   *persistent pulmonary hypertension of newborn (P29.30)*

                 pulmonary hypertension NOS (I27.20)

                 secondary pulmonary arterial hypertension (I27.21)

                 secondary pulmonary hypertension (I27.29)

         DEF: Condition that occurs when pressure within the pulmonary artery is elevated and vascular resistance is observed in the lungs.

     I27.1 **Kyphoscoliotic heart disease**   HCC

☑5th   **I27.2** **Other secondary pulmonary hypertension**

         Code also associated underlying condition

         EXCLUDES 1   *Eisenmenger's syndrome (I27.83)*

         AHA: 2017,4Q,14-15; 2014,4Q,21

         DEF: Condition that occurs when pressure within the pulmonary artery is elevated and vascular resistance is observed in the lungs.

     I27.20 **Pulmonary hypertension, unspecified**   HCC

         Pulmonary hypertension NOS

     I27.21 **Secondary pulmonary arterial hypertension**   HCC

         (Associated) (drug-induced) (toxin-induced) pulmonary arterial hypertension NOS

         (Associated) (drug-induced) (toxin-induced) (secondary) group 1 pulmonary hypertension

         Code also associated conditions if applicable, or adverse effects of drugs or toxins, such as:

           adverse effect of appetite depressants (T50.5X5)

           congenital heart disease (Q20-Q28)

           human immunodeficiency virus [HIV] disease (B20)

           polymyositis (M33.2-)

           portal hypertension (K76.6)

           rheumatoid arthritis (M05.-)

           schistosomiasis (B65.-)

           Sjögren syndrome (M35.0-)

           systemic sclerosis (M34.-)

     I27.22 **Pulmonary hypertension due to left heart disease**   HCC

         Group 2 pulmonary hypertension

         Code also associated left heart disease, if known, such as:

           multiple valve disease (I08.-)

           rheumatic aortic valve diseases (I06.-)

           rheumatic mitral valve diseases (I05.-)

     I27.23 **Pulmonary hypertension due to lung diseases and hypoxia**   HCC

         Group 3 pulmonary hypertension

         Code also associated lung disease, if known, such as:

           ·bronchiectasis (J47.-)

           cystic fibrosis with pulmonary manifestations (E84.0)

           interstitial lung disease (J84.-)

           pleural effusion (J90)

           sleep apnea (G47.3-)

     I27.24 **Chronic thromboembolic pulmonary hypertension**   HCC

         Group 4 pulmonary hypertension

         Code also associated pulmonary embolism, if applicable (I26.-, I27.82)

     I27.29 **Other secondary pulmonary hypertension**   HCC

         Group 5 pulmonary hypertension

         Pulmonary hypertension with unclear multifactorial mechanisms

         Pulmonary hypertension due to hematologic disorders

         Pulmonary hypertension due to metabolic disorders

         Pulmonary hypertension due to other systemic disorders

         Code also other associated disorders, if known, such as:

           chronic myeloid leukemia (C92.10- C92.22)

           essential thrombocythemia (D47.3)

           Gaucher disease (E75.22)

           hypertensive chronic kidney disease with end stage renal disease (I12.0, I13.11, I13.2)

           hyperthyroidism (E05.-)

           hypothyroidism (E00-E03)

           polycythemia vera (D45)

           sarcoidosis (D86.-)

           AHA: 2016,2Q,8

☑5th   **I27.8** **Other specified pulmonary heart diseases**

     I27.81 **Cor pulmonale (chronic)**   HCC

         Cor pulmonale NOS

         EXCLUDES 1   *acute cor pulmonale (I26.0-)*

         AHA: 2014,4Q,21

         DEF: Heart-lung disease appearing in identifiable forms as chronic or acute. The chronic form of this heart-lung disease is marked by dilation, hypertrophy and failure of the right ventricle due to a disease that has affected the function of the lungs, excluding congenital or left heart diseases and is also called chronic cardiopulmonary disease. The acute form is an overload of the right ventricle from a rapid onset of pulmonary hypertension, usually arising from a pulmonary embolism.

     I27.82 **Chronic pulmonary embolism**   HCC

         Use additional code, if applicable, for associated long-term (current) use of anticoagulants (Z79.01)

         EXCLUDES 1   *personal history of pulmonary embolism (Z86.711)*

         DEF: Long-standing condition commonly associated with pulmonary hypertension in which small blood clots travel to the lungs repeatedly over many weeks, months, or years, requiring continuation of established anticoagulant or thrombolytic therapy.

     I27.83 **Eisenmenger's syndrome**   HCC

         Eisenmenger's complex

         (Irreversible) Eisenmenger's disease

         Pulmonary hypertension with right to left shunt related to congenital heart disease

         Code also underlying heart defect, if known, such as:

           atrial septal defect (Q21.1)

           Eisenmenger's defect (Q21.8)

           patent ductus arteriosus (Q25.0)

           ventricular septal defect (Q21.0)

          DEF: Pulmonary hypertension with congenital communication between two circulations resulting in a right to left shunt. This causes reduced oxygen saturation in the arterial blood, leading to cyanosis and organ damage. Once it develops, this life-threating condition is irreversible.

     I27.89 **Other specified pulmonary heart diseases**   HCC

     I27.9 **Pulmonary heart disease, unspecified**   HCC

         Chronic cardiopulmonary disease

☑4th **I28** **Other diseases of pulmonary vessels**

     I28.0 **Arteriovenous fistula of pulmonary vessels**   HCC

         EXCLUDES 1   *congenital arteriovenous fistula (Q25.72)*

☑ Additional Character Required   ☑x7th Placeholder Alert   Manifestation   Unspecified Dx   ►◄ Revised Text   ● New Code   ▲ Revised Code Title

Chapter 9. Diseases of the Circulatory System

I28.1   Aneurysm of pulmonary artery   HCC
    EXCLUDES 1   *congenital aneurysm (Q25.79)*
              congenital arteriovenous aneurysm (Q25.72)

I28.8   Other diseases of pulmonary vessels   HCC
Pulmonary arteritis
Pulmonary endarteritis
Rupture of pulmonary vessels
Stenosis of pulmonary vessels
Stricture of pulmonary vessels

I28.9   Disease of pulmonary vessels, unspecified   HCC

Other forms of heart disease (I30-I52)

✓4ᵗʰ   I30   Acute pericarditis
   INCLUDES   acute mediastinopericarditis
             acute myopericarditis
             acute pericardial effusion
             acute pleuropericarditis
             acute pneumopericarditis
   EXCLUDES 1   *Dressler's syndrome (I24.1)*
             rheumatic pericarditis (acute) (I01.0)
             viral pericarditis due to Coxsakie virus (B33.23)

DEF: Pericarditis: Inflammation affecting the pericardium, the fibroserous membrane that surrounds the heart.

I30.0   Acute **nonspecific idiopathic** pericarditis
I30.1   Infective pericarditis
Pneumococcal pericarditis
Pneumopyopericardium
Purulent pericarditis
Pyopericarditis
Pyopericardium
Pyopneumopericardium
Staphylococcal pericarditis
Streptococcal pericarditis
Suppurative pericarditis
Viral pericarditis
Use additional code (B95-B97) to identify infectious agent

I30.8   Other forms of acute pericarditis
I30.9   Acute pericarditis, unspecified

✓4ᵗʰ   I31   Other diseases of pericardium
     EXCLUDES 1   *diseases of pericardium specified as rheumatic (I09.2)*
               postcardiotomy syndrome (I97.0)
               traumatic injury to pericardium (S26.-)

I31.0   Chronic **adhesive** pericarditis
Accretio cordis
Adherent pericardium
Adhesive mediastinopericarditis

I31.1   Chronic **constrictive** pericarditis
Concretio cordis
Pericardial calcification

I31.2   Hemopericardium, not elsewhere classified
     EXCLUDES 1   *hemopericardium as current complication following acute myocardial infarction (I23.0)*

DEF: Presence of blood in the pericardial sac (pericardium). It can lead to potentially fatal cardiac tamponade if enough blood enters the pericardial cavity.

I31.3   Pericardial effusion (noninflammatory)
Chylopericardium
     EXCLUDES 1   *acute pericardial effusion (I30.9)*

AHA: 2019,1Q,16

TIP: Assign this code for documented malignant pericardial effusion. If the sole reason for admission is to treat the effusion with no treatment rendered for the associated malignancy, this code may be sequenced first.

I31.4   Cardiac tamponade
Code first underlying cause
DEF: Life-threatening condition in which fluid or blood accumulates in the space between the muscle of the heart (myocardium) and the outer sac that covers the heart (pericardium), resulting in compression of the heart.

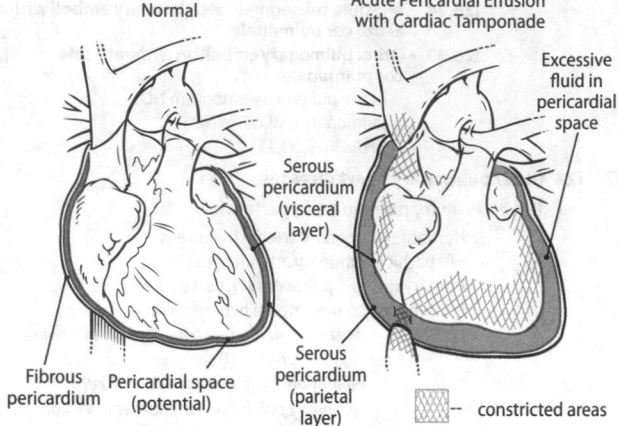

Cardiac Tamponade

Normal   Acute Pericardial Effusion with Cardiac Tamponade

Excessive fluid in pericardial space

Serous pericardium (visceral layer)

Serous pericardium (parietal layer)

Fibrous pericardium   Pericardial space (potential)

╱╱ -- constricted areas

I31.8   Other specified diseases of pericardium
Epicardial plaques
Focal pericardial adhesions

I31.9   Disease of pericardium, unspecified
Pericarditis (chronic) NOS

I32   Pericarditis in diseases classified elsewhere
Code first underlying disease
     EXCLUDES 1   *pericarditis (in):*
              coxsackie (virus) (B33.23)
              gonococcal (A54.83)
              meningococcal (A39.53)
              rheumatoid (arthritis) (M05.31)
              syphilitic (A52.06)
              systemic lupus erythematosus (M32.12)
              tuberculosis (A18.84)

DEF: Pericarditis: Inflammation affecting the pericardium, the fibroserous membrane that surrounds the heart.

✓4ᵗʰ   I33   Acute and subacute endocarditis
     EXCLUDES 1   *acute rheumatic endocarditis (I01.1)*
              endocarditis NOS (I38)

DEF: Endocarditis: Inflammatory disease of the interior lining of the heart chamber and heart valves.

I33.0   Acute and subacute **infective** endocarditis
Bacterial endocarditis (acute) (subacute)
Infective endocarditis (acute) (subacute) NOS
Endocarditis lenta (acute) (subacute)
Malignant endocarditis (acute) (subacute)
Purulent endocarditis (acute) (subacute)
Septic endocarditis (acute) (subacute)
Ulcerative endocarditis (acute) (subacute)
Vegetative endocarditis (acute) (subacute)
Use additional code (B95-B97) to identify infectious agent

I33.9   Acute and subacute endocarditis, unspecified
Acute endocarditis NOS
Acute myoendocarditis NOS
Acute periendocarditis NOS
Subacute endocarditis NOS
Subacute myoendocarditis NOS
Subacute periendocarditis NOS

✓4ᵗʰ **I34 Nonrheumatic mitral valve disorders**

    EXCLUDES 1   *mitral valve disease (I05.9)*
                 mitral valve failure (I05.8)
                 mitral valve stenosis (I05.0)
                 mitral valve disorder of unspecified cause with diseases of aortic and/or tricuspid valve(s) (I08.-)
                 mitral valve disorder of unspecified cause with mitral stenosis or obstruction (I05.0)
                 mitral valve disorder specified as congenital (Q23.2, Q23.9)
                 mitral valve disorder specified as rheumatic (I05.-)

I34.0 Nonrheumatic mitral (valve) insufficiency
    Nonrheumatic mitral (valve) incompetence NOS
    Nonrheumatic mitral (valve) regurgitation NOS

I34.1 Nonrheumatic mitral (valve) prolapse
    Floppy nonrheumatic mitral valve syndrome
    EXCLUDES 1   *Marfan's syndrome (Q87.4-)*

I34.2 Nonrheumatic mitral (valve) stenosis

I34.8 Other nonrheumatic mitral valve disorders

I34.9 Nonrheumatic mitral valve disorder, unspecified

✓4ᵗʰ **I35 Nonrheumatic aortic valve disorders**

    EXCLUDES 1   *aortic valve disorder of unspecified cause but with diseases of mitral and/or tricuspid valve(s) (I08.-)*
                 aortic valve disorder specified as congenital (Q23.0, Q23.1)
                 aortic valve disorder specified as rheumatic (I06.-)
                 hypertrophic subaortic stenosis (I42.1)

I35.0 Nonrheumatic aortic (valve) stenosis

I35.1 Nonrheumatic aortic (valve) insufficiency
    Nonrheumatic aortic (valve) incompetence NOS
    Nonrheumatic aortic (valve) regurgitation NOS

I35.2 Nonrheumatic aortic (valve) stenosis with insufficiency

I35.8 Other nonrheumatic aortic valve disorders

I35.9 Nonrheumatic aortic valve disorder, unspecified

✓4ᵗʰ **I36 Nonrheumatic tricuspid valve disorders**

    EXCLUDES 1   *tricuspid valve disorders of unspecified cause (I07.-)*
                 tricuspid valve disorders specified as congenital (Q22.4, Q22.8, Q22.9)
                 tricuspid valve disorders specified as rheumatic (I07.-)
                 tricuspid valve disorders with aortic and/or mitral valve involvement (I08.-)

I36.0 Nonrheumatic tricuspid (valve) stenosis

I36.1 Nonrheumatic tricuspid (valve) insufficiency
    Nonrheumatic tricuspid (valve) incompetence
    Nonrheumatic tricuspid (valve) regurgitation

I36.2 Nonrheumatic tricuspid (valve) stenosis with insufficiency

I36.8 Other nonrheumatic tricuspid valve disorders

I36.9 Nonrheumatic tricuspid valve disorder, unspecified

✓4ᵗʰ **I37 Nonrheumatic pulmonary valve disorders**

    EXCLUDES 1   *pulmonary valve disorder specified as congenital (Q22.1, Q22.2, Q22.3)*
                 pulmonary valve disorder specified as rheumatic (I09.89)

I37.0 Nonrheumatic pulmonary valve stenosis

I37.1 Nonrheumatic pulmonary valve insufficiency
    Nonrheumatic pulmonary valve incompetence
    Nonrheumatic pulmonary valve regurgitation

I37.2 Nonrheumatic pulmonary valve stenosis with insufficiency

I37.8 Other nonrheumatic pulmonary valve disorders

I37.9 Nonrheumatic pulmonary valve disorder, unspecified

I38 Endocarditis, valve unspecified

    INCLUDES   endocarditis (chronic) NOS
               valvular incompetence NOS
               valvular insufficiency NOS
               valvular regurgitation NOS
               valvular stenosis NOS
               valvulitis (chronic) NOS
    EXCLUDES 1   *congenital insufficiency of cardiac valve NOS (Q24.8)*
                 congenital stenosis of cardiac valve NOS (Q24.8)
                 endocardial fibroelastosis (I42.4)
                 endocarditis specified as rheumatic (I09.1)
    DEF: Endocarditis: Inflammatory disease of the interior lining of the heart chamber and heart valves.

✓4ᵗʰ **I39 Endocarditis and heart valve disorders in diseases classified elsewhere**

    Code first underlying disease, such as:
        Q fever (A78)
    EXCLUDES 1   *endocardial involvement in:*
                    candidiasis (B37.6)
                    gonococcal infection (A54.83)
                    Libman-Sacks disease (M32.11)
                    listerosis (A32.82)
                    meningococcal infection (A39.51)
                    rheumatoid arthritis (M05.31)
                    syphilis (A52.03)
                    tuberculosis (A18.84)
                    typhoid fever (A01.02)
    DEF: Endocarditis: Inflammatory disease of the interior lining of the heart chamber and heart valves.

✓4ᵗʰ **I40 Acute myocarditis**

    INCLUDES   subacute myocarditis
    EXCLUDES 1   *acute rheumatic myocarditis (I01.2)*
    DEF: Myocarditis: Inflammation of the middle layer of the heart, which is composed of muscle tissue.

I40.0 Infective myocarditis
    Septic myocarditis
    Use additional code (B95-B97) to identify infectious agent

I40.1 Isolated myocarditis
    Fiedler's myocarditis
    Giant cell myocarditis
    Idiopathic myocarditis

I40.8 Other acute myocarditis

I40.9 Acute myocarditis, unspecified

✓4ᵗʰ **I41 Myocarditis in diseases classified elsewhere**

    Code first underlying disease, such as:
        typhus (A75.0-A75.9)
    EXCLUDES 1   *myocarditis (in):*
                    Chagas' disease (chronic) (B57.2)
                    acute (B57.0)
                    coxsackie (virus) infection (B33.22)
                    diphtheritic (A36.81)
                    gonococcal (A54.83)
                    influenzal (J09.X9, J10.82, J11.82)
                    meningococcal (A39.52)
                    mumps (B26.82)
                    rheumatoid arthritis (M05.31)
                    sarcoid (D86.85)
                    syphilis (A52.06)
                    toxoplasmosis (B58.81)
                    tuberculous (A18.84)
    DEF: Myocarditis: Inflammation of the middle layer of the heart, which is composed of muscle tissue.

✓4ᵗʰ **I42 Cardiomyopathy**

    INCLUDES   myocardiopathy
    Code first pre-existing cardiomyopathy complicating pregnancy and puerperium (O99.4)
    EXCLUDES 2   *ischemic cardiomyopathy (I25.5)*
                 peripartum cardiomyopathy (O90.3)
                 ventricular hypertrophy (I51.7)

I42.0 Dilated cardiomyopathy   `HCC`
    Congestive cardiomyopathy

I42.1 Obstructive hypertrophic cardiomyopathy   `HCC`
    Hypertrophic subaortic stenosis (idiopathic)
    DEF: Cardiomyopathy marked by left ventricle hypertrophy and an enlarged septum that result in obstructed blood flow, arrhythmias, mitral regurgitation, and sudden cardiac death.
    TIP: When this condition is described as inherited, assign code Q24.8.

I42.2 Other hypertrophic cardiomyopathy   `HCC`
    Nonobstructive hypertrophic cardiomyopathy

I42.3 Endomyocardial (eosinophilic) disease   `HCC`
    Endomyocardial (tropical) fibrosis
    Löffler's endocarditis

I42.4 Endocardial fibroelastosis   `HCC`
    Congenital cardiomyopathy
    Elastomyofibrosis

☑ Additional Character Required   ✓ˣ7ᵗʰ Placeholder Alert   Manifestation   Unspecified Dx   ▶◀ Revised Text   ● New Code   ▲ Revised Code Title

ICD-10-CM 2020   **645**

I42.5 Other **restrictive cardiomyopathy** `HCC`

Constrictive cardiomyopathy NOS

I42.6 Alcoholic **cardiomyopathy** `HCC`

Code also presence of alcoholism (F10.-)

I42.7 **Cardiomyopathy** due to drug and external agent `HCC`

Code first poisoning due to drug or toxin, if applicable (T36-T65 with fifth or sixth character 1-4 or 6)

Use additional code for adverse effect, if applicable, to identify drug (T36-T50 with fifth or sixth character 5)

I42.8 Other **cardiomyopathies** `HCC`

I42.9 **Cardiomyopathy, unspecified** `HCC`

Cardiomyopathy (primary) (secondary) NOS

I43 *Cardiomyopathy in diseases classified elsewhere* `HCC`

Code first underlying disease, such as:
  amyloidosis (E85.-)
  glycogen storage disease (E74.0)
  gout (M10.0-)
  thyrotoxicosis (E05.0-E05.9-)
  `EXCLUDES 1` *cardiomyopathy (in):*
    coxsackie (virus) (B33.24)
    diphtheria (A36.81)
    sarcoidosis (D86.85)
    tuberculosis (A18.84)

`✓4th` **I44** **Atrioventricular and left bundle-branch block**

I44.0 **Atrioventricular block, first degree**

I44.1 **Atrioventricular block, second degree**

Atrioventricular block, type I and II
Möbitz block, type I and II
Second degree block, type I and II
Wenckebach's block

I44.2 **Atrioventricular block, complete** `HCC`

Complete heart block NOS
Third degree block
AHA: 2019,2Q,4

`✓5th` **I44.3** **Other and unspecified atrioventricular block**

Atrioventricular block NOS

I44.30 Unspecified atrioventricular block
I44.39 Other atrioventricular block

I44.4 **Left anterior fascicular block**
I44.5 **Left posterior fascicular block**

`✓5th` **I44.6** **Other and unspecified fascicular block**

I44.60 Unspecified fascicular block
Left bundle-branch hemiblock NOS

I44.69 Other fascicular block

I44.7 **Left bundle-branch block, unspecified**

Conduction Disorders

Sinoatrial node (pacemaker)
Internodal tracts:
  Anterior
  Middle
  Posterior
Atrioventricular node
Atrioventricular bundle (of His)
Atrioventricular block
Accessory bundle (of Kent)
Right bundle branch
Right bundle branch block
Moderator band
Purkinje fibers

Bachmann's bundle
Left bundle branch block
Left bundle branch:
  Anterior fascicle
  Posterior fascicle
Left bundle branch hemiblock

`✓4th` **I45** **Other conduction disorders**

I45.0 **Right fascicular block**

`✓5th` **I45.1** **Other and unspecified right bundle-branch block**

I45.10 Unspecified right bundle-branch block
Right bundle-branch block NOS

I45.19 Other right bundle-branch block

I45.2 **Bifascicular block**
I45.3 **Trifascicular block**
I45.4 **Nonspecific intraventricular block**
Bundle-branch block NOS

I45.5 **Other specified heart block**
Sinoatrial block
Sinoauricular block
`EXCLUDES 1` heart block NOS (I45.9)

I45.6 **Pre-excitation syndrome**
Accelerated atrioventricular conduction
Accessory atrioventricular conduction
Anomalous atrioventricular excitation
Lown-Ganong-Levine syndrome
Pre-excitation atrioventricular conduction
Wolff-Parkinson-White syndrome

`✓5th` **I45.8** **Other specified conduction disorders**

I45.81 Long QT syndrome
DEF: Condition characterized by recurrent syncope, malignant arrhythmias, and sudden death. This syndrome has a characteristic prolonged Q-T interval on an electrocardiogram.

I45.89 Other specified conduction disorders
Atrioventricular [AV] dissociation
Interference dissociation
Isorhythmic dissociation
Nonparoxysmal AV nodal tachycardia
AHA: 2013,2Q,31

I45.9 **Conduction disorder, unspecified**
Heart block NOS
Stokes-Adams syndrome

`✓4th` **I46** **Cardiac arrest**
`EXCLUDES 1` cardiogenic shock (R57.0)
AHA: 2019,2Q,4-5

I46.2 **Cardiac arrest** due to underlying cardiac condition `HCC`
Code first underlying cardiac condition

I46.8 **Cardiac arrest** due to other underlying condition `HCC`
Code first underlying condition

I46.9 **Cardiac arrest, cause unspecified** `HCC`

`✓4th` **I47** **Paroxysmal tachycardia**
Code first tachycardia complicating:
  abortion or ectopic or molar pregnancy (O00-O07, O08.8)
  obstetric surgery and procedures (O75.4)
  `EXCLUDES 1` tachycardia NOS (R00.0)
    sinoauricular tachycardia NOS (R00.0)
    sinus [sinusal] tachycardia NOS (R00.0)

I47.0 **Re-entry ventricular arrhythmia** `HCC`

I47.1 **Supraventricular tachycardia** `HCC`

Atrial (paroxysmal) tachycardia
Atrioventricular [AV] (paroxysmal) tachycardia
Atrioventricular re-entrant (nodal) tachycardia [AVNRT] [AVRT]
Junctional (paroxysmal) tachycardia
Nodal (paroxysmal) tachycardia

I47.2 **Ventricular tachycardia** `HCC`
AHA: 2013,3Q,23

I47.9 **Paroxysmal tachycardia, unspecified** `HCC`
Bouveret (-Hoffman) syndrome

`✓4th` **I48** **Atrial fibrillation and flutter**

I48.0 **Paroxysmal atrial fibrillation** `HCC` `Q`
AHA: 2018,3Q,6

▲ `✓5th` **I48.1** **Persistent atrial fibrillation**
`EXCLUDES 1` ▶permanent atrial fibrillation (I48.21)◀
AHA: 2019,2Q,3; 2018,3Q,6

● **I48.11** Longstanding persistent atrial fibrillation
● **I48.19** Other persistent atrial fibrillation
Chronic persistent atrial fibrillation
Persistent atrial fibrillation, NOS

▲ ✓5ᵗʰ **I48.2** Chronic **atrial fibrillation**
  Permanent atrial fibrillation
  AHA: 2019,2Q,3; 2018,3Q,6

● **I48.20** **Chronic atrial fibrillation, unspecified**
   EXCLUDES 1 *chronic persistent atrial fibrillation (I48.19)*

● **I48.21** **Permanent atrial fibrillation**

I48.3 Typical **atrial flutter** `HCC`
  Type I atrial flutter

I48.4 Atypical **atrial flutter** `HCC`
  Type II atrial flutter

✓5ᵗʰ **I48.9** Unspecified **atrial fibrillation and atrial flutter**

I48.91 **Unspecified atrial fibrillation** `HCC`

I48.92 **Unspecified atrial flutter** `HCC`

✓4ᵗʰ **I49** Other cardiac arrhythmias
  Code first cardiac arrhythmia complicating:
   abortion or ectopic or molar pregnancy (O00–O07, O08.8)
   obstetric surgery and procedures (O75.4)
   EXCLUDES 1 *neonatal dysrhythmia (P29.1-)*
         sinoatrial bradycardia (R00.1)
         sinus bradycardia (R00.1)
         vagal bradycardia (R00.1)
   EXCLUDES 2 *bradycardia NOS (R00.1)*

✓5ᵗʰ **I49.0** Ventricular **fibrillation and flutter**

I49.01 **Ventricular fibrillation** `HCC`

I49.02 **Ventricular flutter** `HCC`

I49.1 Atrial premature **depolarization**
  Atrial premature beats

I49.2 Junctional premature **depolarization** `HCC`

I49.3 Ventricular premature **depolarization**

✓5ᵗʰ **I49.4** Other **and unspecified premature depolarization**

I49.40 **Unspecified premature depolarization**
   Premature beats NOS

I49.49 **Other premature depolarization**
   Ectopic beats
   Extrasystoles
   Extrasystolic arrhythmias
   Premature contractions

I49.5 Sick sinus syndrome `HCC`
  Tachycardia-bradycardia syndrome
  AHA: 2019,1Q,33
  TIP: The presence of a pacemaker controls but does not cure sick sinus syndrome and therefore is considered a reportable chronic condition. When a pacemaker is evaluated by a provider, this code and code Z95.0 Presence of cardiac pacemaker, should be reported, even in the absence of any notable changes or management.

I49.8 Other specified cardiac arrhythmias
  Brugada syndrome
  Coronary sinus rhythm disorder
  Ectopic rhythm disorder
  Nodal rhythm disorder

I49.9 Cardiac arrhythmia, unspecified
  Arrhythmia (cardiac) NOS

✓4ᵗʰ **I50** Heart failure
  Code first:
   heart failure complicating abortion or ectopic or molar pregnancy
    (O00–O07, O08.8)
   heart failure due to hypertension (I11.0)
   heart failure due to hypertension with chronic kidney disease (I13.-)
   heart failure following surgery (I97.13-)
   obstetric surgery and procedures (O75.4)
   rheumatic heart failure (I09.81)
   EXCLUDES 1 *neonatal cardiac failure (P29.0)*
   EXCLUDES 2 *cardiac arrest (I46.-)*
  AHA: 2018,4Q,67; 2018,2Q,9; 2017,1Q,47; 2014,1Q,25; 2013,2Q,33

I50.1 Left ventricular **failure, unspecified** `HCC`
  Cardiac asthma
  Edema of lung with heart disease NOS
  Edema of lung with heart failure
  Left heart failure
  Pulmonary edema with heart disease NOS
  Pulmonary edema with heart failure
  EXCLUDES 1 *edema of lung without heart disease or heart failure*
        (J81.-)
        pulmonary edema without heart disease or failure
        (J81.-)

✓5ᵗʰ **I50.2** Systolic **(congestive) heart failure**
  Heart failure with reduced ejection fraction [HFrEF]
  Systolic left ventricular heart failure
  Code also end stage heart failure, if applicable (I50.84)
  EXCLUDES 1 *combined systolic (congestive) and diastolic*
        (congestive) heart failure (I50.4-)
  AHA: 2017,1Q,46; 2016,1Q,10

I50.20 **Unspecified systolic (congestive) heart** `HCC`
    failure

I50.21 **Acute systolic (congestive) heart failure** `HCC`

I50.22 **Chronic systolic (congestive) heart failure** `HCC`

I50.23 **Acute on chronic systolic (congestive)** `HCC`
    heart failure

✓5ᵗʰ **I50.3** Diastolic **(congestive) heart failure**
  Diastolic left ventricular heart failure
  Heart failure with normal ejection fraction
  Heart failure with preserved ejection fraction [HFpEF]
  Code also end stage heart failure, if applicable (I50.84)
  EXCLUDES 1 *combined systolic (congestive) and diastolic*
        (congestive) heart failure (I50.4-)
  AHA: 2017,1Q,46; 2016,1Q,10

I50.30 **Unspecified diastolic (congestive) heart** `HCC`
    failure

I50.31 **Acute diastolic (congestive) heart failure** `HCC`

I50.32 **Chronic diastolic (congestive) heart failure** `HCC`

I50.33 **Acute on chronic diastolic (congestive)** `HCC`
    heart failure

✓5ᵗʰ **I50.4** Combined systolic **(congestive) and diastolic (congestive)**
  heart failure
  Combined systolic and diastolic left ventricular heart failure
  Heart failure with reduced ejection fraction and diastolic
   dysfunction
  Code also end stage heart failure, if applicable (I50.84)
  AHA: 2017,1Q,46; 2016,1Q,10

I50.40 **Unspecified combined systolic** `HCC`
    (congestive) and diastolic (congestive)
    heart failure

I50.41 **Acute combined systolic (congestive) and** `HCC`
    diastolic (congestive) heart failure

I50.42 **Chronic combined systolic (congestive)** `HCC`
    and diastolic (congestive) heart failure

I50.43 **Acute on chronic combined systolic** `HCC`
    (congestive) and diastolic (congestive)
    heart failure

✓5ᵗʰ **I50.8** Other heart failure
  AHA: 2017,4Q,15-16

✓6ᵗʰ **I50.81** Right **heart failure**
   Right ventricular failure

I50.810 **Right heart failure, unspecified** `HCC`
    Right heart failure without mention of left
     heart failure
    Right ventricular failure NOS

I50.811 Acute right heart failure HCC
Acute isolated right heart failure
Acute (isolated) right ventricular failure

I50.812 Chronic right heart failure HCC
Chronic isolated right heart failure
Chronic (isolated) right ventricular failure

I50.813 Acute on chronic right heart failure HCC
Acute on chronic isolated right heart failure
Acute on chronic (isolated) right ventricular failure
Acute decompensation of chronic (isolated) right ventricular failure
Acute exacerbation of chronic (isolated) right ventricular failure

I50.814 Right heart failure due to left heart failure HCC
Right ventricular failure secondary to left ventricular failure
Code also the type of left ventricular failure, if known (I50.2-I50.43)
EXCLUDES 1   right heart failure with but not due to left heart failure (I50.82)

I50.82 Biventricular heart failure HCC
Code also the type of left ventricular failure as systolic, diastolic, or combined, if known (I50.2-I50.43)

I50.83 High output heart failure HCC
DEF: Occurs when the high demand for blood exceeds the capacity of a normally functioning heart to meet the demand.

I50.84 End stage heart failure HCC
Stage D heart failure
Code also the type of heart failure as systolic, diastolic, or combined, if known (I50.2-I50.43)

I50.89 Other heart failure HCC

I50.9 Heart failure, unspecified HCC
Cardiac, heart or myocardial failure NOS
Congestive heart disease
Congestive heart failure NOS
EXCLUDES 2 ▶fluid overload unrelated to congestive heart failure◀ (E87.70)
AHA: 2017,4Q,15-16; 2017,1Q,45-46; 2014,4Q,21; 2012,4Q,92

✓4ᵗʰ I51 Complications and ill-defined descriptions of heart disease
EXCLUDES 1   any condition in I51.4-I51.9 due to hypertension (I11.-)
any condition in I51.4-I51.9 due to hypertension and chronic kidney disease (I13.-)
heart disease specified as rheumatic (I00-I09)

I51.0 Cardiac septal defect, acquired A
Acquired septal atrial defect (old)
Acquired septal auricular defect (old)
Acquired septal ventricular defect (old)
EXCLUDES 1   cardiac septal defect as current complication following acute myocardial infarction (I23.1, I23.2)
DEF: Abnormal communication between opposite heart chambers due to a defect of the septum. It is not present at birth.

I51.1 Rupture of chordae tendineae, not elsewhere classified HCC
EXCLUDES 1   rupture of chordae tendineae as current complication following acute myocardial infarction (I23.4)

I51.2 Rupture of papillary muscle, not elsewhere classified HCC
EXCLUDES 1   rupture of papillary muscle as current complication following acute myocardial infarction (I23.5)

I51.3 Intracardiac thrombosis, not elsewhere classified
Apical thrombosis (old)
Atrial thrombosis (old)
Auricular thrombosis (old)
Mural thrombosis (old)
Ventricular thrombosis (old)
EXCLUDES 1   intracardiac thrombosis as current complication following acute myocardial infarction (I23.6)
AHA: 2013,1Q,24

I51.4 Myocarditis, unspecified HCC
Chronic (interstitial) myocarditis
Myocardial fibrosis
Myocarditis NOS
EXCLUDES 1   acute or subacute myocarditis (I40.-)
AHA: 2018,4Q,67; 2018,2Q,9

I51.5 Myocardial degeneration HCC
Fatty degeneration of heart or myocardium
Myocardial disease
Senile degeneration of heart or myocardium
AHA: 2018,4Q,67; 2018,2Q,9

I51.7 Cardiomegaly
Cardiac dilatation
Cardiac hypertrophy
Ventricular dilatation
AHA: 2018,4Q,67; 2018,2Q,9

✓5ᵗʰ I51.8 Other ill-defined heart diseases
AHA: 2018,2Q,9

I51.81 Takotsubo syndrome
Reversible left ventricular dysfunction following sudden emotional stress
Stress induced cardiomyopathy
Takotsubo cardiomyopathy
Transient left ventricular apical ballooning syndrome
DEF: Complex of symptoms mimicking myocardial infarct in absence of heart disease, with the majority of cases occurring in postmenopausal women. Heart muscles are temporarily weakened, and a sudden, massive surge of adrenalin stuns the heart, greatly reducing the ability to pump blood.

I51.89 Other ill-defined heart diseases
Carditis (acute)(chronic)
Pancarditis (acute)(chronic)
AHA: 2019,2Q,5; 2018,4Q,67

I51.9 Heart disease, unspecified
AHA: 2018,4Q,67; 2018,2Q,9

I52 Other heart disorders in diseases classified elsewhere
Code first underlying disease, such as:
congenital syphilis (A50.5)
mucopolysaccharidosis (E76.3)
schistosomiasis (B65.0-B65.9)
EXCLUDES 1   heart disease (in):
gonococcal infection (A54.83)
meningococcal infection (A39.50)
rheumatoid arthritis (M05.31)
syphilis (A52.06)

Cerebrovascular diseases (I60-I69)

Use additional code to identify presence of:
alcohol abuse and dependence (F10.-)
exposure to environmental tobacco smoke (Z77.22)
history of tobacco dependence (Z87.891)
hypertension (I10-I16)
occupational exposure to environmental tobacco smoke (Z57.31)
tobacco dependence (F17.-)
tobacco use (Z72.0)
EXCLUDES 1   traumatic intracranial hemorrhage (S06.-)
AHA: 2014,3Q,5; 2012,4Q,91-92

✓4ᵗʰ I60 Nontraumatic subarachnoid hemorrhage
EXCLUDES 1   syphilitic ruptured cerebral aneurysm (A52.05)
EXCLUDES 2   sequelae of subarachnoid hemorrhage (I69.0-)

✓5ᵗʰ I60.0 Nontraumatic subarachnoid hemorrhage from carotid siphon and bifurcation
I60.00 Nontraumatic subarachnoid hemorrhage from unspecified carotid siphon and bifurcation HCC Q
I60.01 Nontraumatic subarachnoid hemorrhage from right carotid siphon and bifurcation HCC Q
I60.02 Nontraumatic subarachnoid hemorrhage from left carotid siphon and bifurcation HCC Q

✓5ᵗʰ I60.1 Nontraumatic subarachnoid hemorrhage from middle cerebral artery
I60.10 Nontraumatic subarachnoid hemorrhage from unspecified middle cerebral artery HCC Q
I60.11 Nontraumatic subarachnoid hemorrhage from right middle cerebral artery HCC Q
I60.12 Nontraumatic subarachnoid hemorrhage from left middle cerebral artery HCC Q

I60.2   **Nontraumatic subarachnoid hemorrhage from anterior communicating artery**   HCC Q

√5ᵗʰ **I60.3**   **Nontraumatic subarachnoid hemorrhage from** posterior communicating artery

     I60.30   **Nontraumatic subarachnoid hemorrhage from unspecified posterior communicating artery**   HCC

     I60.31   **Nontraumatic subarachnoid hemorrhage from** right **posterior communicating artery**   HCC Q

     I60.32   **Nontraumatic subarachnoid hemorrhage from** left **posterior communicating artery**   HCC Q

I60.4   **Nontraumatic subarachnoid hemorrhage from basilar artery**   HCC Q

√5ᵗʰ **I60.5**   **Nontraumatic subarachnoid hemorrhage from** vertebral artery

     I60.50   **Nontraumatic subarachnoid hemorrhage from unspecified vertebral artery**   HCC Q

     I60.51   **Nontraumatic subarachnoid hemorrhage from** right **vertebral artery**   HCC Q

     I60.52   **Nontraumatic subarachnoid hemorrhage from** left **vertebral artery**   HCC Q

I60.6   **Nontraumatic subarachnoid hemorrhage from other intracranial arteries**   HCC Q

I60.7   **Nontraumatic subarachnoid hemorrhage from unspecified intracranial artery**   HCC Q

     Ruptured (congenital) berry aneurysm

     Ruptured (congenital) cerebral aneurysm

     Subarachnoid hemorrhage (nontraumatic) from cerebral artery NOS

     Subarachnoid hemorrhage (nontraumatic) from communicating artery NOS

     EXCLUDES 1   berry aneurysm, nonruptured (I67.1)

I60.8   **Other nontraumatic subarachnoid hemorrhage**   HCC Q

     Meningeal hemorrhage

     Rupture of cerebral arteriovenous malformation

I60.9   **Nontraumatic subarachnoid hemorrhage, unspecified**   HCC Q

√4ᵗʰ **I61**   **Nontraumatic Intracerebral hemorrhage**

     EXCLUDES 2   sequelae of intracerebral hemorrhage (I69.1-)

     AHA: 2017,2Q,9-10

I61.0   **Nontraumatic intracerebral hemorrhage in hemisphere, subcortical**   HCC Q

     Deep intracerebral hemorrhage (nontraumatic)

     AHA: 2016,4Q,27

I61.1   **Nontraumatic intracerebral hemorrhage in hemisphere, cortical**   HCC Q

     Cerebral lobe hemorrhage (nontraumatic)

     Superficial intracerebral hemorrhage (nontraumatic)

I61.2   **Nontraumatic intracerebral hemorrhage in hemisphere, unspecified**   HCC Q

I61.3   **Nontraumatic intracerebral hemorrhage in brain stem**   HCC Q

I61.4   **Nontraumatic intracerebral hemorrhage in cerebellum**   HCC Q

I61.5   **Nontraumatic intracerebral hemorrhage, intraventricular**   HCC Q

I61.6   **Nontraumatic intracerebral hemorrhage,** multiple localized   HCC Q

I61.8   **Other nontraumatic intracerebral hemorrhage**   HCC Q

I61.9   **Nontraumatic intracerebral hemorrhage, unspecified**   HCC Q

√4ᵗʰ **I62**   **Other and unspecified** nontraumatic intracranial **hemorrhage**

     EXCLUDES 2   sequelae of intracranial hemorrhage (I69.2)

√5ᵗʰ **I62.0**   **Nontraumatic** subdural **hemorrhage**

     I62.00   **Nontraumatic subdural hemorrhage, unspecified**   HCC Q

     I62.01   **Nontraumatic** acute **subdural hemorrhage**   HCC Q

     I62.02   **Nontraumatic** subacute **subdural hemorrhage**   HCC Q

     I62.03   **Nontraumatic** chronic **subdural hemorrhage**   HCC Q

I62.1   **Nontraumatic** extradural **hemorrhage**   HCC Q

     Nontraumatic epidural hemorrhage

I62.9   **Nontraumatic intracranial hemorrhage, unspecified**   HCC Q

√4ᵗʰ **I63**   **Cerebral infarction**

     INCLUDES   occlusion and stenosis of cerebral and precerebral arteries, resulting in cerebral infarction

     Use additional code, if applicable, to identify status post administration of tPA (rtPA) in a different facility within the last 24 hours prior to admission to current facility (Z92.82)

     Use additional code, if known, to indicate National Institutes of Health Stroke Scale (NIHSS) score (R29.7-)

     EXCLUDES 2   sequelae of cerebral infarction (I69.3-)

     AHA: 2017,2Q,9-10; 2016,4Q,28,61-62; 2014,1Q,23

     TIP: Weakness on one side of the body documented as secondary to stroke is synonymous with hemiparesis/hemiplegia (G81.-). Weakness of one limb documented as secondary to stroke is synonymous with monoplegia (G83.1-, G83.2-, G83.3-).

√5ᵗʰ **I63.0**   **Cerebral infarction due to** thrombosis of precerebral **arteries**

     I63.00   **Cerebral infarction due to thrombosis of unspecified precerebral artery**   HCC

     √6ᵗʰ **I63.01**   **Cerebral infarction due to thrombosis of** vertebral **artery**

         I63.011   **Cerebral infarction due to thrombosis of** right **vertebral artery**   HCC

         I63.012   **Cerebral infarction due to thrombosis of** left **vertebral artery**   HCC

         I63.013   **Cerebral infarction due to thrombosis of** bilateral **vertebral arteries**   HCC

         I63.019   **Cerebral infarction due to thrombosis of unspecified vertebral artery**   HCC

     I63.02   **Cerebral infarction due to thrombosis of** basilar **artery**   HCC

     √6ᵗʰ **I63.03**   **Cerebral infarction due to thrombosis of** carotid **artery**

         I63.031   **Cerebral infarction due to thrombosis of** right **carotid artery**   HCC

         I63.032   **Cerebral infarction due to thrombosis of** left **carotid artery**   HCC

         I63.033   **Cerebral infarction due to thrombosis of** bilateral **carotid arteries**   HCC

         I63.039   **Cerebral infarction due to thrombosis of unspecified carotid artery**   HCC

     I63.09   **Cerebral infarction due to thrombosis of other precerebral artery**   HCC

√5ᵗʰ **I63.1**   **Cerebral infarction due to** embolism of precerebral **arteries**

     I63.10   **Cerebral infarction due to embolism of unspecified precerebral artery**   HCC

     √6ᵗʰ **I63.11**   **Cerebral infarction due to embolism of** vertebral **artery**

         I63.111   **Cerebral infarction due to embolism of** right **vertebral artery**   HCC

         I63.112   **Cerebral infarction due to embolism of** left **vertebral artery**   HCC

         I63.113   **Cerebral infarction due to embolism of** bilateral **vertebral arteries**   HCC

         I63.119   **Cerebral infarction due to embolism of unspecified vertebral artery**   HCC

     I63.12   **Cerebral infarction due to embolism of** basilar **artery**   HCC

     √6ᵗʰ **I63.13**   **Cerebral infarction due to embolism of** carotid **artery**

         I63.131   **Cerebral infarction due to embolism of** right **carotid artery**   HCC

         I63.132   **Cerebral infarction due to embolism of** left **carotid artery**   HCC

         I63.133   **Cerebral infarction due to embolism of** bilateral **carotid arteries**   HCC

         I63.139   **Cerebral infarction due to embolism of unspecified carotid artery**   HCC

     I63.19   **Cerebral infarction due to embolism of other precerebral artery**   HCC

☑ Additional Character Required   √x7ᵗʰ Placeholder Alert   Manifestation   Unspecified Dx   ▶◀ Revised Text   ● New Code   ▲ Revised Code Title

Chapter 9. Diseases of the Circulatory System

I63.2–I63.49

√5th **I63.2** **Cerebral infarction due to unspecified occlusion or stenosis of precerebral arteries**

     I63.20 **Cerebral infarction due to unspecified occlusion or stenosis of unspecified precerebral arteries** HCC Q

     √6th **I63.21** **Cerebral infarction due to unspecified occlusion or stenosis of vertebral arteries**

         I63.211 **Cerebral infarction due to unspecified occlusion or stenosis of right vertebral artery** HCC Q

         I63.212 **Cerebral infarction due to unspecified occlusion or stenosis of left vertebral artery** HCC Q

         I63.213 **Cerebral infarction due to unspecified occlusion or stenosis of bilateral vertebral arteries** HCC

         I63.219 **Cerebral infarction due to unspecified occlusion or stenosis of unspecified vertebral artery** HCC Q

     I63.22 **Cerebral infarction due to unspecified occlusion or stenosis of basilar artery** HCC Q

     √6th **I63.23** **Cerebral infarction due to unspecified occlusion or stenosis of carotid arteries**

         I63.231 **Cerebral infarction due to unspecified occlusion or stenosis of right carotid arteries** HCC Q

         I63.232 **Cerebral infarction due to unspecified occlusion or stenosis of left carotid arteries** HCC Q

         I63.233 **Cerebral infarction due to unspecified occlusion or stenosis of bilateral carotid arteries** HCC Q

         I63.239 **Cerebral infarction due to unspecified occlusion or stenosis of unspecified carotid artery** HCC Q

     I63.29 **Cerebral infarction due to unspecified occlusion or stenosis of other precerebral arteries** HCC Q

√5th **I63.3** **Cerebral infarction due to thrombosis of cerebral arteries**

     I63.30 **Cerebral infarction due to thrombosis of unspecified cerebral artery** HCC

     √6th **I63.31** **Cerebral infarction due to thrombosis of middle cerebral artery**

         I63.311 **Cerebral infarction due to thrombosis of right middle cerebral artery** HCC

         I63.312 **Cerebral infarction due to thrombosis of left middle cerebral artery** HCC

         I63.313 **Cerebral infarction due to thrombosis of bilateral middle cerebral arteries** HCC

         I63.319 **Cerebral infarction due to thrombosis of unspecified middle cerebral artery** HCC

     √6th **I63.32** **Cerebral infarction due to thrombosis of anterior cerebral artery**

         I63.321 **Cerebral infarction due to thrombosis of right anterior cerebral artery** HCC

         I63.322 **Cerebral infarction due to thrombosis of left anterior cerebral artery** HCC

         I63.323 **Cerebral infarction due to thrombosis of bilateral anterior cerebral arteries** HCC

         I63.329 **Cerebral infarction due to thrombosis of unspecified anterior cerebral artery** HCC

     √6th **I63.33** **Cerebral infarction due to thrombosis of posterior cerebral artery**

         I63.331 **Cerebral infarction due to thrombosis of right posterior cerebral artery** HCC

         I63.332 **Cerebral infarction due to thrombosis of left posterior cerebral artery** HCC

         I63.333 **Cerebral infarction due to thrombosis of bilateral posterior cerebral arteries** HCC

         I63.339 **Cerebral infarction due to thrombosis of unspecified posterior cerebral artery** HCC

     √6th **I63.34** **Cerebral infarction due to thrombosis of cerebellar artery**

         I63.341 **Cerebral infarction due to thrombosis of right cerebellar artery** HCC

         I63.342 **Cerebral infarction due to thrombosis of left cerebellar artery** HCC

         I63.343 **Cerebral infarction due to thrombosis of bilateral cerebellar arteries** HCC

         I63.349 **Cerebral infarction due to thrombosis of unspecified cerebellar artery** HCC

     I63.39 **Cerebral infarction due to thrombosis of other cerebral artery** HCC

√5th **I63.4** **Cerebral infarction due to embolism of cerebral arteries**

     I63.40 **Cerebral infarction due to embolism of unspecified cerebral artery** HCC

     √6th **I63.41** **Cerebral infarction due to embolism of middle cerebral artery**

         I63.411 **Cerebral infarction due to embolism of right middle cerebral artery** HCC

         I63.412 **Cerebral infarction due to embolism of left middle cerebral artery** HCC

         I63.413 **Cerebral infarction due to embolism of bilateral middle cerebral arteries** HCC

         I63.419 **Cerebral infarction due to embolism of unspecified middle cerebral artery** HCC

     √6th **I63.42** **Cerebral infarction due to embolism of anterior cerebral artery**

         I63.421 **Cerebral infarction due to embolism of right anterior cerebral artery** HCC

         I63.422 **Cerebral infarction due to embolism of left anterior cerebral artery** HCC

         I63.423 **Cerebral infarction due to embolism of bilateral anterior cerebral arteries** HCC

         I63.429 **Cerebral infarction due to embolism of unspecified anterior cerebral artery** HCC

     √6th **I63.43** **Cerebral infarction due to embolism of posterior cerebral artery**

         I63.431 **Cerebral infarction due to embolism of right posterior cerebral artery** HCC

         I63.432 **Cerebral infarction due to embolism of left posterior cerebral artery** HCC

         I63.433 **Cerebral infarction due to embolism of bilateral posterior cerebral arteries** HCC

         I63.439 **Cerebral infarction due to embolism of unspecified posterior cerebral artery** HCC

     √6th **I63.44** **Cerebral infarction due to embolism of cerebellar artery**

         I63.441 **Cerebral infarction due to embolism of right cerebellar artery** HCC

         I63.442 **Cerebral infarction due to embolism of left cerebellar artery** HCC

         I63.443 **Cerebral infarction due to embolism of bilateral cerebellar arteries** HCC

         I63.449 **Cerebral infarction due to embolism of unspecified cerebellar artery** HCC

     I63.49 **Cerebral infarction due to embolism of other cerebral artery** HCC

√5ᵗʰ **I63.5** **Cerebral infarction due to unspecified** occlusion or stenosis of cerebral **arteries**

I63.50 **Cerebral infarction due to unspecified occlusion or stenosis of unspecified cerebral artery** `HCC` `Q`

√6ᵗʰ **I63.51** **Cerebral infarction due to unspecified occlusion or stenosis of** middle **cerebral artery**

I63.511 **Cerebral infarction due to unspecified occlusion or stenosis of** right **middle cerebral artery** `HCC` `Q`

I63.512 **Cerebral infarction due to unspecified occlusion or stenosis of** left **middle cerebral artery** `HCC` `Q`

I63.513 **Cerebral infarction due to unspecified occlusion or stenosis of** bilateral **middle cerebral arteries** `HCC` `Q`

I63.519 **Cerebral infarction due to unspecified occlusion or stenosis of unspecified middle cerebral artery** `HCC` `Q`

√6ᵗʰ **I63.52** **Cerebral infarction due to unspecified occlusion or stenosis of** anterior **cerebral artery**

I63.521 **Cerebral infarction due to unspecified occlusion or stenosis of** right **anterior cerebral artery** `HCC` `Q`

I63.522 **Cerebral infarction due to unspecified occlusion or stenosis of** left **anterior cerebral artery** `HCC`

I63.523 **Cerebral infarction due to unspecified occlusion or stenosis of** bilateral **anterior cerebral arteries** `HCC` `Q`

I63.529 **Cerebral infarction due to unspecified occlusion or stenosis of unspecified anterior cerebral artery** `HCC`

√6ᵗʰ **I63.53** **Cerebral infarction due to unspecified occlusion or stenosis of** posterior **cerebral artery**

I63.531 **Cerebral infarction due to unspecified occlusion or stenosis of** right **posterior cerebral artery** `HCC` `Q`

I63.532 **Cerebral infarction due to unspecified occlusion or stenosis of** left **posterior cerebral artery** `HCC` `Q`

I63.533 **Cerebral infarction due to unspecified occlusion or stenosis of** bilateral **posterior cerebral arteries** `HCC` `Q`

I63.539 **Cerebral infarction due to unspecified occlusion or stenosis of unspecified posterior cerebral artery** `HCC` `Q`

√6ᵗʰ **I63.54** **Cerebral infarction due to unspecified occlusion or stenosis of** cerebellar **artery**

I63.541 **Cerebral infarction due to unspecified occlusion or stenosis of** right **cerebellar artery** `HCC`

I63.542 **Cerebral infarction due to unspecified occlusion or stenosis of** left **cerebellar artery** `HCC` `Q`

I63.543 **Cerebral infarction due to unspecified occlusion or stenosis of** bilateral **cerebellar arteries** `HCC` `Q`

I63.549 **Cerebral infarction due to unspecified occlusion or stenosis of unspecified cerebellar artery** `HCC` `Q`

I63.59 **Cerebral infarction due to unspecified occlusion or stenosis of other cerebral artery** `HCC` `Q`

I63.6 **Cerebral infarction due to** cerebral venous **thrombosis, nonpyogenic** `HCC`

√5ᵗʰ **I63.8** **Other cerebral infarction**

AHA: 2018,4Q,16

I63.81 **Other cerebral infarction due to** occlusion or stenosis **of small artery** `HCC`
Lacunar infarction

I63.89 **Other cerebral infarction** `HCC`

I63.9 **Cerebral infarction, unspecified** `HCC`
Stroke NOS

EXCLUDES 2 *transient cerebral ischemic attacks and related syndromes (G45.-)*

AHA: 2015,1Q,25
TIP: When provider documentation does not identify the location of an infarction, imaging reports can be used to pinpoint the location and lead to a more specific infarction code.

√4ᵗʰ **I65** **Occlusion and stenosis of** precerebral **arteries, not resulting in cerebral infarction**

INCLUDES embolism of precerebral artery
narrowing of precerebral artery
obstruction (complete) (partial) of precerebral artery
thrombosis of precerebral artery

EXCLUDES 1 *insufficiency, NOS, of precerebral artery (G45.-)*
insufficiency of precerebral arteries causing cerebral infarction (I63.0-I63.2)

AHA: 2018,2Q,9

√5ᵗʰ **I65.0** **Occlusion and stenosis of** vertebral **artery**

I65.01 **Occlusion and stenosis of** right **vertebral artery** `Q`

I65.02 **Occlusion and stenosis of** left **vertebral artery** `Q`

I65.03 **Occlusion and stenosis of** bilateral **vertebral arteries** `Q`

I65.09 **Occlusion and stenosis of unspecified vertebral artery** `Q`

I65.1 **Occlusion and stenosis of** basilar **artery** `Q`

√5ᵗʰ **I65.2** **Occlusion and stenosis of** carotid **artery**

I65.21 **Occlusion and stenosis of** right **carotid artery** `Q`

I65.22 **Occlusion and stenosis of** left **carotid artery** `Q`

I65.23 **Occlusion and stenosis of** bilateral **carotid arteries** `Q`

I65.29 **Occlusion and stenosis of unspecified carotid artery** `Q`

I65.8 **Occlusion and stenosis of other precerebral arteries** `Q`

I65.9 **Occlusion and stenosis of unspecified precerebral artery** `Q`
Occlusion and stenosis of precerebral artery NOS

√4ᵗʰ **I66** **Occlusion and stenosis of** cerebral **arteries, not resulting in cerebral infarction**

INCLUDES embolism of cerebral artery
narrowing of cerebral artery
obstruction (complete) (partial) of cerebral artery
thrombosis of cerebral artery

EXCLUDES 1 *occlusion and stenosis of cerebral artery causing cerebral infarction (I63.3-I63.5)*

√5ᵗʰ **I66.0** **Occlusion and stenosis of** middle **cerebral artery**

I66.01 **Occlusion and stenosis of** right **middle cerebral artery** `Q`

I66.02 **Occlusion and stenosis of** left **middle cerebral artery** `Q`

I66.03 **Occlusion and stenosis of** bilateral **middle cerebral arteries** `Q`

I66.09 **Occlusion and stenosis of unspecified middle cerebral artery** `Q`

√5ᵗʰ **I66.1** **Occlusion and stenosis of** anterior **cerebral artery**

I66.11 **Occlusion and stenosis of** right **anterior cerebral artery** `Q`

I66.12 **Occlusion and stenosis of** left **anterior cerebral artery** `Q`

I66.13 **Occlusion and stenosis of** bilateral **anterior cerebral arteries** `Q`

I66.19 **Occlusion and stenosis of unspecified anterior cerebral artery** `Q`

√5ᵗʰ **I66.2** **Occlusion and stenosis of** posterior **cerebral artery**

I66.21 **Occlusion and stenosis of** right **posterior cerebral artery** `Q`

✓ Additional Character Required　　√x7ᵗʰ Placeholder Alert　　Manifestation　　Unspecified Dx　　►◄ Revised Text　　● New Code　　▲ Revised Code Title

I66.22   **Occlusion and stenosis of** left **posterior cerebral artery**   Q

I66.23   **Occlusion and stenosis of** bilateral **posterior cerebral arteries**   Q

I66.29   **Occlusion and stenosis of unspecified posterior cerebral artery**   Q

I66.3   **Occlusion and stenosis of** cerebellar **arteries**   Q

I66.8   **Occlusion and stenosis of other cerebral arteries**   Q

Occlusion and stenosis of perforating arteries

I66.9   **Occlusion and stenosis of unspecified cerebral artery**   Q

✓4th **I67   Other cerebrovascular diseases**

   EXCLUDES 2   *sequelae of the listed conditions (I69.8)*

I67.Ø   **Dissection of cerebral arteries, nonruptured**   HCC

   EXCLUDES 1   *ruptured cerebral arteries (I6Ø.7)*

I67.1   **Cerebral aneurysm, nonruptured**

Cerebral aneurysm NOS
Cerebral arteriovenous fistula, acquired
Internal carotid artery aneurysm, intracranial portion
Internal carotid artery aneurysm, NOS

   EXCLUDES 1   *congenital cerebral aneurysm, nonruptured (Q28.-)*
              ruptured cerebral aneurysm (I6Ø.7)

Berry Aneurysm

Berry aneurysms form at the site of a weakness in an arterial wall, often at a junction

Berry aneurysm

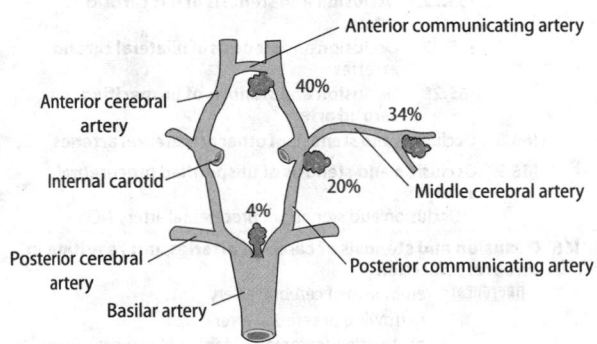

Anterior communicating artery

Anterior cerebral artery   40%

34%

Internal carotid   20%   Middle cerebral artery

4%

Posterior cerebral artery   Posterior communicating artery

Basilar artery

Common sites of berry aneurysms in the circle of Willis arteries

I67.2   **Cerebral atherosclerosis**   Q A

Atheroma of cerebral and precerebral arteries

I67.3   **Progressive vascular leukoencephalopathy**   HCC

Binswanger's disease

I67.4   **Hypertensive encephalopathy**

   EXCLUDES 2   *insufficiency, NOS, of precerebral arteries (G45.2)*

I67.5   **Moyamoya disease**

DEF: Cerebrovascular ischemia. Vessels occlude and rupture, causing tiny hemorrhages at the base of brain. It affects predominantly Japanese people.

I67.6   **Nonpyogenic thrombosis of intracranial venous system**

Nonpyogenic thrombosis of cerebral vein
Nonpyogenic thrombosis of intracranial venous sinus

   EXCLUDES 1   *nonpyogenic thrombosis of intracranial venous system causing infarction (I63.6)*

I67.7   **Cerebral arteritis, not elsewhere classified**

Granulomatous angiitis of the nervous system

   EXCLUDES 1   *allergic granulomatous angiitis (M3Ø.1)*

✓5th I67.8   **Other specified cerebrovascular diseases**

I67.81   **Acute cerebrovascular insufficiency**

Acute cerebrovascular insufficiency unspecified as to location or reversibility

I67.82   **Cerebral ischemia**

Chronic cerebral ischemia

I67.83   **Posterior reversible encephalopathy syndrome**

PRES

✓6th I67.84   **Cerebral vasospasm and vasoconstriction**

I67.841   **Reversible cerebrovascular vasoconstriction syndrome**

Call-Fleming syndrome

Code first underlying condition, if applicable, such as eclampsia (O15.ØØ-O15.9)

I67.848   **Other cerebrovascular vasospasm and vasoconstriction**

✓6th I67.85   **Hereditary cerebrovascular diseases**

AHA: 2018,4Q,17

I67.85Ø   **Cerebral autosomal dominant arteriopathy with subcortical infarcts and leukoencephalopathy**

CADASIL

Code also any associated diagnoses, such as:
epilepsy (G4Ø.-)
stroke (I63.-)
vascular dementia (FØ1.-)

I67.858   **Other hereditary cerebrovascular disease**

I67.89   **Other cerebrovascular disease**

I67.9   **Cerebrovascular disease, unspecified**

✓4th **I68   Cerebrovascular disorders in diseases classified elsewhere**

I68.Ø   *Cerebral amyloid angiopathy*

Code first underlying amyloidosis (E85.-)

I68.2   *Cerebral arteritis in other diseases classified elsewhere*

Code first underlying disease

   EXCLUDES 1   *cerebral arteritis (in):*
             listerosis (A32.89)
             syphilis (A52.Ø4)
             systemic lupus erythematosus (M32.19)
             tuberculosis (A18.89)

I68.8   *Other cerebrovascular disorders in diseases classified elsewhere*

Code first underlying disease

   EXCLUDES 1   *syphilitic cerebral aneurysm (A52.Ø5)*

✓4th **I69   Sequelae of cerebrovascular disease**

NOTE   Category I69 is to be used to indicate conditions in I6Ø-I67 as the cause of sequelae. The "sequelae" include conditions specified as such or as residuals which may occur at any time after the onset of the causal condition

EXCLUDES 1   *personal history of cerebral infarction without residual deficit (Z86.73)*
          personal history of prolonged reversible ischemic neurologic deficit (PRIND) (Z86.73)
          personal history of reversible ischemic neurologcial deficit (RIND) (Z86.73)
          sequelae of traumatic intracranial injury (SØ6.-)

AHA: 2017,1Q,47; 2016,4Q,28; 2015,1Q,25; 2012,4Q,106

TIP: Weakness on one side of the body (unilateral weakness) documented as secondary to old cerebrovascular disease is synonymous with hemiparesis/hemiplegia. Weakness of one limb documented as secondary to old cerebrovascular disease is synonymous with monoplegia.

TIP: For codes describing hemiplegia, hemiparesis, and monoplegia; if the documentation identifies the affected side but not whether it is the dominant or nondominant side, the default is as follows: for ambidextrous patients, the default is dominant; when the left side is affected, the default is nondominant; and when the right side is affected, the default is dominant.

✓5th I69.Ø   **Sequelae of nontraumatic** subarachnoid **hemorrhage**

I69.ØØ   **Unspecified sequelae of nontraumatic subarachnoid hemorrhage**

✓6th I69.Ø1   Cognitive deficits **following nontraumatic subarachnoid hemorrhage**

I69.Ø1Ø   Attention and concentration **deficit following nontraumatic subarachnoid hemorrhage**

I69.Ø11   Memory **deficit following nontraumatic subarachnoid hemorrhage**

    I69.012   **Visuospatial deficit and spatial neglect following nontraumatic subarachnoid hemorrhage**

    I69.013   **Psychomotor deficit following nontraumatic subarachnoid hemorrhage**

    I69.014   **Frontal lobe and executive function deficit following nontraumatic subarachnoid hemorrhage**

    I69.015   **Cognitive social or emotional deficit following nontraumatic subarachnoid hemorrhage**

    I69.018   **Other symptoms and signs involving cognitive functions following nontraumatic subarachnoid hemorrhage**

    I69.019   **Unspecified symptoms and signs involving cognitive functions following nontraumatic subarachnoid hemorrhage**

☑6ᵗʰ   **I69.02**   **Speech and language deficits following nontraumatic subarachnoid hemorrhage**

    I69.020   **Aphasia following nontraumatic subarachnoid hemorrhage**

    I69.021   **Dysphasia following nontraumatic subarachnoid hemorrhage**

    I69.022   **Dysarthria following nontraumatic subarachnoid hemorrhage**

    I69.023   **Fluency disorder following nontraumatic subarachnoid hemorrhage**

        Stuttering following nontraumatic subarachnoid hemorrhage

    I69.028   **Other speech and language deficits following nontraumatic subarachnoid hemorrhage**

☑6ᵗʰ   **I69.03**   **Monoplegia of upper limb following nontraumatic subarachnoid hemorrhage**

    AHA: 2017,1Q,47

    I69.031   **Monoplegia of upper limb following nontraumatic subarachnoid hemorrhage affecting right dominant side**   HCC

    I69.032   **Monoplegia of upper limb following nontraumatic subarachnoid hemorrhage affecting left dominant side**   HCC

    I69.033   **Monoplegia of upper limb following nontraumatic subarachnoid hemorrhage affecting right non-dominant side**   HCC

    I69.034   **Monoplegia of upper limb following nontraumatic subarachnoid hemorrhage affecting left non-dominant side**   HCC

    I69.039   **Monoplegia of upper limb following nontraumatic subarachnoid hemorrhage affecting unspecified side**   HCC

☑6ᵗʰ   **I69.04**   **Monoplegia of lower limb following nontraumatic subarachnoid hemorrhage**

    AHA: 2017,1Q,47

    I69.041   **Monoplegia of lower limb following nontraumatic subarachnoid hemorrhage affecting right dominant side**   HCC

    I69.042   **Monoplegia of lower limb following nontraumatic subarachnoid hemorrhage affecting left dominant side**   HCC

    I69.043   **Monoplegia of lower limb following nontraumatic subarachnoid hemorrhage affecting right non-dominant side**   HCC

    I69.044   **Monoplegia of lower limb following nontraumatic subarachnoid hemorrhage affecting left non-dominant side**   HCC

    I69.049   **Monoplegia of lower limb following nontraumatic subarachnoid hemorrhage affecting unspecified side**   HCC

☑6ᵗʰ   **I69.05**   **Hemiplegia and hemiparesis following nontraumatic subarachnoid hemorrhage**

    AHA: 2015,1Q,25

    I69.051   **Hemiplegia and hemiparesis following nontraumatic subarachnoid hemorrhage affecting right dominant side**   HCC

    I69.052   **Hemiplegia and hemiparesis following nontraumatic subarachnoid hemorrhage affecting left dominant side**   HCC

    I69.053   **Hemiplegia and hemiparesis following nontraumatic subarachnoid hemorrhage affecting right non-dominant side**   HCC

    I69.054   **Hemiplegia and hemiparesis following nontraumatic subarachnoid hemorrhage affecting left non-dominant side**   HCC

    I69.059   **Hemiplegia and hemiparesis following nontraumatic subarachnoid hemorrhage affecting unspecified side**   HCC

☑6ᵗʰ   **I69.06**   **Other paralytic syndrome following nontraumatic subarachnoid hemorrhage**

    Use additional code to identify type of paralytic syndrome, such as:

    locked-in state (G83.5)

    quadriplegia (G82.5-)

    EXCLUDES 1   *hemiplegia/hemiparesis following nontraumatic subarachnoid hemorrhage (I69.05-)*

        monoplegia of lower limb following nontraumatic subarachnoid hemorrhage (I69.04-)

        monoplegia of upper limb following nontraumatic subarachnoid hemorrhage (I69.03-)

    I69.061   **Other paralytic syndrome following nontraumatic subarachnoid hemorrhage affecting right dominant side**   HCC

    I69.062   **Other paralytic syndrome following nontraumatic subarachnoid hemorrhage affecting left dominant side**   HCC

    I69.063   **Other paralytic syndrome following nontraumatic subarachnoid hemorrhage affecting right non-dominant side**   HCC

    I69.064   **Other paralytic syndrome following nontraumatic subarachnoid hemorrhage affecting left non-dominant side**   HCC

    I69.065   **Other paralytic syndrome following nontraumatic subarachnoid hemorrhage, bilateral**   HCC

    I69.069   **Other paralytic syndrome following nontraumatic subarachnoid hemorrhage affecting unspecified side**   HCC

☑6ᵗʰ   **I69.09**   **Other sequelae of nontraumatic subarachnoid hemorrhage**

    I69.090   **Apraxia following nontraumatic subarachnoid hemorrhage**

    I69.091   **Dysphagia following nontraumatic subarachnoid hemorrhage**

        Use additional code to identify the type of dysphagia, if known (R13.1-)

    I69.092   **Facial weakness following nontraumatic subarachnoid hemorrhage**

        Facial droop following nontraumatic subarachnoid hemorrhage

    I69.093   **Ataxia following nontraumatic subarachnoid hemorrhage**

☑ Additional Character Required   ☑x7ᵗʰ Placeholder Alert   Manifestation   Unspecified Dx   ►◄ Revised Text   ● New Code   ▲ Revised Code Title

I69.Ø98 Other sequelae following nontraumatic subarachnoid hemorrhage
Alterations of sensation following nontraumatic subarachnoid hemorrhage
Disturbance of vision following nontraumatic subarachnoid hemorrhage
Use additional code to identify the sequelae

✓5ᵗʰ **I69.1 Sequelae of nontraumatic intracerebral hemorrhage**

I69.10 Unspecified sequelae of nontraumatic intracerebral hemorrhage

✓6ᵗʰ **I69.11 Cognitive deficits following nontraumatic intracerebral hemorrhage**

I69.110 Attention and concentration deficit following nontraumatic intracerebral hemorrhage

I69.111 Memory deficit following nontraumatic intracerebral hemorrhage

I69.112 Visuospatial deficit and spatial neglect following nontraumatic intracerebral hemorrhage

I69.113 Psychomotor deficit following nontraumatic intracerebral hemorrhage

I69.114 Frontal lobe and executive function deficit following nontraumatic intracerebral hemorrhage

I69.115 Cognitive social or emotional deficit following nontraumatic intracerebral hemorrhage

I69.118 Other symptoms and signs involving cognitive functions following nontraumatic intracerebral hemorrhage

I69.119 Unspecified symptoms and signs involving cognitive functions following nontraumatic intracerebral hemorrhage

✓6ᵗʰ **I69.12 Speech and language deficits following nontraumatic intracerebral hemorrhage**

I69.120 Aphasia following nontraumatic intracerebral hemorrhage

I69.121 Dysphasia following nontraumatic intracerebral hemorrhage

I69.122 Dysarthria following nontraumatic intracerebral hemorrhage

I69.123 Fluency disorder following nontraumatic intracerebral hemorrhage
Stuttering following nontraumatic intracerebral hemorrhage

I69.128 Other speech and language deficits following nontraumatic intracerebral hemorrhage

✓6ᵗʰ **I69.13 Monoplegia of upper limb following nontraumatic intracerebral hemorrhage**
AHA: 2017,1Q,47

I69.131 Monoplegia of upper limb following nontraumatic intracerebral hemorrhage affecting right dominant side `HCC`

I69.132 Monoplegia of upper limb following nontraumatic intracerebral hemorrhage affecting left dominant side `HCC`

I69.133 Monoplegia of upper limb following nontraumatic intracerebral hemorrhage affecting right non-dominant side `HCC`

I69.134 Monoplegia of upper limb following nontraumatic intracerebral hemorrhage affecting left non-dominant side `HCC`

I69.139 Monoplegia of upper limb following nontraumatic intracerebral hemorrhage affecting unspecified side `HCC`

✓6ᵗʰ **I69.14 Monoplegia of lower limb following nontraumatic intracerebral hemorrhage**
AHA: 2017,1Q,47

I69.141 Monoplegia of lower limb following nontraumatic intracerebral hemorrhage affecting right dominant side `HCC`

I69.142 Monoplegia of lower limb following nontraumatic intracerebral hemorrhage affecting left dominant side `HCC`

I69.143 Monoplegia of lower limb following nontraumatic intracerebral hemorrhage affecting right non-dominant side `HCC`

I69.144 Monoplegia of lower limb following nontraumatic intracerebral hemorrhage affecting left non-dominant side `HCC`

I69.149 Monoplegia of lower limb following nontraumatic intracerebral hemorrhage affecting unspecified side `HCC`

✓6ᵗʰ **I69.15 Hemiplegia and hemiparesis following nontraumatic intracerebral hemorrhage**
AHA: 2015,1Q,25

I69.151 Hemiplegia and hemiparesis following nontraumatic intracerebral hemorrhage affecting right dominant side `HCC`

I69.152 Hemiplegia and hemiparesis following nontraumatic intracerebral hemorrhage affecting left dominant side `HCC`

I69.153 Hemiplegia and hemiparesis following nontraumatic intracerebral hemorrhage affecting right non-dominant side `HCC`

I69.154 Hemiplegia and hemiparesis following nontraumatic intracerebral hemorrhage affecting left non-dominant side `HCC`

I69.159 Hemiplegia and hemiparesis following nontraumatic intracerebral hemorrhage affecting unspecified side `HCC`

✓6ᵗʰ **I69.16 Other paralytic syndrome following nontraumatic intracerebral hemorrhage**
Use additional code to identify type of paralytic syndrome, such as:
locked-in state (G83.5)
quadriplegia (G82.5-)
EXCLUDES 1 hemiplegia/hemiparesis following nontraumatic intracerebral hemorrhage (I69.15-)
monoplegia of lower limb following nontraumatic intracerebral hemorrhage (I69.14-)
monoplegia of upper limb following nontraumatic intracerebral hemorrhage (I69.13-)

I69.161 Other paralytic syndrome following nontraumatic intracerebral hemorrhage affecting right dominant side `HCC`

I69.162 Other paralytic syndrome following nontraumatic intracerebral hemorrhage affecting left dominant side `HCC`

I69.163 Other paralytic syndrome following nontraumatic intracerebral hemorrhage affecting right non-dominant side `HCC`

I69.164 Other paralytic syndrome following nontraumatic intracerebral hemorrhage affecting left non-dominant side `HCC`

I69.165 Other paralytic syndrome following nontraumatic intracerebral hemorrhage, bilateral `HCC`

I69.169 Other paralytic syndrome following nontraumatic intracerebral hemorrhage affecting unspecified side `HCC`

✓6ᵗʰ **I69.19** **Other sequelae of nontraumatic intracerebral hemorrhage**

I69.190 **Apraxia** following nontraumatic intracerebral hemorrhage

I69.191 **Dysphagia** following nontraumatic intracerebral hemorrhage
Use additional code to identify the type of dysphagia, if known (R13.1-)

I69.192 **Facial weakness** following nontraumatic intracerebral hemorrhage
Facial droop following nontraumatic intracerebral hemorrhage

I69.193 **Ataxia** following nontraumatic intracerebral hemorrhage

I69.198 **Other sequelae of nontraumatic intracerebral hemorrhage**
Alteration of sensations following nontraumatic intracerebral hemorrhage
Disturbance of vision following nontraumatic intracerebral hemorrhage
Use additional code to identify the sequelae

✓5ᵗʰ **I69.2** **Sequelae of other nontraumatic intracranial hemorrhage**

I69.20 **Unspecified sequelae of other nontraumatic intracranial hemorrhage**

✓6ᵗʰ **I69.21** **Cognitive deficits following other nontraumatic intracranial hemorrhage**

I69.210 **Attention and concentration deficit** following other nontraumatic intracranial hemorrhage

I69.211 **Memory deficit** following other nontraumatic intracranial hemorrhage

I69.212 **Visuospatial deficit and spatial neglect** following other nontraumatic intracranial hemorrhage

I69.213 **Psychomotor deficit** following other nontraumatic intracranial hemorrhage

I69.214 **Frontal lobe and executive function deficit** following other nontraumatic intracranial hemorrhage

I69.215 **Cognitive social or emotional deficit** following other nontraumatic intracranial hemorrhage

I69.218 **Other symptoms and signs involving cognitive functions** following other nontraumatic intracranial hemorrhage

I69.219 **Unspecified symptoms and signs involving cognitive functions** following other nontraumatic intracranial hemorrhage

✓6ᵗʰ **I69.22** **Speech and language deficits following other nontraumatic intracranial hemorrhage**

I69.220 **Aphasia** following other nontraumatic intracranial hemorrhage

I69.221 **Dysphasia** following other nontraumatic intracranial hemorrhage

I69.222 **Dysarthria** following other nontraumatic intracranial hemorrhage

I69.223 **Fluency disorder** following other nontraumatic intracranial hemorrhage
Stuttering following other nontraumatic intracranial hemorrhage

I69.228 **Other speech and language deficits** following other nontraumatic intracranial hemorrhage

✓6ᵗʰ **I69.23** **Monoplegia of upper limb following other nontraumatic intracranial hemorrhage**
AHA: 2017,1Q,47

I69.231 **Monoplegia of upper limb following other nontraumatic intracranial hemorrhage affecting right dominant side**   HCC

I69.232 **Monoplegia of upper limb following other nontraumatic intracranial hemorrhage affecting left dominant side**   HCC

I69.233 **Monoplegia of upper limb following other nontraumatic intracranial hemorrhage affecting right non-dominant side**   HCC

I69.234 **Monoplegia of upper limb following other nontraumatic intracranial hemorrhage affecting left non-dominant side**   HCC

I69.239 **Monoplegia of upper limb following other nontraumatic intracranial hemorrhage affecting unspecified side**   HCC

✓6ᵗʰ **I69.24** **Monoplegia of lower limb following other nontraumatic intracranial hemorrhage**
AHA: 2017,1Q,47

I69.241 **Monoplegia of lower limb following other nontraumatic intracranial hemorrhage affecting right dominant side**   HCC

I69.242 **Monoplegia of lower limb following other nontraumatic intracranial hemorrhage affecting left dominant side**   HCC

I69.243 **Monoplegia of lower limb following other nontraumatic intracranial hemorrhage affecting right non-dominant side**   HCC

I69.244 **Monoplegia of lower limb following other nontraumatic intracranial hemorrhage affecting left non-dominant side**   HCC

I69.249 **Monoplegia of lower limb following other nontraumatic intracranial hemorrhage affecting unspecified side**   HCC

✓6ᵗʰ **I69.25** **Hemiplegia and hemiparesis following other nontraumatic intracranial hemorrhage**
AHA: 2015,1Q,25

I69.251 **Hemiplegia and hemiparesis following other nontraumatic intracranial hemorrhage affecting right dominant side**   HCC

I69.252 **Hemiplegia and hemiparesis following other nontraumatic intracranial hemorrhage affecting left dominant side**   HCC

I69.253 **Hemiplegia and hemiparesis following other nontraumatic intracranial hemorrhage affecting right non-dominant side**   HCC

I69.254 **Hemiplegia and hemiparesis following other nontraumatic intracranial hemorrhage affecting left non-dominant side**   HCC

I69.259 **Hemiplegia and hemiparesis following other nontraumatic intracranial hemorrhage affecting unspecified side**   HCC

✓6ᵗʰ **I69.26** **Other paralytic syndrome following other nontraumatic intracranial hemorrhage**
Use additional code to identify type of paralytic syndrome, such as:
locked-in state (G83.5)
quadriplegia (G82.5-)
EXCLUDES 1   *hemiplegia/hemiparesis following other nontraumatic intracranial hemorrhage (I69.25-)*
monoplegia of lower limb following other nontraumatic intracranial hemorrhage (I69.24-)
monoplegia of upper limb following other nontraumatic intracranial hemorrhage (I69.23-)

I69.261 **Other paralytic syndrome following other nontraumatic intracranial hemorrhage affecting right dominant side**   HCC

I69.262 **Other paralytic syndrome following other nontraumatic intracranial hemorrhage affecting left dominant side**   HCC

I69.263 **Other paralytic syndrome following other nontraumatic intracranial hemorrhage affecting right non-dominant side**   HCC

Chapter 9. Diseases of the Circulatory System

I69.264 Other paralytic syndrome following other nontraumatic intracranial hemorrhage affecting left non-dominant side `HCC`

I69.265 Other paralytic syndrome following other nontraumatic intracranial hemorrhage, bilateral `HCC`

I69.269 Other paralytic syndrome following other nontraumatic intracranial hemorrhage affecting unspecified side `HCC`

√6ᵗʰ **I69.29** Other sequelae of other nontraumatic intracranial hemorrhage

I69.290 Apraxia following other nontraumatic intracranial hemorrhage

I69.291 Dysphagia following other nontraumatic intracranial hemorrhage

Use additional code to identify the type of dysphagia, if known (R13.1-)

I69.292 Facial weakness following other nontraumatic intracranial hemorrhage

Facial droop following other nontraumatic intracranial hemorrhage

I69.293 Ataxia following other nontraumatic intracranial hemorrhage

I69.298 Other sequelae of other nontraumatic intracranial hemorrhage

Alteration of sensation following other nontraumatic intracranial hemorrhage

Disturbance of vision following other nontraumatic intracranial hemorrhage

Use additional code to identify the sequelae

√5ᵗʰ **I69.3** Sequelae of cerebral infarction

Sequelae of stroke NOS

AHA: 2013,4Q,127-128; 2012,4Q,92,94

I69.30 Unspecified sequelae of cerebral infarction

√6ᵗʰ **I69.31** Cognitive deficits following cerebral infarction

I69.310 Attention and concentration deficit following cerebral infarction

I69.311 Memory deficit following cerebral infarction

I69.312 Visuospatial deficit and spatial neglect following cerebral infarction

I69.313 Psychomotor deficit following cerebral infarction

I69.314 Frontal lobe and executive function deficit following cerebral infarction

I69.315 Cognitive social or emotional deficit following cerebral infarction

I69.318 Other symptoms and signs involving cognitive functions following cerebral infarction

I69.319 Unspecified symptoms and signs involving cognitive functions following cerebral infarction

I69.32 Speech and language deficits following cerebral infarction

I69.320 Aphasia following cerebral infarction

I69.321 Dysphasia following cerebral infarction

AHA: 2012,4Q,91

I69.322 Dysarthria following cerebral infarction

EXCLUDES 2 transient ischemic attack (TIA) (G45.9)

I69.323 Fluency disorder following cerebral infarction

Stuttering following cerebral infarction

I69.328 Other speech and language deficits following cerebral infarction

√6ᵗʰ **I69.33** Monoplegia of upper limb following cerebral infarction

AHA: 2017,1Q,47

I69.331 Monoplegia of upper limb following cerebral infarction affecting right dominant side `HCC`

I69.332 Monoplegia of upper limb following cerebral infarction affecting left dominant side `HCC`

I69.333 Monoplegia of upper limb following cerebral infarction affecting right non-dominant side `HCC`

I69.334 Monoplegia of upper limb following cerebral infarction affecting left non-dominant side `HCC`

I69.339 Monoplegia of upper limb following cerebral infarction affecting unspecified side `HCC`

√6ᵗʰ **I69.34** Monoplegia of lower limb following cerebral infarction

AHA: 2017,1Q,47

I69.341 Monoplegia of lower limb following cerebral infarction affecting right dominant side `HCC`

I69.342 Monoplegia of lower limb following cerebral infarction affecting left dominant side `HCC`

I69.343 Monoplegia of lower limb following cerebral infarction affecting right non-dominant side `HCC`

I69.344 Monoplegia of lower limb following cerebral infarction affecting left non-dominant side `HCC`

I69.349 Monoplegia of lower limb following cerebral infarction affecting unspecified side `HCC`

√6ᵗʰ **I69.35** Hemiplegia and hemiparesis following cerebral infarction

AHA: 2015,1Q,25

I69.351 Hemiplegia and hemiparesis following cerebral infarction affecting right dominant side `HCC`

EXCLUDES 2 transient ischemic attack (TIA) (G45.9)

I69.352 Hemiplegia and hemiparesis following cerebral infarction affecting left dominant side `HCC`

I69.353 Hemiplegia and hemiparesis following cerebral infarction affecting right non-dominant side `HCC`

I69.354 Hemiplegia and hemiparesis following cerebral infarction affecting left non-dominant side `HCC`

AHA: 2012,4Q,91

I69.359 Hemiplegia and hemiparesis following cerebral infarction affecting unspecified side `HCC`

√6ᵗʰ **I69.36** Other paralytic syndrome following cerebral infarction

Use additional code to identify type of paralytic syndrome, such as:

locked-in state (G83.5)

quadriplegia (G82.5-)

EXCLUDES 1 hemiplegia/hemiparesis following cerebral infarction (I69.35-)

monoplegia of lower limb following cerebral infarction (I69.34-)

monoplegia of upper limb following cerebral infarction (I69.33-)

I69.361 Other paralytic syndrome following cerebral infarction affecting right dominant side `HCC`

I69.362 Other paralytic syndrome following cerebral infarction affecting left dominant side `HCC`

I69.363 Other paralytic syndrome following cerebral infarction affecting right non-dominant side `HCC`

I69.364 Other paralytic syndrome following cerebral infarction affecting left non-dominant side `HCC`

I69.365 Other paralytic syndrome following cerebral infarction, bilateral `HCC`

I69.369 Other paralytic syndrome following cerebral infarction affecting unspecified side `HCC`

☑6ᵗʰ **I69.39** **Other sequelae of cerebral infarction**

    I69.390 **Apraxia** following cerebral infarction

    I69.391 **Dysphagia** following cerebral infarction
        Use additional code to identify the type of dysphagia, if known (R13.1-)

    I69.392 **Facial weakness** following cerebral infarction
        Facial droop following cerebral infarction

    I69.393 **Ataxia** following cerebral infarction

    I69.398 **Other sequelae** of cerebral infarction
        Alteration of sensation following cerebral infarction
        Disturbance of vision following cerebral infarction
        Use additional code to identify the sequelae

☑5ᵗʰ **I69.8** **Sequelae of other cerebrovascular diseases**

    EXCLUDES 1 *sequelae of traumatic intracranial injury (S06.-)*

    I69.80 **Unspecified sequelae of other cerebrovascular disease**

☑6ᵗʰ **I69.81** **Cognitive deficits** following other cerebrovascular disease

    I69.810 **Attention and concentration deficit** following other cerebrovascular disease

    I69.811 **Memory deficit** following other cerebrovascular disease

    I69.812 **Visuospatial deficit and spatial neglect** following other cerebrovascular disease

    I69.813 **Psychomotor deficit** following other cerebrovascular disease

    I69.814 **Frontal lobe and executive function deficit** following other cerebrovascular disease

    I69.815 **Cognitive social or emotional deficit** following other cerebrovascular disease

    I69.818 **Other symptoms and signs involving cognitive functions** following other cerebrovascular disease

    I69.819 **Unspecified symptoms and signs involving cognitive functions** following other cerebrovascular disease

☑6ᵗʰ **I69.82** **Speech and language deficits** following other cerebrovascular disease

    I69.820 **Aphasia** following other cerebrovascular disease

    I69.821 **Dysphasia** following other cerebrovascular disease

    I69.822 **Dysarthria** following other cerebrovascular disease

    I69.823 **Fluency disorder** following other cerebrovascular disease
        Stuttering following other cerebrovascular disease

    I69.828 **Other speech and language deficits** following other cerebrovascular disease

☑6ᵗʰ **I69.83** **Monoplegia of upper limb** following other cerebrovascular disease
    AHA: 2017,1Q,47

    I69.831 **Monoplegia of upper limb** following other cerebrovascular disease affecting **right dominant** side `HCC`

    I69.832 **Monoplegia of upper limb** following other cerebrovascular disease affecting **left dominant** side `HCC`

    I69.833 **Monoplegia of upper limb** following other cerebrovascular disease affecting **right non-dominant** side `HCC`

    I69.834 **Monoplegia of upper limb** following other cerebrovascular disease affecting **left non-dominant** side `HCC`

    I69.839 **Monoplegia of upper limb** following other cerebrovascular disease affecting **unspecified** side `HCC`

☑6ᵗʰ **I69.84** **Monoplegia of lower limb** following other cerebrovascular disease
    AHA: 2017,1Q,47

    I69.841 **Monoplegia of lower limb** following other cerebrovascular disease affecting **right dominant** side `HCC`

    I69.842 **Monoplegia of lower limb** following other cerebrovascular disease affecting **left dominant** side `HCC`

    I69.843 **Monoplegia of lower limb** following other cerebrovascular disease affecting **right non-dominant** side `HCC`

    I69.844 **Monoplegia of lower limb** following other cerebrovascular disease affecting **left non-dominant** side `HCC`

    I69.849 **Monoplegia of lower limb** following other cerebrovascular disease affecting **unspecified** side `HCC`

☑6ᵗʰ **I69.85** **Hemiplegia and hemiparesis** following other cerebrovascular disease
    AHA: 2015,1Q,25

    I69.851 **Hemiplegia and hemiparesis** following other cerebrovascular disease affecting **right dominant** side `HCC`

    I69.852 **Hemiplegia and hemiparesis** following other cerebrovascular disease affecting **left dominant** side `HCC`

    I69.853 **Hemiplegia and hemiparesis** following other cerebrovascular disease affecting **right non-dominant** side `HCC`

    I69.854 **Hemiplegia and hemiparesis** following other cerebrovascular disease affecting **left non-dominant** side `HCC`

    I69.859 **Hemiplegia and hemiparesis** following other cerebrovascular disease affecting **unspecified** side `HCC`

☑6ᵗʰ **I69.86** **Other paralytic syndrome** following other cerebrovascular disease
    Use additional code to identify type of paralytic syndrome, such as:
    locked-in state (G83.5)
    quadriplegia (G82.5-)

    EXCLUDES 1 *hemiplegia/hemiparesis following other cerebrovascular disease (I69.85-)*
        monoplegia of lower limb following other cerebrovascular disease (I69.84-)
        monoplegia of upper limb following other cerebrovascular disease (I69.83-)

    I69.861 **Other paralytic syndrome** following other cerebrovascular disease affecting **right dominant** side `HCC`

    I69.862 **Other paralytic syndrome** following other cerebrovascular disease affecting **left dominant** side `HCC`

    I69.863 **Other paralytic syndrome** following other cerebrovascular disease affecting **right non-dominant** side `HCC`

    I69.864 **Other paralytic syndrome** following other cerebrovascular disease affecting **left non-dominant** side `HCC`

    I69.865 **Other paralytic syndrome** following other cerebrovascular disease, **bilateral** `HCC`

    I69.869 **Other paralytic syndrome** following other cerebrovascular disease affecting **unspecified** side `HCC`

☑6ᵗʰ **I69.89** **Other sequelae of other cerebrovascular disease**

    I69.890 **Apraxia** following other cerebrovascular disease

---

☑ Additional Character Required   ✓x7ᵗʰ Placeholder Alert   Manifestation   Unspecified Dx   ►◄ Revised Text   ● New Code   ▲ Revised Code Title

ICD-10-CM 2020   **657**

Chapter 9. Diseases of the Circulatory System

I69.891–I69.964

I69.891 Dysphagia following other cerebrovascular disease
Use additional code to identify the type of dysphagia, if known (R13.1-)

I69.892 Facial weakness following other cerebrovascular disease
Facial droop following other cerebrovascular disease

I69.893 Ataxia following other cerebrovascular disease

I69.898 Other sequelae of other cerebrovascular disease
Alteration of sensation following other cerebrovascular disease
Disturbance of vision following other cerebrovascular disease
Use additional code to identify the sequelae

✓5ᵗʰ **I69.9 Sequelae of unspecified cerebrovascular diseases**
EXCLUDES 1   sequelae of stroke (I69.3)
sequelae of traumatic intracranial injury (S06.-)

I69.90 Unspecified sequelae of unspecified cerebrovascular disease

✓6ᵗʰ **I69.91 Cognitive deficits following unspecified cerebrovascular disease**

I69.910 Attention and concentration deficit following unspecified cerebrovascular disease

I69.911 Memory deficit following unspecified cerebrovascular disease

I69.912 Visuospatial deficit and spatial neglect following unspecified cerebrovascular disease

I69.913 Psychomotor deficit following unspecified cerebrovascular disease

I69.914 Frontal lobe and executive function deficit following unspecified cerebrovascular disease

I69.915 Cognitive social or emotional deficit following unspecified cerebrovascular disease

I69.918 Other symptoms and signs involving cognitive functions following unspecified cerebrovascular disease

I69.919 Unspecified symptoms and signs involving cognitive functions following unspecified cerebrovascular disease

✓6ᵗʰ **I69.92 Speech and language deficits following unspecified cerebrovascular disease**

I69.920 Aphasia following unspecified cerebrovascular disease

I69.921 Dysphasia following unspecified cerebrovascular disease

I69.922 Dysarthria following unspecified cerebrovascular disease

I69.923 Fluency disorder following unspecified cerebrovascular disease
Stuttering following unspecified cerebrovascular disease

I69.928 Other speech and language deficits following unspecified cerebrovascular disease

✓6ᵗʰ **I69.93 Monoplegia of upper limb following unspecified cerebrovascular disease**
AHA: 2017,1Q,47

I69.931 Monoplegia of upper limb following unspecified cerebrovascular disease affecting right dominant side HCC

I69.932 Monoplegia of upper limb following unspecified cerebrovascular disease affecting left dominant side HCC

I69.933 Monoplegia of upper limb following unspecified cerebrovascular disease affecting right non-dominant side HCC

I69.934 Monoplegia of upper limb following unspecified cerebrovascular disease affecting left non-dominant side HCC

I69.939 Monoplegia of upper limb following unspecified cerebrovascular disease affecting unspecified side HCC

✓6ᵗʰ **I69.94 Monoplegia of lower limb following unspecified cerebrovascular disease**
AHA: 2017,1Q,47

I69.941 Monoplegia of lower limb following unspecified cerebrovascular disease affecting right dominant side HCC

I69.942 Monoplegia of lower limb following unspecified cerebrovascular disease affecting left dominant side HCC

I69.943 Monoplegia of lower limb following unspecified cerebrovascular disease affecting right non-dominant side HCC

I69.944 Monoplegia of lower limb following unspecified cerebrovascular disease affecting left non-dominant side HCC

I69.949 Monoplegia of lower limb following unspecified cerebrovascular disease affecting unspecified side HCC

✓6ᵗʰ **I69.95 Hemiplegia and hemiparesis following unspecified cerebrovascular disease**
AHA: 2015,1Q,25

I69.951 Hemiplegia and hemiparesis following unspecified cerebrovascular disease affecting right dominant side HCC

I69.952 Hemiplegia and hemiparesis following unspecified cerebrovascular disease affecting left dominant side HCC

I69.953 Hemiplegia and hemiparesis following unspecified cerebrovascular disease affecting right non-dominant side HCC

I69.954 Hemiplegia and hemiparesis following unspecified cerebrovascular disease affecting left non-dominant side HCC

I69.959 Hemiplegia and hemiparesis following unspecified cerebrovascular disease affecting unspecified side HCC

✓6ᵗʰ **I69.96 Other paralytic syndrome following unspecified cerebrovascular disease**
Use additional code to identify type of paralytic syndrome, such as:
locked-in state (G83.5)
quadriplegia (G82.5-)
EXCLUDES 1   hemiplegia/hemiparesis following unspecified cerebrovascular disease (I69.95-)
monoplegia of lower limb following unspecified cerebrovascular disease (I69.94-)
monoplegia of upper limb following unspecified cerebrovascular disease (I69.93-)

I69.961 Other paralytic syndrome following unspecified cerebrovascular disease affecting right dominant side HCC

I69.962 Other paralytic syndrome following unspecified cerebrovascular disease affecting left dominant side HCC

I69.963 Other paralytic syndrome following unspecified cerebrovascular disease affecting right non-dominant side HCC

I69.964 Other paralytic syndrome following unspecified cerebrovascular disease affecting left non-dominant side HCC

I69.965 Other paralytic syndrome following unspecified cerebrovascular disease, **bilateral**   HCC

I69.969 Other paralytic syndrome following unspecified cerebrovascular disease **affecting unspecified side**   HCC

✓6ᵗʰ **I69.99** Other sequelae of unspecified cerebrovascular disease

I69.990 **Apraxia** following unspecified cerebrovascular disease

I69.991 **Dysphagia** following unspecified cerebrovascular disease

Use additional code to identify the type of dysphagia, if known (R13.1-)

I69.992 **Facial weakness** following unspecified cerebrovascular disease

Facial droop following unspecified cerebrovascular disease

I69.993 **Ataxia** following unspecified cerebrovascular disease

I69.998 Other sequelae following unspecified cerebrovascular disease

Alteration in sensation following unspecified cerebrovascular disease

Disturbance of vision following unspecified cerebrovascular disease

Use additional code to identify the sequelae

Diseases of arteries, arterioles and capillaries (I70-I79)

✓4ᵗʰ **I70** **Atherosclerosis**

INCLUDES   arterial degeneration
arteriolosclerosis
arteriosclerosis
arteriosclerotic vascular disease
arteriovascular degeneration
atheroma
endarteritis deformans or obliterans
senile arteritis
senile endarteritis
vascular degeneration

Use additional code to identify:
exposure to environmental tobacco smoke (Z77.22)
history of tobacco dependence (Z87.891)
occupational exposure to environmental tobacco smoke (Z57.31)
tobacco dependence (F17.-)
tobacco use (Z72.0)

EXCLUDES 2   *arteriosclerotic cardiovascular disease (I25.1-)*
arteriosclerotic heart disease (I25.1-)
atheroembolism (I75.-)
cerebral atherosclerosis (I67.2)
coronary atherosclerosis (I25.1-)
mesenteric atherosclerosis (K55.1)
precerebral atherosclerosis (I67.2)
primary pulmonary atherosclerosis (I27.0)

I70.0 **Atherosclerosis of aorta**   HCC Q A

I70.1 **Atherosclerosis of renal artery**   HCC Q A

Goldblatt's kidney

EXCLUDES 2   *atherosclerosis of renal arterioles (I12.-)*

✓5ᵗʰ **I70.2** **Atherosclerosis of native arteries of the extremities**

Mönckeberg's (medial) sclerosis

Use additional code, if applicable, to identify chronic total occlusion of artery of extremity (I70.92)

EXCLUDES 2   *atherosclerosis of bypass graft of extremities (I70.30-I70.79)*

AHA: 2018,3Q,4; 2018,2Q,7

✓6ᵗʰ **I70.20** **Unspecified atherosclerosis of native arteries of extremities**

I70.201 Unspecified atherosclerosis of   HCC Q A native arteries of extremities, **right leg**

I70.202 Unspecified atherosclerosis of   HCC Q A native arteries of extremities, **left leg**

I70.203 Unspecified atherosclerosis of   HCC Q A native arteries of extremities, **bilateral legs**

I70.208 Unspecified atherosclerosis of   HCC Q A native arteries of extremities, **other extremity**

I70.209 Unspecified atherosclerosis of   HCC Q A native arteries of extremities, **unspecified extremity**

✓6ᵗʰ **I70.21** **Atherosclerosis of native arteries of extremities with intermittent claudication**

I70.211 **Atherosclerosis of native**   HCC Q A **arteries of extremities with intermittent claudication, right leg**

I70.212 **Atherosclerosis of native**   HCC Q A **arteries of extremities with intermittent claudication, left leg**

I70.213 **Atherosclerosis of native**   HCC Q A **arteries of extremities with intermittent claudication, bilateral legs**

I70.218 **Atherosclerosis of native**   HCC Q A **arteries of extremities with intermittent claudication, other extremity**

I70.219 **Atherosclerosis of native**   HCC Q A **arteries of extremities with intermittent claudication, unspecified extremity**

✓6ᵗʰ **I70.22** **Atherosclerosis of native arteries of extremities with rest pain**

INCLUDES   any condition classifiable to I70.21-

I70.221 **Atherosclerosis of native**   HCC Q A **arteries of extremities with rest pain, right leg**

I70.222 **Atherosclerosis of native**   HCC Q A **arteries of extremities with rest pain, left leg**

I70.223 **Atherosclerosis of native**   HCC Q A **arteries of extremities with rest pain, bilateral legs**

I70.228 **Atherosclerosis of native**   HCC Q A **arteries of extremities with rest pain, other extremity**

I70.229 **Atherosclerosis of native**   HCC Q A **arteries of extremities with rest pain, unspecified extremity**

✓6ᵗʰ **I70.23** **Atherosclerosis of native arteries of right leg with ulceration**

INCLUDES   any condition classifiable to I70.211 and I70.221

Use additional code to identify severity of ulcer (L97.-)

I70.231 **Atherosclerosis of native**   HCC Q A **arteries of right leg with ulceration of thigh**

I70.232 **Atherosclerosis of native**   HCC Q A **arteries of right leg with ulceration of calf**

I70.233 **Atherosclerosis of native**   HCC Q A **arteries of right leg with ulceration of ankle**

I70.234 **Atherosclerosis of native**   HCC Q A **arteries of right leg with ulceration of heel and midfoot**

Atherosclerosis of native arteries of right leg with ulceration of plantar surface of midfoot

I70.235 **Atherosclerosis of native**   HCC Q A **arteries of right leg with ulceration of other part of foot**

Atherosclerosis of native arteries of right leg extremities with ulceration of toe

▲ **I70.238** **Atherosclerosis of native**   HCC Q A **arteries of right leg with ulceration of other part of lower leg**

I70.239 **Atherosclerosis of native**   HCC Q A **arteries of right leg with ulceration of unspecified site**

✔ Additional Character Required   ✓ₓ7ᵗʰ Placeholder Alert   Manifestation   Unspecified Dx   ▶◀ Revised Text   ● New Code   ▲ Revised Code Title

ICD-10-CM 2020   659

√6ᵗʰ **I70.24** **Atherosclerosis of native arteries of left leg with ulceration**

     INCLUDES   any condition classifiable to I70.212 and I70.222

     Use additional code to identify severity of ulcer (L97.-)

I70.241 **Atherosclerosis of native arteries of left leg with ulceration of thigh** HCC Q A

I70.242 **Atherosclerosis of native arteries of left leg with ulceration of calf** HCC Q A

I70.243 **Atherosclerosis of native arteries of left leg with ulceration of ankle** HCC Q A

I70.244 **Atherosclerosis of native arteries of left leg with ulceration of heel and midfoot** HCC Q A

     Atherosclerosis of native arteries of left leg with ulceration of plantar surface of midfoot

I70.245 **Atherosclerosis of native arteries of left leg with ulceration of other part of foot** HCC Q A

     Atherosclerosis of native arteries of left leg extremities with ulceration of toe

I70.248 **Atherosclerosis of native arteries of left leg with ulceration of other part of lower leg** HCC Q A

I70.249 **Atherosclerosis of native arteries of left leg with ulceration of unspecified site** HCC Q A

I70.25 **Atherosclerosis of native arteries of other extremities with ulceration** HCC Q A

     INCLUDES   any condition classifiable to I70.218 and I70.228

     Use additional code to identify the severity of the ulcer (L98.49-)

√6ᵗʰ **I70.26** **Atherosclerosis of native arteries of extremities with gangrene**

     INCLUDES   any condition classifiable to I70.21-, I70.22-, I70.23-, I70.24-, and I70.25-

     Use additional code to identify the severity of any ulcer (L97.-, L98.49-), if applicable

I70.261 **Atherosclerosis of native arteries of extremities with gangrene, right leg** HCC Q A

I70.262 **Atherosclerosis of native arteries of extremities with gangrene, left leg** HCC Q A

I70.263 **Atherosclerosis of native arteries of extremities with gangrene, bilateral legs** HCC Q A

I70.268 **Atherosclerosis of native arteries of extremities with gangrene, other extremity** HCC Q A

I70.269 **Atherosclerosis of native arteries of extremities with gangrene, unspecified extremity** HCC Q A

√6ᵗʰ **I70.29** **Other atherosclerosis of native arteries of extremities**

I70.291 **Other atherosclerosis of native arteries of extremities, right leg** HCC Q A

I70.292 **Other atherosclerosis of native arteries of extremities, left leg** HCC Q A

I70.293 **Other atherosclerosis of native arteries of extremities, bilateral legs** HCC Q A

I70.298 **Other atherosclerosis of native arteries of extremities, other extremity** HCC Q A

I70.299 **Other atherosclerosis of native arteries of extremities, unspecified extremity** HCC Q A

√5ᵗʰ **I70.3** **Atherosclerosis of unspecified type of bypass graft(s) of the extremities**

     Use additional code, if applicable, to identify chronic total occlusion of artery of extremity (I70.92)

     EXCLUDES 1   embolism or thrombus of bypass graft(s) of extremities (T82.8-)

√6ᵗʰ **I70.30** **Unspecified atherosclerosis of unspecified type of bypass graft(s) of the extremities**

I70.301 **Unspecified atherosclerosis of unspecified type of bypass graft(s) of the extremities, right leg** HCC Q A

I70.302 **Unspecified atherosclerosis of unspecified type of bypass graft(s) of the extremities, left leg** HCC Q A

I70.303 **Unspecified atherosclerosis of unspecified type of bypass graft(s) of the extremities, bilateral legs** HCC Q A

I70.308 **Unspecified atherosclerosis of unspecified type of bypass graft(s) of the extremities, other extremity** HCC Q A

I70.309 **Unspecified atherosclerosis of unspecified type of bypass graft(s) of the extremities, unspecified extremity** HCC Q A

√6ᵗʰ **I70.31** **Atherosclerosis of unspecified type of bypass graft(s) of the extremities with intermittent claudication**

I70.311 **Atherosclerosis of unspecified type of bypass graft(s) of the extremities with intermittent claudication, right leg** HCC Q A

I70.312 **Atherosclerosis of unspecified type of bypass graft(s) of the extremities with intermittent claudication, left leg** HCC Q A

I70.313 **Atherosclerosis of unspecified type of bypass graft(s) of the extremities with intermittent claudication, bilateral legs** HCC Q A

I70.318 **Atherosclerosis of unspecified type of bypass graft(s) of the extremities with intermittent claudication, other extremity** HCC Q A

I70.319 **Atherosclerosis of unspecified type of bypass graft(s) of the extremities with intermittent claudication, unspecified extremity** HCC Q A

√6ᵗʰ **I70.32** **Atherosclerosis of unspecified type of bypass graft(s) of the extremities with rest pain**

     INCLUDES   any condition classifiable to I70.31-

I70.321 **Atherosclerosis of unspecified type of bypass graft(s) of the extremities with rest pain, right leg** HCC Q A

I70.322 **Atherosclerosis of unspecified type of bypass graft(s) of the extremities with rest pain, left leg** HCC Q A

I70.323 **Atherosclerosis of unspecified type of bypass graft(s) of the extremities with rest pain, bilateral legs** HCC Q A

I70.328 **Atherosclerosis of unspecified type of bypass graft(s) of the extremities with rest pain, other extremity** HCC Q A

I70.329 **Atherosclerosis of unspecified type of bypass graft(s) of the extremities with rest pain, unspecified extremity** HCC Q A

√6ᵗʰ **I70.33** **Atherosclerosis of unspecified type of bypass graft(s) of the right leg with ulceration**

     INCLUDES   any condition classifiable to I70.311 and I70.321

     Use additional code to identify severity of ulcer (L97.-)

I70.331 **Atherosclerosis of unspecified type of bypass graft(s) of the right leg with ulceration of thigh** HCC Q A

I70.332   **Atherosclerosis of unspecified** HCC Q A **type of bypass graft(s) of the right leg with ulceration of** calf

I70.333   **Atherosclerosis of unspecified** HCC Q A **type of bypass graft(s) of the right leg with ulceration of** ankle

I70.334   **Atherosclerosis of unspecified** HCC Q A **type of bypass graft(s) of the right leg with ulceration of** heel and midfoot

Atherosclerosis of unspecified type of bypass graft(s) of right leg with ulceration of plantar surface of midfoot

I70.335   **Atherosclerosis of unspecified** HCC Q A **type of bypass graft(s) of the right leg with ulceration of other part of foot**

Atherosclerosis of unspecified type of bypass graft(s) of the right leg with ulceration of toe

I70.338   **Atherosclerosis of unspecified** HCC Q A **type of bypass graft(s) of the right leg with ulceration of other part of lower leg**

I70.339   **Atherosclerosis of unspecified** HCC Q A **type of bypass graft(s) of the right leg with ulceration of unspecified site**

✓6ᵗʰ **I70.34**   **Atherosclerosis of unspecified type of bypass graft(s) of the** left leg with ulceration
INCLUDES any condition classifiable to I70.312 and I70.322
Use additional code to identify severity of ulcer (L97.-)

I70.341   **Atherosclerosis of unspecified** HCC Q A **type of bypass graft(s) of the left leg with ulceration of** thigh

I70.342   **Atherosclerosis of unspecified** HCC Q A **type of bypass graft(s) of the left leg with ulceration of** calf

I70.343   **Atherosclerosis of unspecified** HCC Q A **type of bypass graft(s) of the left leg with ulceration of** ankle

I70.344   **Atherosclerosis of unspecified** HCC Q A **type of bypass graft(s) of the left leg with ulceration of** heel and midfoot

Atherosclerosis of unspecified type of bypass graft(s) of left leg with ulceration of plantar surface of midfoot

I70.345   **Atherosclerosis of unspecified** HCC Q A **type of bypass graft(s) of the left leg with ulceration of other part of foot**

Atherosclerosis of unspecified type of bypass graft(s) of the left leg with ulceration of toe

I70.348   **Atherosclerosis of unspecified** HCC Q A **type of bypass graft(s) of the left leg with ulceration of other part of lower leg**

I70.349   **Atherosclerosis of unspecified** HCC Q A **type of bypass graft(s) of the left leg with ulceration of unspecified site**

I70.35   **Atherosclerosis of unspecified type of** HCC Q A **bypass graft(s) of other extremity with** ulceration
INCLUDES any condition classifiable to I70.318 and I70.328
Use additional code to identify severity of ulcer (L98.49-)

✓6ᵗʰ **I70.36**   **Atherosclerosis of unspecified type of bypass graft(s) of the extremities with** gangrene
INCLUDES any condition classifiable to I70.31-, I70.32-, I70.33-, I70.34-, I70.35
Use additional code to identify the severity of any ulcer (L97.-, L98.49-), if applicable

I70.361   **Atherosclerosis of unspecified** HCC Q A **type of bypass graft(s) of the extremities with gangrene,** right leg

I70.362   **Atherosclerosis of unspecified** HCC Q A **type of bypass graft(s) of the extremities with gangrene,** left leg

I70.363   **Atherosclerosis of unspecified** HCC Q A **type of bypass graft(s) of the extremities with gangrene,** bilateral legs

I70.368   **Atherosclerosis of unspecified** HCC Q A **type of bypass graft(s) of the extremities with gangrene, other extremity**

I70.369   **Atherosclerosis of unspecified** HCC Q A **type of bypass graft(s) of the extremities with gangrene, unspecified extremity**

✓6ᵗʰ **I70.39**   **Other atherosclerosis of unspecified type of bypass graft(s) of the extremities**

I70.391   **Other atherosclerosis of** HCC Q A **unspecified type of bypass graft(s) of the extremities,** right leg

I70.392   **Other atherosclerosis of** HCC Q A **unspecified type of bypass graft(s) of the extremities,** left leg

I70.393   **Other atherosclerosis of** HCC Q A **unspecified type of bypass graft(s) of the extremities,** bilateral legs

I70.398   **Other atherosclerosis of** HCC Q A **unspecified type of bypass graft(s) of the extremities, other extremity**

I70.399   **Other atherosclerosis of** HCC Q A **unspecified type of bypass graft(s) of the extremities, unspecified extremity**

✓5ᵗʰ **I70.4**   **Atherosclerosis of** autologous vein bypass graft(s) **of the** extremities
Use additional code, if applicable, to identify chronic total occlusion of artery of extremity (I70.92)

✓6ᵗʰ **I70.40**   **Unspecified atherosclerosis of autologous vein bypass graft(s) of the extremities**

I70.401   **Unspecified atherosclerosis of** HCC Q A **autologous vein bypass graft(s) of the extremities,** right leg

I70.402   **Unspecified atherosclerosis of** HCC Q A **autologous vein bypass graft(s) of the extremities,** left leg

I70.403   **Unspecified atherosclerosis of** HCC Q A **autologous vein bypass graft(s) of the extremities,** bilateral legs

I70.408   **Unspecified atherosclerosis of** HCC Q A **autologous vein bypass graft(s) of the extremities, other extremity**

I70.409   **Unspecified atherosclerosis of** HCC Q A **autologous vein bypass graft(s) of the extremities, unspecified extremity**

✓6ᵗʰ **I70.41**   **Atherosclerosis of autologous vein bypass graft(s) of the extremities with** intermittent claudication

I70.411   **Atherosclerosis of autologous** HCC Q A **vein bypass graft(s) of the extremities with intermittent claudication,** right leg

I70.412   **Atherosclerosis of autologous** HCC Q A **vein bypass graft(s) of the extremities with intermittent claudication,** left leg

I70.413   **Atherosclerosis of autologous** HCC Q A **vein bypass graft(s) of the extremities with intermittent claudication,** bilateral legs

---

☑ Additional Character Required   ✓x7ᵗʰ Placeholder Alert   Manifestation   Unspecified Dx   ▶◀ Revised Text   ● New Code   ▲ Revised Code Title

I70.418 Atherosclerosis of autologous HCC Q A
**vein bypass graft(s) of the
extremities with intermittent
claudication, other extremity**

I70.419 Atherosclerosis of autologous HCC Q A
**vein bypass graft(s) of the
extremities with intermittent
claudication, unspecified
extremity**

✓6ᵗʰ **I70.42 Atherosclerosis of autologous vein bypass graft(s)
of the extremities with rest pain**

INCLUDES   any condition classifiable to I70.41-

I70.421 Atherosclerosis of autologous HCC Q A
**vein bypass graft(s) of the
extremities with rest pain, right
leg**

I70.422 Atherosclerosis of autologous HCC Q A
**vein bypass graft(s) of the
extremities with rest pain, left
leg**

I70.423 Atherosclerosis of autologous HCC Q A
**vein bypass graft(s) of the
extremities with rest pain,
bilateral legs**

I70.428 Atherosclerosis of autologous HCC Q A
**vein bypass graft(s) of the
extremities with rest pain, other
extremity**

I70.429 Atherosclerosis of autologous HCC Q A
**vein bypass graft(s) of the
extremities with rest pain,
unspecified extremity**

✓6ᵗʰ **I70.43 Atherosclerosis of autologous vein bypass graft(s)
of the right leg with ulceration**

INCLUDES   any condition classifiable to I70.411 and
I70.421

Use additional code to identify severity of ulcer (L97.-)

I70.431 Atherosclerosis of autologous HCC Q A
**vein bypass graft(s) of the right
leg with ulceration of thigh**

I70.432 Atherosclerosis of autologous HCC Q A
**vein bypass graft(s) of the right
leg with ulceration of calf**

I70.433 Atherosclerosis of autologous HCC Q A
**vein bypass graft(s) of the right
leg with ulceration of ankle**

I70.434 Atherosclerosis of autologous HCC Q A
**vein bypass graft(s) of the right
leg with ulceration of heel and
midfoot**

Atherosclerosis of autologous vein bypass
graft(s) of right leg with ulceration of
plantar surface of midfoot

I70.435 Atherosclerosis of autologous HCC Q A
**vein bypass graft(s) of the right
leg with ulceration of other part
of foot**

Atherosclerosis of autologous vein bypass
graft(s) of right leg with ulceration of
toe

I70.438 Atherosclerosis of autologous HCC Q A
**vein bypass graft(s) of the right
leg with ulceration of other part
of lower leg**

I70.439 Atherosclerosis of autologous HCC Q A
**vein bypass graft(s) of the right
leg with ulceration of
unspecified site**

✓6ᵗʰ **I70.44 Atherosclerosis of autologous vein bypass graft(s)
of the left leg with ulceration**

INCLUDES   any condition classifiable to I70.412 and
I70.422

Use additional code to identify severity of ulcer (L97.-)

I70.441 Atherosclerosis of autologous HCC Q A
**vein bypass graft(s) of the left
leg with ulceration of thigh**

I70.442 Atherosclerosis of autologous HCC Q A
**vein bypass graft(s) of the left
leg with ulceration of calf**

I70.443 Atherosclerosis of autologous HCC Q A
**vein bypass graft(s) of the left
leg with ulceration of ankle**

I70.444 Atherosclerosis of autologous HCC Q A
**vein bypass graft(s) of the left
leg with ulceration of heel and
midfoot**

Atherosclerosis of autologous vein bypass
graft(s) of left leg with ulceration of
plantar surface of midfoot

I70.445 Atherosclerosis of autologous HCC Q A
**vein bypass graft(s) of the left
leg with ulceration of other part
of foot**

Atherosclerosis of autologous vein bypass
graft(s) of left leg with ulceration of
toe

I70.448 Atherosclerosis of autologous HCC Q A
**vein bypass graft(s) of the left
leg with ulceration of other part
of lower leg**

I70.449 Atherosclerosis of autologous HCC Q A
**vein bypass graft(s) of the left
leg with ulceration of
unspecified site**

I70.45 Atherosclerosis of autologous vein bypass HCC Q A
graft(s) of other extremity with ulceration

INCLUDES   any condition classifiable to I70.418,
I70.428, and I70.438

Use additional code to identify severity of ulcer
(L98.49)

✓6ᵗʰ **I70.46 Atherosclerosis of autologous vein bypass graft(s)
of the extremities with gangrene**

INCLUDES   any condition classifiable to I70.41-,
I70.42-, and I70.43-, I70.44-, I70.45

Use additional code to identify the severity of any
ulcer (L97.-, L98.49-), if applicable

I70.461 Atherosclerosis of autologous HCC Q A
**vein bypass graft(s) of the
extremities with gangrene,
right leg**

I70.462 Atherosclerosis of autologous HCC Q A
**vein bypass graft(s) of the
extremities with gangrene, left
leg**

I70.463 Atherosclerosis of autologous HCC Q A
**vein bypass graft(s) of the
extremities with gangrene,
bilateral legs**

I70.468 Atherosclerosis of autologous HCC Q A
**vein bypass graft(s) of the
extremities with gangrene,
other extremity**

I70.469 Atherosclerosis of autologous HCC Q A
**vein bypass graft(s) of the
extremities with gangrene,
unspecified extremity**

✓6ᵗʰ **I70.49 Other atherosclerosis of autologous vein bypass
graft(s) of the extremities**

I70.491 Other atherosclerosis of HCC Q A
**autologous vein bypass graft(s)
of the extremities, right leg**

I70.492 Other atherosclerosis of HCC Q A
**autologous vein bypass graft(s)
of the extremities, left leg**

I70.493 Other atherosclerosis of HCC Q A
**autologous vein bypass graft(s)
of the extremities, bilateral legs**

I70.498 Other atherosclerosis of HCC Q A
**autologous vein bypass graft(s)
of the extremities, other
extremity**

I70.499 Other atherosclerosis of HCC Q A
**autologous vein bypass graft(s)
of the extremities, unspecified
extremity**

✓5ᵗʰ **I70.5 Atherosclerosis of nonautologous biological bypass graft(s)
of the extremities**

Use additional code, if applicable, to identify chronic total
occlusion of artery of extremity (I70.92)

✓6ᵗʰ **I70.50 Unspecified atherosclerosis of nonautologous
biological bypass graft(s) of the extremities**

I70.501 Unspecified atherosclerosis of HCC Q A
**nonautologous biological
bypass graft(s) of the
extremities, right leg**

I70.502 Unspecified atherosclerosis of nonautologous biological bypass graft(s) of the extremities, left leg HCC Q A

I70.503 Unspecified atherosclerosis of nonautologous biological bypass graft(s) of the extremities, bilateral legs HCC Q A

I70.508 Unspecified atherosclerosis of nonautologous biological bypass graft(s) of the extremities, other extremity HCC Q A

I70.509 Unspecified atherosclerosis of nonautologous biological bypass graft(s) of the extremities, unspecified extremity HCC Q A

✓6ᵗʰ **I70.51** Atherosclerosis of nonautologous biological bypass graft(s) of the extremities intermittent claudication

I70.511 Atherosclerosis of nonautologous biological bypass graft(s) of the extremities with intermittent claudication, right leg HCC Q A

I70.512 Atherosclerosis of nonautologous biological bypass graft(s) of the extremities with intermittent claudication, left leg HCC Q A

I70.513 Atherosclerosis of nonautologous biological bypass graft(s) of the extremities with intermittent claudication, bilateral legs HCC Q A

I70.518 Atherosclerosis of nonautologous biological bypass graft(s) of the extremities with intermittent claudication, other extremity HCC Q A

I70.519 Atherosclerosis of nonautologous biological bypass graft(s) of the extremities with intermittent claudication, unspecified extremity HCC Q A

✓6ᵗʰ **I70.52** Atherosclerosis of nonautologous biological bypass graft(s) of the extremities with rest pain
  INCLUDES   any condition classifiable to I70.51-

I70.521 Atherosclerosis of nonautologous biological bypass graft(s) of the extremities with rest pain, right leg HCC Q A

I70.522 Atherosclerosis of nonautologous biological bypass graft(s) of the extremities with rest pain, left leg HCC Q A

I70.523 Atherosclerosis of nonautologous biological bypass graft(s) of the extremities with rest pain, bilateral legs HCC Q A

I70.528 Atherosclerosis of nonautologous biological bypass graft(s) of the extremities with rest pain, other extremity HCC Q A

I70.529 Atherosclerosis of nonautologous biological bypass graft(s) of the extremities with rest pain, unspecified extremity HCC Q A

✓6ᵗʰ **I70.53** Atherosclerosis of nonautologous biological bypass graft(s) of the right leg with ulceration
  INCLUDES   any condition classifiable to I70.511 and I70.521
  Use additional code to identify severity of ulcer (L97.-)

I70.531 Atherosclerosis of nonautologous biological bypass graft(s) of the right leg with ulceration of thigh HCC Q A

I70.532 Atherosclerosis of nonautologous biological bypass graft(s) of the right leg with ulceration of calf HCC Q A

I70.533 Atherosclerosis of nonautologous biological bypass graft(s) of the right leg with ulceration of ankle HCC Q A

I70.534 Atherosclerosis of nonautologous biological bypass graft(s) of the right leg with ulceration of heel and midfoot HCC Q A
  Atherosclerosis of nonautologous biological bypass graft(s) of right leg with ulceration of plantar surface of midfoot

I70.535 Atherosclerosis of nonautologous biological bypass graft(s) of the right leg with ulceration of other part of foot HCC Q A
  Atherosclerosis of nonautologous biological bypass graft(s) of the right leg with ulceration of toe

I70.538 Atherosclerosis of nonautologous biological bypass graft(s) of the right leg with ulceration of other part of lower leg HCC Q A

I70.539 Atherosclerosis of nonautologous biological bypass graft(s) of the right leg with ulceration of unspecified site HCC Q A

✓6ᵗʰ **I70.54** Atherosclerosis of nonautologous biological bypass graft(s) of the left leg with ulceration
  INCLUDES   any condition classifiable to I70.512 and I70.522
  Use additional code to identify severity of ulcer (L97.-)

I70.541 Atherosclerosis of nonautologous biological bypass graft(s) of the left leg with ulceration of thigh HCC Q A

I70.542 Atherosclerosis of nonautologous biological bypass graft(s) of the left leg with ulceration of calf HCC Q A

I70.543 Atherosclerosis of nonautologous biological bypass graft(s) of the left leg with ulceration of ankle HCC Q A

I70.544 Atherosclerosis of nonautologous biological bypass graft(s) of the left leg with ulceration of heel and midfoot HCC Q A
  Atherosclerosis of nonautologous biological bypass graft(s) of left leg with ulceration of plantar surface of midfoot

I70.545 Atherosclerosis of nonautologous biological bypass graft(s) of the left leg with ulceration of other part of foot HCC Q A
  Atherosclerosis of nonautologous biological bypass graft(s) of the left leg with ulceration of toe

I70.548 Atherosclerosis of nonautologous biological bypass graft(s) of the left leg with ulceration of other part of lower leg HCC Q A

I70.549 Atherosclerosis of nonautologous biological bypass graft(s) of the left leg with ulceration of unspecified site HCC Q A

I70.55 Atherosclerosis of nonautologous biological bypass graft(s) of other extremity with ulceration HCC Q A
  INCLUDES   any condition classifiable to I70.518, I70.528, and I70.538
  Use additional code to identify severity of ulcer (L98.49)

☑ Additional Character Required   ✓ₓ7ᵗʰ Placeholder Alert   Manifestation   Unspecified Dx   ►◄ Revised Text   ● New Code   ▲ Revised Code Title

✓6ᵗʰ **I70.56 Atherosclerosis of nonautologous biological bypass graft(s) of the extremities with gangrene**

> INCLUDES   any condition classifiable to I70.51-, I70.52-, and I70.53-, I70.54-, I70.55
>
> Use additional code to identify the severity of any ulcer (L97.-, L98.49-), if applicable

    I70.561 Atherosclerosis of nonautologous biological bypass graft(s) of the extremities with gangrene, right leg HCC Q A

    I70.562 Atherosclerosis of nonautologous biological bypass graft(s) of the extremities with gangrene, left leg HCC Q A

    I70.563 Atherosclerosis of nonautologous biological bypass graft(s) of the extremities with gangrene, bilateral legs HCC Q A

    I70.568 Atherosclerosis of nonautologous biological bypass graft(s) of the extremities with gangrene, other extremity HCC Q A

    I70.569 Atherosclerosis of nonautologous biological bypass graft(s) of the extremities with gangrene, unspecified extremity HCC Q A

✓6ᵗʰ **I70.59 Other atherosclerosis of nonautologous biological bypass graft(s) of the extremities**

    I70.591 Other atherosclerosis of nonautologous biological bypass graft(s) of the extremities, right leg HCC Q A

    I70.592 Other atherosclerosis of nonautologous biological bypass graft(s) of the extremities, left leg HCC Q A

    I70.593 Other atherosclerosis of nonautologous biological bypass graft(s) of the extremities, bilateral legs HCC Q A

    I70.598 Other atherosclerosis of nonautologous biological bypass graft(s) of the extremities, other extremity HCC Q A

    I70.599 Other atherosclerosis of nonautologous biological bypass graft(s) of the extremities, unspecified extremity HCC Q A

✓5ᵗʰ **I70.6 Atherosclerosis of nonbiological bypass graft(s) of the extremities**

> Use additional code, if applicable, to identify chronic total occlusion of artery of extremity (I70.92)

✓6ᵗʰ **I70.60 Unspecified atherosclerosis of nonbiological bypass graft(s) of the extremities**

    I70.601 Unspecified atherosclerosis of nonbiological bypass graft(s) of the extremities, right leg HCC Q A

    I70.602 Unspecified atherosclerosis of nonbiological bypass graft(s) of the extremities, left leg HCC Q A

    I70.603 Unspecified atherosclerosis of nonbiological bypass graft(s) of the extremities, bilateral legs HCC Q A

    I70.608 Unspecified atherosclerosis of nonbiological bypass graft(s) of the extremities, other extremity HCC Q A

    I70.609 Unspecified atherosclerosis of nonbiological bypass graft(s) of the extremities, unspecified extremity HCC Q A

✓6ᵗʰ **I70.61 Atherosclerosis of nonbiological bypass graft(s) of the extremities with intermittent claudication**

    I70.611 Atherosclerosis of nonbiological bypass graft(s) of the extremities with intermittent claudication, right leg HCC Q A

    I70.612 Atherosclerosis of nonbiological bypass graft(s) of the extremities with intermittent claudication, left leg HCC Q A

    I70.613 Atherosclerosis of nonbiological bypass graft(s) of the extremities with intermittent claudication, bilateral legs HCC Q A

    I70.618 Atherosclerosis of nonbiological bypass graft(s) of the extremities with intermittent claudication, other extremity HCC Q A

    I70.619 Atherosclerosis of nonbiological bypass graft(s) of the extremities with intermittent claudication, unspecified extremity HCC Q A

✓6ᵗʰ **I70.62 Atherosclerosis of nonbiological bypass graft(s) of the extremities with rest pain**

> INCLUDES   any condition classifiable to I70.61-

    I70.621 Atherosclerosis of nonbiological bypass graft(s) of the extremities with rest pain, right leg HCC Q A

    I70.622 Atherosclerosis of nonbiological bypass graft(s) of the extremities with rest pain, left leg HCC Q A

    I70.623 Atherosclerosis of nonbiological bypass graft(s) of the extremities with rest pain, bilateral legs HCC Q A

    I70.628 Atherosclerosis of nonbiological bypass graft(s) of the extremities with rest pain, other extremity HCC Q A

    I70.629 Atherosclerosis of nonbiological bypass graft(s) of the extremities with rest pain, unspecified extremity HCC Q A

✓6ᵗʰ **I70.63 Atherosclerosis of nonbiological bypass graft(s) of the right leg with ulceration**

> INCLUDES   any condition classifiable to I70.611 and I70.621
>
> Use additional code to identify severity of ulcer (L97.-)

    I70.631 Atherosclerosis of nonbiological bypass graft(s) of the right leg with ulceration of thigh HCC Q A

    I70.632 Atherosclerosis of nonbiological bypass graft(s) of the right leg with ulceration of calf HCC Q A

    I70.633 Atherosclerosis of nonbiological bypass graft(s) of the right leg with ulceration of ankle HCC Q A

    I70.634 Atherosclerosis of nonbiological bypass graft(s) of the right leg with ulceration of heel and midfoot HCC Q A

> Atherosclerosis of nonbiological bypass graft(s) of right leg with ulceration of plantar surface of midfoot

    I70.635 Atherosclerosis of nonbiological bypass graft(s) of the right leg with ulceration of other part of foot HCC Q A

> Atherosclerosis of nonbiological bypass graft(s) of the right leg with ulceration of toe

    I70.638 Atherosclerosis of nonbiological bypass graft(s) of the right leg with ulceration of other part of lower leg HCC Q A

    I70.639 Atherosclerosis of nonbiological bypass graft(s) of the right leg with ulceration of unspecified site HCC Q A

✓6ᵗʰ **I70.64 Atherosclerosis of nonbiological bypass graft(s) of the left leg with ulceration**

> INCLUDES   any condition classifiable to I70.612 and I70.622
>
> Use additional code to identify severity of ulcer (L97.-)

    I70.641 Atherosclerosis of nonbiological bypass graft(s) of the left leg with ulceration of thigh HCC Q A

I70.642 Atherosclerosis of nonbiological HCC Q A bypass graft(s) of the left leg with ulceration of calf

I70.643 Atherosclerosis of nonbiological HCC Q A bypass graft(s) of the left leg with ulceration of ankle

I70.644 Atherosclerosis of nonbiological HCC Q A bypass graft(s) of the left leg with ulceration of heel and midfoot

> Atherosclerosis of nonbiological bypass graft(s) of left leg with ulceration of plantar surface of midfoot

I70.645 Atherosclerosis of nonbiological HCC Q A bypass graft(s) of the left leg with ulceration of other part of foot

> Atherosclerosis of nonbiological bypass graft(s) of the left leg with ulceration of toe

I70.648 Atherosclerosis of nonbiological HCC Q A bypass graft(s) of the left leg with ulceration of other part of lower leg

I70.649 Atherosclerosis of nonbiological HCC Q A bypass graft(s) of the left leg with ulceration of unspecified site

I70.65 Atherosclerosis of nonbiological bypass HCC Q A graft(s) of other extremity with ulceration

> INCLUDES   any condition classifiable to I70.618 and I70.628

> Use additional code to identify severity of ulcer (L98.49)

✓6ᵗʰ **I70.66** Atherosclerosis of nonbiological bypass graft(s) of the extremities with gangrene

> INCLUDES   any condition classifiable to I70.61-, I70.62-, I70.63-, I70.64-, I70.65

> Use additional code to identify the severity of any ulcer (L97.-, L98.49-), if applicable

I70.661 Atherosclerosis of nonbiological HCC Q A bypass graft(s) of the extremities with gangrene, right leg

I70.662 Atherosclerosis of nonbiological HCC Q A bypass graft(s) of the extremities with gangrene, left leg

I70.663 Atherosclerosis of nonbiological HCC Q A bypass graft(s) of the extremities with gangrene, bilateral legs

I70.668 Atherosclerosis of nonbiological HCC Q A bypass graft(s) of the extremities with gangrene, other extremity

I70.669 Atherosclerosis of nonbiological HCC Q A bypass graft(s) of the extremities with gangrene, unspecified extremity

✓6ᵗʰ **I70.69** Other atherosclerosis of nonbiological bypass graft(s) of the extremities

I70.691 Other atherosclerosis of HCC Q A nonbiological bypass graft(s) of the extremities, right leg

I70.692 Other atherosclerosis of HCC Q A nonbiological bypass graft(s) of the extremities, left leg

I70.693 Other atherosclerosis of HCC Q A nonbiological bypass graft(s) of the extremities, bilateral legs

I70.698 Other atherosclerosis of HCC Q A nonbiological bypass graft(s) of the extremities, other extremity

I70.699 Other atherosclerosis of HCC Q A nonbiological bypass graft(s) of the extremities, unspecified extremity

✓5ᵗʰ **I70.7** Atherosclerosis of other type of bypass graft(s) of the extremities

> Use additional code, if applicable, to identify chronic total occlusion of artery of extremity (I70.92)

✓6ᵗʰ **I70.70** Unspecified atherosclerosis of other type of bypass graft(s) of the extremities

I70.701 Unspecified atherosclerosis of HCC Q A other type of bypass graft(s) of the extremities, right leg

I70.702 Unspecified atherosclerosis of HCC Q A other type of bypass graft(s) of the extremities, left leg

I70.703 Unspecified atherosclerosis of HCC Q A other type of bypass graft(s) of the extremities, bilateral legs

I70.708 Unspecified atherosclerosis of HCC Q A other type of bypass graft(s) of the extremities, other extremity

I70.709 Unspecified atherosclerosis of HCC Q A other type of bypass graft(s) of the extremities, unspecified extremity

✓6ᵗʰ **I70.71** Atherosclerosis of other type of bypass graft(s) of the extremities with intermittent claudication

I70.711 Atherosclerosis of other type of HCC Q A bypass graft(s) of the extremities with intermittent claudication, right leg

I70.712 Atherosclerosis of other type of HCC Q A bypass graft(s) of the extremities with intermittent claudication, left leg

I70.713 Atherosclerosis of other type of HCC Q A bypass graft(s) of the extremities with intermittent claudication, bilateral legs

I70.718 Atherosclerosis of other type of HCC Q A bypass graft(s) of the extremities with intermittent claudication, other extremity

I70.719 Atherosclerosis of other type of HCC Q A bypass graft(s) of the extremities with intermittent claudication, unspecified extremity

✓6ᵗʰ **I70.72** Atherosclerosis of other type of bypass graft(s) of the extremities with rest pain

> INCLUDES   any condition classifiable to I70.71-

I70.721 Atherosclerosis of other type of HCC Q A bypass graft(s) of the extremities with rest pain, right leg

I70.722 Atherosclerosis of other type of HCC Q A bypass graft(s) of the extremities with rest pain, left leg

I70.723 Atherosclerosis of other type of HCC Q A bypass graft(s) of the extremities with rest pain, bilateral legs

I70.728 Atherosclerosis of other type of HCC Q A bypass graft(s) of the extremities with rest pain, other extremity

I70.729 Atherosclerosis of other type of HCC Q A bypass graft(s) of the extremities with rest pain, unspecified extremity

✓6ᵗʰ **I70.73** Atherosclerosis of other type of bypass graft(s) of the right leg with ulceration

> INCLUDES   any condition classifiable to I70.711 and I70.721

> Use additional code to identify severity of ulcer (L97.-)

I70.731 Atherosclerosis of other type of HCC Q A bypass graft(s) of the right leg with ulceration of thigh

I70.732 Atherosclerosis of other type of HCC Q A bypass graft(s) of the right leg with ulceration of calf

I70.733 Atherosclerosis of other type of HCC Q A bypass graft(s) of the right leg with ulceration of ankle

---

✓ Additional Character Required   ✓x7ᵗʰ Placeholder Alert   Manifestation   Unspecified Dx   ▶◀ Revised Text   ● New Code   ▲ Revised Code Title

ICD-10-CM 2020   665

I70.734 Atherosclerosis of other type of HCC Q A **bypass graft(s) of the right leg with ulceration of** heel and midfoot

Atherosclerosis of other type of bypass graft(s) of right leg with ulceration of plantar surface of midfoot

I70.735 Atherosclerosis of other type of HCC Q A **bypass graft(s) of the right leg with ulceration of other part of foot**

Atherosclerosis of other type of bypass graft(s) of right leg with ulceration of toe

I70.738 Atherosclerosis of other type of HCC Q A **bypass graft(s) of the right leg with ulceration of other part of lower leg**

I70.739 Atherosclerosis of other type of HCC Q A **bypass graft(s) of the right leg with ulceration of unspecified site**

✓6ᵗʰ **I70.74 Atherosclerosis of other type of bypass graft(s) of the** left leg with ulceration

INCLUDES any condition classifiable to I70.712 and I70.722

Use additional code to identify severity of ulcer (L97.-)

I70.741 Atherosclerosis of other type of HCC Q A **bypass graft(s) of the left leg with ulceration of** thigh

I70.742 Atherosclerosis of other type of HCC Q A **bypass graft(s) of the left leg with ulceration of** calf

I70.743 Atherosclerosis of other type of HCC Q A **bypass graft(s) of the left leg with ulceration of** ankle

I70.744 Atherosclerosis of other type of HCC Q A **bypass graft(s) of the left leg with ulceration of** heel and midfoot

Atherosclerosis of other type of bypass graft(s) of left leg with ulceration of plantar surface of midfoot

I70.745 Atherosclerosis of other type of HCC Q A **bypass graft(s) of the left leg with ulceration of other part of foot**

Atherosclerosis of other type of bypass graft(s) of left leg with ulceration of toe

I70.748 Atherosclerosis of other type of HCC Q A **bypass graft(s) of the left leg with ulceration of other part of lower leg**

I70.749 Atherosclerosis of other type of HCC Q A **bypass graft(s) of the left leg with ulceration of unspecified site**

I70.75 Atherosclerosis of other type of bypass HCC Q A **graft(s) of other extremity with** ulceration

INCLUDES any condition classifiable to I70.718 and I70.728

Use additional code to identify severity of ulcer (L98.49)

✓6ᵗʰ **I70.76 Atherosclerosis of other type of bypass graft(s) of the extremities with** gangrene

INCLUDES any condition classifiable to I70.71-, I70.72-, I70.73-, I70.74-, I70.75

Use additional code to identify the severity of any ulcer (L97.-, L98.49-), if applicable

I70.761 Atherosclerosis of other type of HCC Q A **bypass graft(s) of the extremities with gangrene,** right leg

I70.762 Atherosclerosis of other type of HCC Q A **bypass graft(s) of the extremities with gangrene,** left leg

I70.763 Atherosclerosis of other type of HCC Q A **bypass graft(s) of the extremities with gangrene,** bilateral legs

I70.768 Atherosclerosis of other type of HCC Q A **bypass graft(s) of the extremities with gangrene, other extremity**

I70.769 Atherosclerosis of other type of HCC Q A **bypass graft(s) of the extremities with gangrene, unspecified extremity**

✓6ᵗʰ **I70.79 Other atherosclerosis of other type of bypass graft(s) of the extremities**

I70.791 Other atherosclerosis of other HCC Q A **type of bypass graft(s) of the extremities,** right leg

I70.792 Other atherosclerosis of other HCC Q A **type of bypass graft(s) of the extremities,** left leg

I70.793 Other atherosclerosis of other HCC Q A **type of bypass graft(s) of the extremities,** bilateral legs

I70.798 Other atherosclerosis of other HCC Q A **type of bypass graft(s) of the extremities, other extremity**

I70.799 Other atherosclerosis of other HCC A **type of bypass graft(s) of the extremities, unspecified extremity**

I70.8 Atherosclerosis of other arteries Q A

TIP: Arteriosclerosis of the iliac arteries is coded here.

✓5ᵗʰ **I70.9 Other and unspecified atherosclerosis**

I70.90 Unspecified atherosclerosis Q A

I70.91 Generalized atherosclerosis Q A

I70.92 Chronic total occlusion of artery of the HCC Q A **extremities**

Complete occlusion of artery of the extremities

Total occlusion of artery of the extremities

Code first atherosclerosis of arteries of the extremities (I70.2-, I70.3-, I70.4-, I70.5-, I70.6-, I70.7-)

✓4ᵗʰ **I71 Aortic aneurysm and dissection**

EXCLUDES 1 aortic ectasia (I77.81-)

syphilitic aortic aneurysm (A52.01)

traumatic aortic aneurysm (S25.09, S35.09)

✓5ᵗʰ **I71.0 Dissection of aorta**

I71.00 Dissection of unspecified site of aorta HCC

I71.01 Dissection of thoracic **aorta** HCC

I71.02 Dissection of abdominal **aorta** HCC

I71.03 Dissection of thoracoabdominal **aorta** HCC

I71.1 Thoracic aortic aneurysm, ruptured HCC

I71.2 Thoracic aortic aneurysm, without rupture HCC

I71.3 Abdominal aortic aneurysm, ruptured HCC

I71.4 Abdominal aortic aneurysm, without rupture HCC

I71.5 Thoracoabdominal aortic aneurysm, ruptured HCC

I71.6 Thoracoabdominal aortic aneurysm, without rupture HCC

I71.8 Aortic aneurysm of unspecified site, ruptured HCC

Rupture of aorta NOS

I71.9 Aortic aneurysm of unspecified site, without rupture HCC

Aneurysm of aorta

Dilatation of aorta

Hyaline necrosis of aorta

✓4ᵗʰ I72   Other aneurysm

INCLUDES   aneurysm (cirsoid) (false) (ruptured)

EXCLUDES 2   acquired aneurysm (I77.0)
aneurysm (of) aorta (I71.-)
aneurysm (of) arteriovenous NOS (Q27.3-)
carotid artery dissection (I77.71)
cerebral (nonruptured) aneurysm (I67.1)
coronary aneurysm (I25.4)
coronary artery dissection (I25.42)
dissection of artery NEC (I77.79)
dissection of precerebral artery, congenital (nonruptured) (Q28.1)
heart aneurysm (I25.3)
iliac artery dissection (I77.72)
precerebral artery, congenital (nonruptured) (Q28.1)
pulmonary artery aneurysm (I28.1)
renal artery dissection (I77.73)
retinal aneurysm (H35.0)
ruptured cerebral aneurysm (I60.7)
varicose aneurysm (I77.0)
vertebral artery dissection (I77.74)

AHA: 2016,4Q,28-29

Aneurysm

Layers of muscular and elastic tissue

Outer layer

Inner layer

Aneurysm

I72.0   Aneurysm of carotid artery   HCC
Aneurysm of common carotid artery
Aneurysm of external carotid artery
Aneurysm of internal carotid artery, extracranial portion
EXCLUDES 1   aneurysm of internal carotid artery, intracranial portion (I67.1)
aneurysm of internal carotid artery NOS (I67.1)

I72.1   Aneurysm of artery of upper extremity   HCC

I72.2   Aneurysm of renal artery   HCC

I72.3   Aneurysm of iliac artery   HCC

I72.4   Aneurysm of artery of lower extremity   HCC
AHA: 2019,2Q,21

I72.5   Aneurysm of other precerebral arteries   HCC
Aneurysm of basilar artery (trunk)
EXCLUDES 2   aneurysm of carotid artery (I72.0)
aneurysm of vertebral artery (I72.6)
dissection of carotid artery (I77.71)
dissection of other precerebral arteries (I77.75)
dissection of vertebral artery (I77.74)

I72.6   Aneurysm of vertebral artery   HCC
EXCLUDES 2   dissection of vertebral artery (I77.74)

I72.8   Aneurysm of other specified arteries   HCC

I72.9   Aneurysm of unspecified site   HCC

✓4ᵗʰ I73   Other peripheral vascular diseases

EXCLUDES 2   chilblains (T69.1)
frostbite (T33-T34)
immersion hand or foot (T69.0-)
spasm of cerebral artery (G45.9)

AHA: 2018,4Q,87

✓5ᵗʰ I73.0   Raynaud's syndrome
Raynaud's disease
Raynaud's phenomenon (secondary)
DEF: Constriction of the arteries of the digits caused by cold or by nerve or arterial damage and can be prompted by stress or emotion. Blood cannot reach the skin and soft tissues and the skin turns white with blue mottling.

I73.00   Raynaud's syndrome without gangrene

I73.01   Raynaud's syndrome with gangrene   HCC

I73.1   Thromboangiitis obliterans [Buerger's disease]   HCC
DEF: Inflammatory disease of the extremity blood vessels, mainly the lower blood vessels. This disease is associated with heavy tobacco use. The arteries are more affected than veins. It occurs primarily in young men and leads to tissue ischemia and gangrene.

✓5ᵗʰ I73.8   Other specified peripheral vascular diseases
EXCLUDES 1   diabetic (peripheral) angiopathy (E08-E13 with .51-.52)

I73.81   Erythromelalgia   HCC

I73.89   Other specified peripheral vascular diseases   HCC
Acrocyanosis
Erythrocyanosis
Simple acroparesthesia [Schultze's type]
Vasomotor acroparesthesia [Nothnagel's type]

I73.9   Peripheral vascular disease, unspecified   HCC
Intermittent claudication
Peripheral angiopathy NOS
Spasm of artery
EXCLUDES 1   atherosclerosis of the extremities (I70.2-I70.7-)
AHA: 2018,2Q,7

✓4ᵗʰ I74   Arterial embolism and thrombosis

INCLUDES   embolic infarction
embolic occlusion
thrombotic infarction
thrombotic occlusion

Code first:
embolism and thrombosis complicating abortion or ectopic or molar pregnancy (O00-O07, O08.2)
embolism and thrombosis complicating pregnancy, childbirth and the puerperium (O88.-)

EXCLUDES 2   atheroembolism (I75.-)
basilar embolism and thrombosis (I63.0-I63.2, I65.1)
carotid embolism and thrombosis (I63.0-I63.2, I65.2)
cerebral embolism and thrombosis (I63.3-I63.5, I66.-)
coronary embolism and thrombosis (I21-I25)
mesenteric embolism and thrombosis (K55.0-)
ophthalmic embolism and thrombosis (H34.-)
precerebral embolism and thrombosis NOS (I63.0-I63.2, I65.9)
pulmonary embolism and thrombosis (I26.-)
renal embolism and thrombosis (N28.0)
retinal embolism and thrombosis (H34.-)
septic embolism and thrombosis (I76)
vertebral embolism and thrombosis (I63.0-I63.2, I65.0)

✓5ᵗʰ I74.0   Embolism and thrombosis of abdominal aorta

I74.01   Saddle embolus of abdominal aorta   HCC

I74.09   Other arterial embolism and thrombosis of abdominal aorta   HCC
Aortic bifurcation syndrome
Aortoiliac obstruction
Leriche's syndrome

✓5ᵗʰ I74.1   Embolism and thrombosis of other and unspecified parts of aorta

I74.10   Embolism and thrombosis of unspecified parts of aorta   HCC

I74.11   Embolism and thrombosis of thoracic aorta   HCC

I74.19   Embolism and thrombosis of other parts of aorta   HCC

☑ Additional Character Required   ✓x7ᵗʰ Placeholder Alert   Manifestation   Unspecified Dx   ▶◀ Revised Text   ● New Code   ▲ Revised Code Title

CD-10-CM 2020   667

Chapter 9. Diseases of the Circulatory System

I74.2   **Embolism and thrombosis of arteries of the upper extremities** `HCC`

I74.3   **Embolism and thrombosis of arteries of the lower extremities** `HCC`

I74.4   **Embolism and thrombosis of arteries of extremities, unspecified** `HCC`
Peripheral arterial embolism NOS

I74.5   **Embolism and thrombosis of iliac artery** `HCC`

I74.8   **Embolism and thrombosis of other arteries** `HCC`

I74.9   **Embolism and thrombosis of unspecified artery** `HCC`

✓4ᵗʰ **I75 Atheroembolism**

INCLUDES   atherothrombotic microembolism
cholesterol embolism

✓5ᵗʰ **I75.0**   **Atheroembolism of extremities**

✓6ᵗʰ **I75.01**   **Atheroembolism of upper extremity**

I75.011   **Atheroembolism of right upper extremity** `HCC` `Q`

I75.012   **Atheroembolism of left upper extremity** `HCC` `Q`

I75.013   **Atheroembolism of bilateral upper extremities** `HCC` `Q`

I75.019   **Atheroembolism of unspecified upper extremity** `HCC` `Q`

✓6ᵗʰ **I75.02**   **Atheroembolism of lower extremity**

I75.021   **Atheroembolism of right lower extremity** `HCC` `Q`

I75.022   **Atheroembolism of left lower extremity** `HCC` `Q`

I75.023   **Atheroembolism of bilateral lower extremities** `HCC` `Q`

I75.029   **Atheroembolism of unspecified lower extremity** `HCC` `Q`

✓5ᵗʰ **I75.8**   **Atheroembolism of other sites**

I75.81   **Atheroembolism of kidney** `HCC` `Q`
Use additional code for any associated acute kidney failure and chronic kidney disease (N17.-, N18.-)

I75.89   **Atheroembolism of other site** `HCC` `Q`

I76 Septic arterial embolism `HCC`
Code first underlying infection, such as:
   infective endocarditis (I33.0)
   lung abscess (J85.-)
Use additional code to identify the site of the embolism (I74.-)
EXCLUDES 2   septic pulmonary embolism (I26.01, I26.90)

✓4ᵗʰ **I77 Other disorders of arteries and arterioles**

EXCLUDES 2   collagen (vascular) diseases (M30-M36)
hypersensitivity angiitis (M31.0)
pulmonary artery (I28.-)

I77.0   **Arteriovenous fistula, acquired** `HCC`
Aneurysmal varix
Arteriovenous aneurysm, acquired
EXCLUDES 1   arteriovenous aneurysm NOS (Q27.3-)
presence of arteriovenous shunt (fistula) for dialysis (Z99.2)
traumatic — see injury of blood vessel by body region
EXCLUDES 2   cerebral (I67.1)
coronary (I25.4)
DEF: Communication between an artery and vein caused by trauma or invasive procedures.

I77.1   **Stricture of artery** `HCC`
Narrowing of artery

I77.2   **Rupture of artery** `HCC`
Erosion of artery
Fistula of artery
Ulcer of artery
EXCLUDES 1   traumatic rupture of artery — see injury of blood vessel by body region

I77.3   **Arterial fibromuscular dysplasia** `HCC`
Fibromuscular hyperplasia (of) carotid artery
Fibromuscular hyperplasia (of) renal artery

I77.4   **Celiac artery compression syndrome** `HCC`

I77.5   **Necrosis of artery** `HCC`

I77.6   **Arteritis, unspecified** `HCC`
Aortitis NOS
Endarteritis NOS
EXCLUDES 1   arteritis or endarteritis:
aortic arch (M31.4)
cerebral NEC (I67.7)
coronary (I25.89)
deformans (I70.-)
giant cell (M31.5, M31.6)
obliterans (I70.-)
senile (I70.-)

✓5ᵗʰ **I77.7**   **Other arterial dissection**
EXCLUDES 2   dissection of aorta (I71.0-)
dissection of coronary artery (I25.42)
AHA: 2016,4Q,28-29

I77.70   **Dissection of unspecified artery** `HCC`

I77.71   **Dissection of carotid artery** `HCC`

I77.72   **Dissection of iliac artery** `HCC`

I77.73   **Dissection of renal artery** `HCC`

I77.74   **Dissection of vertebral artery** `HCC`
EXCLUDES 2   aneurysm of vertebral artery (I72.6)

I77.75   **Dissection of other precerebral arteries** `HCC`
Dissection of basilar artery (trunk)
EXCLUDES 2   aneurysm of carotid artery (I72.0)
aneurysm of other precerebral arteries (I72.5)
aneurysm of vertebral artery (I72.6)
dissection of carotid artery (I77.71)
dissection of vertebral artery (I77.74)

I77.76   **Dissection of artery of upper extremity** `HCC`

I77.77   **Dissection of artery of lower extremity** `HCC`

I77.79   **Dissection of other specified artery** `HCC`

✓5ᵗʰ **I77.8**   **Other specified disorders of arteries and arterioles**

✓6ᵗʰ **I77.81**   **Aortic ectasia**
Ectasis aorta
EXCLUDES 1   aortic aneurysm and dissection (I71.0-)

I77.810   **Thoracic aortic ectasia** `HCC`

I77.811   **Abdominal aortic ectasia** `HCC`

I77.812   **Thoracoabdominal aortic ectasia** `HCC`

I77.819   **Aortic ectasia, unspecified site** `HCC`

I77.89   **Other specified disorders of arteries and arterioles** `HCC`

I77.9   **Disorder of arteries and arterioles, unspecified** `HCC`
AHA: 2018,2Q,7

✓4ᵗʰ **I78 Diseases of capillaries**

I78.0   **Hereditary hemorrhagic telangiectasia** `HCC`
Rendu-Osler-Weber disease

I78.1   **Nevus, non-neoplastic**
Araneus nevus
Senile nevus
Spider nevus
Stellar nevus
EXCLUDES 1   nevus NOS (D22.-)
vascular NOS (Q82.5)
EXCLUDES 2   blue nevus (D22.-)
flammeus nevus (Q82.5)
hairy nevus (D22.-)
melanocytic nevus (D22.-)
pigmented nevus (D22.-)
portwine nevus (Q82.5)
sanguineous nevus (Q82.5)
strawberry nevus (Q82.5)
verrucous nevus (Q82.5)
AHA: 2019,1Q,21

I78.8   **Other diseases of capillaries**

I78.9   **Disease of capillaries, unspecified**

✓4ᵗʰ **I79 Disorders of arteries, arterioles and capillaries in diseases classified elsewhere**

    I79.0   **Aneurysm of aorta in diseases classified elsewhere**   HCC

        Code first underlying disease

        EXCLUDES 1   syphilitic aneurysm (A52.01)

    I79.1   **Aortitis in diseases classified elsewhere**   HCC

        Code first underlying disease

        EXCLUDES 1   syphilitic aortitis (A52.02)

    I79.8   **Other disorders of arteries, arterioles and capillaries in diseases classified elsewhere**   HCC

        Code first underlying disease, such as:

        amyloidosis (E85.-)

        EXCLUDES 1   diabetic (peripheral) angiopathy (E08-E13 with .51-.52)

                syphilitic endarteritis (A52.09)

                tuberculous endarteritis (A18.89)

Diseases of veins, lymphatic vessels and lymph nodes, not elsewhere classified (I80-I89)

✓4ᵗʰ **I80 Phlebitis and thrombophlebitis**

    INCLUDES   endophlebitis

              inflammation, vein

              periphlebitis

              suppurative phlebitis

    Code first:

    phlebitis and thrombophlebitis complicating abortion, ectopic or molar pregnancy (O00-O07, O08.7)

    phlebitis and thrombophlebitis complicating pregnancy, childbirth and the puerperium (O22.-, O87.-)

    EXCLUDES 1   venous embolism and thrombosis of lower extremities (I82.4-, I82.5-, I82.81-)

    ✓5ᵗʰ **I80.0**   **Phlebitis and thrombophlebitis of superficial vessels of lower extremities**

        Phlebitis and thrombophlebitis of femoropopliteal vein

        I80.00   **Phlebitis and thrombophlebitis of superficial vessels of unspecified lower extremity**

        I80.01   **Phlebitis and thrombophlebitis of superficial vessels of right lower extremity**

        I80.02   **Phlebitis and thrombophlebitis of superficial vessels of left lower extremity**

        I80.03   **Phlebitis and thrombophlebitis of superficial vessels of lower extremities, bilateral**

    ✓5ᵗʰ **I80.1**   **Phlebitis and thrombophlebitis of femoral vein**

        ►Phlebitis and thrombophlebitis of common femoral vein◄

        ►Phlebitis and thrombophlebitis of deep femoral vein◄

        I80.10   **Phlebitis and thrombophlebitis of unspecified femoral vein**   HCC

        I80.11   **Phlebitis and thrombophlebitis of right femoral vein**   HCC

        I80.12   **Phlebitis and thrombophlebitis of left femoral vein**   HCC

        I80.13   **Phlebitis and thrombophlebitis of femoral vein, bilateral**   HCC

    ✓5ᵗʰ **I80.2**   **Phlebitis and thrombophlebitis of other and unspecified deep vessels of lower extremities**

        ✓6ᵗʰ **I80.20**   **Phlebitis and thrombophlebitis of unspecified deep vessels of lower extremities**

            I80.201   **Phlebitis and thrombophlebitis of unspecified deep vessels of right lower extremity**   HCC

            I80.202   **Phlebitis and thrombophlebitis of unspecified deep vessels of left lower extremity**   HCC

            I80.203   **Phlebitis and thrombophlebitis of unspecified deep vessels of lower extremities, bilateral**   HCC

            I80.209   **Phlebitis and thrombophlebitis of unspecified deep vessels of unspecified lower extremity**   HCC

        ✓6ᵗʰ **I80.21**   **Phlebitis and thrombophlebitis of iliac vein**

            ►Phlebitis and thrombophlebitis of common iliac vein◄

            ►Phlebitis and thrombophlebitis of external iliac vein◄

            ►Phlebitis and thrombophlebitis of internal iliac vein◄

            I80.211   **Phlebitis and thrombophlebitis of right iliac vein**   HCC

            I80.212   **Phlebitis and thrombophlebitis of left iliac vein**   HCC

            I80.213   **Phlebitis and thrombophlebitis of iliac vein, bilateral**   HCC

            I80.219   **Phlebitis and thrombophlebitis of unspecified iliac vein**   HCC

    ✓6ᵗʰ **I80.22**   **Phlebitis and thrombophlebitis of popliteal vein**

        I80.221   **Phlebitis and thrombophlebitis of right popliteal vein**   HCC

        I80.222   **Phlebitis and thrombophlebitis of left popliteal vein**   HCC

        I80.223   **Phlebitis and thrombophlebitis of popliteal vein, bilateral**   HCC

        I80.229   **Phlebitis and thrombophlebitis of unspecified popliteal vein**   HCC

    ✓6ᵗʰ **I80.23**   **Phlebitis and thrombophlebitis of tibial vein**

        ►Phlebitis and thrombophlebitis of anterior tibial vein◄

        ►Phlebitis and thrombophlebitis of posterior tibial vein◄

        I80.231   **Phlebitis and thrombophlebitis of right tibial vein**   HCC

        I80.232   **Phlebitis and thrombophlebitis of left tibial vein**   HCC

        I80.233   **Phlebitis and thrombophlebitis of tibial vein, bilateral**   HCC

        I80.239   **Phlebitis and thrombophlebitis of unspecified tibial vein**   HCC

    ●✓6ᵗʰ **I80.24**   **Phlebitis and thrombophlebitis of peroneal vein**

        ●**I80.241**   **Phlebitis and thrombophlebitis of right peroneal vein**

        ●**I80.242**   **Phlebitis and thrombophlebitis of left peroneal vein**

        ●**I80.243**   **Phlebitis and thrombophlebitis of peroneal vein, bilateral**

        ●**I80.249**   **Phlebitis and thrombophlebitis of unspecified peroneal vein**

    ●✓6ᵗʰ **I80.25**   **Phlebitis and thrombophlebitis of calf muscular vein**

        Phlebitis and thrombophlebitis of calf muscular vein, NOS

        Phlebitis and thrombophlebitis of gastrocnemial vein

        Phlebitis and thrombophlebitis of soleal vein

        ●**I80.251**   **Phlebitis and thrombophlebitis of right calf muscular vein**

        ●**I80.252**   **Phlebitis and thrombophlebitis of left calf muscular vein**

        ●**I80.253**   **Phlebitis and thrombophlebitis of calf muscular vein, bilateral**

        ●**I80.259**   **Phlebitis and thrombophlebitis of unspecified calf muscular vein**

    ✓6ᵗʰ **I80.29**   **Phlebitis and thrombophlebitis of other deep vessels of lower extremities**

        I80.291   **Phlebitis and thrombophlebitis of other deep vessels of right lower extremity**   HCC

        I80.292   **Phlebitis and thrombophlebitis of other deep vessels of left lower extremity**   HCC

        I80.293   **Phlebitis and thrombophlebitis of other deep vessels of lower extremity, bilateral**

        I80.299   **Phlebitis and thrombophlebitis of other deep vessels of unspecified lower extremity**   HCC

    I80.3   **Phlebitis and thrombophlebitis of lower extremities, unspecified**

    I80.8   **Phlebitis and thrombophlebitis of other sites**

    I80.9   **Phlebitis and thrombophlebitis of unspecified site**

I81 Portal vein thrombosis

    Portal (vein) obstruction

    EXCLUDES 2   hepatic vein thrombosis (I82.0)

                phlebitis of portal vein (K75.1)

✓ Additional Character Required   ✓x7ᵗʰ Placeholder Alert   Manifestation   Unspecified Dx   ►◄ Revised Text   ● New Code   ▲ Revised Code Title

ICD-10-CM 2020   669

Chapter 9. Diseases of the Circulatory System

I82–I82.499

✓4ᵗʰ **I82 Other venous embolism and thrombosis**

Code first venous embolism and thrombosis complicating:
abortion, ectopic or molar pregnancy (O00-O07, O08.7)
pregnancy, childbirth and the puerperium (O22.-, O87.-)

EXCLUDES 2   venous embolism and thrombosis (of):
     cerebral (I63.6, I67.6)
     coronary (I21-I25)
     intracranial and intraspinal, septic or NOS (G08)
     intracranial, nonpyogenic (I67.6)
     intraspinal, nonpyogenic (G95.1)
     mesenteric (K55.0-)
     portal (I81)
     pulmonary (I26.-)

I82.0 Budd-Chiari syndrome   HCC
Hepatic vein thrombosis
DEF: Thrombosis or other obstruction of the hepatic veins. Symptoms include an enlarged liver, extensive collateral vessels, intractable ascites, and severe portal hypertension.

I82.1 Thrombophlebitis migrans

✓5ᵗʰ **I82.2 Embolism and thrombosis of vena cava and other thoracic veins**

✓6ᵗʰ **I82.21 Embolism and thrombosis of superior vena cava**

I82.210 Acute embolism and thrombosis of superior vena cava   HCC
Embolism and thrombosis of superior vena cava NOS

I82.211 Chronic embolism and thrombosis of superior vena cava   HCC

✓6ᵗʰ **I82.22 Embolism and thrombosis of inferior vena cava**

I82.220 Acute embolism and thrombosis of inferior vena cava   HCC
Embolism and thrombosis of inferior vena cava NOS

I82.221 Chronic embolism and thrombosis of inferior vena cava   HCC

✓6ᵗʰ **I82.29 Embolism and thrombosis of other thoracic veins**
Embolism and thrombosis of brachiocephalic (innominate) vein

I82.290 Acute embolism and thrombosis of other thoracic veins   HCC

I82.291 Chronic embolism and thrombosis of other thoracic veins   HCC

I82.3 Embolism and thrombosis of renal vein   HCC

✓5ᵗʰ **I82.4 Acute embolism and thrombosis of deep veins of lower extremity**

✓6ᵗʰ **I82.40 Acute embolism and thrombosis of unspecified deep veins of lower extremity**
Deep vein thrombosis NOS
DVT NOS

EXCLUDES 1   acute embolism and thrombosis of unspecified deep veins of distal lower extremity (I82.4Z-)
acute embolism and thrombosis of unspecified deep veins of proximal lower extremity (I82.4Y-)

I82.401 Acute embolism and thrombosis of unspecified deep veins of right lower extremity   HCC

I82.402 Acute embolism and thrombosis of unspecified deep veins of left lower extremity   HCC

I82.403 Acute embolism and thrombosis of unspecified deep veins of lower extremity, bilateral   HCC

I82.409 Acute embolism and thrombosis of unspecified deep veins of unspecified lower extremity   HCC

✓6ᵗʰ **I82.41 Acute embolism and thrombosis of femoral vein**
▶Acute embolism and thrombosis of common femoral vein◀
▶Acute embolism and thrombosis of deep femoral vein◀

I82.411 Acute embolism and thrombosis of right femoral vein   HCC

I82.412 Acute embolism and thrombosis of left femoral vein   HCC

I82.413 Acute embolism and thrombosis of femoral vein, bilateral   HCC

I82.419 Acute embolism and thrombosis of unspecified femoral vein   HCC

✓6ᵗʰ **I82.42 Acute embolism and thrombosis of iliac vein**
▶Acute embolism and thrombosis of common iliac vein◀
▶Acute embolism and thrombosis of external iliac vein◀
▶Acute embolism and thrombosis of internal iliac vein◀

I82.421 Acute embolism and thrombosis of right iliac vein   HCC

I82.422 Acute embolism and thrombosis of left iliac vein   HCC

I82.423 Acute embolism and thrombosis of iliac vein, bilateral   HCC

I82.429 Acute embolism and thrombosis of unspecified iliac vein   HCC

✓6ᵗʰ **I82.43 Acute embolism and thrombosis of popliteal vein**

I82.431 Acute embolism and thrombosis of right popliteal vein   HCC

I82.432 Acute embolism and thrombosis of left popliteal vein   HCC

I82.433 Acute embolism and thrombosis of popliteal vein, bilateral   HCC

I82.439 Acute embolism and thrombosis of unspecified popliteal vein   HCC

✓6ᵗʰ **I82.44 Acute embolism and thrombosis of tibial vein**
▶Acute embolism and thrombosis of anterior tibial vein◀
▶Acute embolism and thrombosis of posterior tibial vein◀

I82.441 Acute embolism and thrombosis of right tibial vein   HCC

I82.442 Acute embolism and thrombosis of left tibial vein   HCC

I82.443 Acute embolism and thrombosis of tibial vein, bilateral   HCC

I82.449 Acute embolism and thrombosis of unspecified tibial vein   HCC

✓6ᵗʰ **I82.45 Acute embolism and thrombosis of peroneal vein**

I82.451 Acute embolism and thrombosis of right peroneal vein

I82.452 Acute embolism and thrombosis of left peroneal vein

I82.453 Acute embolism and thrombosis of peroneal vein, bilateral

I82.459 Acute embolism and thrombosis of unspecified peroneal vein

✓6ᵗʰ **I82.46 Acute embolism and thrombosis of calf muscular vein**
Acute embolism and thrombosis of calf muscular vein, NOS
Acute embolism and thrombosis of gastrocnemial vein
Acute embolism and thrombosis of soleal vein

I82.461 Acute embolism and thrombosis of right calf muscular vein

I82.462 Acute embolism and thrombosis of left calf muscular vein

I82.463 Acute embolism and thrombosis of calf muscular vein, bilateral

I82.469 Acute embolism and thrombosis of unspecified calf muscular vein

✓6ᵗʰ **I82.49 Acute embolism and thrombosis of other specified deep vein of lower extremity**

I82.491 Acute embolism and thrombosis of other specified deep vein of right lower extremity   HCC

I82.492 Acute embolism and thrombosis of other specified deep vein of left lower extremity   HCC

I82.493 Acute embolism and thrombosis of other specified deep vein of lower extremity, bilateral   HCC

I82.499 Acute embolism and thrombosis of other specified deep vein of unspecified lower extremity   HCC

√6ᵗʰ **I82.4Y** **Acute embolism and thrombosis of unspecified deep veins of proximal lower extremity**
Acute embolism and thrombosis of deep vein of thigh NOS
Acute embolism and thrombosis of deep vein of upper leg NOS

    I82.4Y1 **Acute embolism and thrombosis of unspecified deep veins of right proximal lower extremity** `HCC`

    I82.4Y2 **Acute embolism and thrombosis of unspecified deep veins of left proximal lower extremity** `HCC`

    I82.4Y3 **Acute embolism and thrombosis of unspecified deep veins of proximal lower extremity, bilateral** `HCC`

    I82.4Y9 **Acute embolism and thrombosis of unspecified deep veins of unspecified proximal lower extremity** `HCC`

√6ᵗʰ **I82.4Z** **Acute embolism and thrombosis of unspecified deep veins of distal lower extremity**
Acute embolism and thrombosis of deep vein of calf NOS
Acute embolism and thrombosis of deep vein of lower leg NOS

    I82.4Z1 **Acute embolism and thrombosis of unspecified deep veins of right distal lower extremity** `HCC`

    I82.4Z2 **Acute embolism and thrombosis of unspecified deep veins of left distal lower extremity** `HCC`

    I82.4Z3 **Acute embolism and thrombosis of unspecified deep veins of distal lower extremity, bilateral** `HCC`

    I82.4Z9 **Acute embolism and thrombosis of unspecified deep veins of unspecified distal lower extremity** `HCC`

√5ᵗʰ **I82.5** **Chronic embolism and thrombosis of deep veins of lower extremity**
Use additional code, if applicable, for associated long-term (current) use of anticoagulants (Z79.01)
    `EXCLUDES 1` *personal history of venous embolism and thrombosis (Z86.718)*

√6ᵗʰ **I82.50** **Chronic embolism and thrombosis of unspecified deep veins of lower extremity**
    `EXCLUDES 1` *chronic embolism and thrombosis of unspecified deep veins of distal lower extremity (I82.5Z-)*
chronic embolism and thrombosis of unspecified deep veins of proximal lower extremity (I82.5Y-)

    I82.501 **Chronic embolism and thrombosis of unspecified deep veins of right lower extremity** `HCC`

    I82.502 **Chronic embolism and thrombosis of unspecified deep veins of left lower extremity** `HCC`

    I82.503 **Chronic embolism and thrombosis of unspecified deep veins of lower extremity, bilateral** `HCC`

    I82.509 **Chronic embolism and thrombosis of unspecified deep veins of unspecified lower extremity** `HCC`

√6ᵗʰ **I82.51** **Chronic embolism and thrombosis of femoral vein**
▶Chronic embolism and thrombosis of common femoral vein◀
▶Chronic embolism and thrombosis of deep femoral vein◀

    I82.511 **Chronic embolism and thrombosis of right femoral vein** `HCC`

    I82.512 **Chronic embolism and thrombosis of left femoral vein** `HCC`

    I82.513 **Chronic embolism and thrombosis of femoral vein, bilateral** `HCC`

    I82.519 **Chronic embolism and thrombosis of unspecified femoral vein** `HCC`

√6ᵗʰ **I82.52** **Chronic embolism and thrombosis of iliac vein**
▶Chronic embolism and thrombosis of common iliac vein◀
▶Chronic embolism and thrombosis of external iliac vein◀
▶Chronic embolism and thrombosis of internal iliac vein◀

    I82.521 **Chronic embolism and thrombosis of right iliac vein** `HCC`

    I82.522 **Chronic embolism and thrombosis of left iliac vein** `HCC`

    I82.523 **Chronic embolism and thrombosis of iliac vein, bilateral** `HCC`

    I82.529 **Chronic embolism and thrombosis of unspecified iliac vein** `HCC`

√6ᵗʰ **I82.53** **Chronic embolism and thrombosis of popliteal vein**

    I82.531 **Chronic embolism and thrombosis of right popliteal vein** `HCC`

    I82.532 **Chronic embolism and thrombosis of left popliteal vein** `HCC`

    I82.533 **Chronic embolism and thrombosis of popliteal vein, bilateral** `HCC`

    I82.539 **Chronic embolism and thrombosis of unspecified popliteal vein** `HCC`

√6ᵗʰ **I82.54** **Chronic embolism and thrombosis of tibial vein**
▶Chronic embolism and thrombosis of anterior tibial vein◀
▶Chronic embolism and thrombosis of posterior tibial vein◀

    I82.541 **Chronic embolism and thrombosis of right tibial vein** `HCC`

    I82.542 **Chronic embolism and thrombosis of left tibial vein** `HCC`

    I82.543 **Chronic embolism and thrombosis of tibial vein, bilateral** `HCC`

    I82.549 **Chronic embolism and thrombosis of unspecified tibial vein** `HCC`

√6ᵗʰ **I82.55** **Chronic embolism and thrombosis of peroneal vein** ●

    I82.551 **Chronic embolism and thrombosis of right peroneal vein** ●

    I82.552 **Chronic embolism and thrombosis of left peroneal vein** ●

    I82.553 **Chronic embolism and thrombosis of peroneal vein, bilateral** ●

    I82.559 **Chronic embolism and thrombosis of unspecified peroneal vein** ●

√6ᵗʰ **I82.56** **Chronic embolism and thrombosis of calf muscular vein** ●
Chronic embolism and thrombosis of calf muscular vein NOS
Chronic embolism and thrombosis of gastrocnemial vein
Chronic embolism and thrombosis of soleal vein

    I82.561 **Chronic embolism and thrombosis of right calf muscular vein** ●

    I82.562 **Chronic embolism and thrombosis of left calf muscular vein** ●

    I82.563 **Chronic embolism and thrombosis of calf muscular vein, bilateral** ●

    I82.569 **Chronic embolism and thrombosis of unspecified calf muscular vein** ●

√6ᵗʰ **I82.59** **Chronic embolism and thrombosis of other specified deep vein of lower extremity**

    I82.591 **Chronic embolism and thrombosis of other specified deep vein of right lower extremity** `HCC`

    I82.592 **Chronic embolism and thrombosis of other specified deep vein of left lower extremity** `HCC`

    I82.593 **Chronic embolism and thrombosis of other specified deep vein of lower extremity, bilateral** `HCC`

I82.599 Chronic embolism and thrombosis of other specified deep vein of unspecified lower extremity   `HCC`

✓6ᵗʰ **I82.5Y** Chronic embolism and thrombosis of unspecified deep veins of proximal lower extremity

Chronic embolism and thrombosis of deep veins of thigh NOS

Chronic embolism and thrombosis of deep veins of upper leg NOS

I82.5Y1 Chronic embolism and thrombosis of unspecified deep veins of right proximal lower extremity   `HCC`

I82.5Y2 Chronic embolism and thrombosis of unspecified deep veins of left proximal lower extremity   `HCC`

I82.5Y3 Chronic embolism and thrombosis of unspecified deep veins of proximal lower extremity, bilateral   `HCC`

I82.5Y9 Chronic embolism and thrombosis of unspecified deep veins of unspecified proximal lower extremity   `HCC`

✓6ᵗʰ **I82.5Z** Chronic embolism and thrombosis of unspecified deep veins of distal lower extremity

Chronic embolism and thrombosis of deep veins of calf NOS

Chronic embolism and thrombosis of deep veins of lower leg NOS

I82.5Z1 Chronic embolism and thrombosis of unspecified deep veins of right distal lower extremity   `HCC`

I82.5Z2 Chronic embolism and thrombosis of unspecified deep veins of left distal lower extremity   `HCC`

I82.5Z3 Chronic embolism and thrombosis of unspecified deep veins of distal lower extremity, bilateral   `HCC`

I82.5Z9 Chronic embolism and thrombosis of unspecified deep veins of unspecified distal lower extremity   `HCC`

✓5ᵗʰ **I82.6** Acute embolism and thrombosis of veins of upper extremity

✓6ᵗʰ **I82.60** Acute embolism and thrombosis of unspecified veins of upper extremity

I82.601 Acute embolism and thrombosis of unspecified veins of right upper extremity

I82.602 Acute embolism and thrombosis of unspecified veins of left upper extremity

I82.603 Acute embolism and thrombosis of unspecified veins of upper extremity, bilateral

I82.609 Acute embolism and thrombosis of unspecified veins of unspecified upper extremity

✓6ᵗʰ **I82.61** Acute embolism and thrombosis of superficial veins of upper extremity

Acute embolism and thrombosis of antecubital vein

Acute embolism and thrombosis of basilic vein

Acute embolism and thrombosis of cephalic vein

I82.611 Acute embolism and thrombosis of superficial veins of right upper extremity

I82.612 Acute embolism and thrombosis of superficial veins of left upper extremity

I82.613 Acute embolism and thrombosis of superficial veins of upper extremity, bilateral

I82.619 Acute embolism and thrombosis of superficial veins of unspecified upper extremity

✓6ᵗʰ **I82.62** Acute embolism and thrombosis of deep veins of upper extremity

Acute embolism and thrombosis of brachial vein

Acute embolism and thrombosis of radial vein

Acute embolism and thrombosis of ulnar vein

I82.621 Acute embolism and thrombosis of deep veins of right upper extremity   `HCC`

I82.622 Acute embolism and thrombosis of deep veins of left upper extremity   `HCC`

I82.623 Acute embolism and thrombosis of deep veins of upper extremity, bilateral   `HCC`

I82.629 Acute embolism and thrombosis of deep veins of unspecified upper extremity   `HCC`

✓5ᵗʰ **I82.7** Chronic embolism and thrombosis of veins of upper extremity

Use additional code, if applicable, for associated long-term (current) use of anticoagulants (Z79.01)

EXCLUDES 1   personal history of venous embolism and thrombosis (Z86.718)

✓6ᵗʰ **I82.70** Chronic embolism and thrombosis of unspecified veins of upper extremity

I82.701 Chronic embolism and thrombosis of unspecified veins of right upper extremity

I82.702 Chronic embolism and thrombosis of unspecified veins of left upper extremity

I82.703 Chronic embolism and thrombosis of unspecified veins of upper extremity, bilateral

I82.709 Chronic embolism and thrombosis of unspecified veins of unspecified upper extremity

✓6ᵗʰ **I82.71** Chronic embolism and thrombosis of superficial veins of upper extremity

Chronic embolism and thrombosis of antecubital vein

Chronic embolism and thrombosis of basilic vein

Chronic embolism and thrombosis of cephalic vein

I82.711 Chronic embolism and thrombosis of superficial veins of right upper extremity

I82.712 Chronic embolism and thrombosis of superficial veins of left upper extremity

I82.713 Chronic embolism and thrombosis of superficial veins of upper extremity, bilateral

I82.719 Chronic embolism and thrombosis of superficial veins of unspecified upper extremity

✓6ᵗʰ **I82.72** Chronic embolism and thrombosis of deep veins of upper extremity

Chronic embolism and thrombosis of brachial vein

Chronic embolism and thrombosis of radial vein

Chronic embolism and thrombosis of ulnar vein

I82.721 Chronic embolism and thrombosis of deep veins of right upper extremity   `HCC`

I82.722 Chronic embolism and thrombosis of deep veins of left upper extremity   `HCC`

I82.723 Chronic embolism and thrombosis of deep veins of upper extremity, bilateral   `HCC`

I82.729 Chronic embolism and thrombosis of deep veins of unspecified upper extremity   `HCC`

✓5ᵗʰ **I82.A** Embolism and thrombosis of axillary vein

✓6ᵗʰ **I82.A1** Acute embolism and thrombosis of axillary vein

I82.A11 Acute embolism and thrombosis of right axillary vein   `HCC`

I82.A12 Acute embolism and thrombosis of left axillary vein   `HCC`

I82.A13 Acute embolism and thrombosis of axillary vein, bilateral   `HCC`

I82.A19 Acute embolism and thrombosis of unspecified axillary vein   `HCC`

✓6ᵗʰ **I82.A2** Chronic embolism and thrombosis of axillary vein

I82.A21 Chronic embolism and thrombosis of right axillary vein   `HCC`

I82.A22 Chronic embolism and thrombosis of **left** axillary vein `HCC`

I82.A23 Chronic embolism and thrombosis of axillary vein, **bilateral** `HCC`

I82.A29 Chronic embolism and thrombosis of unspecified axillary vein `HCC`

✓5ᵗʰ **I82.B** Embolism and thrombosis of subclavian vein

 ✓6ᵗʰ **I82.B1** Acute embolism and thrombosis of subclavian vein

 I82.B11 Acute embolism and thrombosis of **right** subclavian vein `HCC`

 I82.B12 Acute embolism and thrombosis of **left** subclavian vein `HCC`

 I82.B13 Acute embolism and thrombosis of subclavian vein, **bilateral** `HCC`

 I82.B19 Acute embolism and thrombosis of unspecified subclavian vein `HCC`

 ✓6ᵗʰ **I82.B2** Chronic embolism and thrombosis of subclavian vein

 I82.B21 Chronic embolism and thrombosis of **right** subclavian vein `HCC`

 I82.B22 Chronic embolism and thrombosis of **left** subclavian vein `HCC`

 I82.B23 Chronic embolism and thrombosis of subclavian vein, **bilateral** `HCC`

 I82.B29 Chronic embolism and thrombosis of unspecified subclavian vein `HCC`

✓5ᵗʰ **I82.C** Embolism and thrombosis of internal jugular vein

 ✓6ᵗʰ **I82.C1** Acute embolism and thrombosis of internal jugular vein

 I82.C11 Acute embolism and thrombosis of **right** internal jugular vein `HCC`

 I82.C12 Acute embolism and thrombosis of **left** Internal Jugular vein `HCC`

 I82.C13 Acute embolism and thrombosis of internal jugular vein, **bilateral** `HCC`

 I82.C19 Acute embolism and thrombosis of unspecified internal jugular vein `HCC`

 ✓6ᵗʰ **I82.C2** Chronic embolism and thrombosis of internal jugular vein

 I82.C21 Chronic embolism and thrombosis of **right** Internal jugular vein `HCC`

 I82.C22 Chronic embolism and thrombosis of **left** internal jugular vein `HCC`

 I82.C23 Chronic embolism and thrombosis of internal jugular vein, **bilateral** `HCC`

 I82.C29 Chronic embolism and thrombosis of unspecified internal jugular vein `HCC`

✓5ᵗʰ **I82.8** Embolism and thrombosis of other specified veins

 Use additional code, if applicable, for associated long-term (current) use of anticoagulants (Z79.01)

 ✓6ᵗʰ **I82.81** Embolism and thrombosis of superficial veins of lower extremities
 Embolism and thrombosis of saphenous vein (greater) (lesser)

 I82.811 Embolism and thrombosis of superficial veins of **right** lower extremity

 I82.812 Embolism and thrombosis of superficial veins of **left** lower extremity

 I82.813 Embolism and thrombosis of superficial veins of lower extremities, **bilateral**

 I82.819 Embolism and thrombosis of superficial veins of unspecified lower extremity

 ✓6ᵗʰ **I82.89** Embolism and thrombosis of other specified veins

 I82.890 Acute embolism and thrombosis of other specified veins

 I82.891 Chronic embolism and thrombosis of other specified veins

✓5ᵗʰ **I82.9** Embolism and thrombosis of unspecified vein

 I82.90 Acute embolism and thrombosis of unspecified vein
 Embolism of vein NOS
 Thrombosis (vein) NOS

 I82.91 Chronic embolism and thrombosis of unspecified vein

✓4ᵗʰ **I83** Varicose veins of lower extremities

 `EXCLUDES 1` *varicose veins complicating pregnancy (O22.0-)*
 varicose veins complicating the puerperium (O87.4)

 ✓5ᵗʰ **I83.0** Varicose veins of lower extremities with ulcer
 Use additional code to identify severity of ulcer (L97.-)

 ✓6ᵗʰ **I83.00** Varicose veins of unspecified lower extremity with ulcer

 I83.001 Varicose veins of unspecified lower extremity with ulcer of **thigh** `HCC` `A`

 I83.002 Varicose veins of unspecified lower extremity with ulcer of **calf** `HCC` `A`

 I83.003 Varicose veins of unspecified lower extremity with ulcer of **ankle** `HCC` `A`

 I83.004 Varicose veins of unspecified lower extremity with ulcer of **heel and midfoot** `HCC` `A`
 Varicose veins of unspecified lower extremity with ulcer of plantar surface of midfoot

 I83.005 Varicose veins of unspecified lower extremity with ulcer other part of foot `HCC` `A`
 Varicose veins of unspecified lower extremity with ulcer of toe

 I83.008 Varicose veins of unspecified lower extremity with ulcer other part of lower leg `HCC` `A`

 I83.009 Varicose veins of unspecified lower extremity with ulcer of unspecified site `HCC` `A`

 ✓6ᵗʰ **I83.01** Varicose veins of **right** lower extremity with ulcer

 I83.011 Varicose veins of right lower extremity with ulcer of **thigh** `HCC` `A`

 I83.012 Varicose veins of right lower extremity with ulcer of **calf** `HCC` `A`

 I83.013 Varicose veins of right lower extremity with ulcer of **ankle** `HCC` `A`

 I83.014 Varicose veins of right lower extremity with ulcer of **heel and midfoot** `HCC` `A`
 Varicose veins of right lower extremity with ulcer of plantar surface of midfoot

 I83.015 Varicose veins of right lower extremity with ulcer other part of foot `HCC` `A`
 Varicose veins of right lower extremity with ulcer of toe

 I83.018 Varicose veins of right lower extremity with ulcer other part of lower leg `HCC` `A`

 I83.019 Varicose veins of right lower extremity with ulcer of unspecified site `HCC` `A`

 ✓6ᵗʰ **I83.02** Varicose veins of **left** lower extremity with ulcer

 I83.021 Varicose veins of left lower extremity with ulcer of **thigh** `HCC` `A`

 I83.022 Varicose veins of left lower extremity with ulcer of **calf** `HCC` `A`

 I83.023 Varicose veins of left lower extremity with ulcer of **ankle** `HCC` `A`

 I83.024 Varicose veins of left lower extremity with ulcer of **heel and midfoot** `HCC` `A`
 Varicose veins of left lower extremity with ulcer of plantar surface of midfoot

 I83.025 Varicose veins of left lower extremity with ulcer other part of foot `HCC` `A`
 Varicose veins of left lower extremity with ulcer of toe

☑ Additional Character Required   ✓x7ᵗʰ Placeholder Alert   Manifestation   Unspecified Dx   ▶◀ Revised Text   ● New Code   ▲ Revised Code Title

Chapter 9. Diseases of the Circulatory System

I83.Ø28   **Varicose veins of left lower extremity with ulcer other part of lower leg**   HCC A

I83.Ø29   **Varicose veins of left lower extremity with ulcer of unspecified site**   HCC A

√5ᵗʰ **I83.1   Varicose veins of lower extremities with inflammation**

   I83.1Ø   **Varicose veins of unspecified lower extremity with inflammation**   A

   I83.11   **Varicose veins of right lower extremity with inflammation**   A

   I83.12   **Varicose veins of left lower extremity with inflammation**   A

√5ᵗʰ **I83.2   Varicose veins of lower extremities with both ulcer and inflammation**

   Use additional code to identify severity of ulcer (L97.-)

   √6ᵗʰ I83.2Ø   **Varicose veins of unspecified lower extremity with both ulcer and inflammation**

     I83.2Ø1   **Varicose veins of unspecified lower extremity with both ulcer of thigh and inflammation**   HCC A

     I83.2Ø2   **Varicose veins of unspecified lower extremity with both ulcer of calf and inflammation**   HCC A

     I83.2Ø3   **Varicose veins of unspecified lower extremity with both ulcer of ankle and inflammation**   HCC A

     I83.2Ø4   **Varicose veins of unspecified lower extremity with both ulcer of heel and midfoot and inflammation**   HCC A

       Varicose veins of unspecified lower extremity with both ulcer of plantar surface of midfoot and inflammation

     I83.2Ø5   **Varicose veins of unspecified lower extremity with both ulcer of other part of foot and inflammation**   HCC A

       Varicose veins of unspecified lower extremity with both ulcer of toe and inflammation

     I83.2Ø8   **Varicose veins of unspecified lower extremity with both ulcer of other part of lower extremity and inflammation**   HCC A

     I83.2Ø9   **Varicose veins of unspecified lower extremity with both ulcer of unspecified site and inflammation**   HCC A

   √6ᵗʰ I83.21   **Varicose veins of right lower extremity with both ulcer and inflammation**

     I83.211   **Varicose veins of right lower extremity with both ulcer of thigh and inflammation**   HCC A

     I83.212   **Varicose veins of right lower extremity with both ulcer of calf and inflammation**   HCC A

     I83.213   **Varicose veins of right lower extremity with both ulcer of ankle and inflammation**   HCC A

     I83.214   **Varicose veins of right lower extremity with both ulcer of heel and midfoot and inflammation**   HCC A

       Varicose veins of right lower extremity with both ulcer of plantar surface of midfoot and inflammation

     I83.215   **Varicose veins of right lower extremity with both ulcer other part of foot and inflammation**   HCC A

       Varicose veins of right lower extremity with both ulcer of toe and inflammation

     I83.218   **Varicose veins of right lower extremity with both ulcer of other part of lower extremity and inflammation**   HCC A

     I83.219   **Varicose veins of right lower extremity with both ulcer of unspecified site and inflammation**   HCC A

   √6ᵗʰ I83.22   **Varicose veins of left lower extremity with both ulcer and inflammation**

     I83.221   **Varicose veins of left lower extremity with both ulcer of thigh and inflammation**   HCC A

     I83.222   **Varicose veins of left lower extremity with both ulcer of calf and inflammation**   HCC A

     I83.223   **Varicose veins of left lower extremity with both ulcer of ankle and inflammation**   HCC A

     I83.224   **Varicose veins of left lower extremity with both ulcer of heel and midfoot and inflammation**   HCC A

       Varicose veins of left lower extremity with both ulcer of plantar surface of midfoot and inflammation

     I83.225   **Varicose veins of left lower extremity with both ulcer other part of foot and inflammation**   HCC A

       Varicose veins of left lower extremity with both ulcer of toe and inflammation

     I83.228   **Varicose veins of left lower extremity with both ulcer of other part of lower extremity and inflammation**   HCC A

     I83.229   **Varicose veins of left lower extremity with both ulcer of unspecified site and inflammation**   HCC A

√5ᵗʰ **I83.8   Varicose veins of lower extremities with other complications**

   √6ᵗʰ I83.81   **Varicose veins of lower extremities with pain**

     I83.811   **Varicose veins of right lower extremity with pain**   A

     I83.812   **Varicose veins of left lower extremity with pain**   A

     I83.813   **Varicose veins of bilateral lower extremities with pain**   A

     I83.819   **Varicose veins of unspecified lower extremity with pain**   A

   √6ᵗʰ I83.89   **Varicose veins of lower extremities with other complications**

     Varicose veins of lower extremities with edema

     Varicose veins of lower extremities with swelling

     I83.891   **Varicose veins of right lower extremity with other complications**   A

     I83.892   **Varicose veins of left lower extremity with other complications**   A

     I83.893   **Varicose veins of bilateral lower extremities with other complications**   A

     I83.899   **Varicose veins of unspecified lower extremity with other complications**   A

√5ᵗʰ **I83.9   Asymptomatic varicose veins of lower extremities**

   Phlebectasia of lower extremities

   Varicose veins of lower extremities

   Varix of lower extremities

   I83.9Ø   **Asymptomatic varicose veins of unspecified lower extremity**   A

     Varicose veins NOS

   I83.91   **Asymptomatic varicose veins of right lower extremity**   A

   I83.92   **Asymptomatic varicose veins of left lower extremity**   A

   I83.93   **Asymptomatic varicose veins of bilateral lower extremities**   A

√4ᵗʰ **I85   Esophageal varices**

   Use additional code to identify:

     alcohol abuse and dependence (F1Ø.-)

√5ᵗʰ **I85.Ø   Esophageal varices**

   Idiopathic esophageal varices

   Primary esophageal varices

   I85.ØØ   **Esophageal varices without bleeding**   HCC

     Esophageal varices NOS

   I85.Ø1   **Esophageal varices with bleeding**   HCC

✓5ᵗʰ **I85.1** **Secondary esophageal varices**
Esophageal varices secondary to alcoholic liver disease
Esophageal varices secondary to cirrhosis of liver
Esophageal varices secondary to schistosomiasis
Esophageal varices secondary to toxic liver disease
Code first underlying disease

    I85.10 **Secondary esophageal varices** without **bleeding**   HCC

    I85.11 **Secondary esophageal varices** with **bleeding**   HCC

✓4ᵗʰ **I86** **Varicose veins of other sites**
   EXCLUDES 1   varicose veins of unspecified site (I83.9-)
   EXCLUDES 2   retinal varices (H35.0-)

   I86.0 **Sublingual varices**
     DEF: Distended, tortuous veins beneath the tongue.

   I86.1 **Scrotal varices**   ♂
     Varicocele

   I86.2 **Pelvic varices**

   I86.3 **Vulval varices**   ♀
     EXCLUDES 1   vulval varices complicating childbirth and the puerperium (O87.8)
       vulval varices complicating pregnancy (O22.1-)

   I86.4 **Gastric varices**

   I86.8 **Varicose veins of other specified sites**   A
     Varicose ulcer of nasal septum

✓4ᵗʰ **I87** **Other disorders of veins**

✓5ᵗʰ   **I87.0** **Postthrombotic syndrome**
Chronic venous hypertension due to deep vein thrombosis
Postphlebitic syndrome
     EXCLUDES 1   chronic venous hypertension without deep vein thrombosis (I87.3-)

✓6ᵗʰ   **I87.00** **Postthrombotic syndrome** without complications
Asymptomatic postthrombotic syndrome

     I87.001 **Postthrombotic syndrome without complications of** right lower **extremity**

     I87.002 **Postthrombotic syndrome without complications of** left lower **extremity**

     I87.003 **Postthrombotic syndrome without complications of** bilateral lower **extremity**

     I87.009 **Postthrombotic syndrome without complications of unspecified extremity**
Postthrombotic syndrome NOS

✓6ᵗʰ   **I87.01** **Postthrombotic syndrome with** ulcer
Use additional code to specify site and severity of ulcer (L97.-)

     I87.011 **Postthrombotic syndrome with ulcer of** right lower **extremity**   HCC

     I87.012 **Postthrombotic syndrome with ulcer of** left lower **extremity**   HCC

     I87.013 **Postthrombotic syndrome with ulcer of** bilateral lower **extremity**   HCC

     I87.019 **Postthrombotic syndrome with ulcer of unspecified lower extremity**   HCC

✓6ᵗʰ   **I87.02** **Postthrombotic syndrome with** inflammation

     I87.021 **Postthrombotic syndrome with inflammation of** right lower **extremity**

     I87.022 **Postthrombotic syndrome with inflammation of** left lower **extremity**

     I87.023 **Postthrombotic syndrome with inflammation of** bilateral lower **extremity**

     I87.029 **Postthrombotic syndrome with inflammation of unspecified lower extremity**

✓6ᵗʰ   **I87.03** **Postthrombotic syndrome with** ulcer and inflammation
Use additional code to specify site and severity of ulcer (L97.-)

     I87.031 **Postthrombotic syndrome with ulcer and inflammation of** right lower **extremity**   HCC

     I87.032 **Postthrombotic syndrome with ulcer and inflammation of** left lower **extremity**   HCC

     I87.033 **Postthrombotic syndrome with ulcer and inflammation of** bilateral lower **extremity**   HCC

     I87.039 **Postthrombotic syndrome with ulcer and inflammation of unspecified lower extremity**   HCC

✓6ᵗʰ   **I87.09** **Postthrombotic syndrome with other complications**

     I87.091 **Postthrombotic syndrome with other complications of** right lower **extremity**

     I87.092 **Postthrombotic syndrome with other complications of** left lower **extremity**

     I87.093 **Postthrombotic syndrome with other complications of** bilateral lower **extremity**

     I87.099 **Postthrombotic syndrome with other complications of unspecified lower extremity**

   I87.1 **Compression of vein**
Stricture of vein
Vena cava syndrome (inferior) (superior)
     EXCLUDES 2   compression of pulmonary vein (I28.8)

   I87.2 **Venous insufficiency (chronic) (peripheral)**
Stasis dermatitis
     EXCLUDES 1   stasis dermatitis with varicose veins of lower extremities (I83.1-, I83.2-)
     DEF: Insufficient drainage of venous blood in any part of the body that results in edema or dermatosis.

✓5ᵗʰ   **I87.3** **Chronic venous hypertension (idiopathic)**
Stasis edema
     EXCLUDES 1   chronic venous hypertension due to deep vein thrombosis (I87.0-)
       varicose veins of lower extremities (I83.-)

✓6ᵗʰ   **I87.30** **Chronic venous hypertension (idiopathic)** without complications
Asymptomatic chronic venous hypertension (idiopathic)

     I87.301 **Chronic venous hypertension (idiopathic) without complications of** right lower **extremity**

     I87.302 **Chronic venous hypertension (idiopathic) without complications of** left lower **extremity**

     I87.303 **Chronic venous hypertension (idiopathic) without complications of** bilateral lower **extremity**

     I87.309 **Chronic venous hypertension (idiopathic) without complications of unspecified lower extremity**
Chronic venous hypertension NOS

✓6ᵗʰ   **I87.31** **Chronic venous hypertension (idiopathic) with** ulcer
Use additional code to specify site and severity of ulcer (L97.-)

     I87.311 **Chronic venous hypertension (idiopathic) with ulcer of** right lower **extremity**   HCC

     I87.312 **Chronic venous hypertension (idiopathic) with ulcer of** left lower **extremity**   HCC

     I87.313 **Chronic venous hypertension (idiopathic) with ulcer of** bilateral lower **extremity**   HCC

     I87.319 **Chronic venous hypertension (idiopathic) with ulcer of unspecified lower extremity**   HCC

✓6ᵗʰ   **I87.32** **Chronic venous hypertension (idiopathic) with** inflammation

     I87.321 **Chronic venous hypertension (idiopathic) with inflammation of** right lower **extremity**

     I87.322 **Chronic venous hypertension (idiopathic) with inflammation of** left lower **extremity**

     I87.323 **Chronic venous hypertension (idiopathic) with inflammation of** bilateral lower **extremity**

     I87.329 **Chronic venous hypertension (idiopathic) with inflammation of unspecified lower extremity**

✓6ᵗʰ   **I87.33** **Chronic venous hypertension (idiopathic) with** ulcer and inflammation
Use additional code to specify site and severity of ulcer (L97.-)

     I87.331 **Chronic venous hypertension (idiopathic) with ulcer and inflammation of** right lower **extremity**   HCC

☑ Additional Character Required   ✓x7ᵗʰ Placeholder Alert   Manifestation   Unspecified Dx   ►◄ Revised Text   ● New Code   ▲ Revised Code Title

Chapter 9. Diseases of the Circulatory System

I87.332   **Chronic venous hypertension (idiopathic) with ulcer and inflammation of** left lower **extremity**   `HCC`

I87.333   **Chronic venous hypertension (idiopathic) with ulcer and inflammation of** bilateral lower **extremity**   `HCC`

I87.339   **Chronic venous hypertension (idiopathic) with ulcer and inflammation of unspecified lower extremity**   `HCC`

✓6ᵗʰ **I87.39 Chronic venous hypertension (idiopathic) with other complications**

I87.391   **Chronic venous hypertension (idiopathic) with other complications of** right lower **extremity**

I87.392   **Chronic venous hypertension (idiopathic) with other complications of** left lower **extremity**

I87.393   **Chronic venous hypertension (idiopathic) with other complications of** bilateral lower **extremity**

I87.399   **Chronic venous hypertension (idiopathic) with other complications of unspecified lower extremity**

I87.8 Other specified disorders of veins
Phlebosclerosis
Venofibrosis

I87.9 Disorder of vein, unspecified

✓4ᵗʰ **I88 Nonspecific lymphadenitis**
     EXCLUDES 1   acute lymphadenitis, except mesenteric (L04.-)
             enlarged lymph nodes NOS (R59.-)
             human immunodeficiency virus [HIV] disease resulting in generalized lymphadenopathy (B20)

I88.0 Nonspecific mesenteric lymphadenitis
Mesenteric lymphadenitis (acute)(chronic)

I88.1 Chronic lymphadenitis, except mesenteric
Adenitis
Lymphadenitis

I88.8 Other nonspecific lymphadenitis

I88.9 Nonspecific lymphadenitis, unspecified
Lymphadenitis NOS

✓4ᵗʰ **I89 Other noninfective disorders of lymphatic vessels and lymph nodes**
     EXCLUDES 1   chylocele, tunica vaginalis (nonfilarial) NOS (N50.89)
             enlarged lymph nodes NOS (R59.-)
             filarial chylocele (B74.-)
             hereditary lymphedema (Q82.0)

I89.0 Lymphedema, not elsewhere classified
Elephantiasis (nonfilarial) NOS
Lymphangiectasis
Obliteration, lymphatic vessel
Praecox lymphedema
Secondary lymphedema
     EXCLUDES 1   postmastectomy lymphedema (I97.2)

I89.1 Lymphangitis
Chronic lymphangitis
Lymphangitis NOS
Subacute lymphangitis
     EXCLUDES 1   acute lymphangitis (L03.-)

I89.8 Other specified noninfective disorders of lymphatic vessels and lymph nodes
Chylocele (nonfilarial)
Chylous ascites
Chylous cyst
Lipomelanotic reticulosis
Lymph node or vessel fistula
Lymph node or vessel infarction
Lymph node or vessel rupture

I89.9 Noninfective disorder of lymphatic vessels and lymph nodes, unspecified
Disease of lymphatic vessels NOS

Other and unspecified disorders of the circulatory system (I95-I99)

✓4ᵗʰ **I95 Hypotension**
     EXCLUDES 1   cardiovascular collapse (R57.9) (~R57.9)
             maternal hypotension syndrome (O26.5-)
             nonspecific low blood pressure reading NOS (R03.1)

I95.0 Idiopathic hypotension

I95.1 Orthostatic hypotension
Hypotension, postural
     EXCLUDES 1   neurogenic orthostatic hypotension [Shy-Drager] (G90.3)
             orthostatic hypotension due to drugs (I95.2)

I95.2 Hypotension due to drugs
Orthostatic hypotension due to drugs
Use additional code for adverse effect, if applicable, to identify drug (T36-T50 with fifth or sixth character 5)

I95.3 Hypotension of hemodialysis
Intra-dialytic hypotension

✓5ᵗʰ **I95.8 Other hypotension**

I95.81   **Postprocedural hypotension**

I95.89   **Other hypotension**
Chronic hypotension

I95.9 Hypotension, unspecified

I96 Gangrene, not elsewhere classified   `HCC`
Gangrenous cellulitis
     EXCLUDES 1   gangrene in atherosclerosis of native arteries of the extremities (I70.26)
             gangrene in hernia (K40.1, K40.4, K41.1, K41.4, K42.1, K43.1-, K44.1, K45.1, K46.1)
             gangrene in other peripheral vascular diseases (I73.-)
             gangrene of certain specified sites — see Alphabetical Index
             gas gangrene (A48.0)
             pyoderma gangrenosum (L88)
     EXCLUDES 2   gangrene in diabetes mellitus (E08-E13 with .52)
     AHA: 2018,4Q,87; 2018,3Q,3; 2017,3Q,6; 2013,2Q,34

✓4ᵗʰ **I97 Intraoperative and postprocedural complications and disorders of circulatory system, not elsewhere classified**
     EXCLUDES 2   postprocedural shock (T81.1-)
     AHA: 2019,2Q,21

I97.0 Postcardiotomy syndrome

✓5ᵗʰ **I97.1 Other postprocedural cardiac functional disturbances**
     EXCLUDES 2   acute pulmonary insufficiency following thoracic surgery (J95.1)
             intraoperative cardiac functional disturbances (I97.7-)

✓6ᵗʰ **I97.11 Postprocedural cardiac insufficiency**

I97.110   **Postprocedural cardiac insufficiency following** cardiac surgery

I97.111   **Postprocedural cardiac insufficiency following** other surgery

✓6ᵗʰ **I97.12 Postprocedural cardiac arrest**

I97.120   **Postprocedural cardiac arrest following** cardiac surgery

I97.121   **Postprocedural cardiac arrest following** other surgery

✓6ᵗʰ **I97.13 Postprocedural heart failure**
Use additional code to identify the heart failure (I50.-)

I97.130   **Postprocedural heart failure following** cardiac surgery

I97.131   **Postprocedural heart failure following** other surgery

✓6ᵗʰ **I97.19 Other postprocedural cardiac functional disturbances**
Use additional code, if applicable, to further specify disorder

I97.190   **Other postprocedural cardiac functional disturbances following** cardiac surgery
Use additional code, if applicable, for type 4 or type 5 myocardial infarction, to further specify disorder
AHA: 2019,2Q,33

I97.191   **Other postprocedural cardiac functional disturbances following** other surgery

I97.2   **Postmastectomy lymphedema syndrome**   [A]
     Elephantiasis due to mastectomy
     Obliteration of lymphatic vessels

I97.3   **Postprocedural hypertension**

√5ᵗʰ   I97.4   **Intraoperative hemorrhage and hematoma of a circulatory system organ or structure complicating a procedure**
     EXCLUDES 1   *intraoperative hemorrhage and hematoma of a circulatory system organ or structure due to accidental puncture and laceration during a procedure (I97.5-)*
     EXCLUDES 2   *intraoperative cerebrovascular hemorrhage complicating a procedure (G97.3-)*

     √6ᵗʰ   I97.41   **Intraoperative hemorrhage and hematoma of a circulatory system organ or structure complicating a circulatory system procedure**
         I97.410   **Intraoperative hemorrhage and hematoma of a circulatory system organ or structure complicating a cardiac catheterization**
         I97.411   **Intraoperative hemorrhage and hematoma of a circulatory system organ or structure complicating a cardiac bypass**
         I97.418   **Intraoperative hemorrhage and hematoma of a circulatory system organ or structure complicating other circulatory system procedure**

     I97.42   **Intraoperative hemorrhage and hematoma of a circulatory system organ or structure complicating other procedure**

√5ᵗʰ   I97.5   **Accidental puncture and laceration of a circulatory system organ or structure during a procedure**
     EXCLUDES 2   *accidental puncture and laceration of brain during a procedure (G97.4-)*

     I97.51   **Accidental puncture and laceration of a circulatory system organ or structure during a circulatory system procedure**
         AHA: 2019,2Q,24

     I97.52   **Accidental puncture and laceration of a circulatory system organ or structure during other procedure**

√5ᵗʰ   I97.6   **Postprocedural hemorrhage, hematoma and seroma of a circulatory system organ or structure following a procedure**
     EXCLUDES 2   *postprocedural cerebrovascular hemorrhage complicating a procedure (G97.5-)*
     AHA: 2016,4Q,9-10

     √6ᵗʰ   I97.61   **Postprocedural hemorrhage of a circulatory system organ or structure following a circulatory system procedure**
         I97.610   **Postprocedural hemorrhage of a circulatory system organ or structure following a cardiac catheterization**
         I97.611   **Postprocedural hemorrhage of a circulatory system organ or structure following cardiac bypass**
         I97.618   **Postprocedural hemorrhage of a circulatory system organ or structure following other circulatory system procedure**

     √6ᵗʰ   I97.62   **Postprocedural hemorrhage, hematoma and seroma of a circulatory system organ or structure following other procedure**
         I97.620   **Postprocedural hemorrhage of a circulatory system organ or structure following other procedure**
         I97.621   **Postprocedural hematoma of a circulatory system organ or structure following other procedure**
         I97.622   **Postprocedural seroma of a circulatory system organ or structure following other procedure**

     √6ᵗʰ   I97.63   **Postprocedural hematoma of a circulatory system organ or structure following a circulatory system procedure**
         I97.630   **Postprocedural hematoma of a circulatory system organ or structure following a cardiac catheterization**
         I97.631   **Postprocedural hematoma of a circulatory system organ or structure following cardiac bypass**
         I97.638   **Postprocedural hematoma of a circulatory system organ or structure following other circulatory system procedure**

     √6ᵗʰ   I97.64   **Postprocedural seroma of a circulatory system organ or structure following a circulatory system procedure**
         I97.640   **Postprocedural seroma of a circulatory system organ or structure following a cardiac catheterization**
         I97.641   **Postprocedural seroma of a circulatory system organ or structure following cardiac bypass**
         I97.648   **Postprocedural seroma of a circulatory system organ or structure following other circulatory system procedure**

√5ᵗʰ   I97.7   **Intraoperative cardiac functional disturbances**
     EXCLUDES 2   *acute pulmonary insufficiency following thoracic surgery (J95.1)*
         postprocedural cardiac functional disturbances (I97.1-)

     √6ᵗʰ   I97.71   **Intraoperative cardiac arrest**
         I97.710   **Intraoperative cardiac arrest during cardiac surgery**
         I97.711   **Intraoperative cardiac arrest during other surgery**

     √6ᵗʰ   I97.79   **Other intraoperative cardiac functional disturbances**
         Use additional code, if applicable, to further specify disorder
         I97.790   **Other intraoperative cardiac functional disturbances during cardiac surgery**
         I97.791   **Other intraoperative cardiac functional disturbances during other surgery**

√5ᵗʰ   I97.8   **Other intraoperative and postprocedural complications and disorders of the circulatory system, not elsewhere classified**
     Use additional code, if applicable, to further specify disorder

     √6ᵗʰ   I97.81   **Intraoperative cerebrovascular infarction**
         I97.810   **Intraoperative cerebrovascular infarction during cardiac surgery**   HCC
         I97.811   **Intraoperative cerebrovascular infarction during other surgery**   HCC

     √6ᵗʰ   I97.82   **Postprocedural cerebrovascular infarction**
         I97.820   **Postprocedural cerebrovascular infarction following cardiac surgery**   HCC
         I97.821   **Postprocedural cerebrovascular infarction following other surgery**   HCC

     I97.88   **Other intraoperative complications of the circulatory system, not elsewhere classified**

     I97.89   **Other postprocedural complications and disorders of the circulatory system, not elsewhere classified**
         AHA: 2019,2Q,33

√4ᵗʰ   **I99   Other and unspecified disorders of circulatory system**

     I99.8   **Other disorder of circulatory system**

     I99.9   **Unspecified disorder of circulatory system**

☑ Additional Character Required   √x7ᵗʰ Placeholder Alert   Manifestation   Unspecified Dx   ▶◀ Revised Text   ● New Code   ▲ Revised Code Title

Chapter 10. Diseases of the Respiratory System (J00–J99)

Chapter-specific Guidelines with Coding Examples

The chapter-specific guidelines from the ICD-10-CM Official Guidelines for Coding and Reporting have been provided below. Along with these guidelines are coding examples, contained in the shaded boxes, that have been developed to help illustrate the coding and/or sequencing guidance found in these guidelines.

a. Chronic obstructive pulmonary disease [COPD] and asthma

1) Acute exacerbation of chronic obstructive bronchitis and asthma

The codes in categories J44 and J45 distinguish between uncomplicated cases and those in acute exacerbation. An acute exacerbation is a worsening or a decompensation of a chronic condition. An acute exacerbation is not equivalent to an infection superimposed on a chronic condition, though an exacerbation may be triggered by an infection.

Acute streptococcal bronchitis with acute exacerbation of COPD

J20.2   **Acute bronchitis due to streptococcus**

J44.0   **Chronic obstructive pulmonary disease with (acute) lower respiratory infection**

J44.1   **Chronic obstructive pulmonary disease with (acute) exacerbation**

Explanation: ICD-10-CM uses combination codes to create organism-specific classifications for acute bronchitis. Category J44 codes include combination codes with severity components, which differentiate between COPD with acute lower respiratory infection (acute bronchitis), COPD with acute exacerbation, and COPD without mention of a complication (unspecified).

An acute exacerbation is a worsening or a decompensation of a chronic condition. An acute exacerbation is not equivalent to an infection superimposed on a chronic condition, though an exacerbation may be triggered by an infection, as in this example.

Exacerbation of moderate persistent asthma with status asthmaticus

J45.42   **Moderate persistent asthma with status asthmaticus**

Explanation: Category J45 Asthma includes severity-specific subcategories and fifth-character codes to distinguish between uncomplicated cases, those in acute exacerbation, and those with status asthmaticus.

---

b. Acute respiratory failure

1) Acute respiratory failure as principal diagnosis

A code from subcategory J96.0, Acute respiratory failure, or subcategory J96.2, Acute and chronic respiratory failure, may be assigned as a principal diagnosis when it is the condition established after study to be chiefly responsible for occasioning the admission to the hospital, and the selection is supported by the Alphabetic Index and Tabular List. However, chapter-specific coding guidelines (such as obstetrics, poisoning, HIV, newborn) that provide sequencing direction take precedence.

Acute hypoxic respiratory failure due to exacerbation of chronic obstructive bronchitis

J96.01   **Acute respiratory failure with hypoxia**

J44.1   **Chronic obstructive pulmonary disease with (acute) exacerbation**

Explanation: Category J96 classifies respiratory failure with combination codes that designate the severity and the presence of hypoxia and hypercapnia. Code J96.01 is sequenced as the first-listed diagnosis, as the reason for the encounter. Respiratory failure may be assigned as a principal diagnosis when it is the condition established after study to be chiefly responsible for occasioning the encounter and the selection is supported by the Alphabetic Index and Tabular List.

---

2) Acute respiratory failure as secondary diagnosis

Respiratory failure may be listed as a secondary diagnosis if it occurs after admission, or if it is present on admission, but does not meet the definition of principal diagnosis.

Acute respiratory failure due to accidental oxycodone overdose

T40.2X1A   **Poisoning by other opioids, accidental (unintentional), initial encounter**

J96.00   **Acute respiratory failure, unspecified whether with hypoxia or hypercapnia**

Explanation: Respiratory failure may be assigned as a principal diagnosis when it is the condition established after study to be chiefly responsible for occasioning the encounter, and the selection is supported by the Alphabetic Index and Tabular List. However, chapter-specific coding guidelines, such as poisoning, that provide sequencing direction take precedence. When coding a poisoning or reaction to the improper use of a medication (e.g. overdose, wrong substance given or taken in error, wrong route of administration), first assign the appropriate code from categories T36–T50. Use additional code(s) for all manifestations of the poisoning. In this instance, the respiratory failure is a manifestation of the poisoning and is sequenced as a secondary diagnosis.

---

3) Sequencing of acute respiratory failure and another acute condition

When a patient is admitted with respiratory failure and another acute condition, (e.g., myocardial infarction, cerebrovascular accident, aspiration pneumonia), the principal diagnosis will not be the same in every situation. This applies whether the other acute condition is a respiratory or nonrespiratory condition. Selection of the principal diagnosis will be dependent on the circumstances of admission. If both the respiratory failure and the other acute condition are equally responsible for occasioning the admission to the hospital, and there are no chapter-specific sequencing rules, the guideline regarding two or more diagnoses that equally meet the definition for principal diagnosis (*Section II, C.*) may be applied in these situations.

If the documentation is not clear as to whether acute respiratory failure and another condition are equally responsible for occasioning the admission, query the provider for clarification.

Patient presents with acute pneumococcal pneumonia and acute respiratory failure

J96.00   **Acute respiratory failure, unspecified whether with hypoxia or hypercapnia**

J13   **Pneumonia due to Streptococcus pneumoniae**

Explanation: When a patient is seen for respiratory failure and another acute condition, such as a bacterial pneumonia, the principal or first-listed diagnosis is not the same in every situation. This applies whether the other acute condition is a respiratory or nonrespiratory condition. The principal diagnosis depends on the problem chiefly responsible for the encounter.

---

c. Influenza due to certain identified influenza viruses

Code only confirmed cases of influenza due to certain identified influenza viruses (category J09), and due to other identified influenza virus (category J10). This is an exception to the hospital inpatient guideline Section II, H. (Uncertain Diagnosis).

In this context, "confirmation" does not require documentation of positive laboratory testing specific for avian or other novel influenza A or other identified influenza virus. However, coding should be based on the provider's diagnostic statement that the patient has avian influenza, or other novel influenza A, for category J09, or has another particular identified strain of influenza, such as H1N1 or H3N2, but not identified as novel or variant, for category J10.

If the provider records "suspected" or "possible" or "probable" avian influenza, or novel influenza, or other identified influenza, then the appropriate influenza code from category J11, Influenza due to unidentified influenza virus, should be assigned. A code from category J09, Influenza due to certain identified influenza viruses, should not be assigned nor should a code from category J10, Influenza due to other identified influenza virus.

Chapter 10. Diseases of the Respiratory System

Influenza due to avian influenza virus with pneumonia

J09.X1 Influenza due to identified novel influenza A virus with pneumonia

Explanation: Codes in category J09 Influenza due to certain identified influenza viruses should be assigned only for confirmed cases. "Confirmation" does not require positive laboratory testing of a specific influenza virus but does need to be based on the provider's diagnostic statement, which should not include terms such as "possible," "probable," or "suspected."

d. Ventilator associated pneumonia

1) Documentation of ventilator associated pneumonia

As with all procedural or postprocedural complications, code assignment is based on the provider's documentation of the relationship between the condition and the procedure.

Code J95.851, Ventilator associated pneumonia, should be assigned only when the provider has documented ventilator associated pneumonia (VAP). An additional code to identify the organism (e.g., Pseudomonas aeruginosa, code B96.5) should also be assigned. Do not assign an additional code from categories J12-J18 to identify the type of pneumonia.

Code J95.851 should not be assigned for cases where the patient has pneumonia and is on a mechanical ventilator and the provider has not specifically stated that the pneumonia is ventilator-associated pneumonia. If the documentation is unclear as to whether the patient has a pneumonia that is a complication attributable to the mechanical ventilator, query the provider.

2) Ventilator associated pneumonia develops after admission

A patient may be admitted with one type of pneumonia (e.g., code J13, Pneumonia due to Streptococcus pneumonia) and subsequently develop VAP. In this instance, the principal diagnosis would be the appropriate code from categories J12-J18 for the pneumonia diagnosed at the time of admission. Code J95.851, Ventilator associated pneumonia, would be assigned as an additional diagnosis when the provider has also documented the presence of ventilator associated pneumonia.

Chapter 10. Diseases of the Respiratory System (J00-J99)

NOTE   When a respiratory condition is described as occurring in more than one site and is not specifically indexed, it should be classified to the lower anatomic site (e.g., tracheobronchitis to bronchitis in J40).

Use additional code, where applicable, to identify:
- exposure to environmental tobacco smoke (Z77.22)
- exposure to tobacco smoke in the perinatal period (P96.81)
- history of tobacco dependence (Z87.891)
- occupational exposure to environmental tobacco smoke (Z57.31)
- tobacco dependence (F17.-)
- tobacco use (Z72.0)

EXCLUDES 2   *certain conditions originating in the perinatal period (P04-P96)*
certain infectious and parasitic diseases (A00-B99)
complications of pregnancy, childbirth and the puerperium (O00-O9A)
congenital malformations, deformations and chromosomal abnormalities (Q00-Q99)
endocrine, nutritional and metabolic diseases (E00-E88)
injury, poisoning and certain other consequences of external causes (S00-T88)
neoplasms (C00-D49)
smoke inhalation (T59.81-)
symptoms, signs and abnormal clinical and laboratory findings, not elsewhere classified (R00-R94)

This chapter contains the following blocks:
- J00-J06   Acute upper respiratory infections
- J09-J18   Influenza and pneumonia
- J20-J22   Other acute lower respiratory infections
- J30-J39   Other diseases of upper respiratory tract
- J40-J47   Chronic lower respiratory diseases
- J60-J70   Lung diseases due to external agents
- J80-J84   Other respiratory diseases principally affecting the interstitium
- J85-J86   Suppurative and necrotic conditions of the lower respiratory tract
- J90-J94   Other diseases of the pleura
- J95   Intraoperative and postprocedural complications and disorders of respiratory system, not elsewhere classified
- J96-J99   Other diseases of the respiratory system

Acute upper respiratory infections (J00-J06)

EXCLUDES 1   *chronic obstructive pulmonary disease with acute lower respiratory infection (J44.0)*
influenza virus with other respiratory manifestations (J09.X2, J10.1, J11.1)

J00   Acute nasopharyngitis [common cold]
Acute rhinitis
Coryza (acute)
Infective nasopharyngitis NOS
Infective rhinitis
Nasal catarrh, acute
Nasopharyngitis NOS
EXCLUDES 1   *acute pharyngitis (J02.-)*
acute sore throat NOS (J02.9)
pharyngitis NOS (J02.9)
rhinitis NOS (J31.0)
sore throat NOS (J02.9)
EXCLUDES 2   *allergic rhinitis (J30.1-J30.9)*
chronic pharyngitis (J31.2)
chronic rhinitis (J31.0)
chronic sore throat (J31.2)
nasopharyngitis, chronic (J31.1)
vasomotor rhinitis (J30.0)

DEF: Acute inflammation of the mucous membranes that extends from the nares to the pharynx. It is characterized by nasal obstruction, sneezing, runny nose, and sore throat.

J01   Acute sinusitis
INCLUDES   acute abscess of sinus
acute empyema of sinus
acute infection of sinus
acute inflammation of sinus
acute suppuration of sinus
Use additional code (B95-B97) to identify infectious agent
EXCLUDES 1   *sinusitis NOS (J32.9)*
EXCLUDES 2   *chronic sinusitis (J32.0-J32.8)*

J01.0   Acute maxillary sinusitis
Acute antritis
J01.00   Acute maxillary sinusitis, unspecified
J01.01   Acute recurrent maxillary sinusitis

J01.1   Acute frontal sinusitis
J01.10   Acute frontal sinusitis, unspecified
J01.11   Acute recurrent frontal sinusitis

J01.2   Acute ethmoidal sinusitis
J01.20   Acute ethmoidal sinusitis, unspecified
J01.21   Acute recurrent ethmoidal sinusitis

J01.3   Acute sphenoidal sinusitis
J01.30   Acute sphenoidal sinusitis, unspecified
J01.31   Acute recurrent sphenoidal sinusitis

J01.4   Acute pansinusitis
J01.40   Acute pansinusitis, unspecified
J01.41   Acute recurrent pansinusitis

J01.8   Other acute sinusitis
J01.80   Other acute sinusitis
Acute sinusitis involving more than one sinus but not pansinusitis
J01.81   Other acute recurrent sinusitis
Acute recurrent sinusitis involving more than one sinus but not pansinusitis

J01.9   Acute sinusitis, unspecified
J01.90   Acute sinusitis, unspecified
J01.91   Acute recurrent sinusitis, unspecified

J02   Acute pharyngitis
INCLUDES   acute sore throat
EXCLUDES 1   *acute laryngopharyngitis (J06.0)*
peritonsillar abscess (J36)
pharyngeal abscess (J39.1)
retropharyngeal abscess (J39.0)
EXCLUDES 2   *chronic pharyngitis (J31.2)*

J02.0   Streptococcal pharyngitis
Septic pharyngitis
Streptococcal sore throat
EXCLUDES 2   *scarlet fever (A38.-)*

J02.8   Acute pharyngitis due to other specified organisms
Use additional code (B95-B97) to identify infectious agent
EXCLUDES 1   *acute pharyngitis due to coxsackie virus (B08.5)*
acute pharyngitis due to gonococcus (A54.5)
acute pharyngitis due to herpes [simplex] virus (B00.2)
acute pharyngitis due to infectious mononucleosis (B27.-)
enteroviral vesicular pharyngitis (B08.5)

J02.9   Acute pharyngitis, unspecified
Gangrenous pharyngitis (acute)
Infective pharyngitis (acute) NOS
Pharyngitis (acute) NOS
Sore throat (acute) NOS
Suppurative pharyngitis (acute)
Ulcerative pharyngitis (acute)

J03   Acute tonsillitis
EXCLUDES 1   *acute sore throat (J02.-)*
hypertrophy of tonsils (J35.1)
peritonsillar abscess (J36)
sore throat NOS (J02.9)
streptococcal sore throat (J02.0)
EXCLUDES 2   *chronic tonsillitis (J35.0)*

J03.0   Streptococcal tonsillitis
J03.00   Acute streptococcal tonsillitis, unspecified
J03.01   Acute recurrent streptococcal tonsillitis

J03.8   Acute tonsillitis due to other specified organisms
Use additional code (B95-B97) to identify infectious agent
EXCLUDES 1   *diphtheritic tonsillitis (A36.0)*
herpesviral pharyngotonsillitis (B00.2)
streptococcal tonsillitis (J03.0)
tuberculous tonsillitis (A15.8)
Vincent's tonsillitis (A69.1)

J03.80   Acute tonsillitis due to other specified organisms
J03.81   Acute recurrent tonsillitis due to other specified organisms

√5ᵗʰ **J03.9** **Acute tonsillitis, unspecified**
Follicular tonsillitis (acute)
Gangrenous tonsillitis (acute)
Infective tonsillitis (acute)
Tonsillitis (acute) NOS
Ulcerative tonsillitis (acute)

J03.90 **Acute tonsillitis, unspecified**
J03.91 **Acute recurrent tonsillitis, unspecified**

√4ᵗʰ **J04** **Acute laryngitis and tracheitis**
Use additional code (B95-B97) to identify infectious agent
EXCLUDES 1   *acute obstructive laryngitis [croup] and epiglottitis (J05.-)*
EXCLUDES 2   *laryngismus (stridulus) (J38.5)*

J04.0 **Acute laryngitis**
Edematous laryngitis (acute)
Laryngitis (acute) NOS
Subglottic laryngitis (acute)
Suppurative laryngitis (acute)
Ulcerative laryngitis (acute)
EXCLUDES 1   *acute obstructive laryngitis (J05.0)*
EXCLUDES 2   *chronic laryngitis (J37.0)*

√5ᵗʰ **J04.1** **Acute tracheitis**
Acute viral tracheitis
Catarrhal tracheitis (acute)
Tracheitis (acute) NOS
EXCLUDES 2   *chronic tracheitis (J42)*

J04.10 **Acute tracheitis without obstruction**
J04.11 **Acute tracheitis with obstruction**

J04.2 **Acute laryngotracheitis**
Laryngotracheitis NOS
Tracheitis (acute) with laryngitis (acute)
EXCLUDES 1   *acute obstructive laryngotracheitis (J05.0)*
EXCLUDES 2   *chronic laryngotracheitis (J37.1)*

√5ᵗʰ **J04.3** **Supraglottitis, unspecified**
J04.30 **Supraglottitis, unspecified, without obstruction**
J04.31 **Supraglottitis, unspecified, with obstruction**

√4ᵗʰ **J05** **Acute obstructive laryngitis [croup] and epiglottitis**
Use additional code (B95-B97) to identify infectious agent

J05.0 **Acute obstructive laryngitis [croup]**
Obstructive laryngitis (acute) NOS
Obstructive laryngotracheitis NOS
DEF: Acute laryngeal obstruction due to allergies, foreign bodies, or in the majority of cases a viral infection. Symptoms include a harsh, barking cough, hoarseness, and a persistent, high-pitched respiratory sound (stridor).

√5ᵗʰ **J05.1** **Acute epiglottitis**
EXCLUDES 2   *epiglottitis, chronic (J37.0)*

J05.10 **Acute epiglottitis without obstruction**
Epiglottitis NOS
J05.11 **Acute epiglottitis with obstruction**

√4ᵗʰ **J06** **Acute upper respiratory infections of multiple and unspecified sites**
EXCLUDES 1   *acute respiratory infection NOS (J22)*
streptococcal pharyngitis (J02.0)

J06.0 **Acute laryngopharyngitis**
J06.9 **Acute upper respiratory infection, unspecified**
Upper respiratory disease, acute
Upper respiratory infection NOS
▶Use additional code (B95-B97) to identify infectious agent, if known, such as:◀
▶respiratory syncytial virus (RSV) (B97.4)◀

Influenza and pneumonia (J09-J18)

EXCLUDES 2   *allergic or eosinophilic pneumonia (J82)*
aspiration pneumonia NOS (J69.0)
meconium pneumonia (P24.01)
neonatal aspiration pneumonia (P24.-)
pneumonia due to solids and liquids (J69.-)
congenital pneumonia (P23.9)
lipid pneumonia (J69.1)
rheumatic pneumonia (I00)
ventilator associated pneumonia (J95.851)

AHA: 2017,4Q,96
TIP: Documentation of lobar pneumonia or multilobar pneumonia should be coded to J18.1 when the specific organism causing the pneumonia is not identified. When the organism is documented, lobar pneumonia or multilobar pneumonia should be coded using categories J12-J16, depending on the organism that is present.
TIP: Hemoptysis (R04.2) is not customarily associated with pneumonia and may be reported separately.

√4ᵗʰ **J09** **Influenza due to certain identified influenza viruses**
EXCLUDES 1   *influenza A/H1N1 (J10.-)*
influenza due to other identified influenza virus (J10.-)
influenza due to unidentified influenza virus (J11.-)
seasonal influenza due to other identified influenza virus (J10.-)
seasonal influenza due to unidentified influenza virus (J11.-)

√5ᵗʰ **J09.X** **Influenza due to identified novel influenza A virus**
Avian influenza
Bird influenza
Influenza A/H5N1
Influenza of other animal origin, not bird or swine
Swine influenza virus (viruses that normally cause infections in pigs)
AHA: 2016,3Q,10

J09.X1 **Influenza due to identified novel influenza A virus with pneumonia**
Code also, if applicable, associated:
lung abscess (J85.1)
other specified type of pneumonia

J09.X2 **Influenza due to identified novel influenza A virus with other respiratory manifestations**
Influenza due to identified novel influenza A virus NOS
Influenza due to identified novel influenza A virus with laryngitis
Influenza due to identified novel influenza A virus with pharyngitis
Influenza due to identified novel influenza A virus with upper respiratory symptoms
Use additional code, if applicable, for associated:
pleural effusion (J91.8)
sinusitis (J01.-)

J09.X3 **Influenza due to identified novel influenza A virus with gastrointestinal manifestations**
Influenza due to identified novel influenza A virus gastroenteritis
EXCLUDES 1   *'intestinal flu' [viral gastroenteritis] (A08.-)*

J09.X9 **Influenza due to identified novel influenza A virus with other manifestations**
Influenza due to identified novel influenza A virus with encephalopathy
Influenza due to identified novel influenza A virus with myocarditis
Influenza due to identified novel influenza A virus with otitis media
Use additional code to identify manifestation

√4ᵗʰ **J10** **Influenza due to other identified influenza virus**
EXCLUDES 1   *influenza due to avian influenza virus (J09.X-)*
influenza due to swine flu (J09.X-)
influenza due to unidentifed influenza virus (J11.-)

√5ᵗʰ **J10.0** **Influenza due to other identified influenza virus with pneumonia**
Code also associated lung abscess, if applicable (J85.1)

J10.00 **Influenza due to other identified influenza virus with unspecified type of pneumonia**
J10.01 **Influenza due to other identified influenza virus with the same other identified influenza virus pneumonia**

J10.08   **Influenza due to other identified influenza virus with other specified pneumonia**
> Code also other specified type of pneumonia

J10.1   **Influenza due to other identified influenza virus with other respiratory manifestations**
> Influenza due to other identified influenza virus NOS
> Influenza due to other identified influenza virus with laryngitis
> Influenza due to other identified influenza virus with pharyngitis
> Influenza due to other identified influenza virus with upper respiratory symptoms
> Use additional code for associated pleural effusion, if applicable (J91.8)
> Use additional code for associated sinusitis, if applicable (J01.-)
> **AHA:** 2016,3Q,10-11

J10.2   **Influenza due to other identified influenza virus with gastrointestinal manifestations**
> Influenza due to other identified influenza virus gastroenteritis
> EXCLUDES 1   "intestinal flu" [viral gastroenteritis] (A08.-)

✓5ᵗʰ **J10.8**   **Influenza due to other identified influenza virus with other manifestations**

     J10.81   **Influenza due to other identified influenza virus with encephalopathy**

     J10.82   **Influenza due to other identified influenza virus with myocarditis**

     J10.83   **Influenza due to other identified influenza virus with otitis media**
> Use additional code for any associated perforated tympanic membrane (H72.-)

     J10.89   **Influenza due to other identified influenza virus with other manifestations**
> Use additional codes to identify the manifestations

✓4ᵗʰ **J11**   **Influenza due to unidentified influenza virus**

✓5ᵗʰ **J11.0**   **Influenza due to unidentified influenza virus with pneumonia**
> Code also associated lung abscess, if applicable (J85.1)
> **AHA:** 2016,3Q,11

     J11.00   **Influenza due to unidentified influenza virus with unspecified type of pneumonia**
> Influenza with pneumonia NOS

     J11.08   **Influenza due to unidentified influenza virus with specified pneumonia**
> Code also other specified type of pneumonia

J11.1   **Influenza due to unidentified influenza virus with other respiratory manifestations**
> Influenza NOS
> Influenzal laryngitis NOS
> Influenzal pharyngitis NOS
> Influenza with upper respiratory symptoms NOS
> Use additional code for associated pleural effusion, if applicable (J91.8)
> Use additional code for associated sinusitis, if applicable (J01.-)

J11.2   **Influenza due to unidentified influenza virus with gastrointestinal manifestations**
> Influenza gastroenteritis NOS
> EXCLUDES 1   "intestinal flu" [viral gastroenteritis] (A08.-)

✓5ᵗʰ **J11.8**   **Influenza due to unidentified influenza virus with other manifestations**

     J11.81   **Influenza due to unidentified influenza virus with encephalopathy**
> Influenzal encephalopathy NOS

     J11.82   **Influenza due to unidentified influenza virus with myocarditis**
> Influenzal myocarditis NOS

     J11.83   **Influenza due to unidentified influenza virus with otitis media**
> Influenzal otitis media NOS
> Use additional code for any associated perforated tympanic membrane (H72.-)

     J11.89   **Influenza due to unidentified influenza virus with other manifestations**
> Use additional codes to identify the manifestations

✓4ᵗʰ **J12**   **Viral pneumonia, not elsewhere classified**
> INCLUDES   bronchopneumonia due to viruses other than influenza viruses
> Code first associated influenza, if applicable (J09.X1, J10.0-, J11.0-)
> Code also associated abscess, if applicable (J85.1)
> EXCLUDES 1   aspiration pneumonia due to anesthesia during labor and delivery (O74.0)
>   aspiration pneumonia due to anesthesia during pregnancy (O29)
>   aspiration pneumonia due to anesthesia during puerperium (O89.0)
>   aspiration pneumonia due to solids and liquids (J69.-)
>   aspiration pneumonia NOS (J69.0)
>   congenital pneumonia (P23.0)
>   congenital rubella pneumonitis (P35.0)
>   interstitial pneumonia NOS (J84.9)
>   lipid pneumonia (J69.1)
>   neonatal aspiration pneumonia (P24.-)
> **AHA:** 2019,1Q,35; 2018,3Q,24; 2016,3Q,15; 2013,4Q,118

J12.0   **Adenoviral pneumonia**

J12.1   **Respiratory syncytial virus pneumonia**
> ▶RSV pneumonia◄

J12.2   **Parainfluenza virus pneumonia**

J12.3   **Human metapneumovirus pneumonia**

✓5ᵗʰ **J12.8**   **Other viral pneumonia**

     J12.81   **Pneumonia due to SARS-associated coronavirus**
> Severe acute respiratory syndrome NOS
> **DEF:** Severe adult respiratory syndrome caused by the coronavirus, specified as inflammation of the lungs with consolidation.

     J12.89   **Other viral pneumonia**

J12.9   **Viral pneumonia, unspecified**

J13   **Pneumonia due to Streptococcus pneumoniae**   HCC
> Bronchopneumonia due to S. pneumoniae
> Code first associated influenza, if applicable (J09.X1, J10.0-, J11.0-)
> Code also associated abscess, if applicable (J85.1)
> EXCLUDES 1   congenital pneumonia due to S. pneumoniae (P23.6)
>   lobar pneumonia, unspecified organism (J18.1)
>   pneumonia due to other streptococci (J15.3-J15.4)
> **AHA:** 2019,1Q,35; 2018,3Q,24; 2016,3Q,15; 2013,4Q,118

J14   **Pneumonia due to Hemophilus influenzae**   HCC
> Bronchopneumonia due to H. influenzae
> Code first associated influenza, if applicable (J09.X1, J10.0-, J11.0-)
> Code also associated abscess, if applicable (J85.1)
> EXCLUDES 1   congenital pneumonia due to H. influenzae (P23.6)
> **AHA:** 2019,1Q,35; 2018,3Q,24; 2016,3Q,15; 2013,4Q,118

✓4ᵗʰ **J15**   **Bacterial pneumonia, not elsewhere classified**
> INCLUDES   Bronchopneumonia due to bacteria other than S. pneumoniae and H. influenzae
> Code first associated influenza, if applicable (J09.X1, J10.0-, -J11.0-)
> Code also associated abscess, if applicable (J85.1)
> EXCLUDES 1   chlamydial pneumonia (J16.0)
>   congenital pneumonia (P23.-)
>   Legionnaires' disease (A48.1)
>   spirochetal pneumonia (A69.8)
> **AHA:** 2019,1Q,35; 2018,3Q,24; 2016,3Q,15; 2013,4Q,118

J15.0   **Pneumonia due to Klebsiella pneumoniae**   HCC

J15.1   **Pneumonia due to Pseudomonas**   HCC

✓5ᵗʰ **J15.2**   **Pneumonia due to staphylococcus**

     J15.20   **Pneumonia due to staphylococcus, unspecified**   HCC

     ✓6ᵗʰ **J15.21**   **Pneumonia due to Staphylococcus aureus**

         J15.211   **Pneumonia due to methicillin susceptible Staphylococcus aureus**   HCC
> MSSA pneumonia
> Pneumonia due to Staphylococcus aureus NOS

         J15.212   **Pneumonia due to methicillin resistant Staphylococcus aureus**   HCC

     J15.29   **Pneumonia due to other staphylococcus**   HCC

J15.3   **Pneumonia due to streptococcus, group B**   HCC

Chapter 10. Diseases of the Respiratory System

J15.4 Pneumonia due to other streptococci `HCC`
> EXCLUDES 1   *pneumonia due to streptococcus, group B (J15.3)*
> *pneumonia due to Streptococcus pneumoniae (J13)*

J15.5 Pneumonia due to Escherichia coli `HCC`

J15.6 Pneumonia due to other Gram-negative bacteria `HCC`
Pneumonia due to other aerobic Gram-negative bacteria
Pneumonia due to Serratia marcescens

J15.7 Pneumonia due to Mycoplasma pneumoniae

J15.8 Pneumonia due to other specified bacteria `HCC`

J15.9 Unspecified bacterial pneumonia
Pneumonia due to gram-positive bacteria

☑4ᵗʰ **J16 Pneumonia due to other infectious organisms, not elsewhere classified**
Code first associated influenza, if applicable (J09.X1, J10.0-, J11.0-)
Code also associated abscess, if applicable (J85.1)
> EXCLUDES 1   *congenital pneumonia (P23.-)*
> *ornithosis (A70)*
> *pneumocystosis (B59)*
> *pneumonia NOS (J18.9)*

AHA: 2019,1Q,35; 2018,3Q,24; 2016,3Q,15; 2013,4Q,118

J16.0 Chlamydial pneumonia

J16.8 Pneumonia due to other specified infectious organisms

J17 *Pneumonia in diseases classified elsewhere*
Code first underlying disease, such as:
Q fever (A78)
rheumatic fever (I00)
schistosomiasis (B65.0-B65.9)
> EXCLUDES 1   *candidial pneumonia (B37.1)*
> *chlamydial pneumonia (J16.0)*
> *gonorrheal pneumonia (A54.84)*
> *histoplasmosis pneumonia (B39.0-B39.2)*
> *measles pneumonia (B05.2)*
> *nocardiosis pneumonia (A43.0)*
> *pneumocystosis (B59)*
> *pneumonia due to Pneumocystis carinii (B59)*
> *pneumonia due to Pneumocystis jiroveci (B59)*
> *pneumonia in actinomycosis (A42.0)*
> *pneumonia in anthrax (A22.1)*
> *pneumonia in ascariasis (B77.81)*
> *pneumonia in aspergillosis (B44.0-B44.1)*
> *pneumonia in coccidioidomycosis (B38.0-B38.2)*
> *pneumonia in cytomegalovirus disease (B25.0)*
> *pneumonia in toxoplasmosis (B58.3)*
> *rubella pneumonia (B06.81)*
> *salmonella pneumonia (A02.22)*
> *spirochetal infection NEC with pneumonia (A69.8)*
> *tularemia pneumonia (A21.2)*
> *typhoid fever with pneumonia (A01.03)*
> *varicella pneumonia (B01.2)*
> *whooping cough with pneumonia (A37 with fifth character 1)*

AHA: 2019,1Q,35; 2016,3Q,15; 2013,4Q,118

☑4ᵗʰ **J18 Pneumonia, unspecified organism**
Code first associated influenza, if applicable (J09.X1, J10.0-, J11.0-)
> EXCLUDES 1   *abscess of lung with pneumonia (J85.1)*
> *aspiration pneumonia due to anesthesia during labor and delivery (O74.0)*
> *aspiration pneumonia due to anesthesia during pregnancy (O29)*
> *aspiration pneumonia due to anesthesia during puerperium (O89.0)*
> *aspiration pneumonia due to solids and liquids (J69.-)*
> *aspiration pneumonia NOS (J69.0)*
> *congenital pneumonia (P23.0)*
> *drug-induced interstitial lung disorder (J70.2-J70.4)*
> *interstitial pneumonia NOS (J84.9)*
> *lipid pneumonia (J69.1)*
> *neonatal aspiration pneumonia (P24.-)*
> *pneumonitis due to external agents (J67-J70)*
> *pneumonitis due to fumes and vapors (J68.0)*
> *usual interstitial pneumonia (J84.17)*

AHA: 2019,1Q,35; 2016,3Q,15; 2013,4Q,118

J18.0 Bronchopneumonia, unspecified organism
> EXCLUDES 1   *hypostatic bronchopneumonia (J18.2)*
> *lipid pneumonia (J69.1)*
> EXCLUDES 2   *acute bronchiolitis (J21.-)*
> *chronic bronchiolitis (J44.9)*

J18.1 Lobar pneumonia, unspecified organism `HCC`
AHA: 2018,3Q,24
TIP: Use this code for documented lobar pneumonia or multilobar pneumonia when the causal organism is not identified. If the causal organism is identified, codes from categories J12-J16 should be used, depending on the organism that is present.

J18.2 Hypostatic pneumonia, unspecified organism
Hypostatic bronchopneumonia
Passive pneumonia

J18.8 Other pneumonia, unspecified organism

J18.9 Pneumonia, unspecified organism
AHA: 2019,2Q,28; 2014,3Q,4; 2013,4Q,119; 2012,4Q,94

Other acute lower respiratory infections (J20-J22)

> EXCLUDES 2   *chronic obstructive pulmonary disease with acute lower respiratory infection (J44.0)*

☑4ᵗʰ **J20 Acute bronchitis**
> INCLUDES   acute and subacute bronchitis (with) bronchospasm
> acute and subacute bronchitis (with) tracheitis
> acute and subacute bronchitis (with) tracheobronchitis, acute
> acute and subacute fibrinous bronchitis
> acute and subacute membranous bronchitis
> acute and subacute purulent bronchitis
> acute and subacute septic bronchitis
> EXCLUDES 1   *bronchitis NOS (J40)*
> *tracheobronchitis NOS (J40)*
> EXCLUDES 2   *acute bronchitis with bronchiectasis (J47.0)*
> *acute bronchitis with chronic obstructive asthma (J44.0)*
> *acute bronchitis with chronic obstructive pulmonary disease (J44.0)*
> *allergic bronchitis NOS (J45.909-)*
> *bronchitis due to chemicals, fumes and vapors (J68.0)*
> *chronic bronchitis NOS (J42)*
> *chronic mucopurulent bronchitis (J41.1)*
> *chronic obstructive bronchitis (J44.-)*
> *chronic obstructive tracheobronchitis (J44.-)*
> *chronic simple bronchitis (J41.0)*
> *chronic tracheobronchitis (J42)*

AHA: 2019,1Q,35; 2016,3Q,10,16
DEF: Acute inflammation of the main branches of the bronchial tree due to infectious or irritant agents. Symptoms include cough with a varied production of sputum, fever, substernal soreness, and lung rales. Bronchitis usually lasts three to 10 days.

J20.0 Acute bronchitis due to Mycoplasma pneumoniae

J20.1 Acute bronchitis due to Hemophilus influenzae

J20.2 Acute bronchitis due to streptococcus

J20.3 Acute bronchitis due to coxsackievirus

J20.4 Acute bronchitis due to parainfluenza virus

J20.5 **Acute bronchitis due to** respiratory syncytial virus
▶Acute bronchitis due to RSV◀

J20.6 **Acute bronchitis due to** rhinovirus

J20.7 **Acute bronchitis due to** echovirus

J20.8 **Acute bronchitis due to other specified organisms**

J20.9 **Acute bronchitis, unspecified**

✓4ᵗʰ **J21** **Acute bronchiolitis**

    INCLUDES   acute bronchiolitis with bronchospasm

    EXCLUDES 2   *respiratory bronchiolitis interstitial lung disease (J84.115)*

J21.0 **Acute bronchiolitis due to** respiratory syncytial virus
▶Acute bronchiolitis due to RSV◀

J21.1 **Acute bronchiolitis due to** human metapneumovirus

J21.8 **Acute bronchiolitis due to other specified organisms**

J21.9 **Acute bronchiolitis, unspecified**
Bronchiolitis (acute)

    EXCLUDES 1   *chronic bronchiolitis (J44.-)*

J22 **Unspecified acute lower respiratory infection**
Acute (lower) respiratory (tract) infection NOS

    EXCLUDES 1   *upper respiratory infection (acute) (J06.9)*

Other diseases of upper respiratory tract (J30-J39)

✓4ᵗʰ **J30** **Vasomotor and allergic rhinitis**

    INCLUDES   spasmodic rhinorrhea

    EXCLUDES 1   *allergic rhinitis with asthma (bronchial) (J45.909)*
                     rhinitis NOS (J31.0)

J30.0 **Vasomotor rhinitis**
DEF: Noninfectious and nonallergic type of rhinitis for which the cause is often unknown. Symptoms often mimic those of allergic rhinitis with a diagnosis of vasomotor rhinitis typically made after ruling out allergens as the cause.

J30.1 **Allergic rhinitis due to pollen**
Allergy NOS due to pollen
Hay fever
Pollinosis

J30.2 **Other seasonal allergic rhinitis**

J30.5 **Allergic rhinitis due to food**

✓5ᵗʰ **J30.8** **Other allergic rhinitis**

    J30.81 **Allergic rhinitis due to** animal (cat) (dog) hair and dander

    J30.89 **Other allergic rhinitis**
          Perennial allergic rhinitis

J30.9 **Allergic rhinitis, unspecified**

✓4ᵗʰ **J31** **Chronic rhinitis, nasopharyngitis and pharyngitis**
Use additional code to identify:
exposure to environmental tobacco smoke (Z77.22)
exposure to tobacco smoke in the perinatal period (P96.81)
history of tobacco dependence (Z87.891)
occupational exposure to environmental tobacco smoke (Z57.31)
tobacco dependence (F17.-)
tobacco use (Z72.0)

J31.0 **Chronic rhinitis**
Atrophic rhinitis (chronic)
Granulomatous rhinitis (chronic)
Hypertrophic rhinitis (chronic)
Obstructive rhinitis (chronic)
Ozena
Purulent rhinitis (chronic)
Rhinitis (chronic) NOS
Ulcerative rhinitis (chronic)

    EXCLUDES 1   *allergic rhinitis (J30.1-J30.9)*
                     vasomotor rhinitis (J30.0)

DEF: Persistent inflammation of the mucous membranes of the nose, characterized by a postnasal drip.

J31.1 **Chronic nasopharyngitis**

    EXCLUDES 2   *acute nasopharyngitis (J00)*

DEF: Persistent inflammation of the mucous membranes extending from the nares to the pharynx. It is characterized by constant irritation in the nasopharynx and postnasal drip.

J31.2 **Chronic pharyngitis**
Atrophic pharyngitis (chronic)
Chronic sore throat
Granular pharyngitis (chronic)
Hypertrophic pharyngitis (chronic)

    EXCLUDES 2   *acute pharyngitis (J02.9)*

✓4ᵗʰ **J32** **Chronic sinusitis**

    INCLUDES   sinus abscess
              sinus empyema
              sinus infection
              sinus suppuration

Use additional code to identify:
exposure to environmental tobacco smoke (Z77.22)
exposure to tobacco smoke in the perinatal period (P96.81)
history of tobacco dependence (Z87.891)
infectious agent (B95-B97)
occupational exposure to environmental tobacco smoke (Z57.31)
tobacco dependence (F17.-)
tobacco use (Z72.0)

    EXCLUDES 2   *acute sinusitis (J01.-)*

J32.0 **Chronic maxillary sinusitis**
Antritis (chronic)
Maxillary sinusitis NOS

J32.1 **Chronic frontal sinusitis**
Frontal sinusitis NOS

J32.2 **Chronic ethmoidal sinusitis**
Ethmoidal sinusitis NOS

    EXCLUDES 1   *Woakes' ethmoiditis (J33.1)*

J32.3 **Chronic sphenoidal sinusitis**
Sphenoidal sinusitis NOS

J32.4 **Chronic pansinusitis**
Pansinusitis NOS

J32.8 **Other chronic sinusitis**
Sinusitis (chronic) involving more than one sinus but not pansinusitis

J32.9 **Chronic sinusitis, unspecified**
Sinusitis (chronic) NOS

✓4ᵗʰ **J33** **Nasal polyp**
Use additional code to identify:
exposure to environmental tobacco smoke (Z77.22)
exposure to tobacco smoke in the perinatal period (P96.81)
history of tobacco dependence (Z87.891)
occupational exposure to environmental tobacco smoke (Z57.31)
tobacco dependence (F17.-)
tobacco use (Z72.0)

    EXCLUDES 1   *adenomatous polyps (D14.0)*

J33.0 **Polyp of nasal cavity**
Choanal polyp
Nasopharyngeal polyp

J33.1 **Polypoid sinus degeneration**
Woakes' syndrome or ethmoiditis

J33.8 **Other polyp of sinus**
Accessory polyp of sinus
Ethmoidal polyp of sinus
Maxillary polyp of sinus
Sphenoidal polyp of sinus

J33.9 **Nasal polyp, unspecified**

✓4ᵗʰ **J34** **Other and unspecified disorders of nose and nasal sinuses**

    EXCLUDES 2   *varicose ulcer of nasal septum (I86.8)*

J34.0 **Abscess, furuncle and carbuncle of nose**
Cellulitis of nose
Necrosis of nose
Ulceration of nose

J34.1 **Cyst and mucocele of nose and nasal sinus**

J34.2 **Deviated nasal septum**
Deflection or deviation of septum (nasal) (acquired)

    EXCLUDES 1   *congenital deviated nasal septum (Q67.4)*

DEF: Condition in which the nasal septum, a thin wall composed of cartilage and bone that separates the two nostrils, is crooked or displaced from the midline.

J34.3 **Hypertrophy of nasal turbinates**
DEF: Overgrowth of bones within the nasal turbinate, which are ridges of bone and soft tissue that project from the sidewalls of the nasal passages. Hypertrophy can cause obstruction of the nasal passages.

✓ Additional Character Required   ✓×7ᵗʰ Placeholder Alert   Manifestation   Unspecified Dx   ▶◀ Revised Text   ● New Code   ▲ Revised Code Title

Chapter 10. Diseases of the Respiratory System

J34.8–J39.2

✓5ᵗʰ **J34.8 Other specified disorders of nose and nasal sinuses**

  J34.81 Nasal mucositis (ulcerative)
    Code also type of associated therapy, such as:
      antineoplastic and immunosuppressive drugs
      (T45.1X-)
      radiological procedure and radiotherapy (Y84.2)
    EXCLUDES 2 *gastrointestinal mucositis (ulcerative)*
      (K92.81)
      mucositis (ulcerative) of vagina and vulva
      (N76.81)
      oral mucositis (ulcerative) (K12.3-)

  J34.89 Other specified disorders of nose and nasal sinuses
    Perforation of nasal septum NOS
    Rhinolith

J34.9 Unspecified disorder of nose and nasal sinuses

✓4ᵗʰ **J35 Chronic diseases of tonsils and adenoids**
  Use additional code to identify:
    exposure to environmental tobacco smoke (Z77.22)
    exposure to tobacco smoke in the perinatal period (P96.81)
    history of tobacco dependence (Z87.891)
    occupational exposure to environmental tobacco smoke (Z57.31)
    tobacco dependence (F17.-)
    tobacco use (Z72.0)

✓5ᵗʰ **J35.0 Chronic tonsillitis and adenoiditis**
    EXCLUDES 2 *acute tonsillitis (J03.-)*

  J35.01 Chronic tonsillitis
  J35.02 Chronic adenoiditis
  J35.03 Chronic tonsillitis and adenoiditis

J35.1 Hypertrophy of tonsils
  Enlargement of tonsils
  EXCLUDES 1 *hypertrophy of tonsils with tonsillitis (J35.0-)*

J35.2 Hypertrophy of adenoids
  Enlargement of adenoids
  EXCLUDES 1 *hypertrophy of adenoids with adenoiditis (J35.0-)*

J35.3 Hypertrophy of tonsils with hypertrophy of adenoids
  EXCLUDES 1 *hypertrophy of tonsils and adenoids with tonsillitis*
    and adenoiditis (J35.03)

J35.8 Other chronic diseases of tonsils and adenoids
  Adenoid vegetations
  Amygdalolith
  Calculus, tonsil
  Cicatrix of tonsil (and adenoid)
  Tonsillar tag
  Ulcer of tonsil

J35.9 Chronic disease of tonsils and adenoids, unspecified
  Disease (chronic) of tonsils and adenoids NOS

J36 Peritonsillar abscess
  INCLUDES   abscess of tonsil
    peritonsillar cellulitis
    quinsy
  Use additional code (B95-B97) to identify infectious agent
  EXCLUDES 1 *acute tonsillitis (J03.-)*
    chronic tonsillitis (J35.0)
    retropharyngeal abscess (J39.0)
    tonsillitis NOS (J03.9-)

✓4ᵗʰ **J37 Chronic laryngitis and laryngotracheitis**
  Use additional code to identify:
    exposure to environmental tobacco smoke (Z77.22)
    exposure to tobacco smoke in the perinatal period (P96.81)
    history of tobacco dependence (Z87.891)
    infectious agent (B95-B97)
    occupational exposure to environmental tobacco smoke (Z57.31)
    tobacco dependence (F17.-)
    tobacco use (Z72.0)

J37.0 Chronic laryngitis
  Catarrhal laryngitis
  Hypertrophic laryngitis
  Sicca laryngitis
  EXCLUDES 2 *acute laryngitis (J04.0)*
    obstructive (acute) laryngitis (J05.0)

J37.1 Chronic laryngotracheitis
  Laryngitis, chronic, with tracheitis (chronic)
  Tracheitis, chronic, with laryngitis
  EXCLUDES 1 *chronic tracheitis (J42)*
  EXCLUDES 2 *acute laryngotracheitis (J04.2)*
    acute tracheitis (J04.1)

✓4ᵗʰ **J38 Diseases of vocal cords and larynx, not elsewhere classified**
  Use additional code to identify:
    exposure to environmental tobacco smoke (Z77.22)
    exposure to tobacco smoke in the perinatal period (P96.81)
    history of tobacco dependence (Z87.891)
    occupational exposure to environmental tobacco smoke (Z57.31)
    tobacco dependence (F17.-)
    tobacco use (Z72.0)
  EXCLUDES 1 *congenital laryngeal stridor (P28.89)*
    obstructive laryngitis (acute) (J05.0)
    postprocedural subglottic stenosis (J95.5)
    stridor (R06.1)
    ulcerative laryngitis (J04.0)

✓5ᵗʰ **J38.0 Paralysis of vocal cords and larynx**
  Laryngoplegia
  Paralysis of glottis

  J38.00 Paralysis of vocal cords and larynx, unspecified
  J38.01 Paralysis of vocal cords and larynx, unilateral
  J38.02 Paralysis of vocal cords and larynx, bilateral

J38.1 Polyp of vocal cord and larynx
  EXCLUDES 1 *adenomatous polyps (D14.1)*

J38.2 Nodules of vocal cords
  Chorditis (fibrinous)(nodosa)(tuberosa)
  Singer's nodes
  Teacher's nodes

J38.3 Other diseases of vocal cords
  Abscess of vocal cords
  Cellulitis of vocal cords
  Granuloma of vocal cords
  Leukokeratosis of vocal cords
  Leukoplakia of vocal cords

J38.4 Edema of larynx
  Edema (of) glottis
  Subglottic edema
  Supraglottic edema
  EXCLUDES 1 *acute obstructive laryngitis [croup] (J05.0)*
    edematous laryngitis (J04.0)

J38.5 Laryngeal spasm
  Laryngismus (stridulus)

J38.6 Stenosis of larynx

J38.7 Other diseases of larynx
  Abscess of larynx
  Cellulitis of larynx
  Disease of larynx NOS
  Necrosis of larynx
  Pachyderma of larynx
  Perichondritis of larynx
  Ulcer of larynx

✓4ᵗʰ **J39 Other diseases of upper respiratory tract**
  EXCLUDES 1 *acute respiratory infection NOS (J22)*
    acute upper respiratory infection (J06.9)
    upper respiratory inflammation due to chemicals, gases,
    fumes or vapors (J68.2)

J39.0 Retropharyngeal and parapharyngeal abscess
  Peripharyngeal abscess
  EXCLUDES 1 *peritonsillar abscess (J36)*
  DEF: Purulent infection behind the pharynx and the front of the
  precerebral fascia, characterized by neck stiffness, cervical
  lymphadenopathy, sore throat, fever, and stridor.

J39.1 Other abscess of pharynx
  Cellulitis of pharynx
  Nasopharyngeal abscess

J39.2 Other diseases of pharynx
  Cyst of pharynx
  Edema of pharynx
  EXCLUDES 2 *chronic pharyngitis (J31.2)*
    ulcerative pharyngitis (J02.9)

J39.3   **Upper respiratory tract hypersensitivity reaction, site unspecified**

     EXCLUDES 1   *hypersensitivity reaction of upper respiratory tract, such as:*
         extrinsic allergic alveolitis (J67.9)
         pneumoconiosis (J60-J67.9)

J39.8   **Other specified diseases of upper respiratory tract**

J39.9   **Disease of upper respiratory tract, unspecified**

Chronic lower respiratory diseases (J40-J47)

EXCLUDES 1   *bronchitis due to chemicals, gases, fumes and vapors (J68.0)*
EXCLUDES 2   *cystic fibrosis (E84.-)*

J40   **Bronchitis, not specified as acute or chronic**
     Bronchitis NOS
     Bronchitis with tracheitis NOS
     Catarrhal bronchitis
     Tracheobronchitis NOS
     Use additional code to identify:
       exposure to environmental tobacco smoke (Z77.22)
       exposure to tobacco smoke in the perinatal period (P96.81)
       history of tobacco dependence (Z87.891)
       occupational exposure to environmental tobacco smoke (Z57.31)
       tobacco dependence (F17.-)
       tobacco use (Z72.0)

     EXCLUDES 1   *acute bronchitis (J20.-)*
         allergic bronchitis NOS (J45.909-)
         asthmatic bronchitis NOS (J45.9-)
         bronchitis due to chemicals, gases, fumes and vapors (J68.0)

✔4ᵗʰ **J41**   **Simple and mucopurulent chronic bronchitis**
     Use additional code to identify:
       exposure to environmental tobacco smoke (Z77.22)
       exposure to tobacco smoke in the perinatal period (P96.81)
       history of tobacco dependence (Z87.891)
       occupational exposure to environmental tobacco smoke (Z57.31)
       tobacco dependence (F17.-)
       tobacco use (Z72.0)

     EXCLUDES 1   *chronic bronchitis NOS (J42)*
         chronic obstructive bronchitis (J44.-)

J41.0   **Simple chronic bronchitis**   HCC Q

J41.1   **Mucopurulent chronic bronchitis**   HCC Q

J41.8   **Mixed simple and mucopurulent chronic bronchitis**   HCC Q

J42   **Unspecified chronic bronchitis**   HCC Q
     Chronic bronchitis NOS
     Chronic tracheitis
     Chronic tracheobronchitis
     Use additional code to identify:
       exposure to environmental tobacco smoke (Z77.22)
       exposure to tobacco smoke in the perinatal period (P96.81)
       history of tobacco dependence (Z87.891)
       occupational exposure to environmental tobacco smoke (Z57.31)
       tobacco dependence (F17.-)
       tobacco use (Z72.0)

     EXCLUDES 1   *chronic asthmatic bronchitis (J44.-)*
         chronic bronchitis with airways obstruction (J44.-)
         chronic emphysematous bronchitis (J44.-)
         chronic obstructive pulmonary disease NOS (J44.9)
         simple and mucopurulent chronic bronchitis (J41.-)

✔4ᵗʰ **J43**   **Emphysema**
     Use additional code to identify:
       exposure to environmental tobacco smoke (Z77.22)
       history of tobacco dependence (Z87.891)
       occupational exposure to environmental tobacco smoke (Z57.31)
       tobacco dependence (F17.-)
       tobacco use (Z72.0)

     EXCLUDES 1   *compensatory emphysema (J98.3)*
         emphysema due to inhalation of chemicals, gases, fumes or vapors (J68.4)
         emphysema with chronic (obstructive) bronchitis (J44.-)
         emphysematous (obstructive) bronchitis (J44.-)
         interstitial emphysema (J98.2)
         mediastinal emphysema (J98.2)
         neonatal interstitial emphysema (P25.0)
         surgical (subcutaneous) emphysema (T81.82)
         traumatic subcutaneous emphysema (T79.7)

DEF: Pathological condition in which there is destructive enlargement of the air sacs in the lungs resulting in damage and lack of elasticity to the alveolar walls, commonly seen in long-term smokers.

Emphysema — Healthy alveoli: Patent bronchiole, Well-vascularized, Dilated alveoli, Excess mucus. Alveoli w/ Emphysema: Collapsed bronchiole, Enlarged alveoli, Broken/fewer capillaries, Alveolar membranes break down.

J43.0   **Unilateral pulmonary emphysema [MacLeod's syndrome]**   HCC Q
     Swyer-James syndrome
     Unilateral emphysema
     Unilateral hyperlucent lung
     Unilateral pulmonary artery functional hypoplasia
     Unilateral transparency of lung

J43.1   **Panlobular emphysema**   HCC Q
     Panacinar emphysema

J43.2   **Centrilobular emphysema**   HCC Q

J43.8   **Other emphysema**   HCC Q

J43.9   **Emphysema, unspecified**   HCC Q
     Bullous emphysema (lung)(pulmonary)
     Emphysema (lung)(pulmonary) NOS
     Emphysematous bleb
     Vesicular emphysema (lung)(pulmonary)
     AHA: 2019,1Q,34-36; 2017,4Q,97-98

☑️⁴ᵗʰ **J44 Other chronic obstructive pulmonary disease**

     INCLUDES   asthma with chronic obstructive pulmonary disease
                      chronic asthmatic (obstructive) bronchitis
                      chronic bronchitis with airways obstruction
                      chronic bronchitis with emphysema
                      chronic emphysematous bronchitis
                      chronic obstructive asthma
                      chronic obstructive bronchitis
                      chronic obstructive tracheobronchitis

     Code also type of asthma, if applicable (J45.-)
     Use additional code to identify:
        exposure to environmental tobacco smoke (Z77.22)
        history of tobacco dependence (Z87.891)
        occupational exposure to environmental tobacco smoke (Z57.31)
        tobacco dependence (F17.-)
        tobacco use (Z72.0)

     EXCLUDES 1   *bronchiectasis (J47.-)*
                     chronic bronchitis NOS (J42)
                     chronic simple and mucopurulent bronchitis (J41.-)
                     chronic tracheitis (J42)
                     chronic tracheobronchitis (J42)
                     emphysema without chronic bronchitis (J43.-)

     AHA: 2019,1Q,34-36; 2017,4Q,97-98; 2017,1Q,25-26; 2016,3Q,15-16; 2013,4Q,109

▲   **J44.0   Chronic obstructive pulmonary disease with** (acute) **HCC** **Q** **lower respiratory infection**
           Code also to identify the infection
           AHA: 2019,1Q,35; 2017,4Q,96; 2017,1Q,24-25
           TIP: Do not assign when only aspiration pneumonia is present. Aspiration pneumonis is not classified as a respiratory infection.

   J44.1   Chronic obstructive pulmonary disease with (acute) **HCC** **Q** **exacerbation**
          · Decompensated COPD
          Decompensated COPD with (acute) exacerbation
          EXCLUDES 2   *chronic obstructive pulmonary disease [COPD] with acute bronchitis (J44.0)*
                         lung diseases due to external agents (J60-J70)
          AHA: 2019,1Q,34; 2017,4Q,96; 2017,1Q,26; 2016,1Q,36
          TIP: Exacerbation of COPD should not be assumed based upon worsening of a concomitant respiratory disease or when COPD is described as end-stage.
          TIP: Assign J43.9 when COPD exacerbation with emphysema is documented.

   J44.9   Chronic obstructive pulmonary disease, unspecified **HCC** **Q**
          Chronic obstructive airway disease NOS
          Chronic obstructive lung disease NOS
          EXCLUDES 2   *lung diseases due to external agents (J60-J70)*
          AHA: 2019,1Q,36; 2017,4Q,96-97; 2016,1Q,36; 2014,4Q,21; 2013,4Q,109

☑️⁴ᵗʰ **J45 Asthma**

     INCLUDES   allergic (predominantly) asthma
                      allergic bronchitis NOS
                      allergic rhinitis with asthma
                      atopic asthma
                      extrinsic allergic asthma
                      hay fever with asthma
                      idiosyncratic asthma
                      intrinsic nonallergic asthma
                      nonallergic asthma

     Use additional code to identify:
        exposure to environmental tobacco smoke (Z77.22)
        exposure to tobacco smoke in the perinatal period (P96.81)
        history of tobacco dependence (Z87.891)
        occupational exposure to environmental tobacco smoke (Z57.31)
        tobacco dependence (F17.-)
        tobacco use (Z72.0)

     EXCLUDES 1   *detergent asthma (J69.8)*
                     eosinophilic asthma (J82)
                     miner's asthma (J60)
                     wheezing NOS (R06.2)
                     wood asthma (J67.8)

     EXCLUDES 2   *asthma with chronic obstructive pulmonary disease (J44.9)*
                     chronic asthmatic (obstructive) bronchitis (J44.9)
                     chronic obstructive asthma (J44.9)

     AHA: 2019,1Q,36; 2017,1Q,25-26; 2012,4Q,99
     DEF: Status asthmaticus: Severe, intractable episode of asthma that is unresponsive to normal therapeutic measures.

Asthma

Respiratory bronchiole   Smooth muscle fibers   Contraction of smooth muscle fibers

Mucus lining bronchial tubes   Alveoli   Extra mucus secretion in inflamed bronchial tubes   Air trapped within alveoli

Normal alveoli   **Asthmatic alveoli**

☑️⁵ᵗʰ **J45.2   Mild intermittent asthma**

     J45.20   Mild intermittent asthma, uncomplicated
               Mild intermittent asthma NOS
     J45.21   Mild intermittent asthma with (acute) exacerbation
     J45.22   Mild intermittent asthma with status asthmaticus

☑️⁵ᵗʰ **J45.3   Mild persistent asthma**

     J45.30   Mild persistent asthma, uncomplicated
               Mild persistent asthma NOS
     J45.31   Mild persistent asthma with (acute) exacerbation
               AHA: 2016,1Q,35
     J45.32   Mild persistent asthma with status asthmaticus

☑️⁵ᵗʰ **J45.4   Moderate persistent asthma**

     J45.40   Moderate persistent asthma, uncomplicated
               Moderate persistent asthma NOS
     J45.41   Moderate persistent asthma with (acute) exacerbation
               AHA: 2017,1Q,26
     J45.42   Moderate persistent asthma with status asthmaticus

☑️⁵ᵗʰ **J45.5   Severe persistent asthma**

     J45.50   Severe persistent asthma, uncomplicated
               Severe persistent asthma NOS
     J45.51   Severe persistent asthma with (acute) exacerbation
     J45.52   Severe persistent asthma with status asthmaticus

✓5ᵗʰ **J45.9 Other and unspecified asthma**

    ✓6ᵗʰ **J45.90 Unspecified asthma**
        Asthmatic bronchitis NOS
        Childhood asthma NOS
        Late onset asthma
        AHA: 2017,4Q,96; 2017,1Q,25

        J45.901 Unspecified asthma with (acute) exacerbation

        J45.902 Unspecified asthma with status asthmaticus

        J45.909 Unspecified asthma, uncomplicated
           Asthma NOS
           EXCLUDES 2   lung diseases due to external agents (J60-J70)
           AHA: 2017,1Q,25

    ✓6ᵗʰ **J45.99 Other asthma**
        J45.990 Exercise induced bronchospasm
        J45.991 Cough variant asthma
        J45.998 Other asthma

✓4ᵗʰ **J47 Bronchiectasis**
    INCLUDES   bronchiolectasis
    Use additional code to identify:
      exposure to environmental tobacco smoke (Z77.22)
      exposure to tobacco smoke in the perinatal period (P96.81)
      history of tobacco dependence (Z87.891)
      occupational exposure to environmental tobacco smoke (Z57.31)
      tobacco dependence (F17.-)
      tobacco use (Z72.0)
    EXCLUDES 1   congenital bronchiectasis (Q33.4)
                 tuberculous bronchiectasis (current disease) (A15.0)
    DEF: Dilation of the bronchi with mucus production and persistent cough due to infection or chronic conditions that causes diminished lung capacity and frequent infections of the lung.

    J47.0 Bronchiectasis with acute lower respiratory infection HCC
        Bronchiectasis with acute bronchitis
        Use additional code to identify the infection

    J47.1 Bronchiectasis with (acute) exacerbation HCC

    J47.9 Bronchiectasis, uncomplicated HCC
        Bronchiectasis NOS

Lung diseases due to external agents (J60-J70)

EXCLUDES 2   asthma (J45.-)
           malignant neoplasm of bronchus and lung (C34.-)
DEF: Pneumoconiosis: Condition caused by inhaling inorganic dust particles, typically associated with occupations that require regular exposure to mineral dusts. A form of interstitial lung disease that contributes to the inflammation of the air sacs, causing the lung tissue to harden.

J60 Coalworker's pneumoconiosis HCC A
    Anthracosilicosis
    Anthracosis
    Black lung disease
    Coalworker's lung
    EXCLUDES 1   coalworker pneumoconiosis with tuberculosis, any type in A15 (J65)

J61 Pneumoconiosis due to asbestos and other mineral fibers HCC A
    Asbestosis
    EXCLUDES 1   pleural plaque with asbestosis (J92.0)
             pneumoconiosis with tuberculosis, any type in A15 (J65)

✓4ᵗʰ **J62 Pneumoconiosis due to dust containing silica**
    INCLUDES   silicotic fibrosis (massive) of lung
    EXCLUDES 1   pneumoconiosis with tuberculosis, any type in A15 (J65)

    J62.0 Pneumoconiosis due to talc dust HCC

    J62.8 Pneumoconiosis due to other dust containing silica HCC
        Silicosis NOS

✓4ᵗʰ **J63 Pneumoconiosis due to other inorganic dusts**
    EXCLUDES 1   pneumoconiosis with tuberculosis, any type in A15 (J65)

    J63.0 Aluminosis (of lung) HCC
    J63.1 Bauxite fibrosis (of lung) HCC
    J63.2 Berylliosis HCC
    J63.3 Graphite fibrosis (of lung) HCC
    J63.4 Siderosis HCC
    J63.5 Stannosis HCC

    J63.6 Pneumoconiosis due to other specified inorganic dusts HCC

J64 Unspecified pneumoconiosis HCC
    EXCLUDES 1   pneumonoconiosis with tuberculosis, any type in A15 (J65)

J65 Pneumoconiosis associated with tuberculosis HCC
    Any condition in J60-J64 with tuberculosis, any type in A15
    Silicotuberculosis

✓4ᵗʰ **J66 Airway disease due to specific organic dust**
    EXCLUDES 2   allergic alveolitis (J67.-)
             asbestosis (J61)
             bagassosis (J67.1)
             farmer's lung (J67.0)
             hypersensitivity pneumonitis due to organic dust (J67.-)
             reactive airways dysfunction syndrome (J68.3)

    J66.0 Byssinosis HCC
        Airway disease due to cotton dust

    J66.1 Flax-dressers' disease HCC

    J66.2 Cannabinosis HCC

    J66.8 Airway disease due to other specific organic dusts HCC

✓4ᵗʰ **J67 Hypersensitivity pneumonitis due to organic dust**
    INCLUDES   allergic alveolitis and pneumonitis due to inhaled organic dust and particles of fungal, actinomycetic or other origin
    EXCLUDES 1   pneumonitis due to inhalation of chemicals, gases, fumes or vapors (J68.0)

    J67.0 Farmer's lung HCC
        Harvester's lung
        Haymaker's lung
        Moldy hay disease

    J67.1 Bagassosis HCC
        Bagasse disease
        Bagasse pneumonitis

    J67.2 Bird fancier's lung HCC
        Budgerigar fancier's disease or lung
        Pigeon fancier's disease or lung

    J67.3 Suberosis HCC
        Corkhandler's disease or lung
        Corkworker's disease or lung

    J67.4 Maltworker's lung HCC
        Alveolitis due to Aspergillus clavatus

    J67.5 Mushroom-worker's lung HCC

    J67.6 Maple-bark-stripper's lung HCC
        Alveolitis due to Cryptostroma corticale
        Cryptostromosis

    J67.7 Air conditioner and humidifier lung HCC
        Allergic alveolitis due to fungal, thermophilic actinomycetes and other organisms growing in ventilation [air conditioning] systems

    J67.8 Hypersensitivity pneumonitis due to other organic dusts HCC
        Cheese-washer's lung
        Coffee-worker's lung
        Fish-meal worker's lung
        Furrier's lung
        Sequoiosis

    J67.9 Hypersensitivity pneumonitis due to unspecified organic dust HCC
        Allergic alveolitis (extrinsic) NOS
        Hypersensitivity pneumonitis NOS

✓4ᵗʰ **J68 Respiratory conditions due to inhalation of chemicals, gases, fumes and vapors**
    Code first (T51-T65) to identify cause
    Use additional code to identify associated respiratory conditions, such as:
      acute respiratory failure (J96.0-)

    J68.0 Bronchitis and pneumonitis due to chemicals, gases, fumes and vapors HCC
        Chemical bronchitis (acute)
        AHA: 2019,2Q,31

✓ Additional Character Required   ✓x7ᵗʰ Placeholder Alert   Manifestation   Unspecified Dx   ▶◀ Revised Text   ● New Code   ▲ Revised Code Title

ICD-10-CM 2020   689

Chapter 10. Diseases of the Respiratory System

J68.1 **Pulmonary edema** due to chemicals, gases, fumes and vapors   `HCC`

Chemical pulmonary edema (acute) (chronic)

EXCLUDES 1   *pulmonary edema (acute) (chronic) NOS (J81.-)*

J68.2 **Upper respiratory inflammation** due to chemicals, gases, fumes and vapors, not elsewhere classified   `HCC`

J68.3 **Other** acute and subacute respiratory conditions due to chemicals, gases, fumes and vapors   `HCC`

Reactive airways dysfunction syndrome

J68.4 Chronic respiratory conditions due to chemicals, gases, fumes and vapors   `HCC`

Emphysema (diffuse) (chronic) due to inhalation of chemicals, gases, fumes and vapors

Obliterative bronchiolitis (chronic) (subacute) due to inhalation of chemicals, gases, fumes and vapors

Pulmonary fibrosis (chronic) due to inhalation of chemicals, gases, fumes and vapors

EXCLUDES 1   *chronic pulmonary edema due to chemicals, gases, fumes and vapors (J68.1)*

J68.8 **Other respiratory conditions due to chemicals, gases, fumes and vapors**   `HCC`

J68.9 **Unspecified respiratory condition due to chemicals, gases, fumes and vapors**   `HCC`

✓4ᵗʰ **J69 Pneumonitis due to solids and liquids**

EXCLUDES 1   *neonatal aspiration syndromes (P24.-)*
           postprocedural pneumonitis (J95.4)

AHA: 2017,1Q,24

DEF: Pneumonitis: Noninfectious inflammation of the walls of the alveoli in the lung tissue due to inhalation of food, vomit, oils, essences, or other solids or liquids.

J69.0 **Pneumonitis due to** inhalation of food and vomit   `HCC`

Aspiration pneumonia NOS

Aspiration pneumonia (due to) food (regurgitated)

Aspiration pneumonia (due to) gastric secretions

Aspiration pneumonia (due to) milk

Aspiration pneumonia (due to) vomit

Code also any associated foreign body in respiratory tract (T17.-)

EXCLUDES 1   *chemical pneumonitis due to anesthesia (J95.4)*
           obstetric aspiration pneumonitis (O74.0)

AHA: 2019,2Q,6,31

J69.1 **Pneumonitis due to** inhalation of oils and essences   `HCC`

Exogenous lipoid pneumonia

Lipid pneumonia NOS

Code first (T51-T65) to identify substance

EXCLUDES 1   *endogenous lipoid pneumonia (J84.89)*

J69.8 **Pneumonitis due to inhalation of other solids and liquids**   `HCC`

Pneumonitis due to aspiration of blood

Pneumonitis due to aspiration of detergent

Code first (T51-T65) to identify substance

✓4ᵗʰ **J70 Respiratory conditions due to other external agents**

J70.0 **Acute pulmonary manifestations due to** radiation   `HCC`

Radiation pneumonitis

Use additional code (W88-W90, X39.0-) to identify the external cause

J70.1 **Chronic** and other pulmonary manifestations due to radiation   `HCC`

Fibrosis of lung following radiation

Use additional code (W88-W90, X39.0-) to identify the external cause

J70.2 **Acute drug-induced interstitial** lung disorders   `HCC`

Use additional code for adverse effect, if applicable, to identify drug (T36-T50 with fifth or sixth character 5)

EXCLUDES 1   *interstitial pneumonia NOS (J84.9)*
           lymphoid interstitial pneumonia (J84.2)

AHA: 2019,2Q,28

J70.3 **Chronic drug-induced interstitial** lung disorders   `HCC`

Use additional code for adverse effect, if applicable, to identify drug (T36-T50 with fifth or sixth character 5)

EXCLUDES 1   *interstitial pneumonia NOS (J84.9)*
           lymphoid interstitial pneumonia (J84.2)

J70.4 **Drug-induced interstitial lung disorders, unspecified**   `HCC`

Use additional code for adverse effect, if applicable, to identify drug (T36-T50 with fifth or sixth character 5)

EXCLUDES 1   *interstitial pneumonia NOS (J84.9)*
           lymphoid interstitial pneumonia (J84.2)

AHA: 2019,2Q,28

J70.5 **Respiratory conditions due to** smoke inhalation   `HCC`

Smoke inhalation NOS

EXCLUDES 1   *smoke inhalation due to chemicals, gases, fumes and vapors (J68.9)*

AHA: 2013,4Q,121

J70.8 **Respiratory conditions due to other specified external agents**   `HCC`

Code first (T51-T65) to identify the external agent

J70.9 **Respiratory conditions due to unspecified external agent**   `HCC`

Code first (T51-T65) to identify the external agent

Other respiratory diseases principally affecting the interstitium (J80-J84)

J80 Acute respiratory distress syndrome   `HCC`

Acute respiratory distress syndrome in adult or child

Adult hyaline membrane disease

EXCLUDES 1   *respiratory distress syndrome in newborn (perinatal) (P22.0)*

AHA: 2017,1Q,26

DEF: Lung inflammation or injury resulting in a build-up of fluid in the air sacs, preventing the passage of oxygen from the air into the bloodstream.

✓4ᵗʰ **J81 Pulmonary edema**

Use additional code to identify:

exposure to environmental tobacco smoke (Z77.22)

history of tobacco dependence (Z87.891)

occupational exposure to environmental tobacco smoke (Z57.31)

tobacco dependence (F17.-)

tobacco use (Z72.0)

EXCLUDES 1   *chemical (acute) pulmonary edema (J68.1)*
           hypostatic pneumonia (J18.2)
           passive pneumonia (J18.2)
           pulmonary edema due to external agents (J60-J70)
           pulmonary edema with heart disease NOS (I50.1)
           pulmonary edema with heart failure (I50.1)

DEF: Accumulation of fluid in the air sacs of the lungs, making it difficult to breath.

J81.0 **Acute** pulmonary edema   `HCC`

Acute edema of lung

J81.1 **Chronic** pulmonary edema

Pulmonary congestion (chronic) (passive)

Pulmonary edema NOS

J82 Pulmonary eosinophilia, not elsewhere classified   `HCC`

Allergic pneumonia

Eosinophilic asthma

Eosinophilic pneumonia

Löffler's pneumonia

Tropical (pulmonary) eosinophilia NOS

EXCLUDES 1   *pulmonary eosinophilia due to aspergillosis (B44.-)*
           pulmonary eosinophilia due to drugs (J70.2-J70.4)
           pulmonary eosinophilia due to specified parasitic infection (B50-B83)
           pulmonary eosinophilia due to systemic connective tissue disorders (M30-M36)
           pulmonary infiltrate NOS (R91.8)

DEF: Infiltration of eosinophils (white blood cells of the immune system) into the parenchyma of the lungs, resulting in cough, fever, and dyspnea.

✓4ᵗʰ **J84 Other** interstitial pulmonary diseases

EXCLUDES 1   *drug-induced interstitial lung disorders (J70.2-J70.4)*
           interstitial emphysema (J98.2)

EXCLUDES 2   *lung diseases due to external agents (J60-J70)*

DEF: Interstitial: Within the small spaces or gaps occurring in tissue or organs.

✓5ᵗʰ **J84.0** **Alveolar and parieto-alveolar conditions**

J84.01 **Alveolar** proteinosis   `HCC`

DEF: Reduced ventilation due to proteinaceous deposits on alveoli. Symptoms include dyspnea, cough, chest pain, weakness, weight loss, and hemoptysis.

J84.02 **Pulmonary alveolar** microlithiasis   `HCC`

J84.Ø3   *Idiopathic pulmonary hemosiderosis*   HCC

Essential brown induration of lung

Code first underlying disease, such as:

disorders of iron metabolism (E83.1-)

> EXCLUDES 1   *acute idiopathic pulmonary hemorrhage in infants [AIPHI] (RØ4.81)*

DEF: Fibrosis of the alveolar walls marked by abnormal accumulation of iron as hemosiderin in the lungs. It primarily affects children and symptoms include anemia, fluid in the lungs, and blood in the sputum. Etiology is unknown.

J84.Ø9   **Other alveolar and parieto-alveolar conditions**   HCC

✓5ᵗʰ **J84.1**   **Other interstitial pulmonary diseases with fibrosis**

> EXCLUDES 1   *pulmonary fibrosis (chronic) due to inhalation of chemicals, gases, fumes or vapors (J68.4)*
> *pulmonary fibrosis (chronic) following radiation (J7Ø.1)*

J84.1Ø   **Pulmonary fibrosis, unspecified**   HCC

Capillary fibrosis of lung

Cirrhosis of lung (chronic) NOS

Fibrosis of lung (atrophic) (chronic) (confluent) (massive) (perialveolar) (peribronchial) NOS

Induration of lung (chronic) NOS

Postinflammatory pulmonary fibrosis

✓6ᵗʰ **J84.11**   **Idiopathic interstitial pneumonia**

> EXCLUDES 1   *lymphoid interstitial pneumonia (J84.2)*
> *pneumocystis pneumonia (B59)*

J84.111   **Idiopathic interstitial pneumonia, not otherwise specified**   HCC

J84.112   **Idiopathic pulmonary fibrosis**   HCC

Cryptogenic fibrosing alveolitis

Idiopathic fibrosing alveolitis

J84.113   **Idiopathic non-specific interstitial pneumonitis**   HCC

> EXCLUDES 1   *non-specific interstitial pneumonia NOS, or due to known underlying cause (J84.89)*

J84.114   **Acute interstitial pneumonitis**   HCC

Hamman-Rich syndrome

> EXCLUDES 1   *pneumocystis pneumonia (B59)*

J84.115   **Respiratory bronchiolitis interstitial lung disease**   HCC

J84.116   **Cryptogenic organizing pneumonia**   HCC

> EXCLUDES 1   *organizing pneumonia NOS, or due to known underlying cause (J84.89)*

J84.117   **Desquamative interstitial pneumonia**   HCC

J84.17   *Other interstitial pulmonary diseases with fibrosis in diseases classified elsewhere*   HCC

Interstitial pneumonia (nonspecific) (usual) due to collagen vascular disease

Interstitial pneumonia (nonspecific) (usual) in diseases classified elsewhere

Organizing pneumonia due to collagen vascular disease

Organizing pneumonia in diseases classified elsewhere

Code first underlying disease, such as:

progressive systemic sclerosis (M34.Ø)

rheumatoid arthritis (MØ5.ØØ-MØ6.9)

systemic lupus erythematosis (M32.Ø-M32.9)

J84.2   **Lymphoid interstitial pneumonia**   HCC

Lymphoid interstitial pneumonitis

✓5ᵗʰ **J84.8**   **Other specified interstitial pulmonary diseases**

> EXCLUDES 1   *exogenous lipoid pneumonia (J69.1)*
> *unspecified lipoid pneumonia (J69.1)*

J84.81   **Lymphangioleiomyomatosis**   HCC

Lymphangiomyomatosis

J84.82   **Adult pulmonary Langerhans cell histiocytosis**   HCC A

Adult PLCH

J84.83   **Surfactant mutations of the lung**   HCC

DEF: Genetic disorder resulting in insufficient secretion of a complex mixture of phospholipids and proteins that reduce surface tension in the alveoli following the onset of breathing to facilitate lung expansion in the newborn. It is the leading indication for pediatric lung transplantation.

✓6ᵗʰ **J84.84**   **Other interstitial lung diseases of childhood**

J84.841   **Neuroendocrine cell hyperplasia of infancy**   HCC

J84.842   **Pulmonary interstitial glycogenosis**   HCC

J84.843   **Alveolar capillary dysplasia with vein misalignment**   HCC

J84.848   **Other interstitial lung diseases of childhood**   HCC

J84.89   **Other specified interstitial pulmonary diseases**   HCC

Endogenous lipoid pneumonia

Interstitial pneumonitis

Non-specific interstitial pneumonitis NOS

Organizing pneumonia NOS

Code first, if applicable:

poisoning due to drug or toxin (T51-T65 with fifth or sixth character to indicate intent), for toxic pneumonopathy

underlying cause of pneumonopathy, if known

Use additional code, for adverse effect, to identify drug (T36-T5Ø with fifth or sixth character 5), if drug-induced

> EXCLUDES 1   *cryptogenic organizing pneumonia (J84.116)*
> *idiopathic non-specific interstitial pneumonitis (J84.113)*
> *lymphoid interstitial pneumonia (J84.2)*
> *lipoid pneumonia, exogenous or unspecified (J69.1)*

AHA: 2019,2Q,28

J84.9   **Interstitial pulmonary disease, unspecified**   HCC

Interstitial pneumonia NOS

Suppurative and necrotic conditions of the lower respiratory tract (J85-J86)

✓4ᵗʰ **J85**   **Abscess of lung and mediastinum**

Use additional code (B95-B97) to identify infectious agent

J85.Ø   **Gangrene and necrosis of lung**   HCC

J85.1   **Abscess of lung with pneumonia**   HCC

Code also the type of pneumonia

J85.2   **Abscess of lung without pneumonia**   HCC

Abscess of lung NOS

J85.3   **Abscess of mediastinum**   HCC

✓4ᵗʰ **J86**   **Pyothorax**

Use additional code (B95-B97) to identify infectious agent

> EXCLUDES 1   *abscess of lung (J85.-)*
> *pyothorax due to tuberculosis (A15.6)*

DEF: Collection of pus in the pleural space that is commonly caused by an infection that spreads from the lung, such as bacterial pneumonia or a lung abscess.

J86.Ø   **Pyothorax with fistula**   HCC

Bronchocutaneous fistula

Bronchopleural fistula

Hepatopleural fistula

Mediastinal fistula

Pleural fistula

Thoracic fistula

Any condition classifiable to J86.9 with fistula

DEF: Purulent infection of the respiratory cavity, with communication from a cavity to another structure.

✅ Additional Character Required   ✓x7ᵗʰ Placeholder Alert   Manifestation   Unspecified Dx   ▶◀ Revised Text   ● New Code   ▲ Revised Code Title

ICD-10-CM 2020   **691**

J86.9 Pyothorax without fistula   `HCC`

Abscess of pleura
Abscess of thorax
Empyema (chest) (lung) (pleura)
Fibrinopurulent pleurisy
Purulent pleurisy
Pyopneumothorax
Septic pleurisy
Seropurulent pleurisy
Suppurative pleurisy

Other diseases of the pleura (J90-J94)

J90 Pleural effusion, not elsewhere classified

Encysted pleurisy
Pleural effusion NOS
Pleurisy with effusion (exudative) (serous)
> `EXCLUDES 1`   chylous (pleural) effusion (J94.0)
> malignant pleural effusion (J91.0))
> pleurisy NOS (R09.1)
> tuberculous pleural effusion (A15.6)

DEF: Collection of lymph and other fluid within the pleural space.

Pleural Effusion

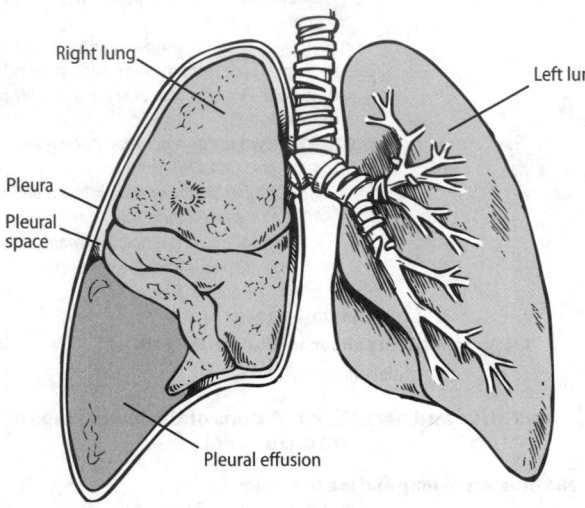

Right lung
Left lung
Pleura
Pleural space
Pleural effusion

√4th J91 Pleural effusion in conditions classified elsewhere

> `EXCLUDES 2`   pleural effusion in heart failure (I50.-)
> pleural effusion in systemic lupus erythematosus (M32.13)

DEF: Collection of lymph and other fluid within the pleural space.

J91.0 *Malignant pleural effusion*

Code first underlying neoplasm

J91.8 *Pleural effusion in other conditions classified elsewhere*

Code first underlying disease, such as:
filariasis (B74.0-B74.9)
influenza (J09.X2, J10.1, J11.1)
AHA: 2015,2Q,15
TIP: Assign this code as a secondary diagnosis to congestive heart failure (I50.-) only if pleural effusion is specifically evaluated or treated.

√4th J92 Pleural plaque

`INCLUDES`   pleural thickening
DEF: Areas of fibrous thickening that form on the parietal or visceral pleura, the membranes that line the ribs and lungs.

J92.0 Pleural plaque with presence of asbestos

J92.9 Pleural plaque without asbestos
Pleural plaque NOS

√4th J93 Pneumothorax and air leak

> `EXCLUDES 1`   congenital or perinatal pneumothorax (P25.1)
> postprocedural air leak (J95.812)
> postprocedural pneumothorax (J95.811)
> pyopneumothorax (J86.-)
> traumatic pneumothorax (S27.0)
> tuberculous (current disease) pneumothorax (A15.-)

DEF: Pneumothorax: Lung displacement due to abnormal leakage of air or gas that is trapped in the pleural space formed by the membrane that encloses the lungs and lines the thoracic cavity.

J93.0 Spontaneous tension pneumothorax
DEF: Leaking air from the lung into the lining, causing collapse.

√5th J93.1 Other spontaneous pneumothorax

J93.11 Primary spontaneous pneumothorax

J93.12 Secondary spontaneous pneumothorax
Code first underlying condition, such as:
catamenial pneumothorax due to endometriosis (N80.8)
cystic fibrosis (E84.-)
eosinophilic pneumonia (J82)
lymphangioleiomyomatosis (J84.81)
malignant neoplasm of bronchus and lung (C34.-)
Marfan's syndrome (Q87.4)
pneumonia due to Pneumocystis carinii (B59)
secondary malignant neoplasm of lung (C78.0-)
spontaneous rupture of the esophagus (K22.3)

√5th J93.8 Other pneumothorax and air leak

J93.81 Chronic pneumothorax

J93.82 Other air leak
Persistent air leak

J93.83 Other pneumothorax
Acute pneumothorax
Spontaneous pneumothorax NOS

J93.9 Pneumothorax, unspecified
Pneumothorax NOS

√4th J94 Other pleural conditions

> `EXCLUDES 1`   pleurisy NOS (R09.1)
> traumatic hemopneumothorax (S27.2)
> traumatic hemothorax (S27.1)
> tuberculous pleural conditions (current disease) (A15.-)

J94.0 Chylous effusion
Chyliform effusion
DEF: Fluid within the pleural space due to the leaking of lymph contents into the space, usually as a result of thoracic duct damage or injury or mediastinal lymphoma.

J94.1 Fibrothorax
DEF: Fibrosis within the pleural lining of the lungs commonly seen as a stiff layer surrounding the lung typically attributed to traumatic hemothorax or pleural effusion.

J94.2 Hemothorax
Hemopneumothorax

J94.8 Other specified pleural conditions
Hydropneumothorax
Hydrothorax

J94.9 Pleural condition, unspecified

Intraoperative and postprocedural complications and disorders of respiratory system, not elsewhere classified (J95)

✓4ᵗʰ J95 Intraoperative and postprocedural complications and disorders of respiratory system, not elsewhere classified

> *EXCLUDES 2*   aspiration pneumonia (J69.-)
> emphysema (subcutaneous) resulting from a procedure (T81.82)
> hypostatic pneumonia (J18.2)
> pulmonary manifestations due to radiation (J70.0-J70.1)

✓5ᵗʰ J95.0 Tracheostomy complications

> **DEF:** Tracheostomy: Formation of a tracheal opening on the neck surface with tube insertion to allow for respiration in cases of obstruction or decreased patency. A tracheostomy may be planned or performed on an emergency basis for temporary or long-term use.

Tracheostomy

Tracheostomy in place

Incision in trachea

Trachea

Tracheostomy tube

J95.00	**Unspecified tracheostomy complication**	HCC
J95.01	**Hemorrhage from tracheostomy stoma**	HCC
J95.02	**Infection of tracheostomy stoma**	HCC

> Use additional code to identify type of infection, such as:
> cellulitis of neck (L03.221)
> sepsis (A40, A41.-)

| J95.03 | **Malfunction of tracheostomy stoma** | HCC |

> Mechanical complication of tracheostomy stoma
> Obstruction of tracheostomy airway
> Tracheal stenosis due to tracheostomy

| J95.04 | **Tracheo-esophageal fistula following tracheostomy** | HCC |
| J95.09 | **Other tracheostomy complication** | HCC |

J95.1 Acute pulmonary insufficiency following thoracic surgery   HCC

> *EXCLUDES 2*   functional disturbances following cardiac surgery (I97.0, I97.1-)

J95.2 Acute pulmonary insufficiency following nonthoracic surgery   HCC

> *EXCLUDES 2*   functional disturbances following cardiac surgery (I97.0, I97.1-)

J95.3 Chronic pulmonary insufficiency following surgery   HCC

> *EXCLUDES 2*   functional disturbances following cardiac surgery (I97.0, I97.1-)

J95.4 Chemical pneumonitis due to anesthesia

> Mendelson's syndrome
> Postprocedural aspiration pneumonia
> Use additional code for adverse effect, if applicable, to identify drug (T41.- with fifth or sixth character 5)

> *EXCLUDES 1*   aspiration pneumonitis due to anesthesia complicating labor and delivery (O74.0)
> aspiration pneumonitis due to anesthesia complicating pregnancy (O29)
> aspiration pneumonitis due to anesthesia complicating the puerperium (O89.01)

J95.5 Postprocedural subglottic stenosis

✓5ᵗʰ J95.6 Intraoperative hemorrhage and hematoma of a respiratory system organ or structure complicating a procedure

> *EXCLUDES 1*   intraoperative hemorrhage and hematoma of a respiratory system organ or structure due to accidental puncture and laceration during procedure (J95.7-)

J95.61 Intraoperative hemorrhage and hematoma of a respiratory system organ or structure complicating a respiratory system procedure

J95.62 Intraoperative hemorrhage and hematoma of a respiratory system organ or structure complicating other procedure

✓5ᵗʰ J95.7 Accidental puncture and laceration of a respiratory system organ or structure during a procedure

> *EXCLUDES 2*   postprocedural pneumothorax (J95.811)

J95.71 Accidental puncture and laceration of a respiratory system organ or structure during a respiratory system procedure

J95.72 Accidental puncture and laceration of a respiratory system organ or structure during other procedure

✓5ᵗʰ J95.8 Other intraoperative and postprocedural complications and disorders of respiratory system, not elsewhere classified

> AHA: 2016,4Q,9-10

✓6ᵗʰ J95.81 Postprocedural pneumothorax and air leak

> **J95.811 Postprocedural pneumothorax**
> **J95.812 Postprocedural air leak**

✓6ᵗʰ J95.82 Postprocedural respiratory failure

> *EXCLUDES 1*   respiratory failure in other conditions (J96.-)

> **J95.821 Acute postprocedural respiratory failure**   HCC
> Postprocedural respiratory failure NOS

> **J95.822 Acute and chronic postprocedural respiratory failure**   HCC

✓6ᵗʰ J95.83 Postprocedural hemorrhage of a respiratory system organ or structure following a procedure

> **J95.830 Postprocedural hemorrhage of a respiratory system organ or structure following a respiratory system procedure**

> **J95.831 Postprocedural hemorrhage of a respiratory system organ or structure following other procedure**

J95.84 Transfusion-related acute lung injury (TRALI)

> **DEF:** Relatively rare, but serious, pulmonary complication of blood transfusion, with acute respiratory distress, noncardiogenic pulmonary edema, cyanosis, hypoxemia, hypotension, fever, and chills.

✓6ᵗʰ J95.85 Complication of respirator [ventilator]

> **J95.850 Mechanical complication of respirator**   HCC

> > *EXCLUDES 1*   encounter for respirator [ventilator] dependence during power failure (Z99.12)

> **J95.851 Ventilator associated pneumonia**   HCC
> Ventilator associated pneumonitis
> Use additional code to identify the organism, if known (B95.-, B96.-, B97.-)

> > *EXCLUDES 1*   ventilator lung in newborn (P27.8)

> > AHA: 2017,1Q,25

> **J95.859 Other complication of respirator [ventilator]**   HCC

☑ Additional Character Required   ✓x7ᵗʰ Placeholder Alert   Manifestation   Unspecified Dx   ▶◀ Revised Text   ● New Code   ▲ Revised Code Title

ICD-10-CM 2020   693

√6ᵗʰ **J95.86** Postprocedural hematoma and seroma of a respiratory system organ or structure following a procedure

     J95.860 Postprocedural hematoma of a respiratory system organ or structure following a respiratory system procedure

     J95.861 Postprocedural hematoma of a respiratory system organ or structure following other procedure

     J95.862 Postprocedural seroma of a respiratory system organ or structure following a respiratory system procedure

     J95.863 Postprocedural seroma of a respiratory system organ or structure following other procedure

J95.88 Other intraoperative complications of respiratory system, not elsewhere classified

J95.89 Other postprocedural complications and disorders of respiratory system, not elsewhere classified

     Use additional code to identify disorder, such as:
         aspiration pneumonia (J69.-)
         bacterial or viral pneumonia (J12-J18)

     EXCLUDES 2   *acute pulmonary insufficiency following thoracic surgery (J95.1)*
         postprocedural subglottic stenosis (J95.5)

Other diseases of the respiratory system (J96-J99)

√4ᵗʰ **J96 Respiratory failure, not elsewhere classified**

     EXCLUDES 1   *acute respiratory distress syndrome (J80)*
         cardiorespiratory failure (R09.2)
         newborn respiratory distress syndrome (P22.0)
         postprocedural respiratory failure (J95.82-)
         respiratory arrest (R09.2)
         respiratory arrest of newborn (P28.81)
         respiratory failure of newborn (P28.5)

√5ᵗʰ **J96.0 Acute respiratory failure**

     J96.00 Acute respiratory failure, unspecified whether with hypoxia or hypercapnia **HCC**
         AHA: 2016,3Q,14; 2013,4Q,121

     J96.01 Acute respiratory failure with hypoxia **HCC**

     J96.02 Acute respiratory failure with hypercapnia **HCC**

√5ᵗʰ **J96.1 Chronic respiratory failure**

     J96.10 Chronic respiratory failure, unspecified whether with hypoxia or hypercapnia **HCC**
         AHA: 2016,1Q,38; 2015,1Q,21

     J96.11 Chronic respiratory failure with hypoxia **HCC**
         AHA: 2013,4Q,129

     J96.12 Chronic respiratory failure with hypercapnia **HCC**

√5ᵗʰ **J96.2 Acute and chronic respiratory failure**

     Acute on chronic respiratory failure

     J96.20 Acute and chronic respiratory failure, unspecified whether with hypoxia or hypercapnia **HCC**

     J96.21 Acute and chronic respiratory failure with hypoxia **HCC**

     J96.22 Acute and chronic respiratory failure with hypercapnia **HCC**

√5ᵗʰ **J96.9 Respiratory failure, unspecified**

     J96.90 Respiratory failure, unspecified, unspecified whether with hypoxia or hypercapnia **HCC**

     J96.91 Respiratory failure, unspecified with hypoxia **HCC**

     J96.92 Respiratory failure, unspecified with hypercapnia **HCC**

√4ᵗʰ **J98 Other respiratory disorders**

     Use additional code to identify:
         exposure to environmental tobacco smoke (Z77.22)
         exposure to tobacco smoke in the perinatal period (P96.81)
         history of tobacco dependence (Z87.891)
         occupational exposure to environmental tobacco smoke (Z57.31)
         tobacco dependence (F17.-)
         tobacco use (Z72.0)

     EXCLUDES 1   *newborn apnea (P28.4)*
         newborn sleep apnea (P28.3)

     EXCLUDES 2   *apnea NOS (R06.81)*
         sleep apnea (G47.3-)

√5ᵗʰ **J98.0 Diseases of bronchus, not elsewhere classified**

     J98.01 Acute bronchospasm

         EXCLUDES 1   *acute bronchiolitis with bronchospasm (J21.-)*
             acute bronchitis with bronchospasm (J20.-)
             asthma (J45.-)
             exercise induced bronchospasm (J45.990)

     J98.09 Other diseases of bronchus, not elsewhere classified

         Broncholithiasis
         Calcification of bronchus
         Stenosis of bronchus
         Tracheobronchial collapse
         Tracheobronchial dyskinesia
         Ulcer of bronchus

√5ᵗʰ **J98.1 Pulmonary collapse**

     EXCLUDES 1   *therapeutic collapse of lung status (Z98.3)*

     J98.11 Atelectasis

         EXCLUDES 1   *newborn atelectasis*
             tuberculous atelectasis (current disease) (A15)

         DEF: Collapse of lung tissue affecting part or all of one lung, preventing normal oxygen absorption to healthy tissues.

     J98.19 Other pulmonary collapse

J98.2 Interstitial emphysema **HCC**

     Mediastinal emphysema

     EXCLUDES 1   *emphysema NOS (J43.9)*
         emphysema in newborn (P25.0)
         surgical emphysema (subcutaneous) (T81.82)
         traumatic subcutaneous emphysema (T79.7)

J98.3 Compensatory emphysema **HCC**

     DEF: Distention of all or part of the lung caused by disease processes or surgical intervention that decreased volume in another part of the lung, causing an overcompensation reaction. Compensatory emphysema occurs in association with pneumonias, pleural effusions, atelectasis, empyema, and pneumothorax.

J98.4 Other disorders of lung

     Calcification of lung
     Cystic lung disease (acquired)
     Lung disease NOS
     Pulmolithiasis

     EXCLUDES 1   *acute interstitial pneumonitis (J84.114)*
         pulmonary insufficiency following surgery (J95.1-J95.2)

√5ᵗʰ **J98.5 Diseases of mediastinum, not elsewhere classified**

     EXCLUDES 2   *abscess of mediastinum (J85.3)*

     AHA: 2016,4Q,29

     J98.51 Mediastinitis

         Code first underlying condition, if applicable, such as postoperative mediastinitis (T81.-)

     J98.59 Other diseases of mediastinum, not elsewhere classified

         Fibrosis of mediastinum
         Hernia of mediastinum
         Retraction of mediastinum

J98.6   **Disorders of diaphragm**
     Diaphragmatitis
     Paralysis of diaphragm
     Relaxation of diaphragm
     EXCLUDES 1   *congenital malformation of diaphragm NEC (Q79.1)*
                   congenital diaphragmatic hernia (Q79.0)
     EXCLUDES 2   *diaphragmatic hernia (K44.-)*

J98.8   **Other specified respiratory disorders**

J98.9   **Respiratory disorder, unspecified**
     Respiratory disease (chronic) NOS

J99   ***Respiratory disorders in diseases classified elsewhere***   HCC

     Code first underlying disease, such as:
       amyloidosis (E85.-)
       ankylosing spondylitis (M45)
       congenital syphilis (A50.5)
       cryoglobulinemia (D89.1)
       early congenital syphilis (A50.0)
       plasminogen deficiency (E88.02)
       schistosomiasis (B65.0-B65.9)
     EXCLUDES 1   *respiratory disorders in:*
            amebiasis (A06.5)
            blastomycosis (B40.0-B40.2)
            candidiasis (B37.1)
            coccidioidomycosis (B38.0-B38.2)
            cystic fibrosis with pulmonary manifestations (E84.0)
            dermatomyositis (M33.01, M33.11)
            histoplasmosis (B39.0-B39.2)
            late syphilis (A52.72, A52.73)
            polymyositis (M33.21)
            sicca syndrome (M35.02)
            systemic lupus erythematosus (M32.13)
            systemic sclerosis (M34.81)
            Wegener's granulomatosis (M31.30-M31.31)

☑ Additional Character Required   √x7ᵗʰ Placeholder Alert   Manifestation   Unspecified Dx   ►◄ Revised Text   ● New Code   ▲ Revised Code Title

Chapter 11. Diseases of the Digestive System (KØØ–K95)

Chapter-specific Guidelines with Coding Examples
Reserved for future guideline expansion.

Chapter 11. Diseases of the Digestive System (K00-K95)

EXCLUDES 2
certain conditions originating in the perinatal period (P04-P96)
certain infectious and parasitic diseases (A00-B99)
complications of pregnancy, childbirth and the puerperium (O00-O9A)
congenital malformations, deformations and chromosomal abnormalities (Q00-Q99)
endocrine, nutritional and metabolic diseases (E00-E88)
injury, poisoning and certain other consequences of external causes (S00-T88)
neoplasms (C00-D49)
symptoms, signs and abnormal clinical and laboratory findings, not elsewhere classified (R00-R94)

This chapter contains the following blocks:
K00-K14   Diseases of oral cavity and salivary glands
K20-K31   Diseases of esophagus, stomach and duodenum
K35-K38   Diseases of appendix
K40-K46   Hernia
K50-K52   Noninfective enteritis and colitis
K55-K64   Other diseases of intestines
K65-K68   Diseases of peritoneum and retroperitoneum
K70-K77   Diseases of liver
K80-K87   Disorders of gallbladder, biliary tract and pancreas
K90-K95   Other diseases of the digestive system

Diseases of oral cavity and salivary glands (K00-K14)

✓4ᵗʰ K00 Disorders of tooth development and eruption

     EXCLUDES 2   embedded and impacted teeth (K01.-)

K00.0 Anodontia
     Hypodontia
     Oligodontia
     EXCLUDES 1   acquired absence of teeth (K08.1-)
     DEF: Partial or complete absence of teeth due to a congenital defect involving the tooth bud.

K00.1 Supernumerary teeth
     Distomolar
     Fourth molar
     Mesiodens
     Paramolar
     Supplementary teeth
     EXCLUDES 2   supernumerary roots (K00.2)

K00.2 Abnormalities of size and form of teeth
     Concrescence of teeth
     Dens evaginatus
     Dens in dente
     Dens invaginatus
     Enamel pearls
     Fusion of teeth
     Gemination of teeth
     Macrodontia
     Microdontia
     Peg-shaped [conical] teeth
     Supernumerary roots
     Taurodontism
     Tuberculum paramolare
     EXCLUDES 1   abnormalities of teeth due to congenital syphilis (A50.5)
               tuberculum Carabelli, which is regarded as a normal variation and should not be coded

K00.3 Mottled teeth
     Dental fluorosis
     Mottling of enamel
     Nonfluoride enamel opacities
     EXCLUDES 2   deposits [accretions] on teeth (K03.6)

K00.4 Disturbances in tooth formation
     Aplasia and hypoplasia of cementum
     Dilaceration of tooth
     Enamel hypoplasia (neonatal) (postnatal) (prenatal)
     Regional odontodysplasia
     Turner's tooth
     EXCLUDES 1   Hutchinson's teeth and mulberry molars in congenital syphilis (A50.5)
     EXCLUDES 2   mottled teeth (K00.3)

K00.5 Hereditary disturbances in tooth structure, not elsewhere classified
     Amelogenesis imperfecta
     Dentinogenesis imperfecta
     Odontogenesis imperfecta
     Dentinal dysplasia
     Shell teeth

K00.6 Disturbances in tooth eruption
     Dentia praecox
     Natal tooth
     Neonatal tooth
     Premature eruption of tooth
     Premature shedding of primary [deciduous] tooth
     Prenatal teeth
     Retained [persistent] primary tooth
     EXCLUDES 2   embedded and impacted teeth (K01.-)

K00.7 Teething syndrome

K00.8 Other disorders of tooth development
     Color changes during tooth formation
     Intrinsic staining of teeth NOS
     EXCLUDES 2   posteruptive color changes (K03.7)

K00.9 Disorder of tooth development, unspecified
     Disorder of odontogenesis NOS

✓4ᵗʰ K01 Embedded and impacted teeth
     EXCLUDES 1   abnormal position of fully erupted teeth (M26.3-)

K01.0 Embedded teeth

K01.1 Impacted teeth

✓4ᵗʰ K02 Dental caries
     INCLUDES   caries of dentine
              dental cavities
              early childhood caries
              pre-eruptive caries
              recurrent caries (dentino enamel junction) (enamel) (to the pulp)
              tooth decay
     DEF: Localized section of tooth decay that begins on the tooth surface with destruction of the calcified enamel, allowing bacterial destruction to continue and form cavities and may extend to the dentin and pulp.

Tooth Anatomy

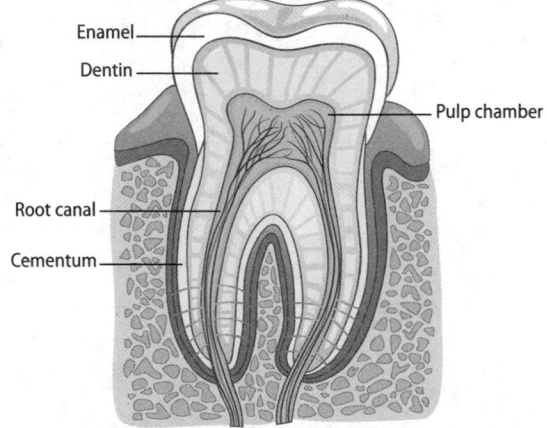

Enamel
Dentin
Pulp chamber
Root canal
Cementum

K02.3 Arrested dental caries
     Arrested coronal and root caries

✓5ᵗʰ K02.5 Dental caries on pit and fissure surface
     Dental caries on chewing surface of tooth
     K02.51 Dental caries on pit and fissure surface limited to enamel
         White spot lesions [initial caries] on pit and fissure surface of tooth
     K02.52 Dental caries on pit and fissure surface penetrating into dentin
         Primary dental caries, cervical origin
     K02.53 Dental caries on pit and fissure surface penetrating into pulp

✓5ᵗʰ **K02.6** **Dental caries on** smooth surface

   K02.61 **Dental caries on smooth surface** limited to enamel
      White spot lesions [initial caries] on smooth surface of tooth

   K02.62 **Dental caries on smooth surface** penetrating into dentin

   K02.63 **Dental caries on smooth surface** penetrating into pulp

  K02.7 **Dental** root **caries**

  K02.9 **Dental caries, unspecified**

✓4ᵗʰ **K03** **Other diseases of hard tissues of teeth**

  EXCLUDES 2 bruxism (F45.8)
           dental caries (K02.-)
           teeth-grinding NOS (F45.8)

  K03.0 **Excessive attrition of teeth**
    Approximal wear of teeth
    Occlusal wear of teeth
    DEF: Attrition: In dentistry, wearing away or erosion of tooth surface from abrasive food or grinding teeth.

  K03.1 **Abrasion of teeth**
    Dentifrice abrasion of teeth
    Habitual abrasion of teeth
    Occupational abrasion of teeth
    Ritual abrasion of teeth
    Traditional abrasion of teeth
    Wedge defect NOS

  K03.2 **Erosion of teeth**
    Erosion of teeth due to diet
    Erosion of teeth due to drugs and medicaments
    Erosion of teeth due to persistent vomiting
    Erosion of teeth NOS
    Idiopathic erosion of teeth
    Occupational erosion of teeth

  K03.3 **Pathological resorption of teeth**
    Internal granuloma of pulp
    Resorption of teeth (external)

  K03.4 **Hypercementosis**
    Cementation hyperplasia

  K03.5 **Ankylosis of teeth**

  K03.6 **Deposits [accretions] on teeth**
    Betel deposits [accretions] on teeth
    Black deposits [accretions] on teeth
    Extrinsic staining of teeth NOS
    Green deposits [accretions] on teeth
    Materia alba deposits [accretions] on teeth
    Orange deposits [accretions] on teeth
    Staining of teeth NOS
    Subgingival dental calculus
    Supragingival dental calculus
    Tobacco deposits [accretions] on teeth

  K03.7 **Posteruptive color changes of dental hard tissues**
    EXCLUDES 2 deposits [accretions] on teeth (K03.6)

✓5ᵗʰ   **K03.8** **Other specified diseases of hard tissues of teeth**

   K03.81 **Cracked tooth**
      EXCLUDES 1 asymptomatic craze lines in enamel - omit code
             broken or fractured tooth due to trauma (S02.5)

   K03.89 **Other specified diseases of hard tissues of teeth**

  K03.9 **Disease of hard tissues of teeth, unspecified**

✓4ᵗʰ **K04** **Diseases of pulp and periapical tissues**
  AHA: 2016,4Q,29-30

✓5ᵗʰ   **K04.0** **Pulpitis**
    Acute pulpitis
    Chronic (hyperplastic) (ulcerative) pulpitis

   K04.01 **Reversible pulpitis**
   K04.02 **Irreversible pulpitis**

  K04.1 **Necrosis of pulp**
    Pulpal gangrene

  K04.2 **Pulp degeneration**
    Denticles
    Pulpal calcifications
    Pulpal stones

  K04.3 **Abnormal hard tissue formation in pulp**
    Secondary or irregular dentine

  K04.4 **Acute apical periodontitis of pulpal origin**
    Acute apical periodontitis NOS
    EXCLUDES 1 acute periodontitis (K05.2-)
    DEF: Severe inflammation of the area surrounding the tip of a tooth's root that is often secondary to infection or trauma.

  K04.5 **Chronic apical periodontitis**
    Apical or periapical granuloma
    Apical periodontitis NOS
    EXCLUDES 1 chronic periodontitis (K05.3-)

  K04.6 **Periapical abscess with sinus**
    Dental abscess with sinus
    Dentoalveolar abscess with sinus

  K04.7 **Periapical abscess without sinus**
    Dental abscess without sinus
    Dentoalveolar abscess without sinus

  K04.8 **Radicular cyst**
    Apical (periodontal) cyst
    Periapical cyst
    Residual radicular cyst
    EXCLUDES 2 lateral periodontal cyst (K09.0)
    DEF: Most common odontogenic cyst in tissue around the tooth apex due to chronic inflammation of dental pulp.

✓5ᵗʰ   **K04.9** **Other and unspecified diseases of pulp and periapical tissues**

   K04.90 **Unspecified diseases of pulp and periapical tissues**
   K04.99 **Other diseases of pulp and periapical tissues**

✓4ᵗʰ **K05** **Gingivitis and periodontal diseases**
  Use additional code to identify:
    alcohol abuse and dependence (F10.-)
    exposure to environmental tobacco smoke (Z77.22)
    exposure to tobacco smoke in the perinatal period (P96.81)
    history of tobacco dependence (Z87.891)
    occupational exposure to environmental tobacco smoke (Z57.31)
    tobacco dependence (F17.-)
    tobacco use (Z72.0)
  AHA: 2016,4Q,29-30

✓5ᵗʰ   **K05.0** **Acute gingivitis**
    EXCLUDES 1 acute necrotizing ulcerative gingivitis (A69.1)
             herpesviral [herpes simplex] gingivostomatitis (B00.2)

   K05.00 **Acute gingivitis,** plaque induced
      Acute gingivitis NOS
      Plaque induced gingival disease

   K05.01 **Acute gingivitis,** non-plaque induced

✓5ᵗʰ   **K05.1** **Chronic gingivitis**
    Desquamative gingivitis (chronic)
    Gingivitis (chronic) NOS
    Hyperplastic gingivitis (chronic)
    Pregnancy associated gingivitis
    Simple marginal gingivitis (chronic)
    Ulcerative gingivitis (chronic)
    Code first, if applicable, diseases of the digestive system complicating pregnacy (O99.61-)

   K05.10 **Chronic gingivitis,** plaque induced
      Chronic gingivitis NOS
      Gingivitis NOS

   K05.11 **Chronic gingivitis,** non-plaque induced

✓5ᵗʰ   **K05.2** **Aggressive periodontitis**
    Acute pericoronitis
    EXCLUDES 1 acute apical periodontitis (K04.4)
           periapical abscess (K04.7)
           periapical abscess with sinus (K04.6)

   K05.20 **Aggressive periodontitis, unspecified**

✓6ᵗʰ   **K05.21** **Aggressive periodontitis,** localized
      Periodontal abscess

    K05.211 **Aggressive periodontitis, localized,** slight
    K05.212 **Aggressive periodontitis, localized,** moderate
    K05.213 **Aggressive periodontitis, localized,** severe
    K05.219 **Aggressive periodontitis, localized, unspecified severity**

✓6ᵗʰ   **K05.22** **Aggressive periodontitis,** generalized

    K05.221 **Aggressive periodontitis, generalized,** slight
    K05.222 **Aggressive periodontitis, generalized,** moderate
    K05.223 **Aggressive periodontitis, generalized,** severe

✓ Additional Character Required   ✓x7ᵗʰ Placeholder Alert   Manifestation   Unspecified Dx   ▶◀ Revised Text   ● New Code   ▲ Revised Code Title

ICD-10-CM 2020   699

K05.229 Aggressive periodontitis, generalized, unspecified severity

✓5ᵗʰ **K05.3 Chronic periodontitis**

Chronic pericoronitis
Complex periodontitis
Periodontitis NOS
Simplex periodontitis
EXCLUDES 1   chronic apical periodontitis (K04.5)

K05.30 Chronic periodontitis, unspecified

✓6ᵗʰ **K05.31 Chronic periodontitis, localized**

K05.311 Chronic periodontitis, localized, slight

K05.312 Chronic periodontitis, localized, moderate

K05.313 Chronic periodontitis, localized, severe

K05.319 Chronic periodontitis, localized, unspecified severity

✓6ᵗʰ **K05.32 Chronic periodontitis, generalized**

K05.321 Chronic periodontitis, generalized, slight

K05.322 Chronic periodontitis, generalized, moderate

K05.323 Chronic periodontitis, generalized, severe

K05.329 Chronic periodontitis, generalized, unspecified

K05.4 Periodontosis
Juvenile periodontosis

K05.5 Other periodontal diseases
Combined periodontic-endodontic lesion
Narrow gingival width (of periodontal soft tissue)
EXCLUDES 2   leukoplakia of gingiva (K13.21)

K05.6 Periodontal disease, unspecified

✓4ᵗʰ **K06 Other disorders of gingiva and edentulous alveolar ridge**

EXCLUDES 2   acute gingivitis (K05.0)
atrophy of edentulous alveolar ridge (K08.2)
chronic gingivitis (K05.1)
gingivitis NOS (K05.1)
AHA: 2016,4Q,29-30

✓5ᵗʰ **K06.0 Gingival recession**

Gingival recession (postinfective) (postprocedural)
AHA: 2017,4Q,16

✓6ᵗʰ **K06.01 Gingival recession, localized**

K06.010 Localized gingival recession, unspecified
Localized gingival recession, NOS

K06.011 Localized gingival recession, minimal
K06.012 Localized gingival recession, moderate
K06.013 Localized gingival recession, severe

✓6ᵗʰ **K06.02 Gingival recession, generalized**

K06.020 Generalized gingival recession, unspecified
Generalized gingival recession, NOS

K06.021 Generalized gingival recession, minimal
K06.022 Generalized gingival recession, moderate
K06.023 Generalized gingival recession, severe

K06.1 Gingival enlargement
Gingival fibromatosis

K06.2 Gingival and edentulous alveolar ridge lesions associated with trauma
Irritative hyperplasia of edentulous ridge [denture hyperplasia]
Use additional code (Chapter 20) to identify external cause or denture status (Z97.2)

K06.3 Horizontal alveolar bone loss

K06.8 Other specified disorders of gingiva and edentulous alveolar ridge
Fibrous epulis
Flabby alveolar ridge
Giant cell epulis
Peripheral giant cell granuloma of gingiva
Pyogenic granuloma of gingiva
Vertical ridge deficiency
EXCLUDES 2   gingival cyst (K09.0)

K06.9 Disorder of gingiva and edentulous alveolar ridge, unspecified

✓4ᵗʰ **K08 Other disorders of teeth and supporting structures**

EXCLUDES 2   dentofacial anomalies [including malocclusion] (M26.-)
disorders of jaw (M27.-)
AHA: 2016,4Q,29-30

K08.0 Exfoliation of teeth due to systemic causes
Code also underlying systemic condition

✓5ᵗʰ **K08.1 Complete loss of teeth**

Acquired loss of teeth, complete
EXCLUDES 1   congenital absence of teeth (K00.0)
exfoliation of teeth due to systemic causes (K08.0)
partial loss of teeth (K08.4-)
DEF: Loss of all teeth as a result of caries, trauma, extraction, periodontal disease, or other specified or unspecified causes.
Synonym(s): complete edentulism

✓6ᵗʰ **K08.10 Complete loss of teeth, unspecified cause**

K08.101 Complete loss of teeth, unspecified cause, class I

K08.102 Complete loss of teeth, unspecified cause, class II

K08.103 Complete loss of teeth, unspecified cause, class III

K08.104 Complete loss of teeth, unspecified cause, class IV

K08.109 Complete loss of teeth, unspecified cause, unspecified class
Edentulism NOS

✓6ᵗʰ **K08.11 Complete loss of teeth due to trauma**

K08.111 Complete loss of teeth due to trauma, class I

K08.112 Complete loss of teeth due to trauma, class II

K08.113 Complete loss of teeth due to trauma, class III

K08.114 Complete loss of teeth due to trauma, class IV

K08.119 Complete loss of teeth due to trauma, unspecified class

✓6ᵗʰ **K08.12 Complete loss of teeth due to periodontal diseases**

K08.121 Complete loss of teeth due to periodontal diseases, class I

K08.122 Complete loss of teeth due to periodontal diseases, class II

K08.123 Complete loss of teeth due to periodontal diseases, class III

K08.124 Complete loss of teeth due to periodontal diseases, class IV

K08.129 Complete loss of teeth due to periodontal diseases, unspecified class

✓6ᵗʰ **K08.13 Complete loss of teeth due to caries**

K08.131 Complete loss of teeth due to caries, class I

K08.132 Complete loss of teeth due to caries, class II

K08.133 Complete loss of teeth due to caries, class III

K08.134 Complete loss of teeth due to caries, class IV

K08.139 Complete loss of teeth due to caries, unspecified class

✓6ᵗʰ **K08.19 Complete loss of teeth due to other specified cause**

K08.191 Complete loss of teeth due to other specified cause, class I

K08.192 Complete loss of teeth due to other specified cause, class II

K08.193 Complete loss of teeth due to other specified cause, class III

K08.194 Complete loss of teeth due to other specified cause, class IV

K08.199 Complete loss of teeth due to other specified cause, unspecified class

✓5ᵗʰ **K08.2 Atrophy of edentulous alveolar ridge**

K08.20 Unspecified atrophy of edentulous alveolar ridge
Atrophy of the mandible NOS
Atrophy of the maxilla NOS

K08.21 Minimal atrophy of the mandible
Minimal atrophy of the edentulous mandible

K08.22 Moderate atrophy of the mandible
Moderate atrophy of the edentulous mandible

K08.23 Severe **atrophy of the** mandible
Severe atrophy of the edentulous mandible

K08.24 Minimal **atrophy of** maxilla
Minimal atrophy of the edentulous maxilla

K08.25 Moderate **atrophy of the** maxilla
Moderate atrophy of the edentulous maxilla

K08.26 Severe **atrophy of the** maxilla
Severe atrophy of the edentulous maxilla

K08.3 **Retained dental root**

√5ᵗʰ **K08.4** **Partial loss of teeth**
Acquired loss of teeth, partial
EXCLUDES 1   *complete loss of teeth (K08.1-)*
    congenital absence of teeth (K00.0)
EXCLUDES 2   *exfoliation of teeth due to systemic causes (K08.0)*

√6ᵗʰ **K08.40** **Partial loss of teeth, unspecified cause**
K08.401 **Partial loss of teeth, unspecified cause,**
class I
K08.402 **Partial loss of teeth, unspecified cause,**
class II
K08.403 **Partial loss of teeth, unspecified cause,**
class III
K08.404 **Partial loss of teeth, unspecified cause,**
class IV
K08.409 **Partial loss of teeth, unspecified cause,**
unspecified class
Tooth extraction status NOS

√6ᵗʰ **K08.41** **Partial loss of teeth due to** trauma
K08.411 **Partial loss of teeth due to trauma,** class
I
K08.412 **Partial loss of teeth due to trauma,** class
II
K08.413 **Partial loss of teeth due to trauma,** class
III
K08.414 **Partial loss of teeth due to trauma,** class
IV
K08.419 **Partial loss of teeth due to trauma,**
unspecified class

√6ᵗʰ **K08.42** **Partial loss of teeth due to** periodontal diseases
K08.421 **Partial loss of teeth due to periodontal**
diseases, class I
K08.422 **Partial loss of teeth due to periodontal**
diseases, class II
K08.423 **Partial loss of teeth due to periodontal**
diseases, class III
K08.424 **Partial loss of teeth due to periodontal**
diseases, class IV
K08.429 **Partial loss of teeth due to periodontal**
diseases, unspecified class

√6ᵗʰ **K08.43** **Partial loss of teeth due to** caries
K08.431 **Partial loss of teeth due to caries,** class I
K08.432 **Partial loss of teeth due to caries,** class II
K08.433 **Partial loss of teeth due to caries,** class III
K08.434 **Partial loss of teeth due to caries,** class IV
K08.439 **Partial loss of teeth due to caries,**
unspecified class

√6ᵗʰ **K08.49** **Partial loss of teeth due to other specified cause**
K08.491 **Partial loss of teeth due to other specified**
cause, class I
K08.492 **Partial loss of teeth due to other specified**
cause, class II
K08.493 **Partial loss of teeth due to other specified**
cause, class III
K08.494 **Partial loss of teeth due to other specified**
cause, class IV
K08.499 **Partial loss of teeth due to other specified**
cause, unspecified class

√5ᵗʰ **K08.5** **Unsatisfactory restoration of tooth**
Defective bridge, crown, filling
Defective dental restoration
EXCLUDES 1   *dental restoration status (Z98.811)*
EXCLUDES 2   *endosseous dental implant failure (M27.6-)*
    unsatisfactory endodontic treatment (M27.5-)

K08.50 **Unsatisfactory restoration of tooth, unspecified**
Defective dental restoration NOS

K08.51 **Open restoration margins of tooth**
Dental restoration failure of marginal integrity
Open margin on tooth restoration
Poor gingival margin to tooth restoration

K08.52 **Unrepairable overhanging of dental restorative**
materials
Overhanging of tooth restoration

√6ᵗʰ **K08.53** **Fractured dental restorative material**
EXCLUDES 1   *cracked tooth (K03.81)*
    traumatic fracture of tooth (S02.5)
K08.530 **Fractured dental restorative material**
without loss of material
K08.531 **Fractured dental restorative material**
with loss of material
K08.539 **Fractured dental restorative material,**
unspecified

K08.54 **Contour of existing restoration of tooth biologically**
incompatible with oral health
Dental restoration failure of periodontal anatomical
integrity
Unacceptable contours of existing restoration of tooth
Unacceptable morphology of existing restoration of
tooth

K08.55 **Allergy to existing dental restorative material**
Use additional code to identify the specific type of
allergy

K08.56 **Poor aesthetic of existing restoration of tooth**
Dental restoration aesthetically inadequate or
displeasing

K08.59 **Other unsatisfactory restoration of tooth**
Other defective dental restoration

√5ᵗʰ **K08.8** **Other specified disorders of teeth and supporting structures**
K08.81 **Primary occlusal trauma**
K08.82 **Secondary occlusal trauma**
K08.89 **Other specified disorders of teeth and supporting**
structures
Enlargement of alveolar ridge NOS
Insufficient anatomic crown height
Insufficient clinical crown length
Irregular alveolar process
Toothache NOS

K08.9 **Disorder of teeth and supporting structures, unspecified**

√4ᵗʰ **K09** **Cysts of oral region, not elsewhere classified**
INCLUDES   lesions showing histological features both of aneurysmal
    cyst and of another fibro-osseous lesion
EXCLUDES 2   *cysts of jaw (M27.0-, M27.4-)*
    radicular cyst (K04.8)

K09.0 **Developmental odontogenic cysts**
Dentigerous cyst
Eruption cyst
Follicular cyst
Gingival cyst
Lateral periodontal cyst
Primordial cyst
EXCLUDES 2   *keratocysts (D16.4, D16.5)*
    odontogenic keratocystic tumors (D16.4, D16.5)

K09.1 **Developmental (nonodontogenic) cysts of oral region**
Cyst (of) incisive canal
Cyst (of) palatine of papilla
Globulomaxillary cyst
Median palatal cyst
Nasoalveolar cyst
Nasolabial cyst
Nasopalatine duct cyst

K09.8 **Other cysts of oral region, not elsewhere classified**
Dermoid cyst
Epidermoid cyst
Lymphoepithelial cyst
Epstein's pearl

K09.9 **Cyst of oral region, unspecified**

√4ᵗʰ **K11** **Diseases of salivary glands**
Use additional code to identify:
alcohol abuse and dependence (F10.-)
exposure to environmental tobacco smoke (Z77.22)
exposure to tobacco smoke in the perinatal period (P96.81)
history of tobacco dependence (Z87.891)
occupational exposure to environmental tobacco smoke (Z57.31)
tobacco dependence (F17.-)
tobacco use (Z72.0)

K11.0 **Atrophy of salivary gland**

☑ Additional Character Required   √×7ᵗʰ Placeholder Alert   Manifestation   Unspecified Dx   ►◄ Revised Text   ● New Code   ▲ Revised Code Title

Chapter 11. Diseases of the Digestive System

K11.1 Hypertrophy of salivary gland
DEF: Overgrowth of or enlarged salivary gland tissue caused by infection, salivary duct blockage, autoimmune diseases, and benign and malignant tumors.

✓5ᵗʰ **K11.2 Sialoadenitis**
Parotitis
EXCLUDES 1   epidemic parotitis (B26.-)
mumps (B26.-)
uveoparotid fever [Heerfordt] (D86.89)
DEF: Inflammation of the salivary gland.

K11.20 Sialoadenitis, unspecified
K11.21 Acute sialoadenitis
EXCLUDES 1   acute recurrent sialoadenitis (K11.22)
K11.22 Acute recurrent sialoadenitis
K11.23 Chronic sialoadenitis

K11.3 Abscess of salivary gland

K11.4 Fistula of salivary gland
EXCLUDES 1   congenital fistula of salivary gland (Q38.4)

K11.5 Sialolithiasis
Calculus of salivary gland or duct
Stone of salivary gland or duct

K11.6 Mucocele of salivary gland
Mucous extravasation cyst of salivary gland
Mucous retention cyst of salivary gland
Ranula

K11.7 Disturbances of salivary secretion
Hypoptyalism
Ptyalism
Xerostomia
EXCLUDES 2   dry mouth NOS (R68.2)

K11.8 Other diseases of salivary glands
Benign lymphoepithelial lesion of salivary gland
Mikulicz' disease
Necrotizing sialometaplasia
Sialectasia
Stenosis of salivary duct
Stricture of salivary duct
EXCLUDES 1   sicca syndrome [Sjögren] (M35.0-)

K11.9 Disease of salivary gland, unspecified
Sialoadenopathy NOS

✓4ᵗʰ **K12 Stomatitis and related lesions**
Use additional code to identify:
alcohol abuse and dependence (F10.-)
exposure to environmental tobacco smoke (Z77.22)
exposure to tobacco smoke in the perinatal period (P96.81)
history of tobacco dependence (Z87.891)
occupational exposure to environmental tobacco smoke (Z57.31)
tobacco dependence (F17.-)
tobacco use (Z72.0)
EXCLUDES 1   cancrum oris (A69.0)
cheilitis (K13.0)
gangrenous stomatitis (A69.0)
herpesviral [herpes simplex] gingivostomatitis (B00.2)
noma (A69.0)

K12.0 Recurrent oral aphthae
Aphthous stomatitis (major) (minor)
Bednar's aphthae
Periadenitis mucosa necrotica recurrens
Recurrent aphthous ulcer
Stomatitis herpetiformis
DEF: Disorder of unknown etiology with small oval or round painful ulcers of the mouth marked by a grayish exudate and a red halo effect.

K12.1 Other forms of stomatitis
Stomatitis NOS
Denture stomatitis
Ulcerative stomatitis
Vesicular stomatitis
EXCLUDES 1   acute necrotizing ulcerative stomatitis (A69.1)
Vincent's stomatitis (A69.1)

K12.2 Cellulitis and abscess of mouth
Cellulitis of mouth (floor)
Submandibular abscess
EXCLUDES 2   abscess of salivary gland (K11.3)
abscess of tongue (K14.0)
periapical abscess (K04.6-K04.7)
periodontal abscess (K05.21)
peritonsillar abscess (J36)

✓5ᵗʰ **K12.3 Oral mucositis (ulcerative)**
Mucositis (oral) (oropharyneal)
EXCLUDES 2   gastrointestinal mucositis (ulcerative) (K92.81)
mucositis (ulcerative) of vagina and vulva (N76.81)
nasal mucositis (ulcerative) (J34.81)

K12.30 Oral mucositis (ulcerative), unspecified
K12.31 Oral mucositis (ulcerative) due to antineoplastic therapy
Use additional code for adverse effect, if applicable, to identify antineoplastic and immunosuppressive drugs (T45.1X5)
Use additional code for other antineoplastic therapy, such as:
radiological procedure and radiotherapy (Y84.2)
K12.32 Oral mucositis (ulcerative) due to other drugs
Use additional code for adverse effect, if applicable, to identify drug (T36-T50 with fifth or sixth character 5)
K12.33 Oral mucositis (ulcerative) due to radiation
Use additional external cause code (W88-W90, X39.0-) to identify cause
K12.39 Other oral mucositis (ulcerative)
Viral oral mucositis (ulcerative)

✓4ᵗʰ **K13 Other diseases of lip and oral mucosa**
INCLUDES   epithelial disturbances of tongue
Use additional code to identify:
alcohol abuse and dependence (F10.-)
exposure to environmental tobacco smoke (Z77.22)
exposure to tobacco smoke in the perinatal period (P96.81)
history of tobacco dependence (Z87.891)
occupational exposure to environmental tobacco smoke (Z57.31)
tobacco dependence (F17.-)
tobacco use (Z72.0)
EXCLUDES 2   certain disorders of gingiva and edentulous alveolar ridge (K05-K06)
cysts of oral region (K09.-)
diseases of tongue (K14.-)
stomatitis and related lesions (K12.-)

K13.0 Diseases of lips
Abscess of lips
Angular cheilitis
Cellulitis of lips
Cheilitis NOS
Cheilodynia
Cheilosis
Exfoliative cheilitis
Fistula of lips
Glandular cheilitis
Hypertrophy of lips
Perlèche NEC
EXCLUDES 1   ariboflavinosis (E53.0)
cheilitis due to radiation-related disorders (L55-L59)
congenital fistula of lips (Q38.0)
congenital hypertrophy of lips (Q18.6)
perlèche due to candidiasis (B37.83)
perlèche due to riboflavin deficiency (E53.0)

K13.1 Cheek and lip biting

☑5ᵗʰ **K13.2 Leukoplakia and other disturbances of oral epithelium, including tongue**
    EXCLUDES 1 *carcinoma in situ of oral epithelium (D00.0-)*
       hairy leukoplakia (K13.3)
    DEF: Leukoplakia: Thickened white patches or lesions appearing on a mucous membrane, such as oral mucosa or tongue.
    K13.21 Leukoplakia of oral mucosa, including tongue
      Leukokeratosis of oral mucosa
      Leukoplakia of gingiva, lips, tongue
      EXCLUDES 1 *hairy leukoplakia (K13.3)*
         leukokeratosis nicotina palati (K13.24)
    K13.22 Minimal keratinized residual ridge mucosa
      Minimal keratinization of alveolar ridge mucosa
    K13.23 Excessive keratinized residual ridge mucosa
      Excessive keratinization of alveolar ridge mucosa
    K13.24 Leukokeratosis nicotina palati
      Smoker's palate
    K13.29 Other disturbances of oral epithelium, including tongue
      Erythroplakia of mouth or tongue
      Focal epithelial hyperplasia of mouth or tongue
      Leukoedema of mouth or tongue
      Other oral epithelium disturbances

K13.3 Hairy leukoplakia

K13.4 Granuloma and granuloma-like lesions of oral mucosa
    Eosinophilic granuloma
    Granuloma pyogenicum
    Verrucous xanthoma

K13.5 Oral submucous fibrosis
    Submucous fibrosis of tongue

K13.6 Irritative hyperplasia of oral mucosa
    EXCLUDES 2 *irritative hyperplasia of edentulous ridge [denture hyperplasia] (K06.2)*

☑5ᵗʰ **K13.7 Other and unspecified lesions of oral mucosa**
    K13.70 Unspecified lesions of oral mucosa
    K13.79 Other lesions of oral mucosa
      Focal oral mucinosis

☑4ᵗʰ **K14 Diseases of tongue**
    Use additional code to identify:
      alcohol abuse and dependence (F10.-)
      exposure to environmental tobacco smoke (Z77.22)
      history of tobacco dependence (Z87.891)
      occupational exposure to environmental tobacco smoke (Z57.31)
      tobacco dependence (F17.-)
      tobacco use (Z72.0)
    EXCLUDES 2 *erythroplakia (K13.29)*
      focal epithelial hyperplasia (K13.29)
      leukedema of tongue (K13.29)
      leukoplakia of tongue (K13.21)
      hairy leukoplakia (K13.3)
      macroglossia (congenital) (Q38.2)
      submucous fibrosis of tongue (K13.5)

K14.0 Glossitis
    Abscess of tongue
    Ulceration (traumatic) of tongue
    EXCLUDES 1 *atrophic glossitis (K14.4)*
    DEF: Inflammation and swelling of the tongue that may be associated with infection, adverse drug reactions, smoking, or injury.

K14.1 Geographic tongue
    Benign migratory glossitis
    Glossitis areata exfoliativa

K14.2 Median rhomboid glossitis

K14.3 Hypertrophy of tongue papillae
    Black hairy tongue
    Coated tongue
    Hypertrophy of foliate papillae
    Lingua villosa nigra

K14.4 Atrophy of tongue papillae
    Atrophic glossitis

K14.5 Plicated tongue
    Fissured tongue
    Furrowed tongue
    Scrotal tongue
    EXCLUDES 1 *fissured tongue, congenital (Q38.3)*

K14.6 Glossodynia
    Glossopyrosis
    Painful tongue

K14.8 Other diseases of tongue
    Atrophy of tongue
    Crenated tongue
    Enlargement of tongue
    Glossocele
    Glossoptosis
    Hypertrophy of tongue

K14.9 Disease of tongue, unspecified
    Glossopathy NOS

Diseases of esophagus, stomach and duodenum (K20-K31)

    EXCLUDES 2 *hiatus hernia (K44.-)*

☑4ᵗʰ **K20 Esophagitis**
    Use additional code to identify:
      alcohol abuse and dependence (F10.-)
    EXCLUDES 1 *erosion of esophagus (K22.1-)*
      esophagitis with gastro-esophageal reflux disease (K21.0)
      reflux esophagitis (K21.0)
      ulcerative esophagitis (K22.1-)
    EXCLUDES 2 *eosinophilic gastritis or gastroenteritis (K52.81)*

K20.0 Eosinophilic esophagitis

K20.8 Other esophagitis
    Abscess of esophagus

K20.9 Esophagitis, unspecified
    Esophagitis NOS

☑4ᵗʰ **K21 Gastro-esophageal reflux disease**
    EXCLUDES 1 *newborn esophageal reflux (P78.83)*

K21.0 Gastro-esophageal reflux disease with esophagitis
    Reflux esophagitis

K21.9 Gastro-esophageal reflux disease without esophagitis
    Esophageal reflux NOS
    AHA: 2016,1Q,18

☑4ᵗʰ **K22 Other diseases of esophagus**
    EXCLUDES 2 *esophageal varices (I85.-)*

K22.0 Achalasia of cardia
    Achalasia NOS
    Cardiospasm
    EXCLUDES 1 *congenital cardiospasm (Q39.5)*
    DEF: Esophageal motility disorder that is caused by absence of the esophageal peristalsis and impaired relaxation of the lower esophageal sphincter. It is characterized by dysphagia, regurgitation, and heartburn.

☑5ᵗʰ **K22.1 Ulcer of esophagus**
    Barrett's ulcer
    Erosion of esophagus
    Fungal ulcer of esophagus
    Peptic ulcer of esophagus
    Ulcer of esophagus due to ingestion of chemicals
    Ulcer of esophagus due to ingestion of drugs and medicaments
    Ulcerative esophagitis
    Code first poisoning due to drug or toxin, if applicable (T36-T65 with fifth or sixth character 1-4 or 6)
    Use additional code for adverse effect, if applicable, to identify drug (T36-T50 with fifth or sixth character 5)
    EXCLUDES 1 *Barrett's esophagus (K22.7-)*
    AHA: 2018,3Q,22; 2017,3Q,27
    TIP: Assign a code for "with bleeding" when an esophageal ulcer and bleeding (hematemesis) are documented. The ICD-10-CM classification assumes the two are related without the provider linking the two conditions. Evidence of bleeding during a procedure is not required.
    TIP: For bleeding ulcers resulting from anticoagulant therapy, code D68.32 Hemorrhagic disorder due to extrinsic circulating anticoagulant, and an adverse-effect code from subcategory T45.5- should also be assigned.
    K22.10 Ulcer of esophagus without bleeding
      Ulcer of esophagus NOS
    K22.11 Ulcer of esophagus with bleeding
      EXCLUDES 2 *bleeding esophageal varices (I85.01, I85.11)*

K22.2   **Esophageal obstruction**
Compression of esophagus
Constriction of esophagus
Stenosis of esophagus
Stricture of esophagus
> **EXCLUDES 1**   *congenital stenosis or stricture of esophagus (Q39.3)*

K22.3   **Perforation of esophagus**
Rupture of esophagus
> **EXCLUDES 1**   *traumatic perforation of (thoracic) esophagus (S27.8-)*

K22.4   **Dyskinesia of esophagus**
Corkscrew esophagus
Diffuse esophageal spasm
Spasm of esophagus
> **EXCLUDES 1**   *cardiospasm (K22.0)*

K22.5   **Diverticulum of esophagus, acquired**
Esophageal pouch, acquired
> **EXCLUDES 1**   *diverticulum of esophagus (congenital) (Q39.6)*

K22.6   **Gastro-esophageal laceration-hemorrhage syndrome**
Mallory-Weiss syndrome

√5ᵗʰ **K22.7**   **Barrett's esophagus**
Barrett's disease
Barrett's syndrome
> **EXCLUDES 1**   *Barrett's ulcer (K22.1)*
>   *malignant neoplasm of esophagus (C15.-)*

DEF: Metaplastic disorder in which specialized columnar epithelial cells replace the normal squamous epithelial cells. Secondary to chronic gastroesophageal reflux damage to the mucosa, this disorder increases the risk of developing adenocarcinoma.

     K22.70   **Barrett's esophagus without dysplasia**   ▣
         Barrett's esophagus NOS

    √6ᵗʰ **K22.71**   **Barrett's esophagus with dysplasia**
         K22.710   **Barrett's esophagus with low grade dysplasia**   ▣
         K22.711   **Barrett's esophagus with high grade dysplasia**   ▣
         K22.719   **Barrett's esophagus with dysplasia, unspecified**   ▣

K22.8   **Other specified diseases of esophagus**
Hemorrhage of esophagus NOS
> **EXCLUDES 2**   *esophageal varices (I85.-)*
>   *Paterson-Kelly syndrome (D50.1)*

K22.9   **Disease of esophagus, unspecified**

K23   ***Disorders of esophagus in diseases classified elsewhere***
Code first underlying disease, such as:
congenital syphilis (A50.5)
> **EXCLUDES 1**   *late syphilis (A52.79)*
>   *megaesophagus due to Chagas' disease (B57.31)*
>   *tuberculosis (A18.83)*

√4ᵗʰ **K25**   **Gastric ulcer**
> **INCLUDES**   erosion (acute) of stomach
>   pylorus ulcer (peptic)
>   stomach ulcer (peptic)

Use additional code to identify:
alcohol abuse and dependence (F10.-)
> **EXCLUDES 1**   *acute gastritis (K29.0-)*
>   *peptic ulcer NOS (K27.-)*

AHA: 2017,3Q,27
TIP: Assign a code for "with hemorrhage" when a gastric ulcer and GI bleeding are documented. The ICD-10-CM classification assumes the two are related without the provider linking the two conditions. Evidence of bleeding during a procedure is not required.
TIP: For bleeding ulcers resulting from anticoagulant therapy, code D68.32 Hemorrhagic disorder due to extrinsic circulating anticoagulant, and an adverse-effect code from subcategory T45.5- should also be assigned.

K25.0   **Acute gastric ulcer with hemorrhage**   ▣
K25.1   **Acute gastric ulcer with perforation**   HCC
K25.2   **Acute gastric ulcer with both hemorrhage and perforation**   HCC ▣
K25.3   **Acute gastric ulcer without hemorrhage or perforation**
K25.4   **Chronic or unspecified gastric ulcer with hemorrhage**   ▣
K25.5   **Chronic or unspecified gastric ulcer with perforation**   HCC
K25.6   **Chronic or unspecified gastric ulcer with both hemorrhage and perforation**   HCC ▣
K25.7   **Chronic gastric ulcer without hemorrhage or perforation**

K25.9   **Gastric ulcer, unspecified as acute or chronic, without hemorrhage or perforation**

Gastrointestinal Ulcers

Esophagus
Esophageal ulcer
Stomach
Duodenal ulcer
Gastric ulcer
Small intestine

√4ᵗʰ **K26**   **Duodenal ulcer**
> **INCLUDES**   erosion (acute) of duodenum
>   duodenum ulcer (peptic)
>   postpyloric ulcer (peptic)

Use additional code to identify:
alcohol abuse and dependence (F10.-)
> **EXCLUDES 1**   *peptic ulcer NOS (K27.-)*

AHA: 2017,3Q,27
TIP: Assign a code for "with hemorrhage" when a duodenal ulcer and GI bleeding are documented. The ICD-10-CM classification assumes the two are related without the provider linking the two conditions. Evidence of bleeding during a procedure is not required.
TIP: For bleeding ulcers resulting from anticoagulant therapy, code D68.32 Hemorrhagic disorder due to extrinsic circulating anticoagulant, and an adverse-effect code from subcategory T45.5- should also be assigned.

K26.0   **Acute duodenal ulcer with hemorrhage**   ▣
K26.1   **Acute duodenal ulcer with perforation**   HCC
K26.2   **Acute duodenal ulcer with both hemorrhage and perforation**   HCC ▣
K26.3   **Acute duodenal ulcer without hemorrhage or perforation**
K26.4   **Chronic or unspecified duodenal ulcer with hemorrhage**   ▣
       AHA: 2016,1Q,14
K26.5   **Chronic or unspecified duodenal ulcer with perforation**   HCC
K26.6   **Chronic or unspecified duodenal ulcer with both hemorrhage and perforation**   HCC ▣
K26.7   **Chronic duodenal ulcer without hemorrhage or perforation**
K26.9   **Duodenal ulcer, unspecified as acute or chronic, without hemorrhage or perforation**

√4ᵗʰ **K27**   **Peptic ulcer, site unspecified**
> **INCLUDES**   gastroduodenal ulcer NOS
>   peptic ulcer NOS

Use additional code to identify:
alcohol abuse and dependence (F10.-)
> **EXCLUDES 1**   *peptic ulcer of newborn (P78.82)*

AHA: 2017,3Q,27
TIP: Assign a code for "with hemorrhage" when a peptic ulcer and GI bleeding are documented. The ICD-10-CM classification assumes the two are related without the provider linking the two conditions. Evidence of bleeding during a procedure is not required.
TIP: For bleeding ulcers resulting from anticoagulant therapy, code D68.32 Hemorrhagic disorder due to extrinsic circulating anticoagulant, and an adverse-effect code from subcategory T45.5- should also be assigned.

K27.0   **Acute peptic ulcer, site unspecified, with hemorrhage**   ▣
K27.1   **Acute peptic ulcer, site unspecified, with perforation**   HCC
K27.2   **Acute peptic ulcer, site unspecified, with both hemorrhage and perforation**   HCC ▣
K27.3   **Acute peptic ulcer, site unspecified, without hemorrhage or perforation**
K27.4   **Chronic or unspecified peptic ulcer, site unspecified, with hemorrhage**   ▣
K27.5   **Chronic or unspecified peptic ulcer, site unspecified, with perforation**   HCC
K27.6   **Chronic or unspecified peptic ulcer, site unspecified, with both hemorrhage and perforation**   HCC ▣

K27.7 Chronic peptic ulcer, site unspecified, without hemorrhage or perforation

K27.9 Peptic ulcer, site unspecified, unspecified as acute or chronic, without hemorrhage or perforation

✓4ᵗʰ **K28** Gastrojejunal ulcer

INCLUDES   anastomotic ulcer (peptic) or erosion
gastrocolic ulcer (peptic) or erosion
gastrointestinal ulcer (peptic) or erosion
gastrojejunal ulcer (peptic) or erosion
jejunal ulcer (peptic) or erosion
marginal ulcer (peptic) or erosion
stomal ulcer (peptic) or erosion

Use additional code to identify:
alcohol abuse and dependence (F10.-)

EXCLUDES 1   *primary ulcer of small intestine (K63.3)*

AHA: 2017,3Q,27

TIP: Assign a code for "with hemorrhage" when a gastrojejunal ulcer and GI bleeding are documented. The ICD-10-CM classification assumes the two are related without the provider linking the two conditions. Evidence of bleeding during a procedure is not required.

TIP: For bleeding ulcers resulting from anticoagulant therapy, code D68.32 Hemorrhagic disorder due to extrinsic circulating anticoagulant, and an adverse-effect code from subcategory T45.5- should also be assigned.

K28.0 Acute gastrojejunal ulcer with hemorrhage   Q

K28.1 Acute gastrojejunal ulcer with perforation   HCC

K28.2 Acute gastrojejunal ulcer with both hemorrhage and perforation   HCC Q

K28.3 Acute gastrojejunal ulcer without hemorrhage or perforation

K28.4 Chronic or unspecified gastrojejunal ulcer with hemorrhage   Q

K28.5 Chronic or unspecified gastrojejunal ulcer with perforation   HCC

K28.6 Chronic or unspecified gastrojejunal ulcer with both hemorrhage and perforation   HCC Q

K28.7 Chronic gastrojejunal ulcer without hemorrhage or perforation

K28.9 Gastrojejunal ulcer, unspecified as acute or chronic, without hemorrhage or perforation

✓4ᵗʰ **K29** Gastritis and duodenitis

EXCLUDES 1   *eosinophilic gastritis or gastroenteritis (K52.81)*
Zollinger-Ellison syndrome (E16.4)

AHA: 2018,3Q,22

TIP: Assign a code for "with bleeding" when gastritis or duodenitis and GI bleeding are documented. The ICD-10-CM classification assumes the two are related without the provider linking the two conditions. Evidence of bleeding during a procedure is not required.

TIP: For bleeding resulting from anticoagulant therapy, code D68.32 Hemorrhagic disorder due to extrinsic circulating anticoagulant, and an adverse-effect code from subcategory T45.5- should also be assigned.

✓5ᵗʰ **K29.0** Acute gastritis

Use additional code to identify:
alcohol abuse and dependence (F10.-)

EXCLUDES 1   *erosion (acute) of stomach (K25.-)*

K29.00 Acute gastritis without bleeding

K29.01 Acute gastritis with bleeding   Q

✓5ᵗʰ **K29.2** Alcoholic gastritis

Use additional code to identify:
alcohol abuse and dependence (F10.-)

K29.20 Alcoholic gastritis without bleeding

K29.21 Alcoholic gastritis with bleeding   Q

✓5ᵗʰ **K29.3** Chronic superficial gastritis

K29.30 Chronic superficial gastritis without bleeding

K29.31 Chronic superficial gastritis with bleeding   Q

✓5ᵗʰ **K29.4** Chronic atrophic gastritis

Gastric atrophy

K29.40 Chronic atrophic gastritis without bleeding

K29.41 Chronic atrophic gastritis with bleeding

✓5ᵗʰ **K29.5** Unspecified chronic gastritis

Chronic antral gastritis
Chronic fundal gastritis

K29.50 Unspecified chronic gastritis without bleeding

K29.51 Unspecified chronic gastritis with bleeding   Q

✓5ᵗʰ **K29.6** Other gastritis

Giant hypertrophic gastritis
Granulomatous gastritis
Ménétrier's disease

K29.60 Other gastritis without bleeding

K29.61 Other gastritis with bleeding   Q

✓5ᵗʰ **K29.7** Gastritis, unspecified

K29.70 Gastritis, unspecified, without bleeding

K29.71 Gastritis, unspecified, with bleeding   Q

✓5ᵗʰ **K29.8** Duodenitis

K29.80 Duodenitis without bleeding

K29.81 Duodenitis with bleeding   Q

✓5ᵗʰ **K29.9** Gastroduodenitis, unspecified

K29.90 Gastroduodenitis, unspecified, without bleeding

K29.91 Gastroduodenitis, unspecified, with bleeding   Q

K30 Functional dyspepsia

Indigestion

EXCLUDES 1   *dyspepsia NOS (R10.13)*
heartburn (R12)
nervous dyspepsia (F45.8)
neurotic dyspepsia (F45.8)
psychogenic dyspepsia (F45.8)

✓4ᵗʰ **K31** Other diseases of stomach and duodenum

INCLUDES   functional disorders of stomach

EXCLUDES 2   *diabetic gastroparesis (E08.43, E09.43, E10.43, E11.43, E13.43)*
diverticulum of duodenum (K57.00-K57.13)

K31.0 Acute dilatation of stomach

Acute distention of stomach

K31.1 Adult hypertrophic pyloric stenosis   A

Pyloric stenosis NOS

EXCLUDES 1   *congenital or infantile pyloric stenosis (Q40.0)*

K31.2 Hourglass stricture and stenosis of stomach

EXCLUDES 1   *congenital hourglass stomach (Q40.2)*
hourglass contraction of stomach (K31.89)

K31.3 Pylorospasm, not elsewhere classified

EXCLUDES 1   *congenital or infantile pylorospasm (Q40.0)*
neurotic pylorospasm (F45.8)
psychogenic pylorospasm (F45.8)

K31.4 Gastric diverticulum

EXCLUDES 1   *congenital diverticulum of stomach (Q40.2)*

K31.5 Obstruction of duodenum

Constriction of duodenum
Duodenal ileus (chronic)
Stenosis of duodenum
Stricture of duodenum
Volvulus of duodenum

EXCLUDES 1   *congenital stenosis of duodenum (Q41.0)*

K31.6 Fistula of stomach and duodenum

Gastrocolic fistula
Gastrojejunocolic fistula

K31.7 Polyp of stomach and duodenum

EXCLUDES 1   *adenomatous polyp of stomach (D13.1)*

✓5ᵗʰ **K31.8** Other specified diseases of stomach and duodenum

✓6ᵗʰ **K31.81** Angiodysplasia of stomach and duodenum

TIP: Assign a code for "with bleeding" when angiodysplasia of the stomach or the duodenum and GI bleeding are documented. The ICD-10-CM classification assumes the two are related without the provider linking the two conditions. Evidence of bleeding during a procedure is not required.

K31.811 Angiodysplasia of stomach and duodenum with bleeding   Q

K31.819 Angiodysplasia of stomach and duodenum without bleeding

Angiodysplasia of stomach and duodenum NOS

K31.82 Dieulafoy lesion (hemorrhagic) of stomach and duodenum

EXCLUDES 2   *Dieulafoy lesion of intestine (K63.81)*

DEF: Abnormally large submucosal artery protruding through a defect in the stomach mucosa or intestines that can cause massive and life-threatening hemorrhaging.

☑ Additional Character Required   ✓ₓ7ᵗʰ Placeholder Alert   Manifestation   Unspecified Dx   ▶◀ Revised Text   ● New Code   ▲ Revised Code Title

ICD-10-CM 2020   705

K31.83   **Achlorhydria**
      DEF: Absence of hydrochloric acid in gastric secretions due to gastric mucosa atrophy. Achlorhydria is unresponsive to histamines.

K31.84   **Gastroparesis**
      Gastroparalysis
      Code first underlying disease, if known, such as:
          anorexia nervosa (F50.0-)
          diabetes mellitus (E08.43, E09.43, E10.43, E11.43, E13.43)
          scleroderma (M34.-)
      AHA: 2013,4Q,114

K31.89   **Other diseases of stomach and duodenum**
      AHA: 2017,1Q,28

K31.9   **Disease of stomach and duodenum, unspecified**

Diseases of appendix (K35-K38)

✓4ᵗʰ **K35**   **Acute appendicitis**
      AHA: 2018,4Q,17-18

✓5ᵗʰ **K35.2**   **Acute appendicitis** with generalized peritonitis
      Appendicitis (acute) with generalized (diffuse) peritonitis following rupture or perforation of appendix

      K35.20   **Acute appendicitis with generalized peritonitis, without abscess**
          (Acute) appendicitis with generalized peritonitis NOS

      K35.21   **Acute appendicitis with generalized peritonitis, with abscess**

✓5ᵗʰ **K35.3**   **Acute appendicitis** with localized peritonitis

      K35.30   **Acute appendicitis with localized peritonitis, without perforation or gangrene**
          Acute appendicitis with localized peritonitis NOS

      K35.31   **Acute appendicitis with localized peritonitis and gangrene, without perforation**

      K35.32   **Acute appendicitis with perforation and localized peritonitis, without abscess**
          (Acute) appendicitis with perforation NOS
          Perforated appendix NOS
          Ruptured appendix (with localized peritonitis) NOS

      K35.33   **Acute appendicitis with perforation and localized peritonitis, with abscess**
          (Acute) appendicitis with (peritoneal) abscess NOS
          Ruptured appendix with localized peritonitis and abscess

✓5ᵗʰ **K35.8**   **Other and unspecified acute appendicitis**

      K35.80   **Unspecified acute appendicitis**
          Acute appendicitis NOS
          Acute appendicitis without (localized) (generalized) peritonitis

      ✓6ᵗʰ **K35.89**   **Other acute appendicitis**

         K35.890   **Other acute appendicitis** without perforation or gangrene

         K35.891   **Other acute appendicitis** without perforation, with gangrene
           (Acute) appendicitis with gangrene NOS

K36   **Other appendicitis**
      Chronic appendicitis
      Recurrent appendicitis

K37   **Unspecified appendicitis**
      EXCLUDES 1   unspecified appendicitis with peritonitis (K35.2-, K35.3-)

✓4ᵗʰ **K38**   **Other diseases of appendix**

      K38.0   **Hyperplasia of appendix**

      K38.1   **Appendicular concretions**
          Fecalith of appendix
          Stercolith of appendix

      K38.2   **Diverticulum of appendix**

      K38.3   **Fistula of appendix**

      K38.8   **Other specified diseases of appendix**
          Intussusception of appendix

      K38.9   **Disease of appendix, unspecified**

Hernia (K40-K46)

NOTE   Hernia with both gangrene and obstruction is classified to hernia with gangrene.

INCLUDES   acquired hernia
          congenital [except diaphragmatic or hiatus] hernia
          recurrent hernia

✓4ᵗʰ **K40**   **Inguinal hernia**

      INCLUDES   bubonocele
          direct inguinal hernia
          double inguinal hernia
          indirect inguinal hernia
          inguinal hernia NOS
          oblique inguinal hernia
          scrotal hernia

      DEF: Within the groin region.

✓5ᵗʰ **K40.0**   **Bilateral inguinal hernia, with obstruction, without gangrene**
      Inguinal hernia (bilateral) causing obstruction without gangrene
      Incarcerated inguinal hernia (bilateral) without gangrene
      Irreducible inguinal hernia (bilateral) without gangrene
      Strangulated inguinal hernia (bilateral) without gangrene

      K40.00   **Bilateral inguinal hernia, with obstruction, without gangrene,** not specified as recurrent
          Bilateral inguinal hernia, with obstruction, without gangrene NOS

      K40.01   **Bilateral inguinal hernia, with obstruction, without gangrene,** recurrent

✓5ᵗʰ **K40.1**   **Bilateral inguinal hernia,** with gangrene

      K40.10   **Bilateral inguinal hernia, with gangrene,** not specified as recurrent
          Bilateral inguinal hernia, with gangrene NOS

      K40.11   **Bilateral inguinal hernia, with gangrene,** recurrent

✓5ᵗʰ **K40.2**   **Bilateral inguinal hernia,** without obstruction or gangrene

      K40.20   **Bilateral inguinal hernia, without obstruction or gangrene,** not specified as recurrent
          Bilateral inguinal hernia NOS

      K40.21   **Bilateral inguinal hernia, without obstruction or gangrene,** recurrent

✓5ᵗʰ **K40.3**   **Unilateral inguinal hernia,** with obstruction, without gangrene
      Inguinal hernia (unilateral) causing obstruction without gangrene
      Incarcerated inguinal hernia (unilateral) without gangrene
      Irreducible inguinal hernia (unilateral) without gangrene
      Strangulated inguinal hernia (unilateral) without gangrene

      K40.30   **Unilateral inguinal hernia, with obstruction, without gangrene,** not specified as recurrent
          Inguinal hernia, with obstruction NOS
          Unilateral inguinal hernia, with obstruction, without gangrene NOS

      K40.31   **Unilateral inguinal hernia, with obstruction, without gangrene,** recurrent

✓5ᵗʰ **K40.4**   **Unilateral inguinal hernia,** with gangrene

      K40.40   **Unilateral inguinal hernia, with gangrene,** not specified as recurrent
          Inguinal hernia with gangrene NOS
          Unilateral inguinal hernia with gangrene NOS

      K40.41   **Unilateral inguinal hernia, with gangrene,** recurrent

✓5ᵗʰ **K40.9**   **Unilateral inguinal hernia,** without obstruction or gangrene

      K40.90   **Unilateral inguinal hernia, without obstruction or gangrene,** not specified as recurrent
          Inguinal hernia NOS
          Unilateral inguinal hernia NOS

    K40.91   **Unilateral inguinal hernia, without obstruction or gangrene, recurrent**

Hernia Sites

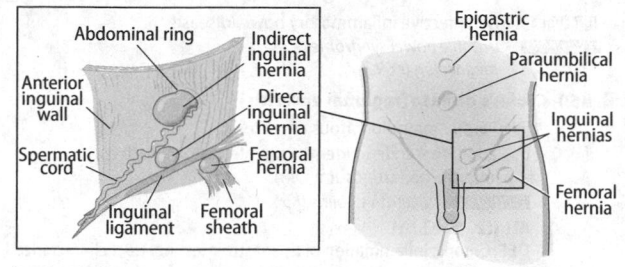

Abdominal ring · Indirect inguinal hernia · Anterior inguinal wall · Direct inguinal hernia · Spermatic cord · Femoral hernia · Inguinal ligament · Femoral sheath · Epigastric hernia · Paraumbilical hernia · Inguinal hernias · Femoral hernia

☑4ᵗʰ **K41**   **Femoral hernia**

☑5ᵗʰ **K41.0**   **Bilateral femoral hernia, with obstruction, without gangrene**

Femoral hernia (bilateral) causing obstruction, without gangrene
Incarcerated femoral hernia (bilateral), without gangrene
Irreducible femoral hernia (bilateral), without gangrene
Strangulated femoral hernia (bilateral), without gangrene

  K41.00   **Bilateral femoral hernia, with obstruction, without gangrene, not specified as recurrent**
    Bilateral femoral hernia, with obstruction, without gangrene NOS

  K41.01   **Bilateral femoral hernia, with obstruction, without gangrene, recurrent**

☑5ᵗʰ **K41.1**   **Bilateral femoral hernia, with gangrene**

  K41.10   **Bilateral femoral hernia, with gangrene, not specified as recurrent**
    Bilateral femoral hernia, with gangrene NOS

  K41.11   **Bilateral femoral hernia, with gangrene, recurrent**

☑5ᵗʰ **K41.2**   **Bilateral femoral hernia, without obstruction or gangrene**

  K41.20   **Bilateral femoral hernia, without obstruction or gangrene, not specified as recurrent**
    Bilateral femoral hernia NOS

  K41.21   **Bilateral femoral hernia, without obstruction or gangrene, recurrent**

☑5ᵗʰ **K41.3**   **Unilateral femoral hernia, with obstruction, without gangrene**

Femoral hernia (unilateral) causing obstruction, without gangrene
Incarcerated femoral hernia (unilateral), without gangrene
Irreducible femoral hernia (unilateral), without gangrene
Strangulated femoral hernia (unilateral), without gangrene

  K41.30   **Unilateral femoral hernia, with obstruction, without gangrene, not specified as recurrent**
    Femoral hernia, with obstruction NOS
    Unilateral femoral hernia, with obstruction NOS

  K41.31   **Unilateral femoral hernia, with obstruction, without gangrene, recurrent**

☑5ᵗʰ **K41.4**   **Unilateral femoral hernia, with gangrene**

  K41.40   **Unilateral femoral hernia, with gangrene, not specified as recurrent**
    Femoral hernia, with gangrene NOS
    Unilateral femoral hernia, with gangrene NOS

  K41.41   **Unilateral femoral hernia, with gangrene, recurrent**

☑5ᵗʰ **K41.9**   **Unilateral femoral hernia, without obstruction or gangrene**

  K41.90   **Unilateral femoral hernia, without obstruction or gangrene, not specified as recurrent**
    Femoral hernia NOS
    Unilateral femoral hernia NOS

  K41.91   **Unilateral femoral hernia, without obstruction or gangrene, recurrent**

☑4ᵗʰ **K42**   **Umbilical hernia**

   INCLUDES   paraumbilical hernia
   EXCLUDES 1   *omphalocele (Q79.2)*

  K42.0   **Umbilical hernia with obstruction, without gangrene**
    Umbilical hernia causing obstruction, without gangrene
    Incarcerated umbilical hernia, without gangrene
    Irreducible umbilical hernia, without gangrene
    Strangulated umbilical hernia, without gangrene

  K42.1   **Umbilical hernia with gangrene**
    Gangrenous umbilical hernia

  K42.9   **Umbilical hernia without obstruction or gangrene**
    Umbilical hernia NOS

☑4ᵗʰ **K43**   **Ventral hernia**

   DEF: Condition in which a loop of bowel protrudes through a weakness in the abdominal wall muscles that may occur as a birth defect, past surgical site (incisional), or form at a stomal site (parastomal).

  K43.0   **Incisional hernia with obstruction, without gangrene**
    Incisional hernia causing obstruction, without gangrene
    Incarcerated incisional hernia, without gangrene
    Irreducible incisional hernia, without gangrene
    Strangulated incisional hernia, without gangrene

  K43.1   **Incisional hernia with gangrene**
    Gangrenous incisional hernia

  K43.2   **Incisional hernia without obstruction or gangrene**
    Incisional hernia NOS

  K43.3   **Parastomal hernia with obstruction, without gangrene**
    Incarcerated parastomal hernia, without gangrene
    Irreducible parastomal hernia, without gangrene
    Parastomal hernia causing obstruction, without gangrene
    Strangulated parastomal hernia, without gangrene

  K43.4   **Parastomal hernia with gangrene**
    Gangrenous parastomal hernia

  K43.5   **Parastomal hernia without obstruction or gangrene**
    Parastomal hernia NOS

  K43.6   **Other and unspecified ventral hernia with obstruction, without gangrene**
    Epigastric hernia causing obstruction, without gangrene
    Hypogastric hernia causing obstruction, without gangrene
    Incarcerated epigastric hernia without gangrene
    Incarcerated hypogastric hernia without gangrene
    Incarcerated midline hernia without gangrene
    Incarcerated spigelian hernia without gangrene
    Incarcerated subxiphoid hernia without gangrene
    Irreducible epigastric hernia without gangrene
    Irreducible hypogastric hernia without gangrene
    Irreducible midline hernia without gangrene
    Irreducible spigelian hernia without gangrene
    Irreducible subxiphoid hernia without gangrene
    Midline hernia causing obstruction, without gangrene
    Spigelian hernia causing obstruction, without gangrene
    Strangulated epigastric hernia without gangrene
    Strangulated hypogastric hernia without gangrene
    Strangulated midline hernia without gangrene
    Strangulated spigelian hernia without gangrene
    Strangulated subxiphoid hernia without gangrene
    Subxiphoid hernia causing obstruction, without gangrene

  K43.7   **Other and unspecified ventral hernia with gangrene**
    Any condition listed under K43.6 specified as gangrenous

  K43.9   **Ventral hernia without obstruction or gangrene**
    Epigastric hernia
    Ventral hernia NOS

☑ Additional Character Required   ✓x7ᵗʰ Placeholder Alert   Manifestation   Unspecified Dx   ►◄ Revised Text   ● New Code   ▲ Revised Code Title

ICD-10-CM 2020   707

✓4ᵗʰ K44 Diaphragmatic hernia

INCLUDES hiatus hernia (esophageal) (sliding)
paraesophageal hernia
EXCLUDES 1 *congenital diaphragmatic hernia (Q79.0)*
congenital hiatus hernia (Q40.1)

DEF: Protrusion of an abdominal organ, usually the stomach, through the esophageal opening within the diaphragm and occurring in two types: the sliding hiatal hernia and the paraesophageal hernia.

Hiatal Hernia

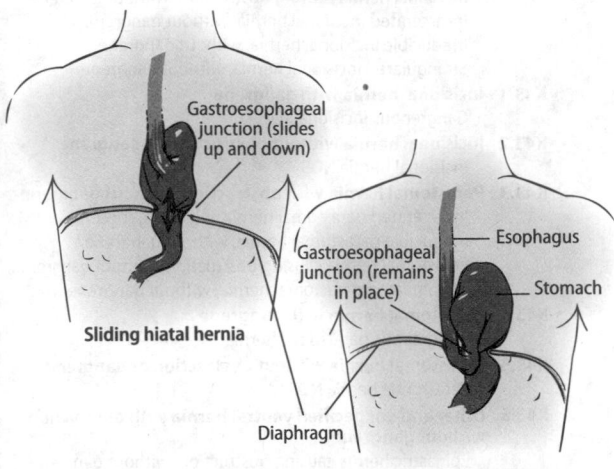

Gastroesophageal junction (slides up and down)

Sliding hiatal hernia

Gastroesophageal junction (remains in place)

Esophagus

Stomach

Diaphragm

Paraesophageal hiatal hernia

K44.0 Diaphragmatic hernia with obstruction, without gangrene
Diaphragmatic hernia causing obstruction
Incarcerated diaphragmatic hernia
Irreducible diaphragmatic hernia
Strangulated diaphragmatic hernia

K44.1 Diaphragmatic hernia with gangrene
Gangrenous diaphragmatic hernia

K44.9 Diaphragmatic hernia without obstruction or gangrene
Diaphragmatic hernia NOS

✓4ᵗʰ K45 Other abdominal hernia

INCLUDES abdominal hernia, specified site NEC
lumbar hernia
obturator hernia
pudendal hernia
retroperitoneal hernia
sciatic hernia

K45.0 Other specified abdominal hernia with obstruction, without gangrene
Other specified abdominal hernia causing obstruction
Other specified incarcerated abdominal hernia
Other specified irreducible abdominal hernia
Other specified strangulated abdominal hernia

K45.1 Other specified abdominal hernia with gangrene
Any condition listed under K45 specified as gangrenous

K45.8 Other specified abdominal hernia without obstruction or gangrene

✓4ᵗʰ K46 Unspecified abdominal hernia

INCLUDES enterocele
epiplocele
hernia NOS
interstitial hernia
intestinal hernia
intra-abdominal hernia
EXCLUDES 1 *vaginal enterocele (N81.5)*

K46.0 Unspecified abdominal hernia with obstruction, without gangrene
Unspecified abdominal hernia causing obstruction
Unspecified incarcerated abdominal hernia
Unspecified irreducible abdominal hernia
Unspecified strangulated abdominal hernia

K46.1 Unspecified abdominal hernia with gangrene
Any condition listed under K46 specified as gangrenous

K46.9 Unspecified abdominal hernia without obstruction or gangrene
Abdominal hernia NOS

Noninfective enteritis and colitis (K50-K52)

INCLUDES noninfective inflammatory bowel disease
EXCLUDES 1 *irritable bowel syndrome (K58.-)*
megacolon (K59.3-)

✓4ᵗʰ K50 Crohn's disease [regional enteritis]

INCLUDES granulomatous enteritis
Use additional code to identify manifestations, such as:
pyoderma gangrenosum (L88)
EXCLUDES 1 *ulcerative colitis (K51.-)*
AHA: 2012,4Q,104
DEF: Chronic inflammation of the gastrointestinal tract characterized by chronic granulomatous disease, most commonly affecting the intestines and the terminal ileum.

✓5ᵗʰ K50.0 Crohn's disease of small intestine

Crohn's disease [regional enteritis] of duodenum
Crohn's disease [regional enteritis] of ileum
Crohn's disease [regional enteritis] of jejunum
Regional ileitis
Terminal ileitis
EXCLUDES 1 *Crohn's disease of both small and large intestine (K50.8-)*

K50.00 Crohn's disease of small intestine without complications HCC

✓6ᵗʰ K50.01 Crohn's disease of small intestine with complications

K50.011 Crohn's disease of small intestine with rectal bleeding HCC

K50.012 Crohn's disease of small intestine with intestinal obstruction HCC

K50.013 Crohn's disease of small intestine with fistula HCC

K50.014 Crohn's disease of small intestine with abscess HCC
AHA: 2012,4Q,104

K50.018 Crohn's disease of small intestine with other complication HCC

K50.019 Crohn's disease of small intestine with unspecified complications HCC

✓5ᵗʰ K50.1 Crohn's disease of large intestine

Crohn's disease [regional enteritis] of colon
Crohn's disease [regional enteritis] of large bowel
Crohn's disease [regional enteritis] of rectum
Granulomatous colitis
Regional colitis
EXCLUDES 1 *Crohn's disease of both small and large intestine (K50.8)*

K50.10 Crohn's disease of large intestine without complications HCC

✓6ᵗʰ K50.11 Crohn's disease of large intestine with complications

K50.111 Crohn's disease of large intestine with rectal bleeding HCC

K50.112 Crohn's disease of large intestine with intestinal obstruction HCC

K50.113 Crohn's disease of large intestine with fistula HCC

K50.114 Crohn's disease of large intestine with abscess HCC

K50.118 Crohn's disease of large intestine with other complication HCC

K50.119 Crohn's disease of large intestine with unspecified complications HCC

✓5ᵗʰ K50.8 Crohn's disease of both small and large intestine

K50.80 Crohn's disease of both small and large intestine without complications HCC

✓6ᵗʰ K50.81 Crohn's disease of both small and large intestine with complications

K50.811 Crohn's disease of both small and large intestine with rectal bleeding HCC

K50.812 Crohn's disease of both small and large intestine with intestinal obstruction HCC

K50.813 Crohn's disease of both small and large intestine with fistula HCC

K50.814 **Crohn's disease of both small and large intestine with** abscess `HCC`

K50.818 **Crohn's disease of both small and large intestine with other complication** `HCC`

K50.819 **Crohn's disease of both small and large intestine with unspecified complications** `HCC`

✓5ᵗʰ **K50.9 Crohn's disease, unspecified**

K50.90 **Crohn's disease, unspecified,** without complications `HCC`
Crohn's disease NOS
Regional enteritis NOS

✓6ᵗʰ K50.91 **Crohn's disease, unspecified,** with complications

K50.911 **Crohn's disease, unspecified, with** rectal bleeding `HCC`

K50.912 **Crohn's disease, unspecified, with** intestinal obstruction `HCC`

K50.913 **Crohn's disease, unspecified, with** fistula `HCC`

K50.914 **Crohn's disease, unspecified, with** abscess `HCC`

K50.918 **Crohn's disease, unspecified, with other complication** `HCC`

K50.919 **Crohn's disease, unspecified, with unspecified complications** `HCC`

✓4ᵗʰ **K51 Ulcerative colitis**

Use additional code to identify manifestations, such as:
pyoderma gangrenosum (L88)

EXCLUDES 1   *Crohn's disease [regional enteritis] (K50.-)*

✓5ᵗʰ **K51.0 Ulcerative (chronic)** pancolitis
Backwash ileitis

K51.00 **Ulcerative (chronic) pancolitis** without complications `HCC`
Ulcerative (chronic) pancolitis NOS

✓6ᵗʰ K51.01 **Ulcerative (chronic) pancolitis** with complications

K51.011 **Ulcerative (chronic) pancolitis with** rectal bleeding `HCC`

K51.012 **Ulcerative (chronic) pancolitis with** intestinal obstruction `HCC`

K51.013 **Ulcerative (chronic) pancolitis with** fistula `HCC`

K51.014 **Ulcerative (chronic) pancolitis with** abscess `HCC`

K51.018 **Ulcerative (chronic) pancolitis with other complication** `HCC`

K51.019 **Ulcerative (chronic) pancolitis with unspecified complications** `HCC`

✓5ᵗʰ **K51.2 Ulcerative (chronic)** proctitis

K51.20 **Ulcerative (chronic) proctitis** without complications `HCC`
Ulcerative (chronic) proctitis NOS

✓6ᵗʰ K51.21 **Ulcerative (chronic) proctitis** with complications

K51.211 **Ulcerative (chronic) proctitis with** rectal bleeding `HCC`

K51.212 **Ulcerative (chronic) proctitis with** intestinal obstruction `HCC`

K51.213 **Ulcerative (chronic) proctitis with** fistula `HCC`

K51.214 **Ulcerative (chronic) proctitis with** abscess `HCC`

K51.218 **Ulcerative (chronic) proctitis with other complication** `HCC`

K51.219 **Ulcerative (chronic) proctitis with unspecified complications** `HCC`

✓5ᵗʰ **K51.3 Ulcerative (chronic)** rectosigmoiditis

K51.30 **Ulcerative (chronic) rectosigmoiditis** without complications `HCC`
Ulcerative (chronic) rectosigmoiditis NOS

✓6ᵗʰ K51.31 **Ulcerative (chronic) rectosigmoiditis with** complications

K51.311 **Ulcerative (chronic) rectosigmoiditis with** rectal bleeding `HCC`

K51.312 **Ulcerative (chronic) rectosigmoiditis with** intestinal obstruction `HCC`

K51.313 **Ulcerative (chronic) rectosigmoiditis with** fistula `HCC`

K51.314 **Ulcerative (chronic) rectosigmoiditis with** abscess `HCC`

K51.318 **Ulcerative (chronic) rectosigmoiditis with other complication** `HCC`

K51.319 **Ulcerative (chronic) rectosigmoiditis with unspecified complications** `HCC`

✓5ᵗʰ **K51.4 Inflammatory polyps of colon**

EXCLUDES 1   *adenomatous polyp of colon (D12.6)*
polyposis of colon (D12.6)
polyps of colon NOS (K63.5)

K51.40 **Inflammatory polyps of colon** without complications `HCC`
Inflammatory polyps of colon NOS

✓6ᵗʰ K51.41 **Inflammatory polyps of colon** with complications

K51.411 **Inflammatory polyps of colon with** rectal bleeding `HCC`

K51.412 **Inflammatory polyps of colon with** intestinal obstruction `HCC`

K51.413 **Inflammatory polyps of colon with** fistula `HCC`

K51.414 **Inflammatory polyps of colon with** abscess `HCC`

K51.418 **Inflammatory polyps of colon with other complication** `HCC`

K51.419 **Inflammatory polyps of colon with unspecified complications** `HCC`

✓5ᵗʰ **K51.5 Left sided colitis**
Left hemicolitis

K51.50 **Left sided colitis** without complications `HCC`
Left sided colitis NOS

✓6ᵗʰ K51.51 **Left sided colitis** with complications

K51.511 **Left sided colitis with** rectal bleeding `HCC`

K51.512 **Left sided colitis with** intestinal obstruction `HCC`

K51.513 **Left sided colitis with** fistula `HCC`

K51.514 **Left sided colitis with** abscess `HCC`

K51.518 **Left sided colitis with other complication** `HCC`

K51.519 **Left sided colitis with unspecified complications** `HCC`

✓5ᵗʰ **K51.8 Other ulcerative colitis**

K51.80 **Other ulcerative colitis** without complications `HCC`

✓6ᵗʰ K51.81 **Other ulcerative colitis** with complications

K51.811 **Other ulcerative colitis with** rectal bleeding `HCC`

K51.812 **Other ulcerative colitis with** intestinal obstruction `HCC`

K51.813 **Other ulcerative colitis with** fistula `HCC`

K51.814 **Other ulcerative colitis with** abscess `HCC`

K51.818 **Other ulcerative colitis with other complication** `HCC`

K51.819 **Other ulcerative colitis with unspecified complications** `HCC`

✓5ᵗʰ **K51.9 Ulcerative colitis, unspecified**

K51.90 **Ulcerative colitis, unspecified,** without complications `HCC`

✓6ᵗʰ K51.91 **Ulcerative colitis, unspecified,** with complications

K51.911 **Ulcerative colitis, unspecified with** rectal bleeding `HCC`

K51.912 **Ulcerative colitis, unspecified with** intestinal obstruction `HCC`

K51.913 **Ulcerative colitis, unspecified with** fistula `HCC`

K51.914 **Ulcerative colitis, unspecified with** abscess `HCC`

K51.918 **Ulcerative colitis, unspecified with other complication** `HCC`

K51.919 **Ulcerative colitis, unspecified with unspecified complications** `HCC`

✓4ᵗʰ **K52 Other and unspecified noninfective gastroenteritis and colitis**
AHA: 2016,4Q,30-31

K52.0 **Gastroenteritis and colitis due to** radiation

☑ Additional Character Required   ✓x7ᵗʰ Placeholder Alert   Manifestation   Unspecified Dx   ▶◀ Revised Text   ● New Code   ▲ Revised Code Title

ICD-10-CM 2020   **709**

Chapter 11. Diseases of the Digestive System

K52.1–K55.1

K52.1 **Toxic** gastroenteritis and colitis
Drug-induced gastroenteritis and colitis
Code first (T51-T65) to identify toxic agent
Use additional code for adverse effect, if applicable, to identify drug (T36-T50 with fifth or sixth character 5)
AHA: 2019,1Q,17

☑5th **K52.2** **Allergic and dietetic** gastroenteritis and colitis
Food hypersensitivity gastroenteritis or colitis
Use additional code to identify type of food allergy (Z91.01-, Z91.02-)
EXCLUDES 2   *allergic eosinophilic colitis (K52.82)*
allergic eosinophilic esophagitis (K20.0)
allergic eosinophilic gastritis (K52.81)
allergic eosinophilic gastroenteritis (K52.81)
food protein-induced proctocolitis (K52.82)
DEF: True immunoglobulin E (IgE)-mediated allergic reaction of the lining of the stomach, intestines, or colon to food proteins. It causes nausea, vomiting, diarrhea, and abdominal cramping.

K52.21 **Food protein-induced** enterocolitis syndrome
FPIES
Use additional code for hypovolemic shock, if present (R57.1)

K52.22 **Food protein-induced** enteropathy

K52.29 **Other allergic and dietetic gastroenteritis and colitis**
Food hypersensitivity gastroenteritis or colitis
Immediate gastrointestinal hypersensitivity

K52.3 **Indeterminate** colitis
Colonic inflammatory bowel disease unclassified (IBDU)
EXCLUDES 1   *unspecified colitis (K52.9)*

☑5th **K52.8** **Other specified noninfective gastroenteritis and colitis**

K52.81 **Eosinophilic gastritis or gastroenteritis**
Eosinophilic enteritis
EXCLUDES 2   *eosinophilic esophagitis (K20.0)*
DEF: Disorder involving the accumulation of eosinophil in the lining of the stomach or multiple levels of the gastrointestinal tract, but without a known cause such as connective tissue disease, drug reaction, malignancy, or parasitic infection.

K52.82 **Eosinophilic colitis**
Allergic proctocolitis
Food-induced eosinophilic proctocolitis
Food protein-induced proctocolitis
Milk protein-induced proctocolitis
DEF: Disorder involving the accumulation of eosinophil in the tissues lining the colon, but without a known cause such as connective tissue disease, drug reaction, malignancy, or parasitic infection. The resultant inflammation may cause extreme abdominal pain, diarrhea, or bloody stool.

☑6th **K52.83** **Microscopic colitis**

K52.831 **Collagenous** colitis
K52.832 **Lymphocytic** colitis
K52.838 **Other microscopic colitis**
K52.839 **Microscopic colitis, unspecified**

K52.89 **Other specified noninfective gastroenteritis and colitis**
AHA: 2019,1Q,20

K52.9 **Noninfective gastroenteritis and colitis, unspecified**
Colitis NOS
Enteritis NOS
Gastroenteritis NOS
Ileitis NOS
Jejunitis NOS
Sigmoiditis NOS
EXCLUDES 1   *diarrhea NOS (R19.7)*
functional diarrhea (K59.1)
infectious gastroenteritis and colitis NOS (A09)
neonatal diarrhea (noninfective) (P78.3)
psychogenic diarrhea (F45.8)

Other diseases of intestines (K55-K64)

☑4th **K55** **Vascular disorders of intestine**
EXCLUDES 1   *necrotizing enterocolitis of newborn (P77.-)*
AHA: 2016,4Q,32

☑5th **K55.0** **Acute vascular disorders of intestine**
Infarction of appendices epiploicae
Mesenteric (artery) (vein) embolism
Mesenteric (artery) (vein) infarction
Mesenteric (artery) (vein) thrombosis

☑6th **K55.01** **Acute (reversible) ischemia of small intestine**

K55.011 **Focal (segmental) acute (reversible) ischemia of small intestine** ᴴᶜᶜ
K55.012 **Diffuse acute (reversible) ischemia of small intestine** ᴴᶜᶜ
K55.019 **Acute (reversible) ischemia of small intestine, extent unspecified** ᴴᶜᶜ

☑6th **K55.02** **Acute infarction of small intestine**
Gangrene of small intestine
Necrosis of small intestine

K55.021 **Focal (segmental) acute infarction of small intestine** ᴴᶜᶜ
K55.022 **Diffuse acute infarction of small intestine** ᴴᶜᶜ
K55.029 **Acute infarction of small intestine, extent unspecified** ᴴᶜᶜ

☑6th **K55.03** **Acute (reversible) ischemia of large intestine**
Acute fulminant ischemic colitis
Subacute ischemic colitis

K55.031 **Focal (segmental) acute (reversible) ischemia of large intestine** ᴴᶜᶜ
K55.032 **Diffuse acute (reversible) ischemia of large intestine** ᴴᶜᶜ
K55.039 **Acute (reversible) ischemia of large intestine, extent unspecified** ᴴᶜᶜ

☑6th **K55.04** **Acute infarction of large intestine**
Gangrene of large intestine
Necrosis of large intestine

K55.041 **Focal (segmental) acute infarction of large intestine** ᴴᶜᶜ
K55.042 **Diffuse acute infarction of large intestine** ᴴᶜᶜ
K55.049 **Acute infarction of large intestine, extent unspecified** ᴴᶜᶜ

☑6th **K55.05** **Acute (reversible) ischemia of intestine, part unspecified**

K55.051 **Focal (segmental) acute (reversible) ischemia of intestine, part unspecified** ᴴᶜᶜ
K55.052 **Diffuse acute (reversible) ischemia of intestine, part unspecified** ᴴᶜᶜ
K55.059 **Acute (reversible) ischemia of intestine, part and extent unspecified** ᴴᶜᶜ

☑6th **K55.06** **Acute infarction of intestine, part unspecified**
Acute intestinal infarction
Gangrene of intestine
Necrosis of intestine

K55.061 **Focal (segmental) acute infarction of intestine, part unspecified** ᴴᶜᶜ
K55.062 **Diffuse acute infarction of intestine, part unspecified** ᴴᶜᶜ
K55.069 **Acute infarction of intestine, part and extent unspecified** ᴴᶜᶜ

K55.1 **Chronic vascular disorders of intestine** ᴴᶜᶜ
Chronic ischemic colitis
Chronic ischemic enteritis
Chronic ischemic enterocolitis
Ischemic stricture of intestine
Mesenteric atherosclerosis
Mesenteric vascular insufficiency

√5ᵗʰ K55.2   Angiodysplasia of colon

     AHA: 2018,3Q,21

     TIP: Assign a code for "with hemorrhage" when angiodysplasia and GI bleeding are documented. The ICD-10-CM classification assumes the two are related without the provider linking the two conditions. Evidence of bleeding during a procedure is not required.

     K55.20   Angiodysplasia of colon without hemorrhage

     K55.21   Angiodysplasia of colon with hemorrhage

        DEF: Small vascular abnormalities due to fragile blood vessels in the colon, resulting in blood loss from the gastrointestinal (GI) tract.

√5ᵗʰ K55.3   Necrotizing enterocolitis

     EXCLUDES 1   *necrotizing enterocolitis of newborn (P77.-)*

     EXCLUDES 2   *necrotizing enterocolitis due to Clostridium difficile (A04.7-)*

     K55.30   Necrotizing enterocolitis, unspecified   HCC

        Necrotizing enterocolitis, NOS

     K55.31   Stage 1 necrotizing enterocolitis   HCC

        Necrotizing enterocolitis without pneumatosis, without perforation

     K55.32   Stage 2 necrotizing enterocolitis   HCC

        Necrotizing enterocolitis with pneumatosis, without perforation

     K55.33   Stage 3 necrotizing enterocolitis   HCC

        Necrotizing enterocolitis with perforation

        Necrotizing enterocolitis with pneumatosis and perforation

K55.8   Other vascular disorders of intestine   HCC

K55.9   Vascular disorder of intestine, unspecified   HCC

     Ischemic colitis

     Ischemic enteritis

     Ischemic enterocolitis

√4ᵗʰ K56   Paralytic ileus and intestinal obstruction without hernia

     EXCLUDES 1   *congenital stricture or stenosis of intestine (Q41-Q42)*

              cystic fibrosis with meconium ileus (E84.11)

              ischemic stricture of intestine (K55.1)

              meconium ileus NOS (P76.0)

              neonatal intestinal obstructions classifiable to P76.-

              obstruction of duodenum (K31.5)

              postprocedural intestinal obstruction (K91.3-)

              stenosis of anus or rectum (K62.4)

K56.0   Paralytic ileus   HCC

     Paralysis of bowel

     Paralysis of colon

     Paralysis of intestine

     EXCLUDES 1   *gallstone ileus (K56.3)*

              ileus NOS (K56.7)

              obstructive ileus NOS (K56.69-)

     DEF: Intestinal obstruction due to paralysis of bowel motility or peristalsis.

K56.1   Intussusception   HCC

     Intussusception or invagination of bowel

     Intussusception or invagination of colon

     Intussusception or invagination of intestine

     Intussusception or invagination of rectum

     EXCLUDES 2   *intussusception of appendix (K38.8)*

     DEF: Intestinal obstruction due to prolapse of a bowel section into an adjacent section. It occurs primarily in children and symptoms include acute abdominal pain, vomiting, and passage of blood and mucus from the rectum.

K56.2   Volvulus   HCC

     Strangulation of colon or intestine

     Torsion of colon or intestine

     Twist of colon or intestine

     EXCLUDES 2   *volvulus of duodenum (K31.5)*

     DEF: Twisting, knotting, or entanglement of the bowel on itself that may quickly compromise oxygen supply to the intestinal tissues. A volvulus usually occurs at the sigmoid and ileocecal areas of the intestines.

Volvulus

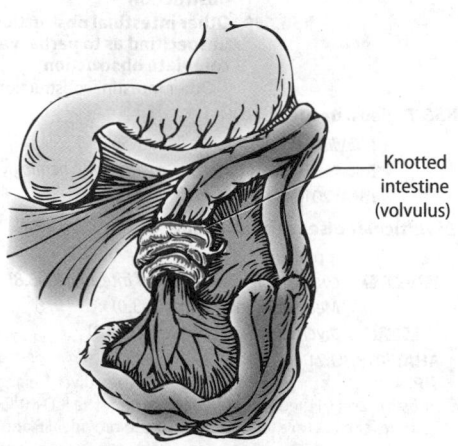

Knotted intestine (volvulus)

K56.3   Gallstone ileus   HCC

     Obstruction of intestine by gallstone

√5ᵗʰ K56.4   Other impaction of intestine

     K56.41   Fecal impaction   HCC

        EXCLUDES 1   *constipation (K59.0-)*

                incomplete defecation (R15.0)

     K56.49   Other impaction of intestine   HCC

√5ᵗʰ K56.5   Intestinal adhesions [bands] with obstruction (postinfection)

     Abdominal hernia due to adhesions with obstruction

     Peritoneal adhesions [bands] with intestinal obstruction (postinfection)

     AHA: 2017,4Q,16-17

     K56.50   Intestinal adhesions [bands], unspecified as to partial versus complete obstruction   HCC

        Intestinal adhesions with obstruction NOS

     K56.51   Intestinal adhesions [bands], with partial obstruction   HCC

        Intestinal adhesions with incomplete obstruction

     K56.52   Intestinal adhesions [bands] with complete obstruction   HCC

√5ᵗʰ K56.6   Other and unspecified intestinal obstruction

     AHA: 2017,4Q,16-17; 2017,2Q,12

     √6ᵗʰ K56.60   Unspecified intestinal obstruction

        EXCLUDES 1   *intestinal obstruction due to specified condition - code to condition*

        K56.600   Partial intestinal obstruction, unspecified as to cause   HCC

           Incomplete intestinal obstruction, NOS

        K56.601   Complete intestinal obstruction, unspecified as to cause   HCC

        K56.609   Unspecified intestinal obstruction, unspecified as to partial versus complete obstruction   HCC

           Intestinal obstruction NOS

☑ Additional Character Required   √x7ᵗʰ Placeholder Alert   Manifestation   Unspecified Dx   ▶◀ Revised Text   ● New Code   ▲ Revised Code Title

ICD-10-CM 2020   711

√6ᵗʰ **K56.69 Other intestinal obstruction**
Enterostenosis NOS
Obstructive ileus NOS
Occlusion of colon or intestine NOS
Stenosis of colon or intestine NOS
Stricture of colon or intestine NOS

> EXCLUDES 1   intestinal obstruction due to specified condition - code to condition

K56.690 Other partial intestinal obstruction   HCC
Other incomplete intestinal obstruction

K56.691 Other complete intestinal obstruction   HCC

K56.699 Other intestinal obstruction unspecified as to partial versus complete obstruction   HCC
Other intestinal obstruction, NEC

K56.7 Ileus, unspecified   HCC

> EXCLUDES 1   obstructive ileus (K56.69-)
> EXCLUDES 2   intestinal obstruction with hernia (K40-K46)

AHA: 2017,1Q,40

√4ᵗʰ **K57 Diverticular disease of intestine**
Code also if applicable peritonitis K65.-

> EXCLUDES 1   congenital diverticulum of intestine (Q43.8)
>   Meckel's diverticulum (Q43.0)
> EXCLUDES 2   diverticulum of appendix (K38.2)

AHA: 2018,3Q,21

TIP: Assign a code for "with bleeding" when diverticular disease of the intestine and GI bleeding are documented. The ICD-10-CM classification assumes the two are related without the provider linking the two conditions. Evidence of bleeding during a procedure is not required.

√5ᵗʰ **K57.0 Diverticulitis of small intestine with perforation and abscess**
Diverticulitis of small intestine with peritonitis

> EXCLUDES 1   diverticulitis of both small and large intestine with perforation and abscess (K57.4-)

K57.00 Diverticulitis of small intestine with perforation and abscess without bleeding

K57.01 Diverticulitis of small intestine with perforation and abscess with bleeding   Q

√5ᵗʰ **K57.1 Diverticular disease of small intestine without perforation or abscess**

> EXCLUDES 1   diverticular disease of both small and large intestine without perforation or abscess (K57.5-)

K57.10 Diverticulosis of small intestine without perforation or abscess without bleeding
Diverticular disease of small intestine NOS

K57.11 Diverticulosis of small intestine without perforation or abscess with bleeding   Q

K57.12 Diverticulitis of small intestine without perforation or abscess without bleeding

K57.13 Diverticulitis of small intestine without perforation or abscess with bleeding   Q

√5ᵗʰ **K57.2 Diverticulitis of large intestine with perforation and abscess**
Diverticulitis of colon with peritonitis

> EXCLUDES 1   diverticulitis of both small and large intestine with perforation and abscess (K57.4-)

K57.20 Diverticulitis of large intestine with perforation and abscess without bleeding

K57.21 Diverticulitis of large intestine with perforation and abscess with bleeding   Q

√5ᵗʰ **K57.3 Diverticular disease of large intestine without perforation or abscess**

> EXCLUDES 1   diverticular disease of both small and large intestine without perforation or abscess (K57.5-)

K57.30 Diverticulosis of large intestine without perforation or abscess without bleeding
Diverticular disease of colon NOS

K57.31 Diverticulosis of large intestine without perforation or abscess with bleeding   Q

K57.32 Diverticulitis of large intestine without perforation or abscess without bleeding

K57.33 Diverticulitis of large intestine without perforation or abscess with bleeding

√5ᵗʰ **K57.4 Diverticulitis of both small and large intestine with perforation and abscess**
Diverticulitis of both small and large intestine with peritonitis

K57.40 Diverticulitis of both small and large intestine with perforation and abscess without bleeding

K57.41 Diverticulitis of both small and large intestine with perforation and abscess with bleeding   Q

√5ᵗʰ **K57.5 Diverticular disease of both small and large intestine without perforation or abscess**

K57.50 Diverticulosis of both small and large intestine without perforation or abscess without bleeding
Diverticular disease of both small and large intestine NOS

K57.51 Diverticulosis of both small and large intestine without perforation or abscess with bleeding   Q

K57.52 Diverticulitis of both small and large intestine without perforation or abscess without bleeding

K57.53 Diverticulitis of both small and large intestine without perforation or abscess with bleeding   Q

√5ᵗʰ **K57.8 Diverticulitis of intestine, part unspecified, with perforation and abscess**
Diverticulitis of intestine NOS with peritonitis

K57.80 Diverticulitis of intestine, part unspecified, with perforation and abscess without bleeding

K57.81 Diverticulitis of intestine, part unspecified, with perforation and abscess with bleeding   Q

√5ᵗʰ **K57.9 Diverticular disease of intestine, part unspecified, without perforation or abscess**

K57.90 Diverticulosis of intestine, part unspecified, without perforation or abscess without bleeding
Diverticular disease of intestine NOS

K57.91 Diverticulosis of intestine, part unspecified, without perforation or abscess with bleeding   Q

K57.92 Diverticulitis of intestine, part unspecified, without perforation or abscess without bleeding

K57.93 Diverticulitis of intestine, part unspecified, without perforation or abscess with bleeding   Q

√4ᵗʰ **K58 Irritable bowel syndrome**

> INCLUDES   irritable colon
>   spastic colon

AHA: 2016,4Q,32-33

K58.0 Irritable bowel syndrome with diarrhea

K58.1 Irritable bowel syndrome with constipation

K58.2 Mixed irritable bowel syndrome

K58.8 Other irritable bowel syndrome

K58.9 Irritable bowel syndrome without diarrhea
Irritable bowel syndrome NOS

√4ᵗʰ **K59 Other functional intestinal disorders**

> EXCLUDES 1   change in bowel habit NOS (R19.4)
>   intestinal malabsorption (K90.-)
>   psychogenic intestinal disorders (F45.8)
> EXCLUDES 2   functional disorders of stomach (K31.-)

√5ᵗʰ **K59.0 Constipation**
~~Use additional code for adverse effect, if applicable, to identify drug (T36-T50 with fifth or sixth character 5)~~

> EXCLUDES 1   fecal impaction (K56.41)
>   incomplete defecation (R15.0)

AHA: 2016,4Q,33

K59.00 Constipation, unspecified

K59.01 Slow transit constipation
DEF: Delay in the transit of fecal material through the colon secondary to smooth muscle dysfunction or decreased peristaltic contractions along the colon.

K59.02 Outlet dysfunction constipation

K59.03 Drug induced constipation
Use additional code for adverse effect, if applicable, to identify drug (T36-T50 with fifth or sixth character 5)

K59.04 Chronic idiopathic constipation
Functional constipation

K59.09 Other constipation
Chronic constipation

K59.1 Functional diarrhea

> EXCLUDES 1   diarrhea NOS (R19.7)
>   irritable bowel syndrome with diarrhea (K58.0)

K59.2 Neurogenic bowel, not elsewhere classified
> **DEF:** Disorder of bowel due to a spinal cord lesion due to injury or as a complication of conditions such as multiple sclerosis (MS) or spina bifida. Loss of bowel control is the primary symptom, manifested as constipation or bowel incontinence.

✓5ᵗʰ **K59.3 Megacolon, not elsewhere classified**
> Dilatation of colon
> Code first, if applicable (T51-T65) to identify toxic agent
>> EXCLUDES 1   congenital megacolon (aganglionic) (Q43.1)
>> megacolon (due to) (in) Chagas' disease (B57.32)
>> megacolon (due to) (in) Clostridium difficile (A04.7-)
>> megacolon (due to) (in) Hirschsprung's disease (Q43.1)
>
> AHA: 2016,4Q,33-34

     K59.31 Toxic megacolon   HCC

     K59.39 Other megacolon
>> Megacolon NOS

K59.4 Anal spasm
> Proctalgia fugax

K59.8 Other specified functional intestinal disorders
> Atony of colon
> Pseudo-obstruction (acute) (chronic) of intestine

K59.9 Functional intestinal disorder, unspecified

✓4ᵗʰ **K60 Fissure and fistula of anal and rectal regions**
>> EXCLUDES 1   fissure and fistula of anal and rectal regions with abscess or cellulitis (K61.-)
>> EXCLUDES 2   anal sphincter tear (healed) (nontraumatic) (old) (K62.81)

K60.0 Acute anal fissure
K60.1 Chronic anal fissure
K60.2 Anal fissure, unspecified
K60.3 Anal fistula
K60.4 Rectal fistula
> Fistula of rectum to skin
>> EXCLUDES 1   rectovaginal fistula (N82.3)
>> vesicorectal fistual (N32.1)

K60.5 Anorectal fistula

✓4ᵗʰ **K61 Abscess of anal and rectal regions**
>> INCLUDES   abscess of anal and rectal regions
>> cellulitis of anal and rectal regions

K61.0 Anal abscess
> Perianal abscess
>> EXCLUDES 2   intrasphincteric abscess (K61.4)

K61.1 Rectal abscess
> Perirectal abscess
>> EXCLUDES 1   ischiorectal abscess (K61.39)
>
> AHA: 2012,4Q,104

K61.2 Anorectal abscess
✓5ᵗʰ **K61.3 Ischiorectal abscess**
> AHA: 2018,4Q,19

     K61.31 Horseshoe abscess

     K61.39 Other ischiorectal abscess
>> Abscess of ischiorectal fossa
>> Ischiorectal abscess, NOS

K61.4 Intrasphincteric abscess
> Intersphincteric abscess

K61.5 Supralevator abscess
> AHA: 2018,4Q,19

✓4ᵗʰ **K62 Other diseases of anus and rectum**
>> INCLUDES   anal canal
>> EXCLUDES 2   colostomy and enterostomy malfunction (K94.0-, K94.1-)
>> fecal incontinence (R15.-)
>> hemorrhoids (K64.-)

K62.0 Anal polyp
K62.1 Rectal polyp
>> EXCLUDES 1   adenomatous polyp (D12.8)
>
> AHA: 2018,1Q,6

K62.2 Anal prolapse
> Prolapse of anal canal

K62.3 Rectal prolapse
> Prolapse of rectal mucosa

K62.4 Stenosis of anus and rectum
> Stricture of anus (sphincter)
> AHA: 2019,2Q,13

K62.5 Hemorrhage of anus and rectum   Q
>> EXCLUDES 1   gastrointestinal bleeding NOS (K92.2)
>> melena (K92.1)
>> neonatal rectal hemorrhage (P54.2)
>
> AHA: 2019,1Q,21

K62.6 Ulcer of anus and rectum
> Solitary ulcer of anus and rectum
> Stercoral ulcer of anus and rectum
>> EXCLUDES 1   fissure and fistula of anus and rectum (K60.-)
>> ulcerative colitis (K51.-)

K62.7 Radiation proctitis
> Use additional code to identify the type of radiation (W90.-)
> AHA: 2019,1Q,21

✓5ᵗʰ **K62.8 Other specified diseases of anus and rectum**
>> EXCLUDES 2   ulcerative proctitis (K51.2)

     K62.81 Anal sphincter tear (healed) (nontraumatic) (old)
>> Tear of anus, nontraumatic
>> Use additional code for any associated fecal incontinence (R15.-)
>>> EXCLUDES 2   anal fissure (K60.-)
>>> anal sphincter tear (healed) (old) complicating delivery (O34.7-)
>>> traumatic tear of anal sphincter (S31.831)

     K62.82 Dysplasia of anus
>> Anal intraepithelial neoplasia I and II (AIN I and II) (histologically confirmed)
>> Dysplasia of anus NOS
>> Mild and moderate dysplasia of anus (histologically confirmed)
>>> EXCLUDES 1   abnormal results from anal cytologic examination without histologic confirmation (R85.61-)
>>> anal intraepithelial neoplasia III (D01.3)
>>> carcinoma in situ of anus (D01.3)
>>> HGSIL of anus (R85.613)
>>> severe dysplasia of anus (D01.3)

     K62.89 Other specified diseases of anus and rectum
>> Proctitis NOS
>> Use additional code for any associated fecal incontinence (R15.-)

K62.9 Disease of anus and rectum, unspecified

✓4ᵗʰ **K63 Other diseases of intestine**

K63.0 Abscess of intestine
>> EXCLUDES 1   abscess of intestine with Crohn's disease (K50.014, K50.114, K50.814, K50.914)
>> abscess of intestine with diverticular disease (K57.0, K57.2, K57.4, K57.8)
>> abscess of intestine with ulcerative colitis (K51.014, K51.214, K51.314, K51.414, K51.514, K51.814, K51.914)
>> EXCLUDES 2   abscess of anal and rectal regions (K61.-)
>> abscess of appendix (K35.3-)

K63.1 Perforation of intestine (nontraumatic)   HCC
> Perforation (nontraumatic) of rectum
>> EXCLUDES 1   perforation (nontraumatic) of duodenum (K26.-)
>> perforation (nontraumatic) of intestine with diverticular disease (K57.0, K57.2, K57.4, K57.8)
>> EXCLUDES 2   perforation (nontraumatic) of appendix (K35.2-, K35.3-)

K63.2 Fistula of intestine
>> EXCLUDES 1   fistula of duodenum (K31.6)
>> fistula of intestine with Crohn's disease (K50.013, K50.113, K50.813, K50.913)
>> fistula of intestine with ulcerative colitis (K51.013, K51.213, K51.313, K51.413, K51.513, K51.813, K51.913)
>> EXCLUDES 2   fistula of anal and rectal regions (K60.-)
>> fistula of appendix (K38.3)
>> intestinal-genital fistula, female (N82.2-N82.4)
>> vesicointestinal fistula (N32.1)
>
> AHA: 2017,3Q,4

✓ Additional Character Required   ✓x7ᵗʰ Placeholder Alert   Manifestation   Unspecified Dx   ►◄ Revised Text   ● New Code   ▲ Revised Code Title

ICD-10-CM 2020   713

K63.3 Ulcer of intestine
Primary ulcer of small intestine
> EXCLUDES 1   *duodenal ulcer (K26.-)*
> *gastrointestinal ulcer (K28.-)*
> *gastrojejunal ulcer (K28.-)*
> *jejunal ulcer (K28.-)*
> *peptic ulcer, site unspecified (K27.-)*
> *ulcer of intestine with perforation (K63.1)*
> *ulcer of anus or rectum (K62.6)*
> *ulcerative colitis (K51.-)*

K63.4 Enteroptosis

K63.5 Polyp of colon
> EXCLUDES 1   *adenomatous polyp of colon ▶(D12.-)◀*
> *inflammatory polyp of colon (K51.4-)*
> *polyposis of colon (D12.6)*

AHA: 2019,1Q,33; 2018,2Q,14; 2017,1Q,15; 2015,2Q,14
TIP: Assign this code when documentation states hyperplastic colon polyp regardless of the site in the colon. Slow-growing, hyperplastic polyps are not precancerous and are classified differently from benign or adenomatous polyps.

✓5ᵗʰ K63.8 Other specified diseases of intestine

K63.81 Dieulafoy lesion of intestine
> EXCLUDES 2   *Dieulafoy lesion of stomach and duodenum (K31.82)*

DEF: Abnormally large submucosal artery protruding through a defect in the stomach mucosa or intestines that can cause massive and life-threatening hemorrhaging.

K63.89 Other specified diseases of intestine
AHA: 2013,2Q,31

K63.9 Disease of intestine, unspecified

✓4ᵗʰ K64 Hemorrhoids and perianal venous thrombosis
> INCLUDES   piles
> EXCLUDES 1   *hemorrhoids complicating childbirth and the puerperium (O87.2)*
> *hemorrhoids complicating pregnancy (O22.4)*

Hemorrhoids

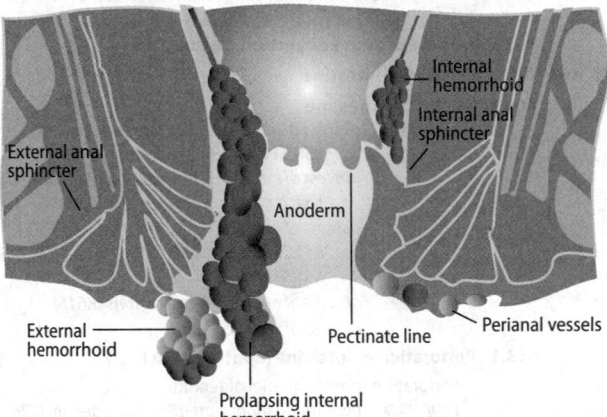

External anal sphincter — Internal hemorrhoid — Internal anal sphincter — Anoderm — External anal sphincter — External hemorrhoid — Pectinate line — Perianal vessels — Prolapsing internal hemorrhoid

K64.0 First degree hemorrhoids
Grade/stage I hemorrhoids
Hemorrhoids (bleeding) without prolapse outside of anal canal

K64.1 Second degree hemorrhoids
Grade/stage II hemorrhoids
Hemorrhoids (bleeding) that prolapse with straining, but retract spontaneously

K64.2 Third degree hemorrhoids
Grade/stage III hemorrhoids
Hemorrhoids (bleeding) that prolapse with straining and require manual replacement back inside anal canal

K64.3 Fourth degree hemorrhoids
Grade/stage IV hemorrhoids
Hemorrhoids (bleeding) with prolapsed tissue that cannot be manually replaced

K64.4 Residual hemorrhoidal skin tags
External hemorrhoids, NOS
Skin tags of anus

K64.5 Perianal venous thrombosis
External hemorrhoids with thrombosis
Perianal hematoma
Thrombosed hemorrhoids NOS

K64.8 Other hemorrhoids
Internal hemorrhoids, without mention of degree
Prolapsed hemorrhoids, degree not specified

K64.9 Unspecified hemorrhoids
Hemorrhoids (bleeding) NOS
Hemorrhoids (bleeding) without mention of degree

Diseases of peritoneum and retroperitoneum (K65-K68)

✓4ᵗʰ K65 Peritonitis
Use additional code (B95-B97), to identify infectious agent, if known
Code also if applicable diverticular disease of intestine (K57.-)
> EXCLUDES 1   *acute appendicitis with generalized peritonitis (K35.2-)*
> *aseptic peritonitis (T81.6)*
> *benign paroxysmal peritonitis (E85.0)*
> *chemical peritonitis (T81.6)*
> *gonococcal peritonitis (A54.85)*
> *neonatal peritonitis (P78.0-P78.1)*
> *pelvic peritonitis, female (N73.3-N73.5)*
> *periodic familial peritonitis (E85.0)*
> *peritonitis due to talc or other foreign substance (T81.6)*
> *peritonitis in chlamydia (A74.81)*
> *peritonitis in diphtheria (A36.89)*
> *peritonitis in syphilis (late) (A52.74)*
> *peritonitis in tuberculosis (A18.31)*
> *peritonitis with or following abortion or ectopic or molar pregnancy (O00-O07, O08.0)*
> *peritonitis with or following appendicitis (K35.-)*
> *puerperal peritonitis (O85)*
> *retroperitoneal infections (K68.-)*

K65.0 Generalized (acute) peritonitis   HCC
Pelvic peritonitis (acute), male
Subphrenic peritonitis (acute)
Suppurative peritonitis (acute)

K65.1 Peritoneal abscess   HCC
Abdominopelvic abscess
Abscess (of) omentum
Abscess (of) peritoneum
Mesenteric abscess
Retrocecal abscess
Subdiaphragmatic abscess
Subhepatic abscess
Subphrenic abscess
AHA: 2019,1Q,15

K65.2 Spontaneous bacterial peritonitis   HCC
> EXCLUDES 1   *bacterial peritonitis NOS (K65.9)*

K65.3 Choleperitonitis   HCC
Peritonitis due to bile
DEF: Inflammation of the peritoneum due to leakage of bile into the peritoneal cavity resulting from rupture of the bile passages or gallbladder.

K65.4 Sclerosing mesenteritis   HCC
Fat necrosis of peritoneum
(Idiopathic) sclerosing mesenteric fibrosis
Mesenteric lipodystrophy
Mesenteric panniculitis
Retractile mesenteritis

K65.8 Other peritonitis   HCC
Chronic proliferative peritonitis
Peritonitis due to urine

K65.9 Peritonitis, unspecified   HCC
Bacterial peritonitis NOS
AHA: 2013,2Q,31

☑4th K66 Other disorders of peritoneum

> EXCLUDES 2   ascites (R18.-)
> peritoneal effusion (chronic) (R18.8)

   K66.0 Peritoneal adhesions (postprocedural) (postinfection)
      Adhesions (of) abdominal (wall)
      Adhesions (of) diaphragm
      Adhesions (of) intestine
      Adhesions (of) male pelvis
      Adhesions (of) omentum
      Adhesions (of) stomach
      Adhesive bands
      Mesenteric adhesions

> EXCLUDES 1   female pelvic adhesions [bands] (N73.6)
> peritoneal adhesions with intestinal obstruction (K56.5-)

   K66.1 Hemoperitoneum

> EXCLUDES 1   traumatic hemoperitoneum (S36.8-)

   K66.8 Other specified disorders of peritoneum
   K66.9 Disorder of peritoneum, unspecified

K67 _Disorders of peritoneum in infectious diseases classified elsewhere_   HCC
      Code first underlying disease, such as:
      congenital syphilis (A50.0)
      helminthiasis (B65.0-B83.9)

> EXCLUDES 1   peritonitis in chlamydia (A74.81)
> peritonitis in diphtheria (A36.89)
> peritonitis in gonococcal (A54.85)
> peritonitis in syphilis (late) (A52.74)
> peritonitis in tuberculosis (A18.31)

☑4th K68 Disorders of retroperitoneum

   ☑5th K68.1 Retroperitoneal abscess

      K68.11 Postprocedural retroperitoneal abscess

> EXCLUDES 2   infection following procedure (T81.4-)

      K68.12 Psoas muscle abscess   HCC

      K68.19 Other retroperitoneal abscess   HCC

       AHA: 2019,1Q,15
       TIP: This code should be used for a diagnosis of internal presacral abscess. If an intra-abdominal abscess is also present, code K65.1 can also be assigned; sequencing depends on the circumstances of admission.

   K68.9 Other disorders of retroperitoneum

Diseases of liver (K70-K77)

> EXCLUDES 1   jaundice NOS (R17)
> EXCLUDES 2   hemochromatosis (E83.11-)
> Reye's syndrome (G93.7)
> viral hepatitis (B15-B19)
> Wilson's disease (E83.0)

☑4th K70 Alcoholic liver disease
      Use additional code to identify:
      alcohol abuse and dependence (F10.-)

   K70.0 Alcoholic fatty liver   A

   ☑5th K70.1 Alcoholic hepatitis

      K70.10 Alcoholic hepatitis without ascites   A

      K70.11 Alcoholic hepatitis with ascites   A

   K70.2 Alcoholic fibrosis and sclerosis of liver   A

   ☑5th K70.3 Alcoholic cirrhosis of liver
      Alcoholic cirrhosis NOS

      K70.30 Alcoholic cirrhosis of liver without ascites   HCC A

      K70.31 Alcoholic cirrhosis of liver with ascites   HCC A
       AHA: 2018,1Q,4

   ☑5th K70.4 Alcoholic hepatic failure
      Acute alcoholic hepatic failure
      Alcoholic hepatic failure NOS
      Chronic alcoholic hepatic failure
      Subacute alcoholic hepatic failure

      K70.40 Alcoholic hepatic failure without coma   HCC A

      K70.41 Alcoholic hepatic failure with coma   HCC A

   K70.9 Alcoholic liver disease, unspecified   HCC A

☑4th K71 Toxic liver disease

> INCLUDES   drug-induced idiosyncratic (unpredictable) liver disease
> drug-induced toxic (predictable) liver disease

      Code first poisoning due to drug or toxin, if applicable (T36-T65 with fifth or sixth character 1-4 or 6)
      Use additional code for adverse effect, if applicable, to identify drug (T36-T50 with fifth or sixth character 5)

> EXCLUDES 2   alcoholic liver disease (K70.-)
> Budd-Chiari syndrome (I82.0)

   K71.0 Toxic liver disease with cholestasis
      Cholestasis with hepatocyte injury
      "Pure" cholestasis

   ☑5th K71.1 Toxic liver disease with hepatic necrosis
      Hepatic failure (acute) (chronic) due to drugs

      K71.10 Toxic liver disease with hepatic necrosis, without coma

      K71.11 Toxic liver disease with hepatic necrosis, with coma   HCC

   K71.2 Toxic liver disease with acute hepatitis
   K71.3 Toxic liver disease with chronic persistent hepatitis
   K71.4 Toxic liver disease with chronic lobular hepatitis

   ☑5th K71.5 Toxic liver disease with chronic active hepatitis
      Toxic liver disease with lupoid hepatitis

      K71.50 Toxic liver disease with chronic active hepatitis without ascites

      K71.51 Toxic liver disease with chronic active hepatitis with ascites
       AHA: 2018,1Q,4

   K71.6 Toxic liver disease with hepatitis, not elsewhere classified
   K71.7 Toxic liver disease with fibrosis and cirrhosis of liver
   K71.8 Toxic liver disease with other disorders of liver
      Toxic liver disease with focal nodular hyperplasia
      Toxic liver disease with hepatic granulomas
      Toxic liver disease with peliosis hepatis
      Toxic liver disease with veno-occlusive disease of liver

   K71.9 Toxic liver disease, unspecified

☑4th K72 Hepatic failure, not elsewhere classified

> INCLUDES   fulminant hepatitis NEC, with hepatic failure
> hepatic encephalopathy NOS
> liver (cell) necrosis with hepatic failure
> malignant hepatitis NEC, with hepatic failure
> yellow liver atrophy or dystrophy

> EXCLUDES 1   alcoholic hepatic failure (K70.4)
> hepatic failure with toxic liver disease (K71.1-)
> icterus of newborn (P55-P59)
> postprocedural hepatic failure (K91.82)

> EXCLUDES 2   hepatic failure complicating abortion or ectopic or molar pregnancy (O00-O07, O08.8)
> hepatic failure complicating pregnancy, childbirth and the puerperium (O26.6-)
> viral hepatitis with hepatic coma (B15-B19)

   AHA: 2017,1Q,41

   ☑5th K72.0 Acute and subacute hepatic failure
      Acute non-viral hepatitis NOS
      AHA: 2015,2Q,17; 2014,2Q,13

      K72.00 Acute and subacute hepatic failure without coma

      K72.01 Acute and subacute hepatic failure with coma   HCC

   ☑5th K72.1 Chronic hepatic failure

      K72.10 Chronic hepatic failure without coma   HCC

      K72.11 Chronic hepatic failure with coma   HCC

   ☑5th K72.9 Hepatic failure, unspecified

      K72.90 Hepatic failure, unspecified without coma   HCC
       AHA: 2018,4Q,20; 2016,2Q,35

      K72.91 Hepatic failure, unspecified with coma   HCC
       Hepatic coma NOS

☑4th K73 Chronic hepatitis, not elsewhere classified

> EXCLUDES 1   alcoholic hepatitis (chronic) (K70.1-)
> drug-induced hepatitis (chronic) (K71.-)
> granulomatous hepatitis (chronic) NEC (K75.3)
> reactive, nonspecific hepatitis (chronic) (K75.2)
> viral hepatitis (chronic) (B15-B19)

   K73.0 Chronic persistent hepatitis, not elsewhere classified   HCC
   K73.1 Chronic lobular hepatitis, not elsewhere classified   HCC

☑ Additional Character Required   ✓x7th Placeholder Alert   Manifestation   Unspecified Dx   ►◄ Revised Text   ● New Code   ▲ Revised Code Title

ICD-10-CM 2020   715

Chapter 11. Diseases of the Digestive System

K73.2   Chronic active hepatitis, not elsewhere classified   `HCC`

K73.8   Other chronic hepatitis, not elsewhere classified   `HCC`

K73.9   Chronic hepatitis, unspecified   `HCC`

`✔4ᵗʰ` **K74**   **Fibrosis and cirrhosis of liver**

    Code also, if applicable, viral hepatitis (acute) (chronic) (B15-B19)

      `EXCLUDES 1`   *alcoholic cirrhosis (of liver) (K70.3)*

           alcoholic fibrosis of liver (K70.2)

           cardiac sclerosis of liver (K76.1)

           cirrhosis (of liver) with toxic liver disease (K71.7)

           congenital cirrhosis (of liver) (P78.81)

           pigmentary cirrhosis (of liver) (E83.110)

K74.0   **Hepatic fibrosis**

K74.1   **Hepatic sclerosis**

K74.2   **Hepatic fibrosis with hepatic sclerosis**

K74.3   **Primary biliary cirrhosis**   `HCC`

    Chronic nonsuppurative destructive cholangitis

    Primary biliary cholangitis

      `EXCLUDES 2`   ▶*primary sclerosing cholangitis*◀ *(K83.01)*

K74.4   **Secondary biliary cirrhosis**   `HCC`

K74.5   **Biliary cirrhosis, unspecified**   `HCC`

`✔5ᵗʰ` **K74.6**   **Other and unspecified cirrhosis of liver**

    K74.60   **Unspecified cirrhosis of liver**   `HCC`

        Cirrhosis (of liver) NOS

        AHA: 2018,1Q,4

    K74.69   **Other cirrhosis of liver**   `HCC`

        Cryptogenic cirrhosis (of liver)

        Macronodular cirrhosis (of liver)

        Micronodular cirrhosis (of liver)

        Mixed type cirrhosis (of liver)

        Portal cirrhosis (of liver)

        Postnecrotic cirrhosis (of liver)

`✔4ᵗʰ` **K75**   **Other inflammatory liver diseases**

      `EXCLUDES 2`   *toxic liver disease (K71.-)*

K75.0   **Abscess of liver**

    Cholangitic hepatic abscess

    Hematogenic hepatic abscess

    Hepatic abscess NOS

    Lymphogenic hepatic abscess

    Pylephlebitic hepatic abscess

      `EXCLUDES 1`   *amebic liver abscess (A06.4)*

           cholangitis without liver abscess (K83.09)

           pylephlebitis without liver abscess (K75.1)

      `EXCLUDES 2`   *acute or subacute hepatitis NOS (B17.9)*

           acute or subacute non-viral hepatitis (K72.0)

           chronic hepatitis NEC (K73.8)

K75.1   **Phlebitis of portal vein**

    Pylephlebitis

      `EXCLUDES 1`   *pylephlebitic liver abscess (K75.0)*

    DEF: Inflammation of the portal vein or branches due to diverticulitis, perforated appendicitis, or peritonitis. Symptoms include fever, chills, jaundice, sweating, and abscess in various body parts.

K75.2   **Nonspecific reactive hepatitis**

      `EXCLUDES 1`   *acute or subacute hepatitis (K72.0-)*

           chronic hepatitis NEC (K73.-)

           viral hepatitis (B15-B19)

K75.3   **Granulomatous hepatitis, not elsewhere classified**

      `EXCLUDES 1`   *acute or subacute hepatitis (K72.0-)*

           chronic hepatitis NEC (K73.-)

           viral hepatitis (B15-B19)

K75.4   **Autoimmune hepatitis**   `HCC`

    Lupoid hepatitis NEC

`✔5ᵗʰ` **K75.8**   **Other specified inflammatory liver diseases**

    K75.81   **Nonalcoholic steatohepatitis (NASH)**

    K75.89   **Other specified inflammatory liver diseases**

K75.9   **Inflammatory liver disease, unspecified**

    Hepatitis NOS

      `EXCLUDES 1`   *acute or subacute hepatitis (K72.0-)*

           chronic hepatitis NEC (K73.-)

           viral hepatitis (B15-B19)

    AHA: 2015,2Q,17

`✔4ᵗʰ` **K76**   **Other diseases of liver**

      `EXCLUDES 2`   *alcoholic liver disease (K70.-)*

           amyloid degeneration of liver (E85.-)

           cystic disease of liver (congenital) (Q44.6)

           hepatic vein thrombosis (I82.0)

           hepatomegaly NOS (R16.0)

           pigmentary cirrhosis (of liver) (E83.110)

           portal vein thrombosis (I81)

           toxic liver disease (K71.-)

K76.0   **Fatty (change of) liver, not elsewhere classified**

    Nonalcoholic fatty liver disease (NAFLD)

      `EXCLUDES 1`   *nonalcoholic steatohepatitis (NASH) (K75.81)*

K76.1   **Chronic passive congestion of liver**

    Cardiac cirrhosis

    Cardiac sclerosis

K76.2   **Central hemorrhagic necrosis of liver**

      `EXCLUDES 1`   *liver necrosis with hepatic failure (K72.-)*

K76.3   **Infarction of liver**

K76.4   **Peliosis hepatis**

    Hepatic angiomatosis

K76.5   **Hepatic veno-occlusive disease**

      `EXCLUDES 1`   *Budd-Chiari syndrome (I82.0)*

K76.6   **Portal hypertension**   `HCC`

    Use additional code for any associated complications, such as:

      portal hypertensive gastropathy (K31.89)

K76.7   **Hepatorenal syndrome**   `HCC`

      `EXCLUDES 1`   *hepatorenal syndrome following labor and delivery (O90.4)*

           postprocedural hepatorenal syndrome (K91.83)

`✔5ᵗʰ` **K76.8**   **Other specified diseases of liver**

    K76.81   **Hepatopulmonary syndrome**   `HCC`

        Code first underlying liver disease, such as:

           alcoholic cirrhosis of liver (K70.3-)

           cirrhosis of liver without mention of alcohol (K74.6-)

    K76.89   **Other specified diseases of liver**

        Cyst (simple) of liver

        Focal nodular hyperplasia of liver

        Hepatoptosis

K76.9   **Liver disease, unspecified**

K77   *Liver disorders in diseases classified elsewhere*

    Code first underlying disease, such as:

    amyloidosis (E85.-)

    congenital syphilis (A50.0, A50.5)

    congenital toxoplasmosis (P37.1)

    schistosomiasis (B65.0-B65.9)

      `EXCLUDES 1`   *alcoholic hepatitis (K70.1-)*

           alcoholic liver disease (K70.-)

           cytomegaloviral hepatitis (B25.1)

           herpesviral [herpes simplex] hepatitis (B00.81)

           infectious mononucleosis with liver disease (B27.0-B27.9 with .9)

           mumps hepatitis (B26.81)

           sarcoidosis with liver disease (D86.89)

           secondary syphilis with liver disease (A51.45)

           syphilis (late) with liver disease (A52.74)

           toxoplasmosis (acquired) hepatitis (B58.1)

           tuberculosis with liver disease (A18.83)

Disorders of gallbladder, biliary tract and pancreas (K80-K87)

✓4ᵗʰ K80 Cholelithiasis

> **EXCLUDES 1** *retained cholelithiasis following cholecystectomy (K91.86)*
>
> **AHA:** 2018,4Q,20
>
> **DEF:** Presence or formation of concretions (calculi or "gallstones") in the gallbladder. The stones contain cholesterol, calcium carbonate, or calcium bilirubinate in pure forms or in various combinations.

Cholelithiasis

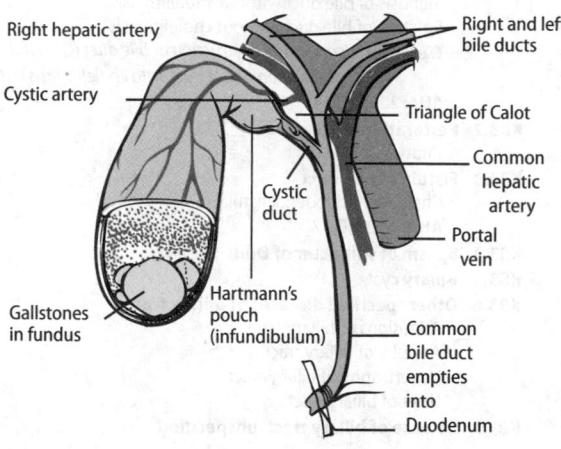

Right hepatic artery — Cystic artery — Right and left bile ducts — Triangle of Calot — Common hepatic artery — Portal vein — Cystic duct — Hartmann's pouch (infundibulum) — Gallstones in fundus — Common bile duct empties into Duodenum

✓5ᵗʰ K80.0 Calculus of gallbladder with acute cholecystitis

> Any condition listed in K80.2 with acute cholecystitis
> Use additional code if applicable for associated gangrene of gallbladder (K82.A1), or perforation of gallbladder (K82.A2)

    K80.00 Calculus of gallbladder with acute cholecystitis without obstruction

    K80.01 Calculus of gallbladder with acute cholecystitis with obstruction

✓5ᵗʰ K80.1 Calculus of gallbladder with other cholecystitis

> Use additional code if applicable for associated gangrene of gallbladder (K82.A1), or perforation of gallbladder (K82.A2)

    K80.10 Calculus of gallbladder with chronic **cholecystitis** without obstruction
    Cholelithiasis with cholecystitis NOS

    K80.11 Calculus of gallbladder with chronic **cholecystitis** with obstruction

    K80.12 Calculus of gallbladder with acute and chronic **cholecystitis** without obstruction

    K80.13 Calculus of gallbladder with acute and chronic **cholecystitis** with obstruction

    K80.18 Calculus of gallbladder with other cholecystitis without obstruction

    K80.19 Calculus of gallbladder with other cholecystitis with obstruction

✓5ᵗʰ K80.2 Calculus of gallbladder without cholecystitis

> Cholecystolithiasis without cholecystitis
> Cholelithiasis (without cholecystitis)
> Colic (recurrent) of gallbladder (without cholecystitis)
> Gallstone (impacted) of cystic duct (without cholecystitis)
> Gallstone (impacted) of gallbladder (without cholecystitis)

    K80.20 Calculus of gallbladder without cholecystitis without obstruction

    K80.21 Calculus of gallbladder without cholecystitis with obstruction

✓5ᵗʰ K80.3 Calculus of bile duct with cholangitis

> Any condition listed in K80.5 with cholangitis
> **DEF:** Cholangitis: Inflammation of the bile ducts.

    K80.30 Calculus of bile duct with cholangitis, unspecified, without obstruction

    K80.31 Calculus of bile duct with cholangitis, unspecified, with obstruction

    K80.32 Calculus of bile duct with acute **cholangitis** without obstruction

    K80.33 Calculus of bile duct with acute **cholangitis** with obstruction

    K80.34 Calculus of bile duct with chronic **cholangitis** without obstruction

    K80.35 Calculus of bile duct with chronic **cholangitis** with obstruction

    K80.36 Calculus of bile duct with acute and chronic **cholangitis** without obstruction

    K80.37 Calculus of bile duct with acute and chronic **cholangitis** with obstruction

✓5ᵗʰ K80.4 Calculus of bile duct with cholecystitis

> Any condition listed in K80.5 with cholecystitis (with cholangitis)
> Use additional code if applicable for associated gangrene of gallbladder (K82.A1), or perforation of gallbladder (K82.A2)
> **AHA:** 2019,1Q,17

    K80.40 Calculus of bile duct with cholecystitis, unspecified, without obstruction

    K80.41 Calculus of bile duct with cholecystitis, unspecified, with obstruction
    AHA: 2019,1Q,17

    K80.42 Calculus of bile duct with acute **cholecystitis** without obstruction

    K80.43 Calculus of bile duct with acute **cholecystitis** with obstruction

    K80.44 Calculus of bile duct with chronic **cholecystitis** without obstruction

    K80.45 Calculus of bile duct with chronic **cholecystitis** with obstruction

    K80.46 Calculus of bile duct with acute and chronic **cholecystitis** without obstruction

    K80.47 Calculus of bile duct with acute and chronic **cholecystitis** with obstruction

✓5ᵗʰ K80.5 Calculus of bile duct without cholangitis or cholecystitis

> Choledocholithiasis (without cholangitis or cholecystitis)
> Gallstone (impacted) of bile duct NOS (without cholangitis or cholecystitis)
> Gallstone (impacted) of common duct (without cholangitis or cholecystitis)
> Gallstone (impacted) of hepatic duct (without cholangitis or cholecystitis)
> Hepatic cholelithiasis (without cholangitis or cholecystitis)
> Hepatic colic (recurrent) (without cholangitis or cholecystitis)
> **DEF:** Cholangitis: Inflammation of the bile ducts.

    K80.50 Calculus of bile duct without cholangitis or cholecystitis without obstruction

    K80.51 Calculus of bile duct without cholangitis or cholecystitis with obstruction

✓5ᵗʰ K80.6 Calculus of gallbladder and bile duct with cholecystitis

> Use additional code if applicable for associated gangrene of gallbladder (K82.A1), or perforation of gallbladder (K82.A2)

    K80.60 Calculus of gallbladder and bile duct with cholecystitis, unspecified, without obstruction

    K80.61 Calculus of gallbladder and bile duct with cholecystitis, unspecified, with obstruction

    K80.62 Calculus of gallbladder and bile duct with acute **cholecystitis** without obstruction

    K80.63 Calculus of gallbladder and bile duct with acute **cholecystitis** with obstruction

    K80.64 Calculus of gallbladder and bile duct with chronic **cholecystitis** without obstruction

    K80.65 Calculus of gallbladder and bile duct with chronic **cholecystitis** with obstruction

    K80.66 Calculus of gallbladder and bile duct with acute and chronic **cholecystitis** without obstruction

    K80.67 Calculus of gallbladder and bile duct with acute and chronic **cholecystitis** with obstruction

✓5ᵗʰ K80.7 Calculus of gallbladder and bile duct without cholecystitis

    K80.70 Calculus of gallbladder and bile duct without cholecystitis without obstruction

    K80.71 Calculus of gallbladder and bile duct without cholecystitis with obstruction

✓5ᵗʰ K80.8 Other cholelithiasis

    K80.80 Other cholelithiasis without obstruction

    K80.81 Other cholelithiasis with obstruction

✓ Additional Character Required   ✓×7ᵗʰ Placeholder Alert   Manifestation   Unspecified Dx   ►◄ Revised Text   ● New Code   ▲ Revised Code Title

ICD-10-CM 2020   **717**

Chapter 11. Diseases of the Digestive System

K81–K85.92

√4ᵗʰ **K81 Cholecystitis**

Use additional code if applicable for associated gangrene of gallbladder (K82.A1), or perforation of gallbladder (K82.A2)

EXCLUDES 1 *cholecystitis with cholelithiasis (K80.-)*

AHA: 2018,4Q,20

K81.0 Acute cholecystitis

Abscess of gallbladder

Angiocholecystitis

Emphysematous (acute) cholecystitis

Empyema of gallbladder

Gangrene of gallbladder

Gangrenous cholecystitis

Suppurative cholecystitis

K81.1 Chronic cholecystitis

K81.2 Acute cholecystitis with chronic cholecystitis

K81.9 Cholecystitis, unspecified

√4ᵗʰ **K82 Other diseases of gallbladder**

EXCLUDES 1 *nonvisualization of gallbladder (R93.2)*

postcholecystectomy syndrome (K91.5)

K82.0 Obstruction of gallbladder

Occlusion of cystic duct or gallbladder without cholelithiasis

Stenosis of cystic duct or gallbladder without cholelithiasis

Stricture of cystic duct or gallbladder without cholelithiasis

EXCLUDES 1 *obstruction of gallbladder with cholelithiasis (K80.-)*

K82.1 Hydrops of gallbladder

Mucocele of gallbladder

K82.2 Perforation of gallbladder

Rupture of cystic duct or gallbladder

EXCLUDES 1 *perforation of gallbladder in cholecystitis (K82.A2)*

K82.3 Fistula of gallbladder

Cholecystocolic fistula

Cholecystoduodenal fistula

K82.4 Cholesterolosis of gallbladder

Strawberry gallbladder

EXCLUDES 1 *cholesterolosis of gallbladder with cholecystitis (K81.-)*

cholesterolosis of gallbladder with cholelithiasis (K80.-)

K82.8 Other specified diseases of gallbladder

Adhesions of cystic duct or gallbladder

Atrophy of cystic duct or gallbladder

Cyst of cystic duct or gallbladder

Dyskinesia of cystic duct or gallbladder

Hypertrophy of cystic duct or gallbladder

Nonfunctioning of cystic duct or gallbladder

Ulcer of cystic duct or gallbladder

K82.9 Disease of gallbladder, unspecified

√5ᵗʰ **K82.A Disorders of gallbladder in diseases classified elsewhere**

Code first the type of cholecystitis (K81.-), or cholelithiasis with cholecystitis (K80.00-K80.19, K80.40-K80.47, K80.60-K80.67)

AHA: 2018,4Q,19-20

K82.A1 Gangrene of gallbladder in cholecystitis

K82.A2 Perforation of gallbladder in cholecystitis

√4ᵗʰ **K83 Other diseases of biliary tract**

EXCLUDES 1 *postcholecystectomy syndrome (K91.5)*

EXCLUDES 2 *conditions involving the gallbladder (K81-K82)*

conditions involving the cystic duct (K81-K82)

√5ᵗʰ **K83.0 Cholangitis**

EXCLUDES 1 *cholangitic liver abscess (K75.0)*

cholangitis with choledocholithiasis (K80.3-, K80.4-)

EXCLUDES 2 *chronic nonsuppurative destructive cholangitis (K74.3)*

primary biliary cholangitis (K74.3)

primary biliary cirrhosis (K74.3)

AHA: 2018,4Q,20

K83.01 Primary sclerosing cholangitis

K83.09 Other cholangitis

Ascending cholangitis

Cholangitis NOS

Primary cholangitis

Recurrent cholangitis

Sclerosing cholangitis

Secondary cholangitis

Stenosing cholangitis

Suppurative cholangitis

K83.1 Obstruction of bile duct

Occlusion of bile duct without cholelithiasis

Stenosis of bile duct without cholelithiasis

Stricture of bile duct without cholelithiasis

EXCLUDES 1 *congenital obstruction of bile duct (Q44.3)*

obstruction of bile duct with cholelithiasis (K80.-)

AHA: 2016,1Q,18

K83.2 Perforation of bile duct

Rupture of bile duct

K83.3 Fistula of bile duct

Choledochoduodenal fistula

AHA: 2019,1Q,17

K83.4 Spasm of sphincter of Oddi

K83.5 Biliary cyst

K83.8 Other specified diseases of biliary tract

Adhesions of biliary tract

Atrophy of biliary tract

Hypertrophy of biliary tract

Ulcer of biliary tract

K83.9 Disease of biliary tract, unspecified

√4ᵗʰ **K85 Acute pancreatitis**

INCLUDES acute (recurrent) pancreatitis

subacute pancreatitis

AHA: 2016,4Q,34

√5ᵗʰ **K85.0 Idiopathic acute pancreatitis**

K85.00 Idiopathic acute pancreatitis without necrosis or infection

K85.01 Idiopathic acute pancreatitis with uninfected necrosis

K85.02 Idiopathic acute pancreatitis with infected necrosis

√5ᵗʰ **K85.1 Biliary acute pancreatitis**

Gallstone pancreatitis

K85.10 Biliary acute pancreatitis without necrosis or infection

K85.11 Biliary acute pancreatitis with uninfected necrosis

K85.12 Biliary acute pancreatitis with infected necrosis

√5ᵗʰ **K85.2 Alcohol induced acute pancreatitis**

EXCLUDES 2 *alcohol induced chronic pancreatitis (K86.0)*

K85.20 Alcohol induced acute pancreatitis without necrosis or infection

K85.21 Alcohol induced acute pancreatitis with uninfected necrosis

K85.22 Alcohol induced acute pancreatitis with infected necrosis

√5ᵗʰ **K85.3 Drug induced acute pancreatitis**

Use additional code for adverse effect, if applicable, to identify drug (T36-T50 with fifth or sixth character 5)

Use additional code to identify drug abuse and dependence (F11.- F17.-)

K85.30 Drug induced acute pancreatitis without necrosis or infection

K85.31 Drug induced acute pancreatitis with uninfected necrosis

K85.32 Drug induced acute pancreatitis with infected necrosis

√5ᵗʰ **K85.8 Other acute pancreatitis**

K85.80 Other acute pancreatitis without necrosis or infection

K85.81 Other acute pancreatitis with uninfected necrosis

K85.82 Other acute pancreatitis with infected necrosis

√5ᵗʰ **K85.9 Acute pancreatitis, unspecified**

Pancreatitis NOS

K85.90 Acute pancreatitis without necrosis or infection, unspecified

K85.91 Acute pancreatitis with uninfected necrosis, unspecified

K85.92 Acute pancreatitis with infected necrosis, unspecified

✓4ᵗʰ **K86 Other diseases of pancreas**

> EXCLUDES 2   *fibrocystic disease of pancreas (E84.-)*
> *islet cell tumor (of pancreas) (D13.7)*
> *pancreatic steatorrhea (K90.3)*

K86.0 Alcohol-induced chronic pancreatitis   HCC

> Use additional code to identify:
> alcohol abuse and dependence (F10.-)
> Code also exocrine pancreatic insufficiency (K86.81)
> EXCLUDES 2   *alcohol induced acute pancreatitis (K85.2-)*

K86.1 Other chronic pancreatitis   HCC

> Chronic pancreatitis NOS
> Infectious chronic pancreatitis
> Recurrent chronic pancreatitis
> Relapsing chronic pancreatitis
> Code also exocrine pancreatic insufficiency (K86.81)

K86.2 Cyst of pancreas

K86.3 Pseudocyst of pancreas

✓5ᵗʰ **K86.8 Other specified diseases of pancreas**

> **AHA:** 2016,4Q,34-35

K86.81 Exocrine pancreatic insufficiency

K86.89 Other specified diseases of pancreas

> Aseptic pancreatic necrosis, unrelated to acute pancreatitis
> Atrophy of pancreas
> Calculus of pancreas
> Cirrhosis of pancreas
> Fibrosis of pancreas
> Pancreatic fat necrosis, unrelated to acute pancreatitis
> Pancreatic infantilism
> Pancreatic necrosis NOS, unrelated to acute pancreatitis

K86.9 Disease of pancreas, unspecified

K87 Disorders of gallbladder, biliary tract and pancreas in diseases classified elsewhere

> Code first underlying disease
> EXCLUDES 1   *cytomegaloviral pancreatitis (B25.2)*
> *mumps pancreatitis (B26.3)*
> *syphilitic gallbladder (A52.74)*
> *syphilitic pancreas (A52.74)*
> *tuberculosis of gallbladder (A18.83)*
> *tuberculosis of pancreas (A18.83)*

Other diseases of the digestive system (K90-K95)

✓4ᵗʰ **K90 Intestinal malabsorption**

> EXCLUDES 1   *intestinal malabsorption following gastrointestinal surgery (K91.2)*

AHA: 2017,4Q,108

K90.0 Celiac disease

> Celiac disease with steatorrhea
> Celiac gluten-sensitive enteropathy
> Nontropical sprue
> Use additional code for associated disorders including:
> dermatitis herpetiformis (L13.0)
> gluten ataxia (G32.81)
> Code also exocrine pancreatic insufficiency (K86.81)
> **DEF:** Malabsorption syndrome due to gluten consumption. Symptoms include fetid, bulky, frothy, oily stools; a distended abdomen; gas; asthenia; electrolyte depletion; and vitamin B, D, and K deficiency.

K90.1 Tropical sprue

> Sprue NOS
> Tropical steatorrhea

K90.2 Blind loop syndrome, not elsewhere classified

> Blind loop syndrome NOS
> EXCLUDES 1   *congenital blind loop syndrome (Q43.8)*
> *postsurgical blind loop syndrome (K91.2)*

K90.3 Pancreatic steatorrhea

✓5ᵗʰ **K90.4 Other malabsorption due to intolerance**

> EXCLUDES 2   *celiac gluten-sensitive enteropathy (K90.0)*
> *lactose intolerance (E73.-)*
> **AHA:** 2016,4Q,35-36

K90.41 Non-celiac gluten sensitivity

> Gluten sensitivity NOS
> Non-celiac gluten sensitive enteropathy

K90.49 Malabsorption due to intolerance, not elsewhere classified

> Malabsorption due to intolerance to carbohydrate
> Malabsorption due to intolerance to fat
> Malabsorption due to intolerance to protein
> Malabsorption due to intolerance to starch

✓5ᵗʰ **K90.8 Other intestinal malabsorption**

K90.81 Whipple's disease

K90.89 Other intestinal malabsorption

K90.9 Intestinal malabsorption, unspecified

✓4ᵗʰ **K91 Intraoperative and postprocedural complications and disorders of digestive system, not elsewhere classified**

> EXCLUDES 2   *complications of artificial opening of digestive system (K94.-)*
> *complications of bariatric procedures (K95.-)*
> *gastrojejunal ulcer (K28.-)*
> *postprocedural (radiation) retroperitoneal abscess (K68.11)*
> *radiation colitis (K52.0)*
> *radiation gastroenteritis (K52.0)*
> *radiation proctitis (K62.7)*

AHA: 2016,4Q,9-10

K91.0 Vomiting following gastrointestinal surgery

K91.1 Postgastric surgery syndromes

> Dumping syndrome
> Postgastrectomy syndrome
> Postvagotomy syndrome

K91.2 Postsurgical malabsorption, not elsewhere classified

> Postsurgical blind loop syndrome
> EXCLUDES 1   *malabsorption osteomalacia in adults (M83.2)*
> *malabsorption osteoporosis, postsurgical (M80.8-, M81.8)*

✓5ᵗʰ **K91.3 Postprocedural intestinal obstruction**

> **AHA:** 2017,4Q,16-17; 2017,1Q,40

K91.30 Postprocedural intestinal obstruction, unspecified as to partial versus complete

> Postprocedural intestinal obstruction NOS

K91.31 Postprocedural partial intestinal obstruction

> Postprocedural incomplete intestinal obstruction

K91.32 Postprocedural complete intestinal obstruction

K91.5 Postcholecystectomy syndrome

✓5ᵗʰ **K91.6 Intraoperative hemorrhage and hematoma of a digestive system organ or structure complicating a procedure**

> EXCLUDES 1   *intraoperative hemorrhage and hematoma of a digestive system organ or structure due to accidental puncture and laceration during a procedure (K91.7-)*

K91.61 Intraoperative hemorrhage and hematoma of a digestive system organ or structure complicating a digestive system procedure

K91.62 Intraoperative hemorrhage and hematoma of a digestive system organ or structure complicating other procedure

✓5ᵗʰ **K91.7 Accidental puncture and laceration of a digestive system organ or structure during a procedure**

K91.71 Accidental puncture and laceration of a digestive system organ or structure during a digestive system procedure

K91.72 Accidental puncture and laceration of a digestive system organ or structure during other procedure

> **AHA:** 2019,2Q,23

✓5ᵗʰ **K91.8 Other intraoperative and postprocedural complications and disorders of digestive system**

K91.81 Other intraoperative complications of digestive system

K91.82 Postprocedural hepatic failure

K91.83 Postprocedural hepatorenal syndrome

✓6ᵗʰ **K91.84 Postprocedural hemorrhage of a digestive system organ or structure following a procedure**

K91.840 Postprocedural hemorrhage of a digestive system organ or structure following a digestive system procedure

> **AHA:** 2016,1Q,15

K91.841 Postprocedural hemorrhage of a digestive system organ or structure following other procedure

---

☑ Additional Character Required   ✓x7ᵗʰ Placeholder Alert   Manifestation   Unspecified Dx   ▶◀ Revised Text   ● New Code   ▲ Revised Code Title

✓6th **K91.85　Complications of** intestinal pouch

K91.850　Pouchitis HCC

Inflammation of internal ileoanal pouch
DEF: Inflammatory complication of an existing surgically created ileoanal pouch, resulting in multiple GI complaints, including diarrhea, abdominal pain, rectal bleeding, fecal urgency, or incontinence.

K91.858　Other complications of intestinal HCC
pouch

AHA: 2019,2Q,13

K91.86　Retained cholelithiasis following cholecystectomy

✓6th **K91.87　Postprocedural hematoma and seroma of a**
digestive system organ or structure following a
procedure

K91.870　Postprocedural hematoma **of a**
digestive system organ or structure following a
digestive system procedure

K91.871　Postprocedural hematoma **of a digestive**
system organ or structure following other
procedure

K91.872　Postprocedural seroma **of a digestive**
system organ or structure following a
digestive system procedure

K91.873　Postprocedural seroma **of a digestive**
system organ or structure following other
procedure

K91.89　Other postprocedural complications and disorders
of digestive system

Use additional code, if applicable, to further specify
disorder

EXCLUDES 2　*postprocedural retroperitoneal abscess*
(K68.11)

AHA: 2017,1Q,40

✓4th **K92　Other diseases of digestive system**

EXCLUDES 1　*neonatal gastrointestinal hemorrhage (P54.0-P54.3)*

K92.0　Hematemesis Q

K92.1　Melena Q

EXCLUDES 1　*occult blood in feces (R19.5)*

K92.2　Gastrointestinal hemorrhage, unspecified Q

Gastric hemorrhage NOS
Intestinal hemorrhage NOS

EXCLUDES 1　*acute hemorrhagic gastritis (K29.01)*
hemorrhage of anus and rectum (K62.5)
angiodysplasia of stomach with hemorrhage
(K31.811)
diverticular disease with hemorrhage (K57.-)
gastritis and duodenitis with hemorrhage (K29.-)
peptic ulcer with hemorrhage (K25-K28)

✓5th **K92.8　Other specified diseases of the digestive system**

K92.81　Gastrointestinal mucositis (ulcerative)

Code also type of associated therapy, such as:
antineoplastic and immunosuppressive drugs
(T45.1X-)
radiological procedure and radiotherapy (Y84.2)

EXCLUDES 2　*mucositis (ulcerative) of vagina and vulva*
(N76.81)
nasal mucositis (ulcerative) (J34.81)
oral mucositis (ulcerative) (K12.3-)

K92.89　Other specified diseases of the digestive system

K92.9　Disease of digestive system, unspecified

✓4th **K94　Complications of artificial openings of the digestive system**

✓5th **K94.0　Colostomy complications**

K94.00　Colostomy complication, unspecified HCC

K94.01　Colostomy hemorrhage HCC

K94.02　Colostomy infection HCC

Use additional code to specify type of infection, such
as:
cellulitis of abdominal wall (L03.311)
sepsis (A40.-, A41.-)

K94.03　Colostomy malfunction HCC

Mechanical complication of colostomy

K94.09　Other complications of colostomy HCC

✓5th **K94.1　Enterostomy complications**

K94.10　Enterostomy complication, unspecified HCC

K94.11　Enterostomy hemorrhage HCC

K94.12　Enterostomy infection HCC

Use additional code to specify type of infection, such
as:
cellulitis of abdominal wall (L03.311)
sepsis (A40.-, A41.-)

K94.13　Enterostomy malfunction HCC

Mechanical complication of enterostomy

K94.19　Other complications of enterostomy HCC

✓5th **K94.2　Gastrostomy complications**

K94.20　Gastrostomy complication, unspecified HCC

K94.21　Gastrostomy hemorrhage HCC

K94.22　Gastrostomy infection HCC

Use additional code to specify type of infection, such
as:
cellulitis of abdominal wall (L03.311)
sepsis (A40.-, A41.-)

K94.23　Gastrostomy malfunction HCC

Mechanical complication of gastrostomy
AHA: 2019,1Q,26

K94.29　Other complications of gastrostomy HCC

✓5th **K94.3　Esophagostomy complications**

K94.30　Esophagostomy complications, unspecified HCC

K94.31　Esophagostomy hemorrhage HCC

K94.32　Esophagostomy infection HCC

Use additional code to identify the infection

K94.33　Esophagostomy malfunction HCC

Mechanical complication of esophagostomy

K94.39　Other complications of esophagostomy HCC

✓4th **K95　Complications of bariatric procedures**

✓5th **K95.0　Complications of** gastric band procedure

K95.01　Infection due to gastric band procedure

Use additional code to specify type of infection or
organism, such as:
bacterial and viral infectious agents (B95.-, B96.-)
cellulitis of abdominal wall (L03.311)
sepsis (A40.-, A41.-)

K95.09　Other complications of gastric band procedure

Use additional code, if applicable, to further specify
complication

✓5th **K95.8　Complications of other bariatric procedure**

EXCLUDES 1　*complications of gastric band surgery (K95.0-)*

K95.81　Infection due to other bariatric procedure

Use additional code to specify type of infection or
organism, such as:
bacterial and viral infectious agents (B95.-, B96.-)
cellulitis of abdominal wall (L03.311)
sepsis (A40.-, A41.-)

K95.89　Other complications of other bariatric procedure

Use additional code, if applicable, to further specify
complication

Chapter 12. Diseases of the Skin and Subcutaneous Tissue (L00–L99)

Chapter-specific Guidelines with Coding Examples

The chapter-specific guidelines from the ICD-10-CM Official Guidelines for Coding and Reporting have been provided below. Along with these guidelines are coding examples, contained in the shaded boxes, that have been developed to help illustrate the coding and/or sequencing guidance found in these guidelines.

a. Pressure ulcer stage codes

1) Pressure ulcer stages

Codes **in** category L89, Pressure ulcer, identify the site **and stage** of the pressure ulcer.

The ICD-10-CM classifies pressure ulcer stages based on severity, which is designated by stages 1-4, **deep tissue pressure injury,** unspecified stage, and unstageable.

Assign as many codes from category L89 as needed to identify all the pressure ulcers the patient has, if applicable.

See Section I.B.14 for pressure ulcer stage documentation by clinicians other than patient's provider.

> Stage 3 pressure ulcer left ankle, 6 x 7 cm that invades the fascia; stage 2 pressure ulcer of left hip
>
> **L89.523**   **Pressure ulcer of left ankle, stage 3**
>
> **L89.222**   **Pressure ulcer of left hip, stage 2**
>
> *Explanation:* Patient has a left ankle pressure ulcer documented as stage 3 and a left hip pressure ulcer documented as stage 2. Combination codes from category L89 Pressure ulcer, identify the site of the pressure ulcer as well as the stage. Assign as many codes from category L89 as needed to identify all the pressure ulcers the patient has.

2) Unstageable pressure ulcers

Assignment of the code for unstageable pressure ulcer (L89.--0) should be based on the clinical documentation. These codes are used for pressure ulcers whose stage cannot be clinically determined (e.g., the ulcer is covered by eschar or has been treated with a skin or muscle graft). This code should not be confused with the codes for unspecified stage (L89.--9). When there is no documentation regarding the stage of the pressure ulcer, assign the appropriate code for unspecified stage (L89.--9).

> Pressure ulcer of the right lower back documented as unstageable due to the presence of thick eschar covering the ulcer
>
> **L89.130**   **Pressure ulcer of right lower back, unstageable**
>
> *Explanation:* Codes for unstageable pressure ulcers are assigned when the stage cannot be clinically determined (e.g., the ulcer is covered by eschar or has been treated with a skin or muscle graft).

3) Documented pressure ulcer stage

Assignment of the pressure ulcer stage code should be guided by clinical documentation of the stage or documentation of the terms found in the Alphabetic Index. For clinical terms describing the stage that are not found in the Alphabetic Index, and there is no documentation of the stage, the provider should be queried.

> Left heel pressure ulcer with partial thickness skin loss involving the dermis
>
> **L89.622**   **Pressure ulcer of left heel, stage 2**
>
> *Explanation:* Code assignment for the pressure ulcer stage should be guided by either the clinical documentation of the stage or the documentation of terms found in the Alphabetic Index. The clinical documentation describing the left heel pressure ulcer "partial thickness skin loss involving the dermis" matches the ICD-10-CM index parenthetical description for stage 2 "(abrasion, blister, partial thickness skin loss involving epidermis and/or dermis)."

4) Patients admitted with pressure ulcers documented as healed

No code is assigned if the documentation states that the pressure ulcer is completely healed **at the time of admission.**

> Patient receiving follow-up examination of a completely healed pressure ulcer of the foot
>
> **Z09**   **Encounter for follow-up examination after completed treatment for conditions other than malignant neoplasm**
>
> **Z87.2**   **Personal history of diseases of the skin and subcutaneous tissue**
>
> *Explanation:* Assign only codes for the reason for the encounter and the personal history of the pressure ulcer. Personal history code Z87.2 includes conditions classifiable to L00–L99 such as pressure ulcer. No code is assigned for a pressure ulcer documented as completely healed.

5) Pressure ulcers documented as healing

Pressure ulcers described as healing should be assigned the appropriate pressure ulcer stage code based on the documentation in the medical record. If the documentation does not provide information about the stage of the healing pressure ulcer, assign the appropriate code for unspecified stage.

If the documentation is unclear as to whether the patient has a current (new) pressure ulcer or if the patient is being treated for a healing pressure ulcer, query the provider.

For ulcers that were present on admission but healed at the time of discharge, assign the code for the site and stage of the pressure ulcer at the time of admission.

6) Patient admitted with pressure ulcer evolving into another stage during the admission

If a patient is admitted to an inpatient hospital with a pressure ulcer at one stage and it progresses to a higher stage, two separate codes should be assigned: one code for the site and stage of the ulcer on admission and a second code for the same ulcer site and the highest stage reported during the stay.

7) Pressure-induced deep tissue damage

For pressure-induced deep tissue damage or deep tissue pressure injury, assign only the appropriate code for pressure-induced deep tissue damage (L89.--6).

b. Non-pressure chronic ulcers

1) Patients admitted with non-pressure ulcers documented as healed

No code is assigned if the documentation states that the non-pressure ulcer is completely healed **at the time of admission.**

2) Non-pressure ulcers documented as healing

Non-pressure ulcers described as healing should be assigned the appropriate non-pressure ulcer code based on the documentation in the medical record. If the documentation does not provide information about the severity of the healing non-pressure ulcer, assign the appropriate code for unspecified severity.

If the documentation is unclear as to whether the patient has a current (new) non-pressure ulcer or if the patient is being treated for a healing non-pressure ulcer, query the provider.

For ulcers that were present on admission but healed at the time of discharge, assign the code for the site and severity of the non-pressure ulcer at the time of admission.

3) Patient admitted with non-pressure ulcer that progresses to another severity level during the admission

If a patient is admitted to an inpatient hospital with a non-pressure ulcer at one severity level and it progresses to a higher severity level, two separate codes should be assigned: one code for the site and severity level of the ulcer on admission and a second code for the same ulcer site and the highest severity level reported during the stay.

See Section I.B.14 for pressure ulcer stage documentation by clinicians other than patient's provider.

Chapter 12. Diseases of the Skin and Subcutaneous Tissue (L00-L99)

EXCLUDES 2   *certain conditions originating in the perinatal period (P04-P96)*
certain infectious and parasitic diseases (A00-B99)
complications of pregnancy, childbirth and the puerperium (O00-O9A)
congenital malformations, deformations, and chromosomal abnormalities (Q00-Q99)
endocrine, nutritional and metabolic diseases (E00-E88)
lipomelanotic reticulosis (I89.8)
neoplasms (C00-D49)
symptoms, signs and abnormal clinical and laboratory findings, not elsewhere classified (R00-R94)
systemic connective tissue disorders (M30-M36)
viral warts (B07.-)

This chapter contains the following blocks:

L00-L08   Infections of the skin and subcutaneous tissue
L10-L14   Bullous disorders
L20-L30   Dermatitis and eczema
L40-L45   Papulosquamous disorders
L49-L54   Urticaria and erythema
L55-L59   Radiation-related disorders of the skin and subcutaneous tissue
L60-L75   Disorders of skin appendages
L76   Intraoperative and postprocedural complications of skin and subcutaneous tissue
L80-L99   Other disorders of the skin and subcutaneous tissue

Infections of the skin and subcutaneous tissue (L00-L08)

Use additional code (B95-B97) to identify infectious agent

EXCLUDES 2   *hordeolum (H00.0)*
infective dermatitis (L30.3)
local infections of skin classified in Chapter 1
lupus panniculitis (L93.2)
panniculitis NOS (M79.3)
panniculitis of neck and back (M54.0-)
perlèche NOS (K13.0)
perlèche due to candidiasis (B37.0)
perlèche due to riboflavin deficiency (E53.0)
pyogenic granuloma (L98.0)
relapsing panniculitis [Weber-Christian] (M35.6)
viral warts (B07.-)
zoster (B02.-)

L00   **Staphylococcal scalded skin syndrome**
Ritter's disease
Use additional code to identify percentage of skin exfoliation (L49.-)

EXCLUDES 1   *bullous impetigo (L01.03)*
pemphigus neonatorum (L01.03)
toxic epidermal necrolysis [Lyell] (L51.2)

DEF: Infectious skin disease of children younger than 5 years marked by eruptions ranging from a few localized blisters to widespread, easily ruptured, fine vesicles and bullae affecting almost the entire body. It results in exfoliation of large planes of skin and leaves raw areas.

✓4ᵗʰ **L01**   **Impetigo**

EXCLUDES 1   *impetigo herpetiformis (L40.1)*

DEF: Acute, superficial, highly contagious skin infection commonly occurring in children. Skin lesions usually appear on the face and consist of vesicles and bullae that burst and form yellow crusts.

✓5ᵗʰ **L01.0**   **Impetigo**

Impetigo contagiosa
Impetigo vulgaris

L01.00   **Impetigo, unspecified**
Impetigo NOS

L01.01   **Non-bullous impetigo**

L01.02   **Bockhart's impetigo**
Impetigo follicularis
Perifolliculitis NOS
Superficial pustular perifolliculitis
DEF: Superficial inflammation of the hair follicles most commonly caused by staph aureus that manifests as rounded, sphere-shaped, pustular eruptions in the areas of the scalp, beard, underarms, extremities, and buttocks.

L01.03   **Bullous impetigo**
Impetigo neonatorum
Pemphigus neonatorum

L01.09   **Other impetigo**
Ulcerative impetigo

L01.1   **Impetiginization of other dermatoses**

✓4ᵗʰ **L02**   **Cutaneous abscess, furuncle and carbuncle**
Use additional code to identify organism (B95-B96)

EXCLUDES 2   *abscess of anus and rectal regions (K61.-)*
abscess of female genital organs (external) (N76.4)
abscess of male genital organs (external) (N48.2, N49.-)

DEF: Carbuncle: Infection of the skin that arises from a collection of interconnected infected boils or furuncles, usually from hair follicles infected by *Staphylococcus.* This condition can produce pus and form drainage cavities.
DEF: Furuncle: Inflamed, painful abscess, cyst, or nodule on the skin caused by bacteria, often *Staphylococcus,* entering along the hair follicle.

✓5ᵗʰ **L02.0**   **Cutaneous abscess, furuncle and carbuncle of face**

EXCLUDES 2   *abscess of ear, external (H60.0)*
abscess of eyelid (H00.0)
abscess of head [any part, except face] (L02.8)
abscess of lacrimal gland (H04.0)
abscess of lacrimal passages (H04.3)
abscess of mouth (K12.2)
abscess of nose (J34.0)
abscess of orbit (H05.0)
submandibular abscess (K12.2)

L02.01   **Cutaneous abscess of face**

L02.02   **Furuncle of face**
Boil of face
Folliculitis of face

L02.03   **Carbuncle of face**

✓5ᵗʰ **L02.1**   **Cutaneous abscess, furuncle and carbuncle of neck**

L02.11   **Cutaneous abscess of neck**

L02.12   **Furuncle of neck**
Boil of neck
Folliculitis of neck

L02.13   **Carbuncle of neck**

✓5ᵗʰ **L02.2**   **Cutaneous abscess, furuncle and carbuncle of trunk**

EXCLUDES 1   *non-newborn omphalitis (L08.82)*
omphalitis of newborn (P38.-)

EXCLUDES 2   *abscess of breast (N61.1)*
abscess of buttocks (L02.3)
abscess of female external genital organs (N76.4)
abscess of hip (L02.4)
abscess of male external genital organs (N48.2, N49.-)

✓6ᵗʰ **L02.21**   **Cutaneous abscess of trunk**

L02.211   **Cutaneous abscess of abdominal wall**
L02.212   **Cutaneous abscess of back [any part, except buttock]**
L02.213   **Cutaneous abscess of chest wall**
L02.214   **Cutaneous abscess of groin**
L02.215   **Cutaneous abscess of perineum**
L02.216   **Cutaneous abscess of umbilicus**
L02.219   **Cutaneous abscess of trunk, unspecified**

✓6ᵗʰ **L02.22**   **Furuncle of trunk**
Boil of trunk
Folliculitis of trunk

L02.221   **Furuncle of abdominal wall**
L02.222   **Furuncle of back [any part, except buttock]**
L02.223   **Furuncle of chest wall**
L02.224   **Furuncle of groin**
L02.225   **Furuncle of perineum**
L02.226   **Furuncle of umbilicus**
L02.229   **Furuncle of trunk, unspecified**

✓6ᵗʰ **L02.23**   **Carbuncle of trunk**

L02.231   **Carbuncle of abdominal wall**
L02.232   **Carbuncle of back [any part, except buttock]**
L02.233   **Carbuncle of chest wall**
L02.234   **Carbuncle of groin**
L02.235   **Carbuncle of perineum**
L02.236   **Carbuncle of umbilicus**
L02.239   **Carbuncle of trunk, unspecified**

✓5ᵗʰ **L02.3**   **Cutaneous abscess, furuncle and carbuncle of buttock**

EXCLUDES 1   *pilonidal cyst with abscess (L05.01)*

L02.31   **Cutaneous abscess of buttock**
Cutaneous abscess of gluteal region

      L02.32   **Furuncle of buttock**
               Boil of buttock
               Folliculitis of buttock
               Furuncle of gluteal region

      L02.33   **Carbuncle of buttock**
               Carbuncle of gluteal region

✓5ᵗʰ L02.4   Cutaneous abscess, furuncle and carbuncle of limb
       EXCLUDES 2   *cutaneous abscess, furuncle and carbuncle of groin (L02.214, L02.224, L02.234)*
                 cutaneous abscess, furuncle and carbuncle of hand (L02.5-)
                 cutaneous abscess, furuncle and carbuncle of foot (L02.6-)

    ✓6ᵗʰ L02.41   Cutaneous abscess of limb
         L02.411   Cutaneous abscess of right axilla
         L02.412   Cutaneous abscess of left axilla
         L02.413   Cutaneous abscess of right upper limb
         L02.414   Cutaneous abscess of left upper limb
         L02.415   Cutaneous abscess of right lower limb
         L02.416   Cutaneous abscess of left lower limb
         L02.419   Cutaneous abscess of limb, unspecified

    ✓6ᵗʰ L02.42   Furuncle of limb
         Boil of limb
         Folliculitis of limb
         L02.421   Furuncle of right axilla
         L02.422   Furuncle of left axilla
         L02.423   Furuncle of right upper limb
         L02.424   Furuncle of left upper limb
         L02.425   Furuncle of right lower limb
         L02.426   Furuncle of left lower limb
         L02.429   Furuncle of limb, unspecified

    ✓6ᵗʰ L02.43   Carbuncle of limb
         L02.431   Carbuncle of right axilla
         L02.432   Carbuncle of left axilla
         L02.433   Carbuncle of right upper limb
         L02.434   Carbuncle of left upper limb
         L02.435   Carbuncle of right lower limb
         L02.436   Carbuncle of left lower limb
         L02.439   Carbuncle of limb, unspecified

✓5ᵗʰ L02.5   Cutaneous abscess, furuncle and carbuncle of hand

    ✓6ᵗʰ L02.51   Cutaneous abscess of hand
         L02.511   Cutaneous abscess of right hand
         L02.512   Cutaneous abscess of left hand
         L02.519   Cutaneous abscess of unspecified hand

    ✓6ᵗʰ L02.52   Furuncle hand
         Boil of hand
         Folliculitis of hand
         L02.521   Furuncle right hand
         L02.522   Furuncle left hand
         L02.529   Furuncle unspecified hand

    ✓6ᵗʰ L02.53   Carbuncle of hand
         L02.531   Carbuncle of right hand
         L02.532   Carbuncle of left hand
         L02.539   Carbuncle of unspecified hand

✓5ᵗʰ L02.6   Cutaneous abscess, furuncle and carbuncle of foot

    ✓6ᵗʰ L02.61   Cutaneous abscess of foot
         L02.611   Cutaneous abscess of right foot
         L02.612   Cutaneous abscess of left foot
         L02.619   Cutaneous abscess of unspecified foot

    ✓6ᵗʰ L02.62   Furuncle of foot
         Boil of foot
         Folliculitis of foot
         L02.621   Furuncle of right foot
         L02.622   Furuncle of left foot
         L02.629   Furuncle of unspecified foot

    ✓6ᵗʰ L02.63   Carbuncle of foot
         L02.631   Carbuncle of right foot
         L02.632   Carbuncle of left foot
         L02.639   Carbuncle of unspecified foot

✓5ᵗʰ L02.8   Cutaneous abscess, furuncle and carbuncle of other sites

    ✓6ᵗʰ L02.81   Cutaneous abscess of other sites
         L02.811   Cutaneous abscess of head [any part, except face]
         L02.818   Cutaneous abscess of other sites

    ✓6ᵗʰ L02.82   Furuncle of other sites
         Boil of other sites
         Folliculitis of other sites
         L02.821   Furuncle of head [any part, except face]
         L02.828   Furuncle of other sites

    ✓6ᵗʰ L02.83   Carbuncle of other sites
         L02.831   Carbuncle of head [any part, except face]
         L02.838   Carbuncle of other sites

✓5ᵗʰ L02.9   Cutaneous abscess, furuncle and carbuncle, unspecified

       L02.91   Cutaneous abscess, unspecified

       L02.92   Furuncle, unspecified
          Boil NOS
          Furunculosis NOS

       L02.93   Carbuncle, unspecified

✓4ᵗʰ L03   Cellulitis and acute lymphangitis

       EXCLUDES 2   *cellulitis of anal and rectal region (K61.-)*
                cellulitis of external auditory canal (H60.1)
                cellulitis of eyelid (H00.0)
                cellulitis of female external genital organs (N76.4)
                cellulitis of lacrimal apparatus (H04.3)
                cellulitis of male external genital organs (N48.2, N49.-)
                cellulitis of mouth (K12.2)
                cellulitis of nose (J34.0)
                eosinophilic cellulitis [Wells] (L98.3)
                febrile neutrophilic dermatosis [Sweet] (L98.2)
                lymphangitis (chronic) (subacute) (I89.1)

       AHA: 2017,4Q,100
       DEF: Cellulitis: Infection of the skin and subcutaneous tissues, most often caused by *Staphylococcus* or *Streptococcus* bacteria secondary to a cutaneous lesion. Progression of the inflammation may lead to abscess and tissue death, or even systemic infection-like bacteremia.
       DEF: Lymphangitis: Inflammation of the lymph channels most often caused by *Streptococcus*.

✓5ᵗʰ L03.0   Cellulitis and acute lymphangitis of finger and toe
       Infection of nail
       Onychia
       Paronychia
       Perionychia

    ✓6ᵗʰ L03.01   Cellulitis of finger
         Felon
         Whitlow
         EXCLUDES 1   *herpetic whitlow (B00.89)*
         DEF: Felon: Superficial bacterial skin infection at the tip of the finger.
         L03.011   Cellulitis of right finger
         L03.012   Cellulitis of left finger
         L03.019   Cellulitis of unspecified finger

    ✓6ᵗʰ L03.02   Acute lymphangitis of finger
         Hangnail with lymphangitis of finger
         L03.021   Acute lymphangitis of right finger
         L03.022   Acute lymphangitis of left finger
         L03.029   Acute lymphangitis of unspecified finger

    ✓6ᵗʰ L03.03   Cellulitis of toe
         L03.031   Cellulitis of right toe
         L03.032   Cellulitis of left toe
         L03.039   Cellulitis of unspecified toe

    ✓6ᵗʰ L03.04   Acute lymphangitis of toe
         Hangnail with lymphangitis of toe
         L03.041   Acute lymphangitis of right toe
         L03.042   Acute lymphangitis of left toe
         L03.049   Acute lymphangitis of unspecified toe

✓5ᵗʰ L03.1   Cellulitis and acute lymphangitis of other parts of limb

    ✓6ᵗʰ L03.11   Cellulitis of other parts of limb
         EXCLUDES 2   *cellulitis of fingers (L03.01-)*
                 cellulitis of toes (L03.03-)
                 groin (L03.314)
         L03.111   Cellulitis of right axilla
         L03.112   Cellulitis of left axilla
         L03.113   Cellulitis of right upper limb
         L03.114   Cellulitis of left upper limb
         L03.115   Cellulitis of right lower limb
         L03.116   Cellulitis of left lower limb
         L03.119   Cellulitis of unspecified part of limb

√6ᵗʰ **L03.12** Acute lymphangitis of other parts of limb

　　EXCLUDES 2　*acute lymphangitis of fingers (L03.2-)*
　　　　　　　acute lymphangitis of groin (L03.324)
　　　　　　　acute lymphangitis of toes (L03.04-)

L03.121 Acute lymphangitis of **right axilla**
L03.122 Acute lymphangitis of **left axilla**
L03.123 Acute lymphangitis of **right upper limb**
L03.124 Acute lymphangitis of **left upper limb**
L03.125 Acute lymphangitis of **right lower limb**
L03.126 Acute lymphangitis of **left lower limb**
L03.129 Acute lymphangitis of **unspecified part of limb**

√5ᵗʰ **L03.2** Cellulitis and acute lymphangitis of **face and neck**

√6ᵗʰ **L03.21** Cellulitis and acute lymphangitis of **face**

L03.211 **Cellulitis of face**

　　EXCLUDES 2　*abscess of orbit (H05.01-)*
　　　　　　　cellulitis of ear (H60.1-)
　　　　　　　cellulitis of eyelid (H00.0-)
　　　　　　　cellulitis of head (L03.81)
　　　　　　　cellulitis of lacrimal apparatus (H04.3)
　　　　　　　cellulitis of lip (K13.0)
　　　　　　　cellulitis of mouth (K12.2)
　　　　　　　cellulitis of nose (internal) (J34.0)
　　　　　　　cellulitis of orbit (H05.01-)
　　　　　　　cellulitis of scalp (L03.81)

　　　　AHA: 2013,4Q,123

L03.212 Acute lymphangitis **of face**
L03.213 **Periorbital cellulitis**
　　　　Preseptal cellulitis
　　　　AHA: 2016,4Q,36

√6ᵗʰ **L03.22** Cellulitis and acute lymphangitis of **neck**

L03.221 **Cellulitis** of **neck**
L03.222 **Acute lymphangitis** of **neck**

√5ᵗʰ **L03.3** Cellulitis and acute lymphangitis of **trunk**

√6ᵗʰ **L03.31** **Cellulitis of trunk**

　　EXCLUDES 2　*cellulitis of anal and rectal regions (K61.-)*
　　　　　　　cellulitis of breast NOS (N61.0)
　　　　　　　cellulitis of female external genital organs (N76.4)
　　　　　　　cellulitis of male external genital organs (N48.2, N49.-)
　　　　　　　omphalitis of newborn (P38.-)
　　　　　　　puerperal cellulitis of breast (O91.2)

L03.311 **Cellulitis of abdominal wall**

　　EXCLUDES 2　*cellulitis of umbilicus (L03.316)*
　　　　　　　cellulitis of groin (L03.314)

L03.312 **Cellulitis of back [any part except buttock]**
L03.313 **Cellulitis of chest wall**
L03.314 **Cellulitis of groin**
L03.315 **Cellulitis of perineum**
L03.316 **Cellulitis of umbilicus**
L03.317 **Cellulitis of buttock**
L03.319 **Cellulitis of trunk, unspecified**

√6ᵗʰ **L03.32** **Acute lymphangitis of trunk**

L03.321 Acute lymphangitis of **abdominal wall**
L03.322 Acute lymphangitis of **back [any part except buttock]**
L03.323 Acute lymphangitis of **chest wall**
L03.324 Acute lymphangitis of **groin**
L03.325 Acute lymphangitis of **perineum**
L03.326 Acute lymphangitis of **umbilicus**
L03.327 Acute lymphangitis of **buttock**
L03.329 Acute lymphangitis of **trunk, unspecified**

√5ᵗʰ **L03.8** Cellulitis and acute lymphangitis of **other sites**

√6ᵗʰ **L03.81** **Cellulitis of other sites**

L03.811 **Cellulitis of head [any part, except face]**
　　　　Cellulitis of scalp
　　　　EXCLUDES 2　*cellulitis of face (L03.211)*
L03.818 **Cellulitis of other sites**

√6ᵗʰ **L03.89** **Acute lymphangitis of other sites**

L03.891 Acute lymphangitis of **head [any part, except face]**

L03.898 Acute lymphangitis of other sites

√5ᵗʰ **L03.9** Cellulitis and acute lymphangitis, unspecified

L03.90 **Cellulitis, unspecified**
L03.91 **Acute lymphangitis, unspecified**

　　EXCLUDES 1　*lymphangitis NOS (I89.1)*

√4ᵗʰ **L04** Acute lymphadenitis

　　INCLUDES　abscess (acute) of lymph nodes, except mesenteric
　　　　　　acute lymphadenitis, except mesenteric
　　EXCLUDES 1　*chronic or subacute lymphadenitis, except mesenteric (I88.1)*
　　　　　　enlarged lymph nodes (R59.-)
　　　　　　human immunodeficiency virus [HIV] disease resulting in generalized lymphadenopathy (B20)
　　　　　　lymphadenitis NOS (I88.9)
　　　　　　nonspecific mesenteric lymphadenitis (I88.0)

　　DEF: Inflammation or enlargement of the lymph nodes.

L04.0 Acute lymphadenitis of **face, head and neck**
L04.1 Acute lymphadenitis of **trunk**
L04.2 Acute lymphadenitis of **upper limb**
　　　Acute lymphadenitis of axilla
　　　Acute lymphadenitis of shoulder
L04.3 Acute lymphadenitis of **lower limb**
　　　Acute lymphadenitis of hip
　　　EXCLUDES 2　*acute lymphadenitis of groin (L04.1)*
L04.8 Acute lymphadenitis of **other sites**
L04.9 Acute lymphadenitis, **unspecified**

√4ᵗʰ **L05** Pilonidal cyst and sinus

　　DEF: Pilonidal cyst: Sac or sinus cavity of trapped epithelial tissues in the sacrococcygeal region, usually associated with ingrown hair.
　　DEF: Pilonidal sinus: Fistula, tract, or channel that extends from an infected area of ingrown hair to another site within the skin or out to the skin surface.

Pilonidal Cyst

Skin
Fistula
Pilonidal cyst
Fat
Bone

√5ᵗʰ **L05.0** **Pilonidal cyst and sinus** with abscess

L05.01 **Pilonidal cyst with abscess**
　　　Pilonidal abscess
　　　Pilonidal dimple with abscess
　　　Postanal dimple with abscess
　　　EXCLUDES 2　*congenital sacral dimple (Q82.6)*
　　　　　　　parasacral dimple (Q82.6)

L05.02 **Pilonidal sinus with abscess**
　　　Coccygeal fistula with abscess
　　　Coccygeal sinus with abscess
　　　Pilonidal fistula with abscess

√5ᵗʰ **L05.9** **Pilonidal cyst and sinus** without abscess

L05.91 **Pilonidal cyst without abscess**
　　　Pilonidal dimple
　　　Postanal dimple
　　　Pilonidal cyst NOS
　　　EXCLUDES 2　*congenital sacral dimple (Q82.6)*
　　　　　　　parasacral dimple (Q82.6)

L05.92 **Pilonidal sinus without abscess**
　　　Coccygeal fistula
　　　Coccygeal sinus without abscess
　　　Pilonidal fistula

☑4ᵗʰ **L08 Other local infections of skin and subcutaneous tissue**

    L08.0 Pyoderma
        Dermatitis gangrenosa
        Purulent dermatitis
        Septic dermatitis
        Suppurative dermatitis
        EXCLUDES 1   *pyoderma gangrenosum (L88)*
                    pyoderma vegetans (L08.81)
        DEF: Any superficial skin disease commonly characterized by the discharging of pus not attributed to another condition.

    L08.1 Erythrasma
        DEF: Chronic, superficial skin infection of brown scaly patches, commonly found in skin folds most prevalent in the overweight or diabetic population.

☑5ᵗʰ   **L08.8 Other specified local infections of the skin and subcutaneous tissue**

        L08.81 Pyoderma vegetans
            EXCLUDES 1   *pyoderma gangrenosum (L88)*
                       pyoderma NOS (L08.0)

        L08.82 Omphalitis not of newborn
            EXCLUDES 1   *omphalitis of newborn (P38.-)*

        L08.89 Other specified local infections of the skin and subcutaneous tissue

    L08.9 Local infection of the skin and subcutaneous tissue, unspecified

Bullous disorders (L10-L14)

EXCLUDES 1   *benign familial pemphigus [Hailey-Hailey] (Q82.8)*
              staphylococcal scalded skin syndrome (L00)
              toxic epidermal necrolysis [Lyell] (L51.2)

☑4ᵗʰ **L10 Pemphigus**

    EXCLUDES 1   *pemphigus neonatorum (L01.03)*

    L10.0 Pemphigus vulgaris
    L10.1 Pemphigus vegetans
    L10.2 Pemphigus foliaceous
    L10.3 Brazilian pemphigus [fogo selvagem]
    L10.4 Pemphigus erythematosus
        Senear-Usher syndrome
    L10.5 Drug-induced pemphigus
        Use additional code for adverse effect, if applicable, to identify drug (T36-T50 with fifth or sixth character 5)

☑5ᵗʰ   **L10.8 Other pemphigus**
        L10.81 Paraneoplastic pemphigus
        L10.89 Other pemphigus
    L10.9 Pemphigus, unspecified

☑4ᵗʰ **L11 Other acantholytic disorders**

    L11.0 Acquired keratosis follicularis
        EXCLUDES 1   *keratosis follicularis (congenital) [Darier-White] (Q82.8)*

    L11.1 Transient acantholytic dermatosis [Grover]
    L11.8 Other specified acantholytic disorders
    L11.9 Acantholytic disorder, unspecified

☑4ᵗʰ **L12 Pemphigoid**

    EXCLUDES 1   *herpes gestationis (O26.4-)*
              impetigo herpetiformis (L40.1)

    L12.0 Bullous pemphigoid
    L12.1 Cicatricial pemphigoid
        Benign mucous membrane pemphigoid
        DEF: Chronic autoimmune disease characterized by subepidermal blistering lesions of the mucosa, including the conjunctiva. It is seen predominantly in the elderly and produces adhesions and scarring.

    L12.2 Chronic bullous disease of childhood   P
        Juvenile dermatitis herpetiformis

☑5ᵗʰ   **L12.3 Acquired epidermolysis bullosa**
        EXCLUDES 1   *epidermolysis bullosa (congenital) (Q81.-)*

        L12.30 Acquired epidermolysis bullosa, unspecified   HCC
        L12.31 Epidermolysis bullosa due to drug   HCC
            Use additional code for adverse effect, if applicable, to identify drug (T36-T50 with fifth or sixth character 5)

        L12.35 Other acquired epidermolysis bullosa   HCC

    L12.8 Other pemphigoid
    L12.9 Pemphigoid, unspecified

☑4ᵗʰ **L13 Other bullous disorders**

    L13.0 Dermatitis herpetiformis
        Duhring's disease
        Hydroa herpetiformis
        EXCLUDES 1   *juvenile dermatitis herpetiformis (L12.2)*
                    senile dermatitis herpetiformis (L12.0)
        DEF: Skin disease to which people are genetically predisposed resulting from an immunological response to gluten. Dermatitis herpetiformis is an extremely pruritic eruption of various lesions that frequently heal, leaving hyperpigmentation or hypopigmentation and occasionally scarring. It is usually associated with asymptomatic gluten-sensitive enteropathy.

    L13.1 Subcorneal pustular dermatitis
        Sneddon-Wilkinson disease
    L13.8 Other specified bullous disorders
    L13.9 Bullous disorder, unspecified

L14   ***Bullous disorders in diseases classified elsewhere***
    Code first underlying disease

Dermatitis and eczema (L20-L30)

NOTE   In this block the terms dermatitis and eczema are used synonymously and interchangeably.

EXCLUDES 2   *chronic (childhood) granulomatous disease (D71)*
              dermatitis gangrenosa (L08.0)
              dermatitis herpetiformis (L13.0)
              dry skin dermatitis (L85.3)
              factitial dermatitis (L98.1)
              perioral dermatitis (L71.0)
              radiation-related disorders of the skin and subcutaneous tissue (L55-L59)
              stasis dermatitis (I87.2)

☑4ᵗʰ **L20 Atopic dermatitis**

    L20.0 Besnier's prurigo

☑5ᵗʰ   **L20.8 Other atopic dermatitis**
        EXCLUDES 2   *circumscribed neurodermatitis (L28.0)*

        L20.81 Atopic neurodermatitis
            Diffuse neurodermatitis
        L20.82 Flexural eczema
        L20.83 Infantile (acute) (chronic) eczema   P
        L20.84 Intrinsic (allergic) eczema
        L20.89 Other atopic dermatitis
    L20.9 Atopic dermatitis, unspecified

☑4ᵗʰ **L21 Seborrheic dermatitis**

    EXCLUDES 2   *infective dermatitis (L30.3)*
              seborrheic keratosis (L82.-)

    L21.0 Seborrhea capitis
        Cradle cap
        AHA: 2018,1Q,6
        TIP: Assign for dandruff in an adult patient.

    L21.1 Seborrheic infantile dermatitis   P
    L21.8 Other seborrheic dermatitis
    L21.9 Seborrheic dermatitis, unspecified
        Seborrhea NOS

L22 Diaper dermatitis
    Diaper erythema
    Diaper rash
    Psoriasiform diaper rash

☑4ᵗʰ **L23 Allergic contact dermatitis**

    EXCLUDES 1   *allergy NOS (T78.40)*
              contact dermatitis NOS (L25.9)
              dermatitis NOS (L30.9)
    EXCLUDES 2   *dermatitis due to substances taken internally (L27.-)*
              dermatitis of eyelid (H01.1-)
              diaper dermatitis (L22)
              eczema of external ear (H60.5-)
              irritant contact dermatitis (L24.-)
              perioral dermatitis (L71.0)
              radiation-related disorders of the skin and subcutaneous tissue (L55-L59)

    L23.0 Allergic contact dermatitis due to metals
        Allergic contact dermatitis due to chromium
        Allergic contact dermatitis due to nickel

    L23.1 Allergic contact dermatitis due to adhesives
    L23.2 Allergic contact dermatitis due to cosmetics

☑ Additional Character Required   ☑ˣ⁷ᵗʰ Placeholder Alert   Manifestation   Unspecified Dx   ▶◀ Revised Text   ● New Code   ▲ Revised Code Title

ICD-10-CM 2020   725

L23.3 **Allergic contact dermatitis due to** drugs in contact with skin
Use additional code for adverse effect, if applicable, to identify drug (T36-T50 with fifth or sixth character 5)
> EXCLUDES 2   *dermatitis due to ingested drugs and medicaments (L27.0-L27.1)*

L23.4 **Allergic contact dermatitis due to** dyes

L23.5 **Allergic contact dermatitis due to other chemical products**
Allergic contact dermatitis due to cement
Allergic contact dermatitis due to insecticide
Allergic contact dermatitis due to plastic
Allergic contact dermatitis due to rubber

L23.6 **Allergic contact dermatitis due to** food in contact with the skin
> EXCLUDES 2   *dermatitis due to ingested food (L27.2)*

L23.7 **Allergic contact dermatitis due to** plants, except food
> EXCLUDES 2   *allergy NOS due to pollen (J30.1)*

✓5ᵗʰ **L23.8** **Allergic contact dermatitis due to other agents**

   L23.81 **Allergic contact dermatitis due to** animal (cat) (dog) dander
Allergic contact dermatitis due to animal (cat) (dog) hair

   L23.89 **Allergic contact dermatitis due to other agents**

L23.9 **Allergic contact dermatitis, unspecified cause**
Allergic contact eczema NOS

✓4ᵗʰ **L24** **Irritant contact** dermatitis
> EXCLUDES 1   *allergy NOS (T78.40)*
> *contact dermatitis NOS (L25.9)*
> *dermatitis NOS (L30.9)*
> EXCLUDES 2   *allergic contact dermatitis (L23.-)*
> *dermatitis due to substances taken internally (L27.-)*
> *dermatitis of eyelid (H01.1-)*
> *diaper dermatitis (L22)*
> *eczema of external ear (H60.5-)*
> *perioral dermatitis (L71.0)*
> *radiation-related disorders of the skin and subcutaneous tissue (L55-L59)*

L24.0 **Irritant contact dermatitis due to** detergents

L24.1 **Irritant contact dermatitis due to** oils and greases

L24.2 **Irritant contact dermatitis due to** solvents
Irritant contact dermatitis due to chlorocompound
Irritant contact dermatitis due to cyclohexane
Irritant contact dermatitis due to ester
Irritant contact dermatitis due to glycol
Irritant contact dermatitis due to hydrocarbon
Irritant contact dermatitis due to ketone

L24.3 **Irritant contact dermatitis due to** cosmetics

L24.4 **Irritant contact dermatitis due to** drugs in contact with skin
Use additional code for adverse effect, if applicable, to identify drug (T36-T50 with fifth or sixth character 5)

L24.5 **Irritant contact dermatitis due to other chemical products**
Irritant contact dermatitis due to cement
Irritant contact dermatitis due to insecticide
Irritant contact dermatitis due to plastic
Irritant contact dermatitis due to rubber

L24.6 **Irritant contact dermatitis due to** food in contact with skin
> EXCLUDES 2   *dermatitis due to ingested food (L27.2)*

L24.7 **Irritant contact dermatitis due to** plants, except food
> EXCLUDES 2   *allergy NOS to pollen (J30.1)*

✓5ᵗʰ **L24.8** **Irritant contact dermatitis due to other agents**

   L24.81 **Irritant contact dermatitis due to** metals
Irritant contact dermatitis due to chromium
Irritant contact dermatitis due to nickel

   L24.89 **Irritant contact dermatitis due to other agents**
Irritant contact dermatitis due to dyes

L24.9 **Irritant contact dermatitis, unspecified cause**
Irritant contact eczema NOS

✓4ᵗʰ **L25** **Unspecified contact dermatitis**
> EXCLUDES 1   *allergic contact dermatitis (L23.-)*
> *allergy NOS (T78.40)*
> *dermatitis NOS (L30.9)*
> *irritant contact dermatitis (L24.-)*
> EXCLUDES 2   *dermatitis due to ingested substances (L27.-)*
> *dermatitis of eyelid (H01.1-)*
> *eczema of external ear (H60.5-)*
> *perioral dermatitis (L71.0)*
> *radiation-related disorders of the skin and subcutaneous tissue (L55-L59)*

L25.0 **Unspecified contact dermatitis due to** cosmetics

L25.1 **Unspecified contact dermatitis due to** drugs in contact with skin
Use additional code for adverse effect, if applicable, to identify drug (T36-T50 with fifth or sixth character 5)
> EXCLUDES 2   *dermatitis due to ingested drugs and medicaments (L27.0-L27.1)*

L25.2 **Unspecified contact dermatitis due to** dyes

L25.3 **Unspecified contact dermatitis due to other chemical products**
Unspecified contact dermatitis due to cement
Unspecified contact dermatitis due to insecticide

L25.4 **Unspecified contact dermatitis due to** food in contact with skin
> EXCLUDES 2   *dermatitis due to ingested food (L27.2)*

L25.5 **Unspecified contact dermatitis due to** plants, except food
> EXCLUDES 1   *nettle rash (L50.9)*
> EXCLUDES 2   *allergy NOS due to pollen (J30.1)*

L25.8 **Unspecified contact dermatitis due to other agents**

L25.9 **Unspecified contact dermatitis, unspecified cause**
Contact dermatitis (occupational) NOS
Contact eczema (occupational) NOS

L26 **Exfoliative** dermatitis
Hebra's pityriasis
> EXCLUDES 1   *Ritter's disease (L00)*

✓4ᵗʰ **L27** **Dermatitis** due to substances taken internally
> EXCLUDES 1   *allergy NOS (T78.40)*
> EXCLUDES 2   *adverse food reaction, except dermatitis (T78.0-T78.1)*
> *contact dermatitis (L23-L25)*
> *drug photoallergic response (L56.1)*
> *drug phototoxic response (L56.0)*
> *urticaria (L50.-)*

L27.0 **Generalized skin eruption due to** drugs and medicaments taken internally
Use additional code for adverse effect, if applicable, to identify drug (T36-T50 with fifth or sixth character 5)

L27.1 **Localized skin eruption due to** drugs and medicaments taken internally
Use additional code for adverse effect, if applicable, to identify drug (T36-T50 with fifth or sixth character 5)

L27.2 **Dermatitis** due to ingested food
> EXCLUDES 2   *dermatitis due to food in contact with skin (L23.6, L24.6, L25.4)*

L27.8 **Dermatitis due to other substances taken internally**

L27.9 **Dermatitis due to unspecified substance taken internally**

✓4ᵗʰ **L28** **Lichen simplex chronicus and prurigo**

L28.0 **Lichen simplex chronicus**
Circumscribed neurodermatitis
Lichen NOS

L28.1 **Prurigo nodularis**

L28.2 **Other prurigo**
Prurigo NOS
Prurigo Hebra
Prurigo mitis
Urticaria papulosa

✓4ᵗʰ **L29** **Pruritus**
> EXCLUDES 1   *neurotic excoriation (L98.1)*
> *psychogenic pruritus (F45.8)*

L29.0 **Pruritus** ani

L29.1 **Pruritus** scroti   ♂

L29.2 **Pruritus** vulvae   ♀

L29.3 **Anogenital** pruritus, unspecified

L29.8 **Other pruritus**

L29.9 Pruritus, unspecified
Itch NOS

☑4ᵗʰ **L30 Other and unspecified dermatitis**
    EXCLUDES 2   contact dermatitis (L23-L25)
                 dry skin dermatitis (L85.3)
                 small plaque parapsoriasis (L41.3)
                 stasis dermatitis (I87.2)

L30.0 Nummular dermatitis

L30.1 Dyshidrosis [pompholyx]

L30.2 Cutaneous autosensitization
Candidid [levurid]
Dermatophytid
Eczematid

L30.3 Infective dermatitis
Infectious eczematoid dermatitis

L30.4 Erythema intertrigo

L30.5 Pityriasis alba
AHA: 2018,1Q,6

L30.8 Other specified dermatitis

L30.9 Dermatitis, unspecified
Eczema NOS

Papulosquamous disorders (L40-L45)

☑4ᵗʰ **L40 Psoriasis**
DEF: Chronic autoimmune condition that speeds up skin cell growth, causing excessive immature skin cells to form raised, rounded erythematous lesions covered by dry, silvery scaling patches. Most commonly found on the scalp, elbows, knees, hands, feet, and genitals, it can also affect the joints with stiffness and swelling.

L40.0 Psoriasis vulgaris
Nummular psoriasis
Plaque psoriasis

L40.1 Generalized pustular psoriasis
Impetigo herpetiformis
Von Zumbusch's disease

L40.2 Acrodermatitis continua

L40.3 Pustulosis palmaris et plantaris

L40.4 Guttate psoriasis

☑5ᵗʰ **L40.5 Arthropathic psoriasis**
  L40.50 Arthropathic psoriasis, unspecified   HCC
  L40.51 Distal interphalangeal psoriatic arthropathy   HCC
  L40.52 Psoriatic arthritis mutilans   HCC
  L40.53 Psoriatic spondylitis   HCC
  L40.54 Psoriatic Juvenile arthropathy   HCC
  L40.59 Other psoriatic arthropathy   HCC

L40.8 Other psoriasis
Flexural psoriasis

L40.9 Psoriasis, unspecified

☑4ᵗʰ **L41 Parapsoriasis**
    EXCLUDES 1   poikiloderma vasculare atrophicans (L94.5)

L41.0 Pityriasis lichenoides et varioliformis acuta
Mucha-Habermann disease

L41.1 Pityriasis lichenoides chronica

L41.3 Small plaque parapsoriasis

L41.4 Large plaque parapsoriasis

L41.5 Retiform parapsoriasis

L41.8 Other parapsoriasis

L41.9 Parapsoriasis, unspecified

L42 Pityriasis rosea

☑4ᵗʰ **L43 Lichen planus**
    EXCLUDES 1   lichen planopilaris (L66.1)

L43.0 Hypertrophic lichen planus

L43.1 Bullous lichen planus

L43.2 Lichenoid drug reaction
Use additional code for adverse effect, if applicable, to identify drug (T36-T50 with fifth or sixth character 5)

L43.3 Subacute (active) lichen planus
Lichen planus tropicus

L43.8 Other lichen planus

L43.9 Lichen planus, unspecified

☑4ᵗʰ **L44 Other papulosquamous disorders**

L44.0 Pityriasis rubra pilaris

L44.1 Lichen nitidus
DEF: Chronic, inflammatory, asymptomatic skin disorder, characterized by numerous glistening, flat-topped, discrete, skin-colored micropapules, most often on the penis, lower abdomen, inner thighs, wrists, forearms, breasts, and buttocks.

L44.2 Lichen striatus

L44.3 Lichen ruber moniliformis

L44.4 Infantile papular acrodermatitis [Gianotti-Crosti]   P

L44.8 Other specified papulosquamous disorders

L44.9 Papulosquamous disorder, unspecified

L45 Papulosquamous disorders in diseases classified elsewhere
Code first underlying disease

Urticaria and erythema (L49-L54)

    EXCLUDES 1   Lyme disease (A69.2-)
                 rosacea (L71.-)

☑4ᵗʰ **L49 Exfoliation due to erythematous conditions according to extent of body surface involved**
Code first erythematous condition causing exfoliation, such as:
Ritter's disease (L00)
▶(Staphylococcal) scalded skin syndrome◀ (L00)
Stevens-Johnson syndrome (L51.1)
Stevens-Johnson syndrome-toxic epidermal necrolysis overlap syndrome (L51.3)
toxic epidermal necrolysis (L51.2)
DEF: Exfoliation: Falling or sloughing off skin in layers.

L49.0 Exfoliation due to erythematous condition involving less than 10 percent of body surface
Exfoliation due to erythematous condition NOS

L49.1 Exfoliation due to erythematous condition involving 10-19 percent of body surface

L49.2 Exfoliation due to erythematous condition involving 20-29 percent of body surface

L49.3 Exfoliation due to erythematous condition involving 30-39 percent of body surface

L49.4 Exfoliation due to erythematous condition involving 40-49 percent of body surface

L49.5 Exfoliation due to erythematous condition involving 50-59 percent of body surface

L49.6 Exfoliation due to erythematous condition involving 60-69 percent of body surface

L49.7 Exfoliation due to erythematous condition involving 70-79 percent of body surface

L49.8 Exfoliation due to erythematous condition involving 80-89 percent of body surface

L49.9 Exfoliation due to erythematous condition involving 90 or more percent of body surface

☑4ᵗʰ **L50 Urticaria**
    EXCLUDES 1   allergic contact dermatitis (L23.-)
                 angioneurotic edema (T78.3)
                 giant urticaria (T78.3)
                 hereditary angio-edema (D84.1)
                 Quincke's edema (T78.3)
                 serum urticaria (T80.6-)
                 solar urticaria (L56.3)
                 urticaria neonatorum (P83.8)
                 urticaria papulosa (L28.2)
                 urticaria pigmentosa ▶(D47.01)◀
DEF: Eruption of itching edema of the skin. **Synonym(s):** hives.

L50.0 Allergic urticaria

L50.1 Idiopathic urticaria

L50.2 Urticaria due to cold and heat
    EXCLUDES 2   familial cold urticaria (M04.2)

L50.3 Dermatographic urticaria

L50.4 Vibratory urticaria

L50.5 Cholinergic urticaria

L50.6 Contact urticaria

L50.8 Other urticaria
Chronic urticaria
Recurrent periodic urticaria

L50.9 Urticaria, unspecified

☑ Additional Character Required   ✓x7ᵗʰ Placeholder Alert   Manifestation   Unspecified Dx   ▶◀ Revised Text   ● New Code   ▲ Revised Code Title

Chapter 12. Diseases of the Skin and Subcutaneous Tissue

L51–L59.9

✓4ᵗʰ L51 Erythema multiforme

Use additional code for adverse effect, if applicable, to identify drug (T36-T50 with fifth or sixth character 5)

Use additional code to identify associated manifestations, such as:
arthropathy associated with dermatological disorders (M14.8-)
conjunctival edema (H11.42)
conjunctivitis (H10.22-)
corneal scars and opacities (H17.-)
corneal ulcer (H16.0-)
edema of eyelid (H02.84-)
inflammation of eyelid (H01.8)
keratoconjunctivitis sicca (H16.22-)
mechanical lagophthalmos (H02.22-)
stomatitis (K12.-)
symblepharon (H11.23-)

Use additional code to identify percentage of skin exfoliation (L49.-)

    EXCLUDES 1   staphylococcal scalded skin syndrome (L00)
              Ritter's disease (L00)

DEF: Acute complex of symptoms with a varied pattern of skin eruptions, such as macular, bullous, popular, nodose, or vesicular lesions on the neck, face, and legs. Erythema (redness of skin and mucous membranes) multiforme (multiple forms) is a hypersensitivity (allergic) reaction that can occur at any age but primarily affects children or young adults.

L51.0 Nonbullous erythema multiforme

L51.1 Stevens-Johnson syndrome   HCC

L51.2 Toxic epidermal necrolysis [Lyell]   HCC

L51.3 Stevens-Johnson syndrome-toxic epidermal necrolysis overlap syndrome   HCC
SJS-TEN overlap syndrome

L51.8 Other erythema multiforme

L51.9 Erythema multiforme, unspecified
Erythema iris
Erythema multiforme major NOS
Erythema multiforme minor NOS
Herpes iris

L52 Erythema nodosum

    EXCLUDES 1   tuberculous erythema nodosum (A18.4)

DEF: Form of panniculitis (inflammation of the fat layer beneath the skin) most often occurring in women. Commonly seen as a hypersensitivity reaction to infections, drugs, sarcoidosis, and specific enteropathies. The acute stage is associated with fever, malaise, and arthralgia. The lesions are pink to blue in color as tender nodules and are found on the front of the legs below the knees.

✓4ᵗʰ L53 Other erythematous conditions

    EXCLUDES 1   erythema ab igne (L59.0)
              erythema due to external agents in contact with skin (L23-L25)
              erythema intertrigo (L30.4)

L53.0 Toxic erythema
Code first poisoning due to drug or toxin, if applicable (T36-T65 with fifth or sixth character 1-4 or 6)
Use additional code for adverse effect, if applicable, to identify drug (T36-T50 with fifth or sixth character 5)

    EXCLUDES 1   neonatal erythema toxicum (P83.1)

L53.1 Erythema annulare centrifugum

L53.2 Erythema marginatum

L53.3 Other chronic figurate erythema

L53.8 Other specified erythematous conditions

L53.9 Erythematous condition, unspecified
Erythema NOS
Erythroderma NOS

L54 Erythema in diseases classified elsewhere
Code first underlying disease

Radiation-related disorders of the skin and subcutaneous tissue (L55-L59)

✓4ᵗʰ L55 Sunburn

L55.0 Sunburn of first degree

L55.1 Sunburn of second degree

L55.2 Sunburn of third degree

L55.9 Sunburn, unspecified

✓4ᵗʰ L56 Other acute skin changes due to ultraviolet radiation

Use additional code to identify the source of the ultraviolet radiation (W89, X32)

L56.0 Drug phototoxic response
Use additional code for adverse effect, if applicable, to identify drug (T36-T50 with fifth or sixth character 5)

L56.1 Drug photoallergic response
Use additional code for adverse effect, if applicable, to identify drug (T36-T50 with fifth or sixth character 5)

L56.2 Photocontact dermatitis [berloque dermatitis]

L56.3 Solar urticaria

L56.4 Polymorphous light eruption

L56.5 Disseminated superficial actinic porokeratosis (DSAP)
DEF: Autosomal dominant skin condition occurring in sun-exposed areas of the skin (particularly the arms and legs), characterized by superficial annular, keratotic, brownish-red spots or thickenings with depressed centers and sharp, ridged borders. It may evolve into squamous cell carcinoma.

L56.8 Other specified acute skin changes due to ultraviolet radiation

L56.9 Acute skin change due to ultraviolet radiation, unspecified

✓4ᵗʰ L57 Skin changes due to chronic exposure to nonionizing radiation

Use additional code to identify the source of the ultraviolet radiation (W89)

L57.0 Actinic keratosis
Keratosis NOS
Senile keratosis
Solar keratosis

L57.1 Actinic reticuloid

L57.2 Cutis rhomboidalis nuchae

L57.3 Poikiloderma of Civatte

L57.4 Cutis laxa senilis
Elastosis senilis

L57.5 Actinic granuloma

L57.8 Other skin changes due to chronic exposure to nonionizing radiation
Farmer's skin
Sailor's skin
Solar dermatitis

L57.9 Skin changes due to chronic exposure to nonionizing radiation, unspecified

✓4ᵗʰ L58 Radiodermatitis

Use additional code to identify the source of the radiation (W88, W90)

L58.0 Acute radiodermatitis

L58.1 Chronic radiodermatitis

L58.9 Radiodermatitis, unspecified

✓4ᵗʰ L59 Other disorders of skin and subcutaneous tissue related to radiation

L59.0 Erythema ab igne [dermatitis ab igne]

L59.8 Other specified disorders of the skin and subcutaneous tissue related to radiation
AHA: 2017,1Q,33

L59.9 Disorder of the skin and subcutaneous tissue related to radiation, unspecified

Disorders of skin appendages (L60-L75)

EXCLUDES1   *congenital malformations of integument (Q84.-)*

✓4ᵗʰ L60 Nail disorders

EXCLUDES2   *clubbing of nails (R68.3)*
           onychia and paronychia (L03.0-)

Nail Disorders

Normal

Koilonychia

Beau's Lines

L60.0   **Ingrowing nail**
L60.1   **Onycholysis**
L60.2   **Onychogryphosis**
L60.3   **Nail dystrophy**
L60.4   **Beau's lines**
L60.5   **Yellow nail syndrome**
L60.8   **Other nail disorders**
L60.9   **Nail disorder, unspecified**

L62 *Nail disorders in diseases classified elsewhere*

Code first underlying disease, such as:
     pachydermoperiostosis (M89.4-)

✓4ᵗʰ L63 Alopecia areata

L63.0   **Alopecia (capitis) totalis**
L63.1   **Alopecia universalis**
L63.2   **Ophiasis**
L63.8   **Other alopecia areata**
L63.9   **Alopecia areata, unspecified**

✓4ᵗʰ L64 Androgenic alopecia

INCLUDES   male-pattern baldness

L64.0   **Drug-induced androgenic alopecia**
     Use additional code for adverse effect, if applicable, to identify drug (T36-T50 with fifth or sixth character 5)
L64.8   **Other androgenic alopecia**
L64.9   **Androgenic alopecia, unspecified**

✓4ᵗʰ L65 Other nonscarring hair loss

Use additional code for adverse effect, if applicable, to identify drug (T36-T50 with fifth or sixth character 5)

EXCLUDES1   *trichotillomania (F63.3)*

L65.0   **Telogen effluvium**
     DEF: Form of nonscarring alopecia characterized by shedding of hair from premature telogen development in follicles due to stress, including shock, childbirth, surgery, drugs, or weight loss.
L65.1   **Anagen effluvium**
L65.2   **Alopecia mucinosa**
L65.8   **Other specified nonscarring hair loss**
L65.9   **Nonscarring hair loss, unspecified**
     Alopecia NOS

✓4ᵗʰ L66 Cicatricial alopecia [scarring hair loss]

L66.0   **Pseudopelade**
L66.1   **Lichen planopilaris**
     Follicular lichen planus
L66.2   **Folliculitis decalvans**
L66.3   **Perifolliculitis capitis abscedens**
L66.4   **Folliculitis ulerythematosa reticulata**

L66.8   **Other cicatricial alopecia**
     AHA: 2015,1Q,19
L66.9   **Cicatricial alopecia, unspecified**

✓4ᵗʰ L67 Hair color and hair shaft abnormalities

EXCLUDES1   *monilethrix (Q84.1)*
           pili annulati (Q84.1)
           telogen effluvium (L65.0)

L67.0   **Trichorrhexis nodosa**
L67.1   **Variations in hair color**
     Canities
     Greyness, hair (premature)
     Heterochromia of hair
     Poliosis circumscripta, acquired
     Poliosis NOS
L67.8   **Other hair color and hair shaft abnormalities**
     Fragilitas crinium
L67.9   **Hair color and hair shaft abnormality, unspecified**

✓4ᵗʰ L68 Hypertrichosis

INCLUDES   excess hair
EXCLUDES1   *congenital hypertrichosis (Q84.2)*
           persistent lanugo (Q84.2)

L68.0   **Hirsutism**
L68.1   **Acquired hypertrichosis lanuginosa**
L68.2   **Localized hypertrichosis**
L68.3   **Polytrichia**
L68.8   **Other hypertrichosis**
L68.9   **Hypertrichosis, unspecified**

✓4ᵗʰ L70 Acne

EXCLUDES2   *acne keloid (L73.0)*

L70.0   **Acne vulgaris**
L70.1   **Acne conglobata**
L70.2   **Acne varioliformis**
     Acne necrotica miliaris
     DEF: Rare form of acne characterized by development of persistent brown papulopustules followed by scar formation. This type of acne usually presents on the brow and temporoparietal part of the scalp.
L70.3   **Acne tropica**
L70.4   **Infantile acne**   P
L70.5   **Acné excoriée**
     Acné excoriée des jeunes filles
     Picker's acne
L70.8   **Other acne**
L70.9   **Acne, unspecified**

✓4ᵗʰ L71 Rosacea

Use additional code for adverse effect, if applicable, to identify drug (T36-T50 with fifth or sixth character 5)

L71.0   **Perioral dermatitis**
L71.1   **Rhinophyma**
L71.8   **Other rosacea**
     AHA: 2018,4Q,15
L71.9   **Rosacea, unspecified**

✓4ᵗʰ L72 Follicular cysts of skin and subcutaneous tissue

L72.0   **Epidermal cyst**
✓5ᵗʰ L72.1   **Pilar and trichodermal cyst**
     L72.11   **Pilar cyst**
     L72.12   **Trichodermal cyst**
           Trichilemmal (proliferating) cyst
L72.2   **Steatocystoma multiplex**
L72.3   **Sebaceous cyst**
     EXCLUDES2   *pilar cyst (L72.11)*
                  trichilemmal (proliferating) cyst (L72.12)
L72.8   **Other follicular cysts of the skin and subcutaneous tissue**
L72.9   **Follicular cyst of the skin and subcutaneous tissue, unspecified**

✓4ᵗʰ L73 Other follicular disorders

L73.0   **Acne keloid**
L73.1   **Pseudofolliculitis barbae**
L73.2   **Hidradenitis suppurativa**
L73.8   **Other specified follicular disorders**
     Sycosis barbae
L73.9   **Follicular disorder, unspecified**

✔ Additional Character Required   ✓x7ᵗʰ Placeholder Alert   Manifestation   Unspecified Dx   ►◄ Revised Text   ● New Code   ▲ Revised Code Title

ICD-10-CM 2020   729

Chapter 12. Diseases of the Skin and Subcutaneous Tissue

L74–L85.9

√4ᵗʰ **L74 Eccrine sweat disorders**

EXCLUDES 2   generalized hyperhidrosis (R61)

DEF: Eccrine sweat glands: Glands found in the dermal and hypodermal layer of the skin throughout the body, particularly on the forehead, scalp, axillae, palms, and soles. These glands produce watery and neutral or slightly acidic sweat.

L74.0 Miliaria rubra

L74.1 Miliaria crystallina

L74.2 Miliaria profunda
Miliaria tropicalis

L74.3 Miliaria, unspecified

L74.4 Anhidrosis
Hypohidrosis
DEF: Inability to sweat normally. When the body can't cool itself through perspiration it can lead to heatstroke, a life-threatening condition.

√5ᵗʰ **L74.5 Focal hyperhidrosis**

√6ᵗʰ **L74.51 Primary focal hyperhidrosis**

L74.510 Primary focal hyperhidrosis, axilla

L74.511 Primary focal hyperhidrosis, face

L74.512 Primary focal hyperhidrosis, palms

L74.513 Primary focal hyperhidrosis, soles

L74.519 Primary focal hyperhidrosis, unspecified

L74.52 Secondary focal hyperhidrosis
Frey's syndrome

L74.8 Other eccrine sweat disorders

L74.9 Eccrine sweat disorder, unspecified
Sweat gland disorder NOS

√4ᵗʰ **L75 Apocrine sweat disorders**

EXCLUDES 1   dyshidrosis (L30.1)
hidradenitis suppurativa (L73.2)

DEF: Apocrine sweat glands: Found in the axilla, areola, and circumanal region, these glands begin to function in puberty and produce viscid milky secretions in response to external stimuli.

L75.0 Bromhidrosis

L75.1 Chromhidrosis

L75.2 Apocrine miliaria
Fox-Fordyce disease
DEF: Chronic, usually pruritic disease evidenced by small follicular papular eruptions, especially in the axillary and pubic areas. Apocrine miliaria develops from the closure and rupture of the affected apocrine glands' intraepidermal portion of the ducts.

L75.8 Other apocrine sweat disorders

L75.9 Apocrine sweat disorder, unspecified

Intraoperative and postprocedural complications of skin and subcutaneous tissue (L76)

√4ᵗʰ **L76 Intraoperative and postprocedural complications of skin and subcutaneous tissue**
AHA: 2016,4Q,9-10

√5ᵗʰ **L76.0 Intraoperative hemorrhage and hematoma of skin and subcutaneous tissue complicating a procedure**

EXCLUDES 1   intraoperative hemorrhage and hematoma of skin and subcutaneous tissue due to accidental puncture and laceration during a procedure (L76.1-)

L76.01 Intraoperative hemorrhage and hematoma of skin and subcutaneous tissue complicating a dermatologic procedure

L76.02 Intraoperative hemorrhage and hematoma of skin and subcutaneous tissue complicating other procedure

√5ᵗʰ **L76.1 Accidental puncture and laceration of skin and subcutaneous tissue during a procedure**

L76.11 Accidental puncture and laceration of skin and subcutaneous tissue during a dermatologic procedure

L76.12 Accidental puncture and laceration of skin and subcutaneous tissue during other procedure

√5ᵗʰ **L76.2 Postprocedural hemorrhage of skin and subcutaneous tissue following a procedure**

L76.21 Postprocedural hemorrhage of skin and subcutaneous tissue following a dermatologic procedure

L76.22 Postprocedural hemorrhage of skin and subcutaneous tissue following other procedure

√5ᵗʰ **L76.3 Postprocedural hematoma and seroma of skin and subcutaneous tissue following a procedure**

L76.31 Postprocedural hematoma of skin and subcutaneous tissue following a dermatologic procedure

L76.32 Postprocedural hematoma of skin and subcutaneous tissue following other procedure

L76.33 Postprocedural seroma of skin and subcutaneous tissue following a dermatologic procedure

L76.34 Postprocedural seroma of skin and subcutaneous tissue following other procedure

√5ᵗʰ **L76.8 Other intraoperative and postprocedural complications of skin and subcutaneous tissue**
Use additional code, if applicable, to further specify disorder

L76.81 Other intraoperative complications of skin and subcutaneous tissue

L76.82 Other postprocedural complications of skin and subcutaneous tissue
AHA: 2017,3Q,6

Other disorders of the skin and subcutaneous tissue (L80-L99)

L80 Vitiligo

EXCLUDES 2   vitiligo of eyelids (H02.73-)
vitiligo of vulva (N90.89)

DEF: Persistent, progressive development of nonpigmented white patches on otherwise normal skin.

√4ᵗʰ **L81 Other disorders of pigmentation**

EXCLUDES 1   birthmark NOS (Q82.5)
Peutz-Jeghers syndrome (Q85.8)

EXCLUDES 2   nevus — see Alphabetical Index

L81.0 Postinflammatory hyperpigmentation

L81.1 Chloasma

L81.2 Freckles

L81.3 Café au lait spots

L81.4 Other melanin hyperpigmentation
Lentigo

L81.5 Leukoderma, not elsewhere classified

L81.6 Other disorders of diminished melanin formation

L81.7 Pigmented purpuric dermatosis
Angioma serpiginosum

L81.8 Other specified disorders of pigmentation
Iron pigmentation
Tattoo pigmentation

L81.9 Disorder of pigmentation, unspecified

√4ᵗʰ **L82 Seborrheic keratosis**

INCLUDES   basal cell papilloma
dermatosis papulosa nigra
Leser-Trélat disease

EXCLUDES 2   seborrheic dermatitis (L21.-)

DEF: Common, benign, noninvasive, lightly pigmented, warty growth composed of basaloid cells that usually appear at middle age as soft, easily crumbling plaques on the face, trunk, and extremities.

L82.0 Inflamed seborrheic keratosis

L82.1 Other seborrheic keratosis
Seborrheic keratosis NOS

L83 Acanthosis nigricans
Confluent and reticulated papillomatosis
DEF: Diffuse, velvety hyperplasia of the spinous skin layer of the axilla and other body folds marked by gray, brown, or black pigmentation. In adult form, it is often associated with malignant acanthosis nigricans in a benign, nevoid form relatively generalized.

L84 Corns and callosities
Callus
Clavus

√4ᵗʰ **L85 Other epidermal thickening**

EXCLUDES 2   hypertrophic disorders of the skin (L91.-)

L85.0 Acquired ichthyosis

EXCLUDES 1   congenital ichthyosis (Q80.-)

L85.1 Acquired keratosis [keratoderma] palmaris et plantaris

EXCLUDES 1   inherited keratosis palmaris et plantaris (Q82.8)

L85.2 Keratosis punctata (palmaris et plantaris)

L85.3 Xerosis cutis
Dry skin dermatitis

L85.8 Other specified epidermal thickening
Cutaneous horn

L85.9 Epidermal thickening, unspecified

L86　Keratoderma in diseases classified elsewhere
　Code first underlying disease, such as:
　　Reiter's disease (M02.3-)
　EXCLUDES 1　gonococcal keratoderma (A54.89)
　　　　gonococcal keratosis (A54.89)
　　　　keratoderma due to vitamin A deficiency (E50.8)
　　　　keratosis due to vitamin A deficiency (E50.8)
　　　　xeroderma due to vitamin A deficiency (E50.8)

√4ᵗʰ **L87　Transepidermal elimination disorders**
　EXCLUDES 1　granuloma annulare (perforating) (L92.0)
　L87.0　Keratosis follicularis et parafollicularis in cutem penetrans
　　Hyperkeratosis follicularis penetrans
　　Kyrle disease
　L87.1　Reactive perforating collagenosis
　L87.2　Elastosis perforans serpiginosa
　L87.8　Other transepidermal elimination disorders
　L87.9　Transepidermal elimination disorder, unspecified

L88　Pyoderma gangrenosum
　Phagedenic pyoderma
　EXCLUDES 1　dermatitis gangrenosa (L08.0)
　DEF: Persistent debilitating skin disease characterized by irregular, boggy, blue-red ulcerations, with central healing and undermined edges.

√4ᵗʰ **L89　Pressure ulcer**
　INCLUDES　bed sore
　　　decubitus ulcer
　　　plaster ulcer
　　　pressure area
　　　pressure sore
　Code first any associated gangrene (I96)
　EXCLUDES 2　decubitus (trophic) ulcer of cervix (uteri) (N86)
　　　diabetic ulcers (E08.621, E08.622, E09.621, E09.622, E10.621, E10.622, E11.621, E11.622, E13.621, E13.622)
　　　non-pressure chronic ulcer of skin (L97.-)
　　　skin infections (L00-L08)
　　　varicose ulcer (I83.0, I83.2)
　AHA: 2018,4Q,69; 2018,3Q,3; 2018,2Q,21; 2017,4Q,109; 2017,1Q,49; 2016,4Q,143
　TIP: The stage of a diagnosed pressure ulcer can be based on documentation from clinicians who are not the patient's provider.

Four Stages of Pressure Ulcer

Stage 1
Persistent focal edema

Stage 2
Abrasion, blister, partial thickness skin loss involving epidermis and/or dermis

Stage 3
Full thickness skin loss involving damage or necrosis of subcutaneous tissue

Stage 4
Necrosis of soft tissues through to underlying muscle, tendon, or bone

√6ᵗʰ **L89.0　Pressure ulcer of elbow**
　√6ᵗʰ **L89.00　Pressure ulcer of unspecified elbow**
　　L89.000　Pressure ulcer of unspecified elbow, unstageable　HCC

L89.001　**Pressure ulcer of unspecified elbow, stage 1**
　Healing pressure ulcer of unspecified elbow, stage 1
　Pressure pre-ulcer skin changes limited to persistent focal edema, unspecified elbow
L89.002　**Pressure ulcer of unspecified elbow, stage 2**　HCC
　Healing pressure ulcer of unspecified elbow, stage 2
　Pressure ulcer with abrasion, blister, partial thickness skin loss involving epidermis and/or dermis, unspecified elbow
L89.003　**Pressure ulcer of unspecified elbow, stage 3**　HCC
　Healing pressure ulcer of unspecified elbow, stage 3
　Pressure ulcer with full thickness skin loss involving damage or necrosis of subcutaneous tissue, unspecified elbow
L89.004　**Pressure ulcer of unspecified elbow, stage 4**　HCC
　Healing pressure ulcer of unspecified elbow, stage 4
　Pressure ulcer with necrosis of soft tissues through to underlying muscle, tendon, or bone, unspecified elbow
● L89.006　**Pressure-induced deep tissue damage of unspecified elbow**
L89.009　**Pressure ulcer of unspecified elbow, unspecified stage**
　Healing pressure ulcer of elbow NOS
　Healing pressure ulcer of unspecified elbow, unspecified stage

√6ᵗʰ **L89.01　Pressure ulcer of right elbow**
L89.010　**Pressure ulcer of right elbow, unstageable**　HCC
L89.011　**Pressure ulcer of right elbow, stage 1**
　Healing pressure ulcer of right elbow, stage 1
　Pressure pre-ulcer skin changes limited to persistent focal edema, right elbow
L89.012　**Pressure ulcer of right elbow, stage 2**　HCC
　Healing pressure ulcer of right elbow, stage 2
　Pressure ulcer with abrasion, blister, partial thickness skin loss involving epidermis and/or dermis, right elbow
L89.013　**Pressure ulcer of right elbow, stage 3**　HCC
　Healing pressure ulcer of right elbow, stage 3
　Pressure ulcer with full thickness skin loss involving damage or necrosis of subcutaneous tissue, right elbow
L89.014　**Pressure ulcer of right elbow, stage 4**　HCC
　Healing pressure ulcer of right elbow, stage 4
　Pressure ulcer with necrosis of soft tissues through to underlying muscle, tendon, or bone, right elbow
● L89.016　**Pressure-induced deep tissue damage of right elbow**
L89.019　**Pressure ulcer of right elbow, unspecified stage**
　Healing pressure right of elbow NOS
　Healing pressure ulcer of right elbow, unspecified stage

√6ᵗʰ **L89.02　Pressure ulcer of left elbow**
L89.020　**Pressure ulcer of left elbow, unstageable**　HCC

☑ Additional Character Required　　√x7ᵗʰ Placeholder Alert　　Manifestation　　Unspecified Dx　　►◄ Revised Text　　● New Code　　▲ Revised Code Title

L89.021　Pressure ulcer of left elbow, stage 1
　　　Healing pressure ulcer of left elbow,
　　　　stage 1
　　　Pressure pre-ulcer skin changes limited to
　　　　persistent focal edema, left elbow

L89.022　Pressure ulcer of left elbow, stage `HCC`
2
　　　Healing pressure ulcer of left elbow,
　　　　stage 2
　　　Pressure ulcer with abrasion, blister, partial
　　　　thickness skin loss involving
　　　　epidermis and/or dermis, left elbow

L89.023　Pressure ulcer of left elbow, `HCC`
stage 3
　　　Healing pressure ulcer of left elbow,
　　　　stage 3
　　　Pressure ulcer with full thickness skin loss
　　　　involving damage or necrosis of
　　　　subcutaneous tissue, left elbow

L89.024　Pressure ulcer of left elbow, `HCC`
stage 4
　　　Healing pressure ulcer of left elbow,
　　　　stage 4
　　　Pressure ulcer with necrosis of soft tissues
　　　　through to underlying muscle,
　　　　tendon, or bone, left elbow

● **L89.026　Pressure-induced deep tissue damage of
left elbow**

**L89.029　Pressure ulcer of left elbow, unspecified
stage**
　　　Healing pressure ulcer of left of elbow NOS
　　　Healing pressure ulcer of left elbow,
　　　　unspecified stage

√5ᵗʰ **L89.1　Pressure ulcer of back**

√6ᵗʰ **L89.10　Pressure ulcer of unspecified part of back**

L89.100　Pressure ulcer of unspecified part `HCC`
of back, unstageable

**L89.101　Pressure ulcer of unspecified part of back,
stage 1**
　　　Healing pressure ulcer of unspecified part
　　　　of back, stage 1
　　　Pressure pre-ulcer skin changes limited to
　　　　persistent focal edema, unspecified
　　　　part of back

L89.102　Pressure ulcer of unspecified part `HCC`
of back, stage 2
　　　Healing pressure ulcer of unspecified part
　　　　of back, stage 2
　　　Pressure ulcer with abrasion, blister, partial
　　　　thickness skin loss involving
　　　　epidermis and/or dermis, unspecified
　　　　part of back

L89.103　Pressure ulcer of unspecified part `HCC`
of back, stage 3
　　　Healing pressure ulcer of unspecified part
　　　　of back, stage 3
　　　Pressure ulcer with full thickness skin loss
　　　　involving damage or necrosis of
　　　　subcutaneous tissue, unspecified part
　　　　of back

L89.104　Pressure ulcer of unspecified part `HCC`
of back, stage 4
　　　Healing pressure ulcer of unspecified part
　　　　of back, stage 4
　　　Pressure ulcer with necrosis of soft tissues
　　　　through to underlying muscle,
　　　　tendon, or bone, unspecified part of
　　　　back

● **L89.106　Pressure-induced deep tissue damage of
unspecified part of back**

**L89.109　Pressure ulcer of unspecified part of back,
unspecified stage**
　　　Healing pressure ulcer of unspecified part
　　　　of back NOS
　　　Healing pressure ulcer of unspecified part
　　　　of back, unspecified stage

√6ᵗʰ **L89.11　Pressure ulcer of right upper back**
　　　Pressure ulcer of right shoulder blade

L89.110　Pressure ulcer of right upper `HCC`
back, unstageable

L89.111　Pressure ulcer of right upper back, stage 1
　　　Healing pressure ulcer of right upper back,
　　　　stage 1
　　　Pressure pre-ulcer skin changes limited to
　　　　persistent focal edema, right upper
　　　　back

L89.112　Pressure ulcer of right upper `HCC`
back, stage 2
　　　Healing pressure ulcer of right upper back,
　　　　stage 2
　　　Pressure ulcer with abrasion, blister, partial
　　　　thickness skin loss involving
　　　　epidermis and/or dermis, right upper
　　　　back

L89.113　Pressure ulcer of right upper `HCC`
back, stage 3
　　　Healing pressure ulcer of right upper back,
　　　　stage 3
　　　Pressure ulcer with full thickness skin loss
　　　　involving damage or necrosis of
　　　　subcutaneous tissue, right upper back

L89.114　Pressure ulcer of right upper `HCC`
back, stage 4
　　　Healing pressure ulcer of right upper back,
　　　　stage 4
　　　Pressure ulcer with necrosis of soft tissues
　　　　through to underlying muscle,
　　　　tendon, or bone, right upper back

● **L89.116　Pressure-induced deep tissue damage of
right upper back**

**L89.119　Pressure ulcer of right upper back,
unspecified stage**
　　　Healing pressure ulcer of right upper back
　　　　NOS
　　　Healing pressure ulcer of right upper back,
　　　　unspecified stage

√6ᵗʰ **L89.12　Pressure ulcer of left upper back**
　　　Pressure ulcer of left shoulder blade

L89.120　Pressure ulcer of left upper back, `HCC`
unstageable

L89.121　Pressure ulcer of left upper back, stage 1
　　　Healing pressure ulcer of left upper back,
　　　　stage 1
　　　Pressure pre-ulcer skin changes limited to
　　　　persistent focal edema, left upper
　　　　back

L89.122　Pressure ulcer of left upper back, `HCC`
stage 2
　　　Healing pressure ulcer of left upper back,
　　　　stage 2
　　　Pressure ulcer with abrasion, blister, partial
　　　　thickness skin loss involving
　　　　epidermis and/or dermis, left upper
　　　　back

L89.123　Pressure ulcer of left upper back, `HCC`
stage 3
　　　Healing pressure ulcer of left upper back,
　　　　stage 3
　　　Pressure ulcer with full thickness skin loss
　　　　involving damage or necrosis of
　　　　subcutaneous tissue, left upper back

L89.124　Pressure ulcer of left upper back, `HCC`
stage 4
　　　Healing pressure ulcer of left upper back,
　　　　stage 4
　　　Pressure ulcer with necrosis of soft tissues
　　　　through to underlying muscle,
　　　　tendon, or bone, left upper back

● **L89.126　Pressure-induced deep tissue damage of
left upper back**

L89.129   **Pressure ulcer of left upper back, unspecified stage**
> Healing pressure ulcer of left upper back NOS
>
> Healing pressure ulcer of left upper back, unspecified stage

√6ᵗʰ   **L89.13**   **Pressure ulcer of right lower back**

L89.130   **Pressure ulcer of right lower back, unstageable**   HCC

L89.131   **Pressure ulcer of right lower back, stage 1**
> Healing pressure ulcer of right lower back, stage 1
>
> Pressure pre-ulcer skin changes limited to persistent focal edema, right lower back

L89.132   **Pressure ulcer of right lower back, stage 2**   HCC
> Healing pressure ulcer of right lower back, stage 2
>
> Pressure ulcer with abrasion, blister, partial thickness skin loss involving epidermis and/or dermis, right lower back

L89.133   **Pressure ulcer of right lower back, stage 3**   HCC
> Healing pressure ulcer of right lower back, stage 3
>
> Pressure ulcer with full thickness skin loss involving damage or necrosis of subcutaneous tissue, right lower back

L89.134   **Pressure ulcer of right lower back, stage 4**   HCC
> Healing pressure ulcer of right lower back, stage 4
>
> Pressure ulcer with necrosis of soft tissues through to underlying muscle, tendon, or bone, right lower back

● **L89.136**   **Pressure-induced deep tissue damage of right lower back**

L89.139   **Pressure ulcer of right lower back, unspecified stage**
> Healing pressure ulcer of right lower back NOS
>
> Healing pressure ulcer of right lower back, unspecified stage

√6ᵗʰ   **L89.14**   **Pressure ulcer of left lower back**

L89.140   **Pressure ulcer of left lower back, unstageable**   HCC

L89.141   **Pressure ulcer of left lower back, stage 1**
> Healing pressure ulcer of left lower back, stage 1
>
> Pressure pre-ulcer skin changes limited to persistent focal edema, left lower back

L89.142   **Pressure ulcer of left lower back, stage 2**   HCC
> Healing pressure ulcer of left lower back, stage 2
>
> Pressure ulcer with abrasion, blister, partial thickness skin loss involving epidermis and/or dermis, left lower back

L89.143   **Pressure ulcer of left lower back, stage 3**   HCC
> Healing pressure ulcer of left lower back, stage 3
>
> Pressure ulcer with full thickness skin loss involving damage or necrosis of subcutaneous tissue, left lower back

L89.144   **Pressure ulcer of left lower back, stage 4**   HCC
> Healing pressure ulcer of left lower back, stage 4
>
> Pressure ulcer with necrosis of soft tissues through to underlying muscle, tendon, or bone, left lower back

● **L89.146**   **Pressure-induced deep tissue damage of left lower back**

L89.149   **Pressure ulcer of left lower back, unspecified stage**
> Healing pressure ulcer of left lower back NOS
>
> Healing pressure ulcer of left lower back, unspecified stage

√6ᵗʰ   **L89.15**   **Pressure ulcer of sacral region**
> Pressure ulcer of coccyx
>
> Pressure ulcer of tailbone

L89.150   **Pressure ulcer of sacral region, unstageable**   HCC

L89.151   **Pressure ulcer of sacral region, stage 1**
> Healing pressure ulcer of sacral region, stage 1
>
> Pressure pre-ulcer skin changes limited to persistent focal edema, sacral region

L89.152   **Pressure ulcer of sacral region, stage 2**   HCC
> Healing pressure ulcer of sacral region, stage 2
>
> Pressure ulcer with abrasion, blister, partial thickness skin loss involving epidermis and/or dermis, sacral region

L89.153   **Pressure ulcer of sacral region, stage 3**   HCC
> Healing pressure ulcer of sacral region, stage 3
>
> Pressure ulcer with full thickness skin loss involving damage or necrosis of subcutaneous tissue, sacral region

L89.154   **Pressure ulcer of sacral region, stage 4**   HCC
> Healing pressure ulcer of sacral region, stage 4
>
> Pressure ulcer with necrosis of soft tissues through to underlying muscle, tendon, or bone, sacral region

● **L89.156**   **Pressure-induced deep tissue damage of sacral region**

L89.159   **Pressure ulcer of sacral region, unspecified stage**
> Healing pressure ulcer of sacral region NOS
>
> Healing pressure ulcer of sacral region, unspecified stage

√5ᵗʰ   **L89.2**   **Pressure ulcer of hip**

√6ᵗʰ   **L89.20**   **Pressure ulcer of unspecified hip**

L89.200   **Pressure ulcer of unspecified hip, unstageable**   HCC

L89.201   **Pressure ulcer of unspecified hip, stage 1**
> Healing pressure ulcer of unspecified hip back, stage 1
>
> Pressure pre-ulcer skin changes limited to persistent focal edema, unspecified hip

L89.202   **Pressure ulcer of unspecified hip, stage 2**   HCC
> Healing pressure ulcer of unspecified hip, stage 2
>
> Pressure ulcer with abrasion, blister, partial thickness skin loss involving epidermis and/or dermis, unspecified hip

L89.203   **Pressure ulcer of unspecified hip, stage 3**   HCC
> Healing pressure ulcer of unspecified hip, stage 3
>
> Pressure ulcer with full thickness skin loss involving damage or necrosis of subcutaneous tissue, unspecified hip

L89.204   **Pressure ulcer of unspecified hip, stage 4**   HCC
> Healing pressure ulcer of unspecified hip, stage 4
>
> Pressure ulcer with necrosis of soft tissues through to underlying muscle, tendon, or bone, unspecified hip

---

☑ Additional Character Required   √x7ᵗʰ Placeholder Alert   Manifestation   Unspecified Dx   ►◄ Revised Text   ● New Code   ▲ Revised Code Title

● **L89.206 Pressure-induced deep tissue damage of unspecified hip**

L89.209 Pressure ulcer of unspecified hip, unspecified stage
Healing pressure ulcer of unspecified hip NOS
Healing pressure ulcer of unspecified hip, unspecified stage

√6ᵗʰ **L89.21 Pressure ulcer of right hip**

L89.210 Pressure ulcer of right hip, unstageable HCC

L89.211 Pressure ulcer of right hip, stage 1
Healing pressure ulcer of right hip back, stage 1
Pressure pre-ulcer skin changes limited to persistent focal edema, right hip

L89.212 Pressure ulcer of right hip, stage 2 HCC
Healing pressure ulcer of right hip, stage 2
Pressure ulcer with abrasion, blister, partial thickness skin loss involving epidermis and/or dermis, right hip

L89.213 Pressure ulcer of right hip, stage 3 HCC
Healing pressure ulcer of right hip, stage 3
Pressure ulcer with full thickness skin loss involving damage or necrosis of subcutaneous tissue, right hip

L89.214 Pressure ulcer of right hip, stage 4 HCC
Healing pressure ulcer of right hip, stage 4
Pressure ulcer with necrosis of soft tissues through to underlying muscle, tendon, or bone, right hip

● **L89.216 Pressure-induced deep tissue damage of right hip**

L89.219 Pressure ulcer of right hip, unspecified stage
Healing pressure ulcer of right hip NOS
Healing pressure ulcer of right hip, unspecified stage

√6ᵗʰ **L89.22 Pressure ulcer of left hip**

L89.220 Pressure ulcer of left hip, unstageable HCC

L89.221 Pressure ulcer of left hip, stage 1
Healing pressure ulcer of left hip back, stage 1
Pressure pre-ulcer skin changes limited to persistent focal edema, left hip

L89.222 Pressure ulcer of left hip, stage 2 HCC
Healing pressure ulcer of left hip, stage 2
Pressure ulcer with abrasion, blister, partial thickness skin loss involving epidermis and/or dermis, left hip

L89.223 Pressure ulcer of left hip, stage 3 HCC
Healing pressure ulcer of left hip, stage 3
Pressure ulcer with full thickness skin loss involving damage or necrosis of subcutaneous tissue, left hip

L89.224 Pressure ulcer of left hip, stage 4 HCC
Healing pressure ulcer of left hip, stage 4
Pressure ulcer with necrosis of soft tissues through to underlying muscle, tendon, or bone, left hip

● **L89.226 Pressure-induced deep tissue damage of left hip**

L89.229 Pressure ulcer of left hip, unspecified stage
Healing pressure ulcer of left hip NOS
Healing pressure ulcer of left hip, unspecified stage

√5ᵗʰ **L89.3 Pressure ulcer of buttock**

√6ᵗʰ **L89.30 Pressure ulcer of unspecified buttock**

L89.300 Pressure ulcer of unspecified buttock, unstageable HCC

L89.301 Pressure ulcer of unspecified buttock, stage 1
Healing pressure ulcer of unspecified buttock, stage 1
Pressure pre-ulcer skin changes limited to persistent focal edema, unspecified buttock

L89.302 Pressure ulcer of unspecified buttock, stage 2 HCC
Healing pressure ulcer of unspecified buttock, stage 2
Pressure ulcer with abrasion, blister, partial thickness skin loss involving epidermis and/or dermis, unspecified buttock

L89.303 Pressure ulcer of unspecified buttock, stage 3 HCC
Healing pressure ulcer of unspecified buttock, stage 3
Pressure ulcer with full thickness skin loss involving damage or necrosis of subcutaneous tissue, unspecified buttock

L89.304 Pressure ulcer of unspecified buttock, stage 4 HCC
Healing pressure ulcer of unspecified buttock, stage 4
Pressure ulcer with necrosis of soft tissues through to underlying muscle, tendon, or bone, unspecified buttock

● **L89.306 Pressure-induced deep tissue damage of unspecified buttock**

L89.309 Pressure ulcer of unspecified buttock, unspecified stage
Healing pressure ulcer of unspecified buttock NOS
Healing pressure ulcer of unspecified buttock, unspecified stage

√6ᵗʰ **L89.31 Pressure ulcer of right buttock**

L89.310 Pressure ulcer of right buttock, unstageable HCC

L89.311 Pressure ulcer of right buttock, stage 1
Healing pressure ulcer of right buttock, stage 1
Pressure pre-ulcer skin changes limited to persistent focal edema, right buttock

L89.312 Pressure ulcer of right buttock, stage 2 HCC
Healing pressure ulcer of right buttock, stage 2
Pressure ulcer with abrasion, blister, partial thickness skin loss involving epidermis and/or dermis, right buttock

L89.313 Pressure ulcer of right buttock, stage 3 HCC
Healing pressure ulcer of right buttock, stage 3
Pressure ulcer with full thickness skin loss involving damage or necrosis of subcutaneous tissue, right buttock

L89.314 Pressure ulcer of right buttock, stage 4 HCC
Healing pressure ulcer of right buttock, stage 4
Pressure ulcer with necrosis of soft tissues through to underlying muscle, tendon, or bone, right buttock

● **L89.316 Pressure-induced deep tissue damage of right buttock**

L89.319 Pressure ulcer of right buttock, unspecified stage
Healing pressure ulcer of right buttock NOS
Healing pressure ulcer of right buttock, unspecified stage

√6ᵗʰ **L89.32 Pressure ulcer of left buttock**

L89.320 Pressure ulcer of left buttock, unstageable HCC

L89.321 **Pressure ulcer of left buttock,** stage 1
     Healing pressure ulcer of left buttock, stage 1
     Pressure pre-ulcer skin changes limited to persistent focal edema, left buttock

L89.322 **Pressure ulcer of left buttock,** HCC **stage 2**
     Healing pressure ulcer of left buttock, stage 2
     Pressure ulcer with abrasion, blister, partial thickness skin loss involving epidermis and/or dermis, left buttock

L89.323 **Pressure ulcer of left buttock,** HCC **stage 3**
     Healing pressure ulcer of left buttock, stage 3
     Pressure ulcer with full thickness skin loss involving damage or necrosis of subcutaneous tissue, left buttock

L89.324 **Pressure ulcer of left buttock,** HCC **stage 4**
     Healing pressure ulcer of left buttock, stage 4
     Pressure ulcer with necrosis of soft tissues through to underlying muscle, tendon, or bone, left buttock

● L89.326 **Pressure-induced** deep tissue damage of **left buttock**

L89.329 **Pressure ulcer of left buttock, unspecified stage**
     Healing pressure ulcer of left buttock NOS
     Healing pressure ulcer of left buttock, unspecified stage

√5th L89.4 **Pressure ulcer of contiguous site of** back, buttock and hip

L89.40 **Pressure ulcer of contiguous site of back, buttock and hip, unspecified stage**
     Healing pressure ulcer of contiguous site of back, buttock and hip NOS
     Healing pressure ulcer of contiguous site of back, buttock and hip, unspecified stage

L89.41 **Pressure ulcer of contiguous site of back, buttock and hip,** stage 1
     Healing pressure ulcer of contiguous site of back, buttock and hip, stage 1
     Pressure pre-ulcer skin changes limited to persistent focal edema, contiguous site of back, buttock and hip

L89.42 **Pressure ulcer of contiguous site of** HCC **back, buttock and hip,** stage 2
     Healing pressure ulcer of contiguous site of back, buttock and hip, stage 2
     Pressure ulcer with abrasion, blister, partial thickness skin loss involving epidermis and/or dermis, contiguous site of back, buttock and hip

L89.43 **Pressure ulcer of contiguous site of** HCC **back, buttock and hip,** stage 3
     Healing pressure ulcer of contiguous site of back, buttock and hip, stage 3
     Pressure ulcer with full thickness skin loss involving damage or necrosis of subcutaneous tissue, contiguous site of back, buttock and hip

L89.44 **Pressure ulcer of contiguous site of** HCC **back, buttock and hip,** stage 4
     Healing pressure ulcer of contiguous site of back, buttock and hip, stage 4
     Pressure ulcer with necrosis of soft tissues through to underlying muscle, tendon, or bone, contiguous site of back, buttock and hip

L89.45 **Pressure ulcer of contiguous site of back,** HCC **buttock and hip,** unstageable

● L89.46 **Pressure-induced** deep tissue damage of **contiguous site of back, buttock and hip**

√5th L89.5 **Pressure ulcer of** ankle

√6th L89.50 **Pressure ulcer of unspecified ankle**

L89.500 **Pressure ulcer of unspecified** HCC **ankle, unstageable**

L89.501 **Pressure ulcer of unspecified ankle,** stage 1
     Healing pressure ulcer of unspecified ankle, stage 1
     Pressure pre-ulcer skin changes limited to persistent focal edema, unspecified ankle

L89.502 **Pressure ulcer of unspecified** HCC **ankle, stage 2**
     Healing pressure ulcer of unspecified ankle, stage 2
     Pressure ulcer with abrasion, blister, partial thickness skin loss involving epidermis and/or dermis, unspecified ankle

L89.503 **Pressure ulcer of unspecified** HCC **ankle, stage 3**
     Healing pressure ulcer of unspecified ankle, stage 3
     Pressure ulcer with full thickness skin loss involving damage or necrosis of subcutaneous tissue, unspecified ankle

L89.504 **Pressure ulcer of unspecified** HCC **ankle, stage 4**
     Healing pressure ulcer of unspecified ankle, stage 4
     Pressure ulcer with necrosis of soft tissues through to underlying muscle, tendon, or bone, unspecified ankle

● L89.506 **Pressure-induced** deep tissue damage of **unspecified ankle**

L89.509 **Pressure ulcer of unspecified ankle, unspecified stage**
     Healing pressure ulcer of unspecified ankle NOS
     Healing pressure ulcer of unspecified ankle, unspecified stage

√6th L89.51 **Pressure ulcer of** right **ankle**

L89.510 **Pressure ulcer of right ankle,** HCC **unstageable**

L89.511 **Pressure ulcer of right ankle,** stage 1
     Healing pressure ulcer of right ankle, stage 1
     Pressure pre-ulcer skin changes limited to persistent focal edema, right ankle

L89.512 **Pressure ulcer of right ankle,** HCC **stage 2**
     Healing pressure ulcer of right ankle, stage 2
     Pressure ulcer with abrasion, blister, partial thickness skin loss involving epidermis and/or dermis, right ankle

L89.513 **Pressure ulcer of right ankle,** HCC **stage 3**
     Healing pressure ulcer of right ankle, stage 3
     Pressure ulcer with full thickness skin loss involving damage or necrosis of subcutaneous tissue, right ankle

L89.514 **Pressure ulcer of right ankle,** HCC **stage 4**
     Healing pressure ulcer of right ankle, stage 4
     Pressure ulcer with necrosis of soft tissues through to underlying muscle, tendon, or bone, right ankle

● L89.516 **Pressure-induced** deep tissue damage of **right ankle**

L89.519 **Pressure ulcer of right ankle, unspecified stage**
     Healing pressure ulcer of right ankle NOS
     Healing pressure ulcer of right ankle, unspecified stage

√6th L89.52 **Pressure ulcer of** left **ankle**

L89.520 **Pressure ulcer of left ankle,** HCC **unstageable**

☑ Additional Character Required   √x7th Placeholder Alert   **Manifestation**   Unspecified Dx   ►◄ Revised Text   ● New Code   ▲ Revised Code Title

L89.521 **Pressure ulcer of left ankle,** stage 1
    Healing pressure ulcer of left ankle, stage 1
    Pressure pre-ulcer skin changes limited to persistent focal edema, left ankle

L89.522 **Pressure ulcer of left ankle,** stage 2   HCC
    Healing pressure ulcer of left ankle, stage 2
    Pressure ulcer with abrasion, blister, partial thickness skin loss involving epidermis and/or dermis, left ankle

L89.523 **Pressure ulcer of left ankle,** stage 3   HCC
    Healing pressure ulcer of left ankle, stage 3
    Pressure ulcer with full thickness skin loss involving damage or necrosis of subcutaneous tissue, left ankle

L89.524 **Pressure ulcer of left ankle,** stage 4   HCC
    Healing pressure ulcer of left ankle, stage 4
    Pressure ulcer with necrosis of soft tissues through to underlying muscle, tendon, or bone, left ankle

● **L89.526** **Pressure-induced** deep tissue damage **of left ankle**

L89.529 **Pressure ulcer of left ankle, unspecified stage**
    Healing pressure ulcer of left ankle NOS
    Healing pressure ulcer of left ankle, unspecified stage

√5ᵗʰ **L89.6** **Pressure ulcer of** heel

  √6ᵗʰ **L89.60** **Pressure ulcer of unspecified heel**

L89.600 **Pressure ulcer of unspecified heel,** unstageable   HCC

L89.601 **Pressure ulcer of unspecified heel,** stage 1
    Healing pressure ulcer of unspecified heel, stage 1
    Pressure pre-ulcer skin changes limited to persistent focal edema, unspecified heel

L89.602 **Pressure ulcer of unspecified heel,** stage 2   HCC
    Healing pressure ulcer of unspecified heel, stage 2
    Pressure ulcer with abrasion, blister, partial thickness skin loss involving epidermis and/or dermis, unspecified heel

L89.603 **Pressure ulcer of unspecified heel,** stage 3   HCC
    Healing pressure ulcer of unspecified heel, stage 3
    Pressure ulcer with full thickness skin loss involving damage or necrosis of subcutaneous tissue, unspecified heel

L89.604 **Pressure ulcer of unspecified heel,** stage 4   HCC
    Healing pressure ulcer of unspecified heel, stage 4
    Pressure ulcer with necrosis of soft tissues through to underlying muscle, tendon, or bone, unspecified heel

● **L89.606** **Pressure-induced** deep tissue damage **of unspecified heel**

L89.609 **Pressure ulcer of unspecified heel, unspecified stage**
    Healing pressure ulcer of unspecified heel NOS
    Healing pressure ulcer of unspecified heel, unspecified stage

  √6ᵗʰ **L89.61** **Pressure ulcer of** right **heel**

L89.610 **Pressure ulcer of right heel,** unstageable   HCC

L89.611 **Pressure ulcer of right heel,** stage 1
    Healing pressure ulcer of right heel, stage 1
    Pressure pre-ulcer skin changes limited to persistent focal edema, right heel

L89.612 **Pressure ulcer of right heel,** stage 2   HCC
    Healing pressure ulcer of right heel, stage 2
    Pressure ulcer with abrasion, blister, partial thickness skin loss involving epidermis and/or dermis, right heel

L89.613 **Pressure ulcer of right heel,** stage 3   HCC
    Healing pressure ulcer of right heel, stage 3
    Pressure ulcer with full thickness skin loss involving damage or necrosis of subcutaneous tissue, right heel

L89.614 **Pressure ulcer of right heel,** stage 4   HCC
    Healing pressure ulcer of right heel, stage 4
    Pressure ulcer with necrosis of soft tissues through to underlying muscle, tendon, or bone, right heel

● **L89.616** **Pressure-induced** deep tissue damage **of right heel**

L89.619 **Pressure ulcer of right heel, unspecified stage**
    Healing pressure ulcer of right heel NOS
    Healing pressure ulcer of right heel, unspecified stage

  √6ᵗʰ **L89.62** **Pressure ulcer of** left **heel**

L89.620 **Pressure ulcer of left heel,** unstageable   HCC

L89.621 **Pressure ulcer of left heel,** stage 1
    Healing pressure ulcer of left heel, stage 1
    Pressure pre-ulcer skin changes limited to persistent focal edema, left heel

L89.622 **Pressure ulcer of left heel,** stage 2   HCC
    Healing pressure ulcer of left heel, stage 2
    Pressure ulcer with abrasion, blister, partial thickness skin loss involving epidermis and/or dermis, left heel

L89.623 **Pressure ulcer of left heel,** stage 3   HCC
    Healing pressure ulcer of left heel, stage 3
    Pressure ulcer with full thickness skin loss involving damage or necrosis of subcutaneous tissue, left heel

L89.624 **Pressure ulcer of left heel,** stage 4   HCC
    Healing pressure ulcer of left heel, stage 4
    Pressure ulcer with necrosis of soft tissues through to underlying muscle, tendon, or bone, left heel

● **L89.626** **Pressure-induced** deep tissue damage **of left heel**

L89.629 **Pressure ulcer of left heel, unspecified stage**
    Healing pressure ulcer of left heel NOS
    Healing pressure ulcer of left heel, unspecified stage

√5ᵗʰ **L89.8** **Pressure ulcer of other site**

  √6ᵗʰ **L89.81** **Pressure ulcer of** head
    Pressure ulcer of face

L89.810 **Pressure ulcer of head,** unstageable   HCC

L89.811 **Pressure ulcer of head,** stage 1
    Healing pressure ulcer of head, stage 1
    Pressure pre-ulcer skin changes limited to persistent focal edema, head

L89.812 **Pressure ulcer of head,** stage 2   HCC
    Healing pressure ulcer of head, stage 2
    Pressure ulcer with abrasion, blister, partial thickness skin loss involving epidermis and/or dermis, head

L89.813 **Pressure ulcer of head,** stage 3   HCC
    Healing pressure ulcer of head, stage 3
    Pressure ulcer with full thickness skin loss involving damage or necrosis of subcutaneous tissue, head

L89.814 Pressure ulcer of head, stage 4   `HCC`
> Healing pressure ulcer of head, stage 4
> Pressure ulcer with necrosis of soft tissues through to underlying muscle, tendon, or bone, head

● **L89.816 Pressure-induced deep tissue damage of head**

L89.819 Pressure ulcer of head, unspecified stage
> Healing pressure ulcer of head NOS
> Healing pressure ulcer of head, unspecified stage

√6ᵗʰ **L89.89 Pressure ulcer of other site**

L89.890 Pressure ulcer of other site, unstageable   `HCC`

L89.891 Pressure ulcer of other site, stage 1
> Healing pressure ulcer of other site, stage 1
> Pressure pre-ulcer skin changes limited to persistent focal edema, other site

L89.892 Pressure ulcer of other site, stage 2   `HCC`
> Healing pressure ulcer of other site, stage 2
> Pressure ulcer with abrasion, blister, partial thickness skin loss involving epidermis and/or dermis, other site

L89.893 Pressure ulcer of other site, stage 3   `HCC`
> Healing pressure ulcer of other site, stage 3
> Pressure ulcer with full thickness skin loss involving damage or necrosis of subcutaneous tissue, other site

L89.894 Pressure ulcer of other site, stage 4   `HCC`
> Healing pressure ulcer of other site, stage 4
> Pressure ulcer with necrosis of soft tissues through to underlying muscle, tendon, or bone, other site

● **L89.896 Pressure-induced deep tissue damage of other site**

L89.899 Pressure ulcer of other site, unspecified stage
> Healing pressure ulcer of other site NOS
> Healing pressure ulcer of other site, unspecified stage

√5ᵗʰ **L89.9 Pressure ulcer of unspecified site**

L89.90 Pressure ulcer of unspecified site, unspecified stage
> Healing pressure ulcer of unspecified site NOS
> Healing pressure ulcer of unspecified site, unspecified stage

L89.91 Pressure ulcer of unspecified site, stage 1
> Healing pressure ulcer of unspecified site, stage 1
> Pressure pre-ulcer skin changes limited to persistent focal edema, unspecified site

L89.92 Pressure ulcer of unspecified site, stage 2   `HCC`
> Healing pressure ulcer of unspecified site, stage 2
> Pressure ulcer with abrasion, blister, partial thickness skin loss involving epidermis and/or dermis, unspecified site

L89.93 Pressure ulcer of unspecified site, stage 3   `HCC`
> Healing pressure ulcer of unspecified site, stage 3
> Pressure ulcer with full thickness skin loss involving damage or necrosis of subcutaneous tissue, unspecified site

L89.94 Pressure ulcer of unspecified site, stage 4   `HCC`
> Healing pressure ulcer of unspecified site, stage 4
> Pressure ulcer with necrosis of soft tissues through to underlying muscle, tendon, or bone, unspecified site

L89.95 Pressure ulcer of unspecified site, unstageable   `HCC`

● **L89.96 Pressure-induced deep tissue damage of unspecified site**

√4ᵗʰ **L90 Atrophic disorders of skin**

L90.0 Lichen sclerosus et atrophicus
> *EXCLUDES 2*   lichen sclerosus of external female genital organs (N90.4)
> lichen sclerosus of external male genital organs (N48.0)

L90.1 Anetoderma of Schweninger-Buzzi

L90.2 Anetoderma of Jadassohn-Pellizzari

L90.3 Atrophoderma of Pasini and Pierini

L90.4 Acrodermatitis chronica atrophicans

L90.5 Scar conditions and fibrosis of skin
> Adherent scar (skin)
> Cicatrix
> Disfigurement of skin due to scar
> Fibrosis of skin NOS
> Scar NOS
> *EXCLUDES 2*   hypertrophic scar (L91.0)
> keloid scar (L91.0)
> **AHA:** 2016,2Q,5; 2015,1Q,19

L90.6 Striae atrophicae

L90.8 Other atrophic disorders of skin

L90.9 Atrophic disorder of skin, unspecified

√4ᵗʰ **L91 Hypertrophic disorders of skin**

L91.0 Hypertrophic scar
> Keloid
> Keloid scar
> *EXCLUDES 2*   acne keloid (L73.0)
> scar NOS (L90.5)
> **DEF:** Overgrowth of scar tissue due to excess amounts of collagen during connective tissue repair, occurring mainly on the upper trunk and face.

L91.8 Other hypertrophic disorders of the skin

L91.9 Hypertrophic disorder of the skin, unspecified

√4ᵗʰ **L92 Granulomatous disorders of skin and subcutaneous tissue**
> *EXCLUDES 2*   actinic granuloma (L57.5)

L92.0 Granuloma annulare
> Perforating granuloma annulare

L92.1 Necrobiosis lipoidica, not elsewhere classified
> *EXCLUDES 1*   necrobiosis lipoidica associated with diabetes mellitus (E08-E13 with .620)

L92.2 Granuloma faciale [eosinophilic granuloma of skin]

L92.3 Foreign body granuloma of the skin and subcutaneous tissue
> Use additional code to identify the type of retained foreign body (Z18.-)

L92.8 Other granulomatous disorders of the skin and subcutaneous tissue

L92.9 Granulomatous disorder of the skin and subcutaneous tissue, unspecified
> *EXCLUDES 2*   umbilical granuloma (P83.81)
> **AHA:** 2017,4Q,21-22

√4ᵗʰ **L93 Lupus erythematosus**
> Use additional code for adverse effect, if applicable, to identify drug (T36-T50 with fifth or sixth character 5)
> *EXCLUDES 1*   lupus exedens (A18.4)
> lupus vulgaris (A18.4)
> scleroderma (M34.-)
> systemic lupus erythematosus (M32.-)
> **DEF:** Inflammatory, autoimmune skin condition in which the body's autoimmune system attacks healthy tissue of the integumentary system.

L93.0 Discoid lupus erythematosus
> Lupus erythematosus NOS

L93.1 Subacute cutaneous lupus erythematosus

L93.2 Other local lupus erythematosus
> Lupus erythematosus profundus
> Lupus panniculitis

√4ᵗʰ **L94 Other localized connective tissue disorders**
> *EXCLUDES 1*   systemic connective tissue disorders (M30-M36)

L94.0 Localized scleroderma [morphea]
> Circumscribed scleroderma

L94.1 Linear scleroderma
> En coup de sabre lesion

L94.2 Calcinosis cutis

L94.3 Sclerodactyly

L94.4 Gottron's papules

L94.5 Poikiloderma vasculare atrophicans

Chapter 12. Diseases of the Skin and Subcutaneous Tissue

L94.6   **Ainhum**

L94.8   **Other specified localized connective tissue disorders**

L94.9   **Localized connective tissue disorder, unspecified**

√4ᵗʰ **L95**   **Vasculitis limited to skin, not elsewhere classified**

EXCLUDES 1   angioma serpiginosum (L81.7)
- Henoch(-Schönlein) purpura (D69.0)
- hypersensitivity angiitis (M31.0)
- lupus panniculitis (L93.2)
- panniculitis NOS (M79.3)
- panniculitis of neck and back (M54.0-)
- polyarteritis nodosa (M30.0)
- relapsing panniculitis (M35.6)
- rheumatoid vasculitis (M05.2)
- serum sickness (T80.6-)
- urticaria (L50.-)
- Wegener's granulomatosis (M31.3-)

L95.0   **Livedoid vasculitis**
- Atrophie blanche (en plaque)

L95.1   **Erythema elevatum diutinum**

L95.8   **Other vasculitis limited to the skin**

L95.9   **Vasculitis limited to the skin, unspecified**

√4ᵗʰ **L97**   **Non-pressure chronic ulcer of lower limb, not elsewhere classified**

INCLUDES   chronic ulcer of skin of lower limb NOS
- non-healing ulcer of skin
- non-infected sinus of skin
- trophic ulcer NOS
- tropical ulcer NOS
- ulcer of skin of lower limb NOS

Code first any associated underlying condition, such as:
- any associated gangrene (I96)
- atherosclerosis of the lower extremities (I70.23-, I70.24-, I70.33-, I70.34-, I70.43-, I70.44-, I70.53-, I70.54-, I70.63-, I70.64-, I70.73-, I70.74-)
- chronic venous hypertension (I87.31-, I87.33-)
- diabetic ulcers (E08.621, E08.622, E09.621, E09.622, E10.621, E10.622, E11.621, E11.622, E13.621, E13.622)
- postphlebitic syndrome (I87.01-, I87.03-)
- postthrombotic syndrome (I87.01-, I87.03-)
- varicose ulcer (I83.0-, I83.2-)

EXCLUDES 2   pressure ulcer (pressure area) (L89.-)
- skin infections (L00-L08)
- specific infections classified to A00-B99

AHA: 2018,4Q,69; 2017,4Q,17

TIP: Assign a code from this category/subcategory for nonpressure ulcers documented as acute.

TIP: The depth and/or severity of a diagnosed nonpressure ulcer can be determined based on medical record documentation from clinicians who are not the patient's provider.

√5ᵗʰ **L97.1**   **Non-pressure chronic ulcer of thigh**

√6ᵗʰ **L97.10**   **Non-pressure chronic ulcer of unspecified thigh**

L97.101   **Non-pressure chronic ulcer of unspecified thigh** limited to breakdown of skin   HCC

L97.102   **Non-pressure chronic ulcer of unspecified thigh** with fat layer exposed   HCC

L97.103   **Non-pressure chronic ulcer of unspecified thigh** with necrosis of muscle   HCC

L97.104   **Non-pressure chronic ulcer of unspecified thigh** with necrosis of bone   HCC

L97.105   **Non-pressure chronic ulcer of unspecified thigh** with muscle involvement without evidence of necrosis   HCC

L97.106   **Non-pressure chronic ulcer of unspecified thigh** with bone involvement without evidence of necrosis   HCC

L97.108   **Non-pressure chronic ulcer of unspecified thigh** with other specified severity   HCC

L97.109   **Non-pressure chronic ulcer of unspecified thigh** with unspecified severity   HCC

√6ᵗʰ **L97.11**   **Non-pressure chronic ulcer of right thigh**

L97.111   **Non-pressure chronic ulcer of right thigh** limited to breakdown of skin   HCC

L97.112   **Non-pressure chronic ulcer of right thigh** with fat layer exposed   HCC

L97.113   **Non-pressure chronic ulcer of right thigh** with necrosis of muscle   HCC

L97.114   **Non-pressure chronic ulcer of right thigh** with necrosis of bone   HCC

L97.115   **Non-pressure chronic ulcer of right thigh** with muscle involvement without evidence of necrosis   HCC

L97.116   **Non-pressure chronic ulcer of right thigh** with bone involvement without evidence of necrosis   HCC

L97.118   **Non-pressure chronic ulcer of right thigh** with other specified severity   HCC

L97.119   **Non-pressure chronic ulcer of right thigh** with unspecified severity   HCC

√6ᵗʰ **L97.12**   **Non-pressure chronic ulcer of left thigh**

L97.121   **Non-pressure chronic ulcer of left thigh** limited to breakdown of skin   HCC

L97.122   **Non-pressure chronic ulcer of left thigh** with fat layer exposed   HCC

L97.123   **Non-pressure chronic ulcer of left thigh** with necrosis of muscle   HCC

L97.124   **Non-pressure chronic ulcer of left thigh** with necrosis of bone   HCC

L97.125   **Non-pressure chronic ulcer of left thigh** with muscle involvement without evidence of necrosis   HCC

L97.126   **Non-pressure chronic ulcer of left thigh** with bone involvement without evidence of necrosis   HCC

L97.128   **Non-pressure chronic ulcer of left thigh** with other specified severity   HCC

L97.129   **Non-pressure chronic ulcer of left thigh** with unspecified severity   HCC

√5ᵗʰ **L97.2**   **Non-pressure chronic ulcer of calf**

√6ᵗʰ **L97.20**   **Non-pressure chronic ulcer of unspecified calf**

L97.201   **Non-pressure chronic ulcer of unspecified calf** limited to breakdown of skin   HCC

L97.202   **Non-pressure chronic ulcer of unspecified calf** with fat layer exposed   HCC

L97.203   **Non-pressure chronic ulcer of unspecified calf** with necrosis of muscle   HCC

L97.204   **Non-pressure chronic ulcer of unspecified calf** with necrosis of bone   HCC

L97.205   **Non-pressure chronic ulcer of unspecified calf** with muscle involvement without evidence of necrosis   HCC

L97.206   **Non-pressure chronic ulcer of unspecified calf** with bone involvement without evidence of necrosis   HCC

L97.208   **Non-pressure chronic ulcer of unspecified calf** with other specified severity   HCC

L97.209   **Non-pressure chronic ulcer of unspecified calf** with unspecified severity   HCC

√6ᵗʰ **L97.21**   **Non-pressure chronic ulcer of right calf**

L97.211   **Non-pressure chronic ulcer of right calf** limited to breakdown of skin   HCC

L97.212   **Non-pressure chronic ulcer of right calf** with fat layer exposed   HCC

L97.213   **Non-pressure chronic ulcer of right calf** with necrosis of muscle   HCC

L97.214 **Non-pressure chronic ulcer of right calf** with necrosis of bone `HCC`

L97.215 **Non-pressure chronic ulcer of right calf** with muscle involvement without evidence of necrosis `HCC`

L97.216 **Non-pressure chronic ulcer of right calf** with bone involvement without evidence of necrosis `HCC`

L97.218 **Non-pressure chronic ulcer of right calf** with other specified severity `HCC`

L97.219 **Non-pressure chronic ulcer of right calf** with unspecified severity `HCC`

✓6th L97.22 **Non-pressure chronic ulcer of** left **calf**

L97.221 **Non-pressure chronic ulcer of left calf** limited to breakdown of skin `HCC`

L97.222 **Non-pressure chronic ulcer of left calf** with fat layer exposed `HCC`

L97.223 **Non-pressure chronic ulcer of left calf** with necrosis of muscle `HCC`

L97.224 **Non-pressure chronic ulcer of left calf** with necrosis of bone `HCC`

L97.225 **Non-pressure chronic ulcer of left calf** with muscle involvement without evidence of necrosis `HCC`

L97.226 **Non-pressure chronic ulcer of left calf** with bone involvement without evidence of necrosis `HCC`

L97.228 **Non-pressure chronic ulcer of left calf** with other specified severity `HCC`

L97.229 **Non-pressure chronic ulcer of left calf** with unspecified severity `HCC`

✓5th L97.3 **Non-pressure chronic ulcer of** ankle

✓6th L97.30 **Non-pressure chronic ulcer of unspecified ankle**

L97.301 **Non-pressure chronic ulcer of unspecified ankle** limited to breakdown of skin `HCC`

L97.302 **Non-pressure chronic ulcer of unspecified ankle** with fat layer exposed `HCC`

L97.303 **Non-pressure chronic ulcer of unspecified ankle** with necrosis of muscle `HCC`

L97.304 **Non-pressure chronic ulcer of unspecified ankle** with necrosis of bone `HCC`

L97.305 **Non-pressure chronic ulcer of unspecified ankle** with muscle involvement without evidence of necrosis `HCC`

L97.306 **Non-pressure chronic ulcer of unspecified ankle** with bone involvement without evidence of necrosis `HCC`

L97.308 **Non-pressure chronic ulcer of unspecified ankle** with other specified severity `HCC`

L97.309 **Non-pressure chronic ulcer of unspecified ankle** with unspecified severity `HCC`

✓6th L97.31 **Non-pressure chronic ulcer of** right **ankle**

L97.311 **Non-pressure chronic ulcer of right ankle** limited to breakdown of skin `HCC`

L97.312 **Non-pressure chronic ulcer of right ankle** with fat layer exposed `HCC`

L97.313 **Non-pressure chronic ulcer of right ankle** with necrosis of muscle `HCC`

L97.314 **Non-pressure chronic ulcer of right ankle** with necrosis of bone `HCC`

L97.315 **Non-pressure chronic ulcer of right ankle** with muscle involvement without evidence of necrosis `HCC`

L97.316 **Non-pressure chronic ulcer of right ankle** with bone involvement without evidence of necrosis `HCC`

L97.318 **Non-pressure chronic ulcer of right ankle with other specified severity** `HCC`

L97.319 **Non-pressure chronic ulcer of right ankle with unspecified severity** `HCC`

✓6th L97.32 **Non-pressure chronic ulcer of** left **ankle**

L97.321 **Non-pressure chronic ulcer of left ankle** limited to breakdown of skin `HCC`

L97.322 **Non-pressure chronic ulcer of left ankle** with fat layer exposed `HCC`

L97.323 **Non-pressure chronic ulcer of left ankle** with necrosis of muscle `HCC`

L97.324 **Non-pressure chronic ulcer of left ankle** with necrosis of bone `HCC`

L97.325 **Non-pressure chronic ulcer of left ankle** with muscle involvement without evidence of necrosis `HCC`

L97.326 **Non-pressure chronic ulcer of left ankle** with bone involvement without evidence of necrosis `HCC`

L97.328 **Non-pressure chronic ulcer of left ankle** with other specified severity `HCC`

L97.329 **Non-pressure chronic ulcer of left ankle with unspecified severity** `HCC`

✓5th L97.4 **Non-pressure chronic ulcer of** heel and midfoot

Non-pressure chronic ulcer of plantar surface of midfoot

✓6th L97.40 **Non-pressure chronic ulcer of unspecified heel and midfoot**

L97.401 **Non-pressure chronic ulcer of unspecified heel and midfoot** limited to breakdown of skin `HCC`

L97.402 **Non-pressure chronic ulcer of unspecified heel and midfoot** with fat layer exposed `HCC`

L97.403 **Non-pressure chronic ulcer of unspecified heel and midfoot** with necrosis of muscle `HCC`

L97.404 **Non-pressure chronic ulcer of unspecified heel and midfoot** with necrosis of bone `HCC`

L97.405 **Non-pressure chronic ulcer of unspecified heel and midfoot** with muscle involvement without evidence of necrosis `HCC`

L97.406 **Non-pressure chronic ulcer of unspecified heel and midfoot** with bone involvement without evidence of necrosis `HCC`

L97.408 **Non-pressure chronic ulcer of unspecified heel and midfoot** with other specified severity `HCC`

L97.409 **Non-pressure chronic ulcer of unspecified heel and midfoot** with unspecified severity `HCC`

✓6th L97.41 **Non-pressure chronic ulcer of** right **heel and midfoot**

L97.411 **Non-pressure chronic ulcer of right heel and midfoot** limited to breakdown of skin `HCC`

L97.412 **Non-pressure chronic ulcer of right heel and midfoot** with fat layer exposed `HCC`

L97.413 **Non-pressure chronic ulcer of right heel and midfoot** with necrosis of muscle `HCC`

L97.414 **Non-pressure chronic ulcer of right heel and midfoot** with necrosis of bone `HCC`

L97.415 **Non-pressure chronic ulcer of right heel and midfoot** with muscle involvement without evidence of necrosis `HCC`

L97.416 **Non-pressure chronic ulcer of right heel and midfoot** with bone involvement without evidence of necrosis `HCC`

L97.418 **Non-pressure chronic ulcer of right heel and midfoot with other specified severity** `HCC`

L97.419 **Non-pressure chronic ulcer of right heel and midfoot with unspecified severity** `HCC`

✓ Additional Character Required   ✓x7th Placeholder Alert   Manifestation   <u>Unspecified Dx</u>   ▶◀ Revised Text   ● New Code   ▲ Revised Code Title

✓6th **L97.42**   **Non-pressure chronic ulcer of** left heel and midfoot

   L97.421   **Non-pressure chronic ulcer of left heel and midfoot** limited to breakdown of skin   HCC
     AHA: 2016,1Q,12

   L97.422   **Non-pressure chronic ulcer of left heel and midfoot** with fat layer exposed   HCC

   L97.423   **Non-pressure chronic ulcer of left heel and midfoot** with necrosis of muscle   HCC

   L97.424   **Non-pressure chronic ulcer of left heel and midfoot** with necrosis of bone   HCC

   L97.425   **Non-pressure chronic ulcer of left heel and midfoot** with muscle involvement without evidence of necrosis   HCC

   L97.426   **Non-pressure chronic ulcer of left heel and midfoot** with bone involvement without evidence of necrosis   HCC

   L97.428   **Non-pressure chronic ulcer of left heel and midfoot with other specified severity**   HCC

   L97.429   **Non-pressure chronic ulcer of left heel and midfoot with unspecified severity**   HCC

✓5th **L97.5**   **Non-pressure chronic ulcer of other part of** foot
    Non-pressure chronic ulcer of toe

   ✓6th **L97.50**   **Non-pressure chronic ulcer of other part of unspecified foot**

     L97.501   **Non-pressure chronic ulcer of other part of unspecified foot** limited to breakdown of skin   HCC

     L97.502   **Non-pressure chronic ulcer of other part of unspecified foot** with fat layer exposed   HCC

     L97.503   **Non-pressure chronic ulcer of other part of unspecified foot** with necrosis of muscle   HCC

     L97.504   **Non-pressure chronic ulcer of other part of unspecified foot** with necrosis of bone   HCC

     L97.505   **Non-pressure chronic ulcer of other part of unspecified foot** with muscle involvement without evidence of necrosis   HCC

     L97.506   **Non-pressure chronic ulcer of other part of unspecified foot** with bone involvement without evidence of necrosis   HCC

     L97.508   **Non-pressure chronic ulcer of other part of unspecified foot with other specified severity**   HCC

     L97.509   **Non-pressure chronic ulcer of other part of unspecified foot with unspecified severity**   HCC

   ✓6th **L97.51**   **Non-pressure chronic ulcer of other part of** right foot

     L97.511   **Non-pressure chronic ulcer of other part of right foot** limited to breakdown of skin   HCC

     L97.512   **Non-pressure chronic ulcer of other part of right foot** with fat layer exposed   HCC

     L97.513   **Non-pressure chronic ulcer of other part of right foot** with necrosis of muscle   HCC

     L97.514   **Non-pressure chronic ulcer of other part of right foot** with necrosis of bone   HCC

     L97.515   **Non-pressure chronic ulcer of other part of right foot** with muscle involvement without evidence of necrosis   HCC

     L97.516   **Non-pressure chronic ulcer of other part of right foot** with bone involvement without evidence of necrosis   HCC

     L97.518   **Non-pressure chronic ulcer of other part of right foot with other specified severity**   HCC

   L97.519   **Non-pressure chronic ulcer of other part of right foot with unspecified severity**   HCC

   ✓6th **L97.52**   **Non-pressure chronic ulcer of other part of** left foot

     L97.521   **Non-pressure chronic ulcer of other part of left foot** limited to breakdown of skin   HCC

     L97.522   **Non-pressure chronic ulcer of other part of left foot** with fat layer exposed   HCC

     L97.523   **Non-pressure chronic ulcer of other part of left foot** with necrosis of muscle   HCC

     L97.524   **Non-pressure chronic ulcer of other part of left foot** with necrosis of bone   HCC

     L97.525   **Non-pressure chronic ulcer of other part of left foot** with muscle involvement without evidence of necrosis   HCC

     L97.526   **Non-pressure chronic ulcer of other part of left foot** with bone involvement without evidence of necrosis   HCC

     L97.528   **Non-pressure chronic ulcer of other part of left foot with other specified severity**   HCC

     L97.529   **Non-pressure chronic ulcer of other part of left foot with unspecified severity**   HCC

✓5th **L97.8**   **Non-pressure chronic ulcer of other part of** lower leg

   ✓6th **L97.80**   **Non-pressure chronic ulcer of other part of unspecified lower leg**

     L97.801   **Non-pressure chronic ulcer of other part of unspecified lower leg** limited to breakdown of skin   HCC

     L97.802   **Non-pressure chronic ulcer of other part of unspecified lower leg** with fat layer exposed   HCC

     L97.803   **Non-pressure chronic ulcer of other part of unspecified lower leg** with necrosis of muscle   HCC

     L97.804   **Non-pressure chronic ulcer of other part of unspecified lower leg** with necrosis of bone   HCC

     L97.805   **Non-pressure chronic ulcer of other part of unspecified lower leg** with muscle involvement without evidence of necrosis   HCC

     L97.806   **Non-pressure chronic ulcer of other part of unspecified lower leg** with bone involvement without evidence of necrosis   HCC

     L97.808   **Non-pressure chronic ulcer of other part of unspecified lower leg with other specified severity**   HCC

     L97.809   **Non-pressure chronic ulcer of other part of unspecified lower leg with unspecified severity**   HCC

   ✓6th **L97.81**   **Non-pressure chronic ulcer of other part of** right lower leg

     L97.811   **Non-pressure chronic ulcer of other part of right lower leg** limited to breakdown of skin   HCC

     L97.812   **Non-pressure chronic ulcer of other part of right lower leg** with fat layer exposed   HCC

     L97.813   **Non-pressure chronic ulcer of other part of right lower leg** with necrosis of muscle   HCC

     L97.814   **Non-pressure chronic ulcer of other part of right lower leg** with necrosis of bone   HCC

     L97.815   **Non-pressure chronic ulcer of other part of right lower leg** with muscle involvement without evidence of necrosis   HCC

     L97.816   **Non-pressure chronic ulcer of other part of right lower leg** with bone involvement without evidence of necrosis   HCC

     L97.818   **Non-pressure chronic ulcer of other part of right lower leg with other specified severity**   HCC

L97.819   **Non-pressure chronic ulcer of other part of right lower leg with unspecified severity** `HCC`

✓6ᵗʰ   L97.82   **Non-pressure chronic ulcer of other part of left lower leg**

L97.821   **Non-pressure chronic ulcer of other part of left lower leg** limited to breakdown of skin `HCC`

L97.822   **Non-pressure chronic ulcer of other part of left lower leg** with fat layer exposed `HCC`

L97.823   **Non-pressure chronic ulcer of other part of left lower leg** with necrosis of muscle `HCC`

L97.824   **Non-pressure chronic ulcer of other part of left lower leg** with necrosis of bone `HCC`

L97.825   **Non-pressure chronic ulcer of other part of left lower leg** with muscle involvement without evidence of necrosis `HCC`

L97.826   **Non-pressure chronic ulcer of other part of left lower leg** with bone involvement without evidence of necrosis `HCC`

L97.828   **Non-pressure chronic ulcer of other part of left lower leg** with other specified severity `HCC`

L97.829   **Non-pressure chronic ulcer of other part of left lower leg** with unspecified severity `HCC`

✓5ᵗʰ   L97.9   **Non-pressure chronic ulcer of unspecified part of** lower leg

✓6ᵗʰ   L97.90   **Non-pressure chronic ulcer of unspecified part of unspecified lower leg**

L97.901   **Non-pressure chronic ulcer of unspecified part of unspecified lower leg** limited to breakdown of skin `HCC`

L97.902   **Non-pressure chronic ulcer of unspecified part of unspecified lower leg** with fat layer exposed `HCC`

L97.903   **Non-pressure chronic ulcer of unspecified part of unspecified lower leg** with necrosis of muscle `HCC`

L97.904   **Non-pressure chronic ulcer of unspecified part of unspecified lower leg** with necrosis of bone `HCC`

L97.905   **Non-pressure chronic ulcer of unspecified part of unspecified lower leg** with muscle involvement without evidence of necrosis `HCC`

L97.906   **Non-pressure chronic ulcer of unspecified part of unspecified lower leg** with bone involvement without evidence of necrosis `HCC`

L97.908   **Non-pressure chronic ulcer of unspecified part of unspecified lower leg** with other specified severity `HCC`

L97.909   **Non-pressure chronic ulcer of unspecified part of unspecified lower leg** with unspecified severity `HCC`

✓6ᵗʰ   L97.91   **Non-pressure chronic ulcer of unspecified part of right lower leg**

L97.911   **Non-pressure chronic ulcer of unspecified part of right lower leg** limited to breakdown of skin `HCC`

L97.912   **Non-pressure chronic ulcer of unspecified part of right lower leg** with fat layer exposed `HCC`

L97.913   **Non-pressure chronic ulcer of unspecified part of right lower leg** with necrosis of muscle `HCC`

L97.914   **Non-pressure chronic ulcer of unspecified part of right lower leg** with necrosis of bone `HCC`

L97.915   **Non-pressure chronic ulcer of unspecified part of right lower leg** with muscle involvement without evidence of necrosis `HCC`

L97.916   **Non-pressure chronic ulcer of unspecified part of right lower leg with bone involvement without evidence of necrosis** `HCC`

L97.918   **Non-pressure chronic ulcer of unspecified part of right lower leg with other specified severity** `HCC`

L97.919   **Non-pressure chronic ulcer of unspecified part of right lower leg with unspecified severity** `HCC`

✓6ᵗʰ   L97.92   **Non-pressure chronic ulcer of unspecified part of left lower leg**

L97.921   **Non-pressure chronic ulcer of unspecified part of left lower leg** limited to breakdown of skin `HCC`

L97.922   **Non-pressure chronic ulcer of unspecified part of left lower leg** with fat layer exposed `HCC`

L97.923   **Non-pressure chronic ulcer of unspecified part of left lower leg** with necrosis of muscle `HCC`

L97.924   **Non-pressure chronic ulcer of unspecified part of left lower leg** with necrosis of bone `HCC`

L97.925   **Non-pressure chronic ulcer of unspecified part of left lower leg** with muscle involvement without evidence of necrosis `HCC`

L97.926   **Non-pressure chronic ulcer of unspecified part of left lower leg** with bone involvement without evidence of necrosis `HCC`

L97.928   **Non-pressure chronic ulcer of unspecified part of left lower leg** with other specified severity `HCC`

L97.929   **Non-pressure chronic ulcer of unspecified part of left lower leg** with unspecified severity `HCC`

✓4ᵗʰ   **L98   Other disorders of skin and subcutaneous tissue, not elsewhere classified**

L98.0   **Pyogenic granuloma**

> `EXCLUDES 2`   *pyogenic granuloma of gingiva (K06.8)*
> *pyogenic granuloma of maxillary alveolar ridge (K04.5)*
> *pyogenic granuloma of oral mucosa (K13.4)*

DEF: Solitary polypoid capillary hemangioma often associated with local irritation, trauma, and superimposed inflammation. Located on the skin and gingival or oral mucosa, they bleed easily and may ulcerate and form crusted sores.

L98.1   **Factitial dermatitis**

Neurotic excoriation

> `EXCLUDES 1`   *excoriation (skin-picking) disorder (F42.4)*

AHA: 2016,4Q,15

DEF: Self-inflicted skin lesions to satisfy an unconscious psychological or emotional need. Methods used to injure the skin include deep excoriations with a sharp instrument, scarification with a knife, or the application of caustic chemicals and burning, sometimes with a cigarette.

L98.2   **Febrile neutrophilic dermatosis [Sweet]**

L98.3   **Eosinophilic cellulitis [Wells]**

✓5ᵗʰ   L98.4   **Non-pressure chronic ulcer of skin, not elsewhere classified**

Chronic ulcer of skin NOS

Tropical ulcer NOS

Ulcer of skin NOS

> `EXCLUDES 2`   *gangrene (I96)*
> *pressure ulcer (pressure area) (L89.-)*
> *skin infections (L00-L08)*
> *specific infections classified to A00-B99*
> *ulcer of lower limb NEC (L97.-)*
> *varicose ulcer (I83.0-I82.2)*

AHA: 2017,4Q,17

TIP: The depth and/or severity of a diagnosed nonpressure ulcer can be determined based on medical record documentation from clinicians who are not the patient's provider.

TIP: Assign a code from this category/subcategory for nonpressure ulcers documented as acute.

✓6ᵗʰ   L98.41   **Non-pressure chronic ulcer of buttock**

L98.411   **Non-pressure chronic ulcer of buttock** limited to breakdown of skin `HCC`

L98.412   **Non-pressure chronic ulcer of buttock** with fat layer exposed `HCC`

☑ Additional Character Required   ✓x7ᵗʰ Placeholder Alert   Manifestation   Unspecified Dx   ▶◀ Revised Text   ● New Code   ▲ Revised Code Title

L98.413 Non-pressure chronic ulcer of buttock with necrosis of muscle `HCC`

L98.414 Non-pressure chronic ulcer of buttock with necrosis of bone `HCC`

L98.415 Non-pressure chronic ulcer of buttock with muscle involvement without evidence of necrosis `HCC`

L98.416 Non-pressure chronic ulcer of buttock with bone involvement without evidence of necrosis `HCC`

L98.418 Non-pressure chronic ulcer of buttock with other specified severity `HCC`

L98.419 Non-pressure chronic ulcer of buttock with unspecified severity `HCC`

✓6ᵗʰ **L98.42 Non-pressure chronic ulcer of back**

L98.421 Non-pressure chronic ulcer of back limited to breakdown of skin `HCC`

L98.422 Non-pressure chronic ulcer of back with fat layer exposed `HCC`

L98.423 Non-pressure chronic ulcer of back with necrosis of muscle `HCC`

L98.424 Non-pressure chronic ulcer of back with necrosis of bone `HCC`

L98.425 Non-pressure chronic ulcer of back with muscle involvement without evidence of necrosis `HCC`

L98.426 Non-pressure chronic ulcer of back with bone involvement without evidence of necrosis `HCC`

L98.428 Non-pressure chronic ulcer of back with other specified severity `HCC`

L98.429 Non-pressure chronic ulcer of back with unspecified severity `HCC`

✓6ᵗʰ **L98.49 Non-pressure chronic ulcer of skin of other sites**

Non-pressure chronic ulcer of skin NOS

L98.491 Non-pressure chronic ulcer of skin of other sites limited to breakdown of skin `HCC`

L98.492 Non-pressure chronic ulcer of skin of other sites with fat layer exposed `HCC`

L98.493 Non-pressure chronic ulcer of skin of other sites with necrosis of muscle `HCC`

L98.494 Non-pressure chronic ulcer of skin of other sites with necrosis of bone `HCC`

L98.495 Non-pressure chronic ulcer of skin of other sites with muscle involvement without evidence of necrosis `HCC`

L98.496 Non-pressure chronic ulcer of skin of other sites with bone involvement without evidence of necrosis `HCC`

L98.498 Non-pressure chronic ulcer of skin of other sites with other specified severity `HCC`

L98.499 Non-pressure chronic ulcer of skin of other sites with unspecified severity `HCC`

L98.5 Mucinosis of the skin
Focal mucinosis
Lichen myxedematosus
Reticular erythematous mucinosis
EXCLUDES 1   *focal oral mucinosis (K13.79)*
                      myxedema (E03.9)

L98.6 Other infiltrative disorders of the skin and subcutaneous tissue
EXCLUDES 1   *hyalinosis cutis et mucosae (E78.89)*

L98.7 Excessive and redundant skin and subcutaneous tissue
Loose or sagging skin, following bariatric surgery weight loss
Loose or sagging skin following dietary weight loss
Loose or sagging skin, NOS
EXCLUDES 2   *acquired excess or redundant skin of eyelid (H02.3-)*
                      congenital excess or redundant skin of eyelid (Q10.3)
                      skin changes due to chronic exposure to nonionizing radiation (L57.-)
AHA: 2016,4Q,36

L98.8 Other specified disorders of the skin and subcutaneous tissue
AHA: 2013,2Q,32

L98.9 Disorder of the skin and subcutaneous tissue, unspecified

L99 *Other disorders of skin and subcutaneous tissue in diseases classified elsewhere*
Code first underlying disease, such as:
amyloidosis (E85.-)
EXCLUDES 1   *skin disorders in diabetes (E08-E13 with .62)*
                      skin disorders in gonorrhea (A54.89)
                      skin disorders in syphilis (A51.31, A52.79)

Chapter 13. Diseases of the Musculoskeletal System and Connective Tissue (M00–M99)

Chapter-specific Guidelines with Coding Examples

The chapter-specific guidelines from the ICD-10-CM Official Guidelines for Coding and Reporting have been provided below. Along with these guidelines are coding examples, contained in the shaded boxes, that have been developed to help illustrate the coding and/or sequencing guidance found in these guidelines.

a. Site and laterality

Most of the codes within Chapter 13 have site and laterality designations. The site represents the bone, joint or the muscle involved. For some conditions where more than one bone, joint or muscle is usually involved, such as osteoarthritis, there is a "multiple sites" code available. For categories where no multiple site code is provided and more than one bone, joint or muscle is involved, multiple codes should be used to indicate the different sites involved.

> Olecranon bursitis of the left elbow
>
> **M70.22**   **Olecranon bursitis, left elbow**
>
> *Explanation:* Most of the codes within chapter 13 have site and laterality designations. The site represents the bone, joint, or the muscle involved.

> Rheumatoid arthritis of multiple sites without rheumatoid factor
>
> **M06.09**   **Rheumatoid arthritis without rheumatoid factor, multiple sites**
>
> *Explanation:* For some conditions where more than one bone, joint or muscle is usually involved, such as osteoarthritis, there is a "multiple sites" code available.

> Adolescent scoliosis in the upper thoracic region and the lumbar vertebrae
>
> **M41.124**   **Adolescent idiopathic scoliosis, thoracic region**
>
> **M41.126**   **Adolescent idiopathic scoliosis, lumbar region**
>
> *Explanation:* For categories without a multiple site code and more than one bone, joint, or muscle is involved, multiple codes should be used to indicate the different sites involved.

1) Bone versus joint

For certain conditions, the bone may be affected at the upper or lower end, (e.g., avascular necrosis of bone, M87, Osteoporosis, M80, M81). Though the portion of the bone affected may be at the joint, the site designation will be the bone, not the joint.

> Idiopathic avascular necrosis of the femoral head of the left hip joint
>
> **M87.052**   **Idiopathic aseptic necrosis of left femur**
>
> *Explanation:* For certain conditions such as avascular necrosis, the bone may be affected at the joint, but the site designation is the bone, not the joint.

b. Acute traumatic versus chronic or recurrent musculoskeletal conditions

Many musculoskeletal conditions are a result of previous injury or trauma to a site, or are recurrent conditions. Bone, joint or muscle conditions that are the result of a healed injury are usually found in chapter 13. Recurrent bone, joint or muscle conditions are also usually found in chapter 13. Any current, acute injury should be coded to the appropriate injury code from chapter 19. Chronic or recurrent conditions should generally be coded with a code from chapter 13. If it is difficult to determine from the documentation in the record which code is best to describe a condition, query the provider.

> Acute traumatic bucket handle tear of right medial meniscus
>
> **S83.211A**   **Bucket-handle tear of medial meniscus, current injury, right knee, initial encounter**
>
> *Explanation:* Any current, acute injury is not coded in chapter 13. It should instead be coded to the appropriate injury code from chapter 19.

> Old bucket handle tear of right medial meniscus
>
> **M23.203**   **Derangement of unspecified medial meniscus due to old tear or injury, right knee**
>
> *Explanation:* Chronic or recurrent conditions should generally be coded with a code from chapter 13.

c. Coding of Pathologic Fractures

7th character A is for use as long as the patient is receiving active treatment for the fracture. Examples of active treatment are: surgical treatment, emergency department encounter, evaluation and continuing treatment by the same or a different physician. While the patient may be seen by a new or different provider over the course of treatment for a pathological fracture, assignment of the 7th character is based on whether the patient is undergoing active treatment and not whether the provider is seeing the patient for the first time.

> Pathologic fracture of left foot, unknown cause, currently under active treatment by a follow-up provider
>
> **M84.475A**   **Pathological fracture, left foot, initial encounter for fracture**
>
> *Explanation:* Seventh character A is for use as long as the patient is receiving active treatment for a pathologic fracture. Examples of active treatment are surgical treatment, emergency department encounter, evaluation, and continuing treatment by the same or a different physician.
>
> The seventh character is based on whether the patient is undergoing active treatment and not whether the provider is seeing the patient for the first time.

7th character D is to be used for encounters after the patient has completed active treatment for the fracture and is receiving routine care for the fracture during the healing or recovery phase. The other 7th characters, listed under each subcategory in the Tabular List, are to be used for subsequent encounters for treatment of problems associated with the healing, such as malunions, nonunions, and sequelae.

Care for complications of surgical treatment for fracture repairs during the healing or recovery phase should be coded with the appropriate complication codes.

See Section I.C.19. Coding of traumatic fractures.

d. Osteoporosis

Osteoporosis is a systemic condition, meaning that all bones of the musculoskeletal system are affected. Therefore, site is not a component of the codes under category M81, Osteoporosis without current pathological fracture. The site codes under category M80, Osteoporosis with current pathological fracture, identify the site of the fracture, not the osteoporosis.

1) Osteoporosis without pathological fracture

Category M81, Osteoporosis without current pathological fracture, is for use for patients with osteoporosis who do not currently have a pathologic fracture due to the osteoporosis, even if they have had a fracture in the past. For patients with a history of osteoporosis fractures, status code Z87.310, Personal history of (healed) osteoporosis fracture, should follow the code from M81.

> Age-related osteoporosis with healed osteoporotic fracture of the lumbar vertebra
>
> **M81.0**   **Age-related osteoporosis without current pathological fracture**
>
> **Z87.310**   **Personal history of (healed) osteoporosis fracture**
>
> *Explanation:* Category M81 is used for patients with osteoporosis who do not currently have a pathologic fracture due to the osteoporosis. To report a previous (healed) fracture, status code Z87.310 Personal history of (healed) osteoporosis fracture, should follow the code from M81.

2) Osteoporosis with current pathological fracture

Category M80, Osteoporosis with current pathological fracture, is for patients who have a current pathologic fracture at the time of an encounter. The codes under M80 identify the site of the fracture. A code from category M80, not a traumatic fracture code, should be used for any patient with known osteoporosis who suffers a fracture, even if the patient had a minor fall or trauma, if that fall or trauma would not usually break a normal, healthy bone.

> Disuse osteoporosis with current fracture of right shoulder sustained lifting a grocery bag, initial encounter
>
> **M80.811A**   **Other osteoporosis with current pathological fracture, right shoulder, initial encounter for fracture**
>
> *Explanation:* A code from category M80, not a traumatic fracture code, should be used for any patient with known osteoporosis who suffers a fracture, even if the patient had a minor fall or trauma, if that fall or trauma would not usually break a normal, healthy bone.

Muscle/Tendon Table

ICD-10-CM categorizes certain muscles and tendons in the upper and lower extremities by their action (e.g., extension, flexion), their anatomical location (e.g., posterior, anterior), and/or whether they are intrinsic or extrinsic to a certain anatomical area. The Muscle/Tendon Table is provided at the beginning of chapters 13 and 19 as a resource to help users when code selection depends on one or more of these characteristics. A **TIP** has been placed at those categories and/or subcategories that relate to this table. Please note that this table is not all-inclusive, and proper code assignment should be based on the provider's documentation.

Body Region	Muscle	Extensor Tendon	Flexor Tendon	Other Tendon
Shoulder				
	Deltoid	Posterior deltoid	Anterior deltoid	
	Rotator cuff			
	Infraspinatus			Infraspinatus
	Subscapularis			Subscapularis
	Supraspinatus			Supraspinatus
	Teres minor			Teres minor
	Teres major	Teres major		
Upper arm				
	Anterior muscles			
	Biceps brachii — long head		Biceps brachii — long head	
	Biceps brachii — short head		Biceps brachii — short head	
	Brachialis		Brachialis	
	Coracobrachialis		Coracobrachialis	
	Posterior muscles			
	Triceps brachii	Triceps brachii		
Forearm				
	Anterior muscles			
	Flexors			
	Deep			
	Flexor digitorum profundus		Flexor digitorum profundus	
	Flexor pollicis longus		Flexor pollicis longus	
	Intermediate			
	Flexor digitorum superficialis		Flexor digitorum superficialis	
	Superficial			
	Flexor carpi radialis		Flexor carpi radialis	
	Flexor carpi ulnaris		Flexor carpi ulnaris	
	Palmaris longus		Palmaris longus	
	Pronators			
	Pronator quadratus			Pronator quadratus
	Pronator teres			Pronator teres
	Posterior muscles			
	Extensors			
	Deep			
	Abductor pollicis longus			Abductor pollicis longus
	Extensor indicis	Extensor indicis		
	Extensor pollicis brevis	Extensor pollicis brevis		
	Extensor pollicis longus	Extensor pollicis longus		
	Superficial			
	Brachioradialis			Brachioradialis
	Extensor carpi radialis brevis	Extensor carpi radialis brevis		
	Extensor carpi radialis longus	Extensor carpi radialis longus		
	Extensor carpi ulnaris	Extensor carpi ulnaris		
	Extensor digiti minimi	Extensor digiti minimi		
	Extensor digitorum	Extensor digitorum		
	Anconeus	Anconeus		
	Supinator			Supinator

Body Region	Muscle	Extensor Tendon	Flexor Tendon	Other Tendon
Hand				
Extrinsic — attach to a site in the forearm as well as a site in the hand with action related to hand movement at the wrist				
	Extensor carpi radialis brevis	Extensor carpi radialis brevis		
	Extensor carpi radialis longus	Extensor carpie radialis longus		
	Extensor carpi ulnaris	Extensor carpi ulnaris		
	Flexor carpi radialis		Flexor carpi radialis	
	Flexor carpi ulnaris		Flexor carpi ulnaris	
	Flexor digitorum superficialis		Flexor digitorum superficialis	
	Palmaris longus		Palmaris longus	
Extrinsic — attach to a site in the forearm as well as a site in the hand with action in the hand related to finger movement				
	Adductor pollicis longus			Adductor pollicis longus
	Extensor digiti minimi	Extensor digiti minimi		
	Extensor digitorum	Extensor digitorum		
	Extensor indicis	Extensor indicis		
	Flexor digitorum profundus		Flexor digitorum profundus	
	Flexor digitorum superficialis		Flexor digitorum superficialis	
Extrinsic — attach to a site in the forearm as well as a site in the hand with action in the hand related to thumb movement				
	Extensor pollicis brevis	Extensor pollicis brevis		
	Extensor pollicis longus	Extensor pollicis longus		
	Flexor pollicis longus		Flexor pollicis longus	
Intrinsic — found within the hand only				
	Adductor pollicis			Adductor pollicis
	Dorsal interossei	Dorsal interossei	Dorsal interossei	
	Lumbricals	Lumbricals	Lumbricals	
	Palmaris brevis			Palmaris brevis
	Palmar interossei	Palmar interossei	Palmar interossei	
	Hypothenar muscles			
	Abductor digiti minimi			Abductor digiti minimi
	Flexor digiti minimi brevis		Flexor digiti minimi brevis	
	Oppenens digiti minimi		Oppenens digiti minimi	
	Thenar muscles			
	Abductor pollicis brevis			Abductor pollicis brevis
	Flexor pollicis brevis		Flexor pollicis brevis	
	Oppenens pollicis		Oppenens pollicis	
Thigh				
	Anterior muscles			
	Iliopsoas		Iliopsoas	
	Pectineus		Pectineus	
	Quadriceps	Quadriceps		
	Rectus femoris	Rectus femoris — Extends knee	Rectus femoris — Flexes hip	
	Vastus intermedius	Vastus intermedius		
	Vastus lateralis	Vastus lateralis		
	Vastus medialis	Vastus medialis		
	Sartorius		Sartorius	
	Medial muscles			
	Adductor brevis			Adductor brevis
	Adductor longus			Adductor longus
	Adductor magnus			Adductor magnus
	Gracilis			Gracilis
	Obturator externus			Obturator externus
	Posterior muscles			
	Hamstring	Hamstring — Extends hip	Hamstring — Flexes knee	
	Biceps femoris	Biceps femoris	Biceps femoris	
	Semimembranosus	Semimembranosus	Semimembranosus	
	Semitendinosus	Semitendinosus	Semitendinosus	

Chapter 13. Diseases of the Musculoskeletal System and Connective Tissue

Body Region	Muscle	Extensor Tendon	Flexor Tendon	Other Tendon
Lower leg				
	Anterior muscles			
	Extensor digitorum longus	Extensor digitorum longus		
	Extensor hallucis longus	Extensor hallucis longus		
	Fibularis (peroneus) tertius	Fibularis (peroneus) tertius		
	Tibialis anterior	Tibialis anterior		Tibialis anterior
	Lateral muscles			
	Fibularis (peroneus) brevis		Fibularis (peroneus) brevis	
	Fibularis (peroneus) longus		Fibularis (peroneus) longus	
	Posterior muscles			
	Deep			
	Flexor digitorum longus		Flexor digitorum longus	
	Flexor hallucis longus		Flexor hallucis longus	
	Popliteus		Popliteus	
	Tibialis posterior		Tibialis posterior	
	Superficial			
	Gastrocnemius		Gastrocnemius	
	Plantaris		Plantaris	
	Soleus		Soleus	
				Calcaneal (Achilles)
Ankle/Foot				
Extrinsic — attach to a site in the lower leg as well as a site in the foot with action related to foot movement at the ankle				
	Plantaris		Plantaris	
	Soleus		Soleus	
	Tibialis anterior	Tibialis anterior		
	Tibialis posterior		Tibialis posterior	
Extrinsic — attach to a site in the lower leg as well as a site in the foot with action in the foot related to toe movement				
	Extensor digitorum longus	Extensor digitorum longus		
	Extensor hallicus longus	Extensor hallicus longus		
	Flexor digitorum longus		Flexor digitorum longus	
	Flexor hallucis longus		Flexor hallucis longus	
Intrinsic — found within the ankle/foot only				
	Dorsal muscles			
	Extensor digitorum brevis	Extensor digitorum brevis		
	Extensor hallucis brevis	Extensor hallucis brevis		
	Plantar muscles			
	Abductor digiti minimi		Abductor digiti minimi	
	Abductor hallucis		Abductor hallucis	
	Dorsal interossei	Dorsal interossei	Dorsal interossei	
	Flexor digiti minimi brevis		Flexor digiti minimi brevis	
	Flexor digitorum brevis		Flexor digitorum brevis	
	Flexor hallucis brevis		Flexor hallucis brevis	
	Lumbricals	Lumbricals	Lumbricals	
	Quadratus plantae		Quadratus plantae	
	Plantar interossei	Plantar interossei	Plantar interossei	

Chapter 13. Diseases of the Musculoskeletal System and Connective Tissue (M00-M99)

NOTE Use an external cause code following the code for the musculoskeletal condition, if applicable, to identify the cause of the musculoskeletal condition

EXCLUDES 2 *arthropathic psoriasis (L40.5-)*
certain conditions originating in the perinatal period (P04-P96)
certain infectious and parasitic diseases (A00-B99)
compartment syndrome (traumatic) (T79.A-)
complications of pregnancy, childbirth and the puerperium (O00-O9A)
congenital malformations, deformations, and chromosomal abnormalities (Q00-Q99)
endocrine, nutritional and metabolic diseases (E00-E88)
injury, poisoning and certain other consequences of external causes (S00-T88)
neoplasms (C00-D49)
symptoms, signs and abnormal clinical and laboratory findings, not elsewhere classified (R00-R94)

This chapter contains the following blocks:

M00-M02	Infectious arthropathies
M04	Autoinflammatory syndromes
M05-M14	Inflammatory polyarthropathies
M15-M19	Osteoarthritis
M20-M25	Other joint disorders
M26-M27	Dentofacial anomalies [including malocclusion] and other disorders of jaw
M30-M36	Systemic connective tissue disorders
M40-M43	Deforming dorsopathies
M45-M49	Spondylopathies
M50-M54	Other dorsopathies
M60-M63	Disorders of muscles
M65-M67	Disorders of synovium and tendon
M70-M79	Other soft tissue disorders
M80-M85	Disorders of bone density and structure
M86-M90	Other osteopathies
M91-M94	Chondropathies
M95	Other disorders of the musculoskeletal system and connective tissue
M96	Intraoperative and postprocedural complications and disorders of musculoskeletal system, not elsewhere classified
M97	Periprosthetic fracture around internal prosthetic joint
M99	Biomechanical lesions, not elsewhere classified

ARTHROPATHIES (M00-M25)

INCLUDES disorders affecting predominantly peripheral (limb) joints

Infectious arthropathies (M00-M02)

NOTE This block comprises arthropathies due to microbiological agents. Distinction is made between the following types of etiological relationship:

a) direct infection of joint, where organisms invade synovial tissue and microbial antigen is present in the joint;

b) indirect infection, which may be of two types: a reactive arthropathy, where microbial infection of the body is established but neither organisms nor antigens can be identified in the joint, and a postinfective arthropathy, where microbial antigen is present but recovery of an organism is inconstant and evidence of local multiplication is lacking.

✓4ᵗʰ M00 Pyogenic arthritis

DEF: Pyogenic: Relating to or involving pus production, often referred to as suppurative or purulent.

✓5ᵗʰ M00.0 Staphylococcal arthritis and polyarthritis

Use additional code (B95.61-B95.8) to identify bacterial agent
EXCLUDES 2 *infection and inflammatory reaction due to internal joint prosthesis (T84.5-)*

M00.00	Staphylococcal arthritis, unspecified joint	HCC

✓6ᵗʰ M00.01 Staphylococcal arthritis, shoulder

M00.011	Staphylococcal arthritis, right shoulder	HCC
M00.012	Staphylococcal arthritis, left shoulder	HCC
M00.019	Staphylococcal arthritis, unspecified shoulder	HCC

✓6ᵗʰ M00.02 Staphylococcal arthritis, elbow

M00.021	Staphylococcal arthritis, right elbow	HCC
M00.022	Staphylococcal arthritis, left elbow	HCC
M00.029	Staphylococcal arthritis, unspecified elbow	HCC

✓6ᵗʰ M00.03 Staphylococcal arthritis, wrist

Staphylococcal arthritis of carpal bones

M00.031	Staphylococcal arthritis, right wrist	HCC
M00.032	Staphylococcal arthritis, left wrist	HCC
M00.039	Staphylococcal arthritis, unspecified wrist	HCC

✓6ᵗʰ M00.04 Staphylococcal arthritis, hand

Staphylococcal arthritis of metacarpus and phalanges

M00.041	Staphylococcal arthritis, right hand	HCC
M00.042	Staphylococcal arthritis, left hand	HCC
M00.049	Staphylococcal arthritis, unspecified hand	HCC

✓6ᵗʰ M00.05 Staphylococcal arthritis, hip

M00.051	Staphylococcal arthritis, right hip	HCC
M00.052	Staphylococcal arthritis, left hip	HCC
M00.059	Staphylococcal arthritis, unspecified hip	HCC

✓6ᵗʰ M00.06 Staphylococcal arthritis, knee

M00.061	Staphylococcal arthritis, right knee	HCC
M00.062	Staphylococcal arthritis, left knee	HCC
M00.069	Staphylococcal arthritis, unspecified knee	HCC

✓6ᵗʰ M00.07 Staphylococcal arthritis, ankle and foot

Staphylococcal arthritis, tarsus, metatarsus and phalanges

M00.071	Staphylococcal arthritis, right ankle and foot	HCC
M00.072	Staphylococcal arthritis, left ankle and foot	HCC
M00.079	Staphylococcal arthritis, unspecified ankle and foot	HCC

M00.08	Staphylococcal arthritis, vertebrae	HCC
M00.09	Staphylococcal polyarthritis	HCC

✓5ᵗʰ M00.1 Pneumococcal arthritis and polyarthritis

M00.10	Pneumococcal arthritis, unspecified joint	HCC

✓6ᵗʰ M00.11 Pneumococcal arthritis, shoulder

M00.111	Pneumococcal arthritis, right shoulder	HCC
M00.112	Pneumococcal arthritis, left shoulder	HCC
M00.119	Pneumococcal arthritis, unspecified shoulder	HCC

✓6ᵗʰ M00.12 Pneumococcal arthritis, elbow

M00.121	Pneumococcal arthritis, right elbow	HCC
M00.122	Pneumococcal arthritis, left elbow	HCC
M00.129	Pneumococcal arthritis, unspecified elbow	HCC

✓6ᵗʰ M00.13 Pneumococcal arthritis, wrist

Pneumococcal arthritis of carpal bones

M00.131	Pneumococcal arthritis, right wrist	HCC
M00.132	Pneumococcal arthritis, left wrist	HCC
M00.139	Pneumococcal arthritis, unspecified wrist	HCC

✓6ᵗʰ M00.14 Pneumococcal arthritis, hand

Pneumococcal arthritis of metacarpus and phalanges

M00.141	Pneumococcal arthritis, right hand	HCC
M00.142	Pneumococcal arthritis, left hand	HCC
M00.149	Pneumococcal arthritis, unspecified hand	HCC

✓6ᵗʰ M00.15 Pneumococcal arthritis, hip

M00.151	Pneumococcal arthritis, right hip	HCC
M00.152	Pneumococcal arthritis, left hip	HCC
M00.159	Pneumococcal arthritis, unspecified hip	HCC

✓6ᵗʰ M00.16 Pneumococcal arthritis, knee

M00.161	Pneumococcal arthritis, right knee	HCC
M00.162	Pneumococcal arthritis, left knee	HCC

✅ Additional Character Required • ✓x7ᵗʰ Placeholder Alert • Manifestation • Unspecified Dx • ▶◀ Revised Text • ● New Code • ▲ Revised Code Title

Chapter 13. Diseases of the Musculoskeletal System and Connective Tissue

        M00.169 **Pneumococcal arthritis, unspecified knee** `HCC`

✓6ᵗʰ M00.17 **Pneumococcal arthritis, ankle and foot**

        Pneumococcal arthritis, tarsus, metatarsus and phalanges

        M00.171 **Pneumococcal arthritis, right ankle and foot** `HCC`

        M00.172 **Pneumococcal arthritis, left ankle and foot** `HCC`

        M00.179 **Pneumococcal arthritis, unspecified ankle and foot** `HCC`

    M00.18 **Pneumococcal arthritis, vertebrae** `HCC`

    M00.19 **Pneumococcal polyarthritis** `HCC`

✓5ᵗʰ M00.2 **Other streptococcal arthritis and polyarthritis**

    Use additional code (B95.0-B95.2, B95.4-B95.5) to identify bacterial agent

    M00.20 **Other streptococcal arthritis, unspecified joint** `HCC`

✓6ᵗʰ M00.21 **Other streptococcal arthritis, shoulder**

        M00.211 **Other streptococcal arthritis, right shoulder** `HCC`

        M00.212 **Other streptococcal arthritis, left shoulder** `HCC`

        M00.219 **Other streptococcal arthritis, unspecified shoulder** `HCC`

✓6ᵗʰ M00.22 **Other streptococcal arthritis, elbow**

        M00.221 **Other streptococcal arthritis, right elbow** `HCC`

        M00.222 **Other streptococcal arthritis, left elbow** `HCC`

        M00.229 **Other streptococcal arthritis, unspecified elbow** `HCC`

✓6ᵗʰ M00.23 **Other streptococcal arthritis, wrist**

        Other streptococcal arthritis of carpal bones

        M00.231 **Other streptococcal arthritis, right wrist** `HCC`

        M00.232 **Other streptococcal arthritis, left wrist** `HCC`

        M00.239 **Other streptococcal arthritis, unspecified wrist** `HCC`

✓6ᵗʰ M00.24 **Other streptococcal arthritis, hand**

        Other streptococcal arthritis metacarpus and phalanges

        M00.241 **Other streptococcal arthritis, right hand** `HCC`

        M00.242 **Other streptococcal arthritis, left hand** `HCC`

        M00.249 **Other streptococcal arthritis, unspecified hand** `HCC`

✓6ᵗʰ M00.25 **Other streptococcal arthritis, hip**

        M00.251 **Other streptococcal arthritis, right hip** `HCC`

        M00.252 **Other streptococcal arthritis, left hip** `HCC`

        M00.259 **Other streptococcal arthritis, unspecified hip** `HCC`

✓6ᵗʰ M00.26 **Other streptococcal arthritis, knee**

        M00.261 **Other streptococcal arthritis, right knee** `HCC`

        M00.262 **Other streptococcal arthritis, left knee** `HCC`

        M00.269 **Other streptococcal arthritis, unspecified knee** `HCC`

✓6ᵗʰ M00.27 **Other streptococcal arthritis, ankle and foot**

        Other streptococcal arthritis, tarsus, metatarsus and phalanges

        M00.271 **Other streptococcal arthritis, right ankle and foot** `HCC`

        M00.272 **Other streptococcal arthritis, left ankle and foot** `HCC`

        M00.279 **Other streptococcal arthritis, unspecified ankle and foot** `HCC`

    M00.28 **Other streptococcal arthritis, vertebrae** `HCC`

    M00.29 **Other streptococcal polyarthritis** `HCC`

✓5ᵗʰ M00.8 **Arthritis and polyarthritis due to other bacteria**

    Use additional code (B96) to identify bacteria

    M00.80 **Arthritis due to other bacteria, unspecified joint** `HCC`

✓6ᵗʰ M00.81 **Arthritis due to other bacteria, shoulder**

        M00.811 **Arthritis due to other bacteria, right shoulder** `HCC`

        M00.812 **Arthritis due to other bacteria, left shoulder** `HCC`

        M00.819 **Arthritis due to other bacteria, unspecified shoulder** `HCC`

✓6ᵗʰ M00.82 **Arthritis due to other bacteria, elbow**

        M00.821 **Arthritis due to other bacteria, right elbow** `HCC`

        M00.822 **Arthritis due to other bacteria, left elbow** `HCC`

        M00.829 **Arthritis due to other bacteria, unspecified elbow** `HCC`

✓6ᵗʰ M00.83 **Arthritis due to other bacteria, wrist**

        Arthritis due to other bacteria, carpal bones

        M00.831 **Arthritis due to other bacteria, right wrist** `HCC`

        M00.832 **Arthritis due to other bacteria, left wrist** `HCC`

        M00.839 **Arthritis due to other bacteria, unspecified wrist** `HCC`

✓6ᵗʰ M00.84 **Arthritis due to other bacteria, hand**

        Arthritis due to other bacteria, metacarpus and phalanges

        M00.841 **Arthritis due to other bacteria, right hand** `HCC`

        M00.842 **Arthritis due to other bacteria, left hand** `HCC`

        M00.849 **Arthritis due to other bacteria, unspecified hand** `HCC`

✓6ᵗʰ M00.85 **Arthritis due to other bacteria, hip**

        M00.851 **Arthritis due to other bacteria, right hip** `HCC`

        M00.852 **Arthritis due to other bacteria, left hip** `HCC`

        M00.859 **Arthritis due to other bacteria, unspecified hip** `HCC`

✓6ᵗʰ M00.86 **Arthritis due to other bacteria, knee**

        M00.861 **Arthritis due to other bacteria, right knee** `HCC`

        M00.862 **Arthritis due to other bacteria, left knee** `HCC`

        M00.869 **Arthritis due to other bacteria, unspecified knee** `HCC`

✓6ᵗʰ M00.87 **Arthritis due to other bacteria, ankle and foot**

        Arthritis due to other bacteria, tarsus, metatarsus, and phalanges

        M00.871 **Arthritis due to other bacteria, right ankle and foot** `HCC`

        M00.872 **Arthritis due to other bacteria, left ankle and foot** `HCC`

        M00.879 **Arthritis due to other bacteria, unspecified ankle and foot** `HCC`

    M00.88 **Arthritis due to other bacteria, vertebrae** `HCC`

    M00.89 **Polyarthritis due to other bacteria** `HCC`

M00.9 **Pyogenic arthritis, unspecified** `HCC`

    Infective arthritis NOS

√4ᵗʰ **M01 Direct infections of joint in infectious and parasitic diseases classified elsewhere**

Code first underlying disease, such as:

leprosy [Hansen's disease] (A30.-)

mycoses (B35-B49)

O'nyong-nyong fever (A92.1)

paratyphoid fever (A01.1-A01.4)

EXCLUDES 1   *arthropathy in Lyme disease (A69.23)*

gonococcal arthritis (A54.42)

meningococcal arthritis (A39.83)

mumps arthritis (B26.85)

postinfective arthropathy (M02.-)

postmeningococcal arthritis (A39.84)

reactive arthritis (M02.3)

rubella arthritis (B06.82)

sarcoidosis arthritis (D86.86)

typhoid fever arthritis (A01.04)

tuberculosis arthritis (A18.01-A18.02)

√5ᵗʰ **M01.X Direct infection of joint in infectious and parasitic diseases classified elsewhere**

M01.X0   *Direct infection of unspecified joint in infectious and parasitic diseases classified elsewhere*   HCC

√6ᵗʰ **M01.X1 Direct infection of shoulder joint in infectious and parasitic diseases classified elsewhere**

M01.X11   *Direct infection of right shoulder in infectious and parasitic diseases classified elsewhere*   HCC

M01.X12   *Direct infection of left shoulder in infectious and parasitic diseases classified elsewhere*   HCC

M01.X19   *Direct infection of unspecified shoulder in infectious and parasitic diseases classified elsewhere*   HCC

√6ᵗʰ **M01.X2 Direct infection of elbow in infectious and parasitic diseases classified elsewhere**

M01.X21   *Direct infection of right elbow in infectious and parasitic diseases classified elsewhere*   HCC

M01.X22   *Direct infection of left elbow in infectious and parasitic diseases classified elsewhere*   HCC

M01.X29   *Direct infection of unspecified elbow in infectious and parasitic diseases classified elsewhere*   HCC

√6ᵗʰ **M01.X3 Direct infection of wrist in infectious and parasitic diseases classified elsewhere**

Direct infection of carpal bones in infectious and parasitic diseases classified elsewhere

M01.X31   *Direct infection of right wrist in infectious and parasitic diseases classified elsewhere*   HCC

M01.X32   *Direct infection of left wrist in infectious and parasitic diseases classified elsewhere*   HCC

M01.X39   *Direct infection of unspecified wrist in infectious and parasitic diseases classified elsewhere*   HCC

√6ᵗʰ **M01.X4 Direct infection of hand in infectious and parasitic diseases classified elsewhere**

Direct infection of metacarpus and phalanges in infectious and parasitic diseases classified elsewhere

M01.X41   *Direct infection of right hand in infectious and parasitic diseases classified elsewhere*   HCC

M01.X42   *Direct infection of left hand in infectious and parasitic diseases classified elsewhere*   HCC

M01.X49   *Direct infection of unspecified hand in infectious and parasitic diseases classified elsewhere*   HCC

√6ᵗʰ **M01.X5 Direct infection of hip in infectious and parasitic diseases classified elsewhere**

M01.X51   *Direct infection of right hip in infectious and parasitic diseases classified elsewhere*   HCC

M01.X52   *Direct infection of left hip in infectious and parasitic diseases classified elsewhere*   HCC

M01.X59   *Direct infection of unspecified hip in infectious and parasitic diseases classified elsewhere*   HCC

√6ᵗʰ **M01.X6 Direct infection of knee in infectious and parasitic diseases classified elsewhere**

M01.X61   *Direct infection of right knee in infectious and parasitic diseases classified elsewhere*   HCC

M01.X62   *Direct infection of left knee in infectious and parasitic diseases classified elsewhere*   HCC

M01.X69   *Direct infection of unspecified knee in infectious and parasitic diseases classified elsewhere*   HCC

√6ᵗʰ **M01.X7 Direct infection of ankle and foot in infectious and parasitic diseases classified elsewhere**

Direct infection of tarsus, metatarsus and phalanges in infectious and parasitic diseases classified elsewhere

M01.X71   *Direct infection of right ankle and foot in infectious and parasitic diseases classified elsewhere*   HCC

M01.X72   *Direct infection of left ankle and foot in infectious and parasitic diseases classified elsewhere*   HCC

M01.X79   *Direct infection of unspecified ankle and foot in infectious and parasitic diseases classified elsewhere*   HCC

M01.X8   *Direct infection of vertebrae in infectious and parasitic diseases classified elsewhere*   HCC

M01.X9   *Direct infection of multiple joints in infectious and parasitic diseases classified elsewhere*   HCC

√4ᵗʰ **M02 Postinfective and reactive arthropathies**

Code first underlying disease, such as:

congenital syphilis [Clutton's joints] (A50.5)

enteritis due to Yersinia enterocolitica (A04.6)

infective endocarditis (I33.0)

viral hepatitis (B15-B19)

EXCLUDES 1   *Behçet's disease (M35.2)*

direct infections of joint in infectious and parasitic diseases classified elsewhere (M01.-)

mumps arthritis (B26.85)

postmeningococcal arthritis (A39.84)

rheumatic fever (I00)

rubella arthritis (B06.82)

syphilis arthritis (late) (A52.77)

tabetic arthropathy [Charcôt's] (A52.16)

√5ᵗʰ **M02.0 Arthropathy following intestinal bypass**

M02.00 Arthropathy following intestinal bypass, unspecified site

√6ᵗʰ **M02.01 Arthropathy following intestinal bypass, shoulder**

M02.011 Arthropathy following intestinal bypass, right shoulder

M02.012 Arthropathy following intestinal bypass, left shoulder

M02.019 Arthropathy following intestinal bypass, unspecified shoulder

√6ᵗʰ **M02.02 Arthropathy following intestinal bypass, elbow**

M02.021 Arthropathy following intestinal bypass, right elbow

M02.022 Arthropathy following intestinal bypass, left elbow

M02.029 Arthropathy following intestinal bypass, unspecified elbow

√6ᵗʰ **M02.03 Arthropathy following intestinal bypass, wrist**

Arthropathy following intestinal bypass, carpal bones

M02.031 Arthropathy following intestinal bypass, right wrist

M02.032 Arthropathy following intestinal bypass, left wrist

M02.039 Arthropathy following intestinal bypass, unspecified wrist

√6ᵗʰ **M02.04 Arthropathy following intestinal bypass, hand**

Arthropathy following intestinal bypass, metacarpals and phalanges

M02.041 Arthropathy following intestinal bypass, right hand

M02.042 Arthropathy following intestinal bypass, left hand

☑ Additional Character Required   √7ᵗʰ Placeholder Alert   Manifestation   Unspecified Dx   ►◄ Revised Text   ● New Code   ▲ Revised Code Title

M02.049 **Arthropathy following intestinal bypass, unspecified hand**

✓6ᵗʰ M02.05 **Arthropathy following intestinal bypass, hip**

  M02.051 **Arthropathy following intestinal bypass, right hip**

  M02.052 **Arthropathy following intestinal bypass, left hip**

  M02.059 **Arthropathy following intestinal bypass, unspecified hip**

✓6ᵗʰ M02.06 **Arthropathy following intestinal bypass, knee**

  M02.061 **Arthropathy following intestinal bypass, right knee**

  M02.062 **Arthropathy following intestinal bypass, left knee**

  M02.069 **Arthropathy following intestinal bypass, unspecified knee**

✓6ᵗʰ M02.07 **Arthropathy following intestinal bypass, ankle and foot**

  Arthropathy following intestinal bypass, tarsus, metatarsus and phalanges

  M02.071 **Arthropathy following intestinal bypass, right ankle and foot**

  M02.072 **Arthropathy following intestinal bypass, left ankle and foot**

  M02.079 **Arthropathy following intestinal bypass, unspecified ankle and foot**

M02.08 **Arthropathy following intestinal bypass, vertebrae**

M02.09 **Arthropathy following intestinal bypass, multiple sites**

✓5ᵗʰ M02.1 **Postdysenteric arthropathy**

  M02.10 **Postdysenteric arthropathy, unspecified site**   HCC

  ✓6ᵗʰ M02.11 **Postdysenteric arthropathy, shoulder**

    M02.111 **Postdysenteric arthropathy, right shoulder**   HCC

    M02.112 **Postdysenteric arthropathy, left shoulder**   HCC

    M02.119 **Postdysenteric arthropathy, unspecified shoulder**   HCC

  ✓6ᵗʰ M02.12 **Postdysenteric arthropathy, elbow**

    M02.121 **Postdysenteric arthropathy, right elbow**   HCC

    M02.122 **Postdysenteric arthropathy, left elbow**   HCC

    M02.129 **Postdysenteric arthropathy, unspecified elbow**   HCC

  ✓6ᵗʰ M02.13 **Postdysenteric arthropathy, wrist**

    Postdysenteric arthropathy, carpal bones

    M02.131 **Postdysenteric arthropathy, right wrist**   HCC

    M02.132 **Postdysenteric arthropathy, left wrist**   HCC

    M02.139 **Postdysenteric arthropathy, unspecified wrist**   HCC

  ✓6ᵗʰ M02.14 **Postdysenteric arthropathy, hand**

    Postdysenteric arthropathy, metacarpus and phalanges

    M02.141 **Postdysenteric arthropathy, right hand**   HCC

    M02.142 **Postdysenteric arthropathy, left hand**   HCC

    M02.149 **Postdysenteric arthropathy, unspecified hand**   HCC

  ✓6ᵗʰ M02.15 **Postdysenteric arthropathy, hip**

    M02.151 **Postdysenteric arthropathy, right hip**   HCC

    M02.152 **Postdysenteric arthropathy, left hip**   HCC

    M02.159 **Postdysenteric arthropathy, unspecified hip**   HCC

  ✓6ᵗʰ M02.16 **Postdysenteric arthropathy, knee**

    M02.161 **Postdysenteric arthropathy, right knee**   HCC

    M02.162 **Postdysenteric arthropathy, left knee**   HCC

    M02.169 **Postdysenteric arthropathy, unspecified knee**   HCC

✓6ᵗʰ M02.17 **Postdysenteric arthropathy, ankle and foot**

  Postdysenteric arthropathy, tarsus, metatarsus and phalanges

  M02.171 **Postdysenteric arthropathy, right ankle and foot**   HCC

  M02.172 **Postdysenteric arthropathy, left ankle and foot**   HCC

  M02.179 **Postdysenteric arthropathy, unspecified ankle and foot**   HCC

M02.18 **Postdysenteric arthropathy, vertebrae**   HCC

M02.19 **Postdysenteric arthropathy, multiple sites**   HCC

✓5ᵗʰ M02.2 **Postimmunization arthropathy**

  M02.20 **Postimmunization arthropathy, unspecified site**

  ✓6ᵗʰ M02.21 **Postimmunization arthropathy, shoulder**

    M02.211 **Postimmunization arthropathy, right shoulder**

    M02.212 **Postimmunization arthropathy, left shoulder**

    M02.219 **Postimmunization arthropathy, unspecified shoulder**

  ✓6ᵗʰ M02.22 **Postimmunization arthropathy, elbow**

    M02.221 **Postimmunization arthropathy, right elbow**

    M02.222 **Postimmunization arthropathy, left elbow**

    M02.229 **Postimmunization arthropathy, unspecified elbow**

  ✓6ᵗʰ M02.23 **Postimmunization arthropathy, wrist**

    Postimmunization arthropathy, carpal bones

    M02.231 **Postimmunization arthropathy, right wrist**

    M02.232 **Postimmunization arthropathy, left wrist**

    M02.239 **Postimmunization arthropathy, unspecified wrist**

  ✓6ᵗʰ M02.24 **Postimmunization arthropathy, hand**

    Postimmunization arthropathy, metacarpus and phalanges

    M02.241 **Postimmunization arthropathy, right hand**

    M02.242 **Postimmunization arthropathy, left hand**

    M02.249 **Postimmunization arthropathy, unspecified hand**

  ✓6ᵗʰ M02.25 **Postimmunization arthropathy, hip**

    M02.251 **Postimmunization arthropathy, right hip**

    M02.252 **Postimmunization arthropathy, left hip**

    M02.259 **Postimmunization arthropathy, unspecified hip**

  ✓6ᵗʰ M02.26 **Postimmunization arthropathy, knee**

    M02.261 **Postimmunization arthropathy, right knee**

    M02.262 **Postimmunization arthropathy, left knee**

    M02.269 **Postimmunization arthropathy, unspecified knee**

  ✓6ᵗʰ M02.27 **Postimmunization arthropathy, ankle and foot**

    Postimmunization arthropathy, tarsus, metatarsus and phalanges

    M02.271 **Postimmunization arthropathy, right ankle and foot**

    M02.272 **Postimmunization arthropathy, left ankle and foot**

    M02.279 **Postimmunization arthropathy, unspecified ankle and foot**

M02.28 **Postimmunization arthropathy, vertebrae**

M02.29 **Postimmunization arthropathy, multiple sites**

✓5ᵗʰ M02.3 **Reiter's disease**

  Reactive arthritis

  DEF: Arthritis, iridocyclitis, and urethritis, sometimes with diarrhea. While symptoms may recur, arthritis is constant.

  M02.30 **Reiter's disease, unspecified site**   HCC

  ✓6ᵗʰ M02.31 **Reiter's disease, shoulder**

    M02.311 **Reiter's disease, right shoulder**   HCC

    M02.312 **Reiter's disease, left shoulder**   HCC

    M02.319 **Reiter's disease, unspecified shoulder**   HCC

  ✓6ᵗʰ M02.32 **Reiter's disease, elbow**

    M02.321 **Reiter's disease, right elbow**   HCC

    M02.322 **Reiter's disease, left elbow**   HCC

     M02.329   Reiter's disease, unspecified elbow   `HCC`

✓6ᵗʰ **M02.33**   Reiter's disease, wrist

     Reiter's disease, carpal bones

     M02.331   Reiter's disease, right wrist   `HCC`

     M02.332   Reiter's disease, left wrist   `HCC`

     M02.339   Reiter's disease, unspecified wrist   `HCC`

✓6ᵗʰ **M02.34**   Reiter's disease, hand

     Reiter's disease, metacarpus and phalanges

     M02.341   Reiter's disease, right hand   `HCC`

     M02.342   Reiter's disease, left hand   `HCC`

     M02.349   Reiter's disease, unspecified hand   `HCC`

✓6ᵗʰ **M02.35**   Reiter's disease, hip

     M02.351   Reiter's disease, right hip   `HCC`

     M02.352   Reiter's disease, left hip   `HCC`

     M02.359   Reiter's disease, unspecified hip   `HCC`

✓6ᵗʰ **M02.36**   Reiter's disease, knee

     M02.361   Reiter's disease, right knee   `HCC`

     M02.362   Reiter's disease, left knee   `HCC`

     M02.369   Reiter's disease, unspecified knee   `HCC`

✓6ᵗʰ **M02.37**   Reiter's disease, ankle and foot

     Reiter's disease, tarsus, metatarsus and phalanges

     M02.371   Reiter's disease, right ankle and foot   `HCC`

     M02.372   Reiter's disease, left ankle and foot   `HCC`

     M02.379   Reiter's disease, unspecified ankle and foot   `HCC`

     M02.38   Reiter's disease, vertebrae   `HCC`

     M02.39   Reiter's disease, multiple sites   `HCC`

✓5ᵗʰ **M02.8**   Other reactive arthropathies

     M02.80   *Other reactive arthropathies, unspecified site*   `HCC`

✓6ᵗʰ **M02.81**   Other reactive arthropathies, shoulder

     M02.811   *Other reactive arthropathies, right shoulder*   `HCC`

     M02.812   *Other reactive arthropathies, left shoulder*   `HCC`

     M02.819   *Other reactive arthropathies, unspecified shoulder*   `HCC`

✓6ᵗʰ **M02.82**   Other reactive arthropathies, elbow

     M02.821   *Other reactive arthropathies, right elbow*   `HCC`

     M02.822   *Other reactive arthropathies, left elbow*   `HCC`

     M02.829   *Other reactive arthropathies, unspecified elbow*   `HCC`

✓6ᵗʰ **M02.83**   Other reactive arthropathies, wrist

     Other reactive arthropathies, carpal bones

     M02.831   *Other reactive arthropathies, right wrist*   `HCC`

     M02.832   *Other reactive arthropathies, left wrist*   `HCC`

     M02.839   *Other reactive arthropathies, unspecified wrist*   `HCC`

✓6ᵗʰ **M02.84**   Other reactive arthropathies, hand

     Other reactive arthropathies, metacarpus and phalanges

     M02.841   *Other reactive arthropathies, right hand*   `HCC`

     M02.842   *Other reactive arthropathies, left hand*   `HCC`

     M02.849   *Other reactive arthropathies, unspecified hand*   `HCC`

✓6ᵗʰ **M02.85**   Other reactive arthropathies, hip

     M02.851   *Other reactive arthropathies, right hip*   `HCC`

     M02.852   *Other reactive arthropathies, left hip*   `HCC`

     M02.859   *Other reactive arthropathies, unspecified hip*   `HCC`

✓6ᵗʰ **M02.86**   Other reactive arthropathies, knee

     M02.861   *Other reactive arthropathies, right knee*   `HCC`

     M02.862   *Other reactive arthropathies, left knee*   `HCC`

     M02.869   *Other reactive arthropathies, unspecified knee*   `HCC`

✓6ᵗʰ **M02.87**   Other reactive arthropathies, ankle and foot

     Other reactive arthropathies, tarsus, metatarsus and phalanges

     M02.871   *Other reactive arthropathies, right ankle and foot*   `HCC`

     M02.872   *Other reactive arthropathies, left ankle and foot*   `HCC`

     M02.879   *Other reactive arthropathies, unspecified ankle and foot*   `HCC`

     M02.88   Other reactive arthropathies, *vertebrae*   `HCC`

     M02.89   Other reactive arthropathies, *multiple sites*   `HCC`

M02.9   Reactive arthropathy, unspecified   `HCC`

Autoinflammatory syndromes (M04)

✓4ᵗʰ **M04**   Autoinflammatory syndromes

     `EXCLUDES 2`   *Crohn's disease (K50.-)*

     AHA: 2016,4Q,37

     M04.1   Periodic fever syndromes   `HCC`

         Familial Mediterranean fever

         Hyperimmunoglobin D syndrome

         Mevalonate kinase deficiency

         Tumor necrosis factor receptor associated periodic syndrome [TRAPS]

     M04.2   Cryopyrin-associated periodic syndromes   `HCC`

         Chronic infantile neurological, cutaneous and articular syndrome [CINCA]

         Familial cold autoinflammatory syndrome

         Familial cold urticaria

         Muckle-Wells syndrome

         Neonatal onset multisystemic inflammatory disorder [NOMID]

     M04.8   Other autoinflammatory syndromes   `HCC`

         Blau syndrome

         Deficiency of interleukin 1 receptor antagonist [DIRA]

         Majeed syndrome

         Periodic fever, aphthous stomatitis, pharyngitis, and adenopathy syndrome [PFAPA]

         Pyogenic arthritis, pyoderma gangrenosum, and acne syndrome [PAPA]

     M04.9   Autoinflammatory syndrome, unspecified   `HCC`

Inflammatory polyarthropathies (M05-M14)

✓4ᵗʰ **M05**   Rheumatoid arthritis with rheumatoid factor

     `EXCLUDES 1`   *rheumatic fever (I00)*

           juvenile rheumatoid arthritis (M08.-)

           rheumatoid arthritis of spine (M45.-)

     DEF: Rheumatoid arthritis: Autoimmune systemic disease that causes chronic inflammation of the joints and other areas of the body, manifested by inflammatory changes in articular structures and synovial membranes, atrophy, and loss in bone density.

✓5ᵗʰ **M05.0**   Felty's syndrome

     Rheumatoid arthritis with splenoadenomegaly and leukopenia

     M05.00   Felty's syndrome, unspecified site   `HCC`

✓6ᵗʰ **M05.01**   Felty's syndrome, shoulder

     M05.011   Felty's syndrome, right shoulder   `HCC`

     M05.012   Felty's syndrome, left shoulder   `HCC`

     M05.019   Felty's syndrome, unspecified shoulder   `HCC`

✓6ᵗʰ **M05.02**   Felty's syndrome, elbow

     M05.021   Felty's syndrome, right elbow   `HCC`

     M05.022   Felty's syndrome, left elbow   `HCC`

     M05.029   Felty's syndrome, unspecified elbow   `HCC`

✓6ᵗʰ **M05.03**   Felty's syndrome, wrist

     Felty's syndrome, carpal bones

     M05.031   Felty's syndrome, right wrist   `HCC`

     M05.032   Felty's syndrome, left wrist   `HCC`

     M05.039   Felty's syndrome, unspecified wrist   `HCC`

✓6ᵗʰ **M05.04**   Felty's syndrome, hand

     Felty's syndrome, metacarpus and phalanges

     M05.041   Felty's syndrome, right hand   `HCC`

✓ Additional Character Required   ✓x7ᵗʰ Placeholder Alert   Manifestation   Unspecified Dx   ►◄ Revised Text   ● New Code   ▲ Revised Code Title

ICD-10-CM 2020   751

M05.042 Felty's syndrome, left hand `HCC`

M05.049 Felty's syndrome, unspecified hand `HCC`

✓6ᵗʰ **M05.05** Felty's syndrome, hip

M05.051 Felty's syndrome, right hip `HCC`

M05.052 Felty's syndrome, left hip `HCC`

M05.059 Felty's syndrome, unspecified hip `HCC`

✓6ᵗʰ **M05.06** Felty's syndrome, knee

M05.061 Felty's syndrome, right knee `HCC`

M05.062 Felty's syndrome, left knee `HCC`

M05.069 Felty's syndrome, unspecified knee `HCC`

✓6ᵗʰ **M05.07** Felty's syndrome, ankle and foot

Felty's syndrome, tarsus, metatarsus and phalanges

M05.071 Felty's syndrome, right ankle and foot `HCC`

M05.072 Felty's syndrome, left ankle and foot `HCC`

M05.079 Felty's syndrome, unspecified ankle and foot `HCC`

M05.09 Felty's syndrome, multiple sites `HCC`

✓5ᵗʰ **M05.1** Rheumatoid lung disease with rheumatoid arthritis

DEF: Lung disorders associated with rheumatoid arthritis.

M05.10 Rheumatoid lung disease with rheumatoid arthritis of unspecified site `HCC`

✓6ᵗʰ **M05.11** Rheumatoid lung disease with rheumatoid arthritis of shoulder

M05.111 Rheumatoid lung disease with rheumatoid arthritis of right shoulder `HCC`

M05.112 Rheumatoid lung disease with rheumatoid arthritis of left shoulder `HCC`

M05.119 Rheumatoid lung disease with rheumatoid arthritis of unspecified shoulder `HCC`

✓6ᵗʰ **M05.12** Rheumatoid lung disease with rheumatoid arthritis of elbow

M05.121 Rheumatoid lung disease with rheumatoid arthritis of right elbow `HCC`

M05.122 Rheumatoid lung disease with rheumatoid arthritis of left elbow `HCC`

M05.129 Rheumatoid lung disease with rheumatoid arthritis of unspecified elbow `HCC`

✓6ᵗʰ **M05.13** Rheumatoid lung disease with rheumatoid arthritis of wrist

Rheumatoid lung disease with rheumatoid arthritis, carpal bones

M05.131 Rheumatoid lung disease with rheumatoid arthritis of right wrist `HCC`

M05.132 Rheumatoid lung disease with rheumatoid arthritis of left wrist `HCC`

M05.139 Rheumatoid lung disease with rheumatoid arthritis of unspecified wrist `HCC`

✓6ᵗʰ **M05.14** Rheumatoid lung disease with rheumatoid arthritis of hand

Rheumatoid lung disease with rheumatoid arthritis, metacarpus and phalanges

M05.141 Rheumatoid lung disease with rheumatoid arthritis of right hand `HCC`

M05.142 Rheumatoid lung disease with rheumatoid arthritis of left hand `HCC`

M05.149 Rheumatoid lung disease with rheumatoid arthritis of unspecified hand `HCC`

✓6ᵗʰ **M05.15** Rheumatoid lung disease with rheumatoid arthritis of hip

M05.151 Rheumatoid lung disease with rheumatoid arthritis of right hip `HCC`

M05.152 Rheumatoid lung disease with rheumatoid arthritis of left hip `HCC`

M05.159 Rheumatoid lung disease with rheumatoid arthritis of unspecified hip `HCC`

✓6ᵗʰ **M05.16** Rheumatoid lung disease with rheumatoid arthritis of knee

M05.161 Rheumatoid lung disease with rheumatoid arthritis of right knee `HCC`

M05.162 Rheumatoid lung disease with rheumatoid arthritis of left knee `HCC`

M05.169 Rheumatoid lung disease with rheumatoid arthritis of unspecified knee `HCC`

✓6ᵗʰ **M05.17** Rheumatoid lung disease with rheumatoid arthritis of ankle and foot

Rheumatoid lung disease with rheumatoid arthritis, tarsus, metatarsus and phalanges

M05.171 Rheumatoid lung disease with rheumatoid arthritis of right ankle and foot `HCC`

M05.172 Rheumatoid lung disease with rheumatoid arthritis of left ankle and foot `HCC`

M05.179 Rheumatoid lung disease with rheumatoid arthritis of unspecified ankle and foot `HCC`

M05.19 Rheumatoid lung disease with rheumatoid arthritis of multiple sites `HCC`

✓5ᵗʰ **M05.2** Rheumatoid vasculitis with rheumatoid arthritis

M05.20 Rheumatoid vasculitis with rheumatoid arthritis of unspecified site `HCC`

✓6ᵗʰ **M05.21** Rheumatoid vasculitis with rheumatoid arthritis of shoulder

M05.211 Rheumatoid vasculitis with rheumatoid arthritis of right shoulder `HCC`

M05.212 Rheumatoid vasculitis with rheumatoid arthritis of left shoulder `HCC`

M05.219 Rheumatoid vasculitis with rheumatoid arthritis of unspecified shoulder `HCC`

✓6ᵗʰ **M05.22** Rheumatoid vasculitis with rheumatoid arthritis of elbow

M05.221 Rheumatoid vasculitis with rheumatoid arthritis of right elbow `HCC`

M05.222 Rheumatoid vasculitis with rheumatoid arthritis of left elbow `HCC`

M05.229 Rheumatoid vasculitis with rheumatoid arthritis of unspecified elbow `HCC`

✓6ᵗʰ **M05.23** Rheumatoid vasculitis with rheumatoid arthritis of wrist

Rheumatoid vasculitis with rheumatoid arthritis, carpal bones

M05.231 Rheumatoid vasculitis with rheumatoid arthritis of right wrist `HCC`

M05.232 Rheumatoid vasculitis with rheumatoid arthritis of left wrist `HCC`

M05.239 Rheumatoid vasculitis with rheumatoid arthritis of unspecified wrist `HCC`

✓6ᵗʰ **M05.24** Rheumatoid vasculitis with rheumatoid arthritis of hand

Rheumatoid vasculitis with rheumatoid arthritis, metacarpus and phalanges

M05.241 Rheumatoid vasculitis with rheumatoid arthritis of right hand `HCC`

M05.242 Rheumatoid vasculitis with rheumatoid arthritis of left hand `HCC`

M05.249 Rheumatoid vasculitis with rheumatoid arthritis of unspecified hand `HCC`

✓6ᵗʰ **M05.25** Rheumatoid vasculitis with rheumatoid arthritis of hip

M05.251 Rheumatoid vasculitis with rheumatoid arthritis of right hip `HCC`

M05.252 Rheumatoid vasculitis with rheumatoid arthritis of left hip `HCC`

M05.259 Rheumatoid vasculitis with rheumatoid arthritis of unspecified hip `HCC`

✓6ᵗʰ **M05.26** Rheumatoid vasculitis with rheumatoid arthritis of knee

M05.261 Rheumatoid vasculitis with rheumatoid arthritis of right knee `HCC`

        M05.262 **Rheumatoid vasculitis with rheumatoid arthritis of left knee** `HCC`

        M05.269 **Rheumatoid vasculitis with rheumatoid arthritis of unspecified knee** `HCC`

✓6ᵗʰ M05.27 **Rheumatoid vasculitis with rheumatoid arthritis of ankle and foot**

    Rheumatoid vasculitis with rheumatoid arthritis, tarsus, metatarsus and phalanges

        M05.271 **Rheumatoid vasculitis with rheumatoid arthritis of right ankle and foot** `HCC`

        M05.272 **Rheumatoid vasculitis with rheumatoid arthritis of left ankle and foot** `HCC`

        M05.279 **Rheumatoid vasculitis with rheumatoid arthritis of unspecified ankle and foot** `HCC`

    M05.29 **Rheumatoid vasculitis with rheumatoid arthritis of multiple sites** `HCC`

✓5ᵗʰ M05.3 **Rheumatoid heart disease with rheumatoid arthritis**

    Rheumatoid carditis
    Rheumatoid endocarditis
    Rheumatoid myocarditis
    Rheumatoid pericarditis

    M05.30 **Rheumatoid heart disease with rheumatoid arthritis of unspecified site** `HCC`

✓6ᵗʰ M05.31 **Rheumatoid heart disease with rheumatoid arthritis of shoulder**

        M05.311 **Rheumatoid heart disease with rheumatoid arthritis of right shoulder** `HCC`

        M05.312 **Rheumatoid heart disease with rheumatoid arthritis of left shoulder** `HCC`

        M05.319 **Rheumatoid heart disease with rheumatoid arthritis of unspecified shoulder** `HCC`

✓6ᵗʰ M05.32 **Rheumatoid heart disease with rheumatoid arthritis of elbow**

        M05.321 **Rheumatoid heart disease with rheumatoid arthritis of right elbow** `HCC`

        M05.322 **Rheumatoid heart disease with rheumatoid arthritis of left elbow** `HCC`

        M05.329 **Rheumatoid heart disease with rheumatoid arthritis of unspecified elbow** `HCC`

✓6ᵗʰ M05.33 **Rheumatoid heart disease with rheumatoid arthritis of wrist**

    Rheumatoid heart disease with rheumatoid arthritis, carpal bones

        M05.331 **Rheumatoid heart disease with rheumatoid arthritis of right wrist** `HCC`

        M05.332 **Rheumatoid heart disease with rheumatoid arthritis of left wrist** `HCC`

        M05.339 **Rheumatoid heart disease with rheumatoid arthritis of unspecified wrist** `HCC`

✓6ᵗʰ M05.34 **Rheumatoid heart disease with rheumatoid arthritis of hand**

    Rheumatoid heart disease with rheumatoid arthritis, metacarpus and phalanges

        M05.341 **Rheumatoid heart disease with rheumatoid arthritis of right hand** `HCC`

        M05.342 **Rheumatoid heart disease with rheumatoid arthritis of left hand** `HCC`

        M05.349 **Rheumatoid heart disease with rheumatoid arthritis of unspecified hand** `HCC`

✓6ᵗʰ M05.35 **Rheumatoid heart disease with rheumatoid arthritis of hip**

        M05.351 **Rheumatoid heart disease with rheumatoid arthritis of right hip** `HCC`

        M05.352 **Rheumatoid heart disease with rheumatoid arthritis of left hip** `HCC`

        M05.359 **Rheumatoid heart disease with rheumatoid arthritis of unspecified hip** `HCC`

✓6ᵗʰ M05.36 **Rheumatoid heart disease with rheumatoid arthritis of knee**

        M05.361 **Rheumatoid heart disease with rheumatoid arthritis of right knee** `HCC`

        M05.362 **Rheumatoid heart disease with rheumatoid arthritis of left knee** `HCC`

        M05.369 **Rheumatoid heart disease with rheumatoid arthritis of unspecified knee** `HCC`

✓6ᵗʰ M05.37 **Rheumatoid heart disease with rheumatoid arthritis of ankle and foot**

    Rheumatoid heart disease with rheumatoid arthritis, tarsus, metatarsus and phalanges

        M05.371 **Rheumatoid heart disease with rheumatoid arthritis of right ankle and foot** `HCC`

        M05.372 **Rheumatoid heart disease with rheumatoid arthritis of left ankle and foot** `HCC`

        M05.379 **Rheumatoid heart disease with rheumatoid arthritis of unspecified ankle and foot** `HCC`

    M05.39 **Rheumatoid heart disease with rheumatoid arthritis of multiple sites** `HCC`

✓5ᵗʰ M05.4 **Rheumatoid myopathy with rheumatoid arthritis**

    M05.40 **Rheumatoid myopathy with rheumatoid arthritis of unspecified site** `HCC`

✓6ᵗʰ M05.41 **Rheumatoid myopathy with rheumatoid arthritis of shoulder**

        M05.411 **Rheumatoid myopathy with rheumatoid arthritis of right shoulder** `HCC`

        M05.412 **Rheumatoid myopathy with rheumatoid arthritis of left shoulder** `HCC`

        M05.419 **Rheumatoid myopathy with rheumatoid arthritis of unspecified shoulder** `HCC`

✓6ᵗʰ M05.42 **Rheumatoid myopathy with rheumatoid arthritis of elbow**

        M05.421 **Rheumatoid myopathy with rheumatoid arthritis of right elbow** `HCC`

        M05.422 **Rheumatoid myopathy with rheumatoid arthritis of left elbow** `HCC`

        M05.429 **Rheumatoid myopathy with rheumatoid arthritis of unspecified elbow** `HCC`

✓6ᵗʰ M05.43 **Rheumatoid myopathy with rheumatoid arthritis of wrist**

    Rheumatoid myopathy with rheumatoid arthritis, carpal bones

        M05.431 **Rheumatoid myopathy with rheumatoid arthritis of right wrist** `HCC`

        M05.432 **Rheumatoid myopathy with rheumatoid arthritis of left wrist** `HCC`

        M05.439 **Rheumatoid myopathy with rheumatoid arthritis of unspecified wrist** `HCC`

✓6ᵗʰ M05.44 **Rheumatoid myopathy with rheumatoid arthritis of hand**

    Rheumatoid myopathy with rheumatoid arthritis, metacarpus and phalanges

        M05.441 **Rheumatoid myopathy with rheumatoid arthritis of right hand** `HCC`

        M05.442 **Rheumatoid myopathy with rheumatoid arthritis of left hand** `HCC`

        M05.449 **Rheumatoid myopathy with rheumatoid arthritis of unspecified hand** `HCC`

✓6ᵗʰ M05.45 **Rheumatoid myopathy with rheumatoid arthritis of hip**

        M05.451 **Rheumatoid myopathy with rheumatoid arthritis of right hip** `HCC`

        M05.452 **Rheumatoid myopathy with rheumatoid arthritis of left hip** `HCC`

        M05.459 **Rheumatoid myopathy with rheumatoid arthritis of unspecified hip** `HCC`

✓6ᵗʰ M05.46 **Rheumatoid myopathy with rheumatoid arthritis of knee**

        M05.461 **Rheumatoid myopathy with rheumatoid arthritis of right knee** `HCC`

        M05.462 **Rheumatoid myopathy with rheumatoid arthritis of left knee** `HCC`

☑ Additional Character Required   ✓x7ᵗʰ Placeholder Alert   Manifestation   Unspecified Dx   ►◄ Revised Text   ● New Code   ▲ Revised Code Title

M05.469 Rheumatoid myopathy with rheumatoid arthritis of unspecified knee `HCC`

✓6ᵗʰ **M05.47** Rheumatoid myopathy with rheumatoid arthritis of ankle and foot

Rheumatoid myopathy with rheumatoid arthritis, tarsus, metatarsus and phalanges

M05.471 Rheumatoid myopathy with rheumatoid arthritis of right ankle and foot `HCC`

M05.472 Rheumatoid myopathy with rheumatoid arthritis of left ankle and foot `HCC`

M05.479 Rheumatoid myopathy with rheumatoid arthritis of unspecified ankle and foot `HCC`

M05.49 Rheumatoid myopathy with rheumatoid arthritis of multiple sites `HCC`

✓5ᵗʰ **M05.5** Rheumatoid polyneuropathy with rheumatoid arthritis

M05.50 Rheumatoid polyneuropathy with rheumatoid arthritis of unspecified site `HCC`

✓6ᵗʰ **M05.51** Rheumatoid polyneuropathy with rheumatoid arthritis of shoulder

M05.511 Rheumatoid polyneuropathy with rheumatoid arthritis of right shoulder `HCC`

M05.512 Rheumatoid polyneuropathy with rheumatoid arthritis of left shoulder `HCC`

M05.519 Rheumatoid polyneuropathy with rheumatoid arthritis of unspecified shoulder `HCC`

✓6ᵗʰ **M05.52** Rheumatoid polyneuropathy with rheumatoid arthritis of elbow

M05.521 Rheumatoid polyneuropathy with rheumatoid arthritis of right elbow `HCC`

M05.522 Rheumatoid polyneuropathy with rheumatoid arthritis of left elbow `HCC`

M05.529 Rheumatoid polyneuropathy with rheumatoid arthritis of unspecified elbow `HCC`

✓6ᵗʰ **M05.53** Rheumatoid polyneuropathy with rheumatoid arthritis of wrist

Rheumatoid polyneuropathy with rheumatoid arthritis, carpal bones

M05.531 Rheumatoid polyneuropathy with rheumatoid arthritis of right wrist `HCC`

M05.532 Rheumatoid polyneuropathy with rheumatoid arthritis of left wrist `HCC`

M05.539 Rheumatoid polyneuropathy with rheumatoid arthritis of unspecified wrist `HCC`

✓6ᵗʰ **M05.54** Rheumatoid polyneuropathy with rheumatoid arthritis of hand

Rheumatoid polyneuropathy with rheumatoid arthritis, metacarpus and phalanges

M05.541 Rheumatoid polyneuropathy with rheumatoid arthritis of right hand `HCC`

M05.542 Rheumatoid polyneuropathy with rheumatoid arthritis of left hand `HCC`

M05.549 Rheumatoid polyneuropathy with rheumatoid arthritis of unspecified hand `HCC`

✓6ᵗʰ **M05.55** Rheumatoid polyneuropathy with rheumatoid arthritis of hip

M05.551 Rheumatoid polyneuropathy with rheumatoid arthritis of right hip `HCC`

M05.552 Rheumatoid polyneuropathy with rheumatoid arthritis of left hip `HCC`

M05.559 Rheumatoid polyneuropathy with rheumatoid arthritis of unspecified hip `HCC`

✓6ᵗʰ **M05.56** Rheumatoid polyneuropathy with rheumatoid arthritis of knee

M05.561 Rheumatoid polyneuropathy with rheumatoid arthritis of right knee `HCC`

M05.562 Rheumatoid polyneuropathy with rheumatoid arthritis of left knee `HCC`

M05.569 Rheumatoid polyneuropathy with rheumatoid arthritis of unspecified knee `HCC`

✓6ᵗʰ **M05.57** Rheumatoid polyneuropathy with rheumatoid arthritis of ankle and foot

Rheumatoid polyneuropathy with rheumatoid arthritis, tarsus, metatarsus and phalanges

M05.571 Rheumatoid polyneuropathy with rheumatoid arthritis of right ankle and foot `HCC`

M05.572 Rheumatoid polyneuropathy with rheumatoid arthritis of left ankle and foot `HCC`

M05.579 Rheumatoid polyneuropathy with rheumatoid arthritis of unspecified ankle and foot `HCC`

M05.59 Rheumatoid polyneuropathy with rheumatoid arthritis of multiple sites `HCC`

✓5ᵗʰ **M05.6** Rheumatoid arthritis with involvement of other organs and systems

M05.60 Rheumatoid arthritis of unspecified site with involvement of other organs and systems `HCC`

✓6ᵗʰ **M05.61** Rheumatoid arthritis of shoulder with involvement of other organs and systems

M05.611 Rheumatoid arthritis of right shoulder with involvement of other organs and systems `HCC`

M05.612 Rheumatoid arthritis of left shoulder with involvement of other organs and systems `HCC`

M05.619 Rheumatoid arthritis of unspecified shoulder with involvement of other organs and systems `HCC`

✓6ᵗʰ **M05.62** Rheumatoid arthritis of elbow with involvement of other organs and systems

M05.621 Rheumatoid arthritis of right elbow with involvement of other organs and systems `HCC`

M05.622 Rheumatoid arthritis of left elbow with involvement of other organs and systems `HCC`

M05.629 Rheumatoid arthritis of unspecified elbow with involvement of other organs and systems `HCC`

✓6ᵗʰ **M05.63** Rheumatoid arthritis of wrist with involvement of other organs and systems

Rheumatoid arthritis of carpal bones with involvement of other organs and systems

M05.631 Rheumatoid arthritis of right wrist with involvement of other organs and systems `HCC`

M05.632 Rheumatoid arthritis of left wrist with involvement of other organs and systems `HCC`

M05.639 Rheumatoid arthritis of unspecified wrist with involvement of other organs and systems `HCC`

✓6ᵗʰ **M05.64** Rheumatoid arthritis of hand with involvement of other organs and systems

Rheumatoid arthritis of metacarpus and phalanges with involvement of other organs and systems

M05.641 Rheumatoid arthritis of right hand with involvement of other organs and systems `HCC`

M05.642 Rheumatoid arthritis of left hand with involvement of other organs and systems `HCC`

M05.649 Rheumatoid arthritis of unspecified hand with involvement of other organs and systems `HCC`

✓6ᵗʰ **M05.65** Rheumatoid arthritis of hip with involvement of other organs and systems

M05.651 Rheumatoid arthritis of right hip with involvement of other organs and systems `HCC`

M05.652 Rheumatoid arthritis of left hip with involvement of other organs and systems `HCC`

M05.659 Rheumatoid arthritis of unspecified hip with involvement of other organs and systems `HCC`

√6ᵗʰ **M05.66** **Rheumatoid arthritis of knee with involvement of other organs and systems**

     M05.661 **Rheumatoid arthritis of right knee with involvement of other organs and systems**   HCC

     M05.662 **Rheumatoid arthritis of left knee with involvement of other organs and systems**   HCC

     M05.669 **Rheumatoid arthritis of unspecified knee with involvement of other organs and systems**   HCC

√6ᵗʰ **M05.67** **Rheumatoid arthritis of ankle and foot with involvement of other organs and systems**

     Rheumatoid arthritis of tarsus, metatarsus and phalanges with involvement of other organs and systems

     M05.671 **Rheumatoid arthritis of right ankle and foot with involvement of other organs and systems**   HCC

     M05.672 **Rheumatoid arthritis of left ankle and foot with involvement of other organs and systems**   HCC

     M05.679 **Rheumatoid arthritis of unspecified ankle and foot with involvement of other organs and systems**   HCC

     M05.69 **Rheumatoid arthritis of multiple sites with involvement of other organs and systems**   HCC

√5ᵗʰ **M05.7** **Rheumatoid arthritis with rheumatoid factor without organ or systems involvement**

     M05.70 **Rheumatoid arthritis with rheumatoid factor of unspecified site without organ or systems involvement**   HCC

√6ᵗʰ **M05.71** **Rheumatoid arthritis with rheumatoid factor of shoulder without organ or systems involvement**

     M05.711 **Rheumatoid arthritis with rheumatoid factor of right shoulder without organ or systems involvement**   HCC

     M05.712 **Rheumatoid arthritis with rheumatoid factor of left shoulder without organ or systems involvement**   HCC

     M05.719 **Rheumatoid arthritis with rheumatoid factor of unspecified shoulder without organ or systems involvement**   HCC

√6ᵗʰ **M05.72** **Rheumatoid arthritis with rheumatoid factor of elbow without organ or systems involvement**

     M05.721 **Rheumatoid arthritis with rheumatoid factor of right elbow without organ or systems involvement**   HCC

     M05.722 **Rheumatoid arthritis with rheumatoid factor of left elbow without organ or systems involvement**   HCC

     M05.729 **Rheumatoid arthritis with rheumatoid factor of unspecified elbow without organ or systems involvement**   HCC

√6ᵗʰ **M05.73** **Rheumatoid arthritis with rheumatoid factor of wrist without organ or systems involvement**

     M05.731 **Rheumatoid arthritis with rheumatoid factor of right wrist without organ or systems involvement**   HCC

     M05.732 **Rheumatoid arthritis with rheumatoid factor of left wrist without organ or systems involvement**   HCC

     M05.739 **Rheumatoid arthritis with rheumatoid factor of unspecified wrist without organ or systems involvement**   HCC

√6ᵗʰ **M05.74** **Rheumatoid arthritis with rheumatoid factor of hand without organ or systems involvement**

     M05.741 **Rheumatoid arthritis with rheumatoid factor of right hand without organ or systems involvement**   HCC

     M05.742 **Rheumatoid arthritis with rheumatoid factor of left hand without organ or systems involvement**   HCC

     M05.749 **Rheumatoid arthritis with rheumatoid factor of unspecified hand without organ or systems involvement**   HCC

√6ᵗʰ **M05.75** **Rheumatoid arthritis with rheumatoid factor of hip without organ or systems involvement**

     M05.751 **Rheumatoid arthritis with rheumatoid factor of right hip without organ or systems involvement**   HCC

     M05.752 **Rheumatoid arthritis with rheumatoid factor of left hip without organ or systems involvement**   HCC

     M05.759 **Rheumatoid arthritis with rheumatoid factor of unspecified hip without organ or systems involvement**   HCC

√6ᵗʰ **M05.76** **Rheumatoid arthritis with rheumatoid factor of knee without organ or systems involvement**

     M05.761 **Rheumatoid arthritis with rheumatoid factor of right knee without organ or systems involvement**   HCC

     M05.762 **Rheumatoid arthritis with rheumatoid factor of left knee without organ or systems involvement**   HCC

     M05.769 **Rheumatoid arthritis with rheumatoid factor of unspecified knee without organ or systems involvement**   HCC

√6ᵗʰ **M05.77** **Rheumatoid arthritis with rheumatoid factor of ankle and foot without organ or systems involvement**

     M05.771 **Rheumatoid arthritis with rheumatoid factor of right ankle and foot without organ or systems involvement**   HCC

     M05.772 **Rheumatoid arthritis with rheumatoid factor of left ankle and foot without organ or systems involvement**   HCC

     M05.779 **Rheumatoid arthritis with rheumatoid factor of unspecified ankle and foot without organ or systems involvement**   HCC

     M05.79 **Rheumatoid arthritis with rheumatoid factor of multiple sites without organ or systems involvement**   HCC

√5ᵗʰ **M05.8** **Other rheumatoid arthritis with rheumatoid factor**

     M05.80 **Other rheumatoid arthritis with rheumatoid factor of unspecified site**   HCC

√6ᵗʰ **M05.81** **Other rheumatoid arthritis with rheumatoid factor of shoulder**

     M05.811 **Other rheumatoid arthritis with rheumatoid factor of right shoulder**   HCC

     M05.812 **Other rheumatoid arthritis with rheumatoid factor of left shoulder**   HCC

     M05.819 **Other rheumatoid arthritis with rheumatoid factor of unspecified shoulder**   HCC

√6ᵗʰ **M05.82** **Other rheumatoid arthritis with rheumatoid factor of elbow**

     M05.821 **Other rheumatoid arthritis with rheumatoid factor of right elbow**   HCC

     M05.822 **Other rheumatoid arthritis with rheumatoid factor of left elbow**   HCC

     M05.829 **Other rheumatoid arthritis with rheumatoid factor of unspecified elbow**   HCC

√6ᵗʰ **M05.83** **Other rheumatoid arthritis with rheumatoid factor of wrist**

     M05.831 **Other rheumatoid arthritis with rheumatoid factor of right wrist**   HCC

     M05.832 **Other rheumatoid arthritis with rheumatoid factor of left wrist**   HCC

     M05.839 **Other rheumatoid arthritis with rheumatoid factor of unspecified wrist**   HCC

☑ Additional Character Required   √x7ᵗʰ Placeholder Alert   Manifestation   Unspecified Dx   ▶◀ Revised Text   ● New Code   ▲ Revised Code Title

ICD-10-CM 2020   755

Chapter 13. Diseases of the Musculoskeletal System and Connective Tissue

✓6th **M05.84** **Other rheumatoid arthritis with rheumatoid factor of hand**

    M05.841 Other rheumatoid arthritis with rheumatoid factor of right hand   HCC

    M05.842 Other rheumatoid arthritis with rheumatoid factor of left hand   HCC

    M05.849 Other rheumatoid arthritis with rheumatoid factor of unspecified hand   HCC

✓6th **M05.85** **Other rheumatoid arthritis with rheumatoid factor of hip**

    M05.851 Other rheumatoid arthritis with rheumatoid factor of right hip   HCC

    M05.852 Other rheumatoid arthritis with rheumatoid factor of left hip   HCC

    M05.859 Other rheumatoid arthritis with rheumatoid factor of unspecified hip   HCC

✓6th **M05.86** **Other rheumatoid arthritis with rheumatoid factor of knee**

    M05.861 Other rheumatoid arthritis with rheumatoid factor of right knee   HCC

    M05.862 Other rheumatoid arthritis with rheumatoid factor of left knee   HCC

    M05.869 Other rheumatoid arthritis with rheumatoid factor of unspecified knee   HCC

✓6th **M05.87** **Other rheumatoid arthritis with rheumatoid factor of ankle and foot**

    M05.871 Other rheumatoid arthritis with rheumatoid factor of right ankle and foot   HCC

    M05.872 Other rheumatoid arthritis with rheumatoid factor of left ankle and foot   HCC

    M05.879 Other rheumatoid arthritis with rheumatoid factor of unspecified ankle and foot   HCC

    M05.89 Other rheumatoid arthritis with rheumatoid factor of multiple sites   HCC

    M05.9 **Rheumatoid arthritis with rheumatoid factor, unspecified**   HCC

✓4th **M06** **Other rheumatoid arthritis**

    DEF: Rheumatoid arthritis: Autoimmune systemic disease that causes chronic inflammation of the joints and other areas of the body, manifested by inflammatory changes in articular structures and synovial membranes, atrophy, and loss in bone density.

✓5th **M06.0** **Rheumatoid arthritis without rheumatoid factor**

    M06.00 Rheumatoid arthritis without rheumatoid factor, unspecified site   HCC

✓6th **M06.01** **Rheumatoid arthritis without rheumatoid factor, shoulder**

    M06.011 Rheumatoid arthritis without rheumatoid factor, right shoulder   HCC

    M06.012 Rheumatoid arthritis without rheumatoid factor, left shoulder   HCC

    M06.019 Rheumatoid arthritis without rheumatoid factor, unspecified shoulder   HCC

✓6th **M06.02** **Rheumatoid arthritis without rheumatoid factor, elbow**

    M06.021 Rheumatoid arthritis without rheumatoid factor, right elbow   HCC

    M06.022 Rheumatoid arthritis without rheumatoid factor, left elbow   HCC

    M06.029 Rheumatoid arthritis without rheumatoid factor, unspecified elbow   HCC

✓6th **M06.03** **Rheumatoid arthritis without rheumatoid factor, wrist**

    M06.031 Rheumatoid arthritis without rheumatoid factor, right wrist   HCC

    M06.032 Rheumatoid arthritis without rheumatoid factor, left wrist   HCC

    M06.039 Rheumatoid arthritis without rheumatoid factor, unspecified wrist   HCC

✓6th **M06.04** **Rheumatoid arthritis without rheumatoid factor, hand**

    M06.041 Rheumatoid arthritis without rheumatoid factor, right hand   HCC

    M06.042 Rheumatoid arthritis without rheumatoid factor, left hand   HCC

    M06.049 Rheumatoid arthritis without rheumatoid factor, unspecified hand   HCC

✓6th **M06.05** **Rheumatoid arthritis without rheumatoid factor, hip**

    M06.051 Rheumatoid arthritis without rheumatoid factor, right hip   HCC

    M06.052 Rheumatoid arthritis without rheumatoid factor, left hip   HCC

    M06.059 Rheumatoid arthritis without rheumatoid factor, unspecified hip   HCC

✓6th **M06.06** **Rheumatoid arthritis without rheumatoid factor, knee**

    M06.061 Rheumatoid arthritis without rheumatoid factor, right knee   HCC

    M06.062 Rheumatoid arthritis without rheumatoid factor, left knee   HCC

    M06.069 Rheumatoid arthritis without rheumatoid factor, unspecified knee   HCC

✓6th **M06.07** **Rheumatoid arthritis without rheumatoid factor, ankle and foot**

    M06.071 Rheumatoid arthritis without rheumatoid factor, right ankle and foot   HCC

    M06.072 Rheumatoid arthritis without rheumatoid factor, left ankle and foot   HCC

    M06.079 Rheumatoid arthritis without rheumatoid factor, unspecified ankle and foot   HCC

    M06.08 Rheumatoid arthritis without rheumatoid factor, vertebrae   HCC

    M06.09 Rheumatoid arthritis without rheumatoid factor, multiple sites   HCC

    M06.1 **Adult-onset Still's disease**   HCC A

     EXCLUDES 1   *Still's disease NOS (M08.2-)*

     DEF: Type of systemic arthritis characterized by a transient rash and spiking fevers. This condition may resolve or develop into a chronic condition and may affect internal organs, as well as joints.

     Synonym(s): *AOSD*

✓5th **M06.2** **Rheumatoid bursitis**

    M06.20 Rheumatoid bursitis, unspecified site   HCC

✓6th **M06.21** **Rheumatoid bursitis, shoulder**

    M06.211 Rheumatoid bursitis, right shoulder   HCC

    M06.212 Rheumatoid bursitis, left shoulder   HCC

    M06.219 Rheumatoid bursitis, unspecified shoulder   HCC

✓6th **M06.22** **Rheumatoid bursitis, elbow**

    M06.221 Rheumatoid bursitis, right elbow   HCC

    M06.222 Rheumatoid bursitis, left elbow   HCC

    M06.229 Rheumatoid bursitis, unspecified elbow   HCC

✓6th **M06.23** **Rheumatoid bursitis, wrist**

    M06.231 Rheumatoid bursitis, right wrist   HCC

    M06.232 Rheumatoid bursitis, left wrist   HCC

    M06.239 Rheumatoid bursitis, unspecified wrist   HCC

✓6th **M06.24** **Rheumatoid bursitis, hand**

    M06.241 Rheumatoid bursitis, right hand   HCC

    M06.242 Rheumatoid bursitis, left hand   HCC

    M06.249 Rheumatoid bursitis, unspecified hand   HCC

✓6th **M06.25** **Rheumatoid bursitis, hip**

    M06.251 Rheumatoid bursitis, right hip   HCC

    M06.252 Rheumatoid bursitis, left hip   HCC

    M06.259 Rheumatoid bursitis, unspecified hip   HCC

✓6th **M06.26** **Rheumatoid bursitis, knee**

    M06.261 Rheumatoid bursitis, right knee   HCC

    M06.262 Rheumatoid bursitis, left knee   HCC

    M06.269 Rheumatoid bursitis, unspecified knee   HCC

√6ᵗʰ **M06.27** **Rheumatoid bursitis**, ankle and foot

    M06.271 **Rheumatoid bursitis**, right ankle and foot   HCC

    M06.272 **Rheumatoid bursitis**, left ankle and foot   HCC

    M06.279 **Rheumatoid bursitis**, unspecified ankle and foot   HCC

M06.28 **Rheumatoid bursitis**, vertebrae   HCC

M06.29 **Rheumatoid bursitis**, multiple sites   HCC

√5ᵗʰ **M06.3** Rheumatoid nodule

    M06.30 **Rheumatoid nodule, unspecified site**   HCC

√6ᵗʰ **M06.31** **Rheumatoid nodule,** shoulder

    M06.311 **Rheumatoid nodule,** right shoulder   HCC

    M06.312 **Rheumatoid nodule,** left shoulder   HCC

    M06.319 **Rheumatoid nodule,** unspecified shoulder   HCC

√6ᵗʰ **M06.32** **Rheumatoid nodule,** elbow

    M06.321 **Rheumatoid nodule,** right elbow   HCC

    M06.322 **Rheumatoid nodule,** left elbow   HCC

    M06.329 **Rheumatoid nodule,** unspecified elbow   HCC

√6ᵗʰ **M06.33** **Rheumatoid nodule,** wrist

    M06.331 **Rheumatoid nodule,** right wrist   HCC

    M06.332 **Rheumatoid nodule,** left wrist   HCC

    M06.339 **Rheumatoid nodule,** unspecified wrist   HCC

√6ᵗʰ **M06.34** **Rheumatoid nodule,** hand

    M06.341 **Rheumatoid nodule,** right hand   HCC

    M06.342 **Rheumatoid nodule,** left hand   HCC

    M06.349 **Rheumatoid nodule,** unspecified hand   HCC

√6ᵗʰ **M06.35** **Rheumatoid nodule,** hip

    M06.351 **Rheumatoid nodule,** right hip   HCC

    M06.352 **Rheumatoid nodule,** left hip   HCC

    M06.359 **Rheumatoid nodule,** unspecified hip   HCC

√6ᵗʰ **M06.36** **Rheumatoid nodule,** knee

    M06.361 **Rheumatoid nodule,** right knee   HCC

    M06.362 **Rheumatoid nodule,** left knee   HCC

    M06.369 **Rheumatoid nodule,** unspecified knee   HCC

√6ᵗʰ **M06.37** **Rheumatoid nodule,** ankle and foot

    M06.371 **Rheumatoid nodule,** right ankle and foot   HCC

    M06.372 **Rheumatoid nodule,** left ankle and foot   HCC

    M06.379 **Rheumatoid nodule,** unspecified ankle and foot   HCC

M06.38 **Rheumatoid nodule,** vertebrae   HCC

M06.39 **Rheumatoid nodule,** multiple sites   HCC

M06.4 **Inflammatory polyarthropathy**   HCC

    EXCLUDES 1   *polyarthritis NOS (M13.0)*

√5ᵗʰ **M06.8** **Other specified rheumatoid arthritis**

    M06.80 **Other specified rheumatoid arthritis, unspecified site**   HCC

√6ᵗʰ **M06.81** **Other specified rheumatoid arthritis,** shoulder

    M06.811 **Other specified rheumatoid arthritis,** right shoulder   HCC

    M06.812 **Other specified rheumatoid arthritis,** left shoulder   HCC

    M06.819 **Other specified rheumatoid arthritis,** unspecified shoulder   HCC

√6ᵗʰ **M06.82** **Other specified rheumatoid arthritis,** elbow

    M06.821 **Other specified rheumatoid arthritis,** right elbow   HCC

    M06.822 **Other specified rheumatoid arthritis,** left elbow   HCC

    M06.829 **Other specified rheumatoid arthritis,** unspecified elbow   HCC

√6ᵗʰ **M06.83** **Other specified rheumatoid arthritis,** wrist

    M06.831 **Other specified rheumatoid arthritis,** right wrist   HCC

    M06.832 **Other specified rheumatoid arthritis,** left wrist   HCC

    M06.839 **Other specified rheumatoid arthritis,** unspecified wrist   HCC

√6ᵗʰ **M06.84** **Other specified rheumatoid arthritis,** hand

    M06.841 **Other specified rheumatoid arthritis,** right hand   HCC

    M06.842 **Other specified rheumatoid arthritis,** left hand   HCC

    M06.849 **Other specified rheumatoid arthritis,** unspecified hand   HCC

√6ᵗʰ **M06.85** **Other specified rheumatoid arthritis,** hip

    M06.851 **Other specified rheumatoid arthritis,** right hip   HCC

    M06.852 **Other specified rheumatoid arthritis,** left hip   HCC

    M06.859 **Other specified rheumatoid arthritis,** unspecified hip   HCC

√6ᵗʰ **M06.86** **Other specified rheumatoid arthritis,** knee

    M06.861 **Other specified rheumatoid arthritis,** right knee   HCC

    M06.862 **Other specified rheumatoid arthritis,** left knee   HCC

    M06.869 **Other specified rheumatoid arthritis,** unspecified knee   HCC

√6ᵗʰ **M06.87** **Other specified rheumatoid arthritis,** ankle and foot

    M06.871 **Other specified rheumatoid arthritis,** right ankle and foot   HCC

    M06.872 **Other specified rheumatoid arthritis,** left ankle and foot   HCC

    M06.879 **Other specified rheumatoid arthritis,** unspecified ankle and foot   HCC

M06.88 **Other specified rheumatoid arthritis,** vertebrae   HCC

M06.89 **Other specified rheumatoid arthritis,** multiple sites   HCC

M06.9 **Rheumatoid arthritis, unspecified**   HCC

√4ᵗʰ **M07** **Enteropathic arthropathies**

    Code also associated enteropathy, such as:
      regional enteritis [Crohn's disease] (K50.-)
      ulcerative colitis (K51.-)

    EXCLUDES 1   *psoriatic arthropathies (L40.5-)*

√5ᵗʰ **M07.6** **Enteropathic arthropathies**

    M07.60 **Enteropathic arthropathies, unspecified site**

√6ᵗʰ **M07.61** **Enteropathic arthropathies,** shoulder

    M07.611 **Enteropathic arthropathies,** right shoulder

    M07.612 **Enteropathic arthropathies,** left shoulder

    M07.619 **Enteropathic arthropathies, unspecified shoulder**

√6ᵗʰ **M07.62** **Enteropathic arthropathies,** elbow

    M07.621 **Enteropathic arthropathies,** right elbow

    M07.622 **Enteropathic arthropathies,** left elbow

    M07.629 **Enteropathic arthropathies, unspecified elbow**

√6ᵗʰ **M07.63** **Enteropathic arthropathies,** wrist

    M07.631 **Enteropathic arthropathies,** right wrist

    M07.632 **Enteropathic arthropathies,** left wrist

    M07.639 **Enteropathic arthropathies, unspecified wrist**

√6ᵗʰ **M07.64** **Enteropathic arthropathies,** hand

    M07.641 **Enteropathic arthropathies,** right hand

    M07.642 **Enteropathic arthropathies,** left hand

    M07.649 **Enteropathic arthropathies, unspecified hand**

√6ᵗʰ **M07.65** **Enteropathic arthropathies,** hip

    M07.651 **Enteropathic arthropathies,** right hip

    M07.652 **Enteropathic arthropathies,** left hip

    M07.659 **Enteropathic arthropathies, unspecified hip**

√6ᵗʰ **M07.66** **Enteropathic arthropathies,** knee

    M07.661 **Enteropathic arthropathies,** right knee

    M07.662 **Enteropathic arthropathies,** left knee

    M07.669 **Enteropathic arthropathies, unspecified knee**

☑ Additional Character Required   √x7ᵗʰ Placeholder Alert   Manifestation   Unspecified Dx   ▶◀ Revised Text   ● New Code   ▲ Revised Code Title

ICD-10-CM 2020   757

Chapter 13. Diseases of the Musculoskeletal System and Connective Tissue

√6ᵗʰ **M07.67 Enteropathic arthropathies, ankle and foot**

     M07.671 Enteropathic arthropathies, right ankle and foot

     M07.672 Enteropathic arthropathies, left ankle and foot

     M07.679 Enteropathic arthropathies, unspecified ankle and foot

M07.68 Enteropathic arthropathies, vertebrae

M07.69 Enteropathic arthropathies, multiple sites

√4ᵗʰ **M08 Juvenile arthritis**

Code also any associated underlying condition, such as:

     regional enteritis [Crohn's disease] (K50.-)

     ulcerative colitis (K51.-)

EXCLUDES 1   arthropathy in Whipple's disease (M14.8)

           Felty's syndrome (M05.0)

           juvenile dermatomyositis (M33.0-)

           psoriatic juvenile arthropathy (L40.54)

√5ᵗʰ **M08.0 Unspecified juvenile rheumatoid arthritis**

Juvenile rheumatoid arthritis with or without rheumatoid factor

M08.00 Unspecified juvenile rheumatoid arthritis of unspecified site HCC

√6ᵗʰ **M08.01 Unspecified juvenile rheumatoid arthritis, shoulder**

     M08.011 Unspecified juvenile rheumatoid arthritis, right shoulder HCC

     M08.012 Unspecified juvenile rheumatoid arthritis, left shoulder HCC

     M08.019 Unspecified juvenile rheumatoid arthritis, unspecified shoulder HCC

√6ᵗʰ **M08.02 Unspecified juvenile rheumatoid arthritis of elbow**

     M08.021 Unspecified juvenile rheumatoid arthritis, right elbow HCC

     M08.022 Unspecified juvenile rheumatoid arthritis, left elbow HCC

     M08.029 Unspecified juvenile rheumatoid arthritis, unspecified elbow HCC

√6ᵗʰ **M08.03 Unspecified juvenile rheumatoid arthritis, wrist**

     M08.031 Unspecified juvenile rheumatoid arthritis, right wrist HCC

     M08.032 Unspecified juvenile rheumatoid arthritis, left wrist HCC

     M08.039 Unspecified juvenile rheumatoid arthritis, unspecified wrist HCC

√6ᵗʰ **M08.04 Unspecified juvenile rheumatoid arthritis, hand**

     M08.041 Unspecified juvenile rheumatoid arthritis, right hand HCC

     M08.042 Unspecified juvenile rheumatoid arthritis, left hand HCC

     M08.049 Unspecified juvenile rheumatoid arthritis, unspecified hand HCC

√6ᵗʰ **M08.05 Unspecified juvenile rheumatoid arthritis, hip**

     M08.051 Unspecified juvenile rheumatoid arthritis, right hip HCC

     M08.052 Unspecified juvenile rheumatoid arthritis, left hip HCC

     M08.059 Unspecified juvenile rheumatoid arthritis, unspecified hip HCC

√6ᵗʰ **M08.06 Unspecified juvenile rheumatoid arthritis, knee**

     M08.061 Unspecified juvenile rheumatoid arthritis, right knee HCC

     M08.062 Unspecified juvenile rheumatoid arthritis, left knee HCC

     M08.069 Unspecified juvenile rheumatoid arthritis, unspecified knee HCC

√6ᵗʰ **M08.07 Unspecified juvenile rheumatoid arthritis, ankle and foot**

     M08.071 Unspecified juvenile rheumatoid arthritis, right ankle and foot HCC

     M08.072 Unspecified juvenile rheumatoid arthritis, left ankle and foot HCC

     M08.079 Unspecified juvenile rheumatoid arthritis, unspecified ankle and foot HCC

M08.08 Unspecified juvenile rheumatoid arthritis, vertebrae HCC

M08.09 Unspecified juvenile rheumatoid arthritis, multiple sites HCC

M08.1 Juvenile ankylosing spondylitis HCC

     EXCLUDES 1   ankylosing spondylitis in adults (M45.0-)

√5ᵗʰ **M08.2 Juvenile rheumatoid arthritis with systemic onset**

Still's disease NOS

EXCLUDES 1   adult-onset Still's disease (M06.1-)

DEF: Systemic juvenile rheumatoid arthritis characterized by a transient rash and spiking fevers that may affect internal organs, as well as joints.

M08.20 Juvenile rheumatoid arthritis with systemic onset, unspecified site HCC

√6ᵗʰ **M08.21 Juvenile rheumatoid arthritis with systemic onset, shoulder**

     M08.211 Juvenile rheumatoid arthritis with systemic onset, right shoulder HCC

     M08.212 Juvenile rheumatoid arthritis with systemic onset, left shoulder HCC

     M08.219 Juvenile rheumatoid arthritis with systemic onset, unspecified shoulder HCC

√6ᵗʰ **M08.22 Juvenile rheumatoid arthritis with systemic onset, elbow**

     M08.221 Juvenile rheumatoid arthritis with systemic onset, right elbow HCC

     M08.222 Juvenile rheumatoid arthritis with systemic onset, left elbow HCC

     M08.229 Juvenile rheumatoid arthritis with systemic onset, unspecified elbow HCC

√6ᵗʰ **M08.23 Juvenile rheumatoid arthritis with systemic onset, wrist**

     M08.231 Juvenile rheumatoid arthritis with systemic onset, right wrist HCC

     M08.232 Juvenile rheumatoid arthritis with systemic onset, left wrist HCC

     M08.239 Juvenile rheumatoid arthritis with systemic onset, unspecified wrist HCC

√6ᵗʰ **M08.24 Juvenile rheumatoid arthritis with systemic onset, hand**

     M08.241 Juvenile rheumatoid arthritis with systemic onset, right hand HCC

     M08.242 Juvenile rheumatoid arthritis with systemic onset, left hand HCC

     M08.249 Juvenile rheumatoid arthritis with systemic onset, unspecified hand HCC

√6ᵗʰ **M08.25 Juvenile rheumatoid arthritis with systemic onset, hip**

     M08.251 Juvenile rheumatoid arthritis with systemic onset, right hip HCC

     M08.252 Juvenile rheumatoid arthritis with systemic onset, left hip HCC

     M08.259 Juvenile rheumatoid arthritis with systemic onset, unspecified hip HCC

√6ᵗʰ **M08.26 Juvenile rheumatoid arthritis with systemic onset, knee**

     M08.261 Juvenile rheumatoid arthritis with systemic onset, right knee HCC

     M08.262 Juvenile rheumatoid arthritis with systemic onset, left knee HCC

     M08.269 Juvenile rheumatoid arthritis with systemic onset, unspecified knee HCC

√6ᵗʰ **M08.27 Juvenile rheumatoid arthritis with systemic onset, ankle and foot**

     M08.271 Juvenile rheumatoid arthritis with systemic onset, right ankle and foot HCC

     M08.272 Juvenile rheumatoid arthritis with systemic onset, left ankle and foot HCC

     M08.279 Juvenile rheumatoid arthritis with systemic onset, unspecified ankle and foot HCC

M08.28 Juvenile rheumatoid arthritis with systemic onset, vertebrae HCC

M08.29 Juvenile rheumatoid arthritis with systemic onset, multiple sites HCC

M08.3 Juvenile rheumatoid polyarthritis (seronegative) HCC

√5ᵗʰ **M08.4 Pauciarticular juvenile rheumatoid arthritis**

M08.40 Pauciarticular juvenile rheumatoid arthritis, unspecified site HCC

√6ᵗʰ **M08.41** Pauciarticular juvenile rheumatoid arthritis, shoulder

    M08.411 Pauciarticular juvenile rheumatoid arthritis, right shoulder `HCC`

    M08.412 Pauciarticular juvenile rheumatoid arthritis, left shoulder `HCC`

    M08.419 Pauciarticular juvenile rheumatoid arthritis, unspecified shoulder `HCC`

√6ᵗʰ **M08.42** Pauciarticular juvenile rheumatoid arthritis, elbow

    M08.421 Pauciarticular juvenile rheumatoid arthritis, right elbow `HCC`

    M08.422 Pauciarticular juvenile rheumatoid arthritis, left elbow `HCC`

    M08.429 Pauciarticular juvenile rheumatoid arthritis, unspecified elbow `HCC`

√6ᵗʰ **M08.43** Pauciarticular juvenile rheumatoid arthritis, wrist

    M08.431 Pauciarticular juvenile rheumatoid arthritis, right wrist `HCC`

    M08.432 Pauciarticular juvenile rheumatoid arthritis, left wrist `HCC`

    M08.439 Pauciarticular juvenile rheumatoid arthritis, unspecified wrist `HCC`

√6ᵗʰ **M08.44** Pauciarticular juvenile rheumatoid arthritis, hand

    M08.441 Pauciarticular juvenile rheumatoid arthritis, right hand `HCC`

    M08.442 Pauciarticular juvenile rheumatoid arthritis, left hand `HCC`

    M08.449 Pauciarticular juvenile rheumatoid arthritis, unspecified hand `HCC`

√6ᵗʰ **M08.45** Pauciarticular juvenile rheumatoid arthritis, hip

    M08.451 Pauciarticular juvenile rheumatoid arthritis, right hip `HCC`

    M08.452 Pauciarticular juvenile rheumatoid arthritis, left hip `HCC`

    M08.459 Pauciarticular juvenile rheumatoid arthritis, unspecified hip `HCC`

√6ᵗʰ **M08.46** Pauciarticular juvenile rheumatoid arthritis, knee

    M08.461 Pauciarticular juvenile rheumatoid arthritis, right knee `HCC`

    M08.462 Pauciarticular juvenile rheumatoid arthritis, left knee `HCC`

    M08.469 Pauciarticular juvenile rheumatoid arthritis, unspecified knee `HCC`

√6ᵗʰ **M08.47** Pauciarticular juvenile rheumatoid arthritis, ankle and foot

    M08.471 Pauciarticular juvenile rheumatoid arthritis, right ankle and foot `HCC`

    M08.472 Pauciarticular juvenile rheumatoid arthritis, left ankle and foot `HCC`

    M08.479 Pauciarticular juvenile rheumatoid arthritis, unspecified ankle and foot `HCC`

  M08.48 Pauciarticular juvenile rheumatoid arthritis, vertebrae `HCC`

√5ᵗʰ **M08.8** Other juvenile arthritis

  M08.80 Other juvenile arthritis, unspecified site `HCC`

√6ᵗʰ **M08.81** Other juvenile arthritis, shoulder

    M08.811 Other juvenile arthritis, right shoulder `HCC`

    M08.812 Other juvenile arthritis, left shoulder `HCC`

    M08.819 Other juvenile arthritis, unspecified shoulder `HCC`

√6ᵗʰ **M08.82** Other juvenile arthritis, elbow

    M08.821 Other juvenile arthritis, right elbow `HCC`

    M08.822 Other juvenile arthritis, left elbow `HCC`

    M08.829 Other juvenile arthritis, unspecified elbow `HCC`

√6ᵗʰ **M08.83** Other juvenile arthritis, wrist

    M08.831 Other juvenile arthritis, right wrist `HCC`

    M08.832 Other juvenile arthritis, left wrist `HCC`

    M08.839 Other juvenile arthritis, unspecified wrist `HCC`

√6ᵗʰ **M08.84** Other juvenile arthritis, hand

    M08.841 Other juvenile arthritis, right hand `HCC`

    M08.842 Other juvenile arthritis, left hand `HCC`

    M08.849 Other juvenile arthritis, unspecified hand `HCC`

√6ᵗʰ **M08.85** Other juvenile arthritis, hip

    M08.851 Other juvenile arthritis, right hip `HCC`

    M08.852 Other juvenile arthritis, left hip `HCC`

    M08.859 Other juvenile arthritis, unspecified hip `HCC`

√6ᵗʰ **M08.86** Other juvenile arthritis, knee

    M08.861 Other juvenile arthritis, right knee `HCC`

    M08.862 Other juvenile arthritis, left knee `HCC`

    M08.869 Other juvenile arthritis, unspecified knee `HCC`

√6ᵗʰ **M08.87** Other juvenile arthritis, ankle and foot

    M08.871 Other juvenile arthritis, right ankle and foot `HCC`

    M08.872 Other juvenile arthritis, left ankle and foot `HCC`

    M08.879 Other juvenile arthritis, unspecified ankle and foot `HCC`

  M08.88 Other juvenile arthritis, other specified site `HCC`

    Other juvenile arthritis, vertebrae

  M08.89 Other juvenile arthritis, multiple sites `HCC`

√5ᵗʰ **M08.9** Juvenile arthritis, unspecified

    EXCLUDES 1 *juvenile rheumatoid arthritis, unspecified (M08.0-)*

  M08.90 Juvenile arthritis, unspecified, unspecified site `HCC`

√6ᵗʰ **M08.91** Juvenile arthritis, unspecified, shoulder

    M08.911 Juvenile arthritis, unspecified, right shoulder `HCC`

    M08.912 Juvenile arthritis, unspecified, left shoulder `HCC`

    M08.919 Juvenile arthritis, unspecified, unspecified shoulder `HCC`

√6ᵗʰ **M08.92** Juvenile arthritis, unspecified, elbow

    M08.921 Juvenile arthritis, unspecified, right elbow `HCC`

    M08.922 Juvenile arthritis, unspecified, left elbow `HCC`

    M08.929 Juvenile arthritis, unspecified, unspecified elbow `HCC`

√6ᵗʰ **M08.93** Juvenile arthritis, unspecified, wrist

    M08.931 Juvenile arthritis, unspecified, right wrist `HCC`

    M08.932 Juvenile arthritis, unspecified, left wrist `HCC`

    M08.939 Juvenile arthritis, unspecified, unspecified wrist `HCC`

√6ᵗʰ **M08.94** Juvenile arthritis, unspecified, hand

    M08.941 Juvenile arthritis, unspecified, right hand `HCC`

    M08.942 Juvenile arthritis, unspecified, left hand `HCC`

    M08.949 Juvenile arthritis, unspecified, unspecified hand `HCC`

√6ᵗʰ **M08.95** Juvenile arthritis, unspecified, hip

    M08.951 Juvenile arthritis, unspecified, right hip `HCC`

    M08.952 Juvenile arthritis, unspecified, left hip `HCC`

    M08.959 Juvenile arthritis, unspecified, unspecified hip `HCC`

√6ᵗʰ **M08.96** Juvenile arthritis, unspecified, knee

    M08.961 Juvenile arthritis, unspecified, right knee `HCC`

    M08.962 Juvenile arthritis, unspecified, left knee `HCC`

☑ Additional Character Required   √×7ᵗʰ Placeholder Alert   Manifestation   Unspecified Dx   ►◄ Revised Text   ● New Code   ▲ Revised Code Title

ICD-10-CM 2020   **759**

M08.969	Juvenile arthritis, unspecified, unspecified knee `HCC`

✓6ᵗʰ **M08.97** Juvenile arthritis, unspecified, ankle and foot

    M08.971 Juvenile arthritis, unspecified, right ankle and foot   `HCC`

    M08.972 Juvenile arthritis, unspecified, left ankle and foot   `HCC`

    M08.979 Juvenile arthritis, unspecified, unspecified ankle and foot   `HCC`

   M08.98 Juvenile arthritis, unspecified, vertebrae   `HCC`

   M08.99 Juvenile arthritis, unspecified, multiple sites   `HCC`

✓4ᵗʰ **M1A Chronic gout**

    Use additional code to identify:

      autonomic neuropathy in diseases classified elsewhere (G99.0)

      calculus of urinary tract in diseases classified elsewhere (N22)

      cardiomyopathy in diseases classified elsewhere (I43)

      disorders of external ear in diseases classified elsewhere (H61.1-, H62.8-)

      disorders of iris and ciliary body in diseases classified elsewhere (H22)

      glomerular disorders in diseases classified elsewhere (N08)

    `EXCLUDES 1`   gout NOS (M10.-)

    `EXCLUDES 2`   acute gout (M10.-)

> The appropriate 7th character is to be added to each code from category M1A.
> 0   without tophus (tophi)
> 1   with tophus (tophi)

✓5ᵗʰ **M1A.0 Idiopathic chronic gout**

    Chronic gouty bursitis

    Primary chronic gout

   ✓x7ᵗʰ **M1A.00** Idiopathic chronic gout, unspecified site

   ✓6ᵗʰ **M1A.01** Idiopathic chronic gout, shoulder

     ✓7ᵗʰ **M1A.011** Idiopathic chronic gout, right shoulder

     ✓7ᵗʰ **M1A.012** Idiopathic chronic gout, left shoulder

     ✓7ᵗʰ **M1A.019** Idiopathic chronic gout, unspecified shoulder

   ✓6ᵗʰ **M1A.02** Idiopathic chronic gout, elbow

     ✓7ᵗʰ **M1A.021** Idiopathic chronic gout, right elbow

     ✓7ᵗʰ **M1A.022** Idiopathic chronic gout, left elbow

     ✓7ᵗʰ **M1A.029** Idiopathic chronic gout, unspecified elbow

   ✓6ᵗʰ **M1A.03** Idiopathic chronic gout, wrist

     ✓7ᵗʰ **M1A.031** Idiopathic chronic gout, right wrist

     ✓7ᵗʰ **M1A.032** Idiopathic chronic gout, left wrist

     ✓7ᵗʰ **M1A.039** Idiopathic chronic gout, unspecified wrist

   ✓6ᵗʰ **M1A.04** Idiopathic chronic gout, hand

     ✓7ᵗʰ **M1A.041** Idiopathic chronic gout, right hand

     ✓7ᵗʰ **M1A.042** Idiopathic chronic gout, left hand

     ✓7ᵗʰ **M1A.049** Idiopathic chronic gout, unspecified hand

   ✓6ᵗʰ **M1A.05** Idiopathic chronic gout, hip

     ✓7ᵗʰ **M1A.051** Idiopathic chronic gout, right hip

     ✓7ᵗʰ **M1A.052** Idiopathic chronic gout, left hip

     ✓7ᵗʰ **M1A.059** Idiopathic chronic gout, unspecified hip

   ✓6ᵗʰ **M1A.06** Idiopathic chronic gout, knee

     ✓7ᵗʰ **M1A.061** Idiopathic chronic gout, right knee

     ✓7ᵗʰ **M1A.062** Idiopathic chronic gout, left knee

     ✓7ᵗʰ **M1A.069** Idiopathic chronic gout, unspecified knee

   ✓6ᵗʰ **M1A.07** Idiopathic chronic gout, ankle and foot

     ✓7ᵗʰ **M1A.071** Idiopathic chronic gout, right ankle and foot

     ✓7ᵗʰ **M1A.072** Idiopathic chronic gout, left ankle and foot

     ✓7ᵗʰ **M1A.079** Idiopathic chronic gout, unspecified ankle and foot

   ✓x7ᵗʰ **M1A.08** Idiopathic chronic gout, vertebrae

   ✓x7ᵗʰ **M1A.09** Idiopathic chronic gout, multiple sites

✓5ᵗʰ **M1A.1 Lead-induced chronic gout**

    Code first toxic effects of lead and its compounds (T56.0-)

   ✓x7ᵗʰ **M1A.10** Lead-induced chronic gout, unspecified site

   ✓6ᵗʰ **M1A.11** Lead-induced chronic gout, shoulder

     ✓7ᵗʰ **M1A.111** Lead-induced chronic gout, right shoulder

     ✓7ᵗʰ **M1A.112** Lead-induced chronic gout, left shoulder

     ✓7ᵗʰ **M1A.119** Lead-induced chronic gout, unspecified shoulder

   ✓6ᵗʰ **M1A.12** Lead-induced chronic gout, elbow

     ✓7ᵗʰ **M1A.121** Lead-induced chronic gout, right elbow

     ✓7ᵗʰ **M1A.122** Lead-induced chronic gout, left elbow

     ✓7ᵗʰ **M1A.129** Lead-induced chronic gout, unspecified elbow

   ✓6ᵗʰ **M1A.13** Lead-induced chronic gout, wrist

     ✓7ᵗʰ **M1A.131** Lead-induced chronic gout, right wrist

     ✓7ᵗʰ **M1A.132** Lead-induced chronic gout, left wrist

     ✓7ᵗʰ **M1A.139** Lead-induced chronic gout, unspecified wrist

   ✓6ᵗʰ **M1A.14** Lead-induced chronic gout, hand

     ✓7ᵗʰ **M1A.141** Lead-induced chronic gout, right hand

     ✓7ᵗʰ **M1A.142** Lead-induced chronic gout, left hand

     ✓7ᵗʰ **M1A.149** Lead-induced chronic gout, unspecified hand

   ✓6ᵗʰ **M1A.15** Lead-induced chronic gout, hip

     ✓7ᵗʰ **M1A.151** Lead-induced chronic gout, right hip

     ✓7ᵗʰ **M1A.152** Lead-induced chronic gout, left hip

     ✓7ᵗʰ **M1A.159** Lead-induced chronic gout, unspecified hip

   ✓6ᵗʰ **M1A.16** Lead-induced chronic gout, knee

     ✓7ᵗʰ **M1A.161** Lead-induced chronic gout, right knee

     ✓7ᵗʰ **M1A.162** Lead-induced chronic gout, left knee

     ✓7ᵗʰ **M1A.169** Lead-induced chronic gout, unspecified knee

   ✓6ᵗʰ **M1A.17** Lead-induced chronic gout, ankle and foot

     ✓7ᵗʰ **M1A.171** Lead-induced chronic gout, right ankle and foot

     ✓7ᵗʰ **M1A.172** Lead-induced chronic gout, left ankle and foot

     ✓7ᵗʰ **M1A.179** Lead-induced chronic gout, unspecified ankle and foot

   ✓x7ᵗʰ **M1A.18** Lead-induced chronic gout, vertebrae

   ✓x7ᵗʰ **M1A.19** Lead-induced chronic gout, multiple sites

✓5ᵗʰ **M1A.2 Drug-induced chronic gout**

    Use additional code for adverse effect, if applicable, to identify drug (T36-T50 with fifth or sixth character 5)

   ✓x7ᵗʰ **M1A.20** Drug-induced chronic gout, unspecified site

   ✓6ᵗʰ **M1A.21** Drug-induced chronic gout, shoulder

     ✓7ᵗʰ **M1A.211** Drug-induced chronic gout, right shoulder

     ✓7ᵗʰ **M1A.212** Drug-induced chronic gout, left shoulder

     ✓7ᵗʰ **M1A.219** Drug-induced chronic gout, unspecified shoulder

   ✓6ᵗʰ **M1A.22** Drug-induced chronic gout, elbow

     ✓7ᵗʰ **M1A.221** Drug-induced chronic gout, right elbow

     ✓7ᵗʰ **M1A.222** Drug-induced chronic gout, left elbow

     ✓7ᵗʰ **M1A.229** Drug-induced chronic gout, unspecified elbow

   ✓6ᵗʰ **M1A.23** Drug-induced chronic gout, wrist

     ✓7ᵗʰ **M1A.231** Drug-induced chronic gout, right wrist

     ✓7ᵗʰ **M1A.232** Drug-induced chronic gout, left wrist

     ✓7ᵗʰ **M1A.239** Drug-induced chronic gout, unspecified wrist

   ✓6ᵗʰ **M1A.24** Drug-induced chronic gout, hand

     ✓7ᵗʰ **M1A.241** Drug-induced chronic gout, right hand

     ✓7ᵗʰ **M1A.242** Drug-induced chronic gout, left hand

     ✓7ᵗʰ **M1A.249** Drug-induced chronic gout, unspecified hand

   ✓6ᵗʰ **M1A.25** Drug-induced chronic gout, hip

     ✓7ᵗʰ **M1A.251** Drug-induced chronic gout, right hip

     ✓7ᵗʰ **M1A.252** Drug-induced chronic gout, left hip

     ✓7ᵗʰ **M1A.259** Drug-induced chronic gout, unspecified hip

   ✓6ᵗʰ **M1A.26** Drug-induced chronic gout, knee

     ✓7ᵗʰ **M1A.261** Drug-induced chronic gout, right knee

     ✓7ᵗʰ **M1A.262** Drug-induced chronic gout, left knee

     ✓7ᵗʰ **M1A.269** Drug-induced chronic gout, unspecified knee

☑6ᵗʰ **M1A.27 Drug-induced chronic gout,** ankle and foot

    ☑7ᵗʰ **M1A.271 Drug-induced chronic gout,** right ankle and foot

    ☑7ᵗʰ **M1A.272 Drug-induced chronic gout,** left ankle and foot

    ☑7ᵗʰ **M1A.279 Drug-induced chronic gout, unspecified** ankle and foot

☑x7ᵗʰ **M1A.28 Drug-induced chronic gout,** vertebrae

☑x7ᵗʰ **M1A.29 Drug-induced chronic gout,** multiple sites

☑5ᵗʰ **M1A.3 Chronic gout** due to renal impairment

    Code first associated renal disease

  ☑x7ᵗʰ **M1A.30 Chronic gout due to renal impairment, unspecified site**

  ☑6ᵗʰ **M1A.31 Chronic gout due to renal impairment,** shoulder

    ☑7ᵗʰ **M1A.311 Chronic gout due to renal impairment, right shoulder**

    ☑7ᵗʰ **M1A.312 Chronic gout due to renal impairment, left shoulder**

    ☑7ᵗʰ **M1A.319 Chronic gout due to renal impairment, unspecified shoulder**

  ☑6ᵗʰ **M1A.32 Chronic gout due to renal impairment,** elbow

    ☑7ᵗʰ **M1A.321 Chronic gout due to renal impairment, right elbow**

    ☑7ᵗʰ **M1A.322 Chronic gout due to renal impairment, left elbow**

    ☑7ᵗʰ **M1A.329 Chronic gout due to renal impairment, unspecified elbow**

  ☑6ᵗʰ **M1A.33 Chronic gout due to renal impairment,** wrist

    ☑7ᵗʰ **M1A.331 Chronic gout due to renal impairment, right wrist**

    ☑7ᵗʰ **M1A.332 Chronic gout due to renal impairment, left wrist**

    ☑7ᵗʰ **M1A.339 Chronic gout due to renal impairment, unspecified wrist**

  ☑6ᵗʰ **M1A.34 Chronic gout due to renal impairment,** hand

    ☑7ᵗʰ **M1A.341 Chronic gout due to renal impairment, right hand**

    ☑7ᵗʰ **M1A.342 Chronic gout due to renal impairment, left hand**

    ☑7ᵗʰ **M1A.349 Chronic gout due to renal impairment, unspecified hand**

  ☑6ᵗʰ **M1A.35 Chronic gout due to renal impairment,** hip

    ☑7ᵗʰ **M1A.351 Chronic gout due to renal impairment, right hip**

    ☑7ᵗʰ **M1A.352 Chronic gout due to renal impairment, left hip**

    ☑7ᵗʰ **M1A.359 Chronic gout due to renal Impairment, unspecified hip**

  ☑6ᵗʰ **M1A.36 Chronic gout due to renal impairment,** knee

    ☑7ᵗʰ **M1A.361 Chronic gout due to renal impairment, right knee**

    ☑7ᵗʰ **M1A.362 Chronic gout due to renal impairment, left knee**

    ☑7ᵗʰ **M1A.369 Chronic gout due to renal impairment, unspecified knee**

  ☑6ᵗʰ **M1A.37 Chronic gout due to renal impairment,** ankle and foot

    ☑7ᵗʰ **M1A.371 Chronic gout due to renal impairment, right ankle and foot**

    ☑7ᵗʰ **M1A.372 Chronic gout due to renal impairment, left ankle and foot**

    ☑7ᵗʰ **M1A.379 Chronic gout due to renal impairment, unspecified ankle and foot**

  ☑x7ᵗʰ **M1A.38 Chronic gout due to renal impairment,** vertebrae

  ☑x7ᵗʰ **M1A.39 Chronic gout due to renal impairment,** multiple sites

☑5ᵗʰ **M1A.4 Other** secondary **chronic gout**

    Code first associated condition

  ☑x7ᵗʰ **M1A.40 Other secondary chronic gout, unspecified site**

  ☑6ᵗʰ **M1A.41 Other secondary chronic gout,** shoulder

    ☑7ᵗʰ **M1A.411 Other secondary chronic gout,** right shoulder

    ☑7ᵗʰ **M1A.412 Other secondary chronic gout,** left shoulder

    ☑7ᵗʰ **M1A.419 Other secondary chronic gout, unspecified shoulder**

  ☑6ᵗʰ **M1A.42 Other secondary chronic gout,** elbow

    ☑7ᵗʰ **M1A.421 Other secondary chronic gout,** right elbow

    ☑7ᵗʰ **M1A.422 Other secondary chronic gout,** left elbow

    ☑7ᵗʰ **M1A.429 Other secondary chronic gout, unspecified elbow**

  ☑6ᵗʰ **M1A.43 Other secondary chronic gout,** wrist

    ☑7ᵗʰ **M1A.431 Other secondary chronic gout,** right wrist

    ☑7ᵗʰ **M1A.432 Other secondary chronic gout,** left wrist

    ☑7ᵗʰ **M1A.439 Other secondary chronic gout, unspecified wrist**

  ☑6ᵗʰ **M1A.44 Other secondary chronic gout,** hand

    ☑7ᵗʰ **M1A.441 Other secondary chronic gout,** right hand

    ☑7ᵗʰ **M1A.442 Other secondary chronic gout,** left hand

    ☑7ᵗʰ **M1A.449 Other secondary chronic gout, unspecified hand**

  ☑6ᵗʰ **M1A.45 Other secondary chronic gout,** hip

    ☑7ᵗʰ **M1A.451 Other secondary chronic gout,** right hip

    ☑7ᵗʰ **M1A.452 Other secondary chronic gout,** left hip

    ☑7ᵗʰ **M1A.459 Other secondary chronic gout, unspecified hip**

  ☑6ᵗʰ **M1A.46 Other secondary chronic gout,** knee

    ☑7ᵗʰ **M1A.461 Other secondary chronic gout,** right knee

    ☑7ᵗʰ **M1A.462 Other secondary chronic gout,** left knee

    ☑7ᵗʰ **M1A.469 Other secondary chronic gout, unspecified knee**

  ☑6ᵗʰ **M1A.47 Other secondary chronic gout,** ankle and foot

    ☑7ᵗʰ **M1A.471 Other secondary chronic gout,** right ankle and foot

    ☑7ᵗʰ **M1A.472 Other secondary chronic gout,** left ankle and foot

    ☑7ᵗʰ **M1A.479 Other secondary chronic gout, unspecified ankle and foot**

  ☑x7ᵗʰ **M1A.48 Other secondary chronic gout,** vertebrae

  ☑x7ᵗʰ **M1A.49 Other secondary chronic gout,** multiple sites

☑x7ᵗʰ **M1A.9 Chronic gout, unspecified**

☑4ᵗʰ **M1Ø Gout**

    Acute gout

    Gout attack

    Gout flare

    Podagra

    Use additional code to identify:

      autonomic neuropathy in diseases classified elsewhere (G99.Ø)

      calculus of urinary tract in diseases classified elsewhere (N22)

      cardiomyopathy in diseases classified elsewhere (I43)

      disorders of external ear in diseases classified elsewhere (H61.1-, H62.8-)

      disorders of iris and ciliary body in diseases classified elsewhere (H22)

      glomerular disorders in diseases classified elsewhere (NØ8)

    EXCLUDES 2   chronic gout (M1A.-)

    DEF: Purine and pyrimidine metabolic disorders, manifested by hyperuricemia and recurrent acute inflammatory arthritis. Monosodium urate or monohydrate crystals may be deposited in and around the joints, leading to joint destruction and severe crippling.

☑5ᵗʰ **M1Ø.Ø Idiopathic gout**

    Gouty bursitis

    Primary gout

  M1Ø.ØØ Idiopathic gout, unspecified site

  ☑6ᵗʰ **M1Ø.Ø1 Idiopathic gout,** shoulder

    M1Ø.Ø11 Idiopathic gout, right shoulder

    M1Ø.Ø12 Idiopathic gout, left shoulder

    M1Ø.Ø19 Idiopathic gout, unspecified shoulder

  ☑6ᵗʰ **M1Ø.Ø2 Idiopathic gout,** elbow

    M1Ø.Ø21 Idiopathic gout, right elbow

    M1Ø.Ø22 Idiopathic gout, left elbow

    M1Ø.Ø29 Idiopathic gout, unspecified elbow

  ☑6ᵗʰ **M1Ø.Ø3 Idiopathic gout,** wrist

    M1Ø.Ø31 Idiopathic gout, right wrist

    M1Ø.Ø32 Idiopathic gout, left wrist

    M1Ø.Ø39 Idiopathic gout, unspecified wrist

  ☑6ᵗʰ **M1Ø.Ø4 Idiopathic gout,** hand

    M1Ø.Ø41 Idiopathic gout, right hand

    M1Ø.Ø42 Idiopathic gout, left hand

    M1Ø.Ø49 Idiopathic gout, unspecified hand

  ☑6ᵗʰ **M1Ø.Ø5 Idiopathic gout,** hip

    M1Ø.Ø51 Idiopathic gout, right hip

    M1Ø.Ø52 Idiopathic gout, left hip

☑ Additional Character Required   ☑x7ᵗʰ Placeholder Alert   Manifestation   Unspecified Dx   ►◄ Revised Text   ● New Code   ▲ Revised Code Title

ICD-10-CM 2020   761

      M10.059 Idiopathic gout, unspecified hip

√6ᵗʰ M10.06 Idiopathic gout, knee

      M10.061 Idiopathic gout, right knee
      M10.062 Idiopathic gout, left knee
      M10.069 Idiopathic gout, unspecified knee

√6ᵗʰ M10.07 Idiopathic gout, ankle and foot

      M10.071 Idiopathic gout, right ankle and foot
      M10.072 Idiopathic gout, left ankle and foot
      M10.079 Idiopathic gout, unspecified ankle and foot

    M10.08 Idiopathic gout, vertebrae
    M10.09 Idiopathic gout, multiple sites

√5ᵗʰ M10.1 Lead-induced gout

    Code first toxic effects of lead and its compounds (T56.0-)

    M10.10 Lead-induced gout, unspecified site

√6ᵗʰ M10.11 Lead-induced gout, shoulder

      M10.111 Lead-induced gout, right shoulder
      M10.112 Lead-induced gout, left shoulder
      M10.119 Lead-induced gout, unspecified shoulder

√6ᵗʰ M10.12 Lead-induced gout, elbow

      M10.121 Lead-induced gout, right elbow
      M10.122 Lead-induced gout, left elbow
      M10.129 Lead-induced gout, unspecified elbow

√6ᵗʰ M10.13 Lead-induced gout, wrist

      M10.131 Lead-induced gout, right wrist
      M10.132 Lead-induced gout, left wrist
      M10.139 Lead-induced gout, unspecified wrist

√6ᵗʰ M10.14 Lead-induced gout, hand

      M10.141 Lead-induced gout, right hand
      M10.142 Lead-induced gout, left hand
      M10.149 Lead-induced gout, unspecified hand

√6ᵗʰ M10.15 Lead-induced gout, hip

      M10.151 Lead-induced gout, right hip
      M10.152 Lead-induced gout, left hip
      M10.159 Lead-induced gout, unspecified hip

√6ᵗʰ M10.16 Lead-induced gout, knee

      M10.161 Lead-induced gout, right knee
      M10.162 Lead-induced gout, left knee
      M10.169 Lead-induced gout, unspecified knee

√6ᵗʰ M10.17 Lead-induced gout, ankle and foot

      M10.171 Lead-induced gout, right ankle and foot
      M10.172 Lead-induced gout, left ankle and foot
      M10.179 Lead-induced gout, unspecified ankle and foot

    M10.18 Lead-induced gout, vertebrae
    M10.19 Lead-induced gout, multiple sites

√5ᵗʰ M10.2 Drug-induced gout

    Use additional code for adverse effect, if applicable, to identify drug (T36-T50 with fifth or sixth character 5)

    M10.20 Drug-induced gout, unspecified site

√6ᵗʰ M10.21 Drug-induced gout, shoulder

      M10.211 Drug-induced gout, right shoulder
      M10.212 Drug-induced gout, left shoulder
      M10.219 Drug-induced gout, unspecified shoulder

√6ᵗʰ M10.22 Drug-induced gout, elbow

      M10.221 Drug-induced gout, right elbow
      M10.222 Drug-induced gout, left elbow
      M10.229 Drug-induced gout, unspecified elbow

√6ᵗʰ M10.23 Drug-induced gout, wrist

      M10.231 Drug-induced gout, right wrist
      M10.232 Drug-induced gout, left wrist
      M10.239 Drug-induced gout, unspecified wrist

√6ᵗʰ M10.24 Drug-induced gout, hand

      M10.241 Drug-induced gout, right hand
      M10.242 Drug-induced gout, left hand
      M10.249 Drug-induced gout, unspecified hand

√6ᵗʰ M10.25 Drug-induced gout, hip

      M10.251 Drug-induced gout, right hip
      M10.252 Drug-induced gout, left hip
      M10.259 Drug-induced gout, unspecified hip

√6ᵗʰ M10.26 Drug-induced gout, knee

      M10.261 Drug-induced gout, right knee
      M10.262 Drug-induced gout, left knee
      M10.269 Drug-induced gout, unspecified knee

√6ᵗʰ M10.27 Drug-induced gout, ankle and foot

      M10.271 Drug-induced gout, right ankle and foot
      M10.272 Drug-induced gout, left ankle and foot
      M10.279 Drug-induced gout, unspecified ankle and foot

    M10.28 Drug-induced gout, vertebrae
    M10.29 Drug-induced gout, multiple sites

√5ᵗʰ M10.3 Gout due to renal impairment

    Code first associated renal disease

    M10.30 Gout due to renal impairment, unspecified site

√6ᵗʰ M10.31 Gout due to renal impairment, shoulder

      M10.311 Gout due to renal impairment, right shoulder
      M10.312 Gout due to renal impairment, left shoulder
      M10.319 Gout due to renal impairment, unspecified shoulder

√6ᵗʰ M10.32 Gout due to renal impairment, elbow

      M10.321 Gout due to renal impairment, right elbow
      M10.322 Gout due to renal impairment, left elbow
      M10.329 Gout due to renal impairment, unspecified elbow

√6ᵗʰ M10.33 Gout due to renal impairment, wrist

      M10.331 Gout due to renal impairment, right wrist
      M10.332 Gout due to renal impairment, left wrist
      M10.339 Gout due to renal impairment, unspecified wrist

√6ᵗʰ M10.34 Gout due to renal impairment, hand

      M10.341 Gout due to renal impairment, right hand
      M10.342 Gout due to renal impairment, left hand
      M10.349 Gout due to renal impairment, unspecified hand

√6ᵗʰ M10.35 Gout due to renal impairment, hip

      M10.351 Gout due to renal impairment, right hip
      M10.352 Gout due to renal impairment, left hip
      M10.359 Gout due to renal impairment, unspecified hip

√6ᵗʰ M10.36 Gout due to renal impairment, knee

      M10.361 Gout due to renal impairment, right knee
      M10.362 Gout due to renal impairment, left knee
      M10.369 Gout due to renal impairment, unspecified knee

√6ᵗʰ M10.37 Gout due to renal impairment, ankle and foot

      M10.371 Gout due to renal impairment, right ankle and foot
      M10.372 Gout due to renal impairment, left ankle and foot
      M10.379 Gout due to renal impairment, unspecified ankle and foot

    M10.38 Gout due to renal impairment, vertebrae
    M10.39 Gout due to renal impairment, multiple sites

√5ᵗʰ M10.4 Other secondary gout

    Code first associated condition

    M10.40 Other secondary gout, unspecified site

√6ᵗʰ M10.41 Other secondary gout, shoulder

      M10.411 Other secondary gout, right shoulder
      M10.412 Other secondary gout, left shoulder
      M10.419 Other secondary gout, unspecified shoulder

√6ᵗʰ M10.42 Other secondary gout, elbow

      M10.421 Other secondary gout, right elbow
      M10.422 Other secondary gout, left elbow
      M10.429 Other secondary gout, unspecified elbow

√6ᵗʰ M10.43 Other secondary gout, wrist

      M10.431 Other secondary gout, right wrist
      M10.432 Other secondary gout, left wrist
      M10.439 Other secondary gout, unspecified wrist

√6ᵗʰ M10.44 Other secondary gout, hand

      M10.441 Other secondary gout, right hand
      M10.442 Other secondary gout, left hand
      M10.449 Other secondary gout, unspecified hand

√6ᵗʰ M10.45 Other secondary gout, hip

      M10.451 Other secondary gout, right hip
      M10.452 Other secondary gout, left hip
      M10.459 Other secondary gout, unspecified hip

✓6ᵗʰ **M10.46** Other secondary gout, knee
     M10.461 Other secondary gout, right knee
     M10.462 Other secondary gout, left knee
     M10.469 Other secondary gout, unspecified knee

✓6ᵗʰ **M10.47** Other secondary gout, ankle and foot
     M10.471 Other secondary gout, right ankle and foot
     M10.472 Other secondary gout, left ankle and foot
     M10.479 Other secondary gout, unspecified ankle and foot

   M10.48 Other secondary gout, vertebrae
   M10.49 Other secondary gout, multiple sites

M10.9 Gout, unspecified
     Gout NOS

✓4ᵗʰ **M11** Other crystal arthropathies

✓5ᵗʰ **M11.0** Hydroxyapatite deposition disease
     DEF: Disease caused by deposits of calcium phosphate crystals in the soft tissues close to the joint (especially tendons) or in the joints. These calcifications can be mono or polyarticular and can cause destruction of the joint involved.

   M11.00 Hydroxyapatite deposition disease, unspecified site

✓6ᵗʰ **M11.01** Hydroxyapatite deposition disease, shoulder
     M11.011 Hydroxyapatite deposition disease, right shoulder
     M11.012 Hydroxyapatite deposition disease, left shoulder
     M11.019 Hydroxyapatite deposition disease, unspecified shoulder

✓6ᵗʰ **M11.02** Hydroxyapatite deposition disease, elbow
     M11.021 Hydroxyapatite deposition disease, right elbow
     M11.022 Hydroxyapatite deposition disease, left elbow
     M11.029 Hydroxyapatite deposition disease, unspecified elbow

✓6ᵗʰ **M11.03** Hydroxyapatite deposition disease, wrist
     M11.031 Hydroxyapatite deposition disease, right wrist
     M11.032 Hydroxyapatite deposition disease, left wrist
     M11.039 Hydroxyapatite deposition disease, unspecified wrist

✓6ᵗʰ **M11.04** Hydroxyapatite deposition disease, hand
     M11.041 Hydroxyapatite deposition disease, right hand
     M11.042 Hydroxyapatite deposition disease, left hand
     M11.049 Hydroxyapatite deposition disease, unspecified hand

✓6ᵗʰ **M11.05** Hydroxyapatite deposition disease, hip
     M11.051 Hydroxyapatite deposition disease, right hip
     M11.052 Hydroxyapatite deposition disease, left hip
     M11.059 Hydroxyapatite deposition disease, unspecified hip

✓6ᵗʰ **M11.06** Hydroxyapatite deposition disease, knee
     M11.061 Hydroxyapatite deposition disease, right knee
     M11.062 Hydroxyapatite deposition disease, left knee
     M11.069 Hydroxyapatite deposition disease, unspecified knee

✓6ᵗʰ **M11.07** Hydroxyapatite deposition disease, ankle and foot
     M11.071 Hydroxyapatite deposition disease, right ankle and foot
     M11.072 Hydroxyapatite deposition disease, left ankle and foot
     M11.079 Hydroxyapatite deposition disease, unspecified ankle and foot

   M11.08 Hydroxyapatite deposition disease, vertebrae
   M11.09 Hydroxyapatite deposition disease, multiple sites

✓5ᵗʰ **M11.1** Familial chondrocalcinosis

   M11.10 Familial chondrocalcinosis, unspecified site

✓6ᵗʰ **M11.11** Familial chondrocalcinosis, shoulder
     M11.111 Familial chondrocalcinosis, right shoulder
     M11.112 Familial chondrocalcinosis, left shoulder
     M11.119 Familial chondrocalcinosis, unspecified shoulder

✓6ᵗʰ **M11.12** Familial chondrocalcinosis, elbow
     M11.121 Familial chondrocalcinosis, right elbow
     M11.122 Familial chondrocalcinosis, left elbow
     M11.129 Familial chondrocalcinosis, unspecified elbow

✓6ᵗʰ **M11.13** Familial chondrocalcinosis, wrist
     M11.131 Familial chondrocalcinosis, right wrist
     M11.132 Familial chondrocalcinosis, left wrist
     M11.139 Familial chondrocalcinosis, unspecified wrist

✓6ᵗʰ **M11.14** Familial chondrocalcinosis, hand
     M11.141 Familial chondrocalcinosis, right hand
     M11.142 Familial chondrocalcinosis, left hand
     M11.149 Familial chondrocalcinosis, unspecified hand

✓6ᵗʰ **M11.15** Familial chondrocalcinosis, hip
     M11.151 Familial chondrocalcinosis, right hip
     M11.152 Familial chondrocalcinosis, left hip
     M11.159 Familial chondrocalcinosis, unspecified hip

✓6ᵗʰ **M11.16** Familial chondrocalcinosis, knee
     M11.161 Familial chondrocalcinosis, right knee
     M11.162 Familial chondrocalcinosis, left knee
     M11.169 Familial chondrocalcinosis, unspecified knee

✓6ᵗʰ **M11.17** Familial chondrocalcinosis, ankle and foot
     M11.171 Familial chondrocalcinosis, right ankle and foot
     M11.172 Familial chondrocalcinosis, left ankle and foot
     M11.179 Familial chondrocalcinosis, unspecified ankle and foot

   M11.18 Familial chondrocalcinosis, vertebrae
   M11.19 Familial chondrocalcinosis, multiple sites

✓5ᵗʰ **M11.2** Other chondrocalcinosis
     Chondrocalcinosis NOS
     AHA: 2018,3Q,20
     TIP: Pseudogout is captured with codes in this subcategory.

   M11.20 Other chondrocalcinosis, unspecified site

✓6ᵗʰ **M11.21** Other chondrocalcinosis, shoulder
     M11.211 Other chondrocalcinosis, right shoulder
     M11.212 Other chondrocalcinosis, left shoulder
     M11.219 Other chondrocalcinosis, unspecified shoulder

✓6ᵗʰ **M11.22** Other chondrocalcinosis, elbow
     M11.221 Other chondrocalcinosis, right elbow
     M11.222 Other chondrocalcinosis, left elbow
     M11.229 Other chondrocalcinosis, unspecified elbow

✓6ᵗʰ **M11.23** Other chondrocalcinosis, wrist
     M11.231 Other chondrocalcinosis, right wrist
     M11.232 Other chondrocalcinosis, left wrist
     M11.239 Other chondrocalcinosis, unspecified wrist

✓6ᵗʰ **M11.24** Other chondrocalcinosis, hand
     M11.241 Other chondrocalcinosis, right hand
     M11.242 Other chondrocalcinosis, left hand
     M11.249 Other chondrocalcinosis, unspecified hand

✓6ᵗʰ **M11.25** Other chondrocalcinosis, hip
     M11.251 Other chondrocalcinosis, right hip
     M11.252 Other chondrocalcinosis, left hip
     M11.259 Other chondrocalcinosis, unspecified hip

✓6ᵗʰ **M11.26** Other chondrocalcinosis, knee
     M11.261 Other chondrocalcinosis, right knee
     M11.262 Other chondrocalcinosis, left knee
     M11.269 Other chondrocalcinosis, unspecified knee

✓6ᵗʰ **M11.27** Other chondrocalcinosis, ankle and foot
     M11.271 Other chondrocalcinosis, right ankle and foot
     M11.272 Other chondrocalcinosis, left ankle and foot
     M11.279 Other chondrocalcinosis, unspecified ankle and foot

   M11.28 Other chondrocalcinosis, vertebrae

M11.29   Other chondrocalcinosis, multiple sites

√5ᵗʰ M11.8   Other specified crystal arthropathies

     M11.80   Other specified crystal arthropathies, unspecified site

√6ᵗʰ M11.81   Other specified crystal arthropathies, shoulder

     M11.811   Other specified crystal arthropathies, right shoulder

     M11.812   Other specified crystal arthropathies, left shoulder

     M11.819   Other specified crystal arthropathies, unspecified shoulder

√6ᵗʰ M11.82   Other specified crystal arthropathies, elbow

     M11.821   Other specified crystal arthropathies, right elbow

     M11.822   Other specified crystal arthropathies, left elbow

     M11.829   Other specified crystal arthropathies, unspecified elbow

√6ᵗʰ M11.83   Other specified crystal arthropathies, wrist

     M11.831   Other specified crystal arthropathies, right wrist

     M11.832   Other specified crystal arthropathies, left wrist

     M11.839   Other specified crystal arthropathies, unspecified wrist

√6ᵗʰ M11.84   Other specified crystal arthropathies, hand

     M11.841   Other specified crystal arthropathies, right hand

     M11.842   Other specified crystal arthropathies, left hand

     M11.849   Other specified crystal arthropathies, unspecified hand

√6ᵗʰ M11.85   Other specified crystal arthropathies, hip

     M11.851   Other specified crystal arthropathies, right hip

     M11.852   Other specified crystal arthropathies, left hip

     M11.859   Other specified crystal arthropathies, unspecified hip

√6ᵗʰ M11.86   Other specified crystal arthropathies, knee

     M11.861   Other specified crystal arthropathies, right knee

     M11.862   Other specified crystal arthropathies, left knee

     M11.869   Other specified crystal arthropathies, unspecified knee

√6ᵗʰ M11.87   Other specified crystal arthropathies, ankle and foot

     M11.871   Other specified crystal arthropathies, right ankle and foot

     M11.872   Other specified crystal arthropathies, left ankle and foot

     M11.879   Other specified crystal arthropathies, unspecified ankle and foot

     M11.88   Other specified crystal arthropathies, vertebrae

     M11.89   Other specified crystal arthropathies, multiple sites

M11.9   Crystal arthropathy, unspecified

√4ᵗʰ **M12**   **Other and unspecified arthropathy**

     EXCLUDES 1   arthrosis (M15-M19)

           cricoarytenoid arthropathy (J38.7)

√5ᵗʰ M12.0   Chronic postrheumatic arthropathy [Jaccoud]

     M12.00   Chronic postrheumatic arthropathy [Jaccoud], unspecified site   HCC

√6ᵗʰ M12.01   Chronic postrheumatic arthropathy [Jaccoud], shoulder

     M12.011   Chronic postrheumatic arthropathy [Jaccoud], right shoulder   HCC

     M12.012   Chronic postrheumatic arthropathy [Jaccoud], left shoulder   HCC

     M12.019   Chronic postrheumatic arthropathy [Jaccoud], unspecified shoulder   HCC

√6ᵗʰ M12.02   Chronic postrheumatic arthropathy [Jaccoud], elbow

     M12.021   Chronic postrheumatic arthropathy [Jaccoud], right elbow   HCC

     M12.022   Chronic postrheumatic arthropathy [Jaccoud], left elbow   HCC

     M12.029   Chronic postrheumatic arthropathy [Jaccoud], unspecified elbow   HCC

√6ᵗʰ M12.03   Chronic postrheumatic arthropathy [Jaccoud], wrist

     M12.031   Chronic postrheumatic arthropathy [Jaccoud], right wrist   HCC

     M12.032   Chronic postrheumatic arthropathy [Jaccoud], left wrist   HCC

     M12.039   Chronic postrheumatic arthropathy [Jaccoud], unspecified wrist   HCC

√6ᵗʰ M12.04   Chronic postrheumatic arthropathy [Jaccoud], hand

     M12.041   Chronic postrheumatic arthropathy [Jaccoud], right hand   HCC

     M12.042   Chronic postrheumatic arthropathy [Jaccoud], left hand   HCC

     M12.049   Chronic postrheumatic arthropathy [Jaccoud], unspecified hand   HCC

√6ᵗʰ M12.05   Chronic postrheumatic arthropathy [Jaccoud], hip

     M12.051   Chronic postrheumatic arthropathy [Jaccoud], right hip   HCC

     M12.052   Chronic postrheumatic arthropathy [Jaccoud], left hip   HCC

     M12.059   Chronic postrheumatic arthropathy [Jaccoud], unspecified hip   HCC

√6ᵗʰ M12.06   Chronic postrheumatic arthropathy [Jaccoud], knee

     M12.061   Chronic postrheumatic arthropathy [Jaccoud], right knee   HCC

     M12.062   Chronic postrheumatic arthropathy [Jaccoud], left knee   HCC

     M12.069   Chronic postrheumatic arthropathy [Jaccoud], unspecified knee   HCC

√6ᵗʰ M12.07   Chronic postrheumatic arthropathy [Jaccoud], ankle and foot

     M12.071   Chronic postrheumatic arthropathy [Jaccoud], right ankle and foot   HCC

     M12.072   Chronic postrheumatic arthropathy [Jaccoud], left ankle and foot   HCC

     M12.079   Chronic postrheumatic arthropathy [Jaccoud], unspecified ankle and foot   HCC

     M12.08   Chronic postrheumatic arthropathy [Jaccoud], other specified site   HCC

         Chronic postrheumatic arthropathy [Jaccoud], vertebrae

     M12.09   Chronic postrheumatic arthropathy [Jaccoud], multiple sites   HCC

√5ᵗʰ M12.1   Kaschin-Beck disease

     Osteochondroarthrosis deformans endemica

     M12.10   Kaschin-Beck disease, unspecified site

√6ᵗʰ M12.11   Kaschin-Beck disease, shoulder

     M12.111   Kaschin-Beck disease, right shoulder

     M12.112   Kaschin-Beck disease, left shoulder

     M12.119   Kaschin-Beck disease, unspecified shoulder

√6ᵗʰ M12.12   Kaschin-Beck disease, elbow

     M12.121   Kaschin-Beck disease, right elbow

     M12.122   Kaschin-Beck disease, left elbow

     M12.129   Kaschin-Beck disease, unspecified elbow

√6ᵗʰ M12.13   Kaschin-Beck disease, wrist

     M12.131   Kaschin-Beck disease, right wrist

     M12.132   Kaschin-Beck disease, left wrist

     M12.139   Kaschin-Beck disease, unspecified wrist

√6ᵗʰ M12.14   Kaschin-Beck disease, hand

     M12.141   Kaschin-Beck disease, right hand

     M12.142   Kaschin-Beck disease, left hand

     M12.149   Kaschin-Beck disease, unspecified hand

√6ᵗʰ M12.15   Kaschin-Beck disease, hip

     M12.151   Kaschin-Beck disease, right hip

     M12.152   Kaschin-Beck disease, left hip

     M12.159   Kaschin-Beck disease, unspecified hip

✓6th **M12.16** **Kaschin-Beck disease,** knee

     M12.161 **Kaschin-Beck disease,** right **knee**

     M12.162 **Kaschin-Beck disease,** left **knee**

     M12.169 **Kaschin-Beck disease, unspecified knee**

✓6th **M12.17** **Kaschin-Beck disease,** ankle and foot

     M12.171 **Kaschin-Beck disease,** right **ankle and foot**

     M12.172 **Kaschin-Beck disease,** left **ankle and foot**

     M12.179 **Kaschin-Beck disease, unspecified ankle and foot**

     M12.18 **Kaschin-Beck disease,** vertebrae

     M12.19 **Kaschin-Beck disease,** multiple sites

✓5th **M12.2** **Villonodular synovitis (pigmented)**

     M12.20 **Villonodular synovitis (pigmented), unspecified site**

✓6th **M12.21** **Villonodular synovitis (pigmented),** shoulder

     M12.211 **Villonodular synovitis (pigmented),** right **shoulder**

     M12.212 **Villonodular synovitis (pigmented),** left **shoulder**

     M12.219 **Villonodular synovitis (pigmented), unspecified shoulder**

✓6th **M12.22** **Villonodular synovitis (pigmented),** elbow

     M12.221 **Villonodular synovitis (pigmented),** right **elbow**

     M12.222 **Villonodular synovitis (pigmented),** left **elbow**

     M12.229 **Villonodular synovitis (pigmented), unspecified elbow**

✓6th **M12.23** **Villonodular synovitis (pigmented),** wrist

     M12.231 **Villonodular synovitis (pigmented),** right **wrist**

     M12.232 **Villonodular synovitis (pigmented),** left **wrist**

     M12.239 **Villonodular synovitis (pigmented), unspecified wrist**

✓6th **M12.24** **Villonodular synovitis (pigmented),** hand

     M12.241 **Villonodular synovitis (pigmented),** right **hand**

     M12.242 **Villonodular synovitis (pigmented),** left **hand**

     M12.249 **Villonodular synovitis (pigmented), unspecified hand**

✓6th **M12.25** **Villonodular synovitis (pigmented),** hip

     M12.251 **Villonodular synovitis (pigmented),** right **hip**

     M12.252 **Villonodular synovitis (pigmented),** left **hip**

     M12.259 **Villonodular synovitis (pigmented), unspecified hip**

✓6th **M12.26** **Villonodular synovitis (pigmented),** knee

     M12.261 **Villonodular synovitis (pigmented),** right **knee**

     M12.262 **Villonodular synovitis (pigmented),** left **knee**

     M12.269 **Villonodular synovitis (pigmented), unspecified knee**

✓6th **M12.27** **Villonodular synovitis (pigmented),** ankle and foot

     M12.271 **Villonodular synovitis (pigmented),** right **ankle and foot**

     M12.272 **Villonodular synovitis (pigmented),** left **ankle and foot**

     M12.279 **Villonodular synovitis (pigmented), unspecified ankle and foot**

     M12.28 **Villonodular synovitis (pigmented), other specified site**

         Villonodular synovitis (pigmented), vertebrae

     M12.29 **Villonodular synovitis (pigmented),** multiple sites

✓5th **M12.3** **Palindromic rheumatism**

     DEF: Sudden and recurring attacks of moderate to severe joint pain and swelling generally occurring in the hands or feet of unknown etiology. After the attack subsides, the joints appear normal again.

     M12.30 **Palindromic rheumatism, unspecified site**

✓6th **M12.31** **Palindromic rheumatism,** shoulder

     M12.311 **Palindromic rheumatism,** right **shoulder**

     M12.312 **Palindromic rheumatism,** left **shoulder**

     M12.319 **Palindromic rheumatism, unspecified shoulder**

✓6th **M12.32** **Palindromic rheumatism,** elbow

     M12.321 **Palindromic rheumatism,** right **elbow**

     M12.322 **Palindromic rheumatism,** left **elbow**

     M12.329 **Palindromic rheumatism, unspecified elbow**

✓6th **M12.33** **Palindromic rheumatism,** wrist

     M12.331 **Palindromic rheumatism,** right **wrist**

     M12.332 **Palindromic rheumatism,** left **wrist**

     M12.339 **Palindromic rheumatism, unspecified wrist**

✓6th **M12.34** **Palindromic rheumatism,** hand

     M12.341 **Palindromic rheumatism,** right **hand**

     M12.342 **Palindromic rheumatism,** left **hand**

     M12.349 **Palindromic rheumatism, unspecified hand**

✓6th **M12.35** **Palindromic rheumatism,** hip

     M12.351 **Palindromic rheumatism,** right **hip**

     M12.352 **Palindromic rheumatism,** left **hip**

     M12.359 **Palindromic rheumatism, unspecified hip**

✓6th **M12.36** **Palindromic rheumatism,** knee

     M12.361 **Palindromic rheumatism,** right **knee**

     M12.362 **Palindromic rheumatism,** left **knee**

     M12.369 **Palindromic rheumatism, unspecified knee**

✓6th **M12.37** **Palindromic rheumatism,** ankle and foot

     M12.371 **Palindromic rheumatism,** right **ankle and foot**

     M12.372 **Palindromic rheumatism,** left **ankle and foot**

     M12.379 **Palindromic rheumatism, unspecified ankle and foot**

     M12.38 **Palindromic rheumatism, other specified site**

         Palindromic rheumatism, vertebrae

     M12.39 **Palindromic rheumatism,** multiple sites

✓5th **M12.4** **Intermittent hydrarthrosis**

     M12.40 **Intermittent hydrarthrosis, unspecified site**

✓6th **M12.41** **Intermittent hydrarthrosis,** shoulder

     M12.411 **Intermittent hydrarthrosis,** right **shoulder**

     M12.412 **Intermittent hydrarthrosis,** left **shoulder**

     M12.419 **Intermittent hydrarthrosis, unspecified shoulder**

✓6th **M12.42** **Intermittent hydrarthrosis,** elbow

     M12.421 **Intermittent hydrarthrosis,** right **elbow**

     M12.422 **Intermittent hydrarthrosis,** left **elbow**

     M12.429 **Intermittent hydrarthrosis, unspecified elbow**

✓6th **M12.43** **Intermittent hydrarthrosis,** wrist

     M12.431 **Intermittent hydrarthrosis,** right **wrist**

     M12.432 **Intermittent hydrarthrosis,** left **wrist**

     M12.439 **Intermittent hydrarthrosis, unspecified wrist**

✓6th **M12.44** **Intermittent hydrarthrosis,** hand

     M12.441 **Intermittent hydrarthrosis,** right **hand**

     M12.442 **Intermittent hydrarthrosis,** left **hand**

     M12.449 **Intermittent hydrarthrosis, unspecified hand**

✓6th **M12.45** **Intermittent hydrarthrosis,** hip

     M12.451 **Intermittent hydrarthrosis,** right **hip**

     M12.452 **Intermittent hydrarthrosis,** left **hip**

     M12.459 **Intermittent hydrarthrosis, unspecified hip**

✓6th **M12.46** **Intermittent hydrarthrosis,** knee

     M12.461 **Intermittent hydrarthrosis,** right **knee**

     M12.462 **Intermittent hydrarthrosis,** left **knee**

     M12.469 **Intermittent hydrarthrosis, unspecified knee**

✓6th **M12.47** **Intermittent hydrarthrosis,** ankle and foot

     M12.471 **Intermittent hydrarthrosis,** right **ankle and foot**

     M12.472 **Intermittent hydrarthrosis,** left **ankle and foot**

     M12.479 **Intermittent hydrarthrosis, unspecified ankle and foot**

     M12.48 **Intermittent hydrarthrosis, other site**

     M12.49 **Intermittent hydrarthrosis,** multiple sites

✓ Additional Character Required   ✓x7th Placeholder Alert   Manifestation   Unspecified Dx   ▶◀ Revised Text   ● New Code   ▲ Revised Code Title

ICD-10-CM 2020   765

√5ᵗʰ **M12.5 Traumatic arthropathy**

    EXCLUDES 1   *current injury–see Alphabetic Index*

        post-traumatic osteoarthritis of first carpometacarpal joint (M18.2-M18.3)

        post-traumatic osteoarthritis of hip (M16.4-M16.5)

        post-traumatic osteoarthritis of knee (M17.2-M17.3)

        post-traumatic osteoarthritis NOS (M19.1-)

        post-traumatic osteoarthritis of other single joints (M19.1-)

    AHA: 2015,1Q,17

    M12.50 Traumatic arthropathy, unspecified site

√6ᵗʰ **M12.51 Traumatic arthropathy, shoulder**

      M12.511 Traumatic arthropathy, right shoulder

      M12.512 Traumatic arthropathy, left shoulder

      M12.519 Traumatic arthropathy, unspecified shoulder

√6ᵗʰ **M12.52 Traumatic arthropathy, elbow**

      M12.521 Traumatic arthropathy, right elbow

      M12.522 Traumatic arthropathy, left elbow

      M12.529 Traumatic arthropathy, unspecified elbow

√6ᵗʰ **M12.53 Traumatic arthropathy, wrist**

      M12.531 Traumatic arthropathy, right wrist

      M12.532 Traumatic arthropathy, left wrist

      M12.539 Traumatic arthropathy, unspecified wrist

√6ᵗʰ **M12.54 Traumatic arthropathy, hand**

      M12.541 Traumatic arthropathy, right hand

      M12.542 Traumatic arthropathy, left hand

      M12.549 Traumatic arthropathy, unspecified hand

√6ᵗʰ **M12.55 Traumatic arthropathy, hip**

      M12.551 Traumatic arthropathy, right hip

      M12.552 Traumatic arthropathy, left hip

      M12.559 Traumatic arthropathy, unspecified hip

√6ᵗʰ **M12.56 Traumatic arthropathy, knee**

      M12.561 Traumatic arthropathy, right knee

      M12.562 Traumatic arthropathy, left knee

      M12.569 Traumatic arthropathy, unspecified knee

√6ᵗʰ **M12.57 Traumatic arthropathy, ankle and foot**

      M12.571 Traumatic arthropathy, right ankle and foot

      M12.572 Traumatic arthropathy, left ankle and foot

      M12.579 Traumatic arthropathy, unspecified ankle and foot

    M12.58 Traumatic arthropathy, other specified site

      Traumatic arthropathy, vertebrae

    M12.59 Traumatic arthropathy, multiple sites

√5ᵗʰ **M12.8 Other specific arthropathies, not elsewhere classified**

    Transient arthropathy

    M12.80 Other specific arthropathies, not elsewhere classified, unspecified site

√6ᵗʰ **M12.81 Other specific arthropathies, not elsewhere classified, shoulder**

      M12.811 Other specific arthropathies, not elsewhere classified, right shoulder

      M12.812 Other specific arthropathies, not elsewhere classified, left shoulder

      M12.819 Other specific arthropathies, not elsewhere classified, unspecified shoulder

√6ᵗʰ **M12.82 Other specific arthropathies, not elsewhere classified, elbow**

      M12.821 Other specific arthropathies, not elsewhere classified, right elbow

      M12.822 Other specific arthropathies, not elsewhere classified, left elbow

      M12.829 Other specific arthropathies, not elsewhere classified, unspecified elbow

√6ᵗʰ **M12.83 Other specific arthropathies, not elsewhere classified, wrist**

      M12.831 Other specific arthropathies, not elsewhere classified, right wrist

      M12.832 Other specific arthropathies, not elsewhere classified, left wrist

      M12.839 Other specific arthropathies, not elsewhere classified, unspecified wrist

√6ᵗʰ **M12.84 Other specific arthropathies, not elsewhere classified, hand**

      M12.841 Other specific arthropathies, not elsewhere classified, right hand

      M12.842 Other specific arthropathies, not elsewhere classified, left hand

      M12.849 Other specific arthropathies, not elsewhere classified, unspecified hand

√6ᵗʰ **M12.85 Other specific arthropathies, not elsewhere classified, hip**

      M12.851 Other specific arthropathies, not elsewhere classified, right hip

      M12.852 Other specific arthropathies, not elsewhere classified, left hip

      M12.859 Other specific arthropathies, not elsewhere classified, unspecified hip

√6ᵗʰ **M12.86 Other specific arthropathies, not elsewhere classified, knee**

      M12.861 Other specific arthropathies, not elsewhere classified, right knee

      M12.862 Other specific arthropathies, not elsewhere classified, left knee

      M12.869 Other specific arthropathies, not elsewhere classified, unspecified knee

√6ᵗʰ **M12.87 Other specific arthropathies, not elsewhere classified, ankle and foot**

      M12.871 Other specific arthropathies, not elsewhere classified, right ankle and foot

      M12.872 Other specific arthropathies, not elsewhere classified, left ankle and foot

      M12.879 Other specific arthropathies, not elsewhere classified, unspecified ankle and foot

    M12.88 Other specific arthropathies, not elsewhere classified, other specified site

      Other specific arthropathies, not elsewhere classified, vertebrae

    M12.89 Other specific arthropathies, not elsewhere classified, multiple sites

M12.9 Arthropathy, unspecified

√4ᵗʰ **M13 Other arthritis**

    EXCLUDES 1   *arthrosis (M15-M19)*

        osteoarthritis (M15-M19)

M13.0 Polyarthritis, unspecified

√5ᵗʰ **M13.1 Monoarthritis, not elsewhere classified**

    M13.10 Monoarthritis, not elsewhere classified, unspecified site

√6ᵗʰ **M13.11 Monoarthritis, not elsewhere classified, shoulder**

      M13.111 Monoarthritis, not elsewhere classified, right shoulder

      M13.112 Monoarthritis, not elsewhere classified, left shoulder

      M13.119 Monoarthritis, not elsewhere classified, unspecified shoulder

√6ᵗʰ **M13.12 Monoarthritis, not elsewhere classified, elbow**

      M13.121 Monoarthritis, not elsewhere classified, right elbow

      M13.122 Monoarthritis, not elsewhere classified, left elbow

      M13.129 Monoarthritis, not elsewhere classified, unspecified elbow

√6ᵗʰ **M13.13 Monoarthritis, not elsewhere classified, wrist**

      M13.131 Monoarthritis, not elsewhere classified, right wrist

      M13.132 Monoarthritis, not elsewhere classified, left wrist

      M13.139 Monoarthritis, not elsewhere classified, unspecified wrist

√6ᵗʰ **M13.14 Monoarthritis, not elsewhere classified, hand**

      M13.141 Monoarthritis, not elsewhere classified, right hand

      M13.142 Monoarthritis, not elsewhere classified, left hand

      M13.149 Monoarthritis, not elsewhere classified, unspecified hand

√6ᵗʰ **M13.15 Monoarthritis, not elsewhere classified, hip**

      M13.151 Monoarthritis, not elsewhere classified, right hip

      M13.152 Monoarthritis, not elsewhere classified, left hip

         M13.159   **Monoarthritis, not elsewhere classified, unspecified hip**

✓6ᵗʰ   M13.16   **Monoarthritis, not elsewhere classified, knee**

     M13.161   **Monoarthritis, not elsewhere classified, right knee**

     M13.162   **Monoarthritis, not elsewhere classified, left knee**

     M13.169   **Monoarthritis, not elsewhere classified, unspecified knee**

✓6ᵗʰ   M13.17   **Monoarthritis, not elsewhere classified, ankle and foot**

     M13.171   **Monoarthritis, not elsewhere classified, right ankle and foot**

     M13.172   **Monoarthritis, not elsewhere classified, left ankle and foot**

     M13.179   **Monoarthritis, not elsewhere classified, unspecified ankle and foot**

✓5ᵗʰ   **M13.8   Other specified arthritis**

     Allergic arthritis

     EXCLUDES 1   *osteoarthritis (M15-M19)*

     M13.80   **Other specified arthritis, unspecified site**

✓6ᵗʰ   M13.81   **Other specified arthritis, shoulder**

     M13.811   **Other specified arthritis, right shoulder**

     M13.812   **Other specified arthritis, left shoulder**

     M13.819   **Other specified arthritis, unspecified shoulder**

✓6ᵗʰ   M13.82   **Other specified arthritis, elbow**

     M13.821   **Other specified arthritis, right elbow**

     M13.822   **Other specified arthritis, left elbow**

     M13.829   **Other specified arthritis, unspecified elbow**

✓6ᵗʰ   M13.83   **Other specified arthritis, wrist**

     M13.831   **Other specified arthritis, right wrist**

     M13.832   **Other specified arthritis, left wrist**

     M13.839   **Other specified arthritis, unspecified wrist**

✓6ᵗʰ   M13.84   **Other specified arthritis, hand**

     M13.841   **Other specified arthritis, right hand**

     M13.842   **Other specified arthritis, left hand**

     M13.849   **Other specified arthritis, unspecified hand**

✓6ᵗʰ   M13.85   **Other specified arthritis, hip**

     M13.851   **Other specified arthritis, right hip**

     M13.852   **Other specified arthritis, left hip**

     M13.859   **Other specified arthritis, unspecified hip**

✓6ᵗʰ   M13.86   **Other specified arthritis, knee**

     M13.861   **Other specified arthritis, right knee**

     M13.862   **Other specified arthritis, left knee**

     M13.869   **Other specified arthritis, unspecified knee**

✓6ᵗʰ   M13.87   **Other specified arthritis, ankle and foot**

     M13.871   **Other specified arthritis, right ankle and foot**

     M13.872   **Other specified arthritis, left ankle and foot**

     M13.879   **Other specified arthritis, unspecified ankle and foot**

     M13.88   **Other specified arthritis, other site**

     M13.89   **Other specified arthritis, multiple sites**

✓4ᵗʰ   **M14   Arthropathies in other diseases classified elsewhere**

     EXCLUDES 1   *arthropathy in:*

         diabetes mellitus (E08-E13 with .61-)

         hematological disorders (M36.2-M36.3)

         hypersensitivity reactions (M36.4)

         neoplastic disease (M36.1)

         neurosyphillis (A52.16)

         sarcoidosis (D86.86)

         enteropathic arthropathies (M07.-)

         juvenile psoriatic arthropathy (L40.54)

         lipoid dermatoarthritis (E78.81)

✓5ᵗʰ   **M14.6   Charcôt's joint**

     Neuropathic arthropathy

     EXCLUDES 1   *Charcôt's joint in diabetes mellitus (E08-E13 with .610)*

         Charcôt's joint in tabes dorsalis (A52.16)

     DEF: Progressive neurologic arthropathy in which chronic degeneration of joints in the weight-bearing areas with peripheral hypertrophy occurs as a complication of a neuropathy disorder. Supporting structures relax from a loss of sensation resulting in chronic joint instability.

     M14.60   **Charcôt's joint, unspecified site**

✓6ᵗʰ   M14.61   **Charcôt's joint, shoulder**

     M14.611   **Charcôt's joint, right shoulder**

     M14.612   **Charcôt's joint, left shoulder**

     M14.619   **Charcôt's joint, unspecified shoulder**

✓6ᵗʰ   M14.62   **Charcôt's joint, elbow**

     M14.621   **Charcôt's joint, right elbow**

     M14.622   **Charcôt's joint, left elbow**

     M14.629   **Charcôt's joint, unspecified elbow**

✓6ᵗʰ   M14.63   **Charcôt's joint, wrist**

     M14.631   **Charcôt's joint, right wrist**

     M14.632   **Charcôt's joint, left wrist**

     M14.639   **Charcôt's joint, unspecified wrist**

✓6ᵗʰ   M14.64   **Charcôt's joint, hand**

     M14.641   **Charcôt's joint, right hand**

     M14.642   **Charcôt's joint, left hand**

     M14.649   **Charcôt's joint, unspecified hand**

✓6ᵗʰ   M14.65   **Charcôt's joint, hip**

     M14.651   **Charcôt's joint, right hip**

     M14.652   **Charcôt's joint, left hip**

     M14.659   **Charcôt's joint, unspecified hip**

✓6ᵗʰ   M14.66   **Charcôt's joint, knee**

     M14.661   **Charcôt's joint, right knee**

     M14.662   **Charcôt's joint, left knee**

     M14.669   **Charcôt's joint, unspecified knee**

✓6ᵗʰ   M14.67   **Charcôt's joint, ankle and foot**

     M14.671   **Charcôt's joint, right ankle and foot**

     M14.672   **Charcôt's joint, left ankle and foot**

     M14.679   **Charcôt's joint, unspecified ankle and foot**

     M14.68   **Charcôt's joint, vertebrae**

     M14.69   **Charcôt's joint, multiple sites**

✓5ᵗʰ   **M14.8   Arthropathies in other specified diseases classified elsewhere**

     Code first underlying disease, such as:

         amyloidosis (E85.-)

         erythema multiforme (L51.-)

         erythema nodosum (L52)

         hemochromatosis (E83.11-)

         hyperparathyroidism (E21.-)

         hypothyroidism (E00-E03)

         sickle-cell disorders (D57.-)

         thyrotoxicosis [hyperthyroidism] (E05.-)

         Whipple's disease (K90.81)

     M14.80   ***Arthropathies in other specified diseases classified elsewhere, unspecified site***

✓6ᵗʰ   M14.81   **Arthropathies in other specified diseases classified elsewhere, shoulder**

     M14.811   ***Arthropathies in other specified diseases classified elsewhere, right shoulder***

     M14.812   ***Arthropathies in other specified diseases classified elsewhere, left shoulder***

     M14.819   ***Arthropathies in other specified diseases classified elsewhere, unspecified shoulder***

☑ Additional Character Required   ✓×7ᵗʰ Placeholder Alert   Manifestation   Unspecified Dx   ▶◀ Revised Text   ● New Code   ▲ Revised Code Title

ICD-10-CM 2020   767

M13.159–M14.819

Chapter 13. Diseases of the Musculoskeletal System and Connective Tissue

✓6th **M14.82** Arthropathies in other specified diseases classified elsewhere, elbow

     M14.821   *Arthropathies in other specified diseases classified elsewhere, right elbow*

     M14.822   *Arthropathies in other specified diseases classified elsewhere, left elbow*

     M14.829   *Arthropathies in other specified diseases classified elsewhere, unspecified elbow*

✓6th **M14.83** Arthropathies in other specified diseases classified elsewhere, wrist

     M14.831   *Arthropathies in other specified diseases classified elsewhere, right wrist*

     M14.832   *Arthropathies in other specified diseases classified elsewhere, left wrist*

     M14.839   *Arthropathies in other specified diseases classified elsewhere, unspecified wrist*

✓6th **M14.84** Arthropathies in other specified diseases classified elsewhere, hand

     M14.841   *Arthropathies in other specified diseases classified elsewhere, right hand*

     M14.842   *Arthropathies in other specified diseases classified elsewhere, left hand*

     M14.849   *Arthropathies in other specified diseases classified elsewhere, unspecified hand*

✓6th **M14.85** Arthropathies in other specified diseases classified elsewhere, hip

     M14.851   *Arthropathies in other specified diseases classified elsewhere, right hip*

     M14.852   *Arthropathies in other specified diseases classified elsewhere, left hip*

     M14.859   *Arthropathies in other specified diseases classified elsewhere, unspecified hip*

✓6th **M14.86** Arthropathies in other specified diseases classified elsewhere, knee

     M14.861   *Arthropathies in other specified diseases classified elsewhere, right knee*

     M14.862   *Arthropathies in other specified diseases classified elsewhere, left knee*

     M14.869   *Arthropathies in other specified diseases classified elsewhere, unspecified knee*

✓6th **M14.87** Arthropathies in other specified diseases classified elsewhere, ankle and foot

     M14.871   *Arthropathies in other specified diseases classified elsewhere, right ankle and foot*

     M14.872   *Arthropathies in other specified diseases classified elsewhere, left ankle and foot*

     M14.879   *Arthropathies in other specified diseases classified elsewhere, unspecified ankle and foot*

     M14.88   *Arthropathies in other specified diseases classified elsewhere, vertebrae*

     M14.89   *Arthropathies in other specified diseases classified elsewhere, multiple sites*

Osteoarthritis (M15-M19)

EXCLUDES 2   *osteoarthritis of spine (M47.-)*

TIP: Assign a primary osteoarthritis code when the type of osteoarthritis—primary, secondary, or generalized—is not specified in the documentation. Primary is considered the default.

✓4th **M15 Polyosteoarthritis**

     INCLUDES   arthritis of multiple sites

     EXCLUDES 1   *bilateral involvement of single joint (M16-M19)*

     M15.0   **Primary generalized (osteo)arthritis**   Q

     M15.1   **Heberden's nodes (with arthropathy)**   Q

         Interphalangeal distal osteoarthritis

     M15.2   **Bouchard's nodes (with arthropathy)**   Q

         Juxtaphalangeal distal osteoarthritis

     M15.3   **Secondary multiple arthritis**   Q

         Post-traumatic polyosteoarthritis

     M15.4   **Erosive (osteo)arthritis**   Q

     M15.8   **Other polyosteoarthritis**   Q

     M15.9   **Polyosteoarthritis, unspecified**   Q

         Generalized osteoarthritis NOS

✓4th **M16 Osteoarthritis of hip**

     AHA: 2016,4Q,146

     M16.0   **Bilateral primary osteoarthritis of hip**   Q

         AHA: 2018,2Q,15

✓5th **M16.1**   Unilateral primary osteoarthritis of hip

     Primary osteoarthritis of hip NOS

     AHA: 2018,2Q,15

     M16.10   **Unilateral primary osteoarthritis, unspecified hip**   Q

     M16.11   **Unilateral primary osteoarthritis, right hip**   Q

     M16.12   **Unilateral primary osteoarthritis, left hip**   Q

     M16.2   **Bilateral osteoarthritis resulting from hip dysplasia**   Q

✓5th **M16.3**   Unilateral osteoarthritis resulting from hip dysplasia

     Dysplastic osteoarthritis of hip NOS

     M16.30   **Unilateral osteoarthritis resulting from hip dysplasia, unspecified hip**   Q

     M16.31   **Unilateral osteoarthritis resulting from hip dysplasia, right hip**   Q

     M16.32   **Unilateral osteoarthritis resulting from hip dysplasia, left hip**   Q

     M16.4   **Bilateral post-traumatic osteoarthritis of hip**   Q

✓5th **M16.5**   Unilateral post-traumatic osteoarthritis of hip

     Post-traumatic osteoarthritis of hip NOS

     M16.50   **Unilateral post-traumatic osteoarthritis, unspecified hip**   Q

     M16.51   **Unilateral post-traumatic osteoarthritis, right hip**   Q

     M16.52   **Unilateral post-traumatic osteoarthritis, left hip**   Q

     M16.6   **Other bilateral secondary osteoarthritis of hip**   Q

     M16.7   **Other unilateral secondary osteoarthritis of hip**   Q

         Secondary osteoarthritis of hip NOS

     M16.9   **Osteoarthritis of hip, unspecified**   Q

✓4th **M17 Osteoarthritis of knee**

     AHA: 2016,4Q,146-147

     M17.0   **Bilateral primary osteoarthritis of knee**   Q

         AHA: 2018,2Q,15

✓5th **M17.1**   Unilateral primary osteoarthritis of knee

     Primary osteoarthritis of knee NOS

     AHA: 2018,2Q,15

     M17.10   **Unilateral primary osteoarthritis, unspecified knee**   Q

     M17.11   **Unilateral primary osteoarthritis, right knee**   Q

     M17.12   **Unilateral primary osteoarthritis, left knee**   Q

     M17.2   **Bilateral post-traumatic osteoarthritis of knee**   Q

✓5th **M17.3**   Unilateral post-traumatic osteoarthritis of knee

     Post-traumatic osteoarthritis of knee NOS

     M17.30   **Unilateral post-traumatic osteoarthritis, unspecified knee**   Q

     M17.31   **Unilateral post-traumatic osteoarthritis, right knee**   Q

     M17.32   **Unilateral post-traumatic osteoarthritis, left knee**   Q

     M17.4   **Other bilateral secondary osteoarthritis of knee**   Q

     M17.5   **Other unilateral secondary osteoarthritis of knee**   Q

         Secondary osteoarthritis of knee NOS

     M17.9   **Osteoarthritis of knee, unspecified**   Q

✓4th **M18 Osteoarthritis of first carpometacarpal joint**

     M18.0   **Bilateral primary osteoarthritis of first carpometacarpal joints**   Q

✓5th **M18.1**   Unilateral primary osteoarthritis of first carpometacarpal joint

     Primary osteoarthritis of first carpometacarpal joint NOS

     M18.10   **Unilateral primary osteoarthritis of first carpometacarpal joint, unspecified hand**   Q

     M18.11   **Unilateral primary osteoarthritis of first carpometacarpal joint, right hand**   Q

     M18.12   **Unilateral primary osteoarthritis of first carpometacarpal joint, left hand**   Q

     M18.2   **Bilateral post-traumatic osteoarthritis of first carpometacarpal joints**   Q

✓5th **M18.3**   Unilateral post-traumatic osteoarthritis of first carpometacarpal joint

     Post-traumatic osteoarthritis of first carpometacarpal joint NOS

     M18.30   **Unilateral post-traumatic osteoarthritis of first carpometacarpal joint, unspecified hand**   Q

M18.31 Unilateral post-traumatic osteoarthritis of first carpometacarpal joint, right hand ▫

M18.32 Unilateral post-traumatic osteoarthritis of first carpometacarpal joint, left hand ▫

M18.4 Other bilateral secondary osteoarthritis of first carpometacarpal joints ▫

✓5th **M18.5** Other unilateral secondary osteoarthritis of first carpometacarpal joint

   Secondary osteoarthritis of first carpometacarpal joint NOS

   M18.50 Other unilateral secondary osteoarthritis of first carpometacarpal joint, unspecified hand ▫

   M18.51 Other unilateral secondary osteoarthritis of first carpometacarpal joint, right hand ▫

   M18.52 Other unilateral secondary osteoarthritis of first carpometacarpal joint, left hand ▫

M18.9 Osteoarthritis of first carpometacarpal joint, unspecified ▫

✓4th **M19** Other and unspecified osteoarthritis

   EXCLUDES 1   polyarthritis (M15.-)
   EXCLUDES 2   arthrosis of spine (M47.-)
                hallux rigidus (M20.2)
                osteoarthritis of spine (M47.-)

✓5th **M19.0** Primary osteoarthritis of other joints

   AHA: 2018,2Q,15; 2016,4Q,145

   ✓6th **M19.01** Primary osteoarthritis, shoulder

      M19.011 Primary osteoarthritis, right shoulder ▫

      M19.012 Primary osteoarthritis, left shoulder ▫

      M19.019 Primary osteoarthritis, unspecified shoulder ▫

   ✓6th **M19.02** Primary osteoarthritis, elbow

      M19.021 Primary osteoarthritis, right elbow ▫

      M19.022 Primary osteoarthritis, left elbow ▫

      M19.029 Primary osteoarthritis, unspecified elbow ▫

   ✓6th **M19.03** Primary osteoarthritis, wrist

      M19.031 Primary osteoarthritis, right wrist ▫

      M19.032 Primary osteoarthritis, left wrist ▫

      M19.039 Primary osteoarthritis, unspecified wrist ▫

   ✓6th **M19.04** Primary osteoarthritis, hand

      EXCLUDES 2   primary osteoarthritis of first carpometacarpal joint (M18.0-, M18.1-)

      M19.041 Primary osteoarthritis, right hand ▫

      M19.042 Primary osteoarthritis, left hand ▫

      M19.049 Primary osteoarthritis, unspecified hand ▫

   ✓6th **M19.07** Primary osteoarthritis ankle and foot

      M19.071 Primary osteoarthritis, right ankle and foot ▫

      M19.072 Primary osteoarthritis, left ankle and foot ▫

      M19.079 Primary osteoarthritis, unspecified ankle and foot ▫

✓5th **M19.1** Post-traumatic osteoarthritis of other joints

   ✓6th **M19.11** Post-traumatic osteoarthritis, shoulder

      M19.111 Post-traumatic osteoarthritis, right shoulder ▫

      M19.112 Post-traumatic osteoarthritis, left shoulder ▫

      M19.119 Post-traumatic osteoarthritis, unspecified shoulder ▫

   ✓6th **M19.12** Post-traumatic osteoarthritis, elbow

      M19.121 Post-traumatic osteoarthritis, right elbow ▫

      M19.122 Post-traumatic osteoarthritis, left elbow ▫

      M19.129 Post-traumatic osteoarthritis, unspecified elbow ▫

   ✓6th **M19.13** Post-traumatic osteoarthritis, wrist

      M19.131 Post-traumatic osteoarthritis, right wrist ▫

M19.132 Post-traumatic osteoarthritis, left wrist ▫

M19.139 Post-traumatic osteoarthritis, unspecified wrist ▫

✓6th **M19.14** Post-traumatic osteoarthritis, hand

   EXCLUDES 2   post-traumatic osteoarthritis of first carpometacarpal joint (M18.2-, M18.3-)

   M19.141 Post-traumatic osteoarthritis, right hand ▫

   M19.142 Post-traumatic osteoarthritis, left hand ▫

   M19.149 Post-traumatic osteoarthritis, unspecified hand ▫

✓6th **M19.17** Post-traumatic osteoarthritis, ankle and foot

   M19.171 Post-traumatic osteoarthritis, right ankle and foot ▫

   M19.172 Post-traumatic osteoarthritis, left ankle and foot ▫

   M19.179 Post-traumatic osteoarthritis, unspecified ankle and foot ▫

✓5th **M19.2** Secondary osteoarthritis of other joints

   ✓6th **M19.21** Secondary osteoarthritis, shoulder

      M19.211 Secondary osteoarthritis, right shoulder ▫

      M19.212 Secondary osteoarthritis, left shoulder ▫

      M19.219 Secondary osteoarthritis, unspecified shoulder ▫

   ✓6th **M19.22** Secondary osteoarthritis, elbow

      M19.221 Secondary osteoarthritis, right elbow ▫

      M19.222 Secondary osteoarthritis, left elbow ▫

      M19.229 Secondary osteoarthritis, unspecified elbow ▫

   ✓6th **M19.23** Secondary osteoarthritis, wrist

      M19.231 Secondary osteoarthritis, right wrist ▫

      M19.232 Secondary osteoarthritis, left wrist ▫

      M19.239 Secondary osteoarthritis, unspecified wrist ▫

   ✓6th **M19.24** Secondary osteoarthritis, hand

      M19.241 Secondary osteoarthritis, right hand ▫

      M19.242 Secondary osteoarthritis, left hand ▫

      M19.249 Secondary osteoarthritis, unspecified hand ▫

   ✓6th **M19.27** Secondary osteoarthritis, ankle and foot

      M19.271 Secondary osteoarthritis, right ankle and foot ▫

      M19.272 Secondary osteoarthritis, left ankle and foot ▫

      M19.279 Secondary osteoarthritis, unspecified ankle and foot ▫

✓5th **M19.9** Osteoarthritis, unspecified site

   M19.90 Unspecified osteoarthritis, unspecified site ▫

      Arthrosis NOS
      Arthritis NOS
      Osteoarthritis NOS
      AHA: 2016,4Q,147

   M19.91 Primary osteoarthritis, unspecified site ▫

      Primary osteoarthritis NOS

   M19.92 Post-traumatic osteoarthritis, unspecified site ▫

      Post-traumatic osteoarthritis NOS

   M19.93 Secondary osteoarthritis, unspecified site ▫

      Secondary osteoarthritis NOS

☑ Additional Character Required   ✓x7th Placeholder Alert   Manifestation   Unspecified Dx   ►◄ Revised Text   ● New Code   ▲ Revised Code Title

Other joint disorders (M20-M25)

EXCLUDES 2   *joints of the spine (M40-M54)*

✓4ᵗʰ M20 Acquired deformities of fingers and toes

  EXCLUDES 1   *acquired absence of fingers and toes (Z89.-)*
          congenital absence of fingers and toes (Q71.3-, Q72.3-)
          congenital deformities and malformations of fingers and toes
            (Q66.-, Q68-Q70, Q74.-)

✓5ᵗʰ M20.0 Deformity of finger(s)

  EXCLUDES 1   *clubbing of fingers (R68.3)*
          palmar fascial fibromatosis [Dupuytren] (M72.0)
          trigger finger (M65.3)

  ✓6ᵗʰ M20.00 Unspecified deformity of finger(s)

    M20.001 Unspecified deformity of right finger(s)
    M20.002 Unspecified deformity of left finger(s)
    M20.009 Unspecified deformity of unspecified finger(s)

  ✓6ᵗʰ M20.01 Mallet finger

    M20.011 Mallet finger of right finger(s)
    M20.012 Mallet finger of left finger(s)
    M20.019 Mallet finger of unspecified finger(s)

  ✓6ᵗʰ M20.02 Boutonnière deformity

    DEF: Deformity of the finger caused by flexion of the proximal interphalangeal joint and hyperextension of the distal joint. The deformity results from rheumatoid arthritis, osteoarthritis, or injury.
    M20.021 Boutonnière deformity of right finger(s)
    M20.022 Boutonnière deformity of left finger(s)
    M20.029 Boutonnière deformity of unspecified finger(s)

  ✓6ᵗʰ M20.03 Swan-neck deformity

    DEF: Flexed distal and hyperextended proximal interphalangeal joint most commonly caused by rheumatoid arthritis.
    M20.031 Swan-neck deformity of right finger(s)
    M20.032 Swan-neck deformity of left finger(s)
    M20.039 Swan-neck deformity of unspecified finger(s)

  ✓6ᵗʰ M20.09 Other deformity of finger(s)

    M20.091 Other deformity of right finger(s)
    M20.092 Other deformity of left finger(s)
    M20.099 Other deformity of finger(s), unspecified finger(s)

✓6ᵗʰ M20.1 Hallux valgus (acquired)

  EXCLUDES 2   *bunion (M21.6-)*
  AHA: 2016,4Q,38
  DEF: Deformity in which the great toe deviates toward the other toes and may even be positioned over or under the second toe.

Hallux Valgus

Hallux valgus

Medial eminence of metatarsal bone

Right foot

  M20.10 Hallux valgus (acquired), unspecified foot
  M20.11 Hallux valgus (acquired), right foot
  M20.12 Hallux valgus (acquired), left foot

✓5ᵗʰ M20.2 Hallux rigidus

  M20.20 Hallux rigidus, unspecified foot
  M20.21 Hallux rigidus, right foot
  M20.22 Hallux rigidus, left foot

✓5ᵗʰ M20.3 Hallux varus (acquired)

  DEF: Deformity in which the great toe deviates away from the other toes.
  M20.30 Hallux varus (acquired), unspecified foot
  M20.31 Hallux varus (acquired), right foot
  M20.32 Hallux varus (acquired), left foot

✓5ᵗʰ M20.4 Other hammer toe(s) (acquired)

  M20.40 Other hammer toe(s) (acquired), unspecified foot
  M20.41 Other hammer toe(s) (acquired), right foot
  M20.42 Other hammer toe(s) (acquired), left foot

✓5ᵗʰ M20.5 Other deformities of toe(s) (acquired)

  ✓6ᵗʰ M20.5X Other deformities of toe(s) (acquired)

    M20.5X1 Other deformities of toe(s) (acquired), right foot
    M20.5X2 Other deformities of toe(s) (acquired), left foot
    M20.5X9 Other deformities of toe(s) (acquired), unspecified foot

✓5ᵗʰ M20.6 Acquired deformities of toe(s), unspecified

  M20.60 Acquired deformities of toe(s), unspecified, unspecified foot
  M20.61 Acquired deformities of toe(s), unspecified, right foot
  M20.62 Acquired deformities of toe(s), unspecified, left foot

✓4ᵗʰ M21 Other acquired deformities of limbs

  EXCLUDES 1   *acquired absence of limb (Z89.-)*
          congenital absence of limbs (Q71-Q73)
          congenital deformities and malformations of limbs (Q65-Q66, Q68-Q74)

  EXCLUDES 2   *acquired deformities of fingers or toes (M20.-)*
          coxa plana (M91.2)

✓5ᵗʰ M21.0 Valgus deformity, not elsewhere classified

  EXCLUDES 1   *metatarsus valgus (Q66.6)*
          talipes calcaneovalgus ▶(Q66.4-)◄

  M21.00 Valgus deformity, not elsewhere classified, unspecified site

  ✓6ᵗʰ M21.02 Valgus deformity, not elsewhere classified, elbow
    Cubitus valgus
    M21.021 Valgus deformity, not elsewhere classified, right elbow
    M21.022 Valgus deformity, not elsewhere classified, left elbow
    M21.029 Valgus deformity, not elsewhere classified, unspecified elbow

  ✓6ᵗʰ M21.05 Valgus deformity, not elsewhere classified, hip
    M21.051 Valgus deformity, not elsewhere classified, right hip
    M21.052 Valgus deformity, not elsewhere classified, left hip
    M21.059 Valgus deformity, not elsewhere classified, unspecified hip

☑6ᵗʰ **M21.06** **Valgus deformity, not elsewhere classified, knee**
Genu valgum
Knock knee
DEF: Genu valga/valgum: Condition in which the thighs slant inward, causing the knees to be angled abnormally close together, leaving the space between the ankles wider than normal.

Genu Valga (knock-knee)

      M21.061 **Valgus deformity, not elsewhere classified, right knee**
      M21.062 **Valgus deformity, not elsewhere classified, left knee**
      M21.069 **Valgus deformity, not elsewhere classified, unspecified knee**

☑6ᵗʰ **M21.07** **Valgus deformity, not elsewhere classified, ankle**
      M21.071 **Valgus deformity, not elsewhere classified, right ankle**
      M21.072 **Valgus deformity, not elsewhere classified, left ankle**
      M21.079 **Valgus deformity, not elsewhere classified, unspecified ankle**

☑5ᵗʰ **M21.1** **Varus deformity, not elsewhere classified**
      EXCLUDES 1   *metatarsus varus* ▶*(Q66.22-)*◀
            tibia vara (M92.5)

      M21.10 **Varus deformity, not elsewhere classified, unspecified site**

☑6ᵗʰ **M21.12** **Varus deformity, not elsewhere classified, elbow**
Cubitus varus, elbow
      M21.121 **Varus deformity, not elsewhere classified, right elbow**
      M21.122 **Varus deformity, not elsewhere classified, left elbow**
      M21.129 **Varus deformity, not elsewhere classified, unspecified elbow**

☑6ᵗʰ **M21.15** **Varus deformity, not elsewhere classified, hip**
      M21.151 **Varus deformity, not elsewhere classified, right hip**
      M21.152 **Varus deformity, not elsewhere classified, left hip**
      M21.159 **Varus deformity, not elsewhere classified, unspecified**

☑6ᵗʰ **M21.16** **Varus deformity, not elsewhere classified, knee**
Bow leg
Genu varum
DEF: Genu varus/varum: Condition in which the thighs and/or legs are bowed in an outward curve with an abnormally increased space between the knees.

Genu Varus (bowleg)

      M21.161 **Varus deformity, not elsewhere classified, right knee**
      M21.162 **Varus deformity, not elsewhere classified, left knee**
      M21.169 **Varus deformity, not elsewhere classified, unspecified knee**

☑6ᵗʰ **M21.17** **Varus deformity, not elsewhere classified, ankle**
      M21.171 **Varus deformity, not elsewhere classified, right ankle**
      M21.172 **Varus deformity, not elsewhere classified, left ankle**
      M21.179 **Varus deformity, not elsewhere classified, unspecified ankle**

☑5ᵗʰ **M21.2** **Flexion deformity**
      M21.20 **Flexion deformity, unspecified site**

☑6ᵗʰ **M21.21** **Flexion deformity, shoulder**
      M21.211 **Flexion deformity, right shoulder**
      M21.212 **Flexion deformity, left shoulder**
      M21.219 **Flexion deformity, unspecified shoulder**

☑6ᵗʰ **M21.22** **Flexion deformity, elbow**
      M21.221 **Flexion deformity, right elbow**
      M21.222 **Flexion deformity, left elbow**
      M21.229 **Flexion deformity, unspecified elbow**

☑6ᵗʰ **M21.23** **Flexion deformity, wrist**
      M21.231 **Flexion deformity, right wrist**
      M21.232 **Flexion deformity, left wrist**
      M21.239 **Flexion deformity, unspecified wrist**

☑6ᵗʰ **M21.24** **Flexion deformity, finger joints**
      M21.241 **Flexion deformity, right finger joints**
      M21.242 **Flexion deformity, left finger joints**
      M21.249 **Flexion deformity, unspecified finger joints**

☑6ᵗʰ **M21.25** **Flexion deformity, hip**
      M21.251 **Flexion deformity, right hip**
      M21.252 **Flexion deformity, left hip**
      M21.259 **Flexion deformity, unspecified hip**

☑6ᵗʰ **M21.26** **Flexion deformity, knee**
      M21.261 **Flexion deformity, right knee**
      M21.262 **Flexion deformity, left knee**
      M21.269 **Flexion deformity, unspecified knee**

☑6ᵗʰ **M21.27** **Flexion deformity, ankle and toes**
      M21.271 **Flexion deformity, right ankle and toes**
      M21.272 **Flexion deformity, left ankle and toes**
      M21.279 **Flexion deformity, unspecified ankle and toes**

☑ Additional Character Required   ☑x7ᵗʰ Placeholder Alert   Manifestation   Unspecified Dx   ▶◀ Revised Text   ● New Code   ▲ Revised Code Title

ICD-10-CM 2020   **771**

✓5th **M21.3** Wrist or foot drop (acquired)

✓6th   **M21.33** Wrist drop (acquired)

     M21.331 Wrist drop, right wrist
     M21.332 Wrist drop, left wrist
     M21.339 Wrist drop, unspecified wrist

✓6th   **M21.37** Foot drop (acquired)

     M21.371 Foot drop, right foot
     M21.372 Foot drop, left foot
     M21.379 Foot drop, unspecified foot

✓5th **M21.4** Flat foot [pes planus] (acquired)

     EXCLUDES 1   *congenital pes planus (Q66.5-)*

    M21.40 Flat foot [pes planus] (acquired), unspecified foot
    M21.41 Flat foot [pes planus] (acquired), right foot
    M21.42 Flat foot [pes planus] (acquired), left foot

✓5th **M21.5** Acquired clawhand, clubhand, clawfoot and clubfoot

     EXCLUDES 1   *clubfoot, not specified as acquired (Q66.89)*

✓6th   **M21.51** Acquired clawhand

     M21.511 Acquired clawhand, right hand
     M21.512 Acquired clawhand, left hand
     M21.519 Acquired clawhand, unspecified hand

✓6th   **M21.52** Acquired clubhand

     M21.521 Acquired clubhand, right hand
     M21.522 Acquired clubhand, left hand
     M21.529 Acquired clubhand, unspecified hand

✓6th   **M21.53** Acquired clawfoot

     DEF: High foot arch with hyperextended toes at the metatarsophalangeal joint and flexed toes at the distal joints.

     M21.531 Acquired clawfoot, right foot
     M21.532 Acquired clawfoot, left foot
     M21.539 Acquired clawfoot, unspecified foot

✓6th   **M21.54** Acquired clubfoot

     DEF: Acquired anomaly of the foot with the heel elevated and rotated outward and the toes pointing inward.

     M21.541 Acquired clubfoot, right foot
     M21.542 Acquired clubfoot, left foot
     M21.549 Acquired clubfoot, unspecified foot

✓5th **M21.6** Other acquired deformities of foot

     EXCLUDES 2   *deformities of toe (acquired) (M20.1-M20.6-)*

     AHA: 2016,4Q,38

✓6th   **M21.61** Bunion

     M21.611 Bunion of right foot
     M21.612 Bunion of left foot
     M21.619 Bunion of unspecified foot

✓6th   **M21.62** Bunionette

     M21.621 Bunionette of right foot
     M21.622 Bunionette of left foot
     M21.629 Bunionette of unspecified foot

✓6th   **M21.6X** Other acquired deformities of foot

     M21.6X1 Other acquired deformities of right foot
     M21.6X2 Other acquired deformities of left foot
     M21.6X9 Other acquired deformities of unspecified foot

✓5th **M21.7** Unequal limb length (acquired)

     NOTE   The site used should correspond to the shorter limb

    M21.70 Unequal limb length (acquired), unspecified site

✓6th   **M21.72** Unequal limb length (acquired), humerus

     M21.721 Unequal limb length (acquired), right humerus
     M21.722 Unequal limb length (acquired), left humerus
     M21.729 Unequal limb length (acquired), unspecified humerus

✓6th   **M21.73** Unequal limb length (acquired), ulna and radius

     M21.731 Unequal limb length (acquired), right ulna
     M21.732 Unequal limb length (acquired), left ulna
     M21.733 Unequal limb length (acquired), right radius
     M21.734 Unequal limb length (acquired), left radius
     M21.739 Unequal limb length (acquired), unspecified ulna and radius

✓6th   **M21.75** Unequal limb length (acquired), femur

     M21.751 Unequal limb length (acquired), right femur
     M21.752 Unequal limb length (acquired), left femur
     M21.759 Unequal limb length (acquired), unspecified femur

✓6th   **M21.76** Unequal limb length (acquired), tibia and fibula

     M21.761 Unequal limb length (acquired), right tibia
     M21.762 Unequal limb length (acquired), left tibia
     M21.763 Unequal limb length (acquired), right fibula
     M21.764 Unequal limb length (acquired), left fibula
     M21.769 Unequal limb length (acquired), unspecified tibia and fibula

✓5th **M21.8** Other specified acquired deformities of limbs

     EXCLUDES 2   *coxa plana (M91.2)*

    M21.80 Other specified acquired deformities of unspecified limb

✓6th   **M21.82** Other specified acquired deformities of upper arm

     M21.821 Other specified acquired deformities of right upper arm
     M21.822 Other specified acquired deformities of left upper arm
     M21.829 Other specified acquired deformities of unspecified upper arm

✓6th   **M21.83** Other specified acquired deformities of forearm

     M21.831 Other specified acquired deformities of right forearm
     M21.832 Other specified acquired deformities of left forearm
     M21.839 Other specified acquired deformities of unspecified forearm

✓6th   **M21.85** Other specified acquired deformities of thigh

     M21.851 Other specified acquired deformities of right thigh
     M21.852 Other specified acquired deformities of left thigh
     M21.859 Other specified acquired deformities of unspecified thigh

✓6th   **M21.86** Other specified acquired deformities of lower leg

     M21.861 Other specified acquired deformities of right lower leg
     M21.862 Other specified acquired deformities of left lower leg
     M21.869 Other specified acquired deformities of unspecified lower leg

✓5th **M21.9** Unspecified acquired deformity of limb and hand

    M21.90 Unspecified acquired deformity of unspecified limb

✓6th   **M21.92** Unspecified acquired deformity of upper arm

     M21.921 Unspecified acquired deformity of right upper arm
     M21.922 Unspecified acquired deformity of left upper arm
     M21.929 Unspecified acquired deformity of unspecified upper arm

✓6th   **M21.93** Unspecified acquired deformity of forearm

     M21.931 Unspecified acquired deformity of right forearm
     M21.932 Unspecified acquired deformity of left forearm
     M21.939 Unspecified acquired deformity of unspecified forearm

✓6th   **M21.94** Unspecified acquired deformity of hand

     M21.941 Unspecified acquired deformity of hand, right hand
     M21.942 Unspecified acquired deformity of hand, left hand
     M21.949 Unspecified acquired deformity of hand, unspecified hand

✓6th   **M21.95** Unspecified acquired deformity of thigh

     M21.951 Unspecified acquired deformity of right thigh
     M21.952 Unspecified acquired deformity of left thigh
     M21.959 Unspecified acquired deformity of unspecified thigh

√6ᵗʰ **M21.96 Unspecified acquired deformity of lower leg**

    M21.961 Unspecified acquired deformity of right lower leg

    M21.962 Unspecified acquired deformity of left lower leg

    M21.969 Unspecified acquired deformity of unspecified lower leg

√4ᵗʰ **M22 Disorder of patella**

    EXCLUDES 1   traumatic dislocation of patella (S83.0-)

√5ᵗʰ **M22.0 Recurrent dislocation of patella**

    M22.00 Recurrent dislocation of patella, unspecified knee

    M22.01 Recurrent dislocation of patella, right knee

    M22.02 Recurrent dislocation of patella, left knee

√5ᵗʰ **M22.1 Recurrent subluxation of patella**

    Incomplete dislocation of patella

    M22.10 Recurrent subluxation of patella, unspecified knee

    M22.11 Recurrent subluxation of patella, right knee

    M22.12 Recurrent subluxation of patella, left knee

√5ᵗʰ **M22.2 Patellofemoral disorders**

    √6ᵗʰ **M22.2X Patellofemoral disorders**

        M22.2X1 Patellofemoral disorders, right knee

        M22.2X2 Patellofemoral disorders, left knee

        M22.2X9 Patellofemoral disorders, unspecified knee

√5ᵗʰ **M22.3 Other derangements of patella**

    √6ᵗʰ **M22.3X Other derangements of patella**

        M22.3X1 Other derangements of patella, right knee

        M22.3X2 Other derangements of patella, left knee

        M22.3X9 Other derangements of patella, unspecified knee

√5ᵗʰ **M22.4 Chondromalacia patellae**

    M22.40 Chondromalacia patellae, unspecified knee

    M22.41 Chondromalacia patellae, right knee

    M22.42 Chondromalacia patellae, left knee

√5ᵗʰ **M22.8 Other disorders of patella**

    √6ᵗʰ **M22.8X Other disorders of patella**

        M22.8X1 Other disorders of patella, right knee

        M22.8X2 Other disorders of patella, left knee

        M22.8X9 Other disorders of patella, unspecified knee

√5ᵗʰ **M22.9 Unspecified disorder of patella**

    M22.90 Unspecified disorder of patella, unspecified knee

    M22.91 Unspecified disorder of patella, right knee

    M22.92 Unspecified disorder of patella, left knee

√4ᵗʰ **M23 Internal derangement of knee**

    EXCLUDES 1   ankylosis (M24.66)

         current injury — see injury of knee and lower leg (S80-S89)

         deformity of knee (M21.-)

         osteochondritis dissecans (M93.2)

         recurrent dislocation or subluxation of joints (M24.4)

         recurrent dislocation or subluxation of patella (M22.0-M22.1)

√5ᵗʰ **M23.0 Cystic meniscus**

    √6ᵗʰ **M23.00 Cystic meniscus, unspecified meniscus**

        Cystic meniscus, unspecified lateral meniscus

        Cystic meniscus, unspecified medial meniscus

        M23.000 Cystic meniscus, unspecified lateral meniscus, right knee

        M23.001 Cystic meniscus, unspecified lateral meniscus, left knee

        M23.002 Cystic meniscus, unspecified lateral meniscus, unspecified knee

        M23.003 Cystic meniscus, unspecified medial meniscus, right knee

        M23.004 Cystic meniscus, unspecified medial meniscus, left knee

        M23.005 Cystic meniscus, unspecified medial meniscus, unspecified knee

        M23.006 Cystic meniscus, unspecified meniscus, right knee

        M23.007 Cystic meniscus, unspecified meniscus, left knee

        M23.009 Cystic meniscus, unspecified meniscus, unspecified knee

√6ᵗʰ **M23.01 Cystic meniscus, anterior horn of medial meniscus**

    M23.011 Cystic meniscus, anterior horn of medial meniscus, right knee

    M23.012 Cystic meniscus, anterior horn of medial meniscus, left knee

    M23.019 Cystic meniscus, anterior horn of medial meniscus, unspecified knee

√6ᵗʰ **M23.02 Cystic meniscus, posterior horn of medial meniscus**

    M23.021 Cystic meniscus, posterior horn of medial meniscus, right knee

    M23.022 Cystic meniscus, posterior horn of medial meniscus, left knee

    M23.029 Cystic meniscus, posterior horn of medial meniscus, unspecified knee

√6ᵗʰ **M23.03 Cystic meniscus, other medial meniscus**

    M23.031 Cystic meniscus, other medial meniscus, right knee

    M23.032 Cystic meniscus, other medial meniscus, left knee

    M23.039 Cystic meniscus, other medial meniscus, unspecified knee

√6ᵗʰ **M23.04 Cystic meniscus, anterior horn of lateral meniscus**

    M23.041 Cystic meniscus, anterior horn of lateral meniscus, right knee

    M23.042 Cystic meniscus, anterior horn of lateral meniscus, left knee

    M23.049 Cystic meniscus, anterior horn of lateral meniscus, unspecified knee

√6ᵗʰ **M23.05 Cystic meniscus, posterior horn of lateral meniscus**

    M23.051 Cystic meniscus, posterior horn of lateral meniscus, right knee

    M23.052 Cystic meniscus, posterior horn of lateral meniscus, left knee

    M23.059 Cystic meniscus, posterior horn of lateral meniscus, unspecified knee

√6ᵗʰ **M23.06 Cystic meniscus, other lateral meniscus**

    M23.061 Cystic meniscus, other lateral meniscus, right knee

    M23.062 Cystic meniscus, other lateral meniscus, left knee

    M23.069 Cystic meniscus, other lateral meniscus, unspecified knee

√5ᵗʰ **M23.2 Derangement of meniscus due to old tear or injury**

    Old bucket-handle tear

    AHA: 2019,2Q,26

Derangement of Meniscus

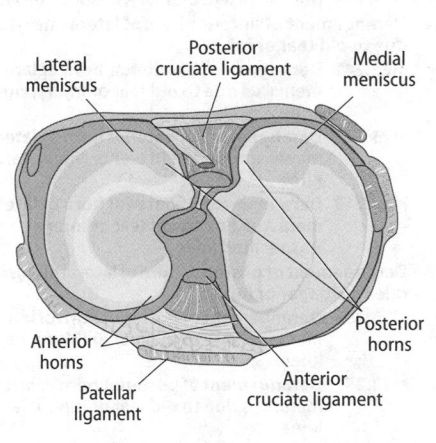

Lateral meniscus   Posterior cruciate ligament   Medial meniscus

Anterior horns   Patellar ligament   Anterior cruciate ligament   Posterior horns

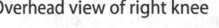

Overhead view of right knee

Bucket handle tear

Radial tear

Meniscus

√6ᵗʰ **M23.20 Derangement of unspecified meniscus due to old tear or injury**

    Derangement of unspecified lateral meniscus due to old tear or injury

    Derangement of unspecified medial meniscus due to old tear or injury

    M23.200 Derangement of unspecified lateral meniscus due to old tear or injury, right knee

✔ Additional Character Required   √x7ᵗʰ Placeholder Alert   Manifestation   Unspecified Dx   ►◄ Revised Text   ● New Code   ▲ Revised Code Title

ICD-10-CM 2020   773

M23.201 **Derangement of unspecified** lateral **meniscus due to old tear or injury,** left **knee**

M23.202 **Derangement of unspecified** lateral **meniscus due to old tear or injury, unspecified knee**

M23.203 **Derangement of unspecified** medial **meniscus due to old tear or injury,** right **knee**

M23.204 **Derangement of unspecified** medial **meniscus due to old tear or injury,** left **knee**

M23.205 **Derangement of unspecified** medial **meniscus due to old tear or injury, unspecified knee**

M23.206 **Derangement of unspecified meniscus due to old tear or injury,** right **knee**

M23.207 **Derangement of unspecified meniscus due to old tear or injury,** left **knee**

M23.209 **Derangement of unspecified meniscus due to old tear or injury, unspecified knee**

√6ᵗʰ M23.21 **Derangement of** anterior horn of medial **meniscus due to old tear or injury**

M23.211 **Derangement of anterior horn of medial meniscus due to old tear or injury,** right **knee**

M23.212 **Derangement of anterior horn of medial meniscus due to old tear or injury,** left **knee**

M23.219 **Derangement of anterior horn of medial meniscus due to old tear or injury, unspecified knee**

√6ᵗʰ M23.22 **Derangement of** posterior horn of medial **meniscus due to old tear or injury**

M23.221 **Derangement of posterior horn of medial meniscus due to old tear or injury,** right **knee**

M23.222 **Derangement of posterior horn of medial meniscus due to old tear or injury,** left **knee**

M23.229 **Derangement of posterior horn of medial meniscus due to old tear or injury, unspecified knee**

√6ᵗʰ M23.23 **Derangement of** other medial **meniscus due to old tear or injury**

M23.231 **Derangement of other medial meniscus due to old tear or injury,** right **knee**

M23.232 **Derangement of other medial meniscus due to old tear or injury,** left **knee**

M23.239 **Derangement of other medial meniscus due to old tear or injury, unspecified knee**

√6ᵗʰ M23.24 **Derangement of** anterior horn of lateral **meniscus due to old tear or injury**

M23.241 **Derangement of anterior horn of lateral meniscus due to old tear or injury,** right **knee**

M23.242 **Derangement of anterior horn of lateral meniscus due to old tear or injury,** left **knee**

M23.249 **Derangement of anterior horn of lateral meniscus due to old tear or injury, unspecified knee**

√6ᵗʰ M23.25 **Derangement of** posterior horn of lateral **meniscus due to old tear or injury**

M23.251 **Derangement of posterior horn of lateral meniscus due to old tear or injury,** right **knee**

M23.252 **Derangement of posterior horn of lateral meniscus due to old tear or injury,** left **knee**

M23.259 **Derangement of posterior horn of lateral meniscus due to old tear or injury, unspecified knee**

√6ᵗʰ M23.26 **Derangement of** other lateral **meniscus due to old tear or injury**

M23.261 **Derangement of other lateral meniscus due to old tear or injury,** right **knee**

M23.262 **Derangement of other lateral meniscus due to old tear or injury,** left **knee**

M23.269 **Derangement of other lateral meniscus due to old tear or injury, unspecified knee**

√5ᵗʰ **M23.3 Other meniscus derangements**

Degenerate meniscus
Detached meniscus
Retained meniscus

√6ᵗʰ M23.30 **Other meniscus derangements, unspecified meniscus**

Other meniscus derangements, unspecified lateral meniscus
Other meniscus derangements, unspecified medial meniscus

M23.300 **Other meniscus derangements, unspecified** lateral **meniscus,** right **knee**

M23.301 **Other meniscus derangements, unspecified** lateral **meniscus,** left **knee**

M23.302 **Other meniscus derangements, unspecified** lateral **meniscus, unspecified knee**

M23.303 **Other meniscus derangements, unspecified** medial **meniscus,** right **knee**

M23.304 **Other meniscus derangements, unspecified** medial **meniscus,** left **knee**

M23.305 **Other meniscus derangements, unspecified** medial **meniscus, unspecified knee**

M23.306 **Other meniscus derangements, unspecified meniscus,** right **knee**

M23.307 **Other meniscus derangements, unspecified meniscus,** left **knee**

M23.309 **Other meniscus derangements, unspecified meniscus, unspecified knee**

√6ᵗʰ M23.31 **Other meniscus derangements,** anterior horn of medial **meniscus**

M23.311 **Other meniscus derangements, anterior horn of medial meniscus,** right **knee**

M23.312 **Other meniscus derangements, anterior horn of medial meniscus,** left **knee**

M23.319 **Other meniscus derangements, anterior horn of medial meniscus, unspecified knee**

√6ᵗʰ M23.32 **Other meniscus derangements,** posterior horn of medial **meniscus**

M23.321 **Other meniscus derangements, posterior horn of medial meniscus,** right **knee**

M23.322 **Other meniscus derangements, posterior horn of medial meniscus,** left **knee**

M23.329 **Other meniscus derangements, posterior horn of medial meniscus, unspecified knee**

√6ᵗʰ M23.33 **Other meniscus derangements,** other medial **meniscus**

M23.331 **Other meniscus derangements, other medial meniscus,** right **knee**

M23.332 **Other meniscus derangements, other medial meniscus,** left **knee**

M23.339 **Other meniscus derangements, other medial meniscus, unspecified knee**

√6ᵗʰ M23.34 **Other meniscus derangements,** anterior horn of lateral **meniscus**

M23.341 **Other meniscus derangements, anterior horn of lateral meniscus,** right **knee**

M23.342 **Other meniscus derangements, anterior horn of lateral meniscus,** left **knee**

M23.349 **Other meniscus derangements, anterior horn of lateral meniscus, unspecified knee**

√6ᵗʰ M23.35 **Other meniscus derangements,** posterior horn of lateral **meniscus**

M23.351 **Other meniscus derangements, posterior horn of lateral meniscus,** right **knee**

M23.352 **Other meniscus derangements, posterior horn of lateral meniscus,** left **knee**

M23.359 **Other meniscus derangements, posterior horn of lateral meniscus, unspecified knee**

√6ᵗʰ M23.36 **Other meniscus derangements,** other lateral **meniscus**

M23.361 **Other meniscus derangements, other lateral meniscus,** right **knee**

M23.362 **Other meniscus derangements, other lateral meniscus,** left **knee**

M23.369 **Other meniscus derangements, other lateral meniscus, unspecified knee**

✓5ᵗʰ M23.4 Loose body in knee

    M23.40 Loose body in knee, unspecified knee
    M23.41 Loose body in knee, right knee
    M23.42 Loose body in knee, left knee

✓5ᵗʰ M23.5 Chronic instability of knee

    M23.50 Chronic instability of knee, unspecified knee
    M23.51 Chronic instability of knee, right knee
    M23.52 Chronic instability of knee, left knee

✓5ᵗʰ M23.6 Other spontaneous disruption of ligament(s) of knee

  ✓6ᵗʰ M23.60 Other spontaneous disruption of unspecified ligament of knee
    M23.601 Other spontaneous disruption of unspecified ligament of right knee
    M23.602 Other spontaneous disruption of unspecified ligament of left knee
    M23.609 Other spontaneous disruption of unspecified ligament of unspecified knee

  ✓6ᵗʰ M23.61 Other spontaneous disruption of anterior cruciate ligament of knee
    M23.611 Other spontaneous disruption of anterior cruciate ligament of right knee
    M23.612 Other spontaneous disruption of anterior cruciate ligament of left knee
    M23.619 Other spontaneous disruption of anterior cruciate ligament of unspecified knee

  ✓6ᵗʰ M23.62 Other spontaneous disruption of posterior cruciate ligament of knee
    M23.621 Other spontaneous disruption of posterior cruciate ligament of right knee
    M23.622 Other spontaneous disruption of posterior cruciate ligament of left knee
    M23.629 Other spontaneous disruption of posterior cruciate ligament of unspecified knee

  ✓6ᵗʰ M23.63 Other spontaneous disruption of medial collateral ligament of knee
    M23.631 Other spontaneous disruption of medial collateral ligament of right knee
    M23.632 Other spontaneous disruption of medial collateral ligament of left knee
    M23.639 Other spontaneous disruption of medial collateral ligament of unspecified knee

  ✓6ᵗʰ M23.64 Other spontaneous disruption of lateral collateral ligament of knee
    M23.641 Other spontaneous disruption of lateral collateral ligament of right knee
    M23.642 Other spontaneous disruption of lateral collateral ligament of left knee
    M23.649 Other spontaneous disruption of lateral collateral ligament of unspecified knee

  ✓6ᵗʰ M23.67 Other spontaneous disruption of capsular ligament of knee
    M23.671 Other spontaneous disruption of capsular ligament of right knee
    M23.672 Other spontaneous disruption of capsular ligament of left knee
    M23.679 Other spontaneous disruption of capsular ligament of unspecified knee

✓5ᵗʰ M23.8 Other internal derangements of knee

    Laxity of ligament of knee
    Snapping knee

  ✓6ᵗʰ M23.8X Other internal derangements of knee
    M23.8X1 Other internal derangements of right knee
    M23.8X2 Other internal derangements of left knee
    M23.8X9 Other internal derangements of unspecified knee

✓5ᵗʰ M23.9 Unspecified internal derangement of knee

    M23.90 Unspecified internal derangement of unspecified knee
    M23.91 Unspecified internal derangement of right knee
    M23.92 Unspecified internal derangement of left knee

✓4ᵗʰ M24 Other specific joint derangements

    EXCLUDES 1 current injury — see injury of joint by body region
    EXCLUDES 2 ganglion (M67.4)
        snapping knee (M23.8-)
        temporomandibular joint disorders (M26.6-)

✓5ᵗʰ M24.0 Loose body in joint

    EXCLUDES 2 loose body in knee (M23.4)

    M24.00 Loose body in unspecified joint

  ✓6ᵗʰ M24.01 Loose body in shoulder
    M24.011 Loose body in right shoulder
    M24.012 Loose body in left shoulder
    M24.019 Loose body in unspecified shoulder

  ✓6ᵗʰ M24.02 Loose body in elbow
    M24.021 Loose body in right elbow
    M24.022 Loose body in left elbow
    M24.029 Loose body in unspecified elbow

  ✓6ᵗʰ M24.03 Loose body in wrist
    M24.031 Loose body in right wrist
    M24.032 Loose body in left wrist
    M24.039 Loose body in unspecified wrist

  ✓6ᵗʰ M24.04 Loose body in finger joints
    M24.041 Loose body in right finger joint(s)
    M24.042 Loose body in left finger joint(s)
    M24.049 Loose body in unspecified finger joint(s)

  ✓6ᵗʰ M24.05 Loose body in hip
    M24.051 Loose body in right hip
    M24.052 Loose body in left hip
    M24.059 Loose body in unspecified hip

  ✓6ᵗʰ M24.07 Loose body in ankle and toe joints
    M24.071 Loose body in right ankle
    M24.072 Loose body in left ankle
    M24.073 Loose body in unspecified ankle
    M24.074 Loose body in right toe joint(s)
    M24.075 Loose body in left toe joint(s)
    M24.076 Loose body in unspecified toe joints

    M24.08 Loose body, other site

✓5ᵗʰ M24.1 Other articular cartilage disorders

    EXCLUDES 2 chondrocalcinosis (M11.1, M11.2-)
        internal derangement of knee (M23.-)
        metastatic calcification (E83.5)
        ochronosis (E70.2)

    M24.10 Other articular cartilage disorders, unspecified site

  ✓6ᵗʰ M24.11 Other articular cartilage disorders, shoulder
    M24.111 Other articular cartilage disorders, right shoulder
    M24.112 Other articular cartilage disorders, left shoulder
    M24.119 Other articular cartilage disorders, unspecified shoulder

  ✓6ᵗʰ M24.12 Other articular cartilage disorders, elbow
    M24.121 Other articular cartilage disorders, right elbow
    M24.122 Other articular cartilage disorders, left elbow
    M24.129 Other articular cartilage disorders, unspecified elbow

  ✓6ᵗʰ M24.13 Other articular cartilage disorders, wrist
    M24.131 Other articular cartilage disorders, right wrist
    M24.132 Other articular cartilage disorders, left wrist
    M24.139 Other articular cartilage disorders, unspecified wrist

  ✓6ᵗʰ M24.14 Other articular cartilage disorders, hand
    M24.141 Other articular cartilage disorders, right hand
    M24.142 Other articular cartilage disorders, left hand
    M24.149 Other articular cartilage disorders, unspecified hand

  ✓6ᵗʰ M24.15 Other articular cartilage disorders, hip
    M24.151 Other articular cartilage disorders, right hip
    M24.152 Other articular cartilage disorders, left hip
    M24.159 Other articular cartilage disorders, unspecified hip

---

✅ Additional Character Required   ✓x7ᵗʰ Placeholder Alert   **Manifestation**   Unspecified Dx   ►◄ Revised Text   ● New Code   ▲ Revised Code Title

✓6ᵗʰ **M24.17** **Other articular cartilage disorders,** ankle and foot

M24.171 **Other articular cartilage disorders,** right ankle

M24.172 **Other articular cartilage disorders,** left ankle

M24.173 **Other articular cartilage disorders, unspecified ankle**

M24.174 **Other articular cartilage disorders,** right foot

M24.175 **Other articular cartilage disorders,** left foot

M24.176 **Other articular cartilage disorders, unspecified foot**

✓5ᵗʰ **M24.2** **Disorder of ligament**

Instability secondary to old ligament injury

Ligamentous laxity NOS

EXCLUDES 1   *familial ligamentous laxity (M35.7)*

EXCLUDES 2   *internal derangement of knee ▶(M23.5-M23.8X9)◀*

M24.20 **Disorder of ligament, unspecified site**

✓6ᵗʰ **M24.21** **Disorder of ligament,** shoulder

M24.211 **Disorder of ligament,** right shoulder

M24.212 **Disorder of ligament,** left shoulder

M24.219 **Disorder of ligament, unspecified shoulder**

✓6ᵗʰ **M24.22** **Disorder of ligament,** elbow

M24.221 **Disorder of ligament,** right elbow

M24.222 **Disorder of ligament,** left elbow

M24.229 **Disorder of ligament, unspecified elbow**

✓6ᵗʰ **M24.23** **Disorder of ligament,** wrist

M24.231 **Disorder of ligament,** right wrist

M24.232 **Disorder of ligament,** left wrist

M24.239 **Disorder of ligament, unspecified wrist**

✓6ᵗʰ **M24.24** **Disorder of ligament,** hand

M24.241 **Disorder of ligament,** right hand

M24.242 **Disorder of ligament,** left hand

M24.249 **Disorder of ligament, unspecified hand**

✓6ᵗʰ **M24.25** **Disorder of ligament,** hip

M24.251 **Disorder of ligament,** right hip

M24.252 **Disorder of ligament,** left hip

M24.259 **Disorder of ligament, unspecified hip**

✓6ᵗʰ **M24.27** **Disorder of ligament,** ankle and foot

M24.271 **Disorder of ligament,** right ankle

M24.272 **Disorder of ligament,** left ankle

M24.273 **Disorder of ligament, unspecified ankle**

M24.274 **Disorder of ligament,** right foot

M24.275 **Disorder of ligament,** left foot

M24.276 **Disorder of ligament, unspecified foot**

M24.28 **Disorder of ligament,** vertebrae

✓5ᵗʰ **M24.3** **Pathological dislocation of joint, not elsewhere classified**

EXCLUDES 1   *congenital dislocation or displacement of joint — see congenital malformations and deformations of the musculoskeletal system (Q65-Q79)*

current injury — see injury of joints and ligaments by body region

recurrent dislocation of joint (M24.4-)

M24.30 **Pathological dislocation of unspecified joint, not elsewhere classified**

✓6ᵗʰ **M24.31** **Pathological dislocation of** shoulder, not elsewhere classified

M24.311 **Pathological dislocation of** right shoulder, not elsewhere classified

M24.312 **Pathological dislocation of** left shoulder, not elsewhere classified

M24.319 **Pathological dislocation of unspecified shoulder, not elsewhere classified**

✓6ᵗʰ **M24.32** **Pathological dislocation of** elbow, not elsewhere classified

M24.321 **Pathological dislocation of** right elbow, not elsewhere classified

M24.322 **Pathological dislocation of** left elbow, not elsewhere classified

M24.329 **Pathological dislocation of unspecified elbow, not elsewhere classified**

✓6ᵗʰ **M24.33** **Pathological dislocation of** wrist, not elsewhere classified

M24.331 **Pathological dislocation of** right wrist, not elsewhere classified

M24.332 **Pathological dislocation of** left wrist, not elsewhere classified

M24.339 **Pathological dislocation of unspecified wrist, not elsewhere classified**

✓6ᵗʰ **M24.34** **Pathological dislocation of** hand, not elsewhere classified

M24.341 **Pathological dislocation of** right hand, not elsewhere classified

M24.342 **Pathological dislocation of** left hand, not elsewhere classified

M24.349 **Pathological dislocation of unspecified hand, not elsewhere classified**

✓6ᵗʰ **M24.35** **Pathological dislocation of** hip, not elsewhere classified

M24.351 **Pathological dislocation of** right hip, not elsewhere classified

M24.352 **Pathological dislocation of** left hip, not elsewhere classified

M24.359 **Pathological dislocation of unspecified hip, not elsewhere classified**

✓6ᵗʰ **M24.36** **Pathological dislocation of** knee, not elsewhere classified

M24.361 **Pathological dislocation of** right knee, not elsewhere classified

M24.362 **Pathological dislocation of** left knee, not elsewhere classified

M24.369 **Pathological dislocation of unspecified knee, not elsewhere classified**

✓6ᵗʰ **M24.37** **Pathological dislocation of** ankle and foot, not elsewhere classified

M24.371 **Pathological dislocation of** right ankle, not elsewhere classified

M24.372 **Pathological dislocation of** left ankle, not elsewhere classified

M24.373 **Pathological dislocation of unspecified ankle, not elsewhere classified**

M24.374 **Pathological dislocation of** right foot, not elsewhere classified

M24.375 **Pathological dislocation of** left foot, not elsewhere classified

M24.376 **Pathological dislocation of unspecified foot, not elsewhere classified**

✓5ᵗʰ **M24.4** **Recurrent dislocation of joint**

Recurrent subluxation of joint

EXCLUDES 2   *recurrent dislocation of patella (M22.0-M22.1)*

recurrent vertebral dislocation (M43.3-, M43.4, M43.5-)

M24.40 **Recurrent dislocation, unspecified joint**

✓6ᵗʰ **M24.41** **Recurrent dislocation,** shoulder

M24.411 **Recurrent dislocation,** right shoulder

M24.412 **Recurrent dislocation,** left shoulder

M24.419 **Recurrent dislocation, unspecified shoulder**

✓6ᵗʰ **M24.42** **Recurrent dislocation,** elbow

M24.421 **Recurrent dislocation,** right elbow

M24.422 **Recurrent dislocation,** left elbow

M24.429 **Recurrent dislocation, unspecified elbow**

✓6ᵗʰ **M24.43** **Recurrent dislocation,** wrist

M24.431 **Recurrent dislocation,** right wrist

M24.432 **Recurrent dislocation,** left wrist

M24.439 **Recurrent dislocation, unspecified wrist**

✓6ᵗʰ **M24.44** **Recurrent dislocation,** hand and finger(s)

M24.441 **Recurrent dislocation,** right hand

M24.442 **Recurrent dislocation,** left hand

M24.443 **Recurrent dislocation, unspecified hand**

M24.444 **Recurrent dislocation,** right finger

M24.445 **Recurrent dislocation,** left finger

M24.446 **Recurrent dislocation, unspecified finger**

✓6ᵗʰ **M24.45** **Recurrent dislocation,** hip

M24.451 **Recurrent dislocation,** right hip

M24.452 **Recurrent dislocation,** left hip

M24.459 **Recurrent dislocation, unspecified hip**

✓6ᵗʰ **M24.46** **Recurrent dislocation,** knee

M24.461 **Recurrent dislocation,** right knee

M24.462 **Recurrent dislocation,** left knee

M24.469 **Recurrent dislocation, unspecified knee**

✓6ᵗʰ **M24.47** **Recurrent dislocation,** ankle, foot and toes

M24.471 **Recurrent dislocation,** right ankle

M24.472 **Recurrent dislocation,** left ankle

M24.473 **Recurrent dislocation, unspecified ankle**

M24.474 **Recurrent dislocation,** right foot

M24.475   **Recurrent dislocation**, left foot
M24.476   **Recurrent dislocation**, unspecified foot
M24.477   **Recurrent dislocation**, right toe(s)
M24.478   **Recurrent dislocation**, left toe(s)
M24.479   **Recurrent dislocation**, unspecified toe(s)

☑5ᵗʰ **M24.5   Contracture of joint**

> EXCLUDES 1   *contracture of muscle without contracture of joint (M62.4-)*
> *contracture of tendon (sheath) without contracture of joint (M62.4-)*
> *Dupuytren's contracture (M72.0)*
> EXCLUDES 2   *acquired deformities of limbs (M20-M21)*

AHA: 2016,2Q,6

M24.50   **Contracture, unspecified joint**
☑6ᵗʰ **M24.51   Contracture, shoulder**
M24.511   **Contracture**, right shoulder
M24.512   **Contracture**, left shoulder
M24.519   **Contracture**, unspecified shoulder
☑6ᵗʰ **M24.52   Contracture, elbow**
M24.521   **Contracture**, right elbow
M24.522   **Contracture**, left elbow
M24.529   **Contracture**, unspecified elbow
☑6ᵗʰ **M24.53   Contracture, wrist**
M24.531   **Contracture**, right wrist
M24.532   **Contracture**, left wrist
M24.539   **Contracture**, unspecified wrist
☑6ᵗʰ **M24.54   Contracture, hand**
M24.541   **Contracture**, right hand
M24.542   **Contracture**, left hand
M24.549   **Contracture**, unspecified hand
☑6ᵗʰ **M24.55   Contracture, hip**
M24.551   **Contracture**, right hip
M24.552   **Contracture**, left hip
M24.559   **Contracture**, unspecified hip
☑6ᵗʰ **M24.56   Contracture, knee**
M24.561   **Contracture**, right knee
M24.562   **Contracture**, left knee
M24.569   **Contracture**, unspecified knee
☑6ᵗʰ **M24.57   Contracture, ankle and foot**
M24.571   **Contracture**, right ankle
M24.572   **Contracture**, left ankle
M24.573   **Contracture**, unspecified ankle
M24.574   **Contracture**, right foot
M24.575   **Contracture**, left foot
M24.576   **Contracture**, unspecified foot

☑5ᵗʰ **M24.6   Ankylosis of joint**

> EXCLUDES 1   *stiffness of joint without ankylosis (M25.6-)*
> EXCLUDES 2   *spine (M43.2-)*

DEF: Ankylosis: Abnormal union or fusion of bones in a joint, which is normally moveable.

M24.60   **Ankylosis, unspecified joint**
☑6ᵗʰ **M24.61   Ankylosis, shoulder**
M24.611   **Ankylosis**, right shoulder
M24.612   **Ankylosis**, left shoulder
M24.619   **Ankylosis**, unspecified shoulder
☑6ᵗʰ **M24.62   Ankylosis, elbow**
M24.621   **Ankylosis**, right elbow
M24.622   **Ankylosis**, left elbow
M24.629   **Ankylosis**, unspecified elbow
☑6ᵗʰ **M24.63   Ankylosis, wrist**
M24.631   **Ankylosis**, right wrist
M24.632   **Ankylosis**, left wrist
M24.639   **Ankylosis**, unspecified wrist
☑6ᵗʰ **M24.64   Ankylosis, hand**
M24.641   **Ankylosis**, right hand
M24.642   **Ankylosis**, left hand
M24.649   **Ankylosis**, unspecified hand
☑6ᵗʰ **M24.65   Ankylosis, hip**
M24.651   **Ankylosis**, right hip
M24.652   **Ankylosis**, left hip
M24.659   **Ankylosis**, unspecified hip
☑6ᵗʰ **M24.66   Ankylosis, knee**
M24.661   **Ankylosis**, right knee
M24.662   **Ankylosis**, left knee
M24.669   **Ankylosis**, unspecified knee

☑6ᵗʰ **M24.67   Ankylosis, ankle and foot**
M24.671   **Ankylosis**, right ankle
M24.672   **Ankylosis**, left ankle
M24.673   **Ankylosis**, unspecified ankle
M24.674   **Ankylosis**, right foot
M24.675   **Ankylosis**, left foot
M24.676   **Ankylosis**, unspecified foot

M24.7   Protrusio acetabuli

> **DEF:** Intrapelvic protrusion of the acetabulum characterized by the sinking of the floor of the acetabulum, causing the femoral head to protrude. It limits hip movement and is of unknown etiology. *Synonym(s):* Otto's pelvis.

☑5ᵗʰ **M24.8   Other specific joint derangements, not elsewhere classified**

> EXCLUDES 2   *iliotibial band syndrome (M76.3)*

M24.80   **Other specific joint derangements of unspecified joint, not elsewhere classified**
☑6ᵗʰ **M24.81   Other specific joint derangements of shoulder, not elsewhere classified**
M24.811   **Other specific joint derangements of** right shoulder, not elsewhere classified
M24.812   **Other specific joint derangements of** left shoulder, not elsewhere classified
M24.819   **Other specific joint derangements of** unspecified shoulder, not elsewhere classified
☑6ᵗʰ **M24.82   Other specific joint derangements of elbow, not elsewhere classified**
M24.821   **Other specific joint derangements of** right elbow, not elsewhere classified
M24.822   **Other specific joint derangements of** left elbow, not elsewhere classified
M24.829   **Other specific joint derangements of** unspecified elbow, not elsewhere classified
☑6ᵗʰ **M24.83   Other specific joint derangements of wrist, not elsewhere classified**
M24.831   **Other specific joint derangements of** right wrist, not elsewhere classified
M24.832   **Other specific joint derangements of** left wrist, not elsewhere classified
M24.839   **Other specific joint derangements of** unspecified wrist, not elsewhere classified
☑6ᵗʰ **M24.84   Other specific joint derangements of hand, not elsewhere classified**
M24.841   **Other specific joint derangements of** right hand, not elsewhere classified
M24.842   **Other specific joint derangements of** left hand, not elsewhere classified
M24.849   **Other specific joint derangements of** unspecified hand, not elsewhere classified
☑6ᵗʰ **M24.85   Other specific joint derangements of hip, not elsewhere classified**
    Irritable hip
M24.851   **Other specific joint derangements of** right hip, not elsewhere classified
M24.852   **Other specific joint derangements of** left hip, not elsewhere classified
M24.859   **Other specific joint derangements of** unspecified hip, not elsewhere classified
☑6ᵗʰ **M24.87   Other specific joint derangements of ankle and foot, not elsewhere classified**
M24.871   **Other specific joint derangements of** right ankle, not elsewhere classified
M24.872   **Other specific joint derangements of** left ankle, not elsewhere classified
M24.873   **Other specific joint derangements of** unspecified ankle, not elsewhere classified
M24.874   **Other specific joint derangements of** right foot, not elsewhere classified
M24.875   **Other specific joint derangements of** left foot, not elsewhere classified
M24.876   **Other specific joint derangements of** unspecified foot, not elsewhere classified

M24.9   Joint derangement, unspecified

☑ Additional Character Required   ☑x7ᵗʰ Placeholder Alert   Manifestation   Unspecified Dx   ►◄ Revised Text   ● New Code   ▲ Revised Code Title

ICD-10-CM 2020   777

✓4th **M25** **Other joint disorder, not elsewhere classified**
　　　EXCLUDES 2　abnormality of gait and mobility (R26.-)
　　　　　　　acquired deformities of limb (M20-M21)
　　　　　　　calcification of bursa (M71.4-)
　　　　　　　calcification of shoulder (joint) (M75.3)
　　　　　　　calcification of tendon (M65.2-)
　　　　　　　difficulty in walking (R26.2)
　　　　　　　temporomandibular joint disorder (M26.6-)

✓5th **M25.0** **Hemarthrosis**
　　　EXCLUDES 1　current injury — see injury of joint by body region
　　　　　　　hemophilic arthropathy (M36.2)

　　　M25.00 Hemarthrosis, unspecified joint
✓6th **M25.01** Hemarthrosis, shoulder
　　　　M25.011 Hemarthrosis, right shoulder
　　　　M25.012 Hemarthrosis, left shoulder
　　　　M25.019 Hemarthrosis, unspecified shoulder
✓6th **M25.02** Hemarthrosis, elbow
　　　　M25.021 Hemarthrosis, right elbow
　　　　M25.022 Hemarthrosis, left elbow
　　　　M25.029 Hemarthrosis, unspecified elbow
✓6th **M25.03** Hemarthrosis, wrist
　　　　M25.031 Hemarthrosis, right wrist
　　　　M25.032 Hemarthrosis, left wrist
　　　　M25.039 Hemarthrosis, unspecified wrist
✓6th **M25.04** Hemarthrosis, hand
　　　　M25.041 Hemarthrosis, right hand
　　　　M25.042 Hemarthrosis, left hand
　　　　M25.049 Hemarthrosis, unspecified hand
✓6th **M25.05** Hemarthrosis, hip
　　　　M25.051 Hemarthrosis, right hip
　　　　M25.052 Hemarthrosis, left hip
　　　　M25.059 Hemarthrosis, unspecified hip
✓6th **M25.06** Hemarthrosis, knee
　　　　M25.061 Hemarthrosis, right knee
　　　　M25.062 Hemarthrosis, left knee
　　　　M25.069 Hemarthrosis, unspecified knee
✓6th **M25.07** Hemarthrosis, ankle and foot
　　　　M25.071 Hemarthrosis, right ankle
　　　　M25.072 Hemarthrosis, left ankle
　　　　M25.073 Hemarthrosis, unspecified ankle
　　　　M25.074 Hemarthrosis, right foot
　　　　M25.075 Hemarthrosis, left foot
　　　　M25.076 Hemarthrosis, unspecified foot
　　　M25.08 Hemarthrosis, other specified site
　　　　Hemarthrosis, vertebrae

✓5th **M25.1** **Fistula of joint**
　　　M25.10 Fistula, unspecified joint
✓6th **M25.11** Fistula, shoulder
　　　　M25.111 Fistula, right shoulder
　　　　M25.112 Fistula, left shoulder
　　　　M25.119 Fistula, unspecified shoulder
✓6th **M25.12** Fistula, elbow
　　　　M25.121 Fistula, right elbow
　　　　M25.122 Fistula, left elbow
　　　　M25.129 Fistula, unspecified elbow
✓6th **M25.13** Fistula, wrist
　　　　M25.131 Fistula, right wrist
　　　　M25.132 Fistula, left wrist
　　　　M25.139 Fistula, unspecified wrist
✓6th **M25.14** Fistula, hand
　　　　M25.141 Fistula, right hand
　　　　M25.142 Fistula, left hand
　　　　M25.149 Fistula, unspecified hand
✓6th **M25.15** Fistula, hip
　　　　M25.151 Fistula, right hip
　　　　M25.152 Fistula, left hip
　　　　M25.159 Fistula, unspecified hip
✓6th **M25.16** Fistula, knee
　　　　M25.161 Fistula, right knee
　　　　M25.162 Fistula, left knee
　　　　M25.169 Fistula, unspecified knee
✓6th **M25.17** Fistula, ankle and foot
　　　　M25.171 Fistula, right ankle
　　　　M25.172 Fistula, left ankle

　　　　M25.173 Fistula, unspecified ankle
　　　　M25.174 Fistula, right foot
　　　　M25.175 Fistula, left foot
　　　　M25.176 Fistula, unspecified foot
　　　M25.18 Fistula, other specified site
　　　　Fistula, vertebrae

✓5th **M25.2** **Flail joint**
　　　DEF: Hinged joint that exhibits an abnormal or excessive degree of range and mobility.
　　　M25.20 Flail joint, unspecified joint
✓6th **M25.21** Flail joint, shoulder
　　　　M25.211 Flail joint, right shoulder
　　　　M25.212 Flail joint, left shoulder
　　　　M25.219 Flail joint, unspecified shoulder
✓6th **M25.22** Flail joint, elbow
　　　　M25.221 Flail joint, right elbow
　　　　M25.222 Flail joint, left elbow
　　　　M25.229 Flail joint, unspecified elbow
✓6th **M25.23** Flail joint, wrist
　　　　M25.231 Flail joint, right wrist
　　　　M25.232 Flail joint, left wrist
　　　　M25.239 Flail joint, unspecified wrist
✓6th **M25.24** Flail joint, hand
　　　　M25.241 Flail joint, right hand
　　　　M25.242 Flail joint, left hand
　　　　M25.249 Flail joint, unspecified hand
✓6th **M25.25** Flail joint, hip
　　　　M25.251 Flail joint, right hip
　　　　M25.252 Flail joint, left hip
　　　　M25.259 Flail joint, unspecified hip
✓6th **M25.26** Flail joint, knee
　　　　M25.261 Flail joint, right knee
　　　　M25.262 Flail joint, left knee
　　　　M25.269 Flail joint, unspecified knee
✓6th **M25.27** Flail joint, ankle and foot
　　　　M25.271 Flail joint, right ankle and foot
　　　　M25.272 Flail joint, left ankle and foot
　　　　M25.279 Flail joint, unspecified ankle and foot
　　　M25.28 Flail joint, other site

✓5th **M25.3** **Other instability of joint**
　　　EXCLUDES 1　instability of joint secondary to old ligament injury (M24.2-)
　　　　　　　instability of joint secondary to removal of joint prosthesis (M96.8-)
　　　EXCLUDES 2　spinal instabilities (M53.2-)
　　　M25.30 Other instability, unspecified joint
✓6th **M25.31** Other instability, shoulder
　　　　M25.311 Other instability, right shoulder
　　　　M25.312 Other instability, left shoulder
　　　　M25.319 Other instability, unspecified shoulder
✓6th **M25.32** Other instability, elbow
　　　　M25.321 Other instability, right elbow
　　　　M25.322 Other instability, left elbow
　　　　M25.329 Other instability, unspecified elbow
✓6th **M25.33** Other instability, wrist
　　　　M25.331 Other instability, right wrist
　　　　M25.332 Other instability, left wrist
　　　　M25.339 Other instability, unspecified wrist
✓6th **M25.34** Other instability, hand
　　　　M25.341 Other instability, right hand
　　　　M25.342 Other instability, left hand
　　　　M25.349 Other instability, unspecified hand
✓6th **M25.35** Other instability, hip
　　　　M25.351 Other instability, right hip
　　　　M25.352 Other instability, left hip
　　　　M25.359 Other instability, unspecified hip
✓6th **M25.36** Other instability, knee
　　　　M25.361 Other instability, right knee
　　　　M25.362 Other instability, left knee
　　　　M25.369 Other instability, unspecified knee
✓6th **M25.37** Other instability, ankle and foot
　　　　M25.371 Other instability, right ankle
　　　　M25.372 Other instability, left ankle
　　　　M25.373 Other instability, unspecified ankle
　　　　M25.374 Other instability, right foot

M25.375   Other instability, left foot
M25.376   Other instability, unspecified foot

✓5th **M25.4   Effusion of joint**

EXCLUDES 1   hydrarthrosis in yaws (A66.6)
intermittent hydrarthrosis (M12.4-)
other infective (teno)synovitis (M65.1-)

M25.40   Effusion, unspecified joint

✓6th **M25.41**   Effusion, shoulder

M25.411   Effusion, right shoulder
M25.412   Effusion, left shoulder
M25.419   Effusion, unspecified shoulder

✓6th **M25.42**   Effusion, elbow

M25.421   Effusion, right elbow
M25.422   Effusion, left elbow
M25.429   Effusion, unspecified elbow

✓6th **M25.43**   Effusion, wrist

M25.431   Effusion, right wrist
M25.432   Effusion, left wrist
M25.439   Effusion, unspecified wrist

✓6th **M25.44**   Effusion, hand

M25.441   Effusion, right hand
M25.442   Effusion, left hand
M25.449   Effusion, unspecified hand

✓6th **M25.45**   Effusion, hip

M25.451   Effusion, right hip
M25.452   Effusion, left hip
M25.459   Effusion, unspecified hip

✓6th **M25.46**   Effusion, knee

M25.461   Effusion, right knee
M25.462   Effusion, left knee
M25.469   Effusion, unspecified knee

✓6th **M25.47**   Effusion, ankle and foot

M25.471   Effusion, right ankle
M25.472   Effusion, left ankle
M25.473   Effusion, unspecified ankle
M25.474   Effusion, right foot
M25.475   Effusion, left foot
M25.476   Effusion, unspecified foot

M25.48   Effusion, other site

✓5th **M25.5   Pain in joint**

EXCLUDES 2   pain in hand (M79.64-)
pain in fingers (M79.64-)
pain in foot (M79.67-)
pain in limb (M79.6-)
pain in toes (M79.67-)

M25.50   Pain in unspecified joint

✓6th **M25.51**   Pain in shoulder

M25.511   Pain in right shoulder
M25.512   Pain in left shoulder
M25.519   Pain in unspecified shoulder

✓6th **M25.52**   Pain in elbow

M25.521   Pain in right elbow
M25.522   Pain in left elbow
M25.529   Pain in unspecified elbow

✓6th **M25.53**   Pain in wrist

M25.531   Pain in right wrist
M25.532   Pain in left wrist
M25.539   Pain in unspecified wrist

✓6th **M25.54**   Pain in joints of hand

AHA: 2016,4Q,38

M25.541   Pain in joints of right hand
M25.542   Pain in joints of left hand
M25.549   Pain in joints of unspecified hand
     Pain in joints of hand NOS

✓6th **M25.55**   Pain in hip

M25.551   Pain in right hip
M25.552   Pain in left hip
M25.559   Pain in unspecified hip

✓6th **M25.56**   Pain in knee

M25.561   Pain in right knee
M25.562   Pain in left knee
M25.569   Pain in unspecified knee

✓6th **M25.57**   Pain in ankle and joints of foot

M25.571   Pain in right ankle and joints of right foot
M25.572   Pain in left ankle and joints of left foot

M25.579   Pain in unspecified ankle and joints of unspecified foot

✓5th **M25.6   Stiffness of joint, not elsewhere classified**

EXCLUDES 1   ankylosis of joint (M24.6-)
contracture of joint (M24.5-)

M25.60   Stiffness of unspecified joint, not elsewhere classified

✓6th **M25.61**   Stiffness of shoulder, not elsewhere classified

M25.611   Stiffness of right shoulder, not elsewhere classified
M25.612   Stiffness of left shoulder, not elsewhere classified
M25.619   Stiffness of unspecified shoulder, not elsewhere classified

✓6th **M25.62**   Stiffness of elbow, not elsewhere classified

M25.621   Stiffness of right elbow, not elsewhere classified
M25.622   Stiffness of left elbow, not elsewhere classified
M25.629   Stiffness of unspecified elbow, not elsewhere classified

✓6th **M25.63**   Stiffness of wrist, not elsewhere classified

M25.631   Stiffness of right wrist, not elsewhere classified
M25.632   Stiffness of left wrist, not elsewhere classified
M25.639   Stiffness of unspecified wrist, not elsewhere classified

✓6th **M25.64**   Stiffness of hand, not elsewhere classified

M25.641   Stiffness of right hand, not elsewhere classified
M25.642   Stiffness of left hand, not elsewhere classified
M25.649   Stiffness of unspecified hand, not elsewhere classified

✓6th **M25.65**   Stiffness of hip, not elsewhere classified

M25.651   Stiffness of right hip, not elsewhere classified
M25.652   Stiffness of left hip, not elsewhere classified
M25.659   Stiffness of unspecified hip, not elsewhere classified

✓6th **M25.66**   Stiffness of knee, not elsewhere classified

M25.661   Stiffness of right knee, not elsewhere classified
M25.662   Stiffness of left knee, not elsewhere classified
M25.669   Stiffness of unspecified knee, not elsewhere classified

✓6th **M25.67**   Stiffness of ankle and foot, not elsewhere classified

M25.671   Stiffness of right ankle, not elsewhere classified
M25.672   Stiffness of left ankle, not elsewhere classified
M25.673   Stiffness of unspecified ankle, not elsewhere classified
M25.674   Stiffness of right foot, not elsewhere classified
M25.675   Stiffness of left foot, not elsewhere classified
M25.676   Stiffness of unspecified foot, not elsewhere classified

✓5th **M25.7   Osteophyte**

M25.70   Osteophyte, unspecified joint

✓6th **M25.71**   Osteophyte, shoulder

M25.711   Osteophyte, right shoulder
M25.712   Osteophyte, left shoulder
M25.719   Osteophyte, unspecified shoulder

✓6th **M25.72**   Osteophyte, elbow

M25.721   Osteophyte, right elbow
M25.722   Osteophyte, left elbow
M25.729   Osteophyte, unspecified elbow

✓6th **M25.73**   Osteophyte, wrist

M25.731   Osteophyte, right wrist
M25.732   Osteophyte, left wrist
M25.739   Osteophyte, unspecified wrist

✓6th **M25.74**   Osteophyte, hand

M25.741   Osteophyte, right hand
M25.742   Osteophyte, left hand

✓ Additional Character Required   ✓x7th Placeholder Alert   Manifestation   Unspecified Dx   ▶◀ Revised Text   ● New Code   ▲ Revised Code Title

Chapter 13. Diseases of the Musculoskeletal System and Connective Tissue

M25.749   Osteophyte, unspecified hand

✓6th M25.75   Osteophyte, hip

    M25.751   Osteophyte, right hip
    M25.752   Osteophyte, left hip
    M25.759   Osteophyte, unspecified hip

✓6th M25.76   Osteophyte, knee

    M25.761   Osteophyte, right knee
    M25.762   Osteophyte, left knee
    M25.769   Osteophyte, unspecified knee

✓6th M25.77   Osteophyte, ankle and foot

    M25.771   Osteophyte, right ankle
    M25.772   Osteophyte, left ankle
    M25.773   Osteophyte, unspecified ankle
    M25.774   Osteophyte, right foot
    M25.775   Osteophyte, left foot
    M25.776   Osteophyte, unspecified foot

    M25.78   Osteophyte, vertebrae

✓5th M25.8   Other specified joint disorders

    M25.80   Other specified joint disorders, unspecified joint

✓6th M25.81   Other specified joint disorders, shoulder

    M25.811   Other specified joint disorders, right shoulder
    M25.812   Other specified joint disorders, left shoulder
    M25.819   Other specified joint disorders, unspecified shoulder

✓6th M25.82   Other specified joint disorders, elbow

    M25.821   Other specified joint disorders, right elbow
    M25.822   Other specified joint disorders, left elbow
    M25.829   Other specified joint disorders, unspecified elbow

✓6th M25.83   Other specified joint disorders, wrist

    M25.831   Other specified joint disorders, right wrist
    M25.832   Other specified joint disorders, left wrist
    M25.839   Other specified joint disorders, unspecified wrist

✓6th M25.84   Other specified joint disorders, hand

    M25.841   Other specified joint disorders, right hand
    M25.842   Other specified joint disorders, left hand
    M25.849   Other specified joint disorders, unspecified hand

✓6th M25.85   Other specified joint disorders, hip

    AHA: 2014,4Q,25
    M25.851   Other specified joint disorders, right hip
    M25.852   Other specified joint disorders, left hip
    M25.859   Other specified joint disorders, unspecified hip

✓6th M25.86   Other specified joint disorders, knee

    M25.861   Other specified joint disorders, right knee
    M25.862   Other specified joint disorders, left knee
    M25.869   Other specified joint disorders, unspecified knee

✓6th M25.87   Other specified joint disorders, ankle and foot

    M25.871   Other specified joint disorders, right ankle and foot
    M25.872   Other specified joint disorders, left ankle and foot
    M25.879   Other specified joint disorders, unspecified ankle and foot

    M25.9   Joint disorder, unspecified

Dentofacial anomalies [including malocclusion] and other disorders of jaw (M26-M27)

EXCLUDES 1   hemifacial atrophy or hypertrophy (Q67.4)
       unilateral condylar hyperplasia or hypoplasia (M27.8)

✓4th **M26**   Dentofacial anomalies [including malocclusion]

✓5th M26.0   Major anomalies of jaw size

    EXCLUDES 1   acromegaly (E22.0)
           Robin's syndrome (Q87.0)

    M26.00   Unspecified anomaly of jaw size
    M26.01   Maxillary hyperplasia
    M26.02   Maxillary hypoplasia
       AHA: 2014,3Q,23
    M26.03   Mandibular hyperplasia
    M26.04   Mandibular hypoplasia

M26.05   Macrogenia
M26.06   Microgenia
M26.07   Excessive tuberosity of jaw
    Entire maxillary tuberosity
M26.09   Other specified anomalies of jaw size

✓5th M26.1   Anomalies of jaw-cranial base relationship

    M26.10   Unspecified anomaly of jaw-cranial base relationship
    M26.11   Maxillary asymmetry
    M26.12   Other jaw asymmetry
    M26.19   Other specified anomalies of jaw-cranial base relationship

✓5th M26.2   Anomalies of dental arch relationship

    M26.20   Unspecified anomaly of dental arch relationship

✓6th M26.21   Malocclusion, Angle's class

    M26.211   Malocclusion, Angle's class I
       Neutro-occlusion
    M26.212   Malocclusion, Angle's class II
       Disto-occlusion Division I
       Disto-occlusion Division II
    M26.213   Malocclusion, Angle's class III
       Mesio-occlusion
    M26.219   Malocclusion, Angle's class, unspecified

✓6th M26.22   Open occlusal relationship

    M26.220   Open anterior occlusal relationship
       Anterior open bite
    M26.221   Open posterior occlusal relationship
       Posterior open bite

    M26.23   Excessive horizontal overlap
       Excessive horizontal overjet
    M26.24   Reverse articulation
       Crossbite (anterior) (posterior)
    M26.25   Anomalies of interarch distance
    M26.29   Other anomalies of dental arch relationship
       Midline deviation of dental arch
       Overbite (excessive) deep
       Overbite (excessive) horizontal
       Overbite (excessive) vertical
       Posterior lingual occlusion of mandibular teeth

✓5th M26.3   Anomalies of tooth position of fully erupted tooth or teeth

    EXCLUDES 2   embedded and impacted teeth (K01.-)

    M26.30   Unspecified anomaly of tooth position of fully erupted tooth or teeth
       Abnormal spacing of fully erupted tooth or teeth NOS
       Displacement of fully erupted tooth or teeth NOS
       Transposition of fully erupted tooth or teeth NOS
    M26.31   Crowding of fully erupted teeth
    M26.32   Excessive spacing of fully erupted teeth
       Diastema of fully erupted tooth or teeth NOS
    M26.33   Horizontal displacement of fully erupted tooth or teeth
       Tipped tooth or teeth
       Tipping of fully erupted tooth
    M26.34   Vertical displacement of fully erupted tooth or teeth
       Extruded tooth
       Infraeruption of tooth or teeth
       Supraeruption of tooth or teeth
    M26.35   Rotation of fully erupted tooth or teeth
    M26.36   Insufficient interocclusal distance of fully erupted teeth (ridge)
       Lack of adequate intermaxillary vertical dimension of fully erupted teeth
    M26.37   Excessive interocclusal distance of fully erupted teeth
       Excessive intermaxillary vertical dimension of fully erupted teeth
       Loss of occlusal vertical dimension of fully erupted teeth
    M26.39   Other anomalies of tooth position of fully erupted tooth or teeth

    M26.4   Malocclusion, unspecified

✓5th M26.5   Dentofacial functional abnormalities

    EXCLUDES 1   bruxism (F45.8)
           teeth-grinding NOS (F45.8)

    M26.50   Dentofacial functional abnormalities, unspecified
    M26.51   Abnormal jaw closure

M26.52 **Limited mandibular range of motion**

M26.53 **Deviation in opening and closing of the mandible**

M26.54 **Insufficient anterior guidance**
Insufficient anterior occlusal guidance

M26.55 **Centric occlusion maximum intercuspation discrepancy**
EXCLUDES 1 *centric occlusion NOS (M26.59)*

M26.56 **Non-working side interference**
Balancing side interference

M26.57 **Lack of posterior occlusal support**

M26.59 **Other dentofacial functional abnormalities**
Centric occlusion (of teeth) NOS
Malocclusion due to abnormal swallowing
Malocclusion due to mouth breathing
Malocclusion due to tongue, lip or finger habits

✓5th **M26.6** **Temporomandibular joint disorders**
EXCLUDES 2 *current temporomandibular joint dislocation (S03.0)*
current temporomandibular joint sprain (S03.4)
AHA: 2016,4Q,38-39

Temporomandibular Joint

Cutaway view of temporomandibular joint (TMJ)

✓6th **M26.60** **Temporomandibular joint disorder, unspecified**

M26.601 **Right** temporomandibular joint disorder, unspecified

M26.602 **Left** temporomandibular joint disorder, unspecified

M26.603 **Bilateral** temporomandibular joint disorder, unspecified

M26.609 **Unspecified** temporomandibular joint disorder, unspecified side
Temporomandibular joint disorder NOS

✓6th **M26.61** **Adhesions and ankylosis of temporomandibular joint**

M26.611 **Adhesions and ankylosis of right** temporomandibular joint

M26.612 **Adhesions and ankylosis of left** temporomandibular joint

M26.613 **Adhesions and ankylosis of bilateral** temporomandibular joint

M26.619 **Adhesions and ankylosis of** temporomandibular joint, unspecified side

✓6th **M26.62** **Arthralgia of temporomandibular joint**

M26.621 **Arthralgia of right** temporomandibular joint

M26.622 **Arthralgia of left** temporomandibular joint

M26.623 **Arthralgia of bilateral** temporomandibular joint

M26.629 **Arthralgia of** temporomandibular joint, unspecified side

✓6th **M26.63** **Articular disc disorder of temporomandibular joint**

M26.631 **Articular disc disorder of right** temporomandibular joint

M26.632 **Articular disc disorder of left** temporomandibular joint

M26.633 **Articular disc disorder of bilateral** temporomandibular joint

M26.639 **Articular disc disorder of** temporomandibular joint, unspecified side

M26.69 **Other specified disorders of temporomandibular joint**

✓5th **M26.7** **Dental alveolar anomalies**

M26.70 **Unspecified alveolar anomaly**

M26.71 **Alveolar maxillary hyperplasia**

M26.72 **Alveolar mandibular hyperplasia**

M26.73 **Alveolar maxillary hypoplasia**

M26.74 **Alveolar mandibular hypoplasia**

M26.79 **Other specified alveolar anomalies**

✓5th **M26.8** **Other dentofacial anomalies**

M26.81 **Anterior soft tissue impingement**
Anterior soft tissue impingement on teeth

M26.82 **Posterior soft tissue impingement**
Posterior soft tissue impingement on teeth

M26.89 **Other dentofacial anomalies**

M26.9 **Dentofacial anomaly, unspecified**

✓4th **M27** **Other diseases of jaws**

M27.0 **Developmental disorders of jaws**
Latent bone cyst of jaw
Stafne's cyst
Torus mandibularis
Torus palatinus

M27.1 **Giant cell granuloma, central**
Giant cell granuloma NOS
EXCLUDES 1 *peripheral giant cell granuloma (K06.8)*

M27.2 **Inflammatory conditions of jaws**
Osteitis of jaw(s)
Osteomyelitis (neonatal) jaw(s)
Osteoradionecrosis jaw(s)
Periostitis jaw(s)
Sequestrum of jaw bone
Use additional code (W88-W90, X39.0) to identify radiation, if radiation-induced
EXCLUDES 2 *osteonecrosis of jaw due to drug (M87.180)*

M27.3 **Alveolitis of jaws**
Alveolar osteitis
Dry socket

✓5th **M27.4** **Other and unspecified cysts of jaw**
EXCLUDES 1 *cysts of oral region (K09.-)*
latent bone cyst of jaw (M27.0)
Stafne's cyst (M27.0)

M27.40 **Unspecified cyst of jaw**
Cyst of jaw NOS

M27.49 **Other cysts of jaw**
Aneurysmal cyst of jaw
Hemorrhagic cyst of jaw
Traumatic cyst of jaw

✓5th **M27.5** **Periradicular pathology associated with previous endodontic treatment**

M27.51 **Perforation of root canal space due to endodontic treatment**

M27.52 **Endodontic overfill**

M27.53 **Endodontic underfill**

M27.59 **Other periradicular pathology associated with previous endodontic treatment**

✓5th **M27.6** **Endosseous dental implant failure**

M27.61 **Osseointegration failure of dental implant**
Hemorrhagic complications of dental implant placement
Iatrogenic osseointegration failure of dental implant
Osseointegration failure of dental implant due to complications of systemic disease
Osseointegration failure of dental implant due to poor bone quality
Pre-integration failure of dental implant NOS
Pre-osseointegration failure of dental implant

M27.62 **Post-osseointegration biological failure of dental implant**
Failure of dental implant due to lack of attached gingiva
Failure of dental implant due to occlusal trauma (caused by poor prosthetic design)
Failure of dental implant due to parafunctional habits
Failure of dental implant due to periodontal infection (peri-implantitis)
Failure of dental implant due to poor oral hygiene
Iatrogenic post-osseointegration failure of dental implant
Post-osseointegration failure of dental implant due to complications of systemic disease

M27.63 **Post-osseointegration mechanical failure of dental implant**
Failure of dental prosthesis causing loss of dental implant
Fracture of dental implant
> EXCLUDES 2   *cracked tooth (KØ3.81)*
> *fractured dental restorative material with loss of material (KØ8.531)*
> *fractured dental restorative material without loss of material (KØ8.530)*
> *fractured tooth (SØ2.5)*

M27.69 **Other endosseous dental implant failure**
Dental implant failure NOS

M27.8 **Other specified diseases of jaws**
Cherubism
Exostosis
Fibrous dysplasia
Unilateral condylar hyperplasia
Unilateral condylar hypoplasia
> EXCLUDES 1   *jaw pain (R68.84)*

M27.9 **Disease of jaws, unspecified**

Systemic connective tissue disorders (M3Ø-M36)

INCLUDES   autoimmune disease NOS
collagen (vascular) disease NOS
systemic autoimmune disease
systemic collagen (vascular) disease
> EXCLUDES 1   *autoimmune disease, single organ or single cell-type-code to relevant condition category*

✓4ᵗʰ **M3Ø** **Polyarteritis nodosa and related conditions**
> EXCLUDES 1   *microscopic polyarteritis (M31.7)*

M3Ø.Ø **Polyarteritis nodosa**   HCC

M3Ø.1 **Polyarteritis with lung involvement [Churg-Strauss]**   HCC
Allergic granulomatous angiitis

M3Ø.2 **Juvenile polyarteritis**   HCC

M3Ø.3 **Mucocutaneous lymph node syndrome [Kawasaki]**   HCC

M3Ø.8 **Other conditions related to polyarteritis nodosa**   HCC
Polyangiitis overlap syndrome

✓4ᵗʰ **M31** **Other necrotizing vasculopathies**

M31.Ø **Hypersensitivity angiitis**   HCC
Goodpasture's syndrome

M31.1 **Thrombotic microangiopathy**   HCC
Thrombotic thrombocytopenic purpura

M31.2 **Lethal midline granuloma**   HCC

✓5ᵗʰ **M31.3** **Wegener's granulomatosis**
Necrotizing respiratory granulomatosis

M31.3Ø **Wegener's granulomatosis without renal involvement**   HCC
Wegener's granulomatosis NOS

M31.31 **Wegener's granulomatosis with renal involvement**   HCC

M31.4 **Aortic arch syndrome [Takayasu]**   HCC

M31.5 **Giant cell arteritis with polymyalgia rheumatica**   HCC

M31.6 **Other giant cell arteritis**   HCC

M31.7 **Microscopic polyangiitis**   HCC
Microscopic polyarteritis
> EXCLUDES 1   *polyarteritis nodosa (M3Ø.Ø)*

M31.8 **Other specified necrotizing vasculopathies**   HCC
Hypocomplementemic vasculitis
Septic vasculitis

M31.9 **Necrotizing vasculopathy, unspecified**   HCC

✓4ᵗʰ **M32** **Systemic lupus erythematosus (SLE)**
> EXCLUDES 1   *lupus erythematosus (discoid) (NOS) (L93.Ø)*

AHA: 2018,3Q,14
TIP: There is no default code for "lupus NOS." Query the provider for the specific type of lupus in order to assign the appropriate code.

M32.Ø **Drug-induced systemic lupus erythematosus**   HCC
Use additional code for adverse effect, if applicable, to identify drug (T36-T5Ø with fifth or sixth character 5)

✓6ᵗʰ **M32.1** **Systemic lupus erythematosus with organ or system involvement**

M32.1Ø **Systemic lupus erythematosus, organ or system involvement unspecified**   HCC

M32.11 **Endocarditis in systemic lupus erythematosus**   HCC
Libman-Sacks disease

M32.12 **Pericarditis in systemic lupus erythematosus**   HCC
Lupus pericarditis

M32.13 **Lung involvement in systemic lupus erythematosus**   HCC
Pleural effusion due to systemic lupus erythematosus

M32.14 **Glomerular disease in systemic lupus erythematosus**   HCC
Lupus renal disease NOS
AHA: 2013,4Q,125

M32.15 **Tubulo-interstitial nephropathy in systemic lupus erythematosus**   HCC

M32.19 **Other organ or system involvement in systemic lupus erythematosus**   HCC

M32.8 **Other forms of systemic lupus erythematosus**   HCC

M32.9 **Systemic lupus erythematosus, unspecified**   HCC
SLE NOS
Systemic lupus erythematosus NOS
Systemic lupus erythematosus without organ involvement

✓4ᵗʰ **M33** **Dermatopolymyositis**
AHA: 2017,4Q,18

✓5ᵗʰ **M33.Ø** **Juvenile dermatomyositis**

M33.ØØ **Juvenile dermatomyositis, organ involvement unspecified**   HCC

M33.Ø1 **Juvenile dermatomyositis with respiratory involvement**   HCC

M33.Ø2 **Juvenile dermatomyositis with myopathy**   HCC

M33.Ø3 **Juvenile dermatomyositis without myopathy**   HCC

M33.Ø9 **Juvenile dermatomyositis with other organ involvement**   HCC

✓5ᵗʰ **M33.1** **Other dermatomyositis**
Adult dermatomyositis

M33.1Ø **Other dermatomyositis, organ involvement unspecified**   HCC

M33.11 **Other dermatomyositis with respiratory involvement**   HCC

M33.12 **Other dermatomyositis with myopathy**   HCC

M33.13 **Other dermatomyositis without myopathy**   HCC
Dermatomyositis NOS

M33.19 **Other dermatomyositis with other organ involvement**   HCC

✓5ᵗʰ **M33.2** **Polymyositis**

M33.2Ø **Polymyositis, organ involvement unspecified**   HCC

M33.21 **Polymyositis with respiratory involvement**   HCC

M33.22 **Polymyositis with myopathy**   HCC

M33.29 **Polymyositis with other organ involvement**   HCC

✓5ᵗʰ **M33.9** **Dermatopolymyositis, unspecified**

M33.9Ø **Dermatopolymyositis, unspecified, organ involvement unspecified**   HCC

M33.91 **Dermatopolymyositis, unspecified with respiratory involvement**   HCC

M33.92 **Dermatopolymyositis, unspecified with myopathy**   HCC

M33.93 **Dermatopolymyositis, unspecified without myopathy**   HCC

M33.99 **Dermatopolymyositis, unspecified with other organ involvement**   HCC

✓4ᵗʰ **M34** **Systemic sclerosis [scleroderma]**
> EXCLUDES 1   *circumscribed scleroderma (L94.Ø)*
> *neonatal scleroderma ▶(P83.88)◀*

M34.Ø **Progressive systemic sclerosis**   HCC

M34.1 **CR(E)ST syndrome**   HCC
Combination of calcinosis, Raynaud's phenomenon, esophageal dysfunction, sclerodactyly, telangiectasia

M34.2 **Systemic sclerosis induced by drug and chemical**   HCC
Code first poisoning due to drug or toxin, if applicable (T36-T65 with fifth or sixth character 1-4 or 6)
Use additional code for adverse effect, if applicable, to identify drug (T36-T5Ø with fifth or sixth character 5)

✓5th **M34.8** **Other forms of systemic sclerosis**

M34.81 **Systemic sclerosis with lung involvement** HCC

M34.82 **Systemic sclerosis with myopathy** HCC

M34.83 **Systemic sclerosis with polyneuropathy** HCC

M34.89 **Other systemic sclerosis** HCC

M34.9 **Systemic sclerosis, unspecified** HCC

✓4th **M35** **Other systemic involvement of connective tissue**

EXCLUDES 1 *reactive perforating collagenosis (L87.1)*

✓5th **M35.0** **Sicca syndrome [Sjögren]**

DEF: Autoimmune disease associated with keratoconjunctivitis, laryngopharyngitis, rhinitis, dry mouth, enlarged parotid gland, and chronic polyarthritis.

M35.00 **Sicca syndrome, unspecified** HCC

M35.01 **Sicca syndrome with keratoconjunctivitis** HCC

M35.02 **Sicca syndrome with lung involvement** HCC

M35.03 **Sicca syndrome with myopathy** HCC

M35.04 **Sicca syndrome with tubulo-interstitial nephropathy** HCC

Renal tubular acidosis in sicca syndrome

M35.09 **Sicca syndrome with other organ involvement** HCC

M35.1 **Other overlap syndromes** HCC

Mixed connective tissue disease

EXCLUDES 1 *polyangiitis overlap syndrome (M30.8)*

M35.2 **Behçet's disease** HCC

M35.3 **Polymyalgia rheumatica** HCC

EXCLUDES 1 *polymyalgia rheumatica with giant cell arteritis (M31.5)*

M35.4 **Diffuse (eosinophilic) fasciitis**

M35.5 **Multifocal fibrosclerosis** HCC

M35.6 **Relapsing panniculitis [Weber-Christian]**

EXCLUDES 1 *lupus panniculitis (L93.2)*
panniculitis NOS (M79.3-)

M35.7 **Hypermobility syndrome**

Familial ligamentous laxity

EXCLUDES 1 *Ehlers-Danlos syndrome ▶(Q79.6-)◀*
ligamentous laxity, NOS (M24.2-)

M35.8 **Other specified systemic involvement of connective tissue** HCC

M35.9 **Systemic involvement of connective tissue, unspecified** HCC

Autoimmune disease (systemic) NOS
Collagen (vascular) disease NOS

✓4th **M36** **Systemic disorders of connective tissue in diseases classified elsewhere**

EXCLUDES 2 *arthropathies in diseases classified elsewhere (M14.-)*

M36.0 *Dermato(poly)myositis in neoplastic disease* HCC

Code first underlying neoplasm (C00-D49)

M36.1 *Arthropathy in neoplastic disease*

Code first underlying neoplasm, such as:
leukemia (C91-C95)
malignant histiocytosis (C96.A)
multiple myeloma (C90.0)

M36.2 *Hemophilic arthropathy*

Hemarthrosis in hemophilic arthropathy
Code first underlying disease, such as:
factor VIII deficiency (D66)
with vascular defect (D68.0)
factor IX deficiency (D67)
hemophilia (classical) (D66)
hemophilia B (D67)
hemophilia C (D68.1)

M36.3 *Arthropathy in other blood disorders*

M36.4 *Arthropathy in hypersensitivity reactions classified elsewhere*

Code first underlying disease, such as:
Henoch (-Schönlein) purpura (D69.0)
serum sickness (T80.6-)

M36.8 *Systemic disorders of connective tissue in other diseases classified elsewhere* HCC

Code first underlying disease, such as:
alkaptonuria (E70.2)
hypogammaglobulinemia (D80.-)
ochronosis (E70.2)

DORSOPATHIES (M40-M54)

Deforming dorsopathies (M40-M43)

✓4th **M40** **Kyphosis and lordosis**

EXCLUDES 1 *congenital kyphosis and lordosis (Q76.4)*
kyphoscoliosis (M41.-)
postprocedural kyphosis and lordosis (M96.-)

Kyphosis and Lordosis

Kyphosis: Excessive convexity in the thoracic region

Lordosis: Excessive concavity in the lumbar region

✓5th **M40.0** **Postural kyphosis**

EXCLUDES 1 *osteochondrosis of spine (M42.-)*

M40.00 **Postural kyphosis, site unspecified**

M40.03 **Postural kyphosis, cervicothoracic region**

M40.04 **Postural kyphosis, thoracic region**

M40.05 **Postural kyphosis, thoracolumbar region**

✓5th **M40.1** **Other secondary kyphosis**

M40.10 **Other secondary kyphosis, site unspecified**

M40.12 **Other secondary kyphosis, cervical region**

M40.13 **Other secondary kyphosis, cervicothoracic region**

M40.14 **Other secondary kyphosis, thoracic region**

M40.15 **Other secondary kyphosis, thoracolumbar region**

✓5th **M40.2** **Other and unspecified kyphosis**

✓6th **M40.20** **Unspecified kyphosis**

M40.202 **Unspecified kyphosis, cervical region**

M40.203 **Unspecified kyphosis, cervicothoracic region**

M40.204 **Unspecified kyphosis, thoracic region**

M40.205 **Unspecified kyphosis, thoracolumbar region**

M40.209 **Unspecified kyphosis, site unspecified**

✓6th **M40.29** **Other kyphosis**

M40.292 **Other kyphosis, cervical region**

M40.293 **Other kyphosis, cervicothoracic region**

M40.294 **Other kyphosis, thoracic region**

M40.295 **Other kyphosis, thoracolumbar region**

M40.299 **Other kyphosis, site unspecified**

✓5th **M40.3** **Flatback syndrome**

M40.30 **Flatback syndrome, site unspecified**

M40.35 **Flatback syndrome, thoracolumbar region**

M40.36 **Flatback syndrome, lumbar region**

M40.37 **Flatback syndrome, lumbosacral region**

✓5th **M40.4** **Postural lordosis**

Acquired lordosis

M40.40 **Postural lordosis, site unspecified**

M40.45 **Postural lordosis, thoracolumbar region**

M40.46 **Postural lordosis, lumbar region**

M40.47 **Postural lordosis, lumbosacral region**

✓5th **M40.5** **Lordosis, unspecified**

M40.50 **Lordosis, unspecified, site unspecified**

M40.55 **Lordosis, unspecified, thoracolumbar region**

M40.56 **Lordosis, unspecified, lumbar region**

M40.57 **Lordosis, unspecified, lumbosacral region**

☑ Additional Character Required ✓x7th Placeholder Alert Manifestation Unspecified Dx ▶◀ Revised Text ● New Code ▲ Revised Code Title

ICD-10-CM 2020 783

✓4ᵗʰ **M41 Scoliosis**

    INCLUDES   kyphoscoliosis
    EXCLUDES 1   *congenital scoliosis due to bony malformation (Q76.3)*
           congenital scoliosis NOS (Q67.5)
           kyphoscoliotic heart disease (I27.1)
           postprocedural scoliosis (M96.-)
           postural congenital scoliosis (Q67.5)

Scoliosis

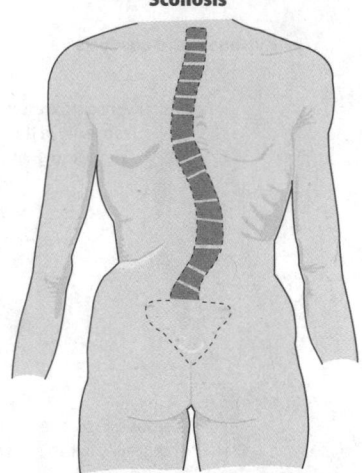

Lateral curvature of spine

✓5ᵗʰ **M41.0 Infantile idiopathic scoliosis**

    AHA: 2014,4Q,26

    M41.00   Infantile idiopathic scoliosis, site unspecified
    M41.02   Infantile idiopathic scoliosis, cervical region
    M41.03   Infantile idiopathic scoliosis, cervicothoracic region
    M41.04   Infantile idiopathic scoliosis, thoracic region
    M41.05   Infantile idiopathic scoliosis, thoracolumbar region
    M41.06   Infantile idiopathic scoliosis, lumbar region
    M41.07   Infantile idiopathic scoliosis, lumbosacral region
    M41.08   Infantile idiopathic scoliosis, sacral and sacrococcygeal region

✓5ᵗʰ **M41.1 Juvenile and adolescent idiopathic scoliosis**

  ✓6ᵗʰ **M41.11 Juvenile idiopathic scoliosis**

    AHA: 2014,4Q,28

    M41.112   Juvenile idiopathic scoliosis, cervical region
    M41.113   Juvenile idiopathic scoliosis, cervicothoracic region
    M41.114   Juvenile idiopathic scoliosis, thoracic region
    M41.115   Juvenile idiopathic scoliosis, thoracolumbar region
    M41.116   Juvenile idiopathic scoliosis, lumbar region
    M41.117   Juvenile idiopathic scoliosis, lumbosacral region
    M41.119   Juvenile idiopathic scoliosis, site unspecified

  ✓6ᵗʰ **M41.12 Adolescent scoliosis**

    M41.122   Adolescent idiopathic scoliosis, cervical region
    M41.123   Adolescent idiopathic scoliosis, cervicothoracic region
    M41.124   Adolescent idiopathic scoliosis, thoracic region
    M41.125   Adolescent idiopathic scoliosis, thoracolumbar region
    M41.126   Adolescent idiopathic scoliosis, lumbar region
    M41.127   Adolescent idiopathic scoliosis, lumbosacral region
    M41.129   Adolescent idiopathic scoliosis, site unspecified

✓5ᵗʰ **M41.2 Other idiopathic scoliosis**

    M41.20   Other idiopathic scoliosis, site unspecified
    M41.22   Other idiopathic scoliosis, cervical region
    M41.23   Other idiopathic scoliosis, cervicothoracic region

    M41.24   Other idiopathic scoliosis, thoracic region
    M41.25   Other idiopathic scoliosis, thoracolumbar region
    M41.26   Other idiopathic scoliosis, lumbar region
    M41.27   Other idiopathic scoliosis, lumbosacral region

✓5ᵗʰ **M41.3 Thoracogenic scoliosis**

    M41.30   Thoracogenic scoliosis, site unspecified
    M41.34   Thoracogenic scoliosis, thoracic region
    M41.35   Thoracogenic scoliosis, thoracolumbar region

✓5ᵗʰ **M41.4 Neuromuscular scoliosis**

    Scoliosis secondary to cerebral palsy, Friedreich's ataxia, poliomyelitis and other neuromuscular disorders
    Code also underlying condition
    AHA: 2014,4Q,27

    M41.40   Neuromuscular scoliosis, site unspecified
    M41.41   Neuromuscular scoliosis, occipito-atlanto-axial region
    M41.42   Neuromuscular scoliosis, cervical region
    M41.43   Neuromuscular scoliosis, cervicothoracic region
    M41.44   Neuromuscular scoliosis, thoracic region
    M41.45   Neuromuscular scoliosis, thoracolumbar region
    M41.46   Neuromuscular scoliosis, lumbar region
    M41.47   Neuromuscular scoliosis, lumbosacral region

✓5ᵗʰ **M41.5 Other secondary scoliosis**

    AHA: 2019,1Q,19

    M41.50   Other secondary scoliosis, site unspecified
    M41.52   Other secondary scoliosis, cervical region
    M41.53   Other secondary scoliosis, cervicothoracic region
    M41.54   Other secondary scoliosis, thoracic region
    M41.55   Other secondary scoliosis, thoracolumbar region
    M41.56   Other secondary scoliosis, lumbar region
    M41.57   Other secondary scoliosis, lumbosacral region

✓5ᵗʰ **M41.8 Other forms of scoliosis**

    M41.80   Other forms of scoliosis, site unspecified
    M41.82   Other forms of scoliosis, cervical region
    M41.83   Other forms of scoliosis, cervicothoracic region
    M41.84   Other forms of scoliosis, thoracic region
    M41.85   Other forms of scoliosis, thoracolumbar region
    M41.86   Other forms of scoliosis, lumbar region
    M41.87   Other forms of scoliosis, lumbosacral region

    M41.9 Scoliosis, unspecified

✓4ᵗʰ **M42 Spinal osteochondrosis**

✓5ᵗʰ **M42.0 Juvenile osteochondrosis of spine**

    Calvé's disease
    Scheuermann's disease
    EXCLUDES 1   *postural kyphosis (M40.0)*

    M42.00   Juvenile osteochondrosis of spine, site unspecified
    M42.01   Juvenile osteochondrosis of spine, occipito-atlanto-axial region
    M42.02   Juvenile osteochondrosis of spine, cervical region
    M42.03   Juvenile osteochondrosis of spine, cervicothoracic region
    M42.04   Juvenile osteochondrosis of spine, thoracic region
    M42.05   Juvenile osteochondrosis of spine, thoracolumbar region
    M42.06   Juvenile osteochondrosis of spine, lumbar region
    M42.07   Juvenile osteochondrosis of spine, lumbosacral region
    M42.08   Juvenile osteochondrosis of spine, sacral and sacrococcygeal region
    M42.09   Juvenile osteochondrosis of spine, multiple sites in spine

✓5ᵗʰ **M42.1 Adult osteochondrosis of spine**

    M42.10   Adult osteochondrosis of spine, site unspecified   Ⓐ
    M42.11   Adult osteochondrosis of spine, occipito-atlanto-axial region   Ⓐ
    M42.12   Adult osteochondrosis of spine, cervical region   Ⓐ
    M42.13   Adult osteochondrosis of spine, cervicothoracic region   Ⓐ
    M42.14   Adult osteochondrosis of spine, thoracic region   Ⓐ
    M42.15   Adult osteochondrosis of spine, thoracolumbar region   Ⓐ
    M42.16   Adult osteochondrosis of spine, lumbar region   Ⓐ

M42.17	**Adult osteochondrosis of spine, lumbosacral region**	▲
M42.18	**Adult osteochondrosis of spine, sacral and sacrococcygeal region**	▲
M42.19	**Adult osteochondrosis of spine, multiple sites in spine**	▲
M42.9	**Spinal osteochondrosis, unspecified**	

✓4ᵗʰ M43 Other deforming dorsopathies

> EXCLUDES 1   *congenital spondylolysis and spondylolisthesis (Q76.2)*
> *hemivertebra (Q76.3-Q76.4)*
> *Klippel-Feil syndrome (Q76.1)*
> *lumbarization and sacralization (Q76.4)*
> *platyspondylisis (Q76.4)*
> *spina bifida occulta (Q76.0)*
> *spinal curvature in osteoporosis (M80.-)*
> *spinal curvature in Paget's disease of bone [osteitis deformans] (M88.-)*

✓5ᵗʰ M43.0 Spondylolysis

> EXCLUDES 1   *congenital spondylolysis (Q76.2)*
> *spondylolisthesis (M43.1)*

M43.00	**Spondylolysis, site unspecified**
M43.01	**Spondylolysis, occipito-atlanto-axial region**
M43.02	**Spondylolysis, cervical region**
M43.03	**Spondylolysis, cervicothoracic region**
M43.04	**Spondylolysis, thoracic region**
M43.05	**Spondylolysis, thoracolumbar region**
M43.06	**Spondylolysis, lumbar region**
M43.07	**Spondylolysis, lumbosacral region**
M43.08	**Spondylolysis, sacral and sacrococcygeal region**
M43.09	**Spondylolysis, multiple sites in spine**

✓5ᵗʰ M43.1 Spondylolisthesis

> EXCLUDES 1   *acute traumatic of lumbosacral region (S33.1)*
> *acute traumatic of sites other than lumbosacral — code to Fracture, vertebra, by region*
> *congenital spondylolisthesis (Q76.2)*

AHA: 2018,3Q,18
TIP: Code also any associated radiculopathy (M54.1-) and/or myelopathy (G99.2)

M43.10	**Spondylolisthesis, site unspecified**
M43.11	**Spondylolisthesis, occipito-atlanto-axial region**
M43.12	**Spondylolisthesis, cervical region**
M43.13	**Spondylolisthesis, cervicothoracic region**
M43.14	**Spondylolisthesis, thoracic region**
M43.15	**Spondylolisthesis, thoracolumbar region**
M43.16	**Spondylolisthesis, lumbar region**
M43.17	**Spondylolisthesis, lumbosacral region**
M43.18	**Spondylolisthesis, sacral and sacrococcygeal region**
M43.19	**Spondylolisthesis, multiple sites in spine**

✓5ᵗʰ M43.2 Fusion of spine

> Ankylosis of spinal joint
> EXCLUDES 1   *ankylosing spondylitis (M45.0-)*
> *congenital fusion of spine (Q76.4)*
> EXCLUDES 2   *arthrodesis status (Z98.1)*
> *pseudoarthrosis after fusion or arthrodesis (M96.0)*

M43.20	**Fusion of spine, site unspecified**
M43.21	**Fusion of spine, occipito-atlanto-axial region**
M43.22	**Fusion of spine, cervical region**
M43.23	**Fusion of spine, cervicothoracic region**
M43.24	**Fusion of spine, thoracic region**
M43.25	**Fusion of spine, thoracolumbar region**
M43.26	**Fusion of spine, lumbar region**
M43.27	**Fusion of spine, lumbosacral region**
M43.28	**Fusion of spine, sacral and sacrococcygeal region**
M43.3	**Recurrent atlantoaxial dislocation with myelopathy**
M43.4	**Other recurrent atlantoaxial dislocation**

✓5ᵗʰ M43.5 Other recurrent vertebral dislocation

> EXCLUDES 1   *biomechanical lesions NEC (M99.-)*

✓6ᵗʰ M43.5X Other recurrent vertebral dislocation

M43.5X2	**Other recurrent vertebral dislocation, cervical region**
M43.5X3	**Other recurrent vertebral dislocation, cervicothoracic region**
M43.5X4	**Other recurrent vertebral dislocation, thoracic region**
M43.5X5	**Other recurrent vertebral dislocation, thoracolumbar region**
M43.5X6	**Other recurrent vertebral dislocation, lumbar region**
M43.5X7	**Other recurrent vertebral dislocation, lumbosacral region**
M43.5X8	**Other recurrent vertebral dislocation, sacral and sacrococcygeal region**
M43.5X9	**Other recurrent vertebral dislocation, site unspecified**

M43.6 Torticollis

> EXCLUDES 1   *congenital (sternomastoid) torticollis (Q68.0)*
> *current injury — see Injury, of spine, by body region*
> *ocular torticollis (R29.891)*
> *psychogenic torticollis (F45.8)*
> *spasmodic torticollis (G24.3)*
> *torticollis due to birth injury (P15.2)*

DEF: Twisted, unnatural position of the neck due to contracted cervical muscles that pull the head to one side.

✓5ᵗʰ M43.8 Other specified deforming dorsopathies

> EXCLUDES 2   *kyphosis and lordosis (M40.-)*
> *scoliosis (M41.-)*

✓6ᵗʰ M43.8X Other specified deforming dorsopathies

M43.8X1	**Other specified deforming dorsopathies, occipito-atlanto-axial region**
M43.8X2	**Other specified deforming dorsopathies, cervical region**
M43.8X3	**Other specified deforming dorsopathies, cervicothoracic region**
M43.8X4	**Other specified deforming dorsopathies, thoracic region**
M43.8X5	**Other specified deforming dorsopathies, thoracolumbar region**
M43.8X6	**Other specified deforming dorsopathies, lumbar region**
M43.8X7	**Other specified deforming dorsopathies, lumbosacral region**
M43.8X8	**Other specified deforming dorsopathies, sacral and sacrococcygeal region**
M43.8X9	**Other specified deforming dorsopathies, site unspecified**
M43.9	**Deforming dorsopathy, unspecified**

> Curvature of spine NOS

Spondylopathies (M45-M49)

✓4ᵗʰ M45 Ankylosing spondylitis

> Rheumatoid arthritis of spine
> EXCLUDES 1   *arthropathy in Reiter's disease (M02.3-)*
> *juvenile (ankylosing) spondylitis (M08.1)*
> EXCLUDES 2   *Behçet's disease (M35.2)*

M45.0	**Ankylosing spondylitis of multiple sites in spine**	HCC
M45.1	**Ankylosing spondylitis of occipito-atlanto-axial region**	HCC
M45.2	**Ankylosing spondylitis of cervical region**	HCC
M45.3	**Ankylosing spondylitis of cervicothoracic region**	HCC
M45.4	**Ankylosing spondylitis of thoracic region**	HCC
M45.5	**Ankylosing spondylitis of thoracolumbar region**	HCC
M45.6	**Ankylosing spondylitis lumbar region**	HCC
M45.7	**Ankylosing spondylitis of lumbosacral region**	HCC
M45.8	**Ankylosing spondylitis sacral and sacrococcygeal region**	HCC
M45.9	**Ankylosing spondylitis of unspecified sites in spine**	HCC

✓4ᵗʰ M46 Other inflammatory spondylopathies

✓5ᵗʰ M46.0 Spinal enthesopathy

> Disorder of ligamentous or muscular attachments of spine

M46.00	**Spinal enthesopathy, site unspecified**	HCC
M46.01	**Spinal enthesopathy, occipito-atlanto-axial region**	HCC
M46.02	**Spinal enthesopathy, cervical region**	HCC
M46.03	**Spinal enthesopathy, cervicothoracic region**	HCC
M46.04	**Spinal enthesopathy, thoracic region**	HCC
M46.05	**Spinal enthesopathy, thoracolumbar region**	HCC
M46.06	**Spinal enthesopathy, lumbar region**	HCC
M46.07	**Spinal enthesopathy, lumbosacral region**	HCC
M46.08	**Spinal enthesopathy, sacral and sacrococcygeal region**	HCC

✓ Additional Character Required   ✓x7ᵗʰ Placeholder Alert   Manifestation   Unspecified Dx   ►◄ Revised Text   ● New Code   ▲ Revised Code Title

M46.Ø9   **Spinal enthesopathy,** multiple sites in spine   `HCC`

M46.1   **Sacroiliitis, not elsewhere classified**   `HCC`

> **DEF:** Inflammation of the sacroiliac joint (situated at the juncture of the sacrum and hip). Symptoms include pain in the buttocks or lower back that can extend down one or both legs.

√5ᵗʰ **M46.2**   **Osteomyelitis of vertebra**

M46.2Ø   **Osteomyelitis of vertebra, site unspecified**   `HCC`

M46.21   **Osteomyelitis of vertebra, occipito-atlanto-axial** region   `HCC`

M46.22   **Osteomyelitis of vertebra, cervical** region   `HCC`

M46.23   **Osteomyelitis of vertebra, cervicothoracic** region   `HCC`

M46.24   **Osteomyelitis of vertebra, thoracic** region   `HCC`

M46.25   **Osteomyelitis of vertebra, thoracolumbar** region   `HCC`

M46.26   **Osteomyelitis of vertebra, lumbar** region   `HCC`

M46.27   **Osteomyelitis of vertebra, lumbosacral** region   `HCC`

M46.28   **Osteomyelitis of vertebra, sacral and sacrococcygeal** region   `HCC`

√5ᵗʰ **M46.3**   **Infection of intervertebral disc (pyogenic)**

> Use additional code (B95-B97) to identify infectious agent

M46.3Ø   **Infection of intervertebral disc (pyogenic), site unspecified**   `HCC`

M46.31   **Infection of intervertebral disc (pyogenic), occipito-atlanto-axial** region   `HCC`

M46.32   **Infection of intervertebral disc (pyogenic), cervical** region   `HCC`

M46.33   **Infection of intervertebral disc (pyogenic), cervicothoracic** region   `HCC`

M46.34   **Infection of intervertebral disc (pyogenic), thoracic** region   `HCC`

M46.35   **Infection of intervertebral disc (pyogenic), thoracolumbar** region   `HCC`

M46.36   **Infection of intervertebral disc (pyogenic), lumbar** region   `HCC`

M46.37   **Infection of intervertebral disc (pyogenic), lumbosacral** region   `HCC`

M46.38   **Infection of intervertebral disc (pyogenic), sacral and sacrococcygeal** region   `HCC`

M46.39   **Infection of intervertebral disc (pyogenic), multiple sites** in spine   `HCC`

√5ᵗʰ **M46.4**   **Discitis, unspecified**

M46.4Ø   **Discitis, unspecified, site unspecified**

M46.41   **Discitis, unspecified, occipito-atlanto-axial** region

M46.42   **Discitis, unspecified, cervical** region

M46.43   **Discitis, unspecified, cervicothoracic** region

M46.44   **Discitis, unspecified, thoracic** region

M46.45   **Discitis, unspecified, thoracolumbar** region

M46.46   **Discitis, unspecified, lumbar** region

M46.47   **Discitis, unspecified, lumbosacral** region

M46.48   **Discitis, unspecified, sacral and sacrococcygeal** region

M46.49   **Discitis, unspecified, multiple sites** in spine

√6ᵗʰ **M46.5**   **Other infective spondylopathies**

M46.5Ø   **Other infective spondylopathies, site unspecified**   `HCC`

M46.51   **Other infective spondylopathies, occipito-atlanto-axial** region   `HCC`

M46.52   **Other infective spondylopathies, cervical** region   `HCC`

M46.53   **Other infective spondylopathies, cervicothoracic** region   `HCC`

M46.54   **Other infective spondylopathies, thoracic** region   `HCC`

M46.55   **Other infective spondylopathies, thoracolumbar** region   `HCC`

M46.56   **Other infective spondylopathies, lumbar** region   `HCC`

M46.57   **Other infective spondylopathies, lumbosacral** region   `HCC`

M46.58   **Other infective spondylopathies, sacral and sacrococcygeal** region   `HCC`

M46.59   **Other infective spondylopathies, multiple sites** in spine   `HCC`

√5ᵗʰ **M46.8**   **Other specified inflammatory spondylopathies**

M46.8Ø   **Other specified inflammatory spondylopathies, site unspecified**   `HCC`

M46.81   **Other specified inflammatory spondylopathies, occipito-atlanto-axial** region   `HCC`

M46.82   **Other specified inflammatory spondylopathies, cervical** region   `HCC`

M46.83   **Other specified inflammatory spondylopathies, cervicothoracic** region   `HCC`

M46.84   **Other specified inflammatory spondylopathies, thoracic** region   `HCC`

M46.85   **Other specified inflammatory spondylopathies, thoracolumbar** region   `HCC`

M46.86   **Other specified inflammatory spondylopathies, lumbar** region   `HCC`

M46.87   **Other specified inflammatory spondylopathies, lumbosacral** region   `HCC`

M46.88   **Other specified inflammatory spondylopathies, sacral and sacrococcygeal** region   `HCC`

M46.89   **Other specified inflammatory spondylopathies, multiple sites** in spine   `HCC`

√5ᵗʰ **M46.9**   **Unspecified inflammatory spondylopathy**

M46.9Ø   **Unspecified inflammatory spondylopathy, site unspecified**   `HCC`

M46.91   **Unspecified inflammatory spondylopathy, occipito-atlanto-axial** region   `HCC`

M46.92   **Unspecified inflammatory spondylopathy, cervical** region   `HCC`

M46.93   **Unspecified inflammatory spondylopathy, cervicothoracic** region   `HCC`

M46.94   **Unspecified inflammatory spondylopathy, thoracic** region   `HCC`

M46.95   **Unspecified inflammatory spondylopathy, thoracolumbar** region   `HCC`

M46.96   **Unspecified inflammatory spondylopathy, lumbar** region   `HCC`

M46.97   **Unspecified inflammatory spondylopathy, lumbosacral** region   `HCC`

M46.98   **Unspecified inflammatory spondylopathy, sacral and sacrococcygeal** region   `HCC`

M46.99   **Unspecified inflammatory spondylopathy, multiple sites** in spine   `HCC`

√4ᵗʰ **M47**   **Spondylosis**

> `INCLUDES`   arthrosis or osteoarthritis of spine
>   degeneration of facet joints

√5ᵗʰ **M47.Ø**   **Anterior spinal and vertebral artery** compression syndromes

√6ᵗʰ **M47.Ø1**   **Anterior spinal artery** compression syndromes

M47.Ø11   **Anterior spinal artery compression syndromes, occipito-atlanto-axial** region

M47.Ø12   **Anterior spinal artery compression syndromes, cervical** region

M47.Ø13   **Anterior spinal artery compression syndromes, cervicothoracic** region

M47.Ø14   **Anterior spinal artery compression syndromes, thoracic** region

M47.Ø15   **Anterior spinal artery compression syndromes, thoracolumbar** region

M47.Ø16   **Anterior spinal artery compression syndromes, lumbar** region

M47.Ø19   **Anterior spinal artery compression syndromes, site unspecified**

√6ᵗʰ **M47.Ø2**   **Vertebral artery** compression syndromes

M47.Ø21   **Vertebral artery compression syndromes, occipito-atlanto-axial** region

M47.Ø22   **Vertebral artery compression syndromes, cervical** region

M47.Ø29   **Vertebral artery compression syndromes, site unspecified**

√5ᵗʰ **M47.1**   **Other spondylosis** with myelopathy

> Spondylogenic compression of spinal cord
> `EXCLUDES 1`   vertebral subluxation ▶*(M43.3-M43.5X9)*◀

M47.1Ø   **Other spondylosis with myelopathy, site unspecified**

M47.11   **Other spondylosis with myelopathy, occipito-atlanto-axial** region

M47.12   **Other spondylosis with myelopathy, cervical** region

M47.13   **Other spondylosis with myelopathy, cervicothoracic** region

M47.14   **Other spondylosis with myelopathy, thoracic** region

M47.15   **Other spondylosis with myelopathy, thoracolumbar** region

M47.16   Other spondylosis with myelopathy, lumbar region

✓5ᵗʰ **M47.2**   **Other spondylosis with radiculopathy**

    M47.20   **Other spondylosis with radiculopathy, site unspecified**

    M47.21   Other spondylosis with radiculopathy, occipito-atlanto-axial region

    M47.22   Other spondylosis with radiculopathy, cervical region

    M47.23   Other spondylosis with radiculopathy, cervicothoracic region

    M47.24   Other spondylosis with radiculopathy, thoracic region

    M47.25   Other spondylosis with radiculopathy, thoracolumbar region

    M47.26   Other spondylosis with radiculopathy, lumbar region

    M47.27   Other spondylosis with radiculopathy, lumbosacral region

    M47.28   Other spondylosis with radiculopathy, sacral and sacrococcygeal region

✓5ᵗʰ **M47.8**   **Other spondylosis**

   ✓6ᵗʰ **M47.81**   **Spondylosis** without myelopathy or radiculopathy

      AHA: 2018,2Q,14

     M47.811   Spondylosis without myelopathy or radiculopathy, occipito-atlanto-axial region

     M47.812   Spondylosis without myelopathy or radiculopathy, cervical region

     M47.813   Spondylosis without myelopathy or radiculopathy, cervicothoracic region

     M47.814   Spondylosis without myelopathy or radiculopathy, thoracic region

     M47.815   Spondylosis without myelopathy or radiculopathy, thoracolumbar region

     M47.816   Spondylosis without myelopathy or radiculopathy, lumbar region

     M47.817   Spondylosis without myelopathy or radiculopathy, lumbosacral region

     M47.818   Spondylosis without myelopathy or radiculopathy, sacral and sacrococcygeal region

     M47.819   Spondylosis without myelopathy or radiculopathy, site unspecified

   ✓6ᵗʰ **M47.89**   **Other spondylosis**

     M47.891   Other spondylosis, occipito-atlanto-axial region

     M47.892   Other spondylosis, cervical region

     M47.893   Other spondylosis, cervicothoracic region

     M47.894   Other spondylosis, thoracic region

     M47.895   Other spondylosis, thoracolumbar region

     M47.896   Other spondylosis, lumbar region

     M47.897   Other spondylosis, lumbosacral region

     M47.898   Other spondylosis, sacral and sacrococcygeal region

     M47.899   Other spondylosis, site unspecified

  M47.9   **Spondylosis, unspecified**

✓4ᵗʰ **M48**   **Other spondylopathies**

  ✓5ᵗʰ **M48.0**   **Spinal stenosis**

     Caudal stenosis

     AHA: 2018,3Q,18-19

     TIP: Code also any associated radiculopathy (M54.1-) and/or myelopathy (G99.2).

    M48.00   Spinal stenosis, site unspecified

    M48.01   Spinal stenosis, occipito-atlanto-axial region

    M48.02   Spinal stenosis, cervical region

    M48.03   Spinal stenosis, cervicothoracic region

    M48.04   Spinal stenosis, thoracic region

    M48.05   Spinal stenosis, thoracolumbar region

   ✓6ᵗʰ **M48.06**   Spinal stenosis, lumbar region

      AHA: 2018,3Q,19; 2017,4Q,18-19

      DEF: Spinal canal narrowing in the lumbar area with nerve root compression, causing muscle pain, fatigue, and weakness during extension of the lumbar spine. Pain is relieved by sitting or bending.

     M48.061   Spinal stenosis, lumbar region without neurogenic claudication

       Spinal stenosis, lumbar region NOS

     M48.062   Spinal stenosis, lumbar region with neurogenic claudication

    M48.07   Spinal stenosis, lumbosacral region

M48.08   Spinal stenosis, sacral and sacrococcygeal region

✓5ᵗʰ **M48.1**   **Ankylosing hyperostosis [Forestier]**

     Diffuse idiopathic skeletal hyperostosis [DISH]

    M48.10   **Ankylosing hyperostosis [Forestier], site unspecified**

    M48.11   Ankylosing hyperostosis [Forestier], occipito-atlanto-axial region

    M48.12   Ankylosing hyperostosis [Forestier], cervical region

    M48.13   Ankylosing hyperostosis [Forestier], cervicothoracic region

    M48.14   Ankylosing hyperostosis [Forestier], thoracic region

    M48.15   Ankylosing hyperostosis [Forestier], thoracolumbar region

    M48.16   Ankylosing hyperostosis [Forestier], lumbar region

    M48.17   Ankylosing hyperostosis [Forestier], lumbosacral region

    M48.18   Ankylosing hyperostosis [Forestier], sacral and sacrococcygeal region

    M48.19   Ankylosing hyperostosis [Forestier], multiple sites in spine

✓5ᵗʰ **M48.2**   **Kissing spine**

    M48.20   **Kissing spine, site unspecified**

    M48.21   Kissing spine, occipito-atlanto-axial region

    M48.22   Kissing spine, cervical region

    M48.23   Kissing spine, cervicothoracic region

    M48.24   Kissing spine, thoracic region

    M48.25   Kissing spine, thoracolumbar region

    M48.26   Kissing spine, lumbar region

    M48.27   Kissing spine, lumbosacral region

✓5ᵗʰ **M48.3**   **Traumatic spondylopathy**

    M48.30   **Traumatic spondylopathy, site unspecified**

    M48.31   Traumatic spondylopathy, occipito-atlanto-axial region

    M48.32   Traumatic spondylopathy, cervical region

    M48.33   Traumatic spondylopathy, cervicothoracic region

    M48.34   Traumatic spondylopathy, thoracic region

    M48.35   Traumatic spondylopathy, thoracolumbar region

    M48.36   Traumatic spondylopathy, lumbar region

    M48.37   Traumatic spondylopathy, lumbosacral region

    M48.38   Traumatic spondylopathy, sacral and sacrococcygeal region

✓5ᵗʰ **M48.4**   **Fatigue fracture of vertebra**

     Stress fracture of vertebra

     EXCLUDES 1   *pathological fracture NOS (M84.4-)*

       pathological fracture of vertebra due to neoplasm (M84.58)

       pathological fracture of vertebra due to osteoporosis (M80.-)

       pathological fracture of vertebra due to other diagnosis (M84.68)

       traumatic fracture of vertebrae (S12.0-S12.3-, S22.0-, S32.0-)

> The appropriate 7th character is to be added to each code from subcategory M48.4.
> A   initial encounter for fracture
> D   subsequent encounter for fracture with routine healing
> G   subsequent encounter for fracture with delayed healing
> S   sequela of fracture

  ✓x7ᵗʰ **M48.40**   **Fatigue fracture of vertebra, site unspecified**   ⑩

  ✓x7ᵗʰ M48.41   Fatigue fracture of vertebra, occipito-atlanto-axial region   ⑩

  ✓x7ᵗʰ M48.42   Fatigue fracture of vertebra, cervical region   ⑩

  ✓x7ᵗʰ M48.43   Fatigue fracture of vertebra, cervicothoracic region   ⑩

  ✓x7ᵗʰ M48.44   Fatigue fracture of vertebra, thoracic region   ⑩

  ✓x7ᵗʰ M48.45   Fatigue fracture of vertebra, thoracolumbar region   ⑩

  ✓x7ᵗʰ M48.46   Fatigue fracture of vertebra, lumbar region   ⑩

  ✓x7ᵗʰ M48.47   Fatigue fracture of vertebra, lumbosacral region   ⑩

  ✓x7ᵗʰ M48.48   Fatigue fracture of vertebra, sacral and sacrococcygeal region   ⑩

☑ Additional Character Required   ✓x7ᵗʰ Placeholder Alert   Manifestation   Unspecified Dx   ▶◀ Revised Text   ● New Code   ▲ Revised Code Title

ICD-10-CM 2020   787

Chapter 13. Diseases of the Musculoskeletal System and Connective Tissue

✓5ᵗʰ **M48.5 Collapsed vertebra, not elsewhere classified**

Collapsed vertebra NOS
Compression fracture of vertebra NOS
Wedging of vertebra NOS

EXCLUDES 1   current injury — see Injury of spine, by body region
fatigue fracture of vertebra (M48.4)
pathological fracture NOS (M84.4-)
pathological fracture of vertebra due to neoplasm
(M84.58)
pathological fracture of vertebra due to osteoporosis
(M8Ø.-)
pathological fracture of vertebra due to other
diagnosis (M84.68)
stress fracture of vertebra (M48.4-)
traumatic fracture of vertebra (S12.-, S22.-, S32.-)

The appropriate 7th character is to be added to each code
from subcategory M48.5.
A   initial encounter for fracture
D   subsequent encounter for fracture with routine healing
G   subsequent encounter for fracture with delayed healing
S   sequela of fracture

1 ✓x 7ᵗʰ **M48.5Ø Collapsed vertebra, not elsewhere classified, site unspecified** HCC

1 ✓x 7ᵗʰ **M48.51 Collapsed vertebra, not elsewhere classified, occipito-atlanto-axial region** HCC

1 ✓x 7ᵗʰ **M48.52 Collapsed vertebra, not elsewhere classified, cervical region** HCC

1 ✓x 7ᵗʰ **M48.53 Collapsed vertebra, not elsewhere classified, cervicothoracic region** HCC

1 ✓x 7ᵗʰ **M48.54 Collapsed vertebra, not elsewhere classified, thoracic region** HCC

1 ✓x 7ᵗʰ **M48.55 Collapsed vertebra, not elsewhere classified, thoracolumbar region** HCC

1 ✓x 7ᵗʰ **M48.56 Collapsed vertebra, not elsewhere classified, lumbar region** HCC

1 ✓x 7ᵗʰ **M48.57 Collapsed vertebra, not elsewhere classified, lumbosacral region** HCC

1 ✓x 7ᵗʰ **M48.58 Collapsed vertebra, not elsewhere classified, sacral and sacrococcygeal region** HCC

✓5ᵗʰ **M48.8 Other specified spondylopathies**

Ossification of posterior longitudinal ligament

✓6ᵗʰ **M48.8X Other specified spondylopathies**

M48.8X1 Other specified spondylopathies, occipito-atlanto-axial region HCC

M48.8X2 Other specified spondylopathies, cervical region HCC

M48.8X3 Other specified spondylopathies, cervicothoracic region HCC

M48.8X4 Other specified spondylopathies, thoracic region HCC

M48.8X5 Other specified spondylopathies, thoracolumbar region HCC

M48.8X6 Other specified spondylopathies, lumbar region HCC

M48.8X7 Other specified spondylopathies, lumbosacral region HCC

M48.8X8 Other specified spondylopathies, sacral and sacrococcygeal region HCC

M48.8X9 Other specified spondylopathies, site unspecified HCC

M48.9 Spondylopathy, unspecified

✓4ᵗʰ **M49 Spondylopathies in diseases classified elsewhere**

INCLUDES   curvature of spine in diseases classified elsewhere
deformity of spine in diseases classified elsewhere
kyphosis in diseases classified elsewhere
scoliosis in diseases classified elsewhere
spondylopathy in diseases classified elsewhere

Code first underlying disease, such as:
brucellosis (A23.-)
Charcôt-Marie-Tooth disease (G6Ø.Ø)
enterobacterial infections (AØ1-AØ4)
osteitis fibrosa cystica (E21.Ø)

EXCLUDES 1   curvature of spine in tuberculosis [Pott's] (A18.Ø1)
enteropathic arthropathies (MØ7.-)
gonococcal spondylitis (A54.41)
neuropathic spondylopathy in syringomyelia (G95.Ø)
neuropathic spondylopathy in tabes dorsalis (A52.11)
neuropathic [tabes dorsalis] spondylitis (A52.11)
nonsyphilitic neuropathic spondylopathy NEC (G98.Ø)
spondylitis in syphilis (acquired) (A52.77)
tuberculous spondylitis (A18.Ø1)
typhoid fever spondylitis (AØ1.Ø5)

✓5ᵗʰ **M49.8 Spondylopathy in diseases classified elsewhere**

M49.8Ø Spondylopathy in diseases classified elsewhere, site unspecified HCC

M49.81 Spondylopathy in diseases classified elsewhere, occipito-atlanto-axial region HCC

M49.82 Spondylopathy in diseases classified elsewhere, cervical region HCC

M49.83 Spondylopathy in diseases classified elsewhere, cervicothoracic region HCC

M49.84 Spondylopathy in diseases classified elsewhere, thoracic region HCC

M49.85 Spondylopathy in diseases classified elsewhere, thoracolumbar region HCC

M49.86 Spondylopathy in diseases classified elsewhere, lumbar region HCC

M49.87 Spondylopathy in diseases classified elsewhere, lumbosacral region HCC

M49.88 Spondylopathy in diseases classified elsewhere, sacral and sacrococcygeal region HCC

M49.89 Spondylopathy in diseases classified elsewhere, multiple sites in spine HCC

Other dorsopathies (M5Ø-M54)

EXCLUDES 1   current injury — see injury of spine by body region
discitis NOS (M46.4-)

✓4ᵗʰ **M5Ø Cervical disc disorders**

NOTE   Code to the most superior level of disorder

INCLUDES   cervicothoracic disc disorders
cervicothoracic disc disorders with cervicalgia

AHA: 2016,4Q,39-40; 2016,1Q,17

✓5ᵗʰ **M5Ø.Ø Cervical disc disorder with myelopathy**

AHA: 2018,3Q,19

M5Ø.ØØ Cervical disc disorder with myelopathy, unspecified cervical region

M5Ø.Ø1 Cervical disc disorder with myelopathy, high cervical region

C2-C3 disc disorder with myelopathy
C3-C4 disc disorder with myelopathy

✓6ᵗʰ **M5Ø.Ø2 Cervical disc disorder with myelopathy, mid-cervical region**

M5Ø.Ø2Ø Cervical disc disorder with myelopathy, mid-cervical region, unspecified level

M5Ø.Ø21 Cervical disc disorder at C4-C5 level with myelopathy

C4-C5 disc disorder with myelopathy

M5Ø.Ø22 Cervical disc disorder at C5-C6 level with myelopathy

C5-C6 disc disorder with myelopathy

M5Ø.Ø23 Cervical disc disorder at C6-C7 level with myelopathy

C6-C7 disc disorder with myelopathy

M5Ø.Ø3 Cervical disc disorder with myelopathy, cervicothoracic region

C7-T1 disc disorder with myelopathy

☑5ᵗʰ **M50.1** **Cervical disc disorder** with radiculopathy

> *EXCLUDES 2*   brachial radiculitis NOS (M54.13)

> **AHA:** 2018,3Q,19

     M50.10   **Cervical disc disorder with radiculopathy, unspecified cervical region**

     M50.11   **Cervical disc disorder with radiculopathy, high cervical region**

> C2-C3 disc disorder with radiculopathy
> C3 radiculopathy due to disc disorder
> C3-C4 disc disorder with radiculopathy
> C4 radiculopathy due to disc disorder

     ☑6ᵗʰ **M50.12**   **Cervical disc disorder with radiculopathy, mid-cervical region**

▲   **M50.120**   **Mid-cervical disc disorder, unspecified level**

         M50.121   **Cervical disc disorder at C4-C5 level with radiculopathy**

> C4-C5 disc disorder with radiculopathy
> C5 radiculopathy due to disc disorder

         M50.122   **Cervical disc disorder at C5-C6 level with radiculopathy**

> C5-C6 disc disorder with radiculopathy
> C6 radiculopathy due to disc disorder

         M50.123   **Cervical disc disorder at C6-C7 level with radiculopathy**

> C6-C7 disc disorder with radiculopathy
> C7 radiculopathy due to disc disorder

     M50.13   **Cervical disc disorder with radiculopathy, cervicothoracic region**

> C7-T1 disc disorder with radiculopathy
> C8 radiculopathy due to disc disorder

☑5ᵗʰ **M50.2** **Other cervical disc** displacement

     M50.20   **Other cervical disc displacement, unspecified cervical region**

     M50.21   **Other cervical disc displacement, high cervical region**

> Other C2-C3 cervical disc displacement
> Other C3-C4 cervical disc displacement

     ☑6ᵗʰ **M50.22**   **Other cervical disc displacement, mid-cervical region**

         M50.220   **Other cervical disc displacement, mid-cervical region, unspecified level**

         M50.221   **Other cervical disc displacement at C4-C5 level**

> Other C4-C5 cervical disc displacement

         M50.222   **Other cervical disc displacement at C5-C6 level**

> Other C5-C6 cervical disc displacement

         M50.223   **Other cervical disc displacement at C6-C7 level**

> Other C6-C7 cervical disc displacement

     M50.23   **Other cervical disc displacement, cervicothoracic region**

> Other C7-T1 cervical disc displacement

☑5ᵗʰ **M50.3** **Other cervical disc** degeneration

     M50.30   **Other cervical disc degeneration, unspecified cervical region**

     M50.31   **Other cervical disc degeneration, high cervical region**

> Other C2-C3 cervical disc degeneration
> Other C3-C4 cervical disc degeneration

     ☑6ᵗʰ **M50.32**   **Other cervical disc degeneration, mid-cervical region**

         M50.320   **Other cervical disc degeneration, mid-cervical region, unspecified level**

         M50.321   **Other cervical disc degeneration at C4-C5 level**

> Other C4-C5 cervical disc degeneration

         M50.322   **Other cervical disc degeneration at C5-C6 level**

> Other C5-C6 cervical disc degeneration

         M50.323   **Other cervical disc degeneration at C6-C7 level**

> Other C6-C7 cervical disc degeneration

     M50.33   **Other cervical disc degeneration, cervicothoracic region**

> Other C7-T1 cervical disc degeneration

☑5ᵗʰ **M50.8** **Other cervical disc disorders**

     M50.80   **Other cervical disc disorders, unspecified cervical region**

     M50.81   **Other cervical disc disorders, high cervical region**

> Other C2-C3 cervical disc disorders
> Other C3-C4 cervical disc disorders

     ☑6ᵗʰ **M50.82**   **Other cervical disc disorders, mid-cervical region**

         M50.820   **Other cervical disc disorders, mid-cervical region, unspecified level**

         M50.821   **Other cervical disc disorders at C4-C5 level**

> Other C4-C5 cervical disc disorders

         M50.822   **Other cervical disc disorders at C5-C6 level**

> Other C5-C6 cervical disc disorders

         M50.823   **Other cervical disc disorders at C6-C7 level**

> Other C6-C7 cervical disc disorders

     M50.83   **Other cervical disc disorders, cervicothoracic region**

> Other C7-T1 cervical disc disorders

☑5ᵗʰ **M50.9** **Cervical disc disorder, unspecified**

     M50.90   **Cervical disc disorder, unspecified, unspecified cervical region**

     M50.91   **Cervical disc disorder, unspecified, high cervical region**

> C2-C3 cervical disc disorder, unspecified
> C3-C4 cervical disc disorder, unspecified

     ☑6ᵗʰ **M50.92**   **Cervical disc disorder, unspecified, mid-cervical region**

         M50.920   **Unspecified cervical disc disorder, mid-cervical region, unspecified level**

         M50.921   **Unspecified cervical disc disorder at C4-C5 level**

> Unspecified C4-C5 cervical disc disorder

         M50.922   **Unspecified cervical disc disorder at C5-C6 level**

> Unspecified C5-C6 cervical disc disorder

         M50.923   **Unspecified cervical disc disorder at C6-C7 level**

> Unspecified C6-C7 cervical disc disorder

     M50.93   **Cervical disc disorder, unspecified, cervicothoracic region**

> C7-T1 cervical disc disorder, unspecified

☑4ᵗʰ **M51** **Thoracic, thoracolumbar, and lumbosacral intervertebral disc disorders**

> *EXCLUDES 2*   cervical and cervicothoracic disc disorders (M50.-)
>   sacral and sacrococcygeal disorders (M53.3)

     ☑5ᵗʰ **M51.0** **Thoracic, thoracolumbar and lumbosacral intervertebral disc disorders** with myelopathy

     M51.04   **Intervertebral disc disorders with myelopathy, thoracic region**

     M51.05   **Intervertebral disc disorders with myelopathy, thoracolumbar region**

     M51.06   **Intervertebral disc disorders with myelopathy, lumbar region**

     ☑5ᵗʰ **M51.1** **Thoracic, thoracolumbar and lumbosacral intervertebral disc disorders** with radiculopathy

> Sciatica due to intervertebral disc disorder

> *EXCLUDES 1*   lumbar radiculitis NOS (M54.16)
>   sciatica NOS (M54.3)

> **AHA:** 2018,3Q,18

     M51.14   **Intervertebral disc disorders with radiculopathy, thoracic region**

     M51.15   **Intervertebral disc disorders with radiculopathy, thoracolumbar region**

     M51.16   **Intervertebral disc disorders with radiculopathy, lumbar region**

     M51.17   **Intervertebral disc disorders with radiculopathy, lumbosacral region**

☑ Additional Character Required   ☑x7ᵗʰ Placeholder Alert   Manifestation   <u>Unspecified Dx</u>   ►◄ Revised Text   ● New Code   ▲ Revised Code Title

Chapter 13. Diseases of the Musculoskeletal System and Connective Tissue

M51.2–M54.32

✓6ᵗʰ **M51.2** **Other thoracic, thoracolumbar and lumbosacral intervertebral disc** displacement
Lumbago due to displacement of intervertebral disc

Displacement Intervertebral Disc

Normal Top View   Herniated Top View

Lamina
Nucleus pulposus
Ligamentum flavum
Disc annulus
Nucleus pulposus
Spinal cord
Herniates through annulus
Spinal nerve

M51.24 **Other intervertebral disc displacement,** thoracic region

M51.25 **Other intervertebral disc displacement,** thoracolumbar **region**

M51.26 **Other intervertebral disc displacement,** lumbar region

M51.27 **Other intervertebral disc displacement,** lumbosacral region

✓5ᵗʰ **M51.3** **Other thoracic, thoracolumbar and lumbosacral intervertebral disc** degeneration
AHA: 2018,2Q,15; 2013,3Q,22

M51.34 **Other intervertebral disc degeneration,** thoracic region

M51.35 **Other intervertebral disc degeneration,** thoracolumbar **region**

M51.36 **Other intervertebral disc degeneration,** lumbar region

M51.37 **Other intervertebral disc degeneration,** lumbosacral **region**

✓5ᵗʰ **M51.4** **Schmorl's nodes**
DEF: Irregular bone defect in the margin of the vertebral body that causes herniation into the end plate of the vertebral body.

M51.44 **Schmorl's nodes,** thoracic **region**

M51.45 **Schmorl's nodes,** thoracolumbar **region**

M51.46 **Schmorl's nodes,** lumbar **region**

M51.47 **Schmorl's nodes,** lumbosacral **region**

✓5ᵗʰ **M51.8** **Other thoracic, thoracolumbar and lumbosacral intervertebral** disc disorders

M51.84 **Other intervertebral disc disorders,** thoracic **region**

M51.85 **Other intervertebral disc disorders,** thoracolumbar **region**

M51.86 **Other intervertebral disc disorders,** lumbar **region**

M51.87 **Other intervertebral disc disorders,** lumbosacral **region**

M51.9 **Unspecified thoracic, thoracolumbar and lumbosacral intervertebral disc disorder**

✓4ᵗʰ **M53** **Other and unspecified dorsopathies, not elsewhere classified**

M53.0 **Cervicocranial syndrome**
Posterior cervical sympathetic syndrome

M53.1 **Cervicobrachial syndrome**
EXCLUDES 2 cervical disc disorder (M50.-)
thoracic outlet syndrome (G54.0)

✓5ᵗʰ **M53.2** **Spinal instabilities**

✓6ᵗʰ **M53.2X** **Spinal** instabilities

M53.2X1 **Spinal instabilities,** occipito-atlanto-axial **region**

M53.2X2 **Spinal instabilities,** cervical **region**

M53.2X3 **Spinal instabilities,** cervicothoracic **region**

M53.2X4 **Spinal instabilities,** thoracic **region**

M53.2X5 **Spinal instabilities,** thoracolumbar **region**

M53.2X6 **Spinal instabilities,** lumbar **region**

M53.2X7 **Spinal instabilities,** lumbosacral **region**

M53.2X8 **Spinal instabilities,** sacral and sacrococcygeal **region**

M53.2X9 **Spinal instabilities,** site unspecified

M53.3 **Sacrococcygeal disorders, not elsewhere classified**
Coccygodynia

✓5ᵗʰ **M53.8** **Other specified** dorsopathies

M53.80 **Other specified dorsopathies, site unspecified**

M53.81 **Other specified dorsopathies,** occipito-atlanto-axial **region**

M53.82 **Other specified dorsopathies,** cervical **region**

M53.83 **Other specified dorsopathies,** cervicothoracic **region**

M53.84 **Other specified dorsopathies,** thoracic **region**

M53.85 **Other specified dorsopathies,** thoracolumbar **region**

M53.86 **Other specified dorsopathies,** lumbar **region**

M53.87 **Other specified dorsopathies,** lumbosacral **region**

M53.88 **Other specified dorsopathies,** sacral and sacrococcygeal **region**

M53.9 **Dorsopathy, unspecified**

✓4ᵗʰ **M54** **Dorsalgia**
EXCLUDES 1 psychogenic dorsalgia (F45.41)

✓5ᵗʰ **M54.0** **Panniculitis affecting regions of neck and back**
EXCLUDES 1 lupus panniculitis (L93.2)
panniculitis NOS (M79.3)
relapsing [Weber-Christian] panniculitis (M35.6)

M54.00 **Panniculitis affecting regions of neck and back, site unspecified**

M54.01 **Panniculitis affecting regions of neck and back,** occipito-atlanto-axial **region**

M54.02 **Panniculitis affecting regions of neck and back,** cervical **region**

M54.03 **Panniculitis affecting regions of neck and back,** cervicothoracic **region**

M54.04 **Panniculitis affecting regions of neck and back,** thoracic **region**

M54.05 **Panniculitis affecting regions of neck and back,** thoracolumbar **region**

M54.06 **Panniculitis affecting regions of neck and back,** lumbar **region**

M54.07 **Panniculitis affecting regions of neck and back,** lumbosacral **region**

M54.08 **Panniculitis affecting regions of neck and back,** sacral and sacrococcygeal **region**

M54.09 **Panniculitis affecting regions, neck and back,** multiple sites **in spine**

✓5ᵗʰ **M54.1** **Radiculopathy**
Brachial neuritis or radiculitis NOS
Lumbar neuritis or radiculitis NOS
Lumbosacral neuritis or radiculitis NOS
Thoracic neuritis or radiculitis NOS
Radiculitis NOS
EXCLUDES 1 neuralgia and neuritis NOS (M79.2)
radiculopathy with cervical disc disorder (M50.1)
radiculopathy with lumbar and other intervertebral disc disorder (M51.1-)
radiculopathy with spondylosis (M47.2-)
AHA: 2018,3Q,18
TIP: A code from this subcategory can be used in addition to a spondylolisthesis code (M43.1-) or a spinal stenosis code (M48.0-) when either condition is documented as the cause of the radiculopathy.

M54.10 **Radiculopathy, site unspecified**

M54.11 **Radiculopathy,** occipito-atlanto-axial **region**

M54.12 **Radiculopathy,** cervical **region**

M54.13 **Radiculopathy,** cervicothoracic **region**

M54.14 **Radiculopathy,** thoracic **region**

M54.15 **Radiculopathy,** thoracolumbar **region**

M54.16 **Radiculopathy,** lumbar **region**

M54.17 **Radiculopathy,** lumbosacral **region**

M54.18 **Radiculopathy,** sacral and sacrococcygeal **region**

M54.2 **Cervicalgia**
EXCLUDES 1 cervicalgia due to intervertebral cervical disc disorder (M50.-)

✓5ᵗʰ **M54.3** **Sciatica**
EXCLUDES 1 lesion of sciatic nerve (G57.0)
sciatica due to intervertebral disc disorder (M51.1-)
sciatica with lumbago (M54.4-)

M54.30 **Sciatica, unspecified side**

M54.31 **Sciatica,** right **side**

M54.32 **Sciatica,** left **side**

√5th **M54.4 Lumbago with sciatica**

> EXCLUDES 1   *lumbago with sciatica due to intervertebral disc disorder (M51.1-)*
>
> **AHA:** 2016,2Q,7

     M54.40 Lumbago with sciatica, unspecified side
     M54.41 Lumbago with sciatica, right side
     M54.42 Lumbago with sciatica, left side

M54.5 Low back pain
     Loin pain
     Lumbago NOS

> EXCLUDES 1   *low back strain (S39.012)*
> *lumbago due to intervertebral disc displacement (M51.2-)*
> *lumbago with sciatica (M54.4-)*

M54.6 Pain in thoracic spine

> EXCLUDES 1   *pain in thoracic spine due to intervertebral disc disorder (M51.-)*

√5th **M54.8 Other dorsalgia**

> EXCLUDES 1   *dorsalgia in thoracic region (M54.6)*
> *low back pain (M54.5)*

     M54.81 Occipital neuralgia
     M54.89 Other dorsalgia

M54.9 Dorsalgia, unspecified
     Backache NOS
     Back pain NOS

SOFT TISSUE DISORDERS (M60-M79)

Disorders of muscles (M60-M63)

> EXCLUDES 1   *dermatopolymyositis (M33.-)*
> *muscular dystrophies and myopathies (G71-G72)*
> *myopathy in amyloidosis (E85.-)*
> *myopathy in polyarteritis nodosa (M30.0)*
> *myopathy in rheumatoid arthritis (M05.32)*
> *myopathy in scleroderma (M34.-)*
> *myopathy in Sjögren's syndrome (M35.03)*
> *myopathy in systemic lupus erythematosus (M32.-)*

√4th **M60 Myositis**

> EXCLUDES 2   *inclusion body myositis [IBM] (G72.41)*

√5th **M60.0 Infective myositis**
     Tropical pyomyositis
     Use additional code (B95-B97) to identify infectious agent

√6th **M60.00 Infective myositis, unspecified site**

     M60.000 Infective myositis, unspecified right arm
         Infective myositis, right upper limb NOS
     M60.001 Infective myositis, unspecified left arm
         Infective myositis, left upper limb NOS
     M60.002 Infective myositis, unspecified arm
         Infective myositis, upper limb NOS
     M60.003 Infective myositis, unspecified right leg
         Infective myositis, right lower limb NOS
     M60.004 Infective myositis, unspecified left leg
         Infective myositis, left lower limb NOS
     M60.005 Infective myositis, unspecified leg
         Infective myositis, lower limb NOS
     M60.009 Infective myositis, unspecified site

√6th **M60.01 Infective myositis, shoulder**

     M60.011 Infective myositis, right shoulder
     M60.012 Infective myositis, left shoulder
     M60.019 Infective myositis, unspecified shoulder

√6th **M60.02 Infective myositis, upper arm**

     M60.021 Infective myositis, right upper arm
     M60.022 Infective myositis, left upper arm
     M60.029 Infective myositis, unspecified upper arm

√6th **M60.03 Infective myositis, forearm**

     M60.031 Infective myositis, right forearm
     M60.032 Infective myositis, left forearm
     M60.039 Infective myositis, unspecified forearm

√6th **M60.04 Infective myositis, hand and fingers**

     M60.041 Infective myositis, right hand
     M60.042 Infective myositis, left hand
     M60.043 Infective myositis, unspecified hand
     M60.044 Infective myositis, right finger(s)
     M60.045 Infective myositis, left finger(s)
     M60.046 Infective myositis, unspecified finger(s)

√6th **M60.05 Infective myositis, thigh**

     M60.051 Infective myositis, right thigh
     M60.052 Infective myositis, left thigh
     M60.059 Infective myositis, unspecified thigh

√6th **M60.06 Infective myositis, lower leg**

     M60.061 Infective myositis, right lower leg
     M60.062 Infective myositis, left lower leg
     M60.069 Infective myositis, unspecified lower leg

√6th **M60.07 Infective myositis, ankle, foot and toes**

     M60.070 Infective myositis, right ankle
     M60.071 Infective myositis, left ankle
     M60.072 Infective myositis, unspecified ankle
     M60.073 Infective myositis, right foot
     M60.074 Infective myositis, left foot
     M60.075 Infective myositis, unspecified foot
     M60.076 Infective myositis, right toe(s)
     M60.077 Infective myositis, left toe(s)
     M60.078 Infective myositis, unspecified toe(s)

     M60.08 Infective myositis, other site
     M60.09 Infective myositis, multiple sites

√5th **M60.1 Interstitial myositis**

     M60.10 Interstitial myositis of unspecified site

√6th **M60.11 Interstitial myositis, shoulder**

     M60.111 Interstitial myositis, right shoulder
     M60.112 Interstitial myositis, left shoulder
     M60.119 Interstitial myositis, unspecified shoulder

√6th **M60.12 Interstitial myositis, upper arm**

     M60.121 Interstitial myositis, right upper arm
     M60.122 Interstitial myositis, left upper arm
     M60.129 Interstitial myositis, unspecified upper arm

√6th **M60.13 Interstitial myositis, forearm**

     M60.131 Interstitial myositis, right forearm
     M60.132 Interstitial myositis, left forearm
     M60.139 Interstitial myositis, unspecified forearm

√6th **M60.14 Interstitial myositis, hand**

     M60.141 Interstitial myositis, right hand
     M60.142 Interstitial myositis, left hand
     M60.149 Interstitial myositis, unspecified hand

√6th **M60.15 Interstitial myositis, thigh**

     M60.151 Interstitial myositis, right thigh
     M60.152 Interstitial myositis, left thigh
     M60.159 Interstitial myositis, unspecified thigh

√6th **M60.16 Interstitial myositis, lower leg**

     M60.161 Interstitial myositis, right lower leg
     M60.162 Interstitial myositis, left lower leg
     M60.169 Interstitial myositis, unspecified lower leg

√6th **M60.17 Interstitial myositis, ankle and foot**

     M60.171 Interstitial myositis, right ankle and foot
     M60.172 Interstitial myositis, left ankle and foot
     M60.179 Interstitial myositis, unspecified ankle and foot

     M60.18 Interstitial myositis, other site
     M60.19 Interstitial myositis, multiple sites

√5th **M60.2 Foreign body granuloma of soft tissue, not elsewhere classified**
     Use additional code to identify the type of retained foreign body (Z18.-)

> EXCLUDES 1   *foreign body granuloma of skin and subcutaneous tissue (L92.3)*

     M60.20 Foreign body granuloma of soft tissue, not elsewhere classified, unspecified site

√6th **M60.21 Foreign body granuloma of soft tissue, not elsewhere classified, shoulder**

     M60.211 Foreign body granuloma of soft tissue, not elsewhere classified, right shoulder
     M60.212 Foreign body granuloma of soft tissue, not elsewhere classified, left shoulder
     M60.219 Foreign body granuloma of soft tissue, not elsewhere classified, unspecified shoulder

√6th **M60.22 Foreign body granuloma of soft tissue, not elsewhere classified, upper arm**

     M60.221 Foreign body granuloma of soft tissue, not elsewhere classified, right upper arm
     M60.222 Foreign body granuloma of soft tissue, not elsewhere classified, left upper arm

✔ Additional Character Required   √x7th Placeholder Alert   Manifestation   Unspecified Dx   ►◄ Revised Text   ● New Code   ▲ Revised Code Title

ICD-10-CM 2020   791

M60.229 Foreign body granuloma of soft tissue, not elsewhere classified, unspecified upper arm

✓6ᵗʰ M60.23 Foreign body granuloma of soft tissue, not elsewhere classified, forearm

M60.231 Foreign body granuloma of soft tissue, not elsewhere classified, right forearm

M60.232 Foreign body granuloma of soft tissue, not elsewhere classified, left forearm

M60.239 Foreign body granuloma of soft tissue, not elsewhere classified, unspecified forearm

✓6ᵗʰ M60.24 Foreign body granuloma of soft tissue, not elsewhere classified, hand

M60.241 Foreign body granuloma of soft tissue, not elsewhere classified, right hand

M60.242 Foreign body granuloma of soft tissue, not elsewhere classified, left hand

M60.249 Foreign body granuloma of soft tissue, not elsewhere classified, unspecified hand

✓6ᵗʰ M60.25 Foreign body granuloma of soft tissue, not elsewhere classified, thigh

M60.251 Foreign body granuloma of soft tissue, not elsewhere classified, right thigh

M60.252 Foreign body granuloma of soft tissue, not elsewhere classified, left thigh

M60.259 Foreign body granuloma of soft tissue, not elsewhere classified, unspecified thigh

✓6ᵗʰ M60.26 Foreign body granuloma of soft tissue, not elsewhere classified, lower leg

M60.261 Foreign body granuloma of soft tissue, not elsewhere classified, right lower leg

M60.262 Foreign body granuloma of soft tissue, not elsewhere classified, left lower leg

M60.269 Foreign body granuloma of soft tissue, not elsewhere classified, unspecified lower leg

✓6ᵗʰ M60.27 Foreign body granuloma of soft tissue, not elsewhere classified, ankle and foot

M60.271 Foreign body granuloma of soft tissue, not elsewhere classified, right ankle and foot

M60.272 Foreign body granuloma of soft tissue, not elsewhere classified, left ankle and foot

M60.279 Foreign body granuloma of soft tissue, not elsewhere classified, unspecified ankle and foot

M60.28 Foreign body granuloma of soft tissue, not elsewhere classified, other site

✓5ᵗʰ M60.8 Other myositis

M60.80 Other myositis, unspecified site

✓6ᵗʰ M60.81 Other myositis, shoulder

M60.811 Other myositis, right shoulder
M60.812 Other myositis, left shoulder
M60.819 Other myositis, unspecified shoulder

✓6ᵗʰ M60.82 Other myositis, upper arm

M60.821 Other myositis, right upper arm
M60.822 Other myositis, left upper arm
M60.829 Other myositis, unspecified upper arm

✓6ᵗʰ M60.83 Other myositis, forearm

M60.831 Other myositis, right forearm
M60.832 Other myositis, left forearm
M60.839 Other myositis, unspecified forearm

✓6ᵗʰ M60.84 Other myositis, hand

M60.841 Other myositis, right hand
M60.842 Other myositis, left hand
M60.849 Other myositis, unspecified hand

✓6ᵗʰ M60.85 Other myositis, thigh

M60.851 Other myositis, right thigh
M60.852 Other myositis, left thigh
M60.859 Other myositis, unspecified thigh

✓6ᵗʰ M60.86 Other myositis, lower leg

M60.861 Other myositis, right lower leg
M60.862 Other myositis, left lower leg
M60.869 Other myositis, unspecified lower leg

✓6ᵗʰ M60.87 Other myositis, ankle and foot

M60.871 Other myositis, right ankle and foot

M60.872 Other myositis, left ankle and foot

M60.879 Other myositis, unspecified ankle and foot

M60.88 Other myositis, other site
M60.89 Other myositis, multiple sites

M60.9 Myositis, unspecified

✓4ᵗʰ M61 Calcification and ossification of muscle

✓5ᵗʰ M61.0 Myositis ossificans traumatica

M61.00 Myositis ossificans traumatica, unspecified site

✓6ᵗʰ M61.01 Myositis ossificans traumatica, shoulder

M61.011 Myositis ossificans traumatica, right shoulder

M61.012 Myositis ossificans traumatica, left shoulder

M61.019 Myositis ossificans traumatica, unspecified shoulder

✓6ᵗʰ M61.02 Myositis ossificans traumatica, upper arm

M61.021 Myositis ossificans traumatica, right upper arm

M61.022 Myositis ossificans traumatica, left upper arm

M61.029 Myositis ossificans traumatica, unspecified upper arm

✓6ᵗʰ M61.03 Myositis ossificans traumatica, forearm

M61.031 Myositis ossificans traumatica, right forearm

M61.032 Myositis ossificans traumatica, left forearm

M61.039 Myositis ossificans traumatica, unspecified forearm

✓6ᵗʰ M61.04 Myositis ossificans traumatica, hand

M61.041 Myositis ossificans traumatica, right hand
M61.042 Myositis ossificans traumatica, left hand
M61.049 Myositis ossificans traumatica, unspecified hand

✓6ᵗʰ M61.05 Myositis ossificans traumatica, thigh

M61.051 Myositis ossificans traumatica, right thigh
M61.052 Myositis ossificans traumatica, left thigh
M61.059 Myositis ossificans traumatica, unspecified thigh

✓6ᵗʰ M61.06 Myositis ossificans traumatica, lower leg

M61.061 Myositis ossificans traumatica, right lower leg

M61.062 Myositis ossificans traumatica, left lower leg

M61.069 Myositis ossificans traumatica, unspecified lower leg

✓6ᵗʰ M61.07 Myositis ossificans traumatica, ankle and foot

M61.071 Myositis ossificans traumatica, right ankle and foot

M61.072 Myositis ossificans traumatica, left ankle and foot

M61.079 Myositis ossificans traumatica, unspecified ankle and foot

M61.08 Myositis ossificans traumatica, other site
M61.09 Myositis ossificans traumatica, multiple sites

✓5ᵗʰ M61.1 Myositis ossificans progressiva

Fibrodysplasia ossificans progressiva

M61.10 Myositis ossificans progressiva, unspecified site

✓6ᵗʰ M61.11 Myositis ossificans progressiva, shoulder

M61.111 Myositis ossificans progressiva, right shoulder

M61.112 Myositis ossificans progressiva, left shoulder

M61.119 Myositis ossificans progressiva, unspecified shoulder

✓6ᵗʰ M61.12 Myositis ossificans progressiva, upper arm

M61.121 Myositis ossificans progressiva, right upper arm

M61.122 Myositis ossificans progressiva, left upper arm

M61.129 Myositis ossificans progressiva, unspecified arm

✓6ᵗʰ M61.13 Myositis ossificans progressiva, forearm

M61.131 Myositis ossificans progressiva, right forearm

M61.132 Myositis ossificans progressiva, left forearm

M61.139 Myositis ossificans progressiva, unspecified forearm

☑6ᵗʰ **M61.14** Myositis ossificans progressiva, hand and finger(s)

M61.141 Myositis ossificans progressiva, right hand

M61.142 Myositis ossificans progressiva, left hand

M61.143 Myositis ossificans progressiva, unspecified hand

M61.144 Myositis ossificans progressiva, right finger(s)

M61.145 Myositis ossificans progressiva, left finger(s)

M61.146 Myositis ossificans progressiva, unspecified finger(s)

☑6ᵗʰ **M61.15** Myositis ossificans progressiva, thigh

M61.151 Myositis ossificans progressiva, right thigh

M61.152 Myositis ossificans progressiva, left thigh

M61.159 Myositis ossificans progressiva, unspecified thigh

☑6ᵗʰ **M61.16** Myositis ossificans progressiva, lower leg

M61.161 Myositis ossificans progressiva, right lower leg

M61.162 Myositis ossificans progressiva, left lower leg

M61.169 Myositis ossificans progressiva, unspecified lower leg

☑6ᵗʰ **M61.17** Myositis ossificans progressiva, ankle, foot and toe(s)

M61.171 Myositis ossificans progressiva, right ankle

M61.172 Myositis ossificans progressiva, left ankle

M61.173 Myositis ossificans progressiva, unspecified ankle

M61.174 Myositis ossificans progressiva, right foot

M61.175 Myositis ossificans progressiva, left foot

M61.176 Myositis ossificans progressiva, unspecified foot

M61.177 Myositis ossificans progressiva, right toe(s)

M61.178 Myositis ossificans progressiva, left toe(s)

M61.179 Myositis ossificans progressiva, unspecified toe(s)

M61.18 Myositis ossificans progressiva, other site

M61.19 Myositis ossificans progressiva, multiple sites

☑5ᵗʰ **M61.2** Paralytic calcification and ossification of muscle

Myositis ossificans associated with quadriplegia or paraplegia

M61.20 Paralytic calcification and ossification of muscle, unspecified site

☑6ᵗʰ **M61.21** Paralytic calcification and ossification of muscle, shoulder

M61.211 Paralytic calcification and ossification of muscle, right shoulder

M61.212 Paralytic calcification and ossification of muscle, left shoulder

M61.219 Paralytic calcification and ossification of muscle, unspecified shoulder

☑6ᵗʰ **M61.22** Paralytic calcification and ossification of muscle, upper arm

M61.221 Paralytic calcification and ossification of muscle, right upper arm

M61.222 Paralytic calcification and ossification of muscle, left upper arm

M61.229 Paralytic calcification and ossification of muscle, unspecified upper arm

☑6ᵗʰ **M61.23** Paralytic calcification and ossification of muscle, forearm

M61.231 Paralytic calcification and ossification of muscle, right forearm

M61.232 Paralytic calcification and ossification of muscle, left forearm

M61.239 Paralytic calcification and ossification of muscle, unspecified forearm

☑6ᵗʰ **M61.24** Paralytic calcification and ossification of muscle, hand

M61.241 Paralytic calcification and ossification of muscle, right hand

M61.242 Paralytic calcification and ossification of muscle, left hand

M61.249 Paralytic calcification and ossification of muscle, unspecified hand

☑6ᵗʰ **M61.25** Paralytic calcification and ossification of muscle, thigh

M61.251 Paralytic calcification and ossification of muscle, right thigh

M61.252 Paralytic calcification and ossification of muscle, left thigh

M61.259 Paralytic calcification and ossification of muscle, unspecified thigh

☑6ᵗʰ **M61.26** Paralytic calcification and ossification of muscle, lower leg

M61.261 Paralytic calcification and ossification of muscle, right lower leg

M61.262 Paralytic calcification and ossification of muscle, left lower leg

M61.269 Paralytic calcification and ossification of muscle, unspecified lower leg

☑6ᵗʰ **M61.27** Paralytic calcification and ossification of muscle, ankle and foot

M61.271 Paralytic calcification and ossification of muscle, right ankle and foot

M61.272 Paralytic calcification and ossification of muscle, left ankle and foot

M61.279 Paralytic calcification and ossification of muscle, unspecified ankle and foot

M61.28 Paralytic calcification and ossification of muscle, other site

M61.29 Paralytic calcification and ossification of muscle, multiple sites

☑5ᵗʰ **M61.3** Calcification and ossification of muscles associated with burns

Myositis ossificans associated with burns

M61.30 Calcification and ossification of muscles associated with burns, unspecified site

☑6ᵗʰ **M61.31** Calcification and ossification of muscles associated with burns, shoulder

M61.311 Calcification and ossification of muscles associated with burns, right shoulder

M61.312 Calcification and ossification of muscles associated with burns, left shoulder

M61.319 Calcification and ossification of muscles associated with burns, unspecified shoulder

☑6ᵗʰ **M61.32** Calcification and ossification of muscles associated with burns, upper arm

M61.321 Calcification and ossification of muscles associated with burns, right upper arm

M61.322 Calcification and ossification of muscles associated with burns, left upper arm

M61.329 Calcification and ossification of muscles associated with burns, unspecified upper arm

☑6ᵗʰ **M61.33** Calcification and ossification of muscles associated with burns, forearm

M61.331 Calcification and ossification of muscles associated with burns, right forearm

M61.332 Calcification and ossification of muscles associated with burns, left forearm

M61.339 Calcification and ossification of muscles associated with burns, unspecified forearm

☑6ᵗʰ **M61.34** Calcification and ossification of muscles associated with burns, hand

M61.341 Calcification and ossification of muscles associated with burns, right hand

M61.342 Calcification and ossification of muscles associated with burns, left hand

M61.349 Calcification and ossification of muscles associated with burns, unspecified hand

☑6ᵗʰ **M61.35** Calcification and ossification of muscles associated with burns, thigh

M61.351 Calcification and ossification of muscles associated with burns, right thigh

M61.352 Calcification and ossification of muscles associated with burns, left thigh

M61.359 Calcification and ossification of muscles associated with burns, unspecified thigh

☑6ᵗʰ **M61.36** Calcification and ossification of muscles associated with burns, lower leg

M61.361 Calcification and ossification of muscles associated with burns, right lower leg

M61.362 Calcification and ossification of muscles associated with burns, left lower leg

☑ Additional Character Required   ☑x7ᵗʰ Placeholder Alert   Manifestation   Unspecified Dx   ►◄ Revised Text   ● New Code   ▲ Revised Code Title

ICD-10-CM 2020   793

M61.369 Calcification and ossification of muscles associated with burns, unspecified lower leg

✓6ᵗʰ **M61.37** Calcification and ossification of muscles associated with burns, ankle and foot

　M61.371 Calcification and ossification of muscles associated with burns, right ankle and foot

　M61.372 Calcification and ossification of muscles associated with burns, left ankle and foot

　M61.379 Calcification and ossification of muscles associated with burns, unspecified ankle and foot

M61.38 Calcification and ossification of muscles associated with burns, other site

M61.39 Calcification and ossification of muscles associated with burns, multiple sites

✓5ᵗʰ **M61.4** Other calcification of muscle

　EXCLUDES 1　calcific tendinitis NOS (M65.2-)

　　　　calcific tendinitis of shoulder (M75.3)

M61.40 Other calcification of muscle, unspecified site

✓6ᵗʰ **M61.41** Other calcification of muscle, shoulder

　M61.411 Other calcification of muscle, right shoulder

　M61.412 Other calcification of muscle, left shoulder

　M61.419 Other calcification of muscle, unspecified shoulder

✓6ᵗʰ **M61.42** Other calcification of muscle, upper arm

　M61.421 Other calcification of muscle, right upper arm

　M61.422 Other calcification of muscle, left upper arm

　M61.429 Other calcification of muscle, unspecified upper arm

✓6ᵗʰ **M61.43** Other calcification of muscle, forearm

　M61.431 Other calcification of muscle, right forearm

　M61.432 Other calcification of muscle, left forearm

　M61.439 Other calcification of muscle, unspecified forearm

✓6ᵗʰ **M61.44** Other calcification of muscle, hand

　M61.441 Other calcification of muscle, right hand

　M61.442 Other calcification of muscle, left hand

　M61.449 Other calcification of muscle, unspecified hand

✓6ᵗʰ **M61.45** Other calcification of muscle, thigh

　M61.451 Other calcification of muscle, right thigh

　M61.452 Other calcification of muscle, left thigh

　M61.459 Other calcification of muscle, unspecified thigh

✓6ᵗʰ **M61.46** Other calcification of muscle, lower leg

　M61.461 Other calcification of muscle, right lower leg

　M61.462 Other calcification of muscle, left lower leg

　M61.469 Other calcification of muscle, unspecified lower leg

✓6ᵗʰ **M61.47** Other calcification of muscle, ankle and foot

　M61.471 Other calcification of muscle, right ankle and foot

　M61.472 Other calcification of muscle, left ankle and foot

　M61.479 Other calcification of muscle, unspecified ankle and foot

M61.48 Other calcification of muscle, other site

M61.49 Other calcification of muscle, multiple sites

✓5ᵗʰ **M61.5** Other ossification of muscle

M61.50 Other ossification of muscle, unspecified site

✓6ᵗʰ **M61.51** Other ossification of muscle, shoulder

　M61.511 Other ossification of muscle, right shoulder

　M61.512 Other ossification of muscle, left shoulder

　M61.519 Other ossification of muscle, unspecified shoulder

✓6ᵗʰ **M61.52** Other ossification of muscle, upper arm

　M61.521 Other ossification of muscle, right upper arm

　M61.522 Other ossification of muscle, left upper arm

　M61.529 Other ossification of muscle, unspecified upper arm

✓6ᵗʰ **M61.53** Other ossification of muscle, forearm

　M61.531 Other ossification of muscle, right forearm

　M61.532 Other ossification of muscle, left forearm

　M61.539 Other ossification of muscle, unspecified forearm

✓6ᵗʰ **M61.54** Other ossification of muscle, hand

　M61.541 Other ossification of muscle, right hand

　M61.542 Other ossification of muscle, left hand

　M61.549 Other ossification of muscle, unspecified hand

✓6ᵗʰ **M61.55** Other ossification of muscle, thigh

　M61.551 Other ossification of muscle, right thigh

　M61.552 Other ossification of muscle, left thigh

　M61.559 Other ossification of muscle, unspecified thigh

✓6ᵗʰ **M61.56** Other ossification of muscle, lower leg

　M61.561 Other ossification of muscle, right lower leg

　M61.562 Other ossification of muscle, left lower leg

　M61.569 Other ossification of muscle, unspecified lower leg

✓6ᵗʰ **M61.57** Other ossification of muscle, ankle and foot

　M61.571 Other ossification of muscle, right ankle and foot

　M61.572 Other ossification of muscle, left ankle and foot

　M61.579 Other ossification of muscle, unspecified ankle and foot

M61.58 Other ossification of muscle, other site

M61.59 Other ossification of muscle, multiple sites

M61.9 Calcification and ossification of muscle, unspecified

✓4ᵗʰ **M62** Other disorders of muscle

　EXCLUDES 1　alcoholic myopathy (G72.1)

　　　　cramp and spasm (R25.2)

　　　　drug-induced myopathy (G72.0)

　　　　myalgia (M79.1-)

　　　　stiff-man syndrome (G25.82)

　EXCLUDES 2　nontraumatic hematoma of muscle (M79.81)

✓5ᵗʰ **M62.0** Separation of muscle (nontraumatic)

　Diastasis of muscle

　EXCLUDES 1　diastasis recti complicating pregnancy, labor and delivery (O71.8)

　　　　traumatic separation of muscle — see strain of muscle by body region

M62.00 Separation of muscle (nontraumatic), unspecified site

✓6ᵗʰ **M62.01** Separation of muscle (nontraumatic), shoulder

　M62.011 Separation of muscle (nontraumatic), right shoulder

　M62.012 Separation of muscle (nontraumatic), left shoulder

　M62.019 Separation of muscle (nontraumatic), unspecified shoulder

✓6ᵗʰ **M62.02** Separation of muscle (nontraumatic), upper arm

　M62.021 Separation of muscle (nontraumatic), right upper arm

　M62.022 Separation of muscle (nontraumatic), left upper arm

　M62.029 Separation of muscle (nontraumatic), unspecified upper arm

✓6ᵗʰ **M62.03** Separation of muscle (nontraumatic), forearm

　M62.031 Separation of muscle (nontraumatic), right forearm

　M62.032 Separation of muscle (nontraumatic), left forearm

　M62.039 Separation of muscle (nontraumatic), unspecified forearm

✓6ᵗʰ **M62.04** Separation of muscle (nontraumatic), hand

　M62.041 Separation of muscle (nontraumatic), right hand

　M62.042 Separation of muscle (nontraumatic), left hand

M62.049 **Separation of muscle (nontraumatic), unspecified hand**

√6th M62.05 **Separation of muscle (nontraumatic),** thigh

    M62.051 **Separation of muscle (nontraumatic), right thigh**

    M62.052 **Separation of muscle (nontraumatic), left thigh**

    M62.059 **Separation of muscle (nontraumatic), unspecified thigh**

√6th M62.06 **Separation of muscle (nontraumatic),** lower leg

    M62.061 **Separation of muscle (nontraumatic), right lower leg**

    M62.062 **Separation of muscle (nontraumatic), left lower leg**

    M62.069 **Separation of muscle (nontraumatic), unspecified lower leg**

√6th M62.07 **Separation of muscle (nontraumatic),** ankle and foot

    M62.071 **Separation of muscle (nontraumatic), right ankle and foot**

    M62.072 **Separation of muscle (nontraumatic), left ankle and foot**

    M62.079 **Separation of muscle (nontraumatic), unspecified ankle and foot**

M62.08 **Separation of muscle (nontraumatic), other site**

√5th M62.1 **Other rupture of muscle (nontraumatic)**

    EXCLUDES 1   *traumatic rupture of muscle — see strain of muscle by body region*

    EXCLUDES 2   *rupture of tendon (M66.-)*

M62.10 **Other rupture of muscle (nontraumatic), unspecified site**

√6th M62.11 **Other rupture of muscle (nontraumatic),** shoulder

    M62.111 **Other rupture of muscle (nontraumatic), right shoulder**

    M62.112 **Other rupture of muscle (nontraumatic), left shoulder**

    M62.119 **Other rupture of muscle (nontraumatic), unspecified shoulder**

√6th M62.12 **Other rupture of muscle (nontraumatic),** upper arm

    M62.121 **Other rupture of muscle (nontraumatic), right upper arm**

    M62.122 **Other rupture of muscle (nontraumatic), left upper arm**

    M62.129 **Other rupture of muscle (nontraumatic), unspecified upper arm**

√6th M62.13 **Other rupture of muscle (nontraumatic),** forearm

    M62.131 **Other rupture of muscle (nontraumatic), right forearm**

    M62.132 **Other rupture of muscle (nontraumatic), left forearm**

    M62.139 **Other rupture of muscle (nontraumatic), unspecified forearm**

√6th M62.14 **Other rupture of muscle (nontraumatic),** hand

    M62.141 **Other rupture of muscle (nontraumatic), right hand**

    M62.142 **Other rupture of muscle (nontraumatic), left hand**

    M62.149 **Other rupture of muscle (nontraumatic), unspecified hand**

√6th M62.15 **Other rupture of muscle (nontraumatic),** thigh

    M62.151 **Other rupture of muscle (nontraumatic), right thigh**

    M62.152 **Other rupture of muscle (nontraumatic), left thigh**

    M62.159 **Other rupture of muscle (nontraumatic), unspecified thigh**

√6th M62.16 **Other rupture of muscle (nontraumatic),** lower leg

    M62.161 **Other rupture of muscle (nontraumatic), right lower leg**

    M62.162 **Other rupture of muscle (nontraumatic), left lower leg**

    M62.169 **Other rupture of muscle (nontraumatic), unspecified lower leg**

√6th M62.17 **Other rupture of muscle (nontraumatic),** ankle and foot

    M62.171 **Other rupture of muscle (nontraumatic), right ankle and foot**

    M62.172 **Other rupture of muscle (nontraumatic), left ankle and foot**

M62.179 **Other rupture of muscle (nontraumatic), unspecified ankle and foot**

M62.18 **Other rupture of muscle (nontraumatic), other site**

√5th M62.2 **Nontraumatic ischemic infarction of muscle**

    EXCLUDES 1   *compartment syndrome (traumatic) (T79.A-)*
        nontraumatic compartment syndrome (M79.A-)
        rhabdomyolysis (M62.82)
        traumatic ischemia of muscle (T79.6)
        Volkmann's ischemic contracture (T79.6)

M62.20 **Nontraumatic ischemic infarction of muscle, unspecified site**

√6th M62.21 **Nontraumatic ischemic infarction of muscle, shoulder**

    M62.211 **Nontraumatic ischemic infarction of muscle, right shoulder**

    M62.212 **Nontraumatic ischemic infarction of muscle, left shoulder**

    M62.219 **Nontraumatic ischemic infarction of muscle, unspecified shoulder**

√6th M62.22 **Nontraumatic ischemic infarction of muscle,** upper arm

    M62.221 **Nontraumatic ischemic infarction of muscle, right upper arm**

    M62.222 **Nontraumatic ischemic infarction of muscle, left upper arm**

    M62.229 **Nontraumatic ischemic infarction of muscle, unspecified upper arm**

√6th M62.23 **Nontraumatic ischemic infarction of muscle, forearm**

    M62.231 **Nontraumatic ischemic infarction of muscle, right forearm**

    M62.232 **Nontraumatic ischemic infarction of muscle, left forearm**

    M62.239 **Nontraumatic ischemic infarction of muscle, unspecified forearm**

√6th M62.24 **Nontraumatic ischemic infarction of muscle,** hand

    M62.241 **Nontraumatic ischemic infarction of muscle, right hand**

    M62.242 **Nontraumatic ischemic infarction of muscle, left hand**

    M62.249 **Nontraumatic ischemic infarction of muscle, unspecified hand**

√6th M62.25 **Nontraumatic ischemic infarction of muscle,** thigh

    M62.251 **Nontraumatic ischemic infarction of muscle, right thigh**

    M62.252 **Nontraumatic ischemic infarction of muscle, left thigh**

    M62.259 **Nontraumatic ischemic infarction of muscle, unspecified thigh**

√6th M62.26 **Nontraumatic ischemic infarction of muscle,** lower leg

    M62.261 **Nontraumatic ischemic infarction of muscle, right lower leg**

    M62.262 **Nontraumatic ischemic infarction of muscle, left lower leg**

    M62.269 **Nontraumatic ischemic infarction of muscle, unspecified lower leg**

√6th M62.27 **Nontraumatic ischemic infarction of muscle,** ankle and foot

    M62.271 **Nontraumatic ischemic infarction of muscle, right ankle and foot**

    M62.272 **Nontraumatic ischemic infarction of muscle, left ankle and foot**

    M62.279 **Nontraumatic ischemic infarction of muscle, unspecified ankle and foot**

M62.28 **Nontraumatic ischemic infarction of muscle, other site**

M62.3 **Immobility syndrome (paraplegic)**

√5th M62.4 **Contracture of muscle**

    Contracture of tendon (sheath)

    EXCLUDES 1   *contracture of joint (M24.5-)*

M62.40 **Contracture of muscle, unspecified site**

√6th M62.41 **Contracture of muscle,** shoulder

    M62.411 **Contracture of muscle, right shoulder**
    M62.412 **Contracture of muscle, left shoulder**
    M62.419 **Contracture of muscle, unspecified shoulder**

√6th M62.42 **Contracture of muscle,** upper arm

    M62.421 **Contracture of muscle, right upper arm**
    M62.422 **Contracture of muscle, left upper arm**

☑ Additional Character Required   √x7th Placeholder Alert   Manifestation   Unspecified Dx   ►◄ Revised Text   ● New Code   ▲ Revised Code Title

ICD-10-CM 2020   **795**

M62.429 Contracture of muscle, unspecified upper arm

✓6ᵗʰ **M62.43** Contracture of muscle, forearm

M62.431 Contracture of muscle, right forearm
M62.432 Contracture of muscle, left forearm
M62.439 Contracture of muscle, unspecified forearm

✓6ᵗʰ **M62.44** Contracture of muscle, hand

M62.441 Contracture of muscle, right hand
M62.442 Contracture of muscle, left hand
M62.449 Contracture of muscle, unspecified hand

✓6ᵗʰ **M62.45** Contracture of muscle, thigh

M62.451 Contracture of muscle, right thigh
M62.452 Contracture of muscle, left thigh
M62.459 Contracture of muscle, unspecified thigh

✓6ᵗʰ **M62.46** Contracture of muscle, lower leg

M62.461 Contracture of muscle, right lower leg
M62.462 Contracture of muscle, left lower leg
M62.469 Contracture of muscle, unspecified lower leg

✓6ᵗʰ **M62.47** Contracture of muscle, ankle and foot

M62.471 Contracture of muscle, right ankle and foot
M62.472 Contracture of muscle, left ankle and foot
M62.479 Contracture of muscle, unspecified ankle and foot

M62.48 Contracture of muscle, other site
M62.49 Contracture of muscle, multiple sites

✓6ᵗʰ **M62.5** Muscle wasting and atrophy, not elsewhere classified

Disuse atrophy NEC

EXCLUDES 1   neuralgic amyotrophy (G54.5)
      progressive muscular atrophy (G12.21)
      sarcopenia (M62.84)

EXCLUDES 2   pelvic muscle wasting (N81.84)

M62.50 Muscle wasting and atrophy, not elsewhere classified, unspecified site

✓6ᵗʰ **M62.51** Muscle wasting and atrophy, not elsewhere classified, shoulder

M62.511 Muscle wasting and atrophy, not elsewhere classified, right shoulder
M62.512 Muscle wasting and atrophy, not elsewhere classified, left shoulder
M62.519 Muscle wasting and atrophy, not elsewhere classified, unspecified shoulder

✓6ᵗʰ **M62.52** Muscle wasting and atrophy, not elsewhere classified, upper arm

M62.521 Muscle wasting and atrophy, not elsewhere classified, right upper arm
M62.522 Muscle wasting and atrophy, not elsewhere classified, left upper arm
M62.529 Muscle wasting and atrophy, not elsewhere classified, unspecified upper arm

✓6ᵗʰ **M62.53** Muscle wasting and atrophy, not elsewhere classified, forearm

M62.531 Muscle wasting and atrophy, not elsewhere classified, right forearm
M62.532 Muscle wasting and atrophy, not elsewhere classified, left forearm
M62.539 Muscle wasting and atrophy, not elsewhere classified, unspecified forearm

✓6ᵗʰ **M62.54** Muscle wasting and atrophy, not elsewhere classified, hand

M62.541 Muscle wasting and atrophy, not elsewhere classified, right hand
M62.542 Muscle wasting and atrophy, not elsewhere classified, left hand
M62.549 Muscle wasting and atrophy, not elsewhere classified, unspecified hand

✓6ᵗʰ **M62.55** Muscle wasting and atrophy, not elsewhere classified, thigh

M62.551 Muscle wasting and atrophy, not elsewhere classified, right thigh
M62.552 Muscle wasting and atrophy, not elsewhere classified, left thigh
M62.559 Muscle wasting and atrophy, not elsewhere classified, unspecified thigh

✓6ᵗʰ **M62.56** Muscle wasting and atrophy, not elsewhere classified, lower leg

M62.561 Muscle wasting and atrophy, not elsewhere classified, right lower leg
M62.562 Muscle wasting and atrophy, not elsewhere classified, left lower leg
M62.569 Muscle wasting and atrophy, not elsewhere classified, unspecified lower leg

✓6ᵗʰ **M62.57** Muscle wasting and atrophy, not elsewhere classified, ankle and foot

M62.571 Muscle wasting and atrophy, not elsewhere classified, right ankle and foot
M62.572 Muscle wasting and atrophy, not elsewhere classified, left ankle and foot
M62.579 Muscle wasting and atrophy, not elsewhere classified, unspecified ankle and foot

M62.58 Muscle wasting and atrophy, not elsewhere classified, other site
M62.59 Muscle wasting and atrophy, not elsewhere classified, multiple sites

✓5ᵗʰ **M62.8** Other specified disorders of muscle

EXCLUDES 2   nontraumatic hematoma of muscle (M79.81)

M62.81 Muscle weakness (generalized)

EXCLUDES 1   muscle weakness in sarcopenia (M62.84)

M62.82 Rhabdomyolysis

EXCLUDES 1   traumatic rhabdomyolysis (T79.6)

AHA: 2019,2Q,12

DEF: Rapid disintegration or destruction of skeletal muscle caused by direct or indirect injury, resulting in the excretion of muscle protein myoglobin into the urine.

✓6ᵗʰ **M62.83** Muscle spasm

M62.830 Muscle spasm of back
M62.831 Muscle spasm of calf

Charley-horse

M62.838 Other muscle spasm

M62.84 Sarcopenia

Age-related sarcopenia
Code first underlying disease, if applicable, such as:
    disorders of myoneural junction and muscle disease in diseases classified elsewhere (G73.-)
    other and unspecified myopathies (G72.-)
    primary disorders of muscles (G71.-)

AHA: 2016,4Q,41

M62.89 Other specified disorders of muscle

Muscle (sheath) hernia

M62.9 Disorder of muscle, unspecified

✓4ᵗʰ **M63** Disorders of muscle in diseases classified elsewhere

Code first underlying disease, such as:
    leprosy (A30.-)
    neoplasm (C49.-, C79.89, D21.-, D48.1)
    schistosomiasis (B65.-)
    trichinellosis (B75)

EXCLUDES 1   myopathy in cysticercosis (B69.81)
      myopathy in endocrine diseases (G73.7)
      myopathy in metabolic diseases (G73.7)
      myopathy in sarcoidosis (D86.87)
      myopathy in secondary syphilis (A51.49)
      myopathy in syphilis (late) (A52.78)
      myopathy in toxoplasmosis (B58.82)
      myopathy in tuberculosis (A18.09)

✓5ᵗʰ **M63.8** Disorders of muscle in diseases classified elsewhere

M63.80 *Disorders of muscle in diseases classified elsewhere, unspecified site*

✓6ᵗʰ **M63.81** Disorders of muscle in diseases classified elsewhere, shoulder

M63.811 *Disorders of muscle in diseases classified elsewhere, right shoulder*
M63.812 *Disorders of muscle in diseases classified elsewhere, left shoulder*
M63.819 *Disorders of muscle in diseases classified elsewhere, unspecified shoulder*

✓6ᵗʰ **M63.82** Disorders of muscle in diseases classified elsewhere, upper arm

M63.821 *Disorders of muscle in diseases classified elsewhere, right upper arm*

M63.822   *Disorders of muscle in diseases classified elsewhere, left upper arm*

M63.829   *Disorders of muscle in diseases classified elsewhere, unspecified upper arm*

√6ᵗʰ   **M63.83**   Disorders of muscle in diseases classified elsewhere, forearm

     M63.831   *Disorders of muscle in diseases classified elsewhere, right forearm*

     M63.832   *Disorders of muscle in diseases classified elsewhere, left forearm*

     M63.839   *Disorders of muscle in diseases classified elsewhere, unspecified forearm*

√6ᵗʰ   **M63.84**   Disorders of muscle in diseases classified elsewhere, hand

     M63.841   *Disorders of muscle in diseases classified elsewhere, right hand*

     M63.842   *Disorders of muscle in diseases classified elsewhere, left hand*

     M63.849   *Disorders of muscle in diseases classified elsewhere, unspecified hand*

√6ᵗʰ   **M63.85**   Disorders of muscle in diseases classified elsewhere, thigh

     M63.851   *Disorders of muscle in diseases classified elsewhere, right thigh*

     M63.852   *Disorders of muscle in diseases classified elsewhere, left thigh*

     M63.859   *Disorders of muscle in diseases classified elsewhere, unspecified thigh*

√6ᵗʰ   **M63.86**   Disorders of muscle in diseases classified elsewhere, lower leg

     M63.861   *Disorders of muscle in diseases classified elsewhere, right lower leg*

     M63.862   *Disorders of muscle in diseases classified elsewhere, left lower leg*

     M63.869   *Disorders of muscle in diseases classified elsewhere, unspecified lower leg*

√6ᵗʰ   **M63.87**   Disorders of muscle in diseases classified elsewhere, ankle and foot

     M63.871   *Disorders of muscle in diseases classified elsewhere, right ankle and foot*

     M63.872   *Disorders of muscle in diseases classified elsewhere, left ankle and foot*

     M63.879   *Disorders of muscle in diseases classified elsewhere, unspecified ankle and foot*

   M63.88   *Disorders of muscle in diseases classified elsewhere, other site*

   M63.89   *Disorders of muscle in diseases classified elsewhere, multiple sites*

Disorders of synovium and tendon (M65-M67)

√4ᵗʰ   **M65**   **Synovitis and tenosynovitis**

     EXCLUDES 1   *chronic crepitant synovitis of hand and wrist (M70.0-)*

          current injury — see injury of ligament or tendon by body region

          soft tissue disorders related to use, overuse and pressure (M70.-)

√5ᵗʰ   **M65.0**   **Abscess of tendon sheath**

     Use additional code (B95-B96) to identify bacterial agent.

     M65.00   **Abscess of tendon sheath, unspecified site**

√6ᵗʰ   **M65.01**   **Abscess of tendon sheath, shoulder**

     M65.011   Abscess of tendon sheath, right shoulder

     M65.012   Abscess of tendon sheath, left shoulder

     M65.019   Abscess of tendon sheath, unspecified shoulder

√6ᵗʰ   **M65.02**   **Abscess of tendon sheath, upper arm**

     M65.021   Abscess of tendon sheath, right upper arm

     M65.022   Abscess of tendon sheath, left upper arm

     M65.029   Abscess of tendon sheath, unspecified upper arm

√6ᵗʰ   **M65.03**   **Abscess of tendon sheath, forearm**

     M65.031   Abscess of tendon sheath, right forearm

     M65.032   Abscess of tendon sheath, left forearm

     M65.039   Abscess of tendon sheath, unspecified forearm

√6ᵗʰ   **M65.04**   **Abscess of tendon sheath, hand**

     M65.041   Abscess of tendon sheath, right hand

     M65.042   Abscess of tendon sheath, left hand

     M65.049   Abscess of tendon sheath, unspecified hand

√6ᵗʰ   **M65.05**   **Abscess of tendon sheath, thigh**

     M65.051   Abscess of tendon sheath, right thigh

     M65.052   Abscess of tendon sheath, left thigh

     M65.059   Abscess of tendon sheath, unspecified thigh

√6ᵗʰ   **M65.06**   **Abscess of tendon sheath, lower leg**

     M65.061   Abscess of tendon sheath, right lower leg

     M65.062   Abscess of tendon sheath, left lower leg

     M65.069   Abscess of tendon sheath, unspecified lower leg

√6ᵗʰ   **M65.07**   **Abscess of tendon sheath, ankle and foot**

     M65.071   Abscess of tendon sheath, right ankle and foot

     M65.072   Abscess of tendon sheath, left ankle and foot

     M65.079   Abscess of tendon sheath, unspecified ankle and foot

   M65.08   Abscess of tendon sheath, other site

√6ᵗʰ   **M65.1**   **Other infective (teno)synovitis**

     M65.10   **Other infective (teno)synovitis, unspecified site**

√6ᵗʰ   **M65.11**   **Other infective (teno)synovitis, shoulder**

     M65.111   Other infective (teno)synovitis, right shoulder

     M65.112   Other infective (teno)synovitis, left shoulder

     M65.119   Other infective (teno)synovitis, unspecified shoulder

√6ᵗʰ   **M65.12**   **Other infective (teno)synovitis, elbow**

     M65.121   Other infective (teno)synovitis, right elbow

     M65.122   Other infective (teno)synovitis, left elbow

     M65.129   Other infective (teno)synovitis, unspecified elbow

√6ᵗʰ   **M65.13**   **Other infective (teno)synovitis, wrist**

     M65.131   Other infective (teno)synovitis, right wrist

     M65.132   Other infective (teno)synovitis, left wrist

     M65.139   Other infective (teno)synovitis, unspecified wrist

√6ᵗʰ   **M65.14**   **Other infective (teno)synovitis, hand**

     M65.141   Other infective (teno)synovitis, right hand

     M65.142   Other infective (teno)synovitis, left hand

     M65.149   Other infective (teno)synovitis, unspecified hand

√6ᵗʰ   **M65.15**   **Other infective (teno)synovitis, hip**

     M65.151   Other infective (teno)synovitis, right hip

     M65.152   Other infective (teno)synovitis, left hip

     M65.159   Other infective (teno)synovitis, unspecified hip

√6ᵗʰ   **M65.16**   **Other infective (teno)synovitis, knee**

     M65.161   Other infective (teno)synovitis, right knee

     M65.162   Other infective (teno)synovitis, left knee

     M65.169   Other infective (teno)synovitis, unspecified knee

√6ᵗʰ   **M65.17**   **Other infective (teno)synovitis, ankle and foot**

     M65.171   Other infective (teno)synovitis, right ankle and foot

     M65.172   Other infective (teno)synovitis, left ankle and foot

     M65.179   Other infective (teno)synovitis, unspecified ankle and foot

   M65.18   Other infective (teno)synovitis, other site

   M65.19   Other infective (teno)synovitis, multiple sites

√5ᵗʰ   **M65.2**   **Calcific tendinitis**

     EXCLUDES 1   *tendinitis as classified in M75-M77*

          calcified tendinitis of shoulder (M75.3)

     M65.20   **Calcific tendinitis, unspecified site**

√6ᵗʰ   **M65.22**   **Calcific tendinitis, upper arm**

     M65.221   Calcific tendinitis, right upper arm

     M65.222   Calcific tendinitis, left upper arm

     M65.229   Calcific tendinitis, unspecified upper arm

√6ᵗʰ   **M65.23**   **Calcific tendinitis, forearm**

     M65.231   Calcific tendinitis, right forearm

     M65.232   Calcific tendinitis, left forearm

     M65.239   Calcific tendinitis, unspecified forearm

√6ᵗʰ   **M65.24**   **Calcific tendinitis, hand**

     M65.241   Calcific tendinitis, right hand

☑ Additional Character Required   √ˣ7ᵗʰ Placeholder Alert   Manifestation   Unspecified Dx   ◄► Revised Text   ● New Code   ▲ Revised Code Title

ICD 10 CM 2020   **797**

M65.242   Calcific tendinitis, left hand
M65.249   Calcific tendinitis, unspecified hand

✓6ᵗʰ   M65.25   Calcific tendinitis, thigh

M65.251   Calcific tendinitis, right thigh
M65.252   Calcific tendinitis, left thigh
M65.259   Calcific tendinitis, unspecified thigh

✓6ᵗʰ   M65.26   Calcific tendinitis, lower leg

M65.261   Calcific tendinitis, right lower leg
M65.262   Calcific tendinitis, left lower leg
M65.269   Calcific tendinitis, unspecified lower leg

✓6ᵗʰ   M65.27   Calcific tendinitis, ankle and foot

M65.271   Calcific tendinitis, right ankle and foot
M65.272   Calcific tendinitis, left ankle and foot
M65.279   Calcific tendinitis, unspecified ankle and foot

M65.28   Calcific tendinitis, other site
M65.29   Calcific tendinitis, multiple sites

✓5ᵗʰ   M65.3   Trigger finger
     Nodular tendinous disease

M65.30   Trigger finger, unspecified finger

✓6ᵗʰ   M65.31   Trigger thumb

M65.311   Trigger thumb, right thumb
M65.312   Trigger thumb, left thumb
M65.319   Trigger thumb, unspecified thumb

✓6ᵗʰ   M65.32   Trigger finger, index finger

M65.321   Trigger finger, right index finger
M65.322   Trigger finger, left index finger
M65.329   Trigger finger, unspecified index finger

✓6ᵗʰ   M65.33   Trigger finger, middle finger

M65.331   Trigger finger, right middle finger
M65.332   Trigger finger, left middle finger
M65.339   Trigger finger, unspecified middle finger

✓6ᵗʰ   M65.34   Trigger finger, ring finger

M65.341   Trigger finger, right ring finger
M65.342   Trigger finger, left ring finger
M65.349   Trigger finger, unspecified ring finger

✓6ᵗʰ   M65.35   Trigger finger, little finger

M65.351   Trigger finger, right little finger
M65.352   Trigger finger, left little finger
M65.359   Trigger finger, unspecified little finger

M65.4   Radial styloid tenosynovitis [de Quervain]

✓5ᵗʰ   M65.8   Other synovitis and tenosynovitis

M65.80   Other synovitis and tenosynovitis, unspecified site

✓6ᵗʰ   M65.81   Other synovitis and tenosynovitis, shoulder

M65.811   Other synovitis and tenosynovitis, right shoulder
M65.812   Other synovitis and tenosynovitis, left shoulder
M65.819   Other synovitis and tenosynovitis, unspecified shoulder

✓6ᵗʰ   M65.82   Other synovitis and tenosynovitis, upper arm

M65.821   Other synovitis and tenosynovitis, right upper arm
M65.822   Other synovitis and tenosynovitis, left upper arm
M65.829   Other synovitis and tenosynovitis, unspecified upper arm

✓6ᵗʰ   M65.83   Other synovitis and tenosynovitis, forearm

M65.831   Other synovitis and tenosynovitis, right forearm
M65.832   Other synovitis and tenosynovitis, left forearm
M65.839   Other synovitis and tenosynovitis, unspecified forearm

✓6ᵗʰ   M65.84   Other synovitis and tenosynovitis, hand

M65.841   Other synovitis and tenosynovitis, right hand
M65.842   Other synovitis and tenosynovitis, left hand
M65.849   Other synovitis and tenosynovitis, unspecified hand

✓6ᵗʰ   M65.85   Other synovitis and tenosynovitis, thigh

M65.851   Other synovitis and tenosynovitis, right thigh
M65.852   Other synovitis and tenosynovitis, left thigh

M65.859   Other synovitis and tenosynovitis, unspecified thigh

✓6ᵗʰ   M65.86   Other synovitis and tenosynovitis, lower leg

M65.861   Other synovitis and tenosynovitis, right lower leg
M65.862   Other synovitis and tenosynovitis, left lower leg
M65.869   Other synovitis and tenosynovitis, unspecified lower leg

✓6ᵗʰ   M65.87   Other synovitis and tenosynovitis, ankle and foot

M65.871   Other synovitis and tenosynovitis, right ankle and foot
M65.872   Other synovitis and tenosynovitis, left ankle and foot
M65.879   Other synovitis and tenosynovitis, unspecified ankle and foot

M65.88   Other synovitis and tenosynovitis, other site
M65.89   Other synovitis and tenosynovitis, multiple sites

M65.9   Synovitis and tenosynovitis, unspecified

✓4ᵗʰ   **M66   Spontaneous rupture of synovium and tendon**

INCLUDES   rupture that occurs when a normal force is applied to tissues that are inferred to have less than normal strength

EXCLUDES 2   rotator cuff syndrome (M75.1-)

     rupture where an abnormal force is applied to normal tissue — see injury of tendon by body region

M66.0   Rupture of popliteal cyst

✓5ᵗʰ   M66.1   Rupture of synovium
     Rupture of synovial cyst

EXCLUDES 2   rupture of popliteal cyst (M66.0)

M66.10   Rupture of synovium, unspecified joint

✓6ᵗʰ   M66.11   Rupture of synovium, shoulder

M66.111   Rupture of synovium, right shoulder
M66.112   Rupture of synovium, left shoulder
M66.119   Rupture of synovium, unspecified shoulder

✓6ᵗʰ   M66.12   Rupture of synovium, elbow

M66.121   Rupture of synovium, right elbow
M66.122   Rupture of synovium, left elbow
M66.129   Rupture of synovium, unspecified elbow

✓6ᵗʰ   M66.13   Rupture of synovium, wrist

M66.131   Rupture of synovium, right wrist
M66.132   Rupture of synovium, left wrist
M66.139   Rupture of synovium, unspecified wrist

✓6ᵗʰ   M66.14   Rupture of synovium, hand and fingers

M66.141   Rupture of synovium, right hand
M66.142   Rupture of synovium, left hand
M66.143   Rupture of synovium, unspecified hand
M66.144   Rupture of synovium, right finger(s)
M66.145   Rupture of synovium, left finger(s)
M66.146   Rupture of synovium, unspecified finger(s)

✓6ᵗʰ   M66.15   Rupture of synovium, hip

M66.151   Rupture of synovium, right hip
M66.152   Rupture of synovium, left hip
M66.159   Rupture of synovium, unspecified hip

✓6ᵗʰ   M66.17   Rupture of synovium, ankle, foot and toes

M66.171   Rupture of synovium, right ankle
M66.172   Rupture of synovium, left ankle
M66.173   Rupture of synovium, unspecified ankle
M66.174   Rupture of synovium, right foot
M66.175   Rupture of synovium, left foot
M66.176   Rupture of synovium, unspecified foot
M66.177   Rupture of synovium, right toe(s)
M66.178   Rupture of synovium, left toe(s)
M66.179   Rupture of synovium, unspecified toe(s)

M66.18   Rupture of synovium, other site

✓5ᵗʰ   M66.2   Spontaneous rupture of extensor tendons

TIP: Refer to the Muscle/Tendon table at the beginning of this chapter.

M66.20   Spontaneous rupture of extensor tendons, unspecified site

✓6ᵗʰ   M66.21   Spontaneous rupture of extensor tendons, shoulder

M66.211   Spontaneous rupture of extensor tendons, right shoulder
M66.212   Spontaneous rupture of extensor tendons, left shoulder

M66.219 Spontaneous rupture of extensor tendons, unspecified shoulder

☑6ᵗʰ **M66.22** Spontaneous rupture of extensor tendons, upper arm

M66.221 Spontaneous rupture of extensor tendons, right upper arm

M66.222 Spontaneous rupture of extensor tendons, left upper arm

M66.229 Spontaneous rupture of extensor tendons, unspecified upper arm

☑6ᵗʰ **M66.23** Spontaneous rupture of extensor tendons, forearm

M66.231 Spontaneous rupture of extensor tendons, right forearm

M66.232 Spontaneous rupture of extensor tendons, left forearm

M66.239 Spontaneous rupture of extensor tendons, unspecified forearm

☑6ᵗʰ **M66.24** Spontaneous rupture of extensor tendons, hand

M66.241 Spontaneous rupture of extensor tendons, right hand

M66.242 Spontaneous rupture of extensor tendons, left hand

M66.249 Spontaneous rupture of extensor tendons, unspecified hand

☑6ᵗʰ **M66.25** Spontaneous rupture of extensor tendons, thigh

M66.251 Spontaneous rupture of extensor tendons, right thigh

M66.252 Spontaneous rupture of extensor tendons, left thigh

M66.259 Spontaneous rupture of extensor tendons, unspecified thigh

☑6ᵗʰ **M66.26** Spontaneous rupture of extensor tendons, lower leg

M66.261 Spontaneous rupture of extensor tendons, right lower leg

M66.262 Spontaneous rupture of extensor tendons, left lower leg

M66.269 Spontaneous rupture of extensor tendons, unspecified lower leg

☑6ᵗʰ **M66.27** Spontaneous rupture of extensor tendons, ankle and foot

M66.271 Spontaneous rupture of extensor tendons, right ankle and foot

M66.272 Spontaneous rupture of extensor tendons, left ankle and foot

M66.279 Spontaneous rupture of extensor tendons, unspecified ankle and foot

M66.28 Spontaneous rupture of extensor tendons, other site

M66.29 Spontaneous rupture of extensor tendons, multiple sites

☑5ᵗʰ **M66.3** Spontaneous rupture of flexor tendons

TIP: Refer to the Muscle/Tendon table at the beginning of this chapter.

M66.30 Spontaneous rupture of flexor tendons, unspecified site

☑6ᵗʰ **M66.31** Spontaneous rupture of flexor tendons, shoulder

M66.311 Spontaneous rupture of flexor tendons, right shoulder

M66.312 Spontaneous rupture of flexor tendons, left shoulder

M66.319 Spontaneous rupture of flexor tendons, unspecified shoulder

☑6ᵗʰ **M66.32** Spontaneous rupture of flexor tendons, upper arm

M66.321 Spontaneous rupture of flexor tendons, right upper arm

M66.322 Spontaneous rupture of flexor tendons, left upper arm

M66.329 Spontaneous rupture of flexor tendons, unspecified upper arm

☑6ᵗʰ **M66.33** Spontaneous rupture of flexor tendons, forearm

M66.331 Spontaneous rupture of flexor tendons, right forearm

M66.332 Spontaneous rupture of flexor tendons, left forearm

M66.339 Spontaneous rupture of flexor tendons, unspecified forearm

☑6ᵗʰ **M66.34** Spontaneous rupture of flexor tendons, hand

M66.341 Spontaneous rupture of flexor tendons, right hand

M66.342 Spontaneous rupture of flexor tendons, left hand

M66.349 Spontaneous rupture of flexor tendons, unspecified hand

☑6ᵗʰ **M66.35** Spontaneous rupture of flexor tendons, thigh

M66.351 Spontaneous rupture of flexor tendons, right thigh

M66.352 Spontaneous rupture of flexor tendons, left thigh

M66.359 Spontaneous rupture of flexor tendons, unspecified thigh

☑6ᵗʰ **M66.36** Spontaneous rupture of flexor tendons, lower leg

M66.361 Spontaneous rupture of flexor tendons, right lower leg

M66.362 Spontaneous rupture of flexor tendons, left lower leg

M66.369 Spontaneous rupture of flexor tendons, unspecified lower leg

☑6ᵗʰ **M66.37** Spontaneous rupture of flexor tendons, ankle and foot

M66.371 Spontaneous rupture of flexor tendons, right ankle and foot

M66.372 Spontaneous rupture of flexor tendons, left ankle and foot

M66.379 Spontaneous rupture of flexor tendons, unspecified ankle and foot

M66.38 Spontaneous rupture of flexor tendons, other site

M66.39 Spontaneous rupture of flexor tendons, multiple sites

☑5ᵗʰ **M66.8** Spontaneous rupture of other tendons

TIP: Refer to the Muscle/Tendon table at the beginning of this chapter.

M66.80 Spontaneous rupture of other tendons, unspecified site

☑6ᵗʰ **M66.81** Spontaneous rupture of other tendons, shoulder

M66.811 Spontaneous rupture of other tendons, right shoulder

M66.812 Spontaneous rupture of other tendons, left shoulder

M66.819 Spontaneous rupture of other tendons, unspecified shoulder

☑6ᵗʰ **M66.82** Spontaneous rupture of other tendons, upper arm

M66.821 Spontaneous rupture of other tendons, right upper arm

M66.822 Spontaneous rupture of other tendons, left upper arm

M66.829 Spontaneous rupture of other tendons, unspecified upper arm

☑6ᵗʰ **M66.83** Spontaneous rupture of other tendons, forearm

M66.831 Spontaneous rupture of other tendons, right forearm

M66.832 Spontaneous rupture of other tendons, left forearm

M66.839 Spontaneous rupture of other tendons, unspecified forearm

☑6ᵗʰ **M66.84** Spontaneous rupture of other tendons, hand

M66.841 Spontaneous rupture of other tendons, right hand

M66.842 Spontaneous rupture of other tendons, left hand

M66.849 Spontaneous rupture of other tendons, unspecified hand

☑6ᵗʰ **M66.85** Spontaneous rupture of other tendons, thigh

M66.851 Spontaneous rupture of other tendons, right thigh

M66.852 Spontaneous rupture of other tendons, left thigh

M66.859 Spontaneous rupture of other tendons, unspecified thigh

☑6ᵗʰ **M66.86** Spontaneous rupture of other tendons, lower leg

M66.861 Spontaneous rupture of other tendons, right lower leg

M66.862 Spontaneous rupture of other tendons, left lower leg

M66.869 Spontaneous rupture of other tendons, unspecified lower leg

☑6ᵗʰ **M66.87** Spontaneous rupture of other tendons, ankle and foot

M66.871 Spontaneous rupture of other tendons, right ankle and foot

☑ Additional Character Required   ☑x7ᵗʰ Placeholder Alert   Manifestation   Unspecified Dx   ►◄ Revised Text   ● New Code   ▲ Revised Code Title

ICD-10-CM 2020   799

           M66.872 **Spontaneous rupture of other tendons, left** ankle and foot

           M66.879 **Spontaneous rupture of other tendons, unspecified ankle and foot**

▲   M66.88 **Spontaneous rupture of other tendons, other sites**

    M66.89 **Spontaneous rupture of other tendons, multiple sites**

   M66.9 **Spontaneous rupture of unspecified tendon**

      Rupture at musculotendinous junction, nontraumatic

✓4th **M67 Other disorders of synovium and tendon**

    EXCLUDES 1   *palmar fascial fibromatosis [Dupuytren] (M72.0)*

            tendinitis NOS (M77.9-)

            xanthomatosis localized to tendons (E78.2)

✓5th **M67.0 Short Achilles tendon (acquired)**

    M67.00 **Short Achilles tendon (acquired), unspecified ankle**

    M67.01 **Short Achilles tendon (acquired), right ankle**

    M67.02 **Short Achilles tendon (acquired), left ankle**

✓5th **M67.2 Synovial hypertrophy, not elsewhere classified**

      EXCLUDES 1   *villonodular synovitis (pigmented) (M12.2-)*

    M67.20 **Synovial hypertrophy, not elsewhere classified, unspecified site**

✓6th   M67.21 **Synovial hypertrophy, not elsewhere classified, shoulder**

       M67.211 **Synovial hypertrophy, not elsewhere classified, right shoulder**

       M67.212 **Synovial hypertrophy, not elsewhere classified, left shoulder**

       M67.219 **Synovial hypertrophy, not elsewhere classified, unspecified shoulder**

✓6th   M67.22 **Synovial hypertrophy, not elsewhere classified, upper arm**

       M67.221 **Synovial hypertrophy, not elsewhere classified, right upper arm**

       M67.222 **Synovial hypertrophy, not elsewhere classified, left upper arm**

       M67.229 **Synovial hypertrophy, not elsewhere classified, unspecified upper arm**

✓6th   M67.23 **Synovial hypertrophy, not elsewhere classified, forearm**

       M67.231 **Synovial hypertrophy, not elsewhere classified, right forearm**

       M67.232 **Synovial hypertrophy, not elsewhere classified, left forearm**

       M67.239 **Synovial hypertrophy, not elsewhere classified, unspecified forearm**

✓6th   M67.24 **Synovial hypertrophy, not elsewhere classified, hand**

       M67.241 **Synovial hypertrophy, not elsewhere classified, right hand**

       M67.242 **Synovial hypertrophy, not elsewhere classified, left hand**

       M67.249 **Synovial hypertrophy, not elsewhere classified, unspecified hand**

✓6th   M67.25 **Synovial hypertrophy, not elsewhere classified, thigh**

       M67.251 **Synovial hypertrophy, not elsewhere classified, right thigh**

       M67.252 **Synovial hypertrophy, not elsewhere classified, left thigh**

       M67.259 **Synovial hypertrophy, not elsewhere classified, unspecified thigh**

✓6th   M67.26 **Synovial hypertrophy, not elsewhere classified, lower leg**

       M67.261 **Synovial hypertrophy, not elsewhere classified, right lower leg**

       M67.262 **Synovial hypertrophy, not elsewhere classified, left lower leg**

       M67.269 **Synovial hypertrophy, not elsewhere classified, unspecified lower leg**

✓6th   M67.27 **Synovial hypertrophy, not elsewhere classified, ankle and foot**

       M67.271 **Synovial hypertrophy, not elsewhere classified, right ankle and foot**

       M67.272 **Synovial hypertrophy, not elsewhere classified, left ankle and foot**

       M67.279 **Synovial hypertrophy, not elsewhere classified, unspecified ankle and foot**

    M67.28 **Synovial hypertrophy, not elsewhere classified, other site**

    M67.29 **Synovial hypertrophy, not elsewhere classified, multiple sites**

✓5th **M67.3 Transient synovitis**

      Toxic synovitis

      EXCLUDES 1   *palindromic rheumatism (M12.3-)*

    M67.30 **Transient synovitis, unspecified site**

✓6th   M67.31 **Transient synovitis, shoulder**

       M67.311 **Transient synovitis, right shoulder**

       M67.312 **Transient synovitis, left shoulder**

       M67.319 **Transient synovitis, unspecified shoulder**

✓6th   M67.32 **Transient synovitis, elbow**

       M67.321 **Transient synovitis, right elbow**

       M67.322 **Transient synovitis, left elbow**

       M67.329 **Transient synovitis, unspecified elbow**

✓6th   M67.33 **Transient synovitis, wrist**

       M67.331 **Transient synovitis, right wrist**

       M67.332 **Transient synovitis, left wrist**

       M67.339 **Transient synovitis, unspecified wrist**

✓6th   M67.34 **Transient synovitis, hand**

       M67.341 **Transient synovitis, right hand**

       M67.342 **Transient synovitis, left hand**

       M67.349 **Transient synovitis, unspecified hand**

✓6th   M67.35 **Transient synovitis, hip**

       M67.351 **Transient synovitis, right hip**

       M67.352 **Transient synovitis, left hip**

       M67.359 **Transient synovitis, unspecified hip**

✓6th   M67.36 **Transient synovitis, knee**

       M67.361 **Transient synovitis, right knee**

       M67.362 **Transient synovitis, left knee**

       M67.369 **Transient synovitis, unspecified knee**

✓6th   M67.37 **Transient synovitis, ankle and foot**

       M67.371 **Transient synovitis, right ankle and foot**

       M67.372 **Transient synovitis, left ankle and foot**

       M67.379 **Transient synovitis, unspecified ankle and foot**

    M67.38 **Transient synovitis, other site**

    M67.39 **Transient synovitis, multiple sites**

✓5th **M67.4 Ganglion**

      Ganglion of joint or tendon (sheath)

      EXCLUDES 1   *ganglion in yaws (A66.6)*

      EXCLUDES 2   *cyst of bursa (M71.2-M71.3)*

            cyst of synovium (M71.2-M71.3)

      DEF: Fluid-filled, benign cyst appearing on a tendon sheath or aponeurosis, frequently connecting to an underlying joint.

    M67.40 **Ganglion, unspecified site**

✓6th   M67.41 **Ganglion, shoulder**

       M67.411 **Ganglion, right shoulder**

       M67.412 **Ganglion, left shoulder**

       M67.419 **Ganglion, unspecified shoulder**

✓6th   M67.42 **Ganglion, elbow**

       M67.421 **Ganglion, right elbow**

       M67.422 **Ganglion, left elbow**

       M67.429 **Ganglion, unspecified elbow**

√6ᵗʰ **M67.43**   **Ganglion,** wrist

Ganglion of Wrist

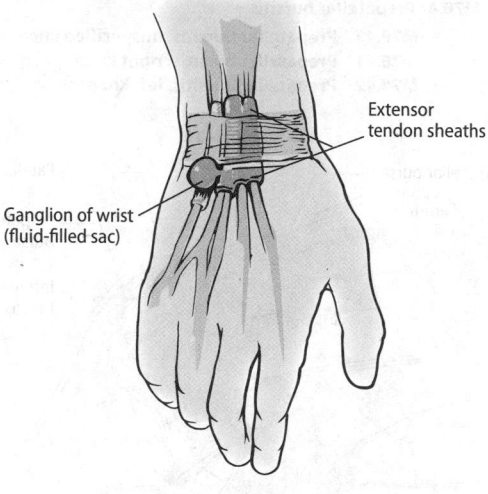

Extensor tendon sheaths

Ganglion of wrist (fluid-filled sac)

M67.431   **Ganglion,** right **wrist**
M67.432   **Ganglion,** left **wrist**
M67.439   **Ganglion,** unspecified **wrist**

√6ᵗʰ **M67.44**   **Ganglion,** hand

M67.441   **Ganglion,** right **hand**
M67.442   **Ganglion,** left **hand**
M67.449   **Ganglion,** unspecified **hand**

√6ᵗʰ **M67.45**   **Ganglion,** hip

M67.451   **Ganglion,** right **hip**
M67.452   **Ganglion,** left **hip**
M67.459   **Ganglion,** unspecified **hip**

√6ᵗʰ **M67.46**   **Ganglion,** knee

M67.461   **Ganglion,** right **knee**
M67.462   **Ganglion,** left **knee**
M67.469   **Ganglion,** unspecified **knee**

√6ᵗʰ **M67.47**   **Ganglion,** ankle and foot

M67.471   **Ganglion,** right **ankle and foot**
M67.472   **Ganglion,** left **ankle and foot**
M67.479   **Ganglion,** unspecified **ankle and foot**

M67.48   **Ganglion, other site**
M67.49   **Ganglion,** multiple sites

√5ᵗʰ **M67.5**   **Plica syndrome**

Plica knee

M67.50   **Plica syndrome,** unspecified **knee**
M67.51   **Plica syndrome,** right **knee**
M67.52   **Plica syndrome,** left **knee**

√5ᵗʰ **M67.8**   **Other specified disorders of synovium and tendon**

M67.80   **Other specified disorders of synovium and tendon, unspecified site**

√6ᵗʰ **M67.81**   **Other specified disorders of synovium and tendon,** shoulder

M67.811   **Other specified disorders of synovium,** right **shoulder**
M67.812   **Other specified disorders of synovium,** left **shoulder**
M67.813   **Other specified disorders of tendon,** right **shoulder**
M67.814   **Other specified disorders of tendon,** left **shoulder**
M67.819   **Other specified disorders of synovium and tendon, unspecified shoulder**

√6ᵗʰ **M67.82**   **Other specified disorders of synovium and tendon,** elbow

M67.821   **Other specified disorders of synovium,** right **elbow**
M67.822   **Other specified disorders of synovium,** left **elbow**
M67.823   **Other specified disorders of tendon,** right **elbow**
M67.824   **Other specified disorders of tendon,** left **elbow**

M67.829   **Other specified disorders of synovium and tendon, unspecified elbow**

√6ᵗʰ **M67.83**   **Other specified disorders of synovium and tendon,** wrist

M67.831   **Other specified disorders of synovium,** right **wrist**
M67.832   **Other specified disorders of synovium,** left **wrist**
M67.833   **Other specified disorders of tendon,** right **wrist**
M67.834   **Other specified disorders of tendon,** left **wrist**
M67.839   **Other specified disorders of synovium and tendon, unspecified wrist**

▲ √6ᵗʰ **M67.84**   **Other specified disorders of synovium and tendon,** hand

M67.841   **Other specified disorders of synovium,** right **hand**
M67.842   **Other specified disorders of synovium,** left **hand**
M67.843   **Other specified disorders of tendon,** right **hand**
M67.844   **Other specified disorders of tendon,** left **hand**
M67.849   **Other specified disorders of synovium and tendon, unspecified hand**

√6ᵗʰ **M67.85**   **Other specified disorders of synovium and tendon,** hip

M67.851   **Other specified disorders of synovium,** right **hip**
M67.852   **Other specified disorders of synovium,** left **hip**
M67.853   **Other specified disorders of tendon,** right **hip**
M67.854   **Other specified disorders of tendon,** left **hip**
M67.859   **Other specified disorders of synovium and tendon, unspecified hip**

√6ᵗʰ **M67.86**   **Other specified disorders of synovium and tendon,** knee

M67.861   **Other specified disorders of synovium,** right **knee**
M67.862   **Other specified disorders of synovium,** left **knee**
M67.863   **Other specified disorders of tendon,** right **knee**
M67.864   **Other specified disorders of tendon,** left **knee**
M67.869   **Other specified disorders of synovium and tendon, unspecified knee**

√6ᵗʰ **M67.87**   **Other specified disorders of synovium and tendon,** ankle and foot

M67.871   **Other specified disorders of synovium,** right **ankle and foot**
M67.872   **Other specified disorders of synovium,** left **ankle and foot**
M67.873   **Other specified disorders of tendon,** right **ankle and foot**
M67.874   **Other specified disorders of tendon,** left **ankle and foot**
M67.879   **Other specified disorders of synovium and tendon, unspecified ankle and foot**

M67.88   **Other specified disorders of synovium and tendon, other site**
M67.89   **Other specified disorders of synovium and tendon,** multiple sites

√5ᵗʰ **M67.9**   **Unspecified disorder of synovium and tendon**

M67.90   **Unspecified disorder of synovium and tendon, unspecified site**

√6ᵗʰ **M67.91**   **Unspecified disorder of synovium and tendon,** shoulder

M67.911   **Unspecified disorder of synovium and tendon,** right **shoulder**
M67.912   **Unspecified disorder of synovium and tendon,** left **shoulder**
M67.919   **Unspecified disorder of synovium and tendon, unspecified shoulder**

√6ᵗʰ **M67.92**   **Unspecified disorder of synovium and tendon,** upper **arm**

M67.921   **Unspecified disorder of synovium and tendon,** right **upper arm**
M67.922   **Unspecified disorder of synovium and tendon,** left **upper arm**

☑ Additional Character Required   √x7ᵗʰ Placeholder Alert   Manifestation   Unspecified Dx   ►◄ Revised Text   ● New Code   ▲ Revised Code Title

M67.929   Unspecified disorder of synovium and tendon, unspecified upper arm

√6ᵗʰ **M67.93**   Unspecified disorder of synovium and tendon, forearm

     M67.931   Unspecified disorder of synovium and tendon, right forearm

     M67.932   Unspecified disorder of synovium and tendon, left forearm

     M67.939   Unspecified disorder of synovium and tendon, unspecified forearm

√6ᵗʰ **M67.94**   Unspecified disorder of synovium and tendon, hand

     M67.941   Unspecified disorder of synovium and tendon, right hand

     M67.942   Unspecified disorder of synovium and tendon, left hand

     M67.949   Unspecified disorder of synovium and tendon, unspecified hand

√6ᵗʰ **M67.95**   Unspecified disorder of synovium and tendon, thigh

     M67.951   Unspecified disorder of synovium and tendon, right thigh

     M67.952   Unspecified disorder of synovium and tendon, left thigh

     M67.959   Unspecified disorder of synovium and tendon, unspecified thigh

√6ᵗʰ **M67.96**   Unspecified disorder of synovium and tendon, lower leg

     M67.961   Unspecified disorder of synovium and tendon, right lower leg

     M67.962   Unspecified disorder of synovium and tendon, left lower leg

     M67.969   Unspecified disorder of synovium and tendon, unspecified lower leg

√6ᵗʰ **M67.97**   Unspecified disorder of synovium and tendon, ankle and foot

     M67.971   Unspecified disorder of synovium and tendon, right ankle and foot

     M67.972   Unspecified disorder of synovium and tendon, left ankle and foot

     M67.979   Unspecified disorder of synovium and tendon, unspecified ankle and foot

M67.98   Unspecified disorder of synovium and tendon, other site

M67.99   Unspecified disorder of synovium and tendon, multiple sites

Other soft tissue disorders (M70-M79)

√4ᵗʰ **M70**   **Soft tissue disorders related to use, overuse and pressure**

   INCLUDES   soft tissue disorders of occupational origin

   Use additional external cause code to identify activity causing disorder (Y93.-)

   EXCLUDES 1   bursitis NOS (M71.9-)

   EXCLUDES 2   bursitis of shoulder (M75.5)

     enthesopathies (M76-M77)

     pressure ulcer (pressure area) (L89.-)

√5ᵗʰ **M70.0**   Crepitant synovitis (acute) (chronic) of hand and wrist

√6ᵗʰ **M70.03**   Crepitant synovitis (acute) (chronic), wrist

     M70.031   Crepitant synovitis (acute) (chronic), right wrist

     M70.032   Crepitant synovitis (acute) (chronic), left wrist

     M70.039   Crepitant synovitis (acute) (chronic), unspecified wrist

√6ᵗʰ **M70.04**   Crepitant synovitis (acute) (chronic), hand

     M70.041   Crepitant synovitis (acute) (chronic), right hand

     M70.042   Crepitant synovitis (acute) (chronic), left hand

     M70.049   Crepitant synovitis (acute) (chronic), unspecified hand

√5ᵗʰ **M70.1**   Bursitis of hand

     M70.10   Bursitis, unspecified hand

     M70.11   Bursitis, right hand

     M70.12   Bursitis, left hand

√5ᵗʰ **M70.2**   Olecranon bursitis

     M70.20   Olecranon bursitis, unspecified elbow

     M70.21   Olecranon bursitis, right elbow

     M70.22   Olecranon bursitis, left elbow

√5ᵗʰ **M70.3**   Other bursitis of elbow

     M70.30   Other bursitis of elbow, unspecified elbow

     M70.31   Other bursitis of elbow, right elbow

     M70.32   Other bursitis of elbow, left elbow

√5ᵗʰ **M70.4**   Prepatellar bursitis

     M70.40   Prepatellar bursitis, unspecified knee

     M70.41   Prepatellar bursitis, right knee

     M70.42   Prepatellar bursitis, left knee

Knee Bursae

Suprapatellar bursa • Femur • Patella • Prepatellar bursa • Infrapatellar bursa • Popliteal bursa • Tibia

√5ᵗʰ **M70.5**   Other bursitis of knee

     M70.50   Other bursitis of knee, unspecified knee

     M70.51   Other bursitis of knee, right knee

     M70.52   Other bursitis of knee, left knee

√5ᵗʰ **M70.6**   Trochanteric bursitis

     Trochanteric tendinitis

     M70.60   Trochanteric bursitis, unspecified hip

     M70.61   Trochanteric bursitis, right hip

     M70.62   Trochanteric bursitis, left hip

√5ᵗʰ **M70.7**   Other bursitis of hip

     Ischial bursitis

     M70.70   Other bursitis of hip, unspecified hip

     M70.71   Other bursitis of hip, right hip

     M70.72   Other bursitis of hip, left hip

√5ᵗʰ **M70.8**   Other soft tissue disorders related to use, overuse and pressure

     M70.80   Other soft tissue disorders related to use, overuse and pressure of unspecified site

√6ᵗʰ **M70.81**   Other soft tissue disorders related to use, overuse and pressure of shoulder

     M70.811   Other soft tissue disorders related to use, overuse and pressure, right shoulder

     M70.812   Other soft tissue disorders related to use, overuse and pressure, left shoulder

     M70.819   Other soft tissue disorders related to use, overuse and pressure, unspecified shoulder

√6ᵗʰ **M70.82**   Other soft tissue disorders related to use, overuse and pressure of upper arm

     M70.821   Other soft tissue disorders related to use, overuse and pressure, right upper arm

     M70.822   Other soft tissue disorders related to use, overuse and pressure, left upper arm

     M70.829   Other soft tissue disorders related to use, overuse and pressure, unspecified upper arms

√6ᵗʰ **M70.83**   Other soft tissue disorders related to use, overuse and pressure of forearm

     M70.831   Other soft tissue disorders related to use, overuse and pressure, right forearm

     M70.832   Other soft tissue disorders related to use, overuse and pressure, left forearm

     M70.839   Other soft tissue disorders related to use, overuse and pressure, unspecified forearm

✓6ᵗʰ **M70.84** Other soft tissue disorders related to use, overuse and pressure of **hand**

    M70.841 Other soft tissue disorders related to use, overuse and pressure, **right** hand

    M70.842 Other soft tissue disorders related to use, overuse and pressure, **left** hand

    M70.849 Other soft tissue disorders related to use, overuse and pressure, unspecified hand

✓6ᵗʰ **M70.85** Other soft tissue disorders related to use, overuse and pressure of **thigh**

    M70.851 Other soft tissue disorders related to use, overuse and pressure, **right** thigh

    M70.852 Other soft tissue disorders related to use, overuse and pressure, **left** thigh

    M70.859 Other soft tissue disorders related to use, overuse and pressure, unspecified thigh

✓6ᵗʰ **M70.86** Other soft tissue disorders related to use, overuse and pressure **lower leg**

    M70.861 Other soft tissue disorders related to use, overuse and pressure, **right** lower leg

    M70.862 Other soft tissue disorders related to use, overuse and pressure, **left** lower leg

    M70.869 Other soft tissue disorders related to use, overuse and pressure, unspecified leg

✓6ᵗʰ **M70.87** Other soft tissue disorders related to use, overuse and pressure of **ankle and foot**

    M70.871 Other soft tissue disorders related to use, overuse and pressure, **right** ankle and foot

    M70.872 Other soft tissue disorders related to use, overuse and pressure, **left** ankle and foot

    M70.879 Other soft tissue disorders related to use, overuse and pressure, unspecified ankle and foot

    M70.88 Other soft tissue disorders related to use, overuse and pressure other site

    M70.89 Other soft tissue disorders related to use, overuse and pressure **multiple sites**

✓5ᵗʰ **M70.9** Unspecified soft tissue disorder related to use, overuse and pressure

    M70.90 Unspecified soft tissue disorder related to use, overuse and pressure of unspecified site

✓6ᵗʰ **M70.91** Unspecified soft tissue disorder related to use, overuse and pressure of **shoulder**

    M70.911 Unspecified soft tissue disorder related to use, overuse and pressure, **right** shoulder

    M70.912 Unspecified soft tissue disorder related to use, overuse and pressure, **left** shoulder

    M70.919 Unspecified soft tissue disorder related to use, overuse and pressure, unspecified shoulder

✓6ᵗʰ **M70.92** Unspecified soft tissue disorder related to use, overuse and pressure of **upper arm**

    M70.921 Unspecified soft tissue disorder related to use, overuse and pressure, **right** upper arm

    M70.922 Unspecified soft tissue disorder related to use, overuse and pressure, **left** upper arm

    M70.929 Unspecified soft tissue disorder related to use, overuse and pressure, unspecified upper arm

✓6ᵗʰ **M70.93** Unspecified soft tissue disorder related to use, overuse and pressure of **forearm**

    M70.931 Unspecified soft tissue disorder related to use, overuse and pressure, **right** forearm

    M70.932 Unspecified soft tissue disorder related to use, overuse and pressure, **left** forearm

    M70.939 Unspecified soft tissue disorder related to use, overuse and pressure, unspecified forearm

✓6ᵗʰ **M70.94** Unspecified soft tissue disorder related to use, overuse and pressure of **hand**

    M70.941 Unspecified soft tissue disorder related to use, overuse and pressure, **right** hand

    M70.942 Unspecified soft tissue disorder related to use, overuse and pressure, **left** hand

    M70.949 Unspecified soft tissue disorder related to use, overuse and pressure, unspecified hand

✓6ᵗʰ **M70.95** Unspecified soft tissue disorder related to use, overuse and pressure of **thigh**

    M70.951 Unspecified soft tissue disorder related to use, overuse and pressure, **right** thigh

    M70.952 Unspecified soft tissue disorder related to use, overuse and pressure, **left** thigh

    M70.959 Unspecified soft tissue disorder related to use, overuse and pressure, unspecified thigh

✓6ᵗʰ **M70.96** Unspecified soft tissue disorder related to use, overuse and pressure **lower leg**

    M70.961 Unspecified soft tissue disorder related to use, overuse and pressure, **right** lower leg

    M70.962 Unspecified soft tissue disorder related to use, overuse and pressure, **left** lower leg

    M70.969 Unspecified soft tissue disorder related to use, overuse and pressure, unspecified lower leg

✓6ᵗʰ **M70.97** Unspecified soft tissue disorder related to use, overuse and pressure of **ankle and foot**

    M70.971 Unspecified soft tissue disorder related to use, overuse and pressure, **right** ankle and foot

    M70.972 Unspecified soft tissue disorder related to use, overuse and pressure, **left** ankle and foot

    M70.979 Unspecified soft tissue disorder related to use, overuse and pressure, unspecified ankle and foot

    M70.98 Unspecified soft tissue disorder related to use, overuse and pressure other

    M70.99 Unspecified soft tissue disorder related to use, overuse and pressure **multiple sites**

✓4ᵗʰ **M71** Other bursopathies

    EXCLUDES 1   bunion (M20.1)

       bursitis related to use, overuse or pressure (M70.-)

       enthesopathies (M76-M77)

✓5ᵗʰ **M71.0** Abscess of bursa

    Use additional code (B95.-, B96.-) to identify causative organism

    M71.00 Abscess of bursa, unspecified site

✓6ᵗʰ **M71.01** Abscess of bursa, **shoulder**

    M71.011 Abscess of bursa, **right** shoulder

    M71.012 Abscess of bursa, **left** shoulder

    M71.019 Abscess of bursa, unspecified shoulder

✓6ᵗʰ **M71.02** Abscess of bursa, **elbow**

    M71.021 Abscess of bursa, **right** elbow

    M71.022 Abscess of bursa, **left** elbow

    M71.029 Abscess of bursa, unspecified elbow

✓6ᵗʰ **M71.03** Abscess of bursa, **wrist**

    M71.031 Abscess of bursa, **right** wrist

    M71.032 Abscess of bursa, **left** wrist

    M71.039 Abscess of bursa, unspecified wrist

✓6ᵗʰ **M71.04** Abscess of bursa, **hand**

    M71.041 Abscess of bursa, **right** hand

    M71.042 Abscess of bursa, **left** hand

    M71.049 Abscess of bursa, unspecified hand

✓6ᵗʰ **M71.05** Abscess of bursa, **hip**

    M71.051 Abscess of bursa, **right** hip

    M71.052 Abscess of bursa, **left** hip

    M71.059 Abscess of bursa, unspecified hip

✓6ᵗʰ **M71.06** Abscess of bursa, **knee**

    M71.061 Abscess of bursa, **right** knee

    M71.062 Abscess of bursa, **left** knee

    M71.069 Abscess of bursa, unspecified knee

✓6ᵗʰ **M71.07** Abscess of bursa, **ankle and foot**

    M71.071 Abscess of bursa, **right** ankle and foot

    M71.072 Abscess of bursa, **left** ankle and foot

    M71.079 Abscess of bursa, unspecified ankle and foot

    M71.08 Abscess of bursa, other site

    M71.09 Abscess of bursa, **multiple sites**

✓5ᵗʰ **M71.1** Other infective bursitis

    Use additional code (B95.-, B96.-) to identify causative organism

    M71.10 Other infective bursitis, unspecified site

✓6ᵗʰ **M71.11** Other infective bursitis, **shoulder**

    M71.111 Other infective bursitis, **right** shoulder

☑ Additional Character Required   ✓x7ᵗʰ Placeholder Alert   Manifestation   Unspecified Dx   ▶◀ Revised Text   ● New Code   ▲ Revised Code Title

ICD-10-CM 2020   803

M71.112   Other infective bursitis, left shoulder
M71.119   Other infective bursitis, unspecified shoulder

✓6ᵗʰ   M71.12   Other infective bursitis, elbow

M71.121   Other infective bursitis, right elbow
M71.122   Other infective bursitis, left elbow
M71.129   Other infective bursitis, unspecified elbow

✓6ᵗʰ   M71.13   Other infective bursitis, wrist

M71.131   Other infective bursitis, right wrist
M71.132   Other infective bursitis, left wrist
M71.139   Other infective bursitis, unspecified wrist

✓6ᵗʰ   M71.14   Other infective bursitis, hand

M71.141   Other infective bursitis, right hand
M71.142   Other infective bursitis, left hand
M71.149   Other infective bursitis, unspecified hand

✓6ᵗʰ   M71.15   Other infective bursitis, hip

M71.151   Other infective bursitis, right hip
M71.152   Other infective bursitis, left hip
M71.159   Other infective bursitis, unspecified hip

✓6ᵗʰ   M71.16   Other infective bursitis, knee

M71.161   Other infective bursitis, right knee
M71.162   Other infective bursitis, left knee
M71.169   Other infective bursitis, unspecified knee

✓6ᵗʰ   M71.17   Other infective bursitis, ankle and foot

M71.171   Other infective bursitis, right ankle and foot
M71.172   Other infective bursitis, left ankle and foot
M71.179   Other infective bursitis, unspecified ankle and foot

M71.18   Other infective bursitis, other site
M71.19   Other infective bursitis, multiple sites

✓5ᵗʰ   M71.2   Synovial cyst of popliteal space [Baker]

EXCLUDES 1   synovial cyst of popliteal space with rupture (M66.0)
DEF: Sac filled with clear synovial fluid in adults, usually secondary to disease inside the joint, located on the back of the knee in the popliteal fossa area. In children, the cyst usually represents a ganglion of one of the tendons in the knee.

Baker's Cyst

Baker's cyst connected to knee joint synovial cavity

M71.20   Synovial cyst of popliteal space [Baker], unspecified knee
M71.21   Synovial cyst of popliteal space [Baker], right knee
M71.22   Synovial cyst of popliteal space [Baker], left knee

✓5ᵗʰ   M71.3   Other bursal cyst

Synovial cyst NOS
EXCLUDES 1   synovial cyst with rupture (M66.1-)

M71.30   Other bursal cyst, unspecified site

✓6ᵗʰ   M71.31   Other bursal cyst, shoulder

M71.311   Other bursal cyst, right shoulder
M71.312   Other bursal cyst, left shoulder
M71.319   Other bursal cyst, unspecified shoulder

✓6ᵗʰ   M71.32   Other bursal cyst, elbow

M71.321   Other bursal cyst, right elbow

M71.322   Other bursal cyst, left elbow
M71.329   Other bursal cyst, unspecified elbow

✓6ᵗʰ   M71.33   Other bursal cyst, wrist

M71.331   Other bursal cyst, right wrist
M71.332   Other bursal cyst, left wrist
M71.339   Other bursal cyst, unspecified wrist

✓6ᵗʰ   M71.34   Other bursal cyst, hand

M71.341   Other bursal cyst, right hand
M71.342   Other bursal cyst, left hand
M71.349   Other bursal cyst, unspecified hand

✓6ᵗʰ   M71.35   Other bursal cyst, hip

M71.351   Other bursal cyst, right hip
M71.352   Other bursal cyst, left hip
M71.359   Other bursal cyst, unspecified hip

✓6ᵗʰ   M71.37   Other bursal cyst, ankle and foot

M71.371   Other bursal cyst, right ankle and foot
M71.372   Other bursal cyst, left ankle and foot
M71.379   Other bursal cyst, unspecified ankle and foot

M71.38   Other bursal cyst, other site
M71.39   Other bursal cyst, multiple sites

✓5ᵗʰ   M71.4   Calcium deposit in bursa

EXCLUDES 2   calcium deposit in bursa of shoulder (M75.3)

M71.40   Calcium deposit in bursa, unspecified site

✓6ᵗʰ   M71.42   Calcium deposit in bursa, elbow

M71.421   Calcium deposit in bursa, right elbow
M71.422   Calcium deposit in bursa, left elbow
M71.429   Calcium deposit in bursa, unspecified elbow

✓6ᵗʰ   M71.43   Calcium deposit in bursa, wrist

M71.431   Calcium deposit in bursa, right wrist
M71.432   Calcium deposit in bursa, left wrist
M71.439   Calcium deposit in bursa, unspecified wrist

✓6ᵗʰ   M71.44   Calcium deposit in bursa, hand

M71.441   Calcium deposit in bursa, right hand
M71.442   Calcium deposit in bursa, left hand
M71.449   Calcium deposit in bursa, unspecified hand

✓6ᵗʰ   M71.45   Calcium deposit in bursa, hip

M71.451   Calcium deposit in bursa, right hip
M71.452   Calcium deposit in bursa, left hip
M71.459   Calcium deposit in bursa, unspecified hip

✓6ᵗʰ   M71.46   Calcium deposit in bursa, knee

M71.461   Calcium deposit in bursa, right knee
M71.462   Calcium deposit in bursa, left knee
M71.469   Calcium deposit in bursa, unspecified knee

✓6ᵗʰ   M71.47   Calcium deposit in bursa, ankle and foot

M71.471   Calcium deposit in bursa, right ankle and foot
M71.472   Calcium deposit in bursa, left ankle and foot
M71.479   Calcium deposit in bursa, unspecified ankle and foot

M71.48   Calcium deposit in bursa, other site
M71.49   Calcium deposit in bursa, multiple sites

✓5ᵗʰ   M71.5   Other bursitis, not elsewhere classified

EXCLUDES 1   bursitis NOS (M71.9-)
EXCLUDES 2   bursitis of shoulder (M75.5)
                 bursitis of tibial collateral [Pellegrini-Stieda] (M76.4-)

M71.50   Other bursitis, not elsewhere classified, unspecified site

✓6ᵗʰ   M71.52   Other bursitis, not elsewhere classified, elbow

M71.521   Other bursitis, not elsewhere classified, right elbow
M71.522   Other bursitis, not elsewhere classified, left elbow
M71.529   Other bursitis, not elsewhere classified, unspecified elbow

✓6ᵗʰ   M71.53   Other bursitis, not elsewhere classified, wrist

M71.531   Other bursitis, not elsewhere classified, right wrist
M71.532   Other bursitis, not elsewhere classified, left wrist
M71.539   Other bursitis, not elsewhere classified, unspecified wrist

✓6th **M71.54** Other bursitis, not elsewhere classified, hand
  M71.541 Other bursitis, not elsewhere classified, right hand
  M71.542 Other bursitis, not elsewhere classified, left hand
  M71.549 Other bursitis, not elsewhere classified, unspecified hand

✓6th **M71.55** Other bursitis, not elsewhere classified, hip
  M71.551 Other bursitis, not elsewhere classified, right hip
  M71.552 Other bursitis, not elsewhere classified, left hip
  M71.559 Other bursitis, not elsewhere classified, unspecified hip

✓6th **M71.56** Other bursitis, not elsewhere classified, knee
  M71.561 Other bursitis, not elsewhere classified, right knee
  M71.562 Other bursitis, not elsewhere classified, left knee
  M71.569 Other bursitis, not elsewhere classified, unspecified knee

✓6th **M71.57** Other bursitis, not elsewhere classified, ankle and foot
  M71.571 Other bursitis, not elsewhere classified, right ankle and foot
  M71.572 Other bursitis, not elsewhere classified, left ankle and foot
  M71.579 Other bursitis, not elsewhere classified, unspecified ankle and foot

  M71.58 Other bursitis, not elsewhere classified, other site

✓5th **M71.8** Other specified bursopathies
  M71.80 Other specified bursopathies, unspecified site

✓6th **M71.81** Other specified bursopathies, shoulder
  M71.811 Other specified bursopathies, right shoulder
  M71.812 Other specified bursopathies, left shoulder
  M71.819 Other specified bursopathies, unspecified shoulder

✓6th **M71.82** Other specified bursopathies, elbow
  M71.821 Other specified bursopathies, right elbow
  M71.822 Other specified bursopathies, left elbow
  M71.829 Other specified bursopathies, unspecified elbow

✓6th **M71.83** Other specified bursopathies, wrist
  M71.831 Other specified bursopathies, right wrist
  M71.832 Other specified bursopathies, left wrist
  M71.839 Other specified bursopathies, unspecified wrist

✓6th **M71.84** Other specified bursopathies, hand
  M71.841 Other specified bursopathies, right hand
  M71.842 Other specified bursopathies, left hand
  M71.849 Other specified bursopathies, unspecified hand

✓6th **M71.85** Other specified bursopathies, hip
  M71.851 Other specified bursopathies, right hip
  M71.852 Other specified bursopathies, left hip
  M71.859 Other specified bursopathies, unspecified hip

✓6th **M71.86** Other specified bursopathies, knee
  M71.861 Other specified bursopathies, right knee
  M71.862 Other specified bursopathies, left knee
  M71.869 Other specified bursopathies, unspecified knee

✓6th **M71.87** Other specified bursopathies, ankle and foot
  M71.871 Other specified bursopathies, right ankle and foot
  M71.872 Other specified bursopathies, left ankle and foot
  M71.879 Other specified bursopathies, unspecified ankle and foot

  M71.88 Other specified bursopathies, other site
  M71.89 Other specified bursopathies, multiple sites

M71.9 Bursopathy, unspecified
  Bursitis NOS

✓4th **M72** **Fibroblastic disorders**
  EXCLUDES 2 retroperitoneal fibromatosis (D48.3)

  M72.0 Palmar fascial fibromatosis [Dupuytren] Ⓐ
    DEF: Dupuytren's contracture: Flexion deformity of a finger, due to shortened, thickened fibrosing of palmar fascia. The cause is unknown, but it is associated with long-standing epilepsy.

  M72.1 Knuckle pads

  M72.2 Plantar fascial fibromatosis
    Plantar fasciitis
    DEF: Rapid-growing and multiplanar nodular swellings and pain in the foot that is not associated with contractures.

  M72.4 Pseudosarcomatous fibromatosis
    Nodular fasciitis

  M72.6 Necrotizing fasciitis HCC
    Use additional code (B95.-, B96.-) to identify causative organism

  M72.8 Other fibroblastic disorders
    Abscess of fascia
    Fasciitis NEC
    Other infective fasciitis
    Use additional code to (B95.-, B96.-) identify causative organism
    EXCLUDES 1 diffuse (eosinophilic) fasciitis (M35.4)
      necrotizing fasciitis (M72.6)
      nodular fasciitis (M72.4)
      perirenal fasciitis NOS (N13.5)
      perirenal fasciitis with infection (N13.6)
      plantar fasciitis (M72.2)

  M72.9 Fibroblastic disorder, unspecified
    Fasciitis NOS
    Fibromatosis NOS

✓4th **M75** **Shoulder lesions**
  EXCLUDES 2 shoulder-hand syndrome (M89.0-)

  ✓5th **M75.0** Adhesive capsulitis of shoulder
    Frozen shoulder
    Periarthritis of shoulder
    AHA: 2015,2Q,23
    M75.00 Adhesive capsulitis of unspecified shoulder
    M75.01 Adhesive capsulitis of right shoulder
    M75.02 Adhesive capsulitis of left shoulder

  ✓5th **M75.1** Rotator cuff tear or rupture, not specified as traumatic
    Rotator cuff syndrome
    Supraspinatus syndrome
    Supraspinatus tear or rupture, not specified as traumatic
    EXCLUDES 1 tear of rotator cuff, traumatic (S46.01-)

    ✓6th **M75.10** Unspecified rotator cuff tear or rupture, not specified as traumatic
      M75.100 Unspecified rotator cuff tear or rupture of unspecified shoulder, not specified as traumatic
      M75.101 Unspecified rotator cuff tear or rupture of right shoulder, not specified as traumatic
      M75.102 Unspecified rotator cuff tear or rupture of left shoulder, not specified as traumatic

    ✓6th **M75.11** Incomplete rotator cuff tear or rupture not specified as traumatic
      M75.110 Incomplete rotator cuff tear or rupture of unspecified shoulder, not specified as traumatic
      M75.111 Incomplete rotator cuff tear or rupture of right shoulder, not specified as traumatic
      M75.112 Incomplete rotator cuff tear or rupture of left shoulder, not specified as traumatic

    ✓6th **M75.12** Complete rotator cuff tear or rupture not specified as traumatic
      M75.120 Complete rotator cuff tear or rupture of unspecified shoulder, not specified as traumatic
      M75.121 Complete rotator cuff tear or rupture of right shoulder, not specified as traumatic
      M75.122 Complete rotator cuff tear or rupture of left shoulder, not specified as traumatic

  ✓5th **M75.2** Bicipital tendinitis
    M75.20 Bicipital tendinitis, unspecified shoulder
    M75.21 Bicipital tendinitis, right shoulder
    M75.22 Bicipital tendinitis, left shoulder

Chapter 13. Diseases of the Musculoskeletal System and Connective Tissue

✓5ᵗʰ **M75.3 Calcific tendinitis of shoulder**
Calcified bursa of shoulder
   M75.30 Calcific tendinitis of unspecified shoulder
   M75.31 Calcific tendinitis of right shoulder
   M75.32 Calcific tendinitis of left shoulder

✓5ᵗʰ **M75.4 Impingement syndrome of shoulder**
   M75.40 Impingement syndrome of unspecified shoulder
   M75.41 Impingement syndrome of right shoulder
   M75.42 Impingement syndrome of left shoulder

✓5ᵗʰ **M75.5 Bursitis of shoulder**
   M75.50 Bursitis of unspecified shoulder
   M75.51 Bursitis of right shoulder
   M75.52 Bursitis of left shoulder

✓5ᵗʰ **M75.8 Other shoulder lesions**
   M75.80 Other shoulder lesions, unspecified shoulder
   M75.81 Other shoulder lesions, right shoulder
   M75.82 Other shoulder lesions, left shoulder

✓5ᵗʰ **M75.9 Shoulder lesion, unspecified**
   M75.90 Shoulder lesion, unspecified, unspecified shoulder
   M75.91 Shoulder lesion, unspecified, right shoulder
   M75.92 Shoulder lesion, unspecified, left shoulder

✓4ᵗʰ **M76 Enthesopathies, lower limb, excluding foot**
   EXCLUDES 2 *bursitis due to use, overuse and pressure (M70.-)*
         enthesopathies of ankle and foot (M77.5-)

✓5ᵗʰ **M76.0 Gluteal tendinitis**
   M76.00 Gluteal tendinitis, unspecified hip
   M76.01 Gluteal tendinitis, right hip
   M76.02 Gluteal tendinitis, left hip

✓5ᵗʰ **M76.1 Psoas tendinitis**
   M76.10 Psoas tendinitis, unspecified hip
   M76.11 Psoas tendinitis, right hip
   M76.12 Psoas tendinitis, left hip

✓5ᵗʰ **M76.2 Iliac crest spur**
   M76.20 Iliac crest spur, unspecified hip
   M76.21 Iliac crest spur, right hip
   M76.22 Iliac crest spur, left hip

✓5ᵗʰ **M76.3 Iliotibial band syndrome**
   M76.30 Iliotibial band syndrome, unspecified leg
   M76.31 Iliotibial band syndrome, right leg
   M76.32 Iliotibial band syndrome, left leg

✓5ᵗʰ **M76.4 Tibial collateral bursitis [Pellegrini-Stieda]**
   M76.40 Tibial collateral bursitis [Pellegrini-Stieda], unspecified leg
   M76.41 Tibial collateral bursitis [Pellegrini-Stieda], right leg
   M76.42 Tibial collateral bursitis [Pellegrini-Stieda], left leg

✓5ᵗʰ **M76.5 Patellar tendinitis**
   M76.50 Patellar tendinitis, unspecified knee
   M76.51 Patellar tendinitis, right knee
   M76.52 Patellar tendinitis, left knee

✓5ᵗʰ **M76.6 Achilles tendinitis**
Achilles bursitis
   M76.60 Achilles tendinitis, unspecified leg
   M76.61 Achilles tendinitis, right leg
   M76.62 Achilles tendinitis, left leg

✓5ᵗʰ **M76.7 Peroneal tendinitis**
   M76.70 Peroneal tendinitis, unspecified leg
   M76.71 Peroneal tendinitis, right leg
   M76.72 Peroneal tendinitis, left leg

✓5ᵗʰ **M76.8 Other specified enthesopathies of lower limb, excluding foot**
   ✓6ᵗʰ **M76.81 Anterior tibial syndrome**
      M76.811 Anterior tibial syndrome, right leg
      M76.812 Anterior tibial syndrome, left leg
      M76.819 Anterior tibial syndrome, unspecified leg
   ✓6ᵗʰ **M76.82 Posterior tibial tendinitis**
      M76.821 Posterior tibial tendinitis, right leg
      M76.822 Posterior tibial tendinitis, left leg
      M76.829 Posterior tibial tendinitis, unspecified leg
   ✓6ᵗʰ **M76.89 Other specified enthesopathies of lower limb, excluding foot**
      M76.891 Other specified enthesopathies of right lower limb, excluding foot
      M76.892 Other specified enthesopathies of left lower limb, excluding foot

   M76.899 Other specified enthesopathies of unspecified lower limb, excluding foot
M76.9 Unspecified enthesopathy, lower limb, excluding foot

✓4ᵗʰ **M77 Other enthesopathies**
   EXCLUDES 1 *bursitis NOS (M71.9-)*
   EXCLUDES 2 *bursitis due to use, overuse and pressure (M70.-)*
         osteophyte (M25.7)
         spinal enthesopathy (M46.0-)

✓5ᵗʰ **M77.0 Medial epicondylitis**
   M77.00 Medial epicondylitis, unspecified elbow
   M77.01 Medial epicondylitis, right elbow
   M77.02 Medial epicondylitis, left elbow

✓5ᵗʰ **M77.1 Lateral epicondylitis**
Tennis elbow
   M77.10 Lateral epicondylitis, unspecified elbow
   M77.11 Lateral epicondylitis, right elbow
   M77.12 Lateral epicondylitis, left elbow

✓5ᵗʰ **M77.2 Periarthritis of wrist**
   M77.20 Periarthritis, unspecified wrist
   M77.21 Periarthritis, right wrist
   M77.22 Periarthritis, left wrist

✓5ᵗʰ **M77.3 Calcaneal spur**
   DEF: Overgrowth of calcaneus bone on the underside of the heel that causes pain on walking. Calcaneal spur is due to a chronic avulsion injury of the plantar fascia from the calcaneus.
   M77.30 Calcaneal spur, unspecified foot
   M77.31 Calcaneal spur, right foot
   M77.32 Calcaneal spur, left foot

✓5ᵗʰ **M77.4 Metatarsalgia**
   EXCLUDES 1 *Morton's metatarsalgia (G57.6)*
   M77.40 Metatarsalgia, unspecified foot
   M77.41 Metatarsalgia, right foot
   M77.42 Metatarsalgia, left foot

▲ ✓5ᵗʰ **M77.5 Other enthesopathy of foot and ankle**
▲   **M77.50 Other enthesopathy of unspecified foot and ankle**
▲   **M77.51 Other enthesopathy of right foot and ankle**
▲   **M77.52 Other enthesopathy of left foot and ankle**

   M77.8 Other enthesopathies, not elsewhere classified
   M77.9 Enthesopathy, unspecified
Bone spur NOS
Capsulitis NOS
Periarthritis NOS
Tendinitis NOS

✓4ᵗʰ **M79 Other and unspecified soft tissue disorders, not elsewhere classified**
   EXCLUDES 1 *psychogenic rheumatism (F45.8)*
         soft tissue pain, psychogenic (F45.41)

   M79.0 Rheumatism, unspecified
   EXCLUDES 1 *fibromyalgia (M79.7)*
         palindromic rheumatism (M12.3-)

✓5ᵗʰ **M79.1 Myalgia**
Myofascial pain syndrome
   EXCLUDES 1 *fibromyalgia (M79.7)*
         myositis (M60.-)
   AHA: 2018,4Q,21
   M79.10 Myalgia, unspecified site
   M79.11 Myalgia of mastication muscle
   M79.12 Myalgia of auxiliary muscles, head and neck
   M79.18 Myalgia, other site

   M79.2 Neuralgia and neuritis, unspecified
   EXCLUDES 1 *brachial radiculitis NOS (M54.1)*
         lumbosacral radiculitis NOS (M54.1)
         mononeuropathies (G56-G58)
         radiculitis NOS (M54.1)
         sciatica (M54.3-M54.4)
   TIP: Assign for documented neuropathic pain.

   M79.3 Panniculitis, unspecified
   EXCLUDES 1 *lupus panniculitis (L93.2)*
         neck and back panniculitis (M54.0-)
         relapsing [Weber-Christian] panniculitis (M35.6)

   M79.4 Hypertrophy of (infrapatellar) fat pad

M79.5   **Residual foreign body in soft tissue**
> *EXCLUDES 1*   foreign body granuloma of skin and subcutaneous
>   tissue (L92.3)
>   foreign body granuloma of soft tissue (M60.2-)

☑5ᵗʰ **M79.6**   **Pain in limb, hand, foot, fingers and toes**
> *EXCLUDES 2*   pain in joint (M25.5-)

   ☑6ᵗʰ **M79.60**   **Pain in limb, unspecified**

     M79.601   **Pain in right arm**
       Pain in right upper limb NOS

     M79.602   **Pain in left arm**
       Pain in left upper limb NOS

     M79.603   **Pain in arm, unspecified**
       Pain in upper limb NOS

     M79.604   **Pain in right leg**
       Pain in right lower limb NOS

     M79.605   **Pain in left leg**
       Pain in left lower limb NOS

     M79.606   **Pain in leg, unspecified**
       Pain in lower limb NOS

     M79.609   **Pain in unspecified limb**
       Pain in limb NOS

   ☑6ᵗʰ **M79.62**   **Pain in upper arm**
     Pain in axillary region

     M79.621   **Pain in right upper arm**
     M79.622   **Pain in left upper arm**
     M79.629   **Pain in unspecified upper arm**

   ☑6ᵗʰ **M79.63**   **Pain in forearm**

     M79.631   **Pain in right forearm**
     M79.632   **Pain in left forearm**
     M79.639   **Pain in unspecified forearm**

   ☑6ᵗʰ **M79.64**   **Pain in hand and fingers**

     M79.641   **Pain in right hand**
     M79.642   **Pain in left hand**
     M79.643   **Pain in unspecified hand**
     M79.644   **Pain in right finger(s)**
     M79.645   **Pain in left finger(s)**
     M79.646   **Pain in unspecified finger(s)**

   ☑6ᵗʰ **M79.65**   **Pain in thigh**

     M79.651   **Pain in right thigh**
     M79.652   **Pain in left thigh**
     M79.659   **Pain in unspecified thigh**

   ☑6ᵗʰ **M79.66**   **Pain in lower leg**

     M79.661   **Pain in right lower leg**
     M79.662   **Pain in left lower leg**
     M79.669   **Pain in unspecified lower leg**

   ☑6ᵗʰ **M79.67**   **Pain in foot and toes**

     M79.671   **Pain in right foot**
     M79.672   **Pain in left foot**
     M79.673   **Pain in unspecified foot**
     M79.674   **Pain in right toe(s)**
     M79.675   **Pain in left toe(s)**
     M79.676   **Pain in unspecified toe(s)**

M79.7   **Fibromyalgia**
   Fibromyositis
   Fibrositis
   Myofibrositis

☑5ᵗʰ **M79.A**   **Nontraumatic compartment syndrome**
   Code first, if applicable, associated postprocedural complication
> *EXCLUDES 1*   compartment syndrome NOS (T79.A-)
>   fibromyalgia (M79.7)
>   nontraumatic ischemic infarction of muscle (M62.2-)
>   traumatic compartment syndrome (T79.A-)

   ☑6ᵗʰ **M79.A1**   **Nontraumatic compartment syndrome of upper extremity**
     Nontraumatic compartment syndrome of shoulder, arm, forearm, wrist, hand, and fingers

     M79.A11   **Nontraumatic compartment syndrome of right upper extremity**
     M79.A12   **Nontraumatic compartment syndrome of left upper extremity**
     M79.A19   **Nontraumatic compartment syndrome of unspecified upper extremity**

   ☑6ᵗʰ **M79.A2**   **Nontraumatic compartment syndrome of lower extremity**
     Nontraumatic compartment syndrome of hip, buttock, thigh, leg, foot, and toes

     M79.A21   **Nontraumatic compartment syndrome of right lower extremity**
     M79.A22   **Nontraumatic compartment syndrome of left lower extremity**
     M79.A29   **Nontraumatic compartment syndrome of unspecified lower extremity**

     M79.A3   **Nontraumatic compartment syndrome of abdomen**
     M79.A9   **Nontraumatic compartment syndrome of other sites**

☑5ᵗʰ **M79.8**   **Other specified soft tissue disorders**

     M79.81   **Nontraumatic hematoma of soft tissue**
       Nontraumatic hematoma of muscle
       Nontraumatic seroma of muscle and soft tissue

     M79.89   **Other specified soft tissue disorders**
       Polyalgia

M79.9   **Soft tissue disorder, unspecified**

OSTEOPATHIES AND CHONDROPATHIES (M80-M94)

Disorders of bone density and structure (M80-M85)

☑4ᵗʰ **M80**   **Osteoporosis with current pathological fracture**
> **INCLUDES**   osteoporosis with current fragility fracture
> Use additional code to identify major osseous defect, if applicable (M89.7-)
> *EXCLUDES 1*   collapsed vertebra NOS (M48.5)
>   pathological fracture NOS (M84.4)
>   wedging of vertebra NOS (M48.5)
> *EXCLUDES 2*   personal history of (healed) osteoporosis fracture (Z87.310)

AHA: 2018,2Q,12
TIP: The site codes in this category identify the site of the fracture, not the site of the osteoporosis.

> The appropriate 7th character is to be added to each code from category M80:
> A   initial encounter for fracture
> D   subsequent encounter for fracture with routine healing
> G   subsequent encounter for fracture with delayed healing
> K   subsequent encounter for fracture with nonunion
> P   subsequent encounter for fracture with malunion
> S   sequela

☑5ᵗʰ **M80.0**   **Age-related osteoporosis with current pathological fracture**
   Involutional osteoporosis with current pathological fracture
   Osteoporosis NOS with current pathological fracture
   Postmenopausal osteoporosis with current pathological fracture
   Senile osteoporosis with current pathological fracture

   ☑x7ᵗʰ **M80.00**   **Age-related osteoporosis with current pathological fracture, unspecified site**   Q A

   ☑6ᵗʰ **M80.01**   **Age-related osteoporosis with current pathological fracture, shoulder**

     ☑7ᵗʰ **M80.011**   **Age-related osteoporosis with current pathological fracture, right shoulder**   Q A

     ☑7ᵗʰ **M80.012**   **Age-related osteoporosis with current pathological fracture, left shoulder**   Q A

     ☑7ᵗʰ **M80.019**   **Age-related osteoporosis with current pathological fracture, unspecified shoulder**   Q A

   ☑6ᵗʰ **M80.02**   **Age-related osteoporosis with current pathological fracture, humerus**

     ☑7ᵗʰ **M80.021**   **Age-related osteoporosis with current pathological fracture, right humerus**   Q A

     ☑7ᵗʰ **M80.022**   **Age-related osteoporosis with current pathological fracture, left humerus**   Q A

     ☑7ᵗʰ **M80.029**   **Age-related osteoporosis with current pathological fracture, unspecified humerus**   Q A

   ☑6ᵗʰ **M80.03**   **Age-related osteoporosis with current pathological fracture, forearm**
     Age-related osteoporosis with current pathological fracture of wrist

     ☑7ᵗʰ **M80.031**   **Age-related osteoporosis with current pathological fracture, right forearm**   Q A

☑ Additional Character Required   ☑x7ᵗʰ Placeholder Alert   Manifestation   Unspecified Dx   ►◄ Revised Text   ● New Code   ▲ Revised Code Title

ICD-10-CM 2020   807

√7th **M80.032 Age-related osteoporosis with current pathological fracture, left forearm** Q A

√7th **M80.039 Age-related osteoporosis with current pathological fracture, unspecified forearm** Q A

√6th **M80.04 Age-related osteoporosis with current pathological fracture, hand**

√7th **M80.041 Age-related osteoporosis with current pathological fracture, right hand** Q A

√7th **M80.042 Age-related osteoporosis with current pathological fracture, left hand** Q A

√7th **M80.049 Age-related osteoporosis with current pathological fracture, unspecified hand** Q A

√6th **M80.05 Age-related osteoporosis with current pathological fracture, femur**
     Age-related osteoporosis with current pathological fracture of hip

1 √7th **M80.051 Age-related osteoporosis with current pathological fracture, right femur** HCC Q A

1 √7th **M80.052 Age-related osteoporosis with current pathological fracture, left femur** HCC Q A

1 √7th **M80.059 Age-related osteoporosis with current pathological fracture, unspecified femur** HCC Q A

√6th **M80.06 Age-related osteoporosis with current pathological fracture, lower leg**

√7th **M80.061 Age-related osteoporosis with current pathological fracture, right lower leg** Q A

√7th **M80.062 Age-related osteoporosis with current pathological fracture, left lower leg** Q A

√7th **M80.069 Age-related osteoporosis with current pathological fracture, unspecified lower leg** Q A

√6th **M80.07 Age-related osteoporosis with current pathological fracture, ankle and foot**

√7th **M80.071 Age-related osteoporosis with current pathological fracture, right ankle and foot** Q A

√7th **M80.072 Age-related osteoporosis with current pathological fracture, left ankle and foot** Q A

√7th **M80.079 Age-related osteoporosis with current pathological fracture, unspecified ankle and foot** Q A

1 √x7th **M80.08 Age-related osteoporosis with current pathological fracture, vertebra(e)** HCC Q A

√5th **M80.8 Other osteoporosis with current pathological fracture**
     Drug-induced osteoporosis with current pathological fracture
     Idiopathic osteoporosis with current pathological fracture
     Osteoporosis of disuse with current pathological fracture
     Postoophorectomy osteoporosis with current pathological fracture
     Postsurgical malabsorption osteoporosis with current pathological fracture
     Post-traumatic osteoporosis with current pathological fracture
     Use additional code for adverse effect, if applicable, to identify drug (T36-T50 with fifth or sixth character 5)

√x7th **M80.80 Other osteoporosis with current pathological fracture, unspecified site** Q

√6th **M80.81 Other osteoporosis with pathological fracture, shoulder**

√7th **M80.811 Other osteoporosis with current pathological fracture, right shoulder** Q

√7th **M80.812 Other osteoporosis with current pathological fracture, left shoulder** Q

√7th **M80.819 Other osteoporosis with current pathological fracture, unspecified shoulder** Q

√6th **M80.82 Other osteoporosis with current pathological fracture, humerus**

√7th **M80.821 Other osteoporosis with current pathological fracture, right humerus** Q

√7th **M80.822 Other osteoporosis with current pathological fracture, left humerus** Q

√7th **M80.829 Other osteoporosis with current pathological fracture, unspecified humerus** Q

√6th **M80.83 Other osteoporosis with current pathological fracture, forearm**
     Other osteoporosis with current pathological fracture of wrist

√7th **M80.831 Other osteoporosis with current pathological fracture, right forearm** Q

√7th **M80.832 Other osteoporosis with current pathological fracture, left forearm** Q

√7th **M80.839 Other osteoporosis with current pathological fracture, unspecified forearm** Q

√6th **M80.84 Other osteoporosis with current pathological fracture, hand**

√7th **M80.841 Other osteoporosis with current pathological fracture, right hand** Q

√7th **M80.842 Other osteoporosis with current pathological fracture, left hand** Q

√7th **M80.849 Other osteoporosis with current pathological fracture, unspecified hand** Q

√6th **M80.85 Other osteoporosis with current pathological fracture, femur**
     Other osteoporosis with current pathological fracture of hip

1 √7th **M80.851 Other osteoporosis with current pathological fracture, right femur** HCC Q

1 √7th **M80.852 Other osteoporosis with current pathological fracture, left femur** HCC Q

1 √7th **M80.859 Other osteoporosis with current pathological fracture, unspecified femur** HCC Q

√6th **M80.86 Other osteoporosis with current pathological fracture, lower leg**

√7th **M80.861 Other osteoporosis with current pathological fracture, right lower leg** Q

√7th **M80.862 Other osteoporosis with current pathological fracture, left lower leg** Q

√7th **M80.869 Other osteoporosis with current pathological fracture, unspecified lower leg** Q

√6th **M80.87 Other osteoporosis with current pathological fracture, ankle and foot**

√7th **M80.871 Other osteoporosis with current pathological fracture, right ankle and foot** Q

√7th **M80.872 Other osteoporosis with current pathological fracture, left ankle and foot** Q

√7th **M80.879 Other osteoporosis with current pathological fracture, unspecified ankle and foot** Q

1 √x7th **M80.88 Other osteoporosis with current pathological fracture, vertebra(e)** HCC Q

√4th **M81 Osteoporosis without current pathological fracture**
     Use additional code to identify:
     major osseous defect, if applicable (M89.7-)
     personal history of (healed) osteoporosis fracture, if applicable (Z87.310)
     EXCLUDES 1 *osteoporosis with current pathological fracture (M80.-)*
         Sudeck's atrophy (M89.0)

M81.0 Age-related osteoporosis without current pathological fracture Q A
     Involutional osteoporosis without current pathological fracture
     Osteoporosis NOS
     Postmenopausal osteoporosis without current pathological fracture
     Senile osteoporosis without current pathological fracture

M81.6 Localized osteoporosis [Lequesne] Q
     EXCLUDES 1 *Sudeck's atrophy (M89.0)*

M81.8 Other osteoporosis without current pathological fracture ▫

  Drug-induced osteoporosis without current pathological fracture

  Idiopathic osteoporosis without current pathological fracture

  Osteoporosis of disuse without current pathological fracture

  Postoophorectomy osteoporosis without current pathological fracture

  Postsurgical malabsorption osteoporosis without current pathological fracture

  Post-traumatic osteoporosis without current pathological fracture

  Use additional code for adverse effect, if applicable, to identify drug (T36-T50 with fifth or sixth character 5)

✓4ᵗʰ M83 Adult osteomalacia

  EXCLUDES 1   infantile and juvenile osteomalacia (E55.0)

      renal osteodystrophy (N25.0)

      rickets (active) (E55.0)

      rickets (active) sequelae (E64.3)

      vitamin D-resistant osteomalacia (E83.3)

      vitamin D-resistant rickets (active) (E83.3)

M83.0 Puerperal osteomalacia   M ♀

M83.1 Senile osteomalacia   A

M83.2 Adult osteomalacia due to malabsorption   A

  Postsurgical malabsorption osteomalacia in adults

M83.3 Adult osteomalacia due to malnutrition   A

M83.4 Aluminum bone disease

M83.5 Other drug-induced osteomalacia in adults   A

  Use additional code for adverse effect, if applicable, to identify drug (T36-T50 with fifth or sixth character 5)

M83.8 Other adult osteomalacia   A

M83.9 Adult osteomalacia, unspecified   A

✓4ᵗʰ M84 Disorder of continuity of bone

  EXCLUDES 2   traumatic fracture of bone-see fracture, by site

✓5ᵗʰ M84.3 Stress fracture

  Fatigue fracture

  March fracture

  Stress fracture NOS

  Stress reaction

  Use additional external cause code(s) to identify the cause of the stress fracture

  EXCLUDES 1   pathological fracture due to osteoporosis (M80.-)

      pathological fracture NOS (M84.4.-)

      traumatic fracture (S12.-, S22.-, S32.-, S42.-, S52.-, S62.-, S72.-, S82.-, S92.-)

  EXCLUDES 2   personal history of (healed) stress (fatigue) fracture (Z87.312)

      stress fracture of vertebra (M48.4-)

The appropriate 7th character is to be added to each code from subcategory M84.3.

A   initial encounter for fracture

D   subsequent encounter for fracture with routine healing

G   subsequent encounter for fracture with delayed healing

K   subsequent encounter for fracture with nonunion

P   subsequent encounter for fracture with malunion

S   sequela

✓x7ᵗʰ M84.30 Stress fracture, unspecified site

✓6ᵗʰ M84.31 Stress fracture, shoulder

  ✓7ᵗʰ M84.311 Stress fracture, right shoulder   ▫

  ✓7ᵗʰ M84.312 Stress fracture, left shoulder   ▫

  ✓7ᵗʰ M84.319 Stress fracture, unspecified shoulder   ▫

✓6ᵗʰ M84.32 Stress fracture, humerus

  ✓7ᵗʰ M84.321 Stress fracture, right humerus   ▫

  ✓7ᵗʰ M84.322 Stress fracture, left humerus   ▫

  ✓7ᵗʰ M84.329 Stress fracture, unspecified humerus   ▫

✓6ᵗʰ M84.33 Stress fracture, ulna and radius

  ✓7ᵗʰ M84.331 Stress fracture, right ulna   ▫

  ✓7ᵗʰ M84.332 Stress fracture, left ulna   ▫

  ✓7ᵗʰ M84.333 Stress fracture, right radius   ▫

  ✓7ᵗʰ M84.334 Stress fracture, left radius   ▫

  ✓7ᵗʰ M84.339 Stress fracture, unspecified ulna and radius   ▫

✓6ᵗʰ M84.34 Stress fracture, hand and fingers

  ✓7ᵗʰ M84.341 Stress fracture, right hand   ▫

  ✓7ᵗʰ M84.342 Stress fracture, left hand   ▫

  ✓7ᵗʰ M84.343 Stress fracture, unspecified hand   ▫

  ✓7ᵗʰ M84.344 Stress fracture, right finger(s)

  ✓7ᵗʰ M84.345 Stress fracture, left finger(s)

  ✓7ᵗʰ M84.346 Stress fracture, unspecified finger(s)

✓6ᵗʰ M84.35 Stress fracture, pelvis and femur

  Stress fracture, hip

  ✓7ᵗʰ M84.350 Stress fracture, pelvis   ▫

  ✓7ᵗʰ M84.351 Stress fracture, right femur   ▫

  ✓7ᵗʰ M84.352 Stress fracture, left femur   ▫

  ✓7ᵗʰ M84.353 Stress fracture, unspecified femur   ▫

  ✓7ᵗʰ M84.359 Stress fracture, hip, unspecified   ▫

✓6ᵗʰ M84.36 Stress fracture, tibia and fibula

  ✓7ᵗʰ M84.361 Stress fracture, right tibia   ▫

  ✓7ᵗʰ M84.362 Stress fracture, left tibia   ▫

  ✓7ᵗʰ M84.363 Stress fracture, right fibula   ▫

  ✓7ᵗʰ M84.364 Stress fracture, left fibula   ▫

  ✓7ᵗʰ M84.369 Stress fracture, unspecified tibia and fibula   ▫

✓6ᵗʰ M84.37 Stress fracture, ankle, foot and toes

  ✓7ᵗʰ M84.371 Stress fracture, right ankle   ▫

  ✓7ᵗʰ M84.372 Stress fracture, left ankle   ▫

  ✓7ᵗʰ M84.373 Stress fracture, unspecified ankle   ▫

  ✓7ᵗʰ M84.374 Stress fracture, right foot   ▫

  ✓7ᵗʰ M84.375 Stress fracture, left foot   ▫

  ✓7ᵗʰ M84.376 Stress fracture, unspecified foot   ▫

  ✓7ᵗʰ M84.377 Stress fracture, right toe(s)

  ✓7ᵗʰ M84.378 Stress fracture, left toe(s)

  ✓7ᵗʰ M84.379 Stress fracture, unspecified toe(s)

✓x7ᵗʰ M84.38 Stress fracture, other site   ▫

  EXCLUDES 2   stress fracture of vertebra (M48.4-)

✓5ᵗʰ M84.4 Pathological fracture, not elsewhere classified

  Chronic fracture

  Pathological fracture NOS

  EXCLUDES 1   collapsed vertebra NEC (M48.5)

      pathological fracture in neoplastic disease (M84.5-)

      pathological fracture in osteoporosis (M80.-)

      pathological fracture in other disease (M84.6-)

      stress fracture (M84.3-)

      traumatic fracture (S12.-, S22.-, S32.-, S42.-, S52.-, S62.-, S72.-, S82.-, S92.-)

  EXCLUDES 2   personal history of (healed) pathological fracture (Z87.311)

The appropriate 7th character is to be added to each code from subcategory M84.4.

A   initial encounter for fracture

D   subsequent encounter for fracture with routine healing

G   subsequent encounter for fracture with delayed healing

K   subsequent encounter for fracture with nonunion

P   subsequent encounter for fracture with malunion

S   sequela

✓x7ᵗʰ M84.40 Pathological fracture, unspecified site

✓6ᵗʰ M84.41 Pathological fracture, shoulder

  ✓7ᵗʰ M84.411 Pathological fracture, right shoulder

  ✓7ᵗʰ M84.412 Pathological fracture, left shoulder

  ✓7ᵗʰ M84.419 Pathological fracture, unspecified shoulder

✓6ᵗʰ M84.42 Pathological fracture, humerus

  ✓7ᵗʰ M84.421 Pathological fracture, right humerus

  ✓7ᵗʰ M84.422 Pathological fracture, left humerus

  ✓7ᵗʰ M84.429 Pathological fracture, unspecified humerus

✓6ᵗʰ M84.43 Pathological fracture, ulna and radius

  ✓7ᵗʰ M84.431 Pathological fracture, right ulna

  ✓7ᵗʰ M84.432 Pathological fracture, left ulna

✔ Additional Character Required   ✓x7ᵗʰ Placeholder Alert   Manifestation   Unspecified Dx   ▶◀ Revised Text   ● New Code   ▲ Revised Code Title

✓7ᵗʰ **M84.433** Pathological fracture, right radius

✓7ᵗʰ **M84.434** Pathological fracture, left radius

✓7ᵗʰ **M84.439** Pathological fracture, unspecified ulna and radius

✓6ᵗʰ **M84.44** Pathological fracture, hand and fingers

  ✓7ᵗʰ **M84.441** Pathological fracture, right hand

  ✓7ᵗʰ **M84.442** Pathological fracture, left hand

  ✓7ᵗʰ **M84.443** Pathological fracture, unspecified hand

  ✓7ᵗʰ **M84.444** Pathological fracture, right finger(s)

  ✓7ᵗʰ **M84.445** Pathological fracture, left finger(s)

  ✓7ᵗʰ **M84.446** Pathological fracture, unspecified finger(s)

✓6ᵗʰ **M84.45** Pathological fracture, femur and pelvis

    AHA: 2016,4Q,43

  ¹ ✓7ᵗʰ **M84.451** Pathological fracture, right femur   HCC

  ¹ ✓7ᵗʰ **M84.452** Pathological fracture, left femur   HCC

  ¹ ✓7ᵗʰ **M84.453** Pathological fracture, unspecified femur   HCC

  ✓7ᵗʰ **M84.454** Pathological fracture, pelvis

  ¹ ✓7ᵗʰ **M84.459** Pathological fracture, hip, unspecified   HCC

✓6ᵗʰ **M84.46** Pathological fracture, tibia and fibula

  ✓7ᵗʰ **M84.461** Pathological fracture, right tibia

  ✓7ᵗʰ **M84.462** Pathological fracture, left tibia

  ✓7ᵗʰ **M84.463** Pathological fracture, right fibula

  ✓7ᵗʰ **M84.464** Pathological fracture, left fibula

  ✓7ᵗʰ **M84.469** Pathological fracture, unspecified tibia and fibula

✓6ᵗʰ **M84.47** Pathological fracture, ankle, foot and toes

  ✓7ᵗʰ **M84.471** Pathological fracture, right ankle

  ✓7ᵗʰ **M84.472** Pathological fracture, left ankle

  ✓7ᵗʰ **M84.473** Pathological fracture, unspecified ankle

  ✓7ᵗʰ **M84.474** Pathological fracture, right foot

  ✓7ᵗʰ **M84.475** Pathological fracture, left foot

  ✓7ᵗʰ **M84.476** Pathological fracture, unspecified foot

  ✓7ᵗʰ **M84.477** Pathological fracture, right toe(s)

  ✓7ᵗʰ **M84.478** Pathological fracture, left toe(s)

  ✓7ᵗʰ **M84.479** Pathological fracture, unspecified toe(s)

✓x7ᵗʰ **M84.48** Pathological fracture, other site

✓5ᵗʰ **M84.5** Pathological fracture in neoplastic disease

    Code also underlying neoplasm

> The appropriate 7th character is to be added to each code from subcategory M84.5.
> A   initial encounter for fracture
> D   subsequent encounter for fracture with routine healing
> G   subsequent encounter for fracture with delayed healing
> K   subsequent encounter for fracture with nonunion
> P   subsequent encounter for fracture with malunion
> S   sequela

✓x7ᵗʰ **M84.50** Pathological fracture in neoplastic disease, unspecified site

✓6ᵗʰ **M84.51** Pathological fracture in neoplastic disease, shoulder

  ✓7ᵗʰ **M84.511** Pathological fracture in neoplastic disease, right shoulder

  ✓7ᵗʰ **M84.512** Pathological fracture in neoplastic disease, left shoulder

  ✓7ᵗʰ **M84.519** Pathological fracture in neoplastic disease, unspecified shoulder

✓6ᵗʰ **M84.52** Pathological fracture in neoplastic disease, humerus

  ✓7ᵗʰ **M84.521** Pathological fracture in neoplastic disease, right humerus

  ✓7ᵗʰ **M84.522** Pathological fracture in neoplastic disease, left humerus

  ✓7ᵗʰ **M84.529** Pathological fracture in neoplastic disease, unspecified humerus

✓6ᵗʰ **M84.53** Pathological fracture in neoplastic disease, ulna and radius

  ✓7ᵗʰ **M84.531** Pathological fracture in neoplastic disease, right ulna

  ✓7ᵗʰ **M84.532** Pathological fracture in neoplastic disease, left ulna

✓7ᵗʰ **M84.533** Pathological fracture in neoplastic disease, right radius

✓7ᵗʰ **M84.534** Pathological fracture in neoplastic disease, left radius

✓7ᵗʰ **M84.539** Pathological fracture in neoplastic disease, unspecified ulna and radius

✓6ᵗʰ **M84.54** Pathological fracture in neoplastic disease, hand

  ✓7ᵗʰ **M84.541** Pathological fracture in neoplastic disease, right hand

  ✓7ᵗʰ **M84.542** Pathological fracture in neoplastic disease, left hand

  ✓7ᵗʰ **M84.549** Pathological fracture in neoplastic disease, unspecified hand

✓6ᵗʰ **M84.55** Pathological fracture in neoplastic disease, pelvis and femur

  ✓7ᵗʰ **M84.550** Pathological fracture in neoplastic disease, pelvis

  ¹ ✓7ᵗʰ **M84.551** Pathological fracture in neoplastic disease, right femur   HCC

  ¹ ✓7ᵗʰ **M84.552** Pathological fracture in neoplastic disease, left femur   HCC

  ¹ ✓7ᵗʰ **M84.553** Pathological fracture in neoplastic disease, unspecified femur   HCC

  ¹ ✓7ᵗʰ **M84.559** Pathological fracture in neoplastic disease, hip, unspecified   HCC

✓6ᵗʰ **M84.56** Pathological fracture in neoplastic disease, tibia and fibula

  ✓7ᵗʰ **M84.561** Pathological fracture in neoplastic disease, right tibia

  ✓7ᵗʰ **M84.562** Pathological fracture in neoplastic disease, left tibia

  ✓7ᵗʰ **M84.563** Pathological fracture in neoplastic disease, right fibula

  ✓7ᵗʰ **M84.564** Pathological fracture in neoplastic disease, left fibula

  ✓7ᵗʰ **M84.569** Pathological fracture in neoplastic disease, unspecified tibia and fibula

✓6ᵗʰ **M84.57** Pathological fracture in neoplastic disease, ankle and foot

  ✓7ᵗʰ **M84.571** Pathological fracture in neoplastic disease, right ankle

  ✓7ᵗʰ **M84.572** Pathological fracture in neoplastic disease, left ankle

  ✓7ᵗʰ **M84.573** Pathological fracture in neoplastic disease, unspecified ankle

  ✓7ᵗʰ **M84.574** Pathological fracture in neoplastic disease, right foot

  ✓7ᵗʰ **M84.575** Pathological fracture in neoplastic disease, left foot

  ✓7ᵗʰ **M84.576** Pathological fracture in neoplastic disease, unspecified foot

✓x7ᵗʰ **M84.58** Pathological fracture in neoplastic disease, other specified site

    Pathological fracture in neoplastic disease, vertebrae

✓5ᵗʰ **M84.6** Pathological fracture in other disease

    Code also underlying condition

    EXCLUDES 1 *pathological fracture in osteoporosis (M80.-)*

> The appropriate 7th character is to be added to each code from subcategory M84.6.
> A   initial encounter for fracture
> D   subsequent encounter for fracture with routine healing
> G   subsequent encounter for fracture with delayed healing
> K   subsequent encounter for fracture with nonunion
> P   subsequent encounter for fracture with malunion
> S   sequela

✓x7ᵗʰ **M84.60** Pathological fracture in other disease, unspecified site

✓6ᵗʰ **M84.61** Pathological fracture in other disease, shoulder

  ✓7ᵗʰ **M84.611** Pathological fracture in other disease, right shoulder

  ✓7ᵗʰ **M84.612** Pathological fracture in other disease, left shoulder

  ✓7ᵗʰ **M84.619** Pathological fracture in other disease, unspecified shoulder

✓6ᵗʰ **M84.62** Pathological fracture in other disease, humerus

  ✓7ᵗʰ **M84.621** Pathological fracture in other disease, right humerus

  ✓7ᵗʰ **M84.622** Pathological fracture in other disease, left humerus

---

HCC CMS-HCC   Q QPP   N Newborn: 0   P Pediatric: 0-17   M Maternity: 12-55   A Adult: 15-124

√7ᵗʰ **M84.629** Pathological fracture in other disease, unspecified humerus

√6ᵗʰ **M84.63** Pathological fracture in other disease, ulna and radius

√7ᵗʰ **M84.631** Pathological fracture in other disease, right ulna

√7ᵗʰ **M84.632** Pathological fracture in other disease, left ulna

√7ᵗʰ **M84.633** Pathological fracture in other disease, right radius

√7ᵗʰ **M84.634** Pathological fracture in other disease, left radius

√7ᵗʰ **M84.639** Pathological fracture in other disease, unspecified ulna and radius

√6ᵗʰ **M84.64** Pathological fracture in other disease, hand

√7ᵗʰ **M84.641** Pathological fracture in other disease, right hand

√7ᵗʰ **M84.642** Pathological fracture in other disease, left hand

√7ᵗʰ **M84.649** Pathological fracture in other disease, unspecified hand

√6ᵗʰ **M84.65** Pathological fracture in other disease, pelvis and femur

√7ᵗʰ **M84.650** Pathological fracture in other disease, pelvis

1 √7ᵗʰ **M84.651** Pathological fracture in other disease, right femur **HCC**

1 √7ᵗʰ **M84.652** Pathological fracture in other disease, left femur **HCC**

1 √7ᵗʰ **M84.653** Pathological fracture in other disease, unspecified femur **HCC**

1 √7ᵗʰ **M84.659** Pathological fracture in other disease, hip, unspecified **HCC**

√6ᵗʰ **M84.66** Pathological fracture in other disease, tibia and fibula

√7ᵗʰ **M84.661** Pathological fracture in other disease, right tibia

√7ᵗʰ **M84.662** Pathological fracture in other disease, left tibia

√7ᵗʰ **M84.663** Pathological fracture in other disease, right fibula

√7ᵗʰ **M84.664** Pathological fracture in other disease, left fibula

√7ᵗʰ **M84.669** Pathological fracture in other disease, unspecified tibia and fibula

√6ᵗʰ **M84.67** Pathological fracture in other disease, ankle and foot

√7ᵗʰ **M84.671** Pathological fracture in other disease, right ankle

√7ᵗʰ **M84.672** Pathological fracture in other disease, left ankle

√7ᵗʰ **M84.673** Pathological fracture in other disease, unspecified ankle

√7ᵗʰ **M84.674** Pathological fracture in other disease, right foot

√7ᵗʰ **M84.675** Pathological fracture in other disease, left foot

√7ᵗʰ **M84.676** Pathological fracture in other disease, unspecified foot

√x7ᵗʰ **M84.68** Pathological fracture in other disease, other site

√5ᵗʰ **M84.7** Nontraumatic fracture, not elsewhere classified

√6ᵗʰ **M84.75** Atypical femoral fracture

AHA: 2016,4Q,41-42

The appropriate 7th character is to be added to each code from M84.75.
A   initial encounter for fracture
D   subsequent encounter for fracture with routine healing
G   subsequent encounter for fracture with delayed healing
K   subsequent encounter for fracture with nonunion
P   subsequent encounter for fracture with malunion
S   sequela

√7ᵗʰ **M84.750** Atypical femoral fracture, unspecified **Q**

√7ᵗʰ **M84.751** Incomplete atypical femoral fracture, right leg **Q**

√7ᵗʰ **M84.752** Incomplete atypical femoral fracture, left leg **Q**

√7ᵗʰ **M84.753** Incomplete atypical femoral fracture, unspecified leg **Q**

1 √7ᵗʰ **M84.754** Complete transverse atypical femoral fracture, right leg **HCC Q**

1 √7ᵗʰ **M84.755** Complete transverse atypical femoral fracture, left leg **HCC Q**

1 √7ᵗʰ **M84.756** Complete transverse atypical femoral fracture, unspecified leg **HCC Q**

1 √7ᵗʰ **M84.757** Complete oblique atypical femoral fracture, right leg **HCC Q**

1 √7ᵗʰ **M84.758** Complete oblique atypical femoral fracture, left leg **HCC**

1 √7ᵗʰ **M84.759** Complete oblique atypical femoral fracture, unspecified leg **HCC Q**

√5ᵗʰ **M84.8** Other disorders of continuity of bone

M84.80 Other disorders of continuity of bone, unspecified site

√6ᵗʰ **M84.81** Other disorders of continuity of bone, shoulder

M84.811 Other disorders of continuity of bone, right shoulder

M84.812 Other disorders of continuity of bone, left shoulder

M84.819 Other disorders of continuity of bone, unspecified shoulder

√6ᵗʰ **M84.82** Other disorders of continuity of bone, humerus

M84.821 Other disorders of continuity of bone, right humerus

M84.822 Other disorders of continuity of bone, left humerus

M84.829 Other disorders of continuity of bone, unspecified humerus

√6ᵗʰ **M84.83** Other disorders of continuity of bone, ulna and radius

M84.831 Other disorders of continuity of bone, right ulna

M84.832 Other disorders of continuity of bone, left ulna

M84.833 Other disorders of continuity of bone, right radius

M84.834 Other disorders of continuity of bone, left radius

M84.839 Other disorders of continuity of bone, unspecified ulna and radius

√6ᵗʰ **M84.84** Other disorders of continuity of bone, hand

M84.841 Other disorders of continuity of bone, right hand

M84.842 Other disorders of continuity of bone, left hand

M84.849 Other disorders of continuity of bone, unspecified hand

√6ᵗʰ **M84.85** Other disorders of continuity of bone, pelvic region and thigh

M84.851 Other disorders of continuity of bone, right pelvic region and thigh

M84.852 Other disorders of continuity of bone, left pelvic region and thigh

M84.859 Other disorders of continuity of bone, unspecified pelvic region and thigh

√6ᵗʰ **M84.86** Other disorders of continuity of bone, tibia and fibula

M84.861 Other disorders of continuity of bone, right tibia

M84.862 Other disorders of continuity of bone, left tibia

M84.863 Other disorders of continuity of bone, right fibula

M84.864 Other disorders of continuity of bone, left fibula

M84.869 Other disorders of continuity of bone, unspecified tibia and fibula

√6ᵗʰ **M84.87** Other disorders of continuity of bone, ankle and foot

M84.871 Other disorders of continuity of bone, right ankle and foot

M84.872 Other disorders of continuity of bone, left ankle and foot

M84.879 Other disorders of continuity of bone, unspecified ankle and foot

M84.88 Other disorders of continuity of bone, other site

M84.9 Disorder of continuity of bone, unspecified

✓ Additional Character Required | √x7ᵗʰ Placeholder Alert | Manifestation | Unspecified Dx | ►◄ Revised Text | ● New Code | ▲ Revised Code Title

✓4th M85 Other disorders of bone density and structure

    EXCLUDES 1   osteogenesis imperfecta (Q78.0)
               osteopetrosis (Q78.2)
               osteopoikilosis (Q78.8)
               polyostotic fibrous dysplasia (Q78.1)

  ✓5th M85.0 Fibrous dysplasia (monostotic)

      EXCLUDES 2   fibrous dysplasia of jaw (M27.8)

    M85.00 Fibrous dysplasia (monostotic), unspecified site

    ✓6th M85.01 Fibrous dysplasia (monostotic), shoulder

        M85.011 Fibrous dysplasia (monostotic), right shoulder
        M85.012 Fibrous dysplasia (monostotic), left shoulder
        M85.019 Fibrous dysplasia (monostotic), unspecified shoulder

    ✓6th M85.02 Fibrous dysplasia (monostotic), upper arm

        M85.021 Fibrous dysplasia (monostotic), right upper arm
        M85.022 Fibrous dysplasia (monostotic), left upper arm
        M85.029 Fibrous dysplasia (monostotic), unspecified upper arm

    ✓6th M85.03 Fibrous dysplasia (monostotic), forearm

        M85.031 Fibrous dysplasia (monostotic), right forearm
        M85.032 Fibrous dysplasia (monostotic), left forearm
        M85.039 Fibrous dysplasia (monostotic), unspecified forearm

    ✓6th M85.04 Fibrous dysplasia (monostotic), hand

        M85.041 Fibrous dysplasia (monostotic), right hand
        M85.042 Fibrous dysplasia (monostotic), left hand
        M85.049 Fibrous dysplasia (monostotic), unspecified hand

    ✓6th M85.05 Fibrous dysplasia (monostotic), thigh

        M85.051 Fibrous dysplasia (monostotic), right thigh
        M85.052 Fibrous dysplasia (monostotic), left thigh
        M85.059 Fibrous dysplasia (monostotic), unspecified thigh

    ✓6th M85.06 Fibrous dysplasia (monostotic), lower leg

        M85.061 Fibrous dysplasia (monostotic), right lower leg
        M85.062 Fibrous dysplasia (monostotic), left lower leg
        M85.069 Fibrous dysplasia (monostotic), unspecified lower leg

    ✓6th M85.07 Fibrous dysplasia (monostotic), ankle and foot

        M85.071 Fibrous dysplasia (monostotic), right ankle and foot
        M85.072 Fibrous dysplasia (monostotic), left ankle and foot
        M85.079 Fibrous dysplasia (monostotic), unspecified ankle and foot

    M85.08 Fibrous dysplasia (monostotic), other site

    M85.09 Fibrous dysplasia (monostotic), multiple sites

  ✓5th M85.1 Skeletal fluorosis

    M85.10 Skeletal fluorosis, unspecified site

    ✓6th M85.11 Skeletal fluorosis, shoulder

        M85.111 Skeletal fluorosis, right shoulder
        M85.112 Skeletal fluorosis, left shoulder
        M85.119 Skeletal fluorosis, unspecified shoulder

    ✓6th M85.12 Skeletal fluorosis, upper arm

        M85.121 Skeletal fluorosis, right upper arm
        M85.122 Skeletal fluorosis, left upper arm
        M85.129 Skeletal fluorosis, unspecified upper arm

    ✓6th M85.13 Skeletal fluorosis, forearm

        M85.131 Skeletal fluorosis, right forearm
        M85.132 Skeletal fluorosis, left forearm
        M85.139 Skeletal fluorosis, unspecified forearm

    ✓6th M85.14 Skeletal fluorosis, hand

        M85.141 Skeletal fluorosis, right hand
        M85.142 Skeletal fluorosis, left hand
        M85.149 Skeletal fluorosis, unspecified hand

    ✓6th M85.15 Skeletal fluorosis, thigh

        M85.151 Skeletal fluorosis, right thigh
        M85.152 Skeletal fluorosis, left thigh
        M85.159 Skeletal fluorosis, unspecified thigh

    ✓6th M85.16 Skeletal fluorosis, lower leg

        M85.161 Skeletal fluorosis, right lower leg
        M85.162 Skeletal fluorosis, left lower leg
        M85.169 Skeletal fluorosis, unspecified lower leg

    ✓6th M85.17 Skeletal fluorosis, ankle and foot

        M85.171 Skeletal fluorosis, right ankle and foot
        M85.172 Skeletal fluorosis, left ankle and foot
        M85.179 Skeletal fluorosis, unspecified ankle and foot

    M85.18 Skeletal fluorosis, other site

    M85.19 Skeletal fluorosis, multiple sites

  M85.2 Hyperostosis of skull

    DEF: Abnormal bone growth on the inner aspect of the cranial bones.

  ✓5th M85.3 Osteitis condensans

    M85.30 Osteitis condensans, unspecified site

    ✓6th M85.31 Osteitis condensans, shoulder

        M85.311 Osteitis condensans, right shoulder
        M85.312 Osteitis condensans, left shoulder
        M85.319 Osteitis condensans, unspecified shoulder

    ✓6th M85.32 Osteitis condensans, upper arm

        M85.321 Osteitis condensans, right upper arm
        M85.322 Osteitis condensans, left upper arm
        M85.329 Osteitis condensans, unspecified upper arm

    ✓6th M85.33 Osteitis condensans, forearm

        M85.331 Osteitis condensans, right forearm
        M85.332 Osteitis condensans, left forearm
        M85.339 Osteitis condensans, unspecified forearm

    ✓6th M85.34 Osteitis condensans, hand

        M85.341 Osteitis condensans, right hand
        M85.342 Osteitis condensans, left hand
        M85.349 Osteitis condensans, unspecified hand

    ✓6th M85.35 Osteitis condensans, thigh

        M85.351 Osteitis condensans, right thigh
        M85.352 Osteitis condensans, left thigh
        M85.359 Osteitis condensans, unspecified thigh

    ✓6th M85.36 Osteitis condensans, lower leg

        M85.361 Osteitis condensans, right lower leg
        M85.362 Osteitis condensans, left lower leg
        M85.369 Osteitis condensans, unspecified lower leg

    ✓6th M85.37 Osteitis condensans, ankle and foot

        M85.371 Osteitis condensans, right ankle and foot
        M85.372 Osteitis condensans, left ankle and foot
        M85.379 Osteitis condensans, unspecified ankle and foot

    M85.38 Osteitis condensans, other site

    M85.39 Osteitis condensans, multiple sites

  ✓5th M85.4 Solitary bone cyst

      EXCLUDES 2   solitary cyst of jaw (M27.4)

    M85.40 Solitary bone cyst, unspecified site

    ✓6th M85.41 Solitary bone cyst, shoulder

        M85.411 Solitary bone cyst, right shoulder
        M85.412 Solitary bone cyst, left shoulder
        M85.419 Solitary bone cyst, unspecified shoulder

    ✓6th M85.42 Solitary bone cyst, humerus

        M85.421 Solitary bone cyst, right humerus
        M85.422 Solitary bone cyst, left humerus
        M85.429 Solitary bone cyst, unspecified humerus

    ✓6th M85.43 Solitary bone cyst, ulna and radius

        M85.431 Solitary bone cyst, right ulna and radius
        M85.432 Solitary bone cyst, left ulna and radius
        M85.439 Solitary bone cyst, unspecified ulna and radius

    ✓6th M85.44 Solitary bone cyst, hand

        M85.441 Solitary bone cyst, right hand
        M85.442 Solitary bone cyst, left hand
        M85.449 Solitary bone cyst, unspecified hand

    ✓6th M85.45 Solitary bone cyst, pelvis

        M85.451 Solitary bone cyst, right pelvis
        M85.452 Solitary bone cyst, left pelvis
        M85.459 Solitary bone cyst, unspecified pelvis

√6ᵗʰ **M85.46** **Solitary bone cyst, tibia and fibula**

     M85.461 Solitary bone cyst, right tibia and fibula
     M85.462 Solitary bone cyst, left tibia and fibula
     M85.469 Solitary bone cyst, unspecified tibia and fibula

√6ᵗʰ **M85.47** **Solitary bone cyst, ankle and foot**

     M85.471 Solitary bone cyst, right ankle and foot
     M85.472 Solitary bone cyst, left ankle and foot
     M85.479 Solitary bone cyst, unspecified ankle and foot

     M85.48 Solitary bone cyst, other site

√5ᵗʰ **M85.5** **Aneurysmal bone cyst**

     EXCLUDES 2   *aneurysmal cyst of jaw (M27.4)*

     DEF: Solitary bone lesion that bulges into the periosteum and is marked by a calcified rim.

     M85.50 Aneurysmal bone cyst, unspecified site

√6ᵗʰ **M85.51** **Aneurysmal bone cyst, shoulder**

     M85.511 Aneurysmal bone cyst, right shoulder
     M85.512 Aneurysmal bone cyst, left shoulder
     M85.519 Aneurysmal bone cyst, unspecified shoulder

√6ᵗʰ **M85.52** **Aneurysmal bone cyst, upper arm**

     M85.521 Aneurysmal bone cyst, right upper arm
     M85.522 Aneurysmal bone cyst, left upper arm
     M85.529 Aneurysmal bone cyst, unspecified upper arm

√6ᵗʰ **M85.53** **Aneurysmal bone cyst, forearm**

     M85.531 Aneurysmal bone cyst, right forearm
     M85.532 Aneurysmal bone cyst, left forearm
     M85.539 Aneurysmal bone cyst, unspecified forearm

√6ᵗʰ **M85.54** **Aneurysmal bone cyst, hand**

     M85.541 Aneurysmal bone cyst, right hand
     M85.542 Aneurysmal bone cyst, left hand
     M85.549 Aneurysmal bone cyst, unspecified hand

√6ᵗʰ **M85.55** **Aneurysmal bone cyst, thigh**

     M85.551 Aneurysmal bone cyst, right thigh
     M85.552 Aneurysmal bone cyst, left thigh
     M85.559 Aneurysmal bone cyst. unspecified thigh

√6ᵗʰ **M85.56** **Aneurysmal bone cyst, lower leg**

     M85.561 Aneurysmal bone cyst, right lower leg
     M85.562 Aneurysmal bone cyst, left lower leg
     M85.569 Aneurysmal bone cyst, unspecified lower leg

√6ᵗʰ **M85.57** **Aneurysmal bone cyst, ankle and foot**

     M85.571 Aneurysmal bone cyst, right ankle and foot
     M85.572 Aneurysmal bone cyst, left ankle and foot
     M85.579 Aneurysmal bone cyst, unspecified ankle and foot

     M85.58 Aneurysmal bone cyst, other site

     M85.59 Aneurysmal bone cyst, multiple sites

√5ᵗʰ **M85.6** **Other cyst of bone**

     EXCLUDES 1   *cyst of jaw NEC (M27.4)*
               osteitis fibrosa cystica generalisata [von Recklinghausen's disease of bone] (E21.0)

     M85.60 Other cyst of bone, unspecified site

√6ᵗʰ **M85.61** **Other cyst of bone, shoulder**

     M85.611 Other cyst of bone, right shoulder
     M85.612 Other cyst of bone, left shoulder
     M85.619 Other cyst of bone, unspecified shoulder

√6ᵗʰ **M85.62** **Other cyst of bone, upper arm**

     M85.621 Other cyst of bone, right upper arm
     M85.622 Other cyst of bone, left upper arm
     M85.629 Other cyst of bone, unspecified upper arm

√6ᵗʰ **M85.63** **Other cyst of bone, forearm**

     M85.631 Other cyst of bone, right forearm
     M85.632 Other cyst of bone, left forearm
     M85.639 Other cyst of bone, unspecified forearm

√6ᵗʰ **M85.64** **Other cyst of bone, hand**

     M85.641 Other cyst of bone, right hand
     M85.642 Other cyst of bone, left hand
     M85.649 Other cyst of bone, unspecified hand

√6ᵗʰ **M85.65** **Other cyst of bone, thigh**

     M85.651 Other cyst of bone, right thigh
     M85.652 Other cyst of bone, left thigh

     M85.659 Other cyst of bone, unspecified thigh

√6ᵗʰ **M85.66** **Other cyst of bone, lower leg**

     M85.661 Other cyst of bone, right lower leg
     M85.662 Other cyst of bone, left lower leg
     M85.669 Other cyst of bone, unspecified lower leg

√6ᵗʰ **M85.67** **Other cyst of bone, ankle and foot**

     M85.671 Other cyst of bone, right ankle and foot
     M85.672 Other cyst of bone, left ankle and foot
     M85.679 Other cyst of bone, unspecified ankle and foot

     M85.68 Other cyst of bone, other site

     M85.69 Other cyst of bone, multiple sites

√5ᵗʰ **M85.8** **Other specified disorders of bone density and structure**

     Hyperostosis of bones, except skull
     Osteosclerosis, acquired

     EXCLUDES 1   *diffuse idiopathic skeletal hyperostosis [DISH] (M48.1)*
               osteosclerosis congenita (Q77.4)
               osteosclerosis fragilitas (generalista) (Q78.2)
               osteosclerosis myelofibrosis (D75.81)

     M85.80 Other specified disorders of bone density and structure, unspecified site

√6ᵗʰ **M85.81** **Other specified disorders of bone density and structure, shoulder**

     M85.811 Other specified disorders of bone density and structure, right shoulder
     M85.812 Other specified disorders of bone density and structure, left shoulder
     M85.819 Other specified disorders of bone density and structure, unspecified shoulder

√6ᵗʰ **M85.82** **Other specified disorders of bone density and structure, upper arm**

     M85.821 Other specified disorders of bone density and structure, right upper arm
     M85.822 Other specified disorders of bone density and structure, left upper arm
     M85.829 Other specified disorders of bone density and structure, unspecified upper arm

√6ᵗʰ **M85.83** **Other specified disorders of bone density and structure, forearm**

     M85.831 Other specified disorders of bone density and structure, right forearm
     M85.832 Other specified disorders of bone density and structure, left forearm
     M85.839 Other specified disorders of bone density and structure, unspecified forearm

√6ᵗʰ **M85.84** **Other specified disorders of bone density and structure, hand**

     M85.841 Other specified disorders of bone density and structure, right hand
     M85.842 Other specified disorders of bone density and structure, left hand
     M85.849 Other specified disorders of bone density and structure, unspecified hand

√6ᵗʰ **M85.85** **Other specified disorders of bone density and structure, thigh**

     M85.851 Other specified disorders of bone density and structure, right thigh
     M85.852 Other specified disorders of bone density and structure, left thigh
     M85.859 Other specified disorders of bone density and structure, unspecified thigh

√6ᵗʰ **M85.86** **Other specified disorders of bone density and structure, lower leg**

     M85.861 Other specified disorders of bone density and structure, right lower leg
     M85.862 Other specified disorders of bone density and structure, left lower leg
     M85.869 Other specified disorders of bone density and structure, unspecified lower leg

√6ᵗʰ **M85.87** **Other specified disorders of bone density and structure, ankle and foot**

     M85.871 Other specified disorders of bone density and structure, right ankle and foot
     M85.872 Other specified disorders of bone density and structure, left ankle and foot
     M85.879 Other specified disorders of bone density and structure, unspecified ankle and foot

     M85.88 Other specified disorders of bone density and structure, other site

     M85.89 Other specified disorders of bone density and structure, multiple sites

✔ Additional Character Required   √x7ᵗʰ Placeholder Alert   Manifestation   Unspecified Dx   ▶◀ Revised Text   ● New Code   ▲ Revised Code Title

ICD-10-CM 2020   813

Chapter 13. Diseases of the Musculoskeletal System and Connective Tissue

M85.9 Disorder of bone density and structure, unspecified

Other osteopathies (M86-M90)

EXCLUDES 1 *postprocedural osteopathies (M96.-)*

√4ᵗʰ **M86 Osteomyelitis**

Use additional code (B95-B97) to identify infectious agent
Use additional code to identify major osseous defect, if applicable (M89.7-)

EXCLUDES 1 *osteomyelitis due to:*
echinococcus (B67.2)
gonococcus (A54.43)
salmonella (A02.24)

EXCLUDES 2 *ostemyelitis of:*
orbit (H05.0-)
petrous bone (H70.2-)
vertebra (M46.2-)

√5ᵗʰ **M86.0** Acute hematogenous osteomyelitis

M86.00 Acute hematogenous osteomyelitis, unspecified site | HCC

√6ᵗʰ **M86.01** Acute hematogenous osteomyelitis, shoulder

M86.011 Acute hematogenous osteomyelitis, right shoulder | HCC

M86.012 Acute hematogenous osteomyelitis, left shoulder | HCC

M86.019 Acute hematogenous osteomyelitis, unspecified shoulder | HCC

√6ᵗʰ **M86.02** Acute hematogenous osteomyelitis, humerus

M86.021 Acute hematogenous osteomyelitis, right humerus | HCC

M86.022 Acute hematogenous osteomyelitis, left humerus | HCC

M86.029 Acute hematogenous osteomyelitis, unspecified humerus | HCC

√6ᵗʰ **M86.03** Acute hematogenous osteomyelitis, radius and ulna

M86.031 Acute hematogenous osteomyelitis, right radius and ulna | HCC

M86.032 Acute hematogenous osteomyelitis, left radius and ulna | HCC

M86.039 Acute hematogenous osteomyelitis, unspecified radius and ulna | HCC

√6ᵗʰ **M86.04** Acute hematogenous osteomyelitis, hand

M86.041 Acute hematogenous osteomyelitis, right hand | HCC

M86.042 Acute hematogenous osteomyelitis, left hand | HCC

M86.049 Acute hematogenous osteomyelitis, unspecified hand | HCC

√6ᵗʰ **M86.05** Acute hematogenous osteomyelitis, femur

M86.051 Acute hematogenous osteomyelitis, right femur | HCC

M86.052 Acute hematogenous osteomyelitis, left femur | HCC

M86.059 Acute hematogenous osteomyelitis, unspecified femur | HCC

√6ᵗʰ **M86.06** Acute hematogenous osteomyelitis, tibia and fibula

M86.061 Acute hematogenous osteomyelitis, right tibia and fibula | HCC

M86.062 Acute hematogenous osteomyelitis, left tibia and fibula | HCC

M86.069 Acute hematogenous osteomyelitis, unspecified tibia and fibula | HCC

√6ᵗʰ **M86.07** Acute hematogenous osteomyelitis, ankle and foot

M86.071 Acute hematogenous osteomyelitis, right ankle and foot | HCC

M86.072 Acute hematogenous osteomyelitis, left ankle and foot | HCC

M86.079 Acute hematogenous osteomyelitis, unspecified ankle and foot | HCC

M86.08 Acute hematogenous osteomyelitis, other sites | HCC

M86.09 Acute hematogenous osteomyelitis, multiple sites | HCC

√5ᵗʰ **M86.1** Other acute osteomyelitis

M86.10 Other acute osteomyelitis, unspecified site | HCC

√6ᵗʰ **M86.11** Other acute osteomyelitis, shoulder

M86.111 Other acute osteomyelitis, right shoulder | HCC

M86.112 Other acute osteomyelitis, left shoulder | HCC

M86.119 Other acute osteomyelitis, unspecified shoulder | HCC

√6ᵗʰ **M86.12** Other acute osteomyelitis, humerus

M86.121 Other acute osteomyelitis, right humerus | HCC

M86.122 Other acute osteomyelitis, left humerus | HCC

M86.129 Other acute osteomyelitis, unspecified humerus | HCC

√6ᵗʰ **M86.13** Other acute osteomyelitis, radius and ulna

M86.131 Other acute osteomyelitis, right radius and ulna | HCC

M86.132 Other acute osteomyelitis, left radius and ulna | HCC

M86.139 Other acute osteomyelitis, unspecified radius and ulna | HCC

√6ᵗʰ **M86.14** Other acute osteomyelitis, hand

M86.141 Other acute osteomyelitis, right hand | HCC

M86.142 Other acute osteomyelitis, left hand | HCC

M86.149 Other acute osteomyelitis, unspecified hand | HCC

√6ᵗʰ **M86.15** Other acute osteomyelitis, femur

M86.151 Other acute osteomyelitis, right femur | HCC

M86.152 Other acute osteomyelitis, left femur | HCC

M86.159 Other acute osteomyelitis, unspecified femur | HCC

√6ᵗʰ **M86.16** Other acute osteomyelitis, tibia and fibula

M86.161 Other acute osteomyelitis, right tibia and fibula | HCC

M86.162 Other acute osteomyelitis, left tibia and fibula | HCC

M86.169 Other acute osteomyelitis, unspecified tibia and fibula | HCC

√6ᵗʰ **M86.17** Other acute osteomyelitis, ankle and foot

M86.171 Other acute osteomyelitis, right ankle and foot | HCC

M86.172 Other acute osteomyelitis, left ankle and foot | HCC

M86.179 Other acute osteomyelitis, unspecified ankle and foot | HCC

M86.18 Other acute osteomyelitis, other site | HCC

M86.19 Other acute osteomyelitis, multiple sites | HCC

√5ᵗʰ **M86.2** Subacute osteomyelitis

M86.20 Subacute osteomyelitis, unspecified site | HCC

√6ᵗʰ **M86.21** Subacute osteomyelitis, shoulder

M86.211 Subacute osteomyelitis, right shoulder | HCC

M86.212 Subacute osteomyelitis, left shoulder | HCC

M86.219 Subacute osteomyelitis, unspecified shoulder | HCC

√6ᵗʰ **M86.22** Subacute osteomyelitis, humerus

M86.221 Subacute osteomyelitis, right humerus | HCC

M86.222 Subacute osteomyelitis, left humerus | HCC

M86.229 Subacute osteomyelitis, unspecified humerus | HCC

√6ᵗʰ **M86.23** Subacute osteomyelitis, radius and ulna

M86.231 Subacute osteomyelitis, right radius and ulna | HCC

M86.232 Subacute osteomyelitis, left radius and ulna | HCC

M86.239 Subacute osteomyelitis, unspecified radius and ulna | HCC

√6ᵗʰ **M86.24** **Subacute osteomyelitis, hand**

    M86.241 **Subacute osteomyelitis, right hand** `HCC`

    M86.242 **Subacute osteomyelitis, left hand** `HCC`

    M86.249 **Subacute osteomyelitis, unspecified hand** `HCC`

√6ᵗʰ **M86.25** **Subacute osteomyelitis, femur**

    M86.251 **Subacute osteomyelitis, right femur** `HCC`

    M86.252 **Subacute osteomyelitis, left femur** `HCC`

    M86.259 **Subacute osteomyelitis, unspecified femur** `HCC`

√6ᵗʰ **M86.26** **Subacute osteomyelitis, tibia and fibula**

    M86.261 **Subacute osteomyelitis, right tibia and fibula** `HCC`

    M86.262 **Subacute osteomyelitis, left tibia and fibula** `HCC`

    M86.269 **Subacute osteomyelitis, unspecified tibia and fibula** `HCC`

√6ᵗʰ **M86.27** **Subacute osteomyelitis, ankle and foot**

    M86.271 **Subacute osteomyelitis, right ankle and foot** `HCC`

    M86.272 **Subacute osteomyelitis, left ankle and foot** `HCC`

    M86.279 **Subacute osteomyelitis, unspecified ankle and foot** `HCC`

    M86.28 **Subacute osteomyelitis, other site** `HCC`

    M86.29 **Subacute osteomyelitis, multiple sites** `HCC`

√5ᵗʰ **M86.3** **Chronic multifocal osteomyelitis**

    M86.30 **Chronic multifocal osteomyelitis, unspecified site** `HCC`

√6ᵗʰ **M86.31** **Chronic multifocal osteomyelitis, shoulder**

    M86.311 **Chronic multifocal osteomyelitis, right shoulder** `HCC`

    M86.312 **Chronic multifocal osteomyelitis, left shoulder** `HCC`

    M86.319 **Chronic multifocal osteomyelitis, unspecified shoulder** `HCC`

√6ᵗʰ **M86.32** **Chronic multifocal osteomyelitis, humerus**

    M86.321 **Chronic multifocal osteomyelitis, right humerus** `HCC`

    M86.322 **Chronic multifocal osteomyelitis, left humerus** `HCC`

    M86.329 **Chronic multifocal osteomyelitis, unspecified humerus** `HCC`

√6ᵗʰ **M86.33** **Chronic multifocal osteomyelitis, radius and ulna**

    M86.331 **Chronic multifocal osteomyelitis, right radius and ulna** `HCC`

    M86.332 **Chronic multifocal osteomyelitis, left radius and ulna** `HCC`

    M86.339 **Chronic multifocal osteomyelitis, unspecified radius and ulna** `HCC`

√6ᵗʰ **M86.34** **Chronic multifocal osteomyelitis, hand**

    M86.341 **Chronic multifocal osteomyelitis, right hand** `HCC`

    M86.342 **Chronic multifocal osteomyelitis, left hand** `HCC`

    M86.349 **Chronic multifocal osteomyelitis, unspecified hand** `HCC`

√6ᵗʰ **M86.35** **Chronic multifocal osteomyelitis, femur**

    M86.351 **Chronic multifocal osteomyelitis, right femur** `HCC`

    M86.352 **Chronic multifocal osteomyelitis, left femur** `HCC`

    M86.359 **Chronic multifocal osteomyelitis, unspecified femur** `HCC`

√6ᵗʰ **M86.36** **Chronic multifocal osteomyelitis, tibia and fibula**

    M86.361 **Chronic multifocal osteomyelitis, right tibia and fibula** `HCC`

    M86.362 **Chronic multifocal osteomyelitis, left tibia and fibula** `HCC`

    M86.369 **Chronic multifocal osteomyelitis, unspecified tibia and fibula** `HCC`

√6ᵗʰ **M86.37** **Chronic multifocal osteomyelitis, ankle and foot**

    M86.371 **Chronic multifocal osteomyelitis, right ankle and foot** `HCC`

    M86.372 **Chronic multifocal osteomyelitis, left ankle and foot** `HCC`

    M86.379 **Chronic multifocal osteomyelitis, unspecified ankle and foot** `HCC`

    M86.38 **Chronic multifocal osteomyelitis, other site** `HCC`

    M86.39 **Chronic multifocal osteomyelitis, multiple sites** `HCC`

√5ᵗʰ **M86.4** **Chronic osteomyelitis with draining sinus**

    M86.40 **Chronic osteomyelitis with draining sinus, unspecified site** `HCC`

√6ᵗʰ **M86.41** **Chronic osteomyelitis with draining sinus, shoulder**

    M86.411 **Chronic osteomyelitis with draining sinus, right shoulder** `HCC`

    M86.412 **Chronic osteomyelitis with draining sinus, left shoulder** `HCC`

    M86.419 **Chronic osteomyelitis with draining sinus, unspecified shoulder** `HCC`

√6ᵗʰ **M86.42** **Chronic osteomyelitis with draining sinus, humerus**

    M86.421 **Chronic osteomyelitis with draining sinus, right humerus** `HCC`

    M86.422 **Chronic osteomyelitis with draining sinus, left humerus** `HCC`

    M86.429 **Chronic osteomyelitis with draining sinus, unspecified humerus** `HCC`

√6ᵗʰ **M86.43** **Chronic osteomyelitis with draining sinus, radius and ulna**

    M86.431 **Chronic osteomyelitis with draining sinus, right radius and ulna** `HCC`

    M86.432 **Chronic osteomyelitis with draining sinus, left radius and ulna** `HCC`

    M86.439 **Chronic osteomyelitis with draining sinus, unspecified radius and ulna** `HCC`

√6ᵗʰ **M86.44** **Chronic osteomyelitis with draining sinus, hand**

    M86.441 **Chronic osteomyelitis with draining sinus, right hand** `HCC`

    M86.442 **Chronic osteomyelitis with draining sinus, left hand** `HCC`

    M86.449 **Chronic osteomyelitis with draining sinus, unspecified hand** `HCC`

√6ᵗʰ **M86.45** **Chronic osteomyelitis with draining sinus, femur**

    M86.451 **Chronic osteomyelitis with draining sinus, right femur** `HCC`

    M86.452 **Chronic osteomyelitis with draining sinus, left femur** `HCC`

    M86.459 **Chronic osteomyelitis with draining sinus, unspecified femur** `HCC`

√6ᵗʰ **M86.46** **Chronic osteomyelitis with draining sinus, tibia and fibula**

    M86.461 **Chronic osteomyelitis with draining sinus, right tibia and fibula** `HCC`

    M86.462 **Chronic osteomyelitis with draining sinus, left tibia and fibula** `HCC`

    M86.469 **Chronic osteomyelitis with draining sinus, unspecified tibia and fibula** `HCC`

√6ᵗʰ **M86.47** **Chronic osteomyelitis with draining sinus, ankle and foot**

    M86.471 **Chronic osteomyelitis with draining sinus, right ankle and foot** `HCC`

    M86.472 **Chronic osteomyelitis with draining sinus, left ankle and foot** `HCC`

    M86.479 **Chronic osteomyelitis with draining sinus, unspecified ankle and foot** `HCC`

    M86.48 **Chronic osteomyelitis with draining sinus, other site** `HCC`

    M86.49 **Chronic osteomyelitis with draining sinus, multiple sites** `HCC`

√5ᵗʰ **M86.5** **Other chronic hematogenous osteomyelitis**

    M86.50 **Other chronic hematogenous osteomyelitis, unspecified site** `HCC`

√6ᵗʰ **M86.51** **Other chronic hematogenous osteomyelitis, shoulder**

    M86.511 **Other chronic hematogenous osteomyelitis, right shoulder** `HCC`

☑ Additional Character Required   √ₓ7ᵗʰ Placeholder Alert   Manifestation   Unspecified Dx   ►◄ Revised Text   ● New Code   ▲ Revised Code Title

M86.512 Other chronic hematogenous osteomyelitis, left shoulder `HCC`

M86.519 Other chronic hematogenous osteomyelitis, unspecified shoulder `HCC`

√6ᵗʰ M86.52 Other chronic hematogenous osteomyelitis, humerus

   M86.521 Other chronic hematogenous osteomyelitis, right humerus `HCC`

   M86.522 Other chronic hematogenous osteomyelitis, left humerus `HCC`

   M86.529 Other chronic hematogenous osteomyelitis, unspecified humerus `HCC`

√6ᵗʰ M86.53 Other chronic hematogenous osteomyelitis, radius and ulna

   M86.531 Other chronic hematogenous osteomyelitis, right radius and ulna `HCC`

   M86.532 Other chronic hematogenous osteomyelitis, left radius and ulna `HCC`

   M86.539 Other chronic hematogenous osteomyelitis, unspecified radius and ulna `HCC`

√6ᵗʰ M86.54 Other chronic hematogenous osteomyelitis, hand

   M86.541 Other chronic hematogenous osteomyelitis, right hand `HCC`

   M86.542 Other chronic hematogenous osteomyelitis, left hand `HCC`

   M86.549 Other chronic hematogenous osteomyelitis, unspecified hand `HCC`

√6ᵗʰ M86.55 Other chronic hematogenous osteomyelitis, femur

   M86.551 Other chronic hematogenous osteomyelitis, right femur `HCC`

   M86.552 Other chronic hematogenous osteomyelitis, left femur `HCC`

   M86.559 Other chronic hematogenous osteomyelitis, unspecified femur `HCC`

√6ᵗʰ M86.56 Other chronic hematogenous osteomyelitis, tibia and fibula

   M86.561 Other chronic hematogenous osteomyelitis, right tibia and fibula `HCC`

   M86.562 Other chronic hematogenous osteomyelitis, left tibia and fibula `HCC`

   M86.569 Other chronic hematogenous osteomyelitis, unspecified tibia and fibula `HCC`

√6ᵗʰ M86.57 Other chronic hematogenous osteomyelitis, ankle and foot

   M86.571 Other chronic hematogenous osteomyelitis, right ankle and foot `HCC`

   M86.572 Other chronic hematogenous osteomyelitis, left ankle and foot `HCC`

   M86.579 Other chronic hematogenous osteomyelitis, unspecified ankle and foot `HCC`

M86.58 Other chronic hematogenous osteomyelitis, other site `HCC`

M86.59 Other chronic hematogenous osteomyelitis, multiple sites `HCC`

√5ᵗʰ M86.6 Other chronic osteomyelitis

   M86.60 Other chronic osteomyelitis, unspecified site `HCC`

   √6ᵗʰ M86.61 Other chronic osteomyelitis, shoulder

      M86.611 Other chronic osteomyelitis, right shoulder `HCC`

      M86.612 Other chronic osteomyelitis, left shoulder `HCC`

      M86.619 Other chronic osteomyelitis, unspecified shoulder `HCC`

   √6ᵗʰ M86.62 Other chronic osteomyelitis, humerus

      M86.621 Other chronic osteomyelitis, right humerus `HCC`

      M86.622 Other chronic osteomyelitis, left humerus `HCC`

      M86.629 Other chronic osteomyelitis, unspecified humerus `HCC`

   √6ᵗʰ M86.63 Other chronic osteomyelitis, radius and ulna

      M86.631 Other chronic osteomyelitis, right radius and ulna `HCC`

M86.632 Other chronic osteomyelitis, left radius and ulna `HCC`

M86.639 Other chronic osteomyelitis, unspecified radius and ulna `HCC`

√6ᵗʰ M86.64 Other chronic osteomyelitis, hand

   M86.641 Other chronic osteomyelitis, right hand `HCC`

   M86.642 Other chronic osteomyelitis, left hand `HCC`

   M86.649 Other chronic osteomyelitis, unspecified hand `HCC`

√6ᵗʰ M86.65 Other chronic osteomyelitis, thigh

   M86.651 Other chronic osteomyelitis, right thigh `HCC`

   M86.652 Other chronic osteomyelitis, left thigh `HCC`

   M86.659 Other chronic osteomyelitis, unspecified thigh `HCC`

√6ᵗʰ M86.66 Other chronic osteomyelitis, tibia and fibula

   M86.661 Other chronic osteomyelitis, right tibia and fibula `HCC`

   M86.662 Other chronic osteomyelitis, left tibia and fibula `HCC`

   M86.669 Other chronic osteomyelitis, unspecified tibia and fibula `HCC`

√6ᵗʰ M86.67 Other chronic osteomyelitis, ankle and foot

   M86.671 Other chronic osteomyelitis, right ankle and foot `HCC`

      AHA: 2016,1Q,13

   M86.672 Other chronic osteomyelitis, left ankle and foot `HCC`

   M86.679 Other chronic osteomyelitis, unspecified ankle and foot `HCC`

M86.68 Other chronic osteomyelitis, other site `HCC`

M86.69 Other chronic osteomyelitis, multiple sites `HCC`

√5ᵗʰ M86.8 Other osteomyelitis

   Brodie's abscess

   √6ᵗʰ M86.8X Other osteomyelitis

      M86.8X0 Other osteomyelitis, multiple sites `HCC`

      M86.8X1 Other osteomyelitis, shoulder `HCC`

      M86.8X2 Other osteomyelitis, upper arm `HCC`

      M86.8X3 Other osteomyelitis, forearm `HCC`

      M86.8X4 Other osteomyelitis, hand `HCC`

      M86.8X5 Other osteomyelitis, thigh `HCC`

      M86.8X6 Other osteomyelitis, lower leg `HCC`

      M86.8X7 Other osteomyelitis, ankle and foot `HCC`

      M86.8X8 Other osteomyelitis, other site `HCC`

      M86.8X9 Other osteomyelitis, unspecified sites `HCC`

M86.9 Osteomyelitis, unspecified `HCC`

   Infection of bone NOS

   Periostitis without osteomyelitis

√4ᵗʰ M87 Osteonecrosis

   `INCLUDES` avascular necrosis of bone

   Use additional code to identify major osseous defect, if applicable (M89.7-)

   `EXCLUDES 1` juvenile osteonecrosis (M91-M92)

      osteochondropathies (M90-M93)

   √5ᵗʰ M87.0 Idiopathic aseptic necrosis of bone

      M87.00 Idiopathic aseptic necrosis of unspecified bone `HCC`

      √6ᵗʰ M87.01 Idiopathic aseptic necrosis of shoulder

         Idiopathic aseptic necrosis of clavicle and scapula

         M87.011 Idiopathic aseptic necrosis of right shoulder `HCC`

         M87.012 Idiopathic aseptic necrosis of left shoulder `HCC`

         M87.019 Idiopathic aseptic necrosis of unspecified shoulder `HCC`

      √6ᵗʰ M87.02 Idiopathic aseptic necrosis of humerus

         M87.021 Idiopathic aseptic necrosis of right humerus `HCC`

         M87.022 Idiopathic aseptic necrosis of left humerus `HCC`

M87.029 **Idiopathic aseptic necrosis of unspecified humerus** `HCC`

✓6ᵗʰ M87.03 **Idiopathic aseptic necrosis of** radius, ulna and carpus

M87.031 **Idiopathic aseptic necrosis of** right radius `HCC`

M87.032 **Idiopathic aseptic necrosis of** left radius `HCC`

M87.033 **Idiopathic aseptic necrosis of unspecified radius** `HCC`

M87.034 **Idiopathic aseptic necrosis of** right ulna `HCC`

M87.035 **Idiopathic aseptic necrosis of** left ulna `HCC`

M87.036 **Idiopathic aseptic necrosis of unspecified ulna** `HCC`

M87.037 **Idiopathic aseptic necrosis of** right carpus `HCC`

M87.038 **Idiopathic aseptic necrosis of** left carpus `HCC`

M87.039 **Idiopathic aseptic necrosis of unspecified carpus** `HCC`

✓6ᵗʰ M87.04 **Idiopathic aseptic necrosis of** hand and fingers

Idiopathic aseptic necrosis of metacarpals and phalanges of hands

M87.041 **Idiopathic aseptic necrosis of** right hand `HCC`

M87.042 **Idiopathic aseptic necrosis of** left hand `HCC`

M87.043 **Idiopathic aseptic necrosis of unspecified hand** `HCC`

M87.044 **Idiopathic aseptic necrosis of** right finger(s) `HCC`

M87.045 **Idiopathic aseptic necrosis of** left finger(s) `HCC`

M87.046 **Idiopathic aseptic necrosis of unspecified finger(s)** `HCC`

✓6ᵗʰ M87.05 **Idiopathic aseptic necrosis of** pelvis and femur

M87.050 **Idiopathic aseptic necrosis of pelvis** `HCC`

M87.051 **Idiopathic aseptic necrosis of** right femur `HCC`

M87.052 **Idiopathic aseptic necrosis of** left femur `HCC`

M87.059 **Idiopathic aseptic necrosis of unspecified femur** `HCC`

✓6ᵗʰ M87.06 **Idiopathic aseptic necrosis of** tibia and fibula

M87.061 **Idiopathic aseptic necrosis of** right tibia `HCC`

M87.062 **Idiopathic aseptic necrosis of** left tibia `HCC`

M87.063 **Idiopathic aseptic necrosis of unspecified tibia** `HCC`

M87.064 **Idiopathic aseptic necrosis of** right fibula `HCC`

M87.065 **Idiopathic aseptic necrosis of** left fibula `HCC`

M87.066 **Idiopathic aseptic necrosis of unspecified fibula** `HCC`

✓6ᵗʰ M87.07 **Idiopathic aseptic necrosis of** ankle, foot and toes

Idiopathic aseptic necrosis of metatarsus, tarsus, and phalanges of toes

M87.071 **Idiopathic aseptic necrosis of** right ankle `HCC`

M87.072 **Idiopathic aseptic necrosis of** left ankle `HCC`

M87.073 **Idiopathic aseptic necrosis of unspecified ankle** `HCC`

M87.074 **Idiopathic aseptic necrosis of** right foot `HCC`

M87.075 **Idiopathic aseptic necrosis of** left foot `HCC`

M87.076 **Idiopathic aseptic necrosis of unspecified foot** `HCC`

M87.077 **Idiopathic aseptic necrosis of** right toe(s) `HCC`

M87.078 **Idiopathic aseptic necrosis of** left toe(s) `HCC`

M87.079 **Idiopathic aseptic necrosis of unspecified toe(s)** `HCC`

M87.08 **Idiopathic aseptic necrosis of bone, other site** `HCC`

M87.09 **Idiopathic aseptic necrosis of bone,** multiple sites `HCC`

✓5ᵗʰ M87.1 **Osteonecrosis** due to drugs

Use additional code for adverse effect, if applicable, to identify drug (T36-T50 with fifth or sixth character 5)

M87.10 **Osteonecrosis due to drugs, unspecified bone** `HCC`

✓6ᵗʰ M87.11 **Osteonecrosis due to drugs,** shoulder

M87.111 **Osteonecrosis due to drugs,** right shoulder `HCC`

M87.112 **Osteonecrosis due to drugs,** left shoulder `HCC`

M87.119 **Osteonecrosis due to drugs, unspecified shoulder** `HCC`

✓6ᵗʰ M87.12 **Osteonecrosis due to drugs,** humerus

M87.121 **Osteonecrosis due to drugs,** right humerus `HCC`

M87.122 **Osteonecrosis due to drugs,** left humerus `HCC`

M87.129 **Osteonecrosis due to drugs, unspecified humerus** `HCC`

✓6ᵗʰ M87.13 **Osteonecrosis due to drugs of** radius, ulna and carpus

M87.131 **Osteonecrosis due to drugs of** right radius `HCC`

M87.132 **Osteonecrosis due to drugs of** left radius `HCC`

M87.133 **Osteonecrosis due to drugs of unspecified radius** `HCC`

M87.134 **Osteonecrosis due to drugs of** right ulna `HCC`

M87.135 **Osteonecrosis due to drugs of** left ulna `HCC`

M87.136 **Osteonecrosis due to drugs of unspecified ulna** `HCC`

M87.137 **Osteonecrosis due to drugs of** right carpus `HCC`

M87.138 **Osteonecrosis due to drugs of** left carpus `HCC`

M87.139 **Osteonecrosis due to drugs of unspecified carpus** `HCC`

✓6ᵗʰ M87.14 **Osteonecrosis due to drugs,** hand and fingers

M87.141 **Osteonecrosis due to drugs,** right hand `HCC`

M87.142 **Osteonecrosis due to drugs,** left hand `HCC`

M87.143 **Osteonecrosis due to drugs, unspecified hand** `HCC`

M87.144 **Osteonecrosis due to drugs,** right finger(s) `HCC`

M87.145 **Osteonecrosis due to drugs,** left finger(s) `HCC`

M87.146 **Osteonecrosis due to drugs, unspecified finger(s)** `HCC`

✓6ᵗʰ M87.15 **Osteonecrosis due to drugs,** pelvis and femur

M87.150 **Osteonecrosis due to drugs, pelvis** `HCC`

M87.151 **Osteonecrosis due to drugs,** right femur `HCC`

M87.152 **Osteonecrosis due to drugs,** left femur `HCC`

M87.159 **Osteonecrosis due to drugs, unspecified femur** `HCC`

✓6ᵗʰ M87.16 **Osteonecrosis due to drugs,** tibia and fibula

M87.161 **Osteonecrosis due to drugs,** right tibia `HCC`

M87.162 **Osteonecrosis due to drugs,** left tibia `HCC`

M87.163 **Osteonecrosis due to drugs, unspecified tibia** `HCC`

M87.164 **Osteonecrosis due to drugs,** right fibula `HCC`

M87.165 **Osteonecrosis due to drugs,** left fibula `HCC`

M87.166 **Osteonecrosis due to drugs, unspecified fibula** `HCC`

✓6ᵗʰ M87.17 **Osteonecrosis due to drugs,** ankle, foot and toes

M87.171 **Osteonecrosis due to drugs,** right ankle `HCC`

M87.172 **Osteonecrosis due to drugs,** left ankle `HCC`

✓ Additional Character Required   ✓x7ᵗʰ Placeholder Alert   Manifestation   Unspecified Dx   ▶◀ Revised Text   ● New Code   ▲ Revised Code Title

	M87.173	Osteonecrosis due to drugs, unspecified ankle	HCC
	M87.174	Osteonecrosis due to drugs, right foot	HCC
	M87.175	Osteonecrosis due to drugs, left foot	HCC
	M87.176	Osteonecrosis due to drugs, unspecified foot	HCC
	M87.177	Osteonecrosis due to drugs, right toe(s)	HCC
	M87.178	Osteonecrosis due to drugs, left toe(s)	HCC
	M87.179	Osteonecrosis due to drugs, unspecified toe(s)	HCC
√6ᵗʰ M87.18		Osteonecrosis due to drugs, other site	
	M87.180	Osteonecrosis due to drugs, jaw	HCC
	M87.188	Osteonecrosis due to drugs, other site	HCC
M87.19		Osteonecrosis due to drugs, multiple sites	HCC

√5ᵗʰ M87.2 Osteonecrosis due to previous trauma

	M87.20	Osteonecrosis due to previous trauma, unspecified bone	HCC
√6ᵗʰ M87.21		Osteonecrosis due to previous trauma, shoulder	
	M87.211	Osteonecrosis due to previous trauma, right shoulder	HCC
	M87.212	Osteonecrosis due to previous trauma, left shoulder	HCC
	M87.219	Osteonecrosis due to previous trauma, unspecified shoulder	HCC
√6ᵗʰ M87.22		Osteonecrosis due to previous trauma, humerus	
	M87.221	Osteonecrosis due to previous trauma, right humerus	HCC
	M87.222	Osteonecrosis due to previous trauma, left humerus	HCC
	M87.229	Osteonecrosis due to previous trauma, unspecified humerus	HCC
√6ᵗʰ M87.23		Osteonecrosis due to previous trauma of radius, ulna and carpus	
	M87.231	Osteonecrosis due to previous trauma of right radius	HCC
	M87.232	Osteonecrosis due to previous trauma of left radius	HCC
	M87.233	Osteonecrosis due to previous trauma of unspecified radius	HCC
	M87.234	Osteonecrosis due to previous trauma of right ulna	HCC
	M87.235	Osteonecrosis due to previous trauma of left ulna	HCC
	M87.236	Osteonecrosis due to previous trauma of unspecified ulna	HCC
	M87.237	Osteonecrosis due to previous trauma of right carpus	HCC
	M87.238	Osteonecrosis due to previous trauma of left carpus	HCC
	M87.239	Osteonecrosis due to previous trauma of unspecified carpus	HCC
√6ᵗʰ M87.24		Osteonecrosis due to previous trauma, hand and fingers	
	M87.241	Osteonecrosis due to previous trauma, right hand	HCC
	M87.242	Osteonecrosis due to previous trauma, left hand	HCC
	M87.243	Osteonecrosis due to previous trauma, unspecified hand	HCC
	M87.244	Osteonecrosis due to previous trauma, right finger(s)	HCC
	M87.245	Osteonecrosis due to previous trauma, left finger(s)	HCC
	M87.246	Osteonecrosis due to previous trauma, unspecified finger(s)	HCC
√6ᵗʰ M87.25		Osteonecrosis due to previous trauma, pelvis and femur	
	M87.250	Osteonecrosis due to previous trauma, pelvis	HCC
	M87.251	Osteonecrosis due to previous trauma, right femur	HCC
	M87.252	Osteonecrosis due to previous trauma, left femur	HCC
	M87.256	Osteonecrosis due to previous trauma, unspecified femur	HCC

√6ᵗʰ M87.26		Osteonecrosis due to previous trauma, tibia and fibula	
	M87.261	Osteonecrosis due to previous trauma, right tibia	HCC
	M87.262	Osteonecrosis due to previous trauma, left tibia	HCC
	M87.263	Osteonecrosis due to previous trauma, unspecified tibia	HCC
	M87.264	Osteonecrosis due to previous trauma, right fibula	HCC
	M87.265	Osteonecrosis due to previous trauma, left fibula	HCC
	M87.266	Osteonecrosis due to previous trauma, unspecified fibula	HCC
√6ᵗʰ M87.27		Osteonecrosis due to previous trauma, ankle, foot and toes	
	M87.271	Osteonecrosis due to previous trauma, right ankle	HCC
	M87.272	Osteonecrosis due to previous trauma, left ankle	HCC
	M87.273	Osteonecrosis due to previous trauma, unspecified ankle	HCC
	M87.274	Osteonecrosis due to previous trauma, right foot	HCC
	M87.275	Osteonecrosis due to previous trauma, left foot	HCC
	M87.276	Osteonecrosis due to previous trauma, unspecified foot	HCC
	M87.277	Osteonecrosis due to previous trauma, right toe(s)	HCC
	M87.278	Osteonecrosis due to previous trauma, left toe(s)	HCC
	M87.279	Osteonecrosis due to previous trauma, unspecified toe(s)	HCC
M87.28		Osteonecrosis due to previous trauma, other site	HCC
M87.29		Osteonecrosis due to previous trauma, multiple sites	HCC

√5ᵗʰ M87.3 Other secondary osteonecrosis

	M87.30	Other secondary osteonecrosis, unspecified bone	HCC
√6ᵗʰ M87.31		Other secondary osteonecrosis, shoulder	
	M87.311	Other secondary osteonecrosis, right shoulder	HCC
	M87.312	Other secondary osteonecrosis, left shoulder	HCC
	M87.319	Other secondary osteonecrosis, unspecified shoulder	HCC
√6ᵗʰ M87.32		Other secondary osteonecrosis, humerus	
	M87.321	Other secondary osteonecrosis, right humerus	HCC
	M87.322	Other secondary osteonecrosis, left humerus	HCC
	M87.329	Other secondary osteonecrosis, unspecified humerus	HCC
√6ᵗʰ M87.33		Other secondary osteonecrosis of radius, ulna and carpus	
	M87.331	Other secondary osteonecrosis of right radius	HCC
	M87.332	Other secondary osteonecrosis of left radius	HCC
	M87.333	Other secondary osteonecrosis of unspecified radius	HCC
	M87.334	Other secondary osteonecrosis of right ulna	HCC
	M87.335	Other secondary osteonecrosis of left ulna	HCC
	M87.336	Other secondary osteonecrosis of unspecified ulna	HCC
	M87.337	Other secondary osteonecrosis of right carpus	HCC
	M87.338	Other secondary osteonecrosis of left carpus	HCC
	M87.339	Other secondary osteonecrosis of unspecified carpus	HCC
√6ᵗʰ M87.34		Other secondary osteonecrosis, hand and fingers	
	M87.341	Other secondary osteonecrosis, right hand	HCC
	M87.342	Other secondary osteonecrosis, left hand	HCC
	M87.343	Other secondary osteonecrosis, unspecified hand	HCC

M87.344 **Other secondary osteonecrosis, right finger(s)** `HCC`

M87.345 **Other secondary osteonecrosis, left finger(s)** `HCC`

M87.346 **Other secondary osteonecrosis, unspecified finger(s)** `HCC`

✓6ᵗʰ M87.35 **Other secondary osteonecrosis, pelvis and femur**

M87.350 **Other secondary osteonecrosis, pelvis** `HCC`

M87.351 **Other secondary osteonecrosis, right femur** `HCC`

M87.352 **Other secondary osteonecrosis, left femur** `HCC`

M87.353 **Other secondary osteonecrosis, unspecified femur** `HCC`

✓6ᵗʰ M87.36 **Other secondary osteonecrosis, tibia and fibula**

M87.361 **Other secondary osteonecrosis, right tibia** `HCC`

M87.362 **Other secondary osteonecrosis, left tibia** `HCC`

M87.363 **Other secondary osteonecrosis, unspecified tibia** `HCC`

M87.364 **Other secondary osteonecrosis, right fibula** `HCC`

M87.365 **Other secondary osteonecrosis, left fibula** `HCC`

M87.366 **Other secondary osteonecrosis, unspecified fibula** `HCC`

✓6ᵗʰ M87.37 **Other secondary osteonecrosis, ankle and foot**

M87.371 **Other secondary osteonecrosis, right ankle** `HCC`

M87.372 **Other secondary osteonecrosis, left ankle** `HCC`

M87.373 **Other secondary osteonecrosis, unspecified ankle** `HCC`

M87.374 **Other secondary osteonecrosis, right foot** `HCC`

M87.375 **Other secondary osteonecrosis, left foot** `HCC`

M87.376 **Other secondary osteonecrosis, unspecified foot** `HCC`

M87.377 **Other secondary osteonecrosis, right toe(s)** `HCC`

M87.378 **Other secondary osteonecrosis, left toe(s)** `HCC`

M87.379 **Other secondary osteonecrosis, unspecified toe(s)** `HCC`

M87.38 **Other secondary osteonecrosis, other site** `HCC`

M87.39 **Other secondary osteonecrosis, multiple sites** `HCC`

✓5ᵗʰ M87.8 **Other osteonecrosis**

M87.80 **Other osteonecrosis, unspecified bone** `HCC`

✓6ᵗʰ M87.81 **Other osteonecrosis, shoulder**

M87.811 **Other osteonecrosis, right shoulder** `HCC`

M87.812 **Other osteonecrosis, left shoulder** `HCC`

M87.819 **Other osteonecrosis, unspecified shoulder** `HCC`

✓6ᵗʰ M87.82 **Other osteonecrosis, humerus**

M87.821 **Other osteonecrosis, right humerus** `HCC`

M87.822 **Other osteonecrosis, left humerus** `HCC`

M87.829 **Other osteonecrosis, unspecified humerus** `HCC`

✓6ᵗʰ M87.83 **Other osteonecrosis of radius, ulna and carpus**

M87.831 **Other osteonecrosis of right radius** `HCC`

M87.832 **Other osteonecrosis of left radius** `HCC`

M87.833 **Other osteonecrosis of unspecified radius** `HCC`

M87.834 **Other osteonecrosis of right ulna** `HCC`

M87.835 **Other osteonecrosis of left ulna** `HCC`

M87.836 **Other osteonecrosis of unspecified ulna** `HCC`

M87.837 **Other osteonecrosis of right carpus** `HCC`

M87.838 **Other osteonecrosis of left carpus** `HCC`

M87.839 **Other osteonecrosis of unspecified carpus** `HCC`

✓6ᵗʰ M87.84 **Other osteonecrosis, hand and fingers**

M87.841 **Other osteonecrosis, right hand** `HCC`

M87.842 **Other osteonecrosis, left hand** `HCC`

M87.843 **Other osteonecrosis, unspecified hand** `HCC`

M87.844 **Other osteonecrosis, right finger(s)** `HCC`

M87.845 **Other osteonecrosis, left finger(s)** `HCC`

M87.849 **Other osteonecrosis, unspecified finger(s)** `HCC`

✓6ᵗʰ M87.85 **Other osteonecrosis, pelvis and femur**

M87.850 **Other osteonecrosis, pelvis** `HCC`

M87.851 **Other osteonecrosis, right femur** `HCC`

M87.852 **Other osteonecrosis, left femur** `HCC`

M87.859 **Other osteonecrosis, unspecified femur** `HCC`

✓6ᵗʰ M87.86 **Other osteonecrosis, tibia and fibula**

M87.861 **Other osteonecrosis, right tibia** `HCC`

M87.862 **Other osteonecrosis, left tibia** `HCC`

M87.863 **Other osteonecrosis, unspecified tibia** `HCC`

M87.864 **Other osteonecrosis, right fibula** `HCC`

M87.865 **Other osteonecrosis, left fibula** `HCC`

M87.869 **Other osteonecrosis, unspecified fibula** `HCC`

✓6ᵗʰ M87.87 **Other osteonecrosis, ankle, foot and toes**

M87.871 **Other osteonecrosis, right ankle** `HCC`

M87.872 **Other osteonecrosis, left ankle** `HCC`

M87.873 **Other osteonecrosis, unspecified ankle** `HCC`

M87.874 **Other osteonecrosis, right foot** `HCC`

M87.875 **Other osteonecrosis, left foot** `HCC`

M87.876 **Other osteonecrosis, unspecified foot** `HCC`

M87.877 **Other osteonecrosis, right toe(s)** `HCC`

M87.878 **Other osteonecrosis, left toe(s)** `HCC`

M87.879 **Other osteonecrosis, unspecified toe(s)** `HCC`

M87.88 **Other osteonecrosis, other site** `HCC`

M87.89 **Other osteonecrosis, multiple sites** `HCC`

M87.9 **Osteonecrosis, unspecified** `HCC`

Necrosis of bone NOS

✓4ᵗʰ **M88 Osteitis deformans [Paget's disease of bone]**

> *EXCLUDES 1*   osteitis deformans in neoplastic disease (M90.6)
>
> **DEF:** Bone disease characterized by numerous cycles of bone resorption by the body. Resorption is followed by accelerated repair attempts, causing bone deformities and bowing, with associated fractures and pain.

M88.0 **Osteitis deformans of skull**

M88.1 **Osteitis deformans of vertebrae**

✓5ᵗʰ M88.8 **Osteitis deformans of other bones**

✓6ᵗʰ M88.81 **Osteitis deformans of shoulder**

M88.811 **Osteitis deformans of right shoulder**

M88.812 **Osteitis deformans of left shoulder**

M88.819 **Osteitis deformans of unspecified shoulder**

✓6ᵗʰ M88.82 **Osteitis deformans of upper arm**

M88.821 **Osteitis deformans of right upper arm**

M88.822 **Osteitis deformans of left upper arm**

M88.829 **Osteitis deformans of unspecified upper arm**

✓6ᵗʰ M88.83 **Osteitis deformans of forearm**

M88.831 **Osteitis deformans of right forearm**

M88.832 **Osteitis deformans of left forearm**

M88.839 **Osteitis deformans of unspecified forearm**

✓6ᵗʰ M88.84 **Osteitis deformans of hand**

M88.841 **Osteitis deformans of right hand**

M88.842 **Osteitis deformans of left hand**

M88.849 **Osteitis deformans of unspecified hand**

✓6ᵗʰ M88.85 **Osteitis deformans of thigh**

M88.851 **Osteitis deformans of right thigh**

M88.852 **Osteitis deformans of left thigh**

M88.859 **Osteitis deformans of unspecified thigh**

☑ Additional Character Required   ✓x7ᵗʰ Placeholder Alert   Manifestation   Unspecified Dx   ▶◀ Revised Text   ● New Code   ▲ Revised Code Title

√6ᵗʰ **M88.86 Osteitis deformans of** lower leg

     M88.861 **Osteitis deformans of** right **lower leg**

     M88.862 **Osteitis deformans of** left **lower leg**

     M88.869 **Osteitis deformans of unspecified lower leg**

√6ᵗʰ **M88.87 Osteitis deformans of** ankle and foot

     M88.871 **Osteitis deformans of** right **ankle and foot**

     M88.872 **Osteitis deformans of** left **ankle and foot**

     M88.879 **Osteitis deformans of unspecified ankle and foot**

M88.88 Osteitis deformans of other bones

     EXCLUDES 2   osteitis deformans of skull (M88.Ø)

                osteitis deformans of vertebrae (M88.1)

M88.89 Osteitis deformans of multiple sites

M88.9 Osteitis deformans of unspecified bone

√4ᵗʰ **M89 Other disorders of bone**

√5ᵗʰ **M89.Ø Algoneurodystrophy**

     Shoulder-hand syndrome

     Sudeck's atrophy

     EXCLUDES 1   causalgia, lower limb (G57.7-)

                causalgia, upper limb (G56.4-)

                complex regional pain syndrome II, lower limb (G57.7-)

                complex regional pain syndrome II, upper limb (G56.4-)

                reflex sympathetic dystrophy (G9Ø.5-)

     M89.ØØ Algoneurodystrophy, unspecified site

√6ᵗʰ **M89.Ø1 Algoneurodystrophy,** shoulder

     M89.Ø11 **Algoneurodystrophy,** right **shoulder**

     M89.Ø12 **Algoneurodystrophy,** left **shoulder**

     M89.Ø19 **Algoneurodystrophy, unspecified shoulder**

√6ᵗʰ **M89.Ø2 Algoneurodystrophy,** upper arm

     M89.Ø21 **Algoneurodystrophy,** right **upper arm**

     M89.Ø22 **Algoneurodystrophy,** left **upper arm**

     M89.Ø29 **Algoneurodystrophy, unspecified upper arm**

√6ᵗʰ **M89.Ø3 Algoneurodystrophy,** forearm

     M89.Ø31 **Algoneurodystrophy,** right **forearm**

     M89.Ø32 **Algoneurodystrophy,** left **forearm**

     M89.Ø39 **Algoneurodystrophy, unspecified forearm**

√6ᵗʰ **M89.Ø4 Algoneurodystrophy,** hand

     M89.Ø41 **Algoneurodystrophy,** right **hand**

     M89.Ø42 **Algoneurodystrophy,** left **hand**

     M89.Ø49 **Algoneurodystrophy, unspecified hand**

√6ᵗʰ **M89.Ø5 Algoneurodystrophy,** thigh

     M89.Ø51 **Algoneurodystrophy,** right **thigh**

     M89.Ø52 **Algoneurodystrophy,** left **thigh**

     M89.Ø59 **Algoneurodystrophy, unspecified thigh**

√6ᵗʰ **M89.Ø6 Algoneurodystrophy,** lower leg

     M89.Ø61 **Algoneurodystrophy,** right **lower leg**

     M89.Ø62 **Algoneurodystrophy,** left **lower leg**

     M89.Ø69 **Algoneurodystrophy, unspecified lower leg**

√6ᵗʰ **M89.Ø7 Algoneurodystrophy,** ankle and foot

     M89.Ø71 **Algoneurodystrophy,** right **ankle and foot**

     M89.Ø72 **Algoneurodystrophy,** left **ankle and foot**

     M89.Ø79 **Algoneurodystrophy, unspecified ankle and foot**

M89.Ø8 Algoneurodystrophy, other site

M89.Ø9 Algoneurodystrophy, multiple sites

√5ᵗʰ **M89.1 Physeal arrest**

     Arrest of growth plate

     Epiphyseal arrest

     Growth plate arrest

√6ᵗʰ **M89.12 Physeal arrest,** humerus

     M89.121 **Complete** physeal arrest, right proximal humerus

     M89.122 **Complete** physeal arrest, left proximal humerus

     M89.123 **Partial** physeal arrest, right proximal humerus

     M89.124 **Partial** physeal arrest, left proximal humerus

     M89.125 **Complete** physeal arrest, right distal humerus

     M89.126 **Complete** physeal arrest, left distal humerus

     M89.127 **Partial** physeal arrest, right distal humerus

     M89.128 **Partial** physeal arrest, left distal humerus

     M89.129 **Physeal arrest, humerus, unspecified**

√6ᵗʰ **M89.13 Physeal arrest,** forearm

     M89.131 **Complete** physeal arrest, right distal radius

     M89.132 **Complete** physeal arrest, left distal radius

     M89.133 **Partial** physeal arrest, right distal radius

     M89.134 **Partial** physeal arrest, left distal radius

     M89.138 **Other physeal arrest of forearm**

     M89.139 **Physeal arrest, forearm, unspecified**

√6ᵗʰ **M89.15 Physeal arrest,** femur

     M89.151 **Complete** physeal arrest, right proximal femur

     M89.152 **Complete** physeal arrest, left proximal femur

     M89.153 **Partial** physeal arrest, right proximal femur

     M89.154 **Partial** physeal arrest, left proximal femur

     M89.155 **Complete** physeal arrest, right distal femur

     M89.156 **Complete** physeal arrest, left distal femur

     M89.157 **Partial** physeal arrest, right distal femur

     M89.158 **Partial** physeal arrest, left distal femur

     M89.159 **Physeal arrest, femur, unspecified**

√6ᵗʰ **M89.16 Physeal arrest,** lower leg

     M89.16Ø **Complete** physeal arrest, right proximal tibia

     M89.161 **Complete** physeal arrest, left proximal tibia

     M89.162 **Partial** physeal arrest, right proximal tibia

     M89.163 **Partial** physeal arrest, left proximal tibia

     M89.164 **Complete** physeal arrest, right distal tibia

     M89.165 **Complete** physeal arrest, left distal tibia

     M89.166 **Partial** physeal arrest, right distal tibia

     M89.167 **Partial** physeal arrest, left distal tibia

     M89.168 **Other physeal arrest of lower leg**

     M89.169 **Physeal arrest, lower leg, unspecified**

M89.18 Physeal arrest, other site

√5ᵗʰ **M89.2 Other disorders of bone development and growth**

     M89.2Ø Other disorders of bone development and growth, unspecified site

√6ᵗʰ **M89.21 Other disorders of bone development and growth,** shoulder

     M89.211 **Other disorders of bone development and growth, right shoulder**

     M89.212 **Other disorders of bone development and growth, left shoulder**

     M89.219 **Other disorders of bone development and growth, unspecified shoulder**

√6ᵗʰ **M89.22 Other disorders of bone development and growth,** humerus

     M89.221 **Other disorders of bone development and growth, right humerus**

     M89.222 **Other disorders of bone development and growth, left humerus**

     M89.229 **Other disorders of bone development and growth, unspecified humerus**

√6ᵗʰ **M89.23 Other disorders of bone development and growth,** ulna and radius

     M89.231 **Other disorders of bone development and growth, right ulna**

     M89.232 **Other disorders of bone development and growth, left ulna**

     M89.233 **Other disorders of bone development and growth, right radius**

     M89.234 **Other disorders of bone development and growth, left radius**

     M89.239 **Other disorders of bone development and growth, unspecified ulna and radius**

√6ᵗʰ **M89.24 Other disorders of bone development and growth,** hand

     M89.241 **Other disorders of bone development and growth, right hand**

     M89.242 **Other disorders of bone development and growth, left hand**

    M89.249 Other disorders of bone development and growth, unspecified hand

✓6ᵗʰ **M89.25** Other disorders of bone development and growth, femur

    M89.251 Other disorders of bone development and growth, right femur

    M89.252 Other disorders of bone development and growth, left femur

    M89.259 Other disorders of bone development and growth, unspecified femur

✓6ᵗʰ **M89.26** Other disorders of bone development and growth, tibia and fibula

    M89.261 Other disorders of bone development and growth, right tibia

    M89.262 Other disorders of bone development and growth, left tibia

    M89.263 Other disorders of bone development and growth, right fibula

    M89.264 Other disorders of bone development and growth, left fibula

    M89.269 Other disorders of bone development and growth, unspecified lower leg

✓6ᵗʰ **M89.27** Other disorders of bone development and growth, ankle and foot

    M89.271 Other disorders of bone development and growth, right ankle and foot

    M89.272 Other disorders of bone development and growth, left ankle and foot

    M89.279 Other disorders of bone development and growth, unspecified ankle and foot

M89.28 Other disorders of bone development and growth, other site

M89.29 Other disorders of bone development and growth, multiple sites

✓5ᵗʰ **M89.3** Hypertrophy of bone

M89.30 Hypertrophy of bone, unspecified site

✓6ᵗʰ **M89.31** Hypertrophy of bone, shoulder

    M89.311 Hypertrophy of bone, right shoulder

    M89.312 Hypertrophy of bone, left shoulder

    M89.319 Hypertrophy of bone, unspecified shoulder

✓6ᵗʰ **M89.32** Hypertrophy of bone, humerus

    M89.321 Hypertrophy of bone, right humerus

    M89.322 Hypertrophy of bone, left humerus

    M89.329 Hypertrophy of bone, unspecified humerus

✓6ᵗʰ **M89.33** Hypertrophy of bone, ulna and radius

    M89.331 Hypertrophy of bone, right ulna

    M89.332 Hypertrophy of bone, left ulna

    M89.333 Hypertrophy of bone, right radius

    M89.334 Hypertrophy of bone, left radius

    M89.339 Hypertrophy of bone, unspecified ulna and radius

✓6ᵗʰ **M89.34** Hypertrophy of bone, hand

    M89.341 Hypertrophy of bone, right hand

    M89.342 Hypertrophy of bone, left hand

    M89.349 Hypertrophy of bone, unspecified hand

✓6ᵗʰ **M89.35** Hypertrophy of bone, femur

    M89.351 Hypertrophy of bone, right femur

    M89.352 Hypertrophy of bone, left femur

    M89.359 Hypertrophy of bone, unspecified femur

✓6ᵗʰ **M89.36** Hypertrophy of bone, tibia and fibula

    M89.361 Hypertrophy of bone, right tibia

    M89.362 Hypertrophy of bone, left tibia

    M89.363 Hypertrophy of bone, right fibula

    M89.364 Hypertrophy of bone, left fibula

    M89.369 Hypertrophy of bone, unspecified tibia and fibula

✓6ᵗʰ **M89.37** Hypertrophy of bone, ankle and foot

    M89.371 Hypertrophy of bone, right ankle and foot

    M89.372 Hypertrophy of bone, left ankle and foot

    M89.379 Hypertrophy of bone, unspecified ankle and foot

M89.38 Hypertrophy of bone, other site

M89.39 Hypertrophy of bone, multiple sites

✓5ᵗʰ **M89.4** Other hypertrophic osteoarthropathy

    Marie-Bamberger disease
    Pachydermoperiostosis

M89.40 Other hypertrophic osteoarthropathy, unspecified site

✓6ᵗʰ **M89.41** Other hypertrophic osteoarthropathy, shoulder

    M89.411 Other hypertrophic osteoarthropathy, right shoulder

    M89.412 Other hypertrophic osteoarthropathy, left shoulder

    M89.419 Other hypertrophic osteoarthropathy, unspecified shoulder

✓6ᵗʰ **M89.42** Other hypertrophic osteoarthropathy, upper arm

    M89.421 Other hypertrophic osteoarthropathy, right upper arm

    M89.422 Other hypertrophic osteoarthropathy, left upper arm

    M89.429 Other hypertrophic osteoarthropathy, unspecified upper arm

✓6ᵗʰ **M89.43** Other hypertrophic osteoarthropathy, forearm

    M89.431 Other hypertrophic osteoarthropathy, right forearm

    M89.432 Other hypertrophic osteoarthropathy, left forearm

    M89.439 Other hypertrophic osteoarthropathy, unspecified forearm

✓6ᵗʰ **M89.44** Other hypertrophic osteoarthropathy, hand

    M89.441 Other hypertrophic osteoarthropathy, right hand

    M89.442 Other hypertrophic osteoarthropathy, left hand

    M89.449 Other hypertrophic osteoarthropathy, unspecified hand

✓6ᵗʰ **M89.45** Other hypertrophic osteoarthropathy, thigh

    M89.451 Other hypertrophic osteoarthropathy, right thigh

    M89.452 Other hypertrophic osteoarthropathy, left thigh

    M89.459 Other hypertrophic osteoarthropathy, unspecified thigh

✓6ᵗʰ **M89.46** Other hypertrophic osteoarthropathy, lower leg

    M89.461 Other hypertrophic osteoarthropathy, right lower leg

    M89.462 Other hypertrophic osteoarthropathy, left lower leg

    M89.469 Other hypertrophic osteoarthropathy, unspecified lower leg

✓6ᵗʰ **M89.47** Other hypertrophic osteoarthropathy, ankle and foot

    M89.471 Other hypertrophic osteoarthropathy, right ankle and foot

    M89.472 Other hypertrophic osteoarthropathy, left ankle and foot

    M89.479 Other hypertrophic osteoarthropathy, unspecified ankle and foot

M89.48 Other hypertrophic osteoarthropathy, other site

M89.49 Other hypertrophic osteoarthropathy, multiple sites

✓5ᵗʰ **M89.5** Osteolysis

    Use additional code to identify major osseous defect, if applicable (M89.7-)

    EXCLUDES 2   periprosthetic osteolysis of internal prosthetic joint (T84.05-)

M89.50 Osteolysis, unspecified site

✓6ᵗʰ **M89.51** Osteolysis, shoulder

    M89.511 Osteolysis, right shoulder

    M89.512 Osteolysis, left shoulder

    M89.519 Osteolysis, unspecified shoulder

✓6ᵗʰ **M89.52** Osteolysis, upper arm

    M89.521 Osteolysis, right upper arm

    M89.522 Osteolysis, left upper arm

    M89.529 Osteolysis, unspecified upper arm

✓6ᵗʰ **M89.53** Osteolysis, forearm

    M89.531 Osteolysis, right forearm

    M89.532 Osteolysis, left forearm

    M89.539 Osteolysis, unspecified forearm

✓6ᵗʰ **M89.54** Osteolysis, hand

    M89.541 Osteolysis, right hand

    M89.542 Osteolysis, left hand

☑ Additional Character Required   ✓ˣ7ᵗʰ Placeholder Alert   Manifestation   Unspecified Dx   ▶◀ Revised Text   ● New Code   ▲ Revised Code Title

ICD-10-CM 2020   821

M89.549 Osteolysis, unspecified hand

✓6th **M89.55 Osteolysis, thigh**

    M89.551 Osteolysis, right thigh

    M89.552 Osteolysis, left thigh

    M89.559 Osteolysis, unspecified thigh

✓6th **M89.56 Osteolysis, lower leg**

    M89.561 Osteolysis, right lower leg

    M89.562 Osteolysis, left lower leg

    M89.569 Osteolysis, unspecified lower leg

✓6th **M89.57 Osteolysis, ankle and foot**

    M89.571 Osteolysis, right ankle and foot

    M89.572 Osteolysis, left ankle and foot

    M89.579 Osteolysis, unspecified ankle and foot

    M89.58 Osteolysis, other site

    M89.59 Osteolysis, multiple sites

✓5th **M89.6 Osteopathy after poliomyelitis**

    Use additional code (B91) to identify previous poliomyelitis

    EXCLUDES 1   *postpolio syndrome (G14)*

    M89.60 Osteopathy after poliomyelitis, unspecified site   HCC

✓6th **M89.61 Osteopathy after poliomyelitis, shoulder**

    M89.611 Osteopathy after poliomyelitis, right shoulder   HCC

    M89.612 Osteopathy after poliomyelitis, left shoulder   HCC

    M89.619 Osteopathy after poliomyelitis, unspecified shoulder   HCC

✓6th **M89.62 Osteopathy after poliomyelitis, upper arm**

    M89.621 Osteopathy after poliomyelitis, right upper arm   HCC

    M89.622 Osteopathy after poliomyelitis, left upper arm   HCC

    M89.629 Osteopathy after poliomyelitis, unspecified upper arm   HCC

✓6th **M89.63 Osteopathy after poliomyelitis, forearm**

    M89.631 Osteopathy after poliomyelitis, right forearm   HCC

    M89.632 Osteopathy after poliomyelitis, left forearm   HCC

    M89.639 Osteopathy after poliomyelitis, unspecified forearm   HCC

✓6th **M89.64 Osteopathy after poliomyelitis, hand**

    M89.641 Osteopathy after poliomyelitis, right hand   HCC

    M89.642 Osteopathy after poliomyelitis, left hand   HCC

    M89.649 Osteopathy after poliomyelitis, unspecified hand   HCC

✓6th **M89.65 Osteopathy after poliomyelitis, thigh**

    M89.651 Osteopathy after poliomyelitis, right thigh   HCC

    M89.652 Osteopathy after poliomyelitis, left thigh   HCC

    M89.659 Osteopathy after poliomyelitis, unspecified thigh   HCC

✓6th **M89.66 Osteopathy after poliomyelitis, lower leg**

    M89.661 Osteopathy after poliomyelitis, right lower leg   HCC

    M89.662 Osteopathy after poliomyelitis, left lower leg   HCC

    M89.669 Osteopathy after poliomyelitis, unspecified lower leg   HCC

✓6th **M89.67 Osteopathy after poliomyelitis, ankle and foot**

    M89.671 Osteopathy after poliomyelitis, right ankle and foot   HCC

    M89.672 Osteopathy after poliomyelitis, left ankle and foot   HCC

    M89.679 Osteopathy after poliomyelitis, unspecified ankle and foot   HCC

    M89.68 Osteopathy after poliomyelitis, other site   HCC

    M89.69 Osteopathy after poliomyelitis, multiple sites   HCC

✓5th **M89.7 Major osseous defect**

    Code first underlying disease, if known, such as:

    aseptic necrosis of bone (M87.-)

    malignant neoplasm of bone (C40.-)

    osteolysis (M89.5)

    osteomyelitis (M86.-)

    osteonecrosis (M87.-)

    osteoporosis (M80.-, M81.-)

    periprosthetic osteolysis (T84.05-)

    M89.70 Major osseous defect, unspecified site

✓6th **M89.71 Major osseous defect, shoulder region**

    Major osseous defect clavicle or scapula

    M89.711 Major osseous defect, right shoulder region

    M89.712 Major osseous defect, left shoulder region

    M89.719 Major osseous defect, unspecified shoulder region

✓6th **M89.72 Major osseous defect, humerus**

    M89.721 Major osseous defect, right humerus

    M89.722 Major osseous defect, left humerus

    M89.729 Major osseous defect, unspecified humerus

✓6th **M89.73 Major osseous defect, forearm**

    Major osseous defect of radius and ulna

    M89.731 Major osseous defect, right forearm

    M89.732 Major osseous defect, left forearm

    M89.739 Major osseous defect, unspecified forearm

✓6th **M89.74 Major osseous defect, hand**

    Major osseous defect of carpus, fingers, metacarpus

    M89.741 Major osseous defect, right hand

    M89.742 Major osseous defect, left hand

    M89.749 Major osseous defect, unspecified hand

✓6th **M89.75 Major osseous defect, pelvic region and thigh**

    Major osseous defect of femur and pelvis

    M89.751 Major osseous defect, right pelvic region and thigh

    M89.752 Major osseous defect, left pelvic region and thigh

    M89.759 Major osseous defect, unspecified pelvic region and thigh

✓6th **M89.76 Major osseous defect, lower leg**

    Major osseous defect of fibula and tibia

    M89.761 Major osseous defect, right lower leg

    M89.762 Major osseous defect, left lower leg

    M89.769 Major osseous defect, unspecified lower leg

✓6th **M89.77 Major osseous defect, ankle and foot**

    Major osseous defect of metatarsus, tarsus, toes

    M89.771 Major osseous defect, right ankle and foot

    M89.772 Major osseous defect, left ankle and foot

    M89.779 Major osseous defect, unspecified ankle and foot

    M89.78 Major osseous defect, other site

    M89.79 Major osseous defect, multiple sites

✓5th **M89.8 Other specified disorders of bone**

    Infantile cortical hyperostoses

    Post-traumatic subperiosteal ossification

✓6th **M89.8X Other specified disorders of bone**

    M89.8X0 Other specified disorders of bone, multiple sites

    M89.8X1 Other specified disorders of bone, shoulder

    M89.8X2 Other specified disorders of bone, upper arm

    M89.8X3 Other specified disorders of bone, forearm

    M89.8X4 Other specified disorders of bone, hand

    M89.8X5 Other specified disorders of bone, thigh

    M89.8X6 Other specified disorders of bone, lower leg

    M89.8X7 Other specified disorders of bone, ankle and foot

    M89.8X8 Other specified disorders of bone, other site

    M89.8X9 Other specified disorders of bone, unspecified site

M89.9   Disorder of bone, unspecified

☑4ᵗʰ **M90**   **Osteopathies in diseases classified elsewhere**

     EXCLUDES 1   osteochondritis, osteomyelitis, and osteopathy (in):
         cryptococcosis (B45.3)
         diabetes mellitus (E08-E13 with .69-)
         gonococcal (A54.43)
         neurogenic syphilis (A52.11)
         renal osteodystrophy (N25.0)
         salmonellosis (A02.24)
         secondary syphilis (A51.46)
         syphilis (late) (A52.77)

☑5ᵗʰ **M90.5**   **Osteonecrosis in diseases classified elsewhere**

     Code first underlying disease, such as:
       caisson disease (T70.3)
       hemoglobinopathy (D50-D64)

     M90.50   *Osteonecrosis in diseases classified elsewhere, unspecified site*   `HCC`

   ☑6ᵗʰ **M90.51**   Osteonecrosis in diseases classified elsewhere, shoulder

       M90.511   *Osteonecrosis in diseases classified elsewhere, right shoulder*   `HCC`

       M90.512   *Osteonecrosis in diseases classified elsewhere, left shoulder*   `HCC`

       M90.519   *Osteonecrosis in diseases classified elsewhere, unspecified shoulder*   `HCC`

   ☑6ᵗʰ **M90.52**   Osteonecrosis in diseases classified elsewhere, upper arm

       M90.521   *Osteonecrosis in diseases classified elsewhere, right upper arm*   `HCC`

       M90.522   *Osteonecrosis in diseases classified elsewhere, left upper arm*   `HCC`

       M90.529   *Osteonecrosis in diseases classified elsewhere, unspecified upper arm*   `HCC`

   ☑6ᵗʰ **M90.53**   Osteonecrosis in diseases classified elsewhere, forearm

       M90.531   *Osteonecrosis in diseases classified elsewhere, right forearm*   `HCC`

       M90.532   *Osteonecrosis in diseases classified elsewhere, left forearm*   `HCC`

       M90.539   *Osteonecrosis in diseases classified elsewhere, unspecified forearm*   `HCC`

   ☑6ᵗʰ **M90.54**   Osteonecrosis in diseases classified elsewhere, hand

       M90.541   *Osteonecrosis in diseases classified elsewhere, right hand*   `HCC`

       M90.542   *Osteonecrosis in diseases classified elsewhere, left hand*   `HCC`

       M90.549   *Osteonecrosis in diseases classified elsewhere, unspecified hand*   `HCC`

   ☑6ᵗʰ **M90.55**   Osteonecrosis in diseases classified elsewhere, thigh

       M90.551   *Osteonecrosis in diseases classified elsewhere, right thigh*   `HCC`

       M90.552   *Osteonecrosis in diseases classified elsewhere, left thigh*   `HCC`

       M90.559   *Osteonecrosis in diseases classified elsewhere, unspecified thigh*   `HCC`

   ☑6ᵗʰ **M90.56**   Osteonecrosis in diseases classified elsewhere, lower leg

       M90.561   *Osteonecrosis in diseases classified elsewhere, right lower leg*   `HCC`

       M90.562   *Osteonecrosis in diseases classified elsewhere, left lower leg*   `HCC`

       M90.569   *Osteonecrosis in diseases classified elsewhere, unspecified lower leg*   `HCC`

   ☑6ᵗʰ **M90.57**   Osteonecrosis in diseases classified elsewhere, ankle and foot

       M90.571   *Osteonecrosis in diseases classified elsewhere, right ankle and foot*   `HCC`

       M90.572   *Osteonecrosis in diseases classified elsewhere, left ankle and foot*   `HCC`

       M90.579   *Osteonecrosis in diseases classified elsewhere, unspecified ankle and foot*   `HCC`

     M90.58   *Osteonecrosis in diseases classified elsewhere, other site*   `HCC`

     M90.59   *Osteonecrosis in diseases classified elsewhere, multiple sites*   `HCC`

☑5ᵗʰ **M90.6**   **Osteitis deformans in neoplastic diseases**

     Osteitis deformans in malignant neoplasm of bone
     Code first the neoplasm (C40.-, C41.-)

     EXCLUDES 1   osteitis deformans [Paget's disease of bone] (M88.-)

     M90.60   *Osteitis deformans in neoplastic diseases, unspecified site*

   ☑6ᵗʰ **M90.61**   Osteitis deformans in neoplastic diseases, shoulder

       M90.611   *Osteitis deformans in neoplastic diseases, right shoulder*

       M90.612   *Osteitis deformans in neoplastic diseases, left shoulder*

       M90.619   *Osteitis deformans in neoplastic diseases, unspecified shoulder*

   ☑6ᵗʰ **M90.62**   Osteitis deformans in neoplastic diseases, upper arm

       M90.621   *Osteitis deformans in neoplastic diseases, right upper arm*

       M90.622   *Osteitis deformans in neoplastic diseases, left upper arm*

       M90.629   *Osteitis deformans in neoplastic diseases, unspecified upper arm*

   ☑6ᵗʰ **M90.63**   Osteitis deformans in neoplastic diseases, forearm

       M90.631   *Osteitis deformans in neoplastic diseases, right forearm*

       M90.632   *Osteitis deformans in neoplastic diseases, left forearm*

       M90.639   *Osteitis deformans in neoplastic diseases, unspecified forearm*

   ☑6ᵗʰ **M90.64**   Osteitis deformans in neoplastic diseases, hand

       M90.641   *Osteitis deformans in neoplastic diseases, right hand*

       M90.642   *Osteitis deformans in neoplastic diseases, left hand*

       M90.649   *Osteitis deformans in neoplastic diseases, unspecified hand*

   ☑6ᵗʰ **M90.65**   Osteitis deformans in neoplastic diseases, thigh

       M90.651   *Osteitis deformans in neoplastic diseases, right thigh*

       M90.652   *Osteitis deformans in neoplastic diseases, left thigh*

       M90.659   *Osteitis deformans in neoplastic diseases, unspecified thigh*

   ☑6ᵗʰ **M90.66**   Osteitis deformans in neoplastic diseases, lower leg

       M90.661   *Osteitis deformans in neoplastic diseases, right lower leg*

       M90.662   *Osteitis deformans in neoplastic diseases, left lower leg*

       M90.669   *Osteitis deformans in neoplastic diseases, unspecified lower leg*

   ☑6ᵗʰ **M90.67**   Osteitis deformans in neoplastic diseases, ankle and foot

       M90.671   *Osteitis deformans in neoplastic diseases, right ankle and foot*

       M90.672   *Osteitis deformans in neoplastic diseases, left ankle and foot*

       M90.679   *Osteitis deformans in neoplastic diseases, unspecified ankle and foot*

     M90.68   *Osteitis deformans in neoplastic diseases, other site*

     M90.69   *Osteitis deformans in neoplastic diseases, multiple sites*

☑5ᵗʰ **M90.8**   **Osteopathy in diseases classified elsewhere**

     Code first underlying disease, such as:
       rickets (E55.0)
       vitamin-D-resistant rickets (E83.3)

     M90.80   *Osteopathy in diseases classified elsewhere, unspecified site*

   ☑6ᵗʰ **M90.81**   Osteopathy in diseases classified elsewhere, shoulder

       M90.811   *Osteopathy in diseases classified elsewhere, right shoulder*

       M90.812   *Osteopathy in diseases classified elsewhere, left shoulder*

       M90.819   *Osteopathy in diseases classified elsewhere, unspecified shoulder*

   ☑6ᵗʰ **M90.82**   Osteopathy in diseases classified elsewhere, upper arm

       M90.821   *Osteopathy in diseases classified elsewhere, right upper arm*

       M90.822   *Osteopathy in diseases classified elsewhere, left upper arm*

☑ Additional Character Required   ☑x7ᵗʰ Placeholder Alert   Manifestation   Unspecified Dx   ▶◀ Revised Text   ● New Code   ▲ Revised Code Title

M90.829 Osteopathy in diseases classified elsewhere, unspecified upper arm

✓6ᵗʰ **M90.83** Osteopathy in diseases classified elsewhere, forearm

M90.831 Osteopathy in diseases classified elsewhere, right forearm

M90.832 Osteopathy in diseases classified elsewhere, left forearm

M90.839 Osteopathy in diseases classified elsewhere, unspecified forearm

✓6ᵗʰ **M90.84** Osteopathy in diseases classified elsewhere, hand

M90.841 Osteopathy in diseases classified elsewhere, right hand

M90.842 Osteopathy in diseases classified elsewhere, left hand

M90.849 Osteopathy in diseases classified elsewhere, unspecified hand

✓6ᵗʰ **M90.85** Osteopathy in diseases classified elsewhere, thigh

M90.851 Osteopathy in diseases classified elsewhere, right thigh

M90.852 Osteopathy in diseases classified elsewhere, left thigh

M90.859 Osteopathy in diseases classified elsewhere, unspecified thigh

✓6ᵗʰ **M90.86** Osteopathy in diseases classified elsewhere, lower leg

M90.861 Osteopathy in diseases classified elsewhere, right lower leg

M90.862 Osteopathy in diseases classified elsewhere, left lower leg

M90.869 Osteopathy in diseases classified elsewhere, unspecified lower leg

✓6ᵗʰ **M90.87** Osteopathy in diseases classified elsewhere, ankle and foot

M90.871 Osteopathy in diseases classified elsewhere, right ankle and foot

M90.872 Osteopathy in diseases classified elsewhere, left ankle and foot

M90.879 Osteopathy in diseases classified elsewhere, unspecified ankle and foot

M90.88 Osteopathy in diseases classified elsewhere, other site

M90.89 Osteopathy in diseases classified elsewhere, multiple sites

Chondropathies (M91-M94)

> EXCLUDES 1   postprocedural chondropathies (M96.-)

✓4ᵗʰ **M91 Juvenile osteochondrosis of hip and pelvis**

> EXCLUDES 1   slipped upper femoral epiphysis (nontraumatic) (M93.0)

M91.0 Juvenile osteochondrosis of pelvis

Osteochondrosis (juvenile) of acetabulum
Osteochondrosis (juvenile) of iliac crest [Buchanan]
Osteochondrosis (juvenile) of ischiopubic synchondrosis [van Neck]
Osteochondrosis (juvenile) of symphysis pubis [Pierson]

✓5ᵗʰ **M91.1** Juvenile osteochondrosis of head of femur [Legg-Calvé-Perthes]

M91.10 Juvenile osteochondrosis of head of femur [Legg-Calvé-Perthes], unspecified leg

M91.11 Juvenile osteochondrosis of head of femur [Legg-Calvé-Perthes], right leg

M91.12 Juvenile osteochondrosis of head of femur [Legg-Calvé-Perthes], left leg

✓5ᵗʰ **M91.2** Coxa plana

Hip deformity due to previous juvenile osteochondrosis

M91.20 Coxa plana, unspecified hip
M91.21 Coxa plana, right hip
M91.22 Coxa plana, left hip

✓5ᵗʰ **M91.3** Pseudocoxalgia

M91.30 Pseudocoxalgia, unspecified hip
M91.31 Pseudocoxalgia, right hip
M91.32 Pseudocoxalgia, left hip

✓5ᵗʰ **M91.4** Coxa magna

M91.40 Coxa magna, unspecified hip
M91.41 Coxa magna, right hip
M91.42 Coxa magna, left hip

✓5ᵗʰ **M91.8** Other juvenile osteochondrosis of hip and pelvis

Juvenile osteochondrosis after reduction of congenital dislocation of hip

M91.80 Other juvenile osteochondrosis of hip and pelvis, unspecified leg

M91.81 Other juvenile osteochondrosis of hip and pelvis, right leg

M91.82 Other juvenile osteochondrosis of hip and pelvis, left leg

✓5ᵗʰ **M91.9** Juvenile osteochondrosis of hip and pelvis, unspecified

M91.90 Juvenile osteochondrosis of hip and pelvis, unspecified, unspecified leg

M91.91 Juvenile osteochondrosis of hip and pelvis, unspecified, right leg

M91.92 Juvenile osteochondrosis of hip and pelvis, unspecified, left leg

✓4ᵗʰ **M92 Other juvenile osteochondrosis**

✓5ᵗʰ **M92.0** Juvenile osteochondrosis of humerus

Osteochondrosis (juvenile) of capitulum of humerus [Panner]
Osteochondrosis (juvenile) of head of humerus [Haas]

M92.00 Juvenile osteochondrosis of humerus, unspecified arm

M92.01 Juvenile osteochondrosis of humerus, right arm

M92.02 Juvenile osteochondrosis of humerus, left arm

✓5ᵗʰ **M92.1** Juvenile osteochondrosis of radius and ulna

Osteochondrosis (juvenile) of lower ulna [Burns]
Osteochondrosis (juvenile) of radial head [Brailsford]

M92.10 Juvenile osteochondrosis of radius and ulna, unspecified arm

M92.11 Juvenile osteochondrosis of radius and ulna, right arm

M92.12 Juvenile osteochondrosis of radius and ulna, left arm

✓5ᵗʰ **M92.2** Juvenile osteochondrosis, hand

✓6ᵗʰ **M92.20** Unspecified juvenile osteochondrosis, hand

M92.201 Unspecified juvenile osteochondrosis, right hand

M92.202 Unspecified juvenile osteochondrosis, left hand

M92.209 Unspecified juvenile osteochondrosis, unspecified hand

✓6ᵗʰ **M92.21** Osteochondrosis (juvenile) of carpal lunate [Kienböck]

M92.211 Osteochondrosis (juvenile) of carpal lunate [Kienböck], right hand

M92.212 Osteochondrosis (juvenile) of carpal lunate [Kienböck], left hand

M92.219 Osteochondrosis (juvenile) of carpal lunate [Kienböck], unspecified hand

✓6ᵗʰ **M92.22** Osteochondrosis (juvenile) of metacarpal heads [Mauclaire]

M92.221 Osteochondrosis (juvenile) of metacarpal heads [Mauclaire], right hand

M92.222 Osteochondrosis (juvenile) of metacarpal heads [Mauclaire], left hand

M92.229 Osteochondrosis (juvenile) of metacarpal heads [Mauclaire], unspecified hand

✓6ᵗʰ **M92.29** Other juvenile osteochondrosis, hand

M92.291 Other juvenile osteochondrosis, right hand

M92.292 Other juvenile osteochondrosis, left hand

M92.299 Other juvenile osteochondrosis, unspecified hand

✓6ᵗʰ **M92.3** Other juvenile osteochondrosis, upper limb

M92.30 Other juvenile osteochondrosis, unspecified upper limb

M92.31 Other juvenile osteochondrosis, right upper limb

M92.32 Other juvenile osteochondrosis, left upper limb

✓5ᵗʰ **M92.4** Juvenile osteochondrosis of patella

Osteochondrosis (juvenile) of primary patellar center [Köhler]
Osteochondrosis (juvenile) of secondary patellar centre [Sinding Larsen]

M92.40 Juvenile osteochondrosis of patella, unspecified knee

M92.41 Juvenile osteochondrosis of patella, right knee

M92.42 Juvenile osteochondrosis of patella, left knee

✓5ᵗʰ **M92.5** **Juvenile osteochondrosis of** tibia and fibula

Osteochondrosis (juvenile) of proximal tibia [Blount]
Osteochondrosis (juvenile) of tibial tubercle [Osgood-Schlatter]
Tibia vara

M92.50 **Juvenile osteochondrosis of tibia and fibula, unspecified leg**

M92.51 **Juvenile osteochondrosis of tibia and fibula,** right **leg**

M92.52 **Juvenile osteochondrosis of tibia and fibula,** left **leg**

✓5ᵗʰ **M92.6** **Juvenile osteochondrosis of** tarsus

Osteochondrosis (juvenile) of calcaneum [Sever]
Osteochondrosis (juvenile) of os tibiale externum [Haglund]
Osteochondrosis (juvenile) of talus [Diaz]
Osteochondrosis (juvenile) of tarsal navicular [Köhler]

M92.60 **Juvenile osteochondrosis of tarsus, unspecified ankle**

M92.61 **Juvenile osteochondrosis of tarsus,** right **ankle**

M92.62 **Juvenile osteochondrosis of tarsus,** left **ankle**

✓5ᵗʰ **M92.7** **Juvenile osteochondrosis of** metatarsus

Osteochondrosis (juvenile) of fifth metatarsus [Iselin]
Osteochondrosis (juvenile) of second metatarsus [Freiberg]

M92.70 **Juvenile osteochondrosis of metatarsus, unspecified foot**

M92.71 **Juvenile osteochondrosis of metatarsus,** right **foot**

M92.72 **Juvenile osteochondrosis of metatarsus,** left **foot**

M92.8 **Other specified juvenile osteochondrosis**

Calcaneal apophysitis

DEF: Calcaneal apophysitis: Inflammation of the calcaneus at the point of Achilles tendon insertion usually occurring in boys ages 8 to 14. Pain, tenderness, and localized swelling are present.

M92.9 **Juvenile osteochondrosis, unspecified**

Juvenile apophysitis NOS
Juvenile epiphysitis NOS
Juvenile osteochondritis NOS
Juvenile osteochondrosis NOS

✓4ᵗʰ **M93** **Other osteochondropathies**

EXCLUDES 2   osteochondrosis of spine (M42.-)

✓5ᵗʰ **M93.0** **Slipped upper femoral epiphysis (nontraumatic)**

Use additional code for associated chondrolysis (M94.3)

✓6ᵗʰ **M93.00** **Unspecified slipped upper femoral epiphysis (nontraumatic)**

M93.001 **Unspecified slipped upper femoral epiphysis (nontraumatic),** right **hip**

M93.002 **Unspecified slipped upper femoral epiphysis (nontraumatic),** left **hip**

M93.003 **Unspecified slipped upper femoral epiphysis (nontraumatic), unspecified hip**

✓6ᵗʰ **M93.01** **Acute slipped upper femoral epiphysis (nontraumatic)**

M93.011 **Acute slipped upper femoral epiphysis (nontraumatic),** right **hip**

M93.012 **Acute slipped upper femoral epiphysis (nontraumatic),** left **hip**

M93.013 **Acute slipped upper femoral epiphysis (nontraumatic), unspecified hip**

✓6ᵗʰ **M93.02** **Chronic slipped upper femoral epiphysis (nontraumatic)**

M93.021 **Chronic slipped upper femoral epiphysis (nontraumatic),** right **hip**

M93.022 **Chronic slipped upper femoral epiphysis (nontraumatic),** left **hip**

M93.023 **Chronic slipped upper femoral epiphysis (nontraumatic), unspecified hip**

✓6ᵗʰ **M93.03** **Acute on chronic slipped upper femoral epiphysis (nontraumatic)**

M93.031 **Acute on chronic slipped upper femoral epiphysis (nontraumatic),** right **hip**

M93.032 **Acute on chronic slipped upper femoral epiphysis (nontraumatic),** left **hip**

M93.033 **Acute on chronic slipped upper femoral epiphysis (nontraumatic), unspecified hip**

M93.1 **Kienböck's disease of adults**   A

Adult osteochondrosis of carpal lunates

✓5ᵗʰ **M93.2** **Osteochondritis dissecans**

DEF: Avascular necrosis caused by lack of blood flow to the bone and cartilage of a joint causing the bone to die. This can result in splinters or pieces of cartilage breaking off in the joint.

M93.20 **Osteochondritis dissecans of unspecified site**

✓6ᵗʰ **M93.21** **Osteochondritis dissecans of** shoulder

M93.211 **Osteochondritis dissecans,** right **shoulder**

M93.212 **Osteochondritis dissecans,** left **shoulder**

M93.219 **Osteochondritis dissecans, unspecified shoulder**

✓6ᵗʰ **M93.22** **Osteochondritis dissecans of** elbow

M93.221 **Osteochondritis dissecans,** right **elbow**

M93.222 **Osteochondritis dissecans,** left **elbow**

M93.229 **Osteochondritis dissecans, unspecified elbow**

✓6ᵗʰ **M93.23** **Osteochondritis dissecans of** wrist

M93.231 **Osteochondritis dissecans,** right **wrist**

M93.232 **Osteochondritis dissecans,** left **wrist**

M93.239 **Osteochondritis dissecans, unspecified wrist**

✓6ᵗʰ **M93.24** **Osteochondritis dissecans of joints of** hand

M93.241 **Osteochondritis dissecans, joints of** right **hand**

M93.242 **Osteochondritis dissecans, joints of** left **hand**

M93.249 **Osteochondritis dissecans, joints of unspecified hand**

✓6ᵗʰ **M93.25** **Osteochondritis dissecans of** hip

M93.251 **Osteochondritis dissecans,** right **hip**

M93.252 **Osteochondritis dissecans,** left **hip**

M93.259 **Osteochondritis dissecans, unspecified hip**

✓6ᵗʰ **M93.26** **Osteochondritis dissecans** knee

M93.261 **Osteochondritis dissecans,** right **knee**

M93.262 **Osteochondritis dissecans,** left **knee**

M93.269 **Osteochondritis dissecans, unspecified knee**

✓6ᵗʰ **M93.27** **Osteochondritis dissecans of** ankle and joints of foot

M93.271 **Osteochondritis dissecans,** right **ankle and joints of** right **foot**

M93.272 **Osteochondritis dissecans,** left **ankle and joints of** left **foot**

M93.279 **Osteochondritis dissecans, unspecified ankle and joints of foot**

M93.28 **Osteochondritis dissecans other site**

M93.29 **Osteochondritis dissecans** multiple sites

✓5ᵗʰ **M93.8** **Other specified osteochondropathies**

M93.80 **Other specified osteochondropathies of unspecified site**

✓6ᵗʰ **M93.81** **Other specified osteochondropathies of** shoulder

M93.811 **Other specified osteochondropathies,** right **shoulder**

M93.812 **Other specified osteochondropathies,** left **shoulder**

M93.819 **Other specified osteochondropathies, unspecified shoulder**

✓6ᵗʰ **M93.82** **Other specified osteochondropathies of** upper arm

M93.821 **Other specified osteochondropathies,** right **upper arm**

M93.822 **Other specified osteochondropathies,** left **upper arm**

M93.829 **Other specified osteochondropathies, unspecified upper arm**

✓6ᵗʰ **M93.83** **Other specified osteochondropathies of** forearm

M93.831 **Other specified osteochondropathies,** right **forearm**

M93.832 **Other specified osteochondropathies,** left **forearm**

M93.839 **Other specified osteochondropathies, unspecified forearm**

✓6ᵗʰ **M93.84** **Other specified osteochondropathies of** hand

M93.841 **Other specified osteochondropathies,** right **hand**

M93.842 **Other specified osteochondropathies,** left **hand**

M93.849 **Other specified osteochondropathies, unspecified hand**

✓6ᵗʰ **M93.85** **Other specified osteochondropathies of** thigh

M93.851 **Other specified osteochondropathies,** right **thigh**

M93.852 **Other specified osteochondropathies,** left **thigh**

☑ Additional Character Required   ✓ˣ7ᵗʰ Placeholder Alert   Manifestation   Unspecified Dx   ►◄ Revised Text   ● New Code   ▲ Revised Code Title

ICD-10-CM 2020   825

        M93.859   **Other specified osteochondropathies, unspecified thigh**

    ✓6ᵗʰ M93.86   **Other specified osteochondropathies** lower leg

        M93.861   **Other specified osteochondropathies, right lower leg**

        M93.862   **Other specified osteochondropathies, left lower leg**

        M93.869   **Other specified osteochondropathies, unspecified lower leg**

    ✓6ᵗʰ M93.87   **Other specified osteochondropathies of** ankle and foot

        M93.871   **Other specified osteochondropathies, right ankle and foot**

        M93.872   **Other specified osteochondropathies, left ankle and foot**

        M93.879   **Other specified osteochondropathies, unspecified ankle and foot**

      M93.88   **Other specified osteochondropathies other site**

      M93.89   **Other specified osteochondropathies** multiple sites

  ✓5ᵗʰ M93.9   **Osteochondropathy, unspecified**

      Apophysitis NOS

      Epiphysitis NOS

      Osteochondritis NOS

      Osteochondrosis NOS

      M93.90   **Osteochondropathy, unspecified of unspecified site**

    ✓6ᵗʰ M93.91   **Osteochondropathy, unspecified of** shoulder

        M93.911   **Osteochondropathy, unspecified, right shoulder**

        M93.912   **Osteochondropathy, unspecified, left shoulder**

        M93.919   **Osteochondropathy, unspecified, unspecified shoulder**

    ✓6ᵗʰ M93.92   **Osteochondropathy, unspecified of** upper arm

        M93.921   **Osteochondropathy, unspecified, right upper arm**

        M93.922   **Osteochondropathy, unspecified, left upper arm**

        M93.929   **Osteochondropathy, unspecified, unspecified upper arm**

    ✓6ᵗʰ M93.93   **Osteochondropathy, unspecified of** forearm

        M93.931   **Osteochondropathy, unspecified, right forearm**

        M93.932   **Osteochondropathy, unspecified, left forearm**

        M93.939   **Osteochondropathy, unspecified, unspecified forearm**

    ✓6ᵗʰ M93.94   **Osteochondropathy, unspecified of** hand

        M93.941   **Osteochondropathy, unspecified, right hand**

        M93.942   **Osteochondropathy, unspecified, left hand**

        M93.949   **Osteochondropathy, unspecified, unspecified hand**

    ✓6ᵗʰ M93.95   **Osteochondropathy, unspecified of** thigh

        M93.951   **Osteochondropathy, unspecified, right thigh**

        M93.952   **Osteochondropathy, unspecified, left thigh**

        M93.959   **Osteochondropathy, unspecified, unspecified thigh**

    ✓6ᵗʰ M93.96   **Osteochondropathy, unspecified** lower leg

        M93.961   **Osteochondropathy, unspecified, right lower leg**

        M93.962   **Osteochondropathy, unspecified, left lower leg**

        M93.969   **Osteochondropathy, unspecified, unspecified lower leg**

    ✓6ᵗʰ M93.97   **Osteochondropathy, unspecified of** ankle and foot

        M93.971   **Osteochondropathy, unspecified, right ankle and foot**

        M93.972   **Osteochondropathy, unspecified, left ankle and foot**

        M93.979   **Osteochondropathy, unspecified, unspecified ankle and foot**

      M93.98   **Osteochondropathy, unspecified other site**

      M93.99   **Osteochondropathy, unspecified** multiple sites

---

✓4ᵗʰ M94   **Other disorders of cartilage**

  M94.0   **Chondrocostal junction syndrome [Tietze]**

      Costochondritis

  M94.1   **Relapsing polychondritis**

  ✓5ᵗʰ M94.2   **Chondromalacia**

      EXCLUDES 1   chondromalacia patellae (M22.4)

      M94.20   **Chondromalacia, unspecified site**

    ✓6ᵗʰ M94.21   **Chondromalacia, shoulder**

        M94.211   **Chondromalacia, right shoulder**

        M94.212   **Chondromalacia, left shoulder**

        M94.219   **Chondromalacia, unspecified shoulder**

    ✓6ᵗʰ M94.22   **Chondromalacia, elbow**

        M94.221   **Chondromalacia, right elbow**

        M94.222   **Chondromalacia, left elbow**

        M94.229   **Chondromalacia, unspecified elbow**

    ✓6ᵗʰ M94.23   **Chondromalacia, wrist**

        M94.231   **Chondromalacia, right wrist**

        M94.232   **Chondromalacia, left wrist**

        M94.239   **Chondromalacia, unspecified wrist**

    ✓6ᵗʰ M94.24   **Chondromalacia, joints of hand**

        M94.241   **Chondromalacia, joints of right hand**

        M94.242   **Chondromalacia, joints of left hand**

        M94.249   **Chondromalacia, joints of unspecified hand**

    ✓6ᵗʰ M94.25   **Chondromalacia, hip**

        M94.251   **Chondromalacia, right hip**

        M94.252   **Chondromalacia, left hip**

        M94.259   **Chondromalacia, unspecified hip**

    ✓6ᵗʰ M94.26   **Chondromalacia, knee**

        M94.261   **Chondromalacia, right knee**

        M94.262   **Chondromalacia, left knee**

        M94.269   **Chondromalacia, unspecified knee**

    ✓6ᵗʰ M94.27   **Chondromalacia, ankle and joints of foot**

        M94.271   **Chondromalacia, right ankle and joints of foot**

        M94.272   **Chondromalacia, left ankle and joints of left foot**

        M94.279   **Chondromalacia, unspecified ankle and joints of foot**

      M94.28   **Chondromalacia, other site**

      M94.29   **Chondromalacia, multiple sites**

  ✓5ᵗʰ M94.3   **Chondrolysis**

      Code first any associated slipped upper femoral epiphysis (nontraumatic) (M93.0-)

    ✓6ᵗʰ M94.35   **Chondrolysis, hip**

        M94.351   **Chondrolysis, right hip**

        M94.352   **Chondrolysis, left hip**

        M94.359   **Chondrolysis, unspecified hip**

  ✓5ᵗʰ M94.8   **Other specified disorders of cartilage**

    ✓6ᵗʰ M94.8X   **Other specified disorders of cartilage**

        M94.8X0   **Other specified disorders of cartilage, multiple sites**

        M94.8X1   **Other specified disorders of cartilage, shoulder**

        M94.8X2   **Other specified disorders of cartilage, upper arm**

        M94.8X3   **Other specified disorders of cartilage, forearm**

        M94.8X4   **Other specified disorders of cartilage, hand**

        M94.8X5   **Other specified disorders of cartilage, thigh**

        M94.8X6   **Other specified disorders of cartilage, lower leg**

        M94.8X7   **Other specified disorders of cartilage, ankle and foot**

        M94.8X8   **Other specified disorders of cartilage, other site**

        M94.8X9   **Other specified disorders of cartilage, unspecified sites**

  M94.9   **Disorder of cartilage, unspecified**

Other disorders of the musculoskeletal system and connective tissue (M95)

☑4ᵗʰ **M95 Other acquired deformities of musculoskeletal system and connective tissue**

     EXCLUDES 2   acquired absence of limbs and organs (Z89-Z90)

           acquired deformities of limbs (M20-M21)

           congenital malformations and deformations of the musculoskeletal system (Q65-Q79)

           deforming dorsopathies (M40-M43)

           dentofacial anomalies [including malocclusion] (M26.-)

           postprocedural musculoskeletal disorders (M96.-)

M95.0 Acquired deformity of nose

     EXCLUDES 2   deviated nasal septum (J34.2)

☑5ᵗʰ **M95.1 Cauliflower ear**

     EXCLUDES 2   other acquired deformities of ear (H61.1)

     DEF: Acquired deformity of the external ear due to injury or subsequent perichondritis.

     M95.10 Cauliflower ear, unspecified ear

     M95.11 Cauliflower ear, right ear

     M95.12 Cauliflower ear, left ear

M95.2 Other acquired deformity of head

M95.3 Acquired deformity of neck

M95.4 Acquired deformity of chest and rib

     AHA: 2014,4Q,26-27

M95.5 Acquired deformity of pelvis

     EXCLUDES 1   maternal care for known or suspected disproportion (O33.-)

M95.8 Other specified acquired deformities of musculoskeletal system

M95.9 Acquired deformity of musculoskeletal system, unspecified

Intraoperative and postprocedural complications and disorders of musculoskeletal system, not elsewhere classified (M96)

☑4ᵗʰ **M96 Intraoperative and postprocedural complications and disorders of musculoskeletal system, not elsewhere classified**

     EXCLUDES 2   arthropathy following intestinal bypass (M02.0-)

           complications of internal orthopedic prosthetic devices, implants and grafts (T84.-)

           disorders associated with osteoporosis (M80)

           periprosthetic fracture around internal prosthetic joint (M97.-)

           presence of functional implants and other devices (Z96-Z97)

M96.0 Pseudarthrosis after fusion or arthrodesis

M96.1 Postlaminectomy syndrome, not elsewhere classified

M96.2 Postradiation kyphosis

M96.3 Postlaminectomy kyphosis

M96.4 Postsurgical lordosis

M96.5 Postradiation scoliosis

☑5ᵗʰ **M96.6 Fracture of bone following insertion of orthopedic implant, joint prosthesis, or bone plate**

     Intraoperative fracture of bone during insertion of orthopedic implant, joint prosthesis, or bone plate

     EXCLUDES 2   complication of internal orthopedic devices, implants or grafts (T84.-)

☑6ᵗʰ **M96.62 Fracture of humerus following insertion of orthopedic implant, joint prosthesis, or bone plate**

     M96.621 Fracture of humerus following insertion of orthopedic implant, joint prosthesis, or bone plate, right arm   HCC

     M96.622 Fracture of humerus following insertion of orthopedic implant, joint prosthesis, or bone plate, left arm   HCC

     M96.629 Fracture of humerus following insertion of orthopedic implant, joint prosthesis, or bone plate, unspecified arm   HCC

☑6ᵗʰ **M96.63 Fracture of radius or ulna following insertion of orthopedic implant, joint prosthesis, or bone plate**

     M96.631 Fracture of radius or ulna following insertion of orthopedic implant, joint prosthesis, or bone plate, right arm   HCC

     M96.632 Fracture of radius or ulna following insertion of orthopedic implant, joint prosthesis, or bone plate, left arm   HCC

     M96.639 Fracture of radius or ulna following insertion of orthopedic implant, joint prosthesis, or bone plate, unspecified arm   HCC

M96.65 Fracture of pelvis following insertion of orthopedic implant, joint prosthesis, or bone plate   HCC

☑6ᵗʰ **M96.66 Fracture of femur following insertion of orthopedic implant, joint prosthesis, or bone plate**

     M96.661 Fracture of femur following insertion of orthopedic implant, joint prosthesis, or bone plate, right leg   HCC

     M96.662 Fracture of femur following insertion of orthopedic implant, joint prosthesis, or bone plate, left leg   HCC

     M96.669 Fracture of femur following insertion of orthopedic implant, joint prosthesis, or bone plate, unspecified leg   HCC

☑6ᵗʰ **M96.67 Fracture of tibia or fibula following insertion of orthopedic implant, joint prosthesis, or bone plate**

     M96.671 Fracture of tibia or fibula following insertion of orthopedic implant, joint prosthesis, or bone plate, right leg   HCC

     M96.672 Fracture of tibia or fibula following insertion of orthopedic implant, joint prosthesis, or bone plate, left leg   HCC

     M96.679 Fracture of tibia or fibula following insertion of orthopedic implant, joint prosthesis, or bone plate, unspecified leg   HCC

M96.69 Fracture of other bone following insertion of orthopedic implant, joint prosthesis, or bone plate   HCC

☑5ᵗʰ **M96.8 Other intraoperative and postprocedural complications and disorders of musculoskeletal system, not elsewhere classified**

     AHA: 2016,4Q,9-10

☑6ᵗʰ **M96.81 Intraoperative hemorrhage and hematoma of a musculoskeletal structure complicating a procedure**

     EXCLUDES 1   intraoperative hemorrhage and hematoma of a musculoskeletal structure due to accidental puncture and laceration during a procedure (M96.82-)

     M96.810 Intraoperative hemorrhage and hematoma of a musculoskeletal structure complicating a musculoskeletal system procedure

     M96.811 Intraoperative hemorrhage and hematoma of a musculoskeletal structure complicating other procedure

☑6ᵗʰ **M96.82 Accidental puncture and laceration of a musculoskeletal structure during a procedure**

     M96.820 Accidental puncture and laceration of a musculoskeletal structure during a musculoskeletal system procedure

     M96.821 Accidental puncture and laceration of a musculoskeletal structure during other procedure

☑6ᵗʰ **M96.83 Postprocedural hemorrhage of a musculoskeletal structure following a procedure**

     M96.830 Postprocedural hemorrhage of a musculoskeletal structure following a musculoskeletal system procedure

     M96.831 Postprocedural hemorrhage of a musculoskeletal structure following other procedure

☑6ᵗʰ **M96.84 Postprocedural hematoma and seroma of a musculoskeletal structure following a procedure**

     M96.840 Postprocedural hematoma of a musculoskeletal structure following a musculoskeletal system procedure

---

☑ Additional Character Required   ☑x7ᵗʰ Placeholder Alert   Manifestation   Unspecified Dx   ▶◀ Revised Text   ● New Code   ▲ Revised Code Title

M96.841 Postprocedural hematoma of a musculoskeletal structure following other procedure
    AHA: 2016,4Q,10

M96.842 Postprocedural seroma of a musculoskeletal structure following a musculoskeletal system procedure

M96.843 Postprocedural seroma of a musculoskeletal structure following other procedure
    AHA: 2018,3Q,6

M96.89 Other intraoperative and postprocedural complications and disorders of the musculoskeletal system
    Instability of joint secondary to removal of joint prosthesis
    Use additional code, if applicable, to further specify disorder

Periprosthetic fractures around internal prosthetic joint (M97)

☑4ᵗʰ **M97** **Periprosthetic fracture around internal prosthetic joint**
    EXCLUDES 2   breakage (fracture) of prosthetic joint (T84.Ø1-)
          fracture of bone following insertion of orthopedic implant, joint prosthesis or bone plate (M96.6-)
    AHA: 2016,4Q,42-43

> The appropriate 7th character is to be added to each code from category M97.
> A   initial encounter
> D   subsequent encounter
> S   sequela

☑5ᵗʰ **M97.Ø** **Periprosthetic fracture around internal prosthetic hip joint**
    AHA: 2018,1Q,21; 2016,4Q,42

   ¹ ☑x7ᵗʰ **M97.Ø1** **Periprosthetic fracture around internal prosthetic right hip joint**   HCC

   ¹ ☑x7ᵗʰ **M97.Ø2** **Periprosthetic fracture around internal prosthetic left hip joint**   HCC

☑5ᵗʰ **M97.1** **Periprosthetic fracture around internal prosthetic knee joint**

   ☑x7ᵗʰ **M97.11** **Periprosthetic fracture around internal prosthetic right knee joint**

   ☑x7ᵗʰ **M97.12** **Periprosthetic fracture around internal prosthetic left knee joint**

☑5ᵗʰ **M97.2** **Periprosthetic fracture around internal prosthetic ankle joint**

   ☑x7ᵗʰ **M97.21** **Periprosthetic fracture around internal prosthetic right ankle joint**

   ☑x7ᵗʰ **M97.22** **Periprosthetic fracture around internal prosthetic left ankle joint**

☑5ᵗʰ **M97.3** **Periprosthetic fracture around internal prosthetic shoulder joint**

   ☑x7ᵗʰ **M97.31** **Periprosthetic fracture around internal prosthetic right shoulder joint**

   ☑x7ᵗʰ **M97.32** **Periprosthetic fracture around internal prosthetic left shoulder joint**

☑5ᵗʰ **M97.4** **Periprosthetic fracture around internal prosthetic elbow joint**

   ☑x7ᵗʰ **M97.41** **Periprosthetic fracture around internal prosthetic right elbow joint**

   ☑x7ᵗʰ **M97.42** **Periprosthetic fracture around internal prosthetic left elbow joint**

☑x7ᵗʰ **M97.8** **Periprosthetic fracture around other internal prosthetic joint**
    Periprosthetic fracture around internal prosthetic finger joint
    Periprosthetic fracture around internal prosthetic spinal joint
    Periprosthetic fracture around internal prosthetic toe joint
    Periprosthetic fracture around internal prosthetic wrist joint
    Use additional code to identify the joint (Z96.6-)

☑x7ᵗʰ **M97.9** **Periprosthetic fracture around unspecified internal prosthetic joint**

Biomechanical lesions, not elsewhere classified (M99)

☑4ᵗʰ **M99** **Biomechanical lesions, not elsewhere classified**
    NOTE   This category should not be used if the condition can be classified elsewhere.

    DEF: Biomechanical lesion: Term used by osteopathic and chiropractic physicians to describe musculoskeletal conditions treated that are not more appropriately classified elsewhere.

☑5ᵗʰ **M99.Ø** **Segmental and somatic dysfunction**

   M99.ØØ **Segmental and somatic dysfunction of head region**

M99.Ø1 **Segmental and somatic dysfunction of cervical region**

M99.Ø2 **Segmental and somatic dysfunction of thoracic region**

M99.Ø3 **Segmental and somatic dysfunction of lumbar region**

M99.Ø4 **Segmental and somatic dysfunction of sacral region**

M99.Ø5 **Segmental and somatic dysfunction of pelvic region**

M99.Ø6 **Segmental and somatic dysfunction of lower extremity**

M99.Ø7 **Segmental and somatic dysfunction of upper extremity**

M99.Ø8 **Segmental and somatic dysfunction of rib cage**

M99.Ø9 **Segmental and somatic dysfunction of abdomen and other regions**

☑5ᵗʰ **M99.1** **Subluxation complex (vertebral)**

M99.1Ø **Subluxation complex (vertebral) of head region**

M99.11 **Subluxation complex (vertebral) of cervical region**

M99.12 **Subluxation complex (vertebral) of thoracic region**

M99.13 **Subluxation complex (vertebral) of lumbar region**

M99.14 **Subluxation complex (vertebral) of sacral region**

M99.15 **Subluxation complex (vertebral) of pelvic region**

M99.16 **Subluxation complex (vertebral) of lower extremity**

M99.17 **Subluxation complex (vertebral) of upper extremity**

M99.18 **Subluxation complex (vertebral) of rib cage**

M99.19 **Subluxation complex (vertebral) of abdomen and other regions**

☑5ᵗʰ **M99.2** **Subluxation stenosis of neural canal**

M99.2Ø **Subluxation stenosis of neural canal of head region**

M99.21 **Subluxation stenosis of neural canal of cervical region**

M99.22 **Subluxation stenosis of neural canal of thoracic region**

M99.23 **Subluxation stenosis of neural canal of lumbar region**

M99.24 **Subluxation stenosis of neural canal of sacral region**

M99.25 **Subluxation stenosis of neural canal of pelvic region**

M99.26 **Subluxation stenosis of neural canal of lower extremity**

M99.27 **Subluxation stenosis of neural canal of upper extremity**

M99.28 **Subluxation stenosis of neural canal of rib cage**

M99.29 **Subluxation stenosis of neural canal of abdomen and other regions**

☑5ᵗʰ **M99.3** **Osseous stenosis of neural canal**

M99.3Ø **Osseous stenosis of neural canal of head region**

M99.31 **Osseous stenosis of neural canal of cervical region**

M99.32 **Osseous stenosis of neural canal of thoracic region**

M99.33 **Osseous stenosis of neural canal of lumbar region**

M99.34 **Osseous stenosis of neural canal of sacral region**

M99.35 **Osseous stenosis of neural canal of pelvic region**

M99.36 **Osseous stenosis of neural canal of lower extremity**

M99.37 **Osseous stenosis of neural canal of upper extremity**

M99.38 **Osseous stenosis of neural canal of rib cage**

M99.39 **Osseous stenosis of neural canal of abdomen and other regions**

☑5ᵗʰ **M99.4** **Connective tissue stenosis of neural canal**

M99.4Ø **Connective tissue stenosis of neural canal of head region**

M99.41 **Connective tissue stenosis of neural canal of cervical region**

M99.42 **Connective tissue stenosis of neural canal of thoracic region**

M99.43 **Connective tissue stenosis of neural canal of lumbar region**

M99.44 **Connective tissue stenosis of neural canal of sacral region**

M99.45 **Connective tissue stenosis of neural canal of pelvic region**

M99.46 **Connective tissue stenosis of neural canal of lower extremity**

M99.47 **Connective tissue stenosis of neural canal of upper extremity**

M99.48 **Connective tissue stenosis of neural canal of rib cage**

M99.49 **Connective tissue stenosis of neural canal of abdomen and other regions**

✓5ᵗʰ **M99.5** **Intervertebral disc stenosis of neural canal**

    M99.50 Intervertebral disc stenosis of neural canal of head region

    M99.51 Intervertebral disc stenosis of neural canal of cervical region

    M99.52 Intervertebral disc stenosis of neural canal of thoracic region

    M99.53 Intervertebral disc stenosis of neural canal of lumbar region

    M99.54 Intervertebral disc stenosis of neural canal of sacral region

    M99.55 Intervertebral disc stenosis of neural canal of pelvic region

    M99.56 Intervertebral disc stenosis of neural canal of lower extremity

    M99.57 Intervertebral disc stenosis of neural canal of upper extremity

    M99.58 Intervertebral disc stenosis of neural canal of rib cage

    M99.59 Intervertebral disc stenosis of neural canal of abdomen and other regions

✓5ᵗʰ **M99.6** **Osseous and subluxation stenosis of intervertebral foramina**

    M99.60 Osseous and subluxation stenosis of intervertebral foramina of head region

    M99.61 Osseous and subluxation stenosis of intervertebral foramina of cervical region

    M99.62 Osseous and subluxation stenosis of intervertebral foramina of thoracic region

    M99.63 Osseous and subluxation stenosis of intervertebral foramina of lumbar region

    M99.64 Osseous and subluxation stenosis of intervertebral foramina of sacral region

    M99.65 Osseous and subluxation stenosis of intervertebral foramina of pelvic region

    M99.66 Osseous and subluxation stenosis of intervertebral foramina of lower extremity

    M99.67 Osseous and subluxation stenosis of intervertebral foramina of upper extremity

    M99.68 Osseous and subluxation stenosis of intervertebral foramina of rib cage

    M99.69 Osseous and subluxation stenosis of intervertebral foramina of abdomen and other regions

✓5ᵗʰ **M99.7** **Connective tissue and disc stenosis of intervertebral foramina**

    M99.70 Connective tissue and disc stenosis of intervertebral foramina of head region

    M99.71 Connective tissue and disc stenosis of intervertebral foramina of cervical region

    M99.72 Connective tissue and disc stenosis of intervertebral foramina of thoracic region

    M99.73 Connective tissue and disc stenosis of intervertebral foramina of lumbar region

    M99.74 Connective tissue and disc stenosis of intervertebral foramina of sacral region

    M99.75 Connective tissue and disc stenosis of intervertebral foramina of pelvic region

    M99.76 Connective tissue and disc stenosis of intervertebral foramina of lower extremity

    M99.77 Connective tissue and disc stenosis of intervertebral foramina of upper extremity

    M99.78 Connective tissue and disc stenosis of intervertebral foramina of rib cage

    M99.79 Connective tissue and disc stenosis of intervertebral foramina of abdomen and other regions

✓5ᵗʰ **M99.8** **Other biomechanical lesions**

    M99.80 Other biomechanical lesions of head region
    M99.81 Other biomechanical lesions of cervical region
    M99.82 Other biomechanical lesions of thoracic region
    M99.83 Other biomechanical lesions of lumbar region
    M99.84 Other biomechanical lesions of sacral region
    M99.85 Other biomechanical lesions of pelvic region
    M99.86 Other biomechanical lesions of lower extremity
    M99.87 Other biomechanical lesions of upper extremity
    M99.88 Other biomechanical lesions of rib cage
    M99.89 Other biomechanical lesions of abdomen and other regions

  M99.9 **Biomechanical lesion, unspecified**

☑ Additional Character Required   ✓ₓ7ᵗʰ Placeholder Alert   Manifestation   Unspecified Dx   ►◄ Revised Text   ● New Code   ▲ Revised Code Title

Chapter 14. Diseases of Genitourinary System (N00–N99)

Chapter-specific Guidelines with Coding Examples

The chapter-specific guidelines from the ICD-10-CM Official Guidelines for Coding and Reporting have been provided below. Along with these guidelines are coding examples, contained in the shaded boxes, that have been developed to help illustrate the coding and/or sequencing guidance found in these guidelines.

a. Chronic kidney disease

1) Stages of chronic kidney disease (CKD)

The ICD-10-CM classifies CKD based on severity. The severity of CKD is designated by stages 1-5. Stage 2, code N18.2, equates to mild CKD; stage 3, code N18.3, equates to moderate CKD; and stage 4, code N18.4, equates to severe CKD. Code N18.6, End stage renal disease (ESRD), is assigned when the provider has documented end-stage renal disease (ESRD).

If both a stage of CKD and ESRD are documented, assign code N18.6 only.

Stage 5 chronic kidney disease with ESRD requiring chronic dialysis

N18.6	End stage renal disease
Z99.2	Dependence on renal dialysis

Explanation: The diagnostic statement indicates the patient has chronic kidney disease, documented both as stage 5 and as ESRD requiring chronic dialysis. Code N18.6 End stage renal disease (ESRD), is assigned when the provider has documented end-stage-renal disease (ESRD). If both a stage of CKD and ESRD are documented, assign code N18.6 only.

---

2) Chronic kidney disease and kidney transplant status

Patients who have undergone kidney transplant may still have some form of chronic kidney disease (CKD) because the kidney transplant may not fully restore kidney function. Therefore, the presence of CKD alone does not constitute a transplant complication. Assign the appropriate N18 code for the patient's stage of CKD and code Z94.0, Kidney transplant status. If a transplant complication such as failure or rejection or other transplant complication is documented, see section I.C.19.g for information on coding complications of a kidney transplant. If the documentation is unclear as to whether the patient has a complication of the transplant, query the provider.

Patient with residual chronic kidney disease stage 1 after kidney transplant

N18.1	Chronic kidney disease, stage 1
Z94.0	Kidney transplant status

Explanation: Patients who have undergone kidney transplant may still have some form of chronic kidney disease (CKD) because the kidney transplant may not fully restore kidney function. The presence of CKD alone does not constitute a transplant complication. Assign the appropriate N18 code for the patient's stage of CKD and code Z94.0 Kidney transplant status.

---

3) Chronic kidney disease with other conditions

Patients with CKD may also suffer from other serious conditions, most commonly diabetes mellitus and hypertension. The sequencing of the CKD code in relationship to codes for other contributing conditions is based on the conventions in the Tabular List.

See I.C.9. Hypertensive chronic kidney disease.

See I.C.19. Chronic kidney disease and kidney transplant complications.

Type 1 diabetic chronic kidney disease, stage 2

E10.22	Type 1 diabetes mellitus with diabetic chronic kidney disease
N18.2	Chronic kidney disease, stage 2 (mild)

Explanation: Patients with CKD may also suffer from other serious conditions such as diabetes mellitus. The sequencing of the CKD code in relationship to codes for other contributing conditions is based on the conventions in the Tabular List. Diabetic CKD code E10.22 includes an instructional note to "Use additional code to identify stage of chronic kidney disease (N18.1–N18.6)," thus providing sequencing direction.

Chapter 14. Diseases of the Genitourinary System (N00-N99)

EXCLUDES 2   *certain conditions originating in the perinatal period (P04-P96)*
certain infectious and parasitic diseases (A00-B99)
complications of pregnancy, childbirth and the puerperium (O00-O9A)
congenital malformations, deformations and chromosomal abnormalities (Q00-Q99)
endocrine, nutritional and metabolic diseases (E00-E88)
injury, poisoning and certain other consequences of external causes (S00-T88)
neoplasms (C00-D49)
symptoms, signs and abnormal clinical and laboratory findings, not elsewhere classified (R00-R94)

This chapter contains the following blocks:

N00-N08	Glomerular diseases
N10-N16	Renal tubulo-interstitial diseases
N17-N19	Acute kidney failure and chronic kidney disease
N20-N23	Urolithiasis
N25-N29	Other disorders of kidney and ureter
N30-N39	Other diseases of the urinary system
N40-N53	Diseases of male genital organs
N60-N65	Disorders of breast
N70-N77	Inflammatory diseases of female pelvic organs
N80-N98	Noninflammatory disorders of female genital tract
N99	Intraoperative and postprocedural complications and disorders of genitourinary system, not elsewhere classified

Glomerular diseases (N00-N08)

Code also any associated kidney failure (N17-N19).

EXCLUDES 1   *hypertensive chronic kidney disease (I12.-)*

DEF: Glomeruli: Clusters of microscopic blood vessels located within the kidneys containing small pores through which waste products are filtered from the blood and urine is formed.
DEF: Glomerulonephritis: Disease of the kidney with diffuse inflammation of the capillary loops of the glomeruli.

√4ᵗʰ **N00 Acute nephritic syndrome**

INCLUDES   acute glomerular disease
acute glomerulonephritis
acute nephritis

EXCLUDES 1   *acute tubulo-interstitial nephritis (N10)*
nephritic syndrome NOS (N05.-)

N00.0 Acute nephritic syndrome with minor glomerular abnormality
Acute nephritic syndrome with minimal change lesion

N00.1 Acute nephritic syndrome with focal and segmental glomerular lesions
Acute nephritic syndrome with focal and segmental hyalinosis
Acute nephritic syndrome with focal and segmental sclerosis
Acute nephritic syndrome with focal glomerulonephritis

N00.2 Acute nephritic syndrome with diffuse membranous glomerulonephritis

N00.3 Acute nephritic syndrome with diffuse mesangial proliferative glomerulonephritis

N00.4 Acute nephritic syndrome with diffuse endocapillary proliferative glomerulonephritis

N00.5 Acute nephritic syndrome with diffuse mesangiocapillary glomerulonephritis
Acute nephritic syndrome with membranoproliferative glomerulonephritis, types 1 and 3, or NOS

N00.6 Acute nephritic syndrome with dense deposit disease
Acute nephritic syndrome with membranoproliferative glomerulonephritis, type 2

N00.7 Acute nephritic syndrome with diffuse crescentic glomerulonephritis
Acute nephritic syndrome with extracapillary glomerulonephritis

N00.8 Acute nephritic syndrome with other morphologic changes
Acute nephritic syndrome with proliferative glomerulonephritis NOS

N00.9 Acute nephritic syndrome with unspecified morphologic changes

√4ᵗʰ **N01 Rapidly progressive nephritic syndrome**

INCLUDES   rapidly progressive glomerular disease
rapidly progressive glomerulonephritis
rapidly progressive nephritis

EXCLUDES 1   *nephritic syndrome NOS (N05.-)*

N01.0 Rapidly progressive nephritic syndrome with minor glomerular abnormality
Rapidly progressive nephritic syndrome with minimal change lesion

N01.1 Rapidly progressive nephritic syndrome with focal and segmental glomerular lesions
Rapidly progressive nephritic syndrome with focal and segmental hyalinosis
Rapidly progressive nephritic syndrome with focal and segmental sclerosis
Rapidly progressive nephritic syndrome with focal glomerulonephritis

N01.2 Rapidly progressive nephritic syndrome with diffuse membranous glomerulonephritis

N01.3 Rapidly progressive nephritic syndrome with diffuse mesangial proliferative glomerulonephritis

N01.4 Rapidly progressive nephritic syndrome with diffuse endocapillary proliferative glomerulonephritis

N01.5 Rapidly progressive nephritic syndrome with diffuse mesangiocapillary glomerulonephritis
Rapidly progressive nephritic syndrome with membranoproliferative glomerulonephritis, types 1 and 3, or NOS

N01.6 Rapidly progressive nephritic syndrome with dense deposit disease
Rapidly progressive nephritic syndrome with membranoproliferative glomerulonephritis, type 2

N01.7 Rapidly progressive nephritic syndrome with diffuse crescentic glomerulonephritis
Rapidly progressive nephritic syndrome with extracapillary glomerulonephritis

N01.8 Rapidly progressive nephritic syndrome with other morphologic changes
Rapidly progressive nephritic syndrome with proliferative glomerulonephritis NOS

N01.9 Rapidly progressive nephritic syndrome with unspecified morphologic changes

√4ᵗʰ **N02 Recurrent and persistent hematuria**

EXCLUDES 1   *acute cystitis with hematuria (N30.01)*
hematuria NOS (R31.9)
hematuria not associated with specified morphologic lesions (R31.-)

N02.0 Recurrent and persistent hematuria with minor glomerular abnormality
Recurrent and persistent hematuria with minimal change lesion

N02.1 Recurrent and persistent hematuria with focal and segmental glomerular lesions
Recurrent and persistent hematuria with focal and segmental hyalinosis
Recurrent and persistent hematuria with focal and segmental sclerosis
Recurrent and persistent hematuria with focal glomerulonephritis

N02.2 Recurrent and persistent hematuria with diffuse membranous glomerulonephritis

N02.3 Recurrent and persistent hematuria with diffuse mesangial proliferative glomerulonephritis

N02.4 Recurrent and persistent hematuria with diffuse endocapillary proliferative glomerulonephritis

N02.5 Recurrent and persistent hematuria with diffuse mesangiocapillary glomerulonephritis
Recurrent and persistent hematuria with membranoproliferative glomerulonephritis, types 1 and 3, or NOS

N02.6 Recurrent and persistent hematuria with dense deposit disease
Recurrent and persistent hematuria with membranoproliferative glomerulonephritis, type 2

N02.7 Recurrent and persistent hematuria with diffuse crescentic glomerulonephritis
Recurrent and persistent hematuria with extracapillary glomerulonephritis

N02.8 **Recurrent and persistent hematuria with other morphologic changes**
Recurrent and persistent hematuria with proliferative glomerulonephritis NOS

N02.9 **Recurrent and persistent hematuria with unspecified morphologic changes**
AHA: 2017,2Q,5

✔4ᵗʰ **N03** **Chronic nephritic syndrome**

INCLUDES chronic glomerular disease
chronic glomerulonephritis
chronic nephritis

EXCLUDES 1 *chronic tubulo-interstitial nephritis (N11.-)*
diffuse sclerosing glomerulonephritis (N05.8-)
nephritic syndrome NOS (N05.-)

DEF: Slow, progressive type of nephritis characterized by inflammation of the capillary loops in the glomeruli of the kidney, which leads to renal failure.

N03.0 **Chronic nephritic syndrome with minor glomerular abnormality**
Chronic nephritic syndrome with minimal change lesion

N03.1 **Chronic nephritic syndrome with focal and segmental glomerular lesions**
Chronic nephritic syndrome with focal and segmental hyalinosis
Chronic nephritic syndrome with focal and segmental sclerosis
Chronic nephritic syndrome with focal glomerulonephritis

N03.2 **Chronic nephritic syndrome with diffuse membranous glomerulonephritis**

N03.3 **Chronic nephritic syndrome with diffuse mesangial proliferative glomerulonephritis**

N03.4 **Chronic nephritic syndrome with diffuse endocapillary proliferative glomerulonephritis**

N03.5 **Chronic nephritic syndrome with diffuse mesangiocapillary glomerulonephritis**
Chronic nephritic syndrome with membranoproliferative glomerulonephritis, types 1 and 3, or NOS

N03.6 **Chronic nephritic syndrome with dense deposit disease**
Chronic nephritic syndrome with membranoproliferative glomerulonephritis, type 2

N03.7 **Chronic nephritic syndrome with diffuse crescentic glomerulonephritis**
Chronic nephritic syndrome with extracapillary glomerulonephritis

N03.8 **Chronic nephritic syndrome with other morphologic changes**
Chronic nephritic syndrome with proliferative glomerulonephritis NOS

N03.9 **Chronic nephritic syndrome with unspecified morphologic changes**

✔4ᵗʰ **N04** **Nephrotic syndrome**

INCLUDES congenital nephrotic syndrome
lipoid nephrosis

N04.0 **Nephrotic syndrome with minor glomerular abnormality**
Nephrotic syndrome with minimal change lesion

N04.1 **Nephrotic syndrome with focal and segmental glomerular lesions**
Nephrotic syndrome with focal and segmental hyalinosis
Nephrotic syndrome with focal and segmental sclerosis
Nephrotic syndrome with focal glomerulonephritis

N04.2 **Nephrotic syndrome with diffuse membranous glomerulonephritis**

N04.3 **Nephrotic syndrome with diffuse mesangial proliferative glomerulonephritis**

N04.4 **Nephrotic syndrome with diffuse endocapillary proliferative glomerulonephritis**

N04.5 **Nephrotic syndrome with diffuse mesangiocapillary glomerulonephritis**
Nephrotic syndrome with membranoproliferative glomerulonephritis, types 1 and 3, or NOS

N04.6 **Nephrotic syndrome with dense deposit disease**
Nephrotic syndrome with membranoproliferative glomerulonephritis, type 2

N04.7 **Nephrotic syndrome with diffuse crescentic glomerulonephritis**
Nephrotic syndrome with extracapillary glomerulonephritis

N04.8 **Nephrotic syndrome with other morphologic changes**
Nephrotic syndrome with proliferative glomerulonephritis NOS

N04.9 **Nephrotic syndrome with unspecified morphologic changes**

✔4ᵗʰ **N05** **Unspecified nephritic syndrome**

INCLUDES glomerular disease NOS
glomerulonephritis NOS
nephritis NOS
nephropathy NOS and renal disease NOS with morphological lesion specified in .0-.8

EXCLUDES 1 *nephropathy NOS with no stated morphological lesion (N28.9)*
renal disease NOS with no stated morphological lesion (N28.9)
tubulo-interstitial nephritis NOS (N12)

N05.0 **Unspecified nephritic syndrome with minor glomerular abnormality**
Unspecified nephritic syndrome with minimal change lesion

N05.1 **Unspecified nephritic syndrome with focal and segmental glomerular lesions**
Unspecified nephritic syndrome with focal and segmental hyalinosis
Unspecified nephritic syndrome with focal and segmental sclerosis
Unspecified nephritic syndrome with focal glomerulonephritis

N05.2 **Unspecified nephritic syndrome with diffuse membranous glomerulonephritis**

N05.3 **Unspecified nephritic syndrome with diffuse mesangial proliferative glomerulonephritis**

N05.4 **Unspecified nephritic syndrome with diffuse endocapillary proliferative glomerulonephritis**

N05.5 **Unspecified nephritic syndrome with diffuse mesangiocapillary glomerulonephritis**
Unspecified nephritic syndrome with membranoproliferative glomerulonephritis, types 1 and 3, or NOS

N05.6 **Unspecified nephritic syndrome with dense deposit disease**
Unspecified nephritic syndrome with membranoproliferative glomerulonephritis, type 2

N05.7 **Unspecified nephritic syndrome with diffuse crescentic glomerulonephritis**
Unspecified nephritic syndrome with extracapillary glomerulonephritis

N05.8 **Unspecified nephritic syndrome with other morphologic changes**
Unspecified nephritic syndrome with proliferative glomerulonephritis NOS

N05.9 **Unspecified nephritic syndrome with unspecified morphologic changes**

✔4ᵗʰ **N06** **Isolated proteinuria with specified morphological lesion**

EXCLUDES 1 *proteinuria not associated with specific morphologic lesions (R80.0)*

N06.0 **Isolated proteinuria with minor glomerular abnormality**
Isolated proteinuria with minimal change lesion

N06.1 **Isolated proteinuria with focal and segmental glomerular lesions**
Isolated proteinuria with focal and segmental hyalinosis
Isolated proteinuria with focal and segmental sclerosis
Isolated proteinuria with focal glomerulonephritis

N06.2 **Isolated proteinuria with diffuse membranous glomerulonephritis**

N06.3 **Isolated proteinuria with diffuse mesangial proliferative glomerulonephritis**

N06.4 **Isolated proteinuria with diffuse endocapillary proliferative glomerulonephritis**

N06.5 **Isolated proteinuria with diffuse mesangiocapillary glomerulonephritis**
Isolated proteinuria with membranoproliferative glomerulonephritis, types 1 and 3, or NOS

N06.6 **Isolated proteinuria with dense deposit disease**
Isolated proteinuria with membranoproliferative glomerulonephritis, type 2

N06.7 **Isolated proteinuria with diffuse crescentic glomerulonephritis**
Isolated proteinuria with extracapillary glomerulonephritis

N06.8 **Isolated proteinuria with other morphologic lesion**
Isolated proteinuria with proliferative glomerulonephritis NOS

N06.9 **Isolated proteinuria with unspecified morphologic lesion**

✔ Additional Character Required   ✔x7ᵗʰ Placeholder Alert   Manifestation   Unspecified Dx   ▶◀ Revised Text   ● New Code   ▲ Revised Code Title

ICD-10-CM 2020   833

Chapter 14. Diseases of the Genitourinary System

☑4ᵗʰ **N07 Hereditary nephropathy, not elsewhere classified**

> EXCLUDES 2 Alport's syndrome (Q87.81-)
> hereditary amyloid nephropathy (E85.-)
> nail patella syndrome (Q87.2)
> non-neuropathic heredofamilial amyloidosis (E85.-)

N07.0 Hereditary nephropathy, not elsewhere classified with minor glomerular abnormality
Hereditary nephropathy, not elsewhere classified with minimal change lesion

N07.1 Hereditary nephropathy, not elsewhere classified with focal and segmental glomerular lesions
Hereditary nephropathy, not elsewhere classified with focal and segmental hyalinosis
Hereditary nephropathy, not elsewhere classified with focal and segmental sclerosis
Hereditary nephropathy, not elsewhere classified with focal glomerulonephritis

N07.2 Hereditary nephropathy, not elsewhere classified with diffuse membranous glomerulonephritis

N07.3 Hereditary nephropathy, not elsewhere classified with diffuse mesangial proliferative glomerulonephritis

N07.4 Hereditary nephropathy, not elsewhere classified with diffuse endocapillary proliferative glomerulonephritis

N07.5 Hereditary nephropathy, not elsewhere classified with diffuse mesangiocapillary glomerulonephritis
Hereditary nephropathy, not elsewhere classified with membranoproliferative glomerulonephritis, types 1 and 3, or NOS

N07.6 Hereditary nephropathy, not elsewhere classified with dense deposit disease
Hereditary nephropathy, not elsewhere classified with membranoproliferative glomerulonephritis, type 2

N07.7 Hereditary nephropathy, not elsewhere classified with diffuse crescentic glomerulonephritis
Hereditary nephropathy, not elsewhere classified with extracapillary glomerulonephritis

N07.8 Hereditary nephropathy, not elsewhere classified with other morphologic lesions
Hereditary nephropathy, not elsewhere classified with proliferative glomerulonephritis NOS

N07.9 Hereditary nephropathy, not elsewhere classified with unspecified morphologic lesions

N08 Glomerular disorders in diseases classified elsewhere
Glomerulonephritis
Nephritis
Nephropathy
Code first underlying disease, such as:
amyloidosis (E85.-)
congenital syphilis (A50.5)
cryoglobulinemia (D89.1)
disseminated intravascular coagulation (D65)
gout (M1A.-, M10.-)
microscopic polyangiitis (M31.7)
multiple myeloma (C90.0-)
sepsis (A40.0-A41.9)
sickle-cell disease (D57.0-D57.8)

> EXCLUDES 1 glomerulonephritis, nephritis and nephropathy (in):
> antiglomerular basement membrane disease (M31.0)
> diabetes (E08-E13 with .21)
> gonococcal (A54.21)
> Goodpasture's syndrome (M31.0)
> hemolytic-uremic syndrome (D59.3)
> lupus (M32.14)
> mumps (B26.83)
> syphilis (A52.75)
> systemic lupus erythematosus (M32.14)
> Wegener's granulomatosis (M31.31)
> pyelonephritis in diseases classified elsewhere (N16)
> renal tubulo-interstitial disorders classified elsewhere (N16)

Renal tubulo-interstitial diseases (N10-N16)

> INCLUDES pyelonephritis
> EXCLUDES 1 pyeloureteritis cystica (N28.85)

N10 Acute pyelonephritis
Acute infectious interstitial nephritis
Acute pyelitis
Acute tubulo-interstitial nephritis
Hemoglobin nephrosis
Myoglobin nephrosis
Use additional code (B95-B97), to identify infectious agent

☑4ᵗʰ **N11 Chronic tubulo-interstitial nephritis**

> INCLUDES chronic infectious interstitial nephritis
> chronic pyelitis
> chronic pyelonephritis
> Use additional code (B95-B97), to identify infectious agent

N11.0 Nonobstructive reflux-associated chronic pyelonephritis
Pyelonephritis (chronic) associated with (vesicoureteral) reflux

> EXCLUDES 1 vesicoureteral reflux NOS (N13.70)

N11.1 Chronic obstructive pyelonephritis
Pyelonephritis (chronic) associated with anomaly of pelviureteric junction
Pyelonephritis (chronic) associated with anomaly of pyel;oureteric junction
Pyelonephritis (chronic) associated with crossing of vessel
Pyelonephritis (chronic) associated with kinking of ureter
Pyelonephritis (chronic) associated with obstruction of ureter
Pyelonephritis (chronic) associated with stricture of pelviureteric junction
Pyelonephritis (chronic) associated with stricture of ureter

> EXCLUDES 1 calculous pyelonephritis (N20.9)
> obstructive uropathy (N13.-)

N11.8 Other chronic tubulo-interstitial nephritis
Nonobstructive chronic pyelonephritis NOS

N11.9 Chronic tubulo-interstitial nephritis, unspecified
Chronic interstitial nephritis NOS
Chronic pyelitis NOS
Chronic pyelonephritis NOS

N12 Tubulo-interstitial nephritis, not specified as acute or chronic
Interstitial nephritis NOS
Pyelitis NOS
Pyelonephritis NOS

> EXCLUDES 1 calculous pyelonephritis (N20.9)

✓4ᵗʰ N13 Obstructive and reflux uropathy

> EXCLUDES 2   *calculus of kidney and ureter without hydronephrosis (N20.-)*
> *congenital obstructive defects of renal pelvis and ureter (Q62.0-Q62.3)*
> *hydronephrosis with ureteropelvic junction obstruction (Q62.11)*
> *obstructive pyelonephritis (N11.1)*

DEF: Hydronephrosis: Distension of the kidney caused by an accumulation of urine that cannot flow out due to an obstruction that may be caused by conditions such as kidney stones or vesicoureteral reflux.

N13.0 Hydronephrosis with ureteropelvic junction obstruction
Hydronephrosis due to acquired occlusion of ureteropelvic junction

> EXCLUDES 2   *hydronephrosis with ureteropelvic junction obstruction due to calculus (N13.2)*

AHA: 2016,4Q,43

Hydronephrosis/UPJ Obstruction

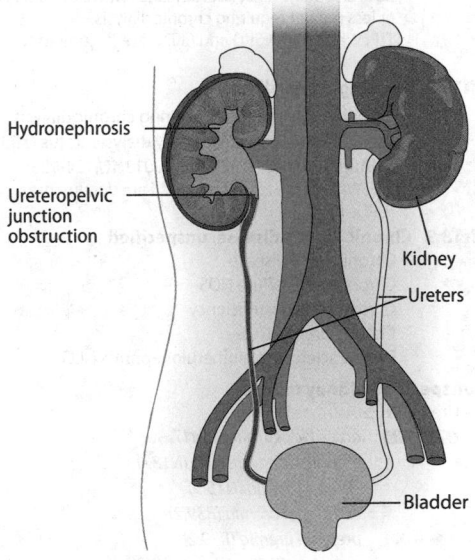

Hydronephrosis

Ureteropelvic junction obstruction

Kidney

Ureters

Bladder

N13.1 Hydronephrosis with ureteral stricture, not elsewhere classified
> EXCLUDES 1   *hydronephrosis with ureteral stricture with infection (N13.6)*

N13.2 Hydronephrosis with renal and ureteral calculous obstruction
> EXCLUDES 1   *hydronephrosis with renal and ureteral calculous obstruction with infection (N13.6)*

✓5ᵗʰ N13.3 Other and unspecified hydronephrosis
> EXCLUDES 1   *hydronephrosis with infection (N13.6)*

     N13.30   Unspecified hydronephrosis
     N13.39   Other hydronephrosis

N13.4 Hydroureter
> EXCLUDES 1   *congenital hydroureter (Q62.3-)*
> *hydroureter with infection (N13.6)*
> *vesicoureteral-reflux with hydroureter (N13.73-)*

DEF: Abnormal enlargement or distension of the ureter with water or urine caused by an obstruction.

N13.5 Crossing vessel and stricture of ureter without hydronephrosis
Kinking and stricture of ureter without hydronephrosis
> EXCLUDES 1   *crossing vessel and stricture of ureter without hydronephrosis with infection (N13.6)*

N13.6 Pyonephrosis
Conditions in N13.0-N13.5 with infection
Obstructive uropathy with infection
Use additional code (B95-B97), to identify infectious agent
AHA: 2018,2Q,21

✓5ᵗʰ N13.7 Vesicoureteral-reflux
> EXCLUDES 1   *reflux-associated pyelonephritis (N11.0)*

DEF: Urine passage from the bladder flows backward up into the ureter and kidneys that can lead to bacterial infection and an increase in hydrostatic pressure, causing kidney damage.

Vesicoureteral Reflux

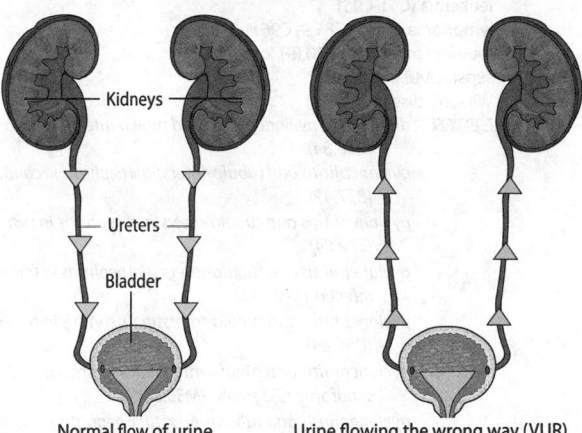

Kidneys

Ureters

Bladder

Normal flow of urine   Urine flowing the wrong way (VUR)

     N13.70   Vesicoureteral-reflux, unspecified
         Vesicoureteral-reflux NOS
     N13.71   Vesicoureteral-reflux without reflux nephropathy
✓6ᵗʰ   **N13.72**   Vesicoureteral-reflux with reflux nephropathy without hydroureter
        N13.721   Vesicoureteral-reflux with reflux nephropathy without hydroureter, unilateral
        N13.722   Vesicoureteral-reflux with reflux nephropathy without hydroureter, bilateral
        N13.729   Vesicoureteral-reflux with reflux nephropathy without hydroureter, unspecified
✓6ᵗʰ   **N13.73**   Vesicoureteral-reflux with reflux nephropathy with hydroureter
        N13.731   Vesicoureteral-reflux with reflux nephropathy with hydroureter, unilateral
        N13.732   Vesicoureteral-reflux with reflux nephropathy with hydroureter, bilateral
        N13.739   Vesicoureteral-reflux with reflux nephropathy with hydroureter, unspecified

N13.8 Other obstructive and reflux uropathy
Urinary tract obstruction due to specified cause
Code first, if applicable, any causal condition, such as:
    enlarged prostate (N40.1)

N13.9 Obstructive and reflux uropathy, unspecified
Urinary tract obstruction NOS

✓4ᵗʰ N14 Drug- and heavy-metal-induced tubulo-interstitial and tubular conditions
Code first poisoning due to drug or toxin, if applicable (T36-T65 with fifth or sixth character 1-4 or 6)
Use additional code for adverse effect, if applicable, to identify drug (T36-T50 with fifth or sixth character 5)

N14.0 Analgesic nephropathy
N14.1 Nephropathy induced by other drugs, medicaments and biological substances
N14.2 Nephropathy induced by unspecified drug, medicament or biological substance
N14.3 Nephropathy induced by heavy metals
N14.4 Toxic nephropathy, not elsewhere classified

✓4ᵗʰ N15 Other renal tubulo-interstitial diseases

N15.0 Balkan nephropathy
Balkan endemic nephropathy
N15.1 Renal and perinephric abscess
N15.8 Other specified renal tubulo-interstitial diseases
N15.9 Renal tubulo-interstitial disease, unspecified
Infection of kidney NOS
> EXCLUDES 1   *urinary tract infection NOS (N39.0)*

☑ Additional Character Required   ✓x7ᵗʰ Placeholder Alert   Manifestation   Unspecified Dx   ▶◀ Revised Text   ● New Code   ▲ Revised Code Title

ICD-10-CM 2020   **835**

N16 Renal tubulo-interstitial disorders in diseases classified elsewhere
Pyelonephritis
Tubulo-interstitial nephritis
Code first underlying disease, such as:
brucellosis (A23.0-A23.9)
cryoglobulinemia (D89.1)
glycogen storage disease (E74.0)
leukemia (C91-C95)
lymphoma (C81.0-C85.9, C96.0-C96.9)
multiple myeloma (C90.0-)
sepsis (A40.0-A41.9)
Wilson's disease (E83.0)

EXCLUDES 1   diphtheritic pyelonephritis and tubulo-interstitial nephritis (A36.84)
pyelonephritis and tubulo-interstitial nephritis in candidiasis (B37.49)
pyelonephritis and tubulo-interstitial nephritis in cystinosis (E72.04)
pyelonephritis and tubulo-interstitial nephritis in salmonella infection (A02.25)
pyelonephritis and tubulo-interstitial nephritis in sarcoidosis (D86.84)
pyelonephritis and tubulo-interstitial nephritis in sicca syndrome [Sjogren's] (M35.04)
pyelonephritis and tubulo-interstitial nephritis in systemic lupus erythematosus (M32.15)
pyelonephritis and tubulo-interstitial nephritis in toxoplasmosis (B58.83)
renal tubular degeneration in diabetes (E08-E13 with .29)
syphilitic pyelonephritis and tubulo-interstitial nephritis (A52.75)

Acute kidney failure and chronic kidney disease (N17-N19)

EXCLUDES 2   congenital renal failure (P96.0)
drug- and heavy-metal-induced tubulo-interstitial and tubular conditions (N14.-)
extrarenal uremia (R39.2)
hemolytic-uremic syndrome (D59.3)
hepatorenal syndrome (K76.7)
postpartum hepatorenal syndrome (O90.4)
posttraumatic renal failure (T79.5)
prerenal uremia (R39.2)
renal failure complicating abortion or ectopic or molar pregnancy (O00-O07, O08.4)
renal failure following labor and delivery (O90.4)
renal failure postprocedural (N99.0)

N17 Acute kidney failure
Code also associated underlying condition
EXCLUDES 1   posttraumatic renal failure (T79.5)
AHA: 2019,2Q,7; 2019,1Q,12; 2013,4Q,124

N17.0 Acute kidney failure with tubular necrosis   HCC
Acute tubular necrosis
Renal tubular necrosis
Tubular necrosis NOS

N17.1 Acute kidney failure with acute cortical necrosis   HCC
Acute cortical necrosis
Cortical necrosis NOS
Renal cortical necrosis

N17.2 Acute kidney failure with medullary necrosis   HCC
Medullary [papillary] necrosis NOS
Acute medullary [papillary] necrosis
Renal medullary [papillary] necrosis

N17.8 Other acute kidney failure   HCC

N17.9 Acute kidney failure, unspecified   HCC
Acute kidney injury (nontraumatic)
EXCLUDES 2   traumatic kidney injury (S37.0-)

N18 Chronic kidney disease (CKD)
Code first any associated:
diabetic chronic kidney disease (E08.22, E09.22, E10.22, E11.22, E13.22)
hypertensive chronic kidney disease (I12.-, I13.-)
Use additional code to identify kidney transplant status, if applicable, (Z94.0)
AHA: 2013,1Q,24
TIP: CKD/ESRD occurring in an individual with a history of kidney transplant should not be assumed to be a transplant complication unless specifically indicated as such by provider documentation.

N18.1 Chronic kidney disease, stage 1

N18.2 Chronic kidney disease, stage 2 (mild)

N18.3 Chronic kidney disease, stage 3 (moderate)   HCC

N18.4 Chronic kidney disease, stage 4 (severe)   HCC

N18.5 Chronic kidney disease, stage 5   HCC
EXCLUDES 1   chronic kidney disease, stage 5 requiring chronic dialysis (N18.6)
DEF: End-stage renal disease (ESRD) with a GFR value of 15 ml/min or less not yet requiring chronic dialysis.
TIP: When both ESRD and CKD 5 are documented, code only for ESRD.

N18.6 End stage renal disease   HCC
Chronic kidney disease requiring chronic dialysis
Use additional code to identify dialysis status (Z99.2)
AHA: 2016,3Q,22; 2016,1Q,12; 2013,4Q,124-125
TIP: When both ESRD and CKD 5 are documented, code only for ESRD.

N18.9 Chronic kidney disease, unspecified
Chronic renal disease
Chronic renal failure NOS
Chronic renal insufficiency
Chronic uremia NOS
Diffuse sclerosing glomerulonephritis NOS

N19 Unspecified kidney failure
Uremia NOS
EXCLUDES 1   acute kidney failure (N17.-)
chronic kidney disease (N18.-)
chronic uremia (N18.9)
extrarenal uremia (R39.2)
prerenal uremia (R39.2)
renal insufficiency (acute) (N28.9)
uremia of newborn (P96.0)

Urolithiasis (N20-N23)

AHA: 2017,1Q,5; 2015,2Q,8
TIP: Codes from this code block can be assigned based on the diagnosis listed in a radiology report when authenticated by a radiologist and available at the time of code assignment.
TIP: Codes from this code block can be assigned based on the diagnosis listed in a radiology report when authenticated by a radiologist and available at the time of code assignment.

N20 Calculus of kidney and ureter
Calculous pyelonephritis
EXCLUDES 1   nephrocalcinosis (E83.5)
that with hydronephrosis (N13.2)

N20.0 Calculus of kidney
Nephrolithiasis NOS
Renal calculus
Renal stone
Staghorn calculus
Stone in kidney

N20.1 Calculus of ureter
Ureteric stone
AHA: 2016,3Q,22

N20.2 Calculus of kidney with calculus of ureter

N20.9 Urinary calculus, unspecified

N21 Calculus of lower urinary tract
INCLUDES   calculus of lower urinary tract with cystitis and urethritis

N21.0 Calculus in bladder
Calculus in diverticulum of bladder
Urinary bladder stone
EXCLUDES 2   staghorn calculus (N20.0)

N21.1 Calculus in urethra
EXCLUDES 2   calculus of prostate (N42.0)

N21.8 Other lower urinary tract calculus

N21.9   **Calculus of lower urinary tract, unspecified**
> **EXCLUDES 1**   *calculus of urinary tract NOS (N20.9)*

N22   *Calculus of urinary tract in diseases classified elsewhere*
> Code first underlying disease, such as:
> gout (M1A.-, M10.-)
> schistosomiasis (B65.0-B65.9)

N23   **Unspecified renal colic**

Other disorders of kidney and ureter (N25-N29)

> **EXCLUDES 2**   *disorders of kidney and ureter with urolithiasis (N20-N23)*

N25   **Disorders resulting from impaired renal tubular function**

     N25.0   **Renal osteodystrophy**
         Azotemic osteodystrophy
         Phosphate-losing tubular disorders
         Renal rickets
         Renal short stature
> **EXCLUDES 2**   *metabolic disorders classifiable to E70-E88*
> **DEF:** Various bone diseases occurring when kidney function is impaired or fails. Abnormal levels of phosphorous and calcium can lead to osteomalacia, osteoporosis, or osteosclerosis.

     N25.1   **Nephrogenic diabetes insipidus**   `HCC`
> **EXCLUDES 1**   *diabetes insipidus NOS (E23.2)*
> **DEF:** Type of diabetes due to the inability of renal tubules to reabsorb water back into the body. It is not responsive to vasopressin (antidiuretic hormone) and it is characterized by excessive thirst and excessive urine production. It may develop into chronic renal insufficiency.

     N25.8   **Other disorders resulting from impaired renal tubular function**

         N25.81   **Secondary hyperparathyroidism of renal origin**   `HCC`
> **EXCLUDES 1**   *secondary hyperparathyroidism, non-renal (E21.1)*
> **EXCLUDES 2**   *metabolic disorders classifiable to E70-E88*
> **DEF:** Parathyroid dysfunction caused by chronic renal failure. Phosphate clearance and vitamin D production is impaired resulting in lowered calcium blood levels and an excessive production of parathyroid hormone.

         N25.89   **Other disorders resulting from impaired renal tubular function**
             Hypokalemic nephropathy
             Lightwood-Albright syndrome
             Renal tubular acidosis NOS

     N25.9   **Disorder resulting from impaired renal tubular function, unspecified**

N26   **Unspecified contracted kidney**
> **EXCLUDES 1**   *contracted kidney due to hypertension (I12.-)*
> *diffuse sclerosing glomerulonephritis (N05.8.-)*
> *hypertensive nephrosclerosis (arteriolar) (arteriosclerotic) (I12.-)*
> *small kidney of unknown cause (N27.-)*

     N26.1   **Atrophy of kidney (terminal)**
     N26.2   **Page kidney**
     N26.9   **Renal sclerosis, unspecified**

N27   **Small kidney of unknown cause**
> **INCLUDES**   oligonephronia

     N27.0   **Small kidney, unilateral**
     N27.1   **Small kidney, bilateral**
     N27.9   **Small kidney, unspecified**

N28   **Other disorders of kidney and ureter, not elsewhere classified**

     N28.0   **Ischemia and infarction of kidney**   `HCC`
         Renal artery embolism
         Renal artery obstruction
         Renal artery occlusion
         Renal artery thrombosis
         Renal infarct
> **EXCLUDES 1**   *atherosclerosis of renal artery (extrarenal part) (I70.1)*
> *congenital stenosis of renal artery (Q27.1)*
> *Goldblatt's kidney (I70.1)*

     N28.1   **Cyst of kidney, acquired**
         Cyst (multiple) (solitary) of kidney (acquired)
> **EXCLUDES 1**   *cystic kidney disease (congenital) (Q61.-)*

N28.8   **Other specified disorders of kidney and ureter**
> **EXCLUDES 1**   *hydroureter (N13.4)*
> *ureteric stricture with hydronephrosis (N13.1)*
> *ureteric stricture without hydronephrosis (N13.5)*

     N28.81   **Hypertrophy of kidney**
     N28.82   **Megaloureter**
     N28.83   **Nephroptosis**
     N28.84   **Pyelitis cystica**
     N28.85   **Pyeloureteritis cystica**
     N28.86   **Ureteritis cystica**
     N28.89   **Other specified disorders of kidney and ureter**

N28.9   **Disorder of kidney and ureter, unspecified**
         Nephropathy NOS
         Renal disease (acute) NOS
         Renal insufficiency (acute)
> **EXCLUDES 1**   *chronic renal insufficiency (N18.9)*
> *unspecified nephritic syndrome (N05.-)*
> **AHA:** 2016, 1Q, 13

N29   *Other disorders of kidney and ureter in diseases classified elsewhere*
> Code first underlying disease, such as:
> amyloidosis (E85.-)
> nephrocalcinosis (E83.5)
> schistosomiasis (B65.0-B65.9)
> **EXCLUDES 1**   *disorders of kidney and ureter in:*
>   *cystinosis (E72.0)*
>   *gonorrhea (A54.21)*
>   *syphilis (A52.75)*
>   *tuberculosis (A18.11)*

Other diseases of the urinary system (N30-N39)

> **EXCLUDES 1**   *urinary infection (complicating):*
> *abortion or ectopic or molar pregnancy (O00-O07, O08.8)*
> *pregnancy, childbirth and the puerperium (O23.-, O75.3, O86.2-)*

N30   **Cystitis**
> Use additional code to identify infectious agent (B95-B97)
> **EXCLUDES 1**   *prostatocystitis (N41.3)*
> **AHA:** 2017, 1Q, 6
> **DEF:** Inflammation of the urinary bladder. Symptoms include dysuria, frequency of urination, urgency, and hematuria.

     N30.0   **Acute cystitis**
> **EXCLUDES 1**   *irradiation cystitis (N30.4-)*
> *trigonitis (N30.3-)*

         N30.00   **Acute cystitis without hematuria**
         N30.01   **Acute cystitis with hematuria**

     N30.1   **Interstitial cystitis (chronic)**
         N30.10   **Interstitial cystitis (chronic) without hematuria**
         N30.11   **Interstitial cystitis (chronic) with hematuria**

     N30.2   **Other chronic cystitis**
         N30.20   **Other chronic cystitis without hematuria**
         N30.21   **Other chronic cystitis with hematuria**

     N30.3   **Trigonitis**
         Urethrotrigonitis
         N30.30   **Trigonitis without hematuria**
         N30.31   **Trigonitis with hematuria**

     N30.4   **Irradiation cystitis**
         N30.40   **Irradiation cystitis without hematuria**
         N30.41   **Irradiation cystitis with hematuria**

     N30.8   **Other cystitis**
         Abscess of bladder
         N30.80   **Other cystitis without hematuria**
         N30.81   **Other cystitis with hematuria**

     N30.9   **Cystitis, unspecified**
         N30.90   **Cystitis, unspecified without hematuria**
         N30.91   **Cystitis, unspecified with hematuria**

N31   **Neuromuscular dysfunction of bladder, not elsewhere classified**
> Use additional code to identify any associated urinary incontinence (N39.3-N39.4-)
> **EXCLUDES 1**   *cord bladder NOS (G95.89)*
> *neurogenic bladder due to cauda equina syndrome (G83.4)*
> *neuromuscular dysfunction due to spinal cord lesion (G95.89)*

     N31.0   **Uninhibited neuropathic bladder, not elsewhere classified**
     N31.1   **Reflex neuropathic bladder, not elsewhere classified**

☑ Additional Character Required   ✔x7ᵗʰ Placeholder Alert   Manifestation   Unspecified Dx   ▶◀ Revised Text   ● New Code   ▲ Revised Code Title

ICD-10-CM 2020   **837**

N31.2   **Flaccid neuropathic bladder, not elsewhere classified**
Atonic (motor) (sensory) neuropathic bladder
Autonomous neuropathic bladder
Nonreflex neuropathic bladder

N31.8   **Other neuromuscular dysfunction of bladder**

N31.9   **Neuromuscular dysfunction of bladder, unspecified**
Neurogenic bladder dysfunction NOS

✓4ᵗʰ **N32**   **Other disorders of bladder**
    EXCLUDES 2   calculus of bladder (N21.0)
              cystocele (N81.1-)
              hernia or prolapse of bladder, female (N81.1-)

N32.0   **Bladder-neck obstruction**
Bladder-neck stenosis (acquired)
    EXCLUDES 1   congenital bladder-neck obstruction (Q64.3-)
DEF: Bladder outlet and vesicourethral obstruction that occurs as a consequence of benign prostatic hypertrophy or prostatic cancer. It may also occur in either sex due to strictures, radiation, cystoscopy, catheterization, injury, infection, blood clots, bladder cancer, impaction, or other disease that compresses the bladder neck.

N32.1   **Vesicointestinal fistula**
Vesicorectal fistula

N32.2   **Vesical fistula, not elsewhere classified**
    EXCLUDES 1   fistula between bladder and female genital tract (N82.0-N82.1)

N32.3   **Diverticulum of bladder**
    EXCLUDES 1   congenital diverticulum of bladder (Q64.6)
              diverticulitis of bladder (N30.8-)

✓5ᵗʰ **N32.8**   **Other specified disorders of bladder**

    N32.81   **Overactive bladder**
       Detrusor muscle hyperactivity
       EXCLUDES 1   frequent urination due to specified bladder condition — code to condition
       DEF: Sudden involuntary contractions of the muscular wall of the bladder that results in a sudden, strong urge to urinate.

    N32.89   **Other specified disorders of bladder**
       Bladder hemorrhage
       Bladder hypertrophy
       Calcified bladder
       Contracted bladder

N32.9   **Bladder disorder, unspecified**

N33   *Bladder disorders in diseases classified elsewhere*
Code first underlying disease, such as:
schistosomiasis (B65.0-B65.9)
    EXCLUDES 1   bladder disorder in syphilis (A52.76)
              bladder disorder in tuberculosis (A18.12)
              candidal cystitis (B37.41)
              chlamydial cystitis (A56.01)
              cystitis in gonorrhea (A54.01)
              cystitis in neurogenic bladder (N31.-)
              diphtheritic cystitis (A36.85)
              neurogenic bladder (N31.-)
              syphilitic cystitis (A52.76)
              trichomonal cystitis (A59.03)

✓4ᵗʰ **N34**   **Urethritis and urethral syndrome**
Use additional code (B95-B97), to identify infectious agent
    EXCLUDES 2   Reiter's disease (M02.3-)
              urethritis in diseases with a predominantly sexual mode of transmission (A50-A64)
              urethrotrigonitis (N30.3-)
AHA: 2017,1Q,6

N34.0   **Urethral abscess**
Abscess (of) Cowper's gland
Abscess (of) Littré's gland
Abscess (of) urethral (gland)
Periurethral abscess
    EXCLUDES 1   urethral caruncle (N36.2)

N34.1   **Nonspecific urethritis**
Nongonococcal urethritis
Nonvenereal urethritis

N34.2   **Other urethritis**
Meatitis, urethral
Postmenopausal urethritis
Ulcer of urethra (meatus)
Urethritis NOS

N34.3   **Urethral syndrome, unspecified**

✓4ᵗʰ **N35**   **Urethral stricture**
    EXCLUDES 1   congenital urethral stricture (Q64.3-)
              postprocedural urethral stricture (N99.1-)
    AHA: 2018,4Q,21-22

✓5ᵗʰ **N35.0**   **Post-traumatic urethral stricture**
Urethral stricture due to injury
    EXCLUDES 1   postprocedural urethral stricture (N99.1-)

    ✓6ᵗʰ **N35.01**   **Post-traumatic urethral stricture, male**

       N35.010   **Post-traumatic urethral stricture, male, meatal**   ♂
       N35.011   **Post-traumatic bulbous urethral stricture**   ♂
       N35.012   **Post-traumatic membranous urethral stricture**   ♂
       N35.013   **Post-traumatic anterior urethral stricture**   ♂
       N35.014   **Post-traumatic urethral stricture, male, unspecified**   ♂
       N35.016   **Post-traumatic urethral stricture, male, overlapping sites**   ♂

    ✓6ᵗʰ **N35.02**   **Post-traumatic urethral stricture, female**

       N35.021   **Urethral stricture due to childbirth**   ♀
       N35.028   **Other post-traumatic urethral stricture, female**   ♀

✓5ᵗʰ **N35.1**   **Postinfective urethral stricture, not elsewhere classified**
    EXCLUDES 1   gonococcal urethral stricture (A54.01)
              syphilitic urethral stricture (A52.76)
              urethral stricture associated with schistosomiasis (B65.-, N29)

    ✓6ᵗʰ **N35.11**   **Postinfective urethral stricture, not elsewhere classified, male**

       N35.111   **Postinfective urethral stricture, not elsewhere classified, male, meatal**   ♂
       N35.112   **Postinfective bulbous urethral stricture, not elsewhere classified, male**   ♂
       N35.113   **Postinfective membranous urethral stricture, not elsewhere classified, male**   ♂
       N35.114   **Postinfective anterior urethral stricture, not elsewhere classified, male**   ♂
       N35.116   **Postinfective urethral stricture, not elsewhere classified, male, overlapping sites**   ♂
       N35.119   **Postinfective urethral stricture, not elsewhere classified, male, unspecified**   ♂

    N35.12   **Postinfective urethral stricture, not elsewhere classified, female**   ♀

✓5ᵗʰ **N35.8**   **Other urethral stricture**
    EXCLUDES 1   postprocedural urethral stricture (N99.1-)

    ✓6ᵗʰ **N35.81**   **Other urethral stricture, male**

       N35.811   **Other urethral stricture, male, meatal**   ♂
       N35.812   **Other urethral bulbous stricture, male**   ♂
       N35.813   **Other membranous urethral stricture, male**   ♂
       N35.814   **Other anterior urethral stricture, male**   ♂
       N35.816   **Other urethral stricture, male, overlapping sites**   ♂
       N35.819   **Other urethral stricture, male, unspecified site**   ♂

    N35.82   **Other urethral stricture, female**   ♀

✓5ᵗʰ **N35.9**   **Urethral stricture, unspecified**

    ✓6ᵗʰ **N35.91**   **Urethral stricture, unspecified, male**

       N35.911   **Unspecified urethral stricture, male, meatal**   ♂

N35.912   **Unspecified bulbous urethral stricture, male**   ♂

N35.913   **Unspecified membranous urethral stricture, male**   ♂

N35.914   **Unspecified anterior urethral stricture, male**   ♂

N35.916   **Unspecified urethral stricture, male, overlapping sites**   ♂

N35.919   **Unspecified urethral stricture, male, unspecified site**   ♂
Pinhole meatus NOS
Urethral stricture NOS

N35.92   **Unspecified urethral stricture, female**   ♀

✓4th **N36**   **Other disorders of urethra**

N36.0   **Urethral fistula**
Urethroperineal fistula
Urethrorectal fistula
Urinary fistula NOS
EXCLUDES 1   urethroscrotal fistula (N50.89)
urethrovaginal fistula (N82.1)
urethrovesicovaginal fistula (N82.1)

N36.1   **Urethral diverticulum**

N36.2   **Urethral caruncle**

✓5th **N36.4**   **Urethral functional and muscular disorders**
Use additional code to identify associated urinary stress incontinence (N39.3)

N36.41   **Hypermobility of urethra**

N36.42   **Intrinsic sphincter deficiency (ISD)**

N36.43   **Combined hypermobility of urethra and intrinsic sphincter deficiency**

N36.44   **Muscular disorders of urethra**
Bladder sphincter dyssynergy

N36.5   **Urethral false passage**

N36.8   **Other specified disorders of urethra**
EXCLUDES 1   congenital urethrocele (Q64.7)
female urethrocele (N81.0)

N36.9   **Urethral disorder, unspecified**

N37   *Urethral disorders in diseases classified elsewhere*
Code first underlying disease
EXCLUDES 1   urethritis (in):
candidal infection (B37.41)
chlamydial (A56.01)
gonorrhea (A54.01)
syphilis (A52.76)
trichomonal infection (A59.03)
tuberculosis (A18.13)

✓4th **N39**   **Other disorders of urinary system**
EXCLUDES 2   hematuria NOS (R31.-)
recurrent or persistent hematuria (N02.-)
recurrent or persistent hematuria with specified morphological lesion (N02.-)
proteinuria NOS (R80.-)

N39.0   **Urinary tract infection, site not specified**
Use additional code (B95-B97), to identify infectious agent
EXCLUDES 1   candidiasis of urinary tract (B37.4-)
neonatal urinary tract infection (P39.3)
▶pyuria (R82.81)◀
urinary tract infection of specified site, such as:
cystitis (N30.-)
urethritis (N34.-)
AHA: 2018,2Q,21,22; 2018,1Q,16; 2017,1Q,6; 2012,4Q,94

N39.3   **Stress incontinence (female) (male)**   Q
Code also any associated overactive bladder (N32.81)
EXCLUDES 1   mixed incontinence (N39.46)

✓5th **N39.4**   **Other specified urinary incontinence**
Code also any associated overactive bladder (N32.81)
EXCLUDES 1   enuresis NOS (R32)
functional urinary incontinence (R39.81)
urinary incontinence associated with cognitive impairment (R39.81)
urinary incontinence NOS (R32)
urinary incontinence of nonorganic origin (F98.0)

N39.41   **Urge incontinence**   Q
EXCLUDES 1   mixed incontinence (N39.46)

N39.42   **Incontinence without sensory awareness**   Q
Insensible (urinary) incontinence

N39.43   **Post-void dribbling**   Q

N39.44   **Nocturnal enuresis**   Q

N39.45   **Continuous leakage**   Q

N39.46   **Mixed incontinence**   Q
Urge and stress incontinence

✓6th **N39.49**   **Other specified urinary incontinence**
AHA: 2016,4Q,44

N39.490   **Overflow incontinence**   Q

N39.491   **Coital incontinence**   Q

N39.492   **Postural (urinary) incontinence**   Q

N39.498   **Other specified urinary incontinence**   Q
Reflex incontinence
Total incontinence

N39.8   **Other specified disorders of urinary system**

N39.9   **Disorder of urinary system, unspecified**

Diseases of male genital organs (N40-N53)

✓4th **N40**   **Benign prostatic hyperplasia**
INCLUDES   adenofibromatous hypertrophy of prostate
benign hypertrophy of the prostate
benign prostatic hypertrophy
BPH
enlarged prostate
nodular prostate
polyp of prostate
EXCLUDES 1   benign neoplasms of prostate (adenoma, benign) (fibroadenoma) (fibroma) (myoma) (D29.1)
EXCLUDES 2   malignant neoplasm of prostate (C61)
DEF: Enlargement of the prostate gland due to an abnormal proliferation of fibrostromal tissue in the paraurethral glands. This condition causes impingement of the urethra resulting in obstructed urinary flow.

N40.0   **Benign prostatic hyperplasia without lower urinary tract symptoms**   A ♂
Enlarged prostate NOS
Enlarged prostate without LUTS

N40.1   **Benign prostatic hyperplasia with lower urinary tract symptoms**   A ♂
Enlarged prostate with LUTS
Use additional code for associated symptoms, when specified:
incomplete bladder emptying (R39.14)
nocturia (R35.1)
straining on urination (R39.16)
urinary frequency (R35.0)
urinary hesitancy (R39.11)
urinary incontinence (N39.4-)
urinary obstruction (N13.8)
urinary retention (R33.8)
urinary urgency (R39.15)
weak urinary stream (R39.12)
AHA: 2018,4Q,55

N40.2   **Nodular prostate without lower urinary tract symptoms**   A ♂
Nodular prostate without LUTS

☑ Additional Character Required   ✓x7th Placeholder Alert   Manifestation   Unspecified Dx   ▶◀ Revised Text   ● New Code   ▲ Revised Code Title

ICD-10-CM 2020   839

Chapter 14. Diseases of the Genitourinary System

N40.3 Nodular **prostate** with lower urinary tract symptoms A ♂
Use additional code for associated symptoms, when specified:
incomplete bladder emptying (R39.14)
nocturia (R35.1)
straining on urination (R39.16)
urinary frequency (R35.0)
urinary hesitancy (R39.11)
urinary incontinence (N39.4-)
urinary obstruction (N13.8)
urinary retention (R33.8)
urinary urgency (R39.15)
weak urinary stream (R39.12)

✓4th **N41 Inflammatory diseases of prostate**
Use additional code (B95-B97), to identify infectious agent

N41.0 **Acute prostatitis** A ♂
N41.1 **Chronic prostatitis** A ♂
N41.2 **Abscess of prostate** A ♂
N41.3 **Prostatocystitis** A ♂
N41.4 **Granulomatous prostatitis** A ♂
N41.8 **Other inflammatory diseases of prostate** A ♂
N41.9 **Inflammatory disease of prostate, unspecified** A ♂
Prostatitis NOS

✓4th **N42 Other and unspecified disorders of prostate**

N42.0 **Calculus of prostate** A ♂
Prostatic stone
DEF: Formation of a small, solid stone often composed of calcium carbonate or calcium phosphate in the prostate gland.

N42.1 **Congestion and hemorrhage of prostate** A ♂
EXCLUDES 1 enlarged prostate (N40.-)
hematuria (R31.-)
hyperplasia of prostate (N40.-)
inflammatory diseases of prostate (N41.-)

✓5th **N42.3** **Dysplasia of prostate**
AHA: 2016,4Q,44

N42.30 **Unspecified dysplasia of prostate** ♂
N42.31 **Prostatic intraepithelial neoplasia** ♂
PIN
Prostatic intraepithelial neoplasia I (PIN I)
Prostatic intraepithelial neoplasia II (PIN II)
EXCLUDES 1 prostatic intraepithelial neoplasia III (PIN III) (D07.5)
DEF: Abnormality of shape and size of the intraepithelial tissues of the prostate. It is a premalignant condition characterized by stalks and absence of a basilar cell layer.

N42.32 **Atypical small acinar proliferation of prostate** ♂
N42.39 **Other dysplasia of prostate** ♂

✓5th **N42.8** **Other specified disorders of prostate**
N42.81 **Prostatodynia syndrome** A ♂
Painful prostate syndrome
N42.82 **Prostatosis syndrome** A ♂
N42.83 **Cyst of prostate** A ♂
N42.89 **Other specified disorders of prostate** A ♂
N42.9 **Disorder of prostate, unspecified** A ♂

✓4th **N43 Hydrocele and spermatocele**
INCLUDES hydrocele of spermatic cord, testis or tunica vaginalis
EXCLUDES 1 congenital hydrocele (P83.5)
DEF: Hydrocele: Serous fluid that collects in the tunica vaginalis of the scrotum along the spermatic cord in males.

N43.0 **Encysted hydrocele** ♂
N43.1 **Infected hydrocele** ♂
Use additional code (B95-B97), to identify infectious agent

N43.2 **Other hydrocele** ♂

Hydrocele

Normal | Noncommunicating hydrocele | Communicating hydrocele | Hydrocele of the cord

N43.3 Hydrocele, unspecified ♂
✓5th **N43.4** Spermatocele of epididymis
Spermatic cyst
DEF: Spermatocele: Noncancerous accumulation of fluid and dead sperm cells normally located at the head of the epididymis that exhibits itself as a hard, smooth scrotal mass and do not normally require treatment unless they become enlarged or cause pain.

N43.40 **Spermatocele of epididymis, unspecified** ♂
N43.41 **Spermatocele of epididymis, single** ♂
N43.42 **Spermatocele of epididymis, multiple** ♂

✓4th **N44 Noninflammatory disorders of testis**
✓5th **N44.0** **Torsion of testis**
N44.00 **Torsion of testis, unspecified** ♂
N44.01 **Extravaginal torsion of spermatic cord** ♂
DEF: Torsion of the spermatic cord just below the tunica vaginalis attachments.
N44.02 **Intravaginal torsion of spermatic cord** ♂
Torsion of spermatic cord NOS
N44.03 **Torsion of appendix testis** ♂
N44.04 **Torsion of appendix epididymis** ♂
N44.1 **Cyst of tunica albuginea testis** ♂
N44.2 **Benign cyst of testis** ♂
N44.8 **Other noninflammatory disorders of the testis** ♂

✓4th **N45 Orchitis and epididymitis**
Use additional code (B95-B97), to identify infectious agent
N45.1 **Epididymitis** ♂
N45.2 **Orchitis** ♂
N45.3 **Epididymo-orchitis** ♂
N45.4 **Abscess of epididymis or testis** ♂

✓4th **N46 Male infertility**
EXCLUDES 1 vasectomy status (Z98.52)
✓5th **N46.0** **Azoospermia**
Absolute male infertility
Male infertility due to germinal (cell) aplasia
Male infertility due to spermatogenic arrest (complete)
DEF: Failure of the development of sperm or the absence of sperm in semen.

N46.01 **Organic azoospermia** A ♂
Azoospermia NOS
✓6th **N46.02** **Azoospermia due to extratesticular causes**
Code also associated cause
N46.021 **Azoospermia due to drug therapy** A ♂
N46.022 **Azoospermia due to infection** A ♂
N46.023 **Azoospermia due to obstruction of efferent ducts** A ♂
N46.024 **Azoospermia due to radiation** A ♂
N46.025 **Azoospermia due to systemic disease** A ♂
N46.029 **Azoospermia due to other extratesticular causes** A ♂

✓5ᵗʰ N46.1 Oligospermia

Male infertility due to germinal cell desquamation
Male infertility due to hypospermatogenesis
Male infertility due to incomplete spermatogenic arrest
DEF: Insufficient production of sperm in semen.

    N46.11 Organic oligospermia   A ♂

         Oligospermia NOS

    ✓6ᵗʰ N46.12 Oligospermia due to extratesticular causes

         Code also associated cause

        N46.121 Oligospermia due to drug therapy   A ♂

        N46.122 Oligospermia due to infection   A ♂

        N46.123 Oligospermia due to obstruction of efferent ducts   A ♂

        N46.124 Oligospermia due to radiation   A ♂

        N46.125 Oligospermia due to systemic disease   A ♂

        N46.129 Oligospermia due to other extratesticular causes   A ♂

    N46.8 Other male infertility   A ♂

    N46.9 Male infertility, unspecified   A ♂

✓4ᵗʰ N47 Disorders of prepuce

    N47.0 Adherent prepuce, newborn   N ♂

    N47.1 Phimosis   ♂

        DEF: Condition in which the foreskin is contracted and cannot be drawn back behind the glans penis.

    N47.2 Paraphimosis   ♂

    N47.3 Deficient foreskin   ♂

    N47.4 Benign cyst of prepuce   ♂

    N47.5 Adhesions of prepuce and glans penis   ♂

    N47.6 Balanoposthitis   ♂

         Use additional code (B95-B97), to identify infectious agent
         EXCLUDES 1   balanitis (N48.1)

    N47.7 Other inflammatory diseases of prepuce   ♂

         Use additional code (B95-B97), to identify infectious agent

    N47.8 Other disorders of prepuce   ♂

✓4ᵗʰ N48 Other disorders of penis

    N48.0 Leukoplakia of penis   ♂

         Balanitis xerotica obliterans
         Kraurosis of penis
         Lichen sclerosus of external male genital organs
         EXCLUDES 1   carcinoma in situ of penis (D07.4)

    N48.1 Balanitis   ♂

         Use additional code (B95-B97), to identify infectious agent
         EXCLUDES 1   amebic balanitis (A06.8)
                   balanitis xerotica obliterans (N48.0)
                   candidal balanitis (B37.42)
                   gonococcal balanitis (A54.23)
                   herpesviral [herpes simplex] balanitis (A60.01)
         DEF: Inflammation of the glans penis, most often affecting uncircumcised males.

    ✓5ᵗʰ N48.2 Other inflammatory disorders of penis

         Use additional code (B95-B97), to identify infectious agent
         EXCLUDES 1   balanitis (N48.1)
                   balanitis xerotica obliterans (N48.0)
                   balanoposthitis (N47.6)

        N48.21 Abscess of corpus cavernosum and penis   ♂

        N48.22 Cellulitis of corpus cavernosum and penis   ♂

        N48.29 Other inflammatory disorders of penis   ♂

    ✓5ᵗʰ N48.3 Priapism

         Painful erection
         Code first underlying cause

        N48.30 Priapism, unspecified   ♂

        N48.31 Priapism due to trauma   ♂

        N48.32 Priapism due to disease classified elsewhere   ♂

        N48.33 Priapism, drug-induced   ♂

        N48.39 Other priapism   ♂

    N48.5 Ulcer of penis   ♂

    N48.6 Induration penis plastica   ♂

         Peyronie's disease
         Plastic induration of penis

    ✓5ᵗʰ N48.8 Other specified disorders of penis

        N48.81 Thrombosis of superficial vein of penis   ♂

        N48.82 Acquired torsion of penis   ♂

              Acquired torsion of penis NOS
              EXCLUDES 1   congenital torsion of penis (Q55.63)

        N48.83 Acquired buried penis   ♂

              EXCLUDES 1   congenital hidden penis (Q55.64)

        N48.89 Other specified disorders of penis   ♂

    N48.9 Disorder of penis, unspecified   ♂

✓4ᵗʰ N49 Inflammatory disorders of male genital organs, not elsewhere classified

     Use additional code (B95-B97), to identify infectious agent
     EXCLUDES 1   inflammation of penis (N48.1, N48.2-)
               orchitis and epididymitis (N45.-)

    N49.0 Inflammatory disorders of seminal vesicle   ♂

         Vesiculitis NOS

    N49.1 Inflammatory disorders of spermatic cord, tunica vaginalis and vas deferens   ♂

         Vasitis

    N49.2 Inflammatory disorders of scrotum   ♂

    N49.3 Fournier gangrene   ♂

    N49.8 Inflammatory disorders of other specified male genital organs   ♂

         Inflammation of multiple sites in male genital organs

    N49.9 Inflammatory disorder of unspecified male genital organ   ♂

         Abscess of unspecified male genital organ
         Boil of unspecified male genital organ
         Carbuncle of unspecified male genital organ
         Cellulitis of unspecified male genital organ

✓4ᵗʰ N50 Other and unspecified disorders of male genital organs

     EXCLUDES 2   torsion of testis (N44.0-)

    N50.0 Atrophy of testis   ♂

    N50.1 Vascular disorders of male genital organs   ♂

         Hematocele, NOS, of male genital organs
         Hemorrhage of male genital organs
         Thrombosis of male genital organs

    N50.3 Cyst of epididymis   ♂

    ✓5ᵗʰ N50.8 Other specified disorders of male genital organs

         AHA: 2016,4Q,45

        ✓6ᵗʰ N50.81 Testicular pain

             N50.811 Right testicular pain   ♂

             N50.812 Left testicular pain   ♂

             N50.819 Testicular pain, unspecified   ♂

        N50.82 Scrotal pain   ♂

        N50.89 Other specified disorders of the male genital organs   ♂

              Atrophy of scrotum, seminal vesicle, spermatic cord, tunica vaginalis and vas deferens
              Chylocele, tunica vaginalis (nonfilarial) NOS
              Edema of scrotum, seminal vesicle, spermatic cord, tunica vaginalis and vas deferens
              Hypertrophy of scrotum, seminal vesicle, spermatic cord, tunica vaginalis and vas deferens
              Stricture of spermatic cord, tunica vaginalis, and vas deferens
              Ulcer of scrotum, seminal vesicle, spermatic cord, testis, tunica vaginalis and vas deferens
              Urethroscrotal fistula

    N50.9 Disorder of male genital organs, unspecified   ♂

✓ Additional Character Required   ✓x7ᵗʰ Placeholder Alert   Manifestation   Unspecified Dx   ►◄ Revised Text   ● New Code   ▲ Revised Code Title

ICD-10-CM 2020   **841**

Chapter 14. Diseases of the Genitourinary System

N51 *Disorders of male genital organs in diseases classified elsewhere* ♂

Code first underlying disease, such as:
filariasis (B74.0-B74.9)

EXCLUDES 1   amebic balanitis (A06.8)
candidal balanitis (B37.42)
gonococcal balanitis (A54.23)
gonococcal prostatitis (A54.22)
herpesviral [herpes simplex] balanitis (A60.01)
trichomonal prostatitis (A59.02)
tuberculous prostatitis (A18.14)

✓4th **N52 Male erectile dysfunction**

EXCLUDES 1   psychogenic impotence (F52.21)

✓5th **N52.0 Vasculogenic erectile dysfunction**

N52.01   **Erectile dysfunction due to arterial insufficiency** A♂

N52.02   **Corporo-venous occlusive erectile dysfunction** A♂

N52.03   **Combined arterial insufficiency and corporo-venous occlusive erectile dysfunction** A♂

N52.1 *Erectile dysfunction due to diseases classified elsewhere* A♂

Code first underlying disease

N52.2 Drug-induced erectile dysfunction A♂

✓5th **N52.3 Postprocedural erectile dysfunction**

AHA: 2016,4Q,45

N52.31   **Erectile dysfunction following radical prostatectomy** A♂

N52.32   **Erectile dysfunction following radical cystectomy** A♂

N52.33   **Erectile dysfunction following urethral surgery** A♂

N52.34   **Erectile dysfunction following simple prostatectomy** A♂

N52.35   **Erectile dysfunction following radiation therapy** A♂

N52.36   **Erectile dysfunction following interstitial seed therapy** A♂

N52.37   **Erectile dysfunction following prostate ablative therapy** A♂

Erectile dysfunction following cryotherapy
Erectile dysfunction following other prostate ablative therapies
Erectile dysfunction following ultrasound ablative therapies

N52.39   **Other and unspecified postprocedural erectile dysfunction** A♂

N52.8 Other male erectile dysfunction A♂

N52.9 Male erectile dysfunction, unspecified A♂

Impotence NOS

✓4th **N53 Other male sexual dysfunction**

EXCLUDES 1   psychogenic sexual dysfunction (F52.-)

✓5th **N53.1 Ejaculatory dysfunction**

EXCLUDES 1   premature ejaculation (F52.4)

N53.11   **Retarded ejaculation** ♂

N53.12   **Painful ejaculation** ♂

N53.13   **Anejaculatory orgasm** ♂

N53.14   **Retrograde ejaculation** ♂

DEF: Form of male sexual dysfunction in which the semen enters the bladder instead of going out through the urethra during ejaculation.

N53.19   **Other ejaculatory dysfunction** ♂

Ejaculatory dysfunction NOS

N53.8 Other male sexual dysfunction ♂

N53.9 Unspecified male sexual dysfunction ♂

Disorders of breast (N60-N65)

EXCLUDES 1   disorders of breast associated with childbirth (O91-O92)

✓4th **N60 Benign mammary dysplasia**

INCLUDES   fibrocystic mastopathy

✓5th **N60.0 Solitary cyst of breast**

Cyst of breast

N60.01   **Solitary cyst of right breast**

N60.02   **Solitary cyst of left breast**

N60.09   **Solitary cyst of unspecified breast**

✓5th **N60.1 Diffuse cystic mastopathy**

Cystic breast
Fibrocystic disease of breast

EXCLUDES 1   diffuse cystic mastopathy with epithelial proliferation (N60.3-)

N60.11   **Diffuse cystic mastopathy of right breast** A

N60.12   **Diffuse cystic mastopathy of left breast** A

N60.19   **Diffuse cystic mastopathy of unspecified breast** A

✓5th **N60.2 Fibroadenosis of breast**

Adenofibrosis of breast

EXCLUDES 2   fibroadenoma of breast (D24.-)

N60.21   **Fibroadenosis of right breast**

N60.22   **Fibroadenosis of left breast**

N60.29   **Fibroadenosis of unspecified breast**

✓5th **N60.3 Fibrosclerosis of breast**

Cystic mastopathy with epithelial proliferation

N60.31   **Fibrosclerosis of right breast**

N60.32   **Fibrosclerosis of left breast**

N60.39   **Fibrosclerosis of unspecified breast**

✓5th **N60.4 Mammary duct ectasia**

N60.41   **Mammary duct ectasia of right breast**

N60.42   **Mammary duct ectasia of left breast**

N60.49   **Mammary duct ectasia of unspecified breast**

✓5th **N60.8 Other benign mammary dysplasias**

N60.81   **Other benign mammary dysplasias of right breast**

N60.82   **Other benign mammary dysplasias of left breast**

N60.89   **Other benign mammary dysplasias of unspecified breast**

✓5th **N60.9 Unspecified benign mammary dysplasia**

N60.91   **Unspecified benign mammary dysplasia of right breast**

N60.92   **Unspecified benign mammary dysplasia of left breast**

N60.99   **Unspecified benign mammary dysplasia of unspecified breast**

✓4th **N61 Inflammatory disorders of breast**

EXCLUDES 1   inflammatory carcinoma of breast (C50.9)
inflammatory disorder of breast associated with childbirth (O91.-)
neonatal infective mastitis (P39.0)
thrombophlebitis of breast [Mondor's disease] (I80.8)

N61.0 Mastitis without abscess

Infective mastitis (acute) (nonpuerperal) (subacute)
Mastitis (acute) (nonpuerperal) (subacute) NOS
Cellulitis (acute) (nonpuerperal) (subacute) of breast NOS
Cellulitis (acute) (nonpuerperal) (subacute) of nipple NOS

N61.1 Abscess of the breast and nipple

Abscess (acute) (chronic) (nonpuerperal) of areola
Abscess (acute) (chronic) (nonpuerperal) of breast
Carbuncle of breast
Mastitis with abscess

N62 Hypertrophy of breast

Gynecomastia
Hypertrophy of breast NOS
Massive pubertal hypertrophy of breast

EXCLUDES 1   breast engorgement of newborn (P83.4)
disproportion of reconstructed breast (N65.1)

✓4th **N63 Unspecified lump in breast**

Nodule(s) NOS in breast

AHA: 2017,4Q,19

N63.0 Unspecified lump in unspecified breast

✓5th **N63.1 Unspecified lump in the right breast**

N63.10   **Unspecified lump in the right breast, unspecified quadrant**

N63.11   **Unspecified lump in the right breast, upper outer quadrant**

N63.12   **Unspecified lump in the right breast, upper inner quadrant**

N63.13   **Unspecified lump in the right breast, lower outer quadrant**

N63.14   **Unspecified lump in the right breast, lower inner quadrant**

●   **N63.15**   Unspecified lump in the right breast, overlapping quadrants

✓5ᵗʰ **N63.2**   Unspecified lump in the left breast

   N63.20   Unspecified lump in the left breast, unspecified quadrant

   N63.21   Unspecified lump in the left breast, upper outer quadrant

   N63.22   Unspecified lump in the left breast, upper inner quadrant

   N63.23   Unspecified lump in the left breast, lower outer quadrant

   N63.24   Unspecified lump in the left breast, lower inner quadrant

●   **N63.25**   Unspecified lump in the left breast, overlapping quadrants

✓5ᵗʰ **N63.3**   Unspecified lump in axillary tail

   N63.31   Unspecified lump in axillary tail of the right breast

   N63.32   Unspecified lump in axillary tail of the left breast

✓5ᵗʰ **N63.4**   Unspecified lump in breast, subareolar

   N63.41   Unspecified lump in right breast, subareolar

   N63.42   Unspecified lump in left breast, subareolar

✓4ᵗʰ **N64**   **Other disorders of breast**

   EXCLUDES 2   mechanical complication of breast prosthesis and implant (T85.4-)

   N64.0   Fissure and fistula of nipple

   N64.1   Fat necrosis of breast

     Fat necrosis (segmental) of breast

     Code first breast necrosis due to breast graft (T85.898)

   N64.2   Atrophy of breast

   N64.3   Galactorrhea not associated with childbirth

   N64.4   Mastodynia

✓5ᵗʰ **N64.5**   Other signs and symptoms in breast

   EXCLUDES 2   abnormal findings on diagnostic imaging of breast (R92.-)

   N64.51   Induration of breast

   N64.52   Nipple discharge

     EXCLUDES 1   abnormal findings in nipple discharge (R89.-)

   N64.53   Retraction of nipple

   N64.59   Other signs and symptoms in breast

✓5ᵗʰ **N64.8**   Other specified disorders of breast

   N64.81   Ptosis of breast   🅐

     EXCLUDES 1   ptosis of native breast in relation to reconstructed breast (N65.1)

   N64.82   Hypoplasia of breast   🅐

     Micromastia

     EXCLUDES 1   congenital absence of breast (Q83.0)

       hypoplasia of native breast in relation to reconstructed breast (N65.1)

   N64.89   Other specified disorders of breast

     Galactocele

     Subinvolution of breast (postlactational)

     AHA: 2019,1Q,32; 2018,1Q,3

   N64.9   Disorder of breast, unspecified

✓4ᵗʰ **N65**   **Deformity and disproportion of reconstructed breast**

   N65.0   Deformity of reconstructed breast   🅐

     Contour irregularity in reconstructed breast

     Excess tissue in reconstructed breast

     Misshapen reconstructed breast

   N65.1   Disproportion of reconstructed breast   🅐

     Breast asymmetry between native breast and reconstructed breast

     Disproportion between native breast and reconstructed breast

Inflammatory diseases of female pelvic organs (N70-N77)

   EXCLUDES 1   inflammatory diseases of female pelvic organs complicating:

     abortion or ectopic or molar pregnancy (O00-O07, O08.0)

     pregnancy, childbirth and the puerperium (O23.-, O75.3, O85, O86.-)

✓4ᵗʰ **N70**   **Salpingitis and oophoritis**

   INCLUDES   abscess (of) fallopian tube

     abscess (of) ovary

     pyosalpinx

     salpingo-oophoritis

     tubo-ovarian abscess

     tubo-ovarian inflammatory disease

   Use additional code (B95-B97), to identify infectious agent

   EXCLUDES 1   gonococcal infection (A54.24)

     tuberculous infection (A18.17)

✓5ᵗʰ **N70.0**   Acute salpingitis and oophoritis

   N70.01   Acute salpingitis   ♀

   N70.02   Acute oophoritis   ♀

   N70.03   Acute salpingitis and oophoritis   ♀

✓5ᵗʰ **N70.1**   Chronic salpingitis and oophoritis

     Hydrosalpinx

   N70.11   Chronic salpingitis   ♀

   N70.12   Chronic oophoritis   ♀

   N70.13   Chronic salpingitis and oophoritis   ♀

✓5ᵗʰ **N70.9**   Salpingitis and oophoritis, unspecified

   N70.91   Salpingitis, unspecified   ♀

   N70.92   Oophoritis, unspecified   ♀

   N70.93   Salpingitis and oophoritis, unspecified   ♀

✓4ᵗʰ **N71**   **Inflammatory disease of uterus, except cervix**

   INCLUDES   endo (myo) metritis

     metritis

     myometritis

     pyometra

     uterine abscess

   Use additional code (B95-B97), to identify infectious agent

   EXCLUDES 1   hyperplastic endometritis (N85.0-)

     infection of uterus following delivery (O85, O86.-)

   N71.0   Acute inflammatory disease of uterus   ♀

   N71.1   Chronic inflammatory disease of uterus   ♀

   N71.9   Inflammatory disease of uterus, unspecified   ♀

N72   **Inflammatory disease of cervix uteri**   ♀

   INCLUDES   cervicitis (with or without erosion or ectropion)

     endocervicitis (with or without erosion or ectropion)

     exocervicitis (with or without erosion or ectropion)

   Use additional code (B95-B97), to identify infectious agent

   EXCLUDES 1   erosion and ectropion of cervix without cervicitis (N86)

✓4ᵗʰ **N73**   **Other female pelvic inflammatory diseases**

   Use additional code (B95-B97), to identify infectious agent

   N73.0   Acute parametritis and pelvic cellulitis   ♀

     Abscess of broad ligament

     Abscess of parametrium

     Pelvic cellulitis, female

     DEF: Parametritis: Inflammation of the parametrium.

   N73.1   Chronic parametritis and pelvic cellulitis   ♀

     Any condition in N73.0 specified as chronic

     EXCLUDES 1   tuberculous parametritis and pelvic cellulitis (A18.17)

   N73.2   Unspecified parametritis and pelvic cellulitis   ♀

     Any condition in N73.0 unspecified whether acute or chronic

   N73.3   Female acute pelvic peritonitis   ♀

   N73.4   Female chronic pelvic peritonitis   ♀

     EXCLUDES 1   tuberculous pelvic (female) peritonitis (A18.17)

   N73.5   Female pelvic peritonitis, unspecified   ♀

   N73.6   Female pelvic peritoneal adhesions (postinfective)   ♀

     EXCLUDES 2   postprocedural pelvic peritoneal adhesions (N99.4)

     AHA: 2014,1Q,6

   N73.8   Other specified female pelvic inflammatory diseases   ♀

   N73.9   Female pelvic inflammatory disease, unspecified   ♀

     Female pelvic infection or inflammation NOS

✔ Additional Character Required   ✓×7ᵗʰ Placeholder Alert   Manifestation   Unspecified Dx   ►◄ Revised Text   ● New Code   ▲ Revised Code Title

ICD-10-CM 2020   843

Chapter 14. Diseases of the Genitourinary System

N74 **Female pelvic inflammatory disorders in diseases classified elsewhere** ♀

Code first underlying disease

EXCLUDES 1
chlamydial cervicitis (A56.02)
chlamydial pelvic inflammatory disease (A56.11)
gonococcal cervicitis (A54.03)
gonococcal pelvic inflammatory disease (A54.24)
herpesviral [herpes simplex] cervicitis (A60.03)
herpesviral [herpes simplex] pelvic inflammatory disease (A60.09)
syphilitic cervicitis (A52.76)
syphilitic pelvic inflammatory disease (A52.76)
trichomonal cervicitis (A59.09)
tuberculous cervicitis (A18.16)
tuberculous pelvic inflammatory disease (A18.17)

√4th **N75 Diseases of Bartholin's gland**

DEF: Bartholin's gland: Mucous-producing gland found in the vestibular bulbs on either side of the vaginal orifice and connected to the mucosal membrane at the opening by a duct.

N75.0 Cyst of Bartholin's gland ♀

N75.1 Abscess of Bartholin's gland ♀

N75.8 Other diseases of Bartholin's gland ♀

Bartholinitis

N75.9 Disease of Bartholin's gland, unspecified ♀

√4th **N76 Other inflammation of vagina and vulva**

Use additional code (B95-B97), to identify infectious agent

EXCLUDES 2
senile (atrophic) vaginitis (N95.2)
vulvar vestibulitis (N94.810)

N76.0 Acute vaginitis ♀

Acute vulvovaginitis
Vaginitis NOS
Vulvovaginitis NOS

N76.1 Subacute and chronic vaginitis ♀

Chronic vulvovaginitis
Subacute vulvovaginitis

N76.2 Acute vulvitis ♀

Vulvitis NOS

N76.3 Subacute and chronic vulvitis ♀

N76.4 Abscess of vulva ♀

Furuncle of vulva

N76.5 Ulceration of vagina ♀

N76.6 Ulceration of vulva ♀

√5th **N76.8 Other specified inflammation of vagina and vulva**

N76.81 Mucositis (ulcerative) of vagina and vulva ♀

Code also type of associated therapy, such as:
antineoplastic and immunosuppressive drugs (T45.1X-)
radiological procedure and radiotherapy (Y84.2)

EXCLUDES 2
gastrointestinal mucositis (ulcerative) (K92.81)
nasal mucositis (ulcerative) (J34.81)
oral mucositis (ulcerative) (K12.3-)

N76.89 Other specified inflammation of vagina and vulva ♀

√4th **N77 Vulvovaginal ulceration and inflammation in diseases classified elsewhere**

N77.0 Ulceration of vulva in diseases classified elsewhere ♀

Code first underlying disease, such as:
Behçet's disease (M35.2)

EXCLUDES 1
ulceration of vulva in gonococcal infection (A54.02)
ulceration of vulva in herpesviral [herpes simplex] infection (A60.04)
ulceration of vulva in syphilis (A51.0)
ulceration of vulva in tuberculosis (A18.18)

N77.1 Vaginitis, vulvitis and vulvovaginitis in diseases classified elsewhere ♀

Code first underlying disease, such as:
pinworm (B80)

EXCLUDES 1
candidal vulvovaginitis (B37.3)
chlamydial vulvovaginitis (A56.02)
gonococcal vulvovaginitis (A54.02)
herpesviral [herpes simplex] vulvovaginitis (A60.04)
trichomonal vulvovaginitis (A59.01)
tuberculous vulvovaginitis (A18.18)
vulvovaginitis in early syphilis (A51.0)
vulvovaginitis in late syphilis (A52.76)

Noninflammatory disorders of female genital tract (N80-N98)

√4th **N80 Endometriosis**

DEF: Aberrant uterine mucosal tissue appearing in areas of the pelvic cavity outside of its normal location, lining the uterus, and inflaming surrounding tissues often resulting in infertility or spontaneous abortion.

N80.0 Endometriosis of uterus ♀

Adenomyosis

EXCLUDES 1
stromal endometriosis (D39.0)

N80.1 Endometriosis of ovary ♀

N80.2 Endometriosis of fallopian tube ♀

N80.3 Endometriosis of pelvic peritoneum ♀

N80.4 Endometriosis of rectovaginal septum and vagina ♀

N80.5 Endometriosis of intestine ♀

N80.6 Endometriosis in cutaneous scar ♀

N80.8 Other endometriosis ♀

Endometriosis of thorax

N80.9 Endometriosis, unspecified ♀

√4th **N81 Female genital prolapse**

EXCLUDES 1
genital prolapse complicating pregnancy, labor or delivery (O34.5-)
prolapse and hernia of ovary and fallopian tube (N83.4-)
prolapse of vaginal vault after hysterectomy (N99.3)

Types of Pelvic Organ Prolapse

Urethrocele
Bladder, Uterus, Rectum, Urethra, Vaginal canal, Urethrocele

Cystocele
Bladder, Uterus, Rectum, Urethra, Vaginal canal, Cystocele

Rectocele
Bladder, Uterus, Rectum, Urethra, Vaginal canal, Rectocele

Enterocele
Bladder, Uterus, Enterocele, Urethra, Terminal ileum, Vaginal canal

N81.0 Urethrocele ♀

EXCLUDES 1
urethrocele with cystocele (N81.1-)
urethrocele with prolapse of uterus (N81.2-N81.4)

√5th **N81.1 Cystocele**

Cystocele with urethrocele
Cystourethrocele

EXCLUDES 1
cystocele with prolapse of uterus (N81.2-N81.4)

N81.10 Cystocele, unspecified ⓪ ♀

Prolapse of (anterior) vaginal wall NOS

N81.11 Cystocele, midline ⓪ ♀

N81.12   **Cystocele, lateral**   ◘ ♀
    Paravaginal cystocele
    DEF: Detachment of the lateral support connections of the vagina at the arcus tendineus fasciae pelvis (ATFP) that results in bladder drop. The bladder herniates into the vagina laterally.

N81.2   **Incomplete uterovaginal prolapse**   ◘ ♀
    First degree uterine prolapse
    Prolapse of cervix NOS
    Second degree uterine prolapse
    EXCLUDES 1   *cervical stump prolapse (N81.85)*

N81.3   **Complete uterovaginal prolapse**   ◘ ♀
    Procidentia (uteri) NOS
    Third degree uterine prolapse

N81.4   **Uterovaginal prolapse, unspecified**   ◘ ♀
    Prolapse of uterus NOS

N81.5   **Vaginal enterocele**   ♀
    EXCLUDES 1   *enterocele with prolapse of uterus (N81.2-N81.4)*

N81.6   **Rectocele**   ♀
    Prolapse of posterior vaginal wall
    Use additional code for any associated fecal incontinence, if applicable (R15.-)
    EXCLUDES 2   *perineocele (N81.81)*
          rectal prolapse (K62.3)
          rectocele with prolapse of uterus (N81.2-N81.4)

✓5ᵗʰ **N81.8**   **Other female genital prolapse**

     N81.81   **Perineocele**   ♀

     N81.82   **Incompetence or weakening of pubocervical tissue**   ♀

     N81.83   **Incompetence or weakening of rectovaginal tissue**   ♀

     N81.84   **Pelvic muscle wasting**   ♀
         Disuse atrophy of pelvic muscles and anal sphincter

     N81.85   **Cervical stump prolapse**   ♀

     N81.89   **Other female genital prolapse**   ◘ ♀
         Deficient perineum
         Old laceration of muscles of pelvic floor

N81.9   **Female genital prolapse, unspecified**   ◘ ♀

✓4ᵗʰ **N82**   **Fistulae involving female genital tract**
     EXCLUDES 1   *vesicointestinal fistulae (N32.1)*

N82.0   **Vesicovaginal fistula**   ♀

N82.1   **Other female urinary-genital tract fistulae**   ♀
    Cervicovesical fistula
    Ureterovaginal fistula
    Urethrovaginal fistula
    Uteroureteric fistula
    Uterovesical fistula
    AHA: 2017,3Q,3

N82.2   **Fistula of vagina to small intestine**   ♀

N82.3   **Fistula of vagina to large intestine**   ♀
    Rectovaginal fistula

N82.4   **Other female intestinal-genital tract fistulae**   ♀
    Intestinouterine fistula

N82.5   **Female genital tract-skin fistulae**   ♀
    Uterus to abdominal wall fistula
    Vaginoperineal fistula

N82.8   **Other female genital tract fistulae**   ♀

N82.9   **Female genital tract fistula, unspecified**   ♀

✓4ᵗʰ **N83**   **Noninflammatory disorders of ovary, fallopian tube and broad ligament**
     EXCLUDES 2   *hydrosalpinx (N70.1-)*
     AHA: 2016,4Q,46

✓5ᵗʰ **N83.0**   **Follicular cyst of ovary**
     Cyst of graafian follicle
     Hemorrhagic follicular cyst (of ovary)

     N83.00   **Follicular cyst of ovary, unspecified side**   ♀

     N83.01   **Follicular cyst of right ovary**   ♀

     N83.02   **Follicular cyst of left ovary**   ♀

✓5ᵗʰ **N83.1**   **Corpus luteum cyst**
     Hemorrhagic corpus luteum cyst

     N83.10   **Corpus luteum cyst of ovary, unspecified side**   ♀

     N83.11   **Corpus luteum cyst of right ovary**   ♀

     N83.12   **Corpus luteum cyst of left ovary**   ♀

✓5ᵗʰ **N83.2**   **Other and unspecified ovarian cysts**
     EXCLUDES 1   *developmental ovarian cyst (Q50.1)*
          neoplastic ovarian cyst (D27.-)
          polycystic ovarian syndrome (E28.2)
          Stein-Leventhal syndrome (E28.2)

     ✓6ᵗʰ **N83.20**   **Unspecified ovarian cysts**

         N83.201   **Unspecified ovarian cyst, right side**   ♀

         N83.202   **Unspecified ovarian cyst, left side**   ♀

         N83.209   **Unspecified ovarian cyst, unspecified side**   ♀
           Ovarian cyst, NOS

     ✓6ᵗʰ **N83.29**   **Other ovarian cysts**
         Retention cyst of ovary
         Simple cyst of ovary

         N83.291   **Other ovarian cyst, right side**   ♀

         N83.292   **Other ovarian cyst, left side**   ♀

         N83.299   **Other ovarian cyst, unspecified side**   ♀

✓5ᵗʰ **N83.3**   **Acquired atrophy of ovary and fallopian tube**

     ✓6ᵗʰ **N83.31**   **Acquired atrophy of ovary**

         N83.311   **Acquired atrophy of right ovary**   ♀

         N83.312   **Acquired atrophy of left ovary**   ♀

         N83.319   **Acquired atrophy of ovary, unspecified side**   ♀
           Acquired atrophy of ovary, NOS

     ✓6ᵗʰ **N83.32**   **Acquired atrophy of fallopian tube**

         N83.321   **Acquired atrophy of right fallopian tube**   ♀

         N83.322   **Acquired atrophy of left fallopian tube**   ♀

         N83.329   **Acquired atrophy of fallopian tube, unspecified side**   ♀
           Acquired atrophy of fallopian tube, NOS

     ✓6ᵗʰ **N83.33**   **Acquired atrophy of ovary and fallopian tube**

         N83.331   **Acquired atrophy of right ovary and fallopian tube**   ♀

         N83.332   **Acquired atrophy of left ovary and fallopian tube**   ♀

         N83.339   **Acquired atrophy of ovary and fallopian tube, unspecified side**   ♀
           Acquired atrophy of ovary and fallopian tube, NOS

✓5ᵗʰ **N83.4**   **Prolapse and hernia of ovary and fallopian tube**

     N83.40   **Prolapse and hernia of ovary and fallopian tube, unspecified side**   ♀
         Prolapse and hernia of ovary and fallopian tube, NOS

     N83.41   **Prolapse and hernia of right ovary and fallopian tube**   ♀

     N83.42   **Prolapse and hernia of left ovary and fallopian tube**   ♀

✓5ᵗʰ **N83.5**   **Torsion of ovary, ovarian pedicle and fallopian tube**
     Torsion of accessory tube

     ✓6ᵗʰ **N83.51**   **Torsion of ovary and ovarian pedicle**

         N83.511   **Torsion of right ovary and ovarian pedicle**   ♀

         N83.512   **Torsion of left ovary and ovarian pedicle**   ♀

         N83.519   **Torsion of ovary and ovarian pedicle, unspecified side**   ♀
           Torsion of ovary and ovarian pedicle, NOS

     ✓6ᵗʰ **N83.52**   **Torsion of fallopian tube**
         Torsion of hydatid of Morgagni

         N83.521   **Torsion of right fallopian tube**   ♀

         N83.522   **Torsion of left fallopian tube**   ♀

         N83.529   **Torsion of fallopian tube, unspecified side**   ♀
           Torsion of fallopian tube, NOS

     N83.53   **Torsion of ovary, ovarian pedicle and fallopian tube**   ♀

☑ Additional Character Required   ✓×7ᵗʰ Placeholder Alert   Manifestation   Unspecified Dx   ▶◀ Revised Text   ● New Code   ▲ Revised Code Title

N83.6   **Hematosalpinx**   ♀

    EXCLUDES 1   *hematosalpinx (with) (in):*
      hematocolpos (N89.7)
      hematometra (N85.7)
      tubal pregnancy (O00.1-)

N83.7   **Hematoma of broad ligament**   ♀

N83.8   **Other noninflammatory disorders of ovary, fallopian tube and broad ligament**   ♀

    Broad ligament laceration syndrome [Allen-Masters]

N83.9   **Noninflammatory disorder of ovary, fallopian tube and broad ligament, unspecified**   ♀

✓4ᵗʰ **N84**   **Polyp of female genital tract**

    EXCLUDES 1   *adenomatous polyp (D28.-)*
      placental polyp (O90.89)

N84.0   **Polyp of corpus uteri**   ♀

    Polyp of endometrium
    Polyp of uterus NOS
    EXCLUDES 1   *polypoid endometrial hyperplasia (N85.0-)*

N84.1   **Polyp of cervix uteri**   ♀

    Mucous polyp of cervix

N84.2   **Polyp of vagina**   ♀

N84.3   **Polyp of vulva**   ♀

    Polyp of labia

N84.8   **Polyp of other parts of female genital tract**   ♀

N84.9   **Polyp of female genital tract, unspecified**   ♀

✓4ᵗʰ **N85**   **Other noninflammatory disorders of uterus, except cervix**

    EXCLUDES 1   *endometriosis (N80.-)*
      inflammatory diseases of uterus (N71.-)
      noninflammatory disorders of cervix, except malposition (N86-N88)
      polyp of corpus uteri (N84.0)
      uterine prolapse (N81.-)

✓5ᵗʰ **N85.0**   **Endometrial hyperplasia**

N85.00   **Endometrial hyperplasia, unspecified**   ♀

    Hyperplasia (adenomatous) (cystic) (glandular) of endometrium
    Hyperplastic endometritis

N85.01   **Benign endometrial hyperplasia**   ♀

    Endometrial hyperplasia (complex) (simple) without atypia

N85.02   **Endometrial intraepithelial neoplasia [EIN]**   ♀

    Endometrial hyperplasia with atypia
    EXCLUDES 1   *malignant neoplasm of endometrium (with endometrial intraepithelial neoplasia [EIN]) (C54.1)*

N85.2   **Hypertrophy of uterus**   ♀

    Bulky or enlarged uterus
    EXCLUDES 1   *puerperal hypertrophy of uterus (O90.89)*

N85.3   **Subinvolution of uterus**   ♀

    EXCLUDES 1   *puerperal subinvolution of uterus (O90.89)*

N85.4   **Malposition of uterus**   ♀

    Anteversion of uterus
    Retroflexion of uterus
    Retroversion of uterus
    EXCLUDES 1   *malposition of uterus complicating pregnancy, labor or delivery (O34.5-, O65.5)*

N85.5   **Inversion of uterus**   ♀

    EXCLUDES 1   *current obstetric trauma (O71.2)*
      postpartum inversion of uterus (O71.2)
    DEF: Abnormality in which the uterus turns inside out.

Inversion of Uterus

Uterus

N85.6   **Intrauterine synechiae**   ♀

N85.7   **Hematometra**   ♀

    Hematosalpinx with hematometra
    EXCLUDES 1   *hematometra with hematocolpos (N89.7)*
    DEF: Accumulation of blood within the uterus.

N85.8   **Other specified noninflammatory disorders of uterus**   ♀

    Atrophy of uterus, acquired
    Fibrosis of uterus NOS

N85.9   **Noninflammatory disorder of uterus, unspecified**   ♀

    Disorder of uterus NOS

N86   **Erosion and ectropion of cervix uteri**   ♀

    Decubitus (trophic) ulcer of cervix
    Eversion of cervix
    EXCLUDES 1   *erosion and ectropion of cervix with cervicitis (N72)*

✓4ᵗʰ **N87**   **Dysplasia of cervix uteri**

    EXCLUDES 1   *abnormal results from cervical cytologic examination without histologic confirmation (R87.61-)*
      carcinoma in situ of cervix uteri (D06.-)
      cervical intraepithelial neoplasia III [CIN III] (D06.-)
      HGSIL of cervix (R87.613)
      severe dysplasia of cervix uteri (D06.-)

N87.0   **Mild cervical dysplasia**   ♀

    Cervical intraepithelial neoplasia I [CIN I]

N87.1   **Moderate cervical dysplasia**   ♀

    Cervical intraepithelial neoplasia II [CIN II]

N87.9   **Dysplasia of cervix uteri, unspecified**   ♀

    Anaplasia of cervix
    Cervical atypism
    Cervical dysplasia NOS

✓4ᵗʰ **N88**   **Other noninflammatory disorders of cervix uteri**

    EXCLUDES 2   *inflammatory disease of cervix (N72)*
      polyp of cervix (N84.1)

N88.0   **Leukoplakia of cervix uteri**   ♀

N88.1   **Old laceration of cervix uteri**   ♀

    Adhesions of cervix
    EXCLUDES 1   *current obstetric trauma (O71.3)*

N88.2   **Stricture and stenosis of cervix uteri**   ♀

    EXCLUDES 1   *stricture and stenosis of cervix uteri complicating labor (O65.5)*

N88.3   **Incompetence of cervix uteri**   ♀

    Investigation and management of (suspected) cervical incompetence in a nonpregnant woman
    EXCLUDES 1   *cervical incompetence complicating pregnancy (O34.3-)*
    DEF: Inadequate functioning of the cervix marked by abnormal widening during pregnancy and causing premature birth or miscarriage.

N88.4   **Hypertrophic elongation of cervix uteri**   ♀

N88.8   **Other specified noninflammatory disorders of cervix uteri** ♀
> EXCLUDES 1   current obstetric trauma (O71.3)

N88.9   **Noninflammatory disorder of cervix uteri, unspecified** ♀

✓4ᵗʰ **N89**   **Other noninflammatory disorders of vagina**
> EXCLUDES 1   abnormal results from vaginal cytologic examination without histologic confirmation (R87.62-)
> carcinoma in situ of vagina (D07.2)
> HGSIL of vagina (R87.623)
> inflammation of vagina (N76.-)
> senile (atrophic) vaginitis (N95.2)
> severe dysplasia of vagina (D07.2)
> trichomonal leukorrhea (A59.00)
> vaginal intraepithelial neoplasia [VAIN], grade III (D07.2)

N89.0   **Mild vaginal dysplasia** ♀
> Vaginal intraepithelial neoplasia [VAIN], grade I

N89.1   **Moderate vaginal dysplasia** ♀
> Vaginal intraepithelial neoplasia [VAIN], grade II

N89.3   **Dysplasia of vagina, unspecified** ♀

N89.4   **Leukoplakia of vagina** ♀

N89.5   **Stricture and atresia of vagina** ♀
> Vaginal adhesions
> Vaginal stenosis
> EXCLUDES 1   congenital atresia or stricture (Q52.4)
> postprocedural adhesions of vagina (N99.2)

N89.6   **Tight hymenal ring** ♀
> Rigid hymen
> Tight introitus
> EXCLUDES 1   imperforate hymen (Q52.3)

N89.7   **Hematocolpos** ♀
> Hematocolpos with hematometra or hematosalpinx
> **AHA:** 2016,4Q,58

N89.8   **Other specified noninflammatory disorders of vagina** ♀
> Leukorrhea NOS
> Old vaginal laceration
> Pessary ulcer of vagina
> EXCLUDES 1   current obstetric trauma (O70.-, O71.4, O71.7-O71.8)
> old laceration involving muscles of pelvic floor (N81.8)

N89.9   **Noninflammatory disorder of vagina, unspecified** ♀

✓4ᵗʰ **N90**   **Other noninflammatory disorders of vulva and perineum**
> EXCLUDES 1   anogenital (venereal) warts (A63.0)
> carcinoma in situ of vulva (D07.1)
> condyloma acuminatum (A63.0)
> current obstetric trauma (O70.-, O71.7-O71.8)
> inflammation of vulva (N76.-)
> severe dysplasia of vulva (D07.1)
> vulvar intraepithelial neoplasm III [VIN III] (D07.1)

N90.0   **Mild vulvar dysplasia** ♀
> Vulvar intraepithelial neoplasia [VIN], grade I

N90.1   **Moderate vulvar dysplasia** ♀
> Vulvar intraepithelial neoplasia [VIN], grade II

N90.3   **Dysplasia of vulva, unspecified** ♀

N90.4   **Leukoplakia of vulva** ♀
> Dystrophy of vulva
> Kraurosis of vulva
> Lichen sclerosus of external female genital organs

N90.5   **Atrophy of vulva** ♀
> Stenosis of vulva

✓5ᵗʰ **N90.6**   **Hypertrophy of vulva**
> **AHA:** 2016,4Q,46

   N90.60   **Unspecified hypertrophy of vulva** ♀
> Unspecified hypertrophy of labia

   N90.61   **Childhood asymmetric labium majus enlargement** ♀
> CALME

   N90.69   **Other specified hypertrophy of vulva** ♀
> Other specified hypertrophy of labia

N90.7   **Vulvar cyst** ♀

✓5ᵗʰ **N90.8**   **Other specified noninflammatory disorders of vulva and perineum**

   ✓6ᵗʰ **N90.81**   **Female genital mutilation status**
> Female genital cutting status

     N90.810   **Female genital mutilation status, unspecified** ♀
> Female genital cutting status, unspecified
> Female genital mutilation status NOS

     N90.811   **Female genital mutilation Type I status** ♀
> Clitorectomy status
> Female genital cutting Type I status

     N90.812   **Female genital mutilation Type II status** ♀
> Clitorectomy with excision of labia minora status
> Female genital cutting Type II status

     N90.813   **Female genital mutilation Type III status** ♀
> Female genital cutting Type III status
> Infibulation status

     N90.818   **Other female genital mutilation status** ♀
> Female genital cutting Type IV status
> Female genital mutilation Type IV status
> Other female genital cutting status

   N90.89   **Other specified noninflammatory disorders of vulva and perineum** ♀
> Adhesions of vulva
> Hypertrophy of clitoris

N90.9   **Noninflammatory disorder of vulva and perineum, unspecified** ♀

✓4ᵗʰ **N91**   **Absent, scanty and rare menstruation**
> EXCLUDES 1   ovarian dysfunction (E28.-)

N91.0   **Primary amenorrhea** ♀

N91.1   **Secondary amenorrhea** ♀

N91.2   **Amenorrhea, unspecified** ♀

N91.3   **Primary oligomenorrhea** ♀

N91.4   **Secondary oligomenorrhea** ♀

N91.5   **Oligomenorrhea, unspecified** ♀
> Hypomenorrhea NOS

✓4ᵗʰ **N92**   **Excessive, frequent and irregular menstruation**
> EXCLUDES 1   postmenopausal bleeding (N95.0)
> precocious puberty (menstruation) (E30.1)

N92.0   **Excessive and frequent menstruation with regular cycle** ♀
> Heavy periods NOS
> Menorrhagia NOS
> Polymenorrhea

N92.1   **Excessive and frequent menstruation with irregular cycle** ♀
> Irregular intermenstrual bleeding
> Irregular, shortened intervals between menstrual bleeding
> Menometrorrhagia
> Metrorrhagia

N92.2   **Excessive menstruation at puberty** P ♀
> Excessive bleeding associated with onset of menstrual periods
> Pubertal menorrhagia
> Puberty bleeding

N92.3   **Ovulation bleeding** ♀
> Regular intermenstrual bleeding

N92.4   **Excessive bleeding in the premenopausal period** ♀
> Climacteric menorrhagia or metrorrhagia
> Menopausal menorrhagia or metrorrhagia
> ▶Perimenopausal bleeding◀
> ▶Perimenopausal menorrhagia or metrorrhagia◀
> Preclimacteric menorrhagia or metrorrhagia
> Premenopausal menorrhagia or metrorrhagia

N92.5   **Other specified irregular menstruation** ♀

☑ Additional Character Required   ✓x7ᵗʰ Placeholder Alert   Manifestation   Unspecified Dx   ▶◀ Revised Text   ● New Code   ▲ Revised Code Title

N92.6 Irregular menstruation, unspecified ♀
Irregular bleeding NOS
Irregular periods NOS
    EXCLUDES 1   irregular menstruation with:
        lengthened intervals or scanty bleeding (N91.3-N91.5)
        shortened intervals or excessive bleeding (N92.1)

✓4th **N93 Other abnormal uterine and vaginal bleeding**
    EXCLUDES 1   neonatal vaginal hemorrhage (P54.6)
        precocious puberty (menstruation) (E30.1)
        pseudomenses (P54.6)

N93.0 Postcoital and contact bleeding ♀

N93.1 Pre-pubertal vaginal bleeding ♀
    AHA: 2016,4Q,47

N93.8 Other specified abnormal uterine and vaginal bleeding ♀
    Dysfunctional or functional uterine or vaginal bleeding NOS

N93.9 Abnormal uterine and vaginal bleeding, unspecified ♀

✓4th **N94 Pain and other conditions associated with female genital organs and menstrual cycle**

N94.0 Mittelschmerz ♀
    DEF: One-sided, lower abdominal pain occurring between menstrual periods that is associated with ovulation.

✓5th **N94.1 Dyspareunia**
    EXCLUDES 1   psychogenic dyspareunia (F52.6)
    AHA: 2016,4Q,47

    N94.10 Unspecified dyspareunia ♀
    N94.11 Superficial (introital) dyspareunia ♀
    N94.12 Deep dyspareunia ♀
    N94.19 Other specified dyspareunia ♀

N94.2 Vaginismus ♀
    EXCLUDES 1   psychogenic vaginismus (F52.5)
    DEF: Spontaneous contractions of the muscles surrounding the vagina, causing it to constrict or close.

N94.3 Premenstrual tension syndrome ♀
    Code also associated menstrual migraine (G43.82-, G43.83-)
    EXCLUDES 1   premenstrual dysphoric disorder (F32.81)

N94.4 Primary dysmenorrhea ♀

N94.5 Secondary dysmenorrhea ♀

N94.6 Dysmenorrhea, unspecified ♀
    EXCLUDES 1   psychogenic dysmenorrhea (F45.8)

✓5th **N94.8 Other specified conditions associated with female genital organs and menstrual cycle**

    ✓6th **N94.81 Vulvodynia**
       N94.810 Vulvar vestibulitis ♀
       N94.818 Other vulvodynia ♀
       N94.819 Vulvodynia, unspecified ♀
         Vulvodynia NOS

    N94.89 Other specified conditions associated with female genital organs and menstrual cycle ♀
       DEF: Hydrocele: Serous fluid that collects in the canal of Nuck in females.

N94.9 Unspecified condition associated with female genital organs and menstrual cycle ♀

✓4th **N95 Menopausal and other perimenopausal disorders**
Menopausal and other perimenopausal disorders due to naturally occurring (age-related) menopause and perimenopause
    EXCLUDES 1   excessive bleeding in the premenopausal period (N92.4)
       menopausal and perimenopausal disorders due to artificial or premature menopause (E89.4-, E28.31-)
       premature menopause (E28.31-)
    EXCLUDES 2   postmenopausal osteoporosis (M81.0-)
       postmenopausal osteoporosis with current pathological fracture (M80.0-)
       postmenopausal urethritis (N34.2)

N95.0 Postmenopausal bleeding ♀

N95.1 Menopausal and female climacteric states ♀
Symptoms such as flushing, sleeplessness, headache, lack of concentration, associated with natural (age-related) menopause
Use additional code for associated symptoms
    EXCLUDES 1   asymptomatic menopausal state (Z78.0)
       symptoms associated with artificial menopause (E89.41)
       symptoms associated with premature menopause (E28.310)

N95.2 Postmenopausal atrophic vaginitis ♀
Senile (atrophic) vaginitis

N95.8 Other specified menopausal and perimenopausal disorders ♀

N95.9 Unspecified menopausal and perimenopausal disorder ♀

N96 Recurrent pregnancy loss ♀
Investigation or care in a nonpregnant woman with history of recurrent pregnancy loss
    EXCLUDES 1   recurrent pregnancy loss with current pregnancy (O26.2-)

✓4th **N97 Female infertility**
    INCLUDES   inability to achieve a pregnancy
       sterility, female NOS
    EXCLUDES 1   female infertility associated with:
       hypopituitarism (E23.0)
       Stein-Leventhal syndrome (E28.2)
    EXCLUDES 2   incompetence of cervix uteri (N88.3)
    DEF: Infertility: Inability to conceive for at least one year with regular intercourse.
    DEF: Primary infertility: Infertility occurring in patients who have never conceived.
    DEF: Secondary infertility: Infertility occurring in patients who have previously conceived.

N97.0 Female infertility associated with anovulation ♀

N97.1 Female infertility of tubal origin ♀
Female infertility associated with congenital anomaly of tube
Female infertility due to tubal block
Female infertility due to tubal occlusion
Female infertility due to tubal stenosis

N97.2 Female infertility of uterine origin ♀
Female infertility associated with congenital anomaly of uterus
Female infertility due to nonimplantation of ovum

N97.8 Female infertility of other origin ♀

N97.9 Female infertility, unspecified ♀

✓4th **N98 Complications associated with artificial fertilization**

N98.0 Infection associated with artificial insemination ♀

N98.1 Hyperstimulation of ovaries ♀
Hyperstimulation of ovaries NOS
Hyperstimulation of ovaries associated with induced ovulation

N98.2 Complications of attempted introduction of fertilized ovum following in vitro fertilization ♀

N98.3 Complications of attempted introduction of embryo in embryo transfer ♀

N98.8 Other complications associated with artificial fertilization ♀

N98.9 Complication associated with artificial fertilization, unspecified ♀

Intraoperative and postprocedural complications and disorders of genitourinary system, not elsewhere classified (N99)

✓4th **N99 Intraoperative and postprocedural complications and disorders of genitourinary system, not elsewhere classified**
    EXCLUDES 2   irradiation cystitis (N30.4-)
       postoophorectomy osteoporosis with current pathological fracture (M80.8-)
       postoophorectomy osteoporosis without current pathological fracture (M81.8)

N99.0 Postprocedural (acute) (chronic) kidney failure
Use additional code to type of kidney disease

√5ᵗʰ **N99.1** **Postprocedural** urethral stricture
      Postcatheterization urethral stricture

  √6ᵗʰ **N99.11** **Postprocedural urethral stricture,** male
      AHA: 2016,4Q,47-48

     N99.110 **Postprocedural urethral stricture, male,** meatal ♂

     N99.111 **Postprocedural** bulbous **urethral stricture, male** ♂

     N99.112 **Postprocedural** membranous **urethral stricture, male** ♂

     N99.113 **Postprocedural** anterior bulbous **urethral stricture, male** ♂

     N99.114 **Postprocedural urethral stricture, male, unspecified** ♂

     N99.115 **Postprocedural** fossa navicularis **urethral stricture** ♂

     N99.116 **Postprocedural urethral stricture, male,** overlapping **sites** ♂

  N99.12 **Postprocedural urethral stricture,** female ♀

N99.2 **Postprocedural** adhesions of vagina ♀

N99.3 Prolapse of vaginal vault **after hysterectomy** ♀

N99.4 **Postprocedural** pelvic peritoneal adhesions
    EXCLUDES 2 *pelvic peritoneal adhesions NOS (N73.6)*
             postinfective pelvic peritoneal adhesions (N73.6)

√5ᵗʰ **N99.5** **Complications of stoma of urinary tract**
    EXCLUDES 2 *mechanical complication of urinary catheter (T83.0-)*
    AHA: 2016,4Q,48

  √6ᵗʰ **N99.51** **Complication of** cystostomy

     N99.510 **Cystostomy** hemorrhage HCC

     N99.511 **Cystostomy** infection HCC

     N99.512 **Cystostomy** malfunction HCC

     N99.518 **Other cystostomy complication** HCC

  √6ᵗʰ **N99.52** **Complication of** incontinent external stoma **of urinary tract**

     N99.520 Hemorrhage **of incontinent external stoma of urinary tract** HCC

     N99.521 Infection **of incontinent external stoma of urinary tract** HCC

     N99.522 Malfunction **of incontinent external stoma of urinary tract** HCC

     N99.523 Herniation **of incontinent stoma of urinary tract** HCC

     N99.524 Stenosis **of incontinent stoma of urinary tract** HCC

     N99.528 **Other complication of incontinent external stoma of urinary tract** HCC

  √6ᵗʰ **N99.53** **Complication of** continent stoma **of urinary tract**

     N99.530 Hemorrhage **of continent stoma of urinary tract** HCC

     N99.531 Infection **of continent stoma of urinary tract** HCC

     N99.532 Malfunction **of continent stoma of urinary tract** HCC

     N99.533 Herniation **of continent stoma of urinary tract** HCC

     N99.534 Stenosis **of continent stoma of urinary tract** HCC

     N99.538 **Other complication of continent stoma of urinary tract** HCC

√5ᵗʰ **N99.6** Intraoperative hemorrhage and hematoma **of a genitourinary system organ or structure complicating a procedure**
    EXCLUDES 1 *intraoperative hemorrhage and hematoma of a genitourinary system organ or structure due to accidental puncture or laceration during a procedure (N99.7-)*

  N99.61 **Intraoperative hemorrhage and hematoma of a genitourinary system organ or structure complicating a** genitourinary system procedure

  N99.62 **Intraoperative hemorrhage and hematoma of a genitourinary system organ or structure complicating** other procedure

√5ᵗʰ **N99.7** Accidental puncture and laceration **of a genitourinary system organ or structure during a procedure**

  N99.71 **Accidental puncture and laceration of a genitourinary system organ or structure during a** genitourinary system procedure

  N99.72 **Accidental puncture and laceration of a genitourinary system organ or structure during** other procedure

√5ᵗʰ **N99.8** **Other intraoperative and postprocedural complications and disorders of genitourinary system**
    AHA: 2016,4Q,9-10

  N99.81 **Other** intraoperative complications **of genitourinary system**

  √6ᵗʰ **N99.82** Postprocedural hemorrhage **of a genitourinary system organ or structure following a procedure**

     N99.820 **Postprocedural hemorrhage of a genitourinary system organ or structure following a** genitourinary system procedure

     N99.821 **Postprocedural hemorrhage of a genitourinary system organ or structure following** other procedure

  N99.83 Residual ovary syndrome ♀

  √6ᵗʰ **N99.84** Postprocedural hematoma and seroma **of a genitourinary system organ or structure following a procedure**

     N99.840 **Postprocedural** hematoma **of a genitourinary system organ or structure following a** genitourinary system procedure

     N99.841 **Postprocedural** hematoma **of a genitourinary system organ or structure following** other procedure

     N99.842 **Postprocedural** seroma **of a genitourinary system organ or structure following a** genitourinary system procedure

     N99.843 **Postprocedural** seroma **of a genitourinary system organ or structure following** other procedure

  N99.85 Post endometrial ablation syndrome

  N99.89 **Other postprocedural complications and disorders of genitourinary system**

Chapter 15. Pregnancy, Childbirth, and the Puerperium (O00–O9A)

Chapter-specific Guidelines with Coding Examples

The chapter-specific guidelines from the ICD-10-CM Official Guidelines for Coding and Reporting have been provided below. Along with these guidelines are coding examples, contained in the shaded boxes, that have been developed to help illustrate the coding and/or sequencing guidance found in these guidelines.

a. General rules for obstetric cases

1) Codes from Chapter 15 and sequencing priority

Obstetric cases require codes from chapter 15, codes in the range O00-O9A, Pregnancy, Childbirth, and the Puerperium. Chapter 15 codes have sequencing priority over codes from other chapters. Additional codes from other chapters may be used in conjunction with chapter 15 codes to further specify conditions. Should the provider document that the pregnancy is incidental to the encounter, then code Z33.1, Pregnant state, incidental, should be used in place of any chapter 15 codes. It is the provider's responsibility to state that the condition being treated is not affecting the pregnancy.

> Bladder abscess in pregnant patient at 25 weeks' gestation
>
> **O23.12** **Infections of bladder in pregnancy, second trimester**
>
> **N30.80** **Other cystitis without hematuria**
>
> **Z3A.25** **25 weeks gestation of pregnancy**
>
> *Explanation:* The documentation does not indicate that the pregnancy is incidental or in any way unaffected by the bladder abscess; therefore, an obstetrics code should be sequenced first. An additional code was provided to identify the specific bladder condition as this information is not called out specifically in the obstetrics code.

2) Chapter 15 codes used only on the maternal record

Chapter 15 codes are to be used only on the maternal record, never on the record of the newborn.

3) Final character for trimester

The majority of codes in Chapter 15 have a final character indicating the trimester of pregnancy. The timeframes for the trimesters are indicated at the beginning of the chapter. If trimester is not a component of a code, it is because the condition always occurs in a specific trimester, or the concept of trimester of pregnancy is not applicable. Certain codes have characters for only certain trimesters because the condition does not occur in all trimesters, but it may occur in more than just one. Assignment of the final character for trimester should be based on the provider's documentation of the trimester (or number of weeks) for the current admission/encounter. This applies to the assignment of trimester for pre-existing conditions as well as those that develop during or are due to the pregnancy. The provider's documentation of the number of weeks may be used to assign the appropriate code identifying the trimester.

Whenever delivery occurs during the current admission, and there is an "in childbirth" option for the obstetric complication being coded, the "in childbirth" code should be assigned.

> Pregnant patient at 21 weeks' gestation admitted with excessive vomiting
>
> **O21.2** **Late vomiting of pregnancy**
>
> **Z3A.21** **21 weeks gestation of pregnancy**
>
> *Explanation:* Category O21 classifies vomiting in pregnancy. Although code selection is based on whether the vomiting is before or after 20 completed weeks, these codes are not further classified by trimester. If vomiting only in the second trimester was documented, the provider should be queried for the specific week of gestation, as this will affect code selection.

4) Selection of trimester for inpatient admissions that encompass more than one trimester

In instances when a patient is admitted to a hospital for complications of pregnancy during one trimester and remains in the hospital into a subsequent trimester, the trimester character for the antepartum complication code should be assigned on the basis of the trimester when the complication developed, not the trimester of the discharge. If the condition developed prior to the current admission/encounter or represents a pre-existing condition, the trimester character for the trimester at the time of the admission/encounter should be assigned.

5) Unspecified trimester

Each category that includes codes for trimester has a code for "unspecified trimester." The "unspecified trimester" code should rarely be used, such as when the documentation in the record is insufficient to determine the trimester and it is not possible to obtain clarification.

6) 7th character for fetus identification

Where applicable, a 7th character is to be assigned for certain categories (O31, O32, O33.3 - O33.6, O35, O36, O40, O41, O60.1, O60.2, O64, and O69) to identify the fetus for which the complication code applies.

Assign 7th character "0":

- For single gestations
- When the documentation in the record is insufficient to determine the fetus affected and it is not possible to obtain clarification.
- When it is not possible to clinically determine which fetus is affected.

> Maternal patient with twin gestations is seen after ultrasound identifies fetus B to be in breech presentation
>
> **O32.1XX2** **Maternal care for breech presentation, fetus 2**
>
> *Explanation:* The documentation indicates that although there are two fetuses, only one fetus is determined to be in breech presentation. Whether fetus 2 or fetus B is used, the coder can assign the seventh character of 2 to identify the second fetus as the one in breech.

b. Selection of OB principal or first-listed diagnosis

1) Routine outpatient prenatal visits

For routine outpatient prenatal visits when no complications are present, a code from category Z34, Encounter for supervision of normal pregnancy, should be used as the first-listed diagnosis. These codes should not be used in conjunction with chapter 15 codes.

2) Supervision of high-risk pregnancy

Codes from category O09, Supervision of high-risk pregnancy, are intended for use only during the prenatal period. For complications during the labor or delivery episode as a result of a high-risk pregnancy, assign the applicable complication codes from Chapter 15. If there are no complications during the labor or delivery episode, assign code O80, Encounter for full-term uncomplicated delivery.

For routine prenatal outpatient visits for patients with high-risk pregnancies, a code from category O09, Supervision of high-risk pregnancy, should be used as the first-listed diagnosis. Secondary chapter 15 codes may be used in conjunction with these codes if appropriate.

> 36-year-old seen in labor with second child at 39 weeks' gestation, delivered a healthy baby, delivery complicated by tear of fourchette that was repaired
>
> **O70.0** **First degree perineal laceration during delivery**
>
> **Z3A.39** **39 weeks gestation of pregnancy**
>
> **Z37.0** **Single live birth**
>
> Explanation: Although this patient is over 35 and having her second child (elderly multigravida), do not append a code from subcategory O09.52-. A code describing the tear of the fourchette, which complicated the delivery, should be used in addition to the applicable Z codes.

3) Episodes when no delivery occurs

In episodes when no delivery occurs, the principal diagnosis should correspond to the principal complication of the pregnancy which necessitated the encounter. Should more than one complication exist, all of which are treated or monitored, any of the complication codes may be sequenced first.

4) When a delivery occurs

When an obstetric patient is admitted and delivers during that admission, the condition that prompted the admission should be sequenced as the principal diagnosis. If multiple conditions prompted the admission, sequence the one most related to the delivery as the principal diagnosis. A code for any complication of the delivery should be assigned as an additional diagnosis. In cases of cesarean delivery, if the patient was admitted with a condition that resulted in the performance of a cesarean procedure, that condition should be selected as the principal diagnosis. If the reason for the admission was unrelated to the condition resulting in the cesarean delivery, the condition related to the reason for the admission should be selected as the principal diagnosis.

Maternal patient with diet-controlled gestational diabetes was seen at 38 weeks' gestation in obstructed labor due to footling presentation; cesarean performed for the malpresentation	
O64.8XX0	**Obstructed labor due to other malposition and malpresentation, not applicable or unspecified**
O24.420	**Gestational diabetes mellitus in childbirth, diet controlled**
Z3A.38	**38 weeks gestation of pregnancy**
Z37.0	**Single live birth**
Explanation: The obstructed labor necessitated the cesarean procedure.	

5) Outcome of delivery

A code from category Z37, Outcome of delivery, should be included on every maternal record when a delivery has occurred. These codes are not to be used on subsequent records or on the newborn record.

c. Pre-existing conditions versus conditions due to the pregnancy

Certain categories in Chapter 15 distinguish between conditions of the mother that existed prior to pregnancy (pre-existing) and those that are a direct result of pregnancy. When assigning codes from Chapter 15, it is important to assess if a condition was pre-existing prior to pregnancy or developed during or due to the pregnancy in order to assign the correct code.

Categories that do not distinguish between pre-existing and pregnancy-related conditions may be used for either. It is acceptable to use codes specifically for the puerperium with codes complicating pregnancy and childbirth if a condition arises postpartum during the delivery encounter.

Type 2 diabetic patient presents at 19 weeks gestation for glucose check. Patient has been taking oral metformin for several years and currently is experiencing no diabetic complications.	
O24.112	**Pre-existing type 2 diabetes mellitus, in pregnancy, second trimester**
E11.9	**Type 2 diabetes mellitus without complications**
Z79.84	**Long term (current) use of oral hypoglycemic drugs**
Explanation: The documentation states that the patient has been on a diabetic medication (oral metformin) for several years, indicating the patient was diabetic prior to becoming pregnant. Reporting pre-existing Type 2 diabetes in a pregnant patient requires two codes to capture the condition, a code from category O24 and a code from category E11. A note at E11 indicates that the code for long-term use of oral hypoglycemic drugs should also be reported.	

d. Pre-existing hypertension in pregnancy

Category O10, Pre-existing hypertension complicating pregnancy, childbirth and the puerperium, includes codes for hypertensive heart and hypertensive chronic kidney disease. When assigning one of the O10 codes that includes hypertensive heart disease or hypertensive chronic kidney disease, it is necessary to add a secondary code from the appropriate hypertension category to specify the type of heart failure or chronic kidney disease.

See Section I.C.9. Hypertension.

e. Fetal conditions affecting the management of the mother

1) Codes from categories O35 and O36

Codes from categories O35, Maternal care for known or suspected fetal abnormality and damage, and O36, Maternal care for other fetal problems, are assigned only when the fetal condition is actually responsible for modifying the management of the mother, i.e., by requiring diagnostic studies, additional observation, special care, or termination of pregnancy. The fact that the fetal condition exists does not justify assigning a code from this series to the mother's record.

A patient with twin gestation is seen for spotting 15 weeks into her pregnancy; the doctors also suspect fetal hydrocephalus. Patient is instructed to return in one week for additional diagnostic testing, sooner if the problem worsens.	
O35.0XX0	**Maternal care for (suspected) central nervous system malformation in fetus, not applicable or unspecified**
O26.852	**Spotting complicating pregnancy, second trimester**
Z3A.15	**15 weeks gestation of pregnancy**
Explanation: Whether the fetal hydrocephalus was suspected or confirmed, an additional code is warranted for this condition since documentation indicates the patient is to return sooner than her routine visit for further testing.	

2) In utero surgery

In cases when surgery is performed on the fetus, a diagnosis code from category O35, Maternal care for known or suspected fetal abnormality and damage, should be assigned identifying the fetal condition. Assign the appropriate procedure code for the procedure performed.

No code from Chapter 16, the perinatal codes, should be used on the mother's record to identify fetal conditions. Surgery performed in utero on a fetus is still to be coded as an obstetric encounter.

f. HIV infection in pregnancy, childbirth and the puerperium

During pregnancy, childbirth or the puerperium, a patient admitted because of an HIV-related illness should receive a principal diagnosis from subcategory O98.7-, Human immunodeficiency [HIV] disease complicating pregnancy, childbirth and the puerperium, followed by the code(s) for the HIV-related illness(es).

Patients with asymptomatic HIV infection status admitted during pregnancy, childbirth, or the puerperium should receive codes of O98.7- and Z21, Asymptomatic human immunodeficiency virus [HIV] infection status.

A previously asymptomatic HIV patient who is 13 weeks pregnant is evaluated for HIV-related candidal bronchitis	
O98.711	**Human immunodeficiency virus [HIV] disease complicating pregnancy, first trimester**
B20	**Human immunodeficiency virus [HIV] disease**
B37.1	**Pulmonary candidiasis**
Z3A.13	**13 weeks gestation of pregnancy**
Explanation: Because candidal bronchitis is an AIDS-related condition, this patient is now considered to have HIV disease. An obstetrics code indicating that HIV is complicating the pregnancy is coded first, followed by B20 for HIV disease as well as a code for the candidal bronchitis.	

g. Diabetes mellitus in pregnancy

Diabetes mellitus is a significant complicating factor in pregnancy. Pregnant women who are diabetic should be assigned a code from category O24, Diabetes mellitus in pregnancy, childbirth, and the puerperium, first, followed by the appropriate diabetes code(s) (E08-E13) from Chapter 4.

h. Long term use of insulin and oral hypoglycemics

See section I.C.4.a.3 for information on the long term use of insulin and oral hypoglycemic.

i. Gestational (pregnancy induced) diabetes

Gestational (pregnancy induced) diabetes can occur during the second and third trimester of pregnancy in women who were not diabetic prior to pregnancy. Gestational diabetes can cause complications in the pregnancy similar to those of pre-existing diabetes mellitus. It also puts the woman at greater risk of developing diabetes after the pregnancy. Codes for gestational diabetes are in subcategory O24.4, Gestational diabetes mellitus. No other code from category O24, Diabetes mellitus in pregnancy, childbirth, and the puerperium, should be used with a code from O24.4.

The codes under subcategory O24.4 include diet controlled, insulin controlled, and controlled by oral hypoglycemic drugs. If a patient with gestational diabetes is treated with both diet and insulin, only the code for insulin-controlled is required. If a patient with gestational diabetes is treated with both diet and oral hypoglycemic medications, only the code for "controlled by oral hypoglycemic drugs" is required. Code Z79.4, Long-term (current) use of insulin or code Z79.84, Long-term (current) use of oral hypoglycemic drugs, should not be assigned with codes from subcategory O24.4.

An abnormal glucose tolerance in pregnancy is assigned a code from subcategory O99.81, Abnormal glucose complicating pregnancy, childbirth, and the puerperium.

j. Sepsis and septic shock complicating abortion, pregnancy, childbirth and the puerperium

When assigning a chapter 15 code for sepsis complicating abortion, pregnancy, childbirth, and the puerperium, a code for the specific type of infection should be assigned as an additional diagnosis. If severe sepsis is present, a code from subcategory R65.2, Severe sepsis, and code(s) for associated organ dysfunction(s) should also be assigned as additional diagnoses.

> Patient is seen several days after a miscarriage with sepsis; cultures return MSSA
>
> | **O03.87** | **Sepsis following complete or unspecified spontaneous abortion** |
> |---|---|
> | **B95.61** | **Methicillin susceptible Staphylococcus aureus infection as the cause of diseases classified elsewhere** |
>
> *Explanation:* The type of infection that caused this patient to become septic was methicillin susceptible *Staphylococcus aureus* (MSSA), which as a secondary code helps capture all aspects related to this patient's septic condition.

k. Puerperal sepsis

Code O85, Puerperal sepsis, should be assigned with a secondary code to identify the causal organism (e.g., for a bacterial infection, assign a code from category B95-B96, Bacterial infections in conditions classified elsewhere). A code from category A40, Streptococcal sepsis, or A41, Other sepsis, should not be used for puerperal sepsis. If applicable, use additional codes to identify severe sepsis (R65.2-) and any associated acute organ dysfunction.

l. Alcohol, tobacco and drug use during pregnancy, childbirth and the puerperium

1) Alcohol use during pregnancy, childbirth and the puerperium

Codes under subcategory O99.31, Alcohol use complicating pregnancy, childbirth, and the puerperium, should be assigned for any pregnancy case when a mother uses alcohol during the pregnancy or postpartum. A secondary code from category F10, Alcohol related disorders, should also be assigned to identify manifestations of the alcohol use.

2) Tobacco use during pregnancy, childbirth and the puerperium

Codes under subcategory O99.33, Smoking (tobacco) complicating pregnancy, childbirth, and the puerperium, should be assigned for any pregnancy case when a mother uses any type of tobacco product during the pregnancy or postpartum. A secondary code from category F17, Nicotine dependence, should also be assigned to identify the type of nicotine dependence.

3) Drug use during pregnancy, childbirth and the puerperium

Codes under subcategory O99.32, Drug use complicating pregnancy, childbirth, and the puerperium, should be assigned for any pregnancy case when a mother uses drugs during the pregnancy or postpartum. This can involve illegal drugs, or inappropriate use or abuse of prescription drugs. Secondary code(s) from categories F11-F16 and F18-F19 should also be assigned to identify manifestations of the drug use.

m. Poisoning, toxic effects, adverse effects and underdosing in a pregnant patient

A code from subcategory O9A.2, Injury, poisoning and certain other consequences of external causes complicating pregnancy, childbirth, and the puerperium, should be sequenced first, followed by the appropriate injury, poisoning, toxic effect, adverse effect or underdosing code, and then the additional code(s) that specifies the condition caused by the poisoning, toxic effect, adverse effect or underdosing.

See Section I.C.19. Adverse effects, poisoning, underdosing and toxic effects.

> Patient treated for accidental carbon monoxide poisoning from a gas heating implement; the patient is 18 weeks' pregnant
>
> | **O9A.212** | **Injury, poisoning and certain other consequences of external causes complicating pregnancy, second trimester** |
> |---|---|
> | **T58.11XA** | **Toxic effect of carbon monoxide from utility gas, accidental (unintentional), initial encounter** |
> | **Z3A.18** | **18 weeks gestation of pregnancy** |
>
> *Explanation:* Although the carbon monoxide poisoning is the reason for the encounter, a code from the obstetrics chapter must be sequenced first. Chapter 15 codes have sequencing priority over codes from other chapters.

n. Normal delivery, code O80

1) Encounter for full term uncomplicated delivery

Code O80 should be assigned when a woman is admitted for a full-term normal delivery and delivers a single, healthy infant without any complications antepartum, during the delivery, or postpartum during the delivery episode. Code O80 is always a principal diagnosis. It is not to be used if any other code from chapter 15 is needed to describe a current complication of the antenatal, delivery, or **postnatal** period. Additional codes from other chapters may be used with code O80 if they are not related to or are in any way complicating the pregnancy.

2) Uncomplicated delivery with resolved antepartum complication

Code O80 may be used if the patient had a complication at some point during the pregnancy, but the complication is not present at the time of the admission for delivery.

> Patient presents in labor at 39 weeks' gestation and delivers a healthy newborn; patient had abnormal glucose levels in her first trimester, which have since resolved
>
> | **O80** | **Encounter for full-term uncomplicated delivery** |
> |---|---|
> | **Z37.0** | **Single live birth** |
>
> *Explanation:* The abnormal glucose levels during the first trimester cannot be coded if they are not affecting the patient's current trimester. Without additional complications associated with the pregnancy, fetus, or mother, code O80 is appropriate.

3) Outcome of delivery for O80

Z37.0, Single live birth, is the only outcome of delivery code appropriate for use with O80.

o. The peripartum and postpartum periods

1) Peripartum and postpartum periods

The postpartum period begins immediately after delivery and continues for six weeks following delivery. The peripartum period is defined as the last month of pregnancy to five months postpartum.

2) Peripartum and postpartum complication

A postpartum complication is any complication occurring within the six-week period.

3) Pregnancy-related complications after 6 week period

Chapter 15 codes may also be used to describe pregnancy-related complications after the peripartum or postpartum period if the provider documents that a condition is pregnancy related.

> Patient referred for varicose veins. She had a baby boy three months ago; the varicose veins started to appear one month ago. The doctor attributes the patient's pregnancy as the cause of the varicose veins, which continue to be painful and bother the patient. She is seeking surgical relief.
>
> | **O87.4** | **Varicose veins of the lower extremity in the puerperium** |
> |---|---|
>
> *Explanation:* Although the varicose veins occurred several months after the delivery of the newborn, the doctor attributed the varicose veins to pregnancy and therefore a code from chapter 15 is appropriate.

4) Admission for routine postpartum care following delivery outside hospital

When the mother delivers outside the hospital prior to admission and is admitted for routine postpartum care and no complications are noted, code Z39.0, Encounter for care and examination of mother immediately after delivery, should be assigned as the principal diagnosis.

5) Pregnancy associated cardiomyopathy

Pregnancy associated cardiomyopathy, code O90.3, is unique in that it may be diagnosed in the third trimester of pregnancy but may continue to progress months after delivery. For this reason, it is referred to as peripartum cardiomyopathy. Code O90.3 is only for use when the cardiomyopathy develops as a result of pregnancy in a woman who did not have pre-existing heart disease.

p. Code O94, Sequelae of complication of pregnancy, childbirth, and the puerperium

1) Code O94

Code O94, Sequelae of complication of pregnancy, childbirth, and the puerperium, is for use in those cases when an initial complication of a pregnancy develops a sequelae requiring care or treatment at a future date.

2) After the initial postpartum period

This code may be used at any time after the initial postpartum period.

3) Sequencing of code O94

This code, like all sequela codes, is to be sequenced following the code describing the sequelae of the complication.

q. Termination of pregnancy and spontaneous abortions

1) Abortion with Liveborn Fetus

When an attempted termination of pregnancy results in a liveborn fetus, assign code Z33.2, Encounter for elective termination of pregnancy and a code from category Z37, Outcome of Delivery.

2) Retained Products of Conception following an abortion

Subsequent encounters for retained products of conception following a spontaneous abortion or elective termination of pregnancy, without complications are assigned O03.4, Incomplete spontaneous abortion without complication, or code O07.4, Failed attempted termination of pregnancy without complication. This advice is appropriate even when

the patient was discharged previously with a discharge diagnosis of complete abortion. If the patient has a specific complication associated with the spontaneous abortion or elective termination of pregnancy in addition to retained products of conception, assign the appropriate complication **code (e.g., O03.-, O04.-, O07.-)** instead of code O03.4 or O07.4.

> Patient was seen two days ago for complete spontaneous abortion but returns today for urinary tract infection (UTI) with ultrasound showing retained products of conception
>
> **O03.38   Urinary tract infection following incomplete spontaneous abortion**
>
> *Explanation:* Although the diagnosis from the patient's previous stay indicated that the patient had a complete abortion, it is now determined that there were actually retained products of conception (POC). An abortion with retained POC is considered incomplete and in this case resulted in the patient developing a UTI.

3) Complications leading to abortion

Codes from Chapter 15 may be used as additional codes to identify any documented complications of the pregnancy in conjunction with codes in categories in O04, O07 and O08.

r. Abuse in a pregnant patient

For suspected or confirmed cases of abuse of a pregnant patient, a code(s) from subcategories O9A.3, Physical abuse complicating pregnancy, childbirth, and the puerperium, O9A.4, Sexual abuse complicating pregnancy, childbirth, and the puerperium, and O9A.5, Psychological abuse complicating pregnancy, childbirth, and the puerperium, should be sequenced first, followed by the appropriate codes (if applicable) to identify any associated current injury due to physical abuse, sexual abuse, and the perpetrator of abuse.

See Section I.C.19. Adult and child abuse, neglect and other maltreatment.

Chapter 15. Pregnancy, Childbirth and the Puerperium (O00–O9A)

> **NOTE**   CODES FROM THIS CHAPTER ARE FOR USE ONLY ON MATERNAL RECORDS, NEVER ON NEWBORN RECORDS
>
> Codes from this chapter are for use for conditions related to or aggravated by the pregnancy, childbirth, or by the puerperium (maternal causes or obstetric causes)

> **NOTE**   Trimesters are counted from the first day of the last menstrual period. They are defined as follows:
>
> 1st trimester- less than 14 weeks Ø days
>
> 2nd trimester- 14 weeks Ø days to less than 28 weeks Ø days
>
> 3rd trimester- 28 weeks Ø days until delivery

Use additional code from category Z3A, Weeks of gestation, to identify the specific week of the pregnancy, if known.

EXCLUDES 1   *supervision of normal pregnancy (Z34.-)*

EXCLUDES 2   *mental and behavioral disorders associated with the puerperium (F53.-)*
obstetrical tetanus (A34)
postpartum necrosis of pituitary gland (E23.Ø)
puerperal osteomalacia (M83.Ø)

AHA: 2016,1Q,3-5; 2014,3Q,17

This chapter contains the following blocks:

O00-O08   Pregnancy with abortive outcome
O09   Supervision of high risk pregnancy
O10-O16   Edema, proteinuria and hypertensive disorders in pregnancy, childbirth and the puerperium
O20-O29   Other maternal disorders predominantly related to pregnancy
O30-O48   Maternal care related to the fetus and amniotic cavity and possible delivery problems
O60-O77   Complications of labor and delivery
O80-O82   Encounter for delivery
O85-O92   Complications predominantly related to the puerperium
O94-O9A   Other obstetric conditions, not elsewhere classified

Pregnancy with abortive outcome (O00-O08)

EXCLUDES 1   *continuing pregnancy in multiple gestation after abortion of one fetus or more (O31.1-, O31.3-)*

TIP: Do not assign a code from category Z3A with codes in this code block.

✓4ᵗʰ O00 Ectopic pregnancy

INCLUDES   ruptured ectopic pregnancy

Use additional code from category O08 to identify any associated complication

AHA: 2016,4Q,48-50; 2014,3Q,17

DEF: Implantation of a fertilized egg outside the uterus, usually in the fallopian tube or abdomen that requires emergency treatment.

Ectopic Pregnancy

Cornual/interstitial
Isthmic
Ampullar
Tubal (fallopian)
Infundibular
Ovarian
Intraligamentous
Abdominal
Cervical
Intramural/mural

✓5ᵗʰ O00.Ø Abdominal pregnancy

EXCLUDES 1   *maternal care for viable fetus in abdominal pregnancy (O36.7-)*

O00.00   **Abdominal pregnancy** without intrauterine pregnancy   Ⓜ♀
Abdominal pregnancy NOS

O00.01   **Abdominal pregnancy** with intrauterine pregnancy   Ⓜ♀

✓5ᵗʰ O00.1 Tubal pregnancy

Fallopian pregnancy
Rupture of (fallopian) tube due to pregnancy
Tubal abortion
AHA: 2017,4Q,20

✓6ᵗʰ O00.1Ø Tubal pregnancy without intrauterine pregnancy

Tubal pregnancy NOS

O00.101   **Right tubal pregnancy without intrauterine pregnancy**   Ⓜ♀

O00.102   **Left tubal pregnancy without intrauterine pregnancy**   Ⓜ♀

O00.109   **Unspecified tubal pregnancy without intrauterine pregnancy**   Ⓜ♀

✓6ᵗʰ O00.11 Tubal pregnancy with intrauterine pregnancy

O00.111   **Right tubal pregnancy with intrauterine pregnancy**   Ⓜ♀

O00.112   **Left tubal pregnancy with intrauterine pregnancy**   Ⓜ♀

O00.119   **Unspecified tubal pregnancy with intrauterine pregnancy**   Ⓜ♀

✓5ᵗʰ O00.2 Ovarian pregnancy

AHA: 2017,4Q,20

✓6ᵗʰ O00.2Ø Ovarian pregnancy without intrauterine pregnancy

Ovarian pregnancy NOS

O00.201   **Right ovarian pregnancy without intrauterine pregnancy**   Ⓜ♀

O00.202   **Left ovarian pregnancy without intrauterine pregnancy**   Ⓜ♀

O00.209   **Unspecified ovarian pregnancy without intrauterine pregnancy**   Ⓜ♀

✓6ᵗʰ O00.21 Ovarian pregnancy with intrauterine pregnancy

O00.211   **Right ovarian pregnancy with intrauterine pregnancy**   Ⓜ♀

O00.212   **Left ovarian pregnancy with intrauterine pregnancy**   Ⓜ♀

O00.219   **Unspecified ovarian pregnancy with intrauterine pregnancy**   Ⓜ♀

✓5ᵗʰ O00.8 Other ectopic pregnancy

Cervical pregnancy
Cornual pregnancy
Intraligamentous pregnancy
Mural pregnancy

O00.80   **Other ectopic pregnancy** without intrauterine pregnancy   ⓆⓂ♀
Other ectopic pregnancy NOS

O00.81   **Other ectopic pregnancy** with intrauterine pregnancy   ⓆⓂ♀

✓5ᵗʰ O00.9 Ectopic pregnancy, unspecified

O00.90   **Unspecified ectopic pregnancy** without intrauterine pregnancy   ⓆⓂ♀
Ectopic pregnancy NOS

O00.91   **Unspecified ectopic pregnancy** with intrauterine pregnancy   ⓆⓂ♀

✓4ᵗʰ O01 Hydatidiform mole

Use additional code from category O08 to identify any associated complication

EXCLUDES 1   *chorioadenoma (destruens) (D39.2)*
malignant hydatidiform mole (D39.2)

AHA: 2014,3Q,17

DEF: Abnormal product of pregnancy, marked by a mass of cysts resembling a bunch of grapes due to chorionic villi proliferation and dissolution. It must be surgically removed.

O01.Ø   **Classical hydatidiform mole**   Ⓜ♀
Complete hydatidiform mole

O01.1   **Incomplete and partial hydatidiform mole**   Ⓜ♀

O01.9   **Hydatidiform mole, unspecified**   Ⓜ♀
Trophoblastic disease NOS
Vesicular mole NOS

☑ Additional Character Required   ✓x7ᵗʰ Placeholder Alert   Manifestation   Unspecified Dx   ▶◀ Revised Text   ● New Code   ▲ Revised Code Title

✓4ᵗʰ **O02 Other abnormal products of conception**

Use additional code from category O08 to identify any associated complication

EXCLUDES 1   *papyraceous fetus (O31.0-)*

AHA: 2014,3Q,17

O02.0 Blighted ovum and nonhydatidiform mole   Ⓜ ♀

Carneous mole
Fleshy mole
Intrauterine mole NOS
Molar pregnancy NEC
Pathological ovum

O02.1 Missed abortion   Ⓠ Ⓜ ♀

Early fetal death, before completion of 20 weeks of gestation, with retention of dead fetus

EXCLUDES 1   *failed induced abortion (O07.-)*
fetal death (intrauterine) (late) (O36.4)
missed abortion with blighted ovum (O02.0)
missed abortion with hydatidiform mole (O01.-)
missed abortion with nonhydatidiform (O02.0)
missed abortion with other abnormal products of conception (O02.8-)
missed delivery (O36.4)
stillbirth (P95)

✓5ᵗʰ **O02.8 Other specified abnormal products of conception**

EXCLUDES 1   *abnormal products of conception with blighted ovum (O02.0)*
abnormal products of conception with hydatidiform mole (O01.-)
abnormal products of conception with nonhydatidiform mole (O02.0)

O02.81 Inappropriate change in quantitative human chorionic gonadotropin (hCG) in early pregnancy   Ⓜ ♀

Biochemical pregnancy
Chemical pregnancy
Inappropriate level of quantitative human chorionic gonadotropin (hCG) for gestational age in early pregnancy

O02.89 Other abnormal products of conception   Ⓜ ♀

O02.9 Abnormal product of conception, unspecified   Ⓜ ♀

✓4ᵗʰ **O03 Spontaneous abortion**

NOTE   Incomplete abortion includes retained products of conception following spontaneous abortion

INCLUDES   miscarriage

O03.0 Genital tract and pelvic infection following incomplete spontaneous abortion   Ⓜ ♀

Endometritis following incomplete spontaneous abortion
Oophoritis following incomplete spontaneous abortion
Parametritis following incomplete spontaneous abortion
Pelvic peritonitis following incomplete spontaneous abortion
Salpingitis following incomplete spontaneous abortion
Salpingo-oophoritis following incomplete spontaneous abortion

EXCLUDES 1   *sepsis following incomplete spontaneous abortion (O03.37)*
urinary tract infection following incomplete spontaneous abortion (O03.38)

O03.1 Delayed or excessive hemorrhage following incomplete spontaneous abortion   Ⓠ Ⓜ ♀

Afibrinogenemia following incomplete spontaneous abortion
Defibrination syndrome following incomplete spontaneous abortion
Hemolysis following incomplete spontaneous abortion
Intravascular coagulation following incomplete spontaneous abortion

O03.2 Embolism following incomplete spontaneous abortion   Ⓜ ♀

Air embolism following incomplete spontaneous abortion
Amniotic fluid embolism following incomplete spontaneous abortion
Blood-clot embolism following incomplete spontaneous abortion
Embolism NOS following incomplete spontaneous abortion
Fat embolism following incomplete spontaneous abortion
Pulmonary embolism following incomplete spontaneous abortion
Pyemic embolism following incomplete spontaneous abortion
Septic or septicopyemic embolism following incomplete spontaneous abortion
Soap embolism following incomplete spontaneous abortion

✓5ᵗʰ **O03.3 Other and unspecified complications following incomplete spontaneous abortion**

O03.30 Unspecified complication following incomplete spontaneous abortion   Ⓜ ♀

O03.31 Shock following incomplete spontaneous abortion   Ⓜ ♀

Circulatory collapse following incomplete spontaneous abortion
Shock (postprocedural) following incomplete spontaneous abortion

EXCLUDES 1   *shock due to infection following incomplete spontaneous abortion (O03.37)*

O03.32 Renal failure following incomplete spontaneous abortion   Ⓜ ♀

Kidney failure (acute) following incomplete spontaneous abortion
Oliguria following incomplete spontaneous abortion
Renal shutdown following incomplete spontaneous abortion
Renal tubular necrosis following incomplete spontaneous abortion
Uremia following incomplete spontaneous abortion

O03.33 Metabolic disorder following incomplete spontaneous abortion   Ⓜ ♀

O03.34 Damage to pelvic organs following incomplete spontaneous abortion   Ⓜ ♀

Laceration, perforation, tear or chemical damage of bladder following incomplete spontaneous abortion
Laceration, perforation, tear or chemical damage of bowel following incomplete spontaneous abortion
Laceration, perforation, tear or chemical damage of broad ligament following incomplete spontaneous abortion
Laceration, perforation, tear or chemical damage of cervix following incomplete spontaneous abortion
Laceration, perforation, tear or chemical damage of periurethral tissue following incomplete spontaneous abortion
Laceration, perforation, tear or chemical damage of uterus following incomplete spontaneous abortion
Laceration, perforation, tear or chemical damage of vagina following incomplete spontaneous abortion

O03.35 Other venous complications following incomplete spontaneous abortion   Ⓜ ♀

O03.36 Cardiac arrest following incomplete spontaneous abortion   Ⓜ ♀

O03.37 Sepsis following incomplete spontaneous abortion   Ⓜ ♀

Use additional code to identify infectious agent (B95-B97)
Use additional code to identify severe sepsis, if applicable (R65.2-)

EXCLUDES 1   *septic or septicopyemic embolism following incomplete spontaneous abortion (O03.2)*

O03.38 **Urinary tract infection following** M ♀
incomplete **spontaneous abortion**
Cystitis following incomplete spontaneous abortion

O03.39 **Incomplete spontaneous abortion with** M ♀
other complications

O03.4 **Incomplete spontaneous abortion without** M ♀
complication

O03.5 **Genital tract and pelvic infection following** M ♀
complete or unspecified spontaneous abortion
Endometritis following complete or unspecified spontaneous
abortion
Oophoritis following complete or unspecified spontaneous
abortion
Parametritis following complete or unspecified spontaneous
abortion
Pelvic peritonitis following complete or unspecified
spontaneous abortion
Salpingitis following complete or unspecified spontaneous
abortion
Salpingo-oophoritis following complete or unspecified
spontaneous abortion
> **EXCLUDES 1** *sepsis following complete or unspecified spontaneous*
> *abortion (O03.87)*
> *urinary tract infection following complete or*
> *unspecified spontaneous abortion (O03.88)*

O03.6 **Delayed or excessive hemorrhage following** ᴼ M ♀
complete or unspecified spontaneous abortion
Afibrinogenemia following complete or unspecified
spontaneous abortion
Defibrination syndrome following complete or unspecified
spontaneous abortion
Hemolysis following complete or unspecified spontaneous
abortion
Intravascular coagulation following complete or unspecified
spontaneous abortion

O03.7 **Embolism following complete or unspecified** M ♀
spontaneous abortion
Air embolism following complete or unspecified spontaneous
abortion
Amniotic fluid embolism following complete or unspecified
spontaneous abortion
Blood-clot embolism following complete or unspecified
spontaneous abortion
Embolism NOS following complete or unspecified spontaneous
abortion
Fat embolism following complete or unspecified spontaneous
abortion
Pulmonary embolism following complete or unspecified
spontaneous abortion
Pyemic embolism following complete or unspecified
spontaneous abortion
Septic or septicopyemic embolism following complete or
unspecified spontaneous abortion
Soap embolism following complete or unspecified spontaneous
abortion

✔5ᵗʰ **O03.8** **Other and unspecified complications following complete or**
unspecified spontaneous abortion
O03.80 **Unspecified complication following** M ♀
complete or unspecified spontaneous
abortion

O03.81 **Shock following complete or unspecified** M ♀
spontaneous abortion
Circulatory collapse following complete or unspecified
spontaneous abortion
Shock (postprocedural) following complete or
unspecified spontaneous abortion
> **EXCLUDES 1** *shock due to infection following complete*
> *or unspecified spontaneous abortion*
> *(O03.87)*

O03.82 **Renal failure following complete or** M ♀
unspecified spontaneous abortion
Kidney failure (acute) following complete or
unspecified spontaneous abortion
Oliguria following complete or unspecified
spontaneous abortion
Renal shutdown following complete or unspecified
spontaneous abortion
Renal tubular necrosis following complete or
unspecified spontaneous abortion
Uremia following complete or unspecified
spontaneous abortion

O03.83 **Metabolic disorder following complete or** M ♀
unspecified spontaneous abortion

O03.84 **Damage to pelvic organs following** M ♀
complete or unspecified spontaneous
abortion
Laceration, perforation, tear or chemical damage of
bladder following complete or unspecified
spontaneous abortion
Laceration, perforation, tear or chemical damage of
bowel following complete or unspecified
spontaneous abortion
Laceration, perforation, tear or chemical damage of
broad ligament following complete or
unspecified spontaneous abortion
Laceration, perforation, tear or chemical damage of
cervix following complete or unspecified
spontaneous abortion
Laceration, perforation, tear or chemical damage of
periurethral tissue following complete or
unspecified spontaneous abortion
Laceration, perforation, tear or chemical damage of
uterus following complete or unspecified
spontaneous abortion
Laceration, perforation, tear or chemical damage of
vagina following complete or unspecified
spontaneous abortion

O03.85 **Other venous complications following** M ♀
complete or unspecified spontaneous
abortion

O03.86 **Cardiac arrest following complete or** M ♀
unspecified spontaneous abortion

O03.87 **Sepsis following complete or unspecified** M ♀
spontaneous abortion
Use additional code to identify infectious agent
(B95-B97)
Use additional code to identify severe sepsis, if
applicable (R65.2-)
> **EXCLUDES 1** *septic or septicopyemic embolism*
> *following complete or unspecified*
> *spontaneous abortion (O03.7)*

O03.88 **Urinary tract infection following complete** M ♀
or unspecified spontaneous abortion
Cystitis following complete or unspecified
spontaneous abortion

O03.89 **Complete or unspecified spontaneous** M ♀
abortion with other complications

O03.9 **Complete or unspecified spontaneous abortion** M ♀
without complication
Miscarriage NOS
Spontaneous abortion NOS

✓4ᵗʰ **O04 Complications following (induced) termination of pregnancy**

    INCLUDES   complications following (induced) termination of pregnancy

    EXCLUDES 1   encounter for elective termination of pregnancy, uncomplicated (Z33.2)

      failed attempted termination of pregnancy (O07.-)

O04.5 Genital tract and pelvic infection following (induced) termination of pregnancy Ⓜ♀

    Endometritis following (induced) termination of pregnancy

    Oophoritis following (induced) termination of pregnancy

    Parametritis following (induced) termination of pregnancy

    Pelvic peritonitis following (induced) termination of pregnancy

    Salpingitis following (induced) termination of pregnancy

    Salpingo-oophoritis following (induced) termination of pregnancy

    EXCLUDES 1   sepsis following (induced) termination of pregnancy (O04.87)

      urinary tract infection following (induced) termination of pregnancy (O04.88)

O04.6 Delayed or excessive hemorrhage following (induced) termination of pregnancy Ⓠ Ⓜ♀

    Afibrinogenemia following (induced) termination of pregnancy

    Defibrination syndrome following (induced) termination of pregnancy

    Hemolysis following (induced) termination of pregnancy

    Intravascular coagulation following (induced) termination of pregnancy

O04.7 Embolism following (induced) termination of pregnancy Ⓜ♀

    Air embolism following (induced) termination of pregnancy

    Amniotic fluid embolism following (induced) termination of pregnancy

    Blood-clot embolism following (induced) termination of pregnancy

    Embolism NOS following (induced) termination of pregnancy

    Fat embolism following (induced) termination of pregnancy

    Pulmonary embolism following (induced) termination of pregnancy

    Pyemic embolism following (induced) termination of pregnancy

    Septic or septicopyemic embolism following (induced) termination of pregnancy

    Soap embolism following (induced) termination of pregnancy

✓5ᵗʰ **O04.8 (Induced) termination of pregnancy with other and unspecified complications**

    O04.80 (Induced) termination of pregnancy with unspecified complications Ⓜ♀

    O04.81 Shock following (induced) termination of pregnancy Ⓜ♀

      Circulatory collapse following (induced) termination of pregnancy

      Shock (postprocedural) following (induced) termination of pregnancy

      EXCLUDES 1   shock due to infection following (induced) termination of pregnancy (O04.87)

    O04.82 Renal failure following (induced) termination of pregnancy Ⓜ♀

      Kidney failure (acute) following (induced) termination of pregnancy

      Oliguria following (induced) termination of pregnancy

      Renal shutdown following (induced) termination of pregnancy

      Renal tubular necrosis following (induced) termination of pregnancy

      Uremia following (induced) termination of pregnancy

    O04.83 Metabolic disorder following (induced) termination of pregnancy Ⓜ♀

O04.84 Damage to pelvic organs following (induced) termination of pregnancy Ⓜ♀

    Laceration, perforation, tear or chemical damage of bladder following (induced) termination of pregnancy

    Laceration, perforation, tear or chemical damage of bowel following (induced) termination of pregnancy

    Laceration, perforation, tear or chemical damage of broad ligament following (induced) termination of pregnancy

    Laceration, perforation, tear or chemical damage of cervix following (induced) termination of pregnancy

    Laceration, perforation, tear or chemical damage of periurethral tissue following (induced) termination of pregnancy

    Laceration, perforation, tear or chemical damage of uterus following (induced) termination of pregnancy

    Laceration, perforation, tear or chemical damage of vagina following (induced) termination of pregnancy

O04.85 Other venous complications following (induced) termination of pregnancy Ⓜ♀

O04.86 Cardiac arrest following (induced) termination of pregnancy Ⓜ♀

O04.87 Sepsis following (induced) termination of pregnancy Ⓜ♀

    Use additional code to identify infectious agent (B95-B97)

    Use additional code to identify severe sepsis, if applicable (R65.2-)

    EXCLUDES 1   septic or septicopyemic embolism following (induced) termination of pregnancy (O04.7)

O04.88 Urinary tract infection following (induced) termination of pregnancy Ⓜ♀

    Cystitis following (induced) termination of pregnancy

O04.89 (Induced) termination of pregnancy with other complications Ⓜ♀

✓4ᵗʰ **O07 Failed attempted termination of pregnancy**

    INCLUDES   failure of attempted induction of termination of pregnancy

      incomplete elective abortion

    EXCLUDES 1   incomplete spontaneous abortion (O03.0-)

O07.0 Genital tract and pelvic infection following failed attempted termination of pregnancy Ⓜ♀

    Endometritis following failed attempted termination of pregnancy

    Oophoritis following failed attempted termination of pregnancy

    Parametritis following failed attempted termination of pregnancy

    Pelvic peritonitis following failed attempted termination of pregnancy

    Salpingitis following failed attempted termination of pregnancy

    Salpingo-oophoritis following failed attempted termination of pregnancy

    EXCLUDES 1   sepsis following failed attempted termination of pregnancy (O07.37)

      urinary tract infection following failed attempted termination of pregnancy (O07.38)

O07.1 Delayed or excessive hemorrhage following failed attempted termination of pregnancy Ⓠ Ⓜ♀

    Afibrinogenemia following failed attempted termination of pregnancy

    Defibrination syndrome following failed attempted termination of pregnancy

    Hemolysis following failed attempted termination of pregnancy

    Intravascular coagulation following failed attempted termination of pregnancy

O07.2 **Embolism following failed attempted termination** Ⓜ ♀
of pregnancy
    Air embolism following failed attempted termination of
      pregnancy
    Amniotic fluid embolism following failed attempted termination
      of pregnancy
    Blood-clot embolism following failed attempted termination
      of pregnancy
    Embolism NOS following failed attempted termination of
      pregnancy
    Fat embolism following failed attempted termination of
      pregnancy
    Pulmonary embolism following failed attempted termination
      of pregnancy
    Pyemic embolism following failed attempted termination of
      pregnancy
    Septic or septicopyemic embolism following failed attempted
      termination of pregnancy
    Soap embolism following failed attempted termination of
      pregnancy

✓5ᵗʰ **O07.3** **Failed attempted termination of pregnancy with other and**
unspecified complications

    O07.30 **Failed attempted termination of** Ⓜ ♀
        pregnancy with unspecified complications

    O07.31 **Shock following failed attempted** Ⓜ ♀
        termination of pregnancy
        Circulatory collapse following failed attempted
          termination of pregnancy
        Shock (postprocedural) following failed attempted
          termination of pregnancy
        EXCLUDES 1   *shock due to infection following failed*
              attempted termination of pregnancy
              (O07.37)

    O07.32 **Renal failure following failed attempted** Ⓜ ♀
        termination of pregnancy
        Kidney failure (acute) following failed attempted
          termination of pregnancy
        Oliguria following failed attempted termination of
          pregnancy
        Renal shutdown following failed attempted
          termination of pregnancy
        Renal tubular necrosis following failed attempted
          termination of pregnancy
        Uremia following failed attempted termination of
          pregnancy

    O07.33 **Metabolic disorder following failed** Ⓜ ♀
        attempted termination of pregnancy

    O07.34 **Damage to pelvic organs following failed** Ⓜ ♀
        attempted termination of pregnancy
        Laceration, perforation, tear or chemical damage of
          bladder following failed attempted termination
          of pregnancy
        Laceration, perforation, tear or chemical damage of
          bowel following failed attempted termination
          of pregnancy
        Laceration, perforation, tear or chemical damage of
          broad ligament following failed attempted
          termination of pregnancy
        Laceration, perforation, tear or chemical damage of
          cervix following failed attempted termination
          of pregnancy
        Laceration, perforation, tear or chemical damage of
          periurethral tissue following failed attempted
          termination of pregnancy
        Laceration, perforation, tear or chemical damage of
          uterus following failed attempted termination
          of pregnancy
        Laceration, perforation, tear or chemical damage of
          vagina following failed attempted termination
          of pregnancy

    O07.35 **Other venous complications following** Ⓜ ♀
        failed attempted termination of
        pregnancy

    O07.36 **Cardiac arrest following failed attempted** Ⓜ ♀
        termination of pregnancy

    O07.37 **Sepsis following failed attempted** Ⓜ ♀
        termination of pregnancy
        Use additional code (B95-B97), to identify infectious
          agent
        Use additional code (R65.2-) to identify severe sepsis,
          if applicable
        EXCLUDES 1   *septic or septicopyemic embolism*
              following failed attempted
              termination of pregnancy (O07.2)

    O07.38 **Urinary tract infection following failed** Ⓜ ♀
        attempted termination of pregnancy
        Cystitis following failed attempted termination of
          pregnancy

    O07.39 **Failed attempted termination of** Ⓜ ♀
        pregnancy with other complications

   O07.4 **Failed attempted termination of pregnancy** without Ⓜ ♀
   complication

✓4ᵗʰ **O08** **Complications following ectopic and molar pregnancy**
   This category is for use with categories O00-O02 to identify any
   associated complications

   O08.0 **Genital tract and pelvic infection following ectopic** Ⓜ ♀
   and molar pregnancy
      Endometritis following ectopic and molar pregnancy
      Oophoritis following ectopic and molar pregnancy
      Parametritis following ectopic and molar pregnancy
      Pelvic peritonitis following ectopic and molar pregnancy
      Salpingitis following ectopic and molar pregnancy
      Salpingo-oophoritis following ectopic and molar pregnancy
      EXCLUDES 1   *sepsis following ectopic and molar pregnancy*
             (O08.82)
            urinary tract infection (O08.83)

   O08.1 **Delayed or excessive hemorrhage following ectopic** ⓞ Ⓜ ♀
   and molar pregnancy
      Afibrinogenemia following ectopic and molar pregnancy
      Defibrination syndrome following ectopic and molar pregnancy
      Hemolysis following ectopic and molar pregnancy
      Intravascular coagulation following ectopic and molar
        pregnancy
      EXCLUDES 1   *delayed or excessive hemorrhage due to incomplete*
             abortion (O03.1)

   O08.2 **Embolism following ectopic and molar pregnancy** Ⓜ ♀
      Air embolism following ectopic and molar pregnancy
      Amniotic fluid embolism following ectopic and molar pregnancy
      Blood-clot embolism following ectopic and molar pregnancy
      Embolism NOS following ectopic and molar pregnancy
      Fat embolism following ectopic and molar pregnancy
      Pulmonary embolism following ectopic and molar pregnancy
      Pyemic embolism following ectopic and molar pregnancy
      Septic or septicopyemic embolism following ectopic and molar
        pregnancy
      Soap embolism following ectopic and molar pregnancy

   O08.3 **Shock following ectopic and molar pregnancy** Ⓜ ♀
      Circulatory collapse following ectopic and molar pregnancy
      Shock (postprocedural) following ectopic and molar pregnancy
      EXCLUDES 1   *shock due to infection following ectopic and molar*
             pregnancy (O08.82)

   O08.4 **Renal failure following ectopic and molar** Ⓜ ♀
   pregnancy
      Kidney failure (acute) following ectopic and molar pregnancy
      Oliguria following ectopic and molar pregnancy
      Renal shutdown following ectopic and molar pregnancy
      Renal tubular necrosis following ectopic and molar pregnancy
      Uremia following ectopic and molar pregnancy

   O08.5 **Metabolic disorders following an ectopic and molar** Ⓜ ♀
   pregnancy

Chapter 15. Pregnancy, Childbirth and the Puerperium

O08.6   **Damage to pelvic organs and tissues following an ectopic and molar pregnancy**   Ⓜ♀

    Laceration, perforation, tear or chemical damage of bladder following an ectopic and molar pregnancy

    Laceration, perforation, tear or chemical damage of bowel following an ectopic and molar pregnancy

    Laceration, perforation, tear or chemical damage of broad ligament following an ectopic and molar pregnancy

    Laceration, perforation, tear or chemical damage of cervix following an ectopic and molar pregnancy

    Laceration, perforation, tear or chemical damage of periurethral tissue following an ectopic and molar pregnancy

    Laceration, perforation, tear or chemical damage of uterus following an ectopic and molar pregnancy

    Laceration, perforation, tear or chemical damage of vagina following an ectopic and molar pregnancy

O08.7   **Other venous complications following an ectopic and molar pregnancy**   Ⓜ♀

√5ᵗʰ **O08.8**   **Other complications following an ectopic and molar pregnancy**

   O08.81   **Cardiac arrest following an ectopic and molar pregnancy**   Ⓜ♀

   O08.82   **Sepsis following ectopic and molar pregnancy**   Ⓜ♀

     Use additional code (B95-B97), to identify infectious agent

     Use additional code (R65.2-) to identify severe sepsis, if applicable

     EXCLUDES 1   *septic or septicopyemic embolism following ectopic and molar pregnancy (O08.2)*

   O08.83   **Urinary tract infection following an ectopic and molar pregnancy**   Ⓜ♀

     Cystitis following an ectopic and molar pregnancy

   O08.89   **Other complications following an ectopic and molar pregnancy**   Ⓜ♀

O08.9   **Unspecified complication following an ectopic and molar pregnancy**   Ⓜ♀

Supervision of high risk pregnancy (O09)

√4ᵗʰ **O09**   **Supervision of high risk pregnancy**

   AHA: 2016,4Q,48-50,150

√5ᵗʰ **O09.0**   **Supervision of pregnancy with history of infertility**

     DEF: Infertility: Inability to conceive for at least one year with regular intercourse.

   O09.00   **Supervision of pregnancy with history of infertility, unspecified trimester**   Ⓜ♀

   O09.01   **Supervision of pregnancy with history of infertility, first trimester**   Ⓜ♀

   O09.02   **Supervision of pregnancy with history of infertility, second trimester**   Ⓜ♀

   O09.03   **Supervision of pregnancy with history of infertility, third trimester**   Ⓜ♀

√5ᵗʰ **O09.1**   **Supervision of pregnancy with history of ectopic pregnancy**

     DEF: Ectopic pregnancy: Implantation of a fertilized egg outside the uterus, usually in the fallopian tube or abdomen that requires emergency treatment.

   O09.10   **Supervision of pregnancy with history of ectopic pregnancy, unspecified trimester**   Ⓜ♀

   O09.11   **Supervision of pregnancy with history of ectopic pregnancy, first trimester**   Ⓜ♀

   O09.12   **Supervision of pregnancy with history of ectopic pregnancy, second trimester**   Ⓜ♀

   O09.13   **Supervision of pregnancy with history of ectopic pregnancy, third trimester**   Ⓜ♀

√5ᵗʰ **O09.A**   **Supervision of pregnancy with history of molar pregnancy**

     DEF: Molar pregnancy: Trophoblastic neoplasm that mimics pregnancy by proliferating from a pathologic ovum and resulting only in a mass of cysts resembling grapes, 80 percent of which are benign, but require surgical removal.

   O09.A0   **Supervision of pregnancy with history of molar pregnancy, unspecified trimester**   Ⓜ♀

   O09.A1   **Supervision of pregnancy with history of molar pregnancy, first trimester**   Ⓜ♀

   O09.A2   **Supervision of pregnancy with history of molar pregnancy, second trimester**   Ⓜ♀

   O09.A3   **Supervision of pregnancy with history of molar pregnancy, third trimester**   Ⓜ♀

√5ᵗʰ **O09.2**   **Supervision of pregnancy with other poor reproductive or obstetric history**

     EXCLUDES 2   *pregnancy care for patient with history of recurrent pregnancy loss (O26.2-)*

√6ᵗʰ **O09.21**   **Supervision of pregnancy with history of pre-term labor**

   O09.211   **Supervision of pregnancy with history of pre-term labor, first trimester**   Ⓜ♀

   O09.212   **Supervision of pregnancy with history of pre-term labor, second trimester**   Ⓜ♀

   O09.213   **Supervision of pregnancy with history of pre-term labor, third trimester**   Ⓜ♀

   O09.219   **Supervision of pregnancy with history of pre-term labor, unspecified trimester**   Ⓜ♀

√6ᵗʰ **O09.29**   **Supervision of pregnancy with other poor reproductive or obstetric history**

     Supervision of pregnancy with history of neonatal death

     Supervision of pregnancy with history of stillbirth

   O09.291   **Supervision of pregnancy with other poor reproductive or obstetric history, first trimester**   Ⓜ♀

   O09.292   **Supervision of pregnancy with other poor reproductive or obstetric history, second trimester**   Ⓜ♀

   O09.293   **Supervision of pregnancy with other poor reproductive or obstetric history, third trimester**   Ⓜ♀

   O09.299   **Supervision of pregnancy with other poor reproductive or obstetric history, unspecified trimester**   Ⓜ♀

√5ᵗʰ **O09.3**   **Supervision of pregnancy with insufficient antenatal care**

     Supervision of concealed pregnancy

     Supervision of hidden pregnancy

   O09.30   **Supervision of pregnancy with insufficient antenatal care, unspecified trimester**   Ⓜ♀

   O09.31   **Supervision of pregnancy with insufficient antenatal care, first trimester**   Ⓜ♀

   O09.32   **Supervision of pregnancy with insufficient antenatal care, second trimester**   Ⓜ♀

   O09.33   **Supervision of pregnancy with insufficient antenatal care, third trimester**   Ⓜ♀

√5ᵗʰ **O09.4**   **Supervision of pregnancy with grand multiparity**

   O09.40   **Supervision of pregnancy with grand multiparity, unspecified trimester**   Ⓜ♀

   O09.41   **Supervision of pregnancy with grand multiparity, first trimester**   Ⓜ♀

   O09.42   **Supervision of pregnancy with grand multiparity, second trimester**   Ⓜ♀

   O09.43   **Supervision of pregnancy with grand multiparity, third trimester**   Ⓜ♀

√5ᵗʰ **O09.5**   **Supervision of elderly primigravida and multigravida**

     Pregnancy for a female 35 years and older at expected date of delivery

√6ᵗʰ **O09.51**   **Supervision of elderly primigravida**

   O09.511   **Supervision of elderly primigravida, first trimester**   Ⓜ♀

   O09.512   **Supervision of elderly primigravida, second trimester**   Ⓜ♀

   O09.513   **Supervision of elderly primigravida, third trimester**   Ⓜ♀

   O09.519   **Supervision of elderly primigravida, unspecified trimester**   Ⓜ♀

√6ᵗʰ **O09.52**   **Supervision of elderly multigravida**

   O09.521   **Supervision of elderly multigravida, first trimester**   Ⓜ♀

   O09.522   **Supervision of elderly multigravida, second trimester**   Ⓜ♀

   O09.523   **Supervision of elderly multigravida, third trimester**   Ⓜ♀

   O09.529   **Supervision of elderly multigravida, unspecified trimester**   Ⓜ♀

☑5ᵗʰ **O09.6 Supervision of** young primigravida and multigravida
    Supervision of pregnancy for a female less than 16 years old at expected date of delivery

  ☑6ᵗʰ **O09.61 Supervision of** young primigravida
      O09.611 Supervision of young primigravida, first trimester   Ⓜ♀
      O09.612 Supervision of young primigravida, second trimester   Ⓜ♀
      O09.613 Supervision of young primigravida, third trimester   Ⓜ♀
      O09.619 Supervision of young primigravida, unspecified trimester   Ⓜ♀

  ☑6ᵗʰ **O09.62 Supervision of** young multigravida
      O09.621 Supervision of young multigravida, first trimester   Ⓜ♀
      O09.622 Supervision of young multigravida, second trimester   Ⓜ♀
      O09.623 Supervision of young multigravida, third trimester   Ⓜ♀
      O09.629 Supervision of young multigravida, unspecified trimester   Ⓜ♀

☑5ᵗʰ **O09.7 Supervision of high risk pregnancy due to** social problems
    O09.70 Supervision of high risk pregnancy due to social problems, unspecified trimester   Ⓜ♀
    O09.71 Supervision of high risk pregnancy due to social problems, first trimester   Ⓜ♀
    O09.72 Supervision of high risk pregnancy due to social problems, second trimester   Ⓜ♀
    O09.73 Supervision of high risk pregnancy due to social problems, third trimester   Ⓜ♀

☑5ᵗʰ **O09.8 Supervision of other high risk pregnancies**
  ☑6ᵗʰ **O09.81 Supervision of pregnancy** resulting from assisted reproductive technology
    Supervision of pregnancy resulting from in-vitro fertilization
    EXCLUDES 2   gestational carrier status (Z33.3)
      O09.811 Supervision of pregnancy resulting from assisted reproductive technology, first trimester   Ⓜ♀
      O09.812 Supervision of pregnancy resulting from assisted reproductive technology, second trimester   Ⓜ♀
      O09.813 Supervision of pregnancy resulting from assisted reproductive technology, third trimester   Ⓜ♀
      O09.819 Supervision of pregnancy resulting from assisted reproductive technology, unspecified trimester   Ⓜ♀

  ☑6ᵗʰ **O09.82 Supervision of pregnancy with** history of in utero procedure during previous pregnancy
      O09.821 Supervision of pregnancy with history of in utero procedure during previous pregnancy, first trimester   Ⓜ♀
      O09.822 Supervision of pregnancy with history of in utero procedure during previous pregnancy, second trimester   Ⓜ♀
      O09.823 Supervision of pregnancy with history of in utero procedure during previous pregnancy, third trimester   Ⓜ♀
      O09.829 Supervision of pregnancy with history of in utero procedure during previous pregnancy, unspecified trimester   Ⓜ♀
        EXCLUDES 1   supervision of pregnancy affected by in utero procedure during current pregnancy (O35.7)

  ☑6ᵗʰ **O09.89 Supervision of other high risk pregnancies**
      O09.891 Supervision of other high risk pregnancies, first trimester   Ⓜ♀
      O09.892 Supervision of other high risk pregnancies, second trimester   Ⓜ♀

      O09.893 Supervision of other high risk pregnancies, third trimester   Ⓜ♀
      O09.899 Supervision of other high risk pregnancies, unspecified trimester   Ⓜ♀

☑5ᵗʰ **O09.9 Supervision of high risk pregnancy, unspecified**
    O09.90 Supervision of high risk pregnancy, unspecified, unspecified trimester   Ⓜ♀
    O09.91 Supervision of high risk pregnancy, unspecified, first trimester   Ⓜ♀
    O09.92 Supervision of high risk pregnancy, unspecified, second trimester   Ⓜ♀
    O09.93 Supervision of high risk pregnancy, unspecified, third trimester   Ⓜ♀

Edema, proteinuria and hypertensive disorders in pregnancy, childbirth and the puerperium (O10-O16)

AHA: 2016,4Q,50

☑4ᵗʰ **O10 Pre-existing** hypertension complicating pregnancy, childbirth and the puerperium
    INCLUDES   pre-existing hypertension with pre-existing proteinuria complicating pregnancy, childbirth and the puerperium
    EXCLUDES 2   pre-existing hypertension with superimposed pre-eclampsia complicating pregnancy, childbirth and the puerperium (O11.-)

  ☑5ᵗʰ **O10.0 Pre-existing** essential hypertension complicating pregnancy, childbirth and the puerperium
    Any condition in I10 specified as a reason for obstetric care during pregnancy, childbirth or the puerperium

    ☑6ᵗʰ **O10.01 Pre-existing essential hypertension complicating** pregnancy
      O10.011 Pre-existing essential hypertension complicating pregnancy, first trimester   Ⓜ♀
      O10.012 Pre-existing essential hypertension complicating pregnancy, second trimester   Ⓜ♀
      O10.013 Pre-existing essential hypertension complicating pregnancy, third trimester   Ⓜ♀
      O10.019 Pre-existing essential hypertension complicating pregnancy, unspecified trimester   Ⓜ♀

    O10.02 Pre-existing essential hypertension complicating childbirth   Ⓜ♀
    O10.03 Pre-existing essential hypertension complicating the puerperium   Ⓜ♀

  ☑5ᵗʰ **O10.1 Pre-existing hypertensive** heart disease **complicating pregnancy, childbirth and the puerperium**
    Any condition in I11 specified as a reason for obstetric care during pregnancy, childbirth or the puerperium
    Use additional code from I11 to identify the type of hypertensive heart disease

    ☑6ᵗʰ **O10.11 Pre-existing hypertensive heart disease complicating** pregnancy
      O10.111 Pre-existing hypertensive heart disease complicating pregnancy, first trimester   Ⓜ♀
      O10.112 Pre-existing hypertensive heart disease complicating pregnancy, second trimester   Ⓜ♀
      O10.113 Pre-existing hypertensive heart disease complicating pregnancy, third trimester   Ⓜ♀
      O10.119 Pre-existing hypertensive heart disease complicating pregnancy, unspecified trimester   Ⓜ♀

    O10.12 Pre-existing hypertensive heart disease complicating childbirth   Ⓜ♀
    O10.13 Pre-existing hypertensive heart disease complicating the puerperium   Ⓜ♀

☑ Additional Character Required   ☑xⓣ Placeholder Alert   Manifestation   Unspecified Dx   ►◄ Revised Text   ● New Code   ▲ Revised Code Title

Chapter 15. Pregnancy, Childbirth and the Puerperium

O10.2–O12.25

√5ᵗʰ **O10.2** **Pre-existing hypertensive** chronic kidney disease **complicating pregnancy, childbirth and the puerperium**
    Any condition in I12 specified as a reason for obstetric care during pregnancy, childbirth or the puerperium
    Use additional code from I12 to identify the type of hypertensive chronic kidney disease

  √6ᵗʰ **O10.21** **Pre-existing hypertensive chronic kidney disease complicating** pregnancy

      O10.211 **Pre-existing hypertensive chronic kidney disease complicating pregnancy, first trimester** Ⓜ♀

      O10.212 **Pre-existing hypertensive chronic kidney disease complicating pregnancy, second trimester** Ⓜ♀

      O10.213 **Pre-existing hypertensive chronic kidney disease complicating pregnancy, third trimester** Ⓜ♀

      O10.219 **Pre-existing hypertensive chronic kidney disease complicating pregnancy, unspecified trimester** Ⓜ♀

    O10.22 **Pre-existing hypertensive chronic kidney disease complicating** childbirth Ⓜ♀

    O10.23 **Pre-existing hypertensive chronic kidney disease complicating the** puerperium Ⓜ♀

√5ᵗʰ **O10.3** **Pre-existing hypertensive** heart and chronic kidney disease **complicating pregnancy, childbirth and the puerperium**
    Any condition in I13 specified as a reason for obstetric care during pregnancy, childbirth or the puerperium
    Use additional code from I13 to identify the type of hypertensive heart and chronic kidney disease

  √6ᵗʰ **O10.31** **Pre-existing hypertensive heart and chronic kidney disease complicating** pregnancy

      O10.311 **Pre-existing hypertensive heart and chronic kidney disease complicating pregnancy, first trimester** Ⓜ♀

      O10.312 **Pre-existing hypertensive heart and chronic kidney disease complicating pregnancy, second trimester** Ⓜ♀

      O10.313 **Pre-existing hypertensive heart and chronic kidney disease complicating pregnancy, third trimester** Ⓜ♀

      O10.319 **Pre-existing hypertensive heart and chronic kidney disease complicating pregnancy, unspecified trimester** Ⓜ♀

    O10.32 **Pre-existing hypertensive heart and chronic kidney disease complicating** childbirth Ⓜ♀

    O10.33 **Pre-existing hypertensive heart and chronic kidney disease complicating the** puerperium Ⓜ♀

√5ᵗʰ **O10.4** **Pre-existing** secondary **hypertension complicating pregnancy, childbirth and the puerperium**
    Any condition in I15 specified as a reason for obstetric care during pregnancy, childbirth or the puerperium
    Use additional code from I15 to identify the type of secondary hypertension

  √6ᵗʰ **O10.41** **Pre-existing secondary hypertension complicating** pregnancy

      O10.411 **Pre-existing secondary hypertension complicating pregnancy, first trimester** Ⓜ♀

      O10.412 **Pre-existing secondary hypertension complicating pregnancy, second trimester** Ⓜ♀

      O10.413 **Pre-existing secondary hypertension complicating pregnancy, third trimester** Ⓜ♀

      O10.419 **Pre-existing secondary hypertension complicating pregnancy, unspecified trimester** Ⓜ♀

    O10.42 **Pre-existing secondary hypertension complicating** childbirth Ⓜ♀

    O10.43 **Pre-existing secondary hypertension complicating the** puerperium Ⓜ♀

√5ᵗʰ **O10.9** **Unspecified pre-existing hypertension complicating pregnancy, childbirth and the puerperium**

  √6ᵗʰ **O10.91** **Unspecified pre-existing hypertension complicating** pregnancy

      O10.911 **Unspecified pre-existing hypertension complicating pregnancy, first trimester** Ⓜ♀

      O10.912 **Unspecified pre-existing hypertension complicating pregnancy, second trimester** Ⓜ♀

      O10.913 **Unspecified pre-existing hypertension complicating pregnancy, third trimester** Ⓜ♀

      O10.919 **Unspecified pre-existing hypertension complicating pregnancy, unspecified trimester** Ⓜ♀

    O10.92 **Unspecified pre-existing hypertension complicating** childbirth Ⓜ♀

    O10.93 **Unspecified pre-existing hypertension complicating the** puerperium Ⓜ♀

√4ᵗʰ **O11** **Pre-existing** hypertension with pre-eclampsia
    INCLUDES   conditions in O10 complicated by pre-eclampsia
          pre-eclampsia superimposed pre-existing in hypertension
    Use additional code from O10 to identify the type of hypertension
    DEF: Complication of pregnancy manifesting in the development of borderline hypertension, protein in the urine, and unresponsive swelling between the 20th week of pregnancy and the end of the first week following birth in mild to moderate cases. Severe preeclampsia presents with hypertension, associated with marked swelling, proteinuria, abdominal pain, and/or visual changes.

  O11.1 **Pre-existing hypertension with pre-eclampsia, first trimester** Ⓜ♀

  O11.2 **Pre-existing hypertension with pre-eclampsia, second trimester** Ⓜ♀

  O11.3 **Pre-existing hypertension with pre-eclampsia, third trimester** Ⓜ♀

  O11.4 **Pre-existing hypertension with pre-eclampsia, complicating** childbirth Ⓜ♀

  O11.5 **Pre-existing hypertension with pre-eclampsia, complicating the** puerperium Ⓜ♀

  O11.9 **Pre-existing hypertension with pre-eclampsia, unspecified trimester** Ⓜ♀

√4ᵗʰ **O12** Gestational [pregnancy-induced] edema and proteinuria without hypertension

  √5ᵗʰ **O12.0** **Gestational** edema

    O12.00 **Gestational edema, unspecified trimester** Ⓜ♀

    O12.01 **Gestational edema, first trimester** Ⓜ♀

    O12.02 **Gestational edema, second trimester** Ⓜ♀

    O12.03 **Gestational edema, third trimester** Ⓜ♀

    O12.04 **Gestational edema, complicating** childbirth Ⓜ♀

    O12.05 **Gestational edema, complicating the** puerperium Ⓜ♀

  √5ᵗʰ **O12.1** **Gestational** proteinuria

    O12.10 **Gestational proteinuria, unspecified trimester** Ⓜ♀

    O12.11 **Gestational proteinuria, first trimester** Ⓜ♀

    O12.12 **Gestational proteinuria, second trimester** Ⓜ♀

    O12.13 **Gestational proteinuria, third trimester** Ⓜ♀

    O12.14 **Gestational proteinuria, complicating** childbirth Ⓜ♀

    O12.15 **Gestational proteinuria, complicating the** puerperium Ⓜ♀

  √5ᵗʰ **O12.2** **Gestational** edema with proteinuria

    O12.20 **Gestational edema with proteinuria, unspecified trimester** Ⓜ♀

    O12.21 **Gestational edema with proteinuria, first trimester** Ⓜ♀

    O12.22 **Gestational edema with proteinuria, second trimester** Ⓜ♀

    O12.23 **Gestational edema with proteinuria, third trimester** Ⓜ♀

    O12.24 **Gestational edema with proteinuria, complicating** childbirth Ⓜ♀

    O12.25 **Gestational edema with proteinuria, complicating the** puerperium Ⓜ♀

✓4th O13 Gestational [pregnancy-induced] hypertension without significant proteinuria

INCLUDES   gestational hypertension NOS
transient hypertension of pregnancy

AHA: 2016,1Q,5

O13.1 Gestational [pregnancy-induced] hypertension without significant proteinuria, first trimester   M ♀

O13.2 Gestational [pregnancy-induced] hypertension without significant proteinuria, second trimester   M ♀

O13.3 Gestational [pregnancy-induced] hypertension without significant proteinuria, third trimester   M ♀

O13.4 Gestational [pregnancy-induced] hypertension without significant proteinuria, complicating childbirth   M ♀

O13.5 Gestational [pregnancy-induced] hypertension without significant proteinuria, complicating the puerperium   M ♀

O13.9 Gestational [pregnancy-induced] hypertension without significant proteinuria, unspecified trimester   M ♀

✓4th O14 Pre-eclampsia

EXCLUDES 1   pre-existing hypertension with pre-eclampsia (O11)

DEF: Complication of pregnancy manifesting in the development of borderline hypertension, protein in the urine, and unresponsive swelling between the 20th week of pregnancy and the end of the first week following birth in mild to moderate cases. Severe preeclampsia presents with hypertension, associated with marked swelling, proteinuria, abdominal pain, and/or visual changes.

✓5th O14.0 Mild to moderate pre-eclampsia

AHA: 2019,2Q,8

O14.00 Mild to moderate pre-eclampsia, unspecified trimester   M ♀

O14.02 Mild to moderate pre-eclampsia, second trimester   M ♀

O14.03 Mild to moderate pre-eclampsia, third trimester   M ♀

O14.04 Mild to moderate pre-eclampsia, complicating childbirth   M ♀

AHA: 2019,2Q,8

O14.05 Mild to moderate pre-eclampsia, complicating the puerperium   M ♀

✓5th O14.1 Severe pre-eclampsia

EXCLUDES 1   HELLP syndrome (O14.2-)

O14.10 Severe pre-eclampsia, unspecified trimester   M ♀

O14.12 Severe pre-eclampsia, second trimester   M ♀

O14.13 Severe pre-eclampsia, third trimester   M ♀

O14.14 Severe pre-eclampsia complicating childbirth   M ♀

O14.15 Severe pre-eclampsia, complicating the puerperium   M ♀

✓5th O14.2 HELLP syndrome

Severe pre-eclampsia with hemolysis, elevated liver enzymes and low platelet count (HELLP)

O14.20 HELLP syndrome (HELLP), unspecified trimester   M ♀

O14.22 HELLP syndrome (HELLP), second trimester   M ♀

O14.23 HELLP syndrome (HELLP), third trimester   M ♀

O14.24 HELLP syndrome, complicating childbirth   M ♀

O14.25 HELLP syndrome, complicating the puerperium   M ♀

✓5th O14.9 Unspecified pre-eclampsia

O14.90 Unspecified pre-eclampsia, unspecified trimester   M ♀

O14.92 Unspecified pre-eclampsia, second trimester   M ♀

O14.93 Unspecified pre-eclampsia, third trimester   M ♀

O14.94 Unspecified pre-eclampsia, complicating childbirth   M ♀

O14.95 Unspecified pre-eclampsia, complicating the puerperium   M ♀

✓4th O15 Eclampsia

INCLUDES   convulsions following conditions in O10-O14 and O16

DEF: Tetany and toxemia producing seizure activity or coma in a pregnant patient who most often has presented with prior preeclampsia (i.e., hypertension, albuminuria, and edema).

✓5th O15.0 Eclampsia complicating pregnancy

O15.00 Eclampsia complicating pregnancy, unspecified trimester   M ♀

O15.02 Eclampsia complicating pregnancy, second trimester   M ♀

O15.03 Eclampsia complicating pregnancy, third trimester   M ♀

O15.1 Eclampsia complicating labor   M ♀

O15.2 Eclampsia complicating the puerperium   M ♀

O15.9 Eclampsia, unspecified as to time period   M ♀

Eclampsia NOS

✓4th O16 Unspecified maternal hypertension

O16.1 Unspecified maternal hypertension, first trimester   M ♀

O16.2 Unspecified maternal hypertension, second trimester   M ♀

O16.3 Unspecified maternal hypertension, third trimester   M ♀

O16.4 Unspecified maternal hypertension, complicating childbirth   M ♀

O16.5 Unspecified maternal hypertension, complicating the puerperium   M ♀

O16.9 Unspecified maternal hypertension, unspecified trimester   M ♀

Other maternal disorders predominantly related to pregnancy (O20-O29)

EXCLUDES 2   maternal care related to the fetus and amniotic cavity and possible delivery problems (O30-O48)
maternal diseases classifiable elsewhere but complicating pregnancy, labor and delivery, and the puerperium (O98-O99)

✓4th O20 Hemorrhage in early pregnancy

INCLUDES   hemorrhage before completion of 20 weeks gestation

EXCLUDES 1   pregnancy with abortive outcome (O00-O08)

O20.0 Threatened abortion   Q M ♀

Hemorrhage specified as due to threatened abortion

DEF: Bloody discharge during pregnancy. The cervix may be dilated and pregnancy threatened, but the pregnancy is not terminated.

O20.8 Other hemorrhage in early pregnancy   Q M ♀

O20.9 Hemorrhage in early pregnancy, unspecified   Q M ♀

✓4th O21 Excessive vomiting in pregnancy

O21.0 Mild hyperemesis gravidarum   M ♀

Hyperemesis gravidarum, mild or unspecified, starting before the end of the 20th week of gestation

O21.1 Hyperemesis gravidarum with metabolic disturbance   M ♀

Hyperemesis gravidarum, starting before the end of the 20th week of gestation, with metabolic disturbance such as carbohydrate depletion

Hyperemesis gravidarum, starting before the end of the 20th week of gestation, with metabolic disturbance such as dehydration

Hyperemesis gravidarum, starting before the end of the 20th week of gestation, with metabolic disturbance such as electrolyte imbalance

O21.2 Late vomiting of pregnancy   M ♀

Excessive vomiting starting after 20 completed weeks of gestation

O21.8 Other vomiting complicating pregnancy   M ♀

Vomiting due to diseases classified elsewhere, complicating pregnancy

Use additional code, to identify cause

O21.9 Vomiting of pregnancy, unspecified   M ♀

☑ Additional Character Required   ✓x7th Placeholder Alert   Manifestation   Unspecified Dx   ►◄ Revised Text   ● New Code   ▲ Revised Code Title

ICD-10-CM 2020   863

O13–O21.9

Chapter 15. Pregnancy, Childbirth and the Puerperium

O22–O23.40

☑4ᵗʰ **O22 Venous complications and hemorrhoids in pregnancy**

EXCLUDES 1   venous complications of:
- abortion NOS (O03.9)
- ectopic or molar pregnancy (O08.7)
- failed attempted abortion (O07.35)
- induced abortion (O04.85)
- spontaneous abortion (O03.89)

EXCLUDES 2   obstetric pulmonary embolism (O88.-)
- venous complications and hemorrhoids of childbirth and the puerperium (O87.-)

☑5ᵗʰ **O22.0 Varicose veins of lower extremity in pregnancy**

Varicose veins NOS in pregnancy

DEF: Distended, tortuous veins of the lower extremities associated with pregnancy.

O22.00	**Varicose veins of lower extremity in pregnancy, unspecified trimester**	Ⓜ♀
O22.01	**Varicose veins of lower extremity in pregnancy,** first trimester	Ⓜ♀
O22.02	**Varicose veins of lower extremity in pregnancy,** second trimester	Ⓜ♀
O22.03	**Varicose veins of lower extremity in pregnancy,** third trimester	Ⓜ♀

☑5ᵗʰ **O22.1 Genital varices in pregnancy**

Perineal varices in pregnancy
Vaginal varices in pregnancy
Vulval varices in pregnancy

O22.10	**Genital varices in pregnancy, unspecified trimester**	Ⓜ♀
O22.11	**Genital varices in pregnancy,** first trimester	Ⓜ♀
O22.12	**Genital varices in pregnancy,** second trimester	Ⓜ♀
O22.13	**Genital varices in pregnancy,** third trimester	Ⓜ♀

☑5ᵗʰ **O22.2 Superficial thrombophlebitis in pregnancy**

Phlebitis in pregnancy NOS
Thrombophlebitis of legs in pregnancy
Thrombosis in pregnancy NOS
Use additional code to identify the superficial thrombophlebitis (I80.0-)

O22.20	**Superficial thrombophlebitis in pregnancy, unspecified trimester**	Ⓜ♀
O22.21	**Superficial thrombophlebitis in pregnancy,** first trimester	Ⓜ♀
O22.22	**Superficial thrombophlebitis in pregnancy,** second trimester	Ⓜ♀
O22.23	**Superficial thrombophlebitis in pregnancy,** third trimester	Ⓜ♀

☑5ᵗʰ **O22.3 Deep phlebothrombosis in pregnancy**

Deep vein thrombosis, antepartum
Use additional code to identify the deep vein thrombosis (I82.4-, I82.5-, I82.62-. I82.72-)
Use additional code, if applicable, for associated long-term (current) use of anticoagulants (Z79.01)

O22.30	**Deep phlebothrombosis in pregnancy, unspecified trimester**	Ⓜ♀
O22.31	**Deep phlebothrombosis in pregnancy,** first trimester	Ⓜ♀
O22.32	**Deep phlebothrombosis in pregnancy,** second trimester	Ⓜ♀
O22.33	**Deep phlebothrombosis in pregnancy,** third trimester	Ⓜ♀

☑5ᵗʰ **O22.4 Hemorrhoids in pregnancy**

O22.40	**Hemorrhoids in pregnancy, unspecified trimester**	Ⓜ♀
O22.41	**Hemorrhoids in pregnancy,** first trimester	Ⓜ♀
O22.42	**Hemorrhoids in pregnancy,** second trimester	Ⓜ♀
O22.43	**Hemorrhoids in pregnancy,** third trimester	Ⓜ♀

☑5ᵗʰ **O22.5 Cerebral venous thrombosis in pregnancy**

Cerebrovenous sinus thrombosis in pregnancy

O22.50	**Cerebral venous thrombosis in pregnancy, unspecified trimester**	Ⓜ♀
O22.51	**Cerebral venous thrombosis in pregnancy,** first trimester	Ⓜ♀
O22.52	**Cerebral venous thrombosis in pregnancy,** second trimester	Ⓜ♀

| O22.53 | **Cerebral venous thrombosis in pregnancy,** third trimester | Ⓜ♀ |

☑5ᵗʰ **O22.8 Other venous complications in pregnancy**

☑6ᵗʰ **O22.8X Other venous complications in pregnancy**

O22.8X1	**Other venous complications in pregnancy,** first trimester	Ⓜ♀
O22.8X2	**Other venous complications in pregnancy,** second trimester	Ⓜ♀
O22.8X3	**Other venous complications in pregnancy,** third trimester	Ⓜ♀
O22.8X9	**Other venous complications in pregnancy, unspecified trimester**	Ⓜ♀

☑5ᵗʰ **O22.9 Venous complication in pregnancy, unspecified**

Gestational phlebitis NOS
Gestational phlebopathy NOS
Gestational thrombosis NOS

O22.90	**Venous complication in pregnancy, unspecified, unspecified trimester**	Ⓜ♀
O22.91	**Venous complication in pregnancy, unspecified,** first trimester	Ⓜ♀
O22.92	**Venous complication in pregnancy, unspecified,** second trimester	Ⓜ♀
O22.93	**Venous complication in pregnancy, unspecified,** third trimester	Ⓜ♀

☑4ᵗʰ **O23 Infections of genitourinary tract in pregnancy**

Use additional code to identify organism (B95.-, B96.-)

EXCLUDES 2   gonococcal infections complicating pregnancy, childbirth and the puerperium (O98.2)
- infections with a predominantly sexual mode of transmission NOS complicating pregnancy, childbirth and the puerperium (O98.3)
- syphilis complicating pregnancy, childbirth and the puerperium (O98.1)
- tuberculosis of genitourinary system complicating pregnancy, childbirth and the puerperium (O98.0)
- venereal disease NOS complicating pregnancy, childbirth and the puerperium (O98.3)

AHA: 2018,2Q,20

☑5ᵗʰ **O23.0 Infections of kidney in pregnancy**

Pyelonephritis in pregnancy

O23.00	**Infections of kidney in pregnancy, unspecified trimester**	Ⓜ♀
O23.01	**Infections of kidney in pregnancy,** first trimester	Ⓜ♀
O23.02	**Infections of kidney in pregnancy,** second trimester	Ⓜ♀
O23.03	**Infections of kidney in pregnancy,** third trimester	Ⓜ♀

☑5ᵗʰ **O23.1 Infections of bladder in pregnancy**

O23.10	**Infections of bladder in pregnancy, unspecified trimester**	Ⓜ♀
O23.11	**Infections of bladder in pregnancy,** first trimester	Ⓜ♀
O23.12	**Infections of bladder in pregnancy,** second trimester	Ⓜ♀
O23.13	**Infections of bladder in pregnancy,** third trimester	Ⓜ♀

☑5ᵗʰ **O23.2 Infections of urethra in pregnancy**

O23.20	**Infections of urethra in pregnancy, unspecified trimester**	Ⓜ♀
O23.21	**Infections of urethra in pregnancy,** first trimester	Ⓜ♀
O23.22	**Infections of urethra in pregnancy,** second trimester	Ⓜ♀
O23.23	**Infections of urethra in pregnancy,** third trimester	Ⓜ♀

☑5ᵗʰ **O23.3 Infections of other parts of urinary tract in pregnancy**

O23.30	**Infections of other parts of urinary tract in pregnancy, unspecified trimester**	Ⓜ♀
O23.31	**Infections of other parts of urinary tract in pregnancy,** first trimester	Ⓜ♀
O23.32	**Infections of other parts of urinary tract in pregnancy,** second trimester	Ⓜ♀
O23.33	**Infections of other parts of urinary tract in pregnancy,** third trimester	Ⓜ♀

☑5ᵗʰ **O23.4 Unspecified infection of urinary tract in pregnancy**

| O23.40 | **Unspecified infection of urinary tract in pregnancy, unspecified trimester** | Ⓜ♀ |

O23.41	**Unspecified infection of urinary tract in pregnancy, first trimester**	M ♀
O23.42	**Unspecified infection of urinary tract in pregnancy, second trimester**	M ♀
O23.43	**Unspecified infection of urinary tract in pregnancy, third trimester**	M ♀

√5ᵗʰ **O23.5** **Infections of the genital tract in pregnancy**

√6ᵗʰ **O23.51** **Infection of cervix in pregnancy**

O23.511	**Infections of cervix in pregnancy, first trimester**	M ♀
O23.512	**Infections of cervix in pregnancy, second trimester**	M ♀
O23.513	**Infections of cervix in pregnancy, third trimester**	M ♀
O23.519	**Infections of cervix in pregnancy, unspecified trimester**	M ♀

√6ᵗʰ **O23.52** **Salpingo-oophoritis in pregnancy**

Oophoritis in pregnancy
Salpingitis in pregnancy

O23.521	**Salpingo-oophoritis in pregnancy, first trimester**	M ♀
O23.522	**Salpingo-oophoritis in pregnancy, second trimester**	M ♀
O23.523	**Salpingo-oophoritis in pregnancy, third trimester**	M ♀
O23.529	**Salpingo-oophoritis in pregnancy, unspecified trimester**	M ♀

√6ᵗʰ **O23.59** **Infection of other part of genital tract in pregnancy**

O23.591	**Infection of other part of genital tract in pregnancy, first trimester**	M ♀
O23.592	**Infection of other part of genital tract in pregnancy, second trimester**	M ♀
O23.593	**Infection of other part of genital tract in pregnancy, third trimester**	M ♀
O23.599	**Infection of other part of genital tract in pregnancy, unspecified trimester**	M ♀

√5ᵗʰ **O23.9** **Unspecified genitourinary tract infection in pregnancy**

Genitourinary tract infection in pregnancy NOS

O23.9Ø	**Unspecified genitourinary tract infection in pregnancy, unspecified trimester**	M ♀
O23.91	**Unspecified genitourinary tract infection in pregnancy, first trimester**	M ♀
O23.92	**Unspecified genitourinary tract infection in pregnancy, second trimester**	M ♀
O23.93	**Unspecified genitourinary tract infection in pregnancy, third trimester**	M ♀

√4ᵗʰ **O24** **Diabetes mellitus in pregnancy, childbirth and the puerperium**

√5ᵗʰ **O24.Ø** **Pre-existing type 1 diabetes mellitus, in pregnancy, childbirth and the puerperium**

Juvenile onset diabetes mellitus, in pregnancy, childbirth and the puerperium
Ketosis-prone diabetes mellitus in pregnancy, childbirth and the puerperium
Use additional code from category E1Ø to further identify any manifestations

√6ᵗʰ **O24.Ø1** **Pre-existing type 1 diabetes mellitus, in pregnancy**

O24.Ø11	**Pre-existing type 1 diabetes mellitus, in pregnancy, first trimester**	Q M ♀
O24.Ø12	**Pre-existing type 1 diabetes mellitus, in pregnancy, second trimester**	Q M ♀
O24.Ø13	**Pre-existing type 1 diabetes mellitus, in pregnancy, third trimester**	Q M ♀
O24.Ø19	**Pre-existing type 1 diabetes mellitus, in pregnancy, unspecified trimester**	Q M ♀
O24.Ø2	**Pre-existing type 1 diabetes mellitus, in childbirth**	Q M ♀
O24.Ø3	**Pre-existing type 1 diabetes mellitus, in the puerperium**	Q M ♀

√5ᵗʰ **O24.1** **Pre-existing type 2 diabetes mellitus, in pregnancy, childbirth and the puerperium**

Insulin-resistant diabetes mellitus in pregnancy, childbirth and the puerperium
Use additional code (for):
from category E11 to further identify any manifestations
long-term (current) use of insulin (Z79.4)

√6ᵗʰ **O24.11** **Pre-existing type 2 diabetes mellitus, in pregnancy**

O24.111	**Pre-existing type 2 diabetes mellitus, in pregnancy, first trimester**	Q M ♀
O24.112	**Pre-existing type 2 diabetes mellitus, in pregnancy, second trimester**	Q M ♀
O24.113	**Pre-existing type 2 diabetes mellitus, in pregnancy, third trimester**	Q M ♀
O24.119	**Pre-existing type 2 diabetes mellitus, in pregnancy, unspecified trimester**	Q M ♀
O24.12	**Pre-existing type 2 diabetes mellitus, in childbirth**	Q M ♀
O24.13	**Pre-existing type 2 diabetes mellitus, in the puerperium**	Q M ♀

√5ᵗʰ **O24.3** **Unspecified pre-existing diabetes mellitus in pregnancy, childbirth and the puerperium**

Use additional code (for):
from category E11 to further identify any manifestation
long-term (current) use of insulin (Z79.4)

√6ᵗʰ **O24.31** **Unspecified pre-existing diabetes mellitus in pregnancy**

O24.311	**Unspecified pre-existing diabetes mellitus in pregnancy, first trimester**	Q M ♀
O24.312	**Unspecified pre-existing diabetes mellitus in pregnancy, second trimester**	Q M ♀
O24.313	**Unspecified pre-existing diabetes mellitus in pregnancy, third trimester**	Q M ♀
O24.319	**Unspecified pre-existing diabetes mellitus in pregnancy, unspecified trimester**	Q M ♀
O24.32	**Unspecified pre-existing diabetes mellitus in childbirth**	Q M ♀
O24.33	**Unspecified pre-existing diabetes mellitus in the puerperium**	Q M ♀

√5ᵗʰ **O24.4** **Gestational diabetes mellitus**

Diabetes mellitus arising in pregnancy
Gestational diabetes mellitus NOS
AHA: 2016,4Q,50; 2015,4Q,34

√6ᵗʰ **O24.41** **Gestational diabetes mellitus in pregnancy**

O24.41Ø	**Gestational diabetes mellitus in pregnancy, diet controlled**	M ♀
O24.414	**Gestational diabetes mellitus in pregnancy, insulin controlled**	M ♀
O24.415	**Gestational diabetes mellitus in pregnancy, controlled by oral hypoglycemic drugs**	M ♀

Gestational diabetes mellitus in pregnancy, controlled by oral antidiabetic drugs

O24.419	**Gestational diabetes mellitus in pregnancy, unspecified control**	M ♀

√6ᵗʰ **O24.42** **Gestational diabetes mellitus in childbirth**

AHA: 2016,1Q,5

O24.42Ø	**Gestational diabetes mellitus in childbirth, diet controlled**	M ♀
O24.424	**Gestational diabetes mellitus in childbirth, insulin controlled**	M ♀
O24.425	**Gestational diabetes mellitus in childbirth, controlled by oral hypoglycemic drugs**	M ♀

Gestational diabetes mellitus in childbirth, controlled by oral antidiabetic drugs

O24.429	**Gestational diabetes mellitus in childbirth, unspecified control**	M ♀

√6ᵗʰ **O24.43** **Gestational diabetes mellitus in the puerperium**

O24.43Ø	**Gestational diabetes mellitus in the puerperium, diet controlled**	M ♀

O24.434   Gestational diabetes mellitus in the puerperium, insulin controlled   M ♀

O24.435   Gestational diabetes mellitus in puerperium, controlled by oral hypoglycemic drugs   M ♀
     Gestational diabetes mellitus in puerperium, controlled by oral antidiabetic drugs

O24.439   Gestational diabetes mellitus in the puerperium, unspecified control   M ♀

✓5th **O24.8**   **Other pre-existing diabetes mellitus in pregnancy, childbirth, and the puerperium**
     Use additional code (for):
       from categories E08, E09 and E13 to further identify any manifestation
     long-term (current) use of insulin (Z79.4)

   ✓6th **O24.81**   Other pre-existing diabetes mellitus in pregnancy

     O24.811   Other pre-existing diabetes mellitus in pregnancy, first trimester   Q M ♀

     O24.812   Other pre-existing diabetes mellitus in pregnancy, second trimester   Q M ♀

     O24.813   Other pre-existing diabetes mellitus in pregnancy, third trimester   Q M ♀

     O24.819   Other pre-existing diabetes mellitus in pregnancy, unspecified trimester   Q M ♀

   O24.82   Other pre-existing diabetes mellitus in childbirth   Q M ♀

   O24.83   Other pre-existing diabetes mellitus in the puerperium   Q M ♀

✓5th **O24.9**   **Unspecified diabetes mellitus in pregnancy, childbirth and the puerperium**
     Use additional code for long-term (current) use of insulin (Z79.4)

   ✓6th **O24.91**   Unspecified diabetes mellitus in pregnancy

     O24.911   Unspecified diabetes mellitus in pregnancy, first trimester   M ♀

     O24.912   Unspecified diabetes mellitus in pregnancy, second trimester   M ♀

     O24.913   Unspecified diabetes mellitus in pregnancy, third trimester   M ♀

     O24.919   Unspecified diabetes mellitus in pregnancy, unspecified trimester   M ♀

   O24.92   Unspecified diabetes mellitus in childbirth   M ♀

   O24.93   Unspecified diabetes mellitus in the puerperium   M ♀

✓4th **O25**   **Malnutrition in pregnancy, childbirth and the puerperium**

   ✓5th **O25.1**   **Malnutrition in pregnancy**

     O25.10   Malnutrition in pregnancy, unspecified trimester   M ♀

     O25.11   Malnutrition in pregnancy, first trimester   M ♀

     O25.12   Malnutrition in pregnancy, second trimester   M ♀

     O25.13   Malnutrition in pregnancy, third trimester   M ♀

   O25.2   **Malnutrition in childbirth**   M ♀

   O25.3   **Malnutrition in the puerperium**   M ♀

✓4th **O26**   **Maternal care for other conditions predominantly related to pregnancy**

   ✓5th **O26.0**   **Excessive weight gain in pregnancy**
       EXCLUDES 2   gestational edema (O12.0, O12.2)

     O26.00   Excessive weight gain in pregnancy, unspecified trimester   M ♀

     O26.01   Excessive weight gain in pregnancy, first trimester   M ♀

     O26.02   Excessive weight gain in pregnancy, second trimester   M ♀

     O26.03   Excessive weight gain in pregnancy, third trimester   M ♀

   ✓5th **O26.1**   **Low weight gain in pregnancy**

     O26.10   Low weight gain in pregnancy, unspecified trimester   M ♀

     O26.11   Low weight gain in pregnancy, first trimester   M ♀

O26.12   Low weight gain in pregnancy, second trimester   M ♀

O26.13   Low weight gain in pregnancy, third trimester   M ♀

✓5th **O26.2**   **Pregnancy care for patient with recurrent pregnancy loss**

   O26.20   Pregnancy care for patient with recurrent pregnancy loss, unspecified trimester   M ♀

   O26.21   Pregnancy care for patient with recurrent pregnancy loss, first trimester   M ♀

   O26.22   Pregnancy care for patient with recurrent pregnancy loss, second trimester   M ♀

   O26.23   Pregnancy care for patient with recurrent pregnancy loss, third trimester   M ♀

✓5th **O26.3**   **Retained intrauterine contraceptive device in pregnancy**

   O26.30   Retained intrauterine contraceptive device in pregnancy, unspecified trimester   M ♀

   O26.31   Retained intrauterine contraceptive device in pregnancy, first trimester   M ♀

   O26.32   Retained intrauterine contraceptive device in pregnancy, second trimester   M ♀

   O26.33   Retained intrauterine contraceptive device in pregnancy, third trimester   M ♀

✓5th **O26.4**   **Herpes gestationis**
     DEF: Rare skin disorder of unknown origin that appears on the abdomen in the second and third trimester as intensely itchy blisters that spread to other sites.

   O26.40   Herpes gestationis, unspecified trimester   M ♀

   O26.41   Herpes gestationis, first trimester   M ♀

   O26.42   Herpes gestationis, second trimester   M ♀

   O26.43   Herpes gestationis, third trimester   M ♀

✓5th **O26.5**   **Maternal hypotension syndrome**
     Supine hypotensive syndrome

   O26.50   Maternal hypotension syndrome, unspecified trimester   M ♀

   O26.51   Maternal hypotension syndrome, first trimester   M ♀

   O26.52   Maternal hypotension syndrome, second trimester   M ♀

   O26.53   Maternal hypotension syndrome, third trimester   M ♀

✓5th **O26.6**   **Liver and biliary tract disorders in pregnancy, childbirth and the puerperium**
     Use additional code to identify the specific disorder
       EXCLUDES 2   hepatorenal syndrome following labor and delivery (O90.4)

   ✓6th **O26.61**   Liver and biliary tract disorders in pregnancy

     O26.611   Liver and biliary tract disorders in pregnancy, first trimester   M ♀

     O26.612   Liver and biliary tract disorders in pregnancy, second trimester   M ♀

     O26.613   Liver and biliary tract disorders in pregnancy, third trimester   M ♀

     O26.619   Liver and biliary tract disorders in pregnancy, unspecified trimester   M ♀

   O26.62   Liver and biliary tract disorders in childbirth   M ♀

   O26.63   Liver and biliary tract disorders in the puerperium   M ♀

✓5th **O26.7**   **Subluxation of symphysis (pubis) in pregnancy, childbirth and the puerperium**
     EXCLUDES 1   traumatic separation of symphysis (pubis) during childbirth (O71.6)

   ✓6th **O26.71**   Subluxation of symphysis (pubis) in pregnancy

     O26.711   Subluxation of symphysis (pubis) in pregnancy, first trimester   M ♀

     O26.712   Subluxation of symphysis (pubis) in pregnancy, second trimester   M ♀

     O26.713   Subluxation of symphysis (pubis) in pregnancy, third trimester   M ♀

     O26.719   Subluxation of symphysis (pubis) in pregnancy, unspecified trimester   M ♀

   O26.72   Subluxation of symphysis (pubis) in childbirth   M ♀

   O26.73   Subluxation of symphysis (pubis) in the puerperium   M ♀

✓5ᵗʰ O26.8 Other specified pregnancy related conditions

✓6ᵗʰ O26.81 Pregnancy related exhaustion and fatigue

O26.811 Pregnancy related exhaustion and fatigue, first trimester Ⓜ♀

O26.812 Pregnancy related exhaustion and fatigue, second trimester Ⓜ♀

O26.813 Pregnancy related exhaustion and fatigue, third trimester Ⓜ♀

O26.819 Pregnancy related exhaustion and fatigue, unspecified trimester Ⓜ♀

✓6ᵗʰ O26.82 Pregnancy related peripheral neuritis

O26.821 Pregnancy related peripheral neuritis, first trimester Ⓜ♀

O26.822 Pregnancy related peripheral neuritis, second trimester Ⓜ♀

O26.823 Pregnancy related peripheral neuritis, third trimester Ⓜ♀

O26.829 Pregnancy related peripheral neuritis, unspecified trimester Ⓜ♀

✓6ᵗʰ O26.83 Pregnancy related renal disease

Use additional code to identify the specific disorder

O26.831 Pregnancy related renal disease, first trimester Ⓜ♀

O26.832 Pregnancy related renal disease, second trimester Ⓜ♀

O26.833 Pregnancy related renal disease, third trimester Ⓜ♀

O26.839 Pregnancy related renal disease, unspecified trimester Ⓜ♀

✓6ᵗʰ O26.84 Uterine size-date discrepancy complicating pregnancy

EXCLUDES 1   *encounter for suspected problem with fetal growth ruled out (Z03.74)*

O26.841 Uterine size-date discrepancy, first trimester Ⓜ♀

O26.842 Uterine size-date discrepancy, second trimester Ⓜ♀

O26.843 Uterine size-date discrepancy, third trimester Ⓜ♀

O26.849 Uterine size-date discrepancy, unspecified trimester Ⓜ♀

✓6ᵗʰ O26.85 Spotting complicating pregnancy

O26.851 Spotting complicating pregnancy, first trimester Ⓜ♀

O26.852 Spotting complicating pregnancy, second trimester Ⓜ♀

O26.853 Spotting complicating pregnancy, third trimester Ⓜ♀

O26.859 Spotting complicating pregnancy, unspecified trimester Ⓜ♀

O26.86 Pruritic urticarial papules and plaques of pregnancy (PUPPP) Ⓜ♀

Polymorphic eruption of pregnancy

✓6ᵗʰ O26.87 Cervical shortening

EXCLUDES 1   *encounter for suspected cervical shortening ruled out (Z03.75)*

DEF: Cervix that has shortened to less than 25 mm before the 24th week of pregnancy. A shortened cervix is a warning sign for impending premature delivery and is treated by cervical cerclage placement or progesterone.

O26.872 Cervical shortening, second trimester Ⓜ♀

O26.873 Cervical shortening, third trimester Ⓜ♀

O26.879 Cervical shortening, unspecified trimester Ⓜ♀

✓6ᵗʰ O26.89 Other specified pregnancy related conditions

AHA: 2015,3Q,40

O26.891 Other specified pregnancy related conditions, first trimester 🄾 Ⓜ♀

O26.892 Other specified pregnancy related conditions, second trimester Ⓜ♀

O26.893 Other specified pregnancy related conditions, third trimester Ⓜ♀

O26.899 Other specified pregnancy related conditions, unspecified trimester 🄾 Ⓜ♀

✓5ᵗʰ O26.9 Pregnancy related conditions, unspecified

O26.90 Pregnancy related conditions, unspecified, unspecified trimester 🄾 Ⓜ♀

O26.91 Pregnancy related conditions, unspecified, first trimester 🄾 Ⓜ♀

O26.92 Pregnancy related conditions, unspecified, second trimester Ⓜ♀

O26.93 Pregnancy related conditions, unspecified, third trimester Ⓜ♀

✓4ᵗʰ O28 Abnormal findings on antenatal screening of mother

EXCLUDES 1   *diagnostic findings classified elsewhere — see Alphabetical Index*

O28.0 Abnormal hematological finding on antenatal screening of mother Ⓜ♀

O28.1 Abnormal biochemical finding on antenatal screening of mother Ⓜ♀

O28.2 Abnormal cytological finding on antenatal screening of mother Ⓜ♀

O28.3 Abnormal ultrasonic finding on antenatal screening of mother Ⓜ♀

O28.4 Abnormal radiological finding on antenatal screening of mother Ⓜ♀

O28.5 Abnormal chromosomal and genetic finding on antenatal screening of mother Ⓜ♀

O28.8 Other abnormal findings on antenatal screening of mother Ⓜ♀

O28.9 Unspecified abnormal findings on antenatal screening of mother Ⓜ♀

✓4ᵗʰ O29 Complications of anesthesia during pregnancy

INCLUDES   maternal complications arising from the administration of a general, regional or local anesthetic, analgesic or other sedation during pregnancy

Use additional code, if necessary, to identify the complication

EXCLUDES 2   *complications of anesthesia during labor and delivery (O74.-)*
    complications of anesthesia during the puerperium (O89.-)

✓5ᵗʰ O29.0 Pulmonary complications of anesthesia during pregnancy

✓6ᵗʰ O29.01 Aspiration pneumonitis due to anesthesia during pregnancy

Inhalation of stomach contents or secretions NOS due to anesthesia during pregnancy

Mendelson's syndrome due to anesthesia during pregnancy

O29.011 Aspiration pneumonitis due to anesthesia during pregnancy, first trimester Ⓜ♀

O29.012 Aspiration pneumonitis due to anesthesia during pregnancy, second trimester Ⓜ♀

O29.013 Aspiration pneumonitis due to anesthesia during pregnancy, third trimester Ⓜ♀

O29.019 Aspiration pneumonitis due to anesthesia during pregnancy, unspecified trimester Ⓜ♀

✓6ᵗʰ O29.02 Pressure collapse of lung due to anesthesia during pregnancy

O29.021 Pressure collapse of lung due to anesthesia during pregnancy, first trimester Ⓜ♀

O29.022 Pressure collapse of lung due to anesthesia during pregnancy, second trimester Ⓜ♀

O29.023 Pressure collapse of lung due to anesthesia during pregnancy, third trimester Ⓜ♀

O29.029 Pressure collapse of lung due to anesthesia during pregnancy, unspecified trimester Ⓜ♀

✓6ᵗʰ O29.09 Other pulmonary complications of anesthesia during pregnancy

O29.091 Other pulmonary complications of anesthesia during pregnancy, first trimester Ⓜ♀

O29.092 Other pulmonary complications of anesthesia during pregnancy, second trimester Ⓜ♀

Chapter 15. Pregnancy, Childbirth and the Puerperium

O26.8–O29.092

O29.Ø93   **Other pulmonary complications of anesthesia during pregnancy, third trimester**   Ⓜ♀

O29.Ø99   **Other pulmonary complications of anesthesia during pregnancy, unspecified trimester**   Ⓜ♀

✓5ᵗʰ **O29.1**   **Cardiac complications of anesthesia during pregnancy**

  ✓6ᵗʰ **O29.11**   Cardiac arrest due to anesthesia during pregnancy

O29.111   **Cardiac arrest due to anesthesia during pregnancy, first trimester**   Ⓜ♀

O29.112   **Cardiac arrest due to anesthesia during pregnancy, second trimester**   Ⓜ♀

O29.113   **Cardiac arrest due to anesthesia during pregnancy, third trimester**   Ⓜ♀

O29.119   **Cardiac arrest due to anesthesia during pregnancy, unspecified trimester**   Ⓜ♀

  ✓6ᵗʰ **O29.12**   Cardiac failure due to anesthesia during pregnancy

O29.121   **Cardiac failure due to anesthesia during pregnancy, first trimester**   Ⓜ♀

O29.122   **Cardiac failure due to anesthesia during pregnancy, second trimester**   Ⓜ♀

O29.123   **Cardiac failure due to anesthesia during pregnancy, third trimester**   Ⓜ♀

O29.129   **Cardiac failure due to anesthesia during pregnancy, unspecified trimester**   Ⓜ♀

  ✓6ᵗʰ **O29.19**   Other cardiac complications of anesthesia during pregnancy

O29.191   **Other cardiac complications of anesthesia during pregnancy, first trimester**   Ⓜ♀

O29.192   **Other cardiac complications of anesthesia during pregnancy, second trimester**   Ⓜ♀

O29.193   **Other cardiac complications of anesthesia during pregnancy, third trimester**   Ⓜ♀

O29.199   **Other cardiac complications of anesthesia during pregnancy, unspecified trimester**   Ⓜ♀

✓5ᵗʰ **O29.2**   **Central nervous system complications of anesthesia during pregnancy**

  ✓6ᵗʰ **O29.21**   Cerebral anoxia due to anesthesia during pregnancy

O29.211   **Cerebral anoxia due to anesthesia during pregnancy, first trimester**   Ⓜ♀

O29.212   **Cerebral anoxia due to anesthesia during pregnancy, second trimester**   Ⓜ♀

O29.213   **Cerebral anoxia due to anesthesia during pregnancy, third trimester**   Ⓜ♀

O29.219   **Cerebral anoxia due to anesthesia during pregnancy, unspecified trimester**   Ⓜ♀

  ✓6ᵗʰ **O29.29**   Other central nervous system complications of anesthesia during pregnancy

O29.291   **Other central nervous system complications of anesthesia during pregnancy, first trimester**   Ⓜ♀

O29.292   **Other central nervous system complications of anesthesia during pregnancy, second trimester**   Ⓜ♀

O29.293   **Other central nervous system complications of anesthesia during pregnancy, third trimester**   Ⓜ♀

O29.299   **Other central nervous system complications of anesthesia during pregnancy, unspecified trimester**   Ⓜ♀

✓5ᵗʰ **O29.3**   **Toxic reaction to local anesthesia during pregnancy**

  ✓6ᵗʰ **O29.3X**   Toxic reaction to local anesthesia during pregnancy

O29.3X1   **Toxic reaction to local anesthesia during pregnancy, first trimester**   Ⓜ♀

O29.3X2   **Toxic reaction to local anesthesia during pregnancy, second trimester**   Ⓜ♀

O29.3X3   **Toxic reaction to local anesthesia during pregnancy, third trimester**   Ⓜ♀

O29.3X9   **Toxic reaction to local anesthesia during pregnancy, unspecified trimester**   Ⓜ♀

✓5ᵗʰ **O29.4**   **Spinal and epidural anesthesia induced headache during pregnancy**

O29.40   **Spinal and epidural anesthesia induced headache during pregnancy, unspecified trimester**   Ⓜ♀

O29.41   **Spinal and epidural anesthesia induced headache during pregnancy, first trimester**   Ⓜ♀

O29.42   **Spinal and epidural anesthesia induced headache during pregnancy, second trimester**   Ⓜ♀

O29.43   **Spinal and epidural anesthesia induced headache during pregnancy, third trimester**   Ⓜ♀

✓5ᵗʰ **O29.5**   **Other complications of spinal and epidural anesthesia during pregnancy**

  ✓6ᵗʰ **O29.5X**   Other complications of spinal and epidural anesthesia during pregnancy

O29.5X1   **Other complications of spinal and epidural anesthesia during pregnancy, first trimester**   Ⓜ♀

O29.5X2   **Other complications of spinal and epidural anesthesia during pregnancy, second trimester**   Ⓜ♀

O29.5X3   **Other complications of spinal and epidural anesthesia during pregnancy, third trimester**   Ⓜ♀

O29.5X9   **Other complications of spinal and epidural anesthesia during pregnancy, unspecified trimester**   Ⓜ♀

✓6ᵗʰ **O29.6**   **Failed or difficult intubation for anesthesia during pregnancy**

O29.60   **Failed or difficult intubation for anesthesia during pregnancy, unspecified trimester**   Ⓜ♀

O29.61   **Failed or difficult intubation for anesthesia during pregnancy, first trimester**   Ⓜ♀

O29.62   **Failed or difficult intubation for anesthesia during pregnancy, second trimester**   Ⓜ♀

O29.63   **Failed or difficult intubation for anesthesia during pregnancy, third trimester**   Ⓜ♀

✓5ᵗʰ **O29.8**   **Other complications of anesthesia during pregnancy**

  ✓6ᵗʰ **O29.8X**   Other complications of anesthesia during pregnancy

O29.8X1   **Other complications of anesthesia during pregnancy, first trimester**   Ⓜ♀

O29.8X2   **Other complications of anesthesia during pregnancy, second trimester**   Ⓜ♀

O29.8X3   **Other complications of anesthesia during pregnancy, third trimester**   Ⓜ♀

O29.8X9   **Other complications of anesthesia during pregnancy, unspecified trimester**   Ⓜ♀

✓5ᵗʰ **O29.9**   **Unspecified complication of anesthesia during pregnancy**

O29.90   **Unspecified complication of anesthesia during pregnancy, unspecified trimester**   Ⓜ♀

O29.91   **Unspecified complication of anesthesia during pregnancy, first trimester**   Ⓜ♀

O29.92   **Unspecified complication of anesthesia during pregnancy, second trimester**   Ⓜ♀

O29.93   **Unspecified complication of anesthesia during pregnancy, third trimester**   Ⓜ♀

Maternal care related to the fetus and amniotic cavity and possible delivery problems (O30-O48)

✓4ᵗʰ **O30 Multiple gestation**
  Code also any complications specific to multiple gestation
  AHA: 2016,4Q,51

✓5ᵗʰ **O30.0 Twin pregnancy**

  ✓6ᵗʰ **O30.00 Twin pregnancy, unspecified number of placenta and unspecified number of amniotic sacs**

  O30.001 Twin pregnancy, unspecified number of placenta and unspecified number of amniotic sacs, first trimester Ⓜ♀

  O30.002 Twin pregnancy, unspecified number of placenta and unspecified number of amniotic sacs, second trimester Ⓜ♀

  O30.003 Twin pregnancy, unspecified number of placenta and unspecified number of amniotic sacs, third trimester Ⓜ♀

  O30.009 Twin pregnancy, unspecified number of placenta and unspecified number of amniotic sacs, unspecified trimester Ⓜ♀

  ✓6ᵗʰ **O30.01 Twin pregnancy, monochorionic/monoamniotic**
    Twin pregnancy, one placenta, one amniotic sac
    EXCLUDES 1 conjoined twins (O30.02-)

Twin Gestation – Monochorionic/Monoamniotic

- 1 Chorionic sac
- 1 Amniotic sac
- 2 Fetuses
- 2 Umbilical cords
- 1 Placenta

  O30.011 Twin pregnancy, monochorionic/monoamniotic, first trimester Ⓜ♀

  O30.012 Twin pregnancy, monochorionic/monoamniotic, second trimester Ⓜ♀

  O30.013 Twin pregnancy, monochorionic/monoamniotic, third trimester Ⓜ♀

  O30.019 Twin pregnancy, monochorionic/monoamniotic, unspecified trimester Ⓜ♀

  ✓6ᵗʰ **O30.02 Conjoined twin pregnancy**

  O30.021 Conjoined twin pregnancy, first trimester Ⓜ♀

  O30.022 Conjoined twin pregnancy, second trimester Ⓜ♀

  O30.023 Conjoined twin pregnancy, third trimester Ⓜ♀

  O30.029 Conjoined twin pregnancy, unspecified trimester Ⓜ♀

  ✓6ᵗʰ **O30.03 Twin pregnancy, monochorionic/diamniotic**
    Twin pregnancy, one placenta, two amniotic sacs

Twin Gestation – Monochorionic/Diamniotic

- 1 Chorionic sac
- 2 Amniotic sacs
- 2 Fetuses
- 2 Umbilical cords
- 1 Placenta

  O30.031 Twin pregnancy, monochorionic/diamniotic, first trimester Ⓜ♀

  O30.032 Twin pregnancy, monochorionic/diamniotic, second trimester Ⓜ♀

  O30.033 Twin pregnancy, monochorionic/diamniotic, third trimester Ⓜ♀

  O30.039 Twin pregnancy, monochorionic/diamniotic, unspecified trimester Ⓜ♀

  ✓6ᵗʰ **O30.04 Twin pregnancy, dichorionic/diamniotic**
    Twin pregnancy, two placentae, two amniotic sacs

Twin Gestation – Dichorionic/Diamniotic

- 2 Chorionic sacs
- 2 Amniotic sacs
- 2 Fetuses
- 2 Umbilical cords
- 2 Placentas

  O30.041 Twin pregnancy, dichorionic/diamniotic, first trimester Ⓜ♀

  O30.042 Twin pregnancy, dichorionic/diamniotic, second trimester Ⓜ♀

  O30.043 Twin pregnancy, dichorionic/diamniotic, third trimester Ⓜ♀

  O30.049 Twin pregnancy, dichorionic/diamniotic, unspecified trimester Ⓜ♀

  ✓6ᵗʰ **O30.09 Twin pregnancy, unable to determine number of placenta and number of amniotic sacs**

  O30.091 Twin pregnancy, unable to determine number of placenta and number of amniotic sacs, first trimester Ⓜ♀

  O30.092 Twin pregnancy, unable to determine number of placenta and number of amniotic sacs, second trimester Ⓜ♀

  O30.093 Twin pregnancy, unable to determine number of placenta and number of amniotic sacs, third trimester Ⓜ♀

✔ Additional Character Required   ✔x7ᵗʰ Placeholder Alert   Manifestation   Unspecified Dx   ►◄ Revised Text   ● New Code   ▲ Revised Code Title

Chapter 15. Pregnancy, Childbirth and the Puerperium

O30.099–O30.299

O30.099	Twin pregnancy, unable to determine number of placenta and number of amniotic sacs, unspecified trimester	Ⓜ ♀

✓5ᵗʰ **O30.1**   Triplet pregnancy

   ✓6ᵗʰ **O30.10**   **Triplet pregnancy, unspecified number of placenta and unspecified number of amniotic sacs**
      AHA: 2016,2Q,8

O30.101	Triplet pregnancy, unspecified number of placenta and unspecified number of amniotic sacs, first trimester	Ⓜ ♀
O30.102	Triplet pregnancy, unspecified number of placenta and unspecified number of amniotic sacs, second trimester	Ⓜ ♀
O30.103	Triplet pregnancy, unspecified number of placenta and unspecified number of amniotic sacs, third trimester	Ⓜ ♀
O30.109	Triplet pregnancy, unspecified number of placenta and unspecified number of amniotic sacs, unspecified trimester	Ⓜ ♀

   ✓6ᵗʰ **O30.11**   **Triplet pregnancy with two or more monochorionic fetuses**

O30.111	Triplet pregnancy with two or more monochorionic fetuses, first trimester	Ⓜ ♀
O30.112	Triplet pregnancy with two or more monochorionic fetuses, second trimester	Ⓜ ♀
O30.113	Triplet pregnancy with two or more monochorionic fetuses, third trimester	Ⓜ ♀
O30.119	Triplet pregnancy with two or more monochorionic fetuses, unspecified trimester	Ⓜ ♀

   ✓6ᵗʰ **O30.12**   **Triplet pregnancy with two or more monoamniotic fetuses**

O30.121	Triplet pregnancy with two or more monoamniotic fetuses, first trimester	Ⓜ ♀
O30.122	Triplet pregnancy with two or more monoamniotic fetuses, second trimester	Ⓜ ♀
O30.123	Triplet pregnancy with two or more monoamniotic fetuses, third trimester	Ⓜ ♀
O30.129	Triplet pregnancy with two or more monoamniotic fetuses, unspecified trimester	Ⓜ ♀

   ✓6ᵗʰ **O30.13**   **Triplet pregnancy, trichorionic/triamniotic**
      AHA: 2018,4Q,22

O30.131	Triplet pregnancy, trichorionic/triamniotic, first trimester	Ⓜ ♀
O30.132	Triplet pregnancy, trichorionic/triamniotic, second trimester	Ⓜ ♀
O30.133	Triplet pregnancy, trichorionic/triamniotic, third trimester	Ⓜ ♀
O30.139	Triplet pregnancy, trichorionic/triamniotic, unspecified trimester	Ⓜ ♀

   ✓6ᵗʰ **O30.19**   **Triplet pregnancy, unable to determine number of placenta and number of amniotic sacs**

O30.191	Triplet pregnancy, unable to determine number of placenta and number of amniotic sacs, first trimester	Ⓜ ♀
O30.192	Triplet pregnancy, unable to determine number of placenta and number of amniotic sacs, second trimester	Ⓜ ♀
O30.193	Triplet pregnancy, unable to determine number of placenta and number of amniotic sacs, third trimester	Ⓜ ♀
O30.199	Triplet pregnancy, unable to determine number of placenta and number of amniotic sacs, unspecified trimester	Ⓜ ♀

✓5ᵗʰ **O30.2**   Quadruplet pregnancy

   ✓6ᵗʰ **O30.20**   **Quadruplet pregnancy, unspecified number of placenta and unspecified number of amniotic sacs**

O30.201	Quadruplet pregnancy, unspecified number of placenta and unspecified number of amniotic sacs, first trimester	Ⓜ ♀
O30.202	Quadruplet pregnancy, unspecified number of placenta and unspecified number of amniotic sacs, second trimester	Ⓜ ♀
O30.203	Quadruplet pregnancy, unspecified number of placenta and unspecified number of amniotic sacs, third trimester	Ⓜ ♀
O30.209	Quadruplet pregnancy, unspecified number of placenta and unspecified number of amniotic sacs, unspecified trimester	Ⓜ ♀

   ✓6ᵗʰ **O30.21**   **Quadruplet pregnancy with two or more monochorionic fetuses**

O30.211	Quadruplet pregnancy with two or more monochorionic fetuses, first trimester	Ⓜ ♀
O30.212	Quadruplet pregnancy with two or more monochorionic fetuses, second trimester	Ⓜ ♀
O30.213	Quadruplet pregnancy with two or more monochorionic fetuses, third trimester	Ⓜ ♀
O30.219	Quadruplet pregnancy with two or more monochorionic fetuses, unspecified trimester	Ⓜ ♀

   ✓6ᵗʰ **O30.22**   **Quadruplet pregnancy with two or more monoamniotic fetuses**

O30.221	Quadruplet pregnancy with two or more monoamniotic fetuses, first trimester	Ⓜ ♀
O30.222	Quadruplet pregnancy with two or more monoamniotic fetuses, second trimester	Ⓜ ♀
O30.223	Quadruplet pregnancy with two or more monoamniotic fetuses, third trimester	Ⓜ ♀
O30.229	Quadruplet pregnancy with two or more monoamniotic fetuses, unspecified trimester	Ⓜ ♀

   ✓6ᵗʰ **O30.23**   **Quadruplet pregnancy, quadrachorionic/quadra-amniotic**
      AHA: 2018,4Q,22

O30.231	Quadruplet pregnancy, quadrachorionic/quadra-amniotic, first trimester	Ⓜ ♀
O30.232	Quadruplet pregnancy, quadrachorionic/quadra-amniotic, second trimester	Ⓜ ♀
O30.233	Quadruplet pregnancy, quadrachorionic/quadra-amniotic, third trimester	Ⓜ ♀
O30.239	Quadruplet pregnancy, quadrachorionic/quadra-amniotic, unspecified trimester	Ⓜ ♀

   ✓6ᵗʰ **O30.29**   **Quadruplet pregnancy, unable to determine number of placenta and number of amniotic sacs**

O30.291	Quadruplet pregnancy, unable to determine number of placenta and number of amniotic sacs, first trimester	Ⓜ ♀
O30.292	Quadruplet pregnancy, unable to determine number of placenta and number of amniotic sacs, second trimester	Ⓜ ♀
O30.293	Quadruplet pregnancy, unable to determine number of placenta and number of amniotic sacs, third trimester	Ⓜ ♀
O30.299	Quadruplet pregnancy, unable to determine number of placenta and number of amniotic sacs, unspecified trimester	Ⓜ ♀

✓5ᵗʰ **O30.8** **Other specified multiple gestation**

Multiple gestation pregnancy greater then quadruplets

✓6ᵗʰ **O30.80** **Other specified multiple gestation, unspecified number of placenta and unspecified number of amniotic sacs**

O30.801 **Other specified multiple gestation, unspecified number of placenta and unspecified number of amniotic sacs, first trimester**   Ⓜ♀

O30.802 **Other specified multiple gestation, unspecified number of placenta and unspecified number of amniotic sacs, second trimester**   Ⓜ♀

O30.803 **Other specified multiple gestation, unspecified number of placenta and unspecified number of amniotic sacs, third trimester**   Ⓜ♀

O30.809 **Other specified multiple gestation, unspecified number of placenta and unspecified number of amniotic sacs, unspecified trimester**   Ⓜ♀

✓6ᵗʰ **O30.81** **Other specified multiple gestation with** two or more monochorionic fetuses

O30.811 **Other specified multiple gestation with two or more monochorionic fetuses, first trimester**   Ⓜ♀

O30.812 **Other specified multiple gestation with two or more monochorionic fetuses, second trimester**   Ⓜ♀

O30.813 **Other specified multiple gestation with two or more monochorionic fetuses, third trimester**   Ⓜ♀

O30.819 **Other specified multiple gestation with two or more monochorionic fetuses, unspecified trimester**   Ⓜ♀

✓6ᵗʰ **O30.82** **Other specified multiple gestation with** two or more monoamniotic fetuses

O30.821 **Other specified multiple gestation with two or more monoamniotic fetuses, first trimester**   Ⓜ♀

O30.822 **Other specified multiple gestation with two or more monoamniotic fetuses, second trimester**   Ⓜ♀

O30.823 **Other specified multiple gestation with two or more monoamniotic fetuses, third trimester**   Ⓜ♀

O30.829 **Other specified multiple gestation with two or more monoamniotic fetuses, unspecified trimester**   Ⓜ♀

✓6ᵗʰ **O30.83** **Other specified multiple gestation,** number of chorions and amnions are both equal to the number of fetuses

Pentachorionic, penta-amniotic pregnancy (quintuplets)

Hexachorionic, hexa-amniotic pregnancy (sextuplets)

Heptachorionic, hepta-amniotic pregnancy (septuplets)

AHA: 2018,4Q,22

O30.831 **Other specified multiple gestation, number of chorions and amnions are both equal to the number of fetuses, first trimester**   Ⓜ♀

O30.832 **Other specified multiple gestation, number of chorions and amnions are both equal to the number of fetuses, second trimester**   Ⓜ♀

O30.833 **Other specified multiple gestation, number of chorions and amnions are both equal to the number of fetuses, third trimester**   Ⓜ♀

O30.839 **Other specified multiple gestation, number of chorions and amnions are both equal to the number of fetuses, unspecified trimester**   Ⓜ♀

✓6ᵗʰ **O30.89** **Other specified multiple gestation,** unable to determine number **of placenta and number of amniotic sacs**

O30.891 **Other specified multiple gestation, unable to determine number of placenta and number of amniotic sacs, first trimester**   Ⓜ♀

O30.892 **Other specified multiple gestation, unable to determine number of placenta and number of amniotic sacs, second trimester**   Ⓜ♀

O30.893 **Other specified multiple gestation, unable to determine number of placenta and number of amniotic sacs, third trimester**   Ⓜ♀

O30.899 **Other specified multiple gestation, unable to determine number of placenta and number of amniotic sacs, unspecified trimester**   Ⓜ♀

✓5ᵗʰ **O30.9** **Multiple gestation, unspecified**

Multiple pregnancy NOS

O30.90 **Multiple gestation, unspecified, unspecified trimester**   Ⓜ♀

O30.91 **Multiple gestation, unspecified, first trimester**   Ⓜ♀

O30.92 **Multiple gestation, unspecified, second trimester**   Ⓜ♀

O30.93 **Multiple gestation, unspecified, third trimester**   Ⓜ♀

✓4ᵗʰ **O31** **Complications specific to multiple gestation**

EXCLUDES 2   *delayed delivery of second twin, triplet, etc. (O63.2)*

malpresentation of one fetus or more (O32.9)

placental transfusion syndromes (O43.0-)

AHA: 2012,4Q,107

One of the following 7th characters is to be assigned to each code under category O31. 7th character 0 is for single gestations and multiple gestations where the fetus is unspecified. 7th characters 1 through 9 are for cases of multiple gestations to identify the fetus for which the code applies. The appropriate code from category O30, Multiple gestation, must also be assigned when assigning a code from category O31 that has a 7th character of 1 through 9.

0   not applicable or unspecified
1   fetus 1
2   fetus 2
3   fetus 3
4   fetus 4
5   fetus 5
9   other fetus

✓5ᵗʰ **O31.0** **Papyraceous fetus**

Fetus compressus

DEF: Fetus that has died, but remains in utero for weeks before delivery, becoming compacted and mummified in appearance, with skin resembling parchment. Occurs most commonly in multigestational pregnancies. *Synonym(s): paper doll fetus.*

✓x7ᵗʰ **O31.00** **Papyraceous fetus, unspecified trimester**   Ⓜ♀

✓x7ᵗʰ **O31.01** **Papyraceous fetus,** first trimester   Ⓜ♀

✓x7ᵗʰ **O31.02** **Papyraceous fetus,** second trimester   Ⓜ♀

✓x7ᵗʰ **O31.03** **Papyraceous fetus,** third trimester   Ⓜ♀

✓5ᵗʰ **O31.1** **Continuing pregnancy** after spontaneous abortion **of one fetus or more**

✓x7ᵗʰ **O31.10** **Continuing pregnancy after spontaneous abortion of one fetus or more, unspecified trimester**   Ⓜ♀

✓x7ᵗʰ **O31.11** **Continuing pregnancy after spontaneous abortion of one fetus or more,** first trimester   Ⓜ♀

✓x7ᵗʰ **O31.12** **Continuing pregnancy after spontaneous abortion of one fetus or more,** second trimester   Ⓜ♀

✓x7ᵗʰ **O31.13** **Continuing pregnancy after spontaneous abortion of one fetus or more,** third trimester   Ⓜ♀

☑ Additional Character Required   ✓x7ᵗʰ Placeholder Alert   Manifestation   Unspecified Dx   ▶◀ Revised Text   ● New Code   ▲ Revised Code Title

ICD-10-CM 2020   871

✓5th **O31.2** **Continuing pregnancy** after intrauterine death **of one fetus or more**
- ✓x7th **O31.20** **Continuing pregnancy after intrauterine death of one fetus or more, unspecified trimester** M ♀
- ✓x7th **O31.21** **Continuing pregnancy after intrauterine death of one fetus or more,** first trimester M ♀
- ✓x7th **O31.22** **Continuing pregnancy after intrauterine death of one fetus or more,** second trimester M ♀
- ✓x7th **O31.23** **Continuing pregnancy after intrauterine death of one fetus or more,** third trimester M ♀

✓5th **O31.3** **Continuing pregnancy after** elective fetal reduction **of one fetus or more**
     Continuing pregnancy after selective termination of one fetus or more
- ✓x7th **O31.30** **Continuing pregnancy after elective fetal reduction of one fetus or more, unspecified trimester** M ♀
- ✓x7th **O31.31** **Continuing pregnancy after elective fetal reduction of one fetus or more,** first trimester M ♀
- ✓x7th **O31.32** **Continuing pregnancy after elective fetal reduction of one fetus or more,** second trimester M ♀
- ✓x7th **O31.33** **Continuing pregnancy after elective fetal reduction of one fetus or more,** third trimester M ♀

✓5th **O31.8** **Other complications specific to multiple gestation**
- ✓6th **O31.8X** **Other complications specific to multiple gestation**
  - ✓7th **O31.8X1** **Other complications specific to multiple gestation,** first trimester M ♀
  - ✓7th **O31.8X2** **Other complications specific to multiple gestation,** second trimester M ♀
  - ✓7th **O31.8X3** **Other complications specific to multiple gestation,** third trimester M ♀
  - ✓7th **O31.8X9** **Other complications specific to multiple gestation, unspecified trimester** M ♀

✓4th **O32** **Maternal care for malpresentation of fetus**
     INCLUDES   the listed conditions as a reason for observation, hospitalization or other obstetric care of the mother, or for cesarean delivery before onset of labor
     EXCLUDES 1   *malpresentation of fetus with obstructed labor (O64.-)*
     AHA: 2012,4Q,107

> One of the following 7th characters is to be assigned to each code under category O32. 7th character 0 is for single gestations and multiple gestations where the fetus is unspecified. 7th characters 1 through 9 are for cases of multiple gestations to identify the fetus for which the code applies. The appropriate code from category O30, Multiple gestation, must also be assigned when assigning a code from category O32 that has a 7th character of 1 through 9.
> 0   not applicable or unspecified
> 1   fetus 1
> 2   fetus 2
> 3   fetus 3
> 4   fetus 4
> 5   fetus 5
> 9   other fetus

- ✓x7th **O32.0** **Maternal care for** unstable lie M ♀
- ✓x7th **O32.1** **Maternal care for** breech presentation M ♀
     Maternal care for buttocks presentation
     Maternal care for complete breech
     Maternal care for frank breech
     EXCLUDES 1   *footling presentation (O32.8)*
                  incomplete breech (O32.8)
     DEF: Fetus presentation in a longitudinal lie with the buttocks or feet closest to birth canal that may require external cephalic version or cesarean delivery.
- ✓x7th **O32.2** **Maternal care for** transverse and oblique lie M ♀
     Maternal care for oblique presentation
     Maternal care for transverse presentation
- ✓x7th **O32.3** **Maternal care for** face, brow and chin presentation M ♀

- ✓x7th **O32.4** **Maternal care for** high head at term M ♀
     Maternal care for failure of head to enter pelvic brim
- ✓x7th **O32.6** **Maternal care for** compound presentation M ♀
- ✓x7th **O32.8** **Maternal care for** other malpresentation of fetus M ♀
     Maternal care for footling presentation
     Maternal care for incomplete breech
- ✓x7th **O32.9** **Maternal care for** malpresentation of fetus, unspecified M ♀

Fetal Malpresentation

Breech   Shoulder (arm prolapse)   Mother's pelvis   Face (mentum)   Compound (extremity together with head)   Oblique

✓4th **O33** **Maternal care for disproportion**
     INCLUDES   the listed conditions as a reason for observation, hospitalization or other obstetric care of the mother, or for cesarean delivery before onset of labor
     EXCLUDES 1   *disproportion with obstructed labor (O65-O66)*

- **O33.0** **Maternal care for disproportion due to** deformity **of maternal pelvic bones** M ♀
     Maternal care for disproportion due to pelvic deformity causing disproportion NOS
- **O33.1** **Maternal care for disproportion due to** generally **contracted pelvis** M ♀
     Maternal care for disproportion due to contracted pelvis NOS causing disproportion
- **O33.2** **Maternal care for disproportion due to** inlet **contraction of pelvis** M ♀
     Maternal care for disproportion due to inlet contraction (pelvis) causing disproportion
- ✓x7th **O33.3** **Maternal care for disproportion due to** outlet **contraction of pelvis** M ♀
     Maternal care for disproportion due to mid-cavity contraction (pelvis)
     Maternal care for disproportion due to outlet contraction (pelvis)

> One of the following 7th characters is to be assigned to code O33.3. 7th character 0 is for single gestations and multiple gestations where the fetus is unspecified. 7th characters 1 through 9 are for cases of multiple gestations to identify the fetus for which the code applies. The appropriate code from category O30, Multiple gestation, must also be assigned when assigning code O33.3 with a 7th character of 1 through 9.
> 0   not applicable or unspecified
> 1   fetus 1
> 2   fetus 2
> 3   fetus 3
> 4   fetus 4
> 5   fetus 5
> 9   other fetus

√x7ᵗʰ O33.4 Maternal care for disproportion of mixed maternal and fetal origin Ⓜ ♀

One of the following 7th characters is to be assigned to code O33.4. 7th character Ø is for single gestations and multiple gestations where the fetus is unspecified. 7th characters 1 through 9 are for cases of multiple gestations to identify the fetus for which the code applies. The appropriate code from category O3Ø, Multiple gestation, must also be assigned when assigning code O33.4 with a 7th character of 1 through 9.
- Ø not applicable or unspecified
- 1 fetus 1
- 2 fetus 2
- 3 fetus 3
- 4 fetus 4
- 5 fetus 5
- 9 other fetus

√x7ᵗʰ O33.5 Maternal care for disproportion due to unusually large fetus Ⓜ ♀

Maternal care for disproportion due to disproportion of fetal origin with normally formed fetus

Maternal care for disproportion due to fetal disproportion NOS

One of the following 7th characters is to be assigned to code O33.5. 7th character Ø is for single gestations and multiple gestations where the fetus is unspecified. 7th characters 1 through 9 are for cases of multiple gestations to identify the fetus for which the code applies. The appropriate code from category O3Ø, Multiple gestation, must also be assigned when assigning code O33.5 with a 7th character of 1 through 9.
- Ø not applicable or unspecified
- 1 fetus 1
- 2 fetus 2
- 3 fetus 3
- 4 fetus 4
- 5 fetus 5
- 9 other fetus

√x7ᵗʰ O33.6 Maternal care for disproportion due to hydrocephalic fetus Ⓜ ♀

One of the following 7th characters is to be assigned to code O33.6. 7th character Ø is for single gestations and multiple gestations where the fetus is unspecified. 7th characters 1 through 9 are for cases of multiple gestations to identify the fetus for which the code applies. The appropriate code from category O3Ø, Multiple gestation, must also be assigned when assigning code O33.6 with a 7th character of 1 through 9.
- Ø not applicable or unspecified
- 1 fetus 1
- 2 fetus 2
- 3 fetus 3
- 4 fetus 4
- 5 fetus 5
- 9 other fetus

√x7ᵗʰ O33.7 Maternal care for disproportion due to other fetal deformities Ⓜ ♀

Maternal care for disproportion due to fetal ascites

Maternal care for disproportion due to fetal hydrops

Maternal care for disproportion due to fetal meningomyelocele

Maternal care for disproportion due to fetal sacral teratoma

Maternal care for disproportion due to fetal tumor

EXCLUDES 1   obstructed labor due to other fetal deformities (O66.3)

AHA: 2016,4Q,51

One of the following 7th characters is to be assigned to code O33.7. 7th character Ø is for single gestations and multiple gestations where the fetus is unspecified. 7th characters 1 through 9 are for cases of multiple gestations to identify the fetus for which the code applies. The appropriate code from category O3Ø, Multiple gestation, must also be assigned when assigning code O33.7 with a 7th character of 1 through 9.
- Ø not applicable or unspecified
- 1 fetus 1
- 2 fetus 2
- 3 fetus 3
- 4 fetus 4
- 5 fetus 5
- 9 other fetus

O33.8 Maternal care for disproportion of other origin Ⓜ ♀

O33.9 Maternal care for disproportion, unspecified Ⓜ ♀

Maternal care for disproportion due to cephalopelvic disproportion NOS

Maternal care for disproportion due to fetopelvic disproportion NOS

√4ᵗʰ O34 Maternal care for abnormality of pelvic organs

INCLUDES   the listed conditions as a reason for hospitalization or other obstetric care of the mother, or for cesarean delivery before onset of labor

Code first any associated obstructed labor (O65.5)

Use additional code for specific condition

√5ᵗʰ O34.Ø Maternal care for congenital malformation of uterus

Maternal care for double uterus

Maternal care for uterus bicornis

O34.ØØ Maternal care for unspecified congenital malformation of uterus, unspecified trimester Ⓜ ♀

O34.Ø1 Maternal care for unspecified congenital malformation of uterus, first trimester Ⓜ ♀

O34.Ø2 Maternal care for unspecified congenital malformation of uterus, second trimester Ⓜ ♀

O34.Ø3 Maternal care for unspecified congenital malformation of uterus, third trimester Ⓜ ♀

√5ᵗʰ O34.1 Maternal care for benign tumor of corpus uteri

EXCLUDES 2   maternal care for benign tumor of cervix (O34.4-)
maternal care for malignant neoplasm of uterus (O9A.1-)

O34.1Ø Maternal care for benign tumor of corpus uteri, unspecified trimester Ⓜ ♀

O34.11 Maternal care for benign tumor of corpus uteri, first trimester Ⓜ ♀

O34.12 Maternal care for benign tumor of corpus uteri, second trimester Ⓜ ♀

O34.13 Maternal care for benign tumor of corpus uteri, third trimester Ⓜ ♀

√5ᵗʰ O34.2 Maternal care due to uterine scar from previous surgery

AHA: 2016,4Q,76

√6ᵗʰ O34.21 Maternal care for scar from previous cesarean delivery

AHA: 2018,3Q,23; 2016,4Q,51-52

O34.211 Maternal care for low transverse scar from previous cesarean delivery Ⓜ ♀

O34.212 Maternal care for vertical scar from previous cesarean delivery Ⓜ ♀

Maternal care for classical scar from previous cesarean delivery

O34.219 Maternal care for unspecified type scar from previous cesarean delivery Ⓜ ♀

O34.29 Maternal care due to uterine scar from other previous surgery Ⓜ ♀

Maternal care due to uterine scar from other transmural uterine incision

√5ᵗʰ O34.3 Maternal care for cervical incompetence

Maternal care for cerclage with or without cervical incompetence

Maternal care for Shirodkar suture with or without cervical incompetence

DEF: Inadequate functioning of the cervix marked by abnormal widening during pregnancy and causing premature birth or miscarriage.

O34.3Ø Maternal care for cervical incompetence, unspecified trimester Ⓜ ♀

O34.31 Maternal care for cervical incompetence, first trimester Ⓜ ♀

O34.32 Maternal care for cervical incompetence, second trimester Ⓜ ♀

O34.33 Maternal care for cervical incompetence, third trimester Ⓜ ♀

√5ᵗʰ O34.4 Maternal care for other abnormalities of cervix

O34.4Ø Maternal care for other abnormalities of cervix, unspecified trimester Ⓜ ♀

O34.41 Maternal care for other abnormalities of cervix, first trimester Ⓜ ♀

O34.42 Maternal care for other abnormalities of cervix, second trimester Ⓜ ♀

O34.43 Maternal care for other abnormalities of cervix, third trimester Ⓜ ♀

☑ Additional Character Required   √x7ᵗʰ Placeholder Alert   Manifestation   Unspecified Dx   ▶◀ Revised Text   ● New Code   ▲ Revised Code Title

ICD-10-CM 2020   873

Chapter 15. Pregnancy, Childbirth and the Puerperium

O34.5–O35.9

√5ᵗʰ **O34.5 Maternal care for** other abnormalities of gravid uterus

√6ᵗʰ **O34.51 Maternal care for** incarceration of gravid uterus

O34.511 Maternal care for incarceration of gravid uterus, first trimester Ⓜ♀

O34.512 Maternal care for incarceration of gravid uterus, second trimester Ⓜ♀

O34.513 Maternal care for incarceration of gravid uterus, third trimester Ⓜ♀

O34.519 Maternal care for incarceration of gravid uterus, unspecified trimester Ⓜ♀

√6ᵗʰ **O34.52 Maternal care for** prolapse of gravid uterus

O34.521 Maternal care for prolapse of gravid uterus, first trimester Ⓜ♀

O34.522 Maternal care for prolapse of gravid uterus, second trimester Ⓜ♀

O34.523 Maternal care for prolapse of gravid uterus, third trimester Ⓜ♀

O34.529 Maternal care for prolapse of gravid uterus, unspecified trimester Ⓜ♀

√6ᵗʰ **O34.53 Maternal care for** retroversion of gravid uterus

O34.531 Maternal care for retroversion of gravid uterus, first trimester Ⓜ♀

O34.532 Maternal care for retroversion of gravid uterus, second trimester Ⓜ♀

O34.533 Maternal care for retroversion of gravid uterus, third trimester Ⓜ♀

O34.539 Maternal care for retroversion of gravid uterus, unspecified trimester Ⓜ♀

√6ᵗʰ **O34.59 Maternal care for other abnormalities of gravid uterus**

O34.591 Maternal care for other abnormalities of gravid uterus, first trimester Ⓜ♀

O34.592 Maternal care for other abnormalities of gravid uterus, second trimester Ⓜ♀

O34.593 Maternal care for other abnormalities of gravid uterus, third trimester Ⓜ♀

O34.599 Maternal care for other abnormalities of gravid uterus, unspecified trimester Ⓜ♀

√5ᵗʰ **O34.6 Maternal care for** abnormality of vagina

EXCLUDES 2   *maternal care for vaginal varices in pregnancy (O22.1-)*

O34.60 Maternal care for abnormality of vagina, unspecified trimester Ⓜ♀

O34.61 Maternal care for abnormality of vagina, first trimester Ⓜ♀

O34.62 Maternal care for abnormality of vagina, second trimester Ⓜ♀

O34.63 Maternal care for abnormality of vagina, third trimester Ⓜ♀

√5ᵗʰ **O34.7 Maternal care for** abnormality of vulva and perineum

EXCLUDES 2   *maternal care for perineal and vulval varices in pregnancy (O22.1-)*

O34.70 Maternal care for abnormality of vulva and perineum, unspecified trimester Ⓜ♀

O34.71 Maternal care for abnormality of vulva and perineum, first trimester Ⓜ♀

O34.72 Maternal care for abnormality of vulva and perineum, second trimester Ⓜ♀

O34.73 Maternal care for abnormality of vulva and perineum, third trimester Ⓜ♀

√5ᵗʰ **O34.8 Maternal care for** other abnormalities of pelvic organs

O34.80 Maternal care for other abnormalities of pelvic organs, unspecified trimester Ⓜ♀

O34.81 Maternal care for other abnormalities of pelvic organs, first trimester Ⓜ♀

O34.82 Maternal care for other abnormalities of pelvic organs, second trimester Ⓜ♀

O34.83 Maternal care for other abnormalities of pelvic organs, third trimester Ⓜ♀

√5ᵗʰ **O34.9 Maternal care for abnormality of pelvic organ, unspecified**

O34.90 Maternal care for abnormality of pelvic organ, unspecified, unspecified trimester Ⓜ♀

O34.91 Maternal care for abnormality of pelvic organ, unspecified, first trimester Ⓜ♀

O34.92 Maternal care for abnormality of pelvic organ, unspecified, second trimester Ⓜ♀

O34.93 Maternal care for abnormality of pelvic organ, unspecified, third trimester Ⓜ♀

√4ᵗʰ **O35 Maternal care for known or suspected fetal abnormality and damage**

INCLUDES   the listed conditions in the fetus as a reason for hospitalization or other obstetric care to the mother, or for termination of pregnancy

Code also any associated maternal condition

EXCLUDES 1   *encounter for suspected maternal and fetal conditions ruled out (Z03.7-)*

One of the following 7th characters is to be assigned to each code under category O35. 7th character Ø is for single gestations and multiple gestations where the fetus is unspecified. 7th characters 1 through 9 are for cases of multiple gestations to identify the fetus for which the code applies. The appropriate code from category O3Ø, Multiple gestation, must also be assigned when assigning a code from category O35 that has a 7th character of 1 through 9.

Ø   not applicable or unspecified
1   fetus 1
2   fetus 2
3   fetus 3
4   fetus 4
5   fetus 5
9   other fetus

√x7ᵗʰ **O35.0 Maternal care for (suspected)** central nervous system malformation in fetus Ⓜ♀
Maternal care for fetal anencephaly
Maternal care for fetal hydrocephalus
Maternal care for fetal spina bifida
EXCLUDES 2   *chromosomal abnormality in fetus (O35.1)*

√x7ᵗʰ **O35.1 Maternal care for (suspected)** chromosomal abnormality in fetus Ⓜ♀

√x7ᵗʰ **O35.2 Maternal care for (suspected)** hereditary disease in fetus Ⓜ♀
EXCLUDES 2   *chromosomal abnormality in fetus (O35.1)*

√x7ᵗʰ **O35.3 Maternal care for (suspected)** damage to fetus from viral disease in mother Ⓜ♀
Maternal care for damage to fetus from maternal cytomegalovirus infection
Maternal care for damage to fetus from maternal rubella

√x7ᵗʰ **O35.4 Maternal care for (suspected)** damage to fetus from alcohol Ⓜ♀

√x7ᵗʰ **O35.5 Maternal care for (suspected)** damage to fetus by drugs Ⓜ♀
Maternal care for damage to fetus from drug addiction

√x7ᵗʰ **O35.6 Maternal care for (suspected)** damage to fetus by radiation Ⓜ♀

√x7ᵗʰ **O35.7 Maternal care for (suspected)** damage to fetus by other medical procedures Ⓜ♀
Maternal care for damage to fetus by amniocentesis
Maternal care for damage to fetus by biopsy procedures
Maternal care for damage to fetus by hematological investigation
Maternal care for damage to fetus by intrauterine contraceptive device
Maternal care for damage to fetus by intrauterine surgery

√x7ᵗʰ **O35.8 Maternal care for other (suspected)** fetal abnormality and damage Ⓜ♀
Maternal care for damage to fetus from maternal listeriosis
Maternal care for damage to fetus from maternal toxoplasmosis

√x7ᵗʰ **O35.9 Maternal care for (suspected)** fetal abnormality and damage, unspecified Ⓜ♀

✓4th O36 Maternal care for other fetal problems

INCLUDES the listed conditions in the fetus as a reason for hospitalization or other obstetric care of the mother, or for termination of pregnancy

EXCLUDES 1 encounter for suspected maternal and fetal conditions ruled out (Z03.7-)

placental transfusion syndromes (O43.0-)

EXCLUDES 2 labor and delivery complicated by fetal stress (O77.-)

AHA: 2015,3Q,40

One of the following 7th characters is to be assigned to each code under category O36. 7th character 0 is for single gestations and multiple gestations where the fetus is unspecified. 7th characters 1 through 9 are for cases of multiple gestations to identify the fetus for which the code applies. The appropriate code from category O30, Multiple gestation, must also be assigned when assigning a code from category O36 that has a 7th character of 1 through 9.

0   not applicable or unspecified
1   fetus 1
2   fetus 2
3   fetus 3
4   fetus 4
5   fetus 5
9   other fetus

✓5th O36.0 Maternal care for rhesus isoimmunization

Maternal care for Rh incompatibility (with hydrops fetalis)

✓6th O36.01 Maternal care for anti-D [Rh] antibodies

AHA: 2014,4Q,17

✓7th **O36.011** Maternal care for anti-D [Rh] antibodies, **first trimester**   Q M ♀

✓7th **O36.012** Maternal care for anti-D [Rh] antibodies, **second trimester**   M ♀

✓7th **O36.013** Maternal care for anti-D [Rh] antibodies, **third trimester**   M ♀

✓7th **O36.019** Maternal care for anti-D [Rh] antibodies, **unspecified trimester**   Q M ♀

✓6th O36.09 Maternal care for other rhesus isoimmunization

✓7th **O36.091** Maternal care for other rhesus isoimmunization, **first trimester**   Q M ♀

✓7th **O36.092** Maternal care for other rhesus isoimmunization, **second trimester**   M ♀

✓7th **O36.093** Maternal care for other rhesus isoimmunization, **third trimester**   M ♀

✓7th **O36.099** Maternal care for other rhesus isoimmunization, **unspecified trimester**   Q M ♀

✓5th O36.1 Maternal care for other isoimmunization

Maternal care for ABO isoimmunization

✓6th O36.11 Maternal care for Anti-A sensitization

Maternal care for isoimmunization NOS (with hydrops fetalis)

✓7th **O36.111** Maternal care for Anti-A sensitization, **first trimester**   M ♀

✓7th **O36.112** Maternal care for Anti-A sensitization, **second trimester**   M ♀

✓7th **O36.113** Maternal care for Anti-A sensitization, **third trimester**   M ♀

✓7th **O36.119** Maternal care for Anti-A sensitization, **unspecified trimester**   M ♀

✓6th O36.19 Maternal care for other isoimmunization

Maternal care for Anti-B sensitization

✓7th **O36.191** Maternal care for other isoimmunization, **first trimester**   M ♀

✓7th **O36.192** Maternal care for other isoimmunization, **second trimester**   M ♀

✓7th **O36.193** Maternal care for other isoimmunization, **third trimester**   M ♀

✓7th **O36.199** Maternal care for other isoimmunization, **unspecified trimester**   M ♀

✓5th O36.2 Maternal care for hydrops fetalis

Maternal care for hydrops fetalis NOS

Maternal care for hydrops fetalis not associated with isoimmunization

EXCLUDES 1 hydrops fetalis associated with ABO isoimmunization (O36.1-)

hydrops fetalis associated with rhesus isoimmunization (O36.0-)

DEF: Hydrops fetalis: Abnormal fluid buildup in at least two of the following fetal organ spaces: the skin (edema), abdomen (ascites), around the heart (pericardia effusion), and around the lung (pleural effusion). Fluid accumulation may also occur in the mother as polyhydramnios and edema of the placenta.

✓x7th **O36.20** Maternal care for hydrops fetalis, **unspecified trimester**   M ♀

✓x7th **O36.21** Maternal care for hydrops fetalis, **first trimester**   M ♀

✓x7th **O36.22** Maternal care for hydrops fetalis, **second trimester**   M ♀

✓x7th **O36.23** Maternal care for hydrops fetalis, **third trimester**   M ♀

✓x7th O36.4 Maternal care for intrauterine death   M ♀

Maternal care for intrauterine fetal death NOS

Maternal care for intrauterine fetal death after completion of 20 weeks of gestation

Maternal care for late fetal death

Maternal care for missed delivery

EXCLUDES 1 missed abortion (O02.1)

stillbirth (P95)

✓5th O36.5 Maternal care for known or suspected poor fetal growth

✓6th O36.51 Maternal care for known or suspected placental insufficiency

✓7th **O36.511** Maternal care for known or suspected placental insufficiency, **first trimester**   M ♀

✓7th **O36.512** Maternal care for known or suspected placental insufficiency, **second trimester**   M ♀

✓7th **O36.513** Maternal care for known or suspected placental insufficiency, **third trimester**   M ♀

✓7th **O36.519** Maternal care for known or suspected placental insufficiency, **unspecified trimester**   M ♀

✓6th O36.59 Maternal care for other known or suspected poor fetal growth

Maternal care for known or suspected light-for-dates NOS

Maternal care for known or suspected small-for-dates NOS

✓7th **O36.591** Maternal care for other known or suspected poor fetal growth, **first trimester**   M ♀

✓7th **O36.592** Maternal care for other known or suspected poor fetal growth, **second trimester**   M ♀

✓7th **O36.593** Maternal care for other known or suspected poor fetal growth, **third trimester**   M ♀

✓7th **O36.599** Maternal care for other known or suspected poor fetal growth, **unspecified trimester**   M ♀

✓5th O36.6 Maternal care for excessive fetal growth

Maternal care for known or suspected large-for-dates

✓x7th **O36.60** Maternal care for excessive fetal growth, **unspecified trimester**   M ♀

✓x7th **O36.61** Maternal care for excessive fetal growth, **first trimester**   M ♀

✓x7th **O36.62** Maternal care for excessive fetal growth, **second trimester**   M ♀

✓x7th **O36.63** Maternal care for excessive fetal growth, **third trimester**   M ♀

✓5th O36.7 Maternal care for viable fetus in abdominal pregnancy

✓x7th **O36.70** Maternal care for viable fetus in abdominal pregnancy, **unspecified trimester**   M ♀

✓x7th **O36.71** Maternal care for viable fetus in abdominal pregnancy, **first trimester**   M ♀

✓x7th **O36.72** Maternal care for viable fetus in abdominal pregnancy, **second trimester**   M ♀

✓ Additional Character Required   ✓x7th Placeholder Alert   Manifestation   Unspecified Dx   ▶◀ Revised Text   ● New Code   ▲ Revised Code Title

ICD-10-CM 2020   875

√x7ᵗʰ **O36.73 Maternal care for viable fetus in abdominal pregnancy,** third trimester Ⓜ♀

√5ᵗʰ **O36.8 Maternal care for other specified fetal problems**

√x7ᵗʰ **O36.80 Pregnancy with inconclusive fetal viability** Ⓜ♀
Encounter to determine fetal viability of pregnancy
AHA: 2019,2Q,29

√6ᵗʰ **O36.81 Decreased fetal movements**

√7ᵗʰ **O36.812 Decreased fetal movements,** second trimester Ⓜ♀

√7ᵗʰ **O36.813 Decreased fetal movements,** third trimester Ⓜ♀

√7ᵗʰ **O36.819 Decreased fetal movements,** unspecified trimester Ⓜ♀

√6ᵗʰ **O36.82 Fetal anemia and thrombocytopenia**

√7ᵗʰ **O36.821 Fetal anemia and thrombocytopenia,** first trimester Ⓜ♀

√7ᵗʰ **O36.822 Fetal anemia and thrombocytopenia,** second trimester Ⓜ♀

√7ᵗʰ **O36.823 Fetal anemia and thrombocytopenia,** third trimester Ⓜ♀

√7ᵗʰ **O36.829 Fetal anemia and thrombocytopenia, unspecified** trimester Ⓜ♀

√6ᵗʰ **O36.83 Maternal care for abnormalities of the fetal heart rate or rhythm**
▶Maternal care for depressed fetal heart rate tones◀
▶Maternal care for fetal bradycardia◀
▶Maternal care for fetal heart rate abnormal variability◀
▶Maternal care for fetal heart rate decelerations◀
▶Maternal care for fetal heart rate irregularity◀
▶Maternal care for fetal tachycardia◀
▶Maternal care for non-reassuring fetal heart rate or rhythm◀
AHA: 2017,4Q,20
TIP: Assign for documented fetal tachycardia, bradycardia, decelerations, or loss of variability detected during antenatal testing.

√7ᵗʰ **O36.831 Maternal care for abnormalities of the fetal heart rate or rhythm, first trimester** Ⓜ♀

√7ᵗʰ **O36.832 Maternal care for abnormalities of the fetal heart rate or rhythm, second trimester** Ⓜ♀

√7ᵗʰ **O36.833 Maternal care for abnormalities of the fetal heart rate or rhythm, third trimester** Ⓜ♀

√7ᵗʰ **O36.839 Maternal care for abnormalities of the fetal heart rate or rhythm, unspecified trimester** Ⓜ♀

√6ᵗʰ **O36.89 Maternal care for other specified fetal problems**

√7ᵗʰ **O36.891 Maternal care for other specified fetal problems,** first trimester Ⓜ♀

√7ᵗʰ **O36.892 Maternal care for other specified fetal problems,** second trimester Ⓜ♀

√7ᵗʰ **O36.893 Maternal care for other specified fetal problems,** third trimester Ⓜ♀

√7ᵗʰ **O36.899 Maternal care for other specified fetal problems,** unspecified trimester Ⓜ♀

√5ᵗʰ **O36.9 Maternal care for fetal problem, unspecified**

√x7ᵗʰ **O36.90 Maternal care for fetal problem, unspecified, unspecified trimester** Ⓜ♀

√x7ᵗʰ **O36.91 Maternal care for fetal problem, unspecified,** first trimester Ⓜ♀

√x7ᵗʰ **O36.92 Maternal care for fetal problem, unspecified,** second trimester Ⓜ♀

√x7ᵗʰ **O36.93 Maternal care for fetal problem, unspecified,** third trimester Ⓜ♀

√4ᵗʰ **O40 Polyhydramnios**
INCLUDES hydramnios
EXCLUDES 1 encounter for suspected maternal and fetal conditions ruled out (Z03.7-)
AHA: 2016,1Q,4
DEF: Excess amniotic fluid surrounding the fetus, typically defined as a total fluid volume of greater than 24.0 cc.

One of the following 7th characters is to be assigned to each code under category O40. 7th character Ø is for single gestations and multiple gestations where the fetus is unspecified. 7th characters 1 through 9 are for cases of multiple gestations to identify the fetus for which the code applies. The appropriate code from category O30, Multiple gestation, must also be assigned when assigning a code from category O40 that has a 7th character of 1 through 9.
Ø not applicable or unspecified
1 fetus 1
2 fetus 2
3 fetus 3
4 fetus 4
5 fetus 5
9 other fetus

√x7ᵗʰ **O40.1 Polyhydramnios,** first trimester Ⓜ♀
√x7ᵗʰ **O40.2 Polyhydramnios,** second trimester Ⓜ♀
√x7ᵗʰ **O40.3 Polyhydramnios,** third trimester Ⓜ♀
√x7ᵗʰ **O40.9 Polyhydramnios,** unspecified trimester Ⓜ♀

√4ᵗʰ **O41 Other disorders of amniotic fluid and membranes**
EXCLUDES 1 encounter for suspected maternal and fetal conditions ruled out (Z03.7-)

One of the following 7th characters is to be assigned to each code under category O41. 7th character Ø is for single gestations and multiple gestations where the fetus is unspecified. 7th characters 1 through 9 are for cases of multiple gestations to identify the fetus for which the code applies. The appropriate code from category O30, Multiple gestation, must also be assigned when assigning a code from category O41 that has a 7th character of 1 through 9.
Ø not applicable or unspecified
1 fetus 1
2 fetus 2
3 fetus 3
4 fetus 4
5 fetus 5
9 other fetus

√5ᵗʰ **O41.0 Oligohydramnios**
Oligohydramnios without rupture of membranes
DEF: Low amniotic fluid, occurring most frequently in the last trimester.

√x7ᵗʰ **O41.00 Oligohydramnios,** unspecified trimester Ⓜ♀
√x7ᵗʰ **O41.01 Oligohydramnios,** first trimester Ⓜ♀
√x7ᵗʰ **O41.02 Oligohydramnios,** second trimester Ⓜ♀
√x7ᵗʰ **O41.03 Oligohydramnios,** third trimester Ⓜ♀

√5ᵗʰ **O41.1 Infection of amniotic sac and membranes**

√6ᵗʰ **O41.10 Infection of amniotic sac and membranes, unspecified**

√7ᵗʰ **O41.101 Infection of amniotic sac and membranes, unspecified,** first trimester Ⓜ♀

√7ᵗʰ **O41.102 Infection of amniotic sac and membranes, unspecified,** second trimester Ⓜ♀

√7ᵗʰ **O41.103 Infection of amniotic sac and membranes, unspecified,** third trimester Ⓜ♀

√7ᵗʰ **O41.109 Infection of amniotic sac and membranes, unspecified,** unspecified trimester Ⓜ♀

√6ᵗʰ **O41.12 Chorioamnionitis**
AHA: 2019,2Q,34

√7ᵗʰ **O41.121 Chorioamnionitis,** first trimester Ⓜ♀
√7ᵗʰ **O41.122 Chorioamnionitis,** second trimester Ⓜ♀
√7ᵗʰ **O41.123 Chorioamnionitis,** third trimester Ⓜ♀
√7ᵗʰ **O41.129 Chorioamnionitis,** unspecified trimester Ⓜ♀

√6ᵗʰ **O41.14 Placentitis**

√7ᵗʰ **O41.141 Placentitis, first trimester** Ⓜ♀

√7ᵗʰ **O41.142 Placentitis, second trimester** Ⓜ♀

√7ᵗʰ **O41.143 Placentitis, third trimester** Ⓜ♀

√7ᵗʰ **O41.149 Placentitis, unspecified trimester** Ⓜ♀

√5ᵗʰ **O41.8 Other specified disorders of amniotic fluid and membranes**

√6ᵗʰ **O41.8X Other specified disorders of amniotic fluid and membranes**

√7ᵗʰ **O41.8X1 Other specified disorders of amniotic fluid and membranes, first trimester** Ⓜ♀

√7ᵗʰ **O41.8X2 Other specified disorders of amniotic fluid and membranes, second trimester** Ⓜ♀

√7ᵗʰ **O41.8X3 Other specified disorders of amniotic fluid and membranes, third trimester** Ⓜ♀

√7ᵗʰ **O41.8X9 Other specified disorders of amniotic fluid and membranes, unspecified trimester** Ⓜ♀

√5ᵗʰ **O41.9 Disorder of amniotic fluid and membranes, unspecified**

√x7ᵗʰ **O41.90 Disorder of amniotic fluid and membranes, unspecified, unspecified trimester** Ⓜ♀

√x7ᵗʰ **O41.91 Disorder of amniotic fluid and membranes, unspecified, first trimester** Ⓜ♀

√x7ᵗʰ **O41.92 Disorder of amniotic fluid and membranes, unspecified, second trimester** Ⓜ♀

√x7ᵗʰ **O41.93 Disorder of amniotic fluid and membranes, unspecified, third trimester** Ⓜ♀

√4ᵗʰ **O42 Premature rupture of membranes**

AHA: 2016,1Q,3

√5ᵗʰ **O42.0 Premature rupture of membranes, onset of labor within 24 hours of rupture**

O42.00 Premature rupture of membranes, onset of labor within 24 hours of rupture, unspecified weeks of gestation Ⓜ♀

√6ᵗʰ **O42.01 Preterm premature rupture of membranes, onset of labor within 24 hours of rupture**

Premature rupture of membranes before 37 completed weeks of gestation

O42.011 Preterm premature rupture of membranes, onset of labor within 24 hours of rupture, first trimester Ⓜ♀

O42.012 Preterm premature rupture of membranes, onset of labor within 24 hours of rupture, second trimester Ⓜ♀

O42.013 Preterm premature rupture of membranes, onset of labor within 24 hours of rupture, third trimester Ⓜ♀

O42.019 Preterm premature rupture of membranes, onset of labor within 24 hours of rupture, unspecified trimester Ⓜ♀

O42.02 Full-term premature rupture of membranes, onset of labor within 24 hours of rupture Ⓜ♀

Premature rupture of membranes at or after 37 completed weeks of gestation, onset of labor within 24 hours of rupture

√5ᵗʰ **O42.1 Premature rupture of membranes, onset of labor more than 24 hours following rupture**

AHA: 2016,1Q,5

O42.10 Premature rupture of membranes, onset of labor more than 24 hours following rupture, unspecified weeks of gestation Ⓜ♀

√6ᵗʰ **O42.11 Preterm premature rupture of membranes, onset of labor more than 24 hours following rupture**

Premature rupture of membranes before 37 completed weeks of gestation

O42.111 Preterm premature rupture of membranes, onset of labor more than 24 hours following rupture, first trimester Ⓜ♀

O42.112 Preterm premature rupture of membranes, onset of labor more than 24 hours following rupture, second trimester Ⓜ♀

O42.113 Preterm premature rupture of membranes, onset of labor more than 24 hours following rupture, third trimester Ⓜ♀

O42.119 Preterm premature rupture of membranes, onset of labor more than 24 hours following rupture, unspecified trimester Ⓜ♀

O42.12 Full-term premature rupture of membranes, onset of labor more than 24 hours following rupture Ⓜ♀

Premature rupture of membranes at or after 37 completed weeks of gestation, onset of labor more than 24 hours following rupture

√5ᵗʰ **O42.9 Premature rupture of membranes, unspecified as to length of time between rupture and onset of labor**

O42.90 Premature rupture of membranes, unspecified as to length of time between rupture and onset of labor, unspecified weeks of gestation Ⓜ♀

√6ᵗʰ **O42.91 Preterm premature rupture of membranes, unspecified as to length of time between rupture and onset of labor**

Premature rupture of membranes before 37 completed weeks of gestation

O42.911 Preterm premature rupture of membranes, unspecified as to length of time between rupture and onset of labor, first trimester Ⓜ♀

O42.912 Preterm premature rupture of membranes, unspecified as to length of time between rupture and onset of labor, second trimester Ⓜ♀

O42.913 Preterm premature rupture of membranes, unspecified as to length of time between rupture and onset of labor, third trimester Ⓜ♀

O42.919 Preterm premature rupture of membranes, unspecified as to length of time between rupture and onset of labor, unspecified trimester Ⓜ♀

O42.92 Full-term premature rupture of membranes, unspecified as to length of time between rupture and onset of labor Ⓜ♀

Premature rupture of membranes at or after 37 completed weeks of gestation, unspecified as to length of time between rupture and onset of labor

√4ᵗʰ **O43 Placental disorders**

EXCLUDES 2 *maternal care for poor fetal growth due to placental insufficiency (O36.5-)*

placenta previa (O44.-)

placental polyp (O90.89)

placentitis (O41.14-)

premature separation of placenta [abruptio placentae] (O45.-)

√5ᵗʰ **O43.0 Placental transfusion syndromes**

√6ᵗʰ **O43.01 Fetomaternal placental transfusion syndrome**

Maternofetal placental transfusion syndrome

O43.011 Fetomaternal placental transfusion syndrome, first trimester Ⓠ Ⓜ♀

O43.012 Fetomaternal placental transfusion syndrome, second trimester Ⓜ♀

O43.013 Fetomaternal placental transfusion syndrome, third trimester Ⓜ♀

O43.019 Fetomaternal placental transfusion syndrome, unspecified trimester Ⓠ Ⓜ♀

☑ Additional Character Required   √x7ᵗʰ Placeholder Alert   Manifestation   Unspecified Dx   ►◄ Revised Text   ● New Code   ▲ Revised Code Title

ICD-10-CM 2020   877

✓6ᵗʰ **O43.02** Fetus-to-fetus placental transfusion syndrome
DEF: Condition in which an imbalance in amniotic fluid occurs due to uneven blood flow between twins sharing a placenta.

Twin to Twin Transfusion Syndrome (TTTS)

Healthy twins   Twins with TTTS

O43.021 Fetus-to-fetus placental transfusion syndrome, first trimester   Ⓜ♀

O43.022 Fetus-to-fetus placental transfusion syndrome, second trimester   Ⓜ♀

O43.023 Fetus-to-fetus placental transfusion syndrome, third trimester   Ⓜ♀

O43.029 Fetus-to-fetus placental transfusion syndrome, unspecified trimester   Ⓜ♀

✓5ᵗʰ **O43.1** Malformation of placenta

  ✓6ᵗʰ **O43.10** Malformation of placenta, unspecified
Abnormal placenta NOS

O43.101 Malformation of placenta, unspecified, first trimester   Ⓜ♀

O43.102 Malformation of placenta, unspecified, second trimester   Ⓜ♀

O43.103 Malformation of placenta, unspecified, third trimester   Ⓜ♀

O43.109 Malformation of placenta, unspecified, unspecified trimester   Ⓜ♀

  ✓6ᵗʰ **O43.11** Circumvallate placenta

O43.111 Circumvallate placenta, first trimester   Ⓜ♀

O43.112 Circumvallate placenta, second trimester   Ⓜ♀

O43.113 Circumvallate placenta, third trimester   Ⓜ♀

O43.119 Circumvallate placenta, unspecified trimester   Ⓜ♀

  ✓6ᵗʰ **O43.12** Velamentous insertion of umbilical cord

O43.121 Velamentous insertion of umbilical cord, first trimester   Ⓜ♀

O43.122 Velamentous insertion of umbilical cord, second trimester   Ⓜ♀

O43.123 Velamentous insertion of umbilical cord, third trimester   Ⓜ♀

O43.129 Velamentous insertion of umbilical cord, unspecified trimester   Ⓜ♀

  ✓6ᵗʰ **O43.19** Other malformation of placenta

O43.191 Other malformation of placenta, first trimester   Ⓜ♀

O43.192 Other malformation of placenta, second trimester   Ⓜ♀

O43.193 Other malformation of placenta, third trimester   Ⓜ♀

O43.199 Other malformation of placenta, unspecified trimester   Ⓜ♀

✓5ᵗʰ **O43.2** Morbidly adherent placenta
Code also associated third stage postpartum hemorrhage, if applicable (O72.0)
  EXCLUDES 1   retained placenta (O73.-)

  ✓6ᵗʰ **O43.21** Placenta accreta
DEF: Condition where the placenta adheres too deeply to the uterine wall; often associated with placenta previa.

O43.211 Placenta accreta, first trimester   Ⓜ♀

O43.212 Placenta accreta, second trimester   Ⓜ♀

O43.213 Placenta accreta, third trimester   Ⓜ♀

O43.219 Placenta accreta, unspecified trimester   Ⓜ♀

  ✓6ᵗʰ **O43.22** Placenta increta
DEF: Condition where the placenta adheres too deeply to the uterine wall and penetrates the muscle; often associated with placenta previa.

O43.221 Placenta increta, first trimester   Ⓜ♀

O43.222 Placenta increta, second trimester   Ⓜ♀

O43.223 Placenta increta, third trimester   Ⓜ♀

O43.229 Placenta increta, unspecified trimester   Ⓜ♀

  ✓6ᵗʰ **O43.23** Placenta percreta
DEF: Condition where the placenta attaches through the uterine muscle and may invade other organs, resulting in antenatal complications, premature delivery, retention of all or a portion of the placenta, or postpartum bleeding.

O43.231 Placenta percreta, first trimester   Ⓜ♀

O43.232 Placenta percreta, second trimester   Ⓜ♀

O43.233 Placenta percreta, third trimester   Ⓜ♀

O43.239 Placenta percreta, unspecified trimester   Ⓜ♀

✓5ᵗʰ **O43.8** Other placental disorders

  ✓6ᵗʰ **O43.81** Placental infarction

O43.811 Placental infarction, first trimester   Ⓜ♀

O43.812 Placental infarction, second trimester   Ⓜ♀

O43.813 Placental infarction, third trimester   Ⓜ♀

O43.819 Placental infarction, unspecified trimester   Ⓜ♀

  ✓6ᵗʰ **O43.89** Other placental disorders
Placental dysfunction

O43.891 Other placental disorders, first trimester   Ⓜ♀

O43.892 Other placental disorders, second trimester   Ⓜ♀

O43.893 Other placental disorders, third trimester   Ⓜ♀

O43.899 Other placental disorders, unspecified trimester   Ⓜ♀

✓5ᵗʰ **O43.9** Unspecified placental disorder

O43.90 Unspecified placental disorder, unspecified trimester   Ⓜ♀

O43.91 Unspecified placental disorder, first trimester   Ⓜ♀

O43.92 Unspecified placental disorder, second trimester   Ⓜ♀

O43.93 Unspecified placental disorder, third trimester   Ⓜ♀

✓4ᵗʰ **O44** Placenta previa
AHA: 2016,4Q,52-53
DEF: Placenta implanted in the lower segment of the uterus, which commonly causes hemorrhage in the last trimester of pregnancy.

✓5ᵗʰ **O44.0** Complete placenta previa NOS or without hemorrhage
Placenta previa NOS

O44.00 Complete placenta previa NOS or without hemorrhage, unspecified trimester   Ⓜ♀

O44.01 Complete placenta previa NOS or without hemorrhage, first trimester   Ⓜ♀

O44.02 Complete placenta previa NOS or without hemorrhage, second trimester   Ⓜ♀

O44.03   Complete placenta previa NOS or without hemorrhage, **third trimester**   M ♀

✓5ᵗʰ O44.1   Complete **placenta previa** with hemorrhage

> **EXCLUDES 1**   *labor and delivery complicated by hemorrhage from vasa previa (O69.4)*

O44.10   Complete placenta previa with hemorrhage, **unspecified trimester**   M ♀

O44.11   Complete placenta previa with hemorrhage, **first trimester**   M ♀

O44.12   Complete placenta previa with hemorrhage, **second trimester**   M ♀

O44.13   Complete placenta previa with hemorrhage, **third trimester**   M ♀

✓5ᵗʰ O44.2   Partial **placenta previa** without hemorrhage

> Marginal placenta previa, NOS or without hemorrhage

O44.20   Partial placenta previa NOS or without hemorrhage, **unspecified trimester**   M ♀

O44.21   Partial placenta previa NOS or without hemorrhage, **first trimester**   M ♀

O44.22   Partial placenta previa NOS or without hemorrhage, **second trimester**   M ♀

O44.23   Partial placenta previa NOS or without hemorrhage, **third trimester**   M ♀

✓5ᵗʰ O44.3   Partial **placenta previa** with hemorrhage

> Marginal placenta previa with hemorrhage

O44.30   Partial placenta previa with hemorrhage, **unspecified trimester**   Q M ♀

O44.31   Partial placenta previa with hemorrhage, **first trimester**   Q M ♀

O44.32   Partial placenta previa with hemorrhage, **second trimester**   M ♀

O44.33   Partial placenta previa with hemorrhage, **third trimester**   M ♀

✓5ᵗʰ O44.4   Low lying **placenta NOS or** without hemorrhage

> Low implantation of placenta NOS or without hemorrhage

O44.40   Low lying placenta NOS or without hemorrhage, **unspecified trimester**   M ♀

O44.41   Low lying placenta NOS or without hemorrhage, **first trimester**   M ♀

O44.42   Low lying placenta NOS or without hemorrhage, **second trimester**   M ♀

O44.43   Low lying placenta NOS or without hemorrhage, **third trimester**   M ♀

✓5ᵗʰ O44.5   Low lying **placenta** with hemorrhage

> Low implantation of placenta with hemorrhage

O44.50   Low lying placenta with hemorrhage, **unspecified trimester**   Q M ♀

O44.51   Low lying placenta with hemorrhage, **first trimester**   Q M ♀

O44.52   Low lying placenta with hemorrhage, **second trimester**   M ♀

O44.53   Low lying placenta with hemorrhage, **third trimester**   M ♀

✓4ᵗʰ O45   **Premature separation of placenta [abruptio placentae]**

✓5ᵗʰ O45.0   Premature separation of placenta with coagulation defect

✓6ᵗʰ O45.00   Premature separation of placenta with coagulation defect, unspecified

O45.001   Premature separation of placenta with coagulation defect, unspecified, **first trimester**   Q M ♀

O45.002   Premature separation of placenta with coagulation defect, unspecified, **second trimester**   M ♀

O45.003   Premature separation of placenta with coagulation defect, unspecified, **third trimester**   M ♀

O45.009   Premature separation of placenta with coagulation defect, unspecified, **unspecified trimester**   Q M ♀

✓6ᵗʰ O45.01   Premature separation of placenta with afibrinogenemia

> Premature separation of placenta with hypofibrinogenemia

O45.011   Premature separation of placenta with afibrinogenemia, **first trimester**   Q M ♀

O45.012   Premature separation of placenta with afibrinogenemia, **second trimester**   M ♀

O45.013   Premature separation of placenta with afibrinogenemia, **third trimester**   M ♀

O45.019   Premature separation of placenta with afibrinogenemia, **unspecified trimester**   Q M ♀

✓6ᵗʰ O45.02   Premature separation of placenta with disseminated intravascular coagulation

O45.021   Premature separation of placenta with disseminated intravascular coagulation, **first trimester**   Q M ♀

O45.022   Premature separation of placenta with disseminated intravascular coagulation, **second trimester**   M ♀

O45.023   Premature separation of placenta with disseminated intravascular coagulation, **third trimester**   M ♀

O45.029   Premature separation of placenta with disseminated intravascular coagulation, **unspecified trimester**   Q M ♀

✓6ᵗʰ O45.09   Premature separation of placenta with other coagulation defect

O45.091   Premature separation of placenta with other coagulation defect, **first trimester**   Q M ♀

O45.092   Premature separation of placenta with other coagulation defect, **second trimester**   M ♀

O45.093   Premature separation of placenta with other coagulation defect, **third trimester**   M ♀

O45.099   Premature separation of placenta with other coagulation defect, **unspecified trimester**   Q M ♀

✓5ᵗʰ O45.8   Other premature separation of placenta

✓6ᵗʰ O45.8X   Other premature separation of placenta

O45.8X1   Other premature separation of placenta, **first trimester**   Q M ♀

O45.8X2   Other premature separation of placenta, **second trimester**   M ♀

O45.8X3   Other premature separation of placenta, **third trimester**   M ♀

O45.8X9   Other premature separation of placenta, **unspecified trimester**   Q M ♀

✓5ᵗʰ O45.9   Premature separation of placenta, unspecified

> Abruptio placentae NOS

O45.90   Premature separation of placenta, unspecified, **unspecified trimester**   Q M ♀

O45.91   Premature separation of placenta, unspecified, **first trimester**   Q M ♀

O45.92   Premature separation of placenta, unspecified, **second trimester**   M ♀

O45.93   Premature separation of placenta, unspecified, **third trimester**   M ♀

✓4ᵗʰ O46   **Antepartum hemorrhage, not elsewhere classified**

> **EXCLUDES 1**   *hemorrhage in early pregnancy (O20.-)*
> *intrapartum hemorrhage NEC (O67.-)*
> *placenta previa (O44.-)*
> *premature separation of placenta [abruptio placentae] (O45.-)*

DEF: Uterine hemorrhage prior to delivery that is not related to placenta previa or abruptio placentae.

✓5ᵗʰ O46.0   Antepartum hemorrhage with coagulation defect

✓6ᵗʰ O46.00   Antepartum hemorrhage with coagulation defect, unspecified

O46.001   Antepartum hemorrhage with coagulation defect, unspecified, **first trimester**   Q M ♀

O46.002   Antepartum hemorrhage with coagulation defect, unspecified, **second trimester**   M ♀

O46.003   Antepartum hemorrhage with coagulation defect, unspecified, **third trimester**   M ♀

✔ Additional Character Required   ✓ₓ7ᵗʰ Placeholder Alert   Manifestation   Unspecified Dx   ▶◀ Revised Text   ● New Code   ▲ Revised Code Title

ICD-10-CM 2020   879

Chapter 15. Pregnancy, Childbirth and the Puerperium

O46.009   **Antepartum hemorrhage with coagulation defect, unspecified, unspecified trimester** ⓞ Ⓜ ♀

√6ᵗʰ   **O46.01**   **Antepartum hemorrhage** with afibrinogenemia

     Antepartum hemorrhage with hypofibrinogenemia

     O46.011   **Antepartum hemorrhage with afibrinogenemia, first trimester** Ⓜ ♀

     O46.012   **Antepartum hemorrhage with afibrinogenemia, second trimester** Ⓜ ♀

     O46.013   **Antepartum hemorrhage with afibrinogenemia, third trimester** Ⓜ ♀

     O46.019   **Antepartum hemorrhage with afibrinogenemia, unspecified trimester** ⓞ Ⓜ ♀

√6ᵗʰ   **O46.02**   **Antepartum hemorrhage** with disseminated intravascular coagulation

     O46.021   **Antepartum hemorrhage with disseminated intravascular coagulation, first trimester** ⓞ Ⓜ ♀

     O46.022   **Antepartum hemorrhage with disseminated intravascular coagulation, second trimester** Ⓜ ♀

     O46.023   **Antepartum hemorrhage with disseminated intravascular coagulation, third trimester** Ⓜ ♀

     O46.029   **Antepartum hemorrhage with disseminated intravascular coagulation, unspecified trimester** ⓞ Ⓜ ♀

√6ᵗʰ   **O46.09**   **Antepartum hemorrhage with other coagulation defect**

     O46.091   **Antepartum hemorrhage with other coagulation defect, first trimester** ⓞ Ⓜ ♀

     O46.092   **Antepartum hemorrhage with other coagulation defect, second trimester** Ⓜ ♀

     O46.093   **Antepartum hemorrhage with other coagulation defect, third trimester** Ⓜ ♀

     O46.099   **Antepartum hemorrhage with other coagulation defect, unspecified trimester** ⓞ Ⓜ ♀

√5ᵗʰ   **O46.8**   **Other antepartum hemorrhage**

√6ᵗʰ   **O46.8X**   **Other antepartum hemorrhage**

     O46.8X1   **Other antepartum hemorrhage, first trimester** ⓞ Ⓜ ♀

     O46.8X2   **Other antepartum hemorrhage, second trimester** Ⓜ ♀

     O46.8X3   **Other antepartum hemorrhage, third trimester** Ⓜ ♀

     O46.8X9   **Other antepartum hemorrhage, unspecified trimester** ⓞ Ⓜ ♀

√5ᵗʰ   **O46.9**   **Antepartum hemorrhage, unspecified**

     O46.90   **Antepartum hemorrhage, unspecified, unspecified trimester** ⓞ Ⓜ ♀

     O46.91   **Antepartum hemorrhage, unspecified, first trimester** ⓞ Ⓜ ♀

     O46.92   **Antepartum hemorrhage, unspecified, second trimester** Ⓜ ♀

     O46.93   **Antepartum hemorrhage, unspecified, third trimester** Ⓜ ♀

√4ᵗʰ   **O47**   **False labor**

     INCLUDES   Braxton Hicks contractions

     threatened labor

     EXCLUDES 1   preterm labor (O60.-)

√5ᵗʰ   **O47.0**   **False labor** before 37 completed weeks of gestation

     O47.00   **False labor before 37 completed weeks of gestation, unspecified trimester** Ⓜ ♀

     O47.02   **False labor before 37 completed weeks of gestation, second trimester** Ⓜ ♀

     O47.03   **False labor before 37 completed weeks of gestation, third trimester** Ⓜ ♀

     O47.1   **False labor** at or after 37 completed weeks of gestation Ⓜ ♀

     O47.9   **False labor, unspecified** Ⓜ ♀

√4ᵗʰ   **O48**   **Late pregnancy**

     O48.0   **Post-term pregnancy** Ⓜ ♀

     Pregnancy over 40 completed weeks to 42 completed weeks gestation

     O48.1   **Prolonged pregnancy** Ⓜ ♀

     Pregnancy which has advanced beyond 42 completed weeks gestation

     AHA: 2016,1Q,5

Complications of labor and delivery (O60-O77)

√4ᵗʰ   **O60**   **Preterm labor**

     INCLUDES   onset (spontaneous) of labor before 37 completed weeks of gestation

     EXCLUDES 1   false labor (O47.0-)

     threatened labor NOS (O47.0-)

√5ᵗʰ   **O60.0**   **Preterm labor** without delivery

     O60.00   **Preterm labor without delivery, unspecified trimester** Ⓜ ♀

     O60.02   **Preterm labor without delivery, second trimester** Ⓜ ♀

     O60.03   **Preterm labor without delivery, third trimester** Ⓜ ♀

√5ᵗʰ   **O60.1**   **Preterm labor** with preterm delivery

     AHA: 2016,2Q,10

> One of the following 7th characters is to be assigned to each code under subcategory O60.1. 7th character Ø is for single gestations and multiple gestations where the fetus is unspecified. 7th characters 1 through 9 are for cases of multiple gestations to identify the fetus for which the code applies. The appropriate code from category O30, Multiple gestation, must also be assigned when assigning a code from subcategory O60.1 that has a 7th character of 1 through 9.
> Ø   not applicable or unspecified
> 1   fetus 1
> 2   fetus 2
> 3   fetus 3
> 4   fetus 4
> 5   fetus 5
> 9   other fetus

     √x7ᵗʰ   **O60.10**   **Preterm labor with preterm delivery, unspecified trimester** Ⓜ ♀

     Preterm labor with delivery NOS

     √x7ᵗʰ   **O60.12**   **Preterm labor** second trimester **with preterm delivery** second trimester Ⓜ ♀

     √x7ᵗʰ   **O60.13**   **Preterm labor** second trimester **with preterm delivery** third trimester Ⓜ ♀

     √x7ᵗʰ   **O60.14**   **Preterm labor** third trimester **with preterm delivery** third trimester Ⓜ ♀

√5ᵗʰ   **O60.2**   **Term delivery with preterm labor**

> One of the following 7th characters is to be assigned to each code under subcategory O60.2. 7th character Ø is for single gestations and multiple gestations where the fetus is unspecified. 7th characters 1 through 9 are for cases of multiple gestations to identify the fetus for which the code applies. The appropriate code from category O30, Multiple gestation, must also be assigned when assigning a code from subcategory O60.2 that has a 7th character of 1 through 9.
> Ø   not applicable or unspecified
> 1   fetus 1
> 2   fetus 2
> 3   fetus 3
> 4   fetus 4
> 5   fetus 5
> 9   other fetus

     √x7ᵗʰ   **O60.20**   **Term delivery with preterm labor, unspecified trimester** Ⓜ ♀

     √x7ᵗʰ   **O60.22**   **Term delivery with preterm labor,** second trimester Ⓜ ♀

     √x7ᵗʰ   **O60.23**   **Term delivery with preterm labor,** third trimester Ⓜ ♀

√4ᵗʰ   **O61**   **Failed induction of labor**

     O61.0   **Failed** medical **induction of labor** Ⓜ ♀

     Failed induction (of labor) by oxytocin

     Failed induction (of labor) by prostaglandins

O61.1   Failed instrumental induction of labor   Ⓜ♀

    Failed mechanical induction (of labor)

    Failed surgical induction (of labor)

O61.8   Other failed induction of labor   Ⓜ♀

O61.9   Failed induction of labor, unspecified   Ⓜ♀

✓4ᵗʰ **O62   Abnormalities of forces of labor**

    DEF: Uterine inertia: Weak or poorly coordinated contractions of the uterus during labor.

O62.0   Primary inadequate contractions   Ⓜ♀

    Failure of cervical dilatation

    Primary hypotonic uterine dysfunction

    Uterine inertia during latent phase of labor

O62.1   Secondary uterine inertia   Ⓜ♀

    Arrested active phase of labor

    Secondary hypotonic uterine dysfunction

O62.2   Other uterine inertia   Ⓜ♀

    Atony of uterus without hemorrhage

    Atony of uterus NOS

    Desultory labor

    Hypotonic uterine dysfunction NOS

    Irregular labor

    Poor contractions

    Slow slope active phase of labor

    Uterine inertia NOS

      EXCLUDES 1   atony of uterus with hemorrhage (postpartum) (O72.1)

                   postpartum atony of uterus without hemorrhage (O75.89)

    DEF: Uterine atony: Failure of the uterine muscles to contract after the fetus and placenta are delivered.

O62.3   Precipitate labor   Ⓜ♀

    DEF: Rapid labor with delivery occurring in three hours or less from the onset of contractions.

O62.4   Hypertonic, incoordinate, and prolonged uterine contractions   Ⓜ♀

    Cervical spasm

    Contraction ring dystocia

    Dyscoordinate labor

    Hour-glass contraction of uterus

    Hypertonic uterine dysfunction

    Incoordinate uterine action

    Tetanic contractions

    Uterine dystocia NOS

    Uterine spasm

      EXCLUDES 1   dystocia (fetal) (maternal) NOS (O66.9)

O62.8   Other abnormalities of forces of labor   Ⓜ♀

O62.9   Abnormality of forces of labor, unspecified   Ⓜ♀

✓4ᵗʰ **O63   Long labor**

O63.0   Prolonged first stage (of labor)   Ⓜ♀

O63.1   Prolonged second stage (of labor)   Ⓜ♀

O63.2   Delayed delivery of second twin, triplet, etc.   Ⓜ♀

O63.9   Long labor, unspecified   Ⓜ♀

    Prolonged labor NOS

✓4ᵗʰ **O64   Obstructed labor due to malposition and malpresentation of fetus**

One of the following 7th characters is to be assigned to each code under category O64. 7th character 0 is for single gestations and multiple gestations where the fetus is unspecified. 7th characters 1 through 9 are for cases of multiple gestations to identify the fetus for which the code applies. The appropriate code from category O30, Multiple gestation, must also be assigned when assigning a code from category O64 that has a 7th character of 1 through 9.

0   not applicable or unspecified

1   fetus 1

2   fetus 2

3   fetus 3

4   fetus 4

5   fetus 5

9   other fetus

Fetal Malposition

Breech

Shoulder (arm prolapse)

Mother's pelvis

Compound (extremity together with head)

Face (mentum)

Oblique

✓x7ᵗʰ **O64.0   Obstructed labor due to incomplete rotation of fetal head**   Ⓜ♀

    Deep transverse arrest

    Obstructed labor due to persistent occipitoiliac (position)

    Obstructed labor due to persistent occipitoposterior (position)

    Obstructed labor due to persistent occipitosacral (position)

    Obstructed labor due to persistent occipitotransverse (position)

✓x7ᵗʰ **O64.1   Obstructed labor due to breech presentation**   Ⓜ♀

    Obstructed labor due to buttocks presentation

    Obstructed labor due to complete breech presentation

    Obstructed labor due to frank breech presentation

✓x7ᵗʰ **O64.2   Obstructed labor due to face presentation**   Ⓜ♀

    Obstructed labor due to chin presentation

✓x7ᵗʰ **O64.3   Obstructed labor due to brow presentation**   Ⓜ♀

✓x7ᵗʰ **O64.4   Obstructed labor due to shoulder presentation**   Ⓜ♀

    Prolapsed arm

      EXCLUDES 1   impacted shoulders (O66.0)

                   shoulder dystocia (O66.0)

✓x7ᵗʰ **O64.5   Obstructed labor due to compound presentation**   ♀

✓x7ᵗʰ **O64.8   Obstructed labor due to other malposition and malpresentation**   Ⓜ♀

    Obstructed labor due to footling presentation

    Obstructed labor due to incomplete breech presentation

✓x7ᵗʰ **O64.9   Obstructed labor due to malposition and malpresentation, unspecified**   Ⓜ♀

✓4ᵗʰ **O65   Obstructed labor due to maternal pelvic abnormality**

O65.0   Obstructed labor due to deformed pelvis   Ⓜ♀

O65.1   Obstructed labor due to generally contracted pelvis   Ⓜ♀

O65.2   Obstructed labor due to pelvic inlet contraction   Ⓜ♀

O65.3   Obstructed labor due to pelvic outlet and mid-cavity contraction   Ⓜ♀

O65.4   Obstructed labor due to fetopelvic disproportion, unspecified   Ⓜ♀

      EXCLUDES 1   dystocia due to abnormality of fetus (O66.2-O66.3)

☑ Additional Character Required   ✓x7ᵗʰ Placeholder Alert   Manifestation   Unspecified Dx   ▶◀ Revised Text   ● New Code   ▲ Revised Code Title

Chapter 15. Pregnancy, Childbirth and the Puerperium

O65.5 **Obstructed labor due to** abnormality of maternal pelvic organs   Ⓜ♀

     Obstructed labor due to conditions listed in O34.-
     Use additional code to identify abnormality of pelvic organs O34.-

O65.8 **Obstructed labor due to other maternal pelvic abnormalities**   Ⓜ♀

O65.9 **Obstructed labor due to maternal pelvic abnormality, unspecified**   Ⓜ♀

✓4ᵗʰ **O66** **Other obstructed labor**

O66.0 **Obstructed labor due to** shoulder dystocia   Ⓜ♀

     Impacted shoulders
     DEF: Obstructed labor due to impacted fetal shoulders. It is an emergency condition that may require cesarean section, forceps delivery, vacuum extraction, or symphysiotomy.

O66.1 **Obstructed labor due to** locked twins   Ⓜ♀

O66.2 **Obstructed labor due to** unusually large fetus   Ⓜ♀

O66.3 **Obstructed labor due to other abnormalities of fetus**   Ⓜ♀

     Dystocia due to fetal ascites
     Dystocia due to fetal hydrops
     Dystocia due to fetal meningomyelocele
     Dystocia due to fetal sacral teratoma
     Dystocia due to fetal tumor
     Dystocia due to hydrocephalic fetus
     Use additional code to identify cause of obstruction

✓5ᵗʰ **O66.4** **Failed trial of labor**

     O66.40 **Failed trial of labor, unspecified**   Ⓜ♀

     O66.41 **Failed** attempted vaginal birth after previous cesarean delivery   Ⓜ♀
         Code first rupture of uterus, if applicable (O71.0-, O71.1)

O66.5 **Attempted application of** vacuum extractor and forceps   Ⓜ♀

     Attempted application of vacuum or forceps, with subsequent delivery by forceps or cesarean delivery

O66.6 **Obstructed labor due to other multiple fetuses**   Ⓜ♀

O66.8 **Other specified obstructed labor**   Ⓜ♀

     Use additional code to identify cause of obstruction

O66.9 **Obstructed labor, unspecified**   Ⓜ♀

     Dystocia NOS
     Fetal dystocia NOS
     Maternal dystocia NOS

✓4ᵗʰ **O67** **Labor and delivery complicated by intrapartum hemorrhage, not elsewhere classified**

     EXCLUDES 1   antepartum hemorrhage NEC (O46.-)
         placenta previa (O44.-)
         premature separation of placenta [abruptio placentae] (O45.-)
     EXCLUDES 2   postpartum hemorrhage (O72.-)

O67.0 **Intrapartum hemorrhage with coagulation defect**   Ⓜ♀

     Intrapartum hemorrhage (excessive) associated with afibrinogenemia
     Intrapartum hemorrhage (excessive) associated with disseminated intravascular coagulation
     Intrapartum hemorrhage (excessive) associated with hyperfibrinolysis
     Intrapartum hemorrhage (excessive) associated with hypofibrinogenemia

O67.8 **Other intrapartum hemorrhage**   Ⓜ♀

     Excessive intrapartum hemorrhage

O67.9 **Intrapartum hemorrhage, unspecified**   Ⓜ♀

O68 **Labor and delivery complicated by abnormality of fetal acid-base balance**   Ⓜ♀

     Fetal acidemia complicating labor and delivery
     Fetal acidosis complicating labor and delivery
     Fetal alkalosis complicating labor and delivery
     Fetal metabolic acidemia complicating labor and delivery

     EXCLUDES 1   fetal stress NOS (O77.9)
         labor and delivery complicated by electrocardiographic evidence of fetal stress (O77.8)
         labor and delivery complicated by ultrasonic evidence of fetal stress (O77.8)

     EXCLUDES 2   abnormality in fetal heart rate or rhythm (O76)
         labor and delivery complicated by meconium in amniotic fluid (O77.0)

✓4ᵗʰ **O69** **Labor and delivery complicated by umbilical cord complications**

     AHA: 2016,1Q,5

     One of the following 7th characters is to be assigned to each code under category O69. 7th character Ø is for single gestations and multiple gestations where the fetus is unspecified. 7th characters 1 through 9 are for cases of multiple gestations to identify the fetus for which the code applies. The appropriate code from category O30, Multiple gestation, must also be assigned when assigning a code from category O69 that has a 7th character of 1 through 9.
     Ø   not applicable or unspecified
     1   fetus 1
     2   fetus 2
     3   fetus 3
     4   fetus 4
     5   fetus 5
     9   other fetus

     ✓x7ᵗʰ **O69.0** **Labor and delivery complicated by** prolapse of cord   Ⓜ♀

         DEF: Abnormal presentation of the fetus marked by a protruding umbilical cord during labor. It can cause fetal death.

     ✓x7ᵗʰ **O69.1** **Labor and delivery complicated by** cord around neck, with compression   Ⓜ♀

         EXCLUDES 1   labor and delivery complicated by cord around neck, without compression (O69.81)

     ✓x7ᵗʰ **O69.2** **Labor and delivery complicated by** other cord entanglement, with compression   Ⓜ♀

         Labor and delivery complicated by compression of cord NOS
         Labor and delivery complicated by entanglement of cords of twins in monoamniotic sac
         Labor and delivery complicated by knot in cord

         EXCLUDES 1   labor and delivery complicated by other cord entanglement, without compression (O69.82)

     ✓x7ᵗʰ **O69.3** **Labor and delivery complicated by** short cord   Ⓜ♀

     ✓x7ᵗʰ **O69.4** **Labor and delivery complicated by** vasa previa   Ⓜ♀

         Labor and delivery complicated by hemorrhage from vasa previa

     ✓x7ᵗʰ **O69.5** **Labor and delivery complicated by** vascular lesion of cord   Ⓜ♀

         Labor and delivery complicated by cord bruising
         Labor and delivery complicated by cord hematoma
         Labor and delivery complicated by thrombosis of umbilical vessels

     ✓5ᵗʰ **O69.8** **Labor and delivery complicated by other cord complications**

         ✓x7ᵗʰ **O69.81** **Labor and delivery complicated by** cord around neck, without compression   Ⓜ♀
             AHA: 2016,1Q,5

         ✓x7ᵗʰ **O69.82** **Labor and delivery complicated by** other cord entanglement, without compression   Ⓜ♀

         ✓x7ᵗʰ **O69.89** **Labor and delivery complicated by other cord complications**   Ⓜ♀

     ✓x7ᵗʰ **O69.9** **Labor and delivery complicated by cord complication, unspecified**   Ⓜ♀

☑4ᵗʰ **O70 Perineal laceration during delivery**

INCLUDES   episiotomy extended by laceration

EXCLUDES 1   *obstetric high vaginal laceration alone (O71.4)*

AHA: 2016,2Q,34; 2016,1Q,3-4,5

O70.0 First degree perineal laceration during delivery   Ⓜ ♀

Perineal laceration, rupture or tear involving fourchette during delivery

Perineal laceration, rupture or tear involving labia during delivery

Perineal laceration, rupture or tear involving skin during delivery

Perineal laceration, rupture or tear involving vagina during delivery

Perineal laceration, rupture or tear involving vulva during delivery

Slight perineal laceration, rupture or tear during delivery

O70.1 Second degree perineal laceration during delivery   Ⓜ ♀

Perineal laceration, rupture or tear during delivery as in O70.0, also involving pelvic floor

Perineal laceration, rupture or tear during delivery as in O70.0, also involving perineal muscles

Perineal laceration, rupture or tear during delivery as in O70.0, also involving vaginal muscles

EXCLUDES 1   *perineal laceration involving anal sphincter (O70.2)*

☑5ᵗʰ **O70.2 Third degree perineal laceration during delivery**

Perineal laceration, rupture or tear during delivery as in O70.1, also involving anal sphincter

Perineal laceration, rupture or tear during delivery as in O70.1, also involving rectovaginal septum

Perineal laceration, rupture or tear during delivery as in O70.1, also involving sphincter NOS

EXCLUDES 1   *anal sphincter tear during delivery without third degree perineal laceration (O70.4)*

perineal laceration involving anal or rectal mucosa (O70.3)

AHA: 2016,4Q,53-54

O70.20 Third degree perineal laceration during delivery, unspecified

O70.21 Third degree perineal laceration during delivery, IIIa   Ⓜ ♀

Third degree perineal laceration during delivery with less than 50% of external anal sphincter (EAS) thickness torn

O70.22 Third degree perineal laceration during delivery, IIIb   Ⓜ ♀

Third degree perineal laceration during delivery with more than 50% external anal sphincter (EAS) thickness torn

O70.23 Third degree perineal laceration during delivery, IIIc   Ⓜ ♀

Third degree perineal laceration during delivery with both external anal sphincter (EAS) and internal anal sphincter (IAS) torn

O70.3 Fourth degree perineal laceration during delivery   Ⓜ ♀

Perineal laceration, rupture or tear during delivery as in O70.2, also involving anal mucosa

Perineal laceration, rupture or tear during delivery as in O70.2, also involving rectal mucosa

O70.4 Anal sphincter tear complicating delivery, not associated with third degree laceration   Ⓜ ♀

EXCLUDES 1   *anal sphincter tear with third degree perineal laceration (O70.2)*

O70.9 Perineal laceration during delivery, unspecified   Ⓜ ♀

☑4ᵗʰ **O71 Other obstetric trauma**

INCLUDES   obstetric damage from instruments

☑5ᵗʰ **O71.0 Rupture of uterus (spontaneous) before onset of labor**

EXCLUDES 1   *disruption of (current) cesarean delivery wound (O90.0)*

laceration of uterus, NEC (O71.81)

O71.00 Rupture of uterus before onset of labor, unspecified trimester   Ⓜ ♀

O71.02 Rupture of uterus before onset of labor, second trimester   Ⓜ ♀

O71.03 Rupture of uterus before onset of labor, third trimester   Ⓜ ♀

O71.1 Rupture of uterus during labor   Ⓜ ♀

Rupture of uterus not stated as occurring before onset of labor

EXCLUDES 1   *disruption of cesarean delivery wound (O90.0)*

laceration of uterus, NEC (O71.81)

O71.2 Postpartum inversion of uterus   Ⓜ ♀

O71.3 Obstetric laceration of cervix   Ⓜ ♀

Annular detachment of cervix

O71.4 Obstetric high vaginal laceration alone   Ⓜ ♀

Laceration of vaginal wall without perineal laceration

EXCLUDES 1   *obstetric high vaginal laceration with perineal laceration (O70.-)*

AHA: 2016,1Q,5

O71.5 Other obstetric injury to pelvic organs   Ⓜ ♀

Obstetric injury to bladder

Obstetric injury to urethra

EXCLUDES 2   *obstetric periurethral trauma (O71.82)*

AHA: 2014,4Q,18

O71.6 Obstetric damage to pelvic joints and ligaments   Ⓜ ♀

Obstetric avulsion of inner symphyseal cartilage

Obstetric damage to coccyx

Obstetric traumatic separation of symphysis (pubis)

O71.7 Obstetric hematoma of pelvis   Ⓜ ♀

Obstetric hematoma of perineum

Obstetric hematoma of vagina

Obstetric hematoma of vulva

☑5ᵗʰ **O71.8 Other specified obstetric trauma**

O71.81 Laceration of uterus, not elsewhere classified   Ⓜ ♀

O71.82 Other specified trauma to perineum and vulva   Ⓜ ♀

Obstetric periurethral trauma

AHA: 2016,1Q,4; 2014,4Q,18

O71.89 Other specified obstetric trauma   Ⓜ ♀

O71.9 Obstetric trauma, unspecified   Ⓜ ♀

☑4ᵗʰ **O72 Postpartum hemorrhage**

INCLUDES   hemorrhage after delivery of fetus or infant

O72.0 Third-stage hemorrhage   Ⓜ ♀

Hemorrhage associated with retained, trapped or adherent placenta

Retained placenta NOS

Code also type of adherent placenta (O43.2-)

O72.1 Other immediate postpartum hemorrhage   Ⓜ ♀

Hemorrhage following delivery of placenta

Postpartum hemorrhage (atonic) NOS

Uterine atony with hemorrhage

EXCLUDES 1   *uterine atony NOS (O62.2)*

uterine atony without hemorrhage (O62.2)

postpartum atony of uterus without hemorrhage (O75.89)

AHA: 2016,1Q,4

DEF: Uterine atony: Failure of the uterine muscles to contract after the fetus and placenta are delivered.

O72.2 Delayed and secondary postpartum hemorrhage   Ⓜ ♀

Hemorrhage associated with retained portions of placenta or membranes after the first 24 hours following delivery of placenta

Retained products of conception NOS, following delivery

O72.3 Postpartum coagulation defects   Ⓜ ♀

Postpartum afibrinogenemia

Postpartum fibrinolysis

☑4ᵗʰ **O73 Retained placenta and membranes, without hemorrhage**

EXCLUDES 1   *placenta accreta (O43.21-)*

placenta increta (O43.22-)

placenta percreta (O43.23-)

DEF: Postpartum condition resulting from failure to expel placental membrane tissues due to failed contractions of the uterine wall.

O73.0 Retained placenta without hemorrhage   Ⓜ ♀

Adherent placenta, without hemorrhage

Trapped placenta without hemorrhage

☑ Additional Character Required   ✗x7ᵗʰ Placeholder Alert   Manifestation   Unspecified Dx   ▶◀ Revised Text   ● New Code   ▲ Revised Code Title

ICD-10-CM 2020   883

O73.1   **Retained** portions of placenta and membranes, without hemorrhage   Ⓜ ♀

Retained products of conception following delivery, without hemorrhage

✓4ᵗʰ **O74**   **Complications of anesthesia during labor and delivery**

> [INCLUDES]   maternal complications arising from the administration of a general, regional or local anesthetic, analgesic or other sedation during labor and delivery

Use additional code, if applicable, to identify specific complication

O74.0   **Aspiration pneumonitis** due to anesthesia during labor and delivery   Ⓜ ♀

Inhalation of stomach contents or secretions NOS due to anesthesia during labor and delivery

Mendelson's syndrome due to anesthesia during labor and delivery

O74.1   **Other** pulmonary **complications of anesthesia during labor and delivery**   Ⓜ ♀

O74.2   **Cardiac complications of anesthesia during labor and delivery**   Ⓜ ♀

O74.3   **Central nervous system complications of anesthesia during labor and delivery**   Ⓜ ♀

O74.4   **Toxic reaction to local anesthesia during labor and delivery**   Ⓜ ♀

O74.5   **Spinal and epidural anesthesia-induced headache during labor and delivery**   Ⓜ ♀

O74.6   **Other complications of** spinal and epidural **anesthesia during labor and delivery**   Ⓜ ♀

O74.7   **Failed or difficult intubation for anesthesia during labor and delivery**   Ⓜ ♀

O74.8   **Other complications of anesthesia during labor and delivery**   Ⓜ ♀

O74.9   **Complication of anesthesia during labor and delivery, unspecified**   Ⓜ ♀

✓4ᵗʰ **O75**   **Other complications of labor and delivery, not elsewhere classified**

> [EXCLUDES 2]   puerperal (postpartum) infection (O86.-)
> puerperal (postpartum) sepsis (O85)

O75.0   **Maternal distress during labor and delivery**   Ⓜ ♀

O75.1   **Shock during or following labor and delivery**   Ⓜ ♀

Obstetric shock following labor and delivery

O75.2   **Pyrexia during labor, not elsewhere classified**   Ⓜ ♀

O75.3   **Other infection during labor**   Ⓜ ♀

Sepsis during labor

Use additional code (B95-B97), to identify infectious agent

O75.4   **Other complications of obstetric surgery and procedures**   Ⓜ ♀

Cardiac arrest following obstetric surgery or procedures

Cardiac failure following obstetric surgery or procedures

Cerebral anoxia following obstetric surgery or procedures

Pulmonary edema following obstetric surgery or procedures

Use additional code to identify specific complication

> [EXCLUDES 2]   complications of anesthesia during labor and delivery (O74.-)
> disruption of obstetrical (surgical) wound (O90.0-O90.1)
> hematoma of obstetrical (surgical) wound (O90.2)
> infection of obstetrical (surgical) wound (O86.0-)

O75.5   **Delayed delivery after artificial rupture of membranes**   Ⓜ ♀

✓5ᵗʰ **O75.8**   **Other specified complications of labor and delivery**

O75.81   **Maternal exhaustion complicating labor and delivery**   Ⓜ ♀

O75.82   **Onset (spontaneous) of labor after 37 completed weeks of gestation but before 39 completed weeks gestation, with delivery by (planned) cesarean section**   Ⓜ ♀

Delivery by (planned) cesarean section occurring after 37 completed weeks of gestation but before 39 completed weeks gestation due to (spontaneous) onset of labor

Code first to specify reason for planned cesarean section such as:

cephalopelvic disproportion (normally formed fetus) (O33.9)

previous cesarean delivery (O34.21)

O75.89   **Other specified complications of labor and delivery**   Ⓜ ♀

O75.9   **Complication of labor and delivery, unspecified**   Ⓜ ♀

O76   **Abnormality in fetal heart rate and rhythm complicating labor and delivery**   Ⓜ ♀

Depressed fetal heart rate tones complicating labor and delivery

Fetal bradycardia complicating labor and delivery

Fetal heart rate decelerations complicating labor and delivery

Fetal heart rate irregularity complicating labor and delivery

Fetal heart rate abnormal variability complicating labor and delivery

Fetal tachycardia complicating labor and delivery

Non-reassuring fetal heart rate or rhythm complicating labor and delivery

> [EXCLUDES 1]   fetal stress NOS (O77.9)
> labor and delivery complicated by electrocardiographic evidence of fetal stress (O77.8)
> labor and delivery complicated by ultrasonic evidence of fetal stress (O77.8)

> [EXCLUDES 2]   fetal metabolic acidemia (O68)
> other fetal stress (O77.0-O77.1)

AHA: 2013,4Q,118

✓4ᵗʰ **O77**   **Other fetal stress complicating labor and delivery**

O77.0   **Labor and delivery complicated by meconium in amniotic fluid**   Ⓜ ♀

AHA: 2013,4Q,117-118

O77.1   **Fetal stress in labor or delivery due to drug administration**   Ⓜ ♀

O77.8   **Labor and delivery complicated by other evidence of fetal stress**   Ⓜ ♀

Labor and delivery complicated by electrocardiographic evidence of fetal stress

Labor and delivery complicated by ultrasonic evidence of fetal stress

> [EXCLUDES 1]   abnormality of fetal acid-base balance (O68)
> abnormality in fetal heart rate or rhythm (O76)
> fetal metabolic acidemia (O68)

O77.9   **Labor and delivery complicated by fetal stress, unspecified**   Ⓜ ♀

> [EXCLUDES 1]   abnormality of fetal acid-base balance (O68)
> abnormality in fetal heart rate or rhythm (O76)
> fetal metabolic acidemia (O68)

Encounter for delivery (O80-O82)

O80   **Encounter for full-term uncomplicated delivery**   Ⓜ ♀

> [NOTE]   Delivery requiring minimal or no assistance, with or without episiotomy, without fetal manipulation [e.g., rotation version] or instrumentation [forceps] of a spontaneous, cephalic, vaginal, full-term, single, live-born infant. This code is for use as a single diagnosis code and is not to be used with any other code from chapter 15.

Use additional code to indicate outcome of delivery (Z37.0)

AHA: 2016,4Q,150; 2014,2Q,9

O82   **Encounter for cesarean delivery without indication**   Ⓜ ♀

Use additional code to indicate outcome of delivery (Z37.0)

Complications predominantly related to the puerperium (O85-O92)

> [EXCLUDES 2]   mental and behavioral disorders associated with the puerperium (F53.-)
> obstetrical tetanus (A34)
> puerperal osteomalacia (M83.0)

O85   **Puerperal sepsis**   Ⓜ ♀

Postpartum sepsis

Puerperal peritonitis

Puerperal pyemia

Use additional code (B95-B97), to identify infectious agent

Use additional code (R65.2-) to identify severe sepsis, if applicable

> [EXCLUDES 1]   fever of unknown origin following delivery (O86.4)
> genital tract infection following delivery (O86.1-)
> obstetric pyemic and septic embolism (O88.3-)
> puerperal septic thrombophlebitis (O86.81)
> urinary tract infection following delivery (O86.2-)

> [EXCLUDES 2]   sepsis during labor (O75.3)

AHA: 2018,4Q,23

☑4ᵗʰ **O86 Other puerperal infections**
    Use additional code (B95-B97), to identify infectious agent
    EXCLUDES 2   *infection during labor (O75.3)*
         obstetrical tetanus (A34)

☑5ᵗʰ **O86.0 Infection of obstetric surgical wound**
    Infected cesarean delivery wound following delivery
    Infected perineal repair following delivery
    EXCLUDES 1   *complications of procedures, not elsewhere classified*
         (T81.4-)
         postprocedural fever NOS (R50.82)
         postprocedural retroperitoneal abscess (K68.11)
    AHA: 2018,4Q,22-23,62

    O86.00 Infection of obstetric surgical wound, unspecified Ⓜ ♀

    O86.01 Infection of obstetric surgical wound, superficial incisional site Ⓜ ♀
        Subcutaneous abscess following an obstetrical procedure
        Stitch abscess following an obstetrical procedure

    O86.02 Infection of obstetric surgical wound, deep incisional site Ⓜ ♀
        Intramuscular abscess following an obstetrical procedure
        ▶Sub-fascial abscess following an obstetrical procedure◀

    O86.03 Infection of obstetric surgical wound, organ and space site Ⓜ ♀
        Intraabdominal abscess following an obstetrical procedure
        Subphrenic abscess following an obstetrical procedure

    O86.04 Sepsis following an obstetrical procedure Ⓜ ♀
        Use additional code to identify the sepsis
        AHA: 2019,2Q,39

    O86.09 Infection of obstetric surgical wound, other surgical site Ⓜ ♀

☑5ᵗʰ **O86.1 Other infection of genital tract following delivery**

    O86.11 Cervicitis following delivery Ⓜ ♀
    O86.12 Endometritis following delivery Ⓜ ♀
    O86.13 Vaginitis following delivery Ⓜ ♀
    O86.19 Other infection of genital tract following delivery Ⓜ ♀

☑5ᵗʰ **O86.2 Urinary tract infection following delivery**

    O86.20 Urinary tract infection following delivery, unspecified Ⓜ ♀
        Puerperal urinary tract infection NOS

    O86.21 Infection of kidney following delivery Ⓜ ♀
    O86.22 Infection of bladder following delivery Ⓜ ♀
        Infection of urethra following delivery

    O86.29 Other urinary tract infection following delivery Ⓜ ♀

    O86.4 Pyrexia of unknown origin following delivery Ⓜ ♀
    Puerperal infection NOS following delivery
    Puerperal pyrexia NOS following delivery
    EXCLUDES 2   *pyrexia during labor (O75.2)*
    DEF: Fever of unknown origin experienced by the mother after childbirth.

☑5ᵗʰ **O86.8 Other specified puerperal infections**

    O86.81 Puerperal septic thrombophlebitis Ⓜ ♀
    O86.89 Other specified puerperal infections Ⓜ ♀

☑4ᵗʰ **O87 Venous complications and hemorrhoids in the puerperium**
    INCLUDES   venous complications in labor, delivery and the puerperium
    EXCLUDES 2   *obstetric embolism (O88.-)*
         puerperal septic thrombophlebitis (O86.81)
         venous complications in pregnancy (O22.-)

    O87.0 Superficial thrombophlebitis in the puerperium Ⓜ ♀
    Puerperal phlebitis NOS
    Puerperal thrombosis NOS

    O87.1 Deep phlebothrombosis in the puerperium Ⓜ ♀
    Deep vein thrombosis, postpartum
    Pelvic thrombophlebitis, postpartum
    Use additional code to identify the deep vein thrombosis (I82.4-, I82.5-, I82.62-. I82.72-)
    Use additional code, if applicable, for associated long-term (current) use of anticoagulants (Z79.01)

    O87.2 Hemorrhoids in the puerperium Ⓜ ♀

    O87.3 Cerebral venous thrombosis in the puerperium Ⓜ ♀
    Cerebrovenous sinus thrombosis in the puerperium

    O87.4 Varicose veins of lower extremity in the puerperium Ⓜ ♀

    O87.8 Other venous complications in the puerperium Ⓜ ♀
    Genital varices in the puerperium

    O87.9 Venous complication in the puerperium, unspecified Ⓜ ♀
    Puerperal phlebopathy NOS

☑4ᵗʰ **O88 Obstetric embolism**
    EXCLUDES 1   *embolism complicating abortion NOS (O03.2)*
         embolism complicating ectopic or molar pregnancy (O08.2)
         embolism complicating failed attempted abortion (O07.2)
         embolism complicating induced abortion (O04.7)
         embolism complicating spontaneous abortion (O03.2, O03.7)

☑5ᵗʰ **O88.0 Obstetric air embolism**
    DEF: Sudden blocking of the pulmonary artery or right ventricle with air or nitrogen bubbles.

    ☑6ᵗʰ **O88.01 Obstetric air embolism in pregnancy**
        O88.011 Air embolism in pregnancy, first trimester Ⓜ ♀
        O88.012 Air embolism in pregnancy, second trimester Ⓜ ♀
        O88.013 Air embolism in pregnancy, third trimester Ⓜ ♀
        O88.019 Air embolism in pregnancy, unspecified trimester Ⓜ ♀

    O88.02 Air embolism in childbirth Ⓜ ♀
    O88.03 Air embolism in the puerperium Ⓜ ♀

☑5ᵗʰ **O88.1 Amniotic fluid embolism**
    Anaphylactoid syndrome in pregnancy

    ☑6ᵗʰ **O88.11 Amniotic fluid embolism in pregnancy**
        O88.111 Amniotic fluid embolism in pregnancy, first trimester Ⓜ ♀
        O88.112 Amniotic fluid embolism in pregnancy, second trimester Ⓜ ♀
        O88.113 Amniotic fluid embolism in pregnancy, third trimester Ⓜ ♀
        O88.119 Amniotic fluid embolism in pregnancy, unspecified trimester Ⓜ ♀

    O88.12 Amniotic fluid embolism in childbirth Ⓜ ♀
    O88.13 Amniotic fluid embolism in the puerperium Ⓜ ♀

☑5ᵗʰ **O88.2 Obstetric thromboembolism**

    ☑6ᵗʰ **O88.21 Thromboembolism in pregnancy**
        Obstetric (pulmonary) embolism NOS
        O88.211 Thromboembolism in pregnancy, first trimester Ⓜ ♀
        O88.212 Thromboembolism in pregnancy, second trimester Ⓜ ♀
        O88.213 Thromboembolism in pregnancy, third trimester Ⓜ ♀
        O88.219 Thromboembolism in pregnancy, unspecified trimester Ⓜ ♀

    O88.22 Thromboembolism in childbirth Ⓜ ♀
    O88.23 Thromboembolism in the puerperium Ⓜ ♀
        Puerperal (pulmonary) embolism NOS

☑5ᵗʰ **O88.3 Obstetric pyemic and septic embolism**

    ☑6ᵗʰ **O88.31 Pyemic and septic embolism in pregnancy**
        O88.311 Pyemic and septic embolism in pregnancy, first trimester Ⓜ ♀
        O88.312 Pyemic and septic embolism in pregnancy, second trimester Ⓜ ♀
        O88.313 Pyemic and septic embolism in pregnancy, third trimester Ⓜ ♀

✔ Additional Character Required   ✔x7ᵗʰ Placeholder Alert   Manifestation   Unspecified Dx   ▶◀ Revised Text   ● New Code   ▲ Revised Code Title

O88.319   **Pyemic and septic embolism in pregnancy, unspecified trimester**   M ♀

O88.32   **Pyemic and septic embolism in** childbirth   M ♀

O88.33   **Pyemic and septic embolism in the** puerperium   M ♀

√5ᵗʰ **O88.8**   **Other obstetric embolism**

Obstetric fat embolism

√6ᵗʰ **O88.81**   **Other embolism in** pregnancy

O88.811   **Other embolism in pregnancy, first trimester**   M ♀

O88.812   **Other embolism in pregnancy, second trimester**   M ♀

O88.813   **Other embolism in pregnancy, third trimester**   M ♀

O88.819   **Other embolism in pregnancy, unspecified trimester**   M ♀

O88.82   **Other embolism in** childbirth   M ♀

O88.83   **Other embolism in the** puerperium   M ♀

√4ᵗʰ **O89**   **Complications of anesthesia during the puerperium**

INCLUDES   maternal complications arising from the administration of a general, regional or local anesthetic, analgesic or other sedation during the puerperium

Use additional code, if applicable, to identify specific complication

√5ᵗʰ **O89.0**   **Pulmonary complications of anesthesia during the puerperium**

O89.01   **Aspiration pneumonitis due to anesthesia during the puerperium**   M ♀

Inhalation of stomach contents or secretions NOS due to anesthesia during the puerperium

Mendelson's syndrome due to anesthesia during the puerperium

O89.09   **Other pulmonary complications of anesthesia during the puerperium**   M ♀

O89.1   **Cardiac complications of anesthesia during the puerperium**   M ♀

O89.2   **Central nervous system complications of anesthesia during the puerperium**   M ♀

O89.3   **Toxic reaction to local anesthesia during the puerperium**   M ♀

O89.4   **Spinal and epidural anesthesia-induced headache during the puerperium**   M ♀

O89.5   **Other complications of spinal and epidural anesthesia during the puerperium**   M ♀

O89.6   **Failed or difficult intubation for anesthesia during the puerperium**   M ♀

O89.8   **Other complications of anesthesia during the puerperium**   M ♀

O89.9   **Complication of anesthesia during the puerperium, unspecified**   M ♀

√4ᵗʰ **O90**   **Complications of the puerperium, not elsewhere classified**

O90.0   **Disruption of cesarean delivery wound**   M ♀

Dehiscence of cesarean delivery wound

EXCLUDES 1   *rupture of uterus (spontaneous) before onset of labor (O71.0-)*

rupture of uterus during labor (O71.1)

O90.1   **Disruption of perineal obstetric wound**   M ♀

Disruption of wound of episiotomy

Disruption of wound of perineal laceration

Secondary perineal tear

O90.2   **Hematoma of obstetric wound**   M ♀

O90.3   **Peripartum cardiomyopathy**   M ♀

Conditions in I42- arising during pregnancy and the puerperium

EXCLUDES 1   *pre-existing heart disease complicating pregnancy and the puerperium (O99.4-)*

DEF: Any structural or functional abnormality of the ventricular myocardium. It is a noninflammatory disease of obscure or unknown etiology with onset during the postpartum period.

O90.4   **Postpartum acute kidney failure**   M ♀

Hepatorenal syndrome following labor and delivery

O90.5   **Postpartum thyroiditis**   M ♀

O90.6   **Postpartum mood disturbance**   Q M ♀

Postpartum blues

Postpartum dysphoria

Postpartum sadness

EXCLUDES 1   *postpartum depression (F53.0)*

puerperal psychosis (F53.1)

√5ᵗʰ **O90.8**   **Other complications of the puerperium, not elsewhere classified**

O90.81   **Anemia of the puerperium**   M ♀

Postpartum anemia NOS

EXCLUDES 1   *pre-existing anemia complicating the puerperium (O99.03)*

O90.89   **Other complications of the puerperium, not elsewhere classified**   M ♀

Placental polyp

O90.9   **Complication of the puerperium, unspecified**   M ♀

√4ᵗʰ **O91**   **Infections of breast associated with pregnancy, the puerperium and lactation**

Use additional code to identify infection

√5ᵗʰ **O91.0**   **Infection of nipple associated with pregnancy, the puerperium and lactation**

√6ᵗʰ **O91.01**   **Infection of nipple associated with** pregnancy

Gestational abscess of nipple

O91.011   **Infection of nipple associated with pregnancy, first trimester**   M ♀

O91.012   **Infection of nipple associated with pregnancy, second trimester**   M ♀

O91.013   **Infection of nipple associated with pregnancy, third trimester**   M ♀

O91.019   **Infection of nipple associated with pregnancy, unspecified trimester**   M ♀

O91.02   **Infection of nipple associated with the** puerperium   M ♀

Puerperal abscess of nipple

O91.03   **Infection of nipple associated with** lactation   M ♀

Abscess of nipple associated with lactation

√5ᵗʰ **O91.1**   **Abscess of breast associated with pregnancy, the puerperium and lactation**

√6ᵗʰ **O91.11**   **Abscess of breast associated with** pregnancy

Gestational mammary abscess

Gestational purulent mastitis

Gestational subareolar abscess

O91.111   **Abscess of breast associated with pregnancy, first trimester**   M ♀

O91.112   **Abscess of breast associated with pregnancy, second trimester**   M ♀

O91.113   **Abscess of breast associated with pregnancy, third trimester**   M ♀

O91.119   **Abscess of breast associated with pregnancy, unspecified trimester**   M ♀

O91.12   **Abscess of breast associated with the** puerperium   M ♀

Puerperal mammary abscess

Puerperal purulent mastitis

Puerperal subareolar abscess

O91.13   **Abscess of breast associated with** lactation   M ♀

Mammary abscess associated with lactation

Purulent mastitis associated with lactation

Subareolar abscess associated with lactation

√5ᵗʰ **O91.2**   **Nonpurulent mastitis associated with pregnancy, the puerperium and lactation**

√6ᵗʰ **O91.21**   **Nonpurulent mastitis associated with** pregnancy

Gestational interstitial mastitis

Gestational lymphangitis of breast

Gestational mastitis NOS

Gestational parenchymatous mastitis

O91.211   **Nonpurulent mastitis associated with pregnancy, first trimester**   M ♀

O91.212   **Nonpurulent mastitis associated with pregnancy, second trimester**   M ♀

O91.213   **Nonpurulent mastitis associated with pregnancy, third trimester**   M ♀

O91.219   **Nonpurulent mastitis associated with pregnancy, unspecified trimester** Ⓜ ♀

O91.22   **Nonpurulent mastitis associated with the puerperium** Ⓜ ♀
Puerperal interstitial mastitis
Puerperal lymphangitis of breast
Puerperal mastitis NOS
Puerperal parenchymatous mastitis

O91.23   **Nonpurulent mastitis associated with lactation** Ⓜ ♀
Interstitial mastitis associated with lactation
Lymphangitis of breast associated with lactation
Mastitis NOS associated with lactation
Parenchymatous mastitis associated with lactation

✓4ᵗʰ **O92   Other disorders of breast and disorders of lactation associated with pregnancy and the puerperium**

✓5ᵗʰ   **O92.0   Retracted nipple associated with pregnancy, the puerperium, and lactation**

✓6ᵗʰ   **O92.01   Retracted nipple associated with pregnancy**

O92.011   **Retracted nipple associated with pregnancy, first trimester** Ⓜ ♀

O92.012   **Retracted nipple associated with pregnancy, second trimester** Ⓜ ♀

O92.013   **Retracted nipple associated with pregnancy, third trimester** Ⓜ ♀

O92.019   **Retracted nipple associated with pregnancy, unspecified trimester** Ⓜ ♀

O92.02   **Retracted nipple associated with the puerperium** Ⓜ ♀

O92.03   **Retracted nipple associated with lactation** Ⓜ ♀

✓5ᵗʰ   **O92.1   Cracked nipple associated with pregnancy, the puerperium, and lactation**
Fissure of nipple, gestational or puerperal

✓6ᵗʰ   **O92.11   Cracked nipple associated with pregnancy**

O92.111   **Cracked nipple associated with pregnancy, first trimester** Ⓜ ♀

O92.112   **Cracked nipple associated with pregnancy, second trimester** Ⓜ ♀

O92.113   **Cracked nipple associated with pregnancy, third trimester** Ⓜ ♀

O92.119   **Cracked nipple associated with pregnancy, unspecified trimester** Ⓜ ♀

O92.12   **Cracked nipple associated with the puerperium** Ⓜ ♀

O92.13   **Cracked nipple associated with lactation** Ⓜ ♀

✓5ᵗʰ   **O92.2   Other and unspecified disorders of breast associated with pregnancy and the puerperium**

O92.20   **Unspecified disorder of breast associated with pregnancy and the puerperium** Ⓜ ♀

O92.29   **Other disorders of breast associated with pregnancy and the puerperium** Ⓜ ♀

O92.3   Agalactia Ⓜ ♀
Primary agalactia
   EXCLUDES 1   elective agalactia (O92.5)
       secondary agalactia (O92.5)
       therapeutic agalactia (O92.5)
DEF: Absence of milk secretion in a female after delivery.

O92.4   Hypogalactia Ⓜ ♀

O92.5   Suppressed lactation Ⓜ ♀
Elective agalactia
Secondary agalactia
Therapeutic agalactia
   EXCLUDES 1   primary agalactia (O92.3)

O92.6   Galactorrhea Ⓜ ♀
DEF: Excessive or persistent milk secretion by the breast that may occur in the absence of nursing.

✓5ᵗʰ   **O92.7   Other and unspecified disorders of lactation**

O92.70   **Unspecified disorders of lactation** Ⓜ ♀

O92.79   **Other disorders of lactation** Ⓜ ♀
Puerperal galactocele

Other obstetric conditions, not elsewhere classified (O94-O9A)

O94   Sequelae of complication of pregnancy, childbirth, and the puerperium Ⓜ ♀
   NOTE   This category is to be used to indicate conditions in O00-O77.-, O85-O94 and O98-O9A.- as the cause of late effects. The sequelae include conditions specified as such, or as late effects, which may occur at any time after the puerperium
Code first condition resulting from (sequela) of complication of pregnancy, childbirth, and the puerperium

✓4ᵗʰ **O98   Maternal infectious and parasitic diseases classifiable elsewhere but complicating pregnancy, childbirth and the puerperium**
   INCLUDES   the listed conditions when complicating the pregnant state, when aggravated by the pregnancy, or as a reason for obstetric care
Use additional code (Chapter 1), to identify specific infectious or parasitic disease
   EXCLUDES 2   herpes gestationis (O26.4-)
       infectious carrier state (O99.82-, O99.83-)
       obstetrical tetanus (A34)
       puerperal infection (O86.-)
       puerperal sepsis (O85)
       when the reason for maternal care is that the disease is known or suspected to have affected the fetus (O35-O36)

✓5ᵗʰ   **O98.0   Tuberculosis complicating pregnancy, childbirth and the puerperium**
Conditions in A15-A19

✓6ᵗʰ   **O98.01   Tuberculosis complicating pregnancy**

O98.011   **Tuberculosis complicating pregnancy, first trimester** Ⓜ ♀

O98.012   **Tuberculosis complicating pregnancy, second trimester** Ⓜ ♀

O98.013   **Tuberculosis complicating pregnancy, third trimester** Ⓜ ♀

O98.019   **Tuberculosis complicating pregnancy, unspecified trimester** Ⓜ ♀

O98.02   **Tuberculosis complicating childbirth** Ⓜ ♀

O98.03   **Tuberculosis complicating the puerperium** Ⓜ ♀

✓5ᵗʰ   **O98.1   Syphilis complicating pregnancy, childbirth and the puerperium**
Conditions in A50-A53

✓6ᵗʰ   **O98.11   Syphilis complicating pregnancy**

O98.111   **Syphilis complicating pregnancy, first trimester** Ⓜ ♀

O98.112   **Syphilis complicating pregnancy, second trimester** Ⓜ ♀

O98.113   **Syphilis complicating pregnancy, third trimester** Ⓜ ♀

O98.119   **Syphilis complicating pregnancy, unspecified trimester** Ⓜ ♀

O98.12   **Syphilis complicating childbirth** Ⓜ ♀

O98.13   **Syphilis complicating the puerperium** Ⓜ ♀

✓5ᵗʰ   **O98.2   Gonorrhea complicating pregnancy, childbirth and the puerperium**
Conditions in A54.-

✓6ᵗʰ   **O98.21   Gonorrhea complicating pregnancy**

O98.211   **Gonorrhea complicating pregnancy, first trimester** Ⓜ ♀

O98.212   **Gonorrhea complicating pregnancy, second trimester** Ⓜ ♀

O98.213   **Gonorrhea complicating pregnancy, third trimester** Ⓜ ♀

O98.219   **Gonorrhea complicating pregnancy, unspecified trimester** Ⓜ ♀

O98.22   **Gonorrhea complicating childbirth** Ⓜ ♀

O98.23   **Gonorrhea complicating the puerperium** Ⓜ ♀

☑ Additional Character Required   ✓x7ᵗʰ Placeholder Alert   Manifestation   Unspecified Dx   ▶◀ Revised Text   ● New Code   ▲ Revised Code Title

√5ᵗʰ **O98.3** **Other infections with a predominantly sexual mode of transmission complicating pregnancy, childbirth and the puerperium**
Conditions in A55-A64

  √6ᵗʰ **O98.31** **Other infections with a predominantly sexual mode of transmission complicating pregnancy**

    O98.311 **Other infections with a predominantly sexual mode of transmission complicating pregnancy, first trimester** Ⓜ♀

    O98.312 **Other infections with a predominantly sexual mode of transmission complicating pregnancy, second trimester** Ⓜ♀

    O98.313 **Other infections with a predominantly sexual mode of transmission complicating pregnancy, third trimester** Ⓜ♀

    O98.319 **Other infections with a predominantly sexual mode of transmission complicating pregnancy, unspecified trimester** Ⓜ♀

  O98.32 **Other infections with a predominantly sexual mode of transmission complicating childbirth** Ⓜ♀

  O98.33 **Other infections with a predominantly sexual mode of transmission complicating the puerperium** Ⓜ♀

√5ᵗʰ **O98.4** **Viral hepatitis complicating pregnancy, childbirth and the puerperium**
Conditions in B15-B19

  √6ᵗʰ **O98.41** **Viral hepatitis complicating pregnancy**

    O98.411 **Viral hepatitis complicating pregnancy, first trimester** Ⓜ♀

    O98.412 **Viral hepatitis complicating pregnancy, second trimester** Ⓜ♀

    O98.413 **Viral hepatitis complicating pregnancy, third trimester** Ⓜ♀

    O98.419 **Viral hepatitis complicating pregnancy, unspecified trimester** Ⓜ♀

  O98.42 **Viral hepatitis complicating childbirth** Ⓜ♀

  O98.43 **Viral hepatitis complicating the puerperium** Ⓜ♀

√5ᵗʰ **O98.5** **Other viral diseases complicating pregnancy, childbirth and the puerperium**
Conditions in A80-B09, B25-B34, R87.81-, R87.82-
    EXCLUDES 1   human immunodeficiency virus [HIV] disease complicating pregnancy, childbirth and the puerperium (O98.7-)

  √6ᵗʰ **O98.51** **Other viral diseases complicating pregnancy**

    O98.511 **Other viral diseases complicating pregnancy, first trimester** Ⓜ♀

    O98.512 **Other viral diseases complicating pregnancy, second trimester** Ⓜ♀

    O98.513 **Other viral diseases complicating pregnancy, third trimester** Ⓜ♀

    O98.519 **Other viral diseases complicating pregnancy, unspecified trimester** Ⓜ♀

  O98.52 **Other viral diseases complicating childbirth** Ⓜ♀

  O98.53 **Other viral diseases complicating the puerperium** Ⓜ♀

√5ᵗʰ **O98.6** **Protozoal diseases complicating pregnancy, childbirth and the puerperium**
Conditions in B50-B64

  √6ᵗʰ **O98.61** **Protozoal diseases complicating pregnancy**

    O98.611 **Protozoal diseases complicating pregnancy, first trimester** Ⓜ♀

    O98.612 **Protozoal diseases complicating pregnancy, second trimester** Ⓜ♀

    O98.613 **Protozoal diseases complicating pregnancy, third trimester** Ⓜ♀

    O98.619 **Protozoal diseases complicating pregnancy, unspecified trimester** Ⓜ♀

  O98.62 **Protozoal diseases complicating childbirth** Ⓜ♀

  O98.63 **Protozoal diseases complicating the puerperium** Ⓜ♀

√5ᵗʰ **O98.7** **Human immunodeficiency virus [HIV] disease complicating pregnancy, childbirth and the puerperium**
Use additional code to identify the type of HIV disease:
acquired immune deficiency syndrome (AIDS) (B20)
asymptomatic HIV status (Z21)
HIV positive NOS (Z21)
symptomatic HIV disease (B20)

  √6ᵗʰ **O98.71** **Human immunodeficiency virus [HIV] disease complicating pregnancy**

    O98.711 **Human immunodeficiency virus [HIV] disease complicating pregnancy, first trimester** Ⓜ♀

    O98.712 **Human immunodeficiency virus [HIV] disease complicating pregnancy, second trimester** Ⓜ♀

    O98.713 **Human immunodeficiency virus [HIV] disease complicating pregnancy, third trimester** Ⓜ♀

    O98.719 **Human immunodeficiency virus [HIV] disease complicating pregnancy, unspecified trimester** Ⓜ♀

  O98.72 **Human immunodeficiency virus [HIV] disease complicating childbirth** Ⓜ♀

  O98.73 **Human immunodeficiency virus [HIV] disease complicating the puerperium** Ⓜ♀

√5ᵗʰ **O98.8** **Other maternal infectious and parasitic diseases complicating pregnancy, childbirth and the puerperium**

  √6ᵗʰ **O98.81** **Other maternal infectious and parasitic diseases complicating pregnancy**

    O98.811 **Other maternal infectious and parasitic diseases complicating pregnancy, first trimester** Ⓜ♀

    O98.812 **Other maternal infectious and parasitic diseases complicating pregnancy, second trimester** Ⓜ♀

    O98.813 **Other maternal infectious and parasitic diseases complicating pregnancy, third trimester** Ⓜ♀

    O98.819 **Other maternal infectious and parasitic diseases complicating pregnancy, unspecified trimester** Ⓜ♀

  O98.82 **Other maternal infectious and parasitic diseases complicating childbirth** Ⓜ♀

  O98.83 **Other maternal infectious and parasitic diseases complicating the puerperium** Ⓜ♀

√5ᵗʰ **O98.9** **Unspecified maternal infectious and parasitic disease complicating pregnancy, childbirth and the puerperium**

  √6ᵗʰ **O98.91** **Unspecified maternal infectious and parasitic disease complicating pregnancy**

    O98.911 **Unspecified maternal infectious and parasitic disease complicating pregnancy, first trimester** Ⓜ♀

    O98.912 **Unspecified maternal infectious and parasitic disease complicating pregnancy, second trimester** Ⓜ♀

    O98.913 **Unspecified maternal infectious and parasitic disease complicating pregnancy, third trimester** Ⓜ♀

    O98.919 **Unspecified maternal infectious and parasitic disease complicating pregnancy, unspecified trimester** Ⓜ♀

  O98.92 **Unspecified maternal infectious and parasitic disease complicating childbirth** Ⓜ♀

  O98.93 **Unspecified maternal infectious and parasitic disease complicating the puerperium** Ⓜ♀

☑4ᵗʰ **O99 Other maternal diseases classifiable elsewhere but complicating pregnancy, childbirth and the puerperium**

INCLUDES   conditions which complicate the pregnant state, are aggravated by the pregnancy or are a main reason for obstetric care

Use additional code to identify specific condition

EXCLUDES 2   when the reason for maternal care is that the condition is known or suspected to have affected the fetus (O35-O36)

☑5ᵗʰ **O99.0 Anemia complicating pregnancy, childbirth and the puerperium**

Conditions in D50-D64

EXCLUDES 1   anemia arising in the puerperium (O90.81)
postpartum anemia NOS (O90.81)

☑6ᵗʰ   **O99.01 Anemia complicating pregnancy**

AHA: 2016,1Q,4

- O99.011 **Anemia complicating pregnancy, first trimester** Ⓜ ♀
- O99.012 **Anemia complicating pregnancy, second trimester** Ⓜ ♀
- O99.013 **Anemia complicating pregnancy, third trimester** Ⓜ ♀
- O99.019 **Anemia complicating pregnancy, unspecified trimester** Ⓜ ♀

  O99.02 **Anemia complicating childbirth** Ⓜ ♀

  O99.03 **Anemia complicating the puerperium** Ⓜ ♀

EXCLUDES 1   postpartum anemia not pre-existing prior to delivery (O90.81)

☑5ᵗʰ **O99.1 Other diseases of the blood and blood-forming organs and certain disorders involving the immune mechanism complicating pregnancy, childbirth and the puerperium**

Conditions in D65-D89

EXCLUDES 1   hemorrhage with coagulation defects (O45.-, O46.0-, O67.0, O72.3)

☑6ᵗʰ   **O99.11 Other diseases of the blood and blood-forming organs and certain disorders involving the immune mechanism complicating pregnancy**

- O99.111 **Other diseases of the blood and blood-forming organs and certain disorders involving the immune mechanism complicating pregnancy, first trimester** Ⓜ ♀
- O99.112 **Other diseases of the blood and blood-forming organs and certain disorders involving the immune mechanism complicating pregnancy, second trimester** Ⓜ ♀
- O99.113 **Other diseases of the blood and blood-forming organs and certain disorders involving the immune mechanism complicating pregnancy, third trimester** Ⓜ ♀
- O99.119 **Other diseases of the blood and blood-forming organs and certain disorders involving the immune mechanism complicating pregnancy, unspecified trimester** Ⓜ ♀

  O99.12 **Other diseases of the blood and blood-forming organs and certain disorders involving the immune mechanism complicating childbirth** Ⓜ ♀

  O99.13 **Other diseases of the blood and blood-forming organs and certain disorders involving the immune mechanism complicating the puerperium** Ⓜ ♀

☑5ᵗʰ **O99.2 Endocrine, nutritional and metabolic diseases complicating pregnancy, childbirth and the puerperium**

Conditions in E00-E88

EXCLUDES 2   diabetes mellitus (O24.-)
malnutrition (O25.-)
postpartum thyroiditis (O90.5)

☑6ᵗʰ   **O99.21 Obesity complicating pregnancy, childbirth, and the puerperium**

Use additional code to identify the type of obesity (E66.-)

AHA: 2018,4Q,80

TIP: Do not assign a BMI code (Z68.-) for obese or overweight patients who are pregnant.

- O99.210 **Obesity complicating pregnancy, unspecified trimester** Ⓜ ♀
- O99.211 **Obesity complicating pregnancy, first trimester** Ⓜ ♀
- O99.212 **Obesity complicating pregnancy, second trimester** Ⓜ ♀
- O99.213 **Obesity complicating pregnancy, third trimester** Ⓜ ♀
- O99.214 **Obesity complicating childbirth** Ⓜ ♀
- O99.215 **Obesity complicating the puerperium** Ⓜ ♀

☑6ᵗʰ   **O99.28 Other endocrine, nutritional and metabolic diseases complicating pregnancy, childbirth and the puerperium**

- O99.280 **Endocrine, nutritional and metabolic diseases complicating pregnancy, unspecified trimester** Ⓜ ♀
- O99.281 **Endocrine, nutritional and metabolic diseases complicating pregnancy, first trimester** Ⓜ ♀
- O99.282 **Endocrine, nutritional and metabolic diseases complicating pregnancy, second trimester** Ⓜ ♀
- O99.283 **Endocrine, nutritional and metabolic diseases complicating pregnancy, third trimester** Ⓜ ♀
- O99.284 **Endocrine, nutritional and metabolic diseases complicating childbirth** Ⓜ ♀
- O99.285 **Endocrine, nutritional and metabolic diseases complicating the puerperium** Ⓜ ♀

☑5ᵗʰ **O99.3 Mental disorders and diseases of the nervous system complicating pregnancy, childbirth and the puerperium**

☑6ᵗʰ   **O99.31 Alcohol use complicating pregnancy, childbirth, and the puerperium**

Use additional code(s) from F10 to identify manifestations of the alcohol use

- O99.310 **Alcohol use complicating pregnancy, unspecified trimester** Ⓜ ♀
- O99.311 **Alcohol use complicating pregnancy, first trimester** Ⓜ ♀
- O99.312 **Alcohol use complicating pregnancy, second trimester** Ⓜ ♀
- O99.313 **Alcohol use complicating pregnancy, third trimester** Ⓜ ♀
- O99.314 **Alcohol use complicating childbirth** Ⓜ ♀
- O99.315 **Alcohol use complicating the puerperium** Ⓜ ♀

☑6ᵗʰ   **O99.32 Drug use complicating pregnancy, childbirth, and the puerperium**

Use additional code(s) from F11-F16 and F18-F19 to identify manifestations of the drug use

AHA: 2018,4Q,69-70; 2018,2Q,10

TIP: When drug use is documented during pregnancy, assign first a code from this subcategory followed by an additional code from F11-F16 and F18-F19 identifying the specific drug use even if not documented as associated with a physical, mental, or behavioral disorder. According to chapter 15 guidelines, it is the provider's responsibility to state that the condition being treated is *not* affecting the pregnancy.

- O99.320 **Drug use complicating pregnancy, unspecified trimester** Ⓜ ♀

☑ Additional Character Required   ☑x7ᵗʰ Placeholder Alert   Manifestation   Unspecified Dx   ▶◀ Revised Text   ● New Code   ▲ Revised Code Title

Chapter 15. Pregnancy, Childbirth and the Puerperium

O99.321–O99.63

    O99.321 Drug use complicating pregnancy, first trimester Ⓜ ♀

    O99.322 Drug use complicating pregnancy, second trimester Ⓜ ♀

    O99.323 Drug use complicating pregnancy, third trimester Ⓜ ♀

    O99.324 Drug use complicating childbirth Ⓜ ♀

    O99.325 Drug use complicating the puerperium Ⓜ ♀

✓6ᵗʰ **O99.33 Tobacco use disorder complicating pregnancy, childbirth, and the puerperium**

Smoking complicating pregnancy, childbirth, and the puerperium

Use additional code from category F17 to identify type of tobacco nicotine dependence

    O99.330 Smoking (tobacco) complicating pregnancy, unspecified trimester Ⓜ ♀

    O99.331 Smoking (tobacco) complicating pregnancy, first trimester Ⓜ ♀

    O99.332 Smoking (tobacco) complicating pregnancy, second trimester Ⓜ ♀

    O99.333 Smoking (tobacco) complicating pregnancy, third trimester Ⓜ ♀

    O99.334 Smoking (tobacco) complicating childbirth Ⓜ ♀

    O99.335 Smoking (tobacco) complicating the puerperium Ⓜ ♀

✓6ᵗʰ **O99.34 Other mental disorders complicating pregnancy, childbirth, and the puerperium**

▶Conditions in F01-F09, F20-F99 and F54-F99◀

EXCLUDES 2   postpartum mood disturbance (O90.6)

     postnatal psychosis (F53.1)

     puerperal psychosis (F53.1)

    O99.340 Other mental disorders complicating pregnancy, unspecified trimester Ⓠ Ⓜ ♀

    O99.341 Other mental disorders complicating pregnancy, first trimester Ⓠ Ⓜ ♀

    O99.342 Other mental disorders complicating pregnancy, second trimester Ⓠ Ⓜ ♀

    O99.343 Other mental disorders complicating pregnancy, third trimester Ⓠ Ⓜ ♀

    O99.344 Other mental disorders complicating childbirth Ⓜ ♀

    O99.345 Other mental disorders complicating the puerperium Ⓠ Ⓜ ♀

    AHA: 2018,4Q,8

✓6ᵗʰ **O99.35 Diseases of the nervous system complicating pregnancy, childbirth, and the puerperium**

Conditions in G00-G99

EXCLUDES 2   pregnancy related peripheral neuritis (O26.8-)

    O99.350 Diseases of the nervous system complicating pregnancy, unspecified trimester Ⓜ ♀

    O99.351 Diseases of the nervous system complicating pregnancy, first trimester Ⓜ ♀

    O99.352 Diseases of the nervous system complicating pregnancy, second trimester Ⓜ ♀

    O99.353 Diseases of the nervous system complicating pregnancy, third trimester Ⓜ ♀

    O99.354 Diseases of the nervous system complicating childbirth Ⓜ ♀

    O99.355 Diseases of the nervous system complicating the puerperium Ⓜ ♀

✓5ᵗʰ **O99.4 Diseases of the circulatory system complicating pregnancy, childbirth and the puerperium**

Conditions in I00-I99

EXCLUDES 1   peripartum cardiomyopathy (O90.3)

EXCLUDES 2   hypertensive disorders (O10-O16)

     obstetric embolism (O88.-)

     venous complications and cerebrovenous sinus thrombosis in labor, childbirth and the puerperium (O87.-)

     venous complications and cerebrovenous sinus thrombosis in pregnancy (O22.-)

    AHA: 2016,2Q,8

✓6ᵗʰ **O99.41 Diseases of the circulatory system complicating pregnancy**

    O99.411 Diseases of the circulatory system complicating pregnancy, first trimester Ⓜ ♀

    O99.412 Diseases of the circulatory system complicating pregnancy, second trimester Ⓜ ♀

    O99.413 Diseases of the circulatory system complicating pregnancy, third trimester Ⓜ ♀

    O99.419 Diseases of the circulatory system complicating pregnancy, unspecified trimester Ⓜ ♀

    O99.42 Diseases of the circulatory system complicating childbirth Ⓜ ♀

    O99.43 Diseases of the circulatory system complicating the puerperium Ⓜ ♀

✓5ᵗʰ **O99.5 Diseases of the respiratory system complicating pregnancy, childbirth and the puerperium**

Conditions in J00-J99

✓6ᵗʰ **O99.51 Diseases of the respiratory system complicating pregnancy**

    O99.511 Diseases of the respiratory system complicating pregnancy, first trimester Ⓜ ♀

    O99.512 Diseases of the respiratory system complicating pregnancy, second trimester Ⓜ ♀

    O99.513 Diseases of the respiratory system complicating pregnancy, third trimester Ⓜ ♀

    O99.519 Diseases of the respiratory system complicating pregnancy, unspecified trimester Ⓜ ♀

    O99.52 Diseases of the respiratory system complicating childbirth Ⓜ ♀

    O99.53 Diseases of the respiratory system complicating the puerperium Ⓜ ♀

✓5ᵗʰ **O99.6 Diseases of the digestive system complicating pregnancy, childbirth and the puerperium**

Conditions in K00-K93

EXCLUDES 2   hemorrhoids in pregnancy (O22.4-)

     liver and biliary tract disorders in pregnancy, childbirth and the puerperium (O26.6-)

✓6ᵗʰ **O99.61 Diseases of the digestive system complicating pregnancy**

    AHA: 2016,1Q,4

    O99.611 Diseases of the digestive system complicating pregnancy, first trimester Ⓜ ♀

    O99.612 Diseases of the digestive system complicating pregnancy, second trimester Ⓜ ♀

    O99.613 Diseases of the digestive system complicating pregnancy, third trimester Ⓜ ♀

    O99.619 Diseases of the digestive system complicating pregnancy, unspecified trimester Ⓜ ♀

    O99.62 Diseases of the digestive system complicating childbirth Ⓜ ♀

    O99.63 Diseases of the digestive system complicating the puerperium Ⓜ ♀

☑5ᵗʰ **O99.7** **Diseases of the** skin and subcutaneous **tissue complicating pregnancy, childbirth and the puerperium**
Conditions in L00-L99

> EXCLUDES 2　herpes gestationis (O26.4)
> pruritic urticarial papules and plaques of pregnancy (PUPPP) (O26.86)

☑6ᵗʰ **O99.71** **Diseases of the skin and subcutaneous tissue complicating** pregnancy

O99.711 **Diseases of the skin and subcutaneous tissue complicating pregnancy,** first **trimester**　Ⓜ♀

O99.712 **Diseases of the skin and subcutaneous tissue complicating pregnancy,** second **trimester**　Ⓜ♀

O99.713 **Diseases of the skin and subcutaneous tissue complicating pregnancy,** third **trimester**　Ⓜ♀

O99.719 **Diseases of the skin and subcutaneous tissue complicating pregnancy, unspecified trimester**　Ⓜ♀

O99.72 **Diseases of the skin and subcutaneous tissue complicating** childbirth　Ⓜ♀

O99.73 **Diseases of the skin and subcutaneous tissue complicating the** puerperium　Ⓜ♀

☑5ᵗʰ **O99.8** **Other specified diseases and conditions complicating pregnancy, childbirth and the puerperium**
Conditions in D00-D48, H00-H95, M00-N99, and Q00-Q99
Use additional code to identify condition

> EXCLUDES 2　genitourinary infections in pregnancy (O23.-)
> infection of genitourinary tract following delivery ▶(O86.1-O86.4)◀
> malignant neoplasm complicating pregnancy, childbirth and the puerperium (O9A.1-)
> maternal care for known or suspected abnormality of maternal pelvic organs (O34.-)
> postpartum acute kidney failure (O90.4)
> traumatic injuries in pregnancy (O9A.2-)

☑6ᵗʰ **O99.81** Abnormal glucose **complicating pregnancy, childbirth and the puerperium**

> EXCLUDES 1　gestational diabetes (O24.4-)

O99.810 **Abnormal glucose complicating** pregnancy　Ⓜ♀

O99.814 **Abnormal glucose complicating** childbirth　Ⓜ♀

O99.815 **Abnormal glucose complicating the** puerperium　Ⓜ♀

☑6ᵗʰ **O99.82** Streptococcus B carrier state **complicating pregnancy, childbirth and the puerperium**

> EXCLUDES 1　carrier of streptococcus group B (GBS) in a nonpregnant woman (Z22.330)

DEF: *Streptococcus* group B colonization: Bacteria normally found in the vagina or lower intestine of many healthy adult women that may infect the fetus during childbirth, causing mental or physical handicaps or death. Women who test positive for *streptococcus* Group B during pregnancy are considered a "colonized" status and are treated with IV antibiotics at the time of delivery and may also be treated with oral antibiotics during the pregnancy.

O99.820 **Streptococcus B carrier state complicating** pregnancy　Ⓜ♀

O99.824 **Streptococcus B carrier state complicating** childbirth　Ⓜ♀
AHA: 2019,2Q,8

O99.825 **Streptococcus B carrier state complicating the** puerperium　Ⓜ♀

☑6ᵗʰ **O99.83** **Other infection carrier state complicating pregnancy, childbirth and the puerperium**
Use additional code to identify the carrier state (Z22.-)

O99.830 **Other infection carrier state complicating** pregnancy　Ⓜ♀

O99.834 **Other infection carrier state complicating** childbirth　Ⓜ♀

O99.835 **Other infection carrier state complicating the** puerperium　Ⓜ♀

☑6ᵗʰ **O99.84** Bariatric surgery status **complicating pregnancy, childbirth and the puerperium**
Gastric banding status complicating pregnancy, childbirth and the puerperium
Gastric bypass status for obesity complicating pregnancy, childbirth and the puerperium
Obesity surgery status complicating pregnancy, childbirth and the puerperium

O99.840 **Bariatric surgery status complicating pregnancy, unspecified trimester**　Ⓜ♀

O99.841 **Bariatric surgery status complicating pregnancy,** first **trimester**　Ⓜ♀

O99.842 **Bariatric surgery status complicating pregnancy,** second **trimester**　Ⓜ♀

O99.843 **Bariatric surgery status complicating pregnancy,** third **trimester**　Ⓜ♀

O99.844 **Bariatric surgery status complicating** childbirth　Ⓜ♀

O99.845 **Bariatric surgery status complicating the** puerperium　Ⓜ♀

O99.89 **Other specified diseases and conditions complicating pregnancy, childbirth and the puerperium**　Ⓜ♀

☑4ᵗʰ **O9A** **Maternal malignant neoplasms, traumatic injuries and abuse classifiable elsewhere but complicating pregnancy, childbirth and the puerperium**

☑5ᵗʰ **O9A.1** Malignant neoplasm **complicating pregnancy, childbirth and the puerperium**
Conditions in C00-C96
Use additional code to identify neoplasm

> EXCLUDES 2　maternal care for benign tumor of corpus uteri (O34.1-)
> maternal care for benign tumor of cervix (O34.4-)

AHA: 2015,3Q,19

☑6ᵗʰ **O9A.11** **Malignant neoplasm complicating** pregnancy

O9A.111 **Malignant neoplasm complicating pregnancy,** first **trimester**　Ⓜ♀

O9A.112 **Malignant neoplasm complicating pregnancy,** second **trimester**　Ⓜ♀

O9A.113 **Malignant neoplasm complicating pregnancy,** third **trimester**　Ⓜ♀

O9A.119 **Malignant neoplasm complicating pregnancy, unspecified trimester**　Ⓜ♀

O9A.12 **Malignant neoplasm complicating** childbirth　Ⓜ♀

O9A.13 **Malignant neoplasm complicating the** puerperium　Ⓜ♀

☑5ᵗʰ **O9A.2** Injury, poisoning and **certain other consequences of** external causes **complicating pregnancy, childbirth and the puerperium**
Conditions in S00-T88, except T74 and T76
Use additional code(s) to identify the injury or poisoning

> EXCLUDES 2　physical, sexual and psychological abuse complicating pregnancy, childbirth and the puerperium (O9A.3-, O9A.4-, O9A.5-)

☑6ᵗʰ **O9A.21** **Injury, poisoning and certain other consequences of external causes complicating** pregnancy

O9A.211 **Injury, poisoning and certain other consequences of external causes complicating pregnancy,** first trimester　Ⓜ♀

O9A.212 **Injury, poisoning and certain other consequences of external causes complicating pregnancy,** second trimester　Ⓜ♀

O9A.213 **Injury, poisoning and certain other consequences of external causes complicating pregnancy,** third trimester　Ⓜ♀

O9A.219 **Injury, poisoning and certain other consequences of external causes complicating pregnancy, unspecified trimester**　Ⓜ♀

☑ Additional Character Required　　☑x7ᵗʰ Placeholder Alert　　Manifestation　　Unspecified Dx　　▶◀ Revised Text　　● New Code　　▲ Revised Code Title

O9A.22 Injury, poisoning and certain other consequences of external causes complicating childbirth Ⓜ ♀

O9A.23 Injury, poisoning and certain other consequences of external causes complicating the puerperium Ⓜ ♀

✓5ᵗʰ **O9A.3 Physical abuse complicating pregnancy, childbirth and the puerperium**

Conditions in T74.11 or T76.11

Use additional code (if applicable):

to identify any associated current injury due to physical abuse

to identify the perpetrator of abuse (Y07.-)

> EXCLUDES 2 *sexual abuse complicating pregnancy, childbirth and the puerperium (O9A.4)*

✓6ᵗʰ **O9A.31 Physical abuse complicating pregnancy**

O9A.311 Physical abuse complicating pregnancy, first trimester Ⓜ ♀

O9A.312 Physical abuse complicating pregnancy, second trimester Ⓜ ♀

O9A.313 Physical abuse complicating pregnancy, third trimester Ⓜ ♀

O9A.319 Physical abuse complicating pregnancy, unspecified trimester Ⓜ ♀

O9A.32 Physical abuse complicating childbirth Ⓜ ♀

O9A.33 Physical abuse complicating the puerperium Ⓜ ♀

✓5ᵗʰ **O9A.4 Sexual abuse complicating pregnancy, childbirth and the puerperium**

Conditions in T74.21 or T76.21

Use additional code (if applicable):

to identify any associated current injury due to sexual abuse

to identify the perpetrator of abuse (Y07.-)

✓6ᵗʰ **O9A.41 Sexual abuse complicating pregnancy**

O9A.411 Sexual abuse complicating pregnancy, first trimester Ⓜ ♀

O9A.412 Sexual abuse complicating pregnancy, second trimester Ⓜ ♀

O9A.413 Sexual abuse complicating pregnancy, third trimester Ⓜ ♀

O9A.419 Sexual abuse complicating pregnancy, unspecified trimester Ⓜ ♀

O9A.42 Sexual abuse complicating childbirth Ⓜ ♀

O9A.43 Sexual abuse complicating the puerperium Ⓜ ♀

✓5ᵗʰ **O9A.5 Psychological abuse complicating pregnancy, childbirth and the puerperium**

Conditions in T74.31 or T76.31

Use additional code to identify the perpetrator of abuse (Y07.-)

✓6ᵗʰ **O9A.51 Psychological abuse complicating pregnancy**

O9A.511 Psychological abuse complicating pregnancy, first trimester Ⓜ ♀

O9A.512 Psychological abuse complicating pregnancy, second trimester Ⓜ ♀

O9A.513 Psychological abuse complicating pregnancy, third trimester Ⓜ ♀

O9A.519 Psychological abuse complicating pregnancy, unspecified trimester Ⓜ ♀

O9A.52 Psychological abuse complicating childbirth Ⓜ ♀

O9A.53 Psychological abuse complicating the puerperium Ⓜ ♀

Chapter 16. Certain Conditions Originating in the Perinatal Period (PØØ–P96)

Chapter-specific Guidelines with Coding Examples

The chapter-specific guidelines from the ICD-10-CM Official Guidelines for Coding and Reporting have been provided below. Along with these guidelines are coding examples, contained in the shaded boxes, that have been developed to help illustrate the coding and/or sequencing guidance found in these guidelines.

For coding and reporting purposes the perinatal period is defined as before birth through the 28th day following birth. The following guidelines are provided for reporting purposes

a. General perinatal rules

1) Use of Chapter 16 codes

Codes in this chapter are <u>never</u> for use on the maternal record. Codes from Chapter 15, the obstetric chapter, are never permitted on the newborn record. Chapter 16 codes may be used throughout the life of the patient if the condition is still present.

2) Principal diagnosis for birth record

When coding the birth episode in a newborn record, assign a code from category Z38, Liveborn infants according to place of birth and type of delivery, as the principal diagnosis. A code from category Z38 is assigned only once, to a newborn at the time of birth. If a newborn is transferred to another institution, a code from category Z38 should not be used at the receiving hospital.

A code from category Z38 is used only on the newborn record, not on the mother's record.

3) Use of codes from other chapters with codes from Chapter 16

Codes from other chapters may be used with codes from chapter 16 if the codes from the other chapters provide more specific detail. Codes for signs and symptoms may be assigned when a definitive diagnosis has not been established. If the reason for the encounter is a perinatal condition, the code from chapter 16 should be sequenced first.

4) Use of Chapter 16 codes after the perinatal period

Should a condition originate in the perinatal period, and continue throughout the life of the patient, the perinatal code should continue to be used regardless of the patient's age.

> A 7-year-old patient with history of birth injury that resulted in Erb's palsy is seen for subscapularis release
>
> **P14.Ø**   **Erb's paralysis due to birth injury**
>
> *Explanation:* Although in this instance Erb's palsy is specifically related to a birth injury, it has not resolved and continues to be a health concern. A perinatal code is appropriate even though this patient is beyond the perinatal period.

5) Birth process or community acquired conditions

If a newborn has a condition that may be either due to the birth process or community acquired and the documentation does not indicate which it is, the default is due to the birth process and the code from Chapter 16 should be used. If the condition is community-acquired, a code from Chapter 16 should not be assigned.

6) Code all clinically significant conditions

All clinically significant conditions noted on routine newborn examination should be coded. A condition is clinically significant if it requires:

clinical evaluation; or

therapeutic treatment; or

diagnostic procedures; or

extended length of hospital stay; or

increased nursing care and/or monitoring; or

has implications for future health care needs

Note: The perinatal guidelines listed above are the same as the general coding guidelines for "additional diagnoses", except for the final point regarding implications for future health care needs. Codes should be assigned for conditions that have been specified by the provider as having implications for future health care needs.

b. Observation and evaluation of newborns for suspected conditions not found

1) Use of ZØ5 codes

Assign a code from category ZØ5, Observation and evaluation of newborns and infants for suspected conditions ruled out, to identify those instances when a healthy newborn is evaluated for a suspected condition that is determined after study not to be present. Do not use a code from category ZØ5 when the patient has identified signs or symptoms of a suspected problem; in such cases code the sign or symptom.

2) ZØ5 on other than the birth record

A code from category ZØ5 may also be assigned as a principal or first-listed code for readmissions or encounters when the code from category Z38 code no longer applies. Codes from category ZØ5 are for use only for healthy newborns and infants for which no condition after study is found to be present.

3) ZØ5 on a birth record

A code from category ZØ5 is to be used as a secondary code after the code from category Z38, Liveborn infants according to place of birth and type of delivery.

> Newborn delivered via vaginal delivery; previous ultrasounds showed what appeared to be an abnormality of the right kidney. Kidney function tests were performed and ultrasounds taken and any genitourinary conditions ruled out.
>
> **Z38.ØØ**   **Single liveborn infant, delivered vaginally**
>
> **ZØ5.6**   **Observation and evaluation of newborn for suspected genitourinary condition ruled out**
>
> *Explanation:* The newborn had no signs or symptoms of kidney or other genitourinary condition but was evaluated after delivery due to the abnormal prenatal ultrasound findings. A Z code describing the type and place of birth should be coded first, followed by a ZØ5 category code for the work performed to rule out a suspected genitourinary condition.

c. Coding additional perinatal diagnoses

1) Assigning codes for conditions that require treatment

Assign codes for conditions that require treatment or further investigation, prolong the length of stay, or require resource utilization.

2) Codes for conditions specified as having implications for future health care needs

Assign codes for conditions that have been specified by the provider as having implications for future health care needs.

Note: This guideline should not be used for adult patients.

> An abnormal noise was heard in the left hip of a post-term newborn during a physical examination. The pediatrician would like to follow the patient after discharge as a hip click can be an early sign of hip dysplasia. The newborn was delivered via cesarean at 41 weeks.
>
> **Z38.Ø1**   **Single liveborn infant, delivered by cesarean**
>
> **PØ8.21**   **Post-term newborn**
>
> **R29.4**   **Clicking hip**
>
> *Explanation:* The abnormal hip noise or click is appended as a secondary diagnosis not only because it is an abnormal finding upon examination, but also due to its potential to be part of a bigger health issue. The hip dysplasia has not yet been diagnosed and does not warrant a code at this time.

d. Prematurity and fetal growth retardation

Providers utilize different criteria in determining prematurity. A code for prematurity should not be assigned unless it is documented. Assignment of codes in categories PØ5, Disorders of newborn related to slow fetal growth and fetal malnutrition, and PØ7, Disorders of newborn related to short gestation and low birth weight, not elsewhere classified, should be based on the recorded birth weight and estimated gestational age.

When both birth weight and gestational age are available, two codes from category PØ7 should be assigned, with the code for birth weight sequenced before the code for gestational age.

Chapter 16. Certain Conditions Originating in the Perinatal Period

e. Low birth weight and immaturity status

Codes from category P07, Disorders of newborn related to short gestation and low birth weight, not elsewhere classified, are for use for a child or adult who was premature or had a low birth weight as a newborn and this is affecting the patient's current health status.

See Section I.C.21. Factors influencing health status and contact with health services, Status.

> A 35-year-old patient, who weighed 659 grams at birth, is seen for heart disease documented as being a consequence of the low birth weight
>
> **I51.9**   **Heart disease, unspecified**
>
> **P07.02**   **Extremely low birth weight newborn, 500–749 grams**
>
> *Explanation:* A code from subcategories P07.0- and P07.1- is appropriate, regardless of the age of the patient, as long as the documentation provides a clear link between the patient's current illness and the low birth weight.

f. Bacterial sepsis of newborn

Category P36, Bacterial sepsis of newborn, includes congenital sepsis. If a perinate is documented as having sepsis without documentation of congenital or community acquired, the default is congenital and a code from category P36 should be assigned. If the P36 code includes the causal organism, an additional code from category B95, Streptococcus, Staphylococcus, and Enterococcus as the cause of diseases classified elsewhere, or B96, Other bacterial agents as the cause of diseases classified elsewhere, should not be assigned. If the P36 code does not include the causal organism, assign an additional code from category B96. If applicable, use additional codes to identify severe sepsis (R65.2-) and any associated acute organ dysfunction.

> A full-term infant develops severe sepsis 24 hours after discharge from the hospital and is readmitted; cultures identified *E. coli* as the infective agent
>
> **P36.4**   **Sepsis of newborn due to Escherichia coli**
>
> **R65.20**   **Severe sepsis without septic shock**
>
> *Explanation:* Even though this newborn was discharged and could have acquired *E. coli* from his/her external environment, due to the lack of documentation specifying specifically how this pathogen was acquired, the default is to code the *E. coli* sepsis as congenital. A code from chapter 1, "Certain Infectious and Parasitic Diseases," is not required because the perinatal sepsis code identifies both the sepsis and the bacteria causing the sepsis.

g. Stillbirth

Code P95, Stillbirth, is only for use in institutions that maintain separate records for stillbirths. No other code should be used with P95. Code P95 should not be used on the mother's record.

Chapter 16. Certain Conditions Originating in the Perinatal Period (P00-P96)

NOTE Codes from this chapter are for use on newborn records only, never on maternal records

INCLUDES conditions that have their origin in the fetal or perinatal period (before birth through the first 28 days after birth) even if morbidity occurs later

EXCLUDES 2 congenital malformations, deformations and chromosomal abnormalities (Q00-Q99)

endocrine, nutritional and metabolic diseases (E00-E88)

injury, poisoning and certain other consequences of external causes (S00-T88)

neoplasms (C00-D49)

tetanus neonatorum (A33)

This chapter contains the following blocks:

P00-P04 Newborn affected by maternal factors and by complications of pregnancy, labor, and delivery

P05-P08 Disorders of newborn related to length of gestation and fetal growth

P09 Abnormal findings on neonatal screening

P10-P15 Birth trauma

P19-P29 Respiratory and cardiovascular disorders specific to the perinatal period

P35-P39 Infections specific to the perinatal period

P50-P61 Hemorrhagic and hematological disorders of newborn

P70-P74 Transitory endocrine and metabolic disorders specific to newborn

P76-P78 Digestive system disorders of newborn

P80-P83 Conditions involving the integument and temperature regulation of newborn

P84 Other problems with newborn

P90-P96 Other disorders originating in the perinatal period

Newborn affected by maternal factors and by complications of pregnancy, labor, and delivery (P00-P04)

NOTE These codes are for use when the listed maternal conditions are specified as the cause of confirmed morbidity or potential morbidity which have their origin in the perinatal period (before birth through the first 28 days after birth).

AHA: 2016,4Q,54-55

✓4ᵗʰ **P00 Newborn affected by maternal conditions that may be unrelated to present pregnancy**

Code first any current condition in newborn

EXCLUDES 2 encounter for observation of newborn for suspected diseases and conditions ruled out (Z05.-)

newborn affected by maternal complications of pregnancy (P01.-)

newborn affected by maternal endocrine and metabolic disorders (P70-P74)

newborn affected by noxious substances transmitted via placenta or breast milk (P04.-)

P00.0 Newborn affected by maternal hypertensive disorders

Newborn affected by maternal conditions classifiable to O10-O11, O13-O16

P00.1 Newborn affected by maternal renal and urinary tract diseases

Newborn affected by maternal conditions classifiable to N00-N39

P00.2 Newborn affected by maternal infectious and parasitic diseases

Newborn affected by maternal infectious disease classifiable to A00-B99, J09 and J10

EXCLUDES 1 maternal genital tract or other localized infections (P00.8)

EXCLUDES 2 infections specific to the perinatal period (P35-P39)

AHA: 2019,2Q,10; 2015,3Q,20

P00.3 Newborn affected by other maternal circulatory and respiratory diseases

Newborn affected by maternal conditions classifiable to I00-I99, J00-J99, Q20-Q34 and not included in P00.0, P00.2

P00.4 Newborn affected by maternal nutritional disorders

Newborn affected by maternal disorders classifiable to E40-E64

Maternal malnutrition NOS

P00.5 Newborn affected by maternal injury

Newborn affected by maternal conditions classifiable to O9A.2-

P00.6 Newborn affected by surgical procedure on mother

Newborn affected by amniocentesis

EXCLUDES 1 Cesarean delivery for present delivery (P03.4)

damage to placenta from amniocentesis, Cesarean delivery or surgical induction (P02.1)

previous surgery to uterus or pelvic organs (P03.89)

EXCLUDES 2 newborn affected by complication of (fetal) intrauterine procedure (P96.5)

P00.7 Newborn affected by other medical procedures on mother, not elsewhere classified

Newborn affected by radiation to mother

EXCLUDES 1 damage to placenta from amniocentesis, cesarean delivery or surgical induction (P02.1)

newborn affected by other complications of labor and delivery (P03.-)

✓5ᵗʰ **P00.8 Newborn affected by other maternal conditions**

P00.81 Newborn affected by periodontal disease in mother

P00.89 Newborn affected by other maternal conditions

Newborn affected by conditions classifiable to T80-T88

Newborn affected by maternal genital tract or other localized infections

Newborn affected by maternal systemic lupus erythematosus

AHA: 2019,2Q,9

P00.9 Newborn affected by unspecified maternal condition

✓4ᵗʰ **P01 Newborn affected by maternal complications of pregnancy**

Code first any current condition in newborn

EXCLUDES 2 encounter for observation of newborn for suspected diseases and conditions ruled out (Z05.-)

P01.0 Newborn affected by incompetent cervix

P01.1 Newborn affected by premature rupture of membranes

P01.2 Newborn affected by oligohydramnios

EXCLUDES 1 oligohydramnios due to premature rupture of membranes (P01.1)

DEF: Oligohydramnios: Low amniotic fluid level, resulting in underdeveloped organs in the fetus.

P01.3 Newborn affected by polyhydramnios

Newborn affected by hydramnios

DEF: Polyhydramnios: Excess amniotic fluid surrounding the fetus, typically defined as a total fluid volume of greater than 24.0 cc.

P01.4 Newborn affected by ectopic pregnancy

Newborn affected by abdominal pregnancy

P01.5 Newborn affected by multiple pregnancy

Newborn affected by triplet (pregnancy)

Newborn affected by twin (pregnancy)

P01.6 Newborn affected by maternal death

P01.7 Newborn affected by malpresentation before labor

Newborn affected by breech presentation before labor

Newborn affected by external version before labor

Newborn affected by face presentation before labor

Newborn affected by transverse lie before labor

Newborn affected by unstable lie before labor

P01.8 Newborn affected by other maternal complications of pregnancy

P01.9 Newborn affected by maternal complication of pregnancy, unspecified

✓4ᵗʰ **P02 Newborn affected by complications of placenta, cord and membranes**

Code first any current condition in newborn

EXCLUDES 2 encounter for observation of newborn for suspected diseases and conditions ruled out (Z05.-)

P02.0 Newborn affected by placenta previa

DEF: Placenta developed in the lower segment of the uterus that can cause hemorrhaging leading to preterm delivery.

P02.1 Newborn affected by other forms of placental separation and hemorrhage

Newborn affected by abruptio placenta

Newborn affected by accidental hemorrhage

Newborn affected by antepartum hemorrhage

Newborn affected by damage to placenta from amniocentesis, cesarean delivery or surgical induction

Newborn affected by maternal blood loss

Newborn affected by premature separation of placenta

✓5ᵗʰ **P02.2 Newborn affected by other and unspecified morphological and functional abnormalities of placenta**

P02.20 Newborn affected by unspecified morphological and functional abnormalities of placenta

✓ Additional Character Required ✓x7ᵗʰ Placeholder Alert Manifestation Unspecified Dx ►◄ Revised Text ● New Code ▲ Revised Code Title

ICD-10-CM 2020 895

Chapter 16. Certain Conditions Originating in the Perinatal Period

P02.29   **Newborn affected by other morphological and functional abnormalities of placenta**
Newborn affected by placental dysfunction
Newborn affected by placental infarction
Newborn affected by placental insufficiency

P02.3   **Newborn affected by placental transfusion syndromes**
Newborn affected by placental and cord abnormalities resulting in twin-to-twin or other transplacental transfusion

P02.4   **Newborn affected by prolapsed cord**

P02.5   **Newborn affected by other compression of umbilical cord**
Newborn affected by umbilical cord (tightly) around neck
Newborn affected by entanglement of umbilical cord
Newborn affected by knot in umbilical cord

✓5ᵗʰ **P02.6**   **Newborn affected by other and unspecified conditions of umbilical cord**

    P02.60   **Newborn affected by unspecified conditions of umbilical cord**

    P02.69   **Newborn affected by other conditions of umbilical cord**
Newborn affected by short umbilical cord
Newborn affected by vasa previa
EXCLUDES 1   *newborn affected by single umbilical artery (Q27.0)*

✓5ᵗʰ **P02.7**   **Newborn affected by chorioamnionitis**
AHA: 2018,4Q,23-24
DEF: Inflammation of the fetal membranes due to maternal infection characterized by fetal tachycardia, respiratory distress, apnea, weak cries, and poor sucking.

    P02.70   **Newborn affected by fetal inflammatory response syndrome**   HCC
Newborn affected by FIRS

    P02.78   **Newborn affected by other conditions from chorioamnionitis**
Newborn affected by amnionitis
Newborn affected by membranitis
Newborn affected by placentitis

P02.8   **Newborn affected by other abnormalities of membranes**

P02.9   **Newborn affected by abnormality of membranes, unspecified**

✓4ᵗʰ **P03**   **Newborn affected by other complications of labor and delivery**
Code first any current condition in newborn
EXCLUDES 2   *encounter for observation of newborn for suspected diseases and conditions ruled out (Z05.-)*

P03.0   **Newborn affected by breech delivery and extraction**

P03.1   **Newborn affected by other malpresentation, malposition and disproportion during labor and delivery**
Newborn affected by contracted pelvis
Newborn affected by conditions classifiable to O64-O66
Newborn affected by persistent occipitoposterior
Newborn affected by transverse lie

P03.2   **Newborn affected by forceps delivery**

Forceps Assisted Birth

Forceps extractor

P03.3   **Newborn affected by delivery by vacuum extractor [ventouse]**

Vacuum Assisted Birth

Vacuum extractor

P03.4   **Newborn affected by Cesarean delivery**

P03.5   **Newborn affected by precipitate delivery**
Newborn affected by rapid second stage

P03.6   **Newborn affected by abnormal uterine contractions**
Newborn affected by conditions classifiable to O62.-, except O62.3
Newborn affected by hypertonic labor
Newborn affected by uterine inertia

✓5ᵗʰ **P03.8**   **Newborn affected by other specified complications of labor and delivery**

    ✓6ᵗʰ **P03.81**   **Newborn affected by abnormality in fetal (intrauterine) heart rate or rhythm**
EXCLUDES 1   *neonatal cardiac dysrhythmia (P29.1-)*

       P03.810   **Newborn affected by abnormality in fetal (intrauterine) heart rate or rhythm before the onset of labor**

       P03.811   **Newborn affected by abnormality in fetal (intrauterine) heart rate or rhythm during labor**

       P03.819   **Newborn affected by abnormality in fetal (intrauterine) heart rate or rhythm, unspecified as to time of onset**

    P03.82   **Meconium passage during delivery**
EXCLUDES 1   *meconium aspiration (P24.00, P24.01)*
meconium staining (P96.83)
DEF: Fetal intestinal activity that increases in response to a fetomaternal distressed state during delivery. The anal sphincter relaxes and meconium is passed into the amniotic fluid.

    P03.89   **Newborn affected by other specified complications of labor and delivery**
Newborn affected by abnormality of maternal soft tissues
Newborn affected by conditions classifiable to O60-O75 and by procedures used in labor and delivery not included in P02.- and P03.0-P03.6
Newborn affected by induction of labor

P03.9   **Newborn affected by complication of labor and delivery, unspecified**

✓4ᵗʰ **P04**   **Newborn affected by noxious substances transmitted via placenta or breast milk**
INCLUDES   nonteratogenic effects of substances transmitted via placenta
EXCLUDES 2   *congenital malformations (Q00-Q99)*
encounter for observation of newborn for suspected diseases and conditions ruled out (Z05.-)
neonatal jaundice from excessive hemolysis due to drugs or toxins transmitted from mother (P58.4)
newborn in contact with and (suspected) exposures hazardous to health not transmitted via placenta or breast milk (Z77.-)

P04.0   **Newborn affected by maternal anesthesia and analgesia in pregnancy, labor and delivery**
Newborn affected by reactions and intoxications from maternal opiates and tranquilizers administered for procedures during pregnancy or labor and delivery
EXCLUDES 2   *newborn affected by other maternal medication (P04.1-)*

☑5ᵗʰ **P04.1 Newborn affected by other maternal medication**

Code first withdrawal symptoms from maternal use of drugs of addiction, if applicable (P96.1)

EXCLUDES 1 dysmorphism due to warfarin (Q86.2)
fetal hydantoin syndrome (Q86.1)

EXCLUDES 2 maternal anesthesia and analgesia in pregnancy, labor and delivery (P04.0)
maternal use of drugs of addiction (P04.4-)

AHA: 2018,4Q,24-25

P04.11 Newborn affected by maternal antineoplastic chemotherapy

P04.12 Newborn affected by maternal cytotoxic drugs

P04.13 Newborn affected by maternal use of anticonvulsants

P04.14 Newborn affected by maternal use of opiates

P04.15 Newborn affected by maternal use of antidepressants

P04.16 Newborn affected by maternal use of amphetamines

P04.17 Newborn affected by maternal use of sedative-hypnotics

P04.1A Newborn affected by maternal use of anxiolytics

P04.18 Newborn affected by other maternal medication

P04.19 Newborn affected by maternal use of unspecified medication

P04.2 Newborn affected by maternal use of tobacco

Newborn affected by exposure in utero to tobacco smoke

EXCLUDES 2 newborn exposure to environmental tobacco smoke (P96.81)

P04.3 Newborn affected by maternal use of alcohol

EXCLUDES 1 fetal alcohol syndrome (Q86.0)

☑5ᵗʰ **P04.4 Newborn affected by maternal use of** drugs of addiction

AHA: 2018,4Q,25

P04.40 Newborn affected by maternal use of unspecified drugs of addiction

P04.41 Newborn affected by maternal use of cocaine
"Crack baby"

P04.42 Newborn affected by maternal use of hallucinogens

EXCLUDES 2 newborn affected by other maternal medication (P04.1-)

P04.49 Newborn affected by maternal use of other drugs of addiction

EXCLUDES 2 newborn affected by maternal anesthesia and analgesia (P04.0)
withdrawal symptoms from maternal use of drugs of addiction (P96.1)

P04.5 Newborn affected by maternal use of nutritional chemical substances

P04.6 Newborn affected by maternal exposure to environmental chemical substances

☑5ᵗʰ **P04.8 Newborn affected by other maternal** noxious substances

AHA: 2018,4Q,25

P04.81 Newborn affected by maternal use of cannabis

P04.89 Newborn affected by other maternal noxious substances

P04.9 Newborn affected by maternal noxious substance, unspecified

Disorders of newborn related to length of gestation and fetal growth (P05-P08)

☑4ᵗʰ **P05 Disorders of newborn related to slow fetal growth and fetal malnutrition**

AHA: 2016,4Q,55-56

☑5ᵗʰ **P05.0 Newborn light for gestational age**

Newborn light-for-dates

Weight below but length above 10th percentile for gestational age

P05.00 Newborn light for gestational age, unspecified weight

P05.01 Newborn light for gestational age, less than 500 grams

P05.02 Newborn light for gestational age, 500-749 grams

P05.03 Newborn light for gestational age, 750-999 grams

P05.04 Newborn light for gestational age, 1000-1249 grams

P05.05 Newborn light for gestational age, 1250-1499 grams

P05.06 Newborn light for gestational age, 1500-1749 grams

P05.07 Newborn light for gestational age, 1750-1999 grams

P05.08 Newborn light for gestational age, 2000-2499 grams

P05.09 Newborn light for gestational age, 2500 grams and over

Newborn light for gestational age, other

☑5ᵗʰ **P05.1 Newborn small for gestational age**

Newborn small-and-light-for-dates

Newborn small-for-dates

Weight and length below 10th percentile for gestational age

P05.10 Newborn small for gestational age, unspecified weight

P05.11 Newborn small for gestational age, less than 500 grams

P05.12 Newborn small for gestational age, 500-749 grams

P05.13 Newborn small for gestational age, 750-999 grams

P05.14 Newborn small for gestational age, 1000-1249 grams

P05.15 Newborn small for gestational age, 1250-1499 grams

P05.16 Newborn small for gestational age, 1500-1749 grams

P05.17 Newborn small for gestational age, 1750-1999 grams

P05.18 Newborn small for gestational age, 2000-2499 grams

P05.19 Newborn small for gestational age, other

Newborn small for gestational age, 2500 grams and over

P05.2 Newborn affected by fetal (intrauterine) malnutrition **not light or small for gestational age**

Infant, not light or small for gestational age, showing signs of fetal malnutrition, such as dry, peeling skin and loss of subcutaneous tissue

EXCLUDES 1 newborn affected by fetal malnutrition with light for gestational age (P05.0-)
newborn affected by fetal malnutrition with small for gestational age (P05.1-)

P05.9 Newborn affected by slow intrauterine growth, unspecified

Newborn affected by fetal growth retardation NOS

☑4ᵗʰ **P07 Disorders of newborn related to short gestation and low birth weight, not elsewhere classified**

NOTE When both birth weight and gestational age of the newborn are available, both should be coded with birth weight sequenced before gestational age

INCLUDES the listed conditions, without further specification, as the cause of morbidity or additional care, in newborn

☑5ᵗʰ **P07.0 Extremely low birth weight newborn**

Newborn birth weight 999 g. or less

EXCLUDES 1 low birth weight due to slow fetal growth and fetal malnutrition (P05.-)

P07.00 Extremely low birth weight newborn, unspecified weight

P07.01 Extremely low birth weight newborn, less than 500 grams

P07.02 Extremely low birth weight newborn, 500-749 grams

P07.03 Extremely low birth weight newborn, 750-999 grams

☑5ᵗʰ **P07.1 Other low birth weight newborn**

Newborn birth weight 1000-2499 g.

EXCLUDES 1 low birth weight due to slow fetal growth and fetal malnutrition (P05.-)

P07.10 Other low birth weight newborn, unspecified weight

P07.14 Other low birth weight newborn, 1000-1249 grams

P07.15 Other low birth weight newborn, 1250-1499 grams

P07.16 Other low birth weight newborn, 1500-1749 grams

P07.17 Other low birth weight newborn, 1750-1999 grams

P07.18 Other low birth weight newborn, 2000-2499 grams

☑ Additional Character Required ☑x7ᵗʰ Placeholder Alert Manifestation Unspecified Dx ▶◀ Revised Text ● New Code ▲ Revised Code Title

ICD-10-CM 2020 897

☑5ᵗʰ **P07.2 Extreme immaturity of newborn**

Less than 28 completed weeks (less than 196 completed days) of gestation.

P07.20 Extreme immaturity of newborn, unspecified weeks of gestation

Gestational age less than 28 completed weeks NOS

P07.21 Extreme immaturity of newborn, gestational age less than 23 completed weeks

Extreme immaturity of newborn, gestational age less than 23 weeks, 0 days

P07.22 Extreme immaturity of newborn, gestational age 23 completed weeks

Extreme immaturity of newborn, gestational age 23 weeks, 0 days through 23 weeks, 6 days

P07.23 Extreme immaturity of newborn, gestational age 24 completed weeks

Extreme immaturity of newborn, gestational age 24 weeks, 0 days through 24 weeks, 6 days

P07.24 Extreme immaturity of newborn, gestational age 25 completed weeks

Extreme immaturity of newborn, gestational age 25 weeks, 0 days through 25 weeks, 6 days

P07.25 Extreme immaturity of newborn, gestational age 26 completed weeks

Extreme immaturity of newborn, gestational age 26 weeks, 0 days through 26 weeks, 6 days

P07.26 Extreme immaturity of newborn, gestational age 27 completed weeks

Extreme immaturity of newborn, gestational age 27 weeks, 0 days through 27 weeks, 6 days

☑5ᵗʰ **P07.3 Preterm [premature] newborn [other]**

28 completed weeks or more but less than 37 completed weeks (196 completed days but less than 259 completed days) of gestation

Prematurity NOS

AHA: 2017,3Q,26

P07.30 Preterm newborn, unspecified weeks of gestation

P07.31 Preterm newborn, gestational age 28 completed weeks

Preterm newborn, gestational age 28 weeks, 0 days through 28 weeks, 6 days

P07.32 Preterm newborn, gestational age 29 completed weeks

Preterm newborn, gestational age 29 weeks, 0 days through 29 weeks, 6 days

P07.33 Preterm newborn, gestational age 30 completed weeks

Preterm newborn, gestational age 30 weeks, 0 days through 30 weeks, 6 days

P07.34 Preterm newborn, gestational age 31 completed weeks

Preterm newborn, gestational age 31 weeks, 0 days through 31 weeks, 6 days

P07.35 Preterm newborn, gestational age 32 completed weeks

Preterm newborn, gestational age 32 weeks, 0 days through 32 weeks, 6 days

P07.36 Preterm newborn, gestational age 33 completed weeks

Preterm newborn, gestational age 33 weeks, 0 days through 33 weeks, 6 days

P07.37 Preterm newborn, gestational age 34 completed weeks

Preterm newborn, gestational age 34 weeks, 0 days through 34 weeks, 6 days

P07.38 Preterm newborn, gestational age 35 completed weeks

Preterm newborn, gestational age 35 weeks, 0 days through 35 weeks, 6 days

P07.39 Preterm newborn, gestational age 36 completed weeks

Preterm newborn, gestational age 36 weeks, 0 days through 36 weeks, 6 days

☑4ᵗʰ **P08 Disorders of newborn related to long gestation and high birth weight**

NOTE When both birth weight and gestational age of the newborn are available, priority of assignment should be given to birth weight

INCLUDES the listed conditions, without further specification, as causes of morbidity or additional care, in newborn

P08.0 Exceptionally large newborn baby

Usually implies a birth weight of 4500 g. or more

EXCLUDES 1 *syndrome of infant of diabetic mother (P70.1)*

syndrome of infant of mother with gestational diabetes (P70.0)

P08.1 Other heavy for gestational age newborn

Other newborn heavy- or large-for-dates regardless of period of gestation

Usually implies a birth weight of 4000 g. to 4499 g.

EXCLUDES 1 *newborn with a birth weight of 4500 or more (P08.0)*

syndrome of infant of diabetic mother (P70.1)

syndrome of infant of mother with gestational diabetes (P70.0).

☑5ᵗʰ **P08.2 Late newborn, not heavy for gestational age**

AHA: 2014,1Q,14

P08.21 Post-term newborn

Newborn with gestation period over 40 completed weeks to 42 completed weeks

P08.22 Prolonged gestation of newborn

Newborn with gestation period over 42 completed weeks (294 days or more), not heavy- or large-for-dates.

Postmaturity NOS

Abnormal findings on neonatal screening (P09)

P09 Abnormal findings on neonatal screening

Use additional code to identify signs, symptoms and conditions associated with the screening

EXCLUDES 2 *nonspecific serologic evidence of human immunodeficiency virus [HIV] (R75)*

Birth trauma (P10-P15)

☑4ᵗʰ **P10 Intracranial laceration and hemorrhage due to birth injury**

EXCLUDES 1 *intracranial hemorrhage of newborn NOS (P52.9)*

intracranial hemorrhage of newborn due to anoxia or hypoxia (P52.-)

nontraumatic intracranial hemorrhage of newborn (P52.-)

P10.0 Subdural hemorrhage due to birth injury

Subdural hematoma (localized) due to birth injury

EXCLUDES 1 *subdural hemorrhage accompanying tentorial tear (P10.4)*

P10.1 Cerebral hemorrhage due to birth injury

P10.2 Intraventricular hemorrhage due to birth injury

P10.3 Subarachnoid hemorrhage due to birth injury

P10.4 Tentorial tear due to birth injury

P10.8 Other intracranial lacerations and hemorrhages due to birth injury

P10.9 Unspecified intracranial laceration and hemorrhage due to birth injury

☑4ᵗʰ **P11 Other birth injuries to central nervous system**

P11.0 Cerebral edema due to birth injury

P11.1 Other specified brain damage due to birth injury

P11.2 Unspecified brain damage due to birth injury

P11.3 Birth injury to facial nerve

Facial palsy due to birth injury

P11.4 Birth injury to other cranial nerves

P11.5 Birth injury to spine and spinal cord

Fracture of spine due to birth injury

P11.9 Birth injury to central nervous system, unspecified

✓4ᵗʰ P12 Birth injury to scalp

Birth Injuries to Scalp

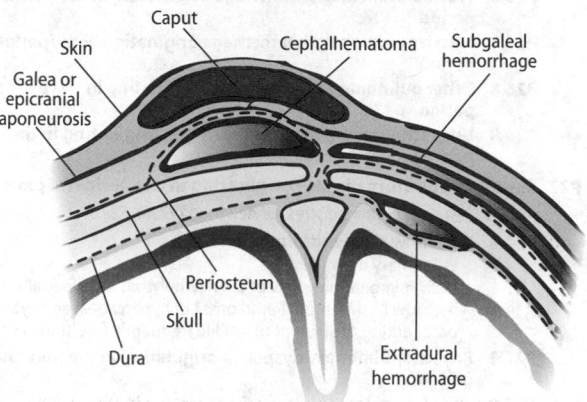

P12.0 Cephalhematoma due to birth injury
   DEF: Condition that occurs in a neonate when blood vessels between the skull and periosteum rupture and blood collects in the subperiosteal space (below the periosteum). It is typically caused by prolonged labor or trauma due to instrument-assisted delivery (e.g., forceps, vacuum extraction), although in rare circumstances, it may indicate a linear skull fracture with intracranial hemorrhage.

P12.1 Chignon (from vacuum extraction) due to birth injury
   DEF: Artificial swelling of the scalp that occurs when a collection of interstitial fluid and blood forms in the area of the scalp where the suction cup was applied during a vacuum-assisted delivery.

P12.2 Epicranial subaponeurotic hemorrhage due to birth injury
   Subgaleal hemorrhage

P12.3 Bruising of scalp due to birth injury

P12.4 Injury of scalp of newborn due to monitoring equipment
   Sampling incision of scalp of newborn
   Scalp clip (electrode) injury of newborn

✓6ᵗʰ P12.8 Other birth injuries to scalp

   P12.81 Caput succedaneum
      DEF: Swelling of the scalp as a result of pressure being exerted on the head from the vaginal walls, uterus, or instrumentation used in assisting a delivery (e.g., vacuum).

   P12.89 Other birth injuries to scalp
P12.9 Birth injury to scalp, unspecified

✓4ᵗʰ P13 Birth injury to skeleton

   EXCLUDES 2   birth injury to spine (P11.5)

   P13.0 Fracture of skull due to birth injury
   P13.1 Other birth injuries to skull
      EXCLUDES 1   cephalhematoma (P12.0)
   P13.2 Birth injury to femur
   P13.3 Birth injury to other long bones
   P13.4 Fracture of clavicle due to birth injury
   P13.8 Birth injuries to other parts of skeleton
   P13.9 Birth injury to skeleton, unspecified

✓4ᵗʰ P14 Birth injury to peripheral nervous system

   P14.0 Erb's paralysis due to birth injury
      DEF: Erb's paralysis: Most common type of brachial plexus (peripheral nerve) injury in a neonate that involves nerve damage at the level of C5-C6. **Synonym(s):** Erb's palsy
   P14.1 Klumpke's paralysis due to birth injury
   P14.2 Phrenic nerve paralysis due to birth injury
   P14.3 Other brachial plexus birth injuries
   P14.8 Birth injuries to other parts of peripheral nervous system
   P14.9 Birth injury to peripheral nervous system, unspecified

✓4ᵗʰ P15 Other birth injuries

   P15.0 Birth injury to liver
      Rupture of liver due to birth injury
   P15.1 Birth injury to spleen
      Rupture of spleen due to birth injury
   P15.2 Sternomastoid injury due to birth injury

P15.3 Birth injury to eye
   Subconjunctival hemorrhage due to birth injury
   Traumatic glaucoma due to birth injury
P15.4 Birth injury to face
   Facial congestion due to birth injury
P15.5 Birth injury to external genitalia
P15.6 Subcutaneous fat necrosis due to birth injury
P15.8 Other specified birth injuries
   TIP: Use for any injury of newborn from scalpel.
P15.9 Birth injury, unspecified

Respiratory and cardiovascular disorders specific to the perinatal period (P19-P29)

✓4ᵗʰ P19 Metabolic acidemia in newborn
   INCLUDES   metabolic acidemia in newborn
   P19.0 Metabolic acidemia in newborn first noted before onset of labor
   P19.1 Metabolic acidemia in newborn first noted during labor
   P19.2 Metabolic acidemia noted at birth
   P19.9 Metabolic acidemia, unspecified

✓4ᵗʰ P22 Respiratory distress of newborn
   EXCLUDES 1   *respiratory arrest of newborn (P28.81)*
        respiratory failure of newborn NOS (P28.5)
   AHA: 2019,2Q,29
   P22.0 Respiratory distress syndrome of newborn
      Cardiorespiratory distress syndrome of newborn
      Hyaline membrane disease
      Idiopathic respiratory distress syndrome [IRDS or RDS] of newborn
      Pulmonary hypoperfusion syndrome
      Respiratory distress syndrome, type I
      EXCLUDES 2 ►*respiratory arrest of newborn (P28.81)*◄
           ►*respiratory failure of newborn NOS (P28.5)*◄
      AHA: 2019,2Q,29
      DEF: Severe chest contractions upon air intake and expiratory grunting. The infant appears blue due to oxygen deficiency and has a rapid respiratory rate, formerly called hyaline membrane disease.
   P22.1 Transient tachypnea of newborn
      Idiopathic tachypnea of newborn
      Respiratory distress syndrome, type II
      Wet lung syndrome
      DEF: Rapid, labored breathing of a newborn. It is a short-term problem that begins after birth and lasts about three days.
   P22.8 Other respiratory distress of newborn
      EXCLUDES 1 ►*respiratory arrest of newborn (P28.81)*◄
           ►*respiratory failure of newborn NOS (P28.5)*◄
   P22.9 Respiratory distress of newborn, unspecified
      EXCLUDES 1 ►*respiratory arrest of newborn (P28.81)*◄
           ►*respiratory failure of newborn NOS (P28.5)*◄

✓4ᵗʰ P23 Congenital pneumonia
   INCLUDES   infective pneumonia acquired in utero or during birth
   EXCLUDES 1   neonatal pneumonia resulting from aspiration (P24.-)
   P23.0 Congenital pneumonia due to viral agent
      Use additional code (B97) to identify organism
      EXCLUDES 1   congenital rubella pneumonitis (P35.0)
   P23.1 Congenital pneumonia due to Chlamydia
   P23.2 Congenital pneumonia due to staphylococcus
   P23.3 Congenital pneumonia due to streptococcus, group B
   P23.4 Congenital pneumonia due to Escherichia coli
   P23.5 Congenital pneumonia due to Pseudomonas
   P23.6 Congenital pneumonia due to other bacterial agents
      Congenital pneumonia due to Hemophilus influenzae
      Congenital pneumonia due to Klebsiella pneumoniae
      Congenital pneumonia due to Mycoplasma
      Congenital pneumonia due to Streptococcus, except group B
      Use additional code (B95-B96) to identify organism
   P23.8 Congenital pneumonia due to other organisms
   P23.9 Congenital pneumonia, unspecified

Caput | Skin | Galea or epicranial aponeurosis | Cephalhematoma | Subgaleal hemorrhage | Periosteum | Skull | Dura | Extradural hemorrhage

Chapter 16. Certain Conditions Originating in the Perinatal Period

P24–P29.2

√4th P24 Neonatal aspiration
    INCLUDES   aspiration in utero and during delivery

  √5th P24.0 Meconium aspiration
      EXCLUDES 1   meconium passage (without aspiration) during delivery (P03.82)
          meconium staining (P96.83)
      DEF: Meconium in the trachea or seen on chest x-ray after birth.

    P24.00 Meconium aspiration without respiratory symptoms
       Meconium aspiration NOS

    P24.01 Meconium aspiration with respiratory symptoms
       Meconium aspiration pneumonia
       Meconium aspiration pneumonitis
       Meconium aspiration syndrome NOS
       Use additional code to identify any secondary pulmonary hypertension, if applicable (I27.2-)
       DEF: Aspiration of fetal intestinal material during or prior to delivery. If is usually a complication of placental insufficiency, causing pneumonitis and bronchial obstruction (inflammatory reaction of lungs).

  √5th P24.1 Neonatal aspiration of (clear) amniotic fluid and mucus
       Neonatal aspiration of liquor (amnii)

    P24.10 Neonatal aspiration of (clear) amniotic fluid and mucus without respiratory symptoms
       Neonatal aspiration of amniotic fluid and mucus NOS

    P24.11 Neonatal aspiration of (clear) amniotic fluid and mucus with respiratory symptoms
       Neonatal aspiration of amniotic fluid and mucus with pneumonia
       Neonatal aspiration of amniotic fluid and mucus with pneumonitis
       Use additional code to identify any secondary pulmonary hypertension, if applicable (I27.2-)

  √5th P24.2 Neonatal aspiration of blood

    P24.20 Neonatal aspiration of blood without respiratory symptoms
       Neonatal aspiration of blood NOS

    P24.21 Neonatal aspiration of blood with respiratory symptoms
       Neonatal aspiration of blood with pneumonia
       Neonatal aspiration of blood with pneumonitis
       Use additional code to identify any secondary pulmonary hypertension, if applicable (I27.2-)

  √5th P24.3 Neonatal aspiration of milk and regurgitated food
       Neonatal aspiration of stomach contents

    P24.30 Neonatal aspiration of milk and regurgitated food without respiratory symptoms
       Neonatal aspiration of milk and regurgitated food NOS

    P24.31 Neonatal aspiration of milk and regurgitated food with respiratory symptoms
       Neonatal aspiration of milk and regurgitated food with pneumonia
       Neonatal aspiration of milk and regurgitated food with pneumonitis
       Use additional code to identify any secondary pulmonary hypertension, if applicable (I27.2-)

  √5th P24.8 Other neonatal aspiration

    P24.80 Other neonatal aspiration without respiratory symptoms
       Neonatal aspiration NEC

    P24.81 Other neonatal aspiration with respiratory symptoms
       Neonatal aspiration pneumonia NEC
       Neonatal aspiration with pneumonitis NEC
       Neonatal aspiration with pneumonia NOS
       Neonatal aspiration with pneumonitis NOS
       Use additional code to identify any secondary pulmonary hypertension, if applicable (I27.2-)

  P24.9 Neonatal aspiration, unspecified

√4th P25 Interstitial emphysema and related conditions originating in the perinatal period

  P25.0 Interstitial emphysema originating in the perinatal period
  P25.1 Pneumothorax originating in the perinatal period
  P25.2 Pneumomediastinum originating in the perinatal period
  P25.3 Pneumopericardium originating in the perinatal period
  P25.8 Other conditions related to interstitial emphysema originating in the perinatal period

√4th P26 Pulmonary hemorrhage originating in the perinatal period
    EXCLUDES 1   acute idiopathic hemorrhage in infants over 28 days old (R04.81)

  P26.0 Tracheobronchial hemorrhage originating in the perinatal period
  P26.1 Massive pulmonary hemorrhage originating in the perinatal period
  P26.8 Other pulmonary hemorrhages originating in the perinatal period
  P26.9 Unspecified pulmonary hemorrhage originating in the perinatal period

√4th P27 Chronic respiratory disease originating in the perinatal period
    EXCLUDES 2   respiratory distress of newborn (P22.0-P22.9)

  P27.0 Wilson-Mikity syndrome
       Pulmonary dysmaturity
       DEF: Pulmonary insufficiency in newborn babies, especially those with low birth weight. Rapid onset of hypercapnia and cyanosis occur during the first month of life frequently resulting in death.

  P27.1 Bronchopulmonary dysplasia originating in the perinatal period
  P27.8 Other chronic respiratory diseases originating in the perinatal period
       Congenital pulmonary fibrosis
       Ventilator lung in newborn
  P27.9 Unspecified chronic respiratory disease originating in the perinatal period

√4th P28 Other respiratory conditions originating in the perinatal period
    EXCLUDES 1   congenital malformations of the respiratory system (Q30-Q34)

  P28.0 Primary atelectasis of newborn
       Primary failure to expand terminal respiratory units
       Pulmonary hypoplasia associated with short gestation
       Pulmonary immaturity NOS

  √5th P28.1 Other and unspecified atelectasis of newborn

    P28.10 Unspecified atelectasis of newborn
       Atelectasis of newborn NOS

    P28.11 Resorption atelectasis without respiratory distress syndrome
      EXCLUDES 1   resorption atelectasis with respiratory distress syndrome (P22.0)

    P28.19 Other atelectasis of newborn
       Partial atelectasis of newborn
       Secondary atelectasis of newborn

  P28.2 Cyanotic attacks of newborn
      EXCLUDES 1   apnea of newborn (P28.3-P28.4)

  P28.3 Primary sleep apnea of newborn
       Central sleep apnea of newborn
       Obstructive sleep apnea of newborn
       Sleep apnea of newborn NOS
       DEF: Unexplained cessation of breathing when a neonate makes no respiratory effort for 20 seconds or longer or when a neonate's breathing cessation is accompanied by cyanosis, bradycardia, or hypotonia.

  P28.4 Other apnea of newborn
       Apnea of prematurity
       Obstructive apnea of newborn
      EXCLUDES 1   obstructive sleep apnea of newborn (P28.3)

  P28.5 Respiratory failure of newborn
      EXCLUDES 1   respiratory arrest of newborn (P28.81)
          respiratory distress of newborn (P22.0-)
       AHA: 2019,2Q,29

  √5th P28.8 Other specified respiratory conditions of newborn

    P28.81 Respiratory arrest of newborn
    P28.89 Other specified respiratory conditions of newborn
       Congenital laryngeal stridor
       Sniffles in newborn
       Snuffles in newborn
      EXCLUDES 1   early congenital syphilitic rhinitis (A50.05)

  P28.9 Respiratory condition of newborn, unspecified
       Respiratory depression in newborn

√4th P29 Cardiovascular disorders originating in the perinatal period
    EXCLUDES 1   congenital malformations of the circulatory system (Q20-Q28)

  P29.0 Neonatal cardiac failure
  √5th P29.1 Neonatal cardiac dysrhythmia

    P29.11 Neonatal tachycardia
    P29.12 Neonatal bradycardia
  P29.2 Neonatal hypertension

✓5ᵗʰ **P29.3**   **Persistent fetal circulation**
> AHA: 2017,4Q,20-21

P29.30   **Pulmonary hypertension of newborn**
> Persistent pulmonary hypertension of newborn
> **DEF:** Condition that occurs when pressure within the pulmonary artery is elevated and vascular resistance is observed in the lungs.

P29.38   **Other persistent fetal circulation**
> Delayed closure of ductus arteriosus

P29.4   **Transient myocardial ischemia in newborn**

✓5ᵗʰ **P29.8**   **Other cardiovascular disorders originating in the perinatal period**

P29.81   **Cardiac arrest of newborn**

P29.89   **Other cardiovascular disorders originating in the perinatal period**
> AHA: 2014,4Q,23

P29.9   **Cardiovascular disorder originating in the perinatal period, unspecified**

Infections specific to the perinatal period (P35-P39)

Infections acquired in utero, during birth via the umbilicus, or during the first 28 days after birth

EXCLUDES 2   *asymptomatic human immunodeficiency virus [HIV] infection status (Z21)*
> *congenital gonococcal infection (A54.-)*
> *congenital pneumonia (P23.-)*
> *congenital syphilis (A50.-)*
> *human immunodeficiency virus [HIV] disease (B20)*
> *infant botulism (A48.51)*
> *infectious diseases not specific to the perinatal period (A00-B99, J09, J10.-)*
> *intestinal infectious disease (A00-A09)*
> *laboratory evidence of human immunodeficiency virus [HIV] (R75)*
> *tetanus neonatorum (A33)*

✓4ᵗʰ **P35**   **Congenital viral diseases**

INCLUDES   infections acquired in utero or during birth

P35.0   **Congenital rubella syndrome**
> Congenital rubella pneumonitis

P35.1   **Congenital cytomegalovirus infection**

P35.2   **Congenital herpesviral [herpes simplex] infection**

P35.3   **Congenital viral hepatitis**

P35.4   **Congenital Zika virus disease**
> Use additional code to identify manifestations of congenital Zika virus disease
> AHA: 2018,4Q,25-26

P35.8   **Other congenital viral diseases**
> Congenital varicella [chickenpox]

P35.9   **Congenital viral disease, unspecified**

✓4ᵗʰ **P36**   **Bacterial sepsis of newborn**

INCLUDES   congenital sepsis
> Use additional code(s), if applicable, to identify severe sepsis (R65.2-) and associated acute organ dysfunction(s)

P36.0   **Sepsis of newborn due to streptococcus, group B**   HCC

✓5ᵗʰ **P36.1**   **Sepsis of newborn due to other and unspecified streptococci**

P36.10   **Sepsis of newborn due to unspecified streptococci**   HCC

P36.19   **Sepsis of newborn due to other streptococci**   HCC

P36.2   **Sepsis of newborn due to Staphylococcus aureus**   HCC

✓5ᵗʰ **P36.3**   **Sepsis of newborn due to other and unspecified staphylococci**

P36.30   **Sepsis of newborn due to unspecified staphylococci**   HCC

P36.39   **Sepsis of newborn due to other staphylococci**   HCC

P36.4   **Sepsis of newborn due to Escherichia coli**   HCC

P36.5   **Sepsis of newborn due to anaerobes**   HCC

P36.8   **Other bacterial sepsis of newborn**   HCC
> Use additional code from category B96 to identify organism

P36.9   **Bacterial sepsis of newborn, unspecified**   HCC

✓4ᵗʰ **P37**   **Other congenital infectious and parasitic diseases**

EXCLUDES 2   *congenital syphilis (A50.-)*
> *infectious neonatal diarrhea (A00-A09)*
> *necrotizing enterocolitis in newborn (P77.-)*
> *noninfectious neonatal diarrhea (P78.3)*
> *ophthalmia neonatorum due to gonococcus (A54.31)*
> *tetanus neonatorum (A33)*

P37.0   **Congenital tuberculosis**

P37.1   **Congenital toxoplasmosis**
> Hydrocephalus due to congenital toxoplasmosis

P37.2   **Neonatal (disseminated) listeriosis**

P37.3   **Congenital falciparum malaria**

P37.4   **Other congenital malaria**

P37.5   **Neonatal candidiasis**

P37.8   **Other specified congenital infectious and parasitic diseases**

P37.9   **Congenital infectious or parasitic disease, unspecified**

✓4ᵗʰ **P38**   **Omphalitis of newborn**

EXCLUDES 1   *omphalitis not of newborn (L08.82)*
> *tetanus omphalitis (A33)*
> *umbilical hemorrhage of newborn (P51.-)*

DEF: Omphalitis: Infection and inflammation of the umbilical stump, often due to bacteria that can spread beyond the umbilical stump to the fascia, muscle, or even the umbilical vessels.

P38.1   **Omphalitis with mild hemorrhage**

P38.9   **Omphalitis without hemorrhage**
> Omphalitis of newborn NOS

✓4ᵗʰ **P39**   **Other infections specific to the perinatal period**
> Use additional code to identify organism or specific infection

P39.0   **Neonatal infective mastitis**

EXCLUDES 1   *breast engorgement of newborn (P83.4)*
> *noninfective mastitis of newborn (P83.4)*

P39.1   **Neonatal conjunctivitis and dacryocystitis**
> Neonatal chlamydial conjunctivitis
> Ophthalmia neonatorum NOS

EXCLUDES 1   *gonococcal conjunctivitis (A54.31)*

P39.2   **Intra-amniotic infection affecting newborn, not elsewhere classified**

P39.3   **Neonatal urinary tract infection**

P39.4   **Neonatal skin infection**
> Neonatal pyoderma

EXCLUDES 1   *pemphigus neonatorum (L00)*
> *staphylococcal scalded skin syndrome (L00)*

P39.8   **Other specified infections specific to the perinatal period**

P39.9   **Infection specific to the perinatal period, unspecified**

Hemorrhagic and hematological disorders of newborn (P50-P61)

EXCLUDES 1   *congenital stenosis and stricture of bile ducts (Q44.3)*
> *Crigler-Najjar syndrome (E80.5)*
> *Dubin-Johnson syndrome (E80.6)*
> *Gilbert syndrome (E80.4)*
> *hereditary hemolytic anemias (D55-D58)*

✓4ᵗʰ **P50**   **Newborn affected by intrauterine (fetal) blood loss**

EXCLUDES 1   *congenital anemia from intrauterine (fetal) blood loss (P61.3)*

P50.0   **Newborn affected by intrauterine (fetal) blood loss from vasa previa**

P50.1   **Newborn affected by intrauterine (fetal) blood loss from ruptured cord**

P50.2   **Newborn affected by intrauterine (fetal) blood loss from placenta**

P50.3   **Newborn affected by hemorrhage into co-twin**

P50.4   **Newborn affected by hemorrhage into maternal circulation**

P50.5   **Newborn affected by intrauterine (fetal) blood loss from cut end of co-twin's cord**

P50.8   **Newborn affected by other intrauterine (fetal) blood loss**

P50.9   **Newborn affected by intrauterine (fetal) blood loss, unspecified**
> Newborn affected by fetal hemorrhage NOS

✓4ᵗʰ **P51**   **Umbilical hemorrhage of newborn**

EXCLUDES 1   *omphalitis with mild hemorrhage (P38.1)*
> *umbilical hemorrhage from cut end of co-twins cord (P50.5)*

P51.0   **Massive umbilical hemorrhage of newborn**

P51.8   **Other umbilical hemorrhages of newborn**
> Slipped umbilical ligature NOS

P51.9   **Umbilical hemorrhage of newborn, unspecified**

Chapter 16. Certain Conditions Originating in the Perinatal Period

P52–P61.3

✓4ᵗʰ **P52 Intracranial nontraumatic hemorrhage of newborn**

    INCLUDES   intracranial hemorrhage due to anoxia or hypoxia

    EXCLUDES 1   *intracranial hemorrhage due to birth injury (P10.-)*

        intracranial hemorrhage due to other injury (S06.-)

  P52.0 Intraventricular (nontraumatic) hemorrhage, grade 1, of newborn

    Subependymal hemorrhage (without intraventricular extension)

    Bleeding into germinal matrix

  P52.1 Intraventricular (nontraumatic) hemorrhage, grade 2, of newborn

    Subependymal hemorrhage with intraventricular extension

    Bleeding into ventricle

✓5ᵗʰ **P52.2 Intraventricular (nontraumatic) hemorrhage, grade 3 and grade 4, of newborn**

    P52.21 Intraventricular (nontraumatic) hemorrhage, grade 3, of newborn

       Subependymal hemorrhage with intraventricular extension with enlargement of ventricle

    P52.22 Intraventricular (nontraumatic) hemorrhage, grade 4, of newborn

       Bleeding into cerebral cortex

       Subependymal hemorrhage with intracerebral extension

  P52.3 Unspecified intraventricular (nontraumatic) hemorrhage of newborn

  P52.4 Intracerebral (nontraumatic) hemorrhage of newborn

  P52.5 Subarachnoid (nontraumatic) hemorrhage of newborn

  P52.6 Cerebellar (nontraumatic) and posterior fossa hemorrhage of newborn

  P52.8 Other intracranial (nontraumatic) hemorrhages of newborn

  P52.9 Intracranial (nontraumatic) hemorrhage of newborn, unspecified

P53 Hemorrhagic disease of newborn

  Vitamin K deficiency of newborn

✓4ᵗʰ **P54 Other neonatal hemorrhages**

    EXCLUDES 1   *newborn affected by (intrauterine) blood loss (P50.-)*

        pulmonary hemorrhage originating in the perinatal period (P26.-)

  P54.0 Neonatal hematemesis

    EXCLUDES 1   *neonatal hematemesis due to swallowed maternal blood (P78.2)*

  P54.1 Neonatal melena

    EXCLUDES 1   *neonatal melena due to swallowed maternal blood (P78.2)*

  P54.2 Neonatal rectal hemorrhage

  P54.3 Other neonatal gastrointestinal hemorrhage

  P54.4 Neonatal adrenal hemorrhage

  P54.5 Neonatal cutaneous hemorrhage

    Neonatal bruising

    Neonatal ecchymoses

    Neonatal petechiae

    Neonatal superficial hematomata

    EXCLUDES 2   *bruising of scalp due to birth injury (P12.3)*

        cephalhematoma due to birth injury (P12.0)

  P54.6 Neonatal vaginal hemorrhage   ♀

    Neonatal pseudomenses

  P54.8 Other specified neonatal hemorrhages

  P54.9 Neonatal hemorrhage, unspecified

✓4ᵗʰ **P55 Hemolytic disease of newborn**

  P55.0 Rh isoimmunization of newborn

    DEF: Incompatible Rh fetal-maternal blood grouping that prematurely destroys red blood cells. Symptoms include jaundice, asphyxia, pulmonary hypertension, edema, respiratory distress, kernicterus, and coagulopathies. It is detected by a Coombs test.

    TIP: A positive Coombs test without documentation of associated Rh isoimmunization should be coded to R79.89 Other specified abnormal findings of blood chemistry.

  P55.1 ABO isoimmunization of newborn

    AHA: 2015,3Q,20

  P55.8 Other hemolytic diseases of newborn

    AHA: 2018,3Q,24

  P55.9 Hemolytic disease of newborn, unspecified

✓4ᵗʰ **P56 Hydrops fetalis due to hemolytic disease**

    EXCLUDES 1   *hydrops fetalis NOS (P83.2)*

  P56.0 Hydrops fetalis due to isoimmunization

✓5ᵗʰ **P56.9 Hydrops fetalis due to other and unspecified hemolytic disease**

    P56.90 Hydrops fetalis due to unspecified hemolytic disease

    P56.99 Hydrops fetalis due to other hemolytic disease

✓4ᵗʰ **P57 Kernicterus**

  P57.0 Kernicterus due to isoimmunization

    DEF: Complication of erythroblastosis fetalis associated with severe neural symptoms, high blood bilirubin levels, and nerve cell destruction. It results in bilirubin-pigmented gray matter of the central nervous system.

  P57.8 Other specified kernicterus

    EXCLUDES 1   *Crigler-Najjar syndrome (E80.5)*

  P57.9 Kernicterus, unspecified

✓4ᵗʰ **P58 Neonatal jaundice due to other excessive hemolysis**

    EXCLUDES 1   *jaundice due to isoimmunization (P55-P57)*

  P58.0 Neonatal jaundice due to bruising

  P58.1 Neonatal jaundice due to bleeding

  P58.2 Neonatal jaundice due to infection

  P58.3 Neonatal jaundice due to polycythemia

✓5ᵗʰ **P58.4 Neonatal jaundice due to drugs or toxins transmitted from mother or given to newborn**

    Code first poisoning due to drug or toxin, if applicable (T36-T65 with fifth or sixth character 1-4 or 6)

    Use additional code for adverse effect, if applicable, to identify drug (T36-T50 with fifth or sixth character 5)

    P58.41 Neonatal jaundice due to drugs or toxins transmitted from mother

    P58.42 Neonatal jaundice due to drugs or toxins given to newborn

  P58.5 Neonatal jaundice due to swallowed maternal blood

  P58.8 Neonatal jaundice due to other specified excessive hemolysis

  P58.9 Neonatal jaundice due to excessive hemolysis, unspecified

✓4ᵗʰ **P59 Neonatal jaundice from other and unspecified causes**

    EXCLUDES 1   *jaundice due to inborn errors of metabolism (E70-E88)*

        kernicterus (P57.-)

  P59.0 Neonatal jaundice associated with preterm delivery

    Hyperbilirubinemia of prematurity

    Jaundice due to delayed conjugation associated with preterm delivery

  P59.1 Inspissated bile syndrome

    DEF: Biliary obstruction in newborn resulting from obstruction of outflow tract.

✓5ᵗʰ **P59.2 Neonatal jaundice from other and unspecified hepatocellular damage**

    EXCLUDES 1   *congenital viral hepatitis (P35.3)*

    P59.20 Neonatal jaundice from unspecified hepatocellular damage

    P59.29 Neonatal jaundice from other hepatocellular damage

       Neonatal giant cell hepatitis

       Neonatal (idiopathic) hepatitis

  P59.3 Neonatal jaundice from breast milk inhibitor

  P59.8 Neonatal jaundice from other specified causes

  P59.9 Neonatal jaundice, unspecified

    Neonatal physiological jaundice (intense)(prolonged) NOS

    AHA: 2015,3Q,20

P60 Disseminated intravascular coagulation of newborn

  Defibrination syndrome of newborn

✓4ᵗʰ **P61 Other perinatal hematological disorders**

    EXCLUDES 1   *transient hypogammaglobulinemia of infancy (D80.7)*

  P61.0 Transient neonatal thrombocytopenia

    Neonatal thrombocytopenia due to exchange transfusion

    Neonatal thrombocytopenia due to idiopathic maternal thrombocytopenia

    Neonatal thrombocytopenia due to isoimmunization

    DEF: Temporary decrease in blood platelets of a newborn that is secondary to placental insufficiency.

  P61.1 Polycythemia neonatorum

    DEF: Abnormal increase of total red blood cells of a newborn that results in hyperviscosity, which slows the flow of blood through small blood vessels.

  P61.2 Anemia of prematurity

  P61.3 Congenital anemia from fetal blood loss

P61.4 **Other congenital anemias, not elsewhere classified**
Congenital anemia NOS

P61.5 **Transient neonatal neutropenia**
> EXCLUDES 1   *congenital neutropenia (nontransient) (D70.0)*
DEF: Low blood neutrophil counts of newborn that occurs due to maternal hypertension, sepsis, twin-twin transfusion, alloimmunization, and hemolytic disease.

P61.6 **Other transient neonatal disorders of coagulation**

P61.8 **Other specified perinatal hematological disorders**

P61.9 **Perinatal hematological disorder, unspecified**

Transitory endocrine and metabolic disorders specific to newborn (P70-P74)

> INCLUDES   transitory endocrine and metabolic disturbances caused by the infant's response to maternal endocrine and metabolic factors, or its adjustment to extrauterine environment

AHA: 2018,2Q,6

☑4ᵗʰ **P70** **Transitory disorders of carbohydrate metabolism specific to newborn**

P70.0 **Syndrome of infant of mother with gestational diabetes**
Newborn (with hypoglycemia) affected by maternal gestational diabetes
> EXCLUDES 1   *newborn (with hypoglycemia) affected by maternal (pre-existing) diabetes mellitus (P70.1)*
> *syndrome of infant of a diabetic mother (P70.1)*

P70.1 **Syndrome of infant of a diabetic mother**
Newborn (with hypoglycemia) affected by maternal (pre-existing) diabetes mellitus
> EXCLUDES 1   *newborn (with hypoglycemia) affected by maternal gestational diabetes (P70.0)*
> *syndrome of infant of mother with gestational diabetes (P70.0)*

P70.2 **Neonatal diabetes mellitus**

P70.3 **Iatrogenic neonatal hypoglycemia**

P70.4 **Other neonatal hypoglycemia**
Transitory neonatal hypoglycemia

P70.8 **Other transitory disorders of carbohydrate metabolism of newborn**

P70.9 **Transitory disorder of carbohydrate metabolism of newborn, unspecified**

☑4ᵗʰ **P71** **Transitory neonatal disorders of calcium and magnesium metabolism**

P71.0 **Cow's milk hypocalcemia in newborn**

P71.1 **Other neonatal hypocalcemia**
> EXCLUDES 1   *neonatal hypoparathyroidism (P71.4)*

P71.2 **Neonatal hypomagnesemia**

P71.3 **Neonatal tetany without calcium or magnesium deficiency**
Neonatal tetany NOS

P71.4 **Transitory neonatal hypoparathyroidism**

P71.8 **Other transitory neonatal disorders of calcium and magnesium metabolism**
AHA: 2016,4Q,54

P71.9 **Transitory neonatal disorder of calcium and magnesium metabolism, unspecified**

☑4ᵗʰ **P72** **Other transitory neonatal endocrine disorders**
> EXCLUDES 1   *congenital hypothyroidism with or without goiter (E03.0-E03.1)*
> *dyshormogenetic goiter (E07.1)*
> *Pendred's syndrome (E07.1)*

P72.0 **Neonatal goiter, not elsewhere classified**
Transitory congenital goiter with normal functioning

P72.1 **Transitory neonatal hyperthyroidism**
Neonatal thyrotoxicosis

P72.2 **Other transitory neonatal disorders of thyroid function, not elsewhere classified**
Transitory neonatal hypothyroidism

P72.8 **Other specified transitory neonatal endocrine disorders**

P72.9 **Transitory neonatal endocrine disorder, unspecified**

☑4ᵗʰ **P74** **Other transitory neonatal electrolyte and metabolic disturbances**
AHA: 2018,4Q,26-27

P74.0 **Late metabolic acidosis of newborn**
> EXCLUDES 1   *(fetal) metabolic acidosis of newborn (P19)*

P74.1 **Dehydration of newborn**

☑5ᵗʰ **P74.2** **Disturbances of sodium balance of newborn**

P74.21 **Hypernatremia of newborn**

P74.22 **Hyponatremia of newborn**

☑5ᵗʰ **P74.3** **Disturbances of potassium balance of newborn**

P74.31 **Hyperkalemia of newborn**

P74.32 **Hypokalemia of newborn**

☑5ᵗʰ **P74.4** **Other transitory electrolyte disturbances of newborn**

P74.41 **Alkalosis of newborn**
Hyperbicarbonatemia

☑6ᵗʰ **P74.42** **Disturbances of chlorine balance of newborn**

P74.421 **Hyperchloremia of newborn**
Hyperchloremic metabolic acidosis
> EXCLUDES 2   *late metabolic acidosis of the newborn ▶(P74.0)◄*

P74.422 **Hypochloremia of newborn**

P74.49 **Other transitory electrolyte disturbance of newborn**

P74.5 **Transitory tyrosinemia of newborn**

P74.6 **Transitory hyperammonemia of newborn**

P74.8 **Other transitory metabolic disturbances of newborn**
Amino-acid metabolic disorders described as transitory

P74.9 **Transitory metabolic disturbance of newborn, unspecified**

Digestive system disorders of newborn (P76-P78)

☑4ᵗʰ **P76** **Other intestinal obstruction of newborn**

P76.0 **Meconium plug syndrome**
Meconium ileus NOS
> EXCLUDES 1   *meconium ileus in cystic fibrosis (E84.11)*
DEF: Meconium obstruction of a newborn's intestines, resulting from unusually thick or hard meconium.

P76.1 **Transitory ileus of newborn**
> EXCLUDES 1   *Hirschsprung's disease (Q43.1)*

P76.2 **Intestinal obstruction due to inspissated milk**

P76.8 **Other specified intestinal obstruction of newborn**
> EXCLUDES 1   *intestinal obstruction classifiable to K56.-*

P76.9 **Intestinal obstruction of newborn, unspecified**

☑4ᵗʰ **P77** **Necrotizing enterocolitis of newborn**
DEF: Serious intestinal infection and inflammation in preterm infants. Severity is measured by stages and may progress to life-threatening perforation or peritonitis. Resection surgical treatment may be necessary.

P77.1 **Stage 1 necrotizing enterocolitis in newborn**
Necrotizing enterocolitis without pneumatosis, without perforation
DEF: Broad-spectrum symptoms with nonspecific signs, including feeding intolerance, abdominal distention, bradycardia, and metabolic abnormalities.

P77.2 **Stage 2 necrotizing enterocolitis in newborn**
Necrotizing enterocolitis with pneumatosis, without perforation
DEF: Radiographic confirmation of necrotizing enterocolitis showing intestinal dilatation, fixed loops of bowels, pneumatosis intestinalis, metabolic acidosis, and thrombocytopenia.

P77.3 **Stage 3 necrotizing enterocolitis in newborn**
Necrotizing enterocolitis with perforation
Necrotizing enterocolitis with pneumatosis and perforation
DEF: Advanced stage in which an infant demonstrates signs of bowel perforation, septic shock, metabolic acidosis, ascites, disseminated intravascular coagulopathy, and neutropenia.

P77.9 **Necrotizing enterocolitis in newborn, unspecified**
Necrotizing enterocolitis in newborn, NOS

☑4ᵗʰ **P78** **Other perinatal digestive system disorders**
> EXCLUDES 1   *cystic fibrosis (E84.0-E84.9)*
> *neonatal gastrointestinal hemorrhages (P54.0-P54.3)*

P78.0 **Perinatal intestinal perforation**
Meconium peritonitis

P78.1 **Other neonatal peritonitis**
Neonatal peritonitis NOS

P78.2 **Neonatal hematemesis and melena due to swallowed maternal blood**

P78.3 **Noninfective neonatal diarrhea**
Neonatal diarrhea NOS

☑5ᵗʰ **P78.8** **Other specified perinatal digestive system disorders**

P78.81 **Congenital cirrhosis (of liver)**

P78.82 **Peptic ulcer of newborn**

P78.83 **Newborn esophageal reflux**
Neonatal esophageal reflux

☑ Additional Character Required   ☑7ᵗʰ Placeholder Alert   Manifestation   Unspecified Dx   ▶◄ Revised Text   ● New Code   ▲ Revised Code Title

ICD-10-CM 2020   **903**

P78.84 Gestational alloimmune liver disease
GALD
Neonatal hemochromatosis
EXCLUDES 1   hemochromatosis (E83.11-)
AHA: 2017,4Q,21
DEF: Severe hepatic injury with onset during fetal development with manifestations beginning during fetal life. It is due to maternal antibodies to fetal hepatic cells (hepatocytes) that cross the placenta into the fetal circulation, causing hepatic cell necrosis.

P78.89 Other specified perinatal digestive system disorders

P78.9 Perinatal digestive system disorder, unspecified

Conditions involving the integument and temperature regulation of newborn (P80-P83)

✓4ᵗʰ P80 Hypothermia of newborn
DEF: Decrease in newborn body temperature due to their larger ratio of surface area to body weight, thin skin with blood vessels close to the surface, and a limited amount of subcutaneous fat.

P80.0 Cold injury syndrome
Severe and usually chronic hypothermia associated with a pink flushed appearance, edema and neurological and biochemical abnormalities.
EXCLUDES 1   mild hypothermia of newborn (P80.8)

P80.8 Other hypothermia of newborn
Mild hypothermia of newborn

P80.9 Hypothermia of newborn, unspecified

✓4ᵗʰ P81 Other disturbances of temperature regulation of newborn

P81.0 Environmental hyperthermia of newborn

P81.8 Other specified disturbances of temperature regulation of newborn

P81.9 Disturbance of temperature regulation of newborn, unspecified
Fever of newborn NOS

✓4ᵗʰ P83 Other conditions of integument specific to newborn
EXCLUDES 1   congenital malformations of skin and integument (Q80-Q84)
hydrops fetalis due to hemolytic disease (P56.-)
neonatal skin infection (P39.4)
staphylococcal scalded skin syndrome (L00)
EXCLUDES 2   cradle cap (L21.0)
diaper [napkin] dermatitis (L22)

P83.0 Sclerema neonatorum
DEF: Diffuse, rapidly progressing white, waxy, nonpitting hardening of tissue, usually of legs and feet that is life-threatening. It is found in preterm or debilitated infants. Etiology is unknown.

P83.1 Neonatal erythema toxicum

P83.2 Hydrops fetalis not due to hemolytic disease
Hydrops fetalis NOS
DEF: Severe, life-threatening problem of a newborn characterized by severe edema of the entire body. It is unrelated to immune response.

✓5ᵗʰ P83.3 Other and unspecified edema specific to newborn

P83.30 Unspecified edema specific to newborn

P83.39 Other edema specific to newborn

P83.4 Breast engorgement of newborn
Noninfective mastitis of newborn

P83.5 Congenital hydrocele ♂
DEF: Hydrocele: Serous fluid that collects in the tunica vaginalis of the scrotum along the spermatic cord in males.

P83.6 Umbilical polyp of newborn

✓5ᵗʰ P83.8 Other specified conditions of integument specific to newborn
AHA: 2017,4Q,21-22

P83.81 Umbilical granuloma
EXCLUDES 2   granulomatous disorder of the skin and subcutaneous tissue, unspecified (L92.9)

P83.88 Other specified conditions of integument specific to newborn
Bronze baby syndrome
Neonatal scleroderma
Urticaria neonatorum

P83.9 Condition of the integument specific to newborn, unspecified

Other problems with newborn (P84)

P84 Other problems with newborn
Acidemia of newborn
Acidosis of newborn
Anoxia of newborn NOS
Asphyxia of newborn NOS
Hypercapnia of newborn
Hypoxemia of newborn
Hypoxia of newborn NOS
Mixed metabolic and respiratory acidosis of newborn
EXCLUDES 1   intracranial hemorrhage due to anoxia or hypoxia (P52.-)
hypoxic ischemic encephalopathy [HIE] (P91.6-)
late metabolic acidosis of newborn (P74.0)

Other disorders originating in the perinatal period (P90-P96)

P90 Convulsions of newborn
EXCLUDES 1   benign myoclonic epilepsy in infancy (G40.3-)
benign neonatal convulsions (familial) (G40.3-)

✓4ᵗʰ P91 Other disturbances of cerebral status of newborn

P91.0 Neonatal cerebral ischemia

P91.1 Acquired periventricular cysts of newborn

P91.2 Neonatal cerebral leukomalacia
Periventricular leukomalacia

P91.3 Neonatal cerebral irritability

P91.4 Neonatal cerebral depression

P91.5 Neonatal coma

✓5ᵗʰ P91.6 Hypoxic ischemic encephalopathy [HIE]
EXCLUDES 1   neonatal cerebral depression (P91.4)
neonatal cerebral irritability (P91.3)
neonatal coma (P91.5)
AHA: 2017,4Q,22

P91.60 Hypoxic ischemic encephalopathy [HIE], unspecified

P91.61 Mild hypoxic ischemic encephalopathy [HIE]

P91.62 Moderate hypoxic ischemic encephalopathy [HIE]

P91.63 Severe hypoxic ischemic encephalopathy [HIE]

✓5ᵗʰ P91.8 Other specified disturbances of cerebral status of newborn
AHA: 2017,4Q,22

✓6ᵗʰ P91.81 Neonatal encephalopathy

P91.811 Neonatal encephalopathy in diseases classified elsewhere
Code first underlying condition, if known, such as:
congenital cirrhosis (of liver) (P78.81)
intracranial nontraumatic hemorrhage of newborn (P52.-)
kernicterus (P57.-)

P91.819 Neonatal encephalopathy, unspecified

P91.88 Other specified disturbances of cerebral status of newborn

P91.9 Disturbance of cerebral status of newborn, unspecified

✓4ᵗʰ P92 Feeding problems of newborn
EXCLUDES 1   eating disorders (F50.-)
feeding problems in child over 28 days old (R63.3)
AHA: 2016,3Q,19
TIP: Continue to assign a code from this category for feeding problems in a patient greater than 28 days old when that feeding problem was initially diagnosed between day 0 and day 28. Do not assign code R63.3.

✓5ᵗʰ P92.0 Vomiting of newborn
EXCLUDES 1   vomiting of child over 28 days old (R11.-)

P92.01 Bilious vomiting of newborn
EXCLUDES 1   bilious vomiting in child over 28 days old (R11.14)

P92.09 Other vomiting of newborn
EXCLUDES 1   regurgitation of food in newborn (P92.1)

P92.1 Regurgitation and rumination of newborn

P92.2 Slow feeding of newborn

P92.3 Underfeeding of newborn

P92.4 Overfeeding of newborn

P92.5 Neonatal difficulty in feeding at breast
AHA: 2017,1Q,28

P92.6 Failure to thrive in newborn
EXCLUDES 1   failure to thrive in child over 28 days old (R62.51)

P92.8 Other feeding problems of newborn

P92.9 Feeding problem of newborn, unspecified

✓4ᵗʰ **P93 Reactions and intoxications due to drugs administered to newborn**

INCLUDES reactions and intoxications due to drugs administered to fetus affecting newborn

EXCLUDES 1 *jaundice due to drugs or toxins transmitted from mother or given to newborn (P58.4-)*

reactions and intoxications from maternal opiates, tranquilizers and other medication (P04.0-P04.1, P04.4-)

withdrawal symptoms from maternal use of drugs of addiction (P96.1)

withdrawal symptoms from therapeutic use of drugs in newborn (P96.2)

P93.0 Grey baby syndrome

Grey syndrome from chloramphenicol administration in newborn

P93.8 Other reactions and intoxications due to drugs administered to newborn

Use additional code for adverse effect, if applicable, to identify drug (T36-T50 with fifth or sixth character 5)

✓4ᵗʰ **P94 Disorders of muscle tone of newborn**

P94.0 Transient neonatal myasthenia gravis

EXCLUDES 1 *myasthenia gravis (G70.0)*

P94.1 Congenital hypertonia

P94.2 Congenital hypotonia

Floppy baby syndrome, unspecified

P94.8 Other disorders of muscle tone of newborn

P94.9 Disorder of muscle tone of newborn, unspecified

P95 Stillbirth

Deadborn fetus NOS

Fetal death of unspecified cause

Stillbirth NOS

EXCLUDES 1 *maternal care for intrauterine death (O36.4)*

missed abortion (O02.1)

outcome of delivery, stillbirth (Z37.1, Z37.3, Z37.4, Z37.7)

✓4ᵗʰ **P96 Other conditions originating in the perinatal period**

P96.0 Congenital renal failure

Uremia of newborn

P96.1 Neonatal withdrawal symptoms from maternal use of drugs of addiction

Drug withdrawal syndrome in infant of dependent mother

Neonatal abstinence syndrome

EXCLUDES 1 *reactions and intoxications from maternal opiates and tranquilizers administered during labor and delivery (P04.0)*

AHA: 2018,4Q,24-25

P96.2 Withdrawal symptoms from therapeutic use of drugs in newborn

P96.3 Wide cranial sutures of newborn

Neonatal craniotabes

P96.5 Complication to newborn due to (fetal) intrauterine procedure

EXCLUDES 2 *newborn affected by amniocentesis (P00.6)*

✓5ᵗʰ **P96.8 Other specified conditions originating in the perinatal period**

P96.81 Exposure to (parental) (environmental) tobacco smoke in the perinatal period

EXCLUDES 2 *newborn affected by in utero exposure to tobacco (P04.2)*

exposure to environmental tobacco smoke after the perinatal period (Z77.22)

P96.82 Delayed separation of umbilical cord

P96.83 Meconium staining

EXCLUDES 1 *meconium aspiration (P24.00, P24.01)*

meconium passage during delivery (P03.82)

DEF: Meconium passed in utero causing discoloration on the fetal skin and nails or on the umbilicus. This staining may be incidental or may be an indicator of significant fetal stress that could affect outcomes.

P96.89 Other specified conditions originating in the perinatal period

Use additional code to specify condition

P96.9 Condition originating in the perinatal period, unspecified

Congenital debility NOS

☑ Additional Character Required ✓x7ᵗʰ Placeholder Alert Manifestation Unspecified Dx ▶◀ Revised Text ● New Code ▲ Revised Code Title

Chapter 17. Congenital Malformations, Deformations, and Chromosomal Abnormalities (Q00–Q99)

Chapter-specific Guidelines with Coding Examples

The chapter-specific guidelines from the ICD-10-CM Official Guidelines for Coding and Reporting have been provided below. Along with these guidelines are coding examples, contained in the shaded boxes, that have been developed to help illustrate the coding and/or sequencing guidance found in these guidelines.

Assign an appropriate code(s) from categories Q00-Q99, Congenital malformations, deformations, and chromosomal abnormalities when a malformation/deformation or chromosomal abnormality is documented. A malformation/deformation/or chromosomal abnormality may be the principal/first-listed diagnosis on a record or a secondary diagnosis.

When a malformation/deformation/or chromosomal abnormality does not have a unique code assignment, assign additional code(s) for any manifestations that may be present.

When the code assignment specifically identifies the malformation/deformation/or chromosomal abnormality, manifestations that are an inherent component of the anomaly should not be coded separately. Additional codes should be assigned for manifestations that are not an inherent component.

8-day-old infant with tetralogy of Fallot and pulmonary stenosis

Q21.3   **Tetralogy of Fallot**

Explanation: Pulmonary stenosis is inherent in the disease process of tetralogy of Fallot. When the code assignment specifically identifies the malformation/deformation/or chromosomal abnormality, manifestations that are inherent components of the anomaly should not be coded separately.

7-month-old infant with Down syndrome and common atrioventricular canal

Q90.9   **Down syndrome, unspecified**

Q21.2   **Atrioventricular septal defect**

Explanation: While a common atrioventricular canal is often associated with patients with Down syndrome, this manifestation is not an inherent component and may be reported separately. When the code assignment specifically identifies the anomaly, manifestations that are inherent components of the condition should not be coded separately. Additional codes should be assigned for manifestations that are not inherent components.

Codes from Chapter 17 may be used throughout the life of the patient. If a congenital malformation or deformity has been corrected, a personal history code should be used to identify the history of the malformation or deformity. Although present at birth, **a** malformation/deformation/or chromosomal abnormality may not be identified until later in life. Whenever the condition is diagnosed by the **provider**, it is appropriate to assign a code from codes Q00-Q99. For the birth admission, the appropriate code from category Z38, Liveborn infants, according to place of birth and type of delivery, should be sequenced as the principal diagnosis, followed by any congenital anomaly codes, Q00- Q99.

Three-year-old with history of corrected ventricular septal defect

Z87.74   **Personal history of (corrected) congenital malformations of heart and circulatory system**

Explanation: If a congenital malformation or deformity has been corrected, a personal history code should be used to identify the history of the malformation or deformity.

Forty-year-old man with headaches diagnosed with congenital arteriovenous malformation of cerebral vessels by brain scan

Q28.2   **Arteriovenous malformation of cerebral vessels**

Explanation: Although present at birth, malformations may not be identified until later in life. Whenever a congenital condition is diagnosed by the physician, it is appropriate to assign a code from the range Q00–Q99.

Newborn with anencephaly delivered vaginally in hospital

Z38.00   **Single liveborn infant, delivered vaginally**

Q00.0   **Anencephaly**

Explanation: For the birth admission, the appropriate code from category Z38 Liveborn infants, according to place of birth and type of delivery, should be sequenced as the principal diagnosis, followed by any congenital anomaly codes, Q00–Q99.

Chapter 17. Congenital Malformations, Deformations and Chromosomal Abnormalities

Chapter 17. Congenital Malformations, Deformations and Chromosomal Abnormalities (Q00-Q99)

> **NOTE**   Codes from this chapter are not for use on maternal records
>
> *EXCLUDES 2*   inborn errors of metabolism (E70-E88)

This chapter contains the following blocks:

Q00-Q07   Congenital malformations of the nervous system
Q10-Q18   Congenital malformations of eye, ear, face and neck
Q20-Q28   Congenital malformations of the circulatory system
Q30-Q34   Congenital malformations of the respiratory system
Q35-Q37   Cleft lip and cleft palate
Q38-Q45   Other congenital malformations of the digestive system
Q50-Q56   Congenital malformations of genital organs
Q60-Q64   Congenital malformations of the urinary system
Q65-Q79   Congenital malformations and deformations of the musculoskeletal system
Q80-Q89   Other congenital malformations
Q90-Q99   Chromosomal abnormalities, not elsewhere classified

Congenital malformations of the nervous system (Q00-Q07)

✓4ᵗʰ **Q00   Anencephaly and similar malformations**

    Q00.0   Anencephaly   HCC

       Acephaly
       Acrania
       Amyelencephaly
       Hemianencephaly
       Hemicephaly

    Q00.1   Craniorachischisis   HCC

    Q00.2   Iniencephaly   HCC

✓4ᵗʰ **Q01   Encephalocele**

    INCLUDES   Arnold-Chiari syndrome, type III
       encephalocystocele
       encephalomyelocele
       hydroencephalocele
       hydromeningocele, cranial
       meningocele, cerebral
       meningoencephalocele

    EXCLUDES 1   Meckel-Gruber syndrome (Q61.9)

    DEF: Congenital protrusion of brain tissue through a defect in the skull.

    Q01.0   Frontal encephalocele   HCC

    Q01.1   Nasofrontal encephalocele   HCC

    Q01.2   Occipital encephalocele   HCC

    Q01.8   Encephalocele of other sites   HCC

    Q01.9   Encephalocele, unspecified   HCC

Q02   Microcephaly   HCC

    INCLUDES   hydromicrocephaly
       micrencephalon

    ▶Code first, if applicable, congenital Zika virus disease◀
    ~~Use additional code, if applicable, to identify congenital Zika virus disease~~

    EXCLUDES 1   Meckel-Gruber syndrome (Q61.9)

    AHA: 2018,4Q,26

    DEF: Congenital disorder in which the head circumference is more than two standard deviations below the mean for age, sex, race, and gestation and associated with a decreased life expectancy.

✓4ᵗʰ **Q03   Congenital hydrocephalus**

    INCLUDES   hydrocephalus in newborn

    EXCLUDES 1   Arnold-Chiari syndrome, type II (Q07.0-)
       acquired hydrocephalus (G91.-)
       hydrocephalus due to congenital toxoplasmosis (P37.1)
       hydrocephalus with spina bifida (Q05.0-Q05.4)

    DEF: Hydrocephalus: Abnormal buildup of cerebrospinal fluid in the brain causing dilation of the ventricles.

Congenital Hydrocephalus

Pressure

Normal ventricles   Hydrocephalic ventricles

    Q03.0   Malformations of aqueduct of Sylvius   HCC

       Anomaly of aqueduct of Sylvius
       Obstruction of aqueduct of Sylvius, congenital
       Stenosis of aqueduct of Sylvius

    Q03.1   Atresia of foramina of Magendie and Luschka   HCC

       Dandy-Walker syndrome

    Q03.8   Other congenital hydrocephalus   HCC

    Q03.9   Congenital hydrocephalus, unspecified   HCC

✓4ᵗʰ **Q04   Other congenital malformations of brain**

    EXCLUDES 1   cyclopia (Q87.0)
       macrocephaly (Q75.3)

    Q04.0   Congenital malformations of corpus callosum   HCC

       Agenesis of corpus callosum

    Q04.1   Arhinencephaly   HCC

    Q04.2   Holoprosencephaly   HCC

    Q04.3   Other reduction deformities of brain   HCC

       Absence of part of brain
       Agenesis of part of brain
       Agyria
       Aplasia of part of brain
       Hydranencephaly
       Hypoplasia of part of brain
       Lissencephaly
       Microgyria
       Pachygyria

    EXCLUDES 1   congenital malformations of corpus callosum (Q04.0)

    Q04.4   Septo-optic dysplasia of brain   HCC

    Q04.5   Megalencephaly   HCC

    Q04.6   Congenital cerebral cysts   HCC

       Porencephaly
       Schizencephaly

    EXCLUDES 1   acquired porencephalic cyst (G93.0)

    Q04.8   Other specified congenital malformations of brain   HCC

       Arnold-Chiari syndrome, type IV
       Macrogyria

    Q04.9   Congenital malformation of brain, unspecified   HCC

       Congenital anomaly NOS of brain
       Congenital deformity NOS of brain
       Congenital disease or lesion NOS of brain
       Multiple anomalies NOS of brain, congenital

✓4th **Q05 Spina bifida**

INCLUDES   hydromeningocele (spinal)
meningocele (spinal)
meningomyelocele
myelocele
myelomeningocele
rachischisis
spina bifida (aperta)(cystica)
syringomyelocele

Use additional code for any associated paraplegia (paraparesis) (G82.2-)

EXCLUDES 1   Arnold-Chiari syndrome, type II (Q07.0-)
spina bifida occulta (Q76.0)

DEF: Lack of closure in the vertebral column with protrusion of the spinal cord through the defect, often in the lumbosacral area. This condition can be recognized by the presence of alpha-fetoproteins in the amniotic fluid.

Spina Bifida

Spina bifida occulta   Meningocele   Myelomeningocele

Q05.0   Cervical spina bifida with hydrocephalus   HCC

Q05.1   Thoracic spina bifida with hydrocephalus   HCC

Dorsal spina bifida with hydrocephalus
Thoracolumbar spina bifida with hydrocephalus

Q05.2   Lumbar spina bifida with hydrocephalus   HCC

Lumbosacral spina bifida with hydrocephalus

Q05.3   Sacral spina bifida with hydrocephalus   HCC

Q05.4   Unspecified spina bifida with hydrocephalus   HCC

Q05.5   Cervical spina bifida without hydrocephalus   HCC

Q05.6   Thoracic spina bifida without hydrocephalus   HCC

Dorsal spina bifida NOS
Thoracolumbar spina bifida NOS

Q05.7   Lumbar spina bifida without hydrocephalus   HCC

Lumbosacral spina bifida NOS

Q05.8   Sacral spina bifida without hydrocephalus   HCC

Q05.9   Spina bifida, unspecified   HCC

✓4th **Q06 Other congenital malformations of spinal cord**

Q06.0   Amyelia   HCC

Q06.1   Hypoplasia and dysplasia of spinal cord   HCC

Atelomyelia
Myelatelia
Myelodysplasia of spinal cord

Q06.2   Diastematomyelia   HCC

DEF: Rare congenital anomaly often associated with spina bifida. The spinal cord is separated into longitudinal halves by a bony, cartilaginous or fibrous septum, each half surrounded by a dural sac.

Q06.3   Other congenital cauda equina malformations   HCC

Q06.4   Hydromyelia   HCC

Hydrorachis

Q06.8   Other specified congenital malformations of spinal cord   HCC

Q06.9   Congenital malformation of spinal cord, unspecified   HCC

Congenital anomaly NOS of spinal cord
Congenital deformity NOS of spinal cord
Congenital disease or lesion NOS of spinal cord

✓4th **Q07 Other congenital malformations of nervous system**

EXCLUDES 2   congenital central alveolar hypoventilation syndrome (G47.35)
familial dysautonomia [Riley-Day] (G90.1)
neurofibromatosis (nonmalignant) (Q85.0-)

✓5th **Q07.0 Arnold-Chiari syndrome**

Arnold-Chiari syndrome, type II

EXCLUDES 1   Arnold-Chiari syndrome, type III (Q01.-)
Arnold-Chiari syndrome, type IV (Q04.8)

DEF: Congenital malformation of the brain in which the cerebellum protrudes through the foramen magnum into the spinal canal.

Q07.00   Arnold-Chiari syndrome without spina bifida or hydrocephalus   HCC

Q07.01   Arnold-Chiari syndrome with spina bifida   HCC

Q07.02   Arnold-Chiari syndrome with hydrocephalus   HCC

Q07.03   Arnold-Chiari syndrome with spina bifida and hydrocephalus   HCC

Q07.8   Other specified congenital malformations of nervous system   HCC

Agenesis of nerve
Displacement of brachial plexus
Jaw-winking syndrome
Marcus Gunn's syndrome

Q07.9   Congenital malformation of nervous system, unspecified   HCC

Congenital anomaly NOS of nervous system
Congenital deformity NOS of nervous system
Congenital disease or lesion NOS of nervous system

Congenital malformations of eye, ear, face and neck (Q10-Q18)

EXCLUDES 2   cleft lip and cleft palate (Q35-Q37)
congenital malformation of cervical spine (Q05.0, Q05.5, Q67.5, Q76.0-Q76.4)
congenital malformation of larynx (Q31.-)
congenital malformation of lip NEC (Q38.0)
congenital malformation of nose (Q30.-)
congenital malformation of parathyroid gland (Q89.2)
congenital malformation of thyroid gland (Q89.2)

✓4th **Q10 Congenital malformations of eyelid, lacrimal apparatus and orbit**

EXCLUDES 1   cryptophthalmos NOS (Q11.2)
cryptophthalmos syndrome (Q87.0)

Q10.0   Congenital ptosis

DEF: Congenital drooping of the eyelid. Ptosis is mostly idiopathic, but may occur genetically.

Q10.1   Congenital ectropion

Q10.2   Congenital entropion

Q10.3   Other congenital malformations of eyelid

Ablepharon
Blepharophimosis, congenital
Coloboma of eyelid
Congenital absence or agenesis of cilia
Congenital absence or agenesis of eyelid
Congenital accessory eyelid
Congenital accessory eye muscle
Congenital malformation of eyelid NOS

Q10.4   Absence and agenesis of lacrimal apparatus

Congenital absence of punctum lacrimale

Q10.5   Congenital stenosis and stricture of lacrimal duct

Q10.6   Other congenital malformations of lacrimal apparatus

Congenital malformation of lacrimal apparatus NOS

Q10.7   Congenital malformation of orbit

✓4th **Q11 Anophthalmos, microphthalmos and macrophthalmos**

Q11.0   Cystic eyeball

Q11.1   Other anophthalmos

Anophthalmos NOS
Agenesis of eye
Aplasia of eye

Q11.2   Microphthalmos

Cryptophthalmos NOS
Dysplasia of eye
Hypoplasia of eye
Rudimentary eye

EXCLUDES 1   cryptophthalmos syndrome (Q87.0)

✓ Additional Character Required   ✓x7th Placeholder Alert   Manifestation   Unspecified Dx   ►◄ Revised Text   ● New Code   ▲ Revised Code Title

ICD-10-CM 2020   **909**

Q11.3 Macrophthalmos
> EXCLUDES 1 *macrophthalmos in congenital glaucoma (Q15.0)*

✓4ᵗʰ **Q12 Congenital lens malformations**

Q12.0 Congenital cataract

Q12.1 Congenital displaced lens

Q12.2 Coloboma of lens

Coloboma of Lens

Coloboma

Q12.3 Congenital aphakia

Q12.4 Spherophakia

Q12.8 Other congenital lens malformations
Microphakia

Q12.9 Congenital lens malformation, unspecified

✓4ᵗʰ **Q13 Congenital malformations of anterior segment of eye**

Q13.0 Coloboma of iris
Coloboma NOS
DEF: Defective or absent section of ocular tissue that may present as mild cupping or a small pit in the ocular disc due to extensive defects in the iris, ciliary body, choroids, and retina.

Q13.1 Absence of iris
Aniridia
Use additional code for associated glaucoma (H42)
DEF: Incompletely formed or absent iris. It affects both eyes and is a dominant trait.

Q13.2 Other congenital malformations of iris
Anisocoria, congenital
Atresia of pupil
Congenital malformation of iris NOS
Corectopia

Q13.3 Congenital corneal opacity

Q13.4 Other congenital corneal malformations
Congenital malformation of cornea NOS
Microcornea
Peter's anomaly

Q13.5 Blue sclera

✓5ᵗʰ **Q13.8 Other congenital malformations of anterior segment of eye**

Q13.81 Rieger's anomaly
Use additional code for associated glaucoma (H42)

Q13.89 Other congenital malformations of anterior segment of eye

Q13.9 Congenital malformation of anterior segment of eye, unspecified

✓4ᵗʰ **Q14 Congenital malformations of posterior segment of eye**
> EXCLUDES 2 *optic nerve hypoplasia (H47.03-)*

Q14.0 Congenital malformation of vitreous humor
Congenital vitreous opacity

Q14.1 Congenital malformation of retina
Congenital retinal aneurysm

Q14.2 Congenital malformation of optic disc
Coloboma of optic disc

Q14.3 Congenital malformation of choroid

Q14.8 Other congenital malformations of posterior segment of eye
Coloboma of the fundus

Q14.9 Congenital malformation of posterior segment of eye, unspecified

✓4ᵗʰ **Q15 Other congenital malformations of eye**
> EXCLUDES 1 *congenital nystagmus (H55.01)*
> *ocular albinism (E70.31-)*
> *optic nerve hypoplasia (H47.03-)*
> *retinitis pigmentosa (H35.52)*

Q15.0 Congenital glaucoma
Axenfeld's anomaly
Buphthalmos
Glaucoma of childhood
Glaucoma of newborn
Hydrophthalmos
Keratoglobus, congenital, with glaucoma
Macrocornea with glaucoma
Macrophthalmos in congenital glaucoma
Megalocornea with glaucoma

Q15.8 Other specified congenital malformations of eye

Q15.9 Congenital malformation of eye, unspecified
Congenital anomaly of eye
Congenital deformity of eye

✓4ᵗʰ **Q16 Congenital malformations of ear causing impairment of hearing**
> EXCLUDES 1 *congenital deafness (H90.-)*

Q16.0 Congenital absence of (ear) auricle

Q16.1 Congenital absence, atresia and stricture of auditory canal (external)
Congenital atresia or stricture of osseous meatus

Q16.2 Absence of eustachian tube

Q16.3 Congenital malformation of ear ossicles
Congenital fusion of ear ossicles

Q16.4 Other congenital malformations of middle ear
Congenital malformation of middle ear NOS

Q16.5 Congenital malformation of inner ear
Congenital anomaly of membranous labyrinth
Congenital anomaly of organ of Corti

Q16.9 Congenital malformation of ear causing impairment of hearing, unspecified
Congenital absence of ear NOS

✓4ᵗʰ **Q17 Other congenital malformations of ear**
> EXCLUDES 1 *congenital malformations of ear with impairment of hearing (Q16.0-Q16.9)*
> *preauricular sinus (Q18.1)*

Q17.0 Accessory auricle
Accessory tragus
Polyotia
Preauricular appendage or tag
Supernumerary ear
Supernumerary lobule

Q17.1 Macrotia
DEF: Birth defect characterized by abnormal enlargement of the pinna of the ear.

Q17.2 Microtia

Q17.3 Other misshapen ear
Pointed ear

Q17.4 Misplaced ear
Low-set ears
> EXCLUDES 1 *cervical auricle (Q18.2)*

Q17.5 Prominent ear
Bat ear

Q17.8 Other specified congenital malformations of ear
Congenital absence of lobe of ear

Q17.9 Congenital malformation of ear, unspecified
Congenital anomaly of ear NOS

✓4ᵗʰ **Q18 Other congenital malformations of face and neck**
> EXCLUDES 1 *cleft lip and cleft palate (Q35-Q37)*
> *conditions classified to Q67.0-Q67.4*
> *congenital malformations of skull and face bones (Q75.-)*
> *cyclopia (Q87.0)*
> *dentofacial anomalies [including malocclusion] (M26.-)*
> *malformation syndromes affecting facial appearance (Q87.0)*
> *persistent thyroglossal duct (Q89.2)*

Q18.0 Sinus, fistula and cyst of branchial cleft
Branchial vestige

Q18.1 Preauricular sinus and cyst
Fistula of auricle, congenital
Cervicoaural fistula

Q18.2 Other branchial cleft malformations
Branchial cleft malformation NOS
Cervical auricle
Otocephaly

Q18.3 Webbing of neck
Pterygium colli
DEF: Congenital malformation characterized by a thick, triangular skinfold that stretches from the lateral side of the neck across the shoulder. It is associated with genetic conditions such as Turner's and Noonan's syndromes.

Q18.4 Macrostomia
DEF: Rare congenital craniofacial bilateral or unilateral anomaly of the mouth due to malformed maxillary and mandibular processes. It results in an abnormally large mouth extending toward the ear.

Q18.5 Microstomia

Q18.6 Macrocheilia
Hypertrophy of lip, congenital

Q18.7 Microcheilia

Q18.8 Other specified congenital malformations of face and neck
Medial cyst of face and neck
Medial fistula of face and neck
Medial sinus of face and neck

Q18.9 Congenital malformation of face and neck, unspecified
Congenital anomaly NOS of face and neck

Congenital malformations of the circulatory system (Q20-Q28)

☑4ᵗʰ Q20 Congenital malformations of cardiac chambers and connections
    EXCLUDES 1   *dextrocardia with situs inversus (Q89.3)*
                        mirror-image atrial arrangement with situs inversus (Q89.3)

Q20.0 Common arterial trunk
Persistent truncus arteriosus
    EXCLUDES 1   *aortic septal defect (Q21.4)*

Q20.1 Double outlet right ventricle
Taussig-Bing syndrome

Q20.2 Double outlet left ventricle

Q20.3 Discordant ventriculoarterial connection
Dextrotransposition of aorta
Transposition of great vessels (complete)

Q20.4 Double inlet ventricle
Common ventricle
Cor triloculare biatriatum
Single ventricle

Q20.5 Discordant atrioventricular connection
Corrected transposition
Levotransposition
Ventricular inversion

Q20.6 Isomerism of atrial appendages
Isomerism of atrial appendages with asplenia or polysplenia

Q20.8 Other congenital malformations of cardiac chambers and connections
Cor binoculare

Q20.9 Congenital malformation of cardiac chambers and connections, unspecified

☑4ᵗʰ Q21 Congenital malformations of cardiac septa
    EXCLUDES 1   *acquired cardiac septal defect (I51.0)*

Q21.0 Ventricular septal defect
Roger's disease

Ventricular Septal Defect

Q21.1 Atrial septal defect
Coronary sinus defect
Patent or persistent foramen ovale
Patent or persistent ostium secundum defect (type II)
Patent or persistent sinus venosus defect

Atrial Septal Defect

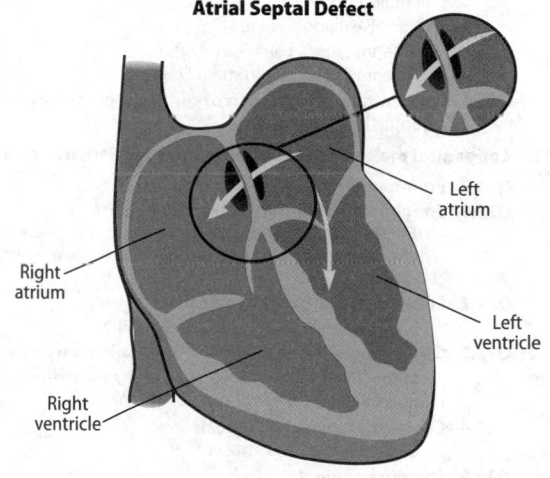

Left atrium

Right atrium

Left ventricle

Right ventricle

☑ Additional Character Required   ✓x7ᵗʰ Placeholder Alert   Manifestation   Unspecified Dx   ▶◀ Revised Text   ● New Code   ▲ Revised Code Title

ICD-10-CM 2020   911

Q21.2 Atrioventricular septal defect
Common atrioventricular canal
Endocardial cushion defect
Ostium primum atrial septal defect (type I)

Atrioventricular Septal Defect

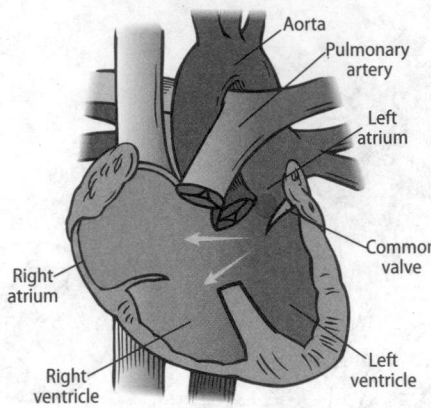

Q21.3 Tetralogy of Fallot
Ventricular septal defect with pulmonary stenosis or atresia, dextroposition of aorta and hypertrophy of right ventricle.
AHA: 2014,3Q,16

Q21.4 Aortopulmonary septal defect
Aortic septal defect
Aortopulmonary window

Q21.8 Other congenital malformations of cardiac septa
Eisenmenger's defect
Pentalogy of Fallot
Code also if applicable:
Eisenmenger's complex (I27.83)
Eisenmenger's syndrome (I27.83)

Q21.9 Congenital malformation of cardiac septum, unspecified
Septal (heart) defect NOS

✓4ᵗʰ **Q22 Congenital malformations of pulmonary and tricuspid valves**

Q22.0 Pulmonary valve atresia

Q22.1 Congenital pulmonary valve stenosis
DEF: Stenosis of the opening between the pulmonary artery and right ventricle, causing obstructed blood outflow from the right ventricle.

Q22.2 Congenital pulmonary valve insufficiency
Congenital pulmonary valve regurgitation

Q22.3 Other congenital malformations of pulmonary valve
Congenital malformation of pulmonary valve NOS
Supernumerary cusps of pulmonary valve

Q22.4 Congenital tricuspid stenosis
Congenital tricuspid atresia

Q22.5 Ebstein's anomaly
DEF: Malformation of the tricuspid valve characterized by septal and posterior leaflets attaching to the wall of the right ventricle. Ebstein's anomaly causes the right ventricle to fuse with the atrium into a large right atrium and a small ventricle and leads to heart failure and abnormal cardiac rhythm.

Q22.6 Hypoplastic right heart syndrome

Q22.8 Other congenital malformations of tricuspid valve

Q22.9 Congenital malformation of tricuspid valve, unspecified

✓4ᵗʰ **Q23 Congenital malformations of aortic and mitral valves**

Q23.0 Congenital stenosis of aortic valve
Congenital aortic atresia
Congenital aortic stenosis NOS
EXCLUDES 1 *congenital stenosis of aortic valve in hypoplastic left heart syndrome (Q23.4)*
congenital subaortic stenosis (Q24.4)
supravalvular aortic stenosis (congenital) (Q25.3)

Q23.1 Congenital insufficiency of aortic valve
Bicuspid aortic valve
Congenital aortic insufficiency

Q23.2 Congenital mitral stenosis
Congenital mitral atresia
DEF: Congenital stenosis of the mitral valve orifice between the left atrium and ventricle, at the supravalvular, valvular, or subvalvular levels, causing obstruction to left ventricular filling.

Q23.3 Congenital mitral insufficiency

Q23.4 Hypoplastic left heart syndrome

Q23.8 Other congenital malformations of aortic and mitral valves

Q23.9 Congenital malformation of aortic and mitral valves, unspecified

✓4ᵗʰ **Q24 Other congenital malformations of heart**
EXCLUDES 1 *endocardial fibroelastosis (I42.4)*

Q24.0 Dextrocardia
EXCLUDES 1 *dextrocardia with situs inversus (Q89.3)*
isomerism of atrial appendages (with asplenia or polysplenia) (Q20.6)
mirror-image atrial arrangement with situs inversus (Q89.3)
DEF: Congenital condition in which the heart is located on the right side of the chest rather than in its normal position on the left.

Q24.1 Levocardia

Q24.2 Cor triatriatum

Q24.3 Pulmonary infundibular stenosis
Subvalvular pulmonic stenosis

Q24.4 Congenital subaortic stenosis
DEF: Congenital heart defect characterized by stenosis of the left ventricular outflow tract due to a fibrous tissue ring or septal hypertrophy below the aortic valve.

Q24.5 Malformation of coronary vessels
Congenital coronary (artery) aneurysm

Q24.6 Congenital heart block

Q24.8 Other specified congenital malformations of heart
Congenital diverticulum of left ventricle
Congenital malformation of myocardium
Congenital malformation of pericardium
Malposition of heart
Uhl's disease

Q24.9 Congenital malformation of heart, unspecified
Congenital anomaly of heart
Congenital disease of heart

✓4ᵗʰ **Q25 Congenital malformations of great arteries**

Q25.0 Patent ductus arteriosus
Patent ductus Botallo
Persistent ductus arteriosus
DEF: Condition in which the normal channel between the pulmonary artery and the aorta fails to close at birth, causing arterial blood to recirculate in the lungs and inhibiting the blood supply to the aorta. **Synonym(s):** *PDA.*

Patent Ductus Arteriosus

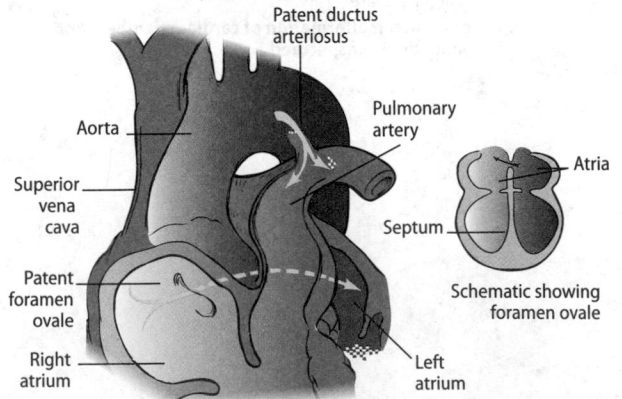

Schematic showing foramen ovale

Q25.1 Coarctation of aorta
Coarctation of aorta (preductal) (postductal)
Stenosis of aorta
AHA: 2016,4Q,56-57

☑5ᵗʰ **Q25.2** **Atresia of aorta**
　　AHA: 2016,4Q,56-57
　　Q25.21 **Interruption of aortic arch**
　　　　Atresia of aortic arch
　　Q25.29 **Other atresia of aorta**
　　　　Atresia of aorta

Q25.3 **Supravalvular aortic stenosis**
　　EXCLUDES 1 *congenital aortic stenosis NOS (Q23.0)*
　　　　　congenital stenosis of aortic valve (Q23.0)

☑5ᵗʰ **Q25.4** **Other congenital malformations of aorta**
　　EXCLUDES 1 *hypoplasia of aorta in hypoplastic left heart*
　　　　　syndrome (Q23.4)
　　AHA: 2016,4Q,57
　　Q25.40 **Congenital malformation of aorta unspecified**
　　Q25.41 **Absence and aplasia of aorta**
　　Q25.42 **Hypoplasia of aorta**
　　Q25.43 **Congenital aneurysm of aorta**
　　　　Congenital aneurysm of aortic root
　　　　Congenital aneurysm of aortic sinus
　　Q25.44 **Congenital dilation of aorta**
　　Q25.45 **Double aortic arch**
　　　　Vascular ring of aorta

Aortic Arch Anomalies

Normal aortic arch

Double aortic arch　　　　Right aortic arch

　　Q25.46 **Tortuous aortic arch**
　　　　Persistent convolutions of aortic arch
　　Q25.47 **Right aortic arch**
　　　　Persistent right aortic arch
　　Q25.48 **Anomalous origin of subclavian artery**
　　Q25.49 **Other congenital malformations of aorta**
　　　　Aortic arch
　　　　Bovine arch

Q25.5 **Atresia of pulmonary artery**
Q25.6 **Stenosis of pulmonary artery**
　　Supravalvular pulmonary stenosis

☑5ᵗʰ **Q25.7** **Other congenital malformations of pulmonary artery**

　　Q25.71 **Coarctation of pulmonary artery**
　　Q25.72 **Congenital pulmonary arteriovenous malformation**
　　　　Congenital pulmonary arteriovenous aneurysm
　　Q25.79 **Other congenital malformations of pulmonary artery**
　　　　Aberrant pulmonary artery
　　　　Agenesis of pulmonary artery
　　　　Congenital aneurysm of pulmonary artery
　　　　Congenital anomaly of pulmonary artery
　　　　Hypoplasia of pulmonary artery

Q25.8 **Other congenital malformations of other great arteries**
Q25.9 **Congenital malformation of great arteries, unspecified**

☑4ᵗʰ **Q26** **Congenital malformations of great veins**

Q26.0 **Congenital stenosis of vena cava**
　　Congenital stenosis of vena cava (inferior)(superior)
Q26.1 **Persistent left superior vena cava**
Q26.2 **Total anomalous pulmonary venous connection**
　　Total anomalous pulmonary venous return [TAPVR],
　　　subdiaphragmatic
　　Total anomalous pulmonary venous return [TAPVR],
　　　supradiaphragmatic
Q26.3 **Partial anomalous pulmonary venous connection**
　　Partial anomalous pulmonary venous return
Q26.4 **Anomalous pulmonary venous connection, unspecified**
Q26.5 **Anomalous portal venous connection**
Q26.6 **Portal vein-hepatic artery fistula**
Q26.8 **Other congenital malformations of great veins**
　　Absence of vena cava (inferior) (superior)
　　Azygos continuation of inferior vena cava
　　Persistent left posterior cardinal vein
　　Scimitar syndrome
Q26.9 **Congenital malformation of great vein, unspecified**
　　Congenital anomaly of vena cava (inferior) (superior) NOS

☑4ᵗʰ **Q27** **Other congenital malformations of peripheral vascular system**
　　EXCLUDES 2 *anomalies of cerebral and precerebral vessels (Q28.0-Q28.3)*
　　　　　anomalies of coronary vessels (Q24.5)
　　　　　anomalies of pulmonary artery (Q25.5-Q25.7)
　　　　　congenital retinal aneurysm (Q14.1)
　　　　　hemangioma and lymphangioma (D18.-)

Q27.0 **Congenital absence and hypoplasia of umbilical artery**
　　Single umbilical artery
Q27.1 **Congenital renal artery stenosis**
Q27.2 **Other congenital malformations of renal artery**
　　Congenital malformation of renal artery NOS
　　Multiple renal arteries

☑5ᵗʰ **Q27.3** **Arteriovenous malformation (peripheral)**
　　Arteriovenous aneurysm
　　EXCLUDES 1 *acquired arteriovenous aneurysm (I77.0)*
　　EXCLUDES 2 *arteriovenous malformation of cerebral vessels*
　　　　　　(Q28.2)
　　　　　arteriovenous malformation of precerebral vessels
　　　　　　(Q28.0)
　　DEF: Arteriovenous malformation: Connecting passage between
　　an artery and a vein.
　　Q27.30 **Arteriovenous malformation, site unspecified**
　　Q27.31 **Arteriovenous malformation of vessel of upper limb**
　　Q27.32 **Arteriovenous malformation of vessel of lower limb**
　　Q27.33 **Arteriovenous malformation of digestive system vessel**
　　　　AHA: 2018,3Q,21
　　Q27.34 **Arteriovenous malformation of renal vessel**
　　Q27.39 **Arteriovenous malformation, other site**

Q27.4 **Congenital phlebectasia**
Q27.8 **Other specified congenital malformations of peripheral vascular system**
　　Absence of peripheral vascular system
　　Atresia of peripheral vascular system
　　Congenital aneurysm (peripheral)
　　Congenital stricture, artery
　　Congenital varix
　　EXCLUDES 1 *arteriovenous malformation (Q27.3-)*
Q27.9 **Congenital malformation of peripheral vascular system, unspecified**
　　Anomaly of artery or vein NOS

☑4ᵗʰ **Q28** **Other congenital malformations of circulatory system**
　　EXCLUDES 1 *congenital aneurysm NOS (Q27.8)*
　　　　　congenital coronary aneurysm (Q24.5)
　　　　　ruptured cerebral arteriovenous malformation (I60.8)
　　　　　ruptured malformation of precerebral vessels (I72.0)
　　EXCLUDES 2 *congenital peripheral aneurysm (Q27.8)*
　　　　　congenital pulmonary aneurysm (Q25.79)
　　　　　congenital retinal aneurysm (Q14.1)

Q28.0 **Arteriovenous malformation of precerebral vessels**
　　Congenital arteriovenous precerebral aneurysm (nonruptured)
Q28.1 **Other malformations of precerebral vessels**
　　Congenital malformation of precerebral vessels NOS
　　Congenital precerebral aneurysm (nonruptured)

☑ Additional Character Required　　☑x7ᵗʰ Placeholder Alert　　Manifestation　　Unspecified Dx　　►◄ Revised Text　　● New Code　　▲ Revised Code Title

Q28.2 Arteriovenous malformation of cerebral vessels
Arteriovenous malformation of brain NOS
Congenital arteriovenous cerebral aneurysm (nonruptured)

Q28.3 Other malformations of cerebral vessels
Congenital cerebral aneurysm (nonruptured)
Congenital malformation of cerebral vessels NOS
Developmental venous anomaly

Q28.8 Other specified congenital malformations of circulatory system
Congenital aneurysm, specified site NEC
Spinal vessel anomaly

Q28.9 Congenital malformation of circulatory system, unspecified

Congenital malformations of the respiratory system (Q30-Q34)

✓4ᵗʰ **Q30 Congenital malformations of nose**
EXCLUDES 1   congenital deviation of nasal septum (Q67.4)

Q30.0 Choanal atresia
Atresia of nares (anterior) (posterior)
Congenital stenosis of nares (anterior) (posterior)

Q30.1 Agenesis and underdevelopment of nose
Congenital absent of nose

Q30.2 Fissured, notched and cleft nose

Q30.3 Congenital perforated nasal septum

Q30.8 Other congenital malformations of nose
Accessory nose
Congenital anomaly of nasal sinus wall

Q30.9 Congenital malformation of nose, unspecified

✓4ᵗʰ **Q31 Congenital malformations of larynx**
EXCLUDES 1   congenital laryngeal stridor NOS (P28.89)

Q31.0 Web of larynx
Glottic web of larynx
Subglottic web of larynx
Web of larynx NOS
DEF: Congenital malformation of the larynx marked by thin, translucent, or thick fibrotic membrane-like structure between the vocal folds. It is characterized by shortness of breath and stridor.

Q31.1 Congenital subglottic stenosis

Q31.2 Laryngeal hypoplasia

Q31.3 Laryngocele

Q31.5 Congenital laryngomalacia

Q31.8 Other congenital malformations of larynx
Absence of larynx
Agenesis of larynx
Atresia of larynx
Congenital cleft thyroid cartilage
Congenital fissure of epiglottis
Congenital stenosis of larynx NEC
Posterior cleft of cricoid cartilage

Q31.9 Congenital malformation of larynx, unspecified

✓4ᵗʰ **Q32 Congenital malformations of trachea and bronchus**
EXCLUDES 1   congenital bronchiectasis (Q33.4)

Q32.0 Congenital tracheomalacia

Q32.1 Other congenital malformations of trachea
Atresia of trachea
Congenital anomaly of tracheal cartilage
Congenital dilatation of trachea
Congenital malformation of trachea
Congenital stenosis of trachea
Congenital tracheocele

Q32.2 Congenital bronchomalacia

Q32.3 Congenital stenosis of bronchus

Q32.4 Other congenital malformations of bronchus
Absence of bronchus
Agenesis of bronchus
Atresia of bronchus
Congenital diverticulum of bronchus
Congenital malformation of bronchus NOS

✓4ᵗʰ **Q33 Congenital malformations of lung**

Q33.0 Congenital cystic lung
Congenital cystic lung disease
Congenital honeycomb lung
Congenital polycystic lung disease
EXCLUDES 1   cystic fibrosis (E84.0)
cystic lung disease, acquired or unspecified (J98.4)

Q33.1 Accessory lobe of lung
Azygos lobe (fissured), lung

Q33.2 Sequestration of lung

Q33.3 Agenesis of lung
Congenital absence of lung (lobe)

Q33.4 Congenital bronchiectasis

Q33.5 Ectopic tissue in lung

Q33.6 Congenital hypoplasia and dysplasia of lung
EXCLUDES 1   pulmonary hypoplasia associated with short gestation (P28.0)

Q33.8 Other congenital malformations of lung

Q33.9 Congenital malformation of lung, unspecified

✓4ᵗʰ **Q34 Other congenital malformations of respiratory system**
EXCLUDES 2   congenital central alveolar hypoventilation syndrome (G47.35)

Q34.0 Anomaly of pleura

Q34.1 Congenital cyst of mediastinum

Q34.8 Other specified congenital malformations of respiratory system
Atresia of nasopharynx

Q34.9 Congenital malformation of respiratory system, unspecified
Congenital absence of respiratory system
Congenital anomaly of respiratory system NOS

Cleft lip and cleft palate (Q35-Q37)

Use additional code to identify associated malformation of the nose (Q30.2)
EXCLUDES 1   Robin's syndrome (Q87.0)

✓4ᵗʰ **Q35 Cleft palate**
INCLUDES   fissure of palate
palatoschisis
EXCLUDES 1   cleft palate with cleft lip (Q37.-)
DEF: Congenital fissure or defect of the roof of the mouth opening to the nasal cavity due to failure of embryonic cells to fuse completely.

Cleft Palate

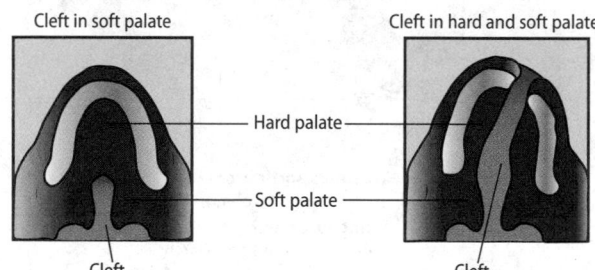

Cleft in soft palate

Cleft in hard and soft palate

Hard palate

Soft palate

Cleft

Cleft

Q35.1 Cleft hard palate

Q35.3 Cleft soft palate

Q35.5 Cleft hard palate with cleft soft palate

Q35.7 Cleft uvula

Q35.9 Cleft palate, unspecified
Cleft palate NOS

✔4ᵗʰ **Q36 Cleft lip**

> INCLUDES   cheiloschisis
> congenital fissure of lip
> harelip
> labium leporinum
> EXCLUDES 1   *cleft lip with cleft palate (Q37.-)*

DEF: Congenital fissure or opening in the upper lip due to failure of embryonic cells to fuse completely.

Cleft Lip

Unilateral incomplete   Unilateral complete   Bilateral complete

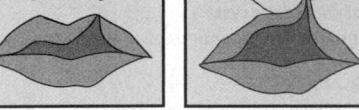

Q36.0 Cleft lip, bilateral
Q36.1 Cleft lip, median
Q36.9 Cleft lip, unilateral
        Cleft lip NOS

✔4ᵗʰ **Q37 Cleft palate with cleft lip**

> INCLUDES   cheilopalatoschisis

Q37.0 Cleft hard palate with bilateral cleft lip
Q37.1 Cleft hard palate with unilateral cleft lip
        Cleft hard palate with cleft lip NOS
Q37.2 Cleft soft palate with bilateral cleft lip
Q37.3 Cleft soft palate with unilateral cleft lip
        Cleft soft palate with cleft lip NOS
Q37.4 Cleft hard and soft palate with bilateral cleft lip
Q37.5 Cleft hard and soft palate with unilateral cleft lip
        Cleft hard and soft palate with cleft lip NOS
Q37.8 Unspecified cleft palate with bilateral cleft lip
Q37.9 Unspecified cleft palate with unilateral cleft lip
        Cleft palate with cleft lip NOS

Other congenital malformations of the digestive system (Q38-Q45)

✔4ᵗʰ **Q38 Other congenital malformations of tongue, mouth and pharynx**

> EXCLUDES 1   *dentofacial anomalies (M26.-)*
> *macrostomia (Q18.4)*
> *microstomia (Q18.5)*

Q38.0 Congenital malformations of lips, not elsewhere classified
        Congenital fistula of lip
        Congenital malformation of lip NOS
        Van der Woude's syndrome
        EXCLUDES 1   *cleft lip (Q36.-)*
                cleft lip with cleft palate (Q37.-)
                macrocheilia (Q18.6)
                microcheilia (Q18.7)
Q38.1 Ankyloglossia
        Tongue tie
Q38.2 Macroglossia
        Congenital hypertrophy of tongue
Q38.3 Other congenital malformations of tongue
        Aglossia
        Bifid tongue
        Congenital adhesion of tongue
        Congenital fissure of tongue
        Congenital malformation of tongue NOS
        Double tongue
        Hypoglossia
        Hypoplasia of tongue
        Microglossia
Q38.4 Congenital malformations of salivary glands and ducts
        Atresia of salivary glands and ducts
        Congenital absence of salivary glands and ducts
        Congenital accessory salivary glands and ducts
        Congenital fistula of salivary gland

Q38.5 Congenital malformations of palate, not elsewhere classified
        Congenital absence of uvula
        Congenital malformation of palate NOS
        Congenital high arched palate
        EXCLUDES 1   *cleft palate (Q35.-)*
                cleft palate with cleft lip (Q37.-)
Q38.6 Other congenital malformations of mouth
        Congenital malformation of mouth NOS
Q38.7 Congenital pharyngeal pouch
        Congenital diverticulum of pharynx
        EXCLUDES 1   *pharyngeal pouch syndrome (D82.1)*
Q38.8 Other congenital malformations of pharynx
        Congenital malformation of pharynx NOS
        Imperforate pharynx

✔4ᵗʰ **Q39 Congenital malformations of esophagus**

Q39.0 Atresia of esophagus without fistula
        Atresia of esophagus NOS
Q39.1 Atresia of esophagus with tracheo-esophageal fistula
        Atresia of esophagus with broncho-esophageal fistula
Q39.2 Congenital tracheo-esophageal fistula without atresia
        Congenital tracheo-esophageal fistula NOS
Q39.3 Congenital stenosis and stricture of esophagus
Q39.4 Esophageal web
Q39.5 Congenital dilatation of esophagus
        Congenital cardiospasm
Q39.6 Congenital diverticulum of esophagus
        Congenital esophageal pouch
Q39.8 Other congenital malformations of esophagus
        Congenital absence of esophagus
        Congenital displacement of esophagus
        Congenital duplication of esophagus
Q39.9 Congenital malformation of esophagus, unspecified

✔4ᵗʰ **Q40 Other congenital malformations of upper alimentary tract**

Q40.0 Congenital hypertrophic pyloric stenosis
        Congenital or infantile constriction
        Congenital or infantile hypertrophy
        Congenital or infantile spasm
        Congenital or infantile stenosis
        Congenital or infantile stricture
Q40.1 Congenital hiatus hernia
        Congenital displacement of cardia through esophageal hiatus
        EXCLUDES 1   *congenital diaphragmatic hernia (Q79.0)*
Q40.2 Other specified congenital malformations of stomach
        Congenital displacement of stomach
        Congenital diverticulum of stomach
        Congenital hourglass stomach
        Congenital duplication of stomach
        Megalogastria
        Microgastria
Q40.3 Congenital malformation of stomach, unspecified
Q40.8 Other specified congenital malformations of upper alimentary tract
Q40.9 Congenital malformation of upper alimentary tract, unspecified
        Congenital anomaly of upper alimentary tract
        Congenital deformity of upper alimentary tract

✔4ᵗʰ **Q41 Congenital absence, atresia and stenosis of small intestine**

> INCLUDES   congenital obstruction, occlusion or stricture of small intestine or intestine NOS
> EXCLUDES 1   *cystic fibrosis with intestinal manifestation (E84.11)*
>   *meconium ileus NOS (without cystic fibrosis) (P76.0)*

Q41.0 Congenital absence, atresia and stenosis of duodenum
Q41.1 Congenital absence, atresia and stenosis of jejunum
        Apple peel syndrome
        Imperforate jejunum
Q41.2 Congenital absence, atresia and stenosis of ileum
Q41.8 Congenital absence, atresia and stenosis of other specified parts of small intestine
Q41.9 Congenital absence, atresia and stenosis of small intestine, part unspecified
        Congenital absence, atresia and stenosis of intestine NOS

✔4ᵗʰ **Q42 Congenital absence, atresia and stenosis of large intestine**

> INCLUDES   congenital obstruction, occlusion and stricture of large intestine

Q42.0 Congenital absence, atresia and stenosis of rectum with fistula

---

✔ Additional Character Required   ✔x7ᵗʰ Placeholder Alert   Manifestation   Unspecified Dx   ▶◀ Revised Text   ● New Code   ▲ Revised Code Title

Q42.1 Congenital absence, atresia and stenosis of rectum without fistula
Imperforate rectum

Q42.2 Congenital absence, atresia and stenosis of anus with fistula

Q42.3 Congenital absence, atresia and stenosis of anus without fistula
Imperforate anus

Q42.8 Congenital absence, atresia and stenosis of other parts of large intestine

Q42.9 Congenital absence, atresia and stenosis of large intestine, part unspecified

✓4ᵗʰ **Q43** Other congenital malformations of intestine

Q43.0 Meckel's diverticulum (displaced) (hypertrophic)
Persistent omphalomesenteric duct
Persistent vitelline duct
DEF: Congenital, abnormal remnant of embryonic digestive system development that leaves a sacculation or outpouching from the wall of the small intestine near the terminal part of the ileum made of acid-secreting tissue as in the stomach.

Q43.1 Hirschsprung's disease
Aganglionosis
Congenital (aganglionic) megacolon
DEF: Congenital enlargement or dilation of the colon, with the absence of nerve cells in a segment of colon distally that causes the inability to defecate.

Q43.2 Other congenital functional disorders of colon
Congenital dilatation of colon

Q43.3 Congenital malformations of intestinal fixation
Congenital omental, anomalous adhesions [bands]
Congenital peritoneal adhesions [bands]
Incomplete rotation of cecum and colon
Insufficient rotation of cecum and colon
Jackson's membrane
Malrotation of colon
Rotation failure of cecum and colon
Universal mesentery

Q43.4 Duplication of intestine

Q43.5 Ectopic anus

Q43.6 Congenital fistula of rectum and anus
EXCLUDES 1 congenital fistula of anus with absence, atresia and stenosis (Q42.2)
congenital fistula of rectum with absence, atresia and stenosis (Q42.0)
congenital rectovaginal fistula (Q52.2)
congenital urethrorectal fistula (Q64.73)
pilonidal fistula or sinus (L05.-)

Q43.7 Persistent cloaca
Cloaca NOS

Q43.8 Other specified congenital malformations of intestine
Congenital blind loop syndrome
Congenital diverticulitis, colon
Congenital diverticulum, intestine
Dolichocolon
Megaloappendix
Megaloduodenum
Microcolon
Transposition of appendix
Transposition of colon
Transposition of intestine
AHA: 2013,2Q,31

Q43.9 Congenital malformation of intestine, unspecified

✓4ᵗʰ **Q44** Congenital malformations of gallbladder, bile ducts and liver

Q44.0 Agenesis, aplasia and hypoplasia of gallbladder
Congenital absence of gallbladder

Q44.1 Other congenital malformations of gallbladder
Congenital malformation of gallbladder NOS
Intrahepatic gallbladder

Q44.2 Atresia of bile ducts

Q44.3 Congenital stenosis and stricture of bile ducts

Q44.4 Choledochal cyst

Q44.5 Other congenital malformations of bile ducts
Accessory hepatic duct
Biliary duct duplication
Congenital malformation of bile duct NOS
Cystic duct duplication

Q44.6 Cystic disease of liver
Fibrocystic disease of liver

Q44.7 Other congenital malformations of liver
Accessory liver
Alagille's syndrome
Congenital absence of liver
Congenital hepatomegaly
Congenital malformation of liver NOS

✓4ᵗʰ **Q45** Other congenital malformations of digestive system
EXCLUDES 2 congenital diaphragmatic hernia (Q79.0)
congenital hiatus hernia (Q40.1)

Q45.0 Agenesis, aplasia and hypoplasia of pancreas
Congenital absence of pancreas

Q45.1 Annular pancreas

Q45.2 Congenital pancreatic cyst

Q45.3 Other congenital malformations of pancreas and pancreatic duct
Accessory pancreas
Congenital malformation of pancreas or pancreatic duct NOS
EXCLUDES 1 congenital diabetes mellitus (E10.-)
cystic fibrosis (E84.0-E84.9)
fibrocystic disease of pancreas (E84.-)
neonatal diabetes mellitus (P70.2)

Q45.8 Other specified congenital malformations of digestive system
Absence (complete) (partial) of alimentary tract NOS
Duplication of digestive system
Malposition, congenital of digestive system

Q45.9 Congenital malformation of digestive system, unspecified
Congenital anomaly of digestive system
Congenital deformity of digestive system

Congenital malformations of genital organs (Q50-Q56)

EXCLUDES 1 androgen insensitivity syndrome (E34.5-)
syndromes associated with anomalies in the number and form of chromosomes (Q90-Q99)

✓4ᵗʰ **Q50** Congenital malformations of ovaries, fallopian tubes and broad ligaments

✓5ᵗʰ **Q50.0** Congenital absence of ovary
EXCLUDES 1 Turner's syndrome (Q96.-)

Q50.01 Congenital absence of ovary, unilateral ♀

Q50.02 Congenital absence of ovary, bilateral ♀

Q50.1 Developmental ovarian cyst ♀

Q50.2 Congenital torsion of ovary ♀

✓5ᵗʰ **Q50.3** Other congenital malformations of ovary

Q50.31 Accessory ovary ♀

Q50.32 Ovarian streak ♀
46, XX with streak gonads

Q50.39 Other congenital malformation of ovary ♀
Congenital malformation of ovary NOS

Q50.4 Embryonic cyst of fallopian tube ♀
Fimbrial cyst

Q50.5 Embryonic cyst of broad ligament ♀
Epoophoron cyst
Parovarian cyst

Q50.6 Other congenital malformations of fallopian tube and broad ligament ♀
Absence of fallopian tube and broad ligament
Accessory fallopian tube and broad ligament
Atresia of fallopian tube and broad ligament
Congenital malformation of fallopian tube or broad ligament NOS

✓4ᵗʰ **Q51** Congenital malformations of uterus and cervix

Q51.0 Agenesis and aplasia of uterus ♀
Congenital absence of uterus

✓5ᵗʰ **Q51.1** Doubling of uterus with doubling of cervix and vagina

Q51.10 Doubling of uterus with doubling of cervix and vagina without obstruction ♀
Doubling of uterus with doubling of cervix and vagina NOS

Q51.11 Doubling of uterus with doubling of cervix and vagina with obstruction ♀

√5ᵗʰ **Q51.2** **Other doubling of uterus**
Doubling of uterus NOS
Septate uterus
AHA: 2018,4Q,27

    Q51.20 **Other doubling of uterus, unspecified** ♀
Septate uterus, unspecified

    Q51.21 **Other complete doubling of uterus** ♀
Complete septate uterus

    Q51.22 **Other partial doubling of uterus** ♀
Partial septate uterus

    Q51.28 **Other doubling of uterus, other specified** ♀
Septate uterus, other specified

Q51.3 **Bicornate uterus** ♀
Bicornate uterus, complete or partial

Q51.4 **Unicornate uterus** ♀
Unicornate uterus with or without a separate uterine horn
Uterus with only one functioning horn

Q51.5 **Agenesis and aplasia of cervix** ♀
Congenital absence of cervix

Q51.6 **Embryonic cyst of cervix** ♀

Q51.7 **Congenital fistulae between uterus and digestive and urinary tracts** ♀

√5ᵗʰ **Q51.8** **Other congenital malformations of uterus and cervix**

    √6ᵗʰ **Q51.81** **Other congenital malformations of uterus**

      Q51.810 **Arcuate uterus** ♀
Arcuatus uterus

      Q51.811 **Hypoplasia of uterus** ♀

      Q51.818 **Other congenital malformations of uterus** ♀
Müllerian anomaly of uterus NEC

    √6ᵗʰ **Q51.82** **Other congenital malformations of cervix**

      Q51.820 **Cervical duplication** ♀

      Q51.821 **Hypoplasia of cervix** ♀

      Q51.828 **Other congenital malformations of cervix** ♀

Q51.9 **Congenital malformation of uterus and cervix, unspecified** ♀

√4ᵗʰ **Q52** **Other congenital malformations of female genitalia**

Q52.0 **Congenital absence of vagina** ♀
Vaginal agenesis, total or partial

√5ᵗʰ **Q52.1** **Doubling of vagina**
EXCLUDES 1 doubling of vagina with doubling of uterus and cervix (Q51.1-)

    Q52.10 **Doubling of vagina, unspecified** ♀
Septate vagina NOS

    Q52.11 **Transverse vaginal septum** ♀

    √6ᵗʰ **Q52.12** **Longitudinal vaginal septum**
AHA: 2016,4Q,58-59

      Q52.120 **Longitudinal vaginal septum, nonobstructing** ♀

      Q52.121 **Longitudinal vaginal septum, obstructing, right side** ♀

      Q52.122 **Longitudinal vaginal septum, obstructing, left side** ♀

      Q52.123 **Longitudinal vaginal septum, microperforate, right side** ♀

      Q52.124 **Longitudinal vaginal septum, microperforate, left side** ♀

      Q52.129 **Other and unspecified longitudinal vaginal septum** ♀

Q52.2 **Congenital rectovaginal fistula** ♀
EXCLUDES 1 cloaca (Q43.7)

Q52.3 **Imperforate hymen** ♀
DEF: Obstructive anomaly of vagina, characterized by complete closure of the membranous fold around the external opening of the vagina, obstructing the vaginal introitus.

Q52.4 **Other congenital malformations of vagina** ♀
Canal of Nuck cyst, congenital
Congenital malformation of vagina NOS
Embryonic vaginal cyst
Gartner's duct cyst

Q52.5 **Fusion of labia** ♀

Q52.6 **Congenital malformation of clitoris** ♀

√5ᵗʰ **Q52.7** **Other and unspecified congenital malformations of vulva**

    Q52.70 **Unspecified congenital malformations of vulva** ♀
Congenital malformation of vulva NOS

    Q52.71 **Congenital absence of vulva** ♀

    Q52.79 **Other congenital malformations of vulva** ♀
Congenital cyst of vulva

Q52.8 **Other specified congenital malformations of female genitalia** ♀

Q52.9 **Congenital malformation of female genitalia, unspecified** ♀

√4ᵗʰ **Q53** **Undescended and ectopic testicle**

√5ᵗʰ **Q53.0** **Ectopic testis**

    Q53.00 **Ectopic testis, unspecified** ♂

    Q53.01 **Ectopic testis, unilateral** ♂

    Q53.02 **Ectopic testes, bilateral** ♂

√5ᵗʰ **Q53.1** **Undescended testicle, unilateral**
AHA: 2017,4Q,22-23

    Q53.10 **Unspecified undescended testicle, unilateral** ♂

    √6ᵗʰ **Q53.11** **Abdominal testis, unilateral**

      Q53.111 **Unilateral intraabdominal testis** ♂

      Q53.112 **Unilateral inguinal testis** ♂

    Q53.12 **Ectopic perineal testis, unilateral** ♂

    Q53.13 **Unilateral high scrotal testis** ♂

√5ᵗʰ **Q53.2** **Undescended testicle, bilateral**
AHA: 2017,4Q,22-23

    Q53.20 **Undescended testicle, unspecified, bilateral** ♂

    √6ᵗʰ **Q53.21** **Abdominal testis, bilateral**

      Q53.211 **Bilateral intraabdominal testes** ♂

      Q53.212 **Bilateral inguinal testes** ♂

    Q53.22 **Ectopic perineal testis, bilateral** ♂

    Q53.23 **Bilateral high scrotal testes** ♂

Q53.9 **Undescended testicle, unspecified** ♂
Cryptorchism NOS

√4ᵗʰ **Q54** **Hypospadias**
EXCLUDES 1 epispadias (Q64.0)
DEF: Abnormal opening of the urethra on the ventral (underside) surface of the penis.

Hypospadias

Balanic (glanular, coronal) hypospadias
Subcoronal hypospadias
Penile hypospadias
Penile raphe
Scrotal hypospadias
Penoscrotal hypospadias
Scrotum
Scrotal raphe
Hypospadias (ventral view)
Perineal hypospadias

Q54.0 **Hypospadias, balanic** ♂
Hypospadias, coronal
Hypospadias, glandular

Q54.1 **Hypospadias, penile** ♂

Q54.2 **Hypospadias, penoscrotal** ♂

Q54.3 **Hypospadias, perineal** ♂

Q54.4 **Congenital chordee** ♂
Chordee without hypospadias

Q54.8 **Other hypospadias** ♂
Hypospadias with intersex state

Q54.9 **Hypospadias, unspecified** ♂

✓4ᵗʰ **Q55 Other congenital malformations of male genital organs**
> EXCLUDES 1   *congenital hydrocele (P83.5)*
> *hypospadias (Q54.-)*

Q55.0 Absence and aplasia of testis   ♂
     Monorchism

Q55.1 Hypoplasia of testis and scrotum   ♂
     Fusion of testes

✓5ᵗʰ **Q55.2 Other and unspecified congenital malformations of testis and scrotum**

     Q55.20 Unspecified congenital malformations of testis and scrotum   ♂
         Congenital malformation of testis or scrotum NOS

     Q55.21 Polyorchism   ♂
         DEF: Congenital anomaly in which there are more than two testes.

     Q55.22 Retractile testis   ♂

     Q55.23 Scrotal transposition   ♂

     Q55.29 Other congenital malformations of testis and scrotum   ♂

Q55.3 Atresia of vas deferens   ♂
     Code first any associated cystic fibrosis (E84.-)

Q55.4 Other congenital malformations of vas deferens, epididymis, seminal vesicles and prostate   ♂
     Absence or aplasia of prostate
     Absence or aplasia of spermatic cord
     Congenital malformation of vas deferens, epididymis, seminal vesicles or prostate NOS

Q55.5 Congenital absence and aplasia of penis   ♂

✓5ᵗʰ **Q55.6 Other congenital malformations of penis**

     Q55.61 Curvature of penis (lateral)   ♂

     Q55.62 Hypoplasia of penis   ♂
         Micropenis

     Q55.63 Congenital torsion of penis   ♂
         EXCLUDES 1   *acquired torsion of penis (N48.82)*

     Q55.64 Hidden penis   ♂
         Buried penis
         Concealed penis
         EXCLUDES 1   *acquired buried penis (N48.83)*

     Q55.69 Other congenital malformation of penis   ♂
         Congenital malformation of penis NOS

Q55.7 Congenital vasocutaneous fistula   ♂

Q55.8 Other specified congenital malformations of male genital organs   ♂

Q55.9 Congenital malformation of male genital organ, unspecified   ♂
     Congenital anomaly of male genital organ
     Congenital deformity of male genital organ

✓4ᵗʰ **Q56 Indeterminate sex and pseudohermaphroditism**
> EXCLUDES 1   *46, XX true hermaphrodite (Q99.1)*
> *androgen insensitivity syndrome (E34.5-)*
> *chimera 46, XX/46, XY true hermaphrodite (Q99.0)*
> *female pseudohermaphroditism with adrenocortical disorder (E25.-)*
> *pseudohermaphroditism with specified chromosomal anomaly (Q96-Q99)*
> *pure gonadal dysgenesis (Q99.1)*

     DEF: Indeterminate sex: External genitalia that is nondescript, lacking the physical appearance specific to either sex.
     DEF: Pseudohermaphroditism: Presence of gonads of one sex and external genitalia of another sex.

Q56.0 Hermaphroditism, not elsewhere classified
     Ovotestis

Q56.1 Male pseudohermaphroditism, not elsewhere classified   ♂
     46, XY with streak gonads
     Male pseudohermaphroditism NOS

Q56.2 Female pseudohermaphroditism, not elsewhere classified   ♀
     Female pseudohermaphroditism NOS

Q56.3 Pseudohermaphroditism, unspecified

Q56.4 Indeterminate sex, unspecified
     Ambiguous genitalia

Congenital malformations of the urinary system (Q60-Q64)

✓4ᵗʰ **Q60 Renal agenesis and other reduction defects of kidney**
> INCLUDES   congenital absence of kidney
> congenital atrophy of kidney
> infantile atrophy of kidney

Q60.0 Renal agenesis, unilateral

Q60.1 Renal agenesis, bilateral

Q60.2 Renal agenesis, unspecified

Q60.3 Renal hypoplasia, unilateral

Q60.4 Renal hypoplasia, bilateral

Q60.5 Renal hypoplasia, unspecified

Q60.6 Potter's syndrome

✓4ᵗʰ **Q61 Cystic kidney disease**
> EXCLUDES 1   *acquired cyst of kidney (N28.1)*
> *Potter's syndrome (Q60.6)*

✓5ᵗʰ **Q61.0 Congenital renal cyst**

     Q61.00 Congenital renal cyst, unspecified
         Cyst of kidney NOS (congenital)

     Q61.01 Congenital single renal cyst

     Q61.02 Congenital multiple renal cysts

✓5ᵗʰ **Q61.1 Polycystic kidney, infantile type**
     Polycystic kidney, autosomal recessive

     Q61.11 Cystic dilatation of collecting ducts

     Q61.19 Other polycystic kidney, infantile type

Q61.2 Polycystic kidney, adult type
     Polycystic kidney, autosomal dominant

Q61.3 Polycystic kidney, unspecified
     AHA: 2016,3Q,22

Q61.4 Renal dysplasia
     Multicystic dysplastic kidney
     Multicystic kidney (development)
     Multicystic kidney disease
     Multicystic renal dysplasia
     EXCLUDES 1   *polycystic kidney disease (Q61.11-Q61.3)*

Q61.5 Medullary cystic kidney
     Nephronopthisis
     Sponge kidney NOS
     DEF: Sponge kidney: Dilated collecting tubules that are usually asymptomatic. Calcinosis in tubules may cause renal insufficiency.

Q61.8 Other cystic kidney diseases
     Fibrocystic kidney
     Fibrocystic renal degeneration or disease

Q61.9 Cystic kidney disease, unspecified
     Meckel-Gruber syndrome

✓4ᵗʰ **Q62 Congenital obstructive defects of renal pelvis and congenital malformations of ureter**

Q62.0 Congenital hydronephrosis

✓5ᵗʰ **Q62.1 Congenital occlusion of ureter**
     Atresia and stenosis of ureter

     Q62.10 Congenital occlusion of ureter, unspecified

     Q62.11 Congenital occlusion of ureteropelvic junction

     Q62.12 Congenital occlusion of ureterovesical orifice

Q62.2 Congenital megaureter
     Congenital dilatation of ureter

✓5ᵗʰ **Q62.3 Other obstructive defects of renal pelvis and ureter**

     Q62.31 Congenital ureterocele, orthotopic

     Q62.32 Cecoureterocele
         Ectopic ureterocele

     Q62.39 Other obstructive defects of renal pelvis and ureter
         Ureteropelvic junction obstruction NOS

Q62.4 Agenesis of ureter
     Congenital absence ureter

Q62.5 Duplication of ureter
     Accessory ureter
     Double ureter

✓5ᵗʰ **Q62.6 Malposition of ureter**

     Q62.60 Malposition of ureter, unspecified

     Q62.61 Deviation of ureter

     Q62.62 Displacement of ureter

     Q62.63 Anomalous implantation of ureter
         Ectopia of ureter
         Ectopic ureter

     Q62.69 Other malposition of ureter

Q62.7 Congenital vesico-uretero-renal reflux

Q62.8 Other congenital malformations of ureter
Anomaly of ureter NOS

√4ᵗʰ **Q63** Other congenital malformations of kidney
> EXCLUDES 1   congenital nephrotic syndrome (N04.-)

Q63.0 Accessory kidney

Q63.1 Lobulated, fused and horseshoe kidney

Q63.2 Ectopic kidney
Congenital displaced kidney
Malrotation of kidney

Q63.3 Hyperplastic and giant kidney
Compensatory hypertrophy of kidney

Q63.8 Other specified congenital malformations of kidney
Congenital renal calculi

Q63.9 Congenital malformation of kidney, unspecified

√4ᵗʰ **Q64** Other congenital malformations of urinary system

Q64.0 Epispadias
> EXCLUDES 1   hypospadias (Q54.-)

Epispadias

Normal external urethral orifice
Glans penis
Foreskin (retracted)
Epispadias

Epispadias (dorsal view)

√5ᵗʰ **Q64.1** Exstrophy of urinary bladder

Q64.10 Exstrophy of urinary bladder, unspecified
Ectopia vesicae

Q64.11 Supravesical fissure of urinary bladder

Q64.12 Cloacal exstrophy of urinary bladder

Q64.19 Other exstrophy of urinary bladder
Extroversion of bladder

Q64.2 Congenital posterior urethral valves

√5ᵗʰ **Q64.3** Other atresia and stenosis of urethra and bladder neck

Q64.31 Congenital bladder neck obstruction
Congenital obstruction of vesicourethral orifice

Q64.32 Congenital stricture of urethra

Q64.33 Congenital stricture of urinary meatus

Q64.39 Other atresia and stenosis of urethra and bladder neck
Atresia and stenosis of urethra and bladder neck NOS

Q64.4 Malformation of urachus
Cyst of urachus
Patent urachus
Prolapse of urachus

Q64.5 Congenital absence of bladder and urethra

Q64.6 Congenital diverticulum of bladder

√5ᵗʰ **Q64.7** Other and unspecified congenital malformations of bladder and urethra
> EXCLUDES 1   congenital prolapse of bladder (mucosa) (Q79.4)

Q64.70 Unspecified congenital malformation of bladder and urethra
Malformation of bladder or urethra NOS

Q64.71 Congenital prolapse of urethra

Q64.72 Congenital prolapse of urinary meatus

Q64.73 Congenital urethrorectal fistula

Q64.74 Double urethra

Q64.75 Double urinary meatus

Q64.79 Other congenital malformations of bladder and urethra

Q64.8 Other specified congenital malformations of urinary system

Q64.9 Congenital malformation of urinary system, unspecified
Congenital anomaly NOS of urinary system
Congenital deformity NOS of urinary system

Congenital malformations and deformations of the musculoskeletal system (Q65-Q79)

√4ᵗʰ **Q65** Congenital deformities of hip
> EXCLUDES 1   clicking hip (R29.4)

√5ᵗʰ **Q65.0** Congenital dislocation of hip, unilateral

Q65.00 Congenital dislocation of unspecified hip, unilateral

Q65.01 Congenital dislocation of right hip, unilateral

Q65.02 Congenital dislocation of left hip, unilateral

Q65.1 Congenital dislocation of hip, bilateral

Q65.2 Congenital dislocation of hip, unspecified

√5ᵗʰ **Q65.3** Congenital partial dislocation of hip, unilateral

Q65.30 Congenital partial dislocation of unspecified hip, unilateral

Q65.31 Congenital partial dislocation of right hip, unilateral

Q65.32 Congenital partial dislocation of left hip, unilateral

Q65.4 Congenital partial dislocation of hip, bilateral

Q65.5 Congenital partial dislocation of hip, unspecified

Q65.6 Congenital unstable hip
Congenital dislocatable hip

√5ᵗʰ **Q65.8** Other congenital deformities of hip

Q65.81 Congenital coxa valga

Q65.82 Congenital coxa vara

Q65.89 Other specified congenital deformities of hip
Anteversion of femoral neck
Congenital acetabular dysplasia

Q65.9 Congenital deformity of hip, unspecified

√4ᵗʰ **Q66** Congenital deformities of feet
> EXCLUDES 1   reduction defects of feet (Q72.-)
> valgus deformities (acquired) (M21.0-)
> varus deformities (acquired) (M21.1-)

▲ √5ᵗʰ **Q66.0** Congenital talipes equinovarus

● **Q66.00** Congenital talipes equinovarus, unspecified foot

● **Q66.01** Congenital talipes equinovarus, right foot

● **Q66.02** Congenital talipes equinovarus, left foot

▲ √5ᵗʰ **Q66.1** Congenital talipes calcaneovarus

● **Q66.10** Congenital talipes calcaneovarus, unspecified foot

● **Q66.11** Congenital talipes calcaneovarus, right foot

● **Q66.12** Congenital talipes calcaneovarus, left foot

√5ᵗʰ **Q66.2** Congenital metatarsus (primus) varus
AHA: 2016,4Q,59

▲ √6ᵗʰ **Q66.21** Congenital metatarsus primus varus

● **Q66.211** Congenital metatarsus primus varus, right foot

● **Q66.212** Congenital metatarsus primus varus, left foot

● **Q66.219** Congenital metatarsus primus varus, unspecified foot

▲ √6ᵗʰ **Q66.22** Congenital metatarsus adductus
Congenital metatarsus varus

● **Q66.221** Congenital metatarsus adductus, right foot

● **Q66.222** Congenital metatarsus adductus, left foot

● **Q66.229** Congenital metatarsus adductus, unspecified foot

▲ √5ᵗʰ **Q66.3** Other congenital varus deformities of feet
Hallux varus, congenital

● **Q66.30** Other congenital varus deformities of feet, unspecified foot

● **Q66.31** Other congenital varus deformities of feet, right foot

● **Q66.32** Other congenital varus deformities of feet, left foot

▲ √5ᵗʰ **Q66.4** Congenital talipes calcaneovalgus

● **Q66.40** Congenital talipes calcaneovalgus, unspecified foot

● **Q66.41** Congenital talipes calcaneovalgus, right foot

● **Q66.42** Congenital talipes calcaneovalgus, left foot

☑ Additional Character Required   √x7ᵗʰ Placeholder Alert   Manifestation   Unspecified Dx   ►◄ Revised Text   ● New Code   ▲ Revised Code Title

ICD-10-CM 2020   **919**

✓5ᵗʰ **Q66.5** **Congenital** pes planus
Congenital flat foot
Congenital rigid flat foot
Congenital spastic (everted) flat foot
　EXCLUDES 1　pes planus, acquired (M21.4)

Q66.50 **Congenital pes planus, unspecified foot**
Q66.51 **Congenital pes planus, right foot**
Q66.52 **Congenital pes planus, left foot**

Q66.6 **Other congenital valgus deformities of feet**
Congenital metatarsus valgus

▲　✓5ᵗʰ **Q66.7** **Congenital** pes cavus
●　　**Q66.70** **Congenital pes cavus, unspecified foot**
●　　**Q66.71** **Congenital pes cavus, right foot**
●　　**Q66.72** **Congenital pes cavus, left foot**

✓5ᵗʰ **Q66.8** **Other congenital deformities of feet**
Q66.80 **Congenital vertical talus deformity, unspecified foot**
Q66.81 **Congenital vertical talus deformity, right foot**
Q66.82 **Congenital vertical talus deformity, left foot**
Q66.89 **Other specified congenital deformities of feet**
Congenital asymmetric talipes
Congenital clubfoot NOS
Congenital talipes NOS
Congenital tarsal coalition
Hammer toe, congenital
DEF: Clubfoot: Congenital anomaly of the foot with the heel elevated and rotated outward and the toes pointing inward.

▲　✓5ᵗʰ **Q66.9** **Congenital deformity of feet, unspecified**
●　　**Q66.90** **Congenital deformity of feet, unspecified, unspecified foot**
●　　**Q66.91** **Congenital deformity of feet, unspecified, right foot**
●　　**Q66.92** **Congenital deformity of feet, unspecified, left foot**

✓4ᵗʰ **Q67** **Congenital musculoskeletal deformities of** head, face, spine and chest
　EXCLUDES 1　congenital malformation syndromes classified to Q87.-
　　Potter's syndrome (Q60.6)

Q67.0 **Congenital** facial asymmetry
Q67.1 **Congenital** compression facies
Q67.2 **Dolichocephaly**
Q67.3 **Plagiocephaly**
Q67.4 **Other congenital deformities of skull, face and jaw**
Congenital depressions in skull
Congenital hemifacial atrophy or hypertrophy
Deviation of nasal septum, congenital
Squashed or bent nose, congenital
　EXCLUDES 1　dentofacial anomalies [including malocclusion] (M26.-)
　　syphilitic saddle nose (A50.5)
DEF: Deviated septum: Condition in which the nasal septum, a thin wall composed of cartilage and bone that separates the two nostrils, is crooked or displaced from the midline.

Q67.5 **Congenital deformity of** spine
Congenital postural scoliosis
Congenital scoliosis NOS
　EXCLUDES 1　infantile idiopathic scoliosis (M41.0)
　　scoliosis due to congenital bony malformation (Q76.3)
AHA: 2014,4Q,26

Q67.6 **Pectus excavatum**
Congenital funnel chest
Q67.7 **Pectus carinatum**
Congenital pigeon chest
Q67.8 **Other congenital deformities of chest**
Congenital deformity of chest wall NOS

✓4ᵗʰ **Q68** **Other congenital musculoskeletal deformities**
　EXCLUDES 1　reduction defects of limb(s) (Q71-Q73)
　EXCLUDES 2　congenital myotonic chondrodystrophy (G71.13)

Q68.0 **Congenital deformity of** sternocleidomastoid muscle
Congenital contracture of sternocleidomastoid (muscle)
Congenital (sternomastoid) torticollis
Sternomastoid tumor (congenital)

Q68.1 **Congenital deformity of** finger(s) and hand
Congenital clubfinger
Spade-like hand (congenital)
Q68.2 **Congenital deformity of** knee
Congenital dislocation of knee
Congenital genu recurvatum
Q68.3 **Congenital bowing of** femur
　EXCLUDES 1　anteversion of femur (neck) (Q65.89)
Q68.4 **Congenital bowing of** tibia and fibula
Q68.5 **Congenital bowing of long bones of leg, unspecified**
Q68.6 **Discoid meniscus**
Q68.8 **Other specified congenital musculoskeletal deformities**
Congenital deformity of clavicle
Congenital deformity of elbow
Congenital deformity of forearm
Congenital deformity of scapula
Congenital deformity of wrist
Congenital dislocation of elbow
Congenital dislocation of shoulder
Congenital dislocation of wrist

✓4ᵗʰ **Q69** **Polydactyly**
Q69.0 **Accessory** finger(s)
Q69.1 **Accessory** thumb(s)
Q69.2 **Accessory** toe(s)
Accessory hallux
Q69.9 **Polydactyly, unspecified**
Supernumerary digit(s) NOS

✓4ᵗʰ **Q70** **Syndactyly**
✓5ᵗʰ **Q70.0** **Fused fingers**
Complex syndactyly of fingers with synostosis
Q70.00 **Fused fingers, unspecified hand**
Q70.01 **Fused fingers, right hand**
Q70.02 **Fused fingers, left hand**
Q70.03 **Fused fingers, bilateral**
✓5ᵗʰ **Q70.1** **Webbed fingers**
Simple syndactyly of fingers without synostosis
Q70.10 **Webbed fingers, unspecified hand**
Q70.11 **Webbed fingers, right hand**
Q70.12 **Webbed fingers, left hand**
Q70.13 **Webbed fingers, bilateral**
✓5ᵗʰ **Q70.2** **Fused toes**
Complex syndactyly of toes with synostosis
Q70.20 **Fused toes, unspecified foot**
Q70.21 **Fused toes, right foot**
Q70.22 **Fused toes, left foot**
Q70.23 **Fused toes, bilateral**
✓5ᵗʰ **Q70.3** **Webbed toes**
Simple syndactyly of toes without synostosis
Q70.30 **Webbed toes, unspecified foot**
Q70.31 **Webbed toes, right foot**
Q70.32 **Webbed toes, left foot**
Q70.33 **Webbed toes, bilateral**
Q70.4 **Polysyndactyly, unspecified**
　EXCLUDES 1　specified syndactyly of hand and feet — code to specified conditions (Q70.0-Q70.3-)
Q70.9 **Syndactyly, unspecified**
Symphalangy NOS

✓4ᵗʰ **Q71** **Reduction defects of** upper limb
✓5ᵗʰ **Q71.0** **Congenital complete absence** of upper limb
Q71.00 **Congenital complete absence of unspecified upper limb**
Q71.01 **Congenital complete absence of right upper limb**
Q71.02 **Congenital complete absence of left upper limb**
Q71.03 **Congenital complete absence of upper limb, bilateral**
✓5ᵗʰ **Q71.1** **Congenital absence of upper arm and forearm with hand present**
Q71.10 **Congenital absence of unspecified upper arm and forearm with hand present**
Q71.11 **Congenital absence of right upper arm and forearm with hand present**
Q71.12 **Congenital absence of left upper arm and forearm with hand present**
Q71.13 **Congenital absence of upper arm and forearm with hand present, bilateral**

√5ᵗʰ **Q71.2** **Congenital** absence of both forearm and hand

     Q71.20 **Congenital absence of both forearm and hand, unspecified upper limb**

     Q71.21 **Congenital absence of both forearm and hand,** right **upper limb**

     Q71.22 **Congenital absence of both forearm and hand,** left **upper limb**

     Q71.23 **Congenital absence of both forearm and hand, bilateral**

√5ᵗʰ **Q71.3** **Congenital** absence of hand and finger

     Q71.30 **Congenital absence of unspecified hand and finger**

     Q71.31 **Congenital absence of** right **hand and finger**

     Q71.32 **Congenital absence of** left **hand and finger**

     Q71.33 **Congenital absence of hand and finger, bilateral**

√5ᵗʰ **Q71.4** **Longitudinal reduction defect of** radius

     Clubhand (congenital)

     Radial clubhand

     Q71.40 **Longitudinal reduction defect of unspecified radius**

     Q71.41 **Longitudinal reduction defect of** right **radius**

     Q71.42 **Longitudinal reduction defect of** left **radius**

     Q71.43 **Longitudinal reduction defect of radius, bilateral**

√5ᵗʰ **Q71.5** **Longitudinal reduction defect of** ulna

     Q71.50 **Longitudinal reduction defect of unspecified ulna**

     Q71.51 **Longitudinal reduction defect of** right **ulna**

     Q71.52 **Longitudinal reduction defect of** left **ulna**

     Q71.53 **Longitudinal reduction defect of ulna, bilateral**

√5ᵗʰ **Q71.6** Lobster-claw hand

     Q71.60 **Lobster-claw hand, unspecified hand**

     Q71.61 **Lobster-claw** right **hand**

     Q71.62 **Lobster-claw** left **hand**

     Q71.63 **Lobster-claw hand,** bilateral

√5ᵗʰ **Q71.8** **Other reduction defects of** upper limb

     √6ᵗʰ **Q71.81** **Congenital** shortening **of upper limb**

         Q71.811 **Congenital shortening of** right **upper limb**

         Q71.812 **Congenital shortening of** left **upper limb**

         Q71.813 **Congenital shortening of upper limb, bilateral**

         Q71.819 **Congenital shortening of unspecified upper limb**

     √6ᵗʰ **Q71.89** **Other reduction defects of upper limb**

         Q71.891 **Other reduction defects of** right **upper limb**

         Q71.892 **Other reduction defects of** left **upper limb**

         Q71.893 **Other reduction defects of upper limb, bilateral**

         Q71.899 **Other reduction defects of unspecified upper limb**

√5ᵗʰ **Q71.9** **Unspecified reduction defect of upper limb**

     Q71.90 **Unspecified reduction defect of unspecified upper limb**

     Q71.91 **Unspecified reduction defect of** right **upper limb**

     Q71.92 **Unspecified reduction defect of** left **upper limb**

     Q71.93 **Unspecified reduction defect of upper limb, bilateral**

√4ᵗʰ **Q72** **Reduction defects of** lower limb

     √5ᵗʰ **Q72.0** **Congenital** complete absence **of lower limb**

         Q72.00 **Congenital complete absence of unspecified lower limb**

         Q72.01 **Congenital complete absence of** right **lower limb**

         Q72.02 **Congenital complete absence of** left **lower limb**

         Q72.03 **Congenital complete absence of lower limb, bilateral**

     √5ᵗʰ **Q72.1** **Congenital** absence of thigh and lower leg with foot present

         Q72.10 **Congenital absence of unspecified thigh and lower leg with foot present**

         Q72.11 **Congenital absence of** right **thigh and lower leg with foot present**

         Q72.12 **Congenital absence of** left **thigh and lower leg with foot present**

         Q72.13 **Congenital absence of thigh and lower leg with foot present, bilateral**

     √5ᵗʰ **Q72.2** **Congenital** absence of both lower leg and foot

         Q72.20 **Congenital absence of both lower leg and foot, unspecified lower limb**

         Q72.21 **Congenital absence of both lower leg and foot,** right **lower limb**

         Q72.22 **Congenital absence of both lower leg and foot,** left **lower limb**

         Q72.23 **Congenital absence of both lower leg and foot,** bilateral

√5ᵗʰ **Q72.3** **Congenital** absence of foot and toe(s)

     Q72.30 **Congenital absence of unspecified foot and toe(s)**

     Q72.31 **Congenital absence of** right **foot and toe(s)**

     Q72.32 **Congenital absence of** left **foot and toe(s)**

     Q72.33 **Congenital absence of foot and toe(s), bilateral**

√5ᵗʰ **Q72.4** **Longitudinal reduction defect of** femur

     Proximal femoral focal deficiency

     Q72.40 **Longitudinal reduction defect of unspecified femur**

     Q72.41 **Longitudinal reduction defect of** right **femur**

     Q72.42 **Longitudinal reduction defect of** left **femur**

     Q72.43 **Longitudinal reduction defect of femur,** bilateral

√5ᵗʰ **Q72.5** **Longitudinal reduction defect of** tibia

     Q72.50 **Longitudinal reduction defect of unspecified tibia**

     Q72.51 **Longitudinal reduction defect of** right **tibia**

     Q72.52 **Longitudinal reduction defect of** left **tibia**

     Q72.53 **Longitudinal reduction defect of tibia,** bilateral

√5ᵗʰ **Q72.6** **Longitudinal reduction defect of** fibula

     Q72.60 **Longitudinal reduction defect of unspecified fibula**

     Q72.61 **Longitudinal reduction defect of** right **fibula**

     Q72.62 **Longitudinal reduction defect of** left **fibula**

     Q72.63 **Longitudinal reduction defect of fibula,** bilateral

√5ᵗʰ **Q72.7** Split foot

     Q72.70 **Split foot, unspecified lower limb**

     Q72.71 **Split foot,** right **lower limb**

     Q72.72 **Split foot,** left **lower limb**

     Q72.73 **Split foot,** bilateral

√5ᵗʰ **Q72.8** **Other reduction defects of** lower limb

     √6ᵗʰ **Q72.81** **Congenital** shortening **of lower limb**

         Q72.811 **Congenital shortening of** right **lower limb**

         Q72.812 **Congenital shortening of** left **lower limb**

         Q72.813 **Congenital shortening of lower limb, bilateral**

         Q72.819 **Congenital shortening of unspecified lower limb**

     √6ᵗʰ **Q72.89** **Other reduction defects of lower limb**

         Q72.891 **Other reduction defects of** right **lower limb**

         Q72.892 **Other reduction defects of** left **lower limb**

         Q72.893 **Other reduction defects of lower limb, bilateral**

         Q72.899 **Other reduction defects of unspecified lower limb**

√5ᵗʰ **Q72.9** **Unspecified reduction defect of lower limb**

     Q72.90 **Unspecified reduction defect of unspecified lower limb**

     Q72.91 **Unspecified reduction defect of** right **lower limb**

     Q72.92 **Unspecified reduction defect of** left **lower limb**

     Q72.93 **Unspecified reduction defect of lower limb,** bilateral

√4ᵗʰ **Q73** **Reduction defects of unspecified limb**

     Q73.0 **Congenital** absence **of unspecified limb(s)**

     Amelia NOS

     Q73.1 Phocomelia, **unspecified limb(s)**

     Phocomelia NOS

     Q73.8 **Other reduction defects of unspecified limb(s)**

     Longitudinal reduction deformity of unspecified limb(s)

     Ectromelia of limb NOS

     Hemimelia of limb NOS

     Reduction defect of limb NOS

☑ Additional Character Required   √x7ᵗʰ Placeholder Alert   Manifestation   Unspecified Dx   ▶◀ Revised Text   ● New Code   ▲ Revised Code Title

Chapter 17. Congenital Malformations, Deformations and Chromosomal Abnormalities

Q74–Q77.9

✓4ᵗʰ **Q74 Other congenital malformations of limb(s)**
    EXCLUDES 1   polydactyly (Q69.-)
          reduction defect of limb (Q71-Q73)
          syndactyly (Q70.-)

Q74.0 Other congenital malformations of upper limb(s), including shoulder girdle
   Accessory carpal bones
   Cleidocranial dysostosis
   Congenital pseudarthrosis of clavicle
   Macrodactylia (fingers)
   Madelung's deformity
   Radioulnar synostosis
   Sprengel's deformity
   Triphalangeal thumb

Q74.1 Congenital malformation of knee
   Congenital absence of patella
   Congenital dislocation of patella
   Congenital genu valgum
   Congenital genu varum
   Rudimentary patella
    EXCLUDES 1   congenital dislocation of knee (Q68.2)
          congenital genu recurvatum (Q68.2)
          nail patella syndrome (Q87.2)

Q74.2 Other congenital malformations of lower limb(s), including pelvic girdle
   Congenital fusion of sacroiliac joint
   Congenital malformation of ankle joint
   Congenital malformation of sacroiliac joint
    EXCLUDES 1   anteversion of femur (neck) (Q65.89)

Q74.3 Arthrogryposis multiplex congenita

Q74.8 Other specified congenital malformations of limb(s)

Q74.9 Unspecified congenital malformation of limb(s)
   Congenital anomaly of limb(s) NOS

✓4ᵗʰ **Q75 Other congenital malformations of skull and face bones**
    EXCLUDES 1   congenital malformation of face NOS (Q18.-)
          congenital malformation syndromes classified to Q87.-
          dentofacial anomalies [including malocclusion] (M26.-)
          musculoskeletal deformities of head and face (Q67.0-Q67.4)
          skull defects associated with congenital anomalies of brain
              such as:
              anencephaly (Q00.0)
              encephalocele (Q01.-)
              hydrocephalus (Q03.-)
              microcephaly (Q02)

Q75.0 Craniosynostosis
   Acrocephaly
   Imperfect fusion of skull
   Oxycephaly
   Trigonocephaly
   DEF: Congenital condition in which one or more of the cranial sutures fuse prematurely, creating a deformed or aberrant head shape.

Q75.1 Craniofacial dysostosis
   Crouzon's disease

Q75.2 Hypertelorism

Q75.3 Macrocephaly

Q75.4 Mandibulofacial dysostosis
   Franceschetti syndrome
   Treacher Collins syndrome

Q75.5 Oculomandibular dysostosis

Q75.8 Other specified congenital malformations of skull and face bones
   Absence of skull bone, congenital
   Congenital deformity of forehead
   Platybasia

Q75.9 Congenital malformation of skull and face bones, unspecified
   Congenital anomaly of face bones NOS
   Congenital anomaly of skull NOS

✓4ᵗʰ **Q76 Congenital malformations of spine and bony thorax**
    EXCLUDES 1   congenital musculoskeletal deformities of spine and chest (Q67.5-Q67.8)

Q76.0 Spina bifida occulta
    EXCLUDES 1   meningocele (spinal) (Q05.-)
          spina bifida (aperta) (cystica) (Q05.-)

Q76.1 Klippel-Feil syndrome
   Cervical fusion syndrome

Q76.2 Congenital spondylolisthesis
   Congenital spondylolysis
    EXCLUDES 1   spondylolisthesis (acquired) (M43.1-)
          spondylolysis (acquired) (M43.0-)

Q76.3 Congenital scoliosis due to congenital bony malformation
   Hemivertebra fusion or failure of segmentation with scoliosis

✓5ᵗʰ **Q76.4 Other congenital malformations of spine, not associated with scoliosis**

  ✓6ᵗʰ **Q76.41 Congenital kyphosis**
     Q76.411 Congenital kyphosis, occipito-atlanto-axial region
     Q76.412 Congenital kyphosis, cervical region
     Q76.413 Congenital kyphosis, cervicothoracic region
     Q76.414 Congenital kyphosis, thoracic region
     Q76.415 Congenital kyphosis, thoracolumbar region
     Q76.419 Congenital kyphosis, unspecified region

  ✓6ᵗʰ **Q76.42 Congenital lordosis**
     Q76.425 Congenital lordosis, thoracolumbar region
     Q76.426 Congenital lordosis, lumbar region
     Q76.427 Congenital lordosis, lumbosacral region
     Q76.428 Congenital lordosis, sacral and sacrococcygeal region
     Q76.429 Congenital lordosis, unspecified region

  Q76.49 Other congenital malformations of spine, not associated with scoliosis
     Congenital absence of vertebra NOS
     Congenital fusion of spine NOS
     Congenital malformation of lumbosacral (joint) (region) NOS
     Congenital malformation of spine NOS
     Hemivertebra NOS
     Malformation of spine NOS
     Platyspondylisis NOS
     Supernumerary vertebra NOS

Q76.5 Cervical rib
   Supernumerary rib in cervical region

Q76.6 Other congenital malformations of ribs
   Accessory rib
   Congenital absence of rib
   Congenital fusion of ribs
   Congenital malformation of ribs NOS
    EXCLUDES 1   short rib syndrome (Q77.2)

Q76.7 Congenital malformation of sternum
   Congenital absence of sternum
   Sternum bifidum

Q76.8 Other congenital malformations of bony thorax

Q76.9 Congenital malformation of bony thorax, unspecified

✓4ᵗʰ **Q77 Osteochondrodysplasia with defects of growth of tubular bones and spine**
    EXCLUDES 1   mucopolysaccharidosis (E76.0-E76.3)
    EXCLUDES 2   congenital myotonic chondrodystrophy (G71.13)

Q77.0 Achondrogenesis
   Hypochondrogenesis

Q77.1 Thanatophoric short stature

Q77.2 Short rib syndrome
   Asphyxiating thoracic dysplasia [Jeune]

Q77.3 Chondrodysplasia punctata
    EXCLUDES 1   Rhizomelic chondrodysplasia punctata (E71.43)

Q77.4 Achondroplasia
   Hypochondroplasia
   Osteosclerosis congenita

Q77.5 Diastrophic dysplasia

Q77.6 Chondroectodermal dysplasia
   Ellis-van Creveld syndrome

Q77.7 Spondyloepiphyseal dysplasia

Q77.8 Other osteochondrodysplasia with defects of growth of tubular bones and spine

Q77.9 Osteochondrodysplasia with defects of growth of tubular bones and spine, unspecified

✓4ᵗʰ Q78 Other osteochondrodysplasias

EXCLUDES 2   *congenital myotonic chondrodystrophy (G71.13)*

Q78.0 Osteogenesis imperfecta
Fragilitas ossium
Osteopsathyrosis

Q78.1 Polyostotic fibrous dysplasia
Albright(-McCune)(-Sternberg) syndrome

Q78.2 Osteopetrosis
Albers-Schönberg syndrome
Osteosclerosis NOS
DEF: Rare congenital condition in which the bones are excessively dense, resulting from a discrepancy in the formation and breakdown of bone.

Q78.3 Progressive diaphyseal dysplasia
Camurati-Engelmann syndrome

Q78.4 Enchondromatosis
Maffucci's syndrome
Ollier's disease

Q78.5 Metaphyseal dysplasia
Pyle's syndrome

Q78.6 Multiple congenital exostoses
Diaphyseal aclasis

Q78.8 Other specified osteochondrodysplasias
Osteopoikilosis

Q78.9 Osteochondrodysplasia, unspecified
Chondrodystrophy NOS
Osteodystrophy NOS

✓4ᵗʰ Q79 Congenital malformations of musculoskeletal system, not elsewhere classified

EXCLUDES 2   *congenital (sternomastoid) torticollis (Q68.0)*

Q79.0 Congenital diaphragmatic hernia
EXCLUDES 1   *congenital hiatus hernia (Q40.1)*

Q79.1 Other congenital malformations of diaphragm
Absence of diaphragm
Congenital malformation of diaphragm NOS
Eventration of diaphragm

Q79.2 Exomphalos
Omphalocele
EXCLUDES 1   *umbilical hernia (K42.-)*

Q79.3 Gastroschisis

Gastroschisis

Herniated small bowel (gastroschisis)
Rectus abdominus m.
Umbilicus
skin
distal
proximal
Defect

Q79.4 Prune belly syndrome
Congenital prolapse of bladder mucosa
Eagle-Barrett syndrome

✓5ᵗʰ Q79.5 Other congenital malformations of abdominal wall

EXCLUDES 1   *umbilical hernia (K42.-)*

Q79.51 Congenital hernia of bladder
Q79.59 Other congenital malformations of abdominal wall

▲ ✓5ᵗʰ **Q79.6 Ehlers-Danlos syndromes**
DEF: Connective tissue disorder that causes hyperextended skin and joints and results in fragile blood vessels with bleeding, poor wound healing, and subcutaneous pseudotumors.

●   **Q79.60 Ehlers-Danlos syndrome, unspecified**

●   **Q79.61 Classical Ehlers-Danlos syndrome**
Classical EDS (cEDS)

   Q79.62 Hypermobile Ehlers-Danlos syndrome
Hypermobile EDS (hEDS)

●   **Q79.63 Vascular Ehlers-Danlos syndrome**
Vascular EDS (vEDS)

●   **Q79.69 Other Ehlers-Danlos syndromes**

Q79.8 Other congenital malformations of musculoskeletal system
Absence of muscle
Absence of tendon
Accessory muscle
Amyotrophia congenita
Congenital constricting bands
Congenital shortening of tendon
Poland syndrome

Q79.9 Congenital malformation of musculoskeletal system, unspecified
Congenital anomaly of musculoskeletal system NOS
Congenital deformity of musculoskeletal system NOS

Other congenital malformations (Q80-Q89)

✓4ᵗʰ Q80 Congenital ichthyosis

EXCLUDES 1   *Refsum's disease (G60.1)*
DEF: Excessive production of skin cells resulting in red, dry, scaly skin.

Q80.0 Ichthyosis vulgaris

Q80.1 X-linked ichthyosis

Q80.2 Lamellar ichthyosis
Collodion baby

Q80.3 Congenital bullous ichthyosiform erythroderma

Q80.4 Harlequin fetus

Q80.8 Other congenital ichthyosis

Q80.9 Congenital ichthyosis, unspecified

✓4ᵗʰ Q81 Epidermolysis bullosa

Q81.0 Epidermolysis bullosa simplex
EXCLUDES 1   *Cockayne's syndrome ▶(Q87.19)◀*

Q81.1 Epidermolysis bullosa letalis
Herlitz' syndrome

Q81.2 Epidermolysis bullosa dystrophica

Q81.8 Other epidermolysis bullosa

Q81.9 Epidermolysis bullosa, unspecified

✓4ᵗʰ Q82 Other congenital malformations of skin

EXCLUDES 1   *acrodermatitis enteropathica (E83.2)*
congenital erythropoietic porphyria (E80.0)
pilonidal cyst or sinus (L05.-)
Sturge-Weber (-Dimitri) syndrome (Q85.8)

Q82.0 Hereditary lymphedema

Q82.1 Xeroderma pigmentosum

Q82.2 Congenital cutaneous mastocytosis
Congenital diffuse cutaneous mastocytosis
Congenital maculopapular cutaneous mastocytosis
Congenital urticaria pigmentosa
EXCLUDES 1   *cutaneous mastocytosis NOS (D47.01)*
diffuse cutaneous mastocytosis (with onset after newborn period) (D47.01)
malignant mastocytosis (C96.2-)
systemic mastocytosis (D47.02)
urticaria pigmentosa (non-congenital) (with onset after newborn period) (D47.01)

AHA: 2017,4Q,5

Q82.3 Incontinentia pigmenti

Q82.4 Ectodermal dysplasia (anhidrotic)
EXCLUDES 1   *Ellis-van Creveld syndrome (Q77.6)*

✓ Additional Character Required   ✓x7ᵗʰ Placeholder Alert   Manifestation   Unspecified Dx   ▶◀ Revised Text   ● New Code   ▲ Revised Code Title

Q82.5 Congenital non-neoplastic nevus
Birthmark NOS
Flammeus Nevus
Portwine Nevus
Sanguineous Nevus
Strawberry Nevus
Vascular Nevus NOS
Verrucous Nevus
EXCLUDES 2   *araneus nevus (I78.1)*
       Café au lait spots (L81.3)
       lentigo (L81.4)
       melanocytic nevus (D22.-)
       nevus NOS (D22.-)
       pigmented nevus (D22.-)
       spider nevus (I78.1)
       stellar nevus (I78.1)

Q82.6 Congenital sacral dimple
Parasacral dimple
EXCLUDES 2   *pilonidal cyst with abscess (L05.01)*
       pilonidal cyst without abscess (L05.91)
AHA: 2016,4Q,60

Q82.8 Other specified congenital malformations of skin
Abnormal palmar creases
Accessory skin tags
Benign familial pemphigus [Hailey-Hailey]
Congenital poikiloderma
Cutis laxa (hyperelastica)
Dermatoglyphic anomalies
Inherited keratosis palmaris et plantaris
Keratosis follicularis [Darier-White]
EXCLUDES 1   *Ehlers-Danlos syndrome ▶(Q79.6-)◀*
AHA: 2016,1Q,17

Q82.9 Congenital malformation of skin, unspecified

√4ᵗʰ Q83 Congenital malformations of breast
EXCLUDES 2   *absence of pectoral muscle (Q79.8)*
       hypoplasia of breast (N64.82)
       micromastia (N64.82)

Q83.0 Congenital absence of breast with absent nipple

Q83.1 Accessory breast
Supernumerary breast

Q83.2 Absent nipple

Q83.3 Accessory nipple
Supernumerary nipple

Q83.8 Other congenital malformations of breast

Q83.9 Congenital malformation of breast, unspecified

√4ᵗʰ Q84 Other congenital malformations of integument

Q84.0 Congenital alopecia
Congenital atrichosis

Q84.1 Congenital morphological disturbances of hair, not elsewhere classified
Beaded hair
Monilethrix
Pili annulati
EXCLUDES 1   *Menkes' kinky hair syndrome (E83.0)*

Q84.2 Other congenital malformations of hair
Congenital hypertrichosis
Congenital malformation of hair NOS
Persistent lanugo

Q84.3 Anonychia
EXCLUDES 1   *nail patella syndrome (Q87.2)*

Q84.4 Congenital leukonychia

Q84.5 Enlarged and hypertrophic nails
Congenital onychauxis
Pachyonychia

Q84.6 Other congenital malformations of nails
Congenital clubnail
Congenital koilonychia
Congenital malformation of nail NOS

Q84.8 Other specified congenital malformations of integument
Aplasia cutis congenita

Q84.9 Congenital malformation of integument, unspecified
Congenital anomaly of integument NOS
Congenital deformity of integument NOS

√4ᵗʰ Q85 Phakomatoses, not elsewhere classified
EXCLUDES 1   *ataxia telangiectasia [Louis-Bar] (G11.3)*
       familial dysautonomia [Riley-Day] (G90.1)

√5ᵗʰ Q85.0 Neurofibromatosis (nonmalignant)

Q85.00 Neurofibromatosis, unspecified   HCC

Q85.01 Neurofibromatosis, type 1   HCC
Von Recklinghausen disease

Q85.02 Neurofibromatosis, type 2   HCC
Acoustic neurofibromatosis
DEF: Inherited condition with cutaneous lesions, benign tumors of peripheral nerves, and bilateral 8th nerve masses.

Q85.03 Schwannomatosis   HCC
DEF: Genetic mutation (SMARCB1/INI1) causing multiple benign tumors along the nerve pathways, except on the 8th cranial (vestibular) nerve.

Q85.09 Other neurofibromatosis   HCC

Q85.1 Tuberous sclerosis   HCC
Bourneville's disease
Epiloia

Q85.8 Other phakomatoses, not elsewhere classified   HCC
Peutz-Jeghers Syndrome
Sturge-Weber(-Dimitri) syndrome
von Hippel-Lindau syndrome
EXCLUDES 1   *Meckel-Gruber syndrome (Q61.9)*

Q85.9 Phakomatosis, unspecified   HCC
Hamartosis NOS

√4ᵗʰ Q86 Congenital malformation syndromes due to known exogenous causes, not elsewhere classified
EXCLUDES 2   *iodine-deficiency-related hypothyroidism (E00-E02)*
       nonteratogenic effects of substances transmitted via placenta or breast milk (P04.-)

Q86.0 Fetal alcohol syndrome (dysmorphic)

Q86.1 Fetal hydantoin syndrome
Meadow's syndrome

Q86.2 Dysmorphism due to warfarin

Q86.8 Other congenital malformation syndromes due to known exogenous causes

√4ᵗʰ Q87 Other specified congenital malformation syndromes affecting multiple systems
Use additional code(s) to identify all associated manifestations

Q87.0 Congenital malformation syndromes predominantly affecting facial appearance
Acrocephalopolysyndactyly
Acrocephalosyndactyly [Apert]
Cryptophthalmos syndrome
Cyclopia
Goldenhar syndrome
Moebius syndrome
Oro-facial-digital syndrome
Robin syndrome
Whistling face

▲ √5ᵗʰ **Q87.1 Congenital malformation syndromes predominantly associated with short stature**
~~Aarskog syndrome~~
~~Cockayne syndrome~~
~~De Lange syndrome~~
~~Dubowitz syndrome~~
~~Noonan syndrome~~
~~Prader-Willi syndrome~~
~~Robinow-Silverman-Smith syndrome~~
~~Russell-Silver syndrome~~
~~Seckel syndrome~~
EXCLUDES 1   *Ellis-van Creveld syndrome (Q77.6)*
       Smith-Lemli-Opitz syndrome (E78.72)

● **Q87.11 Prader-Willi syndrome**

Q87.19 **Other congenital malformation syndromes predominantly associated with short stature**
Aarskog syndrome
Cockayne syndrome
De Lange syndrome
Dubowitz syndrome
Noonan syndrome
Robinow-Silverman-Smith syndrome
Russell-Silver syndrome
Seckel syndrome

Q87.2 **Congenital malformation syndromes predominantly involving limbs**
Holt-Oram syndrome
Klippel-Trenaunay-Weber syndrome
Nail patella syndrome
Rubinstein-Taybi syndrome
Sirenomelia syndrome
Thrombocytopenia with absent radius [TAR] syndrome
VATER syndrome

Q87.3 **Congenital malformation syndromes involving early overgrowth**
Beckwith-Wiedemann syndrome
Sotos syndrome
Weaver syndrome

☑5ᵗʰ **Q87.4** **Marfan's syndrome**
DEF: Disorder that affects the connective tissue of multiple systems, including disproportionly long or abnormal bone structure and eye and cardiovascular complications.

Q87.40 **Marfan's syndrome, unspecified**

☑6ᵗʰ **Q87.41** **Marfan's syndrome with cardiovascular manifestations**
Q87.410 **Marfan's syndrome with aortic dilation**
Q87.418 **Marfan's syndrome with other cardiovascular manifestations**

Q87.42 **Marfan's syndrome with ocular manifestations**

Q87.43 **Marfan's syndrome with skeletal manifestation**

Q87.5 **Other congenital malformation syndromes with other skeletal changes**

☑6ᵗʰ **Q87.8** **Other specified congenital malformation syndromes, not elsewhere classified**
EXCLUDES 1 *Zellweger syndrome (E71.510)*

Q87.81 **Alport syndrome**
Use additional code to identify stage of chronic kidney disease (N18.1-N18.6)

Q87.82 **Arterial tortuosity syndrome**
AHA: 2016,4Q,60-61

Q87.89 **Other specified congenital malformation syndromes, not elsewhere classified**
Laurence-Moon (-Bardet)-Biedl syndrome

☑4ᵗʰ **Q89** **Other congenital malformations, not elsewhere classified**

☑5ᵗʰ **Q89.0** **Congenital absence and malformations of spleen**
EXCLUDES 1 *isomerism of atrial appendages (with asplenia or polysplenia) (Q20.6)*

Q89.01 **Asplenia (congenital)**

Q89.09 **Congenital malformations of spleen**
Congenital splenomegaly

Q89.1 **Congenital malformations of adrenal gland**
EXCLUDES 1 *adrenogenital disorders (E25.-)*
congenital adrenal hyperplasia (E25.0)

Q89.2 **Congenital malformations of other endocrine glands**
Congenital malformation of parathyroid or thyroid gland
Persistent thyroglossal duct
Thyroglossal cyst
EXCLUDES 1 *congenital goiter (E03.0)*
congenital hypothyroidism (E03.1)

Q89.3 **Situs inversus**
Dextrocardia with situs inversus
Mirror-image atrial arrangement with situs inversus
Situs inversus or transversus abdominalis
Situs inversus or transversus thoracis
Transposition of abdominal viscera
Transposition of thoracic viscera
EXCLUDES 1 *dextrocardia NOS (Q24.0)*
DEF: Congenital anomaly in which the internal thoracic and abdominal organs are transposed laterally and found on the opposite side from the normal position.

Q89.4 **Conjoined twins**
Craniopagus
Dicephaly
Pygopagus
Thoracopagus

Q89.7 **Multiple congenital malformations, not elsewhere classified**
Multiple congenital anomalies NOS
Multiple congenital deformities NOS
EXCLUDES 1 *congenital malformation syndromes affecting multiple systems (Q87.-)*

Q89.8 **Other specified congenital malformations**
Use additional code(s) to identify all associated manifestations

Q89.9 **Congenital malformation, unspecified**
Congenital anomaly NOS
Congenital deformity NOS

Chromosomal abnormalities, not elsewhere classified (Q90-Q99)

EXCLUDES 2 *mitochondrial metabolic disorders (E88.4-)*

☑4ᵗʰ **Q90** **Down syndrome**
Use additional code(s) to identify any associated physical conditions and degree of intellectual disabilities (F70-F79)

Q90.0 **Trisomy 21, nonmosaicism (meiotic nondisjunction)**

Q90.1 **Trisomy 21, mosaicism (mitotic nondisjunction)**

Q90.2 **Trisomy 21, translocation**

Q90.9 **Down syndrome, unspecified**
Trisomy 21 NOS

☑4ᵗʰ **Q91** **Trisomy 18 and Trisomy 13**

Q91.0 **Trisomy 18, nonmosaicism (meiotic nondisjunction)**

Q91.1 **Trisomy 18, mosaicism (mitotic nondisjunction)**

Q91.2 **Trisomy 18, translocation**

Q91.3 **Trisomy 18, unspecified**

Q91.4 **Trisomy 13, nonmosaicism (meiotic nondisjunction)**

Q91.5 **Trisomy 13, mosaicism (mitotic nondisjunction)**

Q91.6 **Trisomy 13, translocation**

Q91.7 **Trisomy 13, unspecified**

☑4ᵗʰ **Q92** **Other trisomies and partial trisomies of the autosomes, not elsewhere classified**
INCLUDES unbalanced translocations and insertions
EXCLUDES 1 *trisomies of chromosomes 13, 18, 21 (Q90-Q91)*

Q92.0 **Whole chromosome trisomy, nonmosaicism (meiotic nondisjunction)**

Q92.1 **Whole chromosome trisomy, mosaicism (mitotic nondisjunction)**

Q92.2 **Partial trisomy**
Less than whole arm duplicated
Whole arm or more duplicated
EXCLUDES 1 *partial trisomy due to unbalanced translocation (Q92.5)*

Q92.5 **Duplications with other complex rearrangements**
Partial trisomy due to unbalanced translocations
Code also any associated deletions due to unbalanced translocations, inversions and insertions (Q93.7)

☑5ᵗʰ **Q92.6** **Marker chromosomes**
Trisomies due to dicentrics
Trisomies due to extra rings
Trisomies due to isochromosomes
Individual with marker heterochromatin

Q92.61 **Marker chromosomes in normal individual**

Q92.62 **Marker chromosomes in abnormal individual**

Q92.7 **Triploidy and polyploidy**

Q92.8 **Other specified trisomies and partial trisomies of autosomes**
Duplications identified by fluorescence in situ hybridization (FISH)
Duplications identified by in situ hybridization (ISH)
Duplications seen only at prometaphase

Q92.9 **Trisomy and partial trisomy of autosomes, unspecified**

☑4ᵗʰ **Q93** **Monosomies and deletions from the autosomes, not elsewhere classified**

Q93.0 **Whole chromosome monosomy, nonmosaicism (meiotic nondisjunction)**

Q93.1 **Whole chromosome monosomy, mosaicism (mitotic nondisjunction)**

Q93.2 **Chromosome replaced with ring, dicentric or isochromosome**

☑ Additional Character Required   ☑x7ᵗʰ Placeholder Alert   Manifestation   Unspecified Dx   ►◄ Revised Text   ● New Code   ▲ Revised Code Title

ICD-10-CM 2020   **925**

Q93.3   **Deletion of short arm of chromosome 4**
Wolff-Hirschorn syndrome

Q93.4   **Deletion of short arm of chromosome 5**
Cri-du-chat syndrome

✓5ᵗʰ   **Q93.5**   **Other deletions of part of a chromosome**
AHA: 2018,4Q,28

    Q93.51   **Angelman syndrome**

    Q93.59   **Other deletions of part of a chromosome**

Q93.7   **Deletions with other complex rearrangements**
Deletions due to unbalanced translocations, inversions and insertions
Code also any associated duplications due to unbalanced translocations, inversions and insertions (Q92.5)

✓6ᵗʰ   **Q93.8**   **Other deletions from the autosomes**

    Q93.81   **Velo-cardio-facial syndrome**
Deletion 22q11.2
DEF: Microdeletion syndrome affecting multiple organs characterized by a cleft palate, heart defects, an elongated face with almond-shaped eyes, wide nose, small ears, weak immune system, weak musculature, hypothyroidism, short stature, and scoliosis. The deletion occurs at q11.2 on the long arm of the chromosome 22.

    Q93.82   **Williams syndrome**
AHA: 2018,4Q,28-29

    Q93.88   **Other microdeletions**
Miller-Dieker syndrome
Smith-Magenis syndrome

    Q93.89   **Other deletions from the autosomes**
Deletions identified by fluorescence in situ hybridization (FISH)
Deletions identified by in situ hybridization (ISH)
Deletions seen only at prometaphase

Q93.9   **Deletion from autosomes, unspecified**

✓4ᵗʰ   **Q95**   **Balanced rearrangements and structural markers, not elsewhere classified**
INCLUDES   Robertsonian and balanced reciprocal translocations and insertions

Q95.0   **Balanced translocation and insertion in normal individual**

Q95.1   **Chromosome inversion in normal individual**

Q95.2   **Balanced autosomal rearrangement in abnormal individual**

Q95.3   **Balanced sex/autosomal rearrangement in abnormal individual**

Q95.5   **Individual with autosomal fragile site**

Q95.8   **Other balanced rearrangements and structural markers**

Q95.9   **Balanced rearrangement and structural marker, unspecified**

✓4ᵗʰ   **Q96**   **Turner's syndrome**
EXCLUDES 1   *Noonan syndrome ▶(Q87.19)◀*

Q96.0   **Karyotype 45, X**   ♀

Q96.1   **Karyotype 46, X iso (Xq)**   ♀
Karyotype 46, isochromosome Xq

Q96.2   **Karyotype 46, X with abnormal sex chromosome, except iso (Xq)**   ♀
Karyotype 46, X with abnormal sex chromosome, except isochromosome Xq

Q96.3   **Mosaicism, 45, X/46, XX or XY**   ♀

Q96.4   **Mosaicism, 45, X/other cell line(s) with abnormal sex chromosome**   ♀

Q96.8   **Other variants of Turner's syndrome**   ♀

Q96.9   **Turner's syndrome, unspecified**   ♀

✓4ᵗʰ   **Q97**   **Other sex chromosome abnormalities, female phenotype, not elsewhere classified**
EXCLUDES 1   *Turner's syndrome (Q96.-)*

Q97.0   **Karyotype 47, XXX**   ♀

Q97.1   **Female with more than three X chromosomes**   ♀

Q97.2   **Mosaicism, lines with various numbers of X chromosomes**   ♀

Q97.3   **Female with 46, XY karyotype**   ♀

Q97.8   **Other specified sex chromosome abnormalities, female phenotype**   ♀

Q97.9   **Sex chromosome abnormality, female phenotype, unspecified**   ♀

✓4ᵗʰ   **Q98**   **Other sex chromosome abnormalities, male phenotype, not elsewhere classified**

Q98.0   **Klinefelter syndrome karyotype 47, XXY**   ♂

Q98.1   **Klinefelter syndrome, male with more than two X chromosomes**   ♂

Q98.3   **Other male with 46, XX karyotype**   ♂

Q98.4   **Klinefelter syndrome, unspecified**   ♂

Q98.5   **Karyotype 47, XYY**

Q98.6   **Male with structurally abnormal sex chromosome**

Q98.7   **Male with sex chromosome mosaicism**   ♂

Q98.8   **Other specified sex chromosome abnormalities, male phenotype**   ♂

Q98.9   **Sex chromosome abnormality, male phenotype, unspecified**   ♂

✓4ᵗʰ   **Q99**   **Other chromosome abnormalities, not elsewhere classified**

Q99.0   **Chimera 46, XX/46, XY**
Chimera 46, XX/46, XY true hermaphrodite

Q99.1   **46, XX true hermaphrodite**
46, XX with streak gonads
46, XY with streak gonads
Pure gonadal dysgenesis

Q99.2   **Fragile X chromosome**
Fragile X syndrome

Q99.8   **Other specified chromosome abnormalities**

Q99.9   **Chromosomal abnormality, unspecified**

Chapter 18. Symptoms, Signs, and Abnormal Clinical and Laboratory Findings, Not Elsewhere Classified (R00–R99)

Chapter-specific Guidelines with Coding Examples

The chapter-specific guidelines from the ICD-10-CM Official Guidelines for Coding and Reporting have been provided below. Along with these guidelines are coding examples, contained in the shaded boxes, that have been developed to help illustrate the coding and/or sequencing guidance found in these guidelines.

Chapter 18 includes symptoms, signs, abnormal results of clinical or other investigative procedures, and ill-defined conditions regarding which no diagnosis classifiable elsewhere is recorded. Signs and symptoms that point to a specific diagnosis have been assigned to a category in other chapters of the classification.

a. Use of symptom codes

Codes that describe symptoms and signs are acceptable for reporting purposes when a related definitive diagnosis has not been established (confirmed) by the provider.

> Tenderness and localized pain in the right upper quadrant; based on presentation, probable gallstones
>
> **R10.11**   **Right upper quadrant pain**
>
> **R10.811**   **Right upper quadrant abdominal tenderness**
>
> *Explanation:* Codes that describe symptoms such as abdominal pain are acceptable for reporting purposes when the provider has not established (confirmed) a definitive diagnosis.

b. Use of a symptom code with a definitive diagnosis code

Codes for signs and symptoms may be reported in addition to a related definitive diagnosis when the sign or symptom is not routinely associated with that diagnosis, such as the various signs and symptoms associated with complex syndromes. The definitive diagnosis code should be sequenced before the symptom code.

Signs or symptoms that are associated routinely with a disease process should not be assigned as additional codes, unless otherwise instructed by the classification.

> Pneumonia with hemoptysis
>
> **J18.9**   **Pneumonia, unspecified organism**
>
> **R04.2**   **Hemoptysis**
>
> *Explanation:* Codes for signs and symptoms may be reported in addition to a related definitive diagnosis when the sign or symptom is not routinely associated with that diagnosis.

> Abdominal pain due to acute appendicitis
>
> **K35.80**   **Unspecified acute appendicitis**
>
> *Explanation:* Codes for signs or symptoms routinely associated with a disease process should not be assigned unless the classification instructs otherwise.

c. Combination codes that include symptoms

ICD-10-CM contains a number of combination codes that identify both the definitive diagnosis and common symptoms of that diagnosis. When using one of these combination codes, an additional code should not be assigned for the symptom.

> IBS with diarrhea
>
> **K58.0**   **Irritable bowel syndrome with diarrhea**
>
> *Explanation:* When a combination code identifies both the definitive diagnosis and the symptom, an additional code should not be assigned for the symptom.

d. Repeated falls

Code R29.6, Repeated falls, is for use for encounters when a patient has recently fallen and the reason for the fall is being investigated.

Code Z91.81, History of falling, is for use when a patient has fallen in the past and is at risk for future falls. When appropriate, both codes R29.6 and Z91.81 may be assigned together.

e. Coma scale

The coma scale codes (R40.2-) can be used in conjunction with traumatic brain injury codes, acute cerebrovascular disease or sequelae of cerebrovascular disease codes. These codes are primarily for use by trauma registries, but they may be used in any setting where this information is collected. The coma scale may also be used to assess the status of the central nervous system for other non-trauma conditions, such as monitoring patients in the intensive care unit regardless of medical condition. The coma scale codes should be sequenced after the diagnosis code(s).

These codes, one from each subcategory, are needed to complete the scale. The 7th character indicates when the scale was recorded. The 7th character should match for all three codes.

At a minimum, report the initial score documented on presentation at your facility. This may be a score from the emergency medicine technician (EMT) or in the emergency department. If desired, a facility may choose to capture multiple coma scale scores.

Assign code R40.24, Glasgow coma scale, total score, when only the total score is documented in the medical record and not the individual score(s).

Do not report codes for individual or total Glasgow coma scale scores for a patient with a medically induced coma or a sedated patient.

See Section I.B.14 for coma scale documentation by clinicians other than patient's provider

> 36-year-old man found down after unknown injury with skull fracture and with concussion and loss of consciousness of unknown duration. Upon hospital admission, the patient was evaluated with the following Glasgow coma scores:
>
> Eye-opening response—3: eyes open to speech
>
> Verbal response—3: random speech with no conversational exchange
>
> Motor response—4: pulls limb away from painful stimulus
>
> **S02.0XXA**   **Fracture of vault of skull, initial encounter for closed fracture**
>
> **S06.0X9A**   **Concussion with loss of consciousness of unspecified duration, initial encounter**
>
> **R40.2133**   **Coma scale, eyes open, to sound, at hospital admission**
>
> **R40.2233**   **Coma scale, best verbal response, inappropriate words, at hospital admission**
>
> **R40.2343**   **Coma scale, best motor response, flexion withdrawal, at hospital admission**
>
> *Explanation:* When individual scores for the Glasgow coma scale are documented, one code from each category is needed to complete the scale. The seventh character indicates when the scale was recorded and should match for all three codes. Assign a code from subcategory R40.24- Glasgow coma scale, total score, when only the total and not the individual score(s) is documented.

f. Functional quadriplegia

GUIDELINE HAS BEEN DELETED EFFECTIVE OCTOBER 1, 2017

g. SIRS due to non-infectious process

The systemic inflammatory response syndrome (SIRS) can develop as a result of certain non-infectious disease processes, such as trauma, malignant neoplasm, or pancreatitis. When SIRS is documented with a noninfectious condition, and no subsequent infection is documented, the code for the underlying condition, such as an injury, should be assigned, followed by code R65.10, Systemic inflammatory response syndrome (SIRS) of non-infectious origin without acute organ dysfunction, or code R65.11, Systemic inflammatory response syndrome (SIRS) of non-infectious origin with acute organ dysfunction. If an associated acute organ dysfunction is documented, the appropriate code(s) for the specific type of organ dysfunction(s) should be assigned in addition to code R65.11. If acute organ dysfunction is documented, but it cannot be determined if the acute organ dysfunction is associated with SIRS or due to another condition (e.g., directly due to the trauma), the provider should be queried.

Systemic inflammatory response syndrome (SIRS) due to acute gallstone pancreatitis

K85.1Ø   Biliary acute pancreatitis without necrosis or infection

R65.1Ø   Systemic inflammatory response syndrome [SIRS] of non-infectious origin without acute organ dysfunction

Explanation: When SIRS is documented with a non-infectious condition without subsequent infection documented, the code for the underlying condition such as pancreatitis should be assigned followed by the appropriate code for SIRS of noninfectious origin, either with or without associated organ dysfunction.

h. Death NOS

Code R99, Ill-defined and unknown cause of mortality, is only for use in the very limited circumstance when a patient who has already died is brought into an emergency department or other healthcare facility and is pronounced dead upon arrival. It does not represent the discharge disposition of death.

i. NIHSS stroke scale

The NIH stroke scale (NIHSS) codes (R29.7- -) can be used in conjunction with acute stroke codes (I63) to identify the patient's neurological status and the severity of the stroke. The stroke scale codes should be sequenced after the acute stroke diagnosis code(s).

At a minimum, report the initial score documented. If desired, a facility may choose to capture multiple stroke scale scores.

See Section I.B.14 for NIHSS stroke scale documentation by clinicians other than patient's provider

Chapter 18. Symptoms, Signs and Abnormal Clinical and Laboratory Findings, Not Elsewhere Classified (R00-R99)

NOTE　This chapter includes symptoms, signs, abnormal results of clinical or other investigative procedures, and ill-defined conditions regarding which no diagnosis classifiable elsewhere is recorded.

Signs and symptoms that point rather definitely to a given diagnosis have been assigned to a category in other chapters of the classification. In general, categories in this chapter include the less well-defined conditions and symptoms that, without the necessary study of the case to establish a final diagnosis, point perhaps equally to two or more diseases or to two or more systems of the body. Practically all categories in the chapter could be designated 'not otherwise specified', 'unknown etiology' or 'transient'. The Alphabetical Index should be consulted to determine which symptoms and signs are to be allocated here and which to other chapters. The residual subcategories, numbered .8, are generally provided for other relevant symptoms that cannot be allocated elsewhere in the classification.

The conditions and signs or symptoms included in categories R00-R94 consist of:

(a) cases for which no more specific diagnosis can be made even after all the facts bearing on the case have been investigated;

(b) signs or symptoms existing at the time of initial encounter that proved to be transient and whose causes could not be determined;

(c) provisional diagnosis in a patient who failed to return for further investigation or care;

(d) cases referred elsewhere for investigation or treatment before the diagnosis was made;

(e) cases in which a more precise diagnosis was not available for any other reason;

(f) certain symptoms, for which supplementary information is provided, that represent important problems in medical care in their own right.

EXCLUDES 2　*abnormal findings on antenatal screening of mother (O28.-)*
certain conditions originating in the perinatal period (P04 P96)
signs and symptoms classified in the body system chapters
signs and symptoms of breast (N63, N64.5)

AHA: 2017,1Q,6,7

This chapter contains the following blocks:

R00-R09	Symptoms and signs involving the circulatory and respiratory systems
R10-R19	Symptoms and signs involving the digestive system and abdomen
R20-R23	Symptoms and signs involving the skin and subcutaneous tissue
R25-R29	Symptoms and signs involving the nervous and musculoskeletal systems
R30-R39	Symptoms and signs involving the genitourinary system
R40-R46	Symptoms and signs involving cognition, perception, emotional state and behavior
R47-R49	Symptoms and signs involving speech and voice
R50-R69	General symptoms and signs
R70-R79	Abnormal findings on examination of blood, without diagnosis
R80-R82	Abnormal findings on examination of urine, without diagnosis
R83-R89	Abnormal findings on examination of other body fluids, substances and tissues, without diagnosis
R90-R94	Abnormal findings on diagnostic imaging and in function studies, without diagnosis
R97	Abnormal tumor markers
R99	Ill-defined and unknown cause of mortality

Symptoms and signs involving the circulatory and respiratory systems (R00-R09)

☑4ᵗʰ　**R00　Abnormalities of heart beat**

EXCLUDES 1　*abnormalities originating in the perinatal period (P29.1-)*
EXCLUDES 2　*specified arrhythmias (I47-I49)*

R00.0　Tachycardia, unspecified
Rapid heart beat
Sinoauricular tachycardia NOS
Sinus [sinusal] tachycardia NOS
EXCLUDES 1　*neonatal tachycardia (P29.11)*
paroxysmal tachycardia (I47.-)
DEF: Excessively rapid heart rate of more than 100 beats per minute.

R00.1　Bradycardia, unspecified
Sinoatrial bradycardia
Sinus bradycardia
Slow heart beat
Vagal bradycardia
Use additional code for adverse effect, if applicable, to identify drug (T36-T50 with fifth or sixth character 5)
EXCLUDES 1　*neonatal bradycardia (P29.12)*
DEF: Slowed heartbeat, usually defined as a rate fewer than 60 beats per minute. Heart rhythm may be slow as a result of a congenital defect or an acquired problem.

R00.2　Palpitations
Awareness of heart beat

R00.8　Other abnormalities of heart beat

R00.9　Unspecified abnormalities of heart beat

☑4ᵗʰ　**R01　Cardiac murmurs and other cardiac sounds**

EXCLUDES 1　*cardiac murmurs and sounds originating in the perinatal period (P29.8)*

R01.0　Benign and innocent cardiac murmurs
Functional cardiac murmur

R01.1　Cardiac murmur, unspecified
Cardiac bruit NOS
Heart murmur NOS
Systolic murmur NOS

R01.2　Other cardiac sounds
Cardiac dullness, increased or decreased
Precordial friction

☑4ᵗʰ　**R03　Abnormal blood-pressure reading, without diagnosis**

R03.0　Elevated blood-pressure reading, without diagnosis of hypertension
NOTE　This category is to be used to record an episode of elevated blood pressure in a patient in whom no formal diagnosis of hypertension has been made, or as an isolated incidental finding.

R03.1　Nonspecific low blood-pressure reading
EXCLUDES 1　*hypotension (I95.-)*
maternal hypotension syndrome (O26.5-)
neurogenic orthostatic hypotension (G90.3)

☑4ᵗʰ　**R04　Hemorrhage from respiratory passages**

R04.0　Epistaxis
Hemorrhage from nose
Nosebleed

R04.1　Hemorrhage from throat
EXCLUDES 2　*hemoptysis (R04.2)*

R04.2　Hemoptysis
Blood-stained sputum
Cough with hemorrhage
AHA: 2013,4Q,118

☑5ᵗʰ　**R04.8　Hemorrhage from other sites in respiratory passages**

R04.81　Acute idiopathic pulmonary hemorrhage in infants　P
AIPHI
Acute idiopathic hemorrhage in infants over 28 days old
EXCLUDES 1　*perinatal pulmonary hemorrhage (P26.-)*
von Willebrand's disease (D68.0)

R04.89　Hemorrhage from other sites in respiratory passages
Pulmonary hemorrhage NOS

R04.9　Hemorrhage from respiratory passages, unspecified

R05　Cough
EXCLUDES 1　*cough with hemorrhage (R04.2)*
smoker's cough (J41.0)
AHA: 2016,2Q,33

☑ Additional Character Required　　☑x7ᵗʰ Placeholder Alert　　Manifestation　　Unspecified Dx　　►◄ Revised Text　　● New Code　　▲ Revised Code Title

ICD-10-CM 2020　　　　　　　　　　　　　　　　　　　　　　　　　　　　　　　　929

Chapter 18. Symptoms, Signs and Abnormal Clinical and Laboratory Findings

R06–R09.89

✓4th **R06 Abnormalities of breathing**

> EXCLUDES 1   *acute respiratory distress syndrome (J80)*
> *respiratory arrest (R09.2)*
> *respiratory arrest of newborn (P28.81)*
> *respiratory distress syndrome of newborn (P22.-)*
> *respiratory failure (J96.-)*
> *respiratory failure of newborn (P28.5)*

> ✓5th **R06.0 Dyspnea**
> > EXCLUDES 1   *tachypnea NOS (R06.82)*
> > *transient tachypnea of newborn (P22.1)*
> >
> > **R06.00 Dyspnea, unspecified**
> > AHA: 2017,1Q,26
> > **R06.01 Orthopnea**
> > **R06.02 Shortness of breath**
> > **R06.03 Acute respiratory distress**
> > AHA: 2017,4Q,23
> > **R06.09 Other forms of dyspnea**
>
> **R06.1 Stridor**
> > EXCLUDES 1   *congenital laryngeal stridor (P28.89)*
> > *laryngismus (stridulus) (J38.5)*
> >
> > **DEF:** Certain type of wheezing described as a loud, constant, musical sound produced when breathing with an obstructed airway, like the inspiratory sound heard when laryngeal or esophageal obstruction is present.
>
> **R06.2 Wheezing**
> > EXCLUDES 1   *asthma (J45.-)*
> >
> > AHA: 2016,2Q,33
> > **DEF:** High-pitched whistling sound during breathing due to stenosis of the respiratory passageway. Wheezing is associated with asthma, sleep apnea, bronchiectasis, bronchiolitis, COPD, and pleural effusion.
>
> **R06.3 Periodic breathing**
> > Cheyne-Stokes breathing
>
> **R06.4 Hyperventilation**
> > EXCLUDES 1   *psychogenic hyperventilation (F45.8)*
>
> **R06.5 Mouth breathing**
> > EXCLUDES 2   *dry mouth NOS (R68.2)*
>
> **R06.6 Hiccough**
> > EXCLUDES 1   *psychogenic hiccough (F45.8)*
>
> **R06.7 Sneezing**
> ✓5th **R06.8 Other abnormalities of breathing**
> > **R06.81 Apnea, not elsewhere classified**
> > Apnea NOS
> > > EXCLUDES 1   *apnea (of) newborn (P28.4)*
> > > *sleep apnea (G47.3-)*
> > > *sleep apnea of newborn (primary) (P28.3)*
> >
> > **R06.82 Tachypnea, not elsewhere classified**
> > Tachypnea NOS
> > > EXCLUDES 1   *transitory tachypnea of newborn (P22.1)*
> >
> > **R06.83 Snoring**
> > **R06.89 Other abnormalities of breathing**
> > Breath-holding (spells)
> > Sighing
>
> **R06.9 Unspecified abnormalities of breathing**

✓4th **R07 Pain in throat and chest**

> EXCLUDES 1   *epidemic myalgia (B33.0)*
> EXCLUDES 2   *jaw pain R68.84*
> *pain in breast (N64.4)*

> **R07.0 Pain in throat**
> > EXCLUDES 1   *chronic sore throat (J31.2)*
> > *sore throat (acute) NOS (J02.9)*
> > EXCLUDES 2   *dysphagia (R13.1-)*
> > *pain in neck (M54.2)*
>
> **R07.1 Chest pain on breathing**
> > Painful respiration
>
> **R07.2 Precordial pain**
> > **DEF:** Pain felt in the anterior (front) chest wall over the region of the heart. This type of pain is generally felt slightly to the left of the sternum, but may also extend into the surrounding chest wall region.
>
> ✓5th **R07.8 Other chest pain**
> > **R07.81 Pleurodynia**
> > Pleurodynia NOS
> > > EXCLUDES 1   *epidemic pleurodynia (B33.0)*
> >
> > **R07.82 Intercostal pain**

R07.89 Other chest pain
> Anterior chest-wall pain NOS

R07.9 Chest pain, unspecified

✓4th **R09 Other symptoms and signs involving the circulatory and respiratory system**

> EXCLUDES 1   *acute respiratory distress syndrome (J80)*
> *respiratory arrest of newborn (P28.81)*
> *respiratory distress syndrome of newborn (P22.0)*
> *respiratory failure (J96.-)*
> *respiratory failure of newborn (P28.5)*

> ✓5th **R09.0 Asphyxia and hypoxemia**
> > EXCLUDES 1   *asphyxia due to carbon monoxide (T58.-)*
> > *asphyxia due to foreign body in respiratory tract (T17.-)*
> > *birth (intrauterine) asphyxia (P84)*
> > *hyperventilation (R06.4)*
> > *traumatic asphyxia (T71.-)*
> > EXCLUDES 2   *hypercapnia (R06.89)*
> >
> > **R09.01 Asphyxia**
> > **DEF:** Interference of oxygen intake due to obstruction or injury of airways resulting in a lack of oxygen perfusion to the tissues or excessive carbon dioxide in the blood. Can cause unconsciousness or death.
> >
> > **R09.02 Hypoxemia**
> > **DEF:** Insufficient oxygen in the arterial blood resulting in inadequate delivery of oxygen to the body tissues.
>
> **R09.1 Pleurisy**
> > EXCLUDES 1   *pleurisy with effusion (J90)*
>
> **R09.2 Respiratory arrest**   HCC
> > Cardiorespiratory failure
> > > EXCLUDES 1   *cardiac arrest (I46.-)*
> > > *respiratory arrest of newborn (P28.81)*
> > > *respiratory distress of newborn (P22.0)*
> > > *respiratory failure (J96.-)*
> > > *respiratory failure of newborn (P28.5)*
> > > *respiratory insufficiency (R06.89)*
> > > *respiratory insufficiency of newborn (P28.5)*
>
> **R09.3 Abnormal sputum**
> > Abnormal amount of sputum
> > Abnormal color of sputum
> > Abnormal odor of sputum
> > Excessive sputum
> > > EXCLUDES 1   *blood-stained sputum (R04.2)*
>
> ✓5th **R09.8 Other specified symptoms and signs involving the circulatory and respiratory systems**
> > **R09.81 Nasal congestion**
> > **R09.82 Postnasal drip**
> > **R09.89 Other specified symptoms and signs involving the circulatory and respiratory systems**
> > Abnormal chest percussion
> > Bruit (arterial)
> > Chest tympany
> > Choking sensation
> > Feeling of foreign body in throat
> > Friction sounds in chest
> > Rales
> > Weak pulse
> > > EXCLUDES 2   *foreign body in throat (T17.2-)*
> > > *wheezing (R06.2)*

Symptoms and signs involving the digestive system and abdomen (R10-R19)

EXCLUDES 2   congenital or infantile pylorospasm (Q40.0)
gastrointestinal hemorrhage (K92.0-K92.2)
intestinal obstruction (K56.-)
newborn gastrointestinal hemorrhage (P54.0-P54.3)
newborn intestinal obstruction (P76.-)
pylorospasm (K31.3)
signs and symptoms involving the urinary system (R30-R39)
symptoms referable to female genital organs (N94.-)
symptoms referable to male genital organs (N48-N50)

✓4th **R10 Abdominal and pelvic pain**
   EXCLUDES 1   renal colic (N23)
   EXCLUDES 2   dorsalgia (M54.-)
     flatulence and related conditions (R14.-)

   R10.0 Acute abdomen   🔲
     Severe abdominal pain (generalized) (with abdominal rigidity)
     EXCLUDES 1   abdominal rigidity NOS (R19.3)
       generalized abdominal pain NOS (R10.84)
       localized abdominal pain (R10.1-R10.3-)

✓5th **R10.1 Pain localized to upper abdomen**
     R10.10 Upper abdominal pain, unspecified   🔲
     R10.11 Right upper quadrant pain
     R10.12 Left upper quadrant pain
     R10.13 Epigastric pain   🔲
       Dyspepsia
       EXCLUDES 1   functional dyspepsia (K30)

Abdominal Pain

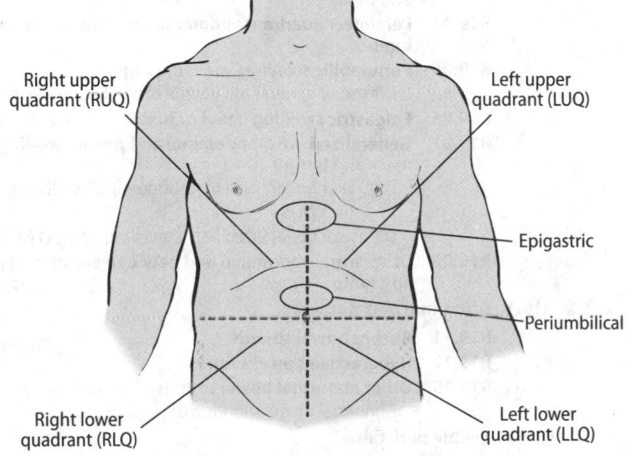

Right upper quadrant (RUQ) — Left upper quadrant (LUQ) — Epigastric — Periumbilical — Right lower quadrant (RLQ) — Left lower quadrant (LLQ)

   R10.2 Pelvic and perineal pain   🔲
     EXCLUDES 1   vulvodynia (N94.81)

✓5th **R10.3 Pain localized to other parts of lower abdomen**
     R10.30 Lower abdominal pain, unspecified   🔲
     R10.31 Right lower quadrant pain   🔲
     R10.32 Left lower quadrant pain   🔲
     R10.33 Periumbilical pain   🔲

✓5th **R10.8 Other abdominal pain**
     ✓6th **R10.81 Abdominal tenderness**
       Abdominal tenderness NOS
       R10.811 Right upper quadrant abdominal tenderness
       R10.812 Left upper quadrant abdominal tenderness
       R10.813 Right lower quadrant abdominal tenderness   🔲
       R10.814 Left lower quadrant abdominal tenderness   🔲
       R10.815 Periumbilic abdominal tenderness   🔲
       R10.816 Epigastric abdominal tenderness   🔲
       R10.817 Generalized abdominal tenderness   🔲

       R10.819 Abdominal tenderness, unspecified site   🔲
     ✓6th **R10.82 Rebound abdominal tenderness**
       R10.821 Right upper quadrant rebound abdominal tenderness
       R10.822 Left upper quadrant rebound abdominal tenderness
       R10.823 Right lower quadrant rebound abdominal tenderness   🔲
       R10.824 Left lower quadrant rebound abdominal tenderness   🔲
       R10.825 Periumbilic rebound abdominal tenderness   🔲
       R10.826 Epigastric rebound abdominal tenderness   🔲
       R10.827 Generalized rebound abdominal tenderness   🔲
       R10.829 Rebound abdominal tenderness, unspecified site   🔲

     R10.83 Colic   🅿
       Colic NOS
       Infantile colic
       EXCLUDES 1   colic in adult and child over 12 months old (R10.84)
       DEF: Inconsolable crying in an otherwise well-fed and healthy infant for more than three hours a day, three days a week, for more than three weeks.
     R10.84 Generalized abdominal pain   🔲
       EXCLUDES 1   generalized abdominal pain associated with acute abdomen (R10.0)

   R10.9 Unspecified abdominal pain   🔲

✓4th **R11 Nausea and vomiting**
   EXCLUDES 1   cyclical vomiting associated with migraine (G43.A-)
     excessive vomiting in pregnancy (O21.-)
     hematemesis (K92.0)
     neonatal hematemesis (P54.0)
     newborn vomiting (P92.0-)
     psychogenic vomiting (F50.89)
     vomiting associated with bulimia nervosa (F50.2)
     vomiting following gastrointestinal surgery (K91.0)

   AHA: 2017,1Q,28
   TIP: Assign a code from this category along with K31.89 Other diseases of stomach and duodenum, to describe cyclical vomiting not due to migraine.

   R11.0 Nausea
     Nausea NOS
     Nausea without vomiting

✓5th **R11.1 Vomiting**
     R11.10 Vomiting, unspecified
       Vomiting NOS
     R11.11 Vomiting without nausea
     R11.12 Projectile vomiting
     R11.13 Vomiting of fecal matter
     R11.14 Bilious vomiting
       Bilious emesis
     R11.15 Cyclical vomiting syndrome unrelated to migraine
       Cyclic vomiting syndrome NOS
       Persistent vomiting
       EXCLUDES 1   cyclical vomiting in migraine (G43.A-)
       EXCLUDES 2   bulimia nervosa (F50.2)
         diabetes mellitus due to underlying condition (E08.-)

   R11.2 Nausea with vomiting, unspecified
     Persistent nausea with vomiting NOS

   R12 Heartburn
     EXCLUDES 1   dyspepsia NOS (R10.13)
       functional dyspepsia (K30)

✓4th **R13 Aphagia and dysphagia**
   R13.0 Aphagia
     Inability to swallow
     EXCLUDES 1   psychogenic aphagia (F50.9)

✓ Additional Character Required   ✓x7th Placeholder Alert   Manifestation   Unspecified Dx   ►◄ Revised Text   ● New Code   ▲ Revised Code Title

ICD-10-CM 2020   931

√5ᵗʰ **R13.1 Dysphagia**

> Code first, if applicable, dysphagia following cerebrovascular disease (I69. with final characters -91)
> *EXCLUDES 1*   *psychogenic dysphagia (F45.8)*

Swallowing Function

Oral phase

Oropharyngeal phase

Pharyngeal phase

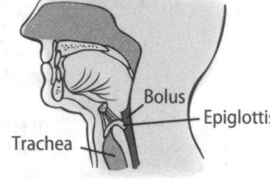

Pharyngoesophageal phase

> **R13.10 Dysphagia, unspecified**
> Difficulty in swallowing NOS
> **R13.11 Dysphagia, oral phase**
> **R13.12 Dysphagia, oropharyngeal phase**
> **R13.13 Dysphagia, pharyngeal phase**
> **R13.14 Dysphagia, pharyngoesophageal phase**
> **R13.19 Other dysphagia**
> Cervical dysphagia
> Neurogenic dysphagia

√4ᵗʰ **R14 Flatulence and related conditions**

> *EXCLUDES 1*   *psychogenic aerophagy (F45.8)*
> **R14.0 Abdominal distension (gaseous)**
> Bloating
> Tympanites (abdominal) (intestinal)
> **R14.1 Gas pain**
> **R14.2 Eructation**
> **R14.3 Flatulence**

√4ᵗʰ **R15 Fecal incontinence**

> *INCLUDES*   encopresis NOS
> *EXCLUDES 1*   *fecal incontinence of nonorganic origin (F98.1)*
> **R15.0 Incomplete defecation**
> *EXCLUDES 1*   *constipation (K59.0-)*
>   *fecal impaction (K56.41)*
> **R15.1 Fecal smearing**
> Fecal soiling
> **R15.2 Fecal urgency**
> **R15.9 Full incontinence of feces**
> Fecal incontinence NOS

√4ᵗʰ **R16 Hepatomegaly and splenomegaly, not elsewhere classified**

> **R16.0 Hepatomegaly, not elsewhere classified**
> Hepatomegaly NOS
> **R16.1 Splenomegaly, not elsewhere classified**
> Splenomegaly NOS
> **R16.2 Hepatomegaly with splenomegaly, not elsewhere classified**
> Hepatosplenomegaly NOS

R17 Unspecified jaundice

> *EXCLUDES 1*   *neonatal jaundice (P55, P57-P59)*

√4ᵗʰ **R18 Ascites**

> *INCLUDES*   fluid in peritoneal cavity
> *EXCLUDES 1*   *ascites in alcoholic cirrhosis (K70.31)*
>   *ascites in alcoholic hepatitis (K70.11)*
>   *ascites in toxic liver disease with chronic active hepatitis (K71.51)*
> **DEF:** Abnormal accumulation of free fluid in the abdominal cavity, causing distention and tightness in addition to shortness of breath as the fluid accumulates. Ascites is usually an underlying disorder and can be a manifestation of any number of diseases.
> **R18.0 Malignant ascites**
> Code first malignancy, such as:
>   malignant neoplasm of ovary (C56.-)
>   secondary malignant neoplasm of retroperitoneum and peritoneum (C78.6)
> **R18.8 Other ascites**
> Ascites NOS
> Peritoneal effusion (chronic)
> **AHA:** 2018,1Q,4

√4ᵗʰ **R19 Other symptoms and signs involving the digestive system and abdomen**

> *EXCLUDES 1*   *acute abdomen (R10.0)*

√5ᵗʰ **R19.0 Intra-abdominal and pelvic swelling, mass and lump**

> *EXCLUDES 1*   *abdominal distension (gaseous) (R14.-)*
>   *ascites (R18.-)*
> **R19.00 Intra-abdominal and pelvic swelling, mass and lump, unspecified site**
> **R19.01 Right upper quadrant abdominal swelling, mass and lump**
> **R19.02 Left upper quadrant abdominal swelling, mass and lump**
> **R19.03 Right lower quadrant abdominal swelling, mass and lump**
> **R19.04 Left lower quadrant abdominal swelling, mass and lump**
> **R19.05 Periumbilic swelling, mass or lump**
> Diffuse or generalized umbilical swelling or mass
> **R19.06 Epigastric swelling, mass or lump**
> **R19.07 Generalized intra-abdominal and pelvic swelling, mass and lump**
> Diffuse or generalized intra-abdominal swelling or mass NOS
> Diffuse or generalized pelvic swelling or mass NOS
> **R19.09 Other intra-abdominal and pelvic swelling, mass and lump**

√5ᵗʰ **R19.1 Abnormal bowel sounds**

> **R19.11 Absent bowel sounds**
> **R19.12 Hyperactive bowel sounds**
> **R19.15 Other abnormal bowel sounds**
> Abnormal bowel sounds NOS

R19.2 Visible peristalsis

> Hyperperistalsis
> **DEF:** Visible movements of muscular attempts to move food through the digestive tract due to pyloric obstruction, stomach obstruction, or intestinal obstruction.

√5ᵗʰ **R19.3 Abdominal rigidity**

> *EXCLUDES 1*   *abdominal rigidity with severe abdominal pain (R10.0)*
> **R19.30 Abdominal rigidity, unspecified site**
> **R19.31 Right upper quadrant abdominal rigidity**
> **R19.32 Left upper quadrant abdominal rigidity**
> **R19.33 Right lower quadrant abdominal rigidity**
> **R19.34 Left lower quadrant abdominal rigidity**
> **R19.35 Periumbilic abdominal rigidity**
> **R19.36 Epigastric abdominal rigidity**
> **R19.37 Generalized abdominal rigidity**

R19.4 Change in bowel habit

> *EXCLUDES 1*   *constipation (K59.0-)*
>   *functional diarrhea (K59.1)*

R19.5 **Other fecal abnormalities**
Abnormal stool color
Bulky stools
Mucus in stools
Occult blood in feces
Occult blood in stools
> EXCLUDES 1   *melena (K92.1)*
>   *neonatal melena (P54.1)*
>
> **AHA:** 2019,1Q,32

R19.6 **Halitosis**

R19.7 **Diarrhea, unspecified**
Diarrhea NOS
> EXCLUDES 1   *functional diarrhea (K59.1)*
>   *neonatal diarrhea (P78.3)*
>   *psychogenic diarrhea (F45.8)*

R19.8 **Other specified symptoms and signs involving the digestive system and abdomen**

Symptoms and signs involving the skin and subcutaneous tissue (R20-R23)

> EXCLUDES 2   *symptoms relating to breast (N64.4-N64.5)*

✓4ᵗʰ **R20** **Disturbances of skin sensation**
> EXCLUDES 1   *dissociative anesthesia and sensory loss (F44.6)*
>   *psychogenic disturbances (F45.8)*

R20.0 **Anesthesia of skin**

R20.1 **Hypoesthesia of skin**

R20.2 **Paresthesia of skin**
Formication
Pins and needles
Tingling skin
> EXCLUDES 1   *acroparesthesia (I73.8)*

R20.3 **Hyperesthesia**

R20.8 **Other disturbances of skin sensation**

R20.9 **Unspecified disturbances of skin sensation**

R21 **Rash and other nonspecific skin eruption**
> INCLUDES   rash NOS
> EXCLUDES 1   *specified type of rash — code to condition*
>   *vesicular eruption (R23.8)*

✓4ᵗʰ **R22** **Localized swelling, mass and lump of skin and subcutaneous tissue**
> INCLUDES   subcutaneous nodules (localized)(superficial)
> EXCLUDES 1   *abnormal findings on diagnostic imaging (R90-R93)*
>   *edema (R60.-)*
>   *enlarged lymph nodes (R59.-)*
>   *localized adiposity (E65)*
>   *swelling of joint (M25.4-)*

R22.0 **Localized swelling, mass and lump, head**

R22.1 **Localized swelling, mass and lump, neck**

R22.2 **Localized swelling, mass and lump, trunk**
> EXCLUDES 1   *intra-abdominal or pelvic mass and lump (R19.0-)*
>   *intra-abdominal or pelvic swelling (R19.0-)*
> EXCLUDES 2   *breast mass and lump (N63)*

✓5ᵗʰ **R22.3** **Localized swelling, mass and lump, upper limb**

     R22.30 **Localized swelling, mass and lump, unspecified upper limb**

     R22.31 **Localized swelling, mass and lump, right upper limb**

     R22.32 **Localized swelling, mass and lump, left upper limb**

     R22.33 **Localized swelling, mass and lump, upper limb, bilateral**

✓5ᵗʰ **R22.4** **Localized swelling, mass and lump, lower limb**

     R22.40 **Localized swelling, mass and lump, unspecified lower limb**

     R22.41 **Localized swelling, mass and lump, right lower limb**

     R22.42 **Localized swelling, mass and lump, left lower limb**

     R22.43 **Localized swelling, mass and lump, lower limb, bilateral**

R22.9 **Localized swelling, mass and lump, unspecified**

✓4ᵗʰ **R23** **Other skin changes**

R23.0 **Cyanosis**
> EXCLUDES 1   *acrocyanosis (I73.8)*
>   *cyanotic attacks of newborn (P28.2)*
>
> **DEF:** Bluish or purplish discoloration of the skin due to an inadequate oxygen blood level.

R23.1 **Pallor**
Clammy skin

R23.2 **Flushing**
Excessive blushing
Code first, if applicable, menopausal and female climacteric states (N95.1)

R23.3 **Spontaneous ecchymoses**
Petechiae
> EXCLUDES 1   *ecchymoses of newborn (P54.5)*
>   *purpura (D69.-)*

R23.4 **Changes in skin texture**
Desquamation of skin
Induration of skin
Scaling of skin
> EXCLUDES 1   *epidermal thickening NOS (L85.9)*

R23.8 **Other skin changes**

R23.9 **Unspecified skin changes**

Symptoms and signs involving the nervous and musculoskeletal systems (R25-R29)

✓4ᵗʰ **R25** **Abnormal involuntary movements**
> EXCLUDES 1   *specific movement disorders (G20-G26)*
>   *stereotyped movement disorders (F98.4)*
>   *tic disorders (F95.-)*

R25.0 **Abnormal head movements**

R25.1 **Tremor, unspecified**
> EXCLUDES 1   *chorea NOS (G25.5)*
>   *essential tremor (G25.0)*
>   *hysterical tremor (F44.4)*
>   *intention tremor (G25.2)*

R25.2 **Cramp and spasm**
> EXCLUDES 2   *carpopedal spasm (R29.0)*
>   *charley-horse (M62.831)*
>   *infantile spasms (G40.4-)*
>   *muscle spasm of back (M62.830)*
>   *muscle spasm of calf (M62.831)*

R25.3 **Fasciculation**
Twitching NOS

R25.8 **Other abnormal involuntary movements**

R25.9 **Unspecified abnormal involuntary movements**

✓4ᵗʰ **R26** **Abnormalities of gait and mobility**
> EXCLUDES 1   *ataxia NOS (R27.0)*
>   *hereditary ataxia (G11.-)*
>   *locomotor (syphilitic) ataxia (A52.11)*
>   *immobility syndrome (paraplegic) (M62.3)*

R26.0 **Ataxic gait**
Staggering gait

R26.1 **Paralytic gait**
Spastic gait

R26.2 **Difficulty in walking, not elsewhere classified**
> EXCLUDES 1   *falling (R29.6)*
>   *unsteadiness on feet (R26.81)*
>
> **AHA:** 2016,2Q,7

✓5ᵗʰ **R26.8** **Other abnormalities of gait and mobility**

     R26.81 **Unsteadiness on feet**

     R26.89 **Other abnormalities of gait and mobility**

R26.9 **Unspecified abnormalities of gait and mobility**

✓4ᵗʰ **R27** **Other lack of coordination**
> EXCLUDES 1   *ataxic gait (R26.0)*
>   *hereditary ataxia (G11.-)*
>   *vertigo NOS (R42)*

R27.0 **Ataxia, unspecified**
> EXCLUDES 1   *ataxia following cerebrovascular disease (I69. with final characters -93)*

R27.8 **Other lack of coordination**

R27.9 **Unspecified lack of coordination**

☑ Additional Character Required   ✓ₓ7ᵗʰ Placeholder Alert   Manifestation   Unspecified Dx   ►◄ Revised Text   ● New Code   ▲ Revised Code Title

ICD-10-CM 2020   933

Chapter 18. Symptoms, Signs and Abnormal Clinical and Laboratory Findings

R29–R31.9

√4th **R29 Other symptoms and signs involving the nervous and musculoskeletal systems**

R29.0 Tetany
Carpopedal spasm
> EXCLUDES 1   *hysterical tetany (F44.5)*
> *neonatal tetany (P71.3)*
> *parathyroid tetany (E20.9)*
> *post-thyroidectomy tetany (E89.2)*

DEF: Calcium or other mineral imbalance causing voluntary muscles such as hands, feet, or larynx to spasm rhythmically.

R29.1 Meningismus

R29.2 Abnormal reflex
> EXCLUDES 2   *abnormal pupillary reflex (H57.0)*
> *hyperactive gag reflex (J39.2)*
> *vasovagal reaction or syncope (R55)*

R29.3 Abnormal posture

R29.4 Clicking hip
> EXCLUDES 1   *congenital deformities of hip (Q65.-)*

R29.5 Transient paralysis
Code first any associated spinal cord injury (S14.0, S14.1-, S24.0, S24.1-, S34.0-, S34.1-)
> EXCLUDES 1   *transient ischemic attack (G45.9)*

R29.6 Repeated falls
Falling
Tendency to fall
> EXCLUDES 2   *at risk for falling (Z91.81)*
> *history of falling (Z91.81)*

AHA: 2016,2Q,6
TIP: Code in addition to Parkinson's disease (G20), when documented.

√5th **R29.7 National Institutes of Health Stroke Scale (NIHSS) score**
Code first the type of cerebral infarction (I63.-)
AHA: 2016,4Q,61-62
TIP: Codes from this subcategory may be assigned based on medical record documentation from clinicians who are not the patient's provider.

√6th **R29.70 NIHSS score 0-9**
R29.700 NIHSS score 0
R29.701 NIHSS score 1
R29.702 NIHSS score 2
R29.703 NIHSS score 3
R29.704 NIHSS score 4
R29.705 NIHSS score 5
R29.706 NIHSS score 6
R29.707 NIHSS score 7
R29.708 NIHSS score 8
R29.709 NIHSS score 9

√6th **R29.71 NIHSS score 10-19**
R29.710 NIHSS score 10
R29.711 NIHSS score 11
R29.712 NIHSS score 12
R29.713 NIHSS score 13
R29.714 NIHSS score 14
R29.715 NIHSS score 15
R29.716 NIHSS score 16
R29.717 NIHSS score 17
R29.718 NIHSS score 18
R29.719 NIHSS score 19

√6th **R29.72 NIHSS score 20-29**
R29.720 NIHSS score 20
R29.721 NIHSS score 21
R29.722 NIHSS score 22
R29.723 NIHSS score 23
R29.724 NIHSS score 24
R29.725 NIHSS score 25
R29.726 NIHSS score 26
R29.727 NIHSS score 27
R29.728 NIHSS score 28
R29.729 NIHSS score 29

√6th **R29.73 NIHSS score 30-39**
R29.730 NIHSS score 30
R29.731 NIHSS score 31
R29.732 NIHSS score 32
R29.733 NIHSS score 33
R29.734 NIHSS score 34
R29.735 NIHSS score 35
R29.736 NIHSS score 36
R29.737 NIHSS score 37
R29.738 NIHSS score 38
R29.739 NIHSS score 39

√6th **R29.74 NIHSS score 40-42**
R29.740 NIHSS score 40
R29.741 NIHSS score 41
R29.742 NIHSS score 42

√5th **R29.8 Other symptoms and signs involving the nervous and musculoskeletal systems**

√6th **R29.81 Other symptoms and signs involving the nervous system**

R29.810 Facial weakness
Facial droop
> EXCLUDES 1   *Bell's palsy (G51.0)*
> *facial weakness following cerebrovascular disease (I69. with final characters -92)*

R29.818 Other symptoms and signs involving the nervous system

√6th **R29.89 Other symptoms and signs involving the musculoskeletal system**
> EXCLUDES 2   *pain in limb (M79.6-)*

R29.890 Loss of height
> EXCLUDES 1   *osteoporosis (M80-M81)*

R29.891 Ocular torticollis
> EXCLUDES 1   *congenital (sternomastoid) torticollis Q68.0*
> *psychogenic torticollis (F45.8)*
> *spasmodic torticollis (G24.3)*
> *torticollis due to birth injury (P15.8)*
> *torticollis NOS M43.6*

DEF: Abnormal head posture as a result of a contracted state of cervical muscles to correct a visual disturbance, either double vision or a visual field defect.

R29.898 Other symptoms and signs involving the musculoskeletal system

√5th **R29.9 Unspecified symptoms and signs involving the nervous and musculoskeletal systems**

R29.90 Unspecified symptoms and signs involving the nervous system

R29.91 Unspecified symptoms and signs involving the musculoskeletal system

Symptoms and signs involving the genitourinary system (R30-R39)

√4th **R30 Pain associated with micturition**
> EXCLUDES 1   *psychogenic pain associated with micturition (F45.8)*

R30.0 Dysuria
Strangury

R30.1 Vesical tenesmus
DEF: Feeling of a full bladder even when there is little or no urine in the bladder.

R30.9 Painful micturition, unspecified
Painful urination NOS

√4th **R31 Hematuria**
> EXCLUDES 1   *hematuria included with underlying conditions, such as:*
> *acute cystitis with hematuria (N30.01)*
> *recurrent and persistent hematuria in glomerular diseases (N02.-)*

AHA: 2017,1Q,17

R31.0 Gross hematuria

R31.1 Benign essential microscopic hematuria

√5th **R31.2 Other microscopic hematuria**
AHA: 2016,4Q,62

R31.21 Asymptomatic microscopic hematuria
AMH

R31.29 Other microscopic hematuria

R31.9 Hematuria, unspecified

R32 Unspecified urinary incontinence

Enuresis NOS

EXCLUDES 1   functional urinary incontinence (R39.81)

nonorganic enuresis (F98.0)

stress incontinence and other specified urinary incontinence (N39.3-N39.4-)

urinary incontinence associated with cognitive impairment (R39.81)

✓4ᵗʰ R33 Retention of urine

EXCLUDES 1   psychogenic retention of urine (F45.8)

R33.0 Drug induced retention of urine

Use additional code for adverse effect, if applicable, to identify drug (T36-T50 with fifth or sixth character 5)

R33.8 Other retention of urine

Code first, if applicable, any causal condition, such as:

enlarged prostate (N40.1)

AHA: 2018,4Q,55

R33.9 Retention of urine, unspecified

R34 Anuria and oliguria

EXCLUDES 1   anuria and oliguria complicating abortion or ectopic or molar pregnancy (O00-O07, O08.4)

anuria and oliguria complicating pregnancy (O26.83-)

anuria and oliguria complicating the puerperium (O90.4)

✓4ᵗʰ R35 Polyuria

Code first, if applicable, any causal condition, such as:

enlarged prostate (N40.1)

EXCLUDES 1   psychogenic polyuria (F45.8)

R35.0 Frequency of micturition

R35.1 Nocturia

R35.8 Other polyuria

Polyuria NOS

✓4ᵗʰ R36 Urethral discharge

R36.0 Urethral discharge without blood

R36.1 Hematospermia   ♂

R36.9 Urethral discharge, unspecified

Penile discharge NOS

Urethrorrhea

R37 Sexual dysfunction, unspecified

✓4ᵗʰ R39 Other and unspecified symptoms and signs involving the genitourinary system

R39.0 Extravasation of urine

✓6ᵗʰ R39.1 Other difficulties with micturition

Code first, if applicable, any causal condition, such as:

enlarged prostate (N40.1)

R39.11 Hesitancy of micturition

R39.12 Poor urinary stream

Weak urinary steam

R39.13 Splitting of urinary stream

R39.14 Feeling of incomplete bladder emptying

R39.15 Urgency of urination

EXCLUDES 1   urge incontinence (N39.41, N39.46)

R39.16 Straining to void

✓6ᵗʰ R39.19 Other difficulties with micturition

AHA: 2016,4Q,63

R39.191 Need to immediately re-void

R39.192 Position dependent micturition

R39.198 Other difficulties with micturition

R39.2 Extrarenal uremia

Prerenal uremia

EXCLUDES 1   uremia NOS (N19)

✓5ᵗʰ R39.8 Other symptoms and signs involving the genitourinary system

AHA: 2017,4Q,22-23

R39.81 Functional urinary incontinence

Urinary incontinence due to cognitive impairment, or severe physical disability or immobility

EXCLUDES 1   stress incontinence and other specified urinary incontinence (N39.3-N39.4-)

urinary incontinence NOS (R32)

R39.82 Chronic bladder pain

AHA: 2016,4Q,64

R39.83 Unilateral non-palpable testicle   ♂

R39.84 Bilateral non-palpable testicles   ♂

R39.89 Other symptoms and signs involving the genitourinary system

R39.9 Unspecified symptoms and signs involving the genitourinary system

Symptoms and signs involving cognition, perception, emotional state and behavior (R40-R46)

EXCLUDES 2   symptoms and signs constituting part of a pattern of mental disorder (F01-F99)

✓4ᵗʰ R40 Somnolence, stupor and coma

EXCLUDES 1   neonatal coma (P91.5)

somnolence, stupor and coma in diabetes (E08-E13)

somnolence, stupor and coma in hepatic failure (K72.-)

somnolence, stupor and coma in hypoglycemia (nondiabetic) (E15)

R40.0 Somnolence

Drowsiness

EXCLUDES 1   coma (R40.2-)

R40.1 Stupor

Catatonic stupor

Semicoma

EXCLUDES 1   catatonic schizophrenia (F20.2)

coma (R40.2-)

depressive stupor (F31-F33)

dissociative stupor (F44.2)

manic stupor (F30.2)

✓5ᵗʰ R40.2 Coma

Code first any associated:

fracture of skull (S02.-)

intracranial injury (S06.-)

NOTE   One code from each subcategory, R40.21-R40.23, is required to complete the coma scale

AHA: 2019,2Q,12; 2018,4Q,70; 2017,4Q,23-25,95; 2015,2Q,17; 2014,1Q,19

TIP: Codes for individual (R40.21-, R40.22, R40.23-) or total (R40.24-) coma scale scores may be assigned based on medical record documentation from clinicians who are not the patient's provider.

TIP: It is not appropriate to assign individual (R40.21-, R40.22-, R40.23-) or total (R40.24-) coma scale score codes for patients who are sedated or in medically induced comas.

R40.20 Unspecified coma   HCC

Coma NOS

Unconsciousness NOS

✓6ᵗʰ R40.21 Coma scale, eyes open

The following appropriate 7th character is to be added to subcategory R40.21-, R40.22-, R40.23-, and R40.24-.

0   unspecified time

1   in the field [EMT or ambulance]

2   at arrival to emergency department

3   at hospital admission

4   24 hours or more after hospital admission

✓7ᵗʰ R40.211 Coma scale, eyes open, never   HCC

Coma scale eye opening score of 1

✓7ᵗʰ R40.212 Coma scale, eyes open, to pain   HCC

Coma scale eye opening score of 2

✓7ᵗʰ R40.213 Coma scale, eyes open, to sound

Coma scale eye opening score of 3

✓7ᵗʰ R40.214 Coma scale, eyes open, spontaneous

Coma scale eye opening score of 4

✓6ᵗʰ R40.22 Coma scale, best verbal response

✓7ᵗʰ R40.221 Coma scale, best verbal response, none   HCC

Coma scale verbal score of 1

✓7ᵗʰ R40.222 Coma scale, best verbal response, incomprehensible words   HCC

Coma scale verbal score of 2

Incomprehensible sounds (2-5 years of age)

Moans/grunts to pain; restless (< 2 years old)

☑ Additional Character Required   ✓x7ᵗʰ Placeholder Alert   Manifestation   Unspecified Dx   ▶◀ Revised Text   ● New Code   ▲ Revised Code Title

√7ᵗʰ **R40.223 Coma scale, best verbal response, inappropriate words**
Coma scale verbal score of 3
Inappropriate crying or screaming (< 2 years of age)
Screaming (2-5 years of age)

√7ᵗʰ **R40.224 Coma scale, best verbal response, confused conversation**
Coma scale verbal score of 4
Inappropriate words (2-5 years of age)
Irritable cries (< 2 years of age)

√7ᵗʰ **R40.225 Coma scale, best verbal response, oriented**
Coma scale verbal score of 5
Cooing or babbling or crying appropriately (< 2 years of age)
Uses appropriate words (2-5 years of age)

√6ᵗʰ **R40.23 Coma scale, best motor response**

√7ᵗʰ **R40.231 Coma scale, best motor response, none**   HCC
Coma scale motor score of 1

√7ᵗʰ **R40.232 Coma scale, best motor response, extension**   HCC
Abnormal extensor posturing to pain or noxious stimuli (< 2 years of age)
Coma scale motor score of 2
Extensor posturing to pain or noxious stimuli (2-5 years of age)

√7ᵗʰ **R40.233 Coma scale, best motor response, abnormal flexion**
Abnormal flexure posturing to pain or noxious stimuli (2-5 years of age)
Coma scale motor score of 3
Flexion/decorticate posturing (< 2 years of age)

√7ᵗʰ **R40.234 Coma scale, best motor response, flexion withdrawal**   HCC
Coma scale motor score of 4
Withdraws from pain or noxious stimuli (2-5 years of age)

√7ᵗʰ **R40.235 Coma scale, best motor response, localizes pain**
Coma scale motor score of 5
Localizes pain (2-5 years of age)
Withdraws to touch (< 2 years of age)

√7ᵗʰ **R40.236 Coma scale, best motor response, obeys commands**
Coma scale motor score of 6
Normal or spontaneous movement (< 2 years of age)
Obeys commands (2-5 years of age)

√6ᵗʰ **R40.24 Glasgow coma scale, total score**

> **NOTE**   Assign a code from subcategory R40.24, when only the total coma score is documented

AHA: 2016,4Q,64-65

√7ᵗʰ **R40.241 Glasgow coma scale score 13-15**

√7ᵗʰ **R40.242 Glasgow coma scale score 9-12**

√7ᵗʰ **R40.243 Glasgow coma scale score 3-8**   HCC

√7ᵗʰ **R40.244 Other coma, without documented Glasgow coma scale score, or with partial score reported**   HCC

R40.3 Persistent vegetative state   HCC
DEF: Persistent wakefulness without consciousness due to a nonfunctioning cerebral cortex.

R40.4 Transient alteration of awareness

√4ᵗʰ **R41 Other symptoms and signs involving cognitive functions and awareness**
EXCLUDES 1   *dissociative [conversion] disorders (F44.-)*
mild cognitive impairment, so stated (G31.84)

R41.0 Disorientation, unspecified
Confusion NOS
Delirium NOS
AHA: 2019,2Q,34

R41.1 Anterograde amnesia

R41.2 Retrograde amnesia

R41.3 Other amnesia
Amnesia NOS
Memory loss NOS
EXCLUDES 1   *amnestic disorder due to known physiologic condition (F04)*
amnestic syndrome due to psychoactive substance use (F10-F19 with 5th character .6)
mild memory disturbance due to known physiological condition (F06.8)
transient global amnesia (G45.4)

R41.4 Neurologic neglect syndrome
Asomatognosia
Hemi-akinesia
Hemi-inattention
Hemispatial neglect
Left-sided neglect
Sensory neglect
Visuospatial neglect
EXCLUDES 1   *visuospatial deficit (R41.842)*

√5ᵗʰ **R41.8 Other symptoms and signs involving cognitive functions and awareness**

R41.81 Age-related cognitive decline   A
Senility NOS

R41.82 Altered mental status, unspecified
Change in mental status NOS
EXCLUDES 1   *altered level of consciousness (R40.-)*
altered mental status due to known condition — code to condition
delirium NOS (R41.0)
AHA: 2012,4Q,97

R41.83 Borderline intellectual functioning
IQ level 71 to 84
EXCLUDES 1   *intellectual disabilities (F70-F79)*

√6ᵗʰ **R41.84 Other specified cognitive deficit**
EXCLUDES 1   *cognitive deficits as sequelae of cerebrovascular disease (I69.01-, I69.11-, I69.21-, I69.31-, I69.81-, I69.91-)*

R41.840 Attention and concentration deficit
EXCLUDES 1   *attention-deficit hyperactivity disorders (F90.-)*

R41.841 Cognitive communication deficit

R41.842 Visuospatial deficit

R41.843 Psychomotor deficit

R41.844 Frontal lobe and executive function deficit

R41.89 Other symptoms and signs involving cognitive functions and awareness
Anosognosia

R41.9 Unspecified symptoms and signs involving cognitive functions and awareness
Unspecified neurocognitive disorder

R42 Dizziness and giddiness   Q
Light-headedness
Vertigo NOS
EXCLUDES 1   *vertiginous syndromes (H81.-)*
vertigo from infrasound (T75.23)

√4ᵗʰ **R43 Disturbances of smell and taste**

R43.0 Anosmia
DEF: Permanent or transient absence of smell that may be congenital or acquired.

R43.1 Parosmia
DEF: Abnormal perception of smell usually triggered by environmental odors.

R43.2 Parageusia
DEF: Abnormal perception of taste.

R43.8 Other disturbances of smell and taste
Mixed disturbance of smell and taste

R43.9 Unspecified disturbances of smell and taste

☑4ᵗʰ **R44 Other symptoms and signs involving general sensations and perceptions**

> **EXCLUDES 1** *alcoholic hallucinations (F1.5)*
> *hallucinations in drug psychosis (F11-F19 with .5)*
> *hallucinations in mood disorders with psychotic symptoms (F30.2, F31.5, F32.3, F33.3)*
> *hallucinations in schizophrenia, schizotypal and delusional disorders (F20-F29)*
>
> **EXCLUDES 2** *disturbances of skin sensation (R20.-)*

R44.0 Auditory hallucinations
R44.1 Visual hallucinations
R44.2 Other hallucinations
R44.3 Hallucinations, unspecified
R44.8 Other symptoms and signs involving general sensations and perceptions
R44.9 Unspecified symptoms and signs involving general sensations and perceptions

☑4ᵗʰ **R45 Symptoms and signs involving emotional state**

R45.0 Nervousness
> Nervous tension
R45.1 Restlessness and agitation
R45.2 Unhappiness
R45.3 Demoralization and apathy
> **EXCLUDES 1** *anhedonia (R45.84)*
R45.4 Irritability and anger
R45.5 Hostility
R45.6 Violent behavior
R45.7 State of emotional shock and stress, unspecified
☑5ᵗʰ **R45.8 Other symptoms and signs involving emotional state**
> **R45.81 Low self-esteem**
> **R45.82 Worries**
> **R45.83 Excessive crying of child, adolescent or adult**
> > **EXCLUDES 1** *excessive crying of infant (baby) R68.11*
> **R45.84 Anhedonia**
> ☑6ᵗʰ **R45.85 Homicidal and suicidal ideations**
> > **EXCLUDES 1** *suicide attempt (T14.91)*
> > **R45.850 Homicidal ideations**
> > **R45.851 Suicidal ideations**
> > > **DEF:** Thoughts of committing suicide but no actual attempt of suicide has been made.
> **R45.86 Emotional lability**
> **R45.87 Impulsiveness**
> **R45.89 Other symptoms and signs involving emotional state**

☑4ᵗʰ **R46 Symptoms and signs involving appearance and behavior**

> **EXCLUDES 1** *appearance and behavior in schizophrenia, schizotypal and delusional disorders (F20-F29)*
> *mental and behavioral disorders (F01-F99)*

R46.0 Very low level of personal hygiene
R46.1 Bizarre personal appearance
R46.2 Strange and inexplicable behavior
R46.3 Overactivity
R46.4 Slowness and poor responsiveness
> **EXCLUDES 1** *stupor (R40.1)*
R46.5 Suspiciousness and marked evasiveness
R46.6 Undue concern and preoccupation with stressful events
R46.7 Verbosity and circumstantial detail obscuring reason for contact
☑5ᵗʰ **R46.8 Other symptoms and signs involving appearance and behavior**
> **R46.81 Obsessive-compulsive behavior**
> > **EXCLUDES 1** *obsessive-compulsive disorder (F42-)*
> **R46.89 Other symptoms and signs involving appearance and behavior**

Symptoms and signs involving speech and voice (R47-R49)

☑4ᵗʰ **R47 Speech disturbances, not elsewhere classified**

> **EXCLUDES 1** *autism (F84.0)*
> *cluttering (F80.81)*
> *specific developmental disorders of speech and language (F80.-)*
> *stuttering (F80.81)*

☑5ᵗʰ **R47.0 Dysphasia and aphasia**
> **R47.01 Aphasia**
> > **EXCLUDES 1** *aphasia following cerebrovascular disease (I69. with final characters -20)*
> > *progressive isolated aphasia (G31.01)*
> **R47.02 Dysphasia**
> > **EXCLUDES 1** *dysphasia following cerebrovascular disease (I69. with final characters -21)*
R47.1 Dysarthria and anarthria
> **EXCLUDES 1** *dysarthria following cerebrovascular disease (I69. with final characters -22)*
☑5ᵗʰ **R47.8 Other speech disturbances**
> **EXCLUDES 1** *dysarthria following cerebrovascular disease (I69. with final characters -28)*
> **R47.81 Slurred speech**
> **R47.82 Fluency disorder in conditions classified elsewhere**
> > Stuttering in conditions classified elsewhere
> > Code first underlying disease or condition, such as:
> > Parkinson's disease (G20)
> > > **EXCLUDES 1** *adult onset fluency disorder (F98.5)*
> > > *childhood onset fluency disorder (F80.81)*
> > > *fluency disorder (stuttering) following cerebrovascular disease (I69. with final characters -23)*
> **R47.89 Other speech disturbances**
R47.9 Unspecified speech disturbances

☑4ᵗʰ **R48 Dyslexia and other symbolic dysfunctions, not elsewhere classified**

> **EXCLUDES 1** *specific developmental disorders of scholastic skills (F81.-)*

R48.0 Dyslexia and alexia
R48.1 Agnosia
> Astereognosia (astereognosis)
> Autotopagnosia
> **EXCLUDES 1** *visual object agnosia (R48.3)*
> **DEF:** Inability to recognize common things such as faces, objects, smells, or voices.
R48.2 Apraxia
> **EXCLUDES 1** *apraxia following cerebrovascular disease (I69. with final characters -90)*
R48.3 Visual agnosia
> Prosopagnosia
> Simultanagnosia (asimultagnosia)
R48.8 Other symbolic dysfunctions
> Acalculia
> Agraphia
> **AHA:** 2017,1Q,27
R48.9 Unspecified symbolic dysfunctions

☑4ᵗʰ **R49 Voice and resonance disorders**

> **EXCLUDES 1** *psychogenic voice and resonance disorders (F44.4)*

R49.0 Dysphonia
> Hoarseness
R49.1 Aphonia
> Loss of voice
☑5ᵗʰ **R49.2 Hypernasality and hyponasality**
> **R49.21 Hypernasality**
> **R49.22 Hyponasality**
R49.8 Other voice and resonance disorders
R49.9 Unspecified voice and resonance disorder
> Change in voice NOS
> Resonance disorder NOS

Chapter 18. Symptoms, Signs and Abnormal Clinical and Laboratory Findings

General symptoms and signs (R50-R69)

☑4ᵗʰ **R50 Fever of other and unknown origin**

EXCLUDES 1   *chills without fever (R68.83)*
febrile convulsions (R56.0-)
fever of unknown origin during labor (O75.2)
fever of unknown origin in newborn (P81.9)
hypothermia due to illness (R68.0)
malignant hyperthermia due to anesthesia (T88.3)
puerperal pyrexia NOS (O86.4)

R50.2   **Drug induced fever**
Use additional code for adverse effect, if applicable, to identify drug (T36-T50 with fifth or sixth character 5)
EXCLUDES 1   *postvaccination (postimmunization) fever (R50.83)*

☑5ᵗʰ R50.8   **Other specified fever**

R50.81   *Fever presenting with conditions classified elsewhere*
Code first underlying condition when associated fever is present, such as with:
leukemia (C91-C95)
neutropenia (D70.-)
sickle-cell disease (D57.-)
AHA: 2014,4Q,22

R50.82   **Postprocedural fever**
EXCLUDES 1   *postprocedural infection (T81.4-)*
posttransfusion fever (R50.84)
postvaccination (postimmunization) fever (R50.83)

R50.83   **Postvaccination fever**
Postimmunization fever

R50.84   **Febrile nonhemolytic transfusion reaction**
FNHTR
Posttransfusion fever

R50.9   **Fever, unspecified**
Fever NOS
Fever of unknown origin [FUO]
Fever with chills
Fever with rigors
Hyperpyrexia NOS
Persistent fever
Pyrexia NOS

R51 Headache   Q
Facial pain NOS
EXCLUDES 1   *atypical face pain (G50.1)*
migraine and other headache syndromes (G43-G44)
trigeminal neuralgia (G50.0)

R52 Pain, unspecified
Acute pain NOS
Generalized pain NOS
Pain NOS
EXCLUDES 1   *acute and chronic pain, not elsewhere classified (G89.-)*
localized pain, unspecified type — code to pain by site, such as:
abdomen pain (R10.-)
back pain (M54.9)
breast pain (N64.4)
chest pain (R07.1-R07.9)
ear pain (H92.0-)
eye pain (H57.1)
headache (R51)
joint pain (M25.5-)
limb pain (M79.6-)
lumbar region pain (M54.5)
pelvic and perineal pain (R10.2)
renal colic (N23)
shoulder pain (M25.51-)
spine pain (M54.-)
throat pain (R07.0)
tongue pain (K14.6)
tooth pain (K08.8)
pain disorders exclusively related to psychological factors (F45.41)

☑4ᵗʰ **R53 Malaise and fatigue**

R53.0   **Neoplastic (malignant) related fatigue**
Code first associated neoplasm

R53.1   **Weakness**
Asthenia NOS
EXCLUDES 1   *age-related weakness (R54)*
muscle weakness (M62.8-)
sarcopenia (M62.84)
senile asthenia (R54)
AHA: 2017,1Q,7; 2015,1Q,25

R53.2   **Functional quadriplegia**   HCC
Complete immobility due to severe physical disability or frailty
EXCLUDES 1   *frailty NOS (R54)*
hysterical paralysis (F44.4)
immobility syndrome (M62.3)
neurologic quadriplegia (G82.5-)
quadriplegia (G82.50)
AHA: 2016,2Q,6
DEF: Inability to move due to a nonphysiological condition, such as dementia. The patient has no mental ability to move independently.

☑5ᵗʰ R53.8   **Other malaise and fatigue**
EXCLUDES 1   *combat exhaustion and fatigue (F43.0)*
congenital debility (P96.9)
exhaustion and fatigue due to excessive exertion (T73.3)
exhaustion and fatigue due to exposure (T73.2)
exhaustion and fatigue due to heat (T67.-)
exhaustion and fatigue due to pregnancy (O26.8-)
exhaustion and fatigue due to recurrent depressive episode (F33)
exhaustion and fatigue due to senile debility (R54)

R53.81   **Other malaise**
Chronic debility
Debility NOS
General physical deterioration
Malaise NOS
Nervous debility
EXCLUDES 1   *age-related physical debility (R54)*

R53.82   **Chronic fatigue, unspecified**
Chronic fatigue syndrome NOS
EXCLUDES 1   *postviral fatigue syndrome (G93.3)*

R53.83   **Other fatigue**
Fatigue NOS
Lack of energy
Lethargy
Tiredness
EXCLUDES 2   *exhaustion and fatigue due to depressive episode (F32.-)*

R54 Age-related physical debility   A
Frailty
Old age
Senescence
Senile asthenia
Senile debility
EXCLUDES 1   *age-related cognitive decline (R41.81)*
sarcopenia (M62.84)
senile psychosis (F03)
senility NOS (R41.81)

R55 Syncope and collapse
Blackout
Fainting
Vasovagal attack
> EXCLUDES 1   cardiogenic shock (R57.0)
> carotid sinus syncope (G90.01)
> heat syncope (T67.1)
> neurocirculatory asthenia (F45.8)
> neurogenic orthostatic hypotension (G90.3)
> orthostatic hypotension (I95.1)
> postprocedural shock (T81.1-)
> psychogenic syncope (F48.8)
> shock NOS (R57.9)
> shock complicating or following abortion or ectopic or molar pregnancy (O00-O07, O08.3)
> shock complicating or following labor and delivery (O75.1)
> Stokes-Adams attack (I45.9)
> unconsciousness NOS (R40.2-)

✓4ᵗʰ R56 Convulsions, not elsewhere classified
> EXCLUDES 1   dissociative convulsions and seizures (F44.5)
> epileptic convulsions and seizures (G40.-)
> newborn convulsions and seizures (P90)

✓5ᵗʰ R56.0 Febrile convulsions

R56.00 Simple febrile convulsions   HCC
Febrile convulsion NOS
Febrile seizure NOS

R56.01 Complex febrile convulsions   HCC
Atypical febrile seizure
Complex febrile seizure
Complicated febrile seizure
> EXCLUDES 1   status epilepticus (G40.901)

R56.1 Post traumatic seizures   HCC
> EXCLUDES 1   post traumatic epilepsy (G40.-)

R56.9 Unspecified convulsions   HCC
Convulsion disorder
Fit NOS
Recurrent convulsions
Seizure(s) (convulsive) NOS
AHA: 2019,1Q,19

✓4ᵗʰ R57 Shock, not elsewhere classified
> EXCLUDES 1   anaphylactic shock NOS (T78.2)
> anaphylactic reaction or shock due to adverse food reaction (T78.0-)
> anaphylactic shock due to adverse effect of correct drug or medicament properly administered (T88.6)
> anaphylactic shock due to serum (T80.5-)
> anesthetic shock (T88.3)
> electric shock (T75.4)
> obstetric shock (O75.1)
> postprocedural shock (T81.1-)
> psychic shock (F43.0)
> shock complicating or following ectopic or molar pregnancy (O00-O07, O08.3)
> shock due to lightning (T75.01)
> traumatic shock (T79.4)
> toxic shock syndrome (A48.3)

R57.0 Cardiogenic shock   HCC
> EXCLUDES 2   septic shock (R65.21)
DEF: Associated with myocardial infarction, cardiac tamponade, and massive pulmonary embolism. Symptoms include mental confusion, reduced blood pressure, tachycardia, pallor, and cold, clammy skin.

R57.1 Hypovolemic shock   HCC
AHA: 2019,2Q,7

R57.8 Other shock   HCC

R57.9 Shock, unspecified   HCC
Failure of peripheral circulation NOS

R58 Hemorrhage, not elsewhere classified
Hemorrhage NOS
> EXCLUDES 1   hemorrhage included with underlying conditions, such as:
> acute duodenal ulcer with hemorrhage (K26.0)
> acute gastritis with bleeding (K29.01)
> ulcerative enterocolitis with rectal bleeding (K51.01)

✓4ᵗʰ R59 Enlarged lymph nodes
> INCLUDES   swollen glands
> EXCLUDES 1   acute lymphadenitis (L04.-)
> chronic lymphadenitis (I88.1)
> lymphadenitis NOS (I88.9)
> mesenteric (acute) (chronic) lymphadenitis (I88.0)

R59.0 Localized enlarged lymph nodes

R59.1 Generalized enlarged lymph nodes
Lymphadenopathy NOS

R59.9 Enlarged lymph nodes, unspecified

✓4ᵗʰ R60 Edema, not elsewhere classified
> EXCLUDES 1   angioneurotic edema (T78.3)
> ascites (R18.-)
> cerebral edema (G93.6)
> cerebral edema due to birth injury (P11.0)
> edema of larynx (J38.4)
> edema of nasopharynx (J39.2)
> edema of pharynx (J39.2)
> gestational edema (O12.0-)
> hereditary edema (Q82.0)
> hydrops fetalis NOS (P83.2)
> hydrothorax (J94.8)
> hydrops fetalis NOS (P83.2)
> newborn edema (P83.3)
> pulmonary edema (J81.-)

R60.0 Localized edema

R60.1 Generalized edema
> EXCLUDES 2   nutritional edema (E40-E46)

R60.9 Edema, unspecified
Fluid retention NOS

R61 Generalized hyperhidrosis
Excessive sweating
Night sweats
Secondary hyperhidrosis
Code first, if applicable, menopausal and female climacteric states (N95.1)
> EXCLUDES 1   focal (primary) (secondary) hyperhidrosis (L74.5-)
> Frey's syndrome (L74.52)
> localized (primary) (secondary) hyperhidrosis (L74.5-)

✓4ᵗʰ R62 Lack of expected normal physiological development in childhood and adults
> EXCLUDES 1   delayed puberty (E30.0)
> gonadal dysgenesis (Q99.1)
> hypopituitarism (E23.0)

R62.0 Delayed milestone in childhood   P
Delayed attainment of expected physiological developmental stage
Late talker
Late walker

✓5ᵗʰ R62.5 Other and unspecified lack of expected normal physiological development in childhood
> EXCLUDES 1   HIV disease resulting in failure to thrive (B20)
> physical retardation due to malnutrition (E45)

R62.50 Unspecified lack of expected normal physiological development in childhood
Infantilism NOS

R62.51 Failure to thrive (child)   P
Failure to gain weight
> EXCLUDES 1   failure to thrive in child under 28 days old (P92.6)
AHA: 2018,4Q,82
DEF: Organic failure to thrive (FTT): Acute or chronic illness that interferes with nutritional intake, absorption, metabolism excretion, and energy requirements.
DEF: Nonorganic failure to thrive (FTT): Symptom of neglect or abuse.

✅ Additional Character Required   ✓x7ᵗʰ Placeholder Alert   Manifestation   Unspecified Dx   ▶◀ Revised Text   ● New Code   ▲ Revised Code Title

Chapter 18. Symptoms, Signs and Abnormal Clinical and Laboratory Findings

R62.52   Short stature (child)
Lack of growth
Physical retardation
Short stature NOS
EXCLUDES 1   *short stature due to endocrine disorder (E34.3)*

R62.59   Other lack of expected normal physiological development in childhood

R62.7   Adult failure to thrive   A

✓4ᵗʰ   R63   Symptoms and signs concerning food and fluid intake
EXCLUDES 1   *bulimia NOS (F50.2)*
      eating disorders of nonorganic origin (F50.-)
      malnutrition (E40-E46)

R63.0   Anorexia
Loss of appetite
EXCLUDES 1   *anorexia nervosa (F50.0-)*
      loss of appetite of nonorganic origin (F50.89)
AHA: 2018,4Q,82
TIP: Assign an additional code from category Z68 when BMI is documented. BMI can be based on documentation from clinicians who are not the patient's provider.

R63.1   Polydipsia
Excessive thirst

R63.2   Polyphagia
Excessive eating
Hyperalimentation NOS

R63.3   Feeding difficulties
Feeding problem (elderly) (infant) NOS
Picky eater
EXCLUDES 1   *eating disorders (F50.-)*
      feeding problems of newborn (P92.-)
      infant feeding disorder of nonorganic origin (F98.2-)
AHA: 2017,1Q,28; 2016,3Q,19
TIP: Do not assign for feeding problems in a patient greater than 28 days old if the feeding problem was initially diagnosed between day 0 and day 28; use a code from category P92 instead.

R63.4   Abnormal weight loss
AHA: 2018,4Q,82
TIP: Assign an additional code from category Z68 when BMI is documented. BMI can be based on documentation from clinicians who are not the patient's provider.

R63.5   Abnormal weight gain
EXCLUDES 1   *excessive weight gain in pregnancy (O26.0-)*
      obesity (E66.-)
AHA: 2018,4Q,82
TIP: Assign an additional code from category Z68 when BMI is documented. BMI can be based on documentation from clinicians who are not the patient's provider.

R63.6   Underweight
Use additional code to identify body mass index (BMI), if known (Z68.-)
EXCLUDES 1   *abnormal weight loss (R63.4)*
      anorexia nervosa (F50.0-)
      malnutrition (E40-E46)
AHA: 2018,4Q,82

R63.8   Other symptoms and signs concerning food and fluid intake

R64   Cachexia   HCC
Wasting syndrome
Code first underlying condition, if known
EXCLUDES 1   *abnormal weight loss (R63.4)*
      nutritional marasmus (E41)
AHA: 2018,4Q,82; 2017,3Q,24
TIP: Assign code E41 when emaciated or emaciation is documented in relation to malnutrition.

✓4ᵗʰ   R65   Symptoms and signs specifically associated with systemic inflammation and infection
AHA: 2019,2Q,38
TIP: When documentation states SIRS with an infection, assign only a code for the infection. ICD-10-CM does not offer a code for SIRS due to infectious process. If sepsis is suspected, query the provider.

✓5ᵗʰ   R65.1   Systemic inflammatory response syndrome [SIRS] of non-infectious origin
Code first underlying condition, such as:
heatstroke ▶(T67.0-)◄
injury and trauma (S00-T88)
EXCLUDES 1   *sepsis — code to infection*
      severe sepsis (R65.2)

R65.10   Systemic inflammatory response syndrome [SIRS] of non-infectious origin without acute organ dysfunction   HCC
Systemic inflammatory response syndrome (SIRS) NOS
AHA: 2019,2Q,24

R65.11   Systemic inflammatory response syndrome [SIRS] of non-infectious origin with acute organ dysfunction   HCC
Use additional code to identify specific acute organ dysfunction, such as:
acute kidney failure (N17.-)
acute respiratory failure (J96.0-)
critical illness myopathy (G72.81)
critical illness polyneuropathy (G62.81)
disseminated intravascular coagulopathy [DIC] (D65)
encephalopathy (metabolic) (septic) (G93.41)
hepatic failure (K72.0-)

✓5ᵗʰ   R65.2   Severe sepsis
Infection with associated acute organ dysfunction
Sepsis with acute organ dysfunction
Sepsis with multiple organ dysfunction
Systemic inflammatory response syndrome due to infectious process with acute organ dysfunction
Code first underlying infection, such as:
infection following a procedure (T81.4-)
infections following infusion, transfusion and therapeutic injection (T80.2-)
puerperal sepsis (O85)
sepsis following complete or unspecified spontaneous abortion (O03.87)
sepsis following ectopic and molar pregnancy (O08.82)
sepsis following incomplete spontaneous abortion (O03.37)
sepsis following (induced) termination of pregnancy (O04.87)
sepsis NOS (A41.9)
Use additional code to identify specific acute organ dysfunction, such as:
acute kidney failure (N17.-)
acute respiratory failure (J96.0-)
critical illness myopathy (G72.81)
critical illness polyneuropathy (G62.81)
disseminated intravascular coagulopathy [DIC] (D65)
encephalopathy (metabolic) (septic) (G93.41)
hepatic failure (K72.0-)
AHA: 2018,4Q,62-63; 2017,4Q,98-99; 2016,3Q,8

R65.20   Severe sepsis without septic shock   HCC
Severe sepsis NOS
AHA: 2016,3Q,14; 2013,4Q,119

R65.21   Severe sepsis with septic shock   HCC
AHA: 2018,4Q,63

✓4ᵗʰ   R68   Other general symptoms and signs

R68.0   Hypothermia, not associated with low environmental temperature
EXCLUDES 1   *hypothermia NOS (accidental) (T68)*
      hypothermia due to anesthesia (T88.51)
      hypothermia due to low environmental temperature (T68)
      newborn hypothermia (P80.-)

☑5ᵗʰ R68.1 Nonspecific symptoms peculiar to infancy
- *EXCLUDES 1*   colic, infantile (R10.83)
- neonatal cerebral irritability (P91.3)
- teething syndrome (K00.7)

R68.11 Excessive crying of infant (baby)   P
- *EXCLUDES 1*   excessive crying of child, adolescent, or adult (R45.83)

R68.12 Fussy infant (baby)   P
- Irritable infant

R68.13 Apparent life threatening event in infant (ALTE)   P
- Apparent life threatening event in newborn
- Brief resolved unexplained event (BRUE)
- Code first confirmed diagnosis, if known
- Use additional code(s) for associated signs and symptoms if no confirmed diagnosis established, or if signs and symptoms are not associated routinely with confirmed diagnosis, or provide additional information for cause of ALTE

R68.19 Other nonspecific symptoms peculiar to infancy   P

R68.2 Dry mouth, unspecified
- *EXCLUDES 1*   dry mouth due to dehydration (E86.0)
- dry mouth due to sicca syndrome [Sjögren] (M35.0-)
- salivary gland hyposecretion (K11.7)

R68.3 Clubbing of fingers
- Clubbing of nails
- *EXCLUDES 1*   congenital clubfinger (Q68.1)
- **DEF:** Enlarged soft tissue of the distal fingers that usually occurs in heart and lung diseases.

☑5ᵗʰ R68.8 Other general symptoms and signs

R68.81 Early satiety
- **DEF:** Premature feeling of being full after eating only a small amount of food. The mechanism of satiety is multifactorial.

R68.82 Decreased libido   A
- Decreased sexual desire

R68.83 Chills (without fever)
- Chills NOS
- *EXCLUDES 1*   chills with fever (R50.9)

R68.84 Jaw pain
- Mandibular pain
- Maxilla pain
- *EXCLUDES 1*   temporomandibular joint arthralgia (M26.62-)

R68.89 Other general symptoms and signs

R69 Illness, unspecified
- Unknown and unspecified cases of morbidity

Abnormal findings on examination of blood, without diagnosis (R70-R79)

EXCLUDES 2   abnormal findings on antenatal screening of mother (O28.-)
- abnormalities of lipids (E78.-)
- abnormalities of platelets and thrombocytes (D69.-)
- abnormalities of white blood cells classified elsewhere (D70-D72)
- coagulation hemorrhagic disorders (D65-D68)
- diagnostic abnormal findings classified elsewhere — see Alphabetical Index
- hemorrhagic and hematological disorders of newborn (P50-P61)

☑4ᵗʰ R70 Elevated erythrocyte sedimentation rate and abnormality of plasma viscosity

R70.0 Elevated erythrocyte sedimentation rate

R70.1 Abnormal plasma viscosity

☑4ᵗʰ R71 Abnormality of red blood cells
- *EXCLUDES 1*   anemias (D50-D64)
- anemia of premature infant (P61.2)
- benign (familial) polycythemia (D75.0)
- congenital anemias (P61.2-P61.4)
- newborn anemia due to isoimmunization (P55.-)
- polycythemia neonatorum (P61.1)
- polycythemia NOS (D75.1)
- polycythemia vera (D45)
- secondary polycythemia (D75.1)

R71.0 Precipitous drop in hematocrit
- Drop (precipitous) in hemoglobin
- Drop in hematocrit

R71.8 Other abnormality of red blood cells
- Abnormal red-cell morphology NOS
- Abnormal red-cell volume NOS
- Anisocytosis
- Poikilocytosis

☑4ᵗʰ R73 Elevated blood glucose level
- *EXCLUDES 1*   diabetes mellitus (E08-E13)
- diabetes mellitus in pregnancy, childbirth and the puerperium (O24.-)
- neonatal disorders (P70.0-P70.2)
- postsurgical hypoinsulinemia (E89.1)

☑5ᵗʰ R73.0 Abnormal glucose
- *EXCLUDES 1*   abnormal glucose in pregnancy (O99.81-)
- diabetes mellitus (E08-E13)
- dysmetabolic syndrome X (E88.81)
- gestational diabetes (O24.4-)
- glycosuria (R81)
- hypoglycemia (E16.2)

R73.01 Impaired fasting glucose
- Elevated fasting glucose

R73.02 Impaired glucose tolerance (oral)
- Elevated glucose tolerance

R73.03 Prediabetes
- Latent diabetes
- **AHA:** 2016,4Q,65

R73.09 Other abnormal glucose
- Abnormal glucose NOS
- Abnormal non-fasting glucose tolerance

R73.9 Hyperglycemia, unspecified

☑4ᵗʰ R74 Abnormal serum enzyme levels

R74.0 Nonspecific elevation of levels of transaminase and lactic acid dehydrogenase [LDH]

R74.8 Abnormal levels of other serum enzymes
- Abnormal level of acid phosphatase
- Abnormal level of alkaline phosphatase
- Abnormal level of amylase
- Abnormal level of lipase [triacylglycerol lipase]
- **AHA:** 2019,2Q,6

R74.9 Abnormal serum enzyme level, unspecified

R75 Inconclusive laboratory evidence of human immunodeficiency virus [HIV]
- Nonconclusive HIV-test finding in infants
- *EXCLUDES 1*   asymptomatic human immunodeficiency virus [HIV] infection status (Z21)
- human immunodeficiency virus [HIV] disease (B20)
- **TIP:** Do not assign for patients previously diagnosed with an HIV-related illness; assign code B20 instead.

☑4ᵗʰ R76 Other abnormal immunological findings in serum

R76.0 Raised antibody titer
- *EXCLUDES 1*   isoimmunization in pregnancy (O36.0-O36.1)
- isoimmunization affecting newborn (P55.-)

☑ Additional Character Required   ☑x7ᵗʰ Placeholder Alert   Manifestation   Unspecified Dx   ►◄ Revised Text   ● New Code   ▲ Revised Code Title

ICD-10-CM 2020   941

R68.1–R76.0

✓5ᵗʰ R76.1 Nonspecific reaction to test for tuberculosis

R76.11 Nonspecific reaction to tuberculin skin test without active tuberculosis
Abnormal result of Mantoux test
PPD positive
Tuberculin (skin test) positive
Tuberculin (skin test) reactor
EXCLUDES 1   nonspecific reaction to cell mediated immunity measurement of gamma interferon antigen response without active tuberculosis (R76.12)

R76.12 Nonspecific reaction to cell mediated immunity measurement of gamma interferon antigen response without active tuberculosis
Nonspecific reaction to QuantiFERON-TB test (QFT) without active tuberculosis
EXCLUDES 1   nonspecific reaction to tuberculin skin test without active tuberculosis (R76.11)
positive tuberculin skin test (R76.11)

R76.8 Other specified abnormal immunological findings in serum
Raised level of immunoglobulins NOS

R76.9 Abnormal immunological finding in serum, unspecified

✓4ᵗʰ R77 Other abnormalities of plasma proteins
EXCLUDES 1   disorders of plasma-protein metabolism (E88.0-)

R77.0 Abnormality of albumin

R77.1 Abnormality of globulin
Hyperglobulinemia NOS

R77.2 Abnormality of alphafetoprotein

R77.8 Other specified abnormalities of plasma proteins

R77.9 Abnormality of plasma protein, unspecified
AHA: 2019,2Q,6

✓4ᵗʰ R78 Findings of drugs and other substances, not normally found in blood
Use additional code to identify the any retained foreign body, if applicable (Z18.-)
EXCLUDES 1   mental or behavioral disorders due to psychoactive substance use (F10-F19)

R78.0 Finding of alcohol in blood
Use additional external cause code (Y90.-), for detail regarding alcohol level

R78.1 Finding of opiate drug in blood

R78.2 Finding of cocaine in blood

R78.3 Finding of hallucinogen in blood

R78.4 Finding of other drugs of addictive potential in blood

R78.5 Finding of other psychotropic drug in blood

R78.6 Finding of steroid agent in blood

✓5ᵗʰ R78.7 Finding of abnormal level of heavy metals in blood

R78.71 Abnormal lead level in blood
EXCLUDES 1   lead poisoning (T56.0-)

R78.79 Finding of abnormal level of heavy metals in blood

✓5ᵗʰ R78.8 Finding of other specified substances, not normally found in blood

R78.81 Bacteremia
EXCLUDES 1   sepsis — code to specified infection
DEF: Laboratory finding of bacteria in the blood in the absence of two or more signs of sepsis. Transient in nature, it can progress to septicemia with a severe infectious process.

R78.89 Finding of other specified substances, not normally found in blood
Finding of abnormal level of lithium in blood

R78.9 Finding of unspecified substance, not normally found in blood

✓4ᵗʰ R79 Other abnormal findings of blood chemistry
Use additional code to identify any retained foreign body, if applicable (Z18.-)
EXCLUDES 1   asymptomatic hyperuricemia (E79.0)
hyperglycemia NOS (R73.9)
hypoglycemia NOS (E16.2)
neonatal hypoglycemia (P70.3-P70.4)
specific findings indicating disorder of amino-acid metabolism (E70-E72)
specific findings indicating disorder of carbohydrate metabolism (E73-E74)
specific findings indicating disorder of lipid metabolism (E75.-)

R79.0 Abnormal level of blood mineral
Abnormal blood level of cobalt
Abnormal blood level of copper
Abnormal blood level of iron
Abnormal blood level of magnesium
Abnormal blood level of mineral NEC
Abnormal blood level of zinc
EXCLUDES 1   abnormal level of lithium (R78.89)
disorders of mineral metabolism (E83.-)
neonatal hypomagnesemia (P71.2)
nutritional mineral deficiency (E58-E61)

R79.1 Abnormal coagulation profile
Abnormal or prolonged bleeding time
Abnormal or prolonged coagulation time
Abnormal or prolonged partial thromboplastin time [PTT]
Abnormal or prolonged prothrombin time [PT]
EXCLUDES 1   coagulation defects (D68.-)
EXCLUDES 2   abnormality of fluid, electrolyte or acid-base balance (E86-E87)

✓5ᵗʰ R79.8 Other specified abnormal findings of blood chemistry

R79.81 Abnormal blood-gas level

R79.82 Elevated C-reactive protein [CRP]

R79.89 Other specified abnormal findings of blood chemistry
AHA: 2019,2Q,6
TIP: Assign for documented abnormal or elevated troponin level when a definitive diagnosis has not been established.
TIP: Assign for positive Coombs test when not further clarified in the documentation.

R79.9 Abnormal finding of blood chemistry, unspecified

Abnormal findings on examination of urine, without diagnosis (R80-R82)

EXCLUDES 1   abnormal findings on antenatal screening of mother (O28.-)
diagnostic abnormal findings classified elsewhere — see Alphabetical Index
specific findings indicating disorder of amino-acid metabolism (E70-E72)
specific findings indicating disorder of carbohydrate metabolism (E73-E74)

✓4ᵗʰ R80 Proteinuria
EXCLUDES 1   gestational proteinuria (O12.1-)

R80.0 Isolated proteinuria
Idiopathic proteinuria
EXCLUDES 1   isolated proteinuria with specific morphological lesion (N06.-)

R80.1 Persistent proteinuria, unspecified

R80.2 Orthostatic proteinuria, unspecified
Postural proteinuria

R80.3 Bence Jones proteinuria

R80.8 Other proteinuria

R80.9 Proteinuria, unspecified
Albuminuria NOS

R81 Glycosuria
EXCLUDES 1   renal glycosuria (E74.8)

✓4ᵗʰ R82 Other and unspecified abnormal findings in urine
INCLUDES   chromoabnormalities in urine
Use additional code to identify any retained foreign body, if applicable (Z18.-)
EXCLUDES 2   hematuria (R31.-)

R82.0 Chyluria
EXCLUDES 1   filarial chyluria (B74.-)

R82.1 Myoglobinuria

R82.2 Biliuria

R82.3 Hemoglobinuria

> EXCLUDES 1   *hemoglobinuria due to hemolysis from external causes NEC (D59.6)*
>
> *hemoglobinuria due to paroxysmal nocturnal [Marchiafava-Micheli] (D59.5)*

DEF: Free hemoglobin in blood due to rapid hemolysis of red blood cells. Causes include burns, crushed injury, sickle cell anemia, thalassemia, parasitic infections, or kidney infections.

R82.4 Acetonuria

Ketonuria

DEF: Excessive excretion of acetone in urine that commonly occurs in diabetic acidosis.

R82.5 Elevated urine levels of drugs, medicaments and biological substances

Elevated urine levels of catecholamines

Elevated urine levels of indoleacetic acid

Elevated urine levels of 17-ketosteroids

Elevated urine levels of steroids

R82.6 Abnormal urine levels of substances chiefly nonmedicinal as to source

Abnormal urine level of heavy metals

☑5ᵗʰ **R82.7 Abnormal findings on microbiological examination of urine**

> EXCLUDES 1   *colonization status (Z22.-)*

AHA: 2016,4Q,65

R82.71 Bacteriuria

R82.79 Other abnormal findings on microbiological examination of urine

Positive culture findings of urine

▲ ☑5ᵗʰ **R82.8 Abnormal findings on cytological and histological examination of urine**

● **R82.81 Pyuria**

Sterile pyuria

● **R82.89 Other abnormal findings on cytological and histological examination of urine**

☑5ᵗʰ **R82.9 Other and unspecified abnormal findings in urine**

R82.90 Unspecified abnormal findings in urine

R82.91 Other chromoabnormalities of urine

Chromoconversion (dipstick)

Idiopathic dipstick converts positive for blood with no cellular forms in sediment

> EXCLUDES 1   *hemoglobinuria (R82.3)*
>
> *myoglobinuria (R82.1)*

☑6ᵗʰ **R82.99 Other abnormal findings in urine**

AHA: 2018,4Q,29-30

R82.991 Hypocitraturia

R82.992 Hyperoxaluria

> EXCLUDES 1   *primary hyperoxaluria (E72.53)*

▲ **R82.993 Hyperuricosuria**

R82.994 Hypercalciuria

Idiopathic hypercalciuria

R82.998 Other abnormal findings in urine

Cells and casts in urine

Crystalluria

Melanuria

Abnormal findings on examination of other body fluids, substances and tissues, without diagnosis (R83-R89)

> EXCLUDES 1   *abnormal findings on antenatal screening of mother (O28.-)*
>
> *diagnostic abnormal findings classified elsewhere — see Alphabetical Index*
>
> EXCLUDES 2   *abnormal findings on examination of blood, without diagnosis (R70-R79)*
>
> *abnormal findings on examination of urine, without diagnosis (R80-R82)*
>
> *abnormal tumor markers (R97.-)*

☑4ᵗʰ **R83 Abnormal findings in cerebrospinal fluid**

Cerebrospinal Fluid

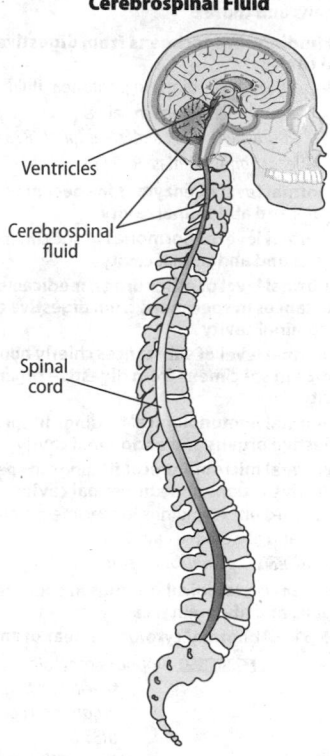

Ventricles

Cerebrospinal fluid

Spinal cord

R83.0 Abnormal level of enzymes in cerebrospinal fluid

R83.1 Abnormal level of hormones in cerebrospinal fluid

R83.2 Abnormal level of other drugs, medicaments and biological substances in cerebrospinal fluid

R83.3 Abnormal level of substances chiefly nonmedicinal as to source in cerebrospinal fluid

R83.4 Abnormal immunological findings in cerebrospinal fluid

R83.5 Abnormal microbiological findings in cerebrospinal fluid

Positive culture findings in cerebrospinal fluid

> EXCLUDES 1   *colonization status (Z22.-)*

R83.6 Abnormal cytological findings in cerebrospinal fluid

R83.8 Other abnormal findings in cerebrospinal fluid

Abnormal chromosomal findings in cerebrospinal fluid

R83.9 Unspecified abnormal finding in cerebrospinal fluid

☑4ᵗʰ **R84 Abnormal findings in specimens from respiratory organs and thorax**

> INCLUDES   abnormal findings in bronchial washings
>
> abnormal findings in nasal secretions
>
> abnormal findings in pleural fluid
>
> abnormal findings in sputum
>
> abnormal findings in throat scrapings
>
> EXCLUDES 1   *blood-stained sputum (R04.2)*

R84.0 Abnormal level of enzymes in specimens from respiratory organs and thorax

R84.1 Abnormal level of hormones in specimens from respiratory organs and thorax

R84.2 Abnormal level of other drugs, medicaments and biological substances in specimens from respiratory organs and thorax

R84.3 Abnormal level of substances chiefly nonmedicinal as to source in specimens from respiratory organs and thorax

R84.4 Abnormal immunological findings in specimens from respiratory organs and thorax

---

☑ Additional Character Required   ✓x7ᵗʰ Placeholder Alert   Manifestation   Unspecified Dx   ►◄ Revised Text   ● New Code   ▲ Revised Code Title

R84.5 Abnormal microbiological findings in specimens from respiratory organs and thorax
Positive culture findings in specimens from respiratory organs and thorax
EXCLUDES 1   colonization status (Z22.-)

R84.6 Abnormal cytological findings in specimens from respiratory organs and thorax

R84.7 Abnormal histological findings in specimens from respiratory organs and thorax

R84.8 Other abnormal findings in specimens from respiratory organs and thorax
Abnormal chromosomal findings in specimens from respiratory organs and thorax

R84.9 Unspecified abnormal finding in specimens from respiratory organs and thorax

✓4ᵗʰ **R85 Abnormal findings in specimens from digestive organs and abdominal cavity**
INCLUDES   abnormal findings in peritoneal fluid
abnormal findings in saliva
EXCLUDES 1   cloudy peritoneal dialysis effluent (R88.0)
fecal abnormalities (R19.5)

R85.0 Abnormal level of enzymes in specimens from digestive organs and abdominal cavity

R85.1 Abnormal level of hormones in specimens from digestive organs and abdominal cavity

R85.2 Abnormal level of other drugs, medicaments and biological substances in specimens from digestive organs and abdominal cavity

R85.3 Abnormal level of substances chiefly nonmedicinal as to source in specimens from digestive organs and abdominal cavity

R85.4 Abnormal immunological findings in specimens from digestive organs and abdominal cavity

R85.5 Abnormal microbiological findings in specimens from digestive organs and abdominal cavity
Positive culture findings in specimens from digestive organs and abdominal cavity
EXCLUDES 1   colonization status (Z22.-)

✓6ᵗʰ **R85.6 Abnormal cytological findings in specimens from digestive organs and abdominal cavity**

✓6ᵗʰ **R85.61 Abnormal cytologic smear of anus**
EXCLUDES 1   abnormal cytological findings in specimens from other digestive organs and abdominal cavity (R85.69)
anal intraepithelial neoplasia I [AIN I] (K62.82)
anal intraepithelial neoplasia II [AIN II] (K62.82)
anal intraepithelial neoplasia III [AIN III] (D01.3)
carcinoma in situ of anus (histologically confirmed) (D01.3)
dysplasia (mild) (moderate) of anus (histologically confirmed) (K62.82)
severe dysplasia of anus (histologically confirmed) (D01.3)
EXCLUDES 2   anal high risk human papillomavirus (HPV) DNA test positive (R85.81)
anal low risk human papillomavirus (HPV) DNA test positive (R85.82)

R85.610 Atypical squamous cells of undetermined significance on cytologic smear of anus [ASC-US]

R85.611 Atypical squamous cells cannot exclude high grade squamous intraepithelial lesion on cytologic smear of anus [ASC-H]

R85.612 Low grade squamous intraepithelial lesion on cytologic smear of anus [LGSIL]

R85.613 High grade squamous intraepithelial lesion on cytologic smear of anus [HGSIL]

R85.614 Cytologic evidence of malignancy on smear of anus

R85.615 Unsatisfactory cytologic smear of anus
Inadequate sample of cytologic smear of anus

R85.616 Satisfactory anal smear but lacking transformation zone

R85.618 Other abnormal cytological findings on specimens from anus

R85.619 Unspecified abnormal cytological findings in specimens from anus
Abnormal anal cytology NOS
Atypical glandular cells of anus NOS

R85.69 Abnormal cytological findings in specimens from other digestive organs and abdominal cavity

R85.7 Abnormal histological findings in specimens from digestive organs and abdominal cavity

✓5ᵗʰ **R85.8 Other abnormal findings in specimens from digestive organs and abdominal cavity**

R85.81 Anal high risk human papillomavirus [HPV] DNA test positive
EXCLUDES 1   anogenital warts due to human papillomavirus (HPV) (A63.0)
condyloma acuminatum (A63.0)

R85.82 Anal low risk human papillomavirus [HPV] DNA test positive
Use additional code for associated human papillomavirus (B97.7)

R85.89 Other abnormal findings in specimens from digestive organs and abdominal cavity
Abnormal chromosomal findings in specimens from digestive organs and abdominal cavity

R85.9 Unspecified abnormal finding in specimens from digestive organs and abdominal cavity

✓4ᵗʰ **R86 Abnormal findings in specimens from male genital organs**
INCLUDES   abnormal findings in prostatic secretions
abnormal findings in semen, seminal fluid
abnormal spermatozoa
EXCLUDES 1   azoospermia (N46.0-)
oligospermia (N46.1-)

R86.0 Abnormal level of enzymes in specimens from male genital organs ♂

R86.1 Abnormal level of hormones in specimens from male genital organs ♂

R86.2 Abnormal level of other drugs, medicaments and biological substances in specimens from male genital organs ♂

R86.3 Abnormal level of substances chiefly nonmedicinal as to source in specimens from male genital organs ♂

R86.4 Abnormal immunological findings in specimens from male genital organs ♂

R86.5 Abnormal microbiological findings in specimens from male genital organs ♂
Positive culture findings in specimens from male genital organs
EXCLUDES 1   colonization status (Z22.-)

R86.6 Abnormal cytological findings in specimens from male genital organs ♂

R86.7 Abnormal histological findings in specimens from male genital organs ♂

R86.8 Other abnormal findings in specimens from male genital organs ♂
Abnormal chromosomal findings in specimens from male genital organs

R86.9 Unspecified abnormal finding in specimens from male genital organs ♂

✓4ᵗʰ **R87 Abnormal findings in specimens from female genital organs**
INCLUDES   abnormal findings in secretion and smears from cervix uteri
abnormal findings in secretion and smears from vagina
abnormal findings in secretion and smears from vulva

R87.0 Abnormal level of enzymes in specimens from female genital organs ♀

R87.1 Abnormal level of hormones in specimens from female genital organs ♀

R87.2 Abnormal level of other drugs, medicaments and biological substances in specimens from female genital organs ♀

R87.3 Abnormal level of substances chiefly nonmedicinal as to source in specimens from female genital organs ♀

R87.4 Abnormal immunological findings in specimens from female genital organs ♀

R87.5 Abnormal microbiological findings in specimens from female genital organs ♀
Positive culture findings in specimens from female genital organs
EXCLUDES 1   colonization status (Z22.-)

✓5ᵗʰ **R87.6** **Abnormal cytological findings in specimens from female genital organs**

✓6ᵗʰ **R87.61** **Abnormal cytological findings in specimens from cervix uteri**

　EXCLUDES 1　*abnormal cytological findings in specimens from other female genital organs (R87.69)*

abnormal cytological findings in specimens from vagina (R87.62-)

carcinoma in situ of cervix uteri (histologically confirmed) (D06.-)

cervical intraepithelial neoplasia I [CIN I] (N87.0)

cervical intraepithelial neoplasia II [CIN II] (N87.1)

cervical intraepithelial neoplasia III [CIN III] (D06.-)

dysplasia (mild) (moderate) of cervix uteri (histologically confirmed) (N87.-)

severe dysplasia of cervix uteri (histologically confirmed) (D06.-)

　EXCLUDES 2　*cervical high risk human papillomavirus (HPV) DNA test positive (R87.810)*

cervical low risk human papillomavirus (HPV) DNA test positive (R87.820)

R87.610 **Atypical squamous cells of undetermined significance on cytologic smear of cervix [ASC-US]** ♀

R87.611 **Atypical squamous cells cannot exclude high grade squamous intraepithelial lesion on cytologic smear of cervix [ASC-H]** ♀

R87.612 **Low grade squamous intraepithelial lesion on cytologic smear of cervix [LGSIL]** ♀

R87.613 **High grade squamous intraepithelial lesion on cytologic smear of cervix [HGSIL]** ♀

R87.614 **Cytologic evidence of malignancy on smear of cervix** ♀

R87.615 **Unsatisfactory cytologic smear of cervix** ♀

Inadequate sample of cytologic smear of cervix

R87.616 **Satisfactory cervical smear but lacking transformation zone** ♀

R87.618 **Other abnormal cytological findings on specimens from cervix uteri** ♀

R87.619 **Unspecified abnormal cytological findings in specimens from cervix uteri** ♀

Abnormal cervical cytology NOS

Abnormal Papanicolaou smear of cervix NOS

Abnormal thin preparation smear of cervix NOS

Atypical endocervial cells of cervix NOS

Atypical endometrial cells of cervix NOS

Atypical glandular cells of cervix NOS

✓6ᵗʰ **R87.62** **Abnormal cytological findings in specimens from vagina**

Use additional code to identify acquired absence of uterus and cervix, if applicable (Z90.71-)

　EXCLUDES 1　*abnormal cytological findings in specimens from cervix uteri (R87.61-)*

abnormal cytological findings in specimens from other female genital organs (R87.69)

carcinoma in situ of vagina (histologically confirmed) (D07.2)

dysplasia (mild) (moderate) of vagina (histologically confirmed) (N89.-)

severe dysplasia of vagina (histologically confirmed) (D07.2)

vaginal intraepithelial neoplasia I [VAIN I] (N89.0)

vaginal intraepithelial neoplasia II [VAIN II] (N89.1)

vaginal intraepithelial neoplasia III [VAIN III] (D07.2)

　EXCLUDES 2　*vaginal high risk human papillomavirus (HPV) DNA test positive (R87.811)*

vaginal low risk human papillomavirus (HPV) DNA test positive (R87.821)

R87.620 **Atypical squamous cells of undetermined significance on cytologic smear of vagina [ASC-US]** ♀

R87.621 **Atypical squamous cells cannot exclude high grade squamous intraepithelial lesion on cytologic smear of vagina [ASC-H]** ♀

R87.622 **Low grade squamous intraepithelial lesion on cytologic smear of vagina [LGSIL]** ♀

R87.623 **High grade squamous intraepithelial lesion on cytologic smear of vagina [HGSIL]** ♀

R87.624 **Cytologic evidence of malignancy on smear of vagina** ♀

R87.625 **Unsatisfactory cytologic smear of vagina** ♀

Inadequate sample of cytologic smear of vagina

R87.628 **Other abnormal cytological findings on specimens from vagina** ♀

R87.629 **Unspecified abnormal cytological findings in specimens from vagina** ♀

Abnormal Papanicolaou smear of vagina NOS

Abnormal thin preparation smear of vagina NOS

Abnormal vaginal cytology NOS

Atypical endocervical cells of vagina NOS

Atypical endometrial cells of vagina NOS

Atypical glandular cells of vagina NOS

R87.69 **Abnormal cytological findings in specimens from other female genital organs** ♀

Abnormal cytological findings in specimens from female genital organs NOS

　EXCLUDES 1　*dysplasia of vulva (histologically confirmed) (N90.0-N90.3)*

☑ Additional Character Required　　✓ₓ7ᵗʰ Placeholder Alert　　Manifestation　　Unspecified Dx　　►◄ Revised Text　　● New Code　　▲ Revised Code Title

Chapter 18. Symptoms, Signs and Abnormal Clinical and Laboratory Findings

R87.7–R93.2

R87.7 **Abnormal histological findings in specimens from female genital organs** ♀

> EXCLUDES 1   *carcinoma in situ (histologically confirmed) of female genital organs (D06-D07.3)*
> *cervical intraepithelial neoplasia I [CIN I] (N87.0)*
> *cervical intraepithelial neoplasia II [CIN II] (N87.1)*
> *cervical intraepithelial neoplasia III [CIN III] (D06.-)*
> *dysplasia (mild) (moderate) of cervix uteri (histologically confirmed) (N87.-)*
> *dysplasia (mild) (moderate) of vagina (histologically confirmed) (N89.-)*
> *severe dysplasia of cervix uteri (histologically confirmed) (D06.-)*
> *severe dysplasia of vagina (histologically confirmed) (D07.2)*
> *vaginal intraepithelial neoplasia I [VAIN I] (N89.0)*
> *vaginal intraepithelial neoplasia II [VAIN II] (N89.1)*
> *vaginal intraepithelial neoplasia III [VAIN III] (D07.2)*

✓5ᵗʰ **R87.8** **Other abnormal findings in specimens from female genital organs**

   ✓6ᵗʰ **R87.81** **High risk human papillomavirus [HPV] DNA test positive from female genital organs**

> EXCLUDES 1   *anogenital warts due to human papillomavirus (HPV) (A63.0)*
> *condyloma acuminatum (A63.0)*

     R87.810 **Cervical high risk human papillomavirus [HPV] DNA test positive** ♀

     R87.811 **Vaginal high risk human papillomavirus [HPV] DNA test positive** ♀

   ✓6ᵗʰ **R87.82** **Low risk human papillomavirus [HPV] DNA test positive from female genital organs**

     Use additional code for associated human papillomavirus (B97.7)

     R87.820 **Cervical low risk human papillomavirus [HPV] DNA test positive** ♀

     R87.821 **Vaginal low risk human papillomavirus [HPV] DNA test positive** ♀

   R87.89 **Other abnormal findings in specimens from female genital organs** ♀

     Abnormal chromosomal findings in specimens from female genital organs

R87.9 **Unspecified abnormal finding in specimens from female genital organs** ♀

✓4ᵗʰ **R88** **Abnormal findings in other body fluids and substances**

R88.0 **Cloudy (hemodialysis) (peritoneal) dialysis effluent**

R88.8 **Abnormal findings in other body fluids and substances**

✓4ᵗʰ **R89** **Abnormal findings in specimens from other organs, systems and tissues**

> INCLUDES   abnormal findings in nipple discharge
> abnormal findings in synovial fluid
> abnormal findings in wound secretions

R89.0 **Abnormal level of enzymes in specimens from other organs, systems and tissues**

R89.1 **Abnormal level of hormones in specimens from other organs, systems and tissues**

R89.2 **Abnormal level of other drugs, medicaments and biological substances in specimens from other organs, systems and tissues**

R89.3 **Abnormal level of substances chiefly nonmedicinal as to source in specimens from other organs, systems and tissues**

R89.4 **Abnormal immunological findings in specimens from other organs, systems and tissues**

R89.5 **Abnormal microbiological findings in specimens from other organs, systems and tissues**

   Positive culture findings in specimens from other organs, systems and tissues

> EXCLUDES 1   *colonization status (Z22.-)*

R89.6 **Abnormal cytological findings in specimens from other organs, systems and tissues**

R89.7 **Abnormal histological findings in specimens from other organs, systems and tissues**

R89.8 **Other abnormal findings in specimens from other organs, systems and tissues**

   Abnormal chromosomal findings in specimens from other organs, systems and tissues

R89.9 **Unspecified abnormal finding in specimens from other organs, systems and tissues**

Abnormal findings on diagnostic imaging and in function studies, without diagnosis (R90-R94)

> INCLUDES   nonspecific abnormal findings on diagnostic imaging by computerized axial tomography [CAT scan]
> nonspecific abnormal findings on diagnostic imaging by magnetic resonance imaging [MRI][NMR]
> nonspecific abnormal findings on diagnostic imaging by positron emission tomography [PET scan]
> nonspecific abnormal findings on diagnostic imaging by thermography
> nonspecific abnormal findings on diagnostic imaging by ultrasound [echogram]
> nonspecific abnormal findings on diagnostic imaging by X-ray examination

> EXCLUDES 1   *abnormal findings on antenatal screening of mother (O28.-)*
> *diagnostic abnormal findings classified elsewhere — see Alphabetical Index*

✓4ᵗʰ **R90** **Abnormal findings on diagnostic imaging of central nervous system**

R90.0 **Intracranial space-occupying lesion found on diagnostic imaging of central nervous system**

✓5ᵗʰ **R90.8** **Other abnormal findings on diagnostic imaging of central nervous system**

   R90.81 **Abnormal echoencephalogram**

   R90.82 **White matter disease, unspecified**

   R90.89 **Other abnormal findings on diagnostic imaging of central nervous system**

     Other cerebrovascular abnormality found on diagnostic imaging of central nervous system

✓4ᵗʰ **R91** **Abnormal findings on diagnostic imaging of lung**

R91.1 **Solitary pulmonary nodule**

   Coin lesion lung
   Solitary pulmonary nodule, subsegmental branch of the bronchial tree

R91.8 **Other nonspecific abnormal finding of lung field**

   Lung mass NOS found on diagnostic imaging of lung
   Pulmonary infiltrate NOS
   Shadow, lung

✓4ᵗʰ **R92** **Abnormal and inconclusive findings on diagnostic imaging of breast**

R92.0 **Mammographic microcalcification found on diagnostic imaging of breast**

> EXCLUDES 2   *mammographic calcification (calculus) found on diagnostic imaging of breast (R92.1)*

   DEF: Calcium and cellular debris deposits in the breast that cannot be felt but can be detected on a mammogram. The deposits can be a sign of cancer, benign conditions, or changes in the breast tissue as a result of inflammation, injury, or an obstructed duct.

R92.1 **Mammographic calcification found on diagnostic imaging of breast**

   Mammographic calculus found on diagnostic imaging of breast

R92.2 **Inconclusive mammogram**

   Dense breasts NOS
   Inconclusive mammogram NEC
   Inconclusive mammography due to dense breasts
   Inconclusive mammography NEC
   AHA: 2015,1Q,24

R92.8 **Other abnormal and inconclusive findings on diagnostic imaging of breast**

✓4ᵗʰ **R93** **Abnormal findings on diagnostic imaging of other body structures**

R93.0 **Abnormal findings on diagnostic imaging of skull and head, not elsewhere classified**

> EXCLUDES 1   *intracranial space-occupying lesion found on diagnostic imaging (R90.0)*

R93.1 **Abnormal findings on diagnostic imaging of heart and coronary circulation**

   Abnormal echocardiogram NOS
   Abnormal heart shadow

R93.2 **Abnormal findings on diagnostic imaging of liver and biliary tract**

   Nonvisualization of gallbladder

R93.3   **Abnormal findings on diagnostic imaging of other parts of digestive tract**

√5th   **R93.4**   **Abnormal findings on diagnostic imaging of urinary organs**
> EXCLUDES 2   hypertrophy of kidney (N28.81)
> AHA: 2016,4Q,66

     R93.41   **Abnormal radiologic findings on diagnostic imaging of renal pelvis, ureter, or bladder**
       Filling defect of bladder found on diagnostic imaging
       Filling defect of renal pelvis found on diagnostic imaging
       Filling defect of ureter found on diagnostic imaging

     √6th   **R93.42**   **Abnormal radiologic findings on diagnostic imaging of kidney**

       R93.421   **Abnormal radiologic findings on diagnostic imaging of right kidney**

       R93.422   **Abnormal radiologic findings on diagnostic imaging of left kidney**

       R93.429   **Abnormal radiologic findings on diagnostic imaging of unspecified kidney**

     R93.49   **Abnormal radiologic findings on diagnostic imaging of other urinary organs**

R93.5   **Abnormal findings on diagnostic imaging of other abdominal regions, including retroperitoneum**

R93.6   **Abnormal findings on diagnostic imaging of limbs**
> EXCLUDES 2   abnormal finding in skin and subcutaneous tissue (R93.8-)

R93.7   **Abnormal findings on diagnostic imaging of other parts of musculoskeletal system**
> EXCLUDES 2   abnormal findings on diagnostic imaging of skull (R93.0)

√5th   **R93.8**   **Abnormal findings on diagnostic imaging of other specified body structures**
> AHA: 2018,4Q,30

     √6th   **R93.81**   **Abnormal radiologic findings on diagnostic imaging of testis**

       R93.811   **Abnormal radiologic findings on diagnostic imaging of right testicle**   ♂

       R93.812   **Abnormal radiologic findings on diagnostic imaging of left testicle**   ♂

       R93.813   **Abnormal radiologic findings on diagnostic imaging of testicles, bilateral**   ♂

       R93.819   **Abnormal radiologic findings on diagnostic imaging of unspecified testicle**   ♂

     R93.89   **Abnormal findings on diagnostic imaging of other specified body structures**
       Abnormal finding by radioisotope localization of placenta
       Abnormal radiological finding in skin and subcutaneous tissue
       Mediastinal shift

R93.9   **Diagnostic imaging inconclusive due to excess body fat of patient**

√4th   **R94**   **Abnormal results of function studies**
> INCLUDES   abnormal results of radionuclide [radioisotope] uptake studies
>   abnormal results of scintigraphy

√5th   **R94.0**   **Abnormal results of function studies of central nervous system**

     R94.01   **Abnormal electroencephalogram [EEG]**

     R94.02   **Abnormal brain scan**

     R94.09   **Abnormal results of other function studies of central nervous system**

√5th   **R94.1**   **Abnormal results of function studies of peripheral nervous system and special senses**

     √6th   **R94.11**   **Abnormal results of function studies of eye**

       R94.110   **Abnormal electro-oculogram [EOG]**

       R94.111   **Abnormal electroretinogram [ERG]**
         Abnormal retinal function study

       R94.112   **Abnormal visually evoked potential [VEP]**

       R94.113   **Abnormal oculomotor study**

       R94.118   **Abnormal results of other function studies of eye**

     √6th   **R94.12**   **Abnormal results of function studies of ear and other special senses**
> AHA: 2016,3Q,17

       R94.120   **Abnormal auditory function study**

       R94.121   **Abnormal vestibular function study**

       R94.128   **Abnormal results of other function studies of ear and other special senses**

     √6th   **R94.13**   **Abnormal results of function studies of peripheral nervous system**

       R94.130   **Abnormal response to nerve stimulation, unspecified**

       R94.131   **Abnormal electromyogram [EMG]**
> EXCLUDES 1   electromyogram of eye (R94.113)

       R94.138   **Abnormal results of other function studies of peripheral nervous system**

R94.2   **Abnormal results of pulmonary function studies**
     Reduced ventilatory capacity
     Reduced vital capacity

√5th   **R94.3**   **Abnormal results of cardiovascular function studies**

     R94.30   **Abnormal result of cardiovascular function study, unspecified**

     R94.31   **Abnormal electrocardiogram [ECG] [EKG]**
> EXCLUDES 1   long QT syndrome (I45.81)

     R94.39   **Abnormal result of other cardiovascular function study**
       Abnormal electrophysiological intracardiac studies
       Abnormal phonocardiogram
       Abnormal vectorcardiogram

R94.4   **Abnormal results of kidney function studies**
     Abnormal renal function test

R94.5   **Abnormal results of liver function studies**

R94.6   **Abnormal results of thyroid function studies**

R94.7   **Abnormal results of other endocrine function studies**
> EXCLUDES 2   abnormal glucose (R73.0-)

R94.8   **Abnormal results of function studies of other organs and systems**
     Abnormal basal metabolic rate [BMR]
     Abnormal bladder function test
     Abnormal splenic function test

Abnormal tumor markers (R97)

√4th   **R97**   **Abnormal tumor markers**
     Elevated tumor associated antigens [TAA]
     Elevated tumor specific antigens [TSA]

R97.0   **Elevated carcinoembryonic antigen [CEA]**

R97.1   **Elevated cancer antigen 125 [CA 125]**

√5th   **R97.2**   **Elevated prostate specific antigen [PSA]**
> AHA: 2016,4Q,66

     R97.20   **Elevated prostate specific antigen [PSA]**   A ♂

     R97.21   **Rising PSA following treatment for malignant neoplasm of prostate**   A ♂

R97.8   **Other abnormal tumor markers**

Ill-defined and unknown cause of mortality (R99)

R99   **Ill-defined and unknown cause of mortality**
     Death (unexplained) NOS
     Unspecified cause of mortality

✔ Additional Character Required   √x7th Placeholder Alert   Manifestation   Unspecified Dx   ▶◀ Revised Text   ● New Code   ▲ Revised Code Title

Chapter 19. Injury, Poisoning, and Certain Other Consequences of External Causes (S00–T88)

Chapter-specific Guidelines with Coding Examples

The chapter-specific guidelines from the ICD-10-CM Official Guidelines for Coding and Reporting have been provided below. Along with these guidelines are coding examples, contained in the shaded boxes, that have been developed to help illustrate the coding and/or sequencing guidance found in these guidelines.

a. Application of 7th characters in Chapter 19

Most categories in chapter 19 have a 7th character requirement for each applicable code. Most categories in this chapter have three 7th character values (with the exception of fractures): A, initial encounter, D, subsequent encounter and S, sequela. Categories for traumatic fractures have additional 7th character values. While the patient may be seen by a new or different provider over the course of treatment for an injury, assignment of the 7th character is based on whether the patient is undergoing active treatment and not whether the provider is seeing the patient for the first time.

For complication codes, active treatment refers to treatment for the condition described by the code, even though it may be related to an earlier precipitating problem. For example, code T84.50XA, Infection and inflammatory reaction due to unspecified internal joint prosthesis, initial encounter, is used when active treatment is provided for the infection, even though the condition relates to the prosthetic device, implant or graft that was placed at a previous encounter.

7th character "A", initial encounter is used for each encounter where the patient is receiving active treatment for the condition.

> Patient evaluated after fall from a skateboard onto the sidewalk, x-rays identify a nondisplaced fracture to the distal pole of the right scaphoid bone. The patient is placed in a cast.
>
> **S62.014A**   **Nondisplaced fracture of distal pole of navicular [scaphoid] bone of right wrist, initial encounter for closed fracture**
>
> **V00.131A**   **Fall from skateboard, initial encounter**
>
> **Y93.51**   **Activity, roller skating (inline) and skateboarding**
>
> **Y92.480**   **Sidewalk as the place of occurrence of the external cause**
>
> **Y99.8**   **Other external cause status**
>
> *Explanation:* This fracture would be coded with a seventh character A for initial encounter because the patient received x-rays to identify the site of the fracture and treatment was rendered; this would be considered active treatment.

7th character "D" subsequent encounter is used for encounters after the patient has completed active treatment of the condition and is receiving routine care for the condition during the healing or recovery phase.

> Patient seen in follow-up after fall from a skateboard onto the sidewalk resulted in casting of the right arm. X-rays are taken to evaluate how well the nondisplaced fracture to the distal pole of the right scaphoid bone is healing. The physician feels the fracture is healing appropriately; no adjustments to the cast are made.
>
> **S62.014D**   **Nondisplaced fracture of distal pole of navicular [scaphoid] bone of right wrist, subsequent encounter for fracture with routine healing**
>
> **V00.131D**   **Fall from skateboard, subsequent encounter**
>
> *Explanation:* This fracture would be coded with a seventh character D for subsequent encounter, whether the same physician who provided the initial cast application or a different physician is now seeing the patient. Although the patient received x-rays, the intent of the x-rays was to assess how the fracture was healing. There was no active treatment rendered and the visit is therefore considered a subsequent encounter.

The aftercare Z codes should not be used for aftercare for conditions such as injuries or poisonings, where 7th characters are provided to identify subsequent care. For example, for aftercare of an injury, assign the acute injury code with the 7th character "D" (subsequent encounter).

7th character "S", sequela, is for use for complications or conditions that arise as a direct result of a condition, such as scar formation after a burn.

The scars are sequelae of the burn. When using 7th character "S", it is necessary to use both the injury code that precipitated the sequela and the code for the sequela itself. The "S" is added only to the injury code, not the sequela code. The 7th character "S" identifies the injury responsible for the sequela. The specific type of sequela (e.g. scar) is sequenced first, followed by the injury code.

See Section I.B.10 Sequelae, (Late Effects)

> Patient with a history of a nondisplaced fracture to the distal pole of the right scaphoid bone due to a fall from a skateboard is seen for evaluation of arthritis to the right wrist that has developed as a consequence of the traumatic fracture.
>
> **M12.531**   **Traumatic arthropathy, right wrist**
>
> **S62.014S**   **Nondisplaced fracture of distal pole of navicular [scaphoid] bone of right wrist, sequela**
>
> **V00.131S**   **Fall from skateboard, sequela**
>
> *Explanation:* The code identifying the specific sequela condition (traumatic arthritis) should be coded first followed by the injury that instigated the development of the sequela (fracture). The scaphoid fracture injury code is given a 7th character S for sequela to represent its role as the inciting injury. The fracture has healed and is not being managed or treated on this admit and therefore is not applicable as a first listed or principal diagnosis. However, it is directly related to the development of the arthritis and should be appended as a secondary code to signify this cause and effect relationship.

b. Coding of injuries

When coding injuries, assign separate codes for each injury unless a combination code is provided, in which case the combination code is assigned. Codes from category T07, Unspecified multiple injuries should not be assigned in the inpatient setting unless information for a more specific code is not available. Traumatic injury codes (S00–T14.9) are not to be used for normal, healing surgical wounds or to identify complications of surgical wounds.

> 11-year-old girl fell from her horse, resulting in a laceration to her right forearm with several large pieces of wooden fragments embedded in the wound as well as abrasions to her right ear; in addition, her right shoulder was dislocated.
>
> **S43.004A**   **Unspecified dislocation of right shoulder joint, initial encounter**
>
> **S51.821A**   **Laceration with foreign body of right forearm, initial encounter**
>
> **S00.411A**   **Abrasion of right ear, initial encounter**
>
> **V80.010A**   **Animal-rider injured by fall from or being thrown from horse in noncollision accident, initial encounter**
>
> **Y93.52**   **Activity, horseback riding**
>
> *Explanation:* Each separate injury should be reported. The patient's injury to the forearm is reported with one combination code that captures both the laceration and the foreign body.

The code for the most serious injury, as determined by the provider and the focus of treatment, is sequenced first.

1) Superficial injuries

Superficial injuries such as abrasions or contusions are not coded when associated with more severe injuries of the same site.

2) Primary injury with damage to nerves/blood vessels

When a primary injury results in minor damage to peripheral nerves or blood vessels, the primary injury is sequenced first with additional code(s) for injuries to nerves and spinal cord (such as category S04), and/or injury to blood vessels (such as category S15). When the primary injury is to the blood vessels or nerves, that injury should be sequenced first.

3) Iatrogenic injuries

Injury codes from Chapter 19 should not be assigned for injuries that occur during, or as a result of, a medical intervention. Assign the appropriate complication code(s).

c. Coding of traumatic fractures

The principles of multiple coding of injuries should be followed in coding fractures. Fractures of specified sites are coded individually by site in accordance with both the provisions within categories S02, S12, S22, S32, S42, S49, S52, S59, S62, S72, S79, S82, S89, S92 and the level of detail furnished by medical record content.

A fracture not indicated as open or closed should be coded to closed. A fracture not indicated whether displaced or not displaced should be coded to displaced.

More specific guidelines are as follows:

1) Initial vs. subsequent encounter for fractures

Traumatic fractures are coded using the appropriate 7th character for initial encounter (A, B, C) for each encounter where the patient is receiving active treatment for the fracture. The appropriate 7th character for initial encounter should also be assigned for a patient who delayed seeking treatment for the fracture or nonunion.

Fractures are coded using the appropriate 7th character for subsequent care for encounters after the patient has completed active treatment of the fracture and is receiving routine care for the fracture during the healing or recovery phase.

Care for complications of surgical treatment for fracture repairs during the healing or recovery phase should be coded with the appropriate complication codes.

Care of complications of fractures, such as malunion and nonunion, should be reported with the appropriate 7th character for subsequent care with nonunion (K, M, N,) or subsequent care with malunion (P, Q, R).

Malunion/nonunion: The appropriate 7th character for initial encounter should also be assigned for a patient who delayed seeking treatment for the fracture or nonunion.

Female patient fell during a forest hiking excursion almost six months ago and until recently did not feel she needed to seek medical attention for her left ankle pain; x-rays show nonunion of lateral malleolus and surgery has been scheduled

S82.62XA	Displaced fracture of lateral malleolus of left fibula, initial encounter for closed fracture
W01.0XXA	Fall on same level from slipping, tripping and stumbling without subsequent striking against object, initial encounter
Y92.821	Forest as place of occurrence of the external cause
Y93.01	Activity, walking, marching and hiking
Y99.8	Other external cause status

Explanation: A seventh character of A is used for the lateral malleolus nonunion fracture to signify that the fracture is receiving active treatment. The delayed care for the fracture has resulted in a nonunion, but capturing the nonunion in the seventh character is trumped by the provision of active care.

The open fracture designations in the assignment of the 7th character for fractures of the forearm, femur and lower leg, including ankle are based on the Gustilo open fracture classification. When the Gustilo classification type is not specified for an open fracture, the 7th character for open fracture type I or II should be assigned (B, E, H, M, Q).

A code from category M80, not a traumatic fracture code, should be used for any patient with known osteoporosis who suffers a fracture, even if the patient had a minor fall or trauma, if that fall or trauma would not usually break a normal, healthy bone.

See Section I.C.13. Osteoporosis.

The aftercare Z codes should not be used for aftercare for traumatic fractures. For aftercare of a traumatic fracture, assign the acute fracture code with the appropriate 7th character.

2) Multiple fractures sequencing

Multiple fractures are sequenced in accordance with the severity of the fracture.

3) Physeal fractures

For physeal fractures, assign only the code identifying the type of physeal fracture. Do not assign a separate code to identify the specific bone that is fractured.

d. Coding of burns and corrosions

The ICD-10-CM makes a distinction between burns and corrosions. The burn codes are for thermal burns, except sunburns, that come from a heat source, such as a fire or hot appliance. The burn codes are also for burns resulting from electricity and radiation. Corrosions are burns due to chemicals. The guidelines are the same for burns and corrosions.

Current burns (T20-T25) are classified by depth, extent and by agent (X code). Burns are classified by depth as first degree (erythema), second degree (blistering), and third degree (full-thickness involvement). Burns of the eye and internal organs (T26-T28) are classified by site, but not by degree.

1) Sequencing of burn and related condition codes

Sequence first the code that reflects the highest degree of burn when more than one burn is present.

a. When the reason for the admission or encounter is for treatment of external multiple burns, sequence first the code that reflects the burn of the highest degree.

b. When a patient has both internal and external burns, the circumstances of admission govern the selection of the principal diagnosis or first-listed diagnosis.

c. When a patient is admitted for burn injuries and other related conditions such as smoke inhalation and/or respiratory failure, the circumstances of admission govern the selection of the principal or first-listed diagnosis.

Patient referred for minor first-degree burns to multiple sites of her right and left hands as well as severe smoke inhalation. While she was sleeping at home, a candle on her dresser lit the bedroom curtains on fire.

T59.811A	Toxic effect of smoke, accidental (unintentional), initial encounter
J70.5	Respiratory conditions due to smoke inhalation
T23.191A	Burn of first degree of multiple sites of right wrist and hand, initial encounter
T23.192A	Burn of first degree of multiple sites of left wrist and hand, initial encounter
X08.8XXA	Exposure to other specified smoke, fire and flames, initial encounter
Y99.8	Other exteranl cause status
Y92.003	Bedroom of unspecified non-institutional (private) residence as the place of occurrence of the external cause
Y93.84	Activity, sleeping

Explanation: Based on the documentation, the inhalation injury is more severe than the first-degree burns and is sequenced first. The burns to the hands are appended as secondary diagnoses.

2) Burns of the same anatomic site

Classify burns of the same anatomic site and on the same side but of different degrees to the subcategory identifying the highest degree recorded in the diagnosis (e.g., for second and third degree burns of right thigh, assign only code T24.311-).

3) Non-healing burns

Non-healing burns are coded as acute burns.

Necrosis of burned skin should be coded as a non-healed burn.

4) Infected burn

For any documented infected burn site, use an additional code for the infection.

5) Assign separate codes for each burn site

When coding burns, assign separate codes for each burn site. Category T30, Burn and corrosion, body region unspecified is extremely vague and should rarely be used.

Codes for burns of "multiple sites" should only be assigned when the medical record documentation does not specify the individual sites.

Patient is treated for third-degree burns of the scalp as well as second-degree burns to the back of the right hand

T20.35XA	Burn of third degree of scalp [any part], initial encounter
T23.261A	Burn of second degree of back of right hand, initial encounter

Explanation: Two codes may be reported as the hand and face represent distinct burn sites.

6) Burns and corrosions classified according to extent of body surface involved

Assign codes from category T31, Burns classified according to extent of body surface involved, or T32, Corrosions classified according to extent of body surface involved, when the site of the burn is not specified or when there is a need for additional data. It is advisable to use category T31 as additional coding when needed to provide data for evaluating burn mortality, such as that needed by burn units. It is also advisable to use category T31 as an additional code for reporting purposes when there is mention of a third-degree burn involving 20 percent or more of the body surface.

Categories T31 and T32 are based on the classic "rule of nines" in estimating body surface involved: head and neck are assigned nine percent, each arm nine percent, each leg 18 percent, the anterior trunk 18 percent, posterior trunk 18 percent, and genitalia one percent. Providers may change these percentage assignments where necessary to accommodate infants and children who have proportionately larger heads than adults, and patients who have large buttocks, thighs, or abdomen that involve burns.

> Patient seen for dressing change after he accidentally spilled acetic acid on himself two days ago. The second-degree burns to his right thigh, covering about 3 percent of his body surface, are healing appropriately.
>
> **T54.2X1D   Toxic effect of corrosive acids and acid-like substances, accidental (unintentional), subsequent encounter**
>
> **T24.611D   Corrosion of second degree of right thigh, subsequent encounter**
>
> **T32.0   Corrosions involving less than 10% of body surface**
>
> *Explanation:* Code T32.0 provides additional information as to how much of the patient's body was affected by the corrosive substance.

7) Encounters for treatment of sequela of burns

Encounters for the treatment of the late effects of burns or corrosions (i.e., scars or joint contractures) should be coded with a burn or corrosion code with the 7th character "S" for sequela.

8) Sequelae with a late effect code and current burn

When appropriate, both a code for a current burn or corrosion with 7th character "A" or "D" and a burn or corrosion code with 7th character "S" may be assigned on the same record (when both a current burn and sequelae of an old burn exist). Burns and corrosions do not heal at the same rate and a current healing wound may still exist with sequela of a healed burn or corrosion.

See Section I.B.10 Sequela (Late Effects)

> Female patient seen for second-degree burn to the left ear; she also has significant scarring on her left elbow from a third-degree burn from childhood
>
> **T20.212A   Burn of second degree of left ear [any part, except ear drum], initial encounter**
>
> **L90.5   Scar conditions and fibrosis of skin**
>
> **T22.322S   Burn of third degree of left elbow, sequela**
>
> *Explanation:* The patient is being seen for management of a current second-degree burn, which is reflected in the code by appending the seventh character of A, indicating active treatment or management of this burn. The elbow scarring is a sequela of a previous third-degree burn. The sequela condition precedes the original burn injury, which is appended with a seventh character of S.

9) Use of an external cause code with burns and corrosions

An external cause code should be used with burns and corrosions to identify the source and intent of the burn, as well as the place where it occurred.

e. Adverse effects, poisoning, underdosing and toxic effects

Codes in categories T36-T65 are combination codes that include the substance that was taken as well as the intent. No additional external cause code is required for poisonings, toxic effects, adverse effects and underdosing codes.

1) Do not code directly from the Table of Drugs

Do not code directly from the Table of Drugs and Chemicals. Always refer back to the Tabular List.

2) Use as many codes as necessary to describe

Use as many codes as necessary to describe completely all drugs, medicinal or biological substances.

3) If the same code would describe the causative agent

If the same code would describe the causative agent for more than one adverse reaction, poisoning, toxic effect or underdosing, assign the code only once.

4) If two or more drugs, medicinal or biological substances

If two or more drugs, medicinal or biological substances are **taken**, code each individually unless a combination code is listed in the Table of Drugs and Chemicals.

If multiple unspecified drugs, medicinal or biological substances were taken, assign the appropriate code from subcategory T50.91, Poisoning by, adverse effect of and underdosing of multiple unspecified drugs, medicaments and biological substances.

5) The occurrence of drug toxicity is classified in ICD-10-CM as follows:

(a) Adverse effect

When coding an adverse effect of a drug that has been correctly prescribed and properly administered, assign the appropriate code for the nature of the adverse effect followed by the appropriate code for the adverse effect of the drug (T36-T50). The code for the drug should have a 5th or 6th character "5" (for example T36.0X5-) Examples of the nature of an adverse effect are tachycardia, delirium, gastrointestinal hemorrhaging, vomiting, hypokalemia, hepatitis, renal failure, or respiratory failure.

> Patient seen for stomach pain and jaundice, indicated by physician as possible side-effects of Inderal, recently started for hypertension. Inderal was discontinued and the patient switched to Atenolol instead.
>
> **R10.9   Unspecified abdominal pain**
>
> **R17   Unspecified jaundice**
>
> **T44.7X5A   Adverse effect of beta-adrenoreceptor antagonists, initial encounter**
>
> **I10   Essential (primary) hypertension**
>
> *Explanation:* The side-effects caused by the drug are listed first, followed by the code for the adverse effect of the drug to capture the specific drug that was used.

(b) Poisoning

When coding a poisoning or reaction to the improper use of a medication (e.g., overdose, wrong substance given or taken in error, wrong route of administration), first assign the appropriate code from categories T36-T50. The poisoning codes have an associated intent as their 5th or 6th character (accidental, intentional self-harm, assault and undetermined. If the intent of the poisoning is unknown or unspecified, code the intent as accidental intent. The undetermined intent is only for use if the documentation in the record specifies that the intent cannot be determined. Use additional code(s) for all manifestations of poisonings.

If there is also a diagnosis of abuse or dependence of the substance, the abuse or dependence is assigned as an additional code.

Examples of poisoning include:

(i)   Error was made in drug prescription
Errors made in drug prescription or in the administration of the drug by provider, nurse, patient, or other person.

(ii)   Overdose of a drug intentionally taken
If an overdose of a drug was intentionally taken or administered and resulted in drug toxicity, it would be coded as a poisoning.

(iii)   Nonprescribed drug taken with correctly prescribed and properly administered drug
If a nonprescribed drug or medicinal agent was taken in combination with a correctly prescribed and properly administered drug, any drug toxicity or other reaction resulting from the interaction of the two drugs would be classified as a poisoning.

(iv)   Interaction of drug(s) and alcohol
When a reaction results from the interaction of a drug(s) and alcohol, this would be classified as poisoning.

See Section I.C.4. if poisoning is the result of insulin pump malfunctions.

(c) Underdosing

Underdosing refers to taking less of a medication than is prescribed by a provider or a manufacturer's instruction. Discontinuing the use of a prescribed medication on the patient's own initiative (not directed by the patient's provider) is also classified as an underdosing. For underdosing, assign the code from categories T36-T50 (fifth or sixth character "6").

Codes for underdosing should never be assigned as principal or first-listed codes. If a patient has a relapse or exacerbation of the medical condition for which the drug is prescribed because of the reduction in dose, then the medical condition itself should be coded.

Noncompliance (Z91.12-, Z91.13- and Z91.14-) or complication of care (Y63.6-Y63.9) codes are to be used with an underdosing code to indicate intent, if known.

> Patient referred for atrial fibrillation with history of chronic atrial fibrillation for which she is prescribed amiodarone. Financial concerns have left the patient unable to pay for her prescriptions and she has been skipping her amiodarone dose every other day to offset the cost.
>
> | I48.20 | Chronic atrial fibrillation, unspecified |
> | T46.2X6A | Underdosing of other antidysrhythmic drugs, initial encounter |
> | Z91.120 | Patient's intentional underdosing of medication regimen due to financial hardship |
>
> *Explanation:* By skipping her amiodarone pill every other day, the patient's atrial fibrillation returned. The condition for which the drug was being taken is reported first, followed by an underdosing code to show that the patient was not adhering to her prescription regiment. The Z code helps elaborate on the patient's social and/or economic circumstances that led to the patient taking less then what she was prescribed.

(d) Toxic effects

When a harmful substance is ingested or comes in contact with a person, this is classified as a toxic effect. The toxic effect codes are in categories T51-T65.

Toxic effect codes have an associated intent: accidental, intentional self-harm, assault and undetermined.

f. Adult and child abuse, neglect and other maltreatment

Sequence first the appropriate code from categories T74.- (Adult and child abuse, neglect and other maltreatment, confirmed) or T76.- (Adult and child abuse, neglect and other maltreatment, suspected) for abuse, neglect and other maltreatment, followed by any accompanying mental health or injury code(s).

If the documentation in the medical record states abuse or neglect it is coded as confirmed (T74.-). It is coded as suspected if it is documented as suspected (T76.-).

For cases of confirmed abuse or neglect an external cause code from the assault section (X92-Y09) should be added to identify the cause of any physical injuries. A perpetrator code (Y07) should be added when the perpetrator of the abuse is known. For suspected cases of abuse or neglect, do not report external cause or perpetrator code.

If a suspected case of abuse, neglect or mistreatment is ruled out during an encounter code Z04.71, Encounter for examination and observation following alleged physical adult abuse, ruled out, or code Z04.72, Encounter for examination and observation following alleged child physical abuse, ruled out, should be used, not a code from T76.

If a suspected case of alleged rape or sexual abuse is ruled out during an encounter code Z04.41, Encounter for examination and observation following alleged adult rape or code Z04.42, Encounter for examination and observation following alleged child rape, should be used, not a code from T76.

If a suspected case of forced sexual exploitation or forced labor exploitation is ruled out during an encounter, code Z04.81, Encounter for examination and observation of victim following forced sexual exploitation, or code Z04.82, Encounter for examination and observation of victim following forced labor exploitation, should be used, not a code from T76.

See Section I.C.15. Abuse in a pregnant patient.

g. Complications of care

1) General guidelines for complications of care

(a) Documentation of complications of care

See Section I.B.16. for information on documentation of complications of care.

2) Pain due to medical devices

Pain associated with devices, implants or grafts left in a surgical site (for example painful hip prosthesis) is assigned to the appropriate code(s) found in Chapter 19, Injury, poisoning, and certain other consequences of

external causes. Specific codes for pain due to medical devices are found in the T code section of the ICD-10-CM. Use additional code(s) from category G89 to identify acute or chronic pain due to presence of the device, implant or graft (G89.18 or G89.28).

> Chronic left breast pain secondary to breast implant
>
> | T85.848A | Pain due to other internal prosthetic devices, implants and grafts, initial encounter |
> | N64.4 | Mastodynia |
> | G89.28 | Other chronic postprocedural pain |
>
> *Explanation:* As the pain is a complication related to the breast implant, the complication code is sequenced first. The T code does not describe the site or type of pain, so additional codes may be appended to indicate that the patient is experiencing chronic pain in the breast.

3) Transplant complications

(a) Transplant complications other than kidney

Codes under category T86, Complications of transplanted organs and tissues, are for use for both complications and rejection of transplanted organs. A transplant complication code is only assigned if the complication affects the function of the transplanted organ. Two codes are required to fully describe a transplant complication: the appropriate code from category T86 and a secondary code that identifies the complication.

Pre-existing conditions or conditions that develop after the transplant are not coded as complications unless they affect the function of the transplanted organs.

See I.C.21. for transplant organ removal status

See I.C.2. for malignant neoplasm associated with transplanted organan.

(b) Kidney transplant complications

Patients who have undergone kidney transplant may still have some form of chronic kidney disease (CKD) because the kidney transplant may not fully restore kidney function. Code T86.1- should be assigned for documented complications of a kidney transplant, such as transplant failure or rejection or other transplant complication. Code T86.1- should not be assigned for post kidney transplant patients who have chronic kidney (CKD) unless a transplant complication such as transplant failure or rejection is documented. If the documentation is unclear as to whether the patient has a complication of the transplant, query the provider.

Conditions that affect the function of the transplanted kidney, other than CKD, should be assigned a code from subcategory T86.1, Complications of transplanted organ, Kidney, and a secondary code that identifies the complication.

For patients with CKD following a kidney transplant, but who do not have a complication such as failure or rejection, *see section I.C.14. Chronic kidney disease and kidney transplant status.*

> Patient seen for chronic kidney disease stage 2; history of successful kidney transplant with no complications identified
>
> | N18.2 | Chronic kidney disease, stage 2 (mild) |
> | Z94.0 | Kidney transplant status |
>
> *Explanation:* This patient's stage 2 CKD is not indicated as being due to the transplanted kidney but instead is just the residual disease the patient had prior to the transplant.

4) Complication codes that include the external cause

As with certain other T codes, some of the complications of care codes have the external cause included in the code. The code includes the nature of the complication as well as the type of procedure that caused the complication. No external cause code indicating the type of procedure is necessary for these codes.

5) Complications of care codes within the body system chapters

Intraoperative and postprocedural complication codes are found within the body system chapters with codes specific to the organs and structures of that body system. These codes should be sequenced first, followed by a code(s) for the specific complication, if applicable.

Complication codes from the body system chapters should be assigned for intraoperative and postprocedural complications (e.g., the appropriate complication code from chapter 9 would be assigned for a vascular intraoperative or postprocedural complication) unless the complication is specifically indexed to a T code in chapter 19.

Muscle/Tendon Table

ICD-10-CM categorizes certain muscles and tendons in the upper and lower extremities by their action (e.g., extension, flexion), their anatomical location (e.g., posterior, anterior), and/or whether they are intrinsic or extrinsic to a certain anatomical area. The Muscle/Tendon Table is provided at the beginning of chapters 13 and 19 as a resource to help users when code selection depends on one or more of these characteristics. A **TIP** has been placed at those categories and/or subcategories that relate to this table. Please note that this table is not all-inclusive, and proper code assignment should be based on the provider's documentation.

Body Region	Muscle	Extensor Tendon	Flexor Tendon	Other Tendon
Shoulder				
	Deltoid	Posterior deltoid	Anterior deltoid	
	Rotator cuff			
	Infraspinatus			Infraspinatus
	Subscapularis			Subscapularis
	Supraspinatus			Supraspinatus
	Teres minor			Teres minor
	Teres major	Teres major		
Upper arm				
	Anterior muscles			
	Biceps brachii — long head		Biceps brachii — long head	
	Biceps brachii — short head		Biceps brachii — short head	
	Brachialis		Brachialis	
	Coracobrachialis		Coracobrachialis	
	Posterior muscles			
	Triceps brachii	Triceps brachii		
Forearm				
	Anterior muscles			
	Flexors			
	Deep			
	Flexor digitorum profundus		Flexor digitorum profundus	
	Flexor pollicis longus		Flexor pollicis longus	
	Intermediate			
	Flexor digitorum superficialis		Flexor digitorum superficialis	
	Superficial			
	Flexor carpi radialis		Flexor carpi radialis	
	Flexor carpi ulnaris		Flexor carpi ulnaris	
	Palmaris longus		Palmaris longus	
	Pronators			
	Pronator quadratus			Pronator quadratus
	Pronator teres			Pronator teres
	Posterior muscles			
	Extensors			
	Deep			
	Abductor pollicis longus			Abductor pollicis longus
	Extensor indicis	Extensor indicis		
	Extensor pollicis brevis	Extensor pollicis brevis		
	Extensor pollicis longus	Extensor pollicis longus		
	Superficial			
	Brachioradialis			Brachioradialis
	Extensor carpi radialis brevis	Extensor carpi radialis brevis		
	Extensor carpi radialis longus	Extensor carpi radialis longus		
	Extensor carpi ulnaris	Extensor carpi ulnaris		
	Extensor digiti minimi	Extensor digiti minimi		
	Extensor digitorum	Extensor digitorum		
	Anconeus	Anconeus		
	Supinator			Supinator

Chapter 19. Injury, Poisoning, and Certain Other Consequences of External Causes

Body Region	Muscle	Extensor Tendon	Flexor Tendon	Other Tendon
Hand				
Extrinsic — attach to a site in the forearm as well as a site in the hand with action related to hand movement at the wrist				
	Extensor carpi radialis brevis	Extensor carpi radialis brevis		
	Extensor carpi radialis longus	Extensor carpie radialis longus		
	Extensor carpi ulnaris	Extensor carpi ulnaris		
	Flexor carpi radialis		Flexor carpi radialis	
	Flexor carpi ulnaris		Flexor carpi ulnaris	
	Flexor digitorum superficialis		Flexor digitorum superficialis	
	Palmaris longus		Palmaris longus	
Extrinsic — attach to a site in the forearm as well as a site in the hand with action in the hand related to finger movement				
	Adductor pollicis longus			Adductor pollicis longus
	Extensor digiti minimi	Extensor digiti minimi		
	Extensor digitorum	Extensor digitorum		
	Extensor indicis	Extensor indicis		
	Flexor digitorum profundus		Flexor digitorum profundus	
	Flexor digitorum superficialis		Flexor digitorum superficialis	
Extrinsic — attach to a site in the forearm as well as a site in the hand with action in the hand related to thumb movement				
	Extensor pollicis brevis	Extensor pollicis brevis		
	Extensor pollicis longus	Extensor pollicis longus		
	Flexor pollicis longus		Flexor pollicis longus	
Intrinsic — found within the hand only				
	Adductor pollicis			Adductor pollicis
	Dorsal interossei	Dorsal interossei	Dorsal interossei	
	Lumbricals	Lumbricals	Lumbricals	
	Palmaris brevis			Palmaris brevis
	Palmar interossei	Palmar interossei	Palmar interossei	
	Hypothenar muscles			
	Abductor digiti minimi			Abductor digiti minimi
	Flexor digiti minimi brevis		Flexor digiti minimi brevis	
	Oppenens digiti minimi		Oppenens digiti minimi	
	Thenar muscles			
	Abductor pollicis brevis			Abductor pollicis brevis
	Flexor pollicis brevis		Flexor pollicis brevis	
	Oppenens pollicis		Oppenens pollicis	
Thigh				
	Anterior muscles			
	Iliopsoas		Iliopsoas	
	Pectineus		Pectineus	
	Quadriceps	Quadriceps		
	Rectus femoris	Rectus femoris — Extends knee	Rectus femoris — Flexes hip	
	Vastus intermedius	Vastus intermedius		
	Vastus lateralis	Vastus lateralis		
	Vastus medialis	Vastus medialis		
	Sartorius		Sartorius	
	Medial muscles			
	Adductor brevis			Adductor brevis
	Adductor longus			Adductor longus
	Adductor magnus			Adductor magnus
	Gracilis			Gracilis
	Obturator externus			Obturator externus
	Posterior muscles			
	Hamstring	Hamstring — Extends hip	Hamstring — Flexes knee	
	Biceps femoris	Biceps femoris	Biceps femoris	
	Semimembranosus	Semimembranosus	Semimembranosus	
	Semitendinosus	Semitendinosus	Semitendinosus	

Body Region	Muscle	Extensor Tendon	Flexor Tendon	Other Tendon
Lower leg				
	Anterior muscles			
	Extensor digitorum longus	Extensor digitorum longus		
	Extensor hallucis longus	Extensor hallucis longus		
	Fibularis (peroneus) tertius	Fibularis (peroneus) tertius		
	Tibialis anterior	Tibialis anterior		Tibialis anterior
	Lateral muscles			
	Fibularis (peroneus) brevis		Fibularis (peroneus) brevis	
	Fibularis (peroneus) longus		Fibularis (peroneus) longus	
	Posterior muscles			
	Deep			
	Flexor digitorum longus		Flexor digitorum longus	
	Flexor hallucis longus		Flexor hallucis longus	
	Popliteus		Popliteus	
	Tibialis posterior		Tibialis posterior	
	Superficial			
	Gastrocnemius		Gastrocnemius	
	Plantaris		Plantaris	
	Soleus		Soleus	
				Calcaneal (Achilles)
Ankle/Foot				
Extrinsic — attach to a site in the lower leg as well as a site in the foot with action related to foot movement at the ankle				
	Plantaris		Plantaris	
	Soleus		Soleus	
	Tibialis anterior	Tibialis anterior		
	Tibialis posterior		Tibialis posterior	
Extrinsic — attach to a site in the lower leg as well as a site in the foot with action in the foot related to toe movement				
	Extensor digitorum longus	Extensor digitorum longus		
	Extensor hallicus longus	Extensor hallicus longus		
	Flexor digitorum longus		Flexor digitorum longus	
	Flexor hallucis longus		Flexor hallucis longus	
Intrinsic — found within the ankle/foot only				
	Dorsal muscles			
	Extensor digitorum brevis	Extensor digitorum brevis		
	Extensor hallucis brevis	Extensor hallucis brevis		
	Plantar muscles			
	Abductor digiti minimi		Abductor digiti minimi	
	Abductor hallucis		Abductor hallucis	
	Dorsal interossei	Dorsal interossei	Dorsal interossei	
	Flexor digiti minimi brevis		Flexor digiti minimi brevis	
	Flexor digitorum brevis		Flexor digitorum brevis	
	Flexor hallucis brevis		Flexor hallucis brevis	
	Lumbricals	Lumbricals	Lumbricals	
	Quadratus plantae		Quadratus plantae	
	Plantar interossei	Plantar interossei	Plantar interossei	

Chapter 19. Injury, Poisoning and Certain Other Consequences of External Causes (S00-T88)

NOTE Use secondary code(s) from Chapter 20, External causes of morbidity, to indicate cause of injury. Codes within the T section that include the external cause do not require an additional external cause code.

Use additional code to identify any retained foreign body, if applicable (Z18.-)

EXCLUDES 1 birth trauma (P10-P15)
obstetric trauma (O70-O71)

NOTE The chapter uses the S-section for coding different types of injuries related to single body regions and the T-section to cover injuries to unspecified body regions as well as poisoning and certain other consequences of external causes.

AHA: 2016,2Q,3-7; 2015,4Q,35-38; 2015,3Q,37-39,40; 2015,2Q,6; 2015,1Q,3-21

TIP: The specific site of an injury can be determined from the radiology report when authenticated by a radiologist and available at the time of code assignment.

TIP: The specific site of an injury can be determined from the radiology report when authenticated by a radiologist and available at the time of code assignment.

This chapter contains the following blocks:

S00-S09	Injuries to the head
S10-S19	Injuries to the neck
S20-S29	Injuries to the thorax
S30-S39	Injuries to the abdomen, lower back, lumbar spine, pelvis and external genitals
S40-S49	Injuries to the shoulder and upper arm
S50-S59	Injuries to the elbow and forearm
S60-S69	Injuries to the wrist, hand and fingers
S70-S79	Injuries to the hip and thigh
S80-S89	Injuries to the knee and lower leg
S90-S99	Injuries to the ankle and foot
T07	Injuries involving multiple body regions
T14	Injury of unspecified body region
T15-T19	Effects of foreign body entering through natural orifice
T20-T25	Burns and corrosions of external body surface, specified by site
T26-T28	Burns and corrosions confined to eye and internal organs
T30-T32	Burns and corrosions of multiple and unspecified body regions
T33-T34	Frostbite
T36-T50	Poisoning by, adverse effect of and underdosing of drugs, medicaments and biological substances
T51-T65	Toxic effects of substances chiefly nonmedicinal as to source
T66-T78	Other and unspecified effects of external causes
T79	Certain early complications of trauma
T80-T88	Complications of surgical and medical care, not elsewhere classified

Injuries to the head (S00-S09)

INCLUDES
injuries of ear
injuries of eye
injuries of face [any part]
injuries of gum
injuries of jaw
injuries of oral cavity
injuries of palate
injuries of periocular area
injuries of scalp
injuries of temporomandibular joint area
injuries of tongue
injuries of tooth

Code also for any associated infection

EXCLUDES 2 burns and corrosions (T20-T32)
effects of foreign body in ear (T16)
effects of foreign body in larynx (T17.3)
effects of foreign body in mouth NOS (T18.0)
effects of foreign body in nose (T17.0-T17.1)
effects of foreign body in pharynx (T17.2)
effects of foreign body on external eye (T15.-)
frostbite (T33-T34)
insect bite or sting, venomous (T63.4)

√4ᵗʰ **S00 Superficial injury of head**

EXCLUDES 1 diffuse cerebral contusion (S06.2-)
focal cerebral contusion (S06.3-)
injury of eye and orbit (S05.-)
open wound of head (S01.-)

The appropriate 7th character is to be added to each code from category S00.
A initial encounter
D subsequent encounter
S sequela

√5ᵗʰ **S00.0 Superficial injury of scalp**

√x7ᵗʰ **S00.00 Unspecified superficial injury of scalp**

√x7ᵗʰ **S00.01 Abrasion of scalp**

√x7ᵗʰ **S00.02 Blister (nonthermal) of scalp**

√x7ᵗʰ **S00.03 Contusion of scalp** 🄾
Bruise of scalp
Hematoma of scalp

√x7ᵗʰ **S00.04 External constriction of part of scalp**

√x7ᵗʰ **S00.05 Superficial foreign body of scalp**
Splinter in the scalp

√x7ᵗʰ **S00.06 Insect bite (nonvenomous) of scalp**

√x7ᵗʰ **S00.07 Other superficial bite of scalp**
EXCLUDES 1 open bite of scalp (S01.05)

√5ᵗʰ **S00.1 Contusion of eyelid and periocular area**
Black eye
EXCLUDES 2 contusion of eyeball and orbital tissues (S05.1)

√x7ᵗʰ **S00.10 Contusion of unspecified eyelid and periocular area**

√x7ᵗʰ **S00.11 Contusion of right eyelid and periocular area**

√x7ᵗʰ **S00.12 Contusion of left eyelid and periocular area**

√5ᵗʰ **S00.2 Other and unspecified superficial injuries of eyelid and periocular area**
EXCLUDES 2 superficial injury of conjunctiva and cornea (S05.0-)

√6ᵗʰ **S00.20 Unspecified superficial injury of eyelid and periocular area**

√7ᵗʰ **S00.201 Unspecified superficial injury of right eyelid and periocular area**

√7ᵗʰ **S00.202 Unspecified superficial injury of left eyelid and periocular area**

√7ᵗʰ **S00.209 Unspecified superficial injury of unspecified eyelid and periocular area**

√6ᵗʰ **S00.21 Abrasion of eyelid and periocular area**

√7ᵗʰ **S00.211 Abrasion of right eyelid and periocular area**

√7ᵗʰ **S00.212 Abrasion of left eyelid and periocular area**

√7ᵗʰ **S00.219 Abrasion of unspecified eyelid and periocular area**

√6ᵗʰ **S00.22 Blister (nonthermal) of eyelid and periocular area**

√7ᵗʰ **S00.221 Blister (nonthermal) of right eyelid and periocular area**

√7ᵗʰ **S00.222 Blister (nonthermal) of left eyelid and periocular area**

√7ᵗʰ **S00.229 Blister (nonthermal) of unspecified eyelid and periocular area**

√6ᵗʰ **S00.24 External constriction of eyelid and periocular area**

√7ᵗʰ **S00.241 External constriction of right eyelid and periocular area**

√7ᵗʰ **S00.242 External constriction of left eyelid and periocular area**

√7ᵗʰ **S00.249 External constriction of unspecified eyelid and periocular area**

√6ᵗʰ **S00.25 Superficial foreign body of eyelid and periocular area**
Splinter of eyelid and periocular area
EXCLUDES 2 retained foreign body in eyelid (H02.81-)

√7ᵗʰ **S00.251 Superficial foreign body of right eyelid and periocular area**

√7ᵗʰ **S00.252 Superficial foreign body of left eyelid and periocular area**

√7ᵗʰ **S00.259 Superficial foreign body of unspecified eyelid and periocular area**

√6ᵗʰ **S00.26 Insect bite (nonvenomous) of eyelid and periocular area**

√7ᵗʰ **S00.261 Insect bite (nonvenomous) of right eyelid and periocular area**

√7ᵗʰ **S00.262 Insect bite (nonvenomous) of left eyelid and periocular area**

√7ᵗʰ **S00.269 Insect bite (nonvenomous) of unspecified eyelid and periocular area**

√6ᵗʰ **S00.27 Other superficial bite of eyelid and periocular area**
EXCLUDES 1 open bite of eyelid and periocular area (S01.15)

√7ᵗʰ **S00.271 Other superficial bite of right eyelid and periocular area**

√7ᵗʰ **S00.272 Other superficial bite of left eyelid and periocular area**

√7ᵗʰ **S00.279 Other superficial bite of unspecified eyelid and periocular area**

√5ᵗʰ **S00.3 Superficial injury of nose**

√x7ᵗʰ **S00.30 Unspecified superficial injury of nose**

√x7ᵗʰ **S00.31 Abrasion of nose**

√x7ᵗʰ **S00.32 Blister (nonthermal) of nose**

√x7ᵗʰ **S00.33** **Contusion** of nose Q
  Bruise of nose
  Hematoma of nose

√x7ᵗʰ **S00.34** **External constriction** of nose

√x7ᵗʰ **S00.35** **Superficial foreign body** of nose
  Splinter in the nose

√x7ᵗʰ **S00.36** **Insect bite (nonvenomous)** of nose

√x7ᵗʰ **S00.37** **Other superficial bite** of nose
  EXCLUDES 1 open bite of nose (S01.25)

√5ᵗʰ **S00.4** **Superficial injury** of ear

  √6ᵗʰ **S00.40** **Unspecified superficial injury** of ear
    √7ᵗʰ **S00.401** Unspecified superficial injury of **right ear**
    √7ᵗʰ **S00.402** Unspecified superficial injury of **left ear**
    √7ᵗʰ **S00.409** Unspecified superficial injury of unspecified ear

  √6ᵗʰ **S00.41** **Abrasion** of ear
    √7ᵗʰ **S00.411** Abrasion of **right ear**
    √7ᵗʰ **S00.412** Abrasion of **left ear**
    √7ᵗʰ **S00.419** Abrasion of unspecified ear

  √6ᵗʰ **S00.42** **Blister (nonthermal)** of ear
    √7ᵗʰ **S00.421** Blister (nonthermal) of **right ear**
    √7ᵗʰ **S00.422** Blister (nonthermal) of **left ear**
    √7ᵗʰ **S00.429** Blister (nonthermal) of unspecified ear

  √6ᵗʰ **S00.43** **Contusion** of ear
    Bruise of ear
    Hematoma of ear
    √7ᵗʰ **S00.431** Contusion of **right** ear Q
    √7ᵗʰ **S00.432** Contusion of **left** ear Q
    √7ᵗʰ **S00.439** Contusion of unspecified ear Q

  √6ᵗʰ **S00.44** **External constriction** of ear
    √7ᵗʰ **S00.441** External constriction of **right** ear
    √7ᵗʰ **S00.442** External constriction of **left** ear
    √7ᵗʰ **S00.449** External constriction of unspecified ear

  √6ᵗʰ **S00.45** **Superficial foreign body** of ear
    Splinter in the ear
    √7ᵗʰ **S00.451** Superficial foreign body of **right** ear
    √7ᵗʰ **S00.452** Superficial foreign body of **left** ear
    √7ᵗʰ **S00.459** Superficial foreign body of unspecified ear

  √6ᵗʰ **S00.46** **Insect bite (nonvenomous)** of ear
    √7ᵗʰ **S00.461** Insect bite (nonvenomous) of **right** ear
    √7ᵗʰ **S00.462** Insect bite (nonvenomous) of **left** ear
    √7ᵗʰ **S00.469** Insect bite (nonvenomous) of unspecified ear

  √6ᵗʰ **S00.47** **Other superficial bite** of ear
    EXCLUDES 1 open bite of ear (S01.35)
    √7ᵗʰ **S00.471** Other superficial bite of **right** ear
    √7ᵗʰ **S00.472** Other superficial bite of **left** ear
    √7ᵗʰ **S00.479** Other superficial bite of unspecified ear

√5ᵗʰ **S00.5** **Superficial injury** of lip and oral cavity

  √6ᵗʰ **S00.50** **Unspecified superficial injury** of lip and oral cavity
    √7ᵗʰ **S00.501** Unspecified superficial injury of **lip**
    √7ᵗʰ **S00.502** Unspecified superficial injury of **oral cavity**

  √6ᵗʰ **S00.51** **Abrasion** of lip and oral cavity
    √7ᵗʰ **S00.511** Abrasion of **lip**
    √7ᵗʰ **S00.512** Abrasion of **oral cavity**

  √6ᵗʰ **S00.52** **Blister (nonthermal)** of lip and oral cavity
    √7ᵗʰ **S00.521** Blister (nonthermal) of **lip**
    √7ᵗʰ **S00.522** Blister (nonthermal) of **oral cavity**

  √6ᵗʰ **S00.53** **Contusion** of lip and oral cavity
    √7ᵗʰ **S00.531** Contusion of **lip** Q
      Bruise of lip
      Hematoma of lip
    √7ᵗʰ **S00.532** Contusion of **oral cavity** Q
      Bruise of oral cavity
      Hematoma of oral cavity

  √6ᵗʰ **S00.54** **External constriction** of lip and oral cavity
    √7ᵗʰ **S00.541** **External constriction** of lip

  √7ᵗʰ **S00.542** **External constriction** of oral cavity

  √6ᵗʰ **S00.55** **Superficial foreign body** of lip and oral cavity
    √7ᵗʰ **S00.551** **Superficial foreign body** of lip
      Splinter of lip and oral cavity
    √7ᵗʰ **S00.552** **Superficial foreign body** of oral cavity
      Splinter of lip and oral cavity

  √6ᵗʰ **S00.56** **Insect bite (nonvenomous)** of lip and oral cavity
    √7ᵗʰ **S00.561** **Insect bite (nonvenomous)** of lip
    √7ᵗʰ **S00.562** **Insect bite (nonvenomous)** of oral cavity

  √6ᵗʰ **S00.57** **Other superficial bite** of lip and oral cavity
    √7ᵗʰ **S00.571** **Other superficial bite** of lip
      EXCLUDES 1 open bite of lip (S01.551)
    √7ᵗʰ **S00.572** **Other superficial bite** of oral cavity
      EXCLUDES 1 open bite of oral cavity (S01.552)

√5ᵗʰ **S00.8** **Superficial injury** of other parts of head
  Superficial injuries of face [any part]

  √x7ᵗʰ **S00.80** **Unspecified superficial injury** of other part of head

  √x7ᵗʰ **S00.81** **Abrasion** of other part of head

  √x7ᵗʰ **S00.82** **Blister (nonthermal)** of other part of head

  √x7ᵗʰ **S00.83** **Contusion** of other part of head Q
    Bruise of other part of head
    Hematoma of other part of head

  √x7ᵗʰ **S00.84** **External constriction** of other part of head

  √x7ᵗʰ **S00.85** **Superficial foreign body** of other part of head
    Splinter in other part of head

  √x7ᵗʰ **S00.86** **Insect bite (nonvenomous)** of other part of head

  √x7ᵗʰ **S00.87** **Other superficial bite** of other part of head
    EXCLUDES 1 open bite of other part of head (S01.85)

√5ᵗʰ **S00.9** **Superficial injury** of unspecified part of head

  √x7ᵗʰ **S00.90** **Unspecified superficial injury** of unspecified part of head

  √x7ᵗʰ **S00.91** **Abrasion** of unspecified part of head

  √x7ᵗʰ **S00.92** **Blister (nonthermal)** of unspecified part of head

  √x7ᵗʰ **S00.93** **Contusion** of unspecified part of head Ш
    Bruise of head
    Hematoma of head

  √x7ᵗʰ **S00.94** **External constriction** of unspecified part of head

  √x7ᵗʰ **S00.95** **Superficial foreign body** of unspecified part of head
    Splinter of head

  √x7ᵗʰ **S00.96** **Insect bite (nonvenomous)** of unspecified part of head

  √x7ᵗʰ **S00.97** **Other superficial bite** of unspecified part of head
    EXCLUDES 1 open bite of head (S01.95)

√4ᵗʰ **S01** **Open wound of head**
  Code also any associated:
    injury of cranial nerve (S04.-)
    injury of muscle and tendon of head (S09.1-)
    intracranial injury (S06.-)
    wound infection
  EXCLUDES 1 open skull fracture (S02.- with 7th character B)
  EXCLUDES 2 injury of eye and orbit (S05.-)
    traumatic amputation of part of head (S08.-)

  The appropriate 7th character is to be added to each code from category S01.
  A initial encounter
  D subsequent encounter
  S sequela

√5ᵗʰ **S01.0** **Open wound of scalp**
  EXCLUDES 1 avulsion of scalp (S08.0)

  √x7ᵗʰ **S01.00** **Unspecified open wound of scalp**

  √x7ᵗʰ **S01.01** **Laceration without foreign body of scalp**

  √x7ᵗʰ **S01.02** **Laceration with foreign body of scalp**

  √x7ᵗʰ **S01.03** **Puncture wound without foreign body of scalp**

  √x7ᵗʰ **S01.04** **Puncture wound with foreign body of scalp**

  √x7ᵗʰ **S01.05** **Open bite** of scalp
    Bite of scalp NOS
    EXCLUDES 1 superficial bite of scalp (S00.06, S00.07-)

S01.1 Open wound of eyelid and periocular area
Open wound of eyelid and periocular area with or without involvement of lacrimal passages

   S01.10 Unspecified open wound of eyelid and periocular area
      S01.101 Unspecified open wound of right eyelid and periocular area
      S01.102 Unspecified open wound of left eyelid and periocular area
      S01.109 Unspecified open wound of unspecified eyelid and periocular area

   S01.11 Laceration without foreign body of eyelid and periocular area
      S01.111 Laceration without foreign body of right eyelid and periocular area
      S01.112 Laceration without foreign body of left eyelid and periocular area
      S01.119 Laceration without foreign body of unspecified eyelid and periocular area

   S01.12 Laceration with foreign body of eyelid and periocular area
      S01.121 Laceration with foreign body of right eyelid and periocular area
      S01.122 Laceration with foreign body of left eyelid and periocular area
      S01.129 Laceration with foreign body of unspecified eyelid and periocular area

   S01.13 Puncture wound without foreign body of eyelid and periocular area
      S01.131 Puncture wound without foreign body of right eyelid and periocular area
      S01.132 Puncture wound without foreign body of left eyelid and periocular area
      S01.139 Puncture wound without foreign body of unspecified eyelid and periocular area

   S01.14 Puncture wound with foreign body of eyelid and periocular area
      S01.141 Puncture wound with foreign body of right eyelid and periocular area
      S01.142 Puncture wound with foreign body of left eyelid and periocular area
      S01.149 Puncture wound with foreign body of unspecified eyelid and periocular area

   S01.15 Open bite of eyelid and periocular area
     Bite of eyelid and periocular area NOS
       EXCLUDES 1   *superficial bite of eyelid and periocular area (S00.26, S00.27)*
      S01.151 Open bite of right eyelid and periocular area
      S01.152 Open bite of left eyelid and periocular area
      S01.159 Open bite of unspecified eyelid and periocular area

S01.2 Open wound of nose
   S01.20 Unspecified open wound of nose
   S01.21 Laceration without foreign body of nose
   S01.22 Laceration with foreign body of nose
   S01.23 Puncture wound without foreign body of nose
   S01.24 Puncture wound with foreign body of nose
   S01.25 Open bite of nose
     Bite of nose NOS
       EXCLUDES 1   *superficial bite of nose (S00.36, S00.37)*

S01.3 Open wound of ear
   S01.30 Unspecified open wound of ear
      S01.301 Unspecified open wound of right ear
      S01.302 Unspecified open wound of left ear
      S01.309 Unspecified open wound of unspecified ear

   S01.31 Laceration without foreign body of ear
      S01.311 Laceration without foreign body of right ear
      S01.312 Laceration without foreign body of left ear
      S01.319 Laceration without foreign body of unspecified ear

   S01.32 Laceration with foreign body of ear
      S01.321 Laceration with foreign body of right ear
      S01.322 Laceration with foreign body of left ear

      S01.329 Laceration with foreign body of unspecified ear

   S01.33 Puncture wound without foreign body of ear
      S01.331 Puncture wound without foreign body of right ear
      S01.332 Puncture wound without foreign body of left ear
      S01.339 Puncture wound without foreign body of unspecified ear

   S01.34 Puncture wound with foreign body of ear
      S01.341 Puncture wound with foreign body of right ear
      S01.342 Puncture wound with foreign body of left ear
      S01.349 Puncture wound with foreign body of unspecified ear

   S01.35 Open bite of ear
     Bite of ear NOS
       EXCLUDES 1   *superficial bite of ear (S00.46, S00.47)*
      S01.351 Open bite of right ear
      S01.352 Open bite of left ear
      S01.359 Open bite of unspecified ear

S01.4 Open wound of cheek and temporomandibular area
   S01.40 Unspecified open wound of cheek and temporomandibular area
      S01.401 Unspecified open wound of right cheek and temporomandibular area
      S01.402 Unspecified open wound of left cheek and temporomandibular area
      S01.409 Unspecified open wound of unspecified cheek and temporomandibular area

   S01.41 Laceration without foreign body of cheek and temporomandibular area
      S01.411 Laceration without foreign body of right cheek and temporomandibular area
      S01.412 Laceration without foreign body of left cheek and temporomandibular area
      S01.419 Laceration without foreign body of unspecified cheek and temporomandibular area

   S01.42 Laceration with foreign body of cheek and temporomandibular area
      S01.421 Laceration with foreign body of right cheek and temporomandibular area
      S01.422 Laceration with foreign body of left cheek and temporomandibular area
      S01.429 Laceration with foreign body of unspecified cheek and temporomandibular area

   S01.43 Puncture wound without foreign body of cheek and temporomandibular area
      S01.431 Puncture wound without foreign body of right cheek and temporomandibular area
      S01.432 Puncture wound without foreign body of left cheek and temporomandibular area
      S01.439 Puncture wound without foreign body of unspecified cheek and temporomandibular area

   S01.44 Puncture wound with foreign body of cheek and temporomandibular area
      S01.441 Puncture wound with foreign body of right cheek and temporomandibular area
      S01.442 Puncture wound with foreign body of left cheek and temporomandibular area
      S01.449 Puncture wound with foreign body of unspecified cheek and temporomandibular area

   S01.45 Open bite of cheek and temporomandibular area
     Bite of cheek and temporomandibular area NOS
       EXCLUDES 2   *superficial bite of cheek and temporomandibular area (S00.86, S00.87)*
      S01.451 Open bite of right cheek and temporomandibular area
      S01.452 Open bite of left cheek and temporomandibular area
      S01.459 Open bite of unspecified cheek and temporomandibular area

√5ᵗʰ **S01.5 Open wound of lip and oral cavity**
> EXCLUDES 2 tooth dislocation (S03.2)
> tooth fracture (S02.5)

√6ᵗʰ **S01.50 Unspecified open wound of lip and oral cavity**
> √7ᵗʰ **S01.501 Unspecified open wound of lip**
> √7ᵗʰ **S01.502 Unspecified open wound of oral cavity**

√6ᵗʰ **S01.51 Laceration of lip and oral cavity without foreign body**
> √7ᵗʰ **S01.511 Laceration without foreign body of lip**
> √7ᵗʰ **S01.512 Laceration without foreign body of oral cavity**

√6ᵗʰ **S01.52 Laceration of lip and oral cavity with foreign body**
> √7ᵗʰ **S01.521 Laceration with foreign body of lip**
> √7ᵗʰ **S01.522 Laceration with foreign body of oral cavity**

√6ᵗʰ **S01.53 Puncture wound of lip and oral cavity without foreign body**
> √7ᵗʰ **S01.531 Puncture wound without foreign body of lip**
> √7ᵗʰ **S01.532 Puncture wound without foreign body of oral cavity**

√6ᵗʰ **S01.54 Puncture wound of lip and oral cavity with foreign body**
> √7ᵗʰ **S01.541 Puncture wound with foreign body of lip**
> √7ᵗʰ **S01.542 Puncture wound with foreign body of oral cavity**

√6ᵗʰ **S01.55 Open bite of lip and oral cavity**
> √7ᵗʰ **S01.551 Open bite of lip**
> > Bite of lip NOS
> > EXCLUDES 1 superficial bite of lip (S00.571)
> √7ᵗʰ **S01.552 Open bite of oral cavity**
> > Bite of oral cavity NOS
> > EXCLUDES 1 superficial bite of oral cavity (S00.572)

√5ᵗʰ **S01.8 Open wound of other parts of head**
> √x7ᵗʰ **S01.80 Unspecified open wound of other part of head**
> √x7ᵗʰ **S01.81 Laceration without foreign body of other part of head**
> √x7ᵗʰ **S01.82 Laceration with foreign body of other part of head**
> √x7ᵗʰ **S01.83 Puncture wound without foreign body of other part of head**
> √x7ᵗʰ **S01.84 Puncture wound with foreign body of other part of head**
> √x7ᵗʰ **S01.85 Open bite of other part of head**
> > Bite of other part of head NOS
> > EXCLUDES 1 superficial bite of other part of head (S00.87)

√5ᵗʰ **S01.9 Open wound of unspecified part of head**
> √x7ᵗʰ **S01.90 Unspecified open wound of unspecified part of head**
> √x7ᵗʰ **S01.91 Laceration without foreign body of unspecified part of head**
> √x7ᵗʰ **S01.92 Laceration with foreign body of unspecified part of head**
> √x7ᵗʰ **S01.93 Puncture wound without foreign body of unspecified part of head**
> √x7ᵗʰ **S01.94 Puncture wound with foreign body of unspecified part of head**
> √x7ᵗʰ **S01.95 Open bite of unspecified part of head**
> > Bite of head NOS
> > EXCLUDES 1 superficial bite of head NOS (S00.97)

√4ᵗʰ **S02 Fracture of skull and facial bones**

> **NOTE**   A fracture not indicated as open or closed should be coded to closed.

> Code also any associated intracranial injury (S06.-)
> **AHA:** 2017,1Q,42; 2016,4Q,66-67

> The appropriate 7th character is to be added to each code from category S02.
> A   initial encounter for closed fracture
> B   initial encounter for open fracture
> D   subsequent encounter for fracture with routine healing
> G   subsequent encounter for fracture with delayed healing
> K   subsequent encounter for fracture with nonunion
> S   sequela

² √x7ᵗʰ **S02.0 Fracture of vault of skull** HCC Q
> Fracture of frontal bone
> Fracture of parietal bone

√5ᵗʰ **S02.1 Fracture of base of skull**
> EXCLUDES 1 orbit NOS (S02.8)
> EXCLUDES 2 ▶lateral orbital wall (S02.84-)◀
> ▶medial orbital wall (S02.83-)◀
> orbital floor (S02.3-)

> √6ᵗʰ **S02.10 Unspecified fracture of base of skull**
> > ² √7ᵗʰ **S02.101 Fracture of base of skull, right side** HCC Q
> > ² √7ᵗʰ **S02.102 Fracture of base of skull, left side** HCC Q
> > ² √7ᵗʰ **S02.109 Fracture of base of skull, unspecified side** HCC Q

> √6ᵗʰ **S02.11 Fracture of occiput**
> > ² √7ᵗʰ **S02.110 Type I occipital condyle fracture, unspecified side** HCC Q
> > ² √7ᵗʰ **S02.111 Type II occipital condyle fracture, unspecified side** HCC Q
> > ² √7ᵗʰ **S02.112 Type III occipital condyle fracture, unspecified side** HCC Q
> > ² √7ᵗʰ **S02.113 Unspecified occipital condyle fracture** HCC Q
> > ² √7ᵗʰ **S02.118 Other fracture of occiput, unspecified side** HCC Q
> > ² √7ᵗʰ **S02.119 Unspecified fracture of occiput** HCC Q
> > ² √7ᵗʰ **S02.11A Type I occipital condyle fracture, right side** HCC Q
> > ² √7ᵗʰ **S02.11B Type I occipital condyle fracture, left side** HCC Q
> > ² √7ᵗʰ **S02.11C Type II occipital condyle fracture, right side** HCC Q
> > ² √7ᵗʰ **S02.11D Type II occipital condyle fracture, left side** HCC Q
> > ² √7ᵗʰ **S02.11E Type III occipital condyle fracture, right side** HCC Q
> > ² √7ᵗʰ **S02.11F Type III occipital condyle fracture, left side** HCC Q
> > ² √7ᵗʰ **S02.11G Other fracture of occiput, right side** HCC Q
> > ² √7ᵗʰ **S02.11H Other fracture of occiput, left side** HCC Q

> √6ᵗʰ **S02.12 Fracture of orbital roof**
> > √7ᵗʰ **S02.121 Fracture of orbital roof, right side**
> > √7ᵗʰ **S02.122 Fracture of orbital roof, left side**
> > √7ᵗʰ **S02.129 Fracture of orbital roof, unspecified side**

> ² √x7ᵗʰ **S02.19 Other fracture of base of skull** HCC Q
> > Fracture of anterior fossa of base of skull
> > Fracture of ethmoid sinus
> > Fracture of frontal sinus
> > Fracture of middle fossa of base of skull
> > ~~Fracture of orbital roof~~
> > Fracture of posterior fossa of base of skull
> > Fracture of sphenoid
> > Fracture of temporal bone

√x7ᵗʰ **S02.2 Fracture of nasal bones** Q

√5ᵗʰ **S02.3 Fracture of orbital floor**
> ▶Fracture of inferior orbital wall◀
> EXCLUDES 1 orbit NOS ▶(S02.85)◀
> EXCLUDES 2 ▶lateral orbital wall (S02.84-)◀
> ▶medial orbital wall (S02.83-)◀
> orbital roof (S02.1-)

> ² √x7ᵗʰ **S02.30 Fracture of orbital floor, unspecified side** HCC Q

☑ Additional Character Required   √x7ᵗʰ Placeholder Alert   Manifestation   Unspecified Dx   ▶◀ Revised Text   ● New Code   ▲ Revised Code Title

² √x7ᵗʰ **S02.31** **Fracture of orbital floor, right side** HCC Q

² √x7ᵗʰ **S02.32** **Fracture of orbital floor, left side** HCC Q

√5ᵗʰ **S02.4** **Fracture of malar, maxillary and zygoma bones**
Fracture of superior maxilla
Fracture of upper jaw (bone)
Fracture of zygomatic process of temporal bone

√6ᵗʰ **S02.40** **Fracture of malar, maxillary and zygoma bones, unspecified**

² √7ᵗʰ **S02.400** **Malar fracture, unspecified side** HCC Q

² √7ᵗʰ **S02.401** **Maxillary fracture, unspecified side** HCC Q

² √7ᵗʰ **S02.402** **Zygomatic fracture, unspecified side** HCC Q

² √7ᵗʰ **S02.40A** **Malar fracture, right side** HCC Q

² √7ᵗʰ **S02.40B** **Malar fracture, left side** HCC Q

² √7ᵗʰ **S02.40C** **Maxillary fracture, right side** HCC Q

² √7ᵗʰ **S02.40D** **Maxillary fracture, left side** HCC Q

² √7ᵗʰ **S02.40E** **Zygomatic fracture, right side** HCC Q

² √7ᵗʰ **S02.40F** **Zygomatic fracture, left side** HCC Q

√6ᵗʰ **S02.41** **LeFort fracture**

DEF: Named for Rene Le Fort, these fractures describe different combinations of multiple fractures that occur from significant force to the midface. A common denominator in all three types of LeFort fractures is fracture of the pterygoid processes, which are two bony plates resembling wings that extend downward from the sphenoid bone.

LeFort Fracture Types

Frontal bone   Nasal bone   Orbital floor
Type III
Type II
Type I
Maxilla
Zygomatic bone (malar) and arch

² √7ᵗʰ **S02.411** **LeFort I fracture** HCC Q

² √7ᵗʰ **S02.412** **LeFort II fracture** HCC Q

² √7ᵗʰ **S02.413** **LeFort III fracture** HCC Q

² √x7ᵗʰ **S02.42** **Fracture of alveolus of maxilla** HCC Q

√x7ᵗʰ **S02.5** **Fracture of tooth (traumatic)**
Broken tooth
EXCLUDES 1   cracked tooth (nontraumatic) (K03.81)

√5ᵗʰ **S02.6** **Fracture of mandible**
Fracture of lower jaw (bone)

√6ᵗʰ **S02.60** **Fracture of mandible, unspecified**

² √7ᵗʰ **S02.600** **Fracture of unspecified part of body of mandible, unspecified side** HCC Q

² √7ᵗʰ **S02.601** **Fracture of unspecified part of body of right mandible** HCC Q

² √7ᵗʰ **S02.602** **Fracture of unspecified part of body of left mandible** HCC Q

² √7ᵗʰ **S02.609** **Fracture of mandible, unspecified** HCC Q

√6ᵗʰ **S02.61** **Fracture of condylar process of mandible**

² √7ᵗʰ **S02.610** **Fracture of condylar process of mandible, unspecified side** HCC Q

² √7ᵗʰ **S02.611** **Fracture of condylar process of right mandible** HCC Q

² √7ᵗʰ **S02.612** **Fracture of condylar process of left mandible** HCC Q

√6ᵗʰ **S02.62** **Fracture of subcondylar process of mandible**

² √7ᵗʰ **S02.620** **Fracture of subcondylar process of mandible, unspecified side** HCC Q

² √7ᵗʰ **S02.621** **Fracture of subcondylar process of right mandible** HCC Q

² √7ᵗʰ **S02.622** **Fracture of subcondylar process of left mandible** HCC Q

√6ᵗʰ **S02.63** **Fracture of coronoid process of mandible**

² √7ᵗʰ **S02.630** **Fracture of coronoid process of mandible, unspecified side** HCC Q

² √7ᵗʰ **S02.631** **Fracture of coronoid process of right mandible** HCC Q

² √7ᵗʰ **S02.632** **Fracture of coronoid process of left mandible** HCC Q

√6ᵗʰ **S02.64** **Fracture of ramus of mandible**

² √7ᵗʰ **S02.640** **Fracture of ramus of mandible, unspecified side** HCC Q

² √7ᵗʰ **S02.641** **Fracture of ramus of right mandible** HCC Q

² √7ᵗʰ **S02.642** **Fracture of ramus of left mandible** HCC Q

√6ᵗʰ **S02.65** **Fracture of angle of mandible**

² √7ᵗʰ **S02.650** **Fracture of angle of mandible, unspecified side** HCC Q

² √7ᵗʰ **S02.651** **Fracture of angle of right mandible** HCC Q

² √7ᵗʰ **S02.652** **Fracture of angle of left mandible** HCC Q

² √x7ᵗʰ **S02.66** **Fracture of symphysis of mandible** HCC Q

√6ᵗʰ **S02.67** **Fracture of alveolus of mandible**

² √7ᵗʰ **S02.670** **Fracture of alveolus of mandible, unspecified side** HCC Q

² √7ᵗʰ **S02.671** **Fracture of alveolus of right mandible** HCC Q

² √7ᵗʰ **S02.672** **Fracture of alveolus of left mandible** HCC Q

² √x7ᵗʰ **S02.69** **Fracture of mandible of other specified site** HCC Q

√5ᵗʰ **S02.8** **Fractures of other specified skull and facial bones**
Fracture of orbit NOS
Fracture of palate
EXCLUDES 1   fracture of orbital floor (S02.3-)
    fracture of orbital roof (S02.1-)
EXCLUDES 2   ▶fracture of orbital floor (S02.3-)◀
    ▶fracture of orbital roof (S02.12-)◀

² √x7ᵗʰ **S02.80** **Fracture of other specified skull and facial bones, unspecified side** HCC Q

² √x7ᵗʰ **S02.81** **Fracture of other specified skull and facial bones, right side** HCC Q

² √x7ᵗʰ **S02.82** **Fracture of other specified skull and facial bones, left side** HCC Q

● √6ᵗʰ **S02.83** **Fracture of medial orbital wall**
EXCLUDES 2   orbital floor (S02.3-)
    orbital roof (S02.12-)

● √7ᵗʰ **S02.831** **Fracture of medial orbital wall, right side**

● √7ᵗʰ **S02.832** **Fracture of medial orbital wall, left side**

● √7ᵗʰ **S02.839** **Fracture of medial orbital wall, unspecified side**

● √6ᵗʰ **S02.84** **Fracture of lateral orbital wall**
EXCLUDES 2   orbital floor (S02.3-)
    orbital roof (S02.12-)

● √7ᵗʰ **S02.841** **Fracture of lateral orbital wall, right side**

● √7ᵗʰ **S02.842** **Fracture of lateral orbital wall, left side**

● √7ᵗʰ **S02.849** **Fracture of lateral orbital wall, unspecified side**

● √x7ᵗʰ **S02.85** **Fracture of orbit, unspecified**
Fracture of orbit NOS
Fracture of orbit wall NOS
EXCLUDES 1   lateral orbital wall (S02.84-)
    medial orbital wall (S02.83-)
    orbital floor (S02.3-)
    orbital roof (S02.12-)

√5ᵗʰ **S02.9** **Fracture of unspecified skull and facial bones**

² √x7ᵗʰ **S02.91** **Unspecified fracture of skull** HCC Q

² √x7ᵗʰ **S02.92** **Unspecified fracture of facial bones** HCC Q

☑4ᵗʰ S03 Dislocation and sprain of joints and ligaments of head

> **INCLUDES** avulsion of joint (capsule) or ligament of head
> laceration of cartilage, joint (capsule) or ligament of head
> sprain of cartilage, joint (capsule) or ligament of head
> traumatic hemarthrosis of joint or ligament of head
> traumatic rupture of joint or ligament of head
> traumatic subluxation of joint or ligament of head
> traumatic tear of joint or ligament of head
> Code also any associated open wound
> **EXCLUDES 2** *strain of muscle or tendon of head (S09.1)*

> The appropriate 7th character is to be added to each code from category S03.
> A   initial encounter
> D   subsequent encounter
> S   sequela

  ☑5ᵗʰ S03.0 Dislocation of jaw

> Dislocation of jaw (cartilage) (meniscus)
> Dislocation of mandible
> Dislocation of temporomandibular (joint)
> **AHA:** 2016,4Q,67

    √x7ᵗʰ S03.00 Dislocation of jaw, unspecified side
    √x7ᵗʰ S03.01 Dislocation of jaw, right side
    √x7ᵗʰ S03.02 Dislocation of jaw, left side
    √x7ᵗʰ S03.03 Dislocation of jaw, bilateral

  √x7ᵗʰ S03.1 Dislocation of septal cartilage of nose
  √x7ᵗʰ S03.2 Dislocation of tooth

  ☑5ᵗʰ S03.4 Sprain of jaw

> Sprain of temporomandibular (joint) (ligament)
> **AHA:** 2016,4Q,67

    √x7ᵗʰ S03.40 Sprain of jaw, unspecified side
    √x7ᵗʰ S03.41 Sprain of jaw, right side
    √x7ᵗʰ S03.42 Sprain of jaw, left side
    √x7ᵗʰ S03.43 Sprain of jaw, bilateral

  √x7ᵗʰ S03.8 Sprain of joints and ligaments of other parts of head
  √x7ᵗʰ S03.9 Sprain of joints and ligaments of unspecified parts of head

☑4ᵗʰ S04 Injury of cranial nerve

> The selection of side should be based on the side of the body being affected
> Code first any associated intracranial injury (S06.-)
> Code also any associated:
>   open wound of head (S01.-)
>   skull fracture (S02.-)

> The appropriate 7th character is to be added to each code from category S04.
> A   initial encounter
> D   subsequent encounter
> S   sequela

  ☑5ᵗʰ S04.0 Injury of optic nerve and pathways

> Use additional code to identify any visual field defect or blindness (H53.4-, H54.-)

    ☑6ᵗʰ S04.01 Injury of optic nerve

> Injury of 2nd cranial nerve

      √7ᵗʰ S04.011 Injury of optic nerve, right eye
      √7ᵗʰ S04.012 Injury of optic nerve, left eye
      √7ᵗʰ S04.019 Injury of optic nerve, unspecified eye

> Injury of optic nerve NOS

    √x7ᵗʰ S04.02 Injury of optic chiasm

    ☑6ᵗʰ S04.03 Injury of optic tract and pathways

> Injury of optic radiation

      √7ᵗʰ S04.031 Injury of optic tract and pathways, right side
      √7ᵗʰ S04.032 Injury of optic tract and pathways, left side
      √7ᵗʰ S04.039 Injury of optic tract and pathways, unspecified side

> Injury of optic tract and pathways NOS

    ☑6ᵗʰ S04.04 Injury of visual cortex

      √7ᵗʰ S04.041 Injury of visual cortex, right side
      √7ᵗʰ S04.042 Injury of visual cortex, left side

      √7ᵗʰ S04.049 Injury of visual cortex, unspecified side

> Injury of visual cortex NOS

  ☑5ᵗʰ S04.1 Injury of oculomotor nerve

> Injury of 3rd cranial nerve

    √x7ᵗʰ S04.10 Injury of oculomotor nerve, unspecified side
    √x7ᵗʰ S04.11 Injury of oculomotor nerve, right side
    √x7ᵗʰ S04.12 Injury of oculomotor nerve, left side

  ☑5ᵗʰ S04.2 Injury of trochlear nerve

> Injury of 4th cranial nerve

    √x7ᵗʰ S04.20 Injury of trochlear nerve, unspecified side
    √x7ᵗʰ S04.21 Injury of trochlear nerve, right side
    √x7ᵗʰ S04.22 Injury of trochlear nerve, left side

  ☑5ᵗʰ S04.3 Injury of trigeminal nerve

> Injury of 5th cranial nerve

    √x7ᵗʰ S04.30 Injury of trigeminal nerve, unspecified side
    √x7ᵗʰ S04.31 Injury of trigeminal nerve, right side
    √x7ᵗʰ S04.32 Injury of trigeminal nerve, left side

  ☑5ᵗʰ S04.4 Injury of abducent nerve

> Injury of 6th cranial nerve

    √x7ᵗʰ S04.40 Injury of abducent nerve, unspecified side
    √x7ᵗʰ S04.41 Injury of abducent nerve, right side
    √x7ᵗʰ S04.42 Injury of abducent nerve, left side

  ☑5ᵗʰ S04.5 Injury of facial nerve

> Injury of 7th cranial nerve

    √x7ᵗʰ S04.50 Injury of facial nerve, unspecified side
    √x7ᵗʰ S04.51 Injury of facial nerve, right side
    √x7ᵗʰ S04.52 Injury of facial nerve, left side

  ☑5ᵗʰ S04.6 Injury of acoustic nerve

> Injury of auditory nerve
> Injury of 8th cranial nerve

    √x7ᵗʰ S04.60 Injury of acoustic nerve, unspecified side
    √x7ᵗʰ S04.61 Injury of acoustic nerve, right side
    √x7ᵗʰ S04.62 Injury of acoustic nerve, left side

  ☑5ᵗʰ S04.7 Injury of accessory nerve

> Injury of 11th cranial nerve

    √x7ᵗʰ S04.70 Injury of accessory nerve, unspecified side
    √x7ᵗʰ S04.71 Injury of accessory nerve, right side
    √x7ᵗʰ S04.72 Injury of accessory nerve, left side

  ☑5ᵗʰ S04.8 Injury of other cranial nerves

    ☑6ᵗʰ S04.81 Injury of olfactory [1st] nerve

      √7ᵗʰ S04.811 Injury of olfactory [1st] nerve, right side
      √7ᵗʰ S04.812 Injury of olfactory [1st] nerve, left side
      √7ᵗʰ S04.819 Injury of olfactory [1st] nerve, unspecified side

    ☑6ᵗʰ S04.89 Injury of other cranial nerves

> Injury of vagus [10th] nerve

      √7ᵗʰ S04.891 Injury of other cranial nerves, right side
      √7ᵗʰ S04.892 Injury of other cranial nerves, left side
      √7ᵗʰ S04.899 Injury of other cranial nerves, unspecified side

  √x7ᵗʰ S04.9 Injury of unspecified cranial nerve

☑4ᵗʰ S05 Injury of eye and orbit

> **INCLUDES** open wound of eye and orbit
> **EXCLUDES 2** *2nd cranial [optic] nerve injury (S04.0-)*
> *3rd cranial [oculomotor] nerve injury (S04.1-)*
> *open wound of eyelid and periocular area (S01.1-)*
> *orbital bone fracture (S02.1-, S02.3-, S02.8-)*
> *superficial injury of eyelid (S00.1-S00.2)*

> The appropriate 7th character is to be added to each code from category S05.
> A   initial encounter
> D   subsequent encounter
> S   sequela

  ☑5ᵗʰ S05.0 Injury of conjunctiva and corneal abrasion without foreign body

> **EXCLUDES 1** *foreign body in conjunctival sac (T15.1)*
> *foreign body in cornea (T15.0)*

    √x7ᵗʰ S05.00 Injury of conjunctiva and corneal abrasion without foreign body, unspecified eye

☑ Additional Character Required   **√x7ᵗʰ** Placeholder Alert   Manifestation   Unspecified Dx   ▶◀ Revised Text   ● New Code   ▲ Revised Code Title

ICD-10-CM 2020   **961**

√x7ᵗʰ **S05.01** Injury of conjunctiva and corneal abrasion without foreign body, **right** eye

√x7ᵗʰ **S05.02** Injury of conjunctiva and corneal abrasion without foreign body, **left** eye

√5ᵗʰ **S05.1** Contusion of eyeball and orbital tissues

Traumatic hyphema

EXCLUDES 2   black eye NOS (S00.1)

                contusion of eyelid and periocular area (S00.1)

√x7ᵗʰ **S05.10** Contusion of eyeball and orbital tissues, unspecified eye

√x7ᵗʰ **S05.11** Contusion of eyeball and orbital tissues, **right** eye

√x7ᵗʰ **S05.12** Contusion of eyeball and orbital tissues, **left** eye

√5ᵗʰ **S05.2** Ocular laceration and rupture with prolapse or loss of intraocular tissue

√x7ᵗʰ **S05.20** Ocular laceration and rupture with prolapse or loss of intraocular tissue, unspecified eye

√x7ᵗʰ **S05.21** Ocular laceration and rupture with prolapse or loss of intraocular tissue, **right** eye

√x7ᵗʰ **S05.22** Ocular laceration and rupture with prolapse or loss of intraocular tissue, **left** eye

√5ᵗʰ **S05.3** Ocular laceration without prolapse or loss of intraocular tissue

Laceration of eye NOS

DEF: Tear in ocular tissue without displacing structures that is due to blunt trauma. It is characterized by pain, redness, and decreased vision.

√x7ᵗʰ **S05.30** Ocular laceration without prolapse or loss of intraocular tissue, unspecified eye

√x7ᵗʰ **S05.31** Ocular laceration without prolapse or loss of intraocular tissue, **right** eye

√x7ᵗʰ **S05.32** Ocular laceration without prolapse or loss of intraocular tissue, **left** eye

√5ᵗʰ **S05.4** Penetrating wound of orbit with or without foreign body

EXCLUDES 2   retained (old) foreign body following penetrating wound in orbit (H05.5-)

√x7ᵗʰ **S05.40** Penetrating wound of orbit with or without foreign body, unspecified eye

√x7ᵗʰ **S05.41** Penetrating wound of orbit with or without foreign body, **right** eye

√x7ᵗʰ **S05.42** Penetrating wound of orbit with or without foreign body, **left** eye

√5ᵗʰ **S05.5** Penetrating wound with foreign body of eyeball

EXCLUDES 2   retained (old) intraocular foreign body (H44.6-, H44.7)

√x7ᵗʰ **S05.50** Penetrating wound with foreign body of unspecified eyeball

√x7ᵗʰ **S05.51** Penetrating wound with foreign body of **right** eyeball

√x7ᵗʰ **S05.52** Penetrating wound with foreign body of **left** eyeball

√5ᵗʰ **S05.6** Penetrating wound without foreign body of eyeball

Ocular penetration NOS

√x7ᵗʰ **S05.60** Penetrating wound without foreign body of unspecified eyeball

√x7ᵗʰ **S05.61** Penetrating wound without foreign body of **right** eyeball

√x7ᵗʰ **S05.62** Penetrating wound without foreign body of **left** eyeball

√5ᵗʰ **S05.7** Avulsion of eye

Traumatic enucleation

√x7ᵗʰ **S05.70** Avulsion of unspecified eye

√x7ᵗʰ **S05.71** Avulsion of **right** eye

√x7ᵗʰ **S05.72** Avulsion of **left** eye

√5ᵗʰ **S05.8** Other injuries of eye and orbit

Lacrimal duct injury

√6ᵗʰ **S05.8X** Other injuries of eye and orbit

√7ᵗʰ **S05.8X1** Other injuries of **right** eye and orbit

√7ᵗʰ **S05.8X2** Other injuries of **left** eye and orbit

√7ᵗʰ **S05.8X9** Other injuries of unspecified eye and orbit

√5ᵗʰ **S05.9** Unspecified injury of eye and orbit

Injury of eye NOS

√x7ᵗʰ **S05.90** Unspecified injury of unspecified eye and orbit

√x7ᵗʰ **S05.91** Unspecified injury of **right** eye and orbit

√x7ᵗʰ **S05.92** Unspecified injury of **left** eye and orbit

√4ᵗʰ **S06** Intracranial injury

NOTE   7th characters D and S do not apply to codes in category S06 with 6th character 7 – death due to brain injury prior to regaining consciousness, or 8 – death due to other cause prior to regaining consciousness.

INCLUDES   traumatic brain injury

Code also any associated:

open wound of head (S01.-)

skull fracture (S02.-)

EXCLUDES 1   head injury NOS (S09.90)

AHA: 2017,4Q,25; 2017,1Q,42; 2015,3Q,37

TIP: Do not assign Z87.820 Personal history of traumatic brain injury, when residual conditions persist after an intracranial injury. The codes for the residual conditions should be first listed, followed by a code from category S06 using seventh character S to identify sequelae.

The appropriate 7th character is to be added to each code from category S06.

A   initial encounter

D   subsequent encounter

S   sequela

√5ᵗʰ **S06.0** Concussion

Commotio cerebri

EXCLUDES 1   concussion with other intracranial injuries classified in subcategories S06.1- to S06.6- , S06.81- and S06.82- — code to specified intracranial injury

AHA: 2016,4Q,67-68

√6ᵗʰ **S06.0X** Concussion

³ √7ᵗʰ **S06.0X0** Concussion without loss of consciousness   HCC Q

³ √7ᵗʰ **S06.0X1** Concussion with loss of consciousness of 30 minutes or less   HCC Q

³ √7ᵗʰ **S06.0X9** Concussion with loss of consciousness of unspecified duration   HCC Q

Concussion NOS

√5ᵗʰ **S06.1** Traumatic cerebral edema

Diffuse traumatic cerebral edema

Focal traumatic cerebral edema

√6ᵗʰ **S06.1X** Traumatic cerebral edema

² √7ᵗʰ **S06.1X0** Traumatic cerebral edema without loss of consciousness   HCC Q

² √7ᵗʰ **S06.1X1** Traumatic cerebral edema with loss of consciousness of 30 minutes or less   HCC Q

² √7ᵗʰ **S06.1X2** Traumatic cerebral edema with loss of consciousness of 31 minutes to 59 minutes   HCC Q

² √7ᵗʰ **S06.1X3** Traumatic cerebral edema with loss of consciousness of 1 hour to 5 hours 59 minutes   HCC Q

² √7ᵗʰ **S06.1X4** Traumatic cerebral edema with loss of consciousness of 6 hours to 24 hours   HCC Q

² √7ᵗʰ **S06.1X5** Traumatic cerebral edema with loss of consciousness greater than 24 hours with return to pre-existing conscious level   HCC

² √7ᵗʰ **S06.1X6** Traumatic cerebral edema with loss of consciousness greater than 24 hours without return to pre-existing conscious level with patient surviving   HCC

√7ᵗʰ **S06.1X7** Traumatic cerebral edema with loss of consciousness of any duration with death due to brain injury prior to regaining consciousness

√7ᵗʰ **S06.1X8** Traumatic cerebral edema with loss of consciousness of any duration with death due to other cause prior to regaining consciousness

² √7ᵗʰ **S06.1X9** Traumatic cerebral edema with loss of consciousness of unspecified duration   HCC Q

Traumatic cerebral edema NOS

√5ᵗʰ **S06.2** **Diffuse traumatic brain injury**

Diffuse axonal brain injury

EXCLUDES 1   traumatic diffuse cerebral edema (S06.1X-)

√6ᵗʰ **S06.2X** Diffuse traumatic brain injury

² √7ᵗʰ **S06.2X0** **Diffuse traumatic brain injury** HCC Q
without loss of consciousness

² √7ᵗʰ **S06.2X1** **Diffuse traumatic brain injury** HCC Q
with loss of consciousness of 30 minutes or less

² √7ᵗʰ **S06.2X2** **Diffuse traumatic brain injury** HCC Q
with loss of consciousness of 31 minutes to 59 minutes

² √7ᵗʰ **S06.2X3** **Diffuse traumatic brain injury** HCC Q
with loss of consciousness of 1 hour to 5 hours 59 minutes

² √7ᵗʰ **S06.2X4** **Diffuse traumatic brain injury** HCC Q
with loss of consciousness of 6 hours to 24 hours

² √7ᵗʰ **S06.2X5** **Diffuse traumatic brain injury** HCC
with loss of consciousness greater than 24 hours with return to pre-existing conscious levels

² √7ᵗʰ **S06.2X6** **Diffuse traumatic brain injury** HCC
with loss of consciousness greater than 24 hours without return to pre-existing conscious level with patient surviving

√7ᵗʰ **S06.2X7** **Diffuse traumatic brain injury with loss of consciousness of any duration with death due to brain injury prior to regaining consciousness**

√7ᵗʰ **S06.2X8** **Diffuse traumatic brain injury with loss of consciousness of any duration with death due to other cause prior to regaining consciousness**

² √7ᵗʰ **S06.2X9** **Diffuse traumatic brain injury** HCC Q
with loss of consciousness of unspecified duration

Diffuse traumatic brain injury NOS

√5ᵗʰ **S06.3** **Focal traumatic brain injury**

EXCLUDES 1   any condition classifiable to S06.4-S06.6
focal cerebral edema (S06.1)

√6ᵗʰ **S06.30** Unspecified focal traumatic brain injury

² √7ᵗʰ **S06.300** **Unspecified focal traumatic brain** HCC Q
injury without loss of consciousness

² √7ᵗʰ **S06.301** **Unspecified focal traumatic brain** HCC Q
injury with loss of consciousness of 30 minutes or less

² √7ᵗʰ **S06.302** **Unspecified focal traumatic brain** HCC Q
injury with loss of consciousness of 31 minutes to 59 minutes

² √7ᵗʰ **S06.303** **Unspecified focal traumatic brain** HCC Q
injury with loss of consciousness of 1 hour to 5 hours 59 minutes

² √7ᵗʰ **S06.304** **Unspecified focal traumatic brain** HCC Q
injury with loss of consciousness of 6 hours to 24 hours

² √7ᵗʰ **S06.305** **Unspecified focal traumatic brain** HCC
injury with loss of consciousness greater than 24 hours with return to pre-existing conscious level

² √7ᵗʰ **S06.306** **Unspecified focal traumatic brain** HCC
injury with loss of consciousness greater than 24 hours without return to pre-existing conscious level with patient surviving

√7ᵗʰ **S06.307** **Unspecified focal traumatic brain injury with loss of consciousness of any duration with death due to brain injury prior to regaining consciousness**

√7ᵗʰ **S06.308** **Unspecified focal traumatic brain injury with loss of consciousness of any duration with death due to other cause prior to regaining consciousness**

² √7ᵗʰ **S06.309** **Unspecified focal traumatic brain** HCC Q
injury with loss of consciousness of unspecified duration

Unspecified focal traumatic brain injury NOS

√6ᵗʰ **S06.31** **Contusion and laceration of right cerebrum**

² √7ᵗʰ **S06.310** **Contusion and laceration of right** HCC
cerebrum without loss of consciousness

² √7ᵗʰ **S06.311** **Contusion and laceration of right** HCC
cerebrum with loss of consciousness of 30 minutes or less

² √7ᵗʰ **S06.312** **Contusion and laceration of right** HCC
cerebrum with loss of consciousness of 31 minutes to 59 minutes

² √7ᵗʰ **S06.313** **Contusion and laceration of right** HCC
cerebrum with loss of consciousness of 1 hour to 5 hours 59 minutes

² √7ᵗʰ **S06.314** **Contusion and laceration of right** HCC
cerebrum with loss of consciousness of 6 hours to 24 hours

² √7ᵗʰ **S06.315** **Contusion and laceration of right** HCC
cerebrum with loss of consciousness greater than 24 hours with return to pre-existing conscious level

² √7ᵗʰ **S06.316** **Contusion and laceration of right** HCC
cerebrum with loss of consciousness greater than 24 hours without return to pre-existing conscious level with patient surviving

√7ᵗʰ **S06.317** **Contusion and laceration of right cerebrum with loss of consciousness of any duration with death due to brain injury prior to regaining consciousness**

√7ᵗʰ **S06.318** **Contusion and laceration of right cerebrum with loss of consciousness of any duration with death due to other cause prior to regaining consciousness**

² √7ᵗʰ **S06.319** **Contusion and laceration of right** HCC
cerebrum with loss of consciousness of unspecified duration

Contusion and laceration of right cerebrum NOS

√6ᵗʰ **S06.32** **Contusion and laceration of left cerebrum**

² √7ᵗʰ **S06.320** **Contusion and laceration of left** HCC
cerebrum without loss of consciousness

² √7ᵗʰ **S06.321** **Contusion and laceration of left** HCC
cerebrum with loss of consciousness of 30 minutes or less

² √7ᵗʰ **S06.322** **Contusion and laceration of left** HCC
cerebrum with loss of consciousness of 31 minutes to 59 minutes

² √7ᵗʰ **S06.323** **Contusion and laceration of left** HCC
cerebrum with loss of consciousness of 1 hour to 5 hours 59 minutes

² √7ᵗʰ **S06.324** **Contusion and laceration of left** HCC
cerebrum with loss of consciousness of 6 hours to 24 hours

² √7ᵗʰ **S06.325** **Contusion and laceration of left** HCC
cerebrum with loss of consciousness greater than 24 hours with return to pre-existing conscious level

² √7ᵗʰ **S06.326** **Contusion and laceration of left** HCC
cerebrum with loss of consciousness greater than 24 hours without return to pre-existing conscious level with patient surviving

√7ᵗʰ **S06.327** **Contusion and laceration of left cerebrum with loss of consciousness of any duration with death due to brain injury prior to regaining consciousness**

√7ᵗʰ **S06.328** **Contusion and laceration of left cerebrum with loss of consciousness of any duration with death due to other cause prior to regaining consciousness**

☑ Additional Character Required   √x7ᵗʰ Placeholder Alert   Manifestation   Unspecified Dx   ▶◀ Revised Text   ● New Code   ▲ Revised Code Title

2 ✓7ᵗʰ **S06.329** **Contusion and laceration of left cerebrum with loss of consciousness of unspecified duration** `HCC`
Contusion and laceration of left cerebrum NOS

✓6ᵗʰ **S06.33** **Contusion and laceration of cerebrum, unspecified**

2 ✓7ᵗʰ **S06.330** **Contusion and laceration of cerebrum, unspecified, without loss of consciousness** `HCC`

2 ✓7ᵗʰ **S06.331** **Contusion and laceration of cerebrum, unspecified, with loss of consciousness of 30 minutes or less** `HCC`

2 ✓7ᵗʰ **S06.332** **Contusion and laceration of cerebrum, unspecified, with loss of consciousness of 31 minutes to 59 minutes** `HCC`

2 ✓7ᵗʰ **S06.333** **Contusion and laceration of cerebrum, unspecified, with loss of consciousness of 1 hour to 5 hours 59 minutes** `HCC`

2 ✓7ᵗʰ **S06.334** **Contusion and laceration of cerebrum, unspecified, with loss of consciousness of 6 hours to 24 hours** `HCC`

2 ✓7ᵗʰ **S06.335** **Contusion and laceration of cerebrum, unspecified, with loss of consciousness greater than 24 hours with return to pre-existing conscious level** `HCC`

2 ✓7ᵗʰ **S06.336** **Contusion and laceration of cerebrum, unspecified, with loss of consciousness greater than 24 hours without return to pre-existing conscious level with patient surviving** `HCC`

✓7ᵗʰ **S06.337** **Contusion and laceration of cerebrum, unspecified, with loss of consciousness of any duration with death due to brain injury prior to regaining consciousness**

✓7ᵗʰ **S06.338** **Contusion and laceration of cerebrum, unspecified, with loss of consciousness of any duration with death due to other cause prior to regaining consciousness**

2 ✓7ᵗʰ **S06.339** **Contusion and laceration of cerebrum, unspecified, with loss of consciousness of unspecified duration** `HCC`
Contusion and laceration of cerebrum NOS

✓6ᵗʰ **S06.34** **Traumatic hemorrhage of right cerebrum**
Traumatic intracerebral hemorrhage and hematoma of right cerebrum

2 ✓7ᵗʰ **S06.340** **Traumatic hemorrhage of right cerebrum without loss of consciousness** `HCC` `Q`

2 ✓7ᵗʰ **S06.341** **Traumatic hemorrhage of right cerebrum with loss of consciousness of 30 minutes or less** `HCC` `Q`

2 ✓7ᵗʰ **S06.342** **Traumatic hemorrhage of right cerebrum with loss of consciousness of 31 minutes to 59 minutes** `HCC` `Q`

2 ✓7ᵗʰ **S06.343** **Traumatic hemorrhage of right cerebrum with loss of consciousness of 1 hours to 5 hours 59 minutes** `HCC` `Q`

2 ✓7ᵗʰ **S06.344** **Traumatic hemorrhage of right cerebrum with loss of consciousness of 6 hours to 24 hours** `HCC` `Q`

2 ✓7ᵗʰ **S06.345** **Traumatic hemorrhage of right cerebrum with loss of consciousness greater than 24 hours with return to pre-existing conscious level** `HCC` `Q`

2 ✓7ᵗʰ **S06.346** **Traumatic hemorrhage of right cerebrum with loss of consciousness greater than 24 hours without return to pre-existing conscious level with patient surviving** `HCC` `Q`

✓7ᵗʰ **S06.347** **Traumatic hemorrhage of right cerebrum with loss of consciousness of any duration with death due to brain injury prior to regaining consciousness** `Q`

✓7ᵗʰ **S06.348** **Traumatic hemorrhage of right cerebrum with loss of consciousness of any duration with death due to other cause prior to regaining consciousness** `Q`

2 ✓7ᵗʰ **S06.349** **Traumatic hemorrhage of right cerebrum with loss of consciousness of unspecified duration** `HCC` `Q`
Traumatic hemorrhage of right cerebrum NOS

✓6ᵗʰ **S06.35** **Traumatic hemorrhage of left cerebrum**
Traumatic intracerebral hemorrhage and hematoma of left cerebrum

2 ✓7ᵗʰ **S06.350** **Traumatic hemorrhage of left cerebrum without loss of consciousness** `HCC` `Q`

2 ✓7ᵗʰ **S06.351** **Traumatic hemorrhage of left cerebrum with loss of consciousness of 30 minutes or less** `HCC` `Q`

2 ✓7ᵗʰ **S06.352** **Traumatic hemorrhage of left cerebrum with loss of consciousness of 31 minutes to 59 minutes** `HCC` `Q`

2 ✓7ᵗʰ **S06.353** **Traumatic hemorrhage of left cerebrum with loss of consciousness of 1 hours to 5 hours 59 minutes** `HCC` `Q`

2 ✓7ᵗʰ **S06.354** **Traumatic hemorrhage of left cerebrum with loss of consciousness of 6 hours to 24 hours** `HCC` `Q`

2 ✓7ᵗʰ **S06.355** **Traumatic hemorrhage of left cerebrum with loss of consciousness greater than 24 hours with return to pre-existing conscious level** `HCC` `Q`

2 ✓7ᵗʰ **S06.356** **Traumatic hemorrhage of left cerebrum with loss of consciousness greater than 24 hours without return to pre-existing conscious level with patient surviving** `HCC` `Q`

✓7ᵗʰ **S06.357** **Traumatic hemorrhage of left cerebrum with loss of consciousness of any duration with death due to brain injury prior to regaining consciousness** `Q`

✓7ᵗʰ **S06.358** **Traumatic hemorrhage of left cerebrum with loss of consciousness of any duration with death due to other cause prior to regaining consciousness** `Q`

2 ✓7ᵗʰ **S06.359** **Traumatic hemorrhage of left cerebrum with loss of consciousness of unspecified duration** `HCC` `Q`
Traumatic hemorrhage of left cerebrum NOS

✓6ᵗʰ **S06.36** **Traumatic hemorrhage of cerebrum, unspecified**
Traumatic intracerebral hemorrhage and hematoma, unspecified

2 ✓7ᵗʰ **S06.360** **Traumatic hemorrhage of cerebrum, unspecified, without loss of consciousness** `HCC` `Q`

2 ✓7ᵗʰ **S06.361** **Traumatic hemorrhage of cerebrum, unspecified, with loss of consciousness of 30 minutes or less** `HCC` `Q`

2 ✓7ᵗʰ **S06.362** **Traumatic hemorrhage of cerebrum, unspecified, with loss of consciousness of 31 minutes to 59 minutes** `HCC` `Q`

2 ✓7ᵗʰ **S06.363** **Traumatic hemorrhage of cerebrum, unspecified, with loss of consciousness of 1 hours to 5 hours 59 minutes** `HCC` `Q`

² ✓7ᵗʰ **S06.364** **Traumatic hemorrhage of cerebrum, unspecified, with loss of consciousness of** 6 hours to 24 hours   HCC Q

² ✓7ᵗʰ **S06.365** **Traumatic hemorrhage of cerebrum, unspecified, with loss of consciousness** greater than 24 hours with return to pre-existing conscious level   HCC Q

² ✓7ᵗʰ **S06.366** **Traumatic hemorrhage of cerebrum, unspecified, with loss of consciousness** greater than 24 hours without return to pre-existing conscious level with patient surviving   HCC Q

✓7ᵗʰ **S06.367** **Traumatic hemorrhage of cerebrum, unspecified, with loss of consciousness of** any duration with death due to brain injury prior to regaining consciousness   Q

✓7ᵗʰ **S06.368** **Traumatic hemorrhage of cerebrum, unspecified, with loss of consciousness of** any duration with death due to **other** cause prior to regaining consciousness   Q

² ✓7ᵗʰ **S06.369** **Traumatic hemorrhage of cerebrum, unspecified, with loss of consciousness of unspecified duration**   HCC Q
    Traumatic hemorrhage of cerebrum NOS

✓6ᵗʰ **S06.37** **Contusion, laceration, and hemorrhage of cerebellum**

² ✓7ᵗʰ **S06.370** **Contusion, laceration, and hemorrhage of cerebellum** without loss of consciousness   HCC Q

² ✓7ᵗʰ **S06.371** **Contusion, laceration, and hemorrhage of cerebellum with loss of consciousness of** 30 minutes or less   HCC Q

² ✓7ᵗʰ **S06.372** **Contusion, laceration, and hemorrhage of cerebellum with loss of consciousness of** 31 minutes to 59 minutes   HCC Q

² ✓7ᵗʰ **S06.373** **Contusion, laceration, and hemorrhage of cerebellum with loss of consciousness of** 1 hour to 5 hours 59 minutes   HCC Q

² ✓7ᵗʰ **S06.374** **Contusion, laceration, and hemorrhage of cerebellum with loss of consciousness of** 6 hours to 24 hours   HCC Q

² ✓7ᵗʰ **S06.375** **Contusion, laceration, and hemorrhage of cerebellum with loss of consciousness** greater than 24 hours with return to pre-existing conscious level   HCC Q

² ✓7ᵗʰ **S06.376** **Contusion, laceration, and hemorrhage of cerebellum with loss of consciousness** greater than 24 hours without return to pre-existing conscious level with patient surviving   HCC Q

✓7ᵗʰ **S06.377** **Contusion, laceration, and hemorrhage of cerebellum with loss of consciousness of** any duration with death due to brain injury prior to regaining consciousness   Q

✓7ᵗʰ **S06.378** **Contusion, laceration, and hemorrhage of cerebellum with loss of consciousness of** any duration with death due to **other** cause prior to regaining consciousness   Q

² ✓7ᵗʰ **S06.379** **Contusion, laceration, and hemorrhage of cerebellum with loss of consciousness of unspecified duration**   HCC Q
    Contusion, laceration, and hemorrhage of cerebellum NOS

✓6ᵗʰ **S06.38** **Contusion, laceration, and hemorrhage of brainstem**

² ✓7ᵗʰ **S06.380** **Contusion, laceration, and hemorrhage of brainstem** without loss of consciousness   HCC Q

² ✓7ᵗʰ **S06.381** **Contusion, laceration, and hemorrhage of brainstem with loss of consciousness of** 30 minutes or less   HCC Q

² ✓7ᵗʰ **S06.382** **Contusion, laceration, and hemorrhage of brainstem with loss of consciousness of** 31 minutes to 59 minutes   HCC Q

² ✓7ᵗʰ **S06.383** **Contusion, laceration, and hemorrhage of brainstem with loss of consciousness of** 1 hour to 5 hours 59 minutes   HCC Q

² ✓7ᵗʰ **S06.384** **Contusion, laceration, and hemorrhage of brainstem with loss of consciousness of** 6 hours to 24 hours   HCC Q

² ✓7ᵗʰ **S06.385** **Contusion, laceration, and hemorrhage of brainstem with loss of consciousness** greater than 24 hours with return to pre-existing conscious level   HCC Q

² ✓7ᵗʰ **S06.386** **Contusion, laceration, and hemorrhage of brainstem with loss of consciousness** greater than 24 hours without return to pre-existing conscious level with patient surviving   HCC Q

✓7ᵗʰ **S06.387** **Contusion, laceration, and hemorrhage of brainstem with loss of consciousness of** any duration with death due to brain injury prior to regaining consciousness   Q

✓7ᵗʰ **S06.388** **Contusion, laceration, and hemorrhage of brainstem with loss of consciousness of** any duration with death due to **other** cause prior to regaining consciousness   Q

² ✓7ᵗʰ **S06.389** **Contusion, laceration, and hemorrhage of brainstem with loss of consciousness of unspecified duration**   HCC Q
    Contusion, laceration, and hemorrhage of brainstem NOS

✓6ᵗʰ **S06.4** **Epidural hemorrhage**
    Extradural hemorrhage NOS
    Extradural hemorrhage (traumatic)
    DEF: Epidural space: Space between the endosteum of the cranium (skull) and the dura mater, the outermost layer of a three-layer membrane that covers the brain.

✓6ᵗʰ **S06.4X** **Epidural hemorrhage**

² ✓7ᵗʰ **S06.4X0** **Epidural hemorrhage** without loss of consciousness   HCC Q

² ✓7ᵗʰ **S06.4X1** **Epidural hemorrhage with loss of consciousness of** 30 minutes or less   HCC Q

² ✓7ᵗʰ **S06.4X2** **Epidural hemorrhage with loss of consciousness of** 31 minutes to 59 minutes   HCC Q

² ✓7ᵗʰ **S06.4X3** **Epidural hemorrhage with loss of consciousness of** 1 hour to 5 hours 59 minutes   HCC Q

² ✓7ᵗʰ **S06.4X4** **Epidural hemorrhage with loss of consciousness of** 6 hours to 24 hours   HCC Q

² ✓7ᵗʰ **S06.4X5** **Epidural hemorrhage with loss of consciousness** greater than 24 hours with return to pre-existing conscious level   HCC Q

² ✓7ᵗʰ **S06.4X6** **Epidural hemorrhage with loss of consciousness** greater than 24 hours without return to pre-existing conscious level with patient surviving   HCC Q

✓7ᵗʰ **S06.4X7** **Epidural hemorrhage with loss of consciousness of** any duration with death due to brain injury prior to regaining consciousness   Q

✓7ᵗʰ **S06.4X8** **Epidural hemorrhage with loss of consciousness of** any duration with death due to **other** causes prior to regaining consciousness   Q

✔ Additional Character Required   ✓x7ᵗʰ Placeholder Alert   Manifestation   Unspecified Dx   ►◄ Revised Text   ● New Code   ▲ Revised Code Title

Chapter 19. Injury, Poisoning and Certain Other Consequences of External Causes

S06.4X9–S06.822

² ✓7ᵗʰ **S06.4X9 Epidural hemorrhage with loss of** HCC Q
consciousness of unspecified
duration
Epidural hemorrhage NOS

✓6ᵗʰ **S06.5 Traumatic subdural hemorrhage**
DEF: Subdural: Potential space between the dura mater and arachnoid membrane around the brain.

✓6ᵗʰ **S06.5X Traumatic subdural hemorrhage**

² ✓7ᵗʰ **S06.5X0 Traumatic subdural hemorrhage** HCC Q
without loss of consciousness

² ✓7ᵗʰ **S06.5X1 Traumatic subdural hemorrhage** HCC Q
with loss of consciousness of 30
minutes or less

² ✓7ᵗʰ **S06.5X2 Traumatic subdural hemorrhage** HCC Q
with loss of consciousness of 31
minutes to 59 minutes

² ✓7ᵗʰ **S06.5X3 Traumatic subdural hemorrhage** HCC Q
with loss of consciousness of 1
hour to 5 hours 59 minutes

² ✓7ᵗʰ **S06.5X4 Traumatic subdural hemorrhage** HCC Q
with loss of consciousness of 6
hours to 24 hours

² ✓7ᵗʰ **S06.5X5 Traumatic subdural hemorrhage** HCC Q
with loss of consciousness greater
than 24 hours with return to
pre-existing conscious level

² ✓7ᵗʰ **S06.5X6 Traumatic subdural hemorrhage** HCC Q
with loss of consciousness greater
than 24 hours without return to
pre-existing conscious level with
patient surviving

✓7ᵗʰ **S06.5X7 Traumatic subdural hemorrhage** Q
with loss of consciousness of any
duration with death due to brain
injury before regaining
consciousness

✓7ᵗʰ **S06.5X8 Traumatic subdural hemorrhage** Q
with loss of consciousness of any
duration with death due to other
cause before regaining
consciousness

² ✓7ᵗʰ **S06.5X9 Traumatic subdural hemorrhage** HCC Q
with loss of consciousness of
unspecified duration
Traumatic subdural hemorrhage NOS

✓5ᵗʰ **S06.6 Traumatic subarachnoid hemorrhage**
DEF: Subarachnoid: Space located between the arachnoid membrane and the pia mater that contains cerebrospinal fluid.

✓6ᵗʰ **S06.6X Traumatic subarachnoid hemorrhage**

² ✓7ᵗʰ **S06.6X0 Traumatic subarachnoid** HCC Q
hemorrhage without loss of
consciousness

² ✓7ᵗʰ **S06.6X1 Traumatic subarachnoid** HCC Q
hemorrhage with loss of
consciousness of 30 minutes or
less

² ✓7ᵗʰ **S06.6X2 Traumatic subarachnoid** HCC Q
hemorrhage with loss of
consciousness of 31 minutes to
59 minutes

² ✓7ᵗʰ **S06.6X3 Traumatic subarachnoid** HCC Q
hemorrhage with loss of
consciousness of 1 hour to 5
hours 59 minutes

² ✓7ᵗʰ **S06.6X4 Traumatic subarachnoid** HCC Q
hemorrhage with loss of
consciousness of 6 hours to 24
hours

² ✓7ᵗʰ **S06.6X5 Traumatic subarachnoid** HCC Q
hemorrhage with loss of
consciousness greater than 24
hours with return to pre-existing
conscious level

² ✓7ᵗʰ **S06.6X6 Traumatic subarachnoid** HCC Q
hemorrhage with loss of
consciousness greater than 24
hours without return to
pre-existing conscious level with
patient surviving

✓7ᵗʰ **S06.6X7 Traumatic subarachnoid** Q
hemorrhage with loss of
consciousness of any duration
with death due to brain injury
prior to regaining consciousness

✓7ᵗʰ **S06.6X8 Traumatic subarachnoid** Q
hemorrhage with loss of
consciousness of any duration
with death due to other cause
prior to regaining consciousness

² ✓7ᵗʰ **S06.6X9 Traumatic subarachnoid** HCC Q
hemorrhage with loss of
consciousness of unspecified
duration
Traumatic subarachnoid hemorrhage NOS

✓5ᵗʰ **S06.8 Other specified intracranial injuries**

✓6ᵗʰ **S06.81 Injury of right internal carotid artery, intracranial**
portion, not elsewhere classified

² ✓7ᵗʰ **S06.810 Injury of right internal carotid** HCC Q
artery, intracranial portion, not
elsewhere classified without loss
of consciousness

² ✓7ᵗʰ **S06.811 Injury of right internal carotid** HCC Q
artery, intracranial portion, not
elsewhere classified with loss of
consciousness of 30 minutes or
less

² ✓7ᵗʰ **S06.812 Injury of right internal carotid** HCC Q
artery, intracranial portion, not
elsewhere classified with loss of
consciousness of 31 minutes to
59 minutes

² ✓7ᵗʰ **S06.813 Injury of right internal carotid** HCC Q
artery, intracranial portion, not
elsewhere classified with loss of
consciousness of 1 hour to 5
hours 59 minutes

² ✓7ᵗʰ **S06.814 Injury of right internal carotid** HCC Q
artery, intracranial portion, not
elsewhere classified with loss of
consciousness of 6 hours to 24
hours

² ✓7ᵗʰ **S06.815 Injury of right internal carotid** HCC
artery, intracranial portion, not
elsewhere classified with loss of
consciousness greater than 24
hours with return to pre-existing
conscious level

² ✓7ᵗʰ **S06.816 Injury of right internal carotid** HCC
artery, intracranial portion, not
elsewhere classified with loss of
consciousness greater than 24
hours without return to
pre-existing conscious level with
patient surviving

✓7ᵗʰ **S06.817 Injury of right internal carotid artery,**
intracranial portion, not elsewhere
classified with loss of consciousness of
any duration with death due to brain
injury prior to regaining consciousness

✓7ᵗʰ **S06.818 Injury of right internal carotid artery,**
intracranial portion, not elsewhere
classified with loss of consciousness of
any duration with death due to other
cause prior to regaining consciousness

² ✓7ᵗʰ **S06.819 Injury of right internal carotid** HCC Q
artery, intracranial portion, not
elsewhere classified with loss of
consciousness of unspecified
duration
Injury of right internal carotid artery,
intracranial portion, not elsewhere
classified NOS

✓6ᵗʰ **S06.82 Injury of left internal carotid artery, intracranial**
portion, not elsewhere classified

² ✓7ᵗʰ **S06.820 Injury of left internal carotid** HCC Q
artery, intracranial portion, not
elsewhere classified without loss
of consciousness

² ✓7ᵗʰ **S06.821 Injury of left internal carotid** HCC Q
artery, intracranial portion, not
elsewhere classified with loss of
consciousness of 30 minutes or
less

² ✓7ᵗʰ **S06.822 Injury of left internal carotid** HCC Q
artery, intracranial portion, not
elsewhere classified with loss of
consciousness of 31 minutes to
59 minutes

² ✓7ᵗʰ **S06.823 Injury of left internal carotid artery, intracranial portion, not elsewhere classified with loss of consciousness of** 1 hour to 5 hours 59 minutes `HCC` `Q`

² ✓7ᵗʰ **S06.824 Injury of left internal carotid artery, intracranial portion, not elsewhere classified with loss of consciousness of** 6 hours to 24 hours `HCC` `Q`

² ✓7ᵗʰ **S06.825 Injury of left internal carotid artery, intracranial portion, not elsewhere classified with loss of consciousness** greater than 24 hours with return to pre-existing conscious level `HCC`

² ✓7ᵗʰ **S06.826 Injury of left internal carotid artery, intracranial portion, not elsewhere classified with loss of consciousness** greater than 24 hours without return to pre-existing conscious level with patient surviving `HCC`

✓7ᵗʰ **S06.827 Injury of left internal carotid artery, intracranial portion, not elsewhere classified with loss of consciousness of** any duration with death due to brain injury prior to regaining consciousness

✓7ᵗʰ **S06.828 Injury of left internal carotid artery, intracranial portion, not elsewhere classified with loss of consciousness of** any duration with death due to other cause prior to regaining consciousness

² ✓7ᵗʰ **S06.829 Injury of left internal carotid artery, intracranial portion, not elsewhere classified with loss of consciousness of unspecified duration** `HCC` `Q`
    Injury of left internal carotid artery, intracranial portion, not elsewhere classified NOS

✓6ᵗʰ **S06.89 Other specified intracranial injury**
    `EXCLUDES 1`   concussion (S06.0X-)

¹ ✓7ᵗʰ **S06.890 Other specified intracranial injury without loss of consciousness** `HCC` `Q`

² ✓7ᵗʰ **S06.891 Other specified intracranial injury with loss of consciousness of** 30 minutes or less `HCC` `Q`

² ✓7ᵗʰ **S06.892 Other specified intracranial injury with loss of consciousness of** 31 minutes to 59 minutes `HCC` `Q`

² ✓7ᵗʰ **S06.893 Other specified intracranial injury with loss of consciousness of** 1 hour to 5 hours 59 minutes `HCC` `Q`

² ✓7ᵗʰ **S06.894 Other specified intracranial injury with loss of consciousness of** 6 hours to 24 hours `HCC` `Q`

² ✓7ᵗʰ **S06.895 Other specified intracranial injury with loss of consciousness** greater than 24 hours with return to pre-existing conscious level `HCC`

² ✓7ᵗʰ **S06.896 Other specified intracranial injury with loss of consciousness** greater than 24 hours without return to pre-existing conscious level with patient surviving `HCC`

✓7ᵗʰ **S06.897 Other specified intracranial injury with loss of consciousness of** any duration with death due to brain injury prior to regaining consciousness

✓7ᵗʰ **S06.898 Other specified intracranial injury with loss of consciousness of** any duration with death due to other cause prior to regaining consciousness

² ✓7ᵗʰ **S06.899 Other specified intracranial injury with loss of consciousness of unspecified duration** `HCC` `Q`

✓5ᵗʰ **S06.9 Unspecified intracranial injury**
    Brain injury NOS
    Head injury NOS with loss of consciousness
    Traumatic brain injury NOS
    `EXCLUDES 1`   conditions classifiable to S06.0- to S06.8- code to specified intracranial injury
        head injury NOS (S09.90)

✓6ᵗʰ **S06.9X Unspecified intracranial injury**

² ✓7ᵗʰ **S06.9X0 Unspecified intracranial injury without loss of consciousness** `HCC` `Q`

² ✓7ᵗʰ **S06.9X1 Unspecified intracranial injury with loss of consciousness of** 30 minutes or less `HCC` `Q`

² ✓7ᵗʰ **S06.9X2 Unspecified intracranial injury with loss of consciousness of** 31 minutes to 59 minutes `HCC` `Q`

² ✓7ᵗʰ **S06.9X3 Unspecified intracranial injury with loss of consciousness of** 1 hour to 5 hours 59 minutes `HCC` `Q`

² ✓7ᵗʰ **S06.9X4 Unspecified intracranial injury with loss of consciousness of** 6 hours to 24 hours `HCC` `Q`

² ✓7ᵗʰ **S06.9X5 Unspecified intracranial injury with loss of consciousness** greater than 24 hours with return to pre-existing conscious level `HCC`

² ✓7ᵗʰ **S06.9X6 Unspecified intracranial injury with loss of consciousness** greater than 24 hours without return to pre-existing conscious level with patient surviving `HCC`

✓7ᵗʰ **S06.9X7 Unspecified intracranial injury with loss of consciousness of** any duration with death due to brain injury prior to regaining consciousness

✓7ᵗʰ **S06.9X8 Unspecified intracranial injury with loss of consciousness of** any duration with death due to other cause prior to regaining consciousness

² ✓7ᵗʰ **S06.9X9 Unspecified intracranial injury with loss of consciousness of unspecified duration** `HCC` `Q`

✓4ᵗʰ **S07 Crushing injury of head**
    Use additional code for all associated injuries, such as:
        intracranial injuries (S06.-)
        skull fractures (S02.-)

    The appropriate 7th character is to be added to each code from category S07.
    A initial encounter
    D subsequent encounter
    S sequela

✓x7ᵗʰ **S07.0 Crushing injury of face**

✓x7ᵗʰ **S07.1 Crushing injury of skull**

✓x7ᵗʰ **S07.8 Crushing injury of other parts of head**

✓x7ᵗʰ **S07.9 Crushing injury of head, part unspecified**

✓4ᵗʰ **S08 Avulsion and traumatic amputation of part of head**
    An amputation not identified as partial or complete should be coded to complete

    The appropriate 7th character is to be added to each code from category S08.
    A initial encounter
    D subsequent encounter
    S sequela

✓x7ᵗʰ **S08.0 Avulsion of scalp**

✓5ᵗʰ **S08.1 Traumatic amputation of ear**

✓6ᵗʰ **S08.11 Complete traumatic amputation of ear**

✓7ᵗʰ **S08.111 Complete traumatic amputation of right ear**

✓7ᵗʰ **S08.112 Complete traumatic amputation of left ear**

✓7ᵗʰ **S08.119 Complete traumatic amputation of unspecified ear**

✓6ᵗʰ **S08.12 Partial traumatic amputation of ear**

✓7ᵗʰ **S08.121 Partial traumatic amputation of right ear**

✓7ᵗʰ **S08.122 Partial traumatic amputation of left ear**

✓7ᵗʰ **S08.129 Partial traumatic amputation of unspecified ear**

✓5ᵗʰ S08.8 Traumatic amputation of other parts of head

    ✓6ᵗʰ S08.81 Traumatic amputation of nose

        ✓7ᵗʰ S08.811 Complete traumatic amputation of nose

        ✓7ᵗʰ S08.812 Partial traumatic amputation of nose

    ✓x7ᵗʰ S08.89 Traumatic amputation of other parts of head

✓4ᵗʰ S09 Other and unspecified injuries of head

The appropriate 7th character is to be added to each code from category S09.
A   initial encounter
D   subsequent encounter
S   sequela

✓x7ᵗʰ S09.0 Injury of blood vessels of head, not elsewhere classified

    EXCLUDES 1   injury of cerebral blood vessels (S06.-)

                  injury of precerebral blood vessels (S15.-)

✓5ᵗʰ S09.1 Injury of muscle and tendon of head

    Code also any associated open wound (S01.-)

    EXCLUDES 2   sprain to joints and ligament of head (S03.9)

    ✓x7ᵗʰ S09.10 Unspecified injury of muscle and tendon of head Q

        Injury of muscle and tendon of head NOS

    ✓x7ᵗʰ S09.11 Strain of muscle and tendon of head Q

    ✓x7ᵗʰ S09.12 Laceration of muscle and tendon of head

    ✓x7ᵗʰ S09.19 Other specified injury of muscle and tendon of head Q

✓5ᵗʰ S09.2 Traumatic rupture of ear drum

    EXCLUDES 1   traumatic rupture of ear drum due to blast injury (S09.31-)

    ✓x7ᵗʰ S09.20 Traumatic rupture of unspecified ear drum

    ✓x7ᵗʰ S09.21 Traumatic rupture of right ear drum

    ✓x7ᵗʰ S09.22 Traumatic rupture of left ear drum

✓5ᵗʰ S09.3 Other specified and unspecified injury of middle and inner ear

    EXCLUDES 1   injury to ear NOS (S09.91-)

    EXCLUDES 2   injury to external ear (S00.4-, S01.3-, S08.1-)

    ✓6ᵗʰ S09.30 Unspecified injury of middle and inner ear

        ✓7ᵗʰ S09.301 Unspecified injury of right middle and inner ear

        ✓7ᵗʰ S09.302 Unspecified injury of left middle and inner ear

        ✓7ᵗʰ S09.309 Unspecified injury of unspecified middle and inner ear

    ✓6ᵗʰ S09.31 Primary blast injury of ear

        Blast injury of ear NOS

        ✓7ᵗʰ S09.311 Primary blast injury of right ear

        ✓7ᵗʰ S09.312 Primary blast injury of left ear

        ✓7ᵗʰ S09.313 Primary blast injury of ear, bilateral

        ✓7ᵗʰ S09.319 Primary blast injury of unspecified ear

    ✓6ᵗʰ S09.39 Other specified injury of middle and inner ear

        Secondary blast injury to ear

        ✓7ᵗʰ S09.391 Other specified injury of right middle and inner ear

        ✓7ᵗʰ S09.392 Other specified injury of left middle and inner ear

        ✓7ᵗʰ S09.399 Other specified injury of unspecified middle and inner ear

✓x7ᵗʰ S09.8 Other specified injuries of head Q

✓5ᵗʰ S09.9 Unspecified injury of face and head

    ✓x7ᵗʰ S09.90 Unspecified injury of head Q

        Head injury NOS

        EXCLUDES 1   brain injury NOS (S06.9-)

                  head injury NOS with loss of consciousness (S06.9-)

                  intracranial injury NOS (S06.9-)

    ✓x7ᵗʰ S09.91 Unspecified injury of ear

        Injury of ear NOS

    ✓x7ᵗʰ S09.92 Unspecified injury of nose Q

        Injury of nose NOS

    ✓x7ᵗʰ S09.93 Unspecified injury of face Q

        Injury of face NOS

        AHA: 2019,2Q,23

Injuries to the neck (S10-S19)

INCLUDES   injuries of nape
              injuries of supraclavicular region
              injuries of throat

EXCLUDES 2   burns and corrosions (T20-T32)
              effects of foreign body in esophagus (T18.1)
              effects of foreign body in larynx (T17.3)
              effects of foreign body in pharynx (T17.2)
              effects of foreign body in trachea (T17.4)
              frostbite (T33-T34)
              insect bite or sting, venomous (T63.4)

✓4ᵗʰ S10 Superficial injury of neck

The appropriate 7th character is to be added to each code from category S10.
A   initial encounter
D   subsequent encounter
S   sequela

✓x7ᵗʰ S10.0 Contusion of throat Q

    Contusion of cervical esophagus

    Contusion of larynx

    Contusion of pharynx

    Contusion of trachea

✓5ᵗʰ S10.1 Other and unspecified superficial injuries of throat

    ✓x7ᵗʰ S10.10 Unspecified superficial injuries of throat

    ✓x7ᵗʰ S10.11 Abrasion of throat

    ✓x7ᵗʰ S10.12 Blister (nonthermal) of throat

    ✓x7ᵗʰ S10.14 External constriction of part of throat

    ✓x7ᵗʰ S10.15 Superficial foreign body of throat

        Splinter in the throat

    ✓x7ᵗʰ S10.16 Insect bite (nonvenomous) of throat

    ✓x7ᵗʰ S10.17 Other superficial bite of throat

        EXCLUDES 1   open bite of throat (S11.85)

✓5ᵗʰ S10.8 Superficial injury of other specified parts of neck

    ✓x7ᵗʰ S10.80 Unspecified superficial injury of other specified part of neck

    ✓x7ᵗʰ S10.81 Abrasion of other specified part of neck

    ✓x7ᵗʰ S10.82 Blister (nonthermal) of other specified part of neck

    ✓x7ᵗʰ S10.83 Contusion of other specified part of neck Q

    ✓x7ᵗʰ S10.84 External constriction of other specified part of neck

    ✓x7ᵗʰ S10.85 Superficial foreign body of other specified part of neck

        Splinter in other specified part of neck

    ✓x7ᵗʰ S10.86 Insect bite of other specified part of neck

    ✓x7ᵗʰ S10.87 Other superficial bite of other specified part of neck

        EXCLUDES 1   open bite of other specified parts of neck (S11.85)

✓5ᵗʰ S10.9 Superficial injury of unspecified part of neck

    ✓x7ᵗʰ S10.90 Unspecified superficial injury of unspecified part of neck

    ✓x7ᵗʰ S10.91 Abrasion of unspecified part of neck

    ✓x7ᵗʰ S10.92 Blister (nonthermal) of unspecified part of neck

    ✓x7ᵗʰ S10.93 Contusion of unspecified part of neck Q

    ✓x7ᵗʰ S10.94 External constriction of unspecified part of neck

    ✓x7ᵗʰ S10.95 Superficial foreign body of unspecified part of neck

    ✓x7ᵗʰ S10.96 Insect bite of unspecified part of neck

    ✓x7ᵗʰ S10.97 Other superficial bite of unspecified part of neck

✓4ᵗʰ S11 Open wound of neck

    Code also any associated:
        spinal cord injury (S14.0, S14.1-)
        wound infection

    EXCLUDES 2   open fracture of vertebra (S12.- with 7th character B)

The appropriate 7th character is to be added to each code from category S11.
A   initial encounter
D   subsequent encounter
S   sequela

✓5ᵗʰ S11.0 Open wound of larynx and trachea

    ✓6ᵗʰ S11.01 Open wound of larynx

        EXCLUDES 2   open wound of vocal cord (S11.03)

        ✓7ᵗʰ S11.011 Laceration without foreign body of larynx

     √7ᵗʰ   **S11.012**   Laceration with foreign body of larynx

     √7ᵗʰ   **S11.013**   Puncture wound without foreign body of larynx

     √7ᵗʰ   **S11.014**   Puncture wound with foreign body of larynx

     √7ᵗʰ   **S11.015**   Open bite of larynx

           Bite of larynx NOS

     √7ᵗʰ   **S11.019**   Unspecified open wound of larynx

   ✓6ᵗʰ   **S11.02**   **Open wound of** trachea

         Open wound of cervical trachea

         Open wound of trachea NOS

         EXCLUDES 2   *open wound of thoracic trachea (S27.5-)*

     √7ᵗʰ   **S11.021**   Laceration without foreign body of trachea

     √7ᵗʰ   **S11.022**   Laceration with foreign body of trachea

     √7ᵗʰ   **S11.023**   Puncture wound without foreign body of trachea

     √7ᵗʰ   **S11.024**   Puncture wound with foreign body of trachea

     √7ᵗʰ   **S11.025**   Open bite of trachea

           Bite of trachea NOS

     √7ᵗʰ   **S11.029**   Unspecified open wound of trachea

   ✓6ᵗʰ   **S11.03**   **Open wound of** vocal cord

     √7ᵗʰ   **S11.031**   Laceration without foreign body of vocal cord

     √7ᵗʰ   **S11.032**   Laceration with foreign body of vocal cord

     √7ᵗʰ   **S11.033**   Puncture wound without foreign body of vocal cord

     √7ᵗʰ   **S11.034**   Puncture wound with foreign body of vocal cord

     √7ᵗʰ   **S11.035**   Open bite of vocal cord

           Bite of vocal cord NOS

     √7ᵗʰ   **S11.039**   Unspecified open wound of vocal cord

✓5ᵗʰ   **S11.1**   **Open wound of** thyroid gland

   √x7ᵗʰ   **S11.10**   Unspecified open wound of thyroid gland

   √x7ᵗʰ   **S11.11**   Laceration without foreign body of thyroid gland

   √x7ᵗʰ   **S11.12**   Laceration with foreign body of thyroid gland

   √x7ᵗʰ   **S11.13**   Puncture wound without foreign body of thyroid gland

   √x7ᵗʰ   **S11.14**   Puncture wound with foreign body of thyroid gland

   √x7ᵗʰ   **S11.15**   Open bite of thyroid gland

         Bite of thyroid gland NOS

✓6ᵗʰ   **S11.2**   **Open wound of** pharynx and cervical esophagus

     EXCLUDES 1   *open wound of esophagus NOS (S27.8-)*

   √x7ᵗʰ   **S11.20**   Unspecified open wound of pharynx and cervical esophagus

   √x7ᵗʰ   **S11.21**   Laceration without foreign body of pharynx and cervical esophagus

   √x7ᵗʰ   **S11.22**   Laceration with foreign body of pharynx and cervical esophagus

   √x7ᵗʰ   **S11.23**   Puncture wound without foreign body of pharynx and cervical esophagus

   √x7ᵗʰ   **S11.24**   Puncture wound with foreign body of pharynx and cervical esophagus

   √x7ᵗʰ   **S11.25**   Open bite of pharynx and cervical esophagus

         Bite of pharynx and cervical esophagus NOS

✓5ᵗʰ   **S11.8**   **Open wound of other specified parts of neck**

   √x7ᵗʰ   **S11.80**   Unspecified open wound of other specified part of neck

   √x7ᵗʰ   **S11.81**   Laceration without foreign body of other specified part of neck

   √x7ᵗʰ   **S11.82**   Laceration with foreign body of other specified part of neck

   √x7ᵗʰ   **S11.83**   Puncture wound without foreign body of other specified part of neck

   √x7ᵗʰ   **S11.84**   Puncture wound with foreign body of other specified part of neck

   √x7ᵗʰ   **S11.85**   Open bite of other specified part of neck

         Bite of other specified part of neck NOS

         EXCLUDES 1   *superficial bite of other specified part of neck (S10.87)*

   √x7ᵗʰ   **S11.89**   Other open wound of other specified part of neck

✓5ᵗʰ   **S11.9**   **Open wound of unspecified part of neck**

   √x7ᵗʰ   **S11.90**   Unspecified open wound of unspecified part of neck

   √x7ᵗʰ   **S11.91**   Laceration without foreign body of unspecified part of neck

   √x7ᵗʰ   **S11.92**   Laceration with foreign body of unspecified part of neck

   √x7ᵗʰ   **S11.93**   Puncture wound without foreign body of unspecified part of neck

   √x7ᵗʰ   **S11.94**   Puncture wound with foreign body of unspecified part of neck

   √x7ᵗʰ   **S11.95**   Open bite of unspecified part of neck

         Bite of neck NOS

         EXCLUDES 1   *superficial bite of neck (S10.97)*

✓4ᵗʰ   **S12**   **Fracture of cervical vertebra and other parts of neck**

     NOTE   A fracture not indicated as displaced or nondisplaced should be coded to displaced.

            A fracture not indicated as open or closed should be coded to closed.

     INCLUDES   fracture of cervical neural arch

            fracture of cervical spine

            fracture of cervical spinous process

            fracture of cervical transverse process

            fracture of cervical vertebral arch

            fracture of neck

Code first any associated cervical spinal cord injury (S14.0, S14.1-)

AHA: 2018,2Q,12; 2015,3Q,37-39

The appropriate 7th character is to be added to all codes from subcategories S12.0-S12.6.

A   initial encounter for closed fracture

B   initial encounter for open fracture

D   subsequent encounter for fracture with routine healing

G   subsequent encounter for fracture with delayed healing

K   subsequent encounter for fracture with nonunion

S   sequela

✓5ᵗʰ   **S12.0**   **Fracture of** first **cervical vertebra**

     Atlas

   ✓6ᵗʰ   **S12.00**   **Unspecified fracture of first cervical vertebra**

     1   √7ᵗʰ   **S12.000**   Unspecified displaced fracture of first cervical vertebra   HCC ⓠ

     1   √7ᵗʰ   **S12.001**   Unspecified nondisplaced fracture of first cervical vertebra   HCC ⓠ

   1   √x7ᵗʰ   **S12.01**   Stable burst fracture of first cervical vertebra   HCC ⓠ

   1   √x7ᵗʰ   **S12.02**   Unstable burst fracture of first cervical vertebra   HCC ⓠ

   ✓6ᵗʰ   **S12.03**   Posterior arch fracture of first cervical vertebra

     1   √7ᵗʰ   **S12.030**   Displaced posterior arch fracture of first cervical vertebra   HCC ⓠ

     1   √7ᵗʰ   **S12.031**   Nondisplaced posterior arch fracture of first cervical vertebra   HCC ⓠ

   ✓6ᵗʰ   **S12.04**   Lateral mass fracture of first cervical vertebra

     1   √7ᵗʰ   **S12.040**   Displaced lateral mass fracture of first cervical vertebra   HCC ⓠ

     1   √7ᵗʰ   **S12.041**   Nondisplaced lateral mass fracture of first cervical vertebra   HCC ⓠ

   ✓6ᵗʰ   **S12.09**   Other fracture of first cervical vertebra

     1   √7ᵗʰ   **S12.090**   Other displaced fracture of first cervical vertebra   HCC ⓠ

     1   √7ᵗʰ   **S12.091**   Other nondisplaced fracture of first cervical vertebra   HCC ⓠ

✓5ᵗʰ   **S12.1**   **Fracture of** second **cervical vertebra**

     Axis

   ✓6ᵗʰ   **S12.10**   Unspecified fracture of second cervical vertebra

     1   √7ᵗʰ   **S12.100**   Unspecified displaced fracture of second cervical vertebra   HCC ⓠ

     1   √7ᵗʰ   **S12.101**   Unspecified nondisplaced fracture of second cervical vertebra   HCC ⓠ

   ✓6ᵗʰ   **S12.11**   Type II dens fracture

     1   √7ᵗʰ   **S12.110**   Anterior displaced Type II dens fracture   HCC ⓠ

     1   √7ᵗʰ   **S12.111**   Posterior displaced Type II dens fracture   HCC ⓠ

     1   √7ᵗʰ   **S12.112**   Nondisplaced Type II dens fracture   HCC ⓠ

   ✓6ᵗʰ   **S12.12**   Other dens fracture

     1   √7ᵗʰ   **S12.120**   Other displaced dens fracture   HCC ⓠ

     1   √7ᵗʰ   **S12.121**   Other nondisplaced dens fracture   HCC ⓠ

✓ Additional Character Required   √x7ᵗʰ Placeholder Alert   Manifestation   Unspecified Dx   ►◄ Revised Text   ● New Code   ▲ Revised Code Title

ICD-10-CM 2020   **969**

✓6ᵗʰ **S12.13** Unspecified traumatic spondylolisthesis of second cervical vertebra

  ¹ ✓7ᵗʰ **S12.130** Unspecified traumatic displaced spondylolisthesis of second cervical vertebra HCC Q

  ¹ ✓7ᵗʰ **S12.131** Unspecified traumatic nondisplaced spondylolisthesis of second cervical vertebra HCC Q

¹ ✓x7ᵗʰ **S12.14** Type III traumatic spondylolisthesis of second cervical vertebra HCC Q

✓6ᵗʰ **S12.15** Other traumatic spondylolisthesis of second cervical vertebra

  ¹ ✓7ᵗʰ **S12.150** Other traumatic displaced spondylolisthesis of second cervical vertebra HCC Q

  ¹ ✓7ᵗʰ **S12.151** Other traumatic nondisplaced spondylolisthesis of second cervical vertebra HCC Q

✓6ᵗʰ **S12.19** Other fracture of second cervical vertebra

  ¹ ✓7ᵗʰ **S12.190** Other displaced fracture of second cervical vertebra HCC Q

  ¹ ✓7ᵗʰ **S12.191** Other nondisplaced fracture of second cervical vertebra HCC Q

✓5ᵗʰ **S12.2** Fracture of third cervical vertebra

  ✓6ᵗʰ **S12.20** Unspecified fracture of third cervical vertebra

    ¹ ✓7ᵗʰ **S12.200** Unspecified displaced fracture of third cervical vertebra HCC Q

    ¹ ✓7ᵗʰ **S12.201** Unspecified nondisplaced fracture of third cervical vertebra HCC Q

  ✓6ᵗʰ **S12.23** Unspecified traumatic spondylolisthesis of third cervical vertebra

    ¹ ✓7ᵗʰ **S12.230** Unspecified traumatic displaced spondylolisthesis of third cervical vertebra HCC Q

    ¹ ✓7ᵗʰ **S12.231** Unspecified traumatic nondisplaced spondylolisthesis of third cervical vertebra HCC Q

  ¹ ✓x7ᵗʰ **S12.24** Type III traumatic spondylolisthesis of third cervical vertebra HCC Q

  ✓6ᵗʰ **S12.25** Other traumatic spondylolisthesis of third cervical vertebra

    ¹ ✓7ᵗʰ **S12.250** Other traumatic displaced spondylolisthesis of third cervical vertebra HCC Q

    ¹ ✓7ᵗʰ **S12.251** Other traumatic nondisplaced spondylolisthesis of third cervical vertebra HCC Q

  ✓6ᵗʰ **S12.29** Other fracture of third cervical vertebra

    ¹ ✓7ᵗʰ **S12.290** Other displaced fracture of third cervical vertebra HCC Q

    ¹ ✓7ᵗʰ **S12.291** Other nondisplaced fracture of third cervical vertebra HCC Q

✓5ᵗʰ **S12.3** Fracture of fourth cervical vertebra

  ✓6ᵗʰ **S12.30** Unspecified fracture of fourth cervical vertebra

    ¹ ✓7ᵗʰ **S12.300** Unspecified displaced fracture of fourth cervical vertebra HCC Q

    ¹ ✓7ᵗʰ **S12.301** Unspecified nondisplaced fracture of fourth cervical vertebra HCC Q

  ✓6ᵗʰ **S12.33** Unspecified traumatic spondylolisthesis of fourth cervical vertebra

    ¹ ✓7ᵗʰ **S12.330** Unspecified traumatic displaced spondylolisthesis of fourth cervical vertebra HCC Q

    ¹ ✓7ᵗʰ **S12.331** Unspecified traumatic nondisplaced spondylolisthesis of fourth cervical vertebra HCC Q

  ¹ ✓x7ᵗʰ **S12.34** Type III traumatic spondylolisthesis of fourth cervical vertebra HCC Q

  ✓6ᵗʰ **S12.35** Other traumatic spondylolisthesis of fourth cervical vertebra

    ¹ ✓7ᵗʰ **S12.350** Other traumatic displaced spondylolisthesis of fourth cervical vertebra HCC Q

    ¹ ✓7ᵗʰ **S12.351** Other traumatic nondisplaced spondylolisthesis of fourth cervical vertebra HCC Q

  ✓6ᵗʰ **S12.39** Other fracture of fourth cervical vertebra

    ¹ ✓7ᵗʰ **S12.390** Other displaced fracture of fourth cervical vertebra HCC Q

    ¹ ✓7ᵗʰ **S12.391** Other nondisplaced fracture of fourth cervical vertebra HCC Q

✓5ᵗʰ **S12.4** Fracture of fifth cervical vertebra

  ✓6ᵗʰ **S12.40** Unspecified fracture of fifth cervical vertebra

    ¹ ✓7ᵗʰ **S12.400** Unspecified displaced fracture of fifth cervical vertebra HCC Q

    ¹ ✓7ᵗʰ **S12.401** Unspecified nondisplaced fracture of fifth cervical vertebra HCC Q

  ✓6ᵗʰ **S12.43** Unspecified traumatic spondylolisthesis of fifth cervical vertebra

    ¹ ✓7ᵗʰ **S12.430** Unspecified traumatic displaced spondylolisthesis of fifth cervical vertebra HCC Q

    ¹ ✓7ᵗʰ **S12.431** Unspecified traumatic nondisplaced spondylolisthesis of fifth cervical vertebra HCC Q

  ¹ ✓x7ᵗʰ **S12.44** Type III traumatic spondylolisthesis of fifth cervical vertebra HCC Q

  ✓6ᵗʰ **S12.45** Other traumatic spondylolisthesis of fifth cervical vertebra

    ¹ ✓7ᵗʰ **S12.450** Other traumatic displaced spondylolisthesis of fifth cervical vertebra HCC Q

    ¹ ✓7ᵗʰ **S12.451** Other traumatic nondisplaced spondylolisthesis of fifth cervical vertebra HCC Q

  ✓6ᵗʰ **S12.49** Other fracture of fifth cervical vertebra

    ¹ ✓7ᵗʰ **S12.490** Other displaced fracture of fifth cervical vertebra HCC Q

    ¹ ✓7ᵗʰ **S12.491** Other nondisplaced fracture of fifth cervical vertebra HCC Q

✓5ᵗʰ **S12.5** Fracture of sixth cervical vertebra

  ✓6ᵗʰ **S12.50** Unspecified fracture of sixth cervical vertebra

    ¹ ✓7ᵗʰ **S12.500** Unspecified displaced fracture of sixth cervical vertebra HCC Q

    ¹ ✓7ᵗʰ **S12.501** Unspecified nondisplaced fracture of sixth cervical vertebra HCC Q

  ✓6ᵗʰ **S12.53** Unspecified traumatic spondylolisthesis of sixth cervical vertebra

    ¹ ✓7ᵗʰ **S12.530** Unspecified traumatic displaced spondylolisthesis of sixth cervical vertebra HCC Q

    ¹ ✓7ᵗʰ **S12.531** Unspecified traumatic nondisplaced spondylolisthesis of sixth cervical vertebra HCC Q

  ¹ ✓x7ᵗʰ **S12.54** Type III traumatic spondylolisthesis of sixth cervical vertebra HCC Q

  ✓6ᵗʰ **S12.55** Other traumatic spondylolisthesis of sixth cervical vertebra

    ¹ ✓7ᵗʰ **S12.550** Other traumatic displaced spondylolisthesis of sixth cervical vertebra HCC Q

    ¹ ✓7ᵗʰ **S12.551** Other traumatic nondisplaced spondylolisthesis of sixth cervical vertebra HCC Q

  ✓6ᵗʰ **S12.59** Other fracture of sixth cervical vertebra

    ¹ ✓7ᵗʰ **S12.590** Other displaced fracture of sixth cervical vertebra HCC Q

    ¹ ✓7ᵗʰ **S12.591** Other nondisplaced fracture of sixth cervical vertebra HCC Q

✓5ᵗʰ **S12.6** Fracture of seventh cervical vertebra

  ✓6ᵗʰ **S12.60** Unspecified fracture of seventh cervical vertebra

    ¹ ✓7ᵗʰ **S12.600** Unspecified displaced fracture of seventh cervical vertebra HCC Q

    ¹ ✓7ᵗʰ **S12.601** Unspecified nondisplaced fracture of seventh cervical vertebra HCC Q

  ✓6ᵗʰ **S12.63** Unspecified traumatic spondylolisthesis of seventh cervical vertebra

    ¹ ✓7ᵗʰ **S12.630** Unspecified traumatic displaced spondylolisthesis of seventh cervical vertebra HCC Q

    ¹ ✓7ᵗʰ **S12.631** Unspecified traumatic nondisplaced spondylolisthesis of seventh cervical vertebra HCC Q

  ¹ ✓x7ᵗʰ **S12.64** Type III traumatic spondylolisthesis of seventh cervical vertebra HCC Q

  ✓6ᵗʰ **S12.65** Other traumatic spondylolisthesis of seventh cervical vertebra

    ¹ ✓7ᵗʰ **S12.650** Other traumatic displaced spondylolisthesis of seventh cervical vertebra HCC Q

¹ ☑7ᵗʰ **S12.651** **Other traumatic nondisplaced spondylolisthesis of seventh cervical vertebra** HCC Q

☑6ᵗʰ **S12.69** **Other fracture of seventh cervical vertebra**

   ¹ ☑7ᵗʰ **S12.690** **Other displaced fracture of seventh cervical vertebra** HCC Q

   ¹ ☑7ᵗʰ **S12.691** **Other nondisplaced fracture of seventh cervical vertebra** HCC Q

¹ ☑x7ᵗʰ **S12.8** **Fracture of other parts of neck** HCC Q

   Hyoid bone
   Larynx
   Thyroid cartilage
   Trachea

> The appropriate 7th character is to be added to code S12.8.
> A   initial encounter
> D   subsequent encounter
> S   sequela

¹ ☑x7ᵗʰ **S12.9** **Fracture of neck, unspecified** HCC Q

   Fracture of neck NOS
   Fracture of cervical spine NOS
   Fracture of cervical vertebra NOS

> The appropriate 7th character is to be added to code S12.9.
> A   initial encounter
> D   subsequent encounter
> S   sequela

☑4ᵗʰ **S13** **Dislocation and sprain of joints and ligaments at neck level**

   INCLUDES   avulsion of joint or ligament at neck level
       laceration of cartilage, joint or ligament at neck level
       sprain of cartilage, joint or ligament at neck level
       traumatic hemarthrosis of joint or ligament at neck level
       traumatic rupture of joint or ligament at neck level
       traumatic subluxation of joint or ligament at neck level
       traumatic tear of joint or ligament at neck level

   Code also any associated open wound
   EXCLUDES 2   strain of muscle or tendon at neck level (S16.1)

> The appropriate 7th character is to be added to each code from category S13.
> A   initial encounter
> D   subsequent encounter
> S   sequela

☑x7ᵗʰ **S13.0** **Traumatic rupture of cervical intervertebral disc**

   EXCLUDES 1   rupture or displacement (nontraumatic) of cervical intervertebral disc NOS (M50.-)

☑5ᵗʰ **S13.1** **Subluxation and dislocation of cervical vertebrae**

   Code also any associated:
       open wound of neck (S11.-)
       spinal cord injury (S14.1-)
   EXCLUDES 2   fracture of cervical vertebrae (S12.0-S12.3-)

  ☑6ᵗʰ **S13.10** **Subluxation and dislocation of unspecified cervical vertebrae**

    ☑7ᵗʰ **S13.100** **Subluxation of unspecified cervical vertebrae**

    ☑7ᵗʰ **S13.101** **Dislocation of unspecified cervical vertebrae**

  ☑6ᵗʰ **S13.11** **Subluxation and dislocation of C0/C1 cervical vertebrae**

    Subluxation and dislocation of atlantooccipital joint
    Subluxation and dislocation of atloidooccipital joint
    Subluxation and dislocation of occipitoatloid joint

    ☑7ᵗʰ **S13.110** **Subluxation of C0/C1 cervical vertebrae**

    ☑7ᵗʰ **S13.111** **Dislocation of C0/C1 cervical vertebrae**

  ☑6ᵗʰ **S13.12** **Subluxation and dislocation of C1/C2 cervical vertebrae**

    Subluxation and dislocation of atlantoaxial joint

    ☑7ᵗʰ **S13.120** **Subluxation of C1/C2 cervical vertebrae**

    ☑7ᵗʰ **S13.121** **Dislocation of C1/C2 cervical vertebrae**

  ☑6ᵗʰ **S13.13** **Subluxation and dislocation of C2/C3 cervical vertebrae**

    ☑7ᵗʰ **S13.130** **Subluxation of C2/C3 cervical vertebrae**

    ☑7ᵗʰ **S13.131** **Dislocation of C2/C3 cervical vertebrae**

  ☑6ᵗʰ **S13.14** **Subluxation and dislocation of C3/C4 cervical vertebrae**

    ☑7ᵗʰ **S13.140** **Subluxation of C3/C4 cervical vertebrae**

    ☑7ᵗʰ **S13.141** **Dislocation of C3/C4 cervical vertebrae**

  ☑6ᵗʰ **S13.15** **Subluxation and dislocation of C4/C5 cervical vertebrae**

    ☑7ᵗʰ **S13.150** **Subluxation of C4/C5 cervical vertebrae**

    ☑7ᵗʰ **S13.151** **Dislocation of C4/C5 cervical vertebrae**

  ☑6ᵗʰ **S13.16** **Subluxation and dislocation of C5/C6 cervical vertebrae**

    ☑7ᵗʰ **S13.160** **Subluxation of C5/C6 cervical vertebrae**

    ☑7ᵗʰ **S13.161** **Dislocation of C5/C6 cervical vertebrae**

  ☑6ᵗʰ **S13.17** **Subluxation and dislocation of C6/C7 cervical vertebrae**

    ☑7ᵗʰ **S13.170** **Subluxation of C6/C7 cervical vertebrae**

    ☑7ᵗʰ **S13.171** **Dislocation of C6/C7 cervical vertebrae**

  ☑6ᵗʰ **S13.18** **Subluxation and dislocation of C7/T1 cervical vertebrae**

    ☑7ᵗʰ **S13.180** **Subluxation of C7/T1 cervical vertebrae**

    ☑7ᵗʰ **S13.181** **Dislocation of C7/T1 cervical vertebrae**

☑5ᵗʰ **S13.2** **Dislocation of other and unspecified parts of neck**

  ☑x7ᵗʰ **S13.20** **Dislocation of unspecified parts of neck**

  ☑x7ᵗʰ **S13.29** **Dislocation of other parts of neck**

☑x7ᵗʰ **S13.4** **Sprain of ligaments of cervical spine**

   Sprain of anterior longitudinal (ligament), cervical
   Sprain of atlanto-axial (joints)
   Sprain of atlanto-occipital (joints)
   Whiplash injury of cervical spine

☑x7ᵗʰ **S13.5** **Sprain of thyroid region**

   Sprain of cricoarytenoid (joint) (ligament)
   Sprain of cricothyroid (joint) (ligament)
   Sprain of thyroid cartilage

☑x7ᵗʰ **S13.8** **Sprain of joints and ligaments of other parts of neck**

☑x7ᵗʰ **S13.9** **Sprain of joints and ligaments of unspecified parts of neck**

☑4ᵗʰ **S14** **Injury of nerves and spinal cord at neck level**

   NOTE   Code to highest level of cervical cord injury

   Code also any associated:
       fracture of cervical vertebra (S12.0- — S12.6.-)
       open wound of neck (S11.-)
       transient paralysis (R29.5)

> The appropriate 7th character is to be added to each code from category S14.
> A   initial encounter
> D   subsequent encounter
> S   sequela

☑x7ᵗʰ **S14.0** **Concussion and edema of cervical spinal cord** HCC

☑5ᵗʰ **S14.1** **Other and unspecified injuries of cervical spinal cord**

  ☑6ᵗʰ **S14.10** **Unspecified injury of cervical spinal cord**

    ☑7ᵗʰ **S14.101** **Unspecified injury at C1 level of cervical spinal cord** HCC

    ☑7ᵗʰ **S14.102** **Unspecified injury at C2 level of cervical spinal cord** HCC

    ☑7ᵗʰ **S14.103** **Unspecified injury at C3 level of cervical spinal cord** HCC

    ☑7ᵗʰ **S14.104** **Unspecified injury at C4 level of cervical spinal cord** HCC

    ☑7ᵗʰ **S14.105** **Unspecified injury at C5 level of cervical spinal cord** HCC

    ☑7ᵗʰ **S14.106** **Unspecified injury at C6 level of cervical spinal cord** HCC

    ☑7ᵗʰ **S14.107** **Unspecified injury at C7 level of cervical spinal cord** HCC

    ☑7ᵗʰ **S14.108** **Unspecified injury at C8 level of cervical spinal cord** HCC

    ☑7ᵗʰ **S14.109** **Unspecified injury at unspecified level of cervical spinal cord** HCC

      Injury of cervical spinal cord NOS

  ☑6ᵗʰ **S14.11** **Complete lesion of cervical spinal cord**

    ☑7ᵗʰ **S14.111** **Complete lesion at C1 level of cervical spinal cord** HCC

    ☑7ᵗʰ **S14.112** **Complete lesion at C2 level of cervical spinal cord** HCC

    ☑7ᵗʰ **S14.113** **Complete lesion at C3 level of cervical spinal cord** HCC

    ☑7ᵗʰ **S14.114** **Complete lesion at C4 level of cervical spinal cord** HCC

    ☑7ᵗʰ **S14.115** **Complete lesion at C5 level of cervical spinal cord** HCC

☑ Additional Character Required   ☑x7ᵗʰ Placeholder Alert   Manifestation   Unspecified Dx   ►◄ Revised Text   ● New Code   ▲ Revised Code Title

√7ᵗʰ **S14.116** **Complete lesion at C6 level of cervical spinal cord** HCC

√7ᵗʰ **S14.117** **Complete lesion at C7 level of cervical spinal cord** HCC

√7ᵗʰ **S14.118** **Complete lesion at C8 level of cervical spinal cord** HCC

√7ᵗʰ **S14.119** **Complete lesion at unspecified level of cervical spinal cord** HCC

√6ᵗʰ **S14.12** Central cord syndrome of cervical spinal cord

√7ᵗʰ **S14.121** **Central cord syndrome at C1 level of cervical spinal cord** HCC

√7ᵗʰ **S14.122** **Central cord syndrome at C2 level of cervical spinal cord** HCC

√7ᵗʰ **S14.123** **Central cord syndrome at C3 level of cervical spinal cord** HCC

√7ᵗʰ **S14.124** **Central cord syndrome at C4 level of cervical spinal cord** HCC

√7ᵗʰ **S14.125** **Central cord syndrome at C5 level of cervical spinal cord** HCC

√7ᵗʰ **S14.126** **Central cord syndrome at C6 level of cervical spinal cord** HCC

√7ᵗʰ **S14.127** **Central cord syndrome at C7 level of cervical spinal cord** HCC

√7ᵗʰ **S14.128** **Central cord syndrome at C8 level of cervical spinal cord** HCC

√7ᵗʰ **S14.129** **Central cord syndrome at unspecified level of cervical spinal cord** HCC

√6ᵗʰ **S14.13** Anterior cord syndrome of cervical spinal cord

√7ᵗʰ **S14.131** **Anterior cord syndrome at C1 level of cervical spinal cord** HCC

√7ᵗʰ **S14.132** **Anterior cord syndrome at C2 level of cervical spinal cord** HCC

√7ᵗʰ **S14.133** **Anterior cord syndrome at C3 level of cervical spinal cord** HCC

√7ᵗʰ **S14.134** **Anterior cord syndrome at C4 level of cervical spinal cord** HCC

√7ᵗʰ **S14.135** **Anterior cord syndrome at C5 level of cervical spinal cord** HCC

√7ᵗʰ **S14.136** **Anterior cord syndrome at C6 level of cervical spinal cord** HCC

√7ᵗʰ **S14.137** **Anterior cord syndrome at C7 level of cervical spinal cord** HCC

√7ᵗʰ **S14.138** **Anterior cord syndrome at C8 level of cervical spinal cord** HCC

√7ᵗʰ **S14.139** **Anterior cord syndrome at unspecified level of cervical spinal cord** HCC

√6ᵗʰ **S14.14** Brown-Séquard syndrome of cervical spinal cord

√7ᵗʰ **S14.141** **Brown-Séquard syndrome at C1 level of cervical spinal cord** HCC

√7ᵗʰ **S14.142** **Brown-Séquard syndrome at C2 level of cervical spinal cord** HCC

√7ᵗʰ **S14.143** **Brown-Séquard syndrome at C3 level of cervical spinal cord** HCC

√7ᵗʰ **S14.144** **Brown-Séquard syndrome at C4 level of cervical spinal cord** HCC

√7ᵗʰ **S14.145** **Brown-Séquard syndrome at C5 level of cervical spinal cord** HCC

√7ᵗʰ **S14.146** **Brown-Séquard syndrome at C6 level of cervical spinal cord** HCC

√7ᵗʰ **S14.147** **Brown-Séquard syndrome at C7 level of cervical spinal cord** HCC

√7ᵗʰ **S14.148** **Brown-Séquard syndrome at C8 level of cervical spinal cord** HCC

√7ᵗʰ **S14.149** **Brown-Séquard syndrome at unspecified level of cervical spinal cord** HCC

√6ᵗʰ **S14.15** Other incomplete lesions of cervical spinal cord

Incomplete lesion of cervical spinal cord NOS
Posterior cord syndrome of cervical spinal cord

√7ᵗʰ **S14.151** **Other incomplete lesion at C1 level of cervical spinal cord** HCC

√7ᵗʰ **S14.152** **Other incomplete lesion at C2 level of cervical spinal cord** HCC

√7ᵗʰ **S14.153** **Other incomplete lesion at C3 level of cervical spinal cord** HCC

√7ᵗʰ **S14.154** **Other incomplete lesion at C4 level of cervical spinal cord** HCC

√7ᵗʰ **S14.155** **Other incomplete lesion at C5 level of cervical spinal cord** HCC

√7ᵗʰ **S14.156** **Other incomplete lesion at C6 level of cervical spinal cord** HCC

√7ᵗʰ **S14.157** **Other incomplete lesion at C7 level of cervical spinal cord** HCC

√7ᵗʰ **S14.158** **Other incomplete lesion at C8 level of cervical spinal cord** HCC

√7ᵗʰ **S14.159** **Other incomplete lesion at unspecified level of cervical spinal cord** HCC

√x7ᵗʰ **S14.2** **Injury of nerve root of cervical spine**

√x7ᵗʰ **S14.3** **Injury of brachial plexus**

√x7ᵗʰ **S14.4** **Injury of peripheral nerves of neck**

√x7ᵗʰ **S14.5** **Injury of cervical sympathetic nerves**

√x7ᵗʰ **S14.8** **Injury of other specified nerves of neck**

√x7ᵗʰ **S14.9** **Injury of unspecified nerves of neck**

√4ᵗʰ **S15** **Injury of blood vessels at neck level**

Code also any associated open wound (S11.-)

The appropriate 7th character is to be added to each code from category S15.
A initial encounter
D subsequent encounter
S sequela

√5ᵗʰ **S15.0** **Injury of carotid artery of neck**

Injury of carotid artery (common) (external) (internal, extracranial portion)
Injury of carotid artery NOS

EXCLUDES 1 *injury of internal carotid artery, intracranial portion (S06.8)*

√6ᵗʰ **S15.00** **Unspecified injury of carotid artery**

√7ᵗʰ **S15.001** **Unspecified injury of right carotid artery**

√7ᵗʰ **S15.002** **Unspecified injury of left carotid artery**

√7ᵗʰ **S15.009** **Unspecified injury of unspecified carotid artery**

√6ᵗʰ **S15.01** Minor laceration of carotid artery

Incomplete transection of carotid artery
Laceration of carotid artery NOS
Superficial laceration of carotid artery

√7ᵗʰ **S15.011** **Minor laceration of right carotid artery**

√7ᵗʰ **S15.012** **Minor laceration of left carotid artery**

√7ᵗʰ **S15.019** **Minor laceration of unspecified carotid artery**

√6ᵗʰ **S15.02** Major laceration of carotid artery

Complete transection of carotid artery
Traumatic rupture of carotid artery

√7ᵗʰ **S15.021** **Major laceration of right carotid artery**

√7ᵗʰ **S15.022** **Major laceration of left carotid artery**

√7ᵗʰ **S15.029** **Major laceration of unspecified carotid artery**

√6ᵗʰ **S15.09** **Other specified injury of carotid artery**

√7ᵗʰ **S15.091** **Other specified injury of right carotid artery**

√7ᵗʰ **S15.092** **Other specified injury of left carotid artery**

√7ᵗʰ **S15.099** **Other specified injury of unspecified carotid artery**

√5ᵗʰ **S15.1** **Injury of vertebral artery**

√6ᵗʰ **S15.10** **Unspecified injury of vertebral artery**

√7ᵗʰ **S15.101** **Unspecified injury of right vertebral artery**

√7ᵗʰ **S15.102** **Unspecified injury of left vertebral artery**

√7ᵗʰ **S15.109** **Unspecified injury of unspecified vertebral artery**

√6ᵗʰ **S15.11** Minor laceration of vertebral artery

Incomplete transection of vertebral artery
Laceration of vertebral artery NOS
Superficial laceration of vertebral artery

√7ᵗʰ **S15.111** **Minor laceration of right vertebral artery**

√7ᵗʰ **S15.112** **Minor laceration of left vertebral artery**

√7ᵗʰ **S15.119** **Minor laceration of unspecified vertebral artery**

√6ᵗʰ **S15.12** Major laceration of vertebral artery

Complete transection of vertebral artery
Traumatic rupture of vertebral artery

√7ᵗʰ **S15.121** **Major laceration of right vertebral artery**

√7ᵗʰ **S15.122** Major laceration of **left** vertebral artery

√7ᵗʰ **S15.129** Major laceration of unspecified vertebral artery

√6ᵗʰ **S15.19** Other specified injury of vertebral artery

    √7ᵗʰ **S15.191** Other specified injury of **right** vertebral artery

    √7ᵗʰ **S15.192** Other specified injury of **left** vertebral artery

    √7ᵗʰ **S15.199** Other specified injury of unspecified vertebral artery

√5ᵗʰ **S15.2** Injury of external jugular vein

    √6ᵗʰ **S15.20** Unspecified injury of external jugular vein

      √7ᵗʰ **S15.201** Unspecified injury of **right** external jugular vein

      √7ᵗʰ **S15.202** Unspecified injury of **left** external jugular vein

      √7ᵗʰ **S15.209** Unspecified injury of unspecified external jugular vein

    √6ᵗʰ **S15.21** Minor laceration of external jugular vein

      Incomplete transection of external jugular vein
      Laceration of external jugular vein NOS
      Superficial laceration of external jugular vein

      √7ᵗʰ **S15.211** Minor laceration of **right** external jugular vein

      √7ᵗʰ **S15.212** Minor laceration of **left** external jugular vein

      √7ᵗʰ **S15.219** Minor laceration of unspecified external jugular vein

    √6ᵗʰ **S15.22** Major laceration of external jugular vein

      Complete transection of external jugular vein
      Traumatic rupture of external jugular vein

      √7ᵗʰ **S15.221** Major laceration of **right** external jugular vein

      √7ᵗʰ **S15.222** Major laceration of **left** external jugular vein

      √7ᵗʰ **S15.229** Major laceration of unspecified external jugular vein

    √6ᵗʰ **S15.29** Other specified injury of external jugular vein

      √7ᵗʰ **S15.291** Other specified injury of **right** external jugular vein

      √7ᵗʰ **S15.292** Other specified injury of **left** external jugular vein

      √7ᵗʰ **S15.299** Other specified injury of unspecified external jugular vein

√5ᵗʰ **S15.3** Injury of internal jugular vein

    √6ᵗʰ **S15.30** Unspecified injury of internal jugular vein

      √7ᵗʰ **S15.301** Unspecified injury of **right** internal jugular vein

      √7ᵗʰ **S15.302** Unspecified injury of **left** internal jugular vein

      √7ᵗʰ **S15.309** Unspecified injury of unspecified internal jugular vein

    √6ᵗʰ **S15.31** Minor laceration of internal jugular vein

      Incomplete transection of internal jugular vein
      Laceration of internal jugular vein NOS
      Superficial laceration of internal jugular vein

      √7ᵗʰ **S15.311** Minor laceration of **right** internal jugular vein

      √7ᵗʰ **S15.312** Minor laceration of **left** internal jugular vein

      √7ᵗʰ **S15.319** Minor laceration of unspecified internal jugular vein

    √6ᵗʰ **S15.32** Major laceration of internal jugular vein

      Complete transection of internal jugular vein
      Traumatic rupture of internal jugular vein

      √7ᵗʰ **S15.321** Major laceration of **right** internal jugular vein

      √7ᵗʰ **S15.322** Major laceration of **left** internal jugular vein

      √7ᵗʰ **S15.329** Major laceration of unspecified internal jugular vein

    √6ᵗʰ **S15.39** Other specified injury of internal jugular vein

      √7ᵗʰ **S15.391** Other specified injury of **right** internal jugular vein

      √7ᵗʰ **S15.392** Other specified injury of **left** internal jugular vein

      √7ᵗʰ **S15.399** Other specified injury of unspecified internal jugular vein

√x7ᵗʰ **S15.8** Injury of other specified blood vessels at neck level

√x7ᵗʰ **S15.9** Injury of unspecified blood vessel at neck level

√4ᵗʰ **S16** Injury of muscle, fascia and tendon at neck level

    Code also any associated open wound (S11.-)

    EXCLUDES 2   *sprain of joint or ligament at neck level (S13.9)*

    The appropriate 7th character is to be added to each code from category S16.
    A   initial encounter
    D   subsequent encounter
    S   sequela

√x7ᵗʰ **S16.1** Strain of muscle, fascia and tendon at neck level

√x7ᵗʰ **S16.2** Laceration of muscle, fascia and tendon at neck level

√x7ᵗʰ **S16.8** Other specified injury of muscle, fascia and tendon at neck level

√x7ᵗʰ **S16.9** Unspecified injury of muscle, fascia and tendon at neck level

√4ᵗʰ **S17** Crushing injury of neck

    Use additional code for all associated injuries, such as:
      injury of blood vessels (S15.-)
      open wound of neck (S11.-)
      spinal cord injury (S14.0, S14.1-)
      vertebral fracture (S12.0- — S12.3-)

    The appropriate 7th character is to be added to each code from category S17.
    A   initial encounter
    D   subsequent encounter
    S   sequela

√x7ᵗʰ **S17.0** Crushing injury of larynx and trachea

√x7ᵗʰ **S17.8** Crushing injury of other specified parts of neck

√x7ᵗʰ **S17.9** Crushing injury of neck, part unspecified

√4ᵗʰ **S19** Other specified and unspecified injuries of neck

    The appropriate 7th character is to be added to each code from category S19.
    A   initial encounter
    D   subsequent encounter
    S   sequela

√5ᵗʰ **S19.8** Other specified injuries of neck

    √x7ᵗʰ **S19.80** Other specified injuries of unspecified part of neck

    √x7ᵗʰ **S19.81** Other specified injuries of larynx

    √x7ᵗʰ **S19.82** Other specified injuries of cervical trachea

      EXCLUDES 2   *other specified injury of thoracic trachea (S27.5-)*

    √x7ᵗʰ **S19.83** Other specified injuries of vocal cord

    √x7ᵗʰ **S19.84** Other specified injuries of thyroid gland

    √x7ᵗʰ **S19.85** Other specified injuries of pharynx and cervical esophagus

    √x7ᵗʰ **S19.89** Other specified injuries of other specified part of neck

√x7ᵗʰ **S19.9** Unspecified injury of neck

Injuries to the thorax (S20-S29)

INCLUDES   injuries of breast
       injuries of chest (wall)
       injuries of interscapular area

EXCLUDES 2   *burns and corrosions (T20-T32)*
       effects of foreign body in bronchus (T17.5)
       effects of foreign body in esophagus (T18.1)
       effects of foreign body in lung (T17.8)
       effects of foreign body in trachea (T17.4)
       frostbite (T33-T34)
       injuries of axilla
       injuries of clavicle
       injuries of scapular region
       injuries of shoulder
       insect bite or sting, venomous (T63.4)

√4ᵗʰ **S20** Superficial injury of thorax

    The appropriate 7th character is to be added to each code from category S20.
    A   initial encounter
    D   subsequent encounter
    S   sequela

√5ᵗʰ **S20.0** Contusion of breast

    √x7ᵗʰ **S20.00** Contusion of breast, unspecified breast

    √x7ᵗʰ **S20.01** Contusion of right breast

☑ Additional Character Required   √x7ᵗʰ Placeholder Alert   Manifestation   Unspecified Dx   ►◄ Revised Text   ● New Code   ▲ Revised Code Title

ICD-10-CM 2020   973

✓x7ᵗʰ **S20.02**   Contusion of left breast

✓5ᵗʰ **S20.1**   **Other and unspecified superficial injuries of breast**

     ✓6ᵗʰ **S20.10**   Unspecified superficial injuries of breast

       ✓7ᵗʰ **S20.101**   Unspecified superficial injuries of breast, right breast

       ✓7ᵗʰ **S20.102**   Unspecified superficial injuries of breast, left breast

       ✓7ᵗʰ **S20.109**   Unspecified superficial injuries of breast, unspecified breast

     ✓6ᵗʰ **S20.11**   Abrasion of breast

       ✓7ᵗʰ **S20.111**   Abrasion of breast, right breast

       ✓7ᵗʰ **S20.112**   Abrasion of breast, left breast

       ✓7ᵗʰ **S20.119**   Abrasion of breast, unspecified breast

     ✓6ᵗʰ **S20.12**   Blister (nonthermal) of breast

       ✓7ᵗʰ **S20.121**   Blister (nonthermal) of breast, right breast

       ✓7ᵗʰ **S20.122**   Blister (nonthermal) of breast, left breast

       ✓7ᵗʰ **S20.129**   Blister (nonthermal) of breast, unspecified breast

     ✓6ᵗʰ **S20.14**   External constriction of part of breast

       ✓7ᵗʰ **S20.141**   External constriction of part of breast, right breast

       ✓7ᵗʰ **S20.142**   External constriction of part of breast, left breast

       ✓7ᵗʰ **S20.149**   External constriction of part of breast, unspecified breast

     ✓6ᵗʰ **S20.15**   Superficial foreign body of breast

       Splinter in the breast

       ✓7ᵗʰ **S20.151**   Superficial foreign body of breast, right breast

       ✓7ᵗʰ **S20.152**   Superficial foreign body of breast, left breast

       ✓7ᵗʰ **S20.159**   Superficial foreign body of breast, unspecified breast

     ✓6ᵗʰ **S20.16**   Insect bite (nonvenomous) of breast

       ✓7ᵗʰ **S20.161**   Insect bite (nonvenomous) of breast, right breast

       ✓7ᵗʰ **S20.162**   Insect bite (nonvenomous) of breast, left breast

       ✓7ᵗʰ **S20.169**   Insect bite (nonvenomous) of breast, unspecified breast

     ✓6ᵗʰ **S20.17**   Other superficial bite of breast

       EXCLUDES 1   *open bite of breast (S21.05-)*

       ✓7ᵗʰ **S20.171**   Other superficial bite of breast, right breast

       ✓7ᵗʰ **S20.172**   Other superficial bite of breast, left breast

       ✓7ᵗʰ **S20.179**   Other superficial bite of breast, unspecified breast

✓5ᵗʰ **S20.2**   **Contusion of thorax**

     ✓x7ᵗʰ **S20.20**   Contusion of thorax, unspecified

     ✓6ᵗʰ **S20.21**   Contusion of front wall of thorax

       ✓7ᵗʰ **S20.211**   Contusion of right front wall of thorax

       ✓7ᵗʰ **S20.212**   Contusion of left front wall of thorax

       ✓7ᵗʰ **S20.219**   Contusion of unspecified front wall of thorax

     ✓6ᵗʰ **S20.22**   Contusion of back wall of thorax

       ✓7ᵗʰ **S20.221**   Contusion of right back wall of thorax

       ✓7ᵗʰ **S20.222**   Contusion of left back wall of thorax

       ✓7ᵗʰ **S20.229**   Contusion of unspecified back wall of thorax

✓5ᵗʰ **S20.3**   **Other and unspecified superficial injuries of front wall of thorax**

     ✓6ᵗʰ **S20.30**   Unspecified superficial injuries of front wall of thorax

       ✓7ᵗʰ **S20.301**   Unspecified superficial injuries of right front wall of thorax

       ✓7ᵗʰ **S20.302**   Unspecified superficial injuries of left front wall of thorax

       ✓7ᵗʰ **S20.309**   Unspecified superficial injuries of unspecified front wall of thorax

     ✓6ᵗʰ **S20.31**   Abrasion of front wall of thorax

       ✓7ᵗʰ **S20.311**   Abrasion of right front wall of thorax

       ✓7ᵗʰ **S20.312**   Abrasion of left front wall of thorax

       ✓7ᵗʰ **S20.319**   Abrasion of unspecified front wall of thorax

     ✓6ᵗʰ **S20.32**   Blister (nonthermal) of front wall of thorax

       ✓7ᵗʰ **S20.321**   Blister (nonthermal) of right front wall of thorax

       ✓7ᵗʰ **S20.322**   Blister (nonthermal) of left front wall of thorax

       ✓7ᵗʰ **S20.329**   Blister (nonthermal) of unspecified front wall of thorax

     ✓6ᵗʰ **S20.34**   External constriction of front wall of thorax

       ✓7ᵗʰ **S20.341**   External constriction of right front wall of thorax

       ✓7ᵗʰ **S20.342**   External constriction of left front wall of thorax

       ✓7ᵗʰ **S20.349**   External constriction of unspecified front wall of thorax

     ✓6ᵗʰ **S20.35**   Superficial foreign body of front wall of thorax

       Splinter in front wall of thorax

       ✓7ᵗʰ **S20.351**   Superficial foreign body of right front wall of thorax

       ✓7ᵗʰ **S20.352**   Superficial foreign body of left front wall of thorax

       ✓7ᵗʰ **S20.359**   Superficial foreign body of unspecified front wall of thorax

     ✓6ᵗʰ **S20.36**   Insect bite (nonvenomous) of front wall of thorax

       ✓7ᵗʰ **S20.361**   Insect bite (nonvenomous) of right front wall of thorax

       ✓7ᵗʰ **S20.362**   Insect bite (nonvenomous) of left front wall of thorax

       ✓7ᵗʰ **S20.369**   Insect bite (nonvenomous) of unspecified front wall of thorax

     ✓6ᵗʰ **S20.37**   Other superficial bite of front wall of thorax

       EXCLUDES 1   *open bite of front wall of thorax (S21.15)*

       ✓7ᵗʰ **S20.371**   Other superficial bite of right front wall of thorax

       ✓7ᵗʰ **S20.372**   Other superficial bite of left front wall of thorax

       ✓7ᵗʰ **S20.379**   Other superficial bite of unspecified front wall of thorax

✓5ᵗʰ **S20.4**   **Other and unspecified superficial injuries of back wall of thorax**

     ✓6ᵗʰ **S20.40**   Unspecified superficial injuries of back wall of thorax

       ✓7ᵗʰ **S20.401**   Unspecified superficial injuries of right back wall of thorax

       ✓7ᵗʰ **S20.402**   Unspecified superficial injuries of left back wall of thorax

       ✓7ᵗʰ **S20.409**   Unspecified superficial injuries of unspecified back wall of thorax

     ✓6ᵗʰ **S20.41**   Abrasion of back wall of thorax

       ✓7ᵗʰ **S20.411**   Abrasion of right back wall of thorax

       ✓7ᵗʰ **S20.412**   Abrasion of left back wall of thorax

       ✓7ᵗʰ **S20.419**   Abrasion of unspecified back wall of thorax

     ✓6ᵗʰ **S20.42**   Blister (nonthermal) of back wall of thorax

       ✓7ᵗʰ **S20.421**   Blister (nonthermal) of right back wall of thorax

       ✓7ᵗʰ **S20.422**   Blister (nonthermal) of left back wall of thorax

       ✓7ᵗʰ **S20.429**   Blister (nonthermal) of unspecified back wall of thorax

     ✓6ᵗʰ **S20.44**   External constriction of back wall of thorax

       ✓7ᵗʰ **S20.441**   External constriction of right back wall of thorax

       ✓7ᵗʰ **S20.442**   External constriction of left back wall of thorax

       ✓7ᵗʰ **S20.449**   External constriction of unspecified back wall of thorax

     ✓6ᵗʰ **S20.45**   Superficial foreign body of back wall of thorax

       Splinter of back wall of thorax

       ✓7ᵗʰ **S20.451**   Superficial foreign body of right back wall of thorax

       ✓7ᵗʰ **S20.452**   Superficial foreign body of left back wall of thorax

       ✓7ᵗʰ **S20.459**   Superficial foreign body of unspecified back wall of thorax

     ✓6ᵗʰ **S20.46**   Insect bite (nonvenomous) of back wall of thorax

       ✓7ᵗʰ **S20.461**   Insect bite (nonvenomous) of right back wall of thorax

       ✓7ᵗʰ **S20.462**   Insect bite (nonvenomous) of left back wall of thorax

✓7ᵗʰ **S20.469** Insect bite (nonvenomous) of unspecified back wall of thorax

✓6ᵗʰ **S20.47** Other superficial bite of back wall of thorax

> **EXCLUDES 1**   open bite of back wall of thorax (S21.25)

✓7ᵗʰ **S20.471** Other superficial bite of right back wall of thorax

✓7ᵗʰ **S20.472** Other superficial bite of left back wall of thorax

✓7ᵗʰ **S20.479** Other superficial bite of unspecified back wall of thorax

✓5ᵗʰ **S20.9** Superficial injury of unspecified parts of thorax

> **EXCLUDES 1**   contusion of thorax NOS (S20.20)

✓x7ᵗʰ **S20.90** Unspecified superficial injury of unspecified parts of thorax

Superficial injury of thoracic wall NOS

✓x7ᵗʰ **S20.91** Abrasion of unspecified parts of thorax

✓x7ᵗʰ **S20.92** Blister (nonthermal) of unspecified parts of thorax

✓x7ᵗʰ **S20.94** External constriction of unspecified parts of thorax

✓x7ᵗʰ **S20.95** Superficial foreign body of unspecified parts of thorax

Splinter in thorax NOS

✓x7ᵗʰ **S20.96** Insect bite (nonvenomous) of unspecified parts of thorax

✓x7ᵗʰ **S20.97** Other superficial bite of unspecified parts of thorax

> **EXCLUDES 1**   open bite of thorax NOS (S21.95)

✓4ᵗʰ **S21** Open wound of thorax

Code also any associated injury, such as:
  injury of heart (S26.-)
  injury of intrathoracic organs (S27.-)
  rib fracture (S22.3-, S22.4-)
  spinal cord injury (S24.0-, S24.1-)
  traumatic hemopneumothorax (S27.3)
  traumatic hemothorax (S27.1)
  traumatic pneumothorax (S27.0)
  wound infection

> **EXCLUDES 1**   traumatic amputation (partial) of thorax (S28.1)

The appropriate 7th character is to be added to each code from category S21.
A   initial encounter
D   subsequent encounter
S   sequela

✓5ᵗʰ **S21.0** Open wound of breast

✓6ᵗʰ **S21.00** Unspecified open wound of breast

✓7ᵗʰ **S21.001** Unspecified open wound of right breast

✓7ᵗʰ **S21.002** Unspecified open wound of left breast

✓7ᵗʰ **S21.009** Unspecified open wound of unspecified breast

✓6ᵗʰ **S21.01** Laceration without foreign body of breast

✓7ᵗʰ **S21.011** Laceration without foreign body of right breast

✓7ᵗʰ **S21.012** Laceration without foreign body of left breast

✓7ᵗʰ **S21.019** Laceration without foreign body of unspecified breast

✓6ᵗʰ **S21.02** Laceration with foreign body of breast

✓7ᵗʰ **S21.021** Laceration with foreign body of right breast

✓7ᵗʰ **S21.022** Laceration with foreign body of left breast

✓7ᵗʰ **S21.029** Laceration with foreign body of unspecified breast

✓6ᵗʰ **S21.03** Puncture wound without foreign body of breast

✓7ᵗʰ **S21.031** Puncture wound without foreign body of right breast

✓7ᵗʰ **S21.032** Puncture wound without foreign body of left breast

✓7ᵗʰ **S21.039** Puncture wound without foreign body of unspecified breast

✓6ᵗʰ **S21.04** Puncture wound with foreign body of breast

✓7ᵗʰ **S21.041** Puncture wound with foreign body of right breast

✓7ᵗʰ **S21.042** Puncture wound with foreign body of left breast

✓7ᵗʰ **S21.049** Puncture wound with foreign body of unspecified breast

✓6ᵗʰ **S21.05** Open bite of breast

Bite of breast NOS

> **EXCLUDES 1**   superficial bite of breast (S20.17)

✓7ᵗʰ **S21.051** Open bite of right breast

✓7ᵗʰ **S21.052** Open bite of left breast

✓7ᵗʰ **S21.059** Open bite of unspecified breast

✓5ᵗʰ **S21.1** Open wound of front wall of thorax without penetration into thoracic cavity

Open wound of chest without penetration into thoracic cavity

✓6ᵗʰ **S21.10** Unspecified open wound of front wall of thorax without penetration into thoracic cavity

✓7ᵗʰ **S21.101** Unspecified open wound of right front wall of thorax without penetration into thoracic cavity

✓7ᵗʰ **S21.102** Unspecified open wound of left front wall of thorax without penetration into thoracic cavity

✓7ᵗʰ **S21.109** Unspecified open wound of unspecified front wall of thorax without penetration into thoracic cavity

✓6ᵗʰ **S21.11** Laceration without foreign body of front wall of thorax without penetration into thoracic cavity

✓7ᵗʰ **S21.111** Laceration without foreign body of right front wall of thorax without penetration into thoracic cavity

✓7ᵗʰ **S21.112** Laceration without foreign body of left front wall of thorax without penetration into thoracic cavity

✓7ᵗʰ **S21.119** Laceration without foreign body of unspecified front wall of thorax without penetration into thoracic cavity

✓6ᵗʰ **S21.12** Laceration with foreign body of front wall of thorax without penetration into thoracic cavity

✓7ᵗʰ **S21.121** Laceration with foreign body of right front wall of thorax without penetration into thoracic cavity

✓7ᵗʰ **S21.122** Laceration with foreign body of left front wall of thorax without penetration into thoracic cavity

✓7ᵗʰ **S21.129** Laceration with foreign body of unspecified front wall of thorax without penetration into thoracic cavity

✓6ᵗʰ **S21.13** Puncture wound without foreign body of front wall of thorax without penetration into thoracic cavity

✓7ᵗʰ **S21.131** Puncture wound without foreign body of right front wall of thorax without penetration into thoracic cavity

✓7ᵗʰ **S21.132** Puncture wound without foreign body of left front wall of thorax without penetration into thoracic cavity

✓7ᵗʰ **S21.139** Puncture wound without foreign body of unspecified front wall of thorax without penetration into thoracic cavity

✓6ᵗʰ **S21.14** Puncture wound with foreign body of front wall of thorax without penetration into thoracic cavity

✓7ᵗʰ **S21.141** Puncture wound with foreign body of right front wall of thorax without penetration into thoracic cavity

✓7ᵗʰ **S21.142** Puncture wound with foreign body of left front wall of thorax without penetration into thoracic cavity

✓7ᵗʰ **S21.149** Puncture wound with foreign body of unspecified front wall of thorax without penetration into thoracic cavity

✓6ᵗʰ **S21.15** Open bite of front wall of thorax without penetration into thoracic cavity

Bite of front wall of thorax NOS

> **EXCLUDES 1**   superficial bite of front wall of thorax (S20.37)

✓7ᵗʰ **S21.151** Open bite of right front wall of thorax without penetration into thoracic cavity

✓7ᵗʰ **S21.152** Open bite of left front wall of thorax without penetration into thoracic cavity

✓7ᵗʰ **S21.159** Open bite of unspecified front wall of thorax without penetration into thoracic cavity

✓5ᵗʰ **S21.2** Open wound of back wall of thorax without penetration into thoracic cavity

✓6ᵗʰ **S21.20** Unspecified open wound of back wall of thorax without penetration into thoracic cavity

✓7ᵗʰ **S21.201** Unspecified open wound of right back wall of thorax without penetration into thoracic cavity

---

✔ Additional Character Required   ✓x7ᵗʰ Placeholder Alert   Manifestation   Unspecified Dx   ►◄ Revised Text   ● New Code   ▲ Revised Code Title

√7th **S21.202** Unspecified open wound of left back wall of thorax without penetration into thoracic cavity

√7th **S21.209** Unspecified open wound of unspecified back wall of thorax without penetration into thoracic cavity

√6th **S21.21** Laceration without foreign body of back wall of thorax without penetration into thoracic cavity

√7th **S21.211** Laceration without foreign body of right back wall of thorax without penetration into thoracic cavity

√7th **S21.212** Laceration without foreign body of left back wall of thorax without penetration into thoracic cavity

√7th **S21.219** Laceration without foreign body of unspecified back wall of thorax without penetration into thoracic cavity

√6th **S21.22** Laceration with foreign body of back wall of thorax without penetration into thoracic cavity

√7th **S21.221** Laceration with foreign body of right back wall of thorax without penetration into thoracic cavity

√7th **S21.222** Laceration with foreign body of left back wall of thorax without penetration into thoracic cavity

√7th **S21.229** Laceration with foreign body of unspecified back wall of thorax without penetration into thoracic cavity

√6th **S21.23** Puncture wound without foreign body of back wall of thorax without penetration into thoracic cavity

√7th **S21.231** Puncture wound without foreign body of right back wall of thorax without penetration into thoracic cavity

√7th **S21.232** Puncture wound without foreign body of left back wall of thorax without penetration into thoracic cavity

√7th **S21.239** Puncture wound without foreign body of unspecified back wall of thorax without penetration into thoracic cavity

√6th **S21.24** Puncture wound with foreign body of back wall of thorax without penetration into thoracic cavity

√7th **S21.241** Puncture wound with foreign body of right back wall of thorax without penetration into thoracic cavity

√7th **S21.242** Puncture wound with foreign body of left back wall of thorax without penetration into thoracic cavity

√7th **S21.249** Puncture wound with foreign body of unspecified back wall of thorax without penetration into thoracic cavity

√6th **S21.25** Open bite of back wall of thorax without penetration into thoracic cavity

Bite of back wall of thorax NOS

EXCLUDES 1   superficial bite of back wall of thorax (S20.47)

√7th **S21.251** Open bite of right back wall of thorax without penetration into thoracic cavity

√7th **S21.252** Open bite of left back wall of thorax without penetration into thoracic cavity

√7th **S21.259** Open bite of unspecified back wall of thorax without penetration into thoracic cavity

√5th **S21.3** Open wound of front wall of thorax with penetration into thoracic cavity

Open wound of chest with penetration into thoracic cavity

√6th **S21.30** Unspecified open wound of front wall of thorax with penetration into thoracic cavity

√7th **S21.301** Unspecified open wound of right front wall of thorax with penetration into thoracic cavity

√7th **S21.302** Unspecified open wound of left front wall of thorax with penetration into thoracic cavity

√7th **S21.309** Unspecified open wound of unspecified front wall of thorax with penetration into thoracic cavity

√6th **S21.31** Laceration without foreign body of front wall of thorax with penetration into thoracic cavity

√7th **S21.311** Laceration without foreign body of right front wall of thorax with penetration into thoracic cavity

√7th **S21.312** Laceration without foreign body of left front wall of thorax with penetration into thoracic cavity

√7th **S21.319** Laceration without foreign body of unspecified front wall of thorax with penetration into thoracic cavity

√6th **S21.32** Laceration with foreign body of front wall of thorax with penetration into thoracic cavity

√7th **S21.321** Laceration with foreign body of right front wall of thorax with penetration into thoracic cavity

√7th **S21.322** Laceration with foreign body of left front wall of thorax with penetration into thoracic cavity

√7th **S21.329** Laceration with foreign body of unspecified front wall of thorax with penetration into thoracic cavity

√6th **S21.33** Puncture wound without foreign body of front wall of thorax with penetration into thoracic cavity

√7th **S21.331** Puncture wound without foreign body of right front wall of thorax with penetration into thoracic cavity

√7th **S21.332** Puncture wound without foreign body of left front wall of thorax with penetration into thoracic cavity

√7th **S21.339** Puncture wound without foreign body of unspecified front wall of thorax with penetration into thoracic cavity

√6th **S21.34** Puncture wound with foreign body of front wall of thorax with penetration into thoracic cavity

√7th **S21.341** Puncture wound with foreign body of right front wall of thorax with penetration into thoracic cavity

√7th **S21.342** Puncture wound with foreign body of left front wall of thorax with penetration into thoracic cavity

√7th **S21.349** Puncture wound with foreign body of unspecified front wall of thorax with penetration into thoracic cavity

√6th **S21.35** Open bite of front wall of thorax with penetration into thoracic cavity

EXCLUDES 1   superficial bite of front wall of thorax (S20.37)

√7th **S21.351** Open bite of right front wall of thorax with penetration into thoracic cavity

√7th **S21.352** Open bite of left front wall of thorax with penetration into thoracic cavity

√7th **S21.359** Open bite of unspecified front wall of thorax with penetration into thoracic cavity

√5th **S21.4** Open wound of back wall of thorax with penetration into thoracic cavity

√6th **S21.40** Unspecified open wound of back wall of thorax with penetration into thoracic cavity

√7th **S21.401** Unspecified open wound of right back wall of thorax with penetration into thoracic cavity

√7th **S21.402** Unspecified open wound of left back wall of thorax with penetration into thoracic cavity

√7th **S21.409** Unspecified open wound of unspecified back wall of thorax with penetration into thoracic cavity

√6th **S21.41** Laceration without foreign body of back wall of thorax with penetration into thoracic cavity

√7th **S21.411** Laceration without foreign body of right back wall of thorax with penetration into thoracic cavity

√7th **S21.412** Laceration without foreign body of left back wall of thorax with penetration into thoracic cavity

√7th **S21.419** Laceration without foreign body of unspecified back wall of thorax with penetration into thoracic cavity

√6th **S21.42** Laceration with foreign body of back wall of thorax with penetration into thoracic cavity

√7th **S21.421** Laceration with foreign body of right back wall of thorax with penetration into thoracic cavity

√7th **S21.422** Laceration with foreign body of left back wall of thorax with penetration into thoracic cavity

√7th **S21.429** Laceration with foreign body of unspecified back wall of thorax with penetration into thoracic cavity

√6ᵗʰ **S21.43** Puncture wound without foreign body of back wall of thorax with penetration into thoracic cavity

     √7ᵗʰ **S21.431** Puncture wound without foreign body of **right** back wall of thorax with penetration into thoracic cavity

     √7ᵗʰ **S21.432** Puncture wound without foreign body of **left** back wall of thorax with penetration into thoracic cavity

     √7ᵗʰ **S21.439** Puncture wound without foreign body of unspecified back wall of thorax with penetration into thoracic cavity

√6ᵗʰ **S21.44** Puncture wound with foreign body of back wall of thorax with penetration into thoracic cavity

     √7ᵗʰ **S21.441** Puncture wound with foreign body of **right** back wall of thorax with penetration into thoracic cavity

     √7ᵗʰ **S21.442** Puncture wound with foreign body of **left** back wall of thorax with penetration into thoracic cavity

     √7ᵗʰ **S21.449** Puncture wound with foreign body of unspecified back wall of thorax with penetration into thoracic cavity

√6ᵗʰ **S21.45** Open bite of back wall of thorax with penetration into thoracic cavity

     Bite of back wall of thorax NOS

     EXCLUDES 1   superficial bite of back wall of thorax (S20.47)

     √7ᵗʰ **S21.451** Open bite of **right** back wall of thorax with penetration into thoracic cavity

     √7ᵗʰ **S21.452** Open bite of **left** back wall of thorax with penetration into thoracic cavity

     √7ᵗʰ **S21.459** Open bite of unspecified back wall of thorax with penetration into thoracic cavity

√5ᵗʰ **S21.9** Open wound of unspecified part of thorax

     Open wound of thoracic wall NOS

     √x7ᵗʰ **S21.90** Unspecified open wound of unspecified part of thorax

     √x7ᵗʰ **S21.91** Laceration without foreign body of unspecified part of thorax

     √x7ᵗʰ **S21.92** Laceration with foreign body of unspecified part of thorax

     √x7ᵗʰ **S21.93** Puncture wound without foreign body of unspecified part of thorax

     √x7ᵗʰ **S21.94** Puncture wound with foreign body of unspecified part of thorax

     √x7ᵗʰ **S21.95** Open bite of unspecified part of thorax

       EXCLUDES 1   superficial bite of thorax (S20.97)

√4ᵗʰ **S22** Fracture of rib(s), sternum and thoracic spine

     NOTE   A fracture not indicated as displaced or nondisplaced should be coded to displaced

       A fracture not indicated as open or closed should be coded to closed

     INCLUDES   fracture of thoracic neural arch

       fracture of thoracic spinous process

       fracture of thoracic transverse process

       fracture of thoracic vertebra

       fracture of thoracic vertebral arch

     Code first any associated:

       injury of intrathoracic organ (S27.-)

       spinal cord injury (S24.0-, S24.1-)

     EXCLUDES 1   transection of thorax (S28.1)

     EXCLUDES 2   fracture of clavicle (S42.0-)

       fracture of scapula (S42.1-)

     AHA: 2018,2Q,12; 2015,3Q,37-39

     The appropriate 7th character is to be added to each code from category S22.

     A   initial encounter for closed fracture

     B   initial encounter for open fracture

     D   subsequent encounter for fracture with routine healing

     G   subsequent encounter for fracture with delayed healing

     K   subsequent encounter for fracture with nonunion

     S   sequela

√5ᵗʰ **S22.0** Fracture of thoracic vertebra

     √6ᵗʰ **S22.00** Fracture of unspecified thoracic vertebra

       1 √7ᵗʰ **S22.000** Wedge compression fracture of unspecified thoracic vertebra   HCC Q

       1 √7ᵗʰ **S22.001** Stable burst fracture of unspecified thoracic vertebra   HCC Q

       1 √7ᵗʰ **S22.002** Unstable burst fracture of unspecified thoracic vertebra   HCC Q

       1 √7ᵗʰ **S22.008** Other fracture of unspecified thoracic vertebra   HCC Q

       1 √7ᵗʰ **S22.009** Unspecified fracture of unspecified thoracic vertebra   HCC Q

     √6ᵗʰ **S22.01** Fracture of first thoracic vertebra

       1 √7ᵗʰ **S22.010** Wedge compression fracture of first thoracic vertebra   HCC Q

       1 √7ᵗʰ **S22.011** Stable burst fracture of first thoracic vertebra   HCC Q

       1 √7ᵗʰ **S22.012** Unstable burst fracture of first thoracic vertebra   HCC Q

       1 √7ᵗʰ **S22.018** Other fracture of first thoracic vertebra   HCC Q

       1 √7ᵗʰ **S22.019** Unspecified fracture of first thoracic vertebra   HCC Q

     √6ᵗʰ **S22.02** Fracture of second thoracic vertebra

       1 √7ᵗʰ **S22.020** Wedge compression fracture of second thoracic vertebra   HCC Q

       1 √7ᵗʰ **S22.021** Stable burst fracture of second thoracic vertebra   HCC Q

       1 √7ᵗʰ **S22.022** Unstable burst fracture of second thoracic vertebra   HCC Q

       1 √7ᵗʰ **S22.028** Other fracture of second thoracic vertebra   HCC Q

       1 √7ᵗʰ **S22.029** Unspecified fracture of second thoracic vertebra   HCC Q

     √6ᵗʰ **S22.03** Fracture of third thoracic vertebra

       1 √7ᵗʰ **S22.030** Wedge compression fracture of third thoracic vertebra   HCC Q

       1 √7ᵗʰ **S22.031** Stable burst fracture of third thoracic vertebra   HCC Q

       1 √7ᵗʰ **S22.032** Unstable burst fracture of third thoracic vertebra   HCC Q

       1 √7ᵗʰ **S22.038** Other fracture of third thoracic vertebra   HCC Q

       1 √7ᵗʰ **S22.039** Unspecified fracture of third thoracic vertebra   HCC Q

     √6ᵗʰ **S22.04** Fracture of fourth thoracic vertebra

       1 √7ᵗʰ **S22.040** Wedge compression fracture of fourth thoracic vertebra   HCC Q

       1 √7ᵗʰ **S22.041** Stable burst fracture of fourth thoracic vertebra   HCC Q

       1 √7ᵗʰ **S22.042** Unstable burst fracture of fourth thoracic vertebra   HCC Q

       1 √7ᵗʰ **S22.048** Other fracture of fourth thoracic vertebra   HCC Q

       1 √7ᵗʰ **S22.049** Unspecified fracture of fourth thoracic vertebra   HCC Q

     √6ᵗʰ **S22.05** Fracture of T5-T6 vertebra

       1 √7ᵗʰ **S22.050** Wedge compression fracture of T5-T6 vertebra   HCC Q

       1 √7ᵗʰ **S22.051** Stable burst fracture of T5-T6 vertebra   HCC Q

       1 √7ᵗʰ **S22.052** Unstable burst fracture of T5-T6 vertebra   HCC Q

       1 √7ᵗʰ **S22.058** Other fracture of T5-T6 vertebra   HCC Q

       1 √7ᵗʰ **S22.059** Unspecified fracture of T5-T6 vertebra   HCC Q

     √6ᵗʰ **S22.06** Fracture of T7-T8 vertebra

       1 √7ᵗʰ **S22.060** Wedge compression fracture of T7-T8 vertebra   HCC Q

       1 √7ᵗʰ **S22.061** Stable burst fracture of T7-T8 vertebra   HCC Q

       1 √7ᵗʰ **S22.062** Unstable burst fracture of T7-T8 vertebra   HCC Q

       1 √7ᵗʰ **S22.068** Other fracture of T7-T8 thoracic vertebra   HCC Q

       1 √7ᵗʰ **S22.069** Unspecified fracture of T7-T8 vertebra   HCC Q

     √6ᵗʰ **S22.07** Fracture of T9-T10 vertebra

       1 √7ᵗʰ **S22.070** Wedge compression fracture of T9-T10 vertebra   HCC Q

       1 √7ᵗʰ **S22.071** Stable burst fracture of T9-T10 vertebra   HCC Q

       1 √7ᵗʰ **S22.072** Unstable burst fracture of T9-T10 vertebra   HCC Q

       1 √7ᵗʰ **S22.078** Other fracture of T9-T10 vertebra   HCC Q

☑ Additional Character Required   √x7ᵗʰ Placeholder Alert   Manifestation   Unspecified Dx   ▶◀ Revised Text   ● New Code   ▲ Revised Code Title

ICD-10-CM 2020   977

Chapter 19. Injury, Poisoning and Certain Other Consequences of External Causes

  ¹ √7ᵗʰ **S22.079** Unspecified fracture of T9-T10 vertebra   HCC Q

  √6ᵗʰ **S22.08** Fracture of T11-T12 vertebra

    ¹ √7ᵗʰ **S22.080** Wedge compression fracture of T11-T12 vertebra   HCC Q

    ¹ √7ᵗʰ **S22.081** Stable burst fracture of T11-T12 vertebra   HCC Q

    ¹ √7ᵗʰ **S22.082** Unstable burst fracture of T11-T12 vertebra   HCC Q

    ¹ √7ᵗʰ **S22.088** Other fracture of T11-T12 vertebra   HCC Q

    ¹ √7ᵗʰ **S22.089** Unspecified fracture of T11-T12 vertebra   HCC Q

  √5ᵗʰ **S22.2** Fracture of sternum

    DEF: Break in flat bone (breast bone) in the anterior thorax caused by blunt trauma to the anterior chest.

    √x7ᵗʰ **S22.20** Unspecified fracture of sternum   Q

    √x7ᵗʰ **S22.21** Fracture of manubrium   Q

    √x7ᵗʰ **S22.22** Fracture of body of sternum   Q

    √x7ᵗʰ **S22.23** Sternal manubrial dissociation   Q

    √x7ᵗʰ **S22.24** Fracture of xiphoid process   Q

  √5ᵗʰ **S22.3** Fracture of one rib

    √x7ᵗʰ **S22.31** Fracture of one rib, right side   Q

    √x7ᵗʰ **S22.32** Fracture of one rib, left side   Q

    √x7ᵗʰ **S22.39** Fracture of one rib, unspecified side   Q

  √5ᵗʰ **S22.4** Multiple fractures of ribs

    Fractures of two or more ribs

    EXCLUDES 1 flail chest (S22.5-)

    √x7ᵗʰ **S22.41** Multiple fractures of ribs, right side   Q

    √x7ᵗʰ **S22.42** Multiple fractures of ribs, left side   Q

    √x7ᵗʰ **S22.43** Multiple fractures of ribs, bilateral   Q

    √x7ᵗʰ **S22.49** Multiple fractures of ribs, unspecified side   Q

  √x7ᵗʰ **S22.5** Flail chest   Q

  √x7ᵗʰ **S22.9** Fracture of bony thorax, part unspecified   Q

√4ᵗʰ **S23** Dislocation and sprain of joints and ligaments of thorax

    INCLUDES avulsion of joint or ligament of thorax
        laceration of cartilage, joint or ligament of thorax
        sprain of cartilage, joint or ligament of thorax
        traumatic hemarthrosis of joint or ligament of thorax
        traumatic rupture of joint or ligament of thorax
        traumatic subluxation of joint or ligament of thorax
        traumatic tear of joint or ligament of thorax

    Code also any associated open wound

    EXCLUDES 2 dislocation, sprain of sternoclavicular joint (S43.2, S43.6)
        strain of muscle or tendon of thorax (S29.01-)

    The appropriate 7th character is to be added to each code from category S23.
    A   initial encounter
    D   subsequent encounter
    S   sequela

  √x7ᵗʰ **S23.0** Traumatic rupture of thoracic intervertebral disc

    EXCLUDES 1 rupture or displacement (nontraumatic) of thoracic intervertebral disc NOS (M51.- with fifth character 4)

  √5ᵗʰ **S23.1** Subluxation and dislocation of thoracic vertebra

    Code also any associated:
      open wound of thorax (S21.-)
      spinal cord injury (S24.0-, S24.1-)
    EXCLUDES 2 fracture of thoracic vertebrae (S22.0-)

    √6ᵗʰ **S23.10** Subluxation and dislocation of unspecified thoracic vertebra

      √7ᵗʰ **S23.100** Subluxation of unspecified thoracic vertebra

      √7ᵗʰ **S23.101** Dislocation of unspecified thoracic vertebra

    √6ᵗʰ **S23.11** Subluxation and dislocation of T1/T2 thoracic vertebra

      √7ᵗʰ **S23.110** Subluxation of T1/T2 thoracic vertebra

      √7ᵗʰ **S23.111** Dislocation of T1/T2 thoracic vertebra

    √6ᵗʰ **S23.12** Subluxation and dislocation of T2/T3-T3/T4 thoracic vertebra

      √7ᵗʰ **S23.120** Subluxation of T2/T3 thoracic vertebra

      √7ᵗʰ **S23.121** Dislocation of T2/T3 thoracic vertebra

      √7ᵗʰ **S23.122** Subluxation of T3/T4 thoracic vertebra

      √7ᵗʰ **S23.123** Dislocation of T3/T4 thoracic vertebra

    √6ᵗʰ **S23.13** Subluxation and dislocation of T4/T5-T5/T6 thoracic vertebra

      √7ᵗʰ **S23.130** Subluxation of T4/T5 thoracic vertebra

      √7ᵗʰ **S23.131** Dislocation of T4/T5 thoracic vertebra

      √7ᵗʰ **S23.132** Subluxation of T5/T6 thoracic vertebra

      √7ᵗʰ **S23.133** Dislocation of T5/T6 thoracic vertebra

    √6ᵗʰ **S23.14** Subluxation and dislocation of T6/T7-T7/T8 thoracic vertebra

      √7ᵗʰ **S23.140** Subluxation of T6/T7 thoracic vertebra

      √7ᵗʰ **S23.141** Dislocation of T6/T7 thoracic vertebra

      √7ᵗʰ **S23.142** Subluxation of T7/T8 thoracic vertebra

      √7ᵗʰ **S23.143** Dislocation of T7/T8 thoracic vertebra

    √6ᵗʰ **S23.15** Subluxation and dislocation of T8/T9-T9/T10 thoracic vertebra

      √7ᵗʰ **S23.150** Subluxation of T8/T9 thoracic vertebra

      √7ᵗʰ **S23.151** Dislocation of T8/T9 thoracic vertebra

      √7ᵗʰ **S23.152** Subluxation of T9/T10 thoracic vertebra

      √7ᵗʰ **S23.153** Dislocation of T9/T10 thoracic vertebra

    √6ᵗʰ **S23.16** Subluxation and dislocation of T10/T11-T11/T12 thoracic vertebra

      √7ᵗʰ **S23.160** Subluxation of T10/T11 thoracic vertebra

      √7ᵗʰ **S23.161** Dislocation of T10/T11 thoracic vertebra

      √7ᵗʰ **S23.162** Subluxation of T11/T12 thoracic vertebra

      √7ᵗʰ **S23.163** Dislocation of T11/T12 thoracic vertebra

    √6ᵗʰ **S23.17** Subluxation and dislocation of T12/L1 thoracic vertebra

      √7ᵗʰ **S23.170** Subluxation of T12/L1 thoracic vertebra

      √7ᵗʰ **S23.171** Dislocation of T12/L1 thoracic vertebra

  √5ᵗʰ **S23.2** Dislocation of other and unspecified parts of thorax

    √x7ᵗʰ **S23.20** Dislocation of unspecified part of thorax

    √x7ᵗʰ **S23.29** Dislocation of other parts of thorax

  √x7ᵗʰ **S23.3** Sprain of ligaments of thoracic spine

  √5ᵗʰ **S23.4** Sprain of ribs and sternum

    √x7ᵗʰ **S23.41** Sprain of ribs

    √6ᵗʰ **S23.42** Sprain of sternum

      √7ᵗʰ **S23.420** Sprain of sternoclavicular (joint) (ligament)

      √7ᵗʰ **S23.421** Sprain of chondrosternal joint

      √7ᵗʰ **S23.428** Other sprain of sternum

      √7ᵗʰ **S23.429** Unspecified sprain of sternum

  √x7ᵗʰ **S23.8** Sprain of other specified parts of thorax

  √x7ᵗʰ **S23.9** Sprain of unspecified parts of thorax

√4ᵗʰ **S24** Injury of nerves and spinal cord at thorax level

    NOTE Code to highest level of thoracic spinal cord injury.

    Injuries to the spinal cord (S24.0 and S24.1) refer to the cord level and not bone level injury, and can affect nerve roots at and below the level given.

    Code also any associated:
      fracture of thoracic vertebra (S22.0-)
      open wound of thorax (S21.-)
      transient paralysis (R29.5)
    EXCLUDES 2 injury of brachial plexus (S14.3)

    The appropriate 7th character is to be added to each code from category S24.
    A   initial encounter
    D   subsequent encounter
    S   sequela

  √x7ᵗʰ **S24.0** Concussion and edema of thoracic spinal cord   HCC

  √5ᵗʰ **S24.1** Other and unspecified injuries of thoracic spinal cord

    √6ᵗʰ **S24.10** Unspecified injury of thoracic spinal cord

      √7ᵗʰ **S24.101** Unspecified injury at T1 level of thoracic spinal cord   HCC

      √7ᵗʰ **S24.102** Unspecified injury at T2-T6 level of thoracic spinal cord   HCC

      √7ᵗʰ **S24.103** Unspecified injury at T7-T10 level of thoracic spinal cord   HCC

      √7ᵗʰ **S24.104** Unspecified injury at T11-T12 level of thoracic spinal cord   HCC

√7ᵗʰ **S24.109 Unspecified injury at unspecified level of thoracic spinal cord**   HCC
  Injury of thoracic spinal cord NOS

√6ᵗʰ **S24.11 Complete lesion of thoracic spinal cord**

  √7ᵗʰ **S24.111 Complete lesion at T1 level of thoracic spinal cord**   HCC

  √7ᵗʰ **S24.112 Complete lesion at T2-T6 level of thoracic spinal cord**   HCC

  √7ᵗʰ **S24.113 Complete lesion at T7-T10 level of thoracic spinal cord**   HCC

  √7ᵗʰ **S24.114 Complete lesion at T11-T12 level of thoracic spinal cord**   HCC

  √7ᵗʰ **S24.119 Complete lesion at unspecified level of thoracic spinal cord**   HCC

√6ᵗʰ **S24.13 Anterior cord syndrome of thoracic spinal cord**

  √7ᵗʰ **S24.131 Anterior cord syndrome at T1 level of thoracic spinal cord**   HCC

  √7ᵗʰ **S24.132 Anterior cord syndrome at T2-T6 level of thoracic spinal cord**   HCC

  √7ᵗʰ **S24.133 Anterior cord syndrome at T7-T10 level of thoracic spinal cord**   HCC

  √7ᵗʰ **S24.134 Anterior cord syndrome at T11-T12 level of thoracic spinal cord**   HCC

  √7ᵗʰ **S24.139 Anterior cord syndrome at unspecified level of thoracic spinal cord**   HCC

√6ᵗʰ **S24.14 Brown-Séquard syndrome of thoracic spinal cord**

  √7ᵗʰ **S24.141 Brown-Séquard syndrome at T1 level of thoracic spinal cord**   HCC

  √7ᵗʰ **S24.142 Brown-Séquard syndrome at T2-T6 level of thoracic spinal cord**   HCC

  √7ᵗʰ **S24.143 Brown-Séquard syndrome at T7-T10 level of thoracic spinal cord**   HCC

  √7ᵗʰ **S24.144 Brown-Séquard syndrome at T11-T12 level of thoracic spinal cord**   HCC

  √7ᵗʰ **S24.149 Brown-Séquard syndrome at unspecified level of thoracic spinal cord**   HCC

√6ᵗʰ **S24.15 Other incomplete lesions of thoracic spinal cord**
  Incomplete lesion of thoracic spinal cord NOS
  Posterior cord syndrome of thoracic spinal cord

  √7ᵗʰ **S24.151 Other incomplete lesion at T1 level of thoracic spinal cord**   HCC

  √7ᵗʰ **S24.152 Other incomplete lesion at T2-T6 level of thoracic spinal cord**   HCC

  √7ᵗʰ **S24.153 Other incomplete lesion at T7-T10 level of thoracic spinal cord**   HCC

  √7ᵗʰ **S24.154 Other incomplete lesion at T11-T12 level of thoracic spinal cord**   HCC

  √7ᵗʰ **S24.159 Other incomplete lesion at unspecified level of thoracic spinal cord**   HCC

√x7ᵗʰ **S24.2 Injury of nerve root of thoracic spine**

√x7ᵗʰ **S24.3 Injury of peripheral nerves of thorax**

√x7ᵗʰ **S24.4 Injury of thoracic sympathetic nervous system**
  Injury of cardiac plexus
  Injury of esophageal plexus
  Injury of pulmonary plexus
  Injury of stellate ganglion
  Injury of thoracic sympathetic ganglion

√x7ᵗʰ **S24.8 Injury of other specified nerves of thorax**

√x7ᵗʰ **S24.9 Injury of unspecified nerve of thorax**

√4ᵗʰ **S25 Injury of blood vessels of thorax**
  Code also any associated open wound (S21.-)

  The appropriate 7th character is to be added to each code from category S25.
    A   initial encounter
    D   subsequent encounter
    S   sequela

√5ᵗʰ **S25.0 Injury of thoracic aorta**
  Injury of aorta NOS

  √x7ᵗʰ **S25.00 Unspecified injury of thoracic aorta**

√x7ᵗʰ **S25.01 Minor laceration of thoracic aorta**
  Incomplete transection of thoracic aorta
  Laceration of thoracic aorta NOS
  Superficial laceration of thoracic aorta

√x7ᵗʰ **S25.02 Major laceration of thoracic aorta**
  Complete transection of thoracic aorta
  Traumatic rupture of thoracic aorta

√x7ᵗʰ **S25.09 Other specified injury of thoracic aorta**

√5ᵗʰ **S25.1 Injury of innominate or subclavian artery**

  √6ᵗʰ **S25.10 Unspecified injury of innominate or subclavian artery**

    √7ᵗʰ **S25.101 Unspecified injury of right innominate or subclavian artery**

    √7ᵗʰ **S25.102 Unspecified injury of left innominate or subclavian artery**

    √7ᵗʰ **S25.109 Unspecified injury of unspecified innominate or subclavian artery**

  √6ᵗʰ **S25.11 Minor laceration of innominate or subclavian artery**
    Incomplete transection of innominate or subclavian artery
    Laceration of innominate or subclavian artery NOS
    Superficial laceration of innominate or subclavian artery

    √7ᵗʰ **S25.111 Minor laceration of right innominate or subclavian artery**

    √7ᵗʰ **S25.112 Minor laceration of left innominate or subclavian artery**

    √7ᵗʰ **S25.119 Minor laceration of unspecified innominate or subclavian artery**

  √6ᵗʰ **S25.12 Major laceration of innominate or subclavian artery**
    Complete transection of innominate or subclavian artery
    Traumatic rupture of innominate or subclavian artery

    √7ᵗʰ **S25.121 Major laceration of right innominate or subclavian artery**

    √7ᵗʰ **S25.122 Major laceration of left innominate or subclavian artery**

    √7ᵗʰ **S25.129 Major laceration of unspecified innominate or subclavian artery**

  √6ᵗʰ **S25.19 Other specified injury of innominate or subclavian artery**

    √7ᵗʰ **S25.191 Other specified injury of right innominate or subclavian artery**

    √7ᵗʰ **S25.192 Other specified injury of left innominate or subclavian artery**

    √7ᵗʰ **S25.199 Other specified injury of unspecified innominate or subclavian artery**

√5ᵗʰ **S25.2 Injury of superior vena cava**
  Injury of vena cava NOS

  √x7ᵗʰ **S25.20 Unspecified injury of superior vena cava**

  √x7ᵗʰ **S25.21 Minor laceration of superior vena cava**
    Incomplete transection of superior vena cava
    Laceration of superior vena cava NOS
    Superficial laceration of superior vena cava

  √x7ᵗʰ **S25.22 Major laceration of superior vena cava**
    Complete transection of superior vena cava
    Traumatic rupture of superior vena cava

  √x7ᵗʰ **S25.29 Other specified injury of superior vena cava**

√5ᵗʰ **S25.3 Injury of innominate or subclavian vein**

  √6ᵗʰ **S25.30 Unspecified injury of innominate or subclavian vein**

    √7ᵗʰ **S25.301 Unspecified injury of right innominate or subclavian vein**

    √7ᵗʰ **S25.302 Unspecified injury of left innominate or subclavian vein**

    √7ᵗʰ **S25.309 Unspecified injury of unspecified innominate or subclavian vein**

  √6ᵗʰ **S25.31 Minor laceration of innominate or subclavian vein**
    Incomplete transection of innominate or subclavian vein
    Laceration of innominate or subclavian vein NOS
    Superficial laceration of innominate or subclavian vein

    √7ᵗʰ **S25.311 Minor laceration of right innominate or subclavian vein**

    √7ᵗʰ **S25.312 Minor laceration of left innominate or subclavian vein**

    √7ᵗʰ **S25.319 Minor laceration of unspecified innominate or subclavian vein**

✔ Additional Character Required   √x7ᵗʰ Placeholder Alert   Manifestation   Unspecified Dx   ▶◀ Revised Text   ● New Code   ▲ Revised Code Title

ICD-10-CM 2020   **979**

Chapter 19. Injury, Poisoning and Certain Other Consequences of External Causes

S25.32–S26.91

√6ᵗʰ **S25.32** Major laceration of innominate or subclavian vein

Complete transection of innominate or subclavian vein

Traumatic rupture of innominate or subclavian vein

√7ᵗʰ **S25.321** Major laceration of right innominate or subclavian vein

√7ᵗʰ **S25.322** Major laceration of left innominate or subclavian vein

√7ᵗʰ **S25.329** Major laceration of unspecified innominate or subclavian vein

√6ᵗʰ **S25.39** Other specified injury of innominate or subclavian vein

√7ᵗʰ **S25.391** Other specified injury of right innominate or subclavian vein

√7ᵗʰ **S25.392** Other specified injury of left innominate or subclavian vein

√7ᵗʰ **S25.399** Other specified injury of unspecified innominate or subclavian vein

√5ᵗʰ **S25.4** Injury of pulmonary blood vessels

√6ᵗʰ **S25.40** Unspecified injury of pulmonary blood vessels

√7ᵗʰ **S25.401** Unspecified injury of right pulmonary blood vessels

√7ᵗʰ **S25.402** Unspecified injury of left pulmonary blood vessels

√7ᵗʰ **S25.409** Unspecified injury of unspecified pulmonary blood vessels

√6ᵗʰ **S25.41** Minor laceration of pulmonary blood vessels

Incomplete transection of pulmonary blood vessels

Laceration of pulmonary blood vessels NOS

Superficial laceration of pulmonary blood vessels

√7ᵗʰ **S25.411** Minor laceration of right pulmonary blood vessels

√7ᵗʰ **S25.412** Minor laceration of left pulmonary blood vessels

√7ᵗʰ **S25.419** Minor laceration of unspecified pulmonary blood vessels

√6ᵗʰ **S25.42** Major laceration of pulmonary blood vessels

Complete transection of pulmonary blood vessels

Traumatic rupture of pulmonary blood vessels

√7ᵗʰ **S25.421** Major laceration of right pulmonary blood vessels

√7ᵗʰ **S25.422** Major laceration of left pulmonary blood vessels

√7ᵗʰ **S25.429** Major laceration of unspecified pulmonary blood vessels

√6ᵗʰ **S25.49** Other specified injury of pulmonary blood vessels

√7ᵗʰ **S25.491** Other specified injury of right pulmonary blood vessels

√7ᵗʰ **S25.492** Other specified injury of left pulmonary blood vessels

√7ᵗʰ **S25.499** Other specified injury of unspecified pulmonary blood vessels

√5ᵗʰ **S25.5** Injury of intercostal blood vessels

√6ᵗʰ **S25.50** Unspecified injury of intercostal blood vessels

√7ᵗʰ **S25.501** Unspecified injury of intercostal blood vessels, right side

√7ᵗʰ **S25.502** Unspecified injury of intercostal blood vessels, left side

√7ᵗʰ **S25.509** Unspecified injury of intercostal blood vessels, unspecified side

√6ᵗʰ **S25.51** Laceration of intercostal blood vessels

√7ᵗʰ **S25.511** Laceration of intercostal blood vessels, right side

√7ᵗʰ **S25.512** Laceration of intercostal blood vessels, left side

√7ᵗʰ **S25.519** Laceration of intercostal blood vessels, unspecified side

√6ᵗʰ **S25.59** Other specified injury of intercostal blood vessels

√7ᵗʰ **S25.591** Other specified injury of intercostal blood vessels, right side

√7ᵗʰ **S25.592** Other specified injury of intercostal blood vessels, left side

√7ᵗʰ **S25.599** Other specified injury of intercostal blood vessels, unspecified side

√5ᵗʰ **S25.8** Injury of other blood vessels of thorax

Injury of azygos vein

Injury of mammary artery or vein

√6ᵗʰ **S25.80** Unspecified injury of other blood vessels of thorax

√7ᵗʰ **S25.801** Unspecified injury of other blood vessels of thorax, right side

√7ᵗʰ **S25.802** Unspecified injury of other blood vessels of thorax, left side

√7ᵗʰ **S25.809** Unspecified injury of other blood vessels of thorax, unspecified side

√6ᵗʰ **S25.81** Laceration of other blood vessels of thorax

√7ᵗʰ **S25.811** Laceration of other blood vessels of thorax, right side

√7ᵗʰ **S25.812** Laceration of other blood vessels of thorax, left side

√7ᵗʰ **S25.819** Laceration of other blood vessels of thorax, unspecified side

√6ᵗʰ **S25.89** Other specified injury of other blood vessels of thorax

√7ᵗʰ **S25.891** Other specified injury of other blood vessels of thorax, right side

√7ᵗʰ **S25.892** Other specified injury of other blood vessels of thorax, left side

√7ᵗʰ **S25.899** Other specified injury of other blood vessels of thorax, unspecified side

√5ᵗʰ **S25.9** Injury of unspecified blood vessel of thorax

√x7ᵗʰ **S25.90** Unspecified injury of unspecified blood vessel of thorax

√x7ᵗʰ **S25.91** Laceration of unspecified blood vessel of thorax

√x7ᵗʰ **S25.99** Other specified injury of unspecified blood vessel of thorax

√4ᵗʰ **S26** Injury of heart

Code also any associated:

open wound of thorax (S21.-)

traumatic hemopneumothorax (S27.2)

traumatic hemothorax (S27.1)

traumatic pneumothorax (S27.0)

The appropriate 7th character is to be added to each code from category S26.

A   initial encounter

D   subsequent encounter

S   sequela

√5ᵗʰ **S26.0** Injury of heart with hemopericardium

√x7ᵗʰ **S26.00** Unspecified injury of heart with hemopericardium

√x7ᵗʰ **S26.01** Contusion of heart with hemopericardium

√6ᵗʰ **S26.02** Laceration of heart with hemopericardium

√7ᵗʰ **S26.020** Mild laceration of heart with hemopericardium

Laceration of heart without penetration of heart chamber

√7ᵗʰ **S26.021** Moderate laceration of heart with hemopericardium

Laceration of heart with penetration of heart chamber

√7ᵗʰ **S26.022** Major laceration of heart with hemopericardium

Laceration of heart with penetration of multiple heart chambers

√x7ᵗʰ **S26.09** Other injury of heart with hemopericardium

√5ᵗʰ **S26.1** Injury of heart without hemopericardium

√x7ᵗʰ **S26.10** Unspecified injury of heart without hemopericardium

√x7ᵗʰ **S26.11** Contusion of heart without hemopericardium

√x7ᵗʰ **S26.12** Laceration of heart without hemopericardium

√x7ᵗʰ **S26.19** Other injury of heart without hemopericardium

√5ᵗʰ **S26.9** Injury of heart, unspecified with or without hemopericardium

√x7ᵗʰ **S26.90** Unspecified injury of heart, unspecified with or without hemopericardium

√x7ᵗʰ **S26.91** Contusion of heart, unspecified with or without hemopericardium

DEF: Bruising within the heart muscle, with no mention of an open wound, usually caused by blunt chest trauma in motor vehicle accidents, falling from great heights, or receiving CPR.

√x7th   **S26.92**   Laceration of heart, unspecified with or without hemopericardium
  Laceration of heart NOS
  AHA: 2019,2Q,24

√7th   **S26.99**   Other injury of heart, unspecified with or without hemopericardium

√4th   **S27**   **Injury of other and unspecified intrathoracic organs**
  Code also any associated open wound of thorax (S21.-)
  EXCLUDES 2   injury of cervical esophagus (S10-S19)
           injury of trachea (cervical) (S10-S19)

> The appropriate 7th character is to be added to each code from category S27.
> A   initial encounter
> D   subsequent encounter
> S   sequela

√x7th   **S27.0**   **Traumatic pneumothorax**
  EXCLUDES 1   spontaneous pneumothorax (J93.-)

√x7th   **S27.1**   **Traumatic hemothorax**

√x7th   **S27.2**   **Traumatic hemopneumothorax**

√5th   **S27.3**   **Other and unspecified injuries of lung**

√6th   **S27.30**   **Unspecified injury of lung**
  √7th   **S27.301**   Unspecified injury of lung, unilateral
  √7th   **S27.302**   Unspecified injury of lung, bilateral
  √7th   **S27.309**   Unspecified injury of lung, unspecified

√6th   **S27.31**   **Primary blast injury of lung**
  Blast injury of lung NOS
  √7th   **S27.311**   Primary blast injury of lung, unilateral
  √7th   **S27.312**   Primary blast injury of lung, bilateral
  √7th   **S27.319**   Primary blast injury of lung, unspecified

√6th   **S27.32**   **Contusion of lung**
  DEF: Bruising of the lung without mention of an open wound.
  √7th   **S27.321**   Contusion of lung, unilateral
  √7th   **S27.322**   Contusion of lung, bilateral
  √7th   **S27.329**   Contusion of lung, unspecified

√6th   **S27.33**   **Laceration of lung**
  √7th   **S27.331**   Laceration of lung, unilateral
  √7th   **S27.332**   Laceration of lung, bilateral
  √7th   **S27.339**   Laceration of lung, unspecified

√6th   **S27.39**   **Other injuries of lung**
  Secondary blast injury of lung
  √7th   **S27.391**   Other injuries of lung, unilateral
  √7th   **S27.392**   Other injuries of lung, bilateral
  √7th   **S27.399**   Other injuries of lung, unspecified

√5th   **S27.4**   **Injury of bronchus**

√6th   **S27.40**   **Unspecified injury of bronchus**
  √7th   **S27.401**   Unspecified injury of bronchus, unilateral
  √7th   **S27.402**   Unspecified injury of bronchus, bilateral
  √7th   **S27.409**   Unspecified injury of bronchus, unspecified

√6th   **S27.41**   **Primary blast injury of bronchus**
  Blast injury of bronchus NOS
  √7th   **S27.411**   Primary blast injury of bronchus, unilateral
  √7th   **S27.412**   Primary blast injury of bronchus, bilateral
  √7th   **S27.419**   Primary blast injury of bronchus, unspecified

√6th   **S27.42**   **Contusion of bronchus**
  √7th   **S27.421**   Contusion of bronchus, unilateral
  √7th   **S27.422**   Contusion of bronchus, bilateral
  √7th   **S27.429**   Contusion of bronchus, unspecified

√6th   **S27.43**   **Laceration of bronchus**
  √7th   **S27.431**   Laceration of bronchus, unilateral
  √7th   **S27.432**   Laceration of bronchus, bilateral
  √7th   **S27.439**   Laceration of bronchus, unspecified

√6th   **S27.49**   **Other injury of bronchus**
  Secondary blast injury of bronchus
  √7th   **S27.491**   Other injury of bronchus, unilateral
  √7th   **S27.492**   Other injury of bronchus, bilateral

√7th   **S27.499**   Other injury of bronchus, unspecified

√5th   **S27.5**   **Injury of thoracic trachea**
  √7th   **S27.50**   Unspecified injury of thoracic trachea
  √7th   **S27.51**   Primary blast injury of thoracic trachea
      Blast injury of thoracic trachea NOS
  √7th   **S27.52**   Contusion of thoracic trachea
  √7th   **S27.53**   Laceration of thoracic trachea
  √7th   **S27.59**   Other injury of thoracic trachea
      Secondary blast injury of thoracic trachea

√5th   **S27.6**   **Injury of pleura**
  √7th   **S27.60**   Unspecified injury of pleura
  √7th   **S27.63**   Laceration of pleura
  √7th   **S27.69**   Other injury of pleura

√5th   **S27.8**   **Injury of other specified intrathoracic organs**

√6th   **S27.80**   **Injury of diaphragm**
  √7th   **S27.802**   Contusion of diaphragm
  √7th   **S27.803**   Laceration of diaphragm
  √7th   **S27.808**   Other injury of diaphragm
  √7th   **S27.809**   Unspecified injury of diaphragm

√6th   **S27.81**   **Injury of esophagus (thoracic part)**
  √7th   **S27.812**   Contusion of esophagus (thoracic part)
  √7th   **S27.813**   Laceration of esophagus (thoracic part)
  √7th   **S27.818**   Other injury of esophagus (thoracic part)
  √7th   **S27.819**   Unspecified injury of esophagus (thoracic part)

√6th   **S27.89**   **Injury of other specified intrathoracic organs**
  Injury of lymphatic thoracic duct
  Injury of thymus gland
  √7th   **S27.892**   Contusion of other specified intrathoracic organs
  √7th   **S27.893**   Laceration of other specified intrathoracic organs
  √7th   **S27.898**   Other injury of other specified intrathoracic organs
  √7th   **S27.899**   Unspecified injury of other specified intrathoracic organs

√x7th   **S27.9**   **Injury of unspecified intrathoracic organ**

√4th   **S28**   **Crushing injury of thorax, and traumatic amputation of part of thorax**

> The appropriate 7th character is to be added to each code from category S28.
> A   initial encounter
> D   subsequent encounter
> S   sequela

√x7th   **S28.0**   **Crushed chest**
  Use additional code for all associated injuries
  EXCLUDES 1   flail chest (S22.5)

√x7th   **S28.1**   **Traumatic amputation (partial) of part of thorax, except breast**

√5th   **S28.2**   **Traumatic amputation of breast**

√6th   **S28.21**   **Complete traumatic amputation of breast**
  Traumatic amputation of breast NOS
  √7th   **S28.211**   Complete traumatic amputation of right breast
  √7th   **S28.212**   Complete traumatic amputation of left breast
  √7th   **S28.219**   Complete traumatic amputation of unspecified breast

√6th   **S28.22**   **Partial traumatic amputation of breast**
  √7th   **S28.221**   Partial traumatic amputation of right breast
  √7th   **S28.222**   Partial traumatic amputation of left breast
  √7th   **S28.229**   Partial traumatic amputation of unspecified breast

---

☑ Additional Character Required   √x7th Placeholder Alert   Manifestation   Unspecified Dx   ►◄ Revised Text   ● New Code   ▲ Revised Code Title

√4ᵗʰ **S29 Other and unspecified injuries of thorax**

    Code also any associated open wound (S21.-)

The appropriate 7th character is to be added to each code from category S29.
- A   initial encounter
- D   subsequent encounter
- S   sequela

√5ᵗʰ **S29.0   Injury of muscle and tendon at thorax level**

    √6ᵗʰ **S29.00   Unspecified injury of muscle and tendon of thorax**

        √7ᵗʰ **S29.001   Unspecified injury of muscle and tendon of front wall of thorax**

        √7ᵗʰ **S29.002   Unspecified injury of muscle and tendon of back wall of thorax**

        √7ᵗʰ **S29.009   Unspecified injury of muscle and tendon of unspecified wall of thorax**

    √6ᵗʰ **S29.01   Strain of muscle and tendon of thorax**

        √7ᵗʰ **S29.011   Strain of muscle and tendon of front wall of thorax**

        √7ᵗʰ **S29.012   Strain of muscle and tendon of back wall of thorax**

        √7ᵗʰ **S29.019   Strain of muscle and tendon of unspecified wall of thorax**

    √6ᵗʰ **S29.02   Laceration of muscle and tendon of thorax**

        √7ᵗʰ **S29.021   Laceration of muscle and tendon of front wall of thorax**

        √7ᵗʰ **S29.022   Laceration of muscle and tendon of back wall of thorax**

        √7ᵗʰ **S29.029   Laceration of muscle and tendon of unspecified wall of thorax**

    √6ᵗʰ **S29.09   Other injury of muscle and tendon of thorax**

        √7ᵗʰ **S29.091   Other injury of muscle and tendon of front wall of thorax**

        √7ᵗʰ **S29.092   Other injury of muscle and tendon of back wall of thorax**

        √7ᵗʰ **S29.099   Other injury of muscle and tendon of unspecified wall of thorax**

√x7ᵗʰ **S29.8   Other specified injuries of thorax**

√x7ᵗʰ **S29.9   Unspecified injury of thorax**

Injuries to the abdomen, lower back, lumbar spine, pelvis and external genitals (S30-S39)

INCLUDES   injuries to the abdominal wall
               injuries to the anus
               injuries to the buttock
               injuries to the external genitalia
               injuries to the flank
               injuries to the groin

EXCLUDES 2   *burns and corrosions (T20-T32)*
               effects of foreign body in anus and rectum (T18.5)
               effects of foreign body in genitourinary tract (T19.-)
               effects of foreign body in stomach, small intestine and colon (T18.2-T18.4)
               frostbite (T33-T34)
               insect bite or sting, venomous (T63.4)

√4ᵗʰ **S30 Superficial injury of abdomen, lower back, pelvis and external genitals**

    EXCLUDES 2   *superficial injury of hip (S70.-)*

The appropriate 7th character is to be added to each code from category S30.
- A   initial encounter
- D   subsequent encounter
- S   sequela

√x7ᵗʰ **S30.0   Contusion of lower back and pelvis**
    Contusion of buttock

√x7ᵗʰ **S30.1   Contusion of abdominal wall**
    Contusion of flank
    Contusion of groin

√5ᵗʰ **S30.2   Contusion of external genital organs**

    √6ᵗʰ **S30.20   Contusion of unspecified external genital organ**

        √7ᵗʰ **S30.201   Contusion of unspecified external genital organ, male**   ♂

        √7ᵗʰ **S30.202   Contusion of unspecified external genital organ, female**   ♀

    √x7ᵗʰ **S30.21   Contusion of penis**   ♂

    √x7ᵗʰ **S30.22   Contusion of scrotum and testes**   ♂

    √x7ᵗʰ **S30.23   Contusion of vagina and vulva**   ♀

√x7ᵗʰ **S30.3   Contusion of anus**

√5ᵗʰ **S30.8   Other superficial injuries of abdomen, lower back, pelvis and external genitals**

    √6ᵗʰ **S30.81   Abrasion of abdomen, lower back, pelvis and external genitals**

        √7ᵗʰ **S30.810   Abrasion of lower back and pelvis**

        √7ᵗʰ **S30.811   Abrasion of abdominal wall**

        √7ᵗʰ **S30.812   Abrasion of penis**   ♂

        √7ᵗʰ **S30.813   Abrasion of scrotum and testes**   ♂

        √7ᵗʰ **S30.814   Abrasion of vagina and vulva**   ♀

        √7ᵗʰ **S30.815   Abrasion of unspecified external genital organs, male**   ♂

        √7ᵗʰ **S30.816   Abrasion of unspecified external genital organs, female**   ♀

        √7ᵗʰ **S30.817   Abrasion of anus**

    √6ᵗʰ **S30.82   Blister (nonthermal) of abdomen, lower back, pelvis and external genitals**

        √7ᵗʰ **S30.820   Blister (nonthermal) of lower back and pelvis**

        √7ᵗʰ **S30.821   Blister (nonthermal) of abdominal wall**

        √7ᵗʰ **S30.822   Blister (nonthermal) of penis**   ♂

        √7ᵗʰ **S30.823   Blister (nonthermal) of scrotum and testes**   ♂

        √7ᵗʰ **S30.824   Blister (nonthermal) of vagina and vulva**   ♀

        √7ᵗʰ **S30.825   Blister (nonthermal) of unspecified external genital organs, male**   ♂

        √7ᵗʰ **S30.826   Blister (nonthermal) of unspecified external genital organs, female**   ♀

        √7ᵗʰ **S30.827   Blister (nonthermal) of anus**

    √6ᵗʰ **S30.84   External constriction of abdomen, lower back, pelvis and external genitals**

        √7ᵗʰ **S30.840   External constriction of lower back and pelvis**

        √7ᵗʰ **S30.841   External constriction of abdominal wall**

        √7ᵗʰ **S30.842   External constriction of penis**   ♂
            Hair tourniquet syndrome of penis
            Use additional cause code to identify the constricting item (W49.0-)

        √7ᵗʰ **S30.843   External constriction of scrotum and testes**   ♂

        √7ᵗʰ **S30.844   External constriction of vagina and vulva**   ♀

        √7ᵗʰ **S30.845   External constriction of unspecified external genital organs, male**   ♂

        √7ᵗʰ **S30.846   External constriction of unspecified external genital organs, female**   ♀

    √6ᵗʰ **S30.85   Superficial foreign body of abdomen, lower back, pelvis and external genitals**
        Splinter in the abdomen, lower back, pelvis and external genitals

        √7ᵗʰ **S30.850   Superficial foreign body of lower back and pelvis**

        √7ᵗʰ **S30.851   Superficial foreign body of abdominal wall**

        √7ᵗʰ **S30.852   Superficial foreign body of penis**   ♂

        √7ᵗʰ **S30.853   Superficial foreign body of scrotum and testes**   ♂

        √7ᵗʰ **S30.854   Superficial foreign body of vagina and vulva**   ♀

        √7ᵗʰ **S30.855   Superficial foreign body of unspecified external genital organs, male**   ♂

        √7ᵗʰ **S30.856   Superficial foreign body of unspecified external genital organs, female**   ♀

        √7ᵗʰ **S30.857   Superficial foreign body of anus**

    √6ᵗʰ **S30.86   Insect bite (nonvenomous) of abdomen, lower back, pelvis and external genitals**

        √7ᵗʰ **S30.860   Insect bite (nonvenomous) of lower back and pelvis**

        √7ᵗʰ **S30.861   Insect bite (nonvenomous) of abdominal wall**

        √7ᵗʰ **S30.862   Insect bite (nonvenomous) of penis**   ♂

√7ᵗʰ **S30.863** **Insect bite** (nonvenomous) of scrotum and testes   ♂

√7ᵗʰ **S30.864** **Insect bite** (nonvenomous) of vagina and vulva   ♀

√7ᵗʰ **S30.865** **Insect bite** (nonvenomous) of **unspecified** external genital organs, male   ♂

√7ᵗʰ **S30.866** **Insect bite** (nonvenomous) of **unspecified** external genital organs, female   ♀

√7ᵗʰ **S30.867** **Insect bite** (nonvenomous) of anus

√6ᵗʰ **S30.87** **Other superficial bite of abdomen, lower back, pelvis and external genitals**

> EXCLUDES 1   *open bite of abdomen, lower back, pelvis and external genitals (S31.05, S31.15, S31.25, S31.35, S31.45, S31.55)*

√7ᵗʰ **S30.870** **Other superficial bite of** lower back and pelvis

√7ᵗʰ **S30.871** **Other superficial bite of** abdominal wall

√7ᵗʰ **S30.872** **Other superficial bite of** penis   ♂

√7ᵗʰ **S30.873** **Other superficial bite of** scrotum and testes   ♂

√7ᵗʰ **S30.874** **Other superficial bite of** vagina and vulva   ♀

√7ᵗʰ **S30.875** **Other superficial bite of** **unspecified** external genital organs, male   ♂

√7ᵗʰ **S30.876** **Other superficial bite of** **unspecified** external genital organs, female   ♀

√7ᵗʰ **S30.877** **Other superficial bite of** anus

√5ᵗʰ **S30.9** **Unspecified superficial injury of abdomen, lower back, pelvis and external genitals**

√x7ᵗʰ **S30.91** **Unspecified superficial injury of** lower back and pelvis

√x7ᵗʰ **S30.92** **Unspecified superficial injury of** abdominal wall

√x7ᵗʰ **S30.93** **Unspecified superficial injury of** penis   ♂

√x7ᵗʰ **S30.94** **Unspecified superficial injury of** scrotum and testes   ♂

√x7ᵗʰ **S30.95** **Unspecified superficial injury of** vagina and vulva   ♀

√x7ᵗʰ **S30.96** **Unspecified superficial injury of** unspecified external genital organs, male   ♂

√x7ᵗʰ **S30.97** **Unspecified superficial injury of** unspecified external genital organs, female   ♀

√x7ᵗʰ **S30.98** **Unspecified superficial injury of** anus

√4ᵗʰ **S31** **Open wound of abdomen, lower back, pelvis and external genitals**

Code also any associated:
   spinal cord injury (S24.0, S24.1-, S34.0-, S34.1-)
   wound infection

> EXCLUDES 1   *traumatic amputation of part of abdomen, lower back and pelvis (S38.2-, S38.3)*

> EXCLUDES 2   *open wound of hip (S71.00-S71.02)*
>   *open fracture of pelvis (S32.1- – S32.9 with 7th character B)*

The appropriate 7th character is to be added to each code from category S31.
A   initial encounter
D   subsequent encounter
S   sequela

√5ᵗʰ **S31.0** **Open wound of** lower back and pelvis

√6ᵗʰ **S31.00** **Unspecified open wound of lower back and pelvis**

√7ᵗʰ **S31.000** **Unspecified open wound of lower back and pelvis** without penetration into retroperitoneum
     Unspecified open wound of lower back and pelvis NOS

√7ᵗʰ **S31.001** **Unspecified open wound of lower back and pelvis** with penetration into retroperitoneum

√6ᵗʰ **S31.01** **Laceration without foreign body of lower back and pelvis**

√7ᵗʰ **S31.010** **Laceration without foreign body of lower back and pelvis** without penetration into retroperitoneum
     Laceration without foreign body of lower back and pelvis NOS

√7ᵗʰ **S31.011** **Laceration without foreign body of lower back and pelvis** with penetration into retroperitoneum

√6ᵗʰ **S31.02** **Laceration with foreign body of lower back and pelvis**

√7ᵗʰ **S31.020** **Laceration with foreign body of lower back and pelvis** without penetration into retroperitoneum
     Laceration with foreign body of lower back and pelvis NOS

√7ᵗʰ **S31.021** **Laceration with foreign body of lower back and pelvis** with penetration into retroperitoneum

√6ᵗʰ **S31.03** **Puncture wound without foreign body of lower back and pelvis**

√7ᵗʰ **S31.030** **Puncture wound without foreign body of lower back and pelvis** without penetration into retroperitoneum
     Puncture wound without foreign body of lower back and pelvis NOS

√7ᵗʰ **S31.031** **Puncture wound without foreign body of lower back and pelvis** with penetration into retroperitoneum

√6ᵗʰ **S31.04** **Puncture wound with foreign body of lower back and pelvis**

√7ᵗʰ **S31.040** **Puncture wound with foreign body of lower back and pelvis** without penetration into retroperitoneum
     Puncture wound with foreign body of lower back and pelvis NOS

√7ᵗʰ **S31.041** **Puncture wound with foreign body of lower back and pelvis** with penetration into retroperitoneum

√6ᵗʰ **S31.05** **Open bite of lower back and pelvis**

Bite of lower back and pelvis NOS

> EXCLUDES 1   *superficial bite of lower back and pelvis (S30.860, S30.870)*

√7ᵗʰ **S31.050** **Open bite of lower back and pelvis** without penetration into retroperitoneum
     Open bite of lower back and pelvis NOS

√7ᵗʰ **S31.051** **Open bite of lower back and pelvis** with penetration into retroperitoneum

√5ᵗʰ **S31.1** **Open wound of** abdominal wall without penetration into peritoneal cavity

Open wound of abdominal wall NOS

> EXCLUDES 2   *open wound of abdominal wall with penetration into peritoneal cavity (S31.6-)*

√6ᵗʰ **S31.10** **Unspecified open wound of abdominal wall without penetration into peritoneal cavity**

√7ᵗʰ **S31.100** **Unspecified open wound of abdominal wall, right upper quadrant** without penetration into peritoneal cavity

√7ᵗʰ **S31.101** **Unspecified open wound of abdominal wall, left upper quadrant** without penetration into peritoneal cavity

√7ᵗʰ **S31.102** **Unspecified open wound of abdominal wall, epigastric region** without penetration into peritoneal cavity

√7ᵗʰ **S31.103** **Unspecified open wound of abdominal wall, right lower quadrant** without penetration into peritoneal cavity

√7ᵗʰ **S31.104** **Unspecified open wound of abdominal wall, left lower quadrant** without penetration into peritoneal cavity

√7ᵗʰ **S31.105** **Unspecified open wound of abdominal wall, periumbilic region** without penetration into peritoneal cavity

√7ᵗʰ **S31.109** **Unspecified open wound of abdominal wall, unspecified quadrant** without penetration into peritoneal cavity
     Unspecified open wound of abdominal wall NOS

√6ᵗʰ **S31.11** **Laceration without foreign body of abdominal wall without penetration into peritoneal cavity**

√7ᵗʰ **S31.110** **Laceration without foreign body of abdominal wall, right upper quadrant** without penetration into peritoneal cavity

√7ᵗʰ **S31.111** **Laceration without foreign body of abdominal wall, left upper quadrant** without penetration into peritoneal cavity

√7ᵗʰ **S31.112** **Laceration without foreign body of abdominal wall, epigastric region** without penetration into peritoneal cavity

---

✅ Additional Character Required   √x7ᵗʰ Placeholder Alert   Manifestation   Unspecified Dx   ►◄ Revised Text   ● New Code   ▲ Revised Code Title

√7ᵗʰ **S31.113** **Laceration without foreign body of abdominal wall, right lower quadrant without penetration into peritoneal cavity**

√7ᵗʰ **S31.114** **Laceration without foreign body of abdominal wall, left lower quadrant without penetration into peritoneal cavity**

√7ᵗʰ **S31.115** **Laceration without foreign body of abdominal wall, periumbilic region without penetration into peritoneal cavity**

√7ᵗʰ **S31.119** **Laceration without foreign body of abdominal wall, unspecified quadrant without penetration into peritoneal cavity**

√6ᵗʰ **S31.12** **Laceration with foreign body of abdominal wall without penetration into peritoneal cavity**

√7ᵗʰ **S31.120** **Laceration of abdominal wall with foreign body, right upper quadrant without penetration into peritoneal cavity**

√7ᵗʰ **S31.121** **Laceration of abdominal wall with foreign body, left upper quadrant without penetration into peritoneal cavity**

√7ᵗʰ **S31.122** **Laceration of abdominal wall with foreign body, epigastric region without penetration into peritoneal cavity**

√7ᵗʰ **S31.123** **Laceration of abdominal wall with foreign body, right lower quadrant without penetration into peritoneal cavity**

√7ᵗʰ **S31.124** **Laceration of abdominal wall with foreign body, left lower quadrant without penetration into peritoneal cavity**

√7ᵗʰ **S31.125** **Laceration of abdominal wall with foreign body, periumbilic region without penetration into peritoneal cavity**

√7ᵗʰ **S31.129** **Laceration of abdominal wall with foreign body, unspecified quadrant without penetration into peritoneal cavity**

√6ᵗʰ **S31.13** **Puncture wound of abdominal wall without foreign body without penetration into peritoneal cavity**

√7ᵗʰ **S31.130** **Puncture wound of abdominal wall without foreign body, right upper quadrant without penetration into peritoneal cavity**

√7ᵗʰ **S31.131** **Puncture wound of abdominal wall without foreign body, left upper quadrant without penetration into peritoneal cavity**

√7ᵗʰ **S31.132** **Puncture wound of abdominal wall without foreign body, epigastric region without penetration into peritoneal cavity**

√7ᵗʰ **S31.133** **Puncture wound of abdominal wall without foreign body, right lower quadrant without penetration into peritoneal cavity**

√7ᵗʰ **S31.134** **Puncture wound of abdominal wall without foreign body, left lower quadrant without penetration into peritoneal cavity**

√7ᵗʰ **S31.135** **Puncture wound of abdominal wall without foreign body, periumbilic region without penetration into peritoneal cavity**

√7ᵗʰ **S31.139** **Puncture wound of abdominal wall without foreign body, unspecified quadrant without penetration into peritoneal cavity**

√6ᵗʰ **S31.14** **Puncture wound of abdominal wall with foreign body without penetration into peritoneal cavity**

√7ᵗʰ **S31.140** **Puncture wound of abdominal wall with foreign body, right upper quadrant without penetration into peritoneal cavity**

√7ᵗʰ **S31.141** **Puncture wound of abdominal wall with foreign body, left upper quadrant without penetration into peritoneal cavity**

√7ᵗʰ **S31.142** **Puncture wound of abdominal wall with foreign body, epigastric region without penetration into peritoneal cavity**

√7ᵗʰ **S31.143** **Puncture wound of abdominal wall with foreign body, right lower quadrant without penetration into peritoneal cavity**

√7ᵗʰ **S31.144** **Puncture wound of abdominal wall with foreign body, left lower quadrant without penetration into peritoneal cavity**

√7ᵗʰ **S31.145** **Puncture wound of abdominal wall with foreign body, periumbilic region without penetration into peritoneal cavity**

√7ᵗʰ **S31.149** **Puncture wound of abdominal wall with foreign body, unspecified quadrant without penetration into peritoneal cavity**

√6ᵗʰ **S31.15** **Open bite of abdominal wall without penetration into peritoneal cavity**
Bite of abdominal wall NOS
EXCLUDES 1   *superficial bite of abdominal wall (S30.871)*

√7ᵗʰ **S31.150** **Open bite of abdominal wall, right upper quadrant without penetration into peritoneal cavity**

√7ᵗʰ **S31.151** **Open bite of abdominal wall, left upper quadrant without penetration into peritoneal cavity**

√7ᵗʰ **S31.152** **Open bite of abdominal wall, epigastric region without penetration into peritoneal cavity**

√7ᵗʰ **S31.153** **Open bite of abdominal wall, right lower quadrant without penetration into peritoneal cavity**

√7ᵗʰ **S31.154** **Open bite of abdominal wall, left lower quadrant without penetration into peritoneal cavity**

√7ᵗʰ **S31.155** **Open bite of abdominal wall, periumbilic region without penetration into peritoneal cavity**

√7ᵗʰ **S31.159** **Open bite of abdominal wall, unspecified quadrant without penetration into peritoneal cavity**

√5ᵗʰ **S31.2** **Open wound of penis**

√x7ᵗʰ **S31.20** **Unspecified open wound of penis**   ♂

√x7ᵗʰ **S31.21** **Laceration without foreign body of penis**   ♂

√x7ᵗʰ **S31.22** **Laceration with foreign body of penis**   ♂

√x7ᵗʰ **S31.23** **Puncture wound without foreign body of penis**   ♂

√x7ᵗʰ **S31.24** **Puncture wound with foreign body of penis**   ♂

√x7ᵗʰ **S31.25** **Open bite of penis**   ♂
Bite of penis NOS
EXCLUDES 1   *superficial bite of penis (S30.862, S30.872)*

√5ᵗʰ **S31.3** **Open wound of scrotum and testes**

√x7ᵗʰ **S31.30** **Unspecified open wound of scrotum and testes**   ♂

√x7ᵗʰ **S31.31** **Laceration without foreign body of scrotum and testes**   ♂

√x7ᵗʰ **S31.32** **Laceration with foreign body of scrotum and testes**   ♂

√x7ᵗʰ **S31.33** **Puncture wound without foreign body of scrotum and testes**   ♂

√x7ᵗʰ **S31.34** **Puncture wound with foreign body of scrotum and testes**   ♂

√x7ᵗʰ **S31.35** **Open bite of scrotum and testes**   ♂
Bite of scrotum and testes NOS
EXCLUDES 1   *superficial bite of scrotum and testes (S30.863, S30.873)*

√5ᵗʰ **S31.4** **Open wound of vagina and vulva**
EXCLUDES 1   *injury to vagina and vulva during delivery (O70.-, O71.4)*

√x7ᵗʰ **S31.40** **Unspecified open wound of vagina and vulva**   ♀

√x7ᵗʰ **S31.41** **Laceration without foreign body of vagina and vulva**   ♀

√x7ᵗʰ **S31.42** **Laceration with foreign body of vagina and vulva**   ♀

√x7ᵗʰ **S31.43** **Puncture wound without foreign body of vagina and vulva**   ♀

√x7ᵗʰ **S31.44** **Puncture wound with foreign body of vagina and vulva**   ♀

√x7ᵗʰ **S31.45** **Open bite of vagina and vulva**   ♀
Bite of vagina and vulva NOS
EXCLUDES 1   *superficial bite of vagina and vulva (S30.864, S30.874)*

✓5th **S31.5** **Open wound of unspecified external genital organs**

> EXCLUDES 1   *traumatic amputation of external genital organs (S38.21, S38.22)*

  ✓6th **S31.50** **Unspecified open wound of unspecified external genital organs**

    ✓7th **S31.501** Unspecified open wound of unspecified external genital organs, male   ♂

    ✓7th **S31.502** Unspecified open wound of unspecified external genital organs, female   ♀

  ✓6th **S31.51** Laceration without foreign body of unspecified external genital organs

    ✓7th **S31.511** Laceration without foreign body of unspecified external genital organs, male   ♂

    ✓7th **S31.512** Laceration without foreign body of unspecified external genital organs, female   ♀

  ✓6th **S31.52** Laceration with foreign body of unspecified external genital organs

    ✓7th **S31.521** Laceration with foreign body of unspecified external genital organs, male   ♂

    ✓7th **S31.522** Laceration with foreign body of unspecified external genital organs, female   ♀

  ✓6th **S31.53** Puncture wound without foreign body of unspecified external genital organs

    ✓7th **S31.531** Puncture wound without foreign body of unspecified external genital organs, male   ♂

    ✓7th **S31.532** Puncture wound without foreign body of unspecified external genital organs, female   ♀

  ✓6th **S31.54** Puncture wound with foreign body of unspecified external genital organs

    ✓7th **S31.541** Puncture wound with foreign body of unspecified external genital organs, male   ♂

    ✓7th **S31.542** Puncture wound with foreign body of unspecified external genital organs, female   ♀

  ✓6th **S31.55** **Open bite of unspecified external genital organs**

> Bite of unspecified external genital organs NOS
>
> EXCLUDES 1   *superficial bite of unspecified external genital organs (S30.865, S30.866, S30.875, S30.876)*

    ✓7th **S31.551** Open bite of unspecified external genital organs, male   ♂

    ✓7th **S31.552** Open bite of unspecified external genital organs, female   ♀

✓5th **S31.6** **Open wound of abdominal wall with penetration into peritoneal cavity**

  ✓6th **S31.60** **Unspecified open wound of abdominal wall with penetration into peritoneal cavity**

    ✓7th **S31.600** Unspecified open wound of abdominal wall, right upper quadrant with penetration into peritoneal cavity

    ✓7th **S31.601** Unspecified open wound of abdominal wall, left upper quadrant with penetration into peritoneal cavity

    ✓7th **S31.602** Unspecified open wound of abdominal wall, epigastric region with penetration into peritoneal cavity

    ✓7th **S31.603** Unspecified open wound of abdominal wall, right lower quadrant with penetration into peritoneal cavity

    ✓7th **S31.604** Unspecified open wound of abdominal wall, left lower quadrant with penetration into peritoneal cavity

    ✓7th **S31.605** Unspecified open wound of abdominal wall, periumbilic region with penetration into peritoneal cavity

    ✓7th **S31.609** Unspecified open wound of abdominal wall, unspecified quadrant with penetration into peritoneal cavity

  ✓6th **S31.61** Laceration without foreign body of abdominal wall with penetration into peritoneal cavity

    ✓7th **S31.610** Laceration without foreign body of abdominal wall, right upper quadrant with penetration into peritoneal cavity

    ✓7th **S31.611** Laceration without foreign body of abdominal wall, left upper quadrant with penetration into peritoneal cavity

    ✓7th **S31.612** Laceration without foreign body of abdominal wall, epigastric region with penetration into peritoneal cavity

    ✓7th **S31.613** Laceration without foreign body of abdominal wall, right lower quadrant with penetration into peritoneal cavity

    ✓7th **S31.614** Laceration without foreign body of abdominal wall, left lower quadrant with penetration into peritoneal cavity

    ✓7th **S31.615** Laceration without foreign body of abdominal wall, periumbilic region with penetration into peritoneal cavity

    ✓7th **S31.619** Laceration without foreign body of abdominal wall, unspecified quadrant with penetration into peritoneal cavity

  ✓6th **S31.62** Laceration with foreign body of abdominal wall with penetration into peritoneal cavity

    ✓7th **S31.620** Laceration with foreign body of abdominal wall, right upper quadrant with penetration into peritoneal cavity

    ✓7th **S31.621** Laceration with foreign body of abdominal wall, left upper quadrant with penetration into peritoneal cavity

    ✓7th **S31.622** Laceration with foreign body of abdominal wall, epigastric region with penetration into peritoneal cavity

    ✓7th **S31.623** Laceration with foreign body of abdominal wall, right lower quadrant with penetration into peritoneal cavity

    ✓7th **S31.624** Laceration with foreign body of abdominal wall, left lower quadrant with penetration into peritoneal cavity

    ✓7th **S31.625** Laceration with foreign body of abdominal wall, periumbilic region with penetration into peritoneal cavity

    ✓7th **S31.629** Laceration with foreign body of abdominal wall, unspecified quadrant with penetration into peritoneal cavity

  ✓6th **S31.63** Puncture wound without foreign body of abdominal wall with penetration into peritoneal cavity

    ✓7th **S31.630** Puncture wound without foreign body of abdominal wall, right upper quadrant with penetration into peritoneal cavity

    ✓7th **S31.631** Puncture wound without foreign body of abdominal wall, left upper quadrant with penetration into peritoneal cavity

    ✓7th **S31.632** Puncture wound without foreign body of abdominal wall, epigastric region with penetration into peritoneal cavity

    ✓7th **S31.633** Puncture wound without foreign body of abdominal wall, right lower quadrant with penetration into peritoneal cavity

    ✓7th **S31.634** Puncture wound without foreign body of abdominal wall, left lower quadrant with penetration into peritoneal cavity

    ✓7th **S31.635** Puncture wound without foreign body of abdominal wall, periumbilic region with penetration into peritoneal cavity

    ✓7th **S31.639** Puncture wound without foreign body of abdominal wall, unspecified quadrant with penetration into peritoneal cavity

  ✓6th **S31.64** Puncture wound with foreign body of abdominal wall with penetration into peritoneal cavity

    ✓7th **S31.640** Puncture wound with foreign body of abdominal wall, right upper quadrant with penetration into peritoneal cavity

    ✓7th **S31.641** Puncture wound with foreign body of abdominal wall, left upper quadrant with penetration into peritoneal cavity

    ✓7th **S31.642** Puncture wound with foreign body of abdominal wall, epigastric region with penetration into peritoneal cavity

    ✓7th **S31.643** Puncture wound with foreign body of abdominal wall, right lower quadrant with penetration into peritoneal cavity

    ✓7th **S31.644** Puncture wound with foreign body of abdominal wall, left lower quadrant with penetration into peritoneal cavity

    ✓7th **S31.645** Puncture wound with foreign body of abdominal wall, periumbilic region with penetration into peritoneal cavity

---

☑ Additional Character Required   ✓x7th Placeholder Alert   Manifestation   Unspecified Dx   ▶◀ Revised Text   ● New Code   ▲ Revised Code Title

√7ᵗʰ **S31.649** **Puncture wound with foreign body of abdominal wall, unspecified quadrant with penetration into peritoneal cavity**

√6ᵗʰ **S31.65** **Open bite** of abdominal wall with penetration into peritoneal cavity
> EXCLUDES 1   *superficial bite of abdominal wall (S30.861, S30.871)*

√7ᵗʰ **S31.650** **Open bite of abdominal wall, right upper quadrant** with penetration into peritoneal cavity

√7ᵗʰ **S31.651** **Open bite of abdominal wall, left upper quadrant** with penetration into peritoneal cavity

√7ᵗʰ **S31.652** **Open bite of abdominal wall, epigastric region** with penetration into peritoneal cavity

√7ᵗʰ **S31.653** **Open bite of abdominal wall, right lower quadrant** with penetration into peritoneal cavity

√7ᵗʰ **S31.654** **Open bite of abdominal wall, left lower quadrant** with penetration into peritoneal cavity

√7ᵗʰ **S31.655** **Open bite of abdominal wall, periumbilic region** with penetration into peritoneal cavity

√7ᵗʰ **S31.659** **Open bite of abdominal wall, unspecified quadrant** with penetration into peritoneal cavity

√5ᵗʰ **S31.8** **Open wound of other parts of abdomen, lower back and pelvis**

√6ᵗʰ **S31.80** **Open wound of unspecified buttock**

√7ᵗʰ **S31.801** **Laceration without foreign body of unspecified buttock**

√7ᵗʰ **S31.802** **Laceration with foreign body of unspecified buttock**

√7ᵗʰ **S31.803** **Puncture wound without foreign body of unspecified buttock**

√7ᵗʰ **S31.804** **Puncture wound with foreign body of unspecified buttock**

√7ᵗʰ **S31.805** **Open bite** of unspecified buttock
> Bite of buttock NOS
> EXCLUDES 1   *superficial bite of buttock (S30.870)*

√7ᵗʰ **S31.809** **Unspecified open wound of unspecified buttock**

√6ᵗʰ **S31.81** **Open wound of right buttock**

√7ᵗʰ **S31.811** **Laceration without foreign body of right buttock**

√7ᵗʰ **S31.812** **Laceration with foreign body of right buttock**

√7ᵗʰ **S31.813** **Puncture wound without foreign body of right buttock**

√7ᵗʰ **S31.814** **Puncture wound with foreign body of right buttock**

√7ᵗʰ **S31.815** **Open bite** of right buttock
> Bite of right buttock NOS
> EXCLUDES 1   *superficial bite of buttock (S30.870)*

√7ᵗʰ **S31.819** **Unspecified open wound of right buttock**

√6ᵗʰ **S31.82** **Open wound of left buttock**

√7ᵗʰ **S31.821** **Laceration without foreign body of left buttock**

√7ᵗʰ **S31.822** **Laceration with foreign body of left buttock**

√7ᵗʰ **S31.823** **Puncture wound without foreign body of left buttock**

√7ᵗʰ **S31.824** **Puncture wound with foreign body of left buttock**

√7ᵗʰ **S31.825** **Open bite** of left buttock
> Bite of left buttock NOS
> EXCLUDES 1   *superficial bite of buttock (S30.870)*

√7ᵗʰ **S31.829** **Unspecified open wound of left buttock**

√6ᵗʰ **S31.83** **Open wound of anus**

√7ᵗʰ **S31.831** **Laceration without foreign body of anus**

√7ᵗʰ **S31.832** **Laceration with foreign body of anus**

√7ᵗʰ **S31.833** **Puncture wound without foreign body of anus**

√7ᵗʰ **S31.834** **Puncture wound with foreign body of anus**

√7ᵗʰ **S31.835** **Open bite** of anus
> Bite of anus NOS
> EXCLUDES 1   *superficial bite of anus (S30.877)*

√7ᵗʰ **S31.839** **Unspecified open wound of anus**

√4ᵗʰ **S32** **Fracture of lumbar spine and pelvis**

> NOTE   A fracture not indicated as displaced or nondisplaced should be coded to displaced.
>
> A fracture not indicated as opened or closed should be coded to closed.

> INCLUDES   fracture of lumbosacral neural arch
> fracture of lumbosacral spinous process
> fracture of lumbosacral transverse process
> fracture of lumbosacral vertebra
> fracture of lumbosacral vertebral arch

Code first any associated spinal cord and spinal nerve injury (S34.-)
> EXCLUDES 1   *transection of abdomen (S38.3)*
> EXCLUDES 2   *fracture of hip NOS (S72.0-)*

AHA: 2018,2Q,12; 2015,3Q,37-39; 2012,4Q,93

> The appropriate 7th character is to be added to each code from category S32.
> A   initial encounter for closed fracture
> B   initial encounter for open fracture
> D   subsequent encounter for fracture with routine healing
> G   subsequent encounter for fracture with delayed healing
> K   subsequent encounter for fracture with nonunion
> S   sequela

√5ᵗʰ **S32.0** **Fracture of lumbar vertebra**
> Fracture of lumbar spine NOS

√6ᵗʰ **S32.00** **Fracture of unspecified lumbar vertebra**

¹ √7ᵗʰ **S32.000** **Wedge compression fracture of unspecified lumbar vertebra** HCC Q

¹ √7ᵗʰ **S32.001** **Stable burst fracture of unspecified lumbar vertebra** HCC Q

¹ √7ᵗʰ **S32.002** **Unstable burst fracture of unspecified lumbar vertebra** HCC Q

¹ √7ᵗʰ **S32.008** **Other fracture of unspecified lumbar vertebra** HCC Q

¹ √7ᵗʰ **S32.009** **Unspecified fracture of unspecified lumbar vertebra** HCC Q

√6ᵗʰ **S32.01** **Fracture of first lumbar vertebra**

¹ √7ᵗʰ **S32.010** **Wedge compression fracture of first lumbar vertebra** HCC Q

¹ √7ᵗʰ **S32.011** **Stable burst fracture of first lumbar vertebra** HCC Q

¹ √7ᵗʰ **S32.012** **Unstable burst fracture of first lumbar vertebra** HCC Q

¹ √7ᵗʰ **S32.018** **Other fracture of first lumbar vertebra** HCC Q

¹ √7ᵗʰ **S32.019** **Unspecified fracture of first lumbar vertebra** HCC Q

√6ᵗʰ **S32.02** **Fracture of second lumbar vertebra**

¹ √7ᵗʰ **S32.020** **Wedge compression fracture of second lumbar vertebra** HCC Q

¹ √7ᵗʰ **S32.021** **Stable burst fracture of second lumbar vertebra** HCC Q

¹ √7ᵗʰ **S32.022** **Unstable burst fracture of second lumbar vertebra** HCC Q

¹ √7ᵗʰ **S32.028** **Other fracture of second lumbar vertebra** HCC Q

¹ √7ᵗʰ **S32.029** **Unspecified fracture of second lumbar vertebra** HCC Q

√6ᵗʰ **S32.03** **Fracture of third lumbar vertebra**

¹ √7ᵗʰ **S32.030** **Wedge compression fracture of third lumbar vertebra** HCC Q

¹ √7ᵗʰ **S32.031** **Stable burst fracture of third lumbar vertebra** HCC Q

¹ √7ᵗʰ **S32.032** **Unstable burst fracture of third lumbar vertebra** HCC Q

¹ √7ᵗʰ **S32.038** **Other fracture of third lumbar vertebra** HCC Q

¹ √7ᵗʰ **S32.039** **Unspecified fracture of third lumbar vertebra** HCC Q

√6ᵗʰ **S32.04** **Fracture of fourth lumbar vertebra**

¹ √7ᵗʰ **S32.040** **Wedge compression fracture of fourth lumbar vertebra** HCC Q

¹ √7ᵗʰ **S32.041** **Stable burst fracture of fourth lumbar vertebra** HCC Q

| HCC CMS-HCC | Q QPP | N Newborn: 0 | P Pediatric: 0-17 | M Maternity: 12-55 | A Adult: 15-124 |

¹ √7ᵗʰ **S32.042** Unstable burst **fracture of fourth lumbar vertebra**   HCC Q

¹ √7ᵗʰ **S32.048** Other fracture of fourth lumbar vertebra   HCC Q

¹ √7ᵗʰ **S32.049** Unspecified fracture of fourth lumbar vertebra   HCC Q

√6ᵗʰ **S32.05** Fracture of **fifth lumbar vertebra**

    ¹ √7ᵗʰ **S32.050** Wedge compression **fracture of fifth lumbar vertebra**   HCC Q

    ¹ √7ᵗʰ **S32.051** Stable burst **fracture of fifth lumbar vertebra**   HCC Q

    ¹ √7ᵗʰ **S32.052** Unstable burst **fracture of fifth lumbar vertebra**   HCC Q

    ¹ √7ᵗʰ **S32.058** Other fracture of fifth lumbar vertebra   HCC Q

    ¹ √7ᵗʰ **S32.059** Unspecified fracture of fifth lumbar vertebra   HCC Q

√5ᵗʰ **S32.1** Fracture of **sacrum**

> **NOTE**   For vertical fractures, code to most medial fracture extension
>
> Use two codes if both a vertical and transverse fracture are present

Code also any associated fracture of pelvic ring (S32.8-)

¹ √x7ᵗʰ **S32.10** Unspecified fracture of sacrum   HCC Q

√6ᵗʰ **S32.11** Zone I **fracture of sacrum**

    Vertical sacral ala fracture of sacrum

Vertical Sacral Fracture Zones

Zones: ① ② ③

    ¹ √7ᵗʰ **S32.110** Nondisplaced Zone I **fracture of sacrum**   HCC Q

    ¹ √7ᵗʰ **S32.111** Minimally displaced Zone I **fracture of sacrum**   HCC Q

    ¹ √7ᵗʰ **S32.112** Severely displaced Zone I **fracture of sacrum**   HCC Q

    ¹ √7ᵗʰ **S32.119** Unspecified Zone I **fracture of sacrum**   HCC Q

√6ᵗʰ **S32.12** Zone II **fracture of sacrum**

    Vertical foraminal region fracture of sacrum

    ¹ √7ᵗʰ **S32.120** Nondisplaced Zone II **fracture of sacrum**   HCC Q

    ¹ √7ᵗʰ **S32.121** Minimally displaced Zone II **fracture of sacrum**   HCC Q

    ¹ √7ᵗʰ **S32.122** Severely displaced Zone II **fracture of sacrum**   HCC Q

    ¹ √7ᵗʰ **S32.129** Unspecified Zone II **fracture of sacrum**   HCC Q

√6ᵗʰ **S32.13** Zone III **fracture of sacrum**

    Vertical fracture into spinal canal region of sacrum

    ¹ √7ᵗʰ **S32.130** Nondisplaced Zone III **fracture of sacrum**   HCC Q

    ¹ √7ᵗʰ **S32.131** Minimally displaced Zone III **fracture of sacrum**   HCC Q

    ¹ √7ᵗʰ **S32.132** Severely displaced Zone III **fracture of sacrum**   HCC Q

---

¹ √7ᵗʰ **S32.139** Unspecified Zone III **fracture of sacrum**   HCC Q

Transverse Sacral Fracture Types

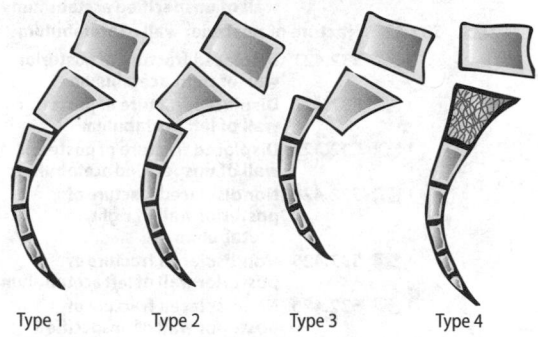

Type 1   Type 2   Type 3   Type 4

¹ √x7ᵗʰ **S32.14** Type 1 **fracture of sacrum**   HCC Q

    Transverse flexion fracture of sacrum without displacement

¹ √x7ᵗʰ **S32.15** Type 2 **fracture of sacrum**   HCC Q

    Transverse flexion fracture of sacrum with posterior displacement

¹ √x7ᵗʰ **S32.16** Type 3 **fracture of sacrum**   HCC Q

    Transverse extension fracture of sacrum with anterior displacement

¹ √x7ᵗʰ **S32.17** Type 4 **fracture of sacrum**   HCC Q

    Transverse segmental comminution of upper sacrum

¹ √x7ᵗʰ **S32.19** Other fracture of sacrum   HCC Q

¹ √x7ᵗʰ **S32.2** Fracture of **coccyx**   HCC Q

√5ᵗʰ **S32.3** Fracture of **ilium**

> **EXCLUDES 1**   *fracture of ilium with associated disruption of pelvic ring (S32.8-)*

√6ᵗʰ **S32.30** Unspecified fracture of ilium

    ¹ √7ᵗʰ **S32.301** Unspecified fracture of right ilium   HCC Q

    ¹ √7ᵗʰ **S32.302** Unspecified fracture of left ilium   HCC Q

    ¹ √7ᵗʰ **S32.309** Unspecified fracture of unspecified ilium   HCC Q

√6ᵗʰ **S32.31** Avulsion **fracture of ilium**

    ¹ √7ᵗʰ **S32.311** Displaced avulsion fracture of right ilium   HCC Q

    ¹ √7ᵗʰ **S32.312** Displaced avulsion fracture of left ilium   HCC Q

    ¹ √7ᵗʰ **S32.313** Displaced avulsion fracture of unspecified ilium   HCC Q

    ¹ √7ᵗʰ **S32.314** Nondisplaced avulsion fracture of right ilium   HCC Q

    ¹ √7ᵗʰ **S32.315** Nondisplaced avulsion fracture of left ilium   HCC Q

    ¹ √7ᵗʰ **S32.316** Nondisplaced avulsion fracture of unspecified ilium   HCC Q

√6ᵗʰ **S32.39** Other fracture of ilium

    ¹ √7ᵗʰ **S32.391** Other fracture of right ilium   HCC Q

    ¹ √7ᵗʰ **S32.392** Other fracture of left ilium   HCC Q

    ¹ √7ᵗʰ **S32.399** Other fracture of unspecified ilium   HCC Q

√5ᵗʰ **S32.4** Fracture of **acetabulum**

    Code also any associated fracture of pelvic ring (S32.8-)

    AHA: 2016,3Q,16

√6ᵗʰ **S32.40** Unspecified fracture of acetabulum

    ¹ √7ᵗʰ **S32.401** Unspecified fracture of right acetabulum   HCC Q

    ¹ √7ᵗʰ **S32.402** Unspecified fracture of left acetabulum   HCC Q

    ¹ √7ᵗʰ **S32.409** Unspecified fracture of unspecified acetabulum   HCC Q

√6ᵗʰ **S32.41** Fracture of **anterior wall** of acetabulum

    ¹ √7ᵗʰ **S32.411** Displaced fracture of anterior wall of right acetabulum   HCC Q

    ¹ √7ᵗʰ **S32.412** Displaced fracture of anterior wall of left acetabulum   HCC Q

    ¹ √7ᵗʰ **S32.413** Displaced fracture of anterior wall of unspecified acetabulum   HCC Q

✔ Additional Character Required   √x7ᵗʰ Placeholder Alert   Manifestation   Unspecified Dx   ►◄ Revised Text   ● New Code   ▲ Revised Code Title

ICD-10-CM 2020   **987**

Chapter 19. Injury, Poisoning and Certain Other Consequences of External Causes

S32.414–S32.609

¹ √7ᵗʰ **S32.414** Nondisplaced fracture of anterior wall of right acetabulum   HCC Q

¹ √7ᵗʰ **S32.415** Nondisplaced fracture of anterior wall of left acetabulum   HCC Q

¹ √7ᵗʰ **S32.416** Nondisplaced fracture of anterior wall of unspecified acetabulum   HCC Q

√6ᵗʰ **S32.42** Fracture of posterior wall of acetabulum

¹ √7ᵗʰ **S32.421** Displaced fracture of posterior wall of right acetabulum   HCC Q

¹ √7ᵗʰ **S32.422** Displaced fracture of posterior wall of left acetabulum   HCC Q

¹ √7ᵗʰ **S32.423** Displaced fracture of posterior wall of unspecified acetabulum   HCC Q

¹ √7ᵗʰ **S32.424** Nondisplaced fracture of posterior wall of right acetabulum   HCC Q

¹ √7ᵗʰ **S32.425** Nondisplaced fracture of posterior wall of left acetabulum   HCC Q

¹ √7ᵗʰ **S32.426** Nondisplaced fracture of posterior wall of unspecified acetabulum   HCC Q

√6ᵗʰ **S32.43** Fracture of anterior column [iliopubic] of acetabulum

¹ √7ᵗʰ **S32.431** Displaced fracture of anterior column [iliopubic] of right acetabulum   HCC Q

¹ √7ᵗʰ **S32.432** Displaced fracture of anterior column [iliopubic] of left acetabulum   HCC Q

¹ √7ᵗʰ **S32.433** Displaced fracture of anterior column [iliopubic] of unspecified acetabulum   HCC Q

¹ √7ᵗʰ **S32.434** Nondisplaced fracture of anterior column [iliopubic] of right acetabulum   HCC Q

¹ √7ᵗʰ **S32.435** Nondisplaced fracture of anterior column [iliopubic] of left acetabulum   HCC Q

¹ √7ᵗʰ **S32.436** Nondisplaced fracture of anterior column [iliopubic] of unspecified acetabulum   HCC Q

√6ᵗʰ **S32.44** Fracture of posterior column [ilioischial] of acetabulum

¹ √7ᵗʰ **S32.441** Displaced fracture of posterior column [ilioischial] of right acetabulum   HCC Q

¹ √7ᵗʰ **S32.442** Displaced fracture of posterior column [ilioischial] of left acetabulum   HCC Q

¹ √7ᵗʰ **S32.443** Displaced fracture of posterior column [ilioischial] of unspecified acetabulum   HCC Q

¹ √7ᵗʰ **S32.444** Nondisplaced fracture of posterior column [ilioischial] of right acetabulum   HCC Q

¹ √7ᵗʰ **S32.445** Nondisplaced fracture of posterior column [ilioischial] of left acetabulum   HCC Q

¹ √7ᵗʰ **S32.446** Nondisplaced fracture of posterior column [ilioischial] of unspecified acetabulum   HCC Q

√6ᵗʰ **S32.45** Transverse fracture of acetabulum

¹ √7ᵗʰ **S32.451** Displaced transverse fracture of right acetabulum   HCC Q

¹ √7ᵗʰ **S32.452** Displaced transverse fracture of left acetabulum   HCC Q

¹ √7ᵗʰ **S32.453** Displaced transverse fracture of unspecified acetabulum   HCC Q

¹ √7ᵗʰ **S32.454** Nondisplaced transverse fracture of right acetabulum   HCC Q

¹ √7ᵗʰ **S32.455** Nondisplaced transverse fracture of left acetabulum   HCC Q

¹ √7ᵗʰ **S32.456** Nondisplaced transverse fracture of unspecified acetabulum   HCC Q

√6ᵗʰ **S32.46** Associated transverse-posterior fracture of acetabulum

¹ √7ᵗʰ **S32.461** Displaced associated transverse-posterior fracture of right acetabulum   HCC Q

¹ √7ᵗʰ **S32.462** Displaced associated transverse-posterior fracture of left acetabulum   HCC Q

¹ √7ᵗʰ **S32.463** Displaced associated transverse-posterior fracture of unspecified acetabulum   HCC Q

¹ √7ᵗʰ **S32.464** Nondisplaced associated transverse-posterior fracture of right acetabulum   HCC Q

¹ √7ᵗʰ **S32.465** Nondisplaced associated transverse-posterior fracture of left acetabulum   HCC Q

¹ √7ᵗʰ **S32.466** Nondisplaced associated transverse-posterior fracture of unspecified acetabulum   HCC Q

√6ᵗʰ **S32.47** Fracture of medial wall of acetabulum

¹ √7ᵗʰ **S32.471** Displaced fracture of medial wall of right acetabulum   HCC Q

¹ √7ᵗʰ **S32.472** Displaced fracture of medial wall of left acetabulum   HCC Q

¹ √7ᵗʰ **S32.473** Displaced fracture of medial wall of unspecified acetabulum   HCC Q

¹ √7ᵗʰ **S32.474** Nondisplaced fracture of medial wall of right acetabulum   HCC Q

¹ √7ᵗʰ **S32.475** Nondisplaced fracture of medial wall of left acetabulum   HCC Q

¹ √7ᵗʰ **S32.476** Nondisplaced fracture of medial wall of unspecified acetabulum   HCC Q

√6ᵗʰ **S32.48** Dome fracture of acetabulum

¹ √7ᵗʰ **S32.481** Displaced dome fracture of right acetabulum   HCC Q

¹ √7ᵗʰ **S32.482** Displaced dome fracture of left acetabulum   HCC Q

¹ √7ᵗʰ **S32.483** Displaced dome fracture of unspecified acetabulum   HCC Q

¹ √7ᵗʰ **S32.484** Nondisplaced dome fracture of right acetabulum   HCC Q

¹ √7ᵗʰ **S32.485** Nondisplaced dome fracture of left acetabulum   HCC Q

¹ √7ᵗʰ **S32.486** Nondisplaced dome fracture of unspecified acetabulum   HCC Q

√6ᵗʰ **S32.49** Other specified fracture of acetabulum

¹ √7ᵗʰ **S32.491** Other specified fracture of right acetabulum   HCC Q

¹ √7ᵗʰ **S32.492** Other specified fracture of left acetabulum   HCC Q

¹ √7ᵗʰ **S32.499** Other specified fracture of unspecified acetabulum   HCC Q

√5ᵗʰ **S32.5** Fracture of pubis

    EXCLUDES 1   *fracture of pubis with associated disruption of pelvic ring (S32.8-)*

√6ᵗʰ **S32.50** Unspecified fracture of pubis

¹ √7ᵗʰ **S32.501** Unspecified fracture of right pubis   HCC Q

¹ √7ᵗʰ **S32.502** Unspecified fracture of left pubis   HCC Q

¹ √7ᵗʰ **S32.509** Unspecified fracture of unspecified pubis   HCC Q

√6ᵗʰ **S32.51** Fracture of superior rim of pubis

¹ √7ᵗʰ **S32.511** Fracture of superior rim of right pubis   HCC Q

¹ √7ᵗʰ **S32.512** Fracture of superior rim of left pubis   HCC Q

¹ √7ᵗʰ **S32.519** Fracture of superior rim of unspecified pubis   HCC Q

√6ᵗʰ **S32.59** Other specified fracture of pubis

¹ √7ᵗʰ **S32.591** Other specified fracture of right pubis   HCC Q

¹ √7ᵗʰ **S32.592** Other specified fracture of left pubis   HCC Q

¹ √7ᵗʰ **S32.599** Other specified fracture of unspecified pubis   HCC Q

√5ᵗʰ **S32.6** Fracture of ischium

    EXCLUDES 1   *fracture of ischium with associated disruption of pelvic ring (S32.8-)*

√6ᵗʰ **S32.60** Unspecified fracture of ischium

¹ √7ᵗʰ **S32.601** Unspecified fracture of right ischium   HCC Q

¹ √7ᵗʰ **S32.602** Unspecified fracture of left ischium   HCC Q

¹ √7ᵗʰ **S32.609** Unspecified fracture of unspecified ischium   HCC Q

√6ᵗʰ **S32.61** Avulsion fracture of ischium

     ¹ √7ᵗʰ **S32.611** **Displaced** avulsion fracture of right ischium   HCC Q

     ¹ √7ᵗʰ **S32.612** **Displaced** avulsion fracture of left ischium   HCC Q

     ¹ √7ᵗʰ **S32.613** **Displaced** avulsion fracture of unspecified ischium   HCC Q

     ¹ √7ᵗʰ **S32.614** **Nondisplaced** avulsion fracture of right ischium   HCC Q

     ¹ √7ᵗʰ **S32.615** **Nondisplaced** avulsion fracture of left ischium   HCC Q

     ¹ √7ᵗʰ **S32.616** **Nondisplaced** avulsion fracture of unspecified ischium   HCC Q

√6ᵗʰ **S32.69** Other specified fracture of ischium

     ¹ √7ᵗʰ **S32.691** **Other specified fracture of right ischium**   HCC Q

     ¹ √7ᵗʰ **S32.692** **Other specified fracture of left ischium**   HCC Q

     ¹ √7ᵗʰ **S32.699** **Other specified fracture of unspecified ischium**   HCC Q

√5ᵗʰ **S32.8** **Fracture of other parts of pelvis**

     Code also any associated:
       fracture of acetabulum (S32.4-)
       sacral fracture (S32.1-)

Fractures Disrupting Pelvic Circle

Pelvic circle — **Stable**

Unstable (two-place fracture)

Iliac crest

Anterior superior iliac spine

Ischial spine

Acetabulum

Femur

Ilium

L5

Sacrum

Coccyx

Pubis

Ischium

Pubic symphysis

Pelvic Bones

√6ᵗʰ **S32.81** **Multiple fractures of pelvis with disruption of pelvic ring**
     Multiple pelvic fractures with disruption of pelvic circle

     ¹ √7ᵗʰ **S32.810** **Multiple fractures of pelvis with stable disruption of pelvic ring**   HCC Q

     ¹ √7ᵗʰ **S32.811** **Multiple fractures of pelvis with unstable disruption of pelvic ring**   HCC Q

¹ √x7ᵗʰ **S32.82** **Multiple fractures of pelvis without disruption of pelvic ring**   HCC Q
     Multiple pelvic fractures without disruption of pelvic circle

¹ √x7ᵗʰ **S32.89** **Fracture of other parts of pelvis**   HCC Q

¹ √x7ᵗʰ **S32.9** **Fracture of unspecified parts of lumbosacral spine and pelvis**   HCC Q
     Fracture of lumbosacral spine NOS
     Fracture of pelvis NOS
     AHA: 2012,4Q,93

√4ᵗʰ **S33** **Dislocation and sprain of joints and ligaments of lumbar spine and pelvis**

     INCLUDES   avulsion of joint or ligament of lumbar spine and pelvis
       laceration of cartilage, joint or ligament of lumbar spine and pelvis
       sprain of cartilage, joint or ligament of lumbar spine and pelvis
       traumatic hemarthrosis of joint or ligament of lumbar spine and pelvis
       traumatic rupture of joint or ligament of lumbar spine and pelvis
       traumatic subluxation of joint or ligament of lumbar spine and pelvis
       traumatic tear of joint or ligament of lumbar spine and pelvis

     Code also any associated open wound
     EXCLUDES 1   nontraumatic rupture or displacement of lumbar intervertebral disc NOS (M51.-)
       obstetric damage to pelvic joints and ligaments (O71.6)
     EXCLUDES 2   dislocation and sprain of joints and ligaments of hip (S73.-)
       strain of muscle of lower back and pelvis (S39.01-)

> The appropriate 7th character is to be added to each code from category S33.
> A   initial encounter
> D   subsequent encounter
> S   sequela

√x7ᵗʰ **S33.0** **Traumatic rupture of lumbar intervertebral disc**
     EXCLUDES 1   rupture or displacement (nontraumatic) of lumbar intervertebral disc NOS (M51.- with fifth character 6)

√5ᵗʰ **S33.1** **Subluxation and dislocation of lumbar vertebra**
     Code also any associated:
       open wound of abdomen, lower back and pelvis (S31)
       spinal cord injury (S24.0, S24.1-, S34.0-, S34.1-)
     EXCLUDES 2   fracture of lumbar vertebrae (S32.0-)

     √6ᵗʰ **S33.10** **Subluxation and dislocation of unspecified lumbar vertebra**

       √7ᵗʰ **S33.100** **Subluxation of unspecified lumbar vertebra**

       √7ᵗʰ **S33.101** **Dislocation of unspecified lumbar vertebra**

     √6ᵗʰ **S33.11** **Subluxation and dislocation of L1/L2 lumbar vertebra**

       √7ᵗʰ **S33.110** **Subluxation of L1/L2 lumbar vertebra**

       √7ᵗʰ **S33.111** **Dislocation of L1/L2 lumbar vertebra**

     √6ᵗʰ **S33.12** **Subluxation and dislocation of L2/L3 lumbar vertebra**

       √7ᵗʰ **S33.120** **Subluxation of L2/L3 lumbar vertebra**

       √7ᵗʰ **S33.121** **Dislocation of L2/L3 lumbar vertebra**

     √6ᵗʰ **S33.13** **Subluxation and dislocation of L3/L4 lumbar vertebra**

       √7ᵗʰ **S33.130** **Subluxation of L3/L4 lumbar vertebra**

       √7ᵗʰ **S33.131** **Dislocation of L3/L4 lumbar vertebra**

     √6ᵗʰ **S33.14** **Subluxation and dislocation of L4/L5 lumbar vertebra**

       √7ᵗʰ **S33.140** **Subluxation of L4/L5 lumbar vertebra**

       √7ᵗʰ **S33.141** **Dislocation of L4/L5 lumbar vertebra**

√x7ᵗʰ **S33.2** **Dislocation of sacroiliac and sacrococcygeal joint**

√5ᵗʰ **S33.3** **Dislocation of other and unspecified parts of lumbar spine and pelvis**

     √x7ᵗʰ **S33.30** **Dislocation of unspecified parts of lumbar spine and pelvis**

     √x7ᵗʰ **S33.39** **Dislocation of other parts of lumbar spine and pelvis**

√x7ᵗʰ **S33.4** **Traumatic rupture of symphysis pubis**

√x7ᵗʰ **S33.5** **Sprain of ligaments of lumbar spine**

√x7ᵗʰ **S33.6** **Sprain of sacroiliac joint**

√x7ᵗʰ **S33.8** **Sprain of other parts of lumbar spine and pelvis**

√x7ᵗʰ **S33.9** **Sprain of unspecified parts of lumbar spine and pelvis**

☑ Additional Character Required   √x7ᵗʰ Placeholder Alert   Manifestation   Unspecified Dx   ►◄ Revised Text   ● New Code   ▲ Revised Code Title

ICD-10-CM 2020   **989**

✓4ᵗʰ **S34 Injury of lumbar and sacral spinal cord and nerves at abdomen, lower back and pelvis level**

NOTE Code to highest level of lumbar cord injury.

Injuries to the spinal cord (S34.0 and S34.1) refer to the cord level and not bone level injury, and can affect nerve roots at and below the level given.

Code also any associated:
fracture of vertebra (S22.0-, S32.0-)
open wound of abdomen, lower back and pelvis (S31.-)
transient paralysis (R29.5)

The appropriate 7th character is to be added to each code from category S34.
A initial encounter
D subsequent encounter
S sequela

✓5ᵗʰ **S34.0 Concussion and edema of lumbar and sacral spinal cord**

  ✓x7ᵗʰ **S34.01 Concussion and edema of lumbar spinal cord** **HCC**

  ✓x7ᵗʰ **S34.02 Concussion and edema of sacral spinal cord** **HCC**

    Concussion and edema of conus medullaris

✓5ᵗʰ **S34.1 Other and unspecified injury of lumbar and sacral spinal cord**

  ✓6ᵗʰ **S34.10 Unspecified injury to lumbar spinal cord**

    ✓7ᵗʰ **S34.101 Unspecified injury to L1 level of lumbar spinal cord** **HCC**

      Unspecified injury to lumbar spinal cord level 1

    ✓7ᵗʰ **S34.102 Unspecified injury to L2 level of lumbar spinal cord** **HCC**

      Unspecified injury to lumbar spinal cord level 2

    ✓7ᵗʰ **S34.103 Unspecified injury to L3 level of lumbar spinal cord** **HCC**

      Unspecified injury to lumbar spinal cord level 3

    ✓7ᵗʰ **S34.104 Unspecified injury to L4 level of lumbar spinal cord** **HCC**

      Unspecified injury to lumbar spinal cord level 4

    ✓7ᵗʰ **S34.105 Unspecified injury to L5 level of lumbar spinal cord** **HCC**

      Unspecified injury to lumbar spinal cord level 5

    ✓7ᵗʰ **S34.109 Unspecified injury to unspecified level of lumbar spinal cord** **HCC**

  ✓6ᵗʰ **S34.11 Complete lesion of lumbar spinal cord**

    ✓7ᵗʰ **S34.111 Complete lesion of L1 level of lumbar spinal cord** **HCC**

      Complete lesion of lumbar spinal cord level 1

    ✓7ᵗʰ **S34.112 Complete lesion of L2 level of lumbar spinal cord** **HCC**

      Complete lesion of lumbar spinal cord level 2

    ✓7ᵗʰ **S34.113 Complete lesion of L3 level of lumbar spinal cord** **HCC**

      Complete lesion of lumbar spinal cord level 3

    ✓7ᵗʰ **S34.114 Complete lesion of L4 level of lumbar spinal cord** **HCC**

      Complete lesion of lumbar spinal cord level 4

    ✓7ᵗʰ **S34.115 Complete lesion of L5 level of lumbar spinal cord** **HCC**

      Complete lesion of lumbar spinal cord level 5

    ✓7ᵗʰ **S34.119 Complete lesion of unspecified level of lumbar spinal cord** **HCC**

  ✓6ᵗʰ **S34.12 Incomplete lesion of lumbar spinal cord**

    ✓7ᵗʰ **S34.121 Incomplete lesion of L1 level of lumbar spinal cord** **HCC**

      Incomplete lesion of lumbar spinal cord level 1

    ✓7ᵗʰ **S34.122 Incomplete lesion of L2 level of lumbar spinal cord** **HCC**

      Incomplete lesion of lumbar spinal cord level 2

    ✓7ᵗʰ **S34.123 Incomplete lesion of L3 level of lumbar spinal cord** **HCC**

      Incomplete lesion of lumbar spinal cord level 3

    ✓7ᵗʰ **S34.124 Incomplete lesion of L4 level of lumbar spinal cord** **HCC**

      Incomplete lesion of lumbar spinal cord level 4

    ✓7ᵗʰ **S34.125 Incomplete lesion of L5 level of lumbar spinal cord** **HCC**

      Incomplete lesion of lumbar spinal cord level 5

    ✓7ᵗʰ **S34.129 Incomplete lesion of unspecified level of lumbar spinal cord** **HCC**

  ✓6ᵗʰ **S34.13 Other and unspecified injury to sacral spinal cord**

    Other injury to conus medullaris

    ✓7ᵗʰ **S34.131 Complete lesion of sacral spinal cord** **HCC**

      Complete lesion of conus medullaris

    ✓7ᵗʰ **S34.132 Incomplete lesion of sacral spinal cord** **HCC**

      Incomplete lesion of conus medullaris

    ✓7ᵗʰ **S34.139 Unspecified injury to sacral spinal cord** **HCC**

      Unspecified injury of conus medullaris

✓5ᵗʰ **S34.2 Injury of nerve root of lumbar and sacral spine**

  ✓x7ᵗʰ **S34.21 Injury of nerve root of lumbar spine**

  ✓x7ᵗʰ **S34.22 Injury of nerve root of sacral spine**

1 ✓x7ᵗʰ **S34.3 Injury of cauda equina** **HCC**

✓x7ᵗʰ **S34.4 Injury of lumbosacral plexus**

✓x7ᵗʰ **S34.5 Injury of lumbar, sacral and pelvic sympathetic nerves**

  Injury of celiac ganglion or plexus
  Injury of hypogastric plexus
  Injury of mesenteric plexus (inferior) (superior)
  Injury of splanchnic nerve

✓x7ᵗʰ **S34.6 Injury of peripheral nerve(s) at abdomen, lower back and pelvis level**

✓x7ᵗʰ **S34.8 Injury of other nerves at abdomen, lower back and pelvis level**

✓x7ᵗʰ **S34.9 Injury of unspecified nerves at abdomen, lower back and pelvis level**

✓4ᵗʰ **S35 Injury of blood vessels at abdomen, lower back and pelvis level**

Code also any associated open wound (S31.-)

The appropriate 7th character is to be added to each code from category S35.
A initial encounter
D subsequent encounter
S sequela

✓5ᵗʰ **S35.0 Injury of abdominal aorta**

  EXCLUDES 1 *injury of aorta NOS (S25.0)*

  ✓x7ᵗʰ **S35.00 Unspecified injury of abdominal aorta**

  ✓x7ᵗʰ **S35.01 Minor laceration of abdominal aorta**

    Incomplete transection of abdominal aorta
    Laceration of abdominal aorta NOS
    Superficial laceration of abdominal aorta

  ✓x7ᵗʰ **S35.02 Major laceration of abdominal aorta**

    Complete transection of abdominal aorta
    Traumatic rupture of abdominal aorta

  ✓x7ᵗʰ **S35.09 Other injury of abdominal aorta**

✓5ᵗʰ **S35.1 Injury of inferior vena cava**

  Injury of hepatic vein

  EXCLUDES 1 *injury of vena cava NOS (S25.2)*

  ✓x7ᵗʰ **S35.10 Unspecified injury of inferior vena cava**

  ✓x7ᵗʰ **S35.11 Minor laceration of inferior vena cava**

    Incomplete transection of inferior vena cava
    Laceration of inferior vena cava NOS
    Superficial laceration of inferior vena cava

  ✓x7ᵗʰ **S35.12 Major laceration of inferior vena cava**

    Complete transection of inferior vena cava
    Traumatic rupture of inferior vena cava

  ✓x7ᵗʰ **S35.19 Other injury of inferior vena cava**

✓5ᵗʰ **S35.2 Injury of celiac or mesenteric artery and branches**

  ✓6ᵗʰ **S35.21 Injury of** celiac artery

    ✓7ᵗʰ **S35.211 Minor laceration of celiac artery**
      Incomplete transection of celiac artery
      Laceration of celiac artery NOS
      Superficial laceration of celiac artery

    ✓7ᵗʰ **S35.212 Major laceration of celiac artery**
      Complete transection of celiac artery
      Traumatic rupture of celiac artery

    ✓7ᵗʰ **S35.218 Other injury of celiac artery**

    ✓7ᵗʰ **S35.219 Unspecified injury of celiac artery**

  ✓6ᵗʰ **S35.22 Injury of** superior mesenteric artery

    ✓7ᵗʰ **S35.221 Minor laceration of superior mesenteric artery**
      Incomplete transection of superior mesenteric artery
      Laceration of superior mesenteric artery NOS
      Superficial laceration of superior mesenteric artery

    ✓7ᵗʰ **S35.222 Major laceration of superior mesenteric artery**
      Complete transection of superior mesenteric artery
      Traumatic rupture of superior mesenteric artery

    ✓7ᵗʰ **S35.228 Other injury of superior mesenteric artery**

    ✓7ᵗʰ **S35.229 Unspecified injury of superior mesenteric artery**

  ✓6ᵗʰ **S35.23 Injury of** inferior mesenteric artery

    ✓7ᵗʰ **S35.231 Minor laceration of inferior mesenteric artery**
      Incomplete transection of inferior mesenteric artery
      Laceration of inferior mesenteric artery NOS
      Superficial laceration of inferior mesenteric artery

    ✓7ᵗʰ **S35.232 Major laceration of inferior mesenteric artery**
      Complete transection of inferior mesenteric artery
      Traumatic rupture of inferior mesenteric artery

    ✓7ᵗʰ **S35.238 Other injury of inferior mesenteric artery**

    ✓7ᵗʰ **S35.239 Unspecified injury of inferior mesenteric artery**

  ✓6ᵗʰ **S35.29 Injury of** branches of celiac and mesenteric artery
      Injury of gastric artery
      Injury of gastroduodenal artery
      Injury of hepatic artery
      Injury of splenic artery

    ✓7ᵗʰ **S35.291 Minor laceration of branches of celiac and mesenteric artery**
      Incomplete transection of branches of celiac and mesenteric artery
      Laceration of branches of celiac and mesenteric artery NOS
      Superficial laceration of branches of celiac and mesenteric artery

    ✓7ᵗʰ **S35.292 Major laceration of branches of celiac and mesenteric artery**
      Complete transection of branches of celiac and mesenteric artery
      Traumatic rupture of branches of celiac and mesenteric artery

    ✓7ᵗʰ **S35.298 Other injury of branches of celiac and mesenteric artery**

    ✓7ᵗʰ **S35.299 Unspecified injury of branches of celiac and mesenteric artery**

✓5ᵗʰ **S35.3 Injury of portal or splenic vein and branches**

  ✓6ᵗʰ **S35.31 Injury of** portal vein

    ✓7ᵗʰ **S35.311 Laceration of portal vein**

    ✓7ᵗʰ **S35.318 Other specified injury of portal vein**

    ✓7ᵗʰ **S35.319 Unspecified injury of portal vein**

  ✓6ᵗʰ **S35.32 Injury of** splenic vein

    ✓7ᵗʰ **S35.321 Laceration of splenic vein**

    ✓7ᵗʰ **S35.328 Other specified injury of splenic vein**

    ✓7ᵗʰ **S35.329 Unspecified injury of splenic vein**

  ✓6ᵗʰ **S35.33 Injury of** superior mesenteric vein

    ✓7ᵗʰ **S35.331 Laceration of superior mesenteric vein**

    ✓7ᵗʰ **S35.338 Other specified injury of superior mesenteric vein**

    ✓7ᵗʰ **S35.339 Unspecified injury of superior mesenteric vein**

  ✓6ᵗʰ **S35.34 Injury of** inferior mesenteric vein

    ✓7ᵗʰ **S35.341 Laceration of inferior mesenteric vein**

    ✓7ᵗʰ **S35.348 Other specified injury of inferior mesenteric vein**

    ✓7ᵗʰ **S35.349 Unspecified injury of inferior mesenteric vein**

✓5ᵗʰ **S35.4 Injury of** renal **blood vessels**

  ✓6ᵗʰ **S35.40 Unspecified injury of renal blood vessel**

    ✓7ᵗʰ **S35.401 Unspecified injury of** right renal artery

    ✓7ᵗʰ **S35.402 Unspecified injury of** left renal artery

    ✓7ᵗʰ **S35.403 Unspecified injury of unspecified renal artery**

    ✓7ᵗʰ **S35.404 Unspecified injury of** right renal vein

    ✓7ᵗʰ **S35.405 Unspecified injury of** left renal vein

    ✓7ᵗʰ **S35.406 Unspecified injury of unspecified renal vein**

  ✓6ᵗʰ **S35.41 Laceration of renal blood vessel**

    ✓7ᵗʰ **S35.411 Laceration of** right renal artery

    ✓7ᵗʰ **S35.412 Laceration of** left renal artery

    ✓7ᵗʰ **S35.413 Laceration of unspecified renal artery**

    ✓7ᵗʰ **S35.414 Laceration of** right renal vein

    ✓7ᵗʰ **S35.415 Laceration of** left renal vein

    ✓7ᵗʰ **S35.416 Laceration of unspecified renal vein**

  ✓6ᵗʰ **S35.49 Other specified injury of renal blood vessel**

    ✓7ᵗʰ **S35.491 Other specified injury of** right renal artery

    ✓7ᵗʰ **S35.492 Other specified injury of** left renal artery

    ✓7ᵗʰ **S35.493 Other specified injury of unspecified renal artery**

    ✓7ᵗʰ **S35.494 Other specified injury of** right renal vein

    ✓7ᵗʰ **S35.495 Other specified injury of** left renal vein

    ✓7ᵗʰ **S35.496 Other specified injury of unspecified renal vein**

✓5ᵗʰ **S35.5 Injury of** iliac **blood vessels**

  ✓x7ᵗʰ **S35.50 Injury of unspecified iliac blood vessel(s)**

  ✓6ᵗʰ **S35.51 Injury of** iliac **artery or vein**
      Injury of hypogastric artery or vein

    ✓7ᵗʰ **S35.511 Injury of** right iliac artery

    ✓7ᵗʰ **S35.512 Injury of** left iliac artery

    ✓7ᵗʰ **S35.513 Injury of unspecified iliac artery**

    ✓7ᵗʰ **S35.514 Injury of** right iliac vein

    ✓7ᵗʰ **S35.515 Injury of** left iliac vein

    ✓7ᵗʰ **S35.516 Injury of unspecified iliac vein**

  ✓6ᵗʰ **S35.53 Injury of** uterine **artery or vein**

    ✓7ᵗʰ **S35.531 Injury of** right uterine artery ♀

    ✓7ᵗʰ **S35.532 Injury of** left uterine artery ♀

    ✓7ᵗʰ **S35.533 Injury of unspecified uterine artery** ♀

    ✓7ᵗʰ **S35.534 Injury of** right uterine vein ♀

    ✓7ᵗʰ **S35.535 Injury of** left uterine vein ♀

    ✓7ᵗʰ **S35.536 Injury of unspecified uterine vein** ♀

  ✓x7ᵗʰ **S35.59 Injury of other iliac blood vessels**

✓5ᵗʰ **S35.8 Injury of other blood vessels at abdomen, lower back and pelvis level**
      Injury of ovarian artery or vein

  ✓6ᵗʰ **S35.8X Injury of other blood vessels at abdomen, lower back and pelvis level**

    ✓7ᵗʰ **S35.8X1 Laceration of other blood vessels at abdomen, lower back and pelvis level**

    ✓7ᵗʰ **S35.8X8 Other specified injury of other blood vessels at abdomen, lower back and pelvis level**

☑ Additional Character Required   ✓x7ᵗʰ Placeholder Alert   Manifestation   Unspecified Dx   ►◄ Revised Text   ● New Code   ▲ Revised Code Title

√7ᵗʰ **S35.8X9** Unspecified injury of other blood vessels at abdomen, lower back and pelvis level

√5ᵗʰ **S35.9** Injury of unspecified blood vessel at abdomen, lower back and pelvis level

√x7ᵗʰ **S35.90** Unspecified injury of unspecified blood vessel at abdomen, lower back and pelvis level

√x7ᵗʰ **S35.91** Laceration of unspecified blood vessel at abdomen, lower back and pelvis level

√x7ᵗʰ **S35.99** Other specified injury of unspecified blood vessel at abdomen, lower back and pelvis level

√4ᵗʰ **S36** Injury of intra-abdominal organs

Code also any associated open wound (S31.-)

The appropriate 7th character is to be added to each code from category S36.
A   initial encounter
D   subsequent encounter
S   sequela

√5ᵗʰ **S36.0** Injury of spleen
AHA: 2015,2Q,36; 2015,1Q,10

√x7ᵗʰ **S36.00** Unspecified injury of spleen

√6ᵗʰ **S36.02** Contusion of spleen

√7ᵗʰ **S36.020** Minor contusion of spleen
Contusion of spleen less than 2 cm

√7ᵗʰ **S36.021** Major contusion of spleen
Contusion of spleen greater than 2 cm

√7ᵗʰ **S36.029** Unspecified contusion of spleen

√6ᵗʰ **S36.03** Laceration of spleen

√7ᵗʰ **S36.030** Superficial (capsular) laceration of spleen
Laceration of spleen less than 1 cm
Minor laceration of spleen

√7ᵗʰ **S36.031** Moderate laceration of spleen
Laceration of spleen 1 to 3 cm

√7ᵗʰ **S36.032** Major laceration of spleen
Avulsion of spleen
Laceration of spleen greater than 3 cm
Massive laceration of spleen
Multiple moderate lacerations of spleen
Stellate laceration of spleen

√7ᵗʰ **S36.039** Unspecified laceration of spleen

√x7ᵗʰ **S36.09** Other injury of spleen

√5ᵗʰ **S36.1** Injury of liver and gallbladder and bile duct

√6ᵗʰ **S36.11** Injury of liver

√7ᵗʰ **S36.112** Contusion of liver

√7ᵗʰ **S36.113** Laceration of liver, unspecified degree

√7ᵗʰ **S36.114** Minor laceration of liver
Laceration involving capsule only, or, without significant involvement of hepatic parenchyma [i.e., less than 1 cm deep]

√7ᵗʰ **S36.115** Moderate laceration of liver
Laceration involving parenchyma but without major disruption of parenchyma [i.e., less than 10 cm long and less than 3 cm deep]

√7ᵗʰ **S36.116** Major laceration of liver
Laceration with significant disruption of hepatic parenchyma [i.e., greater than 10 cm long and 3 cm deep]
Multiple moderate lacerations, with or without hematoma
Stellate laceration of liver

√7ᵗʰ **S36.118** Other injury of liver

√7ᵗʰ **S36.119** Unspecified injury of liver

√6ᵗʰ **S36.12** Injury of gallbladder

√7ᵗʰ **S36.122** Contusion of gallbladder

√7ᵗʰ **S36.123** Laceration of gallbladder

√7ᵗʰ **S36.128** Other injury of gallbladder

√7ᵗʰ **S36.129** Unspecified injury of gallbladder

√x7ᵗʰ **S36.13** Injury of bile duct

√5ᵗʰ **S36.2** Injury of pancreas

√6ᵗʰ **S36.20** Unspecified injury of pancreas

√7ᵗʰ **S36.200** Unspecified injury of head of pancreas

√7ᵗʰ **S36.201** Unspecified injury of body of pancreas

√7ᵗʰ **S36.202** Unspecified injury of tail of pancreas

√7ᵗʰ **S36.209** Unspecified injury of unspecified part of pancreas

√6ᵗʰ **S36.22** Contusion of pancreas

√7ᵗʰ **S36.220** Contusion of head of pancreas

√7ᵗʰ **S36.221** Contusion of body of pancreas

√7ᵗʰ **S36.222** Contusion of tail of pancreas

√7ᵗʰ **S36.229** Contusion of unspecified part of pancreas

√6ᵗʰ **S36.23** Laceration of pancreas, unspecified degree

√7ᵗʰ **S36.230** Laceration of head of pancreas, unspecified degree

√7ᵗʰ **S36.231** Laceration of body of pancreas, unspecified degree

√7ᵗʰ **S36.232** Laceration of tail of pancreas, unspecified degree

√7ᵗʰ **S36.239** Laceration of unspecified part of pancreas, unspecified degree

√6ᵗʰ **S36.24** Minor laceration of pancreas

√7ᵗʰ **S36.240** Minor laceration of head of pancreas

√7ᵗʰ **S36.241** Minor laceration of body of pancreas

√7ᵗʰ **S36.242** Minor laceration of tail of pancreas

√7ᵗʰ **S36.249** Minor laceration of unspecified part of pancreas

√6ᵗʰ **S36.25** Moderate laceration of pancreas

√7ᵗʰ **S36.250** Moderate laceration of head of pancreas

√7ᵗʰ **S36.251** Moderate laceration of body of pancreas

√7ᵗʰ **S36.252** Moderate laceration of tail of pancreas

√7ᵗʰ **S36.259** Moderate laceration of unspecified part of pancreas

√6ᵗʰ **S36.26** Major laceration of pancreas

√7ᵗʰ **S36.260** Major laceration of head of pancreas

√7ᵗʰ **S36.261** Major laceration of body of pancreas

√7ᵗʰ **S36.262** Major laceration of tail of pancreas

√7ᵗʰ **S36.269** Major laceration of unspecified part of pancreas

√6ᵗʰ **S36.29** Other injury of pancreas

√7ᵗʰ **S36.290** Other injury of head of pancreas

√7ᵗʰ **S36.291** Other injury of body of pancreas

√7ᵗʰ **S36.292** Other injury of tail of pancreas

√7ᵗʰ **S36.299** Other injury of unspecified part of pancreas

√5ᵗʰ **S36.3** Injury of stomach

√x7ᵗʰ **S36.30** Unspecified injury of stomach

√x7ᵗʰ **S36.32** Contusion of stomach

√x7ᵗʰ **S36.33** Laceration of stomach

√x7ᵗʰ **S36.39** Other injury of stomach

√5ᵗʰ **S36.4** Injury of small intestine

√6ᵗʰ **S36.40** Unspecified injury of small intestine

√7ᵗʰ **S36.400** Unspecified injury of duodenum

√7ᵗʰ **S36.408** Unspecified injury of other part of small intestine

√7ᵗʰ **S36.409** Unspecified injury of unspecified part of small intestine

√6ᵗʰ **S36.41** Primary blast injury of small intestine
Blast injury of small intestine NOS

√7ᵗʰ **S36.410** Primary blast injury of duodenum

√7ᵗʰ **S36.418** Primary blast injury of other part of small intestine

√7ᵗʰ **S36.419** Primary blast injury of unspecified part of small intestine

√6ᵗʰ **S36.42** Contusion of small intestine

√7ᵗʰ **S36.420** Contusion of duodenum

√7ᵗʰ **S36.428** Contusion of other part of small intestine

√7ᵗʰ **S36.429** Contusion of unspecified part of small intestine

√6ᵗʰ **S36.43** Laceration of small intestine

√7ᵗʰ **S36.430** Laceration of duodenum

√7ᵗʰ **S36.438** Laceration of other part of small intestine

√7ᵗʰ **S36.439** Laceration of unspecified part of small intestine

☑6ᵗʰ **S36.49 Other injury of small intestine**
    ☑7ᵗʰ **S36.490 Other injury of** duodenum
    ☑7ᵗʰ **S36.498 Other injury of other part of small intestine**
    ☑7ᵗʰ **S36.499 Other injury of unspecified part of small intestine**

☑5ᵗʰ **S36.5 Injury of colon**
    EXCLUDES 2   injury of rectum (S36.6-)
    ☑6ᵗʰ **S36.50 Unspecified injury of colon**
      ☑7ᵗʰ **S36.500 Unspecified injury of** ascending [right] colon
      ☑7ᵗʰ **S36.501 Unspecified injury of** transverse colon
      ☑7ᵗʰ **S36.502 Unspecified injury of** descending [left] colon
      ☑7ᵗʰ **S36.503 Unspecified injury of** sigmoid colon
      ☑7ᵗʰ **S36.508 Unspecified injury of other part of colon**
      ☑7ᵗʰ **S36.509 Unspecified injury of unspecified part of colon**
    ☑6ᵗʰ **S36.51 Primary blast injury of colon**
      Blast injury of colon NOS
      ☑7ᵗʰ **S36.510 Primary blast injury of** ascending [right] colon
      ☑7ᵗʰ **S36.511 Primary blast injury of** transverse colon
      ☑7ᵗʰ **S36.512 Primary blast injury of** descending [left] colon
      ☑7ᵗʰ **S36.513 Primary blast injury of** sigmoid colon
      ☑7ᵗʰ **S36.518 Primary blast injury of other part of colon**
      ☑7ᵗʰ **S36.519 Primary blast injury of unspecified part of colon**
    ☑6ᵗʰ **S36.52 Contusion of colon**
      ☑7ᵗʰ **S36.520 Contusion of** ascending [right] colon
      ☑7ᵗʰ **S36.521 Contusion of** transverse colon
      ☑7ᵗʰ **S36.522 Contusion of** descending [left] colon
      ☑7ᵗʰ **S36.523 Contusion of** sigmoid colon
      ☑7ᵗʰ **S36.528 Contusion of other part of colon**
      ☑7ᵗʰ **S36.529 Contusion of unspecified part of colon**
    ☑6ᵗʰ **S36.53 Laceration of colon**
      ☑7ᵗʰ **S36.530 Laceration of** ascending [right] colon
      ☑7ᵗʰ **S36.531 Laceration of** transverse colon
      ☑7ᵗʰ **S36.532 Laceration of** descending [left] colon
      ☑7ᵗʰ **S36.533 Laceration of** sigmoid colon
      ☑7ᵗʰ **S36.538 Laceration of other part of colon**
      ☑7ᵗʰ **S36.539 Laceration of unspecified part of colon**
    ☑6ᵗʰ **S36.59 Other injury of colon**
      Secondary blast injury of colon
      ☑7ᵗʰ **S36.590 Other injury of** ascending [right] colon
      ☑7ᵗʰ **S36.591 Other injury of** transverse colon
      ☑7ᵗʰ **S36.592 Other injury of** descending [left] colon
      ☑7ᵗʰ **S36.593 Other injury of** sigmoid colon
      ☑7ᵗʰ **S36.598 Other injury of other part of colon**
      ☑7ᵗʰ **S36.599 Other injury of unspecified part of colon**

☑5ᵗʰ **S36.6 Injury of** rectum
    ☑x7ᵗʰ **S36.60 Unspecified injury of rectum**
    ☑x7ᵗʰ **S36.61 Primary blast injury of rectum**
      Blast injury of rectum NOS
    ☑x7ᵗʰ **S36.62 Contusion of rectum**
    ☑x7ᵗʰ **S36.63 Laceration of rectum**
    ☑x7ᵗʰ **S36.69 Other injury of rectum**
      Secondary blast injury of rectum

☑5ᵗʰ **S36.8 Injury of other intra-abdominal organs**
    ☑x7ᵗʰ **S36.81 Injury of** peritoneum
    ☑6ᵗʰ **S36.89 Injury of other intra-abdominal organs**
      Injury of retroperitoneum
      ☑7ᵗʰ **S36.892 Contusion of other intra-abdominal organs**
      ☑7ᵗʰ **S36.893 Laceration of other intra-abdominal organs**
      ☑7ᵗʰ **S36.898 Other injury of other intra-abdominal organs**
      ☑7ᵗʰ **S36.899 Unspecified injury of other intra-abdominal organs**

☑5ᵗʰ **S36.9 Injury of unspecified intra-abdominal organ**
    ☑x7ᵗʰ **S36.90 Unspecified injury of unspecified intra-abdominal organ**
    ☑x7ᵗʰ **S36.92 Contusion of unspecified intra-abdominal organ**
    ☑x7ᵗʰ **S36.93 Laceration of unspecified intra-abdominal organ**
    ☑x7ᵗʰ **S36.99 Other injury of unspecified intra-abdominal organ**

☑4ᵗʰ **S37 Injury of urinary and pelvic organs**
    Code also any associated open wound (S31.-)
    EXCLUDES 1   obstetric trauma to pelvic organs (O71.-)
    EXCLUDES 2   injury of peritoneum (S36.81)
                injury of retroperitoneum (S36.89-)

    The appropriate 7th character is to be added to each code from category S37.
    A   initial encounter
    D   subsequent encounter
    S   sequela

☑5ᵗʰ **S37.0 Injury of** kidney
    EXCLUDES 2   acute kidney injury (nontraumatic) (N17.9)
    ☑6ᵗʰ **S37.00 Unspecified injury of kidney**
      ☑7ᵗʰ **S37.001 Unspecified injury of** right kidney
      ☑7ᵗʰ **S37.002 Unspecified injury of** left kidney
      ☑7ᵗʰ **S37.009 Unspecified injury of unspecified kidney**
    ☑6ᵗʰ **S37.01 Minor contusion of kidney**
      Contusion of kidney less than 2 cm
      Contusion of kidney NOS
      ☑7ᵗʰ **S37.011 Minor contusion of** right kidney
      ☑7ᵗʰ **S37.012 Minor contusion of** left kidney
      ☑7ᵗʰ **S37.019 Minor contusion of unspecified kidney**
    ☑6ᵗʰ **S37.02 Major contusion of kidney**
      Contusion of kidney greater than 2 cm
      ☑7ᵗʰ **S37.021 Major contusion of** right kidney
      ☑7ᵗʰ **S37.022 Major contusion of** left kidney
      ☑7ᵗʰ **S37.029 Major contusion of unspecified kidney**
    ☑6ᵗʰ **S37.03 Laceration of kidney, unspecified degree**
      ☑7ᵗʰ **S37.031 Laceration of** right kidney, unspecified degree
      ☑7ᵗʰ **S37.032 Laceration of** left kidney, unspecified degree
      ☑7ᵗʰ **S37.039 Laceration of unspecified kidney, unspecified degree**
    ☑6ᵗʰ **S37.04 Minor laceration of kidney**
      Laceration of kidney less than 1 cm
      ☑7ᵗʰ **S37.041 Minor laceration of** right kidney
      ☑7ᵗʰ **S37.042 Minor laceration of** left kidney
      ☑7ᵗʰ **S37.049 Minor laceration of unspecified kidney**
    ☑6ᵗʰ **S37.05 Moderate laceration of kidney**
      Laceration of kidney 1 to 3 cm
      ☑7ᵗʰ **S37.051 Moderate laceration of** right kidney
      ☑7ᵗʰ **S37.052 Moderate laceration of** left kidney
      ☑7ᵗʰ **S37.059 Moderate laceration of unspecified kidney**
    ☑6ᵗʰ **S37.06 Major laceration of kidney**
      Avulsion of kidney
      Laceration of kidney greater than 3 cm
      Massive laceration of kidney
      Multiple moderate lacerations of kidney
      Stellate laceration of kidney
      ☑7ᵗʰ **S37.061 Major laceration of** right kidney
      ☑7ᵗʰ **S37.062 Major laceration of** left kidney
      ☑7ᵗʰ **S37.069 Major laceration of unspecified kidney**
    ☑6ᵗʰ **S37.09 Other injury of kidney**
      ☑7ᵗʰ **S37.091 Other injury of** right kidney
      ☑7ᵗʰ **S37.092 Other injury of** left kidney
      ☑7ᵗʰ **S37.099 Other injury of unspecified kidney**

☑5ᵗʰ **S37.1 Injury of** ureter
    ☑x7ᵗʰ **S37.10 Unspecified injury of ureter**
    ☑x7ᵗʰ **S37.12 Contusion of ureter**
    ☑x7ᵗʰ **S37.13 Laceration of ureter**
    ☑x7ᵗʰ **S37.19 Other injury of ureter**

☑ Additional Character Required   ☑x7ᵗʰ Placeholder Alert   Manifestation   Unspecified Dx   ►◄ Revised Text   ● New Code   ▲ Revised Code Title

✓5ᵗʰ S37.2 Injury of bladder
- **✓x7ᵗʰ S37.20 Unspecified injury of bladder**
- **✓x7ᵗʰ S37.22 Contusion of bladder**
- **✓x7ᵗʰ S37.23 Laceration of bladder**
- **✓x7ᵗʰ S37.29 Other injury of bladder**

✓5ᵗʰ S37.3 Injury of urethra
- **✓x7ᵗʰ S37.30 Unspecified injury of urethra**
- **✓x7ᵗʰ S37.32 Contusion of urethra**
- **✓x7ᵗʰ S37.33 Laceration of urethra**
- **✓x7ᵗʰ S37.39 Other injury of urethra**

✓5ᵗʰ S37.4 Injury of ovary
- **✓6ᵗʰ S37.40 Unspecified injury of ovary**
  - **✓7ᵗʰ S37.401 Unspecified injury of ovary, unilateral** ♀
  - **✓7ᵗʰ S37.402 Unspecified injury of ovary, bilateral** ♀
  - **✓7ᵗʰ S37.409 Unspecified injury of ovary, unspecified** ♀
- **✓6ᵗʰ S37.42 Contusion of ovary**
  - **✓7ᵗʰ S37.421 Contusion of ovary, unilateral** ♀
  - **✓7ᵗʰ S37.422 Contusion of ovary, bilateral** ♀
  - **✓7ᵗʰ S37.429 Contusion of ovary, unspecified** ♀
- **✓6ᵗʰ S37.43 Laceration of ovary**
  - **✓7ᵗʰ S37.431 Laceration of ovary, unilateral** ♀
  - **✓7ᵗʰ S37.432 Laceration of ovary, bilateral** ♀
  - **✓7ᵗʰ S37.439 Laceration of ovary, unspecified** ♀
- **✓6ᵗʰ S37.49 Other injury of ovary**
  - **✓7ᵗʰ S37.491 Other injury of ovary, unilateral** ♀
  - **✓7ᵗʰ S37.492 Other injury of ovary, bilateral** ♀
  - **✓7ᵗʰ S37.499 Other injury of ovary, unspecified** ♀

✓5ᵗʰ S37.5 Injury of fallopian tube
- **✓6ᵗʰ S37.50 Unspecified injury of fallopian tube**
  - **✓7ᵗʰ S37.501 Unspecified injury of fallopian tube, unilateral** ♀
  - **✓7ᵗʰ S37.502 Unspecified injury of fallopian tube, bilateral** ♀
  - **✓7ᵗʰ S37.509 Unspecified injury of fallopian tube, unspecified** ♀
- **✓6ᵗʰ S37.51 Primary blast injury of fallopian tube**
  - Blast injury of fallopian tube NOS
  - **✓7ᵗʰ S37.511 Primary blast injury of fallopian tube, unilateral** ♀
  - **✓7ᵗʰ S37.512 Primary blast injury of fallopian tube, bilateral** ♀
  - **✓7ᵗʰ S37.519 Primary blast injury of fallopian tube, unspecified** ♀
- **✓6ᵗʰ S37.52 Contusion of fallopian tube**
  - **✓7ᵗʰ S37.521 Contusion of fallopian tube, unilateral** ♀
  - **✓7ᵗʰ S37.522 Contusion of fallopian tube, bilateral** ♀
  - **✓7ᵗʰ S37.529 Contusion of fallopian tube, unspecified** ♀
- **✓6ᵗʰ S37.53 Laceration of fallopian tube**
  - **✓7ᵗʰ S37.531 Laceration of fallopian tube, unilateral** ♀
  - **✓7ᵗʰ S37.532 Laceration of fallopian tube, bilateral** ♀
  - **✓7ᵗʰ S37.539 Laceration of fallopian tube, unspecified** ♀
- **✓6ᵗʰ S37.59 Other injury of fallopian tube**
  - Secondary blast injury of fallopian tube
  - **✓7ᵗʰ S37.591 Other injury of fallopian tube, unilateral** ♀
  - **✓7ᵗʰ S37.592 Other injury of fallopian tube, bilateral** ♀
  - **✓7ᵗʰ S37.599 Other injury of fallopian tube, unspecified** ♀

✓5ᵗʰ S37.6 Injury of uterus
- EXCLUDES 1 injury to gravid uterus (O9A.2-)
  - injury to uterus during delivery (O71.-)
- **✓x7ᵗʰ S37.60 Unspecified injury of uterus** ♀
- **✓x7ᵗʰ S37.62 Contusion of uterus** ♀

✓x7ᵗʰ S37.63 Laceration of uterus ♀
✓x7ᵗʰ S37.69 Other injury of uterus ♀

✓5ᵗʰ S37.8 Injury of other urinary and pelvic organs
- **✓6ᵗʰ S37.81 Injury of adrenal gland**
  - **✓7ᵗʰ S37.812 Contusion of adrenal gland**
  - **✓7ᵗʰ S37.813 Laceration of adrenal gland**
  - **✓7ᵗʰ S37.818 Other injury of adrenal gland**
  - **✓7ᵗʰ S37.819 Unspecified injury of adrenal gland**
- **✓6ᵗʰ S37.82 Injury of prostate**
  - **✓7ᵗʰ S37.822 Contusion of prostate** ♂
  - **✓7ᵗʰ S37.823 Laceration of prostate** ♂
  - **✓7ᵗʰ S37.828 Other injury of prostate** ♂
  - **✓7ᵗʰ S37.829 Unspecified injury of prostate** ♂
- **✓6ᵗʰ S37.89 Injury of other urinary and pelvic organ**
  - **✓7ᵗʰ S37.892 Contusion of other urinary and pelvic organ**
  - **✓7ᵗʰ S37.893 Laceration of other urinary and pelvic organ**
  - **✓7ᵗʰ S37.898 Other injury of other urinary and pelvic organ**
  - **✓7ᵗʰ S37.899 Unspecified injury of other urinary and pelvic organ**

✓5ᵗʰ S37.9 Injury of unspecified urinary and pelvic organ
- **✓x7ᵗʰ S37.90 Unspecified injury of unspecified urinary and pelvic organ**
- **✓x7ᵗʰ S37.92 Contusion of unspecified urinary and pelvic organ**
- **✓x7ᵗʰ S37.93 Laceration of unspecified urinary and pelvic organ**
- **✓x7ᵗʰ S37.99 Other injury of unspecified urinary and pelvic organ**

✓4ᵗʰ S38 Crushing injury and traumatic amputation of abdomen, lower back, pelvis and external genitals

> NOTE An amputation not identified as partial or complete should be coded to complete

> The appropriate 7th character is to be added to each code from category S38.
> A initial encounter
> D subsequent encounter
> S sequela

✓5ᵗʰ S38.0 Crushing injury of external genital organs
- Use additional code for any associated injuries
- **✓6ᵗʰ S38.00 Crushing injury of unspecified external genital organs**
  - **✓7ᵗʰ S38.001 Crushing injury of unspecified external genital organs, male** ♂
  - **✓7ᵗʰ S38.002 Crushing injury of unspecified external genital organs, female** ♀
- **✓x7ᵗʰ S38.01 Crushing injury of penis** ♂
- **✓x7ᵗʰ S38.02 Crushing injury of scrotum and testis** ♂
- **✓x7ᵗʰ S38.03 Crushing injury of vulva** ♀

✓x7ᵗʰ S38.1 Crushing injury of abdomen, lower back, and pelvis
- Use additional code for all associated injuries, such as:
  - fracture of thoracic or lumbar spine and pelvis (S22.0-, S32.-)
  - injury to intra-abdominal organs (S36.-)
  - injury to urinary and pelvic organs (S37.-)
  - open wound of abdominal wall (S31.-)
  - spinal cord injury (S34.0, S34.1-)
  - EXCLUDES 2 crushing injury of external genital organs (S38.0-)

✓5ᵗʰ S38.2 Traumatic amputation of external genital organs
- **✓6ᵗʰ S38.21 Traumatic amputation of female external genital organs**
  - Traumatic amputation of clitoris
  - Traumatic amputation of labium (majus) (minus)
  - Traumatic amputation of vulva
  - **✓7ᵗʰ S38.211 Complete traumatic amputation of female external genital organs** ♀
  - **✓7ᵗʰ S38.212 Partial traumatic amputation of female external genital organs** ♀
- **✓6ᵗʰ S38.22 Traumatic amputation of penis**
  - **✓7ᵗʰ S38.221 Complete traumatic amputation of penis** ♂
  - **✓7ᵗʰ S38.222 Partial traumatic amputation of penis** ♂

☑6ᵗʰ **S38.23** **Traumatic amputation of** scrotum and testis

     ☑7ᵗʰ **S38.231** **Complete** traumatic amputation of scrotum and testis   ♂

     ☑7ᵗʰ **S38.232** **Partial** traumatic amputation of scrotum and testis   ♂

☑×7ᵗʰ **S38.3** **Transection (partial) of abdomen**

☑4ᵗʰ **S39** **Other and unspecified injuries of abdomen, lower back, pelvis and external genitals**

     Code also any associated open wound (S31.-)

     EXCLUDES 2   sprain of joints and ligaments of lumbar spine and pelvis (S33.-)

> The appropriate 7th character is to be added to each code from category S39.
> A   initial encounter
> D   subsequent encounter
> S   sequela

☑5ᵗʰ **S39.0** **Injury of muscle, fascia and tendon of abdomen, lower back and pelvis**

     ☑6ᵗʰ **S39.00** **Unspecified injury of muscle, fascia and tendon of abdomen, lower back and pelvis**

         ☑7ᵗʰ **S39.001** **Unspecified injury of muscle, fascia and tendon of** abdomen

         ☑7ᵗʰ **S39.002** **Unspecified injury of muscle, fascia and tendon of** lower back

         ☑7ᵗʰ **S39.003** **Unspecified injury of muscle, fascia and tendon of** pelvis

     ☑6ᵗʰ **S39.01** **Strain of muscle, fascia and tendon of abdomen, lower back and pelvis**

         ☑7ᵗʰ **S39.011** **Strain of muscle, fascia and tendon of** abdomen

         ☑7ᵗʰ **S39.012** **Strain of muscle, fascia and tendon of** lower back

         ☑7ᵗʰ **S39.013** **Strain of muscle, fascia and tendon of** pelvis

     ☑6ᵗʰ **S39.02** **Laceration of muscle, fascia and tendon of abdomen, lower back and pelvis**

         ☑7ᵗʰ **S39.021** **Laceration of muscle, fascia and tendon of** abdomen

         ☑7ᵗʰ **S39.022** **Laceration of muscle, fascia and tendon of** lower back

         ☑7ᵗʰ **S39.023** **Laceration of muscle, fascia and tendon of** pelvis

     ☑6ᵗʰ **S39.09** **Other injury of muscle, fascia and tendon of abdomen, lower back and pelvis**

         ☑7ᵗʰ **S39.091** **Other injury of muscle, fascia and tendon of** abdomen

         ☑7ᵗʰ **S39.092** **Other injury of muscle, fascia and tendon of** lower back

         ☑7ᵗʰ **S39.093** **Other injury of muscle, fascia and tendon of** pelvis

☑5ᵗʰ **S39.8** **Other specified injuries of abdomen, lower back, pelvis and external genitals**

     ☑×7ᵗʰ **S39.81** **Other specified injuries of** abdomen

     ☑×7ᵗʰ **S39.82** **Other specified injuries of** lower back

     ☑×7ᵗʰ **S39.83** **Other specified injuries of** pelvis

     ☑6ᵗʰ **S39.84** **Other specified injuries of** external genitals

         ☑7ᵗʰ **S39.840** **Fracture of** corpus cavernosum penis   ♂

         ☑7ᵗʰ **S39.848** **Other specified injuries of external genitals**

             TIP: Assign for traumatic rupture of testis.

☑5ᵗʰ **S39.9** **Unspecified injury of abdomen, lower back, pelvis and external genitals**

     ☑×7ᵗʰ **S39.91** **Unspecified injury of** abdomen

     ☑×7ᵗʰ **S39.92** **Unspecified injury of** lower back

     ☑×7ᵗʰ **S39.93** **Unspecified injury of** pelvis

     ☑×7ᵗʰ **S39.94** **Unspecified injury of** external genitals

Injuries to the shoulder and upper arm (S40-S49)

INCLUDES   injuries of axilla
           injuries of scapular region

EXCLUDES 2   burns and corrosions (T20-T32)
           frostbite (T33-T34)
           injuries of elbow (S50-S59)
           insect bite or sting, venomous (T63.4)

☑4ᵗʰ **S40** **Superficial injury of shoulder and upper arm**

> The appropriate 7th character is to be added to each code from category S40.
> A   initial encounter
> D   subsequent encounter
> S   sequela

☑5ᵗʰ **S40.0** **Contusion of shoulder and upper arm**

     ☑6ᵗʰ **S40.01** **Contusion of** shoulder

         ☑7ᵗʰ **S40.011** **Contusion of** right **shoulder**

         ☑7ᵗʰ **S40.012** **Contusion of** left **shoulder**

         ☑7ᵗʰ **S40.019** **Contusion of unspecified shoulder**

     ☑6ᵗʰ **S40.02** **Contusion of** upper arm

         ☑7ᵗʰ **S40.021** **Contusion of** right **upper arm**

         ☑7ᵗʰ **S40.022** **Contusion of** left **upper arm**

         ☑7ᵗʰ **S40.029** **Contusion of unspecified upper arm**

☑5ᵗʰ **S40.2** **Other superficial injuries of** shoulder

     ☑6ᵗʰ **S40.21** **Abrasion** of shoulder

         ☑7ᵗʰ **S40.211** **Abrasion of** right **shoulder**

         ☑7ᵗʰ **S40.212** **Abrasion of** left **shoulder**

         ☑7ᵗʰ **S40.219** **Abrasion of unspecified shoulder**

     ☑6ᵗʰ **S40.22** **Blister (nonthermal) of shoulder**

         ☑7ᵗʰ **S40.221** **Blister (nonthermal) of** right **shoulder**

         ☑7ᵗʰ **S40.222** **Blister (nonthermal) of** left **shoulder**

         ☑7ᵗʰ **S40.229** **Blister (nonthermal) of unspecified shoulder**

     ☑6ᵗʰ **S40.24** **External constriction of shoulder**

         ☑7ᵗʰ **S40.241** **External constriction of** right **shoulder**

         ☑7ᵗʰ **S40.242** **External constriction of** left **shoulder**

         ☑7ᵗʰ **S40.249** **External constriction of unspecified shoulder**

     ☑6ᵗʰ **S40.25** **Superficial foreign body of shoulder**

         Splinter in the shoulder

         ☑7ᵗʰ **S40.251** **Superficial foreign body of** right **shoulder**

         ☑7ᵗʰ **S40.252** **Superficial foreign body of** left **shoulder**

         ☑7ᵗʰ **S40.259** **Superficial foreign body of unspecified shoulder**

     ☑6ᵗʰ **S40.26** **Insect bite (nonvenomous) of shoulder**

         ☑7ᵗʰ **S40.261** **Insect bite (nonvenomous) of** right **shoulder**

         ☑7ᵗʰ **S40.262** **Insect bite (nonvenomous) of** left **shoulder**

         ☑7ᵗʰ **S40.269** **Insect bite (nonvenomous) of unspecified shoulder** ·

     ☑6ᵗʰ **S40.27** **Other superficial bite of shoulder**

         EXCLUDES 1   open bite of shoulder (S41.05)

         ☑7ᵗʰ **S40.271** **Other superficial bite of** right **shoulder**

         ☑7ᵗʰ **S40.272** **Other superficial bite of** left **shoulder**

         ☑7ᵗʰ **S40.279** **Other superficial bite of unspecified shoulder**

☑5ᵗʰ **S40.8** **Other superficial injuries of** upper arm

     ☑6ᵗʰ **S40.81** **Abrasion** of upper arm

         ☑7ᵗʰ **S40.811** **Abrasion of** right **upper arm**

         ☑7ᵗʰ **S40.812** **Abrasion of** left **upper arm**

         ☑7ᵗʰ **S40.819** **Abrasion of unspecified upper arm**

     ☑6ᵗʰ **S40.82** **Blister (nonthermal) of upper arm**

         ☑7ᵗʰ **S40.821** **Blister (nonthermal) of** right **upper arm**

         ☑7ᵗʰ **S40.822** **Blister (nonthermal) of** left **upper arm**

         ☑7ᵗʰ **S40.829** **Blister (nonthermal) of unspecified upper arm**

     ☑6ᵗʰ **S40.84** **External constriction of upper arm**

         ☑7ᵗʰ **S40.841** **External constriction of** right **upper arm**

         ☑7ᵗʰ **S40.842** **External constriction of** left **upper arm**

☑ Additional Character Required   ☑×7ᵗʰ Placeholder Alert   Manifestation   Unspecified Dx   ►◄ Revised Text   ● New Code   ▲ Revised Code Title

ICD-10-CM 2020   995

☑7th **S40.849** External constriction of unspecified upper arm

☑6th **S40.85** Superficial foreign body of upper arm
Splinter in the upper arm

☑7th **S40.851** Superficial foreign body of right upper arm

☑7th **S40.852** Superficial foreign body of left upper arm

☑7th **S40.859** Superficial foreign body of unspecified upper arm

☑6th **S40.86** Insect bite (nonvenomous) of upper arm

☑7th **S40.861** Insect bite (nonvenomous) of right upper arm

☑7th **S40.862** Insect bite (nonvenomous) of left upper arm

☑7th **S40.869** Insect bite (nonvenomous) of unspecified upper arm

☑6th **S40.87** Other superficial bite of upper arm
EXCLUDES 1   open bite of upper arm (S41.14)
EXCLUDES 2   other superficial bite of shoulder (S40.27-)

☑7th **S40.871** Other superficial bite of right upper arm

☑7th **S40.872** Other superficial bite of left upper arm

☑7th **S40.879** Other superficial bite of unspecified upper arm

☑5th **S40.9** Unspecified superficial injury of shoulder and upper arm

☑6th **S40.91** Unspecified superficial injury of shoulder

☑7th **S40.911** Unspecified superficial injury of right shoulder

☑7th **S40.912** Unspecified superficial injury of left shoulder

☑7th **S40.919** Unspecified superficial injury of unspecified shoulder

☑6th **S40.92** Unspecified superficial injury of upper arm

☑7th **S40.921** Unspecified superficial injury of right upper arm

☑7th **S40.922** Unspecified superficial injury of left upper arm

☑7th **S40.929** Unspecified superficial injury of unspecified upper arm

☑4th **S41** **Open wound of shoulder and upper arm**
Code also any associated wound infection
EXCLUDES 1   traumatic amputation of shoulder and upper arm (S48.-)
EXCLUDES 2   open fracture of shoulder and upper arm (S42.- with 7th character B or C)

The appropriate 7th character is to be added to each code from category S41.
A   initial encounter
D   subsequent encounter
S   sequela

☑5th **S41.0** Open wound of shoulder

☑6th **S41.00** Unspecified open wound of shoulder

☑7th **S41.001** Unspecified open wound of right shoulder

☑7th **S41.002** Unspecified open wound of left shoulder

☑7th **S41.009** Unspecified open wound of unspecified shoulder

☑6th **S41.01** Laceration without foreign body of shoulder

☑7th **S41.011** Laceration without foreign body of right shoulder

☑7th **S41.012** Laceration without foreign body of left shoulder

☑7th **S41.019** Laceration without foreign body of unspecified shoulder

☑6th **S41.02** Laceration with foreign body of shoulder

☑7th **S41.021** Laceration with foreign body of right shoulder

☑7th **S41.022** Laceration with foreign body of left shoulder

☑7th **S41.029** Laceration with foreign body of unspecified shoulder

☑6th **S41.03** Puncture wound without foreign body of shoulder

☑7th **S41.031** Puncture wound without foreign body of right shoulder

☑7th **S41.032** Puncture wound without foreign body of left shoulder

☑7th **S41.039** Puncture wound without foreign body of unspecified shoulder

☑6th **S41.04** Puncture wound with foreign body of shoulder

☑7th **S41.041** Puncture wound with foreign body of right shoulder

☑7th **S41.042** Puncture wound with foreign body of left shoulder

☑7th **S41.049** Puncture wound with foreign body of unspecified shoulder

☑6th **S41.05** Open bite of shoulder
Bite of shoulder NOS
EXCLUDES 1   superficial bite of shoulder (S40.27)

☑7th **S41.051** Open bite of right shoulder

☑7th **S41.052** Open bite of left shoulder

☑7th **S41.059** Open bite of unspecified shoulder

☑5th **S41.1** Open wound of upper arm

☑6th **S41.10** Unspecified open wound of upper arm
AHA: 2016,3Q,24

☑7th **S41.101** Unspecified open wound of right upper arm

☑7th **S41.102** Unspecified open wound of left upper arm

☑7th **S41.109** Unspecified open wound of unspecified upper arm

☑6th **S41.11** Laceration without foreign body of upper arm

☑7th **S41.111** Laceration without foreign body of right upper arm

☑7th **S41.112** Laceration without foreign body of left upper arm

☑7th **S41.119** Laceration without foreign body of unspecified upper arm

☑6th **S41.12** Laceration with foreign body of upper arm

☑7th **S41.121** Laceration with foreign body of right upper arm

☑7th **S41.122** Laceration with foreign body of left upper arm

☑7th **S41.129** Laceration with foreign body of unspecified upper arm

☑6th **S41.13** Puncture wound without foreign body of upper arm
AHA: 2016,3Q,24

☑7th **S41.131** Puncture wound without foreign body of right upper arm

☑7th **S41.132** Puncture wound without foreign body of left upper arm

☑7th **S41.139** Puncture wound without foreign body of unspecified upper arm

☑6th **S41.14** Puncture wound with foreign body of upper arm
AHA: 2016,3Q,24

☑7th **S41.141** Puncture wound with foreign body of right upper arm

☑7th **S41.142** Puncture wound with foreign body of left upper arm

☑7th **S41.149** Puncture wound with foreign body of unspecified upper arm

☑6th **S41.15** Open bite of upper arm
Bite of upper arm NOS
EXCLUDES 1   superficial bite of upper arm (S40.87)

☑7th **S41.151** Open bite of right upper arm

☑7th **S41.152** Open bite of left upper arm

☑7th **S41.159** Open bite of unspecified upper arm

✓4th S42 Fracture of shoulder and upper arm

> **NOTE**   A fracture not indicated as displaced or nondisplaced should be coded to displaced
>
> A fracture not indicated as open or closed should be coded to closed

EXCLUDES 1   traumatic amputation of shoulder and upper arm (S48.-)

AHA: 2018,2Q,12; 2015,3Q,37-39

DEF: Diaphysis: Central shaft of a long bone.

DEF: Epiphysis: Proximal and distal rounded ends of a long bone, communicates with the joint.

DEF: Metaphysis: Section of a long bone located between the epiphysis and diaphysis at the proximal and distal ends.

DEF: Physis (growth plate): Narrow zone of cartilaginous tissue between the epiphysis and metaphysis at each end of a long bone. In childhood, proliferation of cells in this zone lengthens the bone. As the bone matures, this area thins, ossification eventually fusing into solid bone and growth stops. *Synonyms: Epiphyseal plate.*

The appropriate 7th character is to be added to all codes from category S42 [unless otherwise indicated].

- A   initial encounter for closed fracture
- B   initial encounter for open fracture
- D   subsequent encounter for fracture with routine healing
- G   subsequent encounter for fracture with delayed healing
- K   subsequent encounter for fracture with nonunion
- P   subsequent encounter for fracture with malunion
- S   sequela

✓5th S42.0 Fracture of clavicle

✓6th S42.00 Fracture of unspecified part of clavicle

- ✓7th **S42.001** Fracture of unspecified part of right clavicle   Q
- ✓7th **S42.002** Fracture of unspecified part of left clavicle   Q
- ✓7th **S42.009** Fracture of unspecified part of unspecified clavicle   Q
  - AHA: 2012,4Q,93

✓6th S42.01 Fracture of sternal end of clavicle

- ✓7th **S42.011** Anterior displaced fracture of sternal end of right clavicle   Q
- ✓7th **S42.012** Anterior displaced fracture of sternal end of left clavicle   Q
- ✓7th **S42.013** Anterior displaced fracture of sternal end of unspecified clavicle   Q
  - Displaced fracture of sternal end of clavicle NOS
- ✓7th **S42.014** Posterior displaced fracture of sternal end of right clavicle   Q
- ✓7th **S42.015** Posterior displaced fracture of sternal end of left clavicle   Q
- ✓7th **S42.016** Posterior displaced fracture of sternal end of unspecified clavicle   Q
- ✓7th **S42.017** Nondisplaced fracture of sternal end of right clavicle   Q
- ✓7th **S42.018** Nondisplaced fracture of sternal end of left clavicle   Q
- ✓7th **S42.019** Nondisplaced fracture of sternal end of unspecified clavicle   Q

✓6th S42.02 Fracture of shaft of clavicle

- ✓7th **S42.021** Displaced fracture of shaft of right clavicle   Q
- ✓7th **S42.022** Displaced fracture of shaft of left clavicle   Q
- ✓7th **S42.023** Displaced fracture of shaft of unspecified clavicle   Q
- ✓7th **S42.024** Nondisplaced fracture of shaft of right clavicle   Q
- ✓7th **S42.025** Nondisplaced fracture of shaft of left clavicle   Q
- ✓7th **S42.026** Nondisplaced fracture of shaft of unspecified clavicle   Q

✓6th S42.03 Fracture of lateral end of clavicle

Fracture of acromial end of clavicle

- ✓7th **S42.031** Displaced fracture of lateral end of right clavicle   Q
- ✓7th **S42.032** Displaced fracture of lateral end of left clavicle   Q
- ✓7th **S42.033** Displaced fracture of lateral end of unspecified clavicle   Q
- ✓7th **S42.034** Nondisplaced fracture of lateral end of right clavicle   Q

- ✓7th **S42.035** Nondisplaced fracture of lateral end of left clavicle   Q
- ✓7th **S42.036** Nondisplaced fracture of lateral end of unspecified clavicle   Q

✓5th S42.1 Fracture of scapula

✓6th S42.10 Fracture of unspecified part of scapula

- ✓7th **S42.101** Fracture of unspecified part of scapula, right shoulder   Q
- ✓7th **S42.102** Fracture of unspecified part of scapula, left shoulder   Q
- ✓7th **S42.109** Fracture of unspecified part of scapula, unspecified shoulder   Q

✓6th S42.11 Fracture of body of scapula

- ✓7th **S42.111** Displaced fracture of body of scapula, right shoulder   Q
- ✓7th **S42.112** Displaced fracture of body of scapula, left shoulder   Q
- ✓7th **S42.113** Displaced fracture of body of scapula, unspecified shoulder   Q
- ✓7th **S42.114** Nondisplaced fracture of body of scapula, right shoulder   Q
- ✓7th **S42.115** Nondisplaced fracture of body of scapula, left shoulder   Q
- ✓7th **S42.116** Nondisplaced fracture of body of scapula, unspecified shoulder   Q

✓6th S42.12 Fracture of acromial process

- ✓7th **S42.121** Displaced fracture of acromial process, right shoulder   Q
- ✓7th **S42.122** Displaced fracture of acromial process, left shoulder   Q
- ✓7th **S42.123** Displaced fracture of acromial process, unspecified shoulder   Q
- ✓7th **S42.124** Nondisplaced fracture of acromial process, right shoulder   Q
- ✓7th **S42.125** Nondisplaced fracture of acromial process, left shoulder   Q
- ✓7th **S42.126** Nondisplaced fracture of acromial process, unspecified shoulder   Q

✓6th S42.13 Fracture of coracoid process

- ✓7th **S42.131** Displaced fracture of coracoid process, right shoulder   Q
- ✓7th **S42.132** Displaced fracture of coracoid process, left shoulder   Q
- ✓7th **S42.133** Displaced fracture of coracoid process, unspecified shoulder   Q
- ✓7th **S42.134** Nondisplaced fracture of coracoid process, right shoulder   Q
- ✓7th **S42.135** Nondisplaced fracture of coracoid process, left shoulder   Q
- ✓7th **S42.136** Nondisplaced fracture of coracoid process, unspecified shoulder   Q

✓6th S42.14 Fracture of glenoid cavity of scapula

- ✓7th **S42.141** Displaced fracture of glenoid cavity of scapula, right shoulder   Q
- ✓7th **S42.142** Displaced fracture of glenoid cavity of scapula, left shoulder   Q
- ✓7th **S42.143** Displaced fracture of glenoid cavity of scapula, unspecified shoulder   Q
- ✓7th **S42.144** Nondisplaced fracture of glenoid cavity of scapula, right shoulder   Q
- ✓7th **S42.145** Nondisplaced fracture of glenoid cavity of scapula, left shoulder   Q
- ✓7th **S42.146** Nondisplaced fracture of glenoid cavity of scapula, unspecified shoulder   Q

✓6th S42.15 Fracture of neck of scapula

- ✓7th **S42.151** Displaced fracture of neck of scapula, right shoulder   Q
- ✓7th **S42.152** Displaced fracture of neck of scapula, left shoulder   Q
- ✓7th **S42.153** Displaced fracture of neck of scapula, unspecified shoulder   Q
- ✓7th **S42.154** Nondisplaced fracture of neck of scapula, right shoulder   Q
- ✓7th **S42.155** Nondisplaced fracture of neck of scapula, left shoulder   Q
- ✓7th **S42.156** Nondisplaced fracture of neck of scapula, unspecified shoulder   Q

☑ Additional Character Required   ✓x7th Placeholder Alert   Manifestation   Unspecified Dx   ▶◀ Revised Text   ● New Code   ▲ Revised Code Title

ICD-10-CM 2020   997

✓6ᵗʰ **S42.19   Fracture of other part of scapula**

   ✓7ᵗʰ **S42.191   Fracture of other part of scapula, right shoulder** Q

   ✓7ᵗʰ **S42.192   Fracture of other part of scapula, left shoulder** Q

   ✓7ᵗʰ **S42.199   Fracture of other part of scapula, unspecified shoulder** Q

✓5ᵗʰ **S42.2   Fracture of upper end of humerus**

Fracture of proximal end of humerus

   EXCLUDES 2   *fracture of shaft of humerus (S42.3-)*

        physeal fracture of upper end of humerus (S49.0-)

✓6ᵗʰ **S42.20   Unspecified fracture of upper end of humerus**

   ✓7ᵗʰ **S42.201   Unspecified fracture of upper end of right humerus** Q

   ✓7ᵗʰ **S42.202   Unspecified fracture of upper end of left humerus** Q

   ✓7ᵗʰ **S42.209   Unspecified fracture of upper end of unspecified humerus** Q

✓6ᵗʰ **S42.21   Unspecified fracture of surgical neck of humerus**

Fracture of neck of humerus NOS

   ✓7ᵗʰ **S42.211   Unspecified displaced fracture of surgical neck of right humerus** Q

   ✓7ᵗʰ **S42.212   Unspecified displaced fracture of surgical neck of left humerus** Q

   ✓7ᵗʰ **S42.213   Unspecified displaced fracture of surgical neck of unspecified humerus** Q

   ✓7ᵗʰ **S42.214   Unspecified nondisplaced fracture of surgical neck of right humerus** Q

   ✓7ᵗʰ **S42.215   Unspecified nondisplaced fracture of surgical neck of left humerus** Q

   ✓7ᵗʰ **S42.216   Unspecified nondisplaced fracture of surgical neck of unspecified humerus** Q

✓6ᵗʰ **S42.22   2-part fracture of surgical neck of humerus**

   ✓7ᵗʰ **S42.221   2-part displaced fracture of surgical neck of right humerus** Q

   ✓7ᵗʰ **S42.222   2-part displaced fracture of surgical neck of left humerus** Q

   ✓7ᵗʰ **S42.223   2-part displaced fracture of surgical neck of unspecified humerus** Q

   ✓7ᵗʰ **S42.224   2-part nondisplaced fracture of surgical neck of right humerus** Q

   ✓7ᵗʰ **S42.225   2-part nondisplaced fracture of surgical neck of left humerus** Q

   ✓7ᵗʰ **S42.226   2-part nondisplaced fracture of surgical neck of unspecified humerus** Q

✓6ᵗʰ **S42.23   3-part fracture of surgical neck of humerus**

   ✓7ᵗʰ **S42.231   3-part fracture of surgical neck of right humerus** Q

   ✓7ᵗʰ **S42.232   3-part fracture of surgical neck of left humerus** Q

   ✓7ᵗʰ **S42.239   3-part fracture of surgical neck of unspecified humerus** Q

✓6ᵗʰ **S42.24   4-part fracture of surgical neck of humerus**

   ✓7ᵗʰ **S42.241   4-part fracture of surgical neck of right humerus** Q

   ✓7ᵗʰ **S42.242   4-part fracture of surgical neck of left humerus** Q

   ✓7ᵗʰ **S42.249   4-part fracture of surgical neck of unspecified humerus** Q

✓6ᵗʰ **S42.25   Fracture of greater tuberosity of humerus**

   ✓7ᵗʰ **S42.251   Displaced fracture of greater tuberosity of right humerus** Q

   ✓7ᵗʰ **S42.252   Displaced fracture of greater tuberosity of left humerus** Q

   ✓7ᵗʰ **S42.253   Displaced fracture of greater tuberosity of unspecified humerus** Q

   ✓7ᵗʰ **S42.254   Nondisplaced fracture of greater tuberosity of right humerus** Q

   ✓7ᵗʰ **S42.255   Nondisplaced fracture of greater tuberosity of left humerus** Q

   ✓7ᵗʰ **S42.256   Nondisplaced fracture of greater tuberosity of unspecified humerus** Q

✓6ᵗʰ **S42.26   Fracture of lesser tuberosity of humerus**

   ✓7ᵗʰ **S42.261   Displaced fracture of lesser tuberosity of right humerus** Q

   ✓7ᵗʰ **S42.262   Displaced fracture of lesser tuberosity of left humerus** Q

   ✓7ᵗʰ **S42.263   Displaced fracture of lesser tuberosity of unspecified humerus** Q

   ✓7ᵗʰ **S42.264   Nondisplaced fracture of lesser tuberosity of right humerus** Q

   ✓7ᵗʰ **S42.265   Nondisplaced fracture of lesser tuberosity of left humerus** Q

   ✓7ᵗʰ **S42.266   Nondisplaced fracture of lesser tuberosity of unspecified humerus** Q

✓6ᵗʰ **S42.27   Torus fracture of upper end of humerus**

> The appropriate 7th character is to be added to all codes in subcategory S42.27
> A   initial encounter for closed fracture
> D   subsequent encounter for fracture with routine healing
> G   subsequent encounter for fracture with delayed healing
> K   subsequent encounter for fracture with nonunion
> P   subsequent encounter for fracture with malunion
> S   sequela

   ✓7ᵗʰ **S42.271   Torus fracture of upper end of right humerus** Q

   ✓7ᵗʰ **S42.272   Torus fracture of upper end of left humerus** Q

   ✓7ᵗʰ **S42.279   Torus fracture of upper end of unspecified humerus** Q

✓6ᵗʰ **S42.29   Other fracture of upper end of humerus**

Fracture of anatomical neck of humerus

Fracture of articular head of humerus

AHA: 2019,1Q,18

   ✓7ᵗʰ **S42.291   Other displaced fracture of upper end of right humerus** Q

   ✓7ᵗʰ **S42.292   Other displaced fracture of upper end of left humerus** Q

   ✓7ᵗʰ **S42.293   Other displaced fracture of upper end of unspecified humerus** Q

   ✓7ᵗʰ **S42.294   Other nondisplaced fracture of upper end of right humerus** Q

   ✓7ᵗʰ **S42.295   Other nondisplaced fracture of upper end of left humerus** Q

   ✓7ᵗʰ **S42.296   Other nondisplaced fracture of upper end of unspecified humerus** Q

✓5ᵗʰ **S42.3   Fracture of shaft of humerus**

Fracture of humerus NOS

Fracture of upper arm NOS

   EXCLUDES 2   *physeal fractures of upper end of humerus (S49.0-)*

        physeal fractures of lower end of humerus (S49.1-)

✓6ᵗʰ **S42.30   Unspecified fracture of shaft of humerus**

   ✓7ᵗʰ **S42.301   Unspecified fracture of shaft of humerus, right arm** Q

   ✓7ᵗʰ **S42.302   Unspecified fracture of shaft of humerus, left arm** Q

   ✓7ᵗʰ **S42.309   Unspecified fracture of shaft of humerus, unspecified arm** Q

✓6ᵗʰ **S42.31   Greenstick fracture of shaft of humerus**

> The appropriate 7th character is to be added to all codes in subcategory S42.31
> A   initial encounter for closed fracture
> D   subsequent encounter for fracture with routine healing
> G   subsequent encounter for fracture with delayed healing
> K   subsequent encounter for fracture with nonunion
> P   subsequent encounter for fracture with malunion
> S   sequela

   ✓7ᵗʰ **S42.311   Greenstick fracture of shaft of humerus, right arm** Q

✓7ᵗʰ **S42.312** Greenstick fracture of shaft of humerus, left arm   Q

✓7ᵗʰ **S42.319** Greenstick fracture of shaft of humerus, unspecified arm   Q

✓6ᵗʰ **S42.32** Transverse fracture of shaft of humerus

✓7ᵗʰ **S42.321** Displaced transverse fracture of shaft of humerus, right arm   Q

✓7ᵗʰ **S42.322** Displaced transverse fracture of shaft of humerus, left arm   Q

✓7ᵗʰ **S42.323** Displaced transverse fracture of shaft of humerus, unspecified arm   Q

✓7ᵗʰ **S42.324** Nondisplaced transverse fracture of shaft of humerus, right arm   Q

✓7ᵗʰ **S42.325** Nondisplaced transverse fracture of shaft of humerus, left arm   Q

✓7ᵗʰ **S42.326** Nondisplaced transverse fracture of shaft of humerus, unspecified arm   Q

✓6ᵗʰ **S42.33** Oblique fracture of shaft of humerus

✓7ᵗʰ **S42.331** Displaced oblique fracture of shaft of humerus, right arm   Q

✓7ᵗʰ **S42.332** Displaced oblique fracture of shaft of humerus, left arm   Q

✓7ᵗʰ **S42.333** Displaced oblique fracture of shaft of humerus, unspecified arm   Q

✓7ᵗʰ **S42.334** Nondisplaced oblique fracture of shaft of humerus, right arm   Q

✓7ᵗʰ **S42.335** Nondisplaced oblique fracture of shaft of humerus, left arm   Q

✓7ᵗʰ **S42.336** Nondisplaced oblique fracture of shaft of humerus, unspecified arm   Q

✓6ᵗʰ **S42.34** Spiral fracture of shaft of humerus

✓7ᵗʰ **S42.341** Displaced spiral fracture of shaft of humerus, right arm   Q

✓7ᵗʰ **S42.342** Displaced spiral fracture of shaft of humerus, left arm   Q

✓7ᵗʰ **S42.343** Displaced spiral fracture of shaft of humerus, unspecified arm   Q

✓7ᵗʰ **S42.344** Nondisplaced spiral fracture of shaft of humerus, right arm   Q

✓7ᵗʰ **S42.345** Nondisplaced spiral fracture of shaft of humerus, left arm   Q

✓7ᵗʰ **S42.346** Nondisplaced spiral fracture of shaft of humerus, unspecified arm   Q

✓6ᵗʰ **S42.35** Comminuted fracture of shaft of humerus

✓7ᵗʰ **S42.351** Displaced comminuted fracture of shaft of humerus, right arm   Q

✓7ᵗʰ **S42.352** Displaced comminuted fracture of shaft of humerus, left arm   Q

✓7ᵗʰ **S42.353** Displaced comminuted fracture of shaft of humerus, unspecified arm   Q

✓7ᵗʰ **S42.354** Nondisplaced comminuted fracture of shaft of humerus, right arm   Q

✓7ᵗʰ **S42.355** Nondisplaced comminuted fracture of shaft of humerus, left arm   Q

✓7ᵗʰ **S42.356** Nondisplaced comminuted fracture of shaft of humerus, unspecified arm   Q

✓6ᵗʰ **S42.36** Segmental fracture of shaft of humerus

✓7ᵗʰ **S42.361** Displaced segmental fracture of shaft of humerus, right arm   Q

✓7ᵗʰ **S42.362** Displaced segmental fracture of shaft of humerus, left arm   Q

✓7ᵗʰ **S42.363** Displaced segmental fracture of shaft of humerus, unspecified arm   Q

✓7ᵗʰ **S42.364** Nondisplaced segmental fracture of shaft of humerus, right arm   Q

✓7ᵗʰ **S42.365** Nondisplaced segmental fracture of shaft of humerus, left arm   Q

✓7ᵗʰ **S42.366** Nondisplaced segmental fracture of shaft of humerus, unspecified arm   Q

✓6ᵗʰ **S42.39** Other fracture of shaft of humerus

✓7ᵗʰ **S42.391** Other fracture of shaft of right humerus   Q

✓7ᵗʰ **S42.392** Other fracture of shaft of left humerus   Q

✓7ᵗʰ **S42.399** Other fracture of shaft of unspecified humerus   Q

✓5ᵗʰ **S42.4** Fracture of lower end of humerus

Fracture of distal end of humerus

EXCLUDES 2   fracture of shaft of humerus (S42.3-)

physeal fracture of lower end of humerus (S49.1-)

✓6ᵗʰ **S42.40** Unspecified fracture of lower end of humerus

Fracture of elbow NOS

✓7ᵗʰ **S42.401** Unspecified fracture of lower end of right humerus   Q

✓7ᵗʰ **S42.402** Unspecified fracture of lower end of left humerus   Q

✓7ᵗʰ **S42.409** Unspecified fracture of lower end of unspecified humerus   Q

✓6ᵗʰ **S42.41** Simple supracondylar fracture without intercondylar fracture of humerus

✓7ᵗʰ **S42.411** Displaced simple supracondylar fracture without intercondylar fracture of right humerus   Q

✓7ᵗʰ **S42.412** Displaced simple supracondylar fracture without intercondylar fracture of left humerus   Q

✓7ᵗʰ **S42.413** Displaced simple supracondylar fracture without intercondylar fracture of unspecified humerus   Q

✓7ᵗʰ **S42.414** Nondisplaced simple supracondylar fracture without intercondylar fracture of right humerus   Q

✓7ᵗʰ **S42.415** Nondisplaced simple supracondylar fracture without intercondylar fracture of left humerus   Q

✓7ᵗʰ **S42.416** Nondisplaced simple supracondylar fracture without intercondylar fracture of unspecified humerus   Q

✓6ᵗʰ **S42.42** Comminuted supracondylar fracture without intercondylar fracture of humerus

✓7ᵗʰ **S42.421** Displaced comminuted supracondylar fracture without intercondylar fracture of right humerus   Q

✓7ᵗʰ **S42.422** Displaced comminuted supracondylar fracture without intercondylar fracture of left humerus   Q

✓7ᵗʰ **S42.423** Displaced comminuted supracondylar fracture without intercondylar fracture of unspecified humerus   Q

✓7ᵗʰ **S42.424** Nondisplaced comminuted supracondylar fracture without intercondylar fracture of right humerus   Q

✓7ᵗʰ **S42.425** Nondisplaced comminuted supracondylar fracture without intercondylar fracture of left humerus   Q

✓7ᵗʰ **S42.426** Nondisplaced comminuted supracondylar fracture without intercondylar fracture of unspecified humerus   Q

✓6ᵗʰ **S42.43** Fracture (avulsion) of lateral epicondyle of humerus

✓7ᵗʰ **S42.431** Displaced fracture (avulsion) of lateral epicondyle of right humerus   Q

✓7ᵗʰ **S42.432** Displaced fracture (avulsion) of lateral epicondyle of left humerus   Q

✓7ᵗʰ **S42.433** Displaced fracture (avulsion) of lateral epicondyle of unspecified humerus   Q

✓7ᵗʰ **S42.434** Nondisplaced fracture (avulsion) of lateral epicondyle of right humerus   Q

✓7ᵗʰ **S42.435** Nondisplaced fracture (avulsion) of lateral epicondyle of left humerus   Q

☑ Additional Character Required   ✓ˣ⁷ᵗʰ Placeholder Alert   Manifestation   Unspecified Dx   ▶◀ Revised Text   ● New Code   ▲ Revised Code Title

Chapter 19. Injury, Poisoning and Certain Other Consequences of External Causes

S42.436–S43.006

√7ᵗʰ **S42.436** Nondisplaced fracture (avulsion) of lateral epicondyle of unspecified humerus Q

√6ᵗʰ **S42.44** Fracture (avulsion) of medial epicondyle of humerus

    √7ᵗʰ **S42.441** Displaced fracture (avulsion) of medial epicondyle of right humerus Q

    √7ᵗʰ **S42.442** Displaced fracture (avulsion) of medial epicondyle of left humerus Q

    √7ᵗʰ **S42.443** Displaced fracture (avulsion) of medial epicondyle of unspecified humerus Q

    √7ᵗʰ **S42.444** Nondisplaced fracture (avulsion) of medial epicondyle of right humerus Q

    √7ᵗʰ **S42.445** Nondisplaced fracture (avulsion) of medial epicondyle of left humerus Q

    √7ᵗʰ **S42.446** Nondisplaced fracture (avulsion) of medial epicondyle of unspecified humerus Q

    √7ᵗʰ **S42.447** Incarcerated fracture (avulsion) of medial epicondyle of right humerus Q

    √7ᵗʰ **S42.448** Incarcerated fracture (avulsion) of medial epicondyle of left humerus Q

    √7ᵗʰ **S42.449** Incarcerated fracture (avulsion) of medial epicondyle of unspecified humerus Q

√6ᵗʰ **S42.45** Fracture of lateral condyle of humerus

    Fracture of capitellum of humerus

    √7ᵗʰ **S42.451** Displaced fracture of lateral condyle of right humerus Q

    √7ᵗʰ **S42.452** Displaced fracture of lateral condyle of left humerus Q

    √7ᵗʰ **S42.453** Displaced fracture of lateral condyle of unspecified humerus Q

    √7ᵗʰ **S42.454** Nondisplaced fracture of lateral condyle of right humerus Q

    √7ᵗʰ **S42.455** Nondisplaced fracture of lateral condyle of left humerus Q

    √7ᵗʰ **S42.456** Nondisplaced fracture of lateral condyle of unspecified humerus Q

√6ᵗʰ **S42.46** Fracture of medial condyle of humerus

    Trochlea fracture of humerus

    √7ᵗʰ **S42.461** Displaced fracture of medial condyle of right humerus Q

    √7ᵗʰ **S42.462** Displaced fracture of medial condyle of left humerus Q

    √7ᵗʰ **S42.463** Displaced fracture of medial condyle of unspecified humerus Q

    √7ᵗʰ **S42.464** Nondisplaced fracture of medial condyle of right humerus Q

    √7ᵗʰ **S42.465** Nondisplaced fracture of medial condyle of left humerus Q

    √7ᵗʰ **S42.466** Nondisplaced fracture of medial condyle of unspecified humerus Q

√6ᵗʰ **S42.47** Transcondylar fracture of humerus

    √7ᵗʰ **S42.471** Displaced transcondylar fracture of right humerus Q

    √7ᵗʰ **S42.472** Displaced transcondylar fracture of left humerus Q

    √7ᵗʰ **S42.473** Displaced transcondylar fracture of unspecified humerus Q

    √7ᵗʰ **S42.474** Nondisplaced transcondylar fracture of right humerus Q

    √7ᵗʰ **S42.475** Nondisplaced transcondylar fracture of left humerus Q

    √7ᵗʰ **S42.476** Nondisplaced transcondylar fracture of unspecified humerus Q

√6ᵗʰ **S42.48** Torus fracture of lower end of humerus

> The appropriate 7th character is to be added to all codes in subcategory S42.48.
> A   initial encounter for closed fracture
> D   subsequent encounter for fracture with routine healing
> G   subsequent encounter for fracture with delayed healing
> K   subsequent encounter for fracture with nonunion
> P   subsequent encounter for fracture with malunion
> S   sequela

    √7ᵗʰ **S42.481** Torus fracture of lower end of right humerus Q

    √7ᵗʰ **S42.482** Torus fracture of lower end of left humerus Q

    √7ᵗʰ **S42.489** Torus fracture of lower end of unspecified humerus Q

√6ᵗʰ **S42.49** Other fracture of lower end of humerus

    √7ᵗʰ **S42.491** Other displaced fracture of lower end of right humerus Q

    √7ᵗʰ **S42.492** Other displaced fracture of lower end of left humerus Q

    √7ᵗʰ **S42.493** Other displaced fracture of lower end of unspecified humerus Q

    √7ᵗʰ **S42.494** Other nondisplaced fracture of lower end of right humerus Q

    √7ᵗʰ **S42.495** Other nondisplaced fracture of lower end of left humerus Q

    √7ᵗʰ **S42.496** Other nondisplaced fracture of lower end of unspecified humerus Q

√5ᵗʰ **S42.9** Fracture of shoulder girdle, part unspecified

    Fracture of shoulder NOS

    √x7ᵗʰ **S42.90** Fracture of unspecified shoulder girdle, part unspecified Q

    √x7ᵗʰ **S42.91** Fracture of right shoulder girdle, part unspecified Q

    √x7ᵗʰ **S42.92** Fracture of left shoulder girdle, part unspecified Q

√4ᵗʰ **S43** Dislocation and sprain of joints and ligaments of shoulder girdle

    INCLUDES   avulsion of joint or ligament of shoulder girdle
    laceration of cartilage, joint or ligament of shoulder girdle
    sprain of cartilage, joint or ligament of shoulder girdle
    traumatic hemarthrosis of joint or ligament of shoulder girdle
    traumatic rupture of joint or ligament of shoulder girdle
    traumatic subluxation of joint or ligament of shoulder girdle
    traumatic tear of joint or ligament of shoulder girdle

    Code also any associated open wound

    EXCLUDES 2   *strain of muscle, fascia and tendon of shoulder and upper arm (S46.-)*

> The appropriate 7th character is to be added to each code from category S43.
> A   initial encounter
> D   subsequent encounter
> S   sequela

√5ᵗʰ **S43.0** Subluxation and dislocation of shoulder joint

    Dislocation of glenohumeral joint
    Subluxation of glenohumeral joint

    √6ᵗʰ **S43.00** Unspecified subluxation and dislocation of shoulder joint

        Dislocation of humerus NOS
        Subluxation of humerus NOS

        √7ᵗʰ **S43.001** Unspecified subluxation of right shoulder joint

        √7ᵗʰ **S43.002** Unspecified subluxation of left shoulder joint

        √7ᵗʰ **S43.003** Unspecified subluxation of unspecified shoulder joint

        √7ᵗʰ **S43.004** Unspecified dislocation of right shoulder joint

        √7ᵗʰ **S43.005** Unspecified dislocation of left shoulder joint

        √7ᵗʰ **S43.006** Unspecified dislocation of unspecified shoulder joint

√6ᵗʰ **S43.01** Anterior subluxation and dislocation of humerus
- √7ᵗʰ **S43.011** Anterior subluxation of right humerus
- √7ᵗʰ **S43.012** Anterior subluxation of left humerus
- √7ᵗʰ **S43.013** Anterior subluxation of unspecified humerus
- √7ᵗʰ **S43.014** Anterior dislocation of right humerus
- √7ᵗʰ **S43.015** Anterior dislocation of left humerus
- √7ᵗʰ **S43.016** Anterior dislocation of unspecified humerus

√6ᵗʰ **S43.02** Posterior subluxation and dislocation of humerus
- √7ᵗʰ **S43.021** Posterior subluxation of right humerus
- √7ᵗʰ **S43.022** Posterior subluxation of left humerus
- √7ᵗʰ **S43.023** Posterior subluxation of unspecified humerus
- √7ᵗʰ **S43.024** Posterior dislocation of right humerus
- √7ᵗʰ **S43.025** Posterior dislocation of left humerus
- √7ᵗʰ **S43.026** Posterior dislocation of unspecified humerus

√6ᵗʰ **S43.03** Inferior subluxation and dislocation of humerus
- √7ᵗʰ **S43.031** Inferior subluxation of right humerus
- √7ᵗʰ **S43.032** Inferior subluxation of left humerus
- √7ᵗʰ **S43.033** Inferior subluxation of unspecified humerus
- √7ᵗʰ **S43.034** Inferior dislocation of right humerus
- √7ᵗʰ **S43.035** Inferior dislocation of left humerus
- √7ᵗʰ **S43.036** Inferior dislocation of unspecified humerus

√6ᵗʰ **S43.08** Other subluxation and dislocation of shoulder joint
- √7ᵗʰ **S43.081** Other subluxation of right shoulder joint
- √7ᵗʰ **S43.082** Other subluxation of left shoulder joint
- √7ᵗʰ **S43.083** Other subluxation of unspecified shoulder joint
- √7ᵗʰ **S43.084** Other dislocation of right shoulder joint
- √7ᵗʰ **S43.085** Other dislocation of left shoulder joint
- √7ᵗʰ **S43.086** Other dislocation of unspecified shoulder joint

√5ᵗʰ **S43.1** Subluxation and dislocation of acromioclavicular joint
√6ᵗʰ **S43.10** Unspecified dislocation of acromioclavicular joint
- √7ᵗʰ **S43.101** Unspecified dislocation of right acromioclavicular joint
- √7ᵗʰ **S43.102** Unspecified dislocation of left acromioclavicular joint
- √7ᵗʰ **S43.109** Unspecified dislocation of unspecified acromioclavicular joint

√6ᵗʰ **S43.11** Subluxation of acromioclavicular joint
- √7ᵗʰ **S43.111** Subluxation of right acromioclavicular joint
- √7ᵗʰ **S43.112** Subluxation of left acromioclavicular joint
- √7ᵗʰ **S43.119** Subluxation of unspecified acromioclavicular joint

√6ᵗʰ **S43.12** Dislocation of acromioclavicular joint, 100%-200% displacement
- √7ᵗʰ **S43.121** Dislocation of right acromioclavicular joint, 100%-200% displacement
- √7ᵗʰ **S43.122** Dislocation of left acromioclavicular joint, 100%-200% displacement
- √7ᵗʰ **S43.129** Dislocation of unspecified acromioclavicular joint, 100%-200% displacement

√6ᵗʰ **S43.13** Dislocation of acromioclavicular joint, greater than 200% displacement
- √7ᵗʰ **S43.131** Dislocation of right acromioclavicular joint, greater than 200% displacement
- √7ᵗʰ **S43.132** Dislocation of left acromioclavicular joint, greater than 200% displacement
- √7ᵗʰ **S43.139** Dislocation of unspecified acromioclavicular joint, greater than 200% displacement

√6ᵗʰ **S43.14** Inferior dislocation of acromioclavicular joint
- √7ᵗʰ **S43.141** Inferior dislocation of right acromioclavicular joint
- √7ᵗʰ **S43.142** Inferior dislocation of left acromioclavicular joint
- √7ᵗʰ **S43.149** Inferior dislocation of unspecified acromioclavicular joint

√6ᵗʰ **S43.15** Posterior dislocation of acromioclavicular joint
- √7ᵗʰ **S43.151** Posterior dislocation of right acromioclavicular joint
- √7ᵗʰ **S43.152** Posterior dislocation of left acromioclavicular joint
- √7ᵗʰ **S43.159** Posterior dislocation of unspecified acromioclavicular joint

√5ᵗʰ **S43.2** Subluxation and dislocation of sternoclavicular joint
√6ᵗʰ **S43.20** Unspecified subluxation and dislocation of sternoclavicular joint
- √7ᵗʰ **S43.201** Unspecified subluxation of right sternoclavicular joint
- √7ᵗʰ **S43.202** Unspecified subluxation of left sternoclavicular joint
- √7ᵗʰ **S43.203** Unspecified subluxation of unspecified sternoclavicular joint
- √7ᵗʰ **S43.204** Unspecified dislocation of right sternoclavicular joint
- √7ᵗʰ **S43.205** Unspecified dislocation of left sternoclavicular joint
- √7ᵗʰ **S43.206** Unspecified dislocation of unspecified sternoclavicular joint

√6ᵗʰ **S43.21** Anterior subluxation and dislocation of sternoclavicular joint
- √7ᵗʰ **S43.211** Anterior subluxation of right sternoclavicular joint
- √7ᵗʰ **S43.212** Anterior subluxation of left sternoclavicular joint
- √7ᵗʰ **S43.213** Anterior subluxation of unspecified sternoclavicular joint
- √7ᵗʰ **S43.214** Anterior dislocation of right sternoclavicular joint
- √7ᵗʰ **S43.215** Anterior dislocation of left sternoclavicular joint
- √7ᵗʰ **S43.216** Anterior dislocation of unspecified sternoclavicular joint

√6ᵗʰ **S43.22** Posterior subluxation and dislocation of sternoclavicular joint
- √7ᵗʰ **S43.221** Posterior subluxation of right sternoclavicular joint
- √7ᵗʰ **S43.222** Posterior subluxation of left sternoclavicular joint
- √7ᵗʰ **S43.223** Posterior subluxation of unspecified sternoclavicular joint
- √7ᵗʰ **S43.224** Posterior dislocation of right sternoclavicular joint
- √7ᵗʰ **S43.225** Posterior dislocation of left sternoclavicular joint
- √7ᵗʰ **S43.226** Posterior dislocation of unspecified sternoclavicular joint

√5ᵗʰ **S43.3** Subluxation and dislocation of other and unspecified parts of shoulder girdle
√6ᵗʰ **S43.30** Subluxation and dislocation of unspecified parts of shoulder girdle
  Dislocation of shoulder girdle NOS
  Subluxation of shoulder girdle NOS
- √7ᵗʰ **S43.301** Subluxation of unspecified parts of right shoulder girdle
- √7ᵗʰ **S43.302** Subluxation of unspecified parts of left shoulder girdle
- √7ᵗʰ **S43.303** Subluxation of unspecified parts of unspecified shoulder girdle
- √7ᵗʰ **S43.304** Dislocation of unspecified parts of right shoulder girdle
- √7ᵗʰ **S43.305** Dislocation of unspecified parts of left shoulder girdle
- √7ᵗʰ **S43.306** Dislocation of unspecified parts of unspecified shoulder girdle

√6ᵗʰ **S43.31** Subluxation and dislocation of scapula
- √7ᵗʰ **S43.311** Subluxation of right scapula
- √7ᵗʰ **S43.312** Subluxation of left scapula
- √7ᵗʰ **S43.313** Subluxation of unspecified scapula
- √7ᵗʰ **S43.314** Dislocation of right scapula
- √7ᵗʰ **S43.315** Dislocation of left scapula
- √7ᵗʰ **S43.316** Dislocation of unspecified scapula

√6ᵗʰ **S43.39** Subluxation and dislocation of other parts of shoulder girdle
- √7ᵗʰ **S43.391** Subluxation of other parts of right shoulder girdle
- √7ᵗʰ **S43.392** Subluxation of other parts of left shoulder girdle

      7ᵗʰ S43.393 Subluxation of other parts of unspecified shoulder girdle

      7ᵗʰ S43.394 Dislocation of other parts of **right** shoulder girdle

      7ᵗʰ S43.395 Dislocation of other parts of **left** shoulder girdle

      7ᵗʰ S43.396 Dislocation of other parts of unspecified shoulder girdle

5ᵗʰ S43.4 Sprain of shoulder joint

    6ᵗʰ S43.40 Unspecified sprain of shoulder joint

      7ᵗʰ S43.401 Unspecified sprain of right shoulder joint

      7ᵗʰ S43.402 Unspecified sprain of left shoulder joint

      7ᵗʰ S43.409 Unspecified sprain of unspecified shoulder joint

    6ᵗʰ S43.41 Sprain of coracohumeral (ligament)

      7ᵗʰ S43.411 Sprain of right coracohumeral (ligament)

      7ᵗʰ S43.412 Sprain of left coracohumeral (ligament)

      7ᵗʰ S43.419 Sprain of unspecified coracohumeral (ligament)

    6ᵗʰ S43.42 Sprain of rotator cuff capsule

      EXCLUDES 1   rotator cuff syndrome (complete) (incomplete), not specified as traumatic (M75.1-)

      EXCLUDES 2   injury of tendon of rotator cuff (S46.0-)

      7ᵗʰ S43.421 Sprain of right rotator cuff capsule

      7ᵗʰ S43.422 Sprain of left rotator cuff capsule

      7ᵗʰ S43.429 Sprain of unspecified rotator cuff capsule

    6ᵗʰ S43.43 Superior glenoid labrum lesion

      SLAP lesion

      AHA: 2019,2Q,26

      DEF: Detachment injury of the superior aspect of the glenoid labrum, which is the ring of fibrocartilage attached to the rim of the glenoid cavity of the scapula.

      7ᵗʰ S43.431 Superior glenoid labrum lesion of right shoulder

      7ᵗʰ S43.432 Superior glenoid labrum lesion of left shoulder

      7ᵗʰ S43.439 Superior glenoid labrum lesion of unspecified shoulder

    6ᵗʰ S43.49 Other sprain of shoulder joint

      7ᵗʰ S43.491 Other sprain of right shoulder joint

      7ᵗʰ S43.492 Other sprain of left shoulder joint

      7ᵗʰ S43.499 Other sprain of unspecified shoulder joint

5ᵗʰ S43.5 Sprain of acromioclavicular joint

    Sprain of acromioclavicular ligament

    x7ᵗʰ S43.50 Sprain of unspecified acromioclavicular joint

    x7ᵗʰ S43.51 Sprain of right acromioclavicular joint

    x7ᵗʰ S43.52 Sprain of left acromioclavicular joint

5ᵗʰ S43.6 Sprain of sternoclavicular joint

    x7ᵗʰ S43.60 Sprain of unspecified sternoclavicular joint

    x7ᵗʰ S43.61 Sprain of right sternoclavicular joint

    x7ᵗʰ S43.62 Sprain of left sternoclavicular joint

5ᵗʰ S43.8 Sprain of other specified parts of shoulder girdle

    x7ᵗʰ S43.80 Sprain of other specified parts of unspecified shoulder girdle

    x7ᵗʰ S43.81 Sprain of other specified parts of right shoulder girdle

    x7ᵗʰ S43.82 Sprain of other specified parts of left shoulder girdle

5ᵗʰ S43.9 Sprain of unspecified parts of shoulder girdle

    x7ᵗʰ S43.90 Sprain of unspecified parts of unspecified shoulder girdle

      Sprain of shoulder girdle NOS

    x7ᵗʰ S43.91 Sprain of unspecified parts of right shoulder girdle

    x7ᵗʰ S43.92 Sprain of unspecified parts of left shoulder girdle

4ᵗʰ S44 Injury of nerves at shoulder and upper arm level

Code also any associated open wound (S41.-)

EXCLUDES 2   injury of brachial plexus (S14.3-)

The appropriate 7th character is to be added to each code from category S44.

A   initial encounter
D   subsequent encounter
S   sequela

5ᵗʰ S44.0 Injury of ulnar nerve at upper arm level

    EXCLUDES 1   ulnar nerve NOS (S54.0)

    x7ᵗʰ S44.00 Injury of ulnar nerve at upper arm level, unspecified arm

    x7ᵗʰ S44.01 Injury of ulnar nerve at upper arm level, right arm

    x7ᵗʰ S44.02 Injury of ulnar nerve at upper arm level, left arm

5ᵗʰ S44.1 Injury of median nerve at upper arm level

    EXCLUDES 1   median nerve NOS (S54.1)

    x7ᵗʰ S44.10 Injury of median nerve at upper arm level, unspecified arm

    x7ᵗʰ S44.11 Injury of median nerve at upper arm level, right arm

    x7ᵗʰ S44.12 Injury of median nerve at upper arm level, left arm

5ᵗʰ S44.2 Injury of radial nerve at upper arm level

    EXCLUDES 1   radial nerve NOS (S54.2)

    x7ᵗʰ S44.20 Injury of radial nerve at upper arm level, unspecified arm

    x7ᵗʰ S44.21 Injury of radial nerve at upper arm level, right arm

    x7ᵗʰ S44.22 Injury of radial nerve at upper arm level, left arm

5ᵗʰ S44.3 Injury of axillary nerve

    x7ᵗʰ S44.30 Injury of axillary nerve, unspecified arm

    x7ᵗʰ S44.31 Injury of axillary nerve, right arm

    x7ᵗʰ S44.32 Injury of axillary nerve, left arm

5ᵗʰ S44.4 Injury of musculocutaneous nerve

    x7ᵗʰ S44.40 Injury of musculocutaneous nerve, unspecified arm

    x7ᵗʰ S44.41 Injury of musculocutaneous nerve, right arm

    x7ᵗʰ S44.42 Injury of musculocutaneous nerve, left arm

5ᵗʰ S44.5 Injury of cutaneous sensory nerve at shoulder and upper arm level

    x7ᵗʰ S44.50 Injury of cutaneous sensory nerve at shoulder and upper arm level, unspecified arm

    x7ᵗʰ S44.51 Injury of cutaneous sensory nerve at shoulder and upper arm level, right arm

    x7ᵗʰ S44.52 Injury of cutaneous sensory nerve at shoulder and upper arm level, left arm

5ᵗʰ S44.8 Injury of other nerves at shoulder and upper arm level

    6ᵗʰ S44.8X Injury of other nerves at shoulder and upper arm level

      7ᵗʰ S44.8X1 Injury of other nerves at shoulder and upper arm level, right arm

      7ᵗʰ S44.8X2 Injury of other nerves at shoulder and upper arm level, left arm

      7ᵗʰ S44.8X9 Injury of other nerves at shoulder and upper arm level, unspecified arm

5ᵗʰ S44.9 Injury of unspecified nerve at shoulder and upper arm level

    x7ᵗʰ S44.90 Injury of unspecified nerve at shoulder and upper arm level, unspecified arm

    x7ᵗʰ S44.91 Injury of unspecified nerve at shoulder and upper arm level, right arm

    x7ᵗʰ S44.92 Injury of unspecified nerve at shoulder and upper arm level, left arm

4ᵗʰ S45 Injury of blood vessels at shoulder and upper arm level

Code also any associated open wound (S41.-)

EXCLUDES 2   injury of subclavian artery (S25.1)
                 injury of subclavian vein (S25.3)

The appropriate 7th character is to be added to each code from category S45.

A   initial encounter
D   subsequent encounter
S   sequela

5ᵗʰ S45.0 Injury of axillary artery

    6ᵗʰ S45.00 Unspecified injury of axillary artery

      7ᵗʰ S45.001 Unspecified injury of axillary artery, right side

      7ᵗʰ S45.002 Unspecified injury of axillary artery, left side

✔7ᵗʰ **S45.009** Unspecified injury of axillary artery, unspecified side

✔6ᵗʰ **S45.01** Laceration of axillary artery

   ✔7ᵗʰ **S45.011** Laceration of axillary artery, right side

   ✔7ᵗʰ **S45.012** Laceration of axillary artery, left side

   ✔7ᵗʰ **S45.019** Laceration of axillary artery, unspecified side

✔6ᵗʰ **S45.09** Other specified injury of axillary artery

   ✔7ᵗʰ **S45.091** Other specified injury of axillary artery, right side

   ✔7ᵗʰ **S45.092** Other specified injury of axillary artery, left side

   ✔7ᵗʰ **S45.099** Other specified injury of axillary artery, unspecified side

✔5ᵗʰ **S45.1** Injury of brachial artery

✔6ᵗʰ **S45.10** Unspecified injury of brachial artery

   ✔7ᵗʰ **S45.101** Unspecified injury of brachial artery, right side

   ✔7ᵗʰ **S45.102** Unspecified injury of brachial artery, left side

   ✔7ᵗʰ **S45.109** Unspecified injury of brachial artery, unspecified side

✔6ᵗʰ **S45.11** Laceration of brachial artery

   ✔7ᵗʰ **S45.111** Laceration of brachial artery, right side

   ✔7ᵗʰ **S45.112** Laceration of brachial artery, left side

   ✔7ᵗʰ **S45.119** Laceration of brachial artery, unspecified side

✔6ᵗʰ **S45.19** Other specified injury of brachial artery

   ✔7ᵗʰ **S45.191** Other specified injury of brachial artery, right side

   ✔7ᵗʰ **S45.192** Other specified injury of brachial artery, left side

   ✔7ᵗʰ **S45.199** Other specified injury of brachial artery, unspecified side

✔5ᵗʰ **S45.2** Injury of axillary or brachial vein

✔6ᵗʰ **S45.20** Unspecified injury of axillary or brachial vein

   ✔7ᵗʰ **S45.201** Unspecified injury of axillary or brachial vein, right side

   ✔7ᵗʰ **S45.202** Unspecified injury of axillary or brachial vein, left side

   ✔7ᵗʰ **S45.209** Unspecified injury of axillary or brachial vein, unspecified side

✔6ᵗʰ **S45.21** Laceration of axillary or brachial vein

   ✔7ᵗʰ **S45.211** Laceration of axillary or brachial vein, right side

   ✔7ᵗʰ **S45.212** Laceration of axillary or brachial vein, left side

   ✔7ᵗʰ **S45.219** Laceration of axillary or brachial vein, unspecified side

✔6ᵗʰ **S45.29** Other specified injury of axillary or brachial vein

   ✔7ᵗʰ **S45.291** Other specified injury of axillary or brachial vein, right side

   ✔7ᵗʰ **S45.292** Other specified injury of axillary or brachial vein, left side

   ✔7ᵗʰ **S45.299** Other specified injury of axillary or brachial vein, unspecified side

✔5ᵗʰ **S45.3** Injury of superficial vein at shoulder and upper arm level

✔6ᵗʰ **S45.30** Unspecified injury of superficial vein at shoulder and upper arm level

   ✔7ᵗʰ **S45.301** Unspecified injury of superficial vein at shoulder and upper arm level, right arm

   ✔7ᵗʰ **S45.302** Unspecified injury of superficial vein at shoulder and upper arm level, left arm

   ✔7ᵗʰ **S45.309** Unspecified injury of superficial vein at shoulder and upper arm level, unspecified arm

✔6ᵗʰ **S45.31** Laceration of superficial vein at shoulder and upper arm level

   ✔7ᵗʰ **S45.311** Laceration of superficial vein at shoulder and upper arm level, right arm

   ✔7ᵗʰ **S45.312** Laceration of superficial vein at shoulder and upper arm level, left arm

   ✔7ᵗʰ **S45.319** Laceration of superficial vein at shoulder and upper arm level, unspecified arm

✔6ᵗʰ **S45.39** Other specified injury of superficial vein at shoulder and upper arm level

   ✔7ᵗʰ **S45.391** Other specified injury of superficial vein at shoulder and upper arm level, right arm

   ✔7ᵗʰ **S45.392** Other specified injury of superficial vein at shoulder and upper arm level, left arm

   ✔7ᵗʰ **S45.399** Other specified injury of superficial vein at shoulder and upper arm level, unspecified arm

✔5ᵗʰ **S45.8** Injury of other specified blood vessels at shoulder and upper arm level

✔6ᵗʰ **S45.80** Unspecified injury of other specified blood vessels at shoulder and upper arm level

   ✔7ᵗʰ **S45.801** Unspecified injury of other specified blood vessels at shoulder and upper arm level, right arm

   ✔7ᵗʰ **S45.802** Unspecified injury of other specified blood vessels at shoulder and upper arm level, left arm

   ✔7ᵗʰ **S45.809** Unspecified injury of other specified blood vessels at shoulder and upper arm level, unspecified arm

✔6ᵗʰ **S45.81** Laceration of other specified blood vessels at shoulder and upper arm level

   ✔7ᵗʰ **S45.811** Laceration of other specified blood vessels at shoulder and upper arm level, right arm

   ✔7ᵗʰ **S45.812** Laceration of other specified blood vessels at shoulder and upper arm level, left arm

   ✔7ᵗʰ **S45.819** Laceration of other specified blood vessels at shoulder and upper arm level, unspecified arm

✔6ᵗʰ **S45.89** Other specified injury of other specified blood vessels at shoulder and upper arm level

   ✔7ᵗʰ **S45.891** Other specified injury of other specified blood vessels at shoulder and upper arm level, right arm

   ✔7ᵗʰ **S45.892** Other specified injury of other specified blood vessels at shoulder and upper arm level, left arm

   ✔7ᵗʰ **S45.899** Other specified injury of other specified blood vessels at shoulder and upper arm level, unspecified arm

✔5ᵗʰ **S45.9** Injury of unspecified blood vessel at shoulder and upper arm level

✔6ᵗʰ **S45.90** Unspecified injury of unspecified blood vessel at shoulder and upper arm level

   ✔7ᵗʰ **S45.901** Unspecified injury of unspecified blood vessel at shoulder and upper arm level, right arm

   ✔7ᵗʰ **S45.902** Unspecified injury of unspecified blood vessel at shoulder and upper arm level, left arm

   ✔7ᵗʰ **S45.909** Unspecified injury of unspecified blood vessel at shoulder and upper arm level, unspecified arm

✔6ᵗʰ **S45.91** Laceration of unspecified blood vessel at shoulder and upper arm level

   ✔7ᵗʰ **S45.911** Laceration of unspecified blood vessel at shoulder and upper arm level, right arm

   ✔7ᵗʰ **S45.912** Laceration of unspecified blood vessel at shoulder and upper arm level, left arm

   ✔7ᵗʰ **S45.919** Laceration of unspecified blood vessel at shoulder and upper arm level, unspecified arm

✔6ᵗʰ **S45.99** Other specified injury of unspecified blood vessel at shoulder and upper arm level

   ✔7ᵗʰ **S45.991** Other specified injury of unspecified blood vessel at shoulder and upper arm level, right arm

   ✔7ᵗʰ **S45.992** Other specified injury of unspecified blood vessel at shoulder and upper arm level, left arm

   ✔7ᵗʰ **S45.999** Other specified injury of unspecified blood vessel at shoulder and upper arm level, unspecified arm

☑ Additional Character Required   ✔x7ᵗʰ Placeholder Alert   Manifestation   Unspecified Dx   ▶◀ Revised Text   ● New Code   ▲ Revised Code Title

ICD-10-CM 2020   1003

✓4ᵗʰ **S46 Injury of muscle, fascia and tendon at shoulder and upper arm level**

Code also any associated open wound (S41.-)

EXCLUDES 2   injury of muscle, fascia and tendon at elbow (S56.-)
sprain of joints and ligaments of shoulder girdle (S43.9)

TIP: Refer to the Muscle/Tendon table at the beginning of this chapter.

The appropriate 7th character is to be added to each code from category S46.
A   initial encounter
D   subsequent encounter
S   sequela

✓5ᵗʰ **S46.0 Injury of muscle(s) and tendon(s) of the** rotator cuff **of shoulder**

✓6ᵗʰ **S46.00 Unspecified injury of muscle(s) and tendon(s) of the rotator cuff of shoulder**

✓7ᵗʰ **S46.001 Unspecified injury of muscle(s) and tendon(s) of the rotator cuff of** right **shoulder**

✓7ᵗʰ **S46.002 Unspecified injury of muscle(s) and tendon(s) of the rotator cuff of** left **shoulder**

✓7ᵗʰ **S46.009 Unspecified injury of muscle(s) and tendon(s) of the rotator cuff of unspecified shoulder**

✓6ᵗʰ **S46.01 Strain of muscle(s) and tendon(s) of the rotator cuff of shoulder**

✓7ᵗʰ **S46.011 Strain of muscle(s) and tendon(s) of the rotator cuff of** right **shoulder**

✓7ᵗʰ **S46.012 Strain of muscle(s) and tendon(s) of the rotator cuff of** left **shoulder**

✓7ᵗʰ **S46.019 Strain of muscle(s) and tendon(s) of the rotator cuff of unspecified shoulder**

✓6ᵗʰ **S46.02 Laceration of muscle(s) and tendon(s) of the rotator cuff of shoulder**

✓7ᵗʰ **S46.021 Laceration of muscle(s) and tendon(s) of the rotator cuff of** right **shoulder**

✓7ᵗʰ **S46.022 Laceration of muscle(s) and tendon(s) of the rotator cuff of** left **shoulder**

✓7ᵗʰ **S46.029 Laceration of muscle(s) and tendon(s) of the rotator cuff of unspecified shoulder**

✓6ᵗʰ **S46.09 Other injury of muscle(s) and tendon(s) of the rotator cuff of shoulder**

✓7ᵗʰ **S46.091 Other injury of muscle(s) and tendon(s) of the rotator cuff of** right **shoulder**

✓7ᵗʰ **S46.092 Other injury of muscle(s) and tendon(s) of the rotator cuff of** left **shoulder**

✓7ᵗʰ **S46.099 Other injury of muscle(s) and tendon(s) of the rotator cuff of unspecified shoulder**

✓5ᵗʰ **S46.1 Injury of muscle, fascia and tendon of** long head of biceps

✓6ᵗʰ **S46.10 Unspecified injury of muscle, fascia and tendon of long head of biceps**

✓7ᵗʰ **S46.101 Unspecified injury of muscle, fascia and tendon of long head of biceps,** right **arm**

✓7ᵗʰ **S46.102 Unspecified injury of muscle, fascia and tendon of long head of biceps,** left **arm**

✓7ᵗʰ **S46.109 Unspecified injury of muscle, fascia and tendon of long head of biceps, unspecified arm**

✓6ᵗʰ **S46.11 Strain of muscle, fascia and tendon of long head of biceps**

AHA: 2019,2Q,27

✓7ᵗʰ **S46.111 Strain of muscle, fascia and tendon of long head of biceps,** right **arm**

✓7ᵗʰ **S46.112 Strain of muscle, fascia and tendon of long head of biceps,** left **arm**

✓7ᵗʰ **S46.119 Strain of muscle, fascia and tendon of long head of biceps, unspecified arm**

✓6ᵗʰ **S46.12 Laceration of muscle, fascia and tendon of long head of biceps**

✓7ᵗʰ **S46.121 Laceration of muscle, fascia and tendon of long head of biceps,** right **arm**

✓7ᵗʰ **S46.122 Laceration of muscle, fascia and tendon of long head of biceps,** left **arm**

✓7ᵗʰ **S46.129 Laceration of muscle, fascia and tendon of long head of biceps, unspecified arm**

✓6ᵗʰ **S46.19 Other injury of muscle, fascia and tendon of long head of biceps**

✓7ᵗʰ **S46.191 Other injury of muscle, fascia and tendon of long head of biceps,** right **arm**

✓7ᵗʰ **S46.192 Other injury of muscle, fascia and tendon of long head of biceps,** left **arm**

✓7ᵗʰ **S46.199 Other injury of muscle, fascia and tendon of long head of biceps, unspecified arm**

✓5ᵗʰ **S46.2 Injury of muscle, fascia and tendon of other parts of biceps**

✓6ᵗʰ **S46.20 Unspecified injury of muscle, fascia and tendon of other parts of biceps**

✓7ᵗʰ **S46.201 Unspecified injury of muscle, fascia and tendon of other parts of biceps,** right **arm**

✓7ᵗʰ **S46.202 Unspecified injury of muscle, fascia and tendon of other parts of biceps,** left **arm**

✓7ᵗʰ **S46.209 Unspecified injury of muscle, fascia and tendon of other parts of biceps, unspecified arm**

✓6ᵗʰ **S46.21 Strain of muscle, fascia and tendon of other parts of biceps**

✓7ᵗʰ **S46.211 Strain of muscle, fascia and tendon of other parts of biceps,** right **arm**

✓7ᵗʰ **S46.212 Strain of muscle, fascia and tendon of other parts of biceps,** left **arm**

✓7ᵗʰ **S46.219 Strain of muscle, fascia and tendon of other parts of biceps, unspecified arm**

✓6ᵗʰ **S46.22 Laceration of muscle, fascia and tendon of other parts of biceps**

✓7ᵗʰ **S46.221 Laceration of muscle, fascia and tendon of other parts of biceps,** right **arm**

✓7ᵗʰ **S46.222 Laceration of muscle, fascia and tendon of other parts of biceps,** left **arm**

✓7ᵗʰ **S46.229 Laceration of muscle, fascia and tendon of other parts of biceps, unspecified arm**

✓6ᵗʰ **S46.29 Other injury of muscle, fascia and tendon of other parts of biceps**

✓7ᵗʰ **S46.291 Other injury of muscle, fascia and tendon of other parts of biceps,** right **arm**

✓7ᵗʰ **S46.292 Other injury of muscle, fascia and tendon of other parts of biceps,** left **arm**

✓7ᵗʰ **S46.299 Other injury of muscle, fascia and tendon of other parts of biceps, unspecified arm**

✓5ᵗʰ **S46.3 Injury of muscle, fascia and tendon of** triceps

✓6ᵗʰ **S46.30 Unspecified injury of muscle, fascia and tendon of triceps**

✓7ᵗʰ **S46.301 Unspecified injury of muscle, fascia and tendon of triceps,** right **arm**

✓7ᵗʰ **S46.302 Unspecified injury of muscle, fascia and tendon of triceps,** left **arm**

✓7ᵗʰ **S46.309 Unspecified injury of muscle, fascia and tendon of triceps, unspecified arm**

✓6ᵗʰ **S46.31 Strain of muscle, fascia and tendon of triceps**

✓7ᵗʰ **S46.311 Strain of muscle, fascia and tendon of triceps,** right **arm**

✓7ᵗʰ **S46.312 Strain of muscle, fascia and tendon of triceps,** left **arm**

✓7ᵗʰ **S46.319 Strain of muscle, fascia and tendon of triceps, unspecified arm**

✓6ᵗʰ **S46.32 Laceration of muscle, fascia and tendon of triceps**

✓7ᵗʰ **S46.321 Laceration of muscle, fascia and tendon of triceps,** right **arm**

✓7ᵗʰ **S46.322 Laceration of muscle, fascia and tendon of triceps,** left **arm**

✓7ᵗʰ **S46.329 Laceration of muscle, fascia and tendon of triceps, unspecified arm**

✓6ᵗʰ **S46.39 Other injury of muscle, fascia and tendon of triceps**

✓7ᵗʰ **S46.391 Other injury of muscle, fascia and tendon of triceps,** right **arm**

✓7ᵗʰ **S46.392 Other injury of muscle, fascia and tendon of triceps,** left **arm**

✓7ᵗʰ **S46.399 Other injury of muscle, fascia and tendon of triceps, unspecified arm**

✓5ᵗʰ **S46.8 Injury of other muscles, fascia and tendons at shoulder and upper arm level**

✓6ᵗʰ **S46.80 Unspecified injury of other muscles, fascia and tendons at shoulder and upper arm level**

✓7ᵗʰ **S46.801 Unspecified injury of other muscles, fascia and tendons at shoulder and upper arm level,** right **arm**

✓7ᵗʰ **S46.802 Unspecified injury of other muscles, fascia and tendons at shoulder and upper arm level,** left **arm**

✓7ᵗʰ **S46.809 Unspecified injury of other muscles, fascia and tendons at shoulder and upper arm level, unspecified arm**

✓6th **S46.81** Strain of other muscles, fascia and tendons at shoulder and upper arm level

    ✓7th **S46.811** Strain of other muscles, fascia and tendons at shoulder and upper arm level, right arm

    ✓7th **S46.812** Strain of other muscles, fascia and tendons at shoulder and upper arm level, left arm

    ✓7th **S46.819** Strain of other muscles, fascia and tendons at shoulder and upper arm level, unspecified arm

✓6th **S46.82** Laceration of other muscles, fascia and tendons at shoulder and upper arm level

    ✓7th **S46.821** Laceration of other muscles, fascia and tendons at shoulder and upper arm level, right arm

    ✓7th **S46.822** Laceration of other muscles, fascia and tendons at shoulder and upper arm level, left arm

    ✓7th **S46.829** Laceration of other muscles, fascia and tendons at shoulder and upper arm level, unspecified arm

✓6th **S46.89** Other injury of other muscles, fascia and tendons at shoulder and upper arm level

    ✓7th **S46.891** Other injury of other muscles, fascia and tendons at shoulder and upper arm level, right arm

    ✓7th **S46.892** Other injury of other muscles, fascia and tendons at shoulder and upper arm level, left arm

    ✓7th **S46.899** Other injury of other muscles, fascia and tendons at shoulder and upper arm level, unspecified arm

✓5th **S46.9** Injury of unspecified muscle, fascia and tendon at shoulder and upper arm level

    ✓6th **S46.90** Unspecified injury of unspecified muscle, fascia and tendon at shoulder and upper arm level

      ✓7th **S46.901** Unspecified injury of unspecified muscle, fascia and tendon at shoulder and upper arm level, right arm

      ✓7th **S46.902** Unspecified injury of unspecified muscle, fascia and tendon at shoulder and upper arm level, left arm

      ✓7th **S46.909** Unspecified injury of unspecified muscle, fascia and tendon at shoulder and upper arm level, unspecified arm

    ✓6th **S46.91** Strain of unspecified muscle, fascia and tendon at shoulder and upper arm level

      ✓7th **S46.911** Strain of unspecified muscle, fascia and tendon at shoulder and upper arm level, right arm

      ✓7th **S46.912** Strain of unspecified muscle, fascia and tendon at shoulder and upper arm level, left arm

      ✓7th **S46.919** Strain of unspecified muscle, fascia and tendon at shoulder and upper arm level, unspecified arm

    ✓6th **S46.92** Laceration of unspecified muscle, fascia and tendon at shoulder and upper arm level

      ✓7th **S46.921** Laceration of unspecified muscle, fascia and tendon at shoulder and upper arm level, right arm

      ✓7th **S46.922** Laceration of unspecified muscle, fascia and tendon at shoulder and upper arm level, left arm

      ✓7th **S46.929** Laceration of unspecified muscle, fascia and tendon at shoulder and upper arm level, unspecified arm

    ✓6th **S46.99** Other injury of unspecified muscle, fascia and tendon at shoulder and upper arm level

      ✓7th **S46.991** Other injury of unspecified muscle, fascia and tendon at shoulder and upper arm level, right arm

      ✓7th **S46.992** Other injury of unspecified muscle, fascia and tendon at shoulder and upper arm level, left arm

      ✓7th **S46.999** Other injury of unspecified muscle, fascia and tendon at shoulder and upper arm level, unspecified arm

✓4th **S47** **Crushing injury** of shoulder and upper arm

    Use additional code for all associated injuries

    EXCLUDES 2   crushing injury of elbow (S57.0-)

    The appropriate 7th character is to be added to each code from category S47.
    A   initial encounter
    D   subsequent encounter
    S   sequela

✓x7th **S47.1** Crushing injury of right shoulder and upper arm

✓x7th **S47.2** Crushing injury of left shoulder and upper arm

✓x7th **S47.9** Crushing injury of shoulder and upper arm, unspecified arm

✓4th **S48** **Traumatic amputation** of shoulder and upper arm

    An amputation not identified as partial or complete should be coded to complete

    EXCLUDES 1   traumatic amputation at elbow level (S58.0)

    The appropriate 7th character is to be added to each code from category S48.
    A   initial encounter
    D   subsequent encounter
    S   sequela

✓5th **S48.0** Traumatic amputation at shoulder joint

    ✓6th **S48.01** Complete traumatic amputation at shoulder joint

      2 ✓7th **S48.011** Complete traumatic amputation at right shoulder joint   HCC

      2 ✓7th **S48.012** Complete traumatic amputation at left shoulder joint   HCC

      2 ✓7th **S48.019** Complete traumatic amputation at unspecified shoulder joint   HCC

    ✓6th **S48.02** Partial traumatic amputation at shoulder joint

      2 ✓7th **S48.021** Partial traumatic amputation at right shoulder joint   HCC

      2 ✓7th **S48.022** Partial traumatic amputation at left shoulder joint   HCC

      2 ✓7th **S48.029** Partial traumatic amputation at unspecified shoulder joint   HCC

✓5th **S48.1** Traumatic amputation at level between shoulder and elbow

    ✓6th **S48.11** Complete traumatic amputation at level between shoulder and elbow

      2 ✓7th **S48.111** Complete traumatic amputation at level between right shoulder and elbow   HCC

      2 ✓7th **S48.112** Complete traumatic amputation at level between left shoulder and elbow   HCC

      2 ✓7th **S48.119** Complete traumatic amputation at level between unspecified shoulder and elbow   HCC

    ✓6th **S48.12** Partial traumatic amputation at level between shoulder and elbow

      2 ✓7th **S48.121** Partial traumatic amputation at level between right shoulder and elbow   HCC

      2 ✓7th **S48.122** Partial traumatic amputation at level between left shoulder and elbow   HCC

      2 ✓7th **S48.129** Partial traumatic amputation at level between unspecified shoulder and elbow   HCC

✓5th **S48.9** Traumatic amputation of shoulder and upper arm, level unspecified

    ✓6th **S48.91** Complete traumatic amputation of shoulder and upper arm, level unspecified

      2 ✓7th **S48.911** Complete traumatic amputation of right shoulder and upper arm, level unspecified   HCC

      2 ✓7th **S48.912** Complete traumatic amputation of left shoulder and upper arm, level unspecified   HCC

      2 ✓7th **S48.919** Complete traumatic amputation of unspecified shoulder and upper arm, level unspecified   HCC

    ✓6th **S48.92** Partial traumatic amputation of shoulder and upper arm, level unspecified

      2 ✓7th **S48.921** Partial traumatic amputation of right shoulder and upper arm, level unspecified   HCC

      2 ✓7th **S48.922** Partial traumatic amputation of left shoulder and upper arm, level unspecified   HCC

✓ Additional Character Required   ✓x7th Placeholder Alert   Manifestation   Unspecified Dx   ▶◀ Revised Text   ● New Code   ▲ Revised Code Title

ICD-10-CM 2020   1005

Chapter 19. Injury, Poisoning and Certain Other Consequences of External Causes

S48.929–S49.92

2 **7ᵗʰ** **S48.929** Partial traumatic amputation of unspecified shoulder and upper arm, level unspecified **HCC**

√4ᵗʰ S49 Other and unspecified injuries of shoulder and upper arm

AHA: 2018,2Q,12; 2018,1Q,3

The appropriate 7th character is to be added to each code from subcategories S49.0 and S49.1.
A   initial encounter for closed fracture
D   subsequent encounter for fracture with routine healing
G   subsequent encounter for fracture with delayed healing
K   subsequent encounter for fracture with nonunion
P   subsequent encounter for fracture with malunion
S   sequela

√5ᵗʰ S49.0 Physeal fracture of upper end of humerus

√6ᵗʰ S49.00 Unspecified physeal fracture of upper end of humerus

7ᵗʰ S49.001 Unspecified physeal fracture of upper end of humerus, right arm **Q**

7ᵗʰ S49.002 Unspecified physeal fracture of upper end of humerus, left arm **Q**

7ᵗʰ S49.009 Unspecified physeal fracture of upper end of humerus, unspecified arm **Q**

√6ᵗʰ S49.01 Salter-Harris Type I physeal fracture of upper end of humerus

7ᵗʰ S49.011 Salter-Harris Type I physeal fracture of upper end of humerus, right arm **Q**

7ᵗʰ S49.012 Salter-Harris Type I physeal fracture of upper end of humerus, left arm **Q**

7ᵗʰ S49.019 Salter-Harris Type I physeal fracture of upper end of humerus, unspecified arm **Q**

√6ᵗʰ S49.02 Salter-Harris Type II physeal fracture of upper end of humerus

7ᵗʰ S49.021 Salter-Harris Type II physeal fracture of upper end of humerus, right arm **Q**

7ᵗʰ S49.022 Salter-Harris Type II physeal fracture of upper end of humerus, left arm **Q**

7ᵗʰ S49.029 Salter-Harris Type II physeal fracture of upper end of humerus, unspecified arm **Q**

√6ᵗʰ S49.03 Salter-Harris Type III physeal fracture of upper end of humerus

7ᵗʰ S49.031 Salter-Harris Type III physeal fracture of upper end of humerus, right arm **Q**

7ᵗʰ S49.032 Salter-Harris Type III physeal fracture of upper end of humerus, left arm **Q**

7ᵗʰ S49.039 Salter-Harris Type III physeal fracture of upper end of humerus, unspecified arm **Q**

√6ᵗʰ S49.04 Salter-Harris Type IV physeal fracture of upper end of humerus

7ᵗʰ S49.041 Salter-Harris Type IV physeal fracture of upper end of humerus, right arm **Q**

7ᵗʰ S49.042 Salter-Harris Type IV physeal fracture of upper end of humerus, left arm **Q**

7ᵗʰ S49.049 Salter-Harris Type IV physeal fracture of upper end of humerus, unspecified arm **Q**

√6ᵗʰ S49.09 Other physeal fracture of upper end of humerus

7ᵗʰ S49.091 Other physeal fracture of upper end of humerus, right arm **Q**

7ᵗʰ S49.092 Other physeal fracture of upper end of humerus, left arm **Q**

7ᵗʰ S49.099 Other physeal fracture of upper end of humerus, unspecified arm **Q**

√5ᵗʰ S49.1 Physeal fracture of lower end of humerus

√6ᵗʰ S49.10 Unspecified physeal fracture of lower end of humerus

7ᵗʰ S49.101 Unspecified physeal fracture of lower end of humerus, right arm **Q**

7ᵗʰ S49.102 Unspecified physeal fracture of lower end of humerus, left arm **Q**

7ᵗʰ S49.109 Unspecified physeal fracture of lower end of humerus, unspecified arm **Q**

√6ᵗʰ S49.11 Salter-Harris Type I physeal fracture of lower end of humerus

7ᵗʰ S49.111 Salter-Harris Type I physeal fracture of lower end of humerus, right arm **Q**

7ᵗʰ S49.112 Salter-Harris Type I physeal fracture of lower end of humerus, left arm **Q**

7ᵗʰ S49.119 Salter-Harris Type I physeal fracture of lower end of humerus, unspecified arm **Q**

√6ᵗʰ S49.12 Salter-Harris Type II physeal fracture of lower end of humerus

7ᵗʰ S49.121 Salter-Harris Type II physeal fracture of lower end of humerus, right arm **Q**

7ᵗʰ S49.122 Salter-Harris Type II physeal fracture of lower end of humerus, left arm **Q**

7ᵗʰ S49.129 Salter-Harris Type II physeal fracture of lower end of humerus, unspecified arm **Q**

√6ᵗʰ S49.13 Salter-Harris Type III physeal fracture of lower end of humerus

7ᵗʰ S49.131 Salter-Harris Type III physeal fracture of lower end of humerus, right arm **Q**

7ᵗʰ S49.132 Salter-Harris Type III physeal fracture of lower end of humerus, left arm **Q**

7ᵗʰ S49.139 Salter-Harris Type III physeal fracture of lower end of humerus, unspecified arm **Q**

√6ᵗʰ S49.14 Salter-Harris Type IV physeal fracture of lower end of humerus

7ᵗʰ S49.141 Salter-Harris Type IV physeal fracture of lower end of humerus, right arm **Q**

7ᵗʰ S49.142 Salter-Harris Type IV physeal fracture of lower end of humerus, left arm **Q**

7ᵗʰ S49.149 Salter-Harris Type IV physeal fracture of lower end of humerus, unspecified arm **Q**

√6ᵗʰ S49.19 Other physeal fracture of lower end of humerus

7ᵗʰ S49.191 Other physeal fracture of lower end of humerus, right arm **Q**

7ᵗʰ S49.192 Other physeal fracture of lower end of humerus, left arm **Q**

7ᵗʰ S49.199 Other physeal fracture of lower end of humerus, unspecified arm **Q**

√5ᵗʰ S49.8 Other specified injuries of shoulder and upper arm

The appropriate 7th character is to be added to each code in subcategory S49.8.
A   initial encounter
D   subsequent encounter
S   sequela

√x7ᵗʰ S49.80 Other specified injuries of shoulder and upper arm, unspecified arm

√x7ᵗʰ S49.81 Other specified injuries of right shoulder and upper arm

√x7ᵗʰ S49.82 Other specified injuries of left shoulder and upper arm

√5ᵗʰ S49.9 Unspecified injury of shoulder and upper arm

The appropriate 7th character is to be added to each code in subcategory S49.9.
A   initial encounter
D   subsequent encounter
S   sequela

√x7ᵗʰ S49.90 Unspecified injury of shoulder and upper arm, unspecified arm

√x7ᵗʰ S49.91 Unspecified injury of right shoulder and upper arm

√x7ᵗʰ S49.92 Unspecified injury of left shoulder and upper arm

Injuries to the elbow and forearm (S50-S59)

EXCLUDES 2   burns and corrosions (T20-T32)
frostbite (T33-T34)
injuries of wrist and hand (S60-S69)
insect bite or sting, venomous (T63.4)

√4th **S50 Superficial injury of elbow and forearm**

EXCLUDES 2   superficial injury of wrist and hand (S60.-)

The appropriate 7th character is to be added to each code from category S50.
A   initial encounter
D   subsequent encounter
S   sequela

√5th **S50.0 Contusion of** elbow

√x7th **S50.00   Contusion of unspecified elbow**

√x7th **S50.01   Contusion of** right **elbow**

√x7th **S50.02   Contusion of** left **elbow**

√5th **S50.1 Contusion of** forearm

√x7th **S50.10   Contusion of unspecified forearm**

√x7th **S50.11   Contusion of** right **forearm**

√x7th **S50.12   Contusion of** left **forearm**

√5th **S50.3 Other superficial injuries of** elbow

√6th **S50.31   Abrasion** of elbow

√7th **S50.311   Abrasion of** right **elbow**

√7th **S50.312   Abrasion of** left **elbow**

√7th **S50.319   Abrasion of unspecified elbow**

√6th **S50.32   Blister (nonthermal) of** elbow

√7th **S50.321   Blister (nonthermal) of** right **elbow**

√7th **S50.322   Blister (nonthermal) of** left **elbow**

√7th **S50.329   Blister (nonthermal) of unspecified elbow**

√6th **S50.34   External constriction** of elbow

√7th **S50.341   External constriction of** right **elbow**

√7th **S50.342   External constriction of** left **elbow**

√7th **S50.349   External constriction of unspecified elbow**

√6th **S50.35   Superficial** foreign body **of elbow**

Splinter in the elbow

√7th **S50.351   Superficial foreign body of** right **elbow**

√7th **S50.352   Superficial foreign body of** left **elbow**

√7th **S50.359   Superficial foreign body of unspecified elbow**

√6th **S50.36   Insect bite (nonvenomous) of** elbow

√7th **S50.361   Insect bite (nonvenomous) of** right **elbow**

√7th **S50.362   Insect bite (nonvenomous) of** left **elbow**

√7th **S50.369   Insect bite (nonvenomous) of unspecified elbow**

√6th **S50.37   Other superficial** bite **of elbow**

EXCLUDES 1   open bite of elbow (S51.05)

√7th **S50.371   Other superficial bite of** right **elbow**

√7th **S50.372   Other superficial bite of** left **elbow**

√7th **S50.379   Other superficial bite of unspecified elbow**

√5th **S50.8 Other superficial injuries of** forearm

√6th **S50.81   Abrasion** of forearm

√7th **S50.811   Abrasion of** right **forearm**

√7th **S50.812   Abrasion of** left **forearm**

√7th **S50.819   Abrasion of unspecified forearm**

√6th **S50.82   Blister (nonthermal) of** forearm

√7th **S50.821   Blister (nonthermal) of** right **forearm**

√7th **S50.822   Blister (nonthermal) of** left **forearm**

√7th **S50.829   Blister (nonthermal) of unspecified forearm**

√6th **S50.84   External constriction** of forearm

√7th **S50.841   External constriction of** right **forearm**

√7th **S50.842   External constriction of** left **forearm**

√7th **S50.849   External constriction of unspecified forearm**

√6th **S50.85   Superficial** foreign body **of forearm**

Splinter in the forearm

√7th **S50.851   Superficial foreign body of** right **forearm**

√7th **S50.852   Superficial foreign body of** left **forearm**

√7th **S50.859   Superficial foreign body of unspecified forearm**

√6th **S50.86   Insect bite (nonvenomous) of** forearm

√7th **S50.861   Insect bite (nonvenomous) of** right **forearm**

√7th **S50.862   Insect bite (nonvenomous) of** left **forearm**

√7th **S50.869   Insect bite (nonvenomous) of unspecified forearm**

√6th **S50.87   Other superficial** bite **of forearm**

EXCLUDES 1   open bite of forearm (S51.85)

√7th **S50.871   Other superficial bite of** right **forearm**

√7th **S50.872   Other superficial bite of** left **forearm**

√7th **S50.879   Other superficial bite of unspecified forearm**

√5th **S50.9 Unspecified superficial injury of elbow and forearm**

√6th **S50.90   Unspecified superficial injury of** elbow

√7th **S50.901   Unspecified superficial injury of** right **elbow**

√7th **S50.902   Unspecified superficial injury of** left **elbow**

√7th **S50.909   Unspecified superficial injury of unspecified elbow**

√6th **S50.91   Unspecified superficial injury of** forearm

√7th **S50.911   Unspecified superficial injury of** right **forearm**

√7th **S50.912   Unspecified superficial injury of** left **forearm**

√7th **S50.919   Unspecified superficial injury of unspecified forearm**

√4th **S51 Open wound of elbow and forearm**

Code also any associated wound infection

EXCLUDES 1   open fracture of elbow and forearm (S52.- with open fracture 7th character)
traumatic amputation of elbow and forearm (S58.-)

EXCLUDES 2   open wound of wrist and hand (S61.-)

The appropriate 7th character is to be added to each code from category S51.
A   initial encounter
D   subsequent encounter
S   sequela

√5th **S51.0 Open wound of** elbow

√6th **S51.00   Unspecified open wound of elbow**

√7th **S51.001   Unspecified open wound of** right **elbow**

AHA: 2012,4Q,108

√7th **S51.002   Unspecified open wound of** left **elbow**

√7th **S51.009   Unspecified open wound of unspecified elbow**

Open wound of elbow NOS

√6th **S51.01   Laceration without foreign body of elbow**

√7th **S51.011   Laceration without foreign body of** right **elbow**

√7th **S51.012   Laceration without foreign body of** left **elbow**

√7th **S51.019   Laceration without foreign body of unspecified elbow**

√6th **S51.02   Laceration with foreign body of elbow**

√7th **S51.021   Laceration with foreign body of** right **elbow**

√7th **S51.022   Laceration with foreign body of** left **elbow**

√7th **S51.029   Laceration with foreign body of unspecified elbow**

√6th **S51.03   Puncture wound without foreign body of elbow**

√7th **S51.031   Puncture wound without foreign body of** right **elbow**

√7th **S51.032   Puncture wound without foreign body of** left **elbow**

√7th **S51.039   Puncture wound without foreign body of unspecified elbow**

√6th **S51.04   Puncture wound with foreign body of elbow**

√7th **S51.041   Puncture wound with foreign body of** right **elbow**

  ☑7ᵗʰ **S51.042** **Puncture wound with foreign body of** left **elbow**

  ☑7ᵗʰ **S51.049** **Puncture wound with foreign body of unspecified elbow**

 ☑6ᵗʰ **S51.05** **Open bite** of elbow

  Bite of elbow NOS

   EXCLUDES 1   superficial bite of elbow (S50.36, S50.37)

  ☑7ᵗʰ **S51.051** **Open bite,** right **elbow**

  ☑7ᵗʰ **S51.052** **Open bite,** left **elbow**

  ☑7ᵗʰ **S51.059** **Open bite, unspecified elbow**

☑5ᵗʰ **S51.8** **Open wound of** forearm

  EXCLUDES 2   open wound of elbow (S51.0-)

 ☑6ᵗʰ **S51.80** **Unspecified open wound of forearm**

  AHA: 2016,3Q,24

  ☑7ᵗʰ **S51.801** **Unspecified open wound of** right **forearm**

  ☑7ᵗʰ **S51.802** **Unspecified open wound of** left **forearm**

  ☑7ᵗʰ **S51.809** **Unspecified open wound of unspecified forearm**

   Open wound of forearm NOS

 ☑6ᵗʰ **S51.81** **Laceration without foreign body of forearm**

  ☑7ᵗʰ **S51.811** **Laceration without foreign body of** right **forearm**

  ☑7ᵗʰ **S51.812** **Laceration without foreign body of** left **forearm**

  ☑7ᵗʰ **S51.819** **Laceration without foreign body of unspecified forearm**

 ☑6ᵗʰ **S51.82** **Laceration with foreign body of forearm**

  ☑7ᵗʰ **S51.821** **Laceration with foreign body of** right **forearm**

  ☑7ᵗʰ **S51.822** **Laceration with foreign body of** left **forearm**

  ☑7ᵗʰ **S51.829** **Laceration with foreign body of unspecified forearm**

 ☑6ᵗʰ **S51.83** **Puncture wound without foreign body** of forearm

  AHA: 2016,3Q,24

  ☑7ᵗʰ **S51.831** **Puncture wound without foreign body of** right **forearm**

  ☑7ᵗʰ **S51.832** **Puncture wound without foreign body of** left **forearm**

  ☑7ᵗʰ **S51.839** **Puncture wound without foreign body of unspecified forearm**

 ☑6ᵗʰ **S51.84** **Puncture wound with foreign body** of forearm

  AHA: 2016,3Q,24

  ☑7ᵗʰ **S51.841** **Puncture wound with foreign body of** right **forearm**

  ☑7ᵗʰ **S51.842** **Puncture wound with foreign body of** left **forearm**

  ☑7ᵗʰ **S51.849** **Puncture wound with foreign body of unspecified forearm**

 ☑6ᵗʰ **S51.85** **Open bite** of forearm

  Bite of forearm NOS

   EXCLUDES 1   superficial bite of forearm (S50.86, S50.87)

  ☑7ᵗʰ **S51.851** **Open bite of** right **forearm**

  ☑7ᵗʰ **S51.852** **Open bite of** left **forearm**

  ☑7ᵗʰ **S51.859** **Open bite of unspecified forearm**

☑4ᵗʰ **S52** **Fracture of forearm**

 NOTE   A fracture not indicated as displaced or nondisplaced should be coded to displaced.

    A fracture not indicated as open or closed should be coded to closed.

    The open fracture designations are based on the Gustilo open fracture classification.

 EXCLUDES 1   traumatic amputation of forearm (S58.-)

 EXCLUDES 2   fracture at wrist and hand level (S62.-)

 AHA: 2018,2Q,12; 2016,1Q,33; 2015,3Q,37-39

 DEF: Diaphysis: Central shaft of a long bone.

 DEF: Epiphysis: Proximal and distal rounded ends of a long bone, communicates with the joint.

 DEF: Metaphysis: Section of a long bone located between the epiphysis and diaphysis at the proximal and distal ends.

 DEF: Physis (growth plate): Narrow zone of cartilaginous tissue between the epiphysis and metaphysis at each end of a long bone. In childhood, proliferation of cells in this zone lengthens the bone. As the bone matures, this area thins, ossification eventually fusing into solid bone and growth stops. *Synonyms: Epiphyseal plate.*

The appropriate 7th character is to be added to all codes from category S52 [unless otherwise indicated].

A   initial encounter for closed fracture

B   initial encounter for open fracture type I or II
  initial encounter for open fracture NOS

C   initial encounter for open fracture type IIIA, IIIB, or IIIC

D   subsequent encounter for closed fracture with routine healing

E   subsequent encounter for open fracture type I or II with routine healing

F   subsequent encounter for open fracture type IIIA, IIIB, or IIIC with routine healing

G   subsequent encounter for closed fracture with delayed healing

H   subsequent encounter for open fracture type I or II with delayed healing

J   subsequent encounter for open fracture type IIIA, IIIB, or IIIC with delayed healing

K   subsequent encounter for closed fracture with nonunion

M   subsequent encounter for open fracture type I or II with nonunion

N   subsequent encounter for open fracture type IIIA, IIIB, or IIIC with nonunion

P   subsequent encounter for closed fracture with malunion

Q   subsequent encounter for open fracture type I or II with malunion

R   subsequent encounter for open fracture type IIIA, IIIB, or IIIC with malunion

S   sequela

☑5ᵗʰ **S52.0** **Fracture of** upper end of ulna

 Fracture of proximal end of ulna

  EXCLUDES 2   fracture of elbow NOS (S42.40-)

      fractures of shaft of ulna (S52.2-)

 ☑6ᵗʰ **S52.00** **Unspecified fracture of upper end of ulna**

  ☑7ᵗʰ **S52.001** **Unspecified fracture of upper end of right ulna** ◻

  ☑7ᵗʰ **S52.002** **Unspecified fracture of upper end of** left **ulna** ◻

  ☑7ᵗʰ **S52.009** **Unspecified fracture of upper end of unspecified ulna** ◻

 ☑6ᵗʰ **S52.01** **Torus fracture of upper end of ulna**

The appropriate 7th character is to be added to all codes in subcategory S52.01

A   initial encounter for closed fracture

D   subsequent encounter for fracture with routine healing

G   subsequent encounter for fracture with delayed healing

K   subsequent encounter for fracture with nonunion

P   subsequent encounter for fracture with malunion

S   sequela

  ☑7ᵗʰ **S52.011** **Torus fracture of upper end of** right **ulna** ◻

  ☑7ᵗʰ **S52.012** **Torus fracture of upper end of** left **ulna** ◻

  ☑7ᵗʰ **S52.019** **Torus fracture of upper end of unspecified ulna** ◻

✓6ᵗʰ **S52.02** **Fracture of** olecranon process without intraarticular extension of ulna

✓7ᵗʰ **S52.021** **Displaced fracture of** olecranon process without intraarticular extension of right ulna   **Q**

✓7ᵗʰ **S52.022** **Displaced fracture of** olecranon process without intraarticular extension of left ulna   **Q**

✓7ᵗʰ **S52.023** **Displaced fracture of** olecranon process without intraarticular extension of unspecified ulna   **Q**

✓7ᵗʰ **S52.024** **Nondisplaced fracture of** olecranon process without intraarticular extension of right ulna   **Q**

✓7ᵗʰ **S52.025** **Nondisplaced fracture of** olecranon process without intraarticular extension of left ulna   **Q**

✓7ᵗʰ **S52.026** **Nondisplaced fracture of** olecranon process without intraarticular extension of unspecified ulna   **Q**

✓6ᵗʰ **S52.03** **Fracture of** olecranon process with intraarticular extension of ulna

✓7ᵗʰ **S52.031** **Displaced fracture of** olecranon process with intraarticular extension of right ulna   **Q**

✓7ᵗʰ **S52.032** **Displaced fracture of** olecranon process with intraarticular extension of left ulna   **Q**

✓7ᵗʰ **S52.033** **Displaced fracture of** olecranon process with intraarticular extension of unspecified ulna   **Q**

✓7ᵗʰ **S52.034** **Nondisplaced fracture of** olecranon process with intraarticular extension of right ulna   **Q**

✓7ᵗʰ **S52.035** **Nondisplaced fracture of** olecranon process with intraarticular extension of left ulna   **Q**

✓7ᵗʰ **S52.036** **Nondisplaced fracture of** olecranon process with intraarticular extension of unspecified ulna   **Q**

✓6ᵗʰ **S52.04** **Fracture of** coronoid process of ulna

✓7ᵗʰ **S52.041** **Displaced fracture of** coronoid process of right ulna   **Q**

✓7ᵗʰ **S52.042** **Displaced fracture of** coronoid process of left ulna   **Q**

✓7ᵗʰ **S52.043** **Displaced fracture of** coronoid process of unspecified ulna   **Q**

✓7ᵗʰ **S52.044** **Nondisplaced fracture of** coronoid process of right ulna   **Q**

✓7ᵗʰ **S52.045** **Nondisplaced fracture of** coronoid process of left ulna   **Q**

✓7ᵗʰ **S52.046** **Nondisplaced fracture of** coronoid process of unspecified ulna   **Q**

✓6ᵗʰ **S52.09** **Other fracture of upper end of ulna**

✓7ᵗʰ **S52.091** **Other fracture of upper end of** right ulna   **Q**

✓7ᵗʰ **S52.092** **Other fracture of upper end of** left ulna   **Q**

✓7ᵗʰ **S52.099** **Other fracture of upper end of** unspecified ulna   **Q**

✓5ᵗʰ **S52.1** **Fracture of** upper end of radius

Fracture of proximal end of radius

EXCLUDES 2   *physeal fractures of upper end of radius (S59.2-)*
fracture of shaft of radius (S52.3-)

✓6ᵗʰ **S52.10** **Unspecified fracture of upper end of radius**

✓7ᵗʰ **S52.101** **Unspecified fracture of upper end of** right radius   **Q**

✓7ᵗʰ **S52.102** **Unspecified fracture of upper end of** left radius   **Q**

✓7ᵗʰ **S52.109** **Unspecified fracture of upper end of** unspecified radius   **Q**

✓6ᵗʰ **S52.11** **Torus fracture of upper end of radius**

The appropriate 7th character is to be added to all codes in subcategory S52.11
A   initial encounter for closed fracture
D   subsequent encounter for fracture with routine healing
G   subsequent encounter for fracture with delayed healing
K   subsequent encounter for fracture with nonunion
P   subsequent encounter for fracture with malunion
S   sequela

✓7ᵗʰ **S52.111** **Torus fracture of upper end of** right radius   **Q**

✓7ᵗʰ **S52.112** **Torus fracture of upper end of** left radius   **Q**

✓7ᵗʰ **S52.119** **Torus fracture of upper end of** unspecified radius   **Q**

✓6ᵗʰ **S52.12** **Fracture of** head of radius

✓7ᵗʰ **S52.121** **Displaced fracture of head of** right radius   **Q**

✓7ᵗʰ **S52.122** **Displaced fracture of head of** left radius   **Q**

✓7ᵗʰ **S52.123** **Displaced fracture of head of** unspecified radius   **Q**

✓7ᵗʰ **S52.124** **Nondisplaced fracture of head of** right radius   **Q**

✓7ᵗʰ **S52.125** **Nondisplaced fracture of head of** left radius   **Q**

✓7ᵗʰ **S52.126** **Nondisplaced fracture of head of** unspecified radius   **Q**

✓6ᵗʰ **S52.13** **Fracture of** neck of radius

✓7ᵗʰ **S52.131** **Displaced fracture of neck of** right radius   **Q**

✓7ᵗʰ **S52.132** **Displaced fracture of neck of** left radius   **Q**

✓7ᵗʰ **S52.133** **Displaced fracture of neck of** unspecified radius   **Q**

✓7ᵗʰ **S52.134** **Nondisplaced fracture of neck of** right radius   **Q**

✓7ᵗʰ **S52.135** **Nondisplaced fracture of neck of** left radius   **Q**

✓7ᵗʰ **S52.136** **Nondisplaced fracture of neck of** unspecified radius   **Q**

✓6ᵗʰ **S52.18** **Other fracture of upper end of radius**

✓7ᵗʰ **S52.181** **Other fracture of upper end of** right radius   **Q**

✓7ᵗʰ **S52.182** **Other fracture of upper end of** left radius   **Q**

✓7ᵗʰ **S52.189** **Other fracture of upper end of** unspecified radius   **Q**

✓5ᵗʰ **S52.2** **Fracture of** shaft of ulna

✓6ᵗʰ **S52.20** **Unspecified fracture of shaft of ulna**

Fracture of ulna NOS

✓7ᵗʰ **S52.201** **Unspecified fracture of shaft of** right ulna   **Q**

✓7ᵗʰ **S52.202** **Unspecified fracture of shaft of** left ulna   **Q**

✓7ᵗʰ **S52.209** **Unspecified fracture of shaft of** unspecified ulna   **Q**

✓6ᵗʰ **S52.21** **Greenstick fracture of shaft of ulna**

The appropriate 7th character is to be added to all codes in subcategory S52.21
A   initial encounter for closed fracture
D   subsequent encounter for fracture with routine healing
G   subsequent encounter for fracture with delayed healing
K   subsequent encounter for fracture with nonunion
P   subsequent encounter for fracture with malunion
S   sequela

✓7ᵗʰ **S52.211** **Greenstick fracture of shaft of** right ulna   **Q**

✓7ᵗʰ **S52.212** **Greenstick fracture of shaft of** left ulna   **Q**

✓ Additional Character Required   ✓x7ᵗʰ Placeholder Alert   Manifestation   Unspecified Dx   ►◄ Revised Text   ● New Code   ▲ Revised Code Title

√7ᵗʰ **S52.219** Greenstick fracture of shaft of unspecified ulna   Q

√6ᵗʰ **S52.22** Transverse fracture of shaft of ulna

  √7ᵗʰ **S52.221** Displaced transverse fracture of shaft of right ulna   Q

  √7ᵗʰ **S52.222** Displaced transverse fracture of shaft of left ulna   Q

  √7ᵗʰ **S52.223** Displaced transverse fracture of shaft of unspecified ulna   Q

  √7ᵗʰ **S52.224** Nondisplaced transverse fracture of shaft of right ulna   Q

  √7ᵗʰ **S52.225** Nondisplaced transverse fracture of shaft of left ulna   Q

  √7ᵗʰ **S52.226** Nondisplaced transverse fracture of shaft of unspecified ulna   Q

√6ᵗʰ **S52.23** Oblique fracture of shaft of ulna

  √7ᵗʰ **S52.231** Displaced oblique fracture of shaft of right ulna   Q

  √7ᵗʰ **S52.232** Displaced oblique fracture of shaft of left ulna   Q

  √7ᵗʰ **S52.233** Displaced oblique fracture of shaft of unspecified ulna   Q

  √7ᵗʰ **S52.234** Nondisplaced oblique fracture of shaft of right ulna   Q

  √7ᵗʰ **S52.235** Nondisplaced oblique fracture of shaft of left ulna   Q

  √7ᵗʰ **S52.236** Nondisplaced oblique fracture of shaft of unspecified ulna   Q

√6ᵗʰ **S52.24** Spiral fracture of shaft of ulna

  √7ᵗʰ **S52.241** Displaced spiral fracture of shaft of ulna, right arm   Q

  √7ᵗʰ **S52.242** Displaced spiral fracture of shaft of ulna, left arm   Q

  √7ᵗʰ **S52.243** Displaced spiral fracture of shaft of ulna, unspecified arm   Q

  √7ᵗʰ **S52.244** Nondisplaced spiral fracture of shaft of ulna, right arm   Q

  √7ᵗʰ **S52.245** Nondisplaced spiral fracture of shaft of ulna, left arm   Q

  √7ᵗʰ **S52.246** Nondisplaced spiral fracture of shaft of ulna, unspecified arm   Q

√6ᵗʰ **S52.25** Comminuted fracture of shaft of ulna

  √7ᵗʰ **S52.251** Displaced comminuted fracture of shaft of ulna, right arm   Q

  √7ᵗʰ **S52.252** Displaced comminuted fracture of shaft of ulna, left arm   Q

  √7ᵗʰ **S52.253** Displaced comminuted fracture of shaft of ulna, unspecified arm   Q

  √7ᵗʰ **S52.254** Nondisplaced comminuted fracture of shaft of ulna, right arm   Q

  √7ᵗʰ **S52.255** Nondisplaced comminuted fracture of shaft of ulna, left arm   Q

  √7ᵗʰ **S52.256** Nondisplaced comminuted fracture of shaft of ulna, unspecified arm   Q

√6ᵗʰ **S52.26** Segmental fracture of shaft of ulna

  √7ᵗʰ **S52.261** Displaced segmental fracture of shaft of ulna, right arm   Q

  √7ᵗʰ **S52.262** Displaced segmental fracture of shaft of ulna, left arm   Q

  √7ᵗʰ **S52.263** Displaced segmental fracture of shaft of ulna, unspecified arm   Q

  √7ᵗʰ **S52.264** Nondisplaced segmental fracture of shaft of ulna, right arm   Q

  √7ᵗʰ **S52.265** Nondisplaced segmental fracture of shaft of ulna, left arm   Q

  √7ᵗʰ **S52.266** Nondisplaced segmental fracture of shaft of ulna, unspecified arm   Q

√6ᵗʰ **S52.27** Monteggia's fracture of ulna

  Fracture of upper shaft of ulna with dislocation of radial head

  √7ᵗʰ **S52.271** Monteggia's fracture of right ulna   Q

  √7ᵗʰ **S52.272** Monteggia's fracture of left ulna   Q

  √7ᵗʰ **S52.279** Monteggia's fracture of unspecified ulna   Q

√6ᵗʰ **S52.28** Bent bone of ulna

  √7ᵗʰ **S52.281** Bent bone of right ulna   Q

  √7ᵗʰ **S52.282** Bent bone of left ulna   Q

  √7ᵗʰ **S52.283** Bent bone of unspecified ulna   Q

√6ᵗʰ **S52.29** Other fracture of shaft of ulna

  √7ᵗʰ **S52.291** Other fracture of shaft of right ulna   Q

  √7ᵗʰ **S52.292** Other fracture of shaft of left ulna   Q

  √7ᵗʰ **S52.299** Other fracture of shaft of unspecified ulna   Q

√5ᵗʰ **S52.3** Fracture of shaft of radius

√6ᵗʰ **S52.30** Unspecified fracture of shaft of radius

  √7ᵗʰ **S52.301** Unspecified fracture of shaft of right radius   Q

  √7ᵗʰ **S52.302** Unspecified fracture of shaft of left radius   Q

  √7ᵗʰ **S52.309** Unspecified fracture of shaft of unspecified radius   Q

√6ᵗʰ **S52.31** Greenstick fracture of shaft of radius

> The appropriate 7th character is to be added to all codes in subcategory S52.31.
> A   initial encounter for closed fracture
> D   subsequent encounter for fracture with routine healing
> G   subsequent encounter for fracture with delayed healing
> K   subsequent encounter for fracture with nonunion
> P   subsequent encounter for fracture with malunion
> S   sequela

  √7ᵗʰ **S52.311** Greenstick fracture of shaft of radius, right arm   Q

  √7ᵗʰ **S52.312** Greenstick fracture of shaft of radius, left arm   Q

  √7ᵗʰ **S52.319** Greenstick fracture of shaft of radius, unspecified arm   Q

√6ᵗʰ **S52.32** Transverse fracture of shaft of radius

  √7ᵗʰ **S52.321** Displaced transverse fracture of shaft of right radius   Q

  √7ᵗʰ **S52.322** Displaced transverse fracture of shaft of left radius   Q

  √7ᵗʰ **S52.323** Displaced transverse fracture of shaft of unspecified radius   Q

  √7ᵗʰ **S52.324** Nondisplaced transverse fracture of shaft of right radius   Q

  √7ᵗʰ **S52.325** Nondisplaced transverse fracture of shaft of left radius   Q

  √7ᵗʰ **S52.326** Nondisplaced transverse fracture of shaft of unspecified radius   Q

√6ᵗʰ **S52.33** Oblique fracture of shaft of radius

  √7ᵗʰ **S52.331** Displaced oblique fracture of shaft of right radius   Q

  √7ᵗʰ **S52.332** Displaced oblique fracture of shaft of left radius   Q

  √7ᵗʰ **S52.333** Displaced oblique fracture of shaft of unspecified radius   Q

  √7ᵗʰ **S52.334** Nondisplaced oblique fracture of shaft of right radius   Q

  √7ᵗʰ **S52.335** Nondisplaced oblique fracture of shaft of left radius   Q

  √7ᵗʰ **S52.336** Nondisplaced oblique fracture of shaft of unspecified radius   Q

√6ᵗʰ **S52.34** Spiral fracture of shaft of radius

  √7ᵗʰ **S52.341** Displaced spiral fracture of shaft of radius, right arm   Q

  √7ᵗʰ **S52.342** Displaced spiral fracture of shaft of radius, left arm   Q

  √7ᵗʰ **S52.343** Displaced spiral fracture of shaft of radius, unspecified arm   Q

  √7ᵗʰ **S52.344** Nondisplaced spiral fracture of shaft of radius, right arm   Q

  √7ᵗʰ **S52.345** Nondisplaced spiral fracture of shaft of radius, left arm   Q

  √7ᵗʰ **S52.346** Nondisplaced spiral fracture of shaft of radius, unspecified arm   Q

√6ᵗʰ **S52.35** Comminuted fracture of shaft of radius

  √7ᵗʰ **S52.351** Displaced comminuted fracture of shaft of radius, right arm   Q

  √7ᵗʰ **S52.352** Displaced comminuted fracture of shaft of radius, left arm   Q

  √7ᵗʰ **S52.353** Displaced comminuted fracture of shaft of radius, unspecified arm   Q

√7ᵗʰ **S52.354** Nondisplaced comminuted fracture of shaft of radius, **right** arm ◫

√7ᵗʰ **S52.355** Nondisplaced comminuted fracture of shaft of radius, **left** arm ◫

√7ᵗʰ **S52.356** Nondisplaced comminuted fracture of shaft of radius, **unspecified** arm ◫

√6ᵗʰ **S52.36** Segmental fracture of shaft of radius

√7ᵗʰ **S52.361** Displaced segmental fracture of shaft of radius, **right** arm ◫

√7ᵗʰ **S52.362** Displaced segmental fracture of shaft of radius, **left** arm ◫

√7ᵗʰ **S52.363** Displaced segmental fracture of shaft of radius, unspecified arm ◫

√7ᵗʰ **S52.364** Nondisplaced segmental fracture of shaft of radius, **right** arm ◫

√7ᵗʰ **S52.365** Nondisplaced segmental fracture of shaft of radius, **left** arm ◫

√7ᵗʰ **S52.366** Nondisplaced segmental fracture of shaft of radius, unspecified arm ◫

√6ᵗʰ **S52.37** Galeazzi's fracture

Fracture of lower shaft of radius with radioulnar joint dislocation

√7ᵗʰ **S52.371** Galeazzi's fracture of **right** radius ◫

√7ᵗʰ **S52.372** Galeazzi's fracture of **left** radius ◫

√7ᵗʰ **S52.379** Galeazzi's fracture of unspecified radius ◫

√6ᵗʰ **S52.38** Bent bone of radius

√7ᵗʰ **S52.381** Bent bone of **right** radius ◫

√7ᵗʰ **S52.382** Bent bone of **left** radius ◫

√7ᵗʰ **S52.389** Bent bone of unspecified radius ◫

√6ᵗʰ **S52.39** Other fracture of shaft of radius

√7ᵗʰ **S52.391** Other fracture of shaft of radius, **right** arm ◫

√7ᵗʰ **S52.392** Other fracture of shaft of radius, **left** arm ◫

√7ᵗʰ **S52.399** Other fracture of shaft of radius, **unspecified** arm ◫

√5ᵗʰ **S52.5** Fracture of lower end of radius

Fracture of distal end of radius

EXCLUDES 2   physeal fractures of lower end of radius (S59.2-)

DEF: Fracture of the distal end of the radius above the wrist, most commonly caused by a fall onto an outstretched hand.

√6ᵗʰ **S52.50** Unspecified fracture of the lower end of radius

√7ᵗʰ **S52.501** Unspecified fracture of the lower end of **right** radius ◫

√7ᵗʰ **S52.502** Unspecified fracture of the lower end of **left** radius ◫

√7ᵗʰ **S52.509** Unspecified fracture of the lower end of unspecified radius ◫

√6ᵗʰ **S52.51** Fracture of radial styloid process

√7ᵗʰ **S52.511** Displaced fracture of **right** radial styloid process ◫

√7ᵗʰ **S52.512** Displaced fracture of **left** radial styloid process ◫

√7ᵗʰ **S52.513** Displaced fracture of unspecified radial styloid process ◫

√7ᵗʰ **S52.514** Nondisplaced fracture of **right** radial styloid process ◫

√7ᵗʰ **S52.515** Nondisplaced fracture of **left** radial styloid process ◫

√7ᵗʰ **S52.516** Nondisplaced fracture of unspecified radial styloid process ◫

√6ᵗʰ **S52.52** Torus fracture of lower end of radius

The appropriate 7th character is to be added to all codes in subcategory S52.52.
A   initial encounter for closed fracture
D   subsequent encounter for fracture with routine healing
G   subsequent encounter for fracture with delayed healing
K   subsequent encounter for fracture with nonunion
P   subsequent encounter for fracture with malunion
S   sequela

√7ᵗʰ **S52.521** Torus fracture of lower end of **right** radius ◫

√7ᵗʰ **S52.522** Torus fracture of lower end of **left** radius ◫

√7ᵗʰ **S52.529** Torus fracture of lower end of unspecified radius ◫

√6ᵗʰ **S52.53** Colles' fracture

AHA: 2016,2Q,4
DEF: Fracture of the radius at the wrist in which the distal fragment is pushed posteriorly. The dorsal angulation of the fragment results in the wrist cocking up.

√7ᵗʰ **S52.531** Colles' fracture of **right** radius ◫

√7ᵗʰ **S52.532** Colles' fracture of **left** radius ◫

√7ᵗʰ **S52.539** Colles' fracture of unspecified radius ◫

√6ᵗʰ **S52.54** Smith's fracture

√7ᵗʰ **S52.541** Smith's fracture of **right** radius ◫

√7ᵗʰ **S52.542** Smith's fracture of **left** radius ◫

√7ᵗʰ **S52.549** Smith's fracture of unspecified radius ◫

√6ᵗʰ **S52.55** Other extraarticular fracture of lower end of radius

√7ᵗʰ **S52.551** Other extraarticular fracture of lower end of **right** radius ◫

√7ᵗʰ **S52.552** Other extraarticular fracture of lower end of **left** radius ◫

√7ᵗʰ **S52.559** Other extraarticular fracture of lower end of unspecified radius ◫

√6ᵗʰ **S52.56** Barton's fracture

√7ᵗʰ **S52.561** Barton's fracture of **right** radius ◫

√7ᵗʰ **S52.562** Barton's fracture of **left** radius ◫

√7ᵗʰ **S52.569** Barton's fracture of unspecified radius ◫

√6ᵗʰ **S52.57** Other intraarticular fracture of lower end of radius

√7ᵗʰ **S52.571** Other intraarticular fracture of lower end of **right** radius ◫

√7ᵗʰ **S52.572** Other intraarticular fracture of lower end of **left** radius ◫

√7ᵗʰ **S52.579** Other intraarticular fracture of lower end of unspecified radius ◫

√6ᵗʰ **S52.59** Other fractures of lower end of radius

√7ᵗʰ **S52.591** Other fractures of lower end of **right** radius ◫

√7ᵗʰ **S52.592** Other fractures of lower end of **left** radius ◫

√7ᵗʰ **S52.599** Other fractures of lower end of unspecified radius ◫

√5ᵗʰ **S52.6** Fracture of lower end of ulna

√6ᵗʰ **S52.60** Unspecified fracture of lower end ulna

√7ᵗʰ **S52.601** Unspecified fracture of lower end of **right** ulna ◫

√7ᵗʰ **S52.602** Unspecified fracture of lower end of **left** ulna ◫

√7ᵗʰ **S52.609** Unspecified fracture of lower end of unspecified ulna ◫

√6ᵗʰ **S52.61** Fracture of ulna styloid process

√7ᵗʰ **S52.611** Displaced fracture of **right** ulna styloid process ◫

√7ᵗʰ **S52.612** Displaced fracture of **left** ulna styloid process ◫

√7ᵗʰ **S52.613** Displaced fracture of unspecified ulna styloid process ◫

√7ᵗʰ **S52.614** Nondisplaced fracture of **right** ulna styloid process ◫

☑ Additional Character Required   √x7ᵗʰ Placeholder Alert   Manifestation   Unspecified Dx   ▶◀ Revised Text   ● New Code   ▲ Revised Code Title

√7ᵗʰ **S52.615** **Nondisplaced** fracture **of left** ulna styloid process ☐ Q

√7ᵗʰ **S52.616** **Nondisplaced** fracture of **unspecified** ulna styloid process ☐ Q

√6ᵗʰ **S52.62** **Torus** fracture of lower end of ulna

> The appropriate 7th character is to be added to all codes in subcategory S52.62.
> A   initial encounter for closed fracture
> D   subsequent encounter for fracture with routine healing
> G   subsequent encounter for fracture with delayed healing
> K   subsequent encounter for fracture with nonunion
> P   subsequent encounter for fracture with malunion
> S   sequela

√7ᵗʰ **S52.621** **Torus fracture of lower end of right** ulna ☐ Q

√7ᵗʰ **S52.622** **Torus fracture of lower end of left** ulna ☐ Q

√7ᵗʰ **S52.629** **Torus fracture of lower end of unspecified** ulna ☐ Q

√6ᵗʰ **S52.69** **Other fracture of lower end of ulna**

√7ᵗʰ **S52.691** **Other fracture of lower end of right** ulna ☐ Q

√7ᵗʰ **S52.692** **Other fracture of lower end of left** ulna ☐ Q

√7ᵗʰ **S52.699** **Other fracture of lower end of unspecified** ulna ☐ Q

√5ᵗʰ **S52.9** **Unspecified fracture of forearm**

√×7ᵗʰ **S52.90** **Unspecified fracture of unspecified forearm** ☐ Q

√×7ᵗʰ **S52.91** **Unspecified fracture of right forearm** ☐ Q

√×7ᵗʰ **S52.92** **Unspecified fracture of left forearm** ☐ Q

√4ᵗʰ **S53** **Dislocation and sprain of joints and ligaments of elbow**

> INCLUDES   avulsion of joint or ligament of elbow
> laceration of cartilage, joint or ligament of elbow
> sprain of cartilage, joint or ligament of elbow
> traumatic hemarthrosis of joint or ligament of elbow
> traumatic rupture of joint or ligament of elbow
> traumatic subluxation of joint or ligament of elbow
> traumatic tear of joint or ligament of elbow

Code also any associated open wound

> EXCLUDES 2   strain of muscle, fascia and tendon at forearm level (S56.-)

> The appropriate 7th character is to be added to each code from category S53.
> A   initial encounter
> D   subsequent encounter
> S   sequela

√5ᵗʰ **S53.0** **Subluxation and dislocation of radial head**

> Dislocation of radiohumeral joint
> Subluxation of radiohumeral joint
> EXCLUDES 1   Monteggia's fracture-dislocation (S52.27-)

√6ᵗʰ **S53.00** **Unspecified subluxation and dislocation of radial head**

√7ᵗʰ **S53.001** **Unspecified subluxation of right radial head**

√7ᵗʰ **S53.002** **Unspecified subluxation of left radial head**

√7ᵗʰ **S53.003** **Unspecified subluxation of unspecified radial head**

√7ᵗʰ **S53.004** **Unspecified dislocation of right radial head**

√7ᵗʰ **S53.005** **Unspecified dislocation of left radial head**

√7ᵗʰ **S53.006** **Unspecified dislocation of unspecified radial head**

√6ᵗʰ **S53.01** **Anterior subluxation and dislocation of radial head**

> Anteriomedial subluxation and dislocation of radial head

√7ᵗʰ **S53.011** **Anterior subluxation of right radial head**

√7ᵗʰ **S53.012** **Anterior subluxation of left radial head**

√7ᵗʰ **S53.013** **Anterior subluxation of unspecified radial head**

√7ᵗʰ **S53.014** **Anterior dislocation of right radial head**

√7ᵗʰ **S53.015** **Anterior dislocation of left radial head**

√7ᵗʰ **S53.016** **Anterior dislocation of unspecified radial head**

√6ᵗʰ **S53.02** **Posterior subluxation and dislocation of radial head**

> Posteriolateral subluxation and dislocation of radial head

√7ᵗʰ **S53.021** **Posterior subluxation of right radial head**

√7ᵗʰ **S53.022** **Posterior subluxation of left radial head**

√7ᵗʰ **S53.023** **Posterior subluxation of unspecified radial head**

√7ᵗʰ **S53.024** **Posterior dislocation of right radial head**

√7ᵗʰ **S53.025** **Posterior dislocation of left radial head**

√7ᵗʰ **S53.026** **Posterior dislocation of unspecified radial head**

√6ᵗʰ **S53.03** **Nursemaid's elbow**

√7ᵗʰ **S53.031** **Nursemaid's elbow, right elbow**

√7ᵗʰ **S53.032** **Nursemaid's elbow, left elbow**

√7ᵗʰ **S53.033** **Nursemaid's elbow, unspecified elbow**

√6ᵗʰ **S53.09** **Other subluxation and dislocation of radial head**

√7ᵗʰ **S53.091** **Other subluxation of right radial head**

√7ᵗʰ **S53.092** **Other subluxation of left radial head**

√7ᵗʰ **S53.093** **Other subluxation of unspecified radial head**

√7ᵗʰ **S53.094** **Other dislocation of right radial head**

√7ᵗʰ **S53.095** **Other dislocation of left radial head**

√7ᵗʰ **S53.096** **Other dislocation of unspecified radial head**

√5ᵗʰ **S53.1** **Subluxation and dislocation of ulnohumeral joint**

> Subluxation and dislocation of elbow NOS
> EXCLUDES 1   dislocation of radial head alone (S53.0-)

√6ᵗʰ **S53.10** **Unspecified subluxation and dislocation of ulnohumeral joint**

√7ᵗʰ **S53.101** **Unspecified subluxation of right ulnohumeral joint**

√7ᵗʰ **S53.102** **Unspecified subluxation of left ulnohumeral joint**

√7ᵗʰ **S53.103** **Unspecified subluxation of unspecified ulnohumeral joint**

√7ᵗʰ **S53.104** **Unspecified dislocation of right ulnohumeral joint**

√7ᵗʰ **S53.105** **Unspecified dislocation of left ulnohumeral joint**

√7ᵗʰ **S53.106** **Unspecified dislocation of unspecified ulnohumeral joint**

√6ᵗʰ **S53.11** **Anterior subluxation and dislocation of ulnohumeral joint**

√7ᵗʰ **S53.111** **Anterior subluxation of right ulnohumeral joint**

√7ᵗʰ **S53.112** **Anterior subluxation of left ulnohumeral joint**

√7ᵗʰ **S53.113** **Anterior subluxation of unspecified ulnohumeral joint**

√7ᵗʰ **S53.114** **Anterior dislocation of right ulnohumeral joint**

> AHA: 2012,4Q,108

√7ᵗʰ **S53.115** **Anterior dislocation of left ulnohumeral joint**

√7ᵗʰ **S53.116** **Anterior dislocation of unspecified ulnohumeral joint**

√6ᵗʰ **S53.12** **Posterior subluxation and dislocation of ulnohumeral joint**

√7ᵗʰ **S53.121** **Posterior subluxation of right ulnohumeral joint**

√7ᵗʰ **S53.122** **Posterior subluxation of left ulnohumeral joint**

√7ᵗʰ **S53.123** **Posterior subluxation of unspecified ulnohumeral joint**

√7ᵗʰ **S53.124** **Posterior dislocation of right ulnohumeral joint**

√7ᵗʰ **S53.125** **Posterior dislocation of left ulnohumeral joint**

√7ᵗʰ **S53.126** **Posterior dislocation of unspecified ulnohumeral joint**

√6ᵗʰ **S53.13** **Medial subluxation and dislocation of ulnohumeral joint**

√7ᵗʰ **S53.131** **Medial subluxation of right ulnohumeral joint**

√7ᵗʰ **S53.132** **Medial subluxation of left ulnohumeral joint**

√7ᵗʰ **S53.133**   **Medial subluxation of unspecified ulnohumeral joint**

√7ᵗʰ **S53.134**   **Medial dislocation of right ulnohumeral joint**

√7ᵗʰ **S53.135**   **Medial dislocation of left ulnohumeral joint**

√7ᵗʰ **S53.136**   **Medial dislocation of unspecified ulnohumeral joint**

√6ᵗʰ **S53.14**   **Lateral subluxation and dislocation of ulnohumeral joint**

√7ᵗʰ **S53.141**   **Lateral subluxation of right ulnohumeral joint**

√7ᵗʰ **S53.142**   **Lateral subluxation of left ulnohumeral joint**

√7ᵗʰ **S53.143**   **Lateral subluxation of unspecified ulnohumeral joint**

√7ᵗʰ **S53.144**   **Lateral dislocation of right ulnohumeral joint**

√7ᵗʰ **S53.145**   **Lateral dislocation of left ulnohumeral joint**

√7ᵗʰ **S53.146**   **Lateral dislocation of unspecified ulnohumeral joint**

√6ᵗʰ **S53.19**   **Other subluxation and dislocation of ulnohumeral joint**

√7ᵗʰ **S53.191**   **Other subluxation of right ulnohumeral joint**

√7ᵗʰ **S53.192**   **Other subluxation of left ulnohumeral joint**

√7ᵗʰ **S53.193**   **Other subluxation of unspecified ulnohumeral joint**

√7ᵗʰ **S53.194**   **Other dislocation of right ulnohumeral joint**

√7ᵗʰ **S53.195**   **Other dislocation of left ulnohumeral joint**

√7ᵗʰ **S53.196**   **Other dislocation of unspecified ulnohumeral joint**

√5ᵗʰ **S53.2**   **Traumatic rupture of radial collateral ligament**

EXCLUDES 1   *sprain of radial collateral ligament NOS (S53.43-)*

√x7ᵗʰ **S53.20**   **Traumatic rupture of unspecified radial collateral ligament**

√x7ᵗʰ **S53.21**   **Traumatic rupture of right radial collateral ligament**

√x7ᵗʰ **S53.22**   **Traumatic rupture of left radial collateral ligament**

√5ᵗʰ **S53.3**   **Traumatic rupture of ulnar collateral ligament**

EXCLUDES 1   *sprain of ulnar collateral ligament (S53.44-)*

√x7ᵗʰ **S53.30**   **Traumatic rupture of unspecified ulnar collateral ligament**

√x7ᵗʰ **S53.31**   **Traumatic rupture of right ulnar collateral ligament**

√x7ᵗʰ **S53.32**   **Traumatic rupture of left ulnar collateral ligament**

√5ᵗʰ **S53.4**   **Sprain of elbow**

EXCLUDES 2   *traumatic rupture of radial collateral ligament (S53.2-)*

traumatic rupture of ulnar collateral ligament (S53.3-)

√6ᵗʰ **S53.40**   **Unspecified sprain of elbow**

√7ᵗʰ **S53.401**   **Unspecified sprain of right elbow**

√7ᵗʰ **S53.402**   **Unspecified sprain of left elbow**

√7ᵗʰ **S53.409**   **Unspecified sprain of unspecified elbow**

Sprain of elbow NOS

√6ᵗʰ **S53.41**   **Radiohumeral (joint) sprain**

√7ᵗʰ **S53.411**   **Radiohumeral (joint) sprain of right elbow**

√7ᵗʰ **S53.412**   **Radiohumeral (joint) sprain of left elbow**

√7ᵗʰ **S53.419**   **Radiohumeral (joint) sprain of unspecified elbow**

√6ᵗʰ **S53.42**   **Ulnohumeral (joint) sprain**

√7ᵗʰ **S53.421**   **Ulnohumeral (joint) sprain of right elbow**

√7ᵗʰ **S53.422**   **Ulnohumeral (joint) sprain of left elbow**

√7ᵗʰ **S53.429**   **Ulnohumeral (joint) sprain of unspecified elbow**

√6ᵗʰ **S53.43**   **Radial collateral ligament sprain**

√7ᵗʰ **S53.431**   **Radial collateral ligament sprain of right elbow**

√7ᵗʰ **S53.432**   **Radial collateral ligament sprain of left elbow**

√7ᵗʰ **S53.439**   **Radial collateral ligament sprain of unspecified elbow**

√6ᵗʰ **S53.44**   **Ulnar collateral ligament sprain**

√7ᵗʰ **S53.441**   **Ulnar collateral ligament sprain of right elbow**

√7ᵗʰ **S53.442**   **Ulnar collateral ligament sprain of left elbow**

√7ᵗʰ **S53.449**   **Ulnar collateral ligament sprain of unspecified elbow**

√6ᵗʰ **S53.49**   **Other sprain of elbow**

√7ᵗʰ **S53.491**   **Other sprain of right elbow**

√7ᵗʰ **S53.492**   **Other sprain of left elbow**

√7ᵗʰ **S53.499**   **Other sprain of unspecified elbow**

√4ᵗʰ **S54**   **Injury of nerves at forearm level**

Code also any associated open wound (S51.-)

EXCLUDES 2   *injury of nerves at wrist and hand level (S64.-)*

The appropriate 7th character is to be added to each code from category S54.
A   initial encounter
D   subsequent encounter
S   sequela

√5ᵗʰ **S54.0**   **Injury of ulnar nerve at forearm level**

Injury of ulnar nerve NOS

√x7ᵗʰ **S54.00**   **Injury of ulnar nerve at forearm level, unspecified arm**

√x7ᵗʰ **S54.01**   **Injury of ulnar nerve at forearm level, right arm**

√x7ᵗʰ **S54.02**   **Injury of ulnar nerve at forearm level, left arm**

√5ᵗʰ **S54.1**   **Injury of median nerve at forearm level**

Injury of median nerve NOS

√x7ᵗʰ **S54.10**   **Injury of median nerve at forearm level, unspecified arm**

√x7ᵗʰ **S54.11**   **Injury of median nerve at forearm level, right arm**

√x7ᵗʰ **S54.12**   **Injury of median nerve at forearm level, left arm**

√5ᵗʰ **S54.2**   **Injury of radial nerve at forearm level**

Injury of radial nerve NOS

√x7ᵗʰ **S54.20**   **Injury of radial nerve at forearm level, unspecified arm**

√x7ᵗʰ **S54.21**   **Injury of radial nerve at forearm level, right arm**

√x7ᵗʰ **S54.22**   **Injury of radial nerve at forearm level, left arm**

√5ᵗʰ **S54.3**   **Injury of cutaneous sensory nerve at forearm level**

√x7ᵗʰ **S54.30**   **Injury of cutaneous sensory nerve at forearm level, unspecified arm**

√x7ᵗʰ **S54.31**   **Injury of cutaneous sensory nerve at forearm level, right arm**

√x7ᵗʰ **S54.32**   **Injury of cutaneous sensory nerve at forearm level, left arm**

√5ᵗʰ **S54.8**   **Injury of other nerves at forearm level**

√6ᵗʰ **S54.8X**   **Injury of other nerves at forearm level**

√7ᵗʰ **S54.8X1**   **Injury of other nerves at forearm level, right arm**

√7ᵗʰ **S54.8X2**   **Injury of other nerves at forearm level, left arm**

√7ᵗʰ **S54.8X9**   **Injury of other nerves at forearm level, unspecified arm**

√5ᵗʰ **S54.9**   **Injury of unspecified nerve at forearm level**

√x7ᵗʰ **S54.90**   **Injury of unspecified nerve at forearm level, unspecified arm**

√x7ᵗʰ **S54.91**   **Injury of unspecified nerve at forearm level, right arm**

√x7ᵗʰ **S54.92**   **Injury of unspecified nerve at forearm level, left arm**

√4ᵗʰ **S55**   **Injury of blood vessels at forearm level**

Code also any associated open wound (S51.-)

EXCLUDES 2   *injury of blood vessels at wrist and hand level (S65.-)*

injury of brachial vessels (S45.1-S45.2)

The appropriate 7th character is to be added to each code from category S55.
A   initial encounter
D   subsequent encounter
S   sequela

√5ᵗʰ **S55.0**   **Injury of ulnar artery at forearm level**

√6ᵗʰ **S55.00**   **Unspecified injury of ulnar artery at forearm level**

√7ᵗʰ **S55.001**   **Unspecified injury of ulnar artery at forearm level, right arm**

√7ᵗʰ **S55.002**   **Unspecified injury of ulnar artery at forearm level, left arm**

☑ Additional Character Required   √x7ᵗʰ Placeholder Alert   Manifestation   Unspecified Dx   ▶◀ Revised Text   ● New Code   ▲ Revised Code Title

ICD-10-CM 2020   1013

√6ᵗʰ **S55.009** Unspecified injury of ulnar artery at forearm level, unspecified arm

√6ᵗʰ **S55.01** Laceration of ulnar artery at forearm level

√7ᵗʰ **S55.011** Laceration of ulnar artery at forearm level, right arm

√7ᵗʰ **S55.012** Laceration of ulnar artery at forearm level, left arm

√7ᵗʰ **S55.019** Laceration of ulnar artery at forearm level, unspecified arm

√6ᵗʰ **S55.09** Other specified injury of ulnar artery at forearm level

√7ᵗʰ **S55.091** Other specified injury of ulnar artery at forearm level, right arm

√7ᵗʰ **S55.092** Other specified injury of ulnar artery at forearm level, left arm

√7ᵗʰ **S55.099** Other specified injury of ulnar artery at forearm level, unspecified arm

√5ᵗʰ **S55.1** Injury of radial artery at forearm level

√6ᵗʰ **S55.10** Unspecified injury of radial artery at forearm level

√7ᵗʰ **S55.101** Unspecified injury of radial artery at forearm level, right arm

√7ᵗʰ **S55.102** Unspecified injury of radial artery at forearm level, left arm

√7ᵗʰ **S55.109** Unspecified injury of radial artery at forearm level, unspecified arm

√6ᵗʰ **S55.11** Laceration of radial artery at forearm level

√7ᵗʰ **S55.111** Laceration of radial artery at forearm level, right arm

√7ᵗʰ **S55.112** Laceration of radial artery at forearm level, left arm

√7ᵗʰ **S55.119** Laceration of radial artery at forearm level, unspecified arm

√6ᵗʰ **S55.19** Other specified injury of radial artery at forearm level

√7ᵗʰ **S55.191** Other specified injury of radial artery at forearm level, right arm

√7ᵗʰ **S55.192** Other specified injury of radial artery at forearm level, left arm

√7ᵗʰ **S55.199** Other specified injury of radial artery at forearm level, unspecified arm

√5ᵗʰ **S55.2** Injury of vein at forearm level

√6ᵗʰ **S55.20** Unspecified injury of vein at forearm level

√7ᵗʰ **S55.201** Unspecified injury of vein at forearm level, right arm

√7ᵗʰ **S55.202** Unspecified injury of vein at forearm level, left arm

√7ᵗʰ **S55.209** Unspecified injury of vein at forearm level, unspecified arm

√6ᵗʰ **S55.21** Laceration of vein at forearm level

√7ᵗʰ **S55.211** Laceration of vein at forearm level, right arm

√7ᵗʰ **S55.212** Laceration of vein at forearm level, left arm

√7ᵗʰ **S55.219** Laceration of vein at forearm level, unspecified arm

√6ᵗʰ **S55.29** Other specified injury of vein at forearm level

√7ᵗʰ **S55.291** Other specified injury of vein at forearm level, right arm

√7ᵗʰ **S55.292** Other specified injury of vein at forearm level, left arm

√7ᵗʰ **S55.299** Other specified injury of vein at forearm level, unspecified arm

√5ᵗʰ **S55.8** Injury of other blood vessels at forearm level

√6ᵗʰ **S55.80** Unspecified injury of other blood vessels at forearm level

√7ᵗʰ **S55.801** Unspecified injury of other blood vessels at forearm level, right arm

√7ᵗʰ **S55.802** Unspecified injury of other blood vessels at forearm level, left arm

√7ᵗʰ **S55.809** Unspecified injury of other blood vessels at forearm level, unspecified arm

√6ᵗʰ **S55.81** Laceration of other blood vessels at forearm level

√7ᵗʰ **S55.811** Laceration of other blood vessels at forearm level, right arm

√7ᵗʰ **S55.812** Laceration of other blood vessels at forearm level, left arm

√7ᵗʰ **S55.819** Laceration of other blood vessels at forearm level, unspecified arm

√6ᵗʰ **S55.89** Other specified injury of other blood vessels at forearm level

√7ᵗʰ **S55.891** Other specified injury of other blood vessels at forearm level, right arm

√7ᵗʰ **S55.892** Other specified injury of other blood vessels at forearm level, left arm

√7ᵗʰ **S55.899** Other specified injury of other blood vessels at forearm level, unspecified arm

√5ᵗʰ **S55.9** Injury of unspecified blood vessel at forearm level

√6ᵗʰ **S55.90** Unspecified injury of unspecified blood vessel at forearm level

√7ᵗʰ **S55.901** Unspecified injury of unspecified blood vessel at forearm level, right arm

√7ᵗʰ **S55.902** Unspecified injury of unspecified blood vessel at forearm level, left arm

√7ᵗʰ **S55.909** Unspecified injury of unspecified blood vessel at forearm level, unspecified arm

√6ᵗʰ **S55.91** Laceration of unspecified blood vessel at forearm level

√7ᵗʰ **S55.911** Laceration of unspecified blood vessel at forearm level, right arm

√7ᵗʰ **S55.912** Laceration of unspecified blood vessel at forearm level, left arm

√7ᵗʰ **S55.919** Laceration of unspecified blood vessel at forearm level, unspecified arm

√6ᵗʰ **S55.99** Other specified injury of unspecified blood vessel at forearm level

√7ᵗʰ **S55.991** Other specified injury of unspecified blood vessel at forearm level, right arm

√7ᵗʰ **S55.992** Other specified injury of unspecified blood vessel at forearm level, left arm

√7ᵗʰ **S55.999** Other specified injury of unspecified blood vessel at forearm level, unspecified arm

√4ᵗʰ **S56** **Injury of muscle, fascia and tendon at forearm level**

Code also any associated open wound (S51.-)

EXCLUDES 2   *injury of muscle, fascia and tendon at or below wrist (S66.-)*
sprain of joints and ligaments of elbow (S53.4-)

TIP: Refer to the Muscle/Tendon table at the beginning of this chapter

The appropriate 7th character is to be added to each code from category S56.
A   initial encounter
D   subsequent encounter
S   sequela

√5ᵗʰ **S56.0** Injury of flexor muscle, fascia and tendon of thumb at forearm level

√6ᵗʰ **S56.00** Unspecified injury of flexor muscle, fascia and tendon of thumb at forearm level

√7ᵗʰ **S56.001** Unspecified injury of flexor muscle, fascia and tendon of right thumb at forearm level

√7ᵗʰ **S56.002** Unspecified injury of flexor muscle, fascia and tendon of left thumb at forearm level

√7ᵗʰ **S56.009** Unspecified injury of flexor muscle, fascia and tendon of unspecified thumb at forearm level

√6ᵗʰ **S56.01** Strain of flexor muscle, fascia and tendon of thumb at forearm level

√7ᵗʰ **S56.011** Strain of flexor muscle, fascia and tendon of right thumb at forearm level

√7ᵗʰ **S56.012** Strain of flexor muscle, fascia and tendon of left thumb at forearm level

√7ᵗʰ **S56.019** Strain of flexor muscle, fascia and tendon of unspecified thumb at forearm level

√6ᵗʰ **S56.02** Laceration of flexor muscle, fascia and tendon of thumb at forearm level

√7ᵗʰ **S56.021** Laceration of flexor muscle, fascia and tendon of right thumb at forearm level

√7ᵗʰ **S56.022** Laceration of flexor muscle, fascia and tendon of left thumb at forearm level

√7ᵗʰ **S56.029** Laceration of flexor muscle, fascia and tendon of unspecified thumb at forearm level

√6ᵗʰ **S56.09** Other injury of flexor muscle, fascia and tendon of thumb at forearm level

√7ᵗʰ **S56.091** Other injury of flexor muscle, fascia and tendon of right thumb at forearm level

√7ᵗʰ **S56.092** Other injury of flexor muscle, fascia and tendon of left thumb at forearm level

√7ᵗʰ **S56.099** Other injury of flexor muscle, fascia and tendon of unspecified thumb at forearm level

√5ᵗʰ **S56.1 Injury of** flexor **muscle, fascia and tendon of other and unspecified** finger **at forearm level**

  √6ᵗʰ **S56.10 Unspecified injury of flexor muscle, fascia and tendon of other and unspecified finger at forearm level**

    √7ᵗʰ **S56.101 Unspecified injury of flexor muscle, fascia and tendon of** right index finger **at forearm level**

    √7ᵗʰ **S56.102 Unspecified injury of flexor muscle, fascia and tendon of** left index finger **at forearm level**

    √7ᵗʰ **S56.103 Unspecified injury of flexor muscle, fascia and tendon of** right middle finger **at forearm level**

    √7ᵗʰ **S56.104 Unspecified injury of flexor muscle, fascia and tendon of** left middle finger **at forearm level**

    √7ᵗʰ **S56.105 Unspecified injury of flexor muscle, fascia and tendon of** right ring finger **at forearm level**

    √7ᵗʰ **S56.106 Unspecified injury of flexor muscle, fascia and tendon of** left ring finger **at forearm level**

    √7ᵗʰ **S56.107 Unspecified injury of flexor muscle, fascia and tendon of** right little finger **at forearm level**

    √7ᵗʰ **S56.108 Unspecified injury of flexor muscle, fascia and tendon of** left little finger **at forearm level**

    √7ᵗʰ **S56.109 Unspecified injury of flexor muscle, fascia and tendon of** unspecified finger **at forearm level**

  √6ᵗʰ **S56.11 Strain of** flexor **muscle, fascia and tendon of other and unspecified finger at forearm level**

    √7ᵗʰ **S56.111 Strain of flexor muscle, fascia and tendon of** right index finger **at forearm level**

    √7ᵗʰ **S56.112 Strain of flexor muscle, fascia and tendon of** left index finger **at forearm level**

    √7ᵗʰ **S56.113 Strain of flexor muscle, fascia and tendon of** right middle finger **at forearm level**

    √7ᵗʰ **S56.114 Strain of flexor muscle, fascia and tendon of** left middle finger **at forearm level**

    √7ᵗʰ **S56.115 Strain of flexor muscle, fascia and tendon of** right ring finger **at forearm level**

    √7ᵗʰ **S56.116 Strain of flexor muscle, fascia and tendon of** left ring finger **at forearm level**

    √7ᵗʰ **S56.117 Strain of flexor muscle, fascia and tendon of** right little finger **at forearm level**

    √7ᵗʰ **S56.118 Strain of flexor muscle, fascia and tendon of** left little finger **at forearm level**

    √7ᵗʰ **S56.119 Strain of flexor muscle, fascia and tendon of finger of** unspecified finger **at forearm level**

  √6ᵗʰ **S56.12 Laceration of** flexor **muscle, fascia and tendon of other and unspecified finger at forearm level**

    √7ᵗʰ **S56.121 Laceration of flexor muscle, fascia and tendon of** right index finger **at forearm level**

    √7ᵗʰ **S56.122 Laceration of flexor muscle, fascia and tendon of** left index finger **at forearm level**

    √7ᵗʰ **S56.123 Laceration of flexor muscle, fascia and tendon of** right middle finger **at forearm level**

    √7ᵗʰ **S56.124 Laceration of flexor muscle, fascia and tendon of** left middle finger **at forearm level**

    √7ᵗʰ **S56.125 Laceration of flexor muscle, fascia and tendon of** right ring finger **at forearm level**

    √7ᵗʰ **S56.126 Laceration of flexor muscle, fascia and tendon of** left ring finger **at forearm level**

    √7ᵗʰ **S56.127 Laceration of flexor muscle, fascia and tendon of** right little finger **at forearm level**

    √7ᵗʰ **S56.128 Laceration of flexor muscle, fascia and tendon of** left little finger **at forearm level**

    √7ᵗʰ **S56.129 Laceration of flexor muscle, fascia and tendon of** unspecified finger **at forearm level**

  √6ᵗʰ **S56.19 Other injury of flexor muscle, fascia and tendon of other and unspecified finger at forearm level**

    √7ᵗʰ **S56.191 Other injury of flexor muscle, fascia and tendon of** right index finger **at forearm level**

    √7ᵗʰ **S56.192 Other injury of flexor muscle, fascia and tendon of** left index finger **at forearm level**

    √7ᵗʰ **S56.193 Other injury of flexor muscle, fascia and tendon of** right middle finger **at forearm level**

    √7ᵗʰ **S56.194 Other injury of flexor muscle, fascia and tendon of** left middle finger **at forearm level**

    √7ᵗʰ **S56.195 Other injury of flexor muscle, fascia and tendon of** right ring finger **at forearm level**

    √7ᵗʰ **S56.196 Other injury of flexor muscle, fascia and tendon of** left ring finger **at forearm level**

    √7ᵗʰ **S56.197 Other injury of flexor muscle, fascia and tendon of** right little finger **at forearm level**

    √7ᵗʰ **S56.198 Other injury of flexor muscle, fascia and tendon of** left little finger **at forearm level**

    √7ᵗʰ **S56.199 Other injury of flexor muscle, fascia and tendon of** unspecified finger **at forearm level**

√5ᵗʰ **S56.2 Injury of other flexor muscle, fascia and tendon at forearm level**

  √6ᵗʰ **S56.20 Unspecified injury of other flexor muscle, fascia and tendon at forearm level**

    √7ᵗʰ **S56.201 Unspecified injury of other flexor muscle, fascia and tendon at forearm level,** right arm

    √7ᵗʰ **S56.202 Unspecified injury of other flexor muscle, fascia and tendon at forearm level,** left arm

    √7ᵗʰ **S56.209 Unspecified injury of other flexor muscle, fascia and tendon at forearm level, unspecified arm**

  √6ᵗʰ **S56.21 Strain of other flexor muscle, fascia and tendon at forearm level**

    √7ᵗʰ **S56.211 Strain of other flexor muscle, fascia and tendon at forearm level,** right arm

    √7ᵗʰ **S56.212 Strain of other flexor muscle, fascia and tendon at forearm level,** left arm

    √7ᵗʰ **S56.219 Strain of other flexor muscle, fascia and tendon at forearm level, unspecified arm**

  √6ᵗʰ **S56.22 Laceration of other flexor muscle, fascia and tendon at forearm level**

    √7ᵗʰ **S56.221 Laceration of other flexor muscle, fascia and tendon at forearm level,** right arm

    √7ᵗʰ **S56.222 Laceration of other flexor muscle, fascia and tendon at forearm level,** left arm

    √7ᵗʰ **S56.229 Laceration of other flexor muscle, fascia and tendon at forearm level, unspecified arm**

  √6ᵗʰ **S56.29 Other injury of other flexor muscle, fascia and tendon at forearm level**

    √7ᵗʰ **S56.291 Other injury of other flexor muscle, fascia and tendon at forearm level,** right arm

    √7ᵗʰ **S56.292 Other injury of other flexor muscle, fascia and tendon at forearm level,** left arm

    √7ᵗʰ **S56.299 Other injury of other flexor muscle, fascia and tendon at forearm level, unspecified arm**

√5ᵗʰ **S56.3 Injury of** extensor or abductor **muscles, fascia and tendons of** thumb **at forearm level**

  √6ᵗʰ **S56.30 Unspecified injury of extensor or abductor muscles, fascia and tendons of thumb at forearm level**

    √7ᵗʰ **S56.301 Unspecified injury of extensor or abductor muscles, fascia and tendons of** right thumb **at forearm level**

    √7ᵗʰ **S56.302 Unspecified injury of extensor or abductor muscles, fascia and tendons of** left thumb **at forearm level**

    √7ᵗʰ **S56.309 Unspecified injury of extensor or abductor muscles, fascia and tendons of unspecified thumb at forearm level**

  √6ᵗʰ **S56.31 Strain of extensor or abductor muscles, fascia and tendons of thumb at forearm level**

    √7ᵗʰ **S56.311 Strain of extensor or abductor muscles, fascia and tendons of** right thumb **at forearm level**

    √7ᵗʰ **S56.312 Strain of extensor or abductor muscles, fascia and tendons of** left thumb **at forearm level**

✅ Additional Character Required   √x7ᵗʰ Placeholder Alert   Manifestation   Unspecified Dx   ▶◀ Revised Text   ● New Code   ▲ Revised Code Title

√7ᵗʰ **S56.319** Strain of extensor or abductor muscles, fascia and tendons of unspecified thumb at forearm level

√6ᵗʰ **S56.32** Laceration of extensor or abductor muscles, fascia and tendons of thumb at forearm level

√7ᵗʰ **S56.321** Laceration of extensor or abductor muscles, fascia and tendons of right thumb at forearm level

√7ᵗʰ **S56.322** Laceration of extensor or abductor muscles, fascia and tendons of left thumb at forearm level

√7ᵗʰ **S56.329** Laceration of extensor or abductor muscles, fascia and tendons of unspecified thumb at forearm level

√6ᵗʰ **S56.39** Other injury of extensor or abductor muscles, fascia and tendons of thumb at forearm level

√7ᵗʰ **S56.391** Other injury of extensor or abductor muscles, fascia and tendons of right thumb at forearm level

√7ᵗʰ **S56.392** Other injury of extensor or abductor muscles, fascia and tendons of left thumb at forearm level

√7ᵗʰ **S56.399** Other injury of extensor or abductor muscles, fascia and tendons of unspecified thumb at forearm level

√5ᵗʰ **S56.4** Injury of extensor muscle, fascia and tendon of other and unspecified finger at forearm level

√6ᵗʰ **S56.40** Unspecified injury of extensor muscle, fascia and tendon of other and unspecified finger at forearm level

√7ᵗʰ **S56.401** Unspecified injury of extensor muscle, fascia and tendon of right index finger at forearm level

√7ᵗʰ **S56.402** Unspecified injury of extensor muscle, fascia and tendon of left index finger at forearm level

√7ᵗʰ **S56.403** Unspecified injury of extensor muscle, fascia and tendon of right middle finger at forearm level

√7ᵗʰ **S56.404** Unspecified injury of extensor muscle, fascia and tendon of left middle finger at forearm level

√7ᵗʰ **S56.405** Unspecified injury of extensor muscle, fascia and tendon of right ring finger at forearm level

√7ᵗʰ **S56.406** Unspecified injury of extensor muscle, fascia and tendon of left ring finger at forearm level

√7ᵗʰ **S56.407** Unspecified injury of extensor muscle, fascia and tendon of right little finger at forearm level

√7ᵗʰ **S56.408** Unspecified injury of extensor muscle, fascia and tendon of left little finger at forearm level

√7ᵗʰ **S56.409** Unspecified injury of extensor muscle, fascia and tendon of unspecified finger at forearm level

√6ᵗʰ **S56.41** Strain of extensor muscle, fascia and tendon of other and unspecified finger at forearm level

√7ᵗʰ **S56.411** Strain of extensor muscle, fascia and tendon of right index finger at forearm level

√7ᵗʰ **S56.412** Strain of extensor muscle, fascia and tendon of left index finger at forearm level

√7ᵗʰ **S56.413** Strain of extensor muscle, fascia and tendon of right middle finger at forearm level

√7ᵗʰ **S56.414** Strain of extensor muscle, fascia and tendon of left middle finger at forearm level

√7ᵗʰ **S56.415** Strain of extensor muscle, fascia and tendon of right ring finger at forearm level

√7ᵗʰ **S56.416** Strain of extensor muscle, fascia and tendon of left ring finger at forearm level

√7ᵗʰ **S56.417** Strain of extensor muscle, fascia and tendon of right little finger at forearm level

√7ᵗʰ **S56.418** Strain of extensor muscle, fascia and tendon of left little finger at forearm level

√7ᵗʰ **S56.419** Strain of extensor muscle, fascia and tendon of finger, unspecified finger at forearm level

√6ᵗʰ **S56.42** Laceration of extensor muscle, fascia and tendon of other and unspecified finger at forearm level

√7ᵗʰ **S56.421** Laceration of extensor muscle, fascia and tendon of right index finger at forearm level

√7ᵗʰ **S56.422** Laceration of extensor muscle, fascia and tendon of left index finger at forearm level

√7ᵗʰ **S56.423** Laceration of extensor muscle, fascia and tendon of right middle finger at forearm level

√7ᵗʰ **S56.424** Laceration of extensor muscle, fascia and tendon of left middle finger at forearm level

√7ᵗʰ **S56.425** Laceration of extensor muscle, fascia and tendon of right ring finger at forearm level

√7ᵗʰ **S56.426** Laceration of extensor muscle, fascia and tendon of left ring finger at forearm level

√7ᵗʰ **S56.427** Laceration of extensor muscle, fascia and tendon of right little finger at forearm level

√7ᵗʰ **S56.428** Laceration of extensor muscle, fascia and tendon of left little finger at forearm level

√7ᵗʰ **S56.429** Laceration of extensor muscle, fascia and tendon of unspecified finger at forearm level

√6ᵗʰ **S56.49** Other injury of extensor muscle, fascia and tendon of other and unspecified finger at forearm level

√7ᵗʰ **S56.491** Other injury of extensor muscle, fascia and tendon of right index finger at forearm level

√7ᵗʰ **S56.492** Other injury of extensor muscle, fascia and tendon of left index finger at forearm level

√7ᵗʰ **S56.493** Other injury of extensor muscle, fascia and tendon of right middle finger at forearm level

√7ᵗʰ **S56.494** Other injury of extensor muscle, fascia and tendon of left middle finger at forearm level

√7ᵗʰ **S56.495** Other injury of extensor muscle, fascia and tendon of right ring finger at forearm level

√7ᵗʰ **S56.496** Other injury of extensor muscle, fascia and tendon of left ring finger at forearm level

√7ᵗʰ **S56.497** Other injury of extensor muscle, fascia and tendon of right little finger at forearm level

√7ᵗʰ **S56.498** Other injury of extensor muscle, fascia and tendon of left little finger at forearm level

√7ᵗʰ **S56.499** Other injury of extensor muscle, fascia and tendon of unspecified finger at forearm level

√5ᵗʰ **S56.5** Injury of other extensor muscle, fascia and tendon at forearm level

√6ᵗʰ **S56.50** Unspecified injury of other extensor muscle, fascia and tendon at forearm level

√7ᵗʰ **S56.501** Unspecified injury of other extensor muscle, fascia and tendon at forearm level, right arm

√7ᵗʰ **S56.502** Unspecified injury of other extensor muscle, fascia and tendon at forearm level, left arm

√7ᵗʰ **S56.509** Unspecified injury of other extensor muscle, fascia and tendon at forearm level, unspecified arm

√6ᵗʰ **S56.51** Strain of other extensor muscle, fascia and tendon at forearm level

√7ᵗʰ **S56.511** Strain of other extensor muscle, fascia and tendon at forearm level, right arm

√7ᵗʰ **S56.512** Strain of other extensor muscle, fascia and tendon at forearm level, left arm

√7ᵗʰ **S56.519** Strain of other extensor muscle, fascia and tendon at forearm level, unspecified arm

√6ᵗʰ **S56.52** Laceration of other extensor muscle, fascia and tendon at forearm level

√7ᵗʰ **S56.521** Laceration of other extensor muscle, fascia and tendon at forearm level, right arm

√7ᵗʰ **S56.522** Laceration of other extensor muscle, fascia and tendon at forearm level, left arm

√7ᵗʰ **S56.529** Laceration of other extensor muscle, fascia and tendon at forearm level, unspecified arm

√6ᵗʰ **S56.59** Other injury of other extensor muscle, fascia and tendon at forearm level

√7ᵗʰ **S56.591** Other injury of other extensor muscle, fascia and tendon at forearm level, right arm

√7ᵗʰ **S56.592** Other injury of other extensor muscle, fascia and tendon at forearm level, left arm

√7ᵗʰ **S56.599** Other injury of other extensor muscle, fascia and tendon at forearm level, unspecified arm

√5ᵗʰ **S56.8** Injury of other muscles, fascia and tendons at forearm level

√6ᵗʰ **S56.80** Unspecified injury of other muscles, fascia and tendons at forearm level

√7ᵗʰ **S56.801** Unspecified injury of other muscles, fascia and tendons at forearm level, right arm

√7ᵗʰ **S56.802** Unspecified injury of other muscles, fascia and tendons at forearm level, left arm

√7ᵗʰ **S56.809** Unspecified injury of other muscles, fascia and tendons at forearm level, unspecified arm

√6ᵗʰ **S56.81** Strain of other muscles, fascia and tendons at forearm level

√7ᵗʰ **S56.811** Strain of other muscles, fascia and tendons at forearm level, right arm

√7ᵗʰ **S56.812** Strain of other muscles, fascia and tendons at forearm level, left arm

√7ᵗʰ **S56.819** Strain of other muscles, fascia and tendons at forearm level, unspecified arm

√6ᵗʰ **S56.82** Laceration of other muscles, fascia and tendons at forearm level

√7ᵗʰ **S56.821** Laceration of other muscles, fascia and tendons at forearm level, right arm

√7ᵗʰ **S56.822** Laceration of other muscles, fascia and tendons at forearm level, left arm

√7ᵗʰ **S56.829** Laceration of other muscles, fascia and tendons at forearm level, unspecified arm

√6ᵗʰ **S56.89** Other injury of other muscles, fascia and tendons at forearm level

√7ᵗʰ **S56.891** Other injury of other muscles, fascia and tendons at forearm level, right arm

√7ᵗʰ **S56.892** Other injury of other muscles, fascia and tendons at forearm level, left arm

√7ᵗʰ **S56.899** Other injury of other muscles, fascia and tendons at forearm level, unspecified arm

√5ᵗʰ **S56.9** Injury of unspecified muscles, fascia and tendons at forearm level

√6ᵗʰ **S56.90** Unspecified injury of unspecified muscles, fascia and tendons at forearm level

√7ᵗʰ **S56.901** Unspecified injury of unspecified muscles, fascia and tendons at forearm level, right arm

√7ᵗʰ **S56.902** Unspecified injury of unspecified muscles, fascia and tendons at forearm level, left arm

√7ᵗʰ **S56.909** Unspecified injury of unspecified muscles, fascia and tendons at forearm level, unspecified arm

√6ᵗʰ **S56.91** Strain of unspecified muscles, fascia and tendons at forearm level

√7ᵗʰ **S56.911** Strain of unspecified muscles, fascia and tendons at forearm level, right arm

√7ᵗʰ **S56.912** Strain of unspecified muscles, fascia and tendons at forearm level, left arm

√7ᵗʰ **S56.919** Strain of unspecified muscles, fascia and tendons at forearm level, unspecified arm

√6ᵗʰ **S56.92** Laceration of unspecified muscles, fascia and tendons at forearm level

√7ᵗʰ **S56.921** Laceration of unspecified muscles, fascia and tendons at forearm level, right arm

√7ᵗʰ **S56.922** Laceration of unspecified muscles, fascia and tendons at forearm level, left arm

√7ᵗʰ **S56.929** Laceration of unspecified muscles, fascia and tendons at forearm level, unspecified arm

√6ᵗʰ **S56.99** Other injury of unspecified muscles, fascia and tendons at forearm level

√7ᵗʰ **S56.991** Other injury of unspecified muscles, fascia and tendons at forearm level, right arm

√7ᵗʰ **S56.992** Other injury of unspecified muscles, fascia and tendons at forearm level, left arm

√7ᵗʰ **S56.999** Other injury of unspecified muscles, fascia and tendons at forearm level, unspecified arm

√4ᵗʰ **S57** Crushing injury of elbow and forearm

Use additional code(s) for all associated injuries

EXCLUDES 2   crushing injury of wrist and hand (S67.-)

The appropriate 7th character is to be added to each code from category S57.
A   initial encounter
D   subsequent encounter
S   sequela

√5ᵗʰ **S57.0** Crushing injury of elbow

√x7ᵗʰ **S57.00** Crushing injury of unspecified elbow

√x7ᵗʰ **S57.01** Crushing injury of right elbow

√x7ᵗʰ **S57.02** Crushing injury of left elbow

√5ᵗʰ **S57.8** Crushing injury of forearm

√x7ᵗʰ **S57.80** Crushing injury of unspecified forearm

√x7ᵗʰ **S57.81** Crushing injury of right forearm

√x7ᵗʰ **S57.82** Crushing injury of left forearm

√4ᵗʰ **S58** Traumatic amputation of elbow and forearm

An amputation not identified as partial or complete should be coded to complete

EXCLUDES 1   traumatic amputation of wrist and hand (S68.-)

The appropriate 7th character is to be added to each code from category S58.
A   initial encounter
D   subsequent encounter
S   sequela

√5ᵗʰ **S58.0** Traumatic amputation at elbow level

√6ᵗʰ **S58.01** Complete traumatic amputation at elbow level

² √7ᵗʰ **S58.011** Complete traumatic amputation at elbow level, right arm   `HCC`

² √7ᵗʰ **S58.012** Complete traumatic amputation at elbow level, left arm   `HCC`

² √7ᵗʰ **S58.019** Complete traumatic amputation at elbow level, unspecified arm   `HCC`

√6ᵗʰ **S58.02** Partial traumatic amputation at elbow level

² √7ᵗʰ **S58.021** Partial traumatic amputation at elbow level, right arm   `HCC`

² √7ᵗʰ **S58.022** Partial traumatic amputation at elbow level, left arm   `HCC`

² √7ᵗʰ **S58.029** Partial traumatic amputation at elbow level, unspecified arm   `HCC`

√5ᵗʰ **S58.1** Traumatic amputation at level between elbow and wrist

√6ᵗʰ **S58.11** Complete traumatic amputation at level between elbow and wrist

² √7ᵗʰ **S58.111** Complete traumatic amputation at level between elbow and wrist, right arm   `HCC`

² √7ᵗʰ **S58.112** Complete traumatic amputation at level between elbow and wrist, left arm   `HCC`

² √7ᵗʰ **S58.119** Complete traumatic amputation at level between elbow and wrist, unspecified arm   `HCC`

√6ᵗʰ **S58.12** Partial traumatic amputation at level between elbow and wrist

² √7ᵗʰ **S58.121** Partial traumatic amputation at level between elbow and wrist, right arm   `HCC`

² √7ᵗʰ **S58.122** Partial traumatic amputation at level between elbow and wrist, left arm   `HCC`

² √7ᵗʰ **S58.129** Partial traumatic amputation at level between elbow and wrist, unspecified arm   `HCC`

✓ Additional Character Required   √x7ᵗʰ Placeholder Alert   Manifestation   Unspecified Dx   ►◄ Revised Text   ● New Code   ▲ Revised Code Title

ICD-10-CM 2020   1017

√5ᵗʰ **S58.9 Traumatic amputation of** forearm, level unspecified

     EXCLUDES 1   *traumatic amputation of wrist (S68.-)*

   √6ᵗʰ   **S58.91 Complete traumatic amputation of forearm, level unspecified**

      2   √7ᵗʰ   **S58.911 Complete traumatic amputation** of right **forearm, level unspecified**   HCC

      2   √7ᵗʰ   **S58.912 Complete traumatic amputation** of left **forearm, level unspecified**   HCC

      2   √7ᵗʰ   **S58.919 Complete traumatic amputation** of unspecified **forearm, level unspecified**   HCC

   √6ᵗʰ   **S58.92 Partial traumatic amputation of forearm, level unspecified**

      2   √7ᵗʰ   **S58.921 Partial traumatic amputation of** right **forearm, level unspecified**   HCC

      2   √7ᵗʰ   **S58.922 Partial traumatic amputation of** left **forearm, level unspecified**   HCC

      2   √7ᵗʰ   **S58.929 Partial traumatic amputation of** unspecified **forearm, level unspecified**   HCC

√4ᵗʰ **S59 Other and unspecified injuries of elbow and forearm**

     EXCLUDES 2   *other and unspecified injuries of wrist and hand (S69.-)*

     AHA: 2018,2Q,12; 2018,1Q,3; 2015,3Q,37-39

> The appropriate 7th character is to be added to each code from subcategories S59.0, S59.1, and S59.2.
> A   initial encounter for closed fracture
> D   subsequent encounter for fracture with routine healing
> G   subsequent encounter for fracture with delayed healing
> K   subsequent encounter for fracture with nonunion
> P   subsequent encounter for fracture with malunion
> S   sequela

   √5ᵗʰ   **S59.0 Physeal fracture of** lower end of ulna

     √6ᵗʰ   **S59.00 Unspecified physeal fracture of lower end of ulna**

       √7ᵗʰ   **S59.001 Unspecified physeal fracture of lower end of ulna,** right **arm**   Q

       √7ᵗʰ   **S59.002 Unspecified physeal fracture of lower end of ulna,** left **arm**   Q

       √7ᵗʰ   **S59.009 Unspecified physeal fracture of lower end of ulna, unspecified arm**   Q

     √6ᵗʰ   **S59.01 Salter-Harris Type I physeal fracture of lower end of ulna**

       √7ᵗʰ   **S59.011 Salter-Harris Type I physeal fracture of lower end of ulna, right arm**   Q

       √7ᵗʰ   **S59.012 Salter-Harris Type I physeal fracture of lower end of ulna,** left **arm**   Q

       √7ᵗʰ   **S59.019 Salter-Harris Type I physeal fracture of lower end of ulna, unspecified arm**   Q

     √6ᵗʰ   **S59.02 Salter-Harris Type II physeal fracture of lower end of ulna**

       √7ᵗʰ   **S59.021 Salter-Harris Type II physeal fracture of lower end of ulna, right arm**   Q

       √7ᵗʰ   **S59.022 Salter-Harris Type II physeal fracture of lower end of ulna,** left **arm**   Q

       √7ᵗʰ   **S59.029 Salter-Harris Type II physeal fracture of lower end of ulna, unspecified arm**   Q

     √6ᵗʰ   **S59.03 Salter-Harris Type III physeal fracture of lower end of ulna**

       √7ᵗʰ   **S59.031 Salter-Harris Type III physeal fracture of lower end of ulna, right arm**   Q

       √7ᵗʰ   **S59.032 Salter-Harris Type III physeal fracture of lower end of ulna,** left **arm**   Q

       √7ᵗʰ   **S59.039 Salter-Harris Type III physeal fracture of lower end of ulna, unspecified arm**   Q

     √6ᵗʰ   **S59.04 Salter-Harris Type IV physeal fracture of lower end of ulna**

       √7ᵗʰ   **S59.041 Salter-Harris Type IV physeal fracture of lower end of ulna, right arm**   Q

       √7ᵗʰ   **S59.042 Salter-Harris Type IV physeal fracture of lower end of ulna,** left **arm**   Q

       √7ᵗʰ   **S59.049 Salter-Harris Type IV physeal fracture of lower end of ulna, unspecified arm**   Q

     √6ᵗʰ   **S59.09 Other physeal fracture of lower end of ulna**

       √7ᵗʰ   **S59.091 Other physeal fracture of lower end of ulna, right arm**   Q

       √7ᵗʰ   **S59.092 Other physeal fracture of lower end of ulna, left arm**   Q

       √7ᵗʰ   **S59.099 Other physeal fracture of lower end of ulna, unspecified arm**   Q

   √5ᵗʰ   **S59.1 Physeal fracture of** upper end of radius

     √6ᵗʰ   **S59.10 Unspecified physeal fracture of upper end of radius**

       √7ᵗʰ   **S59.101 Unspecified physeal fracture of upper end of radius,** right **arm**   Q

       √7ᵗʰ   **S59.102 Unspecified physeal fracture of upper end of radius,** left **arm**   Q

       √7ᵗʰ   **S59.109 Unspecified physeal fracture of upper end of radius, unspecified arm**   Q

     √6ᵗʰ   **S59.11 Salter-Harris Type I physeal fracture of upper end of radius**

       √7ᵗʰ   **S59.111 Salter-Harris Type I physeal fracture of upper end of radius, right arm**   Q

       √7ᵗʰ   **S59.112 Salter-Harris Type I physeal fracture of upper end of radius, left arm**   Q

       √7ᵗʰ   **S59.119 Salter-Harris Type I physeal fracture of upper end of radius, unspecified arm**   Q

     √6ᵗʰ   **S59.12 Salter-Harris Type II physeal fracture of upper end of radius**

       √7ᵗʰ   **S59.121 Salter-Harris Type II physeal fracture of upper end of radius, right arm**   Q

       √7ᵗʰ   **S59.122 Salter-Harris Type II physeal fracture of upper end of radius, left arm**   Q

       √7ᵗʰ   **S59.129 Salter-Harris Type II physeal fracture of upper end of radius, unspecified arm**   Q

     √6ᵗʰ   **S59.13 Salter-Harris Type III physeal fracture of upper end of radius**

       √7ᵗʰ   **S59.131 Salter-Harris Type III physeal fracture of upper end of radius, right arm**   Q

       √7ᵗʰ   **S59.132 Salter-Harris Type III physeal fracture of upper end of radius, left arm**   Q

       √7ᵗʰ   **S59.139 Salter-Harris Type III physeal fracture of upper end of radius, unspecified arm**   Q

     √6ᵗʰ   **S59.14 Salter-Harris Type IV physeal fracture of upper end of radius**

       √7ᵗʰ   **S59.141 Salter-Harris Type IV physeal fracture of upper end of radius, right arm**   Q

       √7ᵗʰ   **S59.142 Salter-Harris Type IV physeal fracture of upper end of radius, left arm**   Q

       √7ᵗʰ   **S59.149 Salter-Harris Type IV physeal fracture of upper end of radius, unspecified arm**   Q

     √6ᵗʰ   **S59.19 Other physeal fracture of upper end of radius**

       √7ᵗʰ   **S59.191 Other physeal fracture of upper end of radius,** right **arm**   Q

       √7ᵗʰ   **S59.192 Other physeal fracture of upper end of radius,** left **arm**   Q

       √7ᵗʰ   **S59.199 Other physeal fracture of upper end of radius, unspecified arm**   Q

   √5ᵗʰ   **S59.2 Physeal fracture of** lower end of radius

     √6ᵗʰ   **S59.20 Unspecified physeal fracture of lower end of radius**

       √7ᵗʰ   **S59.201 Unspecified physeal fracture of lower end of radius,** right **arm**   Q

       √7ᵗʰ   **S59.202 Unspecified physeal fracture of lower end of radius,** left **arm**   Q

       √7ᵗʰ   **S59.209 Unspecified physeal fracture of lower end of radius, unspecified arm**   Q

✓6th **S59.21** Salter-Harris Type I physeal fracture of lower end of radius
- ✓7th **S59.211** Salter-Harris Type I physeal fracture of lower end of radius, right arm   Q
- ✓7th **S59.212** Salter-Harris Type I physeal fracture of lower end of radius, left arm   Q
- ✓7th **S59.219** Salter-Harris Type I physeal fracture of lower end of radius, unspecified arm   Q

✓6th **S59.22** Salter-Harris Type II physeal fracture of lower end of radius
- ✓7th **S59.221** Salter-Harris Type II physeal fracture of lower end of radius, right arm   Q
- ✓7th **S59.222** Salter-Harris Type II physeal fracture of lower end of radius, left arm   Q
- ✓7th **S59.229** Salter-Harris Type II physeal fracture of lower end of radius, unspecified arm   Q

✓6th **S59.23** Salter-Harris Type III physeal fracture of lower end of radius
- ✓7th **S59.231** Salter-Harris Type III physeal fracture of lower end of radius, right arm   Q
- ✓7th **S59.232** Salter-Harris Type III physeal fracture of lower end of radius, left arm   Q
- ✓7th **S59.239** Salter-Harris Type III physeal fracture of lower end of radius, unspecified arm   Q

✓6th **S59.24** Salter-Harris Type IV physeal fracture of lower end of radius
- ✓7th **S59.241** Salter-Harris Type IV physeal fracture of lower end of radius, right arm   Q
- ✓7th **S59.242** Salter-Harris Type IV physeal fracture of lower end of radius, left arm   Q
- ✓7th **S59.249** Salter-Harris Type IV physeal fracture of lower end of radius, unspecified arm   Q

✓6th **S59.29** Other physeal fracture of lower end of radius
- ✓7th **S59.291** Other physeal fracture of lower end of radius, right arm   Q
- ✓7th **S59.292** Other physeal fracture of lower end of radius, left arm   Q
- ✓7th **S59.299** Other physeal fracture of lower end of radius, unspecified arm   Q

✓5th **S59.8** Other specified injuries of elbow and forearm

> The appropriate 7th character is to be added to each code in subcategory S59.8.
> A   initial encounter
> D   subsequent encounter
> S   sequela

✓6th **S59.80** Other specified injuries of elbow
- ✓7th **S59.801** Other specified injuries of right elbow
- ✓7th **S59.802** Other specified injuries of left elbow
- ✓7th **S59.809** Other specified injuries of unspecified elbow

✓6th **S59.81** Other specified injuries of forearm
- ✓7th **S59.811** Other specified injuries right forearm
- ✓7th **S59.812** Other specified injuries left forearm
- ✓7th **S59.819** Other specified injuries unspecified forearm

✓5th **S59.9** Unspecified injury of elbow and forearm

> The appropriate 7th character is to be added to each code in subcategory S59.9.
> A   initial encounter
> D   subsequent encounter
> S   sequela

✓6th **S59.90** Unspecified injury of elbow
- ✓7th **S59.901** Unspecified injury of right elbow
- ✓7th **S59.902** Unspecified injury of left elbow
- ✓7th **S59.909** Unspecified injury of unspecified elbow

✓6th **S59.91** Unspecified injury of forearm
- ✓7th **S59.911** Unspecified injury of right forearm
- ✓7th **S59.912** Unspecified injury of left forearm
- ✓7th **S59.919** Unspecified injury of unspecified forearm

Injuries to the wrist, hand and fingers (S60-S69)

EXCLUDES 2   burns and corrosions (T20-T32)
     frostbite (T33-T34)
     insect bite or sting, venomous (T63.4)

✓4th **S60** Superficial injury of wrist, hand and fingers

> The appropriate 7th character is to be added to each code from category S60.
> A   initial encounter
> D   subsequent encounter
> S   sequela

✓5th **S60.0** Contusion of finger without damage to nail

> EXCLUDES 1   contusion involving nail (matrix) (S60.1)

✓x7th **S60.00** Contusion of unspecified finger without damage to nail
    Contusion of finger(s) NOS

✓6th **S60.01** Contusion of thumb without damage to nail
- ✓7th **S60.011** Contusion of right thumb without damage to nail
- ✓7th **S60.012** Contusion of left thumb without damage to nail
- ✓7th **S60.019** Contusion of unspecified thumb without damage to nail

✓6th **S60.02** Contusion of index finger without damage to nail
- ✓7th **S60.021** Contusion of right index finger without damage to nail
- ✓7th **S60.022** Contusion of left index finger without damage to nail
- ✓7th **S60.029** Contusion of unspecified index finger without damage to nail

✓6th **S60.03** Contusion of middle finger without damage to nail
- ✓7th **S60.031** Contusion of right middle finger without damage to nail
- ✓7th **S60.032** Contusion of left middle finger without damage to nail
- ✓7th **S60.039** Contusion of unspecified middle finger without damage to nail

✓6th **S60.04** Contusion of ring finger without damage to nail
- ✓7th **S60.041** Contusion of right ring finger without damage to nail
- ✓7th **S60.042** Contusion of left ring finger without damage to nail
- ✓7th **S60.049** Contusion of unspecified ring finger without damage to nail

✓6th **S60.05** Contusion of little finger without damage to nail
- ✓7th **S60.051** Contusion of right little finger without damage to nail
- ✓7th **S60.052** Contusion of left little finger without damage to nail
- ✓7th **S60.059** Contusion of unspecified little finger without damage to nail

✓5th **S60.1** Contusion of finger with damage to nail

✓x7th **S60.10** Contusion of unspecified finger with damage to nail

✓6th **S60.11** Contusion of thumb with damage to nail
- ✓7th **S60.111** Contusion of right thumb with damage to nail
- ✓7th **S60.112** Contusion of left thumb with damage to nail
- ✓7th **S60.119** Contusion of unspecified thumb with damage to nail

✓6th **S60.12** Contusion of index finger with damage to nail
- ✓7th **S60.121** Contusion of right index finger with damage to nail
- ✓7th **S60.122** Contusion of left index finger with damage to nail
- ✓7th **S60.129** Contusion of unspecified index finger with damage to nail

✓6th **S60.13** Contusion of middle finger with damage to nail
- ✓7th **S60.131** Contusion of right middle finger with damage to nail
- ✓7th **S60.132** Contusion of left middle finger with damage to nail

---

✓ Additional Character Required   ✓x7th Placeholder Alert   Manifestation   Unspecified Dx   ▶◀ Revised Text   ● New Code   ▲ Revised Code Title

√7th **S60.139** Contusion of unspecified middle finger with damage to nail

√6th **S60.14** Contusion of ring finger with damage to nail

√7th **S60.141** Contusion of right ring finger with damage to nail

√7th **S60.142** Contusion of left ring finger with damage to nail

√7th **S60.149** Contusion of unspecified ring finger with damage to nail

√6th **S60.15** Contusion of little finger with damage to nail

√7th **S60.151** Contusion of right little finger with damage to nail

√7th **S60.152** Contusion of left little finger with damage to nail

√7th **S60.159** Contusion of unspecified little finger with damage to nail

√5th **S60.2** Contusion of wrist and hand

EXCLUDES 2　contusion of fingers (S60.0-, S60.1-)

√6th **S60.21** Contusion of wrist

√7th **S60.211** Contusion of right wrist

√7th **S60.212** Contusion of left wrist

√7th **S60.219** Contusion of unspecified wrist

√6th **S60.22** Contusion of hand

√7th **S60.221** Contusion of right hand

√7th **S60.222** Contusion of left hand

√7th **S60.229** Contusion of unspecified hand

√5th **S60.3** Other superficial injuries of thumb

√6th **S60.31** Abrasion of thumb

√7th **S60.311** Abrasion of right thumb

√7th **S60.312** Abrasion of left thumb

√7th **S60.319** Abrasion of unspecified thumb

√6th **S60.32** Blister (nonthermal) of thumb

√7th **S60.321** Blister (nonthermal) of right thumb

√7th **S60.322** Blister (nonthermal) of left thumb

√7th **S60.329** Blister (nonthermal) of unspecified thumb

√6th **S60.34** External constriction of thumb

Hair tourniquet syndrome of thumb

Use additional cause code to identify the constricting item (W49.0-)

√7th **S60.341** External constriction of right thumb

√7th **S60.342** External constriction of left thumb

√7th **S60.349** External constriction of unspecified thumb

√6th **S60.35** Superficial foreign body of thumb

Splinter in the thumb

√7th **S60.351** Superficial foreign body of right thumb

√7th **S60.352** Superficial foreign body of left thumb

√7th **S60.359** Superficial foreign body of unspecified thumb

√6th **S60.36** Insect bite (nonvenomous) of thumb

√7th **S60.361** Insect bite (nonvenomous) of right thumb

√7th **S60.362** Insect bite (nonvenomous) of left thumb

√7th **S60.369** Insect bite (nonvenomous) of unspecified thumb

√6th **S60.37** Other superficial bite of thumb

EXCLUDES 1　open bite of thumb (S61.05-, S61.15-)

√7th **S60.371** Other superficial bite of right thumb

√7th **S60.372** Other superficial bite of left thumb

√7th **S60.379** Other superficial bite of unspecified thumb

√6th **S60.39** Other superficial injuries of thumb

√7th **S60.391** Other superficial injuries of right thumb

√7th **S60.392** Other superficial injuries of left thumb

√7th **S60.399** Other superficial injuries of unspecified thumb

√5th **S60.4** Other superficial injuries of other fingers

√6th **S60.41** Abrasion of fingers

√7th **S60.410** Abrasion of right index finger

√7th **S60.411** Abrasion of left index finger

√7th **S60.412** Abrasion of right middle finger

√7th **S60.413** Abrasion of left middle finger

√7th **S60.414** Abrasion of right ring finger

√7th **S60.415** Abrasion of left ring finger

√7th **S60.416** Abrasion of right little finger

√7th **S60.417** Abrasion of left little finger

√7th **S60.418** Abrasion of other finger

Abrasion of specified finger with unspecified laterality

√7th **S60.419** Abrasion of unspecified finger

√6th **S60.42** Blister (nonthermal) of fingers

√7th **S60.420** Blister (nonthermal) of right index finger

√7th **S60.421** Blister (nonthermal) of left index finger

√7th **S60.422** Blister (nonthermal) of right middle finger

√7th **S60.423** Blister (nonthermal) of left middle finger

√7th **S60.424** Blister (nonthermal) of right ring finger

√7th **S60.425** Blister (nonthermal) of left ring finger

√7th **S60.426** Blister (nonthermal) of right little finger

√7th **S60.427** Blister (nonthermal) of left little finger

√7th **S60.428** Blister (nonthermal) of other finger

Blister (nonthermal) of specified finger with unspecified laterality

√7th **S60.429** Blister (nonthermal) of unspecified finger

√6th **S60.44** External constriction of fingers

Hair tourniquet syndrome of finger

Use additional cause code to identify the constricting item (W49.0-)

√7th **S60.440** External constriction of right index finger

√7th **S60.441** External constriction of left index finger

√7th **S60.442** External constriction of right middle finger

√7th **S60.443** External constriction of left middle finger

√7th **S60.444** External constriction of right ring finger

√7th **S60.445** External constriction of left ring finger

√7th **S60.446** External constriction of right little finger

√7th **S60.447** External constriction of left little finger

√7th **S60.448** External constriction of other finger

External constriction of specified finger with unspecified laterality

√7th **S60.449** External constriction of unspecified finger

√6th **S60.45** Superficial foreign body of fingers

Splinter in the finger(s)

√7th **S60.450** Superficial foreign body of right index finger

√7th **S60.451** Superficial foreign body of left index finger

√7th **S60.452** Superficial foreign body of right middle finger

√7th **S60.453** Superficial foreign body of left middle finger

√7th **S60.454** Superficial foreign body of right ring finger

√7th **S60.455** Superficial foreign body of left ring finger

√7th **S60.456** Superficial foreign body of right little finger

√7th **S60.457** Superficial foreign body of left little finger

√7th **S60.458** Superficial foreign body of other finger

Superficial foreign body of specified finger with unspecified laterality

√7th **S60.459** Superficial foreign body of unspecified finger

√6th **S60.46** Insect bite (nonvenomous) of fingers

√7th **S60.460** Insect bite (nonvenomous) of right index finger

√7th **S60.461** Insect bite (nonvenomous) of left index finger

√7th **S60.462** Insect bite (nonvenomous) of right middle finger

√7th **S60.463** Insect bite (nonvenomous) of left middle finger

√7th **S60.464** Insect bite (nonvenomous) of right ring finger

√7th **S60.465** Insect bite (nonvenomous) of left ring finger

√7ᵗʰ **S60.466 Insect bite (nonvenomous) of** right little finger

√7ᵗʰ **S60.467 Insect bite (nonvenomous) of** left little finger

√7ᵗʰ **S60.468 Insect bite (nonvenomous) of other finger**
Insect bite (nonvenomous) of specified finger with unspecified laterality

√7ᵗʰ **S60.469 Insect bite (nonvenomous) of unspecified finger**

√6ᵗʰ **S60.47 Other superficial bite of fingers**
EXCLUDES 1   open bite of fingers (S61.25-, S61.35-)

√7ᵗʰ **S60.470 Other superficial bite of** right index **finger**

√7ᵗʰ **S60.471 Other superficial bite of** left index **finger**

√7ᵗʰ **S60.472 Other superficial bite of** right middle **finger**

√7ᵗʰ **S60.473 Other superficial bite of** left middle **finger**

√7ᵗʰ **S60.474 Other superficial bite of** right ring **finger**

√7ᵗʰ **S60.475 Other superficial bite of** left ring **finger**

√7ᵗʰ **S60.476 Other superficial bite of** right little **finger**

√7ᵗʰ **S60.477 Other superficial bite of** left little **finger**

√7ᵗʰ **S60.478 Other superficial bite of other finger**
Other superficial bite of specified finger with unspecified laterality

√7ᵗʰ **S60.479 Other superficial bite of unspecified finger**

√5ᵗʰ **S60.5 Other superficial injuries of** hand
EXCLUDES 2   superficial injuries of fingers (S60.3-, S60.4-)

√6ᵗʰ **S60.51 Abrasion of hand**

√7ᵗʰ **S60.511 Abrasion of** right **hand**

√7ᵗʰ **S60.512 Abrasion of** left **hand**

√7ᵗʰ **S60.519 Abrasion of unspecified hand**

√6ᵗʰ **S60.52 Blister (nonthermal) of hand**

√7ᵗʰ **S60.521 Blister (nonthermal) of** right **hand**

√7ᵗʰ **S60.522 Blister (nonthermal) of** left **hand**

√7ᵗʰ **S60.529 Blister (nonthermal) of unspecified hand**

√6ᵗʰ **S60.54 External constriction of hand**

√7ᵗʰ **S60.541 External constriction of** right **hand**

√7ᵗʰ **S60.542 External constriction of** left **hand**

√7ᵗʰ **S60.549 External constriction of unspecified hand**

√6ᵗʰ **S60.55 Superficial foreign body of hand**
Splinter in the hand

√7ᵗʰ **S60.551 Superficial foreign body of** right **hand**

√7ᵗʰ **S60.552 Superficial foreign body of** left **hand**

√7ᵗʰ **S60.559 Superficial foreign body of unspecified hand**

√6ᵗʰ **S60.56 Insect bite (nonvenomous) of hand**

√7ᵗʰ **S60.561 Insect bite (nonvenomous) of** right **hand**

√7ᵗʰ **S60.562 Insect bite (nonvenomous) of** left **hand**

√7ᵗʰ **S60.569 Insect bite (nonvenomous) of unspecified hand**

√6ᵗʰ **S60.57 Other superficial bite of hand**
EXCLUDES 1   open bite of hand (S61.45-)

√7ᵗʰ **S60.571 Other superficial bite of hand of** right **hand**

√7ᵗʰ **S60.572 Other superficial bite of hand of** left **hand**

√7ᵗʰ **S60.579 Other superficial bite of hand of unspecified hand**

√5ᵗʰ **S60.8 Other superficial injuries of** wrist

√6ᵗʰ **S60.81 Abrasion of wrist**

√7ᵗʰ **S60.811 Abrasion of** right **wrist**

√7ᵗʰ **S60.812 Abrasion of** left **wrist**

√7ᵗʰ **S60.819 Abrasion of unspecified wrist**

√6ᵗʰ **S60.82 Blister (nonthermal) of wrist**

√7ᵗʰ **S60.821 Blister (nonthermal) of** right **wrist**

√7ᵗʰ **S60.822 Blister (nonthermal) of** left **wrist**

√7ᵗʰ **S60.829 Blister (nonthermal) of unspecified wrist**

√6ᵗʰ **S60.84 External constriction of wrist**

√7ᵗʰ **S60.841 External constriction of** right **wrist**

√7ᵗʰ **S60.842 External constriction of** left **wrist**

√7ᵗʰ **S60.849 External constriction of unspecified wrist**

√6ᵗʰ **S60.85 Superficial foreign body of wrist**
Splinter in the wrist

√7ᵗʰ **S60.851 Superficial foreign body of** right **wrist**

√7ᵗʰ **S60.852 Superficial foreign body of** left **wrist**

√7ᵗʰ **S60.859 Superficial foreign body of unspecified wrist**

√6ᵗʰ **S60.86 Insect bite (nonvenomous) of wrist**

√7ᵗʰ **S60.861 Insect bite (nonvenomous) of** right **wrist**

√7ᵗʰ **S60.862 Insect bite (nonvenomous) of** left **wrist**

√7ᵗʰ **S60.869 Insect bite (nonvenomous) of unspecified wrist**

√6ᵗʰ **S60.87 Other superficial bite of wrist**
EXCLUDES 1   open bite of wrist (S61.55)

√7ᵗʰ **S60.871 Other superficial bite of** right **wrist**

√7ᵗʰ **S60.872 Other superficial bite of** left **wrist**

√7ᵗʰ **S60.879 Other superficial bite of unspecified wrist**

√5ᵗʰ **S60.9 Unspecified superficial injury of wrist, hand and fingers**

√6ᵗʰ **S60.91 Unspecified superficial injury of** wrist

√7ᵗʰ **S60.911 Unspecified superficial injury of** right **wrist**

√7ᵗʰ **S60.912 Unspecified superficial injury of** left **wrist**

√7ᵗʰ **S60.919 Unspecified superficial injury of unspecified wrist**

√6ᵗʰ **S60.92 Unspecified superficial injury of** hand

√7ᵗʰ **S60.921 Unspecified superficial injury of** right **hand**

√7ᵗʰ **S60.922 Unspecified superficial injury of** left **hand**

√7ᵗʰ **S60.929 Unspecified superficial injury of unspecified hand**

√6ᵗʰ **S60.93 Unspecified superficial injury of** thumb

√7ᵗʰ **S60.931 Unspecified superficial injury of** right **thumb**

√7ᵗʰ **S60.932 Unspecified superficial injury of** left **thumb**

√7ᵗʰ **S60.939 Unspecified superficial injury of unspecified thumb**

√6ᵗʰ **S60.94 Unspecified superficial injury of other** fingers

√7ᵗʰ **S60.940 Unspecified superficial injury of** right index **finger**

√7ᵗʰ **S60.941 Unspecified superficial injury of** left index **finger**

√7ᵗʰ **S60.942 Unspecified superficial injury of** right middle **finger**

√7ᵗʰ **S60.943 Unspecified superficial injury of** left middle **finger**

√7ᵗʰ **S60.944 Unspecified superficial injury of** right ring **finger**

√7ᵗʰ **S60.945 Unspecified superficial injury of** left ring **finger**

√7ᵗʰ **S60.946 Unspecified superficial injury of** right little **finger**

√7ᵗʰ **S60.947 Unspecified superficial injury of** left little **finger**

√7ᵗʰ **S60.948 Unspecified superficial injury of other finger**
Unspecified superficial injury of specified finger with unspecified laterality

√7ᵗʰ **S60.949 Unspecified superficial injury of unspecified finger**

√4ᵗʰ **S61 Open wound of wrist, hand and fingers**
Code also any associated wound infection
EXCLUDES 1   open fracture of wrist, hand and finger (S62.- with 7th character B)
traumatic amputation of wrist and hand (S68.-)

The appropriate 7th character is to be added to each code from category S61.
A   initial encounter
D   subsequent encounter
S   sequela

√5ᵗʰ **S61.0 Open wound of thumb without damage to nail**
EXCLUDES 1   open wound of thumb with damage to nail (S61.1-)

√6ᵗʰ **S61.00 Unspecified open wound of thumb without damage to nail**

√7ᵗʰ **S61.001 Unspecified open wound of** right **thumb without damage to nail**

✔ Additional Character Required   √ₓ7ᵗʰ Placeholder Alert   Manifestation   Unspecified Dx   ◄► Revised Text   ● New Code   ▲ Revised Code Title

ICD-10-CM 2020   **1021**

Chapter 19. Injury, Poisoning and Certain Other Consequences of External Causes

S61.002–S61.223

√7ᵗʰ **S61.002** Unspecified open wound of **left** thumb without damage to nail

√7ᵗʰ **S61.009** Unspecified open wound of unspecified thumb without damage to nail

√6ᵗʰ **S61.01** Laceration without foreign body of thumb without damage to nail

√7ᵗʰ **S61.011** Laceration without foreign body of **right** thumb without damage to nail

√7ᵗʰ **S61.012** Laceration without foreign body of **left** thumb without damage to nail

√7ᵗʰ **S61.019** Laceration without foreign body of unspecified thumb without damage to nail

√6ᵗʰ **S61.02** Laceration with foreign body of thumb without damage to nail

√7ᵗʰ **S61.021** Laceration with foreign body of **right** thumb without damage to nail

√7ᵗʰ **S61.022** Laceration with foreign body of **left** thumb without damage to nail

√7ᵗʰ **S61.029** Laceration with foreign body of unspecified thumb without damage to nail

√6ᵗʰ **S61.03** Puncture wound without foreign body of thumb without damage to nail

√7ᵗʰ **S61.031** Puncture wound without foreign body of **right** thumb without damage to nail

√7ᵗʰ **S61.032** Puncture wound without foreign body of **left** thumb without damage to nail

√7ᵗʰ **S61.039** Puncture wound without foreign body of unspecified thumb without damage to nail

√6ᵗʰ **S61.04** Puncture wound with foreign body of thumb without damage to nail

√7ᵗʰ **S61.041** Puncture wound with foreign body of **right** thumb without damage to nail

√7ᵗʰ **S61.042** Puncture wound with foreign body of **left** thumb without damage to nail

√7ᵗʰ **S61.049** Puncture wound with foreign body of unspecified thumb without damage to nail

√6ᵗʰ **S61.05** Open bite of thumb without damage to nail

Bite of thumb NOS

EXCLUDES 1   superficial bite of thumb (S60.36-, S60.37-)

√7ᵗʰ **S61.051** Open bite of **right** thumb without damage to nail

√7ᵗʰ **S61.052** Open bite of **left** thumb without damage to nail

√7ᵗʰ **S61.059** Open bite of unspecified thumb without damage to nail

√5ᵗʰ **S61.1** Open wound of thumb with damage to nail

√6ᵗʰ **S61.10** Unspecified open wound of thumb with damage to nail

√7ᵗʰ **S61.101** Unspecified open wound of **right** thumb with damage to nail

√7ᵗʰ **S61.102** Unspecified open wound of **left** thumb with damage to nail

√7ᵗʰ **S61.109** Unspecified open wound of unspecified thumb with damage to nail

√6ᵗʰ **S61.11** Laceration without foreign body of thumb with damage to nail

√7ᵗʰ **S61.111** Laceration without foreign body of **right** thumb with damage to nail

√7ᵗʰ **S61.112** Laceration without foreign body of **left** thumb with damage to nail

√7ᵗʰ **S61.119** Laceration without foreign body of unspecified thumb with damage to nail

√6ᵗʰ **S61.12** Laceration with foreign body of thumb with damage to nail

√7ᵗʰ **S61.121** Laceration with foreign body of **right** thumb with damage to nail

√7ᵗʰ **S61.122** Laceration with foreign body of **left** thumb with damage to nail

√7ᵗʰ **S61.129** Laceration with foreign body of unspecified thumb with damage to nail

√6ᵗʰ **S61.13** Puncture wound without foreign body of thumb with damage to nail

√7ᵗʰ **S61.131** Puncture wound without foreign body of **right** thumb with damage to nail

√7ᵗʰ **S61.132** Puncture wound without foreign body of **left** thumb with damage to nail

√7ᵗʰ **S61.139** Puncture wound without foreign body of unspecified thumb with damage to nail

√6ᵗʰ **S61.14** Puncture wound with foreign body of thumb with damage to nail

√7ᵗʰ **S61.141** Puncture wound with foreign body of **right** thumb with damage to nail

√7ᵗʰ **S61.142** Puncture wound with foreign body of **left** thumb with damage to nail

√7ᵗʰ **S61.149** Puncture wound with foreign body of unspecified thumb with damage to nail

√6ᵗʰ **S61.15** Open bite of thumb with damage to nail

Bite of thumb with damage to nail NOS

EXCLUDES 1   superficial bite of thumb (S60.36-, S60.37-)

√7ᵗʰ **S61.151** Open bite of **right** thumb with damage to nail

√7ᵗʰ **S61.152** Open bite of **left** thumb with damage to nail

√7ᵗʰ **S61.159** Open bite of unspecified thumb with damage to nail

√5ᵗʰ **S61.2** Open wound of other **finger without damage to nail**

EXCLUDES 1   open wound of finger involving nail (matrix) (S61.3-)

EXCLUDES 2   open wound of thumb without damage to nail (S61.0-)

√6ᵗʰ **S61.20** Unspecified open wound of other finger without damage to nail

√7ᵗʰ **S61.200** Unspecified open wound of **right index** finger without damage to nail

√7ᵗʰ **S61.201** Unspecified open wound of **left index** finger without damage to nail

√7ᵗʰ **S61.202** Unspecified open wound of **right middle** finger without damage to nail

√7ᵗʰ **S61.203** Unspecified open wound of **left middle** finger without damage to nail

√7ᵗʰ **S61.204** Unspecified open wound of **right ring** finger without damage to nail

√7ᵗʰ **S61.205** Unspecified open wound of **left ring** finger without damage to nail

√7ᵗʰ **S61.206** Unspecified open wound of **right little** finger without damage to nail

√7ᵗʰ **S61.207** Unspecified open wound of **left little** finger without damage to nail

√7ᵗʰ **S61.208** Unspecified open wound of **other finger** without damage to nail

Unspecified open wound of specified finger with unspecified laterality without damage to nail

√7ᵗʰ **S61.209** Unspecified open wound of unspecified finger without damage to nail

√6ᵗʰ **S61.21** Laceration without foreign body of finger without damage to nail

√7ᵗʰ **S61.210** Laceration without foreign body of **right index** finger without damage to nail

√7ᵗʰ **S61.211** Laceration without foreign body of **left index** finger without damage to nail

√7ᵗʰ **S61.212** Laceration without foreign body of **right middle** finger without damage to nail

√7ᵗʰ **S61.213** Laceration without foreign body of **left middle** finger without damage to nail

√7ᵗʰ **S61.214** Laceration without foreign body of **right ring** finger without damage to nail

√7ᵗʰ **S61.215** Laceration without foreign body of **left ring** finger without damage to nail

√7ᵗʰ **S61.216** Laceration without foreign body of **right little** finger without damage to nail

√7ᵗʰ **S61.217** Laceration without foreign body of **left little** finger without damage to nail

√7ᵗʰ **S61.218** Laceration without foreign body of other finger without damage to nail

Laceration without foreign body of specified finger with unspecified laterality without damage to nail

√7ᵗʰ **S61.219** Laceration without foreign body of unspecified finger without damage to nail

√6ᵗʰ **S61.22** Laceration with foreign body of finger without damage to nail

√7ᵗʰ **S61.220** Laceration with foreign body of **right index** finger without damage to nail

√7ᵗʰ **S61.221** Laceration with foreign body of **left index** finger without damage to nail

√7ᵗʰ **S61.222** Laceration with foreign body of **right middle** finger without damage to nail

√7ᵗʰ **S61.223** Laceration with foreign body of **left middle** finger without damage to nail

✓7ᵗʰ **S61.224** Laceration with foreign body of right ring finger without damage to nail

✓7ᵗʰ **S61.225** Laceration with foreign body of left ring finger without damage to nail

✓7ᵗʰ **S61.226** Laceration with foreign body of right little finger without damage to nail

✓7ᵗʰ **S61.227** Laceration with foreign body of left little finger without damage to nail

✓7ᵗʰ **S61.228** Laceration with foreign body of other finger without damage to nail

　　　Laceration with foreign body of specified finger with unspecified laterality without damage to nail

✓7ᵗʰ **S61.229** Laceration with foreign body of unspecified finger without damage to nail

✓6ᵗʰ **S61.23** Puncture wound without foreign body of finger without damage to nail

✓7ᵗʰ **S61.230** Puncture wound without foreign body of right index finger without damage to nail

✓7ᵗʰ **S61.231** Puncture wound without foreign body of left index finger without damage to nail

✓7ᵗʰ **S61.232** Puncture wound without foreign body of right middle finger without damage to nail

✓7ᵗʰ **S61.233** Puncture wound without foreign body of left middle finger without damage to nail

✓7ᵗʰ **S61.234** Puncture wound without foreign body of right ring finger without damage to nail

✓7ᵗʰ **S61.235** Puncture wound without foreign body of left ring finger without damage to nail

✓7ᵗʰ **S61.236** Puncture wound without foreign body of right little finger without damage to nail

✓7ᵗʰ **S61.237** Puncture wound without foreign body of left little finger without damage to nail

✓7ᵗʰ **S61.238** Puncture wound without foreign body of other finger without damage to nail

　　　Puncture wound without foreign body of specified finger with unspecified laterality without damage to nail

✓7ᵗʰ **S61.239** Puncture wound without foreign body of unspecified finger without damage to nail

✓6ᵗʰ **S61.24** Puncture wound with foreign body of finger without damage to nail

✓7ᵗʰ **S61.240** Puncture wound with foreign body of right index finger without damage to nail

✓7ᵗʰ **S61.241** Puncture wound with foreign body of left index finger without damage to nail

✓7ᵗʰ **S61.242** Puncture wound with foreign body of right middle finger without damage to nail

✓7ᵗʰ **S61.243** Puncture wound with foreign body of left middle finger without damage to nail

✓7ᵗʰ **S61.244** Puncture wound with foreign body of right ring finger without damage to nail

✓7ᵗʰ **S61.245** Puncture wound with foreign body of left ring finger without damage to nail

✓7ᵗʰ **S61.246** Puncture wound with foreign body of right little finger without damage to nail

✓7ᵗʰ **S61.247** Puncture wound with foreign body of left little finger without damage to nail

✓7ᵗʰ **S61.248** Puncture wound with foreign body of other finger without damage to nail

　　　Puncture wound with foreign body of specified finger with unspecified laterality without damage to nail

✓7ᵗʰ **S61.249** Puncture wound with foreign body of unspecified finger without damage to nail

✓6ᵗʰ **S61.25** Open bite of finger without damage to nail

　　　Bite of finger without damage to nail NOS

　　　EXCLUDES 1　*superficial bite of finger (S60.46-, S60.47-)*

✓7ᵗʰ **S61.250** Open bite of right index finger without damage to nail

✓7ᵗʰ **S61.251** Open bite of left index finger without damage to nail

✓7ᵗʰ **S61.252** Open bite of right middle finger without damage to nail

✓7ᵗʰ **S61.253** Open bite of left middle finger without damage to nail

✓7ᵗʰ **S61.254** Open bite of right ring finger without damage to nail

✓7ᵗʰ **S61.255** Open bite of left ring finger without damage to nail

✓7ᵗʰ **S61.256** Open bite of right little finger without damage to nail

✓7ᵗʰ **S61.257** Open bite of left little finger without damage to nail

✓7ᵗʰ **S61.258** Open bite of other finger without damage to nail

　　　Open bite of specified finger with unspecified laterality without damage to nail

✓7ᵗʰ **S61.259** Open bite of unspecified finger without damage to nail

✓5ᵗʰ **S61.3** Open wound of other finger with damage to nail

✓6ᵗʰ **S61.30** Unspecified open wound of finger with damage to nail

✓7ᵗʰ **S61.300** Unspecified open wound of right index finger with damage to nail

✓7ᵗʰ **S61.301** Unspecified open wound of left index finger with damage to nail

✓7ᵗʰ **S61.302** Unspecified open wound of right middle finger with damage to nail

✓7ᵗʰ **S61.303** Unspecified open wound of left middle finger with damage to nail

✓7ᵗʰ **S61.304** Unspecified open wound of right ring finger with damage to nail

✓7ᵗʰ **S61.305** Unspecified open wound of left ring finger with damage to nail

✓7ᵗʰ **S61.306** Unspecified open wound of right little finger with damage to nail

✓7ᵗʰ **S61.307** Unspecified open wound of left little finger with damage to nail

✓7ᵗʰ **S61.308** Unspecified open wound of other finger with damage to nail

　　　Unspecified open wound of specified finger with unspecified laterality with damage to nail

✓7ᵗʰ **S61.309** Unspecified open wound of unspecified finger with damage to nail

✓6ᵗʰ **S61.31** Laceration without foreign body of finger with damage to nail

✓7ᵗʰ **S61.310** Laceration without foreign body of right index finger with damage to nail

✓7ᵗʰ **S61.311** Laceration without foreign body of left index finger with damage to nail

✓7ᵗʰ **S61.312** Laceration without foreign body of right middle finger with damage to nail

✓7ᵗʰ **S61.313** Laceration without foreign body of left middle finger with damage to nail

✓7ᵗʰ **S61.314** Laceration without foreign body of right ring finger with damage to nail

✓7ᵗʰ **S61.315** Laceration without foreign body of left ring finger with damage to nail

✓7ᵗʰ **S61.316** Laceration without foreign body of right little finger with damage to nail

✓7ᵗʰ **S61.317** Laceration without foreign body of left little finger with damage to nail

✓7ᵗʰ **S61.318** Laceration without foreign body of other finger with damage to nail

　　　Laceration without foreign body of specified finger with unspecified laterality with damage to nail

✓7ᵗʰ **S61.319** Laceration without foreign body of unspecified finger with damage to nail

✓6ᵗʰ **S61.32** Laceration with foreign body of finger with damage to nail

✓7ᵗʰ **S61.320** Laceration with foreign body of right index finger with damage to nail

✓7ᵗʰ **S61.321** Laceration with foreign body of left index finger with damage to nail

✓7ᵗʰ **S61.322** Laceration with foreign body of right middle finger with damage to nail

✓7ᵗʰ **S61.323** Laceration with foreign body of left middle finger with damage to nail

✓7ᵗʰ **S61.324** Laceration with foreign body of right ring finger with damage to nail

✓7ᵗʰ **S61.325** Laceration with foreign body of left ring finger with damage to nail

✓7ᵗʰ **S61.326** Laceration with foreign body of right little finger with damage to nail

✓7ᵗʰ **S61.327** Laceration with foreign body of left little finger with damage to nail

☑ Additional Character Required　　✓x7ᵗʰ Placeholder Alert　　Manifestation　　Unspecified Dx　　►◄ Revised Text　　● New Code　　▲ Revised Code Title

ICD-10-CM 2020　　　　　　　　　　　　　　　　　　　　　　　　　　　　　　　　　**1023**

√7ᵗʰ **S61.328 Laceration with foreign body of other finger with damage to nail**
Laceration with foreign body of specified finger with unspecified laterality with damage to nail

√7ᵗʰ **S61.329 Laceration with foreign body of unspecified finger with damage to nail**

√6ᵗʰ **S61.33** Puncture wound without foreign body of finger with damage to nail

√7ᵗʰ **S61.330 Puncture wound without foreign body of right index finger with damage to nail**

√7ᵗʰ **S61.331 Puncture wound without foreign body of left index finger with damage to nail**

√7ᵗʰ **S61.332 Puncture wound without foreign body of right middle finger with damage to nail**

√7ᵗʰ **S61.333 Puncture wound without foreign body of left middle finger with damage to nail**

√7ᵗʰ **S61.334 Puncture wound without foreign body of right ring finger with damage to nail**

√7ᵗʰ **S61.335 Puncture wound without foreign body of left ring finger with damage to nail**

√7ᵗʰ **S61.336 Puncture wound without foreign body of right little finger with damage to nail**

√7ᵗʰ **S61.337 Puncture wound without foreign body of left little finger with damage to nail**

√7ᵗʰ **S61.338 Puncture wound without foreign body of other finger with damage to nail**
Puncture wound without foreign body of specified finger with unspecified laterality with damage to nail

√7ᵗʰ **S61.339 Puncture wound without foreign body of unspecified finger with damage to nail**

√6ᵗʰ **S61.34** Puncture wound with foreign body of finger with damage to nail

√7ᵗʰ **S61.340 Puncture wound with foreign body of right index finger with damage to nail**

√7ᵗʰ **S61.341 Puncture wound with foreign body of left index finger with damage to nail**

√7ᵗʰ **S61.342 Puncture wound with foreign body of right middle finger with damage to nail**

√7ᵗʰ **S61.343 Puncture wound with foreign body of left middle finger with damage to nail**

√7ᵗʰ **S61.344 Puncture wound with foreign body of right ring finger with damage to nail**

√7ᵗʰ **S61.345 Puncture wound with foreign body of left ring finger with damage to nail**

√7ᵗʰ **S61.346 Puncture wound with foreign body of right little finger with damage to nail**

√7ᵗʰ **S61.347 Puncture wound with foreign body of left little finger with damage to nail**

√7ᵗʰ **S61.348 Puncture wound with foreign body of other finger with damage to nail**
Puncture wound with foreign body of specified finger with unspecified laterality with damage to nail

√7ᵗʰ **S61.349 Puncture wound with foreign body of unspecified finger with damage to nail**

√6ᵗʰ **S61.35** Open bite of finger with damage to nail
Bite of finger with damage to nail NOS
EXCLUDES 1 *superficial bite of finger (S60.46-, S60.47-)*

√7ᵗʰ **S61.350 Open bite of right index finger with damage to nail**

√7ᵗʰ **S61.351 Open bite of left index finger with damage to nail**

√7ᵗʰ **S61.352 Open bite of right middle finger with damage to nail**

√7ᵗʰ **S61.353 Open bite of left middle finger with damage to nail**

√7ᵗʰ **S61.354 Open bite of right ring finger with damage to nail**

√7ᵗʰ **S61.355 Open bite of left ring finger with damage to nail**

√7ᵗʰ **S61.356 Open bite of right little finger with damage to nail**

√7ᵗʰ **S61.357 Open bite of left little finger with damage to nail**

√7ᵗʰ **S61.358 Open bite of other finger with damage to nail**
Open bite of specified finger with unspecified laterality with damage to nail

√7ᵗʰ **S61.359 Open bite of unspecified finger with damage to nail**

√5ᵗʰ **S61.4 Open wound of** hand

√6ᵗʰ **S61.40 Unspecified open wound of hand**

√7ᵗʰ **S61.401 Unspecified open wound of right hand**

√7ᵗʰ **S61.402 Unspecified open wound of left hand**

√7ᵗʰ **S61.409 Unspecified open wound of unspecified hand**

√6ᵗʰ **S61.41** Laceration without foreign body of hand

√7ᵗʰ **S61.411 Laceration without foreign body of right hand**

√7ᵗʰ **S61.412 Laceration without foreign body of left hand**

√7ᵗʰ **S61.419 Laceration without foreign body of unspecified hand**

√6ᵗʰ **S61.42** Laceration with foreign body of hand

√7ᵗʰ **S61.421 Laceration with foreign body of right hand**

√7ᵗʰ **S61.422 Laceration with foreign body of left hand**

√7ᵗʰ **S61.429 Laceration with foreign body of unspecified hand**

√6ᵗʰ **S61.43** Puncture wound without foreign body of hand

√7ᵗʰ **S61.431 Puncture wound without foreign body of right hand**

√7ᵗʰ **S61.432 Puncture wound without foreign body of left hand**

√7ᵗʰ **S61.439 Puncture wound without foreign body of unspecified hand**

√6ᵗʰ **S61.44** Puncture wound with foreign body of hand

√7ᵗʰ **S61.441 Puncture wound with foreign body of right hand**

√7ᵗʰ **S61.442 Puncture wound with foreign body of left hand**

√7ᵗʰ **S61.449 Puncture wound with foreign body of unspecified hand**

√6ᵗʰ **S61.45** Open bite of hand
Bite of hand NOS
EXCLUDES 1 *superficial bite of hand (S60.56-, S60.57-)*

√7ᵗʰ **S61.451 Open bite of right hand**

√7ᵗʰ **S61.452 Open bite of left hand**

√7ᵗʰ **S61.459 Open bite of unspecified hand**

√5ᵗʰ **S61.5 Open wound of** wrist

√6ᵗʰ **S61.50 Unspecified open wound of wrist**

√7ᵗʰ **S61.501 Unspecified open wound of right wrist**

√7ᵗʰ **S61.502 Unspecified open wound of left wrist**

√7ᵗʰ **S61.509 Unspecified open wound of unspecified wrist**

√6ᵗʰ **S61.51** Laceration without foreign body of wrist

√7ᵗʰ **S61.511 Laceration without foreign body of right wrist**

√7ᵗʰ **S61.512 Laceration without foreign body of left wrist**

√7ᵗʰ **S61.519 Laceration without foreign body of unspecified wrist**

√6ᵗʰ **S61.52** Laceration with foreign body of wrist

√7ᵗʰ **S61.521 Laceration with foreign body of right wrist**

√7ᵗʰ **S61.522 Laceration with foreign body of left wrist**

√7ᵗʰ **S61.529 Laceration with foreign body of unspecified wrist**

√6ᵗʰ **S61.53** Puncture wound without foreign body of wrist

√7ᵗʰ **S61.531 Puncture wound without foreign body of right wrist**

√7ᵗʰ **S61.532 Puncture wound without foreign body of left wrist**

√7ᵗʰ **S61.539 Puncture wound without foreign body of unspecified wrist**

√6ᵗʰ **S61.54** Puncture wound with foreign body of wrist

√7ᵗʰ **S61.541 Puncture wound with foreign body of right wrist**

√7ᵗʰ **S61.542 Puncture wound with foreign body of left wrist**

√7ᵗʰ **S61.549 Puncture wound with foreign body of unspecified wrist**

✓6ᵗʰ **S61.55** **Open bite** of wrist

Bite of wrist NOS

> **EXCLUDES 1** *superficial bite of wrist (S60.86-, S60.87-)*

✓7ᵗʰ **S61.551** **Open bite of right wrist**

✓7ᵗʰ **S61.552** **Open bite of left wrist**

✓7ᵗʰ **S61.559** **Open bite of unspecified wrist**

✓4ᵗʰ **S62** **Fracture at wrist and hand level**

> **NOTE** A fracture not indicated as displaced or nondisplaced should be coded to displaced
>
> A fracture not indicated as open or closed should be coded to closed

EXCLUDES 1 *traumatic amputation of wrist and hand (S68.-)*

EXCLUDES 2 *fracture of distal parts of ulna and radius (S52.-)*

AHA: 2018,2Q,12; 2015,3Q,37-39

The appropriate 7th character is to be added to each code from category S62.
A   initial encounter for closed fracture
B   initial encounter for open fracture
D   subsequent encounter for fracture with routine healing
G   subsequent encounter for fracture with delayed healing
K   subsequent encounter for fracture with nonunion
P   subsequent encounter for fracture with malunion
S   sequela

✓5ᵗʰ **S62.0** **Fracture of navicular [scaphoid] bone of wrist**

✓6ᵗʰ **S62.00** **Unspecified fracture of navicular [scaphoid] bone of wrist**

✓7ᵗʰ **S62.001** **Unspecified fracture of navicular [scaphoid] bone of right wrist** ◘

✓7ᵗʰ **S62.002** **Unspecified fracture of navicular [scaphoid] bone of left wrist** ◘

AHA: 2012,4Q,106

✓7ᵗʰ **S62.009** **Unspecified fracture of navicular [scaphoid] bone of unspecified wrist** ◘

✓6ᵗʰ **S62.01** **Fracture of distal pole of navicular [scaphoid] bone of wrist**

Fracture of volar tuberosity of navicular [scaphoid] bone of wrist

✓7ᵗʰ **S62.011** **Displaced fracture of distal pole of navicular [scaphoid] bone of right wrist** ◘

✓7ᵗʰ **S62.012** **Displaced fracture of distal pole of navicular [scaphoid] bone of left wrist** ◘

✓7ᵗʰ **S62.013** **Displaced fracture of distal pole of navicular [scaphoid] bone of unspecified wrist** ◘

✓7ᵗʰ **S62.014** **Nondisplaced fracture of distal pole of navicular [scaphoid] bone of right wrist** ◘

✓7ᵗʰ **S62.015** **Nondisplaced fracture of distal pole of navicular [scaphoid] bone of left wrist** ◘

✓7ᵗʰ **S62.016** **Nondisplaced fracture of distal pole of navicular [scaphoid] bone of unspecified wrist** ◘

✓6ᵗʰ **S62.02** **Fracture of middle third of navicular [scaphoid] bone of wrist**

✓7ᵗʰ **S62.021** **Displaced fracture of middle third of navicular [scaphoid] bone of right wrist** ◘

✓7ᵗʰ **S62.022** **Displaced fracture of middle third of navicular [scaphoid] bone of left wrist** ◘

✓7ᵗʰ **S62.023** **Displaced fracture of middle third of navicular [scaphoid] bone of unspecified wrist** ◘

✓7ᵗʰ **S62.024** **Nondisplaced fracture of middle third of navicular [scaphoid] bone of right wrist** ◘

✓7ᵗʰ **S62.025** **Nondisplaced fracture of middle third of navicular [scaphoid] bone of left wrist** ◘

✓7ᵗʰ **S62.026** **Nondisplaced fracture of middle third of navicular [scaphoid] bone of unspecified wrist** ◘

✓6ᵗʰ **S62.03** **Fracture of proximal third of navicular [scaphoid] bone of wrist**

✓7ᵗʰ **S62.031** **Displaced fracture of proximal third of navicular [scaphoid] bone of right wrist** ◘

✓7ᵗʰ **S62.032** **Displaced fracture of proximal third of navicular [scaphoid] bone of left wrist** ◘

✓7ᵗʰ **S62.033** **Displaced fracture of proximal third of navicular [scaphoid] bone of unspecified wrist** ◘

✓7ᵗʰ **S62.034** **Nondisplaced fracture of proximal third of navicular [scaphoid] bone of right wrist** ◘

✓7ᵗʰ **S62.035** **Nondisplaced fracture of proximal third of navicular [scaphoid] bone of left wrist** ◘

✓7ᵗʰ **S62.036** **Nondisplaced fracture of proximal third of navicular [scaphoid] bone of unspecified wrist** ◘

✓5ᵗʰ **S62.1** **Fracture of other and unspecified carpal bone(s)**

> **EXCLUDES 2** *fracture of scaphoid of wrist (S62.0-)*

✓6ᵗʰ **S62.10** **Fracture of unspecified carpal bone**

Fracture of wrist NOS

✓7ᵗʰ **S62.101** **Fracture of unspecified carpal bone, right wrist** ◘

✓7ᵗʰ **S62.102** **Fracture of unspecified carpal bone, left wrist** ◘

AHA: 2012,4Q,95

✓7ᵗʰ **S62.109** **Fracture of unspecified carpal bone, unspecified wrist** ◘

✓6ᵗʰ **S62.11** **Fracture of triquetrum [cuneiform] bone of wrist**

✓7ᵗʰ **S62.111** **Displaced fracture of triquetrum [cuneiform] bone, right wrist** ◘

✓7ᵗʰ **S62.112** **Displaced fracture of triquetrum [cuneiform] bone, left wrist** ◘

✓7ᵗʰ **S62.113** **Displaced fracture of triquetrum [cuneiform] bone, unspecified wrist** ◘

✓7ᵗʰ **S62.114** **Nondisplaced fracture of triquetrum [cuneiform] bone, right wrist** ◘

✓7ᵗʰ **S62.115** **Nondisplaced fracture of triquetrum [cuneiform] bone, left wrist** ◘

✓7ᵗʰ **S62.116** **Nondisplaced fracture of triquetrum [cuneiform] bone, unspecified wrist** ◘

✓6ᵗʰ **S62.12** **Fracture of lunate [semilunar]**

✓7ᵗʰ **S62.121** **Displaced fracture of lunate [semilunar], right wrist** ◘

✓7ᵗʰ **S62.122** **Displaced fracture of lunate [semilunar], left wrist** ◘

✓7ᵗʰ **S62.123** **Displaced fracture of lunate [semilunar], unspecified wrist** ◘

✓7ᵗʰ **S62.124** **Nondisplaced fracture of lunate [semilunar], right wrist** ◘

✓7ᵗʰ **S62.125** **Nondisplaced fracture of lunate [semilunar], left wrist** ◘

✓7ᵗʰ **S62.126** **Nondisplaced fracture of lunate [semilunar], unspecified wrist** ◘

✓6ᵗʰ **S62.13** **Fracture of capitate [os magnum] bone**

✓7ᵗʰ **S62.131** **Displaced fracture of capitate [os magnum] bone, right wrist** ◘

✓7ᵗʰ **S62.132** **Displaced fracture of capitate [os magnum] bone, left wrist** ◘

✓7ᵗʰ **S62.133** **Displaced fracture of capitate [os magnum] bone, unspecified wrist** ◘

✓7ᵗʰ **S62.134** **Nondisplaced fracture of capitate [os magnum] bone, right wrist** ◘

✓7ᵗʰ **S62.135** **Nondisplaced fracture of capitate [os magnum] bone, left wrist** ◘

✓7ᵗʰ **S62.136** **Nondisplaced fracture of capitate [os magnum] bone, unspecified wrist** ◘

✓6ᵗʰ **S62.14** **Fracture of body of hamate [unciform] bone**

Fracture of hamate [unciform] bone NOS

✓7ᵗʰ **S62.141** **Displaced fracture of body of hamate [unciform] bone, right wrist** ◘

☑ Additional Character Required   ✓×7ᵗʰ Placeholder Alert   Manifestation   Unspecified Dx   ►◄ Revised Text   ● New Code   ▲ Revised Code Title

Chapter 19. Injury, Poisoning and Certain Other Consequences of External Causes

S62.142–S62.256

√7ᵗʰ **S62.142** Displaced **fracture of body of hamate [unciform] bone, left wrist** Q

√7ᵗʰ **S62.143** Displaced **fracture of body of hamate [unciform] bone, unspecified wrist** Q

√7ᵗʰ **S62.144** Nondisplaced **fracture of body of hamate [unciform] bone, right wrist** Q

√7ᵗʰ **S62.145** Nondisplaced **fracture of body of hamate [unciform] bone, left wrist** Q

√7ᵗʰ **S62.146** Nondisplaced **fracture of body of hamate [unciform] bone, unspecified wrist** Q

√6ᵗʰ **S62.15** Fracture of **hook process of hamate [unciform] bone**

     Fracture of unciform process of hamate [unciform] bone

√7ᵗʰ **S62.151** Displaced **fracture of hook process of hamate [unciform] bone, right wrist** Q

√7ᵗʰ **S62.152** Displaced **fracture of hook process of hamate [unciform] bone, left wrist** Q

√7ᵗʰ **S62.153** Displaced **fracture of hook process of hamate [unciform] bone, unspecified wrist** Q

√7ᵗʰ **S62.154** Nondisplaced **fracture of hook process of hamate [unciform] bone, right wrist** Q

√7ᵗʰ **S62.155** Nondisplaced **fracture of hook process of hamate [unciform] bone, left wrist** Q

√7ᵗʰ **S62.156** Nondisplaced **fracture of hook process of hamate [unciform] bone, unspecified wrist** Q

√6ᵗʰ **S62.16** Fracture of **pisiform**

√7ᵗʰ **S62.161** Displaced **fracture of pisiform, right wrist** Q

√7ᵗʰ **S62.162** Displaced **fracture of pisiform, left wrist** Q

√7ᵗʰ **S62.163** Displaced **fracture of pisiform, unspecified wrist** Q

√7ᵗʰ **S62.164** Nondisplaced **fracture of pisiform, right wrist** Q

√7ᵗʰ **S62.165** Nondisplaced **fracture of pisiform, left wrist** Q

√7ᵗʰ **S62.166** Nondisplaced **fracture of pisiform, unspecified wrist** Q

√6ᵗʰ **S62.17** Fracture of **trapezium [larger multangular]**

√7ᵗʰ **S62.171** Displaced **fracture of trapezium [larger multangular], right wrist** Q

√7ᵗʰ **S62.172** Displaced **fracture of trapezium [larger multangular], left wrist** Q

√7ᵗʰ **S62.173** Displaced **fracture of trapezium [larger multangular], unspecified wrist** Q

√7ᵗʰ **S62.174** Nondisplaced **fracture of trapezium [larger multangular], right wrist** Q

√7ᵗʰ **S62.175** Nondisplaced **fracture of trapezium [larger multangular], left wrist** Q

√7ᵗʰ **S62.176** Nondisplaced **fracture of trapezium [larger multangular], unspecified wrist** Q

√6ᵗʰ **S62.18** Fracture of **trapezoid [smaller multangular]**

√7ᵗʰ **S62.181** Displaced **fracture of trapezoid [smaller multangular], right wrist** Q

√7ᵗʰ **S62.182** Displaced **fracture of trapezoid [smaller multangular], left wrist** Q

√7ᵗʰ **S62.183** Displaced **fracture of trapezoid [smaller multangular], unspecified wrist** Q

√7ᵗʰ **S62.184** Nondisplaced **fracture of trapezoid [smaller multangular], right wrist** Q

√7ᵗʰ **S62.185** Nondisplaced **fracture of trapezoid [smaller multangular], left wrist** Q

√7ᵗʰ **S62.186** Nondisplaced **fracture of trapezoid [smaller multangular], unspecified wrist** Q

√5ᵗʰ **S62.2** Fracture of **first metacarpal bone**

√6ᵗʰ **S62.20** Unspecified **fracture of first metacarpal bone**

√7ᵗʰ **S62.201** Unspecified **fracture of first metacarpal bone, right hand** Q

√7ᵗʰ **S62.202** Unspecified **fracture of first metacarpal bone, left hand** Q

√7ᵗʰ **S62.209** Unspecified **fracture of first metacarpal bone, unspecified hand** Q

√6ᵗʰ **S62.21** Bennett's **fracture**

     DEF: Intra-articular, two-part fracture at the base of the first metacarpal bone (thumb) on the ulnar side at the carpometacarpal (CMC) joint.

√7ᵗʰ **S62.211** Bennett's **fracture, right hand** Q

√7ᵗʰ **S62.212** Bennett's **fracture, left hand** Q

√7ᵗʰ **S62.213** Bennett's **fracture, unspecified hand** Q

√6ᵗʰ **S62.22** Rolando's **fracture**

     DEF: Comminuted, three part intra-articular fracture at the base of the thumb metacarpal.

√7ᵗʰ **S62.221** Displaced **Rolando's fracture, right hand** Q

√7ᵗʰ **S62.222** Displaced **Rolando's fracture, left hand** Q

√7ᵗʰ **S62.223** Displaced **Rolando's fracture, unspecified hand** Q

√7ᵗʰ **S62.224** Nondisplaced **Rolando's fracture, right hand** Q

√7ᵗʰ **S62.225** Nondisplaced **Rolando's fracture, left hand** Q

√7ᵗʰ **S62.226** Nondisplaced **Rolando's fracture, unspecified hand** Q

√6ᵗʰ **S62.23** Other fracture of **base of first metacarpal bone**

√7ᵗʰ **S62.231** Other displaced **fracture of base of first metacarpal bone, right hand** Q

√7ᵗʰ **S62.232** Other displaced **fracture of base of first metacarpal bone, left hand** Q

√7ᵗʰ **S62.233** Other displaced **fracture of base of first metacarpal bone, unspecified hand** Q

√7ᵗʰ **S62.234** Other nondisplaced **fracture of base of first metacarpal bone, right hand** Q

√7ᵗʰ **S62.235** Other nondisplaced **fracture of base of first metacarpal bone, left hand** Q

√7ᵗʰ **S62.236** Other nondisplaced **fracture of base of first metacarpal bone, unspecified hand** Q

√6ᵗʰ **S62.24** Fracture of **shaft of first metacarpal bone**

√7ᵗʰ **S62.241** Displaced **fracture of shaft of first metacarpal bone, right hand** Q

√7ᵗʰ **S62.242** Displaced **fracture of shaft of first metacarpal bone, left hand** Q

√7ᵗʰ **S62.243** Displaced **fracture of shaft of first metacarpal bone, unspecified hand** Q

√7ᵗʰ **S62.244** Nondisplaced **fracture of shaft of first metacarpal bone, right hand** Q

√7ᵗʰ **S62.245** Nondisplaced **fracture of shaft of first metacarpal bone, left hand** Q

√7ᵗʰ **S62.246** Nondisplaced **fracture of shaft of first metacarpal bone, unspecified hand** Q

√6ᵗʰ **S62.25** Fracture of **neck of first metacarpal bone**

√7ᵗʰ **S62.251** Displaced **fracture of neck of first metacarpal bone, right hand** Q

√7ᵗʰ **S62.252** Displaced **fracture of neck of first metacarpal bone, left hand** Q

√7ᵗʰ **S62.253** Displaced **fracture of neck of first metacarpal bone, unspecified hand** Q

√7ᵗʰ **S62.254** Nondisplaced **fracture of neck of first metacarpal bone, right hand** Q

√7ᵗʰ **S62.255** Nondisplaced **fracture of neck of first metacarpal bone, left hand** Q

√7ᵗʰ **S62.256** Nondisplaced **fracture of neck of first metacarpal bone, unspecified hand** Q

√6ᵗʰ **S62.29 Other fracture of first metacarpal bone**

    √7ᵗʰ **S62.291 Other fracture of first metacarpal bone, right hand** Q

    √7ᵗʰ **S62.292 Other fracture of first metacarpal bone, left hand** Q

    √7ᵗʰ **S62.299 Other fracture of first metacarpal bone, unspecified hand** Q

√5ᵗʰ **S62.3 Fracture of other and unspecified metacarpal bone**

    EXCLUDES 2   *fracture of first metacarpal bone (S62.2-)*

    √6ᵗʰ **S62.30 Unspecified fracture of other metacarpal bone**

       √7ᵗʰ **S62.300 Unspecified fracture of second metacarpal bone, right hand** Q

       √7ᵗʰ **S62.301 Unspecified fracture of second metacarpal bone, left hand** Q

       √7ᵗʰ **S62.302 Unspecified fracture of third metacarpal bone, right hand** Q

       √7ᵗʰ **S62.303 Unspecified fracture of third metacarpal bone, left hand** Q

       √7ᵗʰ **S62.304 Unspecified fracture of fourth metacarpal bone, right hand** Q

       √7ᵗʰ **S62.305 Unspecified fracture of fourth metacarpal bone, left hand** Q

       √7ᵗʰ **S62.306 Unspecified fracture of fifth metacarpal bone, right hand** Q

       √7ᵗʰ **S62.307 Unspecified fracture of fifth metacarpal bone, left hand** Q

       √7ᵗʰ **S62.308 Unspecified fracture of other metacarpal bone** Q
          Unspecified fracture of specified metacarpal bone with unspecified laterality

       √7ᵗʰ **S62.309 Unspecified fracture of unspecified metacarpal bone** Q

    √6ᵗʰ **S62.31 Displaced fracture of base of other metacarpal bone**

       √7ᵗʰ **S62.310 Displaced fracture of base of second metacarpal bone, right hand** Q

       √7ᵗʰ **S62.311 Displaced fracture of base of second metacarpal bone, left hand** Q

       √7ᵗʰ **S62.312 Displaced fracture of base of third metacarpal bone, right hand** Q

       √7ᵗʰ **S62.313 Displaced fracture of base of third metacarpal bone, left hand** Q

       √7ᵗʰ **S62.314 Displaced fracture of base of fourth metacarpal bone, right hand** Q

       √7ᵗʰ **S62.315 Displaced fracture of base of fourth metacarpal bone, left hand** Q

       √7ᵗʰ **S62.316 Displaced fracture of base of fifth metacarpal bone, right hand** Q

       √7ᵗʰ **S62.317 Displaced fracture of base of fifth metacarpal bone, left hand** Q

       √7ᵗʰ **S62.318 Displaced fracture of base of other metacarpal bone** Q
          Displaced fracture of base of specified metacarpal bone with unspecified laterality

       √7ᵗʰ **S62.319 Displaced fracture of base of unspecified metacarpal bone** Q

    √6ᵗʰ **S62.32 Displaced fracture of shaft of other metacarpal bone**

       √7ᵗʰ **S62.320 Displaced fracture of shaft of second metacarpal bone, right hand** Q

       √7ᵗʰ **S62.321 Displaced fracture of shaft of second metacarpal bone, left hand** Q

       √7ᵗʰ **S62.322 Displaced fracture of shaft of third metacarpal bone, right hand** Q

       √7ᵗʰ **S62.323 Displaced fracture of shaft of third metacarpal bone, left hand** Q

       √7ᵗʰ **S62.324 Displaced fracture of shaft of fourth metacarpal bone, right hand** Q

       √7ᵗʰ **S62.325 Displaced fracture of shaft of fourth metacarpal bone, left hand** Q

       √7ᵗʰ **S62.326 Displaced fracture of shaft of fifth metacarpal bone, right hand** Q

       √7ᵗʰ **S62.327 Displaced fracture of shaft of fifth metacarpal bone, left hand** Q

       √7ᵗʰ **S62.328 Displaced fracture of shaft of other metacarpal bone** Q
          Displaced fracture of shaft of specified metacarpal bone with unspecified laterality

       √7ᵗʰ **S62.329 Displaced fracture of shaft of unspecified metacarpal bone** Q

    √6ᵗʰ **S62.33 Displaced fracture of neck of other metacarpal bone**

       √7ᵗʰ **S62.330 Displaced fracture of neck of second metacarpal bone, right hand** Q

       √7ᵗʰ **S62.331 Displaced fracture of neck of second metacarpal bone, left hand** Q

       √7ᵗʰ **S62.332 Displaced fracture of neck of third metacarpal bone, right hand** Q

       √7ᵗʰ **S62.333 Displaced fracture of neck of third metacarpal bone, left hand** Q

       √7ᵗʰ **S62.334 Displaced fracture of neck of fourth metacarpal bone, right hand** Q

       √7ᵗʰ **S62.335 Displaced fracture of neck of fourth metacarpal bone, left hand** Q

       √7ᵗʰ **S62.336 Displaced fracture of neck of fifth metacarpal bone, right hand** Q

       √7ᵗʰ **S62.337 Displaced fracture of neck of fifth metacarpal bone, left hand** Q

       √7ᵗʰ **S62.338 Displaced fracture of neck of other metacarpal bone** Q
          Displaced fracture of neck of specified metacarpal bone with unspecified laterality

       √7ᵗʰ **S62.339 Displaced fracture of neck of unspecified metacarpal bone** Q

    √6ᵗʰ **S62.34 Nondisplaced fracture of base of other metacarpal bone**

       √7ᵗʰ **S62.340 Nondisplaced fracture of base of second metacarpal bone, right hand** Q

       √7ᵗʰ **S62.341 Nondisplaced fracture of base of second metacarpal bone, left hand** Q

       √7ᵗʰ **S62.342 Nondisplaced fracture of base of third metacarpal bone, right hand** Q

       √7ᵗʰ **S62.343 Nondisplaced fracture of base of third metacarpal bone, left hand** Q

       √7ᵗʰ **S62.344 Nondisplaced fracture of base of fourth metacarpal bone, right hand** Q

       √7ᵗʰ **S62.345 Nondisplaced fracture of base of fourth metacarpal bone, left hand** Q

       √7ᵗʰ **S62.346 Nondisplaced fracture of base of fifth metacarpal bone, right hand** Q

       √7ᵗʰ **S62.347 Nondisplaced fracture of base of fifth metacarpal bone, left hand** Q

       √7ᵗʰ **S62.348 Nondisplaced fracture of base of other metacarpal bone** Q
          Nondisplaced fracture of base of specified metacarpal bone with unspecified laterality

       √7ᵗʰ **S62.349 Nondisplaced fracture of base of unspecified metacarpal bone** Q

    √6ᵗʰ **S62.35 Nondisplaced fracture of shaft of other metacarpal bone**

       √7ᵗʰ **S62.350 Nondisplaced fracture of shaft of second metacarpal bone, right hand** Q

       √7ᵗʰ **S62.351 Nondisplaced fracture of shaft of second metacarpal bone, left hand** Q

       √7ᵗʰ **S62.352 Nondisplaced fracture of shaft of third metacarpal bone, right hand** Q

       √7ᵗʰ **S62.353 Nondisplaced fracture of shaft of third metacarpal bone, left hand** Q

       √7ᵗʰ **S62.354 Nondisplaced fracture of shaft of fourth metacarpal bone, right hand** Q

       √7ᵗʰ **S62.355 Nondisplaced fracture of shaft of fourth metacarpal bone, left hand** Q

       √7ᵗʰ **S62.356 Nondisplaced fracture of shaft of fifth metacarpal bone, right hand** Q

       √7ᵗʰ **S62.357 Nondisplaced fracture of shaft of fifth metacarpal bone, left hand** Q

☑ Additional Character Required   √x7ᵗʰ Placeholder Alert   Manifestation   Unspecified Dx   ▶◀ Revised Text   ● New Code   ▲ Revised Code Title

✓7ᵗʰ **S62.358** Nondisplaced fracture of shaft of other metacarpal bone   Q
    Nondisplaced fracture of shaft of specified metacarpal bone with unspecified laterality

✓7ᵗʰ **S62.359** Nondisplaced fracture of shaft of unspecified metacarpal bone   Q

✓6ᵗʰ **S62.36** Nondisplaced fracture of neck of other metacarpal bone

✓7ᵗʰ **S62.360** Nondisplaced fracture of neck of second metacarpal bone, right hand   Q

✓7ᵗʰ **S62.361** Nondisplaced fracture of neck of second metacarpal bone, left hand   Q

✓7ᵗʰ **S62.362** Nondisplaced fracture of neck of third metacarpal bone, right hand   Q

✓7ᵗʰ **S62.363** Nondisplaced fracture of neck of third metacarpal bone, left hand   Q

✓7ᵗʰ **S62.364** Nondisplaced fracture of neck of fourth metacarpal bone, right hand   Q

✓7ᵗʰ **S62.365** Nondisplaced fracture of neck of fourth metacarpal bone, left hand   Q

✓7ᵗʰ **S62.366** Nondisplaced fracture of neck of fifth metacarpal bone, right hand   Q

✓7ᵗʰ **S62.367** Nondisplaced fracture of neck of fifth metacarpal bone, left hand   Q

✓7ᵗʰ **S62.368** Nondisplaced fracture of neck of other metacarpal bone   Q
    Nondisplaced fracture of neck of specified metacarpal bone with unspecified laterality

✓7ᵗʰ **S62.369** Nondisplaced fracture of neck of unspecified metacarpal bone   Q

✓6ᵗʰ **S62.39** Other fracture of other metacarpal bone

✓7ᵗʰ **S62.390** Other fracture of second metacarpal bone, right hand   Q

✓7ᵗʰ **S62.391** Other fracture of second metacarpal bone, left hand   Q

✓7ᵗʰ **S62.392** Other fracture of third metacarpal bone, right hand   Q

✓7ᵗʰ **S62.393** Other fracture of third metacarpal bone, left hand   Q

✓7ᵗʰ **S62.394** Other fracture of fourth metacarpal bone, right hand   Q

✓7ᵗʰ **S62.395** Other fracture of fourth metacarpal bone, left hand   Q

✓7ᵗʰ **S62.396** Other fracture of fifth metacarpal bone, right hand   Q

✓7ᵗʰ **S62.397** Other fracture of fifth metacarpal bone, left hand   Q

✓7ᵗʰ **S62.398** Other fracture of other metacarpal bone   Q
    Other fracture of specified metacarpal bone with unspecified laterality

✓7ᵗʰ **S62.399** Other fracture of unspecified metacarpal bone   Q

✓5ᵗʰ **S62.5** Fracture of thumb

✓6ᵗʰ **S62.50** Fracture of unspecified phalanx of thumb

✓7ᵗʰ **S62.501** Fracture of unspecified phalanx of right thumb

✓7ᵗʰ **S62.502** Fracture of unspecified phalanx of left thumb

✓7ᵗʰ **S62.509** Fracture of unspecified phalanx of unspecified thumb

✓6ᵗʰ **S62.51** Fracture of proximal phalanx of thumb

✓7ᵗʰ **S62.511** Displaced fracture of proximal phalanx of right thumb

✓7ᵗʰ **S62.512** Displaced fracture of proximal phalanx of left thumb

✓7ᵗʰ **S62.513** Displaced fracture of proximal phalanx of unspecified thumb

✓7ᵗʰ **S62.514** Nondisplaced fracture of proximal phalanx of right thumb

✓7ᵗʰ **S62.515** Nondisplaced fracture of proximal phalanx of left thumb

✓7ᵗʰ **S62.516** Nondisplaced fracture of proximal phalanx of unspecified thumb

✓6ᵗʰ **S62.52** Fracture of distal phalanx of thumb

✓7ᵗʰ **S62.521** Displaced fracture of distal phalanx of right thumb

✓7ᵗʰ **S62.522** Displaced fracture of distal phalanx of left thumb

✓7ᵗʰ **S62.523** Displaced fracture of distal phalanx of unspecified thumb

✓7ᵗʰ **S62.524** Nondisplaced fracture of distal phalanx of right thumb

✓7ᵗʰ **S62.525** Nondisplaced fracture of distal phalanx of left thumb

✓7ᵗʰ **S62.526** Nondisplaced fracture of distal phalanx of unspecified thumb

✓5ᵗʰ **S62.6** Fracture of other and unspecified finger(s)

    EXCLUDES 2   fracture of thumb (S62.5-)

✓6ᵗʰ **S62.60** Fracture of unspecified phalanx of finger

✓7ᵗʰ **S62.600** Fracture of unspecified phalanx of right index finger

✓7ᵗʰ **S62.601** Fracture of unspecified phalanx of left index finger

✓7ᵗʰ **S62.602** Fracture of unspecified phalanx of right middle finger

✓7ᵗʰ **S62.603** Fracture of unspecified phalanx of left middle finger

✓7ᵗʰ **S62.604** Fracture of unspecified phalanx of right ring finger

✓7ᵗʰ **S62.605** Fracture of unspecified phalanx of left ring finger

✓7ᵗʰ **S62.606** Fracture of unspecified phalanx of right little finger

✓7ᵗʰ **S62.607** Fracture of unspecified phalanx of left little finger

✓7ᵗʰ **S62.608** Fracture of unspecified phalanx of other finger
    Fracture of unspecified phalanx of specified finger with unspecified laterality

✓7ᵗʰ **S62.609** Fracture of unspecified phalanx of unspecified finger

✓6ᵗʰ **S62.61** Displaced fracture of proximal phalanx of finger

✓7ᵗʰ **S62.610** Displaced fracture of proximal phalanx of right index finger

✓7ᵗʰ **S62.611** Displaced fracture of proximal phalanx of left index finger

✓7ᵗʰ **S62.612** Displaced fracture of proximal phalanx of right middle finger

✓7ᵗʰ **S62.613** Displaced fracture of proximal phalanx of left middle finger

✓7ᵗʰ **S62.614** Displaced fracture of proximal phalanx of right ring finger

✓7ᵗʰ **S62.615** Displaced fracture of proximal phalanx of left ring finger

✓7ᵗʰ **S62.616** Displaced fracture of proximal phalanx of right little finger

✓7ᵗʰ **S62.617** Displaced fracture of proximal phalanx of left little finger

✓7ᵗʰ **S62.618** Displaced fracture of proximal phalanx of other finger
    Displaced fracture of proximal phalanx of specified finger with unspecified laterality

✓7ᵗʰ **S62.619** Displaced fracture of proximal phalanx of unspecified finger

✓6ᵗʰ **S62.62** Displaced fracture of middle phalanx of finger

✓7ᵗʰ **S62.620** Displaced fracture of middle phalanx of right index finger

✓7ᵗʰ **S62.621** Displaced fracture of middle phalanx of left index finger

✓7ᵗʰ **S62.622** Displaced fracture of middle phalanx of right middle finger

✓7ᵗʰ **S62.623** Displaced fracture of middle phalanx of left middle finger

✓7ᵗʰ **S62.624** Displaced fracture of middle phalanx of right ring finger

✓7ᵗʰ **S62.625** Displaced fracture of middle phalanx of left ring finger

✓7ᵗʰ **S62.626** Displaced fracture of middle phalanx of right little finger

✓7ᵗʰ **S62.627** Displaced fracture of middle phalanx of left little finger

✓7ᵗʰ **S62.628 Displaced fracture of middle phalanx of other finger**
Displaced fracture of middle phalanx of specified finger with unspecified laterality

✓7ᵗʰ **S62.629 Displaced fracture of middle phalanx of unspecified finger**

✓6ᵗʰ **S62.63 Displaced fracture of distal phalanx of finger**

✓7ᵗʰ **S62.630 Displaced fracture of distal phalanx of right index finger**

✓7ᵗʰ **S62.631 Displaced fracture of distal phalanx of left index finger**

✓7ᵗʰ **S62.632 Displaced fracture of distal phalanx of right middle finger**

✓7ᵗʰ **S62.633 Displaced fracture of distal phalanx of left middle finger**

✓7ᵗʰ **S62.634 Displaced fracture of distal phalanx of right ring finger**

✓7ᵗʰ **S62.635 Displaced fracture of distal phalanx of left ring finger**

✓7ᵗʰ **S62.636 Displaced fracture of distal phalanx of right little finger**

✓7ᵗʰ **S62.637 Displaced fracture of distal phalanx of left little finger**

✓7ᵗʰ **S62.638 Displaced fracture of distal phalanx of other finger**
Displaced fracture of distal phalanx of specified finger with unspecified laterality

✓7ᵗʰ **S62.639 Displaced fracture of distal phalanx of unspecified finger**

✓6ᵗʰ **S62.64 Nondisplaced fracture of proximal phalanx of finger**

✓7ᵗʰ **S62.640 Nondisplaced fracture of proximal phalanx of right index finger**

✓7ᵗʰ **S62.641 Nondisplaced fracture of proximal phalanx of left index finger**

✓7ᵗʰ **S62.642 Nondisplaced fracture of proximal phalanx of right middle finger**

✓7ᵗʰ **S62.643 Nondisplaced fracture of proximal phalanx of left middle finger**

✓7ᵗʰ **S62.644 Nondisplaced fracture of proximal phalanx of right ring finger**

✓7ᵗʰ **S62.645 Nondisplaced fracture of proximal phalanx of left ring finger**

✓7ᵗʰ **S62.646 Nondisplaced fracture of proximal phalanx of right little finger**

✓7ᵗʰ **S62.647 Nondisplaced fracture of proximal phalanx of left little finger**

✓7ᵗʰ **S62.648 Nondisplaced fracture of proximal phalanx of other finger**
Nondisplaced fracture of proximal phalanx of specified finger with unspecified laterality

✓7ᵗʰ **S62.649 Nondisplaced fracture of proximal phalanx of unspecified finger**

✓6ᵗʰ **S62.65 Nondisplaced fracture of middle phalanx of finger**

✓7ᵗʰ **S62.650 Nondisplaced fracture of middle phalanx of right index finger**

✓7ᵗʰ **S62.651 Nondisplaced fracture of middle phalanx of left index finger**

✓7ᵗʰ **S62.652 Nondisplaced fracture of middle phalanx of right middle finger**

✓7ᵗʰ **S62.653 Nondisplaced fracture of middle phalanx of left middle finger**

✓7ᵗʰ **S62.654 Nondisplaced fracture of middle phalanx of right ring finger**

✓7ᵗʰ **S62.655 Nondisplaced fracture of middle phalanx of left ring finger**

✓7ᵗʰ **S62.656 Nondisplaced fracture of middle phalanx of right little finger**

✓7ᵗʰ **S62.657 Nondisplaced fracture of middle phalanx of left little finger**

✓7ᵗʰ **S62.658 Nondisplaced fracture of middle phalanx of other finger**
Nondisplaced fracture of middle phalanx of specified finger with unspecified laterality

✓7ᵗʰ **S62.659 Nondisplaced fracture of middle phalanx of unspecified finger**

✓6ᵗʰ **S62.66 Nondisplaced fracture of distal phalanx of finger**

✓7ᵗʰ **S62.660 Nondisplaced fracture of distal phalanx of right index finger**

✓7ᵗʰ **S62.661 Nondisplaced fracture of distal phalanx of left index finger**

✓7ᵗʰ **S62.662 Nondisplaced fracture of distal phalanx of right middle finger**

✓7ᵗʰ **S62.663 Nondisplaced fracture of distal phalanx of left middle finger**

✓7ᵗʰ **S62.664 Nondisplaced fracture of distal phalanx of right ring finger**

✓7ᵗʰ **S62.665 Nondisplaced fracture of distal phalanx of left ring finger**

✓7ᵗʰ **S62.666 Nondisplaced fracture of distal phalanx of right little finger**

✓7ᵗʰ **S62.667 Nondisplaced fracture of distal phalanx of left little finger**

✓7ᵗʰ **S62.668 Nondisplaced fracture of distal phalanx of other finger**
Nondisplaced fracture of distal phalanx of specified finger with unspecified laterality

✓7ᵗʰ **S62.669 Nondisplaced fracture of distal phalanx of unspecified finger**

✓5ᵗʰ **S62.9 Unspecified fracture of wrist and hand**

✓x7ᵗʰ **S62.90 Unspecified fracture of unspecified wrist and hand** ⨀

✓x7ᵗʰ **S62.91 Unspecified fracture of right wrist and hand** ⨀

✓x7ᵗʰ **S62.92 Unspecified fracture of left wrist and hand** ⨀

✓4ᵗʰ **S63 Dislocation and sprain of joints and ligaments at wrist and hand level**

INCLUDES   avulsion of joint or ligament at wrist and hand level
laceration of cartilage, joint or ligament at wrist and hand level
sprain of cartilage, joint or ligament at wrist and hand level
traumatic hemarthrosis of joint or ligament at wrist and hand level
traumatic rupture of joint or ligament at wrist and hand level
traumatic subluxation of joint or ligament at wrist and hand level
traumatic tear of joint or ligament at wrist and hand level

Code also any associated open wound

EXCLUDES 2   *strain of muscle, fascia and tendon of wrist and hand (S66.-)*

The appropriate 7th character is to be added to each code from category S63.
A   initial encounter
D   subsequent encounter
S   sequela

✓5ᵗʰ **S63.0 Subluxation and dislocation of wrist and hand joints**

✓6ᵗʰ **S63.00 Unspecified subluxation and dislocation of wrist and hand**
Dislocation of carpal bone NOS
Dislocation of distal end of radius NOS
Subluxation of carpal bone NOS
Subluxation of distal end of radius NOS

✓7ᵗʰ **S63.001 Unspecified subluxation of right wrist and hand**

✓7ᵗʰ **S63.002 Unspecified subluxation of left wrist and hand**

✓7ᵗʰ **S63.003 Unspecified subluxation of unspecified wrist and hand**

✓7ᵗʰ **S63.004 Unspecified dislocation of right wrist and hand**

✓7ᵗʰ **S63.005 Unspecified dislocation of left wrist and hand**

✓7ᵗʰ **S63.006 Unspecified dislocation of unspecified wrist and hand**

✓6ᵗʰ **S63.01 Subluxation and dislocation of distal radioulnar joint**

✓7ᵗʰ **S63.011 Subluxation of distal radioulnar joint of right wrist**

✓7ᵗʰ **S63.012 Subluxation of distal radioulnar joint of left wrist**

✓7ᵗʰ **S63.013 Subluxation of distal radioulnar joint of unspecified wrist**

✓7ᵗʰ **S63.014 Dislocation of distal radioulnar joint of right wrist**

✓7ᵗʰ **S63.015 Dislocation of distal radioulnar joint of left wrist**

✓7ᵗʰ **S63.016 Dislocation of distal radioulnar joint of unspecified wrist**

√6ᵗʰ **S63.02** **Subluxation and dislocation of** radiocarpal **joint**

     √7ᵗʰ **S63.021** **Subluxation of radiocarpal joint of** right **wrist**

     √7ᵗʰ **S63.022** **Subluxation of radiocarpal joint of** left **wrist**

     √7ᵗʰ **S63.023** **Subluxation of radiocarpal joint of** unspecified wrist

     √7ᵗʰ **S63.024** **Dislocation of radiocarpal joint of** right **wrist**

     √7ᵗʰ **S63.025** **Dislocation of radiocarpal joint of** left **wrist**

     √7ᵗʰ **S63.026** **Dislocation of radiocarpal joint of** unspecified wrist

√6ᵗʰ **S63.03** **Subluxation and dislocation of** midcarpal **joint**

     √7ᵗʰ **S63.031** **Subluxation of midcarpal joint of** right **wrist**

     √7ᵗʰ **S63.032** **Subluxation of midcarpal joint of** left **wrist**

     √7ᵗʰ **S63.033** **Subluxation of midcarpal joint of** unspecified wrist

     √7ᵗʰ **S63.034** **Dislocation of midcarpal joint of** right **wrist**

     √7ᵗʰ **S63.035** **Dislocation of midcarpal joint of** left **wrist**

     √7ᵗʰ **S63.036** **Dislocation of midcarpal joint of** unspecified wrist

√6ᵗʰ **S63.04** **Subluxation and dislocation of** carpometacarpal **joint of** thumb

     EXCLUDES 2   *interphalangeal subluxation and dislocation of thumb (S63.1-)*

     √7ᵗʰ **S63.041** **Subluxation of carpometacarpal joint of** right **thumb**

     √7ᵗʰ **S63.042** **Subluxation of carpometacarpal joint of** left **thumb**

     √7ᵗʰ **S63.043** **Subluxation of carpometacarpal joint of** unspecified thumb

     √7ᵗʰ **S63.044** **Dislocation of carpometacarpal joint of** right **thumb**

     √7ᵗʰ **S63.045** **Dislocation of carpometacarpal joint of** left **thumb**

     √7ᵗʰ **S63.046** **Dislocation of carpometacarpal joint of** unspecified thumb

√6ᵗʰ **S63.05** **Subluxation and dislocation of other carpometacarpal joint**

     EXCLUDES 2   *subluxation and dislocation of carpometacarpal joint of thumb (S63.04-)*

     √7ᵗʰ **S63.051** **Subluxation of other carpometacarpal joint of** right **hand**

     √7ᵗʰ **S63.052** **Subluxation of other carpometacarpal joint of** left **hand**

     √7ᵗʰ **S63.053** **Subluxation of other carpometacarpal joint of unspecified hand**

     √7ᵗʰ **S63.054** **Dislocation of other carpometacarpal joint of** right **hand**

     √7ᵗʰ **S63.055** **Dislocation of other carpometacarpal joint of** left **hand**

     √7ᵗʰ **S63.056** **Dislocation of other carpometacarpal joint of unspecified hand**

√6ᵗʰ **S63.06** **Subluxation and dislocation of** metacarpal (bone), **proximal end**

     √7ᵗʰ **S63.061** **Subluxation of metacarpal (bone), proximal end of** right **hand**

     √7ᵗʰ **S63.062** **Subluxation of metacarpal (bone), proximal end of** left **hand**

     √7ᵗʰ **S63.063** **Subluxation of metacarpal (bone), proximal end of unspecified hand**

     √7ᵗʰ **S63.064** **Dislocation of metacarpal (bone), proximal end of** right **hand**

     √7ᵗʰ **S63.065** **Dislocation of metacarpal (bone), proximal end of** left **hand**

     √7ᵗʰ **S63.066** **Dislocation of metacarpal (bone), proximal end of unspecified hand**

√6ᵗʰ **S63.07** **Subluxation and dislocation of** distal end of ulna

     √7ᵗʰ **S63.071** **Subluxation of distal end of** right **ulna**

     √7ᵗʰ **S63.072** **Subluxation of distal end of** left **ulna**

     √7ᵗʰ **S63.073** **Subluxation of distal end of unspecified ulna**

     √7ᵗʰ **S63.074** **Dislocation of distal end of** right **ulna**

     √7ᵗʰ **S63.075** **Dislocation of distal end of** left **ulna**

     √7ᵗʰ **S63.076** **Dislocation of distal end of unspecified ulna**

√6ᵗʰ **S63.09** **Other subluxation and dislocation of wrist and hand**

     √7ᵗʰ **S63.091** **Other** subluxation **of** right **wrist and hand**

     √7ᵗʰ **S63.092** **Other** subluxation **of** left **wrist and hand**

     √7ᵗʰ **S63.093** **Other** subluxation **of unspecified wrist and hand**

     √7ᵗʰ **S63.094** **Other** dislocation **of** right **wrist and hand**

     √7ᵗʰ **S63.095** **Other** dislocation **of** left **wrist and hand**

     √7ᵗʰ **S63.096** **Other** dislocation **of unspecified wrist and hand**

√5ᵗʰ **S63.1** **Subluxation and dislocation of** thumb

     √6ᵗʰ **S63.10** **Unspecified subluxation and dislocation of thumb**

         √7ᵗʰ **S63.101** **Unspecified** subluxation **of** right **thumb**

         √7ᵗʰ **S63.102** **Unspecified** subluxation **of** left **thumb**

         √7ᵗʰ **S63.103** **Unspecified** subluxation **of unspecified thumb**

         √7ᵗʰ **S63.104** **Unspecified** dislocation **of** right **thumb**

         √7ᵗʰ **S63.105** **Unspecified** dislocation **of** left **thumb**

         √7ᵗʰ **S63.106** **Unspecified** dislocation **of unspecified thumb**

     √6ᵗʰ **S63.11** **Subluxation and dislocation of** metacarpophalangeal joint **of thumb**

         √7ᵗʰ **S63.111** **Subluxation of metacarpophalangeal joint of** right **thumb**

         √7ᵗʰ **S63.112** **Subluxation of metacarpophalangeal joint of** left **thumb**

         √7ᵗʰ **S63.113** **Subluxation of metacarpophalangeal joint of unspecified thumb**

         √7ᵗʰ **S63.114** **Dislocation of metacarpophalangeal joint of** right **thumb**

         √7ᵗʰ **S63.115** **Dislocation of metacarpophalangeal joint of** left **thumb**

         √7ᵗʰ **S63.116** **Dislocation of metacarpophalangeal joint of unspecified thumb**

     √6ᵗʰ **S63.12** **Subluxation and dislocation of** interphalangeal joint **of thumb**

         √7ᵗʰ **S63.121** **Subluxation of interphalangeal joint of** right **thumb**

         √7ᵗʰ **S63.122** **Subluxation of interphalangeal joint of** left **thumb**

         √7ᵗʰ **S63.123** **Subluxation of interphalangeal joint of unspecified thumb**

         √7ᵗʰ **S63.124** **Dislocation of interphalangeal joint of** right **thumb**

         √7ᵗʰ **S63.125** **Dislocation of interphalangeal joint of** left **thumb**

         √7ᵗʰ **S63.126** **Dislocation of interphalangeal joint of unspecified thumb**

√5ᵗʰ **S63.2** **Subluxation and dislocation of other** finger(s)

     EXCLUDES 2   *subluxation and dislocation of thumb (S63.1-)*

     √6ᵗʰ **S63.20** **Unspecified subluxation of other finger**

         √7ᵗʰ **S63.200** **Unspecified subluxation of** right **index finger**

         √7ᵗʰ **S63.201** **Unspecified subluxation of** left **index finger**

         √7ᵗʰ **S63.202** **Unspecified subluxation of** right **middle finger**

         √7ᵗʰ **S63.203** **Unspecified subluxation of** left **middle finger**

         √7ᵗʰ **S63.204** **Unspecified subluxation of** right **ring finger**

         √7ᵗʰ **S63.205** **Unspecified subluxation of** left **ring finger**

         √7ᵗʰ **S63.206** **Unspecified subluxation of** right **little finger**

         √7ᵗʰ **S63.207** **Unspecified subluxation of** left **little finger**

         √7ᵗʰ **S63.208** **Unspecified subluxation of other finger**

             Unspecified subluxation of specified finger with unspecified laterality

         √7ᵗʰ **S63.209** **Unspecified subluxation of unspecified finger**

     √6ᵗʰ **S63.21** **Subluxation of** metacarpophalangeal joint **of finger**

         √7ᵗʰ **S63.210** **Subluxation of metacarpophalangeal joint of** right **index finger**

         √7ᵗʰ **S63.211** **Subluxation of metacarpophalangeal joint of** left **index finger**

         √7ᵗʰ **S63.212** **Subluxation of metacarpophalangeal joint of** right **middle finger**

         √7ᵗʰ **S63.213** **Subluxation of metacarpophalangeal joint of** left **middle finger**

√7ᵗʰ **S63.214** **Subluxation of metacarpophalangeal joint of** right ring **finger**

√7ᵗʰ **S63.215** **Subluxation of metacarpophalangeal joint of** left ring **finger**

√7ᵗʰ **S63.216** **Subluxation of metacarpophalangeal joint of** right little **finger**

√7ᵗʰ **S63.217** **Subluxation of metacarpophalangeal joint of** left little **finger**

√7ᵗʰ **S63.218** **Subluxation of metacarpophalangeal joint of other finger**
Subluxation of metacarpophalangeal joint of specified finger with unspecified laterality

√7ᵗʰ **S63.219** **Subluxation of metacarpophalangeal joint of unspecified finger**

√6ᵗʰ **S63.22** **Subluxation of unspecified** interphalangeal **joint of finger**

√7ᵗʰ **S63.220** **Subluxation of unspecified interphalangeal joint of** right index **finger**

√7ᵗʰ **S63.221** **Subluxation of unspecified interphalangeal joint of** left index **finger**

√7ᵗʰ **S63.222** **Subluxation of unspecified interphalangeal joint of** right middle **finger**

√7ᵗʰ **S63.223** **Subluxation of unspecified interphalangeal joint of** left middle **finger**

√7ᵗʰ **S63.224** **Subluxation of unspecified interphalangeal joint of** right ring **finger**

√7ᵗʰ **S63.225** **Subluxation of unspecified interphalangeal joint of** left ring **finger**

√7ᵗʰ **S63.226** **Subluxation of unspecified interphalangeal joint of** right little **finger**

√7ᵗʰ **S63.227** **Subluxation of unspecified interphalangeal joint of** left little **finger**

√7ᵗʰ **S63.228** **Subluxation of unspecified interphalangeal joint of other finger**
Subluxation of unspecified interphalangeal joint of specified finger with unspecified laterality

√7ᵗʰ **S63.229** **Subluxation of unspecified interphalangeal joint of unspecified finger**

√6ᵗʰ **S63.23** **Subluxation of** proximal interphalangeal **joint of finger**

√7ᵗʰ **S63.230** **Subluxation of proximal interphalangeal joint of** right index **finger**

√7ᵗʰ **S63.231** **Subluxation of proximal interphalangeal joint of** left index **finger**

√7ᵗʰ **S63.232** **Subluxation of proximal interphalangeal joint of** right middle **finger**

√7ᵗʰ **S63.233** **Subluxation of proximal interphalangeal joint of** left middle **finger**

√7ᵗʰ **S63.234** **Subluxation of proximal interphalangeal joint of** right ring **finger**

√7ᵗʰ **S63.235** **Subluxation of proximal interphalangeal joint of** left ring **finger**

√7ᵗʰ **S63.236** **Subluxation of proximal interphalangeal joint of** right little **finger**

√7ᵗʰ **S63.237** **Subluxation of proximal interphalangeal joint of** left little **finger**

√7ᵗʰ **S63.238** **Subluxation of proximal interphalangeal joint of other finger**
Subluxation of proximal interphalangeal joint of specified finger with unspecified laterality

√7ᵗʰ **S63.239** **Subluxation of proximal interphalangeal joint of unspecified finger**

√6ᵗʰ **S63.24** **Subluxation of** distal interphalangeal **joint of finger**

√7ᵗʰ **S63.240** **Subluxation of distal interphalangeal joint of** right index **finger**

√7ᵗʰ **S63.241** **Subluxation of distal interphalangeal joint of** left index **finger**

√7ᵗʰ **S63.242** **Subluxation of distal interphalangeal joint of** right middle **finger**

√7ᵗʰ **S63.243** **Subluxation of distal interphalangeal joint of** left middle **finger**

√7ᵗʰ **S63.244** **Subluxation of distal interphalangeal joint of** right ring **finger**

√7ᵗʰ **S63.245** **Subluxation of distal interphalangeal joint of** left ring **finger**

√7ᵗʰ **S63.246** **Subluxation of distal interphalangeal joint of** right little **finger**

√7ᵗʰ **S63.247** **Subluxation of distal interphalangeal joint of** left little **finger**

√7ᵗʰ **S63.248** **Subluxation of distal interphalangeal joint of other finger**
Subluxation of distal interphalangeal joint of specified finger with unspecified laterality

√7ᵗʰ **S63.249** **Subluxation of distal interphalangeal joint of unspecified finger**

√6ᵗʰ **S63.25** **Unspecified dislocation of other finger**

√7ᵗʰ **S63.250** **Unspecified dislocation of** right index **finger**

√7ᵗʰ **S63.251** **Unspecified dislocation of** left index **finger**

√7ᵗʰ **S63.252** **Unspecified dislocation of** right middle **finger**

√7ᵗʰ **S63.253** **Unspecified dislocation of** left middle **finger**

√7ᵗʰ **S63.254** **Unspecified dislocation of** right ring **finger**

√7ᵗʰ **S63.255** **Unspecified dislocation of** left ring **finger**

√7ᵗʰ **S63.256** **Unspecified dislocation of** right little **finger**

√7ᵗʰ **S63.257** **Unspecified dislocation of** left little **finger**

√7ᵗʰ **S63.258** **Unspecified dislocation of other finger**
Unspecified dislocation of specified finger with unspecified laterality

√7ᵗʰ **S63.259** **Unspecified dislocation of unspecified finger**
Unspecified dislocation of unspecified finger with unspecified laterality

√6ᵗʰ **S63.26** **Dislocation of** metacarpophalangeal joint **of finger**

√7ᵗʰ **S63.260** **Dislocation of metacarpophalangeal joint of** right index **finger**

√7ᵗʰ **S63.261** **Dislocation of metacarpophalangeal joint of** left index **finger**

√7ᵗʰ **S63.262** **Dislocation of metacarpophalangeal joint of** right middle **finger**

√7ᵗʰ **S63.263** **Dislocation of metacarpophalangeal joint of** left middle **finger**

√7ᵗʰ **S63.264** **Dislocation of metacarpophalangeal joint of** right ring **finger**

√7ᵗʰ **S63.265** **Dislocation of metacarpophalangeal joint of** left ring **finger**

√7ᵗʰ **S63.266** **Dislocation of metacarpophalangeal joint of** right little **finger**

√7ᵗʰ **S63.267** **Dislocation of metacarpophalangeal joint of** left little **finger**

√7ᵗʰ **S63.268** **Dislocation of metacarpophalangeal joint of other finger**
Dislocation of metacarpophalangeal joint of specified finger with unspecified laterality

√7ᵗʰ **S63.269** **Dislocation of metacarpophalangeal joint of unspecified finger**

√6ᵗʰ **S63.27** **Dislocation of unspecified interphalangeal joint of finger**

√7ᵗʰ **S63.270** **Dislocation of unspecified interphalangeal joint of** right index **finger**

√7ᵗʰ **S63.271** **Dislocation of unspecified interphalangeal joint of** left index **finger**

√7ᵗʰ **S63.272** **Dislocation of unspecified interphalangeal joint of** right middle **finger**

√7ᵗʰ **S63.273** **Dislocation of unspecified interphalangeal joint of** left middle **finger**

√7ᵗʰ **S63.274** **Dislocation of unspecified interphalangeal joint of** right ring **finger**

√7ᵗʰ **S63.275** **Dislocation of unspecified interphalangeal joint of** left ring **finger**

√7ᵗʰ **S63.276** **Dislocation of unspecified interphalangeal joint of** right little **finger**

√7ᵗʰ **S63.277** **Dislocation of unspecified interphalangeal joint of** left little **finger**

√7ᵗʰ **S63.278** **Dislocation of unspecified interphalangeal joint of other finger**
Dislocation of unspecified interphalangeal joint of specified finger with unspecified laterality

---

☑ Additional Character Required   √x7ᵗʰ Placeholder Alert   Manifestation   Unspecified Dx   ►◄ Revised Text   ● New Code   ▲ Revised Code Title

Chapter 19. Injury, Poisoning and Certain Other Consequences of External Causes

S63.279–S63.415

√7ᵗʰ **S63.279** **Dislocation of unspecified interphalangeal joint of unspecified finger**
Dislocation of unspecified interphalangeal joint of unspecified finger without specified laterality

√6ᵗʰ **S63.28** **Dislocation of proximal interphalangeal joint of finger**

√7ᵗʰ **S63.280** **Dislocation of proximal interphalangeal joint of right index finger**

√7ᵗʰ **S63.281** **Dislocation of proximal interphalangeal joint of left index finger**

√7ᵗʰ **S63.282** **Dislocation of proximal interphalangeal joint of right middle finger**

√7ᵗʰ **S63.283** **Dislocation of proximal interphalangeal joint of left middle finger**

√7ᵗʰ **S63.284** **Dislocation of proximal interphalangeal joint of right ring finger**

√7ᵗʰ **S63.285** **Dislocation of proximal interphalangeal joint of left ring finger**

√7ᵗʰ **S63.286** **Dislocation of proximal interphalangeal joint of right little finger**

√7ᵗʰ **S63.287** **Dislocation of proximal interphalangeal joint of left little finger**

√7ᵗʰ **S63.288** **Dislocation of proximal interphalangeal joint of other finger**
Dislocation of proximal interphalangeal joint of specified finger with unspecified laterality

√7ᵗʰ **S63.289** **Dislocation of proximal interphalangeal joint of unspecified finger**

√6ᵗʰ **S63.29** **Dislocation of distal interphalangeal joint of finger**

√7ᵗʰ **S63.290** **Dislocation of distal interphalangeal joint of right index finger**

√7ᵗʰ **S63.291** **Dislocation of distal interphalangeal joint of left index finger**

√7ᵗʰ **S63.292** **Dislocation of distal interphalangeal joint of right middle finger**

√7ᵗʰ **S63.293** **Dislocation of distal interphalangeal joint of left middle finger**

√7ᵗʰ **S63.294** **Dislocation of distal interphalangeal joint of right ring finger**

√7ᵗʰ **S63.295** **Dislocation of distal interphalangeal joint of left ring finger**

√7ᵗʰ **S63.296** **Dislocation of distal interphalangeal joint of right little finger**

√7ᵗʰ **S63.297** **Dislocation of distal interphalangeal joint of left little finger**

√7ᵗʰ **S63.298** **Dislocation of distal interphalangeal joint of other finger**
Dislocation of distal interphalangeal joint of specified finger with unspecified laterality

√7ᵗʰ **S63.299** **Dislocation of distal interphalangeal joint of unspecified finger**

√5ᵗʰ **S63.3** **Traumatic rupture of ligament of wrist**

√6ᵗʰ **S63.30** **Traumatic rupture of unspecified ligament of wrist**

√7ᵗʰ **S63.301** **Traumatic rupture of unspecified ligament of right wrist**

√7ᵗʰ **S63.302** **Traumatic rupture of unspecified ligament of left wrist**

√7ᵗʰ **S63.309** **Traumatic rupture of unspecified ligament of unspecified wrist**

√6ᵗʰ **S63.31** **Traumatic rupture of collateral ligament of wrist**

√7ᵗʰ **S63.311** **Traumatic rupture of collateral ligament of right wrist**

√7ᵗʰ **S63.312** **Traumatic rupture of collateral ligament of left wrist**

√7ᵗʰ **S63.319** **Traumatic rupture of collateral ligament of unspecified wrist**

√6ᵗʰ **S63.32** **Traumatic rupture of radiocarpal ligament**

√7ᵗʰ **S63.321** **Traumatic rupture of right radiocarpal ligament**

√7ᵗʰ **S63.322** **Traumatic rupture of left radiocarpal ligament**

√7ᵗʰ **S63.329** **Traumatic rupture of unspecified radiocarpal ligament**

√6ᵗʰ **S63.33** **Traumatic rupture of ulnocarpal (palmar) ligament**

√7ᵗʰ **S63.331** **Traumatic rupture of right ulnocarpal (palmar) ligament**

√7ᵗʰ **S63.332** **Traumatic rupture of left ulnocarpal (palmar) ligament**

√7ᵗʰ **S63.339** **Traumatic rupture of unspecified ulnocarpal (palmar) ligament**

√6ᵗʰ **S63.39** **Traumatic rupture of other ligament of wrist**

√7ᵗʰ **S63.391** **Traumatic rupture of other ligament of right wrist**

√7ᵗʰ **S63.392** **Traumatic rupture of other ligament of left wrist**

√7ᵗʰ **S63.399** **Traumatic rupture of other ligament of unspecified wrist**

√5ᵗʰ **S63.4** **Traumatic rupture of ligament of finger at metacarpophalangeal and interphalangeal joint(s)**

√6ᵗʰ **S63.40** **Traumatic rupture of unspecified ligament of finger at metacarpophalangeal and interphalangeal joint**

√7ᵗʰ **S63.400** **Traumatic rupture of unspecified ligament of right index finger at metacarpophalangeal and interphalangeal joint**

√7ᵗʰ **S63.401** **Traumatic rupture of unspecified ligament of left index finger at metacarpophalangeal and interphalangeal joint**

√7ᵗʰ **S63.402** **Traumatic rupture of unspecified ligament of right middle finger at metacarpophalangeal and interphalangeal joint**

√7ᵗʰ **S63.403** **Traumatic rupture of unspecified ligament of left middle finger at metacarpophalangeal and interphalangeal joint**

√7ᵗʰ **S63.404** **Traumatic rupture of unspecified ligament of right ring finger at metacarpophalangeal and interphalangeal joint**

√7ᵗʰ **S63.405** **Traumatic rupture of unspecified ligament of left ring finger at metacarpophalangeal and interphalangeal joint**

√7ᵗʰ **S63.406** **Traumatic rupture of unspecified ligament of right little finger at metacarpophalangeal and interphalangeal joint**

√7ᵗʰ **S63.407** **Traumatic rupture of unspecified ligament of left little finger at metacarpophalangeal and interphalangeal joint**

√7ᵗʰ **S63.408** **Traumatic rupture of unspecified ligament of other finger at metacarpophalangeal and interphalangeal joint**
Traumatic rupture of unspecified ligament of specified finger with unspecified laterality at metacarpophalangeal and interphalangeal joint

√7ᵗʰ **S63.409** **Traumatic rupture of unspecified ligament of unspecified finger at metacarpophalangeal and interphalangeal joint**

√6ᵗʰ **S63.41** **Traumatic rupture of collateral ligament of finger at metacarpophalangeal and interphalangeal joint**

√7ᵗʰ **S63.410** **Traumatic rupture of collateral ligament of right index finger at metacarpophalangeal and interphalangeal joint**

√7ᵗʰ **S63.411** **Traumatic rupture of collateral ligament of left index finger at metacarpophalangeal and interphalangeal joint**

√7ᵗʰ **S63.412** **Traumatic rupture of collateral ligament of right middle finger at metacarpophalangeal and interphalangeal joint**

√7ᵗʰ **S63.413** **Traumatic rupture of collateral ligament of left middle finger at metacarpophalangeal and interphalangeal joint**

√7ᵗʰ **S63.414** **Traumatic rupture of collateral ligament of right ring finger at metacarpophalangeal and interphalangeal joint**

√7ᵗʰ **S63.415** **Traumatic rupture of collateral ligament of left ring finger at metacarpophalangeal and interphalangeal joint**

√7ᵗʰ **S63.416** **Traumatic rupture of collateral ligament of right little finger at metacarpophalangeal and interphalangeal joint**

√7ᵗʰ **S63.417** **Traumatic rupture of collateral ligament of left little finger at metacarpophalangeal and interphalangeal joint**

√7ᵗʰ **S63.418** **Traumatic rupture of collateral ligament of other finger at metacarpophalangeal and interphalangeal joint**
Traumatic rupture of collateral ligament of specified finger with unspecified laterality at metacarpophalangeal and interphalangeal joint

√7ᵗʰ **S63.419** **Traumatic rupture of collateral ligament of unspecified finger at metacarpophalangeal and interphalangeal joint**

√6ᵗʰ **S63.42** **Traumatic rupture of palmar ligament of finger at metacarpophalangeal and interphalangeal joint**

√7ᵗʰ **S63.420** **Traumatic rupture of palmar ligament of right index finger at metacarpophalangeal and interphalangeal joint**

√7ᵗʰ **S63.421** **Traumatic rupture of palmar ligament of left index finger at metacarpophalangeal and interphalangeal joint**

√7ᵗʰ **S63.422** **Traumatic rupture of palmar ligament of right middle finger at metacarpophalangeal and interphalangeal joint**

√7ᵗʰ **S63.423** **Traumatic rupture of palmar ligament of left middle finger at metacarpophalangeal and interphalangeal joint**

√7ᵗʰ **S63.424** **Traumatic rupture of palmar ligament of right ring finger at metacarpophalangeal and interphalangeal joint**

√7ᵗʰ **S63.425** **Traumatic rupture of palmar ligament of left ring finger at metacarpophalangeal and interphalangeal joint**

√7ᵗʰ **S63.426** **Traumatic rupture of palmar ligament of right little finger at metacarpophalangeal and interphalangeal joint**

√7ᵗʰ **S63.427** **Traumatic rupture of palmar ligament of left little finger at metacarpophalangeal and interphalangeal joint**

√7ᵗʰ **S63.428** **Traumatic rupture of palmar ligament of other finger at metacarpophalangeal and interphalangeal joint**
Traumatic rupture of palmar ligament of specified finger with unspecified laterality at metacarpophalangeal and interphalangeal joint

√7ᵗʰ **S63.429** **Traumatic rupture of palmar ligament of unspecified finger at metacarpophalangeal and interphalangeal joint**

√6ᵗʰ **S63.43** **Traumatic rupture of volar plate of finger at metacarpophalangeal and interphalangeal joint**

√7ᵗʰ **S63.430** **Traumatic rupture of volar plate of right index finger at metacarpophalangeal and interphalangeal joint**

√7ᵗʰ **S63.431** **Traumatic rupture of volar plate of left index finger at metacarpophalangeal and interphalangeal joint**

√7ᵗʰ **S63.432** **Traumatic rupture of volar plate of right middle finger at metacarpophalangeal and interphalangeal joint**

√7ᵗʰ **S63.433** **Traumatic rupture of volar plate of left middle finger at metacarpophalangeal and interphalangeal joint**

√7ᵗʰ **S63.434** **Traumatic rupture of volar plate of right ring finger at metacarpophalangeal and interphalangeal joint**

√7ᵗʰ **S63.435** **Traumatic rupture of volar plate of left ring finger at metacarpophalangeal and interphalangeal joint**

√7ᵗʰ **S63.436** **Traumatic rupture of volar plate of right little finger at metacarpophalangeal and interphalangeal joint**

√7ᵗʰ **S63.437** **Traumatic rupture of volar plate of left little finger at metacarpophalangeal and interphalangeal joint**

√7ᵗʰ **S63.438** **Traumatic rupture of volar plate of other finger at metacarpophalangeal and interphalangeal joint**
Traumatic rupture of volar plate of specified finger with unspecified laterality at metacarpophalangeal and interphalangeal joint

√7ᵗʰ **S63.439** **Traumatic rupture of volar plate of unspecified finger at metacarpophalangeal and interphalangeal joint**

√6ᵗʰ **S63.49** **Traumatic rupture of other ligament of finger at metacarpophalangeal and interphalangeal joint**

√7ᵗʰ **S63.490** **Traumatic rupture of other ligament of right index finger at metacarpophalangeal and interphalangeal joint**

√7ᵗʰ **S63.491** **Traumatic rupture of other ligament of left index finger at metacarpophalangeal and interphalangeal joint**

√7ᵗʰ **S63.492** **Traumatic rupture of other ligament of right middle finger at metacarpophalangeal and interphalangeal joint**

√7ᵗʰ **S63.493** **Traumatic rupture of other ligament of left middle finger at metacarpophalangeal and interphalangeal joint**

√7ᵗʰ **S63.494** **Traumatic rupture of other ligament of right ring finger at metacarpophalangeal and interphalangeal joint**

√7ᵗʰ **S63.495** **Traumatic rupture of other ligament of left ring finger at metacarpophalangeal and interphalangeal joint**

√7ᵗʰ **S63.496** **Traumatic rupture of other ligament of right little finger at metacarpophalangeal and interphalangeal joint**

√7ᵗʰ **S63.497** **Traumatic rupture of other ligament of left little finger at metacarpophalangeal and interphalangeal joint**

√7ᵗʰ **S63.498** **Traumatic rupture of other ligament of other finger at metacarpophalangeal and interphalangeal joint**
Traumatic rupture of ligament of specified finger with unspecified laterality at metacarpophalangeal and interphalangeal joint

√7ᵗʰ **S63.499** **Traumatic rupture of other ligament of unspecified finger at metacarpophalangeal and interphalangeal joint**

√5ᵗʰ **S63.5** **Other and unspecified sprain of wrist**

√6ᵗʰ **S63.50** **Unspecified sprain of wrist**

√7ᵗʰ **S63.501** **Unspecified sprain of right wrist**

√7ᵗʰ **S63.502** **Unspecified sprain of left wrist**

√7ᵗʰ **S63.509** **Unspecified sprain of unspecified wrist**

√6ᵗʰ **S63.51** **Sprain of carpal (joint)**

√7ᵗʰ **S63.511** **Sprain of carpal joint of right wrist**

√7ᵗʰ **S63.512** **Sprain of carpal joint of left wrist**

√7ᵗʰ **S63.519** **Sprain of carpal joint of unspecified wrist**

√6ᵗʰ **S63.52** **Sprain of radiocarpal joint**

> *EXCLUDES 1*   traumatic rupture of radiocarpal ligament (S63.32-)

√7ᵗʰ **S63.521** **Sprain of radiocarpal joint of right wrist**

√7ᵗʰ **S63.522** **Sprain of radiocarpal joint of left wrist**

√7ᵗʰ **S63.529** **Sprain of radiocarpal joint of unspecified wrist**

√6ᵗʰ **S63.59** **Other specified sprain of wrist**

√7ᵗʰ **S63.591** **Other specified sprain of right wrist**

√7ᵗʰ **S63.592** **Other specified sprain of left wrist**

√7ᵗʰ **S63.599** **Other specified sprain of unspecified wrist**

√5ᵗʰ **S63.6** **Other and unspecified sprain of finger(s)**

> *EXCLUDES 1*   traumatic rupture of ligament of finger at metacarpophalangeal and interphalangeal joint(s) (S63.4-)

√6ᵗʰ **S63.60** **Unspecified sprain of thumb**

√7ᵗʰ **S63.601** **Unspecified sprain of right thumb**

☑ Additional Character Required   √x7ᵗʰ Placeholder Alert   Manifestation   Unspecified Dx   ▶◀ Revised Text   ● New Code   ▲ Revised Code Title

S63.602 Unspecified sprain of left thumb

S63.609 Unspecified sprain of unspecified thumb

√6ᵗʰ **S63.61** Unspecified sprain of other and unspecified finger(s)

     S63.610 Unspecified sprain of right index finger

     S63.611 Unspecified sprain of left index finger

     S63.612 Unspecified sprain of right middle finger

     S63.613 Unspecified sprain of left middle finger

     S63.614 Unspecified sprain of right ring finger

     S63.615 Unspecified sprain of left ring finger

     S63.616 Unspecified sprain of right little finger

     S63.617 Unspecified sprain of left little finger

     S63.618 Unspecified sprain of other finger

         Unspecified sprain of specified finger with unspecified laterality

     S63.619 Unspecified sprain of unspecified finger

√6ᵗʰ **S63.62** Sprain of interphalangeal joint of thumb

     S63.621 Sprain of interphalangeal joint of right thumb

     S63.622 Sprain of interphalangeal joint of left thumb

     S63.629 Sprain of interphalangeal joint of unspecified thumb

√6ᵗʰ **S63.63** Sprain of interphalangeal joint of other and unspecified finger(s)

     S63.630 Sprain of interphalangeal joint of right index finger

     S63.631 Sprain of interphalangeal joint of left index finger

     S63.632 Sprain of interphalangeal joint of right middle finger

     S63.633 Sprain of interphalangeal joint of left middle finger

     S63.634 Sprain of interphalangeal joint of right ring finger

     S63.635 Sprain of interphalangeal joint of left ring finger

     S63.636 Sprain of interphalangeal joint of right little finger

     S63.637 Sprain of interphalangeal joint of left little finger

     S63.638 Sprain of interphalangeal joint of other finger

     S63.639 Sprain of interphalangeal joint of unspecified finger

√6ᵗʰ **S63.64** Sprain of metacarpophalangeal joint of thumb

     S63.641 Sprain of metacarpophalangeal joint of right thumb

     S63.642 Sprain of metacarpophalangeal joint of left thumb

     S63.649 Sprain of metacarpophalangeal joint of unspecified thumb

√6ᵗʰ **S63.65** Sprain of metacarpophalangeal joint of other and unspecified finger(s)

     S63.650 Sprain of metacarpophalangeal joint of right index finger

     S63.651 Sprain of metacarpophalangeal joint of left index finger

     S63.652 Sprain of metacarpophalangeal joint of right middle finger

     S63.653 Sprain of metacarpophalangeal joint of left middle finger

     S63.654 Sprain of metacarpophalangeal joint of right ring finger

     S63.655 Sprain of metacarpophalangeal joint of left ring finger

     S63.656 Sprain of metacarpophalangeal joint of right little finger

     S63.657 Sprain of metacarpophalangeal joint of left little finger

     S63.658 Sprain of metacarpophalangeal joint of other finger

         Sprain of metacarpophalangeal joint of specified finger with unspecified laterality

     S63.659 Sprain of metacarpophalangeal joint of unspecified finger

√6ᵗʰ **S63.68** Other sprain of thumb

     S63.681 Other sprain of right thumb

S63.682 Other sprain of left thumb

S63.689 Other sprain of unspecified thumb

√6ᵗʰ **S63.69** Other sprain of other and unspecified finger(s)

     S63.690 Other sprain of right index finger

     S63.691 Other sprain of left index finger

     S63.692 Other sprain of right middle finger

     S63.693 Other sprain of left middle finger

     S63.694 Other sprain of right ring finger

     S63.695 Other sprain of left ring finger

     S63.696 Other sprain of right little finger

     S63.697 Other sprain of left little finger

     S63.698 Other sprain of other finger

         Other sprain of specified finger with unspecified laterality

     S63.699 Other sprain of unspecified finger

√5ᵗʰ **S63.8** Sprain of other part of wrist and hand

     √6ᵗʰ **S63.8X** Sprain of other part of wrist and hand

         S63.8X1 Sprain of other part of right wrist and hand

         S63.8X2 Sprain of other part of left wrist and hand

         S63.8X9 Sprain of other part of unspecified wrist and hand

√5ᵗʰ **S63.9** Sprain of unspecified part of wrist and hand

     √×7ᵗʰ **S63.90** Sprain of unspecified part of unspecified wrist and hand

     √×7ᵗʰ **S63.91** Sprain of unspecified part of right wrist and hand

     √×7ᵗʰ **S63.92** Sprain of unspecified part of left wrist and hand

√4ᵗʰ **S64** **Injury of nerves at wrist and hand level**

     Code also any associated open wound (S61.-)

     The appropriate 7th character is to be added to each code from category S64.
     A   initial encounter
     D   subsequent encounter
     S   sequela

√5ᵗʰ **S64.0** Injury of ulnar nerve at wrist and hand level

     √×7ᵗʰ **S64.00** Injury of ulnar nerve at wrist and hand level of unspecified arm

     √×7ᵗʰ **S64.01** Injury of ulnar nerve at wrist and hand level of right arm

     √×7ᵗʰ **S64.02** Injury of ulnar nerve at wrist and hand level of left arm

√5ᵗʰ **S64.1** Injury of median nerve at wrist and hand level

     √×7ᵗʰ **S64.10** Injury of median nerve at wrist and hand level of unspecified arm

     √×7ᵗʰ **S64.11** Injury of median nerve at wrist and hand level of right arm

     √×7ᵗʰ **S64.12** Injury of median nerve at wrist and hand level of left arm

√5ᵗʰ **S64.2** Injury of radial nerve at wrist and hand level

     √×7ᵗʰ **S64.20** Injury of radial nerve at wrist and hand level of unspecified arm

     √×7ᵗʰ **S64.21** Injury of radial nerve at wrist and hand level of right arm

     √×7ᵗʰ **S64.22** Injury of radial nerve at wrist and hand level of left arm

√5ᵗʰ **S64.3** Injury of digital nerve of thumb

     √×7ᵗʰ **S64.30** Injury of digital nerve of unspecified thumb

     √×7ᵗʰ **S64.31** Injury of digital nerve of right thumb

     √×7ᵗʰ **S64.32** Injury of digital nerve of left thumb

√5ᵗʰ **S64.4** Injury of digital nerve of other and unspecified finger

     √×7ᵗʰ **S64.40** Injury of digital nerve of unspecified finger

     √6ᵗʰ **S64.49** Injury of digital nerve of other finger

         S64.490 Injury of digital nerve of right index finger

         S64.491 Injury of digital nerve of left index finger

         S64.492 Injury of digital nerve of right middle finger

         S64.493 Injury of digital nerve of left middle finger

         S64.494 Injury of digital nerve of right ring finger

         S64.495 Injury of digital nerve of left ring finger

         S64.496 Injury of digital nerve of right little finger

√7ᵗʰ **S64.497** Injury of digital nerve of left little finger

√7ᵗʰ **S64.498** Injury of digital nerve of other finger

Injury of digital nerve of specified finger with unspecified laterality

√5ᵗʰ **S64.8** Injury of other nerves at wrist and hand level

√6ᵗʰ **S64.8X** Injury of other nerves at wrist and hand level

√7ᵗʰ **S64.8X1** Injury of other nerves at wrist and hand level of right arm

√7ᵗʰ **S64.8X2** Injury of other nerves at wrist and hand level of left arm

√7ᵗʰ **S64.8X9** Injury of other nerves at wrist and hand level of unspecified arm

√5ᵗʰ **S64.9** Injury of unspecified nerve at wrist and hand level

√x7ᵗʰ **S64.90** Injury of unspecified nerve at wrist and hand level of unspecified arm

√x7ᵗʰ **S64.91** Injury of unspecified nerve at wrist and hand level of right arm

√x7ᵗʰ **S64.92** Injury of unspecified nerve at wrist and hand level of left arm

√4ᵗʰ **S65** Injury of blood vessels at wrist and hand level

Code also any associated open wound (S61.-)

The appropriate 7th character is to be added to each code from category S65.
A initial encounter
D subsequent encounter
S sequela

√5ᵗʰ **S65.0** Injury of ulnar artery at wrist and hand level

√6ᵗʰ **S65.00** Unspecified injury of ulnar artery at wrist and hand level

√7ᵗʰ **S65.001** Unspecified injury of ulnar artery at wrist and hand level of right arm

√7ᵗʰ **S65.002** Unspecified injury of ulnar artery at wrist and hand level of left arm

√7ᵗʰ **S65.009** Unspecified injury of ulnar artery at wrist and hand level of unspecified arm

√6ᵗʰ **S65.01** Laceration of ulnar artery at wrist and hand level

√7ᵗʰ **S65.011** Laceration of ulnar artery at wrist and hand level of right arm

√7ᵗʰ **S65.012** Laceration of ulnar artery at wrist and hand level of left arm

√7ᵗʰ **S65.019** Laceration of ulnar artery at wrist and hand level of unspecified arm

√6ᵗʰ **S65.09** Other specified injury of ulnar artery at wrist and hand level

√7ᵗʰ **S65.091** Other specified injury of ulnar artery at wrist and hand level of right arm

√7ᵗʰ **S65.092** Other specified injury of ulnar artery at wrist and hand level of left arm

√7ᵗʰ **S65.099** Other specified injury of ulnar artery at wrist and hand level of unspecified arm

√5ᵗʰ **S65.1** Injury of radial artery at wrist and hand level

√6ᵗʰ **S65.10** Unspecified injury of radial artery at wrist and hand level

√7ᵗʰ **S65.101** Unspecified injury of radial artery at wrist and hand level of right arm

√7ᵗʰ **S65.102** Unspecified injury of radial artery at wrist and hand level of left arm

√7ᵗʰ **S65.109** Unspecified injury of radial artery at wrist and hand level of unspecified arm

√6ᵗʰ **S65.11** Laceration of radial artery at wrist and hand level

√7ᵗʰ **S65.111** Laceration of radial artery at wrist and hand level of right arm

√7ᵗʰ **S65.112** Laceration of radial artery at wrist and hand level of left arm

√7ᵗʰ **S65.119** Laceration of radial artery at wrist and hand level of unspecified arm

√6ᵗʰ **S65.19** Other specified injury of radial artery at wrist and hand level

√7ᵗʰ **S65.191** Other specified injury of radial artery at wrist and hand level of right arm

√7ᵗʰ **S65.192** Other specified injury of radial artery at wrist and hand level of left arm

√7ᵗʰ **S65.199** Other specified injury of radial artery at wrist and hand level of unspecified arm

√5ᵗʰ **S65.2** Injury of superficial palmar arch

√6ᵗʰ **S65.20** Unspecified injury of superficial palmar arch

√7ᵗʰ **S65.201** Unspecified injury of superficial palmar arch of right hand

√7ᵗʰ **S65.202** Unspecified injury of superficial palmar arch of left hand

√7ᵗʰ **S65.209** Unspecified injury of superficial palmar arch of unspecified hand

√6ᵗʰ **S65.21** Laceration of superficial palmar arch

√7ᵗʰ **S65.211** Laceration of superficial palmar arch of right hand

√7ᵗʰ **S65.212** Laceration of superficial palmar arch of left hand

√7ᵗʰ **S65.219** Laceration of superficial palmar arch of unspecified hand

√6ᵗʰ **S65.29** Other specified injury of superficial palmar arch

√7ᵗʰ **S65.291** Other specified injury of superficial palmar arch of right hand

√7ᵗʰ **S65.292** Other specified injury of superficial palmar arch of left hand

√7ᵗʰ **S65.299** Other specified injury of superficial palmar arch of unspecified hand

√5ᵗʰ **S65.3** Injury of deep palmar arch

√6ᵗʰ **S65.30** Unspecified injury of deep palmar arch

√7ᵗʰ **S65.301** Unspecified injury of deep palmar arch of right hand

√7ᵗʰ **S65.302** Unspecified injury of deep palmar arch of left hand

√7ᵗʰ **S65.309** Unspecified injury of deep palmar arch of unspecified hand

√6ᵗʰ **S65.31** Laceration of deep palmar arch

√7ᵗʰ **S65.311** Laceration of deep palmar arch of right hand

√7ᵗʰ **S65.312** Laceration of deep palmar arch of left hand

√7ᵗʰ **S65.319** Laceration of deep palmar arch of unspecified hand

√6ᵗʰ **S65.39** Other specified injury of deep palmar arch

√7ᵗʰ **S65.391** Other specified injury of deep palmar arch of right hand

√7ᵗʰ **S65.392** Other specified injury of deep palmar arch of left hand

√7ᵗʰ **S65.399** Other specified injury of deep palmar arch of unspecified hand

√5ᵗʰ **S65.4** Injury of blood vessel of thumb

√6ᵗʰ **S65.40** Unspecified injury of blood vessel of thumb

√7ᵗʰ **S65.401** Unspecified injury of blood vessel of right thumb

√7ᵗʰ **S65.402** Unspecified injury of blood vessel of left thumb

√7ᵗʰ **S65.409** Unspecified injury of blood vessel of unspecified thumb

√6ᵗʰ **S65.41** Laceration of blood vessel of thumb

√7ᵗʰ **S65.411** Laceration of blood vessel of right thumb

√7ᵗʰ **S65.412** Laceration of blood vessel of left thumb

√7ᵗʰ **S65.419** Laceration of blood vessel of unspecified thumb

√6ᵗʰ **S65.49** Other specified injury of blood vessel of thumb

√7ᵗʰ **S65.491** Other specified injury of blood vessel of right thumb

√7ᵗʰ **S65.492** Other specified injury of blood vessel of left thumb

√7ᵗʰ **S65.499** Other specified injury of blood vessel of unspecified thumb

√5ᵗʰ **S65.5** Injury of blood vessel of other and unspecified finger

√6ᵗʰ **S65.50** Unspecified injury of blood vessel of other and unspecified finger

√7ᵗʰ **S65.500** Unspecified injury of blood vessel of right index finger

√7ᵗʰ **S65.501** Unspecified injury of blood vessel of left index finger

√7ᵗʰ **S65.502** Unspecified injury of blood vessel of right middle finger

√7ᵗʰ **S65.503** Unspecified injury of blood vessel of left middle finger

√7ᵗʰ **S65.504** Unspecified injury of blood vessel of right ring finger

√7ᵗʰ **S65.505** Unspecified injury of blood vessel of left ring finger

√7ᵗʰ **S65.506** Unspecified injury of blood vessel of right little finger

√7ᵗʰ **S65.507** Unspecified injury of blood vessel of left little finger

✔ Additional Character Required   √x7ᵗʰ Placeholder Alert   Manifestation   Unspecified Dx   ▶◀ Revised Text   ● New Code   ▲ Revised Code Title

ICD-10-CM 2020   1035

√7ᵗʰ **S65.508** Unspecified injury of blood vessel of other finger
　Unspecified injury of blood vessel of specified finger with unspecified laterality

√7ᵗʰ **S65.509** Unspecified injury of blood vessel of unspecified finger

√6ᵗʰ **S65.51** Laceration of blood vessel of other and unspecified finger

√7ᵗʰ **S65.510** Laceration of blood vessel of right index finger

√7ᵗʰ **S65.511** Laceration of blood vessel of left index finger

√7ᵗʰ **S65.512** Laceration of blood vessel of right middle finger

√7ᵗʰ **S65.513** Laceration of blood vessel of left middle finger

√7ᵗʰ **S65.514** Laceration of blood vessel of right ring finger

√7ᵗʰ **S65.515** Laceration of blood vessel of left ring finger

√7ᵗʰ **S65.516** Laceration of blood vessel of right little finger

√7ᵗʰ **S65.517** Laceration of blood vessel of left little finger

√7ᵗʰ **S65.518** Laceration of blood vessel of other finger
　Laceration of blood vessel of specified finger with unspecified laterality

√7ᵗʰ **S65.519** Laceration of blood vessel of unspecified finger

√6ᵗʰ **S65.59** Other specified injury of blood vessel of other and unspecified finger

√7ᵗʰ **S65.590** Other specified injury of blood vessel of right index finger

√7ᵗʰ **S65.591** Other specified injury of blood vessel of left index finger

√7ᵗʰ **S65.592** Other specified injury of blood vessel of right middle finger

√7ᵗʰ **S65.593** Other specified injury of blood vessel of left middle finger

√7ᵗʰ **S65.594** Other specified injury of blood vessel of right ring finger

√7ᵗʰ **S65.595** Other specified injury of blood vessel of left ring finger

√7ᵗʰ **S65.596** Other specified injury of blood vessel of right little finger

√7ᵗʰ **S65.597** Other specified injury of blood vessel of left little finger

√7ᵗʰ **S65.598** Other specified injury of blood vessel of other finger
　Other specified injury of blood vessel of specified finger with unspecified laterality

√7ᵗʰ **S65.599** Other specified injury of blood vessel of unspecified finger

√5ᵗʰ **S65.8** Injury of other blood vessels at wrist and hand level

√6ᵗʰ **S65.80** Unspecified injury of other blood vessels at wrist and hand level

√7ᵗʰ **S65.801** Unspecified injury of other blood vessels at wrist and hand level of right arm

√7ᵗʰ **S65.802** Unspecified injury of other blood vessels at wrist and hand level of left arm

√7ᵗʰ **S65.809** Unspecified injury of other blood vessels at wrist and hand level of unspecified arm

√6ᵗʰ **S65.81** Laceration of other blood vessels at wrist and hand level

√7ᵗʰ **S65.811** Laceration of other blood vessels at wrist and hand level of right arm

√7ᵗʰ **S65.812** Laceration of other blood vessels at wrist and hand level of left arm

√7ᵗʰ **S65.819** Laceration of other blood vessels at wrist and hand level of unspecified arm

√6ᵗʰ **S65.89** Other specified injury of other blood vessels at wrist and hand level

√7ᵗʰ **S65.891** Other specified injury of other blood vessels at wrist and hand level of right arm

√7ᵗʰ **S65.892** Other specified injury of other blood vessels at wrist and hand level of left arm

√7ᵗʰ **S65.899** Other specified injury of other blood vessels at wrist and hand level of unspecified arm

√5ᵗʰ **S65.9** Injury of unspecified blood vessel at wrist and hand level

√6ᵗʰ **S65.90** Unspecified injury of unspecified blood vessel at wrist and hand level

√7ᵗʰ **S65.901** Unspecified injury of unspecified blood vessel at wrist and hand level of right arm

√7ᵗʰ **S65.902** Unspecified injury of unspecified blood vessel at wrist and hand level of left arm

√7ᵗʰ **S65.909** Unspecified injury of unspecified blood vessel at wrist and hand level of unspecified arm

√6ᵗʰ **S65.91** Laceration of unspecified blood vessel at wrist and hand level

√7ᵗʰ **S65.911** Laceration of unspecified blood vessel at wrist and hand level of right arm

√7ᵗʰ **S65.912** Laceration of unspecified blood vessel at wrist and hand level of left arm

√7ᵗʰ **S65.919** Laceration of unspecified blood vessel at wrist and hand level of unspecified arm

√6ᵗʰ **S65.99** Other specified injury of unspecified blood vessel at wrist and hand level

√7ᵗʰ **S65.991** Other specified injury of unspecified blood vessel at wrist and hand of right arm

√7ᵗʰ **S65.992** Other specified injury of unspecified blood vessel at wrist and hand of left arm

√7ᵗʰ **S65.999** Other specified injury of unspecified blood vessel at wrist and hand of unspecified arm

√4ᵗʰ **S66** Injury of muscle, fascia and tendon at wrist and hand level

Code also any associated open wound (S61.-)

EXCLUDES 2　sprain of joints and ligaments of wrist and hand (S63.-)

TIP: Refer to the Muscle/Tendon table at the beginning of this chapter.

The appropriate 7th character is to be added to each code from category S66.
A　initial encounter
D　subsequent encounter
S　sequela

√5ᵗʰ **S66.0** Injury of long flexor muscle, fascia and tendon of thumb at wrist and hand level

√6ᵗʰ **S66.00** Unspecified injury of long flexor muscle, fascia and tendon of thumb at wrist and hand level

√7ᵗʰ **S66.001** Unspecified injury of long flexor muscle, fascia and tendon of right thumb at wrist and hand level

√7ᵗʰ **S66.002** Unspecified injury of long flexor muscle, fascia and tendon of left thumb at wrist and hand level

√7ᵗʰ **S66.009** Unspecified injury of long flexor muscle, fascia and tendon of unspecified thumb at wrist and hand level

√6ᵗʰ **S66.01** Strain of long flexor muscle, fascia and tendon of thumb at wrist and hand level

√7ᵗʰ **S66.011** Strain of long flexor muscle, fascia and tendon of right thumb at wrist and hand level

√7ᵗʰ **S66.012** Strain of long flexor muscle, fascia and tendon of left thumb at wrist and hand level

√7ᵗʰ **S66.019** Strain of long flexor muscle, fascia and tendon of unspecified thumb at wrist and hand level

√6ᵗʰ **S66.02** Laceration of long flexor muscle, fascia and tendon of thumb at wrist and hand level

√7ᵗʰ **S66.021** Laceration of long flexor muscle, fascia and tendon of right thumb at wrist and hand level

√7ᵗʰ **S66.022** Laceration of long flexor muscle, fascia and tendon of left thumb at wrist and hand level

√7ᵗʰ **S66.029** Laceration of long flexor muscle, fascia and tendon of unspecified thumb at wrist and hand level

√6ᵗʰ **S66.09** Other specified injury of long flexor muscle, fascia and tendon of thumb at wrist and hand level

√7ᵗʰ **S66.091** Other specified injury of long flexor muscle, fascia and tendon of right thumb at wrist and hand level

√7ᵗʰ **S66.092** Other specified injury of long flexor muscle, fascia and tendon of left thumb at wrist and hand level

√7ᵗʰ **S66.099** Other specified injury of long flexor muscle, fascia and tendon of unspecified thumb at wrist and hand level

√5ᵗʰ **S66.1** Injury of flexor muscle, fascia and tendon of other and unspecified finger at wrist and hand level

    EXCLUDES 2   injury of long flexor muscle, fascia and tendon of thumb at wrist and hand level (S66.0-)

√6ᵗʰ **S66.10** Unspecified injury of flexor muscle, fascia and tendon of other and unspecified finger at wrist and hand level

√7ᵗʰ **S66.100** Unspecified injury of flexor muscle, fascia and tendon of right index finger at wrist and hand level

√7ᵗʰ **S66.101** Unspecified injury of flexor muscle, fascia and tendon of left index finger at wrist and hand level

√7ᵗʰ **S66.102** Unspecified injury of flexor muscle, fascia and tendon of right middle finger at wrist and hand level

√7ᵗʰ **S66.103** Unspecified injury of flexor muscle, fascia and tendon of left middle finger at wrist and hand level

√7ᵗʰ **S66.104** Unspecified injury of flexor muscle, fascia and tendon of right ring finger at wrist and hand level

√7ᵗʰ **S66.105** Unspecified injury of flexor muscle, fascia and tendon of left ring finger at wrist and hand level

√7ᵗʰ **S66.106** Unspecified injury of flexor muscle, fascia and tendon of right little finger at wrist and hand level

√7ᵗʰ **S66.107** Unspecified injury of flexor muscle, fascia and tendon of left little finger at wrist and hand level

√7ᵗʰ **S66.108** Unspecified injury of flexor muscle, fascia and tendon of other finger at wrist and hand level

    Unspecified injury of flexor muscle, fascia and tendon of specified finger with unspecified laterality at wrist and hand level

√7ᵗʰ **S66.109** Unspecified injury of flexor muscle, fascia and tendon of unspecified finger at wrist and hand level

√6ᵗʰ **S66.11** Strain of flexor muscle, fascia and tendon of other and unspecified finger at wrist and hand level

√7ᵗʰ **S66.110** Strain of flexor muscle, fascia and tendon of right index finger at wrist and hand level

√7ᵗʰ **S66.111** Strain of flexor muscle, fascia and tendon of left index finger at wrist and hand level

√7ᵗʰ **S66.112** Strain of flexor muscle, fascia and tendon of right middle finger at wrist and hand level

√7ᵗʰ **S66.113** Strain of flexor muscle, fascia and tendon of left middle finger at wrist and hand level

√7ᵗʰ **S66.114** Strain of flexor muscle, fascia and tendon of right ring finger at wrist and hand level

√7ᵗʰ **S66.115** Strain of flexor muscle, fascia and tendon of left ring finger at wrist and hand level

√7ᵗʰ **S66.116** Strain of flexor muscle, fascia and tendon of right little finger at wrist and hand level

√7ᵗʰ **S66.117** Strain of flexor muscle, fascia and tendon of left little finger at wrist and hand level

√7ᵗʰ **S66.118** Strain of flexor muscle, fascia and tendon of other finger at wrist and hand level

    Strain of flexor muscle, fascia and tendon of specified finger with unspecified laterality at wrist and hand level

√7ᵗʰ **S66.119** Strain of flexor muscle, fascia and tendon of unspecified finger at wrist and hand level

√6ᵗʰ **S66.12** Laceration of flexor muscle, fascia and tendon of other and unspecified finger at wrist and hand level

√7ᵗʰ **S66.120** Laceration of flexor muscle, fascia and tendon of right index finger at wrist and hand level

√7ᵗʰ **S66.121** Laceration of flexor muscle, fascia and tendon of left index finger at wrist and hand level

√7ᵗʰ **S66.122** Laceration of flexor muscle, fascia and tendon of right middle finger at wrist and hand level

√7ᵗʰ **S66.123** Laceration of flexor muscle, fascia and tendon of left middle finger at wrist and hand level

√7ᵗʰ **S66.124** Laceration of flexor muscle, fascia and tendon of right ring finger at wrist and hand level

√7ᵗʰ **S66.125** Laceration of flexor muscle, fascia and tendon of left ring finger at wrist and hand level

√7ᵗʰ **S66.126** Laceration of flexor muscle, fascia and tendon of right little finger at wrist and hand level

√7ᵗʰ **S66.127** Laceration of flexor muscle, fascia and tendon of left little finger at wrist and hand level

√7ᵗʰ **S66.128** Laceration of flexor muscle, fascia and tendon of other finger at wrist and hand level

    Laceration of flexor muscle, fascia and tendon of specified finger with unspecified laterality at wrist and hand level

√7ᵗʰ **S66.129** Laceration of flexor muscle, fascia and tendon of unspecified finger at wrist and hand level

√6ᵗʰ **S66.19** Other injury of flexor muscle, fascia and tendon of other and unspecified finger at wrist and hand level

√7ᵗʰ **S66.190** Other injury of flexor muscle, fascia and tendon of right index finger at wrist and hand level

√7ᵗʰ **S66.191** Other injury of flexor muscle, fascia and tendon of left index finger at wrist and hand level

√7ᵗʰ **S66.192** Other injury of flexor muscle, fascia and tendon of right middle finger at wrist and hand level

√7ᵗʰ **S66.193** Other injury of flexor muscle, fascia and tendon of left middle finger at wrist and hand level

√7ᵗʰ **S66.194** Other injury of flexor muscle, fascia and tendon of right ring finger at wrist and hand level

√7ᵗʰ **S66.195** Other injury of flexor muscle, fascia and tendon of left ring finger at wrist and hand level

√7ᵗʰ **S66.196** Other injury of flexor muscle, fascia and tendon of right little finger at wrist and hand level

√7ᵗʰ **S66.197** Other injury of flexor muscle, fascia and tendon of left little finger at wrist and hand level

√7ᵗʰ **S66.198** Other injury of flexor muscle, fascia and tendon of other finger at wrist and hand level

    Other injury of flexor muscle, fascia and tendon of specified finger with unspecified laterality at wrist and hand level

√7ᵗʰ **S66.199** Other injury of flexor muscle, fascia and tendon of unspecified finger at wrist and hand level

√5ᵗʰ **S66.2** Injury of extensor muscle, fascia and tendon of thumb at wrist and hand level

√6ᵗʰ **S66.20** Unspecified injury of extensor muscle, fascia and tendon of thumb at wrist and hand level

√7ᵗʰ **S66.201** Unspecified injury of extensor muscle, fascia and tendon of right thumb at wrist and hand level

√7ᵗʰ **S66.202** Unspecified injury of extensor muscle, fascia and tendon of left thumb at wrist and hand level

√7ᵗʰ **S66.209** Unspecified injury of extensor muscle, fascia and tendon of unspecified thumb at wrist and hand level

√6ᵗʰ **S66.21** Strain of extensor muscle, fascia and tendon of thumb at wrist and hand level

√7ᵗʰ **S66.211** Strain of extensor muscle, fascia and tendon of right thumb at wrist and hand level

☑ Additional Character Required   √ₓ7ᵗʰ Placeholder Alert   Manifestation   Unspecified Dx   ►◄ Revised Text   ● New Code   ▲ Revised Code Title

ICD-10-CM 2020   1037

√7ᵗʰ **S66.212** Strain of extensor muscle, fascia and tendon of left thumb at wrist and hand level

√7ᵗʰ **S66.219** Strain of extensor muscle, fascia and tendon of unspecified thumb at wrist and hand level

√6ᵗʰ **S66.22** Laceration of extensor muscle, fascia and tendon of thumb at wrist and hand level

√7ᵗʰ **S66.221** Laceration of extensor muscle, fascia and tendon of right thumb at wrist and hand level

√7ᵗʰ **S66.222** Laceration of extensor muscle, fascia and tendon of left thumb at wrist and hand level

√7ᵗʰ **S66.229** Laceration of extensor muscle, fascia and tendon of unspecified thumb at wrist and hand level

√6ᵗʰ **S66.29** Other specified injury of extensor muscle, fascia and tendon of thumb at wrist and hand level

√7ᵗʰ **S66.291** Other specified injury of extensor muscle, fascia and tendon of right thumb at wrist and hand level

√7ᵗʰ **S66.292** Other specified injury of extensor muscle, fascia and tendon of left thumb at wrist and hand level

√7ᵗʰ **S66.299** Other specified injury of extensor muscle, fascia and tendon of unspecified thumb at wrist and hand level

√5ᵗʰ **S66.3** Injury of extensor muscle, fascia and tendon of other and unspecified finger at wrist and hand level

> EXCLUDES 2   injury of extensor muscle, fascia and tendon of thumb at wrist and hand level (S66.2-)

√6ᵗʰ **S66.30** Unspecified injury of extensor muscle, fascia and tendon of other and unspecified finger at wrist and hand level

√7ᵗʰ **S66.300** Unspecified injury of extensor muscle, fascia and tendon of right index finger at wrist and hand level

√7ᵗʰ **S66.301** Unspecified injury of extensor muscle, fascia and tendon of left index finger at wrist and hand level

√7ᵗʰ **S66.302** Unspecified injury of extensor muscle, fascia and tendon of right middle finger at wrist and hand level

√7ᵗʰ **S66.303** Unspecified injury of extensor muscle, fascia and tendon of left middle finger at wrist and hand level

√7ᵗʰ **S66.304** Unspecified injury of extensor muscle, fascia and tendon of right ring finger at wrist and hand level

√7ᵗʰ **S66.305** Unspecified injury of extensor muscle, fascia and tendon of left ring finger at wrist and hand level

√7ᵗʰ **S66.306** Unspecified injury of extensor muscle, fascia and tendon of right little finger at wrist and hand level

√7ᵗʰ **S66.307** Unspecified injury of extensor muscle, fascia and tendon of left little finger at wrist and hand level

√7ᵗʰ **S66.308** Unspecified injury of extensor muscle, fascia and tendon of other finger at wrist and hand level

> Unspecified injury of extensor muscle, fascia and tendon of specified finger with unspecified laterality at wrist and hand level

√7ᵗʰ **S66.309** Unspecified injury of extensor muscle, fascia and tendon of unspecified finger at wrist and hand level

√6ᵗʰ **S66.31** Strain of extensor muscle, fascia and tendon of other and unspecified finger at wrist and hand level

√7ᵗʰ **S66.310** Strain of extensor muscle, fascia and tendon of right index finger at wrist and hand level

√7ᵗʰ **S66.311** Strain of extensor muscle, fascia and tendon of left index finger at wrist and hand level

√7ᵗʰ **S66.312** Strain of extensor muscle, fascia and tendon of right middle finger at wrist and hand level

√7ᵗʰ **S66.313** Strain of extensor muscle, fascia and tendon of left middle finger at wrist and hand level

√7ᵗʰ **S66.314** Strain of extensor muscle, fascia and tendon of right ring finger at wrist and hand level

√7ᵗʰ **S66.315** Strain of extensor muscle, fascia and tendon of left ring finger at wrist and hand level

√7ᵗʰ **S66.316** Strain of extensor muscle, fascia and tendon of right little finger at wrist and hand level

√7ᵗʰ **S66.317** Strain of extensor muscle, fascia and tendon of left little finger at wrist and hand level

√7ᵗʰ **S66.318** Strain of extensor muscle, fascia and tendon of other finger at wrist and hand level

> Strain of extensor muscle, fascia and tendon of specified finger with unspecified laterality at wrist and hand level

√7ᵗʰ **S66.319** Strain of extensor muscle, fascia and tendon of unspecified finger at wrist and hand level

√6ᵗʰ **S66.32** Laceration of extensor muscle, fascia and tendon of other and unspecified finger at wrist and hand level

√7ᵗʰ **S66.320** Laceration of extensor muscle, fascia and tendon of right index finger at wrist and hand level

√7ᵗʰ **S66.321** Laceration of extensor muscle, fascia and tendon of left index finger at wrist and hand level

√7ᵗʰ **S66.322** Laceration of extensor muscle, fascia and tendon of right middle finger at wrist and hand level

√7ᵗʰ **S66.323** Laceration of extensor muscle, fascia and tendon of left middle finger at wrist and hand level

√7ᵗʰ **S66.324** Laceration of extensor muscle, fascia and tendon of right ring finger at wrist and hand level

√7ᵗʰ **S66.325** Laceration of extensor muscle, fascia and tendon of left ring finger at wrist and hand level

√7ᵗʰ **S66.326** Laceration of extensor muscle, fascia and tendon of right little finger at wrist and hand level

√7ᵗʰ **S66.327** Laceration of extensor muscle, fascia and tendon of left little finger at wrist and hand level

√7ᵗʰ **S66.328** Laceration of extensor muscle, fascia and tendon of other finger at wrist and hand level

> Laceration of extensor muscle, fascia and tendon of specified finger with unspecified laterality at wrist and hand level

√7ᵗʰ **S66.329** Laceration of extensor muscle, fascia and tendon of unspecified finger at wrist and hand level

√6ᵗʰ **S66.39** Other injury of extensor muscle, fascia and tendon of other and unspecified finger at wrist and hand level

√7ᵗʰ **S66.390** Other injury of extensor muscle, fascia and tendon of right index finger at wrist and hand level

√7ᵗʰ **S66.391** Other injury of extensor muscle, fascia and tendon of left index finger at wrist and hand level

√7ᵗʰ **S66.392** Other injury of extensor muscle, fascia and tendon of right middle finger at wrist and hand level

√7ᵗʰ **S66.393** Other injury of extensor muscle, fascia and tendon of left middle finger at wrist and hand level

√7ᵗʰ **S66.394** Other injury of extensor muscle, fascia and tendon of right ring finger at wrist and hand level

√7ᵗʰ **S66.395** Other injury of extensor muscle, fascia and tendon of left ring finger at wrist and hand level

√7ᵗʰ **S66.396** Other injury of extensor muscle, fascia and tendon of right little finger at wrist and hand level

√7ᵗʰ **S66.397** Other injury of extensor muscle, fascia and tendon of left little finger at wrist and hand level

√7ᵗʰ **S66.398** Other injury of extensor muscle, fascia and tendon of other finger at wrist and hand level

Other injury of extensor muscle, fascia and tendon of specified finger with unspecified laterality at wrist and hand level

√7ᵗʰ **S66.399** Other injury of extensor muscle, fascia and tendon of unspecified finger at wrist and hand level

√5ᵗʰ **S66.4** Injury of intrinsic muscle, fascia and tendon of thumb at wrist and hand level

√6ᵗʰ **S66.40** Unspecified injury of intrinsic muscle, fascia and tendon of thumb at wrist and hand level

√7ᵗʰ **S66.401** Unspecified injury of intrinsic muscle, fascia and tendon of right thumb at wrist and hand level

√7ᵗʰ **S66.402** Unspecified injury of intrinsic muscle, fascia and tendon of left thumb at wrist and hand level

√7ᵗʰ **S66.409** Unspecified injury of intrinsic muscle, fascia and tendon of unspecified thumb at wrist and hand level

√6ᵗʰ **S66.41** Strain of intrinsic muscle, fascia and tendon of thumb at wrist and hand level

√7ᵗʰ **S66.411** Strain of intrinsic muscle, fascia and tendon of right thumb at wrist and hand level

√7ᵗʰ **S66.412** Strain of intrinsic muscle, fascia and tendon of left thumb at wrist and hand level

√7ᵗʰ **S66.419** Strain of intrinsic muscle, fascia and tendon of unspecified thumb at wrist and hand level

√6ᵗʰ **S66.42** Laceration of intrinsic muscle, fascia and tendon of thumb at wrist and hand level

√7ᵗʰ **S66.421** Laceration of intrinsic muscle, fascia and tendon of right thumb at wrist and hand level

√7ᵗʰ **S66.422** Laceration of intrinsic muscle, fascia and tendon of left thumb at wrist and hand level

√7ᵗʰ **S66.429** Laceration of intrinsic muscle, fascia and tendon of unspecified thumb at wrist and hand level

√6ᵗʰ **S66.49** Other specified injury of intrinsic muscle, fascia and tendon of thumb at wrist and hand level

√7ᵗʰ **S66.491** Other specified injury of intrinsic muscle, fascia and tendon of right thumb at wrist and hand level

√7ᵗʰ **S66.492** Other specified injury of intrinsic muscle, fascia and tendon of left thumb at wrist and hand level

√7ᵗʰ **S66.499** Other specified injury of intrinsic muscle, fascia and tendon of unspecified thumb at wrist and hand level

√5ᵗʰ **S66.5** Injury of intrinsic muscle, fascia and tendon of other and unspecified finger at wrist and hand level

EXCLUDES 2   injury of intrinsic muscle, fascia and tendon of thumb at wrist and hand level (S66.4-)

√6ᵗʰ **S66.50** Unspecified injury of intrinsic muscle, fascia and tendon of other and unspecified finger at wrist and hand level

√7ᵗʰ **S66.500** Unspecified injury of intrinsic muscle, fascia and tendon of right index finger at wrist and hand level

√7ᵗʰ **S66.501** Unspecified injury of intrinsic muscle, fascia and tendon of left index finger at wrist and hand level

√7ᵗʰ **S66.502** Unspecified injury of intrinsic muscle, fascia and tendon of right middle finger at wrist and hand level

√7ᵗʰ **S66.503** Unspecified injury of intrinsic muscle, fascia and tendon of left middle finger at wrist and hand level

√7ᵗʰ **S66.504** Unspecified injury of intrinsic muscle, fascia and tendon of right ring finger at wrist and hand level

√7ᵗʰ **S66.505** Unspecified injury of intrinsic muscle, fascia and tendon of left ring finger at wrist and hand level

√7ᵗʰ **S66.506** Unspecified injury of intrinsic muscle, fascia and tendon of right little finger at wrist and hand level

√7ᵗʰ **S66.507** Unspecified injury of intrinsic muscle, fascia and tendon of left little finger at wrist and hand level

√7ᵗʰ **S66.508** Unspecified injury of intrinsic muscle, fascia and tendon of other finger at wrist and hand level

Unspecified injury of intrinsic muscle, fascia and tendon of specified finger with unspecified laterality at wrist and hand level

√7ᵗʰ **S66.509** Unspecified injury of intrinsic muscle, fascia and tendon of unspecified finger at wrist and hand level

√6ᵗʰ **S66.51** Strain of intrinsic muscle, fascia and tendon of other and unspecified finger at wrist and hand level

√7ᵗʰ **S66.510** Strain of intrinsic muscle, fascia and tendon of right index finger at wrist and hand level

√7ᵗʰ **S66.511** Strain of intrinsic muscle, fascia and tendon of left index finger at wrist and hand level

√7ᵗʰ **S66.512** Strain of intrinsic muscle, fascia and tendon of right middle finger at wrist and hand level

√7ᵗʰ **S66.513** Strain of intrinsic muscle, fascia and tendon of left middle finger at wrist and hand level

√7ᵗʰ **S66.514** Strain of intrinsic muscle, fascia and tendon of right ring finger at wrist and hand level

√7ᵗʰ **S66.515** Strain of intrinsic muscle, fascia and tendon of left ring finger at wrist and hand level

√7ᵗʰ **S66.516** Strain of intrinsic muscle, fascia and tendon of right little finger at wrist and hand level

√7ᵗʰ **S66.517** Strain of intrinsic muscle, fascia and tendon of left little finger at wrist and hand level

√7ᵗʰ **S66.518** Strain of intrinsic muscle, fascia and tendon of other finger at wrist and hand level

Strain of intrinsic muscle, fascia and tendon of specified finger with unspecified laterality at wrist and hand level

√7ᵗʰ **S66.519** Strain of intrinsic muscle, fascia and tendon of unspecified finger at wrist and hand level

√6ᵗʰ **S66.52** Laceration of intrinsic muscle, fascia and tendon of other and unspecified finger at wrist and hand level

√7ᵗʰ **S66.520** Laceration of intrinsic muscle, fascia and tendon of right index finger at wrist and hand level

√7ᵗʰ **S66.521** Laceration of intrinsic muscle, fascia and tendon of left index finger at wrist and hand level

√7ᵗʰ **S66.522** Laceration of intrinsic muscle, fascia and tendon of right middle finger at wrist and hand level

√7ᵗʰ **S66.523** Laceration of intrinsic muscle, fascia and tendon of left middle finger at wrist and hand level

√7ᵗʰ **S66.524** Laceration of intrinsic muscle, fascia and tendon of right ring finger at wrist and hand level

√7ᵗʰ **S66.525** Laceration of intrinsic muscle, fascia and tendon of left ring finger at wrist and hand level

√7ᵗʰ **S66.526** Laceration of intrinsic muscle, fascia and tendon of right little finger at wrist and hand level

√7ᵗʰ **S66.527** Laceration of intrinsic muscle, fascia and tendon of left little finger at wrist and hand level

☑ Additional Character Required   √x7ᵗʰ Placeholder Alert   Manifestation   Unspecified Dx   ►◄ Revised Text   ● New Code   ▲ Revised Code Title

ICD-10-CM 2020   **1039**

√7ᵗʰ **S66.528** Laceration of intrinsic muscle, fascia and tendon of other finger at wrist and hand level

     Laceration of intrinsic muscle, fascia and tendon of specified finger with unspecified laterality at wrist and hand level

√7ᵗʰ **S66.529** Laceration of intrinsic muscle, fascia and tendon of unspecified finger at wrist and hand level

√6ᵗʰ **S66.59** Other injury of intrinsic muscle, fascia and tendon of other and unspecified finger at wrist and hand level

√7ᵗʰ **S66.590** Other injury of intrinsic muscle, fascia and tendon of right index finger at wrist and hand level

√7ᵗʰ **S66.591** Other injury of intrinsic muscle, fascia and tendon of left index finger at wrist and hand level

√7ᵗʰ **S66.592** Other injury of intrinsic muscle, fascia and tendon of right middle finger at wrist and hand level

√7ᵗʰ **S66.593** Other injury of intrinsic muscle, fascia and tendon of left middle finger at wrist and hand level

√7ᵗʰ **S66.594** Other injury of intrinsic muscle, fascia and tendon of right ring finger at wrist and hand level

√7ᵗʰ **S66.595** Other injury of intrinsic muscle, fascia and tendon of left ring finger at wrist and hand level

√7ᵗʰ **S66.596** Other injury of intrinsic muscle, fascia and tendon of right little finger at wrist and hand level

√7ᵗʰ **S66.597** Other injury of intrinsic muscle, fascia and tendon of left little finger at wrist and hand level

√7ᵗʰ **S66.598** Other injury of intrinsic muscle, fascia and tendon of other finger at wrist and hand level

     Other injury of intrinsic muscle, fascia and tendon of specified finger with unspecified laterality at wrist and hand level

√7ᵗʰ **S66.599** Other injury of intrinsic muscle, fascia and tendon of unspecified finger at wrist and hand level

√5ᵗʰ **S66.8** Injury of other specified muscles, fascia and tendons at wrist and hand level

√6ᵗʰ **S66.80** Unspecified injury of other specified muscles, fascia and tendons at wrist and hand level

√7ᵗʰ **S66.801** Unspecified injury of other specified muscles, fascia and tendons at wrist and hand level, right hand

√7ᵗʰ **S66.802** Unspecified injury of other specified muscles, fascia and tendons at wrist and hand level, left hand

√7ᵗʰ **S66.809** Unspecified injury of other specified muscles, fascia and tendons at wrist and hand level, unspecified hand

√6ᵗʰ **S66.81** Strain of other specified muscles, fascia and tendons at wrist and hand level

√7ᵗʰ **S66.811** Strain of other specified muscles, fascia and tendons at wrist and hand level, right hand

√7ᵗʰ **S66.812** Strain of other specified muscles, fascia and tendons at wrist and hand level, left hand

√7ᵗʰ **S66.819** Strain of other specified muscles, fascia and tendons at wrist and hand level, unspecified hand

√6ᵗʰ **S66.82** Laceration of other specified muscles, fascia and tendons at wrist and hand level

√7ᵗʰ **S66.821** Laceration of other specified muscles, fascia and tendons at wrist and hand level, right hand

√7ᵗʰ **S66.822** Laceration of other specified muscles, fascia and tendons at wrist and hand level, left hand

√7ᵗʰ **S66.829** Laceration of other specified muscles, fascia and tendons at wrist and hand level, unspecified hand

√6ᵗʰ **S66.89** Other injury of other specified muscles, fascia and tendons at wrist and hand level

√7ᵗʰ **S66.891** Other injury of other specified muscles, fascia and tendons at wrist and hand level, right hand

√7ᵗʰ **S66.892** Other injury of other specified muscles, fascia and tendons at wrist and hand level, left hand

√7ᵗʰ **S66.899** Other injury of other specified muscles, fascia and tendons at wrist and hand level, unspecified hand

√5ᵗʰ **S66.9** Injury of unspecified muscle, fascia and tendon at wrist and hand level

√6ᵗʰ **S66.90** Unspecified injury of unspecified muscle, fascia and tendon at wrist and hand level

√7ᵗʰ **S66.901** Unspecified injury of unspecified muscle, fascia and tendon at wrist and hand level, right hand

√7ᵗʰ **S66.902** Unspecified injury of unspecified muscle, fascia and tendon at wrist and hand level, left hand

√7ᵗʰ **S66.909** Unspecified injury of unspecified muscle, fascia and tendon at wrist and hand level, unspecified hand

√6ᵗʰ **S66.91** Strain of unspecified muscle, fascia and tendon at wrist and hand level

√7ᵗʰ **S66.911** Strain of unspecified muscle, fascia and tendon at wrist and hand level, right hand

√7ᵗʰ **S66.912** Strain of unspecified muscle, fascia and tendon at wrist and hand level, left hand

√7ᵗʰ **S66.919** Strain of unspecified muscle, fascia and tendon at wrist and hand level, unspecified hand

√6ᵗʰ **S66.92** Laceration of unspecified muscle, fascia and tendon at wrist and hand level

√7ᵗʰ **S66.921** Laceration of unspecified muscle, fascia and tendon at wrist and hand level, right hand

√7ᵗʰ **S66.922** Laceration of unspecified muscle, fascia and tendon at wrist and hand level, left hand

√7ᵗʰ **S66.929** Laceration of unspecified muscle, fascia and tendon at wrist and hand level, unspecified hand

√6ᵗʰ **S66.99** Other injury of unspecified muscle, fascia and tendon at wrist and hand level

√7ᵗʰ **S66.991** Other injury of unspecified muscle, fascia and tendon at wrist and hand level, right hand

√7ᵗʰ **S66.992** Other injury of unspecified muscle, fascia and tendon at wrist and hand level, left hand

√7ᵗʰ **S66.999** Other injury of unspecified muscle, fascia and tendon at wrist and hand level, unspecified hand

√4ᵗʰ **S67** Crushing injury of wrist, hand and fingers

     Use additional code for all associated injuries, such as:
       fracture of wrist and hand (S62.-)
       open wound of wrist and hand (S61.-)

> The appropriate 7th character is to be added to each code from category S67.
> A   initial encounter
> D   subsequent encounter
> S   sequela

√5ᵗʰ **S67.0** Crushing injury of thumb

√x7ᵗʰ **S67.00** Crushing injury of unspecified thumb

√x7ᵗʰ **S67.01** Crushing injury of right thumb

√x7ᵗʰ **S67.02** Crushing injury of left thumb

√5ᵗʰ **S67.1** Crushing injury of other and unspecified finger(s)

     EXCLUDES 2   *crushing injury of thumb (S67.0-)*

√x7ᵗʰ **S67.10** Crushing injury of unspecified finger(s)

√6ᵗʰ **S67.19** Crushing injury of other finger(s)

√7ᵗʰ **S67.190** Crushing injury of right index finger

√7ᵗʰ **S67.191** Crushing injury of left index finger

√7ᵗʰ **S67.192** Crushing injury of right middle finger

√7ᵗʰ **S67.193** Crushing injury of left middle finger

√7ᵗʰ **S67.194** Crushing injury of right ring finger

√7ᵗʰ **S67.195** Crushing injury of left ring finger

√7ᵗʰ **S67.196** Crushing injury of right little finger

√7ᵗʰ **S67.197** Crushing injury of left little finger

√7ᵗʰ **S67.198** Crushing injury of other finger

           Crushing injury of specified finger with unspecified laterality

√5ᵗʰ **S67.2** Crushing injury of hand

     EXCLUDES 2   *crushing injury of fingers (S67.1-)*

                    crushing injury of thumb (S67.0-)

√x7ᵗʰ **S67.20** Crushing injury of unspecified hand

√x7ᵗʰ **S67.21** Crushing injury of right hand

√x7ᵗʰ **S67.22** Crushing injury of left hand

√5ᵗʰ **S67.3** Crushing injury of wrist

√x7ᵗʰ **S67.30** Crushing injury of unspecified wrist

√x7ᵗʰ **S67.31** Crushing injury of right wrist

√x7ᵗʰ **S67.32** Crushing injury of left wrist

√5ᵗʰ **S67.4** Crushing injury of wrist and hand

     EXCLUDES 1   *crushing injury of hand alone (S67.2-)*

                    crushing injury of wrist alone (S67.3-)

     EXCLUDES 2   *crushing injury of fingers (S67.1-)*

                    crushing injury of thumb (S67.0-)

√x7ᵗʰ **S67.40** Crushing injury of unspecified wrist and hand

√x7ᵗʰ **S67.41** Crushing injury of right wrist and hand

√x7ᵗʰ **S67.42** Crushing injury of left wrist and hand

√5ᵗʰ **S67.9** Crushing injury of unspecified part(s) of wrist, hand and fingers

√x7ᵗʰ **S67.90** Crushing injury of unspecified part(s) of unspecified wrist, hand and fingers

√x7ᵗʰ **S67.91** Crushing injury of unspecified part(s) of right wrist, hand and fingers

√x7ᵗʰ **S67.92** Crushing injury of unspecified part(s) of left wrist, hand and fingers

√4ᵗʰ **S68** Traumatic amputation of wrist, hand and fingers

An amputation not identified as partial or complete should be coded to complete.

The appropriate 7th character is to be added to each code from category S68.

A   initial encounter

D   subsequent encounter

S   sequela

√5ᵗʰ **S68.0** Traumatic metacarpophalangeal amputation of thumb

Traumatic amputation of thumb NOS

√6ᵗʰ **S68.01** Complete traumatic metacarpophalangeal amputation of thumb

   3 √7ᵗʰ **S68.011** Complete traumatic metacarpophalangeal amputation of right thumb   HCC

   3 √7ᵗʰ **S68.012** Complete traumatic metacarpophalangeal amputation of left thumb   HCC

   3 √7ᵗʰ **S68.019** Complete traumatic metacarpophalangeal amputation of unspecified thumb   HCC

√6ᵗʰ **S68.02** Partial traumatic metacarpophalangeal amputation of thumb

   3 √7ᵗʰ **S68.021** Partial traumatic metacarpophalangeal amputation of right thumb   HCC

   3 √7ᵗʰ **S68.022** Partial traumatic metacarpophalangeal amputation of left thumb   HCC

   3 √7ᵗʰ **S68.029** Partial traumatic metacarpophalangeal amputation of unspecified thumb   HCC

√5ᵗʰ **S68.1** Traumatic metacarpophalangeal amputation of other and unspecified finger

Traumatic amputation of finger NOS

     EXCLUDES 2   *traumatic metacarpophalangeal amputation of thumb (S68.0-)*

√6ᵗʰ **S68.11** Complete traumatic metacarpophalangeal amputation of other and unspecified finger

   3 √7ᵗʰ **S68.110** Complete traumatic metacarpophalangeal amputation of right index finger   HCC

   3 √7ᵗʰ **S68.111** Complete traumatic metacarpophalangeal amputation of left index finger   HCC

   3 √7ᵗʰ **S68.112** Complete traumatic metacarpophalangeal amputation of right middle finger   HCC

   3 √7ᵗʰ **S68.113** Complete traumatic metacarpophalangeal amputation of left middle finger   HCC

   3 √7ᵗʰ **S68.114** Complete traumatic metacarpophalangeal amputation of right ring finger   HCC

   3 √7ᵗʰ **S68.115** Complete traumatic metacarpophalangeal amputation of left ring finger   HCC

   3 √7ᵗʰ **S68.116** Complete traumatic metacarpophalangeal amputation of right little finger   HCC

   3 √7ᵗʰ **S68.117** Complete traumatic metacarpophalangeal amputation of left little finger   HCC

   3 √7ᵗʰ **S68.118** Complete traumatic metacarpophalangeal amputation of other finger   HCC

         Complete traumatic metacarpophalangeal amputation of specified finger with unspecified laterality

   3 √7ᵗʰ **S68.119** Complete traumatic metacarpophalangeal amputation of unspecified finger   HCC

√6ᵗʰ **S68.12** Partial traumatic metacarpophalangeal amputation of other and unspecified finger

   3 √7ᵗʰ **S68.120** Partial traumatic metacarpophalangeal amputation of right index finger   HCC

   3 √7ᵗʰ **S68.121** Partial traumatic metacarpophalangeal amputation of left index finger   HCC

   3 √7ᵗʰ **S68.122** Partial traumatic metacarpophalangeal amputation of right middle finger   HCC

   3 √7ᵗʰ **S68.123** Partial traumatic metacarpophalangeal amputation of left middle finger   HCC

   3 √7ᵗʰ **S68.124** Partial traumatic metacarpophalangeal amputation of right ring finger   HCC

   3 √7ᵗʰ **S68.125** Partial traumatic metacarpophalangeal amputation of left ring finger   HCC

   3 √7ᵗʰ **S68.126** Partial traumatic metacarpophalangeal amputation of right little finger   HCC

   3 √7ᵗʰ **S68.127** Partial traumatic metacarpophalangeal amputation of left little finger   HCC

   3 √7ᵗʰ **S68.128** Partial traumatic metacarpophalangeal amputation of other finger   HCC

         Partial traumatic metacarpophalangeal amputation of specified finger with unspecified laterality

   3 √7ᵗʰ **S68.129** Partial traumatic metacarpophalangeal amputation of unspecified finger   HCC

√5ᵗʰ **S68.4** Traumatic amputation of hand at wrist level

Traumatic amputation of hand NOS

Traumatic amputation of wrist

√6ᵗʰ **S68.41** Complete traumatic amputation of hand at wrist level

   2 √7ᵗʰ **S68.411** Complete traumatic amputation of right hand at wrist level   HCC

   2 √7ᵗʰ **S68.412** Complete traumatic amputation of left hand at wrist level   HCC

   2 √7ᵗʰ **S68.419** Complete traumatic amputation of unspecified hand at wrist level   HCC

√6ᵗʰ **S68.42** Partial traumatic amputation of hand at wrist level

   2 √7ᵗʰ **S68.421** Partial traumatic amputation of right hand at wrist level   HCC

   2 √7ᵗʰ **S68.422** Partial traumatic amputation of left hand at wrist level   HCC

   2 √7ᵗʰ **S68.429** Partial traumatic amputation of unspecified hand at wrist level   HCC

☑ Additional Character Required   √x7ᵗʰ Placeholder Alert   Manifestation   Unspecified Dx   ▶◀ Revised Text   ● New Code   ▲ Revised Code Title

Chapter 19. Injury, Poisoning and Certain Other Consequences of External Causes

✓5ᵗʰ **S68.5 Traumatic transphalangeal amputation of thumb**
Traumatic interphalangeal joint amputation of thumb

✓6ᵗʰ **S68.51 Complete traumatic transphalangeal amputation of thumb**

³ ✓7ᵗʰ **S68.511 Complete traumatic transphalangeal amputation of right thumb** HCC

³ ✓7ᵗʰ **S68.512 Complete traumatic transphalangeal amputation of left thumb** HCC

³ ✓7ᵗʰ **S68.519 Complete traumatic transphalangeal amputation of unspecified thumb** HCC

✓6ᵗʰ **S68.52 Partial traumatic transphalangeal amputation of thumb**

³ ✓7ᵗʰ **S68.521 Partial traumatic transphalangeal amputation of right thumb** HCC

³ ✓7ᵗʰ **S68.522 Partial traumatic transphalangeal amputation of left thumb** HCC

³ ✓7ᵗʰ **S68.529 Partial traumatic transphalangeal amputation of unspecified thumb** HCC

✓5ᵗʰ **S68.6 Traumatic transphalangeal amputation of other and unspecified finger**

✓6ᵗʰ **S68.61 Complete traumatic transphalangeal amputation of other and unspecified finger(s)**

³ ✓7ᵗʰ **S68.610 Complete traumatic transphalangeal amputation of right index finger** HCC

³ ✓7ᵗʰ **S68.611 Complete traumatic transphalangeal amputation of left index finger** HCC

³ ✓7ᵗʰ **S68.612 Complete traumatic transphalangeal amputation of right middle finger** HCC

³ ✓7ᵗʰ **S68.613 Complete traumatic transphalangeal amputation of left middle finger** HCC

³ ✓7ᵗʰ **S68.614 Complete traumatic transphalangeal amputation of right ring finger** HCC

³ ✓7ᵗʰ **S68.615 Complete traumatic transphalangeal amputation of left ring finger** HCC

³ ✓7ᵗʰ **S68.616 Complete traumatic transphalangeal amputation of right little finger** HCC

³ ✓7ᵗʰ **S68.617 Complete traumatic transphalangeal amputation of left little finger** HCC

³ ✓7ᵗʰ **S68.618 Complete traumatic transphalangeal amputation of other finger** HCC
Complete traumatic transphalangeal amputation of specified finger with unspecified laterality

³ ✓7ᵗʰ **S68.619 Complete traumatic transphalangeal amputation of unspecified finger** HCC

✓6ᵗʰ **S68.62 Partial traumatic transphalangeal amputation of other and unspecified finger**

³ ✓7ᵗʰ **S68.620 Partial traumatic transphalangeal amputation of right index finger** HCC

³ ✓7ᵗʰ **S68.621 Partial traumatic transphalangeal amputation of left index finger** HCC

³ ✓7ᵗʰ **S68.622 Partial traumatic transphalangeal amputation of right middle finger** HCC

³ ✓7ᵗʰ **S68.623 Partial traumatic transphalangeal amputation of left middle finger** HCC

³ ✓7ᵗʰ **S68.624 Partial traumatic transphalangeal amputation of right ring finger** HCC

³ ✓7ᵗʰ **S68.625 Partial traumatic transphalangeal amputation of left ring finger** HCC

³ ✓7ᵗʰ **S68.626 Partial traumatic transphalangeal amputation of right little finger** HCC

³ ✓7ᵗʰ **S68.627 Partial traumatic transphalangeal amputation of left little finger** HCC

³ ✓7ᵗʰ **S68.628 Partial traumatic transphalangeal amputation of other finger** HCC
Partial traumatic transphalangeal amputation of specified finger with unspecified laterality

³ ✓7ᵗʰ **S68.629 Partial traumatic transphalangeal amputation of unspecified finger** HCC

✓5ᵗʰ **S68.7 Traumatic transmetacarpal amputation of hand**

✓6ᵗʰ **S68.71 Complete traumatic transmetacarpal amputation of hand**

² ✓7ᵗʰ **S68.711 Complete traumatic transmetacarpal amputation of right hand** HCC

² ✓7ᵗʰ **S68.712 Complete traumatic transmetacarpal amputation of left hand** HCC

² ✓7ᵗʰ **S68.719 Complete traumatic transmetacarpal amputation of unspecified hand** HCC

✓6ᵗʰ **S68.72 Partial traumatic transmetacarpal amputation of hand**

² ✓7ᵗʰ **S68.721 Partial traumatic transmetacarpal amputation of right hand** HCC

² ✓7ᵗʰ **S68.722 Partial traumatic transmetacarpal amputation of left hand** HCC

² ✓7ᵗʰ **S68.729 Partial traumatic transmetacarpal amputation of unspecified hand** HCC

✓4ᵗʰ **S69 Other and unspecified injuries of wrist, hand and finger(s)**

> The appropriate 7th character is to be added to each code from category S69.
> A initial encounter
> D subsequent encounter
> S sequela

✓5ᵗʰ **S69.8 Other specified injuries of wrist, hand and finger(s)**

✓x7ᵗʰ **S69.80 Other specified injuries of unspecified wrist, hand and finger(s)**

✓x7ᵗʰ **S69.81 Other specified injuries of right wrist, hand and finger(s)**

✓x7ᵗʰ **S69.82 Other specified injuries of left wrist, hand and finger(s)**

✓5ᵗʰ **S69.9 Unspecified injury of wrist, hand and finger(s)**

✓x7ᵗʰ **S69.90 Unspecified injury of unspecified wrist, hand and finger(s)**

✓x7ᵗʰ **S69.91 Unspecified injury of right wrist, hand and finger(s)**

✓x7ᵗʰ **S69.92 Unspecified injury of left wrist, hand and finger(s)**

Injuries to the hip and thigh (S70-S79)

EXCLUDES 2 *burns and corrosions (T20-T32)*
frostbite (T33-T34)
snake bite (T63.0-)
venomous insect bite or sting (T63.4-)

✓4ᵗʰ **S70 Superficial injury of hip and thigh**

> The appropriate 7th character is to be added to each code from category S70.
> A initial encounter
> D subsequent encounter
> S sequela

✓5ᵗʰ **S70.0 Contusion of hip**

✓x7ᵗʰ **S70.00 Contusion of unspecified hip**

✓x7ᵗʰ **S70.01 Contusion of right hip**

✓x7ᵗʰ **S70.02 Contusion of left hip**

✓5ᵗʰ **S70.1 Contusion of thigh**

✓x7ᵗʰ **S70.10 Contusion of unspecified thigh**

✓x7ᵗʰ **S70.11 Contusion of right thigh**

✓x7ᵗʰ **S70.12 Contusion of left thigh**

✓5ᵗʰ **S70.2 Other superficial injuries of hip**

✓6ᵗʰ **S70.21 Abrasion of hip**

✓7ᵗʰ **S70.211 Abrasion, right hip**

✓7ᵗʰ **S70.212 Abrasion, left hip**

✓7ᵗʰ **S70.219 Abrasion, unspecified hip**

✓6ᵗʰ **S70.22 Blister (nonthermal) of hip**

✓7ᵗʰ **S70.221 Blister (nonthermal), right hip**

✓7ᵗʰ **S70.222 Blister (nonthermal), left hip**

✓7ᵗʰ **S70.229 Blister (nonthermal), unspecified hip**

✓6ᵗʰ **S70.24 External constriction of hip**

✓7ᵗʰ **S70.241 External constriction, right hip**

✓7ᵗʰ **S70.242 External constriction, left hip**

✓7ᵗʰ **S70.249 External constriction, unspecified hip**

√6ᵗʰ **S70.25 Superficial foreign body of hip**
Splinter in the hip
- √7ᵗʰ **S70.251 Superficial foreign body, right hip**
- √7ᵗʰ **S70.252 Superficial foreign body, left hip**
- √7ᵗʰ **S70.259 Superficial foreign body, unspecified hip**

√6ᵗʰ **S70.26 Insect bite (nonvenomous) of hip**
- √7ᵗʰ **S70.261 Insect bite (nonvenomous), right hip**
- √7ᵗʰ **S70.262 Insect bite (nonvenomous), left hip**
- √7ᵗʰ **S70.269 Insect bite (nonvenomous), unspecified hip**

√6ᵗʰ **S70.27 Other superficial bite of hip**
- EXCLUDES 1   open bite of hip (S71.05-)
- √7ᵗʰ **S70.271 Other superficial bite of hip, right hip**
- √7ᵗʰ **S70.272 Other superficial bite of hip, left hip**
- √7ᵗʰ **S70.279 Other superficial bite of hip, unspecified hip**

√5ᵗʰ **S70.3 Other superficial injuries of thigh**
√6ᵗʰ **S70.31 Abrasion of thigh**
- √7ᵗʰ **S70.311 Abrasion, right thigh**
- √7ᵗʰ **S70.312 Abrasion, left thigh**
- √7ᵗʰ **S70.319 Abrasion, unspecified thigh**

√6ᵗʰ **S70.32 Blister (nonthermal) of thigh**
- √7ᵗʰ **S70.321 Blister (nonthermal), right thigh**
- √7ᵗʰ **S70.322 Blister (nonthermal), left thigh**
- √7ᵗʰ **S70.329 Blister (nonthermal), unspecified thigh**

√6ᵗʰ **S70.34 External constriction of thigh**
- √7ᵗʰ **S70.341 External constriction, right thigh**
- √7ᵗʰ **S70.342 External constriction, left thigh**
- √7ᵗʰ **S70.349 External constriction, unspecified thigh**

√6ᵗʰ **S70.35 Superficial foreign body of thigh**
Splinter in the thigh
- √7ᵗʰ **S70.351 Superficial foreign body, right thigh**
- √7ᵗʰ **S70.352 Superficial foreign body, left thigh**
- √7ᵗʰ **S70.359 Superficial foreign body, unspecified thigh**

√6ᵗʰ **S70.36 Insect bite (nonvenomous) of thigh**
- √7ᵗʰ **S70.361 Insect bite (nonvenomous), right thigh**
- √7ᵗʰ **S70.362 Insect bite (nonvenomous), left thigh**
- √7ᵗʰ **S70.369 Insect bite (nonvenomous), unspecified thigh**

√6ᵗʰ **S70.37 Other superficial bite of thigh**
- EXCLUDES 1   open bite of thigh (S71.15)
- √7ᵗʰ **S70.371 Other superficial bite of right thigh**
- √7ᵗʰ **S70.372 Other superficial bite of left thigh**
- √7ᵗʰ **S70.379 Other superficial bite of unspecified thigh**

√5ᵗʰ **S70.9 Unspecified superficial injury of hip and thigh**
√6ᵗʰ **S70.91 Unspecified superficial injury of hip**
- √7ᵗʰ **S70.911 Unspecified superficial injury of right hip**
- √7ᵗʰ **S70.912 Unspecified superficial injury of left hip**
- √7ᵗʰ **S70.919 Unspecified superficial injury of unspecified hip**

√6ᵗʰ **S70.92 Unspecified superficial injury of thigh**
- √7ᵗʰ **S70.921 Unspecified superficial injury of right thigh**
- √7ᵗʰ **S70.922 Unspecified superficial injury of left thigh**
- √7ᵗʰ **S70.929 Unspecified superficial injury of unspecified thigh**

√4ᵗʰ **S71 Open wound of hip and thigh**
Code also any associated wound infection
- EXCLUDES 1   open fracture of hip and thigh (S72.-)
     traumatic amputation of hip and thigh (S78.-)
- EXCLUDES 2   bite of venomous animal (T63.-)
     open wound of ankle, foot and toes (S91.-)
     open wound of knee and lower leg (S81.-)

The appropriate 7th character is to be added to each code from category S71.
A   initial encounter
D   subsequent encounter
S   sequela

√5ᵗʰ **S71.0 Open wound of hip**
√6ᵗʰ **S71.00 Unspecified open wound of hip**
- √7ᵗʰ **S71.001 Unspecified open wound, right hip**
- √7ᵗʰ **S71.002 Unspecified open wound, left hip**
- √7ᵗʰ **S71.009 Unspecified open wound, unspecified hip**

√6ᵗʰ **S71.01 Laceration without foreign body of hip**
- √7ᵗʰ **S71.011 Laceration without foreign body, right hip**
- √7ᵗʰ **S71.012 Laceration without foreign body, left hip**
- √7ᵗʰ **S71.019 Laceration without foreign body, unspecified hip**

√6ᵗʰ **S71.02 Laceration with foreign body of hip**
- √7ᵗʰ **S71.021 Laceration with foreign body, right hip**
- √7ᵗʰ **S71.022 Laceration with foreign body, left hip**
- √7ᵗʰ **S71.029 Laceration with foreign body, unspecified hip**

√6ᵗʰ **S71.03 Puncture wound without foreign body of hip**
- √7ᵗʰ **S71.031 Puncture wound without foreign body, right hip**
- √7ᵗʰ **S71.032 Puncture wound without foreign body, left hip**
- √7ᵗʰ **S71.039 Puncture wound without foreign body, unspecified hip**

√6ᵗʰ **S71.04 Puncture wound with foreign body of hip**
- √7ᵗʰ **S71.041 Puncture wound with foreign body, right hip**
- √7ᵗʰ **S71.042 Puncture wound with foreign body, left hip**
- √7ᵗʰ **S71.049 Puncture wound with foreign body, unspecified hip**

√6ᵗʰ **S71.05 Open bite of hip**
Bite of hip NOS
- EXCLUDES 1   superficial bite of hip (S70.26, S70.27)
- √7ᵗʰ **S71.051 Open bite, right hip**
- √7ᵗʰ **S71.052 Open bite, left hip**
- √7ᵗʰ **S71.059 Open bite, unspecified hip**

√5ᵗʰ **S71.1 Open wound of thigh**
√6ᵗʰ **S71.10 Unspecified open wound of thigh**
     AHA: 2016,3Q,24
- √7ᵗʰ **S71.101 Unspecified open wound, right thigh**
- √7ᵗʰ **S71.102 Unspecified open wound, left thigh**
- √7ᵗʰ **S71.109 Unspecified open wound, unspecified thigh**

√6ᵗʰ **S71.11 Laceration without foreign body of thigh**
- √7ᵗʰ **S71.111 Laceration without foreign body, right thigh**
- √7ᵗʰ **S71.112 Laceration without foreign body, left thigh**
- √7ᵗʰ **S71.119 Laceration without foreign body, unspecified thigh**

√6ᵗʰ **S71.12 Laceration with foreign body of thigh**
- √7ᵗʰ **S71.121 Laceration with foreign body, right thigh**
- √7ᵗʰ **S71.122 Laceration with foreign body, left thigh**
- √7ᵗʰ **S71.129 Laceration with foreign body, unspecified thigh**

√6ᵗʰ **S71.13 Puncture wound without foreign body of thigh**
     AHA: 2016,3Q,24
- √7ᵗʰ **S71.131 Puncture wound without foreign body, right thigh**
- √7ᵗʰ **S71.132 Puncture wound without foreign body, left thigh**

√ Additional Character Required   √x7ᵗʰ Placeholder Alert   Manifestation   Unspecified Dx   ▶◀ Revised Text   ● New Code   ▲ Revised Code Title

ICD-10-CM 2020   **1043**

Chapter 19. Injury, Poisoning and Certain Other Consequences of External Causes

S71.139–S72.066

√7ᵗʰ **S71.139 Puncture wound without foreign body, unspecified thigh**

√6ᵗʰ **S71.14 Puncture wound with foreign body of thigh**

    AHA: 2016,3Q,24

√7ᵗʰ **S71.141 Puncture wound with foreign body, right thigh**

√7ᵗʰ **S71.142 Puncture wound with foreign body, left thigh**

√7ᵗʰ **S71.149 Puncture wound with foreign body, unspecified thigh**

√6ᵗʰ **S71.15 Open bite of thigh**

    Bite of thigh NOS

    EXCLUDES 1   superficial bite of thigh (S70.37-)

√7ᵗʰ **S71.151 Open bite, right thigh**

√7ᵗʰ **S71.152 Open bite, left thigh**

√7ᵗʰ **S71.159 Open bite, unspecified thigh**

√4ᵗʰ **S72 Fracture of femur**

    NOTE   A fracture not indicated as displaced or nondisplaced should be coded to displaced.

          A fracture not indicated as open or closed should be coded to closed.

          The open fracture designations are based on the Gustilo open fracture classification.

    EXCLUDES 1   traumatic amputation of hip and thigh (S78.-)

    EXCLUDES 2   fracture of lower leg and ankle (S82.-)

                   fracture of foot (S92.-)

                   periprosthetic fracture of prosthetic implant of hip (M97.0-)

AHA: 2018,2Q,12; 2016,1Q,33; 2015,3Q,37-39; 2015,1Q,17; 2013,4Q,128

DEF: Diaphysis: Central shaft of a long bone.

DEF: Epiphysis: Proximal and distal rounded ends of a long bone communicates with the joint.

DEF: Metaphysis: Section of a long bone located between the epiphysis and diaphysis at the proximal and distal ends.

DEF: Physis (growth plate): Narrow zone of cartilaginous tissue between the epiphysis and metaphysis at each end of a long bone. In childhood, proliferation of cells in this zone lengthens the bone. As the bone matures, this area thins, ossification eventually fusing into solid bone and growth stops. *Synonyms:* Epiphyseal plate.

The appropriate 7th character is to be added to all codes from category S72 [unless otherwise indicated].

A   initial encounter for closed fracture

B   initial encounter for open fracture type I or II

    initial encounter for open fracture NOS

C   initial encounter for open fracture type IIIA, IIIB, or IIIC

D   subsequent encounter for closed fracture with routine healing

E   subsequent encounter for open fracture type I or II with routine healing

F   subsequent encounter for open fracture type IIIA, IIIB, or IIIC with routine healing

G   subsequent encounter for closed fracture with delayed healing

H   subsequent encounter for open fracture type I or II with delayed healing

J   subsequent encounter for open fracture type IIIA, IIIB, or IIIC with delayed healing

K   subsequent encounter for closed fracture with nonunion

M   subsequent encounter for open fracture type I or II with nonunion

N   subsequent encounter for open fracture type IIIA, IIIB, or IIIC with nonunion

P   subsequent encounter for closed fracture with malunion

Q   subsequent encounter for open fracture type I or II with malunion

R   subsequent encounter for open fracture type IIIA, IIIB, or IIIC with malunion

S   sequela

√5ᵗʰ **S72.0 Fracture of head and neck of femur**

    EXCLUDES 2   physeal fracture of upper end of femur (S79.0-)

    AHA: 2016,3Q,16

√6ᵗʰ **S72.00 Fracture of unspecified part of neck of femur**

    Fracture of hip NOS

    Fracture of neck of femur NOS

¹ √7ᵗʰ **S72.001 Fracture of unspecified part of neck of right femur**   HCC Q

¹ √7ᵗʰ **S72.002 Fracture of unspecified part of neck of left femur**   HCC Q

¹ √7ᵗʰ **S72.009 Fracture of unspecified part of neck of unspecified femur**   HCC Q

√6ᵗʰ **S72.01 Unspecified intracapsular fracture of femur**

    Subcapital fracture of femur

¹ √7ᵗʰ **S72.011 Unspecified intracapsular fracture of right femur**   HCC Q

¹ √7ᵗʰ **S72.012 Unspecified intracapsular fracture of left femur**   HCC Q

¹ √7ᵗʰ **S72.019 Unspecified intracapsular fracture of unspecified femur**   HCC Q

√6ᵗʰ **S72.02 Fracture of epiphysis (separation) (upper) of femur**

    Transepiphyseal fracture of femur

    EXCLUDES 1   capital femoral epiphyseal fracture (pediatric) of femur (S79.01-)

                   Salter-Harris Type I physeal fracture of upper end of femur (S79.01-)

¹ √7ᵗʰ **S72.021 Displaced fracture of epiphysis (separation) (upper) of right femur**   HCC Q

¹ √7ᵗʰ **S72.022 Displaced fracture of epiphysis (separation) (upper) of left femur**   HCC Q

¹ √7ᵗʰ **S72.023 Displaced fracture of epiphysis (separation) (upper) of unspecified femur**   HCC Q

¹ √7ᵗʰ **S72.024 Nondisplaced fracture of epiphysis (separation) (upper) of right femur**   HCC Q

¹ √7ᵗʰ **S72.025 Nondisplaced fracture of epiphysis (separation) (upper) of left femur**   HCC Q

¹ √7ᵗʰ **S72.026 Nondisplaced fracture of epiphysis (separation) (upper) of unspecified femur**   HCC Q

√6ᵗʰ **S72.03 Midcervical fracture of femur**

    Transcervical fracture of femur NOS

¹ √7ᵗʰ **S72.031 Displaced midcervical fracture of right femur**   HCC Q

¹ √7ᵗʰ **S72.032 Displaced midcervical fracture of left femur**   HCC Q

¹ √7ᵗʰ **S72.033 Displaced midcervical fracture of unspecified femur**   HCC Q

¹ √7ᵗʰ **S72.034 Nondisplaced midcervical fracture of right femur**   HCC Q

¹ √7ᵗʰ **S72.035 Nondisplaced midcervical fracture of left femur**   HCC Q

¹ √7ᵗʰ **S72.036 Nondisplaced midcervical fracture of unspecified femur**   HCC Q

√6ᵗʰ **S72.04 Fracture of base of neck of femur**

    Cervicotrochanteric fracture of femur

¹ √7ᵗʰ **S72.041 Displaced fracture of base of neck of right femur**   HCC Q

¹ √7ᵗʰ **S72.042 Displaced fracture of base of neck of left femur**   HCC Q

¹ √7ᵗʰ **S72.043 Displaced fracture of base of neck of unspecified femur**   HCC Q

¹ √7ᵗʰ **S72.044 Nondisplaced fracture of base of neck of right femur**   HCC Q

¹ √7ᵗʰ **S72.045 Nondisplaced fracture of base of neck of left femur**   HCC Q

¹ √7ᵗʰ **S72.046 Nondisplaced fracture of base of neck of unspecified femur**   HCC Q

√6ᵗʰ **S72.05 Unspecified fracture of head of femur**

    Fracture of head of femur NOS

¹ √7ᵗʰ **S72.051 Unspecified fracture of head of right femur**   HCC Q

¹ √7ᵗʰ **S72.052 Unspecified fracture of head of left femur**   HCC Q

¹ √7ᵗʰ **S72.059 Unspecified fracture of head of unspecified femur**   HCC Q

√6ᵗʰ **S72.06 Articular fracture of head of femur**

¹ √7ᵗʰ **S72.061 Displaced articular fracture of head of right femur**   HCC Q

¹ √7ᵗʰ **S72.062 Displaced articular fracture of head of left femur**   HCC Q

¹ √7ᵗʰ **S72.063 Displaced articular fracture of head of unspecified femur**   HCC Q

¹ √7ᵗʰ **S72.064 Nondisplaced articular fracture of head of right femur**   HCC Q

¹ √7ᵗʰ **S72.065 Nondisplaced articular fracture of head of left femur**   HCC Q

¹ √7ᵗʰ **S72.066 Nondisplaced articular fracture of head of unspecified femur**   HCC Q

☑6ᵗʰ **S72.09** Other fracture of head and neck of femur

  ¹ ☑7ᵗʰ **S72.091** Other fracture of head and neck of right femur HCC Q

  ¹ ☑7ᵗʰ **S72.092** Other fracture of head and neck of left femur HCC Q

  ¹ ☑7ᵗʰ **S72.099** Other fracture of head and neck of unspecified femur HCC Q

☑5ᵗʰ **S72.1** Pertrochanteric fracture

  AHA: 2016,3Q,16

  ☑6ᵗʰ **S72.10** Unspecified trochanteric fracture of femur

    Fracture of trochanter NOS

    ¹ ☑7ᵗʰ **S72.101** Unspecified trochanteric fracture of right femur HCC Q

    ¹ ☑7ᵗʰ **S72.102** Unspecified trochanteric fracture of left femur HCC Q

    ¹ ☑7ᵗʰ **S72.109** Unspecified trochanteric fracture of unspecified femur HCC Q

  ☑6ᵗʰ **S72.11** Fracture of greater trochanter of femur

    ¹ ☑7ᵗʰ **S72.111** Displaced fracture of greater trochanter of right femur HCC Q

    ¹ ☑7ᵗʰ **S72.112** Displaced fracture of greater trochanter of left femur HCC Q

    ¹ ☑7ᵗʰ **S72.113** Displaced fracture of greater trochanter of unspecified femur HCC Q

    ¹ ☑7ᵗʰ **S72.114** Nondisplaced fracture of greater trochanter of right femur HCC Q

    ¹ ☑7ᵗʰ **S72.115** Nondisplaced fracture of greater trochanter of left femur HCC Q

    ¹ ☑7ᵗʰ **S72.116** Nondisplaced fracture of greater trochanter of unspecified femur HCC Q

  ☑6ᵗʰ **S72.12** Fracture of lesser trochanter of femur

    ¹ ☑7ᵗʰ **S72.121** Displaced fracture of lesser trochanter of right femur HCC Q

    ¹ ☑7ᵗʰ **S72.122** Displaced fracture of lesser trochanter of left femur HCC Q

    ¹ ☑7ᵗʰ **S72.123** Displaced fracture of lesser trochanter of unspecified femur HCC Q

    ¹ ☑7ᵗʰ **S72.124** Nondisplaced fracture of lesser trochanter of right femur HCC Q

    ¹ ☑7ᵗʰ **S72.125** Nondisplaced fracture of lesser trochanter of left femur HCC Q

    ¹ ☑7ᵗʰ **S72.126** Nondisplaced fracture of lesser trochanter of unspecified femur HCC Q

  ☑6ᵗʰ **S72.13** Apophyseal fracture of femur

    EXCLUDES 1   chronic (nontraumatic) slipped upper femoral epiphysis (M93.Ø-)

    ¹ ☑7ᵗʰ **S72.131** Displaced apophyseal fracture of right femur HCC Q

    ¹ ☑7ᵗʰ **S72.132** Displaced apophyseal fracture of left femur HCC Q

    ¹ ☑7ᵗʰ **S72.133** Displaced apophyseal fracture of unspecified femur HCC Q

    ¹ ☑7ᵗʰ **S72.134** Nondisplaced apophyseal fracture of right femur HCC Q

    ¹ ☑7ᵗʰ **S72.135** Nondisplaced apophyseal fracture of left femur HCC Q

    ¹ ☑7ᵗʰ **S72.136** Nondisplaced apophyseal fracture of unspecified femur HCC Q

  ☑6ᵗʰ **S72.14** Intertrochanteric fracture of femur

    ¹ ☑7ᵗʰ **S72.141** Displaced intertrochanteric fracture of right femur HCC Q

    ¹ ☑7ᵗʰ **S72.142** Displaced intertrochanteric fracture of left femur HCC Q

    ¹ ☑7ᵗʰ **S72.143** Displaced intertrochanteric fracture of unspecified femur HCC Q

    ¹ ☑7ᵗʰ **S72.144** Nondisplaced intertrochanteric fracture of right femur HCC Q

    ¹ ☑7ᵗʰ **S72.145** Nondisplaced intertrochanteric fracture of left femur HCC Q

    ¹ ☑7ᵗʰ **S72.146** Nondisplaced intertrochanteric fracture of unspecified femur HCC Q

☑5ᵗʰ **S72.2** Subtrochanteric fracture of femur

  ¹ ☑x7ᵗʰ **S72.21** Displaced subtrochanteric fracture of right femur HCC Q

  ¹ ☑x7ᵗʰ **S72.22** Displaced subtrochanteric fracture of left femur HCC Q

  ¹ ☑x7ᵗʰ **S72.23** Displaced subtrochanteric fracture of unspecified femur HCC Q

  ¹ ☑x7ᵗʰ **S72.24** Nondisplaced subtrochanteric fracture of right femur HCC Q

  ¹ ☑x7ᵗʰ **S72.25** Nondisplaced subtrochanteric fracture of left femur HCC Q

  ¹ ☑x7ᵗʰ **S72.26** Nondisplaced subtrochanteric fracture of unspecified femur HCC Q

☑5ᵗʰ **S72.3** Fracture of shaft of femur

  ☑6ᵗʰ **S72.30** Unspecified fracture of shaft of femur

    ¹ ☑7ᵗʰ **S72.301** Unspecified fracture of shaft of right femur HCC Q

    ¹ ☑7ᵗʰ **S72.302** Unspecified fracture of shaft of left femur HCC Q

    ¹ ☑7ᵗʰ **S72.309** Unspecified fracture of shaft of unspecified femur HCC Q

  ☑6ᵗʰ **S72.32** Transverse fracture of shaft of femur

    ¹ ☑7ᵗʰ **S72.321** Displaced transverse fracture of shaft of right femur HCC Q

    ¹ ☑7ᵗʰ **S72.322** Displaced transverse fracture of shaft of left femur HCC Q

    ¹ ☑7ᵗʰ **S72.323** Displaced transverse fracture of shaft of unspecified femur HCC Q

    ¹ ☑7ᵗʰ **S72.324** Nondisplaced transverse fracture of shaft of right femur HCC Q

    ¹ ☑7ᵗʰ **S72.325** Nondisplaced transverse fracture of shaft of left femur HCC Q

    ¹ ☑7ᵗʰ **S72.326** Nondisplaced transverse fracture of shaft of unspecified femur HCC Q

  ☑6ᵗʰ **S72.33** Oblique fracture of shaft of femur

    ¹ ☑7ᵗʰ **S72.331** Displaced oblique fracture of shaft of right femur HCC Q

    ¹ ☑7ᵗʰ **S72.332** Displaced oblique fracture of shaft of left femur HCC Q

    ¹ ☑7ᵗʰ **S72.333** Displaced oblique fracture of shaft of unspecified femur HCC Q

    ¹ ☑7ᵗʰ **S72.334** Nondisplaced oblique fracture of shaft of right femur HCC Q

    ¹ ☑7ᵗʰ **S72.335** Nondisplaced oblique fracture of shaft of left femur HCC Q

    ¹ ☑7ᵗʰ **S72.336** Nondisplaced oblique fracture of shaft of unspecified femur HCC Q

  ☑6ᵗʰ **S72.34** Spiral fracture of shaft of femur

    ¹ ☑7ᵗʰ **S72.341** Displaced spiral fracture of shaft of right femur HCC Q

    ¹ ☑7ᵗʰ **S72.342** Displaced spiral fracture of shaft of left femur HCC Q

    ¹ ☑7ᵗʰ **S72.343** Displaced spiral fracture of shaft of unspecified femur HCC Q

    ¹ ☑7ᵗʰ **S72.344** Nondisplaced spiral fracture of shaft of right femur HCC Q

    ¹ ☑7ᵗʰ **S72.345** Nondisplaced spiral fracture of shaft of left femur HCC Q

    ¹ ☑7ᵗʰ **S72.346** Nondisplaced spiral fracture of shaft of unspecified femur HCC Q

  ☑6ᵗʰ **S72.35** Comminuted fracture of shaft of femur

    ¹ ☑7ᵗʰ **S72.351** Displaced comminuted fracture of shaft of right femur HCC Q

    ¹ ☑7ᵗʰ **S72.352** Displaced comminuted fracture of shaft of left femur HCC Q

    ¹ ☑7ᵗʰ **S72.353** Displaced comminuted fracture of shaft of unspecified femur HCC Q

    ¹ ☑7ᵗʰ **S72.354** Nondisplaced comminuted fracture of shaft of right femur HCC Q

    ¹ ☑7ᵗʰ **S72.355** Nondisplaced comminuted fracture of shaft of left femur HCC Q

    ¹ ☑7ᵗʰ **S72.356** Nondisplaced comminuted fracture of shaft of unspecified femur HCC Q

  ☑6ᵗʰ **S72.36** Segmental fracture of shaft of femur

    ¹ ☑7ᵗʰ **S72.361** Displaced segmental fracture of shaft of right femur HCC Q

    ¹ ☑7ᵗʰ **S72.362** Displaced segmental fracture of shaft of left femur HCC Q

    ¹ ☑7ᵗʰ **S72.363** Displaced segmental fracture of shaft of unspecified femur HCC Q

    ¹ ☑7ᵗʰ **S72.364** Nondisplaced segmental fracture of shaft of right femur HCC Q

    ¹ ☑7ᵗʰ **S72.365** Nondisplaced segmental fracture of shaft of left femur HCC Q

    ¹ ☑7ᵗʰ **S72.366** Nondisplaced segmental fracture of shaft of unspecified femur HCC Q

  ☑6ᵗʰ **S72.39** Other fracture of shaft of femur

    ¹ ☑7ᵗʰ **S72.391** Other fracture of shaft of right femur HCC Q

☑ Additional Character Required   ☑x7ᵗʰ Placeholder Alert   Manifestation   Unspecified Dx   ►◄ Revised Text   ● New Code   ▲ Revised Code Title

CD-10-CM 2020   1045

¹ √7ᵗʰ **S72.392** **Other fracture of shaft of left femur**   HCC Q

¹ √7ᵗʰ **S72.399** **Other fracture of shaft of unspecified femur**   HCC Q

√5ᵗʰ **S72.4** **Fracture of lower end of femur**

Fracture of distal end of femur

EXCLUDES 2   *fracture of shaft of femur (S72.3-)*

physeal fracture of lower end of femur (S79.1-)

AHA: 2016,4Q,42

√6ᵗʰ **S72.40** **Unspecified fracture of lower end of femur**

AHA: 2018,1Q,21; 2016,4Q,42

¹ √7ᵗʰ **S72.401** **Unspecified fracture of lower end of right femur**   HCC Q

¹ √7ᵗʰ **S72.402** **Unspecified fracture of lower end of left femur**   HCC Q

¹ √7ᵗʰ **S72.409** **Unspecified fracture of lower end of unspecified femur**   HCC Q

√6ᵗʰ **S72.41** **Unspecified condyle fracture of lower end of femur**

Condyle fracture of femur NOS

¹ √7ᵗʰ **S72.411** **Displaced unspecified condyle fracture of lower end of right femur**   HCC Q

¹ √7ᵗʰ **S72.412** **Displaced unspecified condyle fracture of lower end of left femur**   HCC Q

¹ √7ᵗʰ **S72.413** **Displaced unspecified condyle fracture of lower end of unspecified femur**   HCC Q

¹ √7ᵗʰ **S72.414** **Nondisplaced unspecified condyle fracture of lower end of right femur**   HCC Q

¹ √7ᵗʰ **S72.415** **Nondisplaced unspecified condyle fracture of lower end of left femur**   HCC Q

¹ √7ᵗʰ **S72.416** **Nondisplaced unspecified condyle fracture of lower end of unspecified femur**   HCC Q

√6ᵗʰ **S72.42** **Fracture of lateral condyle of femur**

¹ √7ᵗʰ **S72.421** **Displaced fracture of lateral condyle of right femur**   HCC Q

¹ √7ᵗʰ **S72.422** **Displaced fracture of lateral condyle of left femur**   HCC Q

¹ √7ᵗʰ **S72.423** **Displaced fracture of lateral condyle of unspecified femur**   HCC Q

¹ √7ᵗʰ **S72.424** **Nondisplaced fracture of lateral condyle of right femur**   HCC Q

¹ √7ᵗʰ **S72.425** **Nondisplaced fracture of lateral condyle of left femur**   HCC Q

¹ √7ᵗʰ **S72.426** **Nondisplaced fracture of lateral condyle of unspecified femur**   HCC Q

√6ᵗʰ **S72.43** **Fracture of medial condyle of femur**

¹ √7ᵗʰ **S72.431** **Displaced fracture of medial condyle of right femur**   HCC Q

¹ √7ᵗʰ **S72.432** **Displaced fracture of medial condyle of left femur**   HCC Q

¹ √7ᵗʰ **S72.433** **Displaced fracture of medial condyle of unspecified femur**   HCC Q

¹ √7ᵗʰ **S72.434** **Nondisplaced fracture of medial condyle of right femur**   HCC Q

¹ √7ᵗʰ **S72.435** **Nondisplaced fracture of medial condyle of left femur**   HCC Q

¹ √7ᵗʰ **S72.436** **Nondisplaced fracture of medial condyle of unspecified femur**   HCC Q

√6ᵗʰ **S72.44** **Fracture of lower epiphysis (separation) of femur**

EXCLUDES 1   *Salter-Harris Type I physeal fracture of lower end of femur (S79.11-)*

¹ √7ᵗʰ **S72.441** **Displaced fracture of lower epiphysis (separation) of right femur**   HCC Q

¹ √7ᵗʰ **S72.442** **Displaced fracture of lower epiphysis (separation) of left femur**   HCC Q

¹ √7ᵗʰ **S72.443** **Displaced fracture of lower epiphysis (separation) of unspecified femur**   HCC Q

¹ √7ᵗʰ **S72.444** **Nondisplaced fracture of lower epiphysis (separation) of right femur**   HCC Q

¹ √7ᵗʰ **S72.445** **Nondisplaced fracture of lower epiphysis (separation) of left femur**   HCC Q

¹ √7ᵗʰ **S72.446** **Nondisplaced fracture of lower epiphysis (separation) of unspecified femur**   HCC Q

√6ᵗʰ **S72.45** **Supracondylar fracture without intracondylar extension of lower end of femur**

Supracondylar fracture of lower end of femur NOS

EXCLUDES 1   *supracondylar fracture with intracondylar extension of lower end of femur (S72.46-)*

¹ √7ᵗʰ **S72.451** **Displaced supracondylar fracture without intracondylar extension of lower end of right femur**   HCC Q

¹ √7ᵗʰ **S72.452** **Displaced supracondylar fracture without intracondylar extension of lower end of left femur**   HCC Q

¹ √7ᵗʰ **S72.453** **Displaced supracondylar fracture without intracondylar extension of lower end of unspecified femur**   HCC Q

¹ √7ᵗʰ **S72.454** **Nondisplaced supracondylar fracture without intracondylar extension of lower end of right femur**   HCC Q

¹ √7ᵗʰ **S72.455** **Nondisplaced supracondylar fracture without intracondylar extension of lower end of left femur**   HCC Q

¹ √7ᵗʰ **S72.456** **Nondisplaced supracondylar fracture without intracondylar extension of lower end of unspecified femur**   HCC Q

√6ᵗʰ **S72.46** **Supracondylar fracture with intracondylar extension of lower end of femur**

EXCLUDES 1   *supracondylar fracture without intracondylar extension of lower end of femur (S72.45-)*

¹ √7ᵗʰ **S72.461** **Displaced supracondylar fracture with intracondylar extension of lower end of right femur**   HCC Q

¹ √7ᵗʰ **S72.462** **Displaced supracondylar fracture with intracondylar extension of lower end of left femur**   HCC Q

¹ √7ᵗʰ **S72.463** **Displaced supracondylar fracture with intracondylar extension of lower end of unspecified femur**   HCC Q

¹ √7ᵗʰ **S72.464** **Nondisplaced supracondylar fracture with intracondylar extension of lower end of right femur**   HCC Q

¹ √7ᵗʰ **S72.465** **Nondisplaced supracondylar fracture with intracondylar extension of lower end of left femur**   HCC Q

¹ √7ᵗʰ **S72.466** **Nondisplaced supracondylar fracture with intracondylar extension of lower end of unspecified femur**   HCC Q

√6ᵗʰ **S72.47** **Torus fracture of lower end of femur**

The appropriate 7th character is to be added to all codes in subcategory S72.47.
A   initial encounter for closed fracture
D   subsequent encounter for fracture with routine healing
G   subsequent encounter for fracture with delayed healing
K   subsequent encounter for fracture with nonunion
P   subsequent encounter for fracture with malunion
S   sequela

¹ √7ᵗʰ **S72.471** **Torus fracture of lower end of right femur**   HCC Q

¹ √7ᵗʰ **S72.472** **Torus fracture of lower end of left femur**   HCC Q

¹ √7ᵗʰ **S72.479** **Torus fracture of lower end of unspecified femur**   HCC Q

√6ᵗʰ **S72.49** **Other fracture of lower end of femur**

¹ √7ᵗʰ **S72.491** **Other fracture of lower end of right femur**   HCC Q

¹ √7ᵗʰ **S72.492** **Other fracture of lower end of left femur**   HCC Q

¹ √7ᵗʰ **S72.499** **Other fracture of lower end of unspecified femur**   HCC Q

√5ᵗʰ **S72.8 Other fracture of femur**

  √6ᵗʰ **S72.8X Other fracture of femur**

    ¹ √7ᵗʰ **S72.8X1 Other fracture of right femur** `HCC` `Q`

    ¹ √7ᵗʰ **S72.8X2 Other fracture of left femur** `HCC` `Q`

    ¹ √7ᵗʰ **S72.8X9 Other fracture of unspecified femur** `HCC` `Q`

√5ᵗʰ **S72.9 Unspecified fracture of femur**

  Fracture of thigh NOS

  Fracture of upper leg NOS

    EXCLUDES 1   fracture of hip NOS (S72.00-, S72.01-)

  ¹ √x7ᵗʰ **S72.90 Unspecified fracture of unspecified femur** `HCC` `Q`

    AHA: 2012,4Q,93

  ¹ √x7ᵗʰ **S72.91 Unspecified fracture of right femur** `HCC` `Q`

  ¹ √x7ᵗʰ **S72.92 Unspecified fracture of left femur** `HCC` `Q`

√4ᵗʰ **S73 Dislocation and sprain of joint and ligaments of hip**

  INCLUDES   avulsion of joint or ligament of hip

    laceration of cartilage, joint or ligament of hip

    sprain of cartilage, joint or ligament of hip

    traumatic hemarthrosis of joint or ligament of hip

    traumatic rupture of joint or ligament of hip

    traumatic subluxation of joint or ligament of hip

    traumatic tear of joint or ligament of hip

  Code also any associated open wound

    EXCLUDES 2   strain of muscle, fascia and tendon of hip and thigh (S76.-)

> The appropriate 7th character is to be added to each code from category S73.
> A   initial encounter
> D   subsequent encounter
> S   sequela

√5ᵗʰ **S73.0 Subluxation and dislocation of hip**

    EXCLUDES 2   dislocation and subluxation of hip prosthesis (T84.020, T84.021)

  √6ᵗʰ **S73.00 Unspecified subluxation and dislocation of hip**

    Dislocation of hip NOS

    Subluxation of hip NOS

    ¹ √7ᵗʰ **S73.001 Unspecified subluxation of right hip** `HCC`

    ¹ √7ᵗʰ **S73.002 Unspecified subluxation of left hip** `HCC`

    ¹ √7ᵗʰ **S73.003 Unspecified subluxation of unspecified hip** `HCC`

    ¹ √7ᵗʰ **S73.004 Unspecified dislocation of right hip** `HCC`

    ¹ √7ᵗʰ **S73.005 Unspecified dislocation of left hip** `HCC`

    ¹ √7ᵗʰ **S73.006 Unspecified dislocation of unspecified hip** `HCC`

  √6ᵗʰ **S73.01 Posterior subluxation and dislocation of hip**

    ¹ √7ᵗʰ **S73.011 Posterior subluxation of right hip** `HCC`

    ¹ √7ᵗʰ **S73.012 Posterior subluxation of left hip** `HCC`

    ¹ √7ᵗʰ **S73.013 Posterior subluxation of unspecified hip** `HCC`

    ¹ √7ᵗʰ **S73.014 Posterior dislocation of right hip** `HCC`

    ¹ √7ᵗʰ **S73.015 Posterior dislocation of left hip** `HCC`

    ¹ √7ᵗʰ **S73.016 Posterior dislocation of unspecified hip** `HCC`

  √6ᵗʰ **S73.02 Obturator subluxation and dislocation of hip**

    ¹ √7ᵗʰ **S73.021 Obturator subluxation of right hip** `HCC`

    ¹ √7ᵗʰ **S73.022 Obturator subluxation of left hip** `HCC`

    ¹ √7ᵗʰ **S73.023 Obturator subluxation of unspecified hip** `HCC`

    ¹ √7ᵗʰ **S73.024 Obturator dislocation of right hip** `HCC`

    ¹ √7ᵗʰ **S73.025 Obturator dislocation of left hip** `HCC`

    ¹ √7ᵗʰ **S73.026 Obturator dislocation of unspecified hip** `HCC`

  √6ᵗʰ **S73.03 Other anterior subluxation and dislocation of hip**

    ¹ √7ᵗʰ **S73.031 Other anterior subluxation of right hip** `HCC`

    ¹ √7ᵗʰ **S73.032 Other anterior subluxation of left hip** `HCC`

    ¹ √7ᵗʰ **S73.033 Other anterior subluxation of unspecified hip** `HCC`

    ¹ √7ᵗʰ **S73.034 Other anterior dislocation of right hip** `HCC`

    ¹ √7ᵗʰ **S73.035 Other anterior dislocation of left hip** `HCC`

    ¹ √7ᵗʰ **S73.036 Other anterior dislocation of unspecified hip** `HCC`

  √6ᵗʰ **S73.04 Central subluxation and dislocation of hip**

    ¹ √7ᵗʰ **S73.041 Central subluxation of right hip** `HCC`

    ¹ √7ᵗʰ **S73.042 Central subluxation of left hip** `HCC`

    ¹ √7ᵗʰ **S73.043 Central subluxation of unspecified hip** `HCC`

    ¹ √7ᵗʰ **S73.044 Central dislocation of right hip** `HCC`

    ¹ √7ᵗʰ **S73.045 Central dislocation of left hip** `HCC`

    ¹ √7ᵗʰ **S73.046 Central dislocation of unspecified hip** `HCC`

√5ᵗʰ **S73.1 Sprain of hip**

  AHA: 2014,4Q,25

  √6ᵗʰ **S73.10 Unspecified sprain of hip**

    √7ᵗʰ **S73.101 Unspecified sprain of right hip**

    √7ᵗʰ **S73.102 Unspecified sprain of left hip**

    √7ᵗʰ **S73.109 Unspecified sprain of unspecified hip**

  √6ᵗʰ **S73.11 Iliofemoral ligament sprain of hip**

    √7ᵗʰ **S73.111 Iliofemoral ligament sprain of right hip**

    √7ᵗʰ **S73.112 Iliofemoral ligament sprain of left hip**

    √7ᵗʰ **S73.119 Iliofemoral ligament sprain of unspecified hip**

  √6ᵗʰ **S73.12 Ischiocapsular (ligament) sprain of hip**

    √7ᵗʰ **S73.121 Ischiocapsular ligament sprain of right hip**

    √7ᵗʰ **S73.122 Ischiocapsular ligament sprain of left hip**

    √7ᵗʰ **S73.129 Ischiocapsular ligament sprain of unspecified hip**

  √6ᵗʰ **S73.19 Other sprain of hip**

    √7ᵗʰ **S73.191 Other sprain of right hip**

    √7ᵗʰ **S73.192 Other sprain of left hip**

    √7ᵗʰ **S73.199 Other sprain of unspecified hip**

√4ᵗʰ **S74 Injury of nerves at hip and thigh level**

  Code also any associated open wound (S71.-)

    EXCLUDES 2   injury of nerves at ankle and foot level (S94.-)

         injury of nerves at lower leg level (S84.-)

> The appropriate 7th character is to be added to each code from category S74.
> A   initial encounter
> D   subsequent encounter
> S   sequela

√5ᵗʰ **S74.0 Injury of sciatic nerve at hip and thigh level**

  √x7ᵗʰ **S74.00 Injury of sciatic nerve at hip and thigh level, unspecified leg**

  √x7ᵗʰ **S74.01 Injury of sciatic nerve at hip and thigh level, right leg**

  √x7ᵗʰ **S74.02 Injury of sciatic nerve at hip and thigh level, left leg**

√5ᵗʰ **S74.1 Injury of femoral nerve at hip and thigh level**

  √x7ᵗʰ **S74.10 Injury of femoral nerve at hip and thigh level, unspecified leg**

  √x7ᵗʰ **S74.11 Injury of femoral nerve at hip and thigh level, right leg**

  √x7ᵗʰ **S74.12 Injury of femoral nerve at hip and thigh level, left leg**

√5ᵗʰ **S74.2 Injury of cutaneous sensory nerve at hip and thigh level**

  √x7ᵗʰ **S74.20 Injury of cutaneous sensory nerve at hip and thigh level, unspecified leg**

  √x7ᵗʰ **S74.21 Injury of cutaneous sensory nerve at hip and high level, right leg**

  √x7ᵗʰ **S74.22 Injury of cutaneous sensory nerve at hip and thigh level, left leg**

√5ᵗʰ **S74.8 Injury of other nerves at hip and thigh level**

  √6ᵗʰ **S74.8X Injury of other nerves at hip and thigh level**

    √7ᵗʰ **S74.8X1 Injury of other nerves at hip and thigh level, right leg**

    √7ᵗʰ **S74.8X2 Injury of other nerves at hip and thigh level, left leg**

    √7ᵗʰ **S74.8X9 Injury of other nerves at hip and thigh level, unspecified leg**

√5ᵗʰ **S74.9 Injury of unspecified nerve at hip and thigh level**

  √x7ᵗʰ **S74.90 Injury of unspecified nerve at hip and thigh level, unspecified leg**

☑ Additional Character Required   √x7ᵗʰ Placeholder Alert   Manifestation   Unspecified Dx   ▶◀ Revised Text   ● New Code   ▲ Revised Code Title

√×7ᵗʰ **S74.91** Injury of unspecified nerve at hip and thigh level, right leg

√×7ᵗʰ **S74.92** Injury of unspecified nerve at hip and thigh level, left leg

√4ᵗʰ **S75** **Injury of blood vessels at hip and thigh level**

Code also any associated open wound (S71.-)

EXCLUDES 2   injury of blood vessels at lower leg level (S85.-)
            injury of popliteal artery (S85.Ø)

The appropriate 7th character is to be added to each code from category S75.
A   initial encounter
D   subsequent encounter
S   sequela

√5ᵗʰ **S75.Ø** **Injury of femoral artery**

   √6ᵗʰ **S75.ØØ** **Unspecified injury of femoral artery**

      √7ᵗʰ **S75.ØØ1** Unspecified injury of femoral artery, right leg

      √7ᵗʰ **S75.ØØ2** Unspecified injury of femoral artery, left leg

      √7ᵗʰ **S75.ØØ9** Unspecified injury of femoral artery, unspecified leg

   √6ᵗʰ **S75.Ø1** **Minor laceration of femoral artery**

Incomplete transection of femoral artery
Laceration of femoral artery NOS
Superficial laceration of femoral artery

      √7ᵗʰ **S75.Ø11** Minor laceration of femoral artery, right leg

      √7ᵗʰ **S75.Ø12** Minor laceration of femoral artery, left leg

      √7ᵗʰ **S75.Ø19** Minor laceration of femoral artery, unspecified leg

   √6ᵗʰ **S75.Ø2** **Major laceration of femoral artery**

Complete transection of femoral artery
Traumatic rupture of femoral artery

      √7ᵗʰ **S75.Ø21** Major laceration of femoral artery, right leg

      √7ᵗʰ **S75.Ø22** Major laceration of femoral artery, left leg

      √7ᵗʰ **S75.Ø29** Major laceration of femoral artery, unspecified leg

   √6ᵗʰ **S75.Ø9** **Other specified injury of femoral artery**

      √7ᵗʰ **S75.Ø91** Other specified injury of femoral artery, right leg

      √7ᵗʰ **S75.Ø92** Other specified injury of femoral artery, left leg

      √7ᵗʰ **S75.Ø99** Other specified injury of femoral artery, unspecified leg

√5ᵗʰ **S75.1** **Injury of femoral vein at hip and thigh level**

   √6ᵗʰ **S75.1Ø** **Unspecified injury of femoral vein at hip and thigh level**

      √7ᵗʰ **S75.1Ø1** Unspecified injury of femoral vein at hip and thigh level, right leg

      √7ᵗʰ **S75.1Ø2** Unspecified injury of femoral vein at hip and thigh level, left leg

      √7ᵗʰ **S75.1Ø9** Unspecified injury of femoral vein at hip and thigh level, unspecified leg

   √6ᵗʰ **S75.11** **Minor laceration of femoral vein at hip and thigh level**

Incomplete transection of femoral vein at hip and thigh level
Laceration of femoral vein at hip and thigh level NOS
Superficial laceration of femoral vein at hip and thigh level

      √7ᵗʰ **S75.111** Minor laceration of femoral vein at hip and thigh level, right leg

      √7ᵗʰ **S75.112** Minor laceration of femoral vein at hip and thigh level, left leg

      √7ᵗʰ **S75.119** Minor laceration of femoral vein at hip and thigh level, unspecified leg

   √6ᵗʰ **S75.12** **Major laceration of femoral vein at hip and thigh level**

Complete transection of femoral vein at hip and thigh level
Traumatic rupture of femoral vein at hip and thigh level

      √7ᵗʰ **S75.121** Major laceration of femoral vein at hip and thigh level, right leg

      √7ᵗʰ **S75.122** Major laceration of femoral vein at hip and thigh level, left leg

      √7ᵗʰ **S75.129** Major laceration of femoral vein at hip and thigh level, unspecified leg

   √6ᵗʰ **S75.19** **Other specified injury of femoral vein at hip and thigh level**

      √7ᵗʰ **S75.191** Other specified injury of femoral vein at hip and thigh level, right leg

      √7ᵗʰ **S75.192** Other specified injury of femoral vein at hip and thigh level, left leg

      √7ᵗʰ **S75.199** Other specified injury of femoral vein at hip and thigh level, unspecified leg

√5ᵗʰ **S75.2** **Injury of greater saphenous vein at hip and thigh level**

EXCLUDES 1   greater saphenous vein NOS (S85.3)

   √6ᵗʰ **S75.2Ø** **Unspecified injury of greater saphenous vein at hip and thigh level**

      √7ᵗʰ **S75.2Ø1** Unspecified injury of greater saphenous vein at hip and thigh level, right leg

      √7ᵗʰ **S75.2Ø2** Unspecified injury of greater saphenous vein at hip and thigh level, left leg

      √7ᵗʰ **S75.2Ø9** Unspecified injury of greater saphenous vein at hip and thigh level, unspecified leg

   √6ᵗʰ **S75.21** **Minor laceration of greater saphenous vein at hip and thigh level**

Incomplete transection of greater saphenous vein at hip and thigh level
Laceration of greater saphenous vein at hip and thigh level NOS
Superficial laceration of greater saphenous vein at hip and thigh level

      √7ᵗʰ **S75.211** Minor laceration of greater saphenous vein at hip and thigh level, right leg

      √7ᵗʰ **S75.212** Minor laceration of greater saphenous vein at hip and thigh level, left leg

      √7ᵗʰ **S75.219** Minor laceration of greater saphenous vein at hip and thigh level, unspecified leg

   √6ᵗʰ **S75.22** **Major laceration of greater saphenous vein at hip and thigh level**

Complete transection of greater saphenous vein at hip and thigh level
Traumatic rupture of greater saphenous vein at hip and thigh level

      √7ᵗʰ **S75.221** Major laceration of greater saphenous vein at hip and thigh level, right leg

      √7ᵗʰ **S75.222** Major laceration of greater saphenous vein at hip and thigh level, left leg

      √7ᵗʰ **S75.229** Major laceration of greater saphenous vein at hip and thigh level, unspecified leg

   √6ᵗʰ **S75.29** **Other specified injury of greater saphenous vein at hip and thigh level**

      √7ᵗʰ **S75.291** Other specified injury of greater saphenous vein at hip and thigh level, right leg

      √7ᵗʰ **S75.292** Other specified injury of greater saphenous vein at hip and thigh level, left leg

      √7ᵗʰ **S75.299** Other specified injury of greater saphenous vein at hip and thigh level, unspecified leg

√5ᵗʰ **S75.8** **Injury of other blood vessels at hip and thigh level**

   √6ᵗʰ **S75.8Ø** **Unspecified injury of other blood vessels at hip and thigh level**

      √7ᵗʰ **S75.8Ø1** Unspecified injury of other blood vessels at hip and thigh level, right leg

      √7ᵗʰ **S75.8Ø2** Unspecified injury of other blood vessels at hip and thigh level, left leg

      √7ᵗʰ **S75.8Ø9** Unspecified injury of other blood vessels at hip and thigh level, unspecified leg

   √6ᵗʰ **S75.81** **Laceration of other blood vessels at hip and thigh level**

      √7ᵗʰ **S75.811** Laceration of other blood vessels at hip and thigh level, right leg

      √7ᵗʰ **S75.812** Laceration of other blood vessels at hip and thigh level, left leg

      √7ᵗʰ **S75.819** Laceration of other blood vessels at hip and thigh level, unspecified leg

   √6ᵗʰ **S75.89** **Other specified injury of other blood vessels at hip and thigh level**

      √7ᵗʰ **S75.891** Other specified injury of other blood vessels at hip and thigh level, right leg

S75.892   Other specified injury of other blood vessels at hip and thigh level, **left** leg

S75.899   Other specified injury of other blood vessels at hip and thigh level, unspecified leg

S75.9   Injury of unspecified blood vessel at hip and thigh level

   S75.90   Unspecified injury of unspecified blood vessel at hip and thigh level

     S75.901   Unspecified injury of unspecified blood vessel at hip and thigh level, **right** leg

     S75.902   Unspecified injury of unspecified blood vessel at hip and thigh level, **left** leg

     S75.909   Unspecified injury of unspecified blood vessel at hip and thigh level, unspecified leg

   S75.91   Laceration of unspecified blood vessel at hip and thigh level

     S75.911   Laceration of unspecified blood vessel at hip and thigh level, **right** leg

     S75.912   Laceration of unspecified blood vessel at hip and thigh level, **left** leg

     S75.919   Laceration of unspecified blood vessel at hip and thigh level, unspecified leg

   S75.99   Other specified injury of unspecified blood vessel at hip and thigh level

     S75.991   Other specified injury of unspecified blood vessel at hip and thigh level, **right** leg

     S75.992   Other specified injury of unspecified blood vessel at hip and thigh level, **left** leg

     S75.999   Other specified injury of unspecified blood vessel at hip and thigh level, unspecified leg

S76   **Injury of muscle, fascia and tendon at hip and thigh level**

   Code also any associated open wound (S71.-)

   EXCLUDES 2   injury of muscle, fascia and tendon at lower leg level (S86)

           sprain of joint and ligament of hip (S73.1)

   TIP: Refer to the Muscle/Tendon table at the beginning of this chapter.

   The appropriate 7th character is to be added to each code from category S76.
   A   initial encounter
   D   subsequent encounter
   S   sequela

S76.0   Injury of muscle, fascia and tendon of hip

   S76.00   Unspecified injury of muscle, fascia and tendon of hip

     S76.001   Unspecified injury of muscle, fascia and tendon of **right** hip

     S76.002   Unspecified injury of muscle, fascia and tendon of **left** hip

     S76.009   Unspecified injury of muscle, fascia and tendon of unspecified hip

   S76.01   Strain of muscle, fascia and tendon of hip

     S76.011   Strain of muscle, fascia and tendon of **right** hip

     S76.012   Strain of muscle, fascia and tendon of **left** hip

     S76.019   Strain of muscle, fascia and tendon of unspecified hip

   S76.02   Laceration of muscle, fascia and tendon of hip

     S76.021   Laceration of muscle, fascia and tendon of **right** hip

     S76.022   Laceration of muscle, fascia and tendon of **left** hip

     S76.029   Laceration of muscle, fascia and tendon of unspecified hip

   S76.09   Other specified injury of muscle, fascia and tendon of hip

     S76.091   Other specified injury of muscle, fascia and tendon of **right** hip

     S76.092   Other specified injury of muscle, fascia and tendon of **left** hip

     S76.099   Other specified injury of muscle, fascia and tendon of unspecified hip

S76.1   Injury of **quadriceps** muscle, fascia and tendon

   Injury of patellar ligament (tendon)

   S76.10   Unspecified injury of quadriceps muscle, fascia and tendon

     S76.101   Unspecified injury of **right** quadriceps muscle, fascia and tendon

     S76.102   Unspecified injury of **left** quadriceps muscle, fascia and tendon

     S76.109   Unspecified injury of unspecified quadriceps muscle, fascia and tendon

   S76.11   Strain of quadriceps muscle, fascia and tendon

     S76.111   Strain of **right** quadriceps muscle, fascia and tendon

     S76.112   Strain of **left** quadriceps muscle, fascia and tendon

     S76.119   Strain of unspecified quadriceps muscle, fascia and tendon

   S76.12   Laceration of quadriceps muscle, fascia and tendon

     S76.121   Laceration of **right** quadriceps muscle, fascia and tendon

     S76.122   Laceration of **left** quadriceps muscle, fascia and tendon

     S76.129   Laceration of unspecified quadriceps muscle, fascia and tendon

   S76.19   Other specified injury of quadriceps muscle, fascia and tendon

     S76.191   Other specified injury of **right** quadriceps muscle, fascia and tendon

     S76.192   Other specified injury of **left** quadriceps muscle, fascia and tendon

     S76.199   Other specified injury of unspecified quadriceps muscle, fascia and tendon

S76.2   Injury of **adductor** muscle, fascia and tendon of **thigh**

   S76.20   Unspecified injury of adductor muscle, fascia and tendon of thigh

     S76.201   Unspecified injury of adductor muscle, fascia and tendon of **right** thigh

     S76.202   Unspecified injury of adductor muscle, fascia and tendon of **left** thigh

     S76.209   Unspecified injury of adductor muscle, fascia and tendon of unspecified thigh

   S76.21   Strain of adductor muscle, fascia and tendon of thigh

     S76.211   Strain of adductor muscle, fascia and tendon of **right** thigh

     S76.212   Strain of adductor muscle, fascia and tendon of **left** thigh

     S76.219   Strain of adductor muscle, fascia and tendon of unspecified thigh

   S76.22   Laceration of adductor muscle, fascia and tendon of thigh

     S76.221   Laceration of adductor muscle, fascia and tendon of **right** thigh

     S76.222   Laceration of adductor muscle, fascia and tendon of **left** thigh

     S76.229   Laceration of adductor muscle, fascia and tendon of unspecified thigh

   S76.29   Other injury of adductor muscle, fascia and tendon of thigh

     S76.291   Other injury of adductor muscle, fascia and tendon of **right** thigh

     S76.292   Other injury of adductor muscle, fascia and tendon of **left** thigh

     S76.299   Other injury of adductor muscle, fascia and tendon of unspecified thigh

S76.3   Injury of muscle, fascia and tendon of the **posterior muscle group** at thigh level

   S76.30   Unspecified injury of muscle, fascia and tendon of the posterior muscle group at thigh level

     S76.301   Unspecified injury of muscle, fascia and tendon of the posterior muscle group at thigh level, **right** thigh

     S76.302   Unspecified injury of muscle, fascia and tendon of the posterior muscle group at thigh level, **left** thigh

     S76.309   Unspecified injury of muscle, fascia and tendon of the posterior muscle group at thigh level, unspecified thigh

✔ Additional Character Required   ✓x7ᵗʰ Placeholder Alert   Manifestation   Unspecified Dx   ►◄ Revised Text   ● New Code   ▲ Revised Code Title

ICD-10-CM 2020   **1049**

✓6ᵗʰ **S76.31**   Strain of muscle, fascia and tendon of the posterior muscle group at thigh level

    ✓7ᵗʰ **S76.311**   Strain of muscle, fascia and tendon of the posterior muscle group at thigh level, right thigh

    ✓7ᵗʰ **S76.312**   Strain of muscle, fascia and tendon of the posterior muscle group at thigh level, left thigh

    ✓7ᵗʰ **S76.319**   Strain of muscle, fascia and tendon of the posterior muscle group at thigh level, unspecified thigh

✓6ᵗʰ **S76.32**   Laceration of muscle, fascia and tendon of the posterior muscle group at thigh level

    ✓7ᵗʰ **S76.321**   Laceration of muscle, fascia and tendon of the posterior muscle group at thigh level, right thigh

    ✓7ᵗʰ **S76.322**   Laceration of muscle, fascia and tendon of the posterior muscle group at thigh level, left thigh

    ✓7ᵗʰ **S76.329**   Laceration of muscle, fascia and tendon of the posterior muscle group at thigh level, unspecified thigh

✓6ᵗʰ **S76.39**   Other specified injury of muscle, fascia and tendon of the posterior muscle group at thigh level

    ✓7ᵗʰ **S76.391**   Other specified injury of muscle, fascia and tendon of the posterior muscle group at thigh level, right thigh

    ✓7ᵗʰ **S76.392**   Other specified injury of muscle, fascia and tendon of the posterior muscle group at thigh level, left thigh

    ✓7ᵗʰ **S76.399**   Other specified injury of muscle, fascia and tendon of the posterior muscle group at thigh level, unspecified thigh

✓5ᵗʰ **S76.8**   Injury of other specified muscles, fascia and tendons at thigh level

  ✓6ᵗʰ **S76.80**   Unspecified injury of other specified muscles, fascia and tendons at thigh level

    ✓7ᵗʰ **S76.801**   Unspecified injury of other specified muscles, fascia and tendons at thigh level, right thigh

    ✓7ᵗʰ **S76.802**   Unspecified injury of other specified muscles, fascia and tendons at thigh level, left thigh

    ✓7ᵗʰ **S76.809**   Unspecified injury of other specified muscles, fascia and tendons at thigh level, unspecified thigh

  ✓6ᵗʰ **S76.81**   Strain of other specified muscles, fascia and tendons at thigh level

    ✓7ᵗʰ **S76.811**   Strain of other specified muscles, fascia and tendons at thigh level, right thigh

    ✓7ᵗʰ **S76.812**   Strain of other specified muscles, fascia and tendons at thigh level, left thigh

    ✓7ᵗʰ **S76.819**   Strain of other specified muscles, fascia and tendons at thigh level, unspecified thigh

  ✓6ᵗʰ **S76.82**   Laceration of other specified muscles, fascia and tendons at thigh level

    ✓7ᵗʰ **S76.821**   Laceration of other specified muscles, fascia and tendons at thigh level, right thigh

    ✓7ᵗʰ **S76.822**   Laceration of other specified muscles, fascia and tendons at thigh level, left thigh

    ✓7ᵗʰ **S76.829**   Laceration of other specified muscles, fascia and tendons at thigh level, unspecified thigh

  ✓6ᵗʰ **S76.89**   Other injury of other specified muscles, fascia and tendons at thigh level

    ✓7ᵗʰ **S76.891**   Other injury of other specified muscles, fascia and tendons at thigh level, right thigh

    ✓7ᵗʰ **S76.892**   Other injury of other specified muscles, fascia and tendons at thigh level, left thigh

    ✓7ᵗʰ **S76.899**   Other injury of other specified muscles, fascia and tendons at thigh level, unspecified thigh

✓5ᵗʰ **S76.9**   Injury of unspecified muscles, fascia and tendons at thigh level

  ✓6ᵗʰ **S76.90**   Unspecified injury of unspecified muscles, fascia and tendons at thigh level

    ✓7ᵗʰ **S76.901**   Unspecified injury of unspecified muscles, fascia and tendons at thigh level, right thigh

    ✓7ᵗʰ **S76.902**   Unspecified injury of unspecified muscles, fascia and tendons at thigh level, left thigh

    ✓7ᵗʰ **S76.909**   Unspecified injury of unspecified muscles, fascia and tendons at thigh level, unspecified thigh

  ✓6ᵗʰ **S76.91**   Strain of unspecified muscles, fascia and tendons at thigh level

    ✓7ᵗʰ **S76.911**   Strain of unspecified muscles, fascia and tendons at thigh level, right thigh

    ✓7ᵗʰ **S76.912**   Strain of unspecified muscles, fascia and tendons at thigh level, left thigh

    ✓7ᵗʰ **S76.919**   Strain of unspecified muscles, fascia and tendons at thigh level, unspecified thigh

  ✓6ᵗʰ **S76.92**   Laceration of unspecified muscles, fascia and tendons at thigh level

    ✓7ᵗʰ **S76.921**   Laceration of unspecified muscles, fascia and tendons at thigh level, right thigh

    ✓7ᵗʰ **S76.922**   Laceration of unspecified muscles, fascia and tendons at thigh level, left thigh

    ✓7ᵗʰ **S76.929**   Laceration of unspecified muscles, fascia and tendons at thigh level, unspecified thigh

  ✓6ᵗʰ **S76.99**   Other specified injury of unspecified muscles, fascia and tendons at thigh level

    ✓7ᵗʰ **S76.991**   Other specified injury of unspecified muscles, fascia and tendons at thigh level, right thigh

    ✓7ᵗʰ **S76.992**   Other specified injury of unspecified muscles, fascia and tendons at thigh level, left thigh

    ✓7ᵗʰ **S76.999**   Other specified injury of unspecified muscles, fascia and tendons at thigh level, unspecified thigh

✓4ᵗʰ **S77**   Crushing injury of hip and thigh

Use additional code(s) for all associated injuries

EXCLUDES 2   crushing injury of ankle and foot (S97.-)
crushing injury of lower leg (S87.-)

The appropriate 7th character is to be added to each code from category S77.
A   initial encounter
D   subsequent encounter
S   sequela

✓5ᵗʰ **S77.0**   Crushing injury of hip

  ✓x7ᵗʰ **S77.00**   Crushing injury of unspecified hip

  ✓x7ᵗʰ **S77.01**   Crushing injury of right hip

  ✓x7ᵗʰ **S77.02**   Crushing injury of left hip

✓5ᵗʰ **S77.1**   Crushing injury of thigh

  ✓x7ᵗʰ **S77.10**   Crushing injury of unspecified thigh

  ✓x7ᵗʰ **S77.11**   Crushing injury of right thigh

  ✓x7ᵗʰ **S77.12**   Crushing injury of left thigh

✓5ᵗʰ **S77.2**   Crushing injury of hip with thigh

  ✓x7ᵗʰ **S77.20**   Crushing injury of unspecified hip with thigh

  ✓x7ᵗʰ **S77.21**   Crushing injury of right hip with thigh

  ✓x7ᵗʰ **S77.22**   Crushing injury of left hip with thigh

✓4ᵗʰ **S78**   Traumatic amputation of hip and thigh

An amputation not identified as partial or complete should be coded to complete

EXCLUDES 1   traumatic amputation of knee (S88.0-)

The appropriate 7th character is to be added to each code from category S78.
A   initial encounter
D   subsequent encounter
S   sequela

✓5ᵗʰ **S78.0**   Traumatic amputation at hip joint

  ✓6ᵗʰ **S78.01**   Complete traumatic amputation at hip joint

    ✓7ᵗʰ **S78.011**   Complete traumatic amputation at right hip joint   HCC

    ✓7ᵗʰ **S78.012**   Complete traumatic amputation at left hip joint   HCC

    ✓7ᵗʰ **S78.019**   Complete traumatic amputation at unspecified hip joint   HCC

  ✓6ᵗʰ **S78.02**   Partial traumatic amputation at hip joint

    ✓7ᵗʰ **S78.021**   Partial traumatic amputation at right hip joint   HCC

   √7ᵗʰ **S78.022** Partial traumatic amputation at left hip joint   `HCC`

   √7ᵗʰ **S78.029** Partial traumatic amputation at unspecified hip joint   `HCC`

√5ᵗʰ **S78.1** Traumatic amputation at level between hip and knee

   EXCLUDES 1   traumatic amputation of knee (S88.0-)

  √6ᵗʰ **S78.11** Complete traumatic amputation at level between hip and knee

   √7ᵗʰ **S78.111** Complete traumatic amputation at level between right hip and knee   `HCC`

   √7ᵗʰ **S78.112** Complete traumatic amputation at level between left hip and knee   `HCC`

   √7ᵗʰ **S78.119** Complete traumatic amputation at level between unspecified hip and knee   `HCC`

  √6ᵗʰ **S78.12** Partial traumatic amputation at level between hip and knee

   √7ᵗʰ **S78.121** Partial traumatic amputation at level between right hip and knee   `HCC`

   √7ᵗʰ **S78.122** Partial traumatic amputation at level between left hip and knee   `HCC`

   √7ᵗʰ **S78.129** Partial traumatic amputation at level between unspecified hip and knee   `HCC`

√5ᵗʰ **S78.9** Traumatic amputation of hip and thigh, level unspecified

  √6ᵗʰ **S78.91** Complete traumatic amputation of hip and thigh, level unspecified

   √7ᵗʰ **S78.911** Complete traumatic amputation of right hip and thigh, level unspecified   `HCC`

   √7ᵗʰ **S78.912** Complete traumatic amputation of left hip and thigh, level unspecified   `HCC`

   √7ᵗʰ **S78.919** Complete traumatic amputation of unspecified hip and thigh, level unspecified   `HCC`

  √6ᵗʰ **S78.92** Partial traumatic amputation of hip and thigh, level unspecified

   √7ᵗʰ **S78.921** Partial traumatic amputation of right hip and thigh, level unspecified   `HCC`

   √7ᵗʰ **S78.922** Partial traumatic amputation of left hip and thigh, level unspecified   `HCC`

   √7ᵗʰ **S78.929** Partial traumatic amputation of unspecified hip and thigh, level unspecified   `HCC`

√4ᵗʰ **S79** Other and unspecified injuries of hip and thigh

   NOTE   A fracture not indicated as open or closed should be coded to closed

AHA: 2018,2Q,12; 2018,1Q,3; 2015,3Q,37-39

The appropriate 7th character is to be added to each code from subcategories S79.0 and S79.1.
A   initial encounter for closed fracture
D   subsequent encounter for fracture with routine healing
G   subsequent encounter for fracture with delayed healing
K   subsequent encounter for fracture with nonunion
P   subsequent encounter for fracture with malunion
S   sequela

√5ᵗʰ **S79.0** Physeal fracture of upper end of femur

   EXCLUDES 1   apophyseal fracture of upper end of femur (S72.13-)
       nontraumatic slipped upper femoral epiphysis (M93.0-)

  √6ᵗʰ **S79.00** Unspecified physeal fracture of upper end of femur

   ¹ √7ᵗʰ **S79.001** Unspecified physeal fracture of upper end of right femur   `HCC` `Q`

   ¹ √7ᵗʰ **S79.002** Unspecified physeal fracture of upper end of left femur   `HCC` `Q`

   ¹ √7ᵗʰ **S79.009** Unspecified physeal fracture of upper end of unspecified femur   `HCC` `Q`

  √6ᵗʰ **S79.01** Salter-Harris Type I physeal fracture of upper end of femur

   Acute on chronic slipped capital femoral epiphysis (traumatic)
   Acute slipped capital femoral epiphysis (traumatic)
   Capital femoral epiphyseal fracture

   EXCLUDES 1   chronic slipped upper femoral epiphysis (nontraumatic) (M93.02-)

   ¹ √7ᵗʰ **S79.011** Salter-Harris Type I physeal fracture of upper end of right femur   `HCC` `Q`

   ¹ √7ᵗʰ **S79.012** Salter-Harris Type I physeal fracture of upper end of left femur   `HCC` `Q`

   ¹ √7ᵗʰ **S79.019** Salter-Harris Type I physeal fracture of upper end of unspecified femur   `HCC` `Q`

  √6ᵗʰ **S79.09** Other physeal fracture of upper end of femur

   ¹ √7ᵗʰ **S79.091** Other physeal fracture of upper end of right femur   `HCC` `Q`

   ¹ √7ᵗʰ **S79.092** Other physeal fracture of upper end of left femur   `HCC` `Q`

   ¹ √7ᵗʰ **S79.099** Other physeal fracture of upper end of unspecified femur   `HCC` `Q`

√5ᵗʰ **S79.1** Physeal fracture of lower end of femur

  √6ᵗʰ **S79.10** Unspecified physeal fracture of lower end of femur

   ¹ √7ᵗʰ **S79.101** Unspecified physeal fracture of lower end of right femur   `HCC` `Q`

   ¹ √7ᵗʰ **S79.102** Unspecified physeal fracture of lower end of left femur   `HCC` `Q`

   ¹ √7ᵗʰ **S79.109** Unspecified physeal fracture of lower end of unspecified femur   `HCC` `Q`

  √6ᵗʰ **S79.11** Salter-Harris Type I physeal fracture of lower end of femur

   ¹ √7ᵗʰ **S79.111** Salter-Harris Type I physeal fracture of lower end of right femur   `HCC` `Q`

   ¹ √7ᵗʰ **S79.112** Salter-Harris Type I physeal fracture of lower end of left femur   `HCC` `Q`

   ¹ √7ᵗʰ **S79.119** Salter-Harris Type I physeal fracture of lower end of unspecified femur   `HCC` `Q`

  √6ᵗʰ **S79.12** Salter-Harris Type II physeal fracture of lower end of femur

   ¹ √7ᵗʰ **S79.121** Salter-Harris Type II physeal fracture of lower end of right femur   `HCC` `Q`

   ¹ √7ᵗʰ **S79.122** Salter-Harris Type II physeal fracture of lower end of left femur   `HCC` `Q`

   ¹ √7ᵗʰ **S79.129** Salter-Harris Type II physeal fracture of lower end of unspecified femur   `HCC` `Q`

  √6ᵗʰ **S79.13** Salter-Harris Type III physeal fracture of lower end of femur

   ¹ √7ᵗʰ **S79.131** Salter-Harris Type III physeal fracture of lower end of right femur   `HCC` `Q`

   ¹ √7ᵗʰ **S79.132** Salter-Harris Type III physeal fracture of lower end of left femur   `HCC` `Q`

   ¹ √7ᵗʰ **S79.139** Salter-Harris Type III physeal fracture of lower end of unspecified femur   `HCC` `Q`

  √6ᵗʰ **S79.14** Salter-Harris Type IV physeal fracture of lower end of femur

   ¹ √7ᵗʰ **S79.141** Salter-Harris Type IV physeal fracture of lower end of right femur   `HCC` `Q`

   ¹ √7ᵗʰ **S79.142** Salter-Harris Type IV physeal fracture of lower end of left femur   `HCC` `Q`

   ¹ √7ᵗʰ **S79.149** Salter-Harris Type IV physeal fracture of lower end of unspecified femur   `HCC` `Q`

  √6ᵗʰ **S79.19** Other physeal fracture of lower end of femur

   ¹ √7ᵗʰ **S79.191** Other physeal fracture of lower end of right femur   `HCC` `Q`

   ¹ √7ᵗʰ **S79.192** Other physeal fracture of lower end of left femur   `HCC` `Q`

   ¹ √7ᵗʰ **S79.199** Other physeal fracture of lower end of unspecified femur   `HCC` `Q`

✔ Additional Character Required   √x7ᵗʰ Placeholder Alert   Manifestation   Unspecified Dx   ▶◀ Revised Text   ● New Code   ▲ Revised Code Title

Chapter 19. Injury, Poisoning and Certain Other Consequences of External Causes

S79.8–S81.001

✓5ᵗʰ **S79.8** **Other specified injuries of hip and thigh**

> The appropriate 7th character is to be added to each code in subcategory S79.8.
> A   initial encounter
> D   subsequent encounter
> S   sequela

    ✓6ᵗʰ **S79.81** **Other specified injuries of hip**

       ✓7ᵗʰ **S79.811** **Other specified injuries of right hip**

       ✓7ᵗʰ **S79.812** **Other specified injuries of left hip**

       ✓7ᵗʰ **S79.819** **Other specified injuries of unspecified hip**

    ✓6ᵗʰ **S79.82** **Other specified injuries of thigh**

       ✓7ᵗʰ **S79.821** **Other specified injuries of right thigh**

       ✓7ᵗʰ **S79.822** **Other specified injuries of left thigh**

       ✓7ᵗʰ **S79.829** **Other specified injuries of unspecified thigh**

✓5ᵗʰ **S79.9** **Unspecified injury of hip and thigh**

> The appropriate 7th character is to be added to each code in subcategory S79.9.
> A   initial encounter
> D   subsequent encounter
> S   sequela

    ✓6ᵗʰ **S79.91** **Unspecified injury of hip**

       ✓7ᵗʰ **S79.911** **Unspecified injury of right hip**

       ✓7ᵗʰ **S79.912** **Unspecified injury of left hip**

       ✓7ᵗʰ **S79.919** **Unspecified injury of unspecified hip**

    ✓6ᵗʰ **S79.92** **Unspecified injury of thigh**

       ✓7ᵗʰ **S79.921** **Unspecified injury of right thigh**

       ✓7ᵗʰ **S79.922** **Unspecified injury of left thigh**

       ✓7ᵗʰ **S79.929** **Unspecified injury of unspecified thigh**

Injuries to the knee and lower leg (S80-S89)

EXCLUDES 2   *burns and corrosions (T20-T32)*
      frostbite (T33-T34)
      injuries of ankle and foot, except fracture of ankle and malleolus (S90-S99)
      insect bite or sting, venomous (T63.4)

✓4ᵗʰ **S80** **Superficial injury of knee and lower leg**

    EXCLUDES 2   *superficial injury of ankle and foot (S90.-)*

> The appropriate 7th character is to be added to each code from category S80.
> A   initial encounter
> D   subsequent encounter
> S   sequela

    ✓5ᵗʰ **S80.0** **Contusion of knee**

      ✓x7ᵗʰ **S80.00** **Contusion of unspecified knee**

      ✓x7ᵗʰ **S80.01** **Contusion of right knee**

      ✓x7ᵗʰ **S80.02** **Contusion of left knee**

    ✓5ᵗʰ **S80.1** **Contusion of lower leg**

      ✓x7ᵗʰ **S80.10** **Contusion of unspecified lower leg**

      ✓x7ᵗʰ **S80.11** **Contusion of right lower leg**

      ✓x7ᵗʰ **S80.12** **Contusion of left lower leg**

    ✓5ᵗʰ **S80.2** **Other superficial injuries of knee**

      ✓6ᵗʰ **S80.21** **Abrasion of knee**

         ✓7ᵗʰ **S80.211** **Abrasion, right knee**

         ✓7ᵗʰ **S80.212** **Abrasion, left knee**

         ✓7ᵗʰ **S80.219** **Abrasion, unspecified knee**

      ✓6ᵗʰ **S80.22** **Blister (nonthermal) of knee**

         ✓7ᵗʰ **S80.221** **Blister (nonthermal), right knee**

         ✓7ᵗʰ **S80.222** **Blister (nonthermal), left knee**

         ✓7ᵗʰ **S80.229** **Blister (nonthermal), unspecified knee**

      ✓6ᵗʰ **S80.24** **External constriction of knee**

         ✓7ᵗʰ **S80.241** **External constriction, right knee**

         ✓7ᵗʰ **S80.242** **External constriction, left knee**

         ✓7ᵗʰ **S80.249** **External constriction, unspecified knee**

      ✓6ᵗʰ **S80.25** **Superficial foreign body of knee**

        Splinter in the knee

         ✓7ᵗʰ **S80.251** **Superficial foreign body, right knee**

         ✓7ᵗʰ **S80.252** **Superficial foreign body, left knee**

         ✓7ᵗʰ **S80.259** **Superficial foreign body, unspecified knee**

      ✓6ᵗʰ **S80.26** **Insect bite (nonvenomous) of knee**

         ✓7ᵗʰ **S80.261** **Insect bite (nonvenomous), right knee**

         ✓7ᵗʰ **S80.262** **Insect bite (nonvenomous), left knee**

         ✓7ᵗʰ **S80.269** **Insect bite (nonvenomous), unspecified knee**

      ✓6ᵗʰ **S80.27** **Other superficial bite of knee**

         EXCLUDES 1   *open bite of knee (S81.05-)*

         ✓7ᵗʰ **S80.271** **Other superficial bite of right knee**

         ✓7ᵗʰ **S80.272** **Other superficial bite of left knee**

         ✓7ᵗʰ **S80.279** **Other superficial bite of unspecified knee**

    ✓5ᵗʰ **S80.8** **Other superficial injuries of lower leg**

      ✓6ᵗʰ **S80.81** **Abrasion of lower leg**

         ✓7ᵗʰ **S80.811** **Abrasion, right lower leg**

         ✓7ᵗʰ **S80.812** **Abrasion, left lower leg**

         ✓7ᵗʰ **S80.819** **Abrasion, unspecified lower leg**

      ✓6ᵗʰ **S80.82** **Blister (nonthermal) of lower leg**

         ✓7ᵗʰ **S80.821** **Blister (nonthermal), right lower leg**

         ✓7ᵗʰ **S80.822** **Blister (nonthermal), left lower leg**

         ✓7ᵗʰ **S80.829** **Blister (nonthermal), unspecified lower leg**

      ✓6ᵗʰ **S80.84** **External constriction of lower leg**

         ✓7ᵗʰ **S80.841** **External constriction, right lower leg**

         ✓7ᵗʰ **S80.842** **External constriction, left lower leg**

         ✓7ᵗʰ **S80.849** **External constriction, unspecified lower leg**

      ✓6ᵗʰ **S80.85** **Superficial foreign body of lower leg**

        Splinter in the lower leg

         ✓7ᵗʰ **S80.851** **Superficial foreign body, right lower leg**

         ✓7ᵗʰ **S80.852** **Superficial foreign body, left lower leg**

         ✓7ᵗʰ **S80.859** **Superficial foreign body, unspecified lower leg**

      ✓6ᵗʰ **S80.86** **Insect bite (nonvenomous) of lower leg**

         ✓7ᵗʰ **S80.861** **Insect bite (nonvenomous), right lower leg**

         ✓7ᵗʰ **S80.862** **Insect bite (nonvenomous), left lower leg**

         ✓7ᵗʰ **S80.869** **Insect bite (nonvenomous), unspecified lower leg**

      ✓6ᵗʰ **S80.87** **Other superficial bite of lower leg**

         EXCLUDES 1   *open bite of lower leg (S81.85-)*

         ✓7ᵗʰ **S80.871** **Other superficial bite, right lower leg**

         ✓7ᵗʰ **S80.872** **Other superficial bite, left lower leg**

         ✓7ᵗʰ **S80.879** **Other superficial bite, unspecified lower leg**

    ✓5ᵗʰ **S80.9** **Unspecified superficial injury of knee and lower leg**

      ✓6ᵗʰ **S80.91** **Unspecified superficial injury of knee**

         ✓7ᵗʰ **S80.911** **Unspecified superficial injury of right knee**

         ✓7ᵗʰ **S80.912** **Unspecified superficial injury of left knee**

         ✓7ᵗʰ **S80.919** **Unspecified superficial injury of unspecified knee**

      ✓6ᵗʰ **S80.92** **Unspecified superficial injury of lower leg**

         ✓7ᵗʰ **S80.921** **Unspecified superficial injury of right lower leg**

         ✓7ᵗʰ **S80.922** **Unspecified superficial injury of left lower leg**

         ✓7ᵗʰ **S80.929** **Unspecified superficial injury of unspecified lower leg**

✓4ᵗʰ **S81** **Open wound of knee and lower leg**

> Code also any associated wound infection

    EXCLUDES 1   *open fracture of knee and lower leg (S82.-)*
            traumatic amputation of lower leg (S88.-)
    EXCLUDES 2   *open wound of ankle and foot (S91.-)*

> The appropriate 7th character is to be added to each code from category S81.
> A   initial encounter
> D   subsequent encounter
> S   sequela

    ✓5ᵗʰ **S81.0** **Open wound of knee**

      ✓6ᵗʰ **S81.00** **Unspecified open wound of knee**

         ✓7ᵗʰ **S81.001** **Unspecified open wound, right knee**

     ✓7ᵗʰ **S81.002** Unspecified open wound, left knee

     ✓7ᵗʰ **S81.009** Unspecified open wound, unspecified knee

✓6ᵗʰ **S81.01** Laceration without foreign body of knee

     ✓7ᵗʰ **S81.011** Laceration without foreign body, right knee

     ✓7ᵗʰ **S81.012** Laceration without foreign body, left knee

     ✓7ᵗʰ **S81.019** Laceration without foreign body, unspecified knee

✓6ᵗʰ **S81.02** Laceration with foreign body of knee

     ✓7ᵗʰ **S81.021** Laceration with foreign body, right knee

     ✓7ᵗʰ **S81.022** Laceration with foreign body, left knee

     ✓7ᵗʰ **S81.029** Laceration with foreign body, unspecified knee

✓6ᵗʰ **S81.03** Puncture wound without foreign body of knee

     ✓7ᵗʰ **S81.031** Puncture wound without foreign body, right knee

     ✓7ᵗʰ **S81.032** Puncture wound without foreign body, left knee

     ✓7ᵗʰ **S81.039** Puncture wound without foreign body, unspecified knee

✓6ᵗʰ **S81.04** Puncture wound with foreign body of knee

     ✓7ᵗʰ **S81.041** Puncture wound with foreign body, right knee

     ✓7ᵗʰ **S81.042** Puncture wound with foreign body, left knee

     ✓7ᵗʰ **S81.049** Puncture wound with foreign body, unspecified knee

✓6ᵗʰ **S81.05** Open bite of knee

     Bite of knee NOS

     EXCLUDES 1   superficial bite of knee (S80.27-)

     ✓7ᵗʰ **S81.051** Open bite, right knee

     ✓7ᵗʰ **S81.052** Open bite, left knee

     ✓7ᵗʰ **S81.059** Open bite, unspecified knee

✓5ᵗʰ **S81.8** Open wound of lower leg

     ✓6ᵗʰ **S81.80** Unspecified open wound of lower leg

       AHA: 2016,3Q,24

     ✓7ᵗʰ **S81.801** Unspecified open wound, right lower leg

     ✓7ᵗʰ **S81.802** Unspecified open wound, left lower leg

     ✓7ᵗʰ **S81.809** Unspecified open wound, unspecified lower leg

     ✓6ᵗʰ **S81.81** Laceration without foreign body of lower leg

     ✓7ᵗʰ **S81.811** Laceration without foreign body, right lower leg

     ✓7ᵗʰ **S81.812** Laceration without foreign body, left lower leg

     ✓7ᵗʰ **S81.819** Laceration without foreign body, unspecified lower leg

     ✓6ᵗʰ **S81.82** Laceration with foreign body of lower leg

     ✓7ᵗʰ **S81.821** Laceration with foreign body, right lower leg

     ✓7ᵗʰ **S81.822** Laceration with foreign body, left lower leg

     ✓7ᵗʰ **S81.829** Laceration with foreign body, unspecified lower leg

     ✓6ᵗʰ **S81.83** Puncture wound without foreign body of lower leg

       AHA: 2016,3Q,24

     ✓7ᵗʰ **S81.831** Puncture wound without foreign body, right lower leg

     ✓7ᵗʰ **S81.832** Puncture wound without foreign body, left lower leg

     ✓7ᵗʰ **S81.839** Puncture wound without foreign body, unspecified lower leg

     ✓6ᵗʰ **S81.84** Puncture wound with foreign body of lower leg

       AHA: 2016,3Q,24

     ✓7ᵗʰ **S81.841** Puncture wound with foreign body, right lower leg

     ✓7ᵗʰ **S81.842** Puncture wound with foreign body, left lower leg

     ✓7ᵗʰ **S81.849** Puncture wound with foreign body, unspecified lower leg

     ✓6ᵗʰ **S81.85** Open bite of lower leg

     Bite of lower leg NOS

     EXCLUDES 1   superficial bite of lower leg (S80.86-, S80.87-)

     ✓7ᵗʰ **S81.851** Open bite, right lower leg

     ✓7ᵗʰ **S81.852** Open bite, left lower leg

     ✓7ᵗʰ **S81.859** Open bite, unspecified lower leg

✓4ᵗʰ **S82** Fracture of lower leg, including ankle

     NOTE   A fracture not indicated as displaced or nondisplaced should be coded to displaced

       A fracture not indicated as open or closed should be coded to closed

       The open fracture designations are based on the Gustilo open fracture classification.

     INCLUDES   fracture of malleolus

     EXCLUDES 1   traumatic amputation of lower leg (S88.-)

     EXCLUDES 2   fracture of foot, except ankle (S92.-)

       periprosthetic fracture of prosthetic implant of knee (M97.0-)

AHA: 2018,2Q,12; 2016,1Q,33; 2015,3Q,37-39

DEF: Diaphysis: Central shaft of a long bone.

DEF: Epiphysis: Proximal and distal rounded ends of a long bone, communicates with the joint.

DEF: Metaphysis: Section of a long bone located between the epiphysis and diaphysis at the proximal and distal ends.

DEF: Physis (growth plate): Narrow zone of cartilaginous tissue between the epiphysis and metaphysis at each end of a long bone. In childhood, proliferation of cells in this zone lengthens the bone. As the bone matures, this area thins, ossification eventually fusing into solid bone and growth stops. **Synonyms:** Epiphyseal plate.

The appropriate 7th character is to be added to all codes from category S82 [unless otherwise indicated].

A   initial encounter for closed fracture

B   initial encounter for open fracture type I or II
     initial encounter for open fracture NOS

C   initial encounter for open fracture type IIIA, IIIB, or IIIC

D   subsequent encounter for closed fracture with routine healing

E   subsequent encounter for open fracture type I or II with routine healing

F   subsequent encounter for open fracture type IIIA, IIIB, or IIIC with routine healing

G   subsequent encounter for closed fracture with delayed healing

H   subsequent encounter for open fracture type I or II with delayed healing

J   subsequent encounter for open fracture type IIIA, IIIB, or IIIC with delayed healing

K   subsequent encounter for closed fracture with nonunion

M   subsequent encounter for open fracture type I or II with nonunion

N   subsequent encounter for open fracture type IIIA, IIIB, or IIIC with nonunion

P   subsequent encounter for closed fracture with malunion

Q   subsequent encounter for open fracture type I or II with malunion

R   subsequent encounter for open fracture type IIIA, IIIB, or IIIC with malunion

S   sequela

✓5ᵗʰ **S82.0** Fracture of patella

     Knee cap

     ✓6ᵗʰ **S82.00** Unspecified fracture of patella

     ✓7ᵗʰ **S82.001** Unspecified fracture of right patella   Q

     ✓7ᵗʰ **S82.002** Unspecified fracture of left patella   Q

     ✓7ᵗʰ **S82.009** Unspecified fracture of unspecified patella   Q

     ✓6ᵗʰ **S82.01** Osteochondral fracture of patella

     ✓7ᵗʰ **S82.011** Displaced osteochondral fracture of right patella   Q

     ✓7ᵗʰ **S82.012** Displaced osteochondral fracture of left patella   Q

     ✓7ᵗʰ **S82.013** Displaced osteochondral fracture of unspecified patella   Q

     ✓7ᵗʰ **S82.014** Nondisplaced osteochondral fracture of right patella   Q

     ✓7ᵗʰ **S82.015** Nondisplaced osteochondral fracture of left patella   Q

     ✓7ᵗʰ **S82.016** Nondisplaced osteochondral fracture of unspecified patella   Q

     ✓6ᵗʰ **S82.02** Longitudinal fracture of patella

     ✓7ᵗʰ **S82.021** Displaced longitudinal fracture of right patella   Q

     ✓7ᵗʰ **S82.022** Displaced longitudinal fracture of left patella   Q

✓ Additional Character Required   ✓x7ᵗʰ Placeholder Alert   Manifestation   Unspecified Dx   ▶◀ Revised Text   ● New Code   ▲ Revised Code Title

ICD-10-CM 2020   **1053**

√7ᵗʰ **S82.023** Displaced **longitudinal fracture of unspecified patella** Q

√7ᵗʰ **S82.024** Nondisplaced **longitudinal fracture of right patella** Q

√7ᵗʰ **S82.025** Nondisplaced **longitudinal fracture of left patella** Q

√7ᵗʰ **S82.026** Nondisplaced **longitudinal fracture of unspecified patella** Q

√6ᵗʰ **S82.03** **Transverse** fracture of patella

√7ᵗʰ **S82.031** Displaced **transverse fracture of right patella** Q

√7ᵗʰ **S82.032** Displaced **transverse fracture of left patella** Q

√7ᵗʰ **S82.033** Displaced **transverse fracture of unspecified patella** Q

√7ᵗʰ **S82.034** Nondisplaced **transverse fracture of right patella** Q

√7ᵗʰ **S82.035** Nondisplaced **transverse fracture of left patella** Q

√7ᵗʰ **S82.036** Nondisplaced **transverse fracture of unspecified patella** Q

√6ᵗʰ **S82.04** **Comminuted** fracture of patella

√7ᵗʰ **S82.041** Displaced **comminuted fracture of right patella** Q

√7ᵗʰ **S82.042** Displaced **comminuted fracture of left patella** Q

√7ᵗʰ **S82.043** Displaced **comminuted fracture of unspecified patella** Q

√7ᵗʰ **S82.044** Nondisplaced **comminuted fracture of right patella** Q

√7ᵗʰ **S82.045** Nondisplaced **comminuted fracture of left patella** Q

√7ᵗʰ **S82.046** Nondisplaced **comminuted fracture of unspecified patella** Q

√6ᵗʰ **S82.09** **Other fracture of patella**

√7ᵗʰ **S82.091** Other fracture of **right patella** Q

√7ᵗʰ **S82.092** Other fracture of **left patella** Q

√7ᵗʰ **S82.099** Other fracture of **unspecified patella** Q

√5ᵗʰ **S82.1** **Fracture of upper end of tibia**

Fracture of proximal end of tibia

EXCLUDES 2 *fracture of shaft of tibia (S82.2-)*

physeal fracture of upper end of tibia (S89.0-)

√6ᵗʰ **S82.10** **Unspecified fracture of upper end of tibia**

√7ᵗʰ **S82.101** Unspecified fracture of upper end of **right tibia** Q

√7ᵗʰ **S82.102** Unspecified fracture of upper end of **left tibia** Q

√7ᵗʰ **S82.109** Unspecified fracture of upper end of **unspecified tibia** Q

√6ᵗʰ **S82.11** **Fracture of tibial spine**

√7ᵗʰ **S82.111** Displaced fracture of **right tibial spine** Q

√7ᵗʰ **S82.112** Displaced fracture of **left tibial spine** Q

√7ᵗʰ **S82.113** Displaced fracture of **unspecified tibial spine** Q

√7ᵗʰ **S82.114** Nondisplaced fracture of **right tibial spine** Q

√7ᵗʰ **S82.115** Nondisplaced fracture of **left tibial spine** Q

√7ᵗʰ **S82.116** Nondisplaced fracture of **unspecified tibial spine** Q

√6ᵗʰ **S82.12** **Fracture of lateral condyle of tibia**

√7ᵗʰ **S82.121** Displaced fracture of lateral condyle of **right tibia** Q

√7ᵗʰ **S82.122** Displaced fracture of lateral condyle of **left tibia** Q

√7ᵗʰ **S82.123** Displaced fracture of lateral condyle of **unspecified tibia** Q

√7ᵗʰ **S82.124** Nondisplaced fracture of lateral condyle of **right tibia** Q

√7ᵗʰ **S82.125** Nondisplaced fracture of lateral condyle of **left tibia** Q

√7ᵗʰ **S82.126** Nondisplaced fracture of lateral condyle of **unspecified tibia** Q

√6ᵗʰ **S82.13** **Fracture of medial condyle of tibia**

√7ᵗʰ **S82.131** Displaced fracture of medial condyle of **right tibia** Q

√7ᵗʰ **S82.132** Displaced **fracture of medial condyle of left tibia** Q

√7ᵗʰ **S82.133** Displaced **fracture of medial condyle of unspecified tibia** Q

√7ᵗʰ **S82.134** Nondisplaced **fracture of medial condyle of right tibia** Q

√7ᵗʰ **S82.135** Nondisplaced **fracture of medial condyle of left tibia** Q

√7ᵗʰ **S82.136** Nondisplaced **fracture of medial condyle of unspecified tibia** Q

√6ᵗʰ **S82.14** **Bicondylar** fracture of tibia

Fracture of tibial plateau NOS

√7ᵗʰ **S82.141** Displaced **bicondylar fracture of right tibia** Q

√7ᵗʰ **S82.142** Displaced **bicondylar fracture of left tibia** Q

√7ᵗʰ **S82.143** Displaced **bicondylar fracture of unspecified tibia** Q

√7ᵗʰ **S82.144** Nondisplaced **bicondylar fracture of right tibia** Q

√7ᵗʰ **S82.145** Nondisplaced **bicondylar fracture of left tibia** Q

√7ᵗʰ **S82.146** Nondisplaced **bicondylar fracture of unspecified tibia** Q

√6ᵗʰ **S82.15** **Fracture of tibial tuberosity**

√7ᵗʰ **S82.151** Displaced **fracture of right tibial tuberosity** Q

√7ᵗʰ **S82.152** Displaced **fracture of left tibial tuberosity** Q

√7ᵗʰ **S82.153** Displaced **fracture of unspecified tibial tuberosity** Q

√7ᵗʰ **S82.154** Nondisplaced **fracture of right tibial tuberosity** Q

√7ᵗʰ **S82.155** Nondisplaced **fracture of left tibial tuberosity** Q

√7ᵗʰ **S82.156** Nondisplaced **fracture of unspecified tibial tuberosity** Q

√6ᵗʰ **S82.16** **Torus** fracture of upper end of tibia

The appropriate 7th character is to be added to all codes in subcategory S82.16.
A initial encounter for closed fracture
D subsequent encounter for fracture with routine healing
G subsequent encounter for fracture with delayed healing
K subsequent encounter for fracture with nonunion
P subsequent encounter for fracture with malunion
S sequela

√7ᵗʰ **S82.161** Torus fracture of upper end of **right tibia** Q

√7ᵗʰ **S82.162** Torus fracture of upper end of **left tibia** Q

√7ᵗʰ **S82.169** Torus fracture of upper end of **unspecified tibia** Q

√6ᵗʰ **S82.19** **Other fracture of upper end of tibia**

√7ᵗʰ **S82.191** Other fracture of upper end of **right tibia** Q

√7ᵗʰ **S82.192** Other fracture of upper end of **left tibia** Q

√7ᵗʰ **S82.199** Other fracture of upper end of **unspecified tibia** Q

√5ᵗʰ **S82.2** **Fracture of shaft of tibia**

√6ᵗʰ **S82.20** **Unspecified fracture of shaft of tibia**

Fracture of tibia NOS

√7ᵗʰ **S82.201** Unspecified fracture of shaft of **right tibia** Q

√7ᵗʰ **S82.202** Unspecified fracture of shaft of **left tibia** Q

√7ᵗʰ **S82.209** Unspecified fracture of shaft of **unspecified tibia** Q

√6ᵗʰ **S82.22** **Transverse** fracture of shaft of tibia

√7ᵗʰ **S82.221** Displaced **transverse fracture of shaft of right tibia** Q

√7ᵗʰ **S82.222** Displaced **transverse fracture of shaft of left tibia** Q

√7ᵗʰ **S82.223** Displaced **transverse fracture of shaft of unspecified tibia** Q

√7ᵗʰ **S82.224** Nondisplaced **transverse** fracture of shaft of **right** tibia   Q

√7ᵗʰ **S82.225** Nondisplaced **transverse** fracture of shaft of **left** tibia   Q

√7ᵗʰ **S82.226** Nondisplaced **transverse** fracture of shaft of **unspecified** tibia   Q

√6ᵗʰ **S82.23** Oblique **fracture of shaft of tibia**

√7ᵗʰ **S82.231** Displaced **oblique** fracture of shaft of **right** tibia   Q

√7ᵗʰ **S82.232** Displaced **oblique** fracture of shaft of **left** tibia   Q

√7ᵗʰ **S82.233** Displaced **oblique** fracture of shaft of **unspecified** tibia   Q

√7ᵗʰ **S82.234** Nondisplaced **oblique** fracture of shaft of **right** tibia   Q

√7ᵗʰ **S82.235** Nondisplaced **oblique** fracture of shaft of **left** tibia   Q

√7ᵗʰ **S82.236** Nondisplaced **oblique** fracture of shaft of **unspecified** tibia   Q

√6ᵗʰ **S82.24** Spiral **fracture of shaft of tibia**

Toddler fracture

√7ᵗʰ **S82.241** Displaced **spiral** fracture of shaft of **right** tibia   Q

√7ᵗʰ **S82.242** Displaced **spiral** fracture of shaft of **left** tibia   Q

√7ᵗʰ **S82.243** Displaced **spiral** fracture of shaft of **unspecified** tibia   Q

√7ᵗʰ **S82.244** Nondisplaced **spiral** fracture of shaft of **right** tibia   Q

√7ᵗʰ **S82.245** Nondisplaced **spiral** fracture of shaft of **left** tibia   Q

√7ᵗʰ **S82.246** Nondisplaced **spiral** fracture of shaft of **unspecified** tibia   Q

√6ᵗʰ **S82.25** Comminuted **fracture of shaft of tibia**

√7ᵗʰ **S82.251** Displaced **comminuted** fracture of shaft of **right** tibia   Q

√7ᵗʰ **S82.252** Displaced **comminuted** fracture of shaft of **left** tibia   Q

√7ᵗʰ **S82.253** Displaced **comminuted** fracture of shaft of **unspecified** tibia   Q

√7ᵗʰ **S82.254** Nondisplaced **comminuted** fracture of shaft of **right** tibia   Q

√7ᵗʰ **S82.255** Nondisplaced **comminuted** fracture of shaft of **left** tibia   Q

√7ᵗʰ **S82.256** Nondisplaced **comminuted** fracture of shaft of **unspecified** tibia   Q

√6ᵗʰ **S82.26** Segmental **fracture of shaft of tibia**

√7ᵗʰ **S82.261** Displaced **segmental** fracture of shaft of **right** tibia   Q

√7ᵗʰ **S82.262** Displaced **segmental** fracture of shaft of **left** tibia   Q

√7ᵗʰ **S82.263** Displaced **segmental** fracture of shaft of **unspecified** tibia   Q

√7ᵗʰ **S82.264** Nondisplaced **segmental** fracture of shaft of **right** tibia   Q

√7ᵗʰ **S82.265** Nondisplaced **segmental** fracture of shaft of **left** tibia   Q

√7ᵗʰ **S82.266** Nondisplaced **segmental** fracture of shaft of **unspecified** tibia   Q

√6ᵗʰ **S82.29** Other **fracture of shaft of tibia**

√7ᵗʰ **S82.291** Other fracture of shaft of **right** tibia   Q

√7ᵗʰ **S82.292** Other fracture of shaft of **left** tibia   Q

√7ᵗʰ **S82.299** Other fracture of shaft of **unspecified** tibia   Q

√5ᵗʰ **S82.3** Fracture of **lower end of tibia**

EXCLUDES 1   *bimalleolar fracture of lower leg (S82.84-)*
fracture of medial malleolus alone (S82.5-)
Maisonneuve's fracture (S82.86-)
pilon fracture of distal tibia (S82.87-)
trimalleolar fractures of lower leg (S82.85-)

√6ᵗʰ **S82.30** Unspecified **fracture of lower end of tibia**

√7ᵗʰ **S82.301** Unspecified fracture of lower end of **right** tibia   Q

√7ᵗʰ **S82.302** Unspecified fracture of lower end of **left** tibia   Q

√7ᵗʰ **S82.309** Unspecified fracture of lower end of **unspecified** tibia   Q

√6ᵗʰ **S82.31** Torus **fracture of lower end of tibia**

> The appropriate 7th character is to be added to all codes in subcategory S82.31.
> A   initial encounter for closed fracture
> D   subsequent encounter for fracture with routine healing
> G   subsequent encounter for fracture with delayed healing
> K   subsequent encounter for fracture with nonunion
> P   subsequent encounter for fracture with malunion
> S   sequela

√7ᵗʰ **S82.311** Torus fracture of lower end of **right** tibia   Q

√7ᵗʰ **S82.312** Torus fracture of lower end of **left** tibia   Q

√7ᵗʰ **S82.319** Torus fracture of lower end of **unspecified** tibia   Q

√6ᵗʰ **S82.39** Other **fracture of lower end of tibia**

AHA: 2015,1Q,25

√7ᵗʰ **S82.391** Other fracture of lower end of **right** tibia   Q

√7ᵗʰ **S82.392** Other fracture of lower end of **left** tibia   Q

√7ᵗʰ **S82.399** Other fracture of lower end of **unspecified** tibia   Q

√5ᵗʰ **S82.4** Fracture of **shaft of fibula**

EXCLUDES 2   *fracture of lateral malleolus alone (S82.6-)*

√6ᵗʰ **S82.40** Unspecified **fracture of shaft of fibula**

√7ᵗʰ **S82.401** Unspecified fracture of shaft of **right** fibula   Q

√7ᵗʰ **S82.402** Unspecified fracture of shaft of **left** fibula   Q

√7ᵗʰ **S82.409** Unspecified fracture of shaft of **unspecified** fibula   Q

√6ᵗʰ **S82.42** Transverse **fracture of shaft of fibula**

√7ᵗʰ **S82.421** Displaced **transverse** fracture of shaft of **right** fibula   Q

√7ᵗʰ **S82.422** Displaced **transverse** fracture of shaft of **left** fibula   Q

√7ᵗʰ **S82.423** Displaced **transverse** fracture of shaft of **unspecified** fibula   Q

√7ᵗʰ **S82.424** Nondisplaced **transverse** fracture of shaft of **right** fibula   Q

√7ᵗʰ **S82.425** Nondisplaced **transverse** fracture of shaft of **left** fibula   Q

√7ᵗʰ **S82.426** Nondisplaced **transverse** fracture of shaft of **unspecified** fibula   Q

√6ᵗʰ **S82.43** Oblique **fracture of shaft of fibula**

√7ᵗʰ **S82.431** Displaced **oblique** fracture of shaft of **right** fibula   Q

√7ᵗʰ **S82.432** Displaced **oblique** fracture of shaft of **left** fibula   Q

√7ᵗʰ **S82.433** Displaced **oblique** fracture of shaft of **unspecified** fibula   Q

√7ᵗʰ **S82.434** Nondisplaced **oblique** fracture of shaft of **right** fibula   Q

√7ᵗʰ **S82.435** Nondisplaced **oblique** fracture of shaft of **left** fibula   Q

√7ᵗʰ **S82.436** Nondisplaced **oblique** fracture of shaft of **unspecified** fibula   Q

√6ᵗʰ **S82.44** Spiral **fracture of shaft of fibula**

√7ᵗʰ **S82.441** Displaced **spiral** fracture of shaft of **right** fibula   Q

√7ᵗʰ **S82.442** Displaced **spiral** fracture of shaft of **left** fibula   Q

√7ᵗʰ **S82.443** Displaced **spiral** fracture of shaft of **unspecified** fibula   Q

√7ᵗʰ **S82.444** Nondisplaced **spiral** fracture of shaft of **right** fibula   Q

√7ᵗʰ **S82.445** Nondisplaced **spiral** fracture of shaft of **left** fibula   Q

√7ᵗʰ **S82.446** Nondisplaced **spiral** fracture of shaft of **unspecified** fibula   Q

√6ᵗʰ **S82.45** Comminuted **fracture of shaft of fibula**

√7ᵗʰ **S82.451** Displaced **comminuted** fracture of shaft of **right** fibula   Q

√7ᵗʰ **S82.452** Displaced **comminuted** fracture of shaft of **left** fibula   Q

✔ Additional Character Required   √x7ᵗʰ Placeholder Alert   Manifestation   Unspecified Dx   ▶◀ Revised Text   ● New Code   ▲ Revised Code Title

√7ʰ **S82.453** Displaced comminuted fracture of shaft of unspecified fibula   Q

√7ʰ **S82.454** Nondisplaced comminuted fracture of shaft of right fibula   Q

√7ʰ **S82.455** Nondisplaced comminuted fracture of shaft of left fibula   Q

√7ʰ **S82.456** Nondisplaced comminuted fracture of shaft of unspecified fibula   Q

√6ʰ **S82.46** Segmental fracture of shaft of fibula

√7ʰ **S82.461** Displaced segmental fracture of shaft of right fibula   Q

√7ʰ **S82.462** Displaced segmental fracture of shaft of left fibula   Q

√7ʰ **S82.463** Displaced segmental fracture of shaft of unspecified fibula   Q

√7ʰ **S82.464** Nondisplaced segmental fracture of shaft of right fibula   Q

√7ʰ **S82.465** Nondisplaced segmental fracture of shaft of left fibula   Q

√7ʰ **S82.466** Nondisplaced segmental fracture of shaft of unspecified fibula   Q

√6ʰ **S82.49** Other fracture of shaft of fibula

√7ʰ **S82.491** Other fracture of shaft of right fibula   Q

√7ʰ **S82.492** Other fracture of shaft of left fibula   Q

√7ʰ **S82.499** Other fracture of shaft of unspecified fibula   Q

√5ʰ **S82.5** Fracture of medial malleolus

> EXCLUDES 1   *pilon fracture of distal tibia (S82.87-)*
> *Salter-Harris type III of lower end of tibia (S89.13-)*
> *Salter-Harris type IV of lower end of tibia (S89.14-)*

√x7ʰ **S82.51** Displaced fracture of medial malleolus of right tibia   Q

√x7ʰ **S82.52** Displaced fracture of medial malleolus of left tibia   Q

√x7ʰ **S82.53** Displaced fracture of medial malleolus of unspecified tibia   Q

√x7ʰ **S82.54** Nondisplaced fracture of medial malleolus of right tibia   Q

√x7ʰ **S82.55** Nondisplaced fracture of medial malleolus of left tibia   Q

√x7ʰ **S82.56** Nondisplaced fracture of medial malleolus of unspecified tibia   Q

√5ʰ **S82.6** Fracture of lateral malleolus

> EXCLUDES 1   *pilon fracture of distal tibia (S82.87-)*

√x7ʰ **S82.61** Displaced fracture of lateral malleolus of right fibula   Q

√x7ʰ **S82.62** Displaced fracture of lateral malleolus of left fibula   Q

√x7ʰ **S82.63** Displaced fracture of lateral malleolus of unspecified fibula   Q

√x7ʰ **S82.64** Nondisplaced fracture of lateral malleolus of right fibula   Q

√x7ʰ **S82.65** Nondisplaced fracture of lateral malleolus of left fibula   Q

√x7ʰ **S82.66** Nondisplaced fracture of lateral malleolus of unspecified fibula   Q

√5ʰ **S82.8** Other fractures of lower leg

√6ʰ **S82.81** Torus fracture of upper end of fibula

> The appropriate 7th character is to be added to all codes in subcategory S82.81.
> A   initial encounter for closed fracture
> D   subsequent encounter for fracture with routine healing
> G   subsequent encounter for fracture with delayed healing
> K   subsequent encounter for fracture with nonunion
> P   subsequent encounter for fracture with malunion
> S   sequela

√7ʰ **S82.811** Torus fracture of upper end of right fibula   Q

√7ʰ **S82.812** Torus fracture of upper end of left fibula   Q

√7ʰ **S82.819** Torus fracture of upper end of unspecified fibula   Q

√6ʰ **S82.82** Torus fracture of lower end of fibula

> The appropriate 7th character is to be added to all codes in subcategory S82.82.
> A   initial encounter for closed fracture
> D   subsequent encounter for fracture with routine healing
> G   subsequent encounter for fracture with delayed healing
> K   subsequent encounter for fracture with nonunion
> P   subsequent encounter for fracture with malunion
> S   sequela

√7ʰ **S82.821** Torus fracture of lower end of right fibula   Q

√7ʰ **S82.822** Torus fracture of lower end of left fibula   Q

√7ʰ **S82.829** Torus fracture of lower end of unspecified fibula   Q

√6ʰ **S82.83** Other fracture of upper and lower end of fibula

AHA: 2015,1Q,25

√7ʰ **S82.831** Other fracture of upper and lower end of right fibula   Q

√7ʰ **S82.832** Other fracture of upper and lower end of left fibula   Q

√7ʰ **S82.839** Other fracture of upper and lower end of unspecified fibula   Q

√6ʰ **S82.84** Bimalleolar fracture of lower leg

Right Bimalleolar Fracture

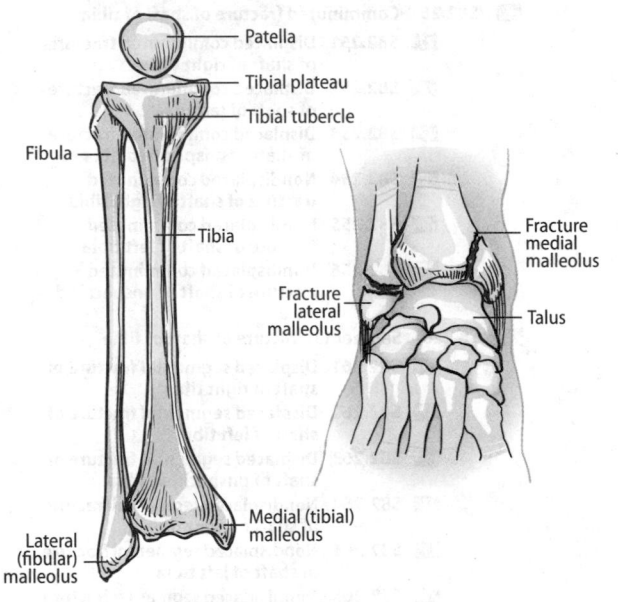

Patella
Tibial plateau
Tibial tubercle
Fibula
Tibia
Fracture lateral malleolus
Fracture medial malleolus
Talus
Lateral (fibular) malleolus
Medial (tibial) malleolus

√7ʰ **S82.841** Displaced bimalleolar fracture of right lower leg   Q

√7ʰ **S82.842** Displaced bimalleolar fracture of left lower leg   Q

√7ʰ **S82.843** Displaced bimalleolar fracture of unspecified lower leg   Q

√7ʰ **S82.844** Nondisplaced bimalleolar fracture of right lower leg   Q

√7ʰ **S82.845** Nondisplaced bimalleolar fracture of left lower leg   Q

√7ʰ **S82.846** Nondisplaced bimalleolar fracture of unspecified lower leg   Q

√6ʰ **S82.85** Trimalleolar fracture of lower leg

√7ʰ **S82.851** Displaced trimalleolar fracture of right lower leg   Q

√7ʰ **S82.852** Displaced trimalleolar fracture of left lower leg   Q

√7ʰ **S82.853** Displaced trimalleolar fracture of unspecified lower leg   Q

√7ʰ **S82.854** Nondisplaced trimalleolar fracture of right lower leg   Q

√7ʰ **S82.855** Nondisplaced trimalleolar fracture of left lower leg   Q

√7ᵗʰ **S82.856** Nondisplaced **trimalleolar** fracture of unspecified lower leg   Q

√6ᵗʰ **S82.86** Maisonneuve's **fracture**

     √7ᵗʰ **S82.861** Displaced **Maisonneuve's fracture** of **right** leg   Q

     √7ᵗʰ **S82.862** Displaced **Maisonneuve's fracture** of **left** leg   Q

     √7ᵗʰ **S82.863** Displaced **Maisonneuve's fracture** of **unspecified** leg   Q

     √7ᵗʰ **S82.864** Nondisplaced **Maisonneuve's fracture** of **right** leg   Q

     √7ᵗʰ **S82.865** Nondisplaced **Maisonneuve's fracture** of **left** leg   Q

     √7ᵗʰ **S82.866** Nondisplaced **Maisonneuve's fracture** of **unspecified** leg   Q

√6ᵗʰ **S82.87** Pilon **fracture of tibia**

     √7ᵗʰ **S82.871** Displaced **pilon fracture of right** tibia   Q

     √7ᵗʰ **S82.872** Displaced **pilon fracture of left** tibia   Q

     √7ᵗʰ **S82.873** Displaced **pilon fracture of unspecified tibia**   Q

     √7ᵗʰ **S82.874** Nondisplaced **pilon fracture of right tibia**   Q

     √7ᵗʰ **S82.875** Nondisplaced **pilon fracture of left tibia**   Q

     √7ᵗʰ **S82.876** Nondisplaced **pilon fracture of unspecified tibia**   Q

√6ᵗʰ **S82.89** Other **fractures of lower leg**

     Fracture of ankle NOS

     √7ᵗʰ **S82.891** Other **fracture of right lower leg**   Q

     √7ᵗʰ **S82.892** Other **fracture of left lower leg**   Q

     √7ᵗʰ **S82.899** Other **fracture of unspecified lower leg**   Q

√5ᵗʰ **S82.9** Unspecified **fracture of lower leg**

     √x7ᵗʰ **S82.90** Unspecified **fracture of unspecified lower leg**   Q

     √x7ᵗʰ **S82.91** Unspecified **fracture of right lower leg**   Q

     √x7ᵗʰ **S82.92** Unspecified **fracture of left lower leg**   Q

√4ᵗʰ **S83** Dislocation and sprain of joints and ligaments of knee

     INCLUDES   avulsion of joint or ligament of knee

         laceration of cartilage, joint or ligament of knee

         sprain of cartilage, joint or ligament of knee

         traumatic hemarthrosis of joint or ligament of knee

         traumatic rupture of joint or ligament of knee

         traumatic subluxation of joint or ligament of knee

         traumatic tear of joint or ligament of knee

     Code also any associated open wound

     EXCLUDES 1   *derangement of patella (M22.0-M22.3)*

         injury of patellar ligament (tendon) (S76.1-)

         internal derangement of knee (M23.-)

         old dislocation of knee (M23.8X)

         pathological dislocation of knee (M24.36)

         recurrent dislocation of knee (M22.0)

     EXCLUDES 2   *strain of muscle, fascia and tendon of lower leg (S86.-)*

     The appropriate 7th character is to be added to each code from category S83.

     A   initial encounter

     D   subsequent encounter

     S   sequela

√5ᵗʰ **S83.0** Subluxation and dislocation of **patella**

     √6ᵗʰ **S83.00** Unspecified **subluxation and dislocation of patella**

         √7ᵗʰ **S83.001** Unspecified **subluxation of right patella**

         √7ᵗʰ **S83.002** Unspecified **subluxation of left patella**

         √7ᵗʰ **S83.003** Unspecified **subluxation of unspecified patella**

         √7ᵗʰ **S83.004** Unspecified **dislocation of right patella**

         √7ᵗʰ **S83.005** Unspecified **dislocation of left patella**

         √7ᵗʰ **S83.006** Unspecified **dislocation of unspecified patella**

     √6ᵗʰ **S83.01** Lateral **subluxation and dislocation of patella**

         √7ᵗʰ **S83.011** Lateral **subluxation of right patella**

         √7ᵗʰ **S83.012** Lateral **subluxation of left patella**

         √7ᵗʰ **S83.013** Lateral **subluxation of unspecified patella**

         √7ᵗʰ **S83.014** Lateral **dislocation of right patella**

√7ᵗʰ **S83.015** Lateral **dislocation of left patella**

√7ᵗʰ **S83.016** Lateral **dislocation of unspecified patella**

√6ᵗʰ **S83.09** Other **subluxation and dislocation of patella**

     √7ᵗʰ **S83.091** Other **subluxation of right patella**

     √7ᵗʰ **S83.092** Other **subluxation of left patella**

     √7ᵗʰ **S83.093** Other **subluxation of unspecified patella**

     √7ᵗʰ **S83.094** Other **dislocation of right patella**

     √7ᵗʰ **S83.095** Other **dislocation of left patella**

     √7ᵗʰ **S83.096** Other **dislocation of unspecified patella**

√5ᵗʰ **S83.1** Subluxation and dislocation of **knee**

     EXCLUDES 2   *instability of knee prosthesis (T84.022, T84.023)*

     √6ᵗʰ **S83.10** Unspecified **subluxation and dislocation of knee**

         √7ᵗʰ **S83.101** Unspecified **subluxation of right knee**

         √7ᵗʰ **S83.102** Unspecified **subluxation of left knee**

         √7ᵗʰ **S83.103** Unspecified **subluxation of unspecified knee**

         √7ᵗʰ **S83.104** Unspecified **dislocation of right knee**

         √7ᵗʰ **S83.105** Unspecified **dislocation of left knee**

         √7ᵗʰ **S83.106** Unspecified **dislocation of unspecified knee**

     √6ᵗʰ **S83.11** Anterior **subluxation and dislocation of proximal end of tibia**

         Posterior subluxation and dislocation of distal end of femur

         √7ᵗʰ **S83.111** Anterior **subluxation of proximal end of tibia, right knee**

         √7ᵗʰ **S83.112** Anterior **subluxation of proximal end of tibia, left knee**

         √7ᵗʰ **S83.113** Anterior **subluxation of proximal end of tibia, unspecified knee**

         √7ᵗʰ **S83.114** Anterior **dislocation of proximal end of tibia, right knee**

         √7ᵗʰ **S83.115** Anterior **dislocation of proximal end of tibia, left knee**

         √7ᵗʰ **S83.116** Anterior **dislocation of proximal end of tibia, unspecified knee**

     √6ᵗʰ **S83.12** Posterior **subluxation and dislocation of proximal end of tibia**

         Anterior dislocation of distal end of femur

         √7ᵗʰ **S83.121** Posterior **subluxation of proximal end of tibia, right knee**

         √7ᵗʰ **S83.122** Posterior **subluxation of proximal end of tibia, left knee**

         √7ᵗʰ **S83.123** Posterior **subluxation of proximal end of tibia, unspecified knee**

         √7ᵗʰ **S83.124** Posterior **dislocation of proximal end of tibia, right knee**

         √7ᵗʰ **S83.125** Posterior **dislocation of proximal end of tibia, left knee**

         √7ᵗʰ **S83.126** Posterior **dislocation of proximal end of tibia, unspecified knee**

     √6ᵗʰ **S83.13** Medial **subluxation and dislocation of proximal end of tibia**

         √7ᵗʰ **S83.131** Medial **subluxation of proximal end of tibia, right knee**

         √7ᵗʰ **S83.132** Medial **subluxation of proximal end of tibia, left knee**

         √7ᵗʰ **S83.133** Medial **subluxation of proximal end of tibia, unspecified knee**

         √7ᵗʰ **S83.134** Medial **dislocation of proximal end of tibia, right knee**

         √7ᵗʰ **S83.135** Medial **dislocation of proximal end of tibia, left knee**

         √7ᵗʰ **S83.136** Medial **dislocation of proximal end of tibia, unspecified knee**

     √6ᵗʰ **S83.14** Lateral **subluxation and dislocation of proximal end of tibia**

         √7ᵗʰ **S83.141** Lateral **subluxation of proximal end of tibia, right knee**

         √7ᵗʰ **S83.142** Lateral **subluxation of proximal end of tibia, left knee**

         √7ᵗʰ **S83.143** Lateral **subluxation of proximal end of tibia, unspecified knee**

         √7ᵗʰ **S83.144** Lateral **dislocation of proximal end of tibia, right knee**

         √7ᵗʰ **S83.145** Lateral **dislocation of proximal end of tibia, left knee**

         √7ᵗʰ **S83.146** Lateral **dislocation of proximal end of tibia, unspecified knee**

☑ Additional Character Required   √x7ᵗʰ Placeholder Alert   Manifestation   Unspecified Dx   ►◄ Revised Text   ● New Code   ▲ Revised Code Title

ICD-10-CM 2020   1057

√6ᵗʰ   **S83.19**   **Other subluxation and dislocation of** knee
- √7ᵗʰ   **S83.191**   **Other** subluxation **of right knee**
- √7ᵗʰ   **S83.192**   **Other** subluxation **of left knee**
- √7ᵗʰ   **S83.193**   **Other** subluxation **of unspecified knee**
- √7ᵗʰ   **S83.194**   **Other** dislocation **of right knee**
- √7ᵗʰ   **S83.195**   **Other** dislocation **of left knee**
- √7ᵗʰ   **S83.196**   **Other** dislocation **of unspecified knee**

√5ᵗʰ   **S83.2**   **Tear of meniscus, current injury**
> EXCLUDES 1   *old bucket-handle tear (M23.2)*
>
> **AHA:** 2019,2Q,26

√6ᵗʰ   **S83.20**   **Tear of unspecified meniscus, current injury**
     Tear of meniscus of knee NOS
- √7ᵗʰ   **S83.200**   **Bucket-handle tear of unspecified meniscus, current injury, right knee**
- √7ᵗʰ   **S83.201**   **Bucket-handle tear of unspecified meniscus, current injury, left knee**
- √7ᵗʰ   **S83.202**   **Bucket-handle tear of unspecified meniscus, current injury, unspecified knee**
- √7ᵗʰ   **S83.203**   **Other tear of unspecified meniscus, current injury, right knee**
- √7ᵗʰ   **S83.204**   **Other tear of unspecified meniscus, current injury, left knee**
- √7ᵗʰ   **S83.205**   **Other tear of unspecified meniscus, current injury, unspecified knee**
- √7ᵗʰ   **S83.206**   **Unspecified tear of unspecified meniscus, current injury, right knee**
- √7ᵗʰ   **S83.207**   **Unspecified tear of unspecified meniscus, current injury, left knee**
- √7ᵗʰ   **S83.209**   **Unspecified tear of unspecified meniscus, current injury, unspecified knee**

√6ᵗʰ   **S83.21**   **Bucket-handle tear of medial meniscus, current injury**
- √7ᵗʰ   **S83.211**   **Bucket-handle tear of medial meniscus, current injury, right knee**
- √7ᵗʰ   **S83.212**   **Bucket-handle tear of medial meniscus, current injury, left knee**
- √7ᵗʰ   **S83.219**   **Bucket-handle tear of medial meniscus, current injury, unspecified knee**

√6ᵗʰ   **S83.22**   **Peripheral tear of medial meniscus, current injury**
- √7ᵗʰ   **S83.221**   **Peripheral tear of medial meniscus, current injury, right knee**
- √7ᵗʰ   **S83.222**   **Peripheral tear of medial meniscus, current injury, left knee**
- √7ᵗʰ   **S83.229**   **Peripheral tear of medial meniscus, current injury, unspecified knee**

√6ᵗʰ   **S83.23**   **Complex tear of medial meniscus, current injury**
- √7ᵗʰ   **S83.231**   **Complex tear of medial meniscus, current injury, right knee**
- √7ᵗʰ   **S83.232**   **Complex tear of medial meniscus, current injury, left knee**
- √7ᵗʰ   **S83.239**   **Complex tear of medial meniscus, current injury, unspecified knee**

√6ᵗʰ   **S83.24**   **Other tear of medial meniscus, current injury**
- √7ᵗʰ   **S83.241**   **Other tear of medial meniscus, current injury, right knee**
- √7ᵗʰ   **S83.242**   **Other tear of medial meniscus, current injury, left knee**
- √7ᵗʰ   **S83.249**   **Other tear of medial meniscus, current injury, unspecified knee**

√6ᵗʰ   **S83.25**   **Bucket-handle tear of lateral meniscus, current injury**
- √7ᵗʰ   **S83.251**   **Bucket-handle tear of lateral meniscus, current injury, right knee**
- √7ᵗʰ   **S83.252**   **Bucket-handle tear of lateral meniscus, current injury, left knee**
- √7ᵗʰ   **S83.259**   **Bucket-handle tear of lateral meniscus, current injury, unspecified knee**

√6ᵗʰ   **S83.26**   **Peripheral tear of lateral meniscus, current injury**
- √7ᵗʰ   **S83.261**   **Peripheral tear of lateral meniscus, current injury, right knee**
- √7ᵗʰ   **S83.262**   **Peripheral tear of lateral meniscus, current injury, left knee**
- √7ᵗʰ   **S83.269**   **Peripheral tear of lateral meniscus, current injury, unspecified knee**

√6ᵗʰ   **S83.27**   **Complex tear of lateral meniscus, current injury**
- √7ᵗʰ   **S83.271**   **Complex tear of lateral meniscus, current injury, right knee**

- √7ᵗʰ   **S83.272**   **Complex tear of lateral meniscus, current injury, left knee**
- √7ᵗʰ   **S83.279**   **Complex tear of lateral meniscus, current injury, unspecified knee**

√6ᵗʰ   **S83.28**   **Other tear of lateral meniscus, current injury**
- √7ᵗʰ   **S83.281**   **Other tear of lateral meniscus, current injury, right knee**
- √7ᵗʰ   **S83.282**   **Other tear of lateral meniscus, current injury, left knee**
- √7ᵗʰ   **S83.289**   **Other tear of lateral meniscus, current injury, unspecified knee**

√5ᵗʰ   **S83.3**   **Tear of articular cartilage of knee, current**
- √×7ᵗʰ   **S83.30**   **Tear of articular cartilage of unspecified knee, current**
- √×7ᵗʰ   **S83.31**   **Tear of articular cartilage of right knee, current**
- √×7ᵗʰ   **S83.32**   **Tear of articular cartilage of left knee, current**

√5ᵗʰ   **S83.4**   **Sprain of collateral ligament of knee**
√6ᵗʰ   **S83.40**   **Sprain of unspecified collateral ligament of knee**
- √7ᵗʰ   **S83.401**   **Sprain of unspecified collateral ligament of right knee**
- √7ᵗʰ   **S83.402**   **Sprain of unspecified collateral ligament of left knee**
- √7ᵗʰ   **S83.409**   **Sprain of unspecified collateral ligament of unspecified knee**

√6ᵗʰ   **S83.41**   **Sprain of medial collateral ligament of knee**
     Sprain of tibial collateral ligament
- √7ᵗʰ   **S83.411**   **Sprain of medial collateral ligament of right knee**
- √7ᵗʰ   **S83.412**   **Sprain of medial collateral ligament of left knee**
- √7ᵗʰ   **S83.419**   **Sprain of medial collateral ligament of unspecified knee**

√6ᵗʰ   **S83.42**   **Sprain of lateral collateral ligament of knee**
     Sprain of fibular collateral ligament
- √7ᵗʰ   **S83.421**   **Sprain of lateral collateral ligament of right knee**
- √7ᵗʰ   **S83.422**   **Sprain of lateral collateral ligament of left knee**
- √7ᵗʰ   **S83.429**   **Sprain of lateral collateral ligament of unspecified knee**

√5ᵗʰ   **S83.5**   **Sprain of cruciate ligament of knee**
> **AHA:** 2016,2Q,3

√6ᵗʰ   **S83.50**   **Sprain of unspecified cruciate ligament of knee**
- √7ᵗʰ   **S83.501**   **Sprain of unspecified cruciate ligament of right knee**
- √7ᵗʰ   **S83.502**   **Sprain of unspecified cruciate ligament of left knee**
- √7ᵗʰ   **S83.509**   **Sprain of unspecified cruciate ligament of unspecified knee**

√6ᵗʰ   **S83.51**   **Sprain of anterior cruciate ligament of knee**
- √7ᵗʰ   **S83.511**   **Sprain of anterior cruciate ligament of right knee**
- √7ᵗʰ   **S83.512**   **Sprain of anterior cruciate ligament of left knee**
- √7ᵗʰ   **S83.519**   **Sprain of anterior cruciate ligament of unspecified knee**

√6ᵗʰ   **S83.52**   **Sprain of posterior cruciate ligament of knee**
- √7ᵗʰ   **S83.521**   **Sprain of posterior cruciate ligament of right knee**
- √7ᵗʰ   **S83.522**   **Sprain of posterior cruciate ligament of left knee**
- √7ᵗʰ   **S83.529**   **Sprain of posterior cruciate ligament of unspecified knee**

√5ᵗʰ   **S83.6**   **Sprain of the superior tibiofibular joint and ligament**
- √×7ᵗʰ   **S83.60**   **Sprain of the superior tibiofibular joint and ligament, unspecified knee**
- √×7ᵗʰ   **S83.61**   **Sprain of the superior tibiofibular joint and ligament, right knee**
- √×7ᵗʰ   **S83.62**   **Sprain of the superior tibiofibular joint and ligament, left knee**

√5ᵗʰ   **S83.8**   **Sprain of other specified parts of knee**
√6ᵗʰ   **S83.8X**   **Sprain of other specified parts of knee**
- √7ᵗʰ   **S83.8X1**   **Sprain of other specified parts of right knee**
- √7ᵗʰ   **S83.8X2**   **Sprain of other specified parts of left knee**
- √7ᵗʰ   **S83.8X9**   **Sprain of other specified parts of unspecified knee**

√5ᵗʰ **S83.9**   Sprain of unspecified site of knee
- √x7ᵗʰ **S83.90**   Sprain of unspecified site of unspecified knee
- √x7ᵗʰ **S83.91**   Sprain of unspecified site of right knee
- √x7ᵗʰ **S83.92**   Sprain of unspecified site of left knee

√4ᵗʰ **S84**   **Injury of nerves at lower leg level**
Code also any associated open wound (S81.-)
EXCLUDES 2   injury of nerves at ankle and foot level (S94.-)

The appropriate 7th character is to be added to each code from category S84.
A   initial encounter
D   subsequent encounter
S   sequela

√5ᵗʰ **S84.0**   Injury of tibial nerve at lower leg level
- √x7ᵗʰ **S84.00**   Injury of tibial nerve at lower leg level, unspecified leg
- √x7ᵗʰ **S84.01**   Injury of tibial nerve at lower leg level, right leg
- √x7ᵗʰ **S84.02**   Injury of tibial nerve at lower leg level, left leg

√5ᵗʰ **S84.1**   Injury of peroneal nerve at lower leg level
- √x7ᵗʰ **S84.10**   Injury of peroneal nerve at lower leg level, unspecified leg
- √x7ᵗʰ **S84.11**   Injury of peroneal nerve at lower leg level, right leg
- √x7ᵗʰ **S84.12**   Injury of peroneal nerve at lower leg level, left leg

√5ᵗʰ **S84.2**   Injury of cutaneous sensory nerve at lower leg level
- √x7ᵗʰ **S84.20**   Injury of cutaneous sensory nerve at lower leg level, unspecified leg
- √x7ᵗʰ **S84.21**   Injury of cutaneous sensory nerve at lower leg level, right leg
- √x7ᵗʰ **S84.22**   Injury of cutaneous sensory nerve at lower leg level, left leg

√5ᵗʰ **S84.8**   Injury of other nerves at lower leg level
- √6ᵗʰ **S84.80**   Injury of other nerves at lower leg level
  - √7ᵗʰ **S84.801**   Injury of other nerves at lower leg level, right leg
  - √7ᵗʰ **S84.802**   Injury of other nerves at lower leg level, left leg
  - √7ᵗʰ **S84.809**   Injury of other nerves at lower leg level, unspecified leg

√5ᵗʰ **S84.9**   Injury of unspecified nerve at lower leg level
- √x7ᵗʰ **S84.90**   Injury of unspecified nerve at lower leg level, unspecified leg
- √x7ᵗʰ **S84.91**   Injury of unspecified nerve at lower leg level, right leg
- √x7ᵗʰ **S84.92**   Injury of unspecified nerve at lower leg level, left leg

√4ᵗʰ **S85**   **Injury of blood vessels at lower leg level**
Code also any associated open wound (S81.-)
EXCLUDES 2   injury of blood vessels at ankle and foot level (S95.-)

The appropriate 7th character is to be added to each code from category S85.
A   initial encounter
D   subsequent encounter
S   sequela

√5ᵗʰ **S85.0**   Injury of popliteal artery
- √6ᵗʰ **S85.00**   Unspecified injury of popliteal artery
  - √7ᵗʰ **S85.001**   Unspecified injury of popliteal artery, right leg
  - √7ᵗʰ **S85.002**   Unspecified injury of popliteal artery, left leg
  - √7ᵗʰ **S85.009**   Unspecified injury of popliteal artery, unspecified leg
- √6ᵗʰ **S85.01**   Laceration of popliteal artery
  - √7ᵗʰ **S85.011**   Laceration of popliteal artery, right leg
  - √7ᵗʰ **S85.012**   Laceration of popliteal artery, left leg
  - √7ᵗʰ **S85.019**   Laceration of popliteal artery, unspecified leg
- √6ᵗʰ **S85.09**   Other specified injury of popliteal artery
  - √7ᵗʰ **S85.091**   Other specified injury of popliteal artery, right leg
  - √7ᵗʰ **S85.092**   Other specified injury of popliteal artery, left leg
  - √7ᵗʰ **S85.099**   Other specified injury of popliteal artery, unspecified leg

√5ᵗʰ **S85.1**   Injury of tibial artery
- √6ᵗʰ **S85.10**   Unspecified injury of unspecified tibial artery
  Injury of tibial artery NOS
  - √7ᵗʰ **S85.101**   Unspecified injury of unspecified tibial artery, right leg
  - √7ᵗʰ **S85.102**   Unspecified injury of unspecified tibial artery, left leg
  - √7ᵗʰ **S85.109**   Unspecified injury of unspecified tibial artery, unspecified leg
- √6ᵗʰ **S85.11**   Laceration of unspecified tibial artery
  - √7ᵗʰ **S85.111**   Laceration of unspecified tibial artery, right leg
  - √7ᵗʰ **S85.112**   Laceration of unspecified tibial artery, left leg
  - √7ᵗʰ **S85.119**   Laceration of unspecified tibial artery, unspecified leg
- √6ᵗʰ **S85.12**   Other specified injury of unspecified tibial artery
  - √7ᵗʰ **S85.121**   Other specified injury of unspecified tibial artery, right leg
  - √7ᵗʰ **S85.122**   Other specified injury of unspecified tibial artery, left leg
  - √7ᵗʰ **S85.129**   Other specified injury of unspecified tibial artery, unspecified leg
- √6ᵗʰ **S85.13**   Unspecified injury of anterior tibial artery
  - √7ᵗʰ **S85.131**   Unspecified injury of anterior tibial artery, right leg
  - √7ᵗʰ **S85.132**   Unspecified injury of anterior tibial artery, left leg
  - √7ᵗʰ **S85.139**   Unspecified injury of anterior tibial artery, unspecified leg
- √6ᵗʰ **S85.14**   Laceration of anterior tibial artery
  - √7ᵗʰ **S85.141**   Laceration of anterior tibial artery, right leg
  - √7ᵗʰ **S85.142**   Laceration of anterior tibial artery, left leg
  - √7ᵗʰ **S85.149**   Laceration of anterior tibial artery, unspecified leg
- √6ᵗʰ **S85.15**   Other specified injury of anterior tibial artery
  - √7ᵗʰ **S85.151**   Other specified injury of anterior tibial artery, right leg
  - √7ᵗʰ **S85.152**   Other specified injury of anterior tibial artery, left leg
  - √7ᵗʰ **S85.159**   Other specified injury of anterior tibial artery, unspecified leg
- √6ᵗʰ **S85.16**   Unspecified injury of posterior tibial artery
  - √7ᵗʰ **S85.161**   Unspecified injury of posterior tibial artery, right leg
  - √7ᵗʰ **S85.162**   Unspecified injury of posterior tibial artery, left leg
  - √7ᵗʰ **S85.169**   Unspecified injury of posterior tibial artery, unspecified leg
- √6ᵗʰ **S85.17**   Laceration of posterior tibial artery
  - √7ᵗʰ **S85.171**   Laceration of posterior tibial artery, right leg
  - √7ᵗʰ **S85.172**   Laceration of posterior tibial artery, left leg
  - √7ᵗʰ **S85.179**   Laceration of posterior tibial artery, unspecified leg
- √6ᵗʰ **S85.18**   Other specified injury of posterior tibial artery
  - √7ᵗʰ **S85.181**   Other specified injury of posterior tibial artery, right leg
  - √7ᵗʰ **S85.182**   Other specified injury of posterior tibial artery, left leg
  - √7ᵗʰ **S85.189**   Other specified injury of posterior tibial artery, unspecified leg

√5ᵗʰ **S85.2**   Injury of peroneal artery
- √6ᵗʰ **S85.20**   Unspecified injury of peroneal artery
  - √7ᵗʰ **S85.201**   Unspecified injury of peroneal artery, right leg
  - √7ᵗʰ **S85.202**   Unspecified injury of peroneal artery, left leg
  - √7ᵗʰ **S85.209**   Unspecified injury of peroneal artery, unspecified leg
- √6ᵗʰ **S85.21**   Laceration of peroneal artery
  - √7ᵗʰ **S85.211**   Laceration of peroneal artery, right leg
  - √7ᵗʰ **S85.212**   Laceration of peroneal artery, left leg
  - √7ᵗʰ **S85.219**   Laceration of peroneal artery, unspecified leg

---

☑ Additional Character Required   √x7ᵗʰ Placeholder Alert   Manifestation   Unspecified Dx   ▶◀ Revised Text   ● New Code   ▲ Revised Code Title

Chapter 19. Injury, Poisoning and Certain Other Consequences of External Causes

S85.29–S86.029

☑6ᵗʰ **S85.29** Other specified injury of peroneal artery

  ☑7ᵗʰ **S85.291** Other specified injury of peroneal artery, **right** leg

  ☑7ᵗʰ **S85.292** Other specified injury of peroneal artery, **left** leg

  ☑7ᵗʰ **S85.299** Other specified injury of peroneal artery, unspecified leg

☑5ᵗʰ **S85.3** Injury of greater saphenous vein at lower leg level

  Injury of greater saphenous vein NOS

  Injury of saphenous vein NOS

  ☑6ᵗʰ **S85.30** Unspecified injury of greater saphenous vein at lower leg level

    ☑7ᵗʰ **S85.301** Unspecified injury of greater saphenous vein at lower leg level, **right** leg

    ☑7ᵗʰ **S85.302** Unspecified injury of greater saphenous vein at lower leg level, **left** leg

    ☑7ᵗʰ **S85.309** Unspecified injury of greater saphenous vein at lower leg level, unspecified leg

  ☑6ᵗʰ **S85.31** Laceration of greater saphenous vein at lower leg level

    ☑7ᵗʰ **S85.311** Laceration of greater saphenous vein at lower leg level, **right** leg

    ☑7ᵗʰ **S85.312** Laceration of greater saphenous vein at lower leg level, **left** leg

    ☑7ᵗʰ **S85.319** Laceration of greater saphenous vein at lower leg level, unspecified leg

  ☑6ᵗʰ **S85.39** Other specified injury of greater saphenous vein at lower leg level

    ☑7ᵗʰ **S85.391** Other specified injury of greater saphenous vein at lower leg level, **right** leg

    ☑7ᵗʰ **S85.392** Other specified injury of greater saphenous vein at lower leg level, **left** leg

    ☑7ᵗʰ **S85.399** Other specified injury of greater saphenous vein at lower leg level, unspecified leg

☑5ᵗʰ **S85.4** Injury of lesser saphenous vein at lower leg level

  ☑6ᵗʰ **S85.40** Unspecified injury of lesser saphenous vein at lower leg level

    ☑7ᵗʰ **S85.401** Unspecified injury of lesser saphenous vein at lower leg level, **right** leg

    ☑7ᵗʰ **S85.402** Unspecified injury of lesser saphenous vein at lower leg level, **left** leg

    ☑7ᵗʰ **S85.409** Unspecified injury of lesser saphenous vein at lower leg level, unspecified leg

  ☑6ᵗʰ **S85.41** Laceration of lesser saphenous vein at lower leg level

    ☑7ᵗʰ **S85.411** Laceration of lesser saphenous vein at lower leg level, **right** leg

    ☑7ᵗʰ **S85.412** Laceration of lesser saphenous vein at lower leg level, **left** leg

    ☑7ᵗʰ **S85.419** Laceration of lesser saphenous vein at lower leg level, unspecified leg

  ☑6ᵗʰ **S85.49** Other specified injury of lesser saphenous vein at lower leg level

    ☑7ᵗʰ **S85.491** Other specified injury of lesser saphenous vein at lower leg level, **right** leg

    ☑7ᵗʰ **S85.492** Other specified injury of lesser saphenous vein at lower leg level, **left** leg

    ☑7ᵗʰ **S85.499** Other specified injury of lesser saphenous vein at lower leg level, unspecified leg

☑5ᵗʰ **S85.5** Injury of popliteal vein

  ☑6ᵗʰ **S85.50** Unspecified injury of popliteal vein

    ☑7ᵗʰ **S85.501** Unspecified injury of popliteal vein, **right** leg

    ☑7ᵗʰ **S85.502** Unspecified injury of popliteal vein, **left** leg

    ☑7ᵗʰ **S85.509** Unspecified injury of popliteal vein, unspecified leg

  ☑6ᵗʰ **S85.51** Laceration of popliteal vein

    ☑7ᵗʰ **S85.511** Laceration of popliteal vein, **right** leg

    ☑7ᵗʰ **S85.512** Laceration of popliteal vein, **left** leg

    ☑7ᵗʰ **S85.519** Laceration of popliteal vein, unspecified leg

  ☑6ᵗʰ **S85.59** Other specified injury of popliteal vein

    ☑7ᵗʰ **S85.591** Other specified injury of popliteal vein, **right** leg

    ☑7ᵗʰ **S85.592** Other specified injury of popliteal vein, **left** leg

    ☑7ᵗʰ **S85.599** Other specified injury of popliteal vein, unspecified leg

☑5ᵗʰ **S85.8** Injury of other blood vessels at lower leg level

  ☑6ᵗʰ **S85.80** Unspecified injury of other blood vessels at lower leg level

    ☑7ᵗʰ **S85.801** Unspecified injury of other blood vessels at lower leg level, **right** leg

    ☑7ᵗʰ **S85.802** Unspecified injury of other blood vessels at lower leg level, **left** leg

    ☑7ᵗʰ **S85.809** Unspecified injury of other blood vessels at lower leg level, unspecified leg

  ☑6ᵗʰ **S85.81** Laceration of other blood vessels at lower leg level

    ☑7ᵗʰ **S85.811** Laceration of other blood vessels at lower leg level, **right** leg

    ☑7ᵗʰ **S85.812** Laceration of other blood vessels at lower leg level, **left** leg

    ☑7ᵗʰ **S85.819** Laceration of other blood vessels at lower leg level, unspecified leg

  ☑6ᵗʰ **S85.89** Other specified injury of other blood vessels at lower leg level

    ☑7ᵗʰ **S85.891** Other specified injury of other blood vessels at lower leg level, **right** leg

    ☑7ᵗʰ **S85.892** Other specified injury of other blood vessels at lower leg level, **left** leg

    ☑7ᵗʰ **S85.899** Other specified injury of other blood vessels at lower leg level, unspecified leg

☑5ᵗʰ **S85.9** Injury of unspecified blood vessel at lower leg level

  ☑6ᵗʰ **S85.90** Unspecified injury of unspecified blood vessel at lower leg level

    ☑7ᵗʰ **S85.901** Unspecified injury of unspecified blood vessel at lower leg level, **right** leg

    ☑7ᵗʰ **S85.902** Unspecified injury of unspecified blood vessel at lower leg level, **left** leg

    ☑7ᵗʰ **S85.909** Unspecified injury of unspecified blood vessel at lower leg level, unspecified leg

  ☑6ᵗʰ **S85.91** Laceration of unspecified blood vessel at lower leg level

    ☑7ᵗʰ **S85.911** Laceration of unspecified blood vessel at lower leg level, **right** leg

    ☑7ᵗʰ **S85.912** Laceration of unspecified blood vessel at lower leg level, **left** leg

    ☑7ᵗʰ **S85.919** Laceration of unspecified blood vessel at lower leg level, unspecified leg

  ☑6ᵗʰ **S85.99** Other specified injury of unspecified blood vessel at lower leg level

    ☑7ᵗʰ **S85.991** Other specified injury of unspecified blood vessel at lower leg level, **right** leg

    ☑7ᵗʰ **S85.992** Other specified injury of unspecified blood vessel at lower leg level, **left** leg

    ☑7ᵗʰ **S85.999** Other specified injury of unspecified blood vessel at lower leg level, unspecified leg

☑4ᵗʰ **S86** Injury of muscle, fascia and tendon at lower leg level

  Code also any associated open wound (S81.-)

  EXCLUDES 2   injury of muscle, fascia and tendon at ankle (S96.-)

           injury of patellar ligament (tendon) (S76.1-)

           sprain of joints and ligaments of knee (S83.-)

  TIP: Refer to the Muscle/Tendon table at the beginning of this chapter.

  The appropriate 7th character is to be added to each code from category S86.

  A   initial encounter

  D   subsequent encounter

  S   sequela

☑5ᵗʰ **S86.0** Injury of Achilles tendon

  ☑6ᵗʰ **S86.00** Unspecified injury of Achilles tendon

    ☑7ᵗʰ **S86.001** Unspecified injury of **right** Achilles tendon

    ☑7ᵗʰ **S86.002** Unspecified injury of **left** Achilles tendon

    ☑7ᵗʰ **S86.009** Unspecified injury of unspecified Achilles tendon

  ☑6ᵗʰ **S86.01** Strain of Achilles tendon

    ☑7ᵗʰ **S86.011** Strain of **right** Achilles tendon

    ☑7ᵗʰ **S86.012** Strain of **left** Achilles tendon

    ☑7ᵗʰ **S86.019** Strain of unspecified Achilles tendon

  ☑6ᵗʰ **S86.02** Laceration of Achilles tendon

    ☑7ᵗʰ **S86.021** Laceration of **right** Achilles tendon

    ☑7ᵗʰ **S86.022** Laceration of **left** Achilles tendon

    ☑7ᵗʰ **S86.029** Laceration of unspecified Achilles tendon

√6ᵗʰ **S86.09** Other specified injury of Achilles tendon

    √7ᵗʰ **S86.091** Other specified injury of right Achilles tendon

    √7ᵗʰ **S86.092** Other specified injury of left Achilles tendon

    √7ᵗʰ **S86.099** Other specified injury of unspecified Achilles tendon

√5ᵗʰ **S86.1** Injury of other muscle(s) and tendon(s) of posterior muscle group at lower leg level

    √6ᵗʰ **S86.10** Unspecified injury of other muscle(s) and tendon(s) of posterior muscle group at lower leg level

      √7ᵗʰ **S86.101** Unspecified injury of other muscle(s) and tendon(s) of posterior muscle group at lower leg level, right leg

      √7ᵗʰ **S86.102** Unspecified injury of other muscle(s) and tendon(s) of posterior muscle group at lower leg level, left leg

      √7ᵗʰ **S86.109** Unspecified injury of other muscle(s) and tendon(s) of posterior muscle group at lower leg level, unspecified leg

    √6ᵗʰ **S86.11** Strain of other muscle(s) and tendon(s) of posterior muscle group at lower leg level

      √7ᵗʰ **S86.111** Strain of other muscle(s) and tendon(s) of posterior muscle group at lower leg level, right leg

      √7ᵗʰ **S86.112** Strain of other muscle(s) and tendon(s) of posterior muscle group at lower leg level, left leg

      √7ᵗʰ **S86.119** Strain of other muscle(s) and tendon(s) of posterior muscle group at lower leg level, unspecified leg

    √6ᵗʰ **S86.12** Laceration of other muscle(s) and tendon(s) of posterior muscle group at lower leg level

      √7ᵗʰ **S86.121** Laceration of other muscle(s) and tendon(s) of posterior muscle group at lower leg level, right leg

      √7ᵗʰ **S86.122** Laceration of other muscle(s) and tendon(s) of posterior muscle group at lower leg level, left leg

      √7ᵗʰ **S86.129** Laceration of other muscle(s) and tendon(s) of posterior muscle group at lower leg level, unspecified leg

    √6ᵗʰ **S86.19** Other injury of other muscle(s) and tendon(s) of posterior muscle group at lower leg level

      √7ᵗʰ **S86.191** Other injury of other muscle(s) and tendon(s) of posterior muscle group at lower leg level, right leg

      √7ᵗʰ **S86.192** Other injury of other muscle(s) and tendon(s) of posterior muscle group at lower leg level, left leg

      √7ᵗʰ **S86.199** Other injury of other muscle(s) and tendon(s) of posterior muscle group at lower leg level, unspecified leg

√5ᵗʰ **S86.2** Injury of muscle(s) and tendon(s) of anterior muscle group at lower leg level

    √6ᵗʰ **S86.20** Unspecified injury of muscle(s) and tendon(s) of anterior muscle group at lower leg level

      √7ᵗʰ **S86.201** Unspecified injury of muscle(s) and tendon(s) of anterior muscle group at lower leg level, right leg

      √7ᵗʰ **S86.202** Unspecified injury of muscle(s) and tendon(s) of anterior muscle group at lower leg level, left leg

      √7ᵗʰ **S86.209** Unspecified injury of muscle(s) and tendon(s) of anterior muscle group at lower leg level, unspecified leg

    √6ᵗʰ **S86.21** Strain of muscle(s) and tendon(s) of anterior muscle group at lower leg level

      √7ᵗʰ **S86.211** Strain of muscle(s) and tendon(s) of anterior muscle group at lower leg level, right leg

      √7ᵗʰ **S86.212** Strain of muscle(s) and tendon(s) of anterior muscle group at lower leg level, left leg

      √7ᵗʰ **S86.219** Strain of muscle(s) and tendon(s) of anterior muscle group at lower leg level, unspecified leg

    √6ᵗʰ **S86.22** Laceration of muscle(s) and tendon(s) of anterior muscle group at lower leg level

      √7ᵗʰ **S86.221** Laceration of muscle(s) and tendon(s) of anterior muscle group at lower leg level, right leg

      √7ᵗʰ **S86.222** Laceration of muscle(s) and tendon(s) of anterior muscle group at lower leg level, left leg

      √7ᵗʰ **S86.229** Laceration of muscle(s) and tendon(s) of anterior muscle group at lower leg level, unspecified leg

    √6ᵗʰ **S86.29** Other injury of muscle(s) and tendon(s) of anterior muscle group at lower leg level

      √7ᵗʰ **S86.291** Other injury of muscle(s) and tendon(s) of anterior muscle group at lower leg level, right leg

      √7ᵗʰ **S86.292** Other injury of muscle(s) and tendon(s) of anterior muscle group at lower leg level, left leg

      √7ᵗʰ **S86.299** Other injury of muscle(s) and tendon(s) of anterior muscle group at lower leg level, unspecified leg

√5ᵗʰ **S86.3** Injury of muscle(s) and tendon(s) of peroneal muscle group at lower leg level

    √6ᵗʰ **S86.30** Unspecified injury of muscle(s) and tendon(s) of peroneal muscle group at lower leg level

      √7ᵗʰ **S86.301** Unspecified injury of muscle(s) and tendon(s) of peroneal muscle group at lower leg level, right leg

      √7ᵗʰ **S86.302** Unspecified injury of muscle(s) and tendon(s) of peroneal muscle group at lower leg level, left leg

      √7ᵗʰ **S86.309** Unspecified injury of muscle(s) and tendon(s) of peroneal muscle group at lower leg level, unspecified leg

    √6ᵗʰ **S86.31** Strain of muscle(s) and tendon(s) of peroneal muscle group at lower leg level

      √7ᵗʰ **S86.311** Strain of muscle(s) and tendon(s) of peroneal muscle group at lower leg level, right leg

      √7ᵗʰ **S86.312** Strain of muscle(s) and tendon(s) of peroneal muscle group at lower leg level, left leg

      √7ᵗʰ **S86.319** Strain of muscle(s) and tendon(s) of peroneal muscle group at lower leg level, unspecified leg

    √6ᵗʰ **S86.32** Laceration of muscle(s) and tendon(s) of peroneal muscle group at lower leg level

      √7ᵗʰ **S86.321** Laceration of muscle(s) and tendon(s) of peroneal muscle group at lower leg level, right leg

      √7ᵗʰ **S86.322** Laceration of muscle(s) and tendon(s) of peroneal muscle group at lower leg level, left leg

      √7ᵗʰ **S86.329** Laceration of muscle(s) and tendon(s) of peroneal muscle group at lower leg level, unspecified leg

    √6ᵗʰ **S86.39** Other injury of muscle(s) and tendon(s) of peroneal muscle group at lower leg level

      √7ᵗʰ **S86.391** Other injury of muscle(s) and tendon(s) of peroneal muscle group at lower leg level, right leg

      √7ᵗʰ **S86.392** Other injury of muscle(s) and tendon(s) of peroneal muscle group at lower leg level, left leg

      √7ᵗʰ **S86.399** Other injury of muscle(s) and tendon(s) of peroneal muscle group at lower leg level, unspecified leg

√5ᵗʰ **S86.8** Injury of other muscles and tendons at lower leg level

    √6ᵗʰ **S86.80** Unspecified injury of other muscles and tendons at lower leg level

      √7ᵗʰ **S86.801** Unspecified injury of other muscle(s) and tendon(s) at lower leg level, right leg

      √7ᵗʰ **S86.802** Unspecified injury of other muscle(s) and tendon(s) at lower leg level, left leg

      √7ᵗʰ **S86.809** Unspecified injury of other muscle(s) and tendon(s) at lower leg level, unspecified leg

    √6ᵗʰ **S86.81** Strain of other muscles and tendons at lower leg level

      √7ᵗʰ **S86.811** Strain of other muscle(s) and tendon(s) at lower leg level, right leg

      √7ᵗʰ **S86.812** Strain of other muscle(s) and tendon(s) at lower leg level, left leg

      √7ᵗʰ **S86.819** Strain of other muscle(s) and tendon(s) at lower leg level, unspecified leg

---

☑ Additional Character Required   √x7ᵗʰ Placeholder Alert   Manifestation   Unspecified Dx   ▶◀ Revised Text   ● New Code   ▲ Revised Code Title

√6ᵗʰ **S86.82 Laceration** of other muscles and tendons at lower leg level

    √7ᵗʰ **S86.821 Laceration** of other muscle(s) and tendon(s) at lower leg level, **right** leg

    √7ᵗʰ **S86.822 Laceration** of other muscle(s) and tendon(s) at lower leg level, **left** leg

    √7ᵗʰ **S86.829 Laceration** of other muscle(s) and tendon(s) at lower leg level, **unspecified** leg

√6ᵗʰ **S86.89 Other injury** of other muscles and tendons at lower leg level

    √7ᵗʰ **S86.891 Other injury** of other muscle(s) and tendon(s) at lower leg level, **right** leg

    √7ᵗʰ **S86.892 Other injury** of other muscle(s) and tendon(s) at lower leg level, **left** leg

    √7ᵗʰ **S86.899 Other injury** of other muscle(s) and tendon(s) at lower leg level, **unspecified** leg

√5ᵗʰ **S86.9 Injury of unspecified muscle and tendon at lower leg level**

    √6ᵗʰ **S86.90 Unspecified injury** of unspecified muscle and tendon at lower leg level

      √7ᵗʰ **S86.901 Unspecified injury** of unspecified muscle(s) and tendon(s) at lower leg level, **right** leg

      √7ᵗʰ **S86.902 Unspecified injury** of unspecified muscle(s) and tendon(s) at lower leg level, **left** leg

      √7ᵗʰ **S86.909 Unspecified injury** of unspecified muscle(s) and tendon(s) at lower leg level, **unspecified** leg

    √6ᵗʰ **S86.91 Strain** of unspecified muscle and tendon at lower leg level

      √7ᵗʰ **S86.911 Strain** of unspecified muscle(s) and tendon(s) at lower leg level, **right** leg

      √7ᵗʰ **S86.912 Strain** of unspecified muscle(s) and tendon(s) at lower leg level, **left** leg

      √7ᵗʰ **S86.919 Strain** of unspecified muscle(s) and tendon(s) at lower leg level, **unspecified** leg

    √6ᵗʰ **S86.92 Laceration** of unspecified muscle and tendon at lower leg level

      √7ᵗʰ **S86.921 Laceration** of unspecified muscle(s) and tendon(s) at lower leg level, **right** leg

      √7ᵗʰ **S86.922 Laceration** of unspecified muscle(s) and tendon(s) at lower leg level, **left** leg

      √7ᵗʰ **S86.929 Laceration** of unspecified muscle(s) and tendon(s) at lower leg level, **unspecified** leg

    √6ᵗʰ **S86.99 Other injury** of unspecified muscle and tendon at lower leg level

      √7ᵗʰ **S86.991 Other injury** of unspecified muscle(s) and tendon(s) at lower leg level, **right** leg

      √7ᵗʰ **S86.992 Other injury** of unspecified muscle(s) and tendon(s) at lower leg level, **left** leg

      √7ᵗʰ **S86.999 Other injury** of unspecified muscle(s) and tendon(s) at lower leg level, **unspecified** leg

√4ᵗʰ **S87 Crushing injury of lower leg**

Use additional code(s) for all associated injuries

EXCLUDES 2   crushing injury of ankle and foot (S97.-)

> The appropriate 7th character is to be added to each code from category S87.
> A   initial encounter
> D   subsequent encounter
> S   sequela

√5ᵗʰ **S87.0 Crushing injury of knee**

    √x7ᵗʰ **S87.00 Crushing injury of unspecified knee**

    √x7ᵗʰ **S87.01 Crushing injury of right knee**

    √x7ᵗʰ **S87.02 Crushing injury of left knee**

√5ᵗʰ **S87.8 Crushing injury of lower leg**

    √x7ᵗʰ **S87.80 Crushing injury of unspecified lower leg**

    √x7ᵗʰ **S87.81 Crushing injury of right lower leg**

    √x7ᵗʰ **S87.82 Crushing injury of left lower leg**

√4ᵗʰ **S88 Traumatic amputation of lower leg**

An amputation not identified as partial or complete should be coded to complete

EXCLUDES 1   traumatic amputation of ankle and foot (S98.-)

> The appropriate 7th character is to be added to each code from category S88.
> A   initial encounter
> D   subsequent encounter
> S   sequela

√5ᵗʰ **S88.0 Traumatic amputation at knee level**

    √6ᵗʰ **S88.01 Complete** traumatic amputation at knee level

      √7ᵗʰ **S88.011 Complete** traumatic amputation at knee level, **right** lower leg   HCC

      √7ᵗʰ **S88.012 Complete** traumatic amputation at knee level, **left** lower leg   HCC

      √7ᵗʰ **S88.019 Complete** traumatic amputation at knee level, **unspecified** lower leg   HCC

    √6ᵗʰ **S88.02 Partial** traumatic amputation at knee level

      √7ᵗʰ **S88.021 Partial** traumatic amputation at knee level, **right** lower leg   HCC

      √7ᵗʰ **S88.022 Partial** traumatic amputation at knee level, **left** lower leg   HCC

      √7ᵗʰ **S88.029 Partial** traumatic amputation at knee level, **unspecified** lower leg   HCC

√5ᵗʰ **S88.1 Traumatic amputation at level between knee and ankle**

    √6ᵗʰ **S88.11 Complete** traumatic amputation at level between knee and ankle

      √7ᵗʰ **S88.111 Complete** traumatic amputation at level between knee and ankle, **right** lower leg   HCC

      √7ᵗʰ **S88.112 Complete** traumatic amputation at level between knee and ankle, **left** lower leg   HCC

      √7ᵗʰ **S88.119 Complete** traumatic amputation at level between knee and ankle, **unspecified** lower leg   HCC

    √6ᵗʰ **S88.12 Partial** traumatic amputation at level between knee and ankle

      √7ᵗʰ **S88.121 Partial** traumatic amputation at level between knee and ankle, **right** lower leg   HCC

      √7ᵗʰ **S88.122 Partial** traumatic amputation at level between knee and ankle, **left** lower leg   HCC

      √7ᵗʰ **S88.129 Partial** traumatic amputation at level between knee and ankle, **unspecified** lower leg   HCC

√5ᵗʰ **S88.9 Traumatic amputation of lower leg, level unspecified**

    √6ᵗʰ **S88.91 Complete** traumatic amputation of lower leg, level unspecified

      √7ᵗʰ **S88.911 Complete** traumatic amputation of **right** lower leg, level unspecified   HCC

      √7ᵗʰ **S88.912 Complete** traumatic amputation of **left** lower leg, level unspecified   HCC

      √7ᵗʰ **S88.919 Complete** traumatic amputation of **unspecified** lower leg, level unspecified   HCC

    √6ᵗʰ **S88.92 Partial** traumatic amputation of lower leg, level unspecified

      √7ᵗʰ **S88.921 Partial** traumatic amputation of **right** lower leg, level unspecified   HCC

      √7ᵗʰ **S88.922 Partial** traumatic amputation of **left** lower leg, level unspecified   HCC

      √7ᵗʰ **S88.929 Partial** traumatic amputation of **unspecified** lower leg, level unspecified   HCC

✓4th **S89 Other and unspecified injuries of lower leg**

> **NOTE**   A fracture not indicated as open or closed should be coded to closed.

> EXCLUDES 2   *other and unspecified injuries of ankle and foot (S99.-)*

> **AHA:** 2018,2Q,12; 2018,1Q,3; 2015,3Q,37-39

> The appropriate 7th character is to be added to each code from subcategories S89.0, S89.1, S89.2, and S89.3.
> A   initial encounter for closed fracture
> D   subsequent encounter for fracture with routine healing
> G   subsequent encounter for fracture with delayed healing
> K   subsequent encounter for fracture with nonunion
> P   subsequent encounter for fracture with malunion
> S   sequela

✓5th **S89.0 Physeal fracture of upper end of tibia**

   ✓6th **S89.00 Unspecified physeal fracture of upper end of tibia**
     ✓7th **S89.001 Unspecified physeal fracture of upper end of right tibia** Q
     ✓7th **S89.002 Unspecified physeal fracture of upper end of left tibia** Q
     ✓7th **S89.009 Unspecified physeal fracture of upper end of unspecified tibia** Q

   ✓6th **S89.01 Salter-Harris Type I physeal fracture of upper end of tibia**
     ✓7th **S89.011 Salter-Harris Type I physeal fracture of upper end of right tibia** Q
     ✓7th **S89.012 Salter-Harris Type I physeal fracture of upper end of left tibia** Q
     ✓7th **S89.019 Salter-Harris Type I physeal fracture of upper end of unspecified tibia** Q

   ✓6th **S89.02 Salter-Harris Type II physeal fracture of upper end of tibia**
     ✓7th **S89.021 Salter-Harris Type II physeal fracture of upper end of right tibia** Q
     ✓7th **S89.022 Salter-Harris Type II physeal fracture of upper end of left tibia** Q
     ✓7th **S89.029 Salter-Harris Type II physeal fracture of upper end of unspecified tibia** Q

   ✓6th **S89.03 Salter-Harris Type III physeal fracture of upper end of tibia**
     ✓7th **S89.031 Salter-Harris Type III physeal fracture of upper end of right tibia** Q
     ✓7th **S89.032 Salter-Harris Type III physeal fracture of upper end of left tibia** Q
     ✓7th **S89.039 Salter-Harris Type III physeal fracture of upper end of unspecified tibia** Q

   ✓6th **S89.04 Salter-Harris Type IV physeal fracture of upper end of tibia**
     ✓7th **S89.041 Salter-Harris Type IV physeal fracture of upper end of right tibia** Q
     ✓7th **S89.042 Salter-Harris Type IV physeal fracture of upper end of left tibia** Q
     ✓7th **S89.049 Salter-Harris Type IV physeal fracture of upper end of unspecified tibia** Q

   ✓6th **S89.09 Other physeal fracture of upper end of tibia**
     ✓7th **S89.091 Other physeal fracture of upper end of right tibia** Q
     ✓7th **S89.092 Other physeal fracture of upper end of left tibia** Q
     ✓7th **S89.099 Other physeal fracture of upper end of unspecified tibia** Q

✓5th **S89.1 Physeal fracture of lower end of tibia**

   ✓6th **S89.10 Unspecified physeal fracture of lower end of tibia**
     ✓7th **S89.101 Unspecified physeal fracture of lower end of right tibia** Q
     ✓7th **S89.102 Unspecified physeal fracture of lower end of left tibia** Q
     ✓7th **S89.109 Unspecified physeal fracture of lower end of unspecified tibia** Q

   ✓6th **S89.11 Salter-Harris Type I physeal fracture of lower end of tibia**
     ✓7th **S89.111 Salter-Harris Type I physeal fracture of lower end of right tibia** Q

     ✓7th **S89.112 Salter-Harris Type I physeal fracture of lower end of left tibia** Q
     ✓7th **S89.119 Salter-Harris Type I physeal fracture of lower end of unspecified tibia** Q

   ✓6th **S89.12 Salter-Harris Type II physeal fracture of lower end of tibia**
     ✓7th **S89.121 Salter-Harris Type II physeal fracture of lower end of right tibia** Q
     ✓7th **S89.122 Salter-Harris Type II physeal fracture of lower end of left tibia** Q
     ✓7th **S89.129 Salter-Harris Type II physeal fracture of lower end of unspecified tibia** Q

   ✓6th **S89.13 Salter-Harris Type III physeal fracture of lower end of tibia**
     EXCLUDES 1   *fracture of medial malleolus (adult) (S82.5-)*
     ✓7th **S89.131 Salter-Harris Type III physeal fracture of lower end of right tibia** Q
     ✓7th **S89.132 Salter-Harris Type III physeal fracture of lower end of left tibia** Q
     ✓7th **S89.139 Salter-Harris Type III physeal fracture of lower end of unspecified tibia** Q

   ✓6th **S89.14 Salter-Harris Type IV physeal fracture of lower end of tibia**
     EXCLUDES 1   *fracture of medial malleolus (adult) (S82.5-)*
     ✓7th **S89.141 Salter-Harris Type IV physeal fracture of lower end of right tibia** Q
     ✓7th **S89.142 Salter-Harris Type IV physeal fracture of lower end of left tibia** Q
     ✓7th **S89.149 Salter-Harris Type IV physeal fracture of lower end of unspecified tibia** Q

   ✓6th **S89.19 Other physeal fracture of lower end of tibia**
     ✓7th **S89.191 Other physeal fracture of lower end of right tibia** Q
     ✓7th **S89.192 Other physeal fracture of lower end of left tibia** Q
     ✓7th **S89.199 Other physeal fracture of lower end of unspecified tibia** Q

✓5th **S89.2 Physeal fracture of upper end of fibula**

   ✓6th **S89.20 Unspecified physeal fracture of upper end of fibula**
     ✓7th **S89.201 Unspecified physeal fracture of upper end of right fibula** Q
     ✓7th **S89.202 Unspecified physeal fracture of upper end of left fibula** Q
     ✓7th **S89.209 Unspecified physeal fracture of upper end of unspecified fibula** Q

   ✓6th **S89.21 Salter-Harris Type I physeal fracture of upper end of fibula**
     ✓7th **S89.211 Salter-Harris Type I physeal fracture of upper end of right fibula** Q
     ✓7th **S89.212 Salter-Harris Type I physeal fracture of upper end of left fibula** Q
     ✓7th **S89.219 Salter-Harris Type I physeal fracture of upper end of unspecified fibula** Q

   ✓6th **S89.22 Salter-Harris Type II physeal fracture of upper end of fibula**
     ✓7th **S89.221 Salter-Harris Type II physeal fracture of upper end of right fibula** Q
     ✓7th **S89.222 Salter-Harris Type II physeal fracture of upper end of left fibula** Q
     ✓7th **S89.229 Salter-Harris Type II physeal fracture of upper end of unspecified fibula** Q

   ✓6th **S89.29 Other physeal fracture of upper end of fibula**
     ✓7th **S89.291 Other physeal fracture of upper end of right fibula** Q
     ✓7th **S89.292 Other physeal fracture of upper end of left fibula** Q
     ✓7th **S89.299 Other physeal fracture of upper end of unspecified fibula** Q

✓5th **S89.3 Physeal fracture of lower end of fibula**

   ✓6th **S89.30 Unspecified physeal fracture of lower end of fibula**
     ✓7th **S89.301 Unspecified physeal fracture of lower end of right fibula** Q

✓ Additional Character Required   ✓x7th Placeholder Alert   Manifestation   Unspecified Dx   ▶◀ Revised Text   ● New Code   ▲ Revised Code Title

√7ᵗʰ **S89.302** Unspecified physeal fracture of lower end of left fibula Q

√7ᵗʰ **S89.309** Unspecified physeal fracture of lower end of unspecified fibula Q

√6ᵗʰ **S89.31** Salter-Harris Type I physeal fracture of lower end of fibula

√7ᵗʰ **S89.311** Salter-Harris Type I physeal fracture of lower end of right fibula Q

√7ᵗʰ **S89.312** Salter-Harris Type I physeal fracture of lower end of left fibula Q

√7ᵗʰ **S89.319** Salter-Harris Type I physeal fracture of lower end of unspecified fibula Q

√6ᵗʰ **S89.32** Salter-Harris Type II physeal fracture of lower end of fibula

√7ᵗʰ **S89.321** Salter-Harris Type II physeal fracture of lower end of right fibula Q

√7ᵗʰ **S89.322** Salter-Harris Type II physeal fracture of lower end of left fibula Q

√7ᵗʰ **S89.329** Salter-Harris Type II physeal fracture of lower end of unspecified fibula Q

√6ᵗʰ **S89.39** Other physeal fracture of lower end of fibula

√7ᵗʰ **S89.391** Other physeal fracture of lower end of right fibula Q

√7ᵗʰ **S89.392** Other physeal fracture of lower end of left fibula Q

√7ᵗʰ **S89.399** Other physeal fracture of lower end of unspecified fibula Q

√5ᵗʰ **S89.8** Other specified injuries of lower leg

The appropriate 7th character is to be added to each code in subcategory S89.8.
A   initial encounter
D   subsequent encounter
S   sequela

√7ᵗʰ **S89.80** Other specified injuries of unspecified lower leg

√7ᵗʰ **S89.81** Other specified injuries of right lower leg

√7ᵗʰ **S89.82** Other specified injuries of left lower leg

√5ᵗʰ **S89.9** Unspecified injury of lower leg

The appropriate 7th character is to be added to each code in subcategory S89.9.
A   initial encounter
D   subsequent encounter
S   sequela

√7ᵗʰ **S89.90** Unspecified injury of unspecified lower leg

√7ᵗʰ **S89.91** Unspecified injury of right lower leg

√7ᵗʰ **S89.92** Unspecified injury of left lower leg

Injuries to the ankle and foot (S90-S99)

EXCLUDES 2   *burns and corrosions (T20-T32)*
fracture of ankle and malleolus (S82.-)
frostbite (T33-T34)
insect bite or sting, venomous (T63.4)

√4ᵗʰ **S90** Superficial injury of ankle, foot and toes

The appropriate 7th character is to be added to each code from category S90.
A   initial encounter
D   subsequent encounter
S   sequela

√5ᵗʰ **S90.0** Contusion of ankle

√7ᵗʰ **S90.00** Contusion of unspecified ankle

√7ᵗʰ **S90.01** Contusion of right ankle

√7ᵗʰ **S90.02** Contusion of left ankle

√5ᵗʰ **S90.1** Contusion of toe without damage to nail

√6ᵗʰ **S90.11** Contusion of great toe without damage to nail

√7ᵗʰ **S90.111** Contusion of right great toe without damage to nail

√7ᵗʰ **S90.112** Contusion of left great toe without damage to nail

√7ᵗʰ **S90.119** Contusion of unspecified great toe without damage to nail

√6ᵗʰ **S90.12** Contusion of lesser toe without damage to nail

√7ᵗʰ **S90.121** Contusion of right lesser toe(s) without damage to nail

√7ᵗʰ **S90.122** Contusion of left lesser toe(s) without damage to nail

√7ᵗʰ **S90.129** Contusion of unspecified lesser toe(s) without damage to nail
Contusion of toe NOS

√5ᵗʰ **S90.2** Contusion of toe with damage to nail

√6ᵗʰ **S90.21** Contusion of great toe with damage to nail

√7ᵗʰ **S90.211** Contusion of right great toe with damage to nail

√7ᵗʰ **S90.212** Contusion of left great toe with damage to nail

√7ᵗʰ **S90.219** Contusion of unspecified great toe with damage to nail

√6ᵗʰ **S90.22** Contusion of lesser toe with damage to nail

√7ᵗʰ **S90.221** Contusion of right lesser toe(s) with damage to nail

√7ᵗʰ **S90.222** Contusion of left lesser toe(s) with damage to nail

√7ᵗʰ **S90.229** Contusion of unspecified lesser toe(s) with damage to nail

√5ᵗʰ **S90.3** Contusion of foot

EXCLUDES 2   *contusion of toes (S90.1-, S90.2-)*

√x7ᵗʰ **S90.30** Contusion of unspecified foot
Contusion of foot NOS

√x7ᵗʰ **S90.31** Contusion of right foot

√x7ᵗʰ **S90.32** Contusion of left foot

√5ᵗʰ **S90.4** Other superficial injuries of toe

√6ᵗʰ **S90.41** Abrasion of toe

√7ᵗʰ **S90.411** Abrasion, right great toe

√7ᵗʰ **S90.412** Abrasion, left great toe

√7ᵗʰ **S90.413** Abrasion, unspecified great toe

√7ᵗʰ **S90.414** Abrasion, right lesser toe(s)

√7ᵗʰ **S90.415** Abrasion, left lesser toe(s)

√7ᵗʰ **S90.416** Abrasion, unspecified lesser toe(s)

√6ᵗʰ **S90.42** Blister (nonthermal) of toe

√7ᵗʰ **S90.421** Blister (nonthermal), right great toe

√7ᵗʰ **S90.422** Blister (nonthermal), left great toe

√7ᵗʰ **S90.423** Blister (nonthermal), unspecified great toe

√7ᵗʰ **S90.424** Blister (nonthermal), right lesser toe(s)

√7ᵗʰ **S90.425** Blister (nonthermal), left lesser toe(s)

√7ᵗʰ **S90.426** Blister (nonthermal), unspecified lesser toe(s)

√6ᵗʰ **S90.44** External constriction of toe
Hair tourniquet syndrome of toe

√7ᵗʰ **S90.441** External constriction, right great toe

√7ᵗʰ **S90.442** External constriction, left great toe

√7ᵗʰ **S90.443** External constriction, unspecified great toe

√7ᵗʰ **S90.444** External constriction, right lesser toe(s)

√7ᵗʰ **S90.445** External constriction, left lesser toe(s)

√7ᵗʰ **S90.446** External constriction, unspecified lesser toe(s)

√6ᵗʰ **S90.45** Superficial foreign body of toe
Splinter in the toe

√7ᵗʰ **S90.451** Superficial foreign body, right great toe

√7ᵗʰ **S90.452** Superficial foreign body, left great toe

√7ᵗʰ **S90.453** Superficial foreign body, unspecified great toe

√7ᵗʰ **S90.454** Superficial foreign body, right lesser toe(s)

√7ᵗʰ **S90.455** Superficial foreign body, left lesser toe(s)

√7ᵗʰ **S90.456** Superficial foreign body, unspecified lesser toe(s)

√6ᵗʰ **S90.46** Insect bite (nonvenomous) of toe

√7ᵗʰ **S90.461** Insect bite (nonvenomous), right great toe

√7ᵗʰ **S90.462** Insect bite (nonvenomous), left great toe

√7ᵗʰ **S90.463** Insect bite (nonvenomous), unspecified great toe

√7ᵗʰ **S90.464** Insect bite (nonvenomous), right lesser toe(s)

√7ᵗʰ **S90.465** Insect bite (nonvenomous), left lesser toe(s)

√7ᵗʰ **S90.466** Insect bite (nonvenomous), unspecified lesser toe(s)

√6ᵗʰ **S90.47** Other superficial bite of toe

    EXCLUDES 1   *open bite of toe (S91.15-, S91.25-)*

√7ᵗʰ **S90.471** Other superficial bite of right great toe

√7ᵗʰ **S90.472** Other superficial bite of left great toe

√7ᵗʰ **S90.473** Other superficial bite of unspecified great toe

√7ᵗʰ **S90.474** Other superficial bite of right lesser toe(s)

√7ᵗʰ **S90.475** Other superficial bite of left lesser toe(s)

√7ᵗʰ **S90.476** Other superficial bite of unspecified lesser toe(s)

√5ᵗʰ **S90.5** Other superficial injuries of ankle

√6ᵗʰ **S90.51** Abrasion of ankle

√7ᵗʰ **S90.511** Abrasion, right ankle

√7ᵗʰ **S90.512** Abrasion, left ankle

√7ᵗʰ **S90.519** Abrasion, unspecified ankle

√6ᵗʰ **S90.52** Blister (nonthermal) of ankle

√7ᵗʰ **S90.521** Blister (nonthermal), right ankle

√7ᵗʰ **S90.522** Blister (nonthermal), left ankle

√7ᵗʰ **S90.529** Blister (nonthermal), unspecified ankle

√6ᵗʰ **S90.54** External constriction of ankle

√7ᵗʰ **S90.541** External constriction, right ankle

√7ᵗʰ **S90.542** External constriction, left ankle

√7ᵗʰ **S90.549** External constriction, unspecified ankle

√6ᵗʰ **S90.55** Superficial foreign body of ankle

    Splinter in the ankle

√7ᵗʰ **S90.551** Superficial foreign body, right ankle

√7ᵗʰ **S90.552** Superficial foreign body, left ankle

√7ᵗʰ **S90.559** Superficial foreign body, unspecified ankle

√6ᵗʰ **S90.56** Insect bite (nonvenomous) of ankle

√7ᵗʰ **S90.561** Insect bite (nonvenomous), right ankle

√7ᵗʰ **S90.562** Insect bite (nonvenomous), left ankle

√7ᵗʰ **S90.569** Insect bite (nonvenomous), unspecified ankle

√6ᵗʰ **S90.57** Other superficial bite of ankle

    EXCLUDES 1   *open bite of ankle (S91.05-)*

√7ᵗʰ **S90.571** Other superficial bite of ankle, right ankle

√7ᵗʰ **S90.572** Other superficial bite of ankle, left ankle

√7ᵗʰ **S90.579** Other superficial bite of ankle, unspecified ankle

√5ᵗʰ **S90.8** Other superficial injuries of foot

√6ᵗʰ **S90.81** Abrasion of foot

√7ᵗʰ **S90.811** Abrasion, right foot

√7ᵗʰ **S90.812** Abrasion, left foot

√7ᵗʰ **S90.819** Abrasion, unspecified foot

√6ᵗʰ **S90.82** Blister (nonthermal) of foot

√7ᵗʰ **S90.821** Blister (nonthermal), right foot

√7ᵗʰ **S90.822** Blister (nonthermal), left foot

√7ᵗʰ **S90.829** Blister (nonthermal), unspecified foot

√6ᵗʰ **S90.84** External constriction of foot

√7ᵗʰ **S90.841** External constriction, right foot

√7ᵗʰ **S90.842** External constriction, left foot

√7ᵗʰ **S90.849** External constriction, unspecified foot

√6ᵗʰ **S90.85** Superficial foreign body of foot

    Splinter in the foot

√7ᵗʰ **S90.851** Superficial foreign body, right foot

√7ᵗʰ **S90.852** Superficial foreign body, left foot

√7ᵗʰ **S90.859** Superficial foreign body, unspecified foot

√6ᵗʰ **S90.86** Insect bite (nonvenomous) of foot

√7ᵗʰ **S90.861** Insect bite (nonvenomous), right foot

√7ᵗʰ **S90.862** Insect bite (nonvenomous), left foot

√7ᵗʰ **S90.869** Insect bite (nonvenomous), unspecified foot

√6ᵗʰ **S90.87** Other superficial bite of foot

    EXCLUDES 1   *open bite of foot (S91.35-)*

√7ᵗʰ **S90.871** Other superficial bite of right foot

√7ᵗʰ **S90.872** Other superficial bite of left foot

√7ᵗʰ **S90.879** Other superficial bite of unspecified foot

√5ᵗʰ **S90.9** Unspecified superficial injury of ankle, foot and toe

√6ᵗʰ **S90.91** Unspecified superficial injury of ankle

√7ᵗʰ **S90.911** Unspecified superficial injury of right ankle

√7ᵗʰ **S90.912** Unspecified superficial injury of left ankle

√7ᵗʰ **S90.919** Unspecified superficial injury of unspecified ankle

√6ᵗʰ **S90.92** Unspecified superficial injury of foot

√7ᵗʰ **S90.921** Unspecified superficial injury of right foot

√7ᵗʰ **S90.922** Unspecified superficial injury of left foot

√7ᵗʰ **S90.929** Unspecified superficial injury of unspecified foot

√6ᵗʰ **S90.93** Unspecified superficial injury of toes

√7ᵗʰ **S90.931** Unspecified superficial injury of right great toe

√7ᵗʰ **S90.932** Unspecified superficial injury of left great toe

√7ᵗʰ **S90.933** Unspecified superficial injury of unspecified great toe

√7ᵗʰ **S90.934** Unspecified superficial injury of right lesser toe(s)

√7ᵗʰ **S90.935** Unspecified superficial injury of left lesser toe(s)

√7ᵗʰ **S90.936** Unspecified superficial injury of unspecified lesser toe(s)

√4ᵗʰ **S91** Open wound of ankle, foot and toes

    Code also any associated wound infection

    EXCLUDES 1   *open fracture of ankle, foot and toes (S92.- with 7th character B)*

            traumatic amputation of ankle and foot (S98.-)

> The appropriate 7th character is to be added to each code from category S91.
> A   initial encounter
> D   subsequent encounter
> S   sequela

√5ᵗʰ **S91.0** Open wound of ankle

√6ᵗʰ **S91.00** Unspecified open wound of ankle

√7ᵗʰ **S91.001** Unspecified open wound, right ankle

√7ᵗʰ **S91.002** Unspecified open wound, left ankle

√7ᵗʰ **S91.009** Unspecified open wound, unspecified ankle

√6ᵗʰ **S91.01** Laceration without foreign body of ankle

√7ᵗʰ **S91.011** Laceration without foreign body, right ankle

√7ᵗʰ **S91.012** Laceration without foreign body, left ankle

√7ᵗʰ **S91.019** Laceration without foreign body, unspecified ankle

√6ᵗʰ **S91.02** Laceration with foreign body of ankle

√7ᵗʰ **S91.021** Laceration with foreign body, right ankle

√7ᵗʰ **S91.022** Laceration with foreign body, left ankle

√7ᵗʰ **S91.029** Laceration with foreign body, unspecified ankle

√6ᵗʰ **S91.03** Puncture wound without foreign body of ankle

√7ᵗʰ **S91.031** Puncture wound without foreign body, right ankle

√7ᵗʰ **S91.032** Puncture wound without foreign body, left ankle

√7ᵗʰ **S91.039** Puncture wound without foreign body, unspecified ankle

√6ᵗʰ **S91.04** Puncture wound with foreign body of ankle

√7ᵗʰ **S91.041** Puncture wound with foreign body, right ankle

√7ᵗʰ **S91.042** Puncture wound with foreign body, left ankle

√7ᵗʰ **S91.049** Puncture wound with foreign body, unspecified ankle

√6ᵗʰ **S91.05** Open bite of ankle

    EXCLUDES 1   *superficial bite of ankle (S90.56-, S90.57-)*

√7ᵗʰ **S91.051** Open bite, right ankle

☑ Additional Character Required   √x7ᵗʰ Placeholder Alert   Manifestation   Unspecified Dx   ►◄ Revised Text   ● New Code   ▲ Revised Code Title

ICD-10-CM 2020   1065

√7ᵗʰ **S91.Ø52** Open bite, left ankle

√7ᵗʰ **S91.Ø59** Open bite, unspecified ankle

√5ᵗʰ **S91.1** Open wound of toe without damage to nail

√6ᵗʰ **S91.1Ø** Unspecified open wound of toe without damage to nail

√7ᵗʰ **S91.1Ø1** Unspecified open wound of right great toe without damage to nail

√7ᵗʰ **S91.1Ø2** Unspecified open wound of left great toe without damage to nail

√7ᵗʰ **S91.1Ø3** Unspecified open wound of unspecified great toe without damage to nail

√7ᵗʰ **S91.1Ø4** Unspecified open wound of right lesser toe(s) without damage to nail

√7ᵗʰ **S91.1Ø5** Unspecified open wound of left lesser toe(s) without damage to nail

√7ᵗʰ **S91.1Ø6** Unspecified open wound of unspecified lesser toe(s) without damage to nail

√7ᵗʰ **S91.1Ø9** Unspecified open wound of unspecified toe(s) without damage to nail

√6ᵗʰ **S91.11** Laceration without foreign body of toe without damage to nail

√7ᵗʰ **S91.111** Laceration without foreign body of right great toe without damage to nail

√7ᵗʰ **S91.112** Laceration without foreign body of left great toe without damage to nail

√7ᵗʰ **S91.113** Laceration without foreign body of unspecified great toe without damage to nail

√7ᵗʰ **S91.114** Laceration without foreign body of right lesser toe(s) without damage to nail

√7ᵗʰ **S91.115** Laceration without foreign body of left lesser toe(s) without damage to nail

√7ᵗʰ **S91.116** Laceration without foreign body of unspecified lesser toe(s) without damage to nail

√7ᵗʰ **S91.119** Laceration without foreign body of unspecified toe without damage to nail

√6ᵗʰ **S91.12** Laceration with foreign body of toe without damage to nail

√7ᵗʰ **S91.121** Laceration with foreign body of right great toe without damage to nail

√7ᵗʰ **S91.122** Laceration with foreign body of left great toe without damage to nail

√7ᵗʰ **S91.123** Laceration with foreign body of unspecified great toe without damage to nail

√7ᵗʰ **S91.124** Laceration with foreign body of right lesser toe(s) without damage to nail

√7ᵗʰ **S91.125** Laceration with foreign body of left lesser toe(s) without damage to nail

√7ᵗʰ **S91.126** Laceration with foreign body of unspecified lesser toe(s) without damage to nail

√7ᵗʰ **S91.129** Laceration with foreign body of unspecified toe(s) without damage to nail

√6ᵗʰ **S91.13** Puncture wound without foreign body of toe without damage to nail

√7ᵗʰ **S91.131** Puncture wound without foreign body of right great toe without damage to nail

√7ᵗʰ **S91.132** Puncture wound without foreign body of left great toe without damage to nail

√7ᵗʰ **S91.133** Puncture wound without foreign body of unspecified great toe without damage to nail

√7ᵗʰ **S91.134** Puncture wound without foreign body of right lesser toe(s) without damage to nail

√7ᵗʰ **S91.135** Puncture wound without foreign body of left lesser toe(s) without damage to nail

√7ᵗʰ **S91.136** Puncture wound without foreign body of unspecified lesser toe(s) without damage to nail

√7ᵗʰ **S91.139** Puncture wound without foreign body of unspecified toe(s) without damage to nail

√6ᵗʰ **S91.14** Puncture wound with foreign body of toe without damage to nail

√7ᵗʰ **S91.141** Puncture wound with foreign body of right great toe without damage to nail

√7ᵗʰ **S91.142** Puncture wound with foreign body of left great toe without damage to nail

√7ᵗʰ **S91.143** Puncture wound with foreign body of unspecified great toe without damage to nail

√7ᵗʰ **S91.144** Puncture wound with foreign body of right lesser toe(s) without damage to nail

√7ᵗʰ **S91.145** Puncture wound with foreign body of left lesser toe(s) without damage to nail

√7ᵗʰ **S91.146** Puncture wound with foreign body of unspecified lesser toe(s) without damage to nail

√7ᵗʰ **S91.149** Puncture wound with foreign body of unspecified toe(s) without damage to nail

√6ᵗʰ **S91.15** Open bite of toe without damage to nail

Bite of toe NOS

EXCLUDES 1   superficial bite of toe (S9Ø.46-, S9Ø.47-)

√7ᵗʰ **S91.151** Open bite of right great toe without damage to nail

√7ᵗʰ **S91.152** Open bite of left great toe without damage to nail

√7ᵗʰ **S91.153** Open bite of unspecified great toe without damage to nail

√7ᵗʰ **S91.154** Open bite of right lesser toe(s) without damage to nail

√7ᵗʰ **S91.155** Open bite of left lesser toe(s) without damage to nail

√7ᵗʰ **S91.156** Open bite of unspecified lesser toe(s) without damage to nail

√7ᵗʰ **S91.159** Open bite of unspecified toe(s) without damage to nail

√5ᵗʰ **S91.2** Open wound of toe with damage to nail

√6ᵗʰ **S91.2Ø** Unspecified open wound of toe with damage to nail

√7ᵗʰ **S91.2Ø1** Unspecified open wound of right great toe with damage to nail

√7ᵗʰ **S91.2Ø2** Unspecified open wound of left great toe with damage to nail

√7ᵗʰ **S91.2Ø3** Unspecified open wound of unspecified great toe with damage to nail

√7ᵗʰ **S91.2Ø4** Unspecified open wound of right lesser toe(s) with damage to nail

√7ᵗʰ **S91.2Ø5** Unspecified open wound of left lesser toe(s) with damage to nail

√7ᵗʰ **S91.2Ø6** Unspecified open wound of unspecified lesser toe(s) with damage to nail

√7ᵗʰ **S91.2Ø9** Unspecified open wound of unspecified toe(s) with damage to nail

√6ᵗʰ **S91.21** Laceration without foreign body of toe with damage to nail

√7ᵗʰ **S91.211** Laceration without foreign body of right great toe with damage to nail

√7ᵗʰ **S91.212** Laceration without foreign body of left great toe with damage to nail

√7ᵗʰ **S91.213** Laceration without foreign body of unspecified great toe with damage to nail

√7ᵗʰ **S91.214** Laceration without foreign body of right lesser toe(s) with damage to nail

√7ᵗʰ **S91.215** Laceration without foreign body of left lesser toe(s) with damage to nail

√7ᵗʰ **S91.216** Laceration without foreign body of unspecified lesser toe(s) with damage to nail

√7ᵗʰ **S91.219** Laceration without foreign body of unspecified toe(s) with damage to nail

√6ᵗʰ **S91.22** Laceration with foreign body of toe with damage to nail

√7ᵗʰ **S91.221** Laceration with foreign body of right great toe with damage to nail

√7ᵗʰ **S91.222** Laceration with foreign body of left great toe with damage to nail

√7ᵗʰ **S91.223** Laceration with foreign body of unspecified great toe with damage to nail

√7ᵗʰ **S91.224** Laceration with foreign body of right lesser toe(s) with damage to nail

√7ᵗʰ **S91.225** Laceration with foreign body of left lesser toe(s) with damage to nail

√7ᵗʰ **S91.226** Laceration with foreign body of unspecified lesser toe(s) with damage to nail

√7ᵗʰ **S91.229** Laceration with foreign body of unspecified toe(s) with damage to nail

√6ᵗʰ **S91.23** Puncture wound without foreign body of toe with damage to nail

√7ᵗʰ **S91.231** Puncture wound without foreign body of right great toe with damage to nail

√7ᵗʰ **S91.232** Puncture wound without foreign body of left great toe with damage to nail

√7ᵗʰ **S91.233** **Puncture wound without foreign body of unspecified great toe with damage to nail**

√7ᵗʰ **S91.234** **Puncture wound without foreign body of right lesser toe(s) with damage to nail**

√7ᵗʰ **S91.235** **Puncture wound without foreign body of left lesser toe(s) with damage to nail**

√7ᵗʰ **S91.236** **Puncture wound without foreign body of unspecified lesser toe(s) with damage to nail**

√7ᵗʰ **S91.239** **Puncture wound without foreign body of unspecified toe(s) with damage to nail**

√6ᵗʰ **S91.24** **Puncture wound with foreign body** of toe with damage to nail

√7ᵗʰ **S91.241** **Puncture wound with foreign body of right great toe with damage to nail**

√7ᵗʰ **S91.242** **Puncture wound with foreign body of left great toe with damage to nail**

√7ᵗʰ **S91.243** **Puncture wound with foreign body of unspecified great toe with damage to nail**

√7ᵗʰ **S91.244** **Puncture wound with foreign body of right lesser toe(s) with damage to nail**

√7ᵗʰ **S91.245** **Puncture wound with foreign body of left lesser toe(s) with damage to nail**

√7ᵗʰ **S91.246** **Puncture wound with foreign body of unspecified lesser toe(s) with damage to nail**

√7ᵗʰ **S91.249** **Puncture wound with foreign body of unspecified toe(s) with damage to nail**

√6ᵗʰ **S91.25** **Open bite** of toe with damage to nail

Bite of toe with damage to nail NOS

EXCLUDES 1   superficial bite of toe (S90.46-, S90.47-)

√7ᵗʰ **S91.251** **Open bite of right great toe with damage to nail**

√7ᵗʰ **S91.252** **Open bite of left great toe with damage to nail**

√7ᵗʰ **S91.253** **Open bite of unspecified great toe with damage to nail**

√7ᵗʰ **S91.254** **Open bite of right lesser toe(s) with damage to nail**

√7ᵗʰ **S91.255** **Open bite of left lesser toe(s) with damage to nail**

√7ᵗʰ **S91.256** **Open bite of unspecified lesser toe(s) with damage to nail**

√7ᵗʰ **S91.259** **Open bite of unspecified toe(s) with damage to nail**

√5ᵗʰ **S91.3** **Open wound** of foot

√6ᵗʰ **S91.30** **Unspecified open wound** of foot

√7ᵗʰ **S91.301** **Unspecified open wound, right foot**

√7ᵗʰ **S91.302** **Unspecified open wound, left foot**

√7ᵗʰ **S91.309** **Unspecified open wound, unspecified foot**

√6ᵗʰ **S91.31** **Laceration without foreign body** of foot

√7ᵗʰ **S91.311** **Laceration without foreign body, right foot**

√7ᵗʰ **S91.312** **Laceration without foreign body, left foot**

√7ᵗʰ **S91.319** **Laceration without foreign body, unspecified foot**

√6ᵗʰ **S91.32** **Laceration with foreign body** of foot

√7ᵗʰ **S91.321** **Laceration with foreign body, right foot**

√7ᵗʰ **S91.322** **Laceration with foreign body, left foot**

√7ᵗʰ **S91.329** **Laceration with foreign body, unspecified foot**

√6ᵗʰ **S91.33** **Puncture wound without foreign body** of foot

√7ᵗʰ **S91.331** **Puncture wound without foreign body, right foot**

√7ᵗʰ **S91.332** **Puncture wound without foreign body, left foot**

√7ᵗʰ **S91.339** **Puncture wound without foreign body, unspecified foot**

√6ᵗʰ **S91.34** **Puncture wound with foreign body** of foot

√7ᵗʰ **S91.341** **Puncture wound with foreign body, right foot**

√7ᵗʰ **S91.342** **Puncture wound with foreign body, left foot**

√7ᵗʰ **S91.349** **Puncture wound with foreign body, unspecified foot**

√6ᵗʰ **S91.35** **Open bite** of foot

EXCLUDES 1   superficial bite of foot (S90.86-, S90.87-)

√7ᵗʰ **S91.351** **Open bite, right foot**

√7ᵗʰ **S91.352** **Open bite, left foot**

√7ᵗʰ **S91.359** **Open bite, unspecified foot**

√4ᵗʰ **S92** **Fracture of foot and toe, except ankle**

NOTE   A fracture not indicated as displaced or nondisplaced should be coded to displaced

A fracture not indicated as open or closed should be coded to closed.

EXCLUDES 1   traumatic amputation of ankle and foot (S98.-)

EXCLUDES 2   fracture of ankle (S82.-)

fracture of malleolus (S82.-)

AHA: 2018,2Q,12; 2015,3Q,37-39

The appropriate 7th character is to be added to each code from category S92.

A   initial encounter for closed fracture

B   initial encounter for open fracture

D   subsequent encounter for fracture with routine healing

G   subsequent encounter for fracture with delayed healing

K   subsequent encounter for fracture with nonunion

P   subsequent encounter for fracture with malunion

S   sequela

√5ᵗʰ **S92.0** **Fracture of** calcaneus

Heel bone

Os calcis

EXCLUDES 2   physeal fracture of calcaneus (S99.0-)

√6ᵗʰ **S92.00** **Unspecified fracture of calcaneus**

√7ᵗʰ **S92.001** **Unspecified fracture of right calcaneus**   Q

√7ᵗʰ **S92.002** **Unspecified fracture of left calcaneus**   Q

√7ᵗʰ **S92.009** **Unspecified fracture of unspecified calcaneus**   Q

√6ᵗʰ **S92.01** **Fracture of** body of calcaneus

√7ᵗʰ **S92.011** **Displaced fracture of body of right calcaneus**   Q

√7ᵗʰ **S92.012** **Displaced fracture of body of left calcaneus**   Q

√7ᵗʰ **S92.013** **Displaced fracture of body of unspecified calcaneus**   Q

√7ᵗʰ **S92.014** **Nondisplaced fracture of body of right calcaneus**   Q

√7ᵗʰ **S92.015** **Nondisplaced fracture of body of left calcaneus**   Q

√7ᵗʰ **S92.016** **Nondisplaced fracture of body of unspecified calcaneus**   Q

√6ᵗʰ **S92.02** **Fracture of** anterior process of calcaneus

√7ᵗʰ **S92.021** **Displaced fracture of anterior process of right calcaneus**   Q

√7ᵗʰ **S92.022** **Displaced fracture of anterior process of left calcaneus**   Q

√7ᵗʰ **S92.023** **Displaced fracture of anterior process of unspecified calcaneus**   Q

√7ᵗʰ **S92.024** **Nondisplaced fracture of anterior process of right calcaneus**   Q

√7ᵗʰ **S92.025** **Nondisplaced fracture of anterior process of left calcaneus**   Q

√7ᵗʰ **S92.026** **Nondisplaced fracture of anterior process of unspecified calcaneus**   Q

√6ᵗʰ **S92.03** **Avulsion fracture of** tuberosity of calcaneus

√7ᵗʰ **S92.031** **Displaced avulsion fracture of tuberosity of right calcaneus**   Q

√7ᵗʰ **S92.032** **Displaced avulsion fracture of tuberosity of left calcaneus**   Q

√7ᵗʰ **S92.033** **Displaced avulsion fracture of tuberosity of unspecified calcaneus**   Q

√7ᵗʰ **S92.034** **Nondisplaced avulsion fracture of tuberosity of right calcaneus**   Q

√7ᵗʰ **S92.035** **Nondisplaced avulsion fracture of tuberosity of left calcaneus**   Q

√7ᵗʰ **S92.036** **Nondisplaced avulsion fracture of tuberosity of unspecified calcaneus**   Q

√6ᵗʰ **S92.04** **Other fracture of** tuberosity of calcaneus

√7ᵗʰ **S92.041** **Displaced other fracture of tuberosity of right calcaneus**   Q

√7ᵗʰ **S92.042** **Displaced other fracture of tuberosity of left calcaneus**   Q

☑ Additional Character Required   √x7ᵗʰ Placeholder Alert   Manifestation   Unspecified Dx   ▶◀ Revised Text   ● New Code   ▲ Revised Code Title

ICD-10-CM 2020   **1067**

Chapter 19. Injury, Poisoning and Certain Other Consequences of External Causes

S92.043–S92.233

- √7ᵗʰ **S92.043** Displaced other fracture of tuberosity of unspecified calcaneus   Q
- √7ᵗʰ **S92.044** Nondisplaced other fracture of tuberosity of right calcaneus   Q
- √7ᵗʰ **S92.045** Nondisplaced other fracture of tuberosity of left calcaneus   Q
- √7ᵗʰ **S92.046** Nondisplaced other fracture of tuberosity of unspecified calcaneus   Q
- √6ᵗʰ **S92.05** Other extraarticular fracture of calcaneus
  - √7ᵗʰ **S92.051** Displaced other extraarticular fracture of right calcaneus   Q
  - √7ᵗʰ **S92.052** Displaced other extraarticular fracture of left calcaneus   Q
  - √7ᵗʰ **S92.053** Displaced other extraarticular fracture of unspecified calcaneus   Q
  - √7ᵗʰ **S92.054** Nondisplaced other extraarticular fracture of right calcaneus   Q
  - √7ᵗʰ **S92.055** Nondisplaced other extraarticular fracture of left calcaneus   Q
  - √7ᵗʰ **S92.056** Nondisplaced other extraarticular fracture of unspecified calcaneus   Q
- √6ᵗʰ **S92.06** Intraarticular fracture of calcaneus
  - √7ᵗʰ **S92.061** Displaced intraarticular fracture of right calcaneus   Q
  - √7ᵗʰ **S92.062** Displaced intraarticular fracture of left calcaneus   Q
  - √7ᵗʰ **S92.063** Displaced intraarticular fracture of unspecified calcaneus   Q
  - √7ᵗʰ **S92.064** Nondisplaced intraarticular fracture of right calcaneus   Q
  - √7ᵗʰ **S92.065** Nondisplaced intraarticular fracture of left calcaneus   Q
  - √7ᵗʰ **S92.066** Nondisplaced intraarticular fracture of unspecified calcaneus   Q
- √5ᵗʰ **S92.1** Fracture of talus
  - Astragalus
  - √6ᵗʰ **S92.10** Unspecified fracture of talus
    - √7ᵗʰ **S92.101** Unspecified fracture of right talus   Q
    - √7ᵗʰ **S92.102** Unspecified fracture of left talus   Q
    - √7ᵗʰ **S92.109** Unspecified fracture of unspecified talus   Q
  - √6ᵗʰ **S92.11** Fracture of neck of talus
    - √7ᵗʰ **S92.111** Displaced fracture of neck of right talus   Q
    - √7ᵗʰ **S92.112** Displaced fracture of neck of left talus   Q
    - √7ᵗʰ **S92.113** Displaced fracture of neck of unspecified talus   Q
    - √7ᵗʰ **S92.114** Nondisplaced fracture of neck of right talus   Q
    - √7ᵗʰ **S92.115** Nondisplaced fracture of neck of left talus   Q
    - √7ᵗʰ **S92.116** Nondisplaced fracture of neck of unspecified talus   Q
  - √6ᵗʰ **S92.12** Fracture of body of talus
    - √7ᵗʰ **S92.121** Displaced fracture of body of right talus   Q
    - √7ᵗʰ **S92.122** Displaced fracture of body of left talus   Q
    - √7ᵗʰ **S92.123** Displaced fracture of body of unspecified talus   Q
    - √7ᵗʰ **S92.124** Nondisplaced fracture of body of right talus   Q
    - √7ᵗʰ **S92.125** Nondisplaced fracture of body of left talus   Q
    - √7ᵗʰ **S92.126** Nondisplaced fracture of body of unspecified talus   Q
  - √6ᵗʰ **S92.13** Fracture of posterior process of talus
    - √7ᵗʰ **S92.131** Displaced fracture of posterior process of right talus   Q
    - √7ᵗʰ **S92.132** Displaced fracture of posterior process of left talus   Q
    - √7ᵗʰ **S92.133** Displaced fracture of posterior process of unspecified talus   Q
    - √7ᵗʰ **S92.134** Nondisplaced fracture of posterior process of right talus   Q
    - √7ᵗʰ **S92.135** Nondisplaced fracture of posterior process of left talus   Q
    - √7ᵗʰ **S92.136** Nondisplaced fracture of posterior process of unspecified talus   Q
  - √6ᵗʰ **S92.14** Dome fracture of talus
    - EXCLUDES 1   osteochondritis dissecans (M93.2)
    - √7ᵗʰ **S92.141** Displaced dome fracture of right talus   Q
    - √7ᵗʰ **S92.142** Displaced dome fracture of left talus   Q
    - √7ᵗʰ **S92.143** Displaced dome fracture of unspecified talus   Q
    - √7ᵗʰ **S92.144** Nondisplaced dome fracture of right talus   Q
    - √7ᵗʰ **S92.145** Nondisplaced dome fracture of left talus   Q
    - √7ᵗʰ **S92.146** Nondisplaced dome fracture of unspecified talus   Q
  - √6ᵗʰ **S92.15** Avulsion fracture (chip fracture) of talus
    - √7ᵗʰ **S92.151** Displaced avulsion fracture (chip fracture) of right talus   Q
    - √7ᵗʰ **S92.152** Displaced avulsion fracture (chip fracture) of left talus   Q
    - √7ᵗʰ **S92.153** Displaced avulsion fracture (chip fracture) of unspecified talus   Q
    - √7ᵗʰ **S92.154** Nondisplaced avulsion fracture (chip fracture) of right talus   Q
    - √7ᵗʰ **S92.155** Nondisplaced avulsion fracture (chip fracture) of left talus   Q
    - √7ᵗʰ **S92.156** Nondisplaced avulsion fracture (chip fracture) of unspecified talus   Q
  - √6ᵗʰ **S92.19** Other fracture of talus
    - √7ᵗʰ **S92.191** Other fracture of right talus   Q
    - √7ᵗʰ **S92.192** Other fracture of left talus   Q
    - √7ᵗʰ **S92.199** Other fracture of unspecified talus   Q
- √5ᵗʰ **S92.2** Fracture of other and unspecified tarsal bone(s)
  - √6ᵗʰ **S92.20** Fracture of unspecified tarsal bone(s)
    - √7ᵗʰ **S92.201** Fracture of unspecified tarsal bone(s) of right foot   Q
    - √7ᵗʰ **S92.202** Fracture of unspecified tarsal bone(s) of left foot   Q
    - √7ᵗʰ **S92.209** Fracture of unspecified tarsal bone(s) of unspecified foot   Q
  - √6ᵗʰ **S92.21** Fracture of cuboid bone
    - √7ᵗʰ **S92.211** Displaced fracture of cuboid bone of right foot   Q
    - √7ᵗʰ **S92.212** Displaced fracture of cuboid bone of left foot   Q
    - √7ᵗʰ **S92.213** Displaced fracture of cuboid bone of unspecified foot   Q
    - √7ᵗʰ **S92.214** Nondisplaced fracture of cuboid bone of right foot   Q
    - √7ᵗʰ **S92.215** Nondisplaced fracture of cuboid bone of left foot   Q
    - √7ᵗʰ **S92.216** Nondisplaced fracture of cuboid bone of unspecified foot   Q
  - √6ᵗʰ **S92.22** Fracture of lateral cuneiform
    - √7ᵗʰ **S92.221** Displaced fracture of lateral cuneiform of right foot   Q
    - √7ᵗʰ **S92.222** Displaced fracture of lateral cuneiform of left foot   Q
    - √7ᵗʰ **S92.223** Displaced fracture of lateral cuneiform of unspecified foot   Q
    - √7ᵗʰ **S92.224** Nondisplaced fracture of lateral cuneiform of right foot   Q
    - √7ᵗʰ **S92.225** Nondisplaced fracture of lateral cuneiform of left foot   Q
    - √7ᵗʰ **S92.226** Nondisplaced fracture of lateral cuneiform of unspecified foot   Q
  - √6ᵗʰ **S92.23** Fracture of intermediate cuneiform
    - √7ᵗʰ **S92.231** Displaced fracture of intermediate cuneiform of right foot   Q
    - √7ᵗʰ **S92.232** Displaced fracture of intermediate cuneiform of left foot   Q
    - √7ᵗʰ **S92.233** Displaced fracture of intermediate cuneiform of unspecified foot   Q

√7ᵗʰ **S92.234** Nondisplaced fracture of intermediate cuneiform of **right** foot   Q

√7ᵗʰ **S92.235** Nondisplaced fracture of intermediate cuneiform of **left** foot   Q

√7ᵗʰ **S92.236** Nondisplaced fracture of intermediate cuneiform of **unspecified** foot   Q

√6ᵗʰ **S92.24** Fracture of medial cuneiform

    √7ᵗʰ **S92.241** Displaced fracture of medial cuneiform of **right** foot   Q

    √7ᵗʰ **S92.242** Displaced fracture of medial cuneiform of **left** foot   Q

    √7ᵗʰ **S92.243** Displaced fracture of medial cuneiform of **unspecified** foot   Q

    √7ᵗʰ **S92.244** Nondisplaced fracture of medial cuneiform of **right** foot   Q

    √7ᵗʰ **S92.245** Nondisplaced fracture of medial cuneiform of **left** foot   Q

    √7ᵗʰ **S92.246** Nondisplaced fracture of medial cuneiform of **unspecified** foot   Q

√6ᵗʰ **S92.25** Fracture of navicular [scaphoid] of foot

    √7ᵗʰ **S92.251** Displaced fracture of navicular [scaphoid] of **right** foot   Q

    √7ᵗʰ **S92.252** Displaced fracture of navicular [scaphoid] of **left** foot   Q

    √7ᵗʰ **S92.253** Displaced fracture of navicular [scaphoid] of **unspecified** foot   Q

    √7ᵗʰ **S92.254** Nondisplaced fracture of navicular [scaphoid] of **right** foot   Q

    √7ᵗʰ **S92.255** Nondisplaced fracture of navicular [scaphoid] of **left** foot   Q

    √7ᵗʰ **S92.256** Nondisplaced fracture of navicular [scaphoid] of **unspecified** foot   Q

√5ᵗʰ **S92.3** Fracture of metatarsal bone(s)

   EXCLUDES 2   *physeal fracture of metatarsal (S99.1-)*

   AHA: 2018,1Q,3

√6ᵗʰ **S92.30** Fracture of unspecified metatarsal bone(s)

    √7ᵗʰ **S92.301** Fracture of unspecified metatarsal bone(s), **right** foot   Q

    √7ᵗʰ **S92.302** Fracture of unspecified metatarsal bone(s), **left** foot   Q

    √7ᵗʰ **S92.309** Fracture of unspecified metatarsal bone(s), **unspecified** foot   Q

√6ᵗʰ **S92.31** Fracture of first metatarsal bone

    √7ᵗʰ **S92.311** Displaced fracture of first metatarsal bone, **right** foot   Q

    √7ᵗʰ **S92.312** Displaced fracture of first metatarsal bone, **left** foot   Q

    √7ᵗʰ **S92.313** Displaced fracture of first metatarsal bone, **unspecified** foot   Q

    √7ᵗʰ **S92.314** Nondisplaced fracture of first metatarsal bone, **right** foot   Q

    √7ᵗʰ **S92.315** Nondisplaced fracture of first metatarsal bone, **left** foot   Q

    √7ᵗʰ **S92.316** Nondisplaced fracture of first metatarsal bone, **unspecified** foot   Q

√6ᵗʰ **S92.32** Fracture of second metatarsal bone

    √7ᵗʰ **S92.321** Displaced fracture of second metatarsal bone, **right** foot   Q

    √7ᵗʰ **S92.322** Displaced fracture of second metatarsal bone, **left** foot   Q

    √7ᵗʰ **S92.323** Displaced fracture of second metatarsal bone, **unspecified** foot   Q

    √7ᵗʰ **S92.324** Nondisplaced fracture of second metatarsal bone, **right** foot   Q

    √7ᵗʰ **S92.325** Nondisplaced fracture of second metatarsal bone, **left** foot   Q

    √7ᵗʰ **S92.326** Nondisplaced fracture of second metatarsal bone, **unspecified** foot   Q

√6ᵗʰ **S92.33** Fracture of third metatarsal bone

    √7ᵗʰ **S92.331** Displaced fracture of third metatarsal bone, **right** foot   Q

    √7ᵗʰ **S92.332** Displaced fracture of third metatarsal bone, **left** foot   Q

    √7ᵗʰ **S92.333** Displaced fracture of third metatarsal bone, **unspecified** foot   Q

    √7ᵗʰ **S92.334** Nondisplaced fracture of third metatarsal bone, **right** foot   Q

√7ᵗʰ **S92.335** Nondisplaced fracture of third metatarsal bone, **left** foot   Q

√7ᵗʰ **S92.336** Nondisplaced fracture of third metatarsal bone, **unspecified** foot   Q

√6ᵗʰ **S92.34** Fracture of fourth metatarsal bone

    √7ᵗʰ **S92.341** Displaced fracture of fourth metatarsal bone, **right** foot   Q

    √7ᵗʰ **S92.342** Displaced fracture of fourth metatarsal bone, **left** foot   Q

    √7ᵗʰ **S92.343** Displaced fracture of fourth metatarsal bone, **unspecified** foot   Q

    √7ᵗʰ **S92.344** Nondisplaced fracture of fourth metatarsal bone, **right** foot   Q

    √7ᵗʰ **S92.345** Nondisplaced fracture of fourth metatarsal bone, **left** foot   Q

    √7ᵗʰ **S92.346** Nondisplaced fracture of fourth metatarsal bone, **unspecified** foot   Q

√6ᵗʰ **S92.35** Fracture of fifth metatarsal bone

    √7ᵗʰ **S92.351** Displaced fracture of fifth metatarsal bone, **right** foot   Q

    √7ᵗʰ **S92.352** Displaced fracture of fifth metatarsal bone, **left** foot   Q

    √7ᵗʰ **S92.353** Displaced fracture of fifth metatarsal bone, **unspecified** foot   Q

    √7ᵗʰ **S92.354** Nondisplaced fracture of fifth metatarsal bone, **right** foot   Q

    √7ᵗʰ **S92.355** Nondisplaced fracture of fifth metatarsal bone, **left** foot   Q

    √7ᵗʰ **S92.356** Nondisplaced fracture of fifth metatarsal bone, **unspecified** foot   Q

√6ᵗʰ **S92.4** Fracture of great toe

   EXCLUDES 2   *physeal fracture of phalanx of toe (S99.2-)*

√6ᵗʰ **S92.40** Unspecified fracture of great toe

    √7ᵗʰ **S92.401** Displaced unspecified fracture of **right** great toe

    √7ᵗʰ **S92.402** Displaced unspecified fracture of **left** great toe

    √7ᵗʰ **S92.403** Displaced unspecified fracture of **unspecified** great toe

    √7ᵗʰ **S92.404** Nondisplaced unspecified fracture of **right** great toe

    √7ᵗʰ **S92.405** Nondisplaced unspecified fracture of **left** great toe

    √7ᵗʰ **S92.406** Nondisplaced unspecified fracture of **unspecified** great toe

√6ᵗʰ **S92.41** Fracture of proximal phalanx of great toe

    √7ᵗʰ **S92.411** Displaced fracture of proximal phalanx of **right** great toe

    √7ᵗʰ **S92.412** Displaced fracture of proximal phalanx of **left** great toe

    √7ᵗʰ **S92.413** Displaced fracture of proximal phalanx of **unspecified** great toe

    √7ᵗʰ **S92.414** Nondisplaced fracture of proximal phalanx of **right** great toe

    √7ᵗʰ **S92.415** Nondisplaced fracture of proximal phalanx of **left** great toe

    √7ᵗʰ **S92.416** Nondisplaced fracture of proximal phalanx of **unspecified** great toe

√6ᵗʰ **S92.42** Fracture of distal phalanx of great toe

    √7ᵗʰ **S92.421** Displaced fracture of distal phalanx of **right** great toe

    √7ᵗʰ **S92.422** Displaced fracture of distal phalanx of **left** great toe

    √7ᵗʰ **S92.423** Displaced fracture of distal phalanx of **unspecified** great toe

    √7ᵗʰ **S92.424** Nondisplaced fracture of distal phalanx of **right** great toe

    √7ᵗʰ **S92.425** Nondisplaced fracture of distal phalanx of **left** great toe

    √7ᵗʰ **S92.426** Nondisplaced fracture of distal phalanx of **unspecified** great toe

√6ᵗʰ **S92.49** Other fracture of great toe

    √7ᵗʰ **S92.491** Other fracture of **right** great toe

    √7ᵗʰ **S92.492** Other fracture of **left** great toe

    √7ᵗʰ **S92.499** Other fracture of **unspecified** great toe

√6ᵗʰ **S92.5** Fracture of lesser toe(s)

   EXCLUDES 2   *physeal fracture of phalanx of toe (S99.2-)*

√6ᵗʰ **S92.50** Unspecified fracture of lesser toe(s)

    √7ᵗʰ **S92.501** Displaced unspecified fracture of **right** lesser toe(s)

☑ Additional Character Required   √x/7ᵗʰ Placeholder Alert   Manifestation   Unspecified Dx   ▶◀ Revised Text   ● New Code   ▲ Revised Code Title

ICD-10-CM 2020   1069

S92.502–S93.131

Chapter 19. Injury, Poisoning and Certain Other Consequences of External Causes

√7th **S92.502** Displaced unspecified fracture of left lesser toe(s)

√7th **S92.503** Displaced unspecified fracture of unspecified lesser toe(s)

√7th **S92.504** Nondisplaced unspecified fracture of right lesser toe(s)

√7th **S92.505** Nondisplaced unspecified fracture of left lesser toe(s)

√7th **S92.506** Nondisplaced unspecified fracture of unspecified lesser toe(s)

√6th **S92.51** Fracture of proximal phalanx of lesser toe(s)

√7th **S92.511** Displaced fracture of proximal phalanx of right lesser toe(s)

√7th **S92.512** Displaced fracture of proximal phalanx of left lesser toe(s)

√7th **S92.513** Displaced fracture of proximal phalanx of unspecified lesser toe(s)

√7th **S92.514** Nondisplaced fracture of proximal phalanx of right lesser toe(s)

√7th **S92.515** Nondisplaced fracture of proximal phalanx of left lesser toe(s))

√7th **S92.516** Nondisplaced fracture of proximal phalanx of unspecified lesser toe(s)

√6th **S92.52** Fracture of middle phalanx of lesser toe(s)

√7th **S92.521** Displaced fracture of middle phalanx of right lesser toe(s)

√7th **S92.522** Displaced fracture of middle phalanx of left lesser toe(s)

√7th **S92.523** Displaced fracture of middle phalanx of unspecified lesser toe(s)

√7th **S92.524** Nondisplaced fracture of middle phalanx of right lesser toe(s)

√7th **S92.525** Nondisplaced fracture of middle phalanx of left lesser toe(s)

√7th **S92.526** Nondisplaced fracture of middle phalanx of unspecified lesser toe(s)

√6th **S92.53** Fracture of distal phalanx of lesser toe(s)

√7th **S92.531** Displaced fracture of distal phalanx of right lesser toe(s)

√7th **S92.532** Displaced fracture of distal phalanx of left lesser toe(s)

√7th **S92.533** Displaced fracture of distal phalanx of unspecified lesser toe(s)

√7th **S92.534** Nondisplaced fracture of distal phalanx of right lesser toe(s)

√7th **S92.535** Nondisplaced fracture of distal phalanx of left lesser toe(s)

√7th **S92.536** Nondisplaced fracture of distal phalanx of unspecified lesser toe(s)

√6th **S92.59** Other fracture of lesser toe(s)

√7th **S92.591** Other fracture of right lesser toe(s)

√7th **S92.592** Other fracture of left lesser toe(s)

√7th **S92.599** Other fracture of unspecified lesser toe(s)

√5th **S92.8** Other fracture of foot, except ankle

√6th **S92.81** Other fracture of foot

Sesamoid fracture of foot
AHA: 2016,4Q,68

√7th **S92.811** Other fracture of right foot   Q

√7th **S92.812** Other fracture of left foot   Q

√7th **S92.819** Other fracture of unspecified foot   Q

√5th **S92.9** Unspecified fracture of foot and toe

√6th **S92.90** Unspecified fracture of foot

√7th **S92.901** Unspecified fracture of right foot   Q

√7th **S92.902** Unspecified fracture of left foot   Q

√7th **S92.909** Unspecified fracture of unspecified foot   Q

√6th **S92.91** Unspecified fracture of toe

√7th **S92.911** Unspecified fracture of right toe(s)

√7th **S92.912** Unspecified fracture of left toe(s)

√7th **S92.919** Unspecified fracture of unspecified toe(s)

√4th **S93 Dislocation and sprain of joints and ligaments at ankle, foot and toe level**

INCLUDES   avulsion of joint or ligament of ankle, foot and toe

laceration of cartilage, joint or ligament of ankle, foot and toe

sprain of cartilage, joint or ligament of ankle, foot and toe

traumatic hemarthrosis of joint or ligament of ankle, foot and toe

traumatic rupture of joint or ligament of ankle, foot and toe

traumatic subluxation of joint or ligament of ankle, foot and toe

traumatic tear of joint or ligament of ankle, foot and toe

Code also any associated open wound

EXCLUDES 2   *strain of muscle and tendon of ankle and foot (S96.-)*

The appropriate 7th character is to be added to each code from category S93.
A   initial encounter
D   subsequent encounter
S   sequela

√5th **S93.0** Subluxation and dislocation of ankle joint

Subluxation and dislocation of astragalus
Subluxation and dislocation of fibula, lower end
Subluxation and dislocation of talus
Subluxation and dislocation of tibia, lower end

√x7th **S93.01** Subluxation of right ankle joint

√x7th **S93.02** Subluxation of left ankle joint

√x7th **S93.03** Subluxation of unspecified ankle joint

√x7th **S93.04** Dislocation of right ankle joint

√x7th **S93.05** Dislocation of left ankle joint

√x7th **S93.06** Dislocation of unspecified ankle joint

√5th **S93.1** Subluxation and dislocation of toe

√6th **S93.10** Unspecified subluxation and dislocation of toe

Dislocation of toe NOS
Subluxation of toe NOS

√7th **S93.101** Unspecified subluxation of right toe(s)

√7th **S93.102** Unspecified subluxation of left toe(s)

√7th **S93.103** Unspecified subluxation of unspecified toe(s)

√7th **S93.104** Unspecified dislocation of right toe(s)

√7th **S93.105** Unspecified dislocation of left toe(s)

√7th **S93.106** Unspecified dislocation of unspecified toe(s)

√6th **S93.11** Dislocation of interphalangeal joint

√7th **S93.111** Dislocation of interphalangeal joint of right great toe

√7th **S93.112** Dislocation of interphalangeal joint of left great toe

√7th **S93.113** Dislocation of interphalangeal joint of unspecified great toe

√7th **S93.114** Dislocation of interphalangeal joint of right lesser toe(s)

√7th **S93.115** Dislocation of interphalangeal joint of left lesser toe(s)

√7th **S93.116** Dislocation of interphalangeal joint of unspecified lesser toe(s)

√7th **S93.119** Dislocation of interphalangeal joint of unspecified toe(s)

√6th **S93.12** Dislocation of metatarsophalangeal joint

√7th **S93.121** Dislocation of metatarsophalangeal joint of right great toe

√7th **S93.122** Dislocation of metatarsophalangeal joint of left great toe

√7th **S93.123** Dislocation of metatarsophalangeal joint of unspecified great toe

√7th **S93.124** Dislocation of metatarsophalangeal joint of right lesser toe(s)

√7th **S93.125** Dislocation of metatarsophalangeal joint of left lesser toe(s)

√7th **S93.126** Dislocation of metatarsophalangeal joint of unspecified lesser toe(s)

√7th **S93.129** Dislocation of metatarsophalangeal joint of unspecified toe(s)

√6th **S93.13** Subluxation of interphalangeal joint

√7th **S93.131** Subluxation of interphalangeal joint of right great toe

√7ᵗʰ **S93.132 Subluxation of interphalangeal joint of left great toe**

√7ᵗʰ **S93.133 Subluxation of interphalangeal joint of unspecified great toe**

√7ᵗʰ **S93.134 Subluxation of interphalangeal joint of right lesser toe(s)**

√7ᵗʰ **S93.135 Subluxation of interphalangeal joint of left lesser toe(s)**

√7ᵗʰ **S93.136 Subluxation of interphalangeal joint of unspecified lesser toe(s)**

√7ᵗʰ **S93.139 Subluxation of interphalangeal joint of unspecified toe(s)**

√6ᵗʰ **S93.14 Subluxation of metatarsophalangeal joint**

√7ᵗʰ **S93.141 Subluxation of metatarsophalangeal joint of right great toe**

√7ᵗʰ **S93.142 Subluxation of metatarsophalangeal joint of left great toe**

√7ᵗʰ **S93.143 Subluxation of metatarsophalangeal joint of unspecified great toe**

√7ᵗʰ **S93.144 Subluxation of metatarsophalangeal joint of right lesser toe(s)**

√7ᵗʰ **S93.145 Subluxation of metatarsophalangeal joint of left lesser toe(s)**

√7ᵗʰ **S93.146 Subluxation of metatarsophalangeal joint of unspecified lesser toe(s)**

√7ᵗʰ **S93.149 Subluxation of metatarsophalangeal joint of unspecified toe(s)**

√5ᵗʰ **S93.3 Subluxation and dislocation of foot**

EXCLUDES 2   *dislocation of toe (S93.1-)*

√6ᵗʰ **S93.30 Unspecified subluxation and dislocation of foot**

Dislocation of foot NOS
Subluxation of foot NOS

√7ᵗʰ **S93.301 Unspecified subluxation of right foot**

√7ᵗʰ **S93.302 Unspecified subluxation of left foot**

√7ᵗʰ **S93.303 Unspecified subluxation of unspecified foot**

√7ᵗʰ **S93.304 Unspecified dislocation of right foot**

√7ᵗʰ **S93.305 Unspecified dislocation of left foot**

√7ᵗʰ **S93.306 Unspecified dislocation of unspecified foot**

√6ᵗʰ **S93.31 Subluxation and dislocation of tarsal joint**

√7ᵗʰ **S93.311 Subluxation of tarsal joint of right foot**

√7ᵗʰ **S93.312 Subluxation of tarsal joint of left foot**

√7ᵗʰ **S93.313 Subluxation of tarsal joint of unspecified foot**

√7ᵗʰ **S93.314 Dislocation of tarsal joint of right foot**

√7ᵗʰ **S93.315 Dislocation of tarsal joint of left foot**

√7ᵗʰ **S93.316 Dislocation of tarsal joint of unspecified foot**

√6ᵗʰ **S93.32 Subluxation and dislocation of tarsometatarsal joint**

√7ᵗʰ **S93.321 Subluxation of tarsometatarsal joint of right foot**

√7ᵗʰ **S93.322 Subluxation of tarsometatarsal joint of left foot**

√7ᵗʰ **S93.323 Subluxation of tarsometatarsal joint of unspecified foot**

√7ᵗʰ **S93.324 Dislocation of tarsometatarsal joint of right foot**

√7ᵗʰ **S93.325 Dislocation of tarsometatarsal joint of left foot**

√7ᵗʰ **S93.326 Dislocation of tarsometatarsal joint of unspecified foot**

√6ᵗʰ **S93.33 Other subluxation and dislocation of foot**

√7ᵗʰ **S93.331 Other subluxation of right foot**

√7ᵗʰ **S93.332 Other subluxation of left foot**

√7ᵗʰ **S93.333 Other subluxation of unspecified foot**

√7ᵗʰ **S93.334 Other dislocation of right foot**

√7ᵗʰ **S93.335 Other dislocation of left foot**

√7ᵗʰ **S93.336 Other dislocation of unspecified foot**

√5ᵗʰ **S93.4 Sprain of ankle**

EXCLUDES 2   *injury of Achilles tendon (S86.0-)*

√6ᵗʰ **S93.40 Sprain of unspecified ligament of ankle**

Sprain of ankle NOS
Sprained ankle NOS

√7ᵗʰ **S93.401 Sprain of unspecified ligament of right ankle**

√7ᵗʰ **S93.402 Sprain of unspecified ligament of left ankle**

√7ᵗʰ **S93.409 Sprain of unspecified ligament of unspecified ankle**

√6ᵗʰ **S93.41 Sprain of calcaneofibular ligament**

√7ᵗʰ **S93.411 Sprain of calcaneofibular ligament of right ankle**

√7ᵗʰ **S93.412 Sprain of calcaneofibular ligament of left ankle**

√7ᵗʰ **S93.419 Sprain of calcaneofibular ligament of unspecified ankle**

√6ᵗʰ **S93.42 Sprain of deltoid ligament**

√7ᵗʰ **S93.421 Sprain of deltoid ligament of right ankle**

√7ᵗʰ **S93.422 Sprain of deltoid ligament of left ankle**

√7ᵗʰ **S93.429 Sprain of deltoid ligament of unspecified ankle**

√6ᵗʰ **S93.43 Sprain of tibiofibular ligament**

√7ᵗʰ **S93.431 Sprain of tibiofibular ligament of right ankle**

√7ᵗʰ **S93.432 Sprain of tibiofibular ligament of left ankle**

√7ᵗʰ **S93.439 Sprain of tibiofibular ligament of unspecified ankle**

√6ᵗʰ **S93.49 Sprain of other ligament of ankle**

Sprain of internal collateral ligament
Sprain of talofibular ligament

√7ᵗʰ **S93.491 Sprain of other ligament of right ankle**

√7ᵗʰ **S93.492 Sprain of other ligament of left ankle**

√7ᵗʰ **S93.499 Sprain of other ligament of unspecified ankle**

√5ᵗʰ **S93.5 Sprain of toe**

√6ᵗʰ **S93.50 Unspecified sprain of toe**

√7ᵗʰ **S93.501 Unspecified sprain of right great toe**

√7ᵗʰ **S93.502 Unspecified sprain of left great toe**

√7ᵗʰ **S93.503 Unspecified sprain of unspecified great toe**

√7ᵗʰ **S93.504 Unspecified sprain of right lesser toe(s)**

√7ᵗʰ **S93.505 Unspecified sprain of left lesser toe(s)**

√7ᵗʰ **S93.506 Unspecified sprain of unspecified lesser toe(s)**

√7ᵗʰ **S93.509 Unspecified sprain of unspecified toe(s)**

√6ᵗʰ **S93.51 Sprain of interphalangeal joint of toe**

√7ᵗʰ **S93.511 Sprain of interphalangeal joint of right great toe**

√7ᵗʰ **S93.512 Sprain of interphalangeal joint of left great toe**

√7ᵗʰ **S93.513 Sprain of interphalangeal joint of unspecified great toe**

√7ᵗʰ **S93.514 Sprain of interphalangeal joint of right lesser toe(s)**

√7ᵗʰ **S93.515 Sprain of interphalangeal joint of left lesser toe(s)**

√7ᵗʰ **S93.516 Sprain of interphalangeal joint of unspecified lesser toe(s)**

√7ᵗʰ **S93.519 Sprain of interphalangeal joint of unspecified toe(s)**

√6ᵗʰ **S93.52 Sprain of metatarsophalangeal joint of toe**

√7ᵗʰ **S93.521 Sprain of metatarsophalangeal joint of right great toe**

√7ᵗʰ **S93.522 Sprain of metatarsophalangeal joint of left great toe**

√7ᵗʰ **S93.523 Sprain of metatarsophalangeal joint of unspecified great toe**

√7ᵗʰ **S93.524 Sprain of metatarsophalangeal joint of right lesser toe(s)**

√7ᵗʰ **S93.525 Sprain of metatarsophalangeal joint of left lesser toe(s)**

√7ᵗʰ **S93.526 Sprain of metatarsophalangeal joint of unspecified lesser toe(s)**

√7ᵗʰ **S93.529 Sprain of metatarsophalangeal joint of unspecified toe(s)**

√5ᵗʰ **S93.6 Sprain of foot**

EXCLUDES 2   *sprain of metatarsophalangeal joint of toe (S93.52-)*
sprain of toe (S93.5-)

√6ᵗʰ **S93.60 Unspecified sprain of foot**

√7ᵗʰ **S93.601 Unspecified sprain of right foot**

√7ᵗʰ **S93.602 Unspecified sprain of left foot**

☑ Additional Character Required   √x7ᵗʰ Placeholder Alert   Manifestation   Unspecified Dx   ▶◀ Revised Text   ● New Code   ▲ Revised Code Title

CD-10-CM 2020   1071

✓7ᵗʰ **S93.609** Unspecified sprain of unspecified foot

✓6ᵗʰ **S93.61** Sprain of tarsal ligament of foot

  ✓7ᵗʰ **S93.611** Sprain of tarsal ligament of right foot

  ✓7ᵗʰ **S93.612** Sprain of tarsal ligament of left foot

  ✓7ᵗʰ **S93.619** Sprain of tarsal ligament of unspecified foot

✓6ᵗʰ **S93.62** Sprain of tarsometatarsal ligament of foot

  ✓7ᵗʰ **S93.621** Sprain of tarsometatarsal ligament of right foot

  ✓7ᵗʰ **S93.622** Sprain of tarsometatarsal ligament of left foot

  ✓7ᵗʰ **S93.629** Sprain of tarsometatarsal ligament of unspecified foot

✓6ᵗʰ **S93.69** Other sprain of foot

  ✓7ᵗʰ **S93.691** Other sprain of right foot

  ✓7ᵗʰ **S93.692** Other sprain of left foot

  ✓7ᵗʰ **S93.699** Other sprain of unspecified foot

✓4ᵗʰ **S94 Injury of nerves at ankle and foot level**

Code also any associated open wound (S91.-)

The appropriate 7th character is to be added to each code from category S94.
- A initial encounter
- D subsequent encounter
- S sequela

✓5ᵗʰ **S94.0** Injury of lateral plantar nerve

  ✓x7ᵗʰ **S94.00** Injury of lateral plantar nerve, unspecified leg

  ✓x7ᵗʰ **S94.01** Injury of lateral plantar nerve, right leg

  ✓x7ᵗʰ **S94.02** Injury of lateral plantar nerve, left leg

✓5ᵗʰ **S94.1** Injury of medial plantar nerve

  ✓x7ᵗʰ **S94.10** Injury of medial plantar nerve, unspecified leg

  ✓x7ᵗʰ **S94.11** Injury of medial plantar nerve, right leg

  ✓x7ᵗʰ **S94.12** Injury of medial plantar nerve, left leg

✓5ᵗʰ **S94.2** Injury of deep peroneal nerve at ankle and foot level

Injury of terminal, lateral branch of deep peroneal nerve

  ✓x7ᵗʰ **S94.20** Injury of deep peroneal nerve at ankle and foot level, unspecified leg

  ✓x7ᵗʰ **S94.21** Injury of deep peroneal nerve at ankle and foot level, right leg

  ✓x7ᵗʰ **S94.22** Injury of deep peroneal nerve at ankle and foot level, left leg

✓5ᵗʰ **S94.3** Injury of cutaneous sensory nerve at ankle and foot level

  ✓x7ᵗʰ **S94.30** Injury of cutaneous sensory nerve at ankle and foot level, unspecified leg

  ✓x7ᵗʰ **S94.31** Injury of cutaneous sensory nerve at ankle and foot level, right leg

  ✓x7ᵗʰ **S94.32** Injury of cutaneous sensory nerve at ankle and foot level, left leg

✓5ᵗʰ **S94.8** Injury of other nerves at ankle and foot level

  ✓6ᵗʰ **S94.8X** Injury of other nerves at ankle and foot level

    ✓7ᵗʰ **S94.8X1** Injury of other nerves at ankle and foot level, right leg

    ✓7ᵗʰ **S94.8X2** Injury of other nerves at ankle and foot level, left leg

    ✓7ᵗʰ **S94.8X9** Injury of other nerves at ankle and foot level, unspecified leg

✓5ᵗʰ **S94.9** Injury of unspecified nerve at ankle and foot level

  ✓x7ᵗʰ **S94.90** Injury of unspecified nerve at ankle and foot level, unspecified leg

  ✓x7ᵗʰ **S94.91** Injury of unspecified nerve at ankle and foot level, right leg

  ✓x7ᵗʰ **S94.92** Injury of unspecified nerve at ankle and foot level, left leg

✓4ᵗʰ **S95 Injury of blood vessels at ankle and foot level**

Code also any associated open wound (S91.-)

EXCLUDES 2   *injury of posterior tibial artery and vein (S85.1-, S85.8-)*

The appropriate 7th character is to be added to each code from category S95.
- A initial encounter
- D subsequent encounter
- S sequela

✓5ᵗʰ **S95.0** Injury of dorsal artery of foot

  ✓6ᵗʰ **S95.00** Unspecified injury of dorsal artery of foot

    ✓7ᵗʰ **S95.001** Unspecified injury of dorsal artery of right foot

    ✓7ᵗʰ **S95.002** Unspecified injury of dorsal artery of left foot

    ✓7ᵗʰ **S95.009** Unspecified injury of dorsal artery of unspecified foot

  ✓6ᵗʰ **S95.01** Laceration of dorsal artery of foot

    ✓7ᵗʰ **S95.011** Laceration of dorsal artery of right foot

    ✓7ᵗʰ **S95.012** Laceration of dorsal artery of left foot

    ✓7ᵗʰ **S95.019** Laceration of dorsal artery of unspecified foot

  ✓6ᵗʰ **S95.09** Other specified injury of dorsal artery of foot

    ✓7ᵗʰ **S95.091** Other specified injury of dorsal artery of right foot

    ✓7ᵗʰ **S95.092** Other specified injury of dorsal artery of left foot

    ✓7ᵗʰ **S95.099** Other specified injury of dorsal artery of unspecified foot

✓5ᵗʰ **S95.1** Injury of plantar artery of foot

  ✓6ᵗʰ **S95.10** Unspecified injury of plantar artery of foot

    ✓7ᵗʰ **S95.101** Unspecified injury of plantar artery of right foot

    ✓7ᵗʰ **S95.102** Unspecified injury of plantar artery of left foot

    ✓7ᵗʰ **S95.109** Unspecified injury of plantar artery of unspecified foot

  ✓6ᵗʰ **S95.11** Laceration of plantar artery of foot

    ✓7ᵗʰ **S95.111** Laceration of plantar artery of right foot

    ✓7ᵗʰ **S95.112** Laceration of plantar artery of left foot

    ✓7ᵗʰ **S95.119** Laceration of plantar artery of unspecified foot

  ✓6ᵗʰ **S95.19** Other specified injury of plantar artery of foot

    ✓7ᵗʰ **S95.191** Other specified injury of plantar artery of right foot

    ✓7ᵗʰ **S95.192** Other specified injury of plantar artery of left foot

    ✓7ᵗʰ **S95.199** Other specified injury of plantar artery of unspecified foot

✓5ᵗʰ **S95.2** Injury of dorsal vein of foot

  ✓6ᵗʰ **S95.20** Unspecified injury of dorsal vein of foot

    ✓7ᵗʰ **S95.201** Unspecified injury of dorsal vein of right foot

    ✓7ᵗʰ **S95.202** Unspecified injury of dorsal vein of left foot

    ✓7ᵗʰ **S95.209** Unspecified injury of dorsal vein of unspecified foot

  ✓6ᵗʰ **S95.21** Laceration of dorsal vein of foot

    ✓7ᵗʰ **S95.211** Laceration of dorsal vein of right foot

    ✓7ᵗʰ **S95.212** Laceration of dorsal vein of left foot

    ✓7ᵗʰ **S95.219** Laceration of dorsal vein of unspecified foot

  ✓6ᵗʰ **S95.29** Other specified injury of dorsal vein of foot

    ✓7ᵗʰ **S95.291** Other specified injury of dorsal vein of right foot

    ✓7ᵗʰ **S95.292** Other specified injury of dorsal vein of left foot

    ✓7ᵗʰ **S95.299** Other specified injury of dorsal vein of unspecified foot

✓5ᵗʰ **S95.8** Injury of other blood vessels at ankle and foot level

  ✓6ᵗʰ **S95.80** Unspecified injury of other blood vessels at ankle and foot level

    ✓7ᵗʰ **S95.801** Unspecified injury of other blood vessels at ankle and foot level, right leg

    ✓7ᵗʰ **S95.802** Unspecified injury of other blood vessels at ankle and foot level, left leg

    ✓7ᵗʰ **S95.809** Unspecified injury of other blood vessels at ankle and foot level, unspecified leg

✓6ᵗʰ **S95.81** Laceration of other blood vessels at ankle and foot level

     ✓7ᵗʰ **S95.811** Laceration of other blood vessels at ankle and foot level, **right leg**

     ✓7ᵗʰ **S95.812** Laceration of other blood vessels at ankle and foot level, **left leg**

     ✓7ᵗʰ **S95.819** Laceration of other blood vessels at ankle and foot level, **unspecified leg**

✓6ᵗʰ **S95.89** Other specified injury of other blood vessels at ankle and foot level

     ✓7ᵗʰ **S95.891** Other specified injury of other blood vessels at ankle and foot level, **right leg**

     ✓7ᵗʰ **S95.892** Other specified injury of other blood vessels at ankle and foot level, **left leg**

     ✓7ᵗʰ **S95.899** Other specified injury of other blood vessels at ankle and foot level, **unspecified leg**

✓5ᵗʰ **S95.9** Injury of unspecified blood vessel at ankle and foot level

     ✓6ᵗʰ **S95.90** Unspecified injury of unspecified blood vessel at ankle and foot level

         ✓7ᵗʰ **S95.901** Unspecified injury of unspecified blood vessel at ankle and foot level, **right leg**

         ✓7ᵗʰ **S95.902** Unspecified injury of unspecified blood vessel at ankle and foot level, **left leg**

         ✓7ᵗʰ **S95.909** Unspecified injury of unspecified blood vessel at ankle and foot level, **unspecified leg**

     ✓6ᵗʰ **S95.91** Laceration of unspecified blood vessel at ankle and foot level

         ✓7ᵗʰ **S95.911** Laceration of unspecified blood vessel at ankle and foot level, **right leg**

         ✓7ᵗʰ **S95.912** Laceration of unspecified blood vessel at ankle and foot level, **left leg**

         ✓7ᵗʰ **S95.919** Laceration of unspecified blood vessel at ankle and foot level, **unspecified leg**

     ✓6ᵗʰ **S95.99** Other specified injury of unspecified blood vessel at ankle and foot level

         ✓7ᵗʰ **S95.991** Other specified injury of unspecified blood vessel at ankle and foot level, **right leg**

         ✓7ᵗʰ **S95.992** Other specified injury of unspecified blood vessel at ankle and foot level, **left leg**

         ✓7ᵗʰ **S95.999** Other specified injury of unspecified blood vessel at ankle and foot level, **unspecified leg**

✓4ᵗʰ **S96 Injury of muscle and tendon at ankle and foot level**

     Code also any associated open wound (S91.-)

     EXCLUDES 2   injury of Achilles tendon (S86.0-)

               sprain of joints and ligaments of ankle and foot (S93.-)

     TIP: Refer to the Muscle/Tendon table at the beginning of this chapter.

> The appropriate 7th character is to be added to each code from category S96.
> A   initial encounter
> D   subsequent encounter
> S   sequela

✓5ᵗʰ **S96.0** Injury of muscle and tendon of long flexor muscle of toe at ankle and foot level

     ✓6ᵗʰ **S96.00** Unspecified injury of muscle and tendon of long flexor muscle of toe at ankle and foot level

         ✓7ᵗʰ **S96.001** Unspecified injury of muscle and tendon of long flexor muscle of toe at ankle and foot level, **right foot**

         ✓7ᵗʰ **S96.002** Unspecified injury of muscle and tendon of long flexor muscle of toe at ankle and foot level, **left foot**

         ✓7ᵗʰ **S96.009** Unspecified injury of muscle and tendon of long flexor muscle of toe at ankle and foot level, **unspecified foot**

     ✓6ᵗʰ **S96.01** Strain of muscle and tendon of long flexor muscle of toe at ankle and foot level

         ✓7ᵗʰ **S96.011** Strain of muscle and tendon of long flexor muscle of toe at ankle and foot level, **right foot**

         ✓7ᵗʰ **S96.012** Strain of muscle and tendon of long flexor muscle of toe at ankle and foot level, **left foot**

         ✓7ᵗʰ **S96.019** Strain of muscle and tendon of long flexor muscle of toe at ankle and foot level, **unspecified foot**

✓6ᵗʰ **S96.02** Laceration of muscle and tendon of long flexor muscle of toe at ankle and foot level

     ✓7ᵗʰ **S96.021** Laceration of muscle and tendon of long flexor muscle of toe at ankle and foot level, **right foot**

     ✓7ᵗʰ **S96.022** Laceration of muscle and tendon of long flexor muscle of toe at ankle and foot level, **left foot**

     ✓7ᵗʰ **S96.029** Laceration of muscle and tendon of long flexor muscle of toe at ankle and foot level, **unspecified foot**

✓6ᵗʰ **S96.09** Other injury of muscle and tendon of long flexor muscle of toe at ankle and foot level

     ✓7ᵗʰ **S96.091** Other injury of muscle and tendon of long flexor muscle of toe at ankle and foot level, **right foot**

     ✓7ᵗʰ **S96.092** Other injury of muscle and tendon of long flexor muscle of toe at ankle and foot level, **left foot**

     ✓7ᵗʰ **S96.099** Other injury of muscle and tendon of long flexor muscle of toe at ankle and foot level, **unspecified foot**

✓5ᵗʰ **S96.1** Injury of muscle and tendon of long extensor muscle of toe at ankle and foot level

     ✓6ᵗʰ **S96.10** Unspecified injury of muscle and tendon of long extensor muscle of toe at ankle and foot level

         ✓7ᵗʰ **S96.101** Unspecified injury of muscle and tendon of long extensor muscle of toe at ankle and foot level, **right foot**

         ✓7ᵗʰ **S96.102** Unspecified injury of muscle and tendon of long extensor muscle of toe at ankle and foot level, **left foot**

         ✓7ᵗʰ **S96.109** Unspecified injury of muscle and tendon of long extensor muscle of toe at ankle and foot level, **unspecified foot**

     ✓6ᵗʰ **S96.11** Strain of muscle and tendon of long extensor muscle of toe at ankle and foot level

         ✓7ᵗʰ **S96.111** Strain of muscle and tendon of long extensor muscle of toe at ankle and foot level, **right foot**

         ✓7ᵗʰ **S96.112** Strain of muscle and tendon of long extensor muscle of toe at ankle and foot level, **left foot**

         ✓7ᵗʰ **S96.119** Strain of muscle and tendon of long extensor muscle of toe at ankle and foot level, **unspecified foot**

     ✓6ᵗʰ **S96.12** Laceration of muscle and tendon of long extensor muscle of toe at ankle and foot level

         ✓7ᵗʰ **S96.121** Laceration of muscle and tendon of long extensor muscle of toe at ankle and foot level, **right foot**

         ✓7ᵗʰ **S96.122** Laceration of muscle and tendon of long extensor muscle of toe at ankle and foot level, **left foot**

         ✓7ᵗʰ **S96.129** Laceration of muscle and tendon of long extensor muscle of toe at ankle and foot level, **unspecified foot**

     ✓6ᵗʰ **S96.19** Other specified injury of muscle and tendon of long extensor muscle of toe at ankle and foot level

         ✓7ᵗʰ **S96.191** Other specified injury of muscle and tendon of long extensor muscle of toe at ankle and foot level, **right foot**

         ✓7ᵗʰ **S96.192** Other specified injury of muscle and tendon of long extensor muscle of toe at ankle and foot level, **left foot**

         ✓7ᵗʰ **S96.199** Other specified injury of muscle and tendon of long extensor muscle of toe at ankle and foot level, **unspecified foot**

✓5ᵗʰ **S96.2** Injury of intrinsic muscle and tendon at ankle and foot level

     ✓6ᵗʰ **S96.20** Unspecified injury of intrinsic muscle and tendon at ankle and foot level

         ✓7ᵗʰ **S96.201** Unspecified injury of intrinsic muscle and tendon at ankle and foot level, **right foot**

         ✓7ᵗʰ **S96.202** Unspecified injury of intrinsic muscle and tendon at ankle and foot level, **left foot**

         ✓7ᵗʰ **S96.209** Unspecified injury of intrinsic muscle and tendon at ankle and foot level, **unspecified foot**

     ✓6ᵗʰ **S96.21** Strain of intrinsic muscle and tendon at ankle and foot level

         ✓7ᵗʰ **S96.211** Strain of intrinsic muscle and tendon at ankle and foot level, **right foot**

         ✓7ᵗʰ **S96.212** Strain of intrinsic muscle and tendon at ankle and foot level, **left foot**

✓ Additional Character Required   ✓x7ᵗʰ Placeholder Alert   Manifestation   Unspecified Dx   ▶◀ Revised Text   ● New Code   ▲ Revised Code Title

ICD-10-CM 2020   1073

√7ᵗʰ **S96.219** Strain of intrinsic muscle and tendon at ankle and foot level, unspecified foot

√6ᵗʰ **S96.22** Laceration of intrinsic muscle and tendon at ankle and foot level

√7ᵗʰ **S96.221** Laceration of intrinsic muscle and tendon at ankle and foot level, right foot

√7ᵗʰ **S96.222** Laceration of intrinsic muscle and tendon at ankle and foot level, left foot

√7ᵗʰ **S96.229** Laceration of intrinsic muscle and tendon at ankle and foot level, unspecified foot

√6ᵗʰ **S96.29** Other specified injury of intrinsic muscle and tendon at ankle and foot level

√7ᵗʰ **S96.291** Other specified injury of intrinsic muscle and tendon at ankle and foot level, right foot

√7ᵗʰ **S96.292** Other specified injury of intrinsic muscle and tendon at ankle and foot level, left foot

√7ᵗʰ **S96.299** Other specified injury of intrinsic muscle and tendon at ankle and foot level, unspecified foot

√5ᵗʰ **S96.8** Injury of other specified muscles and tendons at ankle and foot level

√6ᵗʰ **S96.80** Unspecified injury of other specified muscles and tendons at ankle and foot level

√7ᵗʰ **S96.801** Unspecified injury of other specified muscles and tendons at ankle and foot level, right foot

√7ᵗʰ **S96.802** Unspecified injury of other specified muscles and tendons at ankle and foot level, left foot

√7ᵗʰ **S96.809** Unspecified injury of other specified muscles and tendons at ankle and foot level, unspecified foot

√6ᵗʰ **S96.81** Strain of other specified muscles and tendons at ankle and foot level

√7ᵗʰ **S96.811** Strain of other specified muscles and tendons at ankle and foot level, right foot

√7ᵗʰ **S96.812** Strain of other specified muscles and tendons at ankle and foot level, left foot

√7ᵗʰ **S96.819** Strain of other specified muscles and tendons at ankle and foot level, unspecified foot

√6ᵗʰ **S96.82** Laceration of other specified muscles and tendons at ankle and foot level

√7ᵗʰ **S96.821** Laceration of other specified muscles and tendons at ankle and foot level, right foot

√7ᵗʰ **S96.822** Laceration of other specified muscles and tendons at ankle and foot level, left foot

√7ᵗʰ **S96.829** Laceration of other specified muscles and tendons at ankle and foot level, unspecified foot

√6ᵗʰ **S96.89** Other specified injury of other specified muscles and tendons at ankle and foot level

√7ᵗʰ **S96.891** Other specified injury of other specified muscles and tendons at ankle and foot level, right foot

√7ᵗʰ **S96.892** Other specified injury of other specified muscles and tendons at ankle and foot level, left foot

√7ᵗʰ **S96.899** Other specified injury of other specified muscles and tendons at ankle and foot level, unspecified foot

√5ᵗʰ **S96.9** Injury of unspecified muscle and tendon at ankle and foot level

√6ᵗʰ **S96.90** Unspecified injury of unspecified muscle and tendon at ankle and foot level

√7ᵗʰ **S96.901** Unspecified injury of unspecified muscle and tendon at ankle and foot level, right foot

√7ᵗʰ **S96.902** Unspecified injury of unspecified muscle and tendon at ankle and foot level, left foot

√7ᵗʰ **S96.909** Unspecified injury of unspecified muscle and tendon at ankle and foot level, unspecified foot

√6ᵗʰ **S96.91** Strain of unspecified muscle and tendon at ankle and foot level

√7ᵗʰ **S96.911** Strain of unspecified muscle and tendon at ankle and foot level, right foot

√7ᵗʰ **S96.912** Strain of unspecified muscle and tendon at ankle and foot level, left foot

√7ᵗʰ **S96.919** Strain of unspecified muscle and tendon at ankle and foot level, unspecified foot

√6ᵗʰ **S96.92** Laceration of unspecified muscle and tendon at ankle and foot level

√7ᵗʰ **S96.921** Laceration of unspecified muscle and tendon at ankle and foot level, right foot

√7ᵗʰ **S96.922** Laceration of unspecified muscle and tendon at ankle and foot level, left foot

√7ᵗʰ **S96.929** Laceration of unspecified muscle and tendon at ankle and foot level, unspecified foot

√6ᵗʰ **S96.99** Other specified injury of unspecified muscle and tendon at ankle and foot level

√7ᵗʰ **S96.991** Other specified injury of unspecified muscle and tendon at ankle and foot level, right foot

√7ᵗʰ **S96.992** Other specified injury of unspecified muscle and tendon at ankle and foot level, left foot

√7ᵗʰ **S96.999** Other specified injury of unspecified muscle and tendon at ankle and foot level, unspecified foot

√4ᵗʰ **S97** **Crushing injury of ankle and foot**

Use additional code(s) for all associated injuries

The appropriate 7th character is to be added to each code from category S97.
A   initial encounter
D   subsequent encounter
S   sequela

√5ᵗʰ **S97.0** Crushing injury of ankle

√x7ᵗʰ **S97.00** Crushing injury of unspecified ankle

√x7ᵗʰ **S97.01** Crushing injury of right ankle

√x7ᵗʰ **S97.02** Crushing injury of left ankle

√5ᵗʰ **S97.1** Crushing injury of toe

√6ᵗʰ **S97.10** Crushing injury of unspecified toe(s)

√7ᵗʰ **S97.101** Crushing injury of unspecified right toe(s)

√7ᵗʰ **S97.102** Crushing injury of unspecified left toe(s)

√7ᵗʰ **S97.109** Crushing injury of unspecified toe(s)

Crushing injury of toe NOS

√6ᵗʰ **S97.11** Crushing injury of great toe

√7ᵗʰ **S97.111** Crushing injury of right great toe

√7ᵗʰ **S97.112** Crushing injury of left great toe

√7ᵗʰ **S97.119** Crushing injury of unspecified great toe

√6ᵗʰ **S97.12** Crushing injury of lesser toe(s)

√7ᵗʰ **S97.121** Crushing injury of right lesser toe(s)

√7ᵗʰ **S97.122** Crushing injury of left lesser toe(s)

√7ᵗʰ **S97.129** Crushing injury of unspecified lesser toe(s)

√5ᵗʰ **S97.8** Crushing injury of foot

√x7ᵗʰ **S97.80** Crushing injury of unspecified foot

Crushing injury of foot NOS

√x7ᵗʰ **S97.81** Crushing injury of right foot

√x7ᵗʰ **S97.82** Crushing injury of left foot

√4ᵗʰ **S98** **Traumatic amputation of ankle and foot**

An amputation not identified as partial or complete should be coded to complete

The appropriate 7th character is to be added to each code from category S98.
A   initial encounter
D   subsequent encounter
S   sequela

√5ᵗʰ **S98.0** Traumatic amputation of foot at ankle level

√6ᵗʰ **S98.01** Complete traumatic amputation of foot at ankle level

√7ᵗʰ **S98.011** Complete traumatic amputation of right foot at ankle level   HCC

√7ᵗʰ **S98.012** Complete traumatic amputation of left foot at ankle level   HCC

√7ᵗʰ **S98.019** Complete traumatic amputation of unspecified foot at ankle level   HCC

√6ᵗʰ **S98.02** Partial traumatic amputation of foot at ankle level

√7ᵗʰ **S98.021** Partial traumatic amputation of right foot at ankle level   HCC

√7ᵗʰ **S98.022** Partial traumatic amputation of left foot at ankle level   HCC

✓7ᵗʰ **S98.Ø29** Partial traumatic amputation of unspecified foot at ankle level   HCC

✓5ᵗʰ **S98.1** Traumatic amputation of one toe

   ✓6ᵗʰ **S98.11** Complete traumatic amputation of great toe

     ✓7ᵗʰ **S98.111** Complete traumatic amputation of right great toe   HCC

     ✓7ᵗʰ **S98.112** Complete traumatic amputation of left great toe   HCC

     ✓7ᵗʰ **S98.119** Complete traumatic amputation of unspecified great toe   HCC

   ✓6ᵗʰ **S98.12** Partial traumatic amputation of great toe

     ✓7ᵗʰ **S98.121** Partial traumatic amputation of right great toe   HCC

     ✓7ᵗʰ **S98.122** Partial traumatic amputation of left great toe   HCC

     ✓7ᵗʰ **S98.129** Partial traumatic amputation of unspecified great toe   HCC

   ✓6ᵗʰ **S98.13** Complete traumatic amputation of one lesser toe

     Traumatic amputation of toe NOS

     ✓7ᵗʰ **S98.131** Complete traumatic amputation of one right lesser toe   HCC

     ✓7ᵗʰ **S98.132** Complete traumatic amputation of one left lesser toe   HCC

     ✓7ᵗʰ **S98.139** Complete traumatic amputation of one unspecified lesser toe   HCC

   ✓6ᵗʰ **S98.14** Partial traumatic amputation of one lesser toe

     ✓7ᵗʰ **S98.141** Partial traumatic amputation of one right lesser toe   HCC

     ✓7ᵗʰ **S98.142** Partial traumatic amputation of one left lesser toe   HCC

     ✓7ᵗʰ **S98.149** Partial traumatic amputation of one unspecified lesser toe   HCC

✓5ᵗʰ **S98.2** Traumatic amputation of two or more lesser toes

   ✓6ᵗʰ **S98.21** Complete traumatic amputation of two or more lesser toes

     ✓7ᵗʰ **S98.211** Complete traumatic amputation of two or more right lesser toes   HCC

     ✓7ᵗʰ **S98.212** Complete traumatic amputation of two or more left lesser toes   HCC

     ✓7ᵗʰ **S98.219** Complete traumatic amputation of two or more unspecified lesser toes   HCC

   ✓6ᵗʰ **S98.22** Partial traumatic amputation of two or more lesser toes

     ✓7ᵗʰ **S98.221** Partial traumatic amputation of two or more right lesser toes   HCC

     ✓7ᵗʰ **S98.222** Partial traumatic amputation of two or more left lesser toes   HCC

     ✓7ᵗʰ **S98.229** Partial traumatic amputation of two or more unspecified lesser toes   HCC

✓5ᵗʰ **S98.3** Traumatic amputation of midfoot

   ✓6ᵗʰ **S98.31** Complete traumatic amputation of midfoot

     ✓7ᵗʰ **S98.311** Complete traumatic amputation of right midfoot   HCC

     ✓7ᵗʰ **S98.312** Complete traumatic amputation of left midfoot   HCC

     ✓7ᵗʰ **S98.319** Complete traumatic amputation of unspecified midfoot   HCC

   ✓6ᵗʰ **S98.32** Partial traumatic amputation of midfoot

     ✓7ᵗʰ **S98.321** Partial traumatic amputation of right midfoot   HCC

     ✓7ᵗʰ **S98.322** Partial traumatic amputation of left midfoot   HCC

     ✓7ᵗʰ **S98.329** Partial traumatic amputation of unspecified midfoot   HCC

✓5ᵗʰ **S98.9** Traumatic amputation of foot, level unspecified

   ✓6ᵗʰ **S98.91** Complete traumatic amputation of foot, level unspecified

     ✓7ᵗʰ **S98.911** Complete traumatic amputation of right foot, level unspecified   HCC

     ✓7ᵗʰ **S98.912** Complete traumatic amputation of left foot, level unspecified   HCC

     ✓7ᵗʰ **S98.919** Complete traumatic amputation of unspecified foot, level unspecified   HCC

   ✓6ᵗʰ **S98.92** Partial traumatic amputation of foot, level unspecified

     ✓7ᵗʰ **S98.921** Partial traumatic amputation of right foot, level unspecified   HCC

     ✓7ᵗʰ **S98.922** Partial traumatic amputation of left foot, level unspecified   HCC

     ✓7ᵗʰ **S98.929** Partial traumatic amputation of unspecified foot, level unspecified   HCC

✓4ᵗʰ **S99** Other and unspecified injuries of ankle and foot

   AHA: 2018,2Q,12; 2018,1Q,3; 2016,4Q,68-69

   ✓5ᵗʰ **S99.Ø** Physeal fracture of calcaneus

> The appropriate 7th character is to be added to each code from subcategory S99.Ø.
> A   initial encounter for closed fracture
> B   initial encounter for open fracture
> D   subsequent encounter for fracture with routine healing
> G   subsequent encounter for fracture with delayed healing
> K   subsequent encounter for fracture with nonunion
> P   subsequent encounter for fracture with malunion
> S   sequela

    ✓6ᵗʰ **S99.ØØ** Unspecified physeal fracture of calcaneus

      ✓7ᵗʰ **S99.ØØ1** Unspecified physeal fracture of right calcaneus   Q

      ✓7ᵗʰ **S99.ØØ2** Unspecified physeal fracture of left calcaneus   Q

      ✓7ᵗʰ **S99.ØØ9** Unspecified physeal fracture of unspecified calcaneus   Q

    ✓6ᵗʰ **S99.Ø1** Salter-Harris Type I physeal fracture of calcaneus

      ✓7ᵗʰ **S99.Ø11** Salter-Harris Type I physeal fracture of right calcaneus   Q

      ✓7ᵗʰ **S99.Ø12** Salter-Harris Type I physeal fracture of left calcaneus   Q

      ✓7ᵗʰ **S99.Ø19** Salter-Harris Type I physeal fracture of unspecified calcaneus   Q

    ✓6ᵗʰ **S99.Ø2** Salter-Harris Type II physeal fracture of calcaneus

      ✓7ᵗʰ **S99.Ø21** Salter-Harris Type II physeal fracture of right calcaneus   Q

      ✓7ᵗʰ **S99.Ø22** Salter-Harris Type II physeal fracture of left calcaneus   Q

      ✓7ᵗʰ **S99.Ø29** Salter-Harris Type II physeal fracture of unspecified calcaneus   Q

    ✓6ᵗʰ **S99.Ø3** Salter-Harris Type III physeal fracture of calcaneus

      ✓7ᵗʰ **S99.Ø31** Salter-Harris Type III physeal fracture of right calcaneus   Q

      ✓7ᵗʰ **S99.Ø32** Salter-Harris Type III physeal fracture of left calcaneus   Q

      ✓7ᵗʰ **S99.Ø39** Salter-Harris Type III physeal fracture of unspecified calcaneus   Q

    ✓6ᵗʰ **S99.Ø4** Salter-Harris Type IV physeal fracture of calcaneus

      ✓7ᵗʰ **S99.Ø41** Salter-Harris Type IV physeal fracture of right calcaneus   Q

      ✓7ᵗʰ **S99.Ø42** Salter-Harris Type IV physeal fracture of left calcaneus   Q

      ✓7ᵗʰ **S99.Ø49** Salter-Harris Type IV physeal fracture of unspecified calcaneus   Q

    ✓6ᵗʰ **S99.Ø9** Other physeal fracture of calcaneus

      ✓7ᵗʰ **S99.Ø91** Other physeal fracture of right calcaneus   Q

      ✓7ᵗʰ **S99.Ø92** Other physeal fracture of left calcaneus   Q

      ✓7ᵗʰ **S99.Ø99** Other physeal fracture of unspecified calcaneus   Q

   ✓5ᵗʰ **S99.1** Physeal fracture of metatarsal

> The appropriate 7th character is to be added to each code from subcategory S99.1.
> A   initial encounter for closed fracture
> B   initial encounter for open fracture
> D   subsequent encounter for fracture with routine healing
> G   subsequent encounter for fracture with delayed healing
> K   subsequent encounter for fracture with nonunion
> P   subsequent encounter for fracture with malunion
> S   sequela

    ✓6ᵗʰ **S99.1Ø** Unspecified physeal fracture of metatarsal

      ✓7ᵗʰ **S99.1Ø1** Unspecified physeal fracture of right metatarsal   Q

      ✓7ᵗʰ **S99.1Ø2** Unspecified physeal fracture of left metatarsal   Q

      ✓7ᵗʰ **S99.1Ø9** Unspecified physeal fracture of unspecified metatarsal   Q

☑ Additional Character Required   ✓ₓ7ᵗʰ Placeholder Alert   Manifestation   Unspecified Dx   ▶◀ Revised Text   ● New Code   ▲ Revised Code Title

√6ᵗʰ **S99.11** Salter-Harris Type I physeal fracture of metatarsal

   √7ᵗʰ **S99.111** **Salter-Harris Type I physeal fracture of right metatarsal** Q

   √7ᵗʰ **S99.112** **Salter-Harris Type I physeal fracture of left metatarsal** Q

   √7ᵗʰ **S99.119** **Salter-Harris Type I physeal fracture of unspecified metatarsal** Q

√6ᵗʰ **S99.12** Salter-Harris Type II physeal fracture of metatarsal

   √7ᵗʰ **S99.121** **Salter-Harris Type II physeal fracture of right metatarsal** Q

   √7ᵗʰ **S99.122** **Salter-Harris Type II physeal fracture of left metatarsal** Q

   √7ᵗʰ **S99.129** **Salter-Harris Type II physeal fracture of unspecified metatarsal** Q

√6ᵗʰ **S99.13** Salter-Harris Type III physeal fracture of metatarsal

   √7ᵗʰ **S99.131** **Salter-Harris Type III physeal fracture of right metatarsal** Q

   √7ᵗʰ **S99.132** **Salter-Harris Type III physeal fracture of left metatarsal** Q

   √7ᵗʰ **S99.139** **Salter-Harris Type III physeal fracture of unspecified metatarsal** Q

√6ᵗʰ **S99.14** Salter-Harris Type IV physeal fracture of metatarsal

   √7ᵗʰ **S99.141** **Salter-Harris Type IV physeal fracture of right metatarsal** Q

   √7ᵗʰ **S99.142** **Salter-Harris Type IV physeal fracture of left metatarsal** Q

   √7ᵗʰ **S99.149** **Salter-Harris Type IV physeal fracture of unspecified metatarsal** Q

√6ᵗʰ **S99.19** **Other physeal fracture of metatarsal**

   √7ᵗʰ **S99.191** **Other physeal fracture of right metatarsal** Q

   √7ᵗʰ **S99.192** **Other physeal fracture of left metatarsal** Q

   √7ᵗʰ **S99.199** **Other physeal fracture of unspecified metatarsal** Q

√5ᵗʰ **S99.2** **Physeal fracture of phalanx of toe**

> The appropriate 7th character is to be added to each code from subcategories S99.2.
> A   initial encounter for closed fracture
> B   initial encounter for open fracture
> D   subsequent encounter for fracture with routine healing
> G   subsequent encounter for fracture with delayed healing
> K   subsequent encounter for fracture with nonunion
> P   subsequent encounter for fracture with malunion
> S   sequela

√6ᵗʰ **S99.20** **Unspecified physeal fracture of phalanx of toe**

   √7ᵗʰ **S99.201** **Unspecified physeal fracture of phalanx of right toe**

   √7ᵗʰ **S99.202** **Unspecified physeal fracture of phalanx of left toe**

   √7ᵗʰ **S99.209** **Unspecified physeal fracture of phalanx of unspecified toe**

√6ᵗʰ **S99.21** Salter-Harris Type I physeal fracture of phalanx of toe

   √7ᵗʰ **S99.211** **Salter-Harris Type I physeal fracture of phalanx of right toe**

   √7ᵗʰ **S99.212** **Salter-Harris Type I physeal fracture of phalanx of left toe**

   √7ᵗʰ **S99.219** **Salter-Harris Type I physeal fracture of phalanx of unspecified toe**

√6ᵗʰ **S99.22** Salter-Harris Type II physeal fracture of phalanx of toe

   √7ᵗʰ **S99.221** **Salter-Harris Type II physeal fracture of phalanx of right toe**

   √7ᵗʰ **S99.222** **Salter-Harris Type II physeal fracture of phalanx of left toe**

   √7ᵗʰ **S99.229** **Salter-Harris Type II physeal fracture of phalanx of unspecified toe**

√6ᵗʰ **S99.23** Salter-Harris Type III physeal fracture of phalanx of toe

   √7ᵗʰ **S99.231** **Salter-Harris Type III physeal fracture of phalanx of right toe**

   √7ᵗʰ **S99.232** **Salter-Harris Type III physeal fracture of phalanx of left toe**

   √7ᵗʰ **S99.239** **Salter-Harris Type III physeal fracture of phalanx of unspecified toe**

√6ᵗʰ **S99.24** Salter-Harris Type IV physeal fracture of phalanx of toe

   √7ᵗʰ **S99.241** **Salter-Harris Type IV physeal fracture of phalanx of right toe**

   √7ᵗʰ **S99.242** **Salter-Harris Type IV physeal fracture of phalanx of left toe**

   √7ᵗʰ **S99.249** **Salter-Harris Type IV physeal fracture of phalanx of unspecified toe**

√6ᵗʰ **S99.29** **Other physeal fracture of phalanx of toe**

   √7ᵗʰ **S99.291** **Other physeal fracture of phalanx of right toe**

   √7ᵗʰ **S99.292** **Other physeal fracture of phalanx of left toe**

   √7ᵗʰ **S99.299** **Other physeal fracture of phalanx of unspecified toe**

√5ᵗʰ **S99.8** **Other specified injuries of ankle and foot**

> The appropriate 7th character is to be added to each code from subcategory S99.8.
> A   initial encounter
> D   subsequent encounter
> S   sequela

√6ᵗʰ **S99.81** **Other specified injuries of ankle**

   √7ᵗʰ **S99.811** **Other specified injuries of right ankle**

   √7ᵗʰ **S99.812** **Other specified injuries of left ankle**

   √7ᵗʰ **S99.819** **Other specified injuries of unspecified ankle**

√6ᵗʰ **S99.82** **Other specified injuries of foot**

   √7ᵗʰ **S99.821** **Other specified injuries of right foot**

   √7ᵗʰ **S99.822** **Other specified injuries of left foot**

   √7ᵗʰ **S99.829** **Other specified injuries of unspecified foot**

√5ᵗʰ **S99.9** **Unspecified injury of ankle and foot**

> The appropriate 7th character is to be added to each code from subcategory S99.9.
> A   initial encounter
> D   subsequent encounter
> S   sequela

√6ᵗʰ **S99.91** **Unspecified injury of ankle**

   √7ᵗʰ **S99.911** **Unspecified injury of right ankle**

   √7ᵗʰ **S99.912** **Unspecified injury of left ankle**

   √7ᵗʰ **S99.919** **Unspecified injury of unspecified ankle**

√6ᵗʰ **S99.92** **Unspecified injury of foot**

   √7ᵗʰ **S99.921** **Unspecified injury of right foot**

   √7ᵗʰ **S99.922** **Unspecified injury of left foot**

   √7ᵗʰ **S99.929** **Unspecified injury of unspecified foot**

INJURY, POISONING AND CERTAIN OTHER CONSEQUENCES OF EXTERNAL CAUSES (T07-T88)

Injuries involving multiple body regions (T07)

EXCLUDES 1   *burns and corrosions (T20-T32)*
frostbite (T33-T34)
insect bite or sting, venomous (T63.4)
sunburn (L55.-)

√x7ᵗʰ **T07** **Unspecified multiple injuries**

   EXCLUDES 1   *injury NOS (T14.90)*

   AHA: 2017,4Q,26

> The appropriate 7th character is to be added to code T07.
> A   initial encounter
> D   subsequent encounter
> S   sequela

Injury of unspecified body region (T14)

√4ᵗʰ **T14** **Injury of unspecified body region**

> **EXCLUDES 1**   *multiple unspecified injuries (T07)*

> **AHA:** 2017,4Q,26

> The appropriate 7th character is to be added to each code from category T14.
> A   initial encounter
> D   subsequent encounter
> S   sequela

√x7ᵗʰ **T14.8** **Other injury of unspecified body region**

Abrasion NOS
Contusion NOS
Crush injury NOS
Fracture NOS
Skin injury NOS
Vascular injury NOS
Wound NOS

√5ᵗʰ **T14.9** **Unspecified injury**

√x7ᵗʰ **T14.90** **Injury, unspecified**

Injury NOS

√x7ᵗʰ **T14.91** **Suicide attempt**   HCC

Attempted suicide NOS

Effects of foreign body entering through natural orifice (T15-T19)

> **EXCLUDES 2**   *foreign body accidentally left in operation wound (T81.5-)*
> *foreign body in penetrating wound — see open wound by body region*
> *residual foreign body in soft tissue (M79.5)*
> *splinter, without open wound — see superficial injury by body region*

√4ᵗʰ **T15** **Foreign body on external eye**

> **EXCLUDES 2**   `foreign body in penetrating wound of orbit and eye ball (S05.4-, S05.5-)`
> *open wound of eyelid and periocular area (S01.1-)*
> *retained foreign body in eyelid (H02.8-)*
> *retained (old) foreign body in penetrating wound of orbit and eye ball (H05.5-, H44.6-, H44.7-)*
> *superficial foreign body of eyelid and periocular area (S00.25-)*

> The appropriate 7th character is to be added to each code from category T15.
> A   initial encounter
> D   subsequent encounter
> S   sequela

√5ᵗʰ **T15.0** **Foreign body in cornea**

√x7ᵗʰ **T15.00** **Foreign body in cornea, unspecified eye**

√x7ᵗʰ **T15.01** **Foreign body in cornea, right eye**

√x7ᵗʰ **T15.02** **Foreign body in cornea, left eye**

√5ᵗʰ **T15.1** **Foreign body in conjunctival sac**

√x7ᵗʰ **T15.10** **Foreign body in conjunctival sac, unspecified eye**

√x7ᵗʰ **T15.11** **Foreign body in conjunctival sac, right eye**

√x7ᵗʰ **T15.12** **Foreign body in conjunctival sac, left eye**

√5ᵗʰ **T15.8** **Foreign body in other and multiple parts of external eye**

Foreign body in lacrimal punctum

√x7ᵗʰ **T15.80** **Foreign body in other and multiple parts of external eye, unspecified eye**

√x7ᵗʰ **T15.81** **Foreign body in other and multiple parts of external eye, right eye**

√x7ᵗʰ **T15.82** **Foreign body in other and multiple parts of external eye, left eye**

√5ᵗʰ **T15.9** **Foreign body on external eye, part unspecified**

√x7ᵗʰ **T15.90** **Foreign body on external eye, part unspecified, unspecified eye**

√x7ᵗʰ **T15.91** **Foreign body on external eye, part unspecified, right eye**

√x7ᵗʰ **T15.92** **Foreign body on external eye, part unspecified, left eye**

√4ᵗʰ **T16** **Foreign body in ear**

> **INCLUDES**   foreign body in auditory canal

> The appropriate 7th character is to be added to each code from category T16.
> A   initial encounter
> D   subsequent encounter
> S   sequela

√x7ᵗʰ **T16.1** **Foreign body in right ear**

√x7ᵗʰ **T16.2** **Foreign body in left ear**

√x7ᵗʰ **T16.9** **Foreign body in ear, unspecified ear**

√4ᵗʰ **T17** **Foreign body in respiratory tract**

> The appropriate 7th character is to be added to each code from category T17.
> A   initial encounter
> D   subsequent encounter
> S   sequela

√x7ᵗʰ **T17.0** **Foreign body in nasal sinus**

√x7ᵗʰ **T17.1** **Foreign body in nostril**

Foreign body in nose NOS

√5ᵗʰ **T17.2** **Foreign body in pharynx**

Foreign body in nasopharynx
Foreign body in throat NOS

√6ᵗʰ **T17.20** **Unspecified foreign body in pharynx**

√7ᵗʰ **T17.200** **Unspecified foreign body in pharynx causing asphyxiation**

√7ᵗʰ **T17.208** **Unspecified foreign body in pharynx causing other injury**

√6ᵗʰ **T17.21** **Gastric contents in pharynx**

Aspiration of gastric contents into pharynx
Vomitus in pharynx

√7ᵗʰ **T17.210** **Gastric contents in pharynx causing asphyxiation**

√7ᵗʰ **T17.218** **Gastric contents in pharynx causing other injury**

√6ᵗʰ **T17.22** **Food in pharynx**

Bones in pharynx
Seeds in pharynx

√7ᵗʰ **T17.220** **Food in pharynx causing asphyxiation**

√7ᵗʰ **T17.228** **Food in pharynx causing other injury**

√6ᵗʰ **T17.29** **Other foreign object in pharynx**

√7ᵗʰ **T17.290** **Other foreign object in pharynx causing asphyxiation**

√7ᵗʰ **T17.298** **Other foreign object in pharynx causing other injury**

√5ᵗʰ **T17.3** **Foreign body in larynx**

√6ᵗʰ **T17.30** **Unspecified foreign body in larynx**

√7ᵗʰ **T17.300** **Unspecified foreign body in larynx causing asphyxiation**

√7ᵗʰ **T17.308** **Unspecified foreign body in larynx causing other injury**

√6ᵗʰ **T17.31** **Gastric contents in larynx**

Aspiration of gastric contents into larynx
Vomitus in larynx

√7ᵗʰ **T17.310** **Gastric contents in larynx causing asphyxiation**

√7ᵗʰ **T17.318** **Gastric contents in larynx causing other injury**

√6ᵗʰ **T17.32** **Food in larynx**

Bones in larynx
Seeds in larynx

√7ᵗʰ **T17.320** **Food in larynx causing asphyxiation**

√7ᵗʰ **T17.328** **Food in larynx causing other injury**

√6ᵗʰ **T17.39** **Other foreign object in larynx**

√7ᵗʰ **T17.390** **Other foreign object in larynx causing asphyxiation**

√7ᵗʰ **T17.398** **Other foreign object in larynx causing other injury**

√5ᵗʰ **T17.4** **Foreign body in trachea**

√6ᵗʰ **T17.40** **Unspecified foreign body in trachea**

√7ᵗʰ **T17.400** **Unspecified foreign body in trachea causing asphyxiation**

√7ᵗʰ **T17.408** **Unspecified foreign body in trachea causing other injury**

☑ Additional Character Required   √x7ᵗʰ Placeholder Alert   Manifestation   Unspecified Dx   ▶◀ Revised Text   ● New Code   ▲ Revised Code Title

√6ᵗʰ **T17.41** Gastric contents **in trachea**

    Aspiration of gastric contents into trachea
    Vomitus in trachea

    √7ᵗʰ **T17.410** **Gastric contents in trachea** causing **asphyxiation**

    √7ᵗʰ **T17.418** **Gastric contents in trachea** causing other injury

√6ᵗʰ **T17.42** Food **in trachea**

    Bones in trachea
    Seeds in trachea

    √7ᵗʰ **T17.420** **Food in trachea** causing asphyxiation

    √7ᵗʰ **T17.428** **Food in trachea** causing other injury

√6ᵗʰ **T17.49** Other foreign object **in trachea**

    √7ᵗʰ **T17.490** **Other foreign object in trachea** causing **asphyxiation**

    √7ᵗʰ **T17.498** **Other foreign object in trachea** causing other injury

√5ᵗʰ **T17.5** Foreign body in bronchus

  √6ᵗʰ **T17.50** Unspecified foreign body **in bronchus**

    √7ᵗʰ **T17.500** **Unspecified foreign body in bronchus causing asphyxiation**

    √7ᵗʰ **T17.508** **Unspecified foreign body in bronchus causing other injury**

  √6ᵗʰ **T17.51** Gastric contents **in bronchus**

    Aspiration of gastric contents into bronchus
    Vomitus in bronchus

    √7ᵗʰ **T17.510** **Gastric contents in bronchus** causing **asphyxiation**

    √7ᵗʰ **T17.518** **Gastric contents in bronchus** causing other injury

  √6ᵗʰ **T17.52** Food **in bronchus**

    Bones in bronchus
    Seeds in bronchus

    √7ᵗʰ **T17.520** **Food in bronchus** causing asphyxiation

    √7ᵗʰ **T17.528** **Food in bronchus** causing other injury

  √6ᵗʰ **T17.59** Other foreign object **in bronchus**

    √7ᵗʰ **T17.590** **Other foreign object in bronchus** causing **asphyxiation**

    √7ᵗʰ **T17.598** **Other foreign object in bronchus** causing other injury

√5ᵗʰ **T17.8** Foreign body in other parts of respiratory tract

  Foreign body in bronchioles
  Foreign body in lung

  √6ᵗʰ **T17.80** Unspecified foreign body **in other parts of respiratory tract**

    √7ᵗʰ **T17.800** **Unspecified foreign body in other parts of respiratory tract** causing **asphyxiation**

    √7ᵗʰ **T17.808** **Unspecified foreign body in other parts of respiratory tract** causing other injury

  √6ᵗʰ **T17.81** Gastric contents **in other parts of respiratory tract**

    Aspiration of gastric contents into other parts of respiratory tract
    Vomitus in other parts of respiratory tract

    √7ᵗʰ **T17.810** **Gastric contents in other parts of respiratory tract** causing **asphyxiation**

    √7ᵗʰ **T17.818** **Gastric contents in other parts of respiratory tract** causing other injury

  √6ᵗʰ **T17.82** Food **in other parts of respiratory tract**

    Bones in other parts of respiratory tract
    Seeds in other parts of respiratory tract

    √7ᵗʰ **T17.820** **Food in other parts of respiratory tract** causing **asphyxiation**

    √7ᵗʰ **T17.828** **Food in other parts of respiratory tract** causing other injury

  √6ᵗʰ **T17.89** Other foreign object **in other parts of respiratory tract**

    √7ᵗʰ **T17.890** **Other foreign object in other parts of respiratory tract** causing **asphyxiation**

    √7ᵗʰ **T17.898** **Other foreign object in other parts of respiratory tract** causing other injury

√5ᵗʰ **T17.9** Foreign body in respiratory tract, part unspecified

  √6ᵗʰ **T17.90** Unspecified foreign body **in respiratory tract, part unspecified**

    √7ᵗʰ **T17.900** **Unspecified foreign body in respiratory tract, part unspecified** causing **asphyxiation**

    √7ᵗʰ **T17.908** **Unspecified foreign body in respiratory tract, part unspecified** causing other injury

  √6ᵗʰ **T17.91** Gastric contents **in respiratory tract, part unspecified**

    Aspiration of gastric contents into respiratory tract, part unspecified
    Vomitus in trachea respiratory tract, part unspecified

    √7ᵗʰ **T17.910** **Gastric contents in respiratory tract, part unspecified** causing **asphyxiation**

    √7ᵗʰ **T17.918** **Gastric contents in respiratory tract, part unspecified** causing other injury

  √6ᵗʰ **T17.92** Food **in respiratory tract, part unspecified**

    Bones in respiratory tract, part unspecified
    Seeds in respiratory tract, part unspecified

    √7ᵗʰ **T17.920** **Food in respiratory tract, part unspecified** causing **asphyxiation**

    √7ᵗʰ **T17.928** **Food in respiratory tract, part unspecified** causing other injury

  √6ᵗʰ **T17.99** Other foreign object **in respiratory tract, part unspecified**

    √7ᵗʰ **T17.990** **Other foreign object in respiratory tract, part unspecified** in causing **asphyxiation**

    √7ᵗʰ **T17.998** **Other foreign object in respiratory tract, part unspecified** causing other injury

√4ᵗʰ **T18** **Foreign body in alimentary tract**

  EXCLUDES 2   *foreign body in pharynx (T17.2-)*

  The appropriate 7th character is to be added to each code from category T18.
  A   initial encounter
  D   subsequent encounter
  S   sequela

√x7ᵗʰ **T18.0** **Foreign body in** mouth

√5ᵗʰ **T18.1** **Foreign body in** esophagus

  EXCLUDES 2   *foreign body in respiratory tract (T17.-)*

  √6ᵗʰ **T18.10** Unspecified foreign body **in esophagus**

    √7ᵗʰ **T18.100** **Unspecified foreign body in esophagus causing compression of trachea**
      Unspecified foreign body in esophagus causing obstruction of respiration

    √7ᵗʰ **T18.108** **Unspecified foreign body in esophagus causing other injury**

  √6ᵗʰ **T18.11** Gastric contents **in esophagus**

    Vomitus in esophagus

    √7ᵗʰ **T18.110** **Gastric contents in esophagus** causing **compression of trachea**
      Gastric contents in esophagus causing obstruction of respiration

    √7ᵗʰ **T18.118** **Gastric contents in esophagus** causing other injury

  √6ᵗʰ **T18.12** Food **in esophagus**

    Bones in esophagus
    Seeds in esophagus

    √7ᵗʰ **T18.120** **Food in esophagus** causing **compression of trachea**
      Food in esophagus causing obstruction of respiration

    √7ᵗʰ **T18.128** **Food in esophagus** causing other injury

  √6ᵗʰ **T18.19** Other foreign object **in esophagus**

    AHA: 2015,1Q,23

    √7ᵗʰ **T18.190** **Other foreign object in esophagus causing compression of trachea**
      Other foreign body in esophagus causing obstruction of respiration
      TIP: Any foreign object lodged in the esophagus requires immediate treatment and is considered an injury. Assign this code when there is respiratory compromise or compression.

    √7ᵗʰ **T18.198** **Other foreign object in esophagus causing other injury**
      TIP: Any foreign object lodged in the esophagus requires immediate treatment and is considered an injury. Assign this code when there is no respiratory compromise or compression.

√x7ᵗʰ **T18.2** **Foreign body in** stomach

√x7ᵗʰ **T18.3** **Foreign body in** small intestine

√x7ᵗʰ **T18.4** **Foreign body in** colon

√x7ᵗʰ **T18.5** **Foreign body in** anus and rectum

       Foreign body in rectosigmoid (junction)

√x7ᵗʰ **T18.8** **Foreign body in other parts of alimentary tract**

√x7ᵗʰ **T18.9** **Foreign body of alimentary tract, part unspecified**

       Foreign body in digestive system NOS

       Swallowed foreign body NOS

√4ᵗʰ **T19** **Foreign body in genitourinary tract**

    EXCLUDES 2   *complications due to implanted mesh (T83.7-)*

             mechanical complications of contraceptive device
                 (intrauterine) (vaginal) (T83.3-)

             presence of contraceptive device (intrauterine) (vaginal)
                 (Z97.5)

> The appropriate 7th character is to be added to each code from
> category T19.
> A   initial encounter
> D   subsequent encounter
> S   sequela

√x7ᵗʰ **T19.0** **Foreign body in** urethra

√x7ᵗʰ **T19.1** **Foreign body in** bladder

√x7ᵗʰ **T19.2** **Foreign body in** vulva and vagina   ♀

√x7ᵗʰ **T19.3** **Foreign body in** uterus   ♀

√x7ᵗʰ **T19.4** **Foreign body in** penis   ♂

√x7ᵗʰ **T19.8** **Foreign body in other parts of genitourinary tract**

√x7ᵗʰ **T19.9** **Foreign body in genitourinary tract, part unspecified**

BURNS AND CORROSIONS (T20-T32)

INCLUDES   burns (thermal) from electrical heating appliances

            burns (thermal) from electricity

            burns (thermal) from flame

            burns (thermal) from friction

            burns (thermal) from hot air and hot gases

            burns (thermal) from hot objects

            burns (thermal) from lightning

            burns (thermal) from radiation

            chemical burn [corrosion] (external) (internal)

            scalds

EXCLUDES 2   *erythema [dermatitis] ab igne (L59.0)*

            radiation-related disorders of the skin and subcutaneous tissue
               (L55-L59)

            sunburn (L55.-)

AHA: 2016,2Q,4

Burns and corrosions of external body surface, specified by site (T20-T25)

INCLUDES   burns and corrosions of first degree [erythema]

            burns and corrosions of second degree [blisters] [epidermal loss]

            burns and corrosions of third degree [deep necrosis of underlying
               tissue] [full-thickness skin loss]

Use additional code from category T31 or T32 to identify extent of body surface involved

√4ᵗʰ **T20** **Burn and corrosion of head, face, and neck**

    EXCLUDES 2   *burn and corrosion of ear drum (T28.41, T28.91)*

             burn and corrosion of eye and adnexa (T26.-)

             burn and corrosion of mouth and pharynx (T28.0)

AHA: 2015,1Q,18-19

> The appropriate 7th character is to be added to each code from
> category T20.
> A   initial encounter
> D   subsequent encounter
> S   sequela

√5ᵗʰ **T20.0** **Burn of unspecified degree of head, face, and neck**

       Use additional external cause code to identify the source, place
       and intent of the burn (X00-X19, X75-X77, X96-X98, Y92)

    √x7ᵗʰ **T20.00** **Burn of unspecified degree of head, face, and neck,
unspecified site**

    √6ᵗʰ **T20.01** **Burn of unspecified degree of** ear **[any part, except
ear drum]**

        EXCLUDES 2   *burn of ear drum (T28.41-)*

       √7ᵗʰ **T20.011** **Burn of unspecified degree of** right **ear
[any part, except ear drum]**

       √7ᵗʰ **T20.012** **Burn of unspecified degree of** left **ear [any
part, except ear drum]**

       √7ᵗʰ **T20.019** **Burn of unspecified degree of unspecified
ear [any part, except ear drum]**

√x7ᵗʰ **T20.02** **Burn of unspecified degree of** lip(s)

√x7ᵗʰ **T20.03** **Burn of unspecified degree of** chin

√x7ᵗʰ **T20.04** **Burn of unspecified degree of** nose **(septum)**

√x7ᵗʰ **T20.05** **Burn of unspecified degree of** scalp **[any part]**

√x7ᵗʰ **T20.06** **Burn of unspecified degree of** forehead and cheek

√x7ᵗʰ **T20.07** **Burn of unspecified degree of** neck

√x7ᵗʰ **T20.09** **Burn of unspecified degree of** multiple sites **of head,
face, and neck**

√5ᵗʰ **T20.1** **Burn of** first degree **of head, face, and neck**

       Use additional external cause code to identify the source, place
       and intent of the burn (X00-X19, X75-X77, X96-X98, Y92)

    √x7ᵗʰ **T20.10** **Burn of first degree of head, face, and neck,
unspecified site**

    √6ᵗʰ **T20.11** **Burn of first degree of** ear **[any part, except ear
drum]**

        EXCLUDES 2   *burn of ear drum (T28.41-)*

       √7ᵗʰ **T20.111** **Burn of first degree of** right **ear [any part,
except ear drum]**

       √7ᵗʰ **T20.112** **Burn of first degree of** left **ear [any part,
except ear drum]**

       √7ᵗʰ **T20.119** **Burn of first degree of unspecified ear
[any part, except ear drum]**

√x7ᵗʰ **T20.12** **Burn of first degree of** lip(s)

√x7ᵗʰ **T20.13** **Burn of first degree of** chin

√x7ᵗʰ **T20.14** **Burn of first degree of** nose **(septum)**

√x7ᵗʰ **T20.15** **Burn of first degree of** scalp **[any part]**

√x7ᵗʰ **T20.16** **Burn of first degree of** forehead and cheek

√x7ᵗʰ **T20.17** **Burn of first degree of** neck

√x7ᵗʰ **T20.19** **Burn of first degree of** multiple sites **of head, face,
and neck**

Degree of Burns

Epidermis   Dermis   Subcutaneous   Normal   First Degree Burn

Epidermis   Dermis   Subcutaneous   Second Degree Burn   Third Degree Burn

√5ᵗʰ **T20.2** **Burn of** second degree **of head, face, and neck**

       Use additional external cause code to identify the source, place
       and intent of the burn (X00-X19, X75-X77, X96-X98, Y92)

    √x7ᵗʰ **T20.20** **Burn of second degree of head, face, and neck,
unspecified site**

    √6ᵗʰ **T20.21** **Burn of second degree of** ear **[any part, except ear
drum]**

        EXCLUDES 2   *burn of ear drum (T28.41-)*

       √7ᵗʰ **T20.211** **Burn of second degree of** right **ear [any
part, except ear drum]**

       √7ᵗʰ **T20.212** **Burn of second degree of** left **ear [any
part, except ear drum]**

       √7ᵗʰ **T20.219** **Burn of second degree of unspecified ear
[any part, except ear drum]**

√x7ᵗʰ **T20.22** **Burn of second degree of** lip(s)

√x7ᵗʰ **T20.23** **Burn of second degree of** chin

√x7ᵗʰ **T20.24** **Burn of second degree of** nose **(septum)**

√x7ᵗʰ **T20.25** **Burn of second degree of** scalp **[any part]**

✓ Additional Character Required   √x7ᵗʰ Placeholder Alert   Manifestation   Unspecified Dx   ▶◀ Revised Text   ● New Code   ▲ Revised Code Title

ICD-10-CM 2020   1079

√x7ᵗʰ **T20.26** **Burn of second degree of** forehead and cheek

√x7ᵗʰ **T20.27** **Burn of second degree of** neck

√x7ᵗʰ **T20.29** **Burn of second degree of** multiple sites **of head, face, and neck**

√5ᵗʰ **T20.3** **Burn of** third degree **of head, face, and neck**

Use additional external cause code to identify the source, place and intent of the burn (X00-X19, X75-X77, X96-X98, Y92)

√x7ᵗʰ **T20.30** **Burn of third degree of head, face, and neck, unspecified site**

√6ᵗʰ **T20.31** **Burn of third degree of** ear [any part, except ear drum]

> EXCLUDES 2   *burn of ear drum (T28.41-)*
>
> **AHA:** 2015,1Q,18

√7ᵗʰ **T20.311** **Burn of third degree of** right **ear [any part, except ear drum]**

√7ᵗʰ **T20.312** **Burn of third degree of** left **ear [any part, except ear drum]**

√7ᵗʰ **T20.319** **Burn of third degree of unspecified ear [any part, except ear drum]**

√x7ᵗʰ **T20.32** **Burn of third degree of** lip(s)

√x7ᵗʰ **T20.33** **Burn of third degree of** chin

√x7ᵗʰ **T20.34** **Burn of third degree of** nose (septum)

√x7ᵗʰ **T20.35** **Burn of third degree of** scalp [any part]

√x7ᵗʰ **T20.36** **Burn of third degree of** forehead and cheek

√x7ᵗʰ **T20.37** **Burn of third degree of** neck

√x7ᵗʰ **T20.39** **Burn of third degree of** multiple sites **of head, face, and neck**

√5ᵗʰ **T20.4** **Corrosion of unspecified degree of head, face, and neck**

Code first (T51-T65) to identify chemical and intent
Use additional external cause code to identify place (Y92)

√x7ᵗʰ **T20.40** **Corrosion of unspecified degree of head, face, and neck, unspecified site**

√6ᵗʰ **T20.41** **Corrosion of unspecified degree of** ear [any part, except ear drum]

> EXCLUDES 2   *corrosion of ear drum (T28.91-)*

√7ᵗʰ **T20.411** **Corrosion of unspecified degree of** right **ear [any part, except ear drum]**

√7ᵗʰ **T20.412** **Corrosion of unspecified degree of** left **ear [any part, except ear drum]**

√7ᵗʰ **T20.419** **Corrosion of unspecified degree of unspecified ear [any part, except ear drum]**

√x7ᵗʰ **T20.42** **Corrosion of unspecified degree of** lip(s)

√x7ᵗʰ **T20.43** **Corrosion of unspecified degree of** chin

√x7ᵗʰ **T20.44** **Corrosion of unspecified degree of** nose (septum)

√x7ᵗʰ **T20.45** **Corrosion of unspecified degree of** scalp [any part]

√x7ᵗʰ **T20.46** **Corrosion of unspecified degree of** forehead and cheek

√x7ᵗʰ **T20.47** **Corrosion of unspecified degree of** neck

√x7ᵗʰ **T20.49** **Corrosion of unspecified degree of** multiple sites **of head, face, and neck**

√5ᵗʰ **T20.5** **Corrosion of** first degree **of head, face, and neck**

Code first (T51-T65) to identify chemical and intent
Use additional external cause code to identify place (Y92)

√x7ᵗʰ **T20.50** **Corrosion of first degree of head, face, and neck, unspecified site**

√6ᵗʰ **T20.51** **Corrosion of first degree of** ear [any part, except ear drum]

> EXCLUDES 2   *corrosion of ear drum (T28.91-)*

√7ᵗʰ **T20.511** **Corrosion of first degree of** right **ear [any part, except ear drum]**

√7ᵗʰ **T20.512** **Corrosion of first degree of** left **ear [any part, except ear drum]**

√7ᵗʰ **T20.519** **Corrosion of first degree of unspecified ear [any part, except ear drum]**

√x7ᵗʰ **T20.52** **Corrosion of first degree of** lip(s)

√x7ᵗʰ **T20.53** **Corrosion of first degree of** chin

√x7ᵗʰ **T20.54** **Corrosion of first degree of** nose (septum)

√x7ᵗʰ **T20.55** **Corrosion of first degree of** scalp [any part]

√x7ᵗʰ **T20.56** **Corrosion of first degree of** forehead and cheek

√x7ᵗʰ **T20.57** **Corrosion of first degree of** neck

√x7ᵗʰ **T20.59** **Corrosion of first degree of** multiple sites **of head, face, and neck**

√5ᵗʰ **T20.6** **Corrosion of** second degree **of head, face, and neck**

Code first (T51-T65) to identify chemical and intent
Use additional external cause code to identify place (Y92)

√x7ᵗʰ **T20.60** **Corrosion of second degree of head, face, and neck, unspecified site**

√6ᵗʰ **T20.61** **Corrosion of second degree of** ear [any part, except ear drum]

> EXCLUDES 2   *corrosion of ear drum (T28.91-)*

√7ᵗʰ **T20.611** **Corrosion of second degree of** right **ear [any part, except ear drum]**

√7ᵗʰ **T20.612** **Corrosion of second degree of** left **ear [any part, except ear drum]**

√7ᵗʰ **T20.619** **Corrosion of second degree of unspecified ear [any part, except ear drum]**

√x7ᵗʰ **T20.62** **Corrosion of second degree of** lip(s)

√x7ᵗʰ **T20.63** **Corrosion of second degree of** chin

√x7ᵗʰ **T20.64** **Corrosion of second degree of** nose (septum)

√x7ᵗʰ **T20.65** **Corrosion of second degree of** scalp [any part]

√x7ᵗʰ **T20.66** **Corrosion of second degree of** forehead and cheek

√x7ᵗʰ **T20.67** **Corrosion of second degree of** neck

√x7ᵗʰ **T20.69** **Corrosion of second degree of** multiple sites **of head, face, and neck**

√5ᵗʰ **T20.7** **Corrosion of** third degree **of head, face, and neck**

Code first (T51-T65) to identify chemical and intent
Use additional external cause code to identify place (Y92)

√x7ᵗʰ **T20.70** **Corrosion of third degree of head, face, and neck, unspecified site**

√6ᵗʰ **T20.71** **Corrosion of third degree of** ear [any part, except ear drum]

> EXCLUDES 2   *corrosion of ear drum (T28.91-)*

√7ᵗʰ **T20.711** **Corrosion of third degree of** right **ear [any part, except ear drum]**

√7ᵗʰ **T20.712** **Corrosion of third degree of** left **ear [any part, except ear drum]**

√7ᵗʰ **T20.719** **Corrosion of third degree of unspecified ear [any part, except ear drum]**

√x7ᵗʰ **T20.72** **Corrosion of third degree of** lip(s)

√x7ᵗʰ **T20.73** **Corrosion of third degree of** chin

√x7ᵗʰ **T20.74** **Corrosion of third degree of** nose (septum)

√x7ᵗʰ **T20.75** **Corrosion of third degree of** scalp [any part]

√x7ᵗʰ **T20.76** **Corrosion of third degree of** forehead and cheek

√x7ᵗʰ **T20.77** **Corrosion of third degree of** neck

√x7ᵗʰ **T20.79** **Corrosion of third degree of** multiple sites **of head, face, and neck**

√4ᵗʰ **T21** **Burn and corrosion of trunk**

> INCLUDES   burns and corrosion of hip region
>
> EXCLUDES 2   *burns and corrosion of axilla (T22.- with fifth character 4)*
> *burns and corrosion of scapular region (T22.- with fifth character 6)*
> *burns and corrosion of shoulder (T22.- with fifth character 5)*

The appropriate 7th character is to be added to each code from category T21.
A   initial encounter
D   subsequent encounter
S   sequela

√5ᵗʰ **T21.0** **Burn of unspecified degree of trunk**

Use additional external cause code to identify the source, place and intent of the burn (X00-X19, X75-X77, X96-X98, Y92)

√x7ᵗʰ **T21.00** **Burn of unspecified degree of trunk, unspecified site**

√x7ᵗʰ **T21.01** **Burn of unspecified degree of** chest wall

Burn of unspecified degree of breast

√x7ᵗʰ **T21.02** **Burn of unspecified degree of** abdominal wall

Burn of unspecified degree of flank
Burn of unspecified degree of groin

√x7ᵗʰ **T21.03** **Burn of unspecified degree of** upper back

Burn of unspecified degree of interscapular region

√x7ᵗʰ **T21.04** **Burn of unspecified degree of** lower back

√x7ᵗʰ **T21.05** **Burn of unspecified degree of** buttock

Burn of unspecified degree of anus

√x7ᵗʰ **T21.06** Burn of unspecified degree of male genital region ♂
　　Burn of unspecified degree of penis
　　Burn of unspecified degree of scrotum
　　Burn of unspecified degree of testis

√x7ᵗʰ **T21.07** Burn of unspecified degree of female genital region ♀
　　Burn of unspecified degree of labium (majus) (minus)
　　Burn of unspecified degree of perineum
　　Burn of unspecified degree of vulva
　　EXCLUDES 2　burn of vagina (T28.3)

√x7ᵗʰ **T21.09** Burn of unspecified degree of other site of trunk

√5ᵗʰ **T21.1** Burn of first degree of trunk
　　Use additional external cause code to identify the source, place and intent of the burn (X00-X19, X75-X77, X96-X98, Y92)

√x7ᵗʰ **T21.10** Burn of first degree of trunk, unspecified site

√x7ᵗʰ **T21.11** Burn of first degree of chest wall
　　Burn of first degree of breast

√x7ᵗʰ **T21.12** Burn of first degree of abdominal wall
　　Burn of first degree of flank
　　Burn of first degree of groin

√x7ᵗʰ **T21.13** Burn of first degree of upper back
　　Burn of first degree of interscapular region

√x7ᵗʰ **T21.14** Burn of first degree of lower back

√x7ᵗʰ **T21.15** Burn of first degree of buttock
　　Burn of first degree of anus

√x7ᵗʰ **T21.16** Burn of first degree of male genital region ♂
　　Burn of first degree of penis
　　Burn of first degree of scrotum
　　Burn of first degree of testis

√x7ᵗʰ **T21.17** Burn of first degree of female genital region ♀
　　Burn of first degree of labium (majus) (minus)
　　Burn of first degree of perineum
　　Burn of first degree of vulva
　　EXCLUDES 2　burn of vagina (T28.3)

√x7ᵗʰ **T21.19** Burn of first degree of other site of trunk

√5ᵗʰ **T21.2** Burn of second degree of trunk
　　Use additional external cause code to identify the source, place and intent of the burn (X00-X19, X75-X77, X96-X98, Y92)

√x7ᵗʰ **T21.20** Burn of second degree of trunk, unspecified site

√x7ᵗʰ **T21.21** Burn of second degree of chest wall
　　Burn of second degree of breast

√x7ᵗʰ **T21.22** Burn of second degree of abdominal wall
　　Burn of second degree of flank
　　Burn of second degree of groin

√x7ᵗʰ **T21.23** Burn of second degree of upper back
　　Burn of second degree of interscapular region

√x7ᵗʰ **T21.24** Burn of second degree of lower back

√x7ᵗʰ **T21.25** Burn of second degree of buttock
　　Burn of second degree of anus

√x7ᵗʰ **T21.26** Burn of second degree of male genital region ♂
　　Burn of second degree of penis
　　Burn of second degree of scrotum
　　Burn of second degree of testis

√x7ᵗʰ **T21.27** Burn of second degree of female genital region ♀
　　Burn of second degree of labium (majus) (minus)
　　Burn of second degree of perineum
　　Burn of second degree of vulva
　　EXCLUDES 2　burn of vagina (T28.3)

√x7ᵗʰ **T21.29** Burn of second degree of other site of trunk

√5ᵗʰ **T21.3** Burn of third degree of trunk
　　Use additional external cause code to identify the source, place and intent of the burn (X00-X19, X75-X77, X96-X98, Y92)

√x7ᵗʰ **T21.30** Burn of third degree of trunk, unspecified site

√x7ᵗʰ **T21.31** Burn of third degree of chest wall
　　Burn of third degree of breast
　　AHA: 2016,2Q,5

√x7ᵗʰ **T21.32** Burn of third degree of abdominal wall
　　Burn of third degree of flank
　　Burn of third degree of groin

√x7ᵗʰ **T21.33** Burn of third degree of upper back
　　Burn of third degree of interscapular region

√x7ᵗʰ **T21.34** Burn of third degree of lower back

√x7ᵗʰ **T21.35** Burn of third degree of buttock
　　Burn of third degree of anus

√x7ᵗʰ **T21.36** Burn of third degree of male genital region ♂
　　Burn of third degree of penis
　　Burn of third degree of scrotum
　　Burn of third degree of testis

√x7ᵗʰ **T21.37** Burn of third degree of female genital region ♀
　　Burn of third degree of labium (majus) (minus)
　　Burn of third degree of perineum
　　Burn of third degree of vulva
　　EXCLUDES 2　burn of vagina (T28.3)

√x7ᵗʰ **T21.39** Burn of third degree of other site of trunk

√5ᵗʰ **T21.4** Corrosion of unspecified degree of trunk
　　Code first (T51-T65) to identify chemical and intent
　　Use additional external cause code to identify place (Y92)

√x7ᵗʰ **T21.40** Corrosion of unspecified degree of trunk, unspecified site

√x7ᵗʰ **T21.41** Corrosion of unspecified degree of chest wall
　　Corrosion of unspecified degree of breast

√x7ᵗʰ **T21.42** Corrosion of unspecified degree of abdominal wall
　　Corrosion of unspecified degree of flank
　　Corrosion of unspecified degree of groin

√x7ᵗʰ **T21.43** Corrosion of unspecified degree of upper back
　　Corrosion of unspecified degree of interscapular region

√x7ᵗʰ **T21.44** Corrosion of unspecified degree of lower back

√x7ᵗʰ **T21.45** Corrosion of unspecified degree of buttock
　　Corrosion of unspecified degree of anus

√x7ᵗʰ **T21.46** Corrosion of unspecified degree of male genital region ♂
　　Corrosion of unspecified degree of penis
　　Corrosion of unspecified degree of scrotum
　　Corrosion of unspecified degree of testis

√x7ᵗʰ **T21.47** Corrosion of unspecified degree of female genital region ♀
　　Corrosion of unspecified degree of labium (majus) (minus)
　　Corrosion of unspecified degree of perineum
　　Corrosion of unspecified degree of vulva
　　EXCLUDES 2　corrosion of vagina (T28.8)

√x7ᵗʰ **T21.49** Corrosion of unspecified degree of other site of trunk

√5ᵗʰ **T21.5** Corrosion of first degree of trunk
　　Code first (T51-T65) to identify chemical and intent
　　Use additional external cause code to identify place (Y92)

√x7ᵗʰ **T21.50** Corrosion of first degree of trunk, unspecified site

√x7ᵗʰ **T21.51** Corrosion of first degree of chest wall
　　Corrosion of first degree of breast

√x7ᵗʰ **T21.52** Corrosion of first degree of abdominal wall
　　Corrosion of first degree of flank
　　Corrosion of first degree of groin

√x7ᵗʰ **T21.53** Corrosion of first degree of upper back
　　Corrosion of first degree of interscapular region

√x7ᵗʰ **T21.54** Corrosion of first degree of lower back

√x7ᵗʰ **T21.55** Corrosion of first degree of buttock
　　Corrosion of first degree of anus

√x7ᵗʰ **T21.56** Corrosion of first degree of male genital region ♂
　　Corrosion of first degree of penis
　　Corrosion of first degree of scrotum
　　Corrosion of first degree of testis

√x7ᵗʰ **T21.57** Corrosion of first degree of female genital region ♀
　　Corrosion of first degree of labium (majus) (minus)
　　Corrosion of first degree of perineum
　　Corrosion of first degree of vulva
　　EXCLUDES 2　corrosion of vagina (T28.8)

√x7ᵗʰ **T21.59** Corrosion of first degree of other site of trunk

---

☑ Additional Character Required　√x7ᵗʰ Placeholder Alert　Manifestation　Unspecified Dx　▶◀ Revised Text　● New Code　▲ Revised Code Title

√5ᵗʰ T21.6 Corrosion of second degree of trunk

Code first (T51-T65) to identify chemical and intent
Use additional external cause code to identify place (Y92)

√x7ᵗʰ **T21.60 Corrosion of second degree of trunk, unspecified site**

√x7ᵗʰ **T21.61 Corrosion of second degree of chest wall**

Corrosion of second degree of breast

√x7ᵗʰ **T21.62 Corrosion of second degree of abdominal wall**

Corrosion of second degree of flank
Corrosion of second degree of groin

√x7ᵗʰ **T21.63 Corrosion of second degree of upper back**

Corrosion of second degree of interscapular region

√x7ᵗʰ **T21.64 Corrosion of second degree of lower back**

√x7ᵗʰ **T21.65 Corrosion of second degree of buttock**

Corrosion of second degree of anus

√x7ᵗʰ **T21.66 Corrosion of second degree of male genital region** ♂

Corrosion of second degree of penis
Corrosion of second degree of scrotum
Corrosion of second degree of testis

√x7ᵗʰ **T21.67 Corrosion of second degree of female genital region** ♀

Corrosion of second degree of labium (majus) (minus)
Corrosion of second degree of perineum
Corrosion of second degree of vulva

EXCLUDES 2   corrosion of vagina (T28.8)

√x7ᵗʰ **T21.69 Corrosion of second degree of other site of trunk**

√5ᵗʰ T21.7 Corrosion of third degree of trunk

Code first (T51-T65) to identify chemical and intent
Use additional external cause code to identify place (Y92)

√x7ᵗʰ **T21.70 Corrosion of third degree of trunk, unspecified site**

√x7ᵗʰ **T21.71 Corrosion of third degree of chest wall**

Corrosion of third degree of breast

√x7ᵗʰ **T21.72 Corrosion of third degree of abdominal wall**

Corrosion of third degree of flank
Corrosion of third degree of groin

√x7ᵗʰ **T21.73 Corrosion of third degree of upper back**

Corrosion of third degree of interscapular region

√x7ᵗʰ **T21.74 Corrosion of third degree of lower back**

√x7ᵗʰ **T21.75 Corrosion of third degree of buttock**

Corrosion of third degree of anus

√x7ᵗʰ **T21.76 Corrosion of third degree of male genital region** ♂

Corrosion of third degree of penis
Corrosion of third degree of scrotum
Corrosion of third degree of testis

√x7ᵗʰ **T21.77 Corrosion of third degree of female genital region** ♀

Corrosion of third degree of labium (majus) (minus)
Corrosion of third degree of perineum
Corrosion of third degree of vulva

EXCLUDES 2   corrosion of vagina (T28.8)

√x7ᵗʰ **T21.79 Corrosion of third degree of other site of trunk**

√4ᵗʰ T22 Burn and corrosion of shoulder and upper limb, except wrist and hand

EXCLUDES 2   burn and corrosion of interscapular region (T21.-)
            burn and corrosion of wrist and hand (T23.-)

The appropriate 7th character is to be added to each code from category T22.
A   initial encounter
D   subsequent encounter
S   sequela

√5ᵗʰ T22.0 Burn of unspecified degree of shoulder and upper limb, except wrist and hand

Use additional external cause code to identify the source, place and intent of the burn (X00-X19, X75-X77, X96-X98, Y92)

√x7ᵗʰ **T22.00 Burn of unspecified degree of shoulder and upper limb, except wrist and hand, unspecified site**

√6ᵗʰ **T22.01 Burn of unspecified degree of forearm**

√7ᵗʰ **T22.011 Burn of unspecified degree of right forearm**

√7ᵗʰ **T22.012 Burn of unspecified degree of left forearm**

√7ᵗʰ **T22.019 Burn of unspecified degree of unspecified forearm**

√6ᵗʰ **T22.02 Burn of unspecified degree of elbow**

√7ᵗʰ **T22.021 Burn of unspecified degree of right elbow**

√7ᵗʰ **T22.022 Burn of unspecified degree of left elbow**

√7ᵗʰ **T22.029 Burn of unspecified degree of unspecified elbow**

√6ᵗʰ **T22.03 Burn of unspecified degree of upper arm**

√7ᵗʰ **T22.031 Burn of unspecified degree of right upper arm**

√7ᵗʰ **T22.032 Burn of unspecified degree of left upper arm**

√7ᵗʰ **T22.039 Burn of unspecified degree of unspecified upper arm**

√6ᵗʰ **T22.04 Burn of unspecified degree of axilla**

√7ᵗʰ **T22.041 Burn of unspecified degree of right axilla**

√7ᵗʰ **T22.042 Burn of unspecified degree of left axilla**

√7ᵗʰ **T22.049 Burn of unspecified degree of unspecified axilla**

√6ᵗʰ **T22.05 Burn of unspecified degree of shoulder**

√7ᵗʰ **T22.051 Burn of unspecified degree of right shoulder**

√7ᵗʰ **T22.052 Burn of unspecified degree of left shoulder**

√7ᵗʰ **T22.059 Burn of unspecified degree of unspecified shoulder**

√6ᵗʰ **T22.06 Burn of unspecified degree of scapular region**

√7ᵗʰ **T22.061 Burn of unspecified degree of right scapular region**

√7ᵗʰ **T22.062 Burn of unspecified degree of left scapular region**

√7ᵗʰ **T22.069 Burn of unspecified degree of unspecified scapular region**

√6ᵗʰ **T22.09 Burn of unspecified degree of multiple sites of shoulder and upper limb, except wrist and hand**

√7ᵗʰ **T22.091 Burn of unspecified degree of multiple sites of right shoulder and upper limb, except wrist and hand**

√7ᵗʰ **T22.092 Burn of unspecified degree of multiple sites of left shoulder and upper limb, except wrist and hand**

√7ᵗʰ **T22.099 Burn of unspecified degree of multiple sites of unspecified shoulder and upper limb, except wrist and hand**

√5ᵗʰ T22.1 Burn of first degree of shoulder and upper limb, except wrist and hand

Use additional external cause code to identify the source, place and intent of the burn (X00-X19, X75-X77, X96-X98, Y92)

√x7ᵗʰ **T22.10 Burn of first degree of shoulder and upper limb, except wrist and hand, unspecified site**

√6ᵗʰ **T22.11 Burn of first degree of forearm**

√7ᵗʰ **T22.111 Burn of first degree of right forearm**

√7ᵗʰ **T22.112 Burn of first degree of left forearm**

√7ᵗʰ **T22.119 Burn of first degree of unspecified forearm**

√6ᵗʰ **T22.12 Burn of first degree of elbow**

√7ᵗʰ **T22.121 Burn of first degree of right elbow**

√7ᵗʰ **T22.122 Burn of first degree of left elbow**

√7ᵗʰ **T22.129 Burn of first degree of unspecified elbow**

√6ᵗʰ **T22.13 Burn of first degree of upper arm**

√7ᵗʰ **T22.131 Burn of first degree of right upper arm**

√7ᵗʰ **T22.132 Burn of first degree of left upper arm**

√7ᵗʰ **T22.139 Burn of first degree of unspecified upper arm**

√6ᵗʰ **T22.14 Burn of first degree of axilla**

√7ᵗʰ **T22.141 Burn of first degree of right axilla**

√7ᵗʰ **T22.142 Burn of first degree of left axilla**

√7ᵗʰ **T22.149 Burn of first degree of unspecified axilla**

√6ᵗʰ **T22.15 Burn of first degree of shoulder**

√7ᵗʰ **T22.151 Burn of first degree of right shoulder**

√7ᵗʰ **T22.152 Burn of first degree of left shoulder**

√7ᵗʰ **T22.159 Burn of first degree of unspecified shoulder**

√6ᵗʰ **T22.16 Burn of first degree of scapular region**

√7ᵗʰ **T22.161 Burn of first degree of right scapular region**

√7ᵗʰ **T22.162 Burn of first degree of left scapular region**

√7ᵗʰ **T22.169** Burn of first degree of unspecified scapular region

√6ᵗʰ **T22.19** Burn of first degree of multiple sites of shoulder and upper limb, except wrist and hand

√7ᵗʰ **T22.191** Burn of first degree of multiple sites of right shoulder and upper limb, except wrist and hand

√7ᵗʰ **T22.192** Burn of first degree of multiple sites of left shoulder and upper limb, except wrist and hand

√7ᵗʰ **T22.199** Burn of first degree of multiple sites of unspecified shoulder and upper limb, except wrist and hand

√5ᵗʰ **T22.2 Burn of second degree of shoulder and upper limb, except wrist and hand**

Use additional external cause code to identify the source, place and intent of the burn (X00-X19, X75-X77, X96-X98, Y92)

√x7ᵗʰ **T22.20** Burn of second degree of shoulder and upper limb, except wrist and hand, unspecified site

√6ᵗʰ **T22.21** Burn of second degree of forearm

√7ᵗʰ **T22.211** Burn of second degree of right forearm

√7ᵗʰ **T22.212** Burn of second degree of left forearm

√7ᵗʰ **T22.219** Burn of second degree of unspecified forearm

√6ᵗʰ **T22.22** Burn of second degree of elbow

√7ᵗʰ **T22.221** Burn of second degree of right elbow

√7ᵗʰ **T22.222** Burn of second degree of left elbow

√7ᵗʰ **T22.229** Burn of second degree of unspecified elbow

√6ᵗʰ **T22.23** Burn of second degree of upper arm

√7ᵗʰ **T22.231** Burn of second degree of right upper arm

√7ᵗʰ **T22.232** Burn of second degree of left upper arm

√7ᵗʰ **T22.239** Burn of second degree of unspecified upper arm

√6ᵗʰ **T22.24** Burn of second degree of axilla

√7ᵗʰ **T22.241** Burn of second degree of right axilla

√7ᵗʰ **T22.242** Burn of second degree of left axilla

√7ᵗʰ **T22.249** Burn of second degree of unspecified axilla

√6ᵗʰ **T22.25** Burn of second degree of shoulder

√7ᵗʰ **T22.251** Burn of second degree of right shoulder

√7ᵗʰ **T22.252** Burn of second degree of left shoulder

√7ᵗʰ **T22.259** Burn of second degree of unspecified shoulder

√6ᵗʰ **T22.26** Burn of second degree of scapular region

√7ᵗʰ **T22.261** Burn of second degree of right scapular region

√7ᵗʰ **T22.262** Burn of second degree of left scapular region

√7ᵗʰ **T22.269** Burn of second degree of unspecified scapular region

√6ᵗʰ **T22.29** Burn of second degree of multiple sites of shoulder and upper limb, except wrist and hand

√7ᵗʰ **T22.291** Burn of second degree of multiple sites of right shoulder and upper limb, except wrist and hand

√7ᵗʰ **T22.292** Burn of second degree of multiple sites of left shoulder and upper limb, except wrist and hand

√7ᵗʰ **T22.299** Burn of second degree of multiple sites of unspecified shoulder and upper limb, except wrist and hand

√5ᵗʰ **T22.3 Burn of third degree of shoulder and upper limb, except wrist and hand**

Use additional external cause code to identify the source, place and intent of the burn (X00-X19, X75-X77, X96-X98, Y92)

√x7ᵗʰ **T22.30** Burn of third degree of shoulder and upper limb, except wrist and hand, unspecified site

√6ᵗʰ **T22.31** Burn of third degree of forearm

√7ᵗʰ **T22.311** Burn of third degree of right forearm

√7ᵗʰ **T22.312** Burn of third degree of left forearm

√7ᵗʰ **T22.319** Burn of third degree of unspecified forearm

√6ᵗʰ **T22.32** Burn of third degree of elbow

√7ᵗʰ **T22.321** Burn of third degree of right elbow

√7ᵗʰ **T22.322** Burn of third degree of left elbow

√7ᵗʰ **T22.329** Burn of third degree of unspecified elbow

√6ᵗʰ **T22.33** Burn of third degree of upper arm

√7ᵗʰ **T22.331** Burn of third degree of right upper arm

√7ᵗʰ **T22.332** Burn of third degree of left upper arm

√7ᵗʰ **T22.339** Burn of third degree of unspecified upper arm

√6ᵗʰ **T22.34** Burn of third degree of axilla

√7ᵗʰ **T22.341** Burn of third degree of right axilla

√7ᵗʰ **T22.342** Burn of third degree of left axilla

√7ᵗʰ **T22.349** Burn of third degree of unspecified axilla

√6ᵗʰ **T22.35** Burn of third degree of shoulder

√7ᵗʰ **T22.351** Burn of third degree of right shoulder

√7ᵗʰ **T22.352** Burn of third degree of left shoulder

√7ᵗʰ **T22.359** Burn of third degree of unspecified shoulder

√6ᵗʰ **T22.36** Burn of third degree of scapular region

√7ᵗʰ **T22.361** Burn of third degree of right scapular region

√7ᵗʰ **T22.362** Burn of third degree of left scapular region

√7ᵗʰ **T22.369** Burn of third degree of unspecified scapular region

√6ᵗʰ **T22.39** Burn of third degree of multiple sites of shoulder and upper limb, except wrist and hand

√7ᵗʰ **T22.391** Burn of third degree of multiple sites of right shoulder and upper limb, except wrist and hand

√7ᵗʰ **T22.392** Burn of third degree of multiple sites of left shoulder and upper limb, except wrist and hand

√7ᵗʰ **T22.399** Burn of third degree of multiple sites of unspecified shoulder and upper limb, except wrist and hand

√5ᵗʰ **T22.4 Corrosion of unspecified degree of shoulder and upper limb, except wrist and hand**

Code first (T51-T65) to identify chemical and intent

Use additional external cause code to identify place (Y92)

√x7ᵗʰ **T22.40** Corrosion of unspecified degree of shoulder and upper limb, except wrist and hand, unspecified site

√6ᵗʰ **T22.41** Corrosion of unspecified degree of forearm

√7ᵗʰ **T22.411** Corrosion of unspecified degree of right forearm

√7ᵗʰ **T22.412** Corrosion of unspecified degree of left forearm

√7ᵗʰ **T22.419** Corrosion of unspecified degree of unspecified forearm

√6ᵗʰ **T22.42** Corrosion of unspecified degree of elbow

√7ᵗʰ **T22.421** Corrosion of unspecified degree of right elbow

√7ᵗʰ **T22.422** Corrosion of unspecified degree of left elbow

√7ᵗʰ **T22.429** Corrosion of unspecified degree of unspecified elbow

√6ᵗʰ **T22.43** Corrosion of unspecified degree of upper arm

√7ᵗʰ **T22.431** Corrosion of unspecified degree of right upper arm

√7ᵗʰ **T22.432** Corrosion of unspecified degree of left upper arm

√7ᵗʰ **T22.439** Corrosion of unspecified degree of unspecified upper arm

√6ᵗʰ **T22.44** Corrosion of unspecified degree of axilla

√7ᵗʰ **T22.441** Corrosion of unspecified degree of right axilla

√7ᵗʰ **T22.442** Corrosion of unspecified degree of left axilla

√7ᵗʰ **T22.449** Corrosion of unspecified degree of unspecified axilla

√6ᵗʰ **T22.45** Corrosion of unspecified degree of shoulder

√7ᵗʰ **T22.451** Corrosion of unspecified degree of right shoulder

√7ᵗʰ **T22.452** Corrosion of unspecified degree of left shoulder

√7ᵗʰ **T22.459** Corrosion of unspecified degree of unspecified shoulder

√6ᵗʰ **T22.46** Corrosion of unspecified degree of scapular region

√7ᵗʰ **T22.461** Corrosion of unspecified degree of right scapular region

√7ᵗʰ **T22.462** Corrosion of unspecified degree of left scapular region

☑ Additional Character Required   √x7ᵗʰ Placeholder Alert   Manifestation   Unspecified Dx   ▶◀ Revised Text   ● New Code   ▲ Revised Code Title

ICD-10-CM 2020   1083

Chapter 19. Injury, Poisoning and Certain Other Consequences of External Causes

T22.169–T22.462

√7ᵗʰ **T22.469** Corrosion of unspecified degree of unspecified scapular region

√6ᵗʰ **T22.49** Corrosion of unspecified degree of multiple sites of shoulder and upper limb, except wrist and hand

√7ᵗʰ **T22.491** Corrosion of unspecified degree of multiple sites of right shoulder and upper limb, except wrist and hand

√7ᵗʰ **T22.492** Corrosion of unspecified degree of multiple sites of left shoulder and upper limb, except wrist and hand

√7ᵗʰ **T22.499** Corrosion of unspecified degree of multiple sites of unspecified shoulder and upper limb, except wrist and hand

√5ᵗʰ **T22.5** Corrosion of first degree of shoulder and upper limb, except wrist and hand

Code first (T51-T65) to identify chemical and intent
Use additional external cause code to identify place (Y92)

√7ᵗʰ **T22.50** Corrosion of first degree of shoulder and upper limb, except wrist and hand unspecified site

√6ᵗʰ **T22.51** Corrosion of first degree of forearm

√7ᵗʰ **T22.511** Corrosion of first degree of right forearm

√7ᵗʰ **T22.512** Corrosion of first degree of left forearm

√7ᵗʰ **T22.519** Corrosion of first degree of unspecified forearm

√6ᵗʰ **T22.52** Corrosion of first degree of elbow

√7ᵗʰ **T22.521** Corrosion of first degree of right elbow

√7ᵗʰ **T22.522** Corrosion of first degree of left elbow

√7ᵗʰ **T22.529** Corrosion of first degree of unspecified elbow

√6ᵗʰ **T22.53** Corrosion of first degree of upper arm

√7ᵗʰ **T22.531** Corrosion of first degree of right upper arm

√7ᵗʰ **T22.532** Corrosion of first degree of left upper arm

√7ᵗʰ **T22.539** Corrosion of first degree of unspecified upper arm

√6ᵗʰ **T22.54** Corrosion of first degree of axilla

√7ᵗʰ **T22.541** Corrosion of first degree of right axilla

√7ᵗʰ **T22.542** Corrosion of first degree of left axilla

√7ᵗʰ **T22.549** Corrosion of first degree of unspecified axilla

√6ᵗʰ **T22.55** Corrosion of first degree of shoulder

√7ᵗʰ **T22.551** Corrosion of first degree of right shoulder

√7ᵗʰ **T22.552** Corrosion of first degree of left shoulder

√7ᵗʰ **T22.559** Corrosion of first degree of unspecified shoulder

√6ᵗʰ **T22.56** Corrosion of first degree of scapular region

√7ᵗʰ **T22.561** Corrosion of first degree of right scapular region

√7ᵗʰ **T22.562** Corrosion of first degree of left scapular region

√7ᵗʰ **T22.569** Corrosion of first degree of unspecified scapular region

√6ᵗʰ **T22.59** Corrosion of first degree of multiple sites of shoulder and upper limb, except wrist and hand

√7ᵗʰ **T22.591** Corrosion of first degree of multiple sites of right shoulder and upper limb, except wrist and hand

√7ᵗʰ **T22.592** Corrosion of first degree of multiple sites of left shoulder and upper limb, except wrist and hand

√7ᵗʰ **T22.599** Corrosion of first degree of multiple sites of unspecified shoulder and upper limb, except wrist and hand

√5ᵗʰ **T22.6** Corrosion of second degree of shoulder and upper limb, except wrist and hand

Code first (T51-T65) to identify chemical and intent
Use additional external cause code to identify place (Y92)

√x7ᵗʰ **T22.60** Corrosion of second degree of shoulder and upper limb, except wrist and hand, unspecified site

√6ᵗʰ **T22.61** Corrosion of second degree of forearm

√7ᵗʰ **T22.611** Corrosion of second degree of right forearm

√7ᵗʰ **T22.612** Corrosion of second degree of left forearm

√7ᵗʰ **T22.619** Corrosion of second degree of unspecified forearm

√6ᵗʰ **T22.62** Corrosion of second degree of elbow

√7ᵗʰ **T22.621** Corrosion of second degree of right elbow

√7ᵗʰ **T22.622** Corrosion of second degree of left elbow

√7ᵗʰ **T22.629** Corrosion of second degree of unspecified elbow

√6ᵗʰ **T22.63** Corrosion of second degree of upper arm

√7ᵗʰ **T22.631** Corrosion of second degree of right upper arm

√7ᵗʰ **T22.632** Corrosion of second degree of left upper arm

√7ᵗʰ **T22.639** Corrosion of second degree of unspecified upper arm

√6ᵗʰ **T22.64** Corrosion of second degree of axilla

√7ᵗʰ **T22.641** Corrosion of second degree of right axilla

√7ᵗʰ **T22.642** Corrosion of second degree of left axilla

√7ᵗʰ **T22.649** Corrosion of second degree of unspecified axilla

√6ᵗʰ **T22.65** Corrosion of second degree of shoulder

√7ᵗʰ **T22.651** Corrosion of second degree of right shoulder

√7ᵗʰ **T22.652** Corrosion of second degree of left shoulder

√7ᵗʰ **T22.659** Corrosion of second degree of unspecified shoulder

√6ᵗʰ **T22.66** Corrosion of second degree of scapular region

√7ᵗʰ **T22.661** Corrosion of second degree of right scapular region

√7ᵗʰ **T22.662** Corrosion of second degree of left scapular region

√7ᵗʰ **T22.669** Corrosion of second degree of unspecified scapular region

√6ᵗʰ **T22.69** Corrosion of second degree of multiple sites of shoulder and upper limb, except wrist and hand

√7ᵗʰ **T22.691** Corrosion of second degree of multiple sites of right shoulder and upper limb, except wrist and hand

√7ᵗʰ **T22.692** Corrosion of second degree of multiple sites of left shoulder and upper limb, except wrist and hand

√7ᵗʰ **T22.699** Corrosion of second degree of multiple sites of unspecified shoulder and upper limb, except wrist and hand

√5ᵗʰ **T22.7** Corrosion of third degree of shoulder and upper limb, except wrist and hand

Code first (T51-T65) to identify chemical and intent
Use additional external cause code to identify place (Y92)

√x7ᵗʰ **T22.70** Corrosion of third degree of shoulder and upper limb, except wrist and hand, unspecified site

√6ᵗʰ **T22.71** Corrosion of third degree of forearm

√7ᵗʰ **T22.711** Corrosion of third degree of right forearm

√7ᵗʰ **T22.712** Corrosion of third degree of left forearm

√7ᵗʰ **T22.719** Corrosion of third degree of unspecified forearm

√6ᵗʰ **T22.72** Corrosion of third degree of elbow

√7ᵗʰ **T22.721** Corrosion of third degree of right elbow

√7ᵗʰ **T22.722** Corrosion of third degree of left elbow

√7ᵗʰ **T22.729** Corrosion of third degree of unspecified elbow

√6ᵗʰ **T22.73** Corrosion of third degree of upper arm

√7ᵗʰ **T22.731** Corrosion of third degree of right upper arm

√7ᵗʰ **T22.732** Corrosion of third degree of left upper arm

√7ᵗʰ **T22.739** Corrosion of third degree of unspecified upper arm

√6ᵗʰ **T22.74** Corrosion of third degree of axilla

√7ᵗʰ **T22.741** Corrosion of third degree of right axilla

√7ᵗʰ **T22.742** Corrosion of third degree of left axilla

√7ᵗʰ **T22.749** Corrosion of third degree of unspecified axilla

√6ᵗʰ **T22.75** Corrosion of third degree of shoulder

√7ᵗʰ **T22.751** Corrosion of third degree of right shoulder

√7ᵗʰ **T22.752** Corrosion of third degree of left shoulder

√7ᵗʰ **T22.759** Corrosion of third degree of unspecified shoulder

√6ᵗʰ **T22.76** Corrosion of third degree of scapular region

√7ᵗʰ **T22.761** Corrosion of third degree of right scapular region

√7ᵗʰ **T22.762** Corrosion of third degree of left scapular region

√7ᵗʰ **T22.769** Corrosion of third degree of unspecified scapular region

√6ᵗʰ **T22.79** Corrosion of third degree of multiple sites of shoulder and upper limb, except wrist and hand

√7ᵗʰ **T22.791** Corrosion of third degree of multiple sites of right shoulder and upper limb, except wrist and hand

√7ᵗʰ **T22.792** Corrosion of third degree of multiple sites of left shoulder and upper limb, except wrist and hand

√7ᵗʰ **T22.799** Corrosion of third degree of multiple sites of unspecified shoulder and upper limb, except wrist and hand

✓4ᵗʰ **T23** Burn and corrosion of wrist and hand

AHA: 2015,1Q,19

The appropriate 7th character is to be added to each code from category T23.
A   initial encounter
D   subsequent encounter
S   sequela

√5ᵗʰ **T23.0** Burn of unspecified degree of wrist and hand

Use additional external cause code to identify the source, place and intent of the burn (X00-X19, X75-X77, X96-X98, Y92)

√6ᵗʰ **T23.00** Burn of unspecified degree of hand, unspecified site

√7ᵗʰ **T23.001** Burn of unspecified degree of right hand, unspecified site

√7ᵗʰ **T23.002** Burn of unspecified degree of left hand, unspecified site

√7ᵗʰ **T23.009** Burn of unspecified degree of unspecified hand, unspecified site

√6ᵗʰ **T23.01** Burn of unspecified degree of thumb (nail)

√7ᵗʰ **T23.011** Burn of unspecified degree of right thumb (nail)

√7ᵗʰ **T23.012** Burn of unspecified degree of left thumb (nail)

√7ᵗʰ **T23.019** Burn of unspecified degree of unspecified thumb (nail)

√6ᵗʰ **T23.02** Burn of unspecified degree of single finger (nail) except thumb

√7ᵗʰ **T23.021** Burn of unspecified degree of single right finger (nail) except thumb

√7ᵗʰ **T23.022** Burn of unspecified degree of single left finger (nail) except thumb

√7ᵗʰ **T23.029** Burn of unspecified degree of unspecified single finger (nail) except thumb

√6ᵗʰ **T23.03** Burn of unspecified degree of multiple fingers (nail), not including thumb

√7ᵗʰ **T23.031** Burn of unspecified degree of multiple right fingers (nail), not including thumb

√7ᵗʰ **T23.032** Burn of unspecified degree of multiple left fingers (nail), not including thumb

√7ᵗʰ **T23.039** Burn of unspecified degree of unspecified multiple fingers (nail), not including thumb

√6ᵗʰ **T23.04** Burn of unspecified degree of multiple fingers (nail), including thumb

√7ᵗʰ **T23.041** Burn of unspecified degree of multiple right fingers (nail), including thumb

√7ᵗʰ **T23.042** Burn of unspecified degree of multiple left fingers (nail), including thumb

√7ᵗʰ **T23.049** Burn of unspecified degree of unspecified multiple fingers (nail), including thumb

√6ᵗʰ **T23.05** Burn of unspecified degree of palm

√7ᵗʰ **T23.051** Burn of unspecified degree of right palm

√7ᵗʰ **T23.052** Burn of unspecified degree of left palm

√7ᵗʰ **T23.059** Burn of unspecified degree of unspecified palm

√6ᵗʰ **T23.06** Burn of unspecified degree of back of hand

√7ᵗʰ **T23.061** Burn of unspecified degree of back of right hand

√7ᵗʰ **T23.062** Burn of unspecified degree of back of left hand

√7ᵗʰ **T23.069** Burn of unspecified degree of back of unspecified hand

√6ᵗʰ **T23.07** Burn of unspecified degree of wrist

√7ᵗʰ **T23.071** Burn of unspecified degree of right wrist

√7ᵗʰ **T23.072** Burn of unspecified degree of left wrist

√7ᵗʰ **T23.079** Burn of unspecified degree of unspecified wrist

√6ᵗʰ **T23.09** Burn of unspecified degree of multiple sites of wrist and hand

√7ᵗʰ **T23.091** Burn of unspecified degree of multiple sites of right wrist and hand

√7ᵗʰ **T23.092** Burn of unspecified degree of multiple sites of left wrist and hand

√7ᵗʰ **T23.099** Burn of unspecified degree of multiple sites of unspecified wrist and hand

√5ᵗʰ **T23.1** Burn of first degree of wrist and hand

Use additional external cause code to identify the source, place and intent of the burn (X00-X19, X75-X77, X96-X98, Y92)

√6ᵗʰ **T23.10** Burn of first degree of hand, unspecified site

√7ᵗʰ **T23.101** Burn of first degree of right hand, unspecified site

√7ᵗʰ **T23.102** Burn of first degree of left hand, unspecified site

√7ᵗʰ **T23.109** Burn of first degree of unspecified hand, unspecified site

√6ᵗʰ **T23.11** Burn of first degree of thumb (nail)

√7ᵗʰ **T23.111** Burn of first degree of right thumb (nail)

√7ᵗʰ **T23.112** Burn of first degree of left thumb (nail)

√7ᵗʰ **T23.119** Burn of first degree of unspecified thumb (nail)

√6ᵗʰ **T23.12** Burn of first degree of single finger (nail) except thumb

√7ᵗʰ **T23.121** Burn of first degree of single right finger (nail) except thumb

√7ᵗʰ **T23.122** Burn of first degree of single left finger (nail) except thumb

√7ᵗʰ **T23.129** Burn of first degree of unspecified single finger (nail) except thumb

√6ᵗʰ **T23.13** Burn of first degree of multiple fingers (nail), not including thumb

√7ᵗʰ **T23.131** Burn of first degree of multiple right fingers (nail), not including thumb

√7ᵗʰ **T23.132** Burn of first degree of multiple left fingers (nail), not including thumb

√7ᵗʰ **T23.139** Burn of first degree of unspecified multiple fingers (nail), not including thumb

√6ᵗʰ **T23.14** Burn of first degree of multiple fingers (nail), including thumb

√7ᵗʰ **T23.141** Burn of first degree of multiple right fingers (nail), including thumb

√7ᵗʰ **T23.142** Burn of first degree of multiple left fingers (nail), including thumb

√7ᵗʰ **T23.149** Burn of first degree of unspecified multiple fingers (nail), including thumb

√6ᵗʰ **T23.15** Burn of first degree of palm

√7ᵗʰ **T23.151** Burn of first degree of right palm

√7ᵗʰ **T23.152** Burn of first degree of left palm

√7ᵗʰ **T23.159** Burn of first degree of unspecified palm

√6ᵗʰ **T23.16** Burn of first degree of back of hand

√7ᵗʰ **T23.161** Burn of first degree of back of right hand

√7ᵗʰ **T23.162** Burn of first degree of back of left hand

√7ᵗʰ **T23.169** Burn of first degree of back of unspecified hand

√6ᵗʰ **T23.17** Burn of first degree of wrist

√7ᵗʰ **T23.171** Burn of first degree of right wrist

√7ᵗʰ **T23.172** Burn of first degree of left wrist

√7ᵗʰ **T23.179** Burn of first degree of unspecified wrist

√6ᵗʰ **T23.19** Burn of first degree of multiple sites of wrist and hand

√7ᵗʰ **T23.191** Burn of first degree of multiple sites of right wrist and hand

√7ᵗʰ **T23.192** Burn of first degree of multiple sites of left wrist and hand

√7ᵗʰ **T23.199** Burn of first degree of multiple sites of unspecified wrist and hand

√5ᵗʰ **T23.2** Burn of second degree of wrist and hand

Use additional external cause code to identify the source, place and intent of the burn (X00-X19, X75-X77, X96-X98, Y92)

√6ᵗʰ **T23.20** Burn of second degree of hand, unspecified site

√7ᵗʰ **T23.201** Burn of second degree of right hand, unspecified site

☑ Additional Character Required   √x7ᵗʰ Placeholder Alert   Manifestation   Unspecified Dx   ▶◀ Revised Text   ● New Code   ▲ Revised Code Title

ICD-10-CM 2020

1085

> ✓7th **T23.202** Burn of second degree of left hand, unspecified site
>
> ✓7th **T23.209** Burn of second degree of unspecified hand, unspecified site

✓6th **T23.21** Burn of second degree of thumb (nail)

> ✓7th **T23.211** Burn of second degree of right thumb (nail)
>
> ✓7th **T23.212** Burn of second degree of left thumb (nail)
>
> ✓7th **T23.219** Burn of second degree of unspecified thumb (nail)

✓6th **T23.22** Burn of second degree of single finger (nail) except thumb

> ✓7th **T23.221** Burn of second degree of single right finger (nail) except thumb
>
> ✓7th **T23.222** Burn of second degree of single left finger (nail) except thumb
>
> ✓7th **T23.229** Burn of second degree of unspecified single finger (nail) except thumb

✓6th **T23.23** Burn of second degree of multiple fingers (nail), not including thumb

> ✓7th **T23.231** Burn of second degree of multiple right fingers (nail), not including thumb
>
> ✓7th **T23.232** Burn of second degree of multiple left fingers (nail), not including thumb
>
> ✓7th **T23.239** Burn of second degree of unspecified multiple fingers (nail), not including thumb

✓6th **T23.24** Burn of second degree of multiple fingers (nail), including thumb

> ✓7th **T23.241** Burn of second degree of multiple right fingers (nail), including thumb
>
> ✓7th **T23.242** Burn of second degree of multiple left fingers (nail), including thumb
>
> ✓7th **T23.249** Burn of second degree of unspecified multiple fingers (nail), including thumb

✓6th **T23.25** Burn of second degree of palm

> ✓7th **T23.251** Burn of second degree of right palm
>
> ✓7th **T23.252** Burn of second degree of left palm
>
> ✓7th **T23.259** Burn of second degree of unspecified palm

✓6th **T23.26** Burn of second degree of back of hand

> ✓7th **T23.261** Burn of second degree of back of right hand
>
> ✓7th **T23.262** Burn of second degree of back of left hand
>
> ✓7th **T23.269** Burn of second degree of back of unspecified hand

✓6th **T23.27** Burn of second degree of wrist

> ✓7th **T23.271** Burn of second degree of right wrist
>
> ✓7th **T23.272** Burn of second degree of left wrist
>
> ✓7th **T23.279** Burn of second degree of unspecified wrist

✓6th **T23.29** Burn of second degree of multiple sites of wrist and hand

> ✓7th **T23.291** Burn of second degree of multiple sites of right wrist and hand
>
> ✓7th **T23.292** Burn of second degree of multiple sites of left wrist and hand
>
> ✓7th **T23.299** Burn of second degree of multiple sites of unspecified wrist and hand

✓5th **T23.3** Burn of third degree of wrist and hand

Use additional external cause code to identify the source, place and intent of the burn (X00-X19, X75-X77, X96-X98, Y92)

✓6th **T23.30** Burn of third degree of hand, unspecified site

AHA: 2016,2Q,5

> ✓7th **T23.301** Burn of third degree of right hand, unspecified site
>
> ✓7th **T23.302** Burn of third degree of left hand, unspecified site
>
> ✓7th **T23.309** Burn of third degree of unspecified hand, unspecified site

✓6th **T23.31** Burn of third degree of thumb (nail)

> ✓7th **T23.311** Burn of third degree of right thumb (nail)
>
> ✓7th **T23.312** Burn of third degree of left thumb (nail)
>
> ✓7th **T23.319** Burn of third degree of unspecified thumb (nail)

✓6th **T23.32** Burn of third degree of single finger (nail) except thumb

> ✓7th **T23.321** Burn of third degree of single right finger (nail) except thumb
>
> ✓7th **T23.322** Burn of third degree of single left finger (nail) except thumb
>
> ✓7th **T23.329** Burn of third degree of unspecified single finger (nail) except thumb

✓6th **T23.33** Burn of third degree of multiple fingers (nail), not including thumb

> ✓7th **T23.331** Burn of third degree of multiple right fingers (nail), not including thumb
>
> ✓7th **T23.332** Burn of third degree of multiple left fingers (nail), not including thumb
>
> ✓7th **T23.339** Burn of third degree of unspecified multiple fingers (nail), not including thumb

✓6th **T23.34** Burn of third degree of multiple fingers (nail), including thumb

> ✓7th **T23.341** Burn of third degree of multiple right fingers (nail), including thumb
>
> ✓7th **T23.342** Burn of third degree of multiple left fingers (nail), including thumb
>
> ✓7th **T23.349** Burn of third degree of unspecified multiple fingers (nail), including thumb

✓6th **T23.35** Burn of third degree of palm

> ✓7th **T23.351** Burn of third degree of right palm
>
> ✓7th **T23.352** Burn of third degree of left palm
>
> ✓7th **T23.359** Burn of third degree of unspecified palm

✓6th **T23.36** Burn of third degree of back of hand

> ✓7th **T23.361** Burn of third degree of back of right hand
>
> ✓7th **T23.362** Burn of third degree of back of left hand
>
> ✓7th **T23.369** Burn of third degree of back of unspecified hand

✓6th **T23.37** Burn of third degree of wrist

> ✓7th **T23.371** Burn of third degree of right wrist
>
> ✓7th **T23.372** Burn of third degree of left wrist
>
> ✓7th **T23.379** Burn of third degree of unspecified wrist

✓6th **T23.39** Burn of third degree of multiple sites of wrist and hand

> ✓7th **T23.391** Burn of third degree of multiple sites of right wrist and hand
>
> ✓7th **T23.392** Burn of third degree of multiple sites of left wrist and hand
>
> ✓7th **T23.399** Burn of third degree of multiple sites of unspecified wrist and hand

✓5th **T23.4** Corrosion of unspecified degree of wrist and hand

Code first (T51-T65) to identify chemical and intent
Use additional external cause code to identify place (Y92)

✓6th **T23.40** Corrosion of unspecified degree of hand, unspecified site

> ✓7th **T23.401** Corrosion of unspecified degree of right hand, unspecified site
>
> ✓7th **T23.402** Corrosion of unspecified degree of left hand, unspecified site
>
> ✓7th **T23.409** Corrosion of unspecified degree of unspecified hand, unspecified site

✓6th **T23.41** Corrosion of unspecified degree of thumb (nail)

> ✓7th **T23.411** Corrosion of unspecified degree of right thumb (nail)
>
> ✓7th **T23.412** Corrosion of unspecified degree of left thumb (nail)
>
> ✓7th **T23.419** Corrosion of unspecified degree of unspecified thumb (nail)

✓6th **T23.42** Corrosion of unspecified degree of single finger (nail) except thumb

> ✓7th **T23.421** Corrosion of unspecified degree of single right finger (nail) except thumb
>
> ✓7th **T23.422** Corrosion of unspecified degree of single left finger (nail) except thumb
>
> ✓7th **T23.429** Corrosion of unspecified degree of unspecified single finger (nail) except thumb

✓6th **T23.43** Corrosion of unspecified degree of multiple fingers (nail), not including thumb

> ✓7th **T23.431** Corrosion of unspecified degree of multiple right fingers (nail), not including thumb

√7ᵗʰ **T23.432** Corrosion of unspecified degree of multiple left fingers (nail), not including thumb

√7ᵗʰ **T23.439** Corrosion of unspecified degree of unspecified multiple fingers (nail), not including thumb

√6ᵗʰ **T23.44** Corrosion of unspecified degree of multiple fingers (nail), including thumb

√7ᵗʰ **T23.441** Corrosion of unspecified degree of multiple right fingers (nail), including thumb

√7ᵗʰ **T23.442** Corrosion of unspecified degree of multiple left fingers (nail), including thumb

√7ᵗʰ **T23.449** Corrosion of unspecified degree of unspecified multiple fingers (nail), including thumb

√6ᵗʰ **T23.45** Corrosion of unspecified degree of palm

√7ᵗʰ **T23.451** Corrosion of unspecified degree of right palm

√7ᵗʰ **T23.452** Corrosion of unspecified degree of left palm

√7ᵗʰ **T23.459** Corrosion of unspecified degree of unspecified palm

√6ᵗʰ **T23.46** Corrosion of unspecified degree of back of hand

√7ᵗʰ **T23.461** Corrosion of unspecified degree of back of right hand

√7ᵗʰ **T23.462** Corrosion of unspecified degree of back of left hand

√7ᵗʰ **T23.469** Corrosion of unspecified degree of back of unspecified hand

√6ᵗʰ **T23.47** Corrosion of unspecified degree of wrist

√7ᵗʰ **T23.471** Corrosion of unspecified degree of right wrist

√7ᵗʰ **T23.472** Corrosion of unspecified degree of left wrist

√7ᵗʰ **T23.479** Corrosion of unspecified degree of unspecified wrist

√6ᵗʰ **T23.49** Corrosion of unspecified degree of multiple sites of wrist and hand

√7ᵗʰ **T23.491** Corrosion of unspecified degree of multiple sites of right wrist and hand

√7ᵗʰ **T23.492** Corrosion of unspecified degree of multiple sites of left wrist and hand

√7ᵗʰ **T23.499** Corrosion of unspecified degree of multiple sites of unspecified wrist and hand

√5ᵗʰ **T23.5** Corrosion of first degree of wrist and hand

Code first (T51-T65) to identify chemical and intent
Use additional external cause code to identify place (Y92)

√6ᵗʰ **T23.50** Corrosion of first degree of hand, unspecified site

√7ᵗʰ **T23.501** Corrosion of first degree of right hand, unspecified site

√7ᵗʰ **T23.502** Corrosion of first degree of left hand, unspecified site

√7ᵗʰ **T23.509** Corrosion of first degree of unspecified hand, unspecified site

√6ᵗʰ **T23.51** Corrosion of first degree of thumb (nail)

√7ᵗʰ **T23.511** Corrosion of first degree of right thumb (nail)

√7ᵗʰ **T23.512** Corrosion of first degree of left thumb (nail)

√7ᵗʰ **T23.519** Corrosion of first degree of unspecified thumb (nail)

√6ᵗʰ **T23.52** Corrosion of first degree of single finger (nail) except thumb

√7ᵗʰ **T23.521** Corrosion of first degree of single right finger (nail) except thumb

√7ᵗʰ **T23.522** Corrosion of first degree of single left finger (nail) except thumb

√7ᵗʰ **T23.529** Corrosion of first degree of unspecified single finger (nail) except thumb

√6ᵗʰ **T23.53** Corrosion of first degree of multiple fingers (nail), not including thumb

√7ᵗʰ **T23.531** Corrosion of first degree of multiple right fingers (nail), not including thumb

√7ᵗʰ **T23.532** Corrosion of first degree of multiple left fingers (nail), not including thumb

√7ᵗʰ **T23.539** Corrosion of first degree of unspecified multiple fingers (nail), not including thumb

√6ᵗʰ **T23.54** Corrosion of first degree of multiple fingers (nail), including thumb

√7ᵗʰ **T23.541** Corrosion of first degree of multiple right fingers (nail), including thumb

√7ᵗʰ **T23.542** Corrosion of first degree of multiple left fingers (nail), including thumb

√7ᵗʰ **T23.549** Corrosion of first degree of unspecified multiple fingers (nail), including thumb

√6ᵗʰ **T23.55** Corrosion of first degree of palm

√7ᵗʰ **T23.551** Corrosion of first degree of right palm

√7ᵗʰ **T23.552** Corrosion of first degree of left palm

√7ᵗʰ **T23.559** Corrosion of first degree of unspecified palm

√6ᵗʰ **T23.56** Corrosion of first degree of back of hand

√7ᵗʰ **T23.561** Corrosion of first degree of back of right hand

√7ᵗʰ **T23.562** Corrosion of first degree of back of left hand

√7ᵗʰ **T23.569** Corrosion of first degree of back of unspecified hand

√6ᵗʰ **T23.57** Corrosion of first degree of wrist

√7ᵗʰ **T23.571** Corrosion of first degree of right wrist

√7ᵗʰ **T23.572** Corrosion of first degree of left wrist

√7ᵗʰ **T23.579** Corrosion of first degree of unspecified wrist

√6ᵗʰ **T23.59** Corrosion of first degree of multiple sites of wrist and hand

√7ᵗʰ **T23.591** Corrosion of first degree of multiple sites of right wrist and hand

√7ᵗʰ **T23.592** Corrosion of first degree of multiple sites of left wrist and hand

√7ᵗʰ **T23.599** Corrosion of first degree of multiple sites of unspecified wrist and hand

√5ᵗʰ **T23.6** Corrosion of second degree of wrist and hand

Code first (T51-T65) to identify chemical and intent
Use additional external cause code to identify place (Y92)

√6ᵗʰ **T23.60** Corrosion of second degree of hand, unspecified site

√7ᵗʰ **T23.601** Corrosion of second degree of right hand, unspecified site

√7ᵗʰ **T23.602** Corrosion of second degree of left hand, unspecified site

√7ᵗʰ **T23.609** Corrosion of second degree of unspecified hand, unspecified site

√6ᵗʰ **T23.61** Corrosion of second degree of thumb (nail)

√7ᵗʰ **T23.611** Corrosion of second degree of right thumb (nail)

√7ᵗʰ **T23.612** Corrosion of second degree of left thumb (nail)

√7ᵗʰ **T23.619** Corrosion of second degree of unspecified thumb (nail)

√6ᵗʰ **T23.62** Corrosion of second degree of single finger (nail) except thumb

√7ᵗʰ **T23.621** Corrosion of second degree of single right finger (nail) except thumb

√7ᵗʰ **T23.622** Corrosion of second degree of single left finger (nail) except thumb

√7ᵗʰ **T23.629** Corrosion of second degree of unspecified single finger (nail) except thumb

√6ᵗʰ **T23.63** Corrosion of second degree of multiple fingers (nail), not including thumb

√7ᵗʰ **T23.631** Corrosion of second degree of multiple right fingers (nail), not including thumb

√7ᵗʰ **T23.632** Corrosion of second degree of multiple left fingers (nail), not including thumb

√7ᵗʰ **T23.639** Corrosion of second degree of unspecified multiple fingers (nail), not including thumb

√6ᵗʰ **T23.64** Corrosion of second degree of multiple fingers (nail), including thumb

√7ᵗʰ **T23.641** Corrosion of second degree of multiple right fingers (nail), including thumb

√7ᵗʰ **T23.642** Corrosion of second degree of multiple left fingers (nail), including thumb

√7ᵗʰ **T23.649** Corrosion of second degree of unspecified multiple fingers (nail), including thumb

√6ᵗʰ **T23.65** Corrosion of second degree of palm

√7ᵗʰ **T23.651** Corrosion of second degree of right palm

√7ᵗʰ **T23.652** Corrosion of second degree of left palm

✔ Additional Character Required　　√x7ᵗʰ Placeholder Alert　　Manifestation　　Unspecified Dx　　▶◀ Revised Text　　● New Code　　▲ Revised Code Title

√7ᵗʰ **T23.659** Corrosion of second degree of unspecified palm

√6ᵗʰ **T23.66** Corrosion of second degree of back of hand

√7ᵗʰ **T23.661** Corrosion of second degree back of right hand

√7ᵗʰ **T23.662** Corrosion of second degree back of left hand

√7ᵗʰ **T23.669** Corrosion of second degree back of unspecified hand

√6ᵗʰ **T23.67** Corrosion of second degree of wrist

√7ᵗʰ **T23.671** Corrosion of second degree of right wrist

√7ᵗʰ **T23.672** Corrosion of second degree of left wrist

√7ᵗʰ **T23.679** Corrosion of second degree of unspecified wrist

√6ᵗʰ **T23.69** Corrosion of second degree of multiple sites of wrist and hand

√7ᵗʰ **T23.691** Corrosion of second degree of multiple sites of right wrist and hand

√7ᵗʰ **T23.692** Corrosion of second degree of multiple sites of left wrist and hand

√7ᵗʰ **T23.699** Corrosion of second degree of multiple sites of unspecified wrist and hand

√5ᵗʰ **T23.7** Corrosion of third degree of wrist and hand

Code first (T51-T65) to identify chemical and intent
Use additional external cause code to identify place (Y92)

√6ᵗʰ **T23.70** Corrosion of third degree of hand, unspecified site

√7ᵗʰ **T23.701** Corrosion of third degree of right hand, unspecified site

√7ᵗʰ **T23.702** Corrosion of third degree of left hand, unspecified site

√7ᵗʰ **T23.709** Corrosion of third degree of unspecified hand, unspecified site

√6ᵗʰ **T23.71** Corrosion of third degree of thumb (nail)

√7ᵗʰ **T23.711** Corrosion of third degree of right thumb (nail)

√7ᵗʰ **T23.712** Corrosion of third degree of left thumb (nail)

√7ᵗʰ **T23.719** Corrosion of third degree of unspecified thumb (nail)

√6ᵗʰ **T23.72** Corrosion of third degree of single finger (nail) except thumb

√7ᵗʰ **T23.721** Corrosion of third degree of single right finger (nail) except thumb

√7ᵗʰ **T23.722** Corrosion of third degree of single left finger (nail) except thumb

√7ᵗʰ **T23.729** Corrosion of third degree of unspecified single finger (nail) except thumb

√6ᵗʰ **T23.73** Corrosion of third degree of multiple fingers (nail), not including thumb

√7ᵗʰ **T23.731** Corrosion of third degree of multiple right fingers (nail), not including thumb

√7ᵗʰ **T23.732** Corrosion of third degree of multiple left fingers (nail), not including thumb

√7ᵗʰ **T23.739** Corrosion of third degree of unspecified multiple fingers (nail), not including thumb

√6ᵗʰ **T23.74** Corrosion of third degree of multiple fingers (nail), including thumb

√7ᵗʰ **T23.741** Corrosion of third degree of multiple right fingers (nail), including thumb

√7ᵗʰ **T23.742** Corrosion of third degree of multiple left fingers (nail), including thumb

√7ᵗʰ **T23.749** Corrosion of third degree of unspecified multiple fingers (nail), including thumb

√6ᵗʰ **T23.75** Corrosion of third degree of palm

√7ᵗʰ **T23.751** Corrosion of third degree of right palm

√7ᵗʰ **T23.752** Corrosion of third degree of left palm

√7ᵗʰ **T23.759** Corrosion of third degree of unspecified palm

√6ᵗʰ **T23.76** Corrosion of third degree of back of hand

√7ᵗʰ **T23.761** Corrosion of third degree of back of right hand

√7ᵗʰ **T23.762** Corrosion of third degree of back of left hand

√7ᵗʰ **T23.769** Corrosion of third degree back of unspecified hand

√6ᵗʰ **T23.77** Corrosion of third degree of wrist

√7ᵗʰ **T23.771** Corrosion of third degree of right wrist

√7ᵗʰ **T23.772** Corrosion of third degree of left wrist

√7ᵗʰ **T23.779** Corrosion of third degree of unspecified wrist

√6ᵗʰ **T23.79** Corrosion of third degree of multiple sites of wrist and hand

√7ᵗʰ **T23.791** Corrosion of third degree of multiple sites of right wrist and hand

√7ᵗʰ **T23.792** Corrosion of third degree of multiple sites of left wrist and hand

√7ᵗʰ **T23.799** Corrosion of third degree of multiple sites of unspecified wrist and hand

√4ᵗʰ **T24** Burn and corrosion of lower limb, except ankle and foot

EXCLUDES 2   burn and corrosion of ankle and foot (T25.-)
              burn and corrosion of hip region (T21.-)

The appropriate 7th character is to be added to each code from category T24.
A   initial encounter
D   subsequent encounter
S   sequela

√5ᵗʰ **T24.0** Burn of unspecified degree of lower limb, except ankle and foot

Use additional external cause code to identify the source, place and intent of the burn (X00-X19, X75-X77, X96-X98, Y92)

√6ᵗʰ **T24.00** Burn of unspecified degree of unspecified site of lower limb, except ankle and foot

√7ᵗʰ **T24.001** Burn of unspecified degree of unspecified site of right lower limb, except ankle and foot

√7ᵗʰ **T24.002** Burn of unspecified degree of unspecified site of left lower limb, except ankle and foot

√7ᵗʰ **T24.009** Burn of unspecified degree of unspecified site of unspecified lower limb, except ankle and foot

√6ᵗʰ **T24.01** Burn of unspecified degree of thigh

√7ᵗʰ **T24.011** Burn of unspecified degree of right thigh

√7ᵗʰ **T24.012** Burn of unspecified degree of left thigh

√7ᵗʰ **T24.019** Burn of unspecified degree of unspecified thigh

√6ᵗʰ **T24.02** Burn of unspecified degree of knee

√7ᵗʰ **T24.021** Burn of unspecified degree of right knee

√7ᵗʰ **T24.022** Burn of unspecified degree of left knee

√7ᵗʰ **T24.029** Burn of unspecified degree of unspecified knee

√6ᵗʰ **T24.03** Burn of unspecified degree of lower leg

√7ᵗʰ **T24.031** Burn of unspecified degree of right lower leg

√7ᵗʰ **T24.032** Burn of unspecified degree of left lower leg

√7ᵗʰ **T24.039** Burn of unspecified degree of unspecified lower leg

√6ᵗʰ **T24.09** Burn of unspecified degree of multiple sites of lower limb, except ankle and foot

√7ᵗʰ **T24.091** Burn of unspecified degree of multiple sites of right lower limb, except ankle and foot

√7ᵗʰ **T24.092** Burn of unspecified degree of multiple sites of left lower limb, except ankle and foot

√7ᵗʰ **T24.099** Burn of unspecified degree of multiple sites of unspecified lower limb, except ankle and foot

√5ᵗʰ **T24.1** Burn of first degree of lower limb, except ankle and foot

Use additional external cause code to identify the source, place and intent of the burn (X00-X19, X75-X77, X96-X98, Y92)

√6ᵗʰ **T24.10** Burn of first degree of unspecified site of lower limb, except ankle and foot

√7ᵗʰ **T24.101** Burn of first degree of unspecified site of right lower limb, except ankle and foot

√7ᵗʰ **T24.102** Burn of first degree of unspecified site of left lower limb, except ankle and foot

√7ᵗʰ **T24.109** Burn of first degree of unspecified site of unspecified lower limb, except ankle and foot

√6ᵗʰ **T24.11** Burn of first degree of thigh

√7ᵗʰ **T24.111** Burn of first degree of right thigh

√7ᵗʰ **T24.112** Burn of first degree of left thigh

√7ᵗʰ **T24.119** Burn of first degree of unspecified thigh

√6ᵗʰ **T24.12** Burn of first degree of knee
     √7ᵗʰ **T24.121** Burn of first degree of right knee
     √7ᵗʰ **T24.122** Burn of first degree of left knee
     √7ᵗʰ **T24.129** Burn of first degree of unspecified knee

√6ᵗʰ **T24.13** Burn of first degree of lower leg
     √7ᵗʰ **T24.131** Burn of first degree of right lower leg
     √7ᵗʰ **T24.132** Burn of first degree of left lower leg
     √7ᵗʰ **T24.139** Burn of first degree of unspecified lower leg

√6ᵗʰ **T24.19** Burn of first degree of multiple sites of lower limb, except ankle and foot
     √7ᵗʰ **T24.191** Burn of first degree of multiple sites of right lower limb, except ankle and foot
     √7ᵗʰ **T24.192** Burn of first degree of multiple sites of left lower limb, except ankle and foot
     √7ᵗʰ **T24.199** Burn of first degree of multiple sites of unspecified lower limb, except ankle and foot

√5ᵗʰ **T24.2** Burn of second degree of lower limb, except ankle and foot
     Use additional external cause code to identify the source, place and intent of the burn (X00-X19, X75-X77, X96-X98, Y92)

√6ᵗʰ **T24.20** Burn of second degree of unspecified site of lower limb, except ankle and foot
     √7ᵗʰ **T24.201** Burn of second degree of unspecified site of right lower limb, except ankle and foot
     √7ᵗʰ **T24.202** Burn of second degree of unspecified site of left lower limb, except ankle and foot
     √7ᵗʰ **T24.209** Burn of second degree of unspecified site of unspecified lower limb, except ankle and foot

√6ᵗʰ **T24.21** Burn of second degree of thigh
     √7ᵗʰ **T24.211** Burn of second degree of right thigh
     √7ᵗʰ **T24.212** Burn of second degree of left thigh
     √7ᵗʰ **T24.219** Burn of second degree of unspecified thigh

√6ᵗʰ **T24.22** Burn of second degree of knee
     √7ᵗʰ **T24.221** Burn of second degree of right knee
     √7ᵗʰ **T24.222** Burn of second degree of left knee
     √7ᵗʰ **T24.229** Burn of second degree of unspecified knee

√6ᵗʰ **T24.23** Burn of second degree of lower leg
     √7ᵗʰ **T24.231** Burn of second degree of right lower leg
     √7ᵗʰ **T24.232** Burn of second degree of left lower leg
     √7ᵗʰ **T24.239** Burn of second degree of unspecified lower leg

√6ᵗʰ **T24.29** Burn of second degree of multiple sites of lower limb, except ankle and foot
     √7ᵗʰ **T24.291** Burn of second degree of multiple sites of right lower limb, except ankle and foot
     √7ᵗʰ **T24.292** Burn of second degree of multiple sites of left lower limb, except ankle and foot
     √7ᵗʰ **T24.299** Burn of second degree of multiple sites of unspecified lower limb, except ankle and foot

√5ᵗʰ **T24.3** Burn of third degree of lower limb, except ankle and foot
     Use additional external cause code to identify the source, place and intent of the burn (X00-X19, X75-X77, X96-X98, Y92)

√6ᵗʰ **T24.30** Burn of third degree of unspecified site of lower limb, except ankle and foot
     √7ᵗʰ **T24.301** Burn of third degree of unspecified site of right lower limb, except ankle and foot
     √7ᵗʰ **T24.302** Burn of third degree of unspecified site of left lower limb, except ankle and foot
     √7ᵗʰ **T24.309** Burn of third degree of unspecified site of unspecified lower limb, except ankle and foot

√6ᵗʰ **T24.31** Burn of third degree of thigh
     √7ᵗʰ **T24.311** Burn of third degree of right thigh
     √7ᵗʰ **T24.312** Burn of third degree of left thigh
     √7ᵗʰ **T24.319** Burn of third degree of unspecified thigh

√6ᵗʰ **T24.32** Burn of third degree of knee
     √7ᵗʰ **T24.321** Burn of third degree of right knee
     √7ᵗʰ **T24.322** Burn of third degree of left knee
     √7ᵗʰ **T24.329** Burn of third degree of unspecified knee

√6ᵗʰ **T24.33** Burn of third degree of lower leg
     √7ᵗʰ **T24.331** Burn of third degree of right lower leg

     √7ᵗʰ **T24.332** Burn of third degree of left lower leg
     √7ᵗʰ **T24.339** Burn of third degree of unspecified lower leg

√6ᵗʰ **T24.39** Burn of third degree of multiple sites of lower limb, except ankle and foot
     AHA: 2016,2Q,4
     √7ᵗʰ **T24.391** Burn of third degree of multiple sites of right lower limb, except ankle and foot
     √7ᵗʰ **T24.392** Burn of third degree of multiple sites of left lower limb, except ankle and foot
     √7ᵗʰ **T24.399** Burn of third degree of multiple sites of unspecified lower limb, except ankle and foot

√5ᵗʰ **T24.4** Corrosion of unspecified degree of lower limb, except ankle and foot
     Code first (T51-T65) to identify chemical and intent
     Use additional external cause code to identify place (Y92)

√6ᵗʰ **T24.40** Corrosion of unspecified degree of unspecified site of lower limb, except ankle and foot
     √7ᵗʰ **T24.401** Corrosion of unspecified degree of unspecified site of right lower limb, except ankle and foot
     √7ᵗʰ **T24.402** Corrosion of unspecified degree of unspecified site of left lower limb, except ankle and foot
     √7ᵗʰ **T24.409** Corrosion of unspecified degree of unspecified site of unspecified lower limb, except ankle and foot

√6ᵗʰ **T24.41** Corrosion of unspecified degree of thigh
     √7ᵗʰ **T24.411** Corrosion of unspecified degree of right thigh
     √7ᵗʰ **T24.412** Corrosion of unspecified degree of left thigh
     √7ᵗʰ **T24.419** Corrosion of unspecified degree of unspecified thigh

√6ᵗʰ **T24.42** Corrosion of unspecified degree of knee
     √7ᵗʰ **T24.421** Corrosion of unspecified degree of right knee
     √7ᵗʰ **T24.422** Corrosion of unspecified degree of left knee
     √7ᵗʰ **T24.429** Corrosion of unspecified degree of unspecified knee

√6ᵗʰ **T24.43** Corrosion of unspecified degree of lower leg
     √7ᵗʰ **T24.431** Corrosion of unspecified degree of right lower leg
     √7ᵗʰ **T24.432** Corrosion of unspecified degree of left lower leg
     √7ᵗʰ **T24.439** Corrosion of unspecified degree of unspecified lower leg

√6ᵗʰ **T24.49** Corrosion of unspecified degree of multiple sites of lower limb, except ankle and foot
     √7ᵗʰ **T24.491** Corrosion of unspecified degree of multiple sites of right lower limb, except ankle and foot
     √7ᵗʰ **T24.492** Corrosion of unspecified degree of multiple sites of left lower limb, except ankle and foot
     √7ᵗʰ **T24.499** Corrosion of unspecified degree of multiple sites of unspecified lower limb, except ankle and foot

√5ᵗʰ **T24.5** Corrosion of first degree of lower limb, except ankle and foot
     Code first (T51-T65) to identify chemical and intent
     Use additional external cause code to identify place (Y92)

√6ᵗʰ **T24.50** Corrosion of first degree of unspecified site of lower limb, except ankle and foot
     √7ᵗʰ **T24.501** Corrosion of first degree of unspecified site of right lower limb, except ankle and foot
     √7ᵗʰ **T24.502** Corrosion of first degree of unspecified site of left lower limb, except ankle and foot
     √7ᵗʰ **T24.509** Corrosion of first degree of unspecified site of unspecified lower limb, except ankle and foot

√6ᵗʰ **T24.51** Corrosion of first degree of thigh
     √7ᵗʰ **T24.511** Corrosion of first degree of right thigh
     √7ᵗʰ **T24.512** Corrosion of first degree of left thigh
     √7ᵗʰ **T24.519** Corrosion of first degree of unspecified thigh

√6ᵗʰ **T24.52** Corrosion of first degree of knee
     √7ᵗʰ **T24.521** Corrosion of first degree of right knee

---

☑ Additional Character Required   √x7ᵗʰ Placeholder Alert   Manifestation   Unspecified Dx   ▶◀ Revised Text   ● New Code   ▲ Revised Code Title

√7ᵗʰ **T24.522** Corrosion of first degree of left knee

√7ᵗʰ **T24.529** Corrosion of first degree of unspecified knee

√6ᵗʰ **T24.53** Corrosion of first degree of lower leg

√7ᵗʰ **T24.531** Corrosion of first degree of right lower leg

√7ᵗʰ **T24.532** Corrosion of first degree of left lower leg

√7ᵗʰ **T24.539** Corrosion of first degree of unspecified lower leg

√6ᵗʰ **T24.59** Corrosion of first degree of multiple sites of lower limb, except ankle and foot

√7ᵗʰ **T24.591** Corrosion of first degree of multiple sites of right lower limb, except ankle and foot

√7ᵗʰ **T24.592** Corrosion of first degree of multiple sites of left lower limb, except ankle and foot

√7ᵗʰ **T24.599** Corrosion of first degree of multiple sites of unspecified lower limb, except ankle and foot

√5ᵗʰ **T24.6** Corrosion of second degree of lower limb, except ankle and foot

Code first (T51-T65) to identify chemical and intent
Use additional external cause code to identify place (Y92)

√6ᵗʰ **T24.60** Corrosion of second degree of unspecified site of lower limb, except ankle and foot

√7ᵗʰ **T24.601** Corrosion of second degree of unspecified site of right lower limb, except ankle and foot

√7ᵗʰ **T24.602** Corrosion of second degree of unspecified site of left lower limb, except ankle and foot

√7ᵗʰ **T24.609** Corrosion of second degree of unspecified site of unspecified lower limb, except ankle and foot

√6ᵗʰ **T24.61** Corrosion of second degree of thigh

√7ᵗʰ **T24.611** Corrosion of second degree of right thigh

√7ᵗʰ **T24.612** Corrosion of second degree of left thigh

√7ᵗʰ **T24.619** Corrosion of second degree of unspecified thigh

√6ᵗʰ **T24.62** Corrosion of second degree of knee

√7ᵗʰ **T24.621** Corrosion of second degree of right knee

√7ᵗʰ **T24.622** Corrosion of second degree of left knee

√7ᵗʰ **T24.629** Corrosion of second degree of unspecified knee

√6ᵗʰ **T24.63** Corrosion of second degree of lower leg

√7ᵗʰ **T24.631** Corrosion of second degree of right lower leg

√7ᵗʰ **T24.632** Corrosion of second degree of left lower leg

√7ᵗʰ **T24.639** Corrosion of second degree of unspecified lower leg

√6ᵗʰ **T24.69** Corrosion of second degree of multiple sites of lower limb, except ankle and foot

√7ᵗʰ **T24.691** Corrosion of second degree of multiple sites of right lower limb, except ankle and foot

√7ᵗʰ **T24.692** Corrosion of second degree of multiple sites of left lower limb, except ankle and foot

√7ᵗʰ **T24.699** Corrosion of second degree of multiple sites of unspecified lower limb, except ankle and foot

√5ᵗʰ **T24.7** Corrosion of third degree of lower limb, except ankle and foot

Code first (T51-T65) to identify chemical and intent
Use additional external cause code to identify place (Y92)

√6ᵗʰ **T24.70** Corrosion of third degree of unspecified site of lower limb, except ankle and foot

√7ᵗʰ **T24.701** Corrosion of third degree of unspecified site of right lower limb, except ankle and foot

√7ᵗʰ **T24.702** Corrosion of third degree of unspecified site of left lower limb, except ankle and foot

√7ᵗʰ **T24.709** Corrosion of third degree of unspecified site of unspecified lower limb, except ankle and foot

√6ᵗʰ **T24.71** Corrosion of third degree of thigh

√7ᵗʰ **T24.711** Corrosion of third degree of right thigh

√7ᵗʰ **T24.712** Corrosion of third degree of left thigh

√7ᵗʰ **T24.719** Corrosion of third degree of unspecified thigh

√6ᵗʰ **T24.72** Corrosion of third degree of knee

√7ᵗʰ **T24.721** Corrosion of third degree of right knee

√7ᵗʰ **T24.722** Corrosion of third degree of left knee

√7ᵗʰ **T24.729** Corrosion of third degree of unspecified knee

√6ᵗʰ **T24.73** Corrosion of third degree of lower leg

√7ᵗʰ **T24.731** Corrosion of third degree of right lower leg

√7ᵗʰ **T24.732** Corrosion of third degree of left lower leg

√7ᵗʰ **T24.739** Corrosion of third degree of unspecified lower leg

√6ᵗʰ **T24.79** Corrosion of third degree of multiple sites of lower limb, except ankle and foot

√7ᵗʰ **T24.791** Corrosion of third degree of multiple sites of right lower limb, except ankle and foot

√7ᵗʰ **T24.792** Corrosion of third degree of multiple sites of left lower limb, except ankle and foot

√7ᵗʰ **T24.799** Corrosion of third degree of multiple sites of unspecified lower limb, except ankle and foot

√4ᵗʰ **T25** Burn and corrosion of ankle and foot

The appropriate 7th character is to be added to each code from category T25.
A initial encounter
D subsequent encounter
S sequela

√5ᵗʰ **T25.0** Burn of unspecified degree of ankle and foot

Use additional external cause code to identify the source, place and intent of the burn (X00-X19, X75-X77, X96-X98, Y92)

√6ᵗʰ **T25.01** Burn of unspecified degree of ankle

√7ᵗʰ **T25.011** Burn of unspecified degree of right ankle

√7ᵗʰ **T25.012** Burn of unspecified degree of left ankle

√7ᵗʰ **T25.019** Burn of unspecified degree of unspecified ankle

√6ᵗʰ **T25.02** Burn of unspecified degree of foot

EXCLUDES 2 burn of unspecified degree of toe(s) (nail) (T25.03-)

√7ᵗʰ **T25.021** Burn of unspecified degree of right foot

√7ᵗʰ **T25.022** Burn of unspecified degree of left foot

√7ᵗʰ **T25.029** Burn of unspecified degree of unspecified foot

√6ᵗʰ **T25.03** Burn of unspecified degree of toe(s) (nail)

√7ᵗʰ **T25.031** Burn of unspecified degree of right toe(s) (nail)

√7ᵗʰ **T25.032** Burn of unspecified degree of left toe(s) (nail)

√7ᵗʰ **T25.039** Burn of unspecified degree of unspecified toe(s) (nail)

√6ᵗʰ **T25.09** Burn of unspecified degree of multiple sites of ankle and foot

√7ᵗʰ **T25.091** Burn of unspecified degree of multiple sites of right ankle and foot

√7ᵗʰ **T25.092** Burn of unspecified degree of multiple sites of left ankle and foot

√7ᵗʰ **T25.099** Burn of unspecified degree of multiple sites of unspecified ankle and foot

√5ᵗʰ **T25.1** Burn of first degree of ankle and foot

Use additional external cause code to identify the source, place and intent of the burn (X00-X19, X75-X77, X96-X98, Y92)

√6ᵗʰ **T25.11** Burn of first degree of ankle

√7ᵗʰ **T25.111** Burn of first degree of right ankle

√7ᵗʰ **T25.112** Burn of first degree of left ankle

√7ᵗʰ **T25.119** Burn of first degree of unspecified ankle

√6ᵗʰ **T25.12** Burn of first degree of foot

EXCLUDES 2 burn of first degree of toe(s) (nail) (T25.13-)

√7ᵗʰ **T25.121** Burn of first degree of right foot

√7ᵗʰ **T25.122** Burn of first degree of left foot

√7ᵗʰ **T25.129** Burn of first degree of unspecified foot

√6ᵗʰ **T25.13** Burn of first degree of toe(s) (nail)

√7ᵗʰ **T25.131** Burn of first degree of right toe(s) (nail)

√7ᵗʰ **T25.132** Burn of first degree of left toe(s) (nail)

√7ᵗʰ **T25.139** Burn of first degree of unspecified toe(s) (nail)

√6ᵗʰ **T25.19** Burn of first degree of multiple sites of ankle and foot
- √7ᵗʰ **T25.191** Burn of first degree of multiple sites of right ankle and foot
- √7ᵗʰ **T25.192** Burn of first degree of multiple sites of left ankle and foot
- √7ᵗʰ **T25.199** Burn of first degree of multiple sites of unspecified ankle and foot

√5ᵗʰ **T25.2** Burn of second degree of ankle and foot

Use additional external cause code to identify the source, place and intent of the burn (X00-X19, X75-X77, X96-X98, Y92)

√6ᵗʰ **T25.21** Burn of second degree of ankle
- √7ᵗʰ **T25.211** Burn of second degree of right ankle
- √7ᵗʰ **T25.212** Burn of second degree of left ankle
- √7ᵗʰ **T25.219** Burn of second degree of unspecified ankle

√6ᵗʰ **T25.22** Burn of second degree of foot

EXCLUDES 2   burn of second degree of toe(s) (nail) (T25.23-)
- √7ᵗʰ **T25.221** Burn of second degree of right foot
- √7ᵗʰ **T25.222** Burn of second degree of left foot
- √7ᵗʰ **T25.229** Burn of second degree of unspecified foot

√6ᵗʰ **T25.23** Burn of second degree of toe(s) (nail)
- √7ᵗʰ **T25.231** Burn of second degree of right toe(s) (nail)
- √7ᵗʰ **T25.232** Burn of second degree of left toe(s) (nail)
- √7ᵗʰ **T25.239** Burn of second degree of unspecified toe(s) (nail)

√6ᵗʰ **T25.29** Burn of second degree of multiple sites of ankle and foot
- √7ᵗʰ **T25.291** Burn of second degree of multiple sites of right ankle and foot
- √7ᵗʰ **T25.292** Burn of second degree of multiple sites of left ankle and foot
- √7ᵗʰ **T25.299** Burn of second degree of multiple sites of unspecified ankle and foot

√5ᵗʰ **T25.3** Burn of third degree of ankle and foot

Use additional external cause code to identify the source, place and intent of the burn (X00-X19, X75-X77, X96-X98, Y92)

√6ᵗʰ **T25.31** Burn of third degree of ankle
- √7ᵗʰ **T25.311** Burn of third degree of right ankle
- √7ᵗʰ **T25.312** Burn of third degree of left ankle
- √7ᵗʰ **T25.319** Burn of third degree of unspecified ankle

√6ᵗʰ **T25.32** Burn of third degree of foot

EXCLUDES 2   burn of third degree of toe(s) (nail) (T25.33-)
- √7ᵗʰ **T25.321** Burn of third degree of right foot
- √7ᵗʰ **T25.322** Burn of third degree of left foot
- √7ᵗʰ **T25.329** Burn of third degree of unspecified foot

√6ᵗʰ **T25.33** Burn of third degree of toe(s) (nail)
- √7ᵗʰ **T25.331** Burn of third degree of right toe(s) (nail)
- √7ᵗʰ **T25.332** Burn of third degree of left toe(s) (nail)
- √7ᵗʰ **T25.339** Burn of third degree of unspecified toe(s) (nail)

√6ᵗʰ **T25.39** Burn of third degree of multiple sites of ankle and foot
- √7ᵗʰ **T25.391** Burn of third degree of multiple sites of right ankle and foot
- √7ᵗʰ **T25.392** Burn of third degree of multiple sites of left ankle and foot
- √7ᵗʰ **T25.399** Burn of third degree of multiple sites of unspecified ankle and foot

√5ᵗʰ **T25.4** Corrosion of unspecified degree of ankle and foot

Code first (T51-T65) to identify chemical and intent
Use additional external cause code to identify place (Y92)

√6ᵗʰ **T25.41** Corrosion of unspecified degree of ankle
- √7ᵗʰ **T25.411** Corrosion of unspecified degree of right ankle
- √7ᵗʰ **T25.412** Corrosion of unspecified degree of left ankle
- √7ᵗʰ **T25.419** Corrosion of unspecified degree of unspecified ankle

√6ᵗʰ **T25.42** Corrosion of unspecified degree of foot

EXCLUDES 2   corrosion of unspecified degree of toe(s) (nail) (T25.43-)
- √7ᵗʰ **T25.421** Corrosion of unspecified degree of right foot
- √7ᵗʰ **T25.422** Corrosion of unspecified degree of left foot
- √7ᵗʰ **T25.429** Corrosion of unspecified degree of unspecified foot

√6ᵗʰ **T25.43** Corrosion of unspecified degree of toe(s) (nail)
- √7ᵗʰ **T25.431** Corrosion of unspecified degree of right toe(s) (nail)
- √7ᵗʰ **T25.432** Corrosion of unspecified degree of left toe(s) (nail)
- √7ᵗʰ **T25.439** Corrosion of unspecified degree of unspecified toe(s) (nail)

√6ᵗʰ **T25.49** Corrosion of unspecified degree of multiple sites of ankle and foot
- √7ᵗʰ **T25.491** Corrosion of unspecified degree of multiple sites of right ankle and foot
- √7ᵗʰ **T25.492** Corrosion of unspecified degree of multiple sites of left ankle and foot
- √7ᵗʰ **T25.499** Corrosion of unspecified degree of multiple sites of unspecified ankle and foot

√5ᵗʰ **T25.5** Corrosion of first degree of ankle and foot

Code first (T51-T65) to identify chemical and intent
Use additional external cause code to identify place (Y92)

√6ᵗʰ **T25.51** Corrosion of first degree of ankle
- √7ᵗʰ **T25.511** Corrosion of first degree of right ankle
- √7ᵗʰ **T25.512** Corrosion of first degree of left ankle
- √7ᵗʰ **T25.519** Corrosion of first degree of unspecified ankle

√6ᵗʰ **T25.52** Corrosion of first degree of foot

EXCLUDES 2   corrosion of first degree of toe(s) (nail) (T25.53)
- √7ᵗʰ **T25.521** Corrosion of first degree of right foot
- √7ᵗʰ **T25.522** Corrosion of first degree of left foot
- √7ᵗʰ **T25.529** Corrosion of first degree of unspecified foot

√6ᵗʰ **T25.53** Corrosion of first degree of toe(s) (nail)
- √7ᵗʰ **T25.531** Corrosion of first degree of right toe(s) (nail)
- √7ᵗʰ **T25.532** Corrosion of first degree of left toe(s) (nail)
- √7ᵗʰ **T25.539** Corrosion of first degree of unspecified toe(s) (nail)

√6ᵗʰ **T25.59** Corrosion of first degree of multiple sites of ankle and foot
- √7ᵗʰ **T25.591** Corrosion of first degree of multiple sites of right ankle and foot
- √7ᵗʰ **T25.592** Corrosion of first degree of multiple sites of left ankle and foot
- √7ᵗʰ **T25.599** Corrosion of first degree of multiple sites of unspecified ankle and foot

√5ᵗʰ **T25.6** Corrosion of second degree of ankle and foot

Code first (T51-T65) to identify chemical and intent
Use additional external cause code to identify place (Y92)

√6ᵗʰ **T25.61** Corrosion of second degree of ankle
- √7ᵗʰ **T25.611** Corrosion of second degree of right ankle
- √7ᵗʰ **T25.612** Corrosion of second degree of left ankle
- √7ᵗʰ **T25.619** Corrosion of second degree of unspecified ankle

√6ᵗʰ **T25.62** Corrosion of second degree of foot

EXCLUDES 2   corrosion of second degree of toe(s) (nail) (T25.63-)
- √7ᵗʰ **T25.621** Corrosion of second degree of right foot
- √7ᵗʰ **T25.622** Corrosion of second degree of left foot
- √7ᵗʰ **T25.629** Corrosion of second degree of unspecified foot

√6ᵗʰ **T25.63** Corrosion of second degree of toe(s) (nail)
- √7ᵗʰ **T25.631** Corrosion of second degree of right toe(s) (nail)
- √7ᵗʰ **T25.632** Corrosion of second degree of left toe(s) (nail)
- √7ᵗʰ **T25.639** Corrosion of second degree of unspecified toe(s) (nail)

✔ Additional Character Required   √x7ᵗʰ Placeholder Alert   Manifestation   Unspecified Dx   ▶◀ Revised Text   ● New Code   ▲ Revised Code Title

Chapter 19. Injury, Poisoning and Certain Other Consequences of External Causes

T25.69–T27.7

✓6ᵗʰ **T25.69** Corrosion of second degree of multiple sites of ankle and foot

     ✓7ᵗʰ **T25.691** Corrosion of second degree of right ankle and foot

     ✓7ᵗʰ **T25.692** Corrosion of second degree of left ankle and foot

     ✓7ᵗʰ **T25.699** Corrosion of second degree of unspecified ankle and foot

✓5ᵗʰ **T25.7** Corrosion of third degree of ankle and foot

     Code first (T51-T65) to identify chemical and intent

     Use additional external cause code to identify place (Y92)

     ✓6ᵗʰ **T25.71** Corrosion of third degree of ankle

         ✓7ᵗʰ **T25.711** Corrosion of third degree of right ankle

         ✓7ᵗʰ **T25.712** Corrosion of third degree of left ankle

         ✓7ᵗʰ **T25.719** Corrosion of third degree of unspecified ankle

     ✓6ᵗʰ **T25.72** Corrosion of third degree of foot

         EXCLUDES 2   corrosion of third degree of toe(s) (nail) (T25.73-)

         ✓7ᵗʰ **T25.721** Corrosion of third degree of right foot

         ✓7ᵗʰ **T25.722** Corrosion of third degree of left foot

         ✓7ᵗʰ **T25.729** Corrosion of third degree of unspecified foot

     ✓6ᵗʰ **T25.73** Corrosion of third degree of toe(s) (nail)

         ✓7ᵗʰ **T25.731** Corrosion of third degree of right toe(s) (nail)

         ✓7ᵗʰ **T25.732** Corrosion of third degree of left toe(s) (nail)

         ✓7ᵗʰ **T25.739** Corrosion of third degree of unspecified toe(s) (nail)

     ✓6ᵗʰ **T25.79** Corrosion of third degree of multiple sites of ankle and foot

         ✓7ᵗʰ **T25.791** Corrosion of third degree of multiple sites of right ankle and foot

         ✓7ᵗʰ **T25.792** Corrosion of third degree of multiple sites of left ankle and foot

         ✓7ᵗʰ **T25.799** Corrosion of third degree of multiple sites of unspecified ankle and foot

Burns and corrosions confined to eye and internal organs (T26-T28)

✓4ᵗʰ **T26** **Burn and corrosion confined to eye and adnexa**

     The appropriate 7th character is to be added to each code from category T26.
     A   initial encounter
     D   subsequent encounter
     S   sequela

     ✓5ᵗʰ **T26.0** Burn of eyelid and periocular area

         Use additional external cause code to identify the source, place and intent of the burn (X00-X19, X75-X77, X96-X98, Y92)

         ✓7ᵗʰ **T26.00** Burn of unspecified eyelid and periocular area

         ✓7ᵗʰ **T26.01** Burn of right eyelid and periocular area

         ✓7ᵗʰ **T26.02** Burn of left eyelid and periocular area

     ✓5ᵗʰ **T26.1** Burn of cornea and conjunctival sac

         Use additional external cause code to identify the source, place and intent of the burn (X00-X19, X75-X77, X96-X98, Y92)

         ✓7ᵗʰ **T26.10** Burn of cornea and conjunctival sac, unspecified eye

         ✓7ᵗʰ **T26.11** Burn of cornea and conjunctival sac, right eye

         ✓7ᵗʰ **T26.12** Burn of cornea and conjunctival sac, left eye

     ✓5ᵗʰ **T26.2** Burn with resulting rupture and destruction of eyeball

         Use additional external cause code to identify the source, place and intent of the burn (X00-X19, X75-X77, X96-X98, Y92)

         ✓7ᵗʰ **T26.20** Burn with resulting rupture and destruction of unspecified eyeball

         ✓7ᵗʰ **T26.21** Burn with resulting rupture and destruction of right eyeball

         ✓7ᵗʰ **T26.22** Burn with resulting rupture and destruction of left eyeball

     ✓5ᵗʰ **T26.3** Burns of other specified parts of eye and adnexa

         Use additional external cause code to identify the source, place and intent of the burn (X00-X19, X75-X77, X96-X98, Y92)

         ✓7ᵗʰ **T26.30** Burns of other specified parts of unspecified eye and adnexa

         ✓7ᵗʰ **T26.31** Burns of other specified parts of right eye and adnexa

         ✓7ᵗʰ **T26.32** Burns of other specified parts of left eye and adnexa

     ✓5ᵗʰ **T26.4** Burn of eye and adnexa, part unspecified

         Use additional external cause code to identify the source, place and intent of the burn (X00-X19, X75-X77, X96-X98, Y92)

         ✓7ᵗʰ **T26.40** Burn of unspecified eye and adnexa, part unspecified

         ✓7ᵗʰ **T26.41** Burn of right eye and adnexa, part unspecified

         ✓7ᵗʰ **T26.42** Burn of left eye and adnexa, part unspecified

     ✓5ᵗʰ **T26.5** Corrosion of eyelid and periocular area

         Code first (T51-T65) to identify chemical and intent

         Use additional external cause code to identify place (Y92)

         ✓7ᵗʰ **T26.50** Corrosion of unspecified eyelid and periocular area

         ✓7ᵗʰ **T26.51** Corrosion of right eyelid and periocular area

         ✓7ᵗʰ **T26.52** Corrosion of left eyelid and periocular area

     ✓5ᵗʰ **T26.6** Corrosion of cornea and conjunctival sac

         Code first (T51-T65) to identify chemical and intent

         Use additional external cause code to identify place (Y92)

         ✓7ᵗʰ **T26.60** Corrosion of cornea and conjunctival sac, unspecified eye

         ✓7ᵗʰ **T26.61** Corrosion of cornea and conjunctival sac, right eye

         ✓7ᵗʰ **T26.62** Corrosion of cornea and conjunctival sac, left eye

     ✓5ᵗʰ **T26.7** Corrosion with resulting rupture and destruction of eyeball

         Code first (T51-T65) to identify chemical and intent

         Use additional external cause code to identify place (Y92)

         ✓7ᵗʰ **T26.70** Corrosion with resulting rupture and destruction of unspecified eyeball

         ✓7ᵗʰ **T26.71** Corrosion with resulting rupture and destruction of right eyeball

         ✓7ᵗʰ **T26.72** Corrosion with resulting rupture and destruction of left eyeball

     ✓5ᵗʰ **T26.8** Corrosions of other specified parts of eye and adnexa

         Code first (T51-T65) to identify chemical and intent

         Use additional external cause code to identify place (Y92)

         ✓7ᵗʰ **T26.80** Corrosions of other specified parts of unspecified eye and adnexa

         ✓7ᵗʰ **T26.81** Corrosions of other specified parts of right eye and adnexa

         ✓7ᵗʰ **T26.82** Corrosions of other specified parts of left eye and adnexa

     ✓5ᵗʰ **T26.9** Corrosion of eye and adnexa, part unspecified

         Code first (T51-T65) to identify chemical and intent

         Use additional external cause code to identify place (Y92)

         ✓7ᵗʰ **T26.90** Corrosion of unspecified eye and adnexa, part unspecified

         ✓7ᵗʰ **T26.91** Corrosion of right eye and adnexa, part unspecified

         ✓7ᵗʰ **T26.92** Corrosion of left eye and adnexa, part unspecified

✓4ᵗʰ **T27** **Burn and corrosion of respiratory tract**

     Use additional external cause code to identify the source and intent of the burn (X00-X19, X75-X77, X96-X98)

     Use additional external cause code to identify place (Y92)

     The appropriate 7th character is to be added to each code from category T27.
     A   initial encounter
     D   subsequent encounter
     S   sequela

     ✓7ᵗʰ **T27.0** Burn of larynx and trachea

     ✓7ᵗʰ **T27.1** Burn involving larynx and trachea with lung

     ✓7ᵗʰ **T27.2** Burn of other parts of respiratory tract

         Burn of thoracic cavity

     ✓7ᵗʰ **T27.3** Burn of respiratory tract, part unspecified

     ✓7ᵗʰ **T27.4** Corrosion of larynx and trachea

         Code first (T51-T65) to identify chemical and intent

     ✓7ᵗʰ **T27.5** Corrosion involving larynx and trachea with lung

         ▶Code first (T51-T65) to identify chemical and intent◀

     ✓7ᵗʰ **T27.6** Corrosion of other parts of respiratory tract

         Code first (T51-T65) to identify chemical and intent

     ✓7ᵗʰ **T27.7** Corrosion of respiratory tract, part unspecified

         Code first (T51-T65) to identify chemical and intent

√4ᵗʰ **T28 Burn and corrosion of other internal organs**
  Use additional external cause code to identify the source and intent of the burn (X00-X19, X75-X77, X96-X98)
  Use additional external cause code to identify place (Y92)

  The appropriate 7th character is to be added to each code from category T28.
  A   initial encounter
  D   subsequent encounter
  S   sequela

√x7ᵗʰ **T28.0** Burn of mouth and pharynx
√x7ᵗʰ **T28.1** Burn of esophagus
√x7ᵗʰ **T28.2** Burn of other parts of alimentary tract
√x7ᵗʰ **T28.3** Burn of internal genitourinary organs
√5ᵗʰ **T28.4** Burns of other and unspecified internal organs
    Code first (T51-T65) to identify chemical and intent
  √x7ᵗʰ **T28.40** Burn of unspecified internal organ
  √6ᵗʰ **T28.41** Burn of ear drum
      √7ᵗʰ **T28.411** Burn of right ear drum
      √7ᵗʰ **T28.412** Burn of left ear drum
      √7ᵗʰ **T28.419** Burn of unspecified ear drum
  √x7ᵗʰ **T28.49** Burn of other internal organ
√x7ᵗʰ **T28.5** Corrosion of mouth and pharynx
    Code first (T51-T65) to identify chemical and intent
√x7ᵗʰ **T28.6** Corrosion of esophagus
    Code first (T51-T65) to identify chemical and intent
√x7ᵗʰ **T28.7** Corrosion of other parts of alimentary tract
    Code first (T51-T65) to identify chemical and intent
√x7ᵗʰ **T28.8** Corrosion of internal genitourinary organs
    Code first (T51-T65) to identify chemical and intent
√5ᵗʰ **T28.9** Corrosions of other and unspecified internal organs
    Code first (T51-T65) to identify chemical and intent
  √x7ᵗʰ **T28.90** Corrosions of unspecified internal organs
  √8ᵗʰ **T28.91** Corrosions of ear drum
      √7ᵗʰ **T28.911** Corrosions of right ear drum
      √7ᵗʰ **T28.912** Corrosions of left ear drum
      √7ᵗʰ **T28.919** Corrosions of unspecified ear drum
  √x7ᵗʰ **T28.99** Corrosions of other internal organs

Burns and corrosions of multiple and unspecified body regions (T30-T32)

√4ᵗʰ **T30 Burn and corrosion, body region unspecified**
  T30.0 Burn of unspecified body region, unspecified degree
    This code is not for inpatient use. Code to specified site and degree of burns
    Burn NOS
    Multiple burns NOS
  T30.4 Corrosion of unspecified body region, unspecified degree
    This code is not for inpatient use. Code to specified site and degree of corrosion
    Corrosion NOS
    Multiple corrosion NOS

√4ᵗʰ **T31 Burns classified according to extent of body surface involved**
  NOTE This category is to be used as the primary code only when the site of the burn is unspecified. It should be used as a supplementary code with categories T20-T25 when the site is specified.

  T31.0 Burns involving less than 10% of body surface
√5ᵗʰ **T31.1** Burns involving 10-19% of body surface
  T31.10 Burns involving 10-19% of body surface with 0% to 9% third degree burns
    Burns involving 10-19% of body surface NOS
  T31.11 Burns involving 10-19% of body surface with 10-19% third degree burns HCC
√5ᵗʰ **T31.2** Burns involving 20-29% of body surface
  T31.20 Burns involving 20-29% of body surface with 0% to 9% third degree burns
    Burns involving 20-29% of body surface NOS
  T31.21 Burns involving 20-29% of body surface with 10-19% third degree burns HCC
  T31.22 Burns involving 20-29% of body surface with 20-29% third degree burns HCC

√5ᵗʰ **T31.3** Burns involving 30-39% of body surface
  T31.30 Burns involving 30-39% of body surface with 0% to 9% third degree burns
    Burns involving 30-39% of body surface NOS
  T31.31 Burns involving 30-39% of body surface with 10-19% third degree burns HCC
  T31.32 Burns involving 30-39% of body surface with 20-29% third degree burns HCC
  T31.33 Burns involving 30-39% of body surface with 30-39% third degree burns HCC
√5ᵗʰ **T31.4** Burns involving 40-49% of body surface
  T31.40 Burns involving 40-49% of body surface with 0% to 9% third degree burns
    Burns involving 40-49% of body surface NOS
  T31.41 Burns involving 40-49% of body surface with 10-19% third degree burns HCC
  T31.42 Burns involving 40-49% of body surface with 20-29% third degree burns HCC
  T31.43 Burns involving 40-49% of body surface with 30-39% third degree burns HCC
  T31.44 Burns involving 40-49% of body surface with 40-49% third degree burns HCC
√5ᵗʰ **T31.5** Burns involving 50-59% of body surface
  T31.50 Burns involving 50-59% of body surface with 0% to 9% third degree burns
    Burns involving 50-59% of body surface NOS
  T31.51 Burns involving 50-59% of body surface with 10-19% third degree burns HCC
  T31.52 Burns involving 50-59% of body surface with 20-29% third degree burns HCC
  T31.53 Burns involving 50-59% of body surface with 30-39% third degree burns HCC
  T31.54 Burns involving 50-59% of body surface with 40-49% third degree burns HCC
  T31.55 Burns involving 50-59% of body surface with 50-59% third degree burns HCC
√5ᵗʰ **T31.6** Burns involving 60-69% of body surface
  T31.60 Burns involving 60-69% of body surface with 0% to 9% third degree burns
    Burns involving 60-69% of body surface NOS
  T31.61 Burns involving 60-69% of body surface with 10-19% third degree burns HCC
  T31.62 Burns involving 60-69% of body surface with 20-29% third degree burns HCC
  T31.63 Burns involving 60-69% of body surface with 30-39% third degree burns HCC
  T31.64 Burns involving 60-69% of body surface with 40-49% third degree burns HCC
  T31.65 Burns involving 60-69% of body surface with 50-59% third degree burns HCC
  T31.66 Burns involving 60-69% of body surface with 60-69% third degree burns HCC
√5ᵗʰ **T31.7** Burns involving 70-79% of body surface
  T31.70 Burns involving 70-79% of body surface with 0% to 9% third degree burns
    Burns involving 70-79% of body surface NOS
  T31.71 Burns involving 70-79% of body surface with 10-19% third degree burns HCC
  T31.72 Burns involving 70-79% of body surface with 20-29% third degree burns HCC
  T31.73 Burns involving 70-79% of body surface with 30-39% third degree burns HCC
  T31.74 Burns involving 70-79% of body surface with 40-49% third degree burns HCC
  T31.75 Burns involving 70-79% of body surface with 50-59% third degree burns HCC
  T31.76 Burns involving 70-79% of body surface with 60-69% third degree burns HCC
  T31.77 Burns involving 70-79% of body surface with 70-79% third degree burns HCC
√5ᵗʰ **T31.8** Burns involving 80-89% of body surface
  T31.80 Burns involving 80-89% of body surface with 0% to 9% third degree burns
    Burns involving 80-89% of body surface NOS
  T31.81 Burns involving 80-89% of body surface with 10-19% third degree burns HCC
  T31.82 Burns involving 80-89% of body surface with 20-29% third degree burns HCC
  T31.83 Burns involving 80-89% of body surface with 30-39% third degree burns HCC

T31.84   Burns involving 80-89% of body surface with 40-49% third degree **burns**   `HCC`

T31.85   Burns involving 80-89% of body surface with 50-59% third degree **burns**   `HCC`

T31.86   Burns involving 80-89% of body surface with 60-69% third degree **burns**   `HCC`

T31.87   Burns involving 80-89% of body surface with 70-79% third degree **burns**   `HCC`

T31.88   Burns involving 80-89% of body surface with 80-89% third degree **burns**   `HCC`

√5ᵗʰ **T31.9**   Burns involving 90% or more of body surface

T31.90   Burns involving 90% or more of body surface with 0% to 9% third degree **burns**
Burns involving 90% or more of body surface NOS

T31.91   Burns involving 90% or more of body surface with 10-19% third degree **burns**   `HCC`

T31.92   Burns involving 90% or more of body surface with 20-29% third degree **burns**   `HCC`

T31.93   Burns involving 90% or more of body surface with 30-39% third degree **burns**   `HCC`

T31.94   Burns involving 90% or more of body surface with 40-49% third degree **burns**   `HCC`

T31.95   Burns involving 90% or more of body surface with 50-59% third degree **burns**   `HCC`

T31.96   Burns involving 90% or more of body surface with 60-69% third degree **burns**   `HCC`

T31.97   Burns involving 90% or more of body surface with 70-79% third degree **burns**   `HCC`

T31.98   Burns involving 90% or more of body surface with 80-89% third degree **burns**   `HCC`

T31.99   Burns involving 90% or more of body surface with 90% or more third degree **burns**   `HCC`

Rule of Nines Estimation of Total Body Surface Burned

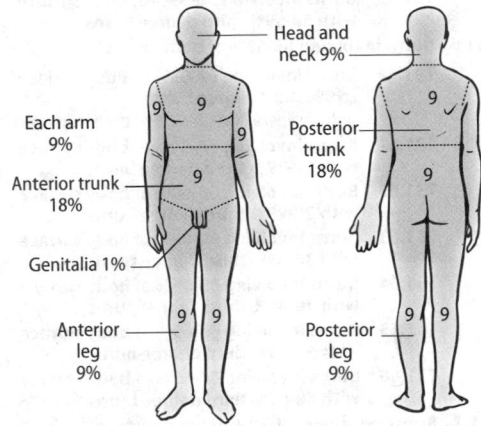

Head and neck 9%

Each arm 9%

Anterior trunk 18%

Genitalia 1%

Anterior leg 9%

Posterior trunk 18%

Posterior leg 9%

√4ᵗʰ **T32**   Corrosions **classified** according to extent of body surface involved

> **NOTE**   This category is to be used as the primary code only when the site of the corrosion is unspecified. It may be used as a supplementary code with categories T20-T25 when the site is specified.

T32.0   Corrosions involving less than 10% of body surface

√5ᵗʰ **T32.1**   Corrosions involving 10-19% of body surface

T32.10   Corrosions involving 10-19% of body surface with 0% to 9% third degree **corrosion**
Corrosions involving 10-19% of body surface NOS

T32.11   Corrosions involving 10-19% of body surface with 10-19% third degree **corrosion**   `HCC`

√5ᵗʰ **T32.2**   Corrosions involving 20-29% of body surface

T32.20   Corrosions involving 20-29% of body surface with 0% to 9% third degree **corrosion**

T32.21   Corrosions involving 20-29% of body surface with 10-19% third degree **corrosion**   `HCC`

T32.22   Corrosions involving 20-29% of body surface with 20-29% third degree **corrosion**   `HCC`

√5ᵗʰ **T32.3**   Corrosions involving 30-39% of body surface

T32.30   Corrosions involving 30-39% of body surface with 0% to 9% third degree **corrosion**

T32.31   Corrosions involving 30-39% of body surface with 10-19% third degree **corrosion**   `HCC`

T32.32   Corrosions involving 30-39% of body surface with 20-29% third degree **corrosion**   `HCC`

T32.33   Corrosions involving 30-39% of body surface with 30-39% third degree **corrosion**   `HCC`

√5ᵗʰ **T32.4**   Corrosions involving 40-49% of body surface

T32.40   Corrosions involving 40-49% of body surface with 0% to 9% third degree **corrosion**

T32.41   Corrosions involving 40-49% of body surface with 10-19% third degree **corrosion**   `HCC`

T32.42   Corrosions involving 40-49% of body surface with 20-29% third degree **corrosion**   `HCC`

T32.43   Corrosions involving 40-49% of body surface with 30-39% third degree **corrosion**   `HCC`

T32.44   Corrosions involving 40-49% of body surface with 40-49% third degree **corrosion**   `HCC`

√5ᵗʰ **T32.5**   Corrosions involving 50-59% of body surface

T32.50   Corrosions involving 50-59% of body surface with 0% to 9% third degree **corrosion**

T32.51   Corrosions involving 50-59% of body surface with 10-19% third degree **corrosion**   `HCC`

T32.52   Corrosions involving 50-59% of body surface with 20-29% third degree **corrosion**   `HCC`

T32.53   Corrosions involving 50-59% of body surface with 30-39% third degree **corrosion**   `HCC`

T32.54   Corrosions involving 50-59% of body surface with 40-49% third degree **corrosion**   `HCC`

T32.55   Corrosions involving 50-59% of body surface with 50-59% third degree **corrosion**   `HCC`

√5ᵗʰ **T32.6**   Corrosions involving 60-69% of body surface

T32.60   Corrosions involving 60-69% of body surface with 0% to 9% third degree **corrosion**

T32.61   Corrosions involving 60-69% of body surface with 10-19% third degree **corrosion**   `HCC`

T32.62   Corrosions involving 60-69% of body surface with 20-29% third degree **corrosion**   `HCC`

T32.63   Corrosions involving 60-69% of body surface with 30-39% third degree **corrosion**   `HCC`

T32.64   Corrosions involving 60-69% of body surface with 40-49% third degree **corrosion**   `HCC`

T32.65   Corrosions involving 60-69% of body surface with 50-59% third degree **corrosion**   `HCC`

T32.66   Corrosions involving 60-69% of body surface with 60-69% third degree **corrosion**   `HCC`

√5ᵗʰ **T32.7**   Corrosions involving 70-79% of body surface

T32.70   Corrosions involving 70-79% of body surface with 0% to 9% third degree **corrosion**

T32.71   Corrosions involving 70-79% of body surface with 10-19% third degree **corrosion**   `HCC`

T32.72   Corrosions involving 70-79% of body surface with 20-29% third degree **corrosion**   `HCC`

T32.73   Corrosions involving 70-79% of body surface with 30-39% third degree **corrosion**   `HCC`

T32.74   Corrosions involving 70-79% of body surface with 40-49% third degree **corrosion**   `HCC`

T32.75   Corrosions involving 70-79% of body surface with 50-59% third degree **corrosion**   `HCC`

T32.76   Corrosions involving 70-79% of body surface with 60-69% third degree **corrosion**   `HCC`

T32.77   Corrosions involving 70-79% of body surface with 70-79% third degree **corrosion**   `HCC`

√5ᵗʰ **T32.8**   Corrosions involving 80-89% of body surface

T32.80   Corrosions involving 80-89% of body surface with 0% to 9% third degree **corrosion**

T32.81   Corrosions involving 80-89% of body surface with 10-19% third degree **corrosion**   `HCC`

T32.82   Corrosions involving 80-89% of body surface with 20-29% third degree **corrosion**   `HCC`

T32.83   Corrosions involving 80-89% of body surface with 30-39% third degree **corrosion**   `HCC`

T32.84   Corrosions involving 80-89% of body surface with 40-49% third degree **corrosion**   `HCC`

T32.85   Corrosions involving 80-89% of body surface with 50-59% third degree **corrosion**   `HCC`

T32.86   Corrosions involving 80-89% of body surface with 60-69% third degree **corrosion**   `HCC`

T32.87   Corrosions involving 80-89% of body surface with 70-79% third degree **corrosion**   `HCC`

T32.88   Corrosions involving 80-89% of body surface with 80-89% third degree **corrosion**   `HCC`

√5th **T32.9** Corrosions involving 90% or more of body surface

T32.90 Corrosions involving 90% or more of body surface with 0% to 9% third degree corrosion

T32.91 Corrosions involving 90% or more of body surface with 10-19% third degree corrosion HCC

T32.92 Corrosions involving 90% or more of body surface with 20-29% third degree corrosion HCC

T32.93 Corrosions involving 90% or more of body surface with 30-39% third degree corrosion HCC

T32.94 Corrosions involving 90% or more of body surface with 40-49% third degree corrosion HCC

T32.95 Corrosions involving 90% or more of body surface with 50-59% third degree corrosion HCC

T32.96 Corrosions involving 90% or more of body surface with 60-69% third degree corrosion HCC

T32.97 Corrosions involving 90% or more of body surface with 70-79% third degree corrosion HCC

T32.98 Corrosions involving 90% or more of body surface with 80-89% third degree corrosion HCC

T32.99 Corrosions involving 90% or more of body surface with 90% or more third degree corrosion HCC

Frostbite (T33-T34)

EXCLUDES 2   hypothermia and other effects of reduced temperature (T68, T69.-)

√4th **T33** **Superficial frostbite**

INCLUDES   frostbite with partial thickness skin loss

The appropriate 7th character is to be added to each code from category T33.
A   initial encounter
D   subsequent encounter
S   sequela

√5th **T33.0** Superficial frostbite of head

√6th **T33.01** Superficial frostbite of ear

√7th **T33.011** Superficial frostbite of right ear

√7th **T33.012** Superficial frostbite of left ear

√7th **T33.019** Superficial frostbite of unspecified ear

√x7th **T33.02** Superficial frostbite of nose

√x7th **T33.09** Superficial frostbite of other part of head

√x7th **T33.1** Superficial frostbite of neck

√x7th **T33.2** Superficial frostbite of thorax

√x7th **T33.3** Superficial frostbite of abdominal wall, lower back and pelvis

√5th **T33.4** Superficial frostbite of arm

EXCLUDES 2   superficial frostbite of wrist and hand (T33.5-)

√x7th **T33.40** Superficial frostbite of unspecified arm

√x7th **T33.41** Superficial frostbite of right arm

√x7th **T33.42** Superficial frostbite of left arm

√5th **T33.5** Superficial frostbite of wrist, hand, and fingers

√6th **T33.51** Superficial frostbite of wrist

√7th **T33.511** Superficial frostbite of right wrist

√7th **T33.512** Superficial frostbite of left wrist

√7th **T33.519** Superficial frostbite of unspecified wrist

√6th **T33.52** Superficial frostbite of hand

EXCLUDES 2   superficial frostbite of fingers (T33.53-)

√7th **T33.521** Superficial frostbite of right hand

√7th **T33.522** Superficial frostbite of left hand

√7th **T33.529** Superficial frostbite of unspecified hand

√6th **T33.53** Superficial frostbite of finger(s)

√7th **T33.531** Superficial frostbite of right finger(s)

√7th **T33.532** Superficial frostbite of left finger(s)

√7th **T33.539** Superficial frostbite of unspecified finger(s)

√5th **T33.6** Superficial frostbite of hip and thigh

√x7th **T33.60** Superficial frostbite of unspecified hip and thigh

√x7th **T33.61** Superficial frostbite of right hip and thigh

√x7th **T33.62** Superficial frostbite of left hip and thigh

√5th **T33.7** Superficial frostbite of knee and lower leg

EXCLUDES 2   superficial frostbite of ankle and foot (T33.8-)

√x7th **T33.70** Superficial frostbite of unspecified knee and lower leg

√x7th **T33.71** Superficial frostbite of right knee and lower leg

√x7th **T33.72** Superficial frostbite of left knee and lower leg

√5th **T33.8** Superficial frostbite of ankle, foot, and toe(s)

√6th **T33.81** Superficial frostbite of ankle

√7th **T33.811** Superficial frostbite of right ankle

√7th **T33.812** Superficial frostbite of left ankle

√7th **T33.819** Superficial frostbite of unspecified ankle

√6th **T33.82** Superficial frostbite of foot

√7th **T33.821** Superficial frostbite of right foot

√7th **T33.822** Superficial frostbite of left foot

√7th **T33.829** Superficial frostbite of unspecified foot

√6th **T33.83** Superficial frostbite of toe(s)

√7th **T33.831** Superficial frostbite of right toe(s)

√7th **T33.832** Superficial frostbite of left toe(s)

√7th **T33.839** Superficial frostbite of unspecified toe(s)

√5th **T33.9** Superficial frostbite of other and unspecified sites

√x7th **T33.90** Superficial frostbite of unspecified sites
Superficial frostbite NOS

√x7th **T33.99** Superficial frostbite of other sites
Superficial frostbite of leg NOS
Superficial frostbite of trunk NOS

√4th **T34** **Frostbite with tissue necrosis**

The appropriate 7th character is to be added to each code from category T34.
A   initial encounter
D   subsequent encounter
S   sequela

√5th **T34.0** Frostbite with tissue necrosis of head

√6th **T34.01** Frostbite with tissue necrosis of ear

√7th **T34.011** Frostbite with tissue necrosis of right ear

√7th **T34.012** Frostbite with tissue necrosis of left ear

√7th **T34.019** Frostbite with tissue necrosis of unspecified ear

√x7th **T34.02** Frostbite with tissue necrosis of nose

√x7th **T34.09** Frostbite with tissue necrosis of other part of head

√x7th **T34.1** Frostbite with tissue necrosis of neck

√x7th **T34.2** Frostbite with tissue necrosis of thorax

√x7th **T34.3** Frostbite with tissue necrosis of abdominal wall, lower back and pelvis

√5th **T34.4** Frostbite with tissue necrosis of arm

EXCLUDES 2   frostbite with tissue necrosis of wrist and hand (T34.5-)

√x7th **T34.40** Frostbite with tissue necrosis of unspecified arm

√x7th **T34.41** Frostbite with tissue necrosis of right arm

√x7th **T34.42** Frostbite with tissue necrosis of left arm

√5th **T34.5** Frostbite with tissue necrosis of wrist, hand, and finger(s)

√6th **T34.51** Frostbite with tissue necrosis of wrist

√7th **T34.511** Frostbite with tissue necrosis of right wrist

√7th **T34.512** Frostbite with tissue necrosis of left wrist

√7th **T34.519** Frostbite with tissue necrosis of unspecified wrist

√6th **T34.52** Frostbite with tissue necrosis of hand

EXCLUDES 2   frostbite with tissue necrosis of finger(s) (T34.53-)

√7th **T34.521** Frostbite with tissue necrosis of right hand

√7th **T34.522** Frostbite with tissue necrosis of left hand

√7th **T34.529** Frostbite with tissue necrosis of unspecified hand

√6th **T34.53** Frostbite with tissue necrosis of finger(s)

√7th **T34.531** Frostbite with tissue necrosis of right finger(s)

√7th **T34.532** Frostbite with tissue necrosis of left finger(s)

√7th **T34.539** Frostbite with tissue necrosis of unspecified finger(s)

√5th **T34.6** Frostbite with tissue necrosis of hip and thigh

√x7th **T34.60** Frostbite with tissue necrosis of unspecified hip and thigh

√x7th **T34.61** Frostbite with tissue necrosis of right hip and thigh

---

√ Additional Character Required   √x7th Placeholder Alert   Manifestation   Unspecified Dx   ►◄ Revised Text   ● New Code   ▲ Revised Code Title

√x 7ᵗʰ **T34.62** **Frostbite with tissue necrosis of** left **hip and thigh**

√5ᵗʰ **T34.7** **Frostbite with tissue necrosis of** knee and lower leg

     EXCLUDES 2   *frostbite with tissue necrosis of ankle and foot (T34.8-)*

     √x 7ᵗʰ **T34.70** **Frostbite with tissue necrosis of unspecified knee and lower leg**

     √x 7ᵗʰ **T34.71** **Frostbite with tissue necrosis of** right **knee and lower leg**

     √x 7ᵗʰ **T34.72** **Frostbite with tissue necrosis of** left **knee and lower leg**

√5ᵗʰ **T34.8** **Frostbite with tissue necrosis of** ankle, foot, and toe(s)

     √6ᵗʰ **T34.81** **Frostbite with tissue necrosis of** ankle

         √7ᵗʰ **T34.811** **Frostbite with tissue necrosis of** right **ankle**

         √7ᵗʰ **T34.812** **Frostbite with tissue necrosis of** left **ankle**

         √7ᵗʰ **T34.819** **Frostbite with tissue necrosis of unspecified ankle**

     √6ᵗʰ **T34.82** **Frostbite with tissue necrosis of** foot

         √7ᵗʰ **T34.821** **Frostbite with tissue necrosis of** right **foot**

         √7ᵗʰ **T34.822** **Frostbite with tissue necrosis of** left **foot**

         √7ᵗʰ **T34.829** **Frostbite with tissue necrosis of unspecified foot**

     √6ᵗʰ **T34.83** **Frostbite with tissue necrosis of** toe(s)

         √7ᵗʰ **T34.831** **Frostbite with tissue necrosis of** right **toe(s)**

         √7ᵗʰ **T34.832** **Frostbite with tissue necrosis of** left **toe(s)**

         √7ᵗʰ **T34.839** **Frostbite with tissue necrosis of unspecified toe(s)**

√5ᵗʰ **T34.9** **Frostbite with tissue necrosis of other and unspecified sites**

     √x 7ᵗʰ **T34.90** **Frostbite with tissue necrosis of unspecified sites**

         Frostbite with tissue necrosis NOS

     √x 7ᵗʰ **T34.99** **Frostbite with tissue necrosis of other sites**

         Frostbite with tissue necrosis of leg NOS

         Frostbite with tissue necrosis of trunk NOS

Poisoning by, adverse effects of and underdosing of drugs, medicaments and biological substances (T36-T50)

INCLUDES   adverse effect of correct substance properly administered

     poisoning by overdose of substance

     poisoning by wrong substance given or taken in error

     underdosing by (inadvertently) (deliberately) taking less substance than prescribed or instructed

Code first, for adverse effects, the nature of the adverse effect, such as:

     adverse effect NOS (T88.7)

     aspirin gastritis (K29.-)

     blood disorders (D56-D76)

     contact dermatitis (L23-L25)

     dermatitis due to substances taken internally (L27.-)

     nephropathy (N14.0-N14.2)

NOTE   The drug giving rise to the adverse effect should be identified by use of codes from categories T36-T50 with fifth or sixth character 5.

Use additional code(s) to specify:

     manifestations of poisoning

     underdosing or failure in dosage during medical and surgical care (Y63.6, Y63.8-Y63.9)

     underdosing of medication regimen (Z91.12-, Z91.13-)

EXCLUDES 1   *toxic reaction to local anesthesia in pregnancy (O29.3-)*

EXCLUDES 2   *abuse and dependence of psychoactive substances (F10-F19)*

     abuse of non-dependence-producing substances (F55.-)

     drug reaction and poisoning affecting newborn (P00-P96)

     pathological drug intoxication (inebriation) (F10-F19)

AHA: 2018,4Q,71; 2016,2Q,8; 2015,3Q,22

√4ᵗʰ **T36** **Poisoning by, adverse effect of and underdosing of systemic antibiotics**

     EXCLUDES 1   *antineoplastic antibiotics (T45.1-)*

         locally applied antibiotic NEC (T49.0)

         topically used antibiotic for ear, nose and throat (T49.6)

         topically used antibiotic for eye (T49.5)

> The appropriate 7th character is to be added to each code from category T36.
> A   initial encounter
> D   subsequent encounter
> S   sequela

√5ᵗʰ **T36.0** **Poisoning by, adverse effect of and underdosing of penicillins**

     √6ᵗʰ **T36.0X** **Poisoning by, adverse effect of and underdosing of** penicillins

         √7ᵗʰ **T36.0X1** **Poisoning by penicillins,** accidental **(unintentional)**

             Poisoning by penicillins NOS

         ² √7ᵗʰ **T36.0X2** **Poisoning by penicillins,** HCC **intentional self-harm**

         √7ᵗʰ **T36.0X3** **Poisoning by penicillins,** assault

         √7ᵗʰ **T36.0X4** **Poisoning by penicillins,** undetermined

         √7ᵗʰ **T36.0X5** **Adverse effect** of penicillins

         √7ᵗʰ **T36.0X6** **Underdosing** of penicillins

√5ᵗʰ **T36.1** **Poisoning by, adverse effect of and underdosing of cephalosporins and other beta-lactam antibiotics**

     √6ᵗʰ **T36.1X** **Poisoning by, adverse effect of and underdosing of** cephalosporins and other beta-lactam antibiotics

         √7ᵗʰ **T36.1X1** **Poisoning by cephalosporins and other beta-lactam antibiotics,** accidental **(unintentional)**

             Poisoning by cephalosporins and other beta-lactam antibiotics NOS

         ² √7ᵗʰ **T36.1X2** **Poisoning by cephalosporins and** HCC **other beta-lactam antibiotics,** intentional self-harm

         √7ᵗʰ **T36.1X3** **Poisoning by cephalosporins and other beta-lactam antibiotics,** assault

         √7ᵗʰ **T36.1X4** **Poisoning by cephalosporins and other beta-lactam antibiotics,** undetermined

         √7ᵗʰ **T36.1X5** **Adverse effect** of cephalosporins and other beta-lactam antibiotics

         √7ᵗʰ **T36.1X6** **Underdosing** of cephalosporins and other beta-lactam antibiotics

√5ᵗʰ **T36.2** **Poisoning by, adverse effect of and underdosing of chloramphenicol group**

     √6ᵗʰ **T36.2X** **Poisoning by, adverse effect of and underdosing of** chloramphenicol group

         √7ᵗʰ **T36.2X1** **Poisoning by chloramphenicol group,** accidental **(unintentional)**

             Poisoning by chloramphenicol group NOS

         ² √7ᵗʰ **T36.2X2** **Poisoning by chloramphenicol** HCC **group, intentional self-harm**

✓7th T36.2X3 Poisoning by chloramphenicol group, assault

✓7th T36.2X4 Poisoning by chloramphenicol group, undetermined

✓7th T36.2X5 Adverse effect of chloramphenicol group

✓7th T36.2X6 Underdosing of chloramphenicol group

✓5th T36.3 Poisoning by, adverse effect of and underdosing of macrolides

  ✓6th T36.3X Poisoning by, adverse effect of and underdosing of macrolides

    ✓7th T36.3X1 Poisoning by macrolides, accidental (unintentional)
      Poisoning by macrolides NOS

    2 ✓7th T36.3X2 Poisoning by macrolides, intentional self-harm   HCC

    ✓7th T36.3X3 Poisoning by macrolides, assault

    ✓7th T36.3X4 Poisoning by macrolides, undetermined

    ✓7th T36.3X5 Adverse effect of macrolides

    ✓7th T36.3X6 Underdosing of macrolides

✓5th T36.4 Poisoning by, adverse effect of and underdosing of tetracyclines

  ✓6th T36.4X Poisoning by, adverse effect of and underdosing of tetracyclines

    ✓7th T36.4X1 Poisoning by tetracyclines, accidental (unintentional)
      Poisoning by tetracyclines NOS

    2 ✓7th T36.4X2 Poisoning by tetracyclines, intentional self-harm   HCC

    ✓7th T36.4X3 Poisoning by tetracyclines, assault

    ✓7th T36.4X4 Poisoning by tetracyclines, undetermined

    ✓7th T36.4X5 Adverse effect of tetracyclines

    ✓7th T36.4X6 Underdosing of tetracyclines

✓5th T36.5 Poisoning by, adverse effect of and underdosing of aminoglycosides
  Poisoning by, adverse effect of and underdosing of streptomycin

  ✓6th T36.5X Poisoning by, adverse effect of and underdosing of aminoglycosides

    ✓7th T36.5X1 Poisoning by aminoglycosides, accidental (unintentional)
      Poisoning by aminoglycosides NOS

    2 ✓7th T36.5X2 Poisoning by aminoglycosides, intentional self-harm   HCC

    ✓7th T36.5X3 Poisoning by aminoglycosides, assault

    ✓7th T36.5X4 Poisoning by aminoglycosides, undetermined

    ✓7th T36.5X5 Adverse effect of aminoglycosides

    ✓7th T36.5X6 Underdosing of aminoglycosides

✓5th T36.6 Poisoning by, adverse effect of and underdosing of rifampicins

  ✓6th T36.6X Poisoning by, adverse effect of and underdosing of rifampicins

    ✓7th T36.6X1 Poisoning by rifampicins, accidental (unintentional)
      Poisoning by rifampicins NOS

    2 ✓7th T36.6X2 Poisoning by rifampicins, intentional self-harm   HCC

    ✓7th T36.6X3 Poisoning by rifampicins, assault

    ✓7th T36.6X4 Poisoning by rifampicins, undetermined

    ✓7th T36.6X5 Adverse effect of rifampicins

    ✓7th T36.6X6 Underdosing of rifampicins

✓5th T36.7 Poisoning by, adverse effect of and underdosing of antifungal antibiotics, systemically used

  ✓6th T36.7X Poisoning by, adverse effect of and underdosing of antifungal antibiotics, systemically used

    ✓7th T36.7X1 Poisoning by antifungal antibiotics, systemically used, accidental (unintentional)
      Poisoning by antifungal antibiotics, systemically used NOS

    2 ✓7th T36.7X2 Poisoning by antifungal antibiotics, systemically used, intentional self-harm   HCC

    ✓7th T36.7X3 Poisoning by antifungal antibiotics, systemically used, assault

    ✓7th T36.7X4 Poisoning by antifungal antibiotics, systemically used, undetermined

    ✓7th T36.7X5 Adverse effect of antifungal antibiotics, systemically used

    ✓7th T36.7X6 Underdosing of antifungal antibiotics, systemically used

✓5th T36.8 Poisoning by, adverse effect of and underdosing of other systemic antibiotics

  ✓6th T36.8X Poisoning by, adverse effect of and underdosing of other systemic antibiotics
    AHA: 2017,1Q,39

    ✓7th T36.8X1 Poisoning by other systemic antibiotics, accidental (unintentional)
      Poisoning by other systemic antibiotics NOS

    2 ✓7th T36.8X2 Poisoning by other systemic antibiotics, intentional self-harm   HCC

    ✓7th T36.8X3 Poisoning by other systemic antibiotics, assault

    ✓7th T36.8X4 Poisoning by other systemic antibiotics, undetermined

    ✓7th T36.8X5 Adverse effect of other systemic antibiotics

    ✓7th T36.8X6 Underdosing of other systemic antibiotics

✓5th T36.9 Poisoning by, adverse effect of and underdosing of unspecified systemic antibiotic

  ✓x7th T36.91 Poisoning by unspecified systemic antibiotic, accidental (unintentional)
    Poisoning by systemic antibiotic NOS

  2 ✓x7th T36.92 Poisoning by unspecified systemic antibiotic, intentional self-harm   HCC

  ✓x7th T36.93 Poisoning by unspecified systemic antibiotic, assault

  ✓x7th T36.94 Poisoning by unspecified systemic antibiotic, undetermined

  ✓x7th T36.95 Adverse effect of unspecified systemic antibiotic

  ✓x7th T36.96 Underdosing of unspecified systemic antibiotic

✓4th T37 Poisoning by, adverse effect of and underdosing of other systemic anti-infectives and antiparasitics

  EXCLUDES 1   *anti-infectives topically used for ear, nose and throat (T49.6-)*
    anti-infectives topically used for eye (T49.5-)
    locally applied anti-infectives NEC (T49.0-)

> The appropriate 7th character is to be added to each code from category T37.
> A   initial encounter
> D   subsequent encounter
> S   sequela

✓5th T37.0 Poisoning by, adverse effect of and underdosing of sulfonamides

  ✓6th T37.0X Poisoning by, adverse effect of and underdosing of sulfonamides

    ✓7th T37.0X1 Poisoning by sulfonamides, accidental (unintentional)
      Poisoning by sulfonamides NOS

    2 ✓7th T37.0X2 Poisoning by sulfonamides, intentional self-harm   HCC

    ✓7th T37.0X3 Poisoning by sulfonamides, assault

    ✓7th T37.0X4 Poisoning by sulfonamides, undetermined

    ✓7th T37.0X5 Adverse effect of sulfonamides

    ✓7th T37.0X6 Underdosing of sulfonamides

✓5th T37.1 Poisoning by, adverse effect of and underdosing of antimycobacterial drugs

  EXCLUDES 1   *rifampicins (T36.6-)*
    streptomycin (T36.5-)

  ✓6th T37.1X Poisoning by, adverse effect of and underdosing of antimycobacterial drugs

    ✓7th T37.1X1 Poisoning by antimycobacterial drugs, accidental (unintentional)
      Poisoning by antimycobacterial drugs NOS

    2 ✓7th T37.1X2 Poisoning by antimycobacterial drugs, intentional self-harm   HCC

    ✓7th T37.1X3 Poisoning by antimycobacterial drugs, assault

    ✓7th T37.1X4 Poisoning by antimycobacterial drugs, undetermined

    ✓7th T37.1X5 Adverse effect of antimycobacterial drugs

    ✓7th T37.1X6 Underdosing of antimycobacterial drugs

☑ Additional Character Required   ✓x7th Placeholder Alert   Manifestation   Unspecified Dx   ►◄ Revised Text   ● New Code   ▲ Revised Code Title

D-10-CM 2020

1097

☑5ᵗʰ **T37.2 Poisoning by, adverse effect of and underdosing of antimalarials and drugs acting on other blood protozoa**
EXCLUDES 1 *hydroxyquinoline derivatives (T37.8-)*

☑6ᵗʰ **T37.2X Poisoning by, adverse effect of and underdosing of antimalarials and drugs acting on other blood protozoa**

☑7ᵗʰ **T37.2X1 Poisoning by antimalarials and drugs acting on other blood protozoa, accidental (unintentional)**
Poisoning by antimalarials and drugs acting on other blood protozoa NOS

² ☑7ᵗʰ **T37.2X2 Poisoning by antimalarials and drugs acting on other blood protozoa, intentional self-harm** HCC

☑7ᵗʰ **T37.2X3 Poisoning by antimalarials and drugs acting on other blood protozoa, assault**

☑7ᵗʰ **T37.2X4 Poisoning by antimalarials and drugs acting on other blood protozoa, undetermined**

☑7ᵗʰ **T37.2X5 Adverse effect of antimalarials and drugs acting on other blood protozoa**

☑7ᵗʰ **T37.2X6 Underdosing of antimalarials and drugs acting on other blood protozoa**

☑5ᵗʰ **T37.3 Poisoning by, adverse effect of and underdosing of other antiprotozoal drugs**

☑6ᵗʰ **T37.3X Poisoning by, adverse effect of and underdosing of other antiprotozoal drugs**

☑7ᵗʰ **T37.3X1 Poisoning by other antiprotozoal drugs, accidental (unintentional)**
Poisoning by other antiprotozoal drugs NOS

² ☑7ᵗʰ **T37.3X2 Poisoning by other antiprotozoal drugs, intentional self-harm** HCC

☑7ᵗʰ **T37.3X3 Poisoning by other antiprotozoal drugs, assault**

☑7ᵗʰ **T37.3X4 Poisoning by other antiprotozoal drugs, undetermined**

☑7ᵗʰ **T37.3X5 Adverse effect of other antiprotozoal drugs**

☑7ᵗʰ **T37.3X6 Underdosing of other antiprotozoal drugs**

☑5ᵗʰ **T37.4 Poisoning by, adverse effect of and underdosing of anthelminthics**

☑6ᵗʰ **T37.4X Poisoning by, adverse effect of and underdosing of anthelminthics**

☑7ᵗʰ **T37.4X1 Poisoning by anthelminthics, accidental (unintentional)**
Poisoning by anthelminthics NOS

² ☑7ᵗʰ **T37.4X2 Poisoning by anthelminthics, intentional self-harm** HCC

☑7ᵗʰ **T37.4X3 Poisoning by anthelminthics, assault**

☑7ᵗʰ **T37.4X4 Poisoning by anthelminthics, undetermined**

☑7ᵗʰ **T37.4X5 Adverse effect of anthelminthics**

☑7ᵗʰ **T37.4X6 Underdosing of anthelminthics**

☑5ᵗʰ **T37.5 Poisoning by, adverse effect of and underdosing of antiviral drugs**
EXCLUDES 1 *amantadine (T42.8-)*
cytarabine (T45.1-)

☑6ᵗʰ **T37.5X Poisoning by, adverse effect of and underdosing of antiviral drugs**

☑7ᵗʰ **T37.5X1 Poisoning by antiviral drugs, accidental (unintentional)**
Poisoning by antiviral drugs NOS

² ☑7ᵗʰ **T37.5X2 Poisoning by antiviral drugs, intentional self-harm** HCC

☑7ᵗʰ **T37.5X3 Poisoning by antiviral drugs, assault**

☑7ᵗʰ **T37.5X4 Poisoning by antiviral drugs, undetermined**

☑7ᵗʰ **T37.5X5 Adverse effect of antiviral drugs**

☑7ᵗʰ **T37.5X6 Underdosing of antiviral drugs**

☑5ᵗʰ **T37.8 Poisoning by, adverse effect of and underdosing of other specified systemic anti-infectives and antiparasitics**
Poisoning by, adverse effect of and underdosing of hydroxyquinoline derivatives
EXCLUDES 1 *antimalarial drugs (T37.2-)*

☑6ᵗʰ **T37.8X Poisoning by, adverse effect of and underdosing of other specified systemic anti-infectives and antiparasitics**

☑7ᵗʰ **T37.8X1 Poisoning by other specified systemic anti-infectives and antiparasitics, accidental (unintentional)**
Poisoning by other specified systemic anti-infectives and antiparasitics NOS

² ☑7ᵗʰ **T37.8X2 Poisoning by other specified systemic anti-infectives and antiparasitics, intentional self-harm** HCC

☑7ᵗʰ **T37.8X3 Poisoning by other specified systemic anti-infectives and antiparasitics, assault**

☑7ᵗʰ **T37.8X4 Poisoning by other specified systemic anti-infectives and antiparasitics, undetermined**

☑7ᵗʰ **T37.8X5 Adverse effect of other specified systemic anti-infectives and antiparasitics**

☑7ᵗʰ **T37.8X6 Underdosing of other specified systemic anti-infectives and antiparasitics**

☑5ᵗʰ **T37.9 Poisoning by, adverse effect of and underdosing of unspecified systemic anti-infective and antiparasitics**

☑×7ᵗʰ **T37.91 Poisoning by unspecified systemic anti-infective and antiparasitics, accidental (unintentional)**
Poisoning by, adverse effect of and underdosing of systemic anti-infective and antiparasitics NOS

² ☑×7ᵗʰ **T37.92 Poisoning by unspecified systemic anti-infective and antiparasitics, intentional self-harm** HCC

☑×7ᵗʰ **T37.93 Poisoning by unspecified systemic anti-infective and antiparasitics, assault**

☑×7ᵗʰ **T37.94 Poisoning by unspecified systemic anti-infective and antiparasitics, undetermined**

☑×7ᵗʰ **T37.95 Adverse effect of unspecified systemic anti-infective and antiparasitic**

☑×7ᵗʰ **T37.96 Underdosing of unspecified systemic anti-infectives and antiparasitics**

☑4ᵗʰ **T38 Poisoning by, adverse effect of and underdosing of hormones and their synthetic substitutes and antagonists, not elsewhere classified**
EXCLUDES 1 *mineralocorticoids and their antagonists (T5Ø.Ø-)*
oxytocic hormones (T48.Ø-)
parathyroid hormones and derivatives (T5Ø.9-)

The appropriate 7th character is to be added to each code from category T38.
A initial encounter
D subsequent encounter
S sequela

☑5ᵗʰ **T38.Ø Poisoning by, adverse effect of and underdosing of glucocorticoids and synthetic analogues**
EXCLUDES 1 *glucocorticoids, topically used (T49.-)*

☑6ᵗʰ **T38.ØX Poisoning by, adverse effect of and underdosing of glucocorticoids and synthetic analogues**

☑7ᵗʰ **T38.ØX1 Poisoning by glucocorticoids and synthetic analogues, accidental (unintentional)**
Poisoning by glucocorticoids and synthetic analogues NOS

² ☑7ᵗʰ **T38.ØX2 Poisoning by glucocorticoids and synthetic analogues, intentional self-harm** HCC

☑7ᵗʰ **T38.ØX3 Poisoning by glucocorticoids and synthetic analogues, assault**

☑7ᵗʰ **T38.ØX4 Poisoning by glucocorticoids and synthetic analogues, undetermined**

☑7ᵗʰ **T38.ØX5 Adverse effect of glucocorticoids and synthetic analogues**

☑7ᵗʰ **T38.ØX6 Underdosing of glucocorticoids and synthetic analogues**

✓5ᵗʰ **T38.1** **Poisoning by, adverse effect of and underdosing of thyroid hormones and substitutes**

     ✓6ᵗʰ **T38.1X** **Poisoning by, adverse effect of and underdosing of** thyroid hormones and substitutes

         ✓7ᵗʰ **T38.1X1** **Poisoning by thyroid hormones and substitutes,** accidental **(unintentional)**
                 Poisoning by thyroid hormones and substitutes NOS

        ² ✓7ᵗʰ **T38.1X2** **Poisoning by thyroid hormones and substitutes,** intentional self-harm   HCC

         ✓7ᵗʰ **T38.1X3** **Poisoning by thyroid hormones and substitutes,** assault

         ✓7ᵗʰ **T38.1X4** **Poisoning by thyroid hormones and substitutes,** undetermined

         ✓7ᵗʰ **T38.1X5** Adverse effect **of thyroid hormones and substitutes**

         ✓7ᵗʰ **T38.1X6** Underdosing **of thyroid hormones and substitutes**

✓5ᵗʰ **T38.2** **Poisoning by, adverse effect of and underdosing of antithyroid drugs**

     ✓6ᵗʰ **T38.2X** **Poisoning by, adverse effect of and underdosing of** antithyroid drugs

         ✓7ᵗʰ **T38.2X1** **Poisoning by antithyroid drugs,** accidental **(unintentional)**
                 Poisoning by antithyroid drugs NOS

        ² ✓7ᵗʰ **T38.2X2** **Poisoning by antithyroid drugs,** intentional self-harm   HCC

         ✓7ᵗʰ **T38.2X3** **Poisoning by antithyroid drugs,** assault

         ✓7ᵗʰ **T38.2X4** **Poisoning by antithyroid drugs,** undetermined

         ✓7ᵗʰ **T38.2X5** Adverse effect **of antithyroid drugs**

         ✓7ᵗʰ **T38.2X6** Underdosing **of antithyroid drugs**

✓5ᵗʰ **T38.3** **Poisoning by, adverse effect of and underdosing of insulin and oral hypoglycemic [antidiabetic] drugs**

     ✓6ᵗʰ **T38.3X** **Poisoning by, adverse effect of and underdosing of** insulin and oral hypoglycemic [antidiabetic] drugs

         ✓7ᵗʰ **T38.3X1** **Poisoning by insulin and oral hypoglycemic [antidiabetic] drugs,** accidental **(unintentional)**
                 Poisoning by insulin and oral hypoglycemic [antidiabetic] drugs NOS

        ² ✓7ᵗʰ **T38.3X2** **Poisoning by insulin and oral hypoglycemic [antidiabetic] drugs,** intentional self-harm   HCC

         ✓7ᵗʰ **T38.3X3** **Poisoning by insulin and oral hypoglycemic [antidiabetic] drugs,** assault

         ✓7ᵗʰ **T38.3X4** **Poisoning by insulin and oral hypoglycemic [antidiabetic] drugs,** undetermined

         ✓7ᵗʰ **T38.3X5** Adverse effect **of insulin and oral hypoglycemic [antidiabetic] drugs**

         ✓7ᵗʰ **T38.3X6** Underdosing **of insulin and oral hypoglycemic [antidiabetic] drugs**

✓5ᵗʰ **T38.4** **Poisoning by, adverse effect of and underdosing of oral contraceptives**
     Poisoning by, adverse effect of and underdosing of multiple- and single-ingredient oral contraceptive preparations

     ✓6ᵗʰ **T38.4X** **Poisoning by, adverse effect of and underdosing of** oral contraceptives

         ✓7ᵗʰ **T38.4X1** **Poisoning by oral contraceptives,** accidental **(unintentional)**
                 Poisoning by oral contraceptives NOS

        ² ✓7ᵗʰ **T38.4X2** **Poisoning by oral contraceptives,** intentional self-harm   HCC

         ✓7ᵗʰ **T38.4X3** **Poisoning by oral contraceptives,** assault

         ✓7ᵗʰ **T38.4X4** **Poisoning by oral contraceptives,** undetermined

         ✓7ᵗʰ **T38.4X5** Adverse effect **of oral contraceptives**

         ✓7ᵗʰ **T38.4X6** Underdosing **of oral contraceptives**

✓5ᵗʰ **T38.5** **Poisoning by, adverse effect of and underdosing of other estrogens and progestogens**
     Poisoning by, adverse effect of and underdosing of estrogens and progestogens mixtures and substitutes

     ✓6ᵗʰ **T38.5X** **Poisoning by, adverse effect of and underdosing of other estrogens and progestogens**

         ✓7ᵗʰ **T38.5X1** **Poisoning by other estrogens and progestogens,** accidental **(unintentional)**
                 Poisoning by other estrogens and progestogens NOS

        ² ✓7ᵗʰ **T38.5X2** **Poisoning by other estrogens and progestogens,** intentional self-harm   HCC

         ✓7ᵗʰ **T38.5X3** **Poisoning by other estrogens and progestogens,** assault

         ✓7ᵗʰ **T38.5X4** **Poisoning by other estrogens and progestogens,** undetermined

         ✓7ᵗʰ **T38.5X5** Adverse effect **of other estrogens and progestogens**

         ✓7ᵗʰ **T38.5X6** Underdosing **of other estrogens and progestogens**

✓5ᵗʰ **T38.6** **Poisoning by, adverse effect of and underdosing of antigonadotrophins, antiestrogens, antiandrogens, not elsewhere classified**
     Poisoning by, adverse effect of and underdosing of tamoxifen

     ✓6ᵗʰ **T38.6X** **Poisoning by, adverse effect of and underdosing of** antigonadotrophins, antiestrogens, antiandrogens, **not elsewhere classified**

         ✓7ᵗʰ **T38.6X1** **Poisoning by antigonadotrophins, antiestrogens, antiandrogens, not elsewhere classified,** accidental **(unintentional)**
                 Poisoning by antigonadotrophins, antiestrogens, antiandrogens, not elsewhere classified NOS

        ² ✓7ᵗʰ **T38.6X2** **Poisoning by antigonadotrophins, antiestrogens, antiandrogens, not elsewhere classified,** intentional self-harm   HCC

         ✓7ᵗʰ **T38.6X3** **Poisoning by antigonadotrophins, antiestrogens, antiandrogens, not elsewhere classified,** assault

         ✓7ᵗʰ **T38.6X4** **Poisoning by antigonadotrophins, antiestrogens, antiandrogens, not elsewhere classified,** undetermined

         ✓7ᵗʰ **T38.6X5** Adverse effect **of antigonadotrophins, antiestrogens, antiandrogens, not elsewhere classified**

         ✓7ᵗʰ **T38.6X6** Underdosing **of antigonadotrophins, antiestrogens, antiandrogens, not elsewhere classified**

✓5ᵗʰ **T38.7** **Poisoning by, adverse effect of and underdosing of androgens and anabolic congeners**

     ✓6ᵗʰ **T38.7X** **Poisoning by, adverse effect of and underdosing of** androgens and anabolic congeners

         ✓7ᵗʰ **T38.7X1** **Poisoning by androgens and anabolic congeners,** accidental **(unintentional)**
                 Poisoning by androgens and anabolic congeners NOS

        ² ✓7ᵗʰ **T38.7X2** **Poisoning by androgens and anabolic congeners,** intentional self-harm   HCC

         ✓7ᵗʰ **T38.7X3** **Poisoning by androgens and anabolic congeners,** assault

         ✓7ᵗʰ **T38.7X4** **Poisoning by androgens and anabolic congeners,** undetermined

         ✓7ᵗʰ **T38.7X5** Adverse effect **of androgens and anabolic congeners**

         ✓7ᵗʰ **T38.7X6** Underdosing **of androgens and anabolic congeners**

✓5ᵗʰ **T38.8** **Poisoning by, adverse effect of and underdosing of other and unspecified hormones and synthetic substitutes**

     ✓6ᵗʰ **T38.80** **Poisoning by, adverse effect of and underdosing of unspecified hormones and synthetic substitutes**

         ✓7ᵗʰ **T38.801** **Poisoning by unspecified hormones and synthetic substitutes,** accidental **(unintentional)**
                 Poisoning by unspecified hormones and synthetic substitutes NOS

        ² ✓7ᵗʰ **T38.802** **Poisoning by unspecified hormones and synthetic substitutes,** intentional self-harm   HCC

☑ Additional Character Required   ✓ⁿ⁷ᵗʰ Placeholder Alert   Manifestation   Unspecified Dx   ►◄ Revised Text   ● New Code   ▲ Revised Code Title

ICD-10-CM 2020   1099

√7ᵗʰ **T38.803** **Poisoning by unspecified hormones and synthetic substitutes,** assault

√7ᵗʰ **T38.804** **Poisoning by unspecified hormones and synthetic substitutes,** undetermined

√7ᵗʰ **T38.805** **Adverse effect of unspecified hormones and synthetic substitutes**

√7ᵗʰ **T38.806** **Underdosing of unspecified hormones and synthetic substitutes**

√6ᵗʰ **T38.81** **Poisoning by, adverse effect of and underdosing of** anterior pituitary [adenohypophyseal] hormones

√7ᵗʰ **T38.811** **Poisoning by anterior pituitary [adenohypophyseal] hormones, accidental (unintentional)**

Poisoning by anterior pituitary [adenohypophyseal] hormones NOS

² √7ᵗʰ **T38.812** **Poisoning by anterior pituitary** ⓗⒸⒸ **[adenohypophyseal] hormones, intentional self-harm**

√7ᵗʰ **T38.813** **Poisoning by anterior pituitary [adenohypophyseal] hormones,** assault

√7ᵗʰ **T38.814** **Poisoning by anterior pituitary [adenohypophyseal] hormones, undetermined**

√7ᵗʰ **T38.815** **Adverse effect of anterior pituitary [adenohypophyseal] hormones**

√7ᵗʰ **T38.816** **Underdosing of anterior pituitary [adenohypophyseal] hormones**

√6ᵗʰ **T38.89** **Poisoning by, adverse effect of and underdosing of other hormones and synthetic substitutes**

√7ᵗʰ **T38.891** **Poisoning by other hormones and synthetic substitutes, accidental (unintentional)**

Poisoning by other hormones and synthetic substitutes NOS

² √7ᵗʰ **T38.892** **Poisoning by other hormones and** ⓗⒸⒸ **synthetic substitutes, intentional self-harm**

√7ᵗʰ **T38.893** **Poisoning by other hormones and synthetic substitutes,** assault

√7ᵗʰ **T38.894** **Poisoning by other hormones and synthetic substitutes, undetermined**

√7ᵗʰ **T38.895** **Adverse effect of other hormones and synthetic substitutes**

√7ᵗʰ **T38.896** **Underdosing of other hormones and synthetic substitutes**

√5ᵗʰ **T38.9** **Poisoning by, adverse effect of and underdosing of other and unspecified hormone antagonists**

√6ᵗʰ **T38.90** **Poisoning by, adverse effect of and underdosing of unspecified hormone antagonists**

√7ᵗʰ **T38.901** **Poisoning by unspecified hormone antagonists, accidental (unintentional)**

Poisoning by unspecified hormone antagonists NOS

² √7ᵗʰ **T38.902** **Poisoning by unspecified** ⓗⒸⒸ **hormone antagonists, intentional self-harm**

√7ᵗʰ **T38.903** **Poisoning by unspecified hormone antagonists,** assault

√7ᵗʰ **T38.904** **Poisoning by unspecified hormone antagonists, undetermined**

√7ᵗʰ **T38.905** **Adverse effect of unspecified hormone antagonists**

√7ᵗʰ **T38.906** **Underdosing of unspecified hormone antagonists**

√6ᵗʰ **T38.99** **Poisoning by, adverse effect of and underdosing of other hormone antagonists**

√7ᵗʰ **T38.991** **Poisoning by other hormone antagonists, accidental (unintentional)**

Poisoning by other hormone antagonists NOS

² √7ᵗʰ **T38.992** **Poisoning by other hormone** ⓗⒸⒸ **antagonists, intentional self-harm**

√7ᵗʰ **T38.993** **Poisoning by other hormone antagonists,** assault

√7ᵗʰ **T38.994** **Poisoning by other hormone antagonists, undetermined**

√7ᵗʰ **T38.995** **Adverse effect of other hormone antagonists**

√7ᵗʰ **T38.996** **Underdosing of other hormone antagonists**

√4ᵗʰ **T39** **Poisoning by, adverse effect of and underdosing of nonopioid analgesics, antipyretics and antirheumatics**

The appropriate 7th character is to be added to each code from category T39.
A   initial encounter
D   subsequent encounter
S   sequela

√5ᵗʰ **T39.0** **Poisoning by, adverse effect of and underdosing of salicylates**

√6ᵗʰ **T39.01** **Poisoning by, adverse effect of and underdosing of aspirin**

Poisoning by, adverse effect of and underdosing of acetylsalicylic acid

√7ᵗʰ **T39.011** **Poisoning by aspirin, accidental (unintentional)**

² √7ᵗʰ **T39.012** **Poisoning by aspirin, intentional** ⓗⒸⒸ **self-harm**

√7ᵗʰ **T39.013** **Poisoning by aspirin,** assault

√7ᵗʰ **T39.014** **Poisoning by aspirin,** undetermined

√7ᵗʰ **T39.015** **Adverse effect of aspirin**

AHA: 2016,1Q,15

√7ᵗʰ **T39.016** **Underdosing of aspirin**

√6ᵗʰ **T39.09** **Poisoning by, adverse effect of and underdosing of other salicylates**

√7ᵗʰ **T39.091** **Poisoning by salicylates, accidental (unintentional)**

Poisoning by salicylates NOS

² √7ᵗʰ **T39.092** **Poisoning by salicylates,** ⓗⒸⒸ **intentional self-harm**

√7ᵗʰ **T39.093** **Poisoning by salicylates,** assault

√7ᵗʰ **T39.094** **Poisoning by salicylates,** undetermined

√7ᵗʰ **T39.095** **Adverse effect of salicylates**

√7ᵗʰ **T39.096** **Underdosing of salicylates**

√5ᵗʰ **T39.1** **Poisoning by, adverse effect of and underdosing of 4-Aminophenol derivatives**

√6ᵗʰ **T39.1X** **Poisoning by, adverse effect of and underdosing of 4-Aminophenol derivatives**

√7ᵗʰ **T39.1X1** **Poisoning by 4-Aminophenol derivatives, accidental (unintentional)**

Poisoning by 4-Aminophenol derivatives NOS

² √7ᵗʰ **T39.1X2** **Poisoning by 4-Aminophenol** ⓗⒸⒸ **derivatives, intentional self-harm**

√7ᵗʰ **T39.1X3** **Poisoning by 4-Aminophenol derivatives, assault**

√7ᵗʰ **T39.1X4** **Poisoning by 4-Aminophenol derivatives, undetermined**

√7ᵗʰ **T39.1X5** **Adverse effect of 4-Aminophenol derivatives**

√7ᵗʰ **T39.1X6** **Underdosing of 4-Aminophenol derivatives**

√5ᵗʰ **T39.2** **Poisoning by, adverse effect of and underdosing of pyrazolone derivatives**

√6ᵗʰ **T39.2X** **Poisoning by, adverse effect of and underdosing of pyrazolone derivatives**

√7ᵗʰ **T39.2X1** **Poisoning by pyrazolone derivatives, accidental (unintentional)**

Poisoning by pyrazolone derivatives NOS

² √7ᵗʰ **T39.2X2** **Poisoning by pyrazolone** ⓗⒸⒸ **derivatives, intentional self-harm**

√7ᵗʰ **T39.2X3** **Poisoning by pyrazolone derivatives, assault**

√7ᵗʰ **T39.2X4** **Poisoning by pyrazolone derivatives, undetermined**

√7ᵗʰ **T39.2X5** **Adverse effect of pyrazolone derivatives**

√7ᵗʰ **T39.2X6** **Underdosing of pyrazolone derivatives**

☑5th **T39.3** **Poisoning by, adverse effect of and underdosing of other nonsteroidal anti-inflammatory drugs [NSAID]**

    ☑6th **T39.31** **Poisoning by, adverse effect of and underdosing of propionic acid derivatives**

        Poisoning by, adverse effect of and underdosing of fenoprofen

        Poisoning by, adverse effect of and underdosing of flurbiprofen

        Poisoning by, adverse effect of and underdosing of ibuprofen

        Poisoning by, adverse effect of and underdosing of ketoprofen

        Poisoning by, adverse effect of and underdosing of naproxen

        Poisoning by, adverse effect of and underdosing of oxaprozin

        ☑7th **T39.311** **Poisoning by propionic acid derivatives, accidental (unintentional)**

        2 ☑7th **T39.312** **Poisoning by propionic acid derivatives, intentional self-harm** `HCC`

        ☑7th **T39.313** **Poisoning by propionic acid derivatives, assault**

        ☑7th **T39.314** **Poisoning by propionic acid derivatives, undetermined**

        ☑7th **T39.315** **Adverse effect of propionic acid derivatives**

        ☑7th **T39.316** **Underdosing of propionic acid derivatives**

    ☑6th **T39.39** **Poisoning by, adverse effect of and underdosing of other nonsteroidal anti-inflammatory drugs [NSAID]**

        ☑7th **T39.391** **Poisoning by other nonsteroidal anti-inflammatory drugs [NSAID], accidental (unintentional)**

        Poisoning by other nonsteroidal anti-inflammatory drugs NOS

        2 ☑7th **T39.392** **Poisoning by other nonsteroidal anti-inflammatory drugs [NSAID], intentional self-harm** `HCC`

        ☑7th **T39.393** **Poisoning by other nonsteroidal anti-inflammatory drugs [NSAID], assault**

        ☑7th **T39.394** **Poisoning by other nonsteroidal anti-inflammatory drugs [NSAID], undetermined**

        ☑7th **T39.395** **Adverse effect of other nonsteroidal anti-inflammatory drugs [NSAID]**

        ☑7th **T39.396** **Underdosing of other nonsteroidal anti-inflammatory drugs [NSAID]**

☑5th **T39.4** **Poisoning by, adverse effect of and underdosing of antirheumatics, not elsewhere classified**

    EXCLUDES 1   poisoning by, adverse effect of and underdosing of glucocorticoids (T38.0-)

          poisoning by, adverse effect of and underdosing of salicylates (T39.0-)

    ☑6th **T39.4X** **Poisoning by, adverse effect of and underdosing of antirheumatics, not elsewhere classified**

        ☑7th **T39.4X1** **Poisoning by antirheumatics, not elsewhere classified, accidental (unintentional)**

        Poisoning by antirheumatics, not elsewhere classified NOS

        2 ☑7th **T39.4X2** **Poisoning by antirheumatics, not elsewhere classified, intentional self-harm** `HCC`

        ☑7th **T39.4X3** **Poisoning by antirheumatics, not elsewhere classified, assault**

        ☑7th **T39.4X4** **Poisoning by antirheumatics, not elsewhere classified, undetermined**

        ☑7th **T39.4X5** **Adverse effect of antirheumatics, not elsewhere classified**

        ☑7th **T39.4X6** **Underdosing of antirheumatics, not elsewhere classified**

☑5th **T39.8** **Poisoning by, adverse effect of and underdosing of other nonopioid analgesics and antipyretics, not elsewhere classified**

    ☑6th **T39.8X** **Poisoning by, adverse effect of and underdosing of other nonopioid analgesics and antipyretics, not elsewhere classified**

        ☑7th **T39.8X1** **Poisoning by other nonopioid analgesics and antipyretics, not elsewhere classified, accidental (unintentional)**

        Poisoning by other nonopioid analgesics and antipyretics, not elsewhere classified NOS

        2 ☑7th **T39.8X2** **Poisoning by other nonopioid analgesics and antipyretics, not elsewhere classified, intentional self-harm** `HCC`

        ☑7th **T39.8X3** **Poisoning by other nonopioid analgesics and antipyretics, not elsewhere classified, assault**

        ☑7th **T39.8X4** **Poisoning by other nonopioid analgesics and antipyretics, not elsewhere classified, undetermined**

        ☑7th **T39.8X5** **Adverse effect of other nonopioid analgesics and antipyretics, not elsewhere classified**

        ☑7th **T39.8X6** **Underdosing of other nonopioid analgesics and antipyretics, not elsewhere classified**

☑5th **T39.9** **Poisoning by, adverse effect of and underdosing of unspecified nonopioid analgesic, antipyretic and antirheumatic**

    ☑x7th **T39.91** **Poisoning by unspecified nonopioid analgesic, antipyretic and antirheumatic, accidental (unintentional)**

        Poisoning by nonopioid analgesic, antipyretic and antirheumatic NOS

    2 ☑x7th **T39.92** **Poisoning by unspecified nonopioid analgesic, antipyretic and antirheumatic, intentional self-harm** `HCC`

    ☑x7th **T39.93** **Poisoning by unspecified nonopioid analgesic, antipyretic and antirheumatic, assault**

    ☑x7th **T39.94** **Poisoning by unspecified nonopioid analgesic, antipyretic and antirheumatic, undetermined**

    ☑x7th **T39.95** **Adverse effect of unspecified nonopioid analgesic, antipyretic and antirheumatic**

    ☑x7th **T39.96** **Underdosing of unspecified nonopioid analgesic, antipyretic and antirheumatic**

☑4th **T40** **Poisoning by, adverse effect of and underdosing of narcotics and psychodysleptics [hallucinogens]**

    EXCLUDES 2   drug dependence and related mental and behavioral disorders due to psychoactive substance use (F10.-F19.-)

    The appropriate 7th character is to be added to each code from category T40.

    A   initial encounter

    D   subsequent encounter

    S   sequela

  ☑5th **T40.0** **Poisoning by, adverse effect of and underdosing of opium**

    ☑6th **T40.0X** **Poisoning by, adverse effect of and underdosing of opium**

        1 ☑7th **T40.0X1** **Poisoning by opium, accidental (unintentional)** `HCC`

        Poisoning by opium NOS

        2 ☑7th **T40.0X2** **Poisoning by opium, intentional self-harm** `HCC`

        ☑7th **T40.0X3** **Poisoning by opium, assault**

        1 ☑7th **T40.0X4** **Poisoning by opium, undetermined** `HCC`

        ☑7th **T40.0X5** **Adverse effect of opium**

        ☑7th **T40.0X6** **Underdosing of opium**

  ☑5th **T40.1** **Poisoning by and adverse effect of heroin**

    ☑6th **T40.1X** **Poisoning by and adverse effect of heroin**

        1 ☑7th **T40.1X1** **Poisoning by heroin, accidental (unintentional)** `HCC`

        Poisoning by heroin NOS

        2 ☑7th **T40.1X2** **Poisoning by heroin, intentional self-harm** `HCC`

        ☑7th **T40.1X3** **Poisoning by heroin, assault**

        1 ☑7th **T40.1X4** **Poisoning by heroin, undetermined** `HCC`

☑ Additional Character Required   ☑x7th Placeholder Alert   Manifestation   Unspecified Dx   ►◄ Revised Text   ● New Code   ▲ Revised Code Title

ICD-10-CM 2020   **1101**

√5ᵗʰ **T40.2** **Poisoning by, adverse effect of and underdosing of other opioids**

√6ᵗʰ   **T40.2X** **Poisoning by, adverse effect of and underdosing of other opioids**

     1 √7ᵗʰ **T40.2X1** **Poisoning by other opioids, accidental (unintentional)**   HCC
       Poisoning by other opioids NOS

     2 √7ᵗʰ **T40.2X2** **Poisoning by other opioids, intentional self-harm**   HCC

     √7ᵗʰ **T40.2X3** **Poisoning by other opioids, assault**

     1 √7ᵗʰ **T40.2X4** **Poisoning by other opioids, undetermined**   HCC

     √7ᵗʰ **T40.2X5** **Adverse effect** of other opioids

     √7ᵗʰ **T40.2X6** **Underdosing** of other opioids

√5ᵗʰ **T40.3** **Poisoning by, adverse effect of and underdosing of methadone**

√6ᵗʰ   **T40.3X** **Poisoning by, adverse effect of and underdosing of methadone**

     1 √7ᵗʰ **T40.3X1** **Poisoning by methadone, accidental (unintentional)**   HCC
       Poisoning by methadone NOS

     2 √7ᵗʰ **T40.3X2** **Poisoning by methadone, intentional self-harm**   HCC

     √7ᵗʰ **T40.3X3** **Poisoning by methadone, assault**

     √7ᵗʰ **T40.3X4** **Poisoning by methadone, undetermined**   HCC

     √7ᵗʰ **T40.3X5** **Adverse effect** of methadone

     √7ᵗʰ **T40.3X6** **Underdosing** of methadone

√5ᵗʰ **T40.4** **Poisoning by, adverse effect of and underdosing of other synthetic narcotics**

√6ᵗʰ   **T40.4X** **Poisoning by, adverse effect of and underdosing of other synthetic narcotics**

     1 √7ᵗʰ **T40.4X1** **Poisoning by other synthetic narcotics, accidental (unintentional)**   HCC
       Poisoning by other synthetic narcotics NOS

     2 √7ᵗʰ **T40.4X2** **Poisoning by other synthetic narcotics, intentional self-harm**   HCC

     √7ᵗʰ **T40.4X3** **Poisoning by other synthetic narcotics, assault**

     1 √7ᵗʰ **T40.4X4** **Poisoning by other synthetic narcotics, undetermined**   HCC

     √7ᵗʰ **T40.4X5** **Adverse effect** of other synthetic narcotics

     √7ᵗʰ **T40.4X6** **Underdosing** of other synthetic narcotics

√5ᵗʰ **T40.5** **Poisoning by, adverse effect of and underdosing of cocaine**

√6ᵗʰ   **T40.5X** **Poisoning by, adverse effect of and underdosing of cocaine**

     1 √7ᵗʰ **T40.5X1** **Poisoning by cocaine, accidental (unintentional)**   HCC
       Poisoning by cocaine NOS
       AHA: 2016,2Q,8

     2 √7ᵗʰ **T40.5X2** **Poisoning by cocaine, intentional self-harm**   HCC

     √7ᵗʰ **T40.5X3** **Poisoning by cocaine, assault**

     1 √7ᵗʰ **T40.5X4** **Poisoning by cocaine, undetermined**   HCC

     √7ᵗʰ **T40.5X5** **Adverse effect** of cocaine

     √7ᵗʰ **T40.5X6** **Underdosing** of cocaine

√5ᵗʰ **T40.6** **Poisoning by, adverse effect of and underdosing of other and unspecified narcotics**

√6ᵗʰ   **T40.60** **Poisoning by, adverse effect of and underdosing of unspecified narcotics**

     1 √7ᵗʰ **T40.601** **Poisoning by unspecified narcotics, accidental (unintentional)**   HCC
       Poisoning by narcotics NOS

     2 √7ᵗʰ **T40.602** **Poisoning by unspecified narcotics, intentional self-harm**   HCC

     √7ᵗʰ **T40.603** **Poisoning by unspecified narcotics, assault**

     1 √7ᵗʰ **T40.604** **Poisoning by unspecified narcotics, undetermined**   HCC

     √7ᵗʰ **T40.605** **Adverse effect** of unspecified narcotics

     √7ᵗʰ **T40.606** **Underdosing** of unspecified narcotics

√6ᵗʰ   **T40.69** **Poisoning by, adverse effect of and underdosing of other narcotics**

     1 √7ᵗʰ **T40.691** **Poisoning by other narcotics, accidental (unintentional)**   HCC
       Poisoning by other narcotics NOS

     2 √7ᵗʰ **T40.692** **Poisoning by other narcotics, intentional self-harm**   HCC

     √7ᵗʰ **T40.693** **Poisoning by other narcotics, assault**

     1 √7ᵗʰ **T40.694** **Poisoning by other narcotics, undetermined**   HCC

     √7ᵗʰ **T40.695** **Adverse effect** of other narcotics

     √7ᵗʰ **T40.696** **Underdosing** of other narcotics

√5ᵗʰ **T40.7** **Poisoning by, adverse effect of and underdosing of cannabis (derivatives)**

√6ᵗʰ   **T40.7X** **Poisoning by, adverse effect of and underdosing of cannabis (derivatives)**

     √7ᵗʰ **T40.7X1** **Poisoning by cannabis (derivatives), accidental (unintentional)**
       Poisoning by cannabis NOS

     2 √7ᵗʰ **T40.7X2** **Poisoning by cannabis (derivatives), intentional self-harm**   HCC

     √7ᵗʰ **T40.7X3** **Poisoning by cannabis (derivatives), assault**

     √7ᵗʰ **T40.7X4** **Poisoning by cannabis (derivatives), undetermined**

     √7ᵗʰ **T40.7X5** **Adverse effect** of cannabis (derivatives)

     √7ᵗʰ **T40.7X6** **Underdosing** of cannabis (derivatives)

√5ᵗʰ **T40.8** **Poisoning by and adverse effect of lysergide [LSD]**

√6ᵗʰ   **T40.8X** **Poisoning by and adverse effect of lysergide [LSD]**

     1 √7ᵗʰ **T40.8X1** **Poisoning by lysergide [LSD], accidental (unintentional)**   HCC
       Poisoning by lysergide [LSD] NOS

     2 √7ᵗʰ **T40.8X2** **Poisoning by lysergide [LSD], intentional self-harm**   HCC

     √7ᵗʰ **T40.8X3** **Poisoning by lysergide [LSD], assault**

     1 √7ᵗʰ **T40.8X4** **Poisoning by lysergide [LSD], undetermined**   HCC

√5ᵗʰ **T40.9** **Poisoning by, adverse effect of and underdosing of other and unspecified psychodysleptics [hallucinogens]**

√6ᵗʰ   **T40.90** **Poisoning by, adverse effect of and underdosing of unspecified psychodysleptics [hallucinogens]**

     1 √7ᵗʰ **T40.901** **Poisoning by unspecified psychodysleptics [hallucinogens], accidental (unintentional)**   HCC

     2 √7ᵗʰ **T40.902** **Poisoning by unspecified psychodysleptics [hallucinogens], intentional self-harm**   HCC

     √7ᵗʰ **T40.903** **Poisoning by unspecified psychodysleptics [hallucinogens], assault**

     1 √7ᵗʰ **T40.904** **Poisoning by unspecified psychodysleptics [hallucinogens], undetermined**   HCC

     √7ᵗʰ **T40.905** **Adverse effect** of unspecified psychodysleptics [hallucinogens]

     √7ᵗʰ **T40.906** **Underdosing** of unspecified psychodysleptics [hallucinogens]

√6ᵗʰ   **T40.99** **Poisoning by, adverse effect of and underdosing of other psychodysleptics [hallucinogens]**

     1 √7ᵗʰ **T40.991** **Poisoning by other psychodysleptics [hallucinogens], accidental (unintentional)**   HCC
       Poisoning by other psychodysleptics [hallucinogens] NOS

     2 √7ᵗʰ **T40.992** **Poisoning by other psychodysleptics [hallucinogens], intentional self-harm**   HCC

     √7ᵗʰ **T40.993** **Poisoning by other psychodysleptics [hallucinogens], assault**

     1 √7ᵗʰ **T40.994** **Poisoning by other psychodysleptics [hallucinogens], undetermined**   HCC

     √7ᵗʰ **T40.995** **Adverse effect** of other psychodysleptics [hallucinogens]

     √7ᵗʰ **T40.996** **Underdosing** of other psychodysleptics [hallucinogens]

☑4ᵗʰ **T41 Poisoning by, adverse effect of and underdosing of anesthetics and therapeutic gases**

EXCLUDES 1   benzodiazepines (T42.4-)
         cocaine (T40.5-)
         complications of anesthesia during labor and delivery (O74.-)
         complications of anesthesia during pregnancy (O29.-)
         complications of anesthesia during the puerperium (O89.-)
         opioids (T40.0-T40.2-)

> The appropriate 7th character is to be added to each code from category T41.
> A   initial encounter
> D   subsequent encounter
> S   sequela

☑5ᵗʰ **T41.0 Poisoning by, adverse effect of and underdosing of inhaled anesthetics**

     EXCLUDES 1   oxygen (T41.5-)

    ☑6ᵗʰ **T41.0X Poisoning by, adverse effect of and underdosing of inhaled anesthetics**

       ☑7ᵗʰ **T41.0X1 Poisoning by inhaled anesthetics, accidental (unintentional)**
          Poisoning by inhaled anesthetics NOS

       ² ☑7ᵗʰ **T41.0X2 Poisoning by inhaled anesthetics, intentional self-harm** HCC

       ☑7ᵗʰ **T41.0X3 Poisoning by inhaled anesthetics, assault**

       ☑7ᵗʰ **T41.0X4 Poisoning by inhaled anesthetics, undetermined**

       ☑7ᵗʰ **T41.0X5 Adverse effect of inhaled anesthetics**

       ☑7ᵗʰ **T41.0X6 Underdosing of inhaled anesthetics**

☑5ᵗʰ **T41.1 Poisoning by, adverse effect of and underdosing of intravenous anesthetics**

    Poisoning by, adverse effect of and underdosing of thiobarbiturates

    ☑6ᵗʰ **T41.1X Poisoning by, adverse effect of and underdosing of intravenous anesthetics**

       ☑7ᵗʰ **T41.1X1 Poisoning by intravenous anesthetics, accidental (unintentional)**
          Poisoning by intravenous anesthetics NOS

       ² ☑7ᵗʰ **T41.1X2 Poisoning by intravenous anesthetics, intentional self-harm** HCC

       ☑7ᵗʰ **T41.1X3 Poisoning by intravenous anesthetics, assault**

       ☑7ᵗʰ **T41.1X4 Poisoning by intravenous anesthetics, undetermined**

       ☑7ᵗʰ **T41.1X5 Adverse effect of intravenous anesthetics**

       ☑7ᵗʰ **T41.1X6 Underdosing of intravenous anesthetics**

☑5ᵗʰ **T41.2 Poisoning by, adverse effect of and underdosing of other and unspecified general anesthetics**

    ☑6ᵗʰ **T41.20 Poisoning by, adverse effect of and underdosing of unspecified general anesthetics**

       ☑7ᵗʰ **T41.201 Poisoning by unspecified general anesthetics, accidental (unintentional)**
          Poisoning by general anesthetics NOS

       ² ☑7ᵗʰ **T41.202 Poisoning by unspecified general anesthetics, intentional self-harm** HCC

       ☑7ᵗʰ **T41.203 Poisoning by unspecified general anesthetics, assault**

       ☑7ᵗʰ **T41.204 Poisoning by unspecified general anesthetics, undetermined**

       ☑7ᵗʰ **T41.205 Adverse effect of unspecified general anesthetics**
          AHA: 2016,4Q,73

       ☑7ᵗʰ **T41.206 Underdosing of unspecified general anesthetics**

    ☑6ᵗʰ **T41.29 Poisoning by, adverse effect of and underdosing of other general anesthetics**

       ☑7ᵗʰ **T41.291 Poisoning by other general anesthetics, accidental (unintentional)**
          Poisoning by other general anesthetics NOS

       ² ☑7ᵗʰ **T41.292 Poisoning by other general anesthetics, intentional self-harm** HCC

       ☑7ᵗʰ **T41.293 Poisoning by other general anesthetics, assault**

       ☑7ᵗʰ **T41.294 Poisoning by other general anesthetics, undetermined**

       ☑7ᵗʰ **T41.295 Adverse effect of other general anesthetics**

       ☑7ᵗʰ **T41.296 Underdosing of other general anesthetics**

☑5ᵗʰ **T41.3 Poisoning by, adverse effect of and underdosing of local anesthetics**

    Cocaine (topical)

     EXCLUDES 2   poisoning by cocaine used as a central nervous system stimulant (T40.5X1-T40.5X4)

    ☑6ᵗʰ **T41.3X Poisoning by, adverse effect of and underdosing of local anesthetics**

       ☑7ᵗʰ **T41.3X1 Poisoning by local anesthetics, accidental (unintentional)**
          Poisoning by local anesthetics NOS

       ² ☑7ᵗʰ **T41.3X2 Poisoning by local anesthetics, intentional self-harm** HCC

       ☑7ᵗʰ **T41.3X3 Poisoning by local anesthetics, assault**

       ☑7ᵗʰ **T41.3X4 Poisoning by local anesthetics, undetermined**

       ☑7ᵗʰ **T41.3X5 Adverse effect of local anesthetics**

       ☑7ᵗʰ **T41.3X6 Underdosing of local anesthetics**

☑5ᵗʰ **T41.4 Poisoning by, adverse effect of and underdosing of unspecified anesthetic**

    ☑×7ᵗʰ **T41.41 Poisoning by unspecified anesthetic, accidental (unintentional)**
       Poisoning by anesthetic NOS

    ² ☑×7ᵗʰ **T41.42 Poisoning by unspecified anesthetic, intentional self-harm** HCC

    ☑×7ᵗʰ **T41.43 Poisoning by unspecified anesthetic, assault**

    ☑×7ᵗʰ **T41.44 Poisoning by unspecified anesthetic, undetermined**

    ☑×7ᵗʰ **T41.45 Adverse effect of unspecified anesthetic**

    ☑×7ᵗʰ **T41.46 Underdosing of unspecified anesthetics**

☑5ᵗʰ **T41.5 Poisoning by, adverse effect of and underdosing of therapeutic gases**

    ☑6ᵗʰ **T41.5X Poisoning by, adverse effect of and underdosing of therapeutic gases**

       ☑7ᵗʰ **T41.5X1 Poisoning by therapeutic gases, accidental (unintentional)**
          Poisoning by therapeutic gases NOS

       ² ☑7ᵗʰ **T41.5X2 Poisoning by therapeutic gases, intentional self-harm** HCC

       ☑7ᵗʰ **T41.5X3 Poisoning by therapeutic gases, assault**

       ☑7ᵗʰ **T41.5X4 Poisoning by therapeutic gases, undetermined**

       ☑7ᵗʰ **T41.5X5 Adverse effect of therapeutic gases**

       ☑7ᵗʰ **T41.5X6 Underdosing of therapeutic gases**

☑4ᵗʰ **T42 Poisoning by, adverse effect of and underdosing of antiepileptic, sedative- hypnotic and antiparkinsonism drugs**

     EXCLUDES 2   drug dependence and related mental and behavioral disorders due to psychoactive substance use (F10.- – F19.-)

> The appropriate 7th character is to be added to each code from category T42.
> A   initial encounter
> D   subsequent encounter
> S   sequela

☑5ᵗʰ **T42.0 Poisoning by, adverse effect of and underdosing of hydantoin derivatives**

    ☑6ᵗʰ **T42.0X Poisoning by, adverse effect of and underdosing of hydantoin derivatives**

       ☑7ᵗʰ **T42.0X1 Poisoning by hydantoin derivatives, accidental (unintentional)**
          Poisoning by hydantoin derivatives NOS

       ² ☑7ᵗʰ **T42.0X2 Poisoning by hydantoin derivatives, intentional self-harm** HCC

       ☑7ᵗʰ **T42.0X3 Poisoning by hydantoin derivatives, assault**

       ☑7ᵗʰ **T42.0X4 Poisoning by hydantoin derivatives, undetermined**

       ☑7ᵗʰ **T42.0X5 Adverse effect of hydantoin derivatives**

       ☑7ᵗʰ **T42.0X6 Underdosing of hydantoin derivatives**

☑5ᵗʰ **T42.1 Poisoning by, adverse effect of and underdosing of iminostilbenes**

    Poisoning by, adverse effect of and underdosing of carbamazepine

    ☑6ᵗʰ **T42.1X Poisoning by, adverse effect of and underdosing of iminostilbenes**

       ☑7ᵗʰ **T42.1X1 Poisoning by iminostilbenes, accidental (unintentional)**
          Poisoning by iminostilbenes NOS

       ² ☑7ᵗʰ **T42.1X2 Poisoning by iminostilbenes, intentional self-harm** HCC

       ☑7ᵗʰ **T42.1X3 Poisoning by iminostilbenes, assault**

☑ Additional Character Required   ☑7ᵗʰ Placeholder Alert   Manifestation   Unspecified Dx   ◄► Revised Text   ● New Code   ▲ Revised Code Title

√7ᵗʰ **T42.1X4** **Poisoning by iminostilbenes, undetermined**

√7ᵗʰ **T42.1X5** **Adverse effect of iminostilbenes**

√7ᵗʰ **T42.1X6** **Underdosing of iminostilbenes**

√5ᵗʰ **T42.2** **Poisoning by, adverse effect of and underdosing of succinimides and oxazolidinediones**

√6ᵗʰ **T42.2X** **Poisoning by, adverse effect of and underdosing of succinimides and oxazolidinediones**

√7ᵗʰ **T42.2X1** **Poisoning by succinimides and oxazolidinediones, accidental (unintentional)**
Poisoning by succinimides and oxazolidinediones NOS

² √7ᵗʰ **T42.2X2** **Poisoning by succinimides and oxazolidinediones, intentional self-harm** ᴴᶜᶜ

√7ᵗʰ **T42.2X3** **Poisoning by succinimides and oxazolidinediones, assault**

√7ᵗʰ **T42.2X4** **Poisoning by succinimides and oxazolidinediones, undetermined**

√7ᵗʰ **T42.2X5** **Adverse effect of succinimides and oxazolidinediones**

√7ᵗʰ **T42.2X6** **Underdosing of succinimides and oxazolidinediones**

√5ᵗʰ **T42.3** **Poisoning by, adverse effect of and underdosing of barbiturates**

EXCLUDES 1   *poisoning by, adverse effect of and underdosing of thiobarbiturates (T41.1-)*

√6ᵗʰ **T42.3X** **Poisoning by, adverse effect of and underdosing of barbiturates**

√7ᵗʰ **T42.3X1** **Poisoning by barbiturates, accidental (unintentional)**
Poisoning by barbiturates NOS

² √7ᵗʰ **T42.3X2** **Poisoning by barbiturates, intentional self-harm** ᴴᶜᶜ

√7ᵗʰ **T42.3X3** **Poisoning by barbiturates, assault**

√7ᵗʰ **T42.3X4** **Poisoning by barbiturates, undetermined**

√7ᵗʰ **T42.3X5** **Adverse effect of barbiturates**

√7ᵗʰ **T42.3X6** **Underdosing of barbiturates**

√5ᵗʰ **T42.4** **Poisoning by, adverse effect of and underdosing of benzodiazepines**

√6ᵗʰ **T42.4X** **Poisoning by, adverse effect of and underdosing of benzodiazepines**

√7ᵗʰ **T42.4X1** **Poisoning by benzodiazepines, accidental (unintentional)**
Poisoning by benzodiazepines NOS

² √7ᵗʰ **T42.4X2** **Poisoning by benzodiazepines, intentional self-harm** ᴴᶜᶜ

√7ᵗʰ **T42.4X3** **Poisoning by benzodiazepines, assault**

√7ᵗʰ **T42.4X4** **Poisoning by benzodiazepines, undetermined**

√7ᵗʰ **T42.4X5** **Adverse effect of benzodiazepines**

√7ᵗʰ **T42.4X6** **Underdosing of benzodiazepines**

√5ᵗʰ **T42.5** **Poisoning by, adverse effect of and underdosing of mixed antiepileptics**

√6ᵗʰ **T42.5X** **Poisoning by, adverse effect of and underdosing of antiepileptics**

√7ᵗʰ **T42.5X1** **Poisoning by mixed antiepileptics, accidental (unintentional)**
Poisoning by mixed antiepileptics NOS

² √7ᵗʰ **T42.5X2** **Poisoning by mixed antiepileptics, intentional self-harm** ᴴᶜᶜ

√7ᵗʰ **T42.5X3** **Poisoning by mixed antiepileptics, assault**

√7ᵗʰ **T42.5X4** **Poisoning by mixed antiepileptics, undetermined**

√7ᵗʰ **T42.5X5** **Adverse effect of mixed antiepileptics**

√7ᵗʰ **T42.5X6** **Underdosing of mixed antiepileptics**

√5ᵗʰ **T42.6** **Poisoning by, adverse effect of and underdosing of other antiepileptic and sedative-hypnotic drugs**
Poisoning by, adverse effect of and underdosing of methaqualone
Poisoning by, adverse effect of and underdosing of valproic acid

EXCLUDES 1   *poisoning by, adverse effect of and underdosing of carbamazepine (T42.1-)*

√6ᵗʰ **T42.6X** **Poisoning by, adverse effect of and underdosing of other antiepileptic and sedative-hypnotic drugs**

√7ᵗʰ **T42.6X1** **Poisoning by other antiepileptic and sedative-hypnotic drugs, accidental (unintentional)**
Poisoning by other antiepileptic and sedative-hypnotic drugs NOS

² √7ᵗʰ **T42.6X2** **Poisoning by other antiepileptic and sedative-hypnotic drugs, intentional self-harm** ᴴᶜᶜ

√7ᵗʰ **T42.6X3** **Poisoning by other antiepileptic and sedative-hypnotic drugs, assault**

√7ᵗʰ **T42.6X4** **Poisoning by other antiepileptic and sedative-hypnotic drugs, undetermined**

√7ᵗʰ **T42.6X5** **Adverse effect of other antiepileptic and sedative-hypnotic drugs**

√7ᵗʰ **T42.6X6** **Underdosing of other antiepileptic and sedative-hypnotic drugs**

√5ᵗʰ **T42.7** **Poisoning by, adverse effect of and underdosing of unspecified antiepileptic and sedative-hypnotic drugs**

√x7ᵗʰ **T42.71** **Poisoning by unspecified antiepileptic and sedative-hypnotic drugs, accidental (unintentional)**
Poisoning by antiepileptic and sedative-hypnotic drugs NOS

² √x7ᵗʰ **T42.72** **Poisoning by unspecified antiepileptic and sedative-hypnotic drugs, intentional self-harm** ᴴᶜᶜ

√x7ᵗʰ **T42.73** **Poisoning by unspecified antiepileptic and sedative-hypnotic drugs, assault**

√x7ᵗʰ **T42.74** **Poisoning by unspecified antiepileptic and sedative-hypnotic drugs, undetermined**

√x7ᵗʰ **T42.75** **Adverse effect of unspecified antiepileptic and sedative-hypnotic drugs**

√x7ᵗʰ **T42.76** **Underdosing of unspecified antiepileptic and sedative-hypnotic drugs**

√5ᵗʰ **T42.8** **Poisoning by, adverse effect of and underdosing of antiparkinsonism drugs and other central muscle-tone depressants**
Poisoning by, adverse effect of and underdosing of amantadine

√6ᵗʰ **T42.8X** **Poisoning by, adverse effect of and underdosing of antiparkinsonism drugs and other central muscle-tone depressants**

√7ᵗʰ **T42.8X1** **Poisoning by antiparkinsonism drugs and other central muscle-tone depressants, accidental (unintentional)**
Poisoning by antiparkinsonism drugs and other central muscle-tone depressants NOS

² √7ᵗʰ **T42.8X2** **Poisoning by antiparkinsonism drugs and other central muscle-tone depressants, intentional self-harm** ᴴᶜᶜ

√7ᵗʰ **T42.8X3** **Poisoning by antiparkinsonism drugs and other central muscle-tone depressants, assault**

√7ᵗʰ **T42.8X4** **Poisoning by antiparkinsonism drugs and other central muscle-tone depressants, undetermined**

√7ᵗʰ **T42.8X5** **Adverse effect of antiparkinsonism drugs and other central muscle-tone depressants**

√7ᵗʰ **T42.8X6** **Underdosing of antiparkinsonism drugs and other central muscle-tone depressants**

✓4ᵗʰ **T43 Poisoning by, adverse effect of and underdosing of psychotropic drugs, not elsewhere classified**

    EXCLUDES 1   appetite depressants (T50.5-)
                    barbiturates (T42.3-)
                    benzodiazepines (T42.4-)
                    methaqualone (T42.6-)
                    psychodysleptics [hallucinogens] (T40.7-T40.9-)

    EXCLUDES 2   drug dependence and related mental and behavioral disorders due to psychoactive substance use (F10.- – F19.-)

> The appropriate 7th character is to be added to each code from category T43.
> A   initial encounter
> D   subsequent encounter
> S   sequela

✓5ᵗʰ **T43.0 Poisoning by, adverse effect of and underdosing of tricyclic and tetracyclic antidepressants**

    ✓6ᵗʰ **T43.01 Poisoning by, adverse effect of and underdosing of tricyclic antidepressants**

       ✓7ᵗʰ **T43.011 Poisoning by tricyclic antidepressants, accidental (unintentional)**
          Poisoning by tricyclic antidepressants NOS

       2 ✓7ᵗʰ **T43.012 Poisoning by tricyclic antidepressants, intentional self-harm**   HCC

       ✓7ᵗʰ **T43.013 Poisoning by tricyclic antidepressants, assault**

       ✓7ᵗʰ **T43.014 Poisoning by tricyclic antidepressants, undetermined**

       ✓7ᵗʰ **T43.015 Adverse effect of tricyclic antidepressants**

       ✓7ᵗʰ **T43.016 Underdosing of tricyclic antidepressants**

    ✓6ᵗʰ **T43.02 Poisoning by, adverse effect of and underdosing of tetracyclic antidepressants**

       ✓7ᵗʰ **T43.021 Poisoning by tetracyclic antidepressants, accidental (unintentional)**
          Poisoning by tetracyclic antidepressants NOS

       2 ✓7ᵗʰ **T43.022 Poisoning by tetracyclic antidepressants, intentional self-harm**   HCC

       ✓7ᵗʰ **T43.023 Poisoning by tetracyclic antidepressants, assault**

       ✓7ᵗʰ **T43.024 Poisoning by tetracyclic antidepressants, undetermined**

       ✓7ᵗʰ **T43.025 Adverse effect of tetracyclic antidepressants**

       ✓7ᵗʰ **T43.026 Underdosing of tetracyclic antidepressants**

✓5ᵗʰ **T43.1 Poisoning by, adverse effect of and underdosing of monoamine-oxidase-inhibitor antidepressants**

    ✓6ᵗʰ **T43.1X Poisoning by, adverse effect of and underdosing of monoamine-oxidase-inhibitor antidepressants**

       ✓7ᵗʰ **T43.1X1 Poisoning by monoamine-oxidase-inhibitor antidepressants, accidental (unintentional)**
          Poisoning by monoamine-oxidase-inhibitor antidepressants NOS

       2 ✓7ᵗʰ **T43.1X2 Poisoning by monoamine-oxidase-inhibitor antidepressants, intentional self-harm**   HCC

       ✓7ᵗʰ **T43.1X3 Poisoning by monoamine-oxidase-inhibitor antidepressants, assault**

       ✓7ᵗʰ **T43.1X4 Poisoning by monoamine-oxidase-inhibitor antidepressants, undetermined**

       ✓7ᵗʰ **T43.1X5 Adverse effect of monoamine-oxidase-inhibitor antidepressants**

       ✓7ᵗʰ **T43.1X6 Underdosing of monoamine-oxidase-inhibitor antidepressants**

✓5ᵗʰ **T43.2 Poisoning by, adverse effect of and underdosing of other and unspecified antidepressants**

    ✓6ᵗʰ **T43.20 Poisoning by, adverse effect of and underdosing of unspecified antidepressants**

       ✓7ᵗʰ **T43.201 Poisoning by unspecified antidepressants, accidental (unintentional)**
          Poisoning by antidepressants NOS

       2 ✓7ᵗʰ **T43.202 Poisoning by unspecified antidepressants, intentional self-harm**   HCC

       ✓7ᵗʰ **T43.203 Poisoning by unspecified antidepressants, assault**

       ✓7ᵗʰ **T43.204 Poisoning by unspecified antidepressants, undetermined**

       ✓7ᵗʰ **T43.205 Adverse effect of unspecified antidepressants**
          Antidepressant discontinuation syndrome

       ✓7ᵗʰ **T43.206 Underdosing of unspecified antidepressants**

    ✓6ᵗʰ **T43.21 Poisoning by, adverse effect of and underdosing of selective serotonin and norepinephrine reuptake inhibitors**
       Poisoning by, adverse effect of and underdosing of SSNRI antidepressants

       ✓7ᵗʰ **T43.211 Poisoning by selective serotonin and norepinephrine reuptake inhibitors, accidental (unintentional)**

       2 ✓7ᵗʰ **T43.212 Poisoning by selective serotonin and norepinephrine reuptake inhibitors, intentional self-harm**   HCC

       ✓7ᵗʰ **T43.213 Poisoning by selective serotonin and norepinephrine reuptake inhibitors, assault**

       ✓7ᵗʰ **T43.214 Poisoning by selective serotonin and norepinephrine reuptake inhibitors, undetermined**

       ✓7ᵗʰ **T43.215 Adverse effect of selective serotonin and norepinephrine reuptake inhibitors**

       ✓7ᵗʰ **T43.216 Underdosing of selective serotonin and norepinephrine reuptake inhibitors**

    ✓6ᵗʰ **T43.22 Poisoning by, adverse effect of and underdosing of selective serotonin reuptake inhibitors**
       Poisoning by, adverse effect of and underdosing of SSRI antidepressants

       ✓7ᵗʰ **T43.221 Poisoning by selective serotonin reuptake inhibitors, accidental (unintentional)**

       2 ✓7ᵗʰ **T43.222 Poisoning by selective serotonin reuptake inhibitors, intentional self-harm**   HCC

       ✓7ᵗʰ **T43.223 Poisoning by selective serotonin reuptake inhibitors, assault**

       ✓7ᵗʰ **T43.224 Poisoning by selective serotonin reuptake inhibitors, undetermined**

       ✓7ᵗʰ **T43.225 Adverse effect of selective serotonin reuptake inhibitors**

       ✓7ᵗʰ **T43.226 Underdosing of selective serotonin reuptake inhibitors**

    ✓6ᵗʰ **T43.29 Poisoning by, adverse effect of and underdosing of other antidepressants**

       ✓7ᵗʰ **T43.291 Poisoning by other antidepressants, accidental (unintentional)**
          Poisoning by other antidepressants NOS

       2 ✓7ᵗʰ **T43.292 Poisoning by other antidepressants, intentional self-harm**   HCC

       ✓7ᵗʰ **T43.293 Poisoning by other antidepressants, assault**

       ✓7ᵗʰ **T43.294 Poisoning by other antidepressants, undetermined**

       ✓7ᵗʰ **T43.295 Adverse effect of other antidepressants**

       ✓7ᵗʰ **T43.296 Underdosing of other antidepressants**

✓5ᵗʰ **T43.3 Poisoning by, adverse effect of and underdosing of phenothiazine antipsychotics and neuroleptics**

    ✓6ᵗʰ **T43.3X Poisoning by, adverse effect of and underdosing of phenothiazine antipsychotics and neuroleptics**

       ✓7ᵗʰ **T43.3X1 Poisoning by phenothiazine antipsychotics and neuroleptics, accidental (unintentional)**
          Poisoning by phenothiazine antipsychotics and neuroleptics NOS

✔ Additional Character Required   ✓x7ᵗʰ Placeholder Alert   Manifestation   Unspecified Dx   ▶◀ Revised Text   ● New Code   ▲ Revised Code Title

ICD-10-CM 2020   1105

² √7ᵗʰ **T43.3X2** **Poisoning by phenothiazine antipsychotics and neuroleptics, intentional self-harm** HCC

√7ᵗʰ **T43.3X3** **Poisoning by phenothiazine antipsychotics and neuroleptics, assault**

√7ᵗʰ **T43.3X4** **Poisoning by phenothiazine antipsychotics and neuroleptics, undetermined**

√7ᵗʰ **T43.3X5** Adverse effect of phenothiazine antipsychotics and neuroleptics

√7ᵗʰ **T43.3X6** Underdosing of phenothiazine antipsychotics and neuroleptics

√5ᵗʰ **T43.4** **Poisoning by, adverse effect of and underdosing of butyrophenone and thiothixene neuroleptics**

√6ᵗʰ **T43.4X** **Poisoning by, adverse effect of and underdosing of butyrophenone and thiothixene neuroleptics**

√7ᵗʰ **T43.4X1** **Poisoning by butyrophenone and thiothixene neuroleptics, accidental (unintentional)**
Poisoning by butyrophenone and thiothixene neuroleptics NOS

² √7ᵗʰ **T43.4X2** **Poisoning by butyrophenone and thiothixene neuroleptics, intentional self-harm** HCC

√7ᵗʰ **T43.4X3** **Poisoning by butyrophenone and thiothixene neuroleptics, assault**

√7ᵗʰ **T43.4X4** **Poisoning by butyrophenone and thiothixene neuroleptics, undetermined**

√7ᵗʰ **T43.4X5** Adverse effect of butyrophenone and thiothixene neuroleptics

√7ᵗʰ **T43.4X6** Underdosing of butyrophenone and thiothixene neuroleptics

√5ᵗʰ **T43.5** **Poisoning by, adverse effect of and underdosing of other and unspecified antipsychotics and neuroleptics**

EXCLUDES 1   poisoning by, adverse effect of and underdosing of rauwolfia (T46.5-)

√6ᵗʰ **T43.50** **Poisoning by, adverse effect of and underdosing of unspecified antipsychotics and neuroleptics**

√7ᵗʰ **T43.501** **Poisoning by unspecified antipsychotics and neuroleptics, accidental (unintentional)**
Poisoning by antipsychotics and neuroleptics NOS

² √7ᵗʰ **T43.502** **Poisoning by unspecified antipsychotics and neuroleptics, intentional self-harm** HCC

√7ᵗʰ **T43.503** **Poisoning by unspecified antipsychotics and neuroleptics, assault**

√7ᵗʰ **T43.504** **Poisoning by unspecified antipsychotics and neuroleptics, undetermined**

√7ᵗʰ **T43.505** Adverse effect of unspecified antipsychotics and neuroleptics

√7ᵗʰ **T43.506** Underdosing of unspecified antipsychotics and neuroleptics

√6ᵗʰ **T43.59** **Poisoning by, adverse effect of and underdosing of other antipsychotics and neuroleptics**
AHA: 2017, 1Q, 40

√7ᵗʰ **T43.591** **Poisoning by other antipsychotics and neuroleptics, accidental (unintentional)**
Poisoning by other antipsychotics and neuroleptics NOS

² √7ᵗʰ **T43.592** **Poisoning by other antipsychotics and neuroleptics, intentional self-harm** HCC

√7ᵗʰ **T43.593** **Poisoning by other antipsychotics and neuroleptics, assault**

√7ᵗʰ **T43.594** **Poisoning by other antipsychotics and neuroleptics, undetermined**

√7ᵗʰ **T43.595** Adverse effect of other antipsychotics and neuroleptics

√7ᵗʰ **T43.596** Underdosing of other antipsychotics and neuroleptics

√5ᵗʰ **T43.6** **Poisoning by, adverse effect of and underdosing of psychostimulants**

EXCLUDES 1   poisoning by, adverse effect of and underdosing of cocaine (T40.5-)

√6ᵗʰ **T43.60** **Poisoning by, adverse effect of and underdosing of unspecified psychostimulant**

¹ √7ᵗʰ **T43.601** **Poisoning by unspecified psychostimulants, accidental (unintentional)** HCC
Poisoning by psychostimulants NOS

² √7ᵗʰ **T43.602** **Poisoning by unspecified psychostimulants, intentional self-harm** HCC

√7ᵗʰ **T43.603** **Poisoning by unspecified psychostimulants, assault**

¹ √7ᵗʰ **T43.604** **Poisoning by unspecified psychostimulants, undetermined** HCC

√7ᵗʰ **T43.605** Adverse effect of unspecified psychostimulants

√7ᵗʰ **T43.606** Underdosing of unspecified psychostimulants

√6ᵗʰ **T43.61** **Poisoning by, adverse effect of and underdosing of caffeine**

¹ √7ᵗʰ **T43.611** **Poisoning by caffeine, accidental (unintentional)** HCC
Poisoning by caffeine NOS

² √7ᵗʰ **T43.612** **Poisoning by caffeine, intentional self-harm** HCC

√7ᵗʰ **T43.613** **Poisoning by caffeine, assault**

¹ √7ᵗʰ **T43.614** **Poisoning by caffeine, undetermined** HCC

√7ᵗʰ **T43.615** Adverse effect of caffeine

√7ᵗʰ **T43.616** Underdosing of caffeine

√6ᵗʰ **T43.62** **Poisoning by, adverse effect of and underdosing of amphetamines**
Poisoning by, adverse effect of and underdosing of methamphetamines

¹ √7ᵗʰ **T43.621** **Poisoning by amphetamines, accidental (unintentional)** HCC
Poisoning by amphetamines NOS

² √7ᵗʰ **T43.622** **Poisoning by amphetamines, intentional self-harm** HCC

√7ᵗʰ **T43.623** **Poisoning by amphetamines, assault**

¹ √7ᵗʰ **T43.624** **Poisoning by amphetamines, undetermined** HCC

√7ᵗʰ **T43.625** Adverse effect of amphetamines

√7ᵗʰ **T43.626** Underdosing of amphetamines

√6ᵗʰ **T43.63** **Poisoning by, adverse effect of and underdosing of methylphenidate**

¹ √7ᵗʰ **T43.631** **Poisoning by methylphenidate, accidental (unintentional)** HCC
Poisoning by methylphenidate NOS

² √7ᵗʰ **T43.632** **Poisoning by methylphenidate, intentional self-harm** HCC

√7ᵗʰ **T43.633** **Poisoning by methylphenidate, assault**

¹ √7ᵗʰ **T43.634** **Poisoning by methylphenidate, undetermined** HCC

√7ᵗʰ **T43.635** Adverse effect of methylphenidate

√7ᵗʰ **T43.636** Underdosing of methylphenidate

√6ᵗʰ **T43.64** **Poisoning by ecstasy**
Poisoning by MDMA
Poisoning by 3,4-methylenedioxymethamphetamine
AHA: 2018, 4Q, 30-31

¹ √7ᵗʰ **T43.641** **Poisoning by ecstasy, accidental (unintentional)** HCC
Poisoning by ecstasy NOS

² √7ᵗʰ **T43.642** **Poisoning by ecstasy, intentional self-harm** HCC

√7ᵗʰ **T43.643** **Poisoning by ecstasy, assault**

¹ √7ᵗʰ **T43.644** **Poisoning by ecstasy, undetermined** HCC

√6ᵗʰ **T43.69** **Poisoning by, adverse effect of and underdosing of other psychostimulants**

¹ √7ᵗʰ **T43.691** **Poisoning by other psychostimulants, accidental (unintentional)** HCC
Poisoning by other psychostimulants NOS

² √7ᵗʰ **T43.692** **Poisoning by other psychostimulants, intentional self-harm** HCC

√7ᵗʰ **T43.693** **Poisoning by other psychostimulants, assault**

¹ √7ᵗʰ **T43.694** **Poisoning by other psychostimulants, undetermined** HCC

√7ᵗʰ **T43.695** Adverse effect of other psychostimulants

√7ᵗʰ **T43.696** Underdosing of other psychostimulants

√5ᵗʰ **T43.8** **Poisoning by, adverse effect of and underdosing of other psychotropic drugs**
√6ᵗʰ **T43.8X** **Poisoning by, adverse effect of and underdosing of other psychotropic drugs**
√7ᵗʰ **T43.8X1** **Poisoning by other psychotropic drugs, accidental (unintentional)**
Poisoning by other psychotropic drugs NOS
² √7ᵗʰ **T43.8X2** **Poisoning by other psychotropic drugs, intentional self-harm** HCC
√7ᵗʰ **T43.8X3** **Poisoning by other psychotropic drugs, assault**
√7ᵗʰ **T43.8X4** **Poisoning by other psychotropic drugs, undetermined**
√7ᵗʰ **T43.8X5** **Adverse effect of other psychotropic drugs**
√7ᵗʰ **T43.8X6** **Underdosing of other psychotropic drugs**
√5ᵗʰ **T43.9** **Poisoning by, adverse effect of and underdosing of unspecified psychotropic drug**
√x7ᵗʰ **T43.91** **Poisoning by unspecified psychotropic drug, accidental (unintentional)**
Poisoning by psychotropic drug NOS
² √x7ᵗʰ **T43.92** **Poisoning by unspecified psychotropic drug, intentional self-harm** HCC
√x7ᵗʰ **T43.93** **Poisoning by unspecified psychotropic drug, assault**
√x7ᵗʰ **T43.94** **Poisoning by unspecified psychotropic drug, undetermined**
√x7ᵗʰ **T43.95** **Adverse effect of unspecified psychotropic drug**
√x7ᵗʰ **T43.96** **Underdosing of unspecified psychotropic drug**

√4ᵗʰ **T44** **Poisoning by, adverse effect of and underdosing of drugs primarily affecting the autonomic nervous system**

The appropriate 7th character is to be added to each code from category T44.
A initial encounter
D subsequent encounter
S sequela

√5ᵗʰ **T44.0** **Poisoning by, adverse effect of and underdosing of anticholinesterase agents**
√6ᵗʰ **T44.0X** **Poisoning by, adverse effect of and underdosing of anticholinesterase agents**
√7ᵗʰ **T44.0X1** **Poisoning by anticholinesterase agents, accidental (unintentional)**
Poisoning by anticholinesterase agents NOS
² √7ᵗʰ **T44.0X2** **Poisoning by anticholinesterase agents, intentional self-harm** HCC
√7ᵗʰ **T44.0X3** **Poisoning by anticholinesterase agents, assault**
√7ᵗʰ **T44.0X4** **Poisoning by anticholinesterase agents, undetermined**
√7ᵗʰ **T44.0X5** **Adverse effect of anticholinesterase agents**
√7ᵗʰ **T44.0X6** **Underdosing of anticholinesterase agents**
√5ᵗʰ **T44.1** **Poisoning by, adverse effect of and underdosing of other parasympathomimetics [cholinergics]**
√6ᵗʰ **T44.1X** **Poisoning by, adverse effect of and underdosing of other parasympathomimetics [cholinergics]**
√7ᵗʰ **T44.1X1** **Poisoning by other parasympathomimetics [cholinergics], accidental (unintentional)**
Poisoning by other parasympathomimetics [cholinergics] NOS
² √7ᵗʰ **T44.1X2** **Poisoning by other parasympathomimetics [cholinergics], intentional self-harm** HCC
√7ᵗʰ **T44.1X3** **Poisoning by other parasympathomimetics [cholinergics], assault**
√7ᵗʰ **T44.1X4** **Poisoning by other parasympathomimetics [cholinergics], undetermined**
√7ᵗʰ **T44.1X5** **Adverse effect of other parasympathomimetics [cholinergics]**
√7ᵗʰ **T44.1X6** **Underdosing of other parasympathomimetics [cholinergics]**

√5ᵗʰ **T44.2** **Poisoning by, adverse effect of and underdosing of ganglionic blocking drugs**
√6ᵗʰ **T44.2X** **Poisoning by, adverse effect of and underdosing of ganglionic blocking drugs**
√7ᵗʰ **T44.2X1** **Poisoning by ganglionic blocking drugs, accidental (unintentional)**
Poisoning by ganglionic blocking drugs NOS
² √7ᵗʰ **T44.2X2** **Poisoning by ganglionic blocking drugs, intentional self-harm** HCC
√7ᵗʰ **T44.2X3** **Poisoning by ganglionic blocking drugs, assault**
√7ᵗʰ **T44.2X4** **Poisoning by ganglionic blocking drugs, undetermined**
√7ᵗʰ **T44.2X5** **Adverse effect of ganglionic blocking drugs**
√7ᵗʰ **T44.2X6** **Underdosing of ganglionic blocking drugs**
√5ᵗʰ **T44.3** **Poisoning by, adverse effect of and underdosing of other parasympatholytics [anticholinergics and antimuscarinics] and spasmolytics**
Poisoning by, adverse effect of and underdosing of papaverine
√6ᵗʰ **T44.3X** **Poisoning by, adverse effect of and underdosing of other parasympatholytics [anticholinergics and antimuscarinics] and spasmolytics**
√7ᵗʰ **T44.3X1** **Poisoning by other parasympatholytics [anticholinergics and antimuscarinics] and spasmolytics, accidental (unintentional)**
Poisoning by other parasympatholytics [anticholinergics and antimuscarinics] and spasmolytics NOS
² √7ᵗʰ **T44.3X2** **Poisoning by other parasympatholytics [anticholinergics and antimuscarinics] and spasmolytics, intentional self-harm** HCC
√7ᵗʰ **T44.3X3** **Poisoning by other parasympatholytics [anticholinergics and antimuscarinics] and spasmolytics, assault**
√7ᵗʰ **T44.3X4** **Poisoning by other parasympatholytics [anticholinergics and antimuscarinics] and spasmolytics, undetermined**
√7ᵗʰ **T44.3X5** **Adverse effect of other parasympatholytics [anticholinergics and antimuscarinics] and spasmolytics**
√7ᵗʰ **T44.3X6** **Underdosing of other parasympatholytics [anticholinergics and antimuscarinics] and spasmolytics**
√5ᵗʰ **T44.4** **Poisoning by, adverse effect of and underdosing of predominantly alpha-adrenoreceptor agonists**
Poisoning by, adverse effect of and underdosing of metaraminol
√6ᵗʰ **T44.4X** **Poisoning by, adverse effect of and underdosing of predominantly alpha-adrenoreceptor agonists**
√7ᵗʰ **T44.4X1** **Poisoning by predominantly alpha-adrenoreceptor agonists, accidental (unintentional)**
Poisoning by predominantly alpha-adrenoreceptor agonists NOS
² √7ᵗʰ **T44.4X2** **Poisoning by predominantly alpha-adrenoreceptor agonists, intentional self-harm** HCC
√7ᵗʰ **T44.4X3** **Poisoning by predominantly alpha-adrenoreceptor agonists, assault**
√7ᵗʰ **T44.4X4** **Poisoning by predominantly alpha-adrenoreceptor agonists, undetermined**
√7ᵗʰ **T44.4X5** **Adverse effect of predominantly alpha-adrenoreceptor agonists**
√7ᵗʰ **T44.4X6** **Underdosing of predominantly alpha-adrenoreceptor agonists**

√5ᵗʰ **T44.5 Poisoning by, adverse effect of and underdosing of predominantly beta-adrenoreceptor agonists**

     EXCLUDES 1   *poisoning by, adverse effect of and underdosing of beta-adrenoreceptor agonists used in asthma therapy (T48.6-)*

   √6ᵗʰ **T44.5X Poisoning by, adverse effect of and underdosing of predominantly beta-adrenoreceptor agonists**

     √7ᵗʰ **T44.5X1 Poisoning by predominantly beta-adrenoreceptor agonists, accidental (unintentional)**

       Poisoning by predominantly beta-adrenoreceptor agonists NOS

     ² √7ᵗʰ **T44.5X2 Poisoning by predominantly beta-adrenoreceptor agonists, intentional self-harm**   HCC

     √7ᵗʰ **T44.5X3 Poisoning by predominantly beta-adrenoreceptor agonists, assault**

     √7ᵗʰ **T44.5X4 Poisoning by predominantly beta-adrenoreceptor agonists, undetermined**

     √7ᵗʰ **T44.5X5 Adverse effect of predominantly beta-adrenoreceptor agonists**

     √7ᵗʰ **T44.5X6 Underdosing of predominantly beta-adrenoreceptor agonists**

√5ᵗʰ **T44.6 Poisoning by, adverse effect of and underdosing of alpha-adrenoreceptor antagonists**

     EXCLUDES 1   *poisoning by, adverse effect of and underdosing of ergot alkaloids (T48.0)*

   √6ᵗʰ **T44.6X Poisoning by, adverse effect of and underdosing of alpha-adrenoreceptor antagonists**

     √7ᵗʰ **T44.6X1 Poisoning by alpha-adrenoreceptor antagonists, accidental (unintentional)**

       Poisoning by alpha-adrenoreceptor antagonists NOS

     ² √7ᵗʰ **T44.6X2 Poisoning by alpha-adrenoreceptor antagonists, intentional self-harm**   HCC

     √7ᵗʰ **T44.6X3 Poisoning by alpha-adrenoreceptor antagonists, assault**

     √7ᵗʰ **T44.6X4 Poisoning by alpha-adrenoreceptor antagonists, undetermined**

     √7ᵗʰ **T44.6X5 Adverse effect of alpha-adrenoreceptor antagonists**

     √7ᵗʰ **T44.6X6 Underdosing of alpha-adrenoreceptor antagonists**

√5ᵗʰ **T44.7 Poisoning by, adverse effect of and underdosing of beta-adrenoreceptor antagonists**

   √6ᵗʰ **T44.7X Poisoning by, adverse effect of and underdosing of beta-adrenoreceptor antagonists**

     √7ᵗʰ **T44.7X1 Poisoning by beta-adrenoreceptor antagonists, accidental (unintentional)**

       Poisoning by beta-adrenoreceptor antagonists NOS

     ² √7ᵗʰ **T44.7X2 Poisoning by beta-adrenoreceptor antagonists, intentional self-harm**   HCC

     √7ᵗʰ **T44.7X3 Poisoning by beta-adrenoreceptor antagonists, assault**

     √7ᵗʰ **T44.7X4 Poisoning by beta-adrenoreceptor antagonists, undetermined**

     √7ᵗʰ **T44.7X5 Adverse effect of beta-adrenoreceptor antagonists**

     √7ᵗʰ **T44.7X6 Underdosing of beta-adrenoreceptor antagonists**

√5ᵗʰ **T44.8 Poisoning by, adverse effect of and underdosing of centrally-acting and adrenergic-neuron- blocking agents**

     EXCLUDES 1   *poisoning by, adverse effect of and underdosing of clonidine (T46.5)*

         poisoning by, adverse effect of and underdosing of guanethidine (T46.5)

   √6ᵗʰ **T44.8X Poisoning by, adverse effect of and underdosing of centrally-acting and adrenergic- neuron-blocking agents**

     √7ᵗʰ **T44.8X1 Poisoning by centrally-acting and adrenergic-neuron-blocking agents, accidental (unintentional)**

       Poisoning by centrally-acting and adrenergic-neuron-blocking agents NOS

     ² √7ᵗʰ **T44.8X2 Poisoning by centrally-acting and adrenergic-neuron-blocking agents, intentional self-harm**   HCC

     √7ᵗʰ **T44.8X3 Poisoning by centrally-acting and adrenergic-neuron-blocking agents, assault**

     √7ᵗʰ **T44.8X4 Poisoning by centrally-acting and adrenergic-neuron-blocking agents, undetermined**

     √7ᵗʰ **T44.8X5 Adverse effect of centrally-acting and adrenergic-neuron-blocking agents**

     √7ᵗʰ **T44.8X6 Underdosing of centrally-acting and adrenergic-neuron-blocking agents**

√5ᵗʰ **T44.9 Poisoning by, adverse effect of and underdosing of other and unspecified drugs primarily affecting the autonomic nervous system**

     Poisoning by, adverse effect of and underdosing of drug stimulating both alpha and beta-adrenoreceptors

   √6ᵗʰ **T44.90 Poisoning by, adverse effect of and underdosing of unspecified drugs primarily affecting the autonomic nervous system**

     √7ᵗʰ **T44.901 Poisoning by unspecified drugs primarily affecting the autonomic nervous system, accidental (unintentional)**

       Poisoning by unspecified drugs primarily affecting the autonomic nervous system NOS

     ² √7ᵗʰ **T44.902 Poisoning by unspecified drugs primarily affecting the autonomic nervous system, intentional self-harm**   HCC

     √7ᵗʰ **T44.903 Poisoning by unspecified drugs primarily affecting the autonomic nervous system, assault**

     √7ᵗʰ **T44.904 Poisoning by unspecified drugs primarily affecting the autonomic nervous system, undetermined**

     √7ᵗʰ **T44.905 Adverse effect of unspecified drugs primarily affecting the autonomic nervous system**

     √7ᵗʰ **T44.906 Underdosing of unspecified drugs primarily affecting the autonomic nervous system**

   √6ᵗʰ **T44.99 Poisoning by, adverse effect of and underdosing of other drugs primarily affecting the autonomic nervous system**

     √7ᵗʰ **T44.991 Poisoning by other drug primarily affecting the autonomic nervous system, accidental (unintentional)**

       Poisoning by other drugs primarily affecting the autonomic nervous system NOS

     ² √7ᵗʰ **T44.992 Poisoning by other drug primarily affecting the autonomic nervous system, intentional self-harm**   HCC

     √7ᵗʰ **T44.993 Poisoning by other drug primarily affecting the autonomic nervous system, assault**

     √7ᵗʰ **T44.994 Poisoning by other drug primarily affecting the autonomic nervous system, undetermined**

     √7ᵗʰ **T44.995 Adverse effect of other drug primarily affecting the autonomic nervous system**

     √7ᵗʰ **T44.996 Underdosing of other drug primarily affecting the autonomic nervous system**

√4ᵗʰ **T45 Poisoning by, adverse effect of and underdosing of primarily systemic and hematological agents, not elsewhere classified**

     The appropriate 7th character is to be added to each code from category T45.
     A   initial encounter
     D   subsequent encounter
     S   sequela

√5ᵗʰ **T45.0 Poisoning by, adverse effect of and underdosing of antiallergic and antiemetic drugs**

     EXCLUDES 1   *poisoning by, adverse effect of and underdosing of phenothiazine-based neuroleptics (T43.3)*

   √6ᵗʰ **T45.0X Poisoning by, adverse effect of and underdosing of antiallergic and antiemetic drugs**

     √7ᵗʰ **T45.0X1 Poisoning by antiallergic and antiemetic drugs, accidental (unintentional)**

       Poisoning by antiallergic and antiemetic drugs NOS

     ² √7ᵗʰ **T45.0X2 Poisoning by antiallergic and antiemetic drugs, intentional self-harm**   HCC

√7th **T45.0X3** **Poisoning** by antiallergic and antiemetic drugs, **assault**

√7th **T45.0X4** **Poisoning** by antiallergic and antiemetic drugs, **undetermined**

√7th **T45.0X5** **Adverse effect** of antiallergic and antiemetic drugs

√7th **T45.0X6** **Underdosing** of antiallergic and antiemetic drugs

√5th **T45.1** **Poisoning by, adverse effect of and underdosing of antineoplastic and immunosuppressive drugs**

EXCLUDES 1   *poisoning by, adverse effect of and underdosing of tamoxifen (T38.6)*

AHA: 2019,1Q,17,20; 2014,4Q,22

√6th **T45.1X** **Poisoning by, adverse effect of and underdosing of** antineoplastic and immunosuppressive drugs

√7th **T45.1X1** **Poisoning** by antineoplastic and immunosuppressive drugs, **accidental (unintentional)**

Poisoning by antineoplastic and immunosuppressive drugs NOS

2 √7th **T45.1X2** **Poisoning** by antineoplastic and immunosuppressive drugs, **intentional self-harm**   HCC

√7th **T45.1X3** **Poisoning** by antineoplastic and immunosuppressive drugs, **assault**

√7th **T45.1X4** **Poisoning** by antineoplastic and immunosuppressive drugs, **undetermined**

√7th **T45.1X5** **Adverse effect** of antineoplastic and immunosuppressive drugs

AHA: 2019,2Q,24,28

√7th **T45.1X6** **Underdosing** of antineoplastic and immunosuppressive drugs

√5th **T45.2** **Poisoning by, adverse effect of and underdosing of vitamins**

EXCLUDES 2   *poisoning by, adverse effect of and underdosing of iron (T45.4)*

poisoning by, adverse effect of and underdosing of nicotinic acid (derivatives) (T46.7)

poisoning by, adverse effect of and underdosing of vitamin K (T45.7)

√6th **T45.2X** **Poisoning by, adverse effect of and underdosing of** vitamins

√7th **T45.2X1** **Poisoning** by vitamins, **accidental (unintentional)**

Poisoning by vitamins NOS

2 √7th **T45.2X2** **Poisoning** by vitamins, **intentional self-harm**   HCC

√7th **T45.2X3** **Poisoning** by vitamins, **assault**

√7th **T45.2X4** **Poisoning** by vitamins, **undetermined**

√7th **T45.2X5** **Adverse effect** of vitamins

√7th **T45.2X6** **Underdosing** of vitamins

EXCLUDES 1   *vitamin deficiencies (E50-E56)*

√5th **T45.3** **Poisoning by, adverse effect of and underdosing of enzymes**

√6th **T45.3X** **Poisoning by, adverse effect of and underdosing of** enzymes

√7th **T45.3X1** **Poisoning** by enzymes, **accidental (unintentional)**

Poisoning by enzymes NOS

2 √7th **T45.3X2** **Poisoning** by enzymes, **intentional self-harm**   HCC

√7th **T45.3X3** **Poisoning** by enzymes, **assault**

√7th **T45.3X4** **Poisoning** by enzymes, **undetermined**

√7th **T45.3X5** **Adverse effect** of enzymes

√7th **T45.3X6** **Underdosing** of enzymes

√5th **T45.4** **Poisoning by, adverse effect of and underdosing of iron and its compounds**

√6th **T45.4X** **Poisoning by, adverse effect of and underdosing of** iron and its compounds

√7th **T45.4X1** **Poisoning** by iron and its compounds, **accidental (unintentional)**

Poisoning by iron and its compounds NOS

2 √7th **T45.4X2** **Poisoning** by iron and its compounds, **intentional self-harm**   HCC

√7th **T45.4X3** **Poisoning** by iron and its compounds, **assault**

√7th **T45.4X4** **Poisoning** by iron and its compounds, **undetermined**

√7th **T45.4X5** **Adverse effect** of iron and its compounds

√7th **T45.4X6** **Underdosing** of iron and its compounds

EXCLUDES 1   *iron deficiency (E61.1)*

√5th **T45.5** **Poisoning by, adverse effect of and underdosing of anticoagulants and antithrombotic drugs**

√6th **T45.51** **Poisoning by, adverse effect of and underdosing of anticoagulants**

√7th **T45.511** **Poisoning** by anticoagulants, **accidental (unintentional)**

Poisoning by anticoagulants NOS

2 √7th **T45.512** **Poisoning** by anticoagulants, **intentional self-harm**   HCC

√7th **T45.513** **Poisoning** by anticoagulants, **assault**

√7th **T45.514** **Poisoning** by anticoagulants, **undetermined**

√7th **T45.515** **Adverse effect** of anticoagulants

AHA: 2016,1Q,14; 2013,2Q,34

√7th **T45.516** **Underdosing** of anticoagulants

√6th **T45.52** **Poisoning by, adverse effect of and underdosing of** antithrombotic drugs

Poisoning by, adverse effect of and underdosing of antiplatelet drugs

EXCLUDES 2   *poisoning by, adverse effect of and underdosing of aspirin (T39.01-)*

poisoning by, adverse effect of and underdosing of acetylsalicylic acid (T39.01-)

√7th **T45.521** **Poisoning** by antithrombotic drugs, **accidental (unintentional)**

Poisoning by antithrombotic drug NOS

2 √7th **T45.522** **Poisoning** by antithrombotic drugs, **intentional self-harm**   HCC

√7th **T45.523** **Poisoning** by antithrombotic drugs, **assault**

√7th **T45.524** **Poisoning** by antithrombotic drugs, **undetermined**

√7th **T45.525** **Adverse effect** of antithrombotic drugs

AHA: 2016,1Q,15

√7th **T45.526** **Underdosing** of antithrombotic drugs

√5th **T45.6** **Poisoning by, adverse effect of and underdosing of fibrinolysis-affecting drugs**

√6th **T45.60** **Poisoning by, adverse effect of and underdosing of unspecified fibrinolysis-affecting drugs**

√7th **T45.601** **Poisoning** by unspecified fibrinolysis-affecting drugs, **accidental (unintentional)**

Poisoning by fibrinolysis-affecting drug NOS

2 √7th **T45.602** **Poisoning** by unspecified fibrinolysis-affecting drugs, **intentional self-harm**   HCC

√7th **T45.603** **Poisoning** by unspecified fibrinolysis-affecting drugs, **assault**

√7th **T45.604** **Poisoning** by unspecified fibrinolysis-affecting drugs, **undetermined**

√7th **T45.605** **Adverse effect** of unspecified fibrinolysis-affecting drugs

√7th **T45.606** **Underdosing** of unspecified fibrinolysis-affecting drugs

√6th **T45.61** **Poisoning by, adverse effect of and underdosing of** thrombolytic drugs

√7th **T45.611** **Poisoning** by thrombolytic drug, **accidental (unintentional)**

Poisoning by thrombolytic drug NOS

2 √7th **T45.612** **Poisoning** by thrombolytic drug, **intentional self-harm**   HCC

√7th **T45.613** **Poisoning** by thrombolytic drug, **assault**

√7th **T45.614** **Poisoning** by thrombolytic drug, **undetermined**

√7th **T45.615** **Adverse effect** of thrombolytic drugs

AHA: 2017,2Q,9

√7th **T45.616** **Underdosing** of thrombolytic drugs

√6th **T45.62** **Poisoning by, adverse effect of and underdosing of** hemostatic drugs

√7th **T45.621** **Poisoning** by hemostatic drug, **accidental (unintentional)**

Poisoning by hemostatic drug NOS

2 √7th **T45.622** **Poisoning** by hemostatic drug, **intentional self-harm**   HCC

✔ Additional Character Required	√x7th Placeholder Alert	Manifestation	Unspecified Dx	◄► Revised Text	● New Code	▲ Revised Code Title

Chapter 19. Injury, Poisoning and Certain Other Consequences of External Causes

T45.623–T46.2X3

√7ᵗʰ **T45.623 Poisoning by hemostatic drug,** assault

√7ᵗʰ **T45.624 Poisoning by hemostatic drug,** undetermined

√7ᵗʰ **T45.625 Adverse effect of hemostatic drug**

√7ᵗʰ **T45.626 Underdosing of hemostatic drugs**

√6ᵗʰ **T45.69 Poisoning by, adverse effect of and underdosing of other fibrinolysis-affecting drugs**

√7ᵗʰ **T45.691 Poisoning by other fibrinolysis-affecting drugs,** accidental (unintentional)
Poisoning by other fibrinolysis-affecting drug NOS

2 √7ᵗʰ **T45.692 Poisoning by other fibrinolysis-affecting drugs,** intentional self-harm   HCC

√7ᵗʰ **T45.693 Poisoning by other fibrinolysis-affecting drugs,** assault

√7ᵗʰ **T45.694 Poisoning by other fibrinolysis-affecting drugs,** undetermined

√7ᵗʰ **T45.695 Adverse effect of other fibrinolysis-affecting drugs**

√7ᵗʰ **T45.696 Underdosing of other fibrinolysis-affecting drugs**

√5ᵗʰ **T45.7 Poisoning by, adverse effect of and underdosing of anticoagulant antagonists, vitamin K and other coagulants**

√6ᵗʰ **T45.7X Poisoning by, adverse effect of and underdosing of anticoagulant antagonists, vitamin K and other coagulants**

√7ᵗʰ **T45.7X1 Poisoning by anticoagulant antagonists, vitamin K and other coagulants,** accidental (unintentional)
Poisoning by anticoagulant antagonists, vitamin K and other coagulants NOS

2 √7ᵗʰ **T45.7X2 Poisoning by anticoagulant antagonists, vitamin K and other coagulants,** intentional self-harm   HCC

√7ᵗʰ **T45.7X3 Poisoning by anticoagulant antagonists, vitamin K and other coagulants,** assault

√7ᵗʰ **T45.7X4 Poisoning by anticoagulant antagonists, vitamin K and other coagulants,** undetermined

√7ᵗʰ **T45.7X5 Adverse effect of anticoagulant antagonists, vitamin K and other coagulants**

√7ᵗʰ **T45.7X6 Underdosing of anticoagulant antagonist, vitamin K and other coagulants**
EXCLUDES 1   vitamin K deficiency (E56.1)

√5ᵗʰ **T45.8 Poisoning by, adverse effect of and underdosing of other primarily systemic and hematological agents**
Poisoning by, adverse effect of and underdosing of liver preparations and other antianemic agents
Poisoning by, adverse effect of and underdosing of natural blood and blood products
Poisoning by, adverse effect of and underdosing of plasma substitute
EXCLUDES 2   poisoning by, adverse effect of and underdosing of immunoglobulin (T50.Z1)
poisoning by, adverse effect of and underdosing of iron (T45.4)
transfusion reactions (T80.-)

√6ᵗʰ **T45.8X Poisoning by, adverse effect of and underdosing of other primarily systemic and hematological agents**

√7ᵗʰ **T45.8X1 Poisoning by other primarily systemic and hematological agents,** accidental (unintentional)
Poisoning by other primarily systemic and hematological agents NOS

2 √7ᵗʰ **T45.8X2 Poisoning by other primarily systemic and hematological agents,** intentional self-harm   HCC

√7ᵗʰ **T45.8X3 Poisoning by other primarily systemic and hematological agents,** assault

√7ᵗʰ **T45.8X4 Poisoning by other primarily systemic and hematological agents,** undetermined

√7ᵗʰ **T45.8X5 Adverse effect of other primarily systemic and hematological agents**
AHA: 2016,4Q,42

√7ᵗʰ **T45.8X6 Underdosing of other primarily systemic and hematological agents**

√5ᵗʰ **T45.9 Poisoning by, adverse effect of and underdosing of unspecified primarily systemic and hematological agent**

√x7ᵗʰ **T45.91 Poisoning by unspecified primarily systemic and hematological agent,** accidental (unintentional)
Poisoning by primarily systemic and hematological agent NOS

2 √x7ᵗʰ **T45.92 Poisoning by unspecified primarily systemic and hematological agent,** intentional self-harm   HCC

√x7ᵗʰ **T45.93 Poisoning by unspecified primarily systemic and hematological agent,** assault

√x7ᵗʰ **T45.94 Poisoning by unspecified primarily systemic and hematological agent,** undetermined

√x7ᵗʰ **T45.95 Adverse effect of unspecified primarily systemic and hematological agent**

√x7ᵗʰ **T45.96 Underdosing of unspecified primarily systemic and hematological agent**

√4ᵗʰ **T46 Poisoning by, adverse effect of and underdosing of agents primarily affecting the cardiovascular system**
EXCLUDES 1   poisoning by, adverse effect of and underdosing of metaraminol (T44.4)

The appropriate 7th character is to be added to each code from category T46.
A   initial encounter
D   subsequent encounter
S   sequela

√5ᵗʰ **T46.0 Poisoning by, adverse effect of and underdosing of cardiac-stimulant glycosides and drugs of similar action**

√6ᵗʰ **T46.0X Poisoning by, adverse effect of and underdosing of cardiac-stimulant glycosides and drugs of similar action**

√7ᵗʰ **T46.0X1 Poisoning by cardiac-stimulant glycosides and drugs of similar action,** accidental (unintentional)
Poisoning by cardiac-stimulant glycosides and drugs of similar action NOS

2 √7ᵗʰ **T46.0X2 Poisoning by cardiac-stimulant glycosides and drugs of similar action,** intentional self-harm   HCC

√7ᵗʰ **T46.0X3 Poisoning by cardiac-stimulant glycosides and drugs of similar action,** assault

√7ᵗʰ **T46.0X4 Poisoning by cardiac-stimulant glycosides and drugs of similar action,** undetermined

√7ᵗʰ **T46.0X5 Adverse effect of cardiac-stimulant glycosides and drugs of similar action**

√7ᵗʰ **T46.0X6 Underdosing of cardiac-stimulant glycosides and drugs of similar action**

√5ᵗʰ **T46.1 Poisoning by, adverse effect of and underdosing of calcium-channel blockers**

√6ᵗʰ **T46.1X Poisoning by, adverse effect of and underdosing of calcium-channel blockers**

√7ᵗʰ **T46.1X1 Poisoning by calcium-channel blockers,** accidental (unintentional)
Poisoning by calcium-channel blockers NOS

2 √7ᵗʰ **T46.1X2 Poisoning by calcium-channel blockers,** intentional self-harm   HCC

√7ᵗʰ **T46.1X3 Poisoning by calcium-channel blockers,** assault

√7ᵗʰ **T46.1X4 Poisoning by calcium-channel blockers,** undetermined

√7ᵗʰ **T46.1X5 Adverse effect of calcium-channel blockers**

√7ᵗʰ **T46.1X6 Underdosing of calcium-channel blockers**

√5ᵗʰ **T46.2 Poisoning by, adverse effect of and underdosing of other antidysrhythmic drugs, not elsewhere classified**
EXCLUDES 1   poisoning by, adverse effect of and underdosing of beta-adrenoreceptor antagonists (T44.7-)

√6ᵗʰ **T46.2X Poisoning by, adverse effect of and underdosing of other antidysrhythmic drugs**

√7ᵗʰ **T46.2X1 Poisoning by other antidysrhythmic drugs,** accidental (unintentional)
Poisoning by other antidysrhythmic drugs NOS

2 √7ᵗʰ **T46.2X2 Poisoning by other antidysrhythmic drugs,** intentional self-harm   HCC

√7ᵗʰ **T46.2X3 Poisoning by other antidysrhythmic drugs,** assault

☑7ᵗʰ **T46.2X4 Poisoning by other antidysrhythmic drugs,** undetermined

☑7ᵗʰ **T46.2X5 Adverse effect** of other antidysrhythmic **drugs**

☑7ᵗʰ **T46.2X6 Underdosing** of other antidysrhythmic **drugs**

☑5ᵗʰ **T46.3 Poisoning by, adverse effect of and underdosing of coronary vasodilators**

Poisoning by, adverse effect of and underdosing of dipyridamole

EXCLUDES 1   *poisoning by, adverse effect of and underdosing of calcium-channel blockers (T46.1)*

☑6ᵗʰ **T46.3X Poisoning by, adverse effect of and underdosing of coronary vasodilators**

☑7ᵗʰ **T46.3X1 Poisoning by coronary vasodilators,** accidental **(unintentional)**

Poisoning by coronary vasodilators NOS

² ☑7ᵗʰ **T46.3X2 Poisoning by coronary**   **HCC** **vasodilators,** intentional **self-harm**

☑7ᵗʰ **T46.3X3 Poisoning by coronary vasodilators,** assault

☑7ᵗʰ **T46.3X4 Poisoning by coronary vasodilators,** undetermined

☑7ᵗʰ **T46.3X5 Adverse effect** of coronary vasodilators

☑7ᵗʰ **T46.3X6 Underdosing** of coronary vasodilators

☑5ᵗʰ **T46.4 Poisoning by, adverse effect of and underdosing of angiotensin-converting-enzyme inhibitors**

☑6ᵗʰ **T46.4X Poisoning by, adverse effect of and underdosing of** angiotensin-converting-enzyme inhibitors

☑7ᵗʰ **T46.4X1 Poisoning by angiotensin-converting-enzyme inhibitors,** accidental **(unintentional)**

Poisoning by angiotensin-converting-enzyme inhibitors NOS

² ☑7ᵗʰ **T46.4X2 Poisoning by**   **HCC** **angiotensin-converting-enzyme inhibitors,** intentional self-harm

☑7ᵗʰ **T46.4X3 Poisoning by angiotensin-converting-enzyme inhibitors,** assault

☑7ᵗʰ **T46.4X4 Poisoning by angiotensin-converting-enzyme inhibitors,** undetermined

☑7ᵗʰ **T46.4X5 Adverse effect** of angiotensin-converting-enzyme inhibitors

☑7ᵗʰ **T46.4X6 Underdosing** of angiotensin-converting-enzyme inhibitors

☑5ᵗʰ **T46.5 Poisoning by, adverse effect of and underdosing of other antihypertensive drugs**

EXCLUDES 2   *poisoning by, adverse effect of and underdosing of beta-adrenoreceptor antagonists (T44.7)*

poisoning by, adverse effect of and underdosing of calcium-channel blockers (T46.1)

poisoning by, adverse effect of and underdosing of diuretics (T50.0-T50.2)

☑6ᵗʰ **T46.5X Poisoning by, adverse effect of and underdosing of other antihypertensive drugs**

☑7ᵗʰ **T46.5X1 Poisoning by other antihypertensive drugs,** accidental **(unintentional)**

Poisoning by other antihypertensive drugs NOS

² ☑7ᵗʰ **T46.5X2 Poisoning by other**   **HCC** **antihypertensive drugs,** intentional self-harm

☑7ᵗʰ **T46.5X3 Poisoning by other antihypertensive drugs,** assault

☑7ᵗʰ **T46.5X4 Poisoning by other antihypertensive drugs,** undetermined

☑7ᵗʰ **T46.5X5 Adverse effect** of other antihypertensive **drugs**

☑7ᵗʰ **T46.5X6 Underdosing** of other antihypertensive **drugs**

☑5ᵗʰ **T46.6 Poisoning by, adverse effect of and underdosing of antihyperlipidemic and antiarteriosclerotic drugs**

☑6ᵗʰ **T46.6X Poisoning by, adverse effect of and underdosing of** antihyperlipidemic and antiarteriosclerotic drugs

☑7ᵗʰ **T46.6X1 Poisoning by antihyperlipidemic and antiarteriosclerotic drugs,** accidental **(unintentional)**

Poisoning by antihyperlipidemic and antiarteriosclerotic drugs NOS

² ☑7ᵗʰ **T46.6X2 Poisoning by antihyperlipidemic**   **HCC** **and antiarteriosclerotic drugs,** intentional self-harm

☑7ᵗʰ **T46.6X3 Poisoning by antihyperlipidemic and antiarteriosclerotic drugs,** assault

☑7ᵗʰ **T46.6X4 Poisoning by antihyperlipidemic and antiarteriosclerotic drugs,** undetermined

☑7ᵗʰ **T46.6X5 Adverse effect** of antihyperlipidemic and antiarteriosclerotic **drugs**

☑7ᵗʰ **T46.6X6 Underdosing** of antihyperlipidemic and antiarteriosclerotic **drugs**

☑5ᵗʰ **T46.7 Poisoning by, adverse effect of and underdosing of peripheral vasodilators**

Poisoning by, adverse effect of and underdosing of nicotinic acid (derivatives)

EXCLUDES 1   *poisoning by, adverse effect of and underdosing of papaverine (T44.3)*

☑6ᵗʰ **T46.7X Poisoning by, adverse effect of and underdosing of** peripheral vasodilators

☑7ᵗʰ **T46.7X1 Poisoning by peripheral vasodilators,** accidental **(unintentional)**

Poisoning by peripheral vasodilators NOS

² ☑7ᵗʰ **T46.7X2 Poisoning by peripheral**   **HCC** **vasodilators,** intentional **self-harm**

☑7ᵗʰ **T46.7X3 Poisoning by peripheral vasodilators,** assault

☑7ᵗʰ **T46.7X4 Poisoning by peripheral vasodilators,** undetermined

☑7ᵗʰ **T46.7X5 Adverse effect** of peripheral vasodilators

☑7ᵗʰ **T46.7X6 Underdosing** of peripheral vasodilators

☑5ᵗʰ **T46.8 Poisoning by, adverse effect of and underdosing of antivaricose drugs, including sclerosing agents**

☑6ᵗʰ **T46.8X Poisoning by, adverse effect of and underdosing of** antivaricose drugs, including sclerosing agents

☑7ᵗʰ **T46.8X1 Poisoning by antivaricose drugs, including sclerosing agents,** accidental **(unintentional)**

Poisoning by antivaricose drugs, including sclerosing agents NOS

² ☑7ᵗʰ **T46.8X2 Poisoning by antivaricose drugs,**   **HCC** **including sclerosing agents,** intentional self-harm

☑7ᵗʰ **T46.8X3 Poisoning by antivaricose drugs, including sclerosing agents,** assault

☑7ᵗʰ **T46.8X4 Poisoning by antivaricose drugs, including sclerosing agents,** undetermined

☑7ᵗʰ **T46.8X5 Adverse effect** of antivaricose drugs, including sclerosing agents

☑7ᵗʰ **T46.8X6 Underdosing** of antivaricose drugs, including sclerosing agents

☑5ᵗʰ **T46.9 Poisoning by, adverse effect of and underdosing of other and unspecified agents primarily affecting the cardiovascular system**

☑6ᵗʰ **T46.9Ø Poisoning by, adverse effect of and underdosing of unspecified agents primarily affecting the cardiovascular system**

☑7ᵗʰ **T46.9Ø1 Poisoning by unspecified agents primarily affecting the cardiovascular system,** accidental **(unintentional)**

² ☑7ᵗʰ **T46.9Ø2 Poisoning by unspecified agents**   **HCC** **primarily affecting the cardiovascular system,** intentional self-harm

☑7ᵗʰ **T46.9Ø3 Poisoning by unspecified agents primarily affecting the cardiovascular system,** assault

☑7ᵗʰ **T46.9Ø4 Poisoning by unspecified agents primarily affecting the cardiovascular system,** undetermined

☑7ᵗʰ **T46.9Ø5 Adverse effect** of unspecified agents primarily affecting the cardiovascular system

☑ Additional Character Required   ✓×7ᵗʰ Placeholder Alert   Manifestation   Unspecified Dx   ▶◀ Revised Text   ● New Code   ▲ Revised Code Title

ICD-10-CM 2020   1111

√7ᵗʰ **T46.906** Underdosing of unspecified agents primarily affecting the cardiovascular system

√6ᵗʰ **T46.99** Poisoning by, adverse effect of and underdosing of other agents primarily affecting the cardiovascular system

√7ᵗʰ **T46.991** Poisoning by other agents primarily affecting the cardiovascular system, accidental (unintentional)

² √7ᵗʰ **T46.992** Poisoning by other agents primarily affecting the cardiovascular system, intentional self-harm   HCC

√7ᵗʰ **T46.993** Poisoning by other agents primarily affecting the cardiovascular system, assault

√7ᵗʰ **T46.994** Poisoning by other agents primarily affecting the cardiovascular system, undetermined

√7ᵗʰ **T46.995** Adverse effect of other agents primarily affecting the cardiovascular system

√7ᵗʰ **T46.996** Underdosing of other agents primarily affecting the cardiovascular system

√4ᵗʰ **T47** Poisoning by, adverse effect of and underdosing of agents primarily affecting the gastrointestinal system

> The appropriate 7th character is to be added to each code from category T47.
> A   initial encounter
> D   subsequent encounter
> S   sequela

√5ᵗʰ **T47.0** Poisoning by, adverse effect of and underdosing of histamine H2-receptor blockers

√6ᵗʰ **T47.0X** Poisoning by, adverse effect of and underdosing of histamine H2-receptor blockers

√7ᵗʰ **T47.0X1** Poisoning by histamine H2-receptor blockers, accidental (unintentional)
Poisoning by histamine H2-receptor blockers NOS

² √7ᵗʰ **T47.0X2** Poisoning by histamine H2-receptor blockers, intentional self-harm   HCC

√7ᵗʰ **T47.0X3** Poisoning by histamine H2-receptor blockers, assault

√7ᵗʰ **T47.0X4** Poisoning by histamine H2-receptor blockers, undetermined

√7ᵗʰ **T47.0X5** Adverse effect of histamine H2-receptor blockers

√7ᵗʰ **T47.0X6** Underdosing of histamine H2-receptor blockers

√5ᵗʰ **T47.1** Poisoning by, adverse effect of and underdosing of other antacids and anti-gastric-secretion drugs

√6ᵗʰ **T47.1X** Poisoning by, adverse effect of and underdosing of other antacids and anti-gastric-secretion drugs

√7ᵗʰ **T47.1X1** Poisoning by other antacids and anti-gastric-secretion drugs, accidental (unintentional)
Poisoning by other antacids and anti-gastric-secretion drugs NOS

² √7ᵗʰ **T47.1X2** Poisoning by other antacids and anti-gastric-secretion drugs, intentional self-harm   HCC

√7ᵗʰ **T47.1X3** Poisoning by other antacids and anti-gastric-secretion drugs, assault

√7ᵗʰ **T47.1X4** Poisoning by other antacids and anti-gastric-secretion drugs, undetermined

√7ᵗʰ **T47.1X5** Adverse effect of other antacids and anti-gastric-secretion drugs

√7ᵗʰ **T47.1X6** Underdosing of other antacids and anti-gastric-secretion drugs

√5ᵗʰ **T47.2** Poisoning by, adverse effect of and underdosing of stimulant laxatives

√6ᵗʰ **T47.2X** Poisoning by, adverse effect of and underdosing of stimulant laxatives

√7ᵗʰ **T47.2X1** Poisoning by stimulant laxatives, accidental (unintentional)
Poisoning by stimulant laxatives NOS

² √7ᵗʰ **T47.2X2** Poisoning by stimulant laxatives, intentional self-harm   HCC

√7ᵗʰ **T47.2X3** Poisoning by stimulant laxatives, assault

√7ᵗʰ **T47.2X4** Poisoning by stimulant laxatives, undetermined

√7ᵗʰ **T47.2X5** Adverse effect of stimulant laxatives

√7ᵗʰ **T47.2X6** Underdosing of stimulant laxatives

√5ᵗʰ **T47.3** Poisoning by, adverse effect of and underdosing of saline and osmotic laxatives

√6ᵗʰ **T47.3X** Poisoning by and adverse effect of saline and osmotic laxatives

√7ᵗʰ **T47.3X1** Poisoning by saline and osmotic laxatives, accidental (unintentional)
Poisoning by saline and osmotic laxatives NOS

² √7ᵗʰ **T47.3X2** Poisoning by saline and osmotic laxatives, intentional self-harm   HCC

√7ᵗʰ **T47.3X3** Poisoning by saline and osmotic laxatives, assault

√7ᵗʰ **T47.3X4** Poisoning by saline and osmotic laxatives, undetermined

√7ᵗʰ **T47.3X5** Adverse effect of saline and osmotic laxatives

√7ᵗʰ **T47.3X6** Underdosing of saline and osmotic laxatives

√5ᵗʰ **T47.4** Poisoning by, adverse effect of and underdosing of other laxatives

√6ᵗʰ **T47.4X** Poisoning by, adverse effect of and underdosing of other laxatives

√7ᵗʰ **T47.4X1** Poisoning by other laxatives, accidental (unintentional)
Poisoning by other laxatives NOS

² √7ᵗʰ **T47.4X2** Poisoning by other laxatives, intentional self-harm   HCC

√7ᵗʰ **T47.4X3** Poisoning by other laxatives, assault

√7ᵗʰ **T47.4X4** Poisoning by other laxatives, undetermined

√7ᵗʰ **T47.4X5** Adverse effect of other laxatives

√7ᵗʰ **T47.4X6** Underdosing of other laxatives

√5ᵗʰ **T47.5** Poisoning by, adverse effect of and underdosing of digestants

√6ᵗʰ **T47.5X** Poisoning by, adverse effect of and underdosing of digestants

√7ᵗʰ **T47.5X1** Poisoning by digestants, accidental (unintentional)
Poisoning by digestants NOS

² √7ᵗʰ **T47.5X2** Poisoning by digestants, intentional self-harm   HCC

√7ᵗʰ **T47.5X3** Poisoning by digestants, assault

√7ᵗʰ **T47.5X4** Poisoning by digestants, undetermined

√7ᵗʰ **T47.5X5** Adverse effect of digestants

√7ᵗʰ **T47.5X6** Underdosing of digestants

√5ᵗʰ **T47.6** Poisoning by, adverse effect of and underdosing of antidiarrheal drugs

> EXCLUDES 2   poisoning by, adverse effect of and underdosing of systemic antibiotics and other anti-infectives (T36-T37)

√6ᵗʰ **T47.6X** Poisoning by, adverse effect of and underdosing of antidiarrheal drugs

√7ᵗʰ **T47.6X1** Poisoning by antidiarrheal drugs, accidental (unintentional)
Poisoning by antidiarrheal drugs NOS

² √7ᵗʰ **T47.6X2** Poisoning by antidiarrheal drugs, intentional self-harm   HCC

√7ᵗʰ **T47.6X3** Poisoning by antidiarrheal drugs, assault

√7ᵗʰ **T47.6X4** Poisoning by antidiarrheal drugs, undetermined

√7ᵗʰ **T47.6X5** Adverse effect of antidiarrheal drugs

√7ᵗʰ **T47.6X6** Underdosing of antidiarrheal drugs

√5ᵗʰ **T47.7** Poisoning by, adverse effect of and underdosing of emetics

√6ᵗʰ **T47.7X** Poisoning by, adverse effect of and underdosing of emetics

√7ᵗʰ **T47.7X1** Poisoning by emetics, accidental (unintentional)
Poisoning by emetics NOS

² √7ᵗʰ **T47.7X2** Poisoning by emetics, intentional self-harm   HCC

√7ᵗʰ **T47.7X3** Poisoning by emetics, assault

√7ᵗʰ **T47.7X4** Poisoning by emetics, undetermined

√7ᵗʰ **T47.7X5** Adverse effect of emetics

√7ᵗʰ **T47.7X6** Underdosing of emetics

✓5ᵗʰ **T47.8 Poisoning by, adverse effect of and underdosing of other agents primarily affecting gastrointestinal system**

  ✓6ᵗʰ **T47.8X Poisoning by, adverse effect of and underdosing of other agents primarily affecting gastrointestinal system**

    ✓7ᵗʰ **T47.8X1 Poisoning by other agents primarily affecting gastrointestinal system, accidental (unintentional)**

        Poisoning by other agents primarily affecting gastrointestinal system NOS

    ² ✓7ᵗʰ **T47.8X2 Poisoning by other agents** HCC **primarily affecting gastrointestinal system, intentional self-harm**

    ✓7ᵗʰ **T47.8X3 Poisoning by other agents primarily affecting gastrointestinal system, assault**

    ✓7ᵗʰ **T47.8X4 Poisoning by other agents primarily affecting gastrointestinal system, undetermined**

    ✓7ᵗʰ **T47.8X5 Adverse effect of other agents primarily affecting gastrointestinal system**

    ✓7ᵗʰ **T47.8X6 Underdosing of other agents primarily affecting gastrointestinal system**

✓5ᵗʰ **T47.9 Poisoning by, adverse effect of and underdosing of unspecified agents primarily affecting the gastrointestinal system**

  ✓x7ᵗʰ **T47.91 Poisoning by unspecified agents primarily affecting the gastrointestinal system, accidental (unintentional)**

        Poisoning by agents primarily affecting the gastrointestinal system NOS

  ² ✓x7ᵗʰ **T47.92 Poisoning by unspecified agents primarily** HCC **affecting the gastrointestinal system, intentional self-harm**

  ✓x7ᵗʰ **T47.93 Poisoning by unspecified agents primarily affecting the gastrointestinal system, assault**

  ✓x7ᵗʰ **T47.94 Poisoning by unspecified agents primarily affecting the gastrointestinal system, undetermined**

  ✓x7ᵗʰ **T47.95 Adverse effect of unspecified agents primarily affecting the gastrointestinal system**

  ✓x7ᵗʰ **T47.96 Underdosing of unspecified agents primarily affecting the gastrointestinal system**

✓4ᵗʰ **T48 Poisoning by, adverse effect of and underdosing of agents primarily acting on smooth and skeletal muscles and the respiratory system**

> The appropriate 7th character is to be added to each code from category T48.
> A   initial encounter
> D   subsequent encounter
> S   sequela

✓5ᵗʰ **T48.0 Poisoning by, adverse effect of and underdosing of oxytocic drugs**

    EXCLUDES 1   *poisoning by, adverse effect of and underdosing of estrogens, progestogens and antagonists (T38.4-T38.6)*

  ✓6ᵗʰ **T48.0X Poisoning by, adverse effect of and underdosing of oxytocic drugs**

    ✓7ᵗʰ **T48.0X1 Poisoning by oxytocic drugs, accidental (unintentional)**

        Poisoning by oxytocic drugs NOS

    ² ✓7ᵗʰ **T48.0X2 Poisoning by oxytocic drugs,** HCC **intentional self-harm**

    ✓7ᵗʰ **T48.0X3 Poisoning by oxytocic drugs, assault**

    ✓7ᵗʰ **T48.0X4 Poisoning by oxytocic drugs, undetermined**

    ✓7ᵗʰ **T48.0X5 Adverse effect of oxytocic drugs**

    ✓7ᵗʰ **T48.0X6 Underdosing of oxytocic drugs**

✓5ᵗʰ **T48.1 Poisoning by, adverse effect of and underdosing of skeletal muscle relaxants [neuromuscular blocking agents]**

  ✓6ᵗʰ **T48.1X Poisoning by, adverse effect of and underdosing of skeletal muscle relaxants [neuromuscular blocking agents]**

    ✓7ᵗʰ **T48.1X1 Poisoning by skeletal muscle relaxants [neuromuscular blocking agents], accidental (unintentional)**

        Poisoning by skeletal muscle relaxants [neuromuscular blocking agents] NOS

    ² ✓7ᵗʰ **T48.1X2 Poisoning by skeletal muscle** HCC **relaxants [neuromuscular blocking agents], intentional self-harm**

    ✓7ᵗʰ **T48.1X3 Poisoning by skeletal muscle relaxants [neuromuscular blocking agents], assault**

    ✓7ᵗʰ **T48.1X4 Poisoning by skeletal muscle relaxants [neuromuscular blocking agents], undetermined**

    ✓7ᵗʰ **T48.1X5 Adverse effect of skeletal muscle relaxants [neuromuscular blocking agents]**

    ✓7ᵗʰ **T48.1X6 Underdosing of skeletal muscle relaxants [neuromuscular blocking agents]**

✓5ᵗʰ **T48.2 Poisoning by, adverse effect of and underdosing of other and unspecified drugs acting on muscles**

  ✓6ᵗʰ **T48.20 Poisoning by, adverse effect of and underdosing of unspecified drugs acting on muscles**

    ✓7ᵗʰ **T48.201 Poisoning by unspecified drugs acting on muscles, accidental (unintentional)**

        Poisoning by unspecified drugs acting on muscles NOS

    ² ✓7ᵗʰ **T48.202 Poisoning by unspecified drugs** HCC **acting on muscles, intentional self-harm**

    ✓7ᵗʰ **T48.203 Poisoning by unspecified drugs acting on muscles, assault**

    ✓7ᵗʰ **T48.204 Poisoning by unspecified drugs acting on muscles, undetermined**

    ✓7ᵗʰ **T48.205 Adverse effect of unspecified drugs acting on muscles**

    ✓7ᵗʰ **T48.206 Underdosing of unspecified drugs acting on muscles**

  ✓6ᵗʰ **T48.29 Poisoning by, adverse effect of and underdosing of other drugs acting on muscles**

    ✓7ᵗʰ **T48.291 Poisoning by other drugs acting on muscles, accidental (unintentional)**

        Poisoning by other drugs acting on muscles NOS

    ² ✓7ᵗʰ **T48.292 Poisoning by other drugs acting** HCC **on muscles, intentional self-harm**

    ✓7ᵗʰ **T48.293 Poisoning by other drugs acting on muscles, assault**

    ✓7ᵗʰ **T48.294 Poisoning by other drugs acting on muscles, undetermined**

    ✓7ᵗʰ **T48.295 Adverse effect of other drugs acting on muscles**

    ✓7ᵗʰ **T48.296 Underdosing of other drugs acting on muscles**

✓5ᵗʰ **T48.3 Poisoning by, adverse effect of and underdosing of antitussives**

  ✓6ᵗʰ **T48.3X Poisoning by, adverse effect of and underdosing of antitussives**

    ✓7ᵗʰ **T48.3X1 Poisoning by antitussives, accidental (unintentional)**

        Poisoning by antitussives NOS

    ² ✓7ᵗʰ **T48.3X2 Poisoning by antitussives,** HCC **intentional self-harm**

    ✓7ᵗʰ **T48.3X3 Poisoning by antitussives, assault**

    ✓7ᵗʰ **T48.3X4 Poisoning by antitussives, undetermined**

    ✓7ᵗʰ **T48.3X5 Adverse effect of antitussives**

    ✓7ᵗʰ **T48.3X6 Underdosing of antitussives**

✓5ᵗʰ **T48.4 Poisoning by, adverse effect of and underdosing of expectorants**

  ✓6ᵗʰ **T48.4X Poisoning by, adverse effect of and underdosing of expectorants**

    ✓7ᵗʰ **T48.4X1 Poisoning by expectorants, accidental (unintentional)**

        Poisoning by expectorants NOS

    ² ✓7ᵗʰ **T48.4X2 Poisoning by expectorants,** HCC **intentional self-harm**

    ✓7ᵗʰ **T48.4X3 Poisoning by expectorants, assault**

    ✓7ᵗʰ **T48.4X4 Poisoning by expectorants, undetermined**

    ✓7ᵗʰ **T48.4X5 Adverse effect of expectorants**

    ✓7ᵗʰ **T48.4X6 Underdosing of expectorants**

☑ Additional Character Required   ✓x7ᵗʰ Placeholder Alert   Manifestation   Unspecified Dx   ▶◀ Revised Text   ● New Code   ▲ Revised Code Title

✓5ᵗʰ **T48.5 Poisoning by, adverse effect of and underdosing of other anti-common-cold drugs**
Poisoning by, adverse effect of and underdosing of decongestants

> EXCLUDES 2 *poisoning by, adverse effect of and underdosing of antipyretics, NEC (T39.9-)*
> *poisoning by, adverse effect of and underdosing of non-steroidal antiinflammatory drugs (T39.3-)*
> *poisoning by, adverse effect of and underdosing of salicylates (T39.Ø-)*

  ✓6ᵗʰ **T48.5X Poisoning by, adverse effect of and underdosing of other anti-common-cold drugs**

    ✓7ᵗʰ **T48.5X1 Poisoning by other anti-common-cold drugs, accidental (unintentional)**
Poisoning by other anti-common-cold drugs NOS

    ² ✓7ᵗʰ **T48.5X2 Poisoning by other anti-common-cold drugs, intentional self-harm** HCC

    ✓7ᵗʰ **T48.5X3 Poisoning by other anti-common-cold drugs, assault**

    ✓7ᵗʰ **T48.5X4 Poisoning by other anti-common-cold drugs, undetermined**

    ✓7ᵗʰ **T48.5X5 Adverse effect of other anti-common-cold drugs**

    ✓7ᵗʰ **T48.5X6 Underdosing of other anti-common-cold drugs**

✓5ᵗʰ **T48.6 Poisoning by, adverse effect of and underdosing of antiasthmatics, not elsewhere classified**
Poisoning by, adverse effect of and underdosing of beta-adrenoreceptor agonists used in asthma therapy

> EXCLUDES 1 *poisoning by, adverse effect of and underdosing of anterior pituitary [adenohypophyseal] hormones (T38.8)*
> *poisoning by, adverse effect of and underdosing of beta-adrenoreceptor agonists not used in asthma therapy (T44.5)*

  ✓6ᵗʰ **T48.6X Poisoning by, adverse effect of and underdosing of antiasthmatics**

    ✓7ᵗʰ **T48.6X1 Poisoning by antiasthmatics, accidental (unintentional)**
Poisoning by antiasthmatics NOS

    ² ✓7ᵗʰ **T48.6X2 Poisoning by antiasthmatics, intentional self-harm** HCC

    ✓7ᵗʰ **T48.6X3 Poisoning by antiasthmatics, assault**

    ✓7ᵗʰ **T48.6X4 Poisoning by antiasthmatics, undetermined**

    ✓7ᵗʰ **T48.6X5 Adverse effect of antiasthmatics**

    ✓7ᵗʰ **T48.6X6 Underdosing of antiasthmatics**

✓5ᵗʰ **T48.9 Poisoning by, adverse effect of and underdosing of other and unspecified agents primarily acting on the respiratory system**

  ✓6ᵗʰ **T48.9Ø Poisoning by, adverse effect of and underdosing of unspecified agents primarily acting on the respiratory system**

    ✓7ᵗʰ **T48.9Ø1 Poisoning by unspecified agents primarily acting on the respiratory system, accidental (unintentional)**

    ² ✓7ᵗʰ **T48.9Ø2 Poisoning by unspecified agents primarily acting on the respiratory system, intentional self-harm** HCC

    ✓7ᵗʰ **T48.9Ø3 Poisoning by unspecified agents primarily acting on the respiratory system, assault**

    ✓7ᵗʰ **T48.9Ø4 Poisoning by unspecified agents primarily acting on the respiratory system, undetermined**

    ✓7ᵗʰ **T48.9Ø5 Adverse effect of unspecified agents primarily acting on the respiratory system**

    ✓7ᵗʰ **T48.9Ø6 Underdosing of unspecified agents primarily acting on the respiratory system**

  ✓6ᵗʰ **T48.99 Poisoning by, adverse effect of and underdosing of other agents primarily acting on the respiratory system**

    ✓7ᵗʰ **T48.991 Poisoning by other agents primarily acting on the respiratory system, accidental (unintentional)**

    ² ✓7ᵗʰ **T48.992 Poisoning by other agents primarily acting on the respiratory system, intentional self-harm** HCC

    ✓7ᵗʰ **T48.993 Poisoning by other agents primarily acting on the respiratory system, assault**

    ✓7ᵗʰ **T48.994 Poisoning by other agents primarily acting on the respiratory system, undetermined**

    ✓7ᵗʰ **T48.995 Adverse effect of other agents primarily acting on the respiratory system**

    ✓7ᵗʰ **T48.996 Underdosing of other agents primarily acting on the respiratory system**

✓4ᵗʰ **T49 Poisoning by, adverse effect of and underdosing of topical agents primarily affecting skin and mucous membrane and ophthalmological, otorhinolaryngological and dental drugs**

> INCLUDES poisoning by, adverse effect of and underdosing of glucocorticoids, topically used

> The appropriate 7th character is to be added to each code from category T49.
> A initial encounter
> D subsequent encounter
> S sequela

✓5ᵗʰ **T49.Ø Poisoning by, adverse effect of and underdosing of local antifungal, anti-infective and anti-inflammatory drugs**

  ✓6ᵗʰ **T49.ØX Poisoning by, adverse effect of and underdosing of local antifungal, anti-infective and anti-inflammatory drugs**

    ✓7ᵗʰ **T49.ØX1 Poisoning by local antifungal, anti-infective and anti-inflammatory drugs, accidental (unintentional)**
Poisoning by local antifungal, anti-infective and anti-inflammatory drugs NOS

    ² ✓7ᵗʰ **T49.ØX2 Poisoning by local antifungal, anti-infective and anti-inflammatory drugs, intentional self-harm** HCC

    ✓7ᵗʰ **T49.ØX3 Poisoning by local antifungal, anti-infective and anti-inflammatory drugs, assault**

    ✓7ᵗʰ **T49.ØX4 Poisoning by local antifungal, anti-infective and anti-inflammatory drugs, undetermined**

    ✓7ᵗʰ **T49.ØX5 Adverse effect of local antifungal, anti-infective and anti-inflammatory drugs**

    ✓7ᵗʰ **T49.ØX6 Underdosing of local antifungal, anti-infective and anti-inflammatory drugs**

✓5ᵗʰ **T49.1 Poisoning by, adverse effect of and underdosing of antipruritics**

  ✓6ᵗʰ **T49.1X Poisoning by, adverse effect of and underdosing of antipruritics**

    ✓7ᵗʰ **T49.1X1 Poisoning by antipruritics, accidental (unintentional)**
Poisoning by antipruritics NOS

    ² ✓7ᵗʰ **T49.1X2 Poisoning by antipruritics, intentional self-harm** HCC

    ✓7ᵗʰ **T49.1X3 Poisoning by antipruritics, assault**

    ✓7ᵗʰ **T49.1X4 Poisoning by antipruritics, undetermined**

    ✓7ᵗʰ **T49.1X5 Adverse effect of antipruritics**

    ✓7ᵗʰ **T49.1X6 Underdosing of antipruritics**

✓5ᵗʰ **T49.2 Poisoning by, adverse effect of and underdosing of local astringents and local detergents**

  ✓6ᵗʰ **T49.2X Poisoning by, adverse effect of and underdosing of local astringents and local detergents**

    ✓7ᵗʰ **T49.2X1 Poisoning by local astringents and local detergents, accidental (unintentional)**
Poisoning by local astringents and local detergents NOS

    ² ✓7ᵗʰ **T49.2X2 Poisoning by local astringents and local detergents, intentional self-harm** HCC

    ✓7ᵗʰ **T49.2X3 Poisoning by local astringents and local detergents, assault**

    ✓7ᵗʰ **T49.2X4 Poisoning by local astringents and local detergents, undetermined**

    ✓7ᵗʰ **T49.2X5 Adverse effect of local astringents and local detergents**

    ✓7ᵗʰ **T49.2X6 Underdosing of local astringents and local detergents**

√5ᵗʰ **T49.3** **Poisoning by, adverse effect of and underdosing of emollients, demulcents and protectants**
    √6ᵗʰ **T49.3X** **Poisoning by, adverse effect of and underdosing of emollients, demulcents and protectants**
        √7ᵗʰ **T49.3X1** **Poisoning by emollients, demulcents and protectants, accidental (unintentional)**
             Poisoning by emollients, demulcents and protectants NOS
        ² √7ᵗʰ **T49.3X2** **Poisoning by emollients, demulcents and protectants, intentional self-harm** `HCC`
        √7ᵗʰ **T49.3X3** **Poisoning by emollients, demulcents and protectants, assault**
        √7ᵗʰ **T49.3X4** **Poisoning by emollients, demulcents and protectants, undetermined**
        √7ᵗʰ **T49.3X5** **Adverse effect of emollients, demulcents and protectants**
        √7ᵗʰ **T49.3X6** **Underdosing of emollients, demulcents and protectants**

√5ᵗʰ **T49.4** **Poisoning by, adverse effect of and underdosing of keratolytics, keratoplastics, and other hair treatment drugs and preparations**
    √6ᵗʰ **T49.4X** **Poisoning by, adverse effect of and underdosing of keratolytics, keratoplastics, and other hair treatment drugs and preparations**
        √7ᵗʰ **T49.4X1** **Poisoning by keratolytics, keratoplastics, and other hair treatment drugs and preparations, accidental (unintentional)**
             Poisoning by keratolytics, keratoplastics, and other hair treatment drugs and preparations NOS
        ² √7ᵗʰ **T49.4X2** **Poisoning by keratolytics, keratoplastics, and other hair treatment drugs and preparations, intentional self-harm** `HCC`
        √7ᵗʰ **T49.4X3** **Poisoning by keratolytics, keratoplastics, and other hair treatment drugs and preparations, assault**
        √7ᵗʰ **T49.4X4** **Poisoning by keratolytics, keratoplastics, and other hair treatment drugs and preparations, undetermined**
        √7ᵗʰ **T49.4X5** **Adverse effect of keratolytics, keratoplastics, and other hair treatment drugs and preparations**
        √7ᵗʰ **T49.4X6** **Underdosing of keratolytics, keratoplastics, and other hair treatment drugs and preparations**

√5ᵗʰ **T49.5** **Poisoning by, adverse effect of and underdosing of ophthalmological drugs and preparations**
    √6ᵗʰ **T49.5X** **Poisoning by, adverse effect of and underdosing of ophthalmological drugs and preparations**
        √7ᵗʰ **T49.5X1** **Poisoning by ophthalmological drugs and preparations, accidental (unintentional)**
             Poisoning by ophthalmological drugs and preparations NOS
        ² √7ᵗʰ **T49.5X2** **Poisoning by ophthalmological drugs and preparations, intentional self-harm** `HCC`
        √7ᵗʰ **T49.5X3** **Poisoning by ophthalmological drugs and preparations, assault**
        √7ᵗʰ **T49.5X4** **Poisoning by ophthalmological drugs and preparations, undetermined**
        √7ᵗʰ **T49.5X5** **Adverse effect of ophthalmological drugs and preparations**
        √7ᵗʰ **T49.5X6** **Underdosing of ophthalmological drugs and preparations**

√5ᵗʰ **T49.6** **Poisoning by, adverse effect of and underdosing of otorhinolaryngological drugs and preparations**
    √6ᵗʰ **T49.6X** **Poisoning by, adverse effect of and underdosing of otorhinolaryngological drugs and preparations**
        √7ᵗʰ **T49.6X1** **Poisoning by otorhinolaryngological drugs and preparations, accidental (unintentional)**
             Poisoning by otorhinolaryngological drugs and preparations NOS
        ² √7ᵗʰ **T49.6X2** **Poisoning by otorhinolaryngological drugs and preparations, intentional self-harm** `HCC`
        √7ᵗʰ **T49.6X3** **Poisoning by otorhinolaryngological drugs and preparations, assault**
        √7ᵗʰ **T49.6X4** **Poisoning by otorhinolaryngological drugs and preparations, undetermined**

        √7ᵗʰ **T49.6X5** **Adverse effect of otorhinolaryngological drugs and preparations**
        √7ᵗʰ **T49.6X6** **Underdosing of otorhinolaryngological drugs and preparations**

√5ᵗʰ **T49.7** **Poisoning by, adverse effect of and underdosing of dental drugs, topically applied**
    √6ᵗʰ **T49.7X** **Poisoning by, adverse effect of and underdosing of dental drugs, topically applied**
        √7ᵗʰ **T49.7X1** **Poisoning by dental drugs, topically applied, accidental (unintentional)**
             Poisoning by dental drugs, topically applied NOS
        ² √7ᵗʰ **T49.7X2** **Poisoning by dental drugs, topically applied, intentional self-harm** `HCC`
        √7ᵗʰ **T49.7X3** **Poisoning by dental drugs, topically applied, assault**
        √7ᵗʰ **T49.7X4** **Poisoning by dental drugs, topically applied, undetermined**
        √7ᵗʰ **T49.7X5** **Adverse effect of dental drugs, topically applied**
        √7ᵗʰ **T49.7X6** **Underdosing of dental drugs, topically applied**

√5ᵗʰ **T49.8** **Poisoning by, adverse effect of and underdosing of other topical agents**
         Poisoning by, adverse effect of and underdosing of spermicides
    √6ᵗʰ **T49.8X** **Poisoning by, adverse effect of and underdosing of other topical agents**
        √7ᵗʰ **T49.8X1** **Poisoning by other topical agents, accidental (unintentional)**
             Poisoning by other topical agents NOS
        ² √7ᵗʰ **T49.8X2** **Poisoning by other topical agents, intentional self-harm** `HCC`
        √7ᵗʰ **T49.8X3** **Poisoning by other topical agents, assault**
        √7ᵗʰ **T49.8X4** **Poisoning by other topical agents, undetermined**
        √7ᵗʰ **T49.8X5** **Adverse effect of other topical agents**
        √7ᵗʰ **T49.8X6** **Underdosing of other topical agents**

√5ᵗʰ **T49.9** **Poisoning by, adverse effect of and underdosing of unspecified topical agent**
    √×7ᵗʰ **T49.91** **Poisoning by unspecified topical agent, accidental (unintentional)**
    ² √×7ᵗʰ **T49.92** **Poisoning by unspecified topical agent, intentional self-harm** `HCC`
    √×7ᵗʰ **T49.93** **Poisoning by unspecified topical agent, assault**
    √×7ᵗʰ **T49.94** **Poisoning by unspecified topical agent, undetermined**
    √×7ᵗʰ **T49.95** **Adverse effect of unspecified topical agent**
    √×7ᵗʰ **T49.96** **Underdosing of unspecified topical agent**

√4ᵗʰ **T50** **Poisoning by, adverse effect of and underdosing of diuretics and other and unspecified drugs, medicaments and biological substances**

> The appropriate 7th character is to be added to each code from category T50.
> A   initial encounter
> D   subsequent encounter
> S   sequela

√5ᵗʰ **T50.0** **Poisoning by, adverse effect of and underdosing of mineralocorticoids and their antagonists**
    √6ᵗʰ **T50.0X** **Poisoning by, adverse effect of and underdosing of mineralocorticoids and their antagonists**
        √7ᵗʰ **T50.0X1** **Poisoning by mineralocorticoids and their antagonists, accidental (unintentional)**
             Poisoning by mineralocorticoids and their antagonists NOS
        ² √7ᵗʰ **T50.0X2** **Poisoning by mineralocorticoids and their antagonists, intentional self-harm** `HCC`
        √7ᵗʰ **T50.0X3** **Poisoning by mineralocorticoids and their antagonists, assault**
        √7ᵗʰ **T50.0X4** **Poisoning by mineralocorticoids and their antagonists, undetermined**
        √7ᵗʰ **T50.0X5** **Adverse effect of mineralocorticoids and their antagonists**
        √7ᵗʰ **T50.0X6** **Underdosing of mineralocorticoids and their antagonists**

√5ᵗʰ **T50.1 Poisoning by, adverse effect of and underdosing of loop [high-ceiling] diuretics**

√6ᵗʰ **T50.1X Poisoning by, adverse effect of and underdosing of loop [high-ceiling] diuretics**

√7ᵗʰ **T50.1X1 Poisoning by loop [high-ceiling] diuretics, accidental (unintentional)**
Poisoning by loop [high-ceiling] diuretics NOS

² √7ᵗʰ **T50.1X2 Poisoning by loop [high-ceiling] diuretics, intentional self-harm** HCC

√7ᵗʰ **T50.1X3 Poisoning by loop [high-ceiling] diuretics, assault**

√7ᵗʰ **T50.1X4 Poisoning by loop [high-ceiling] diuretics, undetermined**

√7ᵗʰ **T50.1X5 Adverse effect of loop [high-ceiling] diuretics**

√7ᵗʰ **T50.1X6 Underdosing of loop [high-ceiling] diuretics**

√5ᵗʰ **T50.2 Poisoning by, adverse effect of and underdosing of carbonic-anhydrase inhibitors, benzothiadiazides and other diuretics**
Poisoning by, adverse effect of and underdosing of acetazolamide

√6ᵗʰ **T50.2X Poisoning by, adverse effect of and underdosing of carbonic-anhydrase inhibitors, benzothiadiazides and other diuretics**

√7ᵗʰ **T50.2X1 Poisoning by carbonic-anhydrase inhibitors, benzothiadiazides and other diuretics, accidental (unintentional)**
Poisoning by carbonic-anhydrase inhibitors, benzothiadiazides and other diuretics NOS

² √7ᵗʰ **T50.2X2 Poisoning by carbonic-anhydrase inhibitors, benzothiadiazides and other diuretics, intentional self-harm** HCC

√7ᵗʰ **T50.2X3 Poisoning by carbonic-anhydrase inhibitors, benzothiadiazides and other diuretics, assault**

√7ᵗʰ **T50.2X4 Poisoning by carbonic-anhydrase inhibitors, benzothiadiazides and other diuretics, undetermined**

√7ᵗʰ **T50.2X5 Adverse effect of carbonic-anhydrase inhibitors, benzothiadiazides and other diuretics**

√7ᵗʰ **T50.2X6 Underdosing of carbonic-anhydrase inhibitors, benzothiadiazides and other diuretics**

√5ᵗʰ **T50.3 Poisoning by, adverse effect of and underdosing of electrolytic, caloric and water-balance agents**
Poisoning by, adverse effect of and underdosing of oral rehydration salts

√6ᵗʰ **T50.3X Poisoning by, adverse effect of and underdosing of electrolytic, caloric and water-balance agents**

√7ᵗʰ **T50.3X1 Poisoning by electrolytic, caloric and water-balance agents, accidental (unintentional)**
Poisoning by electrolytic, caloric and water-balance agents NOS

² √7ᵗʰ **T50.3X2 Poisoning by electrolytic, caloric and water-balance agents, intentional self-harm** HCC

√7ᵗʰ **T50.3X3 Poisoning by electrolytic, caloric and water-balance agents, assault**

√7ᵗʰ **T50.3X4 Poisoning by electrolytic, caloric and water-balance agents, undetermined**

√7ᵗʰ **T50.3X5 Adverse effect of electrolytic, caloric and water-balance agents**

√7ᵗʰ **T50.3X6 Underdosing of electrolytic, caloric and water-balance agents**

√5ᵗʰ **T50.4 Poisoning by, adverse effect of and underdosing of drugs affecting uric acid metabolism**

√6ᵗʰ **T50.4X Poisoning by, adverse effect of and underdosing of drugs affecting uric acid metabolism**

√7ᵗʰ **T50.4X1 Poisoning by drugs affecting uric acid metabolism, accidental (unintentional)**
Poisoning by drugs affecting uric acid metabolism NOS

² √7ᵗʰ **T50.4X2 Poisoning by drugs affecting uric acid metabolism, intentional self-harm** HCC

√7ᵗʰ **T50.4X3 Poisoning by drugs affecting uric acid metabolism, assault**

√7ᵗʰ **T50.4X4 Poisoning by drugs affecting uric acid metabolism, undetermined**

√7ᵗʰ **T50.4X5 Adverse effect of drugs affecting uric acid metabolism**

√7ᵗʰ **T50.4X6 Underdosing of drugs affecting uric acid metabolism**

√5ᵗʰ **T50.5 Poisoning by, adverse effect of and underdosing of appetite depressants**

√6ᵗʰ **T50.5X Poisoning by, adverse effect of and underdosing of appetite depressants**

√7ᵗʰ **T50.5X1 Poisoning by appetite depressants, accidental (unintentional)**
Poisoning by appetite depressants NOS

² √7ᵗʰ **T50.5X2 Poisoning by appetite depressants, intentional self-harm** HCC

√7ᵗʰ **T50.5X3 Poisoning by appetite depressants, assault**

√7ᵗʰ **T50.5X4 Poisoning by appetite depressants, undetermined**

√7ᵗʰ **T50.5X5 Adverse effect of appetite depressants**

√7ᵗʰ **T50.5X6 Underdosing of appetite depressants**

√5ᵗʰ **T50.6 Poisoning by, adverse effect of and underdosing of antidotes and chelating agents**
Poisoning by, adverse effect of and underdosing of alcohol deterrents

√6ᵗʰ **T50.6X Poisoning by, adverse effect of and underdosing of antidotes and chelating agents**

√7ᵗʰ **T50.6X1 Poisoning by antidotes and chelating agents, accidental (unintentional)**
Poisoning by antidotes and chelating agents NOS

² √7ᵗʰ **T50.6X2 Poisoning by antidotes and chelating agents, intentional self-harm** HCC

√7ᵗʰ **T50.6X3 Poisoning by antidotes and chelating agents, assault**

√7ᵗʰ **T50.6X4 Poisoning by antidotes and chelating agents, undetermined**

√7ᵗʰ **T50.6X5 Adverse effect of antidotes and chelating agents**

√7ᵗʰ **T50.6X6 Underdosing of antidotes and chelating agents**

√5ᵗʰ **T50.7 Poisoning by, adverse effect of and underdosing of analeptics and opioid receptor antagonists**

√6ᵗʰ **T50.7X Poisoning by, adverse effect of and underdosing of analeptics and opioid receptor antagonists**

√7ᵗʰ **T50.7X1 Poisoning by analeptics and opioid receptor antagonists, accidental (unintentional)**
Poisoning by analeptics and opioid receptor antagonists NOS

² √7ᵗʰ **T50.7X2 Poisoning by analeptics and opioid receptor antagonists, intentional self-harm** HCC

√7ᵗʰ **T50.7X3 Poisoning by analeptics and opioid receptor antagonists, assault**

√7ᵗʰ **T50.7X4 Poisoning by analeptics and opioid receptor antagonists, undetermined**

√7ᵗʰ **T50.7X5 Adverse effect of analeptics and opioid receptor antagonists**

√7ᵗʰ **T50.7X6 Underdosing of analeptics and opioid receptor antagonists**

√5ᵗʰ **T50.8 Poisoning by, adverse effect of and underdosing of diagnostic agents**

√6ᵗʰ **T50.8X Poisoning by, adverse effect of and underdosing of diagnostic agents**

√7ᵗʰ **T50.8X1 Poisoning by diagnostic agents, accidental (unintentional)**
Poisoning by diagnostic agents NOS

² √7ᵗʰ **T50.8X2 Poisoning by diagnostic agents, intentional self-harm** HCC

√7ᵗʰ **T50.8X3 Poisoning by diagnostic agents, assault**

√7ᵗʰ **T50.8X4 Poisoning by diagnostic agents, undetermined**

√7ᵗʰ **T50.8X5 Adverse effect of diagnostic agents**

√7ᵗʰ **T50.8X6 Underdosing of diagnostic agents**

☑5ᵗʰ **T50.A** **Poisoning by, adverse effect of and underdosing of bacterial vaccines**

  ☑6ᵗʰ **T50.A1** **Poisoning by, adverse effect of and underdosing of** pertussis vaccine, including combinations with a pertussis component

    ☑7ᵗʰ **T50.A11** **Poisoning by pertussis vaccine, including combinations with a pertussis component, accidental (unintentional)**

    ² ☑7ᵗʰ **T50.A12** **Poisoning by pertussis vaccine, including combinations with a pertussis component, intentional self-harm**   HCC

    ☑7ᵗʰ **T50.A13** **Poisoning by pertussis vaccine, including combinations with a pertussis component, assault**

    ☑7ᵗʰ **T50.A14** **Poisoning by pertussis vaccine, including combinations with a pertussis component, undetermined**

    ☑7ᵗʰ **T50.A15** **Adverse effect of pertussis vaccine, including combinations with a pertussis component**

    ☑7ᵗʰ **T50.A16** **Underdosing of pertussis vaccine, including combinations with a pertussis component**

  ☑6ᵗʰ **T50.A2** **Poisoning by, adverse effect of and underdosing of** mixed bacterial vaccines without a pertussis component

    ☑7ᵗʰ **T50.A21** **Poisoning by mixed bacterial vaccines without a pertussis component, accidental (unintentional)**

    ² ☑7ᵗʰ **T50.A22** **Poisoning by mixed bacterial vaccines without a pertussis component, intentional self-harm**   HCC

    ☑7ᵗʰ **T50.A23** **Poisoning by mixed bacterial vaccines without a pertussis component, assault**

    ☑7ᵗʰ **T50.A24** **Poisoning by mixed bacterial vaccines without a pertussis component, undetermined**

    ☑7ᵗʰ **T50.A25** **Adverse effect of mixed bacterial vaccines without a pertussis component**

    ☑7ᵗʰ **T50.A26** **Underdosing of mixed bacterial vaccines without a pertussis component**

  ☑6ᵗʰ **T50.A9** **Poisoning by, adverse effect of and underdosing of other bacterial vaccines**

    ☑7ᵗʰ **T50.A91** **Poisoning by other bacterial vaccines, accidental (unintentional)**

    ² ☑7ᵗʰ **T50.A92** **Poisoning by other bacterial vaccines, intentional self-harm**   HCC

    ☑7ᵗʰ **T50.A93** **Poisoning by other bacterial vaccines, assault**

    ☑7ᵗʰ **T50.A94** **Poisoning by other bacterial vaccines, undetermined**

    ☑7ᵗʰ **T50.A95** **Adverse effect of other bacterial vaccines**

    ☑7ᵗʰ **T50.A96** **Underdosing of other bacterial vaccines**

☑5ᵗʰ **T50.B** **Poisoning by, adverse effect of and underdosing of viral vaccines**

  ☑6ᵗʰ **T50.B1** **Poisoning by, adverse effect of and underdosing of** smallpox vaccines

    ☑7ᵗʰ **T50.B11** **Poisoning by smallpox vaccines, accidental (unintentional)**

    ² ☑7ᵗʰ **T50.B12** **Poisoning by smallpox vaccines, intentional self-harm**   HCC

    ☑7ᵗʰ **T50.B13** **Poisoning by smallpox vaccines, assault**

    ☑7ᵗʰ **T50.B14** **Poisoning by smallpox vaccines, undetermined**

    ☑7ᵗʰ **T50.B15** **Adverse effect of smallpox vaccines**

    ☑7ᵗʰ **T50.B16** **Underdosing of smallpox vaccines**

  ☑6ᵗʰ **T50.B9** **Poisoning by, adverse effect of and underdosing of other viral vaccines**

    ☑7ᵗʰ **T50.B91** **Poisoning by other viral vaccines, accidental (unintentional)**

    ² ☑7ᵗʰ **T50.B92** **Poisoning by other viral vaccines, intentional self-harm**   HCC

    ☑7ᵗʰ **T50.B93** **Poisoning by other viral vaccines, assault**

    ☑7ᵗʰ **T50.B94** **Poisoning by other viral vaccines, undetermined**

    ☑7ᵗʰ **T50.B95** **Adverse effect of other viral vaccines**

    ☑7ᵗʰ **T50.B96** **Underdosing of other viral vaccines**

☑5ᵗʰ **T50.Z** **Poisoning by, adverse effect of and underdosing of other vaccines and biological substances**

  ☑6ᵗʰ **T50.Z1** **Poisoning by, adverse effect of and underdosing of** immunoglobulin

    ☑7ᵗʰ **T50.Z11** **Poisoning by immunoglobulin, accidental (unintentional)**

    ² ☑7ᵗʰ **T50.Z12** **Poisoning by immunoglobulin, intentional self-harm**   HCC

    ☑7ᵗʰ **T50.Z13** **Poisoning by immunoglobulin, assault**

    ☑7ᵗʰ **T50.Z14** **Poisoning by immunoglobulin, undetermined**

    ☑7ᵗʰ **T50.Z15** **Adverse effect of immunoglobulin**

    ☑7ᵗʰ **T50.Z16** **Underdosing of immunoglobulin**

  ☑6ᵗʰ **T50.Z9** **Poisoning by, adverse effect of and underdosing of other vaccines and biological substances**

    ☑7ᵗʰ **T50.Z91** **Poisoning by other vaccines and biological substances, accidental (unintentional)**

    ² ☑7ᵗʰ **T50.Z92** **Poisoning by other vaccines and biological substances, intentional self-harm**   HCC

    ☑7ᵗʰ **T50.Z93** **Poisoning by other vaccines and biological substances, assault**

    ☑7ᵗʰ **T50.Z94** **Poisoning by other vaccines and biological substances, undetermined**

    ☑7ᵗʰ **T50.Z95** **Adverse effect of other vaccines and biological substances**

    ☑7ᵗʰ **T50.Z96** **Underdosing of other vaccines and biological substances**

☑5ᵗʰ **T50.9** **Poisoning by, adverse effect of and underdosing of other and unspecified drugs, medicaments and biological substances**

  AHA: 2016,1Q,38; 2015,1Q,21

  ☑6ᵗʰ **T50.90** **Poisoning by, adverse effect of and underdosing of unspecified drugs, medicaments and biological substances**

    ☑7ᵗʰ **T50.901** **Poisoning by unspecified drugs, medicaments and biological substances, accidental (unintentional)**

    ² ☑7ᵗʰ **T50.902** **Poisoning by unspecified drugs, medicaments and biological substances, intentional self-harm**   HCC

    ☑7ᵗʰ **T50.903** **Poisoning by unspecified drugs, medicaments and biological substances, assault**

    ☑7ᵗʰ **T50.904** **Poisoning by unspecified drugs, medicaments and biological substances, undetermined**

    ☑7ᵗʰ **T50.905** **Adverse effect of unspecified drugs, medicaments and biological substances**

    ☑7ᵗʰ **T50.906** **Underdosing of unspecified drugs, medicaments and biological substances**

  ● ☑6ᵗʰ **T50.91** **Poisoning by, adverse effect of and underdosing of multiple unspecified drugs, medicaments and biological substances**

    Multiple drug ingestion NOS
    Code also any specific drugs, medicaments and biological substances

    ● ☑7ᵗʰ **T50.911** **Poisoning by multiple unspecified drugs, medicaments and biological substances, accidental (unintentional)**

    ● ☑7ᵗʰ **T50.912** **Poisoning by multiple unspecified drugs, medicaments and biological substances, intentional self-harm**

    ● ☑7ᵗʰ **T50.913** **Poisoning by multiple unspecified drugs, medicaments and biological substances, assault**

    ● ☑7ᵗʰ **T50.914** **Poisoning by multiple unspecified drugs, medicaments and biological substances, undetermined**

    ● ☑7ᵗʰ **T50.915** **Adverse effect of multiple unspecified drugs, medicaments and biological substances**

    ● ☑7ᵗʰ **T50.916** **Underdosing of multiple unspecified drugs, medicaments and biological substances**

  ☑6ᵗʰ **T50.99** **Poisoning by, adverse effect of and underdosing of other drugs, medicaments and biological substances**

    ☑7ᵗʰ **T50.991** **Poisoning by other drugs, medicaments and biological substances, accidental (unintentional)**

☑ Additional Character Required   ☑7ᵗʰ Placeholder Alert   Manifestation   Unspecified Dx   ►◄ Revised Text   ● New Code   ▲ Revised Code Title

ICD-10-CM 2020   1117

2 ✓7th **T50.992 Poisoning by other drugs, medicaments and biological substances,** intentional self-harm `HCC`

✓7th **T50.993 Poisoning by other drugs, medicaments and biological substances,** assault

✓7th **T50.994 Poisoning by other drugs, medicaments and biological substances,** undetermined

✓7th **T50.995** Adverse effect **of other drugs, medicaments and biological substances**

✓7th **T50.996** Underdosing **of other drugs, medicaments and biological substances**

Toxic effects of substances chiefly nonmedicinal as to source (T51–T65)

NOTE When no intent is indicated code to accidental. Undetermined intent is only for use when there is specific documentation in the record that the intent of the toxic effect cannot be determined.

Use additional code(s) for all associated manifestations of toxic effect, such as:
personal history of foreign body fully removed (Z87.821)
respiratory conditions due to external agents (J60–J70)
to identify any retained foreign body, if applicable (Z18.-)

EXCLUDES 1 contact with and (suspected) exposure to toxic substances (Z77.-)

AHA: 2017,1Q,39-40

✓4th **T51 Toxic effect of alcohol**

> The appropriate 7th character is to be added to each code from category T51.
> A   initial encounter
> D   subsequent encounter
> S   sequela

✓5th **T51.0 Toxic effect of ethanol**

Toxic effect of ethyl alcohol

EXCLUDES 2 acute alcohol intoxication or "hangover" effects (F10.129, F10.229, F10.929)
drunkenness (F10.129, F10.229, F10.929)
pathological alcohol intoxication (F10.129, F10.229, F10.929)

✓6th **T51.0X Toxic effect of ethanol**

1 ✓7th **T51.0X1 Toxic effect of ethanol,** accidental (unintentional) `HCC`
Toxic effect of ethanol NOS

2 ✓7th **T51.0X2 Toxic effect of ethanol,** intentional self-harm `HCC`

✓7th **T51.0X3 Toxic effect of ethanol,** assault

1 ✓7th **T51.0X4 Toxic effect of ethanol,** undetermined `HCC`

✓5th **T51.1 Toxic effect of methanol**

Toxic effect of methyl alcohol

✓6th **T51.1X Toxic effect of methanol**

✓7th **T51.1X1 Toxic effect of methanol,** accidental (unintentional)
Toxic effect of methanol NOS

2 ✓7th **T51.1X2 Toxic effect of methanol,** intentional self-harm `HCC`

✓7th **T51.1X3 Toxic effect of methanol,** assault

✓7th **T51.1X4 Toxic effect of methanol,** undetermined

✓5th **T51.2 Toxic effect of 2-Propanol**

Toxic effect of isopropyl alcohol

✓6th **T51.2X Toxic effect of 2-Propanol**

✓7th **T51.2X1 Toxic effect of 2-Propanol,** accidental (unintentional)
Toxic effect of 2-Propanol NOS

2 ✓7th **T51.2X2 Toxic effect of 2-Propanol,** intentional self-harm `HCC`

✓7th **T51.2X3 Toxic effect of 2-Propanol,** assault

✓7th **T51.2X4 Toxic effect of 2-Propanol,** undetermined

✓5th **T51.3 Toxic effect of fusel oil**

Toxic effect of amyl alcohol
Toxic effect of butyl [1-butanol] alcohol
Toxic effect of propyl [1-propanol] alcohol

✓6th **T51.3X Toxic effect of fusel oil**

✓7th **T51.3X1 Toxic effect of fusel oil,** accidental (unintentional)
Toxic effect of fusel oil NOS

2 ✓7th **T51.3X2 Toxic effect of fusel oil,** intentional self-harm `HCC`

✓7th **T51.3X3 Toxic effect of fusel oil,** assault

✓7th **T51.3X4 Toxic effect of fusel oil,** undetermined

✓5th **T51.8 Toxic effect of other alcohols**

✓6th **T51.8X Toxic effect of other alcohols**

✓7th **T51.8X1 Toxic effect of other alcohols,** accidental (unintentional)
Toxic effect of other alcohols NOS

2 ✓7th **T51.8X2 Toxic effect of other alcohols,** intentional self-harm `HCC`

✓7th **T51.8X3 Toxic effect of other alcohols,** assault

✓7th **T51.8X4 Toxic effect of other alcohols,** undetermined

✓5th **T51.9 Toxic effect of unspecified alcohol**

✓x7th **T51.91 Toxic effect of unspecified alcohol,** accidental (unintentional)

2 ✓x7th **T51.92 Toxic effect of unspecified alcohol,** intentional self-harm `HCC`

✓x7th **T51.93 Toxic effect of unspecified alcohol,** assault

✓x7th **T51.94 Toxic effect of unspecified alcohol,** undetermined

✓4th **T52 Toxic effect of organic solvents**

EXCLUDES 1 halogen derivatives of aliphatic and aromatic hydrocarbons (T53.-)

> The appropriate 7th character is to be added to each code from category T52.
> A   initial encounter
> D   subsequent encounter
> S   sequela

✓5th **T52.0 Toxic effects of petroleum products**

Toxic effects of ether petroleum
Toxic effects of gasoline [petrol]
Toxic effects of kerosene [paraffin oil]
Toxic effects of naphtha petroleum
Toxic effects of paraffin wax
Toxic effects of spirit petroleum

✓6th **T52.0X Toxic effects of petroleum products**

✓7th **T52.0X1 Toxic effect of petroleum products,** accidental (unintentional)
Toxic effects of petroleum products NOS

2 ✓7th **T52.0X2 Toxic effect of petroleum products,** intentional self-harm `HCC`

✓7th **T52.0X3 Toxic effect of petroleum products,** assault

✓7th **T52.0X4 Toxic effect of petroleum products,** undetermined

✓5th **T52.1 Toxic effects of benzene**

EXCLUDES 1 homologues of benzene (T52.2)
nitroderivatives and aminoderivatives of benzene and its homologues (T65.3)

✓6th **T52.1X Toxic effects of benzene**

✓7th **T52.1X1 Toxic effects of benzene,** accidental (unintentional)
Toxic effects of benzene NOS

2 ✓7th **T52.1X2 Toxic effect of benzene,** intentional self-harm `HCC`

✓7th **T52.1X3 Toxic effect of benzene,** assault

✓7th **T52.1X4 Toxic effect of benzene,** undetermined

✓5th **T52.2 Toxic effects of homologues of benzene**

Toxic effects of toluene [methylbenzene]
Toxic effects of xylene [dimethylbenzene]

✓6th **T52.2X Toxic effects of homologues of benzene**

✓7th **T52.2X1 Toxic effect of homologues of benzene,** accidental (unintentional)
Toxic effects of homologues of benzene NOS

2 ✓7th **T52.2X2 Toxic effect of homologues of benzene,** intentional self-harm `HCC`

✓7th **T52.2X3 Toxic effect of homologues of benzene,** assault

✓7th **T52.2X4 Toxic effect of homologues of benzene,** undetermined

✓5th **T52.3 Toxic effects of glycols**

✓6th **T52.3X Toxic effects of glycols**

✓7th **T52.3X1 Toxic effect of glycols,** accidental (unintentional)
Toxic effects of glycols NOS

2 ✓7th **T52.3X2 Toxic effect of glycols,** intentional self-harm `HCC`

☑️7th T52.3X3 Toxic effect of glycols, assault

☑️7th T52.3X4 Toxic effect of glycols, undetermined

√5th **T52.4 Toxic effects of ketones**

√6th **T52.4X Toxic effects of ketones**

☑️7th **T52.4X1 Toxic effect of ketones, accidental (unintentional)**
Toxic effects of ketones NOS

² ☑️7th **T52.4X2 Toxic effect of ketones, intentional self-harm** HCC

☑️7th **T52.4X3 Toxic effect of ketones, assault**

☑️7th **T52.4X4 Toxic effect of ketones, undetermined**

√5th **T52.8 Toxic effects of other organic solvents**

√6th **T52.8X Toxic effects of other organic solvents**

☑️7th **T52.8X1 Toxic effect of other organic solvents, accidental (unintentional)**
Toxic effects of other organic solvents NOS

² ☑️7th **T52.8X2 Toxic effect of other organic solvents, intentional self-harm** HCC

☑️7th **T52.8X3 Toxic effect of other organic solvents, assault**

☑️7th **T52.8X4 Toxic effect of other organic solvents, undetermined**

√5th **T52.9 Toxic effects of unspecified organic solvent**

√x7th **T52.91 Toxic effect of unspecified organic solvent, accidental (unintentional)**

² √x7th **T52.92 Toxic effect of unspecified organic solvent, intentional self-harm** HCC

√x7th **T52.93 Toxic effect of unspecified organic solvent, assault**

√x7th **T52.94 Toxic effect of unspecified organic solvent, undetermined**

√4th **T53 Toxic effect of halogen derivatives of aliphatic and aromatic hydrocarbons**

The appropriate 7th character is to be added to each code from category T53.
A   initial encounter
D   subsequent encounter
S   sequela

√5th **T53.0 Toxic effects of carbon tetrachloride**
Toxic effects of tetrachloromethane

√6th **T53.0X Toxic effects of carbon tetrachloride**

☑️7th **T53.0X1 Toxic effect of carbon tetrachloride, accidental (unintentional)**
Toxic effects of carbon tetrachloride NOS

² ☑️7th **T53.0X2 Toxic effect of carbon tetrachloride, intentional self-harm** HCC

☑️7th **T53.0X3 Toxic effect of carbon tetrachloride, assault**

☑️7th **T53.0X4 Toxic effect of carbon tetrachloride, undetermined**

√5th **T53.1 Toxic effects of chloroform**
Toxic effects of trichloromethane

√6th **T53.1X Toxic effects of chloroform**

☑️7th **T53.1X1 Toxic effect of chloroform, accidental (unintentional)**
Toxic effects of chloroform NOS

² ☑️7th **T53.1X2 Toxic effect of chloroform, intentional self-harm** HCC

☑️7th **T53.1X3 Toxic effect of chloroform, assault**

☑️7th **T53.1X4 Toxic effect of chloroform, undetermined**

√5th **T53.2 Toxic effects of trichloroethylene**
Toxic effects of trichloroethene

√6th **T53.2X Toxic effects of trichloroethylene**

☑️7th **T53.2X1 Toxic effect of trichloroethylene, accidental (unintentional)**
Toxic effects of trichloroethylene NOS

² ☑️7th **T53.2X2 Toxic effect of trichloroethylene, intentional self-harm** HCC

☑️7th **T53.2X3 Toxic effect of trichloroethylene, assault**

☑️7th **T53.2X4 Toxic effect of trichloroethylene, undetermined**

√5th **T53.3 Toxic effects of tetrachloroethylene**
Toxic effects of perchloroethylene
Toxic effect of tetrachloroethene

√6th **T53.3X Toxic effects of tetrachloroethylene**

☑️7th **T53.3X1 Toxic effect of tetrachloroethylene, accidental (unintentional)**
Toxic effects of tetrachloroethylene NOS

² ☑️7th **T53.3X2 Toxic effect of tetrachloroethylene, intentional self-harm** HCC

☑️7th **T53.3X3 Toxic effect of tetrachloroethylene, assault**

☑️7th **T53.3X4 Toxic effect of tetrachloroethylene, undetermined**

√5th **T53.4 Toxic effects of dichloromethane**
Toxic effects of methylene chloride

√6th **T53.4X Toxic effects of dichloromethane**

☑️7th **T53.4X1 Toxic effect of dichloromethane, accidental (unintentional)**
Toxic effects of dichloromethane NOS

² ☑️7th **T53.4X2 Toxic effect of dichloromethane, intentional self-harm** HCC

☑️7th **T53.4X3 Toxic effect of dichloromethane, assault**

☑️7th **T53.4X4 Toxic effect of dichloromethane, undetermined**

√5th **T53.5 Toxic effects of chlorofluorocarbons**

√6th **T53.5X Toxic effects of chlorofluorocarbons**

☑️7th **T53.5X1 Toxic effect of chlorofluorocarbons, accidental (unintentional)**
Toxic effects of chlorofluorocarbons NOS

² ☑️7th **T53.5X2 Toxic effect of chlorofluorocarbons, intentional self-harm** HCC

☑️7th **T53.5X3 Toxic effect of chlorofluorocarbons, assault**

☑️7th **T53.5X4 Toxic effect of chlorofluorocarbons, undetermined**

√5th **T53.6 Toxic effects of other halogen derivatives of aliphatic hydrocarbons**

√6th **T53.6X Toxic effects of other halogen derivatives of aliphatic hydrocarbons**

☑️7th **T53.6X1 Toxic effect of other halogen derivatives of aliphatic hydrocarbons, accidental (unintentional)**
Toxic effects of other halogen derivatives of aliphatic hydrocarbons NOS

² ☑️7th **T53.6X2 Toxic effect of other halogen derivatives of aliphatic hydrocarbons, intentional self-harm** HCC

☑️7th **T53.6X3 Toxic effect of other halogen derivatives of aliphatic hydrocarbons, assault**

☑️7th **T53.6X4 Toxic effect of other halogen derivatives of aliphatic hydrocarbons, undetermined**

√5th **T53.7 Toxic effects of other halogen derivatives of aromatic hydrocarbons**

√6th **T53.7X Toxic effects of other halogen derivatives of aromatic hydrocarbons**

☑️7th **T53.7X1 Toxic effect of other halogen derivatives of aromatic hydrocarbons, accidental (unintentional)**
Toxic effects of other halogen derivatives of aromatic hydrocarbons NOS

² ☑️7th **T53.7X2 Toxic effect of other halogen derivatives of aromatic hydrocarbons, intentional self-harm** HCC

☑️7th **T53.7X3 Toxic effect of other halogen derivatives of aromatic hydrocarbons, assault**

☑️7th **T53.7X4 Toxic effect of other halogen derivatives of aromatic hydrocarbons, undetermined**

√5th **T53.9 Toxic effects of unspecified halogen derivatives of aliphatic and aromatic hydrocarbons**

√x7th **T53.91 Toxic effect of unspecified halogen derivatives of aliphatic and aromatic hydrocarbons, accidental (unintentional)**

² √x7th **T53.92 Toxic effect of unspecified halogen derivatives of aliphatic and aromatic hydrocarbons, intentional self-harm** HCC

√x7th **T53.93 Toxic effect of unspecified halogen derivatives of aliphatic and aromatic hydrocarbons, assault**

✅ Additional Character Required   √x7th Placeholder Alert   Manifestation   Unspecified Dx   ▶◀ Revised Text   ● New Code   ▲ Revised Code Title

✓x7ʰ **T53.94** Toxic effect of unspecified halogen derivatives of aliphatic and aromatic hydrocarbons, undetermined

✓4ʰ **T54 Toxic effect of corrosive substances**

> The appropriate 7th character is to be added to each code from category T54.
> A   initial encounter
> D   subsequent encounter
> S   sequela

✓5ʰ **T54.0 Toxic effects of phenol and phenol homologues**

✓6ʰ **T54.0X Toxic effects of phenol and phenol homologues**

✓7ʰ **T54.0X1 Toxic effect of phenol and phenol homologues, accidental (unintentional)**
Toxic effects of phenol and phenol homologues NOS

2 ✓7ʰ **T54.0X2 Toxic effect of phenol and phenol homologues, intentional self-harm** HCC

✓7ʰ **T54.0X3 Toxic effect of phenol and phenol homologues, assault**

✓7ʰ **T54.0X4 Toxic effect of phenol and phenol homologues, undetermined**

✓5ʰ **T54.1 Toxic effects of other corrosive organic compounds**

✓6ʰ **T54.1X Toxic effects of other corrosive organic compounds**

✓7ʰ **T54.1X1 Toxic effect of other corrosive organic compounds, accidental (unintentional)**
Toxic effects of other corrosive organic compounds NOS

2 ✓7ʰ **T54.1X2 Toxic effect of other corrosive organic compounds, intentional self-harm** HCC

✓7ʰ **T54.1X3 Toxic effect of other corrosive organic compounds, assault**

✓7ʰ **T54.1X4 Toxic effect of other corrosive organic compounds, undetermined**

✓5ʰ **T54.2 Toxic effects of corrosive acids and acid-like substances**
Toxic effects of hydrochloric acid
Toxic effects of sulfuric acid

✓6ʰ **T54.2X Toxic effects of corrosive acids and acid-like substances**

✓7ʰ **T54.2X1 Toxic effect of corrosive acids and acid-like substances, accidental (unintentional)**
Toxic effects of corrosive acids and acid-like substances NOS

2 ✓7ʰ **T54.2X2 Toxic effect of corrosive acids and acid-like substances, intentional self-harm** HCC

✓7ʰ **T54.2X3 Toxic effect of corrosive acids and acid-like substances, assault**

✓7ʰ **T54.2X4 Toxic effect of corrosive acids and acid-like substances, undetermined**

✓5ʰ **T54.3 Toxic effects of corrosive alkalis and alkali-like substances**
Toxic effects of potassium hydroxide
Toxic effects of sodium hydroxide

✓6ʰ **T54.3X Toxic effects of corrosive alkalis and alkali-like substances**

✓7ʰ **T54.3X1 Toxic effect of corrosive alkalis and alkali-like substances, accidental (unintentional)**
Toxic effects of corrosive alkalis and alkali-like substances NOS

2 ✓7ʰ **T54.3X2 Toxic effect of corrosive alkalis and alkali-like substances, intentional self-harm** HCC

✓7ʰ **T54.3X3 Toxic effect of corrosive alkalis and alkali-like substances, assault**

✓7ʰ **T54.3X4 Toxic effect of corrosive alkalis and alkali-like substances, undetermined**

✓5ʰ **T54.9 Toxic effects of unspecified corrosive substance**

✓x7ʰ **T54.91 Toxic effect of unspecified corrosive substance, accidental (unintentional)**

2 ✓x7ʰ **T54.92 Toxic effect of unspecified corrosive substance, intentional self-harm** HCC

✓x7ʰ **T54.93 Toxic effect of unspecified corrosive substance, assault**

✓x7ʰ **T54.94 Toxic effect of unspecified corrosive substance, undetermined**

✓4ʰ **T55 Toxic effect of soaps and detergents**

> The appropriate 7th character is to be added to each code from category T55.
> A   initial encounter
> D   subsequent encounter
> S   sequela

✓5ʰ **T55.0 Toxic effect of soaps**

✓6ʰ **T55.0X Toxic effect of soaps**

✓7ʰ **T55.0X1 Toxic effect of soaps, accidental (unintentional)**
Toxic effect of soaps NOS

2 ✓7ʰ **T55.0X2 Toxic effect of soaps, intentional self-harm** HCC

✓7ʰ **T55.0X3 Toxic effect of soaps, assault**

✓7ʰ **T55.0X4 Toxic effect of soaps, undetermined**

✓5ʰ **T55.1 Toxic effect of detergents**

✓6ʰ **T55.1X Toxic effect of detergents**

✓7ʰ **T55.1X1 Toxic effect of detergents, accidental (unintentional)**
Toxic effect of detergents NOS

2 ✓7ʰ **T55.1X2 Toxic effect of detergents, intentional self-harm** HCC

✓7ʰ **T55.1X3 Toxic effect of detergents, assault**

✓7ʰ **T55.1X4 Toxic effect of detergents, undetermined**

✓4ʰ **T56 Toxic effect of metals**

> **INCLUDES**   toxic effects of fumes and vapors of metals
> toxic effects of metals from all sources, except medicinal substances
> Use additional code to identify any retained metal foreign body, if applicable (Z18.0-, T18.1-)
> **EXCLUDES 1**   arsenic and its compounds (T57.0)
> manganese and its compounds (T57.2)

> The appropriate 7th character is to be added to each code from category T56.
> A   initial encounter
> D   subsequent encounter
> S   sequela

✓5ʰ **T56.0 Toxic effects of lead and its compounds**

✓6ʰ **T56.0X Toxic effects of lead and its compounds**

✓7ʰ **T56.0X1 Toxic effect of lead and its compounds, accidental (unintentional)**
Toxic effects of lead and its compounds NOS

2 ✓7ʰ **T56.0X2 Toxic effect of lead and its compounds, intentional self-harm** HCC

✓7ʰ **T56.0X3 Toxic effect of lead and its compounds, assault**

✓7ʰ **T56.0X4 Toxic effect of lead and its compounds, undetermined**

✓5ʰ **T56.1 Toxic effects of mercury and its compounds**

✓6ʰ **T56.1X Toxic effects of mercury and its compounds**

✓7ʰ **T56.1X1 Toxic effect of mercury and its compounds, accidental (unintentional)**
Toxic effects of mercury and its compounds NOS

2 ✓7ʰ **T56.1X2 Toxic effect of mercury and its compounds, intentional self-harm** HCC

✓7ʰ **T56.1X3 Toxic effect of mercury and its compounds, assault**

✓7ʰ **T56.1X4 Toxic effect of mercury and its compounds, undetermined**

✓5ʰ **T56.2 Toxic effects of chromium and its compounds**

✓6ʰ **T56.2X Toxic effects of chromium and its compounds**

✓7ʰ **T56.2X1 Toxic effect of chromium and its compounds, accidental (unintentional)**
Toxic effects of chromium and its compounds NOS

2 ✓7ʰ **T56.2X2 Toxic effect of chromium and its compounds, intentional self-harm** HCC

✓7ʰ **T56.2X3 Toxic effect of chromium and its compounds, assault**

✓7ʰ **T56.2X4 Toxic effect of chromium and its compounds, undetermined**

√5ᵗʰ **T56.3** **Toxic effects of cadmium and its compounds**

  √6ᵗʰ **T56.3X** **Toxic effects of cadmium and its compounds**

    √7ᵗʰ **T56.3X1** **Toxic effect of cadmium and its compounds, accidental (unintentional)**
Toxic effects of cadmium and its compounds NOS

    ² √7ᵗʰ **T56.3X2** **Toxic effect of cadmium and its compounds, intentional self-harm** HCC

    √7ᵗʰ **T56.3X3** **Toxic effect of cadmium and its compounds, assault**

    √7ᵗʰ **T56.3X4** **Toxic effect of cadmium and its compounds, undetermined**

√5ᵗʰ **T56.4** **Toxic effects of copper and its compounds**

  √6ᵗʰ **T56.4X** **Toxic effects of copper and its compounds**

    √7ᵗʰ **T56.4X1** **Toxic effect of copper and its compounds, accidental (unintentional)**
Toxic effects of copper and its compounds NOS

    ² √7ᵗʰ **T56.4X2** **Toxic effect of copper and its compounds, intentional self-harm** HCC

    √7ᵗʰ **T56.4X3** **Toxic effect of copper and its compounds, assault**

    √7ᵗʰ **T56.4X4** **Toxic effect of copper and its compounds, undetermined**

√5ᵗʰ **T56.5** **Toxic effects of zinc and its compounds**

  √6ᵗʰ **T56.5X** **Toxic effects of zinc and its compounds**

    √7ᵗʰ **T56.5X1** **Toxic effect of zinc and its compounds, accidental (unintentional)**
Toxic effects of zinc and its compounds NOS

    ² √7ᵗʰ **T56.5X2** **Toxic effect of zinc and its compounds, intentional self-harm** HCC

    √7ᵗʰ **T56.5X3** **Toxic effect of zinc and its compounds, assault**

    √7ᵗʰ **T56.5X4** **Toxic effect of zinc and its compounds, undetermined**

√5ᵗʰ **T56.6** **Toxic effects of tin and its compounds**

  √6ᵗʰ **T56.6X** **Toxic effects of tin and its compounds**

    √7ᵗʰ **T56.6X1** **Toxic effect of tin and its compounds, accidental (unintentional)**
Toxic effects of tin and its compounds NOS

    ² √7ᵗʰ **T56.6X2** **Toxic effect of tin and its compounds, intentional self-harm** HCC

    √7ᵗʰ **T56.6X3** **Toxic effect of tin and its compounds, assault**

    √7ᵗʰ **T56.6X4** **Toxic effect of tin and its compounds, undetermined**

√5ᵗʰ **T56.7** **Toxic effects of beryllium and its compounds**

  √6ᵗʰ **T56.7X** **Toxic effects of beryllium and its compounds**

    √7ᵗʰ **T56.7X1** **Toxic effect of beryllium and its compounds, accidental (unintentional)**
Toxic effects of beryllium and its compounds NOS

    ² √7ᵗʰ **T56.7X2** **Toxic effect of beryllium and its compounds, intentional self-harm** HCC

    √7ᵗʰ **T56.7X3** **Toxic effect of beryllium and its compounds, assault**

    √7ᵗʰ **T56.7X4** **Toxic effect of beryllium and its compounds, undetermined**

√5ᵗʰ **T56.8** **Toxic effects of other metals**

  √6ᵗʰ **T56.81** **Toxic effect of thallium**

    √7ᵗʰ **T56.811** **Toxic effect of thallium, accidental (unintentional)**
Toxic effect of thallium NOS

    ² √7ᵗʰ **T56.812** **Toxic effect of thallium, intentional self-harm** HCC

    √7ᵗʰ **T56.813** **Toxic effect of thallium, assault**

    √7ᵗʰ **T56.814** **Toxic effect of thallium, undetermined**

  √6ᵗʰ **T56.89** **Toxic effects of other metals**

    √7ᵗʰ **T56.891** **Toxic effect of other metals, accidental (unintentional)**
Toxic effects of other metals NOS

    ² √7ᵗʰ **T56.892** **Toxic effect of other metals, intentional self-harm** HCC

    √7ᵗʰ **T56.893** **Toxic effect of other metals, assault**

    √7ᵗʰ **T56.894** **Toxic effect of other metals, undetermined**

√5ᵗʰ **T56.9** **Toxic effects of unspecified metal**

  √x7ᵗʰ **T56.91** **Toxic effect of unspecified metal, accidental (unintentional)**

  ² √x7ᵗʰ **T56.92** **Toxic effect of unspecified metal, intentional self-harm** HCC

  √x7ᵗʰ **T56.93** **Toxic effect of unspecified metal, assault**

  √x7ᵗʰ **T56.94** **Toxic effect of unspecified metal, undetermined**

√4ᵗʰ **T57** **Toxic effect of other inorganic substances**

> The appropriate 7th character is to be added to each code from category T57.
> A   initial encounter
> D   subsequent encounter
> S   sequela

√5ᵗʰ **T57.0** **Toxic effect of arsenic and its compounds**

  √6ᵗʰ **T57.0X** **Toxic effect of arsenic and its compounds**

    √7ᵗʰ **T57.0X1** **Toxic effect of arsenic and its compounds, accidental (unintentional)**
Toxic effect of arsenic and its compounds NOS

    ² √7ᵗʰ **T57.0X2** **Toxic effect of arsenic and its compounds, intentional self-harm** HCC

    √7ᵗʰ **T57.0X3** **Toxic effect of arsenic and its compounds, assault**

    √7ᵗʰ **T57.0X4** **Toxic effect of arsenic and its compounds, undetermined**

√5ᵗʰ **T57.1** **Toxic effect of phosphorus and its compounds**

    EXCLUDES 1   organophosphate insecticides (T60.0)

  √6ᵗʰ **T57.1X** **Toxic effect of phosphorus and its compounds**

    √7ᵗʰ **T57.1X1** **Toxic effect of phosphorus and its compounds, accidental (unintentional)**
Toxic effect of phosphorus and its compounds NOS

    ² √7ᵗʰ **T57.1X2** **Toxic effect of phosphorus and its compounds, intentional self-harm** HCC

    √7ᵗʰ **T57.1X3** **Toxic effect of phosphorus and its compounds, assault**

    √7ᵗʰ **T57.1X4** **Toxic effect of phosphorus and its compounds, undetermined**

√5ᵗʰ **T57.2** **Toxic effect of manganese and its compounds**

  √6ᵗʰ **T57.2X** **Toxic effect of manganese and its compounds**

    √7ᵗʰ **T57.2X1** **Toxic effect of manganese and its compounds, accidental (unintentional)**
Toxic effect of manganese and its compounds NOS

    ² √7ᵗʰ **T57.2X2** **Toxic effect of manganese and its compounds, intentional self-harm** HCC

    √7ᵗʰ **T57.2X3** **Toxic effect of manganese and its compounds, assault**

    √7ᵗʰ **T57.2X4** **Toxic effect of manganese and its compounds, undetermined**

√5ᵗʰ **T57.3** **Toxic effect of hydrogen cyanide**

  √6ᵗʰ **T57.3X** **Toxic effect of hydrogen cyanide**

    √7ᵗʰ **T57.3X1** **Toxic effect of hydrogen cyanide, accidental (unintentional)**
Toxic effect of hydrogen cyanide NOS

    ² √7ᵗʰ **T57.3X2** **Toxic effect of hydrogen cyanide, intentional self-harm** HCC

    √7ᵗʰ **T57.3X3** **Toxic effect of hydrogen cyanide, assault**

    √7ᵗʰ **T57.3X4** **Toxic effect of hydrogen cyanide, undetermined**

√5ᵗʰ **T57.8** **Toxic effect of other specified inorganic substances**

  √6ᵗʰ **T57.8X** **Toxic effect of other specified inorganic substances**

    √7ᵗʰ **T57.8X1** **Toxic effect of other specified inorganic substances, accidental (unintentional)**
Toxic effect of other specified inorganic substances NOS

    ² √7ᵗʰ **T57.8X2** **Toxic effect of other specified inorganic substances, intentional self-harm** HCC

    √7ᵗʰ **T57.8X3** **Toxic effect of other specified inorganic substances, assault**

✓ Additional Character Required   √x7ᵗʰ Placeholder Alert   Manifestation   Unspecified Dx   ►◄ Revised Text   ● New Code   ▲ Revised Code Title

√7ᵗʰ **T57.8X4** **Toxic effect of other specified inorganic substances,** undetermined

√5ᵗʰ **T57.9** **Toxic effect of unspecified inorganic substance**

    √7ᵗʰ **T57.91** **Toxic effect of unspecified inorganic substance, accidental (unintentional)**

    ² √7ᵗʰ **T57.92** **Toxic effect of unspecified inorganic substance,** intentional self-harm   HCC

    √7ᵗʰ **T57.93** **Toxic effect of unspecified inorganic substance,** assault

    √7ᵗʰ **T57.94** **Toxic effect of unspecified inorganic substance,** undetermined

√4ᵗʰ **T58** **Toxic effect of carbon monoxide**

> **INCLUDES**   asphyxiation from carbon monoxide
>   toxic effect of carbon monoxide from all sources

> The appropriate 7th character is to be added to each code from category T58.
> A   initial encounter
> D   subsequent encounter
> S   sequela

√5ᵗʰ **T58.0** **Toxic effect of carbon monoxide** from motor vehicle exhaust

    Toxic effect of exhaust gas from gas engine
    Toxic effect of exhaust gas from motor pump

    √7ᵗʰ **T58.01** **Toxic effect of carbon monoxide from motor vehicle exhaust, accidental (unintentional)**

    ² √7ᵗʰ **T58.02** **Toxic effect of carbon monoxide from motor vehicle exhaust,** intentional self-harm   HCC

    √7ᵗʰ **T58.03** **Toxic effect of carbon monoxide from motor vehicle exhaust,** assault

    √7ᵗʰ **T58.04** **Toxic effect of carbon monoxide from motor vehicle exhaust,** undetermined

√5ᵗʰ **T58.1** **Toxic effect of carbon monoxide** from utility gas

    Toxic effect of acetylene
    Toxic effect of gas NOS used for lighting, heating, cooking
    Toxic effect of water gas

    √7ᵗʰ **T58.11** **Toxic effect of carbon monoxide from utility gas, accidental (unintentional)**

    ² √7ᵗʰ **T58.12** **Toxic effect of carbon monoxide from utility gas,** intentional self-harm   HCC

    √7ᵗʰ **T58.13** **Toxic effect of carbon monoxide from utility gas, assault**

    √7ᵗʰ **T58.14** **Toxic effect of carbon monoxide from utility gas, undetermined**

√5ᵗʰ **T58.2** **Toxic effect of carbon monoxide from incomplete combustion of other domestic fuels**

    Toxic effect of carbon monoxide from incomplete combustion of coal, coke, kerosene, wood

    √6ᵗʰ **T58.2X** **Toxic effect of carbon monoxide** from incomplete combustion of other domestic fuels

        √7ᵗʰ **T58.2X1** **Toxic effect of carbon monoxide from incomplete combustion of other domestic fuels, accidental (unintentional)**

        ² √7ᵗʰ **T58.2X2** **Toxic effect of carbon monoxide from incomplete combustion of other domestic fuels,** intentional self-harm   HCC

        √7ᵗʰ **T58.2X3** **Toxic effect of carbon monoxide from incomplete combustion of other domestic fuels, assault**

        √7ᵗʰ **T58.2X4** **Toxic effect of carbon monoxide from incomplete combustion of other domestic fuels, undetermined**

√5ᵗʰ **T58.8** **Toxic effect of carbon monoxide from other source**

    Toxic effect of carbon monoxide from blast furnace gas
    Toxic effect of carbon monoxide from fuels in industrial use
    Toxic effect of carbon monoxide from kiln vapor

    √6ᵗʰ **T58.8X** **Toxic effect of carbon monoxide from other source**

        √7ᵗʰ **T58.8X1** **Toxic effect of carbon monoxide from other source,** accidental (unintentional)

        ² √7ᵗʰ **T58.8X2** **Toxic effect of carbon monoxide from other source,** intentional self-harm   HCC

        √7ᵗʰ **T58.8X3** **Toxic effect of carbon monoxide from other source,** assault

        √7ᵗʰ **T58.8X4** **Toxic effect of carbon monoxide from other source,** undetermined

√5ᵗʰ **T58.9** **Toxic effect of carbon monoxide from unspecified source**

    √7ᵗʰ **T58.91** **Toxic effect of carbon monoxide from unspecified source,** accidental (unintentional)

---

² √x7ᵗʰ **T58.92** **Toxic effect of carbon monoxide from unspecified source,** intentional self-harm   HCC

√x7ᵗʰ **T58.93** **Toxic effect of carbon monoxide from unspecified source,** assault

√x7ᵗʰ **T58.94** **Toxic effect of carbon monoxide from unspecified source,** undetermined

√4ᵗʰ **T59** **Toxic effect of other gases, fumes and vapors**

> **INCLUDES**   aerosol propellants
> **EXCLUDES 1**   *chlorofluorocarbons (T53.5)*

> The appropriate 7th character is to be added to each code from category T59.
> A   initial encounter
> D   subsequent encounter
> S   sequela

√5ᵗʰ **T59.0** **Toxic effect of nitrogen oxides**

    √6ᵗʰ **T59.0X** **Toxic effect of** nitrogen oxides

        √7ᵗʰ **T59.0X1** **Toxic effect of nitrogen oxides, accidental (unintentional)**
               Toxic effect of nitrogen oxides NOS

        ² √7ᵗʰ **T59.0X2** **Toxic effect of nitrogen oxides,** intentional self-harm   HCC

        √7ᵗʰ **T59.0X3** **Toxic effect of nitrogen oxides, assault**

        √7ᵗʰ **T59.0X4** **Toxic effect of nitrogen oxides, undetermined**

√5ᵗʰ **T59.1** **Toxic effect of sulfur dioxide**

    √6ᵗʰ **T59.1X** **Toxic effect of** sulfur dioxide

        √7ᵗʰ **T59.1X1** **Toxic effect of sulfur dioxide, accidental (unintentional)**
               Toxic effect of sulfur dioxide NOS

        ² √7ᵗʰ **T59.1X2** **Toxic effect of sulfur dioxide,** intentional self-harm   HCC

        √7ᵗʰ **T59.1X3** **Toxic effect of sulfur dioxide, assault**

        √7ᵗʰ **T59.1X4** **Toxic effect of sulfur dioxide, undetermined**

√5ᵗʰ **T59.2** **Toxic effect of formaldehyde**

    √6ᵗʰ **T59.2X** **Toxic effect of** formaldehyde

        √7ᵗʰ **T59.2X1** **Toxic effect of formaldehyde, accidental (unintentional)**
               Toxic effect of formaldehyde NOS

        ² √7ᵗʰ **T59.2X2** **Toxic effect of formaldehyde,** intentional self-harm   HCC

        √7ᵗʰ **T59.2X3** **Toxic effect of formaldehyde, assault**

        √7ᵗʰ **T59.2X4** **Toxic effect of formaldehyde, undetermined**

√5ᵗʰ **T59.3** **Toxic effect of lacrimogenic gas**

    Toxic effect of tear gas

    √6ᵗʰ **T59.3X** **Toxic effect of** lacrimogenic gas

        √7ᵗʰ **T59.3X1** **Toxic effect of lacrimogenic gas, accidental (unintentional)**
               Toxic effect of lacrimogenic gas NOS

        ² √7ᵗʰ **T59.3X2** **Toxic effect of lacrimogenic gas,** intentional self-harm   HCC

        √7ᵗʰ **T59.3X3** **Toxic effect of lacrimogenic gas, assault**

        √7ᵗʰ **T59.3X4** **Toxic effect of lacrimogenic gas, undetermined**

√5ᵗʰ **T59.4** **Toxic effect of chlorine gas**

    √6ᵗʰ **T59.4X** **Toxic effect of** chlorine gas

        √7ᵗʰ **T59.4X1** **Toxic effect of chlorine gas, accidental (unintentional)**
               Toxic effect of chlorine gas NOS

        ² √7ᵗʰ **T59.4X2** **Toxic effect of chlorine gas,** intentional self-harm   HCC

        √7ᵗʰ **T59.4X3** **Toxic effect of chlorine gas, assault**

        √7ᵗʰ **T59.4X4** **Toxic effect of chlorine gas, undetermined**

√5ᵗʰ **T59.5** **Toxic effect of fluorine gas and hydrogen fluoride**

    √6ᵗʰ **T59.5X** **Toxic effect of** fluorine gas and hydrogen fluoride

        √7ᵗʰ **T59.5X1** **Toxic effect of fluorine gas and hydrogen fluoride, accidental (unintentional)**
               Toxic effect of fluorine gas and hydrogen fluoride NOS

        ² √7ᵗʰ **T59.5X2** **Toxic effect of fluorine gas and hydrogen fluoride,** intentional self-harm   HCC

        √7ᵗʰ **T59.5X3** **Toxic effect of fluorine gas and hydrogen fluoride, assault**

☑7ᵗʰ **T59.5X4** Toxic effect of fluorine gas and hydrogen fluoride, undetermined

☑5ᵗʰ **T59.6** Toxic effect of hydrogen sulfide

  ☑6ᵗʰ **T59.6X** Toxic effect of hydrogen sulfide

    ☑7ᵗʰ **T59.6X1** Toxic effect of hydrogen sulfide, accidental (unintentional)
Toxic effect of hydrogen sulfide NOS

    ² ☑7ᵗʰ **T59.6X2** Toxic effect of hydrogen sulfide, intentional self-harm   HCC

    ☑7ᵗʰ **T59.6X3** Toxic effect of hydrogen sulfide, assault

    ☑7ᵗʰ **T59.6X4** Toxic effect of hydrogen sulfide, undetermined

☑5ᵗʰ **T59.7** Toxic effect of carbon dioxide

  ☑6ᵗʰ **T59.7X** Toxic effect of carbon dioxide

    ☑7ᵗʰ **T59.7X1** Toxic effect of carbon dioxide, accidental (unintentional)
Toxic effect of carbon dioxide NOS

    ² ☑7ᵗʰ **T59.7X2** Toxic effect of carbon dioxide, intentional self-harm   HCC

    ☑7ᵗʰ **T59.7X3** Toxic effect of carbon dioxide, assault

    ☑7ᵗʰ **T59.7X4** Toxic effect of carbon dioxide, undetermined

☑5ᵗʰ **T59.8** Toxic effect of other specified gases, fumes and vapors

  ☑6ᵗʰ **T59.81** Toxic effect of smoke
Smoke inhalation
EXCLUDES 2   toxic effect of cigarette (tobacco) smoke (T65.22-)

    ☑7ᵗʰ **T59.811** Toxic effect of smoke, accidental (unintentional)
Toxic effect of smoke NOS
AHA: 2013,4Q,121

    ² ☑7ᵗʰ **T59.812** Toxic effect of smoke, intentional self-harm   HCC

    ☑7ᵗʰ **T59.813** Toxic effect of smoke, assault

    ☑7ᵗʰ **T59.814** Toxic effect of smoke, undetermined

  ☑6ᵗʰ **T59.89** Toxic effect of other specified gases, fumes and vapors

    ☑7ᵗʰ **T59.891** Toxic effect of other specified gases, fumes and vapors, accidental (unintentional)

    ² ☑7ᵗʰ **T59.892** Toxic effect of other specified gases, fumes and vapors, intentional self-harm   HCC

    ☑7ᵗʰ **T59.893** Toxic effect of other specified gases, fumes and vapors, assault

    ☑7ᵗʰ **T59.894** Toxic effect of other specified gases, fumes and vapors, undetermined

☑5ᵗʰ **T59.9** Toxic effect of unspecified gases, fumes and vapors

  ☑x7ᵗʰ **T59.91** Toxic effect of unspecified gases, fumes and vapors, accidental (unintentional)

  ² ☑x7ᵗʰ **T59.92** Toxic effect of unspecified gases, fumes and vapors, intentional self-harm   HCC

  ☑x7ᵗʰ **T59.93** Toxic effect of unspecified gases, fumes and vapors, assault

  ☑x7ᵗʰ **T59.94** Toxic effect of unspecified gases, fumes and vapors, undetermined

☑4ᵗʰ **T60** Toxic effect of pesticides
INCLUDES   toxic effect of wood preservatives

The appropriate 7th character is to be added to each code from category T60.
A   initial encounter
D   subsequent encounter
S   sequela

☑5ᵗʰ **T60.0** Toxic effect of organophosphate and carbamate insecticides

  ☑6ᵗʰ **T60.0X** Toxic effect of organophosphate and carbamate insecticides

    ☑7ᵗʰ **T60.0X1** Toxic effect of organophosphate and carbamate insecticides, accidental (unintentional)
Toxic effect of organophosphate and carbamate insecticides NOS

    ² ☑7ᵗʰ **T60.0X2** Toxic effect of organophosphate and carbamate insecticides, intentional self-harm   HCC

    ☑7ᵗʰ **T60.0X3** Toxic effect of organophosphate and carbamate insecticides, assault

    ☑7ᵗʰ **T60.0X4** Toxic effect of organophosphate and carbamate insecticides, undetermined

☑5ᵗʰ **T60.1** Toxic effect of halogenated insecticides
EXCLUDES 1   chlorinated hydrocarbon (T53.-)

  ☑6ᵗʰ **T60.1X** Toxic effect of halogenated insecticides

    ☑7ᵗʰ **T60.1X1** Toxic effect of halogenated insecticides, accidental (unintentional)
Toxic effect of halogenated insecticides NOS

    ² ☑7ᵗʰ **T60.1X2** Toxic effect of halogenated insecticides, intentional self-harm   HCC

    ☑7ᵗʰ **T60.1X3** Toxic effect of halogenated insecticides, assault

    ☑7ᵗʰ **T60.1X4** Toxic effect of halogenated insecticides, undetermined

☑5ᵗʰ **T60.2** Toxic effect of other insecticides

  ☑6ᵗʰ **T60.2X** Toxic effect of other insecticides

    ☑7ᵗʰ **T60.2X1** Toxic effect of other insecticides, accidental (unintentional)
Toxic effect of other insecticides NOS

    ² ☑7ᵗʰ **T60.2X2** Toxic effect of other insecticides, intentional self-harm   HCC

    ☑7ᵗʰ **T60.2X3** Toxic effect of other insecticides, assault

    ☑7ᵗʰ **T60.2X4** Toxic effect of other insecticides, undetermined

☑5ᵗʰ **T60.3** Toxic effect of herbicides and fungicides

  ☑6ᵗʰ **T60.3X** Toxic effect of herbicides and fungicides

    ☑7ᵗʰ **T60.3X1** Toxic effect of herbicides and fungicides, accidental (unintentional)
Toxic effect of herbicides and fungicides NOS

    ² ☑7ᵗʰ **T60.3X2** Toxic effect of herbicides and fungicides, intentional self-harm   HCC

    ☑7ᵗʰ **T60.3X3** Toxic effect of herbicides and fungicides, assault

    ☑7ᵗʰ **T60.3X4** Toxic effect of herbicides and fungicides, undetermined

☑5ᵗʰ **T60.4** Toxic effect of rodenticides
EXCLUDES 1   strychnine and its salts (T65.1)
thallium (T56.81-)

  ☑6ᵗʰ **T60.4X** Toxic effect of rodenticides

    ☑7ᵗʰ **T60.4X1** Toxic effect of rodenticides, accidental (unintentional)
Toxic effect of rodenticides NOS

    ² ☑7ᵗʰ **T60.4X2** Toxic effect of rodenticides, intentional self-harm   HCC

    ☑7ᵗʰ **T60.4X3** Toxic effect of rodenticides, assault

    ☑7ᵗʰ **T60.4X4** Toxic effect of rodenticides, undetermined

☑5ᵗʰ **T60.8** Toxic effect of other pesticides

  ☑6ᵗʰ **T60.8X** Toxic effect of other pesticides

    ☑7ᵗʰ **T60.8X1** Toxic effect of other pesticides, accidental (unintentional)
Toxic effect of other pesticides NOS

    ² ☑7ᵗʰ **T60.8X2** Toxic effect of other pesticides, intentional self-harm   HCC

    ☑7ᵗʰ **T60.8X3** Toxic effect of other pesticides, assault

    ☑7ᵗʰ **T60.8X4** Toxic effect of other pesticides, undetermined

☑5ᵗʰ **T60.9** Toxic effect of unspecified pesticide

  ☑x7ᵗʰ **T60.91** Toxic effect of unspecified pesticide, accidental (unintentional)

  ² ☑x7ᵗʰ **T60.92** Toxic effect of unspecified pesticide, intentional self-harm   HCC

  ☑x7ᵗʰ **T60.93** Toxic effect of unspecified pesticide, assault

  ☑x7ᵗʰ **T60.94** Toxic effect of unspecified pesticide, undetermined

Chapter 19. Injury, Poisoning and Certain Other Consequences of External Causes

T61–T62.92

√4th **T61 Toxic effect of noxious substances eaten as seafood**

EXCLUDES 1   *allergic reaction to food, such as:*
     anaphylactic reaction or shock due to adverse food reaction (T78.Ø-)
     bacterial foodborne intoxications (AØ5.-)
     dermatitis (L23.6, L25.4, L27.2)
     food protein-induced enterocolitis syndrome (K52.21)
     food protein-induced enteropathy (K52.22)
     gastroenteritis (noninfective) (K52.29)
   toxic effect of aflatoxin and other mycotoxins (T64)
   toxic effect of cyanides (T65.Ø-)
   toxic effect of harmful algae bloom (T65.82-)
   toxic effect of hydrogen cyanide (T57.3-)
   toxic effect of mercury (T56.1-)
   toxic effect of red tide (T65.82-)

The appropriate 7th character is to be added to each code from category T61.
A   initial encounter
D   subsequent encounter
S   sequela

√5th **T61.Ø Ciguatera fish poisoning**

   √x7th **T61.Ø1 Ciguatera fish poisoning, accidental (unintentional)**

   2 √x7th **T61.Ø2 Ciguatera fish poisoning, intentional self-harm**   HCC

   √x7th **T61.Ø3 Ciguatera fish poisoning, assault**

   √x7th **T61.Ø4 Ciguatera fish poisoning, undetermined**

√5th **T61.1 Scombroid fish poisoning**
   Histamine-like syndrome

   √x7th **T61.11 Scombroid fish poisoning, accidental (unintentional)**

   2 √x7th **T61.12 Scombroid fish poisoning, intentional self-harm**   HCC

   √x7th **T61.13 Scombroid fish poisoning, assault**

   √x7th **T61.14 Scombroid fish poisoning, undetermined**

√5th **T61.7 Other fish and shellfish poisoning**

   √6th **T61.77 Other fish poisoning**

     √7th **T61.771 Other fish poisoning, accidental (unintentional)**

     2 √7th **T61.772 Other fish poisoning, intentional self-harm**   HCC

     √7th **T61.773 Other fish poisoning, assault**

     √7th **T61.774 Other fish poisoning, undetermined**

   √6th **T61.78 Other shellfish poisoning**

     √7th **T61.781 Other shellfish poisoning, accidental (unintentional)**

     2 √7th **T61.782 Other shellfish poisoning, intentional self-harm**   HCC

     √7th **T61.783 Other shellfish poisoning, assault**

     √7th **T61.784 Other shellfish poisoning, undetermined**

√5th **T61.8 Toxic effect of other seafood**

   √6th **T61.8X Toxic effect of other seafood**

     √7th **T61.8X1 Toxic effect of other seafood, accidental (unintentional)**

     2 √7th **T61.8X2 Toxic effect of other seafood, intentional self-harm**   HCC

     √7th **T61.8X3 Toxic effect of other seafood, assault**

     √7th **T61.8X4 Toxic effect of other seafood, undetermined**

√5th **T61.9 Toxic effect of unspecified seafood**

   √x7th **T61.91 Toxic effect of unspecified seafood, accidental (unintentional)**

   2 √x7th **T61.92 Toxic effect of unspecified seafood, intentional self-harm**   HCC

   √x7th **T61.93 Toxic effect of unspecified seafood, assault**

   √x7th **T61.94 Toxic effect of unspecified seafood, undetermined**

√4th **T62 Toxic effect of other noxious substances eaten as food**

EXCLUDES 1   *allergic reaction to food, such as:*
     anaphylactic shock (reaction) due to adverse food reaction (T78.Ø-)
     bacterial food borne intoxications (AØ5.-)
     dermatitis (L23.6, L25.4, L27.2)
     food protein-induced enterocolitis syndrome (K52.21)
     food protein-induced enteropathy (K52.22)
     gastroenteritis (noninfective) (K52.29)
   toxic effect of aflatoxin and other mycotoxins (T64)
   toxic effect of cyanides (T65.Ø-)
   toxic effect of hydrogen cyanide (T57.3-)
   toxic effect of mercury (T56.1-)

The appropriate 7th character is to be added to each code from category T62.
A   initial encounter
D   subsequent encounter
S   sequela

√5th **T62.Ø Toxic effect of ingested mushrooms**

   √6th **T62.ØX Toxic effect of ingested mushrooms**

     √7th **T62.ØX1 Toxic effect of ingested mushrooms, accidental (unintentional)**
       Toxic effect of ingested mushrooms NOS

     2 √7th **T62.ØX2 Toxic effect of ingested mushrooms, intentional self-harm**   HCC

     √7th **T62.ØX3 Toxic effect of ingested mushrooms, assault**

     √7th **T62.ØX4 Toxic effect of ingested mushrooms, undetermined**

√5th **T62.1 Toxic effect of ingested berries**

   √6th **T62.1X Toxic effect of ingested berries**

     √7th **T62.1X1 Toxic effect of ingested berries, accidental (unintentional)**
       Toxic effect of ingested berries NOS

     2 √7th **T62.1X2 Toxic effect of ingested berries, intentional self-harm**   HCC

     √7th **T62.1X3 Toxic effect of ingested berries, assault**

     √7th **T62.1X4 Toxic effect of ingested berries, undetermined**

√5th **T62.2 Toxic effect of other ingested (parts of) plant(s)**

   √6th **T62.2X Toxic effect of other ingested (parts of) plant(s)**

     √7th **T62.2X1 Toxic effect of other ingested (parts of) plant(s), accidental (unintentional)**
       Toxic effect of other ingested (parts of) plant(s) NOS

     2 √7th **T62.2X2 Toxic effect of other ingested (parts of) plant(s), intentional self-harm**   HCC

     √7th **T62.2X3 Toxic effect of other ingested (parts of) plant(s), assault**

     √7th **T62.2X4 Toxic effect of other ingested (parts of) plant(s), undetermined**

√5th **T62.8 Toxic effect of other specified noxious substances eaten as food**

   √6th **T62.8X Toxic effect of other specified noxious substances eaten as food**

     √7th **T62.8X1 Toxic effect of other specified noxious substances eaten as food, accidental (unintentional)**
       Toxic effect of other specified substances eaten as food NOS

     2 √7th **T62.8X2 Toxic effect of other specified noxious substances eaten as food, intentional self-harm**   HCC

     √7th **T62.8X3 Toxic effect of other specified noxious substances eaten as food, assault**

     √7th **T62.8X4 Toxic effect of other specified noxious substances eaten as food, undetermined**

√5th **T62.9 Toxic effect of unspecified noxious substance eaten as food**

   √x7th **T62.91 Toxic effect of unspecified noxious substance eaten as food, accidental (unintentional)**
     Toxic effect of unspecified noxious substance eaten as food NOS

   2 √x7th **T62.92 Toxic effect of unspecified noxious substance eaten as food, intentional self-harm**   HCC

√x7ᵗʰ **T62.93** Toxic effect of unspecified noxious substance eaten as food, assault

√x7ᵗʰ **T62.94** Toxic effect of unspecified noxious substance eaten as food, undetermined

√4ᵗʰ **T63** Toxic effect of contact with venomous animals and plants

INCLUDES	bite or touch of venomous animal
	pricked or stuck by thorn or leaf
EXCLUDES 2	ingestion of toxic animal or plant (T61.-, T62.-)

The appropriate 7th character is to be added to each code from category T63.
A   initial encounter
D   subsequent encounter
S   sequela

√5ᵗʰ **T63.0** Toxic effect of snake venom

√6ᵗʰ **T63.00** Toxic effect of unspecified snake venom

√7ᵗʰ **T63.001** Toxic effect of unspecified snake venom, accidental (unintentional)
Toxic effect of unspecified snake venom NOS

² √7ᵗʰ **T63.002** Toxic effect of unspecified snake venom, intentional self-harm HCC

√7ᵗʰ **T63.003** Toxic effect of unspecified snake venom, assault

√7ᵗʰ **T63.004** Toxic effect of unspecified snake venom, undetermined

√6ᵗʰ **T63.01** Toxic effect of rattlesnake venom

√7ᵗʰ **T63.011** Toxic effect of rattlesnake venom, accidental (unintentional)
Toxic effect of rattlesnake venom NOS

² √7ᵗʰ **T63.012** Toxic effect of rattlesnake venom, intentional self-harm HCC

√7ᵗʰ **T63.013** Toxic effect of rattlesnake venom, assault

√7ᵗʰ **T63.014** Toxic effect of rattlesnake venom, undetermined

√6ᵗʰ **T63.02** Toxic effect of coral snake venom

√7ᵗʰ **T63.021** Toxic effect of coral snake venom, accidental (unintentional)
Toxic effect of coral snake venom NOS

² √7ᵗʰ **T63.022** Toxic effect of coral snake venom, intentional self-harm HCC

√7ᵗʰ **T63.023** Toxic effect of coral snake venom, assault

√7ᵗʰ **T63.024** Toxic effect of coral snake venom, undetermined

√6ᵗʰ **T63.03** Toxic effect of taipan venom

√7ᵗʰ **T63.031** Toxic effect of taipan venom, accidental (unintentional)
Toxic effect of taipan venom NOS

² √7ᵗʰ **T63.032** Toxic effect of taipan venom, intentional self-harm HCC

√7ᵗʰ **T63.033** Toxic effect of taipan venom, assault

√7ᵗʰ **T63.034** Toxic effect of taipan venom, undetermined

√6ᵗʰ **T63.04** Toxic effect of cobra venom

√7ᵗʰ **T63.041** Toxic effect of cobra venom, accidental (unintentional)
Toxic effect of cobra venom NOS

² √7ᵗʰ **T63.042** Toxic effect of cobra venom, intentional self-harm HCC

√7ᵗʰ **T63.043** Toxic effect of cobra venom, assault

√7ᵗʰ **T63.044** Toxic effect of cobra venom, undetermined

√6ᵗʰ **T63.06** Toxic effect of venom of other North and South American snake

√7ᵗʰ **T63.061** Toxic effect of venom of other North and South American snake, accidental (unintentional)
Toxic effect of venom of other North and South American snake NOS

² √7ᵗʰ **T63.062** Toxic effect of venom of other North and South American snake, intentional self-harm HCC

√7ᵗʰ **T63.063** Toxic effect of venom of other North and South American snake, assault

√7ᵗʰ **T63.064** Toxic effect of venom of other North and South American snake, undetermined

√6ᵗʰ **T63.07** Toxic effect of venom of other Australian snake

√7ᵗʰ **T63.071** Toxic effect of venom of other Australian snake, accidental (unintentional)
Toxic effect of venom of other Australian snake NOS

² √7ᵗʰ **T63.072** Toxic effect of venom of other Australian snake, intentional self-harm HCC

√7ᵗʰ **T63.073** Toxic effect of venom of other Australian snake, assault

√7ᵗʰ **T63.074** Toxic effect of venom of other Australian snake, undetermined

√6ᵗʰ **T63.08** Toxic effect of venom of other African and Asian snake

√7ᵗʰ **T63.081** Toxic effect of venom of other African and Asian snake, accidental (unintentional)
Toxic effect of venom of other African and Asian snake NOS

² √7ᵗʰ **T63.082** Toxic effect of venom of other African and Asian snake, intentional self-harm HCC

√7ᵗʰ **T63.083** Toxic effect of venom of other African and Asian snake, assault

√7ᵗʰ **T63.084** Toxic effect of venom of other African and Asian snake, undetermined

√6ᵗʰ **T63.09** Toxic effect of venom of other snake

√7ᵗʰ **T63.091** Toxic effect of venom of other snake, accidental (unintentional)
Toxic effect of venom of other snake NOS

² √7ᵗʰ **T63.092** Toxic effect of venom of other snake, intentional self-harm HCC

√7ᵗʰ **T63.093** Toxic effect of venom of other snake, assault

√7ᵗʰ **T63.094** Toxic effect of venom of other snake, undetermined

√5ᵗʰ **T63.1** Toxic effect of venom of other reptiles

√6ᵗʰ **T63.11** Toxic effect of venom of gila monster

√7ᵗʰ **T63.111** Toxic effect of venom of gila monster, accidental (unintentional)
Toxic effect of venom of gila monster NOS

² √7ᵗʰ **T63.112** Toxic effect of venom of gila monster, intentional self-harm HCC

√7ᵗʰ **T63.113** Toxic effect of venom of gila monster, assault

√7ᵗʰ **T63.114** Toxic effect of venom of gila monster, undetermined

√6ᵗʰ **T63.12** Toxic effect of venom of other venomous lizard

√7ᵗʰ **T63.121** Toxic effect of venom of other venomous lizard, accidental (unintentional)
Toxic effect of venom of other venomous lizard NOS

² √7ᵗʰ **T63.122** Toxic effect of venom of other venomous lizard, intentional self-harm HCC

√7ᵗʰ **T63.123** Toxic effect of venom of other venomous lizard, assault

√7ᵗʰ **T63.124** Toxic effect of venom of other venomous lizard, undetermined

√6ᵗʰ **T63.19** Toxic effect of venom of other reptiles

√7ᵗʰ **T63.191** Toxic effect of venom of other reptiles, accidental (unintentional)
Toxic effect of venom of other reptiles NOS

² √7ᵗʰ **T63.192** Toxic effect of venom of other reptiles, intentional self-harm HCC

√7ᵗʰ **T63.193** Toxic effect of venom of other reptiles, assault

√7ᵗʰ **T63.194** Toxic effect of venom of other reptiles, undetermined

√5ᵗʰ **T63.2** Toxic effect of venom of scorpion

√6ᵗʰ **T63.2X** Toxic effect of venom of scorpion

√7ᵗʰ **T63.2X1** Toxic effect of venom of scorpion, accidental (unintentional)
Toxic effect of venom of scorpion NOS

² √7ᵗʰ **T63.2X2** Toxic effect of venom of scorpion, intentional self-harm HCC

√7ᵗʰ **T63.2X3** Toxic effect of venom of scorpion, assault

√7ᵗʰ **T63.2X4** Toxic effect of venom of scorpion, undetermined

Chapter 19. Injury, Poisoning and Certain Other Consequences of External Causes

T63.3–T63.631

√5ᵗʰ **T63.3** **Toxic effect of** venom of spider

  √6ᵗʰ **T63.30** **Toxic effect of unspecified spider venom**

    √7ᵗʰ **T63.301** **Toxic effect of unspecified spider venom, accidental (unintentional)**

    ² √7ᵗʰ **T63.302** **Toxic effect of unspecified spider venom, intentional self-harm** HCC

    √7ᵗʰ **T63.303** **Toxic effect of unspecified spider venom, assault**

    √7ᵗʰ **T63.304** **Toxic effect of unspecified spider venom, undetermined**

  √6ᵗʰ **T63.31** **Toxic effect of venom of** black widow **spider**

    √7ᵗʰ **T63.311** **Toxic effect of venom of black widow spider, accidental (unintentional)**

    ² √7ᵗʰ **T63.312** **Toxic effect of venom of black widow spider, intentional self-harm** HCC

    √7ᵗʰ **T63.313** **Toxic effect of venom of black widow spider, assault**

    √7ᵗʰ **T63.314** **Toxic effect of venom of black widow spider, undetermined**

  √6ᵗʰ **T63.32** **Toxic effect of venom of** tarantula

    √7ᵗʰ **T63.321** **Toxic effect of venom of tarantula, accidental (unintentional)**

    ² √7ᵗʰ **T63.322** **Toxic effect of venom of tarantula, intentional self-harm** HCC

    √7ᵗʰ **T63.323** **Toxic effect of venom of tarantula, assault**

    √7ᵗʰ **T63.324** **Toxic effect of venom of tarantula, undetermined**

  √6ᵗʰ **T63.33** **Toxic effect of venom of** brown recluse **spider**

    √7ᵗʰ **T63.331** **Toxic effect of venom of brown recluse spider, accidental (unintentional)**

    ² √7ᵗʰ **T63.332** **Toxic effect of venom of brown recluse spider, intentional self-harm** HCC

    √7ᵗʰ **T63.333** **Toxic effect of venom of brown recluse spider, assault**

    √7ᵗʰ **T63.334** **Toxic effect of venom of brown recluse spider, undetermined**

  √6ᵗʰ **T63.39** **Toxic effect of venom of other spider**

    √7ᵗʰ **T63.391** **Toxic effect of venom of other spider, accidental (unintentional)**

    ² √7ᵗʰ **T63.392** **Toxic effect of venom of other spider, intentional self-harm** HCC

    √7ᵗʰ **T63.393** **Toxic effect of venom of other spider, assault**

    √7ᵗʰ **T63.394** **Toxic effect of venom of other spider, undetermined**

√5ᵗʰ **T63.4** **Toxic effect of venom of other arthropods**

  √6ᵗʰ **T63.41** **Toxic effect of venom of** centipedes and venomous millipedes

    √7ᵗʰ **T63.411** **Toxic effect of venom of centipedes and venomous millipedes, accidental (unintentional)**

    ² √7ᵗʰ **T63.412** **Toxic effect of venom of centipedes and venomous millipedes, intentional self-harm** HCC

    √7ᵗʰ **T63.413** **Toxic effect of venom of centipedes and venomous millipedes, assault**

    √7ᵗʰ **T63.414** **Toxic effect of venom of centipedes and venomous millipedes, undetermined**

  √6ᵗʰ **T63.42** **Toxic effect of venom of** ants

    √7ᵗʰ **T63.421** **Toxic effect of venom of ants, accidental (unintentional)**

    ² √7ᵗʰ **T63.422** **Toxic effect of venom of ants, intentional self-harm** HCC

    √7ᵗʰ **T63.423** **Toxic effect of venom of ants, assault**

    √7ᵗʰ **T63.424** **Toxic effect of venom of ants, undetermined**

  √6ᵗʰ **T63.43** **Toxic effect of venom of** caterpillars

    √7ᵗʰ **T63.431** **Toxic effect of venom of caterpillars, accidental (unintentional)**

    ² √7ᵗʰ **T63.432** **Toxic effect of venom of caterpillars, intentional self-harm** HCC

    √7ᵗʰ **T63.433** **Toxic effect of venom of caterpillars, assault**

    √7ᵗʰ **T63.434** **Toxic effect of venom of caterpillars, undetermined**

  √6ᵗʰ **T63.44** **Toxic effect of venom of** bees

    √7ᵗʰ **T63.441** **Toxic effect of venom of bees, accidental (unintentional)**

    ² √7ᵗʰ **T63.442** **Toxic effect of venom of bees, intentional self-harm** HCC

    √7ᵗʰ **T63.443** **Toxic effect of venom of bees, assault**

    √7ᵗʰ **T63.444** **Toxic effect of venom of bees, undetermined**

  √6ᵗʰ **T63.45** **Toxic effect of venom of** hornets

    √7ᵗʰ **T63.451** **Toxic effect of venom of hornets, accidental (unintentional)**

    ² √7ᵗʰ **T63.452** **Toxic effect of venom of hornets, intentional self-harm** HCC

    √7ᵗʰ **T63.453** **Toxic effect of venom of hornets, assault**

    √7ᵗʰ **T63.454** **Toxic effect of venom of hornets, undetermined**

  √6ᵗʰ **T63.46** **Toxic effect of venom of** wasps

    Toxic effect of yellow jacket

    √7ᵗʰ **T63.461** **Toxic effect of venom of wasps, accidental (unintentional)**

    ² √7ᵗʰ **T63.462** **Toxic effect of venom of wasps, intentional self-harm** HCC

    √7ᵗʰ **T63.463** **Toxic effect of venom of wasps, assault**

    √7ᵗʰ **T63.464** **Toxic effect of venom of wasps, undetermined**

  √6ᵗʰ **T63.48** **Toxic effect of venom of other arthropod**

    √7ᵗʰ **T63.481** **Toxic effect of venom of other arthropod, accidental (unintentional)**

    ² √7ᵗʰ **T63.482** **Toxic effect of venom of other arthropod, intentional self-harm** HCC

    √7ᵗʰ **T63.483** **Toxic effect of venom of other arthropod, assault**

    √7ᵗʰ **T63.484** **Toxic effect of venom of other arthropod, undetermined**

√5ᵗʰ **T63.5** **Toxic effect of contact with** venomous fish

    EXCLUDES 2   poisoning by ingestion of fish (T61.-)

  √6ᵗʰ **T63.51** **Toxic effect of contact with** stingray

    √7ᵗʰ **T63.511** **Toxic effect of contact with stingray, accidental (unintentional)**

    ² √7ᵗʰ **T63.512** **Toxic effect of contact with stingray, intentional self-harm** HCC

    √7ᵗʰ **T63.513** **Toxic effect of contact with stingray, assault**

    √7ᵗʰ **T63.514** **Toxic effect of contact with stingray, undetermined**

  √6ᵗʰ **T63.59** **Toxic effect of contact with other venomous fish**

    √7ᵗʰ **T63.591** **Toxic effect of contact with other venomous fish, accidental (unintentional)**

    ² √7ᵗʰ **T63.592** **Toxic effect of contact with other venomous fish, intentional self-harm** HCC

    √7ᵗʰ **T63.593** **Toxic effect of contact with other venomous fish, assault**

    √7ᵗʰ **T63.594** **Toxic effect of contact with other venomous fish, undetermined**

√5ᵗʰ **T63.6** **Toxic effect of contact with other venomous marine animals**

    EXCLUDES 1   sea-snake venom (T63.09)

    EXCLUDES 2   poisoning by ingestion of shellfish (T61.78-)

  √6ᵗʰ **T63.61** **Toxic effect of contact with** Portugese Man-o-war

    Toxic effect of contact with bluebottle

    √7ᵗʰ **T63.611** **Toxic effect of contact with Portugese Man-o-war, accidental (unintentional)**

    ² √7ᵗʰ **T63.612** **Toxic effect of contact with Portugese Man-o-war, intentional self-harm** HCC

    √7ᵗʰ **T63.613** **Toxic effect of contact with Portugese Man-o-war, assault**

    √7ᵗʰ **T63.614** **Toxic effect of contact with Portugese Man-o-war, undetermined**

  √6ᵗʰ **T63.62** **Toxic effect of contact with other jellyfish**

    √7ᵗʰ **T63.621** **Toxic effect of contact with other jellyfish, accidental (unintentional)**

    ² √7ᵗʰ **T63.622** **Toxic effect of contact with other jellyfish, intentional self-harm** HCC

    √7ᵗʰ **T63.623** **Toxic effect of contact with other jellyfish, assault**

    √7ᵗʰ **T63.624** **Toxic effect of contact with other jellyfish, undetermined**

  √6ᵗʰ **T63.63** **Toxic effect of contact with** sea anemone

    √7ᵗʰ **T63.631** **Toxic effect of contact with sea anemone, accidental (unintentional)**

² √7ᵗʰ **T63.632** **Toxic effect of contact with sea anemone,** intentional self-harm   HCC

√7ᵗʰ **T63.633** **Toxic effect of contact with sea anemone,** assault

√7ᵗʰ **T63.634** **Toxic effect of contact with sea anemone,** undetermined

√6ᵗʰ **T63.69** **Toxic effect of contact with other venomous marine animals**

√7ᵗʰ **T63.691** **Toxic effect of contact with other venomous marine animals,** accidental (unintentional)

² √7ᵗʰ **T63.692** **Toxic effect of contact with other venomous marine animals,** intentional self-harm   HCC

√7ᵗʰ **T63.693** **Toxic effect of contact with other venomous marine animals,** assault

√7ᵗʰ **T63.694** **Toxic effect of contact with other venomous marine animals,** undetermined

√5ᵗʰ **T63.7** **Toxic effect of contact with** venomous plant

√6ᵗʰ **T63.71** **Toxic effect of contact with venomous** marine plant

√7ᵗʰ **T63.711** **Toxic effect of contact with venomous marine plant,** accidental (unintentional)

² √7ᵗʰ **T63.712** **Toxic effect of contact with venomous marine plant,** intentional self-harm   HCC

√7ᵗʰ **T63.713** **Toxic effect of contact with venomous marine plant,** assault

√7ᵗʰ **T63.714** **Toxic effect of contact with venomous marine plant,** undetermined

√6ᵗʰ **T63.79** **Toxic effect of contact with other venomous plant**

√7ᵗʰ **T63.791** **Toxic effect of contact with other venomous plant,** accidental (unintentional)

² √7ᵗʰ **T63.792** **Toxic effect of contact with other venomous plant,** intentional self-harm   HCC

√7ᵗʰ **T63.793** **Toxic effect of contact with other venomous plant,** assault

√7ᵗʰ **T63.794** **Toxic effect of contact with other venomous plant,** undetermined

√5ᵗʰ **T63.8** **Toxic effect of contact with other venomous animals**

√6ᵗʰ **T63.81** **Toxic effect of contact with venomous** frog

> EXCLUDES 1   *contact with nonvenomous frog (W62.0)*

√7ᵗʰ **T63.811** **Toxic effect of contact with venomous frog,** accidental (unintentional)

² √7ᵗʰ **T63.812** **Toxic effect of contact with venomous frog,** intentional self-harm   HCC

√7ᵗʰ **T63.813** **Toxic effect of contact with venomous frog,** assault

√7ᵗʰ **T63.814** **Toxic effect of contact with venomous frog,** undetermined

√6ᵗʰ **T63.82** **Toxic effect of contact with venomous** toad

> EXCLUDES 1   *contact with nonvenomous toad (W62.1)*

√7ᵗʰ **T63.821** **Toxic effect of contact with venomous toad,** accidental (unintentional)

² √7ᵗʰ **T63.822** **Toxic effect of contact with venomous toad,** intentional self-harm   HCC

√7ᵗʰ **T63.823** **Toxic effect of contact with venomous toad,** assault

√7ᵗʰ **T63.824** **Toxic effect of contact with venomous toad,** undetermined

√6ᵗʰ **T63.83** **Toxic effect of contact with other venomous amphibian**

> EXCLUDES 1   *contact with nonvenomous amphibian (W62.9)*

√7ᵗʰ **T63.831** **Toxic effect of contact with other venomous amphibian,** accidental (unintentional)

² √7ᵗʰ **T63.832** **Toxic effect of contact with other venomous amphibian,** intentional self-harm   HCC

√7ᵗʰ **T63.833** **Toxic effect of contact with other venomous amphibian,** assault

√7ᵗʰ **T63.834** **Toxic effect of contact with other venomous amphibian,** undetermined

√6ᵗʰ **T63.89** **Toxic effect of contact with other venomous animals**

√7ᵗʰ **T63.891** **Toxic effect of contact with other venomous animals,** accidental (unintentional)

² √7ᵗʰ **T63.892** **Toxic effect of contact with other venomous animals,** intentional self-harm   HCC

√7ᵗʰ **T63.893** **Toxic effect of contact with other venomous animals,** assault

√7ᵗʰ **T63.894** **Toxic effect of contact with other venomous animals,** undetermined

√5ᵗʰ **T63.9** **Toxic effect of contact with unspecified venomous animal**

√x7ᵗʰ **T63.91** **Toxic effect of contact with unspecified venomous animal,** accidental (unintentional)

² √x7ᵗʰ **T63.92** **Toxic effect of contact with unspecified venomous animal,** intentional self-harm   HCC

√x7ᵗʰ **T63.93** **Toxic effect of contact with unspecified venomous animal,** assault

√x7ᵗʰ **T63.94** **Toxic effect of contact with unspecified venomous animal,** undetermined

√4ᵗʰ **T64** **Toxic effect of aflatoxin and other mycotoxin food contaminants**

> The appropriate 7th character is to be added to each code from category T64.
> A   initial encounter
> D   subsequent encounter
> S   sequela

√5ᵗʰ **T64.0** **Toxic effect of** aflatoxin

√x7ᵗʰ **T64.01** **Toxic effect of aflatoxin,** accidental (unintentional)

² √x7ᵗʰ **T64.02** **Toxic effect of aflatoxin,** intentional self-harm   HCC

√x7ᵗʰ **T64.03** **Toxic effect of aflatoxin,** assault

√x7ᵗʰ **T64.04** **Toxic effect of aflatoxin,** undetermined

√5ᵗʰ **T64.8** **Toxic effect of other mycotoxin food contaminants**

√x7ᵗʰ **T64.81** **Toxic effect of other mycotoxin food contaminants,** accidental (unintentional)

² √x7ᵗʰ **T64.82** **Toxic effect of other mycotoxin food contaminants,** intentional self-harm   HCC

√x7ᵗʰ **T64.83** **Toxic effect of other mycotoxin food contaminants,** assault

√x7ᵗʰ **T64.84** **Toxic effect of other mycotoxin food contaminants,** undetermined

√4ᵗʰ **T65** **Toxic effect of other and unspecified substances**

> The appropriate 7th character is to be added to each code from category T65.
> A   initial encounter
> D   subsequent encounter
> S   sequela

√5ᵗʰ **T65.0** **Toxic effect of cyanides**

> EXCLUDES 1   *hydrogen cyanide (T57.3-)*

√6ᵗʰ **T65.0X** **Toxic effect of** cyanides

√7ᵗʰ **T65.0X1** **Toxic effect of cyanides,** accidental (unintentional)
     Toxic effect of cyanides NOS

² √7ᵗʰ **T65.0X2** **Toxic effect of cyanides,** intentional self-harm   HCC

√7ᵗʰ **T65.0X3** **Toxic effect of cyanides,** assault

√7ᵗʰ **T65.0X4** **Toxic effect of cyanides,** undetermined

√5ᵗʰ **T65.1** **Toxic effect of strychnine and its salts**

√6ᵗʰ **T65.1X** **Toxic effect of** strychnine and its salts

√7ᵗʰ **T65.1X1** **Toxic effect of strychnine and its salts,** accidental (unintentional)
     Toxic effect of strychnine and its salts NOS

² √7ᵗʰ **T65.1X2** **Toxic effect of strychnine and its salts,** intentional self-harm   HCC

√7ᵗʰ **T65.1X3** **Toxic effect of strychnine and its salts,** assault

√7ᵗʰ **T65.1X4** **Toxic effect of strychnine and its salts,** undetermined

√5ᵗʰ **T65.2** **Toxic effect of tobacco and nicotine**

> EXCLUDES 2   *nicotine dependence (F17.-)*

√6ᵗʰ **T65.21** **Toxic effect of** chewing tobacco

√7ᵗʰ **T65.211** **Toxic effect of chewing tobacco,** accidental (unintentional)
     Toxic effect of chewing tobacco NOS

² √7ᵗʰ **T65.212** **Toxic effect of chewing tobacco,** intentional self-harm   HCC

√7ᵗʰ **T65.213** **Toxic effect of chewing tobacco,** assault

√7ᵗʰ **T65.214** **Toxic effect of chewing tobacco,** undetermined

---

✔ Additional Character Required   √x7ᵗʰ Placeholder Alert   Manifestation   Unspecified Dx   ►◄ Revised Text   ● New Code   ▲ Revised Code Title

Chapter 19. Injury, Poisoning and Certain Other Consequences of External Causes

T65.22–T65.94

√6ᵗʰ **T65.22** **Toxic effect of** tobacco cigarettes

Toxic effect of tobacco smoke

Use additional code for exposure to second hand tobacco smoke (Z57.31, Z77.22)

√7ᵗʰ **T65.221** **Toxic effect of tobacco cigarettes, accidental (unintentional)**

Toxic effect of tobacco cigarettes NOS

2 √7ᵗʰ **T65.222** **Toxic effect of tobacco cigarettes, intentional self-harm**   HCC

√7ᵗʰ **T65.223** **Toxic effect of tobacco cigarettes,** assault

√7ᵗʰ **T65.224** **Toxic effect of tobacco cigarettes, undetermined**

√6ᵗʰ **T65.29** **Toxic effect of other tobacco and nicotine**

√7ᵗʰ **T65.291** **Toxic effect of other tobacco and nicotine, accidental (unintentional)**

Toxic effect of other tobacco and nicotine NOS

2 √7ᵗʰ **T65.292** **Toxic effect of other tobacco and nicotine, intentional self-harm**   HCC

√7ᵗʰ **T65.293** **Toxic effect of other tobacco and nicotine, assault**

√7ᵗʰ **T65.294** **Toxic effect of other tobacco and nicotine, undetermined**

√5ᵗʰ **T65.3** **Toxic effect of nitroderivatives and aminoderivatives of benzene and its homologues**

Toxic effect of anilin [benzenamine]

Toxic effect of nitrobenzene

Toxic effect of trinitrotoluene

√6ᵗʰ **T65.3X** **Toxic effect of** nitroderivatives and aminoderivatives of benzene and its homologues

√7ᵗʰ **T65.3X1** **Toxic effect of nitroderivatives and aminoderivatives of benzene and its homologues, accidental (unintentional)**

Toxic effect of nitroderivatives and aminoderivatives of benzene and its homologues NOS

2 √7ᵗʰ **T65.3X2** **Toxic effect of nitroderivatives and aminoderivatives of benzene and its homologues, intentional self-harm**   HCC

√7ᵗʰ **T65.3X3** **Toxic effect of nitroderivatives and aminoderivatives of benzene and its homologues, assault**

√7ᵗʰ **T65.3X4** **Toxic effect of nitroderivatives and aminoderivatives of benzene and its homologues, undetermined**

√5ᵗʰ **T65.4** **Toxic effect of carbon disulfide**

√6ᵗʰ **T65.4X** **Toxic effect of** carbon disulfide

√7ᵗʰ **T65.4X1** **Toxic effect of carbon disulfide, accidental (unintentional)**

Toxic effect of carbon disulfide NOS

2 √7ᵗʰ **T65.4X2** **Toxic effect of carbon disulfide, intentional self-harm**   HCC

√7ᵗʰ **T65.4X3** **Toxic effect of carbon disulfide,** assault

√7ᵗʰ **T65.4X4** **Toxic effect of carbon disulfide, undetermined**

√5ᵗʰ **T65.5** **Toxic effect of nitroglycerin and other nitric acids and esters**

Toxic effect of 1,2,3-Propanetriol trinitrate

√6ᵗʰ **T65.5X** **Toxic effect of** nitroglycerin and other nitric acids and esters

√7ᵗʰ **T65.5X1** **Toxic effect of nitroglycerin and other nitric acids and esters, accidental (unintentional)**

Toxic effect of nitroglycerin and other nitric acids and esters NOS

2 √7ᵗʰ **T65.5X2** **Toxic effect of nitroglycerin and other nitric acids and esters, intentional self-harm**   HCC

√7ᵗʰ **T65.5X3** **Toxic effect of nitroglycerin and other nitric acids and esters,** assault

√7ᵗʰ **T65.5X4** **Toxic effect of nitroglycerin and other nitric acids and esters, undetermined**

√5ᵗʰ **T65.6** **Toxic effect of paints and dyes, not elsewhere classified**

√6ᵗʰ **T65.6X** **Toxic effect of** paints and dyes, not elsewhere classified

√7ᵗʰ **T65.6X1** **Toxic effect of paints and dyes, not elsewhere classified, accidental (unintentional)**

Toxic effect of paints and dyes NOS

2 √7ᵗʰ **T65.6X2** **Toxic effect of paints and dyes, not elsewhere classified, intentional self-harm**   HCC

√7ᵗʰ **T65.6X3** **Toxic effect of paints and dyes, not elsewhere classified,** assault

√7ᵗʰ **T65.6X4** **Toxic effect of paints and dyes, not elsewhere classified, undetermined**

√5ᵗʰ **T65.8** **Toxic effect of other specified substances**

√6ᵗʰ **T65.81** **Toxic effect of** latex

√7ᵗʰ **T65.811** **Toxic effect of latex, accidental (unintentional)**

Toxic effect of latex NOS

2 √7ᵗʰ **T65.812** **Toxic effect of latex, intentional self-harm**   HCC

√7ᵗʰ **T65.813** **Toxic effect of latex,** assault

√7ᵗʰ **T65.814** **Toxic effect of latex, undetermined**

√6ᵗʰ **T65.82** **Toxic effect of harmful** algae and algae toxins

Toxic effect of (harmful) algae bloom NOS

Toxic effect of blue-green algae bloom

Toxic effect of brown tide

Toxic effect of cyanobacteria bloom

Toxic effect of Florida red tide

Toxic effect of pfiesteria piscicida

Toxic effect of red tide

√7ᵗʰ **T65.821** **Toxic effect of harmful algae and algae toxins, accidental (unintentional)**

Toxic effect of harmful algae and algae toxins NOS

2 √7ᵗʰ **T65.822** **Toxic effect of harmful algae and algae toxins, intentional self-harm**   HCC

√7ᵗʰ **T65.823** **Toxic effect of harmful algae and algae toxins, assault**

√7ᵗʰ **T65.824** **Toxic effect of harmful algae and algae toxins, undetermined**

√6ᵗʰ **T65.83** **Toxic effect of** fiberglass

√7ᵗʰ **T65.831** **Toxic effect of fiberglass, accidental (unintentional)**

Toxic effect of fiberglass NOS

2 √7ᵗʰ **T65.832** **Toxic effect of fiberglass, intentional self-harm**   HCC

√7ᵗʰ **T65.833** **Toxic effect of fiberglass,** assault

√7ᵗʰ **T65.834** **Toxic effect of fiberglass, undetermined**

√6ᵗʰ **T65.89** **Toxic effect of other specified substances**

√7ᵗʰ **T65.891** **Toxic effect of other specified substances, accidental (unintentional)**

Toxic effect of other specified substances NOS

AHA: 2018,1Q,5

2 √7ᵗʰ **T65.892** **Toxic effect of other specified substances, intentional self-harm**   HCC

√7ᵗʰ **T65.893** **Toxic effect of other specified substances, assault**

√7ᵗʰ **T65.894** **Toxic effect of other specified substances, undetermined**

√5ᵗʰ **T65.9** **Toxic effect of unspecified substance**

√x7ᵗʰ **T65.91** **Toxic effect of unspecified substance,** accidental (unintentional)

Poisoning NOS

2 √x7ᵗʰ **T65.92** **Toxic effect of unspecified substance, intentional self-harm**   HCC

√x7ᵗʰ **T65.93** **Toxic effect of unspecified substance,** assault

√x7ᵗʰ **T65.94** **Toxic effect of unspecified substance, undetermined**

Other and unspecified effects of external causes (T66-T78)

✓x7th T66 Radiation sickness, unspecified

> EXCLUDES 1 specified adverse effects of radiation, such as:
>> burns (T20-T31)
>> leukemia (C91-C95)
>> radiation gastroenteritis and colitis (K52.0)
>> radiation pneumonitis (J70.0)
>> radiation related disorders of the skin and subcutaneous tissue (L55-L59)
>> radiation sunburn (L55.-)

> The appropriate 7th character is to be added to code T66.
> A   initial encounter
> D   subsequent encounter
> S   sequela

✓4th T67 Effects of heat and light

> EXCLUDES 1 erythema [dermatitis] ab igne (L59.0)
>> malignant hyperpyrexia due to anesthesia (T88.3)
>> radiation-related disorders of the skin and subcutaneous tissue (L55-L59)
> EXCLUDES 2 burns (T20-T31)
>> sunburn (L55.-)
>> sweat disorder due to heat (L74-L75)

> The appropriate 7th character is to be added to each code from category T67.
> A   initial encounter
> D   subsequent encounter
> S   sequela

✓5th T67.0 Heatstroke and sunstroke

> ~~Heat apoplexy~~
> ~~Heat pyrexia~~
> ~~Siriasis~~
> ~~Thermoplegia~~
> Use additional code(s) to identify any associated complications of heatstroke, such as:
> coma and stupor (R40.-)
> ►rhabdomyolysis (M62.82)◄
> systemic inflammatory response syndrome (R65.1-)
> **DEF:** Headache, vertigo, cramps, and elevated body temperature due to prolonged exposure to high environmental temperatures that requires emergency intervention.

- ✓x7th **T67.01 Heatstroke and sunstroke**
  Heat apoplexy
  Heat pyrexia
  Siriasis
  Thermoplegia
- ✓x7th **T67.02 Exertional heatstroke**
- ✓x7th **T67.09 Other heatstroke and sunstroke**

✓x7th T67.1 Heat syncope
Heat collapse

✓x7th T67.2 Heat cramp

✓x7th T67.3 Heat exhaustion, anhydrotic
Heat prostration due to water depletion
> EXCLUDES 1 heat exhaustion due to salt depletion (T67.4)

✓x7th T67.4 Heat exhaustion due to salt depletion
Heat prostration due to salt (and water) depletion

✓x7th T67.5 Heat exhaustion, unspecified
Heat prostration NOS

✓x7th T67.6 Heat fatigue, transient

✓x7th T67.7 Heat edema

✓x7th T67.8 Other effects of heat and light

✓x7th T67.9 Effect of heat and light, unspecified

✓x7th T68 Hypothermia
Accidental hypothermia
Hypothermia NOS
Use additional code to identify source of exposure:
exposure to excessive cold of man-made origin (W93)
exposure to excessive cold of natural origin (X31)
> EXCLUDES 1 hypothermia following anesthesia (T88.51)
>> hypothermia not associated with low environmental temperature (R68.0)
>> hypothermia of newborn (P80.-)
> EXCLUDES 2 frostbite (T33-T34)

> The appropriate 7th character is to be added to code T68.
> A   initial encounter
> D   subsequent encounter
> S   sequela

✓4th T69 Other effects of reduced temperature
Use additional code to identify source of exposure:
exposure to excessive cold of man-made origin (W93)
exposure to excessive cold of natural origin (X31)
> EXCLUDES 2 frostbite (T33-T34)

> The appropriate 7th character is to be added to each code from category T69.
> A   initial encounter
> D   subsequent encounter
> S   sequela

✓5th T69.0 Immersion hand and foot

✓6th T69.01 Immersion hand
- ✓7th **T69.011 Immersion hand, right hand**
- ✓7th **T69.012 Immersion hand, left hand**
- ✓7th **T69.019 Immersion hand, unspecified hand**

✓6th T69.02 Immersion foot
Trench foot
- ✓7th **T69.021 Immersion foot, right foot**
- ✓7th **T69.022 Immersion foot, left foot**
- ✓7th **T69.029 Immersion foot, unspecified foot**

✓x7th T69.1 Chilblains
> **DEF:** Red, swollen, itchy skin primarily affecting the fingers and toes, nose and ears, and legs. Chilblains follows damp-cold exposure, and can also be associated with pruritus and a burning feeling.

✓x7th T69.8 Other specified effects of reduced temperature

✓x7th T69.9 Effect of reduced temperature, unspecified

✓4th T70 Effects of air pressure and water pressure

> The appropriate 7th character is to be added to each code from category T70.
> A   initial encounter
> D   subsequent encounter
> S   sequela

✓x7th T70.0 Otitic barotrauma
Aero-otitis media
Effects of change in ambient atmospheric pressure or water pressure on ears

✓x7th T70.1 Sinus barotrauma
Aerosinusitis
Effects of change in ambient atmospheric pressure on sinuses

✓5th T70.2 Other and unspecified effects of high altitude
> EXCLUDES 2 polycythemia due to high altitude (D75.1)

✓x7th T70.20 Unspecified effects of high altitude

✓x7th T70.29 Other effects of high altitude
Alpine sickness
Anoxia due to high altitude
Barotrauma NOS
Hypobaropathy
Mountain sickness

✓x7th T70.3 Caisson disease [decompression sickness]
Compressed-air disease
Diver's palsy or paralysis
> **DEF:** Rapid reduction in air pressure while breathing compressed air. Symptoms include skin lesions, joint pains, and respiratory and neurological problems.

☑ Additional Character Required   ✓x7th Placeholder Alert   Manifestation   Unspecified Dx   ►◄ Revised Text   ● New Code   ▲ Revised Code Title

ICD-10-CM 2020   1129

√x7ᵗʰ **T70.4** **Effects of high-pressure fluids**
Hydraulic jet injection (industrial)
Pneumatic jet injection (industrial)
Traumatic jet injection (industrial)

√x7ᵗʰ **T70.8** **Other effects of air pressure and water pressure**

√x7ᵗʰ **T70.9** **Effect of air pressure and water pressure, unspecified**

√4ᵗʰ **T71** **Asphyxiation**
Mechanical suffocation
Traumatic suffocation

> EXCLUDES 1   acute respiratory distress (syndrome) (J80)
> anoxia due to high altitude (T70.2)
> asphyxia NOS (R09.01)
> asphyxia from carbon monoxide (T58.-)
> asphyxia from inhalation of food or foreign body (T17.-)
> asphyxia from other gases, fumes and vapors (T59.-)
> respiratory distress (syndrome) in newborn (P22.-)

> The appropriate 7th character is to be added to each code from category T71.
> A   initial encounter
> D   subsequent encounter
> S   sequela

√5ᵗʰ **T71.1** **Asphyxiation due to mechanical threat to breathing**
Suffocation due to mechanical threat to breathing

√6ᵗʰ **T71.11** **Asphyxiation due to smothering under pillow**

√7ᵗʰ **T71.111** **Asphyxiation due to smothering under pillow, accidental**
Asphyxiation due to smothering under pillow NOS

² √7ᵗʰ **T71.112** **Asphyxiation due to smothering under pillow, intentional self-harm**   HCC

√7ᵗʰ **T71.113** **Asphyxiation due to smothering under pillow, assault**

√7ᵗʰ **T71.114** **Asphyxiation due to smothering under pillow, undetermined**

√6ᵗʰ **T71.12** **Asphyxiation due to plastic bag**

√7ᵗʰ **T71.121** **Asphyxiation due to plastic bag, accidental**
Asphyxiation due to plastic bag NOS

² √7ᵗʰ **T71.122** **Asphyxiation due to plastic bag, intentional self-harm**   HCC

√7ᵗʰ **T71.123** **Asphyxiation due to plastic bag, assault**

√7ᵗʰ **T71.124** **Asphyxiation due to plastic bag, undetermined**

√6ᵗʰ **T71.13** **Asphyxiation due to being trapped in bed linens**

√7ᵗʰ **T71.131** **Asphyxiation due to being trapped in bed linens, accidental**
Asphyxiation due to being trapped in bed linens NOS

² √7ᵗʰ **T71.132** **Asphyxiation due to being trapped in bed linens, intentional self-harm**   HCC

√7ᵗʰ **T71.133** **Asphyxiation due to being trapped in bed linens, assault**

√7ᵗʰ **T71.134** **Asphyxiation due to being trapped in bed linens, undetermined**

√6ᵗʰ **T71.14** **Asphyxiation due to smothering under another person's body (in bed)**

√7ᵗʰ **T71.141** **Asphyxiation due to smothering under another person's body (in bed), accidental**
Asphyxiation due to smothering under another person's body (in bed) NOS

√7ᵗʰ **T71.143** **Asphyxiation due to smothering under another person's body (in bed), assault**

√7ᵗʰ **T71.144** **Asphyxiation due to smothering under another person's body (in bed), undetermined**

√6ᵗʰ **T71.15** **Asphyxiation due to smothering in furniture**

√7ᵗʰ **T71.151** **Asphyxiation due to smothering in furniture, accidental**
Asphyxiation due to smothering in furniture NOS

² √7ᵗʰ **T71.152** **Asphyxiation due to smothering in furniture, intentional self-harm**   HCC

√7ᵗʰ **T71.153** **Asphyxiation due to smothering in furniture, assault**

√7ᵗʰ **T71.154** **Asphyxiation due to smothering in furniture, undetermined**

√6ᵗʰ **T71.16** **Asphyxiation due to hanging**
Hanging by window shade cord
Use additional code for any associated injuries, such as:
crushing injury of neck (S17.-)
fracture of cervical vertebrae (S12.0-S12.2-)
open wound of neck (S11.-)

√7ᵗʰ **T71.161** **Asphyxiation due to hanging, accidental**
Asphyxiation due to hanging NOS
Hanging NOS

² √7ᵗʰ **T71.162** **Asphyxiation due to hanging, intentional self-harm**   HCC

√7ᵗʰ **T71.163** **Asphyxiation due to hanging, assault**

√7ᵗʰ **T71.164** **Asphyxiation due to hanging, undetermined**

√6ᵗʰ **T71.19** **Asphyxiation due to mechanical threat to breathing due to other causes**

√7ᵗʰ **T71.191** **Asphyxiation due to mechanical threat to breathing due to other causes, accidental**
Asphyxiation due to other causes NOS

² √7ᵗʰ **T71.192** **Asphyxiation due to mechanical threat to breathing due to other causes, intentional self-harm**   HCC

√7ᵗʰ **T71.193** **Asphyxiation due to mechanical threat to breathing due to other causes, assault**

√7ᵗʰ **T71.194** **Asphyxiation due to mechanical threat to breathing due to other causes, undetermined**

√5ᵗʰ **T71.2** **Asphyxiation due to systemic oxygen deficiency due to low oxygen content in ambient air**
Suffocation due to systemic oxygen deficiency due to low oxygen content in ambient air

√x7ᵗʰ **T71.20** **Asphyxiation due to systemic oxygen deficiency due to low oxygen content in ambient air due to unspecified cause**

√x7ᵗʰ **T71.21** **Asphyxiation due to cave-in or falling earth**
Use additional code for any associated cataclysm (X34-X38)

√6ᵗʰ **T71.22** **Asphyxiation due to being trapped in a car trunk**

√7ᵗʰ **T71.221** **Asphyxiation due to being trapped in a car trunk, accidental**

² √7ᵗʰ **T71.222** **Asphyxiation due to being trapped in a car trunk, intentional self-harm**   HCC

√7ᵗʰ **T71.223** **Asphyxiation due to being trapped in a car trunk, assault**

√7ᵗʰ **T71.224** **Asphyxiation due to being trapped in a car trunk, undetermined**

√6ᵗʰ **T71.23** **Asphyxiation due to being trapped in a (discarded) refrigerator**

√7ᵗʰ **T71.231** **Asphyxiation due to being trapped in a (discarded) refrigerator, accidental**

² √7ᵗʰ **T71.232** **Asphyxiation due to being trapped in a (discarded) refrigerator, intentional self-harm**   HCC

√7ᵗʰ **T71.233** **Asphyxiation due to being trapped in a (discarded) refrigerator, assault**

√7ᵗʰ **T71.234** **Asphyxiation due to being trapped in a (discarded) refrigerator, undetermined**

√x7ᵗʰ **T71.29** **Asphyxiation due to being trapped in other low oxygen environment**

√x7ᵗʰ **T71.9** **Asphyxiation due to unspecified cause**
Suffocation (by strangulation) due to unspecified cause
Suffocation NOS
Systemic oxygen deficiency due to low oxygen content in ambient air due to unspecified cause
Systemic oxygen deficiency due to mechanical threat to breathing due to unspecified cause
Traumatic asphyxia NOS

✓4ᵗʰ T73 Effects of other deprivation

The appropriate 7th character is to be added to each code from category T73.
A   initial encounter
D   subsequent encounter
S   sequela

✓x7ᵗʰ **T73.0 Starvation**
Deprivation of food

✓x7ᵗʰ **T73.1 Deprivation of water**

✓x7ᵗʰ **T73.2 Exhaustion due to exposure**

✓x7ᵗʰ **T73.3 Exhaustion due to excessive exertion**
Exhaustion due to overexertion

✓x7ᵗʰ **T73.8 Other effects of deprivation**

✓x7ᵗʰ **T73.9 Effect of deprivation, unspecified**

✓4ᵗʰ T74 Adult and child abuse, neglect and other maltreatment, confirmed
Use additional code, if applicable, to identify any associated current injury
Use additional external cause code to identify perpetrator, if known (Y07.-)

EXCLUDES 1   abuse and maltreatment in pregnancy (O9A.3-, O9A.4-, O9A.5-)
adult and child maltreatment, suspected (T76.-)

The appropriate 7th character is to be added to each code from category T74.
A   initial encounter
D   subsequent encounter
S   sequela

✓5ᵗʰ **T74.0 Neglect or abandonment, confirmed**
  ✓x7ᵗʰ **T74.01 Adult neglect or abandonment, confirmed** Ⓐ
  ✓x7ᵗʰ **T74.02 Child neglect or abandonment, confirmed** Ⓟ

✓5ᵗʰ **T74.1 Physical abuse, confirmed**
EXCLUDES 2   sexual abuse (T74.2-)
  ✓x7ᵗʰ **T74.11 Adult physical abuse, confirmed** Ⓐ
  ✓x7ᵗʰ **T74.12 Child physical abuse, confirmed** Ⓟ
    EXCLUDES 2   shaken infant syndrome (T74.4)

✓5ᵗʰ **T74.2 Sexual abuse, confirmed**
Rape, confirmed
Sexual assault, confirmed
  ✓x7ᵗʰ **T74.21 Adult sexual abuse, confirmed** Ⓐ
  ✓x7ᵗʰ **T74.22 Child sexual abuse, confirmed** Ⓟ

✓5ᵗʰ **T74.3 Psychological abuse, confirmed**
Bullying and intimidation, confirmed
Intimidation through social media, confirmed
  ✓x7ᵗʰ **T74.31 Adult psychological abuse, confirmed** Ⓐ
  ✓x7ᵗʰ **T74.32 Child psychological abuse, confirmed** Ⓟ

✓x7ᵗʰ **T74.4 Shaken infant syndrome** Ⓟ

✓5ᵗʰ **T74.5 Forced sexual exploitation, confirmed**
AHA: 2018,4Q,32-33,65
  ✓x7ᵗʰ **T74.51 Adult forced sexual exploitation, confirmed** Ⓐ
  ✓x7ᵗʰ **T74.52 Child sexual exploitation, confirmed** Ⓟ

✓5ᵗʰ **T74.6 Forced labor exploitation, confirmed**
AHA: 2018,4Q,32-33,65
  ✓x7ᵗʰ **T74.61 Adult forced labor exploitation, confirmed** Ⓐ
  ✓x7ᵗʰ **T74.62 Child forced labor exploitation, confirmed** Ⓟ

✓5ᵗʰ **T74.9 Unspecified maltreatment, confirmed**
  ✓x7ᵗʰ **T74.91 Unspecified adult maltreatment, confirmed** Ⓐ
  ✓x7ᵗʰ **T74.92 Unspecified child maltreatment, confirmed** Ⓟ

✓4ᵗʰ T75 Other and unspecified effects of other external causes
EXCLUDES 1   adverse effects NEC (T78.-)
EXCLUDES 2   burns (electric) (T20-T31)

The appropriate 7th character is to be added to each code from category T75.
A   initial encounter
D   subsequent encounter
S   sequela

✓5ᵗʰ **T75.0 Effects of lightning**
Struck by lightning
  ✓x7ᵗʰ **T75.00 Unspecified effects of lightning**
Struck by lightning NOS
  ✓x7ᵗʰ **T75.01 Shock due to being struck by lightning**
  ✓x7ᵗʰ **T75.09 Other effects of lightning**
Use additional code for other effects of lightning

✓x7ᵗʰ **T75.1 Unspecified effects of drowning and nonfatal submersion**
Immersion
EXCLUDES 1   specified effects of drowning — code to effects

✓5ᵗʰ **T75.2 Effects of vibration**
  ✓x7ᵗʰ **T75.20 Unspecified effects of vibration**
  ✓x7ᵗʰ **T75.21 Pneumatic hammer syndrome**
  ✓x7ᵗʰ **T75.22 Traumatic vasospastic syndrome**
  ✓x7ᵗʰ **T75.23 Vertigo from infrasound**
    EXCLUDES 1   vertigo NOS (R42)
  ✓x7ᵗʰ **T75.29 Other effects of vibration**

✓x7ᵗʰ **T75.3 Motion sickness**
Airsickness
Seasickness
Travel sickness
Use additional external cause code to identify vehicle or type of motion (Y92.81-, Y93.5-)

✓x7ᵗʰ **T75.4 Electrocution**
Shock from electric current
Shock from electroshock gun (taser)

✓5ᵗʰ **T75.8 Other specified effects of external causes**
  ✓x7ᵗʰ **T75.81 Effects of abnormal gravitation [G] forces**
  ✓x7ᵗʰ **T75.82 Effects of weightlessness**
  ✓x7ᵗʰ **T75.89 Other specified effects of external causes**

✓4ᵗʰ T76 Adult and child abuse, neglect and other maltreatment, suspected
Use additional code, if applicable, to identify any associated current injury
EXCLUDES 1   adult and child maltreatment, confirmed (T74.-)
suspected abuse and maltreatment in pregnancy (O9A.3-, O9A.4-, O9A.5-)
suspected adult physical abuse, ruled out (Z04.71)
suspected adult sexual abuse, ruled out (Z04.41)
suspected child physical abuse, ruled out (Z04.72)
suspected child sexual abuse, ruled out (Z04.42)
AHA: 2018,4Q,72

The appropriate 7th character is to be added to each code from category T76.
A   initial encounter
D   subsequent encounter
S   sequela

✓5ᵗʰ **T76.0 Neglect or abandonment, suspected**
  ✓x7ᵗʰ **T76.01 Adult neglect or abandonment, suspected** Ⓐ
  ✓x7ᵗʰ **T76.02 Child neglect or abandonment, suspected** Ⓟ

✓5ᵗʰ **T76.1 Physical abuse, suspected**
  ✓x7ᵗʰ **T76.11 Adult physical abuse, suspected** Ⓐ
  ✓x7ᵗʰ **T76.12 Child physical abuse, suspected** Ⓟ
    AHA: 2019,2Q,12

✓5ᵗʰ **T76.2 Sexual abuse, suspected**
Rape, suspected
EXCLUDES 1   alleged abuse, ruled out (Z04.7)
  ✓x7ᵗʰ **T76.21 Adult sexual abuse, suspected** Ⓐ
  ✓x7ᵗʰ **T76.22 Child sexual abuse, suspected** Ⓟ

✓ Additional Character Required   ✓x7ᵗʰ Placeholder Alert   Manifestation   Unspecified Dx   ►◄ Revised Text   ● New Code   ▲ Revised Code Title

ICD-10-CM 2020   1131

Chapter 19. Injury, Poisoning and Certain Other Consequences of External Causes

T76.3–T79.5

√5ᵗʰ **T76.3 Psychological abuse, suspected**
Bullying and intimidation, suspected
Intimidation through social media, suspected

   √x7ᵗʰ **T76.31 Adult psychological abuse, suspected**   Ⓐ

   √x7ᵗʰ **T76.32 Child psychological abuse, suspected**   Ⓟ

√5ᵗʰ **T76.5 Forced sexual exploitation, suspected**
AHA: 2018,4Q,32-33,65

   √x7ᵗʰ **T76.51 Adult forced sexual exploitation, suspected**   Ⓐ

   √x7ᵗʰ **T76.52 Child sexual exploitation, suspected**   Ⓟ

√5ᵗʰ **T76.6 Forced labor exploitation, suspected**
AHA: 2018,4Q,32-33,65

   √x7ᵗʰ **T76.61 Adult forced labor exploitation, suspected**   Ⓐ

   √x7ᵗʰ **T76.62 Child forced labor exploitation, suspected**   Ⓟ

√5ᵗʰ **T76.9 Unspecified maltreatment, suspected**

   √x7ᵗʰ **T76.91 Unspecified adult maltreatment, suspected**   Ⓐ

   √x7ᵗʰ **T76.92 Unspecified child maltreatment, suspected**   Ⓟ

√4ᵗʰ **T78 Adverse effects, not elsewhere classified**

   EXCLUDES 2   complications of surgical and medical care NEC (T80-T88)

> The appropriate 7th character is to be added to each code from category T78.
> A   initial encounter
> D   subsequent encounter
> S   sequela

√5ᵗʰ **T78.0 Anaphylactic reaction due to food**
Anaphylactic reaction due to adverse food reaction
Anaphylactic shock or reaction due to nonpoisonous foods
Anaphylactoid reaction due to food

   √x7ᵗʰ **T78.00 Anaphylactic reaction due to unspecified food**

   √x7ᵗʰ **T78.01 Anaphylactic reaction due to peanuts**

   √x7ᵗʰ **T78.02 Anaphylactic reaction due to shellfish (crustaceans)**

   √x7ᵗʰ **T78.03 Anaphylactic reaction due to other fish**

   √x7ᵗʰ **T78.04 Anaphylactic reaction due to fruits and vegetables**

   √x7ᵗʰ **T78.05 Anaphylactic reaction due to tree nuts and seeds**

      EXCLUDES 2   anaphylactic reaction due to peanuts (T78.01)

   √x7ᵗʰ **T78.06 Anaphylactic reaction due to food additives**

   √x7ᵗʰ **T78.07 Anaphylactic reaction due to milk and dairy products**

   √x7ᵗʰ **T78.08 Anaphylactic reaction due to eggs**

   √x7ᵗʰ **T78.09 Anaphylactic reaction due to other food products**

√x7ᵗʰ **T78.1 Other adverse food reactions, not elsewhere classified**
Use additional code to identify the type of reaction, if applicable

   EXCLUDES 1   anaphylactic reaction or shock due to adverse food reaction (T78.0-)
              anaphylactic reaction due to food (T78.0-)
              bacterial food borne intoxications (A05.-)

   EXCLUDES 2   allergic and dietetic gastroenteritis and colitis (K52.29)
              allergic rhinitis due to food (J30.5)
              dermatitis due to food in contact with skin (L23.6, L24.6, L25.4)
              dermatitis due to ingested food (L27.2)
              food protein-induced enterocolitis syndrome (K52.21)
              food protein-induced enteropathy (K52.22)

√x7ᵗʰ **T78.2 Anaphylactic shock, unspecified**
Allergic shock
Anaphylactic reaction
Anaphylaxis

   EXCLUDES 1   anaphylactic reaction or shock due to adverse effect of correct medicinal substance properly administered (T88.6)
              anaphylactic reaction or shock due to adverse food reaction (T78.0-)
              anaphylactic reaction or shock due to serum (T80.5-)

√x7ᵗʰ **T78.3 Angioneurotic edema**
Allergic angioedema
Giant urticaria
Quincke's edema

   EXCLUDES 1   serum urticaria (T80.6-)
              urticaria (L50.-)

√5ᵗʰ **T78.4 Other and unspecified allergy**

   EXCLUDES 1   specified types of allergic reaction such as:
              allergic diarrhea (K52.29)
              allergic gastroenteritis and colitis (K52.29)
              dermatitis (L23-L25, L27.-)
              food protein-induced enterocolitis syndrome (K52.21)
              food protein-induced enteropathy (K52.22)
              hay fever (J30.1)

   √x7ᵗʰ **T78.40 Allergy, unspecified**
Allergic reaction NOS
Hypersensitivity NOS

   √x7ᵗʰ **T78.41 Arthus phenomenon**
Arthus reaction

   √x7ᵗʰ **T78.49 Other allergy**

√x7ᵗʰ **T78.8 Other adverse effects, not elsewhere classified**

Certain early complications of trauma (T79)

√4ᵗʰ **T79 Certain early complications of trauma, not elsewhere classified**

   EXCLUDES 2   acute respiratory distress syndrome (J80)
              complications occurring during or following medical procedures (T80-T88)
              complications of surgical and medical care NEC (T80-T88)
              newborn respiratory distress syndrome (P22.0)

> The appropriate 7th character is to be added to each code from category T79.
> A   initial encounter
> D   subsequent encounter
> S   sequela

1 √x7ᵗʰ **T79.0 Air embolism (traumatic)**   HCC

   EXCLUDES 1   air embolism complicating abortion or ectopic or molar pregnancy (O00-O07, O08.2)
              air embolism complicating pregnancy, childbirth and the puerperium (O88.0)
              air embolism following infusion, transfusion, and therapeutic injection (T80.0)
              air embolism following procedure NEC (T81.7-)

DEF: Arterial or venous obstruction due to the introduction of air bubbles into the blood vessels following surgery or trauma.

1 √x7ᵗʰ **T79.1 Fat embolism (traumatic)**   HCC

   EXCLUDES 1   fat embolism complicating:
              abortion or ectopic or molar pregnancy (O00-O07, O08.2)
              pregnancy, childbirth and the puerperium (O88.8)

DEF: Arterial blockage due to the entrance of fat into the circulatory system after a fracture of the large bones or administration of corticosteroids.

1 √x7ᵗʰ **T79.2 Traumatic secondary and recurrent hemorrhage and seroma**   HCC

1 √x7ᵗʰ **T79.4 Traumatic shock**   HCC
Shock (immediate) (delayed) following injury

   EXCLUDES 1   anaphylactic shock due to adverse food reaction (T78.0-)
              anaphylactic shock due to correct medicinal substance properly administered (T88.6)
              anaphylactic shock due to serum (T80.5-)
              anaphylactic shock NOS (T78.2)
              anesthetic shock (T88.2)
              electric shock (T75.4)
              nontraumatic shock NEC (R57.-)
              obstetric shock (O75.1)
              postprocedural shock (T81.1-)
              septic shock (R65.21)
              shock complicating abortion or ectopic or molar pregnancy (O00-O07, O08.3)
              shock due to lightning (T75.01)
              shock NOS (R57.9)

1 √x7ᵗʰ **T79.5 Traumatic anuria**   HCC
Crush syndrome
Renal failure following crushing

¹ √x7ᵗʰ **T79.6 Traumatic ischemia of muscle** `HCC`

Traumatic rhabdomyolysis
Volkmann's ischemic contracture

> `EXCLUDES 2`   *anterior tibial syndrome (M76.8)*
> *compartment syndrome (traumatic) (T79.A-)*
> *nontraumatic ischemia of muscle (M62.2-)*

AHA: 2019,2Q,12

¹ √x7ᵗʰ **T79.7 Traumatic subcutaneous emphysema** `HCC`

> `EXCLUDES 1`   *emphysema NOS (J43)*
> *emphysema (subcutaneous) resulting from a procedure (T81.82)*

√5ᵗʰ **T79.A Traumatic compartment syndrome**

> `EXCLUDES 1`   *fibromyalgia (M79.7)*
> *nontraumatic compartment syndrome (M79.A-)*
> ~~traumatic ischemic infarction of muscle (T79.6)~~

> `EXCLUDES 2`   ▶*traumatic ischemic infarction of muscle (T79.6)*◀

DEF: Compression of nerves and blood vessels within an enclosed muscle space due to previous trauma, which leads to impaired blood flow and muscle and nerve damage.

¹ √x7ᵗʰ **T79.A0 Compartment syndrome, unspecified** `HCC`

Compartment syndrome NOS

√6ᵗʰ **T79.A1 Traumatic compartment syndrome of upper extremity**

Traumatic compartment syndrome of shoulder, arm, forearm, wrist, hand, and fingers

¹ √7ᵗʰ **T79.A11 Traumatic compartment syndrome of right upper extremity** `HCC`

¹ √7ᵗʰ **T79.A12 Traumatic compartment syndrome of left upper extremity** `HCC`

¹ √7ᵗʰ **T79.A19 Traumatic compartment syndrome of unspecified upper extremity** `HCC`

√6ᵗʰ **T79.A2 Traumatic compartment syndrome of lower extremity**

Traumatic compartment syndrome of hip, buttock, thigh, leg, foot, and toes

¹ √7ᵗʰ **T79.A21 Traumatic compartment syndrome of right lower extremity** `HCC`

¹ √7ᵗʰ **T79.A22 Traumatic compartment syndrome of left lower extremity** `HCC`

¹ √7ᵗʰ **T79.A29 Traumatic compartment syndrome of unspecified lower extremity** `HCC`

¹ √x7ᵗʰ **T79.A3 Traumatic compartment syndrome of abdomen** `HCC`

¹ √x7ᵗʰ **T79.A9 Traumatic compartment syndrome of other sites** `HCC`

¹ √x7ᵗʰ **T79.8 Other early complications of trauma** `HCC`

¹ √x7ᵗʰ **T79.9 Unspecified early complication of trauma** `HCC`

Complications of surgical and medical care, not elsewhere classified (T80-T88)

Use additional code for adverse effect, if applicable, to identify drug (T36-T50 with fifth or sixth character 5)
Use additional code(s) to identify the specified condition resulting from the complication
Use additional code to identify devices involved and details of circumstances (Y62-Y82)

> `EXCLUDES 2`   *any encounters with medical care for postprocedural conditions in which no complications are present, such as:*
> *artificial opening status (Z93.-)*
> *closure of external stoma (Z43.-)*
> *fitting and adjustment of external prosthetic device (Z44.-)*
> *burns and corrosions from local applications and irradiation (T20-T32)*
> *complications of surgical procedures during pregnancy, childbirth and the puerperium (O00-O9A)*
> *mechanical complication of respirator [ventilator] (J95.850)*
> *poisoning and toxic effects of drugs and chemicals (T36-T65 with fifth or sixth character 1-4 or 6)*
> *postprocedural fever (R50.82)*
> *specified complications classified elsewhere, such as:*
> *cerebrospinal fluid leak from spinal puncture (G97.0)*
> *colostomy malfunction (K94.0-)*
> *disorders of fluid and electrolyte imbalance (E86-E87)*
> *functional disturbances following cardiac surgery (I97.0-I97.1)*
> *intraoperative and postprocedural complications of specified body systems (D78.-, E36.-, E89.-, G97.3-, G97.4, H59.3-, H59.-, H95.2-, H95.3, I97.4-, I97.5, J95.6-, J95.7, K91.6-, L76.-, M96.-, N99.-)*
> *ostomy complications (J95.0-, K94.-, N99.5-)*
> *postgastric surgery syndromes (K91.1)*
> *postlaminectomy syndrome NEC (M96.1)*
> *postmastectomy lymphedema syndrome (I97.2)*
> *postsurgical blind-loop syndrome (K91.2)*
> *ventilator associated pneumonia (J95.851)*

AHA: 2015,1Q,15

√4ᵗʰ **T80 Complications following infusion, transfusion and therapeutic injection**

> `INCLUDES`   complications following perfusion
> `EXCLUDES 2`   *bone marrow transplant rejection (T86.01)*
> *febrile nonhemolytic transfusion reaction (R50.84)*
> *fluid overload due to transfusion (E87.71)*
> *posttransfusion purpura (D69.51)*
> *transfusion associated circulatory overload (TACO) (E87.71)*
> *transfusion (red blood cell) associated hemochromatosis (E83.111)*
> *transfusion related acute lung injury (TRALI) (J95.84)*

The appropriate /th character is to be added to each code from category T80.
A   initial encounter
D   subsequent encounter
S   sequela

√x7ᵗʰ **T80.0 Air embolism following infusion, transfusion and therapeutic injection**

√x7ᵗʰ **T80.1 Vascular complications following infusion, transfusion and therapeutic injection**

Use additional code to identify the vascular complication

> `EXCLUDES 2`   *extravasation of vesicant agent (T80.81-)*
> *infiltration of vesicant agent (T80.81-)*
> *postprocedural vascular complications (T81.7-)*
> *vascular complications specified as due to prosthetic devices, implants and grafts (T82.8-, T83.8-, T84.8-, T85.8-)*

✔ Additional Character Required   √x7ᵗʰ Placeholder Alert   Manifestation   Unspecified Dx   ▶◀ Revised Text   ● New Code   ▲ Revised Code Title

√5ᵗʰ **T80.2** **Infections** following infusion, transfusion and therapeutic injection

Use additional code to identify the specific infection, such as:
sepsis (A41.9)

Use additional code (R65.2-) to identify severe sepsis, if applicable

EXCLUDES 2 *infections specified as due to prosthetic devices, implants and grafts (T82.6-T82.7, T83.5-T83.6, T84.5-T84.7, T85.7)*
postprocedural infections (T81.4-)

AHA: 2018,4Q,62

√6ᵗʰ **T80.21** **Infection** due to central venous catheter

Infection due to pulmonary artery catheter (Swan-Ganz catheter)

AHA: 2019,1Q,13-14

TIP: Only centrally placed catheters are captured with this subcategory. Infections resulting from catheters that are not central lines, including those used for hemodialysis, should be coded to T82.7-.

√7ᵗʰ **T80.211** **Bloodstream infection** due to central venous catheter

Catheter-related bloodstream infection (CRBSI) NOS

Central line-associated bloodstream infection (CLABSI)

Bloodstream infection due to Hickman catheter

Bloodstream infection due to peripherally inserted central catheter (PICC)

Bloodstream infection due to portacath (port-a-cath)

Bloodstream infection due to pulmonary artery catheter

Bloodstream infection due to triple lumen catheter

Bloodstream infection due to umbilical venous catheter

AHA: 2019,1Q,13,14; 2018,4Q,89

√7ᵗʰ **T80.212** **Local infection** due to central venous catheter

Exit or insertion site infection

Local infection due to Hickman catheter

Local infection due to peripherally inserted central catheter (PICC)

Local infection due to portacath (port-a-cath)

Local infection due to pulmonary artery catheter

Local infection due to triple lumen catheter

Local infection due to umbilical venous catheter

Port or reservoir infection

Tunnel infection

√7ᵗʰ **T80.218** **Other infection** due to central venous catheter

Other central line-associated infection

Other infection due to Hickman catheter

Other infection due to peripherally inserted central catheter (PICC)

Other infection due to portacath (port-a-cath)

Other infection due to pulmonary artery catheter

Other infection due to triple lumen catheter

Other infection due to umbilical venous catheter

√7ᵗʰ **T80.219** **Unspecified infection** due to central venous catheter

Central line-associated infection NOS

Unspecified infection due to Hickman catheter

Unspecified infection due to peripherally inserted central catheter (PICC)

Unspecified infection due to portacath (port-a-cath)

Unspecified infection due to pulmonary artery catheter

Unspecified infection due to triple lumen catheter

Unspecified infection due to umbilical venous catheter

√x7ᵗʰ **T80.22** **Acute infection following transfusion, infusion, or injection of blood and blood products**

√x7ᵗʰ **T80.29** **Infection following other infusion, transfusion and therapeutic injection**

√5ᵗʰ **T80.3** **ABO incompatibility** reaction due to transfusion of blood or blood products

EXCLUDES 1 *minor blood group antigens reactions (Duffy) (E) (K) (Kell) (Kidd) (Lewis) (M) (N) (P) (S) (T80.A-)*

√x7ᵗʰ **T80.30** **ABO incompatibility reaction due to transfusion of blood or blood products, unspecified**

ABO incompatibility blood transfusion NOS

Reaction to ABO incompatibility from transfusion NOS

√6ᵗʰ **T80.31** **ABO incompatibility** with hemolytic transfusion reaction

√7ᵗʰ **T80.310** **ABO incompatibility with** acute **hemolytic transfusion reaction**

ABO incompatibility with hemolytic transfusion reaction less than 24 hours after transfusion

Acute hemolytic transfusion reaction (AHTR) due to ABO incompatibility

√7ᵗʰ **T80.311** **ABO incompatibility with** delayed **hemolytic transfusion reaction**

ABO incompatibility with hemolytic transfusion reaction 24 hours or more after transfusion

Delayed hemolytic transfusion reaction (DHTR) due to ABO incompatibility

√7ᵗʰ **T80.319** **ABO incompatibility with hemolytic transfusion reaction, unspecified**

ABO incompatibility with hemolytic transfusion reaction at unspecified time after transfusion

Hemolytic transfusion reaction (HTR) due to ABO incompatibility NOS

√x7ᵗʰ **T80.39** **Other ABO incompatibility reaction due to transfusion of blood or blood products**

Delayed serologic transfusion reaction (DSTR) from ABO incompatibility

Other ABO incompatible blood transfusion

Other reaction to ABO incompatible blood transfusion

√5ᵗʰ **T80.4** **Rh incompatibility** reaction due to transfusion of blood or blood products

Reaction due to incompatibility of Rh antigens (C) (c) (D) (E) (e)

√x7ᵗʰ **T80.40** **Rh incompatibility reaction due to transfusion of blood or blood products, unspecified**

Reaction due to Rh factor in transfusion NOS

Rh incompatible blood transfusion NOS

√6ᵗʰ **T80.41** **Rh incompatibility** with hemolytic transfusion reaction

√7ᵗʰ **T80.410** **Rh incompatibility with** acute **hemolytic transfusion reaction**

Acute hemolytic transfusion reaction (AHTR) due to Rh incompatibility

Rh incompatibility with hemolytic transfusion reaction less than 24 hours after transfusion

√7ᵗʰ **T80.411** **Rh incompatibility with** delayed **hemolytic transfusion reaction**

Delayed hemolytic transfusion reaction (DHTR) due to Rh incompatibility

Rh incompatibility with hemolytic transfusion reaction 24 hours or more after transfusion

√7ᵗʰ **T80.419 Rh incompatibility with hemolytic transfusion reaction, unspecified**

Rh incompatibility with hemolytic transfusion reaction at unspecified time after transfusion

Hemolytic transfusion reaction (HTR) due to Rh incompatibility NOS

√x7ᵗʰ **T80.49 Other Rh incompatibility reaction due to transfusion of blood or blood products**

Delayed serologic transfusion reaction (DSTR) from Rh incompatibility

Other reaction to Rh incompatible blood transfusion

√5ᵗʰ **T80.A Non-ABO incompatibility reaction due to transfusion of blood or blood products**

Reaction due to incompatibility of minor antigens (Duffy) (Kell) (Kidd) (Lewis) (M) (N) (P) (S)

√x7ᵗʰ **T80.A0 Non-ABO incompatibility reaction due to transfusion of blood or blood products, unspecified**

Non-ABO antigen incompatibility reaction from transfusion NOS

√6ᵗʰ **T80.A1 Non-ABO incompatibility with hemolytic transfusion reaction**

√x7ᵗʰ **T80.A10 Non-ABO incompatibility with acute hemolytic transfusion reaction**

Acute hemolytic transfusion reaction (AHTR) due to non-ABO incompatibility

Non-ABO incompatibility with hemolytic transfusion reaction less than 24 hours after transfusion

√x7ᵗʰ **T80.A11 Non-ABO incompatibility with delayed hemolytic transfusion reaction**

Delayed hemolytic transfusion reaction (DHTR) due to non-ABO incompatibility

Non-ABO incompatibility with hemolytic transfusion reaction 24 or more hours after transfusion

√x7ᵗʰ **T80.A19 Non-ABO incompatibility with hemolytic transfusion reaction, unspecified**

Hemolytic transfusion reaction (HTR) due to non-ABO incompatibility NOS

Non-ABO incompatibility with hemolytic transfusion reaction at unspecified time after transfusion

√x7ᵗʰ **T80.A9 Other non-ABO incompatibility reaction due to transfusion of blood or blood products**

Delayed serologic transfusion reaction (DSTR) from non-ABO incompatibility

Other reaction to non-ABO incompatible blood transfusion

√5ᵗʰ **T80.5 Anaphylactic reaction due to serum**

Allergic shock due to serum

Anaphylactic shock due to serum

Anaphylactoid reaction due to serum

Anaphylaxis due to serum

EXCLUDES 1   *ABO incompatibility reaction due to transfusion of blood or blood products (T80.3-)*

allergic reaction or shock NOS (T78.2)

anaphylactic reaction or shock NOS (T78.2)

anaphylactic reaction or shock due to adverse effect of correct medicinal substance properly administered (T88.6)

other serum reaction (T80.6-)

DEF: Life-threatening hypersensitivity to a foreign serum causing respiratory distress, vascular collapse, and shock.

√x7ᵗʰ **T80.51 Anaphylactic reaction due to administration of blood and blood products**

√x7ᵗʰ **T80.52 Anaphylactic reaction due to vaccination**

√x7ᵗʰ **T80.59 Anaphylactic reaction due to other serum**

√5ᵗʰ **T80.6 Other serum reactions**

Intoxication by serum

Protein sickness

Serum rash

Serum sickness

Serum urticaria

EXCLUDES 2   *serum hepatitis (B16-B19)*

DEF: Serum sickness: Hypersensitivity to a foreign serum that causes fever, hives, swelling, and lymphadenopathy.

√x7ᵗʰ **T80.61 Other serum reaction due to administration of blood and blood products**

√x7ᵗʰ **T80.62 Other serum reaction due to vaccination**

√x7ᵗʰ **T80.69 Other serum reaction due to other serum**

Code also, if applicable, arthropathy in hypersensitivity reactions classified elsewhere (M36.4)

√5ᵗʰ **T80.8 Other complications following infusion, transfusion and therapeutic injection**

√6ᵗʰ **T80.81 Extravasation of vesicant agent**

Infiltration of vesicant agent

√7ᵗʰ **T80.810 Extravasation of vesicant antineoplastic chemotherapy**

Infiltration of vesicant antineoplastic chemotherapy

√7ᵗʰ **T80.818 Extravasation of other vesicant agent**

Infiltration of other vesicant agent

√x7ᵗʰ **T80.89 Other complications following infusion, transfusion and therapeutic injection**

Delayed serologic transfusion reaction (DSTR), unspecified incompatibility

Use additional code to identify graft-versus-host reaction, if applicable, (D89.81-)

√5ᵗʰ **T80.9 Unspecified complication following infusion, transfusion and therapeutic injection**

√x7ᵗʰ **T80.90 Unspecified complication following infusion and therapeutic injection**

√6ᵗʰ **T80.91 Hemolytic transfusion reaction, unspecified incompatibility**

EXCLUDES 1   *ABO incompatibility with hemolytic transfusion reaction (T80.31-)*

non-ABO incompatibility with hemolytic transfusion reaction (T80.A1-)

Rh incompatibility with hemolytic transfusion reaction (T80.41-)

√7ᵗʰ **T80.910 Acute hemolytic transfusion reaction, unspecified incompatibility**

√7ᵗʰ **T80.911 Delayed hemolytic transfusion reaction, unspecified incompatibility**

√7ᵗʰ **T80.919 Hemolytic transfusion reaction, unspecified incompatibility, unspecified as acute or delayed**

Hemolytic transfusion reaction NOS

√x7ᵗʰ **T80.92 Unspecified transfusion reaction**

Transfusion reaction NOS

☑ Additional Character Required   √x7ᵗʰ Placeholder Alert   Manifestation   Unspecified Dx   ►◄ Revised Text   ● New Code   ▲ Revised Code Title

ICD-10-CM 2020   1135

T80.419–T80.92

√4ᵗʰ **T81 Complications of procedures, not elsewhere classified**

Use additional code for adverse effect, if applicable, to identify drug (T36-T50 with fifth or sixth character 5)

EXCLUDES 2   *complications following immunization (T88.Ø-T88.1)*
complications following infusion, transfusion and therapeutic injection (T8Ø.-)
complications of transplanted organs and tissue (T86.-)
specified complications classified elsewhere, such as:
    complication of prosthetic devices, implants and grafts (T82-T85)
    dermatitis due to drugs and medicaments (L23.3, L24.4, L25.1, L27.Ø-L27.1)
    endosseous dental implant failure (M27.6-)
    floppy iris syndrome (IFIS) (intraoperative) (H21.81)
    intraoperative and postprocedural complications of specific body system (D78.-, E36.-, E89.-, G97.3-, G97.4, H59.3-, H59.-, H95.2-, H95.3, I97.4-, I97.5, J95, K91.-, L76.-, M96.-, N99.-)
    ostomy complications (J95.Ø-, K94.-, N99.5-)
    plateau iris syndrome (post-iridectomy) (postprocedural) H21.82
    poisoning and toxic effects of drugs and chemicals (T36-T65 with fifth or sixth character 1-4 or 6)

AHA: 2019,2Q,21

> The appropriate 7th character is to be added to each code from category T81.
> A   initial encounter
> D   subsequent encounter
> S   sequela

√5ᵗʰ **T81.1 Postprocedural shock**

Shock during or resulting from a procedure, not elsewhere classified

EXCLUDES 1   *anaphylactic shock due to correct substance properly administered (T88.6)*
anaphylactic shock due to serum (T8Ø.5-)
anaphylactic shock NOS (T78.2)
anesthetic shock (T88.2)
electric shock (T75.4)
obstetric shock (O75.1)
septic shock (R65.21)
shock following abortion or ectopic or molar pregnancy (OØØ-OØ7, OØ8.3)
traumatic shock (T79.4)

√7ᵗʰ **T81.1Ø Postprocedural shock unspecified**

Collapse NOS during or resulting from a procedure, not elsewhere classified
Postprocedural failure of peripheral circulation
Postprocedural shock NOS

1 √7ᵗʰ **T81.11 Postprocedural cardiogenic shock**   HCC

1 √7ᵗʰ **T81.12 Postprocedural septic shock**   HCC

Postprocedural endotoxic shock resulting from a procedure, not elsewhere classified
Postprocedural gram-negative shock resulting from a procedure, not elsewhere classified
Code first underlying infection
Use additional code, to identify any associated acute organ dysfunction, if applicable

AHA: 2018,4Q,63

√7ᵗʰ **T81.19 Other postprocedural shock**

Postprocedural hypovolemic shock

√5ᵗʰ **T81.3 Disruption of wound, not elsewhere classified**

Disruption of any suture materials or other closure methods

EXCLUDES 1   *breakdown (mechanical) of permanent sutures (T85.612)*
displacement of permanent sutures (T85.622)
disruption of cesarean delivery wound (O90.Ø)
disruption of perineal obstetric wound (O90.1)
mechanical complication of permanent sutures NEC (T85.692)

AHA: 2014,1Q,23

√7ᵗʰ **T81.3Ø Disruption of wound, unspecified**

Disruption of wound NOS

√7ᵗʰ **T81.31 Disruption of external operation (surgical) wound, not elsewhere classified**

Dehiscence of operation wound NOS
Disruption of operation wound NOS
Disruption or dehiscence of closure of cornea
Disruption or dehiscence of closure of mucosa
Disruption or dehiscence of closure of skin and subcutaneous tissue
Full-thickness skin disruption or dehiscence
Superficial disruption or dehiscence of operation wound

EXCLUDES 1   *dehiscence of amputation stump (T87.81)*

√7ᵗʰ **T81.32 Disruption of internal operation (surgical) wound, not elsewhere classified**

Deep disruption or dehiscence of operation wound NOS
Disruption or dehiscence of closure of internal organ or other internal tissue
Disruption or dehiscence of closure of muscle or muscle flap
Disruption or dehiscence of closure of ribs or rib cage
Disruption or dehiscence of closure of skull or craniotomy
Disruption or dehiscence of closure of sternum or sternotomy
Disruption or dehiscence of closure of tendon or ligament
Disruption or dehiscence of closure of superficial or muscular fascia

AHA: 2017,3Q,4

√7ᵗʰ **T81.33 Disruption of traumatic injury wound repair**

Disruption or dehiscence of closure of traumatic laceration (external) (internal)

√5ᵗʰ **T81.4 Infection following a procedure**

Wound abscess following a procedure
Use additional code to identify infection
Use additional code (R65.2-) to identify severe sepsis, if applicable

EXCLUDES 2   *bleb associated endophthalmitis (H59.4-)*
infection due to infusion, transfusion and therapeutic injection (T8Ø.2-)
infection due to prosthetic devices, implants and grafts (T82.6-T82.7, T83.5-T83.6, T84.5-T84.7, T85.7)
obstetric surgical wound infection (O86.Ø-)
postprocedural fever NOS (R5Ø.82)
postprocedural retroperitoneal abscess (K68.11)

AHA: 2018,4Q,33-34,62; 2014,1Q,23

√7ᵗʰ **T81.4Ø Infection following a procedure, unspecified**

√7ᵗʰ **T81.41 Infection following a procedure, superficial incisional surgical site**

Subcutaneous abscess following a procedure
Stitch abscess following a procedure

√7ᵗʰ **T81.42 Infection following a procedure, deep incisional surgical site**

Intra-muscular abscess following a procedure

√7ᵗʰ **T81.43 Infection following a procedure, organ and space surgical site**

Intra-abdominal abscess following a procedure
Subphrenic abscess following a procedure

1 √7ᵗʰ **T81.44 Sepsis following a procedure**   HCC

Use additional code to identify the sepsis

√7ᵗʰ **T81.49 Infection following a procedure, other surgical site**

√5ᵗʰ **T81.5 Complications of foreign body accidentally left in body following procedure**

AHA: 2014,4Q,24

√6ᵗʰ **T81.5Ø Unspecified complication of foreign body accidentally left in body following procedure**

√7ᵗʰ **T81.5ØØ Unspecified complication of foreign body accidentally left in body following surgical operation**

√7ᵗʰ **T81.5Ø1 Unspecified complication of foreign body accidentally left in body following infusion or transfusion**

√7ᵗʰ **T81.5Ø2 Unspecified complication of foreign body accidentally left in body following kidney dialysis**   HCC

√7ᵗʰ **T81.503** **Unspecified complication of foreign body accidentally left in body following injection or immunization**

√7ᵗʰ **T81.504** **Unspecified complication of foreign body accidentally left in body following endoscopic examination**

√7ᵗʰ **T81.505** **Unspecified complication of foreign body accidentally left in body following** heart **catheterization**

√7ᵗʰ **T81.506** **Unspecified complication of foreign body accidentally left in body following aspiration, puncture or other catheterization**

√7ᵗʰ **T81.507** **Unspecified complication of foreign body accidentally left in body following removal of catheter or packing**

√7ᵗʰ **T81.508** **Unspecified complication of foreign body accidentally left in body following other procedure**

√7ᵗʰ **T81.509** **Unspecified complication of foreign body accidentally left in body following unspecified procedure**

√6ᵗʰ **T81.51** **Adhesions** **due to foreign body accidentally left in body following procedure**

√7ᵗʰ **T81.510** **Adhesions due to foreign body accidentally left in body following surgical operation**

√7ᵗʰ **T81.511** **Adhesions due to foreign body accidentally left in body following infusion or transfusion**

√7ᵗʰ **T81.512** **Adhesions due to foreign body accidentally left in body following kidney dialysis**   HCC

√7ᵗʰ **T81.513** **Adhesions due to foreign body accidentally left in body following injection or immunization**

√7ᵗʰ **T81.514** **Adhesions due to foreign body accidentally left in body following endoscopic examination**

√7ᵗʰ **T81.515** **Adhesions due to foreign body accidentally left in body following** heart **catheterization**

√7ᵗʰ **T81.516** **Adhesions due to foreign body accidentally left in body following aspiration, puncture or other catheterization**

√7ᵗʰ **T81.517** **Adhesions due to foreign body accidentally left in body following removal of catheter or packing**

√7ᵗʰ **T81.518** **Adhesions due to foreign body accidentally left in body following other procedure**

√7ᵗʰ **T81.519** **Adhesions due to foreign body accidentally left in body following unspecified procedure**

√6ᵗʰ **T81.52** **Obstruction** **due to foreign body accidentally left in body following procedure**

√7ᵗʰ **T81.520** **Obstruction due to foreign body accidentally left in body following surgical operation**

√7ᵗʰ **T81.521** **Obstruction due to foreign body accidentally left in body following infusion or transfusion**

√7ᵗʰ **T81.522** **Obstruction due to foreign body accidentally left in body following kidney dialysis**   HCC

√7ᵗʰ **T81.523** **Obstruction due to foreign body accidentally left in body following injection or immunization**

√7ᵗʰ **T81.524** **Obstruction due to foreign body accidentally left in body following endoscopic examination**

√7ᵗʰ **T81.525** **Obstruction due to foreign body accidentally left in body following** heart **catheterization**

√7ᵗʰ **T81.526** **Obstruction due to foreign body accidentally left in body following aspiration, puncture or other catheterization**

√7ᵗʰ **T81.527** **Obstruction due to foreign body accidentally left in body following removal of catheter or packing**

√7ᵗʰ **T81.528** **Obstruction due to foreign body accidentally left in body following other procedure**

√7ᵗʰ **T81.529** **Obstruction due to foreign body accidentally left in body following unspecified procedure**

√6ᵗʰ **T81.53** **Perforation** **due to foreign body accidentally left in body following procedure**

√7ᵗʰ **T81.530** **Perforation due to foreign body accidentally left in body following surgical operation**

√7ᵗʰ **T81.531** **Perforation due to foreign body accidentally left in body following infusion or transfusion**

√7ᵗʰ **T81.532** **Perforation due to foreign body accidentally left in body following kidney dialysis**   HCC

√7ᵗʰ **T81.533** **Perforation due to foreign body accidentally left in body following injection or immunization**

√7ᵗʰ **T81.534** **Perforation due to foreign body accidentally left in body following endoscopic examination**

√7ᵗʰ **T81.535** **Perforation due to foreign body accidentally left in body following** heart **catheterization**

√7ᵗʰ **T81.536** **Perforation due to foreign body accidentally left in body following aspiration, puncture or other catheterization**

√7ᵗʰ **T81.537** **Perforation due to foreign body accidentally left in body following removal of catheter or packing**

√7ᵗʰ **T81.538** **Perforation due to foreign body accidentally left in body following other procedure**

√7ᵗʰ **T81.539** **Perforation due to foreign body accidentally left in body following unspecified procedure**

√6ᵗʰ **T81.59** **Other complications of foreign body accidentally left in body following procedure**

    EXCLUDES 2   *obstruction or perforation due to prosthetic devices and implants intentionally left in body (T82.0-T82.5, T83.0-T83.4, T83.7, T84.0-T84.4, T85.0-T85.6)*

√7ᵗʰ **T81.590** **Other complications of foreign body accidentally left in body following surgical operation**

√7ᵗʰ **T81.591** **Other complications of foreign body accidentally left in body following infusion or transfusion**

√7ᵗʰ **T81.592** **Other complications of foreign body accidentally left in body following kidney dialysis**   HCC

√7ᵗʰ **T81.593** **Other complications of foreign body accidentally left in body following injection or immunization**

√7ᵗʰ **T81.594** **Other complications of foreign body accidentally left in body following endoscopic examination**

√7ᵗʰ **T81.595** **Other complications of foreign body accidentally left in body following** heart **catheterization**

√7ᵗʰ **T81.596** **Other complications of foreign body accidentally left in body following aspiration, puncture or other catheterization**

√7ᵗʰ **T81.597** **Other complications of foreign body accidentally left in body following removal of catheter or packing**

√7ᵗʰ **T81.598** **Other complications of foreign body accidentally left in body following other procedure**

√7ᵗʰ **T81.599** **Other complications of foreign body accidentally left in body following unspecified procedure**

√5ᵗʰ **T81.6** **Acute reaction to foreign substance accidentally left during a procedure**

    EXCLUDES 2   *complications of foreign body accidentally left in body cavity or operation wound following procedure (T81.5-)*

√x7ᵗʰ **T81.60** **Unspecified acute reaction to foreign substance accidentally left during a procedure**

☑ Additional Character Required   √x7ᵗʰ Placeholder Alert   Manifestation   Unspecified Dx   ▶◀ Revised Text   ● New Code   ▲ Revised Code Title

ICD-10-CM 2020   1137

√x7ᵗʰ **T81.61** Aseptic peritonitis due to foreign substance accidentally left during a procedure
Chemical peritonitis

√x7ᵗʰ **T81.69** Other acute reaction to foreign substance accidentally left during a procedure

√5ᵗʰ **T81.7** Vascular complications following a procedure, not elsewhere classified
Air embolism following procedure NEC
Phlebitis or thrombophlebitis resulting from a procedure

EXCLUDES 1 embolism complicating abortion or ectopic or molar pregnancy (O00–O07, O08.2)
embolism complicating pregnancy, childbirth and the puerperium (O88.-)
traumatic embolism (T79.0)

EXCLUDES 2 embolism due to prosthetic devices, implants and grafts (T82.8-, T83.81, T84.8-, T85.81-)
embolism following infusion, transfusion and therapeutic injection (T80.0)

AHA: 2019,2Q,22

√6ᵗʰ **T81.71** Complication of artery following a procedure, not elsewhere classified

√7ᵗʰ **T81.710** Complication of mesenteric artery following a procedure, not elsewhere classified

√7ᵗʰ **T81.711** Complication of renal artery following a procedure, not elsewhere classified

√7ᵗʰ **T81.718** Complication of other artery following a procedure, not elsewhere classified
AHA: 2019,2Q,21-22

√7ᵗʰ **T81.719** Complication of unspecified artery following a procedure, not elsewhere classified

√x7ᵗʰ **T81.72** Complication of vein following a procedure, not elsewhere classified

√5ᵗʰ **T81.8** Other complications of procedures, not elsewhere classified

EXCLUDES 2 hypothermia following anesthesia (T88.51)
malignant hyperpyrexia due to anesthesia (T88.3)

√x7ᵗʰ **T81.81** Complication of inhalation therapy

√x7ᵗʰ **T81.82** Emphysema (subcutaneous) resulting from a procedure

√x7ᵗʰ **T81.83** Persistent postprocedural fistula
AHA: 2017,3Q,3-4

√x7ᵗʰ **T81.89** Other complications of procedures, not elsewhere classified
Use additional code to specify complication, such as:
postprocedural delirium (F05)
AHA: 2014,1Q,23

√x7ᵗʰ **T81.9** Unspecified complication of procedure

√4ᵗʰ **T82** Complications of cardiac and vascular prosthetic devices, implants and grafts

EXCLUDES 2 failure and rejection of transplanted organs and tissue (T86.-)

The appropriate 7th character is to be added to each code from category T82.
A initial encounter
D subsequent encounter
S sequela

√5ᵗʰ **T82.0** Mechanical complication of heart valve prosthesis
Mechanical complication of artificial heart valve

EXCLUDES 1 mechanical complication of biological heart valve graft (T82.22-)

√x7ᵗʰ **T82.01** Breakdown (mechanical) of heart valve prosthesis

√x7ᵗʰ **T82.02** Displacement of heart valve prosthesis
Malposition of heart valve prosthesis

√x7ᵗʰ **T82.03** Leakage of heart valve prosthesis

√x7ᵗʰ **T82.09** Other mechanical complication of heart valve prosthesis
Obstruction (mechanical) of heart valve prosthesis
Perforation of heart valve prosthesis
Protrusion of heart valve prosthesis

√5ᵗʰ **T82.1** Mechanical complication of cardiac electronic device

√6ᵗʰ **T82.11** Breakdown (mechanical) of cardiac electronic device

√7ᵗʰ **T82.110** Breakdown (mechanical) of cardiac electrode

√7ᵗʰ **T82.111** Breakdown (mechanical) of cardiac pulse generator (battery)

√7ᵗʰ **T82.118** Breakdown (mechanical) of other cardiac electronic device

√7ᵗʰ **T82.119** Breakdown (mechanical) of unspecified cardiac electronic device

√6ᵗʰ **T82.12** Displacement of cardiac electronic device
Malposition of cardiac electronic device

√7ᵗʰ **T82.120** Displacement of cardiac electrode

√7ᵗʰ **T82.121** Displacement of cardiac pulse generator (battery)

√7ᵗʰ **T82.128** Displacement of other cardiac electronic device

√7ᵗʰ **T82.129** Displacement of unspecified cardiac electronic device

√6ᵗʰ **T82.19** Other mechanical complication of cardiac electronic device
Leakage of cardiac electronic device
Obstruction of cardiac electronic device
Perforation of cardiac electronic device
Protrusion of cardiac electronic device

√7ᵗʰ **T82.190** Other mechanical complication of cardiac electrode

√7ᵗʰ **T82.191** Other mechanical complication of cardiac pulse generator (battery)

√7ᵗʰ **T82.198** Other mechanical complication of other cardiac electronic device

√7ᵗʰ **T82.199** Other mechanical complication of unspecified cardiac device

√5ᵗʰ **T82.2** Mechanical complication of coronary artery bypass graft and biological heart valve graft

EXCLUDES 1 mechanical complication of artificial heart valve prosthesis (T82.0-)

√6ᵗʰ **T82.21** Mechanical complication of coronary artery bypass graft

√7ᵗʰ **T82.211** Breakdown (mechanical) of coronary artery bypass graft

√7ᵗʰ **T82.212** Displacement of coronary artery bypass graft
Malposition of coronary artery bypass graft

√7ᵗʰ **T82.213** Leakage of coronary artery bypass graft

√7ᵗʰ **T82.218** Other mechanical complication of coronary artery bypass graft
Obstruction, mechanical of coronary artery bypass graft
Perforation of coronary artery bypass graft
Protrusion of coronary artery bypass graft

√6ᵗʰ **T82.22** Mechanical complication of biological heart valve graft

√7ᵗʰ **T82.221** Breakdown (mechanical) of biological heart valve graft

√7ᵗʰ **T82.222** Displacement of biological heart valve graft
Malposition of biological heart valve graft

√7ᵗʰ **T82.223** Leakage of biological heart valve graft

√7ᵗʰ **T82.228** Other mechanical complication of biological heart valve graft
Obstruction of biological heart valve graft
Perforation of biological heart valve graft
Protrusion of biological heart valve graft

√5ᵗʰ **T82.3** Mechanical complication of other vascular grafts

√6ᵗʰ **T82.31** Breakdown (mechanical) of other vascular grafts

¹√7ᵗʰ **T82.310** Breakdown (mechanical) of aortic (bifurcation) graft (replacement) HCC

¹√7ᵗʰ **T82.311** Breakdown (mechanical) of carotid arterial graft (bypass) HCC

¹√7ᵗʰ **T82.312** Breakdown (mechanical) of femoral arterial graft (bypass) HCC

¹√7ᵗʰ **T82.318** Breakdown (mechanical) of other vascular grafts HCC

¹√7ᵗʰ **T82.319** Breakdown (mechanical) of unspecified vascular grafts HCC

√6ᵗʰ **T82.32** Displacement of other vascular grafts
Malposition of other vascular grafts

¹√7ᵗʰ **T82.320** Displacement of aortic (bifurcation) graft (replacement) HCC

¹√7ᵗʰ **T82.321** Displacement of carotid arterial graft (bypass) HCC

¹√7ᵗʰ **T82.322** Displacement of femoral arterial graft (bypass) HCC

¹√7ᵗʰ **T82.328** Displacement of other vascular grafts HCC

¹ √7ᵗʰ **T82.329 Displacement of unspecified vascular grafts** `HCC`

√6ᵗʰ **T82.33 Leakage** of other vascular grafts

    ¹ √7ᵗʰ **T82.330 Leakage of aortic (bifurcation) graft (replacement)** `HCC`

    ¹ √7ᵗʰ **T82.331 Leakage of carotid arterial graft (bypass)** `HCC`

    ¹ √7ᵗʰ **T82.332 Leakage of femoral arterial graft (bypass)** `HCC`

    ¹ √7ᵗʰ **T82.338 Leakage of other vascular grafts** `HCC`

    ¹ √7ᵗʰ **T82.339 Leakage of unspecified vascular graft** `HCC`

√6ᵗʰ **T82.39 Other mechanical complication of other vascular grafts**

    Obstruction (mechanical) of other vascular grafts

    Perforation of other vascular grafts

    Protrusion of other vascular grafts

    ¹ √7ᵗʰ **T82.390 Other mechanical complication of aortic (bifurcation) graft (replacement)** `HCC`

    ¹ √7ᵗʰ **T82.391 Other mechanical complication of carotid arterial graft (bypass)** `HCC`

    ¹ √7ᵗʰ **T82.392 Other mechanical complication of femoral arterial graft (bypass)** `HCC`

    ¹ √7ᵗʰ **T82.398 Other mechanical complication of other vascular grafts** `HCC`

    ¹ √7ᵗʰ **T82.399 Other mechanical complication of unspecified vascular grafts** `HCC`

√5ᵗʰ **T82.4 Mechanical complication of vascular dialysis catheter**

    Mechanical complication of hemodialysis catheter

    EXCLUDES 1 *mechanical complication of intraperitoneal dialysis catheter (T85.62)*

    √x7ᵗʰ **T82.41 Breakdown (mechanical) of vascular dialysis catheter** `HCC`

    √x7ᵗʰ **T82.42 Displacement of vascular dialysis catheter** `HCC`

      Malposition of vascular dialysis catheter

    √x7ᵗʰ **T82.43 Leakage of vascular dialysis catheter** `HCC`

    √x7ᵗʰ **T82.49 Other complication of vascular dialysis catheter** `HCC`

      Obstruction (mechanical) of vascular dialysis catheter

      Perforation of vascular dialysis catheter

      Protrusion of vascular dialysis catheter

√5ᵗʰ **T82.5 Mechanical complication of other cardiac and vascular devices and implants**

    EXCLUDES 2 *mechanical complication of epidural and subdural infusion catheter (T85.61)*

√6ᵗʰ **T82.51 Breakdown (mechanical) of other cardiac and vascular devices and implants**

    ¹ √7ᵗʰ **T82.510 Breakdown (mechanical) of surgically created arteriovenous fistula** `HCC`

    ¹ √7ᵗʰ **T82.511 Breakdown (mechanical) of surgically created arteriovenous shunt** `HCC`

    √7ᵗʰ **T82.512 Breakdown (mechanical) of artificial heart**

    ¹ √7ᵗʰ **T82.513 Breakdown (mechanical) of balloon (counterpulsation) device** `HCC`

    ¹ √7ᵗʰ **T82.514 Breakdown (mechanical) of infusion catheter** `HCC`

    ¹ √7ᵗʰ **T82.515 Breakdown (mechanical) of umbrella device** `HCC`

    ¹ √7ᵗʰ **T82.518 Breakdown (mechanical) of other cardiac and vascular devices and implants** `HCC`

    √7ᵗʰ **T82.519 Breakdown (mechanical) of unspecified cardiac and vascular devices and implants**

√6ᵗʰ **T82.52 Displacement of other cardiac and vascular devices and implants**

    Malposition of other cardiac and vascular devices and implants

    ¹ √7ᵗʰ **T82.520 Displacement of surgically created arteriovenous fistula** `HCC`

    ¹ √7ᵗʰ **T82.521 Displacement of surgically created arteriovenous shunt** `HCC`

    √7ᵗʰ **T82.522 Displacement of artificial heart**

    ¹ √7ᵗʰ **T82.523 Displacement of balloon (counterpulsation) device** `HCC`

    ¹ √7ᵗʰ **T82.524 Displacement of infusion catheter** `HCC`

    ¹ √7ᵗʰ **T82.525 Displacement of umbrella device** `HCC`

¹ √7ᵗʰ **T82.528 Displacement of other cardiac and vascular devices and implants** `HCC`

    √7ᵗʰ **T82.529 Displacement of unspecified cardiac and vascular devices and implants** `HCC`

√6ᵗʰ **T82.53 Leakage of other cardiac and vascular devices and implants**

    ¹ √7ᵗʰ **T82.530 Leakage of surgically created arteriovenous fistula** `HCC`

    ¹ √7ᵗʰ **T82.531 Leakage of surgically created arteriovenous shunt** `HCC`

    √7ᵗʰ **T82.532 Leakage of artificial heart**

    ¹ √7ᵗʰ **T82.533 Leakage of balloon (counterpulsation) device** `HCC`

    ¹ √7ᵗʰ **T82.534 Leakage of infusion catheter** `HCC`

    ¹ √7ᵗʰ **T82.535 Leakage of umbrella device** `HCC`

    ¹ √7ᵗʰ **T82.538 Leakage of other cardiac and vascular devices and implants** `HCC`

    √7ᵗʰ **T82.539 Leakage of unspecified cardiac and vascular devices and implants**

√6ᵗʰ **T82.59 Other mechanical complication of other cardiac and vascular devices and implants**

    Obstruction (mechanical) of other cardiac and vascular devices and implants

    Perforation of other cardiac and vascular devices and implants

    Protrusion of other cardiac and vascular devices and implants

    ¹ √7ᵗʰ **T82.590 Other mechanical complication of surgically created arteriovenous fistula** `HCC`

    ¹ √7ᵗʰ **T82.591 Other mechanical complication of surgically created arteriovenous shunt** `HCC`

    √7ᵗʰ **T82.592 Other mechanical complication of artificial heart**

    ¹ √7ᵗʰ **T82.593 Other mechanical complication of balloon (counterpulsation) device** `HCC`

    ¹ √7ᵗʰ **T82.594 Other mechanical complication of infusion catheter** `HCC`

    ¹ √7ᵗʰ **T82.595 Other mechanical complication of umbrella device** `HCC`

    ¹ √7ᵗʰ **T82.598 Other mechanical complication of other cardiac and vascular devices and implants** `HCC`

    √7ᵗʰ **T82.599 Other mechanical complication of unspecified cardiac and vascular devices and implants**

¹ √x7ᵗʰ **T82.6 Infection and inflammatory reaction due to cardiac valve prosthesis** `HCC`

    Use additional code to identify infection

¹ √x7ᵗʰ **T82.7 Infection and inflammatory reaction due to other cardiac and vascular devices, implants and grafts** `HCC`

    Use additional code to identify infection

    AHA: 2019,1Q,13-14

    TIP: Assign this code for infections and/or cellulitis resulting from catheters that are not centrally placed (e.g., midline catheters).

√5ᵗʰ **T82.8 Other specified complications of cardiac and vascular prosthetic devices, implants and grafts**

    AHA: 2016,4Q,70

√6ᵗʰ **T82.81 Embolism due to cardiac and vascular prosthetic devices, implants and grafts**

    √7ᵗʰ **T82.817 Embolism due to cardiac prosthetic devices, implants and grafts**

    ¹ √7ᵗʰ **T82.818 Embolism due to vascular prosthetic devices, implants and grafts** `HCC`

√6ᵗʰ **T82.82 Fibrosis due to cardiac and vascular prosthetic devices, implants and grafts**

    √7ᵗʰ **T82.827 Fibrosis due to cardiac prosthetic devices, implants and grafts**

    ¹ √7ᵗʰ **T82.828 Fibrosis due to vascular prosthetic devices, implants and grafts** `HCC`

√6ᵗʰ **T82.83 Hemorrhage due to cardiac and vascular prosthetic devices, implants and grafts**

    √7ᵗʰ **T82.837 Hemorrhage due to cardiac prosthetic devices, implants and grafts**

    ¹ √7ᵗʰ **T82.838 Hemorrhage due to vascular prosthetic devices, implants and grafts** `HCC`

☑ Additional Character Required   √x7ᵗʰ Placeholder Alert   Manifestation   Unspecified Dx   ►◄ Revised Text   ● New Code   ▲ Revised Code Title

ICD-10-CM 2020   **1139**

Chapter 19. Injury, Poisoning and Certain Other Consequences of External Causes

T82.329–T82.838

√6ᵗʰ **T82.84** Pain due to cardiac and vascular prosthetic devices, implants and grafts

√7ᵗʰ **T82.847** Pain due to cardiac prosthetic devices, implants and grafts

¹ √7ᵗʰ **T82.848** Pain due to vascular prosthetic devices, implants and grafts   HCC

√6ᵗʰ **T82.85** Stenosis due to cardiac and vascular prosthetic devices, implants and grafts

√7ᵗʰ **T82.855** Stenosis of coronary artery stent   Q

In-stent stenosis (restenosis) of coronary artery stent

Restenosis of coronary artery stent

¹ √7ᵗʰ **T82.856** Stenosis of peripheral vascular stent   HCC Q

In-stent stenosis (restenosis) of peripheral vascular stent

Restenosis of peripheral vascular stent

√7ᵗʰ **T82.857** Stenosis of other cardiac prosthetic devices, implants and grafts

¹ √7ᵗʰ **T82.858** Stenosis of other vascular prosthetic devices, implants and grafts   HCC

√6ᵗʰ **T82.86** Thrombosis of cardiac and vascular prosthetic devices, implants and grafts

√7ᵗʰ **T82.867** Thrombosis due to cardiac prosthetic devices, implants and grafts

¹ √7ᵗʰ **T82.868** Thrombosis due to vascular prosthetic devices, implants and grafts   HCC

√6ᵗʰ **T82.89** Other specified complication of cardiac and vascular prosthetic devices, implants and grafts

√7ᵗʰ **T82.897** Other specified complication of cardiac prosthetic devices, implants and grafts

AHA: 2019,2Q,33

¹ √7ᵗʰ **T82.898** Other specified complication of vascular prosthetic devices, implants and grafts   HCC

√x7ᵗʰ **T82.9** Unspecified complication of cardiac and vascular prosthetic device, implant and graft

√4ᵗʰ **T83** Complications of genitourinary prosthetic devices, implants and grafts

EXCLUDES 2   *failure and rejection of transplanted organs and tissue (T86.-)*

AHA: 2016,4Q,70-71

The appropriate 7th character is to be added to each code from category T83.

A   initial encounter

D   subsequent encounter

S   sequela

√5ᵗʰ **T83.0** Mechanical complication of urinary catheter

EXCLUDES 2   *complications of stoma of urinary tract (N99.5-)*

√6ᵗʰ **T83.01** Breakdown (mechanical) of urinary catheter

¹ √7ᵗʰ **T83.010** Breakdown (mechanical) of cystostomy catheter   HCC

¹ √7ᵗʰ **T83.011** Breakdown (mechanical) of indwelling urethral catheter   HCC

¹ √7ᵗʰ **T83.012** Breakdown (mechanical) of nephrostomy catheter   HCC

¹ √7ᵗʰ **T83.018** Breakdown (mechanical) of other urinary catheter   HCC

Breakdown (mechanical) of Hopkins catheter

Breakdown (mechanical) of ileostomy catheter

Breakdown (mechanical) urostomy catheter

√6ᵗʰ **T83.02** Displacement of urinary catheter

Malposition of urinary catheter

¹ √7ᵗʰ **T83.020** Displacement of cystostomy catheter   HCC

¹ √7ᵗʰ **T83.021** Displacement of indwelling urethral catheter   HCC

¹ √7ᵗʰ **T83.022** Displacement of nephrostomy catheter   HCC

¹ √7ᵗʰ **T83.028** Displacement of other urinary catheter   HCC

Displacement of Hopkins catheter

Displacement of ileostomy catheter

Displacement of urostomy catheter

√6ᵗʰ **T83.03** Leakage of urinary catheter

¹ √7ᵗʰ **T83.030** Leakage of cystostomy catheter   HCC

¹ √7ᵗʰ **T83.031** Leakage of indwelling urethral catheter   HCC

¹ √7ᵗʰ **T83.032** Leakage of nephrostomy catheter   HCC

¹ √7ᵗʰ **T83.038** Leakage of other urinary catheter   HCC

Leakage of Hopkins catheter

Leakage of ileostomy catheter

Leakage of urostomy catheter

√6ᵗʰ **T83.09** Other mechanical complication of urinary catheter

Obstruction (mechanical) of urinary catheter

Perforation of urinary catheter

Protrusion of urinary catheter

¹ √7ᵗʰ **T83.090** Other mechanical complication of cystostomy catheter   HCC

¹ √7ᵗʰ **T83.091** Other mechanical complication of indwelling urethral catheter   HCC

¹ √7ᵗʰ **T83.092** Other mechanical complication of nephrostomy catheter   HCC

¹ √7ᵗʰ **T83.098** Other mechanical complication of other urinary catheter   HCC

Other mechanical complication of Hopkins catheter

Other mechanical complication of ileostomy catheter

Other mechanical complication of urostomy catheter

√5ᵗʰ **T83.1** Mechanical complication of other urinary devices and implants

√6ᵗʰ **T83.11** Breakdown (mechanical) of other urinary devices and implants

¹ √7ᵗʰ **T83.110** Breakdown (mechanical) of urinary electronic stimulator device   HCC

EXCLUDES 2   *breakdown (mechanical) of electrode (lead) for sacral nerve neurostimulator (T85.111)*

breakdown (mechanical) of implanted electronic sacral neurostimulator, pulse generator or receiver (T85.113)

¹ √7ᵗʰ **T83.111** Breakdown (mechanical) of implanted urinary sphincter   HCC

¹ √7ᵗʰ **T83.112** Breakdown (mechanical) of indwelling ureteral stent   HCC

¹ √7ᵗʰ **T83.113** Breakdown (mechanical) of other urinary stents   HCC

Breakdown (mechanical) of ileal conduit stent

Breakdown (mechanical) of nephroureteral stent

¹ √7ᵗʰ **T83.118** Breakdown (mechanical) of other urinary devices and implants   HCC

√6ᵗʰ **T83.12** Displacement of other urinary devices and implants

Malposition of other urinary devices and implants

¹ √7ᵗʰ **T83.120** Displacement of urinary electronic stimulator device   HCC

EXCLUDES 2   *displacement of electrode (lead) for sacral nerve neurostimulator (T85.121)*

displacement of implanted electronic sacral neurostimulator, pulse generator or receiver (T85.123)

¹ √7ᵗʰ **T83.121** Displacement of implanted urinary sphincter   HCC

¹ √7ᵗʰ **T83.122** Displacement of indwelling ureteral stent   HCC

¹ √7ᵗʰ **T83.123** Displacement of other urinary stents   HCC

Displacement of ileal conduit stent

Displacement of nephroureteral stent

¹ √7ᵗʰ **T83.128** Displacement of other urinary devices and implants   HCC

√6ᵗʰ T83.19 **Other mechanical complication of other urinary devices and implants**
     Leakage of other urinary devices and implants
     Obstruction (mechanical) of other urinary devices and implants
     Perforation of other urinary devices and implants
     Protrusion of other urinary devices and implants

   ¹ **√7ᵗʰ T83.190** **Other mechanical complication of urinary electronic stimulator device**   HCC
      EXCLUDES 2   *other mechanical complication of electrode (lead) for sacral nerve neurostimulator (T85.191)*
          other mechanical complication of implanted electronic sacral neurostimulator, pulse generator or receiver (T85.193)

   ¹ **√7ᵗʰ T83.191** **Other mechanical complication of implanted urinary sphincter**   HCC

   ¹ **√7ᵗʰ T83.192** **Other mechanical complication of indwelling ureteral stent**   HCC

   ¹ **√7ᵗʰ T83.193** **Other mechanical complication of other urinary stent**   HCC
      Other mechanical complication of ileal conduit stent
      Other mechanical complication of nephroureteral stent

   ¹ **√7ᵗʰ T83.198** **Other mechanical complication of other urinary devices and implants**   HCC

√5ᵗʰ T83.2 **Mechanical complication of graft of urinary organ**

   ¹ **√x7ᵗʰ T83.21** **Breakdown (mechanical) of graft of urinary organ**   HCC

   ¹ **√x7ᵗʰ T83.22** **Displacement of graft of urinary organ**   HCC
      Malposition of graft of urinary organ

   ¹ **√x7ᵗʰ T83.23** **Leakage of graft of urinary organ**   HCC

   ¹ **√x7ᵗʰ T83.24** **Erosion of graft of urinary organ**   HCC

   ¹ **√x7ᵗʰ T83.25** **Exposure of graft of urinary organ**   HCC

   ¹ **√x7ᵗʰ T83.29** **Other mechanical complication of graft of urinary organ**   HCC
      Obstruction (mechanical) of graft of urinary organ
      Perforation of graft of urinary organ
      Protrusion of graft of urinary organ

√5ᵗʰ T83.3 **Mechanical complication of intrauterine contraceptive device**

   √x7ᵗʰ T83.31 **Breakdown (mechanical) of intrauterine contraceptive device**   ♀

   √x7ᵗʰ T83.32 **Displacement of intrauterine contraceptive device**   ♀
      Malposition of intrauterine contraceptive device
      Missing string of intrauterine contraceptive device
      AHA: 2018,1Q,5

   √x7ᵗʰ T83.39 **Other mechanical complication of intrauterine contraceptive device**   ♀
      Leakage of intrauterine contraceptive device
      Obstruction (mechanical) of intrauterine contraceptive device
      Perforation of intrauterine contraceptive device
      Protrusion of intrauterine contraceptive device

√5ᵗʰ T83.4 **Mechanical complication of other prosthetic devices, implants and grafts of genital tract**

   √6ᵗʰ T83.41 **Breakdown (mechanical) of other prosthetic devices, implants and grafts of genital tract**

   ¹ **√7ᵗʰ T83.410** **Breakdown (mechanical) of implanted penile prosthesis**   HCC ♂
      Breakdown (mechanical) of penile prosthesis cylinder
      Breakdown (mechanical) of penile prosthesis pump
      Breakdown (mechanical) of penile prosthesis reservoir

   ¹ **√7ᵗʰ T83.411** **Breakdown (mechanical) of implanted testicular prosthesis**   HCC

   ¹ **√7ᵗʰ T83.418** **Breakdown (mechanical) of other prosthetic devices, implants and grafts of genital tract**   HCC

√6ᵗʰ T83.42 **Displacement of other prosthetic devices, implants and grafts of genital tract**
     Malposition of other prosthetic devices, implants and grafts of genital tract

   ¹ **√7ᵗʰ T83.420** **Displacement of implanted penile prosthesis**   HCC ♂
      Displacement of penile prosthesis cylinder
      Displacement of penile prosthesis pump
      Displacement of penile prosthesis reservoir

   ¹ **√7ᵗʰ T83.421** **Displacement of implanted testicular prosthesis**   HCC

   ¹ **√7ᵗʰ T83.428** **Displacement of other prosthetic devices, implants and grafts of genital tract**   HCC
      AHA: 2018,1Q,5

√6ᵗʰ T83.49 **Other mechanical complication of other prosthetic devices, implants and grafts of genital tract**
     Leakage of other prosthetic devices, implants and grafts of genital tract
     Obstruction, mechanical of other prosthetic devices, implants and grafts of genital tract
     Perforation of other prosthetic devices, implants and grafts of genital tract
     Protrusion of other prosthetic devices, implants and grafts of genital tract

   ¹ **√7ᵗʰ T83.490** **Other mechanical complication of implanted penile prosthesis**   HCC ♂
      Other mechanical complication of penile prosthesis cylinder
      Other mechanical complication of penile prosthesis pump
      Other mechanical complication of penile prosthesis reservoir

   ¹ **√7ᵗʰ T83.491** **Other mechanical complication of implanted testicular prosthesis**   HCC

   ¹ **√7ᵗʰ T83.498** **Other mechanical complication of other prosthetic devices, implants and grafts of genital tract**   HCC

√5ᵗʰ T83.5 **Infection and inflammatory reaction due to prosthetic device, implant and graft in urinary system**
     Use additional code to identify infection

   √6ᵗʰ T83.51 **Infection and inflammatory reaction due to urinary catheter**
      EXCLUDES 2   *complications of stoma of urinary tract (N99.5-)*

   ¹ **√7ᵗʰ T83.510** **Infection and inflammatory reaction due to cystostomy catheter**   HCC

   ¹ **√7ᵗʰ T83.511** **Infection and inflammatory reaction due to indwelling urethral catheter**   HCC

   ¹ **√7ᵗʰ T83.512** **Infection and inflammatory reaction due to nephrostomy catheter**   HCC

   ¹ **√7ᵗʰ T83.518** **Infection and inflammatory reaction due to other urinary catheter**   HCC
      Infection and inflammatory reaction due to Hopkins catheter
      Infection and inflammatory reaction due to ileostomy catheter
      Infection and inflammatory reaction due to urostomy catheter

   √6ᵗʰ T83.59 **Infection and inflammatory reaction due to prosthetic device, implant and graft in urinary system**

   ¹ **√7ᵗʰ T83.590** **Infection and inflammatory reaction due to implanted urinary neurostimulation device**   HCC
      EXCLUDES 2   *infection and inflammatory reaction due to electrode lead of sacral nerve neurostimulator (T85.732)*
          infection and inflammatory reaction due to pulse generator or receiver of sacral nerve neurostimulator (T85.734)

☑ Additional Character Required   √x7ᵗʰ Placeholder Alert   Manifestation   Unspecified Dx   ▶◀ Revised Text   ● New Code   ▲ Revised Code Title

Chapter 19. Injury, Poisoning and Certain Other Consequences of External Causes

T83.591–T84.033

1 √7ᵗʰ **T83.591 Infection and inflammatory reaction due to** implanted urinary sphincter   HCC

1 √7ᵗʰ **T83.592 Infection and inflammatory reaction due to** indwelling ureteral stent   HCC

1 √7ᵗʰ **T83.593 Infection and inflammatory reaction due to other urinary stents**   HCC

     Infection and inflammatory reaction due to ileal conduit stents

     Infection and inflammatory reaction due to nephroureteral stent

1 √7ᵗʰ **T83.598 Infection and inflammatory reaction due to other prosthetic device, implant and graft in urinary system**   HCC

√5ᵗʰ **T83.6 Infection and inflammatory reaction due to prosthetic device, implant and graft in** genital tract

     Use additional code to identify infection

1 √x7ᵗʰ **T83.61 Infection and inflammatory reaction due to** implanted penile prosthesis   HCC

     Infection and inflammatory reaction due to penile prosthesis cylinder

     Infection and inflammatory reaction due to penile prosthesis pump

     Infection and inflammatory reaction due to penile prosthesis reservoir

1 √x7ᵗʰ **T83.62 Infection and inflammatory reaction due to** implanted testicular prosthesis   HCC

1 √x7ᵗʰ **T83.69 Infection and inflammatory reaction due to other prosthetic device, implant and graft in genital tract**   HCC

√5ᵗʰ **T83.7 Complications due to** implanted mesh and other prosthetic materials

√6ᵗʰ **T83.71 Erosion of implanted mesh and other prosthetic materials**

1 √7ᵗʰ **T83.711 Erosion of implanted** vaginal mesh to surrounding organ or tissue   HCC ♀

     Erosion of implanted vaginal mesh into pelvic floor muscles

1 √7ᵗʰ **T83.712 Erosion of implanted** urethral mesh to surrounding organ or tissue   HCC

     Erosion of implanted female urethral sling

     Erosion of implanted male urethral sling

     Erosion of implanted urethral mesh into pelvic floor muscles

1 √7ᵗʰ **T83.713 Erosion of implanted** urethral bulking agent to surrounding organ or tissue   HCC

1 √7ᵗʰ **T83.714 Erosion of implanted** ureteral bulking agent to surrounding organ or tissue   HCC

1 √7ᵗʰ **T83.718 Erosion of other implanted mesh to organ or tissue**   HCC

1 √7ᵗʰ **T83.719 Erosion of other prosthetic materials to surrounding organ or tissue**   HCC

√6ᵗʰ **T83.72 Exposure of implanted mesh and other prosthetic materials into surrounding organ or tissue**

     Extrusion of implanted mesh

1 √7ᵗʰ **T83.721 Exposure of implanted** vaginal mesh into vagina   HCC ♀

     Exposure of implanted vaginal mesh through vaginal wall

1 √7ᵗʰ **T83.722 Exposure of implanted** urethral mesh **into** urethra   HCC

     Exposure of implanted female urethral sling

     Exposure of implanted male urethral sling

     Exposure of implanted urethral mesh through urethral wall

1 √7ᵗʰ **T83.723 Exposure of implanted** urethral bulking agent **into** urethra   HCC

1 √7ᵗʰ **T83.724 Exposure of implanted** ureteral bulking agent **into** ureter   HCC

1 √7ᵗʰ **T83.728 Exposure of** other implanted mesh **into organ or tissue**   HCC

1 √7ᵗʰ **T83.729 Exposure of** other prosthetic materials **into organ or tissue**   HCC

1 √x7ᵗʰ **T83.79 Other specified complications due to other genitourinary prosthetic materials**   HCC

√5ᵗʰ **T83.8 Other specified complications of** genitourinary prosthetic devices, implants and grafts

1 √x7ᵗʰ **T83.81 Embolism due to** genitourinary prosthetic devices, implants and grafts   HCC

1 √x7ᵗʰ **T83.82 Fibrosis due to** genitourinary prosthetic devices, implants and grafts

1 √x7ᵗʰ **T83.83 Hemorrhage due to** genitourinary prosthetic devices, implants and grafts   HCC

1 √x7ᵗʰ **T83.84 Pain due to** genitourinary prosthetic devices, implants and grafts   HCC

1 √x7ᵗʰ **T83.85 Stenosis due to** genitourinary prosthetic devices, implants and grafts   HCC

1 √x7ᵗʰ **T83.86 Thrombosis due to** genitourinary prosthetic devices, implants and grafts   HCC

1 √x7ᵗʰ **T83.89 Other specified complication of** genitourinary prosthetic devices, implants and grafts   HCC

1 √x7ᵗʰ **T83.9 Unspecified complication of genitourinary prosthetic device, implant and graft**   HCC

√4ᵗʰ **T84 Complications of internal orthopedic prosthetic devices, implants and grafts**

     EXCLUDES 2   *failure and rejection of transplanted organs and tissues (T86.-)*

         fracture of bone following insertion of orthopedic implant, joint prosthesis or bone plate (M96.6)

The appropriate 7th character is to be added to each code from category T84.

A   initial encounter

D   subsequent encounter

S   sequela

√5ᵗʰ **T84.0 Mechanical complication of** internal joint prosthesis

√6ᵗʰ **T84.01 Broken internal joint prosthesis**

     Breakage (fracture) of prosthetic joint

     Broken prosthetic joint implant

     EXCLUDES 1   *periprosthetic joint implant fracture (M97-)*

     AHA: 2016,4Q,42

1 √7ᵗʰ **T84.010 Broken internal right hip prosthesis**   HCC

1 √7ᵗʰ **T84.011 Broken internal left hip prosthesis**   HCC

1 √7ᵗʰ **T84.012 Broken internal right knee prosthesis**   HCC

1 √7ᵗʰ **T84.013 Broken internal left knee prosthesis**   HCC

1 √7ᵗʰ **T84.018 Broken internal joint prosthesis, other site**   HCC

     Use additional code to identify the joint (Z96.6-)

1 √7ᵗʰ **T84.019 Broken internal joint prosthesis, unspecified site**   HCC

√6ᵗʰ **T84.02 Dislocation of internal joint prosthesis**

     Instability of internal joint prosthesis

     Subluxation of internal joint prosthesis

     AHA: 2019,2Q,27

1 √7ᵗʰ **T84.020 Dislocation of internal** right hip prosthesis   HCC

1 √7ᵗʰ **T84.021 Dislocation of internal** left hip prosthesis   HCC

1 √7ᵗʰ **T84.022 Instability of internal** right knee prosthesis   HCC

1 √7ᵗʰ **T84.023 Instability of internal** left knee prosthesis   HCC

1 √7ᵗʰ **T84.028 Dislocation of other internal joint prosthesis**   HCC

     Use additional code to identify the joint (Z96.6-)

1 √7ᵗʰ **T84.029 Dislocation of unspecified internal joint prosthesis**   HCC

√6ᵗʰ **T84.03 Mechanical loosening of internal prosthetic joint**

     Aseptic loosening of prosthetic joint

1 √7ᵗʰ **T84.030 Mechanical loosening of internal** right hip **prosthetic joint**   HCC

1 √7ᵗʰ **T84.031 Mechanical loosening of internal** left hip **prosthetic joint**   HCC

1 √7ᵗʰ **T84.032 Mechanical loosening of internal** right knee **prosthetic joint**   HCC

1 √7ᵗʰ **T84.033 Mechanical loosening of internal** left knee **prosthetic joint**   HCC

¹ √7ᵗʰ **T84.038** **Mechanical loosening of other internal prosthetic joint** `HCC`
Use additional code to identify the joint (Z96.6-)

¹ √7ᵗʰ **T84.039** **Mechanical loosening of unspecified internal prosthetic joint** `HCC`

√6ᵗʰ **T84.05** **Periprosthetic osteolysis of internal prosthetic joint**
Use additional code to identify major osseous defect, if applicable (M89.7-)

¹ √7ᵗʰ **T84.050** **Periprosthetic osteolysis of internal prosthetic right hip joint** `HCC`

¹ √7ᵗʰ **T84.051** **Periprosthetic osteolysis of internal prosthetic left hip joint** `HCC`

¹ √7ᵗʰ **T84.052** **Periprosthetic osteolysis of internal prosthetic right knee joint** `HCC`

¹ √7ᵗʰ **T84.053** **Periprosthetic osteolysis of internal prosthetic left knee joint** `HCC`

¹ √7ᵗʰ **T84.058** **Periprosthetic osteolysis of other internal prosthetic joint** `HCC`
Use additional code to identify the joint (Z96.6-)

¹ √7ᵗʰ **T84.059** **Periprosthetic osteolysis of unspecified internal prosthetic joint** `HCC`

√6ᵗʰ **T84.06** **Wear of articular bearing surface of internal prosthetic joint**

¹ √7ᵗʰ **T84.060** **Wear of articular bearing surface of internal prosthetic right hip joint** `HCC`

¹ √7ᵗʰ **T84.061** **Wear of articular bearing surface of internal prosthetic left hip joint** `HCC`

¹ √7ᵗʰ **T84.062** **Wear of articular bearing surface of internal prosthetic right knee joint** `HCC`

¹ √7ᵗʰ **T84.063** **Wear of articular bearing surface of internal prosthetic left knee joint** `HCC`

¹ √7ᵗʰ **T84.068** **Wear of articular bearing surface of other internal prosthetic joint** `HCC`
Use additional code to identify the joint (Z96.6-)

¹ √7ᵗʰ **T84.069** **Wear of articular bearing surface of unspecified internal prosthetic joint** `HCC`

√6ᵗʰ **T84.09** **Other mechanical complication of internal joint prosthesis**
Prosthetic joint implant failure NOS
AHA: 2019,1Q,20

¹ √7ᵗʰ **T84.090** **Other mechanical complication of internal right hip prosthesis** `HCC`

¹ √7ᵗʰ **T84.091** **Other mechanical complication of internal left hip prosthesis** `HCC`

¹ √7ᵗʰ **T84.092** **Other mechanical complication of internal right knee prosthesis** `HCC`

¹ √7ᵗʰ **T84.093** **Other mechanical complication of internal left knee prosthesis** `HCC`

¹ √7ᵗʰ **T84.098** **Other mechanical complication of other internal joint prosthesis** `HCC`
Use additional code to identify the joint (Z96.6-)

¹ √7ᵗʰ **T84.099** **Other mechanical complication of unspecified internal joint prosthesis** `HCC`

√5ᵗʰ **T84.1** **Mechanical complication of internal fixation device of bones of limb**
EXCLUDES 2   mechanical complication of internal fixation device of bones of feet (T84.2-)
mechanical complication of internal fixation device of bones of fingers (T84.2-)
mechanical complication of internal fixation device of bones of hands (T84.2-)
mechanical complication of internal fixation device of bones of toes (T84.2-)

√6ᵗʰ **T84.11** **Breakdown (mechanical) of internal fixation device of bones of limb**

¹ √7ᵗʰ **T84.110** **Breakdown (mechanical) of internal fixation device of right humerus** `HCC`

¹ √7ᵗʰ **T84.111** **Breakdown (mechanical) of internal fixation device of left humerus** `HCC`

¹ √7ᵗʰ **T84.112** **Breakdown (mechanical) of internal fixation device of bone of right forearm** `HCC`

¹ √7ᵗʰ **T84.113** **Breakdown (mechanical) of internal fixation device of bone of left forearm** `HCC`

¹ √7ᵗʰ **T84.114** **Breakdown (mechanical) of internal fixation device of right femur** `HCC`

¹ √7ᵗʰ **T84.115** **Breakdown (mechanical) of internal fixation device of left femur** `HCC`

¹ √7ᵗʰ **T84.116** **Breakdown (mechanical) of internal fixation device of bone of right lower leg** `HCC`

¹ √7ᵗʰ **T84.117** **Breakdown (mechanical) of internal fixation device of bone of left lower leg** `HCC`

¹ √7ᵗʰ **T84.119** **Breakdown (mechanical) of internal fixation device of unspecified bone of limb** `HCC`

√6ᵗʰ **T84.12** **Displacement of internal fixation device of bones of limb**
Malposition of internal fixation device of bones of limb

¹ √7ᵗʰ **T84.120** **Displacement of internal fixation device of right humerus** `HCC`

¹ √7ᵗʰ **T84.121** **Displacement of internal fixation device of left humerus** `HCC`

¹ √7ᵗʰ **T84.122** **Displacement of internal fixation device of bone of right forearm** `HCC`

¹ √7ᵗʰ **T84.123** **Displacement of internal fixation device of bone of left forearm** `HCC`

¹ √7ᵗʰ **T84.124** **Displacement of internal fixation device of right femur** `HCC`

¹ √7ᵗʰ **T84.125** **Displacement of internal fixation device of left femur** `HCC`

¹ √7ᵗʰ **T84.126** **Displacement of internal fixation device of bone of right lower leg** `HCC`

¹ √7ᵗʰ **T84.127** **Displacement of internal fixation device of bone of left lower leg** `HCC`

¹ √7ᵗʰ **T84.129** **Displacement of internal fixation device of unspecified bone of limb** `HCC`

√6ᵗʰ **T84.19** **Other mechanical complication of internal fixation device of bones of limb**
Obstruction (mechanical) of internal fixation device of bones of limb
Perforation of internal fixation device of bones of limb
Protrusion of internal fixation device of bones of limb

¹ √7ᵗʰ **T84.190** **Other mechanical complication of internal fixation device of right humerus** `HCC`

¹ √7ᵗʰ **T84.191** **Other mechanical complication of internal fixation device of left humerus** `HCC`

¹ √7ᵗʰ **T84.192** **Other mechanical complication of internal fixation device of bone of right forearm** `HCC`

¹ √7ᵗʰ **T84.193** **Other mechanical complication of internal fixation device of bone of left forearm** `HCC`

¹ √7ᵗʰ **T84.194** **Other mechanical complication of internal fixation device of right femur** `HCC`

¹ √7ᵗʰ **T84.195** **Other mechanical complication of internal fixation device of left femur** `HCC`

¹ √7ᵗʰ **T84.196** **Other mechanical complication of internal fixation device of bone of right lower leg** `HCC`

¹ √7ᵗʰ **T84.197** **Other mechanical complication of internal fixation device of bone of left lower leg** `HCC`

¹ √7ᵗʰ **T84.199** **Other mechanical complication of internal fixation device of unspecified bone of limb** `HCC`

☑ Additional Character Required   √x7ᵗʰ Placeholder Alert   Manifestation   Unspecified Dx   ►◄ Revised Text   ● New Code   ▲ Revised Code Title

ICD-10-CM 2020   1143

√5th **T84.2** **Mechanical complication of** internal fixation device **of** other bones

  √6th **T84.21** Breakdown (mechanical) of internal fixation device of other bones

    1 √7th **T84.210** **Breakdown (mechanical) of internal fixation device of bones of** hand and fingers   HCC

    1 √7th **T84.213** **Breakdown (mechanical) of internal fixation device of bones of** foot and toes   HCC

    1 √7th **T84.216** **Breakdown (mechanical) of internal fixation device of** vertebrae   HCC

    1 √7th **T84.218** **Breakdown (mechanical) of internal fixation device of other bones**   HCC

  √6th **T84.22** Displacement of internal fixation device of other bones

    Malposition of internal fixation device of other bones

    1 √7th **T84.220** **Displacement of internal fixation device of bones of** hand and fingers   HCC

    1 √7th **T84.223** **Displacement of internal fixation device of bones of** foot and toes   HCC

    1 √7th **T84.226** **Displacement of internal fixation device of** vertebrae   HCC

    1 √7th **T84.228** **Displacement of internal fixation device of other bones**   HCC

  √6th **T84.29** Other mechanical complication of internal fixation device of other bones

    Obstruction (mechanical) of internal fixation device of other bones

    Perforation of internal fixation device of other bones

    Protrusion of internal fixation device of other bones

    1 √7th **T84.290** **Other mechanical complication of internal fixation device of bones of** hand and fingers   HCC

    1 √7th **T84.293** **Other mechanical complication of internal fixation device of bones of** foot and toes   HCC

    1 √7th **T84.296** **Other mechanical complication of internal fixation device of** vertebrae   HCC

    1 √7th **T84.298** **Other mechanical complication of internal fixation device of other bones**   HCC

√5th **T84.3** **Mechanical complication of other bone devices, implants and grafts**

  EXCLUDES 2   *other complications of bone graft (T86.83-)*

  √6th **T84.31** Breakdown (mechanical) of other bone devices, implants and grafts

    1 √7th **T84.310** **Breakdown (mechanical) of** electronic bone stimulator   HCC

    1 √7th **T84.318** **Breakdown (mechanical) of other bone devices, implants and grafts**   HCC

  √6th **T84.32** Displacement of other bone devices, implants and grafts

    Malposition of other bone devices, implants and grafts

    1 √7th **T84.320** **Displacement of** electronic bone stimulator   HCC

    1 √7th **T84.328** **Displacement of other bone devices, implants and grafts**   HCC

      AHA: 2014,4Q,28

  √6th **T84.39** Other mechanical complication of other bone devices, implants and grafts

    Obstruction (mechanical) of other bone devices, implants and grafts

    Perforation of other bone devices, implants and grafts

    Protrusion of other bone devices, implants and grafts

    1 √7th **T84.390** **Other mechanical complication of** electronic bone stimulator   HCC

    1 √7th **T84.398** **Other mechanical complication of other bone devices, implants and grafts**   HCC

√5th **T84.4** **Mechanical complication of other internal orthopedic devices, implants and grafts**

  √6th **T84.41** Breakdown (mechanical) of other internal orthopedic devices, implants and grafts

    1 √7th **T84.410** **Breakdown (mechanical) of** muscle and tendon graft   HCC

---

    1 √7th **T84.418** **Breakdown (mechanical) of other internal orthopedic devices, implants and grafts**   HCC

  √6th **T84.42** Displacement of other internal orthopedic devices, implants and grafts

    Malposition of other internal orthopedic devices, implants and grafts

    1 √7th **T84.420** **Displacement of** muscle and tendon graft   HCC

    1 √7th **T84.428** **Displacement of other internal orthopedic devices, implants and grafts**   HCC

  √6th **T84.49** Other mechanical complication of other internal orthopedic devices, implants and grafts

    Mechanical complication of other internal orthopedic devices, implants and grafts NOS

    Obstruction (mechanical) of other internal orthopedic devices, implants and grafts

    Perforation of other internal orthopedic devices, implants and grafts

    Protrusion of other internal orthopedic devices, implants and grafts

    1 √7th **T84.490** **Other mechanical complication of** muscle and tendon graft   HCC

    1 √7th **T84.498** **Other mechanical complication of other internal orthopedic devices, implants and grafts**   HCC

√5th **T84.5** **Infection and inflammatory reaction due to** internal joint prosthesis

  Use additional code to identify infection

  AHA: 2015,1Q,16

  1 √x7th **T84.50** **Infection and inflammatory reaction due to unspecified internal joint prosthesis**   HCC

  1 √x7th **T84.51** **Infection and inflammatory reaction due to internal** right hip **prosthesis**   HCC

  1 √x7th **T84.52** **Infection and inflammatory reaction due to internal** left hip **prosthesis**   HCC

  1 √x7th **T84.53** **Infection and inflammatory reaction due to internal** right knee **prosthesis**   HCC

  1 √x7th **T84.54** **Infection and inflammatory reaction due to internal** left knee **prosthesis**   HCC

  1 √x7th **T84.59** **Infection and inflammatory reaction due to other internal joint prosthesis**   HCC

√5th **T84.6** **Infection and inflammatory reaction due to** internal fixation device

  Use additional code to identify infection

  1 √x7th **T84.60** **Infection and inflammatory reaction due to internal fixation device of unspecified site**   HCC

  √6th **T84.61** Infection and inflammatory reaction due to internal fixation device of arm

    1 √7th **T84.610** **Infection and inflammatory reaction due to internal fixation device of** right humerus   HCC

    1 √7th **T84.611** **Infection and inflammatory reaction due to internal fixation device of** left humerus   HCC

    1 √7th **T84.612** **Infection and inflammatory reaction due to internal fixation device of** right radius   HCC

    1 √7th **T84.613** **Infection and inflammatory reaction due to internal fixation device of** left radius   HCC

    1 √7th **T84.614** **Infection and inflammatory reaction due to internal fixation device of** right ulna   HCC

    1 √7th **T84.615** **Infection and inflammatory reaction due to internal fixation device of** left ulna   HCC

    1 √7th **T84.619** **Infection and inflammatory reaction due to internal fixation device of unspecified bone of arm**   HCC

  √6th **T84.62** Infection and inflammatory reaction due to internal fixation device of leg

    1 √7th **T84.620** **Infection and inflammatory reaction due to internal fixation device of** right femur   HCC

    1 √7th **T84.621** **Infection and inflammatory reaction due to internal fixation device of** left femur   HCC

    1 √7th **T84.622** **Infection and inflammatory reaction due to internal fixation device of** right tibia   HCC

¹ √7ᵗʰ **T84.623 Infection and inflammatory** HCC
reaction due to internal fixation
device of left tibia

¹ √7ᵗʰ **T84.624 Infection and inflammatory** HCC
reaction due to internal fixation
device of right fibula

¹ √7ᵗʰ **T84.625 Infection and inflammatory** HCC
reaction due to internal fixation
device of left fibula

¹ √7ᵗʰ **T84.629 Infection and inflammatory** HCC
reaction due to internal fixation
device of unspecified bone of leg

¹ √x7ᵗʰ **T84.63 Infection and inflammatory reaction due to** HCC
internal fixation device of spine

¹ √x7ᵗʰ **T84.69 Infection and inflammatory reaction due to** HCC
internal fixation device of other site

¹ √x7ᵗʰ **T84.7 Infection and inflammatory reaction due to other** HCC
internal orthopedic prosthetic devices, implants and
grafts

     Use additional code to identify infection

√5ᵗʰ **T84.8 Other specified complications of internal orthopedic**
prosthetic devices, implants and grafts

¹ √x7ᵗʰ **T84.81 Embolism due to internal orthopedic** HCC
prosthetic devices, implants and grafts

¹ √x7ᵗʰ **T84.82 Fibrosis due to internal orthopedic** HCC
prosthetic devices, implants and grafts

¹ √x7ᵗʰ **T84.83 Hemorrhage due to internal orthopedic** HCC
prosthetic devices, implants and grafts

¹ √x7ᵗʰ **T84.84 Pain due to internal orthopedic prosthetic** HCC
devices, implants and grafts

¹ √x7ᵗʰ **T84.85 Stenosis due to internal orthopedic** HCC
prosthetic devices, implants and grafts

¹ √x7ᵗʰ **T84.86 Thrombosis due to internal orthopedic** HCC
prosthetic devices, implants and grafts

¹ √x7ᵗʰ **T84.89 Other specified complication of internal** HCC
orthopedic prosthetic devices, implants and
grafts

¹ √x7ᵗʰ **T84.9 Unspecified complication of internal orthopedic** HCC
prosthetic device, implant and graft

√4ᵗʰ **T85 Complications of other internal prosthetic devices, implants and**
grafts

     EXCLUDES 2   *failure and rejection of transplanted organs and tissue (T86.-)*

     AHA: 2016,4Q,71-72

     The appropriate 7th character is to be added to each code from
     category T85.
     A   initial encounter
     D   subsequent encounter
     S   sequela

√5ᵗʰ **T85.0 Mechanical complication of** ventricular intracranial
(communicating) shunt

¹ √x7ᵗʰ **T85.01 Breakdown (mechanical) of ventricular** HCC
intracranial (communicating) shunt

¹ √x7ᵗʰ **T85.02 Displacement of ventricular intracranial** HCC
(communicating) shunt

     Malposition of ventricular intracranial
     (communicating) shunt

¹ √x7ᵗʰ **T85.03 Leakage of ventricular intracranial** HCC
(communicating) shunt

¹ √x7ᵗʰ **T85.09 Other mechanical complication of** HCC
ventricular intracranial (communicating)
shunt

     Obstruction (mechanical) of ventricular intracranial
     (communicating) shunt
     Perforation of ventricular intracranial
     (communicating) shunt
     Protrusion of ventricular intracranial (communicating)
     shunt

√5ᵗʰ **T85.1 Mechanical complication of** implanted electronic stimulator
of nervous system

√6ᵗʰ **T85.11 Breakdown (mechanical) of implanted electronic**
stimulator of nervous system

¹ √7ᵗʰ **T85.110 Breakdown (mechanical) of** HCC
implanted electronic
neurostimulator of brain
electrode (lead)

¹ √7ᵗʰ **T85.111 Breakdown (mechanical) of** HCC
implanted electronic
neurostimulator of peripheral
nerve electrode (lead)

     Breakdown of electrode (lead) for cranial
     nerve neurostimulators
     Breakdown of electrode (lead) for gastric
     neurostimulator
     Breakdown of electrode (lead) for sacral
     nerve neurostimulator
     Breakdown of electrode (lead) for vagal
     nerve neurostimulators

¹ √7ᵗʰ **T85.112 Breakdown (mechanical) of** HCC
implanted electronic
neurostimulator of spinal cord
electrode (lead)

¹ √7ᵗʰ **T85.113 Breakdown (mechanical) of** HCC
implanted electronic
neurostimulator, generator

     Breakdown (mechanical) of implanted
     electronic neurostimulator generator,
     brain, peripheral, gastric, spinal
     Breakdown (mechanical) of implanted
     electronic sacral neurostimulator,
     pulse generator or receiver

¹ √7ᵗʰ **T85.118 Breakdown (mechanical) of other** HCC
implanted electronic stimulator
of nervous system

√6ᵗʰ **T85.12 Displacement of implanted electronic stimulator**
of nervous system

     Malposition of implanted electronic stimulator of
     nervous system

¹ √7ᵗʰ **T85.120 Displacement of implanted** HCC
electronic neurostimulator of
brain electrode (lead)

¹ √7ᵗʰ **T85.121 Displacement of implanted** HCC
electronic neurostimulator of
peripheral nerve electrode (lead)

     Displacement of electrode (lead) for cranial
     nerve neurostimulators
     Displacement of electrode (lead) for gastric
     neurostimulator
     Displacement of electrode (lead) for sacral
     nerve neurostimulator
     Displacement of electrode (lead) for vagal
     nerve neurostimulators

¹ √7ᵗʰ **T85.122 Displacement of implanted** HCC
electronic neurostimulator of
spinal cord electrode (lead)

¹ √7ᵗʰ **T85.123 Displacement of implanted** HCC
electronic neurostimulator,
generator

     Displacement of implanted electronic
     neurostimulator generator, brain,
     peripheral, gastric, spinal
     Displacement of implanted electronic
     sacral neurostimulator, pulse
     generator or receiver

¹ √7ᵗʰ **T85.128 Displacement of other implanted** HCC
electronic stimulator of nervous
system

√6ᵗʰ **T85.19 Other mechanical complication of implanted**
electronic stimulator of nervous system

     Leakage of implanted electronic stimulator of nervous
     system
     Obstruction (mechanical) of implanted electronic
     stimulator of nervous system
     Perforation of implanted electronic stimulator of
     nervous system
     Protrusion of implanted electronic stimulator of
     nervous system

¹ √7ᵗʰ **T85.190 Other mechanical complication** HCC
of implanted electronic
neurostimulator of brain
electrode (lead)

☑ Additional Character Required   √x7ᵗʰ Placeholder Alert   Manifestation   Unspecified Dx   ►◄ Revised Text   ● New Code   ▲ Revised Code Title

ICD-10-CM 2020   1145

¹ ✓7ᵗʰ **T85.191 Other mechanical complication of implanted electronic neurostimulator** of peripheral nerve electrode (lead)   HCC

Other mechanical complication of electrode (lead) for cranial nerve neurostimulators

Other mechanical complication of electrode (lead) for gastric neurostimulator

Other mechanical complication of electrode (lead) for sacral nerve neurostimulator

Other mechanical complication of electrode (lead) for vagal nerve neurostimulators

¹ ✓7ᵗʰ **T85.192 Other mechanical complication of implanted electronic neurostimulator** of spinal cord electrode (lead)   HCC

¹ ✓7ᵗʰ **T85.193 Other mechanical complication of implanted electronic neurostimulator, generator**   HCC

Other mechanical complication of implanted electronic neurostimulator generator, brain, peripheral, gastric, spinal

Other mechanical complication of implanted electronic sacral neurostimulator, pulse generator or receiver

¹ ✓7ᵗʰ **T85.199 Other mechanical complication of other implanted electronic stimulator of nervous system**   HCC

✓5ᵗʰ **T85.2 Mechanical complication of** intraocular lens

✓x7ᵗʰ **T85.21 Breakdown (mechanical) of intraocular lens**

✓x7ᵗʰ **T85.22 Displacement of intraocular lens**

Malposition of intraocular lens

✓x7ᵗʰ **T85.29 Other mechanical complication of intraocular lens**

Obstruction (mechanical) of intraocular lens

Perforation of intraocular lens

Protrusion of intraocular lens

✓5ᵗʰ **T85.3 Mechanical complication of other ocular prosthetic devices, implants and grafts**

> EXCLUDES 2   other complications of corneal graft (T86.84-)

✓6ᵗʰ **T85.31 Breakdown (mechanical) of other ocular prosthetic devices, implants and grafts**

✓7ᵗʰ **T85.310 Breakdown (mechanical) of prosthetic orbit of** right eye

✓7ᵗʰ **T85.311 Breakdown (mechanical) of prosthetic orbit of** left eye

✓7ᵗʰ **T85.318 Breakdown (mechanical) of other ocular prosthetic devices, implants and grafts**

✓6ᵗʰ **T85.32 Displacement of other ocular prosthetic devices, implants and grafts**

Malposition of other ocular prosthetic devices, implants and grafts

✓7ᵗʰ **T85.320 Displacement of prosthetic orbit of** right eye

✓7ᵗʰ **T85.321 Displacement of prosthetic orbit of** left eye

✓7ᵗʰ **T85.328 Displacement of other ocular prosthetic devices, implants and grafts**

✓6ᵗʰ **T85.39 Other mechanical complication of other ocular prosthetic devices, implants and grafts**

Obstruction (mechanical) of other ocular prosthetic devices, implants and grafts

Perforation of other ocular prosthetic devices, implants and grafts

Protrusion of other ocular prosthetic devices, implants and grafts

✓7ᵗʰ **T85.390 Other mechanical complication of prosthetic orbit of** right eye

✓7ᵗʰ **T85.391 Other mechanical complication of prosthetic orbit of** left eye

✓7ᵗʰ **T85.398 Other mechanical complication of other ocular prosthetic devices, implants and grafts**

✓5ᵗʰ **T85.4 Mechanical complication of** breast prosthesis and implant

✓x7ᵗʰ **T85.41 Breakdown (mechanical) of breast prosthesis and implant**

✓x7ᵗʰ **T85.42 Displacement of breast prosthesis and implant**

Malposition of breast prosthesis and implant

✓x7ᵗʰ **T85.43 Leakage of breast prosthesis and implant**

✓x7ᵗʰ **T85.44 Capsular contracture of breast implant**

✓x7ᵗʰ **T85.49 Other mechanical complication of breast prosthesis and implant**

Obstruction (mechanical) of breast prosthesis and implant

Perforation of breast prosthesis and implant

Protrusion of breast prosthesis and implant

✓5ᵗʰ **T85.5 Mechanical complication of** gastrointestinal prosthetic devices, implants and grafts

✓6ᵗʰ **T85.51 Breakdown (mechanical) of gastrointestinal prosthetic devices, implants and grafts**

✓7ᵗʰ **T85.510 Breakdown (mechanical) of** bile duct prosthesis

✓7ᵗʰ **T85.511 Breakdown (mechanical) of** esophageal anti-reflux device

✓7ᵗʰ **T85.518 Breakdown (mechanical) of other gastrointestinal prosthetic devices, implants and grafts**

✓6ᵗʰ **T85.52 Displacement of gastrointestinal prosthetic devices, implants and grafts**

Malposition of gastrointestinal prosthetic devices, implants and grafts

✓7ᵗʰ **T85.520 Displacement of** bile duct prosthesis

✓7ᵗʰ **T85.521 Displacement of** esophageal anti-reflux device

✓7ᵗʰ **T85.528 Displacement of other gastrointestinal prosthetic devices, implants and grafts**

✓6ᵗʰ **T85.59 Other mechanical complication of gastrointestinal prosthetic devices, implants and**

Obstruction, mechanical of gastrointestinal prosthetic devices, implants and grafts

Perforation of gastrointestinal prosthetic devices, implants and grafts

Protrusion of gastrointestinal prosthetic devices, implants and grafts

✓7ᵗʰ **T85.590 Other mechanical complication of** bile duct prosthesis

✓7ᵗʰ **T85.591 Other mechanical complication of** esophageal anti-reflux device

✓7ᵗʰ **T85.598 Other mechanical complication of other gastrointestinal prosthetic devices, implants and grafts**

✓5ᵗʰ **T85.6 Mechanical complication of other specified internal and external prosthetic devices, implants and grafts**

✓6ᵗʰ **T85.61 Breakdown (mechanical) of other specified internal prosthetic devices, implants and grafts**

✓7ᵗʰ **T85.610 Breakdown (mechanical) of** cranial or spinal infusion catheter

Breakdown (mechanical) of epidural infusion catheter

Breakdown (mechanical) of intrathecal infusion catheter

Breakdown (mechanical) of subarachnoid infusion catheter

Breakdown (mechanical) of subdural infusion catheter

✓7ᵗʰ **T85.611 Breakdown (mechanical) of** intraperitoneal dialysis catheter   HCC

> EXCLUDES 1   mechanical complication of vascular dialysis catheter (T82.4-)

✓7ᵗʰ **T85.612 Breakdown (mechanical) of** permanent sutures

> EXCLUDES 1   mechanical complication of permanent (wire) suture used in bone repair (T84.1-T84.2)

√7th **T85.613** **Breakdown (mechanical) of** artificial skin graft and decellularized allodermis
Failure of artificial skin graft and decellularized allodermis
Non-adherence of artificial skin graft and decellularized allodermis
Poor incorporation of artificial skin graft and decellularized allodermis
Shearing of artificial skin graft and decellularized allodermis

√7th **T85.614** **Breakdown (mechanical) of** insulin pump

1 √7th **T85.615** **Breakdown (mechanical) of other** HCC **nervous system device, implant or graft**
Breakdown (mechanical) of intrathecal infusion pump

√7th **T85.618** **Breakdown (mechanical) of other specified internal prosthetic devices, implants and grafts**

√6th **T85.62** Displacement **of other specified internal prosthetic devices, implants and grafts**
Malposition of other specified internal prosthetic devices, implants and grafts

√7th **T85.620** **Displacement of** cranial or spinal infusion catheter
Displacement of epidural infusion catheter
Displacement of intrathecal infusion catheter
Displacement of subarachnoid infusion catheter
Displacement of subdural infusion catheter

√7th **T85.621** **Displacement of** intraperitoneal HCC dialysis catheter
EXCLUDES 1   *mechanical complication of vascular dialysis catheter (T82.4-)*

√7th **T85.622** **Displacement of** permanent sutures
EXCLUDES 1   *mechanical complication of permanent (wire) suture used in bone repair (T84.1-T84.2)*

√7th **T85.623** **Displacement of** artificial skin graft and decellularized allodermis
Dislodgement of artificial skin graft and decellularized allodermis

√7th **T85.624** **Displacement of** insulin pump

1 √7th **T85.625** **Displacement of other nervous** HCC **system device, implant or graft**
Displacement of intrathecal infusion pump

√7th **T85.628** **Displacement of other specified internal prosthetic devices, implants and grafts**

√6th **T85.63** Leakage **of other specified internal prosthetic devices, implants and grafts**

√7th **T85.630** **Leakage of** cranial or spinal infusion catheter
Leakage of epidural infusion catheter
Leakage of intrathecal infusion catheter infusion catheter
Leakage of subdural infusion catheter
Leakage of subarachnoid infusion catheter

√7th **T85.631** **Leakage of** intraperitoneal HCC dialysis catheter
EXCLUDES 1   *mechanical complication of vascular dialysis catheter (T82.4)*

√7th **T85.633** **Leakage of** insulin pump

1 √7th **T85.635** **Leakage of other nervous system** HCC **device, implant or graft**
Leakage of intrathecal infusion pump

√7th **T85.638** **Leakage of other specified internal prosthetic devices, implants and grafts**

√6th **T85.69** **Other mechanical complication of other specified internal prosthetic devices, implants and grafts**
Obstruction, mechanical of other specified internal prosthetic devices, implants and grafts
Perforation of other specified internal prosthetic devices, implants and grafts
Protrusion of other specified internal prosthetic devices, implants and grafts

√7th **T85.690** **Other mechanical complication of** cranial or spinal infusion catheter
Other mechanical complication of epidural infusion catheter
Other mechanical complication of intrathecal infusion catheter
Other mechanical complication of subarachnoid infusion catheter
Other mechanical complication of subdural infusion catheter

√7th **T85.691** **Other mechanical complication** HCC **of** intraperitoneal dialysis catheter
EXCLUDES 1   *mechanical complication of vascular dialysis catheter (T82.4)*

√7th **T85.692** **Other mechanical complication of** permanent sutures
EXCLUDES 1   *mechanical complication of permanent (wire) suture used in bone repair (T84.1-T84.2)*

√7th **T85.693** **Other mechanical complication of** artificial skin graft and decellularized allodermis

√7th **T85.694** **Other mechanical complication of** insulin pump

1 √7th **T85.695** **Other mechanical complication** HCC **of other nervous system device, implant or graft**
Other mechanical complication of intrathecal infusion pump

√7th **T85.698** **Other mechanical complication of other specified internal prosthetic devices, implants and grafts**
Mechanical complication of nonabsorbable surgical material NOS

√5th **T85.7** Infection and inflammatory reaction **due to other internal prosthetic devices, implants and grafts**
Use additional code to identify infection

√x7th **T85.71** **Infection and inflammatory reaction due to** HCC peritoneal dialysis catheter

1 √x7th **T85.72** **Infection and inflammatory reaction due to** HCC insulin pump

√6th **T85.73** **Infection and inflammatory reaction due to** nervous system **devices, implants and graft**

1 √7th **T85.730** **Infection and inflammatory** HCC **reaction due to** ventricular intracranial (communicating) shunt

1 √7th **T85.731** **Infection and inflammatory** HCC **reaction due to implanted electronic neurostimulator of** brain, electrode (lead)

1 √7th **T85.732** **Infection and inflammatory** HCC **reaction due to implanted electronic neurostimulator of** peripheral nerve, electrode (lead)
Infection and inflammatory reaction due to electrode (lead) for cranial nerve neurostimulators
Infection and inflammatory reaction due to electrode (lead) for gastric neurostimulator
Infection and inflammatory reaction due to electrode (lead) for sacral nerve neurostimulator
Infection and inflammatory reaction due to electrode (lead) for vagal nerve neurostimulators

1 √7th **T85.733** **Infection and inflammatory** HCC **reaction due to implanted electronic neurostimulator of** spinal cord, electrode (lead)

Chapter 19. Injury, Poisoning and Certain Other Consequences of External Causes

T85.734–T86.819

¹ ✓7ᵗʰ **T85.734 Infection and inflammatory reaction due to implanted electronic neurostimulator, generator** HCC
  Generator pocket infection

¹ ✓7ᵗʰ **T85.735 Infection and inflammatory reaction due to cranial or spinal infusion catheter** HCC
  Infection and inflammatory reaction due to epidural catheter
  Infection and inflammatory reaction due to intrathecal infusion catheter
  Infection and inflammatory reaction due to subarachnoid catheter
  Infection and inflammatory reaction due to subdural catheter

¹ ✓7ᵗʰ **T85.738 Infection and inflammatory reaction due to other nervous system device, implant or graft** HCC
  Infection and inflammatory reaction due to intrathecal infusion pump

¹ ✓×7ᵗʰ **T85.79 Infection and inflammatory reaction due to other internal prosthetic devices, implants and grafts** HCC

✓5ᵗʰ **T85.8 Other specified complications of internal prosthetic devices, implants and grafts, not elsewhere classified**

  ✓6ᵗʰ **T85.81 Embolism due to internal prosthetic devices, implants and grafts, not elsewhere classified**

    ¹ ✓7ᵗʰ **T85.810 Embolism due to nervous system prosthetic devices, implants and grafts** HCC

    ✓7ᵗʰ **T85.818 Embolism due to other internal prosthetic devices, implants and grafts**

  ✓6ᵗʰ **T85.82 Fibrosis due to internal prosthetic devices, implants and grafts, not elsewhere classified**

    ¹ ✓7ᵗʰ **T85.820 Fibrosis due to nervous system prosthetic devices, implants and grafts** HCC

    ✓7ᵗʰ **T85.828 Fibrosis due to other internal prosthetic devices, implants and grafts**

  ✓6ᵗʰ **T85.83 Hemorrhage due to internal prosthetic devices, implants and grafts, not elsewhere classified**

    ¹ ✓7ᵗʰ **T85.830 Hemorrhage due to nervous system prosthetic devices, implants and grafts** HCC

    ✓7ᵗʰ **T85.838 Hemorrhage due to other internal prosthetic devices, implants and grafts**

  ✓6ᵗʰ **T85.84 Pain due to internal prosthetic devices, implants and grafts, not elsewhere classified**

    ¹ ✓7ᵗʰ **T85.840 Pain due to nervous system prosthetic devices, implants and grafts** HCC

    ✓7ᵗʰ **T85.848 Pain due to other internal prosthetic devices, implants and grafts**

  ✓6ᵗʰ **T85.85 Stenosis due to internal prosthetic devices, implants and grafts, not elsewhere classified**

    ¹ ✓7ᵗʰ **T85.850 Stenosis due to nervous system prosthetic devices, implants and grafts** HCC

    ✓7ᵗʰ **T85.858 Stenosis due to other internal prosthetic devices, implants and grafts**

  ✓6ᵗʰ **T85.86 Thrombosis due to internal prosthetic devices, implants and grafts, not elsewhere classified**

    ¹ ✓7ᵗʰ **T85.860 Thrombosis due to nervous system prosthetic devices, implants and grafts** HCC

    ✓7ᵗʰ **T85.868 Thrombosis due to other internal prosthetic devices, implants and grafts**

  ✓6ᵗʰ **T85.89 Other specified complication of internal prosthetic devices, implants and grafts, not elsewhere classified**
    Erosion or breakdown of subcutaneous device pocket

    ¹ ✓7ᵗʰ **T85.890 Other specified complication of nervous system prosthetic devices, implants and grafts** HCC

    ✓7ᵗʰ **T85.898 Other specified complication of other internal prosthetic devices, implants and grafts**

✓×7ᵗʰ **T85.9 Unspecified complication of internal prosthetic device, implant and graft**
  Complication of internal prosthetic device, implant and graft NOS

✓4ᵗʰ **T86 Complications of transplanted organs and tissue**
  Use additional code to identify other transplant complications, such as:
  graft-versus-host disease (D89.81-)
  malignancy associated with organ transplant (C80.2)
  · post-transplant lymphoproliferative disorders (PTLD) (D47.Z1)

✓5ᵗʰ **T86.0 Complications of bone marrow transplant**

  T86.00 Unspecified complication of bone marrow transplant HCC

  T86.01 Bone marrow transplant rejection HCC

  T86.02 Bone marrow transplant failure HCC

  T86.03 Bone marrow transplant infection HCC

  T86.09 Other complications of bone marrow transplant HCC

✓5ᵗʰ **T86.1 Complications of kidney transplant**

  T86.10 Unspecified complication of kidney transplant

  T86.11 Kidney transplant rejection

  T86.12 Kidney transplant failure
    AHA: 2013,1Q,24

  T86.13 Kidney transplant infection
    Use additional code to specify infection

  T86.19 Other complication of kidney transplant
    AHA: 2019,2Q,7

✓5ᵗʰ **T86.2 Complications of heart transplant**

    EXCLUDES 1 complication of:
      artificial heart device (T82.5)
      heart-lung transplant (T86.3)

  T86.20 Unspecified complication of heart transplant HCC

  T86.21 Heart transplant rejection HCC

  T86.22 Heart transplant failure HCC

  T86.23 Heart transplant infection HCC
    Use additional code to specify infection

  ✓6ᵗʰ **T86.29 Other complications of heart transplant**

    T86.290 Cardiac allograft vasculopathy HCC

      EXCLUDES 1 atherosclerosis of coronary arteries (I25.75-, I25.76-, I25.81-)

    T86.298 Other complications of heart transplant HCC

✓5ᵗʰ **T86.3 Complications of heart-lung transplant**

  T86.30 Unspecified complication of heart-lung transplant HCC

  T86.31 Heart-lung transplant rejection HCC

  T86.32 Heart-lung transplant failure HCC

  T86.33 Heart-lung transplant infection HCC
    Use additional code to specify infection

  T86.39 Other complications of heart-lung transplant HCC

✓5ᵗʰ **T86.4 Complications of liver transplant**

  T86.40 Unspecified complication of liver transplant HCC

  T86.41 Liver transplant rejection HCC

  T86.42 Liver transplant failure HCC

  T86.43 Liver transplant infection HCC
    Use additional code to identify infection, such as:
    cytomegalovirus (CMV) infection (B25.-)

  T86.49 Other complications of liver transplant HCC

T86.5 Complications of stem cell transplant HCC
    Complications from stem cells from peripheral blood
    Complications from stem cells from umbilical cord

✓5ᵗʰ **T86.8 Complications of other transplanted organs and tissues**

  ✓6ᵗʰ **T86.81 Complications of lung transplant**

    EXCLUDES 1 complication of heart-lung transplant (T86.3-)

    T86.810 Lung transplant rejection HCC

    T86.811 Lung transplant failure HCC

    T86.812 Lung transplant infection HCC
      Use additional code to specify infection

    T86.818 Other complications of lung transplant HCC
      AHA: 2019,2Q,6

    T86.819 Unspecified complication of lung transplant HCC

✓6th   **T86.82**   **Complications of** skin graft **(allograft) (autograft)**

> EXCLUDES 2   complication of artificial skin graft (T85.693)

T86.820   **Skin graft (allograft)** rejection

T86.821   **Skin graft (allograft) (autograft)** failure

T86.822   **Skin graft (allograft) (autograft)** infection
> Use additional code to specify infection

T86.828   **Other complications of skin graft (allograft) (autograft)**

T86.829   **Unspecified complication of skin graft (allograft) (autograft)**

✓6th   **T86.83**   **Complications of** bone graft

> EXCLUDES 2   mechanical complications of bone graft (T84.3-)

T86.830   **Bone graft** rejection

T86.831   **Bone graft** failure

T86.832   **Bone graft** infection
> Use additional code to specify infection

T86.838   **Other complications of bone graft**

T86.839   **Unspecified complication of bone graft**

✓6th   **T86.84**   **Complications of** corneal **transplant**

> EXCLUDES 2   mechanical complications of corneal graft (T85.3-)

T86.840   **Corneal transplant** rejection

T86.841   **Corneal transplant** failure

T86.842   **Corneal transplant** infection   HCC
> Use additional code to specify infection

T86.848   **Other complications of corneal transplant**

T86.849   **Unspecified complication of corneal transplant**

✓6th   **T86.85**   **Complication of** intestine **transplant**

T86.850   **Intestine transplant** rejection   HCC

T86.851   **Intestine transplant** failure   HCC

T86.852   **Intestine transplant** infection   HCC
> Use additional code to specify infection

T86.858   **Other complications of intestine transplant**   HCC

T86.859   **Unspecified complication of intestine transplant**   HCC

✓6th   **T86.89**   **Complications of other transplanted tissue**

> Transplant failure or rejection of pancreas

T86.890   **Other transplanted tissue** rejection

T86.891   **Other transplanted tissue** failure

T86.892   **Other transplanted tissue** infection
> Use additional code to specify infection

T86.898   **Other complications of other transplanted tissue**

T86.899   **Unspecified complication of other transplanted tissue**

✓5th   **T86.9**   **Complication of unspecified transplanted organ and tissue**

T86.90   **Unspecified complication of unspecified transplanted organ and tissue**

T86.91   **Unspecified transplanted organ and tissue** rejection

T86.92   **Unspecified transplanted organ and tissue** failure

T86.93   **Unspecified transplanted organ and tissue** infection
> Use additional code to specify infection

T86.99   **Other complications of unspecified transplanted organ and tissue**

✓4th   **T87**   **Complications peculiar to reattachment and amputation**

✓5th   **T87.0**   **Complications of reattached (part of)** upper extremity

✓6th   **T87.0X**   **Complications of reattached (part of) upper extremity**

T87.0X1   **Complications of reattached (part of)** right **upper extremity**   HCC

T87.0X2   **Complications of reattached (part of)** left **upper extremity**   HCC

T87.0X9   **Complications of reattached (part of) unspecified upper extremity**   HCC

✓5th   **T87.1**   **Complications of reattached (part of)** lower extremity

✓6th   **T87.1X**   **Complications of reattached (part of) lower extremity**

T87.1X1   **Complications of reattached (part of)** right **lower extremity**   HCC

T87.1X2   **Complications of reattached (part of)** left **lower extremity**   HCC

T87.1X9   **Complications of reattached (part of) unspecified lower extremity**   HCC

T87.2   **Complications of other reattached body part**   HCC

✓5th   **T87.3**   **Neuroma of amputation stump**

> **DEF:** Non-neoplastic tumor generated at the proximal end of severed, partially transected, or injured nerve following amputation.

T87.30   **Neuroma of amputation stump, unspecified extremity**   HCC

T87.31   **Neuroma of amputation stump,** right upper **extremity**   HCC

T87.32   **Neuroma of amputation stump,** left upper **extremity**   HCC

T87.33   **Neuroma of amputation stump,** right lower **extremity**   HCC

T87.34   **Neuroma of amputation stump,** left lower **extremity**   HCC

✓5th   **T87.4**   **Infection of amputation stump**

T87.40   **Infection of amputation stump, unspecified extremity**   HCC

T87.41   **Infection of amputation stump,** right upper **extremity**   HCC

T87.42   **Infection of amputation stump,** left upper **extremity**   HCC

T87.43   **Infection of amputation stump,** right lower **extremity**   HCC

T87.44   **Infection of amputation stump,** left lower **extremity**   HCC

✓5th   **T87.5**   **Necrosis of amputation stump**

T87.50   **Necrosis of amputation stump, unspecified extremity**   HCC

T87.51   **Necrosis of amputation stump,** right upper **extremity**   HCC

T87.52   **Necrosis of amputation stump,** left upper **extremity**   HCC

T87.53   **Necrosis of amputation stump,** right lower **extremity**   HCC

T87.54   **Necrosis of amputation stump,** left lower **extremity**   HCC

✓5th   **T87.8**   **Other complications of amputation stump**

T87.81   **Dehiscence of amputation stump**   HCC

T87.89   **Other complications of amputation stump**   HCC
> Amputation stump contracture
> Amputation stump contracture of next proximal joint
> Amputation stump flexion
> Amputation stump edema
> Amputation stump hematoma
> EXCLUDES 2   phantom limb syndrome (G54.6-G54.7)

T87.9   **Unspecified complications of amputation stump**   HCC

✓4th   **T88**   **Other complications of surgical and medical care, not elsewhere classified**

> EXCLUDES 2   complication following infusion, transfusion and therapeutic injection (T80.-)
> complication following procedure NEC (T81.-)
> complications of anesthesia in labor and delivery (O74.-)
> complications of anesthesia in pregnancy (O29.-)
> complications of anesthesia in puerperium (O89.-)
> complications of devices, implants and grafts (T82-T85)
> complications of obstetric surgery and procedure (O75.4)
> dermatitis due to drugs and medicaments (L23.3, L24.4, L25.1, L27.0-L27.1)
> poisoning and toxic effects of drugs and chemicals (T36-T65 with fifth or sixth character 1-4 or 6)
> specified complications classified elsewhere

> The appropriate 7th character is to be added to each code from category T88.
> A   initial encounter
> D   subsequent encounter
> S   sequela

✓7th   **T88.0**   **Infection following immunization**
> Sepsis following immunization
> **AHA:** 2018,4Q,62-63

☑ Additional Character Required   ✓x7th Placeholder Alert   Manifestation   Unspecified Dx   ▶◀ Revised Text   ● New Code   ▲ Revised Code Title

ICD-10-CM 2020   1149

✓x7ᵗʰ T88.1 Other complications following immunization, not elsewhere classified
    Generalized vaccinia
    Rash following immunization
      EXCLUDES 1   *vaccinia not from vaccine (B08.011)*
      EXCLUDES 2   *anaphylactic shock due to serum (T80.5-)*
                other serum reactions (T80.6-)
                postimmunization arthropathy (M02.2)
                postimmunization encephalitis (G04.02)
                postimmunization fever (R50.83)

✓x7ᵗʰ T88.2 Shock due to anesthesia
    Use additional code for adverse effect, if applicable, to identify drug (T41.- with fifth or sixth character 5)
      EXCLUDES 1   *complications of anesthesia (in):*
                labor and delivery (O74.-)
                postprocedural shock NOS (T81.1-)
                pregnancy (O29.-)
                puerperium (O89.-)

✓x7ᵗʰ T88.3 Malignant hyperthermia due to anesthesia
    Use additional code for adverse effect, if applicable, to identify drug (T41.- with fifth or sixth character 5)

✓x7ᵗʰ T88.4 Failed or difficult intubation

✓5ᵗʰ T88.5 Other complications of anesthesia
    Use additional code for adverse effect, if applicable, to identify drug (T41.- with fifth or sixth character 5)

    ✓x7ᵗʰ T88.51 Hypothermia following anesthesia

    ✓x7ᵗʰ T88.52 Failed moderate sedation during procedure
      Failed conscious sedation during procedure
        EXCLUDES 2   *personal history of failed moderate sedation (Z92.83)*

    ✓x7ᵗʰ T88.53 Unintended awareness under general anesthesia during procedure
        EXCLUDES 2   *personal history of unintended awareness under general anesthesia (Z92.84)*
      AHA: 2016,4Q,72-73

    ✓x7ᵗʰ T88.59 Other complications of anesthesia

✓x7ᵗʰ T88.6 Anaphylactic reaction due to adverse effect of correct drug or medicament properly administered
    Anaphylactic shock due to adverse effect of correct drug or medicament properly administered
    Anaphylactoid reaction NOS
    Use additional code for adverse effect, if applicable, to identify drug (T36-T50 with fifth or sixth character 5)
      EXCLUDES 1   *anaphylactic reaction due to serum (T80.5-)*
                anaphylactic shock or reaction due to adverse food reaction (T78.0-)

✓x7ᵗʰ T88.7 Unspecified adverse effect of drug or medicament
    Drug hypersensitivity NOS
    Drug reaction NOS
    Use additional code for adverse effect, if applicable, to identify drug (T36-T50 with fifth or sixth character 5)
      EXCLUDES 1   *specified adverse effects of drugs and medicaments (A00-R94 and T80-T88.6, T88.8)*

✓x7ᵗʰ T88.8 Other specified complications of surgical and medical care, not elsewhere classified
    Use additional code to identify the complication

✓x7ᵗʰ T88.9 Complication of surgical and medical care, unspecified

Chapter 20. External Causes of Morbidity (V00–Y99)

Chapter-specific Guidelines with Coding Examples

The chapter-specific guidelines from the ICD-10-CM Official Guidelines for Coding and Reporting have been provided below. Along with these guidelines are coding examples, contained in the shaded boxes, that have been developed to help illustrate the coding and/or sequencing guidance found in these guidelines.

The external causes of morbidity codes should never be sequenced as the first-listed or principal diagnosis.

External cause codes are intended to provide data for injury research and evaluation of injury prevention strategies. These codes capture how the injury or health condition happened (cause), the intent (unintentional or accidental; or intentional, such as suicide or assault), the place where the event occurred the activity of the patient at the time of the event, and the person's status (e.g., civilian, military).

There is no national requirement for mandatory ICD-10-CM external cause code reporting. Unless a provider is subject to a state-based external cause code reporting mandate or these codes are required by a particular payer, reporting of ICD-10-CM codes in Chapter 20, External Causes of Morbidity, is not required. In the absence of a mandatory reporting requirement, providers are encouraged to voluntarily report external cause codes, as they provide valuable data for injury research and evaluation of injury prevention strategies.

a. General external cause coding guidelines

1) Used with any code in the range of A00.0–T88.9, Z00–Z99

An external cause code may be used with any code in the range of A00.0-T88.9, Z00-Z99, classification that represents a health condition due to an external cause. Though they are most applicable to injuries, they are also valid for use with such things as infections or diseases due to an external source, and other health conditions, such as a heart attack that occurs during strenuous physical activity.

> Actinic reticuloid due to tanning bed use
>
> | **L57.1** | **Actinic reticuloid** |
> |---|---|
> | **W89.1XXA** | **Exposure to tanning bed, initial encounter** |
>
> *Explanation:* An external cause code may be used with any code in the range of A00.0–T88.9, Z00–Z99, classifications that describe health conditions due to an external cause. Code W89.1 Exposure to tanning bed requires a seventh character of A to report this initial encounter, with a placeholder X for the fifth and sixth characters.

2) External cause code used for length of treatment

Assign the external cause code, with the appropriate 7th character (initial encounter, subsequent encounter or sequela) for each encounter for which the injury or condition is being treated.

Most categories in chapter 20 have a 7th character requirement for each applicable code. Most categories in this chapter have three 7th character values: A, initial encounter, D, subsequent encounter and S, sequela. While the patient may be seen by a new or different provider over the course of treatment for an injury or condition, assignment of the 7th character for external cause should match the 7th character of the code assigned for the associated injury or condition for the encounter.

3) Use the full range of external cause codes

Use the full range of external cause codes to completely describe the cause, the intent, the place of occurrence, and if applicable, the activity of the patient at the time of the event, and the patient's status, for all injuries, and other health conditions due to an external cause.

4) Assign as many external cause codes as necessary

Assign as many external cause codes as necessary to fully explain each cause. If only one external code can be recorded, assign the code most related to the principal diagnosis.

5) The selection of the appropriate external cause code

The selection of the appropriate external cause code is guided by the Alphabetic Index of External Causes and by Inclusion and Exclusion notes in the Tabular List.

6) External cause code can never be a principal diagnosis

An external cause code can never be a principal (first-listed) diagnosis.

7) Combination external cause codes

Certain of the external cause codes are combination codes that identify sequential events that result in an injury, such as a fall which results in striking against an object. The injury may be due to either event or both.

The combination external cause code used should correspond to the sequence of events regardless of which caused the most serious injury.

> Toddler tripped and fell while walking and struck his head on an end table, sustaining a scalp contusion
>
> | **S00.03XA** | **Contusion of scalp, initial encounter** |
> |---|---|
> | **W01.190A** | **Fall on same level from slipping, tripping and stumbling with subsequent striking against furniture, initial encounter** |
>
> *Explanation:* Combination external cause codes identify sequential events that result in an injury, such as a fall resulting in striking against an object. The injury may be due to either or both events.

8) No external cause code needed in certain circumstances

No external cause code from Chapter 20 is needed if the external cause and intent are included in a code from another chapter (e.g. T36.0X1- Poisoning by penicillins, accidental (unintentional)).

b. Place of occurrence guideline

Codes from category Y92, Place of occurrence of the external cause, are secondary codes for use after other external cause codes to identify the location of the patient at the time of injury or other condition.

Generally, a place of occurrence code is assigned only once, at the initial encounter for treatment. However, in the rare instance that a new injury occurs during hospitalization, an additional place of occurrence code may be assigned. No 7th characters are used for Y92.

Do not use place of occurrence code Y92.9 if the place is not stated or is not applicable.

> A farmer was working in his barn and sustained a foot contusion when the horse stepped on his left foot
>
> | **S90.32XA** | **Contusion of left foot, initial encounter** |
> |---|---|
> | **W55.19XA** | **Other contact with horse, initial encounter** |
> | **Y92.71** | **Barn as the place of occurrence of the external cause** |
>
> *Explanation:* A place-of-occurrence code from category Y92 is assigned at the initial encounter to identify the location of the patient at the time the injury occurred.

c. Activity code

Assign a code from category Y93, Activity code, to describe the activity of the patient at the time the injury or other health condition occurred.

An activity code is used only once, at the initial encounter for treatment. Only one code from Y93 should be recorded on a medical record.

The activity codes are not applicable to poisonings, adverse effects, misadventures or sequela.

Do not assign Y93.9, Unspecified activity, if the activity is not stated.

A code from category Y93 is appropriate for use with external cause and intent codes if identifying the activity provides additional information about the event.

> Ranch hand who was grooming a horse sustained a foot contusion when the horse stepped on his left foot
>
> | **S90.32XA** | **Contusion of left foot, initial encounter** |
> |---|---|
> | **W55.19XA** | **Other contact with horse, initial encounter** |
> | **Y93.K3** | **Activity, grooming and shearing an animal** |
>
> *Explanation:* One activity code from category Y93 is assigned at the initial encounter only to describe the activity of the patient at the time the injury occurred.

d. Place of occurrence, activity, and status codes used with other external cause code

When applicable, place of occurrence, activity, and external cause status codes are sequenced after the main external cause code(s). Regardless of the number of external cause codes assigned, generally there should be only one place of occurrence code, one activity code, and one external cause status code assigned to an encounter. However, in the rare instance that a new injury occurs during hospitalization, an additional place of occurrence code may be assigned.

e. If the reporting format limits the number of external cause codes

If the reporting format limits the number of external cause codes that can be used in reporting clinical data, report the code for the cause/intent most related to the principal diagnosis. If the format permits capture of additional external cause codes, the cause/intent, including medical misadventures, of the additional events should be reported rather than the codes for place, activity, or external status.

f. Multiple external cause coding guidelines

More than one external cause code is required to fully describe the external cause of an illness or injury. The assignment of external cause codes should be sequenced in the following priority:

If two or more events cause separate injuries, an external cause code should be assigned for each cause. The first-listed external cause code will be selected in the following order:

External codes for child and adult abuse take priority over all other external cause codes.

See Section I.C.19., Child and Adult abuse guidelines.

External cause codes for terrorism events take priority over all other external cause codes except child and adult abuse.

External cause codes for cataclysmic events take priority over all other external cause codes except child and adult abuse and terrorism.

External cause codes for transport accidents take priority over all other external cause codes except cataclysmic events, child and adult abuse and terrorism.

Activity and external cause status codes are assigned following all causal (intent) external cause codes.

The first-listed external cause code should correspond to the cause of the most serious diagnosis due to an assault, accident, or self-harm, following the order of hierarchy listed above..

30-year-old man accidentally discharged his hunting rifle, sustaining an open gunshot wound, with no retained bullet fragments, to the right thigh, which caused him to fall down the stairs, resulting in closed displaced comminuted fracture of his left radial shaft

S71.131A	**Puncture wound without foreign body, right thigh, initial encounter**
W33.02XA	**Accidental discharge of hunting rifle, initial encounter**
S52.352A	**Displaced comminuted fracture of shaft of radius, left arm, initial encounter for closed fracture**
W10.9XXA	**Fall (on) (from) unspecified stairs and steps, initial encounter**

Explanation: If two or more events cause separate injuries, an external cause code should be assigned for each cause.

---

g. Child and adult abuse guideline

Adult and child abuse, neglect and maltreatment are classified as assault. Any of the assault codes may be used to indicate the external cause of any injury resulting from the confirmed abuse.

For confirmed cases of abuse, neglect and maltreatment, when the perpetrator is known, a code from Y07, Perpetrator of maltreatment and neglect, should accompany any other assault codes.

See Section I.C.19. Adult and child abuse, neglect and other maltreatment

h. Unknown or undetermined intent guideline

If the intent (accident, self-harm, assault) of the cause of an injury or other condition is unknown or unspecified, code the intent as accidental intent. All transport accident categories assume accidental intent.

1). Use of undetermined intent

External cause codes for events of undetermined intent are only for use if the documentation in the record specifies that the intent cannot be determined.

i. Sequelae (late effects) of external cause guidelines

1) Sequelae external cause codes

Sequela are reported using the external cause code with the 7th character "S" for sequela. These codes should be used with any report of a late effect or sequela resulting from a previous injury.

See Section I.B.10 Sequela (Late Effects)

2) Sequela external cause code with a related current injury

A sequela external cause code should never be used with a related current nature of injury code.

3) Use of sequela external cause codes for subsequent visits

Use a late effect external cause code for subsequent visits when a late effect of the initial injury is being treated. Do not use a late effect external cause code for subsequent visits for follow-up care (e.g., to assess healing, to receive rehabilitative therapy) of the injury when no late effect of the injury has been documented.

j. Terrorism guidelines

1) Cause of injury identified by the Federal Government (FBI) as terrorism

When the cause of an injury is identified by the Federal Government (FBI) as terrorism, the first-listed external cause code should be a code from category Y38, Terrorism. The definition of terrorism employed by the FBI is found at the inclusion note at the beginning of category Y38. Use additional code for place of occurrence (Y92.-). More than one Y38 code may be assigned if the injury is the result of more than one mechanism of terrorism.

2) Cause of an injury is suspected to be the result of terrorism

When the cause of an injury is suspected to be the result of terrorism a code from category Y38 should not be assigned. Suspected cases should be classified as assault.

3) Code Y38.9, Terrorism, secondary effects

Assign code Y38.9, Terrorism, secondary effects, for conditions occurring subsequent to the terrorist event. This code should not be assigned for conditions that are due to the initial terrorist act.

It is acceptable to assign code Y38.9 with another code from Y38 if there is an injury due to the initial terrorist event and an injury that is a subsequent result of the terrorist event.

k. External cause status

A code from category Y99, External cause status, should be assigned whenever any other external cause code is assigned for an encounter, including an Activity code, except for the events noted below. Assign a code from category Y99, External cause status, to indicate the work status of the person at the time the event occurred. The status code indicates whether the event occurred during military activity, whether a non-military person was at work, whether an individual including a student or volunteer was involved in a non-work activity at the time of the causal event.

A code from Y99, External cause status, should be assigned, when applicable, with other external cause codes, such as transport accidents and falls. The external cause status codes are not applicable to poisonings, adverse effects, misadventures or late effects.

Do not assign a code from category Y99 if no other external cause codes (cause, activity) are applicable for the encounter.

An external cause status code is used only once, at the initial encounter for treatment. Only one code from Y99 should be recorded on a medical record.

Do not assign code Y99.9, Unspecified external cause status, if the status is not stated.

Chapter 20. External Causes of Morbidity (V00-Y99)

NOTE   This chapter permits the classification of environmental events and circumstances as the cause of injury, and other adverse effects. Where a code from this section is applicable, it is intended that it shall be used secondary to a code from another chapter of the Classification indicating the nature of the condition. Most often, the condition will be classifiable to Chapter 19, Injury, poisoning and certain other consequences of external causes (S00-T88). Other conditions that may be stated to be due to external causes are classified in Chapters I to XVIII. For these conditions, codes from Chapter 20 should be used to provide additional information as to the cause of the condition.

AHA: 2018,4Q,58-60

This chapter contains the following blocks:

V00-X58	Accidents
V00-V99	Transport accidents
V00-V09	Pedestrian injured in transport accident
V10-V19	Pedal cycle rider injured in transport accident
V20-V29	Motorcycle rider injured in transport accident
V30-V39	Occupant of three-wheeled motor vehicle injured in transport accident
V40-V49	Car occupant injured in transport accident
V50-V59	Occupant of pick-up truck or van injured in transport accident
V60-V69	Occupant of heavy transport vehicle injured in transport accident
V70-V79	Bus occupant injured in transport accident
V80-V89	Other land transport accidents
V90-V94	Water transport accidents
V95-V97	Air and space transport accidents
V98-V99	Other and unspecified transport accidents
W00-X58	Other external causes of accidental injury
W00-W19	Slipping, tripping, stumbling and falls
W20-W49	Exposure to inanimate mechanical forces
W50-W64	Exposure to animate mechanical forces
W65-W74	Accidental non-transport drowning and submersion
W85-W99	Exposure to electric current, radiation and extreme ambient air temperature and pressure
X00-X08	Exposure to smoke, fire and flames
X10-X19	Contact with heat and hot substances
X30-X39	Exposure to forces of nature
X50	Overexertion and strenuous or repetitive movements
X52-X58	Accidental exposure to other specified factors
X71-X83	Intentional self-harm
X92-Y09	Assault
Y21-Y33	Event of undetermined intent
Y35-Y38	Legal intervention, operations of war, military operations, and terrorism
Y62-Y84	Complications of medical and surgical care
Y62-Y69	Misadventures to patients during surgical and medical care
Y70-Y82	Medical devices associated with adverse incidents in diagnostic and therapeutic use
Y83-Y84	Surgical and other medical procedures as the cause of abnormal reaction of the patient, or of later complication, without mention of misadventure at the time of the procedure
Y90-Y99	Supplementary factors related to causes of morbidity classified elsewhere

ACCIDENTS (V00-X58)

AHA: 2018,2Q,7-8

Transport accidents (V00-V99)

NOTE   This section is structured in 12 groups. Those relating to land transport accidents (V00-V89) reflect the victim's mode of transport and are subdivided to identify the victim's 'counterpart' or the type of event. The vehicle of which the injured person is an occupant is identified in the first two characters since it is seen as the most important factor to identify for prevention purposes. A transport accident is one in which the vehicle involved must be moving or running or in use for transport purposes at the time of the accident.

Use additional code to identify:
airbag injury (W22.1)
type of street or road (Y92.4-)
use of cellular telephone and other electronic equipment at the time of the transport accident (Y93.C-)

EXCLUDES 1   agricultural vehicles in stationary use or maintenance (W31.-)
assault by crashing of motor vehicle (Y03.-)
automobile or motor cycle in stationary use or maintenance — code to type of accident
crashing of motor vehicle, undetermined intent (Y32)
intentional self-harm by crashing of motor vehicle (X82)

EXCLUDES 2   transport accidents due to cataclysm (X34-X38)

NOTE   Definitions related to transport accidents:
(a)   A transport accident (V00-V99) is any accident involving a device designed primarily for, or used at the time primarily for, conveying persons or good from one place to another.

(b)   A public highway [trafficway] or street is the entire width between property lines (or other boundary lines) of land open to the public as a matter of right or custom for purposes of moving persons or property from one place to another. A roadway is that part of the public highway designed, improved and customarily used for vehicular traffic.

(c)   A traffic accident is any vehicle accident occurring on the public highway [i.e. originating on, terminating on, or involving a vehicle partially on the highway]. A vehicle accident is assumed to have occurred on the public highway unless another place is specified, except in the case of accidents involving only off-road motor vehicles, which are classified as nontraffic accidents unless the contrary is stated.

(d)   A nontraffic accident is any vehicle accident that occurs entirely in any place other than a public highway.

(e)   A pedestrian is any person involved in an accident who was not at the time of the accident riding in or on a motor vehicle, railway train, streetcar or animal-drawn or other vehicle, or on a pedal cycle or animal. This includes, a person changing a tire, working on a parked car, or a person on foot. It also includes the user of a pedestrian conveyance such as a baby stroller, ice-skates, skis, sled, roller skates, a skateboard, nonmotorized or motorized wheelchair, motorized mobility scooter, or nonmotorized scooter.

(f)   A driver is an occupant of a transport vehicle who is operating or intending to operate it.

(g)   A passenger is any occupant of a transport vehicle other than the driver, except a person traveling on the outside of the vehicle.

(h)   A person on the outside of a vehicle is any person being transported by a vehicle but not occupying the space normally reserved for the driver or passengers, or the space intended for the transport of property. This includes a person travelling on the bodywork, bumper, fender, roof, running board or step of a vehicle, as well as, hanging on the outside of the vehicle.

(i)   A pedal cycle is any land transport vehicle operated solely by nonmotorized pedals including a bicycle or tricycle.

(j)   A pedal cyclist is any person riding a pedal cycle or in a sidecar or trailer attached to a pedal cycle.

(k)   A motorcycle is a two-wheeled motor vehicle with one or two riding saddles and sometimes with a third wheel for the support of a sidecar. The sidecar is considered part of the motorcycle. This includes a moped, motor scooter, or motorized bicycle.

(l)   A motorcycle rider is any person riding a motorcycle or in a sidecar or trailer attached to the motorcycle.

(m)   A three-wheeled motor vehicle is a motorized tricycle designed primarily for on-road use. This includes a motor-driven tricycle, a motorized rickshaw, or a three-wheeled motor car.

(n)   A car [automobile] is a four-wheeled motor vehicle designed primarily for carrying up to 7 persons. A trailer being towed by the car is considered part of the car. It does not include a van or minivan — see definition (o).

(o)   A pick-up truck or van is a four or six-wheeled motor vehicle designed for carrying passengers as well as property or cargo weighing less than the local limit for classification as a heavy goods vehicle, and not requiring a special driver's license. This includes a minivan and a sport-utility vehicle (SUV).

(p)   A heavy transport vehicle is a motor vehicle designed primarily for carrying property, meeting local criteria for classification as a heavy goods vehicle in terms of weight and requiring a special driver's license.

(q)   A bus (coach) is a motor vehicle designed or adapted primarily for carrying more than 10 passengers, and requiring a special driver's license.

(r)   A railway train or railway vehicle is any device, with or without freight or passenger cars couple to it, designed for traffic on a railway track. This includes subterranean (subways) or elevated trains.

(s)   A streetcar, is a device designed and used primarily for transporting passengers within a municipality, running on rails, usually subject to normal traffic control signals, and operated principally on a right-of-way that forms part of the roadway. This includes a tram or trolley that runs on rails. A trailer being towed by a streetcar is considered part of the streetcar.

(t)   A special vehicle mainly used on industrial premises is a motor vehicle designed primarily for use within the buildings and premises of industrial or commercial establishments. This includes battery-powered airport passenger vehicles or baggage/mail trucks, forklifts, coal-cars in a coal mine, logging cars and trucks used in mines or quarries.

(u)   A special vehicle mainly used in agriculture is a motor vehicle designed specifically for use in farming and agriculture

---

☑ Additional Character Required   ✗x7ᵗʰ Placeholder Alert   Manifestation   Unspecified Dx   ▶◀ Revised Text   ● New Code   ▲ Revised Code Title

ICD-10-CM 2020   1153

(horticulture), to work the land, tend and harvest crops and transport materials on the farm. This includes harvesters, farm machinery and tractor and trailers.

(v) A special construction vehicle is a motor vehicle designed specifically for use on construction and demolition sites. This includes bulldozers, diggers, earth levellers, dump trucks, backhoes, front-end loaders, pavers, and mechanical shovels.

(w) A special all-terrain vehicle is a motor vehicle of special design to enable it to negotiate over rough or soft terrain, snow or sand. Examples of special design are high construction, special wheels and tires, tracks, and support on a cushion of air. This includes snow mobiles, All-terrain vehicles (ATV), and dune buggies. It does not include passenger vehicle designated as Sport Utility Vehicles. (SUV)

(x) A watercraft is any device designed for transporting passengers or goods on water. This includes motor or sailboats, ships, and hovercraft.

(y) An aircraft is any device for transporting passengers or goods in the air. This includes hot-air balloons, gliders, helicopters and airplanes.

(z) A military vehicle is any motorized vehicle operating on a public roadway owned by the military and being operated by a member of the military.

Pedestrian injured in transport accident (V00-V09)

INCLUDES   person changing tire on transport vehicle
    person examining engine of vehicle broken down in (on side of) road

EXCLUDES 1   *fall due to non-transport collision with other person (W03)*
    pedestrian on foot falling (slipping) on ice and snow (W00.-)
    struck or bumped by another person (W51)

The appropriate 7th character is to be added to each code from categories V00-V09.
A initial encounter
D subsequent encounter
S sequela

√4ᵗʰ **V00 Pedestrian conveyance accident**

Use additional place of occurrence and activity external cause codes, if known (Y92.-, Y93.-)

EXCLUDES 1   *collision with another person without fall (W51)*
    fall due to person on foot colliding with another person on foot (W03)
    fall from non-moving wheelchair, nonmotorized scooter and motorized mobility scooter without collision (W05.-)
    pedestrian (conveyance) collision with other land transport vehicle (V01-V09)
    pedestrian on foot falling (slipping) on ice and snow (W00.-)

√5ᵗʰ **V00.0 Pedestrian on foot injured in collision with pedestrian conveyance**

√x7ᵗʰ **V00.01 Pedestrian on foot injured in collision with roller-skater**

√x7ᵗʰ **V00.02 Pedestrian on foot injured in collision with skateboarder**

√x7ᵗʰ **V00.09 Pedestrian on foot injured in collision with other pedestrian conveyance**

√5ᵗʰ **V00.1 Rolling-type pedestrian conveyance accident**

EXCLUDES 1   *accident with baby stroller (V00.82-)*
    accident with motorized mobility scooter (V00.83-)
    accident with wheelchair (powered) (V00.81-)

√6ᵗʰ **V00.11 In-line roller-skate accident**

√7ᵗʰ **V00.111 Fall from in-line roller-skates**

√7ᵗʰ **V00.112 In-line roller-skater colliding with stationary object**

√7ᵗʰ **V00.118 Other in-line roller-skate accident**

EXCLUDES 1   *roller-skater collision with other land transport vehicle (V01-V09 with 5th character 1)*

√6ᵗʰ **V00.12 Non-in-line roller-skate accident**

√7ᵗʰ **V00.121 Fall from non-in-line roller-skates**

√7ᵗʰ **V00.122 Non-in-line roller-skater colliding with stationary object**

√7ᵗʰ **V00.128 Other non-in-line roller-skating accident**

EXCLUDES 1   *roller-skater collision with other land transport vehicle (V01-V09 with 5th character 1)*

√6ᵗʰ **V00.13 Skateboard accident**

√7ᵗʰ **V00.131 Fall from skateboard**

√7ᵗʰ **V00.132 Skateboarder colliding with stationary object**

√7ᵗʰ **V00.138 Other skateboard accident**

EXCLUDES 1   *skateboarder collision with other land transport vehicle (V01-V09 with 5th character 2)*

√6ᵗʰ **V00.14 Scooter (nonmotorized) accident**

EXCLUDES 1   *motor scooter accident (V20-V29)*

√7ᵗʰ **V00.141 Fall from scooter (nonmotorized)**

√7ᵗʰ **V00.142 Scooter (nonmotorized) colliding with stationary object**

√7ᵗʰ **V00.148 Other scooter (nonmotorized) accident**

EXCLUDES 1   *scooter (nonmotorized) collision with other land transport vehicle (V01-V09 with fifth character 9)*

√6ᵗʰ **V00.15 Heelies accident**

Rolling shoe
Wheeled shoe
Wheelies accident

√7ᵗʰ **V00.151 Fall from heelies**

√7ᵗʰ **V00.152 Heelies colliding with stationary object**

√7ᵗʰ **V00.158 Other heelies accident**

√6ᵗʰ **V00.18 Accident on other rolling-type pedestrian conveyance**

√7ᵗʰ **V00.181 Fall from other rolling-type pedestrian conveyance**

√7ᵗʰ **V00.182 Pedestrian on other rolling-type pedestrian conveyance colliding with stationary object**

√7ᵗʰ **V00.188 Other accident on other rolling-type pedestrian conveyance**

√5ᵗʰ **V00.2 Gliding-type pedestrian conveyance accident**

√6ᵗʰ **V00.21 Ice-skates accident**

√7ᵗʰ **V00.211 Fall from ice-skates**

√7ᵗʰ **V00.212 Ice-skater colliding with stationary object**

√7ᵗʰ **V00.218 Other ice-skates accident**

EXCLUDES 1   *ice-skater collision with other land transport vehicle (V01-V09 with 5th character 9)*

√6ᵗʰ **V00.22 Sled accident**

√7ᵗʰ **V00.221 Fall from sled**

√7ᵗʰ **V00.222 Sledder colliding with stationary object**

√7ᵗʰ **V00.228 Other sled accident**

EXCLUDES 1   *sled collision with other land transport vehicle (V01-V09 with 5th character 9)*

√6ᵗʰ **V00.28 Other gliding-type pedestrian conveyance accident**

√7ᵗʰ **V00.281 Fall from other gliding-type pedestrian conveyance**

√7ᵗʰ **V00.282 Pedestrian on other gliding-type pedestrian conveyance colliding with stationary object**

√7ᵗʰ **V00.288 Other accident on other gliding-type pedestrian conveyance**

EXCLUDES 1   *gliding-type pedestrian conveyance collision with other land transport vehicle (V01-V09 with 5th character 9)*

√5ᵗʰ **V00.3 Flat-bottomed pedestrian conveyance accident**

√6ᵗʰ **V00.31 Snowboard accident**

√7ᵗʰ **V00.311 Fall from snowboard**

√7ᵗʰ **V00.312 Snowboarder colliding with stationary object**

✓7ᵗʰ **V00.318 Other snowboard accident**
     EXCLUDES 1   *snowboarder collision with other land transport vehicle (V01-V09 with 5th character 9)*

✓6ᵗʰ **V00.32 Snow-ski accident**

✓7ᵗʰ **V00.321 Fall from snow-skis**

✓7ᵗʰ **V00.322 Snow-skier colliding with stationary object**

✓7ᵗʰ **V00.328 Other snow-ski accident**
     EXCLUDES 1   *snow-skier collision with other land transport vehicle (V01-V09 with 5th character 9)*

✓6ᵗʰ **V00.38 Other flat-bottomed pedestrian conveyance accident**

✓7ᵗʰ **V00.381 Fall from other flat-bottomed pedestrian conveyance**

✓7ᵗʰ **V00.382 Pedestrian on other flat-bottomed pedestrian conveyance colliding with stationary object**

✓7ᵗʰ **V00.388 Other accident on other flat-bottomed pedestrian conveyance**

✓5ᵗʰ **V00.8 Accident on other pedestrian conveyance**

✓6ᵗʰ **V00.81 Accident with wheelchair (powered)**

✓7ᵗʰ **V00.811 Fall from moving wheelchair (powered)**
     EXCLUDES 1   *fall from non-moving wheelchair (W05.0)*

✓7ᵗʰ **V00.812 Wheelchair (powered) colliding with stationary object**

✓7ᵗʰ **V00.818 Other accident with wheelchair (powered)**

✓6ᵗʰ **V00.82 Accident with baby stroller**

✓7ᵗʰ **V00.821 Fall from baby stroller**

✓7ᵗʰ **V00.822 Baby stroller colliding with stationary object**

✓7ᵗʰ **V00.828 Other accident with baby stroller**

✓6ᵗʰ **V00.83 Accident with motorized mobility scooter**

✓7ᵗʰ **V00.831 Fall from motorized mobility scooter**
     EXCLUDES 1   *fall from non-moving motorized mobility scooter (W05.2)*

✓7ᵗʰ **V00.832 Motorized mobility scooter colliding with stationary object**

✓7ᵗʰ **V00.838 Other accident with motorized mobility scooter**

✓6ᵗʰ **V00.89 Accident on other pedestrian conveyance**

✓7ᵗʰ **V00.891 Fall from other pedestrian conveyance**

✓7ᵗʰ **V00.892 Pedestrian on other pedestrian conveyance colliding with stationary object**

✓7ᵗʰ **V00.898 Other accident on other pedestrian conveyance**
     EXCLUDES 1   *other pedestrian (conveyance) collision with other land transport vehicle (V01-V09 with 5th character 9)*

✓4ᵗʰ **V01 Pedestrian injured in collision with pedal cycle**

✓5ᵗʰ **V01.0 Pedestrian injured in collision with pedal cycle in nontraffic accident**

✓x7ᵗʰ **V01.00 Pedestrian on foot injured in collision with pedal cycle in nontraffic accident**
Pedestrian NOS injured in collision with pedal cycle in nontraffic accident

✓x7ᵗʰ **V01.01 Pedestrian on roller-skates injured in collision with pedal cycle in nontraffic accident**

✓x7ᵗʰ **V01.02 Pedestrian on skateboard injured in collision with pedal cycle in nontraffic accident**

✓x7ᵗʰ **V01.09 Pedestrian with other conveyance injured in collision with pedal cycle in nontraffic accident**
Pedestrian with baby stroller injured in collision with pedal cycle in nontraffic accident
Pedestrian on ice-skates injured in collision with pedal cycle in nontraffic accident
Pedestrian on nonmotorized scooter injured in collision with pedal cycle in nontraffic accident
Pedestrian on sled injured in collision with pedal cycle in nontraffic accident
Pedestrian on snowboard injured in collision with pedal cycle in nontraffic accident
Pedestrian on snow-skis injured in collision with pedal cycle in nontraffic accident
Pedestrian in wheelchair (powered) injured in collision with pedal cycle in nontraffic accident
Pedestrian in motorized mobility scooter injured in collision with pedal cycle in nontraffic accident

✓5ᵗʰ **V01.1 Pedestrian injured in collision with pedal cycle in traffic accident**

✓x7ᵗʰ **V01.10 Pedestrian on foot injured in collision with pedal cycle in traffic accident**
Pedestrian NOS injured in collision with pedal cycle in traffic accident

✓x7ᵗʰ **V01.11 Pedestrian on roller-skates injured in collision with pedal cycle in traffic accident**

✓x7ᵗʰ **V01.12 Pedestrian on skateboard injured in collision with pedal cycle in traffic accident**

✓x7ᵗʰ **V01.19 Pedestrian with other conveyance injured in collision with pedal cycle in traffic accident**
Pedestrian with baby stroller injured in collision with pedal cycle in traffic accident
Pedestrian on ice-skates injured in collision with pedal cycle in traffic accident
Pedestrian on nonmotorized scooter injured in collision with pedal cycle in traffic accident
Pedestrian on sled injured in collision with pedal cycle in traffic accident
Pedestrian on snowboard injured in collision with pedal cycle in traffic accident
Pedestrian on snow-skis injured in collision with pedal cycle in traffic accident
Pedestrian in wheelchair (powered) injured in collision with pedal cycle in traffic accident
Pedestrian in motorized mobility scooter injured in collision with pedal cycle in traffic accident

✓5ᵗʰ **V01.9 Pedestrian injured in collision with pedal cycle, unspecified whether traffic or nontraffic accident**

✓x7ᵗʰ **V01.90 Pedestrian on foot injured in collision with pedal cycle, unspecified whether traffic or nontraffic accident**
Pedestrian NOS injured in collision with pedal cycle, unspecified whether traffic or nontraffic accident

✓x7ᵗʰ **V01.91 Pedestrian on roller-skates injured in collision with pedal cycle, unspecified whether traffic or nontraffic accident**

✓x7ᵗʰ **V01.92 Pedestrian on skateboard injured in collision with pedal cycle, unspecified whether traffic or nontraffic accident**

✓ Additional Character Required   ✓x7ᵗʰ Placeholder Alert   Manifestation   Unspecified Dx   ▶◀ Revised Text   ● New Code   ▲ Revised Code Title

☑x7ᵗʰ V01.99 Pedestrian with other conveyance injured in collision with pedal cycle, unspecified whether traffic or nontraffic accident

Pedestrian with baby stroller injured in collision with pedal cycle, unspecified whether traffic or nontraffic accident

Pedestrian on ice-skates injured in collision with pedal cycle unspecified, whether traffic or nontraffic accident

Pedestrian on nonmotorized scooter injured in collision with pedal cycle, unspecified whether traffic or nontraffic accident

Pedestrian on sled injured in collision with pedal cycle unspecified, whether traffic or nontraffic accident

Pedestrian on snowboard injured in collision with pedal cycle, unspecified whether traffic or nontraffic accident

Pedestrian on snow-skis injured in collision with pedal cycle, unspecified whether traffic or nontraffic accident

Pedestrian in wheelchair (powered) injured in collision with pedal cycle, unspecified whether traffic or nontraffic accident

Pedestrian in motorized mobility scooter injured in collision with pedal cycle, unspecified whether traffic or nontraffic accident

☑4ᵗʰ V02 Pedestrian injured in collision with two- or three-wheeled motor vehicle

☑5ᵗʰ V02.0 Pedestrian injured in collision with two- or three-wheeled motor vehicle in nontraffic accident

☑x7ᵗʰ V02.00 Pedestrian on foot injured in collision with two- or three-wheeled motor vehicle in nontraffic accident

Pedestrian NOS injured in collision with two- or three-wheeled motor vehicle in nontraffic accident

☑x7ᵗʰ V02.01 Pedestrian on roller-skates injured in collision with two- or three-wheeled motor vehicle in nontraffic accident

☑x7ᵗʰ V02.02 Pedestrian on skateboard injured in collision with two- or three-wheeled motor vehicle in nontraffic accident

☑x7ᵗʰ V02.09 Pedestrian with other conveyance injured in collision with two- or three-wheeled motor vehicle in nontraffic accident

Pedestrian with baby stroller injured in collision with two- or three-wheeled motor vehicle in nontraffic accident

Pedestrian on ice-skates injured in collision with two- or three-wheeled motor vehicle in nontraffic accident

Pedestrian on nonmotorized scooter injured in collision with two- or three-wheeled motor vehicle in nontraffic accident

Pedestrian on sled injured in collision with two- or three-wheeled motor vehicle in nontraffic accident

Pedestrian on snowboard injured in collision with two- or three-wheeled motor vehicle in nontraffic accident

Pedestrian on snow-skis injured in collision with two- or three-wheeled motor vehicle in nontraffic accident

Pedestrian in wheelchair (powered) injured in collision with two- or three-wheeled motor vehicle in nontraffic accident

Pedestrian in motorized mobility scooter injured in collision with two- or three-wheeled motor vehicle in nontraffic accident

☑5ᵗʰ V02.1 Pedestrian injured in collision with two- or three-wheeled motor vehicle in traffic accident

☑x7ᵗʰ V02.10 Pedestrian on foot injured in collision with two- or three-wheeled motor vehicle in traffic accident

Pedestrian NOS injured in collision with two- or three-wheeled motor vehicle in traffic accident

☑x7ᵗʰ V02.11 Pedestrian on roller-skates injured in collision with two- or three-wheeled motor vehicle in traffic accident

☑x7ᵗʰ V02.12 Pedestrian on skateboard injured in collision with two- or three-wheeled motor vehicle in traffic accident

☑x7ᵗʰ V02.19 Pedestrian with other conveyance injured in collision with two- or three-wheeled motor vehicle in traffic accident

Pedestrian with baby stroller injured in collision with two- or three-wheeled motor vehicle in traffic accident

Pedestrian on ice-skates injured in collision with two- or three-wheeled motor vehicle in traffic accident

Pedestrian on nonmotorized scooter injured in collision with two- or three-wheeled motor vehicle in traffic accident

Pedestrian on sled injured in collision with two- or three-wheeled motor vehicle in traffic accident

Pedestrian on snowboard injured in collision with two- or three-wheeled motor vehicle in traffic accident

Pedestrian on snow-skis injured in collision with two- or three-wheeled motor vehicle in traffic accident

Pedestrian in wheelchair (powered) injured in collision with two- or three-wheeled motor vehicle in traffic accident

Pedestrian in motorized mobility scooter injured in collision with two- or three-wheeled motor vehicle in traffic accident

☑5ᵗʰ V02.9 Pedestrian injured in collision with two- or three-wheeled motor vehicle, unspecified whether traffic or nontraffic accident

☑x7ᵗʰ V02.90 Pedestrian on foot injured in collision with two- or three-wheeled motor vehicle, unspecified whether traffic or nontraffic accident

Pedestrian NOS injured in collision with two- or three-wheeled motor vehicle, unspecified whether traffic or nontraffic accident

☑x7ᵗʰ V02.91 Pedestrian on roller-skates injured in collision with two- or three-wheeled motor vehicle, unspecified whether traffic or nontraffic accident

☑x7ᵗʰ V02.92 Pedestrian on skateboard injured in collision with two- or three-wheeled motor vehicle, unspecified whether traffic or nontraffic accident

☑x7ᵗʰ V02.99 Pedestrian with other conveyance injured in collision with two- or three-wheeled motor vehicle, unspecified whether traffic or nontraffic accident

Pedestrian with baby stroller injured in collision with two- or three-wheeled motor vehicle, unspecified whether traffic or nontraffic accident

Pedestrian on ice-skates injured in collision with two- or three-wheeled motor vehicle, unspecified whether traffic or nontraffic accident

Pedestrian on nonmotorized scooter injured in collision with two- or three-wheeled motor vehicle, unspecified whether traffic or nontraffic accident

Pedestrian on sled injured in collision with two- or three-wheeled motor vehicle, unspecified whether traffic or nontraffic accident

Pedestrian on snowboard injured in collision with two- or three-wheeled motor vehicle, unspecified whether traffic or nontraffic accident

Pedestrian on snow-skis injured in collision with two- or three-wheeled motor vehicle, unspecified whether traffic or nontraffic accident

Pedestrian in wheelchair (powered) injured in collision with two- or three-wheeled motor vehicle, unspecified whether traffic or nontraffic accident

Pedestrian in motorized mobility scooter injured in collision with two- or three wheeled motor vehicle, unspecified whether traffic or nontraffic accident

☑4ᵗʰ V03 Pedestrian injured in collision with car, pick-up truck or van

☑5ᵗʰ V03.0 Pedestrian injured in collision with car, pick-up truck or van in nontraffic accident

☑x7ᵗʰ V03.00 Pedestrian on foot injured in collision with car, pick-up truck or van in nontraffic accident

Pedestrian NOS injured in collision with car, pick-up truck or van in nontraffic accident

☑x7ᵗʰ V03.01 Pedestrian on roller-skates injured in collision with car, pick-up truck or van in nontraffic accident

√x 7ᵗʰ   **V03.02**   **Pedestrian** on skateboard **injured in collision with car, pick-up truck or van in nontraffic accident**

√x 7ᵗʰ   **V03.09**   **Pedestrian with other conveyance injured in collision with car, pick-up truck or van in nontraffic accident**

Pedestrian with baby stroller injured in collision with car, pick-up truck or van in nontraffic accident

Pedestrian on ice-skates injured in collision with car, pick-up truck or van in nontraffic accident

Pedestrian on nonmotorized scooter injured in collision with car, pick-up truck or van in nontraffic accident

Pedestrian on sled injured in collision with car, pick-up truck or van in nontraffic accident

Pedestrian on snowboard injured in collision with car, pick-up truck or van in nontraffic accident

Pedestrian on snow-skis injured in collision with car, pick-up truck or van in nontraffic accident

Pedestrian in wheelchair (powered) injured in collision with car, pick-up truck or van in nontraffic accident

Pedestrian in motorized mobility scooter injured in collision with car, pick-up truck or van in nontraffic accident

√5ᵗʰ   **V03.1**   **Pedestrian injured in collision with car, pick-up truck or van in traffic accident**

√x 7ᵗʰ   **V03.10**   **Pedestrian** on foot **injured in collision with car, pick-up truck or van in traffic accident**

Pedestrian NOS injured in collision with car, pick-up truck or van in traffic accident

√x 7ᵗʰ   **V03.11**   **Pedestrian** on roller-skates **injured in collision with car, pick-up truck or van in traffic accident**

√x 7ᵗʰ   **V03.12**   **Pedestrian** on skateboard **injured in collision with car, pick-up truck or van in traffic accident**

√x 7ᵗʰ   **V03.19**   **Pedestrian with other conveyance injured in collision with car, pick-up truck or van in traffic accident**

Pedestrian with baby stroller injured in collision with car, pick-up truck or van in traffic accident

Pedestrian on ice-skates injured in collision with car, pick-up truck or van in traffic accident

Pedestrian on nonmotorized scooter injured in collision with car, pick-up truck or van in nontraffic accident

Pedestrian on sled injured in collision with car, pick-up truck or van in traffic accident

Pedestrian on snowboard injured in collision with car, plck-up truck or van in traffic accident

Pedestrian on snow-skis injured in collision with car, pick-up truck or van in traffic accident

Pedestrian in wheelchair (powered) injured in collision with car, pick-up truck or van in traffic accident

Pedestrian in motorized mobility scooter injured in collision with car, pick-up truck or van in nontraffic accident

√5ᵗʰ   **V03.9**   **Pedestrian injured in collision with car, pick-up truck or van, unspecified whether traffic or nontraffic accident**

√x 7ᵗʰ   **V03.90**   **Pedestrian** on foot **injured in collision with car, pick-up truck or van, unspecified whether traffic or nontraffic accident**

Pedestrian NOS injured in collision with car, pick-up truck or van, unspecified whether traffic or nontraffic accident

√x 7ᵗʰ   **V03.91**   **Pedestrian** on roller-skates **injured in collision with car, pick-up truck or van, unspecified whether traffic or nontraffic accident**

√x 7ᵗʰ   **V03.92**   **Pedestrian** on skateboard **injured in collision with car, pick-up truck or van, unspecified whether traffic or nontraffic accident**

√x 7ᵗʰ   **V03.99**   **Pedestrian with other conveyance injured in collision with car, pick-up truck or van, unspecified whether traffic or nontraffic accident**

Pedestrian with baby stroller injured in collision with car, pick-up truck or van, unspecified whether traffic or nontraffic accident

Pedestrian on ice-skates injured in collision with car, pick-up truck or van, unspecified whether traffic or nontraffic accident

Pedestrian on nonmotorized scooter injured in collision with car, pick-up truck or van, unspecified whether traffic or nontraffic accident

Pedestrian on sled injured in collision with car, pick-up truck or van in nontraffic accident

Pedestrian on snowboard injured in collision with car, pick-up truck or van, unspecified whether traffic or nontraffic accident

Pedestrian on snow-skis injured in collision with car, pick-up truck or van, unspecified whether traffic or nontraffic accident

Pedestrian in wheelchair (powered) injured in collision with car, pick-up truck or van, unspecified whether traffic or nontraffic accident

Pedestrian in motorized mobility scooter injured in collision with car, pick-up truck or van, unspecified whether traffic or nontraffic accident

√4ᵗʰ   **V04**   **Pedestrian injured in collision with heavy transport vehicle or bus**

EXCLUDES 1   pedestrian injured in collision with military vehicle (V09.01, V09.21)

√5ᵗʰ   **V04.0**   **Pedestrian injured in collision with heavy transport vehicle or bus in nontraffic accident**

√x 7ᵗʰ   **V04.00**   **Pedestrian** on foot **injured in collision with heavy transport vehicle or bus in nontraffic accident**

Pedestrian NOS injured in collision with heavy transport vehicle or bus in nontraffic accident

√x 7ᵗʰ   **V04.01**   **Pedestrian** on roller-skates **injured in collision with heavy transport vehicle or bus in nontraffic accident**

√x 7ᵗʰ   **V04.02**   **Pedestrian** on skateboard **injured in collision with heavy transport vehicle or bus in nontraffic accident**

√x 7ᵗʰ   **V04.09**   **Pedestrian with other conveyance injured in collision with heavy transport vehicle or bus in nontraffic accident**

Pedestrian with baby stroller injured in collision with heavy transport vehicle or bus in nontraffic accident

Pedestrian on ice-skates injured in collision with heavy transport vehicle or bus in nontraffic accident

Pedestrian on nonmotorized scooter injured in collision with heavy transport vehicle or bus in nontraffic accident

Pedestrian on sled injured in collision with heavy transport vehicle or bus in nontraffic accident

Pedestrian on snowboard injured in collision with heavy transport vehicle or bus in nontraffic accident

Pedestrian on snow-skis injured in collision with heavy transport vehicle or bus in nontraffic accident

Pedestrian in wheelchair (powered) injured in collision with heavy transport vehicle or bus in nontraffic accident

Pedestrian in motorized mobility scooter injured in collision with heavy transport vehicle or bus in nontraffic accident

√5ᵗʰ   **V04.1**   **Pedestrian injured in collision with heavy transport vehicle or bus in traffic accident**

√x 7ᵗʰ   **V04.10**   **Pedestrian** on foot **injured in collision with heavy transport vehicle or bus in traffic accident**

Pedestrian NOS injured in collision with heavy transport vehicle or bus in traffic accident

√x 7ᵗʰ   **V04.11**   **Pedestrian** on roller-skates **injured in collision with heavy transport vehicle or bus in traffic accident**

√x 7ᵗʰ   **V04.12**   **Pedestrian** on skateboard **injured in collision with heavy transport vehicle or bus in traffic accident**

☑ Additional Character Required   √x 7ᵗʰ Placeholder Alert   Manifestation   Unspecified Dx   ►◄ Revised Text   ● New Code   ▲ Revised Code Title

ICD-10-CM 2020   1157

√x 7th **V04.19 Pedestrian with other conveyance injured in collision with heavy transport vehicle or bus in traffic accident**

Pedestrian with baby stroller injured in collision with heavy transport vehicle or bus in traffic accident

Pedestrian on ice-skates injured in collision with heavy transport vehicle or bus in traffic accident

Pedestrian on nonmotorized scooter injured in collision with heavy transport vehicle or bus in traffic accident

Pedestrian on sled injured in collision with heavy transport vehicle or bus in traffic accident

Pedestrian on snowboard injured in collision with heavy transport vehicle or bus in traffic accident

Pedestrian on snow-skis injured in collision with heavy transport vehicle or bus in traffic accident

Pedestrian in wheelchair (powered) injured in collision with heavy transport vehicle or bus in traffic accident

Pedestrian in motorized mobility scooter injured in collision with heavy transport vehicle or bus in traffic accident

√5th **V04.9 Pedestrian injured in collision with heavy transport vehicle or bus, unspecified whether traffic or nontraffic accident**

√x 7th **V04.90 Pedestrian on foot injured in collision with heavy transport vehicle or bus, unspecified whether traffic or nontraffic accident**

Pedestrian NOS injured in collision with heavy transport vehicle or bus, unspecified whether traffic or nontraffic accident

√x 7th **V04.91 Pedestrian on roller-skates injured in collision with heavy transport vehicle or bus, unspecified whether traffic or nontraffic accident**

√x 7th **V04.92 Pedestrian on skateboard injured in collision with heavy transport vehicle or bus, unspecified whether traffic or nontraffic accident**

√x 7th **V04.99 Pedestrian with other conveyance injured in collision with heavy transport vehicle or bus, unspecified whether traffic or nontraffic accident**

Pedestrian with baby stroller injured in collision with heavy transport vehicle or bus, unspecified whether traffic or nontraffic accident

Pedestrian on ice-skates injured in collision with heavy transport vehicle or bus, unspecified whether traffic or nontraffic accident

Pedestrian on nonmotorized scooter injured in collision with heavy transport vehicle or bus, unspecified whether traffic or nontraffic accident

Pedestrian on sled injured in collision with heavy transport vehicle or bus, unspecified whether traffic or nontraffic accident

Pedestrian on snowboard injured in collision with heavy transport vehicle or bus, unspecified whether traffic or nontraffic accident

Pedestrian on snow-skis injured in collision with heavy transport vehicle or bus, unspecified whether traffic or nontraffic accident

Pedestrian in wheelchair (powered) injured in collision with heavy transport vehicle or bus, unspecified whether traffic or nontraffic accident

Pedestrian in motorized mobility scooter injured in collision with heavy transport vehicle or bus, unspecified whether traffic or nontraffic accident

√4th **V05 Pedestrian injured in collision with railway train or railway vehicle**

√5th **V05.0 Pedestrian injured in collision with railway train or railway vehicle in nontraffic accident**

√x 7th **V05.00 Pedestrian on foot injured in collision with railway train or railway vehicle in nontraffic accident**

Pedestrian NOS injured in collision with railway train or railway vehicle in nontraffic accident

√x 7th **V05.01 Pedestrian on roller-skates injured in collision with railway train or railway vehicle in nontraffic accident**

√x 7th **V05.02 Pedestrian on skateboard injured in collision with railway train or railway vehicle in nontraffic accident**

√x 7th **V05.09 Pedestrian with other conveyance injured in collision with railway train or railway vehicle in nontraffic accident**

Pedestrian with baby stroller injured in collision with railway train or railway vehicle in nontraffic accident

Pedestrian on ice-skates injured in collision with railway train or railway vehicle in nontraffic accident

Pedestrian on nonmotorized scooter injured in collision with railway train or railway vehicle in nontraffic accident

Pedestrian on sled injured in collision with railway train or railway vehicle in nontraffic accident

Pedestrian on snowboard injured in collision with railway train or railway vehicle in nontraffic accident

Pedestrian on snow-skis injured in collision with railway train or railway vehicle in nontraffic accident

Pedestrian in wheelchair (powered) injured in collision with railway train or railway vehicle in nontraffic accident

Pedestrian in motorized mobility scooter injured in collision with railway train or railway vehicle in nontraffic accident

√5th **V05.1 Pedestrian injured in collision with railway train or railway vehicle in traffic accident**

√x 7th **V05.10 Pedestrian on foot injured in collision with railway train or railway vehicle in traffic accident**

Pedestrian NOS injured in collision with railway train or railway vehicle in traffic accident

√x 7th **V05.11 Pedestrian on roller-skates injured in collision with railway train or railway vehicle in traffic accident**

√x 7th **V05.12 Pedestrian on skateboard injured in collision with railway train or railway vehicle in traffic accident**

√x 7th **V05.19 Pedestrian with other conveyance injured in collision with railway train or railway vehicle in traffic accident**

Pedestrian with baby stroller injured in collision with railway train or railway vehicle in traffic accident

Pedestrian on ice-skates injured in collision with railway train or railway vehicle in traffic accident

Pedestrian on nonmotorized scooter injured in collision with railway train or railway vehicle in traffic accident

Pedestrian on sled injured in collision with railway train or railway vehicle in traffic accident

Pedestrian on snowboard injured in collision with railway train or railway vehicle in traffic accident

Pedestrian on snow-skis injured in collision with railway train or railway vehicle in traffic accident

Pedestrian in wheelchair (powered) injured in collision with railway train or railway vehicle in traffic accident

Pedestrian in motorized mobility scooter injured in collision with railway train or railway vehicle in traffic accident

√5th **V05.9 Pedestrian injured in collision with railway train or railway vehicle, unspecified whether traffic or nontraffic accident**

√x 7th **V05.90 Pedestrian on foot injured in collision with railway train or railway vehicle, unspecified whether traffic or nontraffic accident**

Pedestrian NOS injured in collision with railway train or railway vehicle, unspecified whether traffic or nontraffic accident

√x 7th **V05.91 Pedestrian on roller-skates injured in collision with railway train or railway vehicle, unspecified whether traffic or nontraffic accident**

√x 7th **V05.92 Pedestrian on skateboard injured in collision with railway train or railway vehicle, unspecified whether traffic or nontraffic accident**

√x7ᵗʰ **V05.99** **Pedestrian with other conveyance injured in collision with railway train or railway vehicle, unspecified whether traffic or nontraffic accident**

Pedestrian with baby stroller injured in collision with railway train or railway vehicle, unspecified whether traffic or nontraffic

Pedestrian on ice-skates injured in collision with railway train or railway vehicle, unspecified whether traffic or nontraffic

Pedestrian on nonmotorized scooter injured in collision with railway train or railway vehicle, unspecified whether traffic or nontraffic

Pedestrian on sled injured in collision with railway train or railway vehicle, unspecified whether traffic or nontraffic

Pedestrian on snowboard injured in collision with railway train or railway vehicle, unspecified whether traffic or nontraffic

Pedestrian on snow-skis injured in collision with railway train or railway vehicle, unspecified whether traffic or nontraffic

Pedestrian in wheelchair (powered) injured in collision with railway train or railway vehicle, unspecified whether traffic or nontraffic

Pedestrian in motorized mobility scooter injured in collision with railway train or railway vehicle, unspecified whether traffic or nontraffic

√4ᵗʰ **V06** **Pedestrian injured in collision with other nonmotor vehicle**

INCLUDES   collision with animal-drawn vehicle, animal being ridden, nonpowered streetcar

EXCLUDES 1   *pedestrian injured in collision with pedestrian conveyance (V00.0-)*

√5ᵗʰ **V06.0** **Pedestrian injured in collision with other nonmotor vehicle in nontraffic accident**

√x7ᵗʰ **V06.00** **Pedestrian on foot injured in collision with other nonmotor vehicle in nontraffic accident**

Pedestrian NOS injured in collision with other nonmotor vehicle in nontraffic accident

√x7ᵗʰ **V06.01** **Pedestrian on roller-skates injured in collision with other nonmotor vehicle in nontraffic accident**

√x7ᵗʰ **V06.02** **Pedestrian on skateboard injured in collision with other nonmotor vehicle in nontraffic accident**

√x7ᵗʰ **V06.09** **Pedestrian with other conveyance injured in collision with other nonmotor vehicle in nontraffic accident**

Pedestrian with baby stroller injured in collision with other nonmotor vehicle in nontraffic accident

Pedestrian on ice-skates injured in collision with other nonmotor vehicle in nontraffic accident

Pedestrian on nonmotorized scooter injured in collision with other nonmotor vehicle in nontraffic accident

Pedestrian on sled injured in collision with other nonmotor vehicle in nontraffic accident

Pedestrian on snowboard injured in collision with other nonmotor vehicle in nontraffic accident

Pedestrian on snow-skis injured in collision with other nonmotor vehicle in nontraffic accident

Pedestrian in wheelchair (powered) injured in collision with other nonmotor vehicle in nontraffic accident

Pedestrian in motorized mobility scooter injured in collision with other nonmotor vehicle in nontraffic accident

√5ᵗʰ **V06.1** **Pedestrian injured in collision with other nonmotor vehicle in traffic accident**

√x7ᵗʰ **V06.10** **Pedestrian on foot injured in collision with other nonmotor vehicle in traffic accident**

Pedestrian NOS injured in collision with other nonmotor vehicle in traffic accident

√x7ᵗʰ **V06.11** **Pedestrian on roller-skates injured in collision with other nonmotor vehicle in traffic accident**

√x7ᵗʰ **V06.12** **Pedestrian on skateboard injured in collision with other nonmotor vehicle in traffic accident**

√x7ᵗʰ **V06.19** **Pedestrian with other conveyance injured in collision with other nonmotor vehicle in traffic accident**

Pedestrian with baby stroller injured in collision with other nonmotor vehicle in nontraffic accident

Pedestrian on ice-skates injured in collision with other nonmotor vehicle in traffic accident

Pedestrian on nonmotorized scooter injured in collision with other nonmotor vehicle in traffic accident

Pedestrian on sled injured in collision with other nonmotor vehicle in traffic accident

Pedestrian on snowboard injured in collision with other nonmotor vehicle in traffic accident

Pedestrian on snow-skis injured in collision with other nonmotor vehicle in traffic accident

Pedestrian in wheelchair (powered) injured in collision with other nonmotor vehicle in traffic accident

Pedestrian in motorized mobility scooter injured in collision with other nonmotor vehicle in traffic accident

√5ᵗʰ **V06.9** **Pedestrian injured in collision with other nonmotor vehicle, unspecified whether traffic or nontraffic accident**

√x7ᵗʰ **V06.90** **Pedestrian on foot injured in collision with other nonmotor vehicle, unspecified whether traffic or nontraffic accident**

Pedestrian NOS injured in collision with other nonmotor vehicle, unspecified whether traffic or nontraffic accident

√x7ᵗʰ **V06.91** **Pedestrian on roller-skates injured in collision with other nonmotor vehicle, unspecified whether traffic or nontraffic accident**

√x7ᵗʰ **V06.92** **Pedestrian on skateboard injured in collision with other nonmotor vehicle, unspecified whether traffic or nontraffic accident**

√x7ᵗʰ **V06.99** **Pedestrian with other conveyance injured in collision with other nonmotor vehicle, unspecified whether traffic or nontraffic accident**

Pedestrian with baby stroller injured in collision with other nonmotor vehicle, unspecified whether traffic or nontraffic accident

Pedestrian on ice-skates injured in collision with other nonmotor vehicle, unspecified whether traffic or nontraffic accident

Pedestrian on nonmotorized scooter injured in collision with other nonmotor vehicle, unspecified whether traffic or nontraffic accident

Pedestrian on sled injured in collision with other nonmotor vehicle, unspecified whether traffic or nontraffic accident

Pedestrian on snowboard injured in collision with other nonmotor vehicle, unspecified whether traffic or nontraffic accident

Pedestrian on snow-skis injured in collision with other nonmotor vehicle, unspecified whether traffic or nontraffic accident

Pedestrian in wheelchair (powered) injured in collision with other nonmotor vehicle, unspecified whether traffic or nontraffic accident

Pedestrian in motorized mobility scooter injured in collision with other nonmotorized vehicle, unspecified whether traffic or nontraffic accident

√4ᵗʰ **V09** **Pedestrian injured in other and unspecified transport accidents**

√5ᵗʰ **V09.0** **Pedestrian injured in nontraffic accident involving other and unspecified motor vehicles**

√x7ᵗʰ **V09.00** **Pedestrian injured in nontraffic accident involving unspecified motor vehicles**

√x7ᵗʰ **V09.01** **Pedestrian injured in nontraffic accident involving military vehicle**

√x7ᵗʰ **V09.09** **Pedestrian injured in nontraffic accident involving other motor vehicles**

Pedestrian injured in nontraffic accident by special vehicle

√x7ᵗʰ **V09.1** **Pedestrian injured in unspecified nontraffic accident**

√5ᵗʰ **V09.2** **Pedestrian injured in traffic accident involving other and unspecified motor vehicles**

√x7ᵗʰ **V09.20** **Pedestrian injured in traffic accident involving unspecified motor vehicles**

√x7ᵗʰ **V09.21** **Pedestrian injured in traffic accident involving military vehicle**

☑ Additional Character Required   √x7ᵗʰ Placeholder Alert   Manifestation   Unspecified Dx   ►◄ Revised Text   ● New Code   ▲ Revised Code Title

ICD-10-CM 2020   1159

√x7th **V09.29** Pedestrian injured in traffic accident involving other motor vehicles

√x7th **V09.3** Pedestrian injured in unspecified traffic accident

√x7th **V09.9** Pedestrian injured in unspecified transport accident

Pedal cycle rider injured in transport accident (V10-V19)

INCLUDES any non-motorized vehicle, excluding an animal-drawn vehicle, or a sidecar or trailer attached to the pedal cycle

EXCLUDES 2 rupture of pedal cycle tire (W37.0)

The appropriate 7th character is to be added to each code from categories V10-V19.
A initial encounter
D subsequent encounter
S sequela

√4th **V10** Pedal cycle rider injured in collision with pedestrian or animal

EXCLUDES 1 pedal cycle rider collision with animal-drawn vehicle or animal being ridden (V16.-)

√x7th **V10.0** Pedal cycle driver injured in collision with pedestrian or animal in nontraffic accident

√x7th **V10.1** Pedal cycle passenger injured in collision with pedestrian or animal in nontraffic accident

√x7th **V10.2** Unspecified pedal cyclist injured in collision with pedestrian or animal in nontraffic accident

√x7th **V10.3** Person boarding or alighting a pedal cycle injured in collision with pedestrian or animal

√x7th **V10.4** Pedal cycle driver injured in collision with pedestrian or animal in traffic accident

√x7th **V10.5** Pedal cycle passenger injured in collision with pedestrian or animal in traffic accident

√x7th **V10.9** Unspecified pedal cyclist injured in collision with pedestrian or animal in traffic accident

√4th **V11** Pedal cycle rider injured in collision with other pedal cycle

√x7th **V11.0** Pedal cycle driver injured in collision with other pedal cycle in nontraffic accident

√x7th **V11.1** Pedal cycle passenger injured in collision with other pedal cycle in nontraffic accident

√x7th **V11.2** Unspecified pedal cyclist injured in collision with other pedal cycle in nontraffic accident

√x7th **V11.3** Person boarding or alighting a pedal cycle injured in collision with other pedal cycle

√x7th **V11.4** Pedal cycle driver injured in collision with other pedal cycle in traffic accident

√x7th **V11.5** Pedal cycle passenger injured in collision with other pedal cycle in traffic accident

√x7th **V11.9** Unspecified pedal cyclist injured in collision with other pedal cycle in traffic accident

√4th **V12** Pedal cycle rider injured in collision with two- or three-wheeled motor vehicle

√x7th **V12.0** Pedal cycle driver injured in collision with two- or three-wheeled motor vehicle in nontraffic accident

√x7th **V12.1** Pedal cycle passenger injured in collision with two- or three-wheeled motor vehicle in nontraffic accident

√x7th **V12.2** Unspecified pedal cyclist injured in collision with two- or three-wheeled motor vehicle in nontraffic accident

√x7th **V12.3** Person boarding or alighting a pedal cycle injured in collision with two- or three-wheeled motor vehicle

√x7th **V12.4** Pedal cycle driver injured in collision with two- or three-wheeled motor vehicle in traffic accident

√x7th **V12.5** Pedal cycle passenger injured in collision with two- or three-wheeled motor vehicle in traffic accident

√x7th **V12.9** Unspecified pedal cyclist injured in collision with two- or three-wheeled motor vehicle in traffic accident

√4th **V13** Pedal cycle rider injured in collision with car, pick-up truck or van

√x7th **V13.0** Pedal cycle driver injured in collision with car, pick-up truck or van in nontraffic accident

√x7th **V13.1** Pedal cycle passenger injured in collision with car, pick-up truck or van in nontraffic accident

√x7th **V13.2** Unspecified pedal cyclist injured in collision with car, pick-up truck or van in nontraffic accident

√x7th **V13.3** Person boarding or alighting a pedal cycle injured in collision with car, pick-up truck or van

√x7th **V13.4** Pedal cycle driver injured in collision with car, pick-up truck or van in traffic accident

√x7th **V13.5** Pedal cycle passenger injured in collision with car, pick-up truck or van in traffic accident

√x7th **V13.9** Unspecified pedal cyclist injured in collision with car, pick-up truck or van in traffic accident

√4th **V14** Pedal cycle rider injured in collision with heavy transport vehicle or bus

EXCLUDES 1 pedal cycle rider injured in collision with military vehicle (V19.81)

√x7th **V14.0** Pedal cycle driver injured in collision with heavy transport vehicle or bus in nontraffic accident

√x7th **V14.1** Pedal cycle passenger injured in collision with heavy transport vehicle or bus in nontraffic accident

√x7th **V14.2** Unspecified pedal cyclist injured in collision with heavy transport vehicle or bus in nontraffic accident

√x7th **V14.3** Person boarding or alighting a pedal cycle injured in collision with heavy transport vehicle or bus

√x7th **V14.4** Pedal cycle driver injured in collision with heavy transport vehicle or bus in traffic accident

√x7th **V14.5** Pedal cycle passenger injured in collision with heavy transport vehicle or bus in traffic accident

√x7th **V14.9** Unspecified pedal cyclist injured in collision with heavy transport vehicle or bus in traffic accident

√4th **V15** Pedal cycle rider injured in collision with railway train or railway vehicle

√x7th **V15.0** Pedal cycle driver injured in collision with railway train or railway vehicle in nontraffic accident

√x7th **V15.1** Pedal cycle passenger injured in collision with railway train or railway vehicle in nontraffic accident

√x7th **V15.2** Unspecified pedal cyclist injured in collision with railway train or railway vehicle in nontraffic accident

√x7th **V15.3** Person boarding or alighting a pedal cycle injured in collision with railway train or railway vehicle

√x7th **V15.4** Pedal cycle driver injured in collision with railway train or railway vehicle in traffic accident

√x7th **V15.5** Pedal cycle passenger injured in collision with railway train or railway vehicle in traffic accident

√x7th **V15.9** Unspecified pedal cyclist injured in collision with railway train or railway vehicle in traffic accident

√4th **V16** Pedal cycle rider injured in collision with other nonmotor vehicle

INCLUDES collision with animal-drawn vehicle, animal being ridden, streetcar

√x7th **V16.0** Pedal cycle driver injured in collision with other nonmotor vehicle in nontraffic accident

√x7th **V16.1** Pedal cycle passenger injured in collision with other nonmotor vehicle in nontraffic accident

√x7th **V16.2** Unspecified pedal cyclist injured in collision with other nonmotor vehicle in nontraffic accident

√x7th **V16.3** Person boarding or alighting a pedal cycle injured in collision with other nonmotor vehicle in nontraffic accident

√x7th **V16.4** Pedal cycle driver injured in collision with other nonmotor vehicle in traffic accident

√x7th **V16.5** Pedal cycle passenger injured in collision with other nonmotor vehicle in traffic accident

√x7th **V16.9** Unspecified pedal cyclist injured in collision with other nonmotor vehicle in traffic accident

√4th **V17** Pedal cycle rider injured in collision with fixed or stationary object

√x7th **V17.0** Pedal cycle driver injured in collision with fixed or stationary object in nontraffic accident

√x7th **V17.1** Pedal cycle passenger injured in collision with fixed or stationary object in nontraffic accident

√x7th **V17.2** Unspecified pedal cyclist injured in collision with fixed or stationary object in nontraffic accident

√x7th **V17.3** Person boarding or alighting a pedal cycle injured in collision with fixed or stationary object

√x7th **V17.4** Pedal cycle driver injured in collision with fixed or stationary object in traffic accident

√x7th **V17.5** Pedal cycle passenger injured in collision with fixed or stationary object in traffic accident

√x7th **V17.9** Unspecified pedal cyclist injured in collision with fixed or stationary object in traffic accident

√4th **V18** Pedal cycle rider injured in noncollision transport accident

INCLUDES fall or thrown from pedal cycle (without antecedent collision)
overturning pedal cycle NOS
overturning pedal cycle without collision

√x7th **V18.0** Pedal cycle driver injured in noncollision transport accident in nontraffic accident

√x7th **V18.1** Pedal cycle passenger injured in noncollision transport accident in nontraffic accident

√x7th **V18.2** Unspecified pedal cyclist injured in noncollision transport accident in nontraffic accident

√x7th **V18.3** Person boarding or alighting a pedal cycle injured in noncollision transport accident

✓x7th **V18.4** Pedal cycle driver injured in noncollision transport accident in traffic accident

✓x7th **V18.5** Pedal cycle passenger injured in noncollision transport accident in traffic accident

✓x7th **V18.9** Unspecified pedal cyclist injured in noncollision transport accident in traffic accident

✓4th **V19 Pedal cycle rider injured in other and unspecified transport accidents**

  ✓5th **V19.0** Pedal cycle driver injured in collision with other and unspecified motor vehicles in nontraffic accident

    ✓x7th **V19.00** Pedal cycle driver injured in collision with unspecified motor vehicles in nontraffic accident

    ✓x7th **V19.09** Pedal cycle driver injured in collision with other motor vehicles in nontraffic accident

  ✓5th **V19.1** Pedal cycle passenger injured in collision with other and unspecified motor vehicles in nontraffic accident

    ✓x7th **V19.10** Pedal cycle passenger injured in collision with unspecified motor vehicles in nontraffic accident

    ✓x7th **V19.19** Pedal cycle passenger injured in collision with other motor vehicles in nontraffic accident

  ✓5th **V19.2** Unspecified pedal cyclist injured in collision with other and unspecified motor vehicles in nontraffic accident

    ✓x7th **V19.20** Unspecified pedal cyclist injured in collision with unspecified motor vehicles in nontraffic accident
           Pedal cycle collision NOS, nontraffic

    ✓x7th **V19.29** Unspecified pedal cyclist injured in collision with other motor vehicles in nontraffic accident

  ✓x7th **V19.3** Pedal cyclist (driver) (passenger) injured in unspecified nontraffic accident
          Pedal cycle accident NOS, nontraffic
          Pedal cyclist injured in nontraffic accident NOS

  ✓6th **V19.4** Pedal cycle driver injured in collision with other and unspecified motor vehicles in traffic accident

    ✓x7th **V19.40** Pedal cycle driver injured in collision with unspecified motor vehicles in traffic accident

    ✓x7th **V19.49** Pedal cycle driver injured in collision with other motor vehicles in traffic accident

  ✓6th **V19.5** Pedal cycle passenger injured in collision with other and unspecified motor vehicles in traffic accident

    ✓x7th **V19.50** Pedal cycle passenger injured in collision with unspecified motor vehicles in traffic accident

    ✓x7th **V19.59** Pedal cycle passenger injured in collision with other motor vehicles in traffic accident

  ✓6th **V19.6** Unspecified pedal cyclist injured in collision with other and unspecified motor vehicles in traffic accident

    ✓x7th **V19.60** Unspecified pedal cyclist injured in collision with unspecified motor vehicles in traffic accident
          Pedal cycle collision NOS (traffic)

    ✓x7th **V19.69** Unspecified pedal cyclist injured in collision with other motor vehicles in traffic accident

  ✓5th **V19.8** Pedal cyclist (driver) (passenger) injured in other specified transport accidents

    ✓x7th **V19.81** Pedal cyclist (driver) (passenger) injured in transport accident with military vehicle

    ✓x7th **V19.88** Pedal cyclist (driver) (passenger) injured in other specified transport accidents

  ✓x7th **V19.9** Pedal cyclist (driver) (passenger) injured in unspecified traffic accident
          Pedal cycle accident NOS

Motorcycle rider injured in transport accident (V20-V29)

INCLUDES   moped
            motorcycle with sidecar
            motorized bicycle
            motor scooter

EXCLUDES 1   *three-wheeled motor vehicle (V30-V39)*

The appropriate 7th character is to be added to each code from categories V20-V29.
A   initial encounter
D   subsequent encounter
S   sequela

✓4th **V20 Motorcycle rider injured in collision with pedestrian or animal**

    EXCLUDES 1   *motorcycle rider collision with animal-drawn vehicle or animal being ridden (V26.-)*

  ✓x7th **V20.0** Motorcycle driver injured in collision with pedestrian or animal in nontraffic accident

  ✓x7th **V20.1** Motorcycle passenger injured in collision with pedestrian or animal in nontraffic accident

  ✓x7th **V20.2** Unspecified motorcycle rider injured in collision with pedestrian or animal in nontraffic accident

  ✓x7th **V20.3** Person boarding or alighting a motorcycle injured in collision with pedestrian or animal

  ✓x7th **V20.4** Motorcycle driver injured in collision with pedestrian or animal in traffic accident

  ✓x7th **V20.5** Motorcycle passenger injured in collision with pedestrian or animal in traffic accident

  ✓x7th **V20.9** Unspecified motorcycle rider injured in collision with pedestrian or animal in traffic accident

✓4th **V21 Motorcycle rider injured in collision with pedal cycle**

  ✓x7th **V21.0** Motorcycle driver injured in collision with pedal cycle in nontraffic accident

  ✓x7th **V21.1** Motorcycle passenger injured in collision with pedal cycle in nontraffic accident

  ✓x7th **V21.2** Unspecified motorcycle rider injured in collision with pedal cycle in nontraffic accident

  ✓x7th **V21.3** Person boarding or alighting a motorcycle injured in collision with pedal cycle

  ✓x7th **V21.4** Motorcycle driver injured in collision with pedal cycle in traffic accident

  ✓x7th **V21.5** Motorcycle passenger injured in collision with pedal cycle in traffic accident

  ✓x7th **V21.9** Unspecified motorcycle rider injured in collision with pedal cycle in traffic accident

✓4th **V22 Motorcycle rider injured in collision with two- or three-wheeled motor vehicle**

  ✓x7th **V22.0** Motorcycle driver injured in collision with two- or three-wheeled motor vehicle in nontraffic accident

  ✓x7th **V22.1** Motorcycle passenger injured in collision with two- or three-wheeled motor vehicle in nontraffic accident

  ✓x7th **V22.2** Unspecified motorcycle rider injured in collision with two- or three-wheeled motor vehicle in nontraffic accident

  ✓x7th **V22.3** Person boarding or alighting a motorcycle injured in collision with two- or three-wheeled motor vehicle

  ✓x7th **V22.4** Motorcycle driver injured in collision with two- or three-wheeled motor vehicle in traffic accident

  ✓x7th **V22.5** Motorcycle passenger injured in collision with two- or three-wheeled motor vehicle in traffic accident

  ✓x7th **V22.9** Unspecified motorcycle rider injured in collision with two- or three-wheeled motor vehicle in traffic accident

✓4th **V23 Motorcycle rider injured in collision with car, pick-up truck or van**

  ✓x7th **V23.0** Motorcycle driver injured in collision with car, pick-up truck or van in nontraffic accident

  ✓x7th **V23.1** Motorcycle passenger injured in collision with car, pick-up truck or van in nontraffic accident

  ✓x7th **V23.2** Unspecified motorcycle rider injured in collision with car, pick-up truck or van in nontraffic accident

  ✓x7th **V23.3** Person boarding or alighting a motorcycle injured in collision with car, pick-up truck or van

  ✓x7th **V23.4** Motorcycle driver injured in collision with car, pick-up truck or van in traffic accident

  ✓x7th **V23.5** Motorcycle passenger injured in collision with car, pick-up truck or van in traffic accident

  ✓x7th **V23.9** Unspecified motorcycle rider injured in collision with car, pick-up truck or van in traffic accident

✓4th **V24 Motorcycle rider injured in collision with heavy transport vehicle or bus**

    EXCLUDES 1   *motorcycle rider injured in collision with military vehicle (V29.81)*

  ✓x7th **V24.0** Motorcycle driver injured in collision with heavy transport vehicle or bus in nontraffic accident

  ✓x7th **V24.1** Motorcycle passenger injured in collision with heavy transport vehicle or bus in nontraffic accident

  ✓x7th **V24.2** Unspecified motorcycle rider injured in collision with heavy transport vehicle or bus in nontraffic accident

  ✓x7th **V24.3** Person boarding or alighting a motorcycle injured in collision with heavy transport vehicle or bus

  ✓x7th **V24.4** Motorcycle driver injured in collision with heavy transport vehicle or bus in traffic accident

  ✓x7th **V24.5** Motorcycle passenger injured in collision with heavy transport vehicle or bus in traffic accident

  ✓x7th **V24.9** Unspecified motorcycle rider injured in collision with heavy transport vehicle or bus in traffic accident

✓4th **V25 Motorcycle rider injured in collision with railway train or railway vehicle**

  ✓x7th **V25.0** Motorcycle driver injured in collision with railway train or railway vehicle in nontraffic accident

  ✓x7th **V25.1** Motorcycle passenger injured in collision with railway train or railway vehicle in nontraffic accident

Chapter 20. External Causes of Morbidity

V25.2–V31.0

√x7ᵗʰ **V25.2** Unspecified motorcycle rider injured in collision with railway train or railway vehicle in nontraffic accident

√x7ᵗʰ **V25.3** Person boarding or alighting a motorcycle injured in collision with railway train or railway vehicle

√x7ᵗʰ **V25.4** Motorcycle driver injured in collision with railway train or railway vehicle in traffic accident

√x7ᵗʰ **V25.5** Motorcycle passenger injured in collision with railway train or railway vehicle in traffic accident

√x7ᵗʰ **V25.9** Unspecified motorcycle rider injured in collision with railway train or railway vehicle in traffic accident

√4ᵗʰ **V26** Motorcycle rider injured in collision with other nonmotor vehicle

INCLUDES collision with animal-drawn vehicle, animal being ridden, streetcar

√x7ᵗʰ **V26.0** Motorcycle driver injured in collision with other nonmotor vehicle in nontraffic accident

√x7ᵗʰ **V26.1** Motorcycle passenger injured in collision with other nonmotor vehicle in nontraffic accident

√x7ᵗʰ **V26.2** Unspecified motorcycle rider injured in collision with other nonmotor vehicle in nontraffic accident

√x7ᵗʰ **V26.3** Person boarding or alighting a motorcycle injured in collision with other nonmotor vehicle

√x7ᵗʰ **V26.4** Motorcycle driver injured in collision with other nonmotor vehicle in traffic accident

√x7ᵗʰ **V26.5** Motorcycle passenger injured in collision with other nonmotor vehicle in traffic accident

√x7ᵗʰ **V26.9** Unspecified motorcycle rider injured in collision with other nonmotor vehicle in traffic accident

√4ᵗʰ **V27** Motorcycle rider injured in collision with fixed or stationary object

√x7ᵗʰ **V27.0** Motorcycle driver injured in collision with fixed or stationary object in nontraffic accident

√x7ᵗʰ **V27.1** Motorcycle passenger injured in collision with fixed or stationary object in nontraffic accident

√x7ᵗʰ **V27.2** Unspecified motorcycle rider injured in collision with fixed or stationary object in nontraffic accident

√x7ᵗʰ **V27.3** Person boarding or alighting a motorcycle injured in collision with fixed or stationary object

√x7ᵗʰ **V27.4** Motorcycle driver injured in collision with fixed or stationary object in traffic accident

√x7ᵗʰ **V27.5** Motorcycle passenger injured in collision with fixed or stationary object in traffic accident

√x7ᵗʰ **V27.9** Unspecified motorcycle rider injured in collision with fixed or stationary object in traffic accident

√4ᵗʰ **V28** Motorcycle rider injured in noncollision transport accident

INCLUDES fall or thrown from motorcycle (without antecedent collision)
overturning motorcycle NOS
overturning motorcycle without collision

√x7ᵗʰ **V28.0** Motorcycle driver injured in noncollision transport accident in nontraffic accident

√x7ᵗʰ **V28.1** Motorcycle passenger injured in noncollision transport accident in nontraffic accident

√x7ᵗʰ **V28.2** Unspecified motorcycle rider injured in noncollision transport accident in nontraffic accident

√x7ᵗʰ **V28.3** Person boarding or alighting a motorcycle injured in noncollision transport accident

√x7ᵗʰ **V28.4** Motorcycle driver injured in noncollision transport accident in traffic accident

√x7ᵗʰ **V28.5** Motorcycle passenger injured in noncollision transport accident in traffic accident

√x7ᵗʰ **V28.9** Unspecified motorcycle rider injured in noncollision transport accident in traffic accident

√4ᵗʰ **V29** Motorcycle rider injured in other and unspecified transport accidents

√5ᵗʰ **V29.0** Motorcycle driver injured in collision with other and unspecified motor vehicles in nontraffic accident

√x7ᵗʰ **V29.00** Motorcycle driver injured in collision with unspecified motor vehicles in nontraffic accident

√x7ᵗʰ **V29.09** Motorcycle driver injured in collision with other motor vehicles in nontraffic accident

√5ᵗʰ **V29.1** Motorcycle passenger injured in collision with other and unspecified motor vehicles in nontraffic accident

√x7ᵗʰ **V29.10** Motorcycle passenger injured in collision with unspecified motor vehicles in nontraffic accident

√x7ᵗʰ **V29.19** Motorcycle passenger injured in collision with other motor vehicles in nontraffic accident

√5ᵗʰ **V29.2** Unspecified motorcycle rider injured in collision with other and unspecified motor vehicles in nontraffic accident

√x7ᵗʰ **V29.20** Unspecified motorcycle rider injured in collision with unspecified motor vehicles in nontraffic accident
Motorcycle collision NOS, nontraffic

√x7ᵗʰ **V29.29** Unspecified motorcycle rider injured in collision with other motor vehicles in nontraffic accident

√x7ᵗʰ **V29.3** Motorcycle rider (driver) (passenger) injured in unspecified nontraffic accident
Motorcycle accident NOS, nontraffic
Motorcycle rider injured in nontraffic accident NOS

√5ᵗʰ **V29.4** Motorcycle driver injured in collision with other and unspecified motor vehicles in traffic accident

√x7ᵗʰ **V29.40** Motorcycle driver injured in collision with unspecified motor vehicles in traffic accident

√x7ᵗʰ **V29.49** Motorcycle driver injured in collision with other motor vehicles in traffic accident

√5ᵗʰ **V29.5** Motorcycle passenger injured in collision with other and unspecified motor vehicles in traffic accident

√x7ᵗʰ **V29.50** Motorcycle passenger injured in collision with unspecified motor vehicles in traffic accident

√x7ᵗʰ **V29.59** Motorcycle passenger injured in collision with other motor vehicles in traffic accident

√5ᵗʰ **V29.6** Unspecified motorcycle rider injured in collision with other and unspecified motor vehicles in traffic accident

√x7ᵗʰ **V29.60** Unspecified motorcycle rider injured in collision with unspecified motor vehicles in traffic accident
Motorcycle collision NOS (traffic)

√x7ᵗʰ **V29.69** Unspecified motorcycle rider injured in collision with other motor vehicles in traffic accident

√5ᵗʰ **V29.8** Motorcycle rider (driver) (passenger) injured in other specified transport accidents

√x7ᵗʰ **V29.81** Motorcycle rider (driver) (passenger) injured in transport accident with military vehicle

√x7ᵗʰ **V29.88** Motorcycle rider (driver) (passenger) injured in other specified transport accidents

√x7ᵗʰ **V29.9** Motorcycle rider (driver) (passenger) injured in unspecified traffic accident
Motorcycle accident NOS

Occupant of three-wheeled motor vehicle injured in transport accident (V30-V39)

INCLUDES motorized tricycle
motorized rickshaw
three-wheeled motor car

EXCLUDES 1 all-terrain vehicles (V86.-)
motorcycle with sidecar (V20-V29)
vehicle designed primarily for off-road use (V86.-)

The appropriate 7th character is to be added to each code from categories V30-V39.
A initial encounter
D subsequent encounter
S sequela

√4ᵗʰ **V30** Occupant of three-wheeled motor vehicle injured in collision with pedestrian or animal

EXCLUDES 1 three-wheeled motor vehicle collision with animal-drawn vehicle or animal being ridden (V36.-)

√x7ᵗʰ **V30.0** Driver of three-wheeled motor vehicle injured in collision with pedestrian or animal in nontraffic accident

√x7ᵗʰ **V30.1** Passenger in three-wheeled motor vehicle injured in collision with pedestrian or animal in nontraffic accident

√x7ᵗʰ **V30.2** Person on outside of three-wheeled motor vehicle injured in collision with pedestrian or animal in nontraffic accident

√x7ᵗʰ **V30.3** Unspecified occupant of three-wheeled motor vehicle injured in collision with pedestrian or animal in nontraffic accident

√x7ᵗʰ **V30.4** Person boarding or alighting a three-wheeled motor vehicle injured in collision with pedestrian or animal

√x7ᵗʰ **V30.5** Driver of three-wheeled motor vehicle injured in collision with pedestrian or animal in traffic accident

√x7ᵗʰ **V30.6** Passenger in three-wheeled motor vehicle injured in collision with pedestrian or animal in traffic accident

√x7ᵗʰ **V30.7** Person on outside of three-wheeled motor vehicle injured in collision with pedestrian or animal in traffic accident

√x7ᵗʰ **V30.9** Unspecified occupant of three-wheeled motor vehicle injured in collision with pedestrian or animal in traffic accident

√4ᵗʰ **V31** Occupant of three-wheeled motor vehicle injured in collision with pedal cycle

√x7ᵗʰ **V31.0** Driver of three-wheeled motor vehicle injured in collision with pedal cycle in nontraffic accident

√7th **V31.1** Passenger in three-wheeled motor vehicle injured in collision with pedal cycle in nontraffic accident

√7th **V31.2** Person on outside of three-wheeled motor vehicle injured in collision with pedal cycle in nontraffic accident

√7th **V31.3** Unspecified occupant of three-wheeled motor vehicle injured in collision with pedal cycle in nontraffic accident

√7th **V31.4** Person boarding or alighting a three-wheeled motor vehicle injured in collision with pedal cycle

√7th **V31.5** Driver of three-wheeled motor vehicle injured in collision with pedal cycle in traffic accident

√7th **V31.6** Passenger in three-wheeled motor vehicle injured in collision with pedal cycle in traffic accident

√7th **V31.7** Person on outside of three-wheeled motor vehicle injured in collision with pedal cycle in traffic accident

√7th **V31.9** Unspecified occupant of three-wheeled motor vehicle injured in collision with pedal cycle in traffic accident

√4th **V32** Occupant of three-wheeled motor vehicle injured in collision with two- or three-wheeled motor vehicle

√7th **V32.0** Driver of three-wheeled motor vehicle injured in collision with two- or three-wheeled motor vehicle in nontraffic accident

√7th **V32.1** Passenger in three-wheeled motor vehicle injured in collision with two- or three-wheeled motor vehicle in nontraffic accident

√7th **V32.2** Person on outside of three-wheeled motor vehicle injured in collision with two- or three-wheeled motor vehicle in nontraffic accident

√7th **V32.3** Unspecified occupant of three-wheeled motor vehicle injured in collision with two- or three-wheeled motor vehicle in nontraffic accident

√7th **V32.4** Person boarding or alighting a three-wheeled motor vehicle injured in collision with two- or three-wheeled motor vehicle

√7th **V32.5** Driver of three-wheeled motor vehicle injured in collision with two- or three-wheeled motor vehicle in traffic accident

√7th **V32.6** Passenger in three-wheeled motor vehicle injured in collision with two- or three-wheeled motor vehicle in traffic accident

√7th **V32.7** Person on outside of three-wheeled motor vehicle injured in collision with two- or three-wheeled motor vehicle in traffic accident

√7th **V32.9** Unspecified occupant of three-wheeled motor vehicle injured in collision with two- or three-wheeled motor vehicle in traffic accident

√4th **V33** Occupant of three-wheeled motor vehicle injured in collision with car, pick-up truck or van

√7th **V33.0** Driver of three-wheeled motor vehicle injured in collision with car, pick-up truck or van in nontraffic accident

√7th **V33.1** Passenger in three-wheeled motor vehicle injured in collision with car, pick-up truck or van in nontraffic accident

√7th **V33.2** Person on outside of three-wheeled motor vehicle injured in collision with car, pick-up truck or van in nontraffic accident

√7th **V33.3** Unspecified occupant of three-wheeled motor vehicle injured in collision with car, pick-up truck or van in nontraffic accident

√7th **V33.4** Person boarding or alighting a three-wheeled motor vehicle injured in collision with car, pick-up truck or van

√7th **V33.5** Driver of three-wheeled motor vehicle injured in collision with car, pick-up truck or van in traffic accident

√7th **V33.6** Passenger in three-wheeled motor vehicle injured in collision with car, pick-up truck or van in traffic accident

√7th **V33.7** Person on outside of three-wheeled motor vehicle injured in collision with car, pick-up truck or van in traffic accident

√7th **V33.9** Unspecified occupant of three-wheeled motor vehicle injured in collision with car, pick-up truck or van in traffic accident

√4th **V34** Occupant of three-wheeled motor vehicle injured in collision with heavy transport vehicle or bus

EXCLUDES 1 occupant of three-wheeled motor vehicle injured in collision with military vehicle (V39.81)

√7th **V34.0** Driver of three-wheeled motor vehicle injured in collision with heavy transport vehicle or bus in nontraffic accident

√7th **V34.1** Passenger in three-wheeled motor vehicle injured in collision with heavy transport vehicle or bus in nontraffic accident

√7th **V34.2** Person on outside of three-wheeled motor vehicle injured in collision with heavy transport vehicle or bus in nontraffic accident

√7th **V34.3** Unspecified occupant of three-wheeled motor vehicle injured in collision with heavy transport vehicle or bus in nontraffic accident

√7th **V34.4** Person boarding or alighting a three-wheeled motor vehicle injured in collision with heavy transport vehicle or bus

√7th **V34.5** Driver of three-wheeled motor vehicle injured in collision with heavy transport vehicle or bus in traffic accident

√7th **V34.6** Passenger in three-wheeled motor vehicle injured in collision with heavy transport vehicle or bus in traffic accident

√7th **V34.7** Person on outside of three-wheeled motor vehicle injured in collision with heavy transport vehicle or bus in traffic accident

√7th **V34.9** Unspecified occupant of three-wheeled motor vehicle injured in collision with heavy transport vehicle or bus in traffic accident

√4th **V35** Occupant of three-wheeled motor vehicle injured in collision with railway train or railway vehicle

√7th **V35.0** Driver of three-wheeled motor vehicle injured in collision with railway train or railway vehicle in nontraffic accident

√7th **V35.1** Passenger in three-wheeled motor vehicle injured in collision with railway train or railway vehicle in nontraffic accident

√7th **V35.2** Person on outside of three-wheeled motor vehicle injured in collision with railway train or railway vehicle in nontraffic accident

√7th **V35.3** Unspecified occupant of three-wheeled motor vehicle injured in collision with railway train or railway vehicle in nontraffic accident

√7th **V35.4** Person boarding or alighting a three-wheeled motor vehicle injured in collision with railway train or railway vehicle

√7th **V35.5** Driver of three-wheeled motor vehicle injured in collision with railway train or railway vehicle in traffic accident

√7th **V35.6** Passenger in three-wheeled motor vehicle injured in collision with railway train or railway vehicle in traffic accident

√7th **V35.7** Person on outside of three-wheeled motor vehicle injured in collision with railway train or railway vehicle in traffic accident

√7th **V35.9** Unspecified occupant of three-wheeled motor vehicle injured in collision with railway train or railway vehicle in traffic accident

√4th **V36** Occupant of three-wheeled motor vehicle injured in collision with other nonmotor vehicle

INCLUDES collision with animal-drawn vehicle, animal being ridden, streetcar

√7th **V36.0** Driver of three-wheeled motor vehicle injured in collision with other nonmotor vehicle in nontraffic accident

√7th **V36.1** Passenger in three-wheeled motor vehicle injured in collision with other nonmotor vehicle in nontraffic accident

√7th **V36.2** Person on outside of three-wheeled motor vehicle injured in collision with other nonmotor vehicle in nontraffic accident

√7th **V36.3** Unspecified occupant of three-wheeled motor vehicle injured in collision with other nonmotor vehicle in nontraffic accident

√7th **V36.4** Person boarding or alighting a three-wheeled motor vehicle injured in collision with other nonmotor vehicle

√7th **V36.5** Driver of three-wheeled motor vehicle injured in collision with other nonmotor vehicle in traffic accident

√7th **V36.6** Passenger in three-wheeled motor vehicle injured in collision with other nonmotor vehicle in traffic accident

√7th **V36.7** Person on outside of three-wheeled motor vehicle injured in collision with other nonmotor vehicle in traffic accident

√7th **V36.9** Unspecified occupant of three-wheeled motor vehicle injured in collision with other nonmotor vehicle in traffic accident

√4th **V37** Occupant of three-wheeled motor vehicle injured in collision with fixed or stationary object

√7th **V37.0** Driver of three-wheeled motor vehicle injured in collision with fixed or stationary object in nontraffic accident

√7th **V37.1** Passenger in three-wheeled motor vehicle injured in collision with fixed or stationary object in nontraffic accident

√7th **V37.2** Person on outside of three-wheeled motor vehicle injured in collision with fixed or stationary object in nontraffic accident

√7th **V37.3** Unspecified occupant of three-wheeled motor vehicle injured in collision with fixed or stationary object in nontraffic accident

√7th **V37.4** Person boarding or alighting a three-wheeled motor vehicle injured in collision with fixed or stationary object

√7th **V37.5** Driver of three-wheeled motor vehicle injured in collision with fixed or stationary object in traffic accident

√7th **V37.6** Passenger in three-wheeled motor vehicle injured in collision with fixed or stationary object in traffic accident

√7th **V37.7** Person on outside of three-wheeled motor vehicle injured in collision with fixed or stationary object in traffic accident

√7th **V37.9** Unspecified occupant of three-wheeled motor vehicle injured in collision with fixed or stationary object in traffic accident

☑ Additional Character Required   √7th Placeholder Alert   Manifestation   Unspecified Dx   ►◄ Revised Text   ● New Code   ▲ Revised Code Title

✓4ᵗʰ **V38** **Occupant of three-wheeled motor vehicle injured in noncollision transport accident**

> INCLUDES   fall or thrown from three-wheeled motor vehicle
> overturning of three-wheeled motor vehicle NOS
> overturning of three-wheeled motor vehicle without collision

✓x7ᵗʰ **V38.0** Driver of three-wheeled motor vehicle injured in noncollision transport accident in nontraffic accident

✓x7ᵗʰ **V38.1** Passenger in three-wheeled motor vehicle injured in noncollision transport accident in nontraffic accident

✓x7ᵗʰ **V38.2** Person on outside of three-wheeled motor vehicle injured in noncollision transport accident in nontraffic accident

✓x7ᵗʰ **V38.3** Unspecified occupant of three-wheeled motor vehicle injured in noncollision transport accident in nontraffic accident

✓x7ᵗʰ **V38.4** Person boarding or alighting a three-wheeled motor vehicle injured in noncollision transport accident

✓x7ᵗʰ **V38.5** Driver of three-wheeled motor vehicle injured in noncollision transport accident in traffic accident

✓x7ᵗʰ **V38.6** Passenger in three-wheeled motor vehicle injured in noncollision transport accident in traffic accident

✓x7ᵗʰ **V38.7** Person on outside of three-wheeled motor vehicle injured in noncollision transport accident in traffic accident

✓x7ᵗʰ **V38.9** Unspecified occupant of three-wheeled motor vehicle injured in noncollision transport accident in traffic accident

✓4ᵗʰ **V39** **Occupant of three-wheeled motor vehicle injured in other and unspecified transport accidents**

✓5ᵗʰ **V39.0** Driver of three-wheeled motor vehicle injured in collision with other and unspecified motor vehicles in nontraffic accident

     ✓x7ᵗʰ **V39.00** Driver of three-wheeled motor vehicle injured in collision with unspecified motor vehicles in nontraffic accident

     ✓x7ᵗʰ **V39.09** Driver of three-wheeled motor vehicle injured in collision with other motor vehicles in nontraffic accident

✓5ᵗʰ **V39.1** Passenger in three-wheeled motor vehicle injured in collision with other and unspecified motor vehicles in nontraffic accident

     ✓x7ᵗʰ **V39.10** Passenger in three-wheeled motor vehicle injured in collision with unspecified motor vehicles in nontraffic accident

     ✓x7ᵗʰ **V39.19** Passenger in three-wheeled motor vehicle injured in collision with other motor vehicles in nontraffic accident

✓5ᵗʰ **V39.2** Unspecified occupant of three-wheeled motor vehicle injured in collision with other and unspecified motor vehicles in nontraffic accident

     ✓x7ᵗʰ **V39.20** Unspecified occupant of three-wheeled motor vehicle injured in collision with unspecified motor vehicles in nontraffic accident

> Collision NOS involving three-wheeled motor vehicle, nontraffic

     ✓x7ᵗʰ **V39.29** Unspecified occupant of three-wheeled motor vehicle injured in collision with other motor vehicles in nontraffic accident

✓x7ᵗʰ **V39.3** Occupant (driver) (passenger) of three-wheeled motor vehicle injured in unspecified nontraffic accident

> Accident NOS involving three-wheeled motor vehicle, nontraffic
> Occupant of three-wheeled motor vehicle injured in nontraffic accident NOS

✓5ᵗʰ **V39.4** Driver of three-wheeled motor vehicle injured in collision with other and unspecified motor vehicles in traffic accident

     ✓x7ᵗʰ **V39.40** Driver of three-wheeled motor vehicle injured in collision with unspecified motor vehicles in traffic accident

     ✓x7ᵗʰ **V39.49** Driver of three-wheeled motor vehicle injured in collision with other motor vehicles in traffic accident

✓5ᵗʰ **V39.5** Passenger in three-wheeled motor vehicle injured in collision with other and unspecified motor vehicles in traffic accident

     ✓x7ᵗʰ **V39.50** Passenger in three-wheeled motor vehicle injured in collision with unspecified motor vehicles in traffic accident

     ✓x7ᵗʰ **V39.59** Passenger in three-wheeled motor vehicle injured in collision with other motor vehicles in traffic accident

✓5ᵗʰ **V39.6** Unspecified occupant of three-wheeled motor vehicle injured in collision with other and unspecified motor vehicles in traffic accident

     ✓x7ᵗʰ **V39.60** Unspecified occupant of three-wheeled motor vehicle injured in collision with unspecified motor vehicles in traffic accident

> Collision NOS involving three-wheeled motor vehicle (traffic)

     ✓x7ᵗʰ **V39.69** Unspecified occupant of three-wheeled motor vehicle injured in collision with other motor vehicles in traffic accident

✓5ᵗʰ **V39.8** Occupant (driver) (passenger) of three-wheeled motor vehicle injured in other specified transport accidents

     ✓x7ᵗʰ **V39.81** Occupant (driver) (passenger) of three-wheeled motor vehicle injured in transport accident with military vehicle

     ✓x7ᵗʰ **V39.89** Occupant (driver) (passenger) of three-wheeled motor vehicle injured in other specified transport accidents

✓x7ᵗʰ **V39.9** Occupant (driver) (passenger) of three-wheeled motor vehicle injured in unspecified traffic accident

> Accident NOS involving three-wheeled motor vehicle

Car occupant injured in transport accident (V40-V49)

> INCLUDES   a four-wheeled motor vehicle designed primarily for carrying passengers
> automobile (pulling a trailer or camper)
>
> EXCLUDES 1   bus (V50-V59)
> minibus (V50-V59)
> minivan (V50-V59)
> motorcoach (V70-V79)
> pick-up truck (V50-V59)
> sport utility vehicle (SUV) (V50-V59)

The appropriate 7th character is to be added to each code from categories V40-V49.
A   initial encounter
D   subsequent encounter
S   sequela

✓4ᵗʰ **V40** **Car occupant injured in collision with pedestrian or animal**

> EXCLUDES 1   car collision with animal-drawn vehicle or animal being ridden (V46.-)

✓x7ᵗʰ **V40.0** Car driver injured in collision with pedestrian or animal in nontraffic accident

✓x7ᵗʰ **V40.1** Car passenger injured in collision with pedestrian or animal in nontraffic accident

✓x7ᵗʰ **V40.2** Person on outside of car injured in collision with pedestrian or animal in nontraffic accident

✓x7ᵗʰ **V40.3** Unspecified car occupant injured in collision with pedestrian or animal in nontraffic accident

✓x7ᵗʰ **V40.4** Person boarding or alighting a car injured in collision with pedestrian or animal

✓x7ᵗʰ **V40.5** Car driver injured in collision with pedestrian or animal in traffic accident

✓x7ᵗʰ **V40.6** Car passenger injured in collision with pedestrian or animal in traffic accident

✓x7ᵗʰ **V40.7** Person on outside of car injured in collision with pedestrian or animal in traffic accident

✓x7ᵗʰ **V40.9** Unspecified car occupant injured in collision with pedestrian or animal in traffic accident

✓4ᵗʰ **V41** **Car occupant injured in collision with pedal cycle**

✓x7ᵗʰ **V41.0** Car driver injured in collision with pedal cycle in nontraffic accident

✓x7ᵗʰ **V41.1** Car passenger injured in collision with pedal cycle in nontraffic accident

✓x7ᵗʰ **V41.2** Person on outside of car injured in collision with pedal cycle in nontraffic accident

✓x7ᵗʰ **V41.3** Unspecified car occupant injured in collision with pedal cycle in nontraffic accident

✓x7ᵗʰ **V41.4** Person boarding or alighting a car injured in collision with pedal cycle

✓x7ᵗʰ **V41.5** Car driver injured in collision with pedal cycle in traffic accident

✓x7ᵗʰ **V41.6** Car passenger injured in collision with pedal cycle in traffic accident

✓x7ᵗʰ **V41.7** Person on outside of car injured in collision with pedal cycle in traffic accident

✓x7ᵗʰ **V41.9** Unspecified car occupant injured in collision with pedal cycle in traffic accident

✓4th **V42** **Car occupant injured in collision with two- or three-wheeled motor vehicle**

✓x7th **V42.0** Car driver injured in collision with two- or three-wheeled motor vehicle in nontraffic accident

✓x7th **V42.1** Car passenger injured in collision with two- or three-wheeled motor vehicle in nontraffic accident

✓x7th **V42.2** Person on outside of car injured in collision with two- or three-wheeled motor vehicle in nontraffic accident

✓x7th **V42.3** Unspecified car occupant injured in collision with two- or three-wheeled motor vehicle in nontraffic accident

✓x7th **V42.4** Person boarding or alighting a car injured in collision with two- or three-wheeled motor vehicle

✓x7th **V42.5** Car driver injured in collision with two- or three-wheeled motor vehicle in traffic accident

✓x7th **V42.6** Car passenger injured in collision with two- or three-wheeled motor vehicle in traffic accident

✓x7th **V42.7** Person on outside of car injured in collision with two- or three-wheeled motor vehicle in traffic accident

✓x7th **V42.9** Unspecified car occupant injured in collision with two- or three-wheeled motor vehicle in traffic accident

✓4th **V43** **Car occupant injured in collision with car, pick-up truck or van**

✓5th **V43.0** Car driver injured in collision with car, pick-up truck or van in nontraffic accident

✓x7th **V43.01** Car driver injured in collision with sport utility vehicle in nontraffic accident

✓x7th **V43.02** Car driver injured in collision with other type car in nontraffic accident

✓x7th **V43.03** Car driver injured in collision with pick-up truck in nontraffic accident

✓x7th **V43.04** Car driver injured in collision with van in nontraffic accident

✓5th **V43.1** Car passenger injured in collision with car, pick-up truck or van in nontraffic accident

✓x7th **V43.11** Car passenger injured in collision with sport utility vehicle in nontraffic accident

✓x7th **V43.12** Car passenger injured in collision with other type car in nontraffic accident

✓x7th **V43.13** Car passenger injured in collision with pick-up truck in nontraffic accident

✓x7th **V43.14** Car passenger injured in collision with van in nontraffic accident

✓5th **V43.2** Person on outside of car injured in collision with car, pick-up truck or van in nontraffic accident

✓x7th **V43.21** Person on outside of car injured in collision with sport utility vehicle in nontraffic accident

✓x7th **V43.22** Person on outside of car injured in collision with other type car in nontraffic accident

✓x7th **V43.23** Person on outside of car injured in collision with pick-up truck in nontraffic accident

✓x7th **V43.24** Person on outside of car injured in collision with van in nontraffic accident

✓5th **V43.3** Unspecified car occupant injured in collision with car, pick-up truck or van in nontraffic accident

✓x7th **V43.31** Unspecified car occupant injured in collision with sport utility vehicle in nontraffic accident

✓x7th **V43.32** Unspecified car occupant injured in collision with other type car in nontraffic accident

✓x7th **V43.33** Unspecified car occupant injured in collision with pick-up truck in nontraffic accident

✓x7th **V43.34** Unspecified car occupant injured in collision with van in nontraffic accident

✓5th **V43.4** Person boarding or alighting a car injured in collision with car, pick-up truck or van

✓x7th **V43.41** Person boarding or alighting a car injured in collision with sport utility vehicle

✓x7th **V43.42** Person boarding or alighting a car injured in collision with other type car

✓x7th **V43.43** Person boarding or alighting a car injured in collision with pick-up truck

✓x7th **V43.44** Person boarding or alighting a car injured in collision with van

✓5th **V43.5** Car driver injured in collision with car, pick-up truck or van in traffic accident

✓x7th **V43.51** Car driver injured in collision with sport utility vehicle in traffic accident

✓x7th **V43.52** Car driver injured in collision with other type car in traffic accident

✓x7th **V43.53** Car driver injured in collision with pick-up truck in traffic accident

✓x7th **V43.54** Car driver injured in collision with van in traffic accident

✓5th **V43.6** Car passenger injured in collision with car, pick-up truck or van in traffic accident

✓x7th **V43.61** Car passenger injured in collision with sport utility vehicle in traffic accident

✓x7th **V43.62** Car passenger injured in collision with other type car in traffic accident

✓x7th **V43.63** Car passenger injured in collision with pick-up truck in traffic accident

✓x7th **V43.64** Car passenger injured in collision with van in traffic accident

✓5th **V43.7** Person on outside of car injured in collision with car, pick-up truck or van in traffic accident

✓x7th **V43.71** Person on outside of car injured in collision with sport utility vehicle in traffic accident

✓x7th **V43.72** Person on outside of car injured in collision with other type car in traffic accident

✓x7th **V43.73** Person on outside of car injured in collision with pick-up truck in traffic accident

✓x7th **V43.74** Person on outside of car injured in collision with van in traffic accident

✓5th **V43.9** Unspecified car occupant injured in collision with car, pick-up truck or van in traffic accident

✓x7th **V43.91** Unspecified car occupant injured in collision with sport utility vehicle in traffic accident

✓x7th **V43.92** Unspecified car occupant injured in collision with other type car in traffic accident

✓x7th **V43.93** Unspecified car occupant injured in collision with pick-up truck in traffic accident

✓x7th **V43.94** Unspecified car occupant injured in collision with van in traffic accident

✓4th **V44** **Car occupant injured in collision with heavy transport vehicle or bus**

EXCLUDES 1　car occupant injured in collision with military vehicle (V49.81)

✓x7th **V44.0** Car driver injured in collision with heavy transport vehicle or bus in nontraffic accident

✓x7th **V44.1** Car passenger injured in collision with heavy transport vehicle or bus in nontraffic accident

✓x7th **V44.2** Person on outside of car injured in collision with heavy transport vehicle or bus in nontraffic accident

✓x7th **V44.3** Unspecified car occupant injured in collision with heavy transport vehicle or bus in nontraffic accident

✓x7th **V44.4** Person boarding or alighting a car injured in collision with heavy transport vehicle or bus

✓x7th **V44.5** Car driver injured in collision with heavy transport vehicle or bus in traffic accident

✓x7th **V44.6** Car passenger injured in collision with heavy transport vehicle or bus in traffic accident

✓x7th **V44.7** Person on outside of car injured in collision with heavy transport vehicle or bus in traffic accident

✓x7th **V44.9** Unspecified car occupant injured in collision with heavy transport vehicle or bus in traffic accident

✓4th **V45** **Car occupant injured in collision with railway train or railway vehicle**

✓x7th **V45.0** Car driver injured in collision with railway train or railway vehicle in nontraffic accident

✓x7th **V45.1** Car passenger injured in collision with railway train or railway vehicle in nontraffic accident

✓x7th **V45.2** Person on outside of car injured in collision with railway train or railway vehicle in nontraffic accident

✓x7th **V45.3** Unspecified car occupant injured in collision with railway train or railway vehicle in nontraffic accident

✓x7th **V45.4** Person boarding or alighting a car injured in collision with railway train or railway vehicle

✓x7th **V45.5** Car driver injured in collision with railway train or railway vehicle in traffic accident

✓x7th **V45.6** Car passenger injured in collision with railway train or railway vehicle in traffic accident

✓x7th **V45.7** Person on outside of car injured in collision with railway train or railway vehicle in traffic accident

✓x7th **V45.9** Unspecified car occupant injured in collision with railway train or railway vehicle in traffic accident

✓4th **V46** **Car occupant injured in collision with other nonmotor vehicle**

INCLUDES　collision with animal-drawn vehicle, animal being ridden, streetcar

✓x7th **V46.0** Car driver injured in collision with other nonmotor vehicle in nontraffic accident

✓x7th **V46.1** Car passenger injured in collision with other nonmotor vehicle in nontraffic accident

✓x7th **V46.2** Person on outside of car injured in collision with other nonmotor vehicle in nontraffic accident

---

✓ Additional Character Required　　✓x7th Placeholder Alert　　Manifestation　　Unspecified Dx　　▶◀ Revised Text　　● New Code　　▲ Revised Code Title

Chapter 20. External Causes of Morbidity

✓x7th **V46.3** Unspecified car occupant injured in collision with other nonmotor vehicle **in nontraffic accident**

✓x7th **V46.4** Person boarding or alighting a car injured in collision with other nonmotor vehicle

✓x7th **V46.5** Car driver injured in collision with other nonmotor vehicle in traffic accident

✓x7th **V46.6** Car passenger injured in collision with other nonmotor vehicle in traffic accident

✓x7th **V46.7** Person on outside of car injured in collision with other nonmotor vehicle in traffic accident

✓x7th **V46.9** Unspecified car occupant injured in collision with other nonmotor vehicle in traffic accident

✓4th **V47** Car occupant injured in collision with fixed or stationary object

    AHA: 2016,4Q,73

✓x7th **V47.0** Car driver injured in collision with fixed or stationary object in nontraffic accident

✓x7th **V47.1** Car passenger injured in collision with fixed or stationary object in nontraffic accident

✓x7th **V47.2** Person on outside of car injured in collision with fixed or stationary object in nontraffic accident

✓x7th **V47.3** Unspecified car occupant injured in collision with fixed or stationary object in nontraffic accident

✓x7th **V47.4** Person boarding or alighting a car injured in collision with fixed or stationary object

✓x7th **V47.5** Car driver injured in collision with fixed or stationary object in traffic accident

✓x7th **V47.6** Car passenger injured in collision with fixed or stationary object in traffic accident

✓x7th **V47.7** Person on outside of car injured in collision with fixed or stationary object in traffic accident

✓x7th **V47.9** Unspecified car occupant injured in collision with fixed or stationary object in traffic accident

✓4th **V48** Car occupant injured in noncollision transport accident

    INCLUDES overturning car NOS
                    overturning car without collision

✓x7th **V48.0** Car driver injured in noncollision transport accident in nontraffic accident

✓x7th **V48.1** Car passenger injured in noncollision transport accident in nontraffic accident

✓x7th **V48.2** Person on outside of car injured in noncollision transport accident in nontraffic accident

✓x7th **V48.3** Unspecified car occupant injured in noncollision transport accident in nontraffic accident

✓x7th **V48.4** Person boarding or alighting a car injured in noncollision transport accident

✓x7th **V48.5** Car driver injured in noncollision transport accident in traffic accident

✓x7th **V48.6** Car passenger injured in noncollision transport accident in traffic accident

✓x7th **V48.7** Person on outside of car injured in noncollision transport accident in traffic accident

✓x7th **V48.9** Unspecified car occupant injured in noncollision transport accident in traffic accident

✓4th **V49** Car occupant injured in other and unspecified transport accidents

✓5th **V49.0** Driver injured in collision with other and unspecified motor vehicles in nontraffic accident

    ✓x7th **V49.00** Driver injured in collision with unspecified motor vehicles in nontraffic accident

    ✓x7th **V49.09** Driver injured in collision with other motor vehicles in nontraffic accident

✓5th **V49.1** Passenger injured in collision with other and unspecified motor vehicles in nontraffic accident

    ✓x7th **V49.10** Passenger injured in collision with unspecified motor vehicles in nontraffic accident

    ✓x7th **V49.19** Passenger injured in collision with other motor vehicles in nontraffic accident

✓5th **V49.2** Unspecified car occupant injured in collision with other and unspecified motor vehicles in nontraffic accident

    ✓x7th **V49.20** Unspecified car occupant injured in collision with unspecified motor vehicles in nontraffic accident
        Car collision NOS, nontraffic

    ✓x7th **V49.29** Unspecified car occupant injured in collision with other motor vehicles in nontraffic accident

✓x7th **V49.3** Car occupant (driver) (passenger) injured in unspecified nontraffic accident
    Car accident NOS, nontraffic
    Car occupant injured in nontraffic accident NOS

✓5th **V49.4** Driver injured in collision with other and unspecified motor vehicles in traffic accident

    ✓x7th **V49.40** Driver injured in collision with unspecified motor vehicles in traffic accident

    ✓x7th **V49.49** Driver injured in collision with other motor vehicles in traffic accident

✓5th **V49.5** Passenger injured in collision with other and unspecified motor vehicles in traffic accident

    ✓x7th **V49.50** Passenger injured in collision with unspecified motor vehicles in traffic accident

    ✓x7th **V49.59** Passenger injured in collision with other motor vehicles in traffic accident

✓5th **V49.6** Unspecified car occupant injured in collision with other and unspecified motor vehicles in traffic accident

    ✓x7th **V49.60** Unspecified car occupant injured in collision with unspecified motor vehicles in traffic accident
        Car collision NOS (traffic)

    ✓x7th **V49.69** Unspecified car occupant injured in collision with other motor vehicles in traffic accident

✓5th **V49.8** Car occupant (driver) (passenger) injured in other specified transport accidents

    ✓x7th **V49.81** Car occupant (driver) (passenger) injured in transport accident with military vehicle

    ✓x7th **V49.88** Car occupant (driver) (passenger) injured in other specified transport accidents

✓x7th **V49.9** Car occupant (driver) (passenger) injured in unspecified traffic accident
    Car accident NOS

Occupant of pick-up truck or van injured in transport accident (V50-V59)

    INCLUDES a four or six wheel motor vehicle designed primarily for carrying passengers and property but weighing less than the local limit for classification as a heavy goods vehicle
        minibus
        minivan
        sport utility vehicle (SUV)
        truck
        van
    EXCLUDES 1 heavy transport vehicle (V60-V69)

The appropriate 7th character is to be added to each code from categories V50-V59.
A   initial encounter
D subsequent encounter
S sequela

✓4th **V50** Occupant of pick-up truck or van injured in collision with pedestrian or animal

    EXCLUDES 1 pick-up truck or van collision with animal-drawn vehicle or animal being ridden (V56.-)

✓x7th **V50.0** Driver of pick-up truck or van injured in collision with pedestrian or animal in nontraffic accident

✓x7th **V50.1** Passenger in pick-up truck or van injured in collision with pedestrian or animal in nontraffic accident

✓x7th **V50.2** Person on outside of pick-up truck or van injured in collision with pedestrian or animal in nontraffic accident

✓x7th **V50.3** Unspecified occupant of pick-up truck or van injured in collision with pedestrian or animal in nontraffic accident

✓x7th **V50.4** Person boarding or alighting a pick-up truck or van injured in collision with pedestrian or animal

✓x7th **V50.5** Driver of pick-up truck or van injured in collision with pedestrian or animal in traffic accident

✓x7th **V50.6** Passenger in pick-up truck or van injured in collision with pedestrian or animal in traffic accident

✓x7th **V50.7** Person on outside of pick-up truck or van injured in collision with pedestrian or animal in traffic accident

✓x7th **V50.9** Unspecified occupant of pick-up truck or van injured in collision with pedestrian or animal in traffic accident

✓4th **V51** Occupant of pick-up truck or van injured in collision with pedal cycle

✓x7th **V51.0** Driver of pick-up truck or van injured in collision with pedal cycle in nontraffic accident

✓x7th **V51.1** Passenger in pick-up truck or van injured in collision with pedal cycle in nontraffic accident

✓x7th **V51.2** Person on outside of pick-up truck or van injured in collision with pedal cycle in nontraffic accident

✓x7th **V51.3** Unspecified occupant of pick-up truck or van injured in collision with pedal cycle in nontraffic accident

✓x7th **V51.4** Person boarding or alighting a pick-up truck or van injured in collision with pedal cycle

✓x7th **V51.5** Driver of pick-up truck or van injured in collision with pedal cycle in traffic accident

√x7ᵗʰ **V51.6** Passenger in pick-up truck or van injured in collision with pedal cycle in traffic accident

√x7ᵗʰ **V51.7** Person on outside of pick-up truck or van injured in collision with pedal cycle in traffic accident

√x7ᵗʰ **V51.9** Unspecified occupant of pick-up truck or van injured in collision with pedal cycle in traffic accident

√4ᵗʰ **V52** Occupant of pick-up truck or van injured in collision with two- or three-wheeled motor vehicle

√x7ᵗʰ **V52.0** Driver of pick-up truck or van injured in collision with two- or three-wheeled motor vehicle in nontraffic accident

√x7ᵗʰ **V52.1** Passenger in pick-up truck or van injured in collision with two- or three-wheeled motor vehicle in nontraffic accident

√x7ᵗʰ **V52.2** Person on outside of pick-up truck or van injured in collision with two- or three-wheeled motor vehicle in nontraffic accident

√x7ᵗʰ **V52.3** Unspecified occupant of pick-up truck or van injured in collision with two- or three-wheeled motor vehicle in nontraffic accident

√x7ᵗʰ **V52.4** Person boarding or alighting a pick-up truck or van injured in collision with two- or three-wheeled motor vehicle

√x7ᵗʰ **V52.5** Driver of pick-up truck or van injured in collision with two- or three-wheeled motor vehicle in traffic accident

√x7ᵗʰ **V52.6** Passenger in pick-up truck or van injured in collision with two- or three-wheeled motor vehicle in traffic accident

√x7ᵗʰ **V52.7** Person on outside of pick-up truck or van injured in collision with two- or three-wheeled motor vehicle in traffic accident

√x7ᵗʰ **V52.9** Unspecified occupant of pick-up truck or van injured in collision with two- or three-wheeled motor vehicle in traffic accident

√4ᵗʰ **V53** Occupant of pick-up truck or van injured in collision with car, pick-up truck or van

√x7ᵗʰ **V53.0** Driver of pick-up truck or van injured in collision with car, pick-up truck or van in nontraffic accident

√x7ᵗʰ **V53.1** Passenger in pick-up truck or van injured in collision with car, pick-up truck or van in nontraffic accident

√x7ᵗʰ **V53.2** Person on outside of pick-up truck or van injured in collision with car, pick-up truck or van in nontraffic accident

√x7ᵗʰ **V53.3** Unspecified occupant of pick-up truck or van injured in collision with car, pick-up truck or van in nontraffic accident

√x7ᵗʰ **V53.4** Person boarding or alighting a pick-up truck or van injured in collision with car, pick-up truck or van

√x7ᵗʰ **V53.5** Driver of pick-up truck or van injured in collision with car, pick-up truck or van in traffic accident

√x7ᵗʰ **V53.6** Passenger in pick-up truck or van injured in collision with car, pick-up truck or van in traffic accident

√x7ᵗʰ **V53.7** Person on outside of pick-up truck or van injured in collision with car, pick-up truck or van in traffic accident

√x7ᵗʰ **V53.9** Unspecified occupant of pick-up truck or van injured in collision with car, pick-up truck or van in traffic accident

√4ᵗʰ **V54** Occupant of pick-up truck or van injured in collision with heavy transport vehicle or bus

     EXCLUDES 1   occupant of pick-up truck or van injured in collision with military vehicle (V59.81)

√x7ᵗʰ **V54.0** Driver of pick-up truck or van injured in collision with heavy transport vehicle or bus in nontraffic accident

√x7ᵗʰ **V54.1** Passenger in pick-up truck or van injured in collision with heavy transport vehicle or bus in nontraffic accident

√x7ᵗʰ **V54.2** Person on outside of pick-up truck or van injured in collision with heavy transport vehicle or bus in nontraffic accident

√x7ᵗʰ **V54.3** Unspecified occupant of pick-up truck or van injured in collision with heavy transport vehicle or bus in nontraffic accident

√x7ᵗʰ **V54.4** Person boarding or alighting a pick-up truck or van injured in collision with heavy transport vehicle or bus

√x7ᵗʰ **V54.5** Driver of pick-up truck or van injured in collision with heavy transport vehicle or bus in traffic accident

√x7ᵗʰ **V54.6** Passenger in pick-up truck or van injured in collision with heavy transport vehicle or bus in traffic accident

√x7ᵗʰ **V54.7** Person on outside of pick-up truck or van injured in collision with heavy transport vehicle or bus in traffic accident

√x7ᵗʰ **V54.9** Unspecified occupant of pick-up truck or van injured in collision with heavy transport vehicle or bus in traffic accident

√4ᵗʰ **V55** Occupant of pick-up truck or van injured in collision with railway train or railway vehicle

√x7ᵗʰ **V55.0** Driver of pick-up truck or van injured in collision with railway train or railway vehicle in nontraffic accident

√x7ᵗʰ **V55.1** Passenger in pick-up truck or van injured in collision with railway train or railway vehicle in nontraffic accident

√x7ᵗʰ **V55.2** Person on outside of pick-up truck or van injured in collision with railway train or railway vehicle in nontraffic accident

√x7ᵗʰ **V55.3** Unspecified occupant of pick-up truck or van injured in collision with railway train or railway vehicle in nontraffic accident

√x7ᵗʰ **V55.4** Person boarding or alighting a pick-up truck or van injured in collision with railway train or railway vehicle

√x7ᵗʰ **V55.5** Driver of pick-up truck or van injured in collision with railway train or railway vehicle in traffic accident

√x7ᵗʰ **V55.6** Passenger in pick-up truck or van injured in collision with railway train or railway vehicle in traffic accident

√x7ᵗʰ **V55.7** Person on outside of pick-up truck or van injured in collision with railway train or railway vehicle in traffic accident

√x7ᵗʰ **V55.9** Unspecified occupant of pick-up truck or van injured in collision with railway train or railway vehicle in traffic accident

√4ᵗʰ **V56** Occupant of pick-up truck or van injured in collision with other nonmotor vehicle

     INCLUDES   collision with animal-drawn vehicle, animal being ridden, streetcar

√x7ᵗʰ **V56.0** Driver of pick-up truck or van injured in collision with other nonmotor vehicle in nontraffic accident

√x7ᵗʰ **V56.1** Passenger in pick-up truck or van injured in collision with other nonmotor vehicle in nontraffic accident

√x7ᵗʰ **V56.2** Person on outside of pick-up truck or van injured in collision with other nonmotor vehicle in nontraffic accident

√x7ᵗʰ **V56.3** Unspecified occupant of pick-up truck or van injured in collision with other nonmotor vehicle in nontraffic accident

√x7ᵗʰ **V56.4** Person boarding or alighting a pick-up truck or van injured in collision with other nonmotor vehicle

√x7ᵗʰ **V56.5** Driver of pick-up truck or van injured in collision with other nonmotor vehicle in traffic accident

√x7ᵗʰ **V56.6** Passenger in pick-up truck or van injured in collision with other nonmotor vehicle in traffic accident

√x7ᵗʰ **V56.7** Person on outside of pick-up truck or van injured in collision with other nonmotor vehicle in traffic accident

√x7ᵗʰ **V56.9** Unspecified occupant of pick-up truck or van injured in collision with other nonmotor vehicle in traffic accident

√4ᵗʰ **V57** Occupant of pick-up truck or van injured in collision with fixed or stationary object

√x7ᵗʰ **V57.0** Driver of pick-up truck or van injured in collision with fixed or stationary object in nontraffic accident

√x7ᵗʰ **V57.1** Passenger in pick-up truck or van injured in collision with fixed or stationary object in nontraffic accident

√x7ᵗʰ **V57.2** Person on outside of pick-up truck or van injured in collision with fixed or stationary object in nontraffic accident

√x7ᵗʰ **V57.3** Unspecified occupant of pick-up truck or van injured in collision with fixed or stationary object in nontraffic accident

√x7ᵗʰ **V57.4** Person boarding or alighting a pick-up truck or van injured in collision with fixed or stationary object

√x7ᵗʰ **V57.5** Driver of pick-up truck or van injured in collision with fixed or stationary object in traffic accident

√x7ᵗʰ **V57.6** Passenger in pick-up truck or van injured in collision with fixed or stationary object in traffic accident

√x7ᵗʰ **V57.7** Person on outside of pick-up truck or van injured in collision with fixed or stationary object in traffic accident

√x7ᵗʰ **V57.9** Unspecified occupant of pick-up truck or van injured in collision with fixed or stationary object in traffic accident

√4ᵗʰ **V58** Occupant of pick-up truck or van injured in noncollision transport accident

     INCLUDES   overturning pick-up truck or van NOS
                          overturning pick-up truck or van without collision

√x7ᵗʰ **V58.0** Driver of pick-up truck or van injured in noncollision transport accident in nontraffic accident

√x7ᵗʰ **V58.1** Passenger in pick-up truck or van injured in noncollision transport accident in nontraffic accident

√x7ᵗʰ **V58.2** Person on outside of pick-up truck or van injured in noncollision transport accident in nontraffic accident

√x7ᵗʰ **V58.3** Unspecified occupant of pick-up truck or van injured in noncollision transport accident in nontraffic accident

√x7ᵗʰ **V58.4** Person boarding or alighting a pick-up truck or van injured in noncollision transport accident

√x7ᵗʰ **V58.5** Driver of pick-up truck or van injured in noncollision transport accident in traffic accident

√x7ᵗʰ **V58.6** Passenger in pick-up truck or van injured in noncollision transport accident in traffic accident

√x7ᵗʰ **V58.7** Person on outside of pick-up truck or van injured in noncollision transport accident in traffic accident

√x7ᵗʰ **V58.9** Unspecified occupant of pick-up truck or van injured in noncollision transport accident in traffic accident

---

◂ Additional Character Required   √x7ᵗʰ Placeholder Alert   Manifestation   Unspecified Dx   ▶◀ Revised Text   ● New Code   ▲ Revised Code Title

☑4ᵗʰ **V59** **Occupant of pick-up truck or van injured in other and unspecified transport accidents**

  ☑5ᵗʰ **V59.0** Driver of pick-up truck or van injured in collision with other and unspecified motor vehicles in nontraffic accident

    ✓x7ᵗʰ **V59.00** Driver of pick-up truck or van injured in collision with unspecified motor vehicles in nontraffic accident

    ✓x7ᵗʰ **V59.09** Driver of pick-up truck or van injured in collision with other motor vehicles in nontraffic accident

  ☑5ᵗʰ **V59.1** Passenger in pick-up truck or van injured in collision with other and unspecified motor vehicles in nontraffic accident

    ✓x7ᵗʰ **V59.10** Passenger in pick-up truck or van injured in collision with unspecified motor vehicles in nontraffic accident

    ✓x7ᵗʰ **V59.19** Passenger in pick-up truck or van injured in collision with other motor vehicles in nontraffic accident

  ☑5ᵗʰ **V59.2** Unspecified occupant of pick-up truck or van injured in collision with other and unspecified motor vehicles in nontraffic accident

    ✓x7ᵗʰ **V59.20** Unspecified occupant of pick-up truck or van injured in collision with unspecified motor vehicles in nontraffic accident

        Collision NOS involving pick-up truck or van, nontraffic

    ✓x7ᵗʰ **V59.29** Unspecified occupant of pick-up truck or van injured in collision with other motor vehicles in nontraffic accident

  ✓x7ᵗʰ **V59.3** Occupant (driver) (passenger) of pick-up truck or van injured in unspecified nontraffic accident

        Accident NOS involving pick-up truck or van, nontraffic
        Occupant of pick-up truck or van injured in nontraffic accident NOS

  ☑5ᵗʰ **V59.4** Driver of pick-up truck or van injured in collision with other and unspecified motor vehicles in traffic accident

    ✓x7ᵗʰ **V59.40** Driver of pick-up truck or van injured in collision with unspecified motor vehicles in traffic accident

    ✓x7ᵗʰ **V59.49** Driver of pick-up truck or van injured in collision with other motor vehicles in traffic accident

  ☑5ᵗʰ **V59.5** Passenger in pick-up truck or van injured in collision with other and unspecified motor vehicles in traffic accident

    ✓x7ᵗʰ **V59.50** Passenger in pick-up truck or van injured in collision with unspecified motor vehicles in traffic accident

    ✓x7ᵗʰ **V59.59** Passenger in pick-up truck or van injured in collision with other motor vehicles in traffic accident

  ☑5ᵗʰ **V59.6** Unspecified occupant of pick-up truck or van injured in collision with other and unspecified motor vehicles in traffic accident

    ✓x7ᵗʰ **V59.60** Unspecified occupant of pick-up truck or van injured in collision with unspecified motor vehicles in traffic accident

        Collision NOS involving pick-up truck or van (traffic)

    ✓x7ᵗʰ **V59.69** Unspecified occupant of pick-up truck or van injured in collision with other motor vehicles in traffic accident

  ☑5ᵗʰ **V59.8** Occupant (driver) (passenger) of pick-up truck or van injured in other specified transport accidents

    ✓x7ᵗʰ **V59.81** Occupant (driver) (passenger) of pick-up truck or van injured in transport accident with military vehicle

    ✓x7ᵗʰ **V59.88** Occupant (driver) (passenger) of pick-up truck or van injured in other specified transport accidents

  ✓x7ᵗʰ **V59.9** Occupant (driver) (passenger) of pick-up truck or van injured in unspecified traffic accident

        Accident NOS involving pick-up truck or van

Occupant of heavy transport vehicle injured in transport accident (V60-V69)

INCLUDES   18 wheeler
        armored car
        panel truck
EXCLUDES 1   *bus*
        motorcoach

The appropriate 7th character is to be added to each code from categories V60-V69.
A   initial encounter
D   subsequent encounter
S   sequela

☑4ᵗʰ **V60** **Occupant of heavy transport vehicle injured in collision with pedestrian or animal**

    EXCLUDES 1   *heavy transport vehicle collision with animal-drawn vehicle or animal being ridden (V66.-)*

  ✓x7ᵗʰ **V60.0** Driver of heavy transport vehicle injured in collision with pedestrian or animal in nontraffic accident

  ✓x7ᵗʰ **V60.1** Passenger in heavy transport vehicle injured in collision with pedestrian or animal in nontraffic accident

  ✓x7ᵗʰ **V60.2** Person on outside of heavy transport vehicle injured in collision with pedestrian or animal in nontraffic accident

  ✓x7ᵗʰ **V60.3** Unspecified occupant of heavy transport vehicle injured in collision with pedestrian or animal in nontraffic accident

  ✓x7ᵗʰ **V60.4** Person boarding or alighting a heavy transport vehicle injured in collision with pedestrian or animal

  ✓x7ᵗʰ **V60.5** Driver of heavy transport vehicle injured in collision with pedestrian or animal in traffic accident

  ✓x7ᵗʰ **V60.6** Passenger in heavy transport vehicle injured in collision with pedestrian or animal in traffic accident

  ✓x7ᵗʰ **V60.7** Person on outside of heavy transport vehicle injured in collision with pedestrian or animal in traffic accident

  ✓x7ᵗʰ **V60.9** Unspecified occupant of heavy transport vehicle injured in collision with pedestrian or animal in traffic accident

☑4ᵗʰ **V61** **Occupant of heavy transport vehicle injured in collision with pedal cycle**

  ✓x7ᵗʰ **V61.0** Driver of heavy transport vehicle injured in collision with pedal cycle in nontraffic accident

  ✓x7ᵗʰ **V61.1** Passenger in heavy transport vehicle injured in collision with pedal cycle in nontraffic accident

  ✓x7ᵗʰ **V61.2** Person on outside of heavy transport vehicle injured in collision with pedal cycle in nontraffic accident

  ✓x7ᵗʰ **V61.3** Unspecified occupant of heavy transport vehicle injured in collision with pedal cycle in nontraffic accident

  ✓x7ᵗʰ **V61.4** Person boarding or alighting a heavy transport vehicle injured in collision with pedal cycle while boarding or alighting

  ✓x7ᵗʰ **V61.5** Driver of heavy transport vehicle injured in collision with pedal cycle in traffic accident

  ✓x7ᵗʰ **V61.6** Passenger in heavy transport vehicle injured in collision with pedal cycle in traffic accident

  ✓x7ᵗʰ **V61.7** Person on outside of heavy transport vehicle injured in collision with pedal cycle in traffic accident

  ✓x7ᵗʰ **V61.9** Unspecified occupant of heavy transport vehicle injured in collision with pedal cycle in traffic accident

☑4ᵗʰ **V62** **Occupant of heavy transport vehicle injured in collision with two- or three-wheeled motor vehicle**

  ✓x7ᵗʰ **V62.0** Driver of heavy transport vehicle injured in collision with two- or three-wheeled motor vehicle in nontraffic accident

  ✓x7ᵗʰ **V62.1** Passenger in heavy transport vehicle injured in collision with two- or three-wheeled motor vehicle in nontraffic accident

  ✓x7ᵗʰ **V62.2** Person on outside of heavy transport vehicle injured in collision with two- or three-wheeled motor vehicle in nontraffic accident

  ✓x7ᵗʰ **V62.3** Unspecified occupant of heavy transport vehicle injured in collision with two- or three-wheeled motor vehicle in nontraffic accident

  ✓x7ᵗʰ **V62.4** Person boarding or alighting a heavy transport vehicle injured in collision with two- or three-wheeled motor vehicle

  ✓x7ᵗʰ **V62.5** Driver of heavy transport vehicle injured in collision with two- or three-wheeled motor vehicle in traffic accident

  ✓x7ᵗʰ **V62.6** Passenger in heavy transport vehicle injured in collision with two- or three-wheeled motor vehicle in traffic accident

  ✓x7ᵗʰ **V62.7** Person on outside of heavy transport vehicle injured in collision with two- or three-wheeled motor vehicle in traffic accident

  ✓x7ᵗʰ **V62.9** Unspecified occupant of heavy transport vehicle injured in collision with two- or three-wheeled motor vehicle in traffic accident

☑4ᵗʰ **V63**   **Occupant of heavy transport vehicle injured in collision with car, pick-up truck or van**

✓x7ᵗʰ **V63.0**   Driver of heavy transport vehicle injured in collision with car, pick-up truck or van in nontraffic accident

✓x7ᵗʰ **V63.1**   Passenger in heavy transport vehicle injured in collision with car, pick-up truck or van in nontraffic accident

✓x7ᵗʰ **V63.2**   Person on outside of heavy transport vehicle injured in collision with car, pick-up truck or van in nontraffic accident

✓x7ᵗʰ **V63.3**   Unspecified occupant of heavy transport vehicle injured in collision with car, pick-up truck or van in nontraffic accident

✓x7ᵗʰ **V63.4**   Person boarding or alighting a heavy transport vehicle injured in collision with car, pick-up truck or van

✓x7ᵗʰ **V63.5**   Driver of heavy transport vehicle injured in collision with car, pick-up truck or van in traffic accident

✓x7ᵗʰ **V63.6**   Passenger in heavy transport vehicle injured in collision with car, pick-up truck or van in traffic accident

✓x7ᵗʰ **V63.7**   Person on outside of heavy transport vehicle injured in collision with car, pick-up truck or van in traffic accident

✓x7ᵗʰ **V63.9**   Unspecified occupant of heavy transport vehicle injured in collision with car, pick-up truck or van in traffic accident

☑4ᵗʰ **V64**   **Occupant of heavy transport vehicle injured in collision with heavy transport vehicle or bus**

    EXCLUDES 1   occupant of heavy transport vehicle injured in collision with military vehicle (V69.81)

✓x7ᵗʰ **V64.0**   Driver of heavy transport vehicle injured in collision with heavy transport vehicle or bus in nontraffic accident

✓x7ᵗʰ **V64.1**   Passenger in heavy transport vehicle injured in collision with heavy transport vehicle or bus in nontraffic accident

✓x7ᵗʰ **V64.2**   Person on outside of heavy transport vehicle injured in collision with heavy transport vehicle or bus in nontraffic accident

✓x7ᵗʰ **V64.3**   Unspecified occupant of heavy transport vehicle injured in collision with heavy transport vehicle or bus in nontraffic accident

✓x7ᵗʰ **V64.4**   Person boarding or alighting a heavy transport vehicle injured in collision with heavy transport vehicle or bus while boarding or alighting

✓x7ᵗʰ **V64.5**   Driver of heavy transport vehicle injured in collision with heavy transport vehicle or bus in traffic accident

✓x7ᵗʰ **V64.6**   Passenger in heavy transport vehicle injured in collision with heavy transport vehicle or bus in traffic accident

✓x7ᵗʰ **V64.7**   Person on outside of heavy transport vehicle injured in collision with heavy transport vehicle or bus in traffic accident

✓x7ᵗʰ **V64.9**   Unspecified occupant of heavy transport vehicle injured in collision with heavy transport vehicle or bus in traffic accident

☑4ᵗʰ **V65**   **Occupant of heavy transport vehicle injured in collision with railway train or railway vehicle**

✓x7ᵗʰ **V65.0**   Driver of heavy transport vehicle injured in collision with railway train or railway vehicle in nontraffic accident

✓x7ᵗʰ **V65.1**   Passenger in heavy transport vehicle injured in collision with railway train or railway vehicle in nontraffic accident

✓x7ᵗʰ **V65.2**   Person on outside of heavy transport vehicle injured in collision with railway train or railway vehicle in nontraffic accident

✓x7ᵗʰ **V65.3**   Unspecified occupant of heavy transport vehicle injured in collision with railway train or railway vehicle in nontraffic accident

✓x7ᵗʰ **V65.4**   Person boarding or alighting a heavy transport vehicle injured in collision with railway train or railway vehicle

✓x7ᵗʰ **V65.5**   Driver of heavy transport vehicle injured in collision with railway train or railway vehicle in traffic accident

✓x7ᵗʰ **V65.6**   Passenger in heavy transport vehicle injured in collision with railway train or railway vehicle in traffic accident

✓x7ᵗʰ **V65.7**   Person on outside of heavy transport vehicle injured in collision with railway train or railway vehicle in traffic accident

✓x7ᵗʰ **V65.9**   Unspecified occupant of heavy transport vehicle injured in collision with railway train or railway vehicle in traffic accident

☑4ᵗʰ **V66**   **Occupant of heavy transport vehicle injured in collision with other nonmotor vehicle**

    INCLUDES   collision with animal-drawn vehicle, animal being ridden, streetcar

✓x7ᵗʰ **V66.0**   Driver of heavy transport vehicle injured in collision with other nonmotor vehicle in nontraffic accident

✓x7ᵗʰ **V66.1**   Passenger in heavy transport vehicle injured in collision with other nonmotor vehicle in nontraffic accident

✓x7ᵗʰ **V66.2**   Person on outside of heavy transport vehicle injured in collision with other nonmotor vehicle in nontraffic accident

✓x7ᵗʰ **V66.3**   Unspecified occupant of heavy transport vehicle injured in collision with other nonmotor vehicle in nontraffic accident

✓x7ᵗʰ **V66.4**   Person boarding or alighting a heavy transport vehicle injured in collision with other nonmotor vehicle

✓x7ᵗʰ **V66.5**   Driver of heavy transport vehicle injured in collision with other nonmotor vehicle in traffic accident

✓x7ᵗʰ **V66.6**   Passenger in heavy transport vehicle injured in collision with other nonmotor vehicle in traffic accident

✓x7ᵗʰ **V66.7**   Person on outside of heavy transport vehicle injured in collision with other nonmotor vehicle in traffic accident

✓x7ᵗʰ **V66.9**   Unspecified occupant of heavy transport vehicle injured in collision with other nonmotor vehicle in traffic accident

☑4ᵗʰ **V67**   **Occupant of heavy transport vehicle injured in collision with fixed or stationary object**

✓x7ᵗʰ **V67.0**   Driver of heavy transport vehicle injured in collision with fixed or stationary object in nontraffic accident

✓x7ᵗʰ **V67.1**   Passenger in heavy transport vehicle injured in collision with fixed or stationary object in nontraffic accident

✓x7ᵗʰ **V67.2**   Person on outside of heavy transport vehicle injured in collision with fixed or stationary object in nontraffic accident

✓x7ᵗʰ **V67.3**   Unspecified occupant of heavy transport vehicle injured in collision with fixed or stationary object in nontraffic accident

✓x7ᵗʰ **V67.4**   Person boarding or alighting a heavy transport vehicle injured in collision with fixed or stationary object

✓x7ᵗʰ **V67.5**   Driver of heavy transport vehicle injured in collision with fixed or stationary object in traffic accident

✓x7ᵗʰ **V67.6**   Passenger in heavy transport vehicle injured in collision with fixed or stationary object in traffic accident

✓x7ᵗʰ **V67.7**   Person on outside of heavy transport vehicle injured in collision with fixed or stationary object in traffic accident

✓x7ᵗʰ **V67.9**   Unspecified occupant of heavy transport vehicle injured in collision with fixed or stationary object in traffic accident

☑4ᵗʰ **V68**   **Occupant of heavy transport vehicle injured in noncollision transport accident**

    INCLUDES   overturning heavy transport vehicle NOS
                  overturning heavy transport vehicle without collision

✓x7ᵗʰ **V68.0**   Driver of heavy transport vehicle injured in noncollision transport accident in nontraffic accident

✓x7ᵗʰ **V68.1**   Passenger in heavy transport vehicle injured in noncollision transport accident in nontraffic accident

✓x7ᵗʰ **V68.2**   Person on outside of heavy transport vehicle injured in noncollision transport accident in nontraffic accident

✓x7ᵗʰ **V68.3**   Unspecified occupant of heavy transport vehicle injured in noncollision transport accident in nontraffic accident

✓x7ᵗʰ **V68.4**   Person boarding or alighting a heavy transport vehicle injured in noncollision transport accident

✓x7ᵗʰ **V68.5**   Driver of heavy transport vehicle injured in noncollision transport accident in traffic accident

✓x7ᵗʰ **V68.6**   Passenger in heavy transport vehicle injured in noncollision transport accident in traffic accident

✓x7ᵗʰ **V68.7**   Person on outside of heavy transport vehicle injured in noncollision transport accident in traffic accident

✓x7ᵗʰ **V68.9**   Unspecified occupant of heavy transport vehicle injured in noncollision transport accident in traffic accident

☑4ᵗʰ **V69**   **Occupant of heavy transport vehicle injured in other and unspecified transport accidents**

☑5ᵗʰ **V69.0**   Driver of heavy transport vehicle injured in collision with other and unspecified motor vehicles in nontraffic accident

✓x7ᵗʰ **V69.00**   Driver of heavy transport vehicle injured in collision with unspecified motor vehicles in nontraffic accident

✓x7ᵗʰ **V69.09**   Driver of heavy transport vehicle injured in collision with other motor vehicles in nontraffic accident

☑5ᵗʰ **V69.1**   Passenger in heavy transport vehicle injured in collision with other and unspecified motor vehicles in nontraffic accident

✓x7ᵗʰ **V69.10**   Passenger in heavy transport vehicle injured in collision with unspecified motor vehicles in nontraffic accident

✓x7ᵗʰ **V69.19**   Passenger in heavy transport vehicle injured in collision with other motor vehicles in nontraffic accident

☑5ᵗʰ **V69.2**   Unspecified occupant of heavy transport vehicle injured in collision with other and unspecified motor vehicles in nontraffic accident

✓x7ᵗʰ **V69.20**   Unspecified occupant of heavy transport vehicle injured in collision with unspecified motor vehicles in nontraffic accident

      Collision NOS involving heavy transport vehicle, nontraffic

---

◢ Additional Character Required   ✓x7ᵗʰ Placeholder Alert   Manifestation   Unspecified Dx   ▶◀ Revised Text   ● New Code   ▲ Revised Code Title

√x7ᵗʰ **V69.29** Unspecified occupant of heavy transport vehicle injured in collision with other motor vehicles in nontraffic accident

√5ᵗʰ **V69.3** Occupant (driver) (passenger) of heavy transport vehicle injured in unspecified nontraffic accident

> Accident NOS involving heavy transport vehicle, nontraffic
> Occupant of heavy transport vehicle injured in nontraffic accident NOS

√5ᵗʰ **V69.4** Driver of heavy transport vehicle injured in collision with other and unspecified motor vehicles in traffic accident

    √x7ᵗʰ **V69.40** Driver of heavy transport vehicle injured in collision with unspecified motor vehicles in traffic accident

    √x7ᵗʰ **V69.49** Driver of heavy transport vehicle injured in collision with other motor vehicles in traffic accident

√5ᵗʰ **V69.5** Passenger in heavy transport vehicle injured in collision with other and unspecified motor vehicles in traffic accident

    √x7ᵗʰ **V69.50** Passenger in heavy transport vehicle injured in collision with unspecified motor vehicles in traffic accident

    √x7ᵗʰ **V69.59** Passenger in heavy transport vehicle injured in collision with other motor vehicles in traffic accident

√5ᵗʰ **V69.6** Unspecified occupant of heavy transport vehicle injured in collision with other and unspecified motor vehicles in traffic accident

    √x7ᵗʰ **V69.60** Unspecified occupant of heavy transport vehicle injured in collision with unspecified motor vehicles in traffic accident

> Collision NOS involving heavy transport vehicle (traffic)

    √x7ᵗʰ **V69.69** Unspecified occupant of heavy transport vehicle injured in collision with other motor vehicles in traffic accident

√5ᵗʰ **V69.8** Occupant (driver) (passenger) of heavy transport vehicle injured in other specified transport accidents

    √x7ᵗʰ **V69.81** Occupant (driver) (passenger) of heavy transport vehicle injured in transport accidents with military vehicle

    √x7ᵗʰ **V69.88** Occupant (driver) (passenger) of heavy transport vehicle injured in other specified transport accidents

√x7ᵗʰ **V69.9** Occupant (driver) (passenger) of heavy transport vehicle injured in unspecified traffic accident

> Accident NOS involving heavy transport vehicle

Bus occupant injured in transport accident (V70-V79)

INCLUDES motorcoach
EXCLUDES 1 minibus (V50-V59)

The appropriate 7th character is to be added to each code from categories V70-V79.
A   initial encounter
D   subsequent encounter
S   sequela

√4ᵗʰ **V70** Bus occupant injured in collision with pedestrian or animal

    EXCLUDES 1 bus collision with animal-drawn vehicle or animal being ridden (V76.-)

√x7ᵗʰ **V70.0** Driver of bus injured in collision with pedestrian or animal in nontraffic accident

√x7ᵗʰ **V70.1** Passenger on bus injured in collision with pedestrian or animal in nontraffic accident

√x7ᵗʰ **V70.2** Person on outside of bus injured in collision with pedestrian or animal in nontraffic accident

√x7ᵗʰ **V70.3** Unspecified occupant of bus injured in collision with pedestrian or animal in nontraffic accident

√x7ᵗʰ **V70.4** Person boarding or alighting from bus injured in collision with pedestrian or animal

√x7ᵗʰ **V70.5** Driver of bus injured in collision with pedestrian or animal in traffic accident

√x7ᵗʰ **V70.6** Passenger on bus injured in collision with pedestrian or animal in traffic accident

√x7ᵗʰ **V70.7** Person on outside of bus injured in collision with pedestrian or animal in traffic accident

√x7ᵗʰ **V70.9** Unspecified occupant of bus injured in collision with pedestrian or animal in traffic accident

√4ᵗʰ **V71** Bus occupant injured in collision with pedal cycle

√x7ᵗʰ **V71.0** Driver of bus injured in collision with pedal cycle in nontraffic accident

√x7ᵗʰ **V71.1** Passenger on bus injured in collision with pedal cycle in nontraffic accident

√x7ᵗʰ **V71.2** Person on outside of bus injured in collision with pedal cycle in nontraffic accident

√x7ᵗʰ **V71.3** Unspecified occupant of bus injured in collision with pedal cycle in nontraffic accident

√x7ᵗʰ **V71.4** Person boarding or alighting from bus injured in collision with pedal cycle

√x7ᵗʰ **V71.5** Driver of bus injured in collision with pedal cycle in traffic accident

√x7ᵗʰ **V71.6** Passenger on bus injured in collision with pedal cycle in traffic accident

√x7ᵗʰ **V71.7** Person on outside of bus injured in collision with pedal cycle in traffic accident

√x7ᵗʰ **V71.9** Unspecified occupant of bus injured in collision with pedal cycle in traffic accident

√4ᵗʰ **V72** Bus occupant injured in collision with two- or three-wheeled motor vehicle

√x7ᵗʰ **V72.0** Driver of bus injured in collision with two- or three-wheeled motor vehicle in nontraffic accident

√x7ᵗʰ **V72.1** Passenger on bus injured in collision with two- or three-wheeled motor vehicle in nontraffic accident

√x7ᵗʰ **V72.2** Person on outside of bus injured in collision with two- or three-wheeled motor vehicle in nontraffic accident

√x7ᵗʰ **V72.3** Unspecified occupant of bus injured in collision with two- or three-wheeled motor vehicle in nontraffic accident

√x7ᵗʰ **V72.4** Person boarding or alighting from bus injured in collision with two- or three-wheeled motor vehicle

√x7ᵗʰ **V72.5** Driver of bus injured in collision with two- or three-wheeled motor vehicle in traffic accident

√x7ᵗʰ **V72.6** Passenger on bus injured in collision with two- or three-wheeled motor vehicle in traffic accident

√x7ᵗʰ **V72.7** Person on outside of bus injured in collision with two- or three-wheeled motor vehicle in traffic accident

√x7ᵗʰ **V72.9** Unspecified occupant of bus injured in collision with two- or three-wheeled motor vehicle in traffic accident

√4ᵗʰ **V73** Bus occupant injured in collision with car, pick-up truck or van

√x7ᵗʰ **V73.0** Driver of bus injured in collision with car, pick-up truck or van in nontraffic accident

√x7ᵗʰ **V73.1** Passenger on bus injured in collision with car, pick-up truck or van in nontraffic accident

√x7ᵗʰ **V73.2** Person on outside of bus injured in collision with car, pick-up truck or van in nontraffic accident

√x7ᵗʰ **V73.3** Unspecified occupant of bus injured in collision with car, pick-up truck or van in nontraffic accident

√x7ᵗʰ **V73.4** Person boarding or alighting from bus injured in collision with car, pick-up truck or van

√x7ᵗʰ **V73.5** Driver of bus injured in collision with car, pick-up truck or van in traffic accident

√x7ᵗʰ **V73.6** Passenger on bus injured in collision with car, pick-up truck or van in traffic accident

√x7ᵗʰ **V73.7** Person on outside of bus injured in collision with car, pick-up truck or van in traffic accident

√x7ᵗʰ **V73.9** Unspecified occupant of bus injured in collision with car, pick-up truck or van in traffic accident

√4ᵗʰ **V74** Bus occupant injured in collision with heavy transport vehicle or bus

    EXCLUDES 1 bus occupant injured in collision with military vehicle (V79.81)

√x7ᵗʰ **V74.0** Driver of bus injured in collision with heavy transport vehicle or bus in nontraffic accident

√x7ᵗʰ **V74.1** Passenger on bus injured in collision with heavy transport vehicle or bus in nontraffic accident

√x7ᵗʰ **V74.2** Person on outside of bus injured in collision with heavy transport vehicle or bus in nontraffic accident

√x7ᵗʰ **V74.3** Unspecified occupant of bus injured in collision with heavy transport vehicle or bus in nontraffic accident

√x7ᵗʰ **V74.4** Person boarding or alighting from bus injured in collision with heavy transport vehicle or bus

√x7ᵗʰ **V74.5** Driver of bus injured in collision with heavy transport vehicle or bus in traffic accident

√x7ᵗʰ **V74.6** Passenger on bus injured in collision with heavy transport vehicle or bus in traffic accident

√x7ᵗʰ **V74.7** Person on outside of bus injured in collision with heavy transport vehicle or bus in traffic accident

√x7ᵗʰ **V74.9** Unspecified occupant of bus injured in collision with heavy transport vehicle or bus in traffic accident

√4ᵗʰ **V75** Bus occupant injured in collision with railway train or railway vehicle

√x7ᵗʰ **V75.0** Driver of bus injured in collision with railway train or railway vehicle in nontraffic accident

√x7ᵗʰ **V75.1** Passenger on bus injured in collision with railway train or railway vehicle in nontraffic accident

√x7ᵗʰ **V75.2** Person on outside of bus injured in collision with railway train or railway vehicle in nontraffic accident

√x7th **V75.3** Unspecified occupant of bus injured in collision with railway train or railway vehicle in nontraffic accident

√x7th **V75.4** Person boarding or alighting from bus injured in collision with railway train or railway vehicle

√x7th **V75.5** Driver of bus injured in collision with railway train or railway vehicle in traffic accident

√x7th **V75.6** Passenger on bus injured in collision with railway train or railway vehicle in traffic accident

√x7th **V75.7** Person on outside of bus injured in collision with railway train or railway vehicle in traffic accident

√x7th **V75.9** Unspecified occupant of bus injured in collision with railway train or railway vehicle in traffic accident

√4th **V76 Bus occupant injured in collision with other nonmotor vehicle**

INCLUDES   collision with animal-drawn vehicle, animal being ridden, streetcar

√x7th **V76.Ø** Driver of bus injured in collision with other nonmotor vehicle in nontraffic accident

√x7th **V76.1** Passenger on bus injured in collision with other nonmotor vehicle in nontraffic accident

√x7th **V76.2** Person on outside of bus injured in collision with other nonmotor vehicle in nontraffic accident

√x7th **V76.3** Unspecified occupant of bus injured in collision with other nonmotor vehicle in nontraffic accident

√x7th **V76.4** Person boarding or alighting from bus injured in collision with other nonmotor vehicle

√x7th **V76.5** Driver of bus injured in collision with other nonmotor vehicle in traffic accident

√x7th **V76.6** Passenger on bus injured in collision with other nonmotor vehicle in traffic accident

√x7th **V76.7** Person on outside of bus injured in collision with other nonmotor vehicle in traffic accident

√x7th **V76.9** Unspecified occupant of bus injured in collision with other nonmotor vehicle in traffic accident

√4th **V77 Bus occupant injured in collision with fixed or stationary object**

√x7th **V77.Ø** Driver of bus injured in collision with fixed or stationary object in nontraffic accident

√x7th **V77.1** Passenger on bus injured in collision with fixed or stationary object in nontraffic accident

√x7th **V77.2** Person on outside of bus injured in collision with fixed or stationary object in nontraffic accident

√x7th **V77.3** Unspecified occupant of bus injured in collision with fixed or stationary object in nontraffic accident

√x7th **V77.4** Person boarding or alighting from bus injured in collision with fixed or stationary object

√x7th **V77.5** Driver of bus injured in collision with fixed or stationary object in traffic accident

√x7th **V77.6** Passenger on bus injured in collision with fixed or stationary object in traffic accident

√x7th **V77.7** Person on outside of bus injured in collision with fixed or stationary object in traffic accident

√x7th **V77.9** Unspecified occupant of bus injured in collision with fixed or stationary object in traffic accident

√4th **V78 Bus occupant injured in noncollision transport accident**

INCLUDES   overturning bus NOS
overturning bus without collision

√x7th **V78.Ø** Driver of bus injured in noncollision transport accident in nontraffic accident

√x7th **V78.1** Passenger on bus injured in noncollision transport accident in nontraffic accident

√x7th **V78.2** Person on outside of bus injured in noncollision transport accident in nontraffic accident

√x7th **V78.3** Unspecified occupant of bus injured in noncollision transport accident in nontraffic accident

√x7th **V78.4** Person boarding or alighting from bus injured in noncollision transport accident

√x7th **V78.5** Driver of bus injured in noncollision transport accident in traffic accident

√x7th **V78.6** Passenger on bus injured in noncollision transport accident in traffic accident

√x7th **V78.7** Person on outside of bus injured in noncollision transport accident in traffic accident

√x7th **V78.9** Unspecified occupant of bus injured in noncollision transport accident in traffic accident

√4th **V79 Bus occupant injured in other and unspecified transport accidents**

√5th **V79.Ø** Driver of bus injured in collision with other and unspecified motor vehicles in nontraffic accident

√x7th **V79.ØØ** Driver of bus injured in collision with unspecified motor vehicles in nontraffic accident

√x7th **V79.Ø9** Driver of bus injured in collision with other motor vehicles in nontraffic accident

√5th **V79.1** Passenger on bus injured in collision with other and unspecified motor vehicles in nontraffic accident

√x7th **V79.1Ø** Passenger on bus injured in collision with unspecified motor vehicles in nontraffic accident

√x7th **V79.19** Passenger on bus injured in collision with other motor vehicles in nontraffic accident

√5th **V79.2** Unspecified bus occupant injured in collision with other and unspecified motor vehicles in nontraffic accident

√x7th **V79.2Ø** Unspecified bus occupant injured in collision with unspecified motor vehicles in nontraffic accident
Bus collision NOS, nontraffic

√x7th **V79.29** Unspecified bus occupant injured in collision with other motor vehicles in nontraffic accident

√x7th **V79.3** Bus occupant (driver) (passenger) injured in unspecified nontraffic accident
Bus accident NOS, nontraffic
Bus occupant injured in nontraffic accident NOS

√5th **V79.4** Driver of bus injured in collision with other and unspecified motor vehicles in traffic accident

√x7th **V79.4Ø** Driver of bus injured in collision with unspecified motor vehicles in traffic accident

√x7th **V79.49** Driver of bus injured in collision with other motor vehicles in traffic accident

√5th **V79.5** Passenger on bus injured in collision with other and unspecified motor vehicles in traffic accident

√x7th **V79.5Ø** Passenger on bus injured in collision with unspecified motor vehicles in traffic accident

√x7th **V79.59** Passenger on bus injured in collision with other motor vehicles in traffic accident

√5th **V79.6** Unspecified bus occupant injured in collision with other and unspecified motor vehicles in traffic accident

√x7th **V79.6Ø** Unspecified bus occupant injured in collision with unspecified motor vehicles in traffic accident
Bus collision NOS (traffic)

√x7th **V79.69** Unspecified bus occupant injured in collision with other motor vehicles in traffic accident

√5th **V79.8** Bus occupant (driver) (passenger) injured in other specified transport accidents

√x7th **V79.81** Bus occupant (driver) (passenger) injured in transport accidents with military vehicle

√x7th **V79.88** Bus occupant (driver) (passenger) injured in other specified transport accidents

√x7th **V79.9** Bus occupant (driver) (passenger) injured in unspecified traffic accident
Bus accident NOS

Other land transport accidents (V8Ø-V89)

The appropriate 7th character is to be added to each code from categories V8Ø-V89.
A   initial encounter
D   subsequent encounter
S   sequela

√4th **V8Ø Animal-rider or occupant of animal-drawn vehicle injured in transport accident**

√5th **V8Ø.Ø** Animal-rider or occupant of animal drawn vehicle injured by fall from or being thrown from animal or animal-drawn vehicle in noncollision accident

√6th **V8Ø.Ø1** Animal-rider injured by fall from or being thrown from animal in noncollision accident

√7th **V8Ø.Ø1Ø** Animal-rider injured by fall from or being thrown from horse in noncollision accident

√7th **V8Ø.Ø18** Animal-rider injured by fall from or being thrown from other animal in noncollision accident

√x7th **V8Ø.Ø2** Occupant of animal-drawn vehicle injured by fall from or being thrown from animal-drawn vehicle in noncollision accident
Overturning animal-drawn vehicle NOS
Overturning animal-drawn vehicle without collision

√5th **V8Ø.1** Animal-rider or occupant of animal-drawn vehicle injured in collision with pedestrian or animal

EXCLUDES 1   animal-rider or animal-drawn vehicle collision with animal-drawn vehicle or animal being ridden (V8Ø.7)

√x7th **V8Ø.11** Animal-rider injured in collision with pedestrian or animal

√x7th **V8Ø.12** Occupant of animal-drawn vehicle injured in collision with pedestrian or animal

☑ Additional Character Required   √x7th Placeholder Alert   Manifestation   Unspecified Dx   ►◄ Revised Text   ● New Code   ▲ Revised Code Title

D-10-CM 2020   1171

Chapter 20. External Causes of Morbidity

V80.2–V82.4

√5ᵗʰ **V80.2** **Animal-rider or occupant of animal-drawn vehicle injured in collision with** pedal cycle

  √x7ᵗʰ **V80.21** Animal-rider **injured in collision with pedal cycle**

  √x7ᵗʰ **V80.22** Occupant **of animal-drawn vehicle injured in collision with pedal cycle**

√5ᵗʰ **V80.3** **Animal-rider or occupant of animal-drawn vehicle injured in collision with** two- or three-wheeled motor vehicle

  √x7ᵗʰ **V80.31** Animal-rider **injured in collision with two- or three-wheeled motor vehicle**

  √x7ᵗʰ **V80.32** Occupant **of animal-drawn vehicle injured in collision with two- or three-wheeled motor vehicle**

√5ᵗʰ **V80.4** **Animal-rider or occupant of animal-drawn vehicle injured in collision with** car, pick-up truck, van, heavy transport vehicle or bus

   EXCLUDES 1   *animal-rider injured in collision with military vehicle (V80.910)*

       occupant of animal-drawn vehicle injured in collision with military vehicle (V80.920)

  √x7ᵗʰ **V80.41** Animal-rider **injured in collision with car, pick-up truck, van, heavy transport vehicle or bus**

  √x7ᵗʰ **V80.42** Occupant **of animal-drawn vehicle injured in collision with car, pick-up truck, van, heavy transport vehicle or bus**

√5ᵗʰ **V80.5** **Animal-rider or occupant of animal-drawn vehicle injured in collision with** other specified motor vehicle

  √x7ᵗʰ **V80.51** Animal-rider **injured in collision with other specified motor vehicle**

  √x7ᵗʰ **V80.52** Occupant **of animal-drawn vehicle injured in collision with other specified motor vehicle**

√5ᵗʰ **V80.6** **Animal-rider or occupant of animal-drawn vehicle injured in collision with** railway train or railway vehicle

  √x7ᵗʰ **V80.61** Animal-rider **injured in collision with railway train or railway vehicle**

  √x7ᵗʰ **V80.62** Occupant **of animal-drawn vehicle injured in collision with railway train or railway vehicle**

√5ᵗʰ **V80.7** **Animal-rider or occupant of animal-drawn vehicle injured in collision with** other nonmotor vehicles

  √6ᵗʰ **V80.71** **Animal-rider or occupant of animal-drawn vehicle injured in collision with** animal being ridden

    √7ᵗʰ **V80.710** Animal-rider **injured in collision with other animal being ridden**

    √7ᵗʰ **V80.711** Occupant **of animal-drawn vehicle injured in collision with animal being ridden**

  √6ᵗʰ **V80.72** **Animal-rider or occupant of animal-drawn vehicle injured in collision with** other animal-drawn vehicle

    √7ᵗʰ **V80.720** Animal-rider **injured in collision with animal-drawn vehicle**

    √7ᵗʰ **V80.721** Occupant **of animal-drawn vehicle injured in collision with other animal-drawn vehicle**

  √6ᵗʰ **V80.73** **Animal-rider or occupant of animal-drawn vehicle injured in collision with** streetcar

    √7ᵗʰ **V80.730** Animal-rider **injured in collision with streetcar**

    √7ᵗʰ **V80.731** Occupant **of animal-drawn vehicle injured in collision with streetcar**

  √6ᵗʰ **V80.79** **Animal-rider or occupant of animal-drawn vehicle injured in collision with** other nonmotor vehicles

    √7ᵗʰ **V80.790** Animal-rider **injured in collision with other nonmotor vehicles**

    √7ᵗʰ **V80.791** Occupant **of animal-drawn vehicle injured in collision with other nonmotor vehicles**

√5ᵗʰ **V80.8** **Animal-rider or occupant of animal-drawn vehicle injured in collision with** fixed or stationary object

  √x7ᵗʰ **V80.81** Animal-rider **injured in collision with fixed or stationary object**

  √x7ᵗʰ **V80.82** Occupant **of animal-drawn vehicle injured in collision with fixed or stationary object**

√5ᵗʰ **V80.9** **Animal-rider or occupant of animal-drawn vehicle injured in other and unspecified transport accidents**

  √6ᵗʰ **V80.91** Animal-rider **injured in other and unspecified transport accidents**

    √7ᵗʰ **V80.910** Animal-rider **injured in transport accident with** military vehicle

    √7ᵗʰ **V80.918** Animal-rider **injured in other transport accident**

    √7ᵗʰ **V80.919** Animal-rider **injured in unspecified transport accident**

      Animal rider accident NOS

√6ᵗʰ **V80.92** Occupant **of animal-drawn vehicle injured in other and unspecified transport accidents**

  √7ᵗʰ **V80.920** **Occupant of animal-drawn vehicle injured in transport accident with** military vehicle

  √7ᵗʰ **V80.928** **Occupant of animal-drawn vehicle injured in other transport accident**

  √7ᵗʰ **V80.929** **Occupant of animal-drawn vehicle injured in unspecified transport accident**

    Animal-drawn vehicle accident NOS

√4ᵗʰ **V81** **Occupant of railway train or railway vehicle injured in transport accident**

  INCLUDES   derailment of railway train or railway vehicle

        person on outside of train

  EXCLUDES 1   *streetcar (V82.-)*

√x7ᵗʰ **V81.0** **Occupant of railway train or railway vehicle injured in collision with motor vehicle** in nontraffic accident

  EXCLUDES 1   *occupant of railway train or railway vehicle injured due to collision with military vehicle (V81.83)*

√x7ᵗʰ **V81.1** **Occupant of railway train or railway vehicle injured in collision with motor vehicle** in traffic accident

  EXCLUDES 1   *occupant of railway train or railway vehicle injured due to collision with military vehicle (V81.83)*

√x7ᵗʰ **V81.2** **Occupant of railway train or railway vehicle injured in collision with or** hit by rolling stock

√x7ᵗʰ **V81.3** **Occupant of railway train or railway vehicle injured in collision with other object**

    Railway collision NOS

√x7ᵗʰ **V81.4** **Person injured** while boarding or alighting **from railway train or railway vehicle**

√x7ᵗʰ **V81.5** **Occupant of railway train or railway vehicle injured by** fall in railway train **or railway vehicle**

√x7ᵗʰ **V81.6** **Occupant of railway train or railway vehicle injured by** fall from railway train **or railway vehicle**

√x7ᵗʰ **V81.7** **Occupant of railway train or railway vehicle injured in** derailment without antecedent collision

√5ᵗʰ **V81.8** **Occupant of railway train or railway vehicle injured in other specified railway accidents**

  √x7ᵗʰ **V81.81** **Occupant of railway train or railway vehicle injured due to** explosion or fire **on train**

  √x7ᵗʰ **V81.82** **Occupant of railway train or railway vehicle injured due to** object falling onto **train**

    Occupant of railway train or railway vehicle injured due to falling earth onto train

    Occupant of railway train or railway vehicle injured due to falling rocks onto train

    Occupant of railway train or railway vehicle injured due to falling snow onto train

    Occupant of railway train or railway vehicle injured due to falling trees onto train

  √x7ᵗʰ **V81.83** **Occupant of railway train or railway vehicle injured due to** collision with military vehicle

  √x7ᵗʰ **V81.89** **Occupant of railway train or railway vehicle injured due to other specified railway accident**

√x7ᵗʰ **V81.9** **Occupant of railway train or railway vehicle injured in unspecified railway accident**

    Railway accident NOS

√4ᵗʰ **V82** **Occupant of powered streetcar injured in transport accident**

  INCLUDES   interurban electric car

        person on outside of streetcar

        tram (car)

        trolley (car)

  EXCLUDES 1   *bus (V70-V79)*

        motorcoach (V70-V79)

        nonpowered streetcar (V76.-)

        train (V81.-)

√x7ᵗʰ **V82.0** **Occupant of streetcar injured in collision with motor vehicle in nontraffic accident**

√x7ᵗʰ **V82.1** **Occupant of streetcar injured in collision with motor vehicle in traffic accident**

√x7ᵗʰ **V82.2** **Occupant of streetcar injured in collision with or** hit by rolling stock

√x7ᵗʰ **V82.3** **Occupant of streetcar injured in collision with other object**

  EXCLUDES 1   *collision with animal-drawn vehicle or animal being ridden (V82.8)*

√x7ᵗʰ **V82.4** **Person injured** while boarding or alighting **from streetcar**

√x7ᵗʰ **V82.5 Occupant of streetcar injured by fall in streetcar**
> EXCLUDES 1   *fall in streetcar:*
> > *while boarding or alighting (V82.4)*
> > *with antecedent collision (V82.0–V82.3)*

√x7ᵗʰ **V82.6 Occupant of streetcar injured by fall from streetcar**
> EXCLUDES 1   *fall from streetcar:*
> > *while boarding or alighting (V82.4)*
> > *with antecedent collision (V82.0–V82.3)*

√x7ᵗʰ **V82.7 Occupant of streetcar injured in derailment without antecedent collision**
> EXCLUDES 1   *occupant of streetcar injured in derailment with antecedent collision (V82.0–V82.3)*

√x7ᵗʰ **V82.8 Occupant of streetcar injured in other specified transport accidents**
> Streetcar collision with military vehicle
> Streetcar collision with train or nonmotor vehicles

√x7ᵗʰ **V82.9 Occupant of streetcar injured in unspecified traffic accident**
> Streetcar accident NOS

√4ᵗʰ **V83 Occupant of special vehicle mainly used on industrial premises injured in transport accident**
> INCLUDES   battery-powered airport passenger vehicle
> > battery-powered truck (baggage) (mail)
> > coal-car in mine
> > forklift (truck)
> > logging car
> > self-propelled industrial truck
> > station baggage truck (powered)
> > tram, truck, or tub (powered) in mine or quarry
> EXCLUDES 1   *special construction vehicles (V85.-)*
> > *special industrial vehicle in stationary use or maintenance (W31.-)*

√x7ᵗʰ **V83.0 Driver of special industrial vehicle injured in traffic accident**

√x7ᵗʰ **V83.1 Passenger of special industrial vehicle injured in traffic accident**

√x7ᵗʰ **V83.2 Person on outside of special industrial vehicle injured in traffic accident**

√x7ᵗʰ **V83.3 Unspecified occupant of special industrial vehicle injured in traffic accident**

√x7ᵗʰ **V83.4 Person injured while boarding or alighting from special industrial vehicle**

√x7ᵗʰ **V83.5 Driver of special industrial vehicle injured in nontraffic accident**

√x7ᵗʰ **V83.6 Passenger of special industrial vehicle injured in nontraffic accident**

√x7ᵗʰ **V83.7 Person on outside of special industrial vehicle injured in nontraffic accident**

√x7ᵗʰ **V83.9 Unspecified occupant of special industrial vehicle injured in nontraffic accident**
> Special-industrial-vehicle accident NOS

√4ᵗʰ **V84 Occupant of special vehicle mainly used in agriculture injured in transport accident**
> INCLUDES   self-propelled farm machinery
> > tractor (and trailer)
> EXCLUDES 1   *animal-powered farm machinery accident (W30.8-)*
> > *contact with combine harvester (W30.0)*
> > *special agricultural vehicle in stationary use or maintenance (W30.-)*

√x7ᵗʰ **V84.0 Driver of special agricultural vehicle injured in traffic accident**

√x7ᵗʰ **V84.1 Passenger of special agricultural vehicle injured in traffic accident**

√x7ᵗʰ **V84.2 Person on outside of special agricultural vehicle injured in traffic accident**

√x7ᵗʰ **V84.3 Unspecified occupant of special agricultural vehicle injured in traffic accident**

√x7ᵗʰ **V84.4 Person injured while boarding or alighting from special agricultural vehicle**

√x7ᵗʰ **V84.5 Driver of special agricultural vehicle injured in nontraffic accident**

√x7ᵗʰ **V84.6 Passenger of special agricultural vehicle injured in nontraffic accident**

√x7ᵗʰ **V84.7 Person on outside of special agricultural vehicle injured in nontraffic accident**

√x7ᵗʰ **V84.9 Unspecified occupant of special agricultural vehicle injured in nontraffic accident**
> Special-agricultural vehicle accident NOS

√4ᵗʰ **V85 Occupant of special construction vehicle injured in transport accident**
> INCLUDES   bulldozer
> > digger
> > dump truck
> > earth-leveller
> > mechanical shovel
> > road-roller
> EXCLUDES 1   *special industrial vehicle (V83.-)*
> > *special construction vehicle in stationary use or maintenance (W31.-)*

√x7ᵗʰ **V85.0 Driver of special construction vehicle injured in traffic accident**

√x7ᵗʰ **V85.1 Passenger of special construction vehicle injured in traffic accident**

√x7ᵗʰ **V85.2 Person on outside of special construction vehicle injured in traffic accident**

√x7ᵗʰ **V85.3 Unspecified occupant of special construction vehicle injured in traffic accident**

√x7ᵗʰ **V85.4 Person injured while boarding or alighting from special construction vehicle**

√x7ᵗʰ **V85.5 Driver of special construction vehicle injured in nontraffic accident**

√x7ᵗʰ **V85.6 Passenger of special construction vehicle injured in nontraffic accident**

√x7ᵗʰ **V85.7 Person on outside of special construction vehicle injured in nontraffic accident**

√x7ᵗʰ **V85.9 Unspecified occupant of special construction vehicle injured in nontraffic accident**
> Special-construction-vehicle accident NOS

√4ᵗʰ **V86 Occupant of special all-terrain or other off-road motor vehicle, injured in transport accident**
> EXCLUDES 1   *special all-terrain vehicle in stationary use or maintenance (W31.-)*
> > *sport-utility vehicle (V50-V59)*
> > *three-wheeled motor vehicle designed for on-road use (V30-V39)*
>
> **AHA:** 2017,4Q,26

√5ᵗʰ **V86.0 Driver of special all-terrain or other off-road motor vehicle injured in traffic accident**

> √x7ᵗʰ **V86.01 Driver of ambulance or fire engine injured in traffic accident**

> √x7ᵗʰ **V86.02 Driver of snowmobile injured in traffic accident**

> √x7ᵗʰ **V86.03 Driver of dune buggy injured in traffic accident**

> √x7ᵗʰ **V86.04 Driver of military vehicle injured in traffic accident**

> √x7ᵗʰ **V86.05 Driver of 3- or 4- wheeled all-terrain vehicle (ATV) injured in traffic accident**

> √x7ᵗʰ **V86.06 Driver of dirt bike or motor/cross bike injured in traffic accident**

> √x7ᵗʰ **V86.09 Driver of other special all-terrain or other off-road motor vehicle injured in traffic accident**
> > ~~Driver of dirt bike injured in traffic accident~~
> > Driver of go cart injured in traffic accident
> > Driver of golf cart injured in traffic accident

√5ᵗʰ **V86.1 Passenger of special all-terrain or other off-road motor vehicle injured in traffic accident**

> √x7ᵗʰ **V86.11 Passenger of ambulance or fire engine injured in traffic accident**

> √x7ᵗʰ **V86.12 Passenger of snowmobile injured in traffic accident**

> √x7ᵗʰ **V86.13 Passenger of dune buggy injured in traffic accident**

> √x7ᵗʰ **V86.14 Passenger of military vehicle injured in traffic accident**

> √x7ᵗʰ **V86.15 Passenger of 3- or 4- wheeled all-terrain vehicle (ATV) injured in traffic accident**

> √x7ᵗʰ **V86.16 Passenger of dirt bike or motor/cross bike injured in traffic accident**

> √x7ᵗʰ **V86.19 Passenger of other special all-terrain or other off-road motor vehicle injured in traffic accident**
> > ~~Passenger of dirt bike injured in traffic accident~~
> > Passenger of go cart injured in traffic accident
> > Passenger of golf cart injured in traffic accident

√5ᵗʰ **V86.2 Person on outside of special all-terrain or other off-road motor vehicle injured in traffic accident**

> √x7ᵗʰ **V86.21 Person on outside of ambulance or fire engine injured in traffic accident**

> √x7ᵗʰ **V86.22 Person on outside of snowmobile injured in traffic accident**

> √x7ᵗʰ **V86.23 Person on outside of dune buggy injured in traffic accident**

◀ Additional Character Required	√x7ᵗʰ Placeholder Alert	Manifestation	Unspecified Dx	▶◀ Revised Text	● New Code ▲ Revised Code Title

✓x7ᵗʰ **V86.24** Person on outside of military vehicle injured in traffic accident

✓x7ᵗʰ **V86.25** Person on outside of 3- or 4- wheeled all-terrain vehicle (ATV) injured in traffic accident

✓x7ᵗʰ **V86.26** Person on outside of dirt bike or motor/cross bike injured in traffic accident

✓x7ᵗʰ **V86.29** Person on outside of other special all-terrain or other off-road motor vehicle injured in traffic accident

> Person on outside of dirt bike injured in traffic accident
>
> Person on outside of go cart in traffic accident
>
> Person on outside of golf cart injured in traffic accident

✓5ᵗʰ **V86.3** Unspecified occupant of special all-terrain or other off-road motor vehicle injured in traffic accident

✓x7ᵗʰ **V86.31** Unspecified occupant of ambulance or fire engine injured in traffic accident

✓x7ᵗʰ **V86.32** Unspecified occupant of snowmobile injured in traffic accident

✓x7ᵗʰ **V86.33** Unspecified occupant of dune buggy injured in traffic accident

✓x7ᵗʰ **V86.34** Unspecified occupant of military vehicle injured in traffic accident

✓x7ᵗʰ **V86.35** Unspecified occupant of 3- or 4- wheeled all-terrain vehicle (ATV) injured in traffic accident

✓x7ᵗʰ **V86.36** Unspecified occupant of dirt bike or motor/cross bike injured in traffic accident

✓x7ᵗʰ **V86.39** Unspecified occupant of other special all-terrain or other off-road motor vehicle injured in traffic accident

> Unspecified occupant of dirt bike injured in traffic accident
>
> Unspecified occupant of go cart injured in traffic accident
>
> Unspecified occupant of golf cart injured in traffic accident

✓5ᵗʰ **V86.4** Person injured while boarding or alighting from special all-terrain or other off-road motor vehicle

✓x7ᵗʰ **V86.41** Person injured while boarding or alighting from ambulance or fire engine

✓x7ᵗʰ **V86.42** Person injured while boarding or alighting from snowmobile

✓x7ᵗʰ **V86.43** Person injured while boarding or alighting from dune buggy

✓x7ᵗʰ **V86.44** Person injured while boarding or alighting from military vehicle

✓x7ᵗʰ **V86.45** Person injured while boarding or alighting from a 3- or 4- wheeled all-terrain vehicle (ATV)

✓x7ᵗʰ **V86.46** Person injured while boarding or alighting from a dirt bike or motor/cross bike

✓x7ᵗʰ **V86.49** Person injured while boarding or alighting from other special all-terrain or other off-road motor vehicle

> Person injured while boarding or alighting from dirt bike
>
> Person injured while boarding or alighting from go cart
>
> Person injured while boarding or alighting from golf cart

✓5ᵗʰ **V86.5** Driver of special all-terrain or other off-road motor vehicle injured in nontraffic accident

✓x7ᵗʰ **V86.51** Driver of ambulance or fire engine injured in nontraffic accident

✓x7ᵗʰ **V86.52** Driver of snowmobile injured in nontraffic accident

✓x7ᵗʰ **V86.53** Driver of dune buggy injured in nontraffic accident

✓x7ᵗʰ **V86.54** Driver of military vehicle injured in nontraffic accident

✓x7ᵗʰ **V86.55** Driver of 3- or 4- wheeled all-terrain vehicle (ATV) injured in nontraffic accident

✓x7ᵗʰ **V86.56** Driver of dirt bike or motor/cross bike injured in nontraffic accident

✓x7ᵗʰ **V86.59** Driver of other special all-terrain or other off-road motor vehicle injured in nontraffic accident

> Driver of dirt bike injured in nontraffic accident
>
> Driver of go cart injured in nontraffic accident
>
> Driver of golf cart injured in nontraffic accident

✓5ᵗʰ **V86.6** Passenger of special all-terrain or other off-road motor vehicle injured in nontraffic accident

✓x7ᵗʰ **V86.61** Passenger of ambulance or fire engine injured in nontraffic accident

✓x7ᵗʰ **V86.62** Passenger of snowmobile injured in nontraffic accident

✓x7ᵗʰ **V86.63** Passenger of dune buggy injured in nontraffic accident

✓x7ᵗʰ **V86.64** Passenger of military vehicle injured in nontraffic accident

✓x7ᵗʰ **V86.65** Passenger of 3- or 4- wheeled all-terrain vehicle (ATV) injured in nontraffic accident

✓x7ᵗʰ **V86.66** Passenger of dirt bike or motor/cross bike injured in nontraffic accident

✓x7ᵗʰ **V86.69** Passenger of other special all-terrain or other off-road motor vehicle injured in nontraffic accident

> Passenger of dirt bike injured in nontraffic accident
>
> Passenger of go cart injured in nontraffic accident
>
> Passenger of golf cart injured in nontraffic accident

✓5ᵗʰ **V86.7** Person on outside of special all-terrain or other off-road motor vehicle injured in nontraffic accident

✓x7ᵗʰ **V86.71** Person on outside of ambulance or fire engine injured in nontraffic accident

✓x7ᵗʰ **V86.72** Person on outside of snowmobile injured in nontraffic accident

✓x7ᵗʰ **V86.73** Person on outside of dune buggy injured in nontraffic accident

✓x7ᵗʰ **V86.74** Person on outside of military vehicle injured in nontraffic accident

✓x7ᵗʰ **V86.75** Person on outside of 3- or 4- wheeled all-terrain vehicle (ATV) injured in nontraffic accident

✓x7ᵗʰ **V86.76** Person on outside of dirt bike or motor/cross bike injured in nontraffic accident

✓x7ᵗʰ **V86.79** Person on outside of other special all-terrain or other off-road motor vehicles injured in nontraffic accident

> Person on outside of dirt bike injured in nontraffic accident
>
> Person on outside of go cart injured in nontraffic accident
>
> Person on outside of golf cart injured in nontraffic accident

✓5ᵗʰ **V86.9** Unspecified occupant of special all-terrain or other off-road motor vehicle injured in nontraffic accident

✓x7ᵗʰ **V86.91** Unspecified occupant of ambulance or fire engine injured in nontraffic accident

✓x7ᵗʰ **V86.92** Unspecified occupant of snowmobile injured in nontraffic accident

✓x7ᵗʰ **V86.93** Unspecified occupant of dune buggy injured in nontraffic accident

✓x7ᵗʰ **V86.94** Unspecified occupant of military vehicle injured in nontraffic accident

✓x7ᵗʰ **V86.95** Unspecified occupant of 3- or 4- wheeled all-terrain vehicle (ATV) injured in nontraffic accident

✓x7ᵗʰ **V86.96** Unspecified occupant of dirt bike or motor/cross bike injured in nontraffic accident

✓x7ᵗʰ **V86.99** Unspecified occupant of other special all-terrain or other off-road motor vehicle injured in nontraffic accident

> Off-road motor-vehicle accident NOS
>
> Other motor-vehicle accident NOS
>
> Unspecified occupant of go cart injured in nontraffic accident
>
> Unspecified occupant of golf cart injured in nontraffic accident

✓4ᵗʰ **V87** Traffic accident of specified type but victim's mode of transport unknown

> **EXCLUDES 1**   collision involving:
>
> pedal cycle (V10-V19)
>
> pedestrian (V01-V09)

✓x7ᵗʰ **V87.0** Person injured in collision between car and two- or three-wheeled powered vehicle (traffic)

✓x7ᵗʰ **V87.1** Person injured in collision between other motor vehicle and two- or three-wheeled motor vehicle (traffic)

✓x7ᵗʰ **V87.2** Person injured in collision between car and pick-up truck or van (traffic)

✓x7ᵗʰ **V87.3** Person injured in collision between car and bus (traffic)

✓x7ᵗʰ **V87.4** Person injured in collision between car and heavy transport vehicle (traffic)

✓x7ᵗʰ **V87.5** Person injured in collision between heavy transport vehicle and bus (traffic)

✓x7ᵗʰ **V87.6** Person injured in collision between railway train or railway vehicle and car (traffic)

✓x7ᵗʰ **V87.7** Person injured in collision between other specified motor vehicles (traffic)

√x7ᵗʰ **V87.8** **Person injured in other specified** noncollision **transport accidents** involving motor vehicle **(traffic)**

√x7ᵗʰ **V87.9** **Person injured in other specified (collision)(noncollision) transport accidents** involving nonmotor vehicle **(traffic)**

√4ᵗʰ **V88** **Nontraffic accident of specified type but victim's mode of transport unknown**

     EXCLUDES 1   *collision involving:*
           pedal cycle (V10-V19)
           pedestrian (V01-V09)

√x7ᵗʰ **V88.0** **Person injured in collision between** car and two- or three-wheeled motor vehicle, **nontraffic**

√x7ᵗʰ **V88.1** **Person injured in collision between other** motor vehicle and two- or three-wheeled motor vehicle, **nontraffic**

√x7ᵗʰ **V88.2** **Person injured in collision between** car and pick-up truck or van, **nontraffic**

√x7ᵗʰ **V88.3** **Person injured in collision between** car and bus, **nontraffic**

√x7ᵗʰ **V88.4** **Person injured in collision between** car and heavy transport vehicle, **nontraffic**

√x7ᵗʰ **V88.5** **Person injured in collision between** heavy transport vehicle and bus, **nontraffic**

√x7ᵗʰ **V88.6** **Person injured in collision between** railway train or railway vehicle and car, **nontraffic**

√x7ᵗʰ **V88.7** **Person injured in collision between other specified motor vehicle, nontraffic**

√x7ᵗʰ **V88.8** **Person injured in other specified** noncollision **transport accidents** involving motor vehicle, **nontraffic**

√x7ᵗʰ **V88.9** **Person injured in other specified (collision)(noncollision) transport accidents** involving nonmotor vehicle, **nontraffic**

√4ᵗʰ **V89** **Motor- or nonmotor-vehicle accident, type of vehicle unspecified**

√x7ᵗʰ **V89.0** **Person injured in unspecified** motor-vehicle **accident, nontraffic**
     Motor-vehicle accident NOS, nontraffic

√x7ᵗʰ **V89.1** **Person injured in unspecified** nonmotor-vehicle **accident, nontraffic**
     Nonmotor-vehicle accident NOS (nontraffic)

√x7ᵗʰ **V89.2** **Person injured in unspecified** motor-vehicle **accident, traffic**
     Motor-vehicle accident [MVA] NOS
     Road (traffic) accident [RTA] NOS

√x7ᵗʰ **V89.3** **Person injured in unspecified** nonmotor-vehicle **accident, traffic**
     Nonmotor-vehicle traffic accident NOS

√x7ᵗʰ **V89.9** **Person injured in unspecified vehicle accident**
     Collision NOS

Water transport accidents (V90-V94)

The appropriate 7th character is to be added to each code from categories V90-V94.
A   initial encounter
D   subsequent encounter
S   sequela

√4ᵗʰ **V90** **Drowning and submersion due to accident to watercraft**

     EXCLUDES 1   *civilian water transport accident involving military watercraft (V94.81-)*
           fall into water not from watercraft (W16.-)
           military watercraft accident in military or war operations (Y36.0-, Y37.0-)
           water-transport-related drowning or submersion without accident to watercraft (V92.-)

√5ᵗʰ **V90.0** **Drowning and submersion due to** watercraft overturning

√x7ᵗʰ **V90.00** **Drowning and submersion due to** merchant ship overturning

√x7ᵗʰ **V90.01** **Drowning and submersion due to** passenger ship overturning
     Drowning and submersion due to Ferry-boat overturning
     Drowning and submersion due to Liner overturning

√x7ᵗʰ **V90.02** **Drowning and submersion due to** fishing boat overturning

√x7ᵗʰ **V90.03** **Drowning and submersion due to other** powered watercraft overturning
     Drowning and submersion due to Hovercraft (on open water) overturning
     Drowning and submersion due to Jet ski overturning

√x7ᵗʰ **V90.04** **Drowning and submersion due to** sailboat overturning

√x7ᵗʰ **V90.05** **Drowning and submersion due to** canoe or kayak overturning

√x7ᵗʰ **V90.06** **Drowning and submersion due to (nonpowered)** inflatable craft overturning

√x7ᵗʰ **V90.08** **Drowning and submersion due to other** unpowered watercraft overturning
     Drowning and submersion due to windsurfer overturning

√x7ᵗʰ **V90.09** **Drowning and submersion due to unspecified watercraft overturning**
     Drowning and submersion due to boat NOS overturning
     Drowning and submersion due to ship NOS overturning
     Drowning and submersion due to watercraft NOS overturning

√5ᵗʰ **V90.1** **Drowning and submersion due to** watercraft sinking

√x7ᵗʰ **V90.10** **Drowning and submersion due to** merchant ship sinking

√x7ᵗʰ **V90.11** **Drowning and submersion due to** passenger ship sinking
     Drowning and submersion due to Ferry-boat sinking
     Drowning and submersion due to Liner sinking

√x7ᵗʰ **V90.12** **Drowning and submersion due to** fishing boat sinking

√x7ᵗʰ **V90.13** **Drowning and submersion due to other** powered watercraft sinking
     Drowning and submersion due to Hovercraft (on open water) sinking
     Drowning and submersion due to Jet ski sinking

√x7ᵗʰ **V90.14** **Drowning and submersion due to** sailboat **sinking**

√x7ᵗʰ **V90.15** **Drowning and submersion due to** canoe or kayak sinking

√x7ᵗʰ **V90.16** **Drowning and submersion due to (nonpowered)** inflatable craft **sinking**

√x7ᵗʰ **V90.18** **Drowning and submersion due to other** unpowered watercraft sinking

√x7ᵗʰ **V90.19** **Drowning and submersion due to unspecified watercraft sinking**
     Drowning and submersion due to boat NOS sinking
     Drowning and submersion due to ship NOS sinking
     Drowning and submersion due to watercraft NOS sinking

√5ᵗʰ **V90.2** **Drowning and submersion due to** falling or jumping from burning watercraft

√x7ᵗʰ **V90.20** **Drowning and submersion due to falling or jumping from burning** merchant ship

√x7ᵗʰ **V90.21** **Drowning and submersion due to falling or jumping from burning** passenger ship
     Drowning and submersion due to falling or jumping from burning Ferry-boat
     Drowning and submersion due to falling or jumping from burning Liner

√x7ᵗʰ **V90.22** **Drowning and submersion due to falling or jumping from burning** fishing boat

√x7ᵗʰ **V90.23** **Drowning and submersion due to falling or jumping from other burning** powered watercraft
     Drowning and submersion due to falling and jumping from burning Hovercraft (on open water)
     Drowning and submersion due to falling and jumping from burning Jet ski

√x7ᵗʰ **V90.24** **Drowning and submersion due to falling or jumping from burning** sailboat

√x7ᵗʰ **V90.25** **Drowning and submersion due to falling or jumping from burning** canoe or kayak

√x7ᵗʰ **V90.26** **Drowning and submersion due to falling or jumping from burning (nonpowered)** inflatable craft

√x7ᵗʰ **V90.27** **Drowning and submersion due to falling or jumping from burning** water-skis

√x7ᵗʰ **V90.28** **Drowning and submersion due to falling or jumping from other burning** unpowered watercraft
     Drowning and submersion due to falling and jumping from burning surf-board
     Drowning and submersion due to falling and jumping from burning windsurfer

---

✓ Additional Character Required   √x7ᵗʰ Placeholder Alert   Manifestation   Unspecified Dx   ▶◀ Revised Text   ● New Code   ▲ Revised Code Title

√x7ᵗʰ **V90.29 Drowning and submersion due to falling or jumping from unspecified burning watercraft**

Drowning and submersion due to falling or jumping from burning boat NOS

Drowning and submersion due to falling or jumping from burning ship NOS

Drowning and submersion due to falling or jumping from burning watercraft NOS

√5ᵗʰ **V90.3 Drowning and submersion due to** falling or jumping from crushed watercraft

√x7ᵗʰ **V90.30 Drowning and submersion due to falling or jumping from crushed** merchant ship

√x7ᵗʰ **V90.31 Drowning and submersion due to falling or jumping from crushed** passenger ship

Drowning and submersion due to falling and jumping from crushed Ferry boat

Drowning and submersion due to falling and jumping from crushed Liner

√x7ᵗʰ **V90.32 Drowning and submersion due to falling or jumping from crushed** fishing boat

√x7ᵗʰ **V90.33 Drowning and submersion due to falling or jumping from other crushed** powered **watercraft**

Drowning and submersion due to falling and jumping from crushed Hovercraft

Drowning and submersion due to falling and jumping from crushed Jet ski

√x7ᵗʰ **V90.34 Drowning and submersion due to falling or jumping from crushed** sailboat

√x7ᵗʰ **V90.35 Drowning and submersion due to falling or jumping from crushed** canoe or kayak

√x7ᵗʰ **V90.36 Drowning and submersion due to falling or jumping from crushed (nonpowered)** inflatable craft

√x7ᵗʰ **V90.37 Drowning and submersion due to falling or jumping from crushed** water-skis

√x7ᵗʰ **V90.38 Drowning and submersion due to falling or jumping from other crushed** unpowered **watercraft**

Drowning and submersion due to falling and jumping from crushed surf-board

Drowning and submersion due to falling and jumping from crushed windsurfer

√x7ᵗʰ **V90.39 Drowning and submersion due to falling or jumping from crushed unspecified watercraft**

Drowning and submersion due to falling and jumping from crushed boat NOS

Drowning and submersion due to falling and jumping from crushed ship NOS

Drowning and submersion due to falling and jumping from crushed watercraft NOS

√5ᵗʰ **V90.8 Drowning and submersion due to other accident to watercraft**

√x7ᵗʰ **V90.80 Drowning and submersion due to other accident to** merchant ship

√x7ᵗʰ **V90.81 Drowning and submersion due to other accident to** passenger ship

Drowning and submersion due to other accident to Ferry-boat

Drowning and submersion due to other accident to Liner

√x7ᵗʰ **V90.82 Drowning and submersion due to other accident to** fishing boat

√x7ᵗʰ **V90.83 Drowning and submersion due to other accident to other** powered **watercraft**

Drowning and submersion due to other accident to Hovercraft (on open water)

Drowning and submersion due to other accident to Jet ski

√x7ᵗʰ **V90.84 Drowning and submersion due to other accident to** sailboat

√x7ᵗʰ **V90.85 Drowning and submersion due to other accident to** canoe or kayak

√x7ᵗʰ **V90.86 Drowning and submersion due to other accident to (nonpowered)** inflatable craft

√x7ᵗʰ **V90.87 Drowning and submersion due to other accident to** water-skis

√x7ᵗʰ **V90.88 Drowning and submersion due to other accident to other** unpowered **watercraft**

Drowning and submersion due to other accident to surf-board

Drowning and submersion due to other accident to windsurfer

√x7ᵗʰ **V90.89 Drowning and submersion due to other accident to unspecified watercraft**

Drowning and submersion due to other accident to boat NOS

Drowning and submersion due to other accident to ship NOS

Drowning and submersion due to other accident to watercraft NOS

√4ᵗʰ **V91 Other injury due to accident to watercraft**

INCLUDES   any injury except drowning and submersion as a result of an accident to watercraft

EXCLUDES 1   civilian water transport accident involving military watercraft (V94.81-)

military watercraft accident in military or war operations (Y36, Y37.-)

EXCLUDES 2   drowning and submersion due to accident to watercraft (V90.-)

√5ᵗʰ **V91.0 Burn due to watercraft on fire**

EXCLUDES 1   burn from localized fire or explosion on board ship without accident to watercraft (V93.-)

√x7ᵗʰ **V91.00 Burn due to** merchant ship **on fire**

√x7ᵗʰ **V91.01 Burn due to** passenger ship **on fire**

Burn due to Ferry-boat on fire
Burn due to Liner on fire

√x7ᵗʰ **V91.02 Burn due to** fishing boat **on fire**

√x7ᵗʰ **V91.03 Burn due to other** powered **watercraft on fire**

Burn due to Hovercraft (on open water) on fire
Burn due to Jet ski on fire

√x7ᵗʰ **V91.04 Burn due to** sailboat **on fire**

√x7ᵗʰ **V91.05 Burn due to** canoe or kayak **on fire**

√x7ᵗʰ **V91.06 Burn due to (nonpowered)** inflatable craft **on fire**

√x7ᵗʰ **V91.07 Burn due to** water-skis **on fire**

√x7ᵗʰ **V91.08 Burn due to other** unpowered **watercraft on fire**

√x7ᵗʰ **V91.09 Burn due to unspecified watercraft on fire**

Burn due to boat NOS on fire
Burn due to ship NOS on fire
Burn due to watercraft NOS on fire

√5ᵗʰ **V91.1 Crushed between watercraft and other watercraft or other object due to collision**

Crushed by lifeboat after abandoning ship in a collision

NOTE   Select the specified type of watercraft that the victim was on at the time of the collision

√x7ᵗʰ **V91.10 Crushed between** merchant ship **and other watercraft or other object due to collision**

√x7ᵗʰ **V91.11 Crushed between** passenger ship **and other watercraft or other object due to collision**

Crushed between Ferry-boat and other watercraft or other object due to collision

Crushed between Liner and other watercraft or other object due to collision

√x7ᵗʰ **V91.12 Crushed between** fishing boat **and other watercraft or other object due to collision**

√x7ᵗʰ **V91.13 Crushed between other** powered **watercraft and other watercraft or other object due to collision**

Crushed between Hovercraft (on open water) and other watercraft or other object due to collision

Crushed between Jet ski and other watercraft or other object due to collision

√x7ᵗʰ **V91.14 Crushed between** sailboat **and other watercraft or other object due to collision**

√x7ᵗʰ **V91.15 Crushed between** canoe or kayak **and other watercraft or other object due to collision**

√x7ᵗʰ **V91.16 Crushed between (nonpowered)** inflatable craft **and other watercraft or other object due to collision**

✓x7ᵗʰ **V91.18** **Crushed between other** unpowered **watercraft and other watercraft or other object due to collision**
　　Crushed between surfboard and other watercraft or other object due to collision
　　Crushed between windsurfer and other watercraft or other object due to collision

✓x7ᵗʰ **V91.19** **Crushed between unspecified watercraft and other watercraft or other object due to collision**
　　Crushed between boat NOS and other watercraft or other object due to collision
　　Crushed between ship NOS and other watercraft or other object due to collision
　　Crushed between watercraft NOS and other watercraft or other object due to collision

✓5ᵗʰ **V91.2** **Fall due to collision between watercraft and other watercraft or other object**
　　Fall while remaining on watercraft after collision

> **NOTE** Select the specified type of watercraft that the victim was on at the time of the collision

> **EXCLUDES 1** *crushed between watercraft and other watercraft and other object due to collision (V91.1-)*
> *drowning and submersion due to falling from crushed watercraft (V90.3-)*

✓x7ᵗʰ **V91.20** **Fall due to collision between** merchant ship **and other watercraft or other object**

✓x7ᵗʰ **V91.21** **Fall due to collision between** passenger ship **and other watercraft or other object**
　　Fall due to collision between Ferry-boat and other watercraft or other object
　　Fall due to collision between Liner and other watercraft or other object

✓x7ᵗʰ **V91.22** **Fall due to collision between** fishing boat **and other watercraft or other object**

✓x7ᵗʰ **V91.23** **Fall due to collision between other** powered **watercraft and other watercraft or other object**
　　Fall due to collision between Hovercraft (on open water) and other watercraft or other object
　　Fall due to collision between Jet ski and other watercraft or other object

✓x7ᵗʰ **V91.24** **Fall due to collision between** sailboat **and other watercraft or other object**

✓x7ᵗʰ **V91.25** **Fall due to collision between** canoe or kayak **and other watercraft or other object**

✓x7ᵗʰ **V91.26** **Fall due to collision between (nonpowered)** inflatable craft **and other watercraft or other object**

✓x7ᵗʰ **V91.29** **Fall due to collision between unspecified watercraft and other watercraft or other object**
　　Fall due to collision between boat NOS and other watercraft or other object
　　Fall due to collision between ship NOS and other watercraft or other object
　　Fall due to collision between watercraft NOS and other watercraft or other object

✓5ᵗʰ **V91.3** **Hit or struck by falling object due to accident to watercraft**
　　Hit or struck by falling object (part of damaged watercraft or other object) after falling or jumping from damaged watercraft

> **EXCLUDES 2** *drowning or submersion due to fall or jumping from damaged watercraft (V90.2-, V90.3-)*

✓x7ᵗʰ **V91.30** **Hit or struck by falling object due to accident to** merchant ship

✓x7ᵗʰ **V91.31** **Hit or struck by falling object due to accident to** passenger ship
　　Hit or struck by falling object due to accident to Ferry-boat
　　Hit or struck by falling object due to accident to Liner

✓x7ᵗʰ **V91.32** **Hit or struck by falling object due to accident to** fishing boat

✓x7ᵗʰ **V91.33** **Hit or struck by falling object due to accident to other** powered **watercraft**
　　Hit or struck by falling object due to accident to Hovercraft (on open water)
　　Hit or struck by falling object due to accident to Jet ski

✓x7ᵗʰ **V91.34** **Hit or struck by falling object due to accident to** sailboat

✓x7ᵗʰ **V91.35** **Hit or struck by falling object due to accident to** canoe or kayak

✓x7ᵗʰ **V91.36** **Hit or struck by falling object due to accident to (nonpowered)** inflatable craft

✓x7ᵗʰ **V91.37** **Hit or struck by falling object due to accident to** water-skis
　　Hit by water-skis after jumping off of waterskis

✓x7ᵗʰ **V91.38** **Hit or struck by falling object due to accident to other** unpowered **watercraft**
　　Hit or struck by surf-board after falling off damaged surf-board
　　Hit or struck by object after falling off damaged windsurfer

✓x7ᵗʰ **V91.39** **Hit or struck by falling object due to accident to unspecified watercraft**
　　Hit or struck by falling object due to accident to boat NOS
　　Hit or struck by falling object due to accident to ship NOS
　　Hit or struck by falling object due to accident to watercraft NOS

✓5ᵗʰ **V91.8** **Other injury due to other accident to watercraft**

✓x7ᵗʰ **V91.80** **Other injury due to other accident to** merchant ship

✓x7ᵗʰ **V91.81** **Other injury due to other accident to** passenger ship
　　Other injury due to other accident to Ferry-boat
　　Other injury due to other accident to Liner

✓x7ᵗʰ **V91.82** **Other injury due to other accident to** fishing boat

✓x7ᵗʰ **V91.83** **Other injury due to other accident to other** powered **watercraft**
　　Other injury due to other accident to Hovercraft (on open water)
　　Other injury due to other accident to Jet ski

✓x7ᵗʰ **V91.84** **Other injury due to other accident to** sailboat

✓x7ᵗʰ **V91.85** **Other injury due to other accident to** canoe or kayak

✓x7ᵗʰ **V91.86** **Other injury due to other accident to (nonpowered)** inflatable craft

✓x7ᵗʰ **V91.87** **Other injury due to other accident to** water-skis

✓x7ᵗʰ **V91.88** **Other injury due to other accident to other** unpowered **watercraft**
　　Other injury due to other accident to surf-board
　　Other injury due to other accident to windsurfer

✓x7ᵗʰ **V91.89** **Other injury due to other accident to unspecified watercraft**
　　Other injury due to other accident to boat NOS
　　Other injury due to other accident to ship NOS
　　Other injury due to other accident to watercraft NOS

✓4ᵗʰ **V92** **Drowning and submersion due to accident on board watercraft, without accident to watercraft**

> **EXCLUDES 1** *civilian water transport accident involving military watercraft (V94.81-)*
> *drowning or submersion due to accident to watercraft (V90-V91)*
> *drowning or submersion of diver who voluntarily jumps from boat not involved in an accident (W16.711, W16.721)*
> *fall into water without watercraft (W16.-)*
> *military watercraft accident in military or war operations (Y36, Y37)*

✓5ᵗʰ **V92.Ø** **Drowning and submersion due to** fall off **watercraft**
　　Drowning and submersion due to fall from gangplank of watercraft
　　Drowning and submersion due to fall overboard watercraft

> **EXCLUDES 2** *hitting head on object or bottom of body of water due to fall from watercraft (V94.0-)*

✓x7ᵗʰ **V92.ØØ** **Drowning and submersion due to fall off** merchant ship

✓x7ᵗʰ **V92.Ø1** **Drowning and submersion due to fall off** passenger ship
　　Drowning and submersion due to fall off Ferry-boat
　　Drowning and submersion due to fall off Liner

✓x7ᵗʰ **V92.Ø2** **Drowning and submersion due to fall off** fishing boat

✓x7ᵗʰ **V92.Ø3** **Drowning and submersion due to fall off other** powered **watercraft**
　　Drowning and submersion due to fall off Hovercraft (on open water)
　　Drowning and submersion due to fall off Jet ski

✓x7ᵗʰ **V92.Ø4** **Drowning and submersion due to fall off** sailboat

✓x7ᵗʰ **V92.Ø5** **Drowning and submersion due to fall off** canoe or kayak

√x7ᵗʰ **V92.06** **Drowning and submersion due to fall off (nonpowered)** inflatable craft

√x7ᵗʰ **V92.07** **Drowning and submersion due to fall off** water-skis

EXCLUDES 1   *drowning and submersion due to falling off burning water-skis (V90.27)*
drowning and submersion due to falling off crushed water-skis (V90.37)
hit by boat while water-skiing NOS (V94.X)

√x7ᵗʰ **V92.08** **Drowning and submersion due to fall off other** unpowered **watercraft**

Drowning and submersion due to fall off surf-board
Drowning and submersion due to fall off windsurfer

EXCLUDES 1   *drowning and submersion due to fall off burning unpowered watercraft (V90.28)*
drowning and submersion due to fall off crushed unpowered watercraft (V90.38)
drowning and submersion due to fall off damaged unpowered watercraft (V90.88)
drowning and submersion due to rider of nonpowered watercraft being hit by other watercraft (V94.-)
other injury due to rider of nonpowered watercraft being hit by other watercraft (V94.-)

√x7ᵗʰ **V92.09** **Drowning and submersion due to fall off unspecified watercraft**

Drowning and submersion due to fall off boat NOS
Drowning and submersion due to fall off ship
Drowning and submersion due to fall off watercraft NOS

√5ᵗʰ **V92.1** **Drowning and submersion due to being** thrown overboard **by motion of watercraft**

EXCLUDES 1   *drowning and submersion due to fall off surf-board (V92.08)*
drowning and submersion due to fall off water-skis (V92.07)
drowning and submersion due to fall off windsurfer (V92.08)

√x7ᵗʰ **V92.10** **Drowning and submersion due to being thrown overboard by motion of** merchant ship

√x7ᵗʰ **V92.11** **Drowning and submersion due to being thrown overboard by motion of** passenger ship

Drowning and submersion due to being thrown overboard by motion of Ferry-boat
Drowning and submersion due to being thrown overboard by motion of Liner

√x7ᵗʰ **V92.12** **Drowning and submersion due to being thrown overboard by motion of** fishing boat

√x7ᵗʰ **V92.13** **Drowning and submersion due to being thrown overboard by motion of other** powered **watercraft**

Drowning and submersion due to being thrown overboard by motion of Hovercraft

√x7ᵗʰ **V92.14** **Drowning and submersion due to being thrown overboard by motion of** sailboat

√x7ᵗʰ **V92.15** **Drowning and submersion due to being thrown overboard by motion of** canoe or kayak

√x7ᵗʰ **V92.16** **Drowning and submersion due to being thrown overboard by motion of (nonpowered)** inflatable craft

√x7ᵗʰ **V92.19** **Drowning and submersion due to being thrown overboard by motion of unspecified watercraft**

Drowning and submersion due to being thrown overboard by motion of boat NOS
Drowning and submersion due to being thrown overboard by motion of ship NOS
Drowning and submersion due to being thrown overboard by motion of watercraft NOS

√5ᵗʰ **V92.2** **Drowning and submersion due to being** washed overboard **from watercraft**

Code first any associated cataclysm (X37.0-)

√x7ᵗʰ **V92.20** **Drowning and submersion due to being washed overboard from** merchant ship

√x7ᵗʰ **V92.21** **Drowning and submersion due to being washed overboard from** passenger ship

Drowning and submersion due to being washed overboard from Ferry-boat
Drowning and submersion due to being washed overboard from Liner

√x7ᵗʰ **V92.22** **Drowning and submersion due to being washed overboard from** fishing boat

√x7ᵗʰ **V92.23** **Drowning and submersion due to being washed overboard from other** powered **watercraft**

Drowning and submersion due to being washed overboard from Hovercraft (on open water)
Drowning and submersion due to being washed overboard from Jet ski

√x7ᵗʰ **V92.24** **Drowning and submersion due to being washed overboard from** sailboat

√x7ᵗʰ **V92.25** **Drowning and submersion due to being washed overboard from** canoe or kayak

√x7ᵗʰ **V92.26** **Drowning and submersion due to being washed overboard from (nonpowered)** inflatable craft

√x7ᵗʰ **V92.27** **Drowning and submersion due to being washed overboard from** water-skis

EXCLUDES 1   *drowning and submersion due to fall off water-skis (V92.07)*

√x7ᵗʰ **V92.28** **Drowning and submersion due to being washed overboard from other** unpowered **watercraft**

Drowning and submersion due to being washed overboard from surf-board
Drowning and submersion due to being washed overboard from windsurfer

√x7ᵗʰ **V92.29** **Drowning and submersion due to being washed overboard from unspecified watercraft**

Drowning and submersion due to being washed overboard from boat NOS
Drowning and submersion due to being washed overboard from ship NOS
Drowning and submersion due to being washed overboard from watercraft NOS

√4ᵗʰ **V93** **Other injury due to accident on board watercraft, without accident to watercraft**

EXCLUDES 1   *civilian water transport accident involving military watercraft (V94.81-)*
other injury due to accident to watercraft (V91.-)
military watercraft accident in military or war operations (Y36, Y37.-)

EXCLUDES 2   *drowning and submersion due to accident on board watercraft, without accident to watercraft (V92.-)*

√5ᵗʰ **V93.0** **Burn due to localized fire on board watercraft**

EXCLUDES 1   *burn due to watercraft on fire (V91.0-)*

√x7ᵗʰ **V93.00** **Burn due to localized fire on board** merchant vessel

√x7ᵗʰ **V93.01** **Burn due to localized fire on board** passenger vessel

Burn due to localized fire on board Ferry-boat
Burn due to localized fire on board Liner

√x7ᵗʰ **V93.02** **Burn due to localized fire on board** fishing boat

√x7ᵗʰ **V93.03** **Burn due to localized fire on board other** powered **watercraft**

Burn due to localized fire on board Hovercraft
Burn due to localized fire on board Jet ski

√x7ᵗʰ **V93.04** **Burn due to localized fire on board** sailboat

√x7ᵗʰ **V93.09** **Burn due to localized fire on board unspecified watercraft**

Burn due to localized fire on board boat NOS
Burn due to localized fire on board ship NOS
Burn due to localized fire on board watercraft NOS

√5ᵗʰ **V93.1** **Other burn on board watercraft**

Burn due to source other than fire on board watercraft

EXCLUDES 1   *burn due to watercraft on fire (V91.0-)*

√x7ᵗʰ **V93.10** **Other burn on board** merchant vessel

√x7ᵗʰ **V93.11** **Other burn on board** passenger vessel

Other burn on board Ferry-boat
Other burn on board Liner

√x7ᵗʰ **V93.12** **Other burn on board** fishing boat

√x7ᵗʰ **V93.13** **Other burn on board other** powered **watercraft**

Other burn on board Hovercraft
Other burn on board Jet ski

√x7ᵗʰ **V93.14** **Other burn on board** sailboat

☑7ᵗʰ **V93.19** **Other burn on board unspecified watercraft**
  Other burn on board boat NOS
  Other burn on board ship NOS
  Other burn on board watercraft NOS

☑5ᵗʰ **V93.2** **Heat exposure on board watercraft**
  EXCLUDES 1 *exposure to man-made heat not aboard watercraft (W92)*
      exposure to natural heat while on board watercraft (X30)
      exposure to sunlight while on board watercraft (X32)
  EXCLUDES 2 *burn due to fire on board watercraft (V93.0-)*

☑7ᵗʰ **V93.20** **Heat exposure on board merchant ship**

☑7ᵗʰ **V93.21** **Heat exposure on board passenger ship**
  Heat exposure on board Ferry-boat
  Heat exposure on board Liner

☑7ᵗʰ **V93.22** **Heat exposure on board fishing boat**

☑7ᵗʰ **V93.23** **Heat exposure on board other powered watercraft**
  Heat exposure on board hovercraft

☑7ᵗʰ **V93.24** **Heat exposure on board sailboat**

☑7ᵗʰ **V93.29** **Heat exposure on board unspecified watercraft**
  Heat exposure on board boat NOS
  Heat exposure on board ship NOS
  Heat exposure on board watercraft NOS

☑5ᵗʰ **V93.3** **Fall on board watercraft**
  EXCLUDES 1 *fall due to collision of watercraft (V91.2-)*

☑7ᵗʰ **V93.30** **Fall on board merchant ship**

☑7ᵗʰ **V93.31** **Fall on board passenger ship**
  Fall on board Ferry-boat
  Fall on board Liner

☑7ᵗʰ **V93.32** **Fall on board fishing boat**

☑7ᵗʰ **V93.33** **Fall on board other powered watercraft**
  Fall on board Hovercraft (on open water)
  Fall on board Jet ski

☑7ᵗʰ **V93.34** **Fall on board sailboat**

☑7ᵗʰ **V93.35** **Fall on board canoe or kayak**

☑7ᵗʰ **V93.36** **Fall on board (nonpowered) inflatable craft**

☑7ᵗʰ **V93.38** **Fall on board other unpowered watercraft**

☑7ᵗʰ **V93.39** **Fall on board unspecified watercraft**
  Fall on board boat NOS
  Fall on board ship NOS
  Fall on board watercraft NOS

☑6ᵗʰ **V93.4** **Struck by falling object on board watercraft**
  Hit by falling object on board watercraft
  EXCLUDES 1 *struck by falling object due to accident to watercraft (V91.3)*

☑7ᵗʰ **V93.40** **Struck by falling object on merchant ship**

☑7ᵗʰ **V93.41** **Struck by falling object on passenger ship**
  Struck by falling object on Ferry-boat
  Struck by falling object on Liner

☑7ᵗʰ **V93.42** **Struck by falling object on fishing boat**

☑7ᵗʰ **V93.43** **Struck by falling object on other powered watercraft**
  Struck by falling object on Hovercraft

☑7ᵗʰ **V93.44** **Struck by falling object on sailboat**

☑7ᵗʰ **V93.48** **Struck by falling object on other unpowered watercraft**

☑7ᵗʰ **V93.49** **Struck by falling object on unspecified watercraft**

☑5ᵗʰ **V93.5** **Explosion on board watercraft**
  Boiler explosion on steamship
  EXCLUDES 2 *fire on board watercraft (V93.0-)*

☑7ᵗʰ **V93.50** **Explosion on board merchant ship**

☑7ᵗʰ **V93.51** **Explosion on board passenger ship**
  Explosion on board Ferry-boat
  Explosion on board Liner

☑7ᵗʰ **V93.52** **Explosion on board fishing boat**

☑7ᵗʰ **V93.53** **Explosion on board other powered watercraft**
  Explosion on board Hovercraft
  Explosion on board Jet ski

☑7ᵗʰ **V93.54** **Explosion on board sailboat**

☑7ᵗʰ **V93.59** **Explosion on board unspecified watercraft**
  Explosion on board boat NOS
  Explosion on board ship NOS
  Explosion on board watercraft NOS

☑5ᵗʰ **V93.6** **Machinery accident on board watercraft**
  EXCLUDES 1 *machinery explosion on board watercraft (V93.4-)*
      machinery fire on board watercraft (V93.0-)

☑7ᵗʰ **V93.60** **Machinery accident on board merchant ship**

☑7ᵗʰ **V93.61** **Machinery accident on board passenger ship**
  Machinery accident on board Ferry-boat
  Machinery accident on board Liner

☑7ᵗʰ **V93.62** **Machinery accident on board fishing boat**

☑7ᵗʰ **V93.63** **Machinery accident on board other powered watercraft**
  Machinery accident on board Hovercraft

☑7ᵗʰ **V93.64** **Machinery accident on board sailboat**

☑7ᵗʰ **V93.69** **Machinery accident on board unspecified watercraft**
  Machinery accident on board boat NOS
  Machinery accident on board ship NOS
  Machinery accident on board watercraft NOS

☑5ᵗʰ **V93.8** **Other injury due to other accident on board watercraft**
  Accidental poisoning by gases or fumes on watercraft

☑7ᵗʰ **V93.80** **Other injury due to other accident on board merchant ship**

☑7ᵗʰ **V93.81** **Other injury due to other accident on board passenger ship**
  Other injury due to other accident on board Ferry-boat
  Other injury due to other accident on board Liner

☑7ᵗʰ **V93.82** **Other injury due to other accident on board fishing boat**

☑7ᵗʰ **V93.83** **Other injury due to other accident on board other powered watercraft**
  Other injury due to other accident on board Hovercraft
  Other injury due to other accident on board Jet ski

☑7ᵗʰ **V93.84** **Other injury due to other accident on board sailboat**

☑7ᵗʰ **V93.85** **Other injury due to other accident on board canoe or kayak**

☑7ᵗʰ **V93.86** **Other injury due to other accident on board (nonpowered) inflatable craft**

☑7ᵗʰ **V93.87** **Other injury due to other accident on board water-skis**
  Hit or struck by object while waterskiing

☑7ᵗʰ **V93.88** **Other injury due to other accident on board other unpowered watercraft**
  Hit or struck by object while surfing
  Hit or struck by object while on board windsurfer

☑7ᵗʰ **V93.89** **Other injury due to other accident on board unspecified watercraft**
  Other injury due to other accident on board boat NOS
  Other injury due to other accident on board ship NOS
  Other injury due to other accident on board watercraft NOS

☑4ᵗʰ **V94** **Other and unspecified water transport accidents**
  EXCLUDES 1 *military watercraft accidents in military or war operations (Y36, Y37)*

☑7ᵗʰ **V94.0** **Hitting object or bottom of body of water due to fall from watercraft**
  EXCLUDES 2 *drowning and submersion due to fall from watercraft (V92.0-)*

☑5ᵗʰ **V94.1** **Bather struck by watercraft**
  Swimmer hit by watercraft

☑7ᵗʰ **V94.11** **Bather struck by powered watercraft**

☑7ᵗʰ **V94.12** **Bather struck by nonpowered watercraft**

☑5ᵗʰ **V94.2** **Rider of nonpowered watercraft struck by other watercraft**

☑7ᵗʰ **V94.21** **Rider of nonpowered watercraft struck by other nonpowered watercraft**
  Canoer hit by other nonpowered watercraft
  Surfer hit by other nonpowered watercraft
  Windsurfer hit by other nonpowered watercraft

√x7th **V94.22** **Rider of nonpowered watercraft struck by** powered watercraft

     Canoer hit by motorboat

     Surfer hit by motorboat

     Windsurfer hit by motorboat

√5th **V94.3** **Injury to rider of (inflatable) watercraft being pulled behind other watercraft**

   √x7th **V94.31** **Injury to rider of (inflatable)** recreational **watercraft being pulled behind other watercraft**

      Injury to rider of inner-tube pulled behind motor boat

   √x7th **V94.32** **Injury to rider of** non-recreational **watercraft being pulled behind other watercraft**

      Injury to occupant of dingy being pulled behind boat or ship

      Injury to occupant of life-raft being pulled behind boat or ship

√x7th **V94.4** **Injury to barefoot water-skier**

     Injury to person being pulled behind boat or ship

√5th **V94.8** **Other water transport accident**

   √6th **V94.81** **Water transport accident involving military watercraft**

     √7th **V94.810** **Civilian watercraft involved in water transport accident with military watercraft**

       Passenger on civilian watercraft injured due to accident with military watercraft

     √7th **V94.811** **Civilian in water injured by military watercraft**

     √7th **V94.818** **Other water transport accident involving military watercraft**

   √x7th **V94.89** **Other water transport accident**

√x7th **V94.9** **Unspecified water transport accident**

     Water transport accident NOS

Air and space transport accidents (V95-V97)

EXCLUDES 1   military aircraft accidents in military or war operations (Y36, Y37)

The appropriate 7th character is to be added to each code from categories V95-V97.

A   initial encounter

D   subsequent encounter

S   sequela

√4th **V95** **Accident to powered aircraft causing injury to occupant**

  √5th **V95.0** **Helicopter** accident injuring occupant

   √x7th **V95.00** **Unspecified helicopter accident injuring occupant**

   √x7th **V95.01** **Helicopter** crash **injuring occupant**

   √x7th **V95.02** Forced landing **of helicopter injuring occupant**

   √x7th **V95.03** **Helicopter** collision **injuring occupant**

     Helicopter collision with any object, fixed, movable or moving

   √x7th **V95.04** **Helicopter** fire **injuring occupant**

   √x7th **V95.05** **Helicopter** explosion **injuring occupant**

   √x7th **V95.09** **Other helicopter accident injuring occupant**

  √5th **V95.1** Ultralight, microlight or powered-glider **accident injuring occupant**

   √x7th **V95.10** **Unspecified ultralight, microlight or powered-glider accident injuring occupant**

   √x7th **V95.11** **Ultralight, microlight or powered-glider** crash **injuring occupant**

   √x7th **V95.12** Forced landing **of ultralight, microlight or powered-glider injuring occupant**

   √x7th **V95.13** **Ultralight, microlight or powered-glider** collision **injuring occupant**

     Ultralight, microlight or powered-glider collision with any object, fixed, movable or moving

   √x7th **V95.14** **Ultralight, microlight or powered-glider** fire **injuring occupant**

   √x7th **V95.15** **Ultralight, microlight or powered-glider** explosion **injuring occupant**

   √x7th **V95.19** **Other ultralight, microlight or powered-glider accident injuring occupant**

  √5th **V95.2** **Other private fixed-wing aircraft accident injuring occupant**

   √x7th **V95.20** **Unspecified accident to other private fixed-wing aircraft, injuring occupant**

   √x7th **V95.21** **Other private fixed-wing aircraft crash injuring occupant**

   √x7th **V95.22** Forced landing **of other private fixed-wing aircraft injuring occupant**

   √x7th **V95.23** **Other private fixed-wing aircraft** collision **injuring occupant**

     Other private fixed-wing aircraft collision with any object, fixed, movable or moving

   √x7th **V95.24** **Other private fixed-wing aircraft** fire **injuring occupant**

   √x7th **V95.25** **Other private fixed-wing aircraft** explosion **injuring occupant**

   √x7th **V95.29** **Other accident to other private fixed-wing aircraft injuring occupant**

  √5th **V95.3** Commercial fixed-wing **aircraft accident injuring occupant**

   √x7th **V95.30** **Unspecified accident to commercial fixed-wing aircraft injuring occupant**

   √x7th **V95.31** **Commercial fixed-wing aircraft** crash **injuring occupant**

   √x7th **V95.32** Forced landing **of commercial fixed-wing aircraft injuring occupant**

   √x7th **V95.33** **Commercial fixed-wing aircraft** collision **injuring occupant**

     Commercial fixed-wing aircraft collision with any object, fixed, movable or moving

   √x7th **V95.34** **Commercial fixed-wing aircraft** fire **injuring occupant**

   √x7th **V95.35** **Commercial fixed-wing aircraft** explosion **injuring occupant**

   √x7th **V95.39** **Other accident to commercial fixed-wing aircraft injuring occupant**

  √5th **V95.4** Spacecraft **accident injuring occupant**

   √x7th **V95.40** **Unspecified spacecraft accident injuring occupant**

   √x7th **V95.41** **Spacecraft** crash **injuring occupant**

   √x7th **V95.42** Forced landing **of spacecraft injuring occupant**

   √x7th **V95.43** **Spacecraft** collision **injuring occupant**

     Spacecraft collision with any object, fixed, moveable or moving

   √x7th **V95.44** **Spacecraft** fire **injuring occupant**

   √x7th **V95.45** **Spacecraft** explosion **injuring occupant**

   √x7th **V95.49** **Other spacecraft accident injuring occupant**

  √x7th **V95.8** **Other powered aircraft accidents injuring occupant**

  √x7th **V95.9** **Unspecified aircraft accident injuring occupant**

     Aircraft accident NOS

     Air transport accident NOS

√4th **V96** **Accident to nonpowered aircraft causing injury to occupant**

  √5th **V96.0** Balloon **accident injuring occupant**

   √x7th **V96.00** **Unspecified balloon accident injuring occupant**

   √x7th **V96.01** **Balloon** crash **injuring occupant**

   √x7th **V96.02** Forced landing **of balloon injuring occupant**

   √x7th **V96.03** **Balloon** collision **injuring occupant**

     Balloon collision with any object, fixed, moveable or moving

   √x7th **V96.04** **Balloon** fire **injuring occupant**

   √x7th **V96.05** **Balloon** explosion **injuring occupant**

   √x7th **V96.09** **Other balloon accident injuring occupant**

  √5th **V96.1** Hang-glider **accident injuring occupant**

   √x7th **V96.10** **Unspecified hang-glider accident injuring occupant**

   √x7th **V96.11** **Hang-glider** crash **injuring occupant**

   √x7th **V96.12** Forced landing **of hang-glider injuring occupant**

   √x7th **V96.13** **Hang-glider** collision **injuring occupant**

     Hang-glider collision with any object, fixed, moveable or moving

   √x7th **V96.14** **Hang-glider** fire **injuring occupant**

   √x7th **V96.15** **Hang-glider** explosion **injuring occupant**

   √x7th **V96.19** **Other hang-glider accident injuring occupant**

  √5th **V96.2** **Glider (nonpowered) accident injuring occupant**

   √x7th **V96.20** **Unspecified glider (nonpowered) accident injuring occupant**

   √x7th **V96.21** **Glider (nonpowered)** crash **injuring occupant**

   √x7th **V96.22** Forced landing **of glider (nonpowered) injuring occupant**

√x7ᵗʰ **V96.23** **Glider (nonpowered)** collision **injuring occupant**
> Glider (nonpowered) collision with any object, fixed, moveable or moving

√x7ᵗʰ **V96.24** **Glider (nonpowered)** fire **injuring occupant**

√x7ᵗʰ **V96.25** **Glider (nonpowered)** explosion **injuring occupant**

√x7ᵗʰ **V96.29** **Other glider (nonpowered) accident injuring occupant**

√x7ᵗʰ **V96.8** **Other nonpowered-aircraft accidents injuring occupant**
> Kite carrying a person accident injuring occupant

√x7ᵗʰ **V96.9** **Unspecified nonpowered-aircraft accident injuring occupant**
> Nonpowered-aircraft accident NOS

√4ᵗʰ **V97** **Other specified air transport accidents**

√x7ᵗʰ **V97.0** **Occupant of aircraft injured in other specified air transport accidents**
> Fall in, on or from aircraft in air transport accident
> > EXCLUDES 1   *accident while boarding or alighting aircraft (V97.1)*

√x7ᵗʰ **V97.1** **Person injured while boarding or alighting from aircraft**

√5ᵗʰ **V97.2** **Parachutist accident**

√x7ᵗʰ **V97.21** **Parachutist entangled in object**
> Parachutist landing in tree

√x7ᵗʰ **V97.22** **Parachutist injured on landing**

√x7ᵗʰ **V97.29** **Other parachutist accident**

√5ᵗʰ **V97.3** **Person on ground injured in air transport accident**

√x7ᵗʰ **V97.31** **Hit by object falling from aircraft**
> Hit by crashing aircraft
> Injured by aircraft hitting house
> Injured by aircraft hitting car

√x7ᵗʰ **V97.32** **Injured by rotating propeller**

√x7ᵗʰ **V97.33** **Sucked into jet engine**

√x7ᵗʰ **V97.39** **Other injury to person on ground due to air transport accident**

√5ᵗʰ **V97.8** **Other air transport accidents, not elsewhere classified**
> > EXCLUDES 1   *aircraft accident NOS (V95.9)*
> > *exposure to changes in air pressure during ascent or descent (W94.-)*

√6ᵗʰ **V97.81** **Air transport accident involving military aircraft**

√7ᵗʰ **V97.810** **Civilian aircraft involved in air transport accident with military aircraft**
> Passenger in civilian aircraft injured due to accident with military aircraft

√7ᵗʰ **V97.811** **Civilian injured by military aircraft**

√7ᵗʰ **V97.818** **Other air transport accident involving military aircraft**

√x7ᵗʰ **V97.89** **Other air transport accidents, not elsewhere classified**
> Injury from machinery on aircraft

Other and unspecified transport accidents (V98-V99)

EXCLUDES 1   *vehicle accident, type of vehicle unspecified (V89.-)*

The appropriate 7th character is to be added to each code from categories V98-V99.
A   initial encounter
D   subsequent encounter
S   sequela

√4ᵗʰ **V98** **Other specified transport accidents**

√x7ᵗʰ **V98.0** **Accident to, on or involving** cable-car, **not on rails**
> Caught or dragged by cable-car, not on rails
> Fall or jump from cable-car, not on rails
> Object thrown from or in cable-car, not on rails

√x7ᵗʰ **V98.1** **Accident to, on or involving** land-yacht

√x7ᵗʰ **V98.2** **Accident to, on or involving** ice yacht

√x7ᵗʰ **V98.3** **Accident to, on or involving** ski lift
> Accident to, on or involving ski chair-lift
> Accident to, on or involving ski-lift with gondola

√x7ᵗʰ **V98.8** **Other specified transport accidents**

√x7ᵗʰ **V99** **Unspecified transport accident**

OTHER EXTERNAL CAUSES OF ACCIDENTAL INJURY (W00-X58)

Slipping, tripping, stumbling and falls (W00-W19)

EXCLUDES 1   *assault involving a fall (Y01-Y02)*
> *fall from animal (V80.-)*
> *fall (in) (from) machinery (in operation) (W28-W31)*
> *fall (in) (from) transport vehicle (V01-V99)*
> *intentional self-harm involving a fall (X80-X81)*

EXCLUDES 2   *at risk for fall (history of fall) Z91.81*
> *fall (in) (from) burning building (X00.-)*
> *fall into fire (X00-X04, X08)*

The appropriate 7th character is to be added to each code from categories W00-W19.
A   initial encounter
D   subsequent encounter
S   sequela

√4ᵗʰ **W00** **Fall due to ice and snow**
> INCLUDES   pedestrian on foot falling (slipping) on ice and snow
> EXCLUDES 1   *fall on (from) ice and snow involving pedestrian conveyance (V00.-)*
> > *fall from stairs and steps not due to ice and snow (W10.-)*
> AHA: 2016,2Q,4

√x7ᵗʰ **W00.0** **Fall on** same level **due to ice and snow**

√x7ᵗʰ **W00.1** **Fall from** stairs **and steps due to ice and snow**

√x7ᵗʰ **W00.2** **Other fall from one level to another due to ice and snow**

√x7ᵗʰ **W00.9** **Unspecified fall due to ice and snow**

√4ᵗʰ **W01** **Fall on same level from slipping, tripping and stumbling**
> INCLUDES   fall on moving sidewalk
> EXCLUDES 1   *fall due to bumping (striking) against object (W18.0-)*
> > *fall in shower or bathtub (W18.2-)*
> > *fall on same level NOS (W18.30)*
> > *fall on same level from slipping, tripping and stumbling due to ice or snow (W00.0)*
> > *fall off or from toilet (W18.1-)*
> > *slipping, tripping and stumbling NOS (W18.40)*
> > *slipping, tripping and stumbling without falling (W18.4-)*

√x7ᵗʰ **W01.0** **Fall on same level from slipping, tripping and stumbling** without subsequent striking against object
> Falling over animal

√5ᵗʰ **W01.1** **Fall on same level from slipping, tripping and stumbling** with subsequent striking against object

√x7ᵗʰ **W01.10** **Fall on same level from slipping, tripping and stumbling with subsequent striking against unspecified object**

√6ᵗʰ **W01.11** **Fall on same level from slipping, tripping and stumbling with subsequent striking against** sharp object

√7ᵗʰ **W01.110** **Fall on same level from slipping, tripping and stumbling with subsequent striking against sharp** glass

√7ᵗʰ **W01.111** **Fall on same level from slipping, tripping and stumbling with subsequent striking against** power tool or machine

√7ᵗʰ **W01.118** **Fall on same level from slipping, tripping and stumbling with subsequent striking against other sharp object**

√7ᵗʰ **W01.119** **Fall on same level from slipping, tripping and stumbling with subsequent striking against unspecified sharp object**

√6ᵗʰ **W01.19** **Fall on same level from slipping, tripping and stumbling with subsequent striking against other object**

√7ᵗʰ **W01.190** **Fall on same level from slipping, tripping and stumbling with subsequent striking against** furniture

√7ᵗʰ **W01.198** **Fall on same level from slipping, tripping and stumbling with subsequent striking against other object**

◄ Additional Character Required   √x7ᵗʰ Placeholder Alert   Manifestation   Unspecified Dx   ►◄ Revised Text   ● New Code   ▲ Revised Code Title

ICD-10-CM 2020   1181

✓x7ᵗʰ W03 Other fall on same level due to collision with another person
Fall due to non-transport collision with other person
> EXCLUDES 1   collision with another person without fall (W51)
> crushed or pushed by a crowd or human stampede (W52)
> fall involving pedestrian conveyance (V00-V09)
> fall due to ice or snow (W00)
> fall on same level NOS (W18.30)
AHA: 2012,4Q,108

✓x7ᵗʰ W04 Fall while being carried or supported by other persons
Accidentally dropped while being carried

✓4ᵗʰ W05 Fall from non-moving wheelchair, nonmotorized scooter and motorized mobility scooter
> EXCLUDES 1   fall from moving wheelchair (powered) (V00.811)
> fall from moving motorized mobility scooter (V00.831)
> fall from nonmotorized scooter (V00.141)

✓x7ᵗʰ W05.0 Fall from non-moving wheelchair
AHA: 2019,2Q,27

✓x7ᵗʰ W05.1 Fall from non-moving nonmotorized scooter

✓x7ᵗʰ W05.2 Fall from non-moving motorized mobility scooter

✓x7ᵗʰ W06 Fall from bed

✓x7ᵗʰ W07 Fall from chair

✓x7ᵗʰ W08 Fall from other furniture

✓4ᵗʰ W09 Fall on and from playground equipment
> EXCLUDES 1   fall involving recreational machinery (W31)

✓x7ᵗʰ W09.0 Fall on or from playground slide

✓x7ᵗʰ W09.1 Fall from playground swing

✓x7ᵗʰ W09.2 Fall on or from jungle gym

✓x7ᵗʰ W09.8 Fall on or from other playground equipment

✓4ᵗʰ W10 Fall on and from stairs and steps
> EXCLUDES 1   Fall from stairs and steps due to ice and snow (W00.1)

✓x7ᵗʰ W10.0 Fall (on)(from) escalator

✓x7ᵗʰ W10.1 Fall (on)(from) sidewalk curb

✓x7ᵗʰ W10.2 Fall (on)(from) incline
Fall (on) (from) ramp

✓x7ᵗʰ W10.8 Fall (on) (from) other stairs and steps

✓x7ᵗʰ W10.9 Fall (on) (from) unspecified stairs and steps

✓x7ᵗʰ W11 Fall on and from ladder

✓x7ᵗʰ W12 Fall on and from scaffolding

✓4ᵗʰ W13 Fall from, out of or through building or structure

✓x7ᵗʰ W13.0 Fall from, out of or through balcony
Fall from, out of or through railing

✓x7ᵗʰ W13.1 Fall from, out of or through bridge

✓x7ᵗʰ W13.2 Fall from, out of or through roof

✓x7ᵗʰ W13.3 Fall through floor

✓x7ᵗʰ W13.4 Fall from, out of or through window
> EXCLUDES 2   fall with subsequent striking against sharp glass (W01.110)

✓x7ᵗʰ W13.8 Fall from, out of or through other building or structure
Fall from, out of or through viaduct
Fall from, out of or through wall
Fall from, out of or through flag-pole

✓x7ᵗʰ W13.9 Fall from, out of or through building, not otherwise specified
> EXCLUDES 1   collapse of a building or structure (W20.-)
> fall or jump from burning building or structure (X00.-)

✓x7ᵗʰ W14 Fall from tree

✓x7ᵗʰ W15 Fall from cliff

✓4ᵗʰ W16 Fall, jump or diving into water
> EXCLUDES 1   accidental non-watercraft drowning and submersion not involving fall (W65-W74)
> effects of air pressure from diving (W94.-)
> fall into water from watercraft (V90-V94)
> hitting an object or against bottom when falling from watercraft (V94.0)
> EXCLUDES 2   striking or hitting diving board (W21.4)

✓5ᵗʰ W16.0 Fall into swimming pool
Fall into swimming pool NOS
> EXCLUDES 1   fall into empty swimming pool (W17.3)

✓6ᵗʰ W16.01 Fall into swimming pool striking water surface

✓7ᵗʰ W16.011 Fall into swimming pool striking water surface causing drowning and submersion
> EXCLUDES 1   drowning and submersion while in swimming pool without fall (W67)

✓7ᵗʰ W16.012 Fall into swimming pool striking water surface causing other injury

✓6ᵗʰ W16.02 Fall into swimming pool striking bottom

✓7ᵗʰ W16.021 Fall into swimming pool striking bottom causing drowning and submersion
> EXCLUDES 1   drowning and submersion while in swimming pool without fall (W67)

✓7ᵗʰ W16.022 Fall into swimming pool striking bottom causing other injury

✓6ᵗʰ W16.03 Fall into swimming pool striking wall

✓7ᵗʰ W16.031 Fall into swimming pool striking wall causing drowning and submersion
> EXCLUDES 1   drowning and submersion while in swimming pool without fall (W67)

✓7ᵗʰ W16.032 Fall into swimming pool striking wall causing other injury

✓5ᵗʰ W16.1 Fall into natural body of water
Fall into lake
Fall into open sea
Fall into river
Fall into stream

✓6ᵗʰ W16.11 Fall into natural body of water striking water surface

✓7ᵗʰ W16.111 Fall into natural body of water striking water surface causing drowning and submersion
> EXCLUDES 1   drowning and submersion while in natural body of water without fall (W69)

✓7ᵗʰ W16.112 Fall into natural body of water striking water surface causing other injury

✓6ᵗʰ W16.12 Fall into natural body of water striking bottom

✓7ᵗʰ W16.121 Fall into natural body of water striking bottom causing drowning and submersion
> EXCLUDES 1   drowning and submersion while in natural body of water without fall (W69)

✓7ᵗʰ W16.122 Fall into natural body of water striking bottom causing other injury

✓6ᵗʰ W16.13 Fall into natural body of water striking side

✓7ᵗʰ W16.131 Fall into natural body of water striking side causing drowning and submersion
> EXCLUDES 1   drowning and submersion while in natural body of water without fall (W69)

✓7ᵗʰ W16.132 Fall into natural body of water striking side causing other injury

✓5ᵗʰ W16.2 Fall in (into) filled bathtub or bucket of water

✓6ᵗʰ W16.21 Fall in (into) filled bathtub
> EXCLUDES 1   fall into empty bathtub (W18.2)

✓7ᵗʰ W16.211 Fall in (into) filled bathtub causing drowning and submersion
> EXCLUDES 1   drowning and submersion while in filled bathtub without fall (W65)

✓7ᵗʰ W16.212 Fall in (into) filled bathtub causing other injury

Chapter 20. External Causes of Morbidity

√6ᵗʰ **W16.22 Fall in (into)** bucket of water
   √7ᵗʰ **W16.221 Fall in (into) bucket of water causing** drowning and submersion
   √7ᵗʰ **W16.222 Fall in (into) bucket of water causing** other injury

√5ᵗʰ **W16.3 Fall into other water**
   Fall into fountain
   Fall into reservoir
  √6ᵗʰ **W16.31 Fall into other water** striking water surface
   √7ᵗʰ **W16.311 Fall into other water striking water surface causing** drowning and submersion
     EXCLUDES 1 *drowning and submersion while in other water without fall (W73)*
   √7ᵗʰ **W16.312 Fall into other water striking water surface causing other injury**
  √6ᵗʰ **W16.32 Fall into other water** striking bottom
   √7ᵗʰ **W16.321 Fall into other water striking bottom causing** drowning and submersion
     EXCLUDES 1 *drowning and submersion while in other water without fall (W73)*
   √7ᵗʰ **W16.322 Fall into other water striking bottom causing other injury**
  √6ᵗʰ **W16.33 Fall into other water** striking wall
   √7ᵗʰ **W16.331 Fall into other water striking wall causing** drowning and submersion
     EXCLUDES 1 *drowning and submersion while in other water without fall (W73)*
   √7ᵗʰ **W16.332 Fall into other water striking wall causing other injury**

√5ᵗʰ **W16.4 Fall into unspecified water**
  √x7ᵗʰ **W16.41 Fall into unspecified water causing** drowning and submersion
  √x7ᵗʰ **W16.42 Fall into unspecified water causing other injury**

√5ᵗʰ **W16.5 Jumping or diving into** swimming pool
  √6ᵗʰ **W16.51 Jumping or diving into swimming pool** striking water surface
   √7ᵗʰ **W16.511 Jumping or diving into swimming pool striking water surface causing** drowning and submersion
     EXCLUDES 1 *drowning and submersion while in swimming pool without jumping or diving (W67)*
   √7ᵗʰ **W16.512 Jumping or diving into swimming pool striking water surface causing other injury**
  √6ᵗʰ **W16.52 Jumping or diving into swimming pool** striking bottom
   √7ᵗʰ **W16.521 Jumping or diving into swimming pool striking bottom causing** drowning and submersion
     EXCLUDES 1 *drowning and submersion while in swimming pool without jumping or diving (W67)*
   √7ᵗʰ **W16.522 Jumping or diving into swimming pool striking bottom causing other injury**
  √6ᵗʰ **W16.53 Jumping or diving into swimming pool** striking wall
   √7ᵗʰ **W16.531 Jumping or diving into swimming pool striking wall causing** drowning and submersion
     EXCLUDES 1 *drowning and submersion while in swimming pool without jumping or diving (W67)*
   √7ᵗʰ **W16.532 Jumping or diving into swimming pool striking wall causing other injury**

√5ᵗʰ **W16.6 Jumping or diving into** natural body of water
  Jumping or diving into lake
  Jumping or diving into open sea
  Jumping or diving into river
  Jumping or diving into stream
  √6ᵗʰ **W16.61 Jumping or diving into natural body of water** striking water surface
   √7ᵗʰ **W16.611 Jumping or diving into natural body of water striking water surface causing** drowning and submersion
     EXCLUDES 1 *drowning and submersion while in natural body of water without jumping or diving (W69)*
   √7ᵗʰ **W16.612 Jumping or diving into natural body of water striking water surface causing other injury**
  √6ᵗʰ **W16.62 Jumping or diving into natural body of water** striking bottom
   √7ᵗʰ **W16.621 Jumping or diving into natural body of water striking bottom causing** drowning and submersion
     EXCLUDES 1 *drowning and submersion while in natural body of water without jumping or diving (W69)*
   √7ᵗʰ **W16.622 Jumping or diving into natural body of water striking bottom causing other injury**

√5ᵗʰ **W16.7 Jumping or diving** from boat
  EXCLUDES 1 *fall from boat into water — see watercraft accident (V90-V94)*
  √6ᵗʰ **W16.71 Jumping or diving from boat** striking water surface
   √7ᵗʰ **W16.711 Jumping or diving from boat striking water surface causing** drowning and submersion
   √7ᵗʰ **W16.712 Jumping or diving from boat striking water surface causing other injury**
  √6ᵗʰ **W16.72 Jumping or diving from boat** striking bottom
   √7ᵗʰ **W16.721 Jumping or diving from boat striking bottom causing** drowning and submersion
   √7ᵗʰ **W16.722 Jumping or diving from boat striking bottom causing other injury**

√5ᵗʰ **W16.8 Jumping or diving into other water**
  Jumping or diving into fountain
  Jumping or diving into reservoir
  √6ᵗʰ **W16.81 Jumping or diving into other water** striking water surface
   √7ᵗʰ **W16.811 Jumping or diving into other water striking water surface causing** drowning and submersion
     EXCLUDES 1 *drowning and submersion while in other water without jumping or diving (W73)*
   √7ᵗʰ **W16.812 Jumping or diving into other water striking water surface causing other injury**
  √6ᵗʰ **W16.82 Jumping or diving into other water** striking bottom
   √7ᵗʰ **W16.821 Jumping or diving into other water striking bottom causing** drowning and submersion
     EXCLUDES 1 *drowning and submersion while in other water without jumping or diving (W73)*
   √7ᵗʰ **W16.822 Jumping or diving into other water striking bottom causing other injury**
  √6ᵗʰ **W16.83 Jumping or diving into other water** striking wall
   √7ᵗʰ **W16.831 Jumping or diving into other water striking wall causing** drowning and submersion
     EXCLUDES 1 *drowning and submersion while in other water without jumping or diving (W73)*
   √7ᵗʰ **W16.832 Jumping or diving into other water striking wall causing other injury**

☑5ᵗʰ **W16.9 Jumping or diving into unspecified water**

    ✓x7ᵗʰ **W16.91 Jumping or diving into unspecified water causing drowning and submersion**

    ✓x7ᵗʰ **W16.92 Jumping or diving into unspecified water causing other injury**

☑4ᵗʰ **W17 Other fall from one level to another**

  ✓x7ᵗʰ **W17.0 Fall into well**

  ✓x7ᵗʰ **W17.1 Fall into storm drain or manhole**

  ✓x7ᵗʰ **W17.2 Fall into hole**

    Fall into pit

  ✓x7ᵗʰ **W17.3 Fall into empty swimming pool**

    EXCLUDES 1   *fall into filled swimming pool (W16.0-)*

  ✓x7ᵗʰ **W17.4 Fall from dock**

  ☑5ᵗʰ **W17.8 Other fall from one level to another**

    ✓x7ᵗʰ **W17.81 Fall down embankment (hill)**

    ✓x7ᵗʰ **W17.82 Fall from (out of) grocery cart**

      Fall due to grocery cart tipping over

    ✓x7ᵗʰ **W17.89 Other fall from one level to another**

      Fall from cherry picker

      Fall from lifting device

      Fall from mobile elevated work platform [MEWP]

      Fall from sky lift

      AHA: 2015,2Q,6

☑4ᵗʰ **W18 Other slipping, tripping and stumbling and falls**

  ☑5ᵗʰ **W18.0 Fall due to bumping against object**

    Striking against object with subsequent fall

    EXCLUDES 1   *fall on same level due to slipping, tripping, or stumbling with subsequent striking against object (W01.1-)*

    ✓x7ᵗʰ **W18.00 Striking against unspecified object with subsequent fall**

    ✓x7ᵗʰ **W18.01 Striking against sports equipment with subsequent fall**

    ✓x7ᵗʰ **W18.02 Striking against glass with subsequent fall**

    ✓x7ᵗʰ **W18.09 Striking against other object with subsequent fall**

  ☑5ᵗʰ **W18.1 Fall from or off toilet**

    ✓x7ᵗʰ **W18.11 Fall from or off toilet without subsequent striking against object**

      Fall from (off) toilet NOS

    ✓x7ᵗʰ **W18.12 Fall from or off toilet with subsequent striking against object**

  ✓x7ᵗʰ **W18.2 Fall in (into) shower or empty bathtub**

    EXCLUDES 1   *fall in full bathtub causing drowning or submersion (W16.21-)*

  ☑5ᵗʰ **W18.3 Other and unspecified fall on same level**

    ✓x7ᵗʰ **W18.30 Fall on same level, unspecified**

    ✓x7ᵗʰ **W18.31 Fall on same level due to stepping on an object**

      Fall on same level due to stepping on an animal

      EXCLUDES 1   *slipping, tripping and stumbling without fall due to stepping on animal (W18.41)*

    ✓x7ᵗʰ **W18.39 Other fall on same level**

  ☑5ᵗʰ **W18.4 Slipping, tripping and stumbling without falling**

    EXCLUDES 1   *collision with another person without fall (W51)*

    ✓x7ᵗʰ **W18.40 Slipping, tripping and stumbling without falling, unspecified**

    ✓x7ᵗʰ **W18.41 Slipping, tripping and stumbling without falling due to stepping on object**

      Slipping, tripping and stumbling without falling due to stepping on animal

      EXCLUDES 1   *slipping, tripping and stumbling with fall due to stepping on animal (W18.31)*

    ✓x7ᵗʰ **W18.42 Slipping, tripping and stumbling without falling due to stepping into hole or opening**

    ✓x7ᵗʰ **W18.43 Slipping, tripping and stumbling without falling due to stepping from one level to another**

    ✓x7ᵗʰ **W18.49 Other slipping, tripping and stumbling without falling**

  ✓x7ᵗʰ **W19 Unspecified fall**

    Accidental fall NOS

    AHA: 2012,4Q,95

Exposure to inanimate mechanical forces (W20-W49)

  EXCLUDES 1   *assault (X92-Y09)*

      contact or collision with animals or persons (W50-W64)

      exposure to inanimate mechanical forces involving military or war operations (Y36.-, Y37.-)

      intentional self-harm (X71-X83)

The appropriate 7th character is to be added to each code from categories W20-W49.
A   initial encounter
D   subsequent encounter
S   sequela

☑4ᵗʰ **W20 Struck by thrown, projected or falling object**

  Code first any associated:

    cataclysm (X34-X39)

    lightning strike (T75.00)

    EXCLUDES 1   *falling object in machinery accident (W24, W28-W31)*

      falling object in transport accident (V01-V99)

      object set in motion by explosion (W35-W40)

      object set in motion by firearm (W32-W34)

      struck by thrown sports equipment (W21.-)

  ✓x7ᵗʰ **W20.0 Struck by falling object in cave-in**

    EXCLUDES 2   *asphyxiation due to cave-in (T71.21)*

  ✓x7ᵗʰ **W20.1 Struck by object due to collapse of building**

    EXCLUDES 1   *struck by object due to collapse of burning building (X00.2, X02.2)*

  ✓x7ᵗʰ **W20.8 Other cause of strike by thrown, projected or falling object**

    EXCLUDES 1   *struck by thrown sports equipment (W21.-)*

☑4ᵗʰ **W21 Striking against or struck by sports equipment**

  EXCLUDES 1   *assault with sports equipment (Y08.0-)*

      striking against or struck by sports equipment with subsequent fall (W18.01)

  ☑5ᵗʰ **W21.0 Struck by hit or thrown ball**

    ✓x7ᵗʰ **W21.00 Struck by hit or thrown ball, unspecified type**

    ✓x7ᵗʰ **W21.01 Struck by football**

    ✓x7ᵗʰ **W21.02 Struck by soccer ball**

    ✓x7ᵗʰ **W21.03 Struck by baseball**

    ✓x7ᵗʰ **W21.04 Struck by golf ball**

    ✓x7ᵗʰ **W21.05 Struck by basketball**

    ✓x7ᵗʰ **W21.06 Struck by volleyball**

    ✓x7ᵗʰ **W21.07 Struck by softball**

    ✓x7ᵗʰ **W21.09 Struck by other hit or thrown ball**

  ☑5ᵗʰ **W21.1 Struck by bat, racquet or club**

    ✓x7ᵗʰ **W21.11 Struck by baseball bat**

    ✓x7ᵗʰ **W21.12 Struck by tennis racquet**

    ✓x7ᵗʰ **W21.13 Struck by golf club**

    ✓x7ᵗʰ **W21.19 Struck by other bat, racquet or club**

  ☑5ᵗʰ **W21.2 Struck by hockey stick or puck**

    ☑6ᵗʰ **W21.21 Struck by hockey stick**

      ✓7ᵗʰ **W21.210 Struck by ice hockey stick**

      ✓7ᵗʰ **W21.211 Struck by field hockey stick**

    ☑6ᵗʰ **W21.22 Struck by hockey puck**

      ✓7ᵗʰ **W21.220 Struck by ice hockey puck**

      ✓7ᵗʰ **W21.221 Struck by field hockey puck**

  ☑5ᵗʰ **W21.3 Struck by sports foot wear**

    ✓x7ᵗʰ **W21.31 Struck by shoe cleats**

      Stepped on by shoe cleats

    ✓x7ᵗʰ **W21.32 Struck by skate blades**

      Skated over by skate blades

    ✓x7ᵗʰ **W21.39 Struck by other sports foot wear**

  ✓x7ᵗʰ **W21.4 Striking against diving board**

    Use additional code for subsequent falling into water, if applicable (W16.-)

  ☑5ᵗʰ **W21.8 Striking against or struck by other sports equipment**

    ✓x7ᵗʰ **W21.81 Striking against or struck by football helmet**

    ✓x7ᵗʰ **W21.89 Striking against or struck by other sports equipment**

  ✓x7ᵗʰ **W21.9 Striking against or struck by unspecified sports equipment**

☑4ᵗʰ W22   Striking against or struck by other objects

     EXCLUDES 1   striking against or struck by object with subsequent fall (W18.09)

   ☑5ᵗʰ W22.0   Striking against stationary object

     EXCLUDES 1   striking against stationary sports equipment (W21.8)

     ☑x7ᵗʰ W22.01   Walked into wall

     ☑x7ᵗʰ W22.02   Walked into lamppost

     ☑x7ᵗʰ W22.03   Walked into furniture

     ☑6ᵗʰ W22.04   Striking against wall of swimming pool

       ☑7ᵗʰ W22.041   Striking against wall of swimming pool causing drowning and submersion

         EXCLUDES 1   drowning and submersion while swimming without striking against wall (W67)

       ☑7ᵗʰ W22.042   Striking against wall of swimming pool causing other injury

     ☑x7ᵗʰ W22.09   Striking against other stationary object

   ☑5ᵗʰ W22.1   Striking against or struck by automobile airbag

     ☑x7ᵗʰ W22.10   Striking against or struck by unspecified automobile airbag

     ☑x7ᵗʰ W22.11   Striking against or struck by driver side automobile airbag

     ☑x7ᵗʰ W22.12   Striking against or struck by front passenger side automobile airbag

     ☑x7ᵗʰ W22.19   Striking against or struck by other automobile airbag

   ☑x7ᵗʰ W22.8   Striking against or struck by other objects

     Striking against or struck by object NOS

     EXCLUDES 1   struck by thrown, projected or falling object (W20.-)

☑4ᵗʰ W23   Caught, crushed, jammed or pinched in or between objects

     EXCLUDES 1   injury caused by cutting or piercing instruments (W25-W27)

         injury caused by firearms malfunction (W32.1, W33.1-, W34.1-)

         injury caused by lifting and transmission devices (W24.-)

         injury caused by machinery (W28-W31)

         injury caused by nonpowered hand tools (W27.-)

         injury caused by transport vehicle being used as a means of transportation (V01-V99)

         injury caused by struck by thrown, projected or falling object (W20.-)

   ☑x7ᵗʰ W23.0   Caught, crushed, jammed, or pinched between moving objects

   ☑x7ᵗʰ W23.1   Caught, crushed, jammed, or pinched between stationary objects

☑4ᵗʰ W24   Contact with lifting and transmission devices, not elsewhere classified

     EXCLUDES 1   transport accidents (V01-V99)

   ☑x7ᵗʰ W24.0   Contact with lifting devices, not elsewhere classified

     Contact with chain hoist

     Contact with drive belt

     Contact with pulley (block)

   ☑x7ᵗʰ W24.1   Contact with transmission devices, not elsewhere classified

     Contact with transmission belt or cable

☑x7ᵗʰ W25   Contact with sharp glass

     Code first any associated:

     injury due to flying glass from explosion or firearm discharge (W32-W40)

     transport accident (V00-V99)

     EXCLUDES 1   fall on same level due to slipping, tripping and stumbling with subsequent striking against sharp glass ▶(W01.110)◀

         striking against sharp glass with subsequent fall (W18.02)

     EXCLUDES 2   glass embedded in skin (W45)

☑4ᵗʰ W26   Contact with other sharp objects

     EXCLUDES 2   sharp object(s) embedded in skin (W45)

     AHA: 2016,4Q,73

   ☑x7ᵗʰ W26.0   Contact with knife

     EXCLUDES 1   contact with electric knife (W29.1)

   ☑x7ᵗʰ W26.1   Contact with sword or dagger

   ☑x7ᵗʰ W26.2   Contact with edge of stiff paper

     Paper cut

   ☑x7ᵗʰ W26.8   Contact with other sharp object(s), not elsewhere classified

     Contact with tin can lid

   ☑x7ᵗʰ W26.9   Contact with unspecified sharp object(s)

☑4ᵗʰ W27   Contact with nonpowered hand tool

   ☑x7ᵗʰ W27.0   Contact with workbench tool

     Contact with auger

     Contact with axe

     Contact with chisel

     Contact with handsaw

     Contact with screwdriver

   ☑x7ᵗʰ W27.1   Contact with garden tool

     Contact with hoe

     Contact with nonpowered lawn mower

     Contact with pitchfork

     Contact with rake

   ☑x7ᵗʰ W27.2   Contact with scissors

   ☑x7ᵗʰ W27.3   Contact with needle (sewing)

     EXCLUDES 1   contact with hypodermic needle (W46.-)

   ☑x7ᵗʰ W27.4   Contact with kitchen utensil

     Contact with fork

     Contact with ice-pick

     Contact with can-opener NOS

   ☑x7ᵗʰ W27.5   Contact with paper-cutter

   ☑x7ᵗʰ W27.8   Contact with other nonpowered hand tool

     Contact with nonpowered sewing machine

     Contact with shovel

☑x7ᵗʰ W28   Contact with powered lawn mower

     Powered lawn mower (commercial) (residential)

     EXCLUDES 1   contact with nonpowered lawn mower (W27.1)

     EXCLUDES 2   exposure to electric current (W86.-)

☑4ᵗʰ W29   Contact with other powered hand tools and household machinery

     EXCLUDES 1   contact with commercial machinery (W31.82)

         contact with hot household appliance (X15)

         contact with nonpowered hand tool (W27.-)

         exposure to electric current (W86)

   ☑x7ᵗʰ W29.0   Contact with powered kitchen appliance

     Contact with blender

     Contact with can-opener

     Contact with garbage disposal

     Contact with mixer

   ☑x7ᵗʰ W29.1   Contact with electric knife

   ☑x7ᵗʰ W29.2   Contact with other powered household machinery

     Contact with electric fan

     Contact with powered dryer (clothes) (powered) (spin)

     Contact with washing-machine

     Contact with sewing machine

   ☑x7ᵗʰ W29.3   Contact with powered garden and outdoor hand tools and machinery

     Contact with chainsaw

     Contact with edger

     Contact with garden cultivator (tiller)

     Contact with hedge trimmer

     Contact with other powered garden tool

     EXCLUDES 1   contact with powered lawn mower (W28)

   ☑x7ᵗʰ W29.4   Contact with nail gun

   ☑x7ᵗʰ W29.8   Contact with other powered hand tools and household machinery

     Contact with do-it-yourself tool NOS

☑4ᵗʰ W30   Contact with agricultural machinery

     INCLUDES   animal-powered farm machine

     EXCLUDES 1   agricultural transport vehicle accident (V01-V99)

         explosion of grain store (W40.8)

         exposure to electric current (W86.-)

   ☑x7ᵗʰ W30.0   Contact with combine harvester

     Contact with reaper

     Contact with thresher

   ☑x7ᵗʰ W30.1   Contact with power take-off devices (PTO)

   ☑x7ᵗʰ W30.2   Contact with hay derrick

   ☑x7ᵗʰ W30.3   Contact with grain storage elevator

     EXCLUDES 1   explosion of grain store (W40.8)

Additional Character Required   ☑x7ᵗʰ Placeholder Alert   Manifestation   Unspecified Dx   ▶◀ Revised Text   ● New Code   ▲ Revised Code Title

√5ᵗʰ **W30.8**   **Contact with other specified agricultural machinery**

   √x7ᵗʰ **W30.81**   **Contact with agricultural transport vehicle in stationary use**

     Contact with agricultural transport vehicle under repair, not on public roadway

      EXCLUDES 1   *agricultural transport vehicle accident (V01-V99)*

   √x7ᵗʰ **W30.89**   **Contact with other specified agricultural machinery**

√x7ᵗʰ **W30.9**   **Contact with unspecified agricultural machinery**

     Contact with farm machinery NOS

√4ᵗʰ **W31**   **Contact with other and unspecified machinery**

   EXCLUDES 1   *contact with agricultural machinery (W30.-)*

       contact with machinery in transport under own power or being towed by a vehicle (V01-V99)

       exposure to electric current (W86)

√x7ᵗʰ **W31.0**   **Contact with mining and earth-drilling machinery**

     Contact with bore or drill (land) (seabed)

     Contact with shaft hoist

     Contact with shaft lift

     Contact with undercutter

√x7ᵗʰ **W31.1**   **Contact with metalworking machines**

     Contact with abrasive wheel

     Contact with forging machine

     Contact with lathe

     Contact with mechanical shears

     Contact with metal drilling machine

     Contact with milling machine

     Contact with power press

     Contact with rolling-mill

     Contact with metal sawing machine

√x7ᵗʰ **W31.2**   **Contact with powered woodworking and forming machines**

     Contact with band saw

     Contact with bench saw

     Contact with circular saw

     Contact with molding machine

     Contact with overhead plane

     Contact with powered saw

     Contact with radial saw

     Contact with sander

      EXCLUDES 1   *nonpowered woodworking tools (W27.0)*

√x7ᵗʰ **W31.3**   **Contact with prime movers**

     Contact with gas turbine

     Contact with internal combustion engine

     Contact with steam engine

     Contact with water driven turbine

√5ᵗʰ **W31.8**   **Contact with other specified machinery**

   √x7ᵗʰ **W31.81**   **Contact with recreational machinery**

     Contact with roller coaster

   √x7ᵗʰ **W31.82**   **Contact with other commercial machinery**

     Contact with commercial electric fan

     Contact with commercial kitchen appliances

     Contact with commercial powered dryer (clothes) (powered) (spin)

     Contact with commercial washing-machine

     Contact with commercial sewing machine

      EXCLUDES 1   *contact with household machinery (W29.-)*

            contact with powered lawn mower (W28)

   √x7ᵗʰ **W31.83**   **Contact with special construction vehicle in stationary use**

     Contact with special construction vehicle under repair, not on public roadway

      EXCLUDES 1   *special construction vehicle accident (V01-V99)*

   √x7ᵗʰ **W31.89**   **Contact with other specified machinery**

√x7ᵗʰ **W31.9**   **Contact with unspecified machinery**

     Contact with machinery NOS

√4ᵗʰ **W32**   **Accidental handgun discharge and malfunction**

   INCLUDES   accidental discharge and malfunction of gun for single hand use

       accidental discharge and malfunction of pistol

       accidental discharge and malfunction of revolver

       handgun discharge and malfunction NOS

   EXCLUDES 1   *accidental airgun discharge and malfunction (W34.010, W34.110)*

       accidental BB gun discharge and malfunction (W34.010, W34.110)

       accidental pellet gun discharge and malfunction (W34.010, W34.110)

       accidental shotgun discharge and malfunction (W33.01, W33.11)

       assault by handgun discharge (X93)

       handgun discharge involving legal intervention (Y35.0-)

       handgun discharge involving military or war operations (Y36.4-)

       intentional self-harm by handgun discharge (X72)

       Very pistol discharge and malfunction (W34.09, W34.19)

√x7ᵗʰ **W32.0**   **Accidental handgun discharge**

√x7ᵗʰ **W32.1**   **Accidental handgun malfunction**

     Injury due to explosion of handgun (parts)

     Injury due to malfunction of mechanism or component of handgun

     Injury due to recoil of handgun

     Powder burn from handgun

√4ᵗʰ **W33**   **Accidental rifle, shotgun and larger firearm discharge and malfunction**

   INCLUDES   rifle, shotgun and larger firearm discharge and malfunction NOS

   EXCLUDES 1   *accidental airgun discharge and malfunction (W34.010, W34.110)*

       accidental BB gun discharge and malfunction (W34.010, W34.110)

       accidental handgun discharge and malfunction (W32.-)

       accidental pellet gun discharge and malfunction (W34.010, W34.110)

       assault by rifle, shotgun and larger firearm discharge (X94)

       firearm discharge involving legal intervention (Y35.0-)

       firearm discharge involving military or war operations (Y36.4-)

       intentional self-harm by rifle, shotgun and larger firearm discharge (X73)

√5ᵗʰ **W33.0**   **Accidental rifle, shotgun and larger firearm discharge**

   √x7ᵗʰ **W33.00**   **Accidental discharge of unspecified larger firearm**

     Discharge of unspecified larger firearm NOS

   √x7ᵗʰ **W33.01**   **Accidental discharge of shotgun**

     Discharge of shotgun NOS

   √x7ᵗʰ **W33.02**   **Accidental discharge of hunting rifle**

     Discharge of hunting rifle NOS

   √x7ᵗʰ **W33.03**   **Accidental discharge of machine gun**

     Discharge of machine gun NOS

   √x7ᵗʰ **W33.09**   **Accidental discharge of other larger firearm**

     Discharge of other larger firearm NOS

√5ᵗʰ **W33.1**   **Accidental rifle, shotgun and larger firearm malfunction**

     Injury due to explosion of rifle, shotgun and larger firearm (parts)

     Injury due to malfunction of mechanism or component of rifle, shotgun and larger firearm

     Injury due to piercing, cutting, crushing or pinching due to (by) slide trigger mechanism, scope or other gun part

     Injury due to recoil of rifle, shotgun and larger firearm

     Powder burn from rifle, shotgun and larger firearm

   √x7ᵗʰ **W33.10**   **Accidental malfunction of unspecified larger firearm**

     Malfunction of unspecified larger firearm NOS

   √x7ᵗʰ **W33.11**   **Accidental malfunction of shotgun**

     Malfunction of shotgun NOS

   √x7ᵗʰ **W33.12**   **Accidental malfunction of hunting rifle**

     Malfunction of hunting rifle NOS

   √x7ᵗʰ **W33.13**   **Accidental malfunction of machine gun**

     Malfunction of machine gun NOS

√x7ᵗʰ **W33.19** **Accidental malfunction of other larger firearm**

Malfunction of other larger firearm NOS

√4ᵗʰ **W34** **Accidental discharge and malfunction from other and unspecified firearms and guns**

√5ᵗʰ **W34.0** **Accidental discharge from other and unspecified firearms and guns**

√x7ᵗʰ **W34.00** **Accidental discharge from unspecified firearms or gun**

Discharge from firearm NOS
Gunshot wound NOS
Shot NOS

√6ᵗʰ **W34.01** **Accidental discharge of gas, air or spring-operated guns**

√7ᵗʰ **W34.010** **Accidental discharge of airgun**

Accidental discharge of BB gun
Accidental discharge of pellet gun

√7ᵗʰ **W34.011** **Accidental discharge of paintball gun**

Accidental injury due to paintball discharge

√7ᵗʰ **W34.018** **Accidental discharge of other gas, air or spring-operated gun**

√x7ᵗʰ **W34.09** **Accidental discharge from other specified firearms**

Accidental discharge from Very pistol [flare]

√5ᵗʰ **W34.1** **Accidental malfunction from other and unspecified firearms and guns**

√x7ᵗʰ **W34.10** **Accidental malfunction from unspecified firearms or gun**

Firearm malfunction NOS

√6ᵗʰ **W34.11** **Accidental malfunction of gas, air or spring-operated guns**

√7ᵗʰ **W34.110** **Accidental malfunction of airgun**

Accidental malfunction of BB gun
Accidental malfunction of pellet gun

√7ᵗʰ **W34.111** **Accidental malfunction of paintball gun**

Accidental injury due to paintball gun malfunction

√7ᵗʰ **W34.118** **Accidental malfunction of other gas, air or spring-operated gun**

√x7ᵗʰ **W34.19** **Accidental malfunction from other specified firearms**

Accidental malfunction from Very pistol [flare]

√x7ᵗʰ **W35** **Explosion and rupture of boiler**

> EXCLUDES 1   *explosion and rupture of boiler on watercraft (V93.4)*

√4ᵗʰ **W36** **Explosion and rupture of gas cylinder**

√x7ᵗʰ **W36.1** **Explosion and rupture of aerosol can**

√x7ᵗʰ **W36.2** **Explosion and rupture of air tank**

√x7ᵗʰ **W36.3** **Explosion and rupture of pressurized-gas tank**

√x7ᵗʰ **W36.8** **Explosion and rupture of other gas cylinder**

√x7ᵗʰ **W36.9** **Explosion and rupture of unspecified gas cylinder**

√4ᵗʰ **W37** **Explosion and rupture of pressurized tire, pipe or hose**

√x7ᵗʰ **W37.0** **Explosion of bicycle tire**

√x7ᵗʰ **W37.8** **Explosion and rupture of other pressurized tire, pipe or hose**

√x7ᵗʰ **W38** **Explosion and rupture of other specified pressurized devices**

√x7ᵗʰ **W39** **Discharge of firework**

√4ᵗʰ **W40** **Explosion of other materials**

> EXCLUDES 1   *assault by explosive material (X96)*
> *explosion involving legal intervention (Y35.1-)*
> *explosion involving military or war operations (Y36.0-, Y36.2-)*
> *intentional self-harm by explosive material (X75)*

√x7ᵗʰ **W40.0** **Explosion of blasting material**

Explosion of blasting cap
Explosion of detonator
Explosion of dynamite
Explosion of explosive (any) used in blasting operations

√x7ᵗʰ **W40.1** **Explosion of explosive gases**

Explosion of acetylene
Explosion of butane
Explosion of coal gas
Explosion in mine NOS
Explosion of explosive gas
Explosion of fire damp
Explosion of gasoline fumes
Explosion of methane
Explosion of propane

√x7ᵗʰ **W40.8** **Explosion of other specified explosive materials**

Explosion in dump NOS
Explosion in factory NOS
Explosion in grain store
Explosion in munitions

> EXCLUDES 1   *explosion involving legal intervention (Y35.1-)*
> *explosion involving military or war operations (Y36.0-, Y36.2-)*

√x7ᵗʰ **W40.9** **Explosion of unspecified explosive materials**

Explosion NOS

√4ᵗʰ **W42** **Exposure to noise**

√x7ᵗʰ **W42.0** **Exposure to supersonic waves**

√x7ᵗʰ **W42.9** **Exposure to other noise**

Exposure to sound waves NOS

√4ᵗʰ **W45** **Foreign body or object entering through skin**

> INCLUDES   foreign body or object embedded in skin
> nail embedded in skin

> EXCLUDES 2   *contact with hand tools (nonpowered) (powered) (W27-W29)*
> *contact with other sharp objects (W26.-)*
> *contact with sharp glass (W25.-)*
> *struck by objects (W20-W22)*

√x7ᵗʰ **W45.0** **Nail entering through skin**

√x7ᵗʰ **W45.8** **Other foreign body or object entering through skin**

Splinter in skin NOS

√4ᵗʰ **W46** **Contact with hypodermic needle**

√x7ᵗʰ **W46.0** **Contact with hypodermic needle**

Hypodermic needle stick NOS

√x7ᵗʰ **W46.1** **Contact with contaminated hypodermic needle**

√4ᵗʰ **W49** **Exposure to other inanimate mechanical forces**

> INCLUDES   exposure to abnormal gravitational [G] forces
> exposure to inanimate mechanical forces NEC

> EXCLUDES 1   *exposure to inanimate mechanical forces involving military or war operations (Y36.-, Y37.-)*

√5ᵗʰ **W49.0** **Item causing external constriction**

√x7ᵗʰ **W49.01** **Hair causing external constriction**

√x7ᵗʰ **W49.02** **String or thread causing external constriction**

√x7ᵗʰ **W49.03** **Rubber band causing external constriction**

√x7ᵗʰ **W49.04** **Ring or other jewelry causing external constriction**

√x7ᵗʰ **W49.09** **Other specified item causing external constriction**

√x7ᵗʰ **W49.9** **Exposure to other inanimate mechanical forces**

Exposure to animate mechanical forces (W50-W64)

> EXCLUDES 1   *toxic effect of contact with venomous animals and plants (T63.-)*

The appropriate 7th character is to be added to each code from categories W50-W64.
A   initial encounter
D   subsequent encounter
S   sequela

√4ᵗʰ **W50** **Accidental hit, strike, kick, twist, bite or scratch by another person**

> INCLUDES   hit, strike, kick, twist, bite, or scratch by another person NOS

> EXCLUDES 1   *assault by bodily force (Y04)*
> *struck by objects (W20-W22)*

√x7ᵗʰ **W50.0** **Accidental hit or strike by another person**

Hit or strike by another person NOS

√x7ᵗʰ **W50.1** **Accidental kick by another person**

Kick by another person NOS

√x7ᵗʰ **W50.2** **Accidental twist by another person**

Twist by another person NOS

Additional Character Required   √x7ᵗʰ Placeholder Alert   Manifestation   Unspecified Dx   ►◄ Revised Text   ● New Code   ▲ Revised Code Title

-10-CM 2020   1187

√x7th **W50.3** Accidental bite by another person
     Human bite
     Bite by another person NOS

√x7th **W50.4** Accidental scratch by another person
     Scratch by another person NOS

√x7th **W51** **Accidental striking against or bumped into by another person**
     EXCLUDES 1   assault by striking against or bumping into by another person (Y04.2)
          fall due to collision with another person (W03)

√x7th **W52** **Crushed, pushed or stepped on by crowd or human stampede**
     Crushed, pushed or stepped on by crowd or human stampede with or without fall

√4th **W53** **Contact with rodent**
     INCLUDES   contact with saliva, feces or urine of rodent

   √5th **W53.0** **Contact with mouse**
     √x7th **W53.01** Bitten by mouse
     √x7th **W53.09** Other contact with mouse

   √5th **W53.1** **Contact with rat**
     √x7th **W53.11** Bitten by rat
     √x7th **W53.19** Other contact with rat

   √5th **W53.2** **Contact with squirrel**
     √x7th **W53.21** Bitten by squirrel
     √x7th **W53.29** Other contact with squirrel

   √5th **W53.8** **Contact with other rodent**
     √x7th **W53.81** Bitten by other rodent
     √x7th **W53.89** Other contact with other rodent

√4th **W54** **Contact with dog**
     INCLUDES   contact with saliva, feces or urine of dog

   √x7th **W54.0** Bitten by dog

   √x7th **W54.1** Struck by dog
     Knocked over by dog

   √x7th **W54.8** Other contact with dog

√4th **W55** **Contact with other mammals**
     INCLUDES   contact with saliva, feces or urine of mammal
     EXCLUDES 1   animal being ridden — see transport accidents
          bitten or struck by dog (W54)
          bitten or struck by rodent (W53.-)
          contact with marine mammals (W56.-)

   √5th **W55.0** **Contact with cat**
     √x7th **W55.01** Bitten by cat
     √x7th **W55.03** Scratched by cat
     √x7th **W55.09** Other contact with cat

   √5th **W55.1** **Contact with horse**
     √x7th **W55.11** Bitten by horse
     √x7th **W55.12** Struck by horse
     √x7th **W55.19** Other contact with horse

   √5th **W55.2** **Contact with cow**
     Contact with bull
     √x7th **W55.21** Bitten by cow
     √x7th **W55.22** Struck by cow
        Gored by bull
     √x7th **W55.29** Other contact with cow

   √5th **W55.3** **Contact with other hoof stock**
     Contact with goats
     Contact with sheep
     √x7th **W55.31** Bitten by other hoof stock
     √x7th **W55.32** Struck by other hoof stock
        Gored by goat
        Gored by ram
     √x7th **W55.39** Other contact with other hoof stock

   √5th **W55.4** **Contact with pig**
     √x7th **W55.41** Bitten by pig
     √x7th **W55.42** Struck by pig
     √x7th **W55.49** Other contact with pig

   √5th **W55.5** **Contact with raccoon**
     √x7th **W55.51** Bitten by raccoon

     √x7th **W55.52** Struck by raccoon
     √x7th **W55.59** Other contact with raccoon

   √5th **W55.8** **Contact with other mammals**
     √x7th **W55.81** Bitten by other mammals
     √x7th **W55.82** Struck by other mammals
     √x7th **W55.89** Other contact with other mammals

√4th **W56** **Contact with nonvenomous marine animal**
     EXCLUDES 1   contact with venomous marine animal (T63.-)

   √5th **W56.0** **Contact with dolphin**
     √x7th **W56.01** Bitten by dolphin
     √x7th **W56.02** Struck by dolphin
     √x7th **W56.09** Other contact with dolphin

   √5th **W56.1** **Contact with sea lion**
     √x7th **W56.11** Bitten by sea lion
     √x7th **W56.12** Struck by sea lion
     √x7th **W56.19** Other contact with sea lion

   √5th **W56.2** **Contact with orca**
     Contact with killer whale
     √x7th **W56.21** Bitten by orca
     √x7th **W56.22** Struck by orca
     √x7th **W56.29** Other contact with orca

   √5th **W56.3** **Contact with other marine mammals**
     √x7th **W56.31** Bitten by other marine mammals
     √x7th **W56.32** Struck by other marine mammals
     √x7th **W56.39** Other contact with other marine mammals

   √5th **W56.4** **Contact with shark**
     √x7th **W56.41** Bitten by shark
     √x7th **W56.42** Struck by shark
     √x7th **W56.49** Other contact with shark

   √5th **W56.5** **Contact with other fish**
     √x7th **W56.51** Bitten by other fish
     √x7th **W56.52** Struck by other fish
     √x7th **W56.59** Other contact with other fish

   √5th **W56.8** **Contact with other nonvenomous marine animals**
     √x7th **W56.81** Bitten by other nonvenomous marine animals
     √x7th **W56.82** Struck by other nonvenomous marine animals
     √x7th **W56.89** Other contact with other nonvenomous marine animals

√x7th **W57** **Bitten or stung by nonvenomous insect and other nonvenomous arthropods**
     EXCLUDES 1   contact with venomous insects and arthropods (T63.2-, T63.3-T63.4-)

√4th **W58** **Contact with crocodile or alligator**

   √5th **W58.0** **Contact with alligator**
     √x7th **W58.01** Bitten by alligator
     √x7th **W58.02** Struck by alligator
     √x7th **W58.03** Crushed by alligator
     √x7th **W58.09** Other contact with alligator

   √5th **W58.1** **Contact with crocodile**
     √x7th **W58.11** Bitten by crocodile
     √x7th **W58.12** Struck by crocodile
     √x7th **W58.13** Crushed by crocodile
     √x7th **W58.19** Other contact with crocodile

√4th **W59** **Contact with other nonvenomous reptiles**
     EXCLUDES 1   contact with venomous reptile (T63.0-, T63.1-)

   √5th **W59.0** **Contact with nonvenomous lizards**
     √x7th **W59.01** Bitten by nonvenomous lizards
     √x7th **W59.02** Struck by nonvenomous lizards
     √x7th **W59.09** Other contact with nonvenomous lizards
        Exposure to nonvenomous lizards

   √5th **W59.1** **Contact with nonvenomous snakes**
     √x7th **W59.11** Bitten by nonvenomous snake
     √x7th **W59.12** Struck by nonvenomous snake
     √x7th **W59.13** Crushed by nonvenomous snake
     √x7th **W59.19** Other contact with nonvenomous snake

✓5ᵗʰ **W59.2 Contact with turtles**

> *EXCLUDES 1*   *contact with tortoises (W59.8-)*

    ✓x7ᵗʰ **W59.21 Bitten by turtle**

    ✓x7ᵗʰ **W59.22 Struck by turtle**

    ✓x7ᵗʰ **W59.29 Other contact with turtle**

       Exposure to turtles

✓5ᵗʰ **W59.8 Contact with other nonvenomous reptiles**

    ✓x7ᵗʰ **W59.81 Bitten by other nonvenomous reptiles**

    ✓x7ᵗʰ **W59.82 Struck by other nonvenomous reptiles**

    ✓x7ᵗʰ **W59.83 Crushed by other nonvenomous reptiles**

    ✓x7ᵗʰ **W59.89 Other contact with other nonvenomous reptiles**

✓x7ᵗʰ **W60 Contact with nonvenomous plant thorns and spines and sharp leaves**

> *EXCLUDES 1*   *contact with venomous plants (T63.7-)*

✓4ᵗʰ **W61 Contact with birds (domestic) (wild)**

> **INCLUDES**   contact with excreta of birds

✓5ᵗʰ **W61.0 Contact with parrot**

    ✓x7ᵗʰ **W61.01 Bitten by parrot**

    ✓x7ᵗʰ **W61.02 Struck by parrot**

    ✓x7ᵗʰ **W61.09 Other contact with parrot**

       Exposure to parrots

✓5ᵗʰ **W61.1 Contact with macaw**

    ✓x7ᵗʰ **W61.11 Bitten by macaw**

    ✓x7ᵗʰ **W61.12 Struck by macaw**

    ✓x7ᵗʰ **W61.19 Other contact with macaw**

       Exposure to macaws

✓5ᵗʰ **W61.2 Contact with other psittacines**

    ✓x7ᵗʰ **W61.21 Bitten by other psittacines**

    ✓x7ᵗʰ **W61.22 Struck by other psittacines**

    ✓x7ᵗʰ **W61.29 Other contact with other psittacines**

       Exposure to other psittacines

✓5ᵗʰ **W61.3 Contact with chicken**

    ✓x7ᵗʰ **W61.32 Struck by chicken**

    ✓x7ᵗʰ **W61.33 Pecked by chicken**

    ✓x7ᵗʰ **W61.39 Other contact with chicken**

       Exposure to chickens

✓5ᵗʰ **W61.4 Contact with turkey**

    ✓x7ᵗʰ **W61.42 Struck by turkey**

    ✓x7ᵗʰ **W61.43 Pecked by turkey**

    ✓x7ᵗʰ **W61.49 Other contact with turkey**

✓5ᵗʰ **W61.5 Contact with goose**

    ✓x7ᵗʰ **W61.51 Bitten by goose**

    ✓x7ᵗʰ **W61.52 Struck by goose**

    ✓x7ᵗʰ **W61.59 Other contact with goose**

✓5ᵗʰ **W61.6 Contact with duck**

    ✓x7ᵗʰ **W61.61 Bitten by duck**

    ✓x7ᵗʰ **W61.62 Struck by duck**

    ✓x7ᵗʰ **W61.69 Other contact with duck**

✓5ᵗʰ **W61.9 Contact with other birds**

    ✓x7ᵗʰ **W61.91 Bitten by other birds**

    ✓x7ᵗʰ **W61.92 Struck by other birds**

    ✓x7ᵗʰ **W61.99 Other contact with other birds**

       Contact with bird NOS

✓4ᵗʰ **W62 Contact with nonvenomous amphibians**

> *EXCLUDES 1*   *contact with venomous amphibians (T63.81-R63.83)*

✓x7ᵗʰ **W62.0 Contact with nonvenomous frogs**

✓x7ᵗʰ **W62.1 Contact with nonvenomous toads**

✓x7ᵗʰ **W62.9 Contact with other nonvenomous amphibians**

✓x7ᵗʰ **W64 Exposure to other animate mechanical forces**

> **INCLUDES**   exposure to nonvenomous animal NOS
>
> *EXCLUDES 1*   *contact with venomous animal (T63.-)*

Accidental non-transport drowning and submersion (W65-W74)

> *EXCLUDES 1*   *accidental drowning and submersion due to fall into water (W16.-)*
> *accidental drowning and submersion due to water transport accident (V90.-, V92.-)*
>
> *EXCLUDES 2*   *accidental drowning and submersion due to cataclysm (X34-X39)*

The appropriate 7th character is to be added to each code from categories W65-W74.
A   initial encounter
D   subsequent encounter
S   sequela

✓x7ᵗʰ **W65 Accidental drowning and submersion while in bath-tub**

> *EXCLUDES 1*   *accidental drowning and submersion due to fall in (into) bathtub (W16.211)*

✓x7ᵗʰ **W67 Accidental drowning and submersion while in swimming-pool**

> *EXCLUDES 1*   *accidental drowning and submersion due to fall into swimming pool (W16.011, W16.021, W16.031)*
> *accidental drowning and submersion due to striking into wall of swimming pool (W22.041)*

✓x7ᵗʰ **W69 Accidental drowning and submersion while in natural water**

    Accidental drowning and submersion while in lake
    Accidental drowning and submersion while in open sea
    Accidental drowning and submersion while in river
    Accidental drowning and submersion while in stream

> *EXCLUDES 1*   *accidental drowning and submersion due to fall into natural body of water (W16.111, W16.121, W16.131)*

✓x7ᵗʰ **W73 Other specified cause of accidental non-transport drowning and submersion**

    Accidental drowning and submersion while in quenching tank
    Accidental drowning and submersion while in reservoir

> *EXCLUDES 1*   *accidental drowning and submersion due to fall into other water (W16.311, W16.321, W16.331)*

✓x7ᵗʰ **W74 Unspecified cause of accidental drowning and submersion**

    Drowning NOS

Exposure to electric current, radiation and extreme ambient air temperature and pressure (W85-W99)

> *EXCLUDES 1*   exposure to:
>   *failure in dosage of radiation or temperature during surgical and medical care (Y63.2-Y63.5)*
>   *lightning (T75.0-)*
>   *natural cold (X31)*
>   *natural heat (X30)*
>   *natural radiation NOS (X39)*
>   *radiological procedure and radiotherapy (Y84.2)*
>   *sunlight (X32)*

AHA: 2018,2Q,7-8

The appropriate 7th character is to be added to each code from categories W85-W99.
A   initial encounter
D   subsequent encounter
S   sequela

✓x7ᵗʰ **W85 Exposure to electric transmission lines**

    Broken power line

✓4ᵗʰ **W86 Exposure to other specified electric current**

✓x7ᵗʰ **W86.0 Exposure to domestic wiring and appliances**

✓x7ᵗʰ **W86.1 Exposure to industrial wiring, appliances and electrical machinery**

    Exposure to conductors
    Exposure to control apparatus
    Exposure to electrical equipment and machinery
    Exposure to transformers

✓x7ᵗʰ **W86.8 Exposure to other electric current**

    Exposure to wiring and appliances in or on farm (not farmhouse)
    Exposure to wiring and appliances outdoors
    Exposure to wiring and appliances in or on public building
    Exposure to wiring and appliances in or on residential institutions
    Exposure to wiring and appliances in or on schools

✓4ᵗʰ **W88 Exposure to ionizing radiation**

> *EXCLUDES 1*   *exposure to sunlight (X32)*

✓x7ᵗʰ **W88.0 Exposure to X-rays**

✓x7ᵗʰ **W88.1 Exposure to radioactive isotopes**

Additional Character Required   ✓x7ᵗʰ Placeholder Alert   Manifestation   Unspecified Dx   ▶◀ Revised Text   ● New Code   ▲ Revised Code Title

-10-CM 2020   **1189**

√x7ᵗʰ **W88.8 Exposure to other ionizing radiation**

✓4ᵗʰ **W89 Exposure to man-made visible and ultraviolet light**

INCLUDES exposure to welding light (arc)

EXCLUDES 1 *exposure to sunlight (X32)*

√x7ᵗʰ **W89.0 Exposure to welding light (arc)**

√x7ᵗʰ **W89.1 Exposure to tanning bed**

√x7ᵗʰ **W89.8 Exposure to other man-made visible and ultraviolet light**

√x7ᵗʰ **W89.9 Exposure to unspecified man-made visible and ultraviolet light**

✓4ᵗʰ **W90 Exposure to other nonionizing radiation**

EXCLUDES 1 *exposure to sunlight (X32)*

AHA: 2019,1Q,21

√x7ᵗʰ **W90.0 Exposure to radiofrequency**

√x7ᵗʰ **W90.1 Exposure to infrared radiation**

√x7ᵗʰ **W90.2 Exposure to laser radiation**

√x7ᵗʰ **W90.8 Exposure to other nonionizing radiation**

√x7ᵗʰ **W92 Exposure to excessive heat of man-made origin**

✓4ᵗʰ **W93 Exposure to excessive cold of man-made origin**

√5ᵗʰ **W93.0 Contact with or inhalation of dry ice**

√x7ᵗʰ **W93.01 Contact with dry ice**

√x7ᵗʰ **W93.02 Inhalation of dry ice**

√5ᵗʰ **W93.1 Contact with or inhalation of liquid air**

√x7ᵗʰ **W93.11 Contact with liquid air**

Contact with liquid hydrogen
Contact with liquid nitrogen

√x7ᵗʰ **W93.12 Inhalation of liquid air**

Inhalation of liquid hydrogen
Inhalation of liquid nitrogen

√x7ᵗʰ **W93.2 Prolonged exposure in deep freeze unit or refrigerator**

√x7ᵗʰ **W93.8 Exposure to other excessive cold of man-made origin**

✓4ᵗʰ **W94 Exposure to high and low air pressure and changes in air pressure**

√x7ᵗʰ **W94.0 Exposure to prolonged high air pressure**

√5ᵗʰ **W94.1 Exposure to prolonged low air pressure**

√x7ᵗʰ **W94.11 Exposure to residence or prolonged visit at high altitude**

√x7ᵗʰ **W94.12 Exposure to other prolonged low air pressure**

√5ᵗʰ **W94.2 Exposure to rapid changes in air pressure during ascent**

√x7ᵗʰ **W94.21 Exposure to reduction in atmospheric pressure while surfacing from deep-water diving**

√x7ᵗʰ **W94.22 Exposure to reduction in atmospheric pressure while surfacing from underground**

√x7ᵗʰ **W94.23 Exposure to sudden change in air pressure in aircraft during ascent**

√x7ᵗʰ **W94.29 Exposure to other rapid changes in air pressure during ascent**

√5ᵗʰ **W94.3 Exposure to rapid changes in air pressure during descent**

√x7ᵗʰ **W94.31 Exposure to sudden change in air pressure in aircraft during descent**

√x7ᵗʰ **W94.32 Exposure to high air pressure from rapid descent in water**

√x7ᵗʰ **W94.39 Exposure to other rapid changes in air pressure during descent**

√x7ᵗʰ **W99 Exposure to other man-made environmental factors**

Exposure to smoke, fire and flames (X00-X08)

EXCLUDES 1 *arson (X97)*

EXCLUDES 2 *explosions (W35-W40)*
lightning (T75.0-)
transport accident (V01-V99)

AHA: 2018,2Q,7-8

The appropriate 7th character is to be added to each code from categories X00-X08.

A initial encounter
D subsequent encounter
S sequela

✓4ᵗʰ **X00 Exposure to uncontrolled fire in building or structure**

INCLUDES conflagration in building or structure

Code first any associated cataclysm

EXCLUDES 2 *exposure to ignition or melting of nightwear (X05)*
exposure to ignition or melting of other clothing and apparel (X06.-)
exposure to other specified smoke, fire and flames (X08.-)

AHA: 2016,2Q,5

√x7ᵗʰ **X00.0 Exposure to flames in uncontrolled fire in building or structure**

√x7ᵗʰ **X00.1 Exposure to smoke in uncontrolled fire in building or structure**

√x7ᵗʰ **X00.2 Injury due to collapse of burning building or structure in uncontrolled fire**

EXCLUDES 1 *injury due to collapse of building not on fire (W20.1)*

√x7ᵗʰ **X00.3 Fall from burning building or structure in uncontrolled fire**

√x7ᵗʰ **X00.4 Hit by object from burning building or structure in uncontrolled fire**

AHA: 2016,2Q,4

√x7ᵗʰ **X00.5 Jump from burning building or structure in uncontrolled fire**

√x7ᵗʰ **X00.8 Other exposure to uncontrolled fire in building or structure**

✓4ᵗʰ **X01 Exposure to uncontrolled fire, not in building or structure**

INCLUDES exposure to forest fire

√x7ᵗʰ **X01.0 Exposure to flames in uncontrolled fire, not in building or structure**

√x7ᵗʰ **X01.1 Exposure to smoke in uncontrolled fire, not in building or structure**

√x7ᵗʰ **X01.3 Fall due to uncontrolled fire, not in building or structure**

√x7ᵗʰ **X01.4 Hit by object due to uncontrolled fire, not in building or structure**

√x7ᵗʰ **X01.8 Other exposure to uncontrolled fire, not in building or structure**

✓4ᵗʰ **X02 Exposure to controlled fire in building or structure**

INCLUDES exposure to fire in fireplace
exposure to fire in stove

√x7ᵗʰ **X02.0 Exposure to flames in controlled fire in building or structure**

√x7ᵗʰ **X02.1 Exposure to smoke in controlled fire in building or structure**

√x7ᵗʰ **X02.2 Injury due to collapse of burning building or structure in controlled fire**

EXCLUDES 1 *injury due to collapse of building not on fire (W20.1)*

√x7ᵗʰ **X02.3 Fall from burning building or structure in controlled fire**

√x7ᵗʰ **X02.4 Hit by object from burning building or structure in controlled fire**

√x7ᵗʰ **X02.5 Jump from burning building or structure in controlled fire**

√x7ᵗʰ **X02.8 Other exposure to controlled fire in building or structure**

✓4ᵗʰ **X03 Exposure to controlled fire, not in building or structure**

INCLUDES exposure to bon fire
exposure to camp-fire
exposure to trash fire

√x7ᵗʰ **X03.0 Exposure to flames in controlled fire, not in building or structure**

√x7ᵗʰ **X03.1 Exposure to smoke in controlled fire, not in building or structure**

√x7ᵗʰ **X03.3 Fall due to controlled fire, not in building or structure**

√x7ᵗʰ **X03.4 Hit by object due to controlled fire, not in building or structure**

√x7ᵗʰ **X03.8 Other exposure to controlled fire, not in building or structure**

√x7th **X04** **Exposure to ignition of highly flammable material**

    Exposure to ignition of gasoline
    Exposure to ignition of kerosene
    Exposure to ignition of petrol

    EXCLUDES 2   *exposure to ignition or melting of nightwear (X05)*
                   exposure to ignition or melting of other clothing and apparel (X06)

    AHA: 2016,2Q,4

√x7th **X05** **Exposure to ignition or melting of nightwear**

    EXCLUDES 2   *exposure to uncontrolled fire in building or structure (X00.-)*
                   exposure to uncontrolled fire, not in building or structure (X01.-)
                   exposure to controlled fire in building or structure (X02.-)
                   exposure to controlled fire, not in building or structure (X03.-)
                   exposure to ignition of highly flammable materials (X04.-)

√4th **X06** **Exposure to ignition or melting of other clothing and apparel**

    EXCLUDES 2   *exposure to uncontrolled fire in building or structure (X00.-)*
                   exposure to uncontrolled fire, not in building or structure (X01.-)
                   exposure to controlled fire in building or structure (X02.-)
                   exposure to controlled fire, not in building or structure (X03.-)
                   exposure to ignition of highly flammable materials (X04.-)

√x7th **X06.0** **Exposure to ignition of plastic jewelry**

√x7th **X06.1** **Exposure to melting of plastic jewelry**

√x7th **X06.2** **Exposure to ignition of other clothing and apparel**

√x7th **X06.3** **Exposure to melting of other clothing and apparel**

√4th **X08** **Exposure to other specified smoke, fire and flames**

√5th **X08.0** **Exposure to bed fire**

    Exposure to mattress fire

  √x7th **X08.00** **Exposure to bed fire due to unspecified burning material**

  √x7th **X08.01** **Exposure to bed fire due to burning cigarette**

  √x7th **X08.09** **Exposure to bed fire due to other burning material**

√5th **X08.1** **Exposure to sofa fire**

  √x7th **X08.10** **Exposure to sofa fire due to unspecified burning material**

  √x7th **X08.11** **Exposure to sofa fire due to burning cigarette**

  √x7th **X08.19** **Exposure to sofa fire due to other burning material**

√5th **X08.2** **Exposure to other furniture fire**

  √x7th **X08.20** **Exposure to other furniture fire due to unspecified burning material**

  √x7th **X08.21** **Exposure to other furniture fire due to burning cigarette**

  √x7th **X08.29** **Exposure to other furniture fire due to other burning material**

√x7th **X08.8** **Exposure to other specified smoke, fire and flames**

Contact with heat and hot substances (X10-X19)

    EXCLUDES 1   *exposure to excessive natural heat (X30)*
                   exposure to fire and flames (X00-X08)

    AHA: 2018,2Q,7-8

The appropriate 7th character is to be added to each code from categories X10-X19.
A   initial encounter
D   subsequent encounter
S   sequela

√4th **X10** **Contact with hot drinks, food, fats and cooking oils**

√x7th **X10.0** **Contact with hot drinks**

√x7th **X10.1** **Contact with hot food**

√x7th **X10.2** **Contact with fats and cooking oils**

√4th **X11** **Contact with hot tap-water**

    INCLUDES   contact with boiling tap-water
                contact with boiling water NOS

    EXCLUDES 1   *contact with water heated on stove (X12)*

√x7th **X11.0** **Contact with hot water in bath or tub**

    EXCLUDES 1   *contact with running hot water in bath or tub (X11.1)*

√x7th **X11.1** **Contact with running hot water**

    Contact with hot water running out of hose
    Contact with hot water running out of tap

√x7th **X11.8** **Contact with other hot tap-water**

    Contact with hot water in bucket
    Contact with hot tap-water NOS

√x7th **X12** **Contact with other hot fluids**

    Contact with water heated on stove

    EXCLUDES 1   *hot (liquid) metals (X18)*

√4th **X13** **Contact with steam and other hot vapors**

√x7th **X13.0** **Inhalation of steam and other hot vapors**

√x7th **X13.1** **Other contact with steam and other hot vapors**

√4th **X14** **Contact with hot air and other hot gases**

√x7th **X14.0** **Inhalation of hot air and gases**

√x7th **X14.1** **Other contact with hot air and other hot gases**

√4th **X15** **Contact with hot household appliances**

    EXCLUDES 1   *contact with heating appliances (X16)*
                   contact with powered household appliances (W29.-)
                   exposure to controlled fire in building or structure due to household appliance (X02.8)
                   exposure to household appliances electrical current (W86.0)

√x7th **X15.0** **Contact with hot stove (kitchen)**

√x7th **X15.1** **Contact with hot toaster**

√x7th **X15.2** **Contact with hotplate**

√x7th **X15.3** **Contact with hot saucepan or skillet**

√x7th **X15.8** **Contact with other hot household appliances**

    Contact with cooker
    Contact with kettle
    Contact with light bulbs

√x7th **X16** **Contact with hot heating appliances, radiators and pipes**

    EXCLUDES 1   *contact with powered appliances (W29.-)*
                   exposure to controlled fire in building or structure due to appliance (X02.8)
                   exposure to industrial appliances electrical current (W86.1)

√x7th **X17** **Contact with hot engines, machinery and tools**

    EXCLUDES 1   *contact with hot heating appliances, radiators and pipes (X16)*
                   contact with hot household appliances (X15)

√x7th **X18** **Contact with other hot metals**

    Contact with liquid metal

√x7th **X19** **Contact with other heat and hot substances**

    EXCLUDES 1   *objects that are not normally hot, e.g., an object made hot by a house fire (X00-X08)*

Exposure to forces of nature (X30-X39)

    AHA: 2018,2Q,7-8

The appropriate 7th character is to be added to each code from categories X30-X39.
A   initial encounter
D   subsequent encounter
S   sequela

√x7th **X30** **Exposure to excessive natural heat**

    Exposure to excessive heat as the cause of sunstroke
    Exposure to heat NOS

    EXCLUDES 1   *excessive heat of man-made origin (W92)*
                   exposure to man-made radiation (W89)
                   exposure to sunlight (X32)
                   exposure to tanning bed (W89)

√x7th **X31** **Exposure to excessive natural cold**

    Excessive cold as the cause of chilblains NOS
    Excessive cold as the cause of immersion foot or hand
    Exposure to cold NOS
    Exposure to weather conditions

    EXCLUDES 1   *cold of man-made origin (W93.-)*
                   contact with or inhalation of dry ice (W93.-)
                   contact with or inhalation of liquefied gas (W93.-)

√x7th **X32** **Exposure to sunlight**

    EXCLUDES 1   *man-made radiation (tanning bed) (W89)*

    EXCLUDES 2   *radiation-related disorders of the skin and subcutaneous tissue (L55-L59)*

√x7ᵗʰ **X34 Earthquake**
> EXCLUDES 2   *tidal wave (tsunami) due to earthquake (X37.41)*

√x7ᵗʰ **X35 Volcanic eruption**
> EXCLUDES 2   *tidal wave (tsunami) due to volcanic eruption (X37.41)*

√4ᵗʰ **X36 Avalanche, landslide and other earth movements**
> INCLUDES   victim of mudslide of cataclysmic nature
> EXCLUDES 1   *earthquake (X34)*
> EXCLUDES 2   *transport accident involving collision with avalanche or landslide not in motion (V01-V99)*

  √x7ᵗʰ **X36.0 Collapse of dam or man-made structure causing earth movement**

  √x7ᵗʰ **X36.1 Avalanche, landslide, or mudslide**

√4ᵗʰ **X37 Cataclysmic storm**

  √x7ᵗʰ **X37.0 Hurricane**
> Storm surge
> Typhoon

  √x7ᵗʰ **X37.1 Tornado**
> Cyclone
> Twister

  √x7ᵗʰ **X37.2 Blizzard (snow)(ice)**

  √x7ᵗʰ **X37.3 Dust storm**

  √5ᵗʰ **X37.4 Tidalwave**

    √x7ᵗʰ **X37.41 Tidal wave due to earthquake or volcanic eruption**
> Tidal wave NOS
> Tsunami

    √x7ᵗʰ **X37.42 Tidal wave due to storm**

    √x7ᵗʰ **X37.43 Tidal wave due to landslide**

  √x7ᵗʰ **X37.8 Other cataclysmic storms**
> Cloudburst
> Torrential rain
> EXCLUDES 2   *flood (X38)*

  √x7ᵗʰ **X37.9 Unspecified cataclysmic storm**
> Storm NOS
> EXCLUDES 1   *collapse of dam or man-made structure causing earth movement (X36.0)*

√x7ᵗʰ **X38 Flood**
> Flood arising from remote storm
> Flood of cataclysmic nature arising from melting snow
> Flood resulting directly from storm
> EXCLUDES 1   *collapse of dam or man-made structure causing earth movement (X36.0)*
> *tidal wave NOS (X37.41)*
> *tidal wave caused by storm (X37.42)*

√4ᵗʰ **X39 Exposure to other forces of nature**

  √5ᵗʰ **X39.0 Exposure to natural radiation**
> EXCLUDES 1   *contact with and (suspected) exposure to radon and other naturally occurring radiation (Z77.123)*
> *exposure to man-made radiation (W88-W90)*
> *exposure to sunlight (X32)*

    √x7ᵗʰ **X39.01 Exposure to radon**

    √x7ᵗʰ **X39.08 Exposure to other natural radiation**

  √x7ᵗʰ **X39.8 Other exposure to forces of nature**

Overexertion and strenuous or repetitive movements (X50)

√4ᵗʰ **X50 Overexertion and strenuous or repetitive movements**

AHA: 2018,2Q,7-8; 2016,4Q,73-74

> The appropriate 7th character is to be added to each code from category X50.
> A   initial encounter
> D   subsequent encounter
> S   sequela

  √x7ᵗʰ **X50.0 Overexertion from strenuous movement or load**
> Lifting heavy objects
> Lifting weights

  √x7ᵗʰ **X50.1 Overexertion from prolonged static or awkward postures**
> Prolonged bending
> Prolonged kneeling
> Prolonged reaching
> Prolonged sitting
> Prolonged standing
> Prolonged twisting
> Static bending
> Static kneeling
> Static reaching
> Static sitting
> Static standing
> Static twisting

  √x7ᵗʰ **X50.3 Overexertion from repetitive movements**
> Use of hand as hammer
> EXCLUDES 2   *overuse from prolonged static or awkward postures (X50.1)*

  √x7ᵗʰ **X50.9 Other and unspecified overexertion or strenuous movements or postures**
> Contact pressure
> Contact stress

Accidental exposure to other specified factors (X52-X58)

AHA: 2018,2Q,7-8

> The appropriate 7th character is to be added to each code from categories X52-X58.
> A   initial encounter
> D   subsequent encounter
> S   sequela

√x7ᵗʰ **X52 Prolonged stay in weightless environment**
> Weightlessness in spacecraft (simulator)

√x7ᵗʰ **X58 Exposure to other specified factors**
> Accident NOS
> Exposure NOS

Intentional self-harm (X71-X83)

Purposely self-inflicted injury
Suicide (attempted)

> The appropriate 7th character is to be added to each code from categories X71-X83.
> A   initial encounter
> D   subsequent encounter
> S   sequela

√4ᵗʰ **X71 Intentional self-harm by drowning and submersion**

  √x7ᵗʰ **X71.0 Intentional self-harm by drowning and submersion while in bathtub**   HCC

  √x7ᵗʰ **X71.1 Intentional self-harm by drowning and submersion while in swimming pool**   HCC

  √x7ᵗʰ **X71.2 Intentional self-harm by drowning and submersion after jump into swimming pool**   HCC

  √x7ᵗʰ **X71.3 Intentional self-harm by drowning and submersion in natural water**   HCC

  √x7ᵗʰ **X71.8 Other intentional self-harm by drowning and submersion**   HCC

  √x7ᵗʰ **X71.9 Intentional self-harm by drowning and submersion, unspecified**   HCC

√x7ᵗʰ **X72 Intentional self-harm by handgun discharge**   HCC
> Intentional self-harm by gun for single hand use
> Intentional self-harm by pistol
> Intentional self-harm by revolver
> EXCLUDES 1   *Very pistol (X74.8)*

√4ᵗʰ **X73 Intentional self-harm by rifle, shotgun and larger firearm discharge**
> EXCLUDES 1   *airgun (X74.01)*

  √x7ᵗʰ **X73.0 Intentional self-harm by shotgun discharge**   HCC

  √x7ᵗʰ **X73.1 Intentional self-harm by hunting rifle discharge**   HCC

  √x7ᵗʰ **X73.2 Intentional self-harm by machine gun discharge**   HCC

  √x7ᵗʰ **X73.8 Intentional self-harm by other larger firearm discharge**   HCC

  √x7ᵗʰ **X73.9 Intentional self-harm by unspecified larger firearm discharge**   HCC

√4ᵗʰ **X74 Intentional self-harm by other and unspecified firearm and gun discharge**

  √5ᵗʰ **X74.0 Intentional self-harm by** gas, air or spring-operated guns

    √x7ᵗʰ **X74.01 Intentional self-harm by** airgun   `HCC`

         Intentional self-harm by BB gun discharge
         Intentional self-harm by pellet gun discharge

    √x7ᵗʰ **X74.02 Intentional self-harm by** paintball gun   `HCC`

    √x7ᵗʰ **X74.09 Intentional self-harm by other gas, air or spring-operated gun**   `HCC`

  √x7ᵗʰ **X74.8 Intentional self-harm by other firearm discharge**   `HCC`

       Intentional self-harm by Very pistol [flare] discharge

  √x7ᵗʰ **X74.9 Intentional self-harm by unspecified firearm discharge**   `HCC`

√x7ᵗʰ **X75 Intentional self-harm by explosive material**   `HCC`

√x7ᵗʰ **X76 Intentional self-harm by smoke, fire and flames**   `HCC`

√4ᵗʰ **X77 Intentional self-harm by steam, hot vapors and hot objects**

  √x7ᵗʰ **X77.0 Intentional self-harm by** steam or hot vapors   `HCC`

  √x7ᵗʰ **X77.1 Intentional self-harm by** hot tap water   `HCC`

  √x7ᵗʰ **X77.2 Intentional self-harm by other hot fluids**   `HCC`

  √x7ᵗʰ **X77.3 Intentional self-harm by** hot household appliances   `HCC`

  √x7ᵗʰ **X77.8 Intentional self-harm by other hot objects**   `HCC`

  √x7ᵗʰ **X77.9 Intentional self-harm by unspecified hot objects**   `HCC`

√4ᵗʰ **X78 Intentional self-harm by sharp object**

  √x7ᵗʰ **X78.0 Intentional self-harm by sharp** glass   `HCC`

  √x7ᵗʰ **X78.1 Intentional self-harm by** knife   `HCC`

  √x7ᵗʰ **X78.2 Intentional self-harm by** sword or dagger   `HCC`

  √x7ᵗʰ **X78.8 Intentional self-harm by other sharp object**   `HCC`

  √x7ᵗʰ **X78.9 Intentional self-harm by unspecified sharp object**   `HCC`

√x7ᵗʰ **X79 Intentional self-harm by blunt object**   `HCC`

√x7ᵗʰ **X80 Intentional self-harm by jumping from a high place**   `HCC`

     Intentional fall from one level to another

√4ᵗʰ **X81 Intentional self-harm by jumping or lying in front of moving object**

  √x7ᵗʰ **X81.0 Intentional self-harm by jumping or lying in front of motor vehicle**   `HCC`

  √x7ᵗʰ **X81.1 Intentional self-harm by jumping or lying in front of (subway) train**   `HCC`

  √x7ᵗʰ **X81.8 Intentional self-harm by jumping or lying in front of other moving object**   `HCC`

√4ᵗʰ **X82 Intentional self-harm by crashing of motor vehicle**

  √x7ᵗʰ **X82.0 Intentional collision of motor vehicle with other motor vehicle**   `HCC`

  √x7ᵗʰ **X82.1 Intentional collision of motor vehicle with** train   `HCC`

  √x7ᵗʰ **X82.2 Intentional collision of motor vehicle with** tree   `HCC`

  √x7ᵗʰ **X82.8 Other intentional self-harm by crashing of motor vehicle**   `HCC`

√4ᵗʰ **X83 Intentional self-harm by other specified means**

    `EXCLUDES 1`   *intentional self-harm by poisoning or contact with toxic substance — see Table of Drugs and Chemicals*

  √x7ᵗʰ **X83.0 Intentional self-harm by** crashing of aircraft   `HCC`

  √x7ᵗʰ **X83.1 Intentional self-harm by** electrocution   `HCC`

  √x7ᵗʰ **X83.2 Intentional self-harm by** exposure to extremes of cold   `HCC`

  √x7ᵗʰ **X83.8 Intentional self-harm by other specified means**   `HCC`

Assault (X92–Y09)

`INCLUDES`   homicide
         injuries inflicted by another person with intent to injure or kill, by any means

`EXCLUDES 1`   *injuries due to legal intervention (Y35.-)*
         injuries due to operations of war (Y36.-)
         injuries due to terrorism (Y38.-)

> The appropriate 7th character is to be added to each code from categories X92-Y04 and Y08.
> A   initial encounter
> D   subsequent encounter
> S   sequela

√4ᵗʰ **X92 Assault by drowning and submersion**

  √x7ᵗʰ **X92.0 Assault by drowning and submersion while in** bathtub

√x7ᵗʰ **X92.1 Assault by drowning and submersion while in** swimming pool

√x7ᵗʰ **X92.2 Assault by drowning and submersion** after push into swimming pool

√x7ᵗʰ **X92.3 Assault by drowning and submersion** in natural water

√x7ᵗʰ **X92.8 Other assault by drowning and submersion**

√x7ᵗʰ **X92.9 Assault by drowning and submersion, unspecified**

√x7ᵗʰ **X93 Assault by** handgun discharge

     Assault by discharge of gun for single hand use
     Assault by discharge of pistol
     Assault by discharge of revolver

    `EXCLUDES 1`   *Very pistol (X95.8)*

√4ᵗʰ **X94 Assault by** rifle, shotgun and larger firearm discharge

    `EXCLUDES 1`   *airgun (X95.01)*

  √x7ᵗʰ **X94.0 Assault by** shotgun

  √x7ᵗʰ **X94.1 Assault by** hunting rifle

  √x7ᵗʰ **X94.2 Assault by** machine gun

  √x7ᵗʰ **X94.8 Assault by other larger firearm discharge**

  √x7ᵗʰ **X94.9 Assault by unspecified larger firearm discharge**

√4ᵗʰ **X95 Assault by other and unspecified firearm and gun discharge**

  √5ᵗʰ **X95.0 Assault by** gas, air or spring-operated guns

    √x7ᵗʰ **X95.01 Assault by** airgun discharge

         Assault by BB gun discharge
         Assault by pellet gun discharge

    √x7ᵗʰ **X95.02 Assault by** paintball gun discharge

    √x7ᵗʰ **X95.09 Assault by other gas, air or spring-operated gun**

  √x7ᵗʰ **X95.8 Assault by other firearm discharge**

       Assault by Very pistol [flare] discharge

  √x7ᵗʰ **X95.9 Assault by unspecified firearm discharge**

√4ᵗʰ **X96 Assault by explosive material**

    `EXCLUDES 1`   *incendiary device (X97)*
         terrorism involving explosive material (Y38.2-)

  √x7ᵗʰ **X96.0 Assault by** antipersonnel bomb

    `EXCLUDES 1`   *antipersonnel bomb use in military or war (Y36.2-)*

  √x7ᵗʰ **X96.1 Assault by** gasoline bomb

  √x7ᵗʰ **X96.2 Assault by** letter bomb

  √x7ᵗʰ **X96.3 Assault by** fertilizer bomb

  √x7ᵗʰ **X96.4 Assault by** pipe bomb

  √x7ᵗʰ **X96.8 Assault by other specified explosive**

  √x7ᵗʰ **X96.9 Assault by unspecified explosive**

√x7ᵗʰ **X97 Assault by smoke, fire and flames**

     Assault by arson
     Assault by cigarettes
     Assault by incendiary device

√4ᵗʰ **X98 Assault by steam, hot vapors and hot objects**

  √x7ᵗʰ **X98.0 Assault by** steam or hot vapors

  √x7ᵗʰ **X98.1 Assault by** hot tap water

  √x7ᵗʰ **X98.2 Assault by** hot fluids

  √x7ᵗʰ **X98.3 Assault by** hot household appliances

  √x7ᵗʰ **X98.8 Assault by other hot** objects

  √x7ᵗʰ **X98.9 Assault by unspecified hot objects**

√4ᵗʰ **X99 Assault by sharp object**

    `EXCLUDES 1`   *assault by strike by sports equipment (Y08.0-)*

  √x7ᵗʰ **X99.0 Assault by sharp** glass

  √x7ᵗʰ **X99.1 Assault by** knife

  √x7ᵗʰ **X99.2 Assault by** sword or dagger

  √x7ᵗʰ **X99.8 Assault by other sharp object**

  √x7ᵗʰ **X99.9 Assault by unspecified sharp object**

       Assault by stabbing NOS

√x7ᵗʰ **Y00 Assault by blunt object**

    `EXCLUDES 1`   *assault by strike by sports equipment (Y08.0-)*

√x7ᵗʰ **Y01 Assault by pushing from high place**

√4ᵗʰ **Y02 Assault by pushing or placing victim in front of moving object**

  √x7ᵗʰ **Y02.0 Assault by pushing or placing victim in front of** motor vehicle

√4ᵗʰ Additional Character Required   √x7ᵗʰ Placeholder Alert   Manifestation   Unspecified Dx   ►◄ Revised Text   ● New Code   ▲ Revised Code Title

10-CM 2020   **1193**

✓x7ᵗʰ **Y02.1 Assault by pushing or placing victim in front of (subway) train**

✓x7ᵗʰ **Y02.8 Assault by pushing or placing victim in front of other moving object**

✓4ᵗʰ **Y03 Assault by crashing of motor vehicle**

   ✓x7ᵗʰ **Y03.0 Assault by being hit or run over by motor vehicle**

   ✓x7ᵗʰ **Y03.8 Other assault by crashing of motor vehicle**

✓4ᵗʰ **Y04 Assault by bodily force**

   EXCLUDES 1   assault by:
          submersion (X92.-)
          use of weapon (X93-X95, X99, Y00)

   ✓x7ᵗʰ **Y04.0 Assault by unarmed brawl or fight**

   ✓x7ᵗʰ **Y04.1 Assault by human bite**

   ✓x7ᵗʰ **Y04.2 Assault by strike against or bumped into by another person**

   ✓x7ᵗʰ **Y04.8 Assault by other bodily force**
       Assault by bodily force NOS

✓4ᵗʰ **Y07 Perpetrator of assault, maltreatment and neglect**

   NOTE   Codes from this category are for use only in cases of confirmed abuse (T74.-)

       Selection of the correct perpetrator code is based on the relationship between the perpetrator and the victim

   INCLUDES   perpetrator of abandonment
         perpetrator of emotional neglect
         perpetrator of mental cruelty
         perpetrator of physical abuse
         perpetrator of physical neglect
         perpetrator of sexual abuse
         perpetrator of torture

   ✓5ᵗʰ **Y07.0 Spouse or partner, perpetrator of maltreatment and neglect**
       Spouse or partner, perpetrator of maltreatment and neglect against spouse or partner

       Y07.01 Husband, perpetrator of maltreatment and neglect

       Y07.02 Wife, perpetrator of maltreatment and neglect

       Y07.03 Male partner, perpetrator of maltreatment and neglect

       Y07.04 Female partner, perpetrator of maltreatment and neglect

   ✓5ᵗʰ **Y07.1 Parent (adoptive) (biological), perpetrator of maltreatment and neglect**

       Y07.11 Biological father, perpetrator of maltreatment and neglect

       Y07.12 Biological mother, perpetrator of maltreatment and neglect

       Y07.13 Adoptive father, perpetrator of maltreatment and neglect

       Y07.14 Adoptive mother, perpetrator of maltreatment and neglect

   ✓5ᵗʰ **Y07.4 Other family member, perpetrator of maltreatment and neglect**

     ✓6ᵗʰ **Y07.41 Sibling, perpetrator of maltreatment and neglect**

       EXCLUDES 1   stepsibling, perpetrator of maltreatment and neglect (Y07.435, Y07.436)

       Y07.410 Brother, perpetrator of maltreatment and neglect

       Y07.411 Sister, perpetrator of maltreatment and neglect

     ✓6ᵗʰ **Y07.42 Foster parent, perpetrator of maltreatment and neglect**

       Y07.420 Foster father, perpetrator of maltreatment and neglect

       Y07.421 Foster mother, perpetrator of maltreatment and neglect

     ✓6ᵗʰ **Y07.43 Stepparent or stepsibling, perpetrator of maltreatment and neglect**

       Y07.430 Stepfather, perpetrator of maltreatment and neglect

       Y07.432 Male friend of parent (co-residing in household), perpetrator of maltreatment and neglect

       Y07.433 Stepmother, perpetrator of maltreatment and neglect

       Y07.434 Female friend of parent (co-residing in household), perpetrator of maltreatment and neglect

       Y07.435 Stepbrother, perpetrator or maltreatment and neglect

       Y07.436 Stepsister, perpetrator of maltreatment and neglect

     ✓6ᵗʰ **Y07.49 Other family member, perpetrator of maltreatment and neglect**

       Y07.490 Male cousin, perpetrator of maltreatment and neglect

       Y07.491 Female cousin, perpetrator of maltreatment and neglect

       Y07.499 Other family member, perpetrator of maltreatment and neglect

   ✓5ᵗʰ **Y07.5 Non-family member, perpetrator of maltreatment and neglect**

       Y07.50 Unspecified non-family member, perpetrator of maltreatment and neglect

     ✓6ᵗʰ **Y07.51 Daycare provider, perpetrator of maltreatment and neglect**

       Y07.510 At-home childcare provider, perpetrator of maltreatment and neglect

       Y07.511 Daycare center childcare provider, perpetrator of maltreatment and neglect

       Y07.512 At-home adultcare provider, perpetrator of maltreatment and neglect

       Y07.513 Adultcare center provider, perpetrator of maltreatment and neglect

       Y07.519 Unspecified daycare provider, perpetrator of maltreatment and neglect

     ✓6ᵗʰ **Y07.52 Healthcare provider, perpetrator of maltreatment and neglect**

       Y07.521 Mental health provider, perpetrator of maltreatment and neglect

       Y07.528 Other therapist or healthcare provider, perpetrator of maltreatment and neglect
         Nurse perpetrator of maltreatment and neglect
         Occupational therapist perpetrator of maltreatment and neglect
         Physical therapist perpetrator of maltreatment and neglect
         Speech therapist perpetrator of maltreatment and neglect

       Y07.529 Unspecified healthcare provider, perpetrator of maltreatment and neglect

       Y07.53 Teacher or instructor, perpetrator of maltreatment and neglect
         Coach, perpetrator of maltreatment and neglect

       Y07.59 Other non-family member, perpetrator of maltreatment and neglect

     Y07.6 Multiple perpetrators of maltreatment and neglect
       AHA: 2018,4Q,32

     Y07.9 Unspecified perpetrator of maltreatment and neglect

✓4ᵗʰ **Y08 Assault by other specified means**

   ✓5ᵗʰ **Y08.0 Assault by strike by sport equipment**

     ✓x7ᵗʰ **Y08.01 Assault by strike by hockey stick**

     ✓x7ᵗʰ **Y08.02 Assault by strike by baseball bat**

     ✓x7ᵗʰ **Y08.09 Assault by strike by other specified type of sport equipment**

   ✓5ᵗʰ **Y08.8 Assault by other specified means**

     ✓x7ᵗʰ **Y08.81 Assault by crashing of aircraft**

     ✓x7ᵗʰ **Y08.89 Assault by other specified means**

Y09 Assault by unspecified means
   Assassination (attempted) NOS
   Homicide (attempted) NOS
   Manslaughter (attempted) NOS
   Murder (attempted) NOS

Event of undetermined intent (Y21-Y33)

Undetermined intent is only for use when there is specific documentation in the record that the intent of the injury cannot be determined. If no such documentation is present, code to accidental (unintentional).

The appropriate 7th character is to be added to each code from categories Y21-Y33.
   A   initial encounter
   D   subsequent encounter
   S   sequela

✓4ᵗʰ **Y21 Drowning and submersion, undetermined intent**

   ✓x7ᵗʰ **Y21.0 Drowning and submersion while in bathtub, undetermined intent**

√x7ᵗʰ **Y21.1 Drowning and submersion** after fall into bathtub, **undetermined intent**

√x7ᵗʰ **Y21.2 Drowning and submersion** while in swimming pool, **undetermined intent**

√x7ᵗʰ **Y21.3 Drowning and submersion** after fall into swimming pool, **undetermined intent**

√x7ᵗʰ **Y21.4 Drowning and submersion** in natural water, **undetermined intent**

√x7ᵗʰ **Y21.8 Other drowning and submersion, undetermined intent**

√x7ᵗʰ **Y21.9 Unspecified drowning and submersion, undetermined intent**

√x7ᵗʰ **Y22 Handgun discharge, undetermined intent**
> Discharge of gun for single hand use, undetermined intent
> Discharge of pistol, undetermined intent
> Discharge of revolver, undetermined intent
> EXCLUDES 2   *Very pistol (Y24.8)*

√4ᵗʰ **Y23 Rifle, shotgun and larger firearm discharge, undetermined intent**
> EXCLUDES 2   *airgun (Y24.Ø)*

√x7ᵗʰ **Y23.Ø Shotgun discharge, undetermined intent**

√x7ᵗʰ **Y23.1 Hunting rifle discharge, undetermined intent**

√x7ᵗʰ **Y23.2 Military firearm discharge, undetermined intent**

√x7ᵗʰ **Y23.3 Machine gun discharge, undetermined intent**

√x7ᵗʰ **Y23.8 Other larger firearm discharge, undetermined intent**

√x7ᵗʰ **Y23.9 Unspecified larger firearm discharge, undetermined intent**

√4ᵗʰ **Y24 Other and unspecified firearm discharge, undetermined intent**

√x7ᵗʰ **Y24.Ø Airgun discharge, undetermined intent**
> BB gun discharge, undetermined intent
> Pellet gun discharge, undetermined intent

√x7ᵗʰ **Y24.8 Other firearm discharge, undetermined intent**
> Paintball gun discharge, undetermined intent
> Very pistol [flare] discharge, undetermined intent

√x7ᵗʰ **Y24.9 Unspecified firearm discharge, undetermined intent**

√7ᵗʰ **Y25 Contact with explosive material, undetermined intent**

√x7ᵗʰ **Y26 Exposure to smoke, fire and flames, undetermined intent**

√4ᵗʰ **Y27 Contact with steam, hot vapors and hot objects, undetermined intent**

√x7ᵗʰ **Y27.Ø Contact with steam and hot vapors, undetermined intent**

√x7ᵗʰ **Y27.1 Contact with hot tap water, undetermined intent**

√x7ᵗʰ **Y27.2 Contact with hot fluids, undetermined intent**

√x7ᵗʰ **Y27.3 Contact with hot household appliance, undetermined intent**

√x7ᵗʰ **Y27.8 Contact with other hot objects, undetermined intent**

√x7ᵗʰ **Y27.9 Contact with unspecified hot objects, undetermined intent**

√4ᵗʰ **Y28 Contact with sharp object, undetermined intent**

√x7ᵗʰ **Y28.Ø Contact with sharp glass, undetermined intent**

√x7ᵗʰ **Y28.1 Contact with knife, undetermined intent**

√x7ᵗʰ **Y28.2 Contact with sword or dagger, undetermined intent**

√x7ᵗʰ **Y28.8 Contact with other sharp object, undetermined intent**

√x7ᵗʰ **Y28.9 Contact with unspecified sharp object, undetermined intent**

√x7ᵗʰ **Y29 Contact with blunt object, undetermined intent**

√x7ᵗʰ **Y30 Falling, jumping or pushed from a high place, undetermined intent**
> Victim falling from one level to another, undetermined intent

√x7ᵗʰ **Y31 Falling, lying or running before or into moving object, undetermined intent**

√x7ᵗʰ **Y32 Crashing of motor vehicle, undetermined intent**

√x7ᵗʰ **Y33 Other specified events, undetermined intent**

Legal intervention, operations of war, military operations, and terrorism (Y35-Y38)

> The appropriate 7th character is to be added to each code from categories Y35-Y38.
> A   initial encounter
> D   subsequent encounter
> S   sequela

√4ᵗʰ **Y35 Legal intervention**
> INCLUDES   any injury sustained as a result of an encounter with any law enforcement official, serving in any capacity at the time of the encounter, whether on-duty or off-duty. Includes injury to law enforcement official, suspect and bystander

√5ᵗʰ **Y35.Ø Legal intervention involving firearm discharge**

√6ᵗʰ **Y35.ØØ Legal intervention involving unspecified firearm discharge**
> Legal intervention involving gunshot wound
> Legal intervention involving shot NOS

√7ᵗʰ **Y35.ØØ1 Legal intervention involving unspecified firearm discharge, law enforcement official injured**

√7ᵗʰ **Y35.ØØ2 Legal intervention involving unspecified firearm discharge, bystander injured**

√7ᵗʰ **Y35.ØØ3 Legal intervention involving unspecified firearm discharge, suspect injured**

√7ᵗʰ **Y35.ØØ9 Legal intervention involving unspecified firearm discharge, unspecified person injured**

√6ᵗʰ **Y35.Ø1 Legal intervention involving injury by machine gun**

√7ᵗʰ **Y35.Ø11 Legal intervention involving injury by machine gun, law enforcement official injured**

√7ᵗʰ **Y35.Ø12 Legal intervention involving injury by machine gun, bystander injured**

√7ᵗʰ **Y35.Ø13 Legal intervention involving injury by machine gun, suspect injured**

√7ᵗʰ **Y35.Ø19 Legal intervention involving injury by machine gun, unspecified person injured**

√6ᵗʰ **Y35.Ø2 Legal intervention involving injury by handgun**

√7ᵗʰ **Y35.Ø21 Legal intervention involving injury by handgun, law enforcement official injured**

√7ᵗʰ **Y35.Ø22 Legal intervention involving injury by handgun, bystander injured**

√7ᵗʰ **Y35.Ø23 Legal intervention involving injury by handgun, suspect injured**

√7ᵗʰ **Y35.Ø29 Legal intervention involving injury by handgun, unspecified person injured**

√6ᵗʰ **Y35.Ø3 Legal intervention involving injury by rifle pellet**

√7ᵗʰ **Y35.Ø31 Legal intervention involving injury by rifle pellet, law enforcement official injured**

√7ᵗʰ **Y35.Ø32 Legal intervention involving injury by rifle pellet, bystander injured**

√7ᵗʰ **Y35.Ø33 Legal intervention involving injury by rifle pellet, suspect injured**

√7ᵗʰ **Y35.Ø39 Legal intervention involving injury by rifle pellet, unspecified person injured**

√6ᵗʰ **Y35.Ø4 Legal intervention involving injury by rubber bullet**

√7ᵗʰ **Y35.Ø41 Legal intervention involving injury by rubber bullet, law enforcement official injured**

√7ᵗʰ **Y35.Ø42 Legal intervention involving injury by rubber bullet, bystander injured**

√7ᵗʰ **Y35.Ø43 Legal intervention involving injury by rubber bullet, suspect injured**

√7ᵗʰ **Y35.Ø49 Legal intervention involving injury by rubber bullet, unspecified person injured**

√6ᵗʰ **Y35.Ø9 Legal intervention involving other firearm discharge**

√7ᵗʰ **Y35.Ø91 Legal intervention involving other firearm discharge, law enforcement official injured**

√7ᵗʰ **Y35.Ø92 Legal intervention involving other firearm discharge, bystander injured**

√7ᵗʰ **Y35.Ø93 Legal intervention involving other firearm discharge, suspect injured**

√7ᵗʰ **Y35.Ø99 Legal intervention involving other firearm discharge, unspecified person injured**

Additional Character Required   √x7ᵗʰ Placeholder Alert   Manifestation   Unspecified Dx   ►◄ Revised Text   ● New Code   ▲ Revised Code Title

-10-CM 2020   **1195**

✓5ᵗʰ **Y35.1 Legal intervention involving** explosives

✓6ᵗʰ **Y35.10 Legal intervention involving unspecified explosives**

✓7ᵗʰ **Y35.101 Legal intervention involving unspecified explosives, law enforcement official injured**

✓7ᵗʰ **Y35.102 Legal intervention involving unspecified explosives, bystander injured**

✓7ᵗʰ **Y35.103 Legal intervention involving unspecified explosives, suspect injured**

✓7ᵗʰ **Y35.109 Legal intervention involving unspecified explosives, unspecified person injured**

✓6ᵗʰ **Y35.11 Legal intervention involving injury by** dynamite

✓7ᵗʰ **Y35.111 Legal intervention involving injury by dynamite, law enforcement official injured**

✓7ᵗʰ **Y35.112 Legal intervention involving injury by dynamite, bystander injured**

✓7ᵗʰ **Y35.113 Legal intervention involving injury by dynamite, suspect injured**

✓7ᵗʰ **Y35.119 Legal intervention involving injury by dynamite, unspecified person injured**

✓6ᵗʰ **Y35.12 Legal intervention involving injury by** explosive shell

✓7ᵗʰ **Y35.121 Legal intervention involving injury by explosive shell, law enforcement official injured**

✓7ᵗʰ **Y35.122 Legal intervention involving injury by explosive shell, bystander injured**

✓7ᵗʰ **Y35.123 Legal intervention involving injury by explosive shell, suspect injured**

✓7ᵗʰ **Y35.129 Legal intervention involving injury by explosive shell, unspecified person injured**

✓6ᵗʰ **Y35.19 Legal intervention involving other explosives**

Legal intervention involving injury by grenade
Legal intervention involving injury by mortar bomb

✓7ᵗʰ **Y35.191 Legal intervention involving other explosives, law enforcement official injured**

✓7ᵗʰ **Y35.192 Legal intervention involving other explosives, bystander injured**

✓7ᵗʰ **Y35.193 Legal intervention involving other explosives, suspect injured**

✓7ᵗʰ **Y35.199 Legal intervention involving other explosives, unspecified person injured**

✓5ᵗʰ **Y35.2 Legal intervention involving** gas

Legal intervention involving asphyxiation by gas
Legal intervention involving poisoning by gas

✓6ᵗʰ **Y35.20 Legal intervention involving unspecified gas**

✓7ᵗʰ **Y35.201 Legal intervention involving unspecified gas, law enforcement official injured**

✓7ᵗʰ **Y35.202 Legal intervention involving unspecified gas, bystander injured**

✓7ᵗʰ **Y35.203 Legal intervention involving unspecified gas, suspect injured**

✓7ᵗʰ **Y35.209 Legal intervention involving unspecified gas, unspecified person injured**

✓6ᵗʰ **Y35.21 Legal intervention involving injury by** tear gas

✓7ᵗʰ **Y35.211 Legal intervention involving injury by tear gas, law enforcement official injured**

✓7ᵗʰ **Y35.212 Legal intervention involving injury by tear gas, bystander injured**

✓7ᵗʰ **Y35.213 Legal intervention involving injury by tear gas, suspect injured**

✓7ᵗʰ **Y35.219 Legal intervention involving injury by tear gas, unspecified person injured**

✓6ᵗʰ **Y35.29 Legal intervention involving other gas**

✓7ᵗʰ **Y35.291 Legal intervention involving other gas, law enforcement official injured**

✓7ᵗʰ **Y35.292 Legal intervention involving other gas, bystander injured**

✓7ᵗʰ **Y35.293 Legal intervention involving other gas, suspect injured**

✓7ᵗʰ **Y35.299 Legal intervention involving other gas, unspecified person injured**

✓5ᵗʰ **Y35.3 Legal intervention involving** blunt objects

Legal intervention involving being hit or struck by blunt object

✓6ᵗʰ **Y35.30 Legal intervention involving unspecified blunt objects**

✓7ᵗʰ **Y35.301 Legal intervention involving unspecified blunt objects, law enforcement official injured**

✓7ᵗʰ **Y35.302 Legal intervention involving unspecified blunt objects, bystander injured**

✓7ᵗʰ **Y35.303 Legal intervention involving unspecified blunt objects, suspect injured**

✓7ᵗʰ **Y35.309 Legal intervention involving unspecified blunt objects, unspecified person injured**

✓6ᵗʰ **Y35.31 Legal intervention involving** baton

✓7ᵗʰ **Y35.311 Legal intervention involving baton, law enforcement official injured**

✓7ᵗʰ **Y35.312 Legal intervention involving baton, bystander injured**

✓7ᵗʰ **Y35.313 Legal intervention involving baton, suspect injured**

✓7ᵗʰ **Y35.319 Legal intervention involving baton, unspecified person injured**

✓6ᵗʰ **Y35.39 Legal intervention involving other blunt objects**

✓7ᵗʰ **Y35.391 Legal intervention involving other blunt objects, law enforcement official injured**

✓7ᵗʰ **Y35.392 Legal intervention involving other blunt objects, bystander injured**

✓7ᵗʰ **Y35.393 Legal intervention involving other blunt objects, suspect injured**

✓7ᵗʰ **Y35.399 Legal intervention involving other blunt objects, unspecified person injured**

✓5ᵗʰ **Y35.4 Legal intervention involving** sharp objects

Legal intervention involving being cut by sharp objects
Legal intervention involving being stabbed by sharp objects

✓6ᵗʰ **Y35.40 Legal intervention involving unspecified sharp objects**

✓7ᵗʰ **Y35.401 Legal intervention involving unspecified sharp objects, law enforcement official injured**

✓7ᵗʰ **Y35.402 Legal intervention involving unspecified sharp objects, bystander injured**

✓7ᵗʰ **Y35.403 Legal intervention involving unspecified sharp objects, suspect injured**

✓7ᵗʰ **Y35.409 Legal intervention involving unspecified sharp objects, unspecified person injured**

✓6ᵗʰ **Y35.41 Legal intervention involving** bayonet

✓7ᵗʰ **Y35.411 Legal intervention involving bayonet, law enforcement official injured**

✓7ᵗʰ **Y35.412 Legal intervention involving bayonet, bystander injured**

✓7ᵗʰ **Y35.413 Legal intervention involving bayonet, suspect injured**

✓7ᵗʰ **Y35.419 Legal intervention involving bayonet, unspecified person injured**

✓6ᵗʰ **Y35.49 Legal intervention involving other sharp objects**

✓7ᵗʰ **Y35.491 Legal intervention involving other sharp objects, law enforcement official injured**

✓7ᵗʰ **Y35.492 Legal intervention involving other sharp objects, bystander injured**

✓7ᵗʰ **Y35.493 Legal intervention involving other sharp objects, suspect injured**

✓7ᵗʰ **Y35.499 Legal intervention involving other sharp objects, unspecified person injured**

✓5ᵗʰ **Y35.8 Legal intervention involving other specified means**

✓6ᵗʰ **Y35.81 Legal intervention involving** manhandling

✓7ᵗʰ **Y35.811 Legal intervention involving manhandling, law enforcement official injured**

✓7ᵗʰ **Y35.812 Legal intervention involving manhandling, bystander injured**

✓7ᵗʰ **Y35.813 Legal intervention involving manhandling, suspect injured**

✓7ᵗʰ **Y35.819 Legal intervention involving manhandling, unspecified person injured**

✓6ᵗʰ **Y35.83 Legal intervention involving a** conducted energy device

Electroshock device (taser)
Stun gun

✓7ᵗʰ **Y35.831 Legal intervention involving a conducted energy device, law enforcement official injured**

- ✓7ᵗʰ **Y35.832** **Legal intervention involving a conducted energy device,** bystander **injured**
- ✓7ᵗʰ **Y35.833** **Legal intervention involving a conducted energy device,** suspect **injured**
- ✓7ᵗʰ **Y35.839** **Legal intervention involving a conducted energy device, unspecified person injured**
- ✓6ᵗʰ **Y35.89** **Legal intervention involving other specified means**
  - ✓7ᵗʰ **Y35.891** **Legal intervention involving other specified means,** law enforcement official **injured**
  - ✓7ᵗʰ **Y35.892** **Legal intervention involving other specified means,** bystander **injured**
  - ✓7ᵗʰ **Y35.893** **Legal intervention involving other specified means,** suspect **injured**
    AHA: 2018,1Q,5

✓5ᵗʰ **Y35.9 Legal intervention, means unspecified**
- ✓x7ᵗʰ **Y35.91** **Legal intervention, means unspecified,** law enforcement official **injured**
- ✓x7ᵗʰ **Y35.92** **Legal intervention, means unspecified,** bystander **injured**
- ✓x7ᵗʰ **Y35.93** **Legal intervention, means unspecified,** suspect **injured**
- ✓x7ᵗʰ **Y35.99** **Legal intervention, means unspecified, unspecified person injured**

✓4ᵗʰ **Y36 Operations of war**

> INCLUDES   injuries to military personnel and civilians caused by war, civil insurrection, and peacekeeping missions
>
> EXCLUDES 1   injury to military personnel occurring during peacetime military operations (Y37.-)
> military vehicles involved in transport accidents with non-military vehicle during peacetime (V09.01, V09.21, V19.81, V29.81, V39.81, V49.81, V59.81, V69.81, V79.81)

AHA: 2014,3Q,4

✓5ᵗʰ **Y36.0 War operations involving** explosion of marine weapons
- ✓6ᵗʰ **Y36.00** **War operations involving explosion of unspecified marine weapon**
  War operations involving underwater blast NOS
  - ✓7ᵗʰ **Y36.000** **War operations involving explosion of unspecified marine weapon,** military personnel
  - ✓7ᵗʰ **Y36.001** **War operations involving explosion of unspecified marine weapon,** civilian
- ✓6ᵗʰ **Y36.01** **War operations involving explosion of** depth-charge
  - ✓7ᵗʰ **Y36.010** **War operations involving explosion of depth-charge,** military personnel
  - ✓7ᵗʰ **Y36.011** **War operations involving explosion of depth-charge,** civilian
- ✓6ᵗʰ **Y36.02** **War operations involving explosion of** marine mine
  War operations involving explosion of marine mine, at sea or in harbor
  - ✓7ᵗʰ **Y36.020** **War operations involving explosion of marine mine,** military personnel
  - ✓7ᵗʰ **Y36.021** **War operations involving explosion of marine mine,** civilian
- ✓6ᵗʰ **Y36.03** **War operations involving explosion of** sea-based artillery shell
  - ✓7ᵗʰ **Y36.030** **War operations involving explosion of sea-based artillery shell,** military personnel
  - ✓7ᵗʰ **Y36.031** **War operations involving explosion of sea-based artillery shell,** civilian
- ✓6ᵗʰ **Y36.04** **War operations involving explosion of** torpedo
  - ✓7ᵗʰ **Y36.040** **War operations involving explosion of torpedo,** military personnel
  - ✓7ᵗʰ **Y36.041** **War operations involving explosion of torpedo,** civilian
- ✓6ᵗʰ **Y36.05** **War operations involving** accidental detonation of onboard marine weapons
  - ✓7ᵗʰ **Y36.050** **War operations involving accidental detonation of onboard marine weapons,** military personnel
  - ✓7ᵗʰ **Y36.051** **War operations involving accidental detonation of onboard marine weapons,** civilian
- ✓6ᵗʰ **Y36.09** **War operations involving explosion of other marine weapons**
  - ✓7ᵗʰ **Y36.090** **War operations involving explosion of other marine weapons,** military personnel

- ✓7ᵗʰ **Y36.091** **War operations involving explosion of other marine weapons,** civilian

✓5ᵗʰ **Y36.1 War operations involving** destruction of aircraft
- ✓6ᵗʰ **Y36.10** **War operations involving unspecified destruction of aircraft**
  - ✓7ᵗʰ **Y36.100** **War operations involving unspecified destruction of aircraft,** military personnel
  - ✓7ᵗʰ **Y36.101** **War operations involving unspecified destruction of aircraft,** civilian
- ✓6ᵗʰ **Y36.11** **War operations involving destruction of aircraft due to** enemy fire or explosives
  War operations involving destruction of aircraft due to air to air missile
  War operations involving destruction of aircraft due to explosive placed on aircraft
  War operations involving destruction of aircraft due to rocket propelled grenade [RPG]
  War operations involving destruction of aircraft due to small arms fire
  War operations involving destruction of aircraft due to surface to air missile
  - ✓7ᵗʰ **Y36.110** **War operations involving destruction of aircraft due to enemy fire or explosives,** military personnel
  - ✓7ᵗʰ **Y36.111** **War operations involving destruction of aircraft due to enemy fire or explosives,** civilian
- ✓6ᵗʰ **Y36.12** **War operations involving destruction of aircraft due to** collision with other aircraft
  - ✓7ᵗʰ **Y36.120** **War operations involving destruction of aircraft due to collision with other aircraft,** military personnel
  - ✓7ᵗʰ **Y36.121** **War operations involving destruction of aircraft due to collision with other aircraft,** civilian
- ✓6ᵗʰ **Y36.13** **War operations involving destruction of aircraft due to** onboard fire
  - ✓7ᵗʰ **Y36.130** **War operations involving destruction of aircraft due to onboard fire,** military personnel
  - ✓7ᵗʰ **Y36.131** **War operations involving destruction of aircraft due to onboard fire,** civilian
- ✓6ᵗʰ **Y36.14** **War operations involving destruction of aircraft due to** accidental detonation of onboard munitions and explosives
  - ✓7ᵗʰ **Y36.140** **War operations involving destruction of aircraft due to accidental detonation of onboard munitions and explosives,** military personnel
  - ✓7ᵗʰ **Y36.141** **War operations involving destruction of aircraft due to accidental detonation of onboard munitions and explosives,** civilian
- ✓6ᵗʰ **Y36.19** **War operations involving other destruction of aircraft**
  - ✓7ᵗʰ **Y36.190** **War operations involving other destruction of aircraft,** military personnel
  - ✓7ᵗʰ **Y36.191** **War operations involving other destruction of aircraft,** civilian

✓5ᵗʰ **Y36.2 War operations involving other explosions and fragments**

> EXCLUDES 1   war operations involving explosion of aircraft (Y36.1-)
> war operations involving explosion of marine weapons (Y36.0-)
> war operations involving explosion of nuclear weapons (Y36.5-)
> war operations involving explosion occurring after cessation of hostilities (Y36.8-)

- ✓6ᵗʰ **Y36.20** **War operations involving unspecified explosion and fragments**
  War operations involving air blast NOS
  War operations involving blast NOS
  War operations involving blast fragments NOS
  War operations involving blast wave NOS
  War operations involving blast wind NOS
  War operations involving explosion NOS
  War operations involving explosion of bomb NOS
  - ✓7ᵗʰ **Y36.200** **War operations involving unspecified explosion and fragments,** military personnel
  - ✓7ᵗʰ **Y36.201** **War operations involving unspecified explosion and fragments,** civilian

√6ᵗʰ **Y36.21** **War operations involving explosion of** aerial bomb

     √7ᵗʰ **Y36.210** **War operations involving explosion of aerial bomb, military personnel**

     √7ᵗʰ **Y36.211** **War operations involving explosion of aerial bomb, civilian**

√6ᵗʰ **Y36.22** **War operations involving explosion of** guided missile

     √7ᵗʰ **Y36.220** **War operations involving explosion of guided missile, military personnel**

     √7ᵗʰ **Y36.221** **War operations involving explosion of guided missile, civilian**

√6ᵗʰ **Y36.23** **War operations involving explosion of** improvised explosive device [IED]

     War operations involving explosion of person-borne improvised explosive device [IED]

     War operations involving explosion of vehicle-borne improvised explosive device [IED]

     War operations involving explosion of roadside improvised explosive device [IED]

     √7ᵗʰ **Y36.230** **War operations involving explosion of improvised explosive device [IED], military personnel**

     √7ᵗʰ **Y36.231** **War operations involving explosion of improvised explosive device [IED], civilian**

√6ᵗʰ **Y36.24** **War operations involving explosion due to** accidental detonation and discharge of own munitions or munitions launch device

     √7ᵗʰ **Y36.240** **War operations involving explosion due to accidental detonation and discharge of own munitions or munitions launch device, military personnel**

     √7ᵗʰ **Y36.241** **War operations involving explosion due to accidental detonation and discharge of own munitions or munitions launch device, civilian**

√6ᵗʰ **Y36.25** **War operations involving** fragments from munitions

     √7ᵗʰ **Y36.250** **War operations involving fragments from munitions, military personnel**

     √7ᵗʰ **Y36.251** **War operations involving fragments from munitions, civilian**

√6ᵗʰ **Y36.26** **War operations involving fragments of** improvised explosive device [IED]

     War operations involving fragments of person-borne improvised explosive device [IED]

     War operations involving fragments of vehicle-borne improvised explosive device [IED]

     War operations involving fragments of roadside improvised explosive device [IED]

     √7ᵗʰ **Y36.260** **War operations involving fragments of improvised explosive device [IED], military personnel**

     √7ᵗʰ **Y36.261** **War operations involving fragments of improvised explosive device [IED], civilian**

√6ᵗʰ **Y36.27** **War operations involving** fragments from weapons

     √7ᵗʰ **Y36.270** **War operations involving fragments from weapons, military personnel**

     √7ᵗʰ **Y36.271** **War operations involving fragments from weapons, civilian**

√6ᵗʰ **Y36.29** **War operations involving other explosions and fragments**

     War operations involving explosion of grenade

     War operations involving explosions of land mine

     War operations involving shrapnel NOS

     √7ᵗʰ **Y36.290** **War operations involving other explosions and fragments, military personnel**

     √7ᵗʰ **Y36.291** **War operations involving other explosions and fragments, civilian**

√5ᵗʰ **Y36.3** **War operations involving** fires, conflagrations and hot substances

War operations involving smoke, fumes, and heat from fires, conflagrations and hot substances

     EXCLUDES 1   *war operations involving fires and conflagrations aboard military aircraft (Y36.1-)*

         war operations involving fires and conflagrations aboard military watercraft (Y36.0-)

         war operations involving fires and conflagrations caused indirectly by conventional weapons (Y36.2-)

         war operations involving fires and thermal effects of nuclear weapons (Y36.53-)

√6ᵗʰ **Y36.30** **War operations involving unspecified fire, conflagration and hot substance**

     √7ᵗʰ **Y36.300** **War operations involving unspecified fire, conflagration and hot substance, military personnel**

     √7ᵗʰ **Y36.301** **War operations involving unspecified fire, conflagration and hot substance, civilian**

√6ᵗʰ **Y36.31** **War operations involving** gasoline bomb

     War operations involving incendiary bomb

     War operations involving petrol bomb

     √7ᵗʰ **Y36.310** **War operations involving gasoline bomb, military personnel**

     √7ᵗʰ **Y36.311** **War operations involving gasoline bomb, civilian**

√6ᵗʰ **Y36.32** **War operations involving** incendiary bullet

     √7ᵗʰ **Y36.320** **War operations involving incendiary bullet, military personnel**

     √7ᵗʰ **Y36.321** **War operations involving incendiary bullet, civilian**

√6ᵗʰ **Y36.33** **War operations involving** flamethrower

     √7ᵗʰ **Y36.330** **War operations involving flamethrower, military personnel**

     √7ᵗʰ **Y36.331** **War operations involving flamethrower, civilian**

√6ᵗʰ **Y36.39** **War operations involving other fires, conflagrations and hot substances**

     √7ᵗʰ **Y36.390** **War operations involving other fires, conflagrations and hot substances, military personnel**

     √7ᵗʰ **Y36.391** **War operations involving other fires, conflagrations and hot substances, civilian**

√5ᵗʰ **Y36.4** **War operations involving firearm discharge and other forms of conventional warfare**

√6ᵗʰ **Y36.41** **War operations involving** rubber bullets

     √7ᵗʰ **Y36.410** **War operations involving rubber bullets, military personnel**

     √7ᵗʰ **Y36.411** **War operations involving rubber bullets, civilian**

√6ᵗʰ **Y36.42** **War operations involving** firearms pellets

     √7ᵗʰ **Y36.420** **War operations involving firearms pellets, military personnel**

     √7ᵗʰ **Y36.421** **War operations involving firearms pellets, civilian**

√6ᵗʰ **Y36.43** **War operations involving other firearms discharge**

     War operations involving bullets NOS

     EXCLUDES 1   *war operations involving munitions fragments (Y36.25-)*

         war operations involving incendiary bullets (Y36.32-)

     √7ᵗʰ **Y36.430** **War operations involving other firearm discharge, military personnel**

     √7ᵗʰ **Y36.431** **War operations involving other firearm discharge, civilian**

√6ᵗʰ **Y36.44** **War operations involving** unarmed hand to hand combat

     EXCLUDES 1   *war operations involving combat using blunt or piercing object (Y36.45-)*

         war operations involving intentional restriction of air and airway (Y36.46)

         war operations involving unintentional restriction of air and airway (Y36.47)

     √7ᵗʰ **Y36.440** **War operations involving unarmed hand to hand combat, military personnel**

     √7ᵗʰ **Y36.441** **War operations involving unarmed hand to hand combat, civilian**

√6ᵗʰ **Y36.45** **War operations involving combat using** blunt or piercing object

    √7ᵗʰ **Y36.450** **War operations involving combat using blunt or piercing object,** military personnel

    √7ᵗʰ **Y36.451** **War operations involving combat using blunt or piercing object,** civilian

√6ᵗʰ **Y36.46** **War operations involving** intentional restriction of air and airway

    √7ᵗʰ **Y36.460** **War operations involving intentional restriction of air and airway,** military personnel

    √7ᵗʰ **Y36.461** **War operations involving intentional restriction of air and airway,** civilian

√6ᵗʰ **Y36.47** **War operations involving** unintentional restriction of air and airway

    √7ᵗʰ **Y36.470** **War operations involving unintentional restriction of air and airway,** military personnel

    √7ᵗʰ **Y36.471** **War operations involving unintentional restriction of air and airway,** civilian

√6ᵗʰ **Y36.49** **War operations involving other forms of conventional warfare**

    √7ᵗʰ **Y36.490** **War operations involving other forms of conventional warfare,** military personnel

    √7ᵗʰ **Y36.491** **War operations involving other forms of conventional warfare,** civilian

√5ᵗʰ **Y36.5** **War operations involving** nuclear weapons

    War operations involving dirty bomb NOS

√6ᵗʰ **Y36.50** **War operations involving unspecified effect of nuclear weapon**

    √7ᵗʰ **Y36.500** **War operations involving unspecified effect of nuclear weapon,** military personnel

    √7ᵗʰ **Y36.501** **War operations involving unspecified effect of nuclear weapon,** civilian

√6ᵗʰ **Y36.51** **War operations involving** direct blast **effect of nuclear weapon**

    War operations involving blast pressure of nuclear weapon

    √7ᵗʰ **Y36.510** **War operations involving direct blast effect of nuclear weapon,** military personnel

    √7ᵗʰ **Y36.511** **War operations involving direct blast effect of nuclear weapon,** civilian

√6ᵗʰ **Y36.52** **War operations involving** indirect blast **effect of nuclear weapon**

    War operations involving being thrown by blast of nuclear weapon

    War operations involving being struck or crushed by blast debris of nuclear weapon

    √7ᵗʰ **Y36.520** **War operations involving indirect blast effect of nuclear weapon,** military personnel

    √7ᵗʰ **Y36.521** **War operations involving indirect blast effect of nuclear weapon,** civilian

√6ᵗʰ **Y36.53** **War operations involving** thermal radiation **effect of nuclear weapon**

    War operations involving direct heat from nuclear weapon

    War operation involving fireball effects from nuclear weapon

    √7ᵗʰ **Y36.530** **War operations involving thermal radiation effect of nuclear weapon,** military personnel

    √7ᵗʰ **Y36.531** **War operations involving thermal radiation effect of nuclear weapon,** civilian

√6ᵗʰ **Y36.54** **War operation involving** nuclear radiation **effects of nuclear weapon**

    War operation involving acute radiation exposure from nuclear weapon

    War operation involving exposure to immediate ionizing radiation from nuclear weapon

    War operation involving fallout exposure from nuclear weapon

    War operation involving secondary effects of nuclear weapons

    √7ᵗʰ **Y36.540** **War operation involving nuclear radiation effects of nuclear weapon,** military personnel

    √7ᵗʰ **Y36.541** **War operation involving nuclear radiation effects of nuclear weapon,** civilian

√6ᵗʰ **Y36.59** **War operation involving other effects of nuclear weapons**

    √7ᵗʰ **Y36.590** **War operation involving other effects of nuclear weapons,** military personnel

    √7ᵗʰ **Y36.591** **War operation involving other effects of nuclear weapons,** civilian

√5ᵗʰ **Y36.6** **War operations involving biological weapons**

√6ᵗʰ **Y36.6X** **War operations involving** biological weapons

    √7ᵗʰ **Y36.6X0** **War operations involving biological weapons,** military personnel

    √7ᵗʰ **Y36.6X1** **War operations involving biological weapons,** civilian

√5ᵗʰ **Y36.7** **War operations involving chemical weapons and other forms of unconventional warfare**

    EXCLUDES 1   *war operations involving incendiary devices (Y36.3-, Y36.5-)*

√6ᵗʰ **Y36.7X** **War operations involving** chemical weapons and other forms of unconventional warfare

    √7ᵗʰ **Y36.7X0** **War operations involving chemical weapons and other forms of unconventional warfare,** military personnel

    √7ᵗʰ **Y36.7X1** **War operations involving chemical weapons and other forms of unconventional warfare,** civilian

√5ᵗʰ **Y36.8** **War operations occurring** after cessation of hostilities

    War operations classifiable to categories Y36.0-Y36.8 but occurring after cessation of hostilities

√6ᵗʰ **Y36.81** **Explosion of** mine **placed during war operations but exploding after cessation of hostilities**

    √7ᵗʰ **Y36.810** **Explosion of mine placed during war operations but exploding after cessation of hostilities,** military personnel

    √7ᵗʰ **Y36.811** **Explosion of mine placed during war operations but exploding after cessation of hostilities,** civilian

√6ᵗʰ **Y36.82** **Explosion of** bomb **placed during war operations but exploding after cessation of hostilities**

    √7ᵗʰ **Y36.820** **Explosion of bomb placed during war operations but exploding after cessation of hostilities,** military personnel

    √7ᵗʰ **Y36.821** **Explosion of bomb placed during war operations but exploding after cessation of hostilities,** civilian

√6ᵗʰ **Y36.88** **Other war operations occurring after cessation of hostilities**

    √7ᵗʰ **Y36.880** **Other war operations occurring after cessation of hostilities,** military personnel

    √7ᵗʰ **Y36.881** **Other war operations occurring after cessation of hostilities,** civilian

√6ᵗʰ **Y36.89** **Unspecified war operations occurring after cessation of hostilities**

    √7ᵗʰ **Y36.890** **Unspecified war operations occurring after cessation of hostilities,** military personnel

    √7ᵗʰ **Y36.891** **Unspecified war operations occurring after cessation of hostilities,** civilian

√5ᵗʰ **Y36.9** **Other and unspecified war operations**

√x7ᵗʰ **Y36.90** **War operations, unspecified**

√x7ᵗʰ **Y36.91** **War operations involving unspecified** weapon of mass destruction [WMD]

√x7ᵗʰ **Y36.92** **War operations involving** friendly fire

Additional Character Required   √x7ᵗʰ Placeholder Alert   Manifestation   Unspecified Dx   ▶◀ Revised Text   ● New Code   ▲ Revised Code Title

Chapter 20. External Causes of Morbidity

✓4ᵗʰ **Y37 Military operations**

INCLUDES   injuries to military personnel and civilians occurring during peacetime on military property and during routine military exercises and operations

EXCLUDES 1   *military aircraft involved in aircraft accident with civilian aircraft (V97.81-)*

military vehicles involved in transport accident with civilian vehicle (V09.01, V09.21, V19.81, V29.81, V39.81, V49.81, V59.81, V69.81, V79.81)

military watercraft involved in water transport accident with civilian watercraft (V94.81-)

war operations (Y36.-)

✓5ᵗʰ **Y37.0 Military operations involving** explosion of marine weapons

   ✓6ᵗʰ **Y37.00 Military operations involving explosion of unspecified marine weapon**

     Military operations involving underwater blast NOS

     ✓7ᵗʰ **Y37.000 Military operations involving explosion of unspecified marine weapon, military personnel**

     ✓7ᵗʰ **Y37.001 Military operations involving explosion of unspecified marine weapon, civilian**

   ✓6ᵗʰ **Y37.01 Military operations involving explosion of depth-charge**

     ✓7ᵗʰ **Y37.010 Military operations involving explosion of depth-charge, military personnel**

     ✓7ᵗʰ **Y37.011 Military operations involving explosion of depth-charge, civilian**

   ✓6ᵗʰ **Y37.02 Military operations involving explosion of marine mine**

     Military operations involving explosion of marine mine, at sea or in harbor

     ✓7ᵗʰ **Y37.020 Military operations involving explosion of marine mine, military personnel**

     ✓7ᵗʰ **Y37.021 Military operations involving explosion of marine mine, civilian**

   ✓6ᵗʰ **Y37.03 Military operations involving explosion of sea-based artillery shell**

     ✓7ᵗʰ **Y37.030 Military operations involving explosion of sea-based artillery shell, military personnel**

     ✓7ᵗʰ **Y37.031 Military operations involving explosion of sea-based artillery shell, civilian**

   ✓6ᵗʰ **Y37.04 Military operations involving explosion of torpedo**

     ✓7ᵗʰ **Y37.040 Military operations involving explosion of torpedo, military personnel**

     ✓7ᵗʰ **Y37.041 Military operations involving explosion of torpedo, civilian**

   ✓6ᵗʰ **Y37.05 Military operations involving accidental detonation of onboard marine weapons**

     ✓7ᵗʰ **Y37.050 Military operations involving accidental detonation of onboard marine weapons, military personnel**

     ✓7ᵗʰ **Y37.051 Military operations involving accidental detonation of onboard marine weapons, civilian**

   ✓6ᵗʰ **Y37.09 Military operations involving explosion of other marine weapons**

     ✓7ᵗʰ **Y37.090 Military operations involving explosion of other marine weapons, military personnel**

     ✓7ᵗʰ **Y37.091 Military operations involving explosion of other marine weapons, civilian**

✓5ᵗʰ **Y37.1 Military operations involving** destruction of aircraft

   ✓6ᵗʰ **Y37.10 Military operations involving unspecified destruction of aircraft**

     ✓7ᵗʰ **Y37.100 Military operations involving unspecified destruction of aircraft, military personnel**

     ✓7ᵗʰ **Y37.101 Military operations involving unspecified destruction of aircraft, civilian**

   ✓6ᵗʰ **Y37.11 Military operations involving destruction of aircraft due to enemy fire or explosives**

     Military operations involving destruction of aircraft due to air to air missile

     Military operations involving destruction of aircraft due to explosive placed on aircraft

     Military operations involving destruction of aircraft due to rocket propelled grenade [RPG]

     Military operations involving destruction of aircraft due to small arms fire

     Military operations involving destruction of aircraft due to surface to air missile

     ✓7ᵗʰ **Y37.110 Military operations involving destruction of aircraft due to enemy fire or explosives, military personnel**

     ✓7ᵗʰ **Y37.111 Military operations involving destruction of aircraft due to enemy fire or explosives, civilian**

   ✓6ᵗʰ **Y37.12 Military operations involving destruction of aircraft due to collision with other aircraft**

     ✓7ᵗʰ **Y37.120 Military operations involving destruction of aircraft due to collision with other aircraft, military personnel**

     ✓7ᵗʰ **Y37.121 Military operations involving destruction of aircraft due to collision with other aircraft, civilian**

   ✓6ᵗʰ **Y37.13 Military operations involving destruction of aircraft due to onboard fire**

     ✓7ᵗʰ **Y37.130 Military operations involving destruction of aircraft due to onboard fire, military personnel**

     ✓7ᵗʰ **Y37.131 Military operations involving destruction of aircraft due to onboard fire, civilian**

   ✓6ᵗʰ **Y37.14 Military operations involving destruction of aircraft due to** accidental detonation of onboard munitions and explosives

     ✓7ᵗʰ **Y37.140 Military operations involving destruction of aircraft due to accidental detonation of onboard munitions and explosives, military personnel**

     ✓7ᵗʰ **Y37.141 Military operations involving destruction of aircraft due to accidental detonation of onboard munitions and explosives, civilian**

   ✓6ᵗʰ **Y37.19 Military operations involving other destruction of aircraft**

     ✓7ᵗʰ **Y37.190 Military operations involving other destruction of aircraft, military personnel**

     ✓7ᵗʰ **Y37.191 Military operations involving other destruction of aircraft, civilian**

✓5ᵗʰ **Y37.2 Military operations involving** other explosions and fragments

   EXCLUDES 1   *military operations involving explosion of aircraft (Y37.1-)*

     military operations involving explosion of marine weapons (Y37.0-)

     military operations involving explosion of nuclear weapons (Y37.5-)

   ✓6ᵗʰ **Y37.20 Military operations involving unspecified explosion and fragments**

     Military operations involving air blast NOS

     Military operations involving blast NOS

     Military operations involving blast fragments NOS

     Military operations involving blast wave NOS

     Military operations involving blast wind NOS

     Military operations involving explosion NOS

     Military operations involving explosion of bomb NOS

     ✓7ᵗʰ **Y37.200 Military operations involving unspecified explosion and fragments, military personnel**

     ✓7ᵗʰ **Y37.201 Military operations involving unspecified explosion and fragments, civilian**

   ✓6ᵗʰ **Y37.21 Military operations involving explosion of aerial bomb**

     ✓7ᵗʰ **Y37.210 Military operations involving explosion of aerial bomb, military personnel**

     ✓7ᵗʰ **Y37.211 Military operations involving explosion of aerial bomb, civilian**

   ✓6ᵗʰ **Y37.22 Military operations involving explosion of guided missile**

     ✓7ᵗʰ **Y37.220 Military operations involving explosion of guided missile, military personnel**

☑7ᵗʰ **Y37.221** **Military operations involving explosion of guided missile, civilian**

☑6ᵗʰ **Y37.23** **Military operations involving explosion of improvised explosive device [IED]**

Military operations involving explosion of person-borne improvised explosive device [IED]

Military operations involving explosion of vehicle-borne improvised explosive device [IED]

Military operations involving explosion of roadside improvised explosive device [IED]

☑7ᵗʰ **Y37.230** **Military operations involving explosion of improvised explosive device [IED], military personnel**

☑7ᵗʰ **Y37.231** **Military operations involving explosion of improvised explosive device [IED], civilian**

☑6ᵗʰ **Y37.24** **Military operations involving explosion due to accidental detonation and discharge of own munitions or munitions launch device**

☑7ᵗʰ **Y37.240** **Military operations involving explosion due to accidental detonation and discharge of own munitions or munitions launch device, military personnel**

☑7ᵗʰ **Y37.241** **Military operations involving explosion due to accidental detonation and discharge of own munitions or munitions launch device, civilian**

☑6ᵗʰ **Y37.25** **Military operations involving fragments from munitions**

☑7ᵗʰ **Y37.250** **Military operations involving fragments from munitions, military personnel**

☑7ᵗʰ **Y37.251** **Military operations involving fragments from munitions, civilian**

☑6ᵗʰ **Y37.26** **Military operations involving fragments of improvised explosive device [IED]**

Military operations involving fragments of person-borne improvised explosive device [IED]

Military operations involving fragments of vehicle-borne improvised explosive device [IED]

Military operations involving fragments of roadside improvised explosive device [IED]

☑7ᵗʰ **Y37.260** **Military operations involving fragments of improvised explosive device [IED], military personnel**

☑7ᵗʰ **Y37.261** **Military operations involving fragments of improvised explosive device [IED], civilian**

☑6ᵗʰ **Y37.27** **Military operations involving fragments from weapons**

☑7ᵗʰ **Y37.270** **Military operations involving fragments from weapons, military personnel**

☑7ᵗʰ **Y37.271** **Military operations involving fragments from weapons, civilian**

☑6ᵗʰ **Y37.29** **Military operations involving other explosions and fragments**

Military operations involving explosion of grenade

Military operations involving explosions of land mine

Military operations involving shrapnel NOS

☑7ᵗʰ **Y37.290** **Military operations involving other explosions and fragments, military personnel**

☑7ᵗʰ **Y37.291** **Military operations involving other explosions and fragments, civilian**

☑5ᵗʰ **Y37.3** **Military operations involving fires, conflagrations and hot substances**

Military operations involving smoke, fumes, and heat from fires, conflagrations and hot substances

EXCLUDES 1   *military operations involving fires and conflagrations aboard military aircraft (Y37.1-)*

military operations involving fires and conflagrations aboard military watercraft (Y37.0-)

military operations involving fires and conflagrations caused indirectly by conventional weapons (Y37.2-)

military operations involving fires and thermal effects of nuclear weapons (Y36.53-)

☑6ᵗʰ **Y37.30** **Military operations involving unspecified fire, conflagration and hot substance**

☑7ᵗʰ **Y37.300** **Military operations involving unspecified fire, conflagration and hot substance, military personnel**

☑7ᵗʰ **Y37.301** **Military operations involving unspecified fire, conflagration and hot substance, civilian**

☑6ᵗʰ **Y37.31** **Military operations involving gasoline bomb**

Military operations involving incendiary bomb

Military operations involving petrol bomb

☑7ᵗʰ **Y37.310** **Military operations involving gasoline bomb, military personnel**

☑7ᵗʰ **Y37.311** **Military operations involving gasoline bomb, civilian**

☑6ᵗʰ **Y37.32** **Military operations involving incendiary bullet**

☑7ᵗʰ **Y37.320** **Military operations involving incendiary bullet, military personnel**

☑7ᵗʰ **Y37.321** **Military operations involving incendiary bullet, civilian**

☑6ᵗʰ **Y37.33** **Military operations involving flamethrower**

☑7ᵗʰ **Y37.330** **Military operations involving flamethrower, military personnel**

☑7ᵗʰ **Y37.331** **Military operations involving flamethrower, civilian**

☑6ᵗʰ **Y37.39** **Military operations involving other fires, conflagrations and hot substances**

☑7ᵗʰ **Y37.390** **Military operations involving other fires, conflagrations and hot substances, military personnel**

☑7ᵗʰ **Y37.391** **Military operations involving other fires, conflagrations and hot substances, civilian**

☑5ᵗʰ **Y37.4** **Military operations involving firearm discharge and other forms of conventional warfare**

☑6ᵗʰ **Y37.41** **Military operations involving rubber bullets**

☑7ᵗʰ **Y37.410** **Military operations involving rubber bullets, military personnel**

☑7ᵗʰ **Y37.411** **Military operations involving rubber bullets, civilian**

☑6ᵗʰ **Y37.42** **Military operations involving firearms pellets**

☑7ᵗʰ **Y37.420** **Military operations involving firearms pellets, military personnel**

☑7ᵗʰ **Y37.421** **Military operations involving firearms pellets, civilian**

☑6ᵗʰ **Y37.43** **Military operations involving other firearms discharge**

Military operations involving bullets NOS

EXCLUDES 1   *military operations involving munitions fragments (Y37.25-)*

military operations involving incendiary bullets (Y37.32-)

☑7ᵗʰ **Y37.430** **Military operations involving other firearms discharge, military personnel**

☑7ᵗʰ **Y37.431** **Military operations involving other firearms discharge, civilian**

☑6ᵗʰ **Y37.44** **Military operations involving unarmed hand to hand combat**

EXCLUDES 1   *military operations involving combat using blunt or piercing object (Y37.45-)*

military operations involving intentional restriction of air and airway (Y37.46-)

military operations involving unintentional restriction of air and airway (Y37.47-)

☑7ᵗʰ **Y37.440** **Military operations involving unarmed hand to hand combat, military personnel**

☑7ᵗʰ **Y37.441** **Military operations involving unarmed hand to hand combat, civilian**

☑6ᵗʰ **Y37.45** **Military operations involving combat using blunt or piercing object**

☑7ᵗʰ **Y37.450** **Military operations involving combat using blunt or piercing object, military personnel**

☑7ᵗʰ **Y37.451** **Military operations involving combat using blunt or piercing object, civilian**

☑6ᵗʰ **Y37.46** **Military operations involving intentional restriction of air and airway**

☑7ᵗʰ **Y37.460** **Military operations involving intentional restriction of air and airway, military personnel**

☑7ᵗʰ **Y37.461** **Military operations involving intentional restriction of air and airway, civilian**

◢ Additional Character Required   ☑x7ᵗʰ Placeholder Alert   Manifestation   Unspecified Dx   ▶◀ Revised Text   ● New Code   ▲ Revised Code Title

ICD-10-CM 2020   **1201**

√6ᵗʰ **Y37.47** **Military operations involving unintentional restriction of air and airway**

   √7ᵗʰ **Y37.470** **Military operations involving unintentional restriction of air and airway, military personnel**

   √7ᵗʰ **Y37.471** **Military operations involving unintentional restriction of air and airway, civilian**

√6ᵗʰ **Y37.49** **Military operations involving other forms of conventional warfare**

   √7ᵗʰ **Y37.490** **Military operations involving other forms of conventional warfare, military personnel**

   √7ᵗʰ **Y37.491** **Military operations involving other forms of conventional warfare, civilian**

√5ᵗʰ **Y37.5** **Military operations involving nuclear weapons**

   Military operation involving dirty bomb NOS

√6ᵗʰ **Y37.50** **Military operations involving unspecified effect of nuclear weapon**

   √7ᵗʰ **Y37.500** **Military operations involving unspecified effect of nuclear weapon, military personnel**

   √7ᵗʰ **Y37.501** **Military operations involving unspecified effect of nuclear weapon, civilian**

√6ᵗʰ **Y37.51** **Military operations involving direct blast effect of nuclear weapon**

   Military operations involving blast pressure of nuclear weapon

   √7ᵗʰ **Y37.510** **Military operations involving direct blast effect of nuclear weapon, military personnel**

   √7ᵗʰ **Y37.511** **Military operations involving direct blast effect of nuclear weapon, civilian**

√6ᵗʰ **Y37.52** **Military operations involving indirect blast effect of nuclear weapon**

   Military operations involving being thrown by blast of nuclear weapon

   Military operations involving being struck or crushed by blast debris of nuclear weapon

   √7ᵗʰ **Y37.520** **Military operations involving indirect blast effect of nuclear weapon, military personnel**

   √7ᵗʰ **Y37.521** **Military operations involving indirect blast effect of nuclear weapon, civilian**

√6ᵗʰ **Y37.53** **Military operations involving thermal radiation effect of nuclear weapon**

   Military operations involving direct heat from nuclear weapon

   Military operation involving fireball effects from nuclear weapon

   √7ᵗʰ **Y37.530** **Military operations involving thermal radiation effect of nuclear weapon, military personnel**

   √7ᵗʰ **Y37.531** **Military operations involving thermal radiation effect of nuclear weapon, civilian**

√6ᵗʰ **Y37.54** **Military operation involving nuclear radiation effects of nuclear weapon**

   Military operation involving acute radiation exposure from nuclear weapon

   Military operation involving exposure to immediate ionizing radiation from nuclear weapon

   Military operation involving fallout exposure from nuclear weapon

   Military operation involving secondary effects of nuclear weapons

   √7ᵗʰ **Y37.540** **Military operation involving nuclear radiation effects of nuclear weapon, military personnel**

   √7ᵗʰ **Y37.541** **Military operation involving nuclear radiation effects of nuclear weapon, civilian**

√6ᵗʰ **Y37.59** **Military operation involving other effects of nuclear weapons**

   √7ᵗʰ **Y37.590** **Military operation involving other effects of nuclear weapons, military personnel**

   √7ᵗʰ **Y37.591** **Military operation involving other effects of nuclear weapons, civilian**

√5ᵗʰ **Y37.6** **Military operations involving biological weapons**

√6ᵗʰ **Y37.6X** **Military operations involving biological weapons**

   √7ᵗʰ **Y37.6X0** **Military operations involving biological weapons, military personnel**

   √7ᵗʰ **Y37.6X1** **Military operations involving biological weapons, civilian**

√5ᵗʰ **Y37.7** **Military operations involving chemical weapons and other forms of unconventional warfare**

   EXCLUDES 1 *military operations involving incendiary devices (Y36.3-, Y36.5-)*

√6ᵗʰ **Y37.7X** **Military operations involving chemical weapons and other forms of unconventional warfare**

   √7ᵗʰ **Y37.7X0** **Military operations involving chemical weapons and other forms of unconventional warfare, military personnel**

   √7ᵗʰ **Y37.7X1** **Military operations involving chemical weapons and other forms of unconventional warfare, civilian**

√5ᵗʰ **Y37.9** **Other and unspecified military operations**

   √x7ᵗʰ **Y37.90** **Military operations, unspecified**

   √x7ᵗʰ **Y37.91** **Military operations involving unspecified weapon of mass destruction [WMD]**

   √x7ᵗʰ **Y37.92** **Military operations involving friendly fire**

√4ᵗʰ **Y38** **Terrorism**

NOTE   These codes are for use to identify injuries resulting from the unlawful use of force or violence against persons or property to intimidate or coerce a Government, the civilian population, or any segment thereof, in furtherance of political or social objective

Use additional code for place of occurrence (Y92.-)

√5ᵗʰ **Y38.0** **Terrorism involving explosion of marine weapons**

   Terrorism involving depth-charge

   Terrorism involving marine mine

   Terrorism involving mine NOS, at sea or in harbor

   Terrorism involving sea-based artillery shell

   Terrorism involving torpedo

   Terrorism involving underwater blast

√6ᵗʰ **Y38.0X** **Terrorism involving explosion of marine weapons**

   √7ᵗʰ **Y38.0X1** **Terrorism involving explosion of marine weapons, public safety official injured**

   √7ᵗʰ **Y38.0X2** **Terrorism involving explosion of marine weapons, civilian injured**

   √7ᵗʰ **Y38.0X3** **Terrorism involving explosion of marine weapons, terrorist injured**

√5ᵗʰ **Y38.1** **Terrorism involving destruction of aircraft**

   Terrorism involving aircraft burned

   Terrorism involving aircraft exploded

   Terrorism involving aircraft being shot down

   Terrorism involving aircraft used as a weapon

√6ᵗʰ **Y38.1X** **Terrorism involving destruction of aircraft**

   √7ᵗʰ **Y38.1X1** **Terrorism involving destruction of aircraft, public safety official injured**

   √7ᵗʰ **Y38.1X2** **Terrorism involving destruction of aircraft, civilian injured**

   √7ᵗʰ **Y38.1X3** **Terrorism involving destruction of aircraft, terrorist injured**

√5ᵗʰ **Y38.2** **Terrorism involving other explosions and fragments**

   Terrorism involving antipersonnel (fragments) bomb

   Terrorism involving blast NOS

   Terrorism involving explosion NOS

   Terrorism involving explosion of breech block

   Terrorism involving explosion of cannon block

   Terrorism involving explosion (fragments) of artillery shell

   Terrorism involving explosion (fragments) of bomb

   Terrorism involving explosion (fragments) of grenade

   Terrorism involving explosion (fragments) of guided missile

   Terrorism involving explosion (fragments) of land mine

   Terrorism involving explosion of mortar bomb

   Terrorism involving explosion of munitions

   Terrorism involving explosion (fragments) of rocket

   Terrorism involving explosion (fragments) of shell

   Terrorism involving shrapnel

   Terrorism involving mine NOS, on land

   EXCLUDES 1 *terrorism involving explosion of nuclear weapon (Y38.5)*

      terrorism involving suicide bomber (Y38.81)

√6ᵗʰ **Y38.2X** **Terrorism involving other explosions and fragments**

   √7ᵗʰ **Y38.2X1** **Terrorism involving other explosions and fragments, public safety official injured**

| ✓7ᵗʰ | **Y38.2X2** | **Terrorism involving other explosions and fragments,** civilian **injured** |

✓7ᵗʰ **Y38.2X2** **Terrorism involving other explosions and fragments,** civilian **injured**

✓7ᵗʰ **Y38.2X3** **Terrorism involving other explosions and fragments,** terrorist **injured**

✓5ᵗʰ **Y38.3** **Terrorism involving fires, conflagration and hot substances**

Terrorism involving conflagration NOS
Terrorism involving fire NOS
Terrorism involving petrol bomb

EXCLUDES 1   *terrorism involving fire or heat of nuclear weapon (Y38.5)*

✓6ᵗʰ **Y38.3X** **Terrorism involving fires, conflagration and hot substances**

✓7ᵗʰ **Y38.3X1** **Terrorism involving fires, conflagration and hot substances, public safety official injured**

✓7ᵗʰ **Y38.3X2** **Terrorism involving fires, conflagration and hot substances,** civilian **injured**

✓7ᵗʰ **Y38.3X3** **Terrorism involving fires, conflagration and hot substances,** terrorist **injured**

✓5ᵗʰ **Y38.4** **Terrorism involving firearms**

Terrorism involving carbine bullet
Terrorism involving machine gun bullet
Terrorism involving pellets (shotgun)
Terrorism involving pistol bullet
Terrorism involving rifle bullet
Terrorism involving rubber (rifle) bullet

✓6ᵗʰ **Y38.4X** **Terrorism involving firearms**

✓7ᵗʰ **Y38.4X1** **Terrorism involving firearms, public safety official injured**

✓7ᵗʰ **Y38.4X2** **Terrorism involving firearms,** civilian **injured**

✓7ᵗʰ **Y38.4X3** **Terrorism involving firearms,** terrorist **injured**

✓5ᵗʰ **Y38.5** **Terrorism involving nuclear weapons**

Terrorism involving blast effects of nuclear weapon
Terrorism involving exposure to ionizing radiation from nuclear weapon
Terrorism involving fireball effect of nuclear weapon
Terrorism involving heat from nuclear weapon

✓6ᵗʰ **Y38.5X** **Terrorism involving nuclear weapons**

✓7ᵗʰ **Y38.5X1** **Terrorism involving nuclear weapons, public safety official injured**

✓7ᵗʰ **Y38.5X2** **Terrorism involving nuclear weapons,** civilian **injured**

✓7ᵗʰ **Y38.5X3** **Terrorism involving nuclear weapons,** terrorist **injured**

✓5ᵗʰ **Y38.6** **Terrorism involving biological weapons**

Terrorism involving anthrax
Terrorism involving cholera
Terrorism involving smallpox

✓6ᵗʰ **Y38.6X** **Terrorism involving biological weapons**

✓7ᵗʰ **Y38.6X1** **Terrorism involving biological weapons, public safety official injured**

✓7ᵗʰ **Y38.6X2** **Terrorism involving biological weapons,** civilian **injured**

✓7ᵗʰ **Y38.6X3** **Terrorism involving biological weapons,** terrorist **injured**

✓5ᵗʰ **Y38.7** **Terrorism involving chemical weapons**

Terrorism involving gases, fumes, chemicals
Terrorism involving hydrogen cyanide
Terrorism involving phosgene
Terrorism involving sarin

✓6ᵗʰ **Y38.7X** **Terrorism involving chemical weapons**

✓7ᵗʰ **Y38.7X1** **Terrorism involving chemical weapons, public safety official injured**

✓7ᵗʰ **Y38.7X2** **Terrorism involving chemical weapons,** civilian **injured**

✓7ᵗʰ **Y38.7X3** **Terrorism involving chemical weapons,** terrorist **injured**

✓5ᵗʰ **Y38.8** **Terrorism involving other and unspecified means**

✓x7ᵗʰ **Y38.80** **Terrorism involving unspecified means**
Terrorism NOS

✓6ᵗʰ **Y38.81** **Terrorism involving suicide bomber**

✓7ᵗʰ **Y38.811** **Terrorism involving suicide bomber, public safety official injured**

✓7ᵗʰ **Y38.812** **Terrorism involving suicide bomber,** civilian **injured**

✓6ᵗʰ **Y38.89** **Terrorism involving other means**
Terrorism involving drowning and submersion
Terrorism involving lasers
Terrorism involving piercing or stabbing instruments

✓7ᵗʰ **Y38.891** **Terrorism involving other means, public safety official injured**

✓7ᵗʰ **Y38.892** **Terrorism involving other means,** civilian **injured**

✓7ᵗʰ **Y38.893** **Terrorism involving other means,** terrorist **injured**

✓5ᵗʰ **Y38.9** **Terrorism, secondary effects**

NOTE   This code is for use to identify conditions occurring subsequent to a terrorist attack not those that are due to the initial terrorist attack

✓6ᵗʰ **Y38.9X** **Terrorism, secondary effects**

✓7ᵗʰ **Y38.9X1** **Terrorism, secondary effects, public safety official injured**

✓7ᵗʰ **Y38.9X2** **Terrorism, secondary effects,** civilian **injured**

COMPLICATIONS OF MEDICAL AND SURGICAL CARE (Y62-Y84)

INCLUDES   complications of medical devices
surgical and medical procedures as the cause of abnormal reaction of the patient, or of later complication, without mention of misadventure at the time of the procedure

Misadventures to patients during surgical and medical care (Y62-Y69)

EXCLUDES 1   *surgical and medical procedures as the cause of abnormal reaction of the patient, without mention of misadventure at the time of the procedure (Y83-Y84)*

EXCLUDES 2   *breakdown or malfunctioning of medical device (during procedure) (after implantation) (ongoing use) (Y70-Y82)*

✓4ᵗʰ **Y62** **Failure of sterile precautions during surgical and medical care**

Y62.0 **Failure of sterile precautions during surgical operation**

Y62.1 **Failure of sterile precautions during infusion or transfusion**

Y62.2 **Failure of sterile precautions during kidney dialysis and other perfusion**   **HCC**

Y62.3 **Failure of sterile precautions during injection or immunization**

Y62.4 **Failure of sterile precautions during endoscopic examination**

Y62.5 **Failure of sterile precautions during heart catheterization**

Y62.6 **Failure of sterile precautions during aspiration, puncture and other catheterization**

Y62.8 **Failure of sterile precautions during other surgical and medical care**

Y62.9 **Failure of sterile precautions during unspecified surgical and medical care**

✓4ᵗʰ **Y63** **Failure in dosage during surgical and medical care**

EXCLUDES 2   *accidental overdose of drug or wrong drug given in error (T36-T50)*

Y63.0 **Excessive amount of blood or other fluid given during transfusion or infusion**

Y63.1 **Incorrect dilution of fluid used during infusion**

Y63.2 **Overdose of radiation given during therapy**

Y63.3 **Inadvertent exposure of patient to radiation during medical care**

Y63.4 **Failure in dosage in electroshock or insulin-shock therapy**

Y63.5 **Inappropriate temperature in local application and packing**

Y63.6 **Underdosing and nonadministration of necessary drug, medicament or biological substance**
AHA: 2018,4Q,72

Y63.8 **Failure in dosage during other surgical and medical care**
AHA: 2018,4Q,72

Y63.9 **Failure in dosage during unspecified surgical and medical care**
AHA: 2018,4Q,72

✓4ᵗʰ **Y64** **Contaminated medical or biological substances**

Y64.0 **Contaminated medical or biological substance, transfused or infused**

Y64.1 **Contaminated medical or biological substance, injected or used for immunization**

Y64.8 **Contaminated medical or biological substance administered by other means**

◄ Additional Character Required   ✓x7ᵗʰ Placeholder Alert   Manifestation   Unspecified Dx   ►◄ Revised Text   ● New Code   ▲ Revised Code Title

Y64.9 **Contaminated medical or biological substance administered by unspecified means**

Administered contaminated medical or biological substance NOS

✓4ᵗʰ **Y65** **Other misadventures during surgical and medical care**

Y65.0 **Mismatched blood in transfusion**

Y65.1 **Wrong fluid used in infusion**

Y65.2 **Failure in suture or ligature during surgical operation**

Y65.3 **Endotracheal tube wrongly placed during anesthetic procedure**

Y65.4 **Failure to introduce or to remove other tube or instrument**

✓5ᵗʰ **Y65.5** **Performance of wrong procedure (operation)**

Y65.51 **Performance of wrong procedure (operation) on correct patient**

Wrong device implanted into correct surgical site

EXCLUDES 1　*performance of correct procedure (operation) on wrong side or body part (Y65.53)*

Y65.52 **Performance of procedure (operation) on patient not scheduled for surgery**

Performance of procedure (operation) intended for another patient

Performance of procedure (operation) on wrong patient

Y65.53 **Performance of correct procedure (operation) on wrong side or body part**

Performance of correct procedure (operation) on wrong side

Performance of correct procedure (operation) on wrong site

Y65.8 **Other specified misadventures during surgical and medical care**

AHA: 2019,2Q,23-24

Y66 **Nonadministration of surgical and medical care**

Premature cessation of surgical and medical care

EXCLUDES 1　*DNR status (Z66)*

palliative care (Z51.5)

Y69 **Unspecified misadventure during surgical and medical care**

Medical devices associated with adverse incidents in diagnostic and therapeutic use (Y70-Y82)

INCLUDES　breakdown or malfunction of medical devices (during use) (after implantation) (ongoing use)

EXCLUDES 2　*later complications following use of medical devices without breakdown or malfunctioning of device (Y83-Y84)*

misadventure to patients during surgical and medical care, classifiable to (Y62-Y69)

surgical and other medical procedures as the cause of abnormal reaction of the patient, or of later complication, without mention of misadventure at the time of the procedure (Y83-Y84)

✓4ᵗʰ **Y70** **Anesthesiology devices associated with adverse incidents**

Y70.0 **Diagnostic and monitoring anesthesiology devices associated with adverse incidents**

Y70.1 **Therapeutic (nonsurgical) and rehabilitative anesthesiology devices associated with adverse incidents**

Y70.2 **Prosthetic and other implants, materials and accessory anesthesiology devices associated with adverse incidents**

Y70.3 **Surgical instruments, materials and anesthesiology devices (including sutures) associated with adverse incidents**

Y70.8 **Miscellaneous anesthesiology devices associated with adverse incidents, not elsewhere classified**

✓4ᵗʰ **Y71** **Cardiovascular devices associated with adverse incidents**

Y71.0 **Diagnostic and monitoring cardiovascular devices associated with adverse incidents**

Y71.1 **Therapeutic (nonsurgical) and rehabilitative cardiovascular devices associated with adverse incidents**

Y71.2 **Prosthetic and other implants, materials and accessory cardiovascular devices associated with adverse incidents**

Y71.3 **Surgical instruments, materials and cardiovascular devices (including sutures) associated with adverse incidents**

Y71.8 **Miscellaneous cardiovascular devices associated with adverse incidents, not elsewhere classified**

✓4ᵗʰ **Y72** **Otorhinolaryngological devices associated with adverse incidents**

Y72.0 **Diagnostic and monitoring otorhinolaryngological devices associated with adverse incidents**

Y72.1 **Therapeutic (nonsurgical) and rehabilitative otorhinolaryngological devices associated with adverse incidents**

Y72.2 **Prosthetic and other implants, materials and accessory otorhinolaryngological devices associated with adverse incidents**

Y72.3 **Surgical instruments, materials and otorhinolaryngological devices (including sutures) associated with adverse incidents**

Y72.8 **Miscellaneous otorhinolaryngological devices associated with adverse incidents, not elsewhere classified**

✓4ᵗʰ **Y73** **Gastroenterology and urology devices associated with adverse incidents**

Y73.0 **Diagnostic and monitoring gastroenterology and urology devices associated with adverse incidents**

Y73.1 **Therapeutic (nonsurgical) and rehabilitative gastroenterology and urology devices associated with adverse incidents**

Y73.2 **Prosthetic and other implants, materials and accessory gastroenterology and urology devices associated with adverse incidents**

Y73.3 **Surgical instruments, materials and gastroenterology and urology devices (including sutures) associated with adverse incidents**

Y73.8 **Miscellaneous gastroenterology and urology devices associated with adverse incidents, not elsewhere classified**

✓4ᵗʰ **Y74** **General hospital and personal-use devices associated with adverse incidents**

Y74.0 **Diagnostic and monitoring general hospital and personal-use devices associated with adverse incidents**

Y74.1 **Therapeutic (nonsurgical) and rehabilitative general hospital and personal-use devices associated with adverse incidents**

Y74.2 **Prosthetic and other implants, materials and accessory general hospital and personal-use devices associated with adverse incidents**

Y74.3 **Surgical instruments, materials and general hospital and personal-use devices (including sutures) associated with adverse incidents**

Y74.8 **Miscellaneous general hospital and personal-use devices associated with adverse incidents, not elsewhere classified**

✓4ᵗʰ **Y75** **Neurological devices associated with adverse incidents**

Y75.0 **Diagnostic and monitoring neurological devices associated with adverse incidents**

Y75.1 **Therapeutic (nonsurgical) and rehabilitative neurological devices associated with adverse incidents**

Y75.2 **Prosthetic and other implants, materials and neurological devices associated with adverse incidents**

Y75.3 **Surgical instruments, materials and neurological devices (including sutures) associated with adverse incidents**

Y75.8 **Miscellaneous neurological devices associated with adverse incidents, not elsewhere classified**

✓4ᵗʰ **Y76** **Obstetric and gynecological devices associated with adverse incidents**

Y76.0 **Diagnostic and monitoring obstetric and gynecological devices associated with adverse incidents**　♀

Y76.1 **Therapeutic (nonsurgical) and rehabilitative obstetric and gynecological devices associated with adverse incidents**　♀

Y76.2 **Prosthetic and other implants, materials and accessory obstetric and gynecological devices associated with adverse incidents**　♀

Y76.3 **Surgical instruments, materials and obstetric and gynecological devices (including sutures) associated with adverse incidents**　♀

Y76.8 **Miscellaneous obstetric and gynecological devices associated with adverse incidents, not elsewhere classified**　♀

✓4ᵗʰ **Y77** **Ophthalmic devices associated with adverse incidents**

Y77.0 **Diagnostic and monitoring ophthalmic devices associated with adverse incidents**

Y77.1 **Therapeutic (nonsurgical) and rehabilitative ophthalmic devices associated with adverse incidents**

Y77.2 **Prosthetic and other implants, materials and accessory ophthalmic devices associated with adverse incidents**

Y77.3 **Surgical instruments, materials and ophthalmic devices (including sutures) associated with adverse incidents**

Y77.8 **Miscellaneous ophthalmic devices associated with adverse incidents, not elsewhere classified**

✓4ᵗʰ **Y78** **Radiological devices associated with adverse incidents**

Y78.0 **Diagnostic and monitoring radiological devices associated with adverse incidents**

Y78.1 **Therapeutic (nonsurgical) and rehabilitative radiological devices associated with adverse incidents**

Y78.2 Prosthetic and other implants, materials and accessory radiological devices associated with adverse incidents

Y78.3 Surgical instruments, materials and radiological devices (including sutures) associated with adverse incidents

Y78.8 Miscellaneous radiological devices associated with adverse incidents, not elsewhere classified

✓4ᵗʰ Y79 Orthopedic devices associated with adverse incidents

Y79.0 Diagnostic and monitoring orthopedic devices associated with adverse incidents

Y79.1 Therapeutic (nonsurgical) and rehabilitative orthopedic devices associated with adverse incidents

Y79.2 Prosthetic and other implants, materials and accessory orthopedic devices associated with adverse incidents

Y79.3 Surgical instruments, materials and orthopedic devices (including sutures) associated with adverse incidents

Y79.8 Miscellaneous orthopedic devices associated with adverse incidents, not elsewhere classified

✓4ᵗʰ Y80 Physical medicine devices associated with adverse incidents

Y80.0 Diagnostic and monitoring physical medicine devices associated with adverse incidents

Y80.1 Therapeutic (nonsurgical) and rehabilitative physical medicine devices associated with adverse incidents

Y80.2 Prosthetic and other implants, materials and accessory physical medicine devices associated with adverse incidents

Y80.3 Surgical instruments, materials and physical medicine devices (including sutures) associated with adverse incidents

Y80.8 Miscellaneous physical medicine devices associated with adverse incidents, not elsewhere classified

✓4ᵗʰ Y81 General- and plastic-surgery devices associated with adverse incidents

Y81.0 Diagnostic and monitoring general- and plastic-surgery devices associated with adverse incidents

Y81.1 Therapeutic (nonsurgical) and rehabilitative general- and plastic-surgery devices associated with adverse incidents

Y81.2 Prosthetic and other implants, materials and accessory general- and plastic-surgery devices associated with adverse incidents

Y81.3 Surgical instruments, materials and general- and plastic-surgery devices (including sutures) associated with adverse incidents

Y81.8 Miscellaneous general- and plastic-surgery devices associated with adverse incidents, not elsewhere classified

✓4ᵗʰ Y82 Other and unspecified medical devices associated with adverse incidents

Y82.8 Other medical devices associated with adverse incidents

Y82.9 Unspecified medical devices associated with adverse incidents

Surgical and other medical procedures as the cause of abnormal reaction of the patient, or of later complication, without mention of misadventure at the time of the procedure (Y83-Y84)

EXCLUDES 1   misadventures to patients during surgical and medical care, classifiable to (Y62-Y69)

EXCLUDES 2   breakdown or malfunctioning of medical device (during procedure) (after implantation) (ongoing use) (Y70-Y82)

✓4ᵗʰ Y83 Surgical operation and other surgical procedures as the cause of abnormal reaction of the patient, or of later complication, without mention of misadventure at the time of the procedure

Y83.0 Surgical operation with transplant of whole organ as the cause of abnormal reaction of the patient, or of later complication, without mention of misadventure at the time of the procedure

Y83.1 Surgical operation with implant of artificial internal device as the cause of abnormal reaction of the patient, or of later complication, without mention of misadventure at the time of the procedure

Y83.2 Surgical operation with anastomosis, bypass or graft as the cause of abnormal reaction of the patient, or of later complication, without mention of misadventure at the time of the procedure

Y83.3 Surgical operation with formation of external stoma as the cause of abnormal reaction of the patient, or of later complication, without mention of misadventure at the time of the procedure

Y83.4 Other reconstructive surgery as the cause of abnormal reaction of the patient, or of later complication, without mention of misadventure at the time of the procedure

Y83.5 Amputation of limb(s) as the cause of abnormal reaction of the patient, or of later complication, without mention of misadventure at the time of the procedure

Y83.6 Removal of other organ (partial) (total) as the cause of abnormal reaction of the patient, or of later complication, without mention of misadventure at the time of the procedure

Y83.8 Other surgical procedures as the cause of abnormal reaction of the patient, or of later complication, without mention of misadventure at the time of the procedure

Y83.9 Surgical procedure, unspecified as the cause of abnormal reaction of the patient, or of later complication, without mention of misadventure at the time of the procedure

✓4ᵗʰ Y84 Other medical procedures as the cause of abnormal reaction of the patient, or of later complication, without mention of misadventure at the time of the procedure

Y84.0 Cardiac catheterization as the cause of abnormal reaction of the patient, or of later complication, without mention of misadventure at the time of the procedure

Y84.1 Kidney dialysis as the cause of abnormal reaction of the patient, or of later complication, without mention of misadventure at the time of the procedure

Y84.2 Radiological procedure and radiotherapy as the cause of abnormal reaction of the patient, or of later complication, without mention of misadventure at the time of the procedure
    AHA: 2019,1Q,21; 2017,1Q,33

Y84.3 Shock therapy as the cause of abnormal reaction of the patient, or of later complication, without mention of misadventure at the time of the procedure

Y84.4 Aspiration of fluid as the cause of abnormal reaction of the patient, or of later complication, without mention of misadventure at the time of the procedure

Y84.5 Insertion of gastric or duodenal sound as the cause of abnormal reaction of the patient, or of later complication, without mention of misadventure at the time of the procedure

Y84.6 Urinary catheterization as the cause of abnormal reaction of the patient, or of later complication, without mention of misadventure at the time of the procedure

Y84.7 Blood-sampling as the cause of abnormal reaction of the patient, or of later complication, without mention of misadventure at the time of the procedure

Y84.8 Other medical procedures as the cause of abnormal reaction of the patient, or of later complication, without mention of misadventure at the time of the procedure
    AHA: 2014,4Q,24

Y84.9 Medical procedure, unspecified as the cause of abnormal reaction of the patient, or of later complication, without mention of misadventure at the time of the procedure

Supplementary factors related to causes of morbidity classified elsewhere (Y90-Y99)

NOTE   These categories may be used to provide supplementary information concerning causes of morbidity. They are not to be used for single-condition coding.

✓4ᵗʰ Y90 Evidence of alcohol involvement determined by blood alcohol level
    Code first any associated alcohol related disorders (F10)

Y90.0 Blood alcohol level of less than 20 mg/100 ml

Y90.1 Blood alcohol level of 20-39 mg/100 ml

Y90.2 Blood alcohol level of 40-59 mg/100 ml

Y90.3 Blood alcohol level of 60-79 mg/100 ml

Y90.4 Blood alcohol level of 80-99 mg/100 ml

Y90.5 Blood alcohol level of 100-119 mg/100 ml

Y90.6 Blood alcohol level of 120-199 mg/100 ml

Y90.7 Blood alcohol level of 200-239 mg/100 ml

Y90.8 Blood alcohol level of 240 mg/100 ml or more

Y90.9 Presence of alcohol in blood, level not specified

✓4ᵗʰ Y92   Place of occurrence of the external cause

The following category is for use, when relevant, to identify the place of occurrence of the external cause. Use in conjunction with an activity code.

Place of occurrence should be recorded only at the initial encounter for treatment

✓5ᵗʰ Y92.0   Non-institutional (private) residence as the place of occurrence of the external cause

> *EXCLUDES 1*   abandoned or derelict house (Y92.89)
>
> home under construction but not yet occupied (Y92.6-)
>
> institutional place of residence (Y92.1-)

✓6ᵗʰ Y92.00   Unspecified non-institutional (private) residence as the place of occurrence of the external cause

Y92.000   Kitchen of unspecified non-institutional (private) residence as the place of occurrence of the external cause

Y92.001   Dining room of unspecified non-institutional (private) residence as the place of occurrence of the external cause

Y92.002   Bathroom of unspecified non-institutional (private) residence single-family (private) house as the place of occurrence of the external cause

Y92.003   Bedroom of unspecified non-institutional (private) residence as the place of occurrence of the external cause

Y92.007   Garden or yard of unspecified non-institutional (private) residence as the place of occurrence of the external cause

Y92.008   Other place in unspecified non-institutional (private) residence as the place of occurrence of the external cause

Y92.009   Unspecified place in unspecified non-institutional (private) residence as the place of occurrence of the external cause

Home (NOS) as the place of occurrence of the external cause

✓6ᵗʰ Y92.01   Single-family non-institutional (private) house as the place of occurrence of the external cause

Farmhouse as the place of occurrence of the external cause

> *EXCLUDES 1*   barn (Y92.71)
>
> chicken coop or hen house (Y92.72)
>
> farm field (Y92.73)
>
> orchard (Y92.74)
>
> single family mobile home or trailer (Y92.02-)
>
> slaughter house (Y92.86)

Y92.010   Kitchen of single-family (private) house as the place of occurrence of the external cause

Y92.011   Dining room of single-family (private) house as the place of occurrence of the external cause

Y92.012   Bathroom of single-family (private) house as the place of occurrence of the external cause

Y92.013   Bedroom of single-family (private) house as the place of occurrence of the external cause

Y92.014   Private driveway to single-family (private) house as the place of occurrence of the external cause

Y92.015   Private garage of single-family (private) house as the place of occurrence of the external cause

Y92.016   Swimming-pool in single-family (private) house or garden as the place of occurrence of the external cause

Y92.017   Garden or yard in single-family (private) house as the place of occurrence of the external cause

Y92.018   Other place in single-family (private) house as the place of occurrence of the external cause

Y92.019   Unspecified place in single-family (private) house as the place of occurrence of the external cause

✓6ᵗʰ Y92.02   Mobile home as the place of occurrence of the external cause

Y92.020   Kitchen in mobile home as the place of occurrence of the external cause

Y92.021   Dining room in mobile home as the place of occurrence of the external cause

Y92.022   Bathroom in mobile home as the place of occurrence of the external cause

Y92.023   Bedroom in mobile home as the place of occurrence of the external cause

Y92.024   Driveway of mobile home as the place of occurrence of the external cause

Y92.025   Garage of mobile home as the place of occurrence of the external cause

Y92.026   Swimming-pool of mobile home as the place of occurrence of the external cause

Y92.027   Garden or yard of mobile home as the place of occurrence of the external cause

Y92.028   Other place in mobile home as the place of occurrence of the external cause

Y92.029   Unspecified place in mobile home as the place of occurrence of the external cause

✓6ᵗʰ Y92.03   Apartment as the place of occurrence of the external cause

Condominium as the place of occurrence of the external cause

Co-op apartment as the place of occurrence of the external cause

Y92.030   Kitchen in apartment as the place of occurrence of the external cause

Y92.031   Bathroom in apartment as the place of occurrence of the external cause

Y92.032   Bedroom in apartment as the place of occurrence of the external cause

Y92.038   Other place in apartment as the place of occurrence of the external cause

Y92.039   Unspecified place in apartment as the place of occurrence of the external cause

✓6ᵗʰ Y92.04   Boarding-house as the place of occurrence of the external cause

Y92.040   Kitchen in boarding-house as the place of occurrence of the external cause

Y92.041   Bathroom in boarding-house as the place of occurrence of the external cause

Y92.042   Bedroom in boarding-house as the place of occurrence of the external cause

Y92.043   Driveway of boarding-house as the place of occurrence of the external cause

Y92.044   Garage of boarding-house as the place of occurrence of the external cause

Y92.045   Swimming-pool of boarding-house as the place of occurrence of the external cause

Y92.046   Garden or yard of boarding-house as the place of occurrence of the external cause

Y92.048   Other place in boarding-house as the place of occurrence of the external cause

Y92.049   Unspecified place in boarding-house as the place of occurrence of the external cause

✓6ᵗʰ Y92.09   Other non-institutional residence as the place of occurrence of the external cause

AHA: 2017,2Q,10

Y92.090   Kitchen in other non-institutional residence as the place of occurrence of the external cause

Y92.091   Bathroom in other non-institutional residence as the place of occurrence of the external cause

Y92.092   Bedroom in other non-institutional residence as the place of occurrence of the external cause

Y92.093   Driveway of other non-institutional residence as the place of occurrence of the external cause

Y92.094   Garage of other non-institutional residence as the place of occurrence of the external cause

Y92.095   Swimming-pool of other non-institution residence as the place of occurrence of the external cause

Y92.096   Garden or yard of other non-institution residence as the place of occurrence of the external cause

Y92.Ø98   Other place in other non-institutional residence as the place of occurrence of the external cause

Y92.Ø99   Unspecified place in other non-institutional residence as the place of occurrence of the external cause

☑5ᵗʰ   **Y92.1**   **Institutional (nonprivate) residence as the place of occurrence of the external cause**

Y92.1Ø   Unspecified residential institution as the place of occurrence of the external cause

☑6ᵗʰ   **Y92.11**   Children's home and orphanage as the place of occurrence of the external cause

Y92.11Ø   Kitchen in children's home and orphanage as the place of occurrence of the external cause

Y92.111   Bathroom in children's home and orphanage as the place of occurrence of the external cause

Y92.112   Bedroom in children's home and orphanage as the place of occurrence of the external cause

Y92.113   Driveway of children's home and orphanage as the place of occurrence of the external cause

Y92.114   Garage of children's home and orphanage as the place of occurrence of the external cause

Y92.115   Swimming-pool of children's home and orphanage as the place of occurrence of the external cause

Y92.116   Garden or yard of children's home and orphanage as the place of occurrence of the external cause

Y92.118   Other place in children's home and orphanage as the place of occurrence of the external cause

Y92.119   Unspecified place in children's home and orphanage as the place of occurrence of the external cause

☑6ᵗʰ   **Y92.12**   Nursing home as the place of occurrence of the external cause

Home for the sick as the place of occurrence of the external cause

Hospice as the place of occurrence of the external cause

AHA: 2017,2Q,10

Y92.12Ø   Kitchen in nursing home as the place of occurrence of the external cause

Y92.121   Bathroom in nursing home as the place of occurrence of the external cause

Y92.122   Bedroom in nursing home as the place of occurrence of the external cause

Y92.123   Driveway of nursing home as the place of occurrence of the external cause

Y92.124   Garage of nursing home as the place of occurrence of the external cause

Y92.125   Swimming-pool of nursing home as the place of occurrence of the external cause

Y92.126   Garden or yard of nursing home as the place of occurrence of the external cause

Y92.128   Other place in nursing home as the place of occurrence of the external cause

Y92.129   Unspecified place in nursing home as the place of occurrence of the external cause

☑6ᵗʰ   **Y92.13**   Military base as the place of occurrence of the external cause

EXCLUDES 1   military training grounds (Y92.84)

Y92.13Ø   Kitchen on military base as the place of occurrence of the external cause

Y92.131   Mess hall on military base as the place of occurrence of the external cause

Y92.133   Barracks on military base as the place of occurrence of the external cause

Y92.135   Garage on military base as the place of occurrence of the external cause

Y92.136   Swimming-pool on military base as the place of occurrence of the external cause

Y92.137   Garden or yard on military base as the place of occurrence of the external cause

Y92.138   Other place on military base as the place of occurrence of the external cause

Y92.139   Unspecified place military base as the place of occurrence of the external cause

☑6ᵗʰ   **Y92.14**   Prison as the place of occurrence of the external cause

Y92.14Ø   Kitchen in prison as the place of occurrence of the external cause

Y92.141   Dining room in prison as the place of occurrence of the external cause

Y92.142   Bathroom in prison as the place of occurrence of the external cause

Y92.143   Cell of prison as the place of occurrence of the external cause

Y92.146   Swimming-pool of prison as the place of occurrence of the external cause

Y92.147   Courtyard of prison as the place of occurrence of the external cause

Y92.148   Other place in prison as the place of occurrence of the external cause

Y92.149   Unspecified place in prison as the place of occurrence of the external cause

☑6ᵗʰ   **Y92.15**   Reform school as the place of occurrence of the external cause

Y92.15Ø   Kitchen in reform school as the place of occurrence of the external cause

Y92.151   Dining room in reform school as the place of occurrence of the external cause

Y92.152   Bathroom in reform school as the place of occurrence of the external cause

Y92.153   Bedroom in reform school as the place of occurrence of the external cause

Y92.154   Driveway of reform school as the place of occurrence of the external cause

Y92.155   Garage of reform school as the place of occurrence of the external cause

Y92.156   Swimming-pool of reform school as the place of occurrence of the external cause

Y92.157   Garden or yard of reform school as the place of occurrence of the external cause

Y92.158   Other place in reform school as the place of occurrence of the external cause

Y92.159   Unspecified place in reform school as the place of occurrence of the external cause

☑6ᵗʰ   **Y92.16**   School dormitory as the place of occurrence of the external cause

EXCLUDES 1   reform school as the place of occurrence of the external cause (Y92.15-)

school buildings and grounds as the place of occurrence of the external cause (Y92.2-)

school sports and athletic areas as the place of occurrence of the external cause (Y92.3-)

Y92.16Ø   Kitchen in school dormitory as the place of occurrence of the external cause

Y92.161   Dining room in school dormitory as the place of occurrence of the external cause

Y92.162   Bathroom in school dormitory as the place of occurrence of the external cause

Y92.163   Bedroom in school dormitory as the place of occurrence of the external cause

Y92.168   Other place in school dormitory as the place of occurrence of the external cause

Y92.169   Unspecified place in school dormitory as the place of occurrence of the external cause

☑6ᵗʰ   **Y92.19**   Other specified residential institution as the place of occurrence of the external cause

AHA: 2017,2Q,10

Y92.19Ø   Kitchen in other specified residential institution as the place of occurrence of the external cause

Y92.191   Dining room in other specified residential institution as the place of occurrence of the external cause

Y92.192   Bathroom in other specified residential institution as the place of occurrence of the external cause

Y92.193   Bedroom in other specified residential institution as the place of occurrence of the external cause

Y92.194   Driveway of other specified residential institution as the place of occurrence of the external cause

Additional Character Required   ☑x7ᵗʰ Placeholder Alert   Manifestation   Unspecified Dx   ►◄ Revised Text   ● New Code   ▲ Revised Code Title

-10-CM 2020   1207

Y92.195 **Garage** of other specified residential institution as the place of occurrence of the external cause

Y92.196 **Pool** of other specified residential institution as the place of occurrence of the external cause

Y92.197 **Garden or yard** of other specified residential institution as the place of occurrence of the external cause

Y92.198 **Other place** in other specified residential institution as the place of occurrence of the external cause

Y92.199 **Unspecified place** in other specified residential institution as the place of occurrence of the external cause

✓5ᵗʰ **Y92.2 School, other institution and public administrative area as the place of occurrence of the external cause**

Building and adjacent grounds used by the general public or by a particular group of the public

EXCLUDES 1   *building under construction as the place of occurrence of the external cause (Y92.6)*

residential institution as the place of occurrence of the external cause (Y92.1)

school dormitory as the place of occurrence of the external cause (Y92.16-)

sports and athletics area of schools as the place of occurrence of the external cause (Y92.3-)

✓6ᵗʰ **Y92.21 School (private) (public) (state)** as the place of occurrence of the external cause

Y92.210 **Daycare center** as the place of occurrence of the external cause

Y92.211 **Elementary school** as the place of occurrence of the external cause

Kindergarten as the place of occurrence of the external cause

Y92.212 **Middle school** as the place of occurrence of the external cause

Y92.213 **High school** as the place of occurrence of the external cause

AHA: 2012,4Q,108

Y92.214 **College** as the place of occurrence of the external cause

University as the place of occurrence of the external cause

Y92.215 **Trade school** as the place of occurrence of the external cause

Y92.218 **Other school** as the place of occurrence of the external cause

Y92.219 **Unspecified school** as the place of occurrence of the external cause

Y92.22 **Religious institution** as the place of occurrence of the external cause

Church as the place of occurrence of the external cause

Mosque as the place of occurrence of the external cause

Synagogue as the place of occurrence of the external cause

✓6ᵗʰ **Y92.23 Hospital** as the place of occurrence of the external cause

EXCLUDES 1   *ambulatory (outpatient) health services establishments (Y92.53-)*

home for the sick as the place of occurrence of the external cause (Y92.12-)

hospice as the place of occurrence of the external cause (Y92.12-)

nursing home as the place of occurrence of the external cause (Y92.12-)

Y92.230 **Patient room** in hospital as the place of occurrence of the external cause

Y92.231 **Patient bathroom** in hospital as the place of occurrence of the external cause

Y92.232 **Corridor** of hospital as the place of occurrence of the external cause

Y92.233 **Cafeteria** of hospital as the place of occurrence of the external cause

Y92.234 **Operating room** of hospital as the place of occurrence of the external cause

Y92.238 **Other place** in hospital as the place of occurrence of the external cause

Y92.239 **Unspecified place** in hospital as the place of occurrence of the external cause

✓6ᵗʰ **Y92.24 Public administrative building** as the place of occurrence of the external cause

Y92.240 **Courthouse** as the place of occurrence of the external cause

Y92.241 **Library** as the place of occurrence of the external cause

Y92.242 **Post office** as the place of occurrence of the external cause

Y92.243 **City hall** as the place of occurrence of the external cause

Y92.248 **Other** public administrative building as the place of occurrence of the external cause

✓6ᵗʰ **Y92.25 Cultural building** as the place of occurrence of the external cause

Y92.250 **Art Gallery** as the place of occurrence of the external cause

Y92.251 **Museum** as the place of occurrence of the external cause

Y92.252 **Music hall** as the place of occurrence of the external cause

Y92.253 **Opera house** as the place of occurrence of the external cause

Y92.254 **Theater** (live) as the place of occurrence of the external cause

Y92.258 **Other cultural** public building as the place of occurrence of the external cause

Y92.26 **Movie house or cinema** as the place of occurrence of the external cause

Y92.29 **Other specified public building** as the place of occurrence of the external cause

Assembly hall as the place of occurrence of the external cause

Clubhouse as the place of occurrence of the external cause

✓5ᵗʰ **Y92.3 Sports and athletics area as the place of occurrence of the external cause**

✓6ᵗʰ **Y92.31 Athletic court** as the place of occurrence of the external cause

EXCLUDES 1   *tennis court in private home or garden (Y92.09)*

Y92.310 **Basketball court** as the place of occurrence of the external cause

Y92.311 **Squash court** as the place of occurrence of the external cause

Y92.312 **Tennis court** as the place of occurrence of the external cause

Y92.318 **Other athletic court** as the place of occurrence of the external cause

✓6ᵗʰ **Y92.32 Athletic field** as the place of occurrence of the external cause

Y92.320 **Baseball field** as the place of occurrence of the external cause

Y92.321 **Football field** as the place of occurrence of the external cause

Y92.322 **Soccer field** as the place of occurrence of the external cause

Y92.328 **Other athletic field** as the place of occurrence of the external cause

Cricket field as the place of occurrence of the external cause

Hockey field as the place of occurrence of the external cause

✓6ᵗʰ **Y92.33 Skating rink** as the place of occurrence of the external cause

Y92.330 **Ice skating rink** (indoor) (outdoor) as the place of occurrence of the external cause

Y92.331 **Roller skating rink** as the place of occurrence of the external cause

Y92.34 **Swimming pool** (public) as the place of occurrence of the external cause

EXCLUDES 1   *swimming pool in private home or garden (Y92.016)*

Y92.39 **Other specified sports and athletic area as the place of occurrence of the external cause**
- Golf-course as the place of occurrence of the external cause
- Gymnasium as the place of occurrence of the external cause
- Riding-school as the place of occurrence of the external cause
- Stadium as the place of occurrence of the external cause

√5ᵗʰ **Y92.4** **Street, highway and other paved roadways as the place of occurrence of the external cause**
> EXCLUDES 1   *private driveway of residence (Y92.014, Y92.024, Y92.043, Y92.093, Y92.113, Y92.123, Y92.154, Y92.194)*

√6ᵗʰ **Y92.41** **Street and highway as the place of occurrence of the external cause**
- **Y92.410** **Unspecified street and highway as the place of occurrence of the external cause**
  - Road NOS as the place of occurrence of the external cause
- **Y92.411** **Interstate highway as the place of occurrence of the external cause**
  - Freeway as the place of occurrence of the external cause
  - Motorway as the place of occurrence of the external cause
- **Y92.412** **Parkway as the place of occurrence of the external cause**
- **Y92.413** **State road as the place of occurrence of the external cause**
- **Y92.414** **Local residential or business street as the place of occurrence of the external cause**
- **Y92.415** **Exit ramp or entrance ramp of street or highway as the place of occurrence of the external cause**

√6ᵗʰ **Y92.48** **Other paved roadways as the place of occurrence of the external cause**
- **Y92.480** **Sidewalk as the place of occurrence of the external cause**
- **Y92.481** **Parking lot as the place of occurrence of the external cause**
- **Y92.482** **Bike path as the place of occurrence of the external cause**
- **Y92.488** **Other paved roadways as the place of occurrence of the external cause**

√5ᵗʰ **Y92.5** **Trade and service area as the place of occurrence of the external cause**
> EXCLUDES 1   *garage in private home (Y92.015)*
> *schools and other public administration buildings (Y92.2-)*

√6ᵗʰ **Y92.51** **Private commercial establishments as the place of occurrence of the external cause**
- **Y92.510** **Bank as the place of occurrence of the external cause**
- **Y92.511** **Restaurant or café as the place of occurrence of the external cause**
- **Y92.512** **Supermarket, store or market as the place of occurrence of the external cause**
- **Y92.513** **Shop (commercial) as the place of occurrence of the external cause**

√6ᵗʰ **Y92.52** **Service areas as the place of occurrence of the external cause**
- **Y92.520** **Airport as the place of occurrence of the external cause**
- **Y92.521** **Bus station as the place of occurrence of the external cause**
- **Y92.522** **Railway station as the place of occurrence of the external cause**
- **Y92.523** **Highway rest stop as the place of occurrence of the external cause**
- **Y92.524** **Gas station as the place of occurrence of the external cause**
  - Petroleum station as the place of occurrence of the external cause
  - Service station as the place of occurrence of the external cause

√6ᵗʰ **Y92.53** **Ambulatory health services establishments as the place of occurrence of the external cause**
- **Y92.530** **Ambulatory surgery center as the place of occurrence of the external cause**
  - Outpatient surgery center, including that connected with a hospital as the place of occurrence of the external cause
  - Same day surgery center, including that connected with a hospital as the place of occurrence of the external cause
- **Y92.531** **Health care provider office as the place of occurrence of the external cause**
  - Physician office as the place of occurrence of the external cause
- **Y92.532** **Urgent care center as the place of occurrence of the external cause**
- **Y92.538** **Other ambulatory health services establishments as the place of occurrence of the external cause**
  - AHA: 2019,1Q,21

Y92.59 **Other trade areas as the place of occurrence of the external cause**
- Office building as the place of occurrence of the external cause
- Casino as the place of occurrence of the external cause
- Garage (commercial) as the place of occurrence of the external cause
- Hotel as the place of occurrence of the external cause
- Radio or television station as the place of occurrence of the external cause
- Shopping mall as the place of occurrence of the external cause
- Warehouse as the place of occurrence of the external cause

√5ᵗʰ **Y92.6** **Industrial and construction area as the place of occurrence of the external cause**
- **Y92.61** **Building [any] under construction as the place of occurrence of the external cause**
- **Y92.62** **Dock or shipyard as the place of occurrence of the external cause**
  - Dockyard as the place of occurrence of the external cause
  - Dry dock as the place of occurrence of the external cause
  - Shipyard as the place of occurrence of the external cause
- **Y92.63** **Factory as the place of occurrence of the external cause**
  - Factory building as the place of occurrence of the external cause
  - Factory premises as the place of occurrence of the external cause
  - Industrial yard as the place of occurrence of the external cause
- **Y92.64** **Mine or pit as the place of occurrence of the external cause**
  - Mine as the place of occurrence of the external cause
- **Y92.65** **Oil rig as the place of occurrence of the external cause**
  - Pit (coal) (gravel) (sand) as the place of occurrence of the external cause
- **Y92.69** **Other specified industrial and construction area as the place of occurrence of the external cause**
  - Gasworks as the place of occurrence of the external cause
  - Power-station (coal) (nuclear) (oil) as the place of occurrence of the external cause
  - Tunnel under construction as the place of occurrence of the external cause
  - Workshop as the place of occurrence of the external cause

√5ᵗʰ **Y92.7** **Farm as the place of occurrence of the external cause**
- Ranch as the place of occurrence of the external cause
> EXCLUDES 1   *farmhouse and home premises of farm (Y92.01-)*
- **Y92.71** **Barn as the place of occurrence of the external cause**

Y92.72 **Chicken coop** as the place of occurrence of the external cause

Hen house as the place of occurrence of the external cause

Y92.73 **Farm field** as the place of occurrence of the external cause

Y92.74 **Orchard** as the place of occurrence of the external cause

Y92.79 **Other farm location** as the place of occurrence of the external cause

√6ᵗʰ **Y92.8** **Other places** as the place of occurrence of the external cause

√6ᵗʰ **Y92.81** **Transport vehicle** as the place of occurrence of the external cause

> *EXCLUDES 1*   transport accidents (V00-V99)

Y92.810 **Car** as the place of occurrence of the external cause

Y92.811 **Bus** as the place of occurrence of the external cause

Y92.812 **Truck** as the place of occurrence of the external cause

Y92.813 **Airplane** as the place of occurrence of the external cause

Y92.814 **Boat** as the place of occurrence of the external cause

Y92.815 **Train** as the place of occurrence of the external cause

Y92.816 **Subway car** as the place of occurrence of the external cause

Y92.818 **Other transport vehicle** as the place of occurrence of the external cause

√6ᵗʰ **Y92.82** **Wilderness area**

Y92.820 **Desert** as the place of occurrence of the external cause

Y92.821 **Forest** as the place of occurrence of the external cause

Y92.828 **Other wilderness area** as the place of occurrence of the external cause

Swamp as the place of occurrence of the external cause

Mountain as the place of occurrence of the external cause

Marsh as the place of occurrence of the external cause

Prairie as the place of occurrence of the external cause

√6ᵗʰ **Y92.83** **Recreation area** as the place of occurrence of the external cause

Y92.830 **Public park** as the place of occurrence of the external cause

Y92.831 **Amusement park** as the place of occurrence of the external cause

Y92.832 **Beach** as the place of occurrence of the external cause

Seashore as the place of occurrence of the external cause

Y92.833 **Campsite** as the place of occurrence of the external cause

Y92.834 **Zoological garden (Zoo)** as the place of occurrence of the external cause

Y92.838 **Other recreation area** as the place of occurrence of the external cause

Y92.84 **Military training ground** as the place of occurrence of the external cause

Y92.85 **Railroad track** as the place of occurrence of the external cause

Y92.86 **Slaughter house** as the place of occurrence of the external cause

Y92.89 **Other specified places** as the place of occurrence of the external cause

Derelict house as the place of occurrence of the external cause

Y92.9 **Unspecified place or not applicable**

√4ᵗʰ **Y93** **Activity codes**

> **NOTE**   Category Y93 is provided for use to indicate the activity of the person seeking healthcare for an injury or health condition, such as a heart attack while shoveling snow, which resulted from, or was contributed to, by the activity. These codes are appropriate for use for both acute injuries, such as those from chapter 19, and conditions that are due to the long-term, cumulative effects of an activity, such as those from chapter 13. They are also appropriate for use with external cause codes for cause and intent if identifying the activity provides additional information on the event. These codes should be used in conjunction with codes for external cause status (Y99) and place of occurrence (Y92).

This section contains the following broad activity categories:

Y93.0	Activities involving walking and running
Y93.1	Activities involving water and water craft
Y93.2	Activities involving ice and snow
Y93.3	Activities involving climbing, rappelling, and jumping off
Y93.4	Activities involving dancing and other rhythmic movement
Y93.5	Activities involving other sports and athletics played individually
Y93.6	Activities involving other sports and athletics played as a team or group
Y93.7	Activities involving other specified sports and athletics
Y93.A	Activities involving other cardiorespiratory exercise
Y93.B	Activities involving other muscle strengthening exercises
Y93.C	Activities involving computer technology and electronic devices
Y93.D	Activities involving arts and handcrafts
Y93.E	Activities involving personal hygiene and interior property and clothing maintenance
Y93.F	Activities involving caregiving
Y93.G	Activities involving food preparation, cooking and grilling
Y93.H	Activities involving exterior property and land maintenance, building and construction
Y93.I	Activities involving roller coasters and other types of external motion
Y93.J	Activities involving playing musical instrument
Y93.K	Activities involving animal care
Y93.8	Activities, other specified
Y93.9	Activity, unspecified

√5ᵗʰ **Y93.0** **Activities involving walking and running**

> *EXCLUDES 1*   activity, walking an animal (Y93.K1)
>
> activity, walking or running on a treadmill (Y93.A1)

Y93.01 **Activity, walking, marching and hiking**

Activity, walking, marching and hiking on level or elevated terrain

> *EXCLUDES 1*   activity, mountain climbing (Y93.31)

Y93.02 **Activity, running**

√5ᵗʰ **Y93.1** **Activities involving water and water craft**

> *EXCLUDES 1*   activities involving ice (Y93.2-)

Y93.11 **Activity, swimming**

Y93.12 **Activity, springboard and platform diving**

Y93.13 **Activity, water polo**

Y93.14 **Activity, water aerobics and water exercise**

Y93.15 **Activity, underwater diving and snorkeling**

Activity, SCUBA diving

Y93.16 **Activity, rowing, canoeing, kayaking, rafting and tubing**

Activity, canoeing, kayaking, rafting and tubing in calm and turbulent water

Y93.17 **Activity, water skiing and wake boarding**

Y93.18 **Activity, surfing, windsurfing and boogie boarding**

Activity, water sliding

Y93.19 **Activity, other involving water and watercraft**

Activity involving water NOS

Activity, parasailing

Activity, water survival training and testing

☑5ᵗʰ **Y93.2 Activities involving ice and snow**
> *EXCLUDES 1*   *activity, shoveling ice and snow (Y93.H1)*

Y93.21 Activity, ice skating
Activity, figure skating (singles) (pairs)
Activity, ice dancing
> *EXCLUDES 1*   *activity, ice hockey (Y93.22)*

Y93.22 Activity, ice hockey

Y93.23 Activity, snow (alpine) (downhill) skiing, snowboarding, sledding, tobogganing and snow tubing
> *EXCLUDES 1*   *activity, cross country skiing (Y93.24)*

Y93.24 Activity, cross country skiing
Activity, nordic skiing

Y93.29 Activity, other involving ice and snow
Activity involving ice and snow NOS

☑5ᵗʰ **Y93.3 Activities involving climbing, rappelling and jumping off**
> *EXCLUDES 1*   *activity, hiking on level or elevated terrain (Y93.Ø1)*
>   *activity, jumping rope (Y93.56)*
>   *activity, trampoline jumping (Y93.44)*

Y93.31 Activity, mountain climbing, rock climbing and wall climbing

Y93.32 Activity, rappelling

Y93.33 Activity, BASE jumping
Activity, Building, Antenna, Span, Earth jumping

Y93.34 Activity, bungee jumping

Y93.35 Activity, hang gliding

Y93.39 Activity, other involving climbing, rappelling and jumping off

☑5ᵗʰ **Y93.4 Activities involving dancing and other rhythmic movement**
> *EXCLUDES 1*   *activity, martial arts (Y93.75)*

Y93.41 Activity, dancing
AHA: 2012,4Q,108

Y93.42 Activity, yoga

Y93.43 Activity, gymnastics
Activity, rhythmic gymnastics
> *EXCLUDES 1*   *activity, trampolining (Y93.44)*

Y93.44 Activity, trampolining

Y93.45 Activity, cheerleading

Y93.49 Activity, other involving dancing and other rhythmic movements

☑5ᵗʰ **Y93.5 Activities involving other sports and athletics played individually**
> *EXCLUDES 1*   *activity, dancing (Y93.41)*
>   *activity, gymnastic (Y93.43)*
>   *activity, trampolining (Y93.44)*
>   *activity, yoga (Y93.42)*

Y93.51 Activity, roller skating (inline) and skateboarding

Y93.52 Activity, horseback riding

Y93.53 Activity, golf

Y93.54 Activity, bowling

Y93.55 Activity, bike riding

Y93.56 Activity, jumping rope

Y93.57 Activity, non-running track and field events
> *EXCLUDES 1*   *activity, running (any form) (Y93.Ø2)*

Y93.59 Activity, other involving other sports and athletics played individually
> *EXCLUDES 1*   *activities involving climbing, rappelling, and jumping (Y93.3-)*
>   *activities involving ice and snow (Y93.2-)*
>   *activities involving walking and running (Y93.Ø-)*
>   *activities involving water and watercraft (Y93.1-)*

☑5ᵗʰ **Y93.6 Activities involving other sports and athletics played as a team or group**
> *EXCLUDES 1*   *activity, ice hockey (Y93.22)*
>   *activity, water polo (Y93.13)*

Y93.61 Activity, American tackle football
Activity, football NOS

Y93.62 Activity, American flag or touch football

Y93.63 Activity, rugby

Y93.64 Activity, baseball
Activity, softball

Y93.65 Activity, lacrosse and field hockey

Y93.66 Activity, soccer

Y93.67 Activity, basketball

Y93.68 Activity, volleyball (beach) (court)

Y93.6A Activity, physical games generally associated with school recess, summer camp and children
Activity, capture the flag
Activity, dodge ball
Activity, four square
Activity, kickball

Y93.69 Activity, other involving other sports and athletics played as a team or group
Activity, cricket

☑5ᵗʰ **Y93.7 Activities involving other specified sports and athletics**

Y93.71 Activity, boxing

Y93.72 Activity, wrestling

Y93.73 Activity, racquet and hand sports
Activity, handball
Activity, racquetball
Activity, squash
Activity, tennis

Y93.74 Activity, frisbee
Activity, ultimate frisbee

Y93.75 Activity, martial arts
Activity, combatives

Y93.79 Activity, other specified sports and athletics
> *EXCLUDES 1*   *sports and athletics activities specified in categories Y93.Ø-Y93.6*

☑5ᵗʰ **Y93.A Activities involving other cardiorespiratory exercise**
Activities involving physical training

Y93.A1 Activity, exercise machines primarily for cardiorespiratory conditioning
Activity, elliptical and stepper machines
Activity, stationary bike
Activity, treadmill

Y93.A2 Activity, calisthenics
Activity, jumping jacks
Activity, warm up and cool down

Y93.A3 Activity, aerobic and step exercise

Y93.A4 Activity, circuit training

Y93.A5 Activity, obstacle course
Activity, challenge course
Activity, confidence course

Y93.A6 Activity, grass drills
Activity, guerilla drills

Y93.A9 Activity, other involving cardiorespiratory exercise
> *EXCLUDES 1*   *activities involving cardiorespiratory exercise specified in categories Y93.Ø-Y93.7*

☑5ᵗʰ **Y93.B Activities involving other muscle strengthening exercises**

Y93.B1 Activity, exercise machines primarily for muscle strengthening

Y93.B2 Activity, push-ups, pull-ups, sit-ups

Y93.B3 Activity, free weights
Activity, barbells
Activity, dumbbells

Y93.B4 Activity, pilates

Y93.B9 Activity, other involving muscle strengthening exercises
> *EXCLUDES 1*   *activities involving muscle strengthening specified in categories Y93.Ø-Y93.A*

☑5ᵗʰ **Y93.C Activities involving computer technology and electronic devices**
> *EXCLUDES 1*   *activity, electronic musical keyboard or instruments (Y93.J-)*

Y93.C1 Activity, computer keyboarding
Activity, electronic game playing using keyboard or other stationary device

Y93.C2 Activity, hand held interactive electronic device
Activity, cellular telephone and communication device
Activity, electronic game playing using interactive device
> *EXCLUDES 1*   *activity, electronic game playing using keyboard or other stationary device (Y93.C1)*

Y93.C9 Activity, other involving computer technology and electronic devices

☑5ᵗʰ **Y93.D Activities involving arts and handcrafts**
> *EXCLUDES 1*   *activities involving playing musical instrument (Y93.J-)*

Y93.D1 Activity, knitting and crocheting

☑ Additional Character Required   ☑✗7ᵗʰ Placeholder Alert   Manifestation   Unspecified Dx   ►◄ Revised Text   ● New Code   ▲ Revised Code Title

Y93.D2 **Activity,** sewing

Y93.D3 **Activity,** furniture building and finishing
Activity, furniture repair

Y93.D9 **Activity, other involving arts and handcrafts**

√5ᵗʰ **Y93.E** **Activities involving personal hygiene and interior property and clothing maintenance**
    EXCLUDES 1 *activities involving cooking and grilling (Y93.G-)*
          activities involving exterior property and land maintenance, building and construction (Y93.H-)
          activities involving caregiving (Y93.F-)
          activity, dishwashing (Y93.G1)
          activity, food preparation (Y93.G1)
          activity, gardening (Y93.H2)

Y93.E1 **Activity,** personal bathing and showering

Y93.E2 **Activity,** laundry

Y93.E3 **Activity,** vacuuming

Y93.E4 **Activity,** ironing

Y93.E5 **Activity,** floor mopping and cleaning

Y93.E6 **Activity,** residential relocation
Activity, packing up and unpacking involved in moving to a new residence

Y93.E8 **Activity, other personal hygiene**

Y93.E9 **Activity, other interior property and clothing maintenance**

√5ᵗʰ **Y93.F** **Activities involving** caregiving
Activity involving the provider of caregiving

Y93.F1 **Activity, caregiving,** bathing

Y93.F2 **Activity, caregiving,** lifting

Y93.F9 **Activity, other caregiving**

√5ᵗʰ **Y93.G** **Activities involving food preparation, cooking and grilling**

Y93.G1 **Activity,** food preparation and clean up
Activity, dishwashing

Y93.G2 **Activity,** grilling and smoking food

Y93.G3 **Activity,** cooking and baking
Activity, use of stove, oven and microwave oven

Y93.G9 **Activity, other involving cooking and grilling**

√5ᵗʰ **Y93.H** **Activities involving exterior property and land maintenance, building and construction**

Y93.H1 **Activity,** digging, shoveling and raking
Activity, dirt digging
Activity, raking leaves
Activity, snow shoveling

Y93.H2 **Activity,** gardening and landscaping
Activity, pruning, trimming shrubs, weeding

Y93.H3 **Activity,** building and construction

Y93.H9 **Activity, other involving exterior property and land maintenance, building and construction**

√5ᵗʰ **Y93.I** **Activities involving roller coasters and other types of external motion**

Y93.I1 **Activity,** rollercoaster riding

Y93.I9 **Activity, other involving external motion**

√5ᵗʰ **Y93.J** **Activities involving playing musical instrument**
Activity involving playing electric musical instrument

Y93.J1 **Activity,** piano playing
Activity, musical keyboard (electronic) playing

Y93.J2 **Activity,** drum and other percussion instrument playing

Y93.J3 **Activity,** string instrument playing

Y93.J4 **Activity,** winds and brass instrument playing

√5ᵗʰ **Y93.K** **Activities involving animal care**
    EXCLUDES 1 *activity, horseback riding (Y93.52)*

Y93.K1 **Activity,** walking an animal

Y93.K2 **Activity,** milking an animal

Y93.K3 **Activity,** grooming and shearing an animal

Y93.K9 **Activity, other involving animal care**

√5ᵗʰ **Y93.8** **Activities, other specified**

Y93.81 **Activity,** refereeing a sports activity

Y93.82 **Activity,** spectator at an event

Y93.83 **Activity,** rough housing and horseplay

Y93.84 **Activity,** sleeping

Y93.85 **Activity,** choking game
Activity, blackout game
Activity, fainting game
Activity, pass out game
AHA: 2016,4Q,74-76

Y93.89 **Activity, other specified**

Y93.9 **Activity, unspecified**

Y95 **Nosocomial condition**
AHA: 2013,4Q,119

√4ᵗʰ **Y99** **External cause status**

    NOTE A single code from category Y99 should be used in conjunction with the external cause code(s) assigned to a record to indicate the status of the person at the time the event occurred.

Y99.0 **Civilian activity done for income or pay**
Civilian activity done for financial or other compensation
    EXCLUDES 1 *military activity (Y99.1)*
          volunteer activity (Y99.2)

Y99.1 **Military activity**
    EXCLUDES 1 *activity of off duty military personnel (Y99.8)*

Y99.2 **Volunteer activity**
    EXCLUDES 1 *activity of child or other family member assisting in compensated work of other family member (Y99.8)*

Y99.8 **Other external cause status**
Activity NEC
Activity of child or other family member assisting in compensated work of other family member
Hobby not done for income
Leisure activity
Off-duty activity of military personnel
Recreation or sport not for income or while a student
Student activity
    EXCLUDES 1 *civilian activity done for income or compensation (Y99.0)*
          military activity (Y99.1)
AHA: 2012,4Q,108

Y99.9 **Unspecified external cause status**

Chapter 21. Factors Influencing Health Status and Contact with Health Services (ZØØ–Z99)

Chapter-specific Guidelines with Coding Examples

The chapter-specific guidelines from the ICD-10-CM Official Guidelines for Coding and Reporting have been provided below. Along with these guidelines are coding examples, contained in the shaded boxes, that have been developed to help illustrate the coding and/or sequencing guidance found in these guidelines.

Note: The chapter-specific guidelines provide additional information about the use of Z codes for specified encounters.

a. Use of Z Codes in any healthcare setting

Z codes are for use in any healthcare setting. Z codes may be used as either a first-listed (principal diagnosis code in the inpatient setting) or secondary code, depending on the circumstances of the encounter. Certain Z codes may only be used as first-listed or principal diagnosis.

Patient with middle lobe lung cancer presents for initiation of chemotherapy

Z51.11   **Encounter for antineoplastic chemotherapy**

C34.2   **Malignant neoplasm of middle lobe, bronchus or lung**

Explanation: A Z code can be used as first-listed in this situation based on guidelines in this chapter as well as chapter 2, "Neoplasms."

Patient has chronic lymphocytic leukemia for which the patient had previous chemotherapy and is now in remission

C91.11   **Chronic lymphocytic leukemia of B-cell type in remission**

Z92.21   **Personal history of antineoplastic chemotherapy**

*Explanation:*The personal history Z code is used to describe a secondary (supplementary) diagnosis to identify that this patient has had chemotherapy in the past.

---

b. Z Codes indicate a reason for an encounter

Z codes are not procedure codes. A corresponding procedure code must accompany a Z code to describe any procedure performed.

c. Categories of Z Codes

1) Contact/exposure

Category Z2Ø indicates contact with, and suspected exposure to, communicable diseases. These codes are for patients who do not show any sign or symptom of a disease but are suspected to have been exposed to it by close personal contact with an infected individual or are in an area where a disease is epidemic.

Category Z77, Other contact with and (suspected) exposures hazardous to health, indicates contact with and suspected exposures hazardous to health.

Contact/exposure codes may be used as a first-listed code to explain an encounter for testing, or, more commonly, as a secondary code to identify a potential risk.

2) Inoculations and vaccinations

Code Z23 is for encounters for inoculations and vaccinations. It indicates that a patient is being seen to receive a prophylactic inoculation against a disease. Procedure codes are required to identify the actual administration of the injection and the type(s) of immunizations given. Code Z23 may be used as a secondary code if the inoculation is given as a routine part of preventive health care, such as a well-baby visit.

3) Status

Status codes indicate that a patient is either a carrier of a disease or has the sequelae or residual of a past disease or condition. This includes such things as the presence of prosthetic or mechanical devices resulting from past treatment. A status code is informative, because the status may affect the course of treatment and its outcome. A status code is distinct from a history code. The history code indicates that the patient no longer has the condition.

A status code should not be used with a diagnosis code from one of the body system chapters, if the diagnosis code includes the information provided by the status code. For example, code Z94.1, Heart transplant status, should not be used with a code from subcategory T86.2, Complications of heart transplant. The status code does not provide

additional information. The complication code indicates that the patient is a heart transplant patient.

For encounters for weaning from a mechanical ventilator, assign a code from subcategory J96.1, Chronic respiratory failure, followed by code Z99.11, Dependence on respirator [ventilator] status.

The status Z codes/categories are:

Z14   Genetic carrier

Genetic carrier status indicates that a person carries a gene, associated with a particular disease, which may be passed to offspring who may develop that disease. The person does not have the disease and is not at risk of developing the disease.

Z15   Genetic susceptibility to disease

Genetic susceptibility indicates that a person has a gene that increases the risk of that person developing the disease.

Codes from category Z15 should not be used as principal or first-listed codes. If the patient has the condition to which he/she is susceptible, and that condition is the reason for the encounter, the code for the current condition should be sequenced first. If the patient is being seen for follow-up after completed treatment for this condition, and the condition no longer exists, a follow-up code should be sequenced first, followed by the appropriate personal history and genetic susceptibility codes. If the purpose of the encounter is genetic counseling associated with procreative management, code Z31.5, Encounter for genetic counseling, should be assigned as the first-listed code, followed by a code from category Z15. Additional codes should be assigned for any applicable family or personal history.

Z16   Resistance to antimicrobial drugs

This code indicates that a patient has a condition that is resistant to antimicrobial drug treatment. Sequence the infection code first.

Z17   Estrogen receptor status

Z18   Retained foreign body fragments

Z19   Hormone sensitivity malignancy status

Z21   Asymptomatic HIV infection status

This code indicates that a patient has tested positive for HIV but has manifested no signs or symptoms of the disease.

Z22   Carrier of infectious disease

Carrier status indicates that a person harbors the specific organisms of a disease without manifest symptoms and is capable of transmitting the infection.

Z28.3   Underimmunization status

Z33.1   Pregnant state, incidental

This code is a secondary code only for use when the pregnancy is in no way complicating the reason for visit. Otherwise, a code from the obstetric chapter is required.

Z66   Do not resuscitate

This code may be used when it is documented by the provider that a patient is on do not resuscitate status at any time during the stay.

Z67   Blood type

Z68   Body mass index (BMI)

BMI codes should only be assigned when **there is an associated, reportable diagnosis (such as obesity).** Do not assign BMI codes during pregnancy.

See Section I.B.14 for BMI documentation by clinicians other than the patient's provider.

Patient seen today for chest pain, noncardiac in nature. Nurses notes identify a BMI of 20.5.

RØ7.89   **Other chest pain**

Explanation: Section I.B.14 stipulates that the BMI can be assigned from documentation of someone other than the patient's provider, such as nursing notes, only when the provider has documented that the diagnosis is associated with the BMI. As there is no supporting documentation from the provider linking the BMI to an associated condition, no code is assigned for the BMI.

Z74.Ø1   Bed confinement status

Z76.82   Awaiting organ transplant status

Z78   Other specified health status

Code Z78.1, Physical restraint status, may be used when it is documented by the provider that a patient has been put in restraints during the current encounter. Please note that this code should not be reported when it is documented by the provider that a patient is temporarily restrained during a procedure.

Z79   Long-term (current) drug therapy

Codes from this category indicate a patient's continuous use of a prescribed drug (including such things as aspirin therapy) for the long-term treatment of a condition or for prophylactic use. It is not for use for patients who have addictions to drugs. This subcategory is not for use of medications for detoxification or maintenance programs to prevent withdrawal symptoms in patients with drug dependence (e.g., methadone maintenance for opiate dependence). Assign the appropriate code for the drug dependence instead.

Assign a code from Z79 if the patient is receiving a medication for an extended period as a prophylactic measure (such as for the prevention of deep vein thrombosis) or as treatment of a chronic condition (such as arthritis) or a disease requiring a lengthy course of treatment (such as cancer). Do not assign a code from category Z79 for medication being administered for a brief period of time to treat an acute illness or injury (such as a course of antibiotics to treat acute bronchitis).

Z88   Allergy status to drugs, medicaments and biological substances

Except: Z88.9, Allergy status to unspecified drugs, medicaments and biological substances status

Z89   Acquired absence of limb

Z90   Acquired absence of organs, not elsewhere classified

Z91.0- Allergy status, other than to drugs and biological substances

Z92.82 Status post administration of tPA (rtPA) in a different facility within the last 24 hours prior to admission to a current facility

Assign code Z92.82, Status post administration of tPA (rtPA) in a different facility within the last 24 hours prior to admission to current facility, as a secondary diagnosis when a patient is received by transfer into a facility and documentation indicates they were administered tissue plasminogen activator (tPA) within the last 24 hours prior to admission to the current facility.

This guideline applies even if the patient is still receiving the tPA at the time they are received into the current facility.

The appropriate code for the condition for which the tPA was administered (such as cerebrovascular disease or myocardial infarction) should be assigned first.

Code Z92.82 is only applicable to the receiving facility record and not to the transferring facility record.

Z93   Artificial opening status

Z94   Transplanted organ and tissue status

Z95   Presence of cardiac and vascular implants and grafts

Z96   Presence of other functional implants

Z97   Presence of other devices

Z98   Other postprocedural states

Assign code Z98.85, Transplanted organ removal status, to indicate that a transplanted organ has been previously removed. This code should not be assigned for the encounter in which the transplanted organ is removed. The complication necessitating removal of the transplant organ should be assigned for that encounter.

See section I.C19. for information on the coding of organ transplant complications.

Z99   Dependence on enabling machines and devices, not elsewhere classified

Note: Categories Z89-Z90 and Z93-Z99 are for use only if there are no complications or malfunctions of the organ or tissue replaced, the amputation site or the equipment on which the patient is dependent.

4) History (of)

There are two types of history Z codes, personal and family. Personal history codes explain a patient's past medical condition that no longer exists and is not receiving any treatment, but that has the potential for recurrence, and therefore may require continued monitoring.

Family history codes are for use when a patient has a family member(s) who has had a particular disease that causes the patient to be at higher risk of also contracting the disease.

Personal history codes may be used in conjunction with follow-up codes and family history codes may be used in conjunction with screening codes to explain the need for a test or procedure. History codes are also acceptable on any medical record regardless of the reason for visit. A history of an illness, even if no longer present, is important information that may alter the type of treatment ordered.

The history Z code categories are:

Z80   Family history of primary malignant neoplasm

Z81   Family history of mental and behavioral disorders

Z82   Family history of certain disabilities and chronic diseases (leading to disablement)

Z83   Family history of other specific disorders

Z84   Family history of other conditions

Z85   Personal history of malignant neoplasm

Z86   Personal history of certain other diseases

Z87   Personal history of other diseases and conditions

Z91.4- Personal history of psychological trauma, not elsewhere classified

Z91.5   Personal history of self-harm

Z91.81 History of falling

Z91.82 Personal history of military deployment

Z92   Personal history of medical treatment

Except: Z92.0, Personal history of contraception

Except: Z92.82, Status post administration of tPA (rtPA) in a different facility within the last 24 hours prior to admission to a current facility

5) Screening

Screening is the testing for disease or disease precursors in seemingly well individuals so that early detection and treatment can be provided for those who test positive for the disease (e.g., screening mammogram).

The testing of a person to rule out or confirm a suspected diagnosis because the patient has some sign or symptom is a diagnostic examination, not a screening. In these cases, the sign or symptom is used to explain the reason for the test.

A screening code may be a first-listed code if the reason for the visit is specifically the screening exam. It may also be used as an additional code if the screening is done during an office visit for other health problems. A screening code is not necessary if the screening is inherent to a routine examination, such as a pap smear done during a routine pelvic examination.

Should a condition be discovered during the screening then the code for the condition may be assigned as an additional diagnosis.

Prostate screening of healthy 50-year-old male patient; PSA noted to be elevated but normal digital rectal exam

Z12.5   Encounter for screening for malignant neoplasm of prostate

R97.20   Elevated prostate specific antigen [PSA]

Explanation: The patient had no signs or symptoms of any prostate-related illness prior to coming in for the screening. The screening code is appropriately used as the first-listed code to signify that this was for routine screening. The elevated PSA is reported as a secondary diagnosis to reflect that an abnormal lab value was found as a result of the screening procedure(s).

The Z code indicates that a screening exam is planned. A procedure code is required to confirm that the screening was performed.

The screening Z codes/categories:

Z11   Encounter for screening for infectious and parasitic diseases

Z12   Encounter for screening for malignant neoplasms

Z13   Encounter for screening for other diseases and disorders

Except: Z13.9, Encounter for screening, unspecified

Z36   Encounter for antenatal screening for mother

6) Observation

There are three observation Z code categories. They are for use in very limited circumstances when a person is being observed for a suspected condition that is ruled out. The observation codes are not for use if an injury or illness or any signs or symptoms related to the suspected condition are present. In such cases the diagnosis/symptom code is used with the corresponding external cause code.

The observation codes are to be used as principal diagnosis only. The only exception to this is when the principal diagnosis is required to be a code from category Z38, Liveborn infants according to place of birth and type of delivery. Then a code from category Z05, Encounter for observation and evaluation of newborn for suspected diseases and conditions ruled out, is sequenced after the Z38 code. Additional codes may be used in addition to the observation code but only if they are unrelated to the suspected condition being observed.

Codes from subcategory Z03.7, Encounter for suspected maternal and fetal conditions ruled out, may either be used as a first-listed or as an additional code assignment depending on the case. They are for use in very limited circumstances on a maternal record when an encounter is for a suspected maternal or fetal condition that is ruled out during that encounter (for example, a maternal or fetal condition may be suspected due to an abnormal test result). These codes should not be used when the condition is confirmed. In those cases, the confirmed condition should be coded. In addition, these codes are not for use if an illness or any signs or symptoms related to the suspected condition or problem are present. In such cases the diagnosis/symptom code is used.

Additional codes may be used in addition to the code from subcategory Z03.7, but only if they are unrelated to the suspected condition being evaluated.

Codes from subcategory Z03.7 may not be used for encounters for antenatal screening of mother. *See Section I.C.21. Screening.*

For encounters for suspected fetal condition that are inconclusive following testing and evaluation, assign the appropriate code from category O35, O36, O40 or O41.

The observation Z code categories:

Z03	Encounter for medical observation for suspected diseases and conditions ruled out
Z04	Encounter for examination and observation for other reasons
	Except: Z04.9, Encounter for examination and observation for unspecified reason
Z05	Encounter for observation and evaluation of newborn for suspected diseases and conditions ruled out

7) Aftercare

Aftercare visit codes cover situations when the initial treatment of a disease has been performed and the patient requires continued care during the healing or recovery phase, or for the long-term consequences of the disease. The aftercare Z code should not be used if treatment is directed at a current, acute disease. The diagnosis code is to be used in these cases. Exceptions to this rule are codes Z51.0, Encounter for antineoplastic radiation therapy, and codes from subcategory Z51.1, Encounter for antineoplastic chemotherapy and immunotherapy. These codes are to be first-listed, followed by the diagnosis code when a patient's encounter is solely to receive radiation therapy, chemotherapy, or immunotherapy for the treatment of a neoplasm. If the reason for the encounter is more than one type of antineoplastic therapy, code Z51.0 and a code from subcategory Z51.1 may be assigned together, in which case one of these codes would be reported as a secondary diagnosis.

The aftercare Z codes should also not be used for aftercare for injuries. For aftercare of an injury, assign the acute injury code with the appropriate 7th character (for subsequent encounter).

The aftercare codes are generally first-listed to explain the specific reason for the encounter. An aftercare code may be used as an additional code when some type of aftercare is provided in addition to the reason for admission and no diagnosis code is applicable. An example of this would be the closure of a colostomy during an encounter for treatment of another condition.

Aftercare codes should be used in conjunction with other aftercare codes or diagnosis codes to provide better detail on the specifics of an aftercare encounter visit, unless otherwise directed by the classification. The sequencing of multiple aftercare codes depends on the circumstances of the encounter.

Patient presents for third round of gemcitabine and first dose of antineoplastic radiation therapy for advanced pancreatic carcinoma

Z51.11	**Encounter for antineoplastic chemotherapy**
Z51.0	**Encounter for antineoplastic radiation therapy**
C25.9	**Malignant neoplasm of pancreas, unspecified**

Explanation: Gemcitabine is an antineoplastic chemotherapy. Since the encounter was solely to administer antineoplastic treatment, both forms of treatment are reported and either code can be the first-listed diagnosis, followed by the neoplastic condition code. Aftercare codes are typically not assigned for current treatment of disease; however, Z51.0 and subcategory Z51.1 are an exception to this standard.

Certain aftercare Z code categories need a secondary diagnosis code to describe the resolving condition or sequelae. For others, the condition is included in the code title.

Additional Z code aftercare category terms include fitting and adjustment, and attention to artificial openings.

Status Z codes may be used with aftercare Z codes to indicate the nature of the aftercare. For example code Z95.1, Presence of aortocoronary bypass graft, may be used with code Z48.812, Encounter for surgical aftercare following surgery on the circulatory system, to indicate the surgery for which the aftercare is being performed. A status code should not be used when the aftercare code indicates the type of status, such as using Z43.0, Encounter for attention to tracheostomy, with Z93.0, Tracheostomy status.

The aftercare Z category/codes:

Z42	Encounter for plastic and reconstructive surgery following medical procedure or healed injury
Z43	Encounter for attention to artificial openings
Z44	Encounter for fitting and adjustment of external prosthetic device
Z45	Encounter for adjustment and management of implanted device
Z46	Encounter for fitting and adjustment of other devices
Z47	Orthopedic aftercare
Z48	Encounter for other postprocedural aftercare
Z49	Encounter for care involving renal dialysis
Z51	Encounter for other aftercare and medical care

8) Follow-up

The follow-up codes are used to explain continuing surveillance following completed treatment of a disease, condition, or injury. They imply that the condition has been fully treated and no longer exists. They should not be confused with aftercare codes, or injury codes with a 7th character for subsequent encounter, that explain ongoing care of a healing condition or its sequelae. Follow-up codes may be used in conjunction with history codes to provide the full picture of the healed condition and its treatment. The follow-up code is sequenced first, followed by the history code.

A follow-up code may be used to explain multiple visits. Should a condition be found to have recurred on the follow-up visit, then the diagnosis code for the condition should be assigned in place of the follow-up code.

The follow-up Z code categories:

Z08	Encounter for follow-up examination after completed treatment for malignant neoplasm
Z09	Encounter for follow-up examination after completed treatment for conditions other than malignant neoplasm
Z39	Encounter for maternal postpartum care and examination

Follow-up for patient several months after completing a regime of IV antibiotics for recurrent pneumonia; lungs are clear and pneumonia is resolved

Z09	**Encounter for follow-up examination after completed treatment for conditions other than malignant neoplasm**
Z87.01	**Personal history of pneumonia (recurrent)**

Explanation: Code Z09 identifies the follow-up visit as being unrelated to a malignant neoplasm, and code Z87 describes the condition that has now resolved.

Follow-up for patient several months after completing a regime of IV antibiotics for recurrent pneumonia; pneumonia has recurred, and a new antibiotic regimen has been prescribed

J18.9	**Pneumonia, unspecified organism**

Explanation: Since the follow-up exam for pneumonia determined that the pneumonia was not resolved or recurred, code Z09 Encounter for follow-up examination after completed treatment for conditions other than malignant neoplasm, no longer applies. Instead the first-listed code describes the pneumonia.

9) Donor

Codes in category Z52, Donors of organs and tissues, are used for living individuals who are donating blood or other body tissue. These codes are only for individuals donating for others, not for self-donations. They are not used to identify cadaveric donations.

Chapter 21. Factors Influencing Health Status and Contact with Health Services

10)Counseling

Counseling Z codes are used when a patient or family member receives assistance in the aftermath of an illness or injury, or when support is required in coping with family or social problems.

The counseling Z codes/categories:

Z30.0-	Encounter for general counseling and advice on contraception
Z31.5	Encounter for procreative genetic counseling
Z31.6-	Encounter for general counseling and advice on procreation
Z32.2	Encounter for childbirth instruction
Z32.3	Encounter for childcare instruction
Z69	Encounter for mental health services for victim and perpetrator of abuse
Z70	Counseling related to sexual attitude, behavior and orientation
Z71	Persons encountering health services for other counseling and medical advice, not elsewhere classified

Note: Code Z71.84, Encounter for health counseling related to travel, is to be used for health risk and safety counseling for future travel purposes.

Z76.81	Expectant mother prebirth pediatrician visit

11)Encounters for obstetrical and reproductive services

See Section I.C.15. Pregnancy, Childbirth, and the Puerperium, for further instruction on the use of these codes.

Z codes for pregnancy are for use in those circumstances when none of the problems or complications included in the codes from the Obstetrics chapter exist (a routine prenatal visit or postpartum care). Codes in category Z34, Encounter for supervision of normal pregnancy, are always first-listed and are not to be used with any other code from the OB chapter.

Codes in category Z3A, Weeks of gestation, may be assigned to provide additional information about the pregnancy. Category Z3A codes should not be assigned for pregnancies with abortive outcomes (categories O00-O08), elective termination of pregnancy (code Z33.2), nor for postpartum conditions, as category Z3A is not applicable to these conditions. The date of the admission should be used to determine weeks of gestation for inpatient admissions that encompass more than one gestational week.

The outcome of delivery, category Z37, should be included on all maternal delivery records. It is always a secondary code. Codes in category Z37 should not be used on the newborn record.

Z codes for family planning (contraceptive) or procreative management and counseling should be included on an obstetric record either during the pregnancy or the postpartum stage, if applicable.

Z codes/categories for obstetrical and reproductive services:

Z30	Encounter for contraceptive management
Z31	Encounter for procreative management
Z32.2	Encounter for childbirth instruction
Z32.3	Encounter for childcare instruction
Z33	Pregnant state
Z34	Encounter for supervision of normal pregnancy
Z36	Encounter for antenatal screening of mother
Z3A	Weeks of gestation
Z37	Outcome of delivery
Z39	Encounter for maternal postpartum care and examination
Z76.81	Expectant mother prebirth pediatrician visit

12)Newborns and infants

See Section I.C.16. Newborn (Perinatal) Guidelines, for further instruction on the use of these codes.

Newborn Z codes/categories:

Z76.1	Encounter for health supervision and care of foundling
Z00.1-	Encounter for routine child health examination
Z38	Liveborn infants according to place of birth and type of delivery

13)Routine and administrative examinations

The Z codes allow for the description of encounters for routine examinations, such as, a general check-up, or, examinations for administrative purposes, such as, a pre-employment physical. The codes are not to be used if the examination is for diagnosis of a suspected condition or for treatment purposes. In such cases the diagnosis code is used. During a routine exam, should a diagnosis or condition be discovered, it should be coded as an additional code. Pre-existing and chronic conditions and history codes may also be included as additional codes as long as the examination is for administrative purposes and not focused on any particular condition.

Some of the codes for routine health examinations distinguish between "with" and "without" abnormal findings. Code assignment depends on the information that is known at the time the encounter is being coded. For example, if no abnormal findings were found during the examination, but the encounter is being coded before test results are back, it is acceptable to assign the code for "without abnormal findings." When assigning a code for "with abnormal findings," additional code(s) should be assigned to identify the specific abnormal finding(s).

12-month-old boy presented for well-child visit; pediatrician notices some eczema on the child's scalp and back of the knees

Z00.121	**Encounter for routine child health examination with abnormal findings**
L30.9	**Dermatitis, unspecified**

Explanation: The Z code identifying that this is a routine well-child visit is reported first. Because an abnormal finding (eczema) was documented, a code for this condition may also be appended.

Pre-operative examination and pre-procedural laboratory examination Z codes are for use only in those situations when a patient is being cleared for a procedure or surgery and no treatment is given.

The Z codes/categories for routine and administrative examinations:

Z00	Encounter for general examination without complaint, suspected or reported diagnosis
Z01	Encounter for other special examination without complaint, suspected or reported diagnosis
Z02	Encounter for administrative examination
	Except: Z02.9, Encounter for administrative examinations, unspecified
Z32.0-	Encounter for pregnancy test

14)Miscellaneous Z codes

The miscellaneous Z codes capture a number of other health care encounters that do not fall into one of the other categories. Certain of these codes identify the reason for the encounter; others are for use as additional codes that provide useful information on circumstances that may affect a patient's care and treatment.

Prophylactic organ removal

For encounters specifically for prophylactic removal of an organ (such as prophylactic removal of breasts due to a genetic susceptibility to cancer or a family history of cancer), the principal or first-listed code should be a code from category Z40, Encounter for prophylactic surgery, followed by the appropriate codes to identify the associated risk factor (such as genetic susceptibility or family history).

If the patient has a malignancy of one site and is having prophylactic removal at another site to prevent either a new primary malignancy or metastatic disease, a code for the malignancy should also be assigned in addition to a code from subcategory Z40.0, Encounter for prophylactic surgery for risk factors related to malignant neoplasms. A Z40.0 code should not be assigned if the patient is having organ removal for treatment of a malignancy, such as the removal of the testes for the treatment of prostate cancer.

Miscellaneous Z codes/categories:

Z28	Immunization not carried out
	Except: Z28.3, Underimmunization status
Z29	Encounter for other prophylactic measures
Z40	Encounter for prophylactic surgery
Z41	Encounter for procedures for purposes other than remedying health state
	Except: Z41.9, Encounter for procedure for purposes other than remedying health state, unspecified
Z53	Persons encountering health services for specific procedures and treatment, not carried out
Z55	Problems related to education and literacy
Z56	Problems related to employment and unemployment
Z57	Occupational exposure to risk factors
Z58	Problems related to physical environment
Z59	Problems related to housing and economic circumstances
Z60	Problems related to social environment
Z62	Problems related to upbringing
Z63	Other problems related to primary support group, including family circumstances
Z64	Problems related to certain psychosocial circumstances
Z65	Problems related to other psychosocial circumstances

Z72	Problems related to lifestyle

Note: These codes should be assigned only when the documentation specifies that the patient has an associated problem

Z73	Problems related to life management difficulty
Z74	Problems related to care provider dependency

Except: Z74.01, Bed confinement status

Z75	Problems related to medical facilities and other health care
Z76.0	Encounter for issue of repeat prescription
Z76.3	Healthy person accompanying sick person
Z76.4	Other boarder to healthcare facility
Z76.5	Malingerer [conscious simulation]
Z91.1-	Patient's noncompliance with medical treatment and regimen
Z91.83	Wandering in diseases classified elsewhere
Z91.84-	Oral health risk factors
Z91.89	Other specified personal risk factors, not elsewhere classified

See Section I.B.14 for Z55-Z65 Persons with potential health hazards related to socioeconomic and psychosocial circumstances, documentation by clinicians other than the patient's provider

15) Nonspecific Z codes

Certain Z codes are so non-specific, or potentially redundant with other codes in the classification, that there can be little justification for their use in the inpatient setting. Their use in the outpatient setting should be limited to those instances when there is no further documentation to permit more precise coding. Otherwise, any sign or symptom or any other reason for visit that is captured in another code should be used.

Nonspecific Z codes/categories:

Z02.9	Encounter for administrative examinations, unspecified
Z04.9	Encounter for examination and observation for unspecified reason
Z13.9	Encounter for screening, unspecified
Z41.9	Encounter for procedure for purposes other than remedying health state, unspecified
Z52.9	Donor of unspecified organ or tissue
Z86.59	Personal history of other mental and behavioral disorders
Z88.9	Allergy status to unspecified drugs, medicaments and biological substances status
Z92.0	Personal history of contraception

16) Z codes that may only be principal/first-listed diagnosis

The following Z codes/categories may only be reported as the principal/first-listed diagnosis, except when there are multiple encounters on the same day and the medical records for the encounters are combined:

Z00	Encounter for general examination without complaint, suspected or reported diagnosis

Except: Z00.6

Z01	Encounter for other special examination without complaint, suspected or reported diagnosis

Z02	Encounter for administrative examination
Z03	Encounter for medical observation for suspected diseases and conditions ruled out
Z04	Encounter for examination and observation for other reasons
Z33.2	Encounter for elective termination of pregnancy
Z31.81	Encounter for male factor infertility in female patient
Z31.83	Encounter for assisted reproductive fertility procedure cycle
Z31.84	Encounter for fertility preservation procedure
Z34	Encounter for supervision of normal pregnancy
Z39	Encounter for maternal postpartum care and examination
Z38	Liveborn infants according to place of birth and type of delivery
Z40	Encounter for prophylactic surgery
Z42	Encounter for plastic and reconstructive surgery following medical procedure or healed injury
Z51.0	Encounter for antineoplastic radiation therapy
Z51.1-	Encounter for antineoplastic chemotherapy and immunotherapy
Z52	Donors of organs and tissues

Except: Z52.9, Donor of unspecified organ or tissue

Z76.1	Encounter for health supervision and care of foundling
Z76.2	Encounter for health supervision and care of other healthy infant and child
Z99.12	Encounter for respirator [ventilator] dependence during power failure

---

Female patient seen at 32 weeks' gestation to check the progress of her first pregnancy

Z34.03   **Encounter for supervision of normal first pregnancy, third trimester**

Z3A.32   **32 weeks gestation of pregnancy**

Explanation: Category Z34 is appropriate as a first-listed diagnosis. Category Z3A helps to clarify at which point in the pregnancy the patient was provided supervision.

Chapter 21. Factors Influencing Health Status and Contact With Health Services (Z00–Z99)

NOTE   Z codes represent reasons for encounters. A corresponding procedure code must accompany a Z code if a procedure is performed. Categories Z00–Z99 are provided for occasions when circumstances other than a disease, injury or external cause classifiable to categories A00–Y89 are recorded as "diagnoses" or "problems." This can arise in two main ways:

(a) When a person who may or may not be sick encounters the health services for some specific purpose, such as to receive limited care or service for a current condition, to donate an organ or tissue, to receive prophylactic vaccination (immunization), or to discuss a problem which is in itself not a disease or injury.

(b) When some circumstance or problem is present which influences the person's health status but is not in itself a current illness or injury.

AHA: 2018,4Q,60-61

This chapter contains the following blocks:

Z00-Z13	Persons encountering health services for examinations
Z14-Z15	Genetic carrier and genetic susceptibility to disease
Z16	Resistance to antimicrobial drugs
Z17	Estrogen receptor status
Z18	Retained foreign body fragments
Z19	Hormone sensitivity malignancy status
Z20-Z29	Persons with potential health hazards related to communicable diseases
Z30-Z39	Persons encountering health services in circumstances related to reproduction
Z40-Z53	Encounters for other specific health care
Z55-Z65	Persons with potential health hazards related to socioeconomic and psychosocial circumstances
Z66	Do not resuscitate status
Z67	Blood type
Z68	Body mass index (BMI)
Z69-Z76	Persons encountering health services in other circumstances
Z77-Z99	Persons with potential health hazards related to family and personal history and certain conditions influencing health status

Persons encountering health services for examinations (Z00-Z13)

NOTE   Nonspecific abnormal findings disclosed at the time of these examinations are classified to categories R70-R94.

EXCLUDES 1   *examinations related to pregnancy and reproduction (Z30-Z36, Z39.-)*

√4ᵗʰ **Z00**   **Encounter for general examination without complaint, suspected or reported diagnosis**

     EXCLUDES 1   *encounter for examination for administrative purposes (Z02.-)*

     EXCLUDES 2   *encounter for pre-procedural examinations (Z01.81-)*
                        special screening examinations (Z11-Z13)

     AHA: 2017,4Q,95

√5ᵗʰ **Z00.0**   **Encounter for general** adult medical **examination**

     Encounter for adult periodic examination (annual) (physical) and any associated laboratory and radiologic examinations

         EXCLUDES 1   *encounter for examination of sign or symptom — code to sign or symptom*
                               general health check-up of infant or child (Z00.12.-)

Z00.00   **Encounter for general adult medical**   PDx A
         examination without abnormal findings
         Encounter for adult health check-up NOS
         AHA: 2016,1Q,36

Z00.01   **Encounter for general adult medical**   PDx A
         examination with abnormal findings
         Use additional code to identify abnormal findings
         AHA: 2016,1Q,35-36

√5ᵗʰ **Z00.1**   **Encounter for** newborn, infant and child health **examinations**

√6ᵗʰ   **Z00.11**   **Newborn** health examination

         Health check for child under 29 days old
         Use additional code to identify any abnormal findings

         EXCLUDES 1   *health check for child over 28 days old (Z00.12-)*

Z00.110   **Health examination for**   PDx N
         newborn under 8 days old
         Health check for newborn under 8 days old

Z00.111   **Health examination for**   PDx N
         newborn 8 to 28 days old
         Health check for newborn 8 to 28 days old
         Newborn weight check

√6ᵗʰ   **Z00.12**   **Encounter for** routine child **health examination**

         Health check (routine) for child over 28 days old
         Immunizations appropriate for age
         Routine developmental screening of infant or child
         Routine vison and hearing testing

         EXCLUDES 1   *health check for child under 29 days old (Z00.11-)*
                      health supervision of foundling or other healthy infant or child (Z76.1-Z76.2)
                      newborn health examination (Z00.11-)

         AHA: 2018,4Q,36

Z00.121   **Encounter for routine child**   PDx P
         health examination with abnormal findings
         Use additional code to identify abnormal findings
         AHA: 2016,1Q,34-35

Z00.129   **Encounter for routine child**   PDx P
         health examination without abnormal findings
         Encounter for routine child health examination NOS
         AHA: 2016,1Q,34

Z00.2   **Encounter for examination for** period of rapid growth in childhood   PDx P

Z00.3   **Encounter for examination for** adolescent development **state**   PDx P
     Encounter for puberty development state

Z00.5   **Encounter for examination of** potential donor of organ and tissue   PDx

Z00.6   **Encounter for examination for** normal comparison and control in clinical research program
     Examination of participant or control in clinical research program

√5ᵗʰ **Z00.7**   **Encounter for examination for period of** delayed growth in childhood

Z00.70   **Encounter for examination for period of**   PDx P
     delayed growth in childhood without abnormal findings

Z00.71   **Encounter for examination for period of**   PDx P
     delayed growth in childhood with abnormal findings
     Use additional code to identify abnormal findings

Z00.8   **Encounter for other general examination**   PDx
     Encounter for health examination in population surveys

√4ᵗʰ **Z01**   **Encounter for other** special examination **without complaint, suspected or reported diagnosis**

     INCLUDES   routine examination of specific system

     NOTE   Codes from category Z01 represent the reason for the encounter. A separate procedure code is required to identify any examinations or procedures performed

     EXCLUDES 1   *encounter for examination for administrative purposes (Z02.-)*
                       encounter for examination for suspected conditions, proven not to exist (Z03.-)
                       encounter for laboratory and radiologic examinations as a component of general medical examinations (Z00.0-)
                       encounter for laboratory, radiologic and imaging examinations for sign(s) and symptom(s) — code to the sign(s) or symptom(s)

     EXCLUDES 2   *screening examinations (Z11-Z13)*

√5ᵗʰ **Z01.0**   **Encounter for examination of** eyes and vision

         EXCLUDES 1   *examination for driving license (Z02.4)*

Z01.00   **Encounter for examination of eyes and**   PDx
     vision without abnormal findings
     Encounter for examination of eyes and vision NOS

Z01.01   **Encounter for examination of eyes and**   PDx
     vision with abnormal findings
     Use additional code to identify abnormal findings
     AHA: 2016,4Q,21

HCC CMS-HCC	PDx Primary Dx Only	Q QPP	N Newborn: 0	P Pediatric: 0-17	M Maternity: 12-55	A Adult: 15-1

1218   ICD-10-CM 20

●   √6ᵗʰ **Z01.02 Encounter for examination of eyes and vision following failed vision screening**

> **EXCLUDES 1**   *examination for examination of eyes and vision with abnormal findings (Z01.01)*
>
> *examination for examination of eyes and vision without abnormal findings (Z01.00)*

●   **Z01.020 Encounter for examination of**   PDx
eyes and vision following failed vision screening without abnormal findings

●   **Z01.021 Encounter for examination of**   PDx
eyes and vision following failed vision screening with abnormal findings

> Use additional code to identify abnormal findings

√5ᵗʰ **Z01.1 Encounter for examination of ears and hearing**

     Z01.10 Encounter for examination of ears and   PDx
hearing without abnormal findings

> Encounter for examination of ears and hearing NOS
>
> **AHA:** 2016,4Q,24

     √6ᵗʰ **Z01.11 Encounter for examination of ears and hearing with abnormal findings**

> **AHA:** 2016,3Q,17-18

         Z01.110 Encounter for hearing   PDx
examination following failed hearing screening

         Z01.118 Encounter for examination of   PDx
ears and hearing with other abnormal findings

> Use additional code to identify abnormal findings

     Z01.12 Encounter for hearing conservation and   PDx
treatment

√5ᵗʰ **Z01.2 Encounter for dental examination and cleaning**

     Z01.20 Encounter for dental examination and   PDx
cleaning without abnormal findings

> Encounter for dental examination and cleaning NOS

     Z01.21 Encounter for dental examination and   PDx
cleaning with abnormal findings

> Use additional code to identify abnormal findings

√5ᵗʰ **Z01.3 Encounter for examination of blood pressure**

     Z01.30 Encounter for examination of blood   PDx
pressure without abnormal findings

> Encounter for examination of blood pressure NOS

     Z01.31 Encounter for examination of blood   PDx
pressure with abnormal findings

> Use additional code to identify abnormal findings

√5ᵗʰ **Z01.4 Encounter for gynecological examination**

> **EXCLUDES 2**   *pregnancy examination or test (Z32.0-)*
>
> *routine examination for contraceptive maintenance (Z30.4-)*

     √6ᵗʰ **Z01.41 Encounter for routine gynecological examination**

> Encounter for general gynecological examination with or without cervical smear
>
> Encounter for gynecological examination (general) (routine) NOS
>
> Encounter for pelvic examination (annual) (periodic)
>
> Use additional code:
>
>   for screening for human papillomavirus, if applicable, (Z11.51)
>
>   for screening vaginal pap smear, if applicable (Z12.72)
>
>   to identify acquired absence of uterus, if applicable (Z90.71-)
>
> **EXCLUDES 1**   *gynecologic examination status-post hysterectomy for malignant condition (Z08)*
>
> *screening cervical pap smear not a part of a routine gynecological examination (Z12.4)*

         Z01.411 Encounter for gynecological   PDx ♀
examination (general) (routine) with abnormal findings

> Use additional code to identify abnormal findings

         Z01.419 Encounter for gynecological   PDx ♀
examination (general) (routine) without abnormal findings

     Z01.42 Encounter for cervical smear to confirm   PDx ♀
findings of recent normal smear following initial abnormal smear

√5ᵗʰ **Z01.8 Encounter for other specified special examinations**

     √6ᵗʰ **Z01.81 Encounter for preprocedural examinations**

> Encounter for preoperative examinations
>
> Encounter for radiological and imaging examinations as part of preprocedural examination
>
> **TIP:** Assign a code for the condition necessitating surgery and any findings as additional diagnoses.

         Z01.810 Encounter for preprocedural   PDx
cardiovascular examination

         Z01.811 Encounter for preprocedural   PDx
respiratory examination

         Z01.812 Encounter for preprocedural   PDx
laboratory examination

> Blood and urine tests prior to treatment or procedure

         Z01.818 Encounter for other   PDx
preprocedural examination

> Encounter for preprocedural examination NOS
>
> Encounter for examinations prior to antineoplastic chemotherapy

     Z01.82 Encounter for allergy testing   PDx

> **EXCLUDES 1**   *encounter for antibody response examination (Z01.84)*

     Z01.83 Encounter for blood typing   PDx

> Encounter for Rh typing

     Z01.84 Encounter for antibody response   PDx
examination

> Encounter for immunity status testing
>
> **EXCLUDES 1**   *encounter for allergy testing (Z01.82)*

     Z01.89 Encounter for other specified special   PDx
examinations

√4ᵗʰ **Z02 Encounter for administrative examination**

     Z02.0 Encounter for examination for admission to   PDx
educational institution

> Encounter for examination for admission to preschool (education)
>
> Encounter for examination for re-admission to school following illness or medical treatment

     Z02.1 Encounter for pre-employment examination   PDx

     Z02.2 Encounter for examination for admission to   PDx
residential institution

> **EXCLUDES 1**   *examination for admission to prison (Z02.89)*

     Z02.3 Encounter for examination for recruitment to   PDx
armed forces

     Z02.4 Encounter for examination for driving license   PDx

     Z02.5 Encounter for examination for participation in sport   PDx

> **EXCLUDES 1**   *blood-alcohol and blood-drug test (Z02.83)*

     Z02.6 Encounter for examination for insurance purposes   PDx

√5ᵗʰ **Z02.7 Encounter for issue of medical certificate**

> **EXCLUDES 1**   *encounter for general medical examination (Z00-Z01, Z02.0-Z02.6, Z02.8-Z02.9)*

     Z02.71 Encounter for disability determination   PDx

> Encounter for issue of medical certificate of incapacity
>
> Encounter for issue of medical certificate of invalidity

     Z02.79 Encounter for issue of other medical   PDx
certificate

√5ᵗʰ **Z02.8 Encounter for other administrative examinations**

     Z02.81 Encounter for paternity testing   PDx

     Z02.82 Encounter for adoption services   PDx

     Z02.83 Encounter for blood-alcohol and   PDx
blood-drug test

> Use additional code for findings of alcohol or drugs in blood (R78.-)

◢ Additional Character Required   √x7ᵗʰ Placeholder Alert   Manifestation   Unspecified Dx   ▶◀ Revised Text   ● New Code   ▲ Revised Code Title

Z02.89 Encounter for other administrative examinations `PDx`
- Encounter for examination for admission to prison
- Encounter for examination for admission to summer camp
- Encounter for immigration examination
- Encounter for naturalization examination
- Encounter for premarital examination
  - **EXCLUDES 1** *health supervision of foundling or other healthy infant or child (Z76.1-Z76.2)*

Z02.9 Encounter for administrative examinations, unspecified `PDx`

√4th **Z03** Encounter for medical observation for suspected diseases and conditions ruled out

This category is to be used when a person without a diagnosis is suspected of having an abnormal condition, without signs or symptoms, which requires study, but after examination and observation, is ruled out. This category is also for use for administrative and legal observation status.

EXCLUDES 1 *contact with and (suspected) exposures hazardous to health (Z77.-)*
encounter for observation and evaluation of newborn for suspected diseases and conditions ruled out (Z05.-)
person with feared complaint in whom no diagnosis is made (Z71.1)
signs or symptoms under study — code to signs or symptoms

AHA: 2018,2Q,7-8; 2017,4Q,27

Z03.6 Encounter for observation for suspected toxic effect from ingested substance ruled out `PDx`
- Encounter for observation for suspected adverse effect from drug
- Encounter for observation for suspected poisoning

√5th **Z03.7** Encounter for suspected maternal and fetal conditions ruled out
- Encounter for suspected maternal and fetal conditions not found
  - **EXCLUDES 1** *known or suspected fetal anomalies affecting management of mother, not ruled out (O26.-, O35.-, O36.-, O40.-, O41.-)*

  Z03.71 Encounter for suspected problem with amniotic cavity and membrane ruled out `PDx` `M` ♀
  - Encounter for suspected oligohydramnios ruled out
  - Encounter for suspected polyhydramnios ruled out

  Z03.72 Encounter for suspected placental problem ruled out `PDx` `M` ♀

  Z03.73 Encounter for suspected fetal anomaly ruled out `PDx` `M` ♀

  Z03.74 Encounter for suspected problem with fetal growth ruled out `PDx` `M` ♀

  Z03.75 Encounter for suspected cervical shortening ruled out `PDx` `M` ♀

  Z03.79 Encounter for other suspected maternal and fetal conditions ruled out `PDx` `M` ♀

√5th **Z03.8** Encounter for observation for other suspected diseases and conditions ruled out

  √6th **Z03.81** Encounter for observation for suspected exposure to biological agents ruled out

    Z03.810 Encounter for observation for suspected exposure to anthrax ruled out `PDx`

    Z03.818 Encounter for observation for suspected exposure to other biological agents ruled out `PDx`

  Z03.89 Encounter for observation for other suspected diseases and conditions ruled out `PDx`

√4th **Z04** Encounter for examination and observation for other reasons

INCLUDES encounter for examination for medicolegal reasons

This category is to be used when a person without a diagnosis is suspected of having an abnormal condition, without signs or symptoms, which requires study, but after examination and observation, is ruled-out. This category is also for use for administrative and legal observation status.

AHA: 2018,2Q,7-8

Z04.1 Encounter for examination and observation following transport accident `PDx`
- **EXCLUDES 1** *encounter for examination and observation following work accident (Z04.2)*
- **AHA:** 2019,2Q,11; 2018,2Q,8

Z04.2 Encounter for examination and observation following work accident `PDx`

Z04.3 Encounter for examination and observation following other accident `PDx`

√5th **Z04.4** Encounter for examination and observation following alleged rape
- Encounter for examination and observation of victim following alleged rape
- Encounter for examination and observation of victim following alleged sexual abuse

  Z04.41 Encounter for examination and observation following alleged adult rape `PDx` `A`
  - Suspected adult rape, ruled out
  - Suspected adult sexual abuse, ruled out

  Z04.42 Encounter for examination and observation following alleged child rape `PDx` `P`
  - Suspected child rape, ruled out
  - Suspected child sexual abuse, ruled out

Z04.6 Encounter for general psychiatric examination, requested by authority `PDx`

√5th **Z04.7** Encounter for examination and observation following alleged physical abuse

  Z04.71 Encounter for examination and observation following alleged adult physical abuse `PDx` `A`
  - Suspected adult physical abuse, ruled out
    - **EXCLUDES 1** *confirmed case of adult physical abuse (T74.-)*
    - *encounter for examination and observation following alleged adult sexual abuse (Z04.41)*
    - *suspected case of adult physical abuse, not ruled out (T76.-)*

  Z04.72 Encounter for examination and observation following alleged child physical abuse `PDx` `P`
  - Suspected child physical abuse, ruled out
    - **EXCLUDES 1** *confirmed case of child physical abuse (T74.-)*
    - *encounter for examination and observation following alleged child sexual abuse (Z04.42)*
    - *suspected case of child physical abuse, not ruled out (T76.-)*

√5th **Z04.8** Encounter for examination and observation for other specified reasons
- Encounter for examination and observation for request for expert evidence
- **AHA:** 2018,4Q,32,35,72

  Z04.81 Encounter for examination and observation of victim following forced sexual exploitation `PDx`

  Z04.82 Encounter for examination and observation of victim following forced labor exploitation `PDx`

  Z04.89 Encounter for examination and observation for other specified reasons `PDx`

Z04.9 Encounter for examination and observation for unspecified reason `PDx`
- Encounter for observation NOS

☑️4ᵗʰ **Z05 Encounter for observation and evaluation of newborn for suspected diseases and conditions ruled out**
This category is to be used for newborns, within the neonatal period (the first 28 days of life), who are suspected of having an abnormal condition, but without signs or symptoms, and which, after examination and observation, is ruled out.
AHA: 2017,4Q,27; 2016,4Q,77

Z05.0 Observation and evaluation of newborn for suspected cardiac condition ruled out   N

Z05.1 Observation and evaluation of newborn for suspected infectious condition ruled out   N
AHA: 2019,2Q,10

Z05.2 Observation and evaluation of newborn for suspected neurological condition ruled out   N

Z05.3 Observation and evaluation of newborn for suspected respiratory condition ruled out   N

☑️5ᵗʰ **Z05.4 Observation and evaluation of newborn for suspected genetic, metabolic or immunologic condition ruled out**

    Z05.41 Observation and evaluation of newborn for suspected genetic condition ruled out   N
       AHA: 2016,4Q,55

    Z05.42 Observation and evaluation of newborn for suspected metabolic condition ruled out   N

    Z05.43 Observation and evaluation of newborn for suspected immunologic condition ruled out   N

Z05.5 Observation and evaluation of newborn for suspected gastrointestinal condition ruled out   N

Z05.6 Observation and evaluation of newborn for suspected genitourinary condition ruled out   N

☑️5ᵗʰ **Z05.7 Observation and evaluation of newborn for suspected skin, subcutaneous, musculoskeletal and connective tissue condition ruled out**

    Z05.71 Observation and evaluation of newborn for suspected skin and subcutaneous tissue condition ruled out   N

    Z05.72 Observation and evaluation of newborn for suspected musculoskeletal condition ruled out   N

    Z05.73 Observation and evaluation of newborn for suspected connective tissue condition ruled out   N

Z05.8 Observation and evaluation of newborn for other specified suspected condition ruled out   N

Z05.9 Observation and evaluation of newborn for unspecified suspected condition ruled out   N

Z08 Encounter for follow-up examination after completed treatment for malignant neoplasm
Medical surveillance following completed treatment
Use additional code to identify any acquired absence of organs (Z90.-)
Use additional code to identify the personal history of malignant neoplasm (Z85.-)
EXCLUDES 1   *aftercare following medical care (Z43-Z49, Z51)*

Z09 Encounter for follow-up examination after completed treatment for conditions other than malignant neoplasm
Medical surveillance following completed treatment
Use additional code to identify any applicable history of disease code (Z86.-. Z87.-)
EXCLUDES 1   *aftercare following medical care (Z43-Z49, Z51)*
          surveillance of contraception (Z30.4-)
          surveillance of prosthetic and other medical devices (Z44-Z46)
AHA: 2017,1Q,9; 2015,1Q,8

☑️4ᵗʰ **Z11 Encounter for screening for infectious and parasitic diseases**
Screening is the testing for disease or disease precursors in asymptomatic individuals so that early detection and treatment can be provided for those who test positive for the disease.
EXCLUDES 1   *encounter for diagnostic examination — code to sign or symptom*

Z11.0 Encounter for screening for intestinal infectious diseases

Z11.1 Encounter for screening for respiratory tuberculosis
►Encounter for screening for active tuberculosis disease◄

Z11.2 Encounter for screening for other bacterial diseases

Z11.3 Encounter for screening for infections with a predominantly sexual mode of transmission
EXCLUDES 2   *encounter for screening for human immunodeficiency virus [HIV] (Z11.4)*
          encounter for screening for human papillomavirus (Z11.51)

Z11.4 Encounter for screening for human immunodeficiency virus [HIV]

☑️5ᵗʰ **Z11.5 Encounter for screening for other viral diseases**
EXCLUDES 2   *encounter for screening for viral intestinal disease (Z11.0)*

    Z11.51 Encounter for screening for human papillomavirus (HPV)

    Z11.59 Encounter for screening for other viral diseases

Z11.6 Encounter for screening for other protozoal diseases and helminthiases
EXCLUDES 2   *encounter for screening for protozoal intestinal disease (Z11.0)*

● **Z11.7 Encounter for testing for latent tuberculosis infection**

Z11.8 Encounter for screening for other infectious and parasitic diseases
Encounter for screening for chlamydia
Encounter for screening for rickettsial
Encounter for screening for spirochetal
Encounter for screening for mycoses

Z11.9 Encounter for screening for infectious and parasitic diseases, unspecified

☑️4ᵗʰ **Z12 Encounter for screening for malignant neoplasms**
Screening is the testing for disease or disease precursors in asymptomatic individuals so that early detection and treatment can be provided for those who test positive for the disease.
Use additional code to identify any family history of malignant neoplasm (Z80.-)
EXCLUDES 1   *encounter for diagnostic examination — code to sign or symptom*

Z12.0 Encounter for screening for malignant neoplasm of stomach

☑️5ᵗʰ **Z12.1 Encounter for screening for malignant neoplasm of intestinal tract**
AHA: 2017,1Q,8,9

    Z12.10 Encounter for screening for malignant neoplasm of intestinal tract, unspecified

    Z12.11 Encounter for screening for malignant neoplasm of colon   Q
       Encounter for screening colonoscopy NOS
       AHA: 2019,1Q,32-33; 2018,1Q,6
       TIP: Surveillance colonoscopies are a type of screening exam used to screen for malignancies in those patients with history of polyps and/or cancer (previously removed).

    Z12.12 Encounter for screening for malignant neoplasm of rectum
       AHA: 2018,1Q,6

    Z12.13 Encounter for screening for malignant neoplasm of small intestine

Z12.2 Encounter for screening for malignant neoplasm of respiratory organs

☑️5ᵗʰ **Z12.3 Encounter for screening for malignant neoplasm of breast**

    Z12.31 Encounter for screening mammogram for malignant neoplasm of breast   Q
       EXCLUDES 1   *inconclusive mammogram (R92.2)*
       AHA: 2015,1Q,24

    Z12.39 Encounter for other screening for malignant neoplasm of breast

Z12.4 Encounter for screening for malignant neoplasm of cervix   ♀
Encounter for screening pap smear for malignant neoplasm of cervix
EXCLUDES 1   *when screening is part of general gynecological examination (Z01.4-)*
EXCLUDES 2   *encounter for screening for human papillomavirus (Z11.51)*

Z12.5 Encounter for screening for malignant neoplasm of prostate   ♂

Z12.6 Encounter for screening for malignant neoplasm of bladder

☑️5ᵗʰ **Z12.7 Encounter for screening for malignant neoplasm of other genitourinary organs**

    Z12.71 Encounter for screening for malignant neoplasm of testis   ♂

Z12.72   **Encounter for screening for malignant neoplasm of vagina**   ♀

Vaginal pap smear status-post hysterectomy for non-malignant condition

Use additional code to identify acquired absence of uterus (Z90.71-)

> EXCLUDES 1   *vaginal pap smear status-post hysterectomy for malignant conditions (ZØ8)*

Z12.73   **Encounter for screening for malignant neoplasm of ovary**   ♀

Z12.79   **Encounter for screening for malignant neoplasm of other genitourinary organs**

√5ᵗʰ **Z12.8**   **Encounter for screening for malignant neoplasm of other sites**

Z12.81   **Encounter for screening for malignant neoplasm of oral cavity**

Z12.82   **Encounter for screening for malignant neoplasm of nervous system**

Z12.83   **Encounter for screening for malignant neoplasm of skin**

Z12.89   **Encounter for screening for malignant neoplasm of other sites**

Z12.9   **Encounter for screening for malignant neoplasm, site unspecified**

√4ᵗʰ **Z13**   **Encounter for screening for other diseases and disorders**

Screening is the testing for disease or disease precursors in asymptomatic individuals so that early detection and treatment can be provided for those who test positive for the disease.

> EXCLUDES 1   *encounter for diagnostic examination — code to sign or symptom*

Z13.Ø   **Encounter for screening for diseases of the blood and blood-forming organs and certain disorders involving the immune mechanism**

Z13.1   **Encounter for screening for diabetes mellitus**

√5ᵗʰ **Z13.2**   **Encounter for screening for nutritional, metabolic and other endocrine disorders**

Z13.21   **Encounter for screening for nutritional disorder**

√6ᵗʰ **Z13.22**   **Encounter for screening for metabolic disorder**

Z13.22Ø   **Encounter for screening for lipoid disorders**

Encounter for screening for cholesterol level

Encounter for screening for hypercholesterolemia

Encounter for screening for hyperlipidemia

Z13.228   **Encounter for screening for other metabolic disorders**

Z13.29   **Encounter for screening for other suspected endocrine disorder**

> EXCLUDES 1   *encounter for screening for diabetes mellitus (Z13.1)*

√5ᵗʰ **Z13.3**   **Encounter for screening examination for mental health and behavioral disorders**

AHA: 2018,4Q,35-36

Z13.3Ø   **Encounter for screening examination for mental health and behavioral disorders, unspecified**

Z13.31   **Encounter for screening for depression**

Encounter for screening for depression, adult

Encounter for screening for depression for child or adolescent

Z13.32   **Encounter for screening for maternal depression**   ♀

Encounter for screening for perinatal depression

Z13.39   **Encounter for screening examination for other mental health and behavioral disorders**

Encounter for screening for alcoholism

Encounter for screening for intellectual disabilities

√5ᵗʰ **Z13.4**   **Encounter for screening for certain developmental disorders in childhood**

Encounter for development testing of infant or child

Encounter for screening for developmental handicaps in early childhood

> EXCLUDES 2   *encounter for routine child health examination (ZØØ.12-)*

AHA: 2018,4Q,36

Z13.4Ø   **Encounter for screening for unspecified developmental delays**

Z13.41   **Encounter for autism screening**

Z13.42   **Encounter for screening for global developmental delays (milestones)**

Encounter for screening for developmental handicaps in early childhood

Z13.49   **Encounter for screening for other developmental delays**

Z13.5   **Encounter for screening for eye and ear disorders**

> EXCLUDES 2   *encounter for general hearing examination (ZØ1.1-)*
> *encounter for general vision examination (ZØ1.Ø-)*

AHA: 2016,3Q,17

Z13.6   **Encounter for screening for cardiovascular disorders**

√5ᵗʰ **Z13.7**   **Encounter for screening for genetic and chromosomal anomalies**

> EXCLUDES 1   *genetic testing for procreative management (Z31.4-)*

Z13.71   **Encounter for nonprocreative screening for genetic disease carrier status**

Z13.79   **Encounter for other screening for genetic and chromosomal anomalies**

√5ᵗʰ **Z13.8**   **Encounter for screening for other specified diseases and disorders**

> EXCLUDES 2   *screening for malignant neoplasms (Z12.-)*

√6ᵗʰ **Z13.81**   **Encounter for screening for digestive system disorders**

Z13.81Ø   **Encounter for screening for upper gastrointestinal disorder**

Z13.811   **Encounter for screening for lower gastrointestinal disorder**

> EXCLUDES 1   *encounter for screening for intestinal infectious disease (Z11.Ø)*

Z13.818   **Encounter for screening for other digestive system disorders**

√6ᵗʰ **Z13.82**   **Encounter for screening for musculoskeletal disorder**

Z13.82Ø   **Encounter for screening for osteoporosis**

Z13.828   **Encounter for screening for other musculoskeletal disorder**

Z13.83   **Encounter for screening for respiratory disorder NEC**

> EXCLUDES 1   *encounter for screening for respiratory tuberculosis (Z11.1)*

Z13.84   **Encounter for screening for dental disorders**

√6ᵗʰ **Z13.85**   **Encounter for screening for nervous system disorders**

Z13.85Ø   **Encounter for screening for traumatic brain injury**

Z13.858   **Encounter for screening for other nervous system disorders**

Z13.88   **Encounter for screening for disorder due to exposure to contaminants**

> EXCLUDES 1   *those exposed to contaminants without suspected disorders (Z57.-, Z77.-)*

Z13.89   **Encounter for screening for other disorder**

Encounter for screening for genitourinary disorders

Z13.9   **Encounter for screening, unspecified**

Genetic carrier and genetic susceptibility to disease (Z14-Z15)

√4ᵗʰ **Z14**   **Genetic carrier**

DEF: Individuals carrying a gene mutation associated with a certain disease that typically do not develop the disease but are able to pass the mutated genes to offspring.

√5ᵗʰ **Z14.Ø**   **Hemophilia A carrier**

Z14.Ø1   **Asymptomatic hemophilia A carrier**

Z14.Ø2   **Symptomatic hemophilia A carrier**

Z14.1   **Cystic fibrosis carrier**

Z14.8   **Genetic carrier of other disease**

√4ᵗʰ **Z15**   **Genetic susceptibility to disease**

> INCLUDES   confirmed abnormal gene

Use additional code, if applicable, for any associated family history of the disease (Z8Ø-Z84)

> EXCLUDES 1   *chromosomal anomalies (Q9Ø-Q99)*

√5ᵗʰ **Z15.Ø**   **Genetic susceptibility to malignant neoplasm**

Code first, if applicable, any current malignant neoplasm (CØØ-C75, C81-C96)

Use additional code, if applicable, for any personal history of malignant neoplasm (Z85.-)

Z15.Ø1   **Genetic susceptibility to malignant neoplasm of breast**

Z15.02	**Genetic susceptibility to malignant neoplasm of** ovary	♀
Z15.03	**Genetic susceptibility to malignant neoplasm of** prostate	♂
Z15.04	**Genetic susceptibility to malignant neoplasm of** endometrium	♀
Z15.09	**Genetic susceptibility to other malignant neoplasm**	

✓5ᵗʰ **Z15.8** **Genetic susceptibility to other disease**

Z15.81 **Genetic susceptibility to multiple endocrine neoplasia [MEN]**

> EXCLUDES 1   multiple endocrine neoplasia [MEN] syndromes (E31.2-)

> **DEF:** Group of conditions in which several endocrine glands grow excessively (such as in adenomatous hyperplasia) and/or develop benign or malignant tumors. Tumors and hyperplasia associated with MEN often produce excess hormones, which impede normal physiology. There is no comprehensive cure known for MEN syndrome. Treatment is directed at the hyperplasia or tumors in each individual gland. Tumors are usually surgically removed and oral medications or hormonal injections are used to correct hormone imbalances.

Z15.89 **Genetic susceptibility to other disease**

Resistance to antimicrobial drugs (Z16)

✓4ᵗʰ **Z16** **Resistance to antimicrobial drugs**

> NOTE   The codes in this category are provided for use as additional codes to identify the resistance and non-responsiveness of a condition to antimicrobial drugs.

> Code first the infection

> EXCLUDES 1   Methicillin resistant Staphylococcus aureus infection (A49.02)
> Methicillin resistant Staphylococcus aureus pneumonia (J15.212)
> sepsis due to Methicillin resistant Staphylococcus aureus (A41.02)

✓5ᵗʰ **Z16.1** **Resistance to beta lactam antibiotics**

Z16.10 **Resistance to unspecified beta lactam antibiotics**

Z16.11 **Resistance to penicillins**
Resistance to amoxicillin
Resistance to ampicillin

Z16.12 **Extended spectrum beta lactamase (ESBL) resistance**
> EXCLUDES 2   Methicillin resistant Staphylococcus aureus infection in diseases classified elsewhere (B95.62)

Z16.19 **Resistance to other specified beta lactam antibiotics**
Resistance to cephalosporins

✓5ᵗʰ **Z16.2** **Resistance to other antibiotics**

Z16.20 **Resistance to unspecified antibiotic**
Resistance to antibiotics NOS

Z16.21 **Resistance to vancomycin**

Z16.22 **Resistance to vancomycin related antibiotics**

Z16.23 **Resistance to quinolones and fluoroquinolones**

Z16.24 **Resistance to multiple antibiotics**

Z16.29 **Resistance to other single specified antibiotic**
Resistance to aminoglycosides
Resistance to macrolides
Resistance to sulfonamides
Resistance to tetracyclines

✓5ᵗʰ **Z16.3** **Resistance to other antimicrobial drugs**
> EXCLUDES 1   resistance to antibiotics (Z16.1-, Z16.2-)

Z16.30 **Resistance to unspecified antimicrobial drugs**
Drug resistance NOS

Z16.31 **Resistance to antiparasitic drug(s)**
Resistance to quinine and related compounds

Z16.32 **Resistance to antifungal drug(s)**

Z16.33 **Resistance to antiviral drug(s)**

✓6ᵗʰ **Z16.34** **Resistance to antimycobacterial drug(s)**
Resistance to tuberculostatics

Z16.341 **Resistance to single antimycobacterial drug**
Resistance to antimycobacterial drug NOS

Z16.342 **Resistance to multiple antimycobacterial drugs**

Z16.35 **Resistance to multiple antimicrobial drugs**
> EXCLUDES 1   resistance to multiple antibiotics only (Z16.24)

Z16.39 **Resistance to other specified antimicrobial drug**

Estrogen receptor status (Z17)

✓4ᵗʰ **Z17** **Estrogen receptor status**

Code first malignant neoplasm of breast (C50.-)
DEF: Receptor status of breast cancer cells for the hormone estrogen that is used to help determine treatment and evaluate prognosis. ER+ breast cancer responds to hormone therapies while ER- breast cancer does not.

Z17.0 **Estrogen receptor positive status [ER+]**

Z17.1 **Estrogen receptor negative status [ER-]**

Retained foreign body fragments (Z18)

✓4ᵗʰ **Z18** **Retained foreign body fragments**

> INCLUDES   embedded fragment (status)
> embedded splinter (status)
> retained foreign body status

> EXCLUDES 1   artificial joint prosthesis status (Z96.6-)
> foreign body accidentally left during a procedure (T81.5-)
> foreign body entering through orifice (T15-T19)
> in situ cardiac device (Z95.-)
> organ or tissue replaced by means other than transplant (Z96.-, Z97.-)
> organ or tissue replaced by transplant (Z94.-)
> personal history of retained foreign body fully removed Z87.821
> superficial foreign body (non-embedded splinter) — code to superficial foreign body, by site

> **DEF:** Embedded or retained fragment, splinter, or foreign body, natural or synthetic that can cause infection.

✓5ᵗʰ **Z18.0** **Retained radioactive fragments**

Z18.01 **Retained depleted uranium fragments**

Z18.09 **Other retained radioactive fragments**
Other retained depleted isotope fragments
Retained nontherapeutic radioactive fragments

✓5ᵗʰ **Z18.1** **Retained metal fragments**
> EXCLUDES 1   retained radioactive metal fragments (Z18.01-Z18.09)

Z18.10 **Retained metal fragments, unspecified**
Retained metal fragment NOS

Z18.11 **Retained magnetic metal fragments**

Z18.12 **Retained nonmagnetic metal fragments**

Z18.2 **Retained plastic fragments**
Acrylics fragments
Diethylhexyl phthalates fragments
Isocyanate fragments

✓5ᵗʰ **Z18.3** **Retained organic fragments**

Z18.31 **Retained animal quills or spines**

Z18.32 **Retained tooth**

Z18.33 **Retained wood fragments**

Z18.39 **Other retained organic fragments**

✓5ᵗʰ **Z18.8** **Other specified retained foreign body**

Z18.81 **Retained glass fragments**

Z18.83 **Retained stone or crystalline fragments**
Retained concrete or cement fragments

Z18.89 **Other specified retained foreign body fragments**

Z18.9 **Retained foreign body fragments, unspecified material**

Hormone sensitivity malignancy status (Z19)

✓4ᵗʰ **Z19** **Hormone sensitivity malignancy status**

Code first malignant neoplasm — see Table of Neoplasms, by site, malignant
AHA: 2016,4Q,76

Z19.1 **Hormone sensitive malignancy status**

Z19.2 **Hormone resistant malignancy status**
Castrate resistant prostate malignancy status

◢ Additional Character Required   ✓x7ᵗʰ Placeholder Alert   Manifestation   Unspecified Dx   ▶◀ Revised Text   ● New Code   ▲ Revised Code Title

)-10-CM 2020   **1223**

Persons with potential health hazards related to communicable diseases (Z20-Z29)

✓4ᵗʰ **Z20 Contact with and (suspected) exposure to communicable diseases**

    EXCLUDES 1   carrier of infectious disease (Z22.-)

         diagnosed current infectious or parasitic disease — see Alphabetic Index

    EXCLUDES 2   personal history of infectious and parasitic diseases (Z86.1-)

✓5ᵗʰ **Z20.0 Contact with and (suspected) exposure to intestinal infectious diseases**

    Z20.01 Contact with and (suspected) exposure to intestinal infectious diseases due to Escherichia coli (E. coli)

    Z20.09 Contact with and (suspected) exposure to other intestinal infectious diseases

Z20.1 Contact with and (suspected) exposure to tuberculosis

Z20.2 Contact with and (suspected) exposure to infections with a predominantly sexual mode of transmission

Z20.3 Contact with and (suspected) exposure to rabies

Z20.4 Contact with and (suspected) exposure to rubella

Z20.5 Contact with and (suspected) exposure to viral hepatitis

Z20.6 Contact with and (suspected) exposure to human immunodeficiency virus [HIV]

    EXCLUDES 1   asymptomatic human immunodeficiency virus [HIV] HIV infection status (Z21)

Z20.7 Contact with and (suspected) exposure to pediculosis, acariasis and other infestations

✓5ᵗʰ **Z20.8 Contact with and (suspected) exposure to other communicable diseases**

    ✓6ᵗʰ **Z20.81 Contact with and (suspected) exposure to other bacterial communicable diseases**

        Z20.810 Contact with and (suspected) exposure to anthrax

        Z20.811 Contact with and (suspected) exposure to meningococcus

        Z20.818 Contact with and (suspected) exposure to other bacterial communicable diseases

          AHA: 2019,2Q,10

    ✓6ᵗʰ **Z20.82 Contact with and (suspected) exposure to other viral communicable diseases**

        Z20.820 Contact with and (suspected) exposure to varicella

        Z20.821 Contact with and (suspected) exposure to Zika virus

          AHA: 2018,4Q,35,64

        Z20.828 Contact with and (suspected) exposure to other viral communicable diseases

    Z20.89 Contact with and (suspected) exposure to other communicable diseases

Z20.9 Contact with and (suspected) exposure to unspecified communicable disease

Z21 Asymptomatic human immunodeficiency virus [HIV] infection status   **HCC**

    HIV positive NOS

    Code first human immunodeficiency virus [HIV] disease complicating pregnancy, childbirth and the puerperium, if applicable (O98.7-)

    EXCLUDES 1   acquired immunodeficiency syndrome (B20)

         contact with human immunodeficiency virus [HIV] (Z20.6)

         exposure to human immunodeficiency virus [HIV] (Z20.6)

         human immunodeficiency virus [HIV] disease (B20)

         inconclusive laboratory evidence of human immunodeficiency virus [HIV] (R75)

    AHA: 2019,1Q,8-11

    DEF: Phase of human immunodeficiency virus (HIV) infection with no clinical symptoms. This phase may last for 10 years or more.

✓4ᵗʰ **Z22 Carrier of infectious disease**

    INCLUDES   colonization status

         suspected carrier

    EXCLUDES 2   carrier of viral hepatitis (B18.-)

Z22.0 Carrier of typhoid

Z22.1 Carrier of other intestinal infectious diseases

Z22.2 Carrier of diphtheria

✓5ᵗʰ **Z22.3 Carrier of other specified bacterial diseases**

    Z22.31 Carrier of bacterial disease due to meningococci

    ✓6ᵗʰ **Z22.32 Carrier of bacterial disease due to staphylococci**

        Z22.321 Carrier or suspected carrier of Methicillin susceptible Staphylococcus aureus

          MSSA colonization

        Z22.322 Carrier or suspected carrier of Methicillin resistant Staphylococcus aureus

          MRSA colonization

          DEF: Carriers (colonization) of methicillin resistant Staphylococcus aureus (MRSA) have MRSA on their skin or in their body but do not exhibit signs of infection. These individuals are able to pass MRSA on to others who may develop an infection.

    ✓6ᵗʰ **Z22.33 Carrier of bacterial disease due to streptococci**

        Z22.330 Carrier of Group B streptococcus

          EXCLUDES 1   carrier of streptococcus group B (GBS) complicating pregnancy, childbirth and the puerperium (O99.82-)

        Z22.338 Carrier of other streptococcus

    Z22.39 Carrier of other specified bacterial diseases

Z22.4 Carrier of infections with a predominantly sexual mode of transmission

Z22.6 Carrier of human T-lymphotropic virus type-1 [HTLV-1] infection

Z22.7 Latent tuberculosis

    Latent tuberculosis infection (LTBI)

    EXCLUDES 1   nonspecific reaction to cell mediated immunity measurement of gamma interferon antigen response without active tuberculosis (R76.12)

         nonspecific reaction to tuberculin skin test without active tuberculosis (R76.11)

Z22.8 Carrier of other infectious diseases

Z22.9 Carrier of infectious disease, unspecified

Z23 Encounter for immunization

    Code first any routine childhood examination

    NOTE   Procedure codes are required to identify the types of immunizations given

✓4ᵗʰ **Z28 Immunization not carried out and underimmunization status**

    INCLUDES   vaccination not carried out

✓5ᵗʰ **Z28.0 Immunization not carried out because of contraindication**

    DEF: Contraindication: Situation where a drug, surgery, or other procedure may negatively affect or cause harm to a patient.

    Z28.01 Immunization not carried out because of acute illness of patient

    Z28.02 Immunization not carried out because of chronic illness or condition of patient

    Z28.03 Immunization not carried out because of immune compromised state of patient

    Z28.04 Immunization not carried out because of patient allergy to vaccine or component

    Z28.09 Immunization not carried out because of other contraindication

Z28.1 Immunization not carried out because of patient decision for reasons of belief or group pressure

    Immunization not carried out because of religious belief

✓5ᵗʰ **Z28.2 Immunization not carried out because of patient decision for other and unspecified reason**

    Z28.20 Immunization not carried out because of patient decision for unspecified reason

    Z28.21 Immunization not carried out because of patient refusal

    Z28.29 Immunization not carried out because of patient decision for other reason

Z28.3 Underimmunization status

    Delinquent immunization status

    Lapsed immunization schedule status

✓5ᵗʰ **Z28.8 Immunization not carried out for other reason**

    Z28.81 Immunization not carried out due to patient having had the disease

HCC CMS-HCC   **PDx** Primary Dx Only   **Q** QPP   **N** Newborn: 0   **P** Pediatric: 0-17   **M** Maternity: 12-55   **A** Adult: 15-1

1224   ICD-10-CM 20.

Z28.82   **Immunization not carried out because of** caregiver refusal

Immunization not carried out because of guardian refusal

Immunization not carried out because of parent refusal

> *EXCLUDES 1*   *immunization not carried out because of caregiver refusal because of religious belief (Z28.1)*

Z28.83   **Immunization not carried out due to** unavailability of vaccine

Delay in delivery of vaccine

Lack of availability of vaccine

Manufacturer delay of vaccine

AHA: 2018,4Q,36

Z28.89   **Immunization not carried out for other reason**

Z28.9   **Immunization not carried out for unspecified reason**

✓4ᵗʰ Z29 Encounter for other prophylactic measures

> *EXCLUDES 1*   *desensitization to allergens (Z51.6)*
>
> *prophylactic surgery (Z40.-)*

AHA: 2016,4Q,78-79

✓5ᵗʰ Z29.1   **Encounter for prophylactic immunotherapy**

Encounter for administration of immunoglobulin

Z29.11   **Encounter for prophylactic immunotherapy for** respiratory syncytial virus (RSV)

Z29.12   **Encounter for prophylactic** antivenin

Z29.13   **Encounter for prophylactic** Rho(D) immune globulin

Z29.14   **Encounter for prophylactic** rabies immune globin

Z29.3   **Encounter for prophylactic** fluoride administration

Z29.8   **Encounter for other specified prophylactic measures**

Z29.9   **Encounter for prophylactic measures, unspecified**

Persons encountering health services in circumstances related to reproduction (Z30-Z39)

✓4ᵗʰ Z30 Encounter for contraceptive management

AHA: 2016,4Q,78

DEF: Contraceptive management to prevent pregnancy. Methods include oral medications, intrauterine devices, and surgical procedures for males and females (sterilization).

✓5ᵗʰ Z30.0   **Encounter for general counseling and advice on** contraception

✓6ᵗʰ Z30.01   **Encounter for** initial prescription **of contraceptives**

> *EXCLUDES 1*   *encounter for surveillance of contraceptives (Z30.4-)*

Z30.011   **Encounter for** initial prescription **of contraceptive pills**   ♀

Z30.012   **Encounter for prescription of** emergency **contraception**   ♀

Encounter for postcoital contraception

Z30.013   **Encounter for initial prescription of** injectable **contraceptive**   ♀

Z30.014   **Encounter for initial prescription of** intrauterine **contraceptive device**   ♀

> *EXCLUDES 1*   *encounter for insertion of intrauterine contraceptive device (Z30.430, Z30.432)*

Z30.015   **Encounter for initial prescription of** vaginal ring hormonal **contraceptive**   ♀

Z30.016   **Encounter for initial prescription of** transdermal patch hormonal **contraceptive device**   ♀

Z30.017   **Encounter for initial prescription of** implantable subdermal **contraceptive**   ♀

Z30.018   **Encounter for initial prescription of other contraceptives**   ♀

Encounter for initial prescription of barrier contraception

Encounter for initial prescription of diaphragm

Z30.019   **Encounter for initial prescription of contraceptives, unspecified**   ♀

Z30.02   **Counseling and instruction in** natural family planning **to avoid pregnancy**

Z30.09   **Encounter for other general counseling and advice on contraception**

Encounter for family planning advice NOS

Z30.2   **Encounter for** sterilization

✓5ᵗʰ Z30.4   **Encounter for** surveillance **of contraceptives**

Z30.40   **Encounter for surveillance of contraceptives, unspecified**

Z30.41   **Encounter for surveillance of contraceptive** pills   ♀

Encounter for repeat prescription for contraceptive pill

Z30.42   **Encounter for surveillance of** injectable **contraceptive**   ♀

✓6ᵗʰ Z30.43   **Encounter for surveillance of** intrauterine **contraceptive device**

Z30.430   **Encounter for insertion of intrauterine contraceptive device**   ♀

Z30.431   **Encounter for routine checking of intrauterine contraceptive device**   ♀

Z30.432   **Encounter for removal of intrauterine contraceptive device**   ♀

Z30.433   **Encounter for removal and reinsertion of intrauterine contraceptive device**   ♀

Encounter for replacement of intrauterine contraceptive device

Z30.44   **Encounter for surveillance of** vaginal ring hormonal **contraceptive device**   ♀

Z30.45   **Encounter for surveillance of** transdermal patch hormonal **contraceptive device**   ♀

Z30.46   **Encounter for surveillance of** implantable subdermal **contraceptive**   ♀

Encounter for checking, reinsertion or removal of implantable subdermal contraceptive

Z30.49   **Encounter for surveillance of other contraceptives**   ♀

Encounter for surveillance of barrier contraception

Encounter for surveillance of diaphragm

Z30.8   **Encounter for other contraceptive management**

Encounter for postvasectomy sperm count

Encounter for routine examination for contraceptive maintenance

> *EXCLUDES 1*   *sperm count following sterilization reversal (Z31.42)*
>
> *sperm count for fertility testing (Z31.41)*

Z30.9   **Encounter for contraceptive management, unspecified**

✓4ᵗʰ Z31 Encounter for procreative management

> *EXCLUDES 1*   *complications associated with artificial fertilization (N98.-)*
>
> *female infertility (N97.-)*
>
> *male infertility (N46.-)*

Z31.0   **Encounter for** reversal of previous sterilization

✓5ᵗʰ Z31.4   **Encounter for** procreative investigation and testing

> *EXCLUDES 1*   *postvasectomy sperm count (Z30.8)*

Z31.41   **Encounter for** fertility testing

Encounter for fallopian tube patency testing

Encounter for sperm count for fertility testing

Z31.42   **Aftercare following** sterilization reversal

Sperm count following sterilization reversal

✓6ᵗʰ Z31.43   **Encounter for genetic testing of** female **for procreative management**

Use additional code for recurrent pregnancy loss, if applicable (N96, O26.2-)

> *EXCLUDES 1*   *nonprocreative genetic testing (Z13.7-)*

Z31.430   **Encounter of female for testing for genetic** disease carrier status **for procreative management**   ♀

Z31.438   **Encounter for other genetic testing of female for procreative management**   ♀

✓6ᵗʰ Z31.44   **Encounter for genetic testing of** male **for procreative management**

> *EXCLUDES 1*   *nonprocreative genetic testing (Z13.7-)*

Z31.440   **Encounter of male for testing for genetic** disease carrier status **for procreative management**   ♂

Z31.441   **Encounter for testing of male partner of patient with** recurrent pregnancy loss   Ⓐ ♂

◼ Additional Character Required   **✓x7ᵗʰ** Placeholder Alert   Manifestation   Unspecified Dx   ►◄ Revised Text   ● New Code   ▲ Revised Code Title

◖ ICD-10-CM 2020   **1225**

Chapter 21. Factors Influencing Health Status and Contact With Health Services

Z31.448   **Encounter for other genetic testing of male for procreative management**   A ♂

Z31.49   **Encounter for other procreative investigation and testing**

Z31.5   **Encounter for procreative genetic counseling**
     AHA: 2017,4Q,27

√5ᵗʰ **Z31.6**   **Encounter for general counseling and advice on procreation**

Z31.61   **Procreative counseling and advice using natural family planning**

Z31.62   **Encounter for fertility preservation counseling**
     Encounter for fertility preservation counseling prior to cancer therapy
     Encounter for fertility preservation counseling prior to surgical removal of gonads

Z31.69   **Encounter for other general counseling and advice on procreation**

Z31.7   **Encounter for procreative management and counseling for gestational carrier**   ♀
     EXCLUDES 1   pregnant state, gestational carrier (Z33.3)
     AHA: 2016,4Q,78

√5ᵗʰ **Z31.8**   **Encounter for other procreative management**

Z31.81   **Encounter for male factor infertility in female patient**   PDx ♀

Z31.82   **Encounter for Rh incompatibility status**   ♀
     AHA: 2015,3Q,40; 2014,4Q,17

Z31.83   **Encounter for assisted reproductive fertility procedure cycle**   PDx ♀
     Patient undergoing in vitro fertilization cycle
     Use additional code to identify the type of infertility
     EXCLUDES 1   pre-cycle diagnosis and testing — code to reason for encounter

Z31.84   **Encounter for fertility preservation procedure**   PDx
     Encounter for fertility preservation procedure prior to cancer therapy
     Encounter for fertility preservation procedure prior to surgical removal of gonads

Z31.89   **Encounter for other procreative management**

Z31.9   **Encounter for procreative management, unspecified**

√4ᵗʰ **Z32**   **Encounter for pregnancy test and childbirth and childcare instruction**

√5ᵗʰ **Z32.0**   **Encounter for pregnancy test**

Z32.00   **Encounter for pregnancy test, result unknown**   ♀
     Encounter for pregnancy test NOS

Z32.01   **Encounter for pregnancy test, result positive**   M ♀

Z32.02   **Encounter for pregnancy test, result negative**   ♀

Z32.2   **Encounter for childbirth instruction**

Z32.3   **Encounter for childcare instruction**
     Encounter for prenatal or postpartum childcare instruction

√4ᵗʰ **Z33**   **Pregnant state**

Z33.1   **Pregnant state, incidental**   M ♀
     Pregnant state NOS
     EXCLUDES 1   complications of pregnancy (O00-O9A)
            pregnant state, gestational carrier (Z33.3)

Z33.2   **Encounter for elective termination of pregnancy**   PDx M ♀
     EXCLUDES 1   early fetal death with retention of dead fetus (O02.1)
            late fetal death (O36.4)
            spontaneous abortion (O03)
     TIP: Do not assign a code from category Z3A with this code.

Z33.3   **Pregnant state, gestational carrier**   M ♀
     EXCLUDES 1   encounter for procreative management and counseling for gestational carrier (Z31.7)
     AHA: 2016,4Q,78

√4ᵗʰ **Z34**   **Encounter for supervision of normal pregnancy**
     EXCLUDES 1   any complication of pregnancy (O00-O9A)
            encounter for pregnancy test (Z32.0-)
            encounter for supervision of high risk pregnancy (O09.-)
     AHA: 2014,4Q,17

√5ᵗʰ **Z34.0**   **Encounter for supervision of normal first pregnancy**

Z34.00   **Encounter for supervision of normal first pregnancy, unspecified trimester**   PDx M ♀

Z34.01   **Encounter for supervision of normal first pregnancy, first trimester**   PDx M ♀

Z34.02   **Encounter for supervision of normal first pregnancy, second trimester**   PDx M ♀

Z34.03   **Encounter for supervision of normal first pregnancy, third trimester**   PDx M ♀

√5ᵗʰ **Z34.8**   **Encounter for supervision of other normal pregnancy**

Z34.80   **Encounter for supervision of other normal pregnancy, unspecified trimester**   PDx M ♀

Z34.81   **Encounter for supervision of other normal pregnancy, first trimester**   PDx M ♀

Z34.82   **Encounter for supervision of other normal pregnancy, second trimester**   PDx M ♀

Z34.83   **Encounter for supervision of other normal pregnancy, third trimester**   PDx M ♀

√5ᵗʰ **Z34.9**   **Encounter for supervision of normal pregnancy, unspecified**

Z34.90   **Encounter for supervision of normal pregnancy, unspecified, unspecified trimester**   PDx M ♀

Z34.91   **Encounter for supervision of normal pregnancy, unspecified, first trimester**   PDx M ♀

Z34.92   **Encounter for supervision of normal pregnancy, unspecified, second trimester**   PDx M ♀

Z34.93   **Encounter for supervision of normal pregnancy, unspecified, third trimester**   PDx M ♀

√4ᵗʰ **Z36**   **Encounter for antenatal screening of mother**
     INCLUDES   encounter for placental sample (taken vaginally)
            screening is the testing for disease or disease precursors in asymptomatic individuals so that early detection and treatment can be provided for those who test positive for the disease.
     EXCLUDES 1   diagnostic examination — code to sign or symptom
            encounter for suspected maternal and fetal conditions ruled out (Z03.7-)
            suspected fetal condition affecting management of pregnancy — code to condition in Chapter 15
     EXCLUDES 2   abnormal findings on antenatal screening of mother (O28.-)
            genetic counseling and testing (Z31.43-, Z31.5)
            routine prenatal care (Z34)
     AHA: 2017,4Q,28

Z36.0   **Encounter for antenatal screening for chromosomal anomalies**   M ♀

Z36.1   **Encounter for antenatal screening for raised alphafetoprotein level**   M ♀
     Encounter for antenatal screening for elevated maternal serum alphafetoprotein level
     DEF: High levels of alpha-fetoprotein (AFP) that may indicate a possibility of spina bifida and other neural tube defects, anencephaly, or omphalocele in the fetus.

Z36.2   **Encounter for other antenatal screening follow-up**   M ♀
     Non-visualized anatomy on a previous scan

Z36.3   **Encounter for antenatal screening for malformations**   M ♀
     Screening for a suspected anomaly

Z36.4   **Encounter for antenatal screening for fetal growth retardation**   M ♀
     Intrauterine growth restriction (IUGR)/small-for-dates

Z36.5   **Encounter for antenatal screening for isoimmunization**   M ♀

√5ᵗʰ **Z36.8**   **Encounter for other antenatal screening**

Z36.81   **Encounter for antenatal screening for hydrops fetalis**   M ♀
     DEF: Hydrops fetalis: Abnormal accumulation of fluid in two or more parts of the fetus, such as ascites, effusion of the pleural or pericardial tissues, or edema

Z36.82   **Encounter for antenatal screening for nuchal translucency**   M ♀

Z36.83   **Encounter for fetal screening for congenital cardiac abnormalities**   M ♀

Z36.84   **Encounter for antenatal screening for fetal lung maturity**   M ♀

Z36.85   **Encounter for antenatal screening for Streptococcus B**   M ♀

Z36.86   **Encounter for antenatal screening for cervical length**   M ♀
     Screening for risk of pre-term labor

Z36.87   **Encounter for antenatal screening for uncertain dates**   M ♀

Z36.88   **Encounter for antenatal screening for** fetal macrosomia   Ⓜ♀
     Screening for large-for-dates

Z36.89   **Encounter for other specified antenatal screening**   Ⓜ♀

Z36.8A   **Encounter for antenatal screening for other genetic defects**   Ⓜ♀

Z36.9   **Encounter for antenatal screening, unspecified**   Ⓜ♀

✓4ᵗʰ Z3A Weeks of gestation

NOTE   Codes from category Z3A are for use, only on the maternal record, to indicate the weeks of gestation of the pregnancy, if known.

Code first complications of pregnancy, childbirth and the puerperium (O09-O9A)

AHA: 2019,2Q,11; 2016,2Q,34; 2014,3Q,17; 2014,2Q,9; 2013,2Q,33

TIP: Do not assign a code from this category with codes from categories O00-O08 or code Z33.2.

✓5ᵗʰ **Z3A.0**   **Weeks of gestation of pregnancy,** unspecified or less than 10 weeks

Z3A.00   **Weeks of gestation of pregnancy** not specified   Ⓜ♀

Z3A.01   **Less than 8 weeks gestation of pregnancy**   Ⓜ♀

Z3A.08   **8 weeks gestation of pregnancy**   Ⓜ♀

Z3A.09   **9 weeks gestation of pregnancy**   Ⓜ♀

✓5ᵗʰ **Z3A.1**   **Weeks of gestation of pregnancy, weeks 10-19**

Z3A.10   **10 weeks gestation of pregnancy**   Ⓜ♀

Z3A.11   **11 weeks gestation of pregnancy**   Ⓜ♀

Z3A.12   **12 weeks gestation of pregnancy**   Ⓜ♀

Z3A.13   **13 weeks gestation of pregnancy**   Ⓜ♀

Z3A.14   **14 weeks gestation of pregnancy**   Ⓜ♀

Z3A.15   **15 weeks gestation of pregnancy**   Ⓜ♀

Z3A.16   **16 weeks gestation of pregnancy**   Ⓜ♀

Z3A.17   **17 weeks gestation of pregnancy**   Ⓜ♀

Z3A.18   **18 weeks gestation of pregnancy**   Ⓜ♀

Z3A.19   **19 weeks gestation of pregnancy**   Ⓜ♀

✓5ᵗʰ **Z3A.2**   **Weeks of gestation of pregnancy, weeks 20-29**

Z3A.20   **20 weeks gestation of pregnancy**   Ⓜ♀

Z3A.21   **21 weeks gestation of pregnancy**   Ⓜ♀

Z3A.22   **22 weeks gestation of pregnancy**   Ⓜ♀

Z3A.23   **23 weeks gestation of pregnancy**   Ⓜ♀

Z3A.24   **24 weeks gestation of pregnancy**   Ⓜ♀

Z3A.25   **25 weeks gestation of pregnancy**   Ⓜ♀

Z3A.26   **26 weeks gestation of pregnancy**   Ⓜ♀

Z3A.27   **27 weeks gestation of pregnancy**   Ⓜ♀

Z3A.28   **28 weeks gestation of pregnancy**   Ⓜ♀

Z3A.29   **29 weeks gestation of pregnancy**   Ⓜ♀

✓5ᵗʰ **Z3A.3**   **Weeks of gestation of pregnancy, weeks 30-39**

Z3A.30   **30 weeks gestation of pregnancy**   Ⓜ♀

Z3A.31   **31 weeks gestation of pregnancy**   Ⓜ♀

Z3A.32   **32 weeks gestation of pregnancy**   Ⓜ♀

Z3A.33   **33 weeks gestation of pregnancy**   Ⓜ♀

Z3A.34   **34 weeks gestation of pregnancy**   Ⓜ♀

Z3A.35   **35 weeks gestation of pregnancy**   Ⓜ♀

Z3A.36   **36 weeks gestation of pregnancy**   Ⓜ♀

Z3A.37   **37 weeks gestation of pregnancy**   Ⓜ♀

Z3A.38   **38 weeks gestation of pregnancy**   Ⓜ♀

Z3A.39   **39 weeks gestation of pregnancy**   Ⓜ♀

✓5ᵗʰ **Z3A.4**   **Weeks of gestation of pregnancy, weeks 40 or greater**

AHA: 2014,4Q,23

Z3A.40   **40 weeks gestation of pregnancy**   Ⓜ♀

Z3A.41   **41 weeks gestation of pregnancy**   Ⓜ♀

Z3A.42   **42 weeks gestation of pregnancy**   Ⓜ♀

Z3A.49   **Greater than 42 weeks gestation of pregnancy**   Ⓜ♀

✓4ᵗʰ Z37 Outcome of delivery

This category is intended for use as an additional code to identify the outcome of delivery on the mother's record. It is not for use on the newborn record.

EXCLUDES 1   stillbirth (P95)

Z37.0   **Single live birth**   Ⓜ♀
     AHA: 2016,2Q,34; 2014,2Q,9

Z37.1   **Single stillbirth**   Ⓜ♀

Z37.2   **Twins, both liveborn**   Ⓜ♀

Z37.3   **Twins, one liveborn and one stillborn**   Ⓜ♀

Z37.4   **Twins, both stillborn**   Ⓜ♀

✓5ᵗʰ **Z37.5**   **Other multiple births, all liveborn**

Z37.50   **Multiple births, unspecified, all liveborn**   Ⓜ♀

Z37.51   **Triplets, all liveborn**   Ⓜ♀

Z37.52   **Quadruplets, all liveborn**   Ⓜ♀

Z37.53   **Quintuplets, all liveborn**   Ⓜ♀

Z37.54   **Sextuplets, all liveborn**   Ⓜ♀

Z37.59   **Other multiple births, all liveborn**   Ⓜ♀

✓5ᵗʰ **Z37.6**   **Other multiple births, some liveborn**

Z37.60   **Multiple births, unspecified, some liveborn**   Ⓜ♀

Z37.61   **Triplets, some liveborn**   Ⓜ♀

Z37.62   **Quadruplets, some liveborn**   Ⓜ♀

Z37.63   **Quintuplets, some liveborn**   Ⓜ♀

Z37.64   **Sextuplets, some liveborn**   Ⓜ♀

Z37.69   **Other multiple births, some liveborn**   Ⓜ♀

Z37.7   **Other multiple births, all stillborn**   Ⓜ♀

Z37.9   **Outcome of delivery, unspecified**   Ⓜ♀
     Multiple birth NOS
     Single birth NOS

✓4ᵗʰ Z38 Liveborn infants according to place of birth and type of delivery

This category is for use as the principal code on the initial record of a newborn baby. It is to be used for the initial birth record only. It is not to be used on the mother's record.

AHA: 2017,2Q,5-7; 2016,3Q,18; 2015,2Q,15

TIP: For attending physician services, a code from this category can be reported as first listed every time the physician visits the newborn during the birth admission.

✓5ᵗʰ **Z38.0**   **Single liveborn infant, born in hospital**

Single liveborn infant, born in birthing center or other health care facility

Z38.00   **Single liveborn infant, delivered vaginally**   PDx Ⓝ

Z38.01   **Single liveborn infant, delivered by cesarean**   PDx Ⓝ

Z38.1   **Single liveborn infant, born outside hospital**   PDx Ⓝ

Z38.2   **Single liveborn infant, unspecified as to place of birth**   PDx Ⓝ
     Single liveborn infant NOS

✓5ᵗʰ **Z38.3**   **Twin liveborn infant, born in hospital**

Z38.30   **Twin liveborn infant, delivered vaginally**   PDx Ⓝ

Z38.31   **Twin liveborn infant, delivered by cesarean**   PDx Ⓝ

Z38.4   **Twin liveborn infant, born outside hospital**   PDx Ⓝ

Z38.5   **Twin liveborn infant, unspecified as to place of birth**   PDx Ⓝ

✓5ᵗʰ **Z38.6**   **Other multiple liveborn infant, born in hospital**

Z38.61   **Triplet liveborn infant, delivered vaginally**   PDx Ⓝ

Z38.62   **Triplet liveborn infant, delivered by cesarean**   PDx Ⓝ

Z38.63   **Quadruplet liveborn infant, delivered vaginally**   PDx Ⓝ

Z38.64   **Quadruplet liveborn infant, delivered by cesarean**   PDx Ⓝ

Z38.65   **Quintuplet liveborn infant, delivered vaginally**   PDx Ⓝ

Z38.66   **Quintuplet liveborn infant, delivered by cesarean**   PDx Ⓝ

Z38.68   **Other multiple liveborn infant, delivered vaginally**   PDx Ⓝ

Z38.69   **Other multiple liveborn infant, delivered by cesarean**   PDx Ⓝ

Z38.7   **Other multiple liveborn infant, born outside hospital**   PDx Ⓝ

Additional Character Required   ✓x7ᵗʰ Placeholder Alert   Manifestation   Unspecified Dx   ►◄ Revised Text   ● New Code   ▲ Revised Code Title

-10-CM 2020   1227

Z38.8 Other multiple liveborn infant, unspecified as to place of birth `PDx` `N`

✓4ᵗʰ **Z39** Encounter for maternal postpartum care and examination

Z39.0 Encounter for care and examination of mother immediately after delivery `PDx` `M` ♀
Care and observation in uncomplicated cases when the delivery occurs outside a healthcare facility
EXCLUDES 1　*care for postpartum complication — see Alphabetic Index*

Z39.1 Encounter for care and examination of lactating mother `PDx` `M` ♀
Encounter for supervision of lactation
EXCLUDES 1　*disorders of lactation (O92.-)*

Z39.2 Encounter for routine postpartum follow-up `PDx` `M` ♀

Encounters for other specific health care (Z40-Z53)

Categories Z40-Z53 are intended for use to indicate a reason for care. They may be used for patients who have already been treated for a disease or injury, but who are receiving aftercare or prophylactic care, or care to consolidate the treatment, or to deal with a residual state
EXCLUDES 2　*follow-up examination for medical surveillance after treatment (Z08-Z09)*

✓4ᵗʰ **Z40** Encounter for prophylactic surgery
EXCLUDES 1　*organ donations (Z52.-)*
therapeutic organ removal — code to condition
DEF: Agent or treatment measure intended to prevent or ward off a disease condition.

✓5ᵗʰ **Z40.0** Encounter for prophylactic surgery for risk factors related to malignant neoplasms
Admission for prophylactic organ removal
Use additional code to identify risk factor
AHA: 2017,4Q,28-29

Z40.00 Encounter for prophylactic removal of unspecified organ `PDx`

Z40.01 Encounter for prophylactic removal of breast `PDx`

Z40.02 Encounter for prophylactic removal of ovary(s) `PDx` ♀
Encounter for prophylactic removal of ovary(s) and fallopian tube(s)

Z40.03 Encounter for prophylactic removal of fallopian tube(s) `PDx` ♀

Z40.09 Encounter for prophylactic removal of other organ `PDx`

Z40.8 Encounter for other prophylactic surgery `PDx`

Z40.9 Encounter for prophylactic surgery, unspecified `PDx`

✓4ᵗʰ **Z41** Encounter for procedures for purposes other than remedying health state

Z41.1 Encounter for cosmetic surgery
Encounter for cosmetic breast implant
Encounter for cosmetic procedure
EXCLUDES 1　*encounter for plastic and reconstructive surgery following medical procedure or healed injury (Z42.-)*
encounter for post-mastectomy breast implantation (Z42.1)

Z41.2 Encounter for routine and ritual male circumcision ♂
AHA: 2018,3Q,15
TIP: This code should only be reported when the circumcision is elective (unrelated to a specific diagnosis) and was not performed during the birth admission.

Z41.3 Encounter for ear piercing

Z41.8 Encounter for other procedures for purposes other than remedying health state

Z41.9 Encounter for procedure for purposes other than remedying health state, unspecified

✓4ᵗʰ **Z42** Encounter for plastic and reconstructive surgery following medical procedure or healed injury
EXCLUDES 1　*encounter for cosmetic plastic surgery (Z41.1)*
encounter for plastic surgery for treatment of current injury — code to relevent injury

Z42.1 Encounter for breast reconstruction following mastectomy `PDx` `A`
EXCLUDES 1　*deformity and disproportion of reconstructed breast (N65.1-)*

Z42.8 Encounter for other plastic and reconstructive surgery following medical procedure or healed injury `PDx`
AHA: 2017,1Q,42

✓4ᵗʰ **Z43** Encounter for attention to artificial openings
INCLUDES　closure of artificial openings
passage of sounds or bougies through artificial openings
reforming artificial openings
removal of catheter from artificial openings
toilet or cleansing of artificial openings
EXCLUDES 1　*complications of external stoma (J95.0-, K94.-, N99.5-)*
EXCLUDES 2　*fitting and adjustment of prosthetic and other devices (Z44-Z46)*
AHA: 2019,2Q,33

Z43.0 Encounter for attention to tracheostomy `HCC`

Z43.1 Encounter for attention to gastrostomy `HCC`
EXCLUDES 2　*artificial opening status only, without need for care (Z93.-)*

Z43.2 Encounter for attention to ileostomy `HCC`

Z43.3 Encounter for attention to colostomy `HCC`

Z43.4 Encounter for attention to other artificial openings of digestive tract `HCC`

Z43.5 Encounter for attention to cystostomy `HCC`

Z43.6 Encounter for attention to other artificial openings of urinary tract `HCC`
Encounter for attention to nephrostomy
Encounter for attention to ureterostomy
Encounter for attention to urethrostomy

Z43.7 Encounter for attention to artificial vagina

Z43.8 Encounter for attention to other artificial openings `HCC`

Z43.9 Encounter for attention to unspecified artificial opening `HCC`

✓4ᵗʰ **Z44** Encounter for fitting and adjustment of external prosthetic device
INCLUDES　removal or replacement of external prosthetic device
EXCLUDES 1　*malfunction or other complications of device — see Alphabetical Index*
presence of prosthetic device (Z97.-)

✓5ᵗʰ **Z44.0** Encounter for fitting and adjustment of artificial arm

✓6ᵗʰ **Z44.00** Encounter for fitting and adjustment of unspecified artificial arm

Z44.001 Encounter for fitting and adjustment of unspecified right artificial arm

Z44.002 Encounter for fitting and adjustment of unspecified left artificial arm

Z44.009 Encounter for fitting and adjustment of unspecified artificial arm, unspecified arm

✓6ᵗʰ **Z44.01** Encounter for fitting and adjustment of complete artificial arm

Z44.011 Encounter for fitting and adjustment of complete right artificial arm

Z44.012 Encounter for fitting and adjustment of complete left artificial arm

Z44.019 Encounter for fitting and adjustment of complete artificial arm, unspecified arm

✓6ᵗʰ **Z44.02** Encounter for fitting and adjustment of partial artificial arm

Z44.021 Encounter for fitting and adjustment of partial artificial right arm

Z44.022 Encounter for fitting and adjustment of partial artificial left arm

Z44.029 Encounter for fitting and adjustment of partial artificial arm, unspecified arm

✓5ᵗʰ **Z44.1** Encounter for fitting and adjustment of artificial leg

✓6ᵗʰ **Z44.10** Encounter for fitting and adjustment of unspecified artificial leg

Z44.101 Encounter for fitting and adjustment of unspecified right artificial leg `HCC`

Z44.102 Encounter for fitting and adjustment of unspecified left artificial leg `HCC`

Z44.109 Encounter for fitting and adjustment of unspecified artificial leg, unspecified leg `HCC`

✓6ᵗʰ **Z44.11 Encounter for fitting and adjustment of complete artificial leg**

Z44.111 Encounter for fitting and adjustment of complete right artificial leg `HCC`

Z44.112 Encounter for fitting and adjustment of complete left artificial leg `HCC`

Z44.119 Encounter for fitting and adjustment of complete artificial leg, unspecified leg `HCC`

✓6ᵗʰ **Z44.12 Encounter for fitting and adjustment of partial artificial leg**

Z44.121 Encounter for fitting and adjustment of partial artificial right leg `HCC`

Z44.122 Encounter for fitting and adjustment of partial artificial left leg `HCC`

Z44.129 Encounter for fitting and adjustment of partial artificial leg, unspecified leg `HCC`

✓5ᵗʰ **Z44.2 Encounter for fitting and adjustment of artificial eye**

> *EXCLUDES 1*   mechanical complication of ocular prosthesis (T85.3)

Z44.20 Encounter for fitting and adjustment of artificial eye, unspecified

Z44.21 Encounter for fitting and adjustment of artificial right eye

Z44.22 Encounter for fitting and adjustment of artificial left eye

✓5ᵗʰ **Z44.3 Encounter for fitting and adjustment of external breast prosthesis**

> *EXCLUDES 1*   complications of breast implant (T85.4-)
> encounter for adjustment or removal of breast implant (Z45.81-)
> encounter for initial breast implant insertion for cosmetic breast augmentation (Z41.1)
> encounter for breast reconstruction following mastectomy (Z42.1)

Z44.30 Encounter for fitting and adjustment of external breast prosthesis, unspecified breast

Z44.31 Encounter for fitting and adjustment of external right breast prosthesis

Z44.32 Encounter for fitting and adjustment of external left breast prosthesis

Z44.8 Encounter for fitting and adjustment of other external prosthetic devices

Z44.9 Encounter for fitting and adjustment of unspecified external prosthetic device

✓4ᵗʰ **Z45 Encounter for adjustment and management of implanted device**

`INCLUDES`   removal or replacement of implanted device

EXCLUDES 1   malfunction or other complications of device — see Alphabetical Index

EXCLUDES 2   encounter for fitting and adjustment of non-implanted device (Z46.-)

✓5ᵗʰ **Z45.0 Encounter for adjustment and management of cardiac device**

✓6ᵗʰ **Z45.01 Encounter for adjustment and management of cardiac pacemaker**

Encounter for adjustment and management of cardiac resynchronization therapy pacemaker (CRT-P)

> *EXCLUDES 1*   encounter for adjustment and management of automatic implantable cardiac defibrillator with synchronous cardiac pacemaker (Z45.02)

TIP: Assign an additional code for the condition the pacemaker is controlling (e.g., sick sinus syndrome) only when the interrogation of the pacemaker identifies a problem with this condition.

Z45.010 Encounter for checking and testing of cardiac pacemaker pulse generator [battery]

Encounter for replacing cardiac pacemaker pulse generator [battery]

Z45.018 Encounter for adjustment and management of other part of cardiac pacemaker

> *EXCLUDES 1*   ▶presence of other part of cardiac pacemaker (Z95.0)◀
>
> *EXCLUDES 2*   presence of prosthetic and other devices ▶(Z95.1-Z95.5, Z95.811-Z97)◀

Z45.02 Encounter for adjustment and management of automatic implantable cardiac defibrillator

Encounter for adjustment and management of automatic implantable cardiac defibrillator with synchronous cardiac pacemaker

Encounter for adjustment and management of cardiac resynchronization therapy defibrillator (CRT-D)

Z45.09 Encounter for adjustment and management of other cardiac device

Z45.1 Encounter for adjustment and management of infusion pump

Z45.2 Encounter for adjustment and management of vascular access device

Encounter for adjustment and management of vascular catheters

> *EXCLUDES 1*   encounter for adjustment and management of renal dialysis catheter (Z49.01)

AHA: 2018,3Q,20

✓5ᵗʰ **Z45.3 Encounter for adjustment and management of implanted devices of the special senses**

Z45.31 Encounter for adjustment and management of implanted visual substitution device

✓6ᵗʰ **Z45.32 Encounter for adjustment and management of implanted hearing device**

> *EXCLUDES 1*   encounter for fitting and adjustment of hearing aide (Z46.1)

Z45.320 Encounter for adjustment and management of bone conduction device

Z45.321 Encounter for adjustment and management of cochlear device

Z45.328 Encounter for adjustment and management of other implanted hearing device

✓5ᵗʰ **Z45.4 Encounter for adjustment and management of implanted nervous system device**

Z45.41 Encounter for adjustment and management of cerebrospinal fluid drainage device

Encounter for adjustment and management of cerebral ventricular (communicating) shunt

▲ **Z45.42 Encounter for adjustment and management of neurostimulator**

▶Encounter for adjustment and management of brain neurostimulator◀

▶Encounter for adjustment and management of gastric neurostimulator◀

▶Encounter for adjustment and management of peripheral nerve neurostimulator◀

▶Encounter for adjustment and management of sacral nerve neurostimulator◀

▶Encounter for adjustment and management of spinal cord neurostimulator◀

▶Encounter for adjustment and management of vagus nerve neurostimulator◀

Z45.49 Encounter for adjustment and management of other implanted nervous system device

AHA: 2014,3Q,19

Additional Character Required   ✓x7ᵗʰ Placeholder Alert   Manifestation   Unspecified Dx   ▶◀ Revised Text   ● New Code   ▲ Revised Code Title

-10-CM 2020   1229

Chapter 21. Factors Influencing Health Status and Contact With Health Services

✓5ᵗʰ **Z45.8 Encounter for adjustment and management of other implanted devices**

   ✓6ᵗʰ **Z45.81 Encounter for adjustment or removal of breast implant**

       Encounter for elective implant exchange (different material) (different size)

       ▶Encounter removal of tissue expander with or without synchronous insertion of permanent implant◀

       EXCLUDES 1 *complications of breast implant (T85.4-)*

          encounter for initial breast implant insertion for cosmetic breast augmentation (Z41.1)

          encounter for breast reconstruction following mastectomy (Z42.1)

       Z45.811 Encounter for adjustment or removal of right breast implant

       Z45.812 Encounter for adjustment or removal of left breast implant

       Z45.819 Encounter for adjustment or removal of unspecified breast implant

    Z45.82 Encounter for adjustment or removal of myringotomy device (stent) (tube)

    Z45.89 Encounter for adjustment and management of other implanted devices

       AHA: 2014,4Q,26-28

Z45.9 Encounter for adjustment and management of unspecified implanted device

✓4ᵗʰ **Z46 Encounter for fitting and adjustment of other devices**

    INCLUDES removal or replacement of other device

    EXCLUDES 1 *malfunction or other complications of device — see Alphabetical Index*

    EXCLUDES 2 *encounter for fitting and management of implanted devices (Z45.-)*

       issue of repeat prescription only (Z76.0)

       presence of prosthetic and other devices (Z95-Z97)

Z46.0 Encounter for fitting and adjustment of spectacles and contact lenses

Z46.1 Encounter for fitting and adjustment of hearing aid

    EXCLUDES 1 *encounter for adjustment and management of implanted hearing device (Z45.32-)*

Z46.2 Encounter for fitting and adjustment of other devices related to nervous system and special senses

    EXCLUDES 2 *encounter for adjustment and management of implanted nervous system device (Z45.4-)*

       encounter for adjustment and management of implanted visual substitution device (Z45.31)

Z46.3 Encounter for fitting and adjustment of dental prosthetic device

    Encounter for fitting and adjustment of dentures

Z46.4 Encounter for fitting and adjustment of orthodontic device

✓5ᵗʰ **Z46.5 Encounter for fitting and adjustment of other gastrointestinal appliance and device**

    EXCLUDES 1 *encounter for attention to artificial openings of digestive tract (Z43.1-Z43.4)*

    Z46.51 Encounter for fitting and adjustment of gastric lap band

    Z46.59 Encounter for fitting and adjustment of other gastrointestinal appliance and device

Z46.6 Encounter for fitting and adjustment of urinary device

    EXCLUDES 2 *attention to artificial openings of urinary tract (Z43.5, Z43.6)*

✓5ᵗʰ **Z46.8 Encounter for fitting and adjustment of other specified devices**

    Z46.81 Encounter for fitting and adjustment of insulin pump

       Encounter for insulin pump instruction and training

       Encounter for insulin pump titration

    Z46.82 Encounter for fitting and adjustment of non-vascular catheter

    Z46.89 Encounter for fitting and adjustment of other specified devices

       Encounter for fitting and adjustment of wheelchair

Z46.9 Encounter for fitting and adjustment of unspecified device

✓4ᵗʰ **Z47 Orthopedic aftercare**

    EXCLUDES 1 *aftercare for healing fracture — code to fracture with 7th character D*

Z47.1 Aftercare following joint replacement surgery

    Use additional code to identify the joint (Z96.6-)

Z47.2 Encounter for removal of internal fixation device

    EXCLUDES 1 *encounter for adjustment of internal fixation device for fracture treatment — code to fracture with appropriate 7th character*

       encounter for removal of external fixation device — code to fracture with 7th character D

       infection or inflammatory reaction to internal fixation device (T84.6-)

       mechanical complication of internal fixation device (T84.1-)

✓5ᵗʰ **Z47.3 Aftercare following explantation of joint prosthesis**

    Aftercare following explantation of joint prosthesis, staged procedure

    Encounter for joint prosthesis insertion following prior explantation of joint prosthesis

    AHA: 2015,1Q,16

    Z47.31 Aftercare following explantation of shoulder joint prosthesis

       EXCLUDES 1 *acquired absence of shoulder joint following prior explantation of shoulder joint prosthesis (Z89.23-)*

          shoulder joint prosthesis explantation status (Z89.23-)

    Z47.32 Aftercare following explantation of hip joint prosthesis

       EXCLUDES 1 *acquired absence of hip joint following prior explantation of hip joint prosthesis (Z89.62-)*

          hip joint prosthesis explantation status (Z89.62-)

    Z47.33 Aftercare following explantation of knee joint prosthesis

       EXCLUDES 1 *acquired absence of knee joint following prior explantation of knee prosthesis (Z89.52-)*

          knee joint prosthesis explantation status (Z89.52-)

✓5ᵗʰ **Z47.8 Encounter for other orthopedic aftercare**

    Z47.81 Encounter for orthopedic aftercare following surgical amputation

       Use additional code to identify the limb amputated (Z89.-)

    Z47.82 Encounter for orthopedic aftercare following scoliosis surgery

    Z47.89 Encounter for other orthopedic aftercare

       AHA: 2015,1Q,8

✓4ᵗʰ **Z48 Encounter for other postprocedural aftercare**

    EXCLUDES 1 *encounter for aftercare following injury — code to Injury, by site, with appropriate 7th character for subsequent encounter*

       encounter for follow-up examination after completed treatment (Z08-Z09)

    EXCLUDES 2 *encounter for attention to artificial openings (Z43.-)*

       encounter for fitting and adjustment of prosthetic and other devices (Z44-Z46)

    AHA: 2015,4Q,38; 2015,1Q,6-7

✓5ᵗʰ **Z48.0 Encounter for attention to dressings, sutures and drains**

    EXCLUDES 1 *encounter for planned postprocedural wound closure (Z48.1)*

    Z48.00 Encounter for change or removal of nonsurgical wound dressing

       Encounter for change or removal of wound dressing NOS

    Z48.01 Encounter for change or removal of surgical wound dressing

       AHA: 2019,2Q,33

    Z48.02 Encounter for removal of sutures

       Encounter for removal of staples

    Z48.03 Encounter for change or removal of drains

       AHA: 2019,2Q,33

Z48.1 Encounter for planned postprocedural wound closure

> EXCLUDES 1   encounter for attention to dressings and sutures (Z48.0-)

√5th **Z48.2** Encounter for aftercare following organ transplant

    Z48.21 Encounter for aftercare following heart transplant   HCC

    Z48.22 Encounter for aftercare following kidney transplant

    Z48.23 Encounter for aftercare following liver transplant   HCC

    Z48.24 Encounter for aftercare following lung transplant   HCC

  √6th **Z48.28** Encounter for aftercare following multiple organ transplant

        Z48.280 Encounter for aftercare following heart-lung transplant   HCC

        Z48.288 Encounter for aftercare following multiple organ transplant

  √6th **Z48.29** Encounter for aftercare following other organ transplant

        Z48.290 Encounter for aftercare following bone marrow transplant   HCC

        Z48.298 Encounter for aftercare following other organ transplant

Z48.3 Aftercare following surgery for neoplasm

> Use additional code to identify the neoplasm

√5th **Z48.8** Encounter for other specified postprocedural aftercare

  √6th **Z48.81** Encounter for surgical aftercare following surgery on specified body systems

> These codes identify the body system requiring aftercare. They are for use in conjunction with other aftercare codes to fully explain the aftercare encounter. The condition treated should also be coded if still present.
>
> EXCLUDES 1   aftercare for injury — code the injury with 7th character D
>
> aftercare following surgery for neoplasm (Z48.3)
>
> EXCLUDES 2   aftercare following organ transplant (Z48.2-)
>
> orthopedic aftercare (Z47.-)
>
> AHA: 2015,4Q,38

    Z48.810 Encounter for surgical aftercare following surgery on the sense organs

    Z48.811 Encounter for surgical aftercare following surgery on the nervous system

> EXCLUDES 2   encounter for surgical aftercare following surgery on the sense organs (Z48.810)

    Z48.812 Encounter for surgical aftercare following surgery on the circulatory system

> AHA: 2012,4Q,96

    Z48.813 Encounter for surgical aftercare following surgery on the respiratory system

> AHA: 2019,2Q,33

    Z48.814 Encounter for surgical aftercare following surgery on the teeth or oral cavity

    Z48.815 Encounter for surgical aftercare following surgery on the digestive system

    Z48.816 Encounter for surgical aftercare following surgery on the genitourinary system

> EXCLUDES 1   encounter for aftercare following sterilization reversal (Z31.42)

    Z48.817 Encounter for surgical aftercare following surgery on the skin and subcutaneous tissue

    Z48.89 Encounter for other specified surgical aftercare

√4th **Z49** Encounter for care involving renal dialysis

> Code also associated end stage renal disease (N18.6)

√5th **Z49.0** Preparatory care for renal dialysis

> Encounter for dialysis instruction and training

    Z49.01 Encounter for fitting and adjustment of extracorporeal dialysis catheter   HCC

> Removal or replacement of renal dialysis catheter
>
> Toilet or cleansing of renal dialysis catheter

    Z49.02 Encounter for fitting and adjustment of peritoneal dialysis catheter   HCC

√5th **Z49.3** Encounter for adequacy testing for dialysis

    Z49.31 Encounter for adequacy testing for hemodialysis   HCC

    Z49.32 Encounter for adequacy testing for peritoneal dialysis   HCC

> Encounter for peritoneal equilibration test

√4th **Z51** Encounter for other aftercare and medical care

> Code also condition requiring care
>
> EXCLUDES 1   follow-up examination after treatment (Z08-Z09)

  Z51.0 Encounter for antineoplastic radiation therapy   PDx

> AHA: 2017,4Q,103
>
> TIP: Do not assign when admission is for insertion/implantation of radioactive elements. Assign a code for the malignancy instead. Any complications related to the radioactive elements should be assigned as secondary diagnoses.

√5th **Z51.1** Encounter for antineoplastic chemotherapy and immunotherapy

> EXCLUDES 2   encounter for chemotherapy and immunotherapy for nonneoplastic condition — code to condition

    Z51.11 Encounter for antineoplastic chemotherapy   PDx

> AHA: 2015,3Q,19

    Z51.12 Encounter for antineoplastic immunotherapy   PDx

  Z51.5 Encounter for palliative care

> AHA: 2017,1Q,48

  Z51.6 Encounter for desensitization to allergens

> AHA: 2016,4Q,77

√5th **Z51.8** Encounter for other specified aftercare

> EXCLUDES 1   holiday relief care (Z75.5)

    Z51.81 Encounter for therapeutic drug level monitoring

> Code also any long-term (current) drug therapy (Z79.-)
>
> EXCLUDES 1   encounter for blood-drug test for administrative or medicolegal reasons (Z02.83)
>
> DEF: Drug monitoring: Measurement of the level of a specific drug in the body or measurement of a specific function to assess effectiveness of a drug.

    Z51.89 Encounter for other specified aftercare

> AHA: 2012,4Q,95-97

√4th **Z52** Donors of organs and tissues

> INCLUDES   autologous and other living donors
>
> EXCLUDES 1   cadaveric donor - omit code
>
> examination of potential donor (Z00.5)
>
> AHA: 2012,4Q,99

√5th **Z52.0** Blood donor

  √6th **Z52.00** Unspecified blood donor

        Z52.000 Unspecified donor, whole blood   PDx

        Z52.001 Unspecified donor, stem cells   PDx

        Z52.008 Unspecified donor, other blood   PDx

  √6th **Z52.01** Autologous blood donor

        Z52.010 Autologous donor, whole blood   PDx

        Z52.011 Autologous donor, stem cells   PDx

        Z52.018 Autologous donor, other blood   PDx

  √6th **Z52.09** Other blood donor

> Volunteer donor

        Z52.090 Other blood donor, whole blood   PDx

        Z52.091 Other blood donor, stem cells   PDx

        Z52.098 Other blood donor, other blood   PDx

√5th **Z52.1** Skin donor

    Z52.10 Skin donor, unspecified   PDx

    Z52.11 Skin donor, autologous   PDx

    Z52.19 Skin donor, other   PDx

√5th **Z52.2** Bone donor

    Z52.20 Bone donor, unspecified   PDx

    Z52.21 Bone donor, autologous   PDx

    Z52.29 Bone donor, other   PDx

  Z52.3 Bone marrow donor   PDx

  Z52.4 Kidney donor   PDx

  Z52.5 Cornea donor   PDx

Additional Character Required   √x7th Placeholder Alert   Manifestation   Unspecified Dx   ▶◀ Revised Text   ● New Code   ▲ Revised Code Title

-10-CM 2020   1231

Chapter 21. Factors Influencing Health Status and Contact With Health Services

Z52.6   **Liver** donor   `PDx`

√5ᵗʰ **Z52.8**   **Donor of other specified organs or tissues**

    √6ᵗʰ **Z52.81**   **Egg (Oocyte)** donor

       Z52.810   **Egg (Oocyte)** donor **under age 35, anonymous** recipient   `PDx` ♀
             Egg donor under age 35 NOS

       Z52.811   **Egg (Oocyte)** donor **under age 35, designated** recipient   `PDx` ♀

       Z52.812   **Egg (Oocyte)** donor **age 35 and over, anonymous** recipient   `PDx` ♀
             Egg donor age 35 and over NOS

       Z52.813   **Egg (Oocyte)** donor **age 35 and over, designated** recipient   `PDx` ♀

       Z52.819   **Egg (Oocyte)** donor, **unspecified**   `PDx` ♀

    Z52.89   **Donor of other specified organs or tissues**   `PDx`

Z52.9   **Donor of unspecified organ or tissue**
      Donor NOS

√4ᵗʰ **Z53**   **Persons encountering health services for specific procedures and treatment, not carried out**

√5ᵗʰ **Z53.0**   **Procedure and treatment not carried out because of contraindication**

    Z53.01   **Procedure and treatment not carried out due to patient smoking**

    Z53.09   **Procedure and treatment not carried out because of other contraindication**

Z53.1   **Procedure and treatment not carried out because of patient's decision for** reasons of belief and group pressure

√5ᵗʰ **Z53.2**   **Procedure and treatment not carried out because of patient's decision for other and unspecified reasons**

    Z53.20   **Procedure and treatment not carried out because of patient's decision for unspecified reasons**

    Z53.21   **Procedure and treatment not carried out due to patient** leaving prior to being seen by health care provider

    Z53.29   **Procedure and treatment not carried out because of patient's decision for other reasons**

√5ᵗʰ **Z53.3**   **Procedure converted to open procedure**
      AHA: 2016,4Q,79

    Z53.31   **Laparoscopic** surgical procedure converted to open procedure

    Z53.32   **Thoracoscopic** surgical procedure converted to open procedure

    Z53.33   **Arthroscopic** surgical procedure converted to open procedure

    Z53.39   **Other specified procedure converted to open procedure**

Z53.8   **Procedure and treatment not carried out for other reasons**

Z53.9   **Procedure and treatment not carried out, unspecified reason**

Persons with potential health hazards related to socioeconomic and psychosocial circumstances (Z55-Z65)

AHA: 2018,4Q,58,73; 2018,1Q,18
TIP: Codes from this code block can be assigned based on documentation from clinicians other than the diagnosing provider.

√4ᵗʰ **Z55**   **Problems related to education and literacy**
      EXCLUDES 1   disorders of psychological development (F80-F89)

Z55.0   **Illiteracy and low-level literacy**

Z55.1   **Schooling unavailable and unattainable**

Z55.2   **Failed school examinations**

Z55.3   **Underachievement in school**

Z55.4   **Educational maladjustment and discord with teachers and classmates**

Z55.8   **Other problems related to education and literacy**
      Problems related to inadequate teaching

Z55.9   **Problems related to education and literacy, unspecified**
      Academic problems NOS

√4ᵗʰ **Z56**   **Problems related to employment and unemployment**
      EXCLUDES 2   occupational exposure to risk factors (Z57.-)
             problems related to housing and economic circumstances (Z59.-)

Z56.0   **Unemployment, unspecified**

Z56.1   **Change of job**   `A`

Z56.2   **Threat of job loss**

Z56.3   **Stressful work schedule**

Z56.4   **Discord with boss and workmates**

Z56.5   **Uncongenial work environment**
      Difficult conditions at work

Z56.6   **Other physical and mental strain related to work**

√5ᵗʰ **Z56.8**   **Other problems related to employment**

    Z56.81   **Sexual harassment on the job**

    Z56.82   **Military deployment status**
         Individual (civilian or military) currently deployed in theater or in support of military war, peacekeeping and humanitarian operations

    Z56.89   **Other problems related to employment**

Z56.9   **Unspecified problems related to employment**
      Occupational problems NOS

√4ᵗʰ **Z57**   **Occupational exposure to risk factors**

Z57.0   **Occupational exposure to** noise

Z57.1   **Occupational exposure to** radiation

Z57.2   **Occupational exposure to** dust

√5ᵗʰ **Z57.3**   **Occupational exposure to other air contaminants**

    Z57.31   **Occupational exposure to environmental** tobacco smoke
         EXCLUDES 2   exposure to environmental tobacco smoke (Z77.22)

    Z57.39   **Occupational exposure to other air contaminants**

Z57.4   **Occupational exposure to** toxic agents in agriculture
      Occupational exposure to solids, liquids, gases or vapors in agriculture

Z57.5   **Occupational exposure to** toxic agents in other industries
      Occupational exposure to solids, liquids, gases or vapors in other industries

Z57.6   **Occupational exposure to** extreme temperature

Z57.7   **Occupational exposure to** vibration

Z57.8   **Occupational exposure to other risk factors**

Z57.9   **Occupational exposure to unspecified risk factor**

√4ᵗʰ **Z59**   **Problems related to housing and economic circumstances**
      EXCLUDES 2   problems related to upbringing (Z62.-)

Z59.0   **Homelessness**

Z59.1   **Inadequate housing**
      Lack of heating
      Restriction of space
      Technical defects in home preventing adequate care
      Unsatisfactory surroundings
      EXCLUDES 1   problems related to the natural and physical environment (Z77.1-)

Z59.2   **Discord with neighbors, lodgers and landlord**

Z59.3   **Problems related to living in residential institution**
      Boarding-school resident
      EXCLUDES 1   institutional upbringing (Z62.2)

Z59.4   **Lack of adequate food and safe drinking water**
      Inadequate drinking water supply
      EXCLUDES 1   effects of hunger (T73.0)
             inappropriate diet or eating habits (Z72.4)
             malnutrition (E40-E46)

Z59.5   **Extreme poverty**

Z59.6   **Low income**

Z59.7   **Insufficient social insurance and welfare support**

Z59.8   **Other problems related to housing and economic circumstances**
      Foreclosure on loan
      Isolated dwelling
      Problems with creditors

Z59.9   **Problem related to housing and economic circumstances, unspecified**

√4ᵗʰ **Z60**   **Problems related to social environment**

Z60.0   **Problems of adjustment to life-cycle transitions**
      Empty nest syndrome
      Phase of life problem
      Problem with adjustment to retirement [pension]

Z60.2   **Problems related to living alone**

Z60.3   **Acculturation difficulty**
      Problem with migration
      Problem with social transplantation
      DEF: Problem adapting to a different culture or environment not based on any coexisting mental disorder.

Z60.4   **Social exclusion and rejection**
Exclusion and rejection on the basis of personal characteristics, such as unusual physical appearance, illness or behavior.
> *EXCLUDES 1*   *target of adverse discrimination such as for racial or religious reasons (Z60.5)*

Z60.5   **Target of (perceived) adverse discrimination and persecution**
> *EXCLUDES 1*   *social exclusion and rejection (Z60.4)*

Z60.8   **Other problems related to social environment**

Z60.9   **Problem related to social environment, unspecified**

✓4ᵗʰ **Z62**   **Problems related to upbringing**
> *INCLUDES*   current and past negative life events in childhood
> current and past problems of a child related to upbringing
> *EXCLUDES 2*   *maltreatment syndrome (T74.-)*
> *problems related to housing and economic circumstances (Z59.-)*

Z62.0   **Inadequate parental supervision and control**

Z62.1   **Parental overprotection**

✓5ᵗʰ **Z62.2**   **Upbringing away from parents**
> *EXCLUDES 1*   *problems with boarding school (Z59.3)*

Z62.21   **Child in welfare custody**   **P**
Child in care of non-parental family member
Child in foster care
> *EXCLUDES 2*   *problem for parent due to child in welfare custody (Z63.5)*

Z62.22   **Institutional upbringing**
Child living in orphanage or group home

Z62.29   **Other upbringing away from parents**

Z62.3   **Hostility towards and scapegoating of child**   **P**

Z62.6   **Inappropriate (excessive) parental pressure**

✓5ᵗʰ **Z62.8**   **Other specified problems related to upbringing**

✓6ᵗʰ **Z62.81**   **Personal history of abuse in childhood**

Z62.810   **Personal history of physical and sexual abuse in childhood**
> *EXCLUDES 1*   *current child physical abuse (T74.12, T76.12)*
> *current child sexual abuse (T74.22, T76.22)*

Z62.811   **Personal history of psychological abuse in childhood**
> *EXCLUDES 1*   *current child psychological abuse (T74.32, T76.32)*

Z62.812   **Personal history of neglect in childhood**
> *EXCLUDES 1*   *current child neglect (T74.02, T76.02)*

Z62.813   **Personal history of forced labor or sexual exploitation in childhood**
AHA: 2018,4Q,32,35

Z62.819   **Personal history of unspecified abuse in childhood**
> *EXCLUDES 1*   *current child abuse NOS (T74.92, T76.92)*

✓6ᵗʰ **Z62.82**   **Parent-child conflict**

Z62.820   **Parent-biological child conflict**
Parent-child problem NOS

Z62.821   **Parent-adopted child conflict**

Z62.822   **Parent-foster child conflict**

✓6ᵗʰ **Z62.89**   **Other specified problems related to upbringing**

Z62.890   **Parent-child estrangement NEC**

Z62.891   **Sibling rivalry**

Z62.898   **Other specified problems related to upbringing**

Z62.9   **Problem related to upbringing, unspecified**

✓4ᵗʰ **Z63**   **Other problems related to primary support group, including family circumstances**
> *EXCLUDES 2*   *maltreatment syndrome (T74.-, T76)*
> *parent-child problems (Z62.-)*
> *problems related to negative life events in childhood (Z62.-)*
> *problems related to upbringing (Z62.-)*

Z63.0   **Problems in relationship with spouse or partner**
Relationship distress with spouse or intimate partner
> *EXCLUDES 1*   *counseling for spousal or partner abuse problems (Z69.1)*
> *counseling related to sexual attitude, behavior, and orientation (Z70.-)*

Z63.1   **Problems in relationship with in-laws**

✓5ᵗʰ **Z63.3**   **Absence of family member**
> *EXCLUDES 1*   *absence of family member due to disappearance and death (Z63.4)*
> *absence of family member due to separation and divorce (Z63.5)*

Z63.31   **Absence of family member due to military deployment**
Individual or family affected by other family member being on military deployment
> *EXCLUDES 1*   *family disruption due to return of family member from military deployment (Z63.71)*

Z63.32   **Other absence of family member**

Z63.4   **Disappearance and death of family member**
Assumed death of family member
Bereavement
AHA: 2014,1Q,25

Z63.5   **Disruption of family by separation and divorce**
Marital estrangement

Z63.6   **Dependent relative needing care at home**

✓5ᵗʰ **Z63.7**   **Other stressful life events affecting family and household**

Z63.71   **Stress on family due to return of family member from military deployment**
Individual or family affected by family member having returned from military deployment (current or past conflict)

Z63.72   **Alcoholism and drug addiction in family**

Z63.79   **Other stressful life events affecting family and household**
Anxiety (normal) about sick person in family
Health problems within family
Ill or disturbed family member
Isolated family

Z63.8   **Other specified problems related to primary support group**
Family discord NOS
Family estrangement NOS
High expressed emotional level within family
Inadequate family support NOS
Inadequate or distorted communication within family

Z63.9   **Problem related to primary support group, unspecified**
Relationship disorder NOS

✓4ᵗʰ **Z64**   **Problems related to certain psychosocial circumstances**

Z64.0   **Problems related to unwanted pregnancy**   ♀

Z64.1   **Problems related to multiparity**   ♀

Z64.4   **Discord with counselors**
Discord with probation officer
Discord with social worker

✓4ᵗʰ **Z65**   **Problems related to other psychosocial circumstances**

Z65.0   **Conviction in civil and criminal proceedings without imprisonment**

Z65.1   **Imprisonment and other incarceration**

Z65.2   **Problems related to release from prison**

Z65.3   **Problems related to other legal circumstances**
Arrest
Child custody or support proceedings
Litigation
Prosecution

Z65.4   **Victim of crime and terrorism**
Victim of torture

Z65.5   **Exposure to disaster, war and other hostilities**
> *EXCLUDES 1*   *target of perceived discrimination or persecution (Z60.5)*

Z65.8   **Other specified problems related to psychosocial circumstances**
Religious or spiritual problem

Z65.9   **Problem related to unspecified psychosocial circumstances**

Do not resuscitate status (Z66)

Z66   **Do not resuscitate**
DNR status
DEF: Medical order written by a physician that instructs others not to perform cardiopulmonary resuscitation (CPR), intubation, or advanced life support (ACLS). It prevents unnecessary invasive treatment to prolong life should breathing stop or cardiac arrest occur.

Additional Character Required   ✓x7ᵗʰ Placeholder Alert   Manifestation   Unspecified Dx   ▶◀ Revised Text   ● New Code   ▲ Revised Code Title

-10-CM 2020   1233

Blood type (Z67)

✓4th Z67 Blood type
AHA: 2015,3Q,40

Blood Types

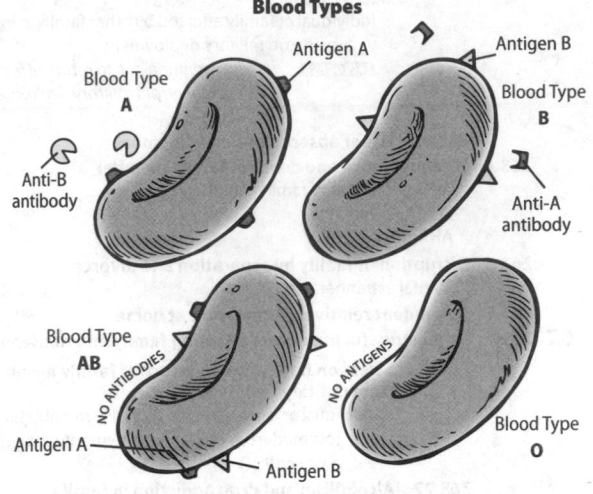

✓5th Z67.1 Type A blood
- Z67.1Ø Type A blood, Rh positive
- Z67.11 Type A blood, Rh negative

✓5th Z67.2 Type B blood
- Z67.2Ø Type B blood, Rh positive
- Z67.21 Type B blood, Rh negative

✓5th Z67.3 Type AB blood
- Z67.3Ø Type AB blood, Rh positive
- Z67.31 Type AB blood, Rh negative

✓5th Z67.4 Type O blood
- Z67.4Ø Type O blood, Rh positive
- Z67.41 Type O blood, Rh negative

✓5th Z67.9 Unspecified blood type
- Z67.9Ø Unspecified blood type, Rh positive
- Z67.91 Unspecified blood type, Rh negative

Body mass index [BMI] (Z68)

✓4th Z68 Body mass index [BMI]
Kilograms per meters squared
> **NOTE** ▶BMI adult codes are for use for persons 2Ø years of age or older◄
> ▶BMI pediatric codes are for use for persons 2-19 years of age.◄
> ▶These percentiles are based on the growth charts published by the Centers for Disease Control and Prevention(CDC)◄

AHA: 2018,4Q,73,77-83; 2017,1Q,39
DEF: Index used to help determine whether an individual is underweight, a healthy weight, overweight, or obese.
TIP: A BMI code may be assigned to support an associated condition based on medical record documentation from clinicians who are not the patient's provider.
TIP: In order to assign a BMI code, the associated condition must meet the definition of a reportable diagnosis for outpatient encounters, per section IV.J of the *ICD-10-CM Official Guidelines for Coding and Reporting.*

- **Z68.1 Body mass index [BMI] 19.9 or less, adult** Ⓐ
- **✓5th Z68.2 Body mass index [BMI] 20-29, adult**
  - Z68.2Ø Body mass index [BMI] 20.0-20.9, adult Ⓐ
  - Z68.21 Body mass index [BMI] 21.0-21.9, adult Ⓐ
  - Z68.22 Body mass index [BMI] 22.0-22.9, adult Ⓐ
  - Z68.23 Body mass index [BMI] 23.0-23.9, adult Ⓐ
  - Z68.24 Body mass index [BMI] 24.0-24.9, adult Ⓐ
  - Z68.25 Body mass index [BMI] 25.0-25.9, adult Ⓐ
  - Z68.26 Body mass index [BMI] 26.0-26.9, adult Ⓐ
  - Z68.27 Body mass index [BMI] 27.0-27.9, adult Ⓐ
  - Z68.28 Body mass index [BMI] 28.0-28.9, adult Ⓐ
  - Z68.29 Body mass index [BMI] 29.0-29.9, adult Ⓐ
- **✓5th Z68.3 Body mass index [BMI] 30-39, adult**
  - Z68.3Ø Body mass index [BMI] 30.0-30.9, adult Ⓐ
  - Z68.31 Body mass index [BMI] 31.0-31.9, adult Ⓐ
  - Z68.32 Body mass index [BMI] 32.0-32.9, adult Ⓐ
  - Z68.33 Body mass index [BMI] 33.0-33.9, adult Ⓐ
  - Z68.34 Body mass index [BMI] 34.0-34.9, adult Ⓐ
  - Z68.35 Body mass index [BMI] 35.0-35.9, adult Ⓐ
  - Z68.36 Body mass index [BMI] 36.0-36.9, adult Ⓐ
  - Z68.37 Body mass index [BMI] 37.0-37.9, adult Ⓐ
  - Z68.38 Body mass index [BMI] 38.0-38.9, adult Ⓐ
  - Z68.39 Body mass index [BMI] 39.0-39.9, adult Ⓐ
- **✓5th Z68.4 Body mass index [BMI] 40 or greater, adult**
  - Z68.41 Body mass index [BMI] 40.0-44.9, adult ᴴᶜᶜ Ⓐ
  - Z68.42 Body mass index [BMI] 45.0-49.9, adult ᴴᶜᶜ Ⓐ
  - Z68.43 Body mass index [BMI] 50.0-59.9, adult ᴴᶜᶜ Ⓐ
  - Z68.44 Body mass index [BMI] 60.0-69.9, adult ᴴᶜᶜ Ⓐ
  - Z68.45 Body mass index [BMI] 70 or greater, adult ᴴᶜᶜ Ⓐ
- **✓5th Z68.5 Body mass index [BMI] pediatric**
  AHA: 2018,4Q,81-82
  - Z68.51 Body mass index [BMI] pediatric, less than 5th percentile for age
  - Z68.52 Body mass index [BMI] pediatric, 5th percentile to less than 85th percentile for age
  - Z68.53 Body mass index [BMI] pediatric, 85th percentile to less than 95th percentile for age
  - Z68.54 Body mass index [BMI] pediatric, greater than or equal to 95th percentile for age

Persons encountering health services in other circumstances (Z69-Z76)

✓4th Z69 Encounter for mental health services for victim and perpetrator of abuse
> **INCLUDES** counseling for victims and perpetrators of abuse

✓5th Z69.Ø Encounter for mental health services for child abuse problems

✓6th Z69.Ø1 Encounter for mental health services for parental child abuse

Z69.Ø1Ø Encounter for mental health services for victim of parental child abuse Ⓟ
> Encounter for mental health services for victim of child abuse by parent
> Encounter for mental health services for victim of child neglect by parent
> Encounter for mental health services for victim of child psychological abuse by parent
> Encounter for mental health services for victim of child sexual abuse by parent

Z69.Ø11 Encounter for mental health services for perpetrator of parental child abuse
> Encounter for mental health services for perpetrator of parental child neglect
> Encounter for mental health services for perpetrator of parental child psychological abuse
> Encounter for mental health services for perpetrator of parental child sexual abuse
> **EXCLUDES 1** encounter for mental health services for non-parental child abuse (Z69.Ø2-)

✓6ᵗʰ **Z69.02** **Encounter for mental health services for non-parental child abuse**

    Z69.020 **Encounter for mental health services for** *victim of* **non-parental child abuse** Ⓟ

        Encounter for mental health services for victim of non-parental child neglect

        Encounter for mental health services for victim of non-parental child psychological abuse

        Encounter for mental health services for victim of non-parental child sexual abuse

    Z69.021 **Encounter for mental health services for** **perpetrator of non-parental child abuse**

        Encounter for mental health services for perpetrator of non-parental child neglect

        Encounter for mental health services for perpetrator of non-parental child psychological abuse

        Encounter for mental health services for perpetrator of non-parental child sexual abuse

✓5ᵗʰ **Z69.1** **Encounter for mental health services for** *spousal or partner* **abuse** **problems**

    Z69.11 **Encounter for mental health services for** *victim of* **spousal or partner abuse**

        Encounter for mental health services for victim of spouse or partner neglect

        Encounter for mental health services for victim of spouse or partner psychological abuse

        Encounter for mental health services for victim of spouse or partner violence, physical

    Z69.12 **Encounter for mental health services for** **perpetrator of spousal or partner abuse**

        Encounter for mental health services for perpetrator of spouse or partner neglect

        Encounter for mental health services for perpetrator of spouse or partner psychological abuse

        Encounter for mental health services for perpetrator of spouse or partner violence, physical

        Encounter for mental health services for perpetrator of spouse or partner violence, sexual

✓5ᵗʰ **Z69.8** **Encounter for mental health services for victim or perpetrator of other abuse**

    Z69.81 **Encounter for mental health services for** *victim of* **other abuse**

        ~~Encounter for mental health services for perpetrator of non-spousal adult abuse~~

        Encounter for mental health services for victim of non-spousal adult abuse

        Encounter for mental health services for victim of spouse or partner violence, sexual

        Encounter for rape victim counseling

    Z69.82 **Encounter for mental health services for** **perpetrator of other abuse**

        ►Encounter for mental health services for perpetrator of non-spousal adult abuse◄

✓4ᵗʰ **Z70** **Counseling related to sexual attitude, behavior and orientation**

    INCLUDES   encounter for mental health services for sexual attitude, behavior and orientation

    EXCLUDES 2   *contraceptive or procreative counseling (Z30-Z31)*

Z70.0 **Counseling related to sexual attitude**

Z70.1 **Counseling related to patient's sexual behavior and orientation**

    Patient concerned regarding impotence

    Patient concerned regarding non-responsiveness

    Patient concerned regarding promiscuity

    Patient concerned regarding sexual orientation

Z70.2 **Counseling related to sexual behavior and orientation of third party**

    Advice sought regarding sexual behavior and orientation of child

    Advice sought regarding sexual behavior and orientation of partner

    Advice sought regarding sexual behavior and orientation of spouse

Z70.3 **Counseling related to combined concerns regarding sexual attitude, behavior and orientation**

Z70.8 **Other sex counseling**

    Encounter for sex education

Z70.9 **Sex counseling, unspecified**

✓4ᵗʰ **Z71** **Persons encountering health services for other counseling and medical advice, not elsewhere classified**

    EXCLUDES 2   *contraceptive or procreation counseling (Z30-Z31)*

                 sex counseling (Z70.-)

Z71.0 **Person encountering health services to consult on behalf of another person**

    Person encountering health services to seek advice or treatment for non-attending third party

    EXCLUDES 2   *anxiety (normal) about sick person in family (Z63.7)*

                 expectant (adoptive) parent(s) pre-birth pediatrician visit (Z76.81)

Z71.1 **Person with feared health complaint in whom no diagnosis is made**

    Person encountering health services with feared condition which was not demonstrated

    Person encountering health services in which problem was normal state

    "Worried well"

    EXCLUDES 1   *medical observation for suspected diseases and conditions proven not to exist (Z03.-)*

Z71.2 **Person consulting for explanation of examination or test findings**

Z71.3 **Dietary counseling and surveillance**

    Use additional code for any associated underlying medical condition

    Use additional code to identify body mass index (BMI), if known (Z68.-)

✓5ᵗʰ **Z71.4** **Alcohol abuse counseling and surveillance**

    Use additional code for alcohol abuse or dependence (F10.-)

    Z71.41 **Alcohol abuse counseling and surveillance of alcoholic**

    Z71.42 **Counseling for family member of alcoholic**

        Counseling for significant other, partner, or friend of alcoholic

✓5ᵗʰ **Z71.5** **Drug abuse counseling and surveillance**

    Use additional code for drug abuse or dependence (F11-F16, F18-F19)

    Z71.51 **Drug abuse counseling and surveillance of drug abuser**

    Z71.52 **Counseling for family member of drug abuser**

        Counseling for significant other, partner, or friend of drug abuser

Z71.6 **Tobacco abuse counseling**

    Use additional code for nicotine dependence (F17.-)

Z71.7 **Human immunodeficiency virus [HIV] counseling**

✓5ᵗʰ **Z71.8** **Other specified counseling**

    EXCLUDES 2   *counseling for contraception (Z30.0-)*

    AHA: 2017,4Q,27

    Z71.81 **Spiritual or religious counseling**

    Z71.82 **Exercise counseling**

    Z71.83 **Encounter for nonprocreative genetic counseling**

        EXCLUDES 1   *counseling for procreative genetics (Z31.5)*

                 counseling for procreative management (Z31.6)

    Z71.84 **Encounter for health counseling related to travel**

        Encounter for health risk and safety counseling for (international) travel

        Code also, if applicable, encounter for immunization (Z23)

        EXCLUDES 2   *encounter for administrative examination (Z02.-)*

                 encounter for other special examination without complaint, suspected or reported diagnosis (Z01.-)

    Z71.89 **Other specified counseling**

Z71.9 **Counseling, unspecified**

    Encounter for medical advice NOS

Additional Character Required   ✓x7ᵗʰ Placeholder Alert   Manifestation   Unspecified Dx   ►◄ Revised Text   ● New Code   ▲ Revised Code Title

-10-CM 2020   1235

Chapter 21. Factors Influencing Health Status and Contact With Health Services

✓4ᵗʰ **Z72 Problems related to lifestyle**

> EXCLUDES 2   *problems related to life-management difficulty (Z73.-)*
>
> *problems related to socioeconomic and psychosocial circumstances (Z55-Z65)*

Z72.0 Tobacco use
Tobacco use NOS

> EXCLUDES 1   *history of tobacco dependence (Z87.891)*
>
> *nicotine dependence (F17.2-)*
>
> *tobacco dependence (F17.2-)*
>
> *tobacco use during pregnancy (O99.33-)*

Z72.3 Lack of physical exercise

Z72.4 Inappropriate diet and eating habits

> EXCLUDES 1   *behavioral eating disorders of infancy or childhood (F98.2-F98.3)*
>
> *eating disorders (F50.-)*
>
> *lack of adequate food (Z59.4)*
>
> *malnutrition and other nutritional deficiencies (E40-E64)*

✓5ᵗʰ **Z72.5 High risk sexual behavior**
Promiscuity

> EXCLUDES 1   *paraphilias (F65)*

Z72.51 High risk heterosexual behavior

Z72.52 High risk homosexual behavior

Z72.53 High risk bisexual behavior

Z72.6 Gambling and betting

> EXCLUDES 1   *compulsive or pathological gambling (F63.0)*

✓5ᵗʰ **Z72.8 Other problems related to lifestyle**

✓6ᵗʰ **Z72.81 Antisocial behavior**

> EXCLUDES 1   *conduct disorders (F91.-)*

Z72.810 Child and adolescent antisocial behavior   P
Antisocial behavior (child) (adolescent) without manifest psychiatric disorder
Delinquency NOS
Group delinquency
Offenses in the context of gang membership
Stealing in company with others
Truancy from school

Z72.811 Adult antisocial behavior   A
Adult antisocial behavior without manifest psychiatric disorder

✓6ᵗʰ **Z72.82 Problems related to sleep**

Z72.820 Sleep deprivation
Lack of adequate sleep

> EXCLUDES 1   *insomnia (G47.0-)*

Z72.821 Inadequate sleep hygiene
Bad sleep habits
Irregular sleep habits
Unhealthy sleep wake schedule

> EXCLUDES 1   *insomnia (F51.0-, G47.0-)*

Z72.89 Other problems related to lifestyle
Self-damaging behavior

Z72.9 Problem related to lifestyle, unspecified

✓4ᵗʰ **Z73 Problems related to life management difficulty**

> EXCLUDES 2   *problems related to socioeconomic and psychosocial circumstances (Z55-Z65)*

DEF: State of emotional, mental, and physical exhaustion causing difficulties in managing personal, school, or work circumstances. It is usually due to prolonged stress or poor interpersonal relationship skills or parenting skills.

Z73.0 Burn-out

Z73.1 Type A behavior pattern

Z73.2 Lack of relaxation and leisure

Z73.3 Stress, not elsewhere classified
Physical and mental strain NOS

> EXCLUDES 1   *stress related to employment or unemployment (Z56.-)*

Z73.4 Inadequate social skills, not elsewhere classified

Z73.5 Social role conflict, not elsewhere classified

Z73.6 Limitation of activities due to disability

> EXCLUDES 1   *care-provider dependency (Z74.-)*

✓5ᵗʰ **Z73.8 Other problems related to life management difficulty**

✓6ᵗʰ **Z73.81 Behavioral insomnia of childhood**

DEF: Behaviors on the part of the child or caregivers that cause negative compliance with a child's sleep schedule resulting in lack of adequate sleep.

Z73.810 Behavioral insomnia of childhood, sleep-onset association type   P

Z73.811 Behavioral insomnia of childhood, limit setting type   P

Z73.812 Behavioral insomnia of childhood, combined type   P

Z73.819 Behavioral insomnia of childhood, unspecified type   P

Z73.82 Dual sensory impairment

Z73.89 Other problems related to life management difficulty

Z73.9 Problem related to life management difficulty, unspecified

✓4ᵗʰ **Z74 Problems related to care provider dependency**

> EXCLUDES 2   *dependence on enabling machines or devices NEC (Z99.-)*

✓5ᵗʰ **Z74.0 Reduced mobility**

Z74.01 Bed confinement status
Bedridden

Z74.09 Other reduced mobility
Chair ridden
Reduced mobility NOS

> EXCLUDES 2   *wheelchair dependence (Z99.3)*

Z74.1 Need for assistance with personal care

Z74.2 Need for assistance at home and no other household member able to render care

Z74.3 Need for continuous supervision

Z74.8 Other problems related to care provider dependency

Z74.9 Problem related to care provider dependency, unspecified

✓4ᵗʰ **Z75 Problems related to medical facilities and other health care**

Z75.0 Medical services not available in home

> EXCLUDES 1   *no other household member able to render care (Z74.2)*

Z75.1 Person awaiting admission to adequate facility elsewhere

Z75.2 Other waiting period for investigation and treatment

Z75.3 Unavailability and inaccessibility of health-care facilities

> EXCLUDES 1   *bed unavailable (Z75.1)*

Z75.4 Unavailability and inaccessibility of other helping agencies

Z75.5 Holiday relief care

Z75.8 Other problems related to medical facilities and other health care

Z75.9 Unspecified problem related to medical facilities and other health care

✓4ᵗʰ **Z76 Persons encountering health services in other circumstances**

Z76.0 Encounter for issue of repeat prescription
Encounter for issue of repeat prescription for appliance
Encounter for issue of repeat prescription for medicaments
Encounter for issue of repeat prescription for spectacles

> EXCLUDES 2   *issue of medical certificate (Z02.7)*
>
> *repeat prescription for contraceptive (Z30.4-)*

Z76.1 Encounter for health supervision and care of foundling   PDx

Z76.2 Encounter for health supervision and care of other healthy infant and child   PDx P
Encounter for medical or nursing care or supervision of healthy infant under circumstances such as adverse socioeconomic conditions at home
Encounter for medical or nursing care or supervision of healthy infant under circumstances such as awaiting foster or adoptive placement
Encounter for medical or nursing care or supervision of healthy infant under circumstances such as maternal illness
Encounter for medical or nursing care or supervision of healthy infant under circumstances such as number of children at home preventing or interfering with normal care

Z76.3 Healthy person accompanying sick person

Z76.4 Other boarder to healthcare facility

> EXCLUDES 1   *homelessness (Z59.0)*

Z76.5 **Malingerer [conscious simulation]**
Person feigning illness (with obvious motivation)
EXCLUDES 1   *factitious disorder (F68.1-, F68.A)*
   peregrinating patient (F68.1-)
DEF: Act of intentionally exaggerating an illness or disability in order to receive personal gain or to avoid punishment or responsibility.

√5ᵗʰ **Z76.8** **Persons encountering health services in other specified circumstances**

Z76.81 **Expectant parent(s) prebirth pediatrician visit**
Pre-adoption pediatrician visit for adoptive parent(s)

Z76.82 **Awaiting organ transplant status**
Patient waiting for organ availability

Z76.89 **Persons encountering health services in other specified circumstances**
Persons encountering health services NOS
AHA: 2014,2Q,10

Persons with potential health hazards related to family and personal history and certain conditions influencing health status (Z77-Z99)

Code also any follow-up examination (Z08-Z09)

√4ᵗʰ **Z77** **Other contact with and (suspected) exposures hazardous to health**
INCLUDES   contact with and (suspected) exposures to potential hazards to health
EXCLUDES 2   *contact with and (suspected) exposure to communicable diseases (Z20.-)*
   exposure to (parental) (environmental) tobacco smoke in the perinatal period (P96.81)
   newborn affected by noxious substances transmitted via placenta or breast milk (P04.-)
   occupational exposure to risk factors (Z57.-)
   retained foreign body (Z18.-)
   retained foreign body fully removed (Z87.821)
   toxic effects of substances chiefly nonmedicinal as to source (T51-T65)

√5ᵗʰ **Z77.0** **Contact with and (suspected) exposure to hazardous, chiefly nonmedicinal, chemicals**

√6ᵗʰ **Z77.01** **Contact with and (suspected) exposure to hazardous metals**

Z77.010 **Contact with and (suspected) exposure to arsenic**

Z77.011 **Contact with and (suspected) exposure to lead**

Z77.012 **Contact with and (suspected) exposure to uranium**
EXCLUDES 1   *retained depleted uranium fragments (Z18.01)*

Z77.018 **Contact with and (suspected) exposure to other hazardous metals**
Contact with and (suspected) exposure to chromium compounds
Contact with and (suspected) exposure to nickel dust

√6ᵗʰ **Z77.02** **Contact with and (suspected) exposure to hazardous aromatic compounds**

Z77.020 **Contact with and (suspected) exposure to aromatic amines**

Z77.021 **Contact with and (suspected) exposure to benzene**

Z77.028 **Contact with and (suspected) exposure to other hazardous aromatic compounds**
Aromatic dyes NOS
Polycyclic aromatic hydrocarbons

√6ᵗʰ **Z77.09** **Contact with and (suspected) exposure to other hazardous, chiefly nonmedicinal, chemicals**

Z77.090 **Contact with and (suspected) exposure to asbestos**

Z77.098 **Contact with and (suspected) exposure to other hazardous, chiefly nonmedicinal, chemicals**
Dyes NOS

√5ᵗʰ **Z77.1** **Contact with and (suspected) exposure to environmental pollution and hazards in the physical environment**

√6ᵗʰ **Z77.11** **Contact with and (suspected) exposure to environmental pollution**

Z77.110 **Contact with and (suspected) exposure to air pollution**

Z77.111 **Contact with and (suspected) exposure to water pollution**

Z77.112 **Contact with and (suspected) exposure to soil pollution**

Z77.118 **Contact with and (suspected) exposure to other environmental pollution**

√6ᵗʰ **Z77.12** **Contact with and (suspected) exposure to hazards in the physical environment**

Z77.120 **Contact with and (suspected) exposure to mold (toxic)**

Z77.121 **Contact with and (suspected) exposure to harmful algae and algae toxins**
Contact with and (suspected) exposure to (harmful) algae bloom NOS
Contact with and (suspected) exposure to blue-green algae bloom
Contact with and (suspected) exposure to brown tide
Contact with and (suspected) exposure to cyanobacteria bloom
Contact with and (suspected) exposure to Florida red tide
Contact with and (suspected) exposure to pfiesteria piscicida
Contact with and (suspected) exposure to red tide

Z77.122 **Contact with and (suspected) exposure to noise**

Z77.123 **Contact with and (suspected) exposure to radon and other naturally occurring radiation**
EXCLUDES 2   *radiation exposure as the cause of a confirmed condition (W88-W90, X39.0-)*
   radiation sickness NOS (T66)

Z77.128 **Contact with and (suspected) exposure to other hazards in the physical environment**

√5ᵗʰ **Z77.2** **Contact with and (suspected) exposure to other hazardous substances**

Z77.21 **Contact with and (suspected) exposure to potentially hazardous body fluids**

Z77.22 **Contact with and (suspected) exposure to environmental tobacco smoke (acute) (chronic)**
Exposure to second hand tobacco smoke (acute) (chronic)
Passive smoking (acute) (chronic)
EXCLUDES 1   *nicotine dependence (F17.-)*
   tobacco use (Z72.0)
EXCLUDES 2   *occupational exposure to environmental tobacco smoke (Z57.31)*

Z77.29 **Contact with and (suspected) exposure to other hazardous substances**
AHA: 2016,2Q,33

Z77.9 **Other contact with and (suspected) exposures hazardous to health**

√4ᵗʰ **Z78** **Other specified health status**
EXCLUDES 2   *asymptomatic human immunodeficiency virus [HIV] infection status (Z21)*
   postprocedural status (Z93-Z99)
   sex reassignment status (Z87.890)

Z78.0 **Asymptomatic menopausal state**   Ⓐ ♀
Menopausal state NOS
Postmenopausal status NOS
EXCLUDES 2   *symptomatic menopausal state (N95.1)*

Z78.1 **Physical restraint status**
EXCLUDES 1   *physical restraint due to a procedure — omit code*
DEF: Application of mechanical restraining devices or manual restraints to limit physical mobility of a patient.

Z78.9 **Other specified health status**

✓4ᵗʰ **Z79 Long term (current) drug therapy**

    INCLUDES   long term (current) drug use for prophylactic purposes

    Code also any therapeutic drug level monitoring (Z51.81)

    EXCLUDES 2   drug abuse and dependence (F11-F19)

        drug use complicating pregnancy, childbirth, and the puerperium (O99.32-)

        long term (current) use of oral antidiabetic drugs (Z79.84)

        long term (current) use of oral hypoglycemic drugs (Z79.84)

✓5ᵗʰ **Z79.0 Long term (current) use of anticoagulants and antithrombotics/antiplatelets**

    EXCLUDES 2   long term (current) use of aspirin (Z79.82)

    Z79.01 Long term (current) use of anticoagulants

    Z79.02 Long term (current) use of antithrombotics/antiplatelets

Z79.1 Long term (current) use of non-steroidal anti-inflammatories (NSAID)

    EXCLUDES 2   long term (current) use of aspirin (Z79.82)

Z79.2 Long term (current) use of antibiotics

Z79.3 Long term (current) use of hormonal contraceptives

    Long term (current) use of birth control pill or patch

Z79.4 Long term (current) use of insulin   **HCC**

    TIP: When both long-term (current) insulin and long-term (current) oral hypoglycemic use is documented, assign only a code for the long-term insulin use.

✓5ᵗʰ **Z79.5 Long term (current) use of steroids**

    Z79.51 Long term (current) use of inhaled steroids

    Z79.52 Long term (current) use of systemic steroids

✓5ᵗʰ **Z79.8 Other long term (current) drug therapy**

    ✓6ᵗʰ **Z79.81 Long term (current) use of agents affecting estrogen receptors and estrogen levels**

       Code first, if applicable:

       malignant neoplasm of breast (C50.-)

       malignant neoplasm of prostate (C61)

       Use additional code, if applicable, to identify:

       estrogen receptor positive status (Z17.0)

       family history of breast cancer (Z80.3)

       genetic susceptibility to malignant neoplasm (cancer) (Z15.0-)

       personal history of breast cancer (Z85.3)

       personal history of prostate cancer (Z85.46)

       postmenopausal status (Z78.0)

       EXCLUDES 1   hormone replacement therapy (Z79.890)

       Z79.810 Long term (current) use of selective estrogen receptor modulators (SERMs)

          Long term (current) use of raloxifene (Evista)

          Long term (current) use of tamoxifen (Nolvadex)

          Long term (current) use of toremifene (Fareston)

       Z79.811 Long term (current) use of aromatase inhibitors

          Long term (current) use of anastrozole (Arimidex)

          Long term (current) use of exemestane (Aromasin)

          Long term (current) use of letrozole (Femara)

       Z79.818 Long term (current) use of other agents affecting estrogen receptors and estrogen levels

          Long term (current) use of estrogen receptor downregulators

          Long term (current) use of fulvestrant (Faslodex)

          Long term (current) use of gonadotropin-releasing hormone (GnRH) agonist

          Long term (current) use of goserelin acetate (Zoladex)

          Long term (current) use of leuprolide acetate (leuprorelin) (Lupron)

          Long term (current) use of megestrol acetate (Megace)

    Z79.82 Long term (current) use of aspirin

    Z79.83 Long term (current) use of bisphosphonates

       AHA: 2016,4Q,42

Z79.84 Long term (current) use of oral hypoglycemic drugs

    Long term (current) use of oral antidiabetic drugs

    EXCLUDES 2   long term (current) use of insulin (Z79.4)

    AHA: 2016,4Q,76

    TIP: When both long-term (current) insulin and long-term (current) oral hypoglycemic use is documented, assign only code Z79.4 for the long-term insulin use.

✓6ᵗʰ **Z79.89 Other long term (current) drug therapy**

    Z79.890 Hormone replacement therapy

    Z79.891 Long term (current) use of opiate analgesic

       Long term (current) use of methadone for pain management

       EXCLUDES 1   methodone use NOS (F11.9-)

          use of methodone for treatment of heroin addiction (F11.2-)

    Z79.899 Other long term (current) drug therapy

       AHA: 2015,4Q,34; 2015,3Q,21

✓4ᵗʰ **Z80 Family history of primary malignant neoplasm**

    Z80.0 Family history of malignant neoplasm of digestive organs

       Conditions classifiable to C15-C26

       AHA: 2018,1Q,6

    Z80.1 Family history of malignant neoplasm of trachea, bronchus and lung

       Conditions classifiable to C33-C34

    Z80.2 Family history of malignant neoplasm of other respiratory and intrathoracic organs

       Conditions classifiable to C30-C32, C37-C39

    Z80.3 Family history of malignant neoplasm of breast

       Conditions classifiable to C50.-

✓5ᵗʰ   **Z80.4 Family history of malignant neoplasm of genital organs**

       Conditions classifiable to C51-C63

    Z80.41 Family history of malignant neoplasm of ovary

    Z80.42 Family history of malignant neoplasm of prostate

    Z80.43 Family history of malignant neoplasm of testis

    Z80.49 Family history of malignant neoplasm of other genital organs

✓5ᵗʰ   **Z80.5 Family history of malignant neoplasm of urinary tract**

       Conditions classifiable to C64-C68

    Z80.51 Family history of malignant neoplasm of kidney

    Z80.52 Family history of malignant neoplasm of bladder

    Z80.59 Family history of malignant neoplasm of other urinary tract organ

    Z80.6 Family history of leukemia

       Conditions classifiable to C91-C95

    Z80.7 Family history of other malignant neoplasms of lymphoid, hematopoietic and related tissues

       Conditions classifiable to C81-C90, C96.-

    Z80.8 Family history of malignant neoplasm of other organs or systems

       Conditions classifiable to C00-C14, C40-C49, C69-C79

    Z80.9 Family history of malignant neoplasm, unspecified

       Conditions classifiable to C80.1

✓4ᵗʰ **Z81 Family history of mental and behavioral disorders**

    Z81.0 Family history of intellectual disabilities

       Conditions classifiable to F70-F79

    Z81.1 Family history of alcohol abuse and dependence

       Conditions classifiable to F10.-

    Z81.2 Family history of tobacco abuse and dependence

       Conditions classifiable to F17.-

    Z81.3 Family history of other psychoactive substance abuse and dependence

       Conditions classifiable to F11-F16, F18-F19

    Z81.4 Family history of other substance abuse and dependence

       Conditions classifiable to F55

    Z81.8 Family history of other mental and behavioral disorders

       Conditions classifiable elsewhere in F01-F99

✓4ᵗʰ **Z82 Family history of certain disabilities and chronic diseases (leading to disablement)**

    Z82.0 Family history of epilepsy and other diseases of the nervous system

       Conditions classifiable to G00-G99

    Z82.1 Family history of blindness and visual loss

       Conditions classifiable to H54.-

HCC CMS-HCC   **PDx** Primary Dx Only   **Q** QPP   **N** Newborn: 0   **P** Pediatric: 0-17   **M** Maternity: 12-55   **A** Adult: 15

1238   ICD-10-CM 2

Z82.2 **Family history of** deafness and hearing loss
Conditions classifiable to H9Ø-H91

Z82.3 **Family history of** stroke
Conditions classifiable to I6Ø-I64

✓5ᵗʰ **Z82.4** **Family history of ischemic heart disease and other diseases of the circulatory system**
Conditions classifiable to IØØ-I52, I65-I99

Z82.41 **Family history of** sudden cardiac death

Z82.49 **Family history of** ischemic heart disease **and other diseases of the circulatory system**

Z82.5 **Family history of** asthma **and other chronic lower respiratory diseases**
Conditions classifiable to J4Ø-J47
EXCLUDES 2   family history of other diseases of the respiratory system (Z83.6)

✓5ᵗʰ **Z82.6** **Family history of arthritis and other diseases of the musculoskeletal system and connective tissue**
Conditions classifiable to MØØ-M99

Z82.61 **Family history of** arthritis

Z82.62 **Family history of** osteoporosis

Z82.69 **Family history of other diseases of the musculoskeletal system and connective tissue**

✓5ᵗʰ **Z82.7** **Family history of congenital malformations, deformations and chromosomal abnormalities**
Conditions classifiable to QØØ-Q99

Z82.71 **Family history of** polycystic kidney

Z82.79 **Family history of other congenital malformations, deformations and chromosomal abnormalities**

Z82.8 **Family history of other disabilities and chronic diseases leading to disablement, not elsewhere classified**

✓4ᵗʰ **Z83** **Family history of other specific disorders**
EXCLUDES 2   contact with and (suspected) exposure to communicable disease in the family (Z2Ø.-)

Z83.Ø **Family history of** human immunodeficiency virus **[HIV] disease**
Conditions classifiable to B2Ø

Z83.1 **Family history of other infectious and parasitic diseases**
Conditions classifiable to AØØ-B19, B25-B94, B99

Z83.2 **Family history of diseases of the** blood and blood-forming organs **and certain disorders involving the immune mechanism**
Conditions classifiable to D5Ø-D89

Z83.3 **Family history of** diabetes mellitus
Conditions classifiable to EØ8-E13

✓6ᵗʰ **Z83.4** **Family history of other endocrine, nutritional and metabolic diseases**
Conditions classifiable to EØØ-EØ7, E15-E88

Z83.41 **Family history of** multiple endocrine neoplasia **[MEN] syndrome**

Z83.42 **Family history of** familial hypercholesterolemia
AHA: 2016,4Q,77

✓6ᵗʰ **Z83.43** **Family history of other disorder of lipoprotein metabolism and other lipidemias**
AHA: 2018,4Q,6,35

Z83.43Ø **Family history of** elevated lipoprotein(a)
Family history of elevated Lp(a)

Z83.438 **Family history of other disorder of lipoprotein metabolism and other lipidemia**
Family history of familial combined hyperlipidemia

Z83.49 **Family history of other endocrine, nutritional and metabolic diseases**

✓5ᵗʰ **Z83.5** **Family history of eye and ear disorders**

✓6ᵗʰ **Z83.51** **Family history of** eye **disorders**
Conditions classifiable to HØØ-H53, H55-H59
EXCLUDES 2   family history of blindness and visual loss (Z82.1)

Z83.511 **Family history of** glaucoma

Z83.518 **Family history of other specified eye disorder**

Z83.52 **Family history of** ear **disorders**
Conditions classifiable to H6Ø-H83, H92-H95
EXCLUDES 2   family history of deafness and hearing loss (Z82.2)

Z83.6 **Family history of other diseases of the** respiratory system
Conditions classifiable to JØØ-J39, J6Ø-J99
EXCLUDES 2   family history of asthma and other chronic lower respiratory diseases (Z82.5)

✓5ᵗʰ **Z83.7** **Family history of diseases of the digestive system**
Conditions classifiable to KØØ-K93

Z83.71 **Family history of** colonic polyps
EXCLUDES 2   family history of malignant neoplasm of digestive organs (Z8Ø.Ø)

Z83.79 **Family history of other diseases of the digestive system**

✓4ᵗʰ **Z84** **Family history of other conditions**

Z84.Ø **Family history of diseases of the** skin and subcutaneous tissue
Conditions classifiable to LØØ-L99

Z84.1 **Family history of disorders of** kidney and ureter
Conditions classifiable to NØØ-N29

Z84.2 **Family history of other diseases of the** genitourinary system
Conditions classifiable to N3Ø-N99

Z84.3 **Family history of** consanguinity

✓5ᵗʰ **Z84.8** **Family history of other specified conditions**

Z84.81 **Family history of carrier of** genetic disease

Z84.82 **Family history of sudden infant death syndrome**
Family history of SIDS
AHA: 2016,4Q,77

Z84.89 **Family history of other specified conditions**

✓4ᵗʰ **Z85** **Personal history of malignant neoplasm**
Code first any follow-up examination after treatment of malignant neoplasm (ZØ8)
Use additional code to identify:
alcohol use and dependence (F1Ø.-)
exposure to environmental tobacco smoke (Z77.22)
history of tobacco dependence (Z87.891)
occupational exposure to environmental tobacco smoke (Z57.31)
tobacco dependence (F17.-)
tobacco use (Z72.Ø)
EXCLUDES 2   personal history of benign neoplasm (Z86.Ø1-)
personal history of carcinoma-in-situ (Z86.ØØ-)
AHA: 2018,4Q,64

✓5ᵗʰ **Z85.Ø** **Personal history of malignant neoplasm of** digestive organs
AHA: 2017,1Q,9

Z85.ØØ **Personal history of malignant neoplasm of unspecified digestive organ**

Z85.Ø1 **Personal history of malignant neoplasm of** esophagus
Conditions classifiable to C15

✓6ᵗʰ **Z85.Ø2** **Personal history of malignant neoplasm of** stomach

Z85.Ø2Ø **Personal history of malignant** carcinoid tumor **of stomach**
Conditions classifiable to C7A.Ø92

Z85.Ø28 **Personal history of other malignant neoplasm of stomach**
Conditions classifiable to C16

✓6ᵗʰ **Z85.Ø3** **Personal history of malignant neoplasm of** large intestine

Z85.Ø3Ø **Personal history of malignant** carcinoid tumor **of large intestine**
Conditions classifiable to C7A.Ø22-C7A.Ø25, C7A.Ø29

Z85.Ø38 **Personal history of other malignant neoplasm of large intestine**
Conditions classifiable to C18

✓6ᵗʰ **Z85.Ø4** **Personal history of malignant neoplasm of** rectum, rectosigmoid junction, and anus

Z85.Ø4Ø **Personal history of malignant** carcinoid tumor **of rectum**
Conditions classifiable to C7A.Ø26

Z85.Ø48 **Personal history of other malignant neoplasm of rectum, rectosigmoid junction, and anus**
Conditions classifiable to C19-C21

Z85.Ø5 **Personal history of malignant neoplasm of** liver
Conditions classifiable to C22

✓6ᵗʰ **Z85.06 Personal history of malignant neoplasm of** small intestine

    Z85.060 Personal history of malignant carcinoid **tumor of small intestine**
        Conditions classifiable to C7A.01-

    Z85.068 Personal history of other malignant neoplasm of small intestine
        Conditions classifiable to C17

Z85.07 Personal history of malignant neoplasm of pancreas
    Conditions classifiable to C25

Z85.09 Personal history of malignant neoplasm of other digestive organs

✓5ᵗʰ **Z85.1 Personal history of malignant neoplasm of** trachea, bronchus and lung

    ✓6ᵗʰ **Z85.11 Personal history of malignant neoplasm of** bronchus and lung

        Z85.110 Personal history of malignant carcinoid **tumor of bronchus and lung**
            Conditions classifiable to C7A.090

        Z85.118 Personal history of other malignant neoplasm of bronchus and lung
            Conditions classifiable to C34

    Z85.12 Personal history of malignant neoplasm of trachea
        Conditions classifiable to C33

✓5ᵗʰ **Z85.2 Personal history of malignant neoplasm of other** respiratory and intrathoracic organs

    Z85.20 Personal history of malignant neoplasm of unspecified respiratory organ

    Z85.21 Personal history of malignant neoplasm of larynx
        Conditions classifiable to C32

    Z85.22 Personal history of malignant neoplasm of nasal cavities, middle ear, and accessory sinuses
        Conditions classifiable to C30-C31

    ✓6ᵗʰ **Z85.23 Personal history of malignant neoplasm of** thymus

        Z85.230 Personal history of malignant carcinoid **tumor of thymus**
            Conditions classifiable to C7A.091

        Z85.238 Personal history of other malignant neoplasm of thymus
            Conditions classifiable to C37

    Z85.29 Personal history of malignant neoplasm of other respiratory and intrathoracic organs

Z85.3 Personal history of malignant neoplasm of breast
    Conditions classifiable to C50.-

✓5ᵗʰ **Z85.4 Personal history of malignant neoplasm of** genital organs
    Conditions classifiable to C51-C63

    Z85.40 Personal history of malignant neoplasm of unspecified female **genital organ** ♀

    Z85.41 Personal history of malignant neoplasm of cervix uteri ♀

    Z85.42 Personal history of malignant neoplasm of other parts of uterus ♀

    Z85.43 Personal history of malignant neoplasm of ovary ♀

    Z85.44 Personal history of malignant neoplasm of other female **genital organs** ♀

    Z85.45 Personal history of malignant neoplasm of unspecified male **genital organ** ♂

    Z85.46 Personal history of malignant neoplasm of prostate ♂

    Z85.47 Personal history of malignant neoplasm of testis ♂

    Z85.48 Personal history of malignant neoplasm of epididymis ♂

    Z85.49 Personal history of malignant neoplasm of other male **genital organs** ♂

✓5ᵗʰ **Z85.5 Personal history of malignant neoplasm of** urinary tract
    Conditions classifiable to C64-C68

    Z85.50 Personal history of malignant neoplasm of unspecified urinary tract organ

    Z85.51 Personal history of malignant neoplasm of bladder

    ✓6ᵗʰ **Z85.52 Personal history of malignant neoplasm of** kidney
        EXCLUDES 1 *personal history of malignant neoplasm of renal pelvis (Z85.53)*

        Z85.520 Personal history of malignant carcinoid **tumor of kidney**
            Conditions classifiable to C7A.093

        Z85.528 Personal history of other malignant neoplasm of kidney
            Conditions classifiable to C64

    Z85.53 Personal history of malignant neoplasm of renal pelvis

    Z85.54 Personal history of malignant neoplasm of ureter

    Z85.59 Personal history of malignant neoplasm of other urinary tract organ

Z85.6 Personal history of leukemia
    Conditions classifiable to C91-C95
    EXCLUDES 1 *leukemia in remission C91.0-C95.9 with 5th character 1*

✓5ᵗʰ **Z85.7 Personal history of other malignant neoplasms of lymphoid, hematopoietic and related tissues**

    Z85.71 Personal history of Hodgkin lymphoma
        Conditions classifiable to C81

    Z85.72 Personal history of non-Hodgkin lymphomas
        Conditions classifiable to C82-C85

    Z85.79 Personal history of other malignant neoplasms of lymphoid, hematopoietic and related tissues
        Conditions classifiable to C88-C90, C96
        EXCLUDES 1 *multiple myeloma in remission (C90.01)*
            plasma cell leukemia in remission (C90.11)
            plasmacytoma in remission (C90.21)

✓5ᵗʰ **Z85.8 Personal history of malignant neoplasms of other organs and systems**
    Conditions classifiable to C00-C14, C40-C49, C69-C75, C7A.098, C76-C79

    ✓6ᵗʰ **Z85.81 Personal history of malignant neoplasm of** lip, oral cavity, and pharynx

        Z85.810 Personal history of malignant neoplasm of tongue

        Z85.818 Personal history of malignant neoplasm of other sites of lip, oral cavity, and pharynx

        Z85.819 Personal history of malignant neoplasm of unspecified site of lip, oral cavity, and pharynx

    ✓6ᵗʰ **Z85.82 Personal history of malignant neoplasm of** skin

        Z85.820 Personal history of malignant melanoma **of skin**
            Conditions classifiable to C43

        Z85.821 Personal history of Merkel cell carcinoma
            Conditions classifiable to C4A

        Z85.828 Personal history of other malignant neoplasm of skin
            Conditions classifiable to C44

    ✓6ᵗʰ **Z85.83 Personal history of malignant neoplasm of** bone and soft tissue

        Z85.830 Personal history of malignant neoplasm of bone

        Z85.831 Personal history of malignant neoplasm of soft tissue
            EXCLUDES 2 *personal history of malignant neoplasm of skin (Z85.82-)*

    ✓6ᵗʰ **Z85.84 Personal history of malignant neoplasm of** eye and nervous tissue

        Z85.840 Personal history of malignant neoplasm of eye

        Z85.841 Personal history of malignant neoplasm of brain

        Z85.848 Personal history of malignant neoplasm of other parts of nervous tissue

    ✓6ᵗʰ **Z85.85 Personal history of malignant neoplasm of** endocrine glands

        Z85.850 Personal history of malignant neoplasm of thyroid

        Z85.858 Personal history of malignant neoplasm of other endocrine glands

    Z85.89 Personal history of malignant neoplasm of other organs and systems

Z85.9 Personal history of malignant neoplasm, unspecified
    Conditions classifiable to C7A.00, C80.1

HCC CMS-HCC   **PD** Primary Dx Only   **Q** QPP   **N** Newborn: 0   **P** Pediatric: 0-17   **M** Maternity: 12-55   **A** Adult: 15

1240

ICD-10-CM

✓4ᵗʰ **Z86 Personal history of certain other diseases**

Code first any follow-up examination after treatment (Z09)

✓5ᵗʰ **Z86.0 Personal history of in-situ and benign neoplasms and neoplasms of uncertain behavior**

EXCLUDES 2   *personal history of malignant neoplasms (Z85.-)*

AHA: 2017,1Q,9

✓6ᵗʰ **Z86.00 Personal history of** in-situ neoplasm

Conditions classifiable to D00-D09

Z86.000 Personal history of in-situ neoplasm of breast

▶Conditions classifiable to D05◀

Z86.001 Personal history of in-situ neoplasm of cervix uteri   ♀

▶Conditions classifiable to D06◀

Personal history of cervical intraepithelial neoplasia III [CIN III]

● **Z86.002 Personal history of in-situ neoplasm of other and unspecified genital organs**

Conditions classifiable to D07

Personal history of high-grade prostatic intraepithelial neoplasia III [HGPIN III]

Personal history of vaginal intraepithelial neoplasia III [VAIN III]

Personal history of vulvar intraepithelial neoplasia III [VIN III]

● **Z86.003 Personal history of in-situ neoplasm of oral cavity, esophagus and stomach**

Conditions classifiable to D00

● **Z86.004 Personal history of in-situ neoplasm of other and unspecified digestive organs**

Conditions classifiable to D01

Personal history of anal intraepithelial neoplasia (AIN III)

● **Z86.005 Personal history of in-situ neoplasm of** middle ear and respiratory system

Conditions classifiable to D02

● **Z86.006 Personal history of** melanoma in-situ

Conditions classifiable to D03

EXCLUDES 2   *sites other than skin — code to personal history of in-situ neoplasm of the site*

● **Z86.007 Personal history of in-situ neoplasm of** skin

Conditions classifiable to D04

Personal history of carcinoma in situ of skin

Z86.008 Personal history of in-situ neoplasm of other site

▶Conditions classifiable to D09◀

~~Personal history of vaginal intraepithelial neoplasia III [VAIN III]~~

~~Personal history of vulvar intraepithelial neoplasia III [VIN III]~~

✓6ᵗʰ **Z86.01 Personal history of** benign neoplasm

Z86.010 Personal history of colonic polyps

AHA: 2017,1Q,14

Z86.011 Personal history of benign neoplasm of the brain

Z86.012 Personal history of benign carcinoid tumor

Z86.018 Personal history of other benign neoplasm

AHA: 2017,1Q,14

Z86.03 Personal history of neoplasm of uncertain behavior

✓5ᵗʰ **Z86.1 Personal history of** infectious and parasitic diseases

Conditions classifiable to A00-B89, B99

EXCLUDES 1   *personal history of infectious diseases specific to a body system*

sequelae of infectious and parasitic diseases (B90-B94)

Z86.11 Personal history of tuberculosis

Z86.12 Personal history of poliomyelitis

Z86.13 Personal history of malaria

Z86.14 Personal history of Methicillin resistant Staphylococcus aureus **infection**

Personal history of MRSA infection

Z86.15 Personal history of latent tuberculosis infection

Z86.19 Personal history of other infectious and parasitic diseases

Z86.2 Personal history of diseases of the blood and blood-forming organs **and certain disorders involving the** immune mechanism

Conditions classifiable to D50-D89

✓5ᵗʰ **Z86.3 Personal history of** endocrine, nutritional and metabolic diseases

Conditions classifiable to E00-E88

Z86.31 Personal history of diabetic foot ulcer

EXCLUDES 2   *current diabetic foot ulcer (E08.621, E09.621, E10.621, E11.621, E13.621)*

Z86.32 Personal history of gestational diabetes   ♀

Personal history of conditions classifiable to O24.4-

EXCLUDES 1   *gestational diabetes mellitus in current pregnancy (O24.4-)*

Z86.39 Personal history of other endocrine, nutritional and metabolic disease

✓5ᵗʰ **Z86.5 Personal history of** mental and behavioral disorders

Conditions classifiable to F40-F59

Z86.51 Personal history of combat and   Ⓐ operational stress reaction

Z86.59 Personal history of other mental and behavioral disorders

✓5ᵗʰ **Z86.6 Personal history of diseases of the** nervous system and sense organs

Conditions classifiable to G00-G99, H00-H95

Z86.61 Personal history of infections of the central nervous system

Personal history of encephalitis

Personal history of meningitis

Z86.69 Personal history of other diseases of the nervous system and sense organs

AHA: 2016,4Q,24

✓5ᵗʰ **Z86.7 Personal history of diseases of the** circulatory system

Conditions classifiable to I00-I99

EXCLUDES 2   *old myocardial infarction (I25.2)*

personal history of anaphylactic shock (Z87.892)

postmyocardial infarction syndrome (I24.1)

✓6ᵗʰ **Z86.71 Personal history of** venous thrombosis and embolism

Z86.711 Personal history of pulmonary **embolism**

Z86.718 Personal history of other venous thrombosis and embolism

Z86.72 Personal history of thrombophlebitis

Z86.73 Personal history of transient ischemic attack **(TIA), and cerebral infarction without residual deficits**

Personal history of prolonged reversible ischemic neurological deficit (PRIND)

Personal history of stroke NOS without residual deficits

EXCLUDES 1   *personal history of traumatic brain injury (Z87.820)*

sequelae of cerebrovascular disease (I69.-)

AHA: 2012,4Q,92

Z86.74 Personal history of sudden cardiac arrest

Personal history of sudden cardiac death successfully resuscitated

Z86.79 Personal history of other diseases of the circulatory system

✓4ᵗʰ **Z87 Personal history of other diseases and conditions**

Code first any follow-up examination after treatment (Z09)

✓5ᵗʰ **Z87.0 Personal history of diseases of the** respiratory system

Conditions classifiable to J00-J99

Z87.01 Personal history of pneumonia (recurrent)

Z87.09 Personal history of other diseases of the respiratory system

✓5ᵗʰ **Z87.1 Personal history of diseases of the** digestive system

Conditions classifiable to K00-K93

Z87.11 Personal history of peptic ulcer **disease**

Z87.19 Personal history of other diseases of the digestive system

AHA: 2017,1Q,14

Z87.2 Personal history of diseases of the skin and subcutaneous tissue

Conditions classifiable to L00-L99

EXCLUDES 2   *personal history of diabetic foot ulcer (Z86.31)*

Additional Character Required   ✓7ᵗʰ Placeholder Alert   Manifestation   Unspecified Dx   ▶◀ Revised Text   ● New Code   ▲ Revised Code Title

10-CM 2020   1241

☑5ᵗʰ **Z87.3** **Personal history of diseases of the** musculoskeletal system and connective tissue

Conditions classifiable to M00-M99

EXCLUDES 2   *personal history of (healed) traumatic fracture (Z87.81)*

☑6ᵗʰ **Z87.31** **Personal history of (healed)** nontraumatic fracture

Z87.310 **Personal history of (healed)** osteoporosis fracture

Personal history of (healed) fragility fracture

Personal history of (healed) collapsed vertebra due to osteoporosis

TIP: Assign for history of osteoporosis fractures that have resolved, even when a code from category M80 indicating current osteoporosis fracture is also reported.

Z87.311 **Personal history of (healed) other pathological fracture**

Personal history of (healed) collapsed vertebra NOS

EXCLUDES 2   *personal history of osteoporosis fracture (Z87.310)*

Z87.312 **Personal history of (healed)** stress fracture

Personal history of (healed) fatigue fracture

Z87.39 **Personal history of other diseases of the musculoskeletal system and connective tissue**

☑5ᵗʰ **Z87.4** **Personal history of diseases of the** genitourinary system

Conditions classifiable to N00-N99

☑6ᵗʰ **Z87.41** **Personal history of** dysplasia of the female genital tract

EXCLUDES 1   *personal history of intraepithelial neoplasia III of female genital tract (Z86.001, Z86.008)*

personal history of malignant neoplasm of female genital tract (Z85.40-Z85.44)

Z87.410 **Personal history of** cervical dysplasia   ♀

Z87.411 **Personal history of** vaginal dysplasia   ♀

Z87.412 **Personal history of** vulvar dysplasia   ♀

Z87.42 **Personal history of other diseases of the** female genital tract   ♀

☑6ᵗʰ **Z87.43** **Personal history of diseases of the** male genital organs

Z87.430 **Personal history of** prostatic dysplasia   ♂

EXCLUDES 1   *personal history of malignant neoplasm of prostate (Z85.46)*

Z87.438 **Personal history of other diseases of** male genital organs   ♂

☑6ᵗʰ **Z87.44** **Personal history of diseases of the** urinary system

EXCLUDES 1   *personal history of malignant neoplasm of cervix uteri (Z85.41)*

Z87.440 **Personal history of** urinary (tract) infections

Z87.441 **Personal history of** nephrotic syndrome

Z87.442 **Personal history of** urinary calculi

Personal history of kidney stones

Z87.448 **Personal history of other diseases of** urinary system

☑5ᵗʰ **Z87.5** **Personal history of complications of** pregnancy, childbirth and the puerperium

Conditions classifiable to O00-O9A

EXCLUDES 2   *recurrent pregnancy loss (N96)*

Z87.51 **Personal history of** pre-term labor   ♀

EXCLUDES 1   *current pregnancy with history of pre-term labor (O09.21-)*

Z87.59 **Personal history of other complications of pregnancy, childbirth and the puerperium**   ♀

Personal history of trophoblastic disease

☑5ᵗʰ **Z87.7** **Personal history of (corrected)** congenital malformations

Conditions classifiable to Q00-Q89 that have been repaired or corrected

EXCLUDES 1   *congenital malformations that have been partially corrected or repair but which still require medical treatment — code to condition*

EXCLUDES 2   *other postprocedural states (Z98.-)*

personal history of medical treatment (Z92.-)

presence of cardiac and vascular implants and grafts (Z95.-)

presence of other devices (Z97.-)

presence of other functional implants (Z96.-)

transplanted organ and tissue status (Z94.-)

☑6ᵗʰ **Z87.71** **Personal history of (corrected) congenital malformations of** genitourinary system

Z87.710 **Personal history of (corrected) hypospadias**   ♂

Z87.718 **Personal history of other specified (corrected) congenital malformations of genitourinary system**

☑6ᵗʰ **Z87.72** **Personal history of (corrected) congenital malformations of** nervous system and sense organs

Z87.720 **Personal history of (corrected) congenital malformations of** eye

Z87.721 **Personal history of (corrected) congenital malformations of** ear

Z87.728 **Personal history of other specified (corrected) congenital malformations of nervous system and sense organs**

☑6ᵗʰ **Z87.73** **Personal history of (corrected) congenital malformations of** digestive system

Z87.730 **Personal history of (corrected)** cleft lip and palate

Z87.738 **Personal history of other specified (corrected) congenital malformations of digestive system**

Z87.74 **Personal history of (corrected) congenital malformations of** heart and circulatory system

Z87.75 **Personal history of (corrected) congenital malformations of** respiratory system

Z87.76 **Personal history of (corrected) congenital malformations of** integument, limbs and musculoskeletal system

☑6ᵗʰ **Z87.79** **Personal history of other (corrected) congenital malformations**

Z87.790 **Personal history of (corrected) congenital malformations of** face and neck

Z87.798 **Personal history of other (corrected) congenital malformations**

☑5ᵗʰ **Z87.8** **Personal history of other specified conditions**

EXCLUDES 2   *personal history of self harm (Z91.5)*

Z87.81 **Personal history of (healed)** traumatic fracture

EXCLUDES 2   *personal history of (healed) nontraumatic fracture (Z87.31-)*

☑6ᵗʰ **Z87.82** **Personal history of other (healed)** physical injury and trauma

Conditions classifiable to S00-T88, except traumatic fractures

Z87.820 **Personal history of** traumatic brain injury

EXCLUDES 1   *personal history of transient ischemic attack (TIA), and cerebral infarction without residual deficits (Z86.73)*

Z87.821 **Personal history of** retained foreign body fully removed

Z87.828 **Personal history of other (healed) physical injury and trauma**

☑6ᵗʰ **Z87.89** **Personal history of other specified conditions**

Z87.890 **Personal history of** sex reassignment

Z87.891 **Personal history of** nicotine dependence

EXCLUDES 1   *current nicotine dependence (F17.2-)*

AHA: 2017,2Q,27

Z87.892 Personal history of anaphylaxis
Code also allergy status such as:
   allergy status to drugs, medicaments and
      biological substances (Z88.-)
   allergy status, other than to drugs and
      biological substances (Z91.0-)
**Z87.898 Personal history of other specified
   conditions**
   AHA: 2013,1Q,21

√4ᵗʰ **Z88 Allergy status to drugs, medicaments and biological substances**
   EXCLUDES 2   allergy status, other than to drugs and biological substances (Z91.0-)
   AHA: 2015,3Q,23
   Z88.0 Allergy status to penicillin
   Z88.1 Allergy status to other antibiotic agents status
   Z88.2 Allergy status to sulfonamides status
   Z88.3 Allergy status to other anti-infective agents status
   Z88.4 Allergy status to anesthetic agent status
   Z88.5 Allergy status to narcotic agent status
   Z88.6 Allergy status to analgesic agent status
   Z88.7 Allergy status to serum and vaccine status
   Z88.8 Allergy status to other drugs, medicaments and biological substances status
   Z88.9 Allergy status to unspecified drugs, medicaments and biological substances status

√4ᵗʰ **Z89 Acquired absence of limb**
   INCLUDES   amputation status
      postprocedural loss of limb
      post-traumatic loss of limb
   EXCLUDES 1   acquired deformities of limbs (M20-M21)
      congenital absence of limbs (Q71-Q73)

   √5ᵗʰ **Z89.0 Acquired absence of thumb and other finger(s)**
      √6ᵗʰ **Z89.01 Acquired absence of thumb**
         Z89.011 Acquired absence of right thumb
         Z89.012 Acquired absence of left thumb
         Z89.019 Acquired absence of unspecified thumb
      √6ᵗʰ **Z89.02 Acquired absence of other finger(s)**
         EXCLUDES 2   acquired absence of thumb (Z89.01-)
         Z89.021 Acquired absence of right finger(s)
         Z89.022 Acquired absence of left finger(s)
         Z89.029 Acquired absence of unspecified finger(s)

   √5ᵗʰ **Z89.1 Acquired absence of hand and wrist**
      √6ᵗʰ **Z89.11 Acquired absence of hand**
         Z89.111 Acquired absence of right hand
         Z89.112 Acquired absence of left hand
         Z89.119 Acquired absence of unspecified hand
      √6ᵗʰ **Z89.12 Acquired absence of wrist**
         Disarticulation at wrist
         Z89.121 Acquired absence of right wrist
         Z89.122 Acquired absence of left wrist
         Z89.129 Acquired absence of unspecified wrist

   √5ᵗʰ **Z89.2 Acquired absence of upper limb above wrist**
      √6ᵗʰ **Z89.20 Acquired absence of upper limb, unspecified level**
         Z89.201 Acquired absence of right upper limb, unspecified level
         Z89.202 Acquired absence of left upper limb, unspecified level
         Z89.209 Acquired absence of unspecified upper limb, unspecified level
            Acquired absence of arm NOS
      √6ᵗʰ **Z89.21 Acquired absence of upper limb below elbow**
         Z89.211 Acquired absence of right upper limb below elbow
         Z89.212 Acquired absence of left upper limb below elbow
         Z89.219 Acquired absence of unspecified upper limb below elbow
      √6ᵗʰ **Z89.22 Acquired absence of upper limb above elbow**
         Disarticulation at elbow
         Z89.221 Acquired absence of right upper limb above elbow
         Z89.222 Acquired absence of left upper limb above elbow
         Z89.229 Acquired absence of unspecified upper limb above elbow

   √6ᵗʰ **Z89.23 Acquired absence of shoulder**
      Acquired absence of shoulder joint following explantation of shoulder joint prosthesis, with or without presence of antibiotic-impregnated cement spacer
      Z89.231 Acquired absence of right shoulder
      Z89.232 Acquired absence of left shoulder
      Z89.239 Acquired absence of unspecified shoulder

   √5ᵗʰ **Z89.4 Acquired absence of toe(s), foot, and ankle**
      √6ᵗʰ **Z89.41 Acquired absence of great toe**
         Z89.411 Acquired absence of right great toe   HCC
         Z89.412 Acquired absence of left great toe   HCC
         Z89.419 Acquired absence of unspecified great toe   HCC
      √6ᵗʰ **Z89.42 Acquired absence of other toe(s)**
         EXCLUDES 2   acquired absence of great toe (Z89.41-)
         Z89.421 Acquired absence of other right toe(s)   HCC
         Z89.422 Acquired absence of other left toe(s)   HCC
         Z89.429 Acquired absence of other toe(s), unspecified side   HCC
      √6ᵗʰ **Z89.43 Acquired absence of foot**
         Z89.431 Acquired absence of right foot   HCC
         Z89.432 Acquired absence of left foot   HCC
         Z89.439 Acquired absence of unspecified foot   HCC
      √6ᵗʰ **Z89.44 Acquired absence of ankle**
         Disarticulation of ankle
         Z89.441 Acquired absence of right ankle   HCC
         Z89.442 Acquired absence of left ankle   HCC
         Z89.449 Acquired absence of unspecified ankle   HCC

   √5ᵗʰ **Z89.5 Acquired absence of leg below knee**
      √6ᵗʰ **Z89.51 Acquired absence of leg below knee**
         Z89.511 Acquired absence of right leg below knee   HCC
         Z89.512 Acquired absence of left leg below knee   HCC
         Z89.519 Acquired absence of unspecified leg below knee   HCC
      √6ᵗʰ **Z89.52 Acquired absence of knee**
         Acquired absence of knee joint following explantation of knee joint prosthesis, with or without presence of antibiotic-impregnated cement spacer
         Z89.521 Acquired absence of right knee
         Z89.522 Acquired absence of left knee
         Z89.529 Acquired absence of unspecified knee

   √5ᵗʰ **Z89.6 Acquired absence of leg above knee**
      √6ᵗʰ **Z89.61 Acquired absence of leg above knee**
         Acquired absence of leg NOS
         Disarticulation at knee
         Z89.611 Acquired absence of right leg above knee   HCC
         Z89.612 Acquired absence of left leg above knee   HCC
         Z89.619 Acquired absence of unspecified leg above knee   HCC
      √6ᵗʰ **Z89.62 Acquired absence of hip**
         Acquired absence of hip joint following explantation of hip joint prosthesis, with or without presence of antibiotic-impregnated cement spacer
         Disarticulation at hip
         Z89.621 Acquired absence of right hip joint
         Z89.622 Acquired absence of left hip joint
         Z89.629 Acquired absence of unspecified hip joint
   Z89.9 Acquired absence of limb, unspecified

√4ᵗʰ **Z90 Acquired absence of organs, not elsewhere classified**
   INCLUDES   postprocedural or post-traumatic loss of body part NEC
   EXCLUDES 1   congenital absence — see Alphabetical Index
   EXCLUDES 2   postprocedural absence of endocrine glands (E89.-)
   √5ᵗʰ **Z90.0 Acquired absence of part of head and neck**
      Z90.01 Acquired absence of eye
      Z90.02 Acquired absence of larynx

Z90.09   **Acquired absence of other part of head and neck**
    Acquired absence of nose
      EXCLUDES 2   teeth (K08.1)

✓5ᵗʰ **Z90.1**   **Acquired absence of breast and nipple**

    Z90.10   **Acquired absence of unspecified breast and nipple**
    Z90.11   **Acquired absence of right breast and nipple**
    Z90.12   **Acquired absence of left breast and nipple**
    Z90.13   **Acquired absence of bilateral breasts and nipples**

Z90.2   **Acquired absence of lung [part of]**
Z90.3   **Acquired absence of stomach [part of]**

✓5ᵗʰ **Z90.4**   **Acquired absence of other specified parts of digestive tract**

    ✓6ᵗʰ **Z90.41**   **Acquired absence of pancreas**
      Code also exocrine pancreatic insufficiency (K86.81)
      Use additional code to identify any associated:
      diabetes mellitus, postpancreatectomy (E13.-)
      insulin use (Z79.4)

      Z90.410   **Acquired total absence of pancreas**
        Acquired absence of pancreas NOS
      Z90.411   **Acquired partial absence of pancreas**

    Z90.49   **Acquired absence of other specified parts of digestive tract**

Z90.5   **Acquired absence of kidney**
Z90.6   **Acquired absence of other parts of urinary tract**
    Acquired absence of bladder

✓5ᵗʰ **Z90.7**   **Acquired absence of genital organ(s)**
    EXCLUDES 1   personal history of sex reassignment (Z87.890)
    EXCLUDES 2   female genital mutilation status (N90.81-)

    ✓6ᵗʰ **Z90.71**   **Acquired absence of cervix and uterus**

      Z90.710   **Acquired absence of both cervix and uterus**   ♀
        Acquired absence of uterus NOS
        Status post total hysterectomy

      Z90.711   **Acquired absence of uterus with remaining cervical stump**   ♀
        Status post partial hysterectomy with remaining cervical stump

      Z90.712   **Acquired absence of cervix with remaining uterus**   ♀

    ✓6ᵗʰ **Z90.72**   **Acquired absence of ovaries**

      Z90.721   **Acquired absence of ovaries, unilateral**   ♀
      Z90.722   **Acquired absence of ovaries, bilateral**   ♀

    Z90.79   **Acquired absence of other genital organ(s)**

✓5ᵗʰ **Z90.8**   **Acquired absence of other organs**

    Z90.81   **Acquired absence of spleen**
    Z90.89   **Acquired absence of other organs**

✓4ᵗʰ **Z91**   **Personal risk factors, not elsewhere classified**
    EXCLUDES 2   contact with and (suspected) exposures hazardous to health (Z77.-)
      exposure to pollution and other problems related to physical environment (Z77.1-)
      female genital mutilation status (N90.81-)
      personal history of physical injury and trauma (Z87.81, Z87.82-)
      occupational exposure to risk factors (Z57.-)

✓5ᵗʰ **Z91.0**   **Allergy status, other than to drugs and biological substances**
    EXCLUDES 2   allergy status to drugs, medicaments, and biological substances (Z88.-)

    ✓6ᵗʰ **Z91.01**   **Food allergy status**
      EXCLUDES 2   food additives allergy status (Z91.02)

      Z91.010   **Allergy to peanuts**
      Z91.011   **Allergy to milk products**
        EXCLUDES 1   lactose intolerance (E73.-)
      Z91.012   **Allergy to eggs**
      Z91.013   **Allergy to seafood**
        Allergy to shellfish
        Allergy to octopus or squid ink
      Z91.018   **Allergy to other foods**
        Allergy to nuts other than peanuts

    Z91.02   **Food additives allergy status**

    ✓6ᵗʰ **Z91.03**   **Insect allergy status**

      Z91.030   **Bee allergy status**
      Z91.038   **Other insect allergy status**

    ✓6ᵗʰ **Z91.04**   **Nonmedicinal substance allergy status**

      Z91.040   **Latex allergy status**
        Latex sensitivity status
      Z91.041   **Radiographic dye allergy status**
        Allergy status to contrast media used for diagnostic X-ray procedure
      Z91.048   **Other nonmedicinal substance allergy status**

    Z91.09   **Other allergy status, other than to drugs and biological substances**

✓5ᵗʰ **Z91.1**   **Patient's noncompliance with medical treatment and regimen**

    Z91.11   **Patient's noncompliance with dietary regimen**

    ✓6ᵗʰ **Z91.12**   **Patient's intentional underdosing of medication regimen**
      Code first underdosing of medication (T36-T50) with fifth or sixth character 6
      EXCLUDES 1   adverse effect of prescribed drug taken as directed — code to adverse effect
        poisoning (overdose) — code to poisoning
      AHA: 2018,4Q,72

      Z91.120   **Patient's intentional underdosing of medication regimen due to financial hardship**
      Z91.128   **Patient's intentional underdosing of medication regimen for other reason**

    ✓6ᵗʰ **Z91.13**   **Patient's unintentional underdosing of medication regimen**
      Code first underdosing of medication (T36-T50) with fifth or sixth character 6
      EXCLUDES 1   adverse effect of prescribed drug taken as directed — code to adverse effect
        poisoning (overdose) — code to poisoning
      AHA: 2018,4Q,72

      Z91.130   **Patient's unintentional underdosing of medication regimen due to age-related debility**
      Z91.138   **Patient's unintentional underdosing of medication regimen for other reason**

    Z91.14   **Patient's other noncompliance with medication regimen**
      Patient's underdosing of medication NOS
      AHA: 2018,4Q,72

    Z91.15   **Patient's noncompliance with renal dialysis**   HCC

    Z91.19   **Patient's noncompliance with other medical treatment and regimen**
      Nonadherence to medical treatment

✓5ᵗʰ **Z91.4**   **Personal history of psychological trauma, not elsewhere classified**

    ✓6ᵗʰ **Z91.41**   **Personal history of adult abuse**
      EXCLUDES 2   personal history of abuse in childhood (Z62.81-)

      Z91.410   **Personal history of adult physical and sexual abuse**   A
        EXCLUDES 1   current adult physical abuse (T74.11, T76.11)
        current adult sexual abuse (T74.21, T76.11)

      Z91.411   **Personal history of adult psychological abuse**
      Z91.412   **Personal history of adult neglect**
        EXCLUDES 1   current adult neglect (T74.01, T76.01)

      Z91.419   **Personal history of unspecified adult abuse**

    Z91.42   **Personal history of forced labor or sexual exploitation**
      AHA: 2018,4Q,32,35

    Z91.49   **Other personal history of psychological trauma, not elsewhere classified**

Z91.5   **Personal history of self-harm**
    Personal history of parasuicide
    Personal history of self-poisoning
    Personal history of suicide attempt

✓5ᵗʰ **Z91.8**   **Other specified personal risk factors, not elsewhere classified**

    Z91.81   **History of falling**
      At risk for falling

Z91.82   **Personal history of military deployment**   A

Individual (civilian or military) with past history of military war, peacekeeping and humanitarian deployment (current or past conflict)

Returned from military deployment

Z91.83   *Wandering in diseases classified elsewhere*

Code first underlying disorder such as:

Alzheimer's disease (G30.-)

autism or pervasive developmental disorder (F84.-)

intellectual disabilities (F70-F79)

unspecified dementia with behavioral disturbance (F03.9-)

✓6th **Z91.84**   **Oral health risk factors**

AHA: 2017,4Q,29

Z91.841   **Risk for dental caries, low**

Z91.842   **Risk for dental caries, moderate**

Z91.843   **Risk for dental caries, high**

Z91.849   **Unspecified risk for dental caries**

Z91.89   **Other specified personal risk factors, not elsewhere classified**

AHA: 2017,1Q,45

✓4th **Z92**   **Personal history of medical treatment**

EXCLUDES 2   postprocedural states (Z98.-)

Z92.0   **Personal history of contraception**

EXCLUDES 1   counseling or management of current contraceptive practices (Z30.-)

long term (current) use of contraception (Z79.3)

presence of (intrauterine) contraceptive device (Z97.5)

✓5th **Z92.2**   **Personal history of drug therapy**

EXCLUDES 2   long term (current) drug therapy (Z79.-)

Z92.21   **Personal history of antineoplastic chemotherapy**

Z92.22   **Personal history of monoclonal drug therapy**

Z92.23   **Personal history of estrogen therapy**

✓6th **Z92.24**   **Personal history of steroid therapy**

Z92.240   **Personal history of inhaled steroid therapy**

Z92.241   **Personal history of systemic steroid therapy**

Personal history of steroid therapy NOS

Z92.25   **Personal history of immunosupression therapy**

EXCLUDES 2   personal history of steroid therapy (Z92.24)

Z92.29   **Personal history of other drug therapy**

Z92.3   **Personal history of irradiation**

Personal history of exposure to therapeutic radiation

EXCLUDES 1   exposure to radiation in the physical environment (Z77.12)

occupational exposure to radiation (Z57.1)

✓5th **Z92.8**   **Personal history of other medical treatment**

Z92.81   **Personal history of extracorporeal membrane oxygenation (ECMO)**

Z92.82   **Status post administration of tPA (rtPA) in a different facility within the last 24 hours prior to admission to current facility**

Code first condition requiring tPA administration, such as:

acute cerebral infarction (I63.-)

acute myocardial infarction (I21.-, I22.-)

AHA: 2013,4Q,124

Z92.83   **Personal history of failed moderate sedation**

Personal history of failed conscious sedation

EXCLUDES 2   failed moderate sedation during procedure (T88.52)

Z92.84   **Personal history of unintended awareness under general anesthesia**

EXCLUDES 2   unintended awareness under general anesthesia during procedure (T88.53)

AHA: 2016,4Q,72-73,77

Z92.89   **Personal history of other medical treatment**

4th **Z93**   **Artificial opening status**

EXCLUDES 1   artificial openings requiring attention or management (Z43.-)

complications of external stoma (J95.0-, K94.-, N99.5-)

Z93.0   **Tracheostomy status**   HCC

AHA: 2013,4Q,129

Z93.1   **Gastrostomy status**   HCC

Z93.2   **Ileostomy status**   HCC

Z93.3   **Colostomy status**   HCC

Z93.4   **Other artificial openings of gastrointestinal tract status**   HCC

✓5th **Z93.5**   **Cystostomy status**

Z93.50   **Unspecified cystostomy status**   HCC

Z93.51   **Cutaneous-vesicostomy status**   HCC

Z93.52   **Appendico-vesicostomy status**   HCC

Z93.59   **Other cystostomy status**   HCC

Z93.6   **Other artificial openings of urinary tract status**   HCC

Nephrostomy status

Ureterostomy status

Urethrostomy status

Z93.8   **Other artificial opening status**   HCC

Z93.9   **Artificial opening status, unspecified**   HCC

✓4th **Z94**   **Transplanted organ and tissue status**

INCLUDES   organ or tissue replaced by heterogenous or homogenous transplant

EXCLUDES 1   complications of transplanted organ or tissue — see Alphabetical Index

EXCLUDES 2   presence of vascular grafts (Z95.-)

Z94.0   **Kidney transplant status**

Z94.1   **Heart transplant status**   HCC

EXCLUDES 1   artificial heart status (Z95.812)

heart-valve replacement status (Z95.2-Z95.4)

Z94.2   **Lung transplant status**   HCC

Z94.3   **Heart and lungs transplant status**   HCC

Z94.4   **Liver transplant status**   HCC

Z94.5   **Skin transplant status**

Autogenous skin transplant status

Z94.6   **Bone transplant status**

Z94.7   **Corneal transplant status**

✓5th **Z94.8**   **Other transplanted organ and tissue status**

Z94.81   **Bone marrow transplant status**   HCC

Z94.82   **Intestine transplant status**   HCC

Z94.83   **Pancreas transplant status**   HCC

Z94.84   **Stem cells transplant status**   HCC

Z94.89   **Other transplanted organ and tissue status**

Z94.9   **Transplanted organ and tissue status, unspecified**

✓4th **Z95**   **Presence of cardiac and vascular implants and grafts**

EXCLUDES 2   complications of cardiac and vascular devices, implants and grafts (T82.-)

Z95.0   **Presence of cardiac pacemaker**

Presence of cardiac resynchronization therapy (CRT-P) pacemaker

EXCLUDES 1   adjustment or management of cardiac device (Z45.0-)

adjustment or management of cardiac pacemaker (Z45.0)

presence of automatic (implantable) cardiac defibrillator with synchronous cardiac pacemaker (Z95.810)

AHA: 2019,1Q,33

Z95.1   **Presence of aortocoronary bypass graft**

Presence of coronary artery bypass graft

Z95.2   **Presence of prosthetic heart valve**

Presence of heart valve NOS

Z95.3   **Presence of xenogenic heart valve**

Z95.4   **Presence of other heart-valve replacement**

Z95.5   **Presence of coronary angioplasty implant and graft**

EXCLUDES 1   coronary angioplasty status without implant and graft (Z98.61)

√5ᵗʰ **Z95.8** **Presence of other cardiac and vascular implants and grafts**

√6ᵗʰ **Z95.81** **Presence of other cardiac implants and grafts**

Z95.810 **Presence of** automatic (implantable) cardiac defibrillator

Presence of automatic (implantable) cardiac defibrillator with synchronous cardiac pacemaker

Presence of cardiac resynchronization therapy defibrillator (CRT-D)

Presence of cardioverter-defibrillator (ICD)

Z95.811 **Presence of** heart assist device   `HCC`

Z95.812 **Presence of** fully implantable artificial heart   `HCC`

Z95.818 **Presence of other cardiac implants and grafts**

√6ᵗʰ **Z95.82** **Presence of other vascular implants and grafts**

Z95.820 **Peripheral** vascular angioplasty status with implants and grafts

`EXCLUDES 1` *peripheral vascular angioplasty without implant and graft (Z98.62)*

Z95.828 **Presence of other vascular implants and grafts**

Presence of intravascular prosthesis NEC

Z95.9 **Presence of cardiac and vascular implant and graft, unspecified**

√4ᵗʰ **Z96** **Presence of other functional implants**

`EXCLUDES 2` *complications of internal prosthetic devices, implants and grafts (T82-T85)*

fitting and adjustment of prosthetic and other devices (Z44-Z46)

Z96.0 **Presence of** urogenital **implants**

Z96.1 **Presence of** intraocular lens

Presence of pseudophakia

√5ᵗʰ **Z96.2** **Presence of** otological and audiological **implants**

Z96.20 **Presence of otological and audiological implant, unspecified**

Z96.21 **Cochlear implant status**

Z96.22 **Myringotomy tube(s) status**

Z96.29 **Presence of other otological and audiological implants**

Presence of bone-conduction hearing device

Presence of eustachian tube stent

Stapes replacement

Z96.3 **Presence of** artificial larynx

√5ᵗʰ **Z96.4** **Presence of** endocrine **implants**

Z96.41 **Presence of** insulin pump (external) (internal)

Z96.49 **Presence of other endocrine implants**

Z96.5 **Presence of** tooth-root and mandibular **implants**

√5ᵗʰ **Z96.6** **Presence of** orthopedic joint **implants**

Z96.60 **Presence of unspecified orthopedic joint implant**

√6ᵗʰ **Z96.61** **Presence of** artificial shoulder joint

Z96.611 **Presence of** right **artificial shoulder joint**

Z96.612 **Presence of** left **artificial shoulder joint**

Z96.619 **Presence of unspecified artificial shoulder joint**

√6ᵗʰ **Z96.62** **Presence of** artificial elbow joint

Z96.621 **Presence of** right **artificial elbow joint**

Z96.622 **Presence of** left **artificial elbow joint**

Z96.629 **Presence of unspecified artificial elbow joint**

√6ᵗʰ **Z96.63** **Presence of** artificial wrist joint

Z96.631 **Presence of** right **artificial wrist joint**

Z96.632 **Presence of** left **artificial wrist joint**

Z96.639 **Presence of unspecified artificial wrist joint**

√6ᵗʰ **Z96.64** **Presence of** artificial hip joint

Hip-joint replacement (partial) (total)

Z96.641 **Presence of** right **artificial hip joint**

Z96.642 **Presence of** left **artificial hip joint**

Z96.643 **Presence of artificial hip joint,** bilateral

Z96.649 **Presence of unspecified artificial hip joint**

√6ᵗʰ **Z96.65** **Presence of** artificial knee joint

Z96.651 **Presence of** right **artificial knee joint**

Z96.652 **Presence of** left **artificial knee joint**

Z96.653 **Presence of artificial knee joint,** bilateral

Z96.659 **Presence of unspecified artificial knee joint**

√6ᵗʰ **Z96.66** **Presence of** artificial ankle joint

Z96.661 **Presence of** right **artificial ankle joint**

Z96.662 **Presence of** left **artificial ankle joint**

Z96.669 **Presence of unspecified artificial ankle joint**

√6ᵗʰ **Z96.69** **Presence of other orthopedic joint implants**

Z96.691 **Finger-joint replacement of** right **hand**

Z96.692 **Finger-joint replacement of** left **hand**

Z96.693 **Finger-joint replacement,** bilateral

Z96.698 **Presence of other orthopedic joint implants**

Z96.7 **Presence of other bone and tendon implants**

Presence of skull plate

√5ᵗʰ **Z96.8** **Presence of other specified functional implants**

Z96.81 **Presence of** artificial skin

Z96.82 **Presence of** neurostimulator

Presence of brain neurostimulator

Presence of gastric neurostimulator

Presence of peripheral nerve neurostimulator

Presence of sacral nerve neurostimulator

Presence of spinal cord neurostimulator

Presence of vagus nerve neurostimulator

Z96.89 **Presence of other specified functional implants**

Z96.9 **Presence of functional implant, unspecified**

√4ᵗʰ **Z97** **Presence of other devices**

`EXCLUDES 1` *complications of internal prosthetic devices, implants and grafts (T82-T85)*

fitting and adjustment of prosthetic and other devices (Z44-Z46)

`EXCLUDES 2` ▶*fitting and adjustment of prosthetic and other devices (Z44-Z46)*◀

presence of cerebrospinal fluid drainage device (Z98.2)

Z97.0 **Presence of** artificial eye

√5ᵗʰ **Z97.1** **Presence of** artificial limb (complete) (partial)

Z97.10 **Presence of artificial limb (complete) (partial), unspecified**

Z97.11 **Presence of artificial** right **arm (complete) (partial)**

Z97.12 **Presence of artificial** left **arm (complete) (partial)**

Z97.13 **Presence of artificial** right **leg (complete) (partial)**

Z97.14 **Presence of artificial** left **leg (complete) (partial)**

Z97.15 **Presence of artificial arms, bilateral (complete) (partial)**

Z97.16 **Presence of artificial legs, bilateral (complete) (partial)**

Z97.2 **Presence of** dental prosthetic device **(complete) (partial)**

Presence of dentures (complete) (partial)

Z97.3 **Presence of** spectacles and contact lenses

Z97.4 **Presence of** external hearing-aid

Z97.5 **Presence of (intrauterine)** contraceptive device

`EXCLUDES 1` *checking, reinsertion or removal of implantable subdermal contraceptive (Z30.46)*

checking, reinsertion or removal of intrauterine contraceptive device (Z30.43-)

Z97.8 **Presence of other specified devices**

√4ᵗʰ **Z98** **Other postprocedural states**

`EXCLUDES 2` *aftercare (Z43-Z49, Z51)*

follow-up medical care (Z08-Z09)

postprocedural complication — see Alphabetical Index

Z98.0 **Intestinal bypass and anastomosis status**

`EXCLUDES 2` *bariatric surgery status (Z98.84)*

gastric bypass status (Z98.84)

obesity surgery status (Z98.84)

Z98.1 **Arthrodesis status**

Z98.2 **Presence of cerebrospinal fluid drainage device**

Presence of CSF shunt

Z98.3 **Post therapeutic collapse of lung status**

Code first underlying disease

√5ᵗʰ **Z98.4** **Cataract extraction status**

Use additional code to identify intraocular lens implant status (Z96.1)

`EXCLUDES 1` *aphakia (H27.0)*

Z98.41 **Cataract extraction status,** right **eye**

Z98.42   **Cataract extraction status, left eye**
Z98.49   **Cataract extraction status, unspecified eye**

√5ᵗʰ **Z98.5 Sterilization status**
> *EXCLUDES 1*   female infertility (N97.-)
> male infertility (N46.-)

Z98.51   **Tubal ligation status**   ♀
Z98.52   **Vasectomy status**   Ⓐ ♂

√5ᵗʰ **Z98.6 Angioplasty status**
Z98.61   **Coronary angioplasty status**
> *EXCLUDES 1*   coronary angioplasty status with implant and graft (Z95.5)

Z98.62   **Peripheral vascular angioplasty status**
> *EXCLUDES 1*   peripheral vascular angioplasty status with implant and graft (Z95.820)

√5ᵗʰ **Z98.8 Other specified postprocedural states**
√6ᵗʰ   Z98.81   **Dental procedure status**

Z98.810   **Dental sealant status**
Z98.811   **Dental restoration status**
> Dental crown status
> Dental fillings status

Z98.818   **Other dental procedure status**

Z98.82   **Breast implant status**
> *EXCLUDES 1*   breast implant removal status (Z98.86)

Z98.83   **Filtering (vitreous) bleb after glaucoma surgery status**
> *EXCLUDES 1*   inflammation (infection) of postprocedural bleb (H59.4-)

Z98.84   **Bariatric surgery status**
> Gastric banding status
> Gastric bypass status for obesity
> Obesity surgery status
> *EXCLUDES 1*   bariatric surgery status complicating pregnancy, childbirth, or the puerperium (O99.84)
> *EXCLUDES 2*   intestinal bypass and anastomosis status (Z98.0)

Z98.85   **Transplanted organ removal status**
> Transplanted organ previously removed due to complication, failure, rejection or infection
> *EXCLUDES 1*   encounter for removal of transplanted organ — code to complication of transplanted organ (T86.-)

Z98.86   **Personal history of breast implant removal**
√6ᵗʰ   Z98.87   **Personal history of in utero procedure**

Z98.870   **Personal history of in utero procedure during pregnancy**   ♀
> *EXCLUDES 2*   complications from in utero procedure for current pregnancy (O35.7)
> supervision of current pregnancy with history of in utero procedure during previous pregnancy (O09.82-)

Z98.871   **Personal history of in utero procedure while a fetus**

√6ᵗʰ   Z98.89   **Other specified postprocedural states**

Z98.890   **Other specified postprocedural states**
> Personal history of surgery, not elsewhere classified

Z98.891   **History of uterine scar from previous surgery**   ♀
> *EXCLUDES 1*   maternal care due to uterine scar from previous surgery (O34.2-)
> **AHA:** 2016,4Q,51-52,76

√4ᵗʰ **Z99 Dependence on enabling machines and devices, not elsewhere classified**
> *EXCLUDES 1*   cardiac pacemaker status (Z95.0)

Z99.0 Dependence on aspirator
√5ᵗʰ **Z99.1 Dependence on respirator**
> Dependence on ventilator

Z99.11   **Dependence on respirator [ventilator] status**   HCC
> **AHA:** 2015,1Q,21

Z99.12   **Encounter for respirator [ventilator] dependence during power failure**   HCC PDx
> *EXCLUDES 1*   mechanical complication of respirator [ventilator] (J95.850)

Z99.2 Dependence on renal dialysis   HCC
> Hemodialysis status
> Peritoneal dialysis status
> Presence of arteriovenous shunt for dialysis
> Renal dialysis status NOS
> *EXCLUDES 1*   encounter for fitting and adjustment of dialysis catheter (Z49.0-)
> *EXCLUDES 2*   noncompliance with renal dialysis (Z91.15)
> **AHA:** 2016,1Q,12; 2013,4Q,125

Z99.3 Dependence on wheelchair
> Wheelchair confinement status
> Code first cause of dependence, such as:
>   muscular dystrophy (G71.0-)
>   obesity (E66.-)

√5ᵗʰ **Z99.8 Dependence on other enabling machines and devices**

Z99.81   **Dependence on supplemental oxygen**
> Dependence on long-term oxygen
> **AHA:** 2013,4Q,129

Z99.89   **Dependence on other enabling machines and devices**
> Dependence on machine or device NOS

Appendix A: Valid 3-character ICD-10-CM Codes

A09	Infectious gastroenteritis and colitis, unspecified
A33	Tetanus neonatorum
A34	Obstetrical tetanus
A35	Other tetanus
A46	Erysipelas
A55	Chlamydial lymphogranuloma (venereum)
A57	Chancroid
A58	Granuloma inguinale
A64	Unspecified sexually transmitted disease
A65	Nonvenereal syphilis
A70	Chlamydia psittaci infections
A78	Q fever
A86	Unspecified viral encephalitis
A89	Unspecified viral infection of central nervous system
A90	Dengue fever [classical dengue]
A91	Dengue hemorrhagic fever
A94	Unspecified arthropod-borne viral fever
A99	Unspecified viral hemorrhagic fever
B03	Smallpox
B04	Monkeypox
B09	Unspecified viral infection characterized by skin and mucous membrane lesions
B20	Human immunodeficiency virus [HIV] disease
B49	Unspecified mycosis
B54	Unspecified malaria
B59	Pneumocystosis
B64	Unspecified protozoal disease
B72	Dracunculiasis
B75	Trichinellosis
B79	Trichuriasis
B80	Enterobiasis
B86	Scabies
B89	Unspecified parasitic disease
B91	Sequelae of poliomyelitis
B92	Sequelae of leprosy
C01	Malignant neoplasm of base of tongue
C07	Malignant neoplasm of parotid gland
C12	Malignant neoplasm of pyriform sinus
C19	Malignant neoplasm of rectosigmoid junction
C20	Malignant neoplasm of rectum
C23	Malignant neoplasm of gallbladder
C33	Malignant neoplasm of trachea
C37	Malignant neoplasm of thymus
C52	Malignant neoplasm of vagina
C55	Malignant neoplasm of uterus, part unspecified
C58	Malignant neoplasm of placenta
C61	Malignant neoplasm of prostate
C73	Malignant neoplasm of thyroid gland
D34	Benign neoplasm of thyroid gland
D45	Polycythemia vera
D62	Acute posthemorrhagic anemia
D65	Disseminated intravascular coagulation [defibrination syndrome]
D66	Hereditary factor VIII deficiency
D67	Hereditary factor IX deficiency
D71	Functional disorders of polymorphonuclear neutrophils
D77	Other disorders of blood and blood-forming organs in diseases classified elsewhere
E02	Subclinical iodine-deficiency hypothyroidism
E15	Nondiabetic hypoglycemic coma
E35	Disorders of endocrine glands in diseases classified elsewhere
E40	Kwashiorkor
E41	Nutritional marasmus
E42	Marasmic kwashiorkor
E43	Unspecified severe protein-calorie malnutrition
E45	Retarded development following protein-calorie malnutrition

E46	Unspecified protein-calorie malnutrition
E52	Niacin deficiency [pellagra]
E54	Ascorbic acid deficiency
E58	Dietary calcium deficiency
E59	Dietary selenium deficiency
E60	Dietary zinc deficiency
E65	Localized adiposity
E68	Sequelae of hyperalimentation
F04	Amnestic disorder due to known physiological condition
F05	Delirium due to known physiological condition
F09	Unspecified mental disorder due to known physiological condition
F21	Schizotypal disorder
F22	Delusional disorders
F23	Brief psychotic disorder
F24	Shared psychotic disorder
F28	Other psychotic disorder not due to a substance or known physiological condition
F29	Unspecified psychosis not due to a substance or known physiological condition
F39	Unspecified mood [affective] disorder
F54	Psychological and behavioral factors associated with disorders or diseases classified elsewhere
F59	Unspecified behavioral syndromes associated with physiological disturbances and physical factors
F66	Other sexual disorders
F69	Unspecified disorder of adult personality and behavior
F70	Mild intellectual disabilities
F71	Moderate intellectual disabilities
F72	Severe intellectual disabilities
F73	Profound intellectual disabilities
F78	Other intellectual disabilities
F79	Unspecified intellectual disabilities
F82	Specific developmental disorder of motor function
F88	Other disorders of psychological development
F89	Unspecified disorder of psychological development
F99	Mental disorder, not otherwise specified
G01	Meningitis in bacterial diseases classified elsewhere
G02	Meningitis in other infectious and parasitic diseases classified elsewhere
G07	Intracranial and intraspinal abscess and granuloma in diseases classified elsewhere
G08	Intracranial and intraspinal phlebitis and thrombophlebitis
G09	Sequelae of inflammatory diseases of central nervous system
G10	Huntington's disease
G14	Postpolio syndrome
G20	Parkinson's disease
G26	Extrapyramidal and movement disorders in diseases classified elsewhere
G35	Multiple sclerosis
G53	Cranial nerve disorders in diseases classified elsewhere
G55	Nerve root and plexus compressions in diseases classified elsewhere
G59	Mononeuropathy in diseases classified elsewhere
G63	Polyneuropathy in diseases classified elsewhere
G64	Other disorders of peripheral nervous system
G92	Toxic encephalopathy
G94	Other disorders of brain in diseases classified elsewhere
H22	Disorders of iris and ciliary body in diseases classified elsewhere
H28	Cataract in diseases classified elsewhere
H32	Chorioretinal disorders in diseases classified elsewhere
H36	Retinal disorders in diseases classified elsewhere
H42	Glaucoma in diseases classified elsewhere
I00	Rheumatic fever without heart involvement
I10	Essential (primary) hypertension
I32	Pericarditis in diseases classified elsewhere
I38	Endocarditis, valve unspecified

I39	Endocarditis and heart valve disorders in diseases classified elsewhere
I41	Myocarditis in diseases classified elsewhere
I43	Cardiomyopathy in diseases classified elsewhere
I52	Other heart disorders in diseases classified elsewhere
I76	Septic arterial embolism
I81	Portal vein thrombosis
I96	Gangrene, not elsewhere classified
J00	Acute nasopharyngitis (common cold)
J13	Pneumonia due to Streptococcus pneumoniae
J14	Pneumonia due to Hemophilus influenzae
J17	Pneumonia in diseases classified elsewhere
J22	Unspecified acute lower respiratory infection
J36	Peritonsillar abscess
J40	Bronchitis, not specified as acute or chronic
J42	Unspecified chronic bronchitis
J60	Coalworker's pneumoconiosis
J61	Pneumoconiosis due to asbestos and other mineral fibers
J64	Unspecified pneumoconiosis
J65	Pneumoconiosis associated with tuberculosis
J80	Acute respiratory distress syndrome
J82	Pulmonary eosinophilia, not elsewhere classified
J90	Pleural effusion, not elsewhere classified
J99	Respiratory disorders in diseases classified elsewhere
K23	Disorders of esophagus in diseases classified elsewhere
K30	Functional dyspepsia
K36	Other appendicitis
K37	Unspecified appendicitis
K67	Disorders of peritoneum in infectious diseases classified elsewhere
K77	Liver disorders in diseases classified elsewhere
K87	Disorders of gallbladder, biliary tract and pancreas in diseases classified elsewhere
L00	Staphylococcal scalded skin syndrome
L14	Bullous disorders in diseases classified elsewhere
L22	Diaper dermatitis
L26	Exfoliative dermatitis
L42	Pityriasis rosea
L45	Papulosquamous disorders in diseases classified elsewhere
L52	Erythema nodosum
L54	Erythema in diseases classified elsewhere
L62	Nail disorders in diseases classified elsewhere
L80	Vitiligo
L83	Acanthosis nigricans
L84	Corns and callosities
L86	Keratoderma in diseases classified elsewhere
L88	Pyoderma gangrenosum
L99	Other disorders of skin and subcutaneous tissue in diseases classified elsewhere
N08	Glomerular disorders in diseases classified elsewhere
N10	Acute tubulo-interstitial nephritis
N12	Tubulo-interstitial nephritis, not specified as acute or chronic
N16	Renal tubulo-interstitial disorders in diseases classified elsewhere
N19	Unspecified kidney failure
N22	Calculus of urinary tract in diseases classified elsewhere
N23	Unspecified renal colic
N29	Other disorders of kidney and ureter in diseases classified elsewhere
N33	Bladder disorders in diseases classified elsewhere
N37	Urethral disorders in diseases classified elsewhere
N51	Disorders of male genital organs in diseases classified elsewhere
N62	Hypertrophy of breast
N72	Inflammatory disease of cervix uteri
N74	Female pelvic inflammatory disorders in diseases classified elsewhere
N86	Erosion and ectropion of cervix uteri
N96	Recurrent pregnancy loss
O68	Labor and delivery complicated by abnormality of fetal acid-base balance
O76	Abnormality in fetal heart rate and rhythm complicating labor and delivery
O80	Encounter for full-term uncomplicated delivery
O82	Encounter for cesarean delivery without indication
O85	Puerperal sepsis
O94	Sequelae of complication of pregnancy, childbirth, and the puerperium
P09	Abnormal findings on neonatal screening
P53	Hemorrhagic disease of newborn
P60	Disseminated intravascular coagulation of newborn
P84	Other problems with newborn
P90	Convulsions of newborn
P95	Stillbirth
Q02	Microcephaly
R05	Cough
R12	Heartburn
R17	Unspecified jaundice
R21	Rash and other nonspecific skin eruption
R32	Unspecified urinary incontinence
R34	Anuria and oliguria
R37	Sexual dysfunction, unspecified
R42	Dizziness and giddiness
R51	Headache
R52	Pain, unspecified
R54	Age-related physical debility
R55	Syncope and collapse
R58	Hemorrhage, not elsewhere classified
R61	Generalized hyperhidrosis
R64	Cachexia
R69	Illness, unspecified
R75	Inconclusive laboratory evidence of human immunodeficiency virus [HIV]
R81	Glycosuria
R99	Ill-defined and unknown cause of mortality
Y09	Assault by unspecified means
Y66	Nonadministration of surgical and medical care
Y69	Unspecified misadventure during surgical and medical care
Y95	Nosocomial condition
Z08	Encounter for follow-up examination after completed treatment for malignant neoplasm
Z09	Encounter for follow-up examination after completed treatment for conditions other than malignant neoplasm
Z21	Asymptomatic human immunodeficiency virus [HIV] infection status
Z23	Encounter for immunization
Z66	Do not resuscitate

Appendix B: Pharmacology List 2020

This section enables the coder to quickly review drugs, drug actions, and indications that are often associated with overlooked or undocumented diagnoses. The coder should review the patient's medication record and know what condition the physician is treating with the prescribed medication based on documentation in the medical record. When documentation is lacking, the coder can reference this section to locate the drug, determine the drug action, confirm drug indications, and when necessary query the physician. When applicable, some of the drugs provided in this resource have also been mapped to their appropriate Z code for long-term drug use.

Drug	Z Code	Drug Action/Classification	Indications
A-Methapred [methylprednisolone sodium succinate]	Z79.52	Corticosteroid	Severe inflammation
Abilify [aripiprazole]		Antipsychotic	Depression, bipolar disorder, schizophrenia, autism symptoms
Abstral [fentanyl citrate]	Z79.891	Analgesic, narcotic	Breakthrough cancer pain
Acarbose [acarbose]	Z79.84	Oral hypoglycemic	Diabetes mellitus
Accupril [quinapril hydrochloride]		ACE inhibitor	Congestive heart failure; hypertension
Acetaminophen with codeine [acetominophen/codeine phosphate]	Z79.891	Analgesic, narcotic	Pain, moderate to severe
Actemra [tocilizumab]		Antirheumatic	Rheumatoid arthritis
Actimmune [interferon gamma-1b]	Z79.899	Antineoplastic interferons; antiviral interferons	Chronic granulomatous disease; malignant osteopetrosis
Activella [estradiol/norethindrone acetate]	Z79.890	Estrogen therapy	Menopause symptoms; vaginal and vulvar atrophy; osteoporosis prevention
Actonel [risedronate sodium]	Z79.83	Biophosphonate	Decrease in bone loss in multiple myeloma patients; Paget's disease; hyperparathyroidism; osteoporosis
Actoplus Met [metformin hydrochloride/pioglitazone hydrochloride]	Z79.84	Oral hypoglycemic	Diabetes mellitus
Actos [pioglitazone hydrochloride]	Z79.84	Oral hypoglycemic	Diabetes mellitus
Aczone [dapsone]		Acne agent, topical	Acne vulgaris
Adalat CC [nifedipine]		Calcium channel blocker	Vasospastic angina; chronic stable angina; hypertension
Adderall XR [amphetamine aspartate and sulfate/dextroamphetamine saccharate and sulfate]		CNS stimulant	Attention deficit hyperactivity disorder (ADHD)
Admelog [insulin lispro]	Z79.4	Insulin	Diabetes mellitus
Advair [fluticasone propionate/salmeterol xinafoate]	Z79.51	Corticosteroid -inhaled; antiasthmatic	Prophylaxis and treatment of asthma and COPD
Advil [ibuprofen]	Z79.1	Nonsteroidal anti-inflammatory drug (NSAID)	Pain or fever relief
Aerospan HFA [flunisolide]	Z79.51	Corticosteroid -inhaled; antiasthmatic	Prophylaxis and treatment of asthma
Afrezza [human insulin recombinant]	Z79.4	Insulin -inhaled	Diabetes mellitus
Aggrastat [tirofiban hydrochloride]	Z79.02	Antiplatelet	Unstable angina; heart attacks
Aggrenox [aspirin/dipyridamole]	Z79.02	Antiplatelet	Lessening of the chance of heart attack or stroke
Aimovig [erenumab-aooe]		Antimigraine	Migraine headache
Airduo Respiclick [fluticasone propionate/salmeterol xinafoate]	Z79.51	Corticosteroid -- inhaled; antiasthmatic	Asthma
Aldactone [spironolactone]		Cardiovascular agent; antihypertensive agent; diuretic; electrolytic and renal agent	Severe heart failure; ascites associated with cirrhosis; hypokalemia
Aleve [naproxen sodium]	Z79.1	Nonsteroidal anti-inflammatory drug (NSAID)	Reduction of temporary aches and pains
Allegra allergy [fexofenadine hydrochloride]		Antihistamine	Seasonal allergic rhinitis
Allopurinol [allopurinol]		Antigout	Gouty arthritis, renal calculus, hyperuricemia, hyperuricemia secondary to leukemia, hyperuricemia secondary to lymphoma
Alora [estradiol]	Z79.890	Estrogen therapy	Menopause symptoms
Alphagan P [brimonidine tartrate]		Antiglaucoma agent (ophthalmic); antihypertensive, ocular	Open angle glaucoma or another condition in which pressure in the eye is too high (ocular hypertension)
Alprazolam [alprazolam]		Antianxiety; sedative/hypnotic	
Altabax [retapamulin]	Z79.2	Antibiotic, topical	Skin infections
Altace [ramipril]		ACE inhibitor	Congestive heart failure; hypertension

Drug	Z Code	Drug Action/Classification	Indications
Altavera [ethinyl estradiol/levonorgestrel]	Z79.3	Contraceptive	Prevention of pregnancy
Alvesco [ciclesonide]	Z79.51	Corticosteroid -inhaled; antiasthmatic	Prophylaxis and treatment of asthma
Alyacen [ethinyl estradiol/norethindrone]	Z79.3	Contraceptive	Prevention of pregnancy
Amaryl [glimepiride]	Z79.84	Oral hypoglycemic	Diabetes mellitus
Ambien [zolpidem tartrate]		CNS depressant; anxiolytic/sedative/hypnotic	Insomnia
Amikacin [amikacin sulfate]	Z79.2	Antibiotic	Gram-negative bacterial infections such as Pseudomonas, Escherichia coli (E. coli), Proteus, Klebsiella-Enterobacter-Serratia
Amitriptyline HCl [amitriptyline hydrochloride]		Antidepressant	Depression
Amoxicillin [amoxicillin]	Z79.2	Antibiotic	Treatment of infections with a broad spectrum of bactericidal activity against many gram-positive and gram-negative micro-organisms; otitis media, gonorrhea, skin, respiratory, gastrointestinal, and genitourinary infections
Ampicillin [ampicillin sodium]	Z79.2	Antibiotic	Bacterial infections
Ampyra [dalfampridine]		Potassium channel blocker	Improvement in walking in patients with multiple sclerosis
Amrix [cyclobenzaprine hydrochloride]		Muscle relaxant	Adjunct to rest and physical therapy for muscle spasms
Anaprox DS [naproxen sodium]	Z79.1	Nonsteroidal anti-inflammatory drug (NSAID)	Pain, inflammation or fever relief
Anastrozole [anastrozole]	Z79.811	Aromatase inhibitor	Postmenopausal breast cancer
Ancef [cefazolin sodium]	Z79.2	Antibiotic	Respiratory tract infections due to Streptococcus pneumoniae, Klebsiella species, Haemophilus influenzae (H. influenzae), Staphylococcus aureus, and group A betahemolytic streptococci; urinary tract infections due to E. coli, Proteus mirabilis, Klebsiella species and some strains of Enterobacter and enterococci; skin and skin structure infections, biliary tract infections, bone and joint infections, genital infections, septicemia, and endocarditis
Androderm [testosterone]	Z79.890	Testosterone therapy -topical	Primary hypogonadism, hypogonadotropic hypogonadism
AndroGel [testosterone]	Z79.890	Testosterone therapy -topical	Primary hypogonadism, hypogonadotropic hypogonadism
Angeliq [drospirenone/estradiol]	Z79.890	Estrogen therapy	Menopause symptoms
Angiomax [bivalirudin]	Z79.01	Anticoagulant	Prevention of blood clots
Antabuse [disulfiram]		Alcohol treatment	Alcoholism
Antineoplastic/chemotherapy	Z79.899	Antineoplastic	Cancer
Apidra [insulin glulisine recombinant]	Z79.4	Insulin	Diabetes mellitus
Aranelle [ethinyl estradiol/norethindrone]	Z79.3	Contraceptive	Prevention of pregnancy; acne
Aranesp [darbepoetin alfa]		Erythropoiesis-stimulating agent (ESA)	Treatment of lower than normal blood cells (anemia) from disorders such as CKD and neoplasms
Argatroban [argatroban]	Z79.01	Anticoagulant	Prophylaxis and treatment of venous thrombosis in thrombocytopenia patients
Aricept [donepezil hydrochloride]		Acetylcholinesterase/cholinesterase inhibitors	Symptoms of mild to moderate Alzheimer's disease; can improve thinking ability in some patients
Arimidex [anastrozole]	Z79.811	Aromatase inhibitor	Postmenopausal breast cancer
Aristospan [triamcinolone hexacetonide]	Z79.52	Corticosteroid	Severe inflammation
Arixtra [fondaparinux sodium]	Z79.01	Anticoagulant	Venous thrombosis and pulmonary embolism
Armonair Respiclick [fluticasone propionate]	Z79.51	Corticosteroid -- inhaled; anitasthmatic	Asthma
Arnuity Ellipta [fluticasone furoate]	Z79.51	Corticosteroid -inhaled; antiasthmatic	Prophylaxis and treatment of asthma
Aromasin [exemestane]	Z79.811	Aromatase inhibitor	Postmenopausal breast cancer
Arthrotec [diclofenac sodium/misoprostol]	Z79.1	Non-steroidal anti-inflammatory drug (NSAID)-prostaglandin combo	Treatment of patients with arthritis who may develop stomach ulcers from taking nonsteroidal anti-inflammatory drugs (NSAIDs) alone; used to help relieve some symptoms of arthritis, such as inflammation, swelling, stiffness, and joint pain
Asacol HD [mesalamine]		Antiinflammatory	Ulcerative colitis

Drug	Z Code	Drug Action/Classification	Indications
Ashlyna [ethinyl estradiol/levonorgestrel]	Z79.3	Contraceptive	Prevention of pregnancy
Asmanex [mometasone furoate]	Z79.51	Corticosteroid -inhaled; antiasthmatic	Prophylaxis and treatment of asthma
Astagraf XL [tacrolimus]	Z79.899	Immunosuppressant	Prophylaxis of organ transplant rejection
Atelvia [risedronate sodium]	Z79.83	Bisphosphonate	Prevention of thinning of the bones (osteoporosis)
Atenolol [atenolol]		Beta blocker	Angina pectoris; hypertension; acute myocardial infarction
Ativan [lorazepam]		Antianxiety; sedative/hypnotic	Anxiety disorder associated with depressive symptoms; controls tension, agitation, irritability, and insomnia
Atripla [efavirenz/emtricitabine/tenofovir disoproxil fumarate]	Z79.899	Antiviral	HIV
Atrovent HFA [ipratropium bromide]		Antiasthmatic/bronchodilator	Chronic bronchitis, emphysema; bronchial asthma
Augmentin [amoxicillin/clavulanate potassium]	Z79.2	Antibiotic	Middle ear, lower respiratory, sinus, skin and skin structures, and urinary tract infections
Avandia [rosiglitazone maleate]	Z79.84	Oral hypoglycemic	Diabetes mellitus
Avapro [irbesartan]		Antihypertensive	Hypertension
Avelox [moxifloxacin hydrochloride]	Z79.2	Antibiotic	Bacterial infections, specifically pneumonia; skin; intra-abdominal; plague; acute sinusitis; acute chronic bronchitis
Aviane-28 [ethinyl estradiol/levonorgestrel]	Z79.3	Contraceptive	Prevention of pregnancy
Avonex [interferon beta-1a]	Z79.899	Antiviral	Treatment of relapsing multiple sclerosis
Axid AR [nizatidine]		Histamine H2-receptor antagonist	Acid/peptic disorder; gastroesophageal reflux; duodenal, gastric, and peptic ulcers
Azactam [aztreonam]	Z79.2	Antibiotic	Severe bacterial infections
Azithromycin [azithromycin]	Z79.2	Antibiotic	Bacterial infections
Bactrim [sulfamethoxazole/trimethoprim]	Z79.2	Antibiotic	Treatment of urinary tract infections, acute otitis media, acute exacerbation of chronic bronchitis, shigellosis, and pneumocystis carinii
Balziva-28 [ethinyl estradiol/norethindrone]	Z79.3	Contraceptive	Prevention of pregnancy
Basaglar [insulin glargine]	Z79.4	Insulin	Diabetes mellitus
Bayer [acetylsalicylic acid]	Z79.82	Aspirin	Prophylaxis and treatment of heart attacks, angina or strokes; reduction of fever, pain and inflammation
Beconase AQ [beclomethasone dipropionate monohydrate]		Corticosteroid -inhaled/nasal	Perennial and seasonal allergies; vasomotor rhinitis
Bekyree [desogestrel/ethinyl estradiol]	Z79.3	Contraceptive	Prevention of pregnancy
Betaseron [interferon beta-1b]	Z79.899	Antiviral	Treatment of relapsing multiple sclerosis
Betoptic [betaxolol hydrochloride]		Beta blocker; ophthalmic glaucoma agent	Lowering of intraocular pressure; also used for treatment of ocular hypertension and chronic open-angle glaucoma
Bevyxxa	Z79.01	Anticoagulant	Prophylaxis of venous thromboembolism
Beyaz [drospirenone/ethinyl estradiol/levomefolate calcium]	Z79.3	Contraceptive	Prevention of pregnancy; acne
Biaxin XL [clarithromycin]	Z79.2	Antibiotic	Acid/peptic disorder or ulcer, acute exacerbation chronic bronchitis, human immunodeficiency virus, lower and upper respiratory tract infection, sinus infection, prophylaxis mycobacterium avium complex, pharyngitis, pneumonia, tonsillitis
Bijuva [estradiol/progesterone]	Z79.890	Estrogen/progesterone therapy	Menopausal symptoms
Biltricide [praziquantel]		Antiparasitic	Infections from Schistosoma species and liver flukes
Binosto [alendronate sodium]	Z79.83	Bisphosphonate	Prevention of thinning of the bones (osteoporosis)
Boniva [ibandronate sodium]	Z79.83	Bisphosphonate	Prevention of thinning of the bones (osteoporosis)
Breo Ellipta [fluticasone furoate/vilanterol trifenatate]	Z79.51	Corticosteroid -- inhaled; anitasthmatic	Maintenance treatment of asthma and COPD
Brevicon 28-day [ethinyl estradiol/norethindrone]	Z79.3	Contraceptive	Prevention of pregnancy; acne
Briellyn [ethinyl estradiol/norethindrone]	Z79.3	Contraceptive	Prevention of pregnancy

Drug	Z Code	Drug Action/Classification	Indications
Brilinta [ticagrelor]	Z79.02	Antiplatelet	Unstable angina; heart attacks; prevention of blood clots
Brisdelle [paroxetine]		Selective serotonin reuptake inhibitor (SSRI)	Vasomotor symptoms related to menopause
Buprenex [buprenorphine hydrochloride]	Z79.891	Analgesic, narcotic	Moderate to severe pain
Buprenorphine HCl and Naloxone HCl [buprenorphine hydrochloride/naloxone hydrochloride]	Z79.891	Analgesic, narcotic	Moderate to severe pain
Buspirone HCl [buspirone hydrochloride]		Antianxiety	Generalized anxiety disorder
Butorphanol tartrate [butorphanol tartrate]	Z79.891	Analgesic, narcotic	Moderate to severe postsurgical pain
Butrans [buprenorphine]	Z79.891	Analgesic, narcotic	Chronic pain
Byetta [exenatide]		Antidiabetic — injectable	Diabetes mellitus
Calan [verapamil hydrochloride]		Calcium channel blocker	Angina pectoris at rest and chronic stable, arrhythmia, atrial fibrillation, atrial flutter, paroxysmal supraventricular tachycardia, ventricular arrhythmia, Hypertension
Caldolor [ibuprofen]	Z79.1	Nonsteroidal anti-inflammatory drug (NSAID)	Pain or fever relief
Cambia [diclofenac potassium]	Z79.1	Nonsteroidal anti-inflammatory drug (NSAID)	Migraine headaches
Camila [norethindrone]	Z79.3	Contraceptive	Prevention of pregnancy; menstrual disorders
Cardizem CD [diltiazem hydrochloride]		Calcium channel blocker	Chronic stable angina, atrial fibrillation, atrial flutter, hypertension, paroxysmal supraventricular tachycardia
Cardura [doxazosin mesylate]		Antihypertensive	Benign prostatic hyperplasia; hypertension
Catapres [clonidine hydrochloride]		Antihypertensive	Hypertension
Cefprozil [cefprozil]	Z79.2	Antibiotic	Acute exacerbation and chronic bronchitis, lower respiratory tract infection, upper respiratory tract infection, pharyngitis, tonsillitis
Ceftriaxone [ceftriaxone sodium]	Z79.2	Antibiotic	Bacterial infections
Celebrex [celecoxib]	Z79.1	Nonsteroidal anti-inflammatory drug (NSAID)	Relief of some symptoms caused by arthritis, such as inflammation, swelling, stiffness, and joint pain
Celestone Soluspan [betamethasone acetate/betamethasone sodium phosphate]	Z79.52	Corticosteroid; antiasthmatic	Asthma; severe inflammation
Celexa [citalopram hydrobromide]		Antidepressant	Depression
Cellcept [mycophenolate mofetil]	Z79.899	Immunosuppressant	Prophylaxis of organ transplant rejection
Centany [mupirocin]	Z79.2	Antibiotic	Skin infections
Cephalexin [cephalexin]	Z79.2	Antibiotic	Bacterial infections
Chantix [varenicline tartrate]		Smoking cessation aid	Nicotine addiction, smoking
Cimduo [lamivudine/tenofovir disoproxil fumarate]	Z79.899	Antiviral	HIV
Cipro [ciprofloxacin hydrochloride]	Z79.2	Antibiotic	Cystitis, infectious diarrhea, gonorrhea, bone and joint infection, gastrointestinal tract infection, lower and upper respiratory tract infection, sinus infection, urinary tract infection, nosocomial pneumonia, chronic prostatitis
Ciprofloxacin [ciprofloxacin]	Z79.2	Antibiotic	Bacterial infections
Clarithromycin [clarithromycin]	Z79.2	Antibiotic	Skin and respiratory bacterial infections
Claritin [loratadine]		Antihistamine	Seasonal allergic rhinitis; chronic idiopathic urticaria
Cleocin [clindamycin phosphate]	Z79.2	Antibiotic	Bacterial infections
Climara [estradiol]	Z79.890	Estrogen therapy	Osteoporosis prevention and to treat menopausal symptoms; vaginal and vulvar atrophy; hypoestrogenism; ovarian failure
Clindamycin [clindamycin phosphate]	Z79.2	Antibiotic	Bacterial infections
Clonazepam [clonazepam]		Anticonvulsant	Absence, akinetic and myoclonic epilepsy, Lennox-Gastaut syndrome
Clonidine HCl [clonidine hydrochloride]		Antihypertensive	Hypertension
Clopidogrel bisulfate [clopidogrel bisulfate]	Z79.02	Antiplatelet	Unstable angina; heart attacks; prevention of blood clots
Codeine [codeine sulfate]	Z79.891	Analgesic, narcotic	Mild to moderate pain

Drug	Z Code	Drug Action/Classification	Indications
Cogentin [benztropine mesylate]		Antiparkinsonism	Parkinson's disease
Colace [docusate sodium]		Gastrointestinal agent; laxative, stool softener	Constipation
Colocort [hydrocortisone]	Z79.52	Corticosteroid	Inflammation of the colon
CombiPatch [ethinyl estradiol/norethindrone acetate]	Z79.890	Estrogen therapy	Menopause symptoms; vaginal and vulvar atrophy; osteoporosis prevention
Combivent respimat [ipratropium bromide/albuterol sulfate]		Antiasthmatic/bronchodilator	Chronic bronchitis, emphysema; bronchial asthma
Compro [prochlorperazine]		Antiemetic; antipsychotic	Nausea, vomiting, and manic phase of bipolar syndrome or schizophrenia
Copaxone [glatiramer acetate]		Immunostimulant	Treatment of relapsing multiple sclerosis
Coreg [carvedilol]		Beta blocker	Hypertension; chronic heart failure; left ventricular dysfunction following myocardial infarction
Coreg CR [carvedilol phosphate]		Beta blocker	Hypertension; chronic heart failure; left ventricular dysfunction following myocardial infarction
Cortef [hydrocortisone]	Z79.52	Corticosteroid	Severe inflammation
Cortenema [hydrocortisone]	Z79.52	Corticosteroid	Inflammation of the colon
Cortifoam [hydrocortisone acetate]	Z79.52	Corticosteroid	Colon and rectum inflammation
Cortisone acetate [cortisone acetate]	Z79.52	Corticosteroid	Inflammation
Cortisporin [hydrocortisone acetate/neomycin sulfate/polymyxin B sulfate]		Topical anti-infective, topical steroid	Dermatosis
Cosentyx [secukinumab]	Z79.899	Immunosuppressant	Plaque psoriasis; psoriatic arthritis; ankylosing spondylitis
Coumadin [warfarin sodium]	Z79.01	Anticoagulant	Prophylaxis and treatment of venous thrombosis, treatment of atrial fibrillation with embolization (pulmonary embolism), arrhythmias, myocardial infarction, and stroke prevention
Cozaar [losartan potassium]		Antihypertensive	Hypertension
Crestor [rosuvastatin calcium]		HMG-CoA reductase inhibitor (statin)	Hypercholesterolemia; hyperlipidemia; hyperproteinemia
Crixivan [indinavir sulfate]	Z79.899	Antiviral	HIV, asymptomatic HIV
Cryselle [ethinyl estradiol/norgestrel]	Z79.3	Contraceptive	Prevention of pregnancy
Cubicin [daptomycin]	Z79.2	Antibiotic	Bacterial skin infections; *Staphylococcus aureus* bloodstream infections
Cyclafem [ethinyl estradiol/norethindrone]	Z79.3	Contraceptive	Prevention of pregnancy
Cyclessa [desogestrel/ethinyl estradiol]	Z79.3	Contraceptive	Prevention of pregnancy
Cyclosporine [cyclosporine]	Z79.899	Immunosuppressant	Prophylaxis of organ transplant rejection
Cyltezo [adalimumab-abdm]	Z79.899	Antirheumatic	Rheumatoid arthritis; juvenile idiopathic arthritis; psoriatic arthritis; Crohn's disease; ulcerative colitis; plaque psoriasis
Cymbalta [duloxetine hydrochloride]		Antidepressant, serotonin and norepinephrine reuptake inhibitor (SNRI)	Major depressive disorder; general anxiety disorder; fibromyalgia; diabetic peripheral neuropathy; chronic musculoskeletal pain
Cytomel [liothyronine sodium]		Thyroid hormone	Hypothyroidism or prevention of euthyroid goiters
Daptomycin [daptomycin]	Z79.2	Antibiotic	Skin and underlying tissue bacterial infections
Dasetta [ethinyl estradiol/norethindrone]	Z79.3	Contraceptive	Prevention of pregnancy
Daypro [oxaprozin]	Z79.1	Nonsteroidal anti-inflammatory drug (NSAID)	Osteoarthritis and rheumatoid arthritis
Daysee [ethinyl estradiol/levonorgestrel]	Z79.3	Contraceptive	Prevention of pregnancy
Delestrogen [estradiol valerate]	Z79.890	Estrogen therapy	Menopause symptoms
Demerol [meperidine hydrochloride]	Z79.891	Analgesic, narcotic	Moderate to severe pain
Depakote [divalproex sodium]		Anticonvulsant	Bipolar affective disorder; complex absence, complex partial and mixed pattern epilepsy; migraine headache
Depo-Medrol [methylprednisolone acetate]	Z79.52	Corticosteroid	Arthritis; joint disorders
Depo-Provera [medroxyprogesterone acetate]	Z79.3, Z79.890	Antineoplastic; contraceptive; progestin	Amenorrhea; carcinoma, endometrium, adjunct; carcinoma, renal; Prevention of pregnancy; hemorrhage

Drug	Z Code	Drug Action/Classification	Indications
Depo-SubQ Provera [medroxyprogesterone acetate]	Z79.3	Contraceptive	Prevention of pregnancy; menstrual disorder pain
Descovy [emtricitabine/tenofovir alafenamide]	Z79.899	Antiretroviral	HIV
Desogen [desogestrel/ethinyl estradiol]	Z79.3	Contraceptive	Prevention of pregnancy
Detrol [tolterodine tartrate]		Muscarinic receptor antagonist	Overactive bladders in patients with urinary frequency, urgency, or urge incontinence
Dexamethasone Intensol [dexamethasone]	Z79.52	Corticosteroid	Arthritis; allergic disorders; breathing disorders; lupus
Dexilant [dexlansoprazole]		Proton pump inhibitor	Healing of erosive esophagitis; relieve of heartburn; treatment of non-erosive gastroesophageal reflux disease
Diabinese [chlorpropamide]	Z79.84	Oral hypoglycemic	Diabetes mellitus
Diaβeta [glyburide]	Z79.84	Oral hypoglycemic	Diabetes mellitus
Diclegis [doxylamine succinate/pyridoxine hydrochloride]		Antiemetic	Nausea/vomiting in pregnancy
Didronel [etidronate disodium]	Z79.83	Bisphosphonate	Paget's disease and irregular bone growth
Dificid [fidaxomicin]	Z79.2	Antibiotic	Clostridium difficile
Diflucan [fluconazole]		Antifungal	Oropharyngeal and esophageal candidiasis and cryptococcal meningitis in AIDS patients
Digoxin [digoxin]		Cardiotonic glycoside	Heart failure, atrial flutter, atrial fibrillation, and supraventricular tachycardia
Dilantin [phenytoin sodium]		Anticonvulsant	Grand mal and psychomotor seizures
Dilaudid [hydromorphone hydrochloride]	Z79.891	Analgesic, narcotic	Moderate to severe pain
Diovan [valsartan]		Angiotensin II receptor blocker	Hypertension
Diskets [methadone hydrochloride]		Opioid agonist	Treatment of opioid addiction
Divigel [estradiol]	Z79.890	Estrogen therapy -topical	Menopause symptoms
Dolophine HCl [methadone hydrochloride]	Z79.891	Analgesic, narcotic; opioid agonist	Pain; treatment of opioid addiction
Doxycycline [doxycycline]	Z79.2	Antibiotic	Bacterial infections; acne
Duavee [bazedoxifene acetate/conjugated estrogens]	Z79.890	Estrogen therapy	Menopause symptoms; osteoporosis prevention
Duetact [glimepiride/pioglitazone hydrochloride]	Z79.84	Oral hypoglycemic	Diabetes mellitus
Duexis [famotidine/ibuprofen]	Z79.1	Nonsteroidal anti-inflammatory drug (NSAID)	Symptomatic treatment of osteoarthritis and rheumatoid arthritis; reduce risk of ulcers
Dulera [formoterol fumarate/mometasone furoate]	Z79.51	Corticosteroid -inhaled; antiasthmatic	Prophylaxis and treatment of asthma
Duragesic [fentanyl]	Z79.891	Analgesic, narcotic	Chronic pain
Duramorph PF [morphine sulfate]	Z79.891	Analgesic, narcotic	Moderate to severe pain
Durlaza [aspirin]	Z79.82	Aspirin	Prevention of heart attack, stroke, angina
Dynacin [minocycline hydrochloride]	Z79.2	Antibiotic	Severe acne treatment
E.E.S. [erythromycin ethylsuccinate]	Z79.2	Antibiotic	Bacterial infections
Effexor XR [venlafaxine hydrochloride]		Antidepressant, serotonin and norepinephrine reuptake inhibitors (SNRIs)	Major depressive disorder; social anxiety disorder; panic disorder
Effient [prasugrel hydrochloride]	Z79.02	Antiplatelet	Lessening of the chance of heart attack or stroke
Elestrin [estradiol]	Z79.890	Estrogen therapy	Menopause symptoms
Eligard [leuprolide acetate]	Z79.818	Agents affecting estrogen receptors and estrogen levels	Palliative treatment of prostate cancer symptoms
Elinest [norgestrel/ethinyl estradiol]	Z79.3	Contraceptive	Prevention of pregnancy
Eliquis [apixaban]	Z79.01	Anticoagulant	Venous thrombosis
Embeda [morphine sulfate/naltrexone hydrochloride]	Z79.891	Analgesic, narcotic	Moderate to severe pain
Emoquette [ethinyl estradiol/desogestrel]	Z79.3	Contraceptive	Prevention of pregnancy

Drug	Z Code	Drug Action/Classification	Indications
Emtriva [emtricitabine]	Z79.899	Antiretroviral	HIV
Enbrel [etanercept]	Z79.899	Antirheumatic	Rheumatoid arthritis; polyarticular juvenile idiopathic arthritis; psoriatic arthritis; ankylosing spondylitis, plaque psoriasis
Enpresse-28 [ethinyl estradiol/levonorgestrel]	Z79.3	Contraceptive	Prevention of pregnancy
Enskyce [desogestrel/ethinyl estradiol]	Z79.3	Contraceptive	Prevention of pregnancy
Entocort EC [budesonide]	Z79.52	Corticosteroid	Crohn's disease; ulcerative colitis
Entresto [sacubitril/valsartan]		Angiotensin II receptor blocker; neprilysin inhibitor	Chronic heart failure
Entyvio [vedolizumab]	Z79.899	Immunosuppressant	Ulcerative colitis; Crohn's disease
Envarsus XR [tacrolimus]	Z79.899	Immunosuppressant	Prophylaxis of organ transplant rejection
Epinephrine [epinephrine]		Bronchodilator, cardiotonic	Most commonly, relief of distress due to bronchospasm and restoration of cardiac rhythm in cardiac arrest
Epivir, Epivir-HBV [lamivudine]	Z79.899	Antiretroviral	HIV, hepatitis B (HBV), asymptomatic HIV
Erelzi [etanercept-szzs]	Z79.899	Antirheumatic	Rheumatoid arthritis; polyarticular juvenile idiopathic arthritis; psoriatic arthritis; ankylosing spondylitis, plaque psoriasis
Errin [norethindrone]	Z79.3	Contraceptive	Prevention of pregnancy
Ertapenem [ertapenem sodium]	Z79.2	Antibiotic	Stomach, urinary tract, pelvis, skin and lung infections
Ery-Tab [erythromycin]	Z79.2	Antibiotic	Bacterial infections
ERYC [erythromycin]	Z79.2	Antibiotic	Respiratory tract infections
Erygel [erythromycin]	Z79.2	Antibiotic, topical	Bacterial skin infections
EryPed [erythromycin ethylsuccinate]	Z79.2	Antibiotic	Bacterial infections; rheumatic fever attacks
Erythrocin [erythromycin lactobionate]	Z79.2	Antibiotic	Bacterial infections
Erythromycin [erythromycin]	Z79.2	Antibiotic	Respiratory tract infections
Estarylla [ethinyl estradiol/norgestimate]	Z79.3	Contraceptive	Prevention of pregnancy
Estrace [estradiol]	Z79.890	Estrogen therapy	Vaginal cream for treatment of vaginal and vulvar atrophy
EstroGel [estradiol]	Z79.890	Estrogen therapy -topical	Menopause symptoms
Estrostep Fe [ethinyl estradiol/norethindrone acetate]	Z79.3	Contraceptive	Prevention of pregnancy
Evista [raloxifene hydrochloride]	Z79.810	Selective estrogen receptor modulator (SERM)	Prevention of thinning of the bones (osteoporosis) only in postmenopausal women
Exalgo [hydromorphone hydrochloride]	Z79.891	Analgesic, narcotic	Moderate to severe pain
Exemestane [exemestane]	Z79.811	Aromatase inhibitor	Postmenopausal breast cancer
Factive [gemifloxacin mesylate]	Z79.2	Antibiotic	Bacterial lung infections
Falmina [ethinyl estradiol/levonorgestrel]	Z79.3	Contraceptive	Prevention of pregnancy
Fareston [toremifene citrate]	Z79.810	Selective estrogen receptor modulator (SERM)	Treatment of metastatic breast cancer in postmenopausal women
Farxiga [dapagliflozin propanediol]	Z79.84	Oral hypoglycemic	Diabetes mellitus
Faslodex [fulvestrant]	Z79.818	Agents affecting estrogen receptors and estrogen levels	Hormone-related breast cancer; metastatic breast cancer
Feldene [piroxicam]	Z79.1	Nonsteroidal anti-inflammatory drug (NSAID)	Treatment of pain and inflammation due to arthritis
Femara [letrozole]	Z79.811	Aromatase inhibitor	Postmenopausal breast cancer
Femcon Fe [ethinyl estradiol/norethindrone]	Z79.3	Contraceptive	Prevention of pregnancy; acne
Femhrt [ethinyl estradiol/norethindrone acetate]	Z79.3, Z79.890	Contraceptive; estrogen therapy	Prevention of pregnancy; menopause symptoms; osteoporosis prevention
Femring [estradiol acetate]	Z79.890	Estrogen therapy	Osteoporosis prevention and to treat menopausal symptoms; hypoestrogenism; ovarian failure
Fentanyl citrate [fentanyl citrate]	Z79.891	Analgesic, narcotic	Postprocedural or chronic pain
Fentora [fentanyl citrate]	Z79.891	Analgesic, narcotic	Breakthrough cancer pain
Fiasp [insulin aspart]	Z79.4	Insulin	Diabetes mellitus

Drug	Z Code	Drug Action/Classification	Indications
Fioricet with codeine [acetaminophen/butalbital/caffeine/codeine phosphate]	Z79.891	Analgesic, narcotic	Tension headaches
Firmagon [degarelix]	Z79.89Ø	Hormone therapy	Prostate cancer
Flagyl [metronidazole]	Z79.2	Antibiotic	Bacterial infections
Flavoxate HCl [flavoxate hydrochloride]		Urinary tract spasmolytic	Relief of dysuria, urgency, nocturia, suprapubic pain, frequency, and incontinence associated with cystitis, prostatitis, urethritis, and urethrocystitis/urethrotrigonitis
Flomax [tamsulosin hydrochloride]		Antiadrenergic	Benign prostatic hyperplasia
Flonase allergy relief [fluticasone propionate]		Corticosteroid -inhaled/nasal	Perennial and seasonal allergic rhinitis
Flovent HFA [fluticasone propionate]	Z79.51	Corticosteroid -inhaled; antiasthmatic	Asthma
Fortamet [metformin hydrochloride]	Z79.84	Oral hypoglycemic	Diabetes mellitus
Fortaz [ceftazidime]	Z79.2	Antibiotic	Pneumonia and lower respiratory infections
Fosamax [alendronate sodium]	Z79.83	Biophosphonate	Osteoporosis; Paget's disease
Fosinopril sodium [fosinopril sodium]		ACE inhibitor	Hypertension
Fosrenol [lanthanum carbonate]		Phosphate binder	End-stage renal disease (ESRD)
Fragmin [dalteparin sodium]	Z79.Ø1	Anticoagulant	Prophylaxis and treatment of blood clots
Gengraf [cyclosporine]	Z79.899	Immunosuppressant	Prophylaxis of organ transplant rejection
Gentamicin sulfate [gentamicin sulfate]	Z79.2	Antibiotic	Severe bacterial infections
Gildagia [ethinyl estradiol/norethindrone]	Z79.3	Contraceptive	Prevention of pregnancy
Gildess [ethinyl estradiol/norethindrone acetate]	Z79.3	Contraceptive	Prevention of pregnancy
Glimepiride [glimepiride]	Z79.84	Oral hypoglycemic	Diabetes mellitus
Glucophage [metformin hydrochloride]	Z79.84	Oral hypoglycemic	Diabetes mellitus
Glucotrol [glipizide]	Z79.84	Oral hypoglycemic	Diabetes mellitus
Glucovance [glyburide/metformin hydrochloride]	Z79.84	Oral hypoglycemic	Diabetes mellitus
Glumetza [metformin hydrochloride]	Z79.84	Oral hypoglycemic	Diabetes mellitus
Glyburide (micronized) [glyburide]	Z79.84	Oral hypoglycemic	Diabetes mellitus
Glynase [glyburide]	Z79.84	Oral hypoglycemic	Diabetes mellitus
Glyset [miglitol]	Z79.84	Oral hypoglycemic	Diabetes mellitus
Harvoni [ledipasvir/sofosbuvir]	Z79.899	Antiviral	Chronic hepatitis C
Heparin sodium [heparin sodium]	Z79.Ø1	Anticoagulant	Prophylaxis and treatment of venous thrombosis, pulmonary embolism; prevention of cerebral thrombosis, and treatment of consumptive coagulopathies
Humalog [insulin lispro recombinant]	Z79.4	Insulin	Diabetes mellitus
Humira [adalimumab]	Z79.899	Antirheumatic	Rheumatoid arthritis; juvenile idiopathic arthritis; psoriatic arthritis; Crohn's disease; ulcerative colitis; plaque psoriasis; hidradenitis suppurativa; uveitis
Humulin R [insulin recombinant]	Z79.4	Insulin	Diabetes mellitus
Hydrochlorothiazide [hydrochlorothiazide]		Diuretic; antihypertensive	Management of hypertension and in adjunctive therapy for edema associated with congestive heart failure; hepatic cirrhosis; corticosteroid, and estrogen therapy
Hydrocodone [acetaminophen/hydrocodone bitartrate]	Z79.891	Analgesic, narcotic	Moderate to severe pain
Hydrocodone bitartrate and acetaminophen [acetaminophen/hydrocodone bitartrate]	Z79.891	Analgesic, narcotic	Pain, moderate to severe
Hydrocortisone [hydrocortisone]	Z79.52	Corticosteroid	Addison's disease; arthritis; immune disorders; allergies; breathing problems
Hydromorphone HCl [hydromorphone hydrochloride]	Z79.891	Analgesic, narcotic	Moderate to severe pain

Drug	Z Code	Drug Action/Classification	Indications
Hyrimoz [adalimumab-adaz]	Z79.899	Antirheumatic	Rheumatoid arthritis; juvenile idiopathic arthritis; psoriatic arthritis; Crohn's disease; ulcerative colitis; plaque psoriasis
Hyzaar [hydrochlorothiazide/ losartan potassium]		Antihypertensive	Hypertension
Ibuprofen [ibuprofen]	Z79.1	Nonsteroidal anti-inflammatory drug (NSAID)	Pain or fever relief
Imitrex [sumatriptan succinate]		Antimigraine	Migraine headache
Imuran [azathioprine]	Z79.899	Immunosuppressant	Rheumatoid arthritis
Inderal [propranolol hydrochloride]		Beta blocker	Angina pectoris; hypertension; cardiac arrhythmias
Indocin [indomethacin]	Z79.1	Nonsteroidal anti-inflammatory drug (NSAID)	Treatment of pain and inflammation
Integrilin [eptifibatide]	Z79.02	Antiplatelet	Unstable angina; heart attacks; prevention of blood clots
Intron A [interferon alfa 2-b]	Z79.899	Antineoplastic interferons; antiviral interferons	Cancer; hepatitis
Introvale [levonorgestrel/ethinyl estradiol]	Z79.3	Contraceptive	Prevention of pregnancy
Invanz [ertapeneum sodium]	Z79.2	Antibiotic	Stomach, urinary tract, pelvis, skin and lung infections
Invokamet [canagliflozin/metformin hydrochloride]	Z79.84	Oral hypoglycemic	Diabetes mellitus
Invokana [canagliflozin]	Z79.84	Oral hypoglycemic	Diabetes mellitus
Isoniazid [isoniazid]	Z79.2	Antibiotic	Tuberculosis
Isopto carpine [pilocarpine hydrochloride]		Cholinergic parasympathomimetic agent	Reduction of intraocular pressure in open-angle glaucoma or ocular hypertension; management of acute angle-closure glaucoma
Isordil [isosorbide dinitrate]		Smooth muscle relaxant	Acute anginal attacks
Isuprel [isoproterenol hydrochloride]		Adrenergic agent	Bronchodilator for asthma, chronic pulmonary emphysema, bronchitis, and other conditions accompanied by bronchospasm; can be used in cardiogenic shock cases
Jantoven [warfarin sodium]	Z79.01	Anticoagulant	Prophylaxis and treatment of venous thrombosis, pulmonary embolism; prevention of cerebral thrombosis, and treatment of consumptive coagulopathies
Janumet [metformin hydrochloride/sitagliptin phosphate]	Z79.84	Oral hypoglycemic	Diabetes mellitus
Januvia [sitagliptin phosphate]	Z79.84	Oral hypoglycemic	Diabetes mellitus
Jencycla [norethindrone]	Z79.3	Contraceptive	Prevention of pregnancy
Jentadueto [linagliptin/metformin hydrochloride]]	Z79.84	Oral hypoglycemic	Diabetes mellitus
Junel [ethinyl estradiol/norethindrone acetate]	Z79.3	Contraceptive	Prevention of pregnancy
K-Tab [potassium chloride]		Replaces potassium and maintains potassium level	Hypokalemia
Kadian [morphine sulfate]	Z79.891	Analgesic, narcotic	Moderate to severe pain
Kariva [desogestrel/ethinyl estradiol]	Z79.3	Contraceptive	Prevention of pregnancy
Kazano [alogliptin benzoate/metformin hydrochloride]	Z79.84	Oral hypoglycemic	Diabetes mellitus
Keflex [cephalexin]	Z79.2	Antibiotic	Bone, middle ear, skin and skin structures, upper respiratory tract and urinary tract infections; acute prostatitis
Kelnor [ethynodiol diacetate/ethinyl estradiol]	Z79.3	Contraceptive	Prevention of pregnancy
Kenalog-10; Kenalog-40 [triamcinolone acetonide]	Z79.52	Corticosteroid	Gouty arthritis; bursitis; tenosynovitis; epicondylitis; rheumatoid arthritis; synovitis; osteoarthritis
Keytruda [pembrolizumab]	Z79.899	Antineoplastic	Cancer
Kimidess [ethinyl estradiol/desogestrel]	Z79.3	Contraceptive	Prevention of pregnancy
Klaron [sulfacetamide sodium]	Z79.2	Antibiotic, topical	Acne vulgaris
Klonopin [clonazepam]		Anticonvulsant; CNS depressant	Epilepsy; seizures; panic disorder
Klor-Con [potassium chloride]		Replaces potassium and maintains potassium level	Hypokalemia

Drug	Z Code	Drug Action/Classification	Indications
Kombiglyze [metformin hydrochloride/saxagliptin hydrochloride]	Z79.84	Oral hypoglycemic	Diabetes mellitus
Kurvelo [ethinyl estradiol/levonorgestrel]	Z79.3	Contraceptive	Prevention of pregnancy; menstrual disorders
Kyleena [levonorgestrel]	Z79.3	Contraceptive	Prevention of pregnancy
Lamisil [terbinafine hydrochloride]		Antifungal	Tinea cruris (jock itch), T. pedis (athlete's foot), T. corporis (ringworm)
Lanoxin [digoxin]		Cardiotonic glycoside	Congestive heart failure
Lantus [insulin glargine recombinant]	Z79.4	Insulin	Diabetes mellitus
Larin [ethinyl estradiol/norethindrone acetate]	Z79.3	Contraceptive	Prevention of pregnancy
Lasix [furosemide]		Antihypertensive; diuretic	Management of edema associated with congestive heart failure, renal disease, including nephrotic syndrome and hypertension
Lazanda [fentanyl citrate]	Z79.891	Analgesics, narcotic	Breakthrough cancer pain
Lescol XL [fluvastatin sodium]	,	HMG-CoA reductase inhibitor (statin)	Hypercholesterolemia; hyperlipidemia; hyperlipoproteinemia
Lessina-28 [ethinyl estradiol/levonorgestrel]	Z79.3	Contraceptive	Prevention of pregnancy
Letrozole [letrozole]	Z79.811	Aromatase inhibitor	Postmenopausal breast cancer
Levemir [insulin detemir recombinant]	Z79.4	Insulin	Diabetes mellitus
Levonest [levonorgestrel/ethinyl estradiol]	Z79.3	Contraceptive	Prevention of pregnancy; menstrual disorders; acne
Levora [levonorgestrel/ethinyl estradiol]	Z79.3	Contraceptive	Prevention of pregnancy
Levothroid [levothyroxine sodium]		Thyroid hormone	Hypothyroidism
Levoxyl [levothyroxine sodium]		Thyroid hormone	Euthyroid goiter; hypothyroidism
Lexapro [escitalopram oxalate]		Antidepressant, selective serotonin reuptake inhibitor (SSRI)	Depression; anxiety
Lialda [mesalamine]		Antiinflammatory	Ulcerative colitis
Librium [chlordiazepoxide hydrochloride]		Antianxiety	Acute withdrawal symptoms, especially from alcohol, or for other anxiety-producing conditions
Lidocaine HCl [lidocaine hydrochloride]		Antiarrhythmic	Management of ventricular arrhythmias or during cardiac manipulation, such as cardiac surgery
Liletta [levonorgestrel]	Z79.3	Contraceptive	Intrauterine device to Prevention of pregnancy
Lincocin [lincocin hydrochloride]	Z79.2	Antibiotic	Severe bacterial infections
Lipitor [atorvastatin calcium]		HMG-CoA reductase inhibitor (statin)	Hypercholesterolemia; hyperlipidemia; hyperproteinemia
Lithium carbonate [lithium carbonate]		Antimanic	Control of manic episodes in bipolar disorders
Lo Loestrin Fe [ethinyl estradiol/norethindrone acetate]	Z79.3	Contraceptive	Prevention of pregnancy
Locoid [hydrocotisone butyrate]	Z79.52	Corticosteroid -topical	Atopic dermatitis; other dermatoses
Loestrin [ethinyl estradiol/norethindrone acetate]	Z79.3	Contraceptive	Prevention of pregnancy
Lomotil [diphenoxylate hydrochloride/atropine sulfate]		Antidiarrheal	Symptoms of chronic and functional diarrhea
Lopid [gemfibrozil]		Lipid regulating agent	Hypercholesterolemia, hyperlipidemia, hyperlipoproteinemia, hypertriglyceridemia
Lopressor [metoprolol tartrate]		Beta blocker	Angina pectoris; hypertension; acute myocardial infarction
Lorazepam [lorazepam]		Antianxiety; sedative/hypnotic	Anxiety disorder associated with depressive symptoms; controls tension, agitation, irritability, and insomnia
Loryna [drospirenone/ethinyl estradiol]	Z79.3	Contraceptive	Prevention of pregnancy
LoSeasonique [ethinyl estradiol/levonorgestrel]	Z79.3	Contraceptive	Prevention of pregnancy
Lotensin [benazepril hydrochloride]		ACE inhibitor	Hypertension
Lotrel [amlodipine besylate/benazepril hydrochloride]		Antihypertensive	Hypertension

Drug	Z Code	Drug Action/Classification	Indications
Lotrisone [clotrimazole/ betamethasone dipropionate]		Antifungal-corticosteroid	Relief of redness, swelling, itching, and other discomfort of fungus infections
Lovastatin [lovastatin]		HMG-CoA reductase inhibitor (statin)	Hypercholesterolemia; hyperlipidemia; hyperlipoproteinemia
Lovenox [enoxaparin sodium]	Z79.01	Anticoagulant	Prophylaxis and treatment of venous thrombosis and pulmonary embolism
Low-Ogestrel-28 [norgestrel/ethinyl estradiol]	Z79.3	Contraceptive	Prevention of pregnancy
Lupron [leuprolide acetate]	Z79.818	Agents affecting estrogen receptors and estrogen levels	Endometriosis symptoms; uterine fibroids
Macrobid [nitrofuantoin]	Z79.2	Antibiotic	Urinary tract infections
Macrodantin [nitrofurantoin]	Z79.2	Antibiotic	Urinary tract infections
Marlissa [ethinyl estradiol/levonorgestrel]	Z79.3	Contraceptive	Prevention of pregnancy
Maxipime [cefepime hydrochloride]	Z79.2	Antibiotic	Bacterial infections
Meclizine hydrochloride [meclizine hydrochloride]		Antihistamine	Nausea and vomiting, and dizziness associated with motion sickness
Medrol [methylprednisolone]	Z79.52	Corticosteroid	Endocrine, rheumatic, hematologic disorders; collagen, dermatological, ophthalmic, respiratory, neoplastic, gastrointestinal, nervous system disorders; allergic and edematous states
Mefoxin [cefoxitin sodium]	Z79.2	Antibiotic	Bacterial infections
Megace ES [megestrol acetate]	Z79.818	Agents affecting estrogen receptors and estrogen levels	Endometrial or advanced breast cancers; weight loss due to AIDS
Menest [esteriefied estrogens]	Z79.890	Estrogen therapy	Menopause symptoms; ovarian failure
Menostar [estradiol]	Z79.890	Estrogen therapy	Menopause symptoms; osteoporosis prevention
Mepron [atovaquone]	Z79.2	Antibiotic	Pneumonia due to penumocystis jiroveci
Merrem [meropenem]	Z79.2	Antibiotic	Bacterial infections of skin or stomach; bacterial meningitis
Metformin [metformin hydrochloride]	Z79.84	Oral hypoglycemic	Diabetes mellitus
Methadone HCl [methadone hydrochloride]	Z79.891	Analgesic, narcotic; opioid agonist	Pain; treatment of opioid addiction
Methadose [methadone hydrochloride]	Z79.891	Analgesic, narcotic	Acute and chronic pain
Methergine [methylergonovine maleate]		Oxytocic agent	Routine management of postpartum hemorrhage after delivery of placenta
Methylprednisolone [methylprednisolone]	Z79.52	Corticosteroid	Inflammatory disorders
Metronidazole [metronidazole]	Z79.2	Antibiotic	Bacterial infections
Miacalcin [calcitonin salmon]		Calcitonin; a peptide hormone	Hypercalcemia, osteoporosis, postmenopausal symptoms, Paget's disease
Microgestin [ethinyl estradiol/norethindrone acetate]	Z79.3	Contraceptive	Prevention of pregnancy
Micronor [norethindrone]	Z79.3	Contraceptive	Prevention of pregnancy
Minastrin [ethinyl estradiol/norethindrone acetate]	Z79.3	Contraceptive	Prevention of pregnancy
Minivelle [estradiol]	Z79.890	Estrogen therapy	Menopause symptoms; osteoporosis prevention
Minocin [minocycline hydrochloride]	Z79.2	Antibiotic	Bacterial infections; acne
Mirena [levonorgestrel]	Z79.3	Contraceptive	Intrauterine device for prevention of pregnancy; menstrual disorders
Mobic [meloxicam]	Z79.1	Nonsteroidal anti-inflammatory drug (NSAID)	Treatment of pain and inflammation due to osteoarthritis and rheumatoid arthritis
Modicon 28 [ethinyl estradiol/norethindrone]	Z79.3	Contraceptive	Prevention of pregnancy
Mono-Linyah [norgestimate/ethinyl estradiol]	Z79.3	Contraceptive	Prevention of pregnancy; menstrual disorders; acne
Monoclonal antibodies	Z79.899	Monoclonal antibodies	Cancer; prophylaxis of organ transplant rejection
Monodox [doxycycline]	Z79.2	Antibiotic	Bacterial infections; acne
Monoket [isosorbide mononitrate]		Antianginal; coronary vasodilator, nitrate	Angina pectoris

Drug	Z Code	Drug Action/Classification	Indications
Monurol [fosfomycin tromethamine]	Z79.2	Antibiotic	Bacterial bladder infections
Morphabond ER [morphine sulfate]	Z79.891	Analgesics, narcotic	Pain
Morphine sulfate [morphine sulfate]	Z79.891	Analgesic, narcotic	Moderate to severe pain
Motrin IB [ibuprofen]	Z79.1	Nonsteroidal anti-inflammatory drug (NSAID)	Pain or fever relief
MS Contin [morphine sulfate]	Z79.891	Analgesic, narcotic	Moderate to severe pain
Multaq [dronedarone hydrochloride]		Cardiac rhythm regulator	Treatment of patients with recent episodes of atrial fibrillation or atrial flutter
Mycobutin [rifabutin]	Z79.2	Antibiotic	Mycobacterium avium complex (MAC) prophylactic in HIV patients
Mytesi [crofelemer]		Antidiarrheal	Diarrhea occurring in HIV/AIDs patient's on anti-retroviral therapy
Myzilra [ethinyl estradiol/levonorgestrel]	Z79.3	Contraceptive	Prevention of pregnancy
Nabumetone [nabumetone]	Z79.1	Non-steroidal anti-inflammatory drug (NSAID)	Osteoarthritis and rheumatoid arthritis
Nalfon [fenoprofen calcium]	Z79.1	Nonsteroidal anti-inflammatory drug (NSAID)	Pain or inflammation relief
Namzaric [memantine/donepezil hydrochlroides]		Acetylcholinesterase/cholinesterase inhibitors	Dementia due to Alzheimer's
Naprelan [naproxen sodium]	Z79.1	Nonsteroidal anti-inflammatory drug (NSAID)	Pain or inflammation relief
Naprosyn [naproxen]	Z79.1	Nonsteroidal anti-inflammatory drug (NSAID)	Rheumatoid, gouty arthritis and osteoarthritis; ankylosing spondylitis; bursitis; dysmenorrhea; pain, mild to moderate; tendonitis
Natazia [estradiol valerate/dienogest]	Z79.3	Contraceptive	Prevention of pregnancy; menstrual disorders
Nebupent [pentamidine isethionate]	Z79.2	Antibiotic	Severe bacterial lung infection in high risk patients with HIV
Nefazodone HCl [nefazodone hydrochloride]		Antidepressant	Depression
Nembutal sodium [pentobarbital sodium]		Sedative/hypnotic	Adjunct medication in diagnostic procedures or for emergency use with convulsive disorders
NeoProfen [ibuprofen lysine]	Z79.1	Nonsteroidal anti-inflammatory drug (NSAID)	Pain or fever relief
Neoral [cyclosporine]	Z79.899	Immunosuppressant	Prophylaxis of organ transplant rejection
Neurontin [gabapentin]		Anticonvulsant	Epilepsy, partial
Nexium [esomeprazole magnesium]		Proton pump inhibitor	Gastroesophageal reflux disease (GERD), erosive esophagitis
Nexplanon [etonogestrel]	Z79.3	Contraceptive	Implantable device used for prevention of pregnancy
Nitrofurantoin [nitrofurantoin]	Z79.2	Antibiotic	Bacterial urinary tract infections
Nitropress [sodium nitroprusside]		Vasodilator	Potent, rapid action in reducing blood pressure in hypertensive crisis or for controlling bleeding during anesthesia by producing controlled hypotension
Nitrostat [nitroglycerin]		Muscle relaxant; antianginal; antihypertensive; coronary vasodilator	Prophylaxis and treatment of angina pectoris; heart failure associated with myocardial infarction; hypertension, perioperative surgery, adjunct
Nor-QD [norethindrone]	Z79.3	Contraceptive	Prevention of pregnancy
Norco [acetaminophen/hydrocodone bitartrate]	Z79.891	Analgesic, narcotic	Moderate to severe pain
Norinyl [mestranol/norethisterone]	Z79.3	Contraceptive	Prevention of pregnancy
Norpace [disopyramide phosphate]		Antiarrhythmic	Coronary artery disease, for prevention, recurrence and control of unifocal, multifocal, and paired PVCs
Nortrel [ethinyl estradiol/norethindrone]	Z79.3	Contraceptive	Prevention of pregnancy
Norvasc [amlodipine besylate]		Calcium channel blocker	Hypertension, chronic stable angina, and vasospastic angina
Novolin [insulin recombinant]	Z79.4	Insulin	Diabetes mellitus
Novolog [insulin aspart recombinant]	Z79.4	Insulin	Diabetes mellitus
Nucynta [tapentadol hydrochloride]	Z79.891	Analgesic, narcotic	Moderate to severe pain
NuvaRing [etonogestrel/ethinyl estradiol]	Z79.3	Contraceptive	Vaginal ring to Prevention of pregnancy
Ogestrel [norgestrel/ethinyl estradiol]	Z79.3	Contraceptive	Prevention of pregnancy

Drug	Z Code	Drug Action/Classification	Indications
Onglyza [saxagliptin hydrochloride]	Z79.84	Oral hypoglycemic	Diabetes mellitus
Opana [oxymorphone hydrochloride]	Z79.891	Analgesic, narcotic	Moderate to severe pain
Oracea [doxycycline]	Z79.2	Antibiotic	Rosacea
Orapred ODT [prednisolone sodium phosphate]	Z79.52	Corticosteroid	Inflammatory disorders
Orbactiv [oritavancin diphosphate]	Z79.2	Antibiotic	Bacterial skin infections
Orencia [abatacept]	Z79.899	Antirheumatic	Rheumatoid arthritis; polyarticular juvenile idiopathic arthritis; psoriatic arthritis
Orilissa [elagolix]	Z79.890	Hormone therapy	Pain associated with endometriosis
Orphenadrine citrate [orphenadrine citrate]		Muscle relaxant	Acute spasms, tension, and post-trauma cases
Orsythia [ethinyl estradiol/levonorgestrel]	Z79.3	Contraceptive	Prevention of pregnancy
Ortho Cyclen-28 [ethinyl estradiol/norgestimate]	Z79.3	Contraceptive	Prevention of pregnancy
Ortho-Novum [norethindrone/ethinyl estradiol]	Z79.3	Contraceptive	Prevention of pregnancy
Ortho-Tri-Cyclen [ethinyl estradiol/norgestimate]	Z79.3	Contraceptive	Prevention of pregnancy
Oseni [alogliptin benzoate/pioglitazone hydrochloride]	Z79.84	Oral hypoglycemic	Diabetes mellitus
Osphena [ospemifene]	Z79.810, Z79.890	Selective estrogen receptor modulator (SERM)	Postmenopausal dyspareunia due to vaginal atrophy; osteoporosis prevention and treatment of menopausal symptoms
Otezla [apremilast]	Z79.899	Antirheumatic	Psoriatic arthritis; plaque psoriasis
Oxazepam [oxazepam]		Antianxiety	Anxiety, tension, and alcohol withdrawal
Oxycodone HCl [oxycodone hydrochloride]	Z79.891	Analgesic, narcotic	Moderate to severe pain
OxyContin [oxycodone hydrochloride]	Z79.891	Analgesic, narcotic	Moderate to severe pain
Ozempic [semaglutide]		Antidiabetic — injectable	Diabetes mellitus
Paxil [paroxetine hydrochloride]		Antidepressant	Anxiety with panic disorder and depression; obsessive-compulsive disorder
PediaPred [prednisolone sodium phosphate]	Z79.52	Corticosteroid	Inflammatory disorders
Pegintron [peginterferon alfa-2b]	Z79.899	Antiviral	Hepatitis C
Penicillin-VK [penicillin V potassium]	Z79.2	Antibiotic	Chorea, prevention; endocarditis, prevention, secondary to tooth extraction; erysipelas; infections of the skin and skin structures, upper respiratory tract; rheumatic fever, prophylaxis; scarlet fever; Vincent's gingivitis; Vincent's pharyngitis
Pentam [pentamidine isethionate]	Z79.2	Antibiotic	Severe bacterial lung infections
Pepcid [famotidine]		Histamine H2-receptor inhibitor	Acid/peptic disorder; adenoma, secretory; gastroesophageal reflux; duodenal and gastric ulcer; Zollinger-Ellison syndrome
Percocet [oxycodone hydrochloride/acetaminophen]	Z79.891	Analgesic, narcotic	Pain, moderate to severe
Persantine [dipyridamole]	Z79.02	Antiplatelet	Therapy for chronic angina pectoris, preventing clots post heart valve surgery
Pfizerpen [penicillin g potassium]	Z79.2	Antibiotic	Severe bacterial infections
Phenobarbital [phenobarbital sodium]		Anticonvulsant	Grand mal epilepsy
Philith [ethinyl estradiol/norethindrone]	Z79.3	Contraceptive	Prevention of pregnancy
Pimtrea [desogestrel/ethinyl estradiol]	Z79.3	Contraceptive	Prevention of pregnancy
Pirmella [ethinyl estradiol/norethindrone]	Z79.3	Contraceptive	Prevention of pregnancy
Pitocin [oxytocin]		Uterotonic	Induction or stimulation of labor at term
Plan B One-Step [levonorgestrel]	Z79.3	Contraceptive	Prevention of pregnancy
Plavix [clopidogrel bisulfate]	Z79.02	Antiplatelet	Lessening of the chance of heart attack or stroke
Ponstel [mefenamic acid]	Z79.1	Nonsteroidal anti-inflammatory drug (NSAID)	Treatment of pain

Drug	Z Code	Drug Action/Classification	Indications
Portia-28 [ethinyl estradiol/levonorgestrel]	Z79.3	Contraceptive	Prevention of pregnancy
Pradaxa [dabigatran etexilate mesylate]	Z79.01	Anticoagulant	Prophylaxis and treatment of blood clots in patients with atrial fibrillation
Prandimet [metformin hydrochloride/repaglinide]	Z79.84	Oral hypoglycemic	Diabetes mellitus
Prandin [repaglinide]	Z79.84	Oral hypoglycemic	Diabetes mellitus
Prasugrel [prasugrel hydrochloride]	Z79.02	Antiplatelet	Lessening the chance of heart attack or stroke
Pravachol [pravastatin sodium]		HMG-CoA reductase inhibitor (statin)	Hypercholesterolemia; hyperlipidemia; hyperlipoproteinemia
Precose [acarbose]	Z79.84	Oral hypoglycemic	Diabetes mellitus
Prednisolone [prednisolone]	Z79.52	Corticosteroid	Inflammatory disorders
Prednisone [prednisone]	Z79.52	Corticosteroid	Used for its immunosuppressant effects and for relief of inflammation; used in arthritis, polymyositis and other systemic diseases
Pregnyl [chorionic gonadotropin]		Gonadotropic hormone	Prepubertal cryptorchidism; hypogonadism; corpus luteum insufficiency and infertility
Prelone [prednisolone]	Z79.52	Corticosteroid	Inflammatory disorders
Prempro [conjugated estrogens/medroxyprogesterone acetate]	Z79.890	Estrogen/progesterone therapy	Menopause; osteoporosis; atrophic vaginitis
Prevacid [lansoprazole]		Proton pump inhibitor	Acid/peptic disorder, erosive esophagitis, duodenal ulcer, Zollinger-Ellison syndrome
Previfem [ethinyl estradiol/norgestimate]	Z79.3	Contraceptive	Prevention of pregnancy
Prezcobix [darunavir/cobicistat]	Z79.899	Antiviral	HIV
Prezista [darunavir ethanolate]	Z79.899	Antiviral	HIV
Priftin [rifapentine]	Z79.2	Antibiotic	Tuberculosis
Prilosec [omeprazole magnesium]		Proton pump inhibitor	Acid/peptic disorder; endocrine adenoma; erosive esophagitis; systemic mastocytosis; gastroesophageal reflux; duodenal, peptic and gastric ulcer; Zollinger-Ellison syndrome
Primaxin [cilastatin sodium/imipenem]	Z79.2	Antibiotic	Skin, stomach, female reproductive organs or lower respiratory tract infections
Prinivil [lisinopril]		ACE inhibitor	Congestive heart failure; hypertension
Pristiq [desvenlafaxine]		Antidepressant; serotonin and norepinephrine reuptake inhibitor (SNRI)	Major depressive disorder
Procardia [nifedipine]		Calcium channel blocker	Management of vasospastic angina and chronic stable angina, hypertension
Prograf [tacrolimus]	Z79.899	Immunosuppressant	Prophylaxis of organ transplant rejection
Prolia [denosumab]	Z79.899	Monoclonal antibody	Treatment and prevention of bone resorption and prevention of bone fracture
Promethazine hydrochloride [promethazine hydrochloride]		Anesthesia, adjunct to; antiemetic; antihistamine; antitussive/expectorant; sedative/hypnotic; vertigo/motion sickness/vomiting	Anesthesia; adjunct; angioedema; conjunctivitis; dermographism; hypersensitivity, motion sickness; pain; perennial, seasonal, and allergic rhinitis; sedation, obstetrical; urticaria
Protonix [pantoprazole]		Proton pump inhibitor	Short-term treatment and maintenance therapy of erosive esophagitis associated with gastroesophageal reflux disease (GERD)
Protopic [tacrolimus]	Z79.899	Immunosuppressant	Atomic dermatitis (eczema)
Proventil-HFA [albuterol sulfate]		Antiasthmatic/bronchodilator	Asthma
Provera [medroxyprogesterone acetate]	Z79.3, Z79.890	Antineoplastic; contraceptive; progestin	Amenorrhea; carcinoma, endometrium, adjunct; carcinoma, renal Prevention of pregnancy; hemorrhage
Prozac [fluoxetine hydrochloride]		Selective serotonin reuptake inhibitor (SSRI)	Bulimia nervosa; depression; obsessive-compulsive disorder
Pulmicort [budesonide]	Z79.51	Corticosteroid -inhaled; antiasthmatic	Prophylaxis and treatment of asthma
Qnasl [beclomethasone dipropionate]		Corticosteroid -inhaled/nasal	Perennial and seasonal allergies; vasomotor rhinitis
Qtern [dapagliflozin propanediol/saxagliptin hydrochloride]	Z79.84	Oral hypoglycemic	Diabetes mellitus

Drug	Z Code	Drug Action/Classification	Indications
Quartette [levonorgestrel/ethinyl estradiol]	Z79.3	Contraceptive	Prevention of pregnancy
Quasense [ethinyl estradiol/levonorgestrel]	Z79.3	Contraceptive	Prevention of pregnancy
Quinidine gluconate [quinidine gluconate]		Antiarrhythmic	Management of cardiac arrhythmias
Qvar [beclomethasone dipropionate]	Z79.51	Corticosteroid -inhaled; antiasthmatic	Prophylaxis and treatment of asthma
Raloxifene HCl [raloxifene hydrochloride]	Z79.810	Selective estrogen receptor modulator (SERM)	Prevention of thinning of the bones (osteoporosis) only in postmenopausal women
Rapaflo [silodosin]		Antiadrenergic	Benign prostatic hyperplasia
Rapamune [sirolimus]	Z79.899	Immunosuppressant	Prophylaxis of organ transplant rejection
Rayos [prednisone]	Z79.52	Corticosteroid; antiasthmatic	Arthritis; blood disorders; allergies; asthma
Rebetol [ribavirin]	Z79.899	Antiviral	Chronic hepatitis C
Rebif [interferon beta-1a]	Z79.899	Antiviral	Treatment of relapsing multiple sclerosis
Reclast [zoledronic acid]	Z79.83	Bisphosphonate	Prevention of thinning of the bones (osteoporosis); Paget's disease; bone cancer
Relenza [zanamivir]		Antiviral	Treat and prevent influenza A and B
Renvela [sevelamer carbonate]		Phosphate binder	Chronic kidney disease (CKD) on dialysis
Repaglinide [repaglinide]	Z79.84	Oral hypoglycemic	Diabetes mellitus
Reprexain [hydrocodone bitartrate/ibuprofen]	Z79.891	Analgesic, narcotic; nonsteroidal anti-inflammatory drug (NSAID)	Pain, inflammation or fever relief
Restasis [cyclosporine ophthalmic emulsion]		Antiinflammatory, ophthalmic	Ocular inflammation due to keratoconjunctivitis sicca
Restoril [temazepam]		Sedative/hypnotic	Insomnia
Retrovir [zidovudine]	Z79.899	Antiretroviral	Indicated in symptomatic HIV infection
Rifadin [rifampin]	Z79.2	Antibiotic	Tuberculosis
Rifamactane [rifampin]	Z79.2	Antibiotic	Tuberculosis
Riomet [metformin hydrochloride]	Z79.84	Oral hypoglycemic	Diabetes mellitus
Risperdal [risperidone]		Antipsychotic/antimanic	Schizophrenia; bipolar I disorder
Ritalin [methylphenidate hydrochloride]		CNS stimulant	Depression; hyperkinetic activity in children
Roxicet [oxycodone hydrochloride/acetaminophen]	Z79.891	Analgesic, narcotic	Pain, moderate to severe
Roxicodone [oxycodone hydrochloride]	Z79.891	Analgesic, narcotic	Pain relief
Ryzodeg [insulin aspart/insulin degludec]	Z79.4	Insulin	Diabetes mellitus
Sabril [vigabatrin]		Anticonvulsant	Refractory complex partial seizures
Safyral [drospirenone/ethinyl estradiol/levomefolate calcium]	Z79.3	Contraceptive	Prevention of pregnancy
Sandimmune [cyclosporine]	Z79.899	Immunosuppressant	Prophylaxis of organ transplant rejection
Sarafem [fluoxetine hydrochloride]		Selective serotonin reuptake inhibitor (SSRI)	Premenstrual dysphoric disorder (PMDD)
Savaysa [edoxaban tosylate]	Z79.01	Anticoagulant	Prophylaxis and treatment of venous thrombosis, pulmonary embolism; prevention of blood clots due to atrial fibrillation
Seasonale [levonorgestrel/ethinyl estradiol]	Z79.3	Contraceptive	Prevention of pregnancy
Seasonique [ethinyl estradiol/levonorgestrel]	Z79.3	Contraceptive	Prevention of pregnancy
Selfemra [fluoxetine hydrochloride]		Selective serotonin reuptake inhibitor (SSRI)	Premenstrual dysphoric disorder (PMDD)
Septra [sulfamethoxazole trimethoprim]	Z79.2	Antibiotic	Urinary tract infections, acute otitis media, acute exacerbations of chronic bronchitis, and shigellosis
Serevent [salmeterol xinafoate]		Bronchodilator	Asthma
Seromycin [cycloserine]	Z79.2	Antibiotic	Tuberculosis; urinary tract infections
Seroquel XR [quetiapine fumarate]		Antipsychotic	Schizophrenia; bipolar disorder; major depressive disorder
Sronyx [ethinyl estradiol/levonorgestrel]	Z79.3	Contraceptive	Prevention of pregnancy

Appendix B: Pharmacology List 2020

Drug	Z Code	Drug Action/Classification	Indications
Silvadene [silver sulfadiazine]	Z79.2	Antibiotic, topical	Wound sepsis due to second/third degree burns
Simulect [basiliximab]	Z79.899	Immunosuppressant	Prophylaxis of organ transplant rejection
Sinemet [carbidopa/levodopa]		Antiparkinsonism	Parkinson's disease
Singulair [montelukast sodium]		Antiasthmatic	Asthma; exercise-induced bronchoconstriction; perennial and seasonal allergic rhinitis
Sirolimus [sirolimus]	Z79.899	Immunosuppressant	Prophylaxis of organ transplant rejection
Sitagliptin [sitagliptin/metformin hydrochloride]	Z79.84	Oral hypoglycemic	Diabetes mellitus
Sivextro [tedizolid phosphate]	Z79.2	Antibiotic	Skin infections including MRSA
Skyla [levonorgestrel]	Z79.3	Contraceptive	Intrauterine device to Prevention of pregnancy
Soliqua [insulin glargine/lixisenatide]	Z79.4	Insulin	Diabetes mellitus
Solodyn [minocycline hydrochloride]	Z79.2	Antibiotic	Bacterial infections
Soltamox [tamoxifen citrate]	Z79.810	Selective estrogen receptor modulator (SERM)	Breast cancer
Solu-Cortef [hydrocortisone sodium succinate]	Z79.52	Corticosteroid; antiasthmatic	Asthma; severe inflammation; allergic reactions
Solu-Medrol [methylprednisolone sodium succinate]	Z79.52	Corticosteroid	Anti-inflammatory and antiallergenic for shock and ulcerative colitis
Spiriva [tiotropium bromide]		Antiasthmatic/bronchodilator	Chronic obstructive pulmonary disease (COPD); asthma
Sprintec [norgestimate/ethinyl estradiol]	Z79.3	Contraceptive	Prevention of pregnancy
Starlix [nateglinide]	Z79.84	Oral hypoglycemic	Diabetes mellitus
Strattera [atomexetine hydrochloride]		CNS stimulant	Attention deficit hyperactivity disorder (ADHD)
Streptomycin sulfate [streptomycin sulfate]	Z79.2	Antibiotic	Severe bacterial infections
Sublimaze preservative free [fentanyl citrate]	Z79.891	Analgesic, narcotic	Pain relief
Supprelin LA [histrelin acetate]	Z79.818	Agents affecting estrogen receptors and estrogen levels	Precocious puberty
Suprax [cefixime]	Z79.2	Antibiotic	Bacterial infections
Sustiva [efavirenz]	Z79.899	Antiviral	HIV/AIDs
Syeda [drospirenone/ethinyl estradiol]	Z79.3	Contraceptive	Prevention of pregnancy
Sylatron [peginterferon alfa-2b]	Z79.899	Antineoplastic interferons; antiviral interferons	Prevention of recurrent malignant melanoma
Symbicort [budesonide/formoterol fumarate dihydrate]	Z79.51	Corticosteroid -inhaled; antiasthmatic	Prophylaxis and treatment of asthma and COPD
Symbyax [olanzapine/fluoxetine]		Antidepressant	Acute depressive episodes associated with bipolar I disorder; treatment resistant depression
Symtuza [darunavir/cobicistat/emtricitabine/tenofovir alafenamide]	Z79.899	Antiretroviral	HIV
Synarel [nafarelin acetate]	Z79.818	Agents affecting estrogen receptors and estrogen levels	Endometriosis symptoms; precocious puberty
Synercid [dalfopristin/quinupristin]	Z79.2	Antibiotic	Severe blood infections
Synjardy [empagliflozin/metformin hydrochloride]	Z79.84	Oral hypoglycemic	Diabetes mellitus
Synthroid [levothyroxine sodium]		Thyroid hormone	Hypothyroidism
Tacrolimus [tacrolimus]	Z79.899	Immunosuppressant	Prophylaxis of organ transplant rejection
Tamiflu [oseltamivir phosphate]		Antiviral	Treatment and prevention of influenza A and B
Tamoxifen citrate [tamoxifen citrate]	Z79.810	Selective estrogen receptor modulator (SERM)	Metastatic breast cancer in postmenopausal women
Tazicef [ceftazidime]	Z79.2	Antibiotic	Confirmed or suspected bacterial infections
Teflaro [ceftaroline fosamil]	Z79.2	Antibiotic	Bacterial skin infections; pneumonia
Tegretol [carbamazepine]		Anticonvulsant; analgesic	Epilepsy, especially with complex symptomatology; specific analgesic for trigeminal neuralgia

Drug	Z Code	Drug Action/Classification	Indications
Tenormin [atenolol]		Beta blocker	Angina pectoris; hypertension; acute myocardial infarction
Terazosin HCl [terazosin hydrochloride]		Antiadrenergic	Benign prostatic hypertrophy; hypertension
Testim [testosterone]	Z79.890	Testosterone therapy -topical	Primary hypogonadism; hypogonadotropic hypogonadism
Tetracycline HCl [tetracycline hydrochloride]	Z79.2	Antibiotic	Bacterial infections
Tiazac [diltiazem hydrochloride]		Calcium channel blocker	Chronic stable angina, atrial fibrillation, atrial flutter, hypertension, paroxysmal supraventricular tachycardia
Tivorbex [indomethacin]	Z79.1	Nonsteroidal anti-inflammatory drug (NSAID)	Treatment of pain, inflammation and joint stiffness
Tobradex [tobramycin/dexamethasone]		Aminoglycoside ocular anti-infective; anti-inflammatory	Infectious conjunctivitis; dermatosis, corticosteroid-responsive with secondary infection; foreign body in eye; corneal inflammation; uveitis
Tobramycin dexamethasone/tobramycin]	Z79.2	Antibiotic	Bacterial eye infections
Topamax [topiramate]		Anticonvulsant	Epilepsy; primary generalized tonic-clonic seizures; seizures associated with Lennox-Gastaut syndrome; migraine headache
Toprol-XL [metoprolol succinate]		Beta blocker	Angina pectoris; hypertension
Toremifene citrate [toremifene citrate]	Z79.810	Selective estrogen receptor modulator (SERM)	Metastatic breast cancer in postmenopausal women
Torisel [temsirolimus]	Z79.899	Antineoplastic	Renal cell carcinoma
Toujeo Solostar [insulin glargine recombinant]	Z79.4	Insulin	Diabetes mellitus
Tradjenta [linagliptin]	Z79.84	Oral hypoglycemic	Diabetes mellitus
Trazodone HCl [trazodone hydrochloride]		Antidepressant	Depression
Trelegy Ellipta [fluticasone furoate/umeclidinium bromide/vilanterol trifenatate]	Z79.51	Corticosteroid -- inhaled; anitasthmatic	COPD
Trelstar [triptorelin pamoate]	Z79.818	Agents affecting estrogen receptors and estrogen levels	Palliative treatment of prostate cancer symptoms
Tresiba [insulin degludec]	Z79.4	Insulin	Diabetes mellitus
Tri-Estarylla [ethinyl estradiol/norgestimate]	Z79.3	Contraceptive	Prevention of pregnancy; acne
Tri-Legest [ethinyl estradiol/norethindrone acetate]	Z79.3	Contraceptive	Prevention of pregnancy
Tri-Linyah [ethinyl estradiol/norgestimate]	Z79.3	Contraceptive	Prevention of pregnancy
Tri-Lo-Estarylla [ethinyl estradiol/norgestimate]	Z79.3	Contraceptive	Prevention of pregnancy
Tri-Lo-Sprintec [ethinyl estradiol/norgestimate]	Z79.3	Contraceptive	Prevention of pregnancy
Tri-Norinyl 28-day [ethinyl estradiol/norethindrone]	Z79.3	Contraceptive	Prevention of pregnancy
Tri-Previfem [ethinyl estradiol/norgestimate]	Z79.3	Contraceptive	Prevention of pregnancy
Tri-Sprintec [ethinyl estradiol/norgestimate]	Z79.3	Contraceptive	Prevention of pregnancy; acne
Triamterene and hydrochlorothiazide [triamterene/ hydrochlorothiazide]		Antihypertensive; diuretic	Edema; hypertension
Trimethoprim [trimethoprim]	Z79.2	Antibiotic	Acute exacerbation chronic bronchitis; travelers' diarrhea; infections of the middle, lower respiratory tract, and urinary tract; pneumonia, pneumocystis; shigellosis
Triptodur [triptorelin]	Z79.818	Agents affecting estrogen receptors and estrogen levels	Precocious puberty
Trivora-28 [ethinyl estradiol/ norgestrel]	Z79.3	Contraceptive	Prevention of pregnancy
Trokendi XR [topiramate]		Anticonvulsant	Epilepsy; primary generalized tonic-clonic seizures; seizures associated with Lennox-Gastaut syndrome; migraine headache

Drug	Z Code	Drug Action/Classification	Indications
Trulicity [dulaglutide]		Antidiabetic -injectable	Diabetes mellitus
Truvada [emtricitabine/ tenofovir disoproxil fumarate]	Z79.899	Antiviral	Treatment and prevention of HIV
Tygacil [tigecycline]	Z79.2	Antibiotic	Bacterial skin or digestive system infections; pneumonia
Tylenol with codeine [acetaminophen/codeine phosphate]	Z79.891	Analgesic, narcotic	Pain and cough
Ultram [tramadol hydrochloride]	Z79.891	Analgesic, non-narcotic (opiate, narcotic-like)	Moderate to severe pain
Unasyn [ampicillin sodium/sulbactam sodium]	Z79.2	Antibiotic	Bacterial infections
Vabomere [meropenem; vaborbactam]	Z79.2	Antibiotic	Complicated urinary tract infections; pyelonephritis
Vagifem [estradiol]	Z79.89Ø	Estrogen therapy	Menopause symptoms
Valium [diazepam]		Antianxiety; muscle relaxant; anticonvulsant	Anxiety, tension, withdrawal from alcohol, muscle spasms and anticonvulsant therapy; epilepsy, generalized tonic-clonic; status epilepticus; stiff-man syndrome; tetanus
Vancocin HCl [vancomycin hydrochloride]	Z79.2	Antibiotic	Severe bacterial infections
Vancomycin HCl [vancomycin hydrochloride]	Z79.2	Antibiotic	Severe bacterial infections
Vantas [histrelin acetate]	Z79.818	Agents affecting estrogen receptors and estrogen levels	Palliative treatment of prostate cancer symptoms
Vasotec [enalaprilat maleate]		ACE inhibitor	Congestive heart failure; hypertension
Velivet [desogestrel/ethinyl estradiol]	Z79.3	Contraceptive	Prevention of pregnancy
Venlafaxine HCl [venlafaxine hydrochloride]		Antidepressant, serotonin and norepinephrine reuptake inhibitor (SNRI)	Major depressive disorder; social anxiety disorder; panic disorder
Ventolin HFA [albuterol sulfate]		Antiasthmatic/bronchodilator	Asthma
Verapamil HCL [verapamil hydrochloride]		Calcium channel blocker	Angina pectoris, chronic stable angina, atrial fibrillation, atrial flutter, paroxysmal supraventricular tachycardia, ventricular arrhythmia, hypertension
Viagra [sildenafil citrate]		Phosphodiesterase-5 (PDE5) inhibitor	Erectile dysfunction
Vibativ [telavancin hydrochloride]	Z79.2	Antibiotic	Pneumonia; severe bacterial skin infections
Vibramycin [doxycycline calcium]	Z79.2	Antibiotic	Bacterial infections
Victoza [liraglutide]		Antidiabetic -injectable	Diabetes mellitus
Vienva [ethinyl estradiol/levonorgestrel]	Z79.3	Contraceptive	Prevention of pregnancy
Viorele [desogestrel/ethinyl estradiol]	Z79.3	Contraceptive	Prevention of pregnancy
Virazole [ribavirin]	Z79.899	Antiviral	Respiratory syncytial virus (RSV)
Viread [tenofovir disoproxil fumarate]	Z79.899	Antiviral	HIV; chronic hepatitis B
Vistaril [hydroxyzine pamoate]		Antianxiety; antiemetic	Treatment of nausea and vomiting, for reducing narcotic requirement in surgery and as tranquilizer for tension, anxiety, agitation states
Vivelle [estradiol]	Z79.89Ø	Estrogen therapy	Menopause symptoms; osteoporosis prevention
Voltaren [diclofenac sodium]	Z79.1	Nonsteroidal anti-inflammatory drug (NSAID)	Treatment of pain, inflammation and joint stiffness due to arthri
Vytorin [ezetimibe/simvastatin]		HMG-CoA reductase inhibitor (statin); cholesterol absorption inhibitor	Hyperlipidemia; hypercholesterolemia
Warfarin [warfarin sodium]	Z79.Ø1	Anticoagulant	Prophylaxis and treatment of venous thrombosis, treatment of atrial fibrillation with embolization (pulmonary embolism), arrhythmias, myocardial infarction, and stroke prevention
Wellbutrin SR, Wellbutrin XL [bupropion hydrochloride]		Antidepressant	Depression
Wera [ethinyl estradiol/norethindrone]	Z79.3	Contraceptive	Prevention of pregnancy
Xalatan [latanoprost]		Prostaglandin F2α analogue	Glaucoma, open-angle; ocular hypertension
Xanax, Xanax XR [alprazolam]		Antianxiety; sedative/hypnotic	Anxiety disorders with panic disorder and depression
Xarelto [rivaraxaban]	Z79.Ø1	Anticoagulant	Prophylaxis and treatment of venous thrombosis, pulmonary embolism; prevention of blood clots due to atrial fibrillation
Xeljanz [tofacitinib citrate]	Z79.899	Antirheumatic	Rheumatoid arthritis; psoriatic arthritis

Drug	Z Code	Drug Action/Classification	Indications
Xgeva [denosumab]	Z79.899	Monoclonal antibody	Treatment and prevention of bone resorption and prevention of bone fracture
...ifaxan [rifaximin]	Z79.2	Antibiotic	E. coli diarrhea
...igduo [dapagliflozin propanediol/metformin hydrochloride]	Z79.84	Oral hypoglycemic	Diabetes mellitus
...ultophy [insulin degludec/liraglutide]	Z79.4	Insulin	Diabetes mellitus
...yrem [sodium oxybate]		CNS depressant; anoxiolytic/sedative/hypnotic	Cataplexy and/or excessive daytime sleepiness in narcolepsy
...yzal [levocetirizine dihydrochloride]		Antihistamine	Perennial allergic rhinitis; chronic idiopathic urticaria
...asmin [drospirenone/ethinyl estradiol]	Z79.3	Contraceptive	Prevention of pregnancy
...az [drospirenone/ethinyl estradiol]	Z79.3	Contraceptive	Prevention of pregnancy; menstrual disorders
...antac [ranitidine hydrochloride]		Histamine H2-receptors inhibitor	Acid/peptic disorder, erosive esophagitis, gastrointestinal hypersecretion, mastocytosis, gastroesophageal reflux, peptic ulcer, Zollinger-Ellison syndrome
...rbaxa [ceftolozane sulfate/tazobactam ...dium]	Z79.2	Antibiotic	Complicated urinary tract and intra-abdominal infections
...storetic ...inopril/hydrochlorothiazide]		ACE inhibitor	Congestive heart failure; hypertension
...stril [lisinopril]		ACE inhibitor	Congestive heart failure; hypertension
...tia [exetimibe]		Antihyperlipidemic	Hypercholesterolemia; sitosterolemia
...c [bisoprolol fumarate/ ...drochlorothiazide]		Antihypertensive	Hypertension
...acef [cefuroxime sodium]	Z79.2	Antibiotic	Bacterial infections
...sor [diclofenac potassium]	Z79.1	Nonsteroidal anti-inflammatory drug (NSAID)	Pain and inflammation relief
...aromax [azithromycin]	Z79.2	Antibiotic	Infections of the cervix, lower respiratory tract, skin and skin structures, urethra, nongonococcal; mycobacterium avium complex; pharyngitis, streptococcal pneumonia; tonsillitis
...or [simvastatin]		HMG-CoA reductase inhibitor (statin)	Hypercholesterolemia; hyperlipidemia; hyperlipoproteinemia; hypertriglyceridemia
...adex [goserelin acetate]	Z79.818	Agents affecting estrogen receptors and estrogen levels	Palliative treatment of prostate cancer and breast cancer symptoms; endometriosis
...oft [sertraline hydrochloride]		Antidepressant	Anxiety with panic disorder and depression; obsessive-compulsive disorder
...eta [zoledronic acid]	Z79.83	Bisphosphonate	Multiple myeloma; Paget's disease
...olex [diclofenac]	Z79.1	Nonsteroidal anti-inflammatory drug (NSAID)	Pain, inflammation or fever relief
...n [piperacillin sodium/tazobactam ...um]	Z79.2	Antibiotic	Bacterial infections
...a [ethynodiol diacetate/ethinyl ...diol]	Z79.3	Contraceptive	Prevention of pregnancy
...rax [acyclovir]		Antiviral	Genital herpes and herpes zoster infections
...olv [buprenorphine/naloxone]		Opioid agonist	Treatment of opioid addiction
...n [bupropion hydrochloride]		Smoking cessation aid	Nicotine addiction, smoking
...[zileuton]		Antiasthmatic	Asthma
...rim [allopurinol]		Antigout	Gouty arthritis, renal calculus, hyperuricemia, hyperuricemia secondary to leukemia, hyperuricemia secondary to lymphoma
...exa [olanzapine]		Antipsychotic/antimanic	Psychotic disorders; schizophrenia
...c allergy [cetirizine hydrochloride]		Antihistamine	Perennial and seasonal allergic rhinitis; chronic urticaria
...x [linezolid]	Z79.2	Antibiotic	Severe bacterial infections

Appendix C: Z Codes for Long-Term Drug Use with Associated Drugs

This resource correlates the Z codes that are used to identify current long-term drug use with a list of drugs that are typically categorized to that class of drug. These lists are not all-inclusive, providing only the more commonly used drugs.

79.01 Long term (current) use of anticoagulants
- Angiomax
- Argatroban
- Arixtra
- Bevyxxa
- Coumadin
- Eliquis
- Fragmin
- Heparin
- Jantoven
- Lovenox
- Pradaxa
- Savaysa
- Warfarin
- Xarelto

9.02 Long term (current) use of antithrombotics/antiplatelets
- Aggrastat
- Aggrenox
- Brilinta
- Clopidogrel bisulfate
- Effient
- Integrilin
- Persantine
- Plavix
- Prasugrel

.1 Long term (current) use of non-steroidal anti-inflammatories (NSAID)
- Advil
- Aleve
- Anaprox DS
- Arthrotec
- Caldolor
- Cambia
- Celebrex
- Daypro
- Duexis
- Feldene
- Ibuprofen
- Indocin
- Mobic
- Motrin IB
- Nabumetone
- Nalfon
- Naprelan
- Naprosyn
- NeoProfen
- Ponstel
- Tivorbex
- Voltaren
- Zipsor
- Zorvolex

Long term (current) use of antibiotics
- Altabax
- Amikacin
- Amoxicillin
- Ampicillin
- Ancef
- Augmentin
- Avelox
- Azactam
- Azithromycin
- Bactrim
- Biaxin XL
- Cefprozil
- Ceftriaxone
- Centany
- Cephalexin
- Cipro
- Ciprofloxacin
- Clarithromycin
- Cleocin
- Clindamycin
- Cubicin
- Daptomycin
- Dificid
- Doxycycline
- Dynacin
- E.E.S.
- Ertapenem
- ERYC
- Erygel
- EryPed
- Ery-Tab
- Erythrocin
- Erythromycin
- Factive
- Flagyl
- Fortaz
- Gentamicin sulfate
- Invanz
- Isoniazid
- Keflex
- Klaron
- Lincocin
- Macrobid
- Macrodantin
- Maxipime
- Mefoxin
- Mepron
- Merrem
- Metronidazole
- Minocin
- Monodox
- Monurol
- Mycobutin
- Nebupent
- Nitrofurantoin
- Oracea
- Orbactiv
- Penicillin-VK
- Pentam
- Pfizerpen
- Priftin
- Primaxin
- Rifadin
- Rimactane
- Septra
- Seromycin
- Silvadene
- Sivextro
- Solodyn
- Streptomycin sulfate
- Suprax
- Synercid
- Tazicef
- Teflaro
- Tetracycline HCl
- Tobramycin
- Trimethoprim
- Tygacil
- Unasyn
- Vabomere
- Vancocin HCl
- Vancomycin HCl
- Vibativ
- Vibramycin
- Xifaxan
- Zerbaxa
- Zinacef
- Zithromax
- Zosyn
- Zyvox

Z79.3 Long term (current) use of hormonal contraceptives
- Altavera
- Alyacen
- Aranelle
- Ashlyna
- Aviane-28
- Balziva-28
- Bekyree
- Beyaz
- Brevicon 28-day
- Briellyn
- Camila
- Cryselle
- Cyclafem
- Cyclessa
- Dasetta
- Daysee
- Depo-Provera
- Depo-SubQ Provera
- Desogen
- Elinest
- Emoquette
- Enpresse-28
- Enskyce
- Errin
- Estarylla
- Estrostep Fe
- Falmina
- Femcon Fe
- Femhrt
- Gildagia
- Gildess
- Introvale
- Jencycla
- Junel
- Kariva
- Kelnor
- Kimidess
- Kurvelo
- Kyleena
- Larin
- Lessina-28
- Levonest
- Levora
- Liletta
- Lo Loestrin Fe

Loestrin
Loryna
LoSeasonique
Low-Ogestrel-28
Marlissa
Microgestin
Micronor
Minastrin
Mirena
Modicon 28
Mono-Linyah
Myzilra
Natazia
Nexplanon
Norinyl
Nor-QD
Nortrel
NuvaRing
Ogestrel
Orsythia
Ortho Cyclen-28
Ortho-Novum
Ortho-Tri-Cyclen
Philith
Pimtrea
Pirmella
Plan B One-Step
Portia-28
Previfem
Provera
Quartette
Quasense
Safyral
Seasonale
Seasonique
Setlakin
Skyla
Sprintec
Syeda
Tri-Estarylla
Tri-Legest
Tri-Linyah
Tri-Lo-Estarylla
Tri-Lo-Sprintec
Tri-Norinyl 28-day
Tri-Previfem
Tri-Sprintec
Trivora-28
Velivet
Vienva
Viorele
Wera
Yasmin
Yaz
Zovia

Z79.4   Long term (current) use of insulin
Admelog
Afrezza
Apidra
Basaglar
Fiasp
Humalog
Humulin R
Lantus
Levemir
Novolin
Novolog

Ryzodeg
Soliqua
Toujeo Solostar
Tresiba
Xultophy

Z79.51   Long term (current) use of inhaled steroids
Advair
Aerospan HFA
Alvesco
Airduo Respiclick
Armonair Respiclick
Arnuity Ellipta
Asmanex
Breo Ellipta
Dulera
Flovent
Pulmicort
Qvar
Symbicort
Trelegy Ellipta

Z79.52   Long term (current) use of systemic steroids
A-Methapred
Aristospan
Celestone Soluspan
Colocort
Cortef
Cortenema
Cortifoam
Cortisone acetate
Depo-Medrol
Dexamethasone Intensol
Entocort EC
Hydrocortisone
Kenalog-1Ø
Kenalog-4Ø
Locoid
Medrol
Methylprednisolone
Orapred ODT
PediaPred
Prednisolone
Prednisone
Prelone
Rayos
Solu-Cortef
Solu-Medrol

Z79.81Ø   Long term (current) use of selective estrogen receptor modulators (SERMs)
Evista
Fareston
Osphena
Raloxifene HCl
Soltamox
Tamoxifen Citrate
Toremifene Citrate

Z79.811   Long term (current) use of aromatase inhibitors
Anastrozole
Arimidex
Aromasin
Exemestane
Femara
Letrozole

Z79.818   Long term (current) use of other agents affecting estrogen receptors and estrogen levels
Eligard
Faslodex
Lupron
Megace ES
Supprelin LA
Synarel
Trelstar
Triptodur
Vantas
Zoladex

Z79.82   Long term (current) use of aspirin
Bayer
Durlaza

Z79.83   Long term (current) use of bisphosphonates
Actonel
Atelvia
Binosto
Boniva
Didronel
Fosamax
Reclast
Zometa

Z79.84   Long term (current) use of oral hypoglycemic drugs
Acarbose
Actoplus Met
Actos
Amaryl
Avandia
Diabinese
DiaBeta
Duetact
Farxiga
Fortamet
Glimepiride
Glucophage
Glucotrol
Glucovance
Glumetza
Glyburide
Glynase
Glyset
Invokamet
Invokana
Janumet
Januvia
Jentadueto
Kazano
Kombiglyze
Metformin
Onglyza
Oseni
PrandiMet
Prandin
Precose
Qtern
Repaglinide
Riomet
Sitagliptin
Starlix
Synjardy
Tradjenta
Xigduo

79.890 Hormone replacement therapy
Activella
Alora
Androderm
AndroGel
Angeliq
Bijuva
Climara
CombiPatch
Delestrogen
Depo-Provera
Divigel
Duavee
Elestrin
Estrace
EstroGel
Femhrt
Femring
Firmagon
Menest
Menostar
Minivelle
Orlissa
Osphena
Prempro
Provera
Testim
Vagifem
Vivelle

.891 Long term (current) use of opiate analgesic
Abstral
Acetaminophen with codeine
Buprenex
Buprenorphine HCl and Naloxone HCl
Butorphanol tartrate
Butrans
Codeine
Demerol
Dilaudid
Dolophine HCl
Duragesic

Duramorph PF
Embeda
Exalgo
Fentanyl Citrate
Fentora
Fioricet with codeine
Hydrocodone
Hydrocodone bitartrate and acetaminophen
Hydromorphone HCl
Kadian
Lazanda
Methadone HCl
Methadose
Morphabond ER
Morphine Sulfate
MS Contin
Norco
Nucynta
Opana
Oxycodone HCl
OxyContin
Percocet
Reprexain
Roxicet
Roxicodone
Sublimaze Preservative Free
Tylenol with codeine
Ultram

Z79.899 Other long term (current) drug therapy
Actimmune
Antineoplastic/chemotherapy
Astagraf XL
Atripla
Avonex
Betaseron
Cellcept
Cimduo
Cosentyx
Crixivan
Cyclosporine

Cyltezo
Descovy
Emtriva
Enbrel
Entyvio
Envarsus XR
Epivir
Erelzi
Gengraf
Harvoni
Humira
Hyrimoz
Imuran
Intron A
Keytruda
Monoclonal antibodies
Neoral
Orencia
Otezla
Pegintron
Prezcobix
Prezista
Prograf
Prolia
Protopic
Rapamune
Rebetol
Rebif
Retrovir
Sandimmune
Simulect
Sirolimus
Sustiva
Sylatron
Symtuza
Tacrolimus
Torisel
Truvada
Virazole
Viread
Xeljanz
Xgeva

Z01.12	Z02.3	Z03.818	Z34.01	Z38.61	Z40.9	Z52.21
Z01.20	Z02.4	Z03.89	Z34.02	Z38.62	Z42.1	Z52.29
Z01.21	Z02.5	Z04.1	Z34.03	Z38.63	Z42.8	Z52.3
Z01.30	Z02.6	Z04.2	Z34.80	Z38.64	Z51.0	Z52.4
Z01.31	Z02.71	Z04.3	Z34.81	Z38.65	Z51.11	Z52.5
Z01.411	Z02.79	Z04.41	Z34.82	Z38.66	Z51.12	Z52.6
Z01.419	Z02.81	Z04.42	Z34.83	Z38.68	Z52.000	Z52.810
Z01.42	Z02.82	Z04.6	Z34.90	Z38.69	Z52.001	Z52.811
Z01.810	Z02.83	Z04.71	Z34.91	Z38.7	Z52.008	Z52.812
Z01.811	Z02.89	Z04.72	Z34.92	Z38.8	Z52.010	Z52.813
Z01.812	Z02.9	Z04.81	Z34.93	Z39.0	Z52.011	Z52.819
Z01.818	Z03.6	Z04.82	Z38.00	Z39.1	Z52.018	Z52.89
Z01.82	Z03.71	Z04.89	Z38.01	Z39.2	Z52.090	Z76.1
Z01.83	Z03.72	Z04.9	Z38.1	Z40.00	Z52.091	Z76.2
Z01.84	Z03.73	Z31.81	Z38.2	Z40.01	Z52.098	Z99.12
Z01.89	Z03.74	Z31.83	Z38.30	Z40.02	Z52.10	
Z02.0	Z03.75	Z31.84	Z38.31	Z40.03	Z52.11	
Z02.1	Z03.79	Z33.2	Z38.4	Z40.09	Z52.19	
Z02.2	Z03.810	Z34.00	Z38.5	Z40.8	Z52.20	

the 1970s, Medicare began demonstration projects that contracted with
ealth maintenance organizations (HMOs) to provide care for Medicare
eneficiaries in exchange for prospective payments. In 1985, this project
anged from demonstration status to a regular part of the Medicare program,
edicare Part C. The Balanced Budget Act (BBA) of 1997 named Medicare's Part C
anaged care program Medicare+Choice, and the Medicare Modernization Act
MA) of 2003 again renamed it to Medicare Advantage (MA).

edicare is one of the world's largest health insurance programs, and about
e-third of the beneficiaries on Medicare are enrolled in a MA private health care
n. Due to the great variance in the health status of Medicare beneficiaries, risk
ustment provides a means of adequately compensating those plans with
ge numbers of seriously ill patients while not overburdening other plans that
ve healthier individuals. Medicare Advantage (MA) plans have been using the
rarchical Condition Category (HCC) risk adjustment model since 2004.

e Risk Adjustment Model

primary purpose of a risk adjustment model is to predict (on average) the
ure health care costs for specific consortiums enrolled in Medicare Advantage
) health plans. CMS is then able to provide capitation payments to these
ate health plans. Capitation payments are an incentive for health plans to
oll not only healthier individuals but those with chronic conditions or who are
re seriously ill by removing some of the financial burden.

MA risk adjustment model uses HCCs to assess the disease burden of its
ollees. HCC diagnostic groupings were created after examining claims data so
enrollees with similar disease processes, and consequently similar health
expenditures, could be pooled into a larger data set in which an average
enditure rate could be determined. The medical conditions included in HCC
gories are those that were determined to most predictably affect the health
us and health care costs of any individual. Several important principles to the
adjustment model and the development of the HCC categories include but
not limited to:

1. The HCC diagnostic categories should be clinically meaningful.
   - Diagnostic categories are well-defined.
   - Clinically specific diseases or medical conditions are grouped to each category.

2. The HCC diagnostic categories should predict medical expenditures.
   - The diagnoses grouped to a specific category should have as close to the same cost burden not only in the current year but also in the future.

3. The HCC diagnostic categories should have adequate sample sizes and discretionary categories excluded to be as accurate and stable in their estimate of costs as possible.
   - A diagnostic category that groups extremely rare diseases or conditions would not be reliably effective in determining current or future costs.
   - Codes that are not credible as cost predictors or may be subject to coding variation should be excluded, when possible.

The HCC diagnostic categories should be both hierarchical and additive.
   - Hierarchical measurement is used within a specific disease process.
   - Disease processes that are unrelated to each other are measured additively.

The diagnostic classification should encourage specificity and should not reward coding proliferation.
   - More diagnosis codes and vague diagnosis codes do not equal greater disease burden.

an 10,000 ICD-10-CM diagnosis codes map to 86 HCCs in the current risk
ment model. Diagnoses are excluded from mapping when they do not
future cost or are vague or variable in diagnosis, coding, or treatment,
symptoms or osteoarthritis. Also excluded are diagnosis codes from
ories, radiology, and home health claims.

Adjustment Factors

S-HCC risk adjustment model uses "risk adjustment factors" to calculate a
re for each member. This score summarizes that particular patient's
d cost of care relative to other members'. Each member's risk score is
n demographic and health status information and is calculated as the

sum of these demographic and health factors weighted by their estimated
marginal contributions to total risk. The model also takes into account where the
patient resides (community or institutional), Medicaid eligibility (full or partial
benefits), the patient's Medicare enrollment status (new or established), age,
disability status, whether the patient is frail or has end-stage renal disease
(ESRD), and even prescription drug use.

No procedure codes, ICD-10-PCS or CPT, are included in the MA risk adjustment
model. The model relies solely on diagnostic and demographic data. Not all
ICD-10-CM diagnoses map to an HCC, and there is no specific code sequencing
involved. The CMS-HCC model is additive as well as hierarchical. The additive
functionality allows a patient to have more than one HCC category assigned,
providing a more complete clinical picture and prediction of resource
consumption. The hierarchical aspect of the model provides a means of ranking
diagnoses that are similar in disease process, by severity. The hierarchy of the
condition categories ensures the patient's conditions are classified to the most
severe condition within the related group. Less severe conditions within a
particular hierarchy are superseded by more severe diagnoses within the same
group. The hierarchy and additive relationship permits this model to characterize
the person's illness level within each disease process, while still allowing the
effects of unrelated disease processes to be counted in the patient's overall score.

Certain combinations of coexisting diagnoses for an individual can increase
medical costs. The CMS-HCC model adjusts for these higher costs by the addition
of "disease interaction" factors. For each patient, multiple HCCs assigned, along
with demographic and disease interaction factors, are used to calculate a single,
combined risk adjustment factor (RAF). The RAF score for an individual member
represents all of the HCCs that have been submitted from all sources for that
member to CMS during the course of an entire calendar year.

There are separate CMS-HCC models for new enrollees and continuing enrollees.
The new enrollee model uses demographic factors only, such as age, sex, and
disability status, and is used when the enrollee has less than 12 months of
medical history. The community model accounts for age, sex, original reason for
Medicare entitlement (age or disability), Medicaid eligibility, and clinical
conditions as measured by HCCs. In the second step, expected costs are adjusted
for outliers based on the member's risk score and whether the patient has ESRD.

Demographic data (age, sex, eligibility) as well as health status (diagnoses codes
submitted on claims to CMS) of an MA population are used to determine the
reimbursement to the health plan to care for their members.

CMS considers a RAF score of 1.0 as the benchmark to indicate the score of the
average healthy patient with the same demographic and diagnostic factors.
These patients are expected to use average or lower-than-average resources.
When the RAF score is higher than 1.0, CMS considers the patient to be sicker
than the average patient with the same criteria and expects
greater-than-average resource utilization.

A low RAF score may accurately indicate a healthier patient, but it may also
falsely indicate a healthier patient due to incomplete or inaccurate coding,
incomplete or insufficient record documentation, or patients who fail to
complete an annual assessment.

A high RAF score may accurately indicate a sicker patient, or it may be falsely
inflated from overcoding due to diagnoses that are reported but not
documented, or from copying and pasting from previous encounters or problem
lists of resolved conditions.

Documentation Requirements

Payment is made per HCC category (not per diagnosis code). No matter how
many times in the year the diagnosis codes are reported, a single payment is
made to the MA plan each year. Each year the list of HCCs and the RAF for each
patient is "reset." This means the annual health assessment is extremely
important, and adequate documentation is critical. Accurate risk adjustment
payment relies on complete medical record documentation and diagnosis
coding. CMS requires that all applicable diagnosis codes be reported and that all
diagnoses be reported to the highest level of specificity and that these be
substantiated by the medical record.

CMS's Guiding Principle:

The risk adjustment diagnosis must be based on clinical medical record
documentation from a face-to-face encounter, coded according to the
ICD-10-CM Guidelines for Coding and Reporting; assigned based on dates of
service within the data collection period, submitted to the MA
organization from an appropriate risk adjustment provider type and an
appropriate risk adjustment physician data source.

A "face-to-face" health service encounter between a patient and healthcare provider describes an encounter between the patient and the provider (MD, DO), including qualified nonphysician practitioners (NPP) (e.g. nurse practitioner or physician's assistant), which is face-to-face with the patient. CMS provides a current listing of acceptable physician specialty types for risk adjustment data submission within the 2012 Regional Technical Assistance Participant Guide. The only exception to the face-to-face encounter requirement is pathology services (professional component only). Currently, CMS does not provide a listing of all services that are considered face-to-face visits for risk adjustment data, but does provide guidance on what types of services are not acceptable for risk adjustment in the Participant Guide. For example, diagnostic radiology does not qualify because diagnostic radiologists typically do not document confirmed diagnoses. Other examples of services that are not acceptable include diagnostic reports that have not been interpreted, such as laboratory reports.

It is essential that the medical record documentation show evidence by provider authentication that the direct face-to-face service was personally furnished by the physician or qualified NPP. Examples of these services include office visits, hospital visits, preoperative anesthesia assessment, and surgical and invasive procedures.

Risk adjustment relies on annual health information. Each enrollee is assigned an individual risk score based on the health status information obtained from the diagnosis codes on the claims. The CMS-HCC model relies on ICD-10-CM coding specificity for accurate risk adjustment by using the most specific code available that is substantiated by the documentation in the medical record. Providers should fully document and accurately code the evaluation and management of all severe and chronic conditions to ensure a full, complete, and accurate clinical record of the patient's condition and reflect the work involved in caring for the patient, particularly those with complex and challenging health issues. All conditions affecting the treatment or management of the patient's health should be documented at least once a year, as applicable to care provided, to accurately describe the true complexity and severity of the patient's health. If the diagnosis coding on the claim is not accurate or complete, the claim may indicate that the provider did much less medical decision-making, evaluation, and management than was actually performed.

Documentation to support or validate risk adjustment conditions may be found anywhere in the note for the face-to-face encounter. It is important to ensure that the note accurately reflects all chronic conditions that affect the health and care of the patient. Each encounter must be unique and reflect only that visit as it occurred. Insufficient documentation influences the assignment of diagnosis codes and directly affects the patient's risk score.

Documentation should properly validate all reported conditions. Each page of progress notes should be properly authenticated and include the patient's name and the date.

Providers should document each clinical diagnosis to the highest degree of specificity per encounter, including all complications and/or manifestations, including clear links to causal conditions. Only confirmed conditions should be documented—no rule-out conditions or abnormal findings without clinical significance. All known conditions, including chronic conditions, that affect the care and treatment of the patient at least once per year should be noted.

Providers should specifically document the condition and clinical significance, and pertinent changes using terminology such as decreased, increased, worsening, improving, or unchanged, or abnormal findings.

Documentation Tips

- Document all cause-and-effect relationships.
- Report the most specific diagnosis code available that is supported by the documentation.
- Include all current diagnoses as part of the current medical decision-making, and document for every visit.
- Identify diagnoses that are current or chronic problems rather than a past medical history or previous resolved condition.
- Document history of heart attack, status codes, etc., that affect the patient's care as "history of" or "PMH" when they no longer exist or are not current conditions.
- Ensure each progress note has the date, signature, and credentials/specialty.
- Document the thought processes used to assess each condition.
- Know high revenue HCCs that are often undiagnosed or undercoded.
- Avoid "unspecified" codes.
- Ensure the codes reported are accurate.

- Ensure each encounter is billed.
- Review rejection reports, and audit reports to assess risks.

Audits

Because reimbursement is by patient, rather than based on an average of the entire population, and is based upon documentation, there is the potential for upcoding. Audits are conducted by the MA plan and CMS recovery auditors.

Initial Validation Audit (IVA)

CMS requires that the MA plan validate HCCs. This is usually performed by an independent auditor working with the plan or a contracted vendor to validate the MA plan's data submitted to CMS.

The MA plan submits the one best medical record that supports each HCC identified for the beneficiary.

Risk Adjustment Data Validation Audit

Risk adjustment data validation (RADV) audits were introduced in 2011 and updated for 2015. They are performed by CMS to validate the integrity and accuracy of risk-adjusted payments by verifying that the diagnosis codes the M plans submit are supported by the medical record documentation for a memb

MA plans can be selected by CMS for RADV audits annually and if chosen are required to submit their members' medical records to CMS. Providers are required to assist the MA plan by providing the medical record documentatio included in the audit. Even though each diagnosis needs to be reported only once in a calendar year, during a RADV audit up to five dates of service may b submitted to support any one HCC.

To be validated, medical record documentation must meet certain criteria an standards. Even if the diagnosis is documented and coded correctly, any deficiency in the documentation can make the encounter and the HCC invali Diagnoses that cannot be validated are considered payment errors. The result the audit are communicated to the MA plan, which then communicates thes results to the provider. Under- and overpayments are subject to payment adjustment. The results of RADV audits can be extrapolated over the MA pla population to calculate potential payment errors and overpayments/ recoupments. Regulations include a RADV appeal process, a document dispu process, and a procedure for obtaining physician-signature attestations.

The following items are reviewed during the validation process:

- The record is for the correct enrollee.
- The record is from the correct calendar year for the payment year bein audited.
- The record is legible.
- The date of service is present on the records and is for a face-to-face v
- The record is from a valid provider type.
- Valid credentials and/or a valid physician specialty are documented o record.
- The record contains a signature from an acceptable type of physician.
- There is a diagnosis on the record.
- The diagnosis supports an HCC.
- The diagnosis supports the submitted HCC.

Mitigate audit risk by coding each reportable diagnosis each time it meets reporting guidelines. Audit regularly to assess areas of risk and in need of improvement and to capture conditions documented but not coded. Chec additional qualifying HCCs. Ensure claims are submitted and that corrected claims are submitted when indicated. There are three claims submission dea January, March, and September. CMS adjusts each member's risk score twi year, with the final reconciliation in August of the year after the plan year.

If providers emphasize correct coding and documentation and perform in audits to determine where the risks are and prepare for audits, incorrect payment is less likely. For additional information on risk adjustment codin Optum360's *Risk Adjustment Coding and HCC Guide.*

2015, in an effort to repeal the faulty Medicare sustainable growth rate (SGR), cus on quality of patient outcomes, and control Medicare spending, Congress ssed the Medicare Access and CHIP Reauthorization Act (MACRA), which cluded sweeping changes for practitioners who provide services reimbursed der the Medicare physician fee schedule (MPFS). MACRA repealed the dicare SGR methodology used for updating the MPFS and replaced it with the ality Payment Program (QPP).

der the QPP, providers who demonstrate success at controlling costs while oviding high-quality care to their patients are eligible to earn increased yments. Clinicians who successfully report on determined criteria receive a ger payment. Those who do not participate at all or do not fulfill the defined uirements receive a negative payment adjustment of 7 percent of Medicare t B reimbursements based on 2019 performance to be applied in 2021; future yment adjustments will rise to as high as +/− 9 percent through the 2020 formance year and will be applied in 2022.

ssage of the Medicare Access and CHIP Reauthorization t of 2015

final rule for implementing MACRA was published November 4, 2016. The l rule primarily provided details on how the QPP was to be implemented, uding requiring the secretary of Health and Human Services (HHS) to sunset value-based (VM) modifier incentive program, the Medicare electronic th record (EHR) incentive program, and the Physician Quality Reporting em (PQRS), and incorporated these incentive programs into the QPP.

olacement of the Sustainable Growth Rate

er the SGR, if overall physician costs were higher than a targeted Medicare enditure, payments were reduced across the board. With the SGR method, nents to clinicians would have resulted in substantial cuts.

use the QPP replaces the SGR methodology, the following revisions were iled in MACRA:

Established conversion factor updates:

- a Medicare physician fee schedule conversion factor adjustment of 0.5 percent in 2016–2019 and a conversion factor adjustment of 0.00 percent for 2020–2025

- the qualifying participant (QP) alternative payment models (APM) conversion factor of 0.75 percent and a nonqualifying provider APM conversion factor of 0.25 percent for 2026 and each subsequent year

r the QPP, the Centers for Medicare and Medicaid Services (CMS) aims to:

Support quality of patient care improvement by focusing on better outcomes for patients, decreasing provider burden, and preserving the independent clinical practice

Promote the adoption of APMs, which align incentives across healthcare stakeholders

Advance existing efforts of delivery system reform, including ensuring a smooth transition to a new system that promotes high-quality, efficient care through unification of CMS legacy programs such as the EHR incentive program

ity Payment Program Established

ACRA final rule established the Quality Payment Program (QPP) effective y 1, 2017. Within the QPP there are two interrelated pathways: advanced tive payment models (APM) and the Merit-based Incentive Payment a (MIPS).

e clinicians (EC) select the track/pathway—MIPS or advanced APMs—they participate in based on the practice size, specialty, location, and patient tion. Unlike previous quality initiatives, a provider does not have to enroll QPP. However, groups wishing to participate in the MIPS program via the ner Assessment of Healthcare Providers and Systems (CAHPS) for MIPS measures or CMS Web Interface (WI) must register by June 30 each year. HPS for MIPS survey is an optional quality measure that groups ating in MIPS can elect to administer.

-based Incentive Payment System

the track for clinicians who opt to participate in traditional Medicare as d to participating through an advanced APM. In doing so, clinicians may ayment adjustment related to evidence-based and practice-specific data. As a result, depending on the degree and success of performance in categories for CY 2019, clinicians receive one of the following:

- Positive payment adjustment in which additional compensation is received; bonuses are also available for meeting the exceptional performance threshold
- Neutral payment adjustment that neither increases nor reduces Medicare payments
- Negative payment adjustment of up to 7 percent of Medicare payment furnished in calendar year (CY) 2021

Participation in the MIPS track is determined based on the amount billed to Medicare and the number of beneficiaries seen per year. The following provider types are eligible for participation if they meet or exceed at least one of the following criteria:

- Medicare billings are equal to or greater than $90,000
- Care is provided for more than 200 covered services
- Care is provided to 200 or more Medicare patients each year

For 2019, the following provider types are considered ECs:

- Physicians (MD, DO, DDS, DMD, DPM, OD, DC)
- Physician assistants (PA)
- Nurse practitioners (NP)
- Clinical nurse specialists (CNS)
- Certified registered nurse anesthetists (CRNA)
- Physical therapist (PT)
- Occupational therapist (OT)
- Qualified speech-language pathologist
- Qualified audiologist
- Clinical psychologist
- Registered dietician or nutrition professionals
- Any clinician group that includes one of the professionals listed above

Anatomy of MIPS

MIPS incorporates pieces of three former Medicare reporting programs:

- Physician Quality Reporting System (PQRS)
- Medicare EHR Incentive Program/meaningful use
- Value-based payment modifier

A measurement-based regime creates a single reporting framework for physicians that comprise four performance categories:

- Quality—replaced the PQRS
- Improvement Activities (IA)—implemented in 2017
- Promoting Interoperability—replaced the Medicare EHR Incentive Program, aka "meaningful use"
- Cost—replaced the value-based modifier

Each of the four performance categories has been weighted, with greatest emphasis placed on the Quality category at 45 percent, Promoting Interoperability is second at 25 percent, IA at 15 percent, and Cost at 15 percent.

The 2019 MIPS performance threshold equates to 30 points out of a possible 100 points. Simply put, eligible clinicians are required to score 30 points to avoid the negative 7 percent payment adjustment.

Quality Performance

Under the MIPS Quality performance category, ECs and groups must select six measures from a listing of more than 250 measures, with at least one of the six measures being an outcome measure. Patient outcomes such as mortality, whether a patient is readmitted to the hospital, and the patient's experience are areas that CMS and the healthcare industry seek to improve. An outcome measure is the way CMS can quantify changes in the health of an individual, groups of individuals, and even certain populations that they can attribute back to a specific intervention or series of interventions.

Quality measures are tools for quantifying, or measuring, healthcare processes and patient outcomes and perceptions, as well as organizational structure and/or systems linked to the ability to provide high-quality healthcare. These measures play an important role under the MIPS. Reporting should be done on a minimum of half of the EC's or group practice's Medicare Part B patients. Each measure is worth up to 10 points and is compared to a national benchmark.

Improvement Activities

The IA category assesses to what degree a clinician participates in activities designed to improve clinical practices. ECs are required to attest that they have participated in a minimum of four improvement activities from an expanded inventory of more than 100 activities across eight subcategories for 90 consecutive days. These eight subcategories include:

- Expanded practice access
- Population management
- Care coordination
- Beneficiary engagement
- Patient safety and practice assessment
- Achieving health equity
- Integrating behavioral and mental health
- Emergency preparedness and response

This category was created with some inherent flexibility; for example, for groups with 15 or fewer participants, nonpatient-facing clinicians (e.g., pathologists), or those ECs in a rural or health professional shortage area (HPSA) are required to declare participation in only up to two activities for at least 90 consecutive days.

Promoting Interoperability

This performance category replaced the Medicare EHR Incentive Program, commonly known as "meaningful use." CMS wants to encourage and promote the use of certified EHR technology (CEHRT) among providers and, in particular, the use of interoperability and sharing of information among clinicians and between providers and patients.

Successful reporting of measures in this category require the EC to report each measure under a single set of objectives and measures based exclusively on the 2015 edition of CEHRT and, as applicable, claim an exclusion. Exclusions are reported by submitting a "0" in addition to the exclusion type that applies to the EC because some measures may be associated with more than one exclusion.

The PI performance category contains four objectives:

- E-Prescribing
- Health Information Exchange
- Provider to Patient Exchange
- Public Health and Clinical Data Exchange

All measures contained within those objectives are required to be reported through the Public Health and Clinical exchange objective. This objective has only five measures in it and therefore the clinician needs to select only two measures, which can be reported to any two registries and do not need to be separate categories (e.g., submitting data to two different clinical data registries).

Cost

In this performance category, CMS determines an EC or group practice's cost score by calculating data from two measures previously included in the value-based payment modifier that involves the total cost of care for attributed beneficiaries and what Medicare spends per beneficiary. This amount is the tot of both Medicare Part A and B payments from three days before through 30 da after a beneficiary has had an inpatient hospitalization episode. CMS then determines which ECs and practices have an adequate number of beneficiaries and hospitalizations associated with them. This number is compared with national benchmarks established for the performance period.

For procedure episodes, the case minimum established is 10 with credit for the episodes going to the clinician who performs the procedure. For acute inpatie medical condition episodes, the case minimum is set at 20, and credit is assign to each clinician who bills the inpatient evaluation and management (E/M) cla lines during a triggered inpatient hospitalization under a TIN that furnishes at least 30 percent of the inpatient E/M claim lines during that particular hospitalization.

Clinicians have no additional submission responsibilities associated with this category as the score is determined from Medicare administrative claims data

The category also has separate benchmarks. The Cost score is determined and compared with those benchmarks with points assigned based on the decile system in a similar manner to the Quality performance category with some differences such as:

- Benchmarks for performance are for the *same* year versus prior year performance.
- Scores are determined once case minimum requirements for each of two measures in this category have been met.

MIPS Scoring

CMS uses scoring to determine an EC's successful participation in the QPP an thereby determine if the clinician's reimbursement will be negative, neutral, positive.

The scoring methodology is a unified approach across all performance categories, allowing eligible clinicians to understand what is expected so the can perform successfully in the MIPS.

For more information and details on QPP, see Optum360's *MACRA Quality Payment Program Guide*.

Chapter 3. Diseases of the Blood and Blood-forming Organs and Certain Disorders Involving the Immune Mechanism (D50–D89)

Red Blood Cells

White Blood Cell

Platelet

Coagulation

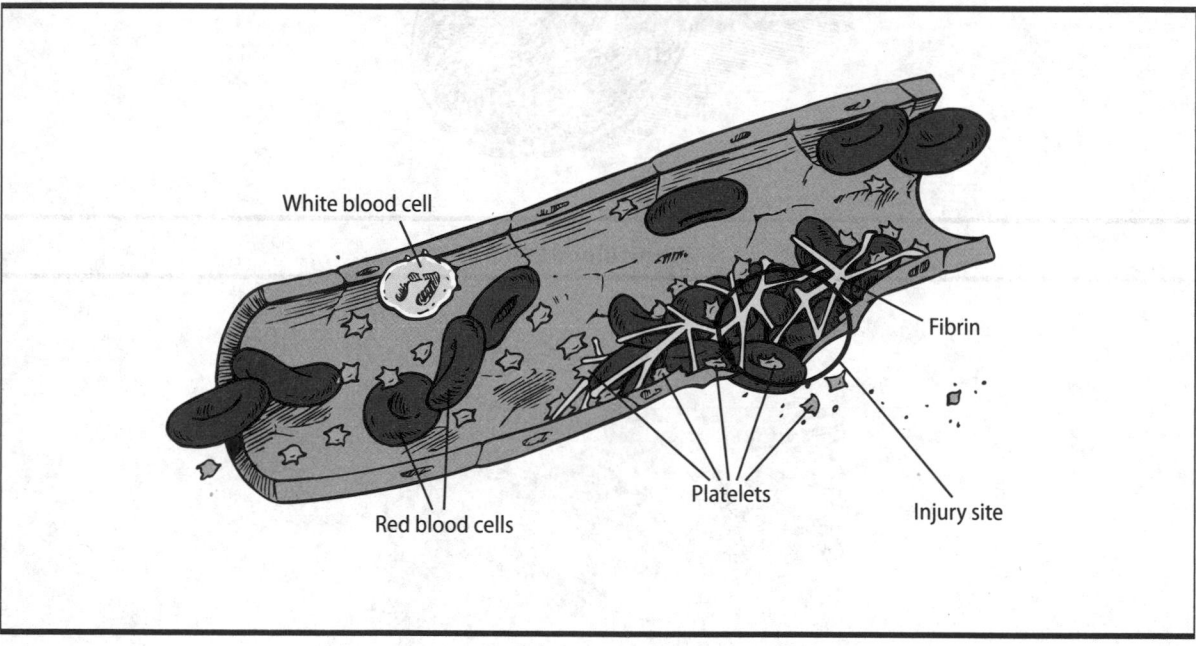

White blood cell

Fibrin

Platelets

Injury site

Red blood cells

Spleen Anatomical Location and External Structures

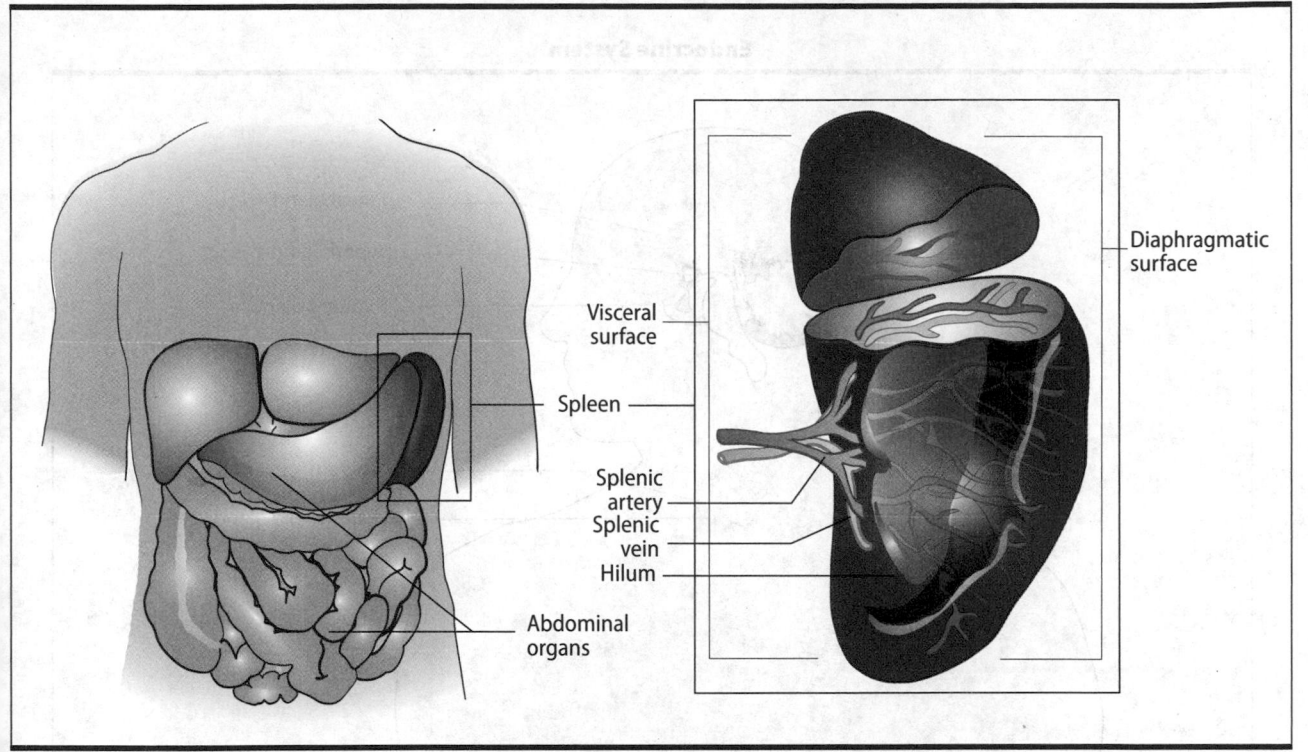

Visceral surface

Spleen

Splenic artery

Splenic vein

Hilum

Abdominal organs

Diaphragmatic surface

Spleen Interior Structures

Capsule

Trabecula

Vascular sinusoid

White pulp

Red pulp

Splenic artery

Splenic vein

Chapter 4. Endocrine, Nutritional and Metabolic Diseases (E00–E89)

Endocrine System

Thyroid

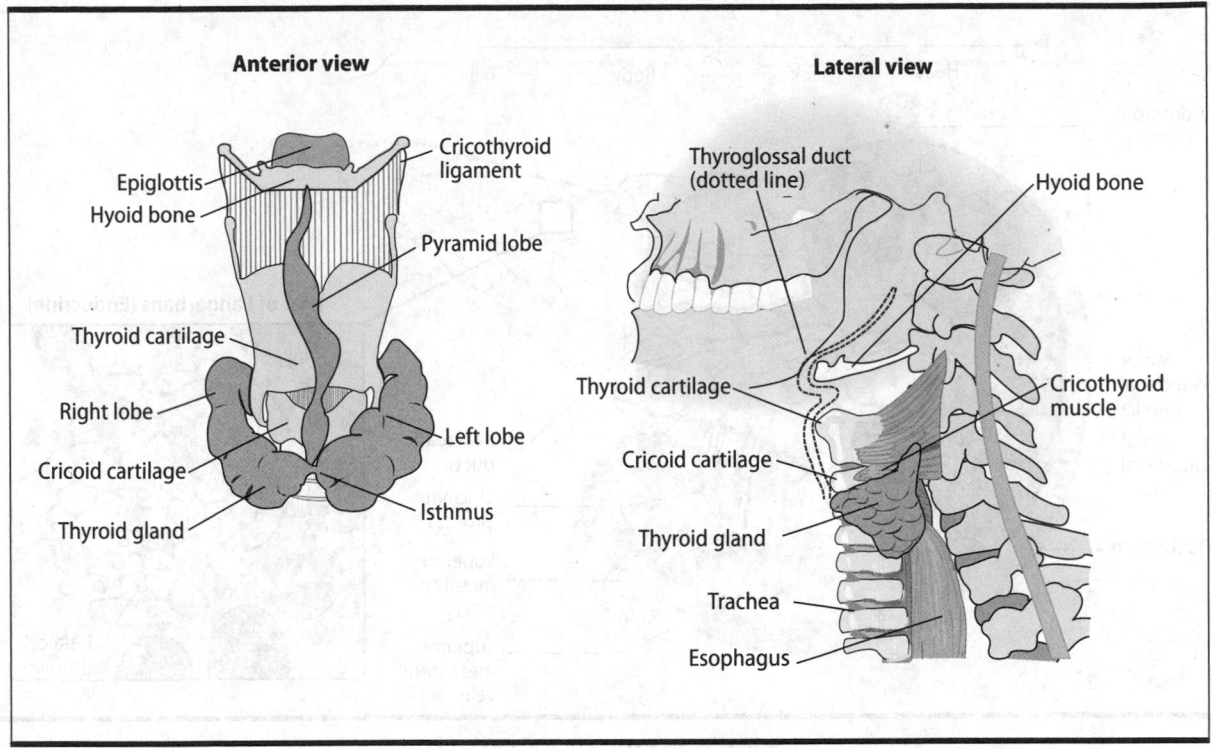

Anterior view

- Epiglottis
- Hyoid bone
- Cricothyroid ligament
- Thyroid cartilage
- Pyramid lobe
- Right lobe
- Left lobe
- Cricoid cartilage
- Isthmus
- Thyroid gland

Lateral view

- Thyroglossal duct (dotted line)
- Hyoid bone
- Thyroid cartilage
- Cricothyroid muscle
- Cricoid cartilage
- Thyroid gland
- Trachea
- Esophagus

Thyroid and Parathyroid Glands

Posterior view

- Epiglottis
- Pharynx
- Thyroid gland
- Parathyroid gland

Pancreas

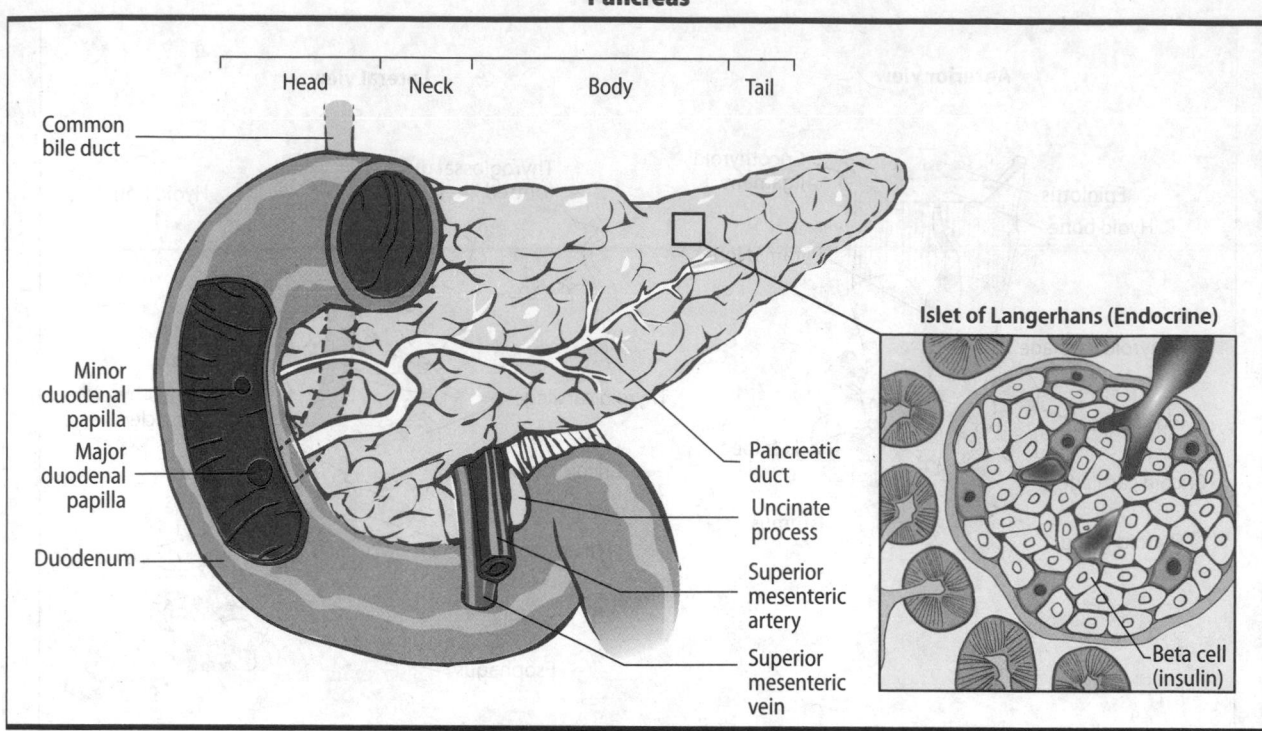

Islet of Langerhans (Endocrine)

Head   Neck   Body   Tail

Common bile duct

Minor duodenal papilla

Major duodenal papilla

Duodenum

Pancreatic duct

Uncinate process

Superior mesenteric artery

Superior mesenteric vein

Beta cell (insulin)

Anatomy of the Adrenal Gland

Adrenal glands

Kidney

Capsule

Cortex

Medulla

Structure of an Ovary

Primordial follicles
Primary follicles
Oocyte
Secondary follicle
Vesicular (graafian) follicle
Corona radiata
Ovulated ovum
Blood vessels
Degenerating corpus luteum (corpus albicans)
Corpus luteum
Developing corpus luteum

Testis and Associated Structures

Spermatic cord
Head of epididymis
Blood vessels and nerves
Efferent ductule
Seminiferous tubule
Rete testis
Septum
Lobule
Ductus deferens
Body of epididymis
Tunica albuginea
Tunica vaginalis
Tail of epididymis

Thymus

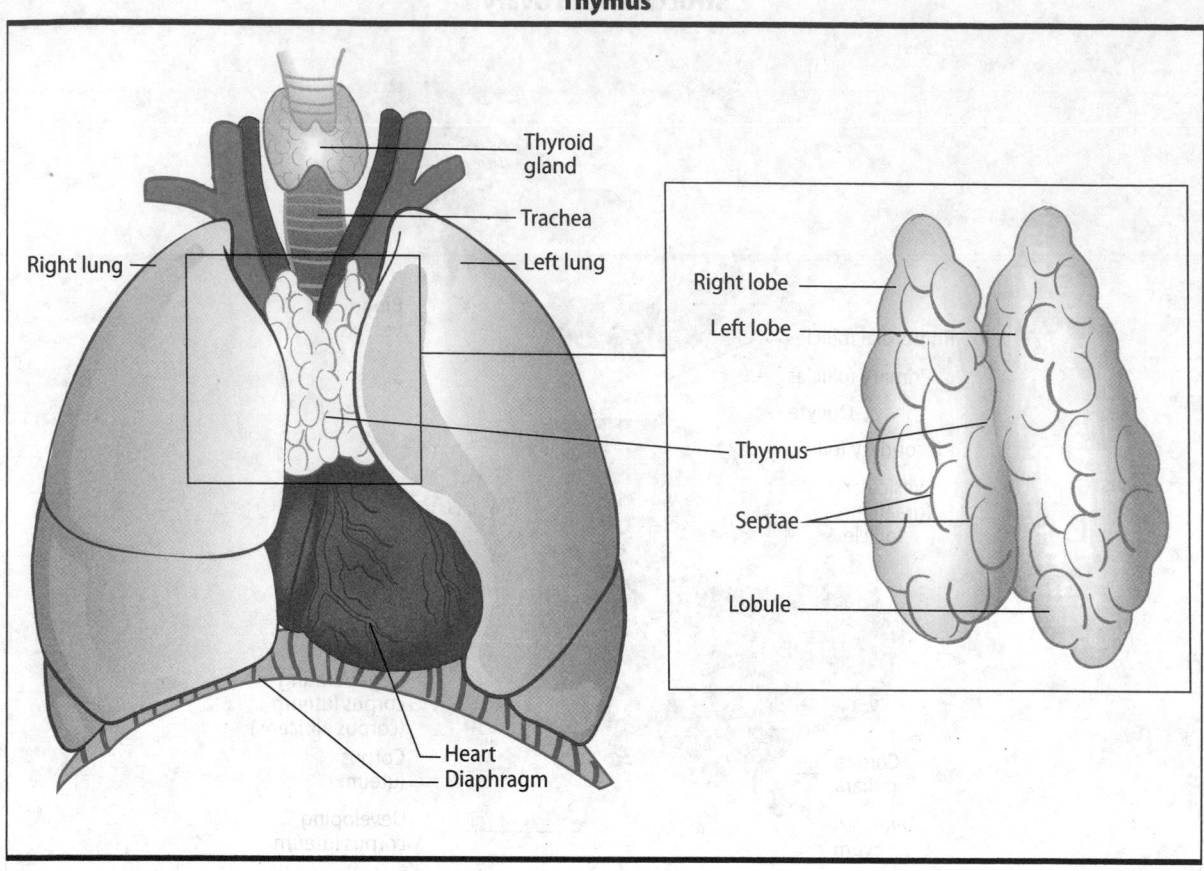

Chapter 6. Diseases of the Nervous System (GØØ–G99)

Brain

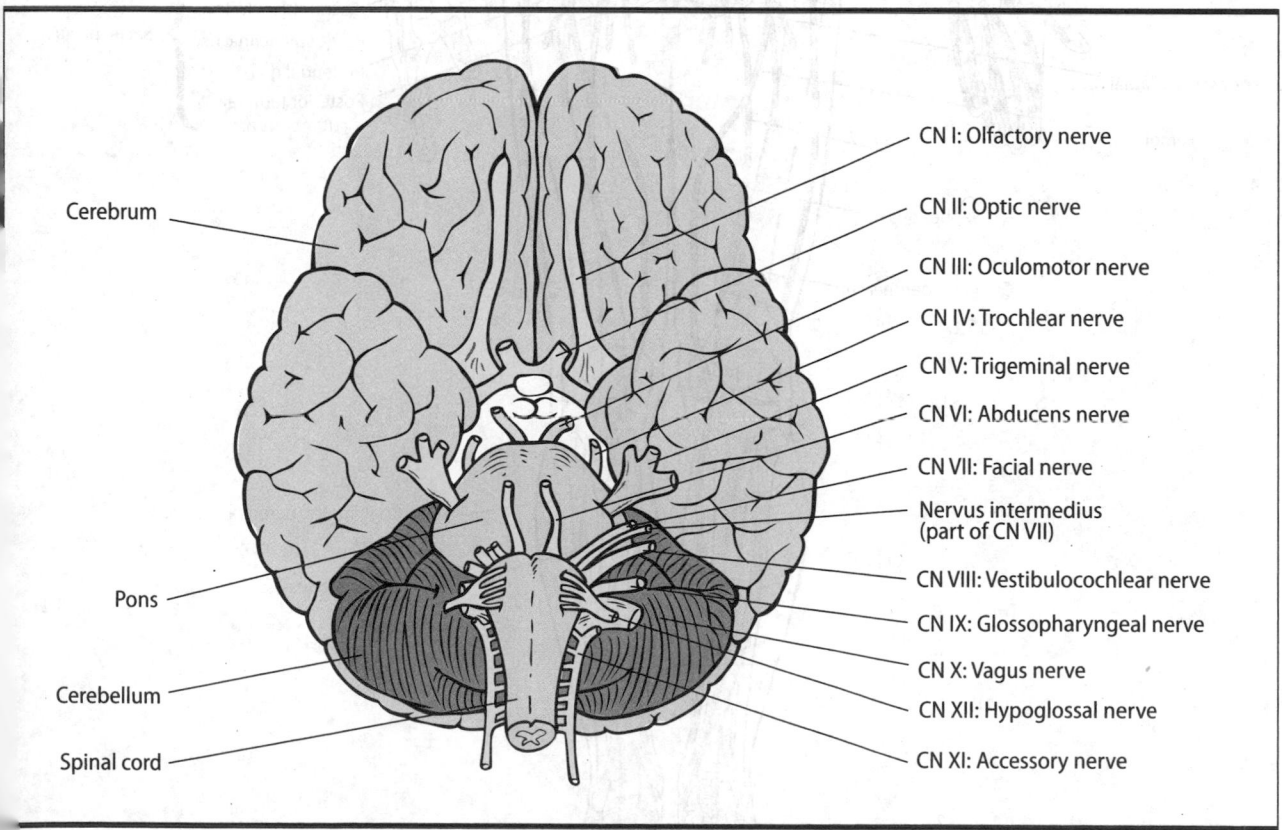

Cranial Nerves

Peripheral Nervous System

Cervical plexus
- Ansa cervicalis
- Transverse cervical n.
- Dorsal scapular n.
- First intercostal n.
- Subclavian n.
- Long thoracic n.

Brachial plexus
- Axillary n.
- Median n.
- Radial n.
- Intercostobrachial n.
- Ulnar n.
- Musculocutaneous n.
- Intercostal nerves

- 12th thoracic n.
- Subcostal n.

- Posterior scrotal/labial n.
- Femoral n.
- Sciatic n.
- Saphenous n.
- Common peroneal n.
- Tibial n.

- Great auricular n.
- Greater occipital n.
- Lesser occipital n.
- Suboccipital n.
- 3rd occipital n.
- L. phrenic n.
- Supraclavicular n.

Cervical plexus

- Subclavian n.
- Axillary n.
- Median n.
- Musculocutaneous n.
- Ulnar n.
- Radial n.
- Thoracic splanchnic n.

- Lumbar splanchnic n.
- Genitofemoral n.
- Iliohypogastric n.
- Ilioinguinal n.
- Obturator n.
- Lateral femoral cutaneous n.
- Accessory obturator n.
- Superior gluteal n.

Lumbar plexus

- Inferior gluteal n.
- Sacral n.
- Sacral splanchnic n.
- Pelvic splanchnic n.
- Pudendal n.
- Posterior femoral cutaneous n.

Sacral plexus

- Superficial fibular (peroneal) n.
- Deep fibular (peroneal) n.

Peripheral Nervous System

Spinal Cord and Spinal Nerves

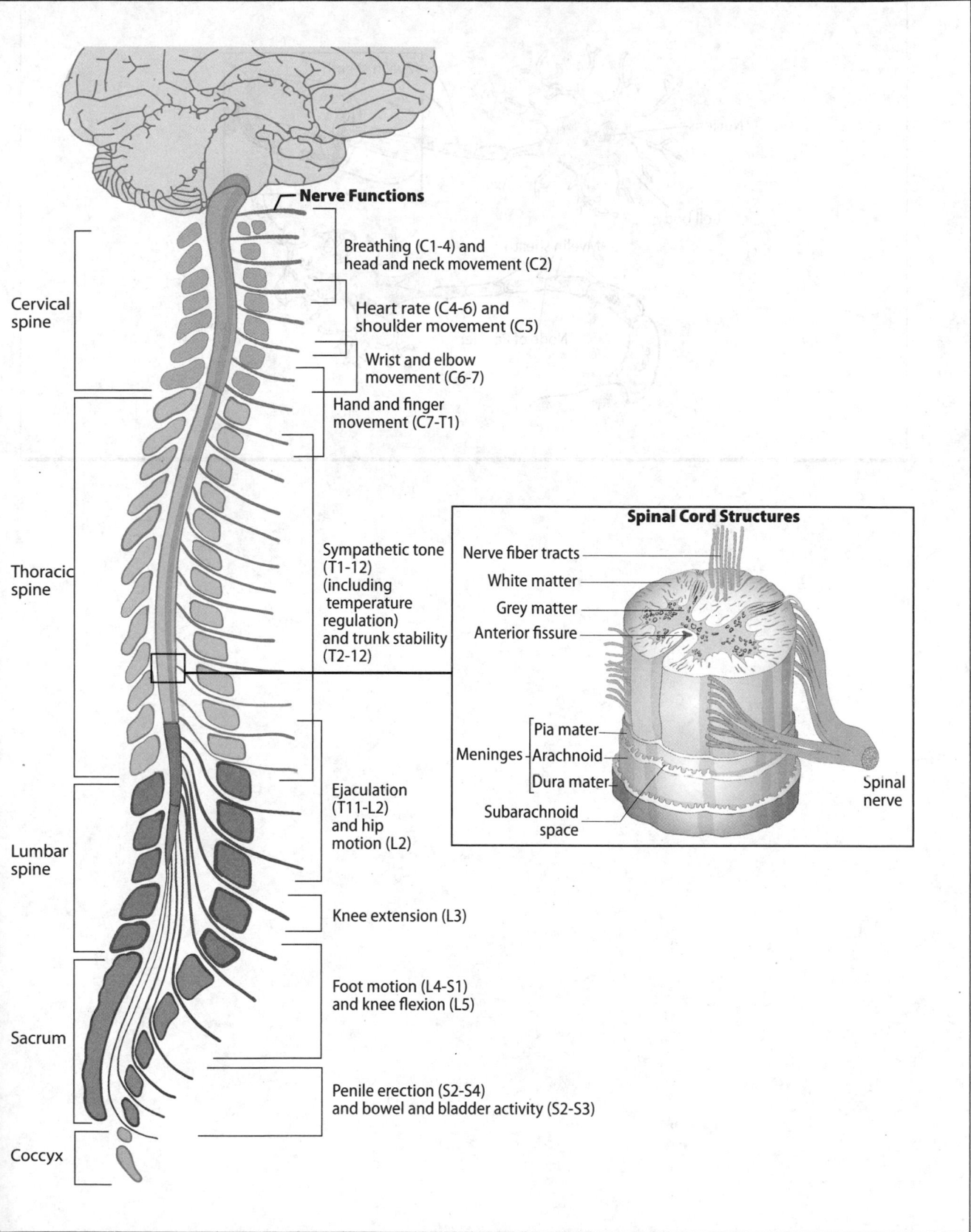

Nerve Functions

Breathing (C1-4) and head and neck movement (C2)

Heart rate (C4-6) and shoulder movement (C5)

Wrist and elbow movement (C6-7)

Hand and finger movement (C7-T1)

Cervical spine

Sympathetic tone (T1-12) (including temperature regulation) and trunk stability (T2-12)

Thoracic spine

Spinal Cord Structures

Nerve fiber tracts
White matter
Grey matter
Anterior fissure

Pia mater
Meninges — Arachnoid
Dura mater

Subarachnoid space

Spinal nerve

Ejaculation (T11-L2) and hip motion (L2)

Lumbar spine

Knee extension (L3)

Foot motion (L4-S1) and knee flexion (L5)

Sacrum

Penile erection (S2-S4) and bowel and bladder activity (S2-S3)

Coccyx

Nerve Cell

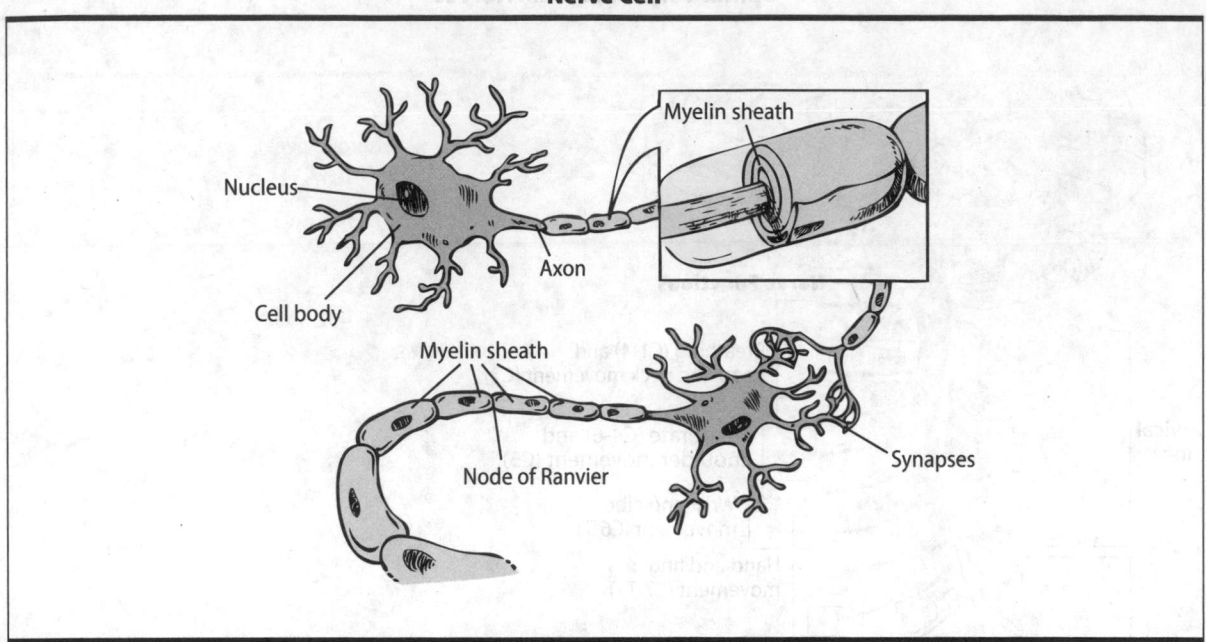

hapter 7. Diseases of the Eye and Adnexa (HØØ–H59)

Eye

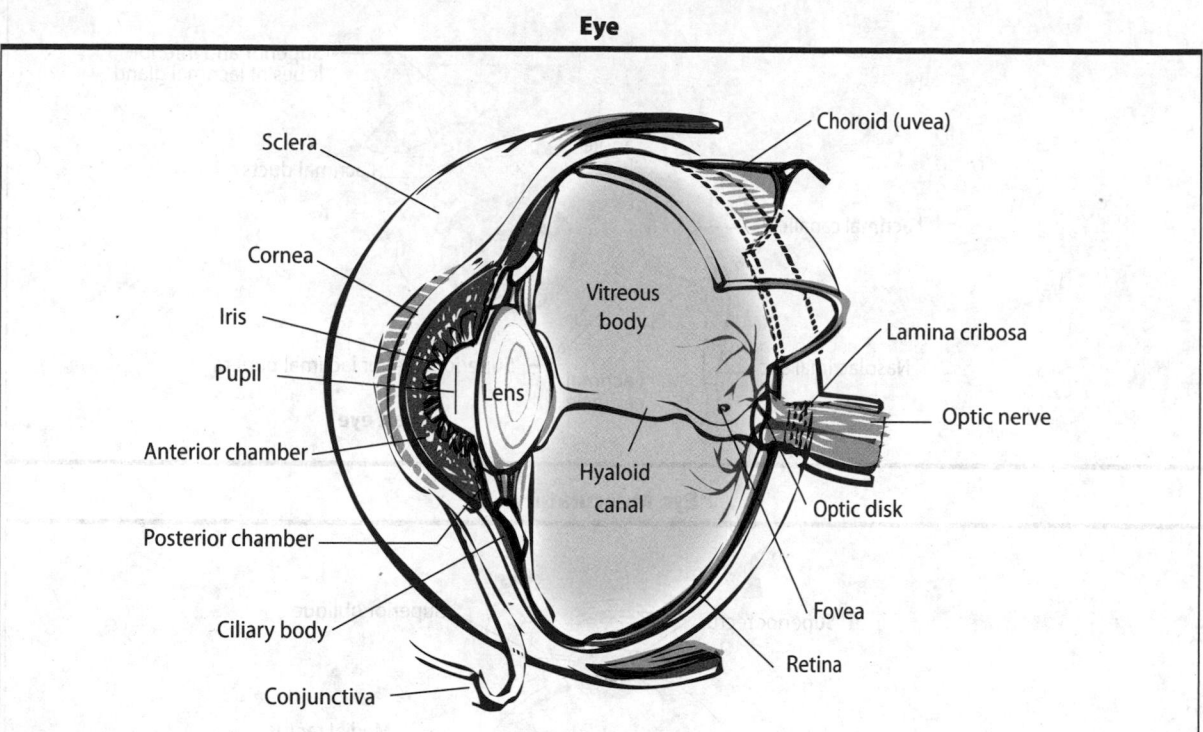

Posterior Pole of Globe/Flow of Aqueous Humor

Lacrimal System

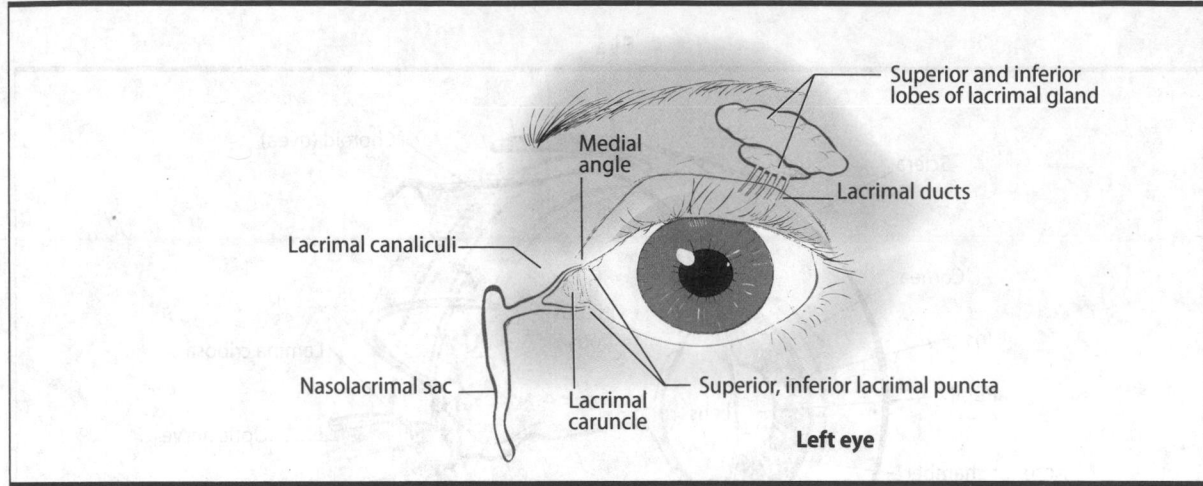

Superior and inferior
lobes of lacrimal gland

Medial
angle

Lacrimal ducts

Lacrimal canaliculi

Lacrimal caruncle

Nasolacrimal sac

Superior, inferior lacrimal puncta

Left eye

Eye Musculature

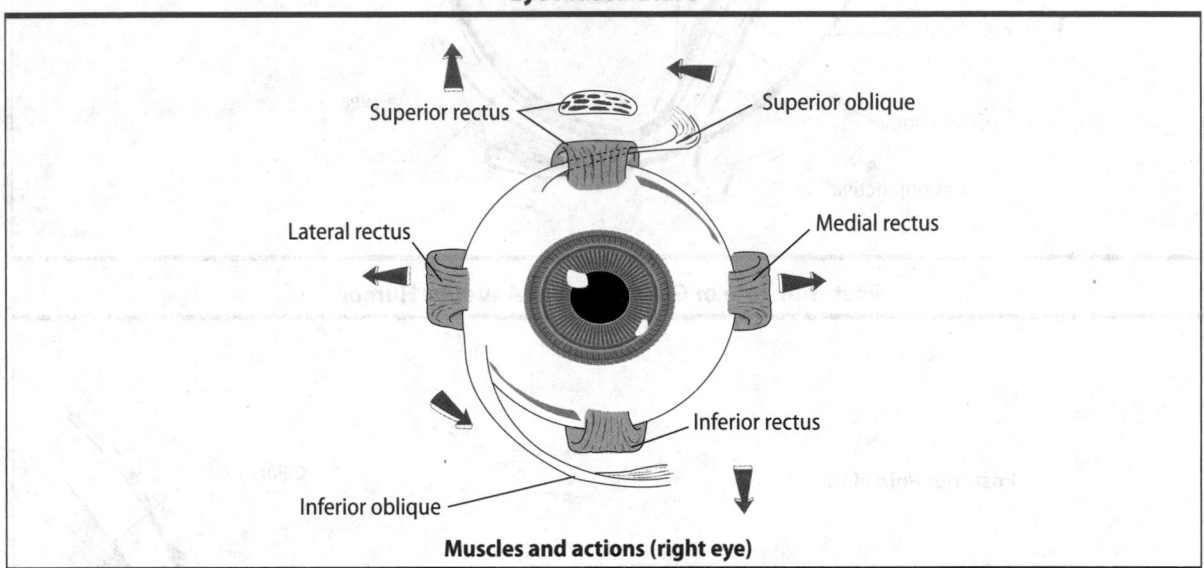

Superior rectus

Superior oblique

Lateral rectus

Medial rectus

Inferior rectus

Inferior oblique

Muscles and actions (right eye)

Eyelid Structures

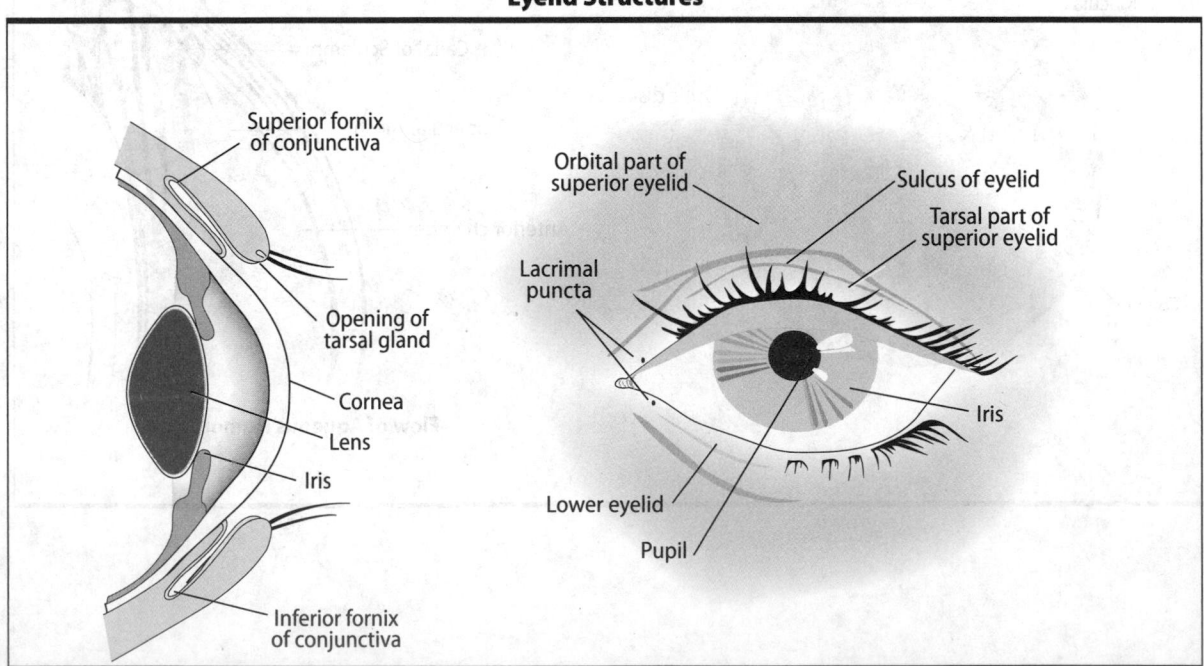

Superior fornix
of conjunctiva

Orbital part of
superior eyelid

Sulcus of eyelid

Tarsal part of
superior eyelid

Lacrimal
puncta

Opening of
tarsal gland

Cornea

Lens

Iris

Iris

Lower eyelid

Pupil

Inferior fornix
of conjunctiva

Chapter 8. Diseases of the Ear and Mastoid Process (H6Ø–H95)

Ear Anatomy

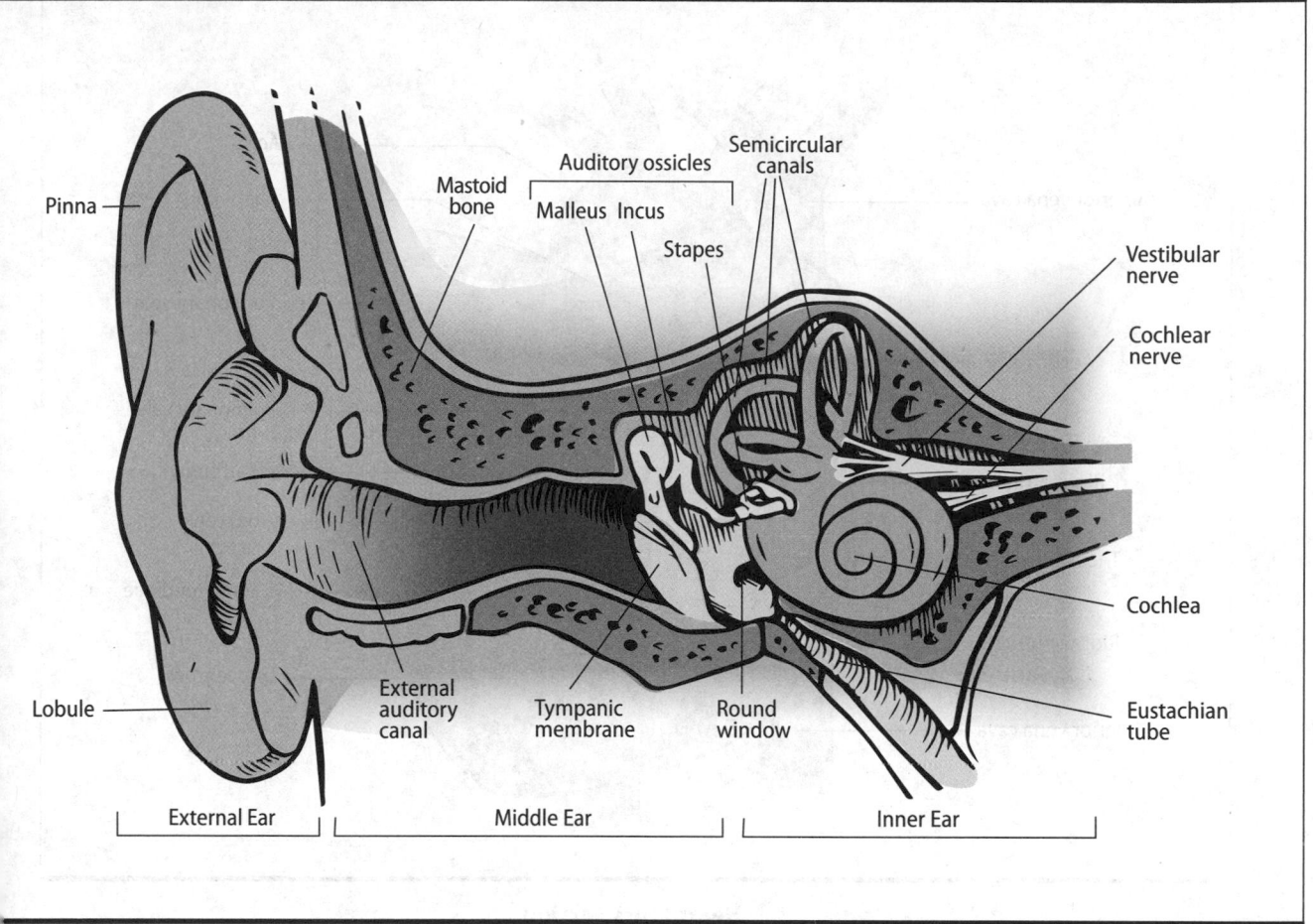

Chapter 9. Diseases of the Circulatory System (I00–I99)

Anatomy of the Heart

Superior vena cava

Aortic valve

Right atrium

Tricuspid valve

Right ventricle

Inferior vena cava

Aorta

Pulmonary artery

Pulmonary vein

Pulmonary valve

Left atrium

Mitral valve

Chorda tendinae

Left ventricle

Heart Cross Section

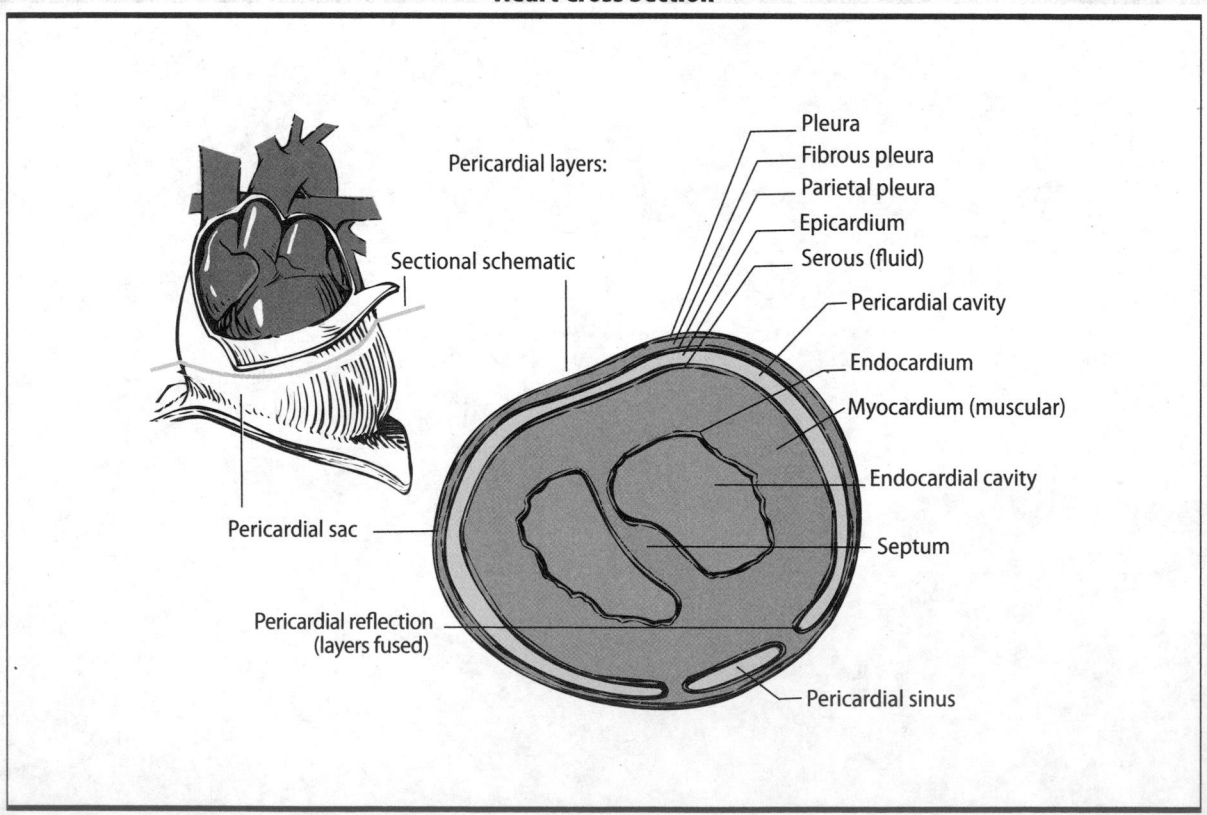

Pericardial layers:

Sectional schematic

Pericardial sac

Pericardial reflection
(layers fused)

Pleura

Fibrous pleura

Parietal pleura

Epicardium

Serous (fluid)

Pericardial cavity

Endocardium

Myocardium (muscular)

Endocardial cavity

Septum

Pericardial sinus

Heart Valves

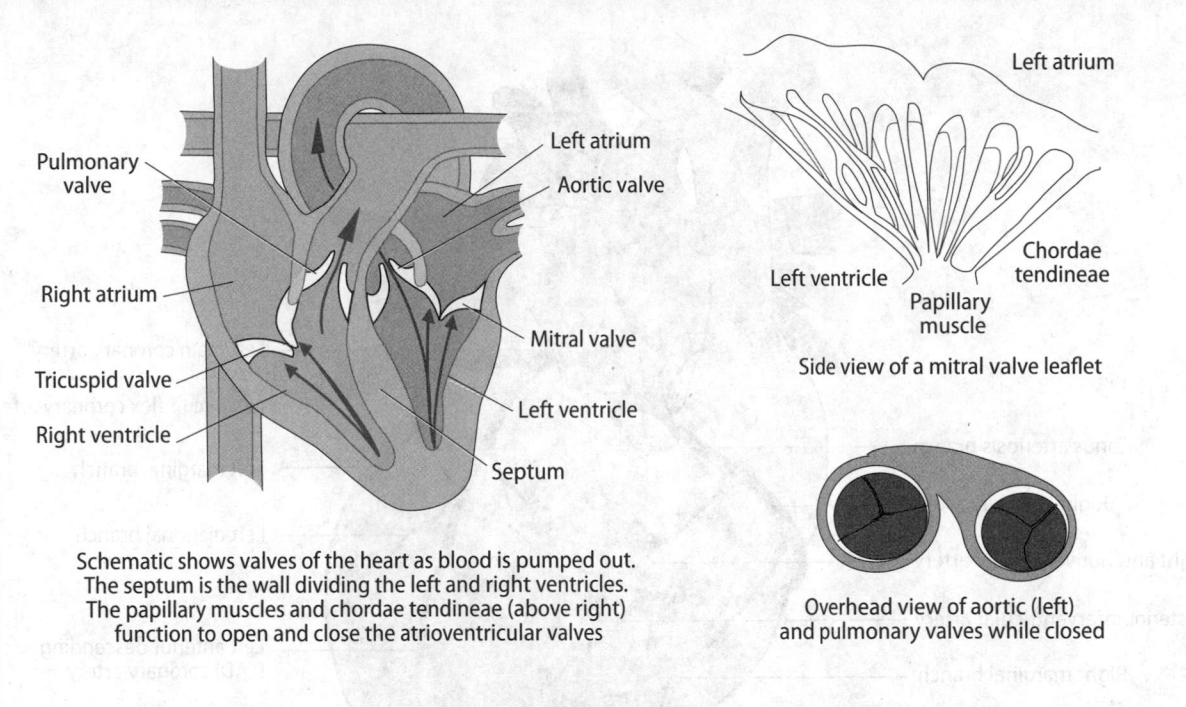

Pulmonary valve

Left atrium

Aortic valve

Right atrium

Mitral valve

Tricuspid valve

Left ventricle

Right ventricle

Septum

Left atrium

Left ventricle

Chordae tendineae

Papillary muscle

Side view of a mitral valve leaflet

Schematic shows valves of the heart as blood is pumped out.
The septum is the wall dividing the left and right ventricles.
The papillary muscles and chordae tendineae (above right)
function to open and close the atrioventricular valves

Overhead view of aortic (left)
and pulmonary valves while closed

Heart Conduction System

Sinoatrial node
(pacemaker)

Atrioventricular node

Atrioventricular bundle
(of His)

Left bundle branch

Right bundle branch

Purkinje fibers

Coronary Arteries

Conus arteriosis branch

Right coronary artery

Right anterior ventricular artery

Posterior interventricular artery

Right marginal branch

Left main coronary artery

Left circumflex coronary artery

Left marginal branch

Left diagonal branch

Left anterior descending (LAD) coronary artery

Anterior interventricular artery

Arteries

Middle temporal a.
Transverse facial a.
Superficial temporal a.
External carotid a.
Internal carotid a.
Common carotid a.
Superior thyroid a.
Inferior thyroid a.
Vertebral a.
Subclavian a.
Innominate a.
Arch of aorta
Ascending aorta
Pulmonary a.
Axillary a.
Internal thoracic a. (mammary)
Descending aorta
Brachial a.
Common hepatic a.
L. gastric a.
Celiac trunk (artery)
Splenic a.
R. gastric a.
Renal a.
Superior mesenteric a.
R. colic a.
Abdominal aorta
L. colic a.
Radial a.
Inferior mesenteric a.
Ulnar a.
Common iliac a.
Internal iliac a.
External iliac a.
Uterine a.
Femoral a.
Popliteal a.
Anterior tibial a.
Peroneal a.
Posterior tibial a.

Veins

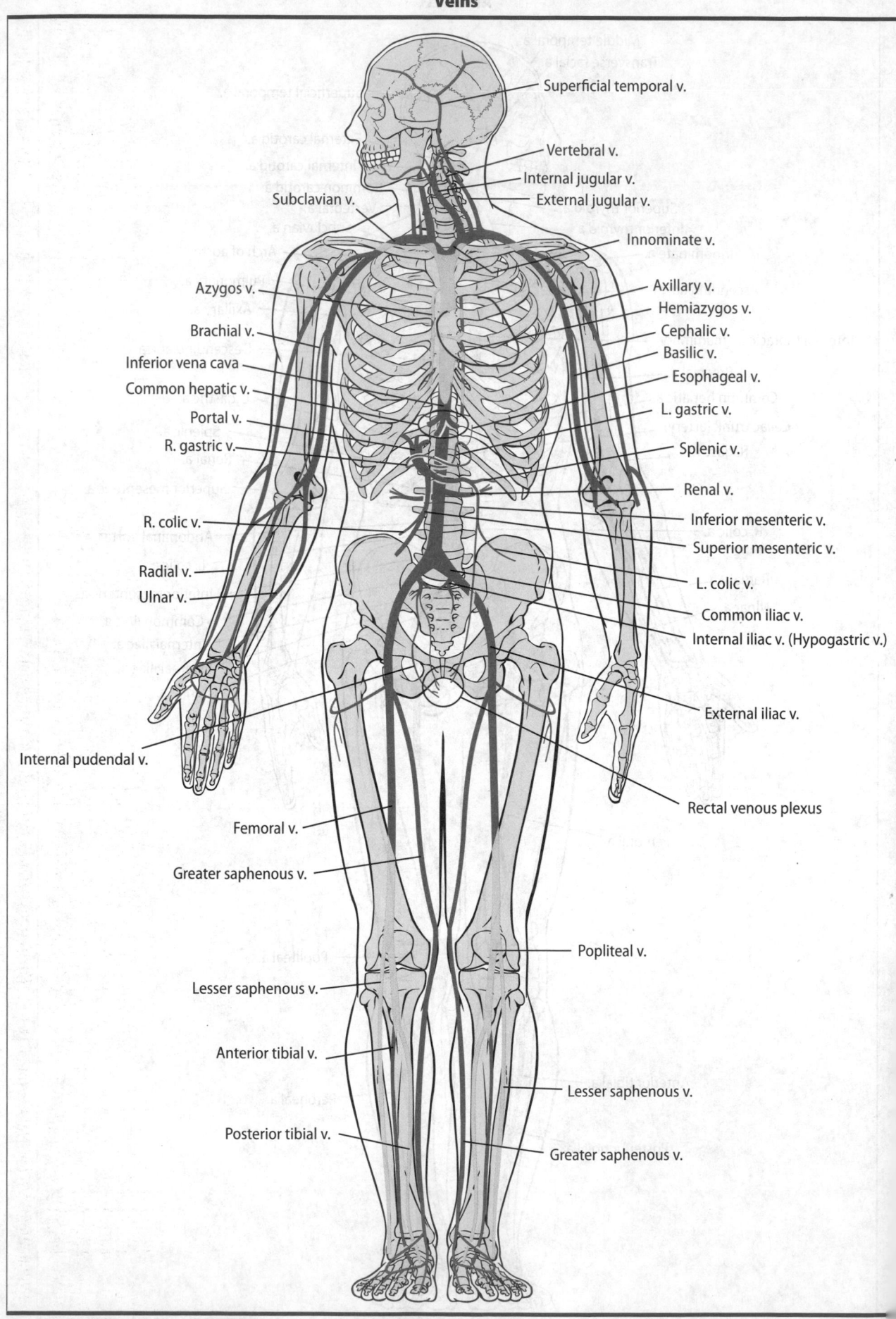

Internal Carotid and Vertebral Arteries and Branches

Side View

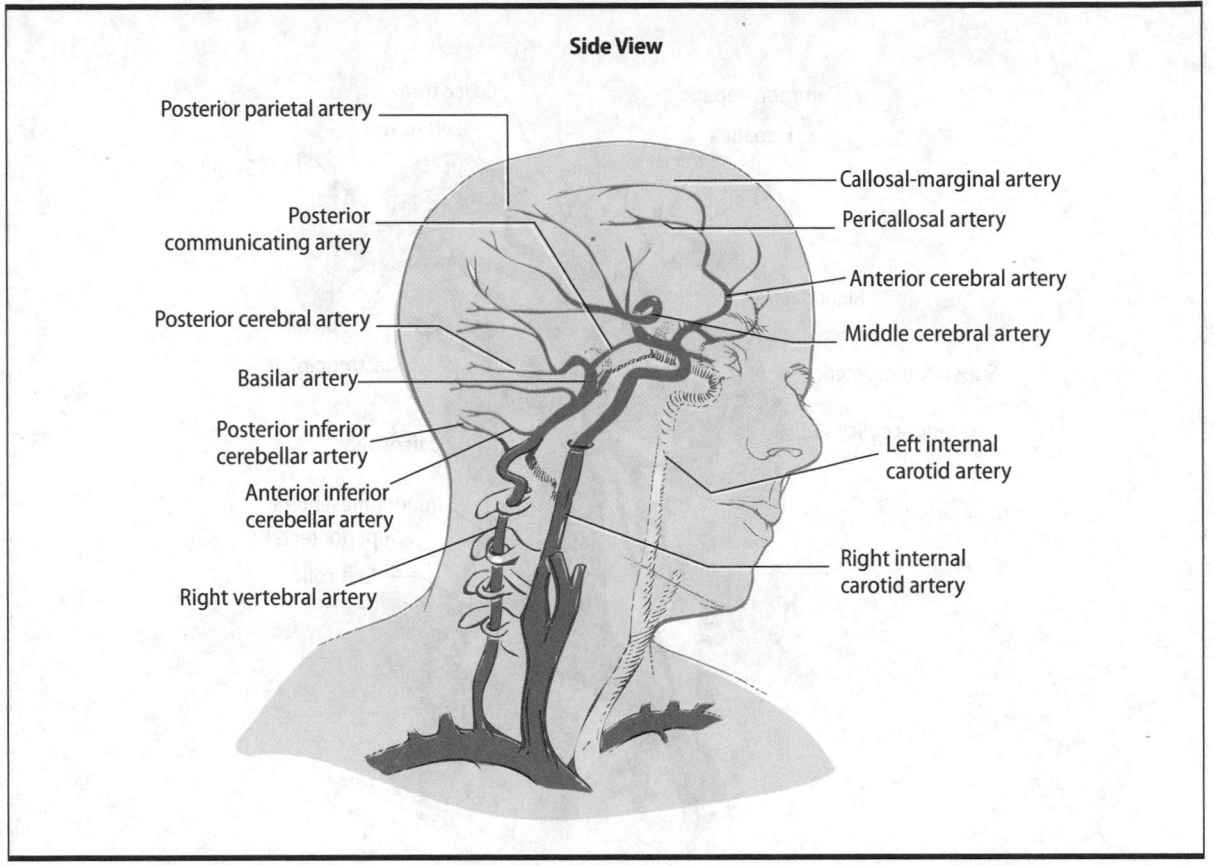

Posterior parietal artery

Posterior communicating artery

Posterior cerebral artery

Basilar artery

Posterior inferior cerebellar artery

Anterior inferior cerebellar artery

Right vertebral artery

Callosal-marginal artery

Pericallosal artery

Anterior cerebral artery

Middle cerebral artery

Left internal carotid artery

Right internal carotid artery

External Carotid Artery and Branches

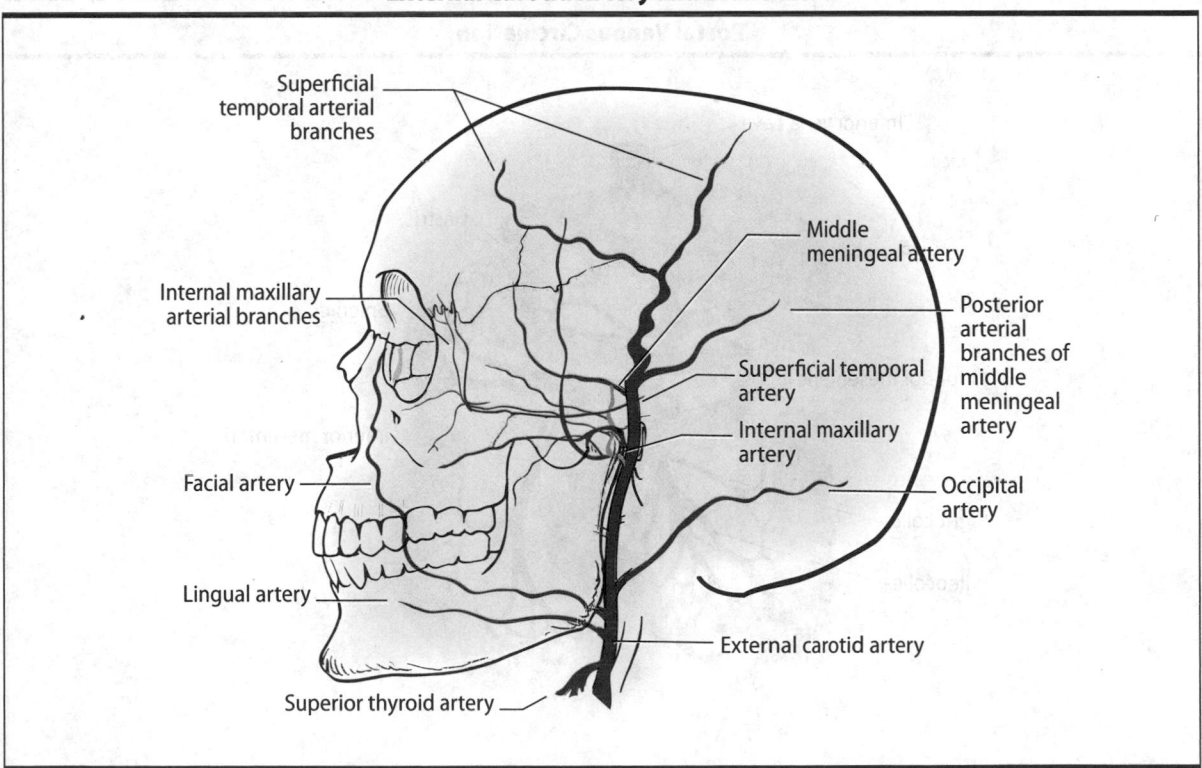

Superficial temporal arterial branches

Internal maxillary arterial branches

Facial artery

Lingual artery

Superior thyroid artery

Middle meningeal artery

Superficial temporal artery

Internal maxillary artery

Posterior arterial branches of middle meningeal artery

Occipital artery

External carotid artery

Branches of Abdominal Aorta

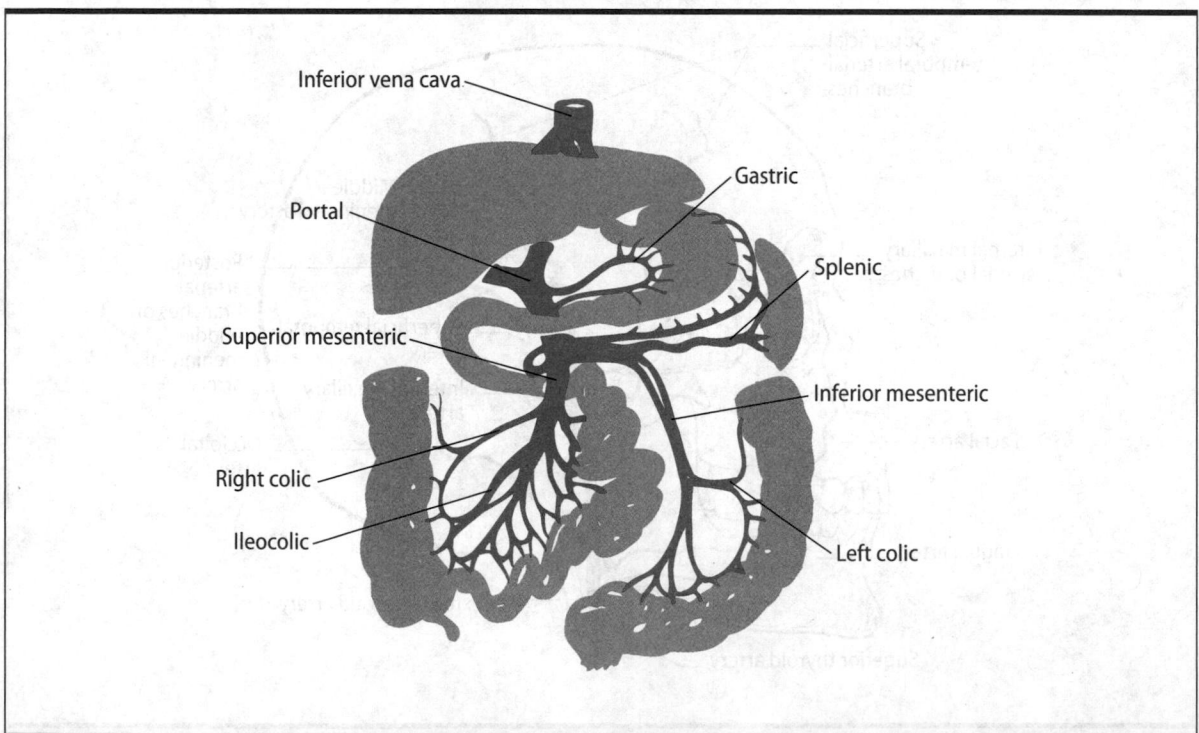

Portal Venous Circulation

Lymphatic System

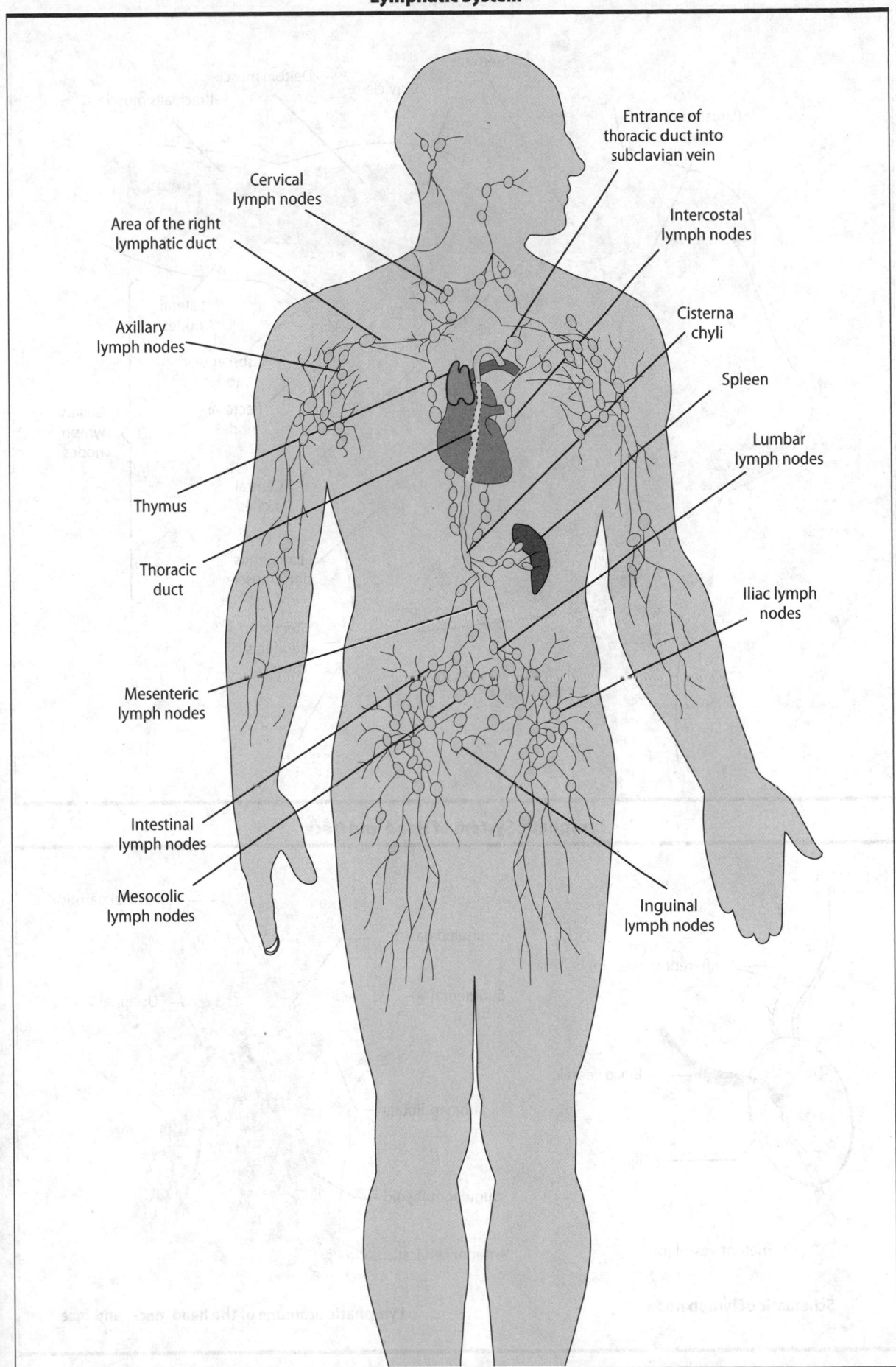

Cervical lymph nodes

Area of the right lymphatic duct

Axillary lymph nodes

Thymus

Thoracic duct

Mesenteric lymph nodes

Intestinal lymph nodes

Mesocolic lymph nodes

Entrance of thoracic duct into subclavian vein

Intercostal lymph nodes

Cisterna chyli

Spleen

Lumbar lymph nodes

Iliac lymph nodes

Inguinal lymph nodes

Axillary Lymph Nodes

Sternum

Clavicle

Deltoid muscle

Brachialis muscle

Parasternal nodes

Lateral nodes

Subscapular nodes

Pectoral nodes

Axillary lymph nodes

Central nodes

Latissimus dorsi muscle

Rectus abdominis muscle

Lymphatic System of Head and Neck

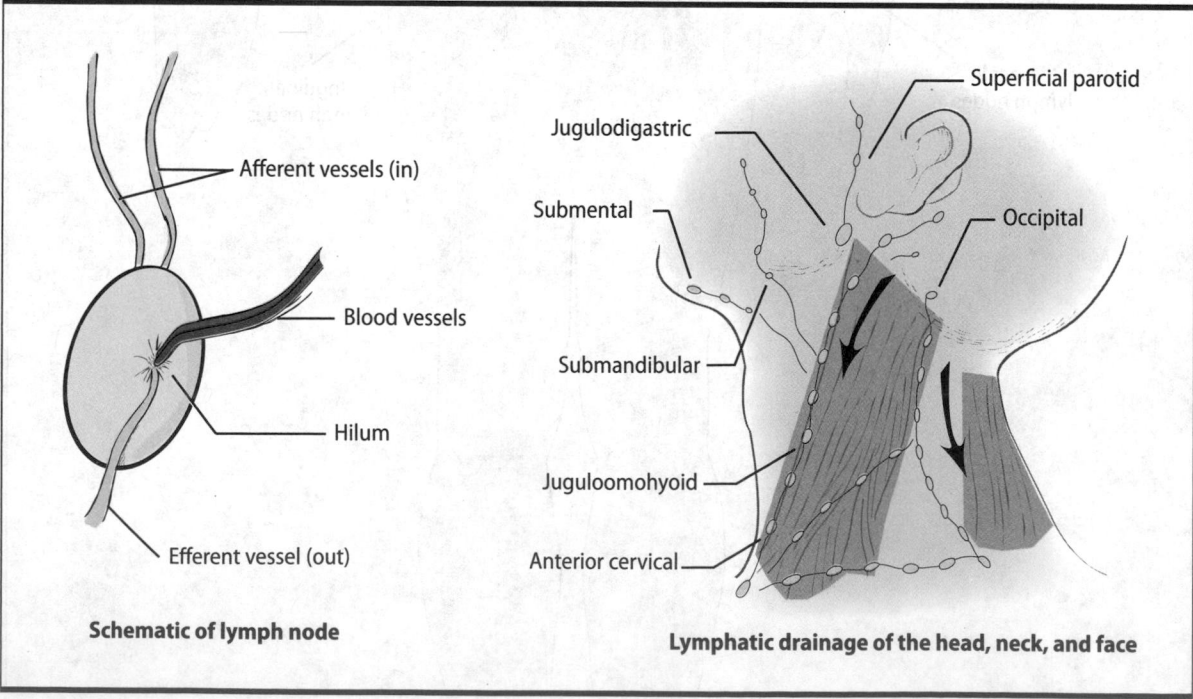

Afferent vessels (in)

Blood vessels

Hilum

Efferent vessel (out)

Schematic of lymph node

Jugulodigastric

Submental

Superficial parotid

Occipital

Submandibular

Juguloomohyoid

Anterior cervical

Lymphatic drainage of the head, neck, and face

Lymphatic Capillaries

Schematic of lymphatic capillaries

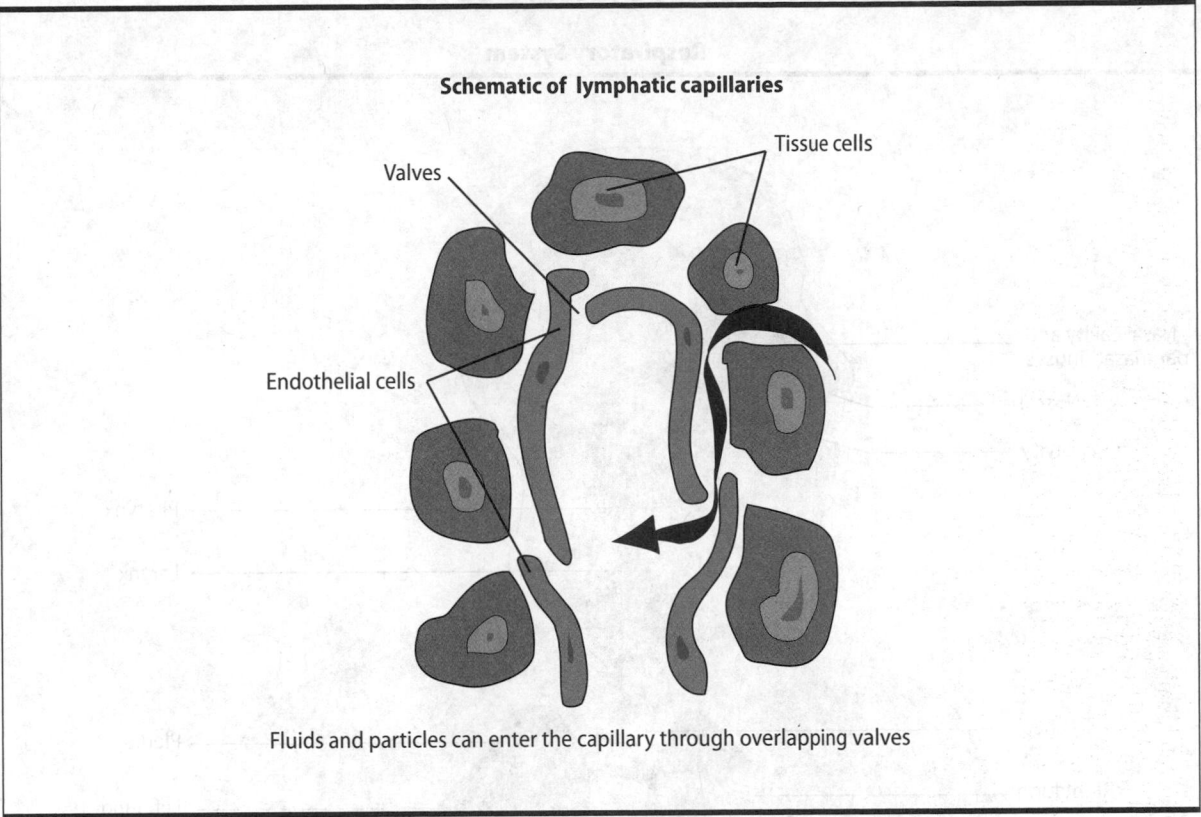

Fluids and particles can enter the capillary through overlapping valves

Lymphatic Drainage

Lymphatic drainage of the colon follows blood supply

Chapter 10. Diseases of the Respiratory System (J00–J99)

Respiratory System

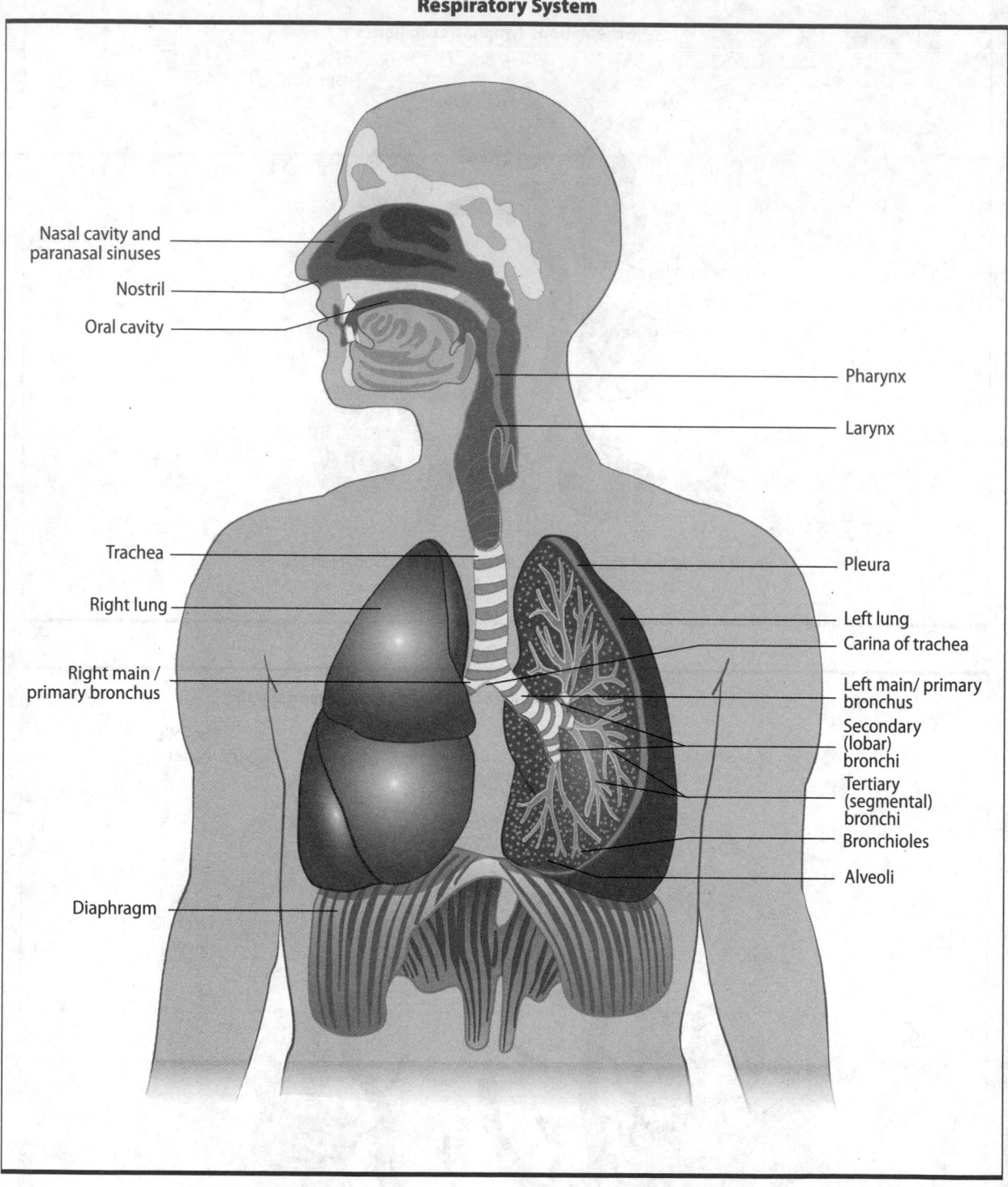

Nasal cavity and
paranasal sinuses

Nostril

Oral cavity

Pharynx

Larynx

Trachea

Pleura

Right lung

Left lung

Carina of trachea

Right main /
primary bronchus

Left main/ primary
bronchus

Secondary
(lobar)
bronchi

Tertiary
(segmental)
bronchi

Bronchioles

Alveoli

Diaphragm

Upper Respiratory System

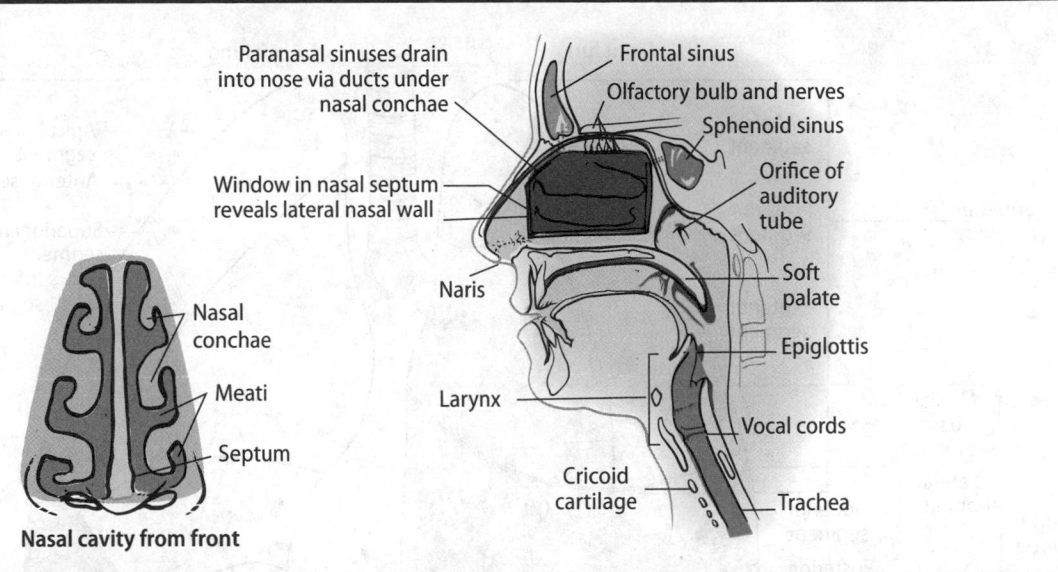

Paranasal sinuses drain into nose via ducts under nasal conchae

Frontal sinus

Olfactory bulb and nerves

Sphenoid sinus

Window in nasal septum reveals lateral nasal wall

Orifice of auditory tube

Naris

Soft palate

Nasal conchae

Meati

Septum

Larynx

Epiglottis

Vocal cords

Cricoid cartilage

Trachea

Nasal cavity from front

Lower Respiratory System

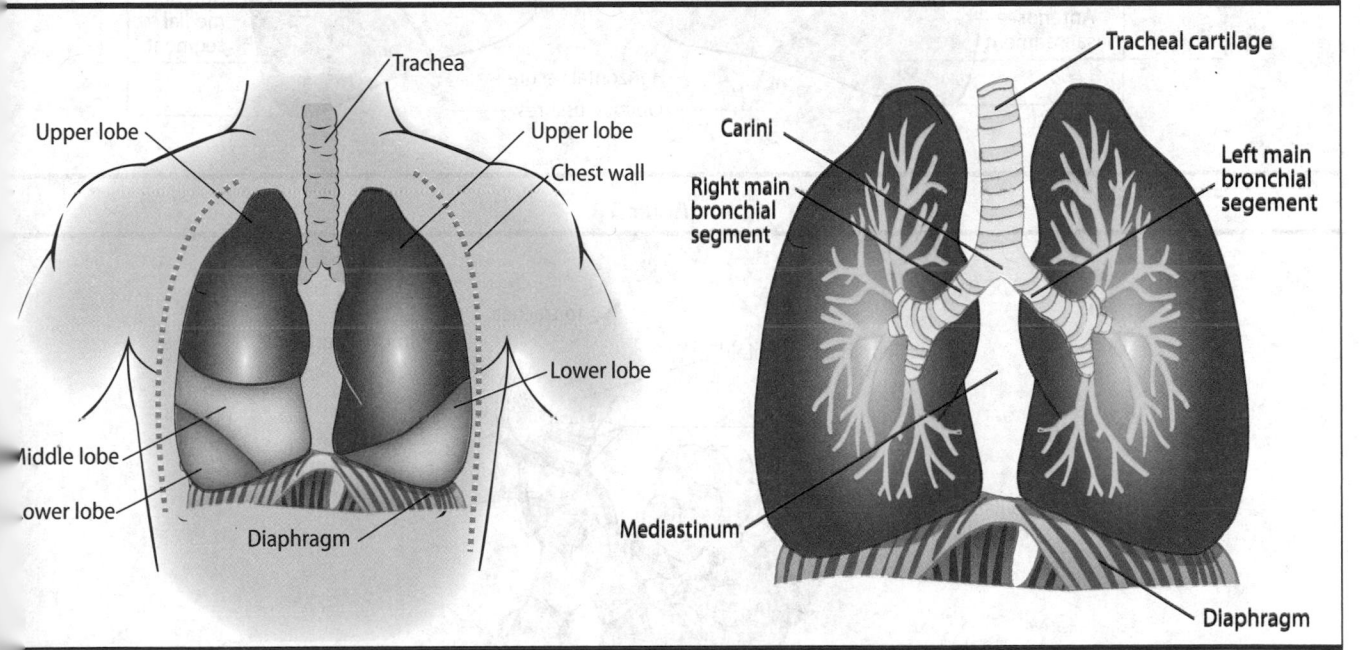

Trachea

Upper lobe

Upper lobe

Chest wall

Middle lobe

Lower lobe

Lower lobe

Diaphragm

Tracheal cartilage

Carini

Right main bronchial segment

Left main bronchial segement

Mediastinum

Diaphragm

Paranasal Sinuses

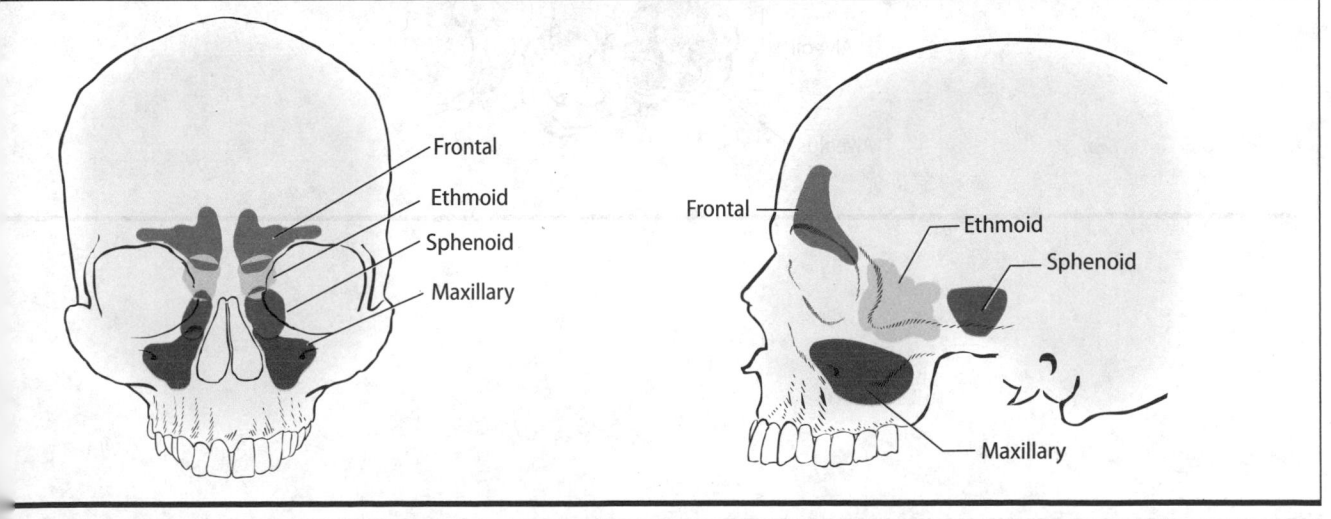

Frontal

Ethmoid

Sphenoid

Maxillary

Frontal

Ethmoid

Sphenoid

Maxillary

Lung Segments

Right lung

Left lung

Apical
segment

Apical-posterior
segment

Anterior segment

Superior
lobe

Posterior
segment

Superior
lobe

Superior lingular
segment

Inferior lingular
segment

Anterior
segment

Medial
basal
segment

Superior
basal
segment

Lateral
segment

Lateral
basal
segment

Superior
segment

Middle
lobe

Posterior
basal
segment

Inferior
lobe

Inferior
lobe

Anterior
basal segment

Anterior
medial
segment

Horizontal fissure

Oblique fissures

Alveoli

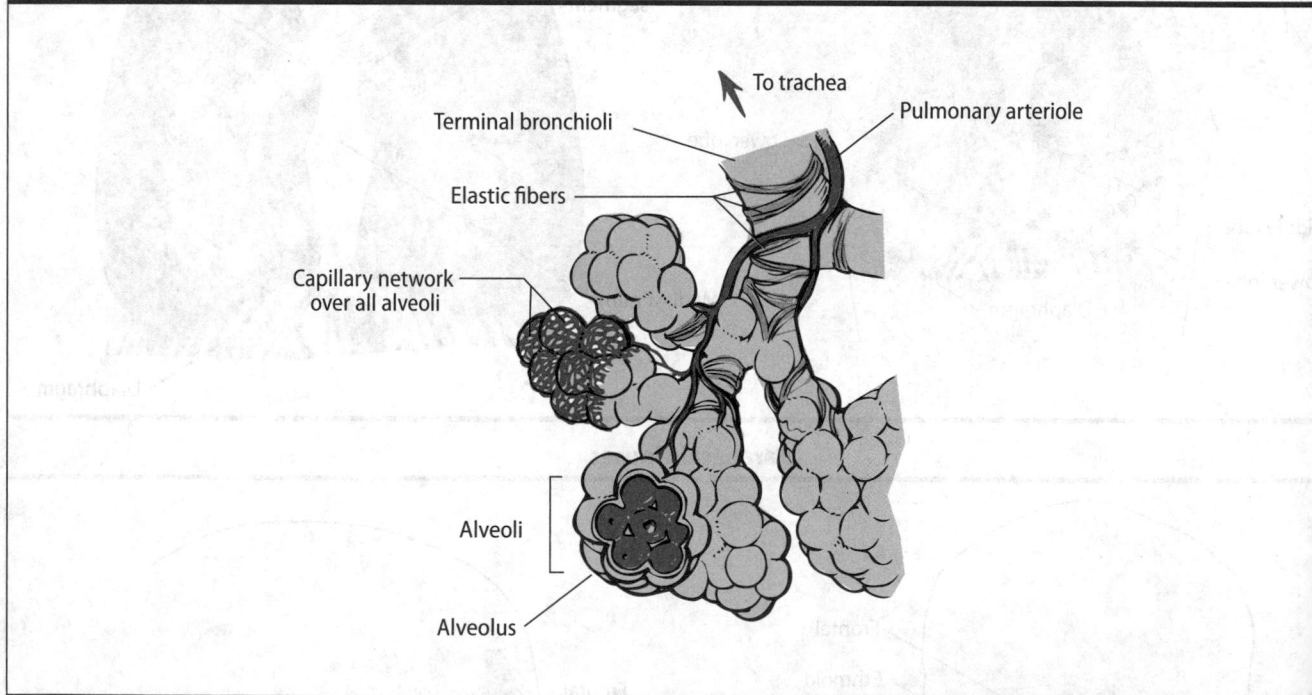

To trachea

Terminal bronchioli

Pulmonary arteriole

Elastic fibers

Capillary network
over all alveoli

Alveoli

Alveolus

apter 11. Diseases of the Digestive System (KØØ–K95)

Digestive System

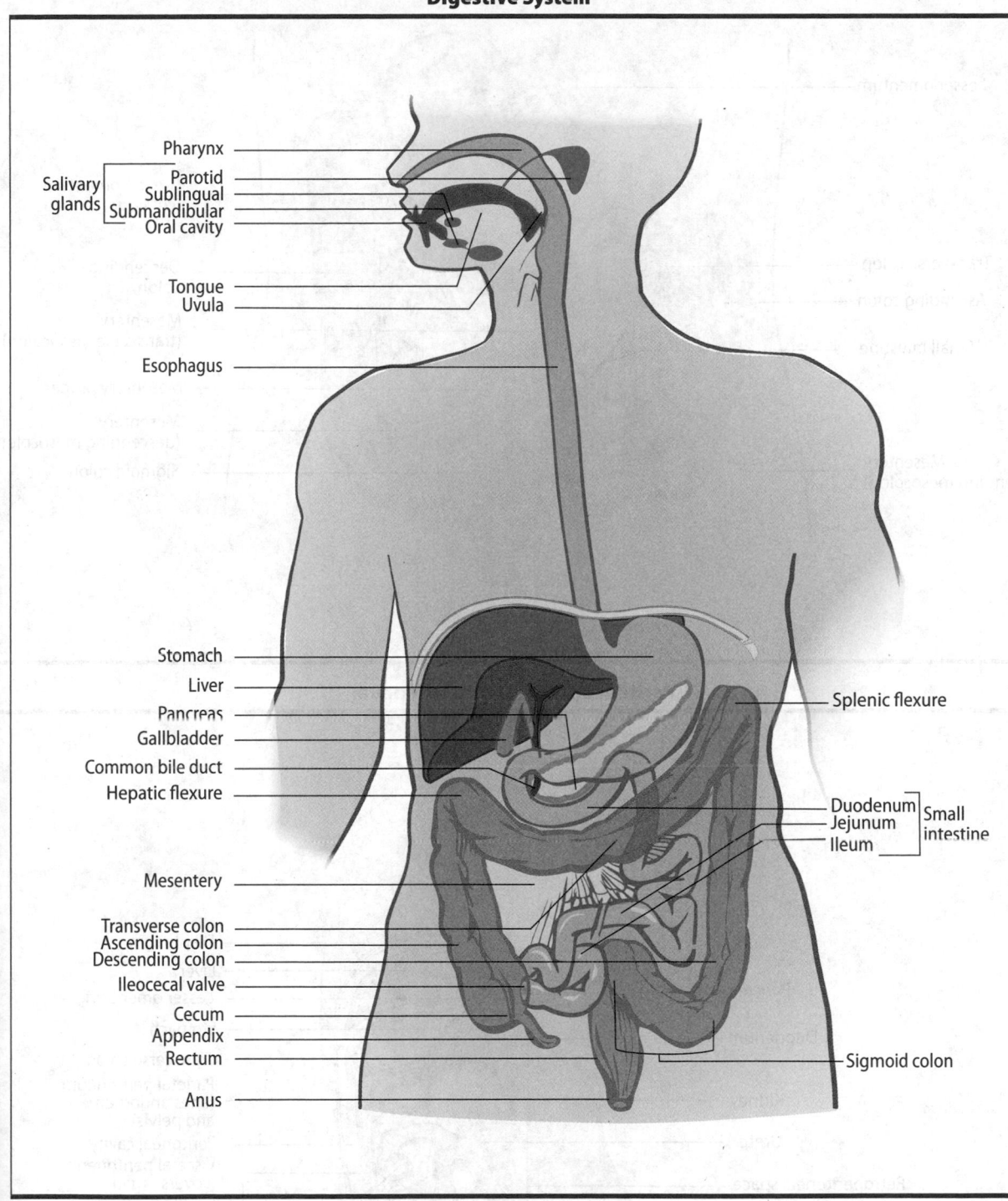

Omentum and Mesentery

Lesser omentum

Greater omentum (cut edge)

Transverse colon

Descending colon

Ascending colon

Mesentery (transverse mesocolon)

Small intestine

Mesentery proper

Mesentery (descending mesocolon)

Mesentery (ascending mesocolon)

Sigmoid colon

Peritoneum and Retroperitoneum

Pancreas

Diaphragm

Liver

Lesser omentum

Duodenum

Stomach

Transverse colon

Kidney

Parietal peritoneum (lines abdomen and pelvis)

Ureter

Peritoneal cavity

Retroperitoneal space

Visceral peritoneum (covers organs)

Small intestine

Mesentery

Greater omentum

Sigmoid colon

Bladder

Rectum

apter 12. Diseases of the Skin and Subcutaneous Tissue (LØØ–L99)

Nail Anatomy

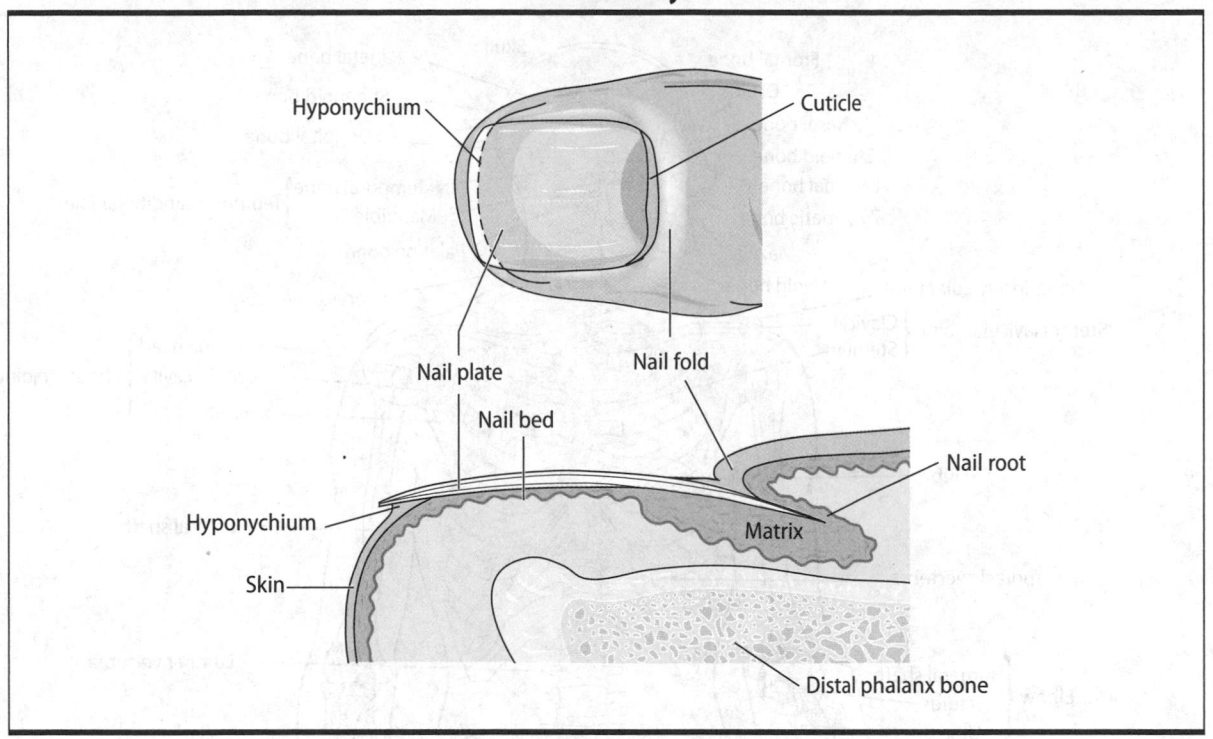

Hyponychium

Cuticle

Nail plate

Nail fold

Nail bed

Hyponychium

Nail root

Matrix

Skin

Distal phalanx bone

Skin and Subcutaneous Tissue

Hair

Basal layer

Layer corneal

Epidermis

Hair shaft

Dermis

Sebaceous gland

Bulb

Hypodermis
(subcutaneous layer)

Hair follicles

Sweat (eccrine gland)

Sensory nerve

Adipose tissue

Blood vessels

Chapter 13. Diseases of the Musculoskeletal System and Connective Tissue (M00–M9

Bones and Joints

Shoulder Anterior View

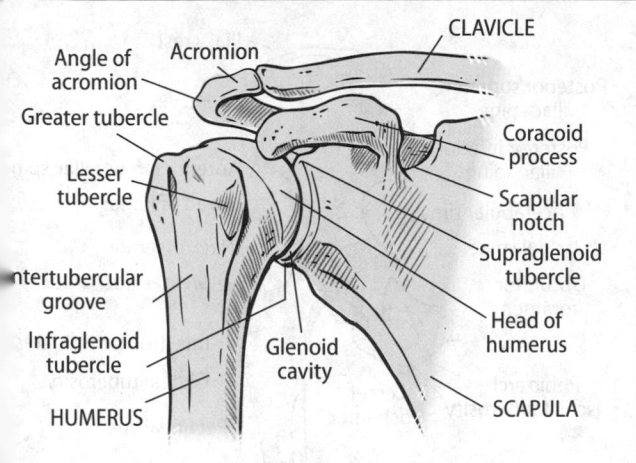

- CLAVICLE
- Acromion
- Angle of acromion
- Greater tubercle
- Lesser tubercle
- Intertubercular groove
- Infraglenoid tubercle
- HUMERUS
- Coracoid process
- Scapular notch
- Supraglenoid tubercle
- Head of humerus
- Glenoid cavity
- SCAPULA

Shoulder Posterior View

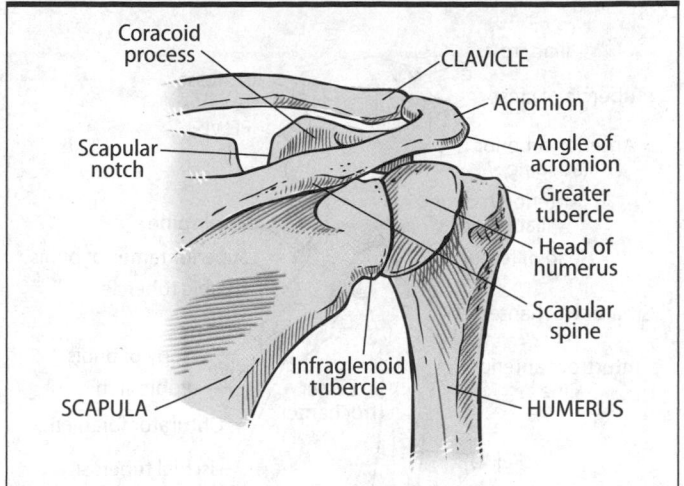

- Coracoid process
- CLAVICLE
- Acromion
- Angle of acromion
- Greater tubercle
- Head of humerus
- Scapular notch
- Scapular spine
- Infraglenoid tubercle
- SCAPULA
- HUMERUS

Elbow Anterior View

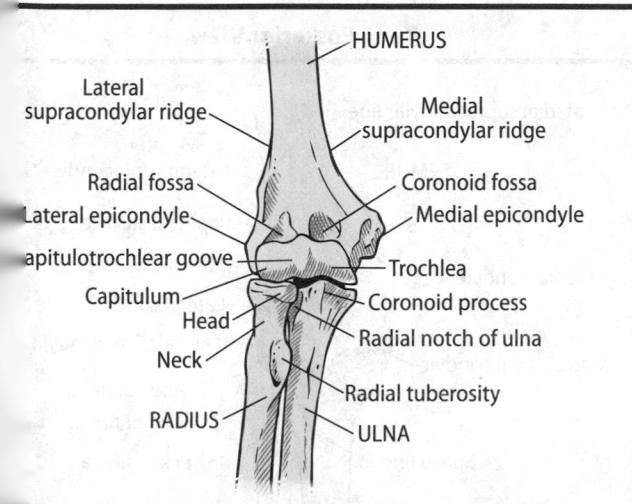

- HUMERUS
- Lateral supracondylar ridge
- Medial supracondylar ridge
- Radial fossa
- Coronoid fossa
- Lateral epicondyle
- Medial epicondyle
- Capitulotrochlear goove
- Trochlea
- Capitulum
- Coronoid process
- Head
- Radial notch of ulna
- Neck
- Radial tuberosity
- RADIUS
- ULNA

Elbow Posterior View

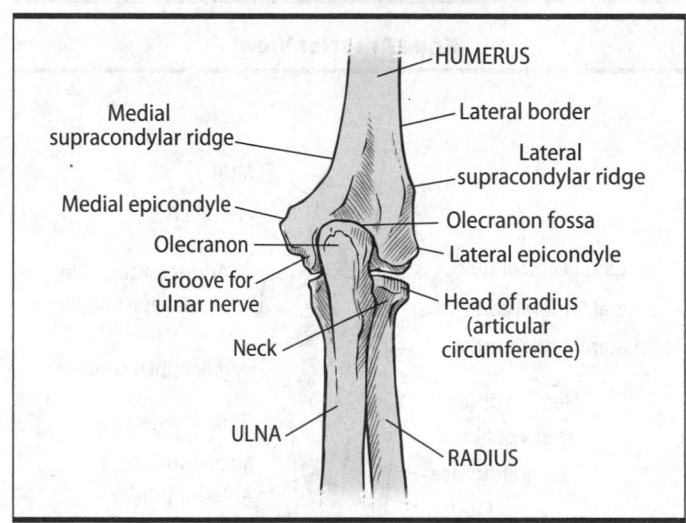

- HUMERUS
- Medial supracondylar ridge
- Lateral border
- Lateral supracondylar ridge
- Medial epicondyle
- Olecranon fossa
- Olecranon
- Lateral epicondyle
- Groove for ulnar nerve
- Head of radius (articular circumference)
- Neck
- ULNA
- RADIUS

Hand

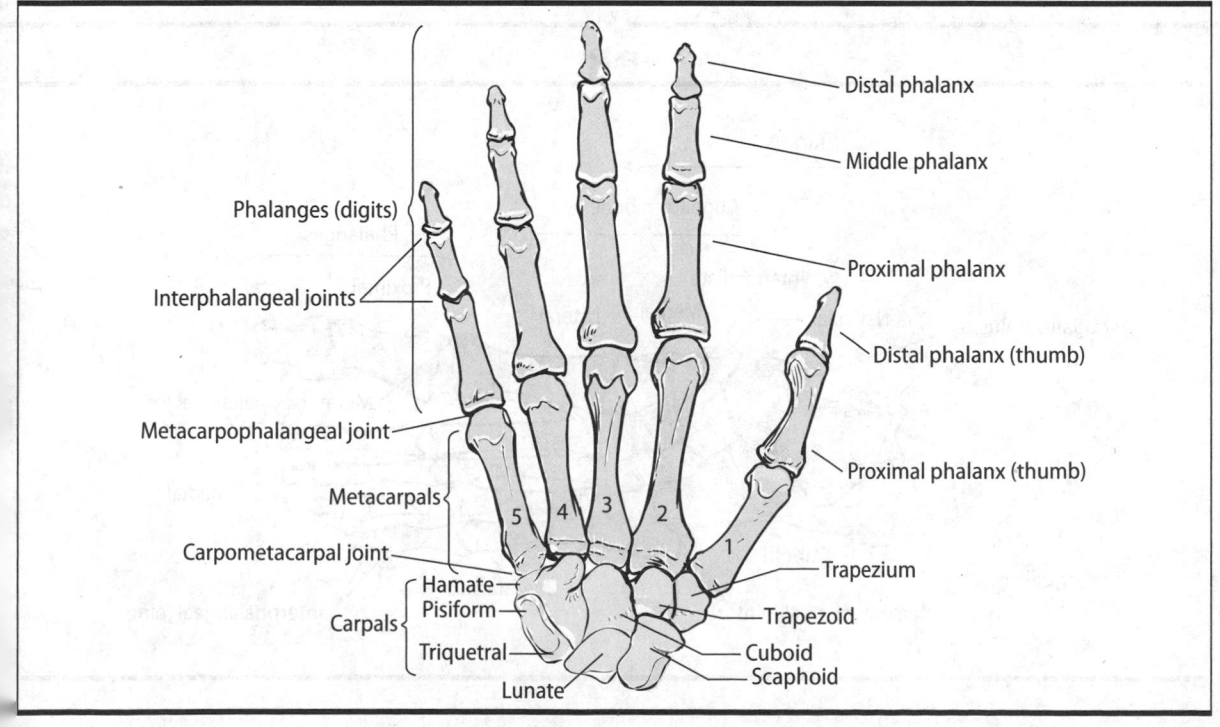

- Distal phalanx
- Middle phalanx
- Phalanges (digits)
- Interphalangeal joints
- Proximal phalanx
- Distal phalanx (thumb)
- Metacarpophalangeal joint
- Proximal phalanx (thumb)
- Metacarpals
- Carpometacarpal joint
- Trapezium
- Hamate
- Pisiform
- Trapezoid
- Carpals
- Triquetral
- Cuboid
- Scaphoid
- Lunate
- 5 4 3 2 1

Hip Anterior View

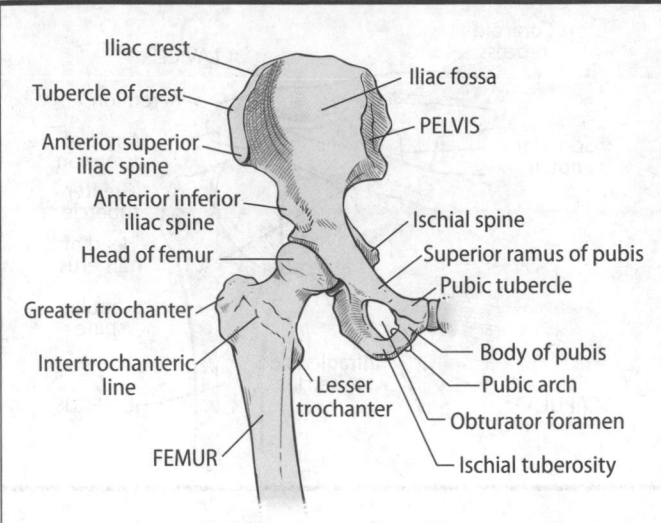

Iliac crest
Tubercle of crest
Anterior superior iliac spine
Anterior inferior iliac spine
Head of femur
Greater trochanter
Intertrochanteric line
FEMUR
Lesser trochanter
Iliac fossa
PELVIS
Ischial spine
Superior ramus of pubis
Pubic tubercle
Body of pubis
Pubic arch
Obturator foramen
Ischial tuberosity

Hip Posterior View

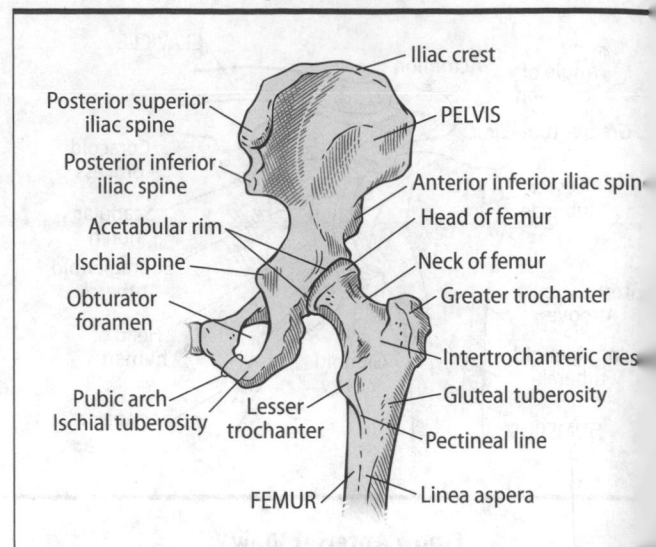

Posterior superior iliac spine
Posterior inferior iliac spine
Acetabular rim
Ischial spine
Obturator foramen
Pubic arch
Ischial tuberosity
Lesser trochanter
Iliac crest
PELVIS
Anterior inferior iliac spin
Head of femur
Neck of femur
Greater trochanter
Intertrochanteric cres
Gluteal tuberosity
Pectineal line
Linea aspera
FEMUR

Knee Anterior View

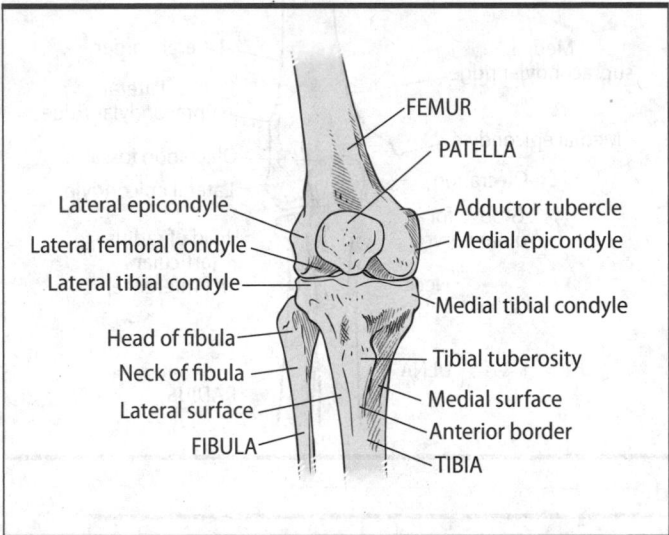

FEMUR
PATELLA
Lateral epicondyle
Lateral femoral condyle
Lateral tibial condyle
Head of fibula
Neck of fibula
Lateral surface
FIBULA
Adductor tubercle
Medial epicondyle
Medial tibial condyle
Tibial tuberosity
Medial surface
Anterior border
TIBIA

Knee Posterior View

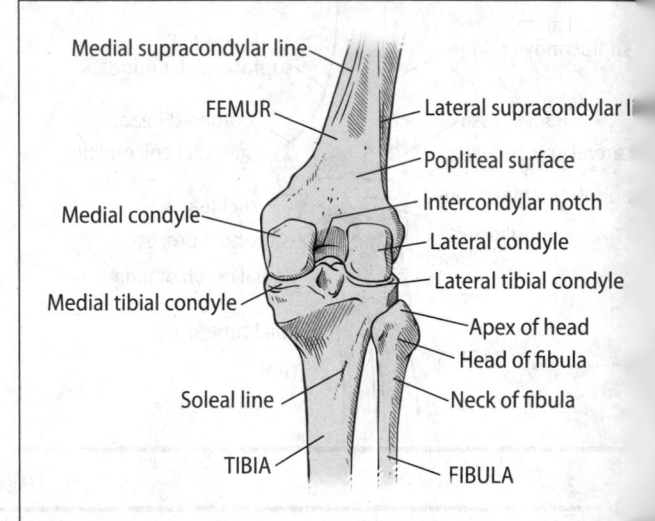

Medial supracondylar line
FEMUR
Medial condyle
Medial tibial condyle
Soleal line
TIBIA
Lateral supracondylar l
Popliteal surface
Intercondylar notch
Lateral condyle
Lateral tibial condyle
Apex of head
Head of fibula
Neck of fibula
FIBULA

Foot

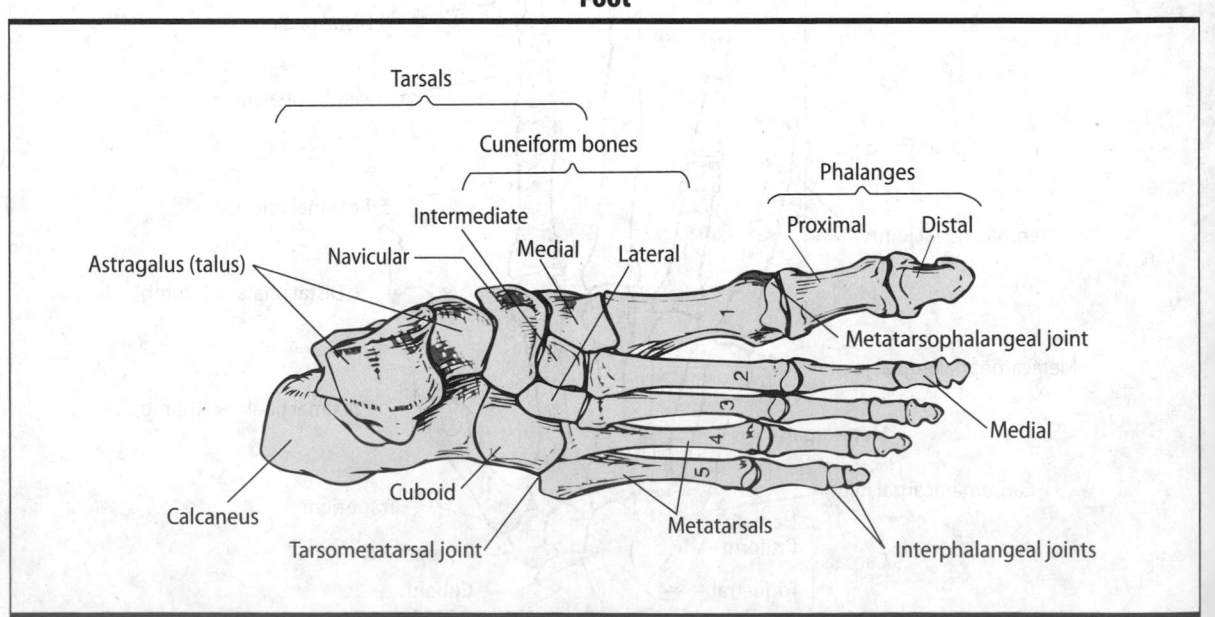

Tarsals
Cuneiform bones
Phalanges
Proximal
Distal
Intermediate
Astragalus (talus)
Navicular
Medial
Lateral
Metatarsophalangeal joint
Medial
Calcaneus
Cuboid
Tarsometatarsal joint
Metatarsals
Interphalangeal joints

Muscles

Temporalis m.

Frontalis m.

Orbicularis oculi m.

Orbicularis oris m.

Depressor labii inferioris m.

Mentalis m.

Masseter m.

Zygomaticus major m.

Splenius m.

Sternocleidomastoid m. (clavicular head)

Omohyoid m.

Sternocleidomastoid m. (sternal head)

Levator scapulae m.

Platysma m.

Deltoid m.

Pectoralis major m.

Latissimus dorsi m.

Coracobrachialis m.

Biceps brachii m. (short head)

Serratus anterior m.

Biceps brachii m. (long head)

Biceps brachii m.

Triceps m.

Linea alba

Brachialis m.

Brachioradialis m.

Rectus abdominis m.

Extensor carpi radialis longus m.

Brachioradialis m.

Bicipital aponeurosis

Pronator teres m.

External oblique m.

Flexor carpi radialis m.

Flexor carpi radialis m.

Extensor carpi radialis longus m.

Palmaris longus m.

Extensor carpi radialis brevis m.

Flexor carpi ulnaris m.

Extensor digitorum m.

exor digitorum superficialis m.

Extensor digiti minimi m.

Extensor retinaculum

Extensor retinaculum

Anterior superior iliac spine

Iliopsoas m.

Pectineus m.

Pubic tubercle

Adductor longus m.

Gracilis m.

Sartorius m.

Tensor fascia latae m.

Rectus femoris m.

Vastus lateralis m.

Tensor fascia latae m.

Vastus medialis m.

Patella

Gastrocnemius m.

Tibia

Tibialis anterior m.

Peroneus longus m.

Soleus m.

Extensor digitorum longus m.

Superior extensor retinaculum

Medial maleolus

Lateral maleolus

Chapter 14. Diseases of the Genitourinary System (NØØ–N99)

Urinary System

Male Genitourinary System

Female Internal Genitalia

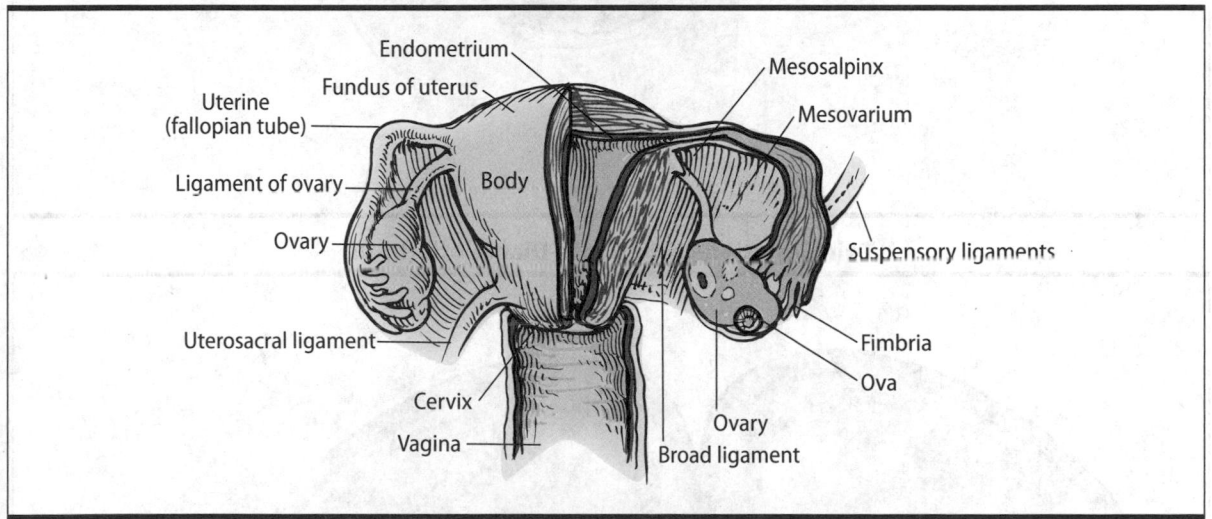

Female Genitourinary Tract Lateral View

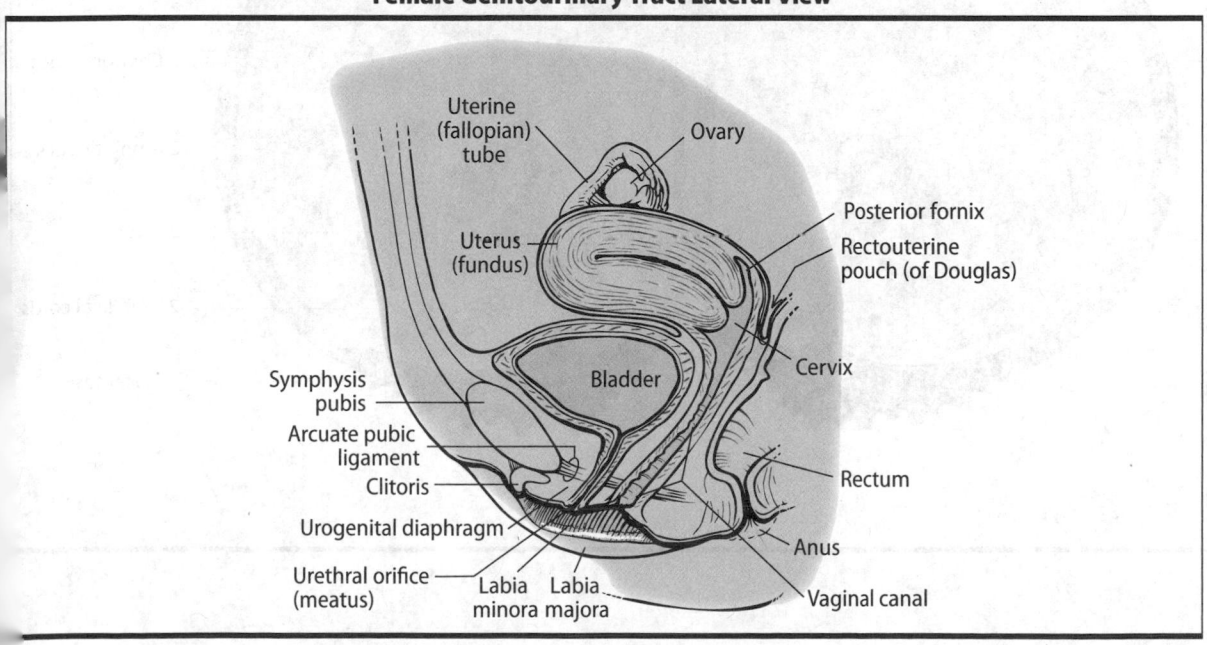

Chapter 15. Pregnancy, Childbirth and the Puerperium (O00–O9A)

Term Pregnancy – Single Gestation

- Placenta
- Umbilical cord
- Amniotic fluid
- Amniotic sac
- Uterus
- Cervix
- Mucous plug
- Vagina
- Pubic bone

Twin Gestation–Dichorionic–Diamniotic (DI-DI)

- 2 Chorionic sacs
- 2 Amniotic sacs
- 2 Fetuses
- 2 Umbilical cords
- 2 Placentas

Twin Gestation–Monochorionic–Diamniotic (MO-DI)

1 Chorionic sac

2 Amniotic sacs

2 Fetuses

2 Umbilical cords

1 Placenta

Twin Gestation–Monochorionic–Monoamniotic (MO-MO)

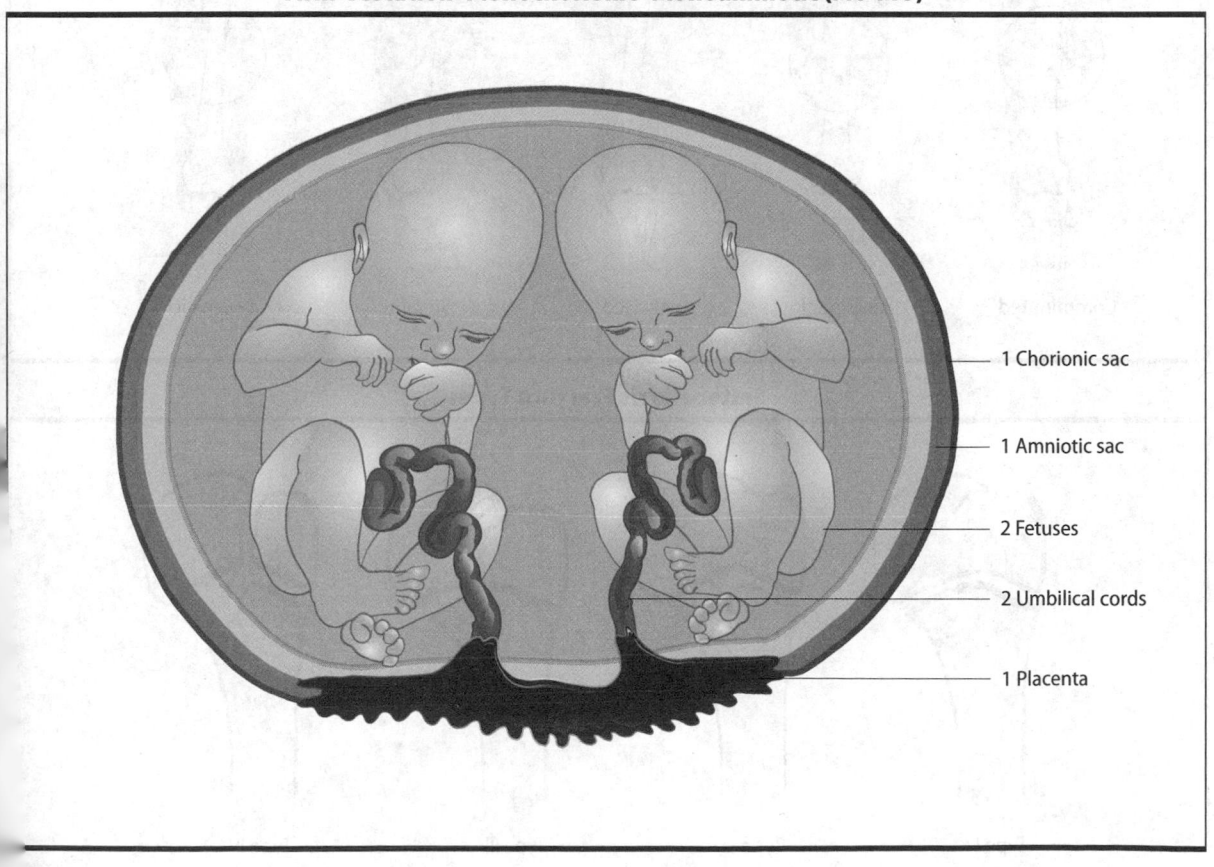

1 Chorionic sac

1 Amniotic sac

2 Fetuses

2 Umbilical cords

1 Placenta

Chapter 19. Injury, Poisoning and Certain Other Consequences of External Causes (S00–T88)

Types of Fractures

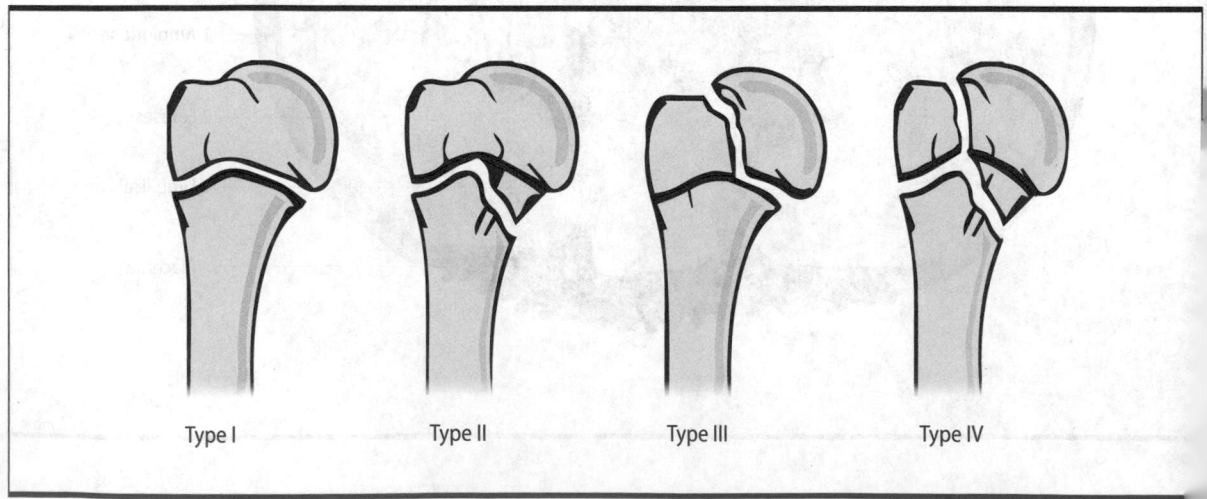

Normal	Transverse	Open/Compound	Oblique	Oblique displaced
Comminuted	Segmental	Avulsed	Spiral	Greenstick

Salter-Harris Fracture Types

Type I	Type II	Type III	Type IV